OPTUM360°™

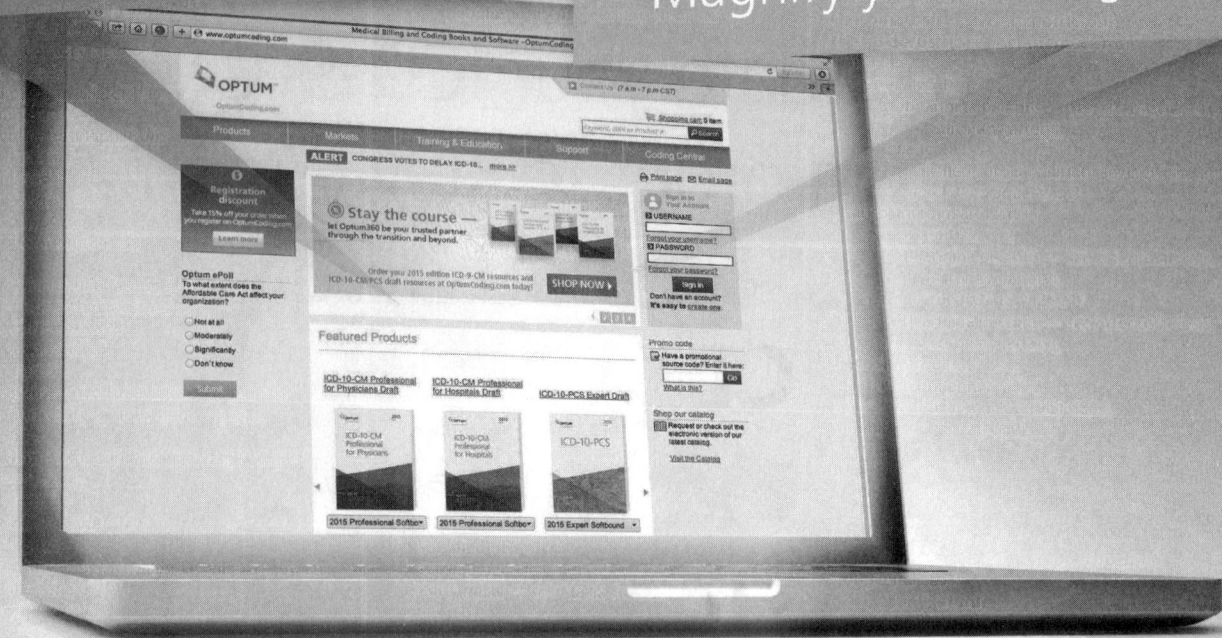

Simplify your ordering.

Magnify your savings.

① Click.

Visit optumcoding.com

- Find the products you need quickly and easily.
- View all available formats and edition years on the same page.
- Chat live with a customer service representative.
- Visit Coding Central for expert resources including articles, *Inside Track to ICD-10* and coding scenarios to test your knowledge.
- View our catalog online. Utilize our interactive online catalog features to view product information quickly and easily.

② Register.

By registering, you'll be able to:

- Enjoy special promotions, discounts and automatic rewards.
- Get recommendations based on your order history.
- Check on shipment status and tracking.
- View order and payment history.
- Pay invoices.
- Manage your address book and ship orders to multiple locations.
- Renew your order with a single click.
- Compile a wish list of the products you want and purchase when you're ready.

③ Save.

Get 15% off your next order

Register for an account and receive a coupon via email for 15% off your next order.

Plus, save even more with our no-cost eRewards program.

OptumCoding.com
eRewards
program

Register for an account and you're automatically enrolled in our eRewards program, where you'll get a $50 coupon for every $500 you spend*. When logged in at optumcoding.com, the eRewards meter keeps track of purchases toward your next reward.

Visit us at optumcoding.com to register today!

ICD-10-CM
Expert for
Hospitals

The Complete Official Draft Code Set

DRAFT

2015

Z codes are secondary except
some chemotherapy Z51-11 can come first
Refer Chap. 21 Guidelines.
malnutrition - also hyper glycemia

Nausea - R11.0
Vomiting - R11.10
N & V - R11.2
diarrhea - R19.7
acute - C91.00

Neoplasm table
has cancer codes.
C-
Diabetes - E08
E09
Type Gio - Type GI E11

Pain -
Convulsions -
metabolic -
Amyloid -
Osteo Arthritis -
rash -
ingrown -
Chondromalacia
Anemia
Osteomyelitis
Examination
New born
Pre term/Infant
Condition New born
Premature Infant
laceration
Gastroenteritis (includes Nausea vomiting)
Candidiasis
Infection/Bacterial/E coli
E coli - Escherichia coli
B 96.20

Main Terms
Seizure
Pneumonia
Abnormal
incontinence
glucose intolerance
Gastrointestinal -
dysphia
Scar
Syncope
Dysfunction
HDS HIV + B20,
Candidiasis
Injection
Carcinoma
Sepsis 41.9, 41.9
Type 1 or 2 diabetes
Malnutrition
Fever
Hypertrophy
Delivery
Overdose
aneurysm
Admission
hernia
Sarcoma
Hypertension
Cystitis
Herpes
cancer - Neoplasm table
Disease -
Overproduction
Depression
alcoholic
dependence

itis - infection inflammation
Lith - calculus
Lith - Kidney
Nephro - Kidney
PED - bad
Pre se rofa
dys/dysphon
(S) dys/dysbol
dot

MRSA - methicillin suscepth
Staphylococcus Aureus
Aureus

Publisher's Notice

The *ICD-10-CM Expert for Hospitals: The Complete Official Draft Code Set* is designed to be an accurate and authoritative source regarding coding and every reasonable effort has been made to ensure accuracy and completeness of the content. However, Optum makes no guarantee, warranty, or representation that this publication is accurate, complete, or without errors. It is understood that Optum is not rendering any legal or other professional services or advice in this publication and that Optum bears no liability for any results or consquences that may arise from the use of this book.

Our Commitment to Accuracy

Optum is committed to producing accurate and reliable materials.

To report corrections, please visit www.optumcoding.com/accuracy or email accuracy@optum.com. You can also reach customer service by calling 1.800.464.3649, option 1.

Acknowledgments

Lauri Gray, RHIT, CPC, AHIMA-Approved ICD-10-CM/PCS Trainer, *Product Manager*
Karen Schmidt, BSN, *Technical Director*
Stacy Perry, *Manager, Desktop Publishing*
Anita Schmidt, BS, RHIT, *Clinical Technical Editor*
Peggy Willard, CCS, AHIMA-Approved ICD-10-CM/PCS Trainer, *Clinical Technical Editor*
Lisa Singley, *Project Manager*
Tracy Betzler, *Senior Desktop Publishing Specialist*
Hope M. Dunn, *Senior Desktop Publishing Specialist*
Katie Russell, *Desktop Publishing Specialist*
Kate Holden, *Editor*

Anita Schmidt, BS, RHIT

Ms. Schmidt has expertise in Level I Adult and Pediatric Trauma hospital coding, specializing in ICD-9-CM, DRG, and CPT coding. Her experience includes analysis of medical record documentation and assignment of ICD-9-CM codes and DRGs, and CPT code assignments for same-day surgery cases. She has conducted coding training and auditing inclusive of DRG validation, conducted electronic health record training, and worked with clinical documentation specialists to identify documentation needs and potential areas for physician education. Ms. Schmidt is an active member of the American Health Information Management Association (AHIMA) and the Minnesota Health Information Management Association (MHIMA).

Karen Schmidt, BSN

Ms. Schmidt has more than 25 years of health care experience beginning with a strong clinical background in critical care nursing and later functioning as director of case management, including the components of quality assurance, utilization management, concurrent coding, case-mix analysis, and discharge planning. Her areas of expertise include ICD-9-CM/DRG coding, outpatient observation, billing compliance, implementation of concurrent coding methodology, and physician documentation education. She is an active member of the American Health Information Management Association (AHIMA).

Peggy Willard, CCS, AHIMA-Approved ICD10-CM/PCS Trainer

Ms. Willard has several years of experience in Level I Adult and Pediatric Trauma hospital coding, specializing in ICD-9-CM, DRG, and CPT coding. She has been extensively trained in ICD-10-CM and PCS. Her recent experience includes in-depth analysis of medical record documentation, ICD-10-CM code assignment, and DRG shifts based on ICD-10-CM code assignment. Ms. Willard's expertise includes conducting coding audits, conducting coding training for coding staff and clinical documentation specialists, and creating internal ICD-10-CM coding guidelines/tips. Ms. Willard is an active member of the American Health Information Management Association (AHIMA) and the Minnesota Health Information Management Association (MHIMA).

Contents

Preface iii

Introduction v
    History and Future of ICD-10-CM v
    ICD-10-CM for Hospitals: The Complete Official Draft Code Set v

How to Use ICD-10-CM for Hospitals (Draft 2015) vi
    Steps to Correct Coding vi
    Organization vi

ICD-10-CM Draft Official Conventions vii
    Format vii
    Punctuation vii
    Abbreviations vii
    General Notes vii

Additional Conventions ix
    Additional Characters Required ix
    Boldface ix
    Color Coding—Medicare Code Edits ix
    Other Notations in the Tabular x
    Other Notations in the Index xii

ICD-10-CM Draft Official Guidelines for
Coding and Reporting .... Coding Guidelines-1

ICD-10-CM Index to Diseases and Injuries 1

ICD-10-CM Neoplasm Table 321

ICD-10-CM Table of Drugs and Chemicals 339

ICD-10-CM Index to External Causes 387

ICD-10-CM Tabular List of Diseases and Injuries 423
    Chapter 1   Certain Infectious and Parasitic Diseases
       (A00-B99) 423
    Chapter 2   Neoplasms (C00-D49) 448
    Chapter 3   Diseases of the Blood and Blood-forming
       Organs (D50-D89) 485
    Chapter 4   Endocrine, Nutritional and Metabolic
       Diseases (E00-E89) 493
    Chapter 5   Mental, Behavioral, and Neurodevelopmental
       Disorders (F01-F99) 510
    Chapter 6   Diseases of the Nervous System (G00-G99) 529
    Chapter 7   Diseases of the Eye and Adnexa (H00-H59) 547
    Chapter 8   Diseases of the Ear and Mastoid Process
       (H60-H95) 580
    Chapter 9   Diseases of the Circulatory System (I00-I99) 591
    Chapter 10 Diseases of the Respiratory System (J00-J99) 628
    Chapter 11 Diseases of the Digestive System (K00-K95) 640
    Chapter 12 Diseases of the Skin and Subcutaneous Tissue
       (L00-L99) 660
    Chapter 13 Diseases of the Musculoskeletal System
       and Connective Tissue (M00-M99) 677
    Chapter 14 Diseases of the Genitourinary System (N00-N99) ... 766
    Chapter 15 Pregnancy, Childbirth and the Puerperium
       (O00-O9A) 781
    Chapter 16 Certain Conditions Originating in the
       Perinatal Period (P00-P96) 814
    Chapter 17 Congenital Malformations, Deformations and
       Chromosomal Abnormalities (Q00-Q99) 825
    Chapter 18 Symptoms, Signs and Abnormal Clinical and
       Laboratory Findings (R00-R99) 841
    Chapter 19 Injury, Poisoning and Certain Other Consequences
       of External Causes (S00-T88) 857
    Chapter 20 External Causes of Morbidity (V00-Y99) 1110
    Chapter 21 Factors Influencing Health Status and Contact
       With Health Services (Z00-Z99) 1175

Illustrations Illustrations-1

Preface

ICD-10-CM Official Preface

This 2015 update of the International Classification of Diseases, 10th revision, Clinical Modification (ICD-10-CM) is being published by the United States government in recognition of its responsibility to promulgate this classification throughout the United States for morbidity coding. The International Statistical Classification of Diseases and Related Health Problems, 10th Revision (ICD-10), published by the World Health Organization (WHO), is the foundation of ICD-10-CM. ICD-10 continues to be the classification used in cause-of-death coding in the United States. The ICD-10-CM is comparable with the ICD-10. The WHO Collaborating Center for the Family of International Classifications in North America, housed at the National Center for Health Statistics (NCHS), has responsibility for the implementation of ICD and other WHO-FIC classifications and serves as a liaison with the WHO, fulfilling international obligations for comparable classifications and the national health data needs of the United States. The historical background of ICD and ICD-10 can be found in the Introduction to the International Classification of Diseases and Related Health Problems (ICD-10), 2008, World Health Organization, Geneva, Switzerland.

ICD-10-CM is the United States' clinical modification of the World Health Organization's ICD-10. The term clinical is used to emphasize the modification's intent: to serve as a useful tool in the area of classification of morbidity data for indexing of medical records, medical care review, and ambulatory and other medical care programs, as well as for basic health statistics. To describe the clinical picture of the patient the codes must be more precise than those needed only for statistical groupings and trend analysis.

Characteristics of ICD-10-CM

ICD-10-CM far exceeds its predecessors in the number of concepts and codes provided. The disease classification has been expanded to include health-related conditions and to provide greater specificity at the 6th and 7th character level. The 6th and 7th characters are not optional and are intended for use in recording the information documented in the clinical record.

must have

7th - encounter of care: D02.62|7   → Here 1 is for right
(chr)   2 is for left
                                    4th character - etiology
                                    5   "   - anatomic site
                                    6   "   - severity
                                    7   "   - encounter of care — A - initial encounter
ICD 10 CM — codes must be **3** min. characters with a decimal   D - subsequent
    | point after that.   S - ~~sequela~~ -
    has only diagnostic codes.   Sequelae
                              ┌ procedure coding system
for Procedures ICD 10 PCS — is intented to replace ICD 9 vol. 3 for facility
                          reporting of inpatient procedures.

current Pro. terminology. CPT — is still used for all outpatient procedures. Also for
                                                           common diagnostic procedure. They a
HCPCS - Health care common procedure coding system. → procedures & medical devices put'c
    ` level II — includes services such as ambulance, med. durable equipment,
                                              prosthetics, orthotics & supplies
Neoplasm Table. Melanoma — also Malignant   when used outside physn's office
                Adenoma — also Benign

Logic based encode — asks sequence or series of questions

PCS - 7 up - 7 characters with NO 'O' & 'I'

Introduction

History and Future of ICD-10-CM

The ICD-10-CM classification system was developed by the National Center for Health Statistics (NCHS) as a clinical modification to the ICD-10 system developed by the World Health Organization (WHO), primarily as a unique system for use in the United States for morbidity and mortality reporting. Although ICD-10-CM has not yet been implemented for use in the United States, ICD-10 has been adopted for use in the coding and classification of mortality data from death certificates. ICD-10 replaced ICD-9 for this purpose as of January 1, 1999. Upon legislative approval, ICD-10-CM is planned as the replacement for ICD-9-CM, volumes 1 and 2.

ICD-10 is the copyrighted product of the World Health Organization (WHO), which has authorized the development of a clinical modification (CM) of ICD-10 for use in the United States. However, all modifications to the ICD-10 must conform to WHO conventions for ICD. The development of ICD-10-CM included comprehensive evaluation by a Technical Advisory Panel and extensive consultation with physician groups, clinical coders, and other industry experts.

The ICD-10-CM draft and crosswalk between ICD-9-CM and ICD-10-CM were made available on the Centers for Medicare and Medicaid Services (CMS) website for public comment. The initial public comment period extended from December 1997 through February 1998. A field test for ICD-10-CM was conducted in the summer of 2003 jointly by The American Hospital Association (AMA) and the American Health Information Management Association (AHIMA). Public comments and suggestions were reviewed and additional modifications to ICD-10-CM were made. Revisions were made to ICD-10-CM based on the established update process for ICD-9-CM (the ICD-9-CM Coordination and Maintenance Committee) and the World Health Organization's ICD-10 (the Update and Revision Committee).

These revisions to ICD-10-CM have included:

- information relevant to ambulatory and managed care encounters
- expanded injury codes
- creation of combination diagnosis/symptom codes to reduce the number of codes needed to fully describe a condition
- the addition of 6th and 7th character classifications
- incorporation of common 4th and 5th character classifications
- classifications specific to laterality
- classification refinement for increased data granularity

This new structure allows for further expansion than was possible with the ICD-9-CM classification system.

This new 2015 draft update release is available for public viewing. ICD-10-CM codes are not currently valid for any purpose or use other than the reporting of mortality data for death certificates.

The Department of Health and Human Services (HHS) published the final rule regarding the adoption of both ICD-10-CM and ICD-10-PCS in the January 16, 2009, Federal Register (45 CFR part 162 [CMS—0013—F]). The initial compliance date for implementation of ICD-10-CM and ICD-10-PCS as a replacement for ICD-9-CM was set at October 1, 2013. On April 17, 2012, the Department of Health and Human Services (HHS) released a notice to postpone the date by which certain health care entities have to comply with International Classification of Diseases, 10th Revision diagnosis and procedure codes (ICD-10). The compliance date for implementation of ICD-10-CM and ICD-10-PCS as a replacement for ICD-9-CM was changed to October 1, 2014. On April 1, 2014, Congress enacted the Protecting Access to Medicare Act of 2014, which contained a provision to delay the implementation of ICD-10-CM/PCS by a least one year. The act prohibits the Department of Health and Human Services (HHS) from adopting the ICD-10-CM/PCS code sets as the mandatory standard until at least October 1, 2015.

ICD-10-CM for Hospitals: The Complete Official Draft Code Set

ICD-10-CM for Hospitals: The Complete Official Draft Code Set 2015 includes many of the enhancements described below in direct response to requests from our subscribers. Many of these enhancements were introduced in the Optum *ICD-9-CM for Hospitals* and users will find many of the conventions, icons, color bars, and other enhancements familiar since many of these features are similar to the hallmark color coding and symbols of our ICD-9-CM code books.

As you review the content, you will find the following:

- Optum Exclusive feature—Check XTension Alert symbol, indicating the need for one or more "filler" x character assignments in the 5th and/or 6th character position to appropriately assign a required character in the 7th character position

- Optum Exclusive feature—Key word differentiation by the use of a green font that highlights the differentiating terms in similar code descriptions in a given category

- Optum Exclusive feature — Exclusive *following* references and Check Additional Character symbol in the indexes. The *following* references (designed and used exclusively by Optum) help coders locate those alphanumeric codes that are out of sequence in the tabular section.

- Optum Exclusive feature — Exclusive shaded guides in the index help users easily follow the indent levels for the subterms under a main term.

- Illustrations at the back of the book feature anatomy and terminology included in the ICD-10-CM classification system

- The complete ICD-10-CM official guidelines for coding and reporting, published by the U.S. Department of Health and Human Services and approved by the cooperating parties (American Health Information Management Association, National Center for Health Statistics, Centers for Medicare and Medicaid Services, American Hospital Association)

- Exclusive color coding, symbols, and footnotes that alert coders to coding and reimbursement issues, including the majority of the Medicare code edits and identification of conditions that significantly affect DRG assignment

- The complication and comorbidity (CC) exclusion list, integrated beneath the applicable codes, which makes it easier to determine complications and comorbidities excluded with a particular principal diagnosis

- All official ICD-10-CM codes, indexes, notes, footnotes, and symbols

- Icons and definitions to differentiate between the two types of Excludes notes

- Check 4th, 5th, 6th, and 7th character symbols identify codes that require the addition of a 4th, 5th, 6th, or 7th character for code specificity and validity

- Color coding and symbol legend at the bottom of each page

Please review "How to Use *ICD-10-CM for Hospitals*" in this manual to learn about the features that will help you assign and report correct codes, ensuring appropriate reimbursement.

How to Use ICD-10-CM for Hospitals (Draft 2015)

This draft of the International Classification of Diseases, 10th Revision, Clinical Modification (ICD-10-CM) is being published by the United States Government in recognition of its responsibility to promulgate this classification throughout the United States for morbidity coding. This code book represents an adaptation of ICD-10 which was created specifically for use in the United States. Future revisions to ICD-10-CM will be made based on the established update process for ICD-9-CM (the ICD-9-CM Coordination and Maintenance Committee) and the World Health Organization's ICD-10 (the Update and Revision Committee). ICD-10-CM has been approved for implementation on October 1, 2015.

Steps to Correct Coding

1. Before beginning to use this code book, review section 1.A., "Conventions for the ICD-10-CM" and section 1.B., "General Coding Guidelines" of the ICD-10-CM Draft Official Guidelines for Coding and Reporting 2014.

2. Look up the main term in the alphabetic index and scan the subterm entries as appropriate. Review continued lines and additional subterms that may appear in the next column or on the next page.

3. Note all parenthetical terms (nonessential modifiers) that help in code selection but do not affect code assignment. Shaded vertical guidelines in the Index are provided to help determine the indentation level for each subterm in relation to the main terms.

4. Pay close attention to the following instructions in the Index:

    – "see," "see also," and "see category" cross-references

    – "with"/"without" notes

    – omit code" notes

    – due to" subterms

    – other instructions found in note boxes, such as "code by site"

    – *Following* references and Check Additional Character symbol in the indexes. The *following* references (designed and used exclusively by Optum) help coders locate those alphanumeric codes that are out of sequence in the tabular section.

5. Do not code from the alphabetic index without verifying the accuracy of the code in the tabular list. Locate the code in the alphanumerically arranged tabular list.

6. To determine the appropriateness of the code selection and proper coding, read all instructional material:

    – "includes" and both types of "excludes" notes

    – "use additional code" and "code first underlying disease"

    – instructions

    – code also"

    – 4th, 5th, and 6thcharacter requirements and 7th character extension requirements

    – CC Exclusions

    – age and sex symbols

7. Consult the official draft ICD-10-CM guidelines, which govern the use of specific codes. These guidelines provide both general and chapter-specific coding guidance.

8. Confirm and assign the correct code.

Organization

This book is organized in the following manner:

Introduction

The introductory material in this book includes the ICD-10-CM Official Preface, the history and future of ICD-10-CM as well as an overview of the classification system.

Draft Official ICD-10-CM Conventions and Guidelines

This section provides an explanation of the conventions and guidelines regulating the appropriate assignment and reporting of ICD-10-CM codes. This coding guidance is presented by the National Center for Health Statistics (NCHS), a governmental agency of the Centers for Disease Control and Prevention (CDC), within the United States Department of Health and Human Services (DHHS).

Alphabetic Index to Diseases

The alphabetic index to diseases is arranged in alphabetic order by disease — by specific illness, injury, eponym, abbreviation, or other descriptive diagnostic term. The Index also lists diagnostic terms for other reasons for encounters with health care professionals.

Neoplasm Table

The Neoplasm Table provides the proper code based upon histology of the neoplasm and site.

Table of Drugs and Chemicals

The Table of Drugs and Chemicals is also included within the Alphabetic Index.

The Table of Drugs and Chemicals lists the drug and the specific codes that identify the drug and the intent. No additional external cause of injury and poisoning code is assigned in ICD-10-CM.

Index to External Causes

The alphabetic index to External Causes of injuries is arranged in alphabetic order by main term indicating the event.

Tabular List of Diseases

ICD-10-CM codes and descriptors are arranged numerically within the tabular list of diseases within 21 separate chapters according to body system or nature of injury and disease. Classifications which were previously considered supplemental to ICD-9-CM (e.g., V codes and E codes) are incorporated into the tabular listing of ICD-10-CM as individual chapters. Chapters 20 External Causes of Morbidity and 21 Factors Influencing Health Status and Contact with Health Services include chapter-specific guidelines.

Illustrations

This section includes illustrations of normal anatomy with ICD-10-CM specific terminology.

Use of Official Sources

The *ICD-10-CM for Hospitals* contains the official U.S. Department of Health and Human Services, Tenth Revision, Clinical Modification (ICD-10-CM) codes, effective for the current year.

The color coding, footnotes, and symbols, which identify coding and reimbursement issues, are derived from official federal government sources, including the Medicare Code Edits (MCE), version 31R.

The ICD-10-CM conventions are general rules for the use of the classification system, independent of the guidelines. These conventions are incorporated within the Index and tabular list as instructional notes and are applicable regardless of the health care setting.

Format

[handwritten: 7 characters, starts with alpha, After 3rd digit there is a decimal]

ICD-10-CM is divided into two main parts: the Index, an alphabetical list of terms and their corresponding code, and the tabular list, a sequential, alphanumeric list of codes divided into chapters based on body system or condition. The Index contains the Index to Diseases and Injuries (main index) and the Index to External Causes of Injury. Also included in the main Index is the Neoplasm Table and a Table of Drugs and Chemicals.

The tabular list contains categories, subcategories, and valid codes.

ICD-10-CM is an alphanumeric classification system. The 1st character of a three-character category is a letter. The 2nd and 3rd characters may be numbers or alpha characters. A three-character category without further subclassification is equivalent to a valid three-character code. Subcategories are either four or five characters. Subcategory characters include either letters or numbers. Codes may be four, five, or six characters in length, in which each level of subdivision after a category is a subcategory. The final level of subdivision is a valid code. The final character in a code may be either a letter or a number.

The ICD-10-CM uses the letter "X" as a place-holder. A placeholder "X" is used as a 5th character place-holder at certain six-character codes to allow for future expansion, without disturbing the 6th character structure. For instance, an initial encounter for accidental poisoning by penicillin is coded to T36.0X1A. The "X" in the 5th character position is a place-holder, or filler character. *[handwritten: correct format]*

Similarly, certain categories have applicable 7th character extensions. In these cases, the 7th character extension is required for all codes within the category, or as otherwise instructed in the tabular list notations. 7th character extensions must always be the last character in the data field. If a code is not a full six characters in length, a dummy place-holder "X" must be used to fill in the empty characters when a 7th character extension is required.

Punctuation

[ ] In the tabular list, brackets are used to enclose synonyms, alternative wording, or explanatory phrases. In the Index, brackets are used to identify manifestation codes.

( ) Parentheses are used in both the Index and tabular list to enclose nonessential modifiers; supplementary words that may be present or absent in the statement of a disease or procedure without affecting the code number to which it is assigned.

: Colons are used in the tabular list after an incomplete term that needs one or more of the modifiers following the colon to make it assignable to a given category.

Abbreviations

NEC

The abbreviation NEC, "Not elsewhere classifiable" represents "other specified" in the ICD-10-CM. An index entry that states NEC directs the coder to an "other specified" code in the tabular list. Codes titled "Other" or "Other specified" in the tabular list (usually a code with a 4th or 6th character 8 and 5th character 9) are for use when the information in the medical record provides detail for which a specific code does not exist.

NOS

The abbreviation NOS, "Not otherwise specified," in the tabular list may be interpreted as "unspecified." Codes in the tabular list with "Unspecified" in the title (usually a code with a 4th or 6th character 9 and 5th character 0) are for use when the information in the medical record is insufficient to assign a more specific code.

Typeface

Boldface

Boldface type is used for main term entries in the alphabetic index, and all codes and descriptions in the tabular list.

Italicized

Italicized type is used for all exclusion notes and to identify manifestation codes, those codes that should not be reported as first-listed (principal) diagnoses.

General Notes

The following conventions and notes appear only in the tabular list of Diseases:

Includes Notes

The word "Includes" appears immediately under certain categories to further define, clarify, or give examples of the content of a code category.

Inclusion Terms

Lists of inclusion terms are included under certain codes. These terms indicate some of the conditions for which that code number may be used. Inclusion terms may be synonyms with the code title, or, in the case of "other specified" codes, the terms may also provide a list of various conditions included within a classification code. The inclusion terms are not exhaustive. The Index may provide additional terms that may also be assigned to a given code.

Excludes Notes

ICD-10-CM has two types of excludes notes. Each note has a different definition for use. However, they are similar in that they both indicate that codes excluded from each other are independent of each other.

Excludes 1

An Excludes 1 note is a "pure" excludes. It means "NOT CODED HERE!" An Excludes 1 note indicates mutually exclusive codes; two conditions that cannot be reported together. For example, a congenital form of a disease may not be reported with the acquired form of the same condition. The code excluded should never be reported with the applicable codes listed above the excludes notation.

Excludes 2

An Excludes 2 note means "NOT INCLUDED HERE." An Excludes 2 note indicates that although the excluded condition is not part of the condition it is excluded from, a patient may have both conditions at the same time. Therefore, when an Excludes 2 note appears under a code, it may be acceptable to use both the code and the excluded code together if supported by the medical documentation.

Default Codes

In the index, the default code is the code listed next to the main term. The default code represents the condition most commonly associated with the main term. This code may be assigned when documentation does not facilitate reporting a more specific code. Alternately, it may provide an unspecified code for the condition.

Syndromes

Follow the alphabetic index guidance when coding syndromes. In the absence of index guidance, assign codes for the documented manifestations of the syndrome.

And

When the term "and" is used in a narrative statement it may be interpreted as "and/or."

With/Without

When "with" and "without" are the two options for the final character of a set of codes, the default is always "without." For five-character codes, a "Ø" as the 5th position character represents "without," and "1" represents "with." For six-character codes, the 6th position character "1" represents "with" and "9" represents "without."

Instructional Notes Used in the Tabular List

In the tabular section, the following instructional notes appear in red type for emphasis:

Code First/Use additional code:

These instructional notes are in red type and provide sequencing instruction. They may appear independently of each other or to designate certain etiology/manifestation paired codes. These instructions signal the coder that an additional code should be reported to provide a more complete picture of that diagnosis.

In etiology/manifestation coding, ICD-10-CM requires the underlying condition to be sequenced first, followed by the manifestation. In these situations, codes with "In diseases classified elsewhere" in the code description are never permitted as a first-listed or principal diagnosis code and must be sequenced following the underlying condition code.

Code Also:

A code also note alerts the coder that more than one code may be required to fully describe the condition. Code sequencing is discretionary. Factors that may determine sequencing include severity and reason for the encounter. These coding notes appear in red type.

Additional Conventions

Color-coding and symbols are included to alert the coder to important reimbursement issues affected by the diagnosis code assignment. Some codes may carry more than one color and/or symbol. For a quick reference to the color codes and their meanings, refer to the color/symbol legend located at the bottom of each page in the tabular listing.

Additional Characters Required

✓4ᵗʰ This symbol indicates that the code requires a 4th character.

✓5ᵗʰ This symbol indicates that the code requires a 5th character.

✓6ᵗʰ This symbol indicates that the code requires a 6th character.

✓7ᵗʰ This symbol indicates that the code requires a 7th character.

✓X7ᵗʰ This symbol indicates that the code requires a 7th character following the placeholder "X". Codes with fewer than six characters that require a 7th character must contain placeholder "X" to fill in the empty character(s).

Boldface

Note
The term "Note" appears enclosed within a red icon and precedes the instructional information. These notes function as an alert, to highlight coding instruction within the text.

Key Word
Green font is used throughout the tabular list of Diseases to differentiate the key words that appear in similar code descriptions in a given category or subcategory.

For example, refer to the list of codes below from category C7A:

C7A.020   Malignant carcinoid tumor of the **appendix**

C7A.021   Malignant carcinoid tumor of the **cecum**

C7A.022   Malignant carcinoid tumor of the **ascending colon**

C7A.023   Malignant carcinoid tumor of the **transverse colon**

C7A.024   Malignant carcinoid tumor of the **descending colon**

C7A.025   Malignant carcinoid tumor of the **sigmoid colon**

C7A.029   Malignant carcinoid tumor of the large intestine, **unspecified portion**

The portion of the code description that appears in bold font above appears in green font in the tabular list, to assist the coder in quickly identifying the key terms and in identifying the correct code. This convention is especially useful when the codes describe laterality, such as the following codes from category H40.22:

H40.221   Chronic angle-closure glaucoma, **right** eye

H40.222   Chronic angle-closure glaucoma, **left** eye

H40.223   Chronic angle-closure glaucoma, **bilateral**

H40.229   Chronic angle-closure glaucoma, **unspecified** eye

The key word convention is only used in those categories in which there are multiple codes with very similar descriptions with only a few words that differentiate them.

Color Coding—Medicare Code Edits
Medicare Administrative Contractors (MACs) and many payers use Medicare code edits to check the coding accuracy on claims. The coding

edit information in this manual is effective from October 1, 2014, to September 30, 2015, and reflects those edits used for acute care hospital inpatient admission. This ICD-10 version of the Medicare Code Editor (MCE) is version 31R. However, the MCE is not intended to be used to process claims because the ICD-10 code set will not be mandated for use until the implementation of ICD-10 beginning no sooner than October 1, 2015.

The Medicare code edits are listed below:

- Invalid diagnosis or procedure code
- External causes of morbidity codes as principal diagnosis
- Duplicate of PDx
- *Age conflict
- *Sex conflict
- *Manifestation code as principal diagnosis
- Nonspecific principal diagnosis (Discontinued as of 10/1/07)
- *Questionable principal diagnosis
- *Unacceptable principal diagnosis
- Nonspecific O.R. procedure (Discontinued as of 10/1/07)
- Noncovered procedure
- Open biopsy check (Discontinued as of 10/1/10)
- Bilateral procedure (Discontinued as of ICD-10 implementation)
- Invalid age
- Invalid sex
- Invalid discharge status
- Limited coverage
- *Wrong procedure performed

Starred edits above that are related to diagnosis issues are identified in this manual by color bars, symbols, or footnotes as described below.

Age and Sex Edit Symbols
The age edits below are used to detect inconsistencies between the patient's age and diagnosis. The following edit symbols appear in the tabular list of diseases to the right of the code description.

Newborn Age: 0   **N**

These diagnoses are intended for newborns and neonates and the patient's age must be 0 years.

Pediatric Age: 0-17   **P**

These diagnoses are intended for children and the patient's age must between 0 and 17 years.

Maternity Age: 12-55   **M**

These diagnoses are intended for childbearing patients between the age of 12 and 55 years.

Adult Age: 15-124   **A**

These diagnoses are intended for the patients between the age of 15 and 124 years.

The sex symbols below are used to detect inconsistencies between the patient's sex and diagnosis. These symbols appear in the tabular list of diseases to the right of the code description.

♂ **Male diagnosis only**

This symbol appears to the right of the code description. This reference appears in the disease and procedure tabular list.

♀ **Female diagnosis only**

This symbol appears to the right of the code description. This reference appears in the disease and procedure tabular list.

Manifestation Code

These codes appear in italic type, with a blue color bar over the title. A manifestation code cannot be reported as a first-listed or principal diagnosis. By definition, a manifestation code represents a demonstration of some aspect of an underlying disease, which is separately classifiable. In the alphabetic index, these codes are listed as the secondary code in brackets. The underlying disease code is listed first.

Unacceptable PDx

These codes will appear with a gray color bar over the code title. These codes do not describe a current illness or injury, but a circumstance which influences a patient's health status. They are considered an unacceptable principal diagnosis for *inpatient* admission.

Questionable admission diagnoses will also appear with a gray color bar over the code title along with a reference to footnote 13. These codes, although not unacceptable as a PDx, may be considered a "questionable admission" when used as PDx in an acute care hospital.

Hospital Acquired Condition (HAC)

These codes will appear with a yellow color bar over the code title. These codes identify conditions that are high cost or high volume or both, are either a complication or comorbidity (CC) or major complication or comorbidity (MCC) that as a secondary diagnosis results in assignment of a case to a higher-paying MS-DRG. These conditions are reasonably preventable through the application of evidence-based guidelines. If the condition is not present on admission (meaning it developed during the hospital admission), the case will not group to the higher-paying MS-DRG based solely upon the reporting of the HAC code. Many of these HACs are conditional, and are based on reporting the specific diagnosis code(s) in combination with certain procedure codes, notated in footnotes.

Wrong Procedure Performed Edit

The Wrong Surgery Edit was created to identify cases in which wrong surgeries occurred. Any claim with a code from the Y65.51-Y65.53 will be denied and returned to the provider. A surgical or other invasive procedure is considered to be a wrong procedure if:

- The procedure was performed on the wrong site
- The procedure was performed on the wrong patient, or
- The incorrect procedure was performed on a patient.

Other Notations in the Tabular

CC Condition

This symbol designates a complication or comorbidity diagnosis that may affect DRG assignment. A complication or comorbidity diagnosis, CC condition, is defined as a significant acute disease, a significant acute manifestation of a chronic disease, an advanced or end stage chronic disease, or a chronic disease associated with systemic physiological decompensation and debility that have consistently greater impact on hospital resources.

A CC icon most often appears to the right of the code description.

MCC Condition

This symbol designates a major complication or comorbidity diagnosis that may affect DRG assignment. An MCC condition meets the same criteria as a CC condition but is associated with a higher acuity level and hospital resource consumption is expected to be higher than that for a CC condition. There are fewer conditions that meet the criteria as an MCC than those for a CC condition.

Similar to a CC icon, an MCC icon appears to the right of the code description.

CC Excludes Notations

Many distinct CC Excludes notations appear directly below the code to which they relate. However, in some cases the CC Excludes information is identical for all codes within a category or subcategory. In those cases, the CC Excludes notation is listed once, at the beginning of the category or subcategory. For example:

G43.6   Persistent migraine aura with cerebral infarction
             CC Excl: For CC codes in subcategory G43.6, unless otherwise noted: G43.601-G43.619, I63.00-I66.9

There are four codes with a CC designation in subcategory G43.6; the CC Excludes notation above applies to all four codes.

Optum ICD-10-CM coding manuals include references to a previously designated CC Excludes notation, and those CC or MCC codes for which there are no excluded conditions. Refer to examples below:

K67   Disorders of peritoneum in infectious diseases classified elsewhere
             CC Excl: See code: K65

A17.83   Tuberculosis neuritis
             CC Excl: No Excl

By definition of being a condition which acts as its own CC or MCC, PDxCC or PDxMCC, the CC exclusion concept (the two conditions being too interrelated) does not apply. However, if a condition carries separate PDxCC/PDxMCC and MCC/CC designations, a CC excludes notation will appear for the CC or MCC designation.

PDx CC PDx MCC PDxCC or PDxMCC Condition

When the MS-DRG system was translated from ICD-9-CM to ICD-10-CM, some significant differences existed. One involved the assignment of two codes in ICD-9-CM, one for an underlying condition, and one for a related acute manifestation. In ICD-10-CM, only one combination code was necessary to replicate the same clinical concept. However, in ICD-9-CM, one of the two codes acted as a CC or MCC for the other. To address this situation, CMS has introduced the concept of certain ICD-10-CM diagnosis codes acting as their own CC or MCC when sequenced as a principal diagnosis. For example, refer to the table below:

ICD-9 PDx	ICD-9 SDx	CC Level	ICD-10 Code with CC or MCC
415.19 Other pulm embolism	415.0 Acute cor pulmonale	MCC	I26.09 Other pulm embolism with acute cor pulmonale

In the ICD-9-CM MS-DRG system, diagnosis code 415.0 acts as an MCC for code 415.19, grouping the case to the highest weighted DRG in its subgroup. In the ICD-10-CM MS-DRG system, the same clinical concept, represented by code I26.09 is sequenced as the principal diagnosis and the code functions as its own MCC. Codes which function as their own CC or MCC when sequenced as a principal diagnosis are designated with the PDxCC or PDxMCC icon to the right of the code description.

HIV HIV

This symbol indicates that the condition is considered a major HIV related diagnosis. When the condition is coded in combination with a diagnosis of human immunodeficiency virus (HIV), code B20, the case will move from MS-DRG 977 to MS-DRGs 974-976.

Bracketed Codes

Some of the ICD-10-CM or ICD-10-PCS referenced codes that appear in this manual use bracketing as a space-saving convention. The numbers or letters within the brackets correspond to all appropriate, valid characters for the character position where the bracket appears. For example:

S04.01[1,2,9] Injury of optic nerve, [right, left, unspecified] eye

The bracketed code above represents three distinct codes:

S04.011	Injury of optic nerve, right eye
S04.012	Injury of optic nerve, left eye
S04.019	Injury of optic nerve, unspecified eye

Similarly, ICD-10-PCS codes may be represented in the same way:

OSU[A,E,R,S] ØBZ Supplement [Right, Left Hip Joint; Acetabular, Femoral Surface] with Resurfacing Device, Open Approach

The bracketed code above represents four distinct codes:

ØSUAØBZ	Supplement Right Hip Joint, Acetabular Surface with Resurfacing Device, Open Approach
ØSUEØBZ	Supplement Left Hip Joint, Acetabular Surface with Resurfacing Device, Open Approach
ØSURØBZ	Supplement Right Hip Joint, Femoral Surface with Resurfacing Device, Open Approach
ØSUSØBZ	Supplement Left Hip Joint, Femoral Surface with Resurfacing Device, Open Approach

Bracketed codes are most often found in CC Excludes notations, as well as in footnotes related to Hospital Acquired Conditions (HACs).

Footnotes

All footnotes are identified by a numerical superscript that appears to the upper left of the code. For example:

[10] I49.01 Ventricular fibrillation

The footnote 10 indicates "MCC = Only if patient is discharged alive." This means that ventricular fibrillation is considered a major complication or comorbidity that may affect DRG assignment only if the patient is discharged alive. Otherwise ventricular fibrillation is assigned as a non-MCC condition.

The following list identifies the meaning of each footnote number in the tabular list of diseases:

1   [HAC 06: Catheter-Associated Urinary Tract Infection (UTI)] This condition represents a hospital acquired condition (HAC) when reported as a secondary diagnosis along with a secondary diagnosis of T83.51XA (Infection and inflammatory reaction due to indwelling urinary catheter, initial encounter) and neither are present on admission.

2   [HAC 11: Surgical Site Infection Following Bariatric Surgery] This condition represents a hospital acquired condition (HAC) when reported as the principal diagnosis along with a secondary diagnosis of K68.11 or K95.01 or K95.81 (surgical site infection) or T81.4XXA (Infection following a procedure, initial encounter) and in combination with one of the following procedure codes, which represent bariatric procedures: ØD16[0,4,8][7,J,K,Z][9,A,B,L] or ØDV64CZ. The secondary diagnosis code is not present on admission.

3   [HAC 10: Deep Vein Thrombosis (DVT)/Pulmonary Embolism (PE) with Total Knee or Hip Replacement] This condition represents a hospital acquired condition (HAC) when reported as a secondary diagnosis in combination with one of the following procedural codes that represent total knee or hip replacement:
ØSR[9,B]0[1,2,3,4,J][9,A,Z]; ØSR[9,B]0[7,K]Z; ØSR[A,E]0[0,1,3,J][9,A,Z]; ØSR[A,E]0[7,K]Z; ØSR[C,D,T,U,V,W]0[7,K]Z; ØSR[C,D,T,U,V,W]0J[9,A,Z]; ØSR[R,S]0[1,3,J][9,A,Z]; ØSR[R,S]0[7,K]Z; ØSU[9,B]ØBZ; ØSU[A,E,R,S]ØBZ. The secondary diagnosis code is not present on admission.

4   [HAC 11: Surgical Site Infection Following Bariatric Surgery] This condition represents a hospital acquired condition (HAC) when reported as a secondary diagnosis along with PDx E66.01 (Morbid obesity) and in combination with one of the following procedure codes, which represent bariatric procedures: ØD16[0,4,8][7,J,K,Z][9,A,B,L] or ØDV64CZ. The secondary diagnosis code is not present on admission.

5   [HAC 08: Surgical Site Infection — Mediastinitis after Coronary Bypass Graft (CABG)] This condition represents a hospital acquired condition (HAC) when reported as a secondary diagnosis in combination with one of the following procedure codes, which represent Coronary Bypass Graft (CABG):
021[0,1,2,3][0,4][9,A,J,K][3,8,9,C,F,W]; 021[0,1,2,3][0,4]Z[3,8,9,C,F]. The secondary diagnosis code is not present on admission.

6   [HAC 12: Surgical Site Infection — Certain Orthopedic Procedures of Spine, Shoulder and Elbow] This condition represents a hospital acquired condition (HAC) when reported as a secondary diagnosis in combination with one of the following procedure codes, which represent spine, shoulder, and elbow procedures:
ØRG[0,1,2,4,6,7,8,A][0,3,4][7,A,J,K,Z][0,1,J]; ØRG[E,F,G,H,J,K][0,3,4][4,7,J,K,Z]Z; ØRG[L,M][0,3,4][4,5,7,J,K,Z]Z; ØRQ[E,F,G,H,J,K,L,M][0,3,4,X]ZZ; ØRU[E,F,G,H,J,K,L,M][0,3,4][7,J,K]Z; ØSG[0,1,3][0,3,4][7,A,J,K,Z][0,1,J]; ØSG[7,8][0,3,4[4,7,J,K,Z]Z. The secondary diagnosis code is not present on admission.

7   This condition represents a hospital acquired condition (HAC) only when reported as the initial encounter (7th character A, B, or C) and the diagnosis is not present upon admission.

8   [HAC 13: Surgical Site Infection (SSI) Following Cardiac Implantable Electronic Device (CIED) Procedures] This condition represents a hospital acquired condition (HAC) when reported as a secondary diagnosis in combination with one of the following procedure codes:
02H43[J,K,M]Z; 02H[6,7]3[J,M]Z; 02H[K,L]3JZ; 02HN[0,3,4][J,M]Z; 02PA[0,3,4]MZ; 02PAXMZ; 02WA[0,3,4]MZ; ØJH[6,8][0,3][4,5,6,7,8,9,P]Z; ØJ[P,W]T[0,3]PZ. The secondary diagnosis is not present upon admission.

9   [HAC 14: Iatrogenic Pneumothorax w/ Venous Catheterization] This condition represents a hospital acquired condition (HAC) when reported as a secondary diagnosis in combination with one of the following procedure codes: 05H[M,N,P,Q]33Z or ØJH63XZ. The secondary diagnosis is not present upon admission.

10 These codes are considered major complication/comorbidity (MCC) conditions and may affect MS-DRG assignment only if the patient is discharged alive.

11 These codes indicate that the wrong procedure was performed on the patient and reimbursement may be affected.

12 This condition represents an unacceptable PDx only when reported as the initial encounter (7th character A).

13 These codes, although not unacceptable as PDx, would be considered questionable as a PDx for acute care hospital admissions.

Other Notations in the Index

Following References

The index includes *following* references to assist in locating "out-of-sequence" codes in the tabular list. "Out-of-sequence" codes contain an alphabetic character (letter) in the 3rd or 4th character position. These codes are placed according to the classification rules — the placement of the codes according to condition — not according to alphabetic or numeric sequencing rules.

Example:

Carcinoma (malignant) (*see also* Neoplasm, by site, malignant)neuroendocrine (*see also* Tumor, neuroendocrine)
    high grade, any site C7A.1 (*following* C75)
    poorly differentiated, any site C7A.1 (*following* C75)

In the tabular rubric, C7A is included after rubric C75 and before C76.

Gout, chronic (*see also* Gout, gouty) M1A.9
    drug-induced M1A.2Ø (*following* MØ8)
      ankle M1A.27-(*following* MØ8)
      elbow M1A.22-(*following* MØ8)

In the tabular rubric, MIA is included after rubric MØ8 and before M1Ø.

ICD-10-CM Draft Official Guidelines for Coding and Reporting 2014

Narrative changes appear in **bold** text.

Items <u>underlined</u> have been moved within the guidelines since the 2013 version.

Italics are used to indicate revisions to heading changes.

The Centers for Medicare and Medicaid Services (CMS) and the National Center for Health Statistics (NCHS), two departments within the U.S. Federal Government's Department of Health and Human Services (DHHS) provide the following guidelines for coding and reporting using the International Classification of Diseases, 10th Revision, Clinical Modification (ICD-10-CM). These guidelines should be used as a companion document to the official version of the ICD-10-CM as published on the NCHS website. The ICD-10-CM is a morbidity classification published by the United States for classifying diagnoses and reason for visits in all health care settings. The ICD-10-CM is based on the ICD-10, the statistical classification of disease published by the World Health Organization (WHO).

These guidelines have been approved by the four organizations that make up the Cooperating Parties for the ICD-10-CM: the American Hospital Association (AHA), the American Health Information Management Association (AHIMA), CMS, and NCHS.

These guidelines are a set of rules that have been developed to accompany and complement the official conventions and instructions provided within the ICD-10-CM itself. The instructions and conventions of the classification take precedence over guidelines. These guidelines are based on the coding and sequencing instructions in the Tabular List and Alphabetic Index of ICD-10-CM, but provide additional instruction. Adherence to these guidelines when assigning ICD-10-CM diagnosis codes is required under the Health Insurance Portability and Accountability Act (HIPAA). The diagnosis codes (Tabular List and Alphabetic Index) have been adopted under HIPAA for all healthcare settings. A joint effort between the healthcare provider and the coder is essential to achieve complete and accurate documentation, code assignment, and reporting of diagnoses and procedures. These guidelines have been developed to assist both the healthcare provider and the coder in identifying those diagnoses and procedures that are to be reported. The importance of consistent, complete documentation in the medical record cannot be overemphasized. Without such documentation accurate coding cannot be achieved. The entire record should be reviewed to determine the specific reason for the encounter and the conditions treated.

The term encounter is used for all settings, including hospital admissions. In the context of these guidelines, the term provider is used throughout the guidelines to mean physician or any qualified health care practitioner who is legally accountable for establishing the patient's diagnosis. Only this set of guidelines, approved by the Cooperating Parties, is official.

The guidelines are organized into sections. Section I includes the structure and conventions of the classification and general guidelines that apply to the entire classification, and chapter-specific guidelines that correspond to the chapters as they are arranged in the classification. Section II includes guidelines for selection of principal diagnosis for non-outpatient settings. Section III includes guidelines for reporting additional diagnoses in non-outpatient settings. Section IV is for outpatient coding and reporting. It is necessary to review all sections of the guidelines to fully understand all of the rules and instructions needed to code properly.

Section I. Conventions, general coding guidelines and chapter specific guidelines 3
- A. Conventions for the ICD-10-CM 3
  1. The Alphabetic Index and Tabular List 3
  2. Format and Structure 3
  3. Use of codes for reporting purposes 3
  4. Placeholder character 3
  5. 7th Characters 3
  6. Abbreviations 3
     a. Alphabetic Index abbreviations 3
     b. Tabular List abbreviations 3
  7. Punctuation 3
  8. Use of "and" 3
  9. Other and Unspecified codes 3
     a. "Other" codes 3
     b. "Unspecified" codes 3
  10. Includes Notes 3
  11. Inclusion Terms 3
  12. Excludes Notes 3
     a. Excludes1 3
     b. Excludes2 3
  13. Etiology/manifestation convention ("code first", "use additional code" and "in diseases classified elsewhere" notes) 3

  14. "And" 4
  15. "With" 4
  16. "See" and "See Also" 4
  17. "Code also note" 4
  18. Default codes 4
- B. General Coding Guidelines 4
  1. Locating a code in the ICD-10-CM 4
  2. Level of Detail in Coding 4
  3. Code or codes from A00.0 through T88.9, Z00-Z99.8 ... 4
  4. Signs and symptoms 4
  5. Conditions that are an integral part of a disease process ... 4
  6. Conditions that are not an integral part of a disease process ... 4
  7. Multiple coding for a single condition 4
  8. Acute and Chronic Conditions 5
  9. Combination Code 5
  10. Sequela (Late Effects) 5
  11. Impending or Threatened Condition 5
  12. Reporting Same Diagnosis Code More than Once 5
  13. Laterality 5
  14. Documentation for BMI, Non-pressure Ulcers and Pressure Ulcer Stages 5
  15. Syndromes 5
  16. Documentation of Complications of Care 5
  17. Borderline Diagnosis 5
  18. Use of Sign/Symptom/Unspecified Codes 5
- C. Chapter-Specific Coding Guidelines 6
  1. Chapter 1: Certain Infectious and Parasitic Diseases (A00-B99) 6
     a. Human immunodeficiency virus (HIV) infections 6
     b. Infectious agents as the cause of diseases classified to other chapters 6
     c. Infections resistant to antibiotics 6
     d. Sepsis, severe sepsis, and septic shock 6
     e. Methicillin resistant *Staphylococcus aureus* (MRSA) conditions 7
  2. Chapter 2: Neoplasms (C00-D49) 8
     a. Treatment directed at the malignancy 8
     b. Treatment of secondary site 8
     c. Coding and sequencing of complications 8
     d. Primary malignancy previously excised 8
     e. Admissions/Encounters involving chemotherapy, immunotherapy and radiation therapy 8
     f. Admission/encounter to determine extent of malignancy 9
     g. Symptoms, signs, and abnormal findings listed in Chapter 18 associated with neoplasms 9
     h. Admission/encounter for pain control/management 9
     i. Malignancy in two or more noncontiguous sites 9
     j. Disseminated malignant neoplasm, unspecified 9
     k. Malignant neoplasm without specification of site 9
     l. Sequencing of neoplasm codes 9
     m. Current malignancy versus personal history of malignancy 9
     n. Leukemia, multiple myeloma, and malignant plasma cell neoplasms in remission versus personal history 9
     o. Aftercare following surgery for neoplasm 9
     p. Follow-up care for completed treatment of a malignancy 9
     q. Prophylactic organ removal for prevention of malignancy 9
     r. Malignant neoplasm associated with transplanted organ 9
  3. Chapter 3: Disease of the Blood and Blood-forming Organs and Certain Disorders Involving the Immune Mechanism (D50-D89) .. 9
  4. Chapter 4: Endocrine, Nutritional, and Metabolic Diseases (E00-E89) 10
     a. Diabetes mellitus 10
  5. Chapter 5: Mental, Behavioral and Neurodevelopmental Disorders (F01 – F99) 10
     a. Pain disorders related to psychological factors 10
     b. Mental and behavioral disorders due to psychoactive substance use 10
  6. Chapter 6: Diseases of Nervous System (G00-G99) 10
     a. Dominant/nondominant side 10
     b. Pain - Category G89 11
  7. Chapter 7: Diseases of Eye and Adnexa (H00-H59) 11
     a. Glaucoma 11
  8. Chapter 8: Diseases of Ear and Mastoid Process (H60-H95) 12
  9. Chapter 9: Diseases of Circulatory System (I00-I99) 12

    a. Hypertension 12
    b. Atherosclerotic coronary artery disease and angina 12
    c. Intraoperative and postprocedural cerebrovascular accident 12
    d. Sequelae of cerebrovascular disease 13
    e. Acute myocardial infarction (AMI) 13
10. Chapter 10: Diseases of *the* Respiratory System (J00-J99) 13
    a. Chronic Obstructive Pulmonary Disease [COPD] and Asthma 13
    b. Acute Respiratory Failure 13
    c. Influenza due to certain identified influenza viruses 13
    d. Ventilator associated pneumonia 13
11. Chapter 11: Diseases of the Digestive System (K00-K95) 14
12. Chapter 12: Diseases of the Skin and Subcutaneous Tissue (L00-L99) 14
    a. Pressure ulcer stage codes 14
13. Chapter 13: Diseases of the Musculoskeletal System and Connective Tissue (M00-M99) 14
    a. Site and laterality 14
    b. Acute traumatic versus chronic or recurrent musculoskeletal conditions 14
    c. Coding of Pathologic Fractures 14
    d. Osteoporosis 14
14. Chapter 14: Diseases of Genitourinary System (N00-N99) 15
    a. Chronic kidney disease 15
15. Chapter 15: Pregnancy, Childbirth, and the Puerperium (O00-O9A) 15
    a. General Rules for Obstetric Cases 15
    b. Selection of OB principal or first-listed diagnosis 15
    c. Pre-existing conditions versus conditions due to the pregnancy 16
    d. Pre-existing hypertension in pregnancy 16
    e. Fetal conditions affecting the management of the mother 16
    f. HIV Infection in pregnancy, childbirth and the puerperium 16
    g. Diabetes mellitus in pregnancy 16
    h. Long term use of insulin 16
    i. Gestational (pregnancy induced) diabetes 16
    j. Sepsis and septic shock complicating abortion, pregnancy, childbirth and the puerperium 16
    k. Puerperal sepsis 16
    l. Alcohol and tobacco use during pregnancy, childbirth and the puerperium 16
    m. Poisoning, toxic effects, adverse effects and underdosing in a pregnant patient 16
    n. Normal delivery, code O80 16
    o. The peripartum and postpartum periods 17
    p. Code O94, Sequelae of complication of pregnancy, childbirth, and the puerperium 17
    q. Termination of Pregnancy and Spontaneous Abortions 17
    r. Abuse in a pregnant patient 17
16. Chapter 16: Certain Conditions Origination in the Perinatal Period (P00-P96) 17
    a. General Perinatal Rules 17
    b. Observation and evaluation of newborns for suspected conditions not found 18
    c. Coding Additional Perinatal Diagnoses 18
    d. Prematurity and fetal growth retardation 18
    e. Low birth weight and immaturity status 18
    f. Bacterial sepsis of newborn 18
    g. Stillbirth 18
17. Chapter 17: Congenital Malformations, Deformations, and Chromosomal Abnormalities (Q00-Q99) 18
18. Chapter 18: Symptoms, Signs, and Abnormal Clinical and Laboratory Findings, Not Elsewhere Classified (R00-R99) 18
    a. Use of symptom codes 18
    b. Use of a symptom code with a definitive diagnosis code 18
    c. Combination codes that include symptoms 18
    d. Repeated falls 18
    e. Coma scale 18
    f. Functional quadriplegia 18
    g. SIRS due to non-infectious process 18
    h. Death NOS 19
19. Chapter 19: Injury, Poisoning, and Certain Other Consequences of External Causes (S00-T88) 19
    a. Application of 7th Characters in Chapter 19 19

    b. Coding of injuries 19
    c. Coding of traumatic fractures 19
    d. Coding of burns and corrosions 19
    e. Adverse effects, poisoning, underdosing and toxic effects 20
    f. Adult and child abuse, neglect and other maltreatment 21
    g. Complications of care 21
20. Chapter 20: External Causes of Morbidity (V00-Y99) 21
    a. General external cause coding guidelines 21
    b. Place of occurrence guideline 22
    c. Activity code 22
    d. Place of occurrence, activity, and status codes used with other external cause code 22
    e. If the reporting format limits the number of external cause codes 22
    f. Multiple external cause coding guidelines 22
    g. Child and adult abuse guideline 22
    h. Unknown or undetermined intent guideline 22
    i. Sequelae (Late Effects) of external cause guidelines 22
    j. Terrorism guidelines 22
    k. External cause status 22
21. Chapter 21: Factors Influencing Health Status and Contact with Health Services (Z00-Z99) 23
    a. Use of Z codes in any healthcare setting 23
    b. Z Codes indicate a reason for an encounter 23
    c. Categories of Z codes 23

Section II. Selection of Principal Diagnosis **27**
  A. Codes for symptoms, signs, and ill-defined conditions 27
  B. Two or more interrelated conditions, each potentially meeting the definition for principal diagnosis 27
  C. Two or more diagnoses that equally meet the definition for principal diagnosis 27
  D. Two or more comparative or contrasting conditions 27
  E. A symptom(s) followed by contrasting/ comparative diagnoses 27
  F. Original treatment plan not carried out 28
  G. Complications of surgery and other medical care 28
  H. Uncertain diagnosis 28
  I. Admission from observation unit 28
    1. Admission Following Medical Observation 28
    2. Admission Following Post-Operative Observation 28
  J. Admission from outpatient surgery 28
  K. Admissions/Encounters for Rehabilitation 28
Section III. Reporting Additional Diagnoses **28**
  A. Previous conditions 28
  B. Abnormal findings 28
  C. Uncertain Diagnosis 28
Section IV. Diagnostic Coding and Reporting Guidelines for Outpatient Services **29**
  A. Selection of first-listed condition 29
    1. Outpatient surgery 29
    2. Observation stay 29
  B. Codes from A00.0 through T88.9, Z00-Z99 29
  C. Accurate reporting of ICD-10-CM diagnosis codes 29
  D. Codes that describe symptoms and signs 29
  E. Encounters for circumstances other than a disease or injury 29
  F. Level of Detail in Coding 29
    1. ICD-10-CM codes with 3, 4, 5, 6 or 7 characters 29
    2. Use of full number of characters required for a code 29
  G. ICD-10-CM code for the diagnosis, condition, problem, or other reason for encounter/visit 29
  H. Uncertain diagnosis 29
  I. Chronic diseases 29
  J. Code all documented conditions that coexist 29
  K. Patients receiving diagnostic services only 29
  L. Patients receiving therapeutic services only 29
  M. Patients receiving preoperative evaluations only 30
  N. Ambulatory surgery 30
  O. Routine outpatient prenatal visits 30
  P. Encounters for general medical examinations with abnormal findings 30
  Q. Encounters for routine health screenings 30
Appendix I. Present on Admission Reporting Guidelines **30**
Categories and Codes Exempt from Diagnosis Present on Admission Requirement **31**

Section I. Conventions, general coding guidelines and chapter specific guidelines

The conventions, general guidelines and chapter-specific guidelines are applicable to all health care settings unless otherwise indicated. The conventions and instructions of the classification take precedence over guidelines.

A. Conventions for the ICD-10-CM

The conventions for the ICD-10-CM are the general rules for use of the classification independent of the guidelines. These conventions are incorporated within the Alphabetic Index and Tabular List of the ICD-10-CM as instructional notes.

1. **The Alphabetic Index and Tabular List**
   The ICD-10-CM is divided into the Alphabetic Index, an alphabetical list of terms and their corresponding code, and the Tabular List, a structured chronological list of codes divided into chapters based on body system or condition. The Alphabetic Index consists of the following parts: the Index of Diseases and Injury, the Index of External Causes of Injury, the Table of Neoplasms and the Table of Drugs and Chemicals.

   See Section I.C2. General guidelines

   See Section I.C.19. Adverse effects, poisoning, underdosing and toxic effects

2. **Format and Structure**
   The ICD-10-CM Tabular List contains categories, subcategories and codes. Characters for categories, subcategories and codes may be either a letter or a number. All categories are 3 characters. A three-character category that has no further subdivision is equivalent to a code. Subcategories are either 4 or 5 characters. Codes may be 3, 4, 5, 6 or 7 characters. That is, each level of subdivision after a category is a subcategory. The final level of subdivision is a code. Codes that have applicable 7th characters are still referred to as codes, not subcategories. A code that has an applicable 7th character is considered invalid without the 7th character.

   The ICD-10-CM uses an indented format for ease in reference.

3. **Use of codes for reporting purposes**
   For reporting purposes only codes are permissible, not categories or subcategories, and any applicable 7th character is required.

4. **Placeholder character**
   The ICD-10-CM utilizes a placeholder character "X". The "X" is used as a placeholder at certain codes to allow for future expansion. An example of this is at the poisoning, adverse effect and underdosing codes, categories T36-T50.

   Where a placeholder exists, the X must be used in order for the code to be considered a valid code.

5. **7th Characters**
   Certain ICD-10-CM categories have applicable 7th characters. The applicable 7th character is required for all codes within the category, or as the notes in the Tabular List instruct. The 7th character must always be the 7th character in the data field. If a code that requires a 7th character is not 6 characters, a placeholder X must be used to fill in the empty characters.

6. **Abbreviations**
   a. **Alphabetic Index abbreviations**
      NEC   "Not elsewhere classifiable"
             This abbreviation in the Alphabetic Index represents "other specified". When a specific code is not available for a condition, the Alphabetic Index directs the coder to the "other specified" code in the Tabular List.
      NOS   "Not otherwise specified"
             This abbreviation is the equivalent of unspecified.
   b. **Tabular List abbreviations**
      NEC   "Not elsewhere classifiable"
             This abbreviation in the Tabular List represents "other specified". When a specific code is not available for a condition the Tabular List includes an NEC entry under a code to identify the code as the "other specified" code.
      NOS   "Not otherwise specified"
             This abbreviation is the equivalent of unspecified.

7. **Punctuation**
   [ ]   Brackets are used in the Tabular List to enclos alternative wording or explanatory phrases. Alphabetic Index to identify manifestation o

   ( )   Parentheses are used in both the Alphabeti to enclose supplementary words that may the statement of a disease or procedure w number to which it is assigned. The terms are referred to as nonessential modifiers. **modifiers in the Alphabetic Index to Diseases apply to subterms following a main term except when a nonessential modifier and a subentry are mutually exclusive, the subentry takes precedence. For example, in the ICD-10-CM Alphabetic Index under the main term Enteritis, "acute" is a nonessential modifier and "chronic" is a subentry. In this case, the nonessential modifier "acute" does not apply to the subentry "chronic".**

   :   Colons are used in the Tabular List after an incomplete term which needs one or more of the modifiers following the colon to make it assignable to a given category.

8. **Use of "and"**
   See Section I.A.14. Use of the term "And"

9. **Other and Unspecified codes**
   a. **"Other" codes**
      Codes titled "other" or "other specified" are for use when the information in the medical record provides detail for which a specific code does not exist. Alphabetic Index entries with NEC in the line designate "other" codes in the Tabular List. These Alphabetic Index entries represent specific disease entities for which no specific code exists so the term is included within an "other" code.

   b. **"Unspecified" codes**
      Codes titled "unspecified" are for use when the information in the medical record is insufficient to assign a more specific code. For those categories for which an unspecified code is not provided, the "other specified" code may represent both other and unspecified.

   See Section I.B.18 Use of Signs/Symptom/Unspecified Codes

10. **Includes Notes**
    This note appears immediately under a three character code title to further define, or give examples of, the content of the category.

11. **Inclusion Terms**
    List of terms is included under some codes. These terms are the conditions for which that code is to be used. The terms may be synonyms of the code title, or, in the case of "other specified" codes, the terms are a list of the various conditions assigned to that code. The inclusion terms are not necessarily exhaustive. Additional terms found only in the Alphabetic Index may also be assigned to a code.

12. **Excludes Notes**
    The ICD-10-CM has two types of excludes notes. Each type of note has a different definition for use but they are all similar in that they indicate that codes excluded from each other are independent of each other.

    a. **Excludes1**
       A type 1 Excludes note is a pure excludes note. It means "NOT CODED HERE!" An Excludes1 note indicates that the code excluded should never be used at the same time as the code above the Excludes1 note. An Excludes1 is used when two conditions cannot occur together, such as a congenital form versus an acquired form of the same condition.

    b. **Excludes2**
       A type 2 Excludes note represents "Not included here". An excludes2 note indicates that the condition excluded is not part of the condition represented by the code, but a patient may have both conditions at the same time. When an Excludes2 note appears under a code, it is acceptable to use both the code and the excluded code together, when appropriate.

13. **Etiology/manifestation convention ("code first", "use additional code" and "in diseases classified elsewhere" notes)**
    Certain conditions have both an underlying etiology and multiple body system manifestations due to the underlying etiology. For such conditions, the ICD-10-CM has a coding convention that requires the underlying condition be sequenced first followed by the manifestation.

ever such a combination exists, there is a "use additional code" e at the etiology code, and a "code first" note at the manifestation ode. These instructional notes indicate the proper sequencing order of the codes, etiology followed by manifestation.

In most cases the manifestation codes will have in the code title, "in diseases classified elsewhere." Codes with this title are a component of the etiology/ manifestation convention. The code title indicates that it is a manifestation code. "In diseases classified elsewhere" codes are never permitted to be used as first-listed or principal diagnosis codes. They must be used in conjunction with an underlying condition code and they must be listed following the underlying condition. See category F02, Dementia in other diseases classified elsewhere, for an example of this convention.

There are manifestation codes that do not have "in diseases classified elsewhere" in the title. For such codes, there is a "use additional code" note at the etiology code and a "code first" note at the manifestation code and the rules for sequencing apply.

In addition to the notes in the Tabular List, these conditions also have a specific Alphabetic Index entry structure. In the Alphabetic Index both conditions are listed together with the etiology code first followed by the manifestation codes in brackets. The code in brackets is always to be sequenced second.

An example of the etiology/manifestation convention is dementia in Parkinson's disease. In the Alphabetic Index, code G20 is listed first, followed by code F02.80 or F02.81 in brackets. Code G20 represents the underlying etiology, Parkinson's disease, and must be sequenced first, whereas codes F02.80 and F02.81 represent the manifestation of dementia in diseases classified elsewhere, with or without behavioral disturbance.

"Code first" and "Use additional code" notes are also used as sequencing rules in the classification for certain codes that are not part of an etiology/ manifestation combination.

See Section I.B.7. Multiple coding for a single condition.

14. "And"

The word "and" should be interpreted to mean either "and" or "or" when it appears in a title.

For example, cases of "tuberculosis of bones", "tuberculosis of joints" and "tuberculosis of bones and joints" are classified to subcategory A18.0, Tuberculosis of bones and joints.

15. "With"

The word "with" should be interpreted to mean "associated with" or "due to" when it appears in a code title, the Alphabetic Index, or an instructional note in the Tabular List.

The word "with" in the Alphabetic Index is sequenced immediately following the main term, not in alphabetical order.

16. "See" and "See Also"

The "see" instruction following a main term in the Alphabetic Index indicates that another term should be referenced. It is necessary to go to the main term referenced with the "see" note to locate the correct code.

A "see also" instruction following a main term in the Alphabetic Index instructs that there is another main term that may also be referenced that may provide additional Alphabetic Index entries that may be useful. It is not necessary to follow the "see also" note when the original main term provides the necessary code.

17. "Code also note"

A "code also" note instructs that two codes may be required to fully describe a condition, but this note does not provide sequencing direction.

18. Default codes

A code listed next to a main term in the ICD-10-CM Alphabetic Index is referred to as a default code. The default code represents that condition that is most commonly associated with the main term, or is the unspecified code for the condition. If a condition is documented in a medical record (for example, appendicitis) without any additional information, such as acute or chronic, the default code should be assigned.

B. General Coding Guidelines

1. Locating a code in the ICD-10-CM

To select a code in the classification that corresponds to a diagnosis or reason for visit documented in a medical record, first locate the term in the Alphabetic Index, and then verify the code in the Tabular List. Read and be guided by instructional notations that appear in both the Alphabetic Index and the Tabular List.

It is essential to use both the Alphabetic Index and Tabular List when locating and assigning a code. The Alphabetic Index does not always provide the full code. Selection of the full code, including laterality and any applicable 7th character can only be done in the Tabular List. A dash (-) at the end of an Alphabetic Index entry indicates that additional characters are required. Even if a dash is not included at the Alphabetic Index entry, it is necessary to refer to the Tabular List to verify that no 7th character is required.

2. Level of Detail in Coding

Diagnosis codes are to be used and reported at their highest number of characters available.

ICD-10-CM diagnosis codes are composed of codes with 3, 4, 5, 6 or 7 characters. Codes with three characters are included in ICD-10-CM as the heading of a category of codes that may be further subdivided by the use of fourth and/or fifth characters and/or sixth characters, which provide greater detail.

A three-character code is to be used only if it is not further subdivided. A code is invalid if it has not been coded to the full number of characters required for that code, including the 7th character, if applicable.

3. Code or codes from A00.0 through T88.9, Z00-Z99.8

The appropriate code or codes from A00.0 through T88.9, Z00-Z99.8 must be used to identify diagnoses, symptoms, conditions, problems, complaints or other reason(s) for the encounter/visit.

4. Signs and symptoms

Codes that describe symptoms and signs, as opposed to diagnoses, are acceptable for reporting purposes when a related definitive diagnosis has not been established (confirmed) by the provider. Chapter 18 of ICD-10-CM, Symptoms, Signs, and Abnormal Clinical and Laboratory Findings, Not Elsewhere Classified (codes R00.0 - R99) contains many, but not all codes for symptoms.

See Section I.B.18 Use of Signs/Symptom/Unspecified Codes

5. Conditions that are an integral part of a disease process

Signs and symptoms that are associated routinely with a disease process should not be assigned as additional codes, unless otherwise instructed by the classification.

6. Conditions that are not an integral part of a disease process

Additional signs and symptoms that may not be associated routinely with a disease process should be coded when present.

7. Multiple coding for a single condition

In addition to the etiology/manifestation convention that requires two codes to fully describe a single condition that affects multiple body systems, there are other single conditions that also require more than one code. "Use additional code" notes are found in the Tabular List at codes that are not part of an etiology/manifestation pair where a secondary code is useful to fully describe a condition. The sequencing rule is the same as the etiology/manifestation pair, "use additional code" indicates that a secondary code should be added.

For example, for bacterial infections that are not included in chapter 1, a secondary code from category B95, Streptococcus, Staphylococcus, and Enterococcus, as the cause of diseases classified elsewhere, or B96, Other bacterial agents as the cause of diseases classified elsewhere, may be required to identify the bacterial organism causing the infection. A "use additional code" note will normally be found at the infectious disease code, indicating a need for the organism code to be added as a secondary code.

"Code first" notes are also under certain codes that are not specifically manifestation codes but may be due to an underlying cause. When there is a "code first" note and an underlying condition is present, the underlying condition should be sequenced first.

"Code, if applicable, any causal condition first", notes indicate that this code may be assigned as a principal diagnosis when the causal condition is unknown or not applicable. If a causal condition is known, then the

without additional info we

code for that condition should be sequenced as the principal or first-listed diagnosis.

Multiple codes may be needed for sequela, complication codes and obstetric codes to more fully describe a condition. See the specific guidelines for these conditions for further instruction.

8. Acute and Chronic Conditions
If the same condition is described as both acute (subacute) and chronic, and separate subentries exist in the Alphabetic Index at the same indentation level, code both and sequence the acute (subacute) code first.

9. Combination Code
A combination code is a single code used to classify:

> Two diagnoses, or
>> A diagnosis with an associated secondary process (manifestation)
>> A diagnosis with an associated complication

Combination codes are identified by referring to subterm entries in the Alphabetic Index and by reading the inclusion and exclusion notes in the Tabular List.

Assign only the combination code when that code fully identifies the diagnostic conditions involved or when the Alphabetic Index so directs. Multiple coding should not be used when the classification provides a combination code that clearly identifies all of the elements documented in the diagnosis. When the combination code lacks necessary specificity in describing the manifestation or complication, an additional code should be used as a secondary code.

10. Sequela (Late Effects)
A sequela is the residual effect (condition produced) after the acute phase of an illness or injury has terminated. There is no time limit on when a sequela code can be used. The residual may be apparent early, such as in cerebral infarction, or it may occur months or years later, such as that due to a previous injury. Coding of sequela generally requires two codes sequenced in the following order: The condition or nature of the sequela is sequenced first. The sequela code is sequenced second.

An exception to the above guidelines are those instances where the code for the sequela is followed by a manifestation code identified in the Tabular List and title, or the sequela code has been expanded (at the fourth, fifth or sixth character levels) to include the manifestation(s). The code for the acute phase of an illness or injury that led to the sequela is never used with a code for the late effect.

See Section I.C.9. Sequelae of cerebrovascular disease

See Section I.C.15. Sequelae of complication of pregnancy, childbirth and the puerperium

See Section I.C.19. Application of 7th characters for Chapter 19

11. Impending or Threatened Condition
Code any condition described at the time of discharge as "impending" or "threatened" as follows:

> If it did occur, code as confirmed diagnosis.
> If it did not occur, reference the Alphabetic Index to determine if the condition has a subentry term for "impending" or "threatened" and also reference main term entries for "Impending" and for "Threatened."
> If the subterms are listed, assign the given code.
> If the subterms are not listed, code the existing underlying condition(s) and not the condition described as impending or threatened.

12. Reporting Same Diagnosis Code more than Once
Each unique ICD-10-CM diagnosis code may be reported only once for an encounter. This applies to bilateral conditions when there are no distinct codes identifying laterality or two different conditions classified to the same ICD-10-CM diagnosis code.

13. Laterality
Some ICD-10-CM codes indicate laterality, specifying whether the condition occurs on the left, right or is bilateral. If no bilateral code is provided and the condition is bilateral, assign separate codes for both

the left and right side. If the side is not identified in the medical record, assign the code for the unspecified side.

14. Documentation for BMI, Non-pressure Ulcers and Pressure Ulcer Stages
For the Body Mass Index (BMI), depth of non-pressure chronic ulcers and pressure ulcer stage codes, code assignment may be based on medical record documentation from clinicians who are not the patient's provider (i.e., physician or other qualified healthcare practitioner legally accountable for establishing the patient's diagnosis), since this information is typically documented by other clinicians involved in the care of the patient (e.g., a dietitian often documents the BMI and nurses often documents the pressure ulcer stages). However, the associated diagnosis (such as overweight, obesity, or pressure ulcer) must be documented by the patient's provider. If there is conflicting medical record documentation, either from the same clinician or different clinicians, the patient's attending provider should be queried for clarification.

The BMI codes should only be reported as secondary diagnoses. As with all other secondary diagnosis codes, the BMI codes should only be assigned when they meet the definition of a reportable additional diagnosis (see Section III, Reporting Additional Diagnoses).

15. Syndromes
Follow the Alphabetic Index guidance when coding syndromes. In the absence of Alphabetic Index guidance, assign codes for the documented manifestations of the syndrome.

Additional codes for manifestations that are not an integral part of the disease process may also be assigned when the condition does not have a unique code.

16. Documentation of Complications of Care
Code assignment is based on the provider's documentation of the relationship between the condition and the care or procedure. The guideline extends to any complications of care, regardless of the chapter the code is located in. It is important to note that not all conditions that occur during or following medical care or surgery are classified as complications. There must be a cause-and-effect relationship between the care provided and the condition, and an indication in the documentation that it is a complication. Query the provider for clarification, if the complication is not clearly documented.

17. Borderline Diagnosis
If the provider documents a "borderline" diagnosis at the time of discharge, the diagnosis is coded as confirmed, unless the classification provides a specific entry (e.g., borderline diabetes). If a borderline condition has a specific index entry in ICD-10-CM, it should be coded as such. Since borderline conditions are not uncertain diagnoses, no distinction is made between the care setting (inpatient versus outpatient). Whenever the documentation is unclear regarding a borderline condition, coders are encouraged to query for clarification.

18. Use of Sign/Symptom/Unspecified Codes
Sign/symptom and "unspecified" codes have acceptable, even necessary, uses. While specific diagnosis codes should be reported when they are supported by the available medical record documentation and clinical knowledge of the patient's health condition, there are instances when signs/symptoms or unspecified codes are the best choices for accurately reflecting the healthcare encounter. Each healthcare encounter should be coded to the level of certainty known for that encounter.

If a definitive diagnosis has not been established by the end of the encounter, it is appropriate to report codes for sign(s) and/or symptom(s) in lieu of a definitive diagnosis. When sufficient clinical information isn't known or available about a particular health condition to assign a more specific code, it is acceptable to report the appropriate "unspecified" code (e.g., a diagnosis of pneumonia has been determined, but not the specific type). Unspecified codes should be reported when they are the codes that most accurately reflects what is known about the patient's condition at the time of that particular encounter. It would be inappropriate to select a specific code that is not supported by the medical record documentation or conduct medically unnecessary diagnostic testing in order to determine a more specific code.

Ruled out – Proven not exist [handwritten note]

C. Chapter-Specific Coding Guidelines

In addition to general coding guidelines, there are guidelines for specific diagnoses and/or conditions in the classification. Unless otherwise indicated, these guidelines apply to all health care settings. Please refer to Section II for guidelines on the selection of principal diagnosis.

1. Chapter 1: Certain Infectious and Parasitic Diseases (A00-B99)

a. Human immunodeficiency virus (HIV) infections

1) Code only confirmed cases

Code only confirmed cases of HIV infection/illness. This is an exception to the hospital inpatient guideline Section II, H.

In this context, "confirmation" does not require documentation of positive serology or culture for HIV; the provider's diagnostic statement that the patient is HIV positive, or has an HIV-related illness is sufficient.

2) Selection and sequencing of HIV codes

(a) Patient admitted for HIV-related condition

If a patient is admitted for an HIV-related condition, the principal diagnosis should be B20, Human immunodeficiency virus [HIV] disease followed by additional diagnosis codes for all reported HIV-related conditions.

(b) Patient with HIV disease admitted for unrelated condition

If a patient with HIV disease is admitted for an unrelated condition (such as a traumatic injury), the code for the unrelated condition (e.g., the nature of injury code) should be the principal diagnosis. Other diagnoses would be B20 followed by additional diagnosis codes for all reported HIV-related conditions.

(c) Whether the patient is newly diagnosed

Whether the patient is newly diagnosed or has had previous admissions/encounters for HIV conditions is irrelevant to the sequencing decision.

(d) Asymptomatic human immunodeficiency virus

Z21, Asymptomatic human immunodeficiency virus [HIV] infection status, is to be applied when the patient without any documentation of symptoms is listed as being "HIV positive," "known HIV," "HIV test positive," or similar terminology. Do not use this code if the term "AIDS" is used or if the patient is treated for any HIV-related illness or is described as having any condition(s) resulting from his/her HIV positive status; use B20 in these cases.

(e) Patients with inconclusive HIV serology

Patients with inconclusive HIV serology, but no definitive diagnosis or manifestations of the illness, may be assigned code R75, Inconclusive laboratory evidence of human immunodeficiency virus [HIV].

(f) Previously diagnosed HIV-related illness

Patients with any known prior diagnosis of an HIV-related illness should be coded to B20. Once a patient has developed an HIV-related illness, the patient should always be assigned code B20 on every subsequent admission/encounter. Patients previously diagnosed with any HIV illness (B20) should never be assigned to R75 or Z21, Asymptomatic human immunodeficiency virus [HIV] infection status.

(g) HIV infection in pregnancy, childbirth and the puerperium

During pregnancy, childbirth or the puerperium, a patient admitted (or presenting for a health care encounter) because of an HIV-related illness should receive a principal diagnosis code of O98.7-, Human immunodeficiency [HIV] disease complicating pregnancy, childbirth and the puerperium, followed by B20 and the code(s) for the HIV-related illness(es). Codes from Chapter 15 always take sequencing priority.

Patients with asymptomatic HIV infection status admitted (or presenting for a health care encounter) during pregnancy, childbirth, or the puerperium should receive codes of O98.7- and Z21.

(h) Encounters for testing for HIV

If a patient is being seen to determine his/her HIV status, use code Z11.4, Encounter for screening for human immunodeficiency virus [HIV]. Use additional codes for any associated high risk behavior.

If a patient with signs or symptoms is being seen for HIV testing, code the signs and symptoms. An additional counseling code Z71.7, Human immunodeficiency virus [HIV] counseling, may be used if counseling is provided during the encounter for the test.

When a patient returns to be informed of his/her HIV test results and the test result is negative, use code Z71.7, Human immunodeficiency virus [HIV] counseling.

If the results are positive, see previous guidelines and assign codes as appropriate.

b. Infectious agents as the cause of diseases classified to other chapters

Certain infections are classified in chapters other than Chapter 1 and no organism is identified as part of the infection code. In these instances, it is necessary to use an additional code from Chapter 1 to identify the organism. A code from category B95, Streptococcus, Staphylococcus, and Enterococcus as the cause of diseases classified to other chapters, B96, Other bacterial agents as the cause of diseases classified to other chapters, or B97, Viral agents as the cause of diseases classified to other chapters, is to be used as an additional code to identify the organism. An instructional note will be found at the infection code advising that an additional organism code is required.

c. Infections resistant to antibiotics

Many bacterial infections are resistant to current antibiotics. It is necessary to identify all infections documented as antibiotic resistant. Assign a code from category Z16, Resistance to antimicrobial drugs, following the infection code only if the infection code does not identify drug resistance.

d. Sepsis, severe sepsis, and septic shock

1) Coding of sepsis and severe sepsis

(a) Sepsis

For a diagnosis of sepsis, assign the appropriate code for the underlying systemic infection. If the type of infection or causal organism is not further specified, assign code A41.9, Sepsis, unspecified organism.

A code from subcategory R65.2, Severe sepsis, should not be assigned unless severe sepsis or an associated acute organ dysfunction is documented.

(i) Negative or inconclusive blood cultures and sepsis
Negative or inconclusive blood cultures do not preclude a diagnosis of sepsis in patients with clinical evidence of the condition, however, the provider should be queried.

(ii) Urosepsis
The term urosepsis is a nonspecific term. It is not to be considered synonymous with sepsis. It has no default code in the Alphabetic Index. Should a provider use this term, he/she must be queried for clarification.

(iii) Sepsis with organ dysfunction
If a patient has sepsis and associated acute organ dysfunction or multiple organ dysfunction (MOD), follow the instructions for coding severe sepsis.

(iv) Acute organ dysfunction that is not clearly associated with the sepsis
If a patient has sepsis and an acute organ dysfunction, but the medical record documentation indicates that the acute organ dysfunction is related to a medical condition other than the sepsis, do not assign a code from subcategory R65.2, Severe sepsis. An acute organ dysfunction must be associated with the sepsis in order to assign the severe sepsis code. If the documentation is not clear as to whether an acute organ dysfunction is related to the sepsis or another medical condition, query the provider.

(b) Severe sepsis

The coding of severe sepsis requires a minimum of 2 codes: first a code for the underlying systemic infection, followed by a code from subcategory R65.2, Severe sepsis. If the causal organism is not documented, assign code A41.9, Sepsis, unspecified organism, for the infection. Additional code(s) for the associated acute organ dysfunction are also required.

Due to the complex nature of severe sepsis, some cases may require querying the provider prior to assignment of the codes.

2) Septic shock

(a) Septic shock generally refers to circulatory failure associated with severe sepsis, and therefore, it represents a type of acute organ dysfunction.

For cases of septic shock, the code for the systemic infection should be sequenced first, followed by code R65.21, Severe sepsis with septic shock or code T81.12, Postprocedural septic shock. Any additional codes for the other acute organ dysfunctions should also be assigned. As noted in the sequencing instructions in the Tabular List, the code for septic shock cannot be assigned as a principal diagnosis.

3) Sequencing of severe sepsis

If severe sepsis is present on admission, and meets the definition of principal diagnosis, the underlying systemic infection should be assigned as principal diagnosis followed by the appropriate code from subcategory R65.2 as required by the sequencing rules in the Tabular List. A code from subcategory R65.2 can never be assigned as a principal diagnosis.

When severe sepsis develops during an encounter (it was not present on admission) the underlying systemic infection and the appropriate code from subcategory R65.2 should be assigned as secondary diagnoses.

Severe sepsis may be present on admission but the diagnosis may not be confirmed until sometime after admission. If the documentation is not clear whether severe sepsis was present on admission, the provider should be queried.

4) Sepsis and severe sepsis with a localized infection

If the reason for admission is both sepsis or severe sepsis and a localized infection, such as pneumonia or cellulitis, a code(s) for the underlying systemic infection should be assigned first and the code for the localized infection should be assigned as a secondary diagnosis. If the patient has severe sepsis, a code from subcategory R65.2 should also be assigned as a secondary diagnosis. If the patient is admitted with a localized infection, such as pneumonia, and sepsis/severe sepsis doesn't develop until after admission, the localized infection should be assigned first, followed by the appropriate sepsis/severe sepsis codes.

5) Sepsis due to a postprocedural infection

(a) Documentation of causal relationship

As with all postprocedural complications, code assignment is based on the provider's documentation of the relationship between the infection and the procedure.

(b) Sepsis due to a postprocedural infection

For such cases, the postprocedural infection code, such as, T80.2, Infections following infusion, transfusion, and therapeutic injection, T81.4, Infection following a procedure, T88.0, Infection following immunization, or O86.0, Infection of obstetric surgical wound, should be coded first, followed by the code for the specific infection. If the patient has severe sepsis the appropriate code from subcategory R65.2 should also be assigned with the additional code(s) for any acute organ dysfunction.

(c) Postprocedural infection and postprocedural septic shock

In cases where a postprocedural infection has occurred and has resulted in severe sepsis and postprocedural septic shock, the code for the precipitating complication such as code T81.4, Infection following a procedure, or O86.0, Infection of obstetrical surgical wound should be coded first followed by

code R65.21, Severe sepsis with septic shock and a code for the systemic infection.

6) Sepsis and severe sepsis associated with a noninfectious process (condition)

In some cases a noninfectious process (condition), such as trauma, may lead to an infection which can result in sepsis or severe sepsis. If sepsis or severe sepsis is documented as associated with a noninfectious condition, such as a burn or serious injury, and this condition meets the definition for principal diagnosis, the code for the noninfectious condition should be sequenced first, followed by the code for the resulting infection. If severe sepsis, is present a code from subcategory R65.2 should also be assigned with any associated organ dysfunction(s) codes. It is not necessary to assign a code from subcategory R65.1, Systemic inflammatory response syndrome (SIRS) of non-infectious origin, for these cases.

If the infection meets the definition of principal diagnosis it should be sequenced before the non-infectious condition. When both the associated non-infectious condition and the infection meet the definition of principal diagnosis either may be assigned as principal diagnosis.

Only one code from category R65, Symptoms and signs specifically associated with systemic inflammation and infection, should be assigned. Therefore, when a non-infectious condition leads to an infection resulting in severe sepsis, assign the appropriate code from subcategory R65.2, Severe sepsis. Do not additionally assign a code from subcategory R65.1, Systemic inflammatory response syndrome (SIRS) of non-infectious origin.

See Section I.C.18. SIRS due to non-infectious process

7) Sepsis and septic shock complicating abortion, pregnancy, childbirth, and the puerperium

See Section I.C.15. Sepsis and septic shock complicating abortion, pregnancy, childbirth and the puerperium

8) Newborn sepsis

See Section I.C.16. f. Bacterial sepsis of Newborn

e. Methicillin resistant *Staphylococcus aureus* (MRSA) conditions

1) Selection and sequencing of MRSA codes

(a) Combination codes for MRSA infection

When a patient is diagnosed with an infection that is due to methicillin resistant *Staphylococcus aureus* (MRSA), and that infection has a combination code that includes the causal organism (e.g., sepsis, pneumonia) assign the appropriate combination code for the condition (e.g., code A41.02, Sepsis due to Methicillin resistant *Staphylococcus aureus* or code J15.212, Pneumonia due to Methicillin resistant *Staphylococcus aureus*). Do not assign code B95.62, Methicillin resistant *Staphylococcus aureus* infection as the cause of diseases classified elsewhere, as an additional code because the combination code includes the type of infection and the MRSA organism. Do not assign a code from subcategory Z16.11, Resistance to penicillins, as an additional diagnosis.

See Section C.1. for instructions on coding and sequencing of sepsis and severe sepsis.

(b) Other codes for MRSA infection

When there is documentation of a current infection (e.g., wound infection, stitch abscess, urinary tract infection) due to MRSA, and that infection does not have a combination code that includes the causal organism, assign the appropriate code to identify the condition along with code B95.62, Methicillin resistant *Staphylococcus aureus* infection as the cause of diseases classified elsewhere for the MRSA infection. Do not assign a code from subcategory Z16.11, Resistance to penicillins.

(c) Methicillin susceptible *Staphylococcus aureus* (MSSA) and MRSA colonization

The condition or state of being colonized or carrying MSSA or MRSA is called colonization or carriage, while an individual person is described as being colonized or being a carrier. Colonization means that MSSA or MSRA is present on or in the body without necessarily causing illness. A positive MRSA colonization test might be documented by the provider as "MRSA screen positive" or "MRSA nasal swab positive".

Assign code Z22.322, Carrier or suspected carrier of Methicillin resistant *Staphylococcus aureus*, for patients documented as having MRSA colonization. Assign code Z22.321, Carrier or suspected carrier of Methicillin susceptible *Staphylococcus aureus*, for patient documented as having MSSA colonization. Colonization is not necessarily indicative of a disease process or as the cause of a specific condition the patient may have unless documented as such by the provider.

(d) MRSA colonization and infection

If a patient is documented as having both MRSA colonization and infection during a hospital admission, code Z22.322, Carrier or suspected carrier of Methicillin resistant *Staphylococcus aureus*, and a code for the MRSA infection may both be assigned.

2. Chapter 2: Neoplasms (C00-D49)

General guidelines

Chapter 2 of the ICD-10-CM contains the codes for most benign and all malignant neoplasms. Certain benign neoplasms, such as prostatic adenomas, may be found in the specific body system chapters. To properly code a neoplasm it is necessary to determine from the record if the neoplasm is benign, in-situ, malignant, or of uncertain histologic behavior. If malignant, any secondary (metastatic) sites should also be determined.

Primary malignant neoplasms overlapping site boundaries

A primary malignant neoplasm that overlaps two or more contiguous (next to each other) sites should be classified to the subcategory/code .8 ('overlapping lesion'), unless the combination is specifically indexed elsewhere. For multiple neoplasms of the same site that are not contiguous such as tumors in different quadrants of the same breast, codes for each site should be assigned.

Malignant neoplasm of ectopic tissue

Malignant neoplasms of ectopic tissue are to be coded to the site of origin mentioned, e.g., ectopic pancreatic malignant neoplasms involving the stomach are coded to pancreas, unspecified (C25.9).

The neoplasm table in the Alphabetic Index should be referenced first. However, if the histological term is documented, that term should be referenced first, rather than going immediately to the Neoplasm Table, in order to determine which column in the Neoplasm Table is appropriate. For example, if the documentation indicates "adenoma," refer to the term in the Alphabetic Index to review the entries under this term and the instructional note to "see also neoplasm, by site, benign." The table provides the proper code based on the type of neoplasm and the site. It is important to select the proper column in the table that corresponds to the type of neoplasm. The Tabular List should then be referenced to verify that the correct code has been selected from the table and that a more specific site code does not exist.

See Section I.C.21. Factors influencing health status and contact with health services, Status, for information regarding Z15.0, codes for genetic susceptibility to cancer.

a. Treatment directed at the malignancy

If the treatment is directed at the malignancy, designate the malignancy as the principal diagnosis.

The only exception to this guideline is if a patient admission/encounter is solely for the administration of chemotherapy, immunotherapy or radiation therapy, assign the appropriate Z51.- code as the first-listed or principal diagnosis, and the diagnosis or problem for which the service is being performed as a secondary diagnosis.

b. Treatment of secondary site

When a patient is admitted because of a primary neoplasm with metastasis and treatment is directed toward the secondary site only, the secondary neoplasm is designated as the principal diagnosis even though the primary malignancy is still present.

c. Coding and sequencing of complications

Coding and sequencing of complications associated with the malignancies or with the therapy thereof are subject to the following guidelines:

1) Anemia associated with malignancy

When admission/encounter is for management of an anemia associated with the malignancy, and the treatment is only for anemia, the appropriate code for the malignancy is sequenced as the principal or first-listed diagnosis followed by the appropriate code for the anemia (such as code D63.0, Anemia in neoplastic disease).

2) Anemia associated with chemotherapy, immunotherapy and radiation therapy

When the admission/encounter is for management of an anemia associated with an adverse effect of the administration of chemotherapy or immunotherapy and the only treatment is for the anemia, the anemia code is sequenced first followed by the appropriate codes for the neoplasm and the adverse effect (T45.1X5, Adverse effect of antineoplastic and immunosuppressive drugs).

When the admission/encounter is for management of an anemia associated with an adverse effect of radiotherapy, the anemia code should be sequenced first, followed by the appropriate neoplasm code and code Y84.2, Radiological procedure and radiotherapy as the cause of abnormal reaction of the patient, or of later complication, without mention of misadventure at the time of the procedure.

3) Management of dehydration due to the malignancy

When the admission/encounter is for management of dehydration due to the malignancy and only the dehydration is being treated (intravenous rehydration), the dehydration is sequenced first, followed by the code(s) for the malignancy.

4) Treatment of a complication resulting from a surgical procedure

When the admission/encounter is for treatment of a complication resulting from a surgical procedure, designate the complication as the principal or first-listed diagnosis if treatment is directed at resolving the complication.

d. Primary malignancy previously excised

When a primary malignancy has been previously excised or eradicated from its site and there is no further treatment directed to that site and there is no evidence of any existing primary malignancy, a code from category Z85, Personal history of malignant neoplasm, should be used to indicate the former site of the malignancy. Any mention of extension, invasion, or metastasis to another site is coded as a secondary malignant neoplasm to that site. The secondary site may be the principal or first-listed with the Z85 code used as a secondary code.

e. Admissions/Encounters involving chemotherapy, immunotherapy and radiation therapy

1) Episode of care involves surgical removal of neoplasm

When an episode of care involves the surgical removal of a neoplasm, primary or secondary site, followed by adjunct chemotherapy or radiation treatment during the same episode of care, the code for the neoplasm should be assigned as principal or first-listed diagnosis.

2) Patient admission/encounter solely for administration of chemotherapy, immunotherapy and radiation therapy

If a patient admission/encounter is solely for the administration of chemotherapy, immunotherapy or radiation therapy assign code Z51.0, Encounter for antineoplastic radiation therapy, or Z51.11, Encounter for antineoplastic chemotherapy, or Z51.12, Encounter for antineoplastic immunotherapy as the first-listed or principal diagnosis. If a patient receives more than one of these therapies during the same admission more than one of these codes may be assigned, in any sequence.

The malignancy for which the therapy is being administered should be assigned as a secondary diagnosis.

3) Patient admitted for radiation therapy, chemotherapy or immunotherapy and develops complications

When a patient is admitted for the purpose of radiotherapy, immunotherapy or chemotherapy and develops complications such as uncontrolled nausea and vomiting or dehydration, the principal or first-listed diagnosis is Z51.0, Encounter for antineoplastic radiation therapy, or Z51.11, Encounter for antineoplastic chemotherapy, or Z51.12, Encounter for antineoplastic immunotherapy followed by any codes for the complications.

f. Admission/encounter to determine extent of malignancy

When the reason for admission/encounter is to determine the extent of the malignancy, or for a procedure such as paracentesis or thoracentesis, the primary malignancy or appropriate metastatic site is designated as the principal or first-listed diagnosis, even though chemotherapy or radiotherapy is administered.

g. Symptoms, signs, and abnormal findings listed in Chapter 18 associated with neoplasms

Symptoms, signs, and ill-defined conditions listed in Chapter 18 characteristic of, or associated with, an existing primary or secondary site malignancy cannot be used to replace the malignancy as principal or first-listed diagnosis, regardless of the number of admissions or encounters for treatment and care of the neoplasm.

See section I.C.21. Factors influencing health status and contact with health services, Encounter for prophylactic organ removal.

h. Admission/encounter for pain control/management

See Section I.C.6. for information on coding admission/encounter for pain control/management.

i. Malignancy in two or more noncontiguous sites

A patient may have more than one malignant tumor in the same organ. These tumors may represent different primaries or metastatic disease, depending on the site. Should the documentation be unclear, the provider should be queried as to the status of each tumor so that the correct codes can be assigned.

j. Disseminated malignant neoplasm, unspecified

Code C80.0, Disseminated malignant neoplasm, unspecified, is for use only in those cases where the patient has advanced metastatic disease and no known primary or secondary sites are specified. It should not be used in place of assigning codes for the primary site and all known secondary sites.

k. Malignant neoplasm without specification of site

Code C80.1, Malignant (primary) neoplasm, unspecified, equates to Cancer, unspecified. This code should only be used when no determination can be made as to the primary site of a malignancy. This code should rarely be used in the inpatient setting.

l. Sequencing of neoplasm codes

1) Encounter for treatment of primary malignancy

If the reason for the encounter is for treatment of a primary malignancy, assign the malignancy as the principal/first-listed diagnosis. The primary site is to be sequenced first, followed by any metastatic sites.

2) Encounter for treatment of secondary malignancy

When an encounter is for a primary malignancy with metastasis and treatment is directed toward the metastatic (secondary) site(s) only, the metastatic site(s) is designated as the principal/first-listed diagnosis. The primary malignancy is coded as an additional code.

3) Malignant neoplasm in a pregnant patient

When a pregnant woman has a malignant neoplasm, a code from subcategory O9A.1-, Malignant neoplasm complicating pregnancy, childbirth, and the puerperium, should be sequenced first, followed by the appropriate code from Chapter 2 to indicate the type of neoplasm.

4) Encounter for complication associated with a neoplasm

When an encounter is for management of a complication associated with a neoplasm, such as dehydration, and the treatment is only for the complication, the complication is coded first, followed by the appropriate code(s) for the neoplasm.

The exception to this guideline is anemia. When the admission/encounter is for management of an anemia associated with the malignancy, and the treatment is only for anemia, the appropriate code for the malignancy is sequenced as the principal or first-listed diagnosis followed by code D63.0, Anemia in neoplastic disease.

5) Complication from surgical procedure for treatment of a neoplasm

When an encounter is for treatment of a complication resulting from a surgical procedure performed for the treatment of the neoplasm, designate the complication as the principal/first-listed diagnosis. See guideline regarding the coding of a current malignancy versus personal history to determine if the code for the neoplasm should also be assigned.

6) Pathologic fracture due to a neoplasm

When an encounter is for a pathological fracture due to a neoplasm, and the focus of treatment is the fracture, a code from subcategory M84.5, Pathological fracture in neoplastic disease, should be sequenced first, followed by the code for the neoplasm.

If the focus of treatment is the neoplasm with an associated pathological fracture, the neoplasm code should be sequenced first, followed by a code from M84.5 for the pathological fracture.

m. Current malignancy versus personal history of malignancy

When a primary malignancy has been excised but further treatment, such as an additional surgery for the malignancy, radiation therapy or chemotherapy is directed to that site, the primary malignancy code should be used until treatment is completed.

When a primary malignancy has been previously excised or eradicated from its site, there is no further treatment (of the malignancy) directed to that site, and there is no evidence of any existing primary malignancy, a code from category Z85, Personal history of malignant neoplasm, should be used to indicate the former site of the malignancy.

See Section I.C.21. Factors influencing health status and contact with health services, History (of)

n. Leukemia, multiple myeloma, and malignant plasma cell neoplasms in remission versus personal history

The categories for leukemia, and category C90, Multiple myeloma and malignant plasma cell neoplasms, have codes indicating whether or not the leukemia has achieved remission. There are also codes Z85.6, Personal history of leukemia, and Z85.79, Personal history of other malignant neoplasms of lymphoid, hematopoietic and related tissues. If the documentation is unclear, as to whether the leukemia has achieved remission, the provider should be queried.

See Section I.C.21. Factors influencing health status and contact with health services, History (of)

o. Aftercare following surgery for neoplasm

See Section I.C.21. Factors influencing health status and contact with health services, Aftercare

p. Follow-up care for completed treatment of a malignancy

See Section I.C.21. Factors influencing health status and contact with health services, Follow-up

q. Prophylactic organ removal for prevention of malignancy

See Section I.C. 21, Factors influencing health status and contact with health services, Prophylactic organ removal

r. Malignant neoplasm associated with transplanted organ

A malignant neoplasm of a transplanted organ should be coded as a transplant complication. Assign first the appropriate code from category T86.-, Complications of transplanted organs and tissue, followed by code C80.2, Malignant neoplasm associated with transplanted organ. Use an additional code for the specific malignancy.

3. Chapter 3: Disease of the Blood and Blood-forming Organs and Certain Disorders Involving the Immune Mechanism (D50-D89)

Reserved for future guideline expansion

4. **Chapter 4: Endocrine, Nutritional, and Metabolic Diseases (E00-E89)**
    a. **Diabetes mellitus**
        The diabetes mellitus codes are combination codes that include the type of diabetes mellitus, the body system affected, and the complications affecting that body system. As many codes within a particular category as are necessary to describe all of the complications of the disease may be used. They should be sequenced based on the reason for a particular encounter. Assign as many codes from categories E08 – E13 as needed to identify all of the associated conditions that the patient has.

        1) **Type of diabetes**
            The age of a patient is not the sole determining factor, though most type 1 diabetics develop the condition before reaching puberty. For this reason type 1 diabetes mellitus is also referred to as juvenile diabetes.

        2) **Type of diabetes mellitus not documented**
            If the type of diabetes mellitus is not documented in the medical record the default is E11.-, Type 2 diabetes mellitus.

        3) **Diabetes mellitus and the use of insulin**
            If the documentation in a medical record does not indicate the type of diabetes but does indicate that the patient uses insulin, code E11, Type 2 diabetes mellitus, should be assigned. Code Z79.4, Long-term (current) use of insulin, should also be assigned to indicate that the patient uses insulin. Code Z79.4 should not be assigned if insulin is given temporarily to bring a type 2 patient's blood sugar under control during an encounter.

        4) **Diabetes mellitus in pregnancy and gestational diabetes**
            See Section I.C.15. Diabetes mellitus in pregnancy.

            See Section I.C.15. Gestational (pregnancy induced) diabetes

        5) **Complications due to insulin pump malfunction**
            (a) **Underdose of insulin due to insulin pump failure**
                An underdose of insulin due to an insulin pump failure should be assigned to a code from subcategory T85.6, Mechanical complication of other specified internal and external prosthetic devices, implants and grafts, that specifies the type of pump malfunction, as the principal or first-listed code, followed by code T38.3x6-, Underdosing of insulin and oral hypoglycemic [antidiabetic] drugs. Additional codes for the type of diabetes mellitus and any associated complications due to the underdosing should also be assigned.

            (b) **Overdose of insulin due to insulin pump failure**
                The principal or first-listed code for an encounter due to an insulin pump malfunction resulting in an overdose of insulin, should also be T85.6-, Mechanical complication of other specified internal and external prosthetic devices, implants and grafts, followed by code T38.3X1-, Poisoning by insulin and oral hypoglycemic [antidiabetic] drugs, accidental (unintentional).

        6) **Secondary diabetes mellitus**
            Codes under categories E08, Diabetes mellitus due to underlying condition, E09, Drug or chemical induced diabetes mellitus, and E13, Other specified diabetes mellitus, identify complications/manifestations associated with secondary diabetes mellitus. Secondary diabetes is always caused by another condition or event (e.g., cystic fibrosis, malignant neoplasm of pancreas, pancreatectomy, adverse effect of drug, or poisoning).

            (a) **Secondary diabetes mellitus and the use of insulin**
                For patients who routinely use insulin, code Z79.4, Long-term (current) use of insulin, should also be assigned. Code Z79.4 should not be assigned if insulin is given temporarily to bring a patient's blood sugar under control during an encounter.

            (b) **Assigning and sequencing secondary diabetes codes and its causes**
                The sequencing of the secondary diabetes codes in relationship to codes for the cause of the diabetes is based on the Tabular List instructions for categories E08, E09 and E13.

            (i) **Secondary diabetes mellitus due to pancreatectomy**
                For postpancreatectomy diabetes mellitus (lack of insulin due to the surgical removal of all or part of the pancreas), assign code E89.1, Postprocedural hypoinsulinemia. Assign a code from category E13 and a code from subcategory Z90.41-, Acquired absence of pancreas, as additional codes.

            (ii) **Secondary diabetes due to drugs**
                Secondary diabetes may be caused by an adverse effect of correctly administered medications, poisoning or sequela of poisoning.
                See section I.C.19.e for coding of adverse effects and poisoning, and section I.C.20 for external cause code reporting.

5. **Chapter 5: Mental, Behavioral and Neurodevelopmental Disorders (F01 – F99)**
    a. **Pain disorders related to psychological factors**
        Assign code F45.41, for pain that is exclusively related to psychological disorders. As indicated by the Excludes 1 note under category G89, a code from category G89 should not be assigned with code F45.41

        Code F45.42, Pain disorders with related psychological factors, should be used with a code from category G89, Pain, not elsewhere classified, if there is documentation of a psychological component for a patient with acute or chronic pain.
        See Section I.C.6. Pain

    b. **Mental and behavioral disorders due to psychoactive substance use**
        1) **In remission**
            Selection of codes for "in remission" for categories F10-F19, Mental and behavioral disorders due to psychoactive substance use (categories F10-F19 with -.21) requires the provider's clinical judgment. The appropriate codes for "in remission" are assigned only on the basis of provider documentation (as defined in the Official Guidelines for Coding and Reporting).

        2) **Psychoactive substance use, abuse and dependence**
            When the provider documentation refers to use, abuse and dependence of the same substance (e.g. alcohol, opioid, cannabis, etc.), only one code should be assigned to identify the pattern of use based on the following hierarchy:

            *   If both use and abuse are documented, assign only the code for abuse
            *   If both abuse and dependence are documented, assign only the code for dependence
            *   If use, abuse and dependence are all documented, assign only the code for dependence
            *   If both use and dependence are documented, assign only the code for dependence.

        3) **Psychoactive substance use**
            As with all other diagnoses, the codes for psychoactive substance use (F10.9-, F11.9-, F12.9-, F13.9-, F14.9-, F15.9-, F16.9-) should only be assigned based on provider documentation and when they meet the definition of a reportable diagnosis (see Section III, Reporting Additional Diagnoses). The codes are to be used only when the psychoactive substance use is associated with a mental or behavioral disorder, and such a relationship is documented by the provider.

6. **Chapter 6: Diseases of Nervous System (G00-G99)**
    a. **Dominant/nondominant side**
        Codes from category G81, Hemiplegia and hemiparesis, and subcategories, G83.1, Monoplegia of lower limb, G83.2, Monoplegia of upper limb, and G83.3, Monoplegia, unspecified, identify whether the dominant or nondominant side is affected. Should the affected side be documented, but not specified as dominant or nondominant, and the classification system does not indicate a default, code selection is as follows:

        *   For ambidextrous patients, the default should be dominant.
        *   If the left side is affected, the default is non-dominant.

- If the right side is affected, the default is dominant.

b. Pain - Category G89

1) General coding information

Codes in category G89, Pain, not elsewhere classified, may be used in conjunction with codes from other categories and chapters to provide more detail about acute or chronic pain and neoplasm-related pain, unless otherwise indicated below.

If the pain is not specified as acute or chronic, post-thoracotomy, postprocedural, or neoplasm-related, do not assign codes from category G89.

A code from category G89 should not be assigned if the underlying (definitive) diagnosis is known, unless the reason for the encounter is pain control/ management and not management of the underlying condition.

When an admission or encounter is for a procedure aimed at treating the underlying condition (e.g., spinal fusion, kyphoplasty), a code for the underlying condition (e.g., vertebral fracture, spinal stenosis) should be assigned as the principal diagnosis. No code from category G89 should be assigned.

(a) Category G89 codes as principal or first-listed diagnosis

Category G89 codes are acceptable as principal diagnosis or the first-listed code:

- When pain control or pain management is the reason for the admission/encounter (e.g., a patient with displaced intervertebral disc, nerve impingement and severe back pain presents for injection of steroid into the spinal canal). The underlying cause of the pain should be reported as an additional diagnosis, if known.

- When a patient is admitted for the insertion of a neurostimulator for pain control, assign the appropriate pain code as the principal or first-listed diagnosis. When an admission or encounter is for a procedure aimed at treating the underlying condition and a neurostimulator is inserted for pain control during the same admission/encounter, a code for the underlying condition should be assigned as the principal diagnosis and the appropriate pain code should be assigned as a secondary diagnosis.

(b) Use of category G89 codes in conjunction with site specific pain codes

(i) Assigning category G89 and site-specific pain codes

Codes from category G89 may be used in conjunction with codes that identify the site of pain (including codes from chapter 18) if the category G89 code provides additional information. For example, if the code describes the site of the pain, but does not fully describe whether the pain is acute or chronic, then both codes should be assigned.

(ii) Sequencing of category G89 codes with site-specific pain codes

The sequencing of category G89 codes with site-specific pain codes (including chapter 18 codes), is dependent on the circumstances of the encounter/admission as follows:

- If the encounter is for pain control or pain management, assign the code from category G89 followed by the code identifying the specific site of pain (e.g., encounter for pain management for acute neck pain from trauma is assigned code G89.11, Acute pain due to trauma, followed by code M54.2, Cervicalgia, to identify the site of pain).

- If the encounter is for any other reason except pain control or pain management, and a related definitive diagnosis has not been established (confirmed) by the provider, assign the code for the specific site of pain first, followed by the appropriate code from category G89.

2) Pain due to devices, implants and grafts

See Section I.C.19. Pain due to medical devices

3) Postoperative pain

The provider's documentation should be used to guide the coding of postoperative pain, as well as *Section III. Reporting Additional Diagnoses* and *Section IV. Diagnostic Coding and Reporting in the Outpatient Setting.*

The default for post-thoracotomy and other postoperative pain not specified as acute or chronic is the code for the acute form.

Routine or expected postoperative pain immediately after surgery should not be coded.

(a) Postoperative pain not associated with specific postoperative complication

Postoperative pain not associated with a specific postoperative complication is assigned to the appropriate postoperative pain code in category G89.

(b) Postoperative pain associated with specific postoperative complication

Postoperative pain associated with a specific postoperative complication (such as painful wire sutures) is assigned to the appropriate code(s) found in Chapter 19, Injury, poisoning, and certain other consequences of external causes. If appropriate, use additional code(s) from category G89 to identify acute or chronic pain (G89.18 or G89.28).

4) Chronic pain

Chronic pain is classified to subcategory G89.2. There is no time frame defining when pain becomes chronic pain. The provider's documentation should be used to guide use of these codes.

5) Neoplasm related pain

Code G89.3 is assigned to pain documented as being related, associated or due to cancer, primary or secondary malignancy, or tumor. This code is assigned regardless of whether the pain is acute or chronic.

This code may be assigned as the principal or first-listed code when the stated reason for the admission/encounter is documented as pain control/pain management. The underlying neoplasm should be reported as an additional diagnosis.

When the reason for the admission/encounter is management of the neoplasm and the pain associated with the neoplasm is also documented, code G89.3 may be assigned as an additional diagnosis. It is not necessary to assign an additional code for the site of the pain.

See Section I.C.2 for instructions on the sequencing of neoplasms for all other stated reasons for the admission/encounter (except for pain control/pain management).

6) Chronic pain syndrome

Central pain syndrome (G89.0) and chronic pain syndrome (G89.4) are different than the term "chronic pain," and therefore codes should only be used when the provider has specifically documented this condition.

See Section I.C.5. Pain disorders related to psychological factors

7. Chapter 7: Diseases of Eye and Adnexa (H00-H59)

a. Glaucoma

1) Assigning glaucoma codes

Assign as many codes from category H40, Glaucoma, as needed to identify the type of glaucoma, the affected eye, and the glaucoma stage.

2) Bilateral glaucoma with same type and stage

When a patient has bilateral glaucoma and both eyes are documented as being the same type and stage, and there is a code for bilateral glaucoma, report only the code for the type of glaucoma, bilateral, with the seventh character for the stage.

When a patient has bilateral glaucoma and both eyes are documented as being the same type and stage, and the classification does not provide a code for bilateral glaucoma (i.e. subcategories H40.10, H40.11 and H40.20) report only one code for the type of glaucoma with the appropriate seventh character for the stage.

3) Bilateral glaucoma stage with different types or stages

When a patient has bilateral glaucoma and each eye is documented as having a different type or stage, and the classification distinguishes laterality, assign the appropriate code for each eye rather than the code for bilateral glaucoma.

When a patient has bilateral glaucoma and each eye is documented as having a different type, and the classification does not distinguish laterality (i.e. subcategories H40.10, H40.11 and H40.20), assign one code for each type of glaucoma with the appropriate seventh character for the stage.

When a patient has bilateral glaucoma and each eye is documented as having the same type, but different stage, and the classification does not distinguish laterality (i.e. subcategories H40.10, H40.11 and H40.20), assign a code for the type of glaucoma for each eye with the seventh character for the specific glaucoma stage documented for each eye.

4) Patient admitted with glaucoma and stage evolves during the admission

If a patient is admitted with glaucoma and the stage progresses during the admission, assign the code for highest stage documented.

5) Indeterminate stage glaucoma

Assignment of the seventh character "4" for "indeterminate stage" should be based on the clinical documentation. The seventh character "4" is used for glaucomas whose stage cannot be clinically determined. This seventh character should not be confused with the seventh character "0", unspecified, which should be assigned when there is no documentation regarding the stage of the glaucoma.

8. Chapter 8: Diseases of Ear and Mastoid Process (H60-H95)

Reserved for future guideline expansion

9. Chapter 9: Diseases of Circulatory System (I00-I99)

a. Hypertension

1) Hypertension with heart disease

Heart conditions classified to I50.- or I51.4-I51.9, are assigned to, a code from category I11, Hypertensive heart disease, when a causal relationship is stated (due to hypertension) or implied (hypertensive). Use an additional code from category I50, Heart failure, to identify the type of heart failure in those patients with heart failure.

The same heart conditions (I50.-, I51.4-I51.9) with hypertension, but without a stated causal relationship, are coded separately. Sequence according to the circumstances of the admission/encounter.

2) Hypertensive chronic kidney disease

Assign codes from category I12, Hypertensive chronic kidney disease, when both hypertension and a condition classifiable to category N18, Chronic kidney disease (CKD), are present. Unlike hypertension with heart disease, ICD-10-CM presumes a cause-and-effect relationship and classifies chronic kidney disease with hypertension as hypertensive chronic kidney disease.

The appropriate code from category N18 should be used as a secondary code with a code from category I12 to identify the stage of chronic kidney disease.

See Section I.C.14. Chronic kidney disease.

If a patient has hypertensive chronic kidney disease and acute renal failure, an additional code for the acute renal failure is required.

3) Hypertensive heart and chronic kidney disease

Assign codes from combination category I13, Hypertensive heart and chronic kidney disease, when both hypertensive kidney disease and hypertensive heart disease are stated in the diagnosis. Assume a relationship between the hypertension and the chronic kidney disease, whether or not the condition is so designated. If heart failure is present, assign an additional code from category I50 to identify the type of heart failure.

The appropriate code from category N18, Chronic kidney disease, should be used as a secondary code with a code from category I13 to identify the stage of chronic kidney disease.

See Section I.C.14. Chronic kidney disease.

The codes in category I13, Hypertensive heart and chronic kidney disease, are combination codes that include hypertension, heart disease and chronic kidney disease. The Includes note at I13 specifies that the conditions included at I11 and I12 are included together in I13. If a patient has hypertension, heart disease and chronic kidney disease then a code from I13 should be used, not individual codes for hypertension, heart disease and chronic kidney disease, or codes from I11 or I12.

For patients with both acute renal failure and chronic kidney disease an additional code for acute renal failure is required.

4) Hypertensive cerebrovascular disease

For hypertensive cerebrovascular disease, first assign the appropriate code from categories I60-I69, followed by the appropriate hypertension code.

5) Hypertensive retinopathy

Subcategory H35.0, Background retinopathy and retinal vascular changes, should be used with a code from category I10 – I15, Hypertensive disease to include the systemic hypertension. The sequencing is based on the reason for the encounter.

6) Hypertension, secondary

Secondary hypertension is due to an underlying condition. Two codes are required: one to identify the underlying etiology and one from category I15 to identify the hypertension. Sequencing of codes is determined by the reason for admission/encounter.

7) Hypertension, transient

Assign code R03.0, Elevated blood pressure reading without diagnosis of hypertension, unless patient has an established diagnosis of hypertension. Assign code O13.-, Gestational [pregnancy-induced] hypertension without significant proteinuria, or O14.-, Pre-eclampsia, for transient hypertension of pregnancy.

8) Hypertension, controlled

This diagnostic statement usually refers to an existing state of hypertension under control by therapy. Assign the appropriate code from categories I10-I15, Hypertensive diseases.

9) Hypertension, uncontrolled

Uncontrolled hypertension may refer to untreated hypertension or hypertension not responding to current therapeutic regimen. In either case, assign the appropriate code from categories I10-I15, Hypertensive diseases.

b. Atherosclerotic coronary artery disease and angina

ICD-10-CM has combination codes for atherosclerotic heart disease with angina pectoris. The subcategories for these codes are I25.11, Atherosclerotic heart disease of native coronary artery with angina pectoris and I25.7, Atherosclerosis of coronary artery bypass graft(s) and coronary artery of transplanted heart with angina pectoris.

When using one of these combination codes it is not necessary to use an additional code for angina pectoris. A causal relationship can be assumed in a patient with both atherosclerosis and angina pectoris, unless the documentation indicates the angina is due to something other than the atherosclerosis.

If a patient with coronary artery disease is admitted due to an acute myocardial infarction (AMI), the AMI should be sequenced before the coronary artery disease.

See Section I.C.9. Acute myocardial infarction (AMI)

c. Intraoperative and postprocedural cerebrovascular accident

Medical record documentation should clearly specify the cause-and-effect relationship between the medical intervention and the cerebrovascular accident in order to assign a code for intraoperative or postprocedural cerebrovascular accident.

Proper code assignment depends on whether it was an infarction or hemorrhage and whether it occurred intraoperatively or postoperatively. If it was a cerebral hemorrhage, code assignment depends on the type of procedure performed.

d. Sequelae of cerebrovascular disease

1) Category I69, sequelae of cerebrovascular disease

Category I69 is used to indicate conditions classifiable to categories I60-I67 as the causes of sequela (neurologic deficits), themselves classified elsewhere. These "late effects" include neurologic deficits that persist after initial onset of conditions classifiable to categories I60-I67. The neurologic deficits caused by cerebrovascular disease may be present from the onset or may arise at any time after the onset of the condition classifiable to categories I60-I67.

Codes from category I69, Sequelae of cerebrovascular disease, that specify hemiplegia, hemiparesis and monoplegia identify whether the dominant or nondominant side is affected. Should the affected side be documented, but not specified as dominant or nondominant, and the classification system does not indicate a default, code selection is as follows:

- For ambidextrous patients, the default should be dominant.
- If the left side is affected, the default is non-dominant.
- If the right side is affected, the default is dominant.

2) Codes from category I69 with codes from I60-I67

Codes from category I69 may be assigned on a health care record with codes from I60-I67, if the patient has a current cerebrovascular disease and deficits from an old cerebrovascular disease.

3) Codes from category I69 and Personal history of transient ischemic attack (TIA) and cerebral infarction (Z86.73)

Codes from category I69 should not be assigned if the patient does not have neurologic deficits.

See Section I.C.21. 4. History (of) for use of personal history codes

e. Acute myocardial infarction (AMI)

1) ST elevation myocardial infarction (STEMI) and non ST elevation myocardial infarction (NSTEMI)

The ICD-10-CM codes for acute myocardial infarction (AMI) identify the site, such as anterolateral wall or true posterior wall. Subcategories I21.0-I21.2 and code I21.3 are used for ST elevation myocardial infarction (STEMI). Code I21.4, Non-ST elevation (NSTEMI) myocardial infarction, is used for non ST elevation myocardial infarction (NSTEMI) and nontransmural MIs.

If NSTEMI evolves to STEMI, assign the STEMI code. If STEMI converts to NSTEMI due to thrombolytic therapy, it is still coded as STEMI.

For encounters occurring while the myocardial infarction is equal to, or less than, four weeks old, including transfers to another acute setting or a postacute setting, and the patient requires continued care for the myocardial infarction, codes from category I21 may continue to be reported. For encounters after the 4 week time frame and the patient is still receiving care related to the myocardial infarction, the appropriate aftercare code should be assigned, rather than a code from category I21. For old or healed myocardial infarctions not requiring further care, code I25.2, Old myocardial infarction, may be assigned.

2) Acute myocardial infarction, unspecified

Code I21.3, ST elevation (STEMI) myocardial infarction of unspecified site, is the default for the unspecified term acute myocardial infarction. If only STEMI or transmural MI without the site is documented, query the provider as to the site, or assign code I21.3.

3) AMI documented as nontransmural or subendocardial but site provided

If an AMI is documented as nontransmural or subendocardial, but the site is provided, it is still coded as a subendocardial AMI.

See Section I.C.21.3 for information on coding status post administration of tPA in a different facility within the last 24 hrs.

4) Subsequent acute myocardial infarction

A code from category I22, Subsequent ST elevation (STEMI) and non ST elevation (NSTEMI) myocardial infarction, is to be used when a patient who has suffered an AMI has a new AMI within the 4 week time frame of the initial AMI. A code from category I22 must be used in conjunction with a code from category I21.

The sequencing of the I22 and I21 codes depends on the circumstances of the encounter.

10. Chapter 10: Diseases of the Respiratory System (J00-J99)

a. Chronic Obstructive Pulmonary Disease [COPD] and Asthma

1) Acute exacerbation of chronic obstructive bronchitis and asthma

The codes in categories J44 and J45 distinguish between uncomplicated cases and those in acute exacerbation. An acute exacerbation is a worsening or a decompensation of a chronic condition. An acute exacerbation is not equivalent to an infection superimposed on a chronic condition, though an exacerbation may be triggered by an infection.

b. Acute Respiratory Failure

1) Acute respiratory failure as principal diagnosis

A code from subcategory J96.0, Acute respiratory failure, or subcategory J96.2, Acute and chronic respiratory failure, may be assigned as a principal diagnosis when it is the condition established after study to be chiefly responsible for occasioning the admission to the hospital, and the selection is supported by the Alphabetic Index and Tabular List. However, chapter-specific coding guidelines (such as obstetrics, poisoning, HIV, newborn) that provide sequencing direction take precedence.

2) Acute respiratory failure as secondary diagnosis

Respiratory failure may be listed as a secondary diagnosis if it occurs after admission, or if it is present on admission, but does not meet the definition of principal diagnosis.

3) Sequencing of acute respiratory failure and another acute condition

When a patient is admitted with respiratory failure and another acute condition, (e.g., myocardial infarction, cerebrovascular accident, aspiration pneumonia), the principal diagnosis will not be the same in every situation. This applies whether the other acute condition is a respiratory or nonrespiratory condition. Selection of the principal diagnosis will be dependent on the circumstances of admission. If both the respiratory failure and the other acute condition are equally responsible for occasioning the admission to the hospital, and there are no chapter-specific sequencing rules, the guideline regarding two or more diagnoses that equally meet the definition for principal diagnosis (Section II, C.) may be applied in these situations.

If the documentation is not clear as to whether acute respiratory failure and another condition are equally responsible for occasioning the admission, query the provider for clarification.

c. Influenza due to certain identified influenza viruses

Code only confirmed cases of influenza due to certain identified influenza viruses (category J09), and due to other identified influenza virus (category J10). This is an exception to the hospital inpatient guideline Section II, H. (Uncertain Diagnosis).

In this context, "confirmation" does not require documentation of positive laboratory testing specific for avian or other novel influenza A or other identified influenza virus. However, coding should be based on the provider's diagnostic statement that the patient has avian influenza, or other novel influenza A, for category J09, or has another particular identified strain of influenza, such as H1N1 or H3N2, but not identified as novel or variant, for category J10.

If the provider records "suspected" or "possible" or "probable" avian influenza, or novel influenza, or other identified influenza, then the appropriate influenza code from category J11, Influenza due to unidentified influenza virus, should be assigned. A code from category J09, Influenza due to certain identified influenza viruses, should not be assigned nor should a code from category J10, Influenza due to other identified influenza virus.

d. Ventilator associated pneumonia

1) Documentation of ventilator associated pneumonia

As with all procedural or postprocedural complications, code assignment is based on the provider's documentation of the relationship between the condition and the procedure.

Code J95.851, Ventilator associated pneumonia, should be assigned only when the provider has documented ventilator associated pneumonia (VAP). An additional code to identify the organism (e.g., Pseudomonas aeruginosa, code B96.5) should also be assigned. Do not assign an additional code from categories J12-J18 to identify the type of pneumonia.

Code J95.851 should not be assigned for cases where the patient has pneumonia and is on a mechanical ventilator and the provider has not specifically stated that the pneumonia is ventilator-associated pneumonia. If the documentation is unclear as to whether the patient has a pneumonia that is a complication attributable to the mechanical ventilator, query the provider.

2) Ventilator associated pneumonia develops after admission
A patient may be admitted with one type of pneumonia (e.g., code J13, Pneumonia due to Streptococcus pneumonia) and subsequently develop VAP. In this instance, the principal diagnosis would be the appropriate code from categories J12-J18 for the pneumonia diagnosed at the time of admission. Code J95.851, Ventilator associated pneumonia, would be assigned as an additional diagnosis when the provider has also documented the presence of ventilator associated pneumonia.

11. Chapter 11: Diseases of the Digestive System (K00-K95)
Reserved for future guideline expansion

12. Chapter 12: Diseases of the Skin and Subcutaneous Tissue (L00-L99)
a. Pressure ulcer stage codes
1) Pressure ulcer stages
Codes from category L89, Pressure ulcer, are combination codes that identify the site of the pressure ulcer as well as the stage of the ulcer.

The ICD-10-CM classifies pressure ulcer stages based on severity, which is designated by stages 1-4, unspecified stage and unstageable.

Assign as many codes from category L89 as needed to identify all the pressure ulcers the patient has, if applicable.

2) Unstageable pressure ulcers
Assignment of the code for unstageable pressure ulcer (L89.--0) should be based on the clinical documentation. These codes are used for pressure ulcers whose stage cannot be clinically determined (e.g., the ulcer is covered by eschar or has been treated with a skin or muscle graft) and pressure ulcers that are documented as deep tissue injury but not documented as due to trauma. This code should not be confused with the codes for unspecified stage (L89.--9). When there is no documentation regarding the stage of the pressure ulcer, assign the appropriate code for unspecified stage (L89.--9).

3) Documented pressure ulcer stage
Assignment of the pressure ulcer stage code should be guided by clinical documentation of the stage or documentation of the terms found in the Alphabetic Index. For clinical terms describing the stage that are not found in the Alphabetic Index, and there is no documentation of the stage, the provider should be queried.

4) Patients admitted with pressure ulcers documented as healed
No code is assigned if the documentation states that the pressure ulcer is completely healed.

5) Patients admitted with pressure ulcers documented as healing
Pressure ulcers described as healing should be assigned the appropriate pressure ulcer stage code based on the documentation in the medical record. If the documentation does not provide information about the stage of the healing pressure ulcer, assign the appropriate code for unspecified stage.

If the documentation is unclear as to whether the patient has a current (new) pressure ulcer or if the patient is being treated for a healing pressure ulcer, query the provider.

6) Patient admitted with pressure ulcer evolving into another stage during the admission
If a patient is admitted with a pressure ulcer at one stage and it progresses to a higher stage, assign the code for the highest stage reported for that site.

13. Chapter 13: Diseases of the Musculoskeletal System and Connective Tissue (M00-M99)
a. Site and laterality
Most of the codes within Chapter 13 have site and laterality designations. The site represents the bone, joint or the muscle involved. For some conditions where more than one bone, joint or muscle is usually involved, such as osteoarthritis, there is a "multiple sites" code available. For categories where no multiple site code is provided and more than one bone, joint or muscle is involved, multiple codes should be used to indicate the different sites involved.

1) Bone versus joint
For certain conditions, the bone may be affected at the upper or lower end, (e.g., avascular necrosis of bone, M87, Osteoporosis, M80, M81). Though the portion of the bone affected may be at the joint, the site designation will be the bone, not the joint.

b. Acute traumatic versus chronic or recurrent musculoskeletal conditions
Many musculoskeletal conditions are a result of previous injury or trauma to a site, or are recurrent conditions. Bone, joint or muscle conditions that are the result of a healed injury are usually found in chapter 13. Recurrent bone, joint or muscle conditions are also usually found in chapter 13. Any current, acute injury should be coded to the appropriate injury code from chapter 19. Chronic or recurrent conditions should generally be coded with a code from chapter 13. If it is difficult to determine from the documentation in the record which code is best to describe a condition, query the provider.

c. Coding of Pathologic Fractures
7th character A is for use as long as the patient is receiving active treatment for the fracture. Examples of active treatment are: surgical treatment, emergency department encounter, evaluation and treatment by a new physician. 7th character, D is to be used for encounters after the patient has completed active treatment. The other 7th characters, listed under each subcategory in the Tabular List, are to be used for subsequent encounters for treatment of problems associated with the healing, such as malunions, nonunions, and sequelae.

Care for complications of surgical treatment for fracture repairs during the healing or recovery phase should be coded with the appropriate complication codes.

See Section I.C.19. Coding of traumatic fractures.

d. Osteoporosis
Osteoporosis is a systemic condition, meaning that all bones of the musculoskeletal system are affected. Therefore, site is not a component of the codes under category M81, Osteoporosis without current pathological fracture. The site codes under category M80, Osteoporosis with current pathological fracture, identify the site of the fracture, not the osteoporosis.

1) Osteoporosis without pathological fracture
Category M81, Osteoporosis without current pathological fracture, is for use for patients with osteoporosis who do not currently have a pathologic fracture due to the osteoporosis, even if they have had a fracture in the past. For patients with a history of osteoporosis fractures, status code Z87.310, Personal history of (healed) osteoporosis fracture, should follow the code from M81.

2) Osteoporosis with current pathological fracture
Category M80, Osteoporosis with current pathological fracture, is for patients who have a current pathologic fracture at the time of an encounter. The codes under M80 identify the site of the fracture. A code from category M80, not a traumatic fracture code, should be used for any patient with known osteoporosis who suffers a fracture, even if the patient had a minor fall or trauma, if that fall or trauma would not usually break a normal, healthy bone.

14. **Chapter 14: Diseases of Genitourinary System (NØØ-N99)**

a. **Chronic kidney disease**

1) **Stages of chronic kidney disease (CKD)**

The ICD-1Ø-CM classifies CKD based on severity. The severity of CKD is designated by stages 1-5. Stage 2, code N18.2, equates to mild CKD; stage 3, code N18.3, equates to moderate CKD; and stage 4, code N18.4, equates to severe CKD. Code N18.6, End stage renal disease (ESRD), is assigned when the provider has documented end-stage-renal disease (ESRD).

If both a stage of CKD and ESRD are documented, assign code N18.6 only.

2) **Chronic kidney disease and kidney transplant status**

Patients who have undergone kidney transplant may still have some form of chronic kidney disease (CKD) because the kidney transplant may not fully restore kidney function. Therefore, the presence of CKD alone does not constitute a transplant complication. Assign the appropriate N18 code for the patient's stage of CKD and code Z94.Ø, Kidney transplant status. If a transplant complication such as failure or rejection or other transplant complication is documented, see section I.C.19.g for information on coding complications of a kidney transplant. If the documentation is unclear as to whether the patient has a complication of the transplant, query the provider.

3) **Chronic kidney disease with other conditions**

Patients with CKD may also suffer from other serious conditions, most commonly diabetes mellitus and hypertension. The sequencing of the CKD code in relationship to codes for other contributing conditions is based on the conventions in the Tabular List.

See I.C.9. Hypertensive chronic kidney disease.

See I.C.19. Chronic kidney disease and kidney transplant complications.

15. **Chapter 15: Pregnancy, Childbirth, and the Puerperium (OØØ-O9A)**

a. **General Rules for Obstetric Cases**

1) **Codes from chapter 15 and sequencing priority**

Obstetric cases require codes from chapter 15, codes in the range OØØ-O9A, Pregnancy, Childbirth, and the Puerperium. Chapter 15 codes have sequencing priority over codes from other chapters. Additional codes from other chapters may be used in conjunction with chapter 15 codes to further specify conditions. Should the provider document that the pregnancy is incidental to the encounter, then code Z33.1, Pregnant state, incidental, should be used in place of any chapter 15 codes. It is the provider's responsibility to state that the condition being treated is not affecting the pregnancy.

2) **Chapter 15 codes used only on the maternal record**

Chapter 15 codes are to be used only on the maternal record, never on the record of the newborn.

3) **Final character for trimester**

The majority of codes in Chapter 15 have a final character indicating the trimester of pregnancy. The timeframes for the trimesters are indicated at the beginning of the chapter. If trimester is not a component of a code it is because the condition always occurs in a specific trimester, or the concept of trimester of pregnancy is not applicable. Certain codes have characters for only certain trimesters because the condition does not occur in all trimesters, but it may occur in more than just one.

Assignment of the final character for trimester should be based on the provider's documentation of the trimester (or number of weeks) for the current admission/encounter. This applies to the assignment of trimester for pre-existing conditions as well as those that develop during or are due to the pregnancy. The provider's documentation of the number of weeks may be used to assign the appropriate code identifying the trimester.

Whenever delivery occurs during the current admission, and there is an "in childbirth" option for the obstetric complication being coded, the "in childbirth" code should be assigned.

4) **Selection of trimester for inpatient admissions that encompass more than one trimesters**

In instances when a patient is admitted to a hospital for complications of pregnancy during one trimester and remains in the hospital into a subsequent trimester, the trimester character for the antepartum complication code should be assigned on the basis of the trimester when the complication developed, not the trimester of the discharge. If the condition developed prior to the current admission/encounter or represents a pre-existing condition, the trimester character for the trimester at the time of the admission/encounter should be assigned.

5) **Unspecified trimester**

Each category that includes codes for trimester has a code for "unspecified trimester." The "unspecified trimester" code should rarely be used, such as when the documentation in the record is insufficient to determine the trimester and it is not possible to obtain clarification.

6) **7th character for fetus identification**

Where applicable, a 7th character is to be assigned for certain categories (O31, O32, O33.3 - O33.6, O35, O36, O4Ø, O41, O6Ø.1, O6Ø.2, O64, and O69) to identify the fetus for which the complication code applies.

Assign 7th character "Ø":

- For single gestations
- When the documentation in the record is insufficient to determine the fetus affected and it is not possible to obtain clarification.
- When it is not possible to clinically determine which fetus is affected.

b. **Selection of OB principal or first-listed diagnosis**

1) **Routine outpatient prenatal visits**

For routine outpatient prenatal visits when no complications are present, a code from category Z34, Encounter for supervision of normal pregnancy, should be used as the first-listed diagnosis. These codes should not be used in conjunction with chapter 15 codes.

2) **Prenatal outpatient visits for high-risk patients**

For routine prenatal outpatient visits for patients with high-risk pregnancies, a code from category OØ9, Supervision of high-risk pregnancy, should be used as the first-listed diagnosis. Secondary chapter 15 codes may be used in conjunction with these codes if appropriate.

3) **Episodes when no delivery occurs**

In episodes when no delivery occurs, the principal diagnosis should correspond to the principal complication of the pregnancy which necessitated the encounter. Should more than one complication exist, all of which are treated or monitored, any of the complications codes may be sequenced first.

4) **When a delivery occurs**

When a delivery occurs, the principal diagnosis should correspond to the main circumstances or complication of the delivery. In cases of cesarean delivery, the selection of the principal diagnosis should be the condition established after study that was responsible for the patient's admission. If the patient was admitted with a condition that resulted in the performance of a cesarean procedure, that condition should be selected as the principal diagnosis. If the reason for the admission/encounter was unrelated to the condition resulting in the cesarean delivery, the condition related to the reason for the admission/encounter should be selected as the principal diagnosis.

5) **Outcome of delivery**

A code from category Z37, Outcome of delivery, should be included on every maternal record when a delivery has occurred. These codes are not to be used on subsequent records or on the newborn record.

Gretia Plena church

c. **Pre-existing conditions versus conditions due to the pregnancy**

Certain categories in Chapter 15 distinguish between conditions of the mother that existed prior to pregnancy (pre-existing) and those that are a direct result of pregnancy. When assigning codes from Chapter 15, it is important to assess if a condition was pre-existing prior to pregnancy or developed during or due to the pregnancy in order to assign the correct code.

Categories that do not distinguish between pre-existing and pregnancy-related conditions may be used for either. It is acceptable to use codes specifically for the puerperium with codes complicating pregnancy and childbirth if a condition arises postpartum during the delivery encounter.

d. **Pre-existing hypertension in pregnancy**

Category O10, Pre-existing hypertension complicating pregnancy, childbirth and the puerperium, includes codes for hypertensive heart and hypertensive chronic kidney disease. When assigning one of the O10 codes that includes hypertensive heart disease or hypertensive chronic kidney disease, it is necessary to add a secondary code from the appropriate hypertension category to specify the type of heart failure or chronic kidney disease.

See Section I.C.9. Hypertension.

e. **Fetal conditions affecting the management of the mother**

1) **Codes from categories O35 and O36**

Codes from categories O35, Maternal care for known or suspected fetal abnormality and damage, and O36, Maternal care for other fetal problems, are assigned only when the fetal condition is actually responsible for modifying the management of the mother, i.e., by requiring diagnostic studies, additional observation, special care, or termination of pregnancy. The fact that the fetal condition exists does not justify assigning a code from this series to the mother's record.

2) **In utero surgery**

In cases when surgery is performed on the fetus, a diagnosis code from category O35, Maternal care for known or suspected fetal abnormality and damage, should be assigned identifying the fetal condition. Assign the appropriate procedure code for the procedure performed.

No code from Chapter 16, the perinatal codes, should be used on the mother's record to identify fetal conditions. Surgery performed in utero on a fetus is still to be coded as an obstetric encounter.

f. **HIV Infection in pregnancy, childbirth and the puerperium**

During pregnancy, childbirth or the puerperium, a patient admitted because of an HIV-related illness should receive a principal diagnosis from subcategory O98.7-, Human immunodeficiency [HIV] disease complicating pregnancy, childbirth and the puerperium, followed by the code(s) for the HIV-related illness(es).

Patients with asymptomatic HIV infection status admitted during pregnancy, childbirth, or the puerperium should receive codes of O98.7- and Z21, Asymptomatic human immunodeficiency virus [HIV] infection status.

g. **Diabetes mellitus in pregnancy**

Diabetes mellitus is a significant complicating factor in pregnancy. Pregnant women who are diabetic should be assigned a code from category O24, Diabetes mellitus in pregnancy, childbirth, and the puerperium, first, followed by the appropriate diabetes code(s) (E08-E13) from Chapter 4.

h. **Long term use of insulin**

Code Z79.4, Long-term (current) use of insulin, should also be assigned if the diabetes mellitus is being treated with insulin.

i. **Gestational (pregnancy induced) diabetes**

Gestational (pregnancy induced) diabetes can occur during the second and third trimester of pregnancy in women who were not diabetic prior to pregnancy. Gestational diabetes can cause complications in the pregnancy similar to those of pre-existing diabetes mellitus. It also puts the woman at greater risk of developing diabetes after the pregnancy. Codes for gestational diabetes are in subcategory O24.4, Gestational diabetes mellitus. No

other code from category O24, Diabetes mellitus in pregnancy, childbirth, and the puerperium, should be used with a code from O24.4.

The codes under subcategory O24.4 include diet controlled and insulin controlled. If a patient with gestational diabetes is treated with both diet and insulin, only the code for insulin-controlled is required.

Code Z79.4, Long-term (current) use of insulin, should not be assigned with codes from subcategory O24.4.

An abnormal glucose tolerance in pregnancy is assigned a code from subcategory O99.81, Abnormal glucose complicating pregnancy, childbirth, and the puerperium.

j. **Sepsis and septic shock complicating abortion, pregnancy, childbirth and the puerperium**

When assigning a chapter 15 code for sepsis complicating abortion, pregnancy, childbirth, and the puerperium, a code for the specific type of infection should be assigned as an additional diagnosis. If severe sepsis is present, a code from subcategory R65.2, Severe sepsis, and code(s) for associated organ dysfunction(s) should also be assigned as additional diagnoses.

k. **Puerperal sepsis**

Code O85, Puerperal sepsis, should be assigned with a secondary code to identify the causal organism (e.g., for a bacterial infection, assign a code from category B95-B96, Bacterial infections in conditions classified elsewhere). A code from category A40, Streptococcal sepsis, or A41, Other sepsis, should not be used for puerperal sepsis. If applicable, use additional codes to identify severe sepsis (R65.2-) and any associated acute organ dysfunction.

l. **Alcohol and tobacco use during pregnancy, childbirth and the puerperium**

1) **Alcohol use during pregnancy, childbirth and the puerperium**

Codes under subcategory O99.31, Alcohol use complicating pregnancy, childbirth, and the puerperium, should be assigned for any pregnancy case when a mother uses alcohol during the pregnancy or postpartum. A secondary code from category F10, Alcohol related disorders, should also be assigned to identify manifestations of the alcohol use.

2) **Tobacco use during pregnancy, childbirth and the puerperium**

Codes under subcategory O99.33, Smoking (tobacco) complicating pregnancy, childbirth, and the puerperium, should be assigned for any pregnancy case when a mother uses any type of tobacco product during the pregnancy or postpartum. A secondary code from category F17, Nicotine dependence, or code Z72.0, Tobacco use, should also be assigned to identify the type of nicotine dependence.

m. **Poisoning, toxic effects, adverse effects and underdosing in a pregnant patient**

A code from subcategory O9A.2, Injury, poisoning and certain other consequences of external causes complicating pregnancy, childbirth, and the puerperium, should be sequenced first, followed by the appropriate injury, poisoning, toxic effect, adverse effect or underdosing code, and then the additional code(s) that specifies the condition caused by the poisoning, toxic effect, adverse effect or underdosing.

See Section I.C.19. Adverse effects, poisoning, underdosing and toxic effects.

n. **Normal delivery, code O80**

1) **Encounter for full term uncomplicated delivery**

Code O80 should be assigned when a woman is admitted for a full-term normal delivery and delivers a single, healthy infant without any complications antepartum, during the delivery, or postpartum during the delivery episode. Code O80 is always a principal diagnosis. It is not to be used if any other code from chapter 15 is needed to describe a current complication of the antenatal, delivery, or perinatal period. Additional codes from other chapters may be used with code O80 if they are not related to or are in any way complicating the pregnancy.

2) Uncomplicated delivery with resolved antepartum complication
Code O80 may be used if the patient had a complication at some point during the pregnancy, but the complication is not present at the time of the admission for delivery.

3) Outcome of delivery for O80
Z37.0, Single live birth, is the only outcome of delivery code appropriate for use with O80.

o. The peripartum and postpartum periods

1) Peripartum and postpartum periods
The postpartum period begins immediately after delivery and continues for six weeks following delivery. The peripartum period is defined as the last month of pregnancy to five months postpartum.

2) Peripartum and postpartum complication
A postpartum complication is any complication occurring within the six-week period.

3) Pregnancy-related complications after 6 week period
Chapter 15 codes may also be used to describe pregnancy-related complications after the peripartum or postpartum period if the provider documents that a condition is pregnancy related.

4) Admission for routine postpartum care following delivery outside hospital
When the mother delivers outside the hospital prior to admission and is admitted for routine postpartum care and no complications are noted, code Z39.0, Encounter for care and examination of mother immediately after delivery, should be assigned as the principal diagnosis.

5) Pregnancy associated cardiomyopathy
Pregnancy associated cardiomyopathy, code O90.3, is unique in that it may be diagnosed in the third trimester of pregnancy but may continue to progress months after delivery. For this reason, it is referred to as peripartum cardiomyopathy. Code O90.3 is only for use when the cardiomyopathy develops as a result of pregnancy in a woman who did not have pre-existing heart disease.

p. Code O94, Sequelae of complication of pregnancy, childbirth, and the puerperium

1) Code O94
Code O94, Sequelae of complication of pregnancy, childbirth, and the puerperium, is for use in those cases when an initial complication of a pregnancy develops a sequelae requiring care or treatment at a future date.

2) After the initial postpartum period
This code may be used at any time after the initial postpartum period.

3) Sequencing of code O94
This code, like all late effect codes, is to be sequenced following the code describing the sequelae of the complication.

q. Termination of Pregnancy and Spontaneous Abortions

1) Abortion with liveborn fetus
When an attempted termination of pregnancy results in a liveborn fetus, assign code Z33.2, Encounter for elective termination of pregnancy and a code from category Z37, Outcome of Delivery.

2) Retained products of conception following an abortion
Subsequent encounters for retained products of conception following a spontaneous abortion or elective termination of pregnancy are assigned the appropriate code from category O03, Spontaneous abortion, or codes O07.4, Failed attempted termination of pregnancy without complication and Z33.2, Encounter for elective termination of pregnancy. This advice is appropriate even when the patient was discharged previously with a discharge diagnosis of complete abortion.

3) Complications leading to abortion
Codes from Chapter 15 may be used as additional codes to identify any documented complications of the pregnancy in conjunction with codes in categories in O07 and O08.

r. Abuse in a pregnant patient
For suspected or confirmed cases of abuse of a pregnant patient, a code(s) from subcategories O9A.3, Physical abuse complicating pregnancy, childbirth, and the puerperium, O9A.4, Sexual abuse complicating pregnancy, childbirth, and the puerperium, and O9A.5, Psychological abuse complicating pregnancy, childbirth, and the puerperium, should be sequenced first, followed by the appropriate codes (if applicable) to identify any associated current injury due to physical abuse, sexual abuse, and the perpetrator of abuse.

See Section I.C.19.f. Adult and child abuse, neglect and other maltreatment.

16. Chapter 16: Certain Conditions Origination in the Perinatal Period (P00-P96)
For coding and reporting purposes the perinatal period is defined as before birth through the 28th day following birth. The following guidelines are provided for reporting purposes

a. General Perinatal Rules

1) Use of Chapter 16 codes
Codes in this chapter are never for use on the maternal record. Codes from Chapter 15, the obstetric chapter, are never permitted on the newborn record. Chapter 16 codes may be used throughout the life of the patient if the condition is still present.

2) Principal diagnosis for birth record
When coding the birth episode in a newborn record, assign a code from category Z38, Liveborn infants according to place of birth and type of delivery, as the principal diagnosis. A code from category Z38 is assigned only once, to a newborn at the time of birth. If a newborn is transferred to another institution, a code from category Z38 should not be used at the receiving hospital.

A code from category Z38 is used only on the newborn record, not on the mother's record.

3) Use of codes from other chapters with codes from Chapter 16
Codes from other chapters may be used with codes from chapter 16 if the codes from the other chapters provide more specific detail. Codes for signs and symptoms may be assigned when a definitive diagnosis has not been established. If the reason for the encounter is a perinatal condition, the code from chapter 16 should be sequenced first.

4) Use of Chapter 16 codes after the perinatal period
Should a condition originate in the perinatal period, and continue throughout the life of the patient, the perinatal code should continue to be used regardless of the patient's age.

5) Birth process or community acquired conditions
If a newborn has a condition that may be either due to the birth process or community acquired and the documentation does not indicate which it is, the default is due to the birth process and the code from Chapter 16 should be used. If the condition is community-acquired, a code from Chapter 16 should not be assigned.

6) Code all clinically significant conditions
All clinically significant conditions noted on routine newborn examination should be coded. A condition is clinically significant if it requires:

- clinical evaluation; or
- therapeutic treatment; or
- diagnostic procedures; or
- extended length of hospital stay; or
- increased nursing care and/or monitoring; or
- has implications for future health care needs

Note: The perinatal guidelines listed above are the same as the general coding guidelines for "additional diagnoses", except for the final point regarding implications for future health care needs. Codes should be assigned for conditions that have been specified by the provider as having implications for future health care needs.

b. **Observation and evaluation of newborns for suspected conditions not found**
   Reserved for future expansion

c. **Coding Additional Perinatal Diagnoses**

   1) **Assigning codes for conditions that require treatment**
      Assign codes for conditions that require treatment or further investigation, prolong the length of stay, or require resource utilization.

   2) **Codes for conditions specified as having implications for future health care needs**
      Assign codes for conditions that have been specified by the provider as having implications for future health care needs.

      Note: This guideline should not be used for adult patients.

d. **Prematurity and fetal growth retardation**
   Providers utilize different criteria in determining prematurity. A code for prematurity should not be assigned unless it is documented. Assignment of codes in categories P05, Disorders of newborn related to slow fetal growth and fetal malnutrition, and P07, Disorders of newborn related to short gestation and low birth weight, not elsewhere classified, should be based on the recorded birth weight and estimated gestational age. Codes from category P05 should not be assigned with codes from category P07.

   When both birth weight and gestational age are available, two codes from category P07 should be assigned, with the code for birth weight sequenced before the code for gestational age.

e. **Low birth weight and immaturity status**
   Codes from category P07, Disorders of newborn related to short gestation and low birth weight, not elsewhere classified, are for use for a child or adult who was premature or had a low birth weight as a newborn and this is affecting the patient's current health status.

   See Section I.C.21. Factors influencing health status and contact with health services, Status.

f. **Bacterial sepsis of newborn**
   Category P36, Bacterial sepsis of newborn, includes congenital sepsis. If a perinate is documented as having sepsis without documentation of congenital or community acquired, the default is congenital and a code from category P36 should be assigned. If the P36 code includes the causal organism, an additional code from category B95, Streptococcus, Staphylococcus, and Enterococcus as the cause of diseases classified elsewhere, or B96, Other bacterial agents as the cause of diseases classified elsewhere, should not be assigned. If the P36 code does not include the causal organism, assign an additional code from category B96. If applicable, use additional codes to identify severe sepsis (R65.2-) and any associated acute organ dysfunction.

g. **Stillbirth**
   Code P95, Stillbirth, is only for use in institutions that maintain separate records for stillbirths. No other code should be used with P95. Code P95 should not be used on the mother's record.

17. **Chapter 17: Congenital Malformations, Deformations, and Chromosomal Abnormalities (Q00-Q99)**
    Assign an appropriate code(s) from categories Q00-Q99, Congenital malformations, deformations, and chromosomal abnormalities when a malformation/deformation or chromosomal abnormality is documented. A malformation/deformation/or chromosomal abnormality may be the principal/first-listed diagnosis on a record or a secondary diagnosis.

    When a malformation/deformation/or chromosomal abnormality does not have a unique code assignment, assign additional code(s) for any manifestations that may be present.

    When the code assignment specifically identifies the malformation/deformation/or chromosomal abnormality, manifestations that are an inherent component of the anomaly should not be coded separately. Additional codes should be assigned for manifestations that are not an inherent component.

    Codes from Chapter 17 may be used throughout the life of the patient. If a congenital malformation or deformity has been corrected, a personal history code should be used to identify the history of the malformation or deformity. Although present at birth, malformation/deformation/or chromosomal abnormality may not be identified until later in life.

Whenever the condition is diagnosed by the physician, it is appropriate to assign a code from codes Q00-Q99.

For the birth admission, the appropriate code from category Z38, Liveborn infants, according to place of birth and type of delivery, should be sequenced as the principal diagnosis, followed by any congenital anomaly codes, Q00-Q99.

18. **Chapter 18: Symptoms, Signs, and Abnormal Clinical and Laboratory Findings, Not Elsewhere Classified (R00-R99)**
    Chapter 18 includes symptoms, signs, abnormal results of clinical or other investigative procedures, and ill-defined conditions regarding which no diagnosis classifiable elsewhere is recorded. Signs and symptoms that point to a specific diagnosis have been assigned to a category in other chapters of the classification.

a. **Use of symptom codes**
   Codes that describe symptoms and signs are acceptable for reporting purposes when a related definitive diagnosis has not been established (confirmed) by the provider.

b. **Use of a symptom code with a definitive diagnosis code**
   Codes for signs and symptoms may be reported in addition to a related definitive diagnosis when the sign or symptom is not routinely associated with that diagnosis, such as the various signs and symptoms associated with complex syndromes. The definitive diagnosis code should be sequenced before the symptom code.

   Signs or symptoms that are associated routinely with a disease process should not be assigned as additional codes, unless otherwise instructed by the classification.

c. **Combination codes that include symptoms**
   ICD-10-CM contains a number of combination codes that identify both the definitive diagnosis and common symptoms of that diagnosis. When using one of these combination codes, an additional code should not be assigned for the symptom.

d. **Repeated falls**
   Code R29.6, Repeated falls, is for use for encounters when a patient has recently fallen and the reason for the fall is being investigated.

   Code Z91.81, History of falling, is for use when a patient has fallen in the past and is at risk for future falls. When appropriate, both codes R29.6 and Z91.81 may be assigned together.

e. **Coma scale**
   The coma scale codes (R40.2-) can be used in conjunction with traumatic brain injury codes, acute cerebrovascular disease or sequelae of cerebrovascular disease codes. These codes are primarily for use by trauma registries, but they may be used in any setting where this information is collected. The coma scale codes should be sequenced after the diagnosis code(s).

   These codes, one from each subcategory, are needed to complete the scale. The 7th character indicates when the scale was recorded. The 7th character should match for all three codes.

   At a minimum, report the initial score documented on presentation at your facility. This may be a score from the emergency medicine technician (EMT) or in the emergency department. If desired, a facility may choose to capture multiple Glasgow coma scale scores.

   Assign code R40.24, Glasgow coma scale, total score, when only the total score is documented in the medical record and not the individual score(s).

f. **Functional quadriplegia**
   Functional quadriplegia (code R53.2) is the lack of ability to use one's limbs or to ambulate due to extreme debility. It is not associated with neurologic deficit or injury, and code R53.2 should not be used for cases of neurologic quadriplegia. It should only be assigned if functional quadriplegia is specifically documented in the medical record.

g. **SIRS due to non-infectious process**
   The systemic inflammatory response syndrome (SIRS) can develop as a result of certain non-infectious disease processes, such as trauma, malignant neoplasm, or pancreatitis. When SIRS is documented with a noninfectious condition, and no subsequent infection is documented, the code for the underlying condition, such as an injury, should be assigned, followed by code R65.10, Systemic inflammatory response syndrome (SIRS) of non-infectious origin without acute organ dysfunction, or code R65.11, Systemic inflammatory response syndrome (SIRS) of non-infectious origin

with acute organ dysfunction. If an associated acute organ dysfunction is documented, the appropriate code(s) for the specific type of organ dysfunction(s) should be assigned in addition to code R65.11. If acute organ dysfunction is documented, but it cannot be determined if the acute organ dysfunction is associated with SIRS or due to another condition (e.g., directly due to the trauma), the provider should be queried.

h. Death NOS
Code R99, Ill-defined and unknown cause of mortality, is only for use in the very limited circumstance when a patient who has already died is brought into an emergency department or other healthcare facility and is pronounced dead upon arrival. It does not represent the discharge disposition of death.

19. Chapter 19: Injury, Poisoning, and Certain Other Consequences of External Causes (S00-T88)

a. Application of 7th Characters in Chapter 19
Most categories in chapter 19 have a 7th character requirement for each applicable code. Most categories in this chapter have three 7th character values (with the exception of fractures): A, initial encounter, D, subsequent encounter and S, sequela. Categories for traumatic fractures have additional 7th character values.

7th character "A", initial encounter is used while the patient is receiving active treatment for the condition. Examples of active treatment are: surgical treatment, emergency department encounter, and evaluation and treatment by a new physician.

7th character "D" subsequent encounter is used for encounters after the patient has received active treatment of the condition and is receiving routine care for the condition during the healing or recovery phase. Examples of subsequent care are: cast change or removal, removal of external or internal fixation device, medication adjustment, other aftercare and follow up visits following treatment of the injury or condition.

The aftercare Z codes should not be used for aftercare for conditions such as injuries or poisonings, where 7th characters are provided to identify subsequent care. For example, for aftercare of an injury, assign the acute injury code with the 7th character "D" (subsequent encounter).

7th character "S", sequela, is for use for complications or conditions that arise as a direct result of a condition, such as scar formation after a burn. The scars are sequelae of the burn. When using 7th character "S", it is necessary to use both the injury code that precipitated the sequela and the code for the sequela itself. The "S" is added only to the injury code, not the sequela code. The 7th character "S" identifies the injury responsible for the sequela. The specific type of sequela (e.g. scar) is sequenced first, followed by the injury code.

b. Coding of injuries
When coding injuries, assign separate codes for each injury unless a combination code is provided, in which case the combination code is assigned. Code T07, Unspecified multiple injuries should not be assigned in the inpatient setting unless information for a more specific code is not available. Traumatic injury codes (S00-T14.9) are not to be used for normal, healing surgical wounds or to identify complications of surgical wounds.

The code for the most serious injury, as determined by the provider and the focus of treatment, is sequenced first.

1) Superficial injuries
Superficial injuries such as abrasions or contusions are not coded when associated with more severe injuries of the same site.

2) Primary injury with damage to nerves/blood vessels
When a primary injury results in minor damage to peripheral nerves or blood vessels, the primary injury is sequenced first with additional code(s) for injuries to nerves and spinal cord (such as category S04), and/or injury to blood vessels (such as category S15). When the primary injury is to the blood vessels or nerves, that injury should be sequenced first.

c. Coding of traumatic fractures
The principles of multiple coding of injuries should be followed in coding fractures. Fractures of specified sites are coded individually by site in accordance with both the provisions within categories S02, S12, S22, S32, S42, S49, S52, S59, S62, S72, S79, S82, S89, S92 and the level of detail furnished by medical record content.

A fracture not indicated as open or closed should be coded to closed. A fracture not indicated whether displaced or not displaced should be coded to displaced.

More specific guidelines are as follows:

1) Initial vs. subsequent encounter for fractures
Traumatic fractures are coded using the appropriate 7th character extension for initial encounter (A, B, C) while the patient is receiving active treatment for the fracture. Examples of active treatment are: surgical treatment, emergency department encounter, and evaluation and treatment by a new physician. The appropriate 7th character for initial encounter should also be assigned for a patient who delayed seeking treatment for the fracture or nonunion.

Fractures are coded using the appropriate 7th character extension for subsequent care for encounters after the patient has completed active treatment of the fracture and is receiving routine care for the fracture during the healing or recovery phase. Examples of fracture aftercare are: cast change or removal, removal of external or internal fixation device, medication adjustment, and follow-up visits following fracture treatment.

Care for complications of surgical treatment for fracture repairs during the healing or recovery phase should be coded with the appropriate complication codes.

Care of complications of fractures, such as malunion and nonunion, should be reported with the appropriate 7th character extensions for subsequent care with nonunion (K, M, N,) or subsequent care with malunion (P, Q, R).

A code from category M80, not a traumatic fracture code, should be used for any patient with known osteoporosis who suffers a fracture, even if the patient had a minor fall or trauma, if that fall or trauma would not usually break a normal, healthy bone.

See Section I.C.13. Osteoporosis.

The aftercare Z codes should not be used for aftercare for traumatic fractures. For aftercare of a traumatic fracture, assign the acute fracture code with the appropriate 7th character.

2) Multiple fractures sequencing
Multiple fractures are sequenced in accordance with the severity of the fracture.

d. Coding of burns and corrosions
The ICD-10-CM makes a distinction between burns and corrosions. The burn codes are for thermal burns, except sunburns, that come from a heat source, such as a fire or hot appliance. The burn codes are also for burns resulting from electricity and radiation. Corrosions are burns due to chemicals. The guidelines are the same for burns and corrosions.

Current burns (T20-T25) are classified by depth, extent and by agent (X code). Burns are classified by depth as first degree (erythema), second degree (blistering), and third degree (full-thickness involvement). Burns of the eye and internal organs (T26-T28) are classified by site, but not by degree.

1) Sequencing of burn and related condition codes
Sequence first the code that reflects the highest degree of burn when more than one burn is present.

a. When the reason for the admission or encounter is for treatment of external multiple burns, sequence first the code that reflects the burn of the highest degree.

b. When a patient has both internal and external burns, the circumstances of admission govern the selection of the principal diagnosis or first-listed diagnosis.

c. When a patient is admitted for burn injuries and other related conditions such as smoke inhalation and/or respiratory failure, the circumstances of admission govern the selection of the principal or first-listed diagnosis.

2) Burns of the same local site

Classify burns of the same local site (three-character category level, T20-T28) but of different degrees to the subcategory identifying the highest degree recorded in the diagnosis.

3) Non-healing burns

Non-healing burns are coded as acute burns.

Necrosis of burned skin should be coded as a non-healed burn.

4) Infected burn

For any documented infected burn site, use an additional code for the infection.

5) Assign separate codes for each burn site

When coding burns, assign separate codes for each burn site. Category T30, Burn and corrosion, body region unspecified is extremely vague and should rarely be used.

6) Burns and corrosions classified according to extent of body surface involved

Assign codes from category T31, Burns classified according to extent of body surface involved, or T32, Corrosions classified according to extent of body surface involved, when the site of the burn is not specified or when there is a need for additional data. It is advisable to use category T31 as additional coding when needed to provide data for evaluating burn mortality, such as that needed by burn units. It is also advisable to use category T31 as an additional code for reporting purposes when there is mention of a third-degree burn involving 20 percent or more of the body surface.

Categories T31 and T32 are based on the classic "rule of nines" in estimating body surface involved: head and neck are assigned nine percent, each arm nine percent, each leg 18 percent, the anterior trunk 18 percent, posterior trunk 18 percent, and genitalia one percent. Providers may change these percentage assignments where necessary to accommodate infants and children who have proportionately larger heads than adults, and patients who have large buttocks, thighs, or abdomen that involve burns.

7) Encounters for treatment of sequela of burns

Encounters for the treatment of the late effects of burns or corrosions (i.e., scars or joint contractures) should be coded with a burn or corrosion code with the 7th character "S" for sequela.

8) Sequelae with a late effect code and current burn

When appropriate, both a code for a current burn or corrosion with 7th character "A" or "D" and a burn or corrosion code with 7th character "S" may be assigned on the same record (when both a current burn and sequelae of an old burn exist). Burns and corrosions do not heal at the same rate and a current healing wound may still exist with sequela of a healed burn or corrosion.

9) Use of an external cause code with burns and corrosions

An external cause code should be used with burns and corrosions to identify the source and intent of the burn, as well as the place where it occurred.

e. Adverse effects, poisoning, underdosing and toxic effects

Codes in categories T36-T65 are combination codes that include the substance that was taken as well as the intent. No additional external cause code is required for poisonings, toxic effects, adverse effects and underdosing codes.

1) Do not code directly from the Table of Drugs

Do not code directly from the Table of Drugs and Chemicals. Always refer back to the Tabular List.

2) Use as many codes as necessary to describe

Use as many codes as necessary to describe completely all drugs, medicinal or biological substances.

3) If the same code would describe the causative agent

If the same code would describe the causative agent for more than one adverse reaction, poisoning, toxic effect or underdosing, assign the code only once.

4) If two or more drugs, medicinal or biological substances

If two or more drugs, medicinal or biological substances are reported, code each individually unless a combination code is listed in the Table of Drugs and Chemicals.

5) The occurrence of drug toxicity is classified in ICD-10-CM as follows:

(a) Adverse effect

When coding an adverse effect of a drug that has been correctly prescribed and properly administered, assign the appropriate code for the nature of the adverse effect followed by the appropriate code for the adverse effect of the drug (T36-T50). The code for the drug should have a 5th or 6th character "5" (for example T36.0X5-) Examples of the nature of an adverse effect are tachycardia, delirium, gastrointestinal hemorrhaging, vomiting, hypokalemia, hepatitis, renal failure, or respiratory failure.

(b) Poisoning

When coding a poisoning or reaction to the improper use of a medication (e.g., overdose, wrong substance given or taken in error, wrong route of administration), first assign the appropriate code from categories T36-T50. The poisoning codes have an associated intent as their 5th or 6th character (accidental, intentional self-harm, assault and undetermined. Use additional code(s) for all manifestations of poisonings.

If there is also a diagnosis of abuse or dependence of the substance, the abuse or dependence is assigned as an additional code.

Examples of poisoning include:

(i) Error was made in drug prescription

Errors made in drug prescription or in the administration of the drug by provider, nurse, patient, or other person.

(ii) Overdose of a drug intentionally taken

If an overdose of a drug was intentionally taken or administered and resulted in drug toxicity, it would be coded as a poisoning.

(iii) Nonprescribed drug taken with correctly prescribed and properly administered drug

If a nonprescribed drug or medicinal agent was taken in combination with a correctly prescribed and properly administered drug, any drug toxicity or other reaction resulting from the interaction of the two drugs would be classified as a poisoning.

(iv) Interaction of drug(s) and alcohol

When a reaction results from the interaction of a drug(s) and alcohol, this would be classified as poisoning.

See Section I.C.4. if poisoning is the result of insulin pump malfunctions.

(c) Underdosing

Underdosing refers to taking less of a medication than is prescribed by a provider or a manufacturer's instruction. For underdosing, assign the code from categories T36-T50 (fifth or sixth character "6").

Codes for underdosing should never be assigned as principal or first-listed codes. If a patient has a relapse or exacerbation of the medical condition for which the drug is prescribed because of the reduction in dose, then the medical condition itself should be coded.

Noncompliance (Z91.12-, Z91.13-) or complication of care (Y63.6-Y63.9) codes are to be used with an underdosing code to indicate intent, if known.

(d) Toxic effects

When a harmful substance is ingested or comes in contact with a person, this is classified as a toxic effect. The toxic effect codes are in categories T51-T65.

Toxic effect codes have an associated intent: accidental, intentional self-harm, assault and undetermined.

f. Adult and child abuse, neglect and other maltreatment

Sequence first the appropriate code from categories T74.- (Adult and child abuse, neglect and other maltreatment, confirmed) or T76.- (Adult and child abuse, neglect and other maltreatment, suspected) for abuse, neglect and other maltreatment, followed by any accompanying mental health or injury code(s).

If the documentation in the medical record states abuse or neglect it is coded as confirmed (T74.-). It is coded as suspected if it is documented as suspected (T76.-).

For cases of confirmed abuse or neglect an external cause code from the assault section (X92-Y08) should be added to identify the cause of any physical injuries. A perpetrator code (Y07) should be added when the perpetrator of the abuse is known. For suspected cases of abuse or neglect, do not report external cause or perpetrator code.

If a suspected case of abuse, neglect or mistreatment is ruled out during an encounter code Z04.71, Encounter for examination and observation following alleged physical adult abuse, ruled out, or code Z04.72, Encounter for examination and observation following alleged child physical abuse, ruled out, should be used, not a code from T76.

If a suspected case of alleged rape or sexual abuse is ruled out during an encounter code Z04.41, Encounter for examination and observation following alleged physical adult abuse, ruled out, or code Z04.42, Encounter for examination and observation following alleged rape or sexual abuse, ruled out, should be used, not a code from T76.

See Section I.C.15. Abuse in a pregnant patient.

g. Complications of care

1) General guidelines for complications of care

(a) Documentation of complications of care

See Section I.B.16. for information on documentation of complications of care.

2) Pain due to medical devices

Pain associated with devices, implants or grafts left in a surgical site (for example painful hip prosthesis) is assigned to the appropriate code(s) found in Chapter 19, Injury, poisoning, and certain other consequences of external causes. Specific codes for pain due to medical devices are found in the T code section of the ICD-10-CM. Use additional code(s) from category G89 to identify acute or chronic pain due to presence of the device, implant or graft (G89.18 or G89.28).

3) Transplant complications

(a) Transplant complications other than kidney

Codes under category T86, Complications of transplanted organs and tissues, are for use for both complications and rejection of transplanted organs. A transplant complication code is only assigned if the complication affects the function of the transplanted organ. Two codes are required to fully describe a transplant complication: the appropriate code from category T86 and a secondary code that identifies the complication.

Pre-existing conditions or conditions that develop after the transplant are not coded as complications unless they affect the function of the transplanted organs.

See I.C.21. for transplant organ removal status

See I.C.2. for malignant neoplasm associated with transplanted organ.

(b) Kidney transplant complications

Patients who have undergone kidney transplant may still have some form of chronic kidney disease (CKD) because the kidney transplant may not fully restore kidney function. Code T86.1- should be assigned for documented complications of a kidney transplant, such as transplant failure or rejection or other transplant complication. Code T86.1- should not be assigned for post kidney transplant patients who have chronic kidney (CKD) unless a transplant complication such as transplant failure or rejection is documented. If the documentation is unclear as to whether the patient has a complication of the transplant, query the provider.

Conditions that affect the function of the transplanted kidney, other than CKD, should be assigned a code from subcategory T86.1, Complications of transplanted organ, Kidney, and a secondary code that identifies the complication.

For patients with CKD following a kidney transplant, but who do not have a complication such as failure or rejection, *see section I.C.14. Chronic kidney disease and kidney transplant status.*

4) Complication codes that include the external cause

As with certain other T codes, some of the complications of care codes have the external cause included in the code. The code includes the nature of the complication as well as the type of procedure that caused the complication. No external cause code indicating the type of procedure is necessary for these codes.

5) Complications of care codes within the body system chapters

Intraoperative and postprocedural complication codes are found within the body system chapters with codes specific to the organs and structures of that body system. These codes should be sequenced first, followed by a code(s) for the specific complication, if applicable.

20. Chapter 20: External Causes of Morbidity (V00-Y99)
The external causes of morbidity codes should never be sequenced as the first-listed or principal diagnosis.

External cause codes are intended to provide data for injury research and evaluation of injury prevention strategies. These codes capture how the injury or health condition happened (cause), the intent (unintentional or accidental; or intentional, such as suicide or assault), the place where the event occurred the activity of the patient at the time of the event, and the person's status (e.g., civilian, military).

There is no national requirement for mandatory ICD-10-CM external cause code reporting. Unless a provider is subject to a state-based external cause code reporting mandate or these codes are required by a particular payer, reporting of ICD-10-CM codes in Chapter 20, External Causes of Morbidity, is not required. In the absence of a mandatory reporting requirement, providers are encouraged to voluntarily report external cause codes, as they provide valuable data for injury research and evaluation of injury prevention strategies.

a. General external cause coding guidelines

1) Used with any code in the range of A00.0-T88.9, Z00-Z99

An external cause code may be used with any code in the range of A00.0-T88.9, Z00-Z99, classification that is a health condition due to an external cause. Though they are most applicable to injuries, they are also valid for use with such things as infections or diseases due to an external source, and other health conditions, such as a heart attack that occurs during strenuous physical activity.

2) External cause code used for length of treatment

Assign the external cause code, with the appropriate 7th character (initial encounter, subsequent encounter or sequela) for each encounter for which the injury or condition is being treated.

3) Use the full range of external cause codes

Use the full range of external cause codes to completely describe the cause, the intent, the place of occurrence, and if applicable, the activity of the patient at the time of the event, and the patient's status, for all injuries, and other health conditions due to an external cause.

4) Assign as many external cause codes as necessary

Assign as many external cause codes as necessary to fully explain each cause. If only one external code can be recorded, assign the code most related to the principal diagnosis.

5) The selection of the appropriate external cause code

The selection of the appropriate external cause code is guided by the Alphabetic Index of External Causes and by Inclusion and Exclusion notes in the Tabular List.

6) External cause code can never be a principal diagnosis
An external cause code can never be a principal (first-listed) diagnosis.

7) Combination external cause codes
Certain of the external cause codes are combination codes that identify sequential events that result in an injury, such as a fall which results in striking against an object. The injury may be due to either event or both. The combination external cause code used should correspond to the sequence of events regardless of which caused the most serious injury.

8) No external cause code needed in certain circumstances
No external cause code from Chapter 20 is needed if the external cause and intent are included in a code from another chapter (e.g. T36.0x1- Poisoning by penicillins, accidental (unintentional)).

b. Place of occurrence guideline
Codes from category Y92, Place of occurrence of the external cause, are secondary codes for use after other external cause codes to identify the location of the patient at the time of injury or other condition.

A place of occurrence code is used only once, at the initial encounter for treatment. No 7th characters are used for Y92. Only one code from Y92 should be recorded on a medical record.

Do not use place of occurrence code Y92.9 if the place is not stated or is not applicable.

c. Activity code
Assign a code from category Y93, Activity code, to describe the activity of the patient at the time the injury or other health condition occurred.

An activity code is used only once, at the initial encounter for treatment. Only one code from Y93 should be recorded on a medical record.

The activity codes are not applicable to poisonings, adverse effects, misadventures or sequela.

Do not assign Y93.9, Unspecified activity, if the activity is not stated.

A code from category Y93 is appropriate for use with external cause and intent codes if identifying the activity provides additional information about the event.

d. Place of occurrence, activity, and status codes used with other external cause code
When applicable, place of occurrence, activity, and external cause status codes are sequenced after the main external cause code(s). Regardless of the number of external cause codes assigned, there should be only one place of occurrence code, one activity code, and one external cause status code assigned to an encounter.

e. If the reporting format limits the number of external cause codes
If the reporting format limits the number of external cause codes that can be used in reporting clinical data, report the code for the cause/intent most related to the principal diagnosis. If the format permits capture of additional external cause codes, the cause/intent, including medical misadventures, of the additional events should be reported rather than the codes for place, activity, or external status.

f. Multiple external cause coding guidelines
More than one external cause code is required to fully describe the external cause of an illness or injury. The assignment of external cause codes should be sequenced in the following priority:

If two or more events cause separate injuries, an external cause code should be assigned for each cause. The first-listed external cause code will be selected in the following order:

External codes for child and adult abuse take priority over all other external cause codes.

See Section I.C.19., Child and Adult abuse guidelines.

External cause codes for terrorism events take priority over all other external cause codes except child and adult abuse.

External cause codes for cataclysmic events take priority over all other external cause codes except child and adult abuse and terrorism.

External cause codes for transport accidents take priority over all other external cause codes except cataclysmic events, child and adult abuse and terrorism.

Activity and external cause status codes are assigned following all causal (intent) external cause codes.

The first-listed external cause code should correspond to the cause of the most serious diagnosis due to an assault, accident, or self-harm, following the order of hierarchy listed above.

g. Child and adult abuse guideline
Adult and child abuse, neglect and maltreatment are classified as assault. Any of the assault codes may be used to indicate the external cause of any injury resulting from the confirmed abuse.

For confirmed cases of abuse, neglect and maltreatment, when the perpetrator is known, a code from Y07, Perpetrator of maltreatment and neglect, should accompany any other assault codes.

See Section I.C.19. Adult and child abuse, neglect and other maltreatment

h. Unknown or undetermined intent guideline
If the intent (accident, self-harm, assault) of the cause of an injury or other condition is unknown or unspecified, code the intent as accidental intent. All transport accident categories assume accidental intent.

1) Use of undetermined intent
External cause codes for events of undetermined intent are only for use if the documentation in the record specifies that the intent cannot be determined.

i. Sequelae (Late Effects) of external cause guidelines
1) Sequelae external cause codes
Sequela are reported using the external cause code with the 7th character extension "S" for sequela. These codes should be used with any report of a late effect or sequela resulting from a previous injury.

2) Sequela external cause code with a related current injury
A sequela external cause code should never be used with a related current nature of injury code.

3) Use of sequela external cause codes for subsequent visits
Use a late effect external cause code for subsequent visits when a late effect of the initial injury is being treated. Do not use a late effect external cause code for subsequent visits for follow-up care (e.g., to assess healing, to receive rehabilitative therapy) of the injury when no late effect of the injury has been documented.

j. Terrorism guidelines
1) Cause of injury identified by the Federal Government (FBI) as terrorism
When the cause of an injury is identified by the Federal Government (FBI) as terrorism, the first-listed external cause code should be a code from category Y38, Terrorism. The definition of terrorism employed by the FBI is found at the inclusion note at the beginning of category Y38. Use additional code for place of occurrence (Y92.-). More than one Y38 code may be assigned if the injury is the result of more than one mechanism of terrorism.

2) Cause of an injury is suspected to be the result of terrorism
When the cause of an injury is suspected to be the result of terrorism a code from category Y38 should not be assigned. Suspected cases should be classified as assault.

3) Code Y38.9, terrorism, secondary effects
Assign code Y38.9, Terrorism, secondary effects, for conditions occurring subsequent to the terrorist event. This code should not be assigned for conditions that are due to the initial terrorist act.

It is acceptable to assign code Y38.9 with another code from Y38 if there is an injury due to the initial terrorist event and an injury that is a subsequent result of the terrorist event.

k. External cause status
A code from category Y99, External cause status, should be assigned whenever any other external cause code is assigned for an encounter, including an Activity code, except for the events noted below. Assign a code from category Y99, External cause status, to

indicate the work status of the person at the time the event occurred. The status code indicates whether the event occurred during military activity, whether a non-military person was at work, whether an individual including a student or volunteer was involved in a non-work activity at the time of the causal event.

A code from Y99, External cause status, should be assigned, when applicable, with other external cause codes, such as transport accidents and falls. The external cause status codes are not applicable to poisonings, adverse effects, misadventures or late effects.

Do not assign a code from category Y99 if no other external cause codes (cause, activity) are applicable for the encounter.

An external cause status code is used only once, at the initial encounter for treatment. Only one code from Y99 should be recorded on a medical record.

Do not assign code Y99.9, Unspecified external cause status, if the status is not stated.

21. **Chapter 21: Factors Influencing Health Status and Contact with Health Services (Z00-Z99)**
Note: The chapter specific guidelines provide additional information about the use of Z codes for specified encounters.

a. **Use of Z codes in any healthcare setting**
Z codes are for use in any healthcare setting. Z codes may be used as either a first-listed (principal diagnosis code in the inpatient setting) or secondary code, depending on the circumstances of the encounter. Certain Z codes may only be used as first-listed or principal diagnosis.

b. **Z Codes indicate a reason for an encounter**
Z codes are not procedure codes. A corresponding procedure code must accompany a Z code to describe any procedure performed.

c. **Categories of Z codes**

1) **Contact/exposure**
Category Z20 indicates contact with, and suspected exposure to, communicable diseases. These codes are for patients who do not show any sign or symptom of a disease but are suspected to have been exposed to it by close personal contact with an infected individual or are in an area where a disease is epidemic.

Category Z77, indicates contact with and suspected exposures hazardous to health.

Contact/exposure codes may be used as a first-listed code to explain an encounter for testing, or, more commonly, as a secondary code to identify a potential risk.

2) **Inoculations and vaccinations**
Code Z23 is for encounters for inoculations and vaccinations. It indicates that a patient is being seen to receive a prophylactic inoculation against a disease. Procedure codes are required to identify the actual administration of the injection and the type(s) of immunizations given. Code Z23 may be used as a secondary code if the inoculation is given as a routine part of preventive health care, such as a well-baby visit.

3) **Status**
Status codes indicate that a patient is either a carrier of a disease or has the sequelae or residual of a past disease or condition. This includes such things as the presence of prosthetic or mechanical devices resulting from past treatment. A status code is informative, because the status may affect the course of treatment and its outcome. A status code is distinct from a history code. The history code indicates that the patient no longer has the condition.

A status code should not be used with a diagnosis code from one of the body system chapters, if the diagnosis code includes the information provided by the status code. For example, code Z94.1, Heart transplant status, should not be used with a code from subcategory T86.2, Complications of heart transplant. The status code does not provide additional information. The complication code indicates that the patient is a heart transplant patient.

For encounters for weaning from a mechanical ventilator, assign a code from subcategory J96.1, Chronic respiratory

failure, followed by code Z99.11, Dependence on respirator [ventilator] status.

The status Z codes/categories are:

Z14   Genetic carrier

Genetic carrier status indicates that a person carries a gene, associated with a particular disease, which may be passed to offspring who may develop that disease. The person does not have the disease and is not at risk of developing the disease.

Z15   Genetic susceptibility to disease

Genetic susceptibility indicates that a person has a gene that increases the risk of that person developing the disease.

Codes from category Z15 should not be used as principal or first-listed codes. If the patient has the condition to which he/she is susceptible, and that condition is the reason for the encounter, the code for the current condition should be sequenced first. If the patient is being seen for follow-up after completed treatment for this condition, and the condition no longer exists, a follow-up code should be sequenced first, followed by the appropriate personal history and genetic susceptibility codes. If the purpose of the encounter is genetic counseling associated with procreative management, code Z31.5, Encounter for genetic counseling, should be assigned as the first-listed code, followed by a code from category Z15. Additional codes should be assigned for any applicable family or personal history.

Z16   Resistance to antimicrobial drugs

This code indicates that a patient has a condition that is resistant to antimicrobial drug treatment. Sequence the infection code first.

Z17   Estrogen receptor status

Z18   Retained foreign body fragments

Z21   Asymptomatic HIV infection status

This code indicates that a patient has tested positive for HIV but has manifested no signs or symptoms of the disease.

Z22   Carrier of infectious disease

Carrier status indicates that a person harbors the specific organisms of a disease without manifest symptoms and is capable of transmitting the infection.

Z28.3   Underimmunization status

Z33.1   Pregnant state, incidental

This code is a secondary code only for use when the pregnancy is in no way complicating the reason for visit. Otherwise, a code from the obstetric chapter is required.

Z66   Do not resuscitate

This code may be used when it is documented by the provider that a patient is on do not resuscitate status at any time during the stay.

Z67   Blood type

Z68   Body mass index (BMI)

Z74.01 Bed confinement status

Z76.82 Awaiting organ transplant status

Z78   Other specified health status

Code Z78.1, Physical restraint status, may be used when it is documented by the provider that a patient has been put in restraints during the current encounter. Please note that this code should not be reported when it is documented by the provider that a patient is temporarily restrained during a procedure.

Z79   Long-term (current) drug therapy

Codes from this category indicate a patient's continuous use of a prescribed drug (including such things as aspirin therapy) for the long-term treatment of a condition or for prophylactic use. It is not for use for patients who have addictions to drugs. This subcategory is not for use of medications for detoxification or maintenance programs to prevent withdrawal symptoms in patients with drug dependence (e.g., methadone maintenance for opiate dependence). Assign the appropriate code for the drug dependence instead.

Assign a code from Z79 if the patient is receiving a medication for an extended period as a prophylactic measure (such as for the prevention of deep vein thrombosis) or as treatment of a chronic condition (such as arthritis) or a disease requiring a lengthy course of treatment (such as cancer). Do not assign a code from category Z79 for medication being administered for a brief period of time to treat an acute illness or injury (such as a course of antibiotics to treat acute bronchitis).

Z88 Allergy status to drugs, medicaments and biological substances

Except: Z88.9, Allergy status to unspecified drugs, medicaments and biological substances status

Z89 Acquired absence of limb

Z90 Acquired absence of organs, not elsewhere classified

Z91.0- Allergy status, other than to drugs and biological substances

Z92.82 Status post administration of tPA (rtPA) in a different facility within the last 24 hours prior to admission to a current facility

Assign code Z92.82, Status post administration of tPA (rtPA) in a different facility within the last 24 hours prior to admission to current facility, as a secondary diagnosis when a patient is received by transfer into a facility and documentation indicates they were administered tissue plasminogen activator (tPA) within the last 24 hours prior to admission to the current facility.

This guideline applies even if the patient is still receiving the tPA at the time they are received into the current facility.

The appropriate code for the condition for which the tPA was administered (such as cerebrovascular disease or myocardial infarction) should be assigned first.

Code Z92.82 is only applicable to the receiving facility record and not to the transferring facility record.

Z93 Artificial opening status

Z94 Transplanted organ and tissue status

Z95 Presence of cardiac and vascular implants and grafts

Z96 Presence of other functional implants

Z97 Presence of other devices

Z98 Other postprocedural states

Assign code Z98.85, Transplanted organ removal status, to indicate that a transplanted organ has been previously removed. This code should not be assigned for the encounter in which the transplanted organ is removed. The complication necessitating removal of the transplant organ should be assigned for that encounter.

See section I.C19.g.3. for information on the coding of organ transplant complications.

Z99 Dependence on enabling machines and devices, not elsewhere classified

Note: Categories Z89-Z90 and Z93-Z99 are for use only if there are no complications or malfunctions of the organ or tissue replaced, the amputation site or the equipment on which the patient is dependent.

4) **History (of)**
There are two types of history Z codes, personal and family. Personal history codes explain a patient's past medical condition that no longer exists and is not receiving any treatment, but that has the potential for recurrence, and therefore may require continued monitoring.

Family history codes are for use when a patient has a family member(s) who has had a particular disease that causes the patient to be at higher risk of also contracting the disease.

Personal history codes may be used in conjunction with follow-up codes and family history codes may be used in conjunction with screening codes to explain the need for a test or procedure. History codes are also acceptable on any medical record regardless of the reason for visit. A history of an illness, even if no longer present, is important information that may alter the type of treatment ordered.

The history Z code categories are:

Z80 Family history of primary malignant neoplasm

Z81 Family history of mental and behavioral disorders

Z82 Family history of certain disabilities and chronic diseases (leading to disablement)

Z83 Family history of other specific disorders

Z84 Family history of other conditions

Z85 Personal history of malignant neoplasm

Z86 Personal history of certain other diseases

Z87 Personal history of other diseases and conditions

Z91.4- Personal history of psychological trauma, not elsewhere classified

Z91.5 Personal history of self-harm

Z91.8- Other specified personal risk factors, not elsewhere classified

Exception: Z91.83, Wandering in diseases classified elsewhere

Z92 Personal history of medical treatment

Except: Z92.0, Personal history of contraception

Except: Z92.82, Status post administration of tPA (rtPA) in a different facility within the last 24 hours prior to admission to a current facility

5) **Screening**
Screening is the testing for disease or disease precursors in seemingly well individuals so that early detection and treatment can be provided for those who test positive for the disease (e.g., screening mammogram).

The testing of a person to rule out or confirm a suspected diagnosis because the patient has some sign or symptom is a diagnostic examination, not a screening. In these cases, the sign or symptom is used to explain the reason for the test.

A screening code may be a first-listed code if the reason for the visit is specifically the screening exam. It may also be used as an additional code if the screening is done during an office visit for other health problems. A screening code is not necessary if the screening is inherent to a routine examination, such as a pap smear done during a routine pelvic examination.

Should a condition be discovered during the screening then the code for the condition may be assigned as an additional diagnosis.

The Z code indicates that a screening exam is planned. A procedure code is required to confirm that the screening was performed.

The screening Z codes/categories:

Z11 Encounter for screening for infectious and parasitic diseases

Z12 Encounter for screening for malignant neoplasms

Z13 Encounter for screening for other diseases and disorders

Except: Z13.9, Encounter for screening, unspecified

Z36 Encounter for antenatal screening for mother

6) **Observation**
There are two observation Z code categories. They are for use in very limited circumstances when a person is being observed for a suspected condition that is ruled out. The observation codes are not for use if an injury or illness or any signs or symptoms

related to the suspected condition are present. In such cases the diagnosis/symptom code is used with the corresponding external cause code.

The observation codes are to be used as principal diagnosis only. Additional codes may be used in addition to the observation code but only if they are unrelated to the suspected condition being observed.

Codes from subcategory Z03.7, Encounter for suspected maternal and fetal conditions ruled out, may either be used as a first-listed or as an additional code assignment depending on the case. They are for use in very limited circumstances on a maternal record when an encounter is for a suspected maternal or fetal condition that is ruled out during that encounter (for example, a maternal or fetal condition may be suspected due to an abnormal test result). These codes should not be used when the condition is confirmed. In those cases, the confirmed condition should be coded. In addition, these codes are not for use if an illness or any signs or symptoms related to the suspected condition or problem are present. In such cases the diagnosis/symptom code is used.

Additional codes may be used in addition to the code from subcategory Z03.7, but only if they are unrelated to the suspected condition being evaluated.

Codes from subcategory Z03.7 may not be used for encounters for antenatal screening of mother. *See Section I.C.21.c.5, Screening.*

For encounters for suspected fetal condition that are inconclusive following testing and evaluation, assign the appropriate code from category O35, O36, O40 or O41.

The observation Z code categories:

Z03   Encounter for medical observation for suspected diseases and conditions ruled out

Z04   Encounter for examination and observation for other reasons

     Except: Z04.9, Encounter for examination and observation for unspecified reason

7) Aftercare

Aftercare visit codes cover situations when the initial treatment of a disease has been performed and the patient requires continued care during the healing or recovery phase, or for the long-term consequences of the disease. The aftercare Z code should not be used if treatment is directed at a current, acute disease. The diagnosis code is to be used in these cases. Exceptions to this rule are codes Z51.0, Encounter for antineoplastic radiation therapy, and codes from subcategory Z51.1, Encounter for antineoplastic chemotherapy and immunotherapy. These codes are to be first-listed, followed by the diagnosis code when a patient's encounter is solely to receive radiation therapy, chemotherapy, or immunotherapy for the treatment of a neoplasm. If the reason for the encounter is more than one type of antineoplastic therapy, code Z51.0 and a code from subcategory Z51.1 may be assigned together, in which case one of these codes would be reported as a secondary diagnosis.

The aftercare Z codes should also not be used for aftercare for injuries. For aftercare of an injury, assign the acute injury code with the appropriate 7th character (for subsequent encounter).

The aftercare codes are generally first-listed to explain the specific reason for the encounter. An aftercare code may be used as an additional code when some type of aftercare is provided in addition to the reason for admission and no diagnosis code is applicable. An example of this would be the closure of a colostomy during an encounter for treatment of another condition.

Aftercare codes should be used in conjunction with other aftercare codes or diagnosis codes to provide better detail on the specifics of an aftercare encounter visit, unless otherwise directed by the classification. Should a patient receive multiple types of antineoplastic therapy during the same encounter, code Z51.0, Encounter for antineoplastic radiation therapy, and codes from subcategory Z51.1, Encounter for antineoplastic

chemotherapy and immunotherapy, may be used together on a record. The sequencing of multiple aftercare codes depends on the circumstances of the encounter.

Certain aftercare Z code categories need a secondary diagnosis code to describe the resolving condition or sequelae. For others, the condition is included in the code title.

Additional Z code aftercare category terms include fitting and adjustment, and attention to artificial openings.

Status Z codes may be used with aftercare Z codes to indicate the nature of the aftercare. For example code Z95.1, Presence of aortocoronary bypass graft, may be used with code Z48.812, Encounter for surgical aftercare following surgery on the circulatory system, to indicate the surgery for which the aftercare is being performed. A status code should not be used when the aftercare code indicates the type of status, such as using Z43.0, Encounter for attention to tracheostomy, with Z93.0, Tracheostomy status.

The aftercare Z category/codes:

Z42   Encounter for plastic and reconstructive surgery following medical procedure or healed injury

Z43   Encounter for attention to artificial openings

Z44   Encounter for fitting and adjustment of external prosthetic device

Z45   Encounter for adjustment and management of implanted device

Z46   Encounter for fitting and adjustment of other devices

Z47   Orthopedic aftercare

Z48   Encounter for other postprocedural aftercare

Z49   Encounter for care involving renal dialysis

Z51   Encounter for other aftercare

8) Follow-up

The follow-up codes are used to explain continuing surveillance following completed treatment of a disease, condition, or injury. They imply that the condition has been fully treated and no longer exists. They should not be confused with aftercare codes, or injury codes with a 7th character for subsequent encounter, that explain ongoing care of a healing condition or its sequelae. Follow-up codes may be used in conjunction with history codes to provide the full picture of the healed condition and its treatment. The follow-up code is sequenced first, followed by the history code.

A follow-up code may be used to explain multiple visits. Should a condition be found to have recurred on the follow-up visit, then the diagnosis code for the condition should be assigned in place of the follow-up code.

The follow-up Z code categories:

Z08   Encounter for follow-up examination after completed treatment for malignant neoplasm

Z09   Encounter for follow-up examination after completed treatment for conditions other than malignant neoplasm

Z39   Encounter for maternal postpartum care and examination

9) Donor

Codes in category Z52, Donors of organs and tissues, are used for living individuals who are donating blood or other body tissue. These codes are only for individuals donating for others, not for self-donations. They are not used to identify cadaveric donations.

10) Counseling

Counseling Z codes are used when a patient or family member receives assistance in the aftermath of an illness or injury, or when support is required in coping with family or social problems. They are not used in conjunction with a diagnosis code when the counseling component of care is considered integral to standard treatment.

The counseling Z codes/categories:

Z30.0-   Encounter for general counseling and advice on contraception

Z31.5   Encounter for genetic counseling

Z31.6-   Encounter for general counseling and advice on procreation

Z32.2   Encounter for childbirth instruction

Z32.3   Encounter for childcare instruction

Z69   Encounter for mental health services for victim and perpetrator of abuse

Z70   Counseling related to sexual attitude, behavior and orientation

Z71   Persons encountering health services for other counseling and medical advice, not elsewhere classified

Z76.81   Expectant mother prebirth pediatrician visit

11) Encounters for obstetrical and reproductive services

See Section I.C.15. Pregnancy, Childbirth, and the Puerperium, for further instruction on the use of these codes.

Z codes for pregnancy are for use in those circumstances when none of the problems or complications included in the codes from the Obstetrics chapter exist (a routine prenatal visit or postpartum care). Codes in category Z34, Encounter for supervision of normal pregnancy, are always first-listed and are not to be used with any other code from the OB chapter.

Codes in category Z3A, Weeks of gestation, may be assigned to provide additional information about the pregnancy. **The date of the admission should be used to determine weeks of gestation for inpatient admissions that encompass more than one gestational week.**

The outcome of delivery, category Z37, should be included on all maternal delivery records. It is always a secondary code. Codes in category Z37 should not be used on the newborn record.

Z codes for family planning (contraceptive) or procreative management and counseling should be included on an obstetric record either during the pregnancy or the postpartum stage, if applicable.

Z codes/categories for obstetrical and reproductive services:

Z30   Encounter for contraceptive management

Z31   Encounter for procreative management

Z32.2   Encounter for childbirth instruction

Z32.3   Encounter for childcare instruction

Z33   Pregnant state

Z34   Encounter for supervision of normal pregnancy

Z36   Encounter for antenatal screening of mother

Z3A   Weeks of gestation

Z37   Outcome of delivery

Z39   Encounter for maternal postpartum care and examination

Z76.81   Expectant mother prebirth pediatrician visit

12) Newborns and Infants

See Section I.C.16. Newborn (Perinatal) Guidelines, for further instruction on the use of these codes.

Newborn Z codes/categories:

Z76.1   Encounter for health supervision and care of foundling

Z00.1-   Encounter for routine child health examination

Z38   Liveborn infants according to place of birth and type of delivery

13) Routine and administrative examinations

The Z codes allow for the description of encounters for routine examinations, such as, a general check-up, or, examinations for administrative purposes, such as, a pre-employment physical. The codes are not to be used if the examination is for diagnosis of a suspected condition or for treatment purposes. In such cases the diagnosis code is used. During a routine exam, should a diagnosis or condition be discovered, it should be coded as an additional code. Pre-existing and chronic conditions and history codes may also be included as additional codes as long as the examination is for administrative purposes and not focused on any particular condition.

Some of the codes for routine health examinations distinguish between "with" and "without" abnormal findings. Code assignment depends on the information that is known at the time the encounter is being coded. For example, if no abnormal findings were found during the examination, but the encounter is being coded before test results are back, it is acceptable to assign the code for "without abnormal findings." When assigning a code for "with abnormal findings," additional code(s) should be assigned to identify the specific abnormal finding(s).

Pre-operative examination and pre-procedural laboratory examination Z codes are for use only in those situations when a patient is being cleared for a procedure or surgery and no treatment is given.

The Z codes/categories for routine and administrative examinations:

Z00   Encounter for general examination without complaint, suspected or reported diagnosis

Z01   Encounter for other special examination without complaint, suspected or reported diagnosis

Z02   Encounter for administrative examination

Except: Z02.9, Encounter for administrative examinations, unspecified

Z32.0-   Encounter for pregnancy test

14) Miscellaneous Z codes

The miscellaneous Z codes capture a number of other health care encounters that do not fall into one of the other categories. Certain of these codes identify the reason for the encounter; others are for use as additional codes that provide useful information on circumstances that may affect a patient's care and treatment.

Prophylactic Organ Removal

For encounters specifically for prophylactic removal of an organ (such as prophylactic removal of breasts due to a genetic susceptibility to cancer or a family history of cancer), the principal or first-listed code should be a code from category Z40, Encounter for prophylactic surgery, followed by the appropriate codes to identify the associated risk factor (such as genetic susceptibility or family history).

If the patient has a malignancy of one site and is having prophylactic removal at another site to prevent either a new primary malignancy or metastatic disease, a code for the malignancy should also be assigned in addition to a code from subcategory Z40.0, Encounter for prophylactic surgery for risk factors related to malignant neoplasms. A Z40.0 code should not be assigned if the patient is having organ removal for treatment of a malignancy, such as the removal of the testes for the treatment of prostate cancer.

Miscellaneous Z codes/categories:

Z28   Immunization not carried out

Except: Z28.3, Underimmunization status

Z40   Encounter for prophylactic surgery

Z41   Encounter for procedures for purposes other than remedying health state

Except: Z41.9, Encounter for procedure for purposes other than remedying health state, unspecified

Z53   Persons encountering health services for specific procedures and treatment, not carried out

Z55   Problems related to education and literacy

Z56   Problems related to employment and unemployment

Z57   Occupational exposure to risk factors

Z58   Problems related to physical environment

Z59   Problems related to housing and economic circumstances

Z60   Problems related to social environment

Z62   Problems related to upbringing

Z63   Other problems related to primary support group, including family circumstances

Z64	Problems related to certain psychosocial circumstances	
Z65	Problems related to other psychosocial circumstances	
Z72	Problems related to lifestyle	
Z73	Problems related to life management difficulty	
Z74	Problems related to care provider dependency	
	Except: Z74.01, Bed confinement status	
Z75	Problems related to medical facilities and other health care	
Z76.0	Encounter for issue of repeat prescription	
Z76.3	Healthy person accompanying sick person	
Z76.4	Other boarder to healthcare facility	
Z76.5	Malingerer [conscious simulation]	
Z91.1-	Patient's noncompliance with medical treatment and regimen	
Z91.83	Wandering in diseases classified elsewhere	
Z91.89	Other specified personal risk factors, not elsewhere classified	

15) Nonspecific Z codes

Certain Z codes are so non-specific, or potentially redundant with other codes in the classification, that there can be little justification for their use in the inpatient setting. Their use in the outpatient setting should be limited to those instances when there is no further documentation to permit more precise coding. Otherwise, any sign or symptom or any other reason for visit that is captured in another code should be used.

Nonspecific Z codes/categories:

Z02.9	Encounter for administrative examinations, unspecified
Z04.9	Encounter for examination and observation for unspecified reason
Z13.9	Encounter for screening, unspecified
Z41.9	Encounter for procedure for purposes other than remedying health state, unspecified
Z52.9	Donor of unspecified organ or tissue
Z86.59	Personal history of other mental and behavioral disorders
Z88.9	Allergy status to unspecified drugs, medicaments and biological substances status
Z92.0	Personal history of contraception

16) Z codes that may only be principal/first-listed diagnosis

The following Z codes/categories may only be reported as the principal/first-listed diagnosis, except when there are multiple encounters on the same day and the medical records for the encounters are combined:

Z00	Encounter for general examination without complaint, suspected or reported diagnosis
Z01	Encounter for other special examination without complaint, suspected or reported diagnosis
Z02	Encounter for administrative examination
Z03	Encounter for medical observation for suspected diseases and conditions ruled out
Z04	Encounter for examination and observation for other reasons
Z31.81	Encounter for male factor infertility in female patient
Z31.82	Encounter for Rh incompatibility status
Z31.83	Encounter for assisted reproductive fertility procedure cycle
Z31.84	Encounter for fertility preservation procedure
Z33.2	Encounter for elective termination of pregnancy
Z34	Encounter for supervision of normal pregnancy
Z38	Liveborn infants according to place of birth and type of delivery
Z39	Encounter for maternal postpartum care and examination
Z42	Encounter for plastic and reconstructive surgery following medical procedure or healed injury
Z51.0	Encounter for antineoplastic radiation therapy

Z51.1-	Encounter for antineoplastic chemotherapy and immunotherapy
Z52	Donors of organs and tissues
	Except: Z52.9, Donor of unspecified organ or tissue
Z76.1	Encounter for health supervision and care of foundling
Z76.2	Encounter for health supervision and care of other healthy infant and child
Z99.12	Encounter for respirator [ventilator] dependence during power failure

Section II. Selection of Principal Diagnosis

The circumstances of inpatient admission always govern the selection of principal diagnosis. The principal diagnosis is defined in the Uniform Hospital Discharge Data Set (UHDDS) as "that condition established after study to be chiefly responsible for occasioning the admission of the patient to the hospital for care."

The UHDDS definitions are used by hospitals to report inpatient data elements in a standardized manner. These data elements and their definitions can be found in the July 31, 1985, Federal Register (Vol. 50, No, 147), pp. 31038-40.

Since that time the application of the UHDDS definitions has been expanded to include all non-outpatient settings (acute care, short term, long term care and psychiatric hospitals; home health agencies; rehab facilities; nursing homes, etc).

In determining principal diagnosis the coding conventions in the ICD-10-CM, the Tabular List and Alphabetic Index take precedence over these official coding guidelines.

(See Section I.A., Conventions for the ICD-10-CM)

The importance of consistent, complete documentation in the medical record cannot be overemphasized. Without such documentation the application of all coding guidelines is a difficult, if not impossible, task.

A. Codes for symptoms, signs, and ill-defined conditions

Codes for symptoms, signs, and ill-defined conditions from Chapter 18 are not to be used as principal diagnosis when a related definitive diagnosis has been established.

B. Two or more interrelated conditions, each potentially meeting the definition for principal diagnosis

When there are two or more interrelated conditions (such as diseases in the same ICD-10-CM chapter or manifestations characteristically associated with a certain disease) potentially meeting the definition of principal diagnosis, either condition may be sequenced first, unless the circumstances of the admission, the therapy provided, the Tabular List, or the Alphabetic Index indicate otherwise.

C. Two or more diagnoses that equally meet the definition for principal diagnosis

In the unusual instance when two or more diagnoses equally meet the criteria for principal diagnosis as determined by the circumstances of admission, diagnostic workup and/or therapy provided, and the Alphabetic Index, Tabular List, or another coding guidelines does not provide sequencing direction, any one of the diagnoses may be sequenced first.

D. Two or more comparative or contrasting conditions

In those rare instances when two or more contrasting or comparative diagnoses are documented as "either/or" (or similar terminology), they are coded as if the diagnoses were confirmed and the diagnoses are sequenced according to the circumstances of the admission. If no further determination can be made as to which diagnosis should be principal, either diagnosis may be sequenced first.

E. A symptom(s) followed by contrasting/ comparative diagnoses

When a symptom(s) is followed by contrasting/comparative diagnoses, the symptom code is sequenced first. **However, if the symptom code is integral to the conditions listed, no code for the symptom is reported.** All the contrasting/comparative diagnoses should be coded as additional diagnoses.

F. Original treatment plan not carried out
Sequence as the principal diagnosis the condition, which after study occasioned the admission to the hospital, even though treatment may not have been carried out due to unforeseen circumstances.

G. Complications of surgery and other medical care
When the admission is for treatment of a complication resulting from surgery or other medical care, the complication code is sequenced as the principal diagnosis. If the complication is classified to the T80-T88 series and the code lacks the necessary specificity in describing the complication, an additional code for the specific complication should be assigned.

H. Uncertain diagnosis
If the diagnosis documented at the time of discharge is qualified as "probable", "suspected", "likely", "questionable", "possible", or "still to be ruled out", or other similar terms indicating uncertainty, code the condition as if it existed or was established. The bases for these guidelines are the diagnostic workup, arrangements for further workup or observation, and initial therapeutic approach that correspond most closely with the established diagnosis.

Note: This guideline is applicable only to inpatient admissions to short-term, acute, long-term care and psychiatric hospitals.

I. Admission from observation unit

1. **Admission Following Medical Observation**
   When a patient is admitted to an observation unit for a medical condition, which either worsens or does not improve, and is subsequently admitted as an inpatient of the same hospital for this same medical condition, the principal diagnosis would be the medical condition which led to the hospital admission.

2. **Admission Following Post-Operative Observation**
   When a patient is admitted to an observation unit to monitor a condition (or complication) that develops following outpatient surgery, and then is subsequently admitted as an inpatient of the same hospital, hospitals should apply the Uniform Hospital Discharge Data Set (UHDDS) definition of principal diagnosis as "that condition established after study to be chiefly responsible for occasioning the admission of the patient to the hospital for care."

J. Admission from outpatient surgery
When a patient receives surgery in the hospital's outpatient surgery department and is subsequently admitted for continuing inpatient care at the same hospital, the following guidelines should be followed in selecting the principal diagnosis for the inpatient admission:

- If the reason for the inpatient admission is a complication, assign the complication as the principal diagnosis.
- If no complication, or other condition, is documented as the reason for the inpatient admission, assign the reason for the outpatient surgery as the principal diagnosis.
- If the reason for the inpatient admission is another condition unrelated to the surgery, assign the unrelated condition as the principal diagnosis.

K. Admissions/Encounters for Rehabilitation
When the purpose for the admission/encounter is rehabilitation, sequence first the code for the condition for which the service is being performed. For example, for an admission/encounter for rehabilitation for right-sided dominant hemiplegia following a cerebrovascular infarction, report code I69.351, Hemiplegia and hemiparesis following cerebral infarction affecting right dominant side, as the first-listed or principal diagnosis.

If the condition for which the rehabilitation service is no longer present, report the appropriate aftercare code as the first-listed or principal diagnosis. For example, if a patient with severe degenerative osteoarthritis of the hip, underwent hip replacement and the current encounter/admission is for rehabilitation, report code Z47.1, Aftercare following joint replacement surgery, as the first-listed or principal diagnosis.

See Section I.C.21.c.7, Factors influencing health states and contact with health services, Aftercare.

Section III. Reporting Additional Diagnoses

GENERAL RULES FOR OTHER (ADDITIONAL) DIAGNOSES
For reporting purposes the definition for "other diagnoses" is interpreted as additional conditions that affect patient care in terms of requiring:

- clinical evaluation; or
- therapeutic treatment; or
- diagnostic procedures; or
- extended length of hospital stay; or
- increased nursing care and/or monitoring.

The UHDDS item #11-b defines Other Diagnoses as "all conditions that coexist at the time of admission, that develop subsequently, or that affect the treatment received and/or the length of stay. Diagnoses that relate to an earlier episode which have no bearing on the current hospital stay are to be excluded." UHDDS definitions apply to inpatients in acute care, short-term, long term care and psychiatric hospital setting. The UHDDS definitions are used by acute care short-term hospitals to report inpatient data elements in a standardized manner. These data elements and their definitions can be found in the July 31, 1985, Federal Register (Vol. 5Ø, No, 147), pp. 31Ø38-4Ø.

Since that time the application of the UHDDS definitions has been expanded to include all non-outpatient settings (acute care, short term, long term care and psychiatric hospitals; home health agencies; rehab facilities; nursing homes, etc).

The following guidelines are to be applied in designating "other diagnoses" when neither the Alphabetic Index nor the Tabular List in ICD-10-CM provide direction. The listing of the diagnoses in the patient record is the responsibility of the attending provider.

A. Previous conditions
If the provider has included a diagnosis in the final diagnostic statement, such as the discharge summary or the face sheet, it should ordinarily be coded. Some providers include in the diagnostic statement resolved conditions or diagnoses and status-post procedures from previous admission that have no bearing on the current stay. Such conditions are not to be reported and are coded only if required by hospital policy.

However, history codes (categories Z80-Z87) may be used as secondary codes if the historical condition or family history has an impact on current care or influences treatment.

B. Abnormal findings
Abnormal findings (laboratory, x-ray, pathologic, and other diagnostic results) are not coded and reported unless the provider indicates their clinical significance. if the findings are outside the normal range and the attending provider has ordered other tests to evaluate the condition or prescribed treatment, it is appropriate to ask the provider whether the abnormal finding should be added.

Please note: This differs from the coding practices in the outpatient setting for coding encounters for diagnostic tests that have been interpreted by a provider.

C. Uncertain Diagnosis
If the diagnosis documented at the time of discharge is qualified as "probable", "suspected", "likely", "questionable", "possible", or "still to be ruled out" or other similar terms indicating uncertainty, code the condition as if it existed or was established. The bases for these guidelines are the diagnostic workup, arrangements for further workup or observation, and initial therapeutic approach that correspond most closely with the established diagnosis.

Note: This guideline is applicable only to inpatient admissions to short-term, acute, long-term care and psychiatric hospitals.

Section IV. Diagnostic Coding and Reporting Guidelines for Outpatient Services

These coding guidelines for outpatient diagnoses have been approved for use by hospitals/ providers in coding and reporting hospital-based outpatient services and provider-based office visits.

Information about the use of certain abbreviations, punctuation, symbols, and other conventions used in the ICD-10-CM Tabular List (code numbers and titles), can be found in Section IA of these guidelines, under "Conventions Used in the Tabular List." **Section I.B. contains general guidelines that apply to the entire classification. Section I.C. contains chapter-specific guidelines that correspond to the chapters as they are arranged in the classification.** Information about the correct sequence to use in finding a code is also described in Section I.

The terms encounter and visit are often used interchangeably in describing outpatient service contacts and, therefore, appear together in these guidelines without distinguishing one from the other.

Though the conventions and general guidelines apply to all settings, coding guidelines for outpatient and provider reporting of diagnoses will vary in a number of instances from those for inpatient diagnoses, recognizing that:

> The Uniform Hospital Discharge Data Set (UHDDS) definition of principal diagnosis applies only to inpatients in acute, short-term, long-term care and psychiatric hospitals.

> Coding guidelines for inconclusive diagnoses (probable, suspected, rule out, etc.) were developed for inpatient reporting and do not apply to outpatients.

A. Selection of first-listed condition

In the outpatient setting, the term first-listed diagnosis is used in lieu of principal diagnosis.

In determining the first-listed diagnosis the coding conventions of ICD-10-CM, as well as the general and disease specific guidelines take precedence over the outpatient guidelines.

Diagnoses often are not established at the time of the initial encounter/visit. It may take two or more visits before the diagnosis is confirmed.

The most critical rule involves beginning the search for the correct code assignment through the Alphabetic Index. Never begin searching initially in the Tabular List as this will lead to coding errors.

1. Outpatient surgery

When a patient presents for outpatient surgery (same day surgery), code the reason for the surgery as the first-listed diagnosis (reason for the encounter), even if the surgery is not performed due to a contraindication.

2. Observation stay

When a patient is admitted for observation for a medical condition, assign a code for the medical condition as the first-listed diagnosis.

When a patient presents for outpatient surgery and develops complications requiring admission to observation, code the reason for the surgery as the first reported diagnosis (reason for the encounter), followed by codes for the complications as secondary diagnoses.

B. Codes from A00.0 through T88.9, Z00-Z99

The appropriate code(s) from A00.0 through T88.9, Z00-Z99 must be used to identify diagnoses, symptoms, conditions, problems, complaints, or other reason(s) for the encounter/visit.

C. Accurate reporting of ICD-10-CM diagnosis codes

For accurate reporting of ICD-10-CM diagnosis codes, the documentation should describe the patient's condition, using terminology which includes specific diagnoses as well as symptoms, problems, or reasons for the encounter. There are ICD-10-CM codes to describe all of these.

D. Codes that describe symptoms and signs

Codes that describe symptoms and signs, as opposed to diagnoses, are acceptable for reporting purposes when a diagnosis has not been established (confirmed) by the provider. Chapter 18 of ICD-10-CM, Symptoms, Signs, and Abnormal Clinical and Laboratory Findings Not Elsewhere Classified (codes R00-R99) contain many, but not all codes for symptoms.

E. Encounters for circumstances other than a disease or injury

ICD-10-CM provides codes to deal with encounters for circumstances other than a disease or injury. The Factors Influencing Health Status and Contact with Health Services codes (Z00-Z99) are provided to deal with occasions when circumstances other than a disease or injury are recorded as diagnosis or problems.

See Section I.C.21. Factors influencing health status and contact with health services.

F. Level of Detail in Coding

1. ICD-10-CM codes with 3, 4, 5, 6 or 7 characters

ICD-10-CM is composed of codes with 3, 4, 5, 6 or 7 characters. Codes with three characters are included in ICD-10-CM as the heading of a category of codes that may be further subdivided by the use of fourth, fifth, sixth or seventh characters to provide greater specificity.

2. Use of full number of characters required for a code

A three-character code is to be used only if it is not further subdivided. A code is invalid if it has not been coded to the full number of characters required for that code, including the 7th character extension, if applicable.

G. ICD-10-CM code for the diagnosis, condition, problem, or other reason for encounter/visit

List first the ICD-10-CM code for the diagnosis, condition, problem, or other reason for encounter/visit shown in the medical record to be chiefly responsible for the services provided. List additional codes that describe any coexisting conditions. In some cases the first-listed diagnosis may be a symptom when a diagnosis has not been established (confirmed) by the physician.

H. Uncertain diagnosis

Do not code diagnoses documented as "probable", "suspected," "questionable," "rule out," or "working diagnosis" or other similar terms indicating uncertainty. Rather, code the condition(s) to the highest degree of certainty for that encounter/visit, such as symptoms, signs, abnormal test results, or other reason for the visit.

Please note: This differs from the coding practices used by short-term, acute care, long-term care and psychiatric hospitals.

I. Chronic diseases

Chronic diseases treated on an ongoing basis may be coded and reported as many times as the patient receives treatment and care for the condition(s)

J. Code all documented conditions that coexist

Code all documented conditions that coexist at the time of the encounter/visit, and require or affect patient care treatment or management. Do not code conditions that were previously treated and no longer exist. However, history codes (categories Z80-Z87) may be used as secondary codes if the historical condition or family history has an impact on current care or influences treatment.

K. Patients receiving diagnostic services only

For patients receiving diagnostic services only during an encounter/visit, sequence first the diagnosis, condition, problem, or other reason for encounter/visit shown in the medical record to be chiefly responsible for the outpatient services provided during the encounter/visit. Codes for other diagnoses (e.g., chronic conditions) may be sequenced as additional diagnoses.

For encounters for routine laboratory/radiology testing in the absence of any signs, symptoms, or associated diagnosis, assign Z01.89, Encounter for other specified special examinations. If routine testing is performed during the same encounter as a test to evaluate a sign, symptom, or diagnosis, it is appropriate to assign both the Z code and the code describing the reason for the non-routine test.

For outpatient encounters for diagnostic tests that have been interpreted by a physician, and the final report is available at the time of coding, code any confirmed or definitive diagnosis(es) documented in the interpretation. Do not code related signs and symptoms as additional diagnoses.

Please note: This differs from the coding practice in the hospital inpatient setting regarding abnormal findings on test results.

L. Patients receiving therapeutic services only

For patients receiving therapeutic services only during an encounter/visit, sequence first the diagnosis, condition, problem, or other reason for encounter/visit shown in the medical record to be chiefly responsible for the outpatient services provided during the encounter/visit. Codes for other diagnoses (e.g., chronic conditions) may be sequenced as additional diagnoses.

The only exception to this rule is that when the primary reason for the admission/encounter is chemotherapy or radiation therapy, the appropriate Z code for the service is listed first, and the diagnosis or problem for which the service is being performed listed second.

M. Patients receiving preoperative evaluations only
For patients receiving preoperative evaluations only, sequence first a code from subcategory Z01.81, Encounter for pre-procedural examinations, to describe the pre-op consultations. Assign a code for the condition to describe the reason for the surgery as an additional diagnosis. Code also any findings related to the pre-op evaluation.

N. Ambulatory surgery
For ambulatory surgery, code the diagnosis for which the surgery was performed. If the postoperative diagnosis is known to be different from the preoperative diagnosis at the time the diagnosis is confirmed, select the postoperative diagnosis for coding, since it is the most definitive.

O. Routine outpatient prenatal visits
See Section I.C.15. Routine outpatient prenatal visits.

P. Encounters for general medical examinations with abnormal findings
The subcategories for encounters for general medical examinations, Z00.0-, provide codes for with and without abnormal findings. Should a general medical examination result in an abnormal finding, the code for general medical examination with abnormal finding should be assigned as the first-listed diagnosis. A secondary code for the abnormal finding should also be coded.

Q. Encounters for routine health screenings
See Section I.C.21. Factors influencing health status and contact with health services, Screening

Appendix I. Present on Admission Reporting Guidelines

Introduction
These guidelines are to be used as a supplement to the *ICD-10-CM Official Guidelines for Coding and Reporting* to facilitate the assignment of the Present on Admission (POA) indicator for each diagnosis and external cause of injury code reported on claim forms (UB-04 and 837 Institutional).

These guidelines are not intended to replace any guidelines in the main body of the *ICD-10-CM Official Guidelines for Coding and Reporting*. The POA guidelines are not intended to provide guidance on when a condition should be coded, but rather, how to apply the POA indicator to the final set of diagnosis codes that have been assigned in accordance with Sections I, II, and III of the official coding guidelines. Subsequent to the assignment of the ICD-10-CM codes, the POA indicator should then be assigned to those conditions that have been coded.

As stated in the Introduction to the *ICD-10-CM Official Guidelines for Coding and Reporting*, a joint effort between the healthcare provider and the coder is essential to achieve complete and accurate documentation, code assignment, and reporting of diagnoses and procedures. The importance of consistent, complete documentation in the medical record cannot be overemphasized. Medical record documentation from any provider involved in the care and treatment of the patient may be used to support the determination of whether a condition was present on admission or not. In the context of the official coding guidelines, the term "provider" means a physician or any qualified healthcare practitioner who is legally accountable for establishing the patient's diagnosis.

These guidelines are not a substitute for the provider's clinical judgment as to the determination of whether a condition was/was not present on admission. The provider should be queried regarding issues related to the linking of signs/symptoms, timing of test results, and the timing of findings.

General Reporting Requirements
All claims involving inpatient admissions to general acute care hospitals or other facilities that are subject to a law or regulation mandating collection of present on admission information.

Present on admission is defined as present at the time the order for inpatient admission occurs -- conditions that develop during an

outpatient encounter, including emergency department, observation, or outpatient surgery, are considered as present on admission.

POA indicator is assigned to principal and secondary diagnoses (as defined in Section II of the Official Guidelines for Coding and Reporting) and the external cause of injury codes.

Issues related to inconsistent, missing, conflicting or unclear documentation must still be resolved by the provider.

If a condition would not be coded and reported based on UHDDS definitions and current official coding guidelines, then the POA indicator would not be reported.

Reporting Options

    Y – Yes

    N – No

    U – Unknown

    W – Clinically undetermined

    Unreported/Not used (or "1" for Medicare usage) – (Exempt from POA reporting)

Reporting Definitions

    Y – present at the time of inpatient admission

    N – not present at the time of inpatient admission

    U – documentation is insufficient to determine if condition is present on admission

    W – provider is unable to clinically determine whether condition was present on admission or not

Timeframe for POA Identification and Documentation
There is no required timeframe as to when a provider (per the definition of "provider" used in these guidelines) must identify or document a condition to be present on admission. In some clinical situations, it may not be possible for a provider to make a definitive diagnosis (or a condition may not be recognized or reported by the patient) for a period of time after admission. In some cases it may be several days before the provider arrives at a definitive diagnosis. This does not mean that the condition was not present on admission. Determination of whether the condition was present on admission or not will be based on the applicable POA guideline as identified in this document, or on the provider's best clinical judgment.

If at the time of code assignment the documentation is unclear as to whether a condition was present on admission or not, it is appropriate to query the provider for clarification.

Assigning the POA Indicator

Condition is on the "Exempt from Reporting" list
Leave the "present on admission" field blank if the condition is on the list of ICD-10-CM codes for which this field is not applicable. This is the only circumstance in which the field may be left blank.

POA Explicitly Documented
Assign "Y" for any condition the provider explicitly documents as being present on admission.

Assign "N" for any condition the provider explicitly documents as not present at the time of admission.

Conditions diagnosed prior to inpatient admission
Assign "Y" for conditions that were diagnosed prior to admission (example: hypertension, diabetes mellitus, asthma).

Conditions diagnosed during the admission but clearly present before admission
Assign "Y" for conditions diagnosed during the admission that were clearly present but not diagnosed until after admission occurred.

Diagnoses subsequently confirmed after admission are considered present on admission if at the time of admission they are documented as suspected, possible, rule out, differential diagnosis, or constitute an underlying cause of a symptom that is present at the time of admission.

Condition develops during outpatient encounter prior to inpatient admission
Assign "Y" for any condition that develops during an outpatient encounter prior to a written order for inpatient admission.

Documentation does not indicate whether condition was present on admission

Assign "U" when the medical record documentation is unclear as to whether the condition was present on admission. "U" should not be routinely assigned and used only in very limited circumstances. Coders are encouraged to query the providers when the documentation is unclear.

Documentation states that it cannot be determined whether the condition was or was not present on admission

Assign "W" when the medical record documentation indicates that it cannot be clinically determined whether or not the condition was present on admission.

Chronic condition with acute exacerbation during the admission

If a single code identifies both the chronic condition and the acute exacerbation, see POA guidelines pertaining to combination codes.

If a single code only identifies the chronic condition and not the acute exacerbation (e.g., acute exacerbation of chronic leukemia), assign "Y."

Conditions documented as possible, probable, suspected, or rule out at the time of discharge

If the final diagnosis contains a possible, probable, suspected, or rule out diagnosis, and this diagnosis was based on signs, symptoms or clinical findings suspected at the time of inpatient admission, assign "Y."

If the final diagnosis contains a possible, probable, suspected, or rule out diagnosis, and this diagnosis was based on signs, symptoms or clinical findings that were not present on admission, assign "N."

Conditions documented as impending or threatened at the time of discharge

If the final diagnosis contains an impending or threatened diagnosis, and this diagnosis is based on symptoms or clinical findings that were present on admission, assign "Y".

If the final diagnosis contains an impending or threatened diagnosis, and this diagnosis is based on symptoms or clinical findings that were not present on admission, assign "N".

Acute and Chronic Conditions

Assign "Y" for acute conditions that are present at time of admission and N for acute conditions that are not present at time of admission.

Assign "Y" for chronic conditions, even though the condition may not be diagnosed until after admission.

If a single code identifies both an acute and chronic condition, see the POA guidelines for combination codes.

Combination Codes

Assign "N" if any part of the combination code was not present on admission (e.g., COPD with acute exacerbation and the exacerbation was not present on admission; gastric ulcer that does not start bleeding until after admission; asthma patient develops status asthmaticus after admission).

Assign "Y" if all parts of the combination code were present on admission (e.g., patient with acute prostatitis admitted with hematuria).

If the final diagnosis includes comparative or contrasting diagnoses, and both were present, or suspected, at the time of admission, assign "Y".

For infection codes that include the causal organism, assign "Y" if the infection (or signs of the infection) was present on admission, even though the culture results may not be known until after admission (e.g., patient is admitted with pneumonia and the provider documents pseudomonas as the causal organism a few days later).

Same Diagnosis Code for Two or More Conditions

When the same ICD-10-CM diagnosis code applies to two or more conditions during the same encounter (e.g. two separate conditions classified to the same ICD-10-CM diagnosis code):

> Assign "Y" if all conditions represented by the single ICD-10-CM code were present on admission (e.g. bilateral unspecified age-related cataracts).

Assign "N" if any of the conditions represented by the single ICD-10-CM code was not present on admission (e.g. traumatic secondary and recurrent hemorrhage and seroma is assigned to a single code T79.2, but only one of the conditions was present on admission).

Obstetrical conditions

Whether or not the patient delivers during the current hospitalization does not affect assignment of the POA indicator. The determining factor for POA assignment is whether the pregnancy complication or obstetrical condition described by the code was present at the time of admission or not.

If the pregnancy complication or obstetrical condition was present on admission (e.g., patient admitted in preterm labor), assign "Y".

If the pregnancy complication or obstetrical condition was not present on admission (e.g., 2nd degree laceration during delivery, postpartum hemorrhage that occurred during current hospitalization, fetal distress develops after admission), assign "N".

If the obstetrical code includes more than one diagnosis and any of the diagnoses identified by the code were not present on admission assign "N". (e.g., Category O11, Pre-existing hypertension with pre-eclampsia).

Perinatal conditions

Newborns are not considered to be admitted until after birth. Therefore, any condition present at birth or that developed in utero is considered present at admission and should be assigned "Y". This includes conditions that occur during delivery (e.g., injury during delivery, meconium aspiration, exposure to streptococcus B in the vaginal canal).

Congenital conditions and anomalies

Assign "Y" for congenital conditions and anomalies except for categories Q00-Q99, Congenital anomalies, which are on the exempt list. Congenital conditions are always considered present on admission.

External cause of injury codes

Assign "Y" for any external cause code representing an external cause of morbidity that occurred prior to inpatient admission (e.g., patient fell out of bed at home, patient fell out of bed in emergency room prior to admission).

Assign "N" for any external cause code representing an external cause of morbidity that occurred during inpatient hospitalization (e.g., patient fell out of hospital bed during hospital stay, patient experienced an adverse reaction to a medication administered after inpatient admission).

Categories and Codes Exempt from Diagnosis Present on Admission Requirement

Note: "Diagnosis present on admission" for these code categories are exempt because they represent circumstances regarding the healthcare encounter or factors influencing health status that do not represent a current disease or injury or are always present on admission.

B90–B94	Sequelae of infectious and parasitic diseases
E64	Sequelae of malnutrition and other nutritional deficiencies
I25.2	Old myocardial infarction
I69	Sequelae of cerebrovascular disease
O09	Supervision of high risk pregnancy
O66.5	Attempted application of vacuum extractor and forceps
O80	Encounter for full-term uncomplicated delivery
O94	Sequelae of complication of pregnancy, childbirth, and the puerperium
P00	Newborn (suspected to be) affected by maternal conditions that may be unrelated to present pregnancy
Q00 – Q99	Congenital malformations, deformations and chromosomal abnormalities
S00-T88.9	Injury, poisoning and certain other consequences of external causes with 7th character representing subsequent encounter or sequela
V00- V09	Pedestrian injured in transport accident
	Except: V00.81-, Accident with wheelchair (powered)
	V00.83-, Accident with motorized mobility scooter
V10-V19	Pedal cycle rider injured in transport accident
V20-V29	Motorcycle rider injured in transport accident

V30-V39	Occupant of three-wheeled motor vehicle injured in transport accident	Z08	Encounter for follow-up examination following completed treatment for malignant neoplasm
V40-V49	Car occupant injured in transport accident	Z09	Encounter for follow-up examination after completed treatment for conditions other than malignant neoplasm
V50-V59	Occupant of pick-up truck or van injured in transport accident	Z11	Encounter for screening for infectious and parasitic diseases
V60-V69	Occupant of heavy transport vehicle injured in transport accident	Z11.8	Encounter for screening for other infectious and parasitic diseases
V70-V79	Bus occupant injured in transport accident	Z12	Encounter for screening for malignant neoplasms
V80-V89	Other land transport accidents	Z13	Encounter for screening for other diseases and disorders
V90-V94	Water transport accidents	Z13.4	Encounter for screening for certain developmental disorders in childhood
V95-V97	Air and space transport accidents		
V98-V99	Other and unspecified transport accidents	Z13.5	Encounter for screening for eye and ear disorders
W09	Fall on and from playground equipment	Z13.6	Encounter for screening for cardiovascular disorders
W14	Fall from tree	Z13.83	Encounter for screening for respiratory disorder NEC
W15	Fall from cliff	Z13.89	Encounter for screening for other disorder
W17.0	Fall into well	Z14	Genetic carrier
W17.1	Fall into storm drain or manhole	Z15	Genetic susceptibility to disease
W18.01	Striking against sports equipment with subsequent fall	Z17	Estrogen receptor status
W21	Striking against or struck by sports equipment	Z18	Retained foreign body fragments
W30	Contact with agricultural machinery	Z22	Carrier of infectious disease
W31	Contact with other and unspecified machinery	Z23	Encounter for immunization
W32-W34	Accidental handgun discharge and malfunction	Z28	Immunization not carried out and underimmunization status
W35-W40	Exposure to inanimate mechanical forces	Z28.3	Underimmunization status
W52	Crushed, pushed or stepped on by crowd or human stampede	Z30	Encounter for contraceptive management
W56	Contact with nonvenomous marine animal	Z31	Encounter for procreative management
W58	Contact with crocodile or alligator	Z34	Encounter for supervision of normal pregnancy
W61	Contact with birds (domestic) (wild)	Z36	Encounter for antenatal screening of mother
W62	Contact with nonvenomous amphibians	Z37	Outcome of delivery
W89	Exposure to man-made visible and ultraviolet light	Z38	Liveborn infants according to place of birth and type of delivery
X02	Exposure to controlled fire in building or structure	Z39	Encounter for maternal postpartum care and examination
X03	Exposure to controlled fire, not in building or structure	Z41	Encounter for procedures for purposes other than remedying health state
X04	Exposure to ignition of highly flammable material		
X52	Prolonged stay in weightless environment	Z42	Encounter for plastic and reconstructive surgery following medical procedure or healed injury
X71	Intentional self-harm by drowning and submersion		
	Except: X71.0-, Intentional self-harm by drowning and submersion while in bath tub	Z43	Encounter for attention to artificial openings
		Z44	Encounter for fitting and adjustment of external prosthetic device
X72	Intentional self-harm by handgun discharge	Z45	Encounter for adjustment and management of implanted device
X73	Intentional self-harm by rifle, shotgun and larger firearm discharge	Z46	Encounter for fitting and adjustment of other devices
X74	Intentional self-harm by other and unspecified firearm and gun discharge	Z47.8	Encounter for other orthopedic aftercare
		Z49	Encounter for care involving renal dialysis
X75	Intentional self-harm by explosive material	Z51	Encounter for other aftercare
X76	Intentional self-harm by smoke, fire and flames	Z51.5	Encounter for palliative care
X77	Intentional self-harm by steam, hot vapors and hot objects	Z51.8	Encounter for other specified aftercare
X81	Intentional self-harm by jumping or lying in front of moving object	Z52	Donors of organs and tissues
		Z59	Problems related to housing and economic circumstances
X82	Intentional self-harm by crashing of motor vehicle	Z63	Other problems related to primary support groupincluding family circumstances
X83	Intentional self-harm by other specified means		
Y03	**Assault by crashing of motor vehicle**	Z65	Problems related to other psychosocial circumstances
Y07	**Perpetrator of assault, maltreatment and neglect**	Z65.8	Other specified problems related to psychosocial circumstances
Y08.8	**Assault by strike by sports equipment**	Z67.1-Z67.9	Blood type
Y21	Drowning and submersion, undetermined intent	Z68	Body mass index (BMI)
Y22	Handgun discharge, undetermined intent	Z72	Problems related to lifestyle
Y23	Rifle, shotgun and larger firearm discharge, undetermined intent	Z74.01	Bed confinement status
Y24	Other and unspecified firearm discharge, undetermined intent	Z76	Persons encountering health services in other circumstances
Y30	Falling, jumping or pushed from a high place, undetermined intent	Z77.110- Z77.128	Environmental pollution and hazards in the physical environment
Y32	**Assault by crashing of motor vehicle, undetermined intent**	Z78	Other specified health status
Y36	Operations of war	Z79	Long term (current) drug therapy
Y37	Military operations	Z80	Family history of primary malignant neoplasm
Y92	Place of occurrence of the external cause	Z81	Family history of mental and behavioral disorders
Y93	Activity code	Z82	Family history of certain disabilities and chronic diseases (leading to disablement)
Y99	External cause status		
Z00	Encounter for general examination without complaint, suspected or reported diagnosis	Z83	Family history of other specific disorders
		Z84	Family history of other conditions
Z01	Encounter for other special examination without complaint, suspected or reported diagnosis	Z85	Personal history of primary malignant neoplasm
		Z86	Personal history of certain other diseases
Z02	Encounter for administrative examination	Z87	Personal history of other diseases and conditions
Z03	Encounter for medical observation for suspected diseases and conditions ruled out	Z87.828	Personal history of other (healed) physical injury and trauma
		Z87.891	Personal history of nicotine dependence

Z88	Allergy status to drugs, medicaments and biological substances	Z92	Personal history of medical treatment
Z89	Acquired absence of limb	Z93	Artificial opening status
Z90.710	Acquired absence of both cervix and uterus	Z94	Transplanted organ and tissue status
Z91.0	Allergy status, other than to drugs and biological substances	Z95	Presence of cardiac and vascular implants and grafts
Z91.4	Personal history of psychological trauma, not elsewhere classified	Z97	Presence of other devices
Z91.5	Personal history of self-harm	Z98	Other postprocedural states
Z91.8	Other specified risk factors, not elsewhere classified	Z99	Dependence on enabling machines and devices, not elsewhere classified

Tabular list will
show if there is any
add on codes for

For Exam certain conditions.
2 codes if there is more than
* Check in the conditions.
the second one always
no matter cola

Always read this & check your code in the back (handwritten annotation)

A

Aarskog's syndrome Q87.1
Abandonment — *see* Maltreatment
Abasia (-astasia) (hysterical) F44.4
Abderhalden-Kaufmann-Lignac syndrome (cystinosis) E72.04
Abdomen, abdominal (*see also* condition)
  acute R10.0
  angina K55.1
  muscle deficiency syndrome Q79.4
Abdominalgia — *see* Pain, abdominal
Abduction contracture, hip or other joint — *see* Contraction, joint
Aberrant (congenital) (*see also* Malposition, congenital)
  adrenal gland Q89.1
  artery (peripheral) Q27.8
    basilar NEC Q28.1
    cerebral Q28.3
    coronary Q24.5
    digestive system Q27.8
    eye Q15.8
    lower limb Q27.8
    precerebral Q28.1
    pulmonary Q25.79
    renal Q27.2
    retina Q14.1
    specified site NEC Q27.8
    subclavian Q27.8
    upper limb Q27.8
    vertebral Q28.1
  breast Q83.8
  endocrine gland NEC Q89.2
  hepatic duct Q44.5
  pancreas Q45.3
  parathyroid gland Q89.2
  pituitary gland Q89.2
  sebaceous glands, mucous membrane, mouth, congenital Q38.6
  spleen Q89.09
  subclavian artery Q27.8
  thymus (gland) Q89.2
  thyroid gland Q89.2
  vein (peripheral) NEC Q27.8
    cerebral Q28.3
    digestive system Q27.8
    lower limb Q27.8
    precerebral Q28.1
    specified site NEC Q27.8
    upper limb Q27.8
Aberration
  distantal — *see* Disturbance, visual
  mental F99
Abetalipoproteinemia E78.6
Abiotrophy R68.89
Ablatio, ablation
  retinae — *see* Detachment, retina
Ablepharia, ablepharon Q10.3
Abnormal, abnormality, abnormalities (*see also* Anomaly)
  acid-base balance (mixed) E87.4
  albumin R77.0
  alphafetoprotein R77.2
  alveolar ridge K08.9
  anatomical relationship Q89.9
  apertures, congenital, diaphragm Q79.1
  auditory perception H93.29- ☑
    diplacusis — *see* Diplacusis
    hyperacusis — *see* Hyperacusis
    recruitment — *see* Recruitment, auditory
    threshold shift — *see* Shift, auditory threshold
  autosomes Q99.9
    fragile site Q95.5
  basal metabolic rate R94.8
  biosynthesis, testicular androgen E29.1
  bleeding time R79.1
  blood level (of)
    cobalt R79.0
    copper R79.0
    iron R79.0
    lithium R78.89

Abnormal, abnormality, abnormalities — *continued*
  blood level — *continued*
    magnesium R79.0
    mineral NEC R79.0
    zinc R79.0
  blood pressure
    elevated R03.0
    low reading (nonspecific) R03.1
  blood sugar R73.09
  blood-gas level R79.81
  bowel sounds R19.15
    absent R19.11
    hyperactive R19.12
  brain scan R94.02
  breathing R06.9
  caloric test R94.138
  cerebrospinal fluid R83.9
    cytology R83.6
    drug level R83.2
    enzyme level R83.0
    hormones R83.1
    immunology R83.4
    microbiology R83.5
    nonmedicinal level R83.3
    specified type NEC R83.8
  chemistry, blood R79.9
    C-reactive protein R79.82
    drugs — *see* Findings, abnormal, in blood
    gas level R79.81
    minerals R79.0
    pancytopenia D61.818
    PTT R79.1
    specified NEC R79.89
    toxins — *see* Findings, abnormal, in blood
  chest sounds (friction) (rales) R09.89
  chromosome, chromosomal Q99.9
    with more than three X chromosomes, female Q97.1
    analysis result R89.8
      bronchial washings R84.8
      cerebrospinal fluid R83.8
      cervix uteri NEC R87.89
      nasal secretions R84.8
      nipple discharge R89.8
      peritoneal fluid R85.89
      pleural fluid R84.8
      prostatic secretions R86.8
      saliva R85.89
      seminal fluid R86.8
      sputum R84.8
      synovial fluid R89.8
      throat scrapings R84.8
      vagina R87.89
      vulva R87.89
      wound secretions R89.8
    dicentric replacement Q93.2
    ring replacement Q93.2
    sex Q99.8
      female phenotype Q97.9
        specified NEC Q97.8
      male phenotype Q98.9
        specified NEC Q98.8
      structural male Q98.6
    specified NEC Q99.8
  clinical findings NEC R68.89
  coagulation D68.9
    newborn, transient P61.6
    profile R79.1
    time R79.1
  communication — *see* Fistula
  conjunctiva, vascular H11.41- ☑
  coronary artery Q24.5
  cortisol-binding globulin E27.8
  course, eustachian tube Q17.8
  creatinine clearance R94.4
  cytology
    anus R85.619
      atypical squamous cells cannot exclude high grade squamous intraepithelial lesion (ASC-H) R85.611
      atypical squamous cells of undetermined significance (ASC-US) R85.610

Abnormal, abnormality, abnormalities — *continued*
  cytology — *continued*
    anus — *continued*
      cytologic evidence of malignancy R85.614
      high grade squamous intraepithelial lesion (HGSIL) R85.613
      human papillomavirus (HPV) DNA test
        high risk positive R85.81
        low risk postive R85.82
      inadequate smear R85.615
      low grade squamous intraepithelial lesion (LGSIL) R85.612
      satisfactory anal smear but lacking transformation zone R85.616
      specified NEC R85.618
      unsatisfactory smear R85.615
    female genital organs — *see* Abnormal, Papanicolaou (smear)
  dark adaptation curve H53.61
  dentofacial NEC — *see* Anomaly, dentofacial
  development, developmental Q89.9
    central nervous system Q07.9
  diagnostic imaging
    abdomen, abdominal region NEC R93.5
    biliary tract R93.2
    breast R92.8
    central nervous system NEC R90.89
    cerebrovascular NEC R90.89
    coronary circulation R93.1
    digestive tract NEC R93.3
    gastrointestinal (tract) R93.3
    genitourinary organs R93.8
    head R93.0
    heart R93.1
    intrathoracic organ NEC R93.8
    limbs R93.6
    liver R93.2
    lung (field) R91.8
    musculoskeletal system NEC R93.7
    retroperitoneum R93.5
    site specified NEC R93.8
    skin and subcutaneous tissue R93.8
    skull R93.0
    urinary organs R93.4
  direction, teeth, fully erupted M26.30
  ear ossicles, acquired NEC H74.39- ☑
    ankylosis — *see* Ankylosis, ear ossicles
    discontinuity — *see* Discontinuity, ossicles, ear
    partial loss — *see* Loss, ossicles, ear (partial)
  Ebstein Q22.5
  echocardiogram R93.1
  echoencephalogram R90.81
  echogram — *see* Abnormal, diagnostic imaging
  electrocardiogram [ECG] [EKG] R94.31
  electroencephalogram [EEG] R94.01
  electrolyte — *see* Imbalance, electrolyte
  electromyogram [EMG] R94.131
  electro-oculogram [EOG] R94.110
  electrophysiological intracardiac studies R94.39
  electroretinogram [ERG] R94.111
  erythrocytes
    congenital, with perinatal jaundice D58.9
  feces (color) (contents) (mucus) R19.5
  finding — *see* Findings, abnormal, without diagnosis
  fluid
    amniotic — *see* Abnormal, specimen, specified
    cerebrospinal — *see* Abnormal, cerebrospinal fluid
    peritoneal — *see* Abnormal, specimen, digestive organs
    pleural — *see* Abnormal, specimen, respiratory organs
    synovial — *see* Abnormal, specimen, specified
    thorax (bronchial washings) (pleural fluid) — *see* Abnormal, specimen, respiratory organs
    vaginal — *see* Abnormal, specimen, female genital organs
  form
    teeth K00.2
    uterus — *see* Anomaly, uterus
  function studies
    auditory R94.120
    bladder R94.8

Abnormal, abnormality, abnormalities —
    continued
    function studies — *continued*
      brain R94.09
      cardiovascular R94.30
      ear R94.128
      endocrine NEC R94.7
      eye NEC R94.118
      kidney R94.4
      liver R94.5
      nervous system
        central NEC R94.09
        peripheral NEC R94.138
      pancreas R94.8
      placenta R94.8
      pulmonary R94.2
      special senses NEC R94.128
      spleen R94.8
      thyroid R94.6
      vestibular R94.121
    gait — *see* Gait
      hysterical F44.4
    gastrin secretion E16.4
    globulin R77.1
      cortisol-binding E27.8
      thyroid-binding E07.89
    glomerular, minor (*see also* N00-N07 with fourth
        character .0) N05.0
    glucagon secretion E16.3
    glucose tolerance (test) (non-fasting) R73.09
    gravitational (G) forces or states (effect of) T75.81 ☑
    hair (color) (shaft) L67.9
      specified NEC L67.8
    hard tissue formation in pulp (dental) K04.3
    head movement R25.0
    heart
      rate R00.9
        specified NEC R00.8
      shadow R93.1
      sounds NEC R01.2
    hemoglobin (disease) (*see also* Disease, hemoglobin)
        D58.2
      trait — *see* Trait, hemoglobin, abnormal
    histology NEC R89.7
    immunological findings R89.4
      in serum R76.9
        specified NEC R76.8
    increase in appetite R63.2
    involuntary movement — *see* Abnormal, movement,
        involuntary
    jaw closure M26.51
    karyotype R89.8
    kidney function test R94.4
    knee jerk R29.2
    leukocyte (cell) (differential) NEC D72.9
    liver
    loss of
      height R29.890
      weight R63.4
    mammogram NEC R92.8
      calcification (calculus) R92.1
      microcalcification R92.0
    Mantoux test R76.11
    movement (disorder) (*see also* Disorder, movement)
      head R25.0
      involuntary R25.9
        fasciculation R25.3
        of head R25.0
        spasm R25.2
        specified type NEC R25.8
        tremor R25.1
    myoglobin (Aberdeen) (Annapolis) R89.7
    neonatal screening P09
    oculomotor study R94.113
    palmar creases Q82.8
    Papanicolaou (smear)
      anus R85.619
        atypical squamous cells cannot exclude high
          grade squamous intraepithelial lesion
          (ASC-H) R85.611
        atypical squamous cells of undetermined signif-
          icance (ASC-US) R85.610
        cytologic evidence of malignancy R85.614
        high grade squamous intraepithelial lesion
          (HGSIL) R85.613
        human papillomavirus (HPV) DNA test
          high risk positive R85.81
          low risk postive R85.82

Abnormal, abnormality, abnormalities —
    continued
    Papanicolaou — *continued*
      anus — *continued*
        inadequate smear R85.615
        low grade squamous intraepithelial lesion
          (LGSIL) R85.612
        satisfactory anal smear but lacking transforma-
          tion zone R85.616
        specified NEC R85.618
        unsatisfactory smear R85.615
      bronchial washings R84.6
      cerebrospinal fluid R83.6
      cervix R87.619
        atypical squamous cells cannot exclude high
          grade squamous intraepithelial lesion
          (ASC-H) R87.611
        atypical squamous cells of undetermined signif-
          icance (ASC-US) R87.610
        cytologic evidence of malignancy R87.614
        high grade squamous intraepithelial lesion
          (HGSIL) R87.613
        inadequate smear R87.615
        low grade squamous intraepithelial lesion
          (LGSIL) R87.612
        non-atypical endometrial cells R87.618
        satisfactory cervical smear but lacking transfor-
          mation zone R87.616
        specified NEC R87.618
        thin preparaton R87.619
        unsatisfactory smear R87.615
      nasal secretions R84.6
      nipple discharge R89.6
      peritoneal fluid R85.69
      pleural fluid R84.6
      prostatic secretions R86.6
      saliva R85.69
      seminal fluid R86.6
      sites NEC R89.6
      sputum R84.6
      synovial fluid R89.6
      throat scrapings R84.6
      vagina R87.629
        atypical squamous cells cannot exclude high
          grade squamous intraepithelial lesion
          (ASC-H) R87.621
        atypical squamous cells of undetermined signif-
          icance (ASC-US) R87.620
        cytologic evidence of malignancy R87.624
        high grade squamous intraepithelial lesion
          (HGSIL) R87.623
        inadequate smear R87.625
        low grade squamous intraepithelial lesion
          (LGSIL) R87.622
        specified NEC R87.628
        thin preparation R87.629
        unsatisfactory smear R87.625
      vulva R87.69
      wound secretions R89.6
    partial thromboplastin time (PTT) R79.1
    pelvis (bony) — *see* Deformity, pelvis
    percussion, chest (tympany) R09.89
    periods (grossly) — *see* Menstruation
    phonocardiogram R94.39
    plantar reflex R29.2
    plasma
      protein R77.9
        specified NEC R77.8
      viscosity R70.1
    pleural (folds) Q34.0
    posture R29.3
    product of conception O02.9
      specified type NEC O02.89
    prothrombin time (PT) R79.1
    pulmonary
      artery, congenital Q25.79
      function, newborn P28.89
      test results R94.2
    pulsations in neck R00.2
    pupillary H21.56- ☑
      function (reaction) (reflex) — *see* Anomaly, pupil,
        function
    radiological examination — *see* Abnormal, diagnostic
      imaging
    red blood cell(s) (morphology) (volume) R71.8
    reflex — *see* Reflex
    renal function test R94.4
    response to nerve stimulation R94.130

Abnormal, abnormality, abnormalities —
    continued
    retinal correspondence H53.31
    retinal function study R94.111
    rhythm, heart (*see also* Arrhythmia)
    saliva — *see* Abnormal, specimen, digestive organs
    scan
      kidney R94.4
      liver R93.2
      thyroid R94.6
    secretion
      gastrin E16.4
      glucagon E16.3
    semen, seminal fluid — *see* Abnormal, specimen, male
      genital organs
    serum level (of)
      acid phosphatase R74.8
      alkaline phosphatase R74.8
      amylase R74.8
      enzymes R74.9
        specified NEC R74.8
      lipase R74.8
      triacylglycerol lipase R74.8
    shape
      gravid uterus — *see* Anomaly, uterus
    sinus venosus Q21.1
    size, tooth, teeth K00.2
    spacing, tooth, teeth, fully erupted M26.30
    specimen
      digestive organs (peritoneal fluid) (saliva) R85.9
        cytology R85.69
        drug level R85.2
        enzyme level R85.0
        histology R85.7
        hormones R85.1
        immunology R85.4
        microbiology R85.5
        nonmedicinal level R85.3
        specified type NEC R85.89
      female genital organs (secretions) (smears) R87.9
        cytology R87.69
          cervix R87.619
            human papillomavirus (HPV) DNA test
              high risk positive R87.810
              low risk positive R87.820
            inadequate (unsatisfactory) smear
              R87.615
            non-atypical endometrial cells R87.618
            specified NEC R87.618
          vagina R87.629
            human papillomavirus (HPV) DNA test
              high risk positive R87.811
              low risk positive R87.821
            inadequate (unsatisfactory) smear
              R87.625
          vulva R87.69
        drug level R87.2
        enzyme level R87.0
        histological R87.7
        hormones R87.1
        immunology R87.4
        microbiology R87.5
        nonmedicinal level R87.3
        specified type NEC R87.89
      male genital organs (prostatic secretions) (semen)
        R86.9
        cytology R86.6
        drug level R86.2
        enzyme level R86.0
        histological R86.7
        hormones R86.1
        immunology R86.4
        microbiology R86.5
        nonmedicinal level R86.3
        specified type NEC R86.8
      nipple discharge — *see* Abnormal, specimen,
        specified
      respiratory organs (bronchial washings) (nasal se-
        cretions) (pleural fluid) (sputum) R84.9
        cytology R84.6
        drug level R84.2
        enzyme level R84.0
        histology R84.7
        hormones R84.1
        immunology R84.4
        microbiology R84.5
        nonmedicinal level R84.3
        specified type NEC R84.8

Abnormal, abnormality, abnormalities — *continued*
- specimen — *continued*
  - specified organ, system and tissue NOS R89.9
    - cytology R89.6
    - drug level R89.2
    - enzyme level R89.0
    - histology R89.7
    - hormones R89.1
    - immunology R89.4
    - microbiology R89.5
    - nonmedicinal level R89.3
    - specified type NEC R89.8
  - synovial fluid — *see* Abnormal, specimen, specified
  - thorax (bronchial washings) (pleural fluids) — *see* Abnormal, specimen, respiratory organs
  - vagina (secretion) (smear) R87.629
  - vulva (secretion) (smear) R87.69
  - wound secretion — *see* Abnormal, specimen, specified
- spermatozoa — *see* Abnormal, specimen, male genital organs
- sputum (amount) (color) (odor) R09.3
- stool (color) (contents) (mucus) R19.5
  - bloody K92.1
  - guaiac positive R19.5
- synchondrosis Q78.8
- thermography (*see also* Abnormal, diagnostic imaging) R93.8
- thyroid-binding globulin E07.89
- tooth, teeth (form) (size) K00.2
- toxicology (findings) R78.9
- transport protein E88.09
- tumor marker NEC R97.8
- ultrasound results — *see* Abnormal, diagnostic imaging
- umbilical cord complicating delivery O69.9 ☑
- urination NEC R39.19
- urine (constituents) R82.90
  - bile R82.2
  - cytological examination R82.8
  - drugs R82.5
  - fat R82.0
  - glucose R81
  - heavy metals R82.6
  - hemoglobin R82.3
  - histological examination R82.8
  - ketones R82.4
  - microbiological examination (culture) R82.7
  - myoglobin R82.1
  - positive culture R82.7
  - protein — *see* Proteinuria
  - specified substance NEC R82.99
    - chromoabnormality NEC R82.91
  - substances nonmedical R82.6
- uterine hemorrhage — *see* Hemorrhage, uterus
- vectorcardiogram R94.39
- visually evoked potential (VEP) R94.112
- white blood cells D72.9
  - specified NEC D72.89
- X-ray examination — *see* Abnormal, diagnostic imaging

Abnormity (any organ or part) — *see* Anomaly
Abocclusion M26.29
- hemolytic disease (newborn) P55.1
- incompatibility reaction ABO — *see* Complication(s), transfusion, incompatibility reaction, ABO

Abolition, language R48.8
Aborter, habitual or recurrent — *see* Loss (of), pregnancy, recurrent
Abortion (complete) (spontaneous) O03.9
- with
  - retained products of conception — *see* Abortion, incomplete
- attempted (elective) (failed) O07.4
  - complicated by O07.30
    - afibrinogenemia O07.1
    - cardiac arrest O07.36
    - chemical damage of pelvic organ(s) O07.34
    - circulatory collapse O07.31
    - cystitis O07.38
    - defibrination syndrome O07.1
    - electrolyte imbalance O07.33
    - embolism (air) (amniotic fluid) (blood clot) (fat) (pulmonary) (septic) (soap) O07.2
    - endometritis O07.0
    - genital tract and pelvic infection O07.0
    - hemolysis O07.1

Abortion — *continued*
- attempted — *continued*
  - complicated by — *continued*
    - hemorrhage (delayed) (excessive) O07.1
    - infection
      - genital tract or pelvic O07.0
      - urinary tract tract O07.38
    - intravascular coagulation O07.1
    - laceration of pelvic organ(s) O07.34
    - metabolic disorder O07.33
    - oliguria O07.32
    - oophoritis O07.0
    - parametritis O07.0
    - pelvic peritonitis O07.0
    - perforation of pelvic organ(s) O07.34
    - renal failure or shutdown O07.32
    - salpingitis or salpingo-oophoritis O07.0
    - sepsis O07.37
    - shock O07.31
    - specified condition NEC O07.39
    - tubular necrosis (renal) O07.32
    - uremia O07.32
    - urinary tract infection O07.38
    - venous complication NEC O07.35
      - embolism (air) (amniotic fluid) (blood clot) (fat) (pulmonary) (septic) (soap) O07.2
- complicated (by) (following) O03.80
  - afibrinogenemia O03.6
  - cardiac arrest O03.86
  - chemical damage of pelvic organ(s) O03.84
  - circulatory collapse O03.81
  - cystitis O03.88
  - defibrination syndrome O03.6
  - electrolyte imbalance O03.83
  - embolism (air) (amniotic fluid) (blood clot) (fat) (pulmonary) (septic) (soap) O03.7
  - endometritis O03.5
  - genital tract and pelvic infection O03.5
  - hemolysis O03.6
  - hemorrhage (delayed) (excessive) O03.6
  - infection
    - genital tract or pelvic O03.5
    - urinary tract O03.88
  - intravascular coagulation O03.6
  - laceration of pelvic organ(s) O03.84
  - metabolic disorder O03.83
  - oliguria O03.82
  - oophoritis O03.5
  - parametritis O03.5
  - pelvic peritonitis O03.5
  - perforation of pelvic organ(s) O03.84
  - renal failure or shutdown O03.82
  - salpingitis or salpingo-oophoritis O03.5
  - sepsis O03.87
  - shock O03.81
  - specified condition NEC O03.89
  - tubular necrosis (renal) O03.82
  - uremia O03.82
  - urinary tract infection O03.88
  - venous complication NEC O03.85
    - embolism (air) (amniotic fluid) (blood clot) (fat) (pulmonary) (septic) (soap) O03.7
- failed — *see* Abortion, attempted
- habitual or recurrent N96
  - with current abortion — *see* categories O03-O06
  - without current pregnancy N96
  - care in current pregnancy O26.2- ☑
- incomplete (spontaneous) O03.4
  - complicated (by) (following) O03.30
    - afibrinogenemia O03.1
    - cardiac arrest O03.36
    - chemical damage of pelvic organ(s) O03.34
    - circulatory collapse O03.31
    - cystitis O03.38
    - defibrination syndrome O03.1
    - electrolyte imbalance O03.33
    - embolism (air) (amniotic fluid) (blood clot) (fat) (pulmonary) (septic) (soap) O03.2
    - endometritis O03.0
    - genital tract and pelvic infection O03.0
    - hemolysis O03.1
    - hemorrhage (delayed) (excessive) O03.1
    - infection
      - genital tract or pelvic O03.0
      - urinary tract O03.38
    - intravascular coagulation O03.1
    - laceration of pelvic organ(s) O03.34
    - metabolic disorder O03.33

Abortion — *continued*
- incomplete — *continued*
  - complicated — *continued*
    - oliguria O03.32
    - oophoritis O03.0
    - parametritis O03.0
    - pelvic peritonitis O03.0
    - perforation of pelvic organ(s) O03.34
    - renal failure or shutdown O03.32
    - salpingitis or salpingo-oophoritis O03.0
    - sepsis O03.37
    - shock O03.31
    - specified condition NEC O03.39
    - tubular necrosis (renal) O03.32
    - uremia O03.32
    - urinary infection O03.38
    - venous complication NEC O03.35
      - embolism (air) (amniotic fluid) (blood clot) (fat) (pulmonary) (septic) (soap) O03.2
- induced (encounter for) Z33.2
  - complicated by O04.80
    - afibrinogenemia O04.6
    - cardiac arrest O04.86
    - chemical damage of pelvic organ(s) O04.84
    - circulatory collapse O04.81
    - cystitis O04.88
    - defibrination syndrome O04.6
    - electrolyte imbalance O04.83
    - embolism (air) (amniotic fluid) (blood clot) (fat) (pulmonary) (septic) (soap) O04.7
    - endometritis O04.5
    - genital tract and pelvic infection O04.5
    - hemolysis O04.6
    - hemorrhage (delayed) (excessive) O04.6
    - infection
      - genital tract or pelvic O04.5
      - urinary tract O04.88
    - intravascular coagulation O04.6
    - laceration of pelvic organ(s) O04.84
    - metabolic disorder O04.83
    - oliguria O04.82
    - oophoritis O04.5
    - parametritis O04.5
    - pelvic peritonitis O04.5
    - perforation of pelvic organ(s) O04.84
    - renal failure or shutdown O04.82
    - salpingitis or salpingo-oophoritis O04.5
    - sepsis O04.87
    - shock O04.81
    - specified condition NEC O04.89
    - tubular necrosis (renal) O04.82
    - uremia O04.82
    - urinary tract infection O04.88
    - venous complication NEC O04.85
      - embolism (air) (amniotic fluid) (blood clot) (fat) (pulmonary) (septic) (soap) O04.7
- missed O02.1
- spontaneous — *see* Abortion (complete) (spontaneous)
  - threatened O20.0
- threatened (spontaneous) O20.0
- tubal O00.1

Abortus fever A23.1
Aboulomania F60.7
Abrami's disease D59.8
Abramov-Fiedler myocarditis (acute isolated myocarditis) I40.1
Abrasion T14.8
- abdomen, abdominal (wall) S30.811 ☑
- alveolar process S00.512 ☑
- ankle S90.51- ☑
- antecubital space — *see* Abrasion, elbow
- anus S30.817 ☑
- arm (upper) S40.81- ☑
- auditory canal — *see* Abrasion, ear
- auricle — *see* Abrasion, ear
- axilla — *see* Abrasion, arm
- back, lower S30.810 ☑
- breast S20.11- ☑
- brow S00.81 ☑
- buttock S30.810 ☑
- calf — *see* Abrasion, leg
- canthus — *see* Abrasion, eyelid
- cheek S00.81 ☑
  - internal S00.512 ☑
- chest wall — *see* Abrasion, thorax
- chin S00.81 ☑
- clitoris S30.814 ☑

Abrasion — continued
cornea S05.0-☑
costal region — see Abrasion, thorax
dental K03.1
digit(s)
  foot — see Abrasion, toe
  hand — see Abrasion, finger
ear S00.41-☑
elbow S50.31-☑
epididymis S30.813 ☑
epigastric region S30.811 ☑
epiglottis S10.11 ☑
esophagus (thoracic) S27.818 ☑
  cervical S10.11 ☑
eyebrow — see Abrasion, eyelid
eyelid S00.21-☑
face S00.81 ☑
finger(s) S60.41-☑
  index S60.41-☑
  little S60.41-☑
  middle S60.41-☑
  ring S60.41-☑
flank S30.811 ☑
foot (except toe(s) alone) S90.81-☑
  toe — see Abrasion, toe
forearm S50.81-☑
  elbow only — see Abrasion, elbow
forehead S00.81 ☑
genital organs, external
  female S30.816 ☑
  male S30.815 ☑
groin S30.811 ☑
gum S00.512 ☑
hand S60.51-☑
head S00.91 ☑
  ear — see Abrasion, ear
  eyelid — see Abrasion, eyelid
  lip S00.511 ☑
  nose S00.31 ☑
  oral cavity S00.512 ☑
  scalp S00.01 ☑
  specified site NEC S00.81 ☑
heel — see Abrasion, foot
hip S70.21-☑
inguinal region S30.811 ☑
interscapular region S20.419 ☑
jaw S00.81 ☑
knee S80.21-☑
labium (majus) (minus) S30.814 ☑
larynx S10.11 ☑
leg (lower) S80.81-☑
  knee — see Abrasion, knee
  upper — see Abrasion, thigh
lip S00.511 ☑
lower back S30.810 ☑
lumbar region S30.810 ☑
malar region S00.81 ☑
mammary — see Abrasion, breast
mastoid region S00.81 ☑
mouth S00.512 ☑
nail
  finger — see Abrasion, finger
  toe — see Abrasion, toe
nape S10.81 ☑
nasal S00.31 ☑
neck S10.91 ☑
  specified site NEC S10.81 ☑
  throat S10.11 ☑
nose S00.31 ☑
occipital region S00.01 ☑
oral cavity S00.512 ☑
orbital region — see Abrasion, eyelid
palate S00.512 ☑
palm — see Abrasion, hand
parietal region S00.01 ☑
pelvis S30.810 ☑
penis S30.812 ☑
perineum
  female S30.814 ☑
  male S30.810 ☑
periocular area — see Abrasion, eyelid
phalanges
  finger — see Abrasion, finger
  toe — see Abrasion, toe
pharynx S10.11 ☑
pinna — see Abrasion, ear

Abrasion — continued
popliteal space — see Abrasion, knee
prepuce S30.812 ☑
pubic region S30.810 ☑
pudendum
  female S30.816 ☑
  male S30.815 ☑
sacral region S30.810 ☑
scalp S00.01 ☑
scapular region — see Abrasion, shoulder
scrotum S30.813 ☑
shin — see Abrasion, leg
shoulder S40.21-☑
skin NEC T14.8
sternal region S20.319 ☑
submaxillary region S00.81 ☑
submental region S00.81 ☑
subungual
  finger(s) — see Abrasion, finger
  toe(s) — see Abrasion, toe
supraclavicular fossa S10.81 ☑
supraorbital S00.81 ☑
temple S00.81 ☑
temporal region S00.81 ☑
testis S30.813 ☑
thigh S70.31-☑
thorax, thoracic (wall) S20.91 ☑
  back S20.41-☑
  front S20.31-☑
throat S10.11 ☑
thumb S60.31-☑
toe(s) (lesser) S90.416 ☑
  great S90.41-☑
tongue S00.512 ☑
tooth, teeth (dentifrice) (habitual) (hard tissues) (occupational) (ritual) (traditional) K03.1
trachea S10.11 ☑
tunica vaginalis S30.813 ☑
tympanum, tympanic membrane — see Abrasion, ear
uvula S00.512 ☑
vagina S30.814 ☑
vocal cords S10.11 ☑
vulva S30.814 ☑
wrist S60.81-☑
Abrism — see Poisoning, food, noxious, plant
Abruptio placentae O45.9-☑
  with
    afibrinogenemia O45.01-☑
    coagulation defect O45.00-☑
      specified NEC O45.09-☑
    disseminated intravascular coagulation O45.02-☑
    hypofibrinogenemia O45.01-☑
  specified NEC O45.8-☑
Abruption, placenta — see Abruptio placentae
Abscess (connective tissue) (embolic) (fistulous) (infective) (metastatic) (multiple) (pernicious) (pyogenic) (septic) L02.91
  with
    diverticular disease (intestine) K57.80
      with bleeding K57.81
      large intestine K57.20
        with
          bleeding K57.21
          small intestine K57.40
            with bleeding K57.41
      small intestine K57.00
        with
          bleeding K57.01
          large intestine K57.40
            with bleeding K57.41
    lymphangitis — code by site under Abscess
  abdomen, abdominal
    cavity K65.1
    wall L02.211
  abdominopelvic K65.1
  accessory sinus — see Sinusitis
  adrenal (capsule) (gland) E27.8
  alveolar K04.7
    with sinus K04.6
  amebic A06.4
    brain (and liver or lung abscess) A06.6
    genitourinary tract A06.82
    liver (without mention of brain or lung abscess) A06.4
    lung (and liver) (without mention of brain abscess) A06.5
    specified site NEC A06.89

Abscess — continued
  amebic — continued
    spleen A06.89
  anerobic A48.0
  ankle — see Abscess, lower limb
  anorectal K61.2
  antecubital space — see Abscess, upper limb
  antrum (chronic) (Highmore) — see Sinusitis, maxillary
  anus K61.0
  apical (tooth) K04.7
    with sinus (alveolar) K04.6
  appendix K35.3
  areola (acute) (chronic) (nonpuerperal) N61
    puerperal, postpartum or gestational — see Infection, nipple
  arm (any part) — see Abscess, upper limb
  artery (wall) I77.89
  atheromatous I77.2
  auricle, ear — see Abscess, ear, external
  axilla (region) L02.41-☑
    lymph gland or node L04.2
  back (any part, except buttock) L02.212
  Bartholin's gland N75.1
    with
      abortion — see Abortion, by type complicated by, sepsis
      ectopic or molar pregnancy O08.0
    following ectopic or molar pregnancy O08.0
  Bezold's — see Mastoiditis, acute
  bilharziasis B65.1
  bladder (wall) — see Cystitis, specified type NEC
  bone (subperiosteal) (see also Osteomyelitis, specified type NEC)
    accessory sinus (chronic) — see Sinusitis
    chronic or old — see Osteomyelitis, chronic
    jaw (lower) (upper) M27.2
    mastoid — see Mastoiditis, acute, subperiosteal
    petrous — see Petrositis
    spinal (tuberculous) A18.01
      nontuberculous — see Osteomyelitis, vertebra
  bowel K63.0
  brain (any part) (cystic) (otogenic) G06.0
    amebic (with abscess of any other site) A06.6
    gonococcal A54.82
    pheomycotic (chromomycotic) B43.1
    tuberculous A17.81
  breast (acute) (chronic) (nonpuerperal) N61
    newborn P39.0
    puerperal, postpartum, gestational — see Mastitis, obstetric, purulent
  broad ligament N73.2
    acute N73.0
    chronic N73.1
  Brodie's (localized) (chronic) M86.8X-☑
  bronchi J98.09
  buccal cavity K12.2
  bulbourethral gland N34.0
  bursa M71.00
    ankle M71.07-☑
    elbow M71.02-☑
    foot M71.07-☑
    hand M71.04-☑
    hip M71.05-☑
    knee M71.06-☑
    multiple sites M71.09
    pharyngeal J39.1
    shoulder M71.01-☑
    specified site NEC M71.08
    wrist M71.03-☑
  buttock L02.31
  canthus — see Blepharoconjunctivitis
  cartilage — see Disorder, cartilage, specified type NEC
  cecum K35.3
  cerebellum, cerebellar G06.0
    sequelae G09
  cerebral (embolic) G06.0
    sequelae G09
  cervical (meaning neck) L02.11
    lymph gland or node L04.0
  cervix (stump) (uteri) — see Cervicitis
  cheek (external) L02.01
    inner K12.2
  chest J86.9
    with fistula J86.0
    wall L02.213
  chin L02.01
  choroid — see Inflammation, chorioretinal

Abscess — *continued*
circumtonsillar J36
cold (lung) (tuberculous) (*see also* Tuberculosis, abscess, lung)
  articular — *see* Tuberculosis, joint
colon (wall) K63.0
colostomy K94.02
conjunctiva — *see* Conjunctivitis, acute
cornea H16.31- ☑
corpus
  cavernosum N48.21
  luteum — *see* Oophoritis
Cowper's gland N34.0
cranium G06.0
cul-de-sac (Douglas') (posterior) — *see* Peritonitis, pelvic, female
cutaneous — *see* Abscess, by site
dental K04.7
  with sinus (alveolar) K04.6
dentoalveolar K04.7
  with sinus K04.6
diaphragm, diaphragmatic K65.1
Douglas' cul-de-sac or pouch — *see* Peritonitis, pelvic, female
Dubois A50.59
ear (middle) (*see also* Otitis, media, suppurative)
  acute — *see* Otitis, media, suppurative, acute
  external H60.0- ☑
entamebic — *see* Abscess, amebic
enterostomy K94.12
epididymis N45.4
epidural G06.2
  brain G06.0
  spinal cord G06.1
epiglottis J38.7
epiploon, epiploic K65.1
erysipelatous — *see* Erysipelas
esophagus K20.8
ethmoid (bone) (chronic) (sinus) J32.2
external auditory canal — *see* Abscess, ear, external
extradural G06.2
  brain G06.0
    sequelae G09
  spinal cord G06.1
extraperitoneal K68.19
eye — *see* Endophthalmitis, purulent
eyelid H00.03- ☑
face (any part, except ear, eye and nose) L02.01
fallopian tube — *see* Salpingitis
fascia M72.8
fauces J39.1
fecal K63.0
femoral (region) — *see* Abscess, lower limb
filaria, filarial — *see* Infestation, filarial
finger (any) (*see also* Abscess, hand)
  nail — *see* Cellulitis, finger
foot L02.61- ☑
forehead L02.01
frontal sinus (chronic) J32.1
gallbladder K81.0
genital organ or tract
  female (external) N76.4
  male N49.9
    multiple sites N49.8
    specified NEC N49.8
gestational mammary O91.11- ☑
gestational subareolar O91.11- ☑
gingival K05.21
gland, glandular (lymph) (acute) — *see* Lymphadenitis, acute
gluteal (region) L02.31
gonorrheal — *see* Gonococcus
groin L02.214
gum K05.21
hand L02.51- ☑
head NEC L02.811
  face (any part, except ear, eye and nose) L02.01
heart — *see* Carditis
heel — *see* Abscess, foot
helminthic — *see* Infestation, helminth
hepatic (cholangitic) (hematogenic) (lymphogenic) (pylephlebitic) K75.0
  amebic A06.4
hip (region) — *see* Abscess, lower limb
ileocecal K35.3
ileostomy (bud) K94.12
iliac (region) L02.214

Abscess — *continued*
iliac — *continued*
  fossa K35.3
infraclavicular (fossa) — *see* Abscess, upper limb
inguinal (region) L02.214
  lymph gland or node L04.1
intestine, intestinal NEC K63.0
  rectal K61.1
intra-abdominal (*see also* Abscess, peritoneum) K65.1
  postoperative T81.4 ☑
    retroperitoneal K68.11
intracranial G06.0
intramammary — *see* Abscess, breast
intraorbital — *see* Abscess, orbit
intraperitoneal K65.1
intrasphincteric (anus) K61.4
intraspinal G06.1
intratonsillar J36
ischiorectal (fossa) K61.3
jaw (bone) (lower) (upper) M27.2
joint — *see* Arthritis, pyogenic or pyemic
  spine (tuberculous) A18.01
    nontuberculous — *see* Spondylopathy, infective
kidney N15.1
  with calculus N20.0
    with hydronephrosis N13.6
  puerperal (postpartum) O86.21
knee (*see also* Abscess, lower limb)
  joint M00.9
labium (majus) (minus) N76.4
lacrimal
  caruncle — *see* Inflammation, lacrimal, passages, acute
  gland — *see* Dacryoadenitis
  passages (duct) (sac) — *see* Inflammation, lacrimal, passages, acute
lacunar N34.0
larynx J38.7
lateral (alveolar) K04.7
  with sinus K04.6
leg (any part) — *see* Abscess, lower limb
lens H27.8
lingual K14.0
  tonsil J36
lip K13.0
Littre's gland N34.0
liver (cholangitic) (hematogenic) (lymphogenic) (pylephlebitic) (pyogenic) K75.0
  amebic (due to Entamoeba histolytica) (dysenteric) (tropical) A06.4
  with
    brain abscess (and liver or lung abscess) A06.6
    lung abscess A06.5
loin (region) L02.211
lower limb L02.41- ☑
lumbar (tuberculous) A18.01
  nontuberculous L02.212
lung (miliary) (putrid) J85.2
  with pneumonia J85.1
    due to specified organism (see Pneumonia, in (due to))
  amebic (with liver abscess) A06.5
  with
    brain abscess A06.6
    pneumonia A06.5
lymph, lymphatic, gland or node (acute) (*see also* Lymphadenitis, acute)
  mesentery I88.0
malar M27.2
mammary gland — *see* Abscess, breast
marginal, anus K61.0
mastoid — *see* Mastoiditis, acute
maxilla, maxillary M27.2
  molar (tooth) K04.7
    with sinus K04.6
  premolar K04.7
  sinus (chronic) J32.0
mediastinum J85.3
meibomian gland — *see* Hordeolum
meninges G06.2
mesentery, mesenteric K65.1
mesosalpinx — *see* Salpingitis
mons pubis L02.215
mouth (floor) K12.2
muscle — *see* Myositis, infective
myocardium I40.0

Abscess — *continued*
nabothian (follicle) — *see* Cervicitis
nasal J32.9
nasopharyngeal J39.1
navel L02.216
  newborn P38.9
    with mild hemorrhage P38.1
    without hemorrhage P38.9
neck (region) L02.11
  lymph gland or node L04.0
nephritic — *see* Abscess, kidney
nipple N61
  associated with
    lactation — *see* Pregnancy, complicated by,
    pregnancy — *see* Pregnancy, complicated by
nose (external) (fossa) (septum) J34.0
  sinus (chronic) — *see* Sinusitis
omentum K65.1
operative wound T81.4 ☑
orbit, orbital — *see* Cellulitis, orbit
otogenic G06.0
ovary, ovarian (corpus luteum) — *see* Oophoritis
oviduct — *see* Oophoritis
palate (soft) K12.2
  hard M27.2
palmar (space) — *see* Abscess, hand
pancreas (duct) — *see* Pancreatitis, acute
parafrenal N48.21
parametric, parametrium N73.2
  acute N73.0
  chronic N73.1
paranephric N15.1
parapancreatic — *see* Pancreatitis, acute
parapharyngeal J39.0
pararectal K61.1
parasinus — *see* Sinusitis
parauterine (*see also* Disease, pelvis, inflammatory) N73.2
paravaginal — *see* Vaginitis
parietal region (scalp) L02.811
parodontal K05.21
parotid (duct) (gland) K11.3
  region K12.2
pectoral (region) L02.213
pelvis, pelvic
  female — *see* Disease, pelvis, inflammatory
  male, peritoneal K65.1
penis N48.21
  gonococcal (accessory gland) (periurethral) A54.1
perianal K61.0
periapical K04.7
  with sinus (alveolar) K04.6
periappendicular K35.3
pericardial I30.1
pericecal K35.3
pericemental K05.21
pericholecystic — *see* Cholecystitis, acute
pericoronal K05.21
peridental K05.21
perimetric (*see also* Disease, pelvis, inflammatory) N73.2
perinephric, perinephritic — *see* Abscess, kidney
perineum, perineal (superficial) L02.215
  urethra N34.0
periodontal (parietal) K05.21
  apical K04.7
periosteum, periosteal (*see also* Osteomyelitis, specified type NEC)
  with osteomyelitis (*see also* Osteomyelitis, specified type NEC)
    acute — *see* Osteomyelitis, acute
    chronic — *see* Osteomyelitis, chronic
peripharyngeal J39.0
peripleuritic J86.9
  with fistula J86.0
periprostatic N41.2
perirectal K61.1
perirenal (tissue) — *see* Abscess, kidney
perisinuous (nose) — *see* Sinusitis
peritoneum, peritoneal (perforated) (ruptured) K65.1
  with appendicitis K35.3
  pelvic
    female — *see* Peritonitis, pelvic, female
    male K65.1
  postoperative T81.4 ☑
  puerperal, postpartum, childbirth O85
  tuberculous A18.31
peritonsillar J36

Abscess — *continued*
- perityphlic K35.3
- periureteral N28.89
- periurethral N34.0
  - gonococcal (accessory gland) (periurethral) A54.1
- periuterine (*see also* Disease, pelvis, inflammatory) N73.2
- perivesical — *see* Cystitis, specified type NEC
- petrous bone — *see* Petrositis
- phagedenic NOS L02.91
  - chancroid A57
- pharynx, pharyngeal (lateral) J39.1
- pilonidal L05.01
- pituitary (gland) E23.6
- pleura J86.9
  - with fistula J86.0
- popliteal — *see* Abscess, lower limb
- postcecal K35.3
- postlaryngeal J38.7
- postnasal J34.0
- postoperative (any site) T81.4 ☑
  - retroperitoneal K68.11
- postpharyngeal J39.0
- posttonsillar J36
- post-typhoid A01.09
- pouch of Douglas — *see* Peritonitis, pelvic, female
- premammary — *see* Abscess, breast
- prepatellar — *see* Abscess, lower limb
- prostate N41.2
  - gonococcal (acute) (chronic) A54.22
- psoas muscle K68.12
- puerperal — *code by* site under Puerperal, abscess
- pulmonary — *see* Abscess, lung
- pulp, pulpal (dental) K04.0
- rectovaginal septum K63.0
- rectovesical — *see* Cystitis, specified type NEC
- rectum K61.1
- renal — *see* Abscess, kidney
- retina — *see* Inflammation, chorioretinal
- retrobulbar — *see* Abscess, orbit
- retrocecal K65.1
- retrolaryngeal J38.7
- retromammary — *see* Abscess, breast
- retroperitoneal NEC K68.19
  - postprocedural K68.11
- retropharyngeal J39.0
- retrouterine — *see* Peritonitis, pelvic, female
- retrovesical — *see* Cystitis, specified type NEC
- root, tooth K04.7
  - with sinus (alveolar) K04.6
- round ligament (*see also* Disease, pelvis, inflammatory) N73.2
- rupture (spontaneous) NOS L02.91
- sacrum (tuberculous) A18.01
  - nontuberculous M46.28
- salivary (duct) (gland) K11.3
- scalp (any part) L02.811
- scapular — *see* Osteomyelitis, specified type NEC
- sclera — *see* Scleritis
- scrofulous (tuberculous) A18.2
- scrotum N49.2
- seminal vesicle N49.0
- septal, dental K04.7
  - with sinus (alveolar) K04.6
- serous — *see* Periostitis
- shoulder (region) — *see* Abscess, upper limb
- sigmoid K63.0
- sinus (accessory) (chronic) (nasal) (*see also* Sinusitis)
  - intracranial venous (any) G06.0
- Skene's duct or gland N34.0
- skin — *see* Abscess, by site
- specified site NEC L02.818
- spermatic cord N49.1
- sphenoidal (sinus) (chronic) J32.3
- spinal cord (any part) (staphylococcal) G06.1
  - tuberculous A17.81
- spine (column) (tuberculous) A18.01
  - epidural G06.1
  - nontuberculous — *see* Osteomyelitis, vertebra
- spleen D73.3
  - amebic A06.89
- stitch T81.4 ☑
- subarachnoid G06.2
  - brain G06.0
  - spinal cord G06.1
- subareolar — *see* Abscess, breast
- subcecal K35.3
- subcutaneous (*see also* Abscess, by site)

Abscess — *continued*
- subcutaneous (*see also* Abscess, by site) — *continued*
  - pheomycotic (chromomycotic) B43.2
- subdiaphragmatic K65.1
- subdural G06.2
  - brain G06.0
    - sequelae G09
  - spinal cord G06.1
- subgaleal L02.811
- subhepatic K65.1
- sublingual K12.2
  - gland K11.3
- submammary — *see* Abscess, breast
- submandibular (region) (space) (triangle) K12.2
  - gland K11.3
- submaxillary (region) L02.01
  - gland K11.3
- submental L02.01
  - gland K11.3
- subperiosteal — *see* Osteomyelitis, specified type NEC
- subphrenic K65.1
  - postoperative T81.4 ☑
- suburethral N34.0
- sudoriparous L75.8
- supraclavicular (fossa) — *see* Abscess, upper limb
- suprapelvic, acute N73.0
- suprarenal (capsule) (gland) E27.8
- sweat gland L74.8
- tear duct — *see* Inflammation, lacrimal, passages, acute
- temple L02.01
- temporal region L02.01
- temporosphenoidal G06.0
- tendon (sheath) M65.00
  - ankle M65.07- ☑
  - foot M65.07- ☑
  - forearm M65.03- ☑
  - hand M65.04- ☑
  - lower leg M65.06- ☑
  - pelvic region M65.05- ☑
  - shoulder region M65.01- ☑
  - specified site NEC M65.08
  - thigh M65.05- ☑
  - upper arm M65.02- ☑
- testis N45.4
- thigh — *see* Abscess, lower limb
- thorax J86.9
  - with fistula J86.0
- throat J39.1
- thumb (*see also* Abscess, hand)
  - nail — *see* Cellulitis, finger
- thymus (gland) E32.1
- thyroid (gland) E06.0
- toe (any) (*see also* Abscess, foot)
  - nail — *see* Cellulitis, toe
- tongue (staphylococcal) K14.0
- tonsil(s) (lingual) J36
- tonsillopharyngeal J36
- tooth, teeth (root) K04.7
  - with sinus (alveolar) K04.6
  - supporting structures NEC K05.21
- trachea J39.8
- trunk L02.219
  - abdominal wall L02.211
  - back L02.212
  - chest wall L02.213
  - groin L02.214
  - perineum L02.215
  - umbilicus L02.216
- tubal — *see* Salpingitis
- tuberculous — *see* Tuberculosis, abscess
- tubo-ovarian — *see* Salpingo-oophoritis
- tunica vaginalis N49.1
- umbilicus L02.216
- upper
  - limb L02.41- ☑
  - respiratory J39.8
- urethral (gland) N34.0
- urinary N34.0
- uterus, uterine (wall) (*see also* Endometritis)
  - ligament (*see also* Disease, pelvis, inflammatory) N73.2
  - neck — *see* Cervicitis
- uvula K12.2
- vagina (wall) — *see* Vaginitis
- vaginorectal — *see* Vaginitis

Abscess — *continued*
- vas deferens N49.1
- vermiform appendix K35.3
- vertebra (column) (tuberculous) A18.01
  - nontuberculous — *see* Osteomyelitis, vertebra
- vesical — *see* Cystitis, specified type NEC
- vesico-uterine pouch — *see* Peritonitis, pelvic, female
- vitreous (humor) — *see* Endophthalmitis, purulent
- vocal cord J38.3
- von Bezold's — *see* Mastoiditis, acute
- vulva N76.4
- vulvovaginal gland N75.1
- web space — *see* Abscess, hand
- wound T81.4 ☑
- wrist — *see* Abscess, upper limb

Absence (of) (organ or part) (complete or partial)
- adrenal (gland) (congenital) Q89.1
  - acquired E89.6
- albumin in blood E88.09
- alimentary tract (congenital) Q45.8
  - upper Q40.8
- alveolar process (acquired) — *see* Anomaly, alveolar
- ankle (acquired) Z89.44- ☑
- anus (congenital) Q42.3
  - with fistula Q42.2
- aorta (congenital) Q25.4
- appendix, congenital Q42.8
- arm (acquired) Z89.20- ☑
  - above elbow Z89.22- ☑
    - congenital (with hand present) — *see* Agenesis, arm, with hand present
    - and hand — *see* Agenesis, forearm, and hand
  - below elbow Z89.21- ☑
    - congenital (with hand present) — *see* Agenesis, arm, with hand present
    - and hand — *see* Agenesis, forearm, and hand
  - congenital — *see* Defect, reduction, upper limb
  - shoulder (following explantation of shoulder joint prosthesis) (joint) (with or without presence of antibiotic-impregnated cement spacer) Z89.23- ☑
    - congenital (with hand present) — *see* Agenesis, arm, with hand present
- artery (congenital) (peripheral) Q27.8
  - brain Q28.3
  - coronary Q24.5
  - pulmonary Q25.79
  - specified NEC Q27.8
  - umbilical Q27.0
- atrial septum (congenital) Q21.1
- auditory canal (congenital) (external) Q16.1
- auricle (ear), congenital Q16.0
- bile, biliary duct, congenital Q44.5
- bladder (acquired) Z90.6
  - congenital Q64.5
- bowel sounds R19.11
- brain Q00.0
  - part of Q04.3
- breast(s) (and nipple(s)) (acquired) Z90.1- ☑
  - congenital Q83.8
- broad ligament Q50.6
- bronchus (congenital) Q32.4
- canaliculus lacrimalis, congenital Q10.4
- cerebellum (vermis) Q04.3
- cervix (acquired) (with uterus) Z90.710
  - with remaining uterus Z90.712
  - congenital Q51.5
- chin, congenital Q18.8
- cilia (congenital) Q10.3
  - acquired — *see* Madarosis
- clitoris (congenital) Q52.6
- coccyx, congenital Q76.49
- cold sense R20.8
- congenital
  - lumen — *see* Atresia
  - organ or site NEC — *see* Agenesis
  - septum — *see* Imperfect, closure
- corpus callosum Q04.0
- cricoid cartilage, congenital Q31.8
- diaphragm (with hernia), congenital Q79.1
- digestive organ(s) or tract, congenital Q45.8
  - acquired NEC Z90.49
  - upper Q40.8
- ductus arteriosus Q28.8
- duodenum (acquired) Z90.49
  - congenital Q41.0

Absence — continued

ear, congenital Q16.9
  acquired H93.8- ☑
  auricle Q16.0
  external Q16.0
  inner Q16.5
  lobe, lobule Q17.8
  middle, except ossicles Q16.4
    ossicles Q16.3
  ossicles Q16.3
ejaculatory duct (congenital) Q55.4
endocrine gland (congenital) NEC Q89.2
  acquired E89.89
epididymis (congenital) Q55.4
  acquired Z90.79
epiglottis, congenital Q31.8
esophagus (congenital) Q39.8
  acquired (partial) Z90.49
eustachian tube (congenital) Q16.2
extremity (acquired) Z89.9
  congenital Q73.0
  knee (following explanation of knee joint prosthesis) (joint) (with or without presence of antibiotic-impregnated cement spacer) Z89.52- ☑
  lower (above knee) Z89.619
    below knee Z89.51- ☑
  upper — see Absence, arm
eye (acquired) Z90.01
  congenital Q11.1
  muscle (congenital) Q10.3
eyeball (acquired) Z90.01
  congenital Q11.1
eyelid (fold) (congenital) Q10.3
  acquired Z90.01
face, specified part NEC Q18.8
fallopian tube(s) (acquired) Z90.79
  congenital Q50.6
family member (causing problem in home) NEC (see also Disruption, family) Z63.32
femur, congenital — see Defect, reduction, lower limb, longitudinal, femur
fibrinogen (congenital) D68.2
  acquired D65
finger(s) (acquired) Z89.02- ☑
  congenital — see Agenesis, hand
foot (acquired) Z89.43- ☑
  congenital — see Agenesis, foot
forearm (acquired) — see Absence, arm, below elbow
gallbladder (acquired) Z90.49
  congenital Q44.0
gamma globulin in blood D80.1
  hereditary D80.0
genital organs
  acquired (female) (male) Z90.79
  female, congenital Q52.8
    external Q52.71
    internal NEC Q52.8
  male, congenital Q55.8
genitourinary organs, congenital NEC
  female Q52.8
  male Q55.8
globe (acquired) Z90.01
  congenital Q11.1
glottis, congenital Q31.8
hand and wrist (acquired) Z89.11- ☑
  congenital — see Agenesis, hand
head, part (acquired) NEC Z90.09
heat sense R20.8
hip (following explanation of hip joint prosthesis) (joint) (with or without presence of antibiotic-impregnated cement spacer) Z89.62- ☑
hymen (congenital) Q52.4
ileum (acquired) Z90.49
  congenital Q41.2
immunoglobulin, isolated NEC D80.3
  IgA D80.2
  IgG D80.3
  IgM D80.4
incus (acquired) — see Loss, ossicles, ear
  congenital Q16.3
inner ear, congenital Q16.5
intestine (acquired) (small) Z90.49
  congenital Q41.9
    specified NEC Q41.8
  large Z90.49
    congenital Q42.9
      specified NEC Q42.8
iris, congenital Q13.1

Absence — continued

jejunum (acquired) Z90.49
  congenital Q41.1
joint
  acquired
    hip (following explanation of hip joint prosthesis) (with or without presence of antibiotic-impregnated cement spacer) Z89.62- ☑
    knee (following explanation of knee joint prosthesis) (with or without presence of antibiotic-impregnated cement spacer) Z89.52- ☑
    shoulder (following explanation of shoulder joint prosthesis) (with or without presence of antibiotic-impregnated cement spacer) Z89.23- ☑
  congenital NEC Q74.8
kidney(s) (acquired) Z90.5
  congenital Q60.2
    bilateral Q60.1
    unilateral Q60.0
knee (following explanation of knee joint prosthesis) (joint) (with or without presence of antibiotic-impregnated cement spacer) Z89.52- ☑
labyrinth, membranous Q16.5
larynx (congenital) Q31.8
  acquired Z90.02
leg (acquired) (above knee) Z89.61- ☑
  below knee (acquired) Z89.51- ☑
  congenital — see Defect, reduction, lower limb
lens (acquired) (see also Aphakia)
  congenital Q12.3
  post cataract extraction Z98.4- ☑
limb (acquired) — see Absence, extremity
lip Q38.6
liver (congenital) Q44.7
lung (fissure) (lobe) (bilateral) (unilateral) (congenital) Q33.3
  acquired (any part) Z90.2
menstruation -– see Amenorrhea
muscle (congenital) (pectoral) Q79.8
  ocular Q10.3
neck, part Q18.8
neutrophil — see Agranulocytosis
nipple(s) (with breast(s)) (acquired) Z90.1- ☑
  congenital Q83.2
nose (congenital) Q30.1
  acquired Z90.09
organ
  of Corti, congenital Q16.5
  or site, congenital NEC Q89.8
    acquired NEC Z90.89
osseous meatus (ear) Q16.4
ovary (acquired)
  bilateral Z90.722
  congenital
    bilateral Q50.02
    unilateral Q50.01
  unilateral Z90.721
oviduct (acquired)
  bilateral Z90.722
  congenital Q50.6
  unilateral Z90.721
pancreas (congenital) Q45.0
  acquired Z90.410
    complete Z90.410
    partial Z90.411
    total Z90.410
parathyroid gland (acquired) E89.2
  congenital Q89.2
patella, congenital Q74.1
penis (congenital) Q55.5
  acquired Z90.79
pericardium (congenital) Q24.8
pituitary gland (congenital) Q89.2
  acquired E89.3
prostate (acquired) Z90.79
  congenital Q55.4
pulmonary valve Q22.0
punctum lacrimale (congenital) Q10.4
radius, congenital — see Defect, reduction, upper limb, longitudinal, radius
rectum (congenital) Q42.1
  with fistula Q42.0
  acquired Z90.49
respiratory organ NOS Q34.9
rib (acquired) Z90.89

Absence — continued

rib — continued
  congenital Q76.6
sacrum, congenital Q76.49
salivary gland(s), congenital Q38.4
scrotum, congenital Q55.29
seminal vesicles (congenital) Q55.4
  acquired Z90.79
septum
  atrial (congenital) Q21.1
  between aorta and pulmonary artery Q21.4
  ventricular (congenital) Q20.4
sex chromosome
  female phenotype Q97.8
  male phenotype Q98.8
skull bone (congenital) Q75.8
  with
    anencephaly Q00.0
    encephalocele — see Encephalocele
    hydrocephalus Q03.9
      with spina bifida — see Spina bifida, by site, with hydrocephalus
    microcephaly Q02
spermatic cord, congenital Q55.4
spine, congenital Q76.49
spleen (congenital) Q89.01
  acquired Z90.81
sternum, congenital Q76.7
stomach (acquired) (partial) Z90.3
  congenital Q40.2
superior vena cava, congenital Q26.8
teeth, tooth (congenital) K00.0
  acquired (complete) K08.109
    class I K08.101
    class II K08.102
    class III K08.103
    class IV K08.104
  due to
    caries K08.139
      class I K08.131
      class II K08.132
      class III K08.133
      class IV K08.134
    periodontal disease K08.129
      class I K08.121
      class II K08.122
      class III K08.123
      class IV K08.124
    specified NEC K08.199
      class I K08.191
      class II K08.192
      class III K08.193
      class IV K08.194
    trauma K08.119
      class I K08.111
      class II K08.112
      class III K08.113
      class IV K08.114
  partial K08.409
    class I K08.401
    class II K08.402
    class III K08.403
    class IV K08.404
  due to
    caries K08.439
      class I K08.431
      class II K08.432
      class III K08.433
      class IV K08.434
    periodontal disease K08.429
      class I K08.421
      class II K08.422
      class III K08.423
      class IV K08.424
    specified NEC K08.499
      class I K08.491
      class II K08.492
      class III K08.493
      class IV K08.494
    trauma K08.419
      class I K08.411
      class II K08.412
      class III K08.413
      class IV K08.414
tendon (congenital) Q79.8
testis (congenital) Q55.0
  acquired Z90.79
thumb (acquired) Z89.01- ☑

Index

Absence — *continued*
  thumb — *continued*
    congenital — *see* Agenesis, hand
  thymus gland Q89.2
  thyroid (gland) (acquired) E89.0
    cartilage, congenital Q31.8
    congenital E03.1
  toe(s) (acquired) Z89.42- ☑
    with foot — *see* Absence, foot and ankle
    congenital — *see* Agenesis, foot
    great Z89.41- ☑
  tongue, congenital Q38.3
  trachea (cartilage), congenital Q32.1
  transverse aortic arch, congenital Q25.4
  tricuspid valve Q22.4
  umbilical artery, congenital Q27.0
  upper arm and forearm with hand present, congenital
        — *see* Agenesis, arm, with hand present
  ureter (congenital) Q62.4
    acquired Z90.6
  urethra, congenital Q64.5
  uterus (acquired) Z90.710
    with cervix Z90.710
    with remaining cervical stump Z90.711
    congenital Q51.0
  uvula, congenital Q38.5
  vagina, congenital Q52.0
  vas deferens (congenital) Q55.4
    acquired Z90.79
  vein (peripheral) congenital NEC Q27.8
    cerebral Q28.3
    digestive system Q27.8
    great Q26.8
    lower limb Q27.8
    portal Q26.5
    precerebral Q28.1
    specified site NEC Q27.8
    upper limb Q27.8
  vena cava (inferior) (superior), congenital Q26.8
  ventricular septum Q20.4
  vertebra, congenital Q76.49
  vulva, congenital Q52.71
  wrist (acquired) Z89.12- ☑
Absorbent system disease I87.8
Absorption
  carbohydrate, disturbance K90.4
  chemical — *see* Table of Drugs and Chemicals
    through placenta (newborn) P04.9
      environmental substance P04.6
      nutritional substance P04.5
      obstetric anesthetic or analgesic drug P04.0
  drug NEC — *see* Table of Drugs and Chemicals
    addictive
      through placenta (newborn) P04.49
        cocaine P04.41
    medicinal
      through placenta (newborn) P04.1
    through placenta (newborn) P04.1
      obstetric anesthetic or analgesic drug P04.0
  fat, disturbance K90.4
    pancreatic K90.3
  noxious substance — *see* Table of Drugs and Chemicals
  protein, disturbance K90.4
  starch, disturbance K90.4
  toxic substance — *see* Table of Drugs and Chemicals
  uremic — *see* Uremia
Abstinence symptoms, syndrome
  alcohol F10.239
    with delirium F10.231
  cocaine F14.23
  neonatal P96.1
  nicotine — *see* Dependence, drug, nicotine, with, withdrawal
  opioid F11.93
    with dependence F11.23
  psychoactive NEC F19.939
    with
      delirium F19.931
      dependence F19.239
        with
          delirium F19.231
          perceptual disturbance F19.232
        uncomplicated F19.230
      perceptual disturbance F19.932
    uncomplicated F19.930
  sedative F13.939

Abstinence symptoms, syndrome — *continued*
  sedative — *continued*
    with
      delirium F13.931
      dependence F13.239
        with
          delirium F13.231
          perceptual disturbance F13.232
        uncomplicated F13.230
      perceptual disturbance F13.932
    uncomplicated F13.930
  stimulant NEC F15.93
    with dependence F15.23
Abulia R68.89
Abulomania F60.7
Abuse
  adult — *see* Maltreatment, adult
    as reason for
      couple seeking advice (including offender)
          Z63.0
  alcohol (non-dependent) F10.10
    with
      anxiety disorder F10.180
      intoxication F10.129
        with delirium F10.121
        uncomplicated F10.120
      mood disorder F10.14
      other specified disorder F10.188
      psychosis F10.159
        delusions F10.150
        hallucinations F10.151
      sexual dysfunction F10.181
      sleep disorder F10.182
      unspecified disorder F10.19
    counseling and surveillance Z71.41
  amphetamine (or related substance) — *see* Abuse,
      drug, stimulant NEC
  analgesics (non-prescribed) (over the counter) F55.8
  antacids F55.0
  antidepressants — *see* Abuse, drug, psychoactive NEC
  anxiolytic — *see* Abuse, drug, sedative
  barbiturates — *see* Abuse, drug, sedative
  caffeine — *see* Abuse, drug, stimulant NEC
  cannabis, cannabinoids — *see* Abuse, drug, cannabis
  child — *see* Maltreatment, child
  cocaine — *see* Abuse, drug, cocaine
  drug NEC (non-dependent) F19.10
    with sleep disorder F19.182
    amphetamine type — *see* Abuse, drug, stimulant
        NEC
    analgesics (non-prescribed) (over the counter)
        F55.8
    antacids F55.0
    antidepressants — *see* Abuse, drug, psychoactive
        NEC
    anxiolytics — *see* Abuse, drug, sedative
    barbiturates — *see* Abuse, drug, sedative
    caffeine — *see* Abuse, drug, stimulant NEC
    cannabis F12.10
      with
        anxiety disorder F12.180
        intoxication F12.129
          with
            delirium F12.121
            perceptual disturbance F12.122
          uncomplicated F12.120
        other specified disorder F12.188
        psychosis F12.159
          delusions F12.150
          hallucinations F12.151
        unspecified disorder F12.19
    cocaine F14.10
      with
        anxiety disorder F14.180
        intoxication F14.129
          with
            delirium F14.121
            perceptual disturbance F14.122
          uncomplicated F14.120
        mood disorder F14.14
        other specified disorder F14.188
        psychosis F14.159
          delusions F14.150
          hallucinations F14.151
        sexual dysfunction F14.181
        sleep disorder F14.182
        unspecified disorder F14.19
      counseling and surveillance Z71.51

Abuse — *continued*
  drug — *continued*
    hallucinogen F16.10
      with
        anxiety disorder F16.180
        flashbacks F16.183
        intoxication F16.129
          with
            delirium F16.121
            perceptual disturbance F16.122
          uncomplicated F16.120
        mood disorder F16.14
        other specified disorder F16.188
        perception disorder, persisting F16.183
        psychosis F16.159
          delusions F16.150
          hallucinations F16.151
        unspecified disorder F16.19
    hashish — *see* Abuse, drug, cannabis
    herbal or folk remedies F55.1
    hormones F55.3
    hypnotics — *see* Abuse, drug, sedative
    inhalant F18.10
      with
        anxiety disorder F18.180
        dementia, persisting F18.17
        intoxication F18.129
          with delirium F18.121
          uncomplicated F18.120
        mood disorder F18.14
        other specified disorder F18.188
        psychosis F18.159
          delusions F18.150
          hallucinations F18.151
        unspecified disorder F18.19
    laxatives F55.2
    LSD — *see* Abuse, drug, hallucinogen
    marihuana — *see* Abuse, drug, cannabis
    morphine type (opioids) — *see* Abuse, drug, opioid
    opioid F11.10
      with
        intoxication F11.129
          with
            delirium F11.121
            perceptual disturbance F11.122
          uncomplicated F11.120
        mood disorder F11.14
        other specified disorder F11.188
        psychosis F11.159
          delusions F11.150
          hallucinations F11.151
        sexual dysfunction F11.181
        sleep disorder F11.182
        unspecified disorder F11.19
    PCP (phencyclidine) (or related substance) — *see*
        Abuse, drug, hallucinogen
    psychoactive NEC F19.10
      with
        amnestic disorder F19.16
        anxiety disorder F19.180
        dementia F19.17
        intoxication F19.129
          with
            delirium F19.121
            perceptual disturbance F19.122
          uncomplicated F19.120
        mood disorder F19.14
        other specified disorder F19.188
        psychosis F19.159
          delusions F19.150
          hallucinations F19.151
        sexual dysfunction F19.181
        sleep disorder F19.182
        unspecified disorder F19.19
    sedative, hypnotic or anxiolytic F13.10
      with
        anxiety disorder F13.180
        intoxication F13.129
          with delirium F13.121
          uncomplicated F13.120
        mood disorder F13.14
        other specified disorder F13.188
        psychosis F13.159
          delusions F13.150
          hallucinations F13.151
        sexual dysfunction F13.181
        sleep disorder F13.182
        unspecified disorder F13.19

Absence — Abuse

Index

Abuse — *continued*
  drug — *continued*
    solvent — *see* Abuse, drug, inhalant
    steroids F55.3
    stimulant NEC F15.10
      with
        anxiety disorder F15.180
        intoxication F15.129
          with
            delirium F15.121
            perceptual disturbance F15.122
          uncomplicated F15.120
        mood disorder F15.14
        other specified disorder F15.188
        psychosis F15.159
          delusions F15.150
          hallucinations F15.151
        sexual dysfunction F15.181
        sleep disorder F15.182
        unspecified disorder F15.19
    tranquilizers — *see* Abuse, drug, sedative
    vitamins F55.4
  hallucinogens — *see* Abuse, drug, hallucinogen
  hashish — *see* Abuse, drug, cannabis
  herbal or folk remedies F55.1
  hormones F55.3
  hypnotic — *see* Abuse, drug, sedative
  inhalant — *see* Abuse, drug, inhalant
  laxatives F55.2
  LSD — *see* Abuse, drug, hallucinogen
  marihuana — *see* Abuse, drug, cannabis
  morphine type (opioids) — *see* Abuse, drug, opioid
  non-psychoactive substance NEC F55.8
    antacids F55.0
    folk remedies F55.1
    herbal remedies F55.1
    hormones F55.3
    laxatives F55.2
    steroids F55.3
    vitamins F55.4
  opioids — *see* Abuse, drug, opioid
  PCP (phencyclidine) (or related substance) — *see* Abuse, drug, hallucinogen
  physical (adult) (child) — *see* Maltreatment
  psychoactive substance — *see* Abuse, drug, psychoactive NEC
  psychological (adult) (child) — *see* Maltreatment
  sedative — *see* Abuse, drug, sedative
  sexual — *see* Maltreatment
  solvent — *see* Abuse, drug, inhalant
  steroids F55.3
  vitamins F55.4
Acalculia R48.8
  developmental F81.2
Acanthamebiasis (with) B60.10
  conjunctiva B60.12
  keratoconjunctivitis B60.13
  meningoencephalitis B60.11
  other specified B60.19
Acanthocephaliasis B83.8
Acanthocheilonemiasis B74.4
Acanthocytosis E78.6
Acantholysis L11.9
Acanthosis (acquired) (nigricans) L83
  benign Q82.8
  congenital Q82.8
  seborrheic L82.1
    inflamed L82.0
  tongue K14.3
Acapnia E87.3
Acarbia E87.2
Acardia, acardius Q89.8
Acardiacus amorphus Q89.8
Acardiotrophia I51.4
Acariasis B88.0
  scabies B86
Acarodermatitis (urticarioides) B88.0
Acarophobia F40.218
Acatalasemia, acatalasia E80.3
Acathisia (drug induced) G25.71
Accelerated atrioventricular conduction I45.6
Accentuation of personality traits (type A) Z73.1
Accessory (congenital)
  adrenal gland Q89.1
  anus Q43.4
  appendix Q43.4
  atrioventricular conduction I45.6

Accessory — *continued*
  auditory ossicles Q16.3
  auricle (ear) Q17.0
  biliary duct or passage Q44.5
  bladder Q64.79
  blood vessels NEC Q27.9
    coronary Q24.5
  bone NEC Q79.8
  breast tissue, axilla Q83.1
  carpal bones Q74.0
  cecum Q43.4
  chromosome(s) NEC (nonsex) Q92.9
    with complex rearrangements NEC Q92.5
      seen only at prometaphase Q92.8
    13 — *see* Trisomy, 13
    18 — *see* Trisomy, 18
    21 — *see* Trisomy, 21
    partial Q92.9
    sex
      female phenotype Q97.8
  coronary artery Q24.5
  cusp(s), heart valve NEC Q24.8
    pulmonary Q22.3
  cystic duct Q44.5
  digit(s) Q69.9
  ear (auricle) (lobe) Q17.0
  endocrine gland NEC Q89.2
  eye muscle Q10.3
  eyelid Q10.3
  face bone(s) Q75.8
  fallopian tube (fimbria) (ostium) Q50.6
  finger(s) Q69.0
  foreskin N47.8
  frontonasal process Q75.8
  gallbladder Q44.1
  genital organ(s)
    female Q52.8
      external Q52.79
      internal NEC Q52.8
    male Q55.8
  genitourinary organs NEC Q89.8
    female Q52.8
    male Q55.8
  hallux Q69.2
  heart Q24.8
    valve NEC Q24.8
      pulmonary Q22.3
  hepatic ducts Q44.5
  hymen Q52.4
  intestine (large) (small) Q43.4
  kidney Q63.0
  lacrimal canal Q10.6
  leaflet, heart valve NEC Q24.8
  ligament, broad Q50.6
  liver Q44.7
    duct Q44.5
  lobule (ear) Q17.0
  lung (lobe) Q33.1
  muscle Q79.8
  navicular of carpus Q74.0
  nervous system, part NEC Q07.8
  nipple Q83.3
  nose Q30.8
  organ or site not listed — *see* Anomaly, by site
  ovary Q50.31
  oviduct Q50.6
  pancreas Q45.3
  parathyroid gland Q89.2
  parotid gland (and duct) Q38.4
  pituitary gland Q89.2
  preauricular appendage Q17.0
  prepuce N47.8
  renal arteries (multiple) Q27.2
  rib Q76.6
    cervical Q76.5
  roots (teeth) K00.2
  salivary gland Q38.4
  sesamoid bones Q74.8
    foot Q74.2
    hand Q74.0
  skin tags Q82.8
  spleen Q89.09
  sternum Q76.7
  submaxillary gland Q38.4
  tarsal bones Q74.2
  teeth, tooth K00.1
  tendon Q79.8
  thumb Q69.1

Accessory — *continued*
  thymus gland Q89.2
  thyroid gland Q89.2
  toes Q69.2
  tongue Q38.3
  tooth, teeth K00.1
  tragus Q17.0
  ureter Q62.5
  urethra Q64.79
  urinary organ or tract NEC Q64.8
  uterus Q51.2
  vagina Q52.10
  valve, heart NEC Q24.8
    pulmonary Q22.3
  vertebra Q76.49
  vocal cords Q31.8
  vulva Q52.79
Accident
  birth — *see* Birth, injury
  cardiac — *see* Infarct, myocardium
  cerebral I63.9
  cerebrovascular (embolic) (ischemic) (thrombotic) I63.9
    aborted I63.9
    hemorrhagic — *see* Hemorrhage, intracranial, intracerebral
    old (without sequelae) Z86.73
      with sequelae (of) — *see* Sequelae, infarction, cerebral
  coronary — *see* Infarct, myocardium
  craniovascular I63.9
  vascular, brain I63.9
Accidental — *see* condition
Accommodation (disorder) (*see also* condition)
  hysterical paralysis of F44.89
  insufficiency of H52.4
  paresis — *see* Paresis, of accommodation
  spasm — *see* Spasm, of accommodation
Accouchement — *see* Delivery
Accreta placenta O43.21- ☑
Accretio cordis (nonrheumatic) I31.0
Accretions, tooth, teeth K03.6
Acculturation difficulty Z60.3
Accumulation secretion, prostate N42.89
Acephalia, acephalism, acephalus, acephaly Q00.0
Acephalobrachia monster Q89.8
Acephalochirus monster Q89.8
Acephalogaster Q89.8
Acephalostomus monster Q89.8
Acephalothorax Q89.8
Acerophobia F40.298
Acetonemia R79.89
  in Type 1 diabetes E10.10
    with coma E10.11
Acetonuria R82.4
Achalasia (cardia) (esophagus) K22.0
  congenital Q39.5
  pylorus Q40.0
  sphincteral NEC K59.8
Ache(s) — *see* Pain
Acheilia Q38.6
Achillobursitis — *see* Tendinitis, Achilles
Achillodynia — *see* Tendinitis, Achilles
Achlorhydria, achlorhydric (neurogenic) K31.83
  anemia D50.8
  diarrhea K31.83
  psychogenic F45.8
  secondary to vagotomy K91.1
Achluophobia F40.228
Acholia K82.8
Acholuric jaundice (familial) (splenomegalic) (*see also* Spherocytosis)
  acquired D59.8
Achondrogenesis Q77.0
Achondroplasia (osteosclerosis congenita) Q77.4
Achroma, cutis L80
Achromat (ism), achromatopsia (acquired) (congenital) H53.51
Achromia, congenital — *see* Albinism
Achromia parasitica B36.0
Achylia gastrica K31.89
  psychogenic F45.8
Acid
  burn — *see* Corrosion
  deficiency
    amide nicotinic E52
    ascorbic E54
    folic E53.8

Abuse — Acid

Acid — continued
  deficiency — continued
    nicotinic E52
    pantothenic E53.8
  intoxication E87.2
  peptic disease K30
  phosphatase deficiency E83.39
  stomach K30
    psychogenic F45.8
Acidemia E87.2
  argininosuccinic E72.22
  isovaleric E71.110
  metabolic (newborn) P19.9
    first noted before onset of labor P19.0
    first noted during labor P19.1
    noted at birth P19.2
  methylmalonic E71.120
  pipecolic E72.3
  propionic E71.121
Acidity, gastric (high) K30
  psychogenic F45.8
Acidocytopenia — see Agranulocytosis
Acidocytosis D72.1
Acidopenia — see Agranulocytosis
Acidosis (lactic) (respiratory) E87.2
  in Type 1 diabetes E10.10
    with coma E10.11
  kidney, tubular N25.89
  lactic E87.2
  metabolic NEC E87.2
    with respiratory acidosis E87.4
    late, of newborn P74.0
  mixed metabolic and respiratory, newborn P84
  newborn P84
  renal (hyperchloremic) (tubular) N25.89
  respiratory E87.2
    complicated by
      metabolic
        acidosis E87.4
        alkalosis E87.4
Aciduria
  argininosuccinic E72.22
  glutaric (type I) E72.3
    type II E71.313
    type III E71.5- ☑
  orotic (congenital) (hereditary) (pyrimidine deficiency) E79.8
    anemia D53.0
Acladiosis (skin) B36.0
Aclasis, diaphyseal Q78.6
Acleistocardia Q21.1
Aclusion — see Anomaly, dentofacial, malocclusion
Acne L70.9
  artificialis L70.8
  atrophica L70.2
  cachecticorum (Hebra) L70.8
  conglobata L70.1
  cystic L70.0
  decalvans L66.2
  excoriée des jeunes filles L70.5
  frontalis L70.2
  indurata L70.0
  infantile L70.4
  keloid L73.0
  lupoid L70.2
  necrotic, necrotica (miliaris) L70.2
  neonatal L70.4
  nodular L70.0
  occupational L70.8
  picker's L70.5
  pustular L70.0
  rodens L70.2
  rosacea L71.9
  specified NEC L70.8
  tropica L70.3
  varioliformis L70.2
  vulgaris L70.0
Acnitis (primary) A18.4
Acosta's disease T70.29 ☑
Acoustic — see condition
Acousticophobia F40.298
Acquired (see also condition)
  immunodeficiency syndrome (AIDS) B20
Acrania Q00.0
Acroangiodermatitis I78.9
Acroasphyxia, chronic I73.89
Acrobystitis N47.7
Acrocephalopolysyndactyly Q87.0

Acrocephalosyndactyly Q87.0
Acrocephaly Q75.0
Acrochondrohyperplasia — see Syndrome, Marfan's
Acrocyanosis I73.8 ☑
  newborn P28.2
    meaning transient blue hands and feet — omit code
Acrodermatitis L30.8
  atrophicans (chronica) L90.4
  continua (Hallopeau) L40.2
  enteropathica (hereditary) E83.2
  Hallopeau's L40.2
  infantile papular L44.4
  perstans L40.2
  pustulosa continua L40.2
  recalcitrant pustular L40.2
Acrodynia — see Poisoning, mercury
Acromegaly, acromegalia E22.0
Acromelalgia I73.81
Acromicria, acromikria Q79.8
Acronyx L60.0
Acropachy, thyroid — see Thyrotoxicosis
Acroparesthesia (simple) (vasomotor) I73.89
Acropathy, thyroid — see Thyrotoxicosis
Acrophobia F40.241
Acroposthitis N47.7
Acroscleriasis, acroscleroderma, acrosclerosis — see Sclerosis, systemic
Acrosphacelus I96
Acrospiroma, eccrine — see Neoplasm, skin, benign
Acrostealgia — see Osteochondropathy
Acrotrophodynia — see Immersion
ACTH ectopic syndrome E24.3
Actinic — see condition
Actinobacillosis, actinobacillus A28.8
  mallei A24.0
  muris A25.1
Actinomyces israelii (infection) — see Actinomycosis
Actinomycetoma (foot) B47.1
Actinomycosis, actinomycotic A42.9
  with pneumonia A42.0
  abdominal A42.1
  cervicofacial A42.2
  cutaneous A42.89
  gastrointestinal A42.1
  pulmonary A42.0
  sepsis A42.7
  specified site NEC A42.89
Actinoneuritis G62.82
Action, heart
  disorder I49.9
  irregular I49.9
    psychogenic F45.8
Activated protein C resistance D68.51
Active — see condition
Acute (see also condition)
  abdomen R10.0
  gallbladder — see Cholecystitis, acute
Acyanotic heart disease (congenital) Q24.9
Acystia Q64.5
Adair-Dighton syndrome (brittle bones and blue sclera, deafness) Q78.0
Adamantinoblastoma — see Ameloblastoma
Adamantinoma (see also Cyst, calcifying odontogenic)
  long bones C40.90
    lower limb C40.2- ☑
    upper limb C40.0- ☑
  malignant C41.1
    jaw (bone) (lower) C41.1
      upper C41.0
  tibial C40.2- ☑
Adamantoblastoma — see Ameloblastoma
Adams-Stokes (-Morgagni) disease or syndrome I45.9
Adaption reaction — see Disorder, adjustment
Addiction (see also Dependence) F19.20
  alcohol, alcoholic (ethyl) (methyl) (wood) (without remission) F10.20
    with remission F10.21
  drug — see Dependence, drug
  ethyl alcohol (without remission) F10.20
    with remission F10.21
  heroin — see Dependence, drug, opioid
  methyl alcohol (without remission) F10.20
    with remission F10.21
  methylated spirit (without remission) F10.20
    with remission F10.21

Addiction — continued
  morphine (-like substances) — see Dependence, drug, opioid
  nicotine — see Dependence, drug, nicotine
  opium and opioids — see Dependence, drug, opioid
  tobacco — see Dependence, drug, nicotine
Addison-Biermer anemia (pernicious) D51.0
Addisonian crisis E27.2
Addison's
  anemia (pernicious) D51.0
  disease (bronze) or syndrome E27.1
    tuberculous A18.7
  keloid L94.0
Addison-Schilder complex E71.528
Additional (see also Accessory)
  chromosome(s) Q99.8
    21 — see Trisomy, 21
    sex — see Abnormal, chromosome, sex
Adduction contracture, hip or other joint — see Contraction, joint
Adenitis (see also Lymphadenitis)
  acute, unspecified site L04.9
  axillary I88.9
    acute L04.2
    chronic or subacute I88.1
  Bartholin's gland N75.8
  bulbourethral gland — see Urethritis
  cervical I88.9
    acute L04.0
    chronic or subacute I88.1
  chancroid (Hemophilus ducreyi) A57
  chronic, unspecified site I88.1
  Cowper's gland — see Urethritis
  due to Pasteurella multocida (p. septica) A28.0
  epidemic, acute B27.09
  gangrenous L04.9
  gonorrheal NEC A54.89
  groin I88.9
    acute L04.1
    chronic or subacute I88.1
  infectious (acute) (epidemic) B27.09
  inguinal I88.9
    acute L04.1
    chronic or subacute I88.1
  lymph gland or node, except mesenteric I88.9
    acute — see Lymphadenitis, acute
    chronic or subacute I88.1
  mesenteric (acute) (chronic) (nonspecific) (subacute) I88.0
  parotid gland (suppurative) — see Sialoadenitis
  salivary gland (any) (suppurative) — see Sialoadenitis
  scrofulous (tuberculous) A18.2
  Skene's duct or gland — see Urethritis
  strumous, tuberculous A18.2
  subacute, unspecified site I88.1
  sublingual gland (suppurative) — see Sialoadenitis
  submandibular gland (suppurative) — see Sialoadenitis
  submaxillary gland (suppurative) — see Sialoadenitis
  tuberculous — see Tuberculosis, lymph gland
  urethral gland — see Urethritis
  Wharton's duct (suppurative) — see Sialoadenitis
Adenoacanthoma — see Neoplasm, malignant, by site
Adenoameloblastoma — see Cyst, calcifying odontogenic
Adenocarcinoid (tumor) — see Neoplasm, malignant, by site
Adenocarcinoma (see also Neoplasm, malignant, by site)
  acidophil
    specified site — see Neoplasm, malignant, by site
    unspecified site C75.1
  adrenal cortical C74.0- ☑
  alveolar — see Neoplasm, lung, malignant
  apocrine
    breast — see Neoplasm, breast, malignant
    in situ
      breast D05.8- ☑
      specified site NEC — see Neoplasm, skin, in situ
      unspecified site D04.9
    specified site NEC — see Neoplasm, skin, malignant
    unspecified site C44.99
  basal cell
    specified site — see Neoplasm, skin, malignant
    unspecified site C08.9
  basophil
    specified site — see Neoplasm, malignant, by site

Adenocarcinoma — *continued*
  basophil — *continued*
    unspecified site C75.1
  bile duct type C22.1
    liver C22.1
    specified site NEC — *see* Neoplasm, malignant, by site
    unspecified site C22.1
  bronchiolar — *see* Neoplasm, lung, malignant
  bronchioloalveolar — *see* Neoplasm, lung, malignant
  ceruminous C44.29- ☑
  cervix, in situ (*see also* Carcinoma, cervix uteri, in situ) D06.9
  chromophobe
    specified site — *see* Neoplasm, malignant, by site
    unspecified site C75.1
  diffuse type
    specified site — *see* Neoplasm, malignant, by site
    unspecified site C16.9
  duct
    infiltrating
      with Paget's disease — *see* Neoplasm, breast, malignant
      specified site — *see* Neoplasm, malignant, by site
      unspecified site (female) C50.91- ☑
        male C50.92-
    specified site –- *see* Neoplasm, malignant, by site
    unspecified site
      female C56.9
      male C61
  eosinophil
    specified site — *see* Neoplasm, malignant, by site
    unspecified site C75.1
  follicular
    with papillary C73
    moderately differentiated C73
    specified site — *see* Neoplasm, malignant, by site
    trabecular C73
    unspecified site C73
    well differentiated C73
  Hurthle cell C73
  in
    adenomatous
      polyposis coli C18.9
  infiltrating duct
    with Paget's disease — *see* Neoplasm, breast, malignant
    specified site — *see* Neoplasm, by site, malignant
    unspecified site (female) C50.91- ☑
      male C50.92- ☑
  inflammatory
    specified site — *see* Neoplasm, by site, malignant
    unspecified site (female) C50.91- ☑
      male C50.92- ☑
  intestinal type
    specified site — *see* Neoplasm, by site, malignant
    unspecified site C16.9
  intracystic papillary
  intraductal
    breast D05.1- ☑
    noninfiltrating
      breast D05.1- ☑
      papillary
        with invasion
          specified site — *see* Neoplasm, by site, malignant
          unspecified site (female) C50.91- ☑
            male C50.92- ☑
        breast D05.1- ☑
        specified site NEC — *see* Neoplasm, in situ, by site
        unspecified site D05.1- ☑
    specified site NEC — *see* Neoplasm, in situ, by site
    unspecified site D05.1- ☑
  papillary
    with invasion
      specified site — *see* Neoplasm, malignant, by site
      unspecified site (female) C50.91- ☑
        male C50.92- ☑
    breast D05.1- ☑
    specified site — *see* Neoplasm, in situ, by site
    unspecified site D05.1- ☑
  specified site NEC — *see* Neoplasm, in situ, by site
  unspecified site D05.1- ☑

Adenocarcinoma — *continued*
  islet cell
    with exocrine, mixed
      specified site — *see* Neoplasm, malignant, by site
      unspecified site C25.9
    pancreas C25.4
    specified site NEC — *see* Neoplasm, malignant, by site
    unspecified site C25.4
  lobular
    in situ
      breast D05.0- ☑
      specified site NEC — *see* Neoplasm, in situ, by site
      unspecified site D05.0- ☑
    specified site — *see* Neoplasm, malignant, by site
    unspecified site (female) C50.91- ☑
      male C50.92- ☑
  mucoid (*see also* Neoplasm, malignant, by site)
    cell
      specified site — *see* Neoplasm, malignant, by site
      unspecified site C75.1
  nonencapsulated sclerosing C73
  papillary
    with follicular C73
    follicular variant C73
    intraductal (noninfiltrating)
      with invasion
        specified site — *see* Neoplasm, malignant, by site
        unspecified site (female) C50.91- ☑
          male C50.92- ☑
      breast D05.1- ☑
      specified site NEC — *see* Neoplasm, in situ, by site
      unspecified site D05.1- ☑
    serous
      specified site — *see* Neoplasm, malignant, by site
      unspecified site C56.9
  papillocystic
    specified site — *see* Neoplasm, malignant, by site
    unspecified site C56.9
  pseudomucinous
    specified site — *see* Neoplasm, malignant, by site
    unspecified site C56.9
  renal cell C64- ☑
  sebaceous — *see* Neoplasm, skin, malignant
  serous (*see also* Neoplasm, malignant, by site)
    papillary
      specified site — *see* Neoplasm, malignant, by site
      unspecified site C56.9
  sweat gland — *see* Neoplasm, skin, malignant
  water-clear cell C75.0
Adenocarcinoma-in-situ (*see also* Neoplasm, in situ, by site)
  breast D05.9- ☑
Adenofibroma
  clear cell — *see* Neoplasm, benign, by site
  endometrioid D27.9
    borderline malignancy D39.10
    malignant C56- ☑
  mucinous
    specified site — *see* Neoplasm, benign, by site
    unspecified site D27.9
  papillary
    specified site — *see* Neoplasm, benign, by site
    unspecified site D27.9
  prostate — *see* Enlargement, enlarged, prostate
  serous
    specified site — *see* Neoplasm, benign, by site
    unspecified site D27.9
  specified site — *see* Neoplasm, benign, by site
  unspecified site D27.9
Adenofibrosis
  breast — *see* Fibroadenosis, breast
  endometrioid N80.0
Adenoiditis (chronic) J35.02
  with tonsillitis J35.03
  acute J03.90
    recurrent J03.91
    specified organism NEC J03.80
      recurrent J03.81
    staphylococcal J03.80

Adenoiditis — *continued*
  acute — *continued*
    staphylococcal — *continued*
      recurrent J03.81
    streptococcal J03.00
      recurrent J03.01
Adenoids — *see* condition
Adenolipoma — *see* Neoplasm, benign, by site
Adenolipomatosis, Launois-Bensaude E88.89
Adenolymphoma
  specified site — *see* Neoplasm, benign, by site
  unspecified site D11.9
Adenoma (*see also* Neoplasm, benign, by site)
  acidophil
    specified site — *see* Neoplasm, benign, by site
    unspecified site D35.2
  acidophil-basophil, mixed
    specified site — *see* Neoplasm, benign, by site
    unspecified site D35.2
  adrenal (cortical) D35.00
    clear cell D35.00
    compact cell D35.00
    glomerulosa cell D35.00
    heavily pigmented variant D35.00
    mixed cell D35.00
  alpha-cell
    pancreas D13.7
    specified site NEC — *see* Neoplasm, benign, by site
    unspecified site D13.7
  alveolar D14.30
  apocrine
    breast D24- ☑
    specified site NEC — *see* Neoplasm, skin, benign, by site
    unspecified site D23.9
  basal cell D11.9
  basophil
    specified site — *see* Neoplasm, benign, by site
    unspecified site D35.2
  basophil-acidophil, mixed
    specified site — *see* Neoplasm, benign, by site
    unspecified site D35.2
  beta-cell
    pancreas D13.7
    specified site NEC — *see* Neoplasm, benign, by site
    unspecified site D13.7
  bile duct D13.4
    common D13.5
    extrahepatic D13.5
    intrahepatic D13.4
    specified site NEC — *see* Neoplasm, benign, by site
    unspecified site D13.4
  black D35.00
  bronchial D38.1
    cylindroid type — *see* Neoplasm, lung, malignant
  ceruminous D23.2- ☑
  chief cell D35.1
  chromophobe
    specified site — *see* Neoplasm, benign, by site
    unspecified site D35.2
  colloid
    specified site — *see* Neoplasm, benign, by site
    unspecified site D34
  duct
  eccrine, papillary — *see* Neoplasm, skin, benign
  endocrine, multiple
    single specified site — *see* Neoplasm, uncertain behavior, by site
    two or more specified sites D44- ☑
    unspecified site D44.9
  endometrioid (*see also* Neoplasm, benign)
    borderline malignancy — *see* Neoplasm, uncertain behavior, by site
  eosinophil
    specified site — *see* Neoplasm, benign, by site
    unspecified site D35.2
  fetal
    specified site — *see* Neoplasm, benign, by site
    unspecified site D34
  follicular
    specified site — *see* Neoplasm, benign, by site
    unspecified site D34
  hepatocelluiar D13.4
  Hurthle cell D34
  islet cell
    pancreas D13.7
    specified site NEC — *see* Neoplasm, benign, by site
    unspecified site D13.7

Adenoma — continued
  liver cell D13.4
  macrofollicular
    specified site — see Neoplasm, benign, by site
    unspecified site D34
  malignant, malignum — see Neoplasm, malignant, by site
  microcystic
    pancreas D13.7
    specified site NEC — see Neoplasm, benign, by site
    unspecified site D13.7
  microfollicular
    specified site — see Neoplasm, benign, by site
    unspecified site D34
  mucoid cell
    specified site — see Neoplasm, benign, by site
    unspecified site D35.2
  multiple endocrine
    single specified site — see Neoplasm, uncertain behavior, by site
    two or more specified sites D44- ☑
    unspecified site D44.9
  nipple D24- ☑
  papillary (see also Neoplasm, benign, by site)
    eccrine — see Neoplasm, skin, benign, by site
  Pick's tubular
    specified site — see Neoplasm, benign, by site
    unspecified site
      female D27.9
      male D29.20
  pleomorphic
    carcinoma in — see Neoplasm, salivary gland, malignant
      specified site — see Neoplasm, malignant, by site
      unspecified site C08.9
  polypoid (see also Neoplasm, benign)
    adenocarcinoma in — see Neoplasm, malignant, by site
    adenocarcinoma in situ — see Neoplasm, in situ, by site
  prostate — see Neoplasm, benign, prostate
  rete cell D29.20
  sebaceous — see Neoplasm, skin, benign
  Sertoli cell
    specified site — see Neoplasm, benign, by site
    unspecified site
      female D27.9
      male D29.20
  skin appendage — see Neoplasm, skin, benign
  sudoriferous gland — see Neoplasm, skin, benign
  sweat gland — see Neoplasm, skin, benign
  testicular
    specified site — see Neoplasm, benign, by site
    unspecified site
      female D27.9
      male D29.20
  tubular (see also Neoplasm, benign, by site)
    adenocarcinoma in — see Neoplasm, malignant, by site
    adenocarcinoma in situ — see Neoplasm, in situ, by site
    Pick's
      specified site — see Neoplasm, benign, by site
      unspecified site
        female D27.9
        male D29.20
  tubulovillous (see also Neoplasm, benign, by site)
    adenocarcinoma in — see Neoplasm, malignant, by site
    adenocarcinoma in situ — see Neoplasm, in situ, by site
  villous — see Neoplasm, uncertain behavior, by site
    adenocarcinoma in — see Neoplasm, malignant, by site
    adenocarcinoma in situ — see Neoplasm, in situ, by site
  water-clear cell D35.1
Adenomatosis
  endocrine (multiple) E31.20
    single specified site — see Neoplasm, uncertain behavior, by site
  erosive of nipple D24- ☑
  pluriendocrine — see Adenomatosis, endocrine
  pulmonary D38.1
    malignant — see Neoplasm, lung, malignant
  specified site — see Neoplasm, benign, by site

Adenomatosis — continued
  unspecified site D12.6
Adenomatous
  goiter (nontoxic) E04.9
    with hyperthyroidism — see Hyperthyroidism, with, goiter, nodular
    toxic — see Hyperthyroidism, with, goiter, nodular
Adenomyoma (see also Neoplasm, benign, by site)
  prostate — see Enlarged, prostate
Adenomyometritis N80.0
Adenomyosis N80.0
Adenopathy (lymph gland) R59.9
  generalized R59.1
  inguinal R59.0
  localized R59.0
  mediastinal R59.0
  mesentery R59.0
  syphilitic (secondary) A51.49
  tracheobronchial R59.0
    tuberculous A15.4
      primary (progressive) A15.7
  tuberculous (see also Tuberculosis, lymph gland)
    tracheobronchial A15.4
      primary (progressive) A15.7
Adenosalpingitis — see Salpingitis
Adenosarcoma — see Neoplasm, malignant, by site
Adenosclerosis I88.8
Adenosis (sclerosing) breast — see Fibroadenosis, breast
Adenovirus, as cause of disease classified elsewhere
  B97.0
Adentia (complete) (partial) — see Absence, teeth
Adherent (see also Adhesions)
  labia (minora) N90.89
  pericardium (nonrheumatic) I31.0
    rheumatic I09.2
  placenta (with hemorrhage) O72.0
    without hemorrhage O73.0
  prepuce, newborn N47.0
  scar (skin) L90.5
  tendon in scar L90.5
Adhesions, adhesive (postinfective) K66.0
  with intestinal obstruction K56.5
  abdominal (wall) — see Adhesions, peritoneum
  appendix K38.8
  bile duct (common) (hepatic) K83.8
  bladder (sphincter) N32.89
  bowel — see Adhesions, peritoneum
  cardiac I31.0
    rheumatic I09.2
  cecum — see Adhesions, peritoneum
  cervicovaginal N88.1
    congenital Q52.8
    postpartal O90.89
    old N88.1
  cervix N88.1
  ciliary body NEC — see Adhesions, iris
  clitoris N90.89
  colon — see Adhesions, peritoneum
  common duct K83.8
  congenital (see also Anomaly, by site)
    fingers — see Syndactylism, complex, fingers
    omental, anomalous Q43.3
    peritoneal Q43.3
    tongue (to gum or roof of mouth) Q38.3
  conjunctiva (acquired) H11.21- ☑
    congenital Q15.8
  cystic duct K82.8
  diaphragm — see Adhesions, peritoneum
  due to foreign body — see Foreign body
  duodenum — see Adhesions, peritoneum
  ear
    middle H74.1- ☑
  epididymis N50.8
  epidural — see Adhesions, meninges
  epiglottis J38.7
  eyelid H02.59
  female pelvis N73.6
  gallbladder K82.8
  globe H44.89
  heart I31.0
    rheumatic I09.2
  ileocecal (coil) — see Adhesions, peritoneum
  ileum — see Adhesions, peritoneum
  intestine (see also Adhesions, peritoneum)
    with obstruction K56.5
  intra-abdominal — see Adhesions, peritoneum
  iris H21.50- ☑

Adhesions, adhesive — continued
  iris — continued
    anterior H21.51- ☑
    goniosynechiae H21.52- ☑
    posterior H21.54- ☑
    to corneal graft T85.89 ☑
  joint — see Ankylosis
    knee M23.8X ☑
    temporomandibular M26.61
  labium (majus) (minus), congenital Q52.5
  liver — see Adhesions, peritoneum
  lung J98.4
  mediastinum J98.5
  meninges (cerebral) (spinal) G96.12
    congenital Q07.8
    tuberculous (cerebral) (spinal) A17.0
  mesenteric — see Adhesions, peritoneum
  nasal (septum) (to turbinates) J34.89
  ocular muscle — see Strabismus, mechanical
  omentum — see Adhesions, peritoneum
  ovary N73.6
    congenital (to cecum, kidney or omentum) Q50.39
  paraovarian N73.6
  pelvic (peritoneal)
    female N73.6
      postprocedural N99.4
    male — see Adhesions, peritoneum
    postpartal (old) N73.6
    tuberculous A18.17
  penis to scrotum (congenital) Q55.8
  periappendiceal (see also Adhesions, peritoneum)
  pericardium (nonrheumatic) I31.0
    focal I31.8
    rheumatic I09.2
    tuberculous A18.84
  pericholecystic K82.8
  perigastric — see Adhesions, peritoneum
  periovarian N73.6
  periprostatic N42.89
  perirectal — see Adhesions, peritoneum
  perirenal N28.89
  peritoneum, peritoneal (postinfective) (postprocedural) K66.0
    with obstruction (intestinal) K56.5
    congenital Q43.3
    pelvic, female N73.6
      postprocedural N99.4
    postpartal, pelvic N73.6
    to uterus N73.6
  peritubal N73.6
  periureteral N28.89
  periuterine N73.6
  perivesical N32.89
  perivesicular (seminal vesicle) N50.8
  pleura, pleuritic J94.8
    tuberculous NEC A15.6
  pleuropericardial J94.8
  postoperative (gastrointestinal tract) K66.0
    with obstruction K91.3
    due to foreign body accidentally left in wound — see Foreign body, accidentally left during a procedure
    pelvic peritoneal N99.4
    urethra — see Stricture, urethra, postprocedural
    vagina N99.2
  postpartal, old (vulva or perineum) N90.89
  preputial, prepuce N47.5
  pulmonary J98.4
  pylorus — see Adhesions, peritoneum
  sciatic nerve — see Lesion, nerve, sciatic
  seminal vesicle N50.8
  shoulder (joint) — see Capsulitis, adhesive
  sigmoid flexure — see Adhesions, peritoneum
  spermatic cord (acquired) N50.8
    congenital Q55.4
  spinal canal G96.12
  stomach — see Adhesions, peritoneum
  subscapular — see Capsulitis, adhesive
  temporomandibular M26.61
  tendinitis (see also Tenosynovitis, specified type NEC)
    shoulder — see Capsulitis, adhesive
  testis N44.8
  tongue, congenital (to gum or roof of mouth) Q38.3
    acquired K14.8
  trachea J39.8
  tubo-ovarian N73.6
  tunica vaginalis N44.8
  uterus N73.6

☑ Additional Character Required — Refer to the Tabular List for Character Selection   ▽ Subterms under main terms may continue to next column or page

Adhesions, adhesive — *continued*
  uterus — *continued*
    internal N85.6
    to abdominal wall N73.6
  vagina (chronic) N89.5
    postoperative N99.2
  vitromacular H43.82- ☑
  vitreous H43.89
  vulva N90.89
Adiaspiromycosis B48.8
Adie (-Holmes) **pupil or syndrome** — *see* Anomaly,
  pupil, function, tonic pupil
Adiponecrosis neonatorum P83.8
Adiposis (*see also* Obesity)
  cerebralis E23.6
  dolorosa E88.2
Adiposity (*see also* Obesity)
  heart — *see* Degeneration, myocardial
  localized E65
Adiposogenital dystrophy E23.6
Adjustment
  disorder — *see* Disorder, adjustment
  implanted device — *see* Encounter (for), adjustment
    (of)
  prosthesis, external — *see* Fitting
  reaction — *see* Disorder, adjustment
Administration of tPA (rtPA) in a different facility within
  the last 24 hours prior to admission to current facility Z92.82
Admission (for) (*see also* Encounter (for))
  adjustment (of)
    artificial
      arm Z44.00- ☑
        complete Z44.01- ☑
        partial Z44.02- ☑
      eye Z44.2 ☑
      leg Z44.10- ☑
        complete Z44.11- ☑
        partial Z44.12- ☑
    brain neuropacemaker Z46.2
      implanted Z45.42
    breast
      implant Z45.81 ☑
      prosthesis (external) Z44.3 ☑
    colostomy belt Z46.89
    contact lenses Z46.0
    cystostomy device Z46.6
    dental prosthesis Z46.3
    device NEC
      abdominal Z46.89
      implanted Z45.89
        cardiac Z45.09
          defibrillator (with synchronous cardiac
            pacemaker) Z45.02
          pacemaker Z45.018
            pulse generator Z45.010
        hearing device Z45.328
          bone conduction Z45.320
          cochlear Z45.321
        infusion pump Z45.1
        nervous system Z45.49
          CSF drainage Z45.41
          hearing device — *see* Admission, adjust-
            ment, device, implanted, hearing
            device
          neuropacemaker Z45.42
          visual substitution Z45.31
        specified NEC Z45.89
        vascular access Z45.2
        visual substitution Z45.31
      nervous system Z46.2
        implanted — *see* Admission, adjustment,
          device, implanted, nervous system
    orthodontic Z46.4
    prosthetic Z44.9
      arm — *see* Admission, adjustment, artificial,
        arm
      breast Z44.3 ☑
      dental Z46.3
      eye Z44.2 ☑
      leg — *see* Admission, adjustment, artificial,
        leg
      specified type NEC Z44.8
    substitution
      auditory Z46.2

Admission — *continued*
  adjustment — *continued*
    device — *continued*
      substitution — *continued*
        auditory — *continued*
          implanted — *see* Admission, adjust-
            ment, device, implanted, hearing
            device
        nervous system Z46.2
          implanted — *see* Admission, adjust-
            ment, device, implanted, nervous
            system
        visual Z46.2
          implanted Z45.31
    urinary Z46.6
    hearing aid Z46.1
      implanted — *see* Admission, adjustment, de-
        vice, implanted, hearing device
    ileostomy device Z46.89
    intestinal appliance or device NEC Z46.89
    neuropacemaker (brain) (peripheral nerve) (spinal
      cord) Z46.2
      implanted Z45.42
    orthodontic device Z46.4
    orthopedic (brace) (cast) (device) (shoes) Z46.89
    pacemaker
      cardiac Z45.018
        pulse generator Z45.010
      nervous system Z46.2
        implanted Z45.42
    portacath (port-a-cath) Z45.2
    prosthesis Z44.9
      arm — *see* Admission, adjustment, artificial,
        arm
      breast Z44.3 ☑
      dental Z46.3
      eye Z44.2 ☑
      leg — *see* Admission, adjustment, artificial, leg
      specified NEC Z44.8
    spectacles Z46.0
  aftercare (*see also* Aftercare) Z51.89
    postpartum
      immediately after delivery Z39.0
      routine follow-up Z39.2
    radiation therapy (antineoplastic) Z51.0
  attention to artificial opening (of) Z43.9
    artificial vagina Z43.7
    colostomy Z43.3
    cystostomy Z43.5
    enterostomy Z43.4
    gastrostomy Z43.1
    ileostomy Z43.2
    jejunostomy Z43.4
    nephrostomy Z43.6
    specified site NEC Z43.8
      intestinal tract Z43.4
      urinary tract Z43.6
    tracheostomy Z43.0
    ureterostomy Z43.6
    urethrostomy Z43.6
  breast augmentation or reduction Z41.1
  breast reconstruction following mastectomy Z42.1
  change of
    dressing (nonsurgical) Z48.00
    neuropacemaker device (brain) (peripheral nerve)
      (spinal cord) Z46.2
      implanted Z45.42
    surgical dressing Z48.01
  circumcision, ritual or routine (in absence of diagnosis)
    Z41.2
  clinical research investigation (control) (normal com-
    parison) (participant) Z00.6
  contraceptive management Z30.9
  cosmetic surgery NEC Z41.1
  counseling (*see also* Counseling)
    dietary Z71.3
    HIV Z71.7
    human immunodeficiency virus Z71.7
    nonattending third party Z71.0
    procreative management NEC Z31.69
  delivery, full-term, uncomplicated O80
    cesarean, without indication O82
  dietary surveillance and counseling Z71.3
  ear piercing Z41.3
  examination at health care facility (adult) (*see also*
    Examination) Z00.00
    with abnormal findings Z00.01

Admission — *continued*
  examination at health care facility (*see also* Examina-
    tion) — *continued*
    clinical research investigation (control) (normal
      comparison) (participant) Z00.6
    dental Z01.20
      with abnormal findings Z01.21
    donor (potential) Z00.5
    ear Z01.10
      with abnormal findings NEC Z01.118
    eye Z01.00
      with abnormal findings Z01.01
    general, specified reason NEC Z00.8
    hearing Z01.10
      with abnormal findings NEC Z01.118
    postpartum checkup Z39.2
    psychiatric (general) Z00.8
      requested by authority Z04.6
    vision Z01.00
      with abnormal findings Z01.01
  fitting (of)
    artificial
      arm — *see* Admission, adjustment, artificial,
        arm
      eye Z44.2 ☑
      leg — *see* Admission, adjustment, artificial, leg
    brain neuropacemaker Z46.2
      implanted Z45.42
    breast prosthesis (external) Z44.3 ☑
    colostomy belt Z46.89
    contact lenses Z46.0
    cystostomy device Z46.6
    dental prosthesis Z46.3
    dentures Z46.3
    device NEC
      abdominal Z46.89
      nervous system Z46.2
        implanted — *see* Admission, adjustment,
          device, implanted, nervous system
      orthodontic Z46.4
      prosthetic Z44.9
        breast Z44.3 ☑
        dental Z46.3
        eye Z44.2 ☑
      substitution
        auditory Z46.2
          implanted — *see* Admission, adjust-
            ment, device, implanted, hearing
            device
        nervous system Z46.2
          implanted — *see* Admission, adjust-
            ment, device, implanted, nervous
            system
        visual Z46.2
          implanted Z45.31
    hearing aid Z46.1
    ileostomy device Z46.89
    intestinal appliance or device NEC Z46.89
    neuropacemaker (brain) (peripheral nerve) (spinal
      cord) Z46.2
      implanted Z45.42
    orthodontic device Z46.4
    orthopedic device (brace) (cast) (shoes) Z46.89
    prosthesis Z44.9
      arm — *see* Admission, adjustment, artificial,
        arm
      breast Z44.3 ☑
      dental Z46.3
      eye Z44.2 ☑
      leg — *see* Admission, adjustment, artificial, leg
      specified type NEC Z44.8
    spectacles Z46.0
  follow-up examination Z09
  intrauterine device management Z30.431
    initial prescription Z30.014
  mental health evaluation Z00.8
    requested by authority Z04.6
  observation — *see* Observation
  Papanicolaou smear, cervix Z12.4
    for suspected malignant neoplasm Z12.4
  plastic and reconstructive surgery following medical
    procedure or healed injury NEC Z42.8
  plastic surgery, cosmetic NEC Z41.1
  postpartum observation
    immediately after delivery Z39.0
    routine follow-up Z39.2
  poststerilization (for restoration) Z31.0
    aftercare Z31.42

Admission — *continued*
  procreative management Z31.9
  prophylactic (measure)
    organ removal Z40.00
      breast Z40.01
      ovary Z40.02
      specified organ NEC Z40.09
      testes Z40.09
    vaccination Z23
  psychiatric examination (general) Z00.8
    requested by authority Z04.6
  radiation therapy (antineoplastic) Z51.0
  reconstructive surgery following medical procedure
    or healed injury NEC Z42.8
  removal of
    cystostomy catheter Z43.5
    drains Z48.03
    dressing (nonsurgical) Z48.00
    intrauterine contraceptive device Z30.432
    neuropacemaker (brain) (peripheral nerve) (spinal
      cord) Z46.2
      implanted Z45.42
    staples Z48.02
    surgical dressing Z48.01
    sutures Z48.02
    ureteral stent Z46.6
  respirator [ventilator] use during power failure Z99.12
  restoration of organ continuity (poststerilization) Z31.0
    aftercare Z31.42
  sensitivity test (*see also* Test, skin)
    allergy NEC Z01.82
    Mantoux Z11.1
  tuboplasty following previous sterilization Z31.0
    aftercare Z31.42
  vasoplasty following previous sterilization Z31.0
    aftercare Z31.42
  vision examination Z01.00
    with abnormal findings Z01.01
  waiting period for admission to other facility Z75.1
Adnexitis (suppurative) — *see* Salpingo-oophoritis
Adolescent X-linked adrenoleukodystrophy E71.521
Adrenal (gland) — *see* condition
Adrenalism, tuberculous A18.7
Adrenalitis, adrenitis E27.8
  autoimmune E27.1
  meningococcal, hemorrhagic A39.1
Adrenarche, premature E27.0
Adrenocortical syndrome — *see* Cushing's, syndrome
Adrenogenital syndrome E25.9
  acquired E25.8
  congenital E25.0
  salt loss E25.0
Adrenogenitalism, congenital E25.0
Adrenoleukodystrophy E71.529
  neonatal E71.511
  X-linked E71.529
    Addison only phenotype E71.528
    Addison-Schilder E71.528
    adolescent E71.521
    adrenomyeloneuropathy E71.522
    childhood cerebral E71.520
    other specified E71.528
Adrenomyeloneuropathy E71.522
Adventitious bursa — *see* Bursopathy, specified type
  NEC
Adverse effect — *see* Table of Drugs and Chemicals,
  categories T36-T50, with 6th character 5
Advice — *see* Counseling
Adynamia (episodica) (hereditary) (periodic) G72.3
Aeration lung imperfect, newborn — *see* Atelectasis
Aerobullosis T70.3 ☑
Aerocele — *see* Embolism, air
Aerodermectasia
  subcutaneous (traumatic) T79.7 ☑
Aerodontalgia T70.29 ☑
Aeroembolism T70.3 ☑
Aerogenes capsulatus infection A48.0
Aero-otitis media T70.0 ☑
Aerophagy, aerophagia (psychogenic) F45.8
Aerophobia F40.228
Aerosinusitis T70.1 ☑
Aerotitis T70.0 ☑
Affection — *see* Disease
Afibrinogenemia (*see also* Defect, coagulation) D68.8
  acquired D65
  congenital D68.2
  following ectopic or molar pregnancy O08.1

Afibrinogenemia — *continued*
  in abortion — *see* Abortion, by type, complicated by,
    afibrinogenemia
  puerperal O72.3
African
  sleeping sickness B56.9
  tick fever A68.1
  trypanosomiasis B56.9
    gambian B56.0
    rhodesian B56.1
Aftercare (*see also* Care) Z51.89
  following surgery (for) (on)
    amputation Z47.81
    attention to
      drains Z48.03
      dressings (nonsurgical) Z48.00
        surgical Z48.01
      sutures Z48.02
    circulatory system Z48.812
    delayed (planned) wound closure Z48.1
    digestive system Z48.815
    explantation of joint prosthesis (staged procedure)
      hip Z47.32
      knee Z47.33
      shoulder Z47.31
    genitourinary system Z48.816
    joint replacement Z47.1
    neoplasm Z48.3
    nervous system Z48.811
    oral cavity Z48.814
    organ transplant
      bone marrow Z48.290
      heart Z48.21
      heart-lung Z48.280
      kidney Z48.22
      liver Z48.23
      lung Z48.24
      multiple organs NEC Z48.288
      specified NEC Z48.298
    orthopedic NEC Z47.89
    planned wound closure Z48.1
    removal of internal fixation device Z47.2
    respiratory system Z48.813
    scoliosis Z47.82
    sense organs Z48.810
    skin and subcutaneous tissue Z48.817
    specified body system
      circulatory Z48.812
      digestive Z48.815
      genitourinary Z48.816
      nervous Z48.811
      oral cavity Z48.814
      respiratory Z48.813
      sense organs Z48.810
      skin and subcutaneous tissue Z48.817
      teeth Z48.814
    specified NEC Z48.89
    spinal Z48.89
    teeth Z48.814
  fracture — *code to* fracture with seventh character D
  involving
    removal of
      drains Z48.03
      dressings (nonsurgical) Z48.00
      staples Z48.02
      surgical dressings Z48.01
      sutures Z48.02
    neuropacemaker (brain) (peripheral nerve) (spinal
      cord) Z46.2
      implanted Z45.42
  orthopedic NEC Z47.89
  postprocedural — *see* Aftercare, following surgery
After-cataract — *see* Cataract, secondary
Agalactia (primary) O92.3
  elective, secondary or therapeutic O92.5
Agammaglobulinemia (acquired (secondary)) (nonfamilial) D80.1
  with
    immunoglobulin-bearing B-lymphocytes D80.1
    lymphopenia D81.9
  autosomal recessive (Swiss type) D80.0
  Bruton's X-linked D80.0
  common variable (CVAgamma) D80.1
  congenital sex-linked D80.0
  hereditary D80.0
  lymphopenic D81.9
  Swiss type (autosomal recessive) D80.0

Agammaglobulinemia — *continued*
  X-linked (with growth hormone deficiency)(Bruton)
    D80.0
Aganglionosis (bowel) (colon) Q43.1
Age (old) — *see* Senility
Agenesis
  adrenal (gland) Q89.1
  alimentary tract (complete) (partial) NEC Q45.8
    upper Q40.8
  anus, anal (canal) Q42.3
    with fistula Q42.2
  aorta Q25.4
  appendix Q42.8
  arm (complete) Q71.0- ☑
    with hand present Q71.1- ☑
  artery (peripheral) Q27.9
    brain Q28.3
    coronary Q24.5
    pulmonary Q25.79
    specified NEC Q27.8
    umbilical Q27.0
  auditory (canal) (external) Q16.1
  auricle (ear) Q16.0
  bile duct or passage Q44.5
  bladder Q64.5
  bone Q79.9
  brain Q00.0
    part of Q04.3
  breast (with nipple present) Q83.8
    with absent nipple Q83.0
  bronchus Q32.4
  canaliculus lacrimalis Q10.4
  carpus — *see* Agenesis, hand
  cartilage Q79.9
  cecum Q42.8
  cerebellum Q04.3
  cervix Q51.5
  chin Q18.8
  cilia Q10.3
  circulatory system, part NOS Q28.9
  clavicle Q74.0
  clitoris Q52.6
  coccyx Q76.49
  colon Q42.9
    specified NEC Q42.8
  corpus callosum Q04.0
  cricoid cartilage Q31.8
  diaphragm (with hernia) Q79.1
  digestive organ(s) or tract (complete) (partial) NEC
    Q45.8
    upper Q40.8
  ductus arteriosus Q28.8
  duodenum Q41.0
  ear Q16.9
    auricle Q16.0
    lobe Q17.8
  ejaculatory duct Q55.4
  endocrine (gland) NEC Q89.2
  epiglottis Q31.8
  esophagus Q39.8
  eustachian tube Q16.2
  eye Q11.1
    adnexa Q15.8
  eyelid (fold) Q10.3
  face
    bones NEC Q75.8
    specified part NEC Q18.8
  fallopian tube Q50.6
  femur — *see* Defect, reduction, lower limb, longitudi-
    nal, femur
  fibula — *see* Defect, reduction, lower limb, longitudi-
    nal, fibula
  finger (complete) (partial) — *see* Agenesis, hand
  foot (and toes) (complete) (partial) Q72.3- ☑
  forearm (with hand present) — *see* Agenesis, arm,
    with hand present
    and hand Q71.2- ☑
  gallbladder Q44.0
  gastric Q40.2
  genitalia, genital (organ(s))
    female Q52.8
      external Q52.71
      internal NEC Q52.8
    male Q55.8
  glottis Q31.8
  hair Q84.0
  hand (and fingers) (complete) (partial) Q71.3- ☑
  heart Q24.8

Agenesis — *continued*
  heart — *continued*
    valve NEC Q24.8
      pulmonary Q22.0
  hepatic Q44.7
  humerus — *see* Defect, reduction, upper limb
  hymen Q52.4
  ileum Q41.2
  incus Q16.3
  intestine (small) Q41.9
    large Q42.9
      specified NEC Q42.8
  iris (dilator fibers) Q13.1
  jaw M26.09
  jejunum Q41.1
  kidney(s) (partial) Q60.2
    bilateral Q60.1
    unilateral Q60.0
  labium (majus) (minus) Q52.71
  labyrinth, membranous Q16.5
  lacrimal apparatus Q10.4
  larynx Q31.8
  leg (complete) Q72.0- ☑
    with foot present Q72.1- ☑
    lower leg (with foot present) — *see* Agenesis, leg,
        with foot present
      and foot Q72.2- ☑
  lens Q12.3
  limb (complete) Q73.0
    lower — *see* Agenesis, leg
    upper — *see* Agenesis, arm
  lip Q38.0
  liver Q44.7
  lung (fissure) (lobe) (bilateral) (unilateral) Q33.3
  mandible, maxilla M26.09
  metacarpus — *see* Agenesis, hand
  metatarsus — *see* Agenesis, foot
  muscle Q79.8
    eyelid Q10.3
    ocular Q15.8
  musculoskeletal system NEC Q79.8
  nail(s) Q84.3
  neck, part Q18.8
  nerve Q07.8
  nervous system, part NEC Q07.8
  nipple Q83.2
  nose Q30.1
  nuclear Q07.8
  organ
    of Corti Q16.5
    or site not listed — *see* Anomaly, by site
  osseous meatus (ear) Q16.1
  ovary
    bilateral Q50.02
    unilateral Q50.01
  oviduct Q50.6
  pancreas Q45.0
  parathyroid (gland) Q89.2
  parotid gland(s) Q38.4
  patella Q74.1
  pelvic girdle (complete) (partial) Q74.2
  penis Q55.5
  pericardium Q24.8
  pituitary (gland) Q89.2
  prostate Q55.4
  punctum lacrimale Q10.4
  radioulnar — *see* Defect, reduction, upper limb
  radius — *see* Defect, reduction, upper limb, longitudi-
      nal, radius
  rectum Q42.1
    with fistula Q42.0
  renal Q60.2
    bilateral Q60.1
    unilateral Q60.0
  respiratory organ NEC Q34.8
  rib Q76.6
  roof of orbit Q75.8
  round ligament Q52.8
  sacrum Q76.49
  salivary gland Q38.4
  scapula Q74.0
  scrotum Q55.29
  seminal vesicles Q55.4
  septum
    atrial Q21.1
    between aorta and pulmonary artery Q21.4
    ventricular Q20.4
  shoulder girdle (complete) (partial) Q74.0

Agenesis — *continued*
  skull (bone) Q75.8
    with
      anencephaly Q00.0
      encephalocele — *see* Encephalocele
      hydrocephalus Q03.9
        with spina bifida — *see* Spina bifida, by site,
            with hydrocephalus
      microcephaly Q02
  spermatic cord Q55.4
  spinal cord Q06.0
  spine Q76.49
  spleen Q89.01
  sternum Q76.7
  stomach Q40.2
  submaxillary gland(s) (congenital) Q38.4
  tarsus — *see* Agenesis, foot
  tendon Q79.8
  testicle Q55.0
  thymus (gland) Q89.2
  thyroid (gland) E03.1
    cartilage Q31.8
  tibia — *see* Defect, reduction, lower limb, longitudinal,
      tibia
  tibiofibular — *see* Defect, reduction, lower limb,
      specified type NEC
  toe (and foot) (complete) (partial) — *see* Agenesis,
      foot
  tongue Q38.3
  trachea (cartilage) Q32.1
  ulna — *see* Defect, reduction, upper limb, longitudinal,
      ulna
  upper limb — *see* Agenesis, arm
  ureter Q62.4
  urethra Q64.5
  urinary tract NEC Q64.8
  uterus Q51.0
  uvula Q38.5
  vagina Q52.0
  vas deferens Q55.4
  vein(s) (peripheral) Q27.9
    brain Q28.3
    great NEC Q26.8
    portal Q26.5
  vena cava (inferior) (superior) Q26.8
  vermis of cerebellum Q04.3
  vertebra Q76.49
  vulva Q52.71
Ageusia R43.2
Agitated — *see* condition
Agitation R45.1
Aglossia (congenital) Q38.3
Aglossia-adactylia syndrome Q87.0
Aglycogenosis E74.00
Agnosia (body image) (other senses) (tactile) R48.1
  developmental F88
  verbal R48.1
    auditory R48.1
      developmental F80.2
    developmental F80.2
  visual (object) R48.3
Agoraphobia F40.00
  with panic disorder F40.01
  without panic disorder F40.02
Agrammatism R48.8
Agranulocytopenia — *see* Agranulocytosis
Agranulocytosis (chronic) (cyclical) (genetic) (infantile)
    (periodic) (pernicious) (*see also* Neutropenia) D70.9
  congenital D70.0
  cytoreductive cancer chemotherapy sequela D70.1
  drug-induced D70.2
    due to cytoreductive cancer chemotherapy D70.1
  due to infection D70.3
  secondary D70.4
    drug-induced D70.2
      due to cytoreductive cancer chemotherapy
          D70.1
Agraphia (absolute) R48.8
  with alexia R48.0
  developmental F81.81
Ague (dumb) — *see* Malaria
Agyria Q04.3
Ahumada-del Castillo syndrome E23.0
Aichomophobia F40.298
AIDS (related complex) B20
Ailment heart — *see* Disease, heart
Ailurophobia F40.218
Ainhum (disease) L94.6

AIPHI (acute idiopathic pulmonary hemorrhage in infants
    (over 28 days old)) R04.81
Air
  anterior mediastinum J98.2
  compressed, disease T70.3 ☑
  conditioner lung or pneumonitis J67.7
  embolism (artery) (cerebral) (any site) T79.0 ☑
    with ectopic or molar pregnancy O08.2
    due to implanted device NEC — *see* Complications,
        by site and type, specified NEC
    following
      abortion — *see* Abortion by type, complicated
          by, embolism
      ectopic or molar pregnancy O08.2
    infusion, therapeutic injection or transfusion
        T80.0 ☑
    in pregnancy, childbirth or puerperium — *see*
        Embolism, obstetric
    traumatic T79.0 ☑
  hunger, psychogenic F45.8
  rarefied, effects of — *see* Effect, adverse, high altitude
  sickness T75.3 ☑
Airplane sickness T75.3 ☑
Akathisia (drug-induced) (treatment-induced) G25.71
  neuroleptic induced (acute) G25.71
Akinesia R29.898
Akinetic mutism R41.89
Akureyri's disease G93.3
Alactasia, congenital E73.0
Alagille's syndrome Q44.7
Alastrim B03
Albers-Schönberg syndrome Q78.2
Albert's syndrome — *see* Tendinitis, Achilles
Albinism, albino E70.30
  with hematologic abnormality E70.339
    Chédiak-Higashi syndrome E70.330
    Hermansky-Pudlak syndrome E70.331
    other specified E70.338
  I E70.320
  II E70.321
  ocular E70.319
    autosomal recessive E70.311
    other specified E70.318
    X-linked E70.310
  oculocutaneous E70.329
    other specified E70.328
    tyrosinase (ty) negative E70.320
    tyrosinase (ty) positive E70.321
  other specified E70.39
Albinismus E70.30
Albright (-McCune)(-Sternberg) syndrome Q78.1
Albuminous — *see* condition
Albuminuria, albuminuric (acute) (chronic) (subacute)
    (*see also* Proteinuria) R80.9
  complicating pregnancy — *see* Proteinuria, gestational
  with
      gestational hypertension — *see* Pre-eclampsia
      pre-existing hypertension — *see* Hypertension,
          complicating pregnancy, pre-existing,
          with, pre-eclampsia
  gestational — *see* Proteinuria, gestational
  with
      gestational hypertension — *see* Pre-eclampsia
      pre-existing hypertension — *see* Hypertension,
          complicating pregnancy, pre-existing,
          with, pre-eclampsia
  orthostatic R80.2
  postural R80.2
  pre-eclamptic — *see* Pre-eclampsia
  scarlatinal A38.8
Albuminurophobia F40.298
Alcaptonuria E70.29
Alcohol, alcoholic, alcohol-induced
  addiction (without remission) F10.20
    with remission F10.21
  amnestic disorder, persisting F10.96
    with dependence F10.26
  brain syndrome, chronic F10.97
    with dependence F10.27
  cardiopathy I42.6
  counseling and surveillance Z71.41
    family member Z71.42
  delirium (acute) (tremens) (withdrawal) F10.231
    with intoxication F10.921
      in
        abuse F10.121
        dependence F10.221

Alcohol, alcoholic, alcohol-induced — *continued*
- dementia F10.97
  - with dependence F10.27
- deterioration F10.97
  - with dependence F10.27
- hallucinosis (acute) F10.951
  - in
    - abuse F10.151
    - dependence F10.251
- insanity F10.959
- intoxication (acute) (without dependence) F10.129
  - with
    - delirium F10.121
    - dependence F10.229
      - with delirium F10.221
      - uncomplicated F10.220
    - uncomplicated F10.120
- jealousy F10.988
- Korsakoff's, Korsakov's, Korsakow's F10.26
- liver K70.9
  - acute — *see* Disease, liver, alcoholic, hepatitis
- mania (acute) (chronic) F10.959
- paranoia, paranoid (type) psychosis F10.950
- pellagra E52
- poisoning, accidental (acute) NEC — *see* Table of Drugs and Chemicals, alcohol, poisoning
- psychosis — *see* Psychosis, alcoholic
- withdrawal (without convulsions) F10.239
  - with delirium F10.231

Alcoholism (chronic) (without remission) F10.20
- with
  - psychosis — *see* Psychosis, alcoholic
  - remission F10.21
  - Korsakov's F10.96
    - with dependence F10.26

Alder (-Reilly) **anomaly or syndrome** (leukocyte granulation) D72.0

Aldosteronism E26.9
- familial (type I) E26.02
- glucocorticoid-remediable E26.02
- primary (due to) (bilateral) adrenal hyperplasia) E26.09
- primary NEC E26.09
- secondary E26.1
- specified NEC E26.89

Aldosteronoma D44.10

Aldrich (-Wiskott) **syndrome** (eczema-thrombocytopenia) D82.0

Alektorophobia F40.218

Aleppo boil B55.1

Aleukemic — *see* condition

Aleukia
- congenital D70.0
- hemorrhagica D61.9
  - congenital D61.09
- splenica D73.1

Alexia R48.0
- developmental F81.0
- secondary to organic lesion R48.0

Algoneurodystrophy M89.00
- ankle M89.07- ☑
- foot M89.07- ☑
- forearm M89.03- ☑
- hand M89.04- ☑
- lower leg M89.06- ☑
- multiple sites M89.0- ☑
- shoulder M89.01- ☑
- specified site NEC M89.08
- thigh M89.05- ☑
- upper arm M89.02- ☑

Algophobia F40.298

Alienation, mental — *see* Psychosis

Alkalemia E87.3

Alkalosis E87.3
- metabolic E87.3
  - with respiratory acidosis E87.4
- respiratory E87.3

Alkaptonuria E70.29

Allen-Masters syndrome N83.8

Allergy, allergic (reaction) (to) T78.40 ☑
- air-borne substance NEC (rhinitis) J30.89
- alveolitis (extrinsic) J67.9
  - due to
    - Aspergillus clavatus J67.4
    - Cryptostroma corticale J67.6
    - organisms (fungal, thermophilic actinomycete) growing in ventilation (air conditioning) systems J67.7

Allergy, allergic — *continued*
- alveolitis — *continued*
  - specified type NEC J67.8
- anaphylactic reaction or shock T78.2 ☑
- angioneurotic edema T78.3 ☑
- animal (dander) (epidermal) (hair) (rhinitis) J30.81
- bee sting (anaphylactic shock) — *see* Toxicity, venom, arthropod, bee
- biological — *see* Allergy, drug
- colitis K52.2
- dander (animal) (rhinitis) J30.81
- dandruff (rhinitis) J30.81
- dental restorative material (existing) K08.55
- dermatitis — *see* Dermatitis, contact, allergic
- diathesis — *see* History, allergy
- drug, medicament & biological (any) (external) (internal) T78.40 ☑
  - correct substance properly administered — *see* Table of Drugs and Chemicals, by drug, adverse effect
  - wrong substance given or taken NEC (by accident) — *see* Table of Drugs and Chemicals, by drug, poisoning
- due to pollen J30.1
- dust (house) (stock) (rhinitis) J30.89
  - with asthma — *see* Asthma, allergic extrinsic
- eczema — *see* Dermatitis, contact, allergic
- epidermal (animal) (rhinitis) J30.81
- feathers (rhinitis) J30.89
- food (any) (ingested) NEC T78.1 ☑
  - anaphylactic shock — *see* Shock, anaphylactic, due to food
  - dermatitis — *see* Dermatitis, due to, food
  - dietary counseling and surveillance Z71.3
  - in contact with skin L23.6
  - rhinitis J30.5
  - status (without reaction) Z91.018
    - eggs Z91.012
    - milk products Z91.011
    - peanuts Z91.010
    - seafood Z91.013
    - specified NEC Z91.018
- gastrointestinal K52.2
- grain J30.1
- grass (hay fever) (pollen) J30.1
  - asthma — *see* Asthma, allergic extrinsic
- hair (animal) (rhinitis) J30.81
- history (of) — *see* History, allergy
- horse serum — *see* Allergy, serum
- inhalant (rhinitis) J30.89
  - pollen J30.1
- kapok (rhinitis) J30.89
- medicine — *see* Allergy, drug
- milk protein K52.2
- nasal, seasonal due to pollen J30.1
- pneumonia J82
- pollen (any) (hay fever) J30.1
  - asthma — *see* Asthma, allergic extrinsic
- primrose J30.1
- primula J30.1
- purpura D69.0
- ragweed (hay fever) (pollen) J30.1
  - asthma — *see* Asthma, allergic extrinsic
- rose (pollen) J30.1
- seasonal NEC J30.2
- Senecio jacobae (pollen) J30.1
- serum (*see also* Reaction, serum) T80.69 ☑
  - anaphylactic shock T80.59 ☑
- shock (anaphylactic) T78.2 ☑
  - due to
    - administration of blood and blood products T80.51 ☑
    - adverse effect of correct medicinal substance properly administered T88.6 ☑
    - immunization T80.52 ☑
    - serum NEC T80.59 ☑
    - vaccination T80.52 ☑
- specific NEC T78.49 ☑
- tree (any) (hay fever) (pollen) J30.1
  - asthma — *see* Asthma, allergic extrinsic
- upper respiratory J30.9
- urticaria L50.0
- vaccine — *see* Allergy, serum
- wheat — *see* Allergy, food

Allescheriasis B48.2

Alligator skin disease Q80.9

Allocheiria, allochiria R20.8

Almeida's disease — *see* Paracoccidioidomycosis

Alopecia (hereditaria) (seborrheica) L65.9
- androgenic L64.9
  - drug-induced L64.0
  - specified NEC L64.8
- areata L63.9
  - ophiasis L63.2
  - specified NEC L63.8
  - totalis L63.0
  - universalis L63.1
- cicatricial L66.9
  - specified NEC L66.8
- circumscripta L63.9
- congenital, congenitalis Q84.0
- due to cytotoxic drugs NEC L65.8
- mucinosa L65.2
- postinfective NEC L65.8
- postpartum L65.0
- premature L64.8
- specific (syphilitic) A51.32
- specified NEC L65.8
- syphilitic (secondary) A51.32
- totalis (capitis) L63.0
- universalis (entire body) L63.1
- X-ray L58.1

Alpers' disease G31.81

Alpine sickness T70.29 ☑

Alport syndrome Q87.81

ALTE (apparent life threatening event) **in newborn and infant** R68.13

Alteration (of), **Altered**
- awareness, transient R40.4
- mental status R41.82
- pattern of family relationships affecting child Z62.898
- sensation
  - following
    - cerebrovascular disease I69.998
      - cerebral infarction I69.398
      - intracerebral hemorrhage I69.198
      - nontraumatic intracranial hemorrhage NEC I69.298
    - specified disease NEC I69.898
    - subarachnoid hemorrhage I69.098

Alternating — *see* condition

Altitude, high (effects) — *see* Effect, adverse, high altitude

Aluminosis (of lung) J63.0

Alveolitis
- allergic (extrinsic) — *see* Pneumonitis, hypersensitivity
- due to
  - Aspergillus clavatus J67.4
  - Cryptostroma corticale J67.6
- fibrosing (cryptogenic) (idiopathic) J84.112
- jaw M27.3
- sicca dolorosa M27.3

Alveolus, alveolar — *see* condition

Alymphocytosis D72.810
- thymic (with immunodeficiency) D82.1

Alymphoplasia, thymic D82.1

Alzheimer's disease or sclerosis — *see* Disease, Alzheimer's

Amastia (with nipple present) Q83.8
- with absent nipple Q83.0

Amathophobia F40.228

Amaurosis (acquired) (congenital) (*see also* Blindness)
- fugax G45.3
- hysterical F44.6
- Leber's congenital H35.50
- uremic — *see* Uremia

Amaurotic idiocy (infantile) (juvenile) (late) E75.4

Amaxophobia F40.248

Ambiguous genitalia Q56.4

Amblyopia (congenital) (ex anopsia) (partial) (suppression) H53.00- ☑
- anisometropic — *see* Amblyopia, refractive
- deprivation H53.01- ☑
- hysterical F44.6
- nocturnal (*see also* Blindness, night)
  - vitamin A deficiency E50.5
- refractive H53.02- ☑
- strabismic H53.03- ☑
- tobacco H53.8
- toxic NEC H53.8
- uremic — *see* Uremia

Ameba, amebic (histolytica) (*see also* Amebiasis)
- abscess (liver) A06.4

Amebiasis A06.9

Amebiasis — *continued*
with abscess — *see* Abscess, amebic
acute A06.0
chronic (intestine) A06.1
with abscess — *see* Abscess, amebic
cutaneous A06.7
cutis A06.7
cystitis A06.81
genitourinary tract NEC A06.82
hepatic — *see* Abscess, liver, amebic
intestine A06.0
nondysenteric colitis A06.2
skin A06.7
specified site NEC A06.89
Ameboma (of intestine) A06.3
Amelia Q73.0
lower limb — *see* Agenesis, leg
upper limb — *see* Agenesis, arm
Ameloblastoma (*see also* Cyst, calcifying odontogenic)
long bones C40.9-
lower limb C40.2- ☑
upper limb C40.0- ☑
malignant C41.1
jaw (bone) (lower) C41.1
upper C41.0
tibial C40.2- ☑
Amelogenesis imperfecta K00.5
nonhereditaria (segmentalis) K00.4
Amenorrhea N91.2
hyperhormonal E28.8
primary N91.0
secondary N91.1
Amentia — *see* Disability, intellectual
Meynert's (nonalcoholic) F04
American
leishmaniasis B55.2
mountain tick fever A93.2
Ametropia — *see* Disorder, refraction
Amianthosis J61
Amimia R48.8
Amino-acid disorder E72.9
anemia D53.0
Aminoacidopathy E72.9
Aminoaciduria E72.9
Amnesia R41.3
anterograde R41.1
auditory R48.8
dissociative F44.0
hysterical F44.0
postictal in epilepsy — *see* Epilepsy
psychogenic F44.0
retrograde R41.2
transient global G45.4
Amnes(t)ic syndrome (post-traumatic) F04
induced by
alcohol F10.96
with dependence F10.26
psychoactive NEC F19.96
with
abuse F19.16
dependence F19.26
sedative F13.96
with dependence F13.26
Amnion, amniotic — *see* condition
Amnionitis — *see* Pregnancy, complicated by
Amok F68.8
Amoral traits F60.89
Ampulla
lower esophagus K22.8
phrenic K22.8
Amputation (*see also* Absence, by site, acquired)
neuroma (postoperative) (traumatic) — *see* Complications, amputation stump, neuroma
stump (surgical)
abnormal, painful, or with complication (late) — *see* Complications, amputation stump
healed or old NOS Z89.9
traumatic (complete) (partial)
arm (upper) (complete) S48.91- ☑
at
elbow S58.01- ☑
partial S58.02- ☑
shoulder joint (complete) S48.01- ☑
partial S48.02- ☑
between
elbow and wrist (complete) S58.11- ☑
partial S58.12- ☑

Amputation — *continued*
traumatic — *continued*
arm — *continued*
between — *continued*
shoulder and elbow (complete) S48.11- ☑
partial S48.12- ☑
partial S48.92- ☑
breast (complete) S28.21- ☑
partial S28.22- ☑
clitoris (complete) S38.211- ☑
partial S38.212- ☑
ear (complete) S08.11- ☑
partial S08.12- ☑
finger (complete) (metacarpophalangeal)
S68.11- ☑
index S68.11- ☑
little S68.11- ☑
middle S68.11- ☑
partial S68.12- ☑
index S68.12- ☑
little S68.12- ☑
middle S68.12- ☑
ring S68.12- ☑
ring S68.11- ☑
thumb — *see* Amputation, traumatic, thumb
transphalangeal (complete) S68.61- ☑
index S68.61- ☑
little S68.61- ☑
middle S68.61- ☑
partial S68.62- ☑
index S68.62- ☑
little S68.62- ☑
middle S68.62- ☑
ring S68.62- ☑
ring S68.61- ☑
foot (complete) S98.91- ☑
at ankle level S98.01- ☑
partial S98.02- ☑
midfoot S98.31- ☑
partial S98.32- ☑
partial S98.92- ☑
forearm (complete) S58.91- ☑
at elbow level (complete) S58.01- ☑
partial S58.02- ☑
between elbow and wrist (complete) S58.11- ☑
partial S58.12- ☑
partial S58.92- ☑
genital organ(s) (external)
female (complete) S38.211 ☑
partial S38.212 ☑
male
penis (complete) S38.221 ☑
partial S38.222 ☑
scrotum (complete) S38.231 ☑
partial S38.232 ☑
testes (complete) S38.231 ☑
partial S38.232 ☑
hand (complete) (wrist level) S68.41- ☑
finger(s) alone — *see* Amputation, traumatic, finger
partial S68.42- ☑
thumb alone — *see* Amputation, traumatic, thumb
transmetacarpal (complete) S68.71- ☑
partial S68.72- ☑
head
ear — *see* Amputation, traumatic, ear
nose (partial) S08.812 ☑
complete S08.811 ☑
part S08.89 ☑
scalp S08.0 ☑
hip (and thigh) (complete) S78.91- ☑
at hip joint (complete) S78.01- ☑
partial S78.02- ☑
between hip and knee (complete) S78.11- ☑
partial S78.12- ☑
partial S78.92- ☑
labium (majus) (minus) (complete) S38.21- ☑
partial S38.21- ☑
leg (lower) S88.91- ☑
at knee level S88.01- ☑
partial S88.02- ☑
between knee and ankle S88.11- ☑
partial S88.12- ☑
partial S88.92- ☑
nose (partial) S08.812 ☑

Amputation — *continued*
traumatic — *continued*
nose — *continued*
complete S08.811 ☑
penis (complete) S38.221 ☑
partial S38.222 ☑
scrotum (complete) S38.231 ☑
partial S38.232 ☑
shoulder — *see* Amputation, traumatic, arm
at shoulder joint — *see* Amputation, traumatic, arm, at shoulder joint
testes (complete) S38.231 ☑
partial S38.232 ☑
thigh — *see* Amputation, traumatic, hip
thorax, part of S28.1 ☑
breast — *see* Amputation, traumatic, breast
thumb (complete) (metacarpophalangeal)
S68.01- ☑
partial S68.02- ☑
transphalangeal (complete) S68.51- ☑
partial S68.52- ☑
toe (lesser) S98.13- ☑
great S98.11- ☑
partial S98.12- ☑
more than one S98.21- ☑
partial S98.22- ☑
partial S98.14- ☑
vulva (complete) S38.211 ☑
partial S38.212 ☑
Amputee (bilateral) (old) Z89.9
Amsterdam dwarfism Q87.1
Amusia R48.8
developmental F80.89
Amyelencephalus, amyelencephaly Q00.0
Amyelia Q06.0
Amygdalitis — *see* Tonsillitis
Amygdalolith J35.8
Amyloid heart (disease) E85.4 [I43]
Amyloidosis (generalized) (primary) E85.9
with lung involvement E85.4 [J99]
familial E85.2
genetic E85.2
heart E85.4 [I43]
hemodialysis-associated E85.3
liver E85.4 [K77]
localized E85.4
neuropathic heredofamilial E85.1
non-neuropathic heredofamilial E85.0
organ limited E85.4
Portuguese E85.1
pulmonary E85.4 [J99]
secondary systemic E85.3
skin (lichen) (macular) E85.4 [L99]
specified NEC E85.8
subglottic E85.4 [J99]
Amylopectinosis (brancher enzyme deficiency) E74.03
Amylophagia — *see* Pica
Amyoplasia congenita Q79.8
Amyotonia M62.89
congenita G70.2
Amyotrophia, amyotrophy, amyotrophic G71.8
congenita Q79.8
diabetic — *see* Diabetes, amyotrophy
lateral sclerosis G12.21
neuralgic G54.5
spinal progressive G12.21
Anacidity, gastric K31.83
psychogenic F45.8
Anaerosis of newborn P28.89
Analbuminemia E88.09
Analgesia — *see* Anesthesia
Analphalipoproteinemia E78.6
Anaphylactic
purpura D69.0
shock or reaction — *see* Shock, anaphylactic
Anaphylactoid shock or reaction — *see* Shock, anaphylactic
Anaphylactoid syndrome of pregnancy O88.01- ☑
Anaphylaxis — *see* Shock, anaphylactic
Anaplasia cervix (*see also* Dysplasia, cervix) N87.9
Anaplasmosis, human A77.49
Anarthria R47.1
Anasarca R60.1
cardiac — *see* Failure, heart, congestive
lung J18.2
newborn P83.2
nutritional E43

Anasarca — continued
  pulmonary J18.2
  renal N04.9
Anastomosis
  aneurysmal — see Aneurysm
  arteriovenous ruptured brain I60.8
  intestinal K63.89
    complicated NEC K91.89
      involving urinary tract N99.89
  retinal and choroidal vessels (congenital) Q14.8
Anatomical narrow angle H40.03- ☑
Ancylostoma, ancylostomiasis (braziliense) (caninum)
  (ceylanicum) (duodenale) B76.0
  Necator americanus B76.1
Andersen's disease (glycogen storage) E74.09
Anderson-Fabry disease E75.21
Andes disease T70.29 ☑
Andrews' disease (bacterid) L08.89
Androblastoma
  benign
    specified site — see Neoplasm, benign, by site
    unspecified site
      female D27.9
      male D29.20
  malignant
    specified site — see Neoplasm, malignant, by site
    unspecified site
      female C56.9
      male C62.90
  specified site — see Neoplasm, uncertain behavior,
    by site
  tubular
    with lipid storage
      specified site — see Neoplasm, benign, by site
      unspecified site
        female D27.9
        male D29.20
    specified site — see Neoplasm, benign, by site
    unspecified site
      female D27.9
      male D29.20
  unspecified site
    female D39.10
    male D40.10
Androgen insensitivity syndrome (see also Syndrome,
  androgen insensitivity) E34.50
Androgen resistance syndrome (see also Syndrome,
  androgen insensitivity) E34.50
Android pelvis Q74.2
  with disproportion (fetopelvic) O33.3 ☑
    causing obstructed labor O65.3
Androphobia F40.290
Anectasis, pulmonary (newborn) — see Atelectasis
Anemia (essential) (general) (hemoglobin deficiency)
  (infantile) (primary) (profound) D64.9
  with (due to) (in)
    disorder of
      anaerobic glycolysis D55.2
      pentose phosphate pathway D55.1
    koilonychia D50.9
  achlorhydric D50.8
  achrestic D53.1
  Addison (-Biermer) (pernicious) D51.0
  agranulocytic — see Agranulocytosis
  amino-acid-deficiency D53.0
  aplastic D61.9
    congenital D61.09
    drug-induced D61.1
    due to
      drugs D61.1
      external agents NEC D61.2
      infection D61.2
      radiation D61.2
    idiopathic D61.3
    red cell (pure) D60.9
      chronic D60.0
      congenital D61.01
      specified type NEC D60.8
      transient D60.1
    specified type NEC D61.89
    toxic D61.2
  aregenerative
    congenital D61.09
  asiderotic D50.9
  atypical (primary) D64.9
  Baghdad spring D55.0
  Balantidium coli A07.0
  Biermer's (pernicious) D51.0

Anemia — continued
  blood loss (chronic) D50.0
    acute D62
  bothriocephalus B70.0 [D63.8]
  brickmaker's B76.9 [D63.8]
  cerebral I67.89
  childhood D58.9
  chlorotic D50.8
  chronic
    blood loss D50.0
    hemolytic D58.9
      idiopathic D59.9
    simple D53.9
  chronica congenita aregenerativa D61.09
  combined system disease NEC D51.0 [G32.0]
    due to dietary vitamin B12 deficiency D51.3 [G32.0]
  complicating pregnancy, childbirth or puerperium —
    see Pregnancy, complicated by (management
    affected by), anemia
  congenital P61.4
    aplastic D61.09
    due to isoimmunization NOS P55.9
    dyserythropoietic, dyshematopoietic D64.4
    following fetal blood loss P61.3
    Heinz body D58.2
    hereditary hemolytic NOS D58.9
    pernicious D51.0
    spherocytic D58.0
  Cooley's (erythroblastic) D56.1
  cytogenic D51.0
  deficiency D53.9
    6-PGD D55.1
    2, 3 diphosphoglycurate mutase D55.2
    2, 3 PG D55.2
    6 phosphogluconate dehydrogenase D55.1
    amino-acid D53.0
    combined B12 and folate D53.1
    enzyme D55.9
      drug-induced (hemolytic) D59.2
      glucose-6-phosphate dehydrogenase (G6PD)
        D55.0
      glycolytic D55.2
      nucleotide metabolism D55.3
      related to hexose monophosphate (HMP) shunt
        pathway NEC D55.1
      specified type NEC D55.8
    erythrocytic glutathione D55.1
    folate D52.9
      dietary D52.0
      drug-induced D52.1
    folic acid D52.9
      dietary D52.0
      drug-induced D52.1
    G SH D55.1
    G6PD D55.0
    GGS-R D55.1
    glucose-6-phosphate dehydrogenase D55.0
    glutathione reductase D55.1
    glyceraldehyde phosphate dehydrogenase D55.2
    hexokinase D55.2
    iron D50.9
      secondary to blood loss (chronic) D50.0
    nutritional D53.9
      with
        poor iron absorption D50.8
        specified deficiency NEC D53.8
    phosphofructo-aldolase D55.2
    phosphoglycerate kinase D55.2
    PK D55.2
    protein D53.0
    pyruvate kinase D55.2
    transcobalamin II D51.2
    triose-phosphate isomerase D55.2
    vitamin B12 NOS D51.9
      dietary D51.3
      due to
        intrinsic factor deficiency D51.0
        selective vitamin B12 malabsorption with
          proteinuria D51.1
      pernicious D51.0
      specified type NEC D51.8
  Diamond-Blackfan (congenital hypoplastic) D61.01
  dibothriocephalus B70.0 [D63.8]
  dimorphic D53.1
  diphasic D53.1
  Diphyllobothrium (Dibothriocephalus) B70.0 [D63.8]
  due to (in) (with)
    antineoplastic chemotherapy D64.81

Anemia — continued
  due to — continued
    blood loss (chronic) D50.0
      acute D62
    chemotherapy, antineoplastic D64.81
    chronic disease classified elsewhere NEC D63.8
    chronic kidney disease D63.1
    deficiency
      amino-acid D53.0
      copper D53.8
      folate (folic acid) D52.9
        dietary D52.0
        drug-induced D52.1
      molybdenum D53.8
      protein D53.0
      zinc D53.8
    dietary vitamin B12 deficiency D51.3
    disorder of
      glutathione metabolism D55.1
      nucleotide metabolism D55.3
    drug — see Anemia, by type (see also Table of
      Drugs and Chemicals)
    end stage renal disease D63.1
    enzyme disorder D55.9
    fetal blood loss P61.3
    fish tapeworm (D.latum) infestation B70.0 [D63.8]
    hemorrhage (chronic) D50.0
      acute D62
    impaired absorption D50.9
    loss of blood (chronic) D50.0
      acute D62
    myxedema E03.9 [D63.8]
    Necator americanus B76.1 [D63.8]
    prematurity P61.2
    selective vitamin B12 malabsorption with protein-
      uria D51.1
    transcobalamin II deficiency D51.2
  Dyke-Young type (secondary) (symptomatic) D59.1
  dyserythropoietic (congenital) D64.4
  dyshematopoietic (congenital) D64.4
  Egyptian B76.9 [D63.8]
  elliptocytosis — see Elliptocytosis
  enzyme-deficiency, drug-induced D59.2
  epidemic (see also Ancylostomiasis) B76.9 [D63.8]
  erythroblastic
    familial D56.1
    newborn (see also Disease, hemolytic) P55.9
    of childhood D56.1
  erythrocytic glutathione deficiency D55.1
  erythropoietin-resistant anemia (EPO resistant anemia)
    D63.1
  Faber's (achlorhydric anemia) D50.9
  factitious (self-induced blood letting) D50.0
  familial erythroblastic D56.1
  Fanconi's (congenital pancytopenia) D61.09
  favism D55.0
  fish tapeworm (D. latum) infestation B70.0 [D63.8]
  folate (folic acid) deficiency D52.9
  glucose-6-phosphate dehydrogenase (G6PD) deficien-
    cy D55.0
  glutathione-reductase deficiency D55.1
  goat's milk D52.0
  granulocytic — see Agranulocytosis
  Heinz body, congenital D58.2
  hemolytic D58.9
    acquired D59.9
      with hemoglobinuria NEC D59.6
      autoimmune NEC D59.1
      infectious D59.4
      specified type NEC D59.8
      toxic D59.4
    acute D59.9
      due to enzyme deficiency specified type NEC
        D55.8
      Lederer's D59.1
    autoimmune D59.1
      drug-induced D59.0
    chronic D58.9
      idiopathic D59.9
    cold type (secondary) (symptomatic) D59.1
    congenital (spherocytic) — see Spherocytosis
    due to
      cardiac conditions D59.4
      drugs (nonautoimmune) D59.2
        autoimmune D59.0
      enzyme disorder D55.9
        drug-induced D59.2

Anemia — *continued*
  hemolytic — *continued*
    due to — *continued*
      presence of shunt or other internal prosthetic
          device D59.4
      familial D58.9
      hereditary D58.9
        due to enzyme disorder D55.9
          specified type NEC D55.8
        specified type NEC D58.8
      idiopathic (chronic) D59.9
      mechanical D59.4
      microangiopathic D59.4
      nonautoimmune D59.4
        drug-induced D59.2
      nonspherocytic
        congenital or hereditary NEC D55.8
          glucose-6-phosphate dehydrogenase defi-
              ciency D55.0
          pyruvate kinase deficiency D55.2
          type
            I D55.1
            II D55.2
          type
            I D55.1
            II D55.2
      secondary D59.4
        autoimmune D59.1
      specified (hereditary) type NEC D58.8
      Stransky-Regala type (*see also* Hemoglobinopathy)
          D58.8
      symptomatic D59.4
        autoimmune D59.1
      toxic D59.4
      warm type (secondary) (symptomatic) D59.1
    hemorrhagic (chronic) D50.0
      acute D62
    Herrick's D57.1
    hexokinase deficiency D55.2
    hookworm B76.9 [D63.8]
    hypochromic (idiopathic) (microcytic) (normoblastic)
        D50.9
      due to blood loss (chronic) D50.0
        acute D62
      familial sex-linked D64.0
      pyridoxine-responsive D64.3
      sideroblastic, sex-linked D64.0
    hypoplasia, red blood cells D61.9
      congenital or familial D61.01
    hypoplastic (idiopathic) D61.9
      congenital or familial (of childhood) D61.01
    hypoproliferative (refractive) D61.9
    idiopathic D64.9
      aplastic D61.3
      hemolytic, chronic D59.9
    in (due to) (with)
      chronic kidney disease D63.1
      end stage renal disease D63.1
      failure, kidney (renal) D63.1
      neoplastic disease (*see also* Neoplasm) D63.0
    intertropical (*see also* Ancylostomiasis) D63.8
    iron deficiency D50.9
      secondary to blood loss (chronic) D50.0
        acute D62
      specified type NEC D50.8
    Joseph-Diamond-Blackfan (congenital hypoplastic)
        D61.01
    Lederer's (hemolytic) D59.1
    leukoerythroblastic D61.82
    macrocytic D53.9
      nutritional D52.0
      tropical D52.8
    malarial (*see also* Malaria) B54 [D63.8]
    malignant (progressive) D51.0
    malnutrition D53.9
    marsh (*see also* Malaria) B54 [D63.8]
    Mediterranean (with other hemoglobinopathy) D56.9
    megaloblastic D53.1
      combined B12 and folate deficiency D53.1
      hereditary D51.1
      nutritional D52.0
      orotic aciduria D53.0
      refractory D53.1
      specified type NEC D53.1
    megalocytic D53.1
    microcytic (hypochromic) D50.9
      due to blood loss (chronic) D50.0
        acute D62

Anemia — *continued*
  microcytic — *continued*
    familial D56.8
    microdrepanocytosis D57.40
    microelliptopoikilocytic (Rietti-Greppi- Micheli) D56.9
    miner's B76.9 [D63.8]
    myelodysplastic D46.9
    myelofibrosis D75.81
    myelogenous D64.89
    myelopathic D64.89
    myelophthisic D61.82
    myeloproliferative D47.Z9 (*following* D47.4)
    newborn P61.4
      due to
        ABO (antibodies, isoimmunization, maternal/fe-
            tal incompatibility) P55.1
        Rh (antibodies, isoimmunization, maternal/fetal
            incompatibility) P55.0
      following fetal blood loss P61.3
      posthemorrhagic (fetal) P61.3
    nonspherocytic hemolytic — *see* Anemia, hemolytic,
        nonspherocytic
    normocytic (infectional) D64.9
      due to blood loss (chronic) D50.0
        acute D62
      myelophthisic D61.82
    nutritional (deficiency) D53.9
      with
        poor iron absorption D50.8
        specified deficiency NEC D53.8
      megaloblastic D52.0
    of prematurity P61.2
    orotaciduric (congenital) (hereditary) D53.0
    osteosclerotic D64.89
    ovalocytosis (hereditary) — *see* Elliptocytosis
    paludal (*see also* Malaria) B54 [D63.8]
    pernicious (congenital) (malignant) (progressive) D51.0
    pleochromic D64.89
      of sprue D52.8
    posthemorrhagic (chronic) D50.0
      acute D62
      newborn P61.3
    postoperative (postprocedural)
      due to (acute) blood loss D62
        chronic blood loss D50.0
      specified NEC D64.9
    postpartum O90.81
    pressure D64.89
    progressive D64.9
      malignant D51.0
      pernicious D51.0
    protein-deficiency D53.0
    pseudoleukemica infantum D64.89
    pure red cell D60.9
      congenital D61.01
    pyridoxine-responsive D64.3
    pyruvate kinase deficiency D55.2
    refractory D46.4
      with
        excess of blasts D46.20
          1 (RAEB 1) D46.21
          2 (RAEB 2) D46.22
          in transformation (RAEB T) — *see* Leukemia,
              acute myeloblastic
        hemochromatosis D46.1
        sideroblasts (ring) (RARS) D46.1
      without ring sideroblasts, so stated D46.0
      without sideroblasts without excess of blasts D46.0
      megaloblastic D53.1
      sideroblastic D46.1
      sideropenic D50.9
    Rietti-Greppi-Micheli D56.9
    scorbutic D53.2
    secondary to
      blood loss (chronic) D50.0
        acute D62
      hemorrhage (chronic) D50.0
        acute D62
    semiplastic D61.89
    sickle-cell — *see* Disease, sickle-cell
    sideroblastic D64.3
      hereditary D64.0
      hypochromic, sex-linked D64.0
      pyridoxine-responsive NEC D64.3
      refractory D46.1
      secondary (due to)
        disease D64.1
        drugs and toxins D64.2

Anemia — *continued*
  sideroblastic — *continued*
    specified type NEC D64.3
  sideropenic (refractory) D50.9
    due to blood loss (chronic) D50.0
      acute D62
  simple chronic D53.9
  specified type NEC D64.89
  spherocytic (hereditary) — *see* Spherocytosis
  splenic D64.89
  splenomegalic D64.89
  stomatocytosis D58.8
  syphilitic (acquired) (late) A52.79 [D63.8]
  target cell D64.89
  thalassemia D56.9
  thrombocytopenic — *see* Thrombocytopenia
  toxic D61.2
  tropical B76.9 [D63.8]
    macrocytic D52.8
  tuberculous A18.89 [D63.8]
  vegan D51.3
  vitamin
    B6-responsive D64.3
    B12 deficiency (dietary) pernicious D51.0
  von Jaksch's D64.89
  Witts' (achlorhydric anemia) D50.8
Anemophobia F40.228
Anencephalus, anencephaly Q00.0
Anergasia — *see* Psychosis, organic
Anesthesia, anesthetic R20.0
  complication or reaction NEC (*see also* Complications,
      anesthesia) T88.59 ☑
    due to
      correct substance properly administered — *see*
          Table of Drugs and Chemicals, by drug,
          adverse effect
      overdose or wrong substance given — *see* Ta-
          ble of Drugs and Chemicals, by drug,
          poisoning
  cornea H18.81- ☑
  dissociative F44.6
  functional (hysterical) F44.6
  hyperesthetic, thalamic G89.0
  hysterical F44.6
  local skin lesion R20.0
  sexual (psychogenic) F52.1
  shock (due to) T88.2 ☑
  skin R20.0
  testicular N50.9
Anetoderma (maculosum) (of) L90.8
  Jadassohn-Pellizzari L90.2
  Schweniger-Buzzi L90.1
Aneurin deficiency E51.9
Aneurysm (anastomotic) (artery) (cirsoid) (diffuse) (false)
    (fusiform) (multiple) (saccular) I72.9
  abdominal (aorta) I71.4
    ruptured I71.3
    syphilitic A52.01
  aorta, aortic (nonsyphilitic) I71.9
    abdominal I71.4
      ruptured I71.3
    arch I71.2
      ruptured I71.1
    arteriosclerotic I71.9
      ruptured I71.8
    ascending I71.2
      ruptured I71.1
    congenital Q25.4
    descending I71.9
      abdominal I71.4
        ruptured I71.3
      ruptured I71.8
      thoracic I71.2
        ruptured I71.1
    ruptured I71.8
    sinus, congenital Q25.4
    syphilitic A52.01
    thoracic I71.2
      ruptured I71.1
    thoracoabdominal I71.6
      ruptured I71.5
    thorax, thoracic (arch) I71.2
      ruptured I71.1
    transverse I71.2
      ruptured I71.1
    valve (heart) (*see also* Endocarditis, aortic) I35.8
  arteriosclerotic I72.9
    cerebral I67.1

Aneurysm — *continued*
  arteriosclerotic — *continued*
    cerebral — *continued*
      ruptured — *see* Hemorrhage, intracranial,
        subarachnoid
    arteriovenous (congenital) (*see also* Malformation, ar-
        teriovenous)
      acquired I77.0
        brain I67.1
        coronary I25.41
        pulmonary I28.0
      brain Q28.2
        ruptured I60.8
      peripheral — *see* Malformation, arteriovenous,
        peripheral
      precerebral vessels Q28.0
      specified site NEC (*see also* Malformation, arteriove-
        nous)
        acquired I77.0
  basal — *see* Aneurysm, brain
  berry (congenital) (nonruptured) I67.1
    ruptured I60.7
  brain I67.1
    arteriosclerotic I67.1
      ruptured — *see* Hemorrhage, intracranial,
        subarachnoid
    arteriovenous (congenital) (nonruptured) Q28.2
      acquired I67.1
        ruptured I60.8
      ruptured I60.8
    berry (congenital) (nonruptured) I67.1
      ruptured (*see also* Hemorrhage, intracranial,
        subarachnoid) I60.7
    congenital Q28.3
      ruptured I60.7
    meninges I67.1
      ruptured I60.8
    miliary (congenital) (nonruptured) I67.1
      ruptured (*see also* Hemorrhage, intracranial,
        subarachnoid) I60.7
    mycotic I33.0
    ruptured — *see* Hemorrhage, intracranial, subarach-
      noid
    syphilitic (hemorrhage) A52.05
  cardiac (false) (*see also* Aneurysm, heart) I25.3
  carotid artery (common) (external) I72.0
    internal (intracranial) I67.1
      extracranial portion I72.0
      ruptured into brain I60.0- ☑
    syphilitic A52.09
      intracranial A52.05
  cavernous sinus I67.1
    arteriovenous (congenital) (nonruptured) Q28.3
      ruptured I60.8
  celiac I72.8
  central nervous system, syphilitic A52.05
  cerebral — *see* Aneurysm, brain
  chest — *see* Aneurysm, thorax
  circle of Willis I67.1
    congenital Q28.3
      ruptured I60.6
    ruptured I60.6
  common iliac artery I72.3
  congenital (peripheral) Q27.8
    brain Q28.3
      ruptured I60.7
    coronary Q24.5
    digestive system Q27.8
    lower limb Q27.8
    pulmonary Q25.79
    retina Q14.1
    specified site NEC Q27.8
    upper limb Q27.8
  conjunctiva — *see* Abnormality, conjunctiva, vascular
  conus arteriosus — *see* Aneurysm, heart
  coronary (arteriosclerotic) (artery) I25.41
    arteriovenous, congenital Q24.5
    congenital Q24.5
    ruptured — *see* Infarct, myocardium
    syphilitic A52.06
    vein I25.89
  cylindroid (aorta) I71.9
    ruptured I71.8
    syphilitic A52.01
  ductus arteriosus Q25.0
  endocardial, infective (any valve) I33.0
  femoral (artery) (ruptured) I72.4
  gastroduodenal I72.8

Aneurysm — *continued*
  gastroepiploic I72.8
  heart (wall) (chronic or with a stated duration of over
    4 weeks) I25.3
    valve — *see* Endocarditis
  hepatic I72.8
  iliac (common) (artery) (ruptured) I72.3
  infective I72.9
    endocardial (any valve) I33.0
  innominate (nonsyphilitic) I72.8
    syphilitic A52.09
  interauricular septum — *see* Aneurysm, heart
  interventricular septum — *see* Aneurysm, heart
  intrathoracic (nonsyphilitic) I71.2
    ruptured I71.1
    syphilitic A52.01
  lower limb I72.4
  lung (pulmonary artery) I28.1
  mediastinal (nonsyphilitic) I72.8
    syphilitic A52.09
  miliary (congenital) I67.1
    ruptured — *see* Hemorrhage, intracerebral, sub-
      arachnoid, intracranial
  mitral (heart) (valve) I34.8
  mural — *see* Aneurysm, heart
  mycotic I72.9
    endocardial (any valve) I33.0
    ruptured, brain — *see* Hemorrhage, intracerebral,
      subarachnoid
  myocardium — *see* Aneurysm, heart
  neck I72.0
  pancreaticoduodenal I72.8
  patent ductus arteriosus Q25.0
  peripheral NEC I72.8
    congenital Q27.8
      digestive system Q27.8
      lower limb Q27.8
      specified site NEC Q27.8
      upper limb Q27.8
  popliteal (artery) (ruptured) I72.4
  precerebral, congenital (nonruptured) Q28.1
  pulmonary I28.1
    arteriovenous Q25.72
      acquired I28.0
    syphilitic A52.09
    valve (heart) — *see* Endocarditis, pulmonary
  racemose (peripheral) I72.9
    congenital — *see* Aneurysm, congenital
  radial I72.1
  Rasmussen NEC A15.0
  renal (artery) I72.2
  retina (*see also* Disorder, retina, microaneurysms)
    congenital Q14.1
    diabetic — *see* Diabetes, microaneurysms, retinal
  sinus of Valsalva Q25.4
  specified NEC I72.8
  spinal (cord) I72.8
    syphilitic (hemorrhage) A52.09
  splenic I72.8
  subclavian (artery) (ruptured) I72.8
    syphilitic A52.09
  superior mesenteric I72.8
  syphilitic (aorta) A52.01
    central nervous system A52.05
    congenital (late) A50.54 [I79.0]
    spine, spinal A52.09
  thoracoabdominal (aorta) I71.6
    ruptured I71.5
    syphilitic A52.01
  thorax, thoracic (aorta) (arch) (nonsyphilitic) I71.2
    ruptured I71.1
    syphilitic A52.01
  traumatic (complication) (early), specified site — *see*
    Injury, blood vessel
  tricuspid (heart) (valve) I07.8
  ulnar I72.1
  upper limb (ruptured) I72.1
  valve, valvular — *see* Endocarditis
  venous (*see also* Varix) I86.8
    congenital Q27.8
      digestive system Q27.8
      lower limb Q27.8
      specified site NEC Q27.8
      upper limb Q27.8
  ventricle — *see* Aneurysm, heart
  visceral NEC I72.8

Angelman syndrome Q93.5
Anger R45.4

Angiectasis, angiectopia I99.8
Angiitis I77.6
  allergic granulomatous M30.1
  hypersensitivity M31.0
  necrotizing M31.9
    specified NEC M31.8
  nervous system, granulomatous I67.7
Angina (attack) (cardiac) (chest) (heart) (pectoris) (syn-
    drome) (vasomotor) I20.9
  with
    atherosclerotic heart disease — *see* Arteriosclerosis,
      coronary (artery),
    documented spasm I20.1
  abdominal K55.1
  accelerated — *see* Angina, unstable
  agranulocytic — *see* Agranulocytosis
  angiospastic — *see* Angina, with documented spasm
  aphthous B08.5
  crescendo — *see* Angina, unstable
  croupous J05.0
  cruris I73.9
  de novo effort — *see* Angina, unstable
  diphtheritic, membranous A36.0
  equivalent I20.8
  exudative, chronic J37.0
  following acute myocardial infarction I23.7
  gangrenous diphtheritic A36.0
  intestinal K55.1
  Ludovici K12.2
  Ludwig's K12.2
  malignant diphtheritic A36.0
  membranous J05.0
    diphtheritic A36.0
    Vincent's A69.1
  mesenteric K55.1
  monocytic — *see* Mononucleosis, infectious
  of effort — *see* Angina, specified NEC
  phlegmonous J36
    diphtheritic A36.0
  post-infarctional I23.7
  pre-infarctional — *see* Angina, unstable
  Prinzmetal — *see* Angina, with documented spasm
  progressive — *see* Angina, unstable
  pseudomembranous A69.1
  pultaceous, diphtheritic A36.0
  spasm-induced — *see* Angina, with documented
    spasm
  specified NEC I20.8
  stable I20.9
  stenocardia — *see* Angina, specified NEC
  stridulous, diphtheritic A36.2
  tonsil J36
  trachealis J05.0
  unstable I20.0
  variant — *see* Angina, with documented spasm
  Vincent's A69.1
  worsening effort — *see* Angina, unstable
Angioblastoma — *see* Neoplasm, connective tissue,
    uncertain behavior
Angiocholecystitis — *see* Cholecystitis, acute
Angiocholitis (*see also* Cholecystitis, acute) K83.0
Angiodysgenesis spinalis G95.19
Angiodysplasia (cecum) (colon) K55.20
  with bleeding K55.21
  duodenum (and stomach) K31.819
    with bleeding K31.811
  stomach (and duodenum) K31.819
    with bleeding K31.811
Angioedema (allergic) (any site) (with urticaria) T78.3 ☑
  hereditary D84.1
Angioendothelioma — *see* Neoplasm, uncertain behav-
    ior, by site
  benign D18.00
    intra-abdominal D18.03
    intracranial D18.02
    skin D18.01
    specified site NEC D18.09
  bone — *see* Neoplasm, bone, malignant
  Ewing's — *see* Neoplasm, bone, malignant
Angioendotheliomatosis C85.8- ☑
Angiofibroma (*see also* Neoplasm, benign, by site)
  juvenile
    specified site — *see* Neoplasm, benign, by site
    unspecified site D10.6
Angiohemophilia (A) (B) D68.0
Angioid streaks (choroid) (macula) (retina) H35.33
Angiokeratoma — *see* Neoplasm, skin, benign

Angiokeratoma — *continued*
  corporis diffusum E75.21
Angioleiomyoma — *see* Neoplasm, connective tissue,
  benign
Angiolipoma (*see also* Lipoma)
  infiltrating — *see* Lipoma
Angioma (*see also* Hemangioma, by site)
  capillary I78.1
  hemorrhagicum hereditaria I78.0
  intra-abdominal D18.03
  intracranial D18.02
  malignant — *see* Neoplasm, connective tissue, malig-
    nant
  plexiform D18.00
    intra-abdominal D18.03
    intracranial D18.02
    skin D18.01
    specified site NEC D18.09
  senile I78.1
  serpiginosum L81.7
  skin D18.01
  specified site NEC D18.09
  spider I78.1
  stellate I78.1
  venous Q28.3
Angiomatosis Q82.8
  bacillary A79.89
  encephalotrigeminal Q85.8
  hemorrhagic familial I78.0
  hereditary familial I78.0
  liver K76.4
Angiomyolipoma — *see* Lipoma
Angiomyoliposarcoma — *see* Neoplasm, connective
  tissue, malignant
Angiomyoma — *see* Neoplasm, connective tissue, benign
Angiomyosarcoma — *see* Neoplasm, connective tissue,
  malignant
Angiomyxoma — *see* Neoplasm, connective tissue, uncertain behavior
Angioneurosis F45.8
Angioneurotic edema (allergic) (any site) (with urticaria)
  T78.3 ☑
  hereditary D84.1
Angiopathia, angiopathy I99.9
  cerebral I67.9
    amyloid E85.4 [I68.0]
  diabetic (peripheral) — *see* Diabetes, angiopathy
  peripheral I73.9
    diabetic — *see* Diabetes, angiopathy
    specified type NEC I73.89
  retinae syphilitica A52.05
  retinalis (juvenilis)
    diabetic — *see* Diabetes, retinopathy
    proliferative — *see* Retinopathy, proliferative
Angiosarcoma (*see also* Neoplasm, connective tissue,
  malignant)
  liver C22.3
Angiosclerosis — *see* Arteriosclerosis
Angiospasm (peripheral) (traumatic) (vessel) I73.9
  brachial plexus G54.0
  cerebral G45.9
  cervical plexus G54.2
  nerve
    arm — *see* Mononeuropathy, upper limb
      axillary G54.0
      median — *see* Lesion, nerve, median
      ulnar — *see* Lesion, nerve, ulnar
    axillary G54.0
    leg — *see* Mononeuropathy, lower limb
    median — *see* Lesion, nerve, median
    plantar — *see* Lesion, nerve, plantar
    ulnar — *see* Lesion, nerve, ulnar
Angiospastic disease or edema I73.9
Angiostrongyliasis
  due to
    Parastrongylus
      cantonensis B83.2
      costaricensis B81.3
    intestinal B81.3
Anguillulosis — *see* Strongyloidiasis
Angulation
  cecum — *see* Obstruction, intestine
  coccyx (acquired) (*see also* subcategory) M43.8 ☑
    congenital NEC Q76.49
  femur (acquired) (*see also* Deformity, limb, specified
    type NEC, thigh)

Angulation — *continued*
  femur (*see also* Deformity, limb, specified type, thigh)
    — *continued*
    congenital Q74.2
  intestine (large) (small) — *see* Obstruction, intestine
  sacrum (acquired) (*see also* subcategory) M43.8 ☑
    congenital NEC Q76.49
  sigmoid (flexure) — *see* Obstruction, intestine
  spine — *see* Dorsopathy, deforming, specified NEC
  tibia (acquired) (*see also* Deformity, limb, specified
    type NEC, lower leg)
    congenital Q74.2
  ureter N13.5
    with infection N13.6
  wrist (acquired) (*see also* Deformity, limb, specified
    type NEC, forearm)
    congenital Q74.0
Angulus infectiosus (lips) K13.0
Anhedonia R45.84
Anhidrosis L74.4
Anhydration, anhydremia E86.0
  with
    hypernatremia E87.0
    hyponatremia E87.1
Anhydremia E86.0
  with
    hypernatremia E87.0
    hyponatremia E87.1
Anidrosis L74.4
Aniridia (congenital) Q13.1
Anisakiasis (infection) (infestation) B81.0
Anisakis larvae infestation B81.0
Aniseikonia H52.32
Anisocoria (pupil) H57.02
  congenital Q13.2
Anisocytosis R71.8
Anisometropia (congenital) H52.31
Ankle — *see* condition
Ankyloblepharon (eyelid) (acquired) (*see also* Blepharophimosis)
  filiforme (adnatum) (congenital) Q10.3
  total Q10.3
Ankyloglossia Q38.1
Ankylosis (fibrous) (osseous) (joint) M24.60
  ankle M24.67- ☑
  arthrodesis status Z98.1
  cricoarytenoid (cartilage) (joint) (larynx) J38.7
  dental K03.5
  ear ossicles H74.31- ☑
  elbow M24.62- ☑
  foot M24.67- ☑
  hand M24.64- ☑
  hip M24.65- ☑
  incostapedial joint (infectional) — *see* Ankylosis, ear
    ossicles
  jaw (temporomandibular) M26.61
  knee M24.66- ☑
  lumbosacral (joint) M43.27
  postoperative (status) Z98.1
  produced by surgical fusion, status Z98.1
  sacro-iliac (joint) M43.28
  shoulder M24.61- ☑
  spine (joint) (*see also* Fusion, spine)
    spondylitic — *see* Spondylitis, ankylosing
  surgical Z98.1
  temporomandibular M26.61
  tooth, teeth (hard tissues) K03.5
  wrist M24.63- ☑
Ankylostoma — *see* Ancylostoma
Ankylostomiasis — *see* Ancylostomiasis
Ankylurethria — *see* Stricture, urethra
Annular (*see also* condition)
  detachment, cervix N88.8
  organ or site, congenital NEC — *see* Distortion
  pancreas (congenital) Q45.1
Anodontia (complete) (partial) (vera) K00.0
  acquired K08.10 ☑
Anomaly, anomalous (congenital) (unspecified type)
  Q89.9
  abdominal wall NEC Q79.59
  acoustic nerve Q07.8
  adrenal (gland) Q89.1
  Alder (-Reilly) (leukocyte granulation) D72.0
  alimentary tract Q45.9
    upper Q40.9
  alveolar M26.70
    hyperplasia M26.79

Anomaly, anomalous — *continued*
  alveolar — *continued*
    hyperplasia — *continued*
      mandibular M26.72
      maxillary M26.71
    hypoplasia M26.79
      mandibular M26.74
      maxillary M26.73
    ridge (process) M26.79
    specified NEC M26.79
  ankle (joint) Q74.2
  anus Q43.9
  aorta (arch) NEC Q25.4
    coarctation (preductal) (postductal) Q25.1
  aortic cusp or valve Q23.9
  appendix Q43.8
  apple peel syndrome Q41.1
  aqueduct of Sylvius Q03.0
    with spina bifida — *see* Spina bifida, with hydro-
      cephalus
  arm Q74.0
  arteriovenous NEC
    coronary Q24.5
    gastrointestinal Q27.33
      acquired — *see* Angiodysplasia
  artery (peripheral) Q27.9
    basilar NEC Q28.1
    cerebral Q28.3
    coronary Q24.5
    digestive system Q27.8
    eye Q15.8
    great Q25.9
      specified NEC Q25.8
    lower limb Q27.8
    peripheral Q27.9
      specified NEC Q27.8
    pulmonary NEC Q25.79
    renal Q27.2
    retina Q14.1
    specified site NEC Q27.8
    subclavian Q27.8
    umbilical Q27.0
    upper limb Q27.8
    vertebral NEC Q28.1
  aryteno-epiglottic folds Q31.8
  atrial
    bands or folds Q20.8
    septa Q21.1
  atrioventricular
    excitation I45.6
    septum Q21.0
  auditory canal Q17.8
  auricle
    ear Q17.8
      causing impairment of hearing Q16.9
    heart Q20.8
  Axenfeld's Q15.0
  back Q89.9
  band
    atrial Q20.8
    heart Q24.8
    ventricular Q24.8
  Bartholin's duct Q38.4
  biliary duct or passage Q44.5
  bladder Q64.70
    absence Q64.5
    diverticulum Q64.6
    exstrophy Q64.10
      cloacal Q64.12
      extroversion Q64.19
      specified type NEC Q64.19
      supravesical fissure Q64.11
    neck obstruction Q64.31
    specified type NEC Q64.79
  bone Q79.9
    arm Q74.0
    face Q75.9
    leg Q74.2
    pelvic girdle Q74.2
    shoulder girdle Q74.0
    skull Q75.9
      with
        anencephaly Q00.0
        encephalocele — *see* Encephalocele
        hydrocephalus Q03.9
          with spina bifida — *see* Spina bifida, by
            site, with hydrocephalus
        microcephaly Q02

Anomaly, anomalous — *continued*
brain (multiple) Q04.9
  vessel Q28.3
breast Q83.9
broad ligament Q50.6
bronchus Q32.4
bulbus cordis Q21.9
bursa Q79.9
canal of Nuck Q52.4
canthus Q10.3
capillary Q27.9
cardiac Q24.9
  chambers Q20.9
    specified NEC Q20.8
  septal closure Q21.9
    specified NEC Q21.8
  valve NEC Q24.8
    pulmonary Q22.3
cardiovascular system Q28.8
carpus Q74.0
caruncle, lacrimal Q10.6
cascade stomach Q40.2
cauda equina Q06.3
cecum Q43.9
cerebral Q04.9
  vessels Q28.3
cervix Q51.9
Chédiak-Higashi (-Steinbrinck) (congenital gigantism of peroxidase granules) E70.330
cheek Q18.9
chest wall Q67.8
  bones Q76.9
chin Q18.9
chordae tendineae Q24.8
choroid Q14.3
  plexus Q07.8
chromosomes, chromosomal Q99.9
  D (1) — *see* condition, chromosome 13
  E (3) — *see* condition, chromosome 18
  G — *see* condition, chromosome 21
  sex
    female phenotype Q97.8
    gonadal dysgenesis (pure) Q99.1
    Klinefelter's Q98.4
    male phenotype Q98.9
    Turner's Q96.9
  specified NEC Q99.8
cilia Q10.3
circulatory system Q28.9
clavicle Q74.0
clitoris Q52.6
coccyx Q76.49
colon Q43.9
common duct Q44.5
communication
  coronary artery Q24.5
  left ventricle with right atrium Q21.0
concha (ear) Q17.3
connection
  portal vein Q26.5
  pulmonary venous Q26.4
    partial Q26.3
    total Q26.2
  renal artery with kidney Q27.2
cornea (shape) Q13.4
coronary artery or vein Q24.5
cranium — *see* Anomaly, skull
cricoid cartilage Q31.8
cystic duct Q44.5
dental
  alveolar — *see* Anomaly, alveolar
  arch relationship M26.20
    specified NEC M26.29
dentofacial M26.9
  alveolar — *see* Anomaly, alveolar
  dental arch relationship M26.20
    specified NEC M26.29
  functional M26.50
    specified NEC M26.59
  jaw size M26.00
    macrogenia M26.05
    mandibular
      hyperplasia M26.03
      hypoplasia M26.04
    maxillary
      hyperplasia M26.01
      hypoplasia M26.02
    microgenia M26.06

Anomaly, anomalous — *continued*
dentofacial — *continued*
  jaw size — *continued*
    specified type NEC M26.09
  jaw-cranial base relationship M26.10
    asymmetry M26.12
      maxillary M26.11
    specified type NEC M26.19
  malocclusion M26.4
    dental arch relationship NEC M26.29
    jaw size — *see* Anomaly, dentofacial, jaw size
    jaw-cranial base relationship — *see* Anomaly, dentofacial, jaw-cranial base relationship
  specified type NEC M26.89
  temporomandibular joint M26.60
    adhesions M26.61
    ankylosis M26.61
    arthralgia M26.62
    articular disc M26.63
    specified type NEC M26.69
  tooth position, fully erupted M26.30
    specified NEC M26.39
dermatoglyphic Q82.8
diaphragm (apertures) NEC Q79.1
digestive organ(s) or tract Q45.9
  lower Q43.9
  upper Q40.9
distance, interarch (excessive) (inadequate) M26.25
distribution, coronary artery Q24.5
ductus
  arteriosus Q25.0
  botalli Q25.0
duodenum Q43.9
dura (brain) Q04.9
  spinal cord Q06.9
ear (external) Q17.9
  causing impairment of hearing Q16.9
  inner Q16.5
  middle (causing impairment of hearing) Q16.4
    ossicles Q16.3
Ebstein's (heart) (tricuspid valve) Q22.5
ectodermal Q82.9
Eisenmenger's (ventricular septal defect) Q21.8
ejaculatory duct Q55.4
elbow Q74.0
endocrine gland NEC Q89.2
epididymis Q55.4
epiglottis Q31.8
esophagus Q39.9
eustachian tube Q17.8
eye Q15.9
  anterior segment Q13.9
    specified NEC Q13.89
  posterior segment Q14.9
    specified NEC Q14.8
  ptosis (eyelid) Q10.0
  specified NEC Q15.8
eyebrow Q18.8
eyelid Q10.3
  ptosis Q10.0
face Q18.9
  bone(s) Q75.9
fallopian tube Q50.6
fascia Q79.9
femur NEC Q74.2
fibula NEC Q74.2
finger Q74.0
fixation, intestine Q43.3
flexion (joint) NOS Q74.9
  hip or thigh Q65.89
foot NEC Q74.2
  varus (congenital) Q66.3
foramen
  Botalli Q21.1
  ovale Q21.1
forearm Q74.0
forehead Q75.8
form, teeth K00.2
fovea centralis Q14.1
frontal bone — *see* Anomaly, skull
gallbladder (position) (shape) (size) Q44.1
Gartner's duct Q52.4
gastrointestinal tract Q45.9
genitalia, genital organ(s) or system
  female Q52.9
    external Q52.70
    internal NOS Q52.9
  male Q55.9

Anomaly, anomalous — *continued*
genitalia, genital organ(s) or system — *continued*
  male — *continued*
    hydrocele P83.5
    specified NEC Q55.8
genitourinary NEC
  female Q52.9
  male Q55.9
Gerbode Q21.0
glottis Q31.8
granulation or granulocyte, genetic (constitutional) (leukocyte) D72.0
gum Q38.6
gyri Q07.9
hair Q84.2
hand Q74.0
hard tissue formation in pulp K04.3
head — *see* Anomaly, skull
heart Q24.9
  auricle Q20.8
  bands or folds Q24.8
  fibroelastosis cordis I42.4
  obstructive NEC Q22.6
  patent ductus arteriosus (Botalli) Q25.0
  septum Q21.9
    auricular Q21.1
    interatrial Q21.1
    interventricular Q21.0
      with pulmonary stenosis or atresia, dextraposition of aorta and hypertrophy of right ventricle Q21.3
    specified NEC Q21.8
    ventricular Q21.0
      with pulmonary stenosis or atresia, dextraposition of aorta and hypertrophy of right ventricle Q21.3
  tetralogy of Fallot Q21.3
  valve NEC Q24.8
    aortic
      bicuspid valve Q23.1
      insufficiency Q23.1
      stenosis Q23.0
        subaortic Q24.4
    mitral
      insufficiency Q23.3
      stenosis Q23.2
    pulmonary Q22.3
      atresia Q22.0
      insufficiency Q22.2
      stenosis Q22.1
        infundibular Q24.3
        subvalvular Q24.3
    tricuspid
      atresia Q22.4
      stenosis Q22.4
  ventricle Q20.8
heel NEC Q74.2
Hegglin's D72.0
hemianencephaly Q00.0
hemicephaly Q00.0
hemicrania Q00.0
hepatic duct Q44.5
hip NEC Q74.2
hourglass stomach Q40.2
humerus Q74.0
hydatid of Morgagni
  female Q50.5
  male (epididymal) Q55.4
    testicular Q55.29
hymen Q52.4
hypersegmentation of neutrophils, hereditary D72.0
hypophyseal Q89.2
ileocecal (coil) (valve) Q43.9
ileum Q43.9
ilium NEC Q74.2
integument Q84.9
  specified NEC Q84.8
interarch distance (excessive) (inadequate) M26.25
intervertebral cartilage or disc Q76.49
intestine (large) (small) Q43.9
  with anomalous adhesions, fixation or malrotation Q43.3
iris Q13.2
ischium NEC Q74.2
jaw — *see* Anomaly, dentofacial
  alveolar — *see* Anomaly, alveolar
jaw-cranial base relationship — *see* Anomaly, dentofacial, jaw-cranial base relationship

☑ **Additional Character Required** — Refer to the Tabular List for Character Selection   ▽ Subterms under main terms may continue to next column or page

Anomaly, anomalous — *continued*
  jejunum Q43.8
  joint Q74.9
    specified NEC Q74.8
  Jordan's D72.0
  kidney(s) (calyx) (pelvis) Q63.9
    artery Q27.2
    specified NEC Q63.8
  Klippel-Feil (brevicollis) Q76.1
  knee Q74.1
  labium (majus) (minus) Q52.70
  labyrinth, membranous Q16.5
  lacrimal apparatus or duct Q10.6
  larynx, laryngeal (muscle) Q31.9
    web (bed) Q31.0
  lens Q12.9
  leukocytes, genetic D72.0
    granulation (constitutional) D72.0
  lid (fold) Q10.3
  ligament Q79.9
    broad Q50.6
    round Q52.8
  limb Q74.9
    lower NEC Q74.2
      reduction deformity — *see* Defect, reduction,
          lower limb
    upper Q74.0
  lip Q38.0
  liver Q44.7
    duct Q44.5
  lower limb NEC Q74.2
  lumbosacral (joint) (region) Q76.49
    kyphosis — *see* Kyphosis, congenital
    lordosis — *see* Lordosis, congenital
  lung (fissure) (lobe) Q33.9
  mandible — *see* Anomaly, dentofacial
  maxilla — *see* Anomaly, dentofacial
  May (-Hegglin) D72.0
  meatus urinarius NEC Q64.79
  meningeal bands or folds Q07.9
    constriction of Q07.8
    spinal Q06.9
  meninges Q07.9
    cerebral Q04.8
    spinal Q06.9
  meningocele Q05.9
  mesentery Q45.9
  metacarpus Q74.0
  metatarsus NEC Q74.2
  middle ear Q16.4
    ossicles Q16.3
  mitral (leaflets) (valve) Q23.9
    insufficiency Q23.3
    specified NEC Q23.8
    stenosis Q23.2
  mouth Q38.6
  Müllerian (*see also* Anomaly, by site)
    uterus NEC Q51.818
  multiple NEC Q89.7
  muscle Q79.9
    eyelid Q10.3
  musculoskeletal system, except limbs Q79.9
  myocardium Q24.8
  nail Q84.6
  narrowness, eyelid Q10.3
  nasal sinus (wall) Q30.8
  neck (any part) Q18.9
  nerve Q07.9
    acoustic Q07.8
    optic Q07.8
  nervous system (central) Q07.9
  nipple Q83.9
  nose, nasal (bones) (cartilage) (septum) (sinus) Q30.9
    specified NEC Q30.8
  ocular muscle Q15.8
  omphalomesenteric duct Q43.0
  opening, pulmonary veins Q26.4
  optic
    disc Q14.2
    nerve Q07.8
  opticociliary vessels Q13.2
  orbit (eye) Q10.7
  organ Q89.9
    of Corti Q16.5
  origin
    artery
      innominate Q25.8
      pulmonary Q25.79

Anomaly, anomalous — *continued*
  origin — *continued*
    artery — *continued*
      renal Q27.2
      subclavian Q25.8
  osseous meatus (ear) Q16.1
  ovary Q50.39
  oviduct Q50.6
  palate (hard) (soft) NEC Q38.5
  pancreas or pancreatic duct Q45.3
  papillary muscles Q24.8
  parathyroid gland Q89.2
  paraurethral ducts Q64.79
  parotid (gland) Q38.4
  patella Q74.1
  Pelger-Huët (hereditary hyposegmentation) D72.0
  pelvic girdle NEC Q74.2
  pelvis (bony) NEC Q74.2
    rachitic E64.3
  penis (glans) Q55.69
  pericardium Q24.8
  peripheral vascular system Q27.9
  Peter's Q13.4
  pharynx Q38.8
  pigmentation L81.9
    congenital Q82.8
  pituitary (gland) Q89.2
  pleural (folds) Q34.0
  portal vein Q26.5
    connection Q26.5
  position, tooth, teeth, fully erupted M26.30
    specified NEC M26.39
  precerebral vessel Q28.1
  prepuce Q55.69
  prostate Q55.4
  pulmonary Q33.9
    artery NEC Q25.79
    valve Q22.3
      atresia Q22.0
      insufficiency Q22.2
      specified type NEC Q22.3
      stenosis Q22.1
        infundibular Q24.3
        subvalvular Q24.3
    venous connection Q26.4
      partial Q26.3
      total Q26.2
  pupil Q13.2
    function H57.00
      anisocoria H57.02
      Argyll Robertson pupil H57.01
      miosis H57.03
      mydriasis H57.04
      specified type NEC H57.09
      tonic pupil H57.05- ☑
  pylorus Q40.3
  radius Q74.0
  rectum Q43.9
  reduction (extremity) (limb)
    femur (longitudinal) — *see* Defect, reduction,
        lower limb, longitudinal, femur
    fibula (longitudinal) — *see* Defect, reduction, lower
        limb, longitudinal, fibula
    lower limb — *see* Defect, reduction, lower limb
    radius (longitudinal) — *see* Defect, reduction, up-
        per limb, longitudinal, radius
    tibia (longitudinal) — *see* Defect, reduction, lower
        limb, longitudinal, tibia
    ulna (longitudinal) — *see* Defect, reduction, upper
        limb, longitudinal, ulna
    upper limb — *see* Defect, reduction, upper limb
  refraction — *see* Disorder, refraction
  renal Q63.9
    artery Q27.2
    pelvis Q63.9
      specified NEC Q63.8
  respiratory system Q34.9
    specified NEC Q34.8
  retina Q14.1
  rib Q76.6
    cervical Q76.5
  Rieger's Q13.81
  rotation — *see* Malrotation
    hip or thigh Q65.89
  round ligament Q52.8
  sacroiliac (joint) NEC Q74.2
  sacrum NEC Q76.49
    kyphosis — *see* Kyphosis, congenital

Anomaly, anomalous — *continued*
  sacrum — *continued*
    lordosis — *see* Lordosis, congenital
  saddle nose, syphilitic A50.57
  salivary duct or gland Q38.4
  scapula Q74.0
  scrotum — *see* Malformation, testis and scrotum
  sebaceous gland Q82.9
  seminal vesicles Q55.4
  sense organs NEC Q07.8
  sex chromosomes NEC (*see also* Anomaly, chromo-
      somes)
    female phenotype Q97.8
    male phenotype Q98.9
  shoulder (girdle) (joint) Q74.0
  sigmoid (flexure) Q43.9
  simian crease Q82.8
  sinus of Valsalva Q25.4
  skeleton generalized Q78.9
  skin (appendage) Q82.9
  skull Q75.9
    with
      anencephaly Q00.0
      encephalocele — *see* Encephalocele
      hydrocephalus Q03.9
        with spina bifida — *see* Spina bifida, by site,
            with hydrocephalus
      microcephaly Q02
  specified organ or site NEC Q89.8
  spermatic cord Q55.4
  spine, spinal NEC Q76.49
    column NEC Q76.49
      kyphosis — *see* Kyphosis, congenital
      lordosis — *see* Lordosis, congenital
    cord Q06.9
    nerve root Q07.8
  spleen Q89.09
    agenesis Q89.01
  stenonian duct Q38.4
  sternum NEC Q76.7
  stomach Q40.3
  submaxillary gland Q38.4
  tarsus NEC Q74.2
  tendon Q79.9
  testis — *see* Malformation, testis and scrotum
  thigh NEC Q74.2
  thorax (wall) Q67.8
    bony Q76.9
  throat Q38.8
  thumb Q74.0
  thymus gland Q89.2
  thyroid (gland) Q89.2
    cartilage Q31.8
  tibia NEC Q74.2
    saber A50.56
  toe Q74.2
  tongue Q38.3
  tooth, teeth K00.9
    eruption K00.6
    position, fully erupted M26.30
    spacing, fully erupted M26.30
  trachea (cartilage) Q32.1
  tragus Q17.9
  tricuspid (leaflet) (valve) Q22.9
    atresia or stenosis Q22.4
    Ebstein's Q22.5
  Uhl's (hypoplasia of myocardium, right ventricle) Q24.8
  ulna Q74.0
  umbilical artery Q27.0
  union
    cricoid cartilage and thyroid cartilage Q31.8
    thyroid cartilage and hyoid bone Q31.8
    trachea with larynx Q31.8
  upper limb Q74.0
  urachus Q64.4
  ureter Q62.8
    obstructive NEC Q62.39
      cecoureterocele Q62.32
      orthotopic ureterocele Q62.31
  urethra Q64.70
    absence Q64.5
    double Q64.74
    fistula to rectum Q64.73
    obstructive Q64.39
      stricture Q64.32
    prolapse Q64.71
    specified type NEC Q64.79
  urinary tract Q64.9

Anomaly, anomalous — Aphthae, aphthous

Anomaly, anomalous — *continued*
  uterus Q51.9
    with only one functioning horn Q51.4
  uvula Q38.5
  vagina Q52.4
  valleculae Q31.8
  valve (heart) NEC Q24.8
    coronary sinus Q24.5
    inferior vena cava Q24.8
    pulmonary Q22.3
    sinus coronario Q24.5
    venae cavae inferioris Q24.8
  vas deferens Q55.4
  vascular Q27.9
    brain Q28.3
    ring Q25.4
  vein(s) (peripheral) Q27.9
    brain Q28.3
    cerebral Q28.3
    coronary Q24.5
    developmental Q28.3
    great Q26.9
      specified NEC Q26.8
  vena cava (inferior) (superior) Q26.9
  venous — *see* Anomaly, vein(s)
  venous return Q26.8
  ventricular
    bands or folds Q24.8
    septa Q21.0
  vertebra Q76.49
    kyphosis — *see* Kyphosis, congenital
    lordosis — *see* Lordosis, congenital
  vesicourethral orifice Q64.79
  vessel(s) Q27.9
    optic papilla Q14.2
    precerebral Q28.1
  vitelline duct Q43.0
  vitreous body or humor Q14.0
  vulva Q52.70
  wrist (joint) Q74.0
Anomia R48.8
Anonychia (congenital) Q84.3
  acquired L60.8
Anophthalmos, anophthalmus (congenital) (globe) Q11.1
  acquired Z90.01
Anopia, anopsia H53.46- ☑
  quadrant H53.46- ☑
Anorchia, anorchism, anorchidism Q55.0
Anorexia R63.0
  hysterical F44.89
  nervosa F50.00
    atypical F50.9
    binge-eating type F50.2
      with purging F50.02
    restricting type F50.01
Anorgasmy, psychogenic (female) F52.31
  male F52.32
Anosmia R43.0
  hysterical F44.6
  postinfectional J39.8
Anosognosia R41.89
Anosteoplasia Q78.9
Anovulatory cycle N97.0
Anoxemia R09.02
  newborn P84
Anoxia (pathological) R09.02
  altitude T70.29 ☑
  cerebral G93.1
    complicating
      anesthesia (general) (local) or other sedation T88.59 ☑
        in labor and delivery O74.3
        in pregnancy O29.21- ☑
        postpartum, puerperal O89.2
      delivery (cesarean) (instrumental) O75.4
    during a procedure G97.81
    newborn P84
    resulting from a procedure G97.82
  due to
    drowning T75.1 ☑
    high altitude T70.29 ☑
  heart — *see* Insufficiency, coronary
  intrauterine P84
  myocardial — *see* Insufficiency, coronary
  newborn P84
  spinal cord G95.11

Anoxia — *continued*
  systemic (by suffocation) (low content in atmosphere) — *see* Asphyxia, traumatic
Anteflexion — *see* Anteversion
Antenatal
  care (normal pregnancy) Z34.90
  screening (encounter for) of mother Z36
Antepartum — *see* condition
Anterior — *see* condition
Antero-occlusion M26.220
Anteversion
  cervix — *see* Anteversion, uterus
  femur (neck), congenital Q65.89
  uterus, uterine (cervix) (postinfectional) (postpartal, old) N85.4
    congenital Q51.818
    in pregnancy or childbirth — *see* Pregnancy, complicated by
Anthophobia F40.228
Anthracosilicosis J60
Anthracosis (lung) (occupational) J60
  lingua K14.3
Anthrax A22.9
  with pneumonia A22.1
  cerebral A22.8
  colitis A22.2
  cutaneous A22.0
  gastrointestinal A22.2
  inhalation A22.1
  intestinal A22.2
  meningitis A22.8
  pulmonary A22.1
  respiratory A22.1
  sepsis A22.7
  specified manifestation NEC A22.8
Anthropoid pelvis Q74.2
  with disproportion (fetopelvic) O33.0
Anthropophobia F40.10
  generalized F40.11
Antibodies, maternal (blood group) — *see* Isoimmunization, affecting management of pregnancy
  anti-D — *see* Isoimmunization, affecting management of pregnancy, Rh
  newborn P55.0
Antibody
  anticardiolipin R76.0
    with
      hemorrhagic disorder D68.312
      hypercoagulable state D68.61
  antiphosphatidylglycerol R76.0
    with
      hemorrhagic disorder D68.312
      hypercoagulable state D68.61
  antiphosphatidylinositol R76.0
    with
      hemorrhagic disorder D68.312
      hypercoagulable state D68.61
  antiphosphatidylserine R76.0
    with
      hemorrhagic disorder D68.312
      hypercoagulable state D68.61
  antiphospholipid R76.0
    with
      hemorrhagic disorder D68.312
      hypercoagulable state D68.61
Anticardiolipin syndrome D68.61
Anticoagulant, circulating (intrinsic) (*see also* Disorder, hemorrhagic) D68.318
  drug-induced (extrinsic) (*see also* Disorder, hemorrhagic) D68.32
Antidiuretic hormone syndrome E22.2
Antimonial cholera — *see* Poisoning, antimony
Antiphospholipid
  antibody
    with hemorrhagic disorder D68.312
    syndrome D68.61
Antisocial personality F60.2
Antithrombinemia — *see* Circulating anticoagulants
Antithromboplastinemia D68.318
Antithromboplastinogenemia D68.318
Antitoxin complication or reaction — *see* Complications, vaccination
Antlophobia F40.228
Antritis J32.0
  maxilla J32.0
    acute J01.00
      recurrent J01.01
  stomach K29.60

Antritis — *continued*
  stomach — *continued*
    with bleeding K29.61
Antrum, antral — *see* condition
Anuria R34
  calculous (impacted) (recurrent) (*see also* Calculus, urinary) N20.9
  following
    abortion — *see* Abortion by type complicated by, renal failure
    ectopic or molar pregnancy O08.4
  newborn P96.0
  postprocedural N99.0
  postrenal N13.8
  traumatic (following crushing) T79.5 ☑
Anus, anal — *see* condition
Anusitis K62.89
Anxiety F41.9
  depression F41.8
  episodic paroxysmal F41.0
  generalized F41.1
  hysteria F41.8
  neurosis F41.1
  panic type F41.0
  reaction F41.1
  separation, abnormal (of childhood) F93.0
  specified NEC F41.8
  state F41.1
Aorta, aortic — *see* condition
Aortectasia — *see* Ectasia, aorta
  with aneurysm — *see* Aneurysm, aorta
Aortitis (nonsyphilitic) (calcific) I77.6
  arteriosclerotic I70.0
  Doehle-Heller A52.02
  luetic A52.02
  rheumatic — *see* Endocarditis, acute, rheumatic
  specific (syphilitic) A52.02
  syphilitic A52.02
    congenital A50.54 [I79.1]
Apathetic thyroid storm — *see* Thyrotoxicosis
Apathy R45.3
Apeirophobia F40.228
Apepsia K30
  psychogenic F45.8
Aperistalsis, esophagus K22.0
Apertognathia M26.29
Apert's syndrome Q87.0
Aphagia R13.0
  psychogenic F50.9
Aphakia (acquired) (postoperative) H27.0- ☑
  congenital Q12.3
Aphasia (amnestic) (global) (nominal) (semantic) (syntactic) R47.01
  acquired, with epilepsy (Landau-Kleffner syndrome) — *see* Epilepsy, specified NEC
  auditory (developmental) F80.2
  developmental (receptive type) F80.2
    expressive type F80.1
    Wernicke's F80.2
  following
    cerebrovascular disease I69.920
      cerebral infarction I69.320
      intracerebral hemorrhage I69.120
      nontraumatic intracranial hemorrhage NEC I69.220
      specified disease NEC I69.820
      subarachnoid hemorrhage I69.020
  primary progressive G31.01 [F02.80]
    with behavioral disturbance G31.01 [F02.81]
  progressive isolated G31.01 [F02.80]
    with behavioral disturbance G31.01 [F02.81]
  sensory F80.2
  syphilis, tertiary A52.19
  Wernicke's (developmental) F80.2
Aphonia (organic) R49.1
  hysterical F44.4
  psychogenic F44.4
Aphthae, aphthous (*see also* condition)
  Bednar's K12.0
  cachectic K14.0
  epizootic B08.8
  fever B08.8
  oral (recurrent) K12.0
  stomatitis (major) (minor) K12.0
  thrush B37.0
  ulcer (oral) (recurrent) K12.0
    genital organ(s) NEC
      female N76.6

Aphthae, aphthous — *continued*
  ulcer — *continued*
    genital organ(s) — *continued*
      male N50.8
    larynx J38.7
Apical — *see* condition
Apiphobia F40.218
Aplasia (*see also* Agenesis)
  abdominal muscle syndrome Q79.4
  alveolar process (acquired) — *see* Anomaly, alveolar
    congenital Q38.6
  aorta (congenital) Q25.4
  axialis extracorticalis (congenita) E75.29
  bone marrow (myeloid) D61.9
    congenital D61.01
  brain Q00.0
    part of Q04.3
  bronchus Q32.4
  cementum K00.4
  cerebellum Q04.3
  cervix (congenital) Q51.5
  congenital pure red cell D61.01
  corpus callosum Q04.0
  cutis congenita Q84.8
  erythrocyte congenital D61.01
  extracortical axial E75.29
  eye Q11.1
  fovea centralis (congenital) Q14.1
  gallbladder, congenital Q44.0
  iris Q13.1
  labyrinth, membranous Q16.5
  limb (congenital) Q73.8
    lower — *see* Defect, reduction, lower limb
    upper — *see* Agenesis, arm
  lung, congenital (bilateral) (unilateral) Q33.3
  pancreas Q45.0
  parathyroid-thymic D82.1
  Pelizaeus-Merzbacher E75.29
  penis Q55.5
  prostate Q55.4
  red cell (with thymoma) D60.9
    acquired D60.9
      due to drugs D60.9
    adult D60.9
    chronic D60.0
    congenital D61.01
    constitutional D61.01
    due to drugs D60.9
    hereditary D61.01
    of infants D61.01
    primary D61.01
    pure D61.01
      due to drugs D60.9
    specified type NEC D60.8
    transient D60.1
  round ligament Q52.8
  skin Q84.8
  spermatic cord Q55.4
  spleen Q89.01
  testicle Q55.0
  thymic, with immunodeficiency D82.1
  thyroid (congenital) (with myxedema) E03.1
  uterus Q51.0
  ventral horn cell Q06.1
Apnea, apneic (of) (spells) R06.81
  newborn NEC P28.4
    obstructive P28.4
    sleep (central) (obstructive) (primary) P28.3
  prematurity P28.4
  sleep G47.30
    central (primary) G47.31
      in conditions classified elsewhere G47.37
    obstructive (adult) (pediatric) G47.33
    primary central G47.31
    specified NEC G47.39
Apneumatosis, newborn P28.0
Apocrine metaplasia (breast) — *see* Dysplasia, mammary, specified type NEC
Apophysitis (bone) (*see also* Osteochondropathy)
  calcaneus M92.8
  juvenile M92.9
Apoplectiform convulsions (cerebral ischemia) I67.82
Apoplexia, apoplexy, apoplectic
  adrenal A39.1
  heart (auricle) (ventricle) — *see* Infarct, myocardium
  heat T67.0 ☑
  hemorrhagic (stroke) — *see* Hemorrhage, intracranial

Apoplexia, apoplexy, apoplectic — *continued*
  meninges, hemorrhagic — *see* Hemorrhage, intracranial, subarachnoid
  uremic N18.9 [I68.8]
Appearance
  bizarre R46.1
  specified NEC R46.89
  very low level of personal hygiene R46.0
Appendage
  epididymal (organ of Morgagni) Q55.4
  intestine (epiploic) Q43.8
  preauricular Q17.0
  testicular (organ of Morgagni) Q55.29
Appendicitis (pneumococcal) (retrocecal) K37
  with
    perforation or rupture K35.2
    peritoneal abscess K35.3
    peritonitis NEC K35.3
      generalized (with perforation or rupture) K35.2
      localized (with perforation or rupture) K35.3
  acute (catarrhal) (fulminating) (gangrenous) (obstructive) (retrocecal) (suppurative) K35.80
    with
      peritoneal abscess K35.3
      peritonitis NEC K35.3
        generalized (with perforation or rupture) K35.2
        localized (with perforation or rupture) K35.3
    specified NEC K35.89
  amebic A06.89
  chronic (recurrent) K36
  exacerbation — *see* Appendicitis, acute
  gangrenous — *see* Appendicitis, acute
  healed (obliterative) K36
  interval K36
  neurogenic K36
  obstructive K36
  recurrent K36
  relapsing K36
  subacute (adhesive) K36
  subsiding K36
  suppurative — *see* Appendicitis, acute
  tuberculous A18.32
Appendicopathia oxyurica B80
Appendix, appendicular (*see also* condition)
  epididymis Q55.4
  Morgagni
    female Q50.5
    male (epididymal) Q55.4
      testicular Q55.29
  testis Q55.29
Appetite
  depraved — *see* Pica
  excessive R63.2
  lack or loss (*see also* Anorexia) R63.0
    nonorganic origin F50.8
    psychogenic F50.8
  perverted (hysterical) — *see* Pica
Apple peel syndrome Q41.1
Apprehension state F41.1
Apprehensiveness, abnormal F41.9
Approximal wear K03.0
Apraxia (classic) (ideational) (ideokinetic) (ideomotor) (motor) (verbal) R48.2
  following
    cerebrovascular disease I69.990
      cerebral infarction I69.390
      intracerebral hemorrhage I69.190
      nontraumatic intracranial hemorrhage NEC I69.290
      specified disease NEC I69.890
      subarachnoid hemorrhage I69.090
  oculomotor, congenital H51.8
Aptyalism K11.7
Apudoma — *see* Neoplasm, uncertain behavior, by site
Aqueous misdirection H40.83- ☑
Arabicum elephantiasis — *see* Infestation, filarial
Arachnitis — *see* Meningitis
Arachnodactyly — *see* Syndrome, Marfan's
Arachnoiditis (acute) (adhesive) (basal) (brain) (cerebrospinal) — *see* Meningitis
Arachnophobia F40.210
Arboencephalitis, Australian A83.4
Arborization block (heart) I45.5
ARC (AIDS-related complex) B20
Arches — *see* condition
Arcuate uterus Q51.810

Arcuatus uterus Q51.810
Arcus (cornea) senilis — *see* Degeneration, cornea, senile
Arc-welder's lung J63.4
Areflexia R29.2
Areola — *see* condition
Argentaffinoma (*see also* Neoplasm, uncertain behavior, by site)
  malignant — *see* Neoplasm, malignant, by site
  syndrome E34.0
Argininemia E72.21
Arginosuccinic aciduria E72.22
Argyll Robertson phenomenon, pupil or syndrome (syphilitic) A52.19
  atypical H57.09
  nonsyphilitic H57.09
Argyria, argyriasis
  conjunctival H11.13- ☑
  from drug or medicament — *see* Table of Drugs and Chemicals, by substance
Argyrosis, conjunctival H11.13- ☑
Arhinencephaly Q04.1
Ariboflavinosis E53.0
Arm — *see* condition
Arnold-Chiari disease, obstruction or syndrome (type II) Q07.00
  with
    hydrocephalus Q07.02
      with spina bifida Q07.03
    spina bifida Q07.01
      with hydrocephalus Q07.03
  type III — *see* Encephalocele
  type IV Q04.8
Aromatic amino-acid metabolism disorder E70.9
  specified NEC E70.8
Arousals, confusional G47.51
Arrest, arrested
  cardiac I46.9
    complicating
      abortion — *see* Abortion, by type, complicated by, cardiac arrest
      anesthesia (general) (local) or other sedation — *see* Table of Drugs and Chemicals, by drug
        in labor and delivery O74.2
        in pregnancy O29.11- ☑
        postpartum, puerperal O89.1
      delivery (cesarean) (instrumental) O75.4
    due to
      cardiac condition I46.2
      specified condition NEC I46.8
    intraoperative I97.71- ☑
    newborn P29.81
    postprocedural I97.12- ☑
      obstetric procedure O75.4
  cardiorespiratory — *see* Arrest, cardiac
  circulatory — *see* Arrest, cardiac
  deep transverse O64.0 ☑
  development or growth
    bone — *see* Disorder, bone, development or growth
    child R62.50
    tracheal rings Q32.1
  epiphyseal
    complete
      femur M89.15- ☑
      humerus M89.12- ☑
      tibia M89.16- ☑
      ulna M89.13- ☑
    forearm M89.13- ☑
      specified NEC M89.13- ☑
      ulna — *see* Arrest, epiphyseal, by type, ulna
    lower leg M89.16- ☑
      specified NEC M89.168
      tibia — *see* Arrest, epiphyseal, by type, tibia
    partial
      femur M89.15- ☑
      humerus M89.12- ☑
      tibia M89.16- ☑
      ulna M89.13- ☑
    specified NEC M89.18
  granulopoiesis — *see* Agranulocytosis
  growth plate — *see* Arrest, epiphyseal
  heart — *see* Arrest, cardiac
  legal, anxiety concerning Z65.3
  physeal — *see* Arrest, epiphyseal
  respiratory R09.2
    newborn P28.81

Arrest, arrested — continued
- sinus I45.5
- spermatogenesis (complete) — see Azoospermia
  - incomplete — see Oligospermia
- transverse (deep) O64.0 ☑

Arrhenoblastoma
- benign
  - specified site — see Neoplasm, benign, by site
  - unspecified site
    - female D27.9
    - male D29.20
- malignant
  - specified site — see Neoplasm, malignant, by site
  - unspecified site
    - female C56.9
    - male C62.90
- specified site — see Neoplasm, uncertain behavior, by site
- unspecified site
  - female D39.10
  - male D40.10

Arrhythmia (auricle) (cardiac) (juvenile) (nodal) (reflex) (sinus) (supraventricular) (transitory) (ventricle) I49.9
- block I45.9
- extrasystolic I49.49
- newborn
  - bradycardia P29.12
  - occurring before birth P03.819
    - before onset of labor P03.810
    - during labor P03.811
  - tachycardia P29.11
- psychogenic F45.8
- specified NEC I49.8
- vagal R55
- ventricular re-entry I47.0

Arrillaga-Ayerza syndrome (pulmonary sclerosis with pulmonary hypertension) I27.0

Arsenical pigmentation L81.8
- from drug or medicament — see Table of Drugs and Chemicals

Arsenism — see Poisoning, arsenic

Arterial — see condition

Arteriofibrosis — see Arteriosclerosis

Arteriolar sclerosis — see Arteriosclerosis

Arteriolith — see Arteriosclerosis

Arteriolitis I77.6
- necrotizing, kidney I77.5
- renal — see Hypertension, kidney

Arteriolosclerosis — see Arteriosclerosis

Arterionephrosclerosis — see Hypertension, kidney

Arteriopathy I77.9

Arteriosclerosis, arteriosclerotic (diffuse) (obliterans) (of) (senile) (with calcification) I70.90
- aorta I70.0
- arteries of extremities — see Arteriosclerosis, extremities
- brain I67.2
- bypass graft
  - coronary — see Arteriosclerosis, coronary, bypass graft
  - extremities — see Arteriosclerosis, extremities, bypass graft
- cardiac — see Disease, heart, ischemic, atherosclerotic
- cardiopathy — see Disease, heart, ischemic, atherosclerotic
- cardiorenal — see Hypertension, cardiorenal
- cardiovascular — see Disease, heart, ischemic, atherosclerotic
- carotid (see also Occlusion, artery, carotid) I65.2- ☑
- central nervous system I67.2
- cerebral I67.2
- cerebrovascular I67.2
- coronary (artery) I25.10
  - bypass graft I25.810
    - with
      - angina pectoris I25.709
        - with documented spasm I25.701
        - specified type NEC I25.708
        - unstable I25.700
      - ischemic chest pain I25.709
    - autologous artery I25.810
      - with
        - angina pectoris I25.729
          - with documented spasm I25.721
          - specified type I25.728
          - unstable I25.720
        - ischemic chest pain I25.729
    - autologous vein I25.810

Arteriosclerosis, arteriosclerotic — continued
- coronary — continued
  - bypass graft — continued
    - autologous vein — continued
      - with
        - angina pectoris I25.719
          - with documented spasm I25.711
          - specified type I25.718
          - unstable I25.710
        - ischemic chest pain I25.719
      - nonautologous biological I25.810
        - with
          - angina pectoris I25.739
            - with documented spasm I25.731
            - specified type I25.738
            - unstable I25.730
          - ischemic chest pain I25.739
      - specified type NEC I25.810
        - with
          - angina pectoris I25.799
            - with documented spasm I25.791
            - specified type I25.798
            - unstable I25.790
          - ischemic chest pain I25.799
  - due to
    - calcified coronary lesion (severely) I25.84
    - lipid rich plaque I25.83
  - native vessel
    - with
      - angina pectoris I25.119
        - with documented spasm I25.111
        - specified type NEC I25.118
        - unstable I25.110
      - ischemic chest pain I25.119
  - transplanted heart I25.811
    - bypass graft I25.812
      - with
        - angina pectoris I25.769
          - with documented spasm I25.761
          - specified type I25.768
          - unstable I25.760
        - ischemic chest pain I25.769
    - native coronary artery I25.811
      - with
        - angina pectoris I25.759
          - with documented spasm I25.751
          - specified type I25.758
          - unstable I25.750
        - ischemic chest pain I25.759
- extremities (native arteries) I70.209
  - bypass graft I70.309
    - autologous vein graft I70.409
      - leg I70.409
        - with
          - gangrene (and intermittent claudication, rest pain and ulcer) I70.469
          - intermittent claudication I70.419
          - rest pain (and intermittent claudication) I70.429
        - bilateral I70.403
          - with
            - gangrene (and intermittent claudication, rest pain and ulcer) I70.463
            - intermittent claudication I70.463
            - rest pain (and intermittent claudication) I70.423
            - specified type NEC I70.493
        - left I70.402
          - with
            - gangrene (and intermittent claudication, rest pain and ulcer) I70.462
            - intermittent claudication I70.412
            - rest pain (and intermittent claudication) I70.422
            - ulceration (and intermittent claudication and rest pain) I70.449
              - ankle I70.443
              - calf I70.442
              - foot site NEC I70.445
              - heel I70.444
              - lower leg NEC I70.448
              - midfoot I70.444
              - thigh I70.441
            - specified type NEC I70.492

Arteriosclerosis, arteriosclerotic — continued
- extremities — continued
  - bypass graft — continued
    - autologous vein graft — continued
      - leg — continued
        - right I70.401
          - with
            - gangrene (and intermittent claudication, rest pain and ulcer) I70.461
            - intermittent claudication I70.411
            - rest pain (and intermittent claudication) I70.421
            - ulceration (and intermittent claudication and rest pain) I70.439
              - ankle I70.433
              - calf I70.432
              - foot site NEC I70.435
              - heel I70.434
              - lower leg NEC I70.438
              - midfoot I70.434
              - thigh I70.431
            - specified type NEC I70.491
        - specified type NEC I70.499
      - specified NEC I70.408
        - with
          - gangrene (and intermittent claudication, rest pain and ulcer) I70.468
          - intermittent claudication I70.418
          - rest pain (and intermittent claudication) I70.428
          - ulceration (and intermittent claudication and rest pain) I70.45
          - specified type NEC I70.498
  - leg I70.309
    - with
      - gangrene (and intermittent claudication, rest pain and ulcer) I70.369
      - intermittent claudication I70.319
      - rest pain (and intermittent claudication) I70.329
    - bilateral I70.303
      - with
        - gangrene (and intermittent claudication, rest pain and ulcer) I70.363
        - intermittent claudication I70.313
        - rest pain (and intermittent claudication) I70.323
        - specified type NEC I70.393
    - left I70.302
      - with
        - gangrene (and intermittent claudication, rest pain and ulcer) I70.362
        - intermittent claudication I70.312
        - rest pain (and intermittent claudication) I70.322
        - ulceration (and intermittent claudication and rest pain) I70.349
          - ankle I70.343
          - calf I70.342
          - foot site NEC I70.345
          - heel I70.344
          - lower leg NEC I70.348
          - midfoot I70.344
          - thigh I70.341
        - specified type NEC I70.392
    - right I70.301
      - with
        - gangrene (and intermittent claudication, rest pain and ulcer) I70.361
        - intermittent claudication I70.311
        - rest pain (and intermittent claudication) I70.321
        - ulceration (and intermittent claudication and rest pain) I70.339
          - ankle I70.333
          - calf I70.332
          - foot site NEC I70.335
          - heel I70.334
          - lower leg NEC I70.338
          - midfoot I70.334
          - thigh I70.331
        - specified type NEC I70.391

Arteriosclerosis, arteriosclerotic — *continued*
  extremities — *continued*
    bypass graft — *continued*
      leg — *continued*
        specified type NEC I70.399
      nonautologous biological graft I70.509
        leg I70.509
          with
            gangrene (and intermittent claudication, rest pain and ulcer) I70.569
            intermittent claudication I70.519
            rest pain (and intermittent claudication) I70.529
          bilateral I70.503
            with
              gangrene (and intermittent claudication, rest pain and ulcer) I70.563
              intermittent claudication I70.513
              rest pain (and intermittent claudication) I70.523
              specified type NEC I70.593
          left I70.502
            with
              gangrene (and intermittent claudication, rest pain and ulcer) I70.562
              intermittent claudication I70.512
              rest pain (and intermittent claudication) I70.522
              ulceration (and intermittent claudication and rest pain) I70.549
              ankle I70.543
              calf I70.542
              foot site NEC I70.545
              heel I70.544
              lower leg NEC I70.548
              midfoot I70.544
              thigh I70.541
              specified type NEC I70.592
          right I70.501
            with
              gangrene (and intermittent claudication, rest pain and ulcer) I70.561
              intermittent claudication I70.511
              rest pain (and intermittent claudication) I70.521
              ulceration (and intermittent claudication and rest pain) I70.539
              ankle I70.533
              calf I70.532
              foot site NEC I70.535
              heel I70.534
              lower leg NEC I70.538
              midfoot I70.534
              thigh I70.531
              specified type NEC I70.591
          specified type NEC I70.599
        specified NEC I70.508
          with
            gangrene (and intermittent claudication, rest pain and ulcer) I70.568
            intermittent claudication I70.518
            rest pain (and intermittent claudication) I70.528
            ulceration (and intermittent claudication and rest pain) I70.55
          specified type NEC I70.598
      nonbiological graft I70.609
        leg I70.609
          with
            gangrene (and intermittent claudication, rest pain and ulcer) I70.669
            intermittent claudication I70.619
            rest pain (and intermittent claudication) I70.629
          bilateral I70.603
            with
              gangrene (and intermittent claudication, rest pain and ulcer) I70.663
              intermittent claudication I70.613

Arteriosclerosis, arteriosclerotic — *continued*
  extremities — *continued*
    bypass graft — *continued*
      nonbiological graft — *continued*
        leg — *continued*
          bilateral — *continued*
            with — *continued*
              rest pain (and intermittent claudication) I70.623
              specified type NEC I70.693
          left I70.602
            with
              gangrene (and intermittent claudication, rest pain and ulcer) I70.662
              intermittent claudication I70.612
              rest pain (and intermittent claudication) I70.622
              ulceration (and intermittent claudication and rest pain) I70.649
              ankle I70.643
              calf I70.642
              foot site NEC I70.645
              heel I70.644
              lower leg NEC I70.648
              midfoot I70.644
              thigh I70.641
              specified type NEC I70.692
          right I70.601
            with
              gangrene (and intermittent claudication, rest pain and ulcer) I70.661
              intermittent claudication I70.611
              rest pain (and intermittent claudication) I70.621
              ulceration (and intermittent claudication and rest pain) I70.639
              ankle I70.633
              calf I70.632
              foot site NEC I70.635
              heel I70.634
              lower leg NEC I70.638
              midfoot I70.634
              thigh I70.631
              specified type NEC I70.691
          specified type NEC I70.699
        specified NEC I70.608
          with
            gangrene (and intermittent claudication, rest pain and ulcer) I70.668
            intermittent claudication I70.618
            rest pain (and intermittent claudication) I70.628
            ulceration (and intermittent claudication and rest pain) I70.65
          specified type NEC I70.698
      specified graft NEC I70.709
        leg I70.709
          with
            gangrene (and intermittent claudication, rest pain and ulcer) I70.769
            intermittent claudication I70.719
            rest pain (and intermittent claudication) I70.729
          bilateral I70.703
            with
              gangrene (and intermittent claudication, rest pain and ulcer) I70.763
              intermittent claudication I70.713
              rest pain (and intermittent claudication) I70.723
              specified type NEC I70.793
          left I70.702
            with
              gangrene (and intermittent claudication, rest pain and ulcer) I70.762
              intermittent claudication I70.712
              rest pain (and intermittent claudication) I70.722

Arteriosclerosis, arteriosclerotic — *continued*
  extremities — *continued*
    bypass graft — *continued*
      specified graft — *continued*
        leg — *continued*
          left — *continued*
            with — *continued*
              ulceration (and intermittent claudication and rest pain) I70.749
              ankle I70.743
              calf I70.742
              foot site NEC I70.745
              heel I70.744
              lower leg NEC I70.748
              midfoot I70.744
              thigh I70.741
              specified type NEC I70.792
          right I70.701
            with
              gangrene (and intermittent claudication, rest pain and ulcer) I70.761
              intermittent claudication I70.711
              rest pain (and intermittent claudication) I70.721
              ulceration (and intermittent claudication and rest pain) I70.739
              ankle I70.733
              calf I70.732
              foot site NEC I70.735
              heel I70.734
              lower leg NEC I70.738
              midfoot I70.734
              thigh I70.731
              specified type NEC I70.791
          specified type NEC I70.799
        specified NEC I70.708
          with
            gangrene (and intermittent claudication, rest pain and ulcer) I70.768
            intermittent claudication I70.718
            rest pain (and intermittent claudication) I70.728
            ulceration (and intermittent claudication and rest pain) I70.75
          specified type NEC I70.798
      specified NEC I70.308
        with
          gangrene (and intermittent claudication, rest pain and ulcer) I70.368
          intermittent claudication I70.318
          rest pain (and intermittent claudication) I70.328
          ulceration (and intermittent claudication and rest pain) I70.35
        specifiec type NEC I70.398
    leg I70.209
      with
        gangrene (and intermittent claudication, rest pain and ulcer) I70.269
        intermittent claudication I70.219
        rest pain (and intermittent claudication) I70.229
      bilateral I70.203
        with
          gangrene (and intermittent claudication, rest pain and ulcer) I70.263
          intermittent claudication I70.213
          rest pain (and intermittent claudication) I70.223
          specified type NEC I70.293
      left I70.202
        with
          gangrene (and intermittent claudication, rest pain and ulcer) I70.262
          intermittent claudication I70.212
          rest pain (and intermittent claudication) I70.222
          ulceration (and intermittent claudication and rest pain) I70.249
          ankle I70.243
          calf I70.242
          foot site NEC I70.245
          heel I70.244
          lower leg NEC I70.248

Arteriosclerosis, arteriosclerotic — *continued*
  extremities — *continued*
    leg — *continued*
      left — *continued*
        with — *continued*
          ulceration — *continued*
            midfoot I70.244
            thigh I70.241
          specified type NEC I70.292
      right I70.201
        with
          gangrene (and intermittent claudication, rest pain and ulcer) I70.261
          intermittent claudication I70.211
          rest pain (and intermittent claudication) I70.221
          ulceration (and intermittent claudication and rest pain) I70.239
            ankle I70.233
            calf I70.232
            foot site NEC I70.235
            heel I70.234
            lower leg NEC I70.238
            midfoot I70.234
            thigh I70.231
          specified type NEC I70.291
        specified type NEC I70.299
      specified site NEC I70.208
        with
          gangrene (and intermittent claudication, rest pain and ulcer) I70.268
          intermittent claudication I70.218
          rest pain (and intermittent claudication) I70.228
          ulceration (and intermittent claudication and rest pain) I70.25
        specified type NEC I70.298
  generalized I70.91
  heart (disease) — *see* Arteriosclerosis, coronary (artery),
  kidney — *see* Hypertension, kidney
  medial — *see* Arteriosclerosis, extremities
  mesenteric (artery) K55.1
  Mönckeberg's — *see* Arteriosclerosis, extremities
  myocarditis I51.4
  peripheral (of extremities) — *see* Arteriosclerosis, extremities
  pulmonary (idiopathic) I27.0
  renal (arterioles) (*see also* Hypertension, kidney) artery I70.1
  retina (vascular) I70.8 [H35.0-] ☑
  specified artery NEC I70.8
  spinal (cord) G95.19
  vertebral (artery) I67.2
Arteriospasm I73.9
Arteriovenous — *see* condition
Arteritis I77.6
  allergic M31.0
  aorta (nonsyphilitic) I77.6
    syphilitic A52.02
  aortic arch M31.4
  brachiocephalic M31.4
  brain I67.7
    syphilitic A52.04
  cerebral I67.7
    in systemic lupus erythematosus M32.19
    listerial A32.89
    syphilitic A52.04
    tuberculous A18.89
  coronary (artery) I25.89
    rheumatic I01.8
      chronic I09.89
    syphilitic A52.06
  cranial (left) (right), giant cell M31.6
  deformans — *see* Arteriosclerosis
  giant cell NEC M31.6
    with polymyalgia rheumatica M31.5
  necrosing or necrotizing M31.9
    specified NEC M31.8
  nodosa M30.0
  obliterans — *see* Arteriosclerosis
  pulmonary I28.8
  rheumatic — *see* Fever, rheumatic
  senile — *see* Arteriosclerosis
  suppurative I77.2
  syphilitic (general) A52.09
    brain A52.04
    coronary A52.06

Arteritis — *continued*
  syphilitic — *continued*
    spinal A52.09
  temporal, giant cell M31.6
  young female aortic arch syndrome M31.4
Artery, arterial (*see also* condition)
  abscess I77.89
  single umbilical Q27.0
Arthralgia (allergic) (*see also* Pain, joint)
  in caisson disease T70.3 ☑
  temporomandibular M26.62
Arthritis, arthritic (acute) (chronic) (nonpyogenic) (subacute) M19.90
  allergic — *see* Arthritis, specified form NEC
  ankylosing (crippling) (spine) (*see also* Spondylitis, ankylosing)
    sites other than spine — *see* Arthritis, specified form NEC
  atrophic — *see* Osteoarthritis
    spine — *see* Spondylitis, ankylosing
  back — *see* Spondylopathy, inflammatory
  blennorrhagic (gonococcal) A54.42
  Charcot's — *see* Arthropathy, neuropathic
    diabetic — *see* Diabetes, arthropathy, neuropathic
    syringomyelic G95.0
  chylous (filarial) (*see also* category M01) B74.9
  climacteric (any site) NEC — *see* Arthritis, specified form NEC
  crystal (-induced) — *see* Arthritis, in, crystals
  deformans — *see* Osteoarthritis
  degenerative — *see* Osteoarthritis
  due to or associated with
    acromegaly E22.0
    brucellosis — *see* Brucellosis
    caisson disease T70.3 ☑
    diabetes — *see* Diabetes, arthropathy
    dracontiasis (*see also* category M01) B72
    enteritis NEC
      regional — *see* Enteritis, regional
    erysipelas (*see also* category M01) A46
    erythema
      epidemic A25.1
      nodosum L52
    filariasis NOS B74.9
    glanders A24.0
    helminthiasis (*see also* category M01) B83.9
    hemophilia D66 [M36.2]
    Henoch- (Schönlein) purpura D69.0 [M36.4]
    human parvovirus (*see also* category M01) B97.6
    infectious disease NEC M01 ☑
    leprosy (see also category M01) (*see also* Leprosy) A30.9
    Lyme disease A69.23
    mycobacteria (*see also* category M01) A31.8
    parasitic disease NEC (*see also* category M01) B89
    paratyphoid fever (see also category M01) (*see also* Fever, paratyphoid) A01.4
    rat bite fever (*see also* category M01) A25.1
    regional enteritis — *see* Enteritis, regional
    respiratory disorder NOS J98.9
    serum sickness (*see also* Reaction, serum) T80.69 ☑
    syringomyelia G95.0
    typhoid fever A01.04
  epidemic erythema A25.1
  febrile — *see* Fever, rheumatic
  gonococcal A54.42
  gouty (acute) — *see* Gout, idiopathic
  in (due to)
    acromegaly (*see also* subcategory M14.8-) E22.0
    amyloidosis (*see also* subcategory M14.8-) E85.4
    bacterial disease (*see also* subcategory M01) A49.9
    Behçet's syndrome M35.2
    caisson disease (*see also* subcategory M14.8-) T70.3 ☑
    coliform bacilli (Escherichia coli) — *see* Arthritis, in, pyogenic organism NEC
    crystals M11.9
      dicalcium phosphate — *see* Arthritis, in, crystals, specified type NEC
      hydroxyapatite M11.0- ☑
      pyrophosphate — *see* Arthritis, in, crystals, specified type NEC
      specified type NEC M11.80
        ankle M11.87- ☑
        elbow M11.82- ☑
        foot joint M11.87- ☑
        hand joint M11.84- ☑

Arthritis, arthritic — *continued*
  in — *continued*
    crystals — *continued*
      specified type — *continued*
        hip M11.85- ☑
        knee M11.86- ☑
        multiple sites M11.8- ☑
        shoulder M11.81- ☑
        vertebrae M11.88
        wrist M11.83- ☑
    dermatoarthritis, lipoid E78.81
    dracontiasis (dracunculiasis) (*see also* category M01) B72
    endocrine disorder NEC (*see also* subcategory M14.8-) E34.9
    enteritis, infectious NEC (*see also* category M01) A09
      specified organism NEC (*see also* category M01) A08.8
    erythema
      multiforme (*see also* subcategory M14.8-) L51.9
      nodosum (*see also* subcategory M14.8-) L52
    gout — *see* Gout, idiopathic
    helminthiasis NEC (*see also* category M01) B83.9
    hemochromatosis (*see also* subcategory M14.8-) E83.118
    hemoglobinopathy NEC D58.2 [M36.3]
    hemophilia NEC D66 [M36.2]
    Hemophilus influenzae M00.8- ☑ [B96.3]
    Henoch (-Schönlein) purpura D69.0 [M36.4]
    hyperparathyroidism NEC (*see also* subcategory M14.8-) E21.3
    hypersensitivity reaction NEC T78.49 ☑ [M36.4]
    hypogammaglobulinemia (*see also* subcategory M14.8-) D80.1
    hypothyroidism NEC (*see also* subcategory M14.8-) E03.9
    infection — *see* Arthritis, pyogenic or pyemic
      spine — *see* Spondylopathy, infective
    infectious disease NEC M01 ☑
    leprosy (*see also* category M01) A30.9
    leukemia NEC C95.9- ☑ [M36.1]
    lipoid dermatoarthritis E78.81
    Lyme disease A69.23
    Mediterranean fever, familial (*see also* subcategory M14.8-) E85.0
    Meningococcus A39.83
    metabolic disorder NEC (*see also* subcategory M14.8-) E88.9
    multiple myelomatosis C90.0- ☑ [M36.1]
    mumps B26.85
    mycosis NEC (*see also* category M01) B49
    myelomatosis (multiple) C90.0- ☑ [M36.1]
    neurological disorder NEC G98.0
    ochronosis (*see also* subcategory M14.8-) E70.29
    O'nyong-nyong (*see also* category M01) A92.1
    parasitic disease NEC (*see also* category M01) B89
    paratyphoid fever (*see also* category M01) A01.4
    Pseudomonas — *see* Arthritis, pyogenic, bacterial NEC
    psoriasis L40.50
    pyogenic organism NEC — *see* Arthritis, pyogenic, bacterial NEC
    Reiter's disease — *see* Reiter's disease
    respiratory disorder NEC (*see also* subcategory M14.8-) J98.9
    reticulosis, malignant (*see also* subcategory M14.8-) C86.0
    rubella B06.82
    Salmonella (arizonae) (cholerae-suis) (enteritidis) (typhimurium) A02.23
    sarcoidosis D86.86
    specified bacteria NEC — *see* Arthritis, pyogenic, bacterial NEC
    sporotrichosis B42.82
    syringomyelia G95.0
    thalassemia NEC D56.9 [M36.3]
    tuberculosis — *see* Tuberculosis, arthritis
    typhoid fever A01.04
    urethritis, Reiter's — *see* Reiter's disease
    viral disease NEC (*see also* category M01) B34.9
  infectious or infective (*see also* Arthritis, pyogenic or pyemic)
    spine — *see* Spondylopathy, infective
  juvenile M08.90
    with systemic onset — *see* Still's disease
    ankle M08.97- ☑

Arthritis, arthritic — *continued*
  juvenile — *continued*
    elbow M08.92- ☑
    foot joint M08.97- ☑
    hand joint M08.94- ☑
    hip M08.95- ☑
    knee M08.96- ☑
    multiple site M08.99
    pauciarticular M08.40
      ankle M08.47- ☑
      elbow M08.42- ☑
      foot joint M08.47- ☑
      hand joint M08.44- ☑
      hip M08.45- ☑
      knee M08.46- ☑
      shoulder M08.41- ☑
      vertebrae M08.48
      wrist M08.43- ☑
    psoriatic L40.54
    rheumatoid — *see* Arthritis, rheumatoid, juvenile
    shoulder M08.91- ☑
    specified type NEC M08.80
      ankle M08.87- ☑
      elbow M08.82- ☑
      foot joint M08.87- ☑
      hand joint M08.84- ☑
      hip M08.85- ☑
      knee M08.86- ☑
      multiple site M08.89
      shoulder M08.81- ☑
      specified joint NEC M08.88
      vertebrae M08.88
      wrist M08.83- ☑
    wrist M08.93- ☑
  meaning osteoarthritis — *see* Osteoarthritis
  meningococcal A39.83
  menopausal (any site) NEC — *see* Arthritis, specified form NEC
  mutilans (psoriatic) L40.52
  mycotic NEC (*see also* category M01) B49
  neuropathic (Charcot) — *see* Arthropathy, neuropathic
    diabetic — *see* Diabetes, arthropathy, neuropathic
    nonsyphilitic NEC G98.0
    syringomyelic G95.0
  ochronotic (*see also* subcategory M14.8-) E70.29
  palindromic (any site) — *see* Rheumatism, palindromic
  pneumococcal M00.10
    ankle M00.17- ☑
    elbow M00.12- ☑
    foot joint — *see* Arthritis, pneumococcal, ankle
    hand joint M00.14- ☑
    hip M00.15- ☑
    knee M00.16- ☑
    multiple site M00.19
    shoulder M00.11- ☑
    vertebra M00.18
    wrist M00.13- ☑
  postdysenteric — *see* Arthropathy, postdysenteric
  postmeningococcal A39.84
  postrheumatic, chronic — *see* Arthropathy, postrheumatic, chronic
  primary progressive (*see also* Arthritis, specified form NEC)
    spine — *see* Spondylitis, ankylosing
  psoriatic L40.50
  purulent (any site except spine) — *see* Arthritis, pyogenic or pyemic
    spine — *see* Spondylopathy, infective
  pyogenic or pyemic (any site except spine) M00.9
    bacterial NEC M00.80
      ankle M00.87- ☑
      elbow M00.82- ☑
      foot joint — *see* Arthritis, pyogenic, bacterial NEC, ankle
      hand joint M00.84- ☑
      hip M00.85- ☑
      knee M00.86- ☑
      multiple site M00.89
      shoulder M00.81- ☑
      vertebra M00.88
      wrist M00.83- ☑
    pneumococcal — *see* Arthritis, pneumococcal
    spine — *see* Spondylopathy, infective
    staphylococcal — *see* Arthritis, staphylococcal
    streptococcal — *see* Arthritis, streptococcal NEC
      pneumococcal — *see* Arthritis, pneumococcal

Arthritis, arthritic — *continued*
  reactive — *see* Reiter's disease
  rheumatic (*see also* Arthritis, rheumatoid)
    acute or subacute — *see* Fever, rheumatic
  rheumatoid M06.9
    with
      carditis — *see* Rheumatoid, carditis
      endocarditis — *see* Rheumatoid, carditis
      heart involvement NEC — *see* Rheumatoid, carditis
      lung involvement — *see* Rheumatoid, lung
      myocarditis — *see* Rheumatoid, carditis
      myopathy — *see* Rheumatoid, myopathy
      pericarditis — *see* Rheumatoid, carditis
      polyneuropathy — *see* Rheumatoid, polyneuropathy
      rheumatoid factor — *see* Arthritis, rheumatoid, seropositive
      splenoadenomegaly and leukopenia — *see* Felty's syndrome
      vasculitis — *see* Rheumatoid, vasculitis
      visceral involvement NEC — *see* Rheumatoid, arthritis, with involvement of organs NEC
    juvenile (with or without rheumatoid factor) M08.00
      ankle M08.07- ☑
      elbow M08.02- ☑
      foot joint M08.07- ☑
      hand joint M08.04- ☑
      hip M08.05- ☑
      knee M08.06- ☑
      multiple site M08.09
      shoulder M08.01- ☑
      vertebra M08.08
      wrist M08.03- ☑
    seronegative M06.00
      ankle M06.07- ☑
      elbow M06.02- ☑
      foot joint M06.07- ☑
      hand joint M06.04- ☑
      hip M06.05- ☑
      knee M06.06- ☑
      multiple site M06.09
      shoulder M06.01- ☑
      vertebra M06.08
      wrist M06.03- ☑
    seropositive M05.9
      without organ involvement M05.70
        ankle M05.77- ☑
        elbow M05.72- ☑
        foot joint M05.77- ☑
        hand joint M05.74- ☑
        hip M05.75- ☑
        knee M05.76- ☑
        multiple sites M05.79
        shoulder M05.71- ☑
        vertebra — *see* Spondylitis, ankylosing
        wrist M05.73- ☑
      specified NEC M05.80
        ankle M05.87- ☑
        elbow M05.82- ☑
        foot joint M05.87- ☑
        hand joint M05.84- ☑
        hip M05.85- ☑
        knee M05.86- ☑
        multiple sites M05.89
        shoulder M05.81- ☑
        vertebra — *see* Spondylitis, ankylosing
        wrist M05.83- ☑
    specified type NEC M06.80
      ankle M06.87- ☑
      elbow M06.82- ☑
      foot joint M06.87- ☑
      hand joint M06.84- ☑
      hip M06.85- ☑
      knee M06.86- ☑
      multiple site M06.89
      shoulder M06.81- ☑
      vertebra M06.88
      wrist M06.83- ☑
    spine — *see* Spondylitis, ankylosing
  rubella B06.82
  scorbutic (*see also* subcategory M14.8-) E54
  senile or senescent — *see* Osteoarthritis
  septic (any site except spine) — *see* Arthritis, pyogenic or pyemic

Arthritis, arthritic — *continued*
  septic — *see* Arthritis, pyogenic or pyemic — *continued*
    spine — *see* Spondylopathy, infective
  serum (nontherapeutic) (therapeutic) — *see* Arthropathy, postimmunization
  specified form NEC M13.80
    ankle M13.87- ☑
    elbow M13.82- ☑
    foot joint M13.87- ☑
    hand joint M13.84- ☑
    hip M13.85- ☑
    knee M13.86- ☑
    multiple site M13.89
    shoulder M13.81- ☑
    specified joint NEC M13.88
    wrist M13.83- ☑
  spine (*see also* Spondylopathy, inflammatory)
    infectious or infective NEC — *see* Spondylopathy, infective
    Marie-Strümpell — *see* Spondylitis, ankylosing
    pyogenic — *see* Spondylopathy, infective
    rheumatoid — *see* Spondylitis, ankylosing
    traumatic (old) — *see* Spondylopathy, traumatic
    tuberculous A18.01
  staphylococcal M00.00
    ankle M00.07- ☑
    elbow M00.02- ☑
    foot joint — *see* Arthritis, staphylococcal, ankle
    hand joint M00.04- ☑
    hip M00.05- ☑
    knee M00.06- ☑
    multiple site M00.09
    shoulder M00.01- ☑
    vertebra M00.08
    wrist M00.03- ☑
  streptococcal NEC M00.20
    ankle M00.27- ☑
    elbow M00.22- ☑
    foot joint — *see* Arthritis, streptococcal, ankle
    hand joint M00.24- ☑
    hip M00.25- ☑
    knee M00.26- ☑
    multiple site M00.29
    shoulder M00.21- ☑
    vertebra M00.28
    wrist M00.23- ☑
  suppurative — *see* Arthritis, pyogenic or pyemic
  syphilitic (late) A52.16
    congenital A50.55 [M12.80]
  syphilitica deformans (Charcot) A52.16
  temporomandibular M26.69
  toxic of menopause (any site) — *see* Arthritis, specified form NEC
  transient — *see* Arthropathy, specified form NEC
  traumatic (chronic) — *see* Arthropathy, traumatic
  tuberculous A18.02
    spine A18.01
  uratic — *see* Gout, idiopathic
  urethritica (Reiter's) — *see* Reiter's disease
  vertebral — *see* Spondylopathy, inflammatory
  villous (any site) — *see* Arthropathy, specified form NEC

Arthrocele — *see* Effusion, joint
Arthrodesis status Z98.1
Arthrodynia (*see also* Pain, joint)
Arthrodysplasia Q74.9
Arthrofibrosis, joint — *see* Ankylosis
Arthrogryposis (congenital) Q68.8
  multiplex congenita Q74.3
Arthrokatadysis M24.7
Arthropathy (*see also* Arthritis) M12.9
  Charcot's — *see* Arthropathy, neuropathic
    diabetic — *see* Diabetes, arthropathy, neuropathic
    syringomyelic G95.0
  cricoarytenoid J38.7
  crystal (-induced) — *see* Arthritis, in, crystals
  diabetic NEC — *see* Diabetes, arthropathy
  distal interphalangeal, psoriatic L40.51
  enteropathic M07.60
    ankle M07.67- ☑
    elbow M07.62- ☑
    foot joint M07.67- ☑
    hand joint M07.64- ☑
    hip M07.65- ☑
    knee M07.66- ☑

Arthropathy — *continued*
enteropathic — *continued*
multiple site M07.69
shoulder M07.61- ☑
vertebra M07.68
wrist M07.63- ☑
following intestinal bypass M02.00
ankle M02.07- ☑
elbow M02.02- ☑
foot joint M02.07- ☑
hand joint M02.04- ☑
hip M02.05- ☑
knee M02.06- ☑
multiple site M02.09
shoulder M02.01- ☑
vertebra M02.08
wrist M02.03- ☑
gouty (*see also* Gout, idiopathic)
in (due to)
Lesch-Nyhan syndrome E79.1 [M14.8-] ☑
sickle-cell disorders D57- ☑ [M14.8-] ☑
hemophilic NEC D66 [M36.2]
in (due to)
hyperparathyroidism NEC E21.3 [M14.8-] ☑
metabolic disease NOS E88.9 [M14.8-] ☑
in (due to)
acromegaly E22.0 [M14.8-] ☑
amyloidosis E85.4 [M14.8-] ☑
blood disorder NOS D75.9 [M36.3]
diabetes — *see* Diabetes, arthropathy
endocrine disease NOS E34.9 [M14.8-] ☑
erythema
multiforme L51.9 [M14.8-] ☑
nodosum L52 [M14.8-] ☑
hemochromatosis E83.118 [M14.8-] ☑
hemoglobinopathy NEC D58.2 [M36.3]
hemophilia NEC D66 [M36.2]
Henoch-Schönlein purpura D69.0 [M36.4]
hyperthyroidism E05.90 [M14.8-] ☑
hypothyroidism E03.9 [M14.8-] ☑
infective endocarditis I33.0 [M12.80]
leukemia NEC C95.9- ☑ [M36.1]
malignant histiocytosis C96.A [M36.1]
metabolic disease NOS E88.9 [M14.8-] ☑
multiple myeloma C90.0- ☑ [M36.1]
neoplastic disease NOS (*see also* Neoplasm) D49.9 [M36.1]
nutritional deficiency (*see also* subcategory M14.8-) E63.9
psoriasis NOS L40.50
sarcoidosis D86.86
syphilis (late) A52.77
congenital A50.55 [M12.80]
thyrotoxicosis (*see also* subcategory M14.8-) E05.90
ulcerative colitis K51.90 [M07.60]
viral hepatitis (postinfectious) NEC B19.9 [M12.80]
Whipple's disease (*see also* subcategory M14.8-) K90.81
Jaccoud — *see* Arthropathy, postrheumatic, chronic
juvenile — *see* Arthritis, juvenile
psoriatic L40.54
mutilans (psoriatic) L40.52
neuropathic (Charcot) M14.60
ankle M14.67- ☑
diabetic — *see* Diabetes, arthropathy, neuropathic
elbow M14.62- ☑
foot joint M14.67- ☑
hand joint M14.64- ☑
hip M14.65- ☑
knee M14.66- ☑
multiple site M14.69
nonsyphilitic NEC G98.0
shoulder M14.61- ☑
syringomyelic G95.0
vertebra M14.68
wrist M14.63- ☑
osteopulmonary — *see* Osteoarthropathy, hypertrophic, specified NEC
postdysenteric M02.10
ankle M02.17- ☑
elbow M02.12- ☑
foot joint M02.17- ☑
hand joint M02.14- ☑
hip M02.15- ☑
knee M02.16- ☑
multiple site M02.19
shoulder M02.11- ☑

Arthropathy — *continued*
postdysenteric — *continued*
vertebra M02.18
wrist M02.13- ☑
postimmunization M02.20
ankle M02.27- ☑
elbow M02.22- ☑
foot joint M02.27- ☑
hand joint M02.24- ☑
hip M02.25- ☑
knee M02.26- ☑
multiple site M02.29
shoulder M02.21- ☑
vertebra M02.28
wrist M02.23- ☑
postinfectious NEC B99 [M12.80]
in (due to)
enteritis due to Yersinia enterocolitica A04.6 [M12.80]
syphilis A52.77
viral hepatitis NEC B19.9 [M12.80]
postrheumatic, chronic (Jaccoud) M12.00
ankle M12.07- ☑
elbow M12.02- ☑
foot joint M12.07- ☑
hand joint M12.04- ☑
hip M12.05- ☑
knee M12.06- ☑
multiple site M12.09
shoulder M12.01- ☑
specified joint NEC M12.08
vertebra M12.08
wrist M12.03- ☑
psoriatic NEC L40.59
interphalangeal, distal L40.51
reactive M02.9
in (due to)
infective endocarditis I33.0 [M02.9]
specified type NEC M02.80
ankle M02.87- ☑
elbow M02.82- ☑
foot joint M02.87- ☑
hand joint M02.84- ☑
hip M02.85- ☑
knee M02.86- ☑
multiple site M02.89
shoulder M02.81- ☑
vertebra M02.88
wrist M02.83- ☑
specified form NEC M12.80
ankle M12.87- ☑
elbow M12.82- ☑
foot joint M12.87- ☑
hand joint M12.84- ☑
hip M12.85- ☑
knee M12.86- ☑
multiple site M12.89
shoulder M12.81- ☑
specified joint NEC M12.88
vertebrae M12.88
wrist M12.83- ☑
syringomyelic G95.0
tabes dorsalis A52.16
tabetic A52.16
transient — *see* Arthropathy, specified form NEC
traumatic M12.50
ankle M12.57- ☑
elbow M12.52- ☑
foot joint M12.57- ☑
hand joint M12.54- ☑
hip M12.55- ☑
knee M12.56- ☑
multiple site M12.59
shoulder M12.51- ☑
specified joint NEC M12.58
vertebrae M12.58
wrist M12.53- ☑
Arthropyosis — *see* Arthritis, pyogenic or pyemic
Arthrosis (deformans) (degenerative) (localized) (*see also* Osteoarthritis) M19.90
spine — *see* Spondylosis
Arthus' phenomenon or reaction T78.41 ☑
due to
drug — *see* Table of Drugs and Chemicals, by drug
Articular — *see* condition
Articulation, reverse (teeth) M26.24

Artificial
insemination complication — *see* Complications, artificial, fertilization
opening status (functioning) (without complication) Z93.9
anus (colostomy) Z93.3
colostomy Z93.3
cystostomy Z93.50
appendico-vesicostomy Z93.52
cutaneous Z93.51
specified NEC Z93.59
enterostomy Z93.4
gastrostomy Z93.1
ileostomy Z93.2
intestinal tract NEC Z93.4
jejunostomy Z93.4
nephrostomy Z93.6
specified site NEC Z93.8
tracheostomy Z93.0
ureterostomy Z93.6
urethrostomy Z93.6
urinary tract NEC Z93.6
vagina Z93.8
vagina status Z93.8
Arytenoid — *see* condition
Asbestosis (occupational) J61
Ascariasis B77.9
with
complications NEC B77.89
intestinal complications B77.0
pneumonia, pneumonitis B77.81
Ascaridosis, ascariasis — *see* Ascariasis
Ascaris (infection) (infestation) (lumbricoides) — *see* Ascariasis
Ascending — *see* condition
ASC-H (atypical squamous cells cannot exclude high grade squamous intraepithelial lesion on cytologic smear)
anus R85.611
cervix R87.611
vagina R87.621
Aschoff's bodies — *see* Myocarditis, rheumatic
Ascites (abdominal) R18.8
cardiac I50.9
chylous (nonfilarial) I89.8
filarial — *see* Infestation, filarial
due to
cirrhosis, alcoholic K70.31
hepatitis
alcoholic K70.11
chronic active K71.51
S. japonicum B65.2
heart I50.9
malignant R18.0
pseudochylous R18.8
syphilitic A52.74
tuberculous A18.31
ASC-US (atypical squamous cells of undetermined significance on cytologic smear)
anus R85.610
cervix R87.610
vagina R87.620
Aseptic — *see* condition
Asherman's syndrome N85.6
Asialia K11.7
Asiatic cholera — *see* Cholera
Asimultagnosia (simultanagnosia) R48.3
Askin's tumor — *see* Neoplasm, connective tissue, malignant
Asocial personality F60.2
Asomatognosia R41.4
Aspartylglucosaminuria E77.1
Asperger's disease or syndrome F84.5
Aspergilloma — *see* Aspergillosis
Aspergillosis (with pneumonia) B44.9
bronchopulmonary, allergic B44.81
disseminated B44.7
generalized B44.7
pulmonary NEC B44.1
allergic B44.81
invasive B44.0
specified NEC B44.89
tonsillar B44.2
Aspergillus (flavus) (fumigatus) (infection) (terreus) — *see* Aspergillosis
Aspermatogenesis — *see* Azoospermia
Aspermia (testis) — *see* Azoospermia
Asphyxia, asphyxiation (by) R09.01

☑ **Additional Character Required** — Refer to the Tabular List for Character Selection · Subterms under main terms may continue to next column or page

Asphyxia, asphyxiation — *continued*
antenatal P84
birth P84
bunny bag — *see* Asphyxia, due to, mechanical threat to breathing, trapped in bed clothes
crushing S28.0 ☑
drowning T75.1 ☑
gas, fumes, or vapor — *see* Table of Drugs and Chemicals
inhalation — *see* Inhalation
intrauterine P84
local I73.00
   with gangrene I73.01
mucus (*see also* Foreign body, respiratory tract, causing asphyxia)
newborn P84
pathological R09.01
postnatal P84
   mechanical — *see* Asphyxia, due to, mechanical threat to breathing
prenatal P84
reticularis R23.1
strangulation — *see* Asphyxia, due to, mechanical threat to breathing
submersion T75.1 ☑
traumatic T71.9 ☑
   due to
      crushed chest S28.0 ☑
      foreign body (in) — *see* Foreign body, respiratory tract, causing asphyxia
      low oxygen content of ambient air T71.20 ☑
         due to
            being trapped in
               low oxygen environment T71.29 ☑
               in car trunk T71.221 ☑
                  circumstances undetermined T71.224 ☑
                  done with intent to harm by
                     another person T71.223 ☑
                     self T71.222 ☑
               in refrigerator T71.231 ☑
                  circumstances undetermined T71.234 ☑
                  done with intent to harm by
                     another person T71.233 ☑
                     self T71.232 ☑
      cave-in T71.21 ☑
      mechanical threat to breathing (accidental) T71.191 ☑
         circumstances undetermined T71.194 ☑
         done with intent to harm by
           another person T71.193 ☑
           self T71.192 ☑
      hanging T71.161 ☑
         circumstances undetermined T71.164 ☑
         done with intent to harm by
           another person T71.163 ☑
           self T71.162 ☑
      plastic bag T71.121 ☑
         circumstances undetermined T71.124 ☑
         done with intent to harm by
           another person T71.123 ☑
           self T71.122 ☑
      smothering
         in furniture T71.151 ☑
            circumstances undetermined T71.154 ☑
            done with intent to harm by
              another person T71.153 ☑
              self T71.152 ☑
         under
           another person's body T71.141 ☑
              circumstances undetermined T71.144 ☑
              done with intent to harm T71.143 ☑
           pillow T71.111 ☑
              circumstances undetermined T71.114 ☑
              done with intent to harm by
                 another person T71.113 ☑
                 self T71.112 ☑
      trapped in bed clothes T71.131 ☑
         circumstances undetermined T71.134 ☑
         done with intent to harm by
           another person T71.133 ☑
           self T71.132 ☑

Asphyxia, asphyxiation — *continued*
vomiting, vomitus — *see* Foreign body, respiratory tract, causing asphyxia
Aspiration
amniotic (clear) fluid (newborn) P24.10
   with
      pneumonia (pneumonitis) P24.11
      respiratory symptoms P24.11
blood
   newborn (without respiratory symptoms) P24.20
      with
         pneumonia (pneumonitis) P24.21
         respiratory symptoms P24.21
      specified age NEC — *see* Foreign body, respiratory tract
bronchitis J69.0
food or foreign body (with asphyxiation) — *see* Asphyxia, food
liquor (amnii) (newborn) P24.10
   with
      pneumonia (pneumonitis) P24.11
      respiratory symptoms P24.11
meconium (newborn) (without respiratory symptoms) P24.00
   with
      pneumonitis (pneumonitis) P24.01
      respiratory symptoms P24.01
milk (newborn) (without respiratory symptoms) P24.30
   with
      pneumonia (pneumonitis) P24.31
      respiratory symptoms P24.31
   specified age NEC — *see* Foreign body, respiratory tract
mucus (*see also* Foreign body, by site, causing asphyxia)
   newborn P24.10
      with
         pneumonia (pneumonitis) P24.11
         respiratory symptoms P24.11
neonatal P24.9
   specific NEC (without respiratory symptoms) P24.80
      with
         pneumonia (pneumonitis) P24.81
         respiratory symptoms P24.81
newborn P24.9
   specific NEC (without respiratory symptoms) P24.80
      with
         pneumonia (pneumonitis) P24.81
         respiratory symptoms P24.81
pneumonia J69.0
pneumonitis J69.0
syndrome of newborn — *see* Aspiration, by substance, with pneumonia
vernix caseosa (newborn) P24.80
   with
      pneumonia (pneumonitis) P24.81
      respiratory symptoms P24.81
vomitus (*see also* Foreign body, respiratory tract)
   newborn (without respiratory symptoms) P24.30
      with
         pneumonia (pneumonitis) P24.31
         respiratory symptoms P24.31
Asplenia (congenital) Q89.01
postsurgical Z90.81
Assam fever B55.0
Assault, sexual — *see* Maltreatment
Assmann's focus NEC A15.0
Astasia (-abasia) (hysterical) F44.4
Asteatosis cutis L85.3
Astereognosia, astereognosis R48.1
Asterixis R27.8
   in liver disease K71.3
Asteroid hyalitis — *see* Deposit, crystalline
Asthenia, asthenic R53.1
cardiac (*see also* Failure, heart) I50.9
   psychogenic F45.8
cardiovascular (*see also* Failure, heart) I50.9
   psychogenic F45.8
heart (*see also* Failure, heart) I50.9
   psychogenic F45.8
hysterical F44.4
myocardial (*see also* Failure, heart) I50.9
   psychogenic F45.8
nervous F48.8
neurocirculatory F45.8
neurotic F48.8
psychogenic F48.8
psychoneurotic F48.8

Asthenia, asthenic — *continued*
psychophysiologic F48.8
reaction (psychophysiologic) F48.8
senile R54
Asthenopia (*see also* Discomfort, visual)
hysterical F44.6
psychogenic F44.6
Asthenospermia — *see* Abnormal, specimen, male genital organs
Asthma, asthmatic (bronchial) (catarrh) (spasmodic) J45.909
with
   chronic obstructive bronchitis J44.9
      with
         acute lower respiratory infection J44.0
         exacerbation (acute) J44.1
   chronic obstructive pulmonary disease J44.9
      with
         acute lower respiratory infection J44.0
         exacerbation (acute) J44.1
   exacerbation (acute) J45.901
   hay fever — *see* Asthma, allergic extrinsic
   rhinitis, allergic — *see* Asthma, allergic extrinsic
   status asthmaticus J45.902
allergic extrinsic J45.909
   with
      exacerbation (acute) J45.901
      status asthmaticus J45.902
atopic — *see* Asthma, allergic extrinsic
cardiac — *see* Failure, ventricular, left
cardiobronchial I50.1
childhood J45.909
   with
      exacerbation (acute) J45.901
      status asthmaticus J45.902
chronic obstructive J44.9
   with
      acute lower respiratory infection J44.0
      exacerbation (acute) J44.1
collier's J60
cough variant J45.991
detergent J69.8
due to
   detergent J69.8
   inhalation of fumes J68.3
eosinophilic J82
extrinsic, allergic — *see* Asthma, allergic extrinsic
grinder's J62.8
hay — *see* Asthma, allergic extrinsic
heart I50.9
idiosyncratic — *see* Asthma, nonallergic
intermittent (mild) J45.20
   with
      exacerbation (acute) J45.21
      status asthmaticus J45.22
intrinsic, nonallergic — *see* Asthma, nonallergic
Kopp's E32.8
late-onset J45.909
   with
      exacerbation (acute) J45.901
      status asthmaticus J45.902
mild intermittent J45.20
   with
      exacerbation (acute) J45.21
      status asthmaticus J45.22
mild persistent J45.30
   with
      exacerbation (acute) J45.31
      status asthmaticus J45.32
Millar's (laryngismus stridulus) J38.5
miner's J60
mixed J45.909
   with
      exacerbation (acute) J45.901
      status asthmaticus J45.902
moderate persistent J45.40
   with
      exacerbation (acute) J45.41
      status asthmaticus J45.42
nervous — *see* Asthma, nonallergic
nonallergic (intrinsic) J45.909
   with
      exacerbation (acute) J45.901
      status asthmaticus J45.902
persistent
   mild J45.30
      with
         exacerbation (acute) J45.31

Asthma, asthmatic — *continued*
  persistent — *continued*
    mild — *continued*
      with — *continued*
        status asthmaticus J45.32
    moderate J45.40
      with
        exacerbation (acute) J45.41
        status asthmaticus J45.42
    severe J45.50
      with
        exacerbation (acute) J45.51
        status asthmaticus J45.52
  platinum J45.998
  pneumoconiotic NEC J64
  potter's J62.8
  predominantly allergic J45.909
  psychogenic F54
  pulmonary eosinophilic J82
  red cedar J67.8
  Rostan's I50.1
  sandblaster's J62.8
  sequoiosis J67.8
  severe persistent J45.50
    with
      exacerbation (acute) J45.51
      status asthmaticus J45.52
  specified NEC J45.998
  stonemason's J62.8
  thymic E32.8
  tuberculous — *see* Tuberculosis, pulmonary
  Wichmann's (laryngismus stridulus) J38.5
  wood J67.8
Astigmatism (compound) (congenital) H52.20- ☑
  irregular H52.21- ☑
  regular H52.22- ☑
Astraphobia F40.220
Astroblastoma
  specified site — *see* Neoplasm, malignant, by site
  unspecified site C71.9
Astrocytoma (cystic)
  anaplastic
    specified site — *see* Neoplasm, malignant, by site
    unspecified site C71.9
  fibrillary
    specified site — *see* Neoplasm, malignant, by site
    unspecified site C71.9
  fibrous
    specified site — *see* Neoplasm, malignant, by site
    unspecified site C71.9
  gemistocytic
    specified site — *see* Neoplasm, malignant, by site
    unspecified site C71.9
  juvenile
    specified site — *see* Neoplasm, malignant, by site
    unspecified site C71.9
  pilocytic
    specified site — *see* Neoplasm, malignant, by site
    unspecified site C71.9
  piloid
    specified site — *see* Neoplasm, malignant, by site
    unspecified site C71.9
  protoplasmic
    specified site — *see* Neoplasm, malignant, by site
    unspecified site C71.9
  specified site NEC — *see* Neoplasm, malignant, by site
  subependymal D43.2
    giant cell
      specified site — *see* Neoplasm, uncertain behavior, by site
      unspecified site D43.2
    specified site — *see* Neoplasm, uncertain behavior, by site
    unspecified site D43.2
  unspecified site C71.9
Astroglioma
  specified site — *see* Neoplasm, malignant, by site
  unspecified site C71.9
Asymbolia R48.8
Asymmetry (*see also* Distortion)
  between native and reconstructed breast N65.1
  face Q67.0
  jaw (lower) — *see* Anomaly, dentofacial, jaw-cranial base relationship, asymmetry
Asynergia, asynergy R27.8
  ventricular I51.89
Asystole (heart) — *see* Arrest, cardiac

At risk
  for falling Z91.81
Ataxia, ataxy, ataxic R27.0
  acute R27.8
  brain (hereditary) G11.9
  cerebellar (hereditary) G11.9
    with defective DNA repair G11.3
    alcoholic G31.2
    early-onset G11.1
    in
      alcoholism G31.2
      myxedema E03.9 [G13.2]
      neoplastic disease (*see also* Neoplasm) D49.9 [G13.1]
      specified disease NEC G32.81
    late-onset (Marie's) G11.2
  cerebral (hereditary) G11.9
  congenital nonprogressive G11.0
  family, familial — *see* Ataxia, hereditary
  following
    cerebrovascular disease I69.993
      cerebral infarction I69.393
      intracerebral hemorrhage I69.193
      nontraumatic intracranial hemorrhage NEC I69.293
      specified disease NEC I69.893
      subarachnoid hemorrhage I69.093
  Friedreich's (heredofamilial) (cerebellar) (spinal) G11.1
  gait R26.0
    hysterical F44.4
  general R27.8
  gluten M35.9 [G32.81]
    with celiac disease K90.0 [G32.81]
  hereditary G11.9
    with neuropathy G60.2
    cerebellar — *see* Ataxia, cerebellar
    spastic G11.4
    specified NEC G11.8
    spinal (Friedreich's) G11.1
  heredofamilial — *see* Ataxia, hereditary
  Hunt's G11.1
  hysterical F44.4
  locomotor (progressive) (syphilitic) (partial) (spastic) A52.11
    diabetic — *see* Diabetes, ataxia
  Marie's (cerebellar) (heredofamilial) (late-onset) G11.2
  nonorganic origin F44.4
  nonprogressive, congenital G11.0
  psychogenic F44.4
  Roussy-Lévy G60.0
  Sanger-Brown's (hereditary) G11.2
  spastic hereditary G11.4
  spinal
    hereditary (Friedreich's) G11.1
    progressive (syphilitic) A52.11
  spinocerebellar, X-linked recessive G11.1
  telangiectasia (Louis-Bar) G11.3
Ataxia-telangiectasia (Louis-Bar) G11.3
Atelectasis (massive) (partial) (pressure) (pulmonary) J98.11
  newborn P28.10
    due to resorption P28.11
    partial P28.19
    primary P28.0
    secondary P28.19
  primary (newborn) P28.0
  tuberculous — *see* Tuberculosis, pulmonary
Atelocardia Q24.9
Atelomyelia Q06.1
Atheroembolism
  of
    extremities
      lower I75.02- ☑
      upper I75.01- ☑
    kidney I75.81
    specified NEC I75.89
Atheroma, atheromatous (*see also* Arteriosclerosis) I70.90
  aorta, aortic I70.0
    valve (*see also* Endocarditis, aortic) I35.8
  aorto-iliac I70.0
  artery — *see* Arteriosclerosis
  basilar (artery) I67.2
  carotid (artery) (common) (internal) I67.2
  cerebral (arteries) I67.2
  coronary (artery) I25.10
    with angina pectoris — *see* Arteriosclerosis, coronary (artery),

Atheroma, atheromatous — *continued*
  degeneration — *see* Arteriosclerosis
  heart, cardiac — *see* Disease, heart, ischemic, atherosclerotic
  mitral (valve) I34.8
  myocardium, myocardial — *see* Disease, heart, ischemic, atherosclerotic
  pulmonary valve (heart) (*see also* Endocarditis, pulmonary) I37.8
  tricuspid (heart) (valve) I36.8
  valve, valvular — *see* Endocarditis
  vertebral (artery) I67.2
Atheromatosis — *see* Arteriosclerosis
Atherosclerosis (*see also* Arteriosclerosis)
  coronary
    artery I25.10
      with angina pectoris — *see* Arteriosclerosis, coronary (artery),
      due to
        calcified coronary lesion (severely) I25.84
        lipid rich plaque I25.83
    transplanted heart I25.811
      bypass graft I25.812
        with angina pectoris — *see* Arteriosclerosis, coronary (artery),
      native coronary artery I25.811
        with angina pectoris — *see* Arteriosclerosis, coronary (artery),
Athetosis (acquired) R25.8
  bilateral (congenital) G80.3
  congenital (bilateral) (double) G80.3
  double (congenital) G80.3
  unilateral R25.8
Athlete's
  foot B35.3
  heart I51.7
Athrepsia E41
Athyrea (acquired) (*see also* Hypothyroidism)
  congenital E03.1
Atonia, atony, atonic
  bladder (sphincter) (neurogenic) N31.2
  capillary I78.8
  cecum K59.8
    psychogenic F45.8
  colon — *see* Atony, intestine
  congenital P94.2
  esophagus K22.8
  intestine K59.8
    psychogenic F45.8
  stomach K31.89
    neurotic or psychogenic F45.8
  uterus (during labor) O62.2
    with hemorrhage (postpartum) O72.1
    postpartum (with hemorrhage) O72.1
      without hemorrhage O75.89
Atopy — *see* History, allergy
Atransferrinemia, congenital E88.09
Atresia, atretic
  alimentary organ or tract NEC Q45.8
    upper Q40.8
  ani, anus, anal (canal) Q42.3
    with fistula Q42.2
  aorta (arch) (ring) Q25.2
  aortic (orifice) (valve) Q23.0
    arch Q25.2
    congenital with hypoplasia of ascending aorta and defective development of left ventricle (with mitral stenosis) Q23.4
    in hypoplastic left heart syndrome Q23.4
  aqueduct of Sylvius Q03.0
    with spina bifida — *see* Spina bifida, with hydrocephalus
  artery NEC Q27.8
    cerebral Q28.3
    coronary Q24.5
    digestive system Q27.8
    eye Q15.8
    lower limb Q27.8
    pulmonary Q25.5
    specified site NEC Q27.8
    umbilical Q27.0
    upper limb Q27.8
  auditory canal (external) Q16.1
  bile duct (common) (congenital) (hepatic) Q44.2
    acquired — *see* Obstruction, bile duct
  bladder (neck) Q64.39
    obstruction Q64.31
  bronchus Q32.4

Atresia, atretic — *continued*
- cecum Q42.8
- cervix (acquired) N88.2
  - congenital Q51.828
  - in pregnancy or childbirth — *see* Anomaly, cervix, in pregnancy or childbirth
    - causing obstructed labor O65.5
- choana Q30.0
- colon Q42.9
  - specified NEC Q42.8
- common duct Q44.2
- cricoid cartilage Q31.8
- cystic duct Q44.2
  - acquired K82.8
    - with obstruction K82.0
- digestive organs NEC Q45.8
- duodenum Q41.0
- ear canal Q16.1
- ejaculatory duct Q55.4
- epiglottis Q31.8
- esophagus Q39.0
  - with tracheoesophageal fistula Q39.1
- eustachian tube Q17.8
- fallopian tube (congenital) Q50.6
  - acquired N97.1
- follicular cyst N83.0
- foramen of
  - Luschka Q03.1
    - with spina bifida — *see* Spina bifida, with hydrocephalus
  - Magendie Q03.1
    - with spina bifida — *see* Spina bifida, with hydrocephalus
- gallbladder Q44.1
- genital organ
  - external
    - female Q52.79
    - male Q55.8
  - internal
    - female Q52.8
    - male Q55.8
- glottis Q31.8
- gullet Q39.0
  - with tracheoesophageal fistula Q39.1
- heart valve NEC Q24.8
  - pulmonary Q22.0
  - tricuspid Q22.4
- hymen Q52.3
  - acquired (postinfective) N89.6
- ileum Q41.2
- intestine (small) Q41.9
  - large Q42.9
    - specified NEC Q42.8
- iris, filtration angle Q15.0
- jejunum Q41.1
- lacrimal apparatus Q10.4
- larynx Q31.8
- meatus urinarius Q64.33
- mitral valve Q23.2
  - in hypoplastic left heart syndrome Q23.4
- nares (anterior) (posterior) Q30.0
- nasopharynx Q34.8
- nose, nostril Q30.0
  - acquired J34.89
- organ or site NEC Q89.8
- osseous meatus (ear) Q16.1
- oviduct (congenital) Q50.6
  - acquired N97.1
- parotid duct Q38.4
  - acquired K11.8
- pulmonary (artery) Q25.5
  - valve Q22.0
- pulmonic Q22.0
- pupil Q13.2
- rectum Q42.1
  - with fistula Q42.0
- salivary duct Q38.4
  - acquired K11.8
- sublingual duct Q38.4
  - acquired K11.8
- submandibular duct Q38.4
  - acquired K11.8
- submaxillary duct Q38.4
  - acquired K11.8
- thyroid cartilage Q31.8
- trachea Q32.1
- tricuspid valve Q22.4
- ureter Q62.10

Atresia, atretic — *continued*
- ureter — *continued*
  - pelvic junction Q62.11
  - vesical orifice Q62.12
- ureteropelvic junction Q62.11
- ureterovesical orifice Q62.12
- urethra (valvular) Q64.39
  - stricture Q64.32
- urinary tract NEC Q64.8
- uterus Q51.818
  - acquired N85.8
- vagina (congenital) Q52.4
  - acquired (postinfectional) (senile) N89.5
- vas deferens Q55.3
- vascular NEC Q27.8
  - cerebral Q28.3
  - digestive system Q27.8
  - lower limb Q27.8
  - specified site NEC Q27.8
  - upper limb Q27.8
- vein NEC Q27.8
  - digestive system Q27.8
  - great Q26.8
  - lower limb Q27.8
  - portal Q26.5
  - pulmonary Q26.3
  - specified site NEC Q27.8
  - upper limb Q27.8
- vena cava (inferior) (superior) Q26.8
- vesicourethral orifice Q64.31
- vulva Q52.79
  - acquired N90.5

Atrichia, atrichosis — *see* Alopecia

Atrophia (*see also* Atrophy)
- cutis senilis L90.8
  - due to radiation L57.8
- gyrata of choroid and retina H31.23
- senilis R54
  - dermatological L90.8
    - due to radiation (nonionizing) (solar) L57.8
- unguium L60.3
  - congenita Q84.6

Atrophie blanche (en plaque) (de Milian) L95.0

Atrophoderma, atrophodermia (of) L90.9
- diffusum (idiopathic) L90.4
- maculatum L90.8
  - et striatum L90.8
    - due to syphilis A52.79
  - syphilitic A51.39
- neuriticum L90.8
- Pasini and Pierini L90.3
- pigmentosum Q82.1
- reticulatum symmetricum faciei L66.4
- senile L90.8
  - due to radiation (nonionizing) (solar) L57.8
- vermiculata (cheeks) L66.4

Atrophy, atrophic (of)
- adrenal (capsule) (gland) E27.49
  - primary (autoimmune) E27.1
- alveolar process or ridge (edentulous) K08.20
- anal sphincter (disuse) N81.84
- appendix K38.8
- arteriosclerotic — *see* Arteriosclerosis
- bile duct (common) (hepatic) K83.8
- bladder N32.89
  - neurogenic N31.8
- blanche (en plaque) (of Milian) L95.0
- bone (senile) NEC (*see also* Disorder, bone, specified type NEC)
  - due to
    - tabes dorsalis (neurogenic) A52.11
- brain (cortex) (progressive) G31.9
  - frontotemporal circumscribed G31.01 [F02.80]
    - with behavioral disturbance G31.01 [F02.81]
  - senile NEC G31.1
- breast N64.2
  - obstetric — *see* Disorder, breast, specified type NEC
- buccal cavity K13.79
- cardiac — *see* Degeneration, myocardial
- cartilage (infectional) (joint) — *see* Disorder, cartilage, specified NEC
- cerebellar — *see* Atrophy, brain
- cerebral — *see* Atrophy, brain
- cervix (mucosa) (senile) (uteri) N88.8
  - menopausal N95.8
- Charcot-Marie-Tooth G60.0
- choroid (central) (macular) (myopic) (retina) H31.10- ☑

Atrophy, atrophic — *continued*
- choroid — *continued*
  - diffuse secondary H31.12- ☑
  - gyrate H31.23
  - senile H31.11- ☑
- ciliary body — *see* Atrophy, iris
- conjunctiva (senile) H11.89
- corpus cavernosum N48.89
- cortical — *see* Atrophy, brain
- cystic duct K82.8
- Déjérine-Thomas G23.8
- disuse NEC — *see* Atrophy, muscle
- Duchenne-Aran G12.21
- ear H93.8- ☑
- edentulous alveolar ridge K08.20
- endometrium (senile) N85.8
  - cervix N88.8
- enteric K63.89
- epididymis N50.8
- eyeball — *see* Disorder, globe, degenerated condition, atrophy
- eyelid (senile) — *see* Disorder, eyelid, degenerative
- facial (skin) L90.9
- fallopian tube (senile) N83.32
  - with ovary N83.33
- fascioscapulohumeral (Landouzy- Déjérine) G71.0
- fatty, thymus (gland) E32.8
- gallbladder K82.8
- gastric K29.40
  - with bleeding K29.41
- gastrointestinal K63.89
- glandular I89.8
- globe H44.52- ☑
- gum K06.0
- hair L67.8
- heart (brown) — *see* Degeneration, myocardial
- hemifacial Q67.4
  - Romberg G51.8
- infantile E41
  - paralysis, acute — *see* Poliomyelitis, paralytic
- intestine K63.89
- iris (essential) (progressive) H21.26- ☑
  - specified NEC H21.29
- kidney (senile) (terminal) (*see also* Sclerosis, renal) N26.1
  - congenital or infantile Q60.5
    - bilateral Q60.4
    - unilateral Q60.3
  - hydronephrotic — *see* Hydronephrosis
- lacrimal gland (primary) H04.14- ☑
  - secondary H04.15- ☑
- Landouzy-Déjérine G71.0
- laryngitis, infective J37.0
- larynx J38.7
- Leber's optic (hereditary) H47.22
- lip K13.0
- liver (yellow) K72.90
  - with coma K72.91
  - acute, subacute K72.00
    - with coma K72.01
  - chronic K72.10
    - with coma K72.11
- lung (senile) J98.4
- macular (dermatological) L90.8
  - syphilitic, skin A51.39
    - striated A52.79
- mandible (edentulous) K08.20
  - minimal K08.21
  - moderate K08.22
  - severe K08.23
- maxilla K08.20
  - minimal K08.24
  - moderate K08.25
  - severe K08.26
- muscle, muscular (diffuse) (general) (idiopathic) (primary) M62.50
  - ankle M62.57- ☑
  - Duchenne-Aran G12.21
  - foot M62.57- ☑
  - forearm M62.53- ☑
  - hand M62.54- ☑
  - infantile spinal G12.0
  - lower leg M62.56- ☑
  - multiple sites M62.59
  - myelopathic — *see* Atrophy, muscle, spinal
  - myotonic G71.11
  - neuritic G58.9
  - neuropathic (peroneal) (progressive) G60.0

Atrophy, atrophic — *continued*
  muscle, muscular — *continued*
    pelvic (disuse) N81.84
    peroneal G60.0
    progressive (bulbar) G12.21
      adult G12.1
      infantile (spinal) G12.0
      spinal G12.9
        adult G12.1
        infantile G12.0
    pseudohypertrophic G71.0
    shoulder region M62.51- ☑
    specified site NEC M62.58
    spinal G12.9
      adult form G12.1
      Aran-Duchenne G12.21
      childhood form, type II G12.1
      distal G12.1
      hereditary NEC G12.1
      infantile, type I (Werdnig-Hoffmann) G12.0
      juvenile form, type III (Kugelberg- Welander) G12.1
      progressive G12.21
      scapuloperoneal form G12.1
      specified NEC G12.8
    syphilitic A52.78
    thigh M62.55- ☑
    upper arm M62.52- ☑
  myocardium — *see* Degeneration, myocardial
  myometrium (senile) N85.8
    cervix N88.8
  myopathic NEC — *see* Atrophy, muscle
  myotonia G71.11
  nail L60.3
  nasopharynx J31.1
  nerve (*see also* Disorder, nerve)
    abducens — *see* Strabismus, paralytic, sixth nerve
    accessory G52.8
    acoustic or auditory H93.3 ☑
    cranial G52.9
      eighth (auditory) H93.3 ☑
      eleventh (accessory) G52.8
      fifth (trigeminal) G50.8
      first (olfactory) G52.0
      fourth (trochlear) — *see* Strabismus, paralytic, fourth nerve
      second (optic) H47.20
      sixth (abducens) — *see* Strabismus, paralytic, sixth nerve
      tenth (pneumogastric) (vagus) G52.2
      third (oculomotor) — *see* Strabismus, paralytic, third nerve
      twelfth (hypoglossal) G52.3
    hypoglossal G52.3
    oculomotor — *see* Strabismus, paralytic, third nerve
    olfactory G52.0
    optic (papillomacular bundle)
      syphilitic (late) A52.15
        congenital A50.44
    pneumogastric G52.2
    trigeminal G50.8
    trochlear — *see* Strabismus, paralytic, fourth nerve
    vagus (pneumogastric) G52.2
  neurogenic, bone, tabetic A52.11
  nutritional E41
  old age R54
  olivopontocerebellar G23.8
  optic (nerve) H47.20
    glaucomatous H47.23- ☑
    hereditary H47.22
    primary H47.21- ☑
    specified type NEC H47.29- ☑
    syphilitic (late) A52.15
      congenital A50.44
  orbit H05.31- ☑
  ovary (senile) N83.31
    with fallopian tube N83.33
  oviduct (senile) — *see* Atrophy, fallopian tube
  palsy, diffuse (progressive) G12.22
  pancreas (duct) (senile) K86.8
  parotid gland K11.0
  pelvic muscle N81.84
  penis N48.89
  pharynx J39.2
  pluriglandular E31.8
    autoimmune E31.0
  polyarthritis M15.9

Atrophy, atrophic — *continued*
  prostate N42.89
  pseudohypertrophic (muscle) G71.0
  renal (*see also* Sclerosis, renal) N26.1
  retina, retinal (postinfectional) H35.89
  rhinitis J31.0
  salivary gland K11.0
  scar L90.5
  sclerosis, lobar (of brain) G31.09 [F02.80]
    with behavioral disturbance G31.09 [F02.81]
  scrotum N50.8
  seminal vesicle N50.8
  senile R54
    due to radiation (nonionizing) (solar) L57.8
  skin (patches) (spots) L90.9
    degenerative (senile) L90.8
    due to radiation (nonionizing) (solar) L57.8
    senile L90.8
  spermatic cord N50.8
  spinal (acute) (cord) G95.89
    muscular — *see* Atrophy, muscle, spinal
    paralysis G12.20
      acute — *see* Poliomyelitis, paralytic
      meaning progressive muscular atrophy G12.21
  spine (column) — *see* Spondylopathy, specified NEC
  spleen (senile) D73.0
  stomach K29.40
    with bleeding K29.41
  striate (skin) L90.6
    syphilitic A52.79
  subcutaneous L90.9
  sublingual gland K11.0
  submandibular gland K11.0
  submaxillary gland K11.0
  Sudeck's — *see* Algoneurodystrophy
  suprarenal (capsule) (gland) E27.49
    primary E27.1
  systemic affecting central nervous system in
      myxedema E03.9 [G13.2]
      neoplastic disease (*see also* Neoplasm) D49.9 [G13.1]
      specified disease NEC G13.8
  tarso-orbital fascia, congenital Q10.3
  testis N50.0
  thenar, partial — *see* Syndrome, carpal tunnel
  thymus (fatty) E32.8
  thyroid (gland) (acquired) E03.4
    with cretinism E03.1
    congenital (with myxedema) E03.1
  tongue (senile) K14.8
    papillae K14.4
  trachea J39.8
  tunica vaginalis N50.8
  turbinate J34.89
  tympanic membrane (nonflaccid) H73.82- ☑
    flaccid H73.81- ☑
  upper respiratory tract J39.8
  uterus, uterine (senile) N85.8
    cervix N88.8
    due to radiation (intended effect) N85.8
      adverse effect or misadventure N99.89
  vagina (senile) N95.2
  vas deferens N50.8
  vascular I99.8
  vertebra (senile) — *see* Spondylopathy, specified NEC
  vulva (senile) N90.5
  Werdnig-Hoffmann G12.0
  yellow — *see* Failure, hepatic
Attack, attacks
  with alteration of consciousness (with automatisms) — *see* Epilepsy, localization-related, symptomatic, with complex partial seizures
  without alteration of consciousness — *see* Epilepsy, localization-related, symptomatic, with simple partial seizures
  Adams-Stokes I45.9
  akinetic — *see* Epilepsy, generalized, specified NEC
  angina — *see* Angina
  atonic — *see* Epilepsy, generalized, specified NEC
  benign shuddering G25.83
  cataleptic — *see* Catalepsy
  coronary — *see* Infarct, myocardium
  cyanotic, newborn P28.2
  drop NEC R55
  epileptic — *see* Epilepsy
  heart — *see* infarct, myocardium
  hysterical F44.9

Attack, attacks — *continued*
  jacksonian — *see* Epilepsy, localization-related, symptomatic, with simple partial seizures
  myocardium, myocardial — *see* Infarct, myocardium
  myoclonic — *see* Epilepsy, generalized, specified NEC
  panic F41.0
  psychomotor — *see* Epilepsy, localization-related, symptomatic, with complex partial seizures
  salaam — *see* Epilepsy, spasms
  schizophreniform, brief F23
  shuddering, benign G25.83
  Stokes-Adams I45.9
  syncope R55
  transient ischemic (TIA) G45.9
    specified NEC G45.8
  unconsciousness R55
    hysterical F44.89
  vasomotor R55
  vasovagal (paroxysmal) (idiopathic) R55
Attention (to)
  artificial
    opening (of) Z43.9
      digestive tract NEC Z43.4
        colon Z43.3
        ilium Z43.2
        stomach Z43.1
      specified NEC Z43.8
      trachea Z43.0
      urinary tract NEC Z43.6
        cystostomy Z43.5
        nephrostomy Z43.6
        ureterostomy Z43.6
        urethrostomy Z43.6
      vagina Z43.7
  colostomy Z43.3
  cystostomy Z43.5
  deficit disorder or syndrome F98.8
    with hyperactivity — *see* Disorder, attention-deficit hyperactivity
  gastrostomy Z43.1
  ileostomy Z43.2
  jejunostomy Z43.4
  nephrostomy Z43.6
  surgical dressings Z48.01
  sutures Z48.02
  tracheostomy Z43.0
  ureterostomy Z43.6
  urethrostomy Z43.6
Attrition
  gum K06.0
  tooth, teeth (excessive) (hard tissues) K03.0
Atypical, atypism (*see also* condition)
  cells (on cytolgocial smear) (endocervical) (endometrial) (glandular)
    cervix R87.619
    vagina R87.629
  cervical N87.9
  endometrium N85.9
    hyperplasia N85.00
  parenting situation Z62.9
Auditory — *see* condition
Aujeszky's disease B33.8
Aurantiasis, cutis E67.1
Auricle, auricular (*see also* condition)
  cervical Q18.2
Auriculotemporal syndrome G50.8
Austin Flint murmur (aortic insufficiency) I35.1
Australian
  Q fever A78
  X disease A83.4
Autism, autistic (childhood) (infantile) F84.0
  atypical F84.9
Autodigestion R68.89
Autoerythrocyte sensitization (syndrome) D69.2
Autographism L50.3
Autoimmune
  disease (systemic) M35.9
  inhibitors to clotting factors D68.311
  lymphoproliferative syndrome [ALPS] D89.82
  thyroiditis E06.3
Autointoxication R68.89
Automatism G93.89
  with temporal sclerosis G93.81
  epileptic — *see* Epilepsy, localization-related, symptomatic, with complex partial seizures
  paroxysmal, idiopathic — *see* Epilepsy, localization-related, symptomatic, with complex partial seizures

Autonomic, autonomous
bladder (neurogenic) N31.2
hysteria seizure F44.5
Autosensitivity, erythrocyte D69.2
Autosensitization, cutaneous L30.2
Autosome — *see* condition by chromosome involved
Autotopagnosia R48.1
Autotoxemia R68.89
Autumn — *see* condition
Avellis' syndrome G46.8
Aversion
oral R63.3
newborn P92.- ☑
nonorganic origin F98.2 ☑
sexual F52.1
Aviator's
disease or sickness — *see* Effect, adverse, high altitude
ear T70.0 ☑
Avitaminosis (multiple) (*see also* Deficiency, vitamin) E56.9
B E53.9
with
beriberi E51.11
pellagra E52
B2 E53.0
B6 E53.1
B12 E53.8
D E55.9
with rickets E55.0
G E53.0
K E56.1
nicotinic acid E52
AVNRT (atrioventricular nodal re-entrant tachycardia) I47.1
AVRT (atrioventricular nodal re-entrant tachycardia) I47.1
Avulsion (traumatic)
blood vessel — *see* Injury, blood vessel
bone — *see* Fracture, by site
cartilage (*see also* Dislocation, by site)
symphyseal (inner), complicating delivery O71.6
external site other than limb — *see* Wound, open, by site
eye S05.7- ☑
head (intracranial)
external site NEC S08.89 ☑
scalp S08.0 ☑
internal organ or site — *see* Injury, by site
joint (*see also* Dislocation, by site)
capsule — *see* Sprain, by site
kidney S37.06- ☑
ligament — *see* Sprain, by site
limb (*see also* Amputation, traumatic, by site)
skin and subcutaneous tissue — *see* Wound, open, by site
muscle — *see* Injury, muscle
nerve (root) — *see* Injury, nerve
scalp S08.0 ☑
skin and subcutaneous tissue — *see* Wound, open, by site
spleen S36.032 ☑
symphyseal cartilage (inner), complicating delivery O71.6
tendon — *see* Injury, muscle
tooth S03.2 ☑
Awareness of heart beat R00.2
Axenfeld's
anomaly or syndrome Q15.0
degeneration (calcareous) Q13.4
Axilla, axillary (*see also* condition)
breast Q83.1
Axonotmesis — *see* Injury, nerve
Ayerza's disease or syndrome (pulmonary artery sclerosis with pulmonary hypertension) I27.0
Azoospermia (organic) N46.01
due to
drug therapy N46.021
efferent duct obstruction N46.023
infection N46.022
radiation N46.024
specified cause NEC N46.029
systemic disease N46.025
Azotemia R79.89
meaning uremia N19
Aztec ear Q17.3
Azygos
continuation inferior vena cava Q26.8
lobe (lung) Q33.1

B

Baastrup's disease — *see* Kissing spine
Babesiosis B60.0
Babington's disease (familial hemorrhagic telangiectasia) I78.0
Babinski's syndrome A52.79
Baby
crying constantly R68.11
floppy (syndrome) P94.2
Bacillary — *see* condition
Bacilluria N39.0
Bacillus (*see also* Infection, bacillus)
abortus infection A23.1
anthracis infection A22.9
coli infection (*see also* Escherichia coli) B96.20
Flexner's A03.1
mallei infection A24.0
Shiga's A03.0
suipestifer infection — *see* Infection, salmonella
Back — *see* condition
Backache (postural) M54.9
sacroiliac M53.3
specified NEC M54.89
Backflow — *see* Reflux
Backward reading (dyslexia) F81.0
Bacteremia R78.81
with sepsis — *see* Sepsis
Bactericholia — *see* Cholecystitis, acute
Bacterid, bacteride (pustular) L40.3
Bacterium, bacteria, bacterial
agent NEC, as cause of disease classified elsewhere B96.89
in blood — *see* Bacteremia
in urine — *see* Bacteriuria
Bacteriuria, bacteruria N39.0
asymptomatic N39.0
Bacteroides
fragilis, as cause of disease classified elsewhere B96.6
Bad
heart — *see* Disease, heart
trip
due to drug abuse — *see* Abuse, drug, hallucinogen
due to drug dependence — *see* Dependence, drug, hallucinogen
Baelz's disease (cheilitis glandularis apostematosa) K13.0
Baerensprung's disease (eczema marginatum) B35.6
Bagasse disease or pneumonitis J67.1
Bagassosis J67.1
Baker's cyst — *see* Cyst, Baker's
Bakwin-Krida syndrome (craniometaphyseal dysplasia) Q78.5
Balancing side interference M26.56
Balanitis (circinata) (erosiva) (gangrenosa) (phagedenic) (vulgaris) N48.1
amebic A06.82
candidal B37.42
due to Haemophilus ducreyi A57
gonococcal (acute) (chronic) A54.09
xerotica obliterans N48.0
Balanoposthitis N47.6
gonococcal (acute) (chronic) A54.09
ulcerative (specific) A63.8
Balanorrhagia — *see* Balanitis
Balantidiasis, balantidiosis A07.0
Bald tongue K14.4
Baldness (*see also* Alopecia)
male-pattern — *see* Alopecia, androgenic
Balkan grippe A78
Balloon disease — *see* Effect, adverse, high altitude
Balo's disease (concentric sclerosis) G37.5
Bamberger-Marie disease — *see* Osteoarthropathy, hypertrophic, specified type NEC
Bancroft's filariasis B74.0
Band(s)
adhesive — *see* Adhesions, peritoneum
anomalous or congenital (*see also* Anomaly, by site)
heart (atrial) (ventricular) Q24.8
intestine Q43.3
omentum Q43.3
cervix N88.1
constricting, congenital Q79.8
gallbladder (congenital) Q44.1
intestinal (adhesive) — *see* Adhesions, peritoneum

Band(s) — *continued*
obstructive
intestine K56.5
peritoneum K56.5
periappendiceal, congenital Q43.3
peritoneal (adhesive) — *see* Adhesions, peritoneum
uterus N73.6
internal N85.6
vagina N89.5
Bandemia D72.825
Bandl's ring (contraction), complicating delivery O62.4
Bangkok hemorrhagic fever A91
Bang's disease (brucella abortus) A23.1
Bankruptcy, anxiety concerning Z59.8
Bannister's disease T78.3 ☑
hereditary D84.1
Banti's disease or syndrome (with cirrhosis) (with portal hypertension) K76.6
Bar, median, prostate — *see* Enlargement, enlarged, prostate
Barcoo disease or rot — *see* Ulcer, skin
Barlow's disease E54
Barodontalgia T70.29 ☑
Baron Münchausen syndrome — *see* Disorder, factitious
Barosinusitis T70.1 ☑
Barotitis T70.0 ☑
Barotrauma T70.29 ☑
odontalgia T70.29 ☑
otitic T70.0 ☑
sinus T70.1 ☑
Barraquer (-Simons) disease or syndrome (progressive lipodystrophy) E88.1
Barré-Guillain disease or syndrome G61.0
Barrel chest M95.4
Barré-Liéou syndrome (posterior cervical sympathetic) M53.0
Barrett's
disease — *see* Barrett's, esophagus
esophagus K22.70
with dysplasia K22.719
high grade K22.711
low grade K22.710
without dysplasia K22.70
syndrome — *see* Barrett's, esophagus
ulcer K22.10
with bleeding K22.11
without bleeding K22.10
Bársony (-Polgár) (-Teschendorf) syndrome (corkscrew esophagus) K22.4
Barth syndrome E78.71
Bartholinitis (suppurating) N75.8
gonococcal (acute) (chronic) (with abscess) A54.1
Bartonellosis A44.9
cutaneous A44.1
mucocutaneous A44.1
specified NEC A44.8
systemic A44.0
Barton's fracture S52.56- ☑
Bartter's syndrome E26.81
Basal — *see* condition
Basan's (hidrotic) ectodermal dysplasia Q82.4
Baseball finger — *see* Dislocation, finger
Basedow's disease (exophthalmic goiter) — *see* Hyperthyroidism, with, goiter
Basic — *see* condition
Basilar — *see* condition
Bason's (hidrotic) ectodermal dysplasia Q82.4
Basopenia — *see* Agranulocytosis
Basophilia D72.824
Basophilism (cortico-adrenal) (Cushing's) (pituitary) E24.0
Bassen-Kornzweig disease or syndrome E78.6
Bat ear Q17.5
Bateman's
disease B08.1
purpura (senile) D69.2
Bathing cramp T75.1 ☑
Bathophobia F40.248
Batten (-Mayou) disease E75.4
retina E75.4 [H36]
Batten-Steinert syndrome G71.11
Battered — *see* Maltreatment
Battey Mycobacterium infection A31.0
Battle exhaustion F43.0
Battledore placenta O43.19- ☑

Baumgarten-Cruveilhier cirrhosis, disease or syndrome K74.69
Bauxite fibrosis (of lung) J63.1
Bayle's disease (general paresis) A52.17
Bazin's disease (primary) (tuberculous) A18.4
Beach ear — see Swimmer's, ear
Beaded hair (congenital) Q84.1
Béal conjunctivitis or syndrome B30.2
Beard's disease (neurasthenia) F48.8
Beat(s)
  atrial, premature I49.1
  ectopic I49.49
  elbow — see Bursitis, elbow
  escaped, heart I49.49
  hand — see Bursitis, hand
  knee — see Bursitis, knee
  premature I49.40
    atrial I49.1
    auricular I49.1
    supraventricular I49.1
Beau's
  disease or syndrome — see Degeneration, myocardial
  lines (transverse furrows on fingernails) L60.4
Bechterev's syndrome — see Spondylitis, ankylosing
Becker's
  cardiomyopathy I42.8
  disease
    idiopathic mural endomyocardial disease I42.3
    myotonia congenita, recessive form G71.12
  dystrophy G71.0
  pigmented hairy nevus D22.5
Beck's syndrome (anterior spinal artery occlusion) I65.8
Beckwith-Wiedemann syndrome Q87.3
Bed confinement status Z74.01
Bed sore — see Ulcer, pressure, by site
Bedbug bite(s) — see Bite(s), by site, superficial, insect
Bedclothes, asphyxiation or suffocation by — see Asphyxia, traumatic, due to, mechanical, trapped
Bednar's
  aphthae K12.0
  tumor — see Neoplasm, malignant, by site
Bedridden Z74.01
Bedsore — see Ulcer, pressure, by site
Bedwetting — see Enuresis
Bee sting (with allergic or anaphylactic shock) — see Toxicity, venom, arthropod, bee
Beer drinker's heart (disease) I42.6
Begbie's disease (exophthalmic goiter) — see Hyperthyroidism, with, goiter
Behavior
  antisocial
    adult Z72.811
    child or adolescent Z72.810
  disorder, disturbance — see Disorder, conduct
  disruptive — see Disorder, conduct
  drug seeking Z72.89
  inexplicable R46.2
  marked evasiveness R46.5
  obsessive-compulsive R46.81
  overactivity R46.3
  poor responsiveness R46.4
  self-damaging (life-style) Z72.89
  sleep-incompatible Z72.821
  slowness R46.4
  specified NEC R46.89
  strange (and inexplicable) R46.2
  suspiciousness R46.5
  type A pattern Z73.1
  undue concern or preoccupation with stressful events R46.6
  verbosity and circumstantial detail obscuring reason for contact R46.7
Behçet's disease or syndrome M35.2
Behr's disease — see Degeneration, macula
Beigel's disease or morbus (white piedra) B36.2
Bejel A65
Bekhterev's syndrome — see Spondylitis, ankylosing
Belching — see Eructation
Bell's
  mania F30.8
  palsy, paralysis G51.0
    infant or newborn P11.3
  spasm G51.3
Bence Jones albuminuria or proteinuria NEC R80.3
Bends T70.3 ☑
Benedikt's paralysis or syndrome G46.3

Benign (see also condition)
  prostatic hyperplasia — see Hyperplasia, prostate
Bennett's fracture (displaced) S62.21- ☑
Benson's disease — see Deposit, crystalline
Bent
  back (hysterical) F44.4
  nose M95.0
    congenital Q67.4
Bereavement (uncomplicated) Z63.4
Bergeron's disease (hysterical chorea) F44.4
Berger's disease — see Nephropathy, IgA
Beriberi (dry) E51.11
  heart (disease) E51.12
  polyneuropathy E51.11
  wet E51.12
    involving circulatory system E51.11
Berlin's disease or edema (traumatic) S05.8X- ☑
Berlock (berloque) **dermatitis** L56.2
Bernard-Horner syndrome G90.2
Bernard-Soulier disease or thrombopathia D69.1
Bernhardt (-Roth) **disease** — see Mononeuropathy, lower limb, meralgia paresthetica
Bernheim's syndrome — see Failure, heart, congestive
Bertielliasis B71.8
Berylliosis (lung) J63.2
Besnier-Boeck (-Schaumann) **disease** — see Sarcoidosis
Besnier's
  lupus pernio D86.3
  prurigo L20.0
Bestiality F65.89
Best's disease H35.50
Betalipoproteinemia, broad or floating E78.2
Beta-mercaptolactate-cysteine disulfiduria E72.09
Betting and gambling Z72.6
  pathological (compulsive) F63.0
Bezoar T18.9 ☑
  intestine T18.3 ☑
  stomach T18.2 ☑
Bezold's abscess — see Mastoiditis, acute
Bianchi's syndrome R48.8
Bicornate or bicornis uterus Q51.3
  in pregnancy or childbirth O34.59- ☑
    causing obstructed labor O65.5
Bicuspid aortic valve Q23.1
Biedl-Bardet syndrome Q87.89
Bielschowsky (-Jansky) **disease** E75.4
Biermer's (pernicious) anemia or disease D51.0
Biett's disease L93.0
Bifid (congenital)
  apex, heart Q24.8
  clitoris Q52.6
  kidney Q63.8
  nose Q30.2
  patella Q74.1
  scrotum Q55.29
  toe NEC Q74.2
  tongue Q38.3
  ureter Q62.8
  uterus Q51.3
  uvula Q35.7
Biforis uterus (suprasimplex) Q51.3
Bifurcation (congenital)
  gallbladder Q44.1
  kidney pelvis Q63.8
  renal pelvis Q63.8
  rib Q76.6
  tongue, congenital Q38.3
  trachea Q32.1
  ureter Q62.8
  urethra Q64.74
  vertebra Q76.49
Big spleen syndrome D73.1
Bigeminal pulse R00.8
Bilateral — see condition
Bile
  duct — see condition
  pigments in urine R82.2
Bilharziasis (see also Schistosomiasis)
  chyluria B65.0
  cutaneous B65.3
  galacturia B65.0
  hematochyluria B65.0
  intestinal B65.1
  lipemia B65.9
  lipuria B65.0
  oriental B65.2
  piarhemia B65.9

Bilharziasis — continued
  pulmonary NOS B65.9 [J99]
    pneumonia B65.9 [J17]
  tropical hematuria B65.0
  vesical B65.0
Biliary — see condition
Bilirubin metabolism disorder E80.7
  specified NEC E80.6
Bilirubinemia, familial nonhemolytic E80.4
Bilirubinuria R82.2
Biliuria R82.2
Bilocular stomach K31.2
Binswanger's disease I67.3
Biparta, bipartite
  carpal scaphoid Q74.0
  patella Q74.1
  vagina Q52.10
Bird
  face Q75.8
  fancier's disease or lung J67.2
Birth
  complications in mother — see Delivery, complicated
  compression during NOS P15.9
  defect — see Anomaly
  immature (less than 37 completed weeks) — see Preterm, newborn
    extremely (less than 28 completed weeks) — see Immaturity, extreme
  inattention, at or after — see Maltreatment, child, neglect
  injury NOS P15.9
    basal ganglia P11.1
    brachial plexus NEC P14.3
    brain (compression) (pressure) P11.2
    central nervous system NOS P11.9
    cerebellum P11.1
    cerebral hemorrhage P10.1
    external genitalia P15.5
    eye P15.3
    face P15.4
    fracture
      bone P13.9
        specified NEC P13.8
      clavicle P13.4
      femur P13.2
      humerus P13.3
      long bone, except femur P13.3
      radius and ulna P13.3
      skull P13.0
      spine P11.5
      tibia and fibula P13.3
    intracranial P11.2
      laceration or hemorrhage P10.9
        specified NEC P10.8
    intraventricular hemorrhage P10.2
    laceration
      brain P10.1
      by scalpel P15.8
      peripheral nerve P14.9
    liver P15.0
    meninges
      brain P11.1
      spinal cord P11.5
    nerve
      brachial plexus P14.3
      cranial NEC (except facial) P11.4
      facial P11.3
      peripheral P14.9
      phrenic (paralysis) P14.2
    paralysis
      facial nerve P11.3
      spinal P11.5
    penis P15.5
    rupture
      spinal cord P11.5
    scalp P12.9
    scalpel wound P15.8
    scrotum P15.5
    skull NEC P13.1
      fracture P13.0
    specified type NEC P15.8
    spinal cord P11.5
    spine P11.5
    spleen P15.1
    sternomastoid (hematoma) P15.2
    subarachnoid hemorrhage P10.3
    subcutaneous fat necrosis P15.6
    subdural hemorrhage P10.0

Birth — *continued*
 injury — *continued*
  tentorial tear P10.4
  testes P15.5
  vulva P15.5
 lack of care, at or after — *see* Maltreatment, child, neglect
 neglect, at or after — *see* Maltreatment, child, neglect
 palsy or paralysis, newborn, NOS (birth injury) P14.9
 premature (infant) — *see* Preterm, newborn
 shock, newborn P96.89
 trauma — *see* Birth, injury
 weight
  4000 grams to 4499 grams P08.1
  4500 grams or more P08.0
  low (2499 grams or less) — *see* Low, birthweight
   extremely (999 grams or less) — *see* Low, birthweight, extreme
Birthmark Q82.5
Birt-Hogg-Dube syndrome Q87.89
Bisalbuminemia E88.09
Biskra's button B55.1
Bite(s) (animal) (human)
 abdomen, abdominal
  wall S31.159 ☑
   with penetration into peritoneal cavity S31.659 ☑
   epigastric region S31.152 ☑
    with penetration into peritoneal cavity S31.652 ☑
   left
    lower quadrant S31.154 ☑
     with penetration into peritoneal cavity S31.654 ☑
    upper quadrant S31.151 ☑
     with penetration into peritoneal cavity S31.651 ☑
   periumbilic region S31.155 ☑
    with penetration into peritoneal cavity S31.655 ☑
   right
    lower quadrant S31.153 ☑
     with penetration into peritoneal cavity S31.653 ☑
    upper quadrant S31.150 ☑
     with penetration into peritoneal cavity S31.650 ☑
   superficial NEC S30.871 ☑
    insect S30.861 ☑
 alveolar (process) — *see* Bite, oral cavity
 amphibian (venomous) — *see* Venom, bite, amphibian
 animal (*see also* Bite, by site)
  venomous — *see* Venom
 ankle S91.05- ☑
  superficial NEC S90.57- ☑
   insect S90.56- ☑
 antecubital space — *see* Bite, elbow
 anus S31.835 ☑
  superficial NEC S30.877 ☑
   insect S30.867 ☑
 arm (upper) S41.15- ☑
  lower — *see* Bite, forearm
  superficial NEC S40.87- ☑
   insect S40.86- ☑
 arthropod NEC — *see* Venom, bite, arthropod
 auditory canal (external) (meatus) — *see* Bite, ear
 auricle, ear — *see* Bite, ear
 axilla — *see* Bite, arm
 back (*see also* Bite, thorax, back)
  lower S31.050 ☑
   with penetration into retroperitoneal space S31.051 ☑
   superficial NEC S30.870 ☑
    insect S30.860 ☑
 bedbug — *see* Bite(s), by site, superficial, insect
 breast S21.05- ☑
  superficial NEC S20.17- ☑
   insect S20.16- ☑
 brow — *see* Bite, head, specified site NEC
 buttock S31.805 ☑
  left S31.825 ☑
  right S31.815 ☑
  superficial NEC S30.870 ☑
   insect S30.860 ☑
 calf — *see* Bite, leg
 canaliculus lacrimalis — *see* Bite, eyelid

Bite(s) — *continued*
 canthus, eye — *see* Bite, eyelid
 centipede — *see* Toxicity, venom, arthropod, centipede
 cheek (external) S01.45- ☑
  internal — *see* Bite, oral cavity
  superficial NEC S00.87 ☑
   insect S00.86 ☑
 chest wall — *see* Bite, thorax
 chigger B88.0
 chin — *see* Bite, head, specified site NEC
 clitoris — *see* Bite, vulva
 costal region — *see* Bite, thorax
 digit(s)
  hand — *see* Bite, finger
  toe — *see* Bite, toe
 ear (canal) (external) S01.35- ☑
  superficial NEC S00.47- ☑
   insect S00.46- ☑
 elbow S51.05- ☑
  superficial NEC S50.37- ☑
   insect S50.36- ☑
 epididymis — *see* Bite, testis
 epigastric region — *see* Bite, abdomen
 epiglottis — *see* Bite, neck, specified site NEC
 esophagus, cervical S11.25 ☑
  superficial NEC S10.17 ☑
   insect S10.16 ☑
 eyebrow — *see* Bite, eyelid
 eyelid S01.15- ☑
  superficial NEC S00.27- ☑
   insect S00.26- ☑
 face NEC — *see* Bite, head, specified site NEC
 finger(s) S61.259 ☑
  with
   damage to nail S61.359 ☑
  index S61.258 ☑
   with
    damage to nail S61.358 ☑
   left S61.251 ☑
    with
     damage to nail S61.351 ☑
   right S61.250 ☑
    with
     damage to nail S61.350 ☑
   superficial NEC S60.478 ☑
    insect S60.46- ☑
  little S61.25- ☑
   with
    damage to nail S61.35- ☑
   superficial NEC S60.47- ☑
    insect S60.46- ☑
  middle S61.25- ☑
   with
    damage to nail S61.35- ☑
   superficial NEC S60.47- ☑
    insect S60.46- ☑
  ring S61.25- ☑
   with
    damage to nail S61.35- ☑
   superficial NEC S60.47- ☑
    insect S60.46- ☑
  superficial NEC S60.479 ☑
   insect S60.469 ☑
  thumb — *see* Bite, thumb
 flank — *see* Bite, abdomen, wall
 flea — *see* Bite, by site, superficial, insect
 foot (except toe(s) alone) S91.35- ☑
  superficial NEC S90.87- ☑
   insect S90.86- ☑
  toe — *see* Bite, toe
 forearm S51.85- ☑
  elbow only — *see* Bite, elbow
  superficial NEC S50.87- ☑
   insect S50.86- ☑
 forehead — *see* Bite, head, specified site NEC
 genital organs, external
  female S30.552 ☑
   superficial NEC S30.876 ☑
    insect S30.866 ☑
   vagina and vulva — *see* Bite, vulva
  male S31.551 ☑
   penis — *see* Bite, penis
   scrotum — *see* Bite, scrotum
   superficial NEC S30.875 ☑
    insect S30.865 ☑

Bite(s) — *continued*
 genital organs, external — *continued*
  male — *continued*
   testes — *see* Bite, testis
 groin — *see* Bite, abdomen, wall
 gum — *see* Bite, oral cavity
 hand S61.45- ☑
  finger — *see* Bite, finger
  superficial NEC S60.57- ☑
   insect S60.56- ☑
  thumb — *see* Bite, thumb
 head S01.95 ☑
  cheek — *see* Bite, cheek
  ear — *see* Bite, ear
  eyelid — *see* Bite, eyelid
  lip — *see* Bite, lip
  nose — *see* Bite, nose
  oral cavity — *see* Bite, oral cavity
  scalp — *see* Bite, scalp
  specified site NEC S01.85 ☑
   superficial NEC S00.87 ☑
    insect S00.86 ☑
  superficial NEC S00.97 ☑
   insect S00.96 ☑
  temporomandibular area — *see* Bite, cheek
 heel — *see* Bite, foot
 hip S71.05- ☑
  superficial NEC S70.27- ☑
   insect S70.26- ☑
 hymen S31.45 ☑
 hypochondrium — *see* Bite, abdomen, wall
 hypogastric region — *see* Bite, abdomen, wall
 inguinal region — *see* Bite, abdomen, wall
 insect — *see* Bite, by site, superficial, insect
 instep — *see* Bite, foot
 interscapular region — *see* Bite, thorax, back
 jaw — *see* Bite, head, specified site NEC
 knee S81.05- ☑
  superficial NEC S80.27- ☑
   insect S80.26- ☑
 labium (majus) (minus) — *see* Bite, vulva
 lacrimal duct — *see* Bite, eyelid
 larynx S11.015 ☑
  superficial NEC S10.17 ☑
   insect S10.16 ☑
 leg (lower) S81.85- ☑
  ankle — *see* Bite, ankle
  foot — *see* Bite, foot
  knee — *see* Bite, knee
  superficial NEC S80.87- ☑
   insect S80.86- ☑
  toe — *see* Bite, toe
  upper — *see* Bite, thigh
 lip S01.551 ☑
  superficial NEC S00.571 ☑
   insect S00.561 ☑
 lizard (venomous) — *see* Venom, bite, reptile
 loin — *see* Bite, abdomen, wall
 lower back — *see* Bite, back, lower
 lumbar region — *see* Bite, back, lower
 malar region — *see* Bite, head, specified site NEC
 mammary — *see* Bite, breast
 marine animals (venomous) — *see* Toxicity, venom, marine animal
 mastoid region — *see* Bite, head, specified site NEC
 mouth — *see* Bite, oral cavity
 nail
  finger — *see* Bite, finger
  toe — *see* Bite, toe
 nape — *see* Bite, neck, specified site NEC
 nasal (septum) (sinus) — *see* Bite, nose
 nasopharynx — *see* Bite, head, specified site NEC
 neck S11.95 ☑
  involving
   cervical esophagus — *see* Bite, esophagus, cervical
   larynx — *see* Bite, larynx
   pharynx — *see* Bite, pharynx
   thyroid gland S11.15 ☑
   trachea — *see* Bite, trachea
  specified site NEC S11.85 ☑
   superficial NEC S10.87 ☑
    insect S10.86 ☑
  superficial NEC S10.97 ☑
   insect S10.96 ☑
  throat S11.85 ☑

Index

Birth — Bite

Bite(s) — *continued*
neck — *continued*
    throat — *continued*
        superficial NEC S10.17 ☑
            insect S10.16 ☑
    nose (septum) (sinus) S01.25 ☑
        superficial NEC S00.37 ☑
            insect S00.36 ☑
    occipital region — *see* Bite, scalp
    oral cavity S01.552 ☑
        superficial NEC S00.572 ☑
            insect S00.562 ☑
    orbital region — *see* Bite, eyelid
    palate — *see* Bite, oral cavity
    palm — *see* Bite, hand
    parietal region — *see* Bite, scalp
    pelvis S31.050 ☑
        with penetration into retroperitoneal space
            S31.051 ☑
        superficial NEC S30.870 ☑
            insect S30.860 ☑
    penis S31.25 ☑
        superficial NEC S30.872 ☑
            insect S30.862 ☑
    perineum
        female — *see* Bite, vulva
        male — *see* Bite, pelvis
    periocular area (with or without lacrimal passages) —
        see Bite, eyelid
    phalanges
        finger — *see* Bite, finger
        toe — *see* Bite, toe
    pharynx S11.25 ☑
        superficial NEC S10.17 ☑
            insect S10.16 ☑
    pinna — *see* Bite, ear
    poisonous — *see* Venom
    popliteal space — *see* Bite, knee
    prepuce — *see* Bite, penis
    pubic region — *see* Bite, abdomen, wall
    rectovaginal septum — *see* Bite, vulva
    red bug B88.0
    reptile NEC (*see also* Venom, bite, reptile)
        nonvenomous — *see* Bite, by site
        snake — *see* Venom, bite, snake
    sacral region — *see* Bite, back, lower
    sacroiliac region — *see* Bite, back, lower
    salivary gland — *see* Bite, oral cavity
    scalp S01.05 ☑
        superficial NEC S00.07 ☑
            insect S00.06 ☑
    scapular region — *see* Bite, shoulder
    scrotum S31.35 ☑
        superficial NEC S30.873 ☑
            insect S30.863 ☑
    sea-snake (venomous) — *see* Toxicity, venom, snake,
        sea snake
    shin — *see* Bite, leg
    shoulder S41.05- ☑
        superficial NEC S40.27- ☑
            insect S40.26- ☑
    snake (*see also* Venom, bite, snake)
        nonvenomous — *see* Bite, by site
    spermatic cord — *see* Bite, testis
    spider (venomous) — *see* Toxicity, venom, spider
        nonvenomous — *see* Bite, by site, superficial, insect
    sternal region — *see* Bite, thorax, front
    submaxillary region — *see* Bite, head, specified site
        NEC
    submental region — *see* Bite, head, specified site NEC
    subungual
        finger(s) — *see* Bite, finger
        toe — *see* Bite, toe
    superficial — *see* Bite, by site, superficial
    supraclavicular fossa S11.85 ☑
    supraorbital — *see* Bite, head, specified site NEC
    temple, temporal region — *see* Bite, head, specified
        site NEC
    temporomandibular area — *see* Bite, cheek
    testis S31.35 ☑
        superficial NEC S30.873 ☑
            insect S30.863 ☑
    thigh S71.15- ☑
        superficial NEC S70.37- ☑
            insect S70.36- ☑
    thorax, thoracic (wall) S21.95 ☑

Bite(s) — *continued*
thorax, thoracic — *continued*
    back S21.25- ☑
        with penetration into thoracic cavity S21.45- ☑
    breast — *see* Bite, breast
    front S21.15- ☑
        with penetration into thoracic cavity S21.35- ☑
    superficial NEC S20.97 ☑
        back S20.47- ☑
        front S20.37- ☑
        insect S20.96 ☑
            back S20.46- ☑
            front S20.36- ☑
throat — *see* Bite, neck, throat
thumb S61.05- ☑
    with
        damage to nail S61.15- ☑
    superficial NEC S60.37- ☑
        insect S60.36- ☑
thyroid S11.15 ☑
    superficial NEC S10.87 ☑
        insect S10.86 ☑
toe(s) S91.15- ☑
    with
        damage to nail S91.25- ☑
    great S91.15- ☑
        with
            damage to nail S91.25- ☑
    lesser S91.15- ☑
        with
            damage to nail S91.25- ☑
    superficial NEC S90.47- ☑
        great S90.47- ☑
        insect S90.46- ☑
            great S90.46- ☑
tongue S01.552 ☑
trachea S11.025 ☑
    superficial NEC S10.17 ☑
        insect S10.16 ☑
tunica vaginalis — *see* Bite, testis
tympanum, tympanic membrane — *see* Bite, ear
umbilical region S31.155 ☑
uvula — *see* Bite, oral cavity
vagina — *see* Bite, vulva
venomous — *see* Venom
vocal cords S11.035 ☑
    superficial NEC S10.17 ☑
        insect S10.16 ☑
vulva S31.45 ☑
    superficial NEC S30.874 ☑
        insect S30.864 ☑
wrist S61.55- ☑
    superficial NEC S60.87- ☑
        insect S60.86- ☑
Biting, cheek or lip K13.1
Biventricular failure (heart) I50.9
Björck (-Thorson) **syndrome** (malignant carcinoid) E34.0
Black
death A20.9
eye S00.1- ☑
hairy tongue K14.3
heel (foot) S90.3- ☑
lung (disease) J60
palm (hand) S60.22- ☑
Blackfan-Diamond anemia or syndrome (congenital
    hypoplastic anemia) D61.01
Blackhead L70.0
Blackout R55
Bladder — *see* condition
Blast (air) (hydraulic) (immersion) (underwater)
blindness S05.8X- ☑
injury
    abdomen or thorax — *see* Injury, by site
    ear (acoustic nerve trauma) — *see* Injury, nerve,
        acoustic, specified type NEC
    syndrome NEC T70.8
Blastoma — *see* Neoplasm, malignant, by site
pulmonary — *see* Neoplasm, lung, malignant
Blastomycosis, blastomycotic B40.9
Brazilian — *see* Paracoccidioidomycosis
cutaneous B40.3
disseminated B40.7
European — *see* Cryptococcosis
generalized B40.7
keloidal B48.0
North American B40.9

Blastomycosis, blastomycotic — *continued*
primary pulmonary B40.0
pulmonary B40.2
    acute B40.0
    chronic B40.1
skin B40.3
South American — *see* Paracoccidioidomycosis
specified NEC B40.89
Bleb(s) R23.8
emphysematous (lung) (solitary) J43.9
endophthalmitis H59.43
filtering (vitreous), after glaucoma surgery Z98.83
inflamed (infected), postprocedural H59.40
    stage 1 H59.41
    stage 2 H59.42
    stage 3 H59.43
lung (ruptured) J43.9
    congenital — *see* Atelectasis
    newborn P25.8
subpleural (emphysematous) J43.9
Blebitis, postprocedural H59.40
stage 1 H59.41
stage 2 H59.42
stage 3 H59.43
Bleeder (familial) (hereditary) — *see* Hemophilia
Bleeding (*see also* Hemorrhage)
anal K62.5
anovulatory N97.0
atonic, following delivery O72.1
capillary I78.8
    puerperal O72.2
contact (postcoital) N93.0
due to uterine subinvolution N85.3
ear — *see* Otorrhagia
excessive, associated with menopausal onset N92.4
familial — *see* Defect, coagulation
following intercourse N93.0
gastrointestinal K92.2
hemorrhoids — *see* Hemorrhoids
intermenstrual (regular) N92.3
    irregular N92.1
intraoperative — *see* Complication, intraoperative,
    hemorrhage
irregular N92.6
menopausal N92.4
newborn, intraventricular — *see* Newborn, affected
    by, hemorrhage, intraventricular
nipple N64.59
nose R04.0
ovulation N92.3
postclimacteric N95.0
postcoital N93.0
postmenopausal N95.0
postoperative — *see* Complication, postprocedural,
    hemorrhage
preclimacteric N92.4
puberty (excessive, with onset of menstrual periods)
    N92.2
rectum, rectal K62.5
    newborn P54.2
tendencies — *see* Defect, coagulation
throat R04.1
tooth socket (post-extraction) K91.840
umbilical stump P51.9
uterus, uterine NEC N93.9
    climacteric N92.4
    dysfunctional of functional N93.8
    menopausal N92.4
    preclimacteric or premenopausal N92.4
    unrelated to menstrual cycle N93.9
vagina, vaginal (abnormal) N93.9
    dysfunctional or functional N93.8
    newborn P54.6
vicarious N94.89
Blennorrhagia, blennorrhagic — *see* Gonorrhea
Blennorrhea (acute) (chronic) (*see also* Gonorrhea)
inclusion (neonatal) (newborn) P39.1
lower genitourinary tract (gonococcal) A54.00
neonatorum (gonococcal ophthalmia) A54.31
Blepharelosis — *see* Entropion
Blepharitis (angularis) (ciliaris) (eyelid) (marginal)
    (nonulcerative) H01.009
herpes zoster B02.39
left H01.006
    lower H01.005
    upper H01.004
right H01.003
    lower H01.002

☑ **Additional Character Required — Refer to the Tabular List for Character Selection**   ▽ **Subterms under main terms may continue to next column or page**

Blepharitis — *continued*
right — *continued*
upper H01.001
squamous H01.029
left H01.026
lower H01.025
upper H01.024
right H01.023
lower H01.022
upper H01.021
ulcerative H01.019
left H01.016
lower H01.015
upper H01.014
right H01.013
lower H01.012
upper H01.011
Blepharochalasis H02.30
congenital Q10.0
left H02.36
lower H02.35
upper H02.34
right H02.33
lower H02.32
upper H02.31
Blepharoclonus H02.59
Blepharoconjunctivitis H10.50- ☑
angular H10.52- ☑
contact H10.53- ☑
ligneous H10.51- ☑
Blepharophimosis (eyelid) H02.529
congenital Q10.3
left H02.526
lower H02.525
upper H02.524
right H02.523
lower H02.522
upper H02.521
Blepharoptosis H02.40- ☑
congenital Q10.0
mechanical H02.41- ☑
myogenic H02.42- ☑
neurogenic H02.43- ☑
paralytic H02.43- ☑
Blepharopyorrhea, gonococcal A54.39
Blepharospasm G24.5
drug induced G24.01
Blighted ovum O02.0
Blind (*see also* Blindness)
bronchus (congenital) Q32.4
loop syndrome K90.2
congenital Q43.8
sac, fallopian tube (congenital) Q50.6
spot, enlarged — *see* Defect, visual field, localized, scotoma, blind spot area
tract or tube, congenital NEC — *see* Atresia, by site
Blindness (acquired) (congenital) (both eyes) H54.0
blast S05.8X- ☑
color — *see* Deficiency, color vision
concussion S05.8X- ☑
cortical H47.619
left brain H47.612
right brain H47.611
day H53.11
due to injury (current episode) S05.9- ☑
sequelae — *code to* injury with seventh character S
eclipse (total) — *see* Retinopathy, solar
emotional (hysterical) F44.6
face H53.16
hysterical F44.6
legal (both eyes) (USA definition) H54.8
mind R48.8
night H53.60
abnormal dark adaptation curve H53.61
acquired H53.62
congenital H53.63
specified type NEC H53.69
vitamin A deficiency E50.5
one eye (other eye normal) H54.40
left (normal vision on right) H54.42
low vision on right H54.12
low vision, other eye H54.10
right (normal vision on left) H54.41
low vision on left H54.11
psychic R48.8
river B73.01
snow — *see* Photokeratitis

Blindness — *continued*
sun, solar — *see* Retinopathy, solar
transient — *see* Disturbance, vision, subjective, loss, transient
traumatic (current episode) S05.9- ☑
word (developmental) F81.0
acquired R48.0
secondary to organic lesion R48.0
Blister (nonthermal)
abdominal wall S30.821 ☑
alveolar process S00.522 ☑
ankle S90.52- ☑
antecubital space — *see* Blister, elbow
anus S30.827 ☑
arm (upper) S40.82- ☑
auditory canal — *see* Blister, ear
auricle — *see* Blister, ear
axilla — *see* Blister, arm
back, lower S30.820 ☑
beetle dermatitis L24.89
breast S20.12- ☑
brow S00.82 ☑
calf — *see* Blister, leg
canthus — *see* Blister, eyelid
cheek S00.82 ☑
internal S00.522 ☑
chest wall — *see* Blister, thorax
chin S00.82 ☑
costal region — *see* Blister, thorax
digit(s)
foot — *see* Blister, toe
hand — *see* Blister, finger
due to burn — *see* Burn, by site, second degree
ear S00.42- ☑
elbow S50.32- ☑
epiglottis S10.12 ☑
esophagus, cervical S10.12 ☑
eyebrow — *see* Blister, eyelid
eyelid S00.22- ☑
face S00.82 ☑
fever B00.1
finger(s) S60.429 ☑
index S60.42- ☑
little S60.42- ☑
middle S60.42- ☑
ring S60.42- ☑
foot (except toe(s) alone) S90.82- ☑
toe — *see* Blister, toe
forearm S50.82- ☑
elbow only — *see* Blister, elbow
forehead S00.82 ☑
fracture — *omit code*
genital organ
female S30.826 ☑
male S30.825 ☑
gum S00.522 ☑
hand S60.52- ☑
head S00.92 ☑
ear — *see* Blister, ear
eyelid — *see* Blister, eyelid
lip S00.521 ☑
nose S00.32 ☑
oral cavity S00.522 ☑
scalp S00.02 ☑
specified site NEC S00.82 ☑
heel — *see* Blister, foot
hip S70.22- ☑
interscapular region S20.429 ☑
jaw S00.82 ☑
knee S80.22- ☑
larynx S10.12 ☑
leg (lower) S80.82- ☑
knee — *see* Blister, knee
upper — *see* Blister, thigh
lip S00.521 ☑
malar region S00.82 ☑
mammary — *see* Blister, breast
mastoid region S00.82 ☑
mouth S00.522 ☑
multiple, skin, nontraumatic R23.8
nail
finger — *see* Blister, finger
toe — *see* Blister, toe
nasal S00.32 ☑
neck S10.92 ☑
specified site NEC S10.82 ☑

Blister — *continued*
neck — *continued*
throat S10.12 ☑
nose S00.32 ☑
occipital region S00.02 ☑
oral cavity S00.522 ☑
orbital region — *see* Blister, eyelid
palate S00.522 ☑
palm — *see* Blister, hand
parietal region S00.02 ☑
pelvis S30.820 ☑
penis S30.822 ☑
periocular area — *see* Blister, eyelid
phalanges
finger — *see* Blister, finger
toe — *see* Blister, toe
pharynx S10.12 ☑
pinna — *see* Blister, ear
popliteal space — *see* Blister, knee
scalp S00.02 ☑
scapular region — *see* Blister, shoulder
scrotum S30.823 ☑
shin — *see* Blister, leg
shoulder S40.22- ☑
sternal region S20.329 ☑
submaxillary region S00.82 ☑
submental region S00.82 ☑
subungual
finger(s) — *see* Blister, finger
toe(s) — *see* Blister, toe
supraclavicular fossa S10.82 ☑
supraorbital S00.82 ☑
temple S00.82 ☑
temporal region S00.82 ☑
testis S30.823 ☑
thermal — *see* Burn, second degree, by site
thigh S70.32- ☑
thorax, thoracic (wall) S20.92 ☑
back S20.42- ☑
front S20.32- ☑
throat S10.12 ☑
thumb S60.32- ☑
toe(s) S90.42- ☑
great S90.42- ☑
tongue S00.522 ☑
trachea S10.12 ☑
tympanum, tympanic membrane — *see* Blister, ear
upper arm — *see* Blister, arm (upper)
uvula S00.522 ☑
vagina S30.824 ☑
vocal cords S10.12 ☑
vulva S30.824 ☑
wrist S60.82- ☑
Bloating R14.0
Bloch-Sulzberger disease or syndrome Q82.3
Block, blocked
alveolocapillary J84.10
arborization (heart) I45.5
arrhythmic I45.9
atrioventricular (incomplete) (partial) I44.30
with atrioventricular dissociation I44.2
complete I44.2
congenital Q24.6
congenital Q24.6
first degree I44.0
second degree (types I and II) I44.1
specified NEC I44.39
third degree I44.2
types I and II I44.1
auriculoventricular — *see* Block, atrioventricular
bifascicular (cardiac) I45.2
bundle-branch (complete) (false) (incomplete) I45.4
bilateral I45.2
left I44.7
with right bundle branch block I45.2
hemiblock I44.60
anterior I44.4
posterior I44.5
incomplete I44.7
with right bundle branch block I45.2
right I45.10
with
left bundle branch block I45.2
left fascicular block I45.2
specified NEC I45.19
Wilson's type I45.19
cardiac I45.9

▽ Subterms under main terms may continue to next column or page   ☑ Additional Character Required — Refer to the Tabular List for Character Selection   39

Blepharitis — Block, blocked

Block, blocked — continued
  conduction I45.9
    complete I44.2
  fascicular (left) I44.60
    anterior I44.4
    posterior I44.5
    right I45.0
    specified NEC I44.69
  foramen Magendie (acquired) G91.1
    congenital Q03.1
      with spina bifida — see Spina bifida, by site, with hydrocephalus
  heart I45.9
    bundle branch I45.4
      bilateral I45.2
    complete (atrioventricular) I44.2
    congenital Q24.6
    first degree (atrioventricular) I44.0
    second degree (atrioventricular) I44.1
    specified type NEC I45.5
    third degree (atrioventricular) I44.2
  hepatic vein I82.0
  intraventricular (nonspecific) I45.4
    bundle branch
      bilateral I45.2
  kidney N28.9
    postcystoscopic or postprocedural N99.0
  Mobitz (types I and II) I44.1
  myocardial — see Block, heart
  nodal I45.5
  organ or site, congenital NEC — see Atresia, by site
  portal (vein) I81
  second degree (types I and II) I44.1
  sinoatrial I45.5
  sinoauricular I45.5
  third degree I44.2
  trifascicular I45.3
  tubal N97.1
  vein NOS I82.90
  Wenckebach (types I and II) I44.1
Blockage — see Obstruction
Blocq's disease F44.4
Blood
  constituents, abnormal R78.9
  disease D75.9
  donor — see Donor, blood
  dyscrasia D75.9
    with
      abortion — see Abortion, by type, complicated by hemorrhage
      ectopic pregnancy O08.1
      molar pregnancy O08.1
    following ectopic or molar pregnancy O08.1
    newborn P61.9
    puerperal, postpartum O72.3
  flukes NEC — see Schistosomiasis
  in
    feces K92.1
      occult R19.5
    urine — see Hematuria
  mole O02.0
  occult in feces R19.5
  pressure
    decreased, due to shock following injury T79.4 ☑
    examination only Z01.30
    fluctuating I99.8
    high — see Hypertension
      borderline R03.0
      incidental reading, without diagnosis of hypertension R03.0
    low (see also Hypotension)
      incidental reading, without diagnosis of hypotension R03.1
  spitting — see Hemoptysis
  staining cornea — see Pigmentation, cornea, stromal
  transfusion
    reaction or complication — see Complications, transfusion
  type
    A (Rh positive) Z67.10
      Rh negative Z67.11
    AB (Rh positive) Z67.30
      Rh negative Z67.31
    B (Rh positive) Z67.20
      Rh negative Z67.21
    O (Rh positive) Z67.40
      Rh negative Z67.41
    Rh (positive) Z67.90

Blood — continued
  type — continued
    Rh — continued
      negative Z67.91
  vessel rupture — see Hemorrhage
  vomiting — see Hematemesis
Blood-forming organs, disease D75.9
Bloodgood's disease — see Mastopathy, cystic
Bloom (-Machacek)(-Torre) **syndrome** Q82.8
Blount's disease or osteochondrosis — see Osteochondrosis, juvenile, tibia
Blue
  baby Q24.9
  diaper syndrome E72.09
  dome cyst (breast) — see Cyst, breast
  dot cataract Q12.0
  nevus D22.9
  sclera Q13.5
    with fragility of bone and deafness Q78.0
  toe syndrome I75.02- ☑
Blueness — see Cyanosis
Blues, postpartal O90.6
  baby O90.6
Blurring, visual H53.8
Blushing (abnormal) (excessive) R23.2
BMI — see Body, mass index
Boarder, hospital NEC Z76.4
  accompanying sick person Z76.3
  healthy infant or child Z76.2
    foundling Z76.1
Bockhart's impetigo L01.02
Bodechtel-Guttman disease (subacute sclerosing panencephalitis) A81.1
Boder-Sedgwick syndrome (ataxia-telangiectasia) G11.3
Body, bodies
  Aschoff's — see Myocarditis, rheumatic
  asteroid, vitreous — see Deposit, crystalline
  cytoid (retina) — see Occlusion, artery, retina
  drusen (degenerative) (macula) (retinal) (see also Degeneration, macula, drusen)
    optic disc — see Drusen, optic disc
  foreign — see Foreign body
  loose
    joint, except knee — see Loose, body, joint
      knee M23.4- ☑
    sheath, tendon — see Disorder, tendon, specified type NEC
  mass index (BMI)
    adult
      19 or less Z68.1
      20.0-20.9 Z68.20
      21.0-21.9 Z68.21
      22.0-22.9 Z68.22
      23.0-23.9 Z68.23
      24.0-24.9 Z68.24
      25.0-25.9 Z68.25
      26.0-26.9 Z68.26
      27.0-27.9 Z68.27
      28.0-28.9 Z68.28
      29.0-29.9 Z68.29
      30.0-30.9 Z68.30
      31.0-31.9 Z68.31
      32.0-32.9 Z68.32
      33.0-33.9 Z68.33
      34.0-34.9 Z68.34
      35.0-35.9 Z68.35
      36.0-36.9 Z68.36
      37.0-37.9 Z68.37
      38.0-38.9 Z68.38
      39.0-39.9 Z68.39
      40.0-44.9 Z68.41
      45.0-49.9 Z68.42
      50.0-59.9 Z68.43
      60.0-69.9 Z68.44
      70 and over Z68.45
    pediatric
      5th percentile to less than 85th percentile for age Z68.52
      85th percentile to less than 95th percentile for age Z68.53
      less than fifth percentile for age Z68.51
      greater than or equal to ninety-fifth percentile for age Z68.54
  Mooser's A75.2
  rice (see also Loose, body, joint)
    knee M23.4- ☑
  rocking F98.4

Boeck's
  disease or sarcoid — see Sarcoidosis
  lupoid (miliary) D86.3
Boerhaave's syndrome (spontaneous esophageal rupture) K22.3
Boggy
  cervix N88.8
  uterus N85.8
Boil (see also Furuncle, by site)
  Aleppo B55.1
  Baghdad B55.1
  Delhi B55.1
  lacrimal
    gland — see Dacryoadenitis
    passages (duct) (sac) — see Inflammation, lacrimal, passages, acute
  Natal B55.1
  orbit, orbital — see Abscess, orbit
  tropical B55.1
Bold hives — see Urticaria
Bombé, iris — see Membrane, pupillary
Bone — see condition
Bonnevie-Ullrich syndrome Q87.1
Bonnier's syndrome H81.8 ☑
Bonvale dam fever T73.3 ☑
Bony block of joint — see Ankylosis
BOOP (bronchiolitis obliterans organized pneumonia) J84.89
Borderline
  diabetes mellitus R73.09
  hypertension R03.0
  osteopenia M85.8- ☑
  pelvis, with obstruction during labor O65.1
  personality F60.3
Borna disease A83.9
Bornholm disease B33.0
Boston exanthem A88.0
Botalli, ductus (patent) (persistent) Q25.0
Bothriocephalus latus infestation B70.0
Botulism (foodborne intoxication) A05.1
  infant A48.51
  non-foodborne A48.52
  wound A48.52
Bouba — see Yaws
Bouchard's nodes (with arthropathy) M15.2
Bouffée délirante F23
Bouillaud's disease or syndrome (rheumatic heart disease) I01.9
Bourneville's disease Q85.1
Boutonniere deformity (finger) — see Deformity, finger, boutonniere
Bouveret (-Hoffmann) **syndrome** (paroxysmal tachycardia) I47.9
Bovine heart — see Hypertrophy, cardiac
Bowel — see condition
Bowen's
  dermatosis (precancerous) — see Neoplasm, skin, in situ
  disease — see Neoplasm, skin, in situ
  epithelioma — see Neoplasm, skin, in situ
  type
    epidermoid carcinoma-in-situ — see Neoplasm, skin, in situ
    intraepidermal squamous cell carcinoma — see Neoplasm, skin, in situ
Bowing
  femur (see also Deformity, limb, specified type NEC, thigh)
    congenital Q68.3
  fibula (see also Deformity, limb, specified type NEC, lower leg)
    congenital Q68.4
  forearm — see Deformity, limb, specified type NEC, forearm
  leg(s), long bones, congenital Q68.5
  radius — see Deformity, limb, specified type NEC, forearm
  tibia (see also Deformity, limb, specified type NEC, lower leg)
    congenital Q68.4
Bowleg(s) (acquired) M21.16- ☑
  congenital Q68.5
  rachitic E64.3
Boyd's dysentery A03.2
Brachial — see condition
Brachycardia R00.1
Brachycephaly Q75.0

Bradley's disease A08.19
Bradyarrhythmia, cardiac I49.8
Bradycardia (sinoatrial) (sinus) (vagal) R00.1
  neonatal P29.12
  reflex G90.09
  tachycardia syndrome I49.5
Bradykinesia R25.8
Bradypnea R06.89
Bradytachycardia I49.5
Brailsford's disease or osteochondrosis — *see* Osteochondrosis, juvenile, radius
Brain (*see also* condition)
  death G93.82
  syndrome — *see* Syndrome, brain
Branched-chain amino-acid disorder E71.2
Branchial — *see* condition
  cartilage, congenital Q18.2
Branchiogenic remnant (in neck) Q18.0
Brandt's syndrome (acrodermatitis enteropathica) E83.2
Brash (water) R12
Bravais-jacksonian epilepsy — *see* Epilepsy, localization-related, symptomatic, with simple partial seizures
Braxton Hicks contractions — *see* False, labor
Brazilian leishmaniasis B55.2
BRBPR K62.5
Break, retina (without detachment) H33.30- ☑
  with retinal detachment — *see* Detachment, retina
  horseshoe tear H33.31- ☑
  multiple H33.33- ☑
  round hole H33.32- ☑
Breakdown
  device, graft or implant (*see also* Complications, by site and type, mechanical) T85.618 ☑
    arterial graft NEC — *see* Complication, cardiovascular device, mechanical, vascular
    breast (implant) T85.41 ☑
    catheter NEC T85.618 ☑
      cystostomy T83.010 ☑
      dialysis (renal) T82.41 ☑
        intraperitoneal T85.611 ☑
      infusion NEC T82.514 ☑
        spinal (epidural) (subdural) T85.610 ☑
      urinary (indwelling) T83.018 ☑
    electronic (electrode) (pulse generator) (stimulator)
      bone T84.310 ☑
      cardiac T82.119 ☑
        electrode T82.110 ☑
        pulse generator T82.111 ☑
        specified type NEC T82.118 ☑
      nervous system — *see* Complication, prosthetic device, mechanical, electronic nervous system stimulator
      urinary — *see* Complication, genitourinary, device, urinary, mechanical
    fixation, internal (orthopedic) NEC — *see* Complication, fixation device, mechanical
    gastrointestinal — *see* Complications, prosthetic device, mechanical, gastrointestinal device
    genital NEC T83.418 ☑
      intrauterine contraceptive device T83.31 ☑
      penile prosthesis T83.410 ☑
    heart NEC — *see* Complication, cardiovascular device, mechanical
    joint prosthesis — *see* Complications..., joint prosthesis, internal, mechanical, by site
    ocular NEC — *see* Complications, prosthetic device, mechanical, ocular device
    orthopedic NEC — *see* Complication, orthopedic, device, mechanical
    specified NEC T85.618 ☑
    sutures, permanent T85.612 ☑
      used in bone repair — *see* Complications, fixation device, internal (orthopedic), mechanical
    urinary NEC (*see also* Complication, genitourinary, device, urinary, mechanical)
      graft T83.21 ☑
    vascular NEC — *see* Complication, cardiovascular device, mechanical
    ventricular intracranial shunt T85.01 ☑
  nervous F48.8
  perineum O90.1
  respirator J95.850
    specified NEC J95.859
  ventilator J95.850

Breakdown — *continued*
  ventilator — *continued*
    specified NEC J95.859
Breast (*see also* condition)
  buds E30.1
    in newborn P96.89
  dense R92.2
  nodule N63
Breath
  foul R19.6
  holder, child R06.89
  holding spell R06.89
  shortness R06.02
Breathing
  labored — *see* Hyperventilation
  mouth R06.5
    causing malocclusion M26.5 ☑
  periodic R06.3
    high altitude G47.32
Breathlessness R06.81
Breda's disease — *see* Yaws
Breech presentation (mother) O32.1 ☑
  causing obstructed labor O64.1 ☑
  footling O32.8 ☑
    causing obstructed labor O64.8 ☑
  incomplete O32.8 ☑
    causing obstructed labor O64.8 ☑
Breisky's disease N90.4
Brennemann's syndrome I88.0
Brenner
  tumor (benign) D27.9
    borderline malignancy D39.1- ☑
    malignant C56 ☑
    proliferating D39.1- ☑
Bretonneau's disease or angina A36.0
Breus' mole O02.0
Brevicollis Q76.49
Brickmakers' anemia B76.9 [D63.8]
Bridge, myocardial Q24.5
Bright red blood per rectum (BRBPR) K62.5
Bright's disease (*see also* Nephritis)
  arteriosclerotic — *see* Hypertension, kidney
Brill (-Zinsser) **disease** (recrudescent typhus) A75.1
  flea-borne A75.2
  louse-borne A75.1
Brill-Symmers' disease C82.90
Brion-Kayser disease — *see* Fever, parathyroid
Briquet's disorder or syndrome F45.0
Brissaud's
  infantilism or dwarfism E23.0
  motor-verbal tic F95.2
Brittle
  bones disease Q78.0
  nails L60.3
    congenital Q84.6
Broad (*see also* condition)
  beta disease E78.2
  ligament laceration syndrome N83.8
Broad- or floating-betalipoproteinemia E78.2
Brock's syndrome (atelectasis due to enlarged lymph nodes) J98.19
Brocq-Duhring disease (dermatitis herpetiformis) L13.0
Brodie's abscess or disease M86.8X- ☑
Broken
  arches (*see also* Deformity, limb, flat foot)
  arm (meaning upper limb) — *see* Fracture, arm
  back — *see* Fracture, vertebra
  bone — *see* Fracture
  implant or internal device — *see* Complications, by site and type, mechanical
  leg (meaning lower limb) — *see* Fracture, leg
  nose S02.2 ☑
  tooth, teeth — *see* Fracture, tooth
Bromhidrosis, bromidrosis L75.0
Bromidism, bromism G92
  chronic (dependence) F13.20
  due to
    correct substance properly administered — *see* Table of Drugs and Chemicals, by drug, adverse effect
    overdose or wrong substance given or taken — *see* Table of Drugs and Chemicals, by drug, poisoning
Bromidrosiphobia F40.298
Bronchi, bronchial — *see* condition
Bronchiectasis (cylindrical) (diffuse) (fusiform) (localized) (saccular) J47.9

Bronchiectasis — *continued*
  with
    acute
      bronchitis J47.0
      lower respiratory infection J47.0
    exacerbation (acute) J47.1
  congenital Q33.4
  tuberculous NEC — *see* Tuberculosis, pulmonary
Bronchiolectasis — *see* Bronchiectasis
Bronchiolitis (acute) (infective) (subacute) J21.9
  with
    bronchospasm or obstruction J21.9
    influenza, flu or grippe — *see* Influenza, with, respiratory manifestations NEC
  chemical (chronic) J68.4
    acute J68.0
  chronic (fibrosing) (obliterative) J44.9
  due to
    external agent — *see* Bronchitis, acute, due to
    human metapneumovirus J21.1
    respiratory syncytial virus J21.0
    specified organism NEC J21.8
  fibrosa obliterans J44.9
  influenzal — *see* Influenza, with, respiratory manifestations NEC
  obliterans J42
    with organizing pneumonia (BOOP) J84.89
  obliterative (chronic) (subacute) J44.9
    due to chemicals, gases, fumes or vapors (inhalation) J68.4
    due to fumes or vapors J68.4
  respiratory, interstitial lung disease J84.115
Bronchitis (diffuse) (fibrinous) (hypostatic) (infective) (membranous) J40
  with
    influenza, flu or grippe — *see* Influenza, with, respiratory manifestations NEC
    obstruction (airway) (lung) J44.9
    tracheitis (15 years of age and above) J40
      acute or subacute J20.9
      chronic J42
      under 15 years of age J20.9
  acute or subacute (with bronchospasm or obstruction) J20.9
    with
      bronchiectasis J47.0
      chronic obstructive pulmonary disease J44.0
    chemical (due to gases, fumes or vapors) J68.0
    due to
      fumes or vapors J68.0
      Haemophilus influenzae J20.1
      Mycoplasma pneumoniae J20.0
      radiation J70.0
      specified organism NEC J20.8
      Streptococcus J20.2
      virus
        coxsackie J20.3
        echovirus J20.7
        parainfluenzae J20.4
        respiratory syncytial J20.5
        rhinovirus J20.6
    viral NEC J20.8
  allergic (acute) J45.909
    with
      exacerbation (acute) J45.901
      status asthmaticus J45.902
  arachidic T17.528 ☑
  aspiration (due to fumes or vapors) J68.0
  asthmatic J45.9 ☑
    chronic J44.9
      with
        acute lower respiratory infection J44.0
        exacerbation (acute) J44.1
  capillary — *see* Pneumonia, broncho
  caseous (tuberculous) A15.5
  Castellani's A69.8
  catarrhal (15 years of age and above) J40
    acute — *see* Bronchitis, acute
    chronic J41.0
    under 15 years of age J20.9
  chemical (acute) (subacute) J68.0
    chronic J68.4
    due to fumes or vapors J68.0
      chronic J68.4
  chronic J42
    with
      airways obstruction J44.9
      tracheitis (chronic) J42

Bradley's disease — Bronchitis

▽ Subterms under main terms may continue to next column or page   ☑ Additional Character Required — Refer to the Tabular List for Character Selection   41

Bronchitis — *continued*
  chronic — *continued*
    asthmatic (obstructive) J44.9
    catarrhal J41.0
    chemical (due to fumes or vapors) J68.4
    due to
      chemicals, gases, fumes or vapors (inhalation) J68.4
      radiation J70.1
      tobacco smoking J41.0
    emphysematous J44.9
    mucopurulent J41.1
    non-obstructive J41.0
    obliterans J44.9
    obstructive J44.9
    purulent J41.1
    simple J41.0
  croupous — *see* Bronchitis, acute
  due to gases, fumes or vapors (chemical) J68.0
  emphysematous (obstructive) J44.9
  exudative — *see* Bronchitis, acute
  fetid J41.1
  grippal — *see* Influenza, with, respiratory manifestations NEC
  in those under 15 years age — *see* Bronchitis, acute
    chronic — *see* Bronchitis, chronic
  influenzal — *see* Influenza, with, respiratory manifestations NEC
  mixed simple and mucopurulent J41.8
  moulder's J62.8
  mucopurulent (chronic) (recurrent) J41.1
    acute or subacute J20.9
    simple (mixed) J41.8
  obliterans (chronic) J44.9
  obstructive (chronic) (diffuse) J44.9
  pituitous J41.1
  pneumococcal, acute or subacute J20.2
  pseudomembranous, acute or subacute — *see* Bronchitis, acute
  purulent (chronic) (recurrent) J41.1
    acute or subacute — *see* Bronchitis, acute
  putrid J41.1
  senile (chronic) J42
  simple and mucopurulent (mixed) J41.8
  smokers' J41.0
  spirochetal NEC A69.8
  subacute — *see* Bronchitis, acute
  suppurative (chronic) J41.1
    acute or subacute — *see* Bronchitis, acute
  tuberculous A15.5
  under 15 years of age — *see* Bronchitis, acute
    chronic — *see* Bronchitis, chronic
  viral NEC, acute or subacute (*see also* Bronchitis, acute) J20.8
Bronchoalveolitis J18.0
Bronchoaspergillosis B44.1
Bronchocele meaning goiter E04.0
Broncholithiasis J98.09
  tuberculous NEC A15.5
Bronchomalacia J98.09
  congenital Q32.2
Bronchomycosis NOS B49 [J99]
  candidal B37.1
Bronchopleuropneumonia — *see* Pneumonia, broncho
Bronchopneumonia — *see* Pneumonia, broncho
Bronchopneumonitis — *see* Pneumonia, broncho
Bronchopulmonary — *see* condition
Bronchopulmonitis — *see* Pneumonia, broncho
Bronchorrhagia (see Hemoptysis)
Bronchorrhea J98.09
  acute J20.9
  chronic (infective) (purulent) J42
Bronchospasm (acute) J98.01
  with
    bronchiolitis, acute J21.9
    bronchitis, acute (conditions in J20) — *see* Bronchitis, acute
    due to external agent — *see* condition, respiratory, acute, due to
  exercise induced J45.990
Bronchospirochetosis A69.8
  Castellani A69.8
Bronchostenosis J98.09
Bronchus — *see* condition
Brontophobia F40.220
Bronze baby syndrome P83.8
Brooke's tumor — *see* Neoplasm, skin, benign

Brown enamel of teeth (hereditary) K00.5
Brown's sheath syndrome H50.61- ☑
Brown-Séquard disease, paralysis or syndrome G83.81
Bruce sepsis A23.0
Brucellosis (infection) A23.9
  abortus A23.1
  canis A23.3
  dermatitis A23.9
  melitensis A23.0
  mixed A23.8
  sepsis A23.9
    melitensis A23.0
    specified NEC A23.8
  suis A23.2
Bruck-de Lange disease Q87.1
Bruck's disease — *see* Deformity, limb
Brugsch's syndrome Q82.8
Bruise (skin surface intact) (*see also* Contusion)
  with
    open wound — *see* Wound, open
  internal organ — *see* Injury, by site
  newborn P54.5
  scalp, due to birth injury, newborn P12.3
  umbilical cord O69.5 ☑
Bruit (arterial) R09.89
  cardiac R01.1
Brush burn — *see* Abrasion, by site
Bruton's X-linked agammaglobulinemia D80.0
Bruxism
  psychogenic F45.8
  sleep related G47.63
Bubbly lung syndrome P27.0
Bubo I88.8
  blennorrhagic (gonococcal) A54.89
  chancroidal A57
  climatic A55
  due to Haemophilus ducreyi A57
  gonococcal A54.89
  indolent (nonspecific) I88.8
  inguinal (nonspecific) I88.8
    chancroidal A57
    climatic A55
    due to H. ducreyi A57
    infective I88.8
  scrofulous (tuberculous) A18.2
  soft chancre A57
  suppurating — *see* Lymphadenitis, acute
  syphilitic (primary) A51.0
    congenital A50.07
  tropical A55
  virulent (chancroidal) A57
Bubonic plague A20.0
Bubonocele — *see* Hernia, inguinal
Buccal — *see* condition
Buchanan's disease or osteochondrosis M91.0
Buchem's syndrome (hyperostosis corticalis) M85.2
Bucket-handle fracture or tear (semilunar cartilage) — *see* Tear, meniscus
Budd-Chiari syndrome (hepatic vein thrombosis) I82.0
Budgerigar fancier's disease or lung J67.2
Buds
  breast E30.1
    in newborn P96.89
Buerger's disease (thromboangiitis obliterans) I73.1
Bulbar — *see* condition
Bulbus cordis (left ventricle) (persistent) Q21.8
Bulimia (nervosa) F50.2
  atypical F50.9
  normal weight F50.9
Bulky
  stools R19.5
  uterus N85.2
Bulla (e) R23.8
  lung (emphysematous) (solitary) J43.9
    newborn P25.8
Bullet wound (*see also* Wound, open)
  fracture — *code as* Fracture, by site
  internal organ — *see* Injury, by site
Bundle
  branch block (complete) (false) (incomplete) — *see* Block, bundle-branch
  of His — *see* condition
Bunion — *see* Deformity, toe, hallux valgus
Buphthalmia, buphthalmos (congenital) Q15.0
Burdwan fever B55.0
Bürger-Grütz disease or syndrome E78.3

Buried
  penis (congenital) Q55.64
    acquired N48.83
  roots K08.3
Burke's syndrome K86.8
Burkitt
  cell leukemia C91.0- ☑
  lymphoma (malignant) C83.7- ☑
    small noncleaved, diffuse C83.7- ☑
    spleen C83.77
    undifferentiated C83.7- ☑
  tumor C83.7- ☑
  type
    acute lymphoblastic leukemia C91.0- ☑
    undifferentiated C83.7- ☑
Burn (electricity) (flame) (hot gas, liquid or hot object) (radiation) (steam) (thermal) T30.0
  abdomen, abdominal (muscle) (wall) T21.02 ☑
    first degree T21.12 ☑
    second degree T21.22 ☑
    third degree T21.32 ☑
  above elbow T22.039 ☑
    first degree T22.139 ☑
    left T22.032 ☑
      first degree T22.132 ☑
      second degree T22.232 ☑
      third degree T22.332 ☑
    right T22.031 ☑
      first degree T22.131 ☑
      second degree T22.231 ☑
      third degree T22.331 ☑
    second degree T22.239 ☑
    third degree T22.339 ☑
  acid (caustic) (external) (internal) — *see* Corrosion, by site
  alimentary tract NEC T28.2 ☑
    esophagus T28.1 ☑
    mouth T28.0 ☑
    pharynx T28.0 ☑
  alkaline (caustic) (external) (internal) — *see* Corrosion, by site
  ankle T25.019 ☑
    first degree T25.119 ☑
    left T25.012 ☑
      first degree T25.112 ☑
      second degree T25.212 ☑
      third degree T25.312 ☑
    multiple with foot — *see* Burn, lower, limb, multiple, ankle and foot
    right T25.011 ☑
      first degree T25.111 ☑
      second degree T25.211 ☑
      third degree T25.311 ☑
    second degree T25.219 ☑
    third degree T25.319 ☑
  anus — *see* Burn, buttock
  arm (lower) (upper) — *see* Burn, upper, limb
  axilla T22.049 ☑
    first degree T22.149 ☑
    left T22.042 ☑
      first degree T22.142 ☑
      second degree T22.242 ☑
      third degree T22.342 ☑
    right T22.041 ☑
      first degree T22.141 ☑
      second degree T22.241 ☑
      third degree T22.341 ☑
    second degree T22.249 ☑
    third degree T22.349 ☑
  back (lower) T21.04 ☑
    first degree T21.14 ☑
    second degree T21.24 ☑
    third degree T21.34 ☑
    upper T21.03 ☑
      first degree T21.13 ☑
      second degree T21.23 ☑
      third degree T21.33 ☑
  blisters — *code as* Burn, second degree, by site
  breast(s) — *see* Burn, chest wall
  buttock(s) T21.05 ☑
    first degree T21.15 ☑
    second degree T21.25 ☑
    third degree T21.35 ☑
  calf T24.039 ☑
    first degree T24.139 ☑
    left T24.032 ☑

☑ Additional Character Required — Refer to the Tabular List for Character Selection   ▽ Subterms under main terms may continue to next column or page

Burn — *continued*
calf — *continued*
left — *continued*
first degree T24.132 ✓
second degree T24.232 ✓
third degree T24.332 ✓
right T24.031 ✓
first degree T24.131 ✓
second degree T24.231 ✓
third degree T24.331 ✓
second degree T24.239 ✓
third degree T24.339 ✓
canthus (eye) — *see* Burn, eyelid
caustic acid or alkaline — *see* Corrosion, by site
cervix T28.3 ✓
cheek T20.06 ✓
first degree T20.16 ✓
second degree T20.26 ✓
third degree T20.36 ✓
chemical (acids) (alkalines) (caustics) (external) (internal) — *see* Corrosion, by site
chest wall T21.01 ✓
first degree T21.11 ✓
second degree T21.21 ✓
third degree T21.31 ✓
chin T20.03 ✓
first degree T20.13 ✓
second degree T20.23 ✓
third degree T20.33 ✓
colon T28.2 ✓
conjunctiva (and cornea) — *see* Burn, cornea
cornea (and conjunctiva) T26.1- ✓
chemical — *see* Corrosion, cornea
corrosion (external) (internal) — *see* Corrosion, by site
deep necrosis of underlying tissue — *code as* Burn, third degree, by site
dorsum of hand T23.069 ✓
first degree T23.169 ✓
left T23.062 ✓
first degree T23.162 ✓
second degree T23.262 ✓
third degree T23.362 ✓
right T23.061 ✓
first degree T23.161 ✓
second degree T23.261 ✓
third degree T23.361 ✓
second degree T23.269 ✓
third degree T23.369 ✓
due to ingested chemical agent — *see* Corrosion, by site
ear (auricle) (external) (canal) T20.01 ✓
first degree T20.11 ✓
second degree T20.21 ✓
third degree T20.31 ✓
elbow T22.029 ✓
first degree T22.129 ✓
left T22.022 ✓
first degree T22.122 ✓
second degree T22.222 ✓
third degree T22.322 ✓
right T22.021 ✓
first degree T22.121 ✓
second degree T22.221 ✓
third degree T22.321 ✓
second degree T22.229 ✓
third degree T22.329 ✓
epidermal loss — *code as* Burn, second degree, by site
erythema, erythematous — *code as* Burn, first degree, by site
esophagus T28.1 ✓
extent (percentage of body surface)
less than 10 percent T31.0
10-19 percent T31.10
with 0-9 percent third degree burns T31.10
with 10-19 percent third degree burns T31.11
20-29 percent T31.20
with 0-9 percent third degree burns T31.20
with 10-19 percent third degree burns T31.21
with 20-29 percent third degree burns T31.22
30-39 percent T31.30
with 0-9 percent third degree burns T31.30
with 10-19 percent third degree burns T31.31
with 20-29 percent third degree burns T31.32
with 30-39 percent third degree burns T31.33
40-49 percent T31.40
with 0-9 percent third degree burns T31.40

Burn — *continued*
extent — *continued*
40-49 percent — *continued*
with 10-19 percent third degree burns T31.41
with 20-29 percent third degree burns T31.42
with 30-39 percent third degree burns T31.43
with 40-49 percent third degree burns T31.44
50-59 percent T31.50
with 0-9 percent third degree burns T31.50
with 10-19 percent third degree burns T31.51
with 20-29 percent third degree burns T31.52
with 30-39 percent third degree burns T31.53
with 40-49 percent third degree burns T31.54
with 50-59 percent third degree burns T31.55
60-69 percent T31.60
with 0-9 percent third degree burns T31.60
with 10-19 percent third degree burns T31.61
with 20-29 percent third degree burns T31.62
with 30-39 percent third degree burns T31.63
with 40-49 percent third degree burns T31.64
with 50-59 percent third degree burns T31.65
with 60-69 percent third degree burns T31.66
70-79 percent T31.70
with 0-9 percent third degree burns T31.70
with 10-19 percent third degree burns T31.71
with 20-29 percent third degree burns T31.72
with 30-39 percent third degree burns T31.73
with 40-49 percent third degree burns T31.74
with 50-59 percent third degree burns T31.75
with 60-69 percent third degree burns T31.76
with 70-79 percent third degree burns T31.77
80-89 percent T31.80
with 0-9 percent third degree burns T31.80
with 10-19 percent third degree burns T31.81
with 20-29 percent third degree burns T31.82
with 30-39 percent third degree burns T31.83
with 40-49 percent third degree burns T31.84
with 50-59 percent third degree burns T31.85
with 60-69 percent third degree burns T31.86
with 70-79 percent third degree burns T31.87
with 80-89 percent third degree burns T31.88
90 percent or more T31.90
with 0-9 percent third degree burns T31.90
with 10-19 percent third degree burns T31.91
with 20-29 percent third degree burns T31.92
with 30-39 percent third degree burns T31.93
with 40-49 percent third degree burns T31.94
with 50-59 percent third degree burns T31.95
with 60-69 percent third degree burns T31.96
with 70-79 percent third degree burns T31.97
with 80-89 percent third degree burns T31.98
with 90 percent or more third degree burns T31.99
extremity — *see* Burn, limb
eye(s) and adnexa T26.4- ✓
with resulting rupture and destruction of eyeball T26.2- ✓
conjunctival sac — *see* Burn, cornea
cornea — *see* Burn, cornea
lid — *see* Burn, eyelid
periocular area — *see* Burn, eyelid
specified site NEC T26.3- ✓
eyeball — *see* Burn, eye
eyelid(s) T26.0- ✓
chemical — *see* Corrosion, eyelid
face — *see* Burn, head
finger T23.029 ✓
first degree T23.129 ✓
left T23.022 ✓
first degree T23.122 ✓
second degree T23.222 ✓
third degree T23.322 ✓
multiple sites (without thumb) T23.039 ✓
with thumb T23.049 ✓
first degree T23.149 ✓
left T23.042 ✓
first degree T23.142 ✓
second degree T23.242 ✓
third degree T23.342 ✓
right T23.041 ✓
first degree T23.141 ✓
second degree T23.241 ✓
third degree T23.341 ✓
second degree T23.249 ✓
third degree T23.349 ✓
first degree T23.139 ✓
left T23.032 ✓

Burn — *continued*
finger — *continued*
multiple sites — *continued*
left — *continued*
first degree T23.132 ✓
second degree T23.232 ✓
third degree T23.332 ✓
right T23.031 ✓
first degree T23.131 ✓
second degree T23.231 ✓
third degree T23.331 ✓
second degree T23.239 ✓
third degree T23.339 ✓
right T23.021 ✓
first degree T23.121 ✓
second degree T23.221 ✓
third degree T23.321 ✓
second degree T23.229 ✓
third degree T23.329 ✓
flank — *see* Burn, abdominal wall
foot T25.029 ✓
first degree T25.129 ✓
left T25.022 ✓
first degree T25.122 ✓
second degree T25.222 ✓
third degree T25.322 ✓
multiple with ankle — *see* Burn, lower, limb, multiple, ankle and foot
right T25.021 ✓
first degree T25.121 ✓
second degree T25.221 ✓
third degree T25.321 ✓
second degree T25.229 ✓
third degree T25.329 ✓
forearm T22.019 ✓
first degree T22.119 ✓
left T22.012 ✓
first degree T22.112 ✓
second degree T22.212 ✓
third degree T22.312 ✓
right T22.011 ✓
first degree T22.111 ✓
second degree T22.211 ✓
third degree T22.311 ✓
second degree T22.219 ✓
third degree T22.319 ✓
forehead T20.06 ✓
first degree T20.16 ✓
second degree T20.26 ✓
third degree T20.36 ✓
fourth degree — *code as* Burn, third degree, by site
friction — *see* Burn, by site
from swallowing caustic or corrosive substance NEC — *see* Corrosion, by site
full thickness skin loss — *code as* Burn, third degree, by site
gastrointestinal tract NEC T28.2 ✓
from swallowing caustic or corrosive substance T28.7 ✓
genital organs
external
female T21.07 ✓
first degree T21.17 ✓
second degree T21.27 ✓
third degree T21.37 ✓
male T21.06 ✓
first degree T21.16 ✓
second degree T21.26 ✓
third degree T21.36 ✓
internal T28.3 ✓
from caustic or corrosive substance T28.8 ✓
groin — *see* Burn, abdominal wall
hand(s) T23.009 ✓
back — *see* Burn, dorsum of hand
finger — *see* Burn, finger
first degree T23.109 ✓
left T23.002 ✓
first degree T23.102 ✓
second degree T23.202 ✓
third degree T23.302 ✓
multiple sites with wrist T23.099 ✓
first degree T23.199 ✓
left T23.092 ✓
first degree T23.192 ✓
second degree T23.292 ✓
third degree T23.392 ✓

Burn — *continued*
- hand(s) — *continued*
  - multiple sites with wrist — *continued*
    - right T23.091 ☑
      - first degree T23.191 ☑
        - second degree T23.291 ☑
        - third degree T23.391 ☑
    - second degree T23.299 ☑
    - third degree T23.399 ☑
  - palm — *see* Burn, palm
  - right T23.001 ☑
    - first degree T23.101 ☑
    - second degree T23.201 ☑
    - third degree T23.301 ☑
  - second degree T23.209 ☑
  - third degree T23.309 ☑
  - thumb — *see* Burn, thumb
- head (and face) (and neck) T20.00 ☑
  - cheek — *see* Burn, cheek
  - chin — *see* Burn, chin
  - ear — *see* Burn, ear
  - eye(s) only — *see* Burn, eye
  - first degree T20.10 ☑
  - forehead — *see* Burn, forehead
  - lip — *see* Burn, lip
  - multiple sites T20.09 ☑
    - first degree T20.19 ☑
    - second degree T20.29 ☑
    - third degree T20.39 ☑
  - neck — *see* Burn, neck
  - nose — *see* Burn, nose
  - scalp — *see* Burn, scalp
  - second degree T20.20 ☑
  - third degree T20.30 ☑
- hip(s) — *see* Burn, lower, limb
- inhalation — *see* Burn, respiratory tract
  - caustic or corrosive substance (fumes) — *see* Corrosion, respiratory tract
- internal organ(s) T28.40 ☑
  - alimentary tract T28.2 ☑
    - esophagus T28.1 ☑
  - eardrum T28.41 ☑
  - esophagus T28.1 ☑
  - from caustic or corrosive substance (swallowing) NEC — *see* Corrosion, by site
  - genitourinary T28.3 ☑
  - mouth T28.0 ☑
  - pharynx T28.0 ☑
  - respiratory tract — *see* Burn, respiratory tract
  - specified organ NEC T28.49 ☑
- interscapular region — *see* Burn, back, upper
- intestine (large) (small) T28.2 ☑
- knee T24.029 ☑
  - first degree T24.129 ☑
  - left T24.022 ☑
    - first degree T24.122 ☑
    - second degree T24.222 ☑
    - third degree T24.322 ☑
  - right T24.021 ☑
    - first degree T24.121 ☑
    - second degree T24.221 ☑
    - third degree T24.321 ☑
  - second degree T24.229 ☑
  - third degree T24.329 ☑
- labium (majus) (minus) — *see* Burn, genital organs, external, female
- lacrimal apparatus, duct, gland or sac — *see* Burn, eye, specified site NEC
- larynx T27.0 ☑
  - with lung T27.1 ☑
- leg(s) (lower) (upper) — *see* Burn, lower, limb
- lightning — *see* Burn, by site
- limb(s)
  - lower (except ankle or foot alone) — *see* Burn, lower, limb
  - upper — *see* Burn, upper limb
- lip(s) T20.02 ☑
  - first degree T20.12 ☑
  - second degree T20.22 ☑
  - third degree T20.32 ☑
- lower
  - back — *see* Burn, back
  - limb T24.009 ☑
    - ankle — *see* Burn, ankle
    - calf — *see* Burn, calf
    - first degree T24.109 ☑

Burn — *continued*
- lower — *continued*
  - limb — *continued*
    - foot — *see* Burn, foot
    - hip — *see* Burn, thigh
    - knee — *see* Burn, knee
    - left T24.002 ☑
      - first degree T24.102 ☑
      - second degree T24.202 ☑
      - third degree T24.302 ☑
    - multiple sites, except ankle and foot T24.099 ☑
      - ankle and foot T25.099 ☑
        - first degree T25.199 ☑
        - left T25.092 ☑
          - first degree T25.192 ☑
          - second degree T25.292 ☑
          - third degree T25.392 ☑
        - right T25.091 ☑
          - first degree T25.191 ☑
          - second degree T25.291 ☑
          - third degree T25.391 ☑
        - second degree T25.299 ☑
        - third degree T25.399 ☑
      - first degree T24.199 ☑
      - left T24.092 ☑
        - first degree T24.192 ☑
        - second degree T24.292 ☑
        - third degree T24.392 ☑
      - right T24.091 ☑
        - first degree T24.191 ☑
        - second degree T24.291 ☑
        - third degree T24.391 ☑
      - second degree T24.299 ☑
      - third degree T24.399 ☑
    - right T24.001 ☑
      - first degree T24.101 ☑
      - second degree T24.201 ☑
      - third degree T24.301 ☑
    - second degree T24.209 ☑
    - thigh — *see* Burn, thigh
    - third degree T24.309 ☑
    - toe — *see* Burn, toe
- lung (with larynx and trachea) T27.1 ☑
- mouth T28.0 ☑
- neck T20.07 ☑
  - first degree T20.17 ☑
  - second degree T20.27 ☑
  - third degree T20.37 ☑
- nose (septum) T20.04 ☑
  - first degree T20.14 ☑
  - second degree T20.24 ☑
  - third degree T20.34 ☑
- ocular adnexa — *see* Burn, eye
- orbit region — *see* Burn, eyelid
- palm T23.059 ☑
  - first degree T23.159 ☑
  - left T23.052 ☑
    - first degree T23.152 ☑
    - second degree T23.252 ☑
    - third degree T23.352 ☑
  - right T23.051 ☑
    - first degree T23.151 ☑
    - second degree T23.251 ☑
    - third degree T23.351 ☑
  - second degree T23.259 ☑
  - third degree T23.359 ☑
- partial thickness — *code as* Burn, unspecified degree, by site
- pelvis — *see* Burn, trunk
- penis — *see* Burn, genital organs, external, male
- perineum
  - female — *see* Burn, genital organs, external, female
  - male — *see* Burn, genital organs, external, male
- periocular area — *see* Burn, eyelid
- pharynx T28.0 ☑
- rectum T28.2 ☑
- respiratory tract T27.3 ☑
  - larynx — *see* Burn, larynx
  - specified part NEC T27.2 ☑
  - trachea — *see* Burn, trachea
- sac, lacrimal — *see* Burn, eye, specified site NEC
- scalp T20.05 ☑
  - first degree T20.15 ☑
  - second degree T20.25 ☑
  - third degree T20.35 ☑

Burn — *continued*
- scapular region T22.069 ☑
  - first degree T22.169 ☑
  - left T22.062 ☑
    - first degree T22.162 ☑
    - second degree T22.262 ☑
    - third degree T22.362 ☑
  - right T22.061 ☑
    - first degree T22.161 ☑
    - second degree T22.261 ☑
    - third degree T22.361 ☑
  - second degree T22.269 ☑
  - third degree T22.369 ☑
- sclera — *see* Burn, eye, specified site NEC
- scrotum — *see* Burn, genital organs, external, male
- shoulder T22.059 ☑
  - first degree T22.159 ☑
  - left T22.052 ☑
    - first degree T22.152 ☑
    - second degree T22.252 ☑
    - third degree T22.352 ☑
  - right T22.051 ☑
    - first degree T22.151 ☑
    - second degree T22.251 ☑
    - third degree T22.351 ☑
  - second degree T22.259 ☑
  - third degree T22.359 ☑
- stomach T28.2 ☑
- temple — *see* Burn, head
- testis — *see* Burn, genital organs, external, male
- thigh T24.019 ☑
  - first degree T24.119 ☑
  - left T24.012 ☑
    - first degree T24.112 ☑
    - second degree T24.212 ☑
    - third degree T24.312 ☑
  - right T24.011 ☑
    - first degree T24.111 ☑
    - second degree T24.211 ☑
    - third degree T24.311 ☑
  - second degree T24.219 ☑
  - third degree T24.319 ☑
- thorax (external) — *see* Burn, trunk
- throat (meaning pharynx) T28.0 ☑
- thumb(s) T23.019 ☑
  - first degree T23.119 ☑
  - left T23.012 ☑
    - first degree T23.112 ☑
    - second degree T23.212 ☑
    - third degree T23.312 ☑
  - multiple sites with fingers T23.049 ☑
    - first degree T23.149 ☑
    - left T23.042 ☑
      - first degree T23.142 ☑
      - second degree T23.242 ☑
      - third degree T23.342 ☑
    - right T23.041 ☑
      - first degree T23.141 ☑
      - second degree T23.241 ☑
      - third degree T23.341 ☑
    - second degree T23.249 ☑
    - third degree T23.349 ☑
  - right T23.011 ☑
    - first degree T23.111 ☑
    - second degree T23.211 ☑
    - third degree T23.311 ☑
  - second degree T23.219 ☑
  - third degree T23.319 ☑
- toe T25.039 ☑
  - first degree T25.139 ☑
  - left T25.032 ☑
    - first degree T25.132 ☑
    - second degree T25.232 ☑
    - third degree T25.332 ☑
  - right T25.031 ☑
    - first degree T25.131 ☑
    - second degree T25.231 ☑
    - third degree T25.331 ☑
  - second degree T25.239 ☑
  - third degree T25.339 ☑
- tongue T28.0 ☑
- tonsil(s) T28.0 ☑
- trachea T27.0 ☑
  - with lung T27.1 ☑
- trunk T21.00 ☑

Burn — continued
   trunk — continued
      abdominal wall — see Burn, abdominal wall
      anus — see Burn, buttock
      axilla — see Burn, upper limb
      back — see Burn, back
      breast — see Burn, chest wall
      buttock — see Burn, buttock
      chest wall — see Burn, chest wall
      first degree T21.10 ☑
      flank — see Burn, abdominal wall
      genital
         female — see Burn, genital organs, external,
            female
         male — see Burn, genital organs, external, male
      groin — see Burn, abdominal wall
      interscapular region — see Burn, back, upper
      labia — see Burn, genital organs, external, female
      lower back — see Burn, back
      penis — see Burn, genital organs, external, male
      perineum
         female — see Burn, genital organs, external,
            female
         male — see Burn, genital organs, external, male
      scapula region — see Burn, scapular region
      scrotum — see Burn, genital organs, external, male
      second degree T21.20 ☑
      specified site NEC T21.09 ☑
         first degree T21.19 ☑
         second degree T21.29 ☑
         third degree T21.39 ☑
      testes — see Burn, genital organs, external, male
      third degree T21.30 ☑
      upper back — see Burn, back, upper
      vulva — see Burn, genital organs, external, female
   unspecified site with extent of body surface involved
      specified
      less than 10 percent T31.0
      10-19 percent (0-9 percent third degree) T31.10
         with 10-19 percent third degree T31.11
      20-29 percent (0-9 percent third degree) T31.20
         with
            10-19 percent third degree T31.21
            20-29 percent third degree T31.22
      30-39 percent (0-9 percent third degree) T31.30
         with
            10-19 percent third degree T31.31
            20-29 percent third degree T31.32
            30-39 percent third degree T31.33
      40-49 percent (0-9 percent third degree) T31.40
         with
            10-19 percent third degree T31.41
            20-29 percent third degree T31.42
            30-39 percent third degree T31.43
            40-49 percent third degree T31.44
      50-59 percent (0-9 percent third degree) T31.50
         with
            10-19 percent third degree T31.51
            20-29 percent third degree T31.52
            30-39 percent third degree T31.53
            40-49 percent third degree T31.54
            50-59 percent third degree T31.55
      60-69 percent (0-9 percent third degree) T31.60
         with
            10-19 percent third degree T31.61
            20-29 percent third degree T31.62
            30-39 percent third degree T31.63
            40-49 percent third degree T31.64
            50-59 percent third degree T31.65
            60-69 percent third degree T31.66
      70-79 percent (0-9 percent third degree) T31.70
         with
            10-19 percent third degree T31.71
            20-29 percent third degree T31.72
            30-39 percent third degree T31.73
            40-49 percent third degree T31.74
            50-59 percent third degree T31.75
            60-69 percent third degree T31.76
            70-79 percent third degree T31.77
      80-89 percent (0-9 percent third degree) T31.80
         with
            10-19 percent third degree T31.81
            20-29 percent third degree T31.82
            30-39 percent third degree T31.83
            40-49 percent third degree T31.84
            50-59 percent third degree T31.85
            60-69 percent third degree T31.86
            70-79 percent third degree T31.87

Burn — continued
   unspecified site with extent of body surface involved
      specified — continued
      80-89 percent — continued
         with — continued
            80-89 percent third degree T31.88
      90 percent or more (0-9 percent third degree)
         T31.90
         with
            10-19 percent third degree T31.91
            20-29 percent third degree T31.92
            30-39 percent third degree T31.93
            40-49 percent third degree T31.94
            50-59 percent third degree T31.95
            60-69 percent third degree T31.96
            70-79 percent third degree T31.97
            80-89 percent third degree T31.98
            90-99 percent third degree T31.99
   upper limb T22.00 ☑
      above elbow — see Burn, above elbow
      axilla — see Burn, axilla
      elbow — see Burn, elbow
      first degree T22.10 ☑
      forearm — see Burn, forearm
      hand — see Burn, hand
      interscapular region — see Burn, back, upper
      multiple sites T22.099 ☑
         first degree T22.199 ☑
         left T22.092 ☑
            first degree T22.192 ☑
            second degree T22.292 ☑
            third degree T22.392 ☑
         right T22.091 ☑
            first degree T22.191 ☑
            second degree T22.291 ☑
            third degree T22.391 ☑
         second degree T22.299 ☑
         third degree T22.399 ☑
      scapular region — see Burn, scapular region
      second degree T22.20 ☑
      shoulder — see Burn, shoulder
      third degree T22.30 ☑
      wrist — see Burn, wrist
   uterus T28.3 ☑
   vagina T28.3 ☑
   vulva — see Burn, genital organs, external, female
   wrist T23.079 ☑
      first degree T23.179 ☑
      left T23.072 ☑
         first degree T23.172 ☑
         second degree T23.272 ☑
         third degree T23.372 ☑
      multiple sites with hand T23.099 ☑
         first degree T23.199 ☑
         left T23.092 ☑
            first degree T23.192 ☑
            second degree T23.292 ☑
            third degree T23.392 ☑
         right T23.091 ☑
            first degree T23.191 ☑
            second degree T23.291 ☑
            third degree T23.391 ☑
         second degree T23.299 ☑
         third degree T23.399 ☑
      right T23.071 ☑
         first degree T23.171 ☑
         second degree T23.271 ☑
         third degree T23.371 ☑
      second degree T23.279 ☑
      third degree T23.379 ☑

Burnett's syndrome E83.52
Burning
   feet syndrome E53.9
   sensation R20.8
   tongue K14.6
Burn-out (state) Z73.0
Burns' disease or osteochondrosis — see Osteochondrosis, juvenile, ulna
Bursa — see condition
Bursitis M71.9
   Achilles — see Tendinitis, Achilles
   adhesive — see Bursitis, specified NEC
   ankle — see Enthesopathy, lower limb, ankle, specified
      type NEC
   calcaneal — see Enthesopathy, foot, specified type
      NEC

Bursitis — continued
   collateral ligament, tibial — see Bursitis, tibial collateral
   due to use, overuse, pressure (see also Disorder, soft
      tissue, due to use, specified type NEC)
      specified NEC — see Disorder, soft tissue, due to
         use, specified NEC
   Duplay's M75.0 ☑
   elbow NEC M70.3- ☑
      olecranon M70.2- ☑
   finger — see Disorder, soft tissue, due to use, specified
      type NEC, hand
   foot — see Enthesopathy, foot, specified type NEC
   gonococcal A54.49
   gouty — see Gout, idiopathic
   hand M70.1- ☑
   hip NEC M70.7- ☑
      trochanteric M70.6- ☑
   infective NEC M71.10
      abscess — see Abscess, bursa
      ankle M71.17- ☑
      elbow M71.12- ☑
      foot M71.17- ☑
      hand M71.14- ☑
      hip M71.15- ☑
      knee M71.16- ☑
      multiple sites M71.19
      shoulder M71.11- ☑
      specified site NEC M71.18
      wrist M71.13- ☑
   ischial — see Bursitis, hip
   knee NEC M70.5- ☑
      prepatellar M70.4- ☑
   occupational NEC (see also Disorder, soft tissue, due
      to, use)
   olecranon — see Bursitis, elbow, olecranon
   pharyngeal J39.1
   popliteal — see Bursitis, knee
   prepatellar M70.4- ☑
   radiohumeral M77.8
   rheumatoid M06.20
      ankle M06.27- ☑
      elbow M06.22- ☑
      foot joint M06.27- ☑
      hand joint M06.24- ☑
      hip M06.25- ☑
      knee M06.26- ☑
      multiple site M06.29
      shoulder M06.21- ☑
      vertebra M06.28
      wrist M06.23- ☑
   scapulohumeral — see Bursitis, shoulder
   semimembranous muscle (knee) — see Bursitis, knee
   shoulder M75.5- ☑
      adhesive — see Capsulitis, adhesive
   specified NEC M71.50
      ankle M71.57- ☑
      due to use, overuse or pressure — see Disorder,
         soft tissue, due to, use
      elbow M71.52- ☑
      foot M71.57- ☑
      hand M71.54- ☑
      hip M71.55- ☑
      knee M71.56- ☑
      shoulder — see Bursitis, shoulder
      specified site NEC M71.58
      tibial collateral M76.4- ☑
      wrist M71.53- ☑
   subacromial — see Bursitis, shoulder
   subcoracoid — see Bursitis, shoulder
   subdeltoid — see Bursitis, shoulder
   syphilitic A52.78
   Thornwaldt, Tornwaldt J39.2
   tibial collateral — see Bursitis, tibial collateral
   toe — see Enthesopathy, foot, specified type NEC
   trochanteric (area) — see Bursitis, hip, trochanteric
   wrist — see Bursitis, hand
Bursopathy M71.9
   specified type NEC M71.80
      ankle M71.87- ☑
      elbow M71.82- ☑
      foot M71.87- ☑
      hand M71.84- ☑
      hip M71.85- ☑
      knee M71.86- ☑
      multiple sites M71.89
      shoulder M71.81- ☑

Bursopathy — *continued*
  specified type — *continued*
    specified site NEC M71.88
    wrist M71.83- ☑
Burst stitches or sutures (complication of surgery)
  T81.31 ☑
  external operation wound T81.31 ☑
  internal operation wound T81.32 ☑
Buruli ulcer A31.1
Bury's disease L95.1
Buschke's
  disease B45.3
  scleredema — *see* Sclerosis, systemic
Busse-Buschke disease B45.3
Buttock — *see* condition
Button
  Biskra B55.1
  Delhi B55.1
  oriental B55.1
Buttonhole deformity (finger) — *see* Deformity, finger, boutonniere
Bwamba fever A92.8
Byssinosis J66.0
Bywaters' syndrome T79.5 ☑

C

Cachexia R64
  cancerous R64
  cardiac — *see* Disease, heart
  dehydration E86.0
    with
      hypernatremia E87.0
      hyponatremia E87.1
  due to malnutrition R64
  exophthalmic — *see* Hyperthyroidism
  heart — *see* Disease, heart
  hypophyseal E23.0
  hypopituitary E23.0
  lead — *see* Poisoning, lead
  malignant R64
  marsh — *see* Malaria
  nervous F48.8
  old age R54
  paludal — *see* Malaria
  pituitary E23.0
  renal N28.9
  saturnine — *see* Poisoning, lead
  senile R54
  Simmonds' E23.0
  splenica D73.0
  strumipriva E03.4
  tuberculous NEC — *see* Tuberculosis
Café, au lait spots L81.3
Caffey's syndrome Q78.8
Caisson disease T70.3 ☑
Cake kidney Q63.1
Caked breast (puerperal, postpartum) O92.79
Calabar swelling B74.3
Calcaneal spur — *see* Spur, bone, calcaneal
Calcaneo-apophysitis M92.8
Calcareous — *see* condition
Calcicosis J62.8
Calciferol (vitamin D) deficiency E55.9
  with rickets E55.0
Calcification
  adrenal (capsule) (gland) E27.49
    tuberculous E35 [B90.8]
  aorta I70.0
  artery (annular) — *see* Arteriosclerosis
  auricle (ear) — *see* Disorder, pinna, specified type NEC
  basal ganglia G23.8
  bladder N32.89
    due to Schistosoma hematobium B65.0
  brain (cortex) — *see* Calcification, cerebral
  bronchus J98.09
  bursa M71.40
    ankle M71.47- ☑
    elbow M71.42- ☑
    foot M71.47- ☑
    hand M71.44- ☑
    hip M71.45- ☑
    knee M71.46- ☑
    multiple sites M71.49
    shoulder M75.3- ☑
    specified site NEC M71.48
    wrist M71.43- ☑

Calcification — *continued*
  cardiac — *see* Degeneration, myocardial
  cerebral (cortex) G93.89
    artery I67.2
  cervix (uteri) N88.8
  choroid plexus G93.89
  conjunctiva — *see* Concretion, conjunctiva
  corpora cavernosa (penis) N48.89
  cortex (brain) — *see* Calcification, cerebral
  dental pulp (nodular) K04.2
  dentinal papilla K00.4
  fallopian tube N83.8
  falx cerebri G96.19
  gallbladder K82.8
  general E83.59
  heart (*see also* Degeneration, myocardial)
    valve — *see* Endocarditis
  idiopathic infantile arterial (IIAC) Q28.8
  intervertebral cartilage or disc (postinfective) — *see* Disorder, disc, specified NEC
  intracranial — *see* Calcification, cerebral
  joint — *see* Disorder, joint, specified type NEC
  kidney N28.89
    tuberculous N29 [B90.1]
  larynx (senile) J38.7
  lens — *see* Cataract, specified NEC
  lung (active) (postinfectional) J98.4
    tuberculous B90.9
  lymph gland or node (postinfectional) I89.8
    tuberculous (*see also* Tuberculosis, lymph gland) B90.8
  mammographic R92.1
  massive (paraplegic) — *see* Myositis, ossificans, in, quadriplegia
  medial — *see* Arteriosclerosis, extremities
  meninges (cerebral) (spinal) G96.19
  metastatic E83.59
  Mönckeberg's — *see* Arteriosclerosis, extremities
  muscle M61.9
    due to burns — *see* Myositis, ossificans, in, burns
    paralytic — *see* Myositis, ossificans, in, quadriplegia
    specified type NEC M61.40
      ankle M61.47- ☑
      foot M61.47- ☑
      forearm M61.43- ☑
      hand M61.44- ☑
      lower leg M61.46- ☑
      multiple sites M61.49
      pelvic region M61.45- ☑
      shoulder region M61.41- ☑
      specified site NEC M61.48
      thigh M61.45- ☑
      upper arm M61.42- ☑
  myocardium, myocardial — *see* Degeneration, myocardial
  ovary N83.8
  pancreas K86.8
  penis N48.89
  periarticular — *see* Disorder, joint, specified type NEC
  pericardium (*see also* Pericarditis) I31.1
  pineal gland E34.8
  pleura J94.8
    postinfectional J94.8
    tuberculous NEC B90.9
  pulpal (dental) (nodular) K04.2
  sclera H15.89
  spleen D73.89
  subcutaneous L94.2
  suprarenal (capsule) (gland) E27.49
  tendon (sheath) (*see also* Tenosynovitis, specified type NEC)
    with bursitis, synovitis or tenosynovitis — *see* Tendinitis, calcific
  trachea J39.8
  ureter N28.89
  uterus N85.8
  vitreous — *see* Deposit, crystalline
Calcified — *see* Calcification
Calcinosis (interstitial) (tumoral) (universalis) E83.59
  with Raynaud's phenomenon, esophageal dysfunction, sclerodactyly, telangiectasia (CREST syndrome) M34.1
  circumscripta (skin) L94.2
  cutis L94.2
Calciphylaxis (*see also* Calcification, by site) E83.59
Calcium
  deposits — *see* Calcification, by site

Calcium — *continued*
  metabolism disorder E83.50
  salts or soaps in vitreous — *see* Deposit, crystalline
Calciuria R82.99
Calculi — *see* Calculus
Calculosis, intrahepatic — *see* Calculus, bile duct
Calculus, calculi, calculous
  ampulla of Vater — *see* Calculus, bile duct
  anuria (impacted) (recurrent) (*see also* Calculus, urinary) N20.9
  appendix K38.1
  bile duct (common) (hepatic) K80.50
    with
      calculus of gallbladder —- *see* Calculus, gallbladder and bile duct
      cholangitis K80.30
        with
          cholecystitis — *see* Calculus, bile duct, with cholecystitis
          obstruction K80.31
        acute K80.32
          with
            chronic cholangitis K80.36
              with obstruction K80.37
            obstruction K80.33
        chronic K80.34
          with
            acute cholangitis K80.36
              with obstruction K80.37
            obstruction K80.35
      cholecystitis (with cholangitis) K80.40
        with obstruction K80.41
        acute K80.42
          with
            chronic cholecystitis K80.46
              with obstruction K80.47
            obstruction K80.43
        chronic K80.44
          with
            acute cholecystitis K80.46
              with obstruction K80.47
            obstruction K80.45
      obstruction K80.51
  biliary (*see also* Calculus, gallbladder)
    specified NEC K80.80
      with obstruction K80.81
  bilirubin, multiple — *see* Calculus, gallbladder
  bladder (encysted) (impacted) (urinary) (diverticulum) N21.0
  bronchus J98.09
  calyx (kidney) (renal) — *see* Calculus, kidney
  cholesterol (pure) (solitary) — *see* Calculus, gallbladder
  common duct (bile) — *see* Calculus, bile duct
  conjunctiva — *see* Concretion, conjunctiva
  cystic N21.0
    duct — *see* Calculus, gallbladder
  dental (subgingival) (supragingival) K03.6
  diverticulum
    bladder N21.0
    kidney N20.0
  epididymis N50.8
  gallbladder K80.20
    with
      bile duct calculus — *see* Calculus, gallbladder and bile duct
      cholecystitis K80.10
        with obstruction K80.11
        acute K80.00
          with
            chronic cholecystitis K80.12
              with obstruction K80.13
            obstruction K80.01
        chronic K80.10
          with
            acute cholecystitis K80.12
              with obstruction K80.13
            obstruction K80.11
      specified NEC K80.18
        with obstruction K80.19
      obstruction K80.21
  gallbladder and bile duct K80.70
    with
      cholecystitis K80.60
        with obstruction K80.61
        acute K80.62
          with
            chronic cholecystitis K80.66
              with obstruction K80.67

Calculus, calculi, calculous — *continued*
　gallbladder and bile duct — *continued*
　　with — *continued*
　　　cholecystitis — *continued*
　　　　acute — *continued*
　　　　　with — *continued*
　　　　　　obstruction K80.63
　　　　chronic K80.64
　　　　　with
　　　　　　acute cholecystitis K80.66
　　　　　　　with obstruction K80.67
　　　　　　obstruction K80.65
　　　　obstruction K80.71
　hepatic (duct) — *see* Calculus, bile duct
　ileal conduit N21.8
　intestinal (impaction) (obstruction) K56.49
　kidney (impacted) (multiple) (pelvis) (recurrent)
　　　(staghorn) N20.0
　　with calculus, ureter N20.2
　　congenital Q63.8
　lacrimal passages — *see* Dacryolith
　liver (impacted) — *see* Calculus, bile duct
　lung J98.4
　mammographic R92.1
　nephritic (impacted) (recurrent) — *see* Calculus, kidney
　nose J34.89
　pancreas (duct) K86.8
　parotid duct or gland K11.5
　pelvis, encysted — *see* Calculus, kidney
　prostate N42.0
　pulmonary J98.4
　pyelitis (impacted) (recurrent) N20.0
　　with hydronephrosis N13.2
　pyelonephritis (impacted) (recurrent) N20 ☑
　　with hydronephrosis N13.2
　renal (impacted) (recurrent) — *see* Calculus, kidney
　salivary (duct) (gland) K11.5
　seminal vesicle N50.8
　staghorn — *see* Calculus, kidney
　Stensen's duct K11.5
　stomach K31.89
　sublingual duct or gland K11.5
　　congenital Q38.4
　submandibular duct, gland or region K11.5
　submaxillary duct, gland or region K11.5
　suburethral N21.8
　tonsil J35.8
　tooth, teeth (subgingival) (supragingival) K03.6
　tunica vaginalis N50.8
　ureter (impacted) (recurrent) N20.1
　　with calculus, kidney N20.2
　　　with hydronephrosis N13.2
　　　　with infection N13.6
　urethra (impacted) N21.1
　urinary (duct) (impacted) (passage) (tract) N20.9
　　with hydronephrosis N13.2
　　　with infection N13.6
　　in (due to)
　　　lower N21.9
　　　　specified NEC N21.8
　vagina N89.8
　vesical (impacted) N21.0
　Wharton's duct K11.5
　xanthine E79.8 [N22]
Calicectasis N28.89
Caliectasis N28.89
California
　disease B38.9
　encephalitis A83.5
Caligo cornea — *see* Opacity, cornea, central
Callositas, callosity (infected) L84
Callus (infected) L84
　bone — *see* Osteophyte
　excessive, following fracture — *code as* Sequelae
　　of fracture
Calorie deficiency or malnutrition (see also Malnutrition) E46
Calvé-Perthes disease — *see* Legg-Calvé-Perthes disease
Calvé's disease — *see* Osteochondrosis, juvenile, spine
Calvities — *see* Alopecia, androgenic
Cameroon fever — *see* Malaria
Camptocormia (hysterical) F44.4
Camurati-Engelmann syndrome Q78.3
Canal (see also condition)
　atrioventricular common Q21.2
Canaliculitis (lacrimal) (acute) (subacute) H04.33- ☑
　Actinomyces A42.89

Canaliculitis — *continued*
　chronic H04.42- ☑
Canavan's disease E75.29
Canceled procedure (surgical) Z53.9
　because of
　　contraindication Z53.09
　　　smoking Z53.01
　　left against medical advice (AMA) Z53.21
　　patient's decision Z53.20
　　　for reasons of belief or group pressure Z53.1
　　　specified reason NEC Z53.29
　　specified reason NEC Z53.8
Cancer (see also Neoplasm, by site, malignant)
　bile duct type liver C22.1
　blood — *see* Leukemia
　breast (see also Neoplasm, breast, malignant)
　　C50.91- ☑
　hepatocellular C22.0
　lung (see also Neoplasm, lung, malignant) C34.90
　ovarian (see also Neoplasm ovary, malignant) C56.9
　unspecified site (primary) C80.1
Cancer (o)**phobia** F45.29
Cancerous — *see* Neoplasm, malignant, by site
Cancrum oris A69.0
Candidiasis, candidal B37.9
　balanitis B37.42
　bronchitis B37.1
　cheilitis B37.83
　congenital P37.5
　cystitis B37.41
　disseminated B37.7
　endocarditis B37.6
　enteritis B37.82
　esophagitis B37.81
　intertrigo B37.2
　lung B37.1
　meningitis B37.5
　mouth B37.0
　nails B37.2
　neonatal P37.5
　onychia B37.2
　oral B37.0
　osteomyelitis B37.89
　otitis externa B37.84
　paronychia B37.2
　perionyxis B37.2
　pneumonia B37.1
　proctitis B37.82
　pulmonary B37.1
　pyelonephritis B37.49
　sepsis B37.7
　skin B37.2
　specified site NEC B37.89
　stomatitis B37.0
　systemic B37.7
　urethritis B37.41
　urogenital site NEC B37.49
　vagina B37.3
　vulva B37.3
　vulvovaginitis B37.3
Candidid L30.2
Candidosis — *see* Candidiasis
Candiru infection or infestation B88.8
Canities (premature) L67.1
　congenital Q84.2
Canker (mouth) (sore) K12.0
　rash A38.9
Cannabinosis J66.2
Canton fever A75.9
Cantrell's syndrome Q87.89
Capillariasis (intestinal) B81.1
　hepatic B83.8
Capillary — *see* condition
Caplan's syndrome — *see* Rheumatoid, lung
Capsule — *see* condition
Capsulitis (joint) (see also Enthesopathy)
　adhesive (shoulder) M75.0- ☑
　hepatic K65.8
　labyrinthine — *see* Otosclerosis, specified NEC
　thyroid E06.9
Caput
　crepitus Q75.8
　medusae I86.8
　succedaneum P12.81
Car sickness T75.3 ☑
Carapata (disease) A68.0
Carate — *see* Pinta

Carbon lung J60
Carbuncle L02.93
　abdominal wall L02.231
　anus K61.0
　auditory canal, external — *see* Abscess, ear, external
　auricle ear — *see* Abscess, ear, external
　axilla L02.43- ☑
　back (any part) L02.232
　breast N61
　buttock L02.33
　cheek (external) L02.03
　chest wall L02.233
　chin L02.03
　corpus cavernosum N48.21
　ear (any part) (external) (middle) — *see* Abscess, ear, external
　external auditory canal — *see* Abscess, ear, external
　eyelid — *see* Abscess, eyelid
　face NEC L02.03
　femoral (region) — *see* Carbuncle, lower limb
　finger — *see* Carbuncle, hand
　flank L02.231
　foot L02.63- ☑
　forehead L02.03
　genital — *see* Abscess, genital
　gluteal (region) L02.33
　groin L02.234
　hand L02.53- ☑
　head NEC L02.831
　heel — *see* Carbuncle, foot
　hip — *see* Carbuncle, lower limb
　kidney — *see* Abscess, kidney
　knee — *see* Carbuncle, lower limb
　labium (majus) (minus) N76.4
　lacrimal
　　gland — *see* Dacryoadenitis
　　passages (duct) (sac) — *see* Inflammation, lacrimal, passages, acute
　leg — *see* Carbuncle, lower limb
　lower limb L02.43- ☑
　malignant A22.0
　navel L02.236
　neck L02.13
　nose (external) (septum) J34.0
　orbit, orbital — *see* Abscess, orbit
　palmar (space) — *see* Carbuncle, hand
　partes posteriores L02.33
　pectoral region L02.233
　penis N48.21
　perineum L02.235
　pinna — *see* Abscess, ear, external
　popliteal — *see* Carbuncle, lower limb
　scalp L02.831
　seminal vesicle N49.0
　shoulder — *see* Carbuncle, upper limb
　specified site NEC L02.838
　temple (region) L02.03
　thumb — *see* Carbuncle, hand
　toe — *see* Carbuncle, foot
　trunk L02.239
　　abdominal wall L02.231
　　back L02.232
　　chest wall L02.233
　　groin L02.234
　　perineum L02.235
　　umbilicus L02.236
　umbilicus L02.236
　upper limb L02.43- ☑
　urethra N34.0
　vulva N76.4
Carbunculus — *see* Carbuncle
Carcinoid (tumor) — *see* Tumor, carcinoid
Carcinoidosis E34.0
Carcinoma (malignant) (see also Neoplasm, by site, malignant)
　acidophil
　　specified site — *see* Neoplasm, malignant, by site
　　unspecified site C75.1
　acidophil-basophil, mixed
　　specified site — *see* Neoplasm, malignant, by site
　　unspecified site C75.1
　adnexal (skin) — *see* Neoplasm, skin, malignant
　adrenal cortical C74.0- ☑
　alveolar — *see* Neoplasm, lung, malignant
　　cell — *see* Neoplasm, lung, malignant
　ameloblastic C41.1
　　upper jaw (bone) C41.0

Carcinoma — *continued*
apocrine
breast — *see* Neoplasm, breast, malignant
specified site NEC — *see* Neoplasm, skin, malignant
unspecified site C44.99
basal cell (pigmented) (*see also* Neoplasm, skin, malignant) C44.91
fibro-epithelial — *see* Neoplasm, skin, malignant
morphea — *see* Neoplasm, skin, malignant
multicentric — *see* Neoplasm, skin, malignant
basaloid
basal-squamous cell, mixed — *see* Neoplasm, skin, malignant
basophil
specified site — *see* Neoplasm, malignant, by site
unspecified site C75.1
basophil-acidophil, mixed
specified site — *see* Neoplasm, malignant, by site
unspecified site C75.1
basosquamous — *see* Neoplasm, skin, malignant
bile duct
with hepatocellular, mixed C22.0
liver C22.1
specified site NEC — *see* Neoplasm, malignant, by site
unspecified site C22.1
branchial or branchiogenic C10.4
bronchial or bronchogenic — *see* Neoplasm, lung, malignant
bronchiolar — *see* Neoplasm, lung, malignant
bronchioloalveolar — *see* Neoplasm, lung, malignant
C cell
specified site — *see* Neoplasm, malignant, by site
unspecified site C73
ceruminous C44.29- ☑
cervix uteri
in situ D06.9
endocervix D06.0
exocervix D06.1
specified site NEC D06.7
chorionic
specified site — *see* Neoplasm, malignant, by site
unspecified site
female C58
male C62.90
chromophobe
specified site — *see* Neoplasm, malignant, by site
unspecified site C75.1
cloacogenic
specified site — *see* Neoplasm, malignant, by site
unspecified site C21.2
diffuse type
specified site — *see* Neoplasm, malignant, by site
unspecified site C16.9
duct (cell)
with Paget's disease — *see* Neoplasm, breast, malignant
infiltrating
with lobular carcinoma (in situ)
specified site — *see* Neoplasm, malignant, by site
unspecified site (female) C50.91- ☑
male C50.92- ☑
specified site — *see* Neoplasm, malignant, by site
unspecified site (female) C50.91- ☑
male C50.92- ☑
ductal
with lobular
specified site — *see* Neoplasm, malignant, by site
unspecified site (female) C50.91- ☑
male C50.92- ☑
ductular, infiltrating
specified site — *see* Neoplasm, malignant, by site
unspecified site (female) C50.91- ☑
male C50.92- ☑
embryonal
liver C22.7
endometrioid
specified site — *see* Neoplasm, malignant, by site
unspecified site
female C56.9
male C61
eosinophil
specified site — *see* Neoplasm, malignant, by site
unspecified site C75.1

Carcinoma — *continued*
epidermoid (*see also* Neoplasm, skin, malignant)
in situ, Bowen's type — *see* Neoplasm, skin, in situ
fibroepithelial, basal cell — *see* Neoplasm, skin, malignant
follicular
with papillary (mixed) C73
moderately differentiated C73
pure follicle C73
specified site — *see* Neoplasm, malignant, by site
trabecular C73
unspecified site C73
well differentiated C73
generalized, with unspecified primary site C80.0
glycogen-rich — *see* Neoplasm, breast, malignant
granulosa cell C56- ☑
hepatic cell C22.0
hepatocellular C22.0
with bile duct, mixed C22.0
fibrolamellar C22.0
hepatocholangiolitic C22.0
Hurthle cell C73
in
adenomatous
polyposis coli C18.9
pleomorphic adenoma — *see* Neoplasm, salivary glands, malignant
situ — *see* Carcinoma-in-situ
infiltrating
duct
with lobular
specified site — *see* Neoplasm, malignant, by site
unspecified site (female) C50.91- ☑
male C50.92- ☑
with Paget's disease — *see* Neoplasm, breast, malignant
specified site — *see* Neoplasm, malignant
unspecified site (female) C50.91- ☑
male C50.92- ☑
ductular
specified site — *see* Neoplasm, malignant
unspecified site (female) C50.91- ☑
male C50.92- ☑
lobular
specified site — *see* Neoplasm, malignant
unspecified site (female) C50.91- ☑
male C50.92- ☑
inflammatory
specified site — *see* Neoplasm, malignant
unspecified site (female) C50.91- ☑
male C50.92- ☑
intestinal type
specified site — *see* Neoplasm, malignant, by site
unspecified site C16.9
intracystic
noninfiltrating — *see* Neoplasm, in situ, by site
intraductal (noninfiltrating)
with Paget's disease — *see* Neoplasm, breast, malignant
breast D05.1- ☑
papillary
with invasion
specified site — *see* Neoplasm, malignant, by site
unspecified site (female) C50.91- ☑
male C50.92- ☑
breast D05.1- ☑
specified site NEC — *see* Neoplasm, in situ, by site
unspecified site (female) D05.1- ☑
specified site NEC — *see* Neoplasm, in situ, by site
unspecified site (female) D05.1- ☑
intraepidermal — *see* Neoplasm, in situ
squamous cell, Bowen's type — *see* Neoplasm, skin, in situ
intraepithelial — *see* Neoplasm, in situ, by site
squamous cell — *see* Neoplasm, in situ, by site
intraosseous C41.1
upper jaw (bone) C41.0
islet cell
with exocrine, mixed
specified site — *see* Neoplasm, malignant, by site
unspecified site C25.9
pancreas C25.4

Carcinoma — *continued*
islet cell — *continued*
specified site NEC — *see* Neoplasm, malignant, by site
unspecified site C25.4
juvenile, breast — *see* Neoplasm, breast, malignant
large cell
small cell
specified site — *see* Neoplasm, malignant, by site
unspecified site C34.90
Leydig cell (testis)
specified site — *see* Neoplasm, malignant, by site
unspecified site
female C56.9
male C62.90
lipid-rich (female) C50.91- ☑
male C50.92- ☑
liver cell C22.0
liver NEC C22.7
lobular (infiltrating)
with intraductal
specified site — *see* Neoplasm, malignant, by site
unspecified site (female) C50.91- ☑
male C50.92- ☑
noninfiltrating
breast D05.0- ☑
specified site NEC — *see* Neoplasm, in situ, by site
unspecified site D05.0- ☑
specified site — *see* Neoplasm, malignant, by site
unspecified site (female) C50.91- ☑
male C50.92- ☑
medullary
with
amyloid stroma
specified site — *see* Neoplasm, malignant, by site
unspecified site C73
lymphoid stroma
specified site — *see* Neoplasm, malignant, by site
unspecified site (female) C50.91- ☑
male C50.92- ☑
Merkel cell C4A.9 (*following* C43)
anal margin C4A.51 (*following* C43)
anal skin C4A.51 (*following* C43)
canthus C4A.1- ☑ (*following* C43)
ear and external auricular canal C4A.2- ☑ (*following* C43)
external auricular canal C4A.2- ☑ (*following* C43)
eyelid, including canthus C4A.1- ☑ (*following* C43)
face C4A.30 (*following* C43)
specified NEC C4A.39 (*following* C43)
hip C4A.7- ☑ (*following* C43)
lip C4A.0 (*following* C43)
lower limb, including hip C4A.7- ☑ (*following* C43)
neck C4A.4 (*following* C43)
nodal presentation C7B.1 (*following* C75)
nose C4A.31 (*following* C43)
overlapping sites C4A.8 (*following* C43)
perianal skin C4A.51 (*following* C43)
scalp C4A.4 (*following* C43)
secondary C7B.1 (*following* C75)
shoulder C4A.6- ☑ (*following* C43)
skin of breast C4A.52 (*following* C43)
trunk NEC C4A.59 (*following* C43)
upper limb, including shoulder C4A.6- ☑ (*following* C43)
visceral metastatic C7B.1 (*following* C75)
metastatic — *see* Neoplasm, secondary, by site
metatypical — *see* Neoplasm, skin, malignant
morphea, basal cell — *see* Neoplasm, skin, malignant
mucoid
cell
specified site — *see* Neoplasm, malignant, by site
unspecified site C75.1
neuroendocrine (*see also* Tumor, neuroendocrine)
high grade, any site C7A.1 (*following* C75)
poorly differentiated, any site C7A.1 (*following* C75)
nonencapsulated sclerosing C73
noninfiltrating
intracystic — *see* Neoplasm, in situ, by site
intraductal
breast D05.1- ☑

☑ **Additional Character Required — Refer to the Tabular List for Character Selection**   ▽ **Subterms under main terms may continue to next column or page**

Carcinoma — *continued*
  noninfiltrating — *continued*
    intraductal — *continued*
      papillary
        breast D05.1- ☑
        specified site NEC — *see* Neoplasm, in situ, by site
        unspecified site D05.1- ☑
      specified site — *see* Neoplasm, in situ, by site
      unspecified site D05.1- ☑
      lobular
        breast D05.0- ☑
        specified site NEC — *see* Neoplasm, in situ, by site
        unspecified site (female) D05.0- ☑
  oat cell
    specified site — *see* Neoplasm, malignant, by site
    unspecified site C34.90
  odontogenic C41.1
    upper jaw (bone) C41.0
  papillary
    with follicular (mixed) C73
    follicular variant C73
    intraductal (noninfiltrating)
      with invasion
        specified site — *see* Neoplasm, malignant, by site
        unspecified site (female) C50.91- ☑
          male C50.92- ☑
      breast D05.1- ☑
      specified site NEC — *see* Neoplasm, in situ, by site
      unspecified site D05.1- ☑
    serous
      specified site — *see* Neoplasm, malignant, by site
    surface
      specified site — *see* Neoplasm, malignant, by site
      unspecified site C56.9
    unspecified site C56.9
  papillocystic
    specified site — *see* Neoplasm, malignant, by site
    unspecified site C56.9
  parafollicular cell
    specified site — *see* Neoplasm, malignant, by site
    unspecified site C73
  pilomatrix — *see* Neoplasm, skin, malignant
  pseudomucinous
    specified site — *see* Neoplasm, malignant, by site
    unspecified site C56.9
  renal cell C64- ☑
  Schmincke — *see* Neoplasm, nasopharynx, malignant
  Schneiderian
    specified site — *see* Neoplasm, malignant, by site
    unspecified site C30.0
  sebaceous — *see* Neoplasm, skin, malignant
  secondary (*see also* Neoplasm, secondary, by site)
    Merkel cell C7B.1 (*following* C75)
  secretory, breast — *see* Neoplasm, breast, malignant
  serous
    papillary
      specified site — *see* Neoplasm, malignant, by site
      unspecified site C56.9
    surface, papillary
      specified site — *see* Neoplasm, malignant, by site
      unspecified site C56.9
  Sertoli cell
    specified site — *see* Neoplasm, malignant, by site
    unspecified site C62.90
      female C56.9
      male C62.90
  skin appendage — *see* Neoplasm, skin, malignant
  small cell
    fusiform cell
      specified site — *see* Neoplasm, malignant, by site
      unspecified site C34.90
    intermediate cell
      specified site — *see* Neoplasm, malignant, by site
      unspecified site C34.90
    large cell
      specified site — *see* Neoplasm, malignant, by site

Carcinoma — *continued*
  small cell — *continued*
    large cell — *continued*
      unspecified site C34.90
    solid
      with amyloid stroma
        specified site — *see* Neoplasm, malignant, by site
        unspecified site C73
    microinvasive
      specified site — *see* Neoplasm, malignant, by site
      unspecified site C53.9
    sweat gland — *see* Neoplasm, skin, malignant
    theca cell C56.- ☑
    thymic C37
    unspecified site (primary) C80.1
    water-clear cell C75.0
Carcinoma-in-situ (*see also* Neoplasm, in situ, by site)
  breast NOS D05.9- ☑
    specified type NEC D05.8- ☑
  epidermoid (*see also* Neoplasm, in situ, by site)
    with questionable stromal invasion
      cervix D06.9
      specified site NEC — *see* Neoplasm, in situ, by site
      unspecified site D06.9
    Bowen's type — *see* Neoplasm, skin, in situ
  intraductal
    breast D05.1- ☑
    specified site NEC — *see* Neoplasm, in situ, by site
    unspecified site D05.1- ☑
  lobular
    with
      infiltrating duct
        breast (female) C50.91- ☑
          male C50.92- ☑
        specified site NEC — *see* Neoplasm, malignant
        unspecified site (female) C50.91- ☑
          male C50.92- ☑
      intraductal
        breast D05.8- ☑
        specified site NEC — *see* Neoplasm, in situ, by site
        unspecified site (female) D05.8- ☑
    breast D05.0- ☑
    specified site NEC — *see* Neoplasm, in situ, by site
    unspecified site D05.0- ☑
  squamous cell (*see also* Neoplasm, in situ, by site)
    with questionable stromal invasion
      cervix D06.9
      specified site NEC — *see* Neoplasm, in situ, by site
      unspecified site D06.9
Carcinomaphobia F45.29
Carcinomatosis C80.0
  peritonei C78.6
  unspecified site (primary) (secondary) C80.0
Carcinosarcoma — *see* Neoplasm, malignant, by site
  embryonal — *see* Neoplasm, malignant, by site
Cardia, cardial — *see* condition
Cardiac (*see also* condition)
  death, sudden — *see* Arrest, cardiac
  pacemaker
    in situ Z95.0
    management or adjustment Z45.018
  tamponade I31.4
Cardialgia — *see* Pain, precordial
Cardiectasis — *see* Hypertrophy, cardiac
Cardiochalasia K21.9
Cardiomalacia I51.5
Cardiomegalia glycogenica diffusa E74.02 [I43]
Cardiomegaly (*see also* Hypertrophy, cardiac)
  congenital Q24.8
  glycogen E74.02 [I43]
  idiopathic I51.7
Cardiomyoliposis I51.5
Cardiomyopathy (familial) (idiopathic) I42.9
  alcoholic I42.6
  amyloid E85.4 [I43]
  arteriosclerotic — *see* Disease, heart, ischemic, atherosclerotic
  beriberi E51.12
  cobalt-beer I42.6
  congenital I42.4
  congestive I42.0

Cardiomyopathy — *continued*
  constrictive NOS I42.5
  dilated I42.0
  due to
    alcohol I42.6
    beriberi E51.12
    cardiac glycogenosis E74.02 [I43]
    drugs I42.7
    external agents NEC I42.7
    Friedreich's ataxia G11.1
    myotonia atrophica G71.11 [I43]
    progressive muscular dystrophy G71.0
  glycogen storage E74.02 [I43]
  hypertensive — *see* Hypertension, heart
  hypertrophic (nonobstructive) I42.2
    obstructive I42.1
      congenital Q24.8
  in
    Chagas' disease (chronic) B57.2
      acute B57.0
    sarcoidosis D86.85
  ischemic I25.5
  metabolic E88.9 [I43]
    thyrotoxic E05.90 [I43]
      with thyroid storm E05.91 [I43]
  newborn I42.8
    congenital I42.4
  nutritional E63.9 [I43]
    beriberi E51.12
  obscure of Africa I42.8
  peripartum O90.3
  postpartum O90.3
  restrictive NEC I42.5
  rheumatic I09.0
  secondary I42.9
  stress induced I51.81
  takotsubo I51.81
  thyrotoxic E05.90 [I43]
    with thyroid storm E05.91 [I43]
  toxic NEC I42.7
  tuberculous A18.84
  viral B33.24
Cardionephritis — *see* Hypertension, cardiorenal
Cardionephropathy — *see* Hypertension, cardiorenal
Cardionephrosis — *see* Hypertension, cardiorenal
Cardiopathia nigra I27.0
Cardiopathy (*see also* Disease, heart) I51.9
  idiopathic I42.9
  mucopolysaccharidosis E76.3 [I52]
Cardiopericarditis — *see* Pericarditis
Cardiophobia F45.29
Cardiorenal — *see* condition
Cardiorrhexis — *see* Infarct, myocardium
Cardiosclerosis — *see* Disease, heart, ischemic, atherosclerotic
Cardiosis — *see* Disease, heart
Cardiospasm (esophagus) (reflex) (stomach) K22.0
  congenital Q39.5
  with megaesophagus Q39.5
Cardiostenosis — *see* Disease, heart
Cardiosymphysis I31.0
Cardiovascular — *see* condition
Carditis (acute) (bacterial) (chronic) (subacute) I51.89
  meningococcal A39.50
  rheumatic — *see* Disease, heart, rheumatic
  rheumatoid — *see* Rheumatoid, carditis
  viral B33.20
Care (of) (for) (following)
  child (routine) Z76.2
  family member (handicapped) (sick)
    creating problem for family Z63.6
    provided away from home for holiday relief Z75.5
    unavailable, due to
      absence (person rendering care) (sufferer) Z74.2
      inability (any reason) of person rendering care Z74.2
  foundling Z76.1
  holiday relief Z75.5
  improper — *see* Maltreatment
  lack of (at or after birth) (infant) — *see* Maltreatment, child, neglect
  lactating mother Z39.1
  palliative Z51.5
  postpartum
    immediately after delivery Z39.0
    routine follow-up Z39.2
  respite Z75.5

Carcinoma — Care

Care — continued
unavailable, due to
absence of person rendering care Z74.2
inability (any reason) of person rendering care Z74.2
well-baby Z76.2
Caries
bone NEC A18.03
dental K02.9
arrested (coronal) (root) K02.3
chewing surface
limited to enamel K02.51
penetrating into dentin K02.52
penetrating into pulp K02.53
coronal surface
chewing surface
limited to enamel K02.51
penetrating into dentin K02.52
penetrating into pulp K02.53
pit and fissure surface
limited to enamel K02.51
penetrating into dentin K02.52
penetrating into pulp K02.53
smooth surface
limited to enamel K02.61
penetrating into dentin K02.62
penetrating into pulp K02.63
pit and fissure surface
limited to enamel K02.51
penetrating into dentin K02.52
penetrating into pulp K02.53
root K02.7
smooth surface
limited to enamel K02.61
penetrating into dentin K02.62
penetrating into pulp K02.63
external meatus — see Disorder, ear, external, specified type NEC
hip (tuberculous) A18.02
initial (tooth)
chewing surface K02.51
pit and fissure surface K02.51
smooth surface K02.61
knee (tuberculous) A18.02
labyrinth H83.8 ☑
limb NEC (tuberculous) A18.03
mastoid process (chronic) — see Mastoiditis, chronic
tuberculous A18.03
middle ear H74.8 ☑
nose (tuberculous) A18.03
orbit (tuberculous) A18.03
ossicles, ear — see Abnormal, ear ossicles
petrous bone — see Petrositis
root (dental) (tooth) K02.7
sacrum (tuberculous) A18.01
spine, spinal (column) (tuberculous) A18.01
syphilitic A52.77
congenital (early) A50.02 [M90.80]
tooth, teeth — see Caries, dental
tuberculous A18.03
vertebra (column) (tuberculous) A18.01
Carious teeth — see Caries, dental
Carneous mole O02.0
Carnitine insufficiency E71.40
Carotid body or sinus syndrome G90.01
Carotidynia G90.01
Carotinemia (dietary) E67.1
Carotinosis (cutis) (skin) E67.1
Carpal tunnel syndrome — see Syndrome, carpal tunnel
Carpenter's syndrome Q87.0
Carpopedal spasm — see Tetany
Carr-Barr-Plunkett syndrome Q97.1
Carrier (suspected) of
amebiasis Z22.1
bacterial disease NEC Z22.39
diphtheria Z22.2
intestinal infectious NEC Z22.1
typhoid Z22.0
meningococcal Z22.31
sexually transmitted Z22.4
specified NEC Z22.39
staphylococcal (Methicillin susceptible) Z22.321
Methicillin resistant Z22.322
streptococcal Z22.338
group B Z22.330
typhoid Z22.0
cholera Z22.1
diphtheria Z22.2

Carrier of — continued
gastrointestinal pathogens NEC Z22.1
genetic Z14.8
cystic fibrosis Z14.1
hemophilia A (asymptomatic) Z14.01
symptomatic Z14.02
gonorrhea Z22.4
HAA (hepatitis Australian-antigen) Z22.59
HB (c)(s)-AG Z22.51
hepatitis (viral) Z22.50
Australia-antigen (HAA) Z22.59
B surface antigen (HBsAg) Z22.51
with acute delta- (super)infection B17.0
C Z22.52
specified NEC Z22.59
human T-cell lymphotropic virus type-1 (HTLV-1) infection Z22.6
infectious organism Z22.9
specified NEC Z22.8
meningococci Z22.31
Salmonella typhosa Z22.0
serum hepatitis — see Carrier, hepatitis
staphylococci (Methicillin susceptible) Z22.321
Methicillin resistant Z22.322
streptococci Z22.338
group B Z22.330
syphilis Z22.4
typhoid Z22.0
venereal disease NEC Z22.4
Carrion's disease A44.0
Carter's relapsing fever (Asiatic) A68.1
Cartilage — see condition
Caruncle (inflamed)
conjunctiva (acute) — see Conjunctivitis, acute
labium (majus) (minus) N90.89
lacrimal — see Inflammation, lacrimal, passages
myrtiform N89.8
urethral (benign) N36.2
Cascade stomach K31.2
Caseation lymphatic gland (tuberculous) A18.2
Cassidy (-Scholte) syndrome (malignant carcinoid) E34.0
Castellani's disease A69.8
Castration, traumatic, male S38.231 ☑
Casts in urine R82.99
Cat
cry syndrome Q93.4
ear Q17.3
eye syndrome Q92.8
Catabolism, senile R54
Catalepsy (hysterical) F44.2
schizophrenic F20.2
Cataplexy (idiopathic) — see Narcolepsy
Cataract (cortical) (immature) (incipient) H26.9
with
neovascularization — see Cataract, complicated
age-related — see Cataract, senile
anterior
and posterior axial embryonal Q12.0
pyramidal Q12.0
associated with
galactosemia E74.21 [H28]
myotonic disorders G71.19 [H28]
blue Q12.0
central Q12.0
cerulean Q12.0
complicated H26.20
with
neovascularization H26.21- ☑
ocular disorder H26.22- ☑
glaucomatous flecks H26.23- ☑
congenital Q12.0
coraliform Q12.0
coronary Q12.0
crystalline Q12.0
diabetic — see Diabetes, cataract
drug-induced H26.3- ☑
due to
ocular disorder — see Cataract, complicated
radiation H26.8
electric H26.8
extraction status Z98.4- ☑
glass-blower's H26.8
heat ray H26.8
heterochromic — see Cataract, complicated
hypermature — see Cataract, senile, morgagnian type
in (due to)
chronic iridocyclitis — see Cataract, complicated

Cataract — continued
in — continued
diabetes — see Diabetes, cataract
endocrine disease E34.9 [H28]
eye disease — see Cataract, complicated
hypoparathyroidism E20.9 [H28]
malnutrition-dehydration E46 [H28]
metabolic disease E88.9 [H28]
myotonic disorders G71.19 [H28]
nutritional disease E63.9 [H28]
infantile — see Cataract, presenile
irradiational — see Cataract, specified NEC
juvenile — see Cataract, presenile
malnutrition-dehydration E46 [H28]
morgagnian — see Cataract, senile, morgagnian type
myotonic G71.19 [H28]
myxedema E03.9 [H28]
nuclear
embryonal Q12.0
sclerosis — see Cataract, senile, nuclear
presenile H26.00- ☑
combined forms H26.06- ☑
cortical H26.01- ☑
lamellar — see Cataract, presenile, cortical
nuclear H26.03- ☑
specified NEC H26.09
subcapsular polar (anterior) H26.04- ☑
posterior H26.05- ☑
zonular — see Cataract, presenile, cortical
secondary H26.40
Soemmering's ring H26.41- ☑
specified NEC H26.49- ☑
to eye disease — see Cataract, complicated
senile H25.9
brunescens — see Cataract, senile, nuclear
combined forms H25.81- ☑
coronary — see Cataract, senile, incipient
cortical H25.01- ☑
hypermature — see Cataract, senile, morgagnian type
incipient (mature) (total) H25.09- ☑
cortical — see Cataract, senile, cortical
subcapsular — see Cataract, senile, subcapsular
morgagnian type (hypermature) H25.2- ☑
nuclear (sclerosis) H25.1- ☑
polar subcapsular (anterior) (posterior) — see Cataract, senile, incipient
punctate — see Cataract, senile, incipient
specified NEC H25.89
subcapsular polar (anterior) H25.03- ☑
posterior H25.04- ☑
snowflake — see Diabetes, cataract
specified NEC H26.8
toxic — see Cataract, drug-induced
traumatic H26.10- ☑
localized H26.11- ☑
partially resolved H26.12- ☑
total H26.13- ☑
zonular (perinuclear) Q12.0
Cataracta (see also Cataract)
brunescens — see Cataract, senile, nuclear
centralis pulverulenta Q12.0
cerulea Q12.0
complicata — see Cataract, complicated
congenita Q12.0
coralliformis Q12.0
coronaria Q12.0
diabetic — see Diabetes, cataract
membranacea
accreta — see Cataract, secondary
congenita Q12.0
nigra — see Cataract, senile, nuclear
sunflower — see Cataract, complicated
Catarrh, catarrhal (acute) (febrile) (infectious) (inflammation) (see also condition) J00
bronchial — see Bronchitis
chest — see Bronchitis
chronic J31.0
due to congenital syphilis A50.03
enteric — see Enteritis
eustachian H68.009
fauces — see Pharyngitis
gastrointestinal — see Enteritis
gingivitis K05.00
nonplaque induced K05.01
plaque induced K05.00
hay — see Fever, hay

Catarrh, catarrhal — *continued*
  intestinal — *see* Enteritis
  larynx, chronic J37.0
  liver B15.9
    with hepatic coma B15.0
  lung — *see* Bronchitis
  middle ear, chronic — *see* Otitis, media, nonsuppurative, chronic, serous
  mouth K12.1
  nasal (chronic) — *see* Rhinitis
  nasobronchial J31.1
  nasopharyngeal (chronic) J31.1
    acute J00
  pulmonary — *see* Bronchitis
  spring (eye) (vernal) — *see* Conjunctivitis, acute, atopic
  summer (hay) — *see* Fever, hay
  throat J31.2
  tubotympanal (*see also* Otitis, media, nonsuppurative)
    chronic — *see* Otitis, media, nonsuppurative, chronic, serous
Catatonia (schizophrenic) F20.2
Catatonic
  disorder due to known physiologic condition F06.1
  schizophrenia F20.2
  stupor R40.1
Cat-scratch (*see also* Abrasion)
  disease or fever A28.1
Cauda equina — *see* condition
Cauliflower ear M95.1- ☑
Causalgia (upper limb) G56.4- ☑
  lower limb G57.7- ☑
Cause
  external, general effects T75.89 ☑
Caustic burn — *see* Corrosion, by site
Cavare's disease (familial periodic paralysis) G72.3
Cave-in, injury
  crushing (severe) — *see* Crush
  suffocation — *see* Asphyxia, traumatic, due to low oxygen, due to cave-in
Cavernitis (penis) N48.29
Cavernositis N48.29
Cavernous — *see* condition
Cavitation of lung (*see also* Tuberculosis, pulmonary)
  nontuberculous J98.4
Cavities, dental — *see* Caries, dental
Cavity
  lung — *see* Cavitation of lung
  optic papilla Q14.2
  pulmonary — *see* Cavitation of lung
Cavovarus foot, congenital Q66.1
Cavus foot (congenital) Q66.7
  acquired — *see* Deformity, limb, foot, specified NEC
Cazenave's disease L10.2
Cecitis K52.9
  with perforation, peritonitis, or rupture K65.8
Cecum — *see* condition
Celiac
  artery compression syndrome I77.4
  disease K90.0
  infantilism K90.0
Cell(s), **cellular** (*see also* condition)
  in urine R82.99
Cellulitis (diffuse) (phlegmonous) (septic) (suppurative) L03.90
  abdominal wall L03.311
  anaerobic A48.0
  ankle — *see* Cellulitis, lower limb
  anus K61.0
  arm — *see* Cellulitis, upper limb
  auricle (ear) — *see* Cellulitis, ear
  axilla L03.11- ☑
  back (any part) L03.312
  broad ligament
    acute N73.0
  buttock L03.317
  cervical (meaning neck) L03.221
  cervix (uteri) — *see* Cervicitis
  cheek (external) L03.211
    internal K12.2
  chest wall L03.313
  chronic L03.90
  clostridial A48.0
  corpus cavernosum N48.22
  digit
    finger — *see* Cellulitis, finger
    toe — *see* Cellulitis, toe

Cellulitis — *continued*
  Douglas' cul-de-sac or pouch
    acute N73.0
  drainage site (following operation) T81.4 ☑
  ear (external) H60.1- ☑
  eosinophilic (granulomatous) L98.3
  erysipelatous — *see* Erysipelas
  external auditory canal — *see* Cellulitis, ear
  eyelid — *see* Abscess, eyelid
  face NEC L03.211
  finger (intrathecal) (periosteal) (subcutaneous) (subcuticular) L03.01- ☑
  foot — *see* Cellulitis, lower limb
  gangrenous — *see* Gangrene
  genital organ NEC
    female (external) N76.4
    male N49.9
      multiple sites N49.8
      specified NEC N49.8
  gluteal (region) L03.317
  gonococcal A54.89
  groin L03.314
  hand — *see* Cellulitis, upper limb
  head NEC L03.811
    face (any part, except ear, eye and nose) L03.211
  heel — *see* Cellulitis, lower limb
  hip — *see* Cellulitis, lower limb
  jaw (region) L03.211
  knee — *see* Cellulitis, lower limb
  labium (majus) (minus) — *see* Vulvitis
  lacrimal passages — *see* Inflammation, lacrimal, passages
  larynx J38.7
  leg — *see* Cellulitis, lower limb
  lip K13.0
  lower limb L03.11- ☑
    toe — *see* Cellulitis, toe
  mouth (floor) K12.2
  multiple sites, so stated L03.90
  nasopharynx J39.1
  navel L03.316
    newborn P38.9
      with mild hemorrhage P38.1
      without hemorrhage P38.9
  neck (region) L03.221
  nose (septum) (external) J34.0
  orbit, orbital H05.01- ☑
  palate (soft) K12.2
  pectoral (region) L03.313
  pelvis, pelvic (chronic)
    female (*see also* Disease, pelvis, inflammatory) N73.2
      acute N73.0
      following ectopic or molar pregnancy O08.0
    male K65.0
  penis N48.22
  perineal, perineum L03.315
  perirectal K61.1
  peritonsillar J36
  periurethral N34.0
  periuterine (*see also* Disease, pelvis, inflammatory) N73.2
    acute N73.0
  pharynx J39.1
  rectum K61.1
  retroperitoneal K68.9
  round ligament
    acute N73.0
  scalp (any part) L03.811
  scrotum N49.2
  seminal vesicle N49.0
  shoulder — *see* Cellulitis, upper limb
  specified site NEC L03.818
  submandibular (region) (space) (triangle) K12.2
    gland K11.3
  submaxillary (region) K12.2
    gland K11.3
  thigh — *see* Cellulitis, lower limb
  thumb (intrathecal) (periosteal) (subcutaneous) (subcuticular) — *see* Cellulitis, finger
  toe (intrathecal) (periosteal) (subcutaneous) (subcuticular) L03.03- ☑
  tonsil J36
  trunk L03.319
    abdominal wall L03.311
    back (any part) L03.312
    buttock L03.317
    chest wall L03.313

Cellulitis — *continued*
  trunk — *continued*
    groin L03.314
    perineal, perineum L03.315
    umbilicus L03.316
  tuberculous (primary) A18.4
  umbilicus L03.316
  upper limb L03.11- ☑
    axilla — *see* Cellulitis, axilla
    finger — *see* Cellulitis, finger
    thumb — *see* Cellulitis, finger
  vaccinal T88.0 ☑
  vocal cord J38.3
  vulva — *see* Vulvitis
  wrist — *see* Cellulitis, upper limb
Cementoblastoma, benign — *see* Cyst, calcifying odontogenic
Cementoma — *see* Cyst, calcifying odontogenic
Cementoperiostitis — *see* Periodontitis
Cementosis K03.4
Central auditory processing disorder H93.25
Central pain syndrome G89.0
Cephalematocele, cephal (o)hematocele
  newborn P52.8
    birth injury P10.8
  traumatic — *see* Hematoma, brain
Cephalematoma, cephalhematoma (calcified)
  newborn (birth injury) P12.0
  traumatic — *see* Hematoma, brain
Cephalgia, cephalalgia (*see also* Headache)
  histamine G44.009
    intractable G44.001
    not intractable G44.009
  trigeminal autonomic (TAC) NEC G44.099
    intractable G44.091
    not intractable G44.099
Cephalic — *see* condition
Cephalitis — *see* Encephalitis
Cephalocele — *see* Encephalocele
Cephalomenia N94.89
Cephalopelvic — *see* condition
Cerclage (with cervical incompetence) in pregnancy — *see* Incompetence, cervix, in pregnancy
Cerebellitis — *see* Encephalitis
Cerebellum, cerebellar — *see* condition
Cerebral — *see* condition
Cerebritis — *see* Encephalitis
Cerebro-hepato-renal syndrome Q87.89
Cerebromalacia — *see* Softening, brain
  sequelae of cerebrovascular disease I69.398
Cerebroside lipidosis E75.22
Cerebrospasticity (congenital) G80.1
Cerebrospinal — *see* condition
Cerebrum — *see* condition
Ceroid-lipofuscinosis, neuronal E75.4
Cerumen (accumulation) (impacted) H61.2- ☑
Cervical (*see also* condition)
  auricle Q18.2
  dysplasia in pregnancy — *see* Abnormal, cervix, in pregnancy or childbirth
  erosion in pregnancy — *see* Abnormal, cervix, in pregnancy or childbirth
  fibrosis in pregnancy — *see* Abnormal, cervix, in pregnancy or childbirth
  fusion syndrome Q76.1
  rib Q76.5
  shortening (complicating pregnancy) O26.87- ☑
Cervicalgia M54.2
Cervicitis (acute) (chronic) (nonvenereal) (senile (atrophic)) (subacute) (with ulceration) N72
  with
    abortion — *see* Abortion, by type complicated by genital tract and pelvic infection
    ectopic pregnancy O08.0
    molar pregnancy O08.0
  chlamydial A56.09
  gonococcal A54.03
  herpesviral A60.03
  puerperal (postpartum) O86.11
  syphilitic A52.76
  trichomonal A59.09
  tuberculous A18.16
Cervicocolpitis (emphysematosa) (see also Cervicitis) N72
Cervix — *see* condition
Cesarean delivery, previous, affecting management of pregnancy O34.21

Céstan

ICD-10-CM Draft (2015)

Index

Céstan — Chlorosis

Céstan (-Chenais) paralysis or syndrome G46.3
Céstan-Raymond syndrome I65.8
Cestode infestation B71.9
  specified type NEC B71.8
Cestodiasis B71.9
Chabert's disease A22.9
Chacaleh E53.8
Chafing L30.4
Chagas' (-Mazza) disease (chronic) B57.2
  with
    cardiovascular involvement NEC B57.2
    digestive system involvement B57.30
      megacolon B57.32
      megaesophagus B57.31
      other specified B57.39
    megacolon B57.32
    megaesophagus B57.31
    myocarditis B57.2
    nervous system involvement B57.40
      meningitis B57.41
      meningoencephalitis B57.42
      other specified B57.49
    specified organ involvement NEC B57.5
  acute (with) B57.1
    cardiovascular NEC B57.0
    myocarditis B57.0
Chagres fever B50.9
Chairridden Z74.09
Chalasia (cardiac sphincter) K21.9
Chalazion H00.19
  left H00.16
    lower H00.15
    upper H00.14
  right H00.13
    lower H00.12
    upper H00.11
Chalcosis (see also Disorder, globe, degenerative, chalcosis)
  cornea — see Deposit, cornea
  crystalline lens — see Cataract, complicated
  retina H35.89
Chalicosis (pulmonum) J62.8
Chancre (any genital site) (hard) (hunterian) (mixed) (primary) (seronegative) (seropositive) (syphilitic) A51.0
  congenital A50.07
  conjunctiva NEC A51.2
  Ducrey's A57
  extragenital A51.2
  eyelid A51.2
  lip A51.2
  nipple A51.2
  Nisbet's A57
  of
    carate A67.0
    pinta A67.0
    yaws A66.0
  palate, soft A51.2
  phagedenic A57
  simple A57
  soft A57
    bubo A57
    palate A51.2
  urethra A51.0
  yaws A66.0
Chancroid (anus) (genital) (penis) (perineum) (rectum) (urethra) (vulva) A57
Chandler's disease (osteochondritis dissecans, hip) — see Osteochondritis, dissecans, hip
Change(s) (in) (of) (see also Removal)
  arteriosclerotic — see Arteriosclerosis
  bone (see also Disorder, bone)
    diabetic — see Diabetes, bone change
  bowel habit R19.4
  cardiorenal (vascular) — see Hypertension, cardiorenal
  cardiovascular — see Disease, cardiovascular
  circulatory I99.9
  cognitive (mild) (organic) R41.89
  color, tooth, teeth
    during formation K00.8
    posteruptive K03.7
  contraceptive device Z30.433
  corneal membrane H18.30
    Bowman's membrane fold or rupture H18.31- ☑
    Descemet's membrane
      fold H18.32- ☑
      rupture H18.33- ☑
  coronary — see Disease, heart, ischemic

Change(s) — continued
  degenerative, spine or vertebra — see Spondylosis
  dental pulp, regressive K04.2
  dressing (nonsurgical) Z48.00
    surgical Z48.01
  heart — see Disease, heart
  hip joint — see Derangement, joint, hip
  hyperplastic larynx J38.7
  hypertrophic
    nasal sinus J34.89
    turbinate, nasal J34.3
    upper respiratory tract J39.8
  indwelling catheter Z46.6
  inflammatory (see also Inflammation)
    sacroiliac M46.1
  job, anxiety concerning Z56.1
  joint — see Derangement, joint
  life — see Menopause
  mental status R41.82
  minimal (glomerular) (see also N00-N07 with fourth character .0) N05.0
  myocardium, myocardial — see Degeneration, myocardial
  of life — see Menopause
  pacemaker Z45.018
    pulse generator Z45.010
  personality (enduring) F68.8
    due to (secondary to)
      general medical condition F07.0
      secondary (nonspecific) F60.89
  regressive, dental pulp K04.2
  renal — see Disease, renal
  retina H35.9
    myopic H44.2- ☑
  sacroiliac joint M53.3
  senile (see also condition) R54
  sensory R20.8
  skin R23.9
    acute, due to ultraviolet radiation L56.9
      specified NEC L56.8
    chronic, due to nonionizing radiation L57.9
      specified NEC L57.8
    cyanosis R23.0
    flushing R23.2
    pallor R23.1
    petechiae R23.3
    specified change NEC R23.8
    swelling — see Mass, localized
    texture R23.4
  trophic
    arm — see Mononeuropathy, upper limb
    leg — see Mononeuropathy, lower limb
  vascular I99.9
  vasomotor I73.9
  voice R49.9
    psychogenic F44.4
    specified NEC R49.8
Changing sleep-work schedule, affecting sleep G47.26
Changuinola fever A93.1
Chapping skin T69.8 ☑
Charcot-Marie-Tooth disease, paralysis or syndrome G60.0
Charcot's
  arthropathy — see Arthropathy, neuropathic
  cirrhosis K74.3
  disease (tabetic arthropathy) A52.16
  joint (disease) (tabetic) A52.16
    diabetic — see Diabetes, with, arthropathy
    syringomyelic G95.0
  syndrome (intermittent claudication) I73.9
CHARGE association Q89.8
Charley-horse (quadriceps) M62.831
  traumatic (quadriceps) S76.11- ☑
Charlouis' disease — see Yaws
Cheadle's disease E54
Checking (of)
  cardiac pacemaker (battery) (electrode(s)) Z45.018
    pulse generator Z45.010
  intrauterine contraceptive device Z30.431
Check-up — see Examination
Chédiak-Higashi (-Steinbrinck) **syndrome** (congenital gigantism of peroxidase granules) E70.330
Cheek — see condition
Cheese itch B88.0
Cheese-washer's lung J67.8
Cheese-worker's lung J67.8

Cheilitis (acute) (angular) (catarrhal) (chronic) (exfoliative) (gangrenous) (glandular) (infectional) (suppurative) (ulcerative) (vesicular) K13.0
  actinic (due to sun) L56.8
    other than from sun L59.8
  candidal B37.83
Cheilodynia K13.0
Cheiloschisis — see Cleft, lip
Cheilosis (angular) K13.0
  with pellagra E52
  due to
    vitamin B2 (riboflavin) deficiency E53.0
Cheiromegaly M79.89
Cheiropompholyx L30.1
Cheloid — see Keloid
Chemical burn — see Corrosion, by site
Chemodectoma — see Paraganglioma, nonchromaffin
Chemosis, conjunctiva — see Edema, conjunctiva
Chemotherapy (session) (for)
  cancer Z51.11
  neoplasm Z51.11
Cherubism M27.8
Chest — see condition
Cheyne-Stokes breathing (respiration) R06.3
Chiari's
  disease or syndrome (hepatic vein thrombosis) I82.0
  malformation
    type I G93.5
    type II — see Spina bifida
    net Q24.8
Chicago disease B40.9
Chickenpox — see Varicella
Chiclero ulcer or sore B55.1
Chigger (infestation) B88.0
Chignon (disease) B36.8
  newborn (from vacuum extraction) (birth injury) P12.1
Chilaiditi's syndrome (subphrenic displacement, colon) Q43.3
Chilblain(s) (lupus) T69.1 ☑
Child
  custody dispute Z65.3
Childbirth — see Delivery
Childhood
  cerebral X-linked adrenoleukodystrophy E71.520
  period of rapid growth Z00.2
Chill(s) R68.83
  with fever R50.9
  without fever R68.83
  congestive in malarial regions B54
Chilomastigiasis A07.8
Chimera 46,XX/46,XY Q99.0
Chin — see condition
Chinese dysentery A03.9
Chionophobia F40.228
Chitral fever A93.1
Chlamydia, chlamydial A74.9
  cervicitis A56.09
  conjunctivitis A74.0
  cystitis A56.01
  endometritis A56.11
  epididymitis A56.19
  female
    pelvic inflammatory disease A56.11
    pelviperitonitis A56.11
  orchitis A56.19
  peritonitis A74.81
  pharyngitis A56.4
  proctitis A56.3
  psittaci (infection) A70
  salpingitis A56.11
  sexually-transmitted infection NEC A56.8
  specified NEC A74.89
  urethritis A56.01
  vulvovaginitis A56.02
Chlamydiosis — see Chlamydia
Chloasma (skin) (idiopathic) (symptomatic) L81.1
  eyelid H02.719
    hyperthyroid E05.90 [H02.719]
      with thyroid storm E05.91 [H02.719]
    left H02.716
      lower H02.715
      upper H02.714
    right H02.713
      lower H02.712
      upper H02.711
Chloroma C92.3- ☑
Chlorosis D50.9

52   ☑ Additional Character Required — Refer to the Tabular List for Character Selection   ▽ Subterms under main terms may continue to next column or page

Chlorosis — *continued*
  Egyptian B76.9 [D63.8]
  miner's B76.9 [D63.8]
Chlorotic anemia D50.8
Chocolate cyst (ovary) N80.1
Choked
  disc or disk — *see* Papilledema
  on food, phlegm, or vomitus NOS — *see* Foreign body, by site
  while vomiting NOS — *see* Foreign body, by site
Chokes (resulting from bends) T70.3 ☑
Choking sensation R09.89
Cholangiectasis K83.8
Cholangiocarcinoma
  with hepatocellular carcinoma, combined C22.0
  liver C22.1
  specified site NEC — *see* Neoplasm, malignant, by site
  unspecified site C22.1
Cholangiohepatitis K83.8
  due to fluke infestation B66.1
Cholangiohepatoma C22.0
Cholangiolitis (acute) (chronic) (extrahepatic) (gangrenous) (intrahepatic) K83.0
  paratyphoidal — *see* Fever, paratyphoid
  typhoidal A01.09
Cholangioma D13.4
  malignant — *see* Cholangiocarcinoma
Cholangitis (ascending) (primary) (recurrent) (sclerosing) (secondary) (stenosing) (suppurative) K83.0
  with calculus, bile duct — *see* Calculus, bile duct, with cholangitis
  chronic nonsuppurative destructive K74.3
Cholecystectasia K82.8
Cholecystitis K81.9
  with
    calculus, stones in
      bile duct (common) (hepatic) — *see* Calculus, bile duct, with cholecystitis
      cystic duct — *see* Calculus, gallbladder, with cholecystitis
      gallbladder — *see* Calculus, gallbladder, with cholecystitis
      choledocholithiasis — *see* Calculus, bile duct, with cholecystitis
      cholelithiasis — *see* Calculus, gallbladder, with cholecystitis
  acute (emphysematous) (gangrenous) (suppurative) K81.0
    with
      calculus, stones in
        cystic duct — *see* Calculus, gallbladder, with cholecystitis, acute
        gallbladder — *see* Calculus, gallbladder, with cholecystitis, acute
        choledocholithiasis — *see* Calculus, bile duct, with cholecystitis, acute
        cholelithiasis — *see* Calculus, gallbladder, with cholecystitis, acute
    chronic cholecystitis K81.2
      with gallbladder calculus K80.12
        with obstruction K80.13
  chronic K81.1
    with acute cholecystitis K81.2
      with gallbladder calculus K80.12
        with obstruction K80.13
  emphysematous (acute) — *see* Cholecystitis, acute
  gangrenous — *see* Cholecystitis, acute
  paratyphoidal, current A01.4
  suppurative — *see* Cholecystitis, acute
  typhoidal A01.09
Cholecystolithiasis — *see* Calculus, gallbladder
Choledochitis (suppurative) K83.0
Choledocholith — *see* Calculus, bile duct
Choledocholithiasis (common duct) (hepatic duct) — *see* Calculus, bile duct
  cystic — *see* Calculus, gallbladder
  typhoidal A01.09
Cholelithiasis (cystic duct) (gallbladder) (impacted) (multiple) — *see* Calculus, gallbladder
  bile duct (common) (hepatic) — *see* Calculus, bile duct
  hepatic duct — *see* Calculus, bile duct
  specified NEC K80.80
    with obstruction K80.81
Cholemia (*see also* Jaundice)
  familial (simple) (congenital) E80.4
  Gilbert's E80.4
Choleperitoneum, choleperitonitis K65.3

Cholera (Asiatic) (epidemic) (malignant) A00.9
  antimonial — *see* Poisoning, antimony
  classical A00.0
  due to Vibrio cholerae 01 A00.9
    biovar cholerae A00.0
    biovar eltor A00.1
    el tor A00.1
  el tor A00.1
Cholerine — *see* Cholera
Cholestasis NEC K83.1
  with hepatocyte injury K71.0
  due to total parenteral nutrition (TPN) K76.89
  pure K71.0
Cholesteatoma (ear) (middle) (with reaction) H71.9- ☑
  attic H71.0- ☑
  external ear (canal) H60.4- ☑
  mastoid H71.2- ☑
  postmastoidectomy cavity (recurrent) — *see* Complications, postmastoidectomy, recurrent cholesteatoma
  recurrent (postmastoidectomy) — *see* Complications, postmastoidectomy, recurrent cholesteatoma
  tympanum H71.1- ☑
Cholesteatosis, diffuse H71.3- ☑
Cholesteremia E78.0
Cholesterin in vitreous — *see* Deposit, crystalline
Cholesterol
  deposit
    retina H35.89
    vitreous — *see* Deposit, crystalline
  elevated (high) E78.0
    with elevated (high) triglycerides E78.2
    screening for Z13.220
  imbibition of gallbladder K82.4
Cholesterolemia (essential) (familial) (hereditary) (pure) E78.0
Cholesterolosis, cholesterosis (gallbladder) K82.4
  cerebrotendinous E75.5
Cholocolic fistula K82.3
Choluria R82.2
Chondritis M94.8X9
  aurical H61.03- ☑
  costal (Tietze's) M94.0
  external ear H61.03- ☑
  patella, posttraumatic — *see* Chondromalacia, patella
  pinna H61.03- ☑
  purulent M94.8X- ☑
  tuberculous NEC A18.02
    intervertebral A18.01
Chondroblastoma (*see also* Neoplasm, bone, benign)
  malignant — *see* Neoplasm, bone, malignant
Chondrocalcinosis M11.20
  ankle M11.27- ☑
  elbow M11.22- ☑
  familial M11.10
    ankle M11.17- ☑
    elbow M11.12- ☑
    foot joint M11.17- ☑
    hand joint M11.14- ☑
    hip M11.15- ☑
    knee M11.16- ☑
    multiple site M11.19
    shoulder M11.11- ☑
    vertebrae M11.18
    wrist M11.13- ☑
  foot joint M11.27- ☑
  hand joint M11.24- ☑
  hip M11.25- ☑
  knee M11.26- ☑
  multiple site M11.29
  shoulder M11.21- ☑
  specified type NEC M11.20
    ankle M11.27- ☑
    elbow M11.22- ☑
    foot joint M11.27- ☑
    hand joint M11.24- ☑
    hip M11.25- ☑
    knee M11.26- ☑
    multiple site M11.29
    shoulder M11.21- ☑
    vertebrae M11.28
    wrist M11.23- ☑
  vertebrae M11.28
  wrist M11.23- ☑
Chondrodermatitis nodularis helicis or anthelicis — *see* Perichondritis, ear

Chondrodysplasia Q78.9
  with hemangioma Q78.4
  calcificans congenita Q77.3
  fetalis Q77.4
  metaphyseal (Jansen's) (McKusick's) (Schmid's) Q78.5
  punctata Q77.3
Chondrodystrophy, chondrodystrophia (familial) (fetalis) (hypoplastic) Q78.9
  calcificans congenita Q77.3
  myotonic (congenital) G71.13
  punctata Q77.3
Chondroectodermal dysplasia Q77.6
Chondrogenesis imperfecta Q77.4
Chondrolysis M94.35- ☑
Chondroma (*see also* Neoplasm, cartilage, benign)
  juxtacortical — *see* Neoplasm, bone, benign
  periosteal — *see* Neoplasm, bone, benign
Chondromalacia (systemic) M94.20
  acromioclavicular joint M94.21- ☑
  ankle M94.27- ☑
  elbow M94.22- ☑
  foot joint M94.27- ☑
  glenohumeral joint M94.21- ☑
  hand joint M94.24- ☑
  hip M94.25- ☑
  knee M94.26- ☑
    patella M22.4- ☑
  multiple sites M94.29
  patella M22.4- ☑
  rib M94.28
  sacroiliac joint M94.259
  shoulder M94.21- ☑
  sternoclavicular joint M94.21- ☑
  vertebral joint M94.28
  wrist M94.23- ☑
Chondromatosis (*see also* Neoplasm, cartilage, uncertain behavior)
  internal Q78.4
Chondromyxosarcoma — *see* Neoplasm, cartilage, malignant
Chondro-osteodysplasia (Morquio-Brailsford type) E76.219
Chondro-osteodystrophy E76.29
Chondro-osteoma — *see* Neoplasm, bone, benign
Chondropathia tuberosa M94.0
Chondrosarcoma — *see* Neoplasm, cartilage, malignant
  juxtacortical — *see* Neoplasm, bone, malignant
  mesenchymal — *see* Neoplasm, connective tissue, malignant
  myxoid — *see* Neoplasm, cartilage, malignant
Chordee (nonvenereal) N48.89
  congenital Q54.4
  gonococcal A54.09
Chorditis (fibrinous) (nodosa) (tuberosa) J38.2
Chordoma — *see* Neoplasm, vertebral (column), malignant
Chorea (chronic) (gravis) (posthemiplegic) (senile) (spasmodic) G25.5
  with
    heart involvement I02.0
      active or acute (conditions in I01-) I02.0
        rheumatic I02.9
          with valvular disorder I02.0
      rheumatic heart disease (chronic) (inactive)(quiescent) — *code to* rheumatic heart condition involved
  drug-induced G25.4
  habit F95.8
  hereditary G10
  Huntington's G10
  hysterical F44.4
  minor I02.9
    with heart involvement I02.0
  progressive G25.5
    hereditary G10
  rheumatic (chronic) I02.9
    with heart involvement I02.0
  Sydenham's I02.9
    with heart involvement — *see* Chorea, with rheumatic heart disease
    nonrheumatic G25.5
Choreoathetosis (paroxysmal) G25.5
Chorioadenoma (destruens) D39.2
Chorioamnionitis O41.12- ☑
Chorioangioma D26.7
Choriocarcinoma — *see* Neoplasm, malignant, by site
  combined with

Choriocarcinoma — *continued*
    combined with — *continued*
        embryonal carcinoma — *see* Neoplasm, malignant, by site
        other germ cell elements — *see* Neoplasm, malignant, by site
        teratoma — *see* Neoplasm, malignant, by site
    specified site — *see* Neoplasm, malignant, by site
    unspecified site
        female C58
        male C62.90
Chorioencephalitis (acute) (lymphocytic) (serous) A87.2
Chorioepithelioma — *see* Choriocarcinoma
Choriomeningitis (acute) (lymphocytic) (serous) A87.2
Chorionepithelioma — *see* Choriocarcinoma
Chorioretinitis (*see also* Inflammation, chorioretinal)
    disseminated (*see also* Inflammation, chorioretinal, disseminated)
        in neurosyphilis A52.19
    Egyptian B76.9 [D63.8]
    focal (*see also* Inflammation, chorioretinal, focal)
    histoplasmic B39.9 [H32]
    in (due to)
        histoplasmosis B39.9 [H32]
        syphilis (secondary) A51.43
            late A52.71
        toxoplasmosis (acquired) B58.01
            congenital (active) P37.1 [H32]
        tuberculosis A18.53
    juxtapapillary, juxtapapillaris — *see* Inflammation, chorioretinal, focal, juxtapapillary
    leprous A30.9 [H32]
    miner's B76.9 [D63.8]
    progressive myopia (degeneration) H44.2- ☑
    syphilitic (secondary) A51.43
        congenital (early) A50.01 [H32]
            late A50.32
        late A52.71
    tuberculous A18.53
Chorioretinopathy, central serous H35.71- ☑
Choroid — *see* condition
Choroideremia H31.21
Choroiditis — *see* Chorioretinitis
Choroidopathy — *see* Disorder, choroid
Choroidoretinitis — *see* Chorioretinitis
Choroidoretinopathy, central serous — *see* Chorioretinopathy, central serous
Christian-Weber disease M35.6
Christmas disease D67
Chromaffinoma (*see also* Neoplasm, benign, by site)
    malignant — *see* Neoplasm, malignant, by site
Chromatopsia — *see* Deficiency, color vision
Chromhidrosis, chromidrosis L75.1
Chromoblastomycosis — *see* Chromomycosis
Chromoconversion R82.91
Chromomycosis B43.9
    brain abscess B43.1
    cerebral B43.1
    cutaneous B43.0
    skin B43.0
    specified NEC B43.8
    subcutaneous abscess or cyst B43.2
Chromophytosis B36.0
Chromosome — *see* Anomaly, by chromosome involved
    D (1) — *see* Anomaly, chromosome 13
    E (3) — *see* Anomaly, chromosome 18
    G — *see* Anomaly, chromosome 21
Chromotrichomycosis B36.8
Chronic — *see* condition
    fracture — *see* Fracture, pathological
Churg-Strauss syndrome M30.1
Chyle cyst, mesentery I89.8
Chylocele (nonfilarial) I89.8
    filarial (*see also* Infestation, filarial) B74.9 [N51]
    tunica vaginalis N50.8
        filarial (*see also* Infestation, filarial) B74.9 [N51]
Chylomicronemia (fasting) (with hyperprebetalipoproteinemia) E78.3
Chylopericardium I31.3
    acute I30.9
Chylothorax (nonfilarial) I89.8
    filarial (*see also* Infestation, filarial) B74.9 [J91.8]
Chylous — *see* condition
Chyluria (nonfilarial) R82.0
    due to
        bilharziasis B65.0
        Brugia (malayi) B74.1

Chyluria — *continued*
    due to — *continued*
        Brugia — *continued*
            timori B74.2
        schistosomiasis (bilharziasis) B65.0
        Wuchereria (bancrofti) B74.0
    filarial — *see* Infestation, filarial
Cicatricial (deformity) — *see* Cicatrix
Cicatrix (adherent) (contracted) (painful) (vicious) (*see also* Scar) L90.5
    adenoid (and tonsil) J35.8
    alveolar process M26.79
    anus K62.89
    auricle — *see* Disorder, pinna, specified type NEC
    bile duct (common) (hepatic) K83.8
    bladder N32.89
    bone — *see* Disorder, bone, specified type NEC
    brain G93.89
    cervix (postoperative) (postpartal) N88.1
    common duct K83.8
    cornea H17.9
        tuberculous A18.59
    duodenum (bulb), obstructive K31.5
    esophagus K22.2
    eyelid — *see* Disorder, eyelid function
    hypopharynx J39.2
    lacrimal passages — *see* Obstruction, lacrimal
    larynx J38.7
    lung J98.4
    middle ear H74.8 ☑
    mouth K13.79
    muscle M62.89
        with contracture — *see* Contraction, muscle NEC
    nasopharynx J39.2
    palate (soft) K13.79
    penis N48.89
    pharynx J39.2
    prostate N42.89
    rectum K62.89
    retina — *see* Scar, chorioretinal
    semilunar cartilage — *see* Derangement, meniscus
    seminal vesicle N50.8
    skin L90.5
        infected L08.89
        postinfective L90.5
        tuberculous B90.8
    specified site NEC L90.5
    throat J39.2
    tongue K14.8
    tonsil (and adenoid) J35.8
    trachea J39.8
    tuberculous NEC B90.9
    urethra N36.8
    uterus N85.8
    vagina N89.8
        postoperative N99.2
    vocal cord J38.3
    wrist, constricting (annular) L90.5
CIDP (chronic inflammatory demyelinating polyneuropathy) G61.81
CIN — *see* Neoplasia, intraepithelial, cervix
Cinchonism — *see* Deafness, ototoxic
    correct substance properly administered — *see* Table of Drugs and Chemicals, by drug, adverse effect
    overdose or wrong substance given or taken — *see* Table of Drugs and Chemicals, by drug, poisoning
Circle of Willis — *see* condition
Circular — *see* condition
Circulating anticoagulants (*see also* Disorder, hemorrhagic) D68.318
    due to drugs (*see also* Disorder, hemorrhagic) D68.32
    following childbirth O72.3
Circulation
    collateral, any site I99.8
    defective (lower extremity) I99.8
        congenital Q28.9
    embryonic Q28.9
    failure (peripheral) R57.9
        newborn P29.89
    fetal, persistent P29.3
    heart, incomplete Q28.9
Circulatory system — *see* condition
Circulus senilis (cornea) — *see* Degeneration, cornea, senile
Circumcision (in absence of medical indication) (ritual) (routine) Z41.2
Circumscribed — *see* condition

Circumvallate placenta O43.11- ☑
Cirrhosis, cirrhotic (hepatic) (liver) K74.60
    alcoholic K70.30
        with ascites K70.31
    atrophic — *see* Cirrhosis, liver
    Baumgarten-Cruveilhier K74.69
    biliary (cholangiolitic) (cholangitic) (hypertrophic) (obstructive) (pericholangiolitic) K74.5
        due to
            Clonorchiasis B66.1
            flukes B66.3
        primary K74.3
        secondary K74.4
    cardiac (of liver) K76.1
    Charcot's K74.3
    cholangiolitic, cholangitic, cholostatic (primary) K74.3
    congestive K76.1
    Cruveilhier-Baumgarten K74.69
    cryptogenic (liver) K74.69
    due to
        hepatolenticular degeneration E83.01
        Wilson's disease E83.01
        xanthomatosis E78.2
    fatty K76.0
        alcoholic K70.0
    Hanot's (hypertrophic) K74.3
    hepatic — *see* Cirrhosis, liver
    hypertrophic K74.3
    Indian childhood K74.69
    kidney — *see* Sclerosis, renal
    Laennec's K70.30
        with ascites K70.31
        alcoholic K70.30
            with ascites K70.31
        nonalcoholic K74.69
    liver K74.60
        alcoholic K70.30
            with ascites K70.31
            fatty K70.0
        congenital P78.81
        syphilitic A52.74
    lung (chronic) J84.10
    macronodular K74.69
        alcoholic K70.30
            with ascites K70.31
    micronodular K74.69
        alcoholic K70.30
            with ascites K70.31
    mixed type K74.69
    monolobular K74.3
    nephritis — *see* Sclerosis, renal
    nutritional K74.69
        alcoholic K70.30
            with ascites K70.31
    obstructive — *see* Cirrhosis, biliary
    ovarian N83.8
    pancreas (duct) K86.8
    pigmentary E83.110
    portal K74.69
        alcoholic K70.30
            with ascites K70.31
    postnecrotic K74.69
        alcoholic K70.30
            with ascites K70.31
    pulmonary J84.10
    renal — *see* Sclerosis, renal
    spleen D73.2
    stasis K76.1
    Todd's K74.3
    unilobar K74.3
    xanthomatous (biliary) K74.5
        due to xanthomatosis (familial) (metabolic) (primary) E78.2
Cistern, subarachnoid R93.0
Citrullinemia E72.23
Citrullinuria E72.23
Civatte's disease or poikiloderma L57.3
Clam digger's itch B65.3
Clammy skin R23.1
Clap — *see* Gonorrhea
Clarke-Hadfield syndrome (pancreatic infantilism) K86.8
Clark's paralysis G80.9
Clastothrix L67.8
Claude Bernard-Horner syndrome G90.2
    traumatic — *see* Injury, nerve, cervical sympathetic
Claude's disease or syndrome G46.3
Claudicatio venosa intermittens I87.8

Claudication, intermittent I73.9
  cerebral (artery) G45.9
  spinal cord (arteriosclerotic) G95.19
    syphilitic A52.09
  venous (axillary) I87.8
Claustrophobia F40.240
Clavus (infected) L84
Clawfoot (congenital) Q66.89
  acquired — see Deformity, limb, clawfoot
Clawhand (acquired) (see also Deformity, limb, clawhand)
  congenital Q68.1
Clawtoe (congenital) Q66.89
  acquired — see Deformity, toe, specified NEC
Clay eating — see Pica
Cleansing of artificial opening — see Attention to, artificial, opening
Cleft (congenital) (see also Imperfect, closure)
  alveolar process M26.79
  branchial (cyst) (persistent) Q18.2
  cricoid cartilage, posterior Q31.8
  lip (unilateral) Q36.9
    with cleft palate Q37.9
      hard Q37.1
        with soft Q37.5
      soft Q37.3
        with hard Q37.5
    bilateral Q36.0
      with cleft palate Q37.8
        hard Q37.0
          with soft Q37.4
        soft Q37.2
          with hard Q37.4
    median Q36.1
  nose Q30.2
  palate Q35.9
    with cleft lip (unilateral) Q37.9
      bilateral Q37.8
    hard Q35.1
      with
        cleft lip (unilateral) Q37.1
          bilateral Q37.0
        soft Q35.5
          with cleft lip (unilateral) Q37.5
            bilateral Q37.4
    medial Q35.5
    soft Q35.3
      with
        cleft lip (unilateral) Q37.3
          bilateral Q37.2
      hard Q35.5
        with cleft lip (unilateral) Q37.5
          bilateral Q37.4
  penis Q55.69
  scrotum Q55.29
  thyroid cartilage Q31.8
  uvula Q35.7
Cleidocranial dysostosis Q74.0
Cleptomania F63.2
Clicking hip (newborn) R29.4
Climacteric (female) (see also Menopause)
  arthritis (any site) NEC — see Arthritis, specified form NEC
  depression (single episode) F32.8
  male (symptoms) (syndrome) NEC N50.8
  paranoid state F22
  polyarthritis NEC — see Arthritis, specified form NEC
  symptoms (female) N95.1
Clinical research investigation (clinical trial) (control subject) (normal comparison) (participant) Z00.6
Clitoris — see condition
Cloaca (persistent) Q43.7
Clonorchiasis, clonorchis infection (liver) B66.1
Clonus R25.8
Closed bite M26.29
Clostridium (C.) **perfringens, as cause of disease classified elsewhere** B96.7
Closure
  congenital, nose Q30.0
  cranial sutures, premature Q75.0
  defective or imperfect NEC — see Imperfect, closure
  fistula, delayed — see Fistula
  foramen ovale, imperfect Q21.1
  hymen N89.6
  interauricular septum, defective Q21.1
  interventricular septum, defective Q21.0
  lacrimal duct (see also Stenosis, lacrimal, duct)
    congenital Q10.5
  nose (congenital) Q30.0

Closure — continued
  nose — continued
    acquired M95.0
  of artificial opening — see Attention to, artificial, opening
  vagina N89.5
  valve — see Endocarditis
  vulva N90.5
Clot (blood) (see also Embolism)
  artery (obstruction) (occlusion) — see Embolism
  bladder N32.89
  brain (intradural or extradural) — see Occlusion, artery, cerebral
  circulation I74.9
  heart (see also Infarct, myocardium)
    not resulting in infarction I24.0
  vein — see Thrombosis
Clouded state R40.1
  epileptic — see Epilepsy, specified NEC
  paroxysmal — see Epilepsy, specified NEC
Cloudy antrum, antra J32.0
Clouston's (hidrotic) **ectodermal dysplasia** Q82.4
Clubbed nail pachydermoperiostosis M89.40 [L62]
Clubbing of finger(s) (nails) R68.3
Clubfinger R68.3
  congenital Q68.1
Clubfoot (congenital) Q66.89
  acquired — see Deformity, limb, clubfoot
  equinovarus Q66.0
  paralytic — see Deformity, limb, clubfoot
Clubhand (congenital) (radial) Q71.4- ☑
  acquired — see Deformity, limb, clubhand
Clubnail R68.3
  congenital Q84.6
Clump, kidney Q63.1
Clumsiness, clumsy child syndrome F82
Cluttering F80.81
Clutton's joints A50.51 [M12.80]
Coagulation, intravascular (diffuse) (disseminated) (see also Defibrination syndrome)
  complicating abortion — see Abortion, by type, complicated by, intravascular coagulation
  following ectopic or molar pregnancy O08.1
Coagulopathy (see also Defect, coagulation)
  consumption D65
  intravascular D65
    newborn P60
Coalition
  calcaneo-scaphoid Q66.89
  tarsal Q66.89
Coalminer's
  elbow — see Bursitis, elbow, olecranon
  lung or pneumoconiosis J60
Coalworker's lung or pneumoconiosis J60
Coarctation
  aorta (preductal) (postductal) Q25.1
  pulmonary artery Q25.71
Coated tongue K14.3
Coats' disease (exudative retinopathy) — see Retinopathy, exudative
Cocainism — see Dependence, drug, cocaine
Coccidioidomycosis B38.9
  cutaneous B38.3
  disseminated B38.7
  generalized B38.7
  meninges B38.4
  prostate B38.81
  pulmonary B38.2
    acute B38.0
    chronic B38.1
  skin B38.3
  specified NEC B38.89
Coccidioidosis — see Coccidioidomycosis
Coccidiosis (intestinal) A07.3
Coccydynia, coccygodynia M53.3
Coccyx — see condition
Cochin-China diarrhea K90.1
Cockayne's syndrome Q87.1
Cocked up toe — see Deformity, toe, specified NEC
Cock's peculiar tumor L72.3
Codman's tumor — see Neoplasm, bone, benign
Coenurosis B71.8
Coffee-worker's lung J67.8
Cogan's syndrome H16.32- ☑
  oculomotor apraxia H51.8
Coitus, painful (female) N94.1
  male N53.12

Coitus, painful — continued
  psychogenic F52.6
Cold J00
  with influenza, flu, or grippe — see Influenza, with, respiratory manifestations NEC
  agglutinin disease or hemoglobinuria (chronic) D59.1
  bronchial — see Bronchitis
  chest — see Bronchitis
  common (head) J00
  effects of T69.9 ☑
    specified effect NEC T69.8 ☑
  excessive, effects of T69.9 ☑
    specified effect NEC T69.8 ☑
  exhaustion from T69.8 ☑
  exposure to T69.9 ☑
    specified effect NEC T69.8 ☑
  head J00
  injury syndrome (newborn) P80.0
  on lung — see Bronchitis
  rose J30.1
  sensitivity, auto-immune D59.1
  virus J00
Coldsore B00.1
Colibacillosis A49.8
  as the cause of other disease (see also Escherichia coli) B96.20
  generalized A41.50
Colic (bilious) (infantile) (intestinal) (recurrent) (spasmodic) R10.83
  abdomen R10.83
    psychogenic F45.8
  appendix, appendicular K38.8
  bile duct — see Calculus, bile duct
  biliary — see Calculus, bile duct
  common duct — see Calculus, bile duct
  cystic duct — see Calculus, gallbladder
  Devonshire NEC — see Poisoning, lead
  gallbladder — see Calculus, gallbladder
  gallstone — see Calculus, gallbladder
    gallbladder or cystic duct — see Calculus, gallbladder
  hepatic (duct) — see Calculus, bile duct
  hysterical F45.8
  kidney N23
  lead NEC — see Poisoning, lead
  mucous K58.9
    with diarrhea K58.0
    psychogenic F54
  nephritic N23
  painter's NEC — see Poisoning, lead
  pancreas K86.8
  psychogenic F45.8
  renal N23
  saturnine NEC — see Poisoning, lead
  ureter N23
  urethral N36.8
    due to calculus N21.1
  uterus NEC N94.89
    menstrual — see Dysmenorrhea
  worm NOS B83.9
Colicystitis — see Cystitis
Colitis (acute) (catarrhal) (chronic) (noninfective) (hemorrhagic) (see also Enteritis) K52.9
  allergic K52.2
  amebic (acute) (see also Amebiasis) A06.0
    nondysenteric A06.2
  anthrax A22.2
  bacillary — see Infection, Shigella
  balantidial A07.0
  Clostridium difficile A04.7
  coccidial A07.3
  collagenous K52.89
  cystica superficialis K52.89
  dietary counseling and surveillance (for) Z71.3
  dietetic K52.2
  drug-induced K52.1
  due to radiation K52.0
  eosinophilic K52.82
  food hypersensitivity K52.2
  giardial A07.1
  granulomatous — see Enteritis, regional, large intestine
  infectious — see Enteritis, infectious
  ischemic K55.9
    acute (fulminant) (subacute) K55.0
    chronic K55.1
    due to mesenteric artery insufficiency K55.1

Colitis — *continued*
  ischemic — *continued*
    fulminant (acute) K55.0
    left sided K51.50
      with
        abscess K51.514
        complication K51.519
          specified NEC K51.518
        fistula K51.513
        obstruction K51.512
        rectal bleeding K51.511
  lymphocytic K52.89
  membranous
    psychogenic F54
  microscopic (collagenous) (lymphocytic) K52.89
  mucous — *see* Syndrome, irritable, bowel
    psychogenic F54
  noninfective K52.9
    specified NEC K52.89
  polyposa — *see* Polyp, colon, inflammatory
  protozoal A07.9
  pseudomembranous A04.7
  pseudomucinous — *see* Syndrome, irritable, bowel
  regional — *see* Enteritis, regional, large intestine
  segmental — *see* Enteritis, regional, large intestine
  septic — *see* Enteritis, infectious
  spastic K58.9
    with diarrhea K58.0
    psychogenic F54
  staphylococcal A04.8
    foodborne A05.0
  subacute ischemic K55.0
  thromboulcerative K55.0
  toxic NEC K52.1
    due to Clostridium difficile A04.7
  transmural — *see* Enteritis, regional, large intestine
  trichomonal A07.8
  tuberculous (ulcerative) A18.32
  ulcerative (chronic) K51.90
    with
      complication K51.919
        abscess K51.914
        fistula K51.913
        obstruction K51.912
        rectal bleeding K51.911
        specified complication NEC K51.918
    enterocolitis — *see* Enterocolitis, ulcerative
    ileocolitis — *see* Ileocolitis, ulcerative
    mucosal proctocolitis — *see* Proctocolitis, mucosal
    proctitis — *see* Proctitis, ulcerative
    pseudopolyposis — *see* Polyp, colon, inflammatory
    psychogenic F54
    rectosigmoiditis — *see* Rectosigmoiditis, ulcerative
    specified type NEC K51.80
      with
        complication K51.819
          abscess K51.814
          fistula K51.813
          obstruction K51.812
          rectal bleeding K51.811
          specified complication NEC K51.818

Collagenosis, collagen disease (nonvascular) (vascular) M35.9
  cardiovascular I42.8
  reactive perforating L87.1
  specified NEC M35.8

Collapse R55
  adrenal E27.2
  cardiorespiratory R57.0
  cardiovascular R57.0
    newborn P29.89
  circulatory (peripheral) R57.9
    during or after labor and delivery O75.1
    following ectopic or molar pregnancy O08.3
    newborn P29.89
  during or
    after labor and delivery O75.1
    resulting from a procedure, not elsewhere classified T81.10 ☑
  external ear canal — *see* Stenosis, external ear canal
  general R55
  heart — *see* Disease, heart
  heat T67.1 ☑
  hysterical F44.89
  labyrinth, membranous (congenital) Q16.5
  lung (massive) (*see also* Atelectasis) J98.19
    pressure due to anesthesia (general) (local) or other sedation T88.2 ☑

Collapse — *continued*
  lung (*see also* Atelectasis) — *continued*
    pressure due to anesthesia or other sedation — *continued*
      during labor and delivery O74.1
      in pregnancy O29.02-
      postpartum, puerperal O89.09
  myocardial — *see* Disease, heart
  nervous F48.8
  neurocirculatory F45.8
  nose M95.0
  postoperative T81.10 ☑
  pulmonary (*see also* Atelectasis) J98.19
    newborn — *see* Atelectasis
  trachea J39.8
  tracheobronchial J98.09
  valvular — *see* Endocarditis
  vascular (peripheral) R57.9
    during or after labor and delivery O75.1
    following ectopic or molar pregnancy O08.3
    newborn P29.89
  vertebra M48.50- ☑
    cervical region M48.52- ☑
    cervicothoracic region M48.53- ☑
    in (due to)
      metastasis — *see* Collapse, vertebra, in, specified disease NEC
      osteoporosis (*see also* Osteoporosis) M80.88 ☑
        cervical region M80.88 ☑
        cervicothoracic region M80.88 ☑
        lumbar region M80.88 ☑
        lumbosacral region M80.88 ☑
        multiple sites M80.88 ☑
        occipito-atlanto-axial region M80.88 ☑
        sacrococcygeal region M80.88 ☑
        thoracic region M80.88 ☑
        thoracolumbar region M80.88 ☑
      specified disease NEC M48.50- ☑
        cervical region M48.52- ☑
        cervicothoracic region M48.53- ☑
        lumbar region M48.56- ☑
        lumbosacral region M48.57- ☑
        occipito-atlanto-axial region M48.51- ☑
        sacrococcygeal region M48.58- ☑
        thoracic region M48.54- ☑
        thoracolumbar region M48.55- ☑
    lumbar region M48.56- ☑
    lumbosacral region M48.57- ☑
    occipito-atlanto-axial region M48.51- ☑
    sacrococcygeal region M48.58- ☑
    thoracic region M48.54- ☑
    thoracolumbar region M48.55- ☑

Collateral (*see also* condition)
  circulation (venous) I87.8
  dilation, veins I87.8

Colles' fracture S52.53- ☑

Collet (-Sicard) syndrome G52.7

Collier's asthma or lung J60

Collodion baby Q80.2

Colloid nodule (of thyroid) (cystic) E04.1

Coloboma (iris) Q13.0
  eyelid Q10.3
  fundus Q14.8
  lens Q12.2
  optic disc (congenital) Q14.2
    acquired H47.31- ☑

Coloenteritis — *see* Enteritis

Colon — *see* condition

Colonization
  MRSA (Methicillin resistant Staphylococcus aureus) Z22.322
  MSSA (Methicillin susceptible Staphylococcus aureus) Z22.321
  status — *see* Carrier (suspected) of

Coloptosis K63.4

Color blindness — *see* Deficiency, color vision

Colostomy
  attention to Z43.3
  fitting or adjustment Z46.89
  malfunctioning K94.03
  status Z93.3

Colpitis (acute) — *see* Vaginitis

Colpocele N81.5

Colpocystitis — *see* Vaginitis

Colpospasm N94.2

Column, spinal, vertebral — *see* condition

Coma R40.20
  with
    motor response (none) R40.231 ☑
      abnormal R40.233 ☑
      extension R40.232 ☑
      flexion withdrawal R40.234 ☑
      localizes pain R40.235 ☑
      obeys commands R40.236 ☑
    opening of eyes (never) R40.211 ☑
      in response to
        pain R40.212 ☑
        sound R40.213 ☑
      spontaneous R40.214 ☑
    verbal response (none) R40.221 ☑
      confused conversation R40.224 ☑
      inappropriate words R40.223 ☑
      incomprehensible words R40.222 ☑
      oriented R40.225 ☑
  eclamptic — *see* Eclampsia
  epileptic — *see* Epilepsy
  Glasgow, scale score — *see* Glasgow coma scale
  hepatic — *see* Failure, hepatic, by type, with coma
  hyperglycemic (diabetic) — *see* Diabetes, coma
  hyperosmolar (diabetic) — *see* Diabetes, coma
  hypoglycemic (diabetic) — *see* Diabetes, coma, hypoglycemic
    nondiabetic E15
  in diabetes — *see* Diabetes, coma
  insulin-induced — *see* Coma, hypoglycemic
  myxedematous E03.5
  newborn P91.5
  persistent vegetative state R40.3
  specified NEC, without documented Glasgow coma scale score, or with partial Glasgow coma scale score reported R40.244

Comatose — *see* Coma

Combat fatigue F43.0

Combined — *see* condition

Comedo, comedones (giant) L70.0

Comedocarcinoma (*see also* Neoplasm, breast, malignant)
  noninfiltrating
    breast D05.8- ☑
    specified site — *see* Neoplasm, in situ, by site
    unspecified site D05.8- ☑

Comedomastitis — *see* Ectasia, mammary duct

Comminuted fracture — *code as* Fracture, closed

Common
  arterial trunk Q20.0
  atrioventricular canal Q21.2
  atrium Q21.1
  cold (head) J00
  truncus (arteriosus) Q20.0
  variable immunodeficiency — *see* Immunodeficiency, common variable
  ventricle Q20.4

Commotio, commotion (current)
  brain — *see* Injury, intracranial, concussion
  cerebri — *see* Injury, intracranial, concussion
  retinae S05.8X- ☑
  spinal cord — *see* Injury, spinal cord, by region
  spinalis — *see* Injury, spinal cord, by region

Communication
  between
    base of aorta and pulmonary artery Q21.4
    left ventricle and right atrium Q20.5
    pericardial sac and pleural sac Q34.8
    pulmonary artery and pulmonary vein, congenital Q25.72
  congenital between uterus and digestive or urinary tract Q51.7

Compartment syndrome (deep) (posterior) (traumatic) T79.A0 ☑ (*following* T79.7)
  abdomen T79.A3 ☑ (*following* T79.7)
  lower extremity (hip, buttock, thigh, leg, foot, toes) T79.A2 ☑ (*following* T79.7)
  nontraumatic
    abdomen M79.A3 (*following* M79.7)
    lower extremity (hip, buttock, thigh, leg, foot, toes) M79.A2- ☑ (*following* M79.7)
    specified site NEC M79.A9 (*following* M79.7)
    upper extremity (shoulder, arm, forearm, wrist, hand, fingers) M79.A1- ☑ (*following* M79.7)
  specified site NEC T79.A9 ☑ (*following* T79.7)
  upper extremity (shoulder, arm, forearm, wrist, hand, fingers) T79.A1- ☑ (*following* T79.7)

☑ **Additional Character Required** — **Refer to the Tabular List for Character Selection**
▽ **Subterms under main terms may continue to next column or page**

Compensation
failure — *see* Disease, heart
neurosis, psychoneurosis — *see* Disorder, factitious

Complaint (*see also* Disease)
bowel, functional K59.9
psychogenic F45.8
intestine, functional K59.9
psychogenic F45.8
kidney — *see* Disease, renal
miners' J60

Complete — *see* condition

Complex
Addison-Schilder E71.528
cardiorenal — *see* Hypertension, cardiorenal
Costen's M26.69
disseminated mycobacterium avium- intracellulare (DMAC) A31.2
Eisenmenger's (ventricular septal defect) I27.89
hypersexual F52.8
jumped process, spine — *see* Dislocation, vertebra
primary, tuberculous A15.7
Schilder-Addison E71.528
subluxation (vertebral) M99.19
abdomen M99.19
acromioclavicular M99.17
cervical region M99.11
cervicothoracic M99.11
costochondral M99.18
costovertebral M99.18
head region M99.10
hip M99.15
lower extremity M99.16
lumbar region M99.13
lumbosacral M99.13
occipitocervical M99.10
pelvic region M99.15
pubic M99.15
rib cage M99.18
sacral region M99.14
sacrococcygeal M99.14
sacroiliac M99.14
specified NEC M99.19
sternochondral M99.18
sternoclavicular M99.17
thoracic region M99.12
thoracolumbar M99.12
upper extremity M99.17
Taussig-Bing (transposition, aorta and overriding pulmonary artery) Q20.1

Complication(s) (from) (of)
accidental puncture or laceration during a procedure (of) — *see* Complications, intraoperative (intraprocedural), puncture or laceration
amputation stump (surgical) (late) NEC T87.9
dehiscence T87.81
infection or inflammation T87.40
lower limb T87.4- ☑
upper limb T87.4- ☑
necrosis T87.50
lower limb T87.5- ☑
upper limb T87.5- ☑
neuroma T87.30
lower limb T87.3- ☑
upper limb T87.3- ☑
specified type NEC T87.89
anastomosis (and bypass) (*see also* Complications, prosthetic device or implant)
intestinal (internal) NEC K91.89
involving urinary tract N99.89
urinary tract (involving intestinal tract) N99.89
vascular — *see* Complications, cardiovascular device or implant
anesthesia, anesthetic (*see also* Anesthesia, complication) T88.59
brain, postpartum, puerperal O89.2
cardiac
in
labor and delivery O74.2
pregnancy O29.19- ☑
postpartum, puerperal O89.1
central nervous system
in
labor and delivery O74.3
pregnancy O29.29- ☑
postpartum, puerperal O89.2
difficult or failed intubation T88.4 ☑
in pregnancy O29.6- ☑

Complication(s) — *continued*
anesthesia, anesthetic (*see also* Anesthesia, complication) — *continued*
failed sedation (conscious) (moderate) during procedure T88.52
hyperthermia, malignant T88.3 ☑
hypothermia T88.51 ☑
intubation failure T88.4 ☑
malignant hyperthermia T88.3 ☑
pulmonary
in
labor and delivery O74.1
pregnancy NEC O29.09- ☑
postpartum, puerperal O89.09
shock T88.2 ☑
spinal and epidural
in
labor and delivery NEC O74.6
headache O74.5
pregnancy NEC O29.5X- ☑
postpartum, puerperal NEC O89.5
headache O89.4
anti-reflux device — *see* Complications, esophageal anti-reflux device
aortic (bifurcation) graft — *see* Complications, graft, vascular
aortocoronary (bypass) graft — *see* Complications, coronary artery (bypass) graft
aortofemoral (bypass) graft — *see* Complications, extremity artery (bypass) graft
arteriovenous
fistula, surgically created T82.9 ☑
embolism T82.818 ☑
fibrosis T82.828 ☑
hemorrhage T82.838 ☑
infection or inflammation T82.7 ☑
mechanical
breakdown T82.510 ☑
displacement T82.520 ☑
leakage T82.530 ☑
malposition T82.520 ☑
obstruction T82.590 ☑
perforation T82.590 ☑
protrusion T82.590 ☑
pain T82.848 ☑
specified type NEC T82.898 ☑
stenosis T82.858 ☑
thrombosis T82.868 ☑
shunt, surgically created T82.9 ☑
embolism T82.818 ☑
fibrosis T82.828 ☑
hemorrhage T82.838 ☑
infection or inflammation T82.7 ☑
mechanical
breakdown T82.511 ☑
displacement T82.521 ☑
leakage T82.531 ☑
malposition T82.521 ☑
obstruction T82.591 ☑
perforation T82.591 ☑
protrusion T82.591 ☑
pain T82.848 ☑
specified type NEC T82.898 ☑
stenosis T82.858 ☑
thrombosis T82.868 ☑
arthroplasty — *see* Complications, joint prosthesis
artificial
fertilization or insemination N98.9
attempted introduction (of)
embryo in embryo transfer N98.3
ovum following in vitro fertilization N98.2
hyperstimulation of ovaries N98.1
infection N98.0
specified NEC N98.8
heart T82.9 ☑
embolism T82.817 ☑
fibrosis T82.827 ☑
hemorrhage T82.837 ☑
infection or inflammation T82.7 ☑
mechanical
breakdown T82.512 ☑
displacement T82.522 ☑
leakage T82.532 ☑
malposition T82.522 ☑
obstruction T82.592 ☑
perforation T82.592 ☑

Complication(s) — *continued*
artificial — *continued*
heart — *continued*
mechanical — *continued*
protrusion T82.592 ☑
pain T82.847 ☑
specified type NEC T82.897 ☑
stenosis T82.857 ☑
thrombosis T82.867 ☑
opening
cecostomy — *see* Complications, colostomy
colostomy — *see* Complications, colostomy
cystostomy — *see* Complications, cystostomy
enterostomy — *see* Complications, enterostomy
gastrostomy — *see* Complications, gastrostomy
ileostomy — *see* Complications, enterostomy
jejunostomy — *see* Complications, enterostomy
nephrostomy — *see* Complications, stoma, urinary tract
tracheostomy — *see* Complications, tracheostomy
ureterostomy — *see* Complications, stoma, urinary tract
urethrostomy — *see* Complications, stoma, urinary tract
balloon implant or device
gastrointestinal T85.9 ☑
embolism T85.81 ☑
fibrosis T85.82 ☑
hemorrhage T85.83 ☑
infection and inflammation T85.79 ☑
pain T85.84 ☑
specified type NEC T85.89 ☑
stenosis T85.85 ☑
thrombosis T85.86 ☑
vascular (counterpulsation) T82.9 ☑
embolism T82.818 ☑
fibrosis T82.828 ☑
hemorrhage T82.838 ☑
infection or inflammation T82.7 ☑
mechanical
breakdown T82.513 ☑
displacement T82.523 ☑
leakage T82.533 ☑
malposition T82.523 ☑
obstruction T82.593 ☑
perforation T82.593 ☑
protrusion T82.593 ☑
pain T82.848 ☑
specified type NEC T82.898 ☑
stenosis T82.858 ☑
thrombosis T82.868 ☑
bariatric procedure
gastric band procedure K95.09
infection K95.01
specified procedure NEC K95.89
infection K95.81
bile duct implant (prosthetic) T85.9 ☑
embolism T85.81 ☑
fibrosis T85.82 ☑
hemorrhage T85.83 ☑
infection and inflammation T85.79 ☑
mechanical
breakdown T85.510 ☑
displacement T85.520 ☑
malfunction T85.510 ☑
malposition T85.520 ☑
obstruction T85.590 ☑
perforation T85.590 ☑
protrusion T85.590 ☑
specified NEC T85.590 ☑
pain T85.84 ☑
specified type NEC T85.89 ☑
stenosis T85.85 ☑
thrombosis T85.86 ☑
bladder device (auxiliary) — *see* Complications, genitourinary, device or implant, urinary system
bleeding (postoperative) — *see* Complication, postoperative, hemorrhage
intraoperative — *see* Complication, intraoperative, hemorrhage
blood vessel graft — *see* Complications, graft, vascular
bone
device NEC T84.9 ☑
embolism T84.81 ☑

Complication(s) — *continued*
bone — *continued*
  device — *continued*
    fibrosis T84.82 ☑
    hemorrhage T84.83 ☑
    infection or inflammation T84.7 ☑
    mechanical
      breakdown T84.318 ☑
      displacement T84.328 ☑
      malposition T84.328 ☑
      obstruction T84.398 ☑
      perforation T84.398 ☑
      protrusion T84.398 ☑
    pain T84.84 ☑
    specified type NEC T84.89 ☑
    stenosis T84.85 ☑
    thrombosis T84.86 ☑
  graft — *see* Complications, graft, bone
  growth stimulator (electrode) — *see* Complications, electronic stimulator device, bone
  marrow transplant — *see* Complications, transplant, bone, marrow
brain neurostimulator (electrode) — *see* Complications, electronic stimulator device, brain
breast implant (prosthetic) T85.9 ☑
  capsular contracture T85.44 ☑
  embolism T85.81 ☑
  fibrosis T85.82 ☑
  hemorrhage T85.83 ☑
  infection and inflammation T85.79 ☑
  mechanical
    breakdown T85.41 ☑
    displacement T85.42 ☑
    leakage T85.43 ☑
    malposition T85.42 ☑
    obstruction T85.49 ☑
    perforation T85.49 ☑
    protrusion T85.49 ☑
    specified NEC T85.49 ☑
  pain T85.84 ☑
  specified type NEC T85.89 ☑
  stenosis T85.85 ☑
  thrombosis T85.86 ☑
bypass (*see also* Complications, prosthetic device or implant)
  aortocoronary — *see* Complications, coronary artery (bypass) graft
  arterial (*see also* Complications, graft, vascular)
    extremity — *see* Complications, extremity artery (bypass) graft
cardiac (*see also* Disease, heart)
  device, implant or graft T82.9 ☑
    embolism T82.817 ☑
    fibrosis T82.827 ☑
    hemorrhage T82.837 ☑
    infection or inflammation T82.7 ☑
      valve prosthesis T82.6 ☑
    mechanical
      breakdown T82.519 ☑
        specified device NEC T82.518 ☑
      displacement T82.529 ☑
        specified device NEC T82.528 ☑
      leakage T82.539 ☑
        specified device NEC T82.538 ☑
      malposition T82.529 ☑
        specified device NEC T82.528 ☑
      obstruction T82.599 ☑
        specified device NEC T82.598 ☑
      perforation T82.599 ☑
        specified device NEC T82.598 ☑
      protrusion T82.599 ☑
        specified device NEC T82.598 ☑
    pain T82.847 ☑
    specified type NEC T82.897 ☑
    stenosis T82.857 ☑
    thrombosis T82.867 ☑
cardiovascular device, graft or implant T82.9 ☑
  aortic graft — *see* Complications, graft, vascular
  arteriovenous
    fistula, artificial — *see* Complication, arteriovenous, fistula, surgically created
    shunt — *see* Complication, arteriovenous, shunt, surgically created
  artificial heart — *see* Complication, artificial, heart
  balloon (counterpulsation) device — *see* Complication, balloon implant, vascular

Complication(s) — *continued*
cardiovascular device, graft or implant — *continued*
  carotid artery graft — *see* Complications, graft, vascular
  coronary bypass graft — *see* Complication, coronary artery (bypass) graft
  dialysis catheter (vascular) — *see* Complication, catheter, dialysis
  electronic T82.9 ☑
    electrode T82.9 ☑
      embolism T82.817 ☑
      fibrosis T82.827 ☑
      hemorrhage T82.837 ☑
      infection T82.7 ☑
      mechanical
        breakdown T82.110 ☑
        displacement T82.120 ☑
        leakage T82.190 ☑
        obstruction T82.190 ☑
        perforation T82.190 ☑
        protrusion T82.190 ☑
        specified type NEC T82.190 ☑
      pain T82.847 ☑
      specified NEC T82.897 ☑
      stenosis T82.857 ☑
      thrombosis T82.867 ☑
    embolism T82.817 ☑
    fibrosis T82.827 ☑
    hemorrhage T82.837 ☑
    infection T82.7 ☑
    mechanical
      breakdown T82.119 ☑
      displacement T82.129 ☑
      leakage T82.199 ☑
      obstruction T82.199 ☑
      perforation T82.199 ☑
      protrusion T82.199 ☑
      specified type NEC T82.199 ☑
    pain T82.847 ☑
    pulse generator T82.9 ☑
      embolism T82.817 ☑
      fibrosis T82.827 ☑
      hemorrhage T82.837 ☑
      infection T82.7 ☑
      mechanical
        breakdown T82.111 ☑
        displacement T82.121 ☑
        leakage T82.191 ☑
        obstruction T82.191 ☑
        perforation T82.191 ☑
        protrusion T82.191 ☑
        specified type NEC T82.191 ☑
      pain T82.847 ☑
      specified NEC T82.897 ☑
      stenosis T82.857 ☑
      thrombosis T82.867 ☑
    specified condition NEC T82.897 ☑
    specified device NEC T82.9 ☑
      embolism T82.817 ☑
      fibrosis T82.827 ☑
      hemorrhage T82.837 ☑
      infection T82.7 ☑
      mechanical
        breakdown T82.118 ☑
        displacement T82.128 ☑
        leakage T82.198 ☑
        obstruction T82.198 ☑
        perforation T82.198 ☑
        protrusion T82.198 ☑
        specified type NEC T82.198 ☑
      pain T82.847 ☑
      specified NEC T82.897 ☑
      stenosis T82.857 ☑
      thrombosis T82.867 ☑
    stenosis T82.857 ☑
    thrombosis T82.867 ☑
  extremity artery graft — *see* Complication, extremity artery (bypass) graft
  femoral artery graft — *see* Complication, extremity artery (bypass) graft
  heart
    transplant — *see* Complication, transplant, heart
    valve — *see* Complication, prosthetic device, heart valve

Complication(s) — *continued*
cardiovascular device, graft or implant — *continued*
  heart — *continued*
    valve — *see* Complication, prosthetic device, heart valve — *continued*
      graft — *see* Complication, heart, valve, graft
    heart-lung transplant — *see* Complication, transplant, heart, with lung
    infection or inflammation T82.7 ☑
    umbrella device — *see* Complication, umbrella device, vascular
    vascular graft (or anastomosis) — *see* Complication, graft, vascular
  carotid artery (bypass) graft — *see* Complications, graft, vascular
  catheter (device) NEC (*see also* Complications, prosthetic device or implant)
    cystostomy T83.9 ☑
      embolism T83.81 ☑
      fibrosis T83.82 ☑
      hemorrhage T83.83 ☑
      infection and inflammation T83.59 ☑
      mechanical
        breakdown T83.010 ☑
        displacement T83.020 ☑
        leakage T83.030 ☑
        malposition T83.020 ☑
        obstruction T83.090 ☑
        perforation T83.090 ☑
        protrusion T83.090 ☑
        specified NEC T83.090 ☑
      pain T83.84 ☑
      specified type NEC T83.89 ☑
      stenosis T83.85 ☑
      thrombosis T83.86 ☑
    dialysis (vascular) T82.9 ☑
      embolism T82.818 ☑
      fibrosis T82.828 ☑
      hemorrhage T82.838 ☑
      infection and inflammation T82.7 ☑
      intraperitoneal — *see* Complications, catheter, intraperitoneal
      mechanical
        breakdown T82.41 ☑
        displacement T82.42 ☑
        leakage T82.43 ☑
        malposition T82.42 ☑
        obstruction T82.49 ☑
        perforation T82.49 ☑
        protrusion T82.49 ☑
      pain T82.848 ☑
      specified type NEC T82.898 ☑
      stenosis T82.858 ☑
      thrombosis T82.868 ☑
    epidural infusion T85.9 ☑
      embolism T85.81 ☑
      fibrosis T85.82 ☑
      hemorrhage T85.83 ☑
      infection and inflammation T85.79 ☑
      mechanical
        breakdown T85.610 ☑
        displacement T85.620 ☑
        leakage T85.630 ☑
        malfunction T85.610 ☑
        malposition T85.620 ☑
        obstruction T85.690 ☑
        perforation T85.690 ☑
        protrusion T85.690 ☑
        specified NEC T85.690 ☑
      pain T85.84 ☑
      specified type NEC T85.89 ☑
      stenosis T85.85 ☑
      thrombosis T85.86 ☑
    intraperitoneal dialysis T85.9 ☑
      embolism T85.81 ☑
      fibrosis T85.82 ☑
      hemorrhage T85.83 ☑
      infection and inflammation T85.71 ☑
      mechanical
        breakdown T85.611 ☑
        displacement T85.621 ☑
        leakage T85.631 ☑
        malfunction T85.611 ☑
        malposition T85.621 ☑
        obstruction T85.691 ☑

58

☑ **Additional Character Required** — Refer to the Tabular List for Character Selection   ▽ **Subterms under main terms may continue to next column or page**

Index

Complication — Complication

Complication(s) — *continued*
  catheter (*see also* Complications, prosthetic device or implant) — *continued*
    intraperitoneal dialysis — *continued*
      mechanical — *continued*
        perforation T85.691 ☑
        protrusion T85.691 ☑
        specified NEC T85.691 ☑
      pain T85.84 ☑
      specified type NEC T85.89 ☑
      stenosis T85.85 ☑
      thrombosis T85.86 ☑
    intravenous infusion T82.9 ☑
      embolism T82.818 ☑
      fibrosis T82.828 ☑
      hemorrhage T82.838 ☑
      infection or inflammation T82.7 ☑
      mechanical
        breakdown T82.514 ☑
        displacement T82.524 ☑
        leakage T82.534 ☑
        malposition T82.524 ☑
        obstruction T82.594 ☑
        perforation T82.594 ☑
        protrusion T82.594 ☑
      pain T82.848 ☑
      specified type NEC T82.898 ☑
      stenosis T82.858 ☑
      thrombosis T82.868 ☑
    subdural infusion T85.9 ☑
      embolism T85.81 ☑
      fibrosis T85.82 ☑
      hemorrhage T85.83 ☑
      infection and inflammation T85.79 ☑
      mechanical
        breakdown T85.610 ☑
        displacement T85.620 ☑
        leakage T85.630 ☑
        malfunction T85.610 ☑
        malposition T85.620 ☑
        obstruction T85.690 ☑
        perforation T85.690 ☑
        protrusion T85.690 ☑
        specified NEC T85.690 ☑
      pain T85.84 ☑
      specified type NEC T85.89 ☑
      stenosis T85.85 ☑
      thrombosis T85.86 ☑
    urethral, indwelling T83.9 ☑
      displacement T83.028 ☑
      embolism T83.81 ☑
      fibrosis T83.82 ☑
      hemorrhage T83.83 ☑
      infection and inflammation T83.51 ☑
      leakage T83.038 ☑
      malposition T83.028 ☑
      mechanical
        breakdown T83.018 ☑
      obstruction (mechanical) T83.098 ☑
      pain T83.84 ☑
      perforation T83.098 ☑
      protrusion T83.098 ☑
      specified type NEC T83.098 ☑
      stenosis T83.85 ☑
      thrombosis T83.86 ☑
    urinary (indwelling) — *see* Complications, catheter, urethral, indwelling
  cecostomy (stoma) — *see* Complications, colostomy
  cesarean delivery wound NEC O90.89
    disruption O90.0
    hematoma O90.2
    infection (following delivery) O86.0
  chemotherapy (antineoplastic) NEC T88.7 ☑
  chin implant (prosthetic) — *see* Complication, prosthetic device or implant, specified NEC
  circulatory system I99.8
    intraoperative I97.88
    postprocedural I97.89
      following cardiac surgery I97.19- ☑
        postcardiotomy syndrome I97.0
      hypertension I97.3
      lymphedema after mastectomy I97.2
      postcardiotomy syndrome I97.0
      specified NEC I97.89
  colostomy (stoma) K94.00
    hemorrhage K94.01

Complication(s) — *continued*
  colostomy — *continued*
    infection K94.02
    malfunction K94.03
    mechanical K94.03
    specified complication NEC K94.09
  contraceptive device, intrauterine — *see* Complications, intrauterine, contraceptive device
  cord (umbilical) — *see* Complications, umbilical cord
  corneal graft — *see* Complications, graft, cornea
  coronary artery (bypass) graft T82.9 ☑
    atherosclerosis — *see* Arteriosclerosis, coronary (artery),
    embolism T82.818 ☑
    fibrosis T82.828 ☑
    hemorrhage T82.838 ☑
    infection and inflammation T82.7 ☑
    mechanical
      breakdown T82.211 ☑
      displacement T82.212 ☑
      leakage T82.213 ☑
      malposition T82.212 ☑
      obstruction T82.218 ☑
      perforation T82.218 ☑
      protrusion T82.218 ☑
      specified NEC T82.218 ☑
    pain T82.848 ☑
    specified type NEC T82.897 ☑
    stenosis T82.858 ☑
    thrombosis T82.868 ☑
  counterpulsation device (balloon), intra- aortic — *see* Complications, balloon implant, vascular
  cystostomy (stoma) N99.518
    catheter — *see* Complications, catheter, cystostomy
    hemorrhage N99.510
    infection N99.511
    malfunction N99.512
    specified type NEC N99.518
  delivery (*see also* Complications, obstetric) O75.9
    procedure (instrumental) (manual) (surgical) O75.4
    specified NEC O75.89
  dialysis (peritoneal) (renal) (*see also* Complications, infusion)
    catheter (vascular) — *see* Complication, catheter, dialysis
      peritoneal, intraperitoneal — *see* Complications, catheter, intraperitoneal
  dorsal column (spinal) neurostimulator — *see* Complications, electronic stimulator device, spinal cord
  drug NEC T88.7 ☑
  ear procedure (*see also* Disorder, ear)
    intraoperative H95.88
      hematoma — *see* Complications, intraoperative, hemorrhage (hematoma) (of), ear
      hemorrhage — *see* Complications, intraoperative, hemorrhage (hematoma) (of), ear
      laceration — *see* Complications, intraoperative, puncture or laceration..., ear
      specified NEC H95.88
    postoperative H95.89
      external ear canal stenosis H95.81- ☑
      hematoma — *see* Complications, postprocedural, hemorrhage (hematoma) (of), ear
      hemorrhage — *see* Complications, postprocedural, hemorrhage (hematoma) (of), ear
      postmastoidectomy — *see* Complications, postmastoidectomy
      specified NEC H95.89
  ectopic pregnancy O08.9
    damage to pelvic organs O08.6
    embolism O08.2
    genital infection O08.0
    hemorrhage (delayed) (excessive) O08.1
    metabolic disorder O08.5
    renal failure O08.4
    shock O08.3
    specified type NEC O08.0
    venous complication NEC O08.7
  electronic stimulator device
    bladder (urinary) — *see* Complications, electronic stimulator device, urinary
    bone T84.9 ☑
      breakdown T84.310 ☑
      displacement T84.320 ☑
      embolism T84.81 ☑
      fibrosis T84.82 ☑

Complication(s) — *continued*
  electronic stimulator device — *continued*
    bone — *continued*
      hemorrhage T84.83 ☑
      infection or inflammation T84.7 ☑
      malfunction T84.310 ☑
      malposition T84.320 ☑
      mechanical NEC T84.390 ☑
      obstruction T84.390 ☑
      pain T84.84 ☑
      perforation T84.390 ☑
      protrusion T84.390 ☑
      specified type NEC T84.89 ☑
      stenosis T84.85 ☑
      thrombosis T84.86 ☑
    brain T85.9 ☑
      embolism T85.81 ☑
      fibrosis T85.82 ☑
      hemorrhage T85.83 ☑
      infection and inflammation T85.79 ☑
      mechanical
        breakdown T85.110 ☑
        displacement T85.120 ☑
        leakage T85.190 ☑
        malposition T85.120 ☑
        obstruction T85.190 ☑
        perforation T85.190 ☑
        protrusion T85.190 ☑
        specified NEC T85.190 ☑
      pain T85.84 ☑
      specified type NEC T85.89 ☑
      stenosis T85.85 ☑
      thrombosis T85.86 ☑
    cardiac (defibrillator) (pacemaker) — *see* Complications, cardiovascular device or implant, electronic
    muscle T84.9 ☑
      breakdown T84.418 ☑
      displacement T84.428 ☑
      embolism T84.81 ☑
      fibrosis T84.82 ☑
      hemorrhage T84.83 ☑
      infection or inflammation T84.7 ☑
      mechanical NEC T84.498 ☑
      pain T84.84 ☑
      specified type NEC T84.89 ☑
      stenosis T84.85 ☑
      thrombosis T84.86 ☑
    nervous system T85.9 ☑
      brain — *see* Complications, electronic stimulator device, brain
      embolism T85.81 ☑
      fibrosis T85.82 ☑
      hemorrhage T85.83 ☑
      infection and inflammation T85.79 ☑
      mechanical
        breakdown T85.118 ☑
        displacement T85.128 ☑
        leakage T85.199 ☑
        malposition T85.128 ☑
        obstruction T85.199 ☑
        perforation T85.199 ☑
        protrusion T85.199 ☑
        specified NEC T85.199 ☑
      pain T85.84 ☑
      peripheral nerve — *see* Complications, electronic stimulator device, peripheral nerve
      specified type NEC T85.89 ☑
      spinal cord — *see* Complications, electronic stimulator device, spinal cord
      stenosis T85.85 ☑
      thrombosis T85.86 ☑
    peripheral nerve T85.9 ☑
      embolism T85.81 ☑
      fibrosis T85.82 ☑
      hemorrhage T85.83 ☑
      infection and inflammation T85.79 ☑
      mechanical
        breakdown T85.111 ☑
        displacement T85.121 ☑
        leakage T85.191 ☑
        malposition T85.121 ☑
        obstruction T85.191 ☑
        perforation T85.191 ☑
        protrusion T85.191 ☑
        specified NEC T85.191 ☑

Complication(s) — *continued*
electronic stimulator device — *continued*
  peripheral nerve — *continued*
    pain T85.84 ☑
    specified type NEC T85.89 ☑
    stenosis T85.85 ☑
    thrombosis T85.86 ☑
  spinal cord T85.9 ☑
    embolism T85.81 ☑
    fibrosis T85.82 ☑
    hemorrhage T85.83 ☑
    infection and inflammation T85.79 ☑
    mechanical
      breakdown T85.112 ☑
      displacement T85.122 ☑
      leakage T85.192 ☑
      malposition T85.122 ☑
      obstruction T85.192 ☑
      perforation T85.192 ☑
      protrusion T85.192 ☑
      specified NEC T85.192 ☑
    pain T85.84 ☑
    specified type NEC T85.89 ☑
    stenosis T85.85 ☑
    thrombosis T85.86 ☑
  urinary T83.9 ☑
    embolism T83.81 ☑
    fibrosis T83.82 ☑
    hemorrhage T83.83 ☑
    infection and inflammation T83.59 ☑
    mechanical
      breakdown T83.110 ☑
      displacement T83.120 ☑
      malposition T83.120 ☑
      perforation T83.190 ☑
      protrusion T83.190 ☑
      specified NEC T83.190 ☑
    pain T83.84 ☑
    specified type NEC T83.89 ☑
    stenosis T83.85 ☑
    thrombosis T83.86 ☑
electroshock therapy T88.9 ☑
  specified NEC T88.8 ☑
endocrine E34.9
  postprocedural
    adrenal hypofunction E89.6
    hypoinsulinemia E89.1
    hypoparathyroidism E89.2
    hypopituitarism E89.3
    hypothyroidism E89.0
    ovarian failure E89.40
      asymptomatic E89.40
      symptomatic E89.41
    specified NEC E89.89
    testicular hypofunction E89.5
endodontic treatment NEC M27.59
enterostomy (stoma) K94.10
  hemorrhage K94.11
  infection K94.12
  malfunction K94.13
  mechanical K94.13
  specified complication NEC K94.19
episiotomy, disruption O90.1
esophageal anti-reflux device T85.9 ☑
  embolism T85.81 ☑
  fibrosis T85.82 ☑
  hemorrhage T85.83 ☑
  infection and inflammation T85.79 ☑
  mechanical
    breakdown T85.511 ☑
    displacement T85.521 ☑
    malfunction T85.511 ☑
    malposition T85.521 ☑
    obstruction T85.591 ☑
    perforation T85.591 ☑
    protrusion T85.591 ☑
    specified NEC T85.591 ☑
  pain T85.84 ☑
  specified type NEC T85.89 ☑
  stenosis T85.85 ☑
  thrombosis T85.86 ☑
esophagostomy K94.30
  hemorrhage K94.31
  infection K94.32
  malfunction K94.33
  mechanical K94.33

Complication(s) — *continued*
esophagostomy — *continued*
  specified complication NEC K94.39
extracorporeal circulation T80.90 ☑
extremity artery (bypass) graft T82.9 ☑
  arteriosclerosis — *see* Arteriosclerosis, extremities, bypass graft
  embolism T82.818 ☑
  fibrosis T82.828 ☑
  hemorrhage T82.838 ☑
  infection and inflammation T82.7 ☑
  mechanical
    breakdown T82.318 ☑
      femoral artery T82.312 ☑
    displacement T82.328 ☑
      femoral artery T82.322 ☑
    leakage T82.338 ☑
      femoral artery T82.332 ☑
    malposition T82.328 ☑
      femoral artery T82.322 ☑
    obstruction T82.398 ☑
      femoral artery T82.392 ☑
    perforation T82.398 ☑
      femoral artery T82.392 ☑
    protrusion T82.398 ☑
      femoral artery T82.392 ☑
  pain T82.848 ☑
  specified type NEC T82.898 ☑
  stenosis T82.858 ☑
  thrombosis T82.868 ☑
eye H57.9
  corneal graft — *see* Complications, graft, cornea
  implant (prosthetic) T85.9 ☑
    embolism T85.81 ☑
    fibrosis T85.82 ☑
    hemorrhage T85.83 ☑
    infection and inflammation T85.79 ☑
    mechanical
      breakdown T85.318 ☑
      displacement T85.328 ☑
      leakage T85.398 ☑
      malposition T85.328 ☑
      obstruction T85.398 ☑
      perforation T85.398 ☑
      protrusion T85.398 ☑
      specified NEC T85.398 ☑
    pain T85.84 ☑
    specified type NEC T85.89 ☑
    stenosis T85.85 ☑
    thrombosis T85.86 ☑
  intraocular lens — *see* Complications, intraocular lens
  orbital prosthesis — *see* Complications, orbital prosthesis
female genital N94.9
  device, implant or graft NEC — *see* Complications, genitourinary, device or implant, genital tract
femoral artery (bypass) graft — *see* Complication, extremity artery (bypass) graft
fixation device, internal (orthopedic) T84.9 ☑
  infection and inflammation T84.60 ☑
    arm T84.61- ☑
      humerus T84.61- ☑
      radius T84.61- ☑
      ulna T84.61- ☑
    leg T84.629 ☑
      femur T84.62- ☑
      fibula T84.62- ☑
      tibia T84.62- ☑
    specified site NEC T84.89 ☑
    spine T84.63 ☑
  mechanical
    breakdown
      limb T84.119 ☑
        carpal T84.210 ☑
        femur T84.11- ☑
        fibula T84.11- ☑
        humerus T84.11- ☑
        metacarpal T84.210 ☑
        metatarsal T84.213 ☑
        phalanx
          foot T84.213 ☑
          hand T84.210 ☑
        radius T84.11- ☑
        tarsal T84.213 ☑
        tibia T84.11- ☑

Complication(s) — *continued*
fixation device, internal — *continued*
  mechanical — *continued*
    breakdown — *continued*
      limb — *continued*
        ulna T84.11- ☑
      specified bone NEC T84.218 ☑
      spine T84.216 ☑
    displacement
      limb T84.129 ☑
        carpal T84.220 ☑
        femur T84.12- ☑
        fibula T84.12- ☑
        humerus T84.12- ☑
        metacarpal T84.220 ☑
        metatarsal T84.223 ☑
        phalanx
          foot T84.223 ☑
          hand T84.220 ☑
        radius T84.12- ☑
        tarsal T84.223 ☑
        tibia T84.12- ☑
        ulna T84.12- ☑
      specified bone NEC T84.228 ☑
      spine T84.226 ☑
    malposition — *see* Complications, fixation device, internal, mechanical, displacement
    obstruction — *see* Complications, fixation device, internal, mechanical, specified type NEC
    perforation — *see* Complications, fixation device, internal, mechanical, specified type NEC
    protrusion — *see* Complications, fixation device, internal, mechanical, specified type NEC
    specified type NEC
      limb T84.199 ☑
        carpal T84.290 ☑
        femur T84.19- ☑
        fibula T84.19- ☑
        humerus T84.19- ☑
        metacarpal T84.290 ☑
        metatarsal T84.293 ☑
        phalanx
          foot T84.293 ☑
          hand T84.290 ☑
        radius T84.19- ☑
        tarsal T84.293 ☑
        tibia T84.19- ☑
        ulna T84.19- ☑
      specified bone NEC T84.298 ☑
      vertebra T84.296 ☑
  specified type NEC T84.89 ☑
    embolism T84.81 ☑
    fibrosis T84.82 ☑
    hemorrhage T84.83 ☑
    pain T84.84 ☑
    specified complication NEC T84.89 ☑
    stenosis T84.85 ☑
    thrombosis T84.86 ☑
following
  acute myocardial infarction NEC I23.8
    aneurysm (false) (of cardiac wall) (of heart wall) (ruptured) I23.3
    angina I23.7
    atrial
      septal defect I23.1
      thrombosis I23.6
    cardiac wall rupture I23.3
    chordae tendinae rupture I23.4
    defect
      septal
        atrial (heart) I23.1
        ventricular (heart) I23.2
    hemopericardium I23.0
    papillary muscle rupture I23.5
    rupture
      cardiac wall I23.3
        with hemopericardium I23.0
      chordae tendineae I23.4
      papillary muscle I23.5
    specified NEC I23.8
    thrombosis
      atrium I23.6
      auricular appendage I23.6
      ventricle (heart) I23.6

☑ **Additional Character Required — Refer to the Tabular List for Character Selection**   ▽ **Subterms under main terms may continue to next column or page**

Complication(s) — *continued*
　following — *continued*
　　acute myocardial infarction — *continued*
　　　ventricular
　　　　septal defect I23.2
　　　　thrombosis I23.6
　　ectopic or molar pregnancy O08.9
　　　cardiac arrest O08.81
　　　sepsis O08.82
　　　specified type NEC O08.89
　　　urinary tract infection O08.83
　　termination of pregnancy — *see* Abortion
　gastrointestinal K92.9
　　bile duct prosthesis — *see* Complications, bile duct implant
　　esophageal anti-reflux device — *see* Complications, esophageal anti-reflux device
　　postoperative
　　　colostomy — *see* Complications, colostomy
　　　dumping syndrome K91.1
　　　enterostomy — *see* Complications, enterostomy
　　　gastrostomy — *see* Complications, gastrostomy
　　　malabsorption NEC K91.2
　　　obstruction K91.3
　　　postcholecystectomy syndrome K91.5
　　　specified NEC K91.89
　　　vomiting after GI surgery K91.0
　　prosthetic device or implant
　　　bile duct prosthesis — *see* Complications, bile duct implant
　　　esophageal anti-reflux device — *see* Complications, esophageal anti-reflux device
　　　specified type NEC
　　　　embolism T85.81 ☑
　　　　fibrosis T85.82 ☑
　　　　hemorrhage T85.83 ☑
　　　　mechanical
　　　　　breakdown T85.518 ☑
　　　　　displacement T85.528 ☑
　　　　　malfunction T85.518 ☑
　　　　　malposition T85.528 ☑
　　　　　obstruction T85.598 ☑
　　　　　perforation T85.598 ☑
　　　　　protrusion T85.598 ☑
　　　　　specified NEC T85.598 ☑
　　　　pain T85.84 ☑
　　　　specified complication NEC T85.89 ☑
　　　　stenosis T85.85 ☑
　　　　thrombosis T85.86 ☑
　gastrostomy (stoma) K94.20
　　hemorrhage K94.21
　　infection K94.22
　　malfunction K94.23
　　mechanical K94.23
　　specified complication NEC K94.29
　genitourinary
　　device or implant T83.9 ☑
　　　genital tract T83.9 ☑
　　　　infection or inflammation T83.6 ☑
　　　　intrauterine contraceptive device — *see* Complications, intrauterine, contraceptive device
　　　　mechanical — *see* Complications, by device, mechanical
　　　　mesh — *see* Complications, mesh
　　　　penile prosthesis — *see* Complications, prosthetic device, penile
　　　　specified type NEC T83.89 ☑
　　　　　embolism T83.81 ☑
　　　　　fibrosis T83.82 ☑
　　　　　hemorrhage T83.83 ☑
　　　　　pain T83.84 ☑
　　　　　specified complication NEC T83.89 ☑
　　　　　stenosis T83.85 ☑
　　　　　thrombosis T83.86 ☑
　　　　vaginal mesh — *see* Complications, mesh
　　　urinary system T83.9 ☑
　　　　cystostomy catheter — *see* Complication, catheter, cystostomy
　　　　electronic stimulator — *see* Complications, electronic stimulator device, urinary
　　　　indwelling urethral catheter — *see* Complications, catheter, urethral, indwelling
　　　　infection or inflammation T83.59 ☑
　　　　　indwelling urinary catheter T83.51 ☑

Complication(s) — *continued*
　genitourinary — *continued*
　　device or implant — *continued*
　　　urinary system — *continued*
　　　　kidney transplant — *see* Complication, transplant, kidney
　　　　organ graft — *see* Complication, graft, urinary organ
　　　　specified type NEC T83.89 ☑
　　　　　embolism T83.81 ☑
　　　　　fibrosis T83.82 ☑
　　　　　hemorrhage T83.83 ☑
　　　　　mechanical T83.198 ☑
　　　　　　breakdown T83.118 ☑
　　　　　　displacement T83.128 ☑
　　　　　　malfunction T83.118 ☑
　　　　　　malposition T83.128 ☑
　　　　　　obstruction T83.198 ☑
　　　　　　perforation T83.198 ☑
　　　　　　protrusion T83.198 ☑
　　　　　　specified NEC T83.198 ☑
　　　　　pain T83.84 ☑
　　　　　specified complication NEC T83.89 ☑
　　　　　stenosis T83.85 ☑
　　　　　thrombosis T83.86 ☑
　　　　sphincter implant — *see* Complications, implant, urinary sphincter
　　postprocedural
　　　pelvic peritoneal adhesions N99.4
　　　renal failure N99.0
　　　specified NEC N99.89
　　　stoma — *see* Complications, stoma, urinary tract
　　　urethral stricture — *see* Stricture, urethra, postprocedural
　　　vaginal
　　　　adhesions N99.2
　　　　vault prolapse N99.3
　graft (bypass) (patch) (*see also* Complications, prosthetic device or implant)
　　aorta — *see* Complications, graft, vascular
　　arterial — *see* Complication, graft, vascular
　　bone T86.839
　　　failure T86.831
　　　infection T86.832
　　　mechanical T84.318 ☑
　　　　breakdown T84.318 ☑
　　　　displacement T84.328 ☑
　　　　protrusion T84.398 ☑
　　　　specified type NEC T84.398 ☑
　　　rejection T86.830
　　　specified type NEC T86.838
　　carotid artery — *see* Complications, graft, vascular
　　cornea T86.849
　　　failure T86.841
　　　infection T86.842
　　　mechanical T85.398 ☑
　　　　breakdown T85.318 ☑
　　　　displacement T85.328 ☑
　　　　protrusion T85.398 ☑
　　　　specified type NEC T85.398 ☑
　　　rejection T86.840
　　　retroprosthetic membrane T85.398 ☑
　　　specified type NEC T86.848
　　femoral artery (bypass) — *see* Complication, extremity artery (bypass) graft
　　genital organ or tract — *see* Complications, genitourinary, device or implant, genital tract
　　muscle T84.9 ☑
　　　breakdown T84.410 ☑
　　　displacement T84.420 ☑
　　　embolism T84.81 ☑
　　　fibrosis T84.82 ☑
　　　hemorrhage T84.83 ☑
　　　infection and inflammation T84.7 ☑
　　　mechanical NEC T84.490 ☑
　　　pain T84.84 ☑
　　　specified type NEC T84.89 ☑
　　　stenosis T84.85 ☑
　　　thrombosis T84.86 ☑
　　nerve — *see* Complication, prosthetic device or implant, specified NEC
　　skin — *see* Complications, prosthetic device or implant, skin graft
　　tendon T84.9 ☑
　　　breakdown T84.410 ☑

Complication(s) — *continued*
　graft (*see also* Complications, prosthetic device or implant) — *continued*
　　tendon — *continued*
　　　displacement T84.420 ☑
　　　embolism T84.81 ☑
　　　fibrosis T84.82 ☑
　　　hemorrhage T84.83 ☑
　　　infection and inflammation T84.7 ☑
　　　mechanical NEC T84.490 ☑
　　　pain T84.84 ☑
　　　specified type NEC T84.89 ☑
　　　stenosis T84.85 ☑
　　　thrombosis T84.86 ☑
　　urinary organ T83.9 ☑
　　　embolism T83.81 ☑
　　　fibrosis T83.82 ☑
　　　hemorrhage T83.83 ☑
　　　infection and inflammation T83.59 ☑
　　　　indwelling urinary catheter T83.51 ☑
　　　mechanical
　　　　breakdown T83.21 ☑
　　　　displacement T83.22 ☑
　　　　leakage T83.23 ☑
　　　　malposition T83.22 ☑
　　　　obstruction T83.29 ☑
　　　　perforation T83.29 ☑
　　　　protrusion T83.29 ☑
　　　　specified NEC T83.29 ☑
　　　pain T83.84 ☑
　　　specified type NEC T83.89 ☑
　　　stenosis T83.85 ☑
　　　thrombosis T83.86 ☑
　　vascular T82.9 ☑
　　　embolism T82.818 ☑
　　　femoral artery — *see* Complication, extremity artery (bypass) graft
　　　fibrosis T82.828 ☑
　　　hemorrhage T82.838 ☑
　　　mechanical
　　　　breakdown T82.319 ☑
　　　　　aorta (bifurcation) T82.310 ☑
　　　　　carotid artery T82.311 ☑
　　　　　specified vessel NEC T82.318 ☑
　　　　displacement T82.329 ☑
　　　　　aorta (bifurcation) T82.320 ☑
　　　　　carotid artery T82.321 ☑
　　　　　specified vessel NEC T82.328 ☑
　　　　leakage T82.339 ☑
　　　　　aorta (bifurcation) T82.330 ☑
　　　　　carotid artery T82.331 ☑
　　　　　specified vessel NEC T82.338 ☑
　　　　malposition T82.329 ☑
　　　　　aorta (bifurcation) T82.320 ☑
　　　　　carotid artery T82.321 ☑
　　　　　specified vessel NEC T82.328 ☑
　　　　obstruction T82.399 ☑
　　　　　aorta (bifurcation) T82.390 ☑
　　　　　carotid artery T82.391 ☑
　　　　　specified vessel NEC T82.398 ☑
　　　　perforation T82.399 ☑
　　　　　aorta (bifurcation) T82.390 ☑
　　　　　carotid artery T82.391 ☑
　　　　　specified vessel NEC T82.398 ☑
　　　　protrusion T82.399 ☑
　　　　　aorta (bifurcation) T82.390 ☑
　　　　　carotid artery T82.391 ☑
　　　　　specified vessel NEC T82.398 ☑
　　　pain T82.848 ☑
　　　specified complication NEC T82.898 ☑
　　　stenosis T82.858 ☑
　　　thrombosis T82.868 ☑
　heart I51.9
　　assist device
　　　infection and inflammation T82.7 ☑
　　following acute myocardial infarction — *see* Complications, following, acute myocardial infarction
　　postoperative — *see* Complications, circulatory system
　　transplant — *see* Complication, transplant, heart and lung(s) — *see* Complications, transplant, heart, with lung
　　valve
　　　graft (biological) T82.9 ☑
　　　　embolism T82.817 ☑

Complication(s) — *continued*
- heart — *continued*
  - valve — *continued*
    - graft — *continued*
      - fibrosis T82.827 ☑
      - hemorrhage T82.837 ☑
      - infection and inflammation T82.7 ☑
      - mechanical T82.228 ☑
        - breakdown T82.221 ☑
        - displacement T82.222 ☑
        - leakage T82.223 ☑
        - malposition T82.222 ☑
        - obstruction T82.228 ☑
        - perforation T82.228 ☑
        - protrusion T82.228 ☑
      - pain T82.847 ☑
      - specified type NEC T82.897 ☑
      - stenosis T82.857 ☑
      - thrombosis T82.867 ☑
    - prosthesis T82.9 ☑
      - embolism T82.817 ☑
      - fibrosis T82.827 ☑
      - hemorrhage T82.837 ☑
      - infection or inflammation T82.6 ☑
      - mechanical T82.09 ☑
        - breakdown T82.01 ☑
        - displacement T82.02 ☑
        - leakage T82.03 ☑
        - malposition T82.02 ☑
        - obstruction T82.09 ☑
        - perforation T82.09 ☑
        - protrusion T82.09 ☑
      - pain T82.847 ☑
      - specified type NEC T82.897 ☑
        - mechanical T82.09 ☑
      - stenosis T82.857 ☑
      - thrombosis T82.867 ☑
- hematoma
  - intraoperative — *see* Complication, intraoperative, hemorrhage
  - postprocedural — *see* Complication, postprocedural, hemorrhage
- hemodialysis — *see* Complications, dialysis
- hemorrhage
  - intraoperative — *see* Complication, intraoperative, hemorrhage
  - postprocedural — *see* Complication, postprocedural, hemorrhage
- ileostomy (stoma) — *see* Complications, enterostomy
- immunization (procedure) — *see* Complications, vaccination
- implant (*see also* Complications, by site and type)
  - urinary sphincter T83.9 ☑
    - embolism T83.81 ☑
    - fibrosis T83.82 ☑
    - hemorrhage T83.83 ☑
    - infection and inflammation T83.59 ☑
    - mechanical
      - breakdown T83.111 ☑
      - displacement T83.121 ☑
      - leakage T83.191 ☑
      - malposition T83.121 ☑
      - obstruction T83.191 ☑
      - perforation T83.191 ☑
      - protrusion T83.191 ☑
      - specified NEC T83.191 ☑
    - pain T83.84 ☑
    - specified type NEC T83.89 ☑
    - stenosis T83.85 ☑
    - thrombosis T83.86 ☑
- infusion (procedure) T80.90 ☑
  - air embolism T80.0 ☑
  - blood — *see* Complications, transfusion
  - catheter — *see* Complications, catheter
  - infection T80.29 ☑
  - pump — *see* Complications, cardiovascular, device or implant
  - sepsis T80.29 ☑
  - serum reaction (*see also* Reaction, serum) T80.69 ☑
    - anaphylactic shock (*see also* Shock, anaphylactic) T80.59 ☑
  - specified type NEC T80.89 ☑
- inhalation therapy NEC T81.81 ☑
- injection (procedure) T80.90 ☑
  - drug reaction — *see* Reaction, drug
  - infection T80.29 ☑

Complication(s) — *continued*
- injection — *continued*
  - sepsis T80.29 ☑
  - serum (prophylactic) (therapeutic) — *see* Complications, vaccination
  - specified type NEC T80.89 ☑
  - vaccine (any) — *see* Complications, vaccination
- inoculation (any) — *see* Complications, vaccination
- insulin pump
  - infection and inflammation T85.72 ☑
  - mechanical
    - breakdown T85.614 ☑
    - displacement T85.624 ☑
    - leakage T85.633 ☑
    - malposition T85.624 ☑
    - obstruction T85.694 ☑
    - perforation T85.694 ☑
    - protrusion T85.694 ☑
    - specified NEC T85.694 ☑
- intestinal pouch NEC K91.858
- intraocular lens (prosthetic) T85.9 ☑
  - embolism T85.81 ☑
  - fibrosis T85.82 ☑
  - hemorrhage T85.83 ☑
  - infection and inflammation T85.79 ☑
  - mechanical
    - breakdown T85.21 ☑
    - displacement T85.22 ☑
    - malposition T85.22 ☑
    - obstruction T85.29 ☑
    - perforation T85.29 ☑
    - protrusion T85.29 ☑
    - specified NEC T85.29 ☑
  - pain T85.84 ☑
  - specified type NEC T85.89 ☑
  - stenosis T85.85 ☑
  - thrombosis T85.86 ☑
- intraoperative (intraprocedural)
  - cardiac arrest
    - during cardiac surgery I97.710 ☑
    - during other surgery I97.711 ☑
  - cardiac functional disturbance NEC
    - during cardiac surgery I97.790 ☑
    - during other surgery I97.791 ☑
  - hemorrhage (hematoma) (of)
    - circulatory system organ or structure
      - during cardiac bypass I97.411
      - during cardiac catheterization I97.410
      - during other circulatory system procedure I97.418
      - during other procedure I97.42
    - digestive system organ
      - during procedure on digestive system K91.61
      - during procedure on other organ K91.62
    - ear
      - during procedure on ear and mastoid process H95.21
      - during procedure on other organ H95.22
    - endocrine system organ or structure
      - during procedure on endocrine system organ or structure E36.01
      - during procedure on other organ E36.02
    - eye and adnexa
      - during ophthalmic procedure H59.11- ☑
      - during other procedure H59.12- ☑
    - genitourinary organ or structure
      - during procedure on genitourinary organ or structure N99.61
      - during procedure on other organ N99.62
    - mastoid process
      - during procedure on ear and mastoid process H95.21
      - during procedure on other organ H95.22
    - musculoskeletal structure
      - during musculoskeletal surgery M96.810
      - during non-orthopedic surgery M96.811
      - during orthopedic surgery M96.810
    - nervous system
      - during a nervous system procedure G97.31
      - during other procedure G97.32
    - respiratory system
      - during other procedure J95.62
      - during procedure on respiratory system organ or structure J95.61
    - skin and subcutaneous tissue
      - during a dermatologic procedure L76.01

Complication(s) — *continued*
- intraoperative — *continued*
  - hemorrhage — *continued*
    - skin and subcutaneous tissue — *continued*
      - during a procedure on other organ L76.02
    - spleen
      - during a procedure on other organ D78.02
      - during a procedure on the spleen D78.01
  - puncture or laceration (accidental) (unintentional) (of)
    - brain
      - during a nervous system procedure G97.48
      - during other procedure G97.49
    - circulatory system organ or structure
      - during circulatory system procedure I97.51
      - during other procedure I97.52
    - digestive system
      - during procedure on digestive system K91.71
      - during procedure on other organ K91.72
    - ear
      - during procedure on ear and mastoid process H95.31
      - during procedure on other organ H95.32
    - endocrine system organ or structure
      - during procedure on endocrine system organ or structure E36.11
      - during procedure on other organ E36.12
    - eye and adnexa
      - during ophthalmic procedure H59.21- ☑
      - during other procedure H59.22- ☑
    - genitourinary organ or structure
      - during procedure on genitourinary organ or structure N99.71
      - during procedure on other organ N99.72
    - mastoid process
      - during procedure on ear and mastoid process H95.31
      - during procedure on other organ H95.32
    - musculoskeletal structure
      - during musculoskeletal surgery M96.820
      - during non-orthopedic surgery M96.821
      - during orthopedic surgery M96.820
    - nervous system
      - during a nervous system procedure G97.48
      - during other procedure G97.49
    - respiratory system
      - during other procedure J95.72
      - during procedure on respiratory system organ or structure J95.71
    - skin and subcutaneous tissue
      - during a dermatologic procedure L76.11
      - during a procedure on other organ L76.12
    - spleen
      - during a procedure on other organ D78.12
      - during a procedure on the spleen D78.11
  - specified NEC
    - circulatory system I97.88
    - digestive system K91.81
    - ear H95.88
    - endocrine system E36.8
    - eye and adnexa H59.88
    - genitourinary system N99.81
    - mastoid process H95.88
    - musculoskeletal structure M96.89
    - nervous system G97.81
    - respiratory system J95.88
    - skin and subcutaneous tissue L76.81
    - spleen D78.81
- intraperitoneal catheter (dialysis) (infusion) — *see* Complications, catheter, intraperitoneal
- intrauterine
  - contraceptive device
    - embolism T83.81 ☑
    - fibrosis T83.82 ☑
    - hemorrhage T83.83 ☑
    - infection and inflammation T83.6 ☑
    - mechanical
      - breakdown T83.31 ☑
      - displacement T83.32 ☑
      - malposition T83.32 ☑
      - obstruction T83.39 ☑
      - perforation T83.39 ☑
      - protrusion T83.39 ☑
      - specified NEC T83.39 ☑
    - pain T83.84 ☑
    - specified type NEC T83.89 ☑
    - stenosis T83.85 ☑

62

☑ Additional Character Required — Refer to the Tabular List for Character Selection ▽ Subterms under main terms may continue to next column or page

Complication(s) — *continued*
 intrauterine — *continued*
  contraceptive device — *continued*
   thrombosis T83.86 ☑
  procedure (fetal), to newborn P96.5
 jejunostomy (stoma) — *see* Complications, enterostomy
 joint prosthesis, internal T84.9 ☑
  breakage (fracture) T84.01- ☑
  dislocation T84.02- ☑
  fracture T84.01- ☑
  infection or inflammation T84.50 ☑
   hip T84.5- ☑
   knee T84.5- ☑
   specified joint NEC T84.59 ☑
  instability T84.02- ☑
  malposition — *see* Complications, joint prosthesis, mechanical, displacement
  mechanical
   breakage, broken T84.01- ☑
   dislocation T84.02- ☑
   fracture T84.01- ☑
   instability T84.02- ☑
   leakage — *see* Complications, joint prosthesis, mechanical, specified NEC
   loosening T84.039 ☑
    hip T84.03- ☑
    knee T84.03- ☑
    specified joint NEC T84.038 ☑
   obstruction — *see* Complications, joint prosthesis, mechanical, specified NEC
   perforation — *see* Complications, joint prosthesis, mechanical, specified NEC
   periprosthetic
    fracture T84.049 ☑
     hip T84.04- ☑
     knee T84.04- ☑
     other specified joint T84.048 ☑
    osteolysis T84.059 ☑
     hip T84.05- ☑
     knee T84.05- ☑
     other specified joint T84.058 ☑
   protrusion — *see* Complications, joint prosthesis, mechanical, specified NEC
   specified complication NEC T84.099 ☑
    hip T84.09- ☑
    knee T84.09- ☑
    other specified joint T84.098 ☑
   subluxation T84.02- ☑
   wear of articular bearing surface T84.069 ☑
    hip T84.06- ☑
    knee T84.06- ☑
    other specified joint T84.068 ☑
  specified joint NEC T84.89 ☑
   embolism T84.81 ☑
   fibrosis T84.82 ☑
   hemorrhage T84.83 ☑
   pain T84.84 ☑
   specified complication NEC T84.89 ☑
   stenosis T84.85 ☑
   thrombosis T84.86 ☑
  subluxation T84.02- ☑
 kidney transplant — *see* Complications, transplant, kidney
 labor O75.9
  specified NEC O75.89
 liver transplant (immune or nonimmune) — *see* Complications, transplant, liver
 lumbar puncture G97.1
  cerebrospinal fluid leak G97.0
  headache or reaction G97.1
 lung transplant — *see* Complications, transplant, lung and heart — *see* Complications, transplant, lung, with heart
 male genital N50.9
  device, implant or graft — *see* Complications, genitourinary, device or implant, genital tract
  postprocedural or postoperative — *see* Complications, genitourinary, postprocedural
   specified NEC N99.89
 mastoid (process) procedure
  intraoperative H95.88
   hematoma — *see* Complications, intraoperative, hemorrhage (hematoma) (of), mastoid process

Complication(s) — *continued*
 mastoid procedure — *continued*
  intraoperative — *continued*
   hemorrhage — *see* Complications, intraoperative, hemorrhage (hematoma) (of), mastoid process
   laceration — *see* Complications, intraoperative, puncture or laceration, mastoid process
   specified NEC H95.88
  postmastoidectomy — *see* Complications, postmastoidectomy
  postoperative H95.89
   external ear canal stenosis H95.81 ☑
   hematoma — *see* Complications, postprocedural, hemorrhage (hematoma) (of), mastoid process
   hemorrhage — *see* Complications, postprocedural, hemorrhage (hematoma) (of), mastoid process
   postmastoidectomy — *see* Complications, postmastoidectomy
   specified NEC H95.89
 mastoidectomy cavity — *see* Complications, postmastoidectomy
 mechanical — *see* Complications, by site and type, mechanical
 medical procedures (*see also* Complication(s), intraoperative) T88.9 ☑
 metabolic E88.9
  postoperative E89.89
   specified NEC E89.89
 molar pregnancy NOS O08.9
  damage to pelvic organs O08.6
  embolism O08.2
  genital infection O08.0
  hemorrhage (delayed) (excessive) O08.1
  metabolic disorder O08.5
  renal failure O08.4
  shock O08.3
  specified type NEC O08.0
  venous complication NEC O08.7
 musculoskeletal system (*see also* Complication, intraoperative (intraprocedural), by site)
  device, implant or graft NEC — *see* Complications, orthopedic, device or implant
  internal fixation (nail) (plate) (rod) — *see* Complications, fixation device, internal
  joint prosthesis — *see* Complications, joint prosthesis
  post radiation M96.89
   kyphosis M96.3
   scoliosis M96.5
   specified complication NEC M96.89
  postoperative (postprocedural) M96.89
   with osteoporosis — *see* Osteoporosis
   fracture following insertion of device — *see* Fracture, following insertion of orthopedic implant, joint prosthesis or bone plate
   joint instability after prosthesis removal M96.89
   lordosis M96.4
   postlaminectomy syndrome NEC M96.1
    kyphosis M96.3
   pseudarthrosis M96.0
   specified complication NEC M96.89
 nephrostomy (stoma) — *see* Complications, stoma, urinary tract, external NEC
 nervous system G98.8
  central G96.9
  device, implant or graft (*see also* Complication, prosthetic device or implant, specified NEC)
   electronic stimulator (electrode(s)) — *see* Complications, electronic stimulator device
   ventricular shunt — *see* Complications, ventricular shunt
  electronic stimulator (electrode(s)) — *see* Complications, electronic stimulator device
  postprocedural G97.82
   intracranial hypotension G97.2
   specified NEC G97.82
   spinal fluid leak G97.0
 newborn, due to intrauterine (fetal) procedure P96.5
 nonabsorbable (permanent) sutures — *see* Complication, sutures, permanent
 obstetric O75.9
  procedure (instrumental) (manual) (surgical)
   specified NEC O75.4
  specified NEC O75.89

Complication(s) — *continued*
 obstetric — *continued*
  surgical wound NEC O90.89
   hematoma O90.2
   infection O86.0
  ocular lens implant — *see* Complications, intraocular lens
  ophthalmologic
   postprocedural bleb — *see* Blebitis
  orbital prosthesis T85.9 ☑
   embolism T85.81 ☑
   fibrosis T85.82 ☑
   hemorrhage T85.83 ☑
   infection and inflammation T85.79 ☑
   mechanical
    breakdown T85.31- ☑
    displacement T85.32- ☑
    malposition T85.32- ☑
    obstruction T85.39- ☑
    perforation T85.39- ☑
    protrusion T85.39- ☑
    specified NEC T85.39- ☑
   pain T85.84 ☑
   specified type NEC T85.89 ☑
   stenosis T85.85 ☑
   thrombosis T85.86 ☑
  organ or tissue transplant (partial) (total) — *see* Complications, transplant
  orthopedic (*see also* Disorder, soft tissue)
   device or implant T84.9 ☑
    bone
     device or implant — *see* Complication, bone, device NEC
     graft — *see* Complication, graft, bone
    breakdown T84.418 ☑
    displacement T84.428 ☑
    electronic bone stimulator — *see* Complications, electronic stimulator device, bone
    embolism T84.81 ☑
    fibrosis T84.82 ☑
    fixation device — *see* Complication, fixation device, internal
    hemorrhage T84.83 ☑
    infection or inflammation T84.7 ☑
    joint prosthesis — *see* Complication, joint prosthesis, internal
    malfunction T84.418 ☑
    malposition T84.428 ☑
    mechanical NEC T84.498 ☑
    muscle graft — *see* Complications, graft, muscle
    obstruction T84.498 ☑
    pain T84.84 ☑
    perforation T84.498 ☑
    protrusion T84.498 ☑
    specified complication NEC T84.89 ☑
    stenosis T84.85 ☑
    tendon graft — *see* Complications, graft, tendon
    thrombosis T84.86 ☑
   fracture (following insertion of device) — *see* Fracture, following insertion of orthopedic implant, joint prosthesis or bone plate
   postprocedural M96.89
    fracture — *see* Fracture, following insertion of orthopedic implant, joint prosthesis or bone plate
    postlaminectomy syndrome NEC M96.1
     kyphosis M96.3
     lordosis M96.4
    postradiation
     kyphosis M96.2
     scoliosis M96.5
    pseudarthrosis post-fusion M96.0
    specified type NEC M96.89
  pacemaker (cardiac) — *see* Complications, cardiovascular device or implant, electronic
  pancreas transplant — *see* Complications, transplant, pancreas
  penile prosthesis (implant) — *see* Complications, prosthetic device, penile
  perfusion NEC T80.90 ☑
  perineal repair (obstetrical) NEC O90.89
   disruption O90.1
   hematoma O90.2
   infection (following delivery) O86.0
  phototherapy T88.9 ☑
   specified NEC T88.8 ☑

Index

Complication — Complication

Complication(s) — *continued*
- postmastoidectomy NEC H95.19- ☑
  - cyst, mucosal H95.13- ☑
  - granulation H95.12- ☑
  - inflammation, chronic H95.11- ☑
  - recurrent cholesteatoma H95.0- ☑
- postoperative — *see* Complications, postprocedural
  - circulatory — *see* Complications, circulatory system
  - ear — *see* Complications, ear
  - endocrine — *see* Complications, endocrine
  - eye — *see* Complications, eye
  - lumbar puncture G97.1
    - cerebrospinal fluid leak G97.0
  - nervous system (central) (peripheral) — *see* Complications, nervous
  - respiratory system — *see* Complications, respiratory system
- postprocedural (*see also* Complications, surgical procedure)
  - cardiac arrest
    - following cardiac surgery I97.120
    - following other surgery I97.121
  - cardiac functional disturbance NEC
    - following cardiac surgery I97.190
    - following other surgery I97.191
  - cardiac insufficiency
    - following cardiac surgery I97.110
    - following other surgery I97.111
  - chorioretinal scars following retinal surgery H59.81- ☑
  - following cataract surgery
    - cataract (lens) fragments H59.02- ☑
    - cystoid macular edema H59.03- ☑
    - specified NEC H59.09- ☑
    - vitreous (touch) syndrome H59.01- ☑
  - heart failure
    - following cardiac surgery I97.130
    - following other surgery I97.131
  - hemorrhage (hematoma) (of)
    - circulatory system organ or structure
      - following a cardiac bypass I97.611
      - following a cardiac catheterization I97.610
      - following other circulatory system procedure I97.618
      - following other procedure I97.62
    - digestive system
      - following procedure on digestive system K91.840
      - following procedure on other organ K91.841
    - ear
      - following other procedure H95.42
      - following procedure on ear and mastoid process H95.41
    - endocrine system
      - following endocrine system procedure E89.810
      - following other procedure E89.811
    - eye and adnexa
      - following ophthalmic procedure H59.31- ☑
      - following other procedure H59.32- ☑
    - genitourinary organ or structure
      - following procedure on genitourinary organ or structure N99.820
      - following procedure on other organ N99.821
    - mastoid process
      - following other procedure H95.42
      - following procedure on ear and mastoid process H95.41
    - musculoskeletal structure
      - following musculoskeletal surgery M96.830
      - following non-orthopedic surgery M96.831
      - following orthopedic surgery M96.830
    - nervous system
      - following a nervous system procedure G97.51
      - following other procedure G97.52
    - respiratory system
      - following a respiratory system procedure J95.830
      - following other procedure J95.831
    - skin and subcutaneous tissue
      - following a dermatologic procedure L76.21
      - following a procedure on other organ L76.22
    - spleen
      - following procedure on other organ D78.22
      - following procedure on the spleen D78.21

Complication(s) — *continued*
- postprocedural (*see also* Complications, surgical procedure) — *continued*
  - specified NEC
    - circulatory system I97.89
    - digestive K91.89
    - ear H95.89
    - endocrine E89.89
    - eye and adnexa H59.89
    - genitourinary N99.89
    - mastoid process H95.89
    - metabolic E89.89
    - musculoskeletal structure M96.89
    - nervous system G97.82
    - respiratory system J95.89
    - skin and subcutaneous tissue L76.82
    - spleen D78.89
- pregnancy NEC — *see* Pregnancy, complicated by
- prosthetic device or implant T85.9 ☑
  - bile duct — *see* Complications, bile duct implant
  - breast — *see* Complications, breast implant
  - cardiac and vascular NEC — *see* Complications, cardiovascular device or implant
  - corneal transplant — *see* Complications, graft, cornea
  - electronic nervous system stimulator — *see* Complications, electronic stimulator device
  - epidural infusion catheter — *see* Complications, catheter, epidural
  - esophageal anti-reflux device — *see* Complications, esophageal anti-reflux device
  - genital organ or tract — *see* Complications, genitourinary, device or implant, genital tract
  - heart valve — *see* Complications, heart, valve, prosthesis
  - infection or inflammation T85.79 ☑
    - intestine transplant T86.892
    - liver transplant T86.43
    - lung transplant T86.812
    - pancreas transplant T86.892
    - skin graft T86.822
  - intraocular lens — *see* Complications, intraocular lens
  - intraperitoneal (dialysis) catheter — *see* Complications, catheter, intraperitoneal
  - joint — *see* Complications, joint prosthesis, internal
  - mechanical NEC T85.698 ☑
    - dialysis catheter (vascular) (*see also* Complication, catheter, dialysis, mechanical)
      - peritoneal — *see* Complication, catheter, intraperitoneal, mechanical
    - gastrointestinal device T85.598 ☑
    - ocular device T85.398 ☑
    - subdural (infusion) catheter T85.690 ☑
    - suture, permanent T85.692 ☑
      - that for bone repair — *see* Complications, fixation device, internal (orthopedic), mechanical
    - ventricular shunt
      - breakdown T85.01 ☑
      - displacement T85.02 ☑
      - leakage T85.03 ☑
      - malposition T85.02 ☑
      - obstruction T85.09 ☑
      - perforation T85.09 ☑
      - protrusion T85.09 ☑
      - specified NEC T85.09 ☑
  - mesh
    - erosion (to surrounding organ or tissue) T83.718 ☑
      - vaginal (into pelvic floor muscles) T83.711 ☑
    - exposure (into surrounding organ or tissue) T83.728 ☑
      - vaginal (into vagina) (through vaginal wall) T83.721 ☑
  - orbital — *see* Complications, orbital prosthesis
  - penile T83.9 ☑
    - embolism T83.81 ☑
    - fibrosis T83.82 ☑
    - hemorrhage T83.83 ☑
    - infection and inflammation T83.6 ☑
    - mechanical
      - breakdown T83.410 ☑
      - displacement T83.420 ☑
      - leakage T83.490 ☑
      - malposition T83.420 ☑

Complication(s) — *continued*
- prosthetic device or implant — *continued*
  - penile — *continued*
    - mechanical — *continued*
      - obstruction T83.490 ☑
      - perforation T83.490 ☑
      - protrusion T83.490 ☑
      - specified NEC T83.490 ☑
    - pain T83.84 ☑
    - specified type NEC T83.89 ☑
    - stenosis T83.85 ☑
    - thrombosis T83.86 ☑
  - prosthetic materials NEC
    - erosion (to surrounding organ or tissue) T83.718 ☑
      - vaginal (into pelvic floor muscles) T83.711 ☑
    - exposure (into surrounding organ or tissue) T83.728 ☑
      - vaginal (into vagina) (through vaginal wall) T83.721 ☑
  - skin graft T86.829
    - artificial skin or decellularized allodermis
      - embolism T85.81 ☑
      - fibrosis T85.82 ☑
      - hemorrhage T85.83 ☑
      - infection and inflammation T85.79 ☑
      - mechanical
        - breakdown T85.613 ☑
        - displacement T85.623 ☑
        - malfunction T85.613 ☑
        - malposition T85.623 ☑
        - obstruction T85.693 ☑
        - perforation T85.693 ☑
        - protrusion T85.693 ☑
        - specified NEC T85.693 ☑
      - pain T85.84 ☑
      - specified type NEC T85.89 ☑
      - stenosis T85.85 ☑
      - thrombosis T85.86 ☑
    - failure T86.821
    - infection T86.822
    - rejection T86.820
    - specified NEC T86.828
  - specified NEC T85.9 ☑
    - embolism T85.81 ☑
    - fibrosis T85.82 ☑
    - hemorrhage T85.83 ☑
    - infection and inflammation T85.79 ☑
    - mechanical
      - breakdown T85.618 ☑
      - displacement T85.628 ☑
      - leakage T85.638 ☑
      - malfunction T85.618 ☑
      - malposition T85.628 ☑
      - obstruction T85.698 ☑
      - perforation T85.698 ☑
      - protrusion T85.698 ☑
      - specified NEC T85.698 ☑
    - pain T85.84 ☑
    - specified type NEC T85.89 ☑
    - stenosis T85.85 ☑
    - thrombosis T85.86 ☑
  - subdural infusion catheter — *see* Complications, catheter, subdural
  - sutures — *see* Complications, sutures
  - urinary organ or tract NEC — *see* Complications, genitourinary, device or implant, urinary system
  - vascular — *see* Complications, cardiovascular device or implant
  - ventricular shunt — *see* Complications, ventricular shunt (device)
- puerperium — *see* Puerperal
- puncture, spinal G97.1
  - cerebrospinal fluid leak G97.0
  - headache or reaction G97.1
- pyelogram N99.89
- radiation
  - kyphosis M96.2
  - scoliosis M96.5
- reattached
  - extremity (infection) (rejection)
    - lower T87.1X- ☑
    - upper T87.0X- ☑
  - specified body part NEC T87.2

Complication(s) — *continued*
reconstructed breast
asymmetry between native and reconstructed breast N65.1
deformity N65.0
disproportion between native and reconstructed breast N65.1
excess tissue N65.0
misshappen N65.0
reimplant NEC (*see also* Complications, prosthetic device or implant)
limb (infection) (rejection) — *see* Complications, reattached, extremity
organ (partial) (total) — *see* Complications, transplant
prosthetic device NEC — *see* Complications, prosthetic device
renal N28.9
allograft — *see* Complications, transplant, kidney
dialysis — *see* Complications, dialysis
respirator
mechancial J95.850
specified NEC J95.859
respiratory system J98.9
device, implant or graft — *see* Complication, prosthetic device or implant, specified NEC
lung transplant — *see* Complications, prosthetic device or implant, lung transplant
postoperative J95.89
air leak J95.812
Mendelson's syndrome (chemical pneumonitis) J95.4
pneumothorax J95.811
pulmonary insufficiency (acute) (after nonthoracic surgery) J95.2
chronic J95.3
following thoracic surgery J95.1
respiratory failure (acute) J95.821
acute and chronic J95.822
specified NEC J95.89
subglottic stenosis J95.5
tracheostomy complication — *see* Complications, tracheostomy
therapy T81.89
sedation during labor and delivery O74.9
cardiac O74.2
central nervous system O74.3
pulmonary NEC O74.1
shunt (*see also* Complications, prosthetic device or implant)
arteriovenous — *see* Complications, arteriovenous, shunt
ventricular (communicating) — *see* Complications, ventricular shunt
skin
graft T86.829
failure T86.821
infection T86.822
rejection T86.820
specified type NEC T86.828
spinal
anesthesia — *see* Complications, anesthesia, spinal
catheter (epidural) (subdural) — *see* Complications, catheter
puncture or tap G97.1
cerebrospinal fluid leak G97.0
headache or reaction G97.1
stent
bile duct — *see* Complications, bile duct prosthesis
urinary T83.9 ☑
embolism T83.81 ☑
fibrosis T83.82 ☑
hemorrhage T83.83 ☑
infection and inflammation T83.59 ☑
mechanical
breakdown T83.112 ☑
displacement T83.122 ☑
leakage T83.192 ☑
malposition T83.122 ☑
obstruction T83.192 ☑
perforation T83.192 ☑
protrusion T83.192 ☑
specified NEC T83.192 ☑
pain T83.84 ☑
specified type NEC T83.89 ☑
stenosis T83.85 ☑
thrombosis T83.86 ☑

Complication(s) — *continued*
stoma
digestive tract
colostomy — *see* Complications, colostomy
enterostomy — *see* Complications, enterostomy
esophagostomy — *see* Complications, esophagostomy
gastrostomy — *see* Complications, gastrostomy
urinary tract N99.538
cystostomy — *see* Complications, cystostomy
external NOS N99.528
hemorrhage N99.520
infection N99.521
malfunction N99.522
specified type NEC N99.528
hemorrhage N99.530
infection N99.531
malfunction N99.532
specified type NEC N99.538
stomach banding — *see* Complication(s), bariatric procedure
stomach stapling — *see* Complication(s), bariatric procedure
surgical material, nonabsorbable — *see* Complication, suture, permanent
surgical procedure (on) T81.9 ☑
amputation stump (late) — *see* Complications, amputation stump
cardiac — *see* Complications, circulatory system
cholesteatoma, recurrent — *see* Complications, postmastoidectomy, recurrent cholesteatoma
circulatory (early) — *see* Complications, circulatory system
digestive system — *see* Complications, gastrointestinal
dumping syndrome (postgastrectomy) K91.1
ear — *see* Complications, ear
elephantiasis or lymphedema I97.89
postmastectomy I97.2
emphysema (surgical) T81.82 ☑
endocrine — *see* Complications, endocrine
eye — *see* Complications, eye
fistula (persistent postoperative) T81.83 ☑
foreign body inadvertently left in wound (sponge) (suture) (swab) — *see* Foreign body, accidentally left during a procedure
gastrointestinal — *see* Complications, gastrointestinal
genitourinary NEC N99.89
hematoma
intraoperative — *see* Complication, intraoperative, hemorrhage
postprocedural — *see* Complication, postprocedural, hemorrhage
hemorrhage
intraoperative — *see* Complication, intraoperative, hemorrhage
postprocedural — *see* Complication, postprocedural, hemorrhage
hepatic failure K91.82
hyperglycemia (postpancreatectomy) E89.1
hypoinsulinemia (postpancreatectomy) E89.1
hypoparathyroidism (postparathyroidectomy) E89.2
hypopituitarism (posthypophysectomy) E89.3
hypothyroidism (post-thyroidectomy) E89.0
intestinal obstruction K91.3
intracranial hypotension following ventricular shunting (ventriculostomy) G97.2
lymphedema I97.89
postmastectomy I97.2
malabsorption (postsurgical) NEC K91.2
osteoporosis — *see* Osteoporosis, postsurgical malabsorption
mastoidectomy cavity NEC — *see* Complications, postmastoidectomy
metabolic E89.89
specified NEC E89.89
musculoskeletal — *see* Complications, musculoskeletal system
nervous system (central) (peripheral) — *see* Complications, nervous system
ovarian failure E89.40
asymptomatic E89.40
symptomatic E89.41

Complication(s) — *continued*
surgical procedure — *continued*
peripheral vascular — *see* Complications, surgical procedure, vascular
postcardiotomy syndrome I97.0
postcholecystectomy syndrome K91.5
postcommissurotomy syndrome I97.0
postgastrectomy dumping syndrome K91.1
postlaminectomy syndrome NEC M96.1
kyphosis M96.3
postmastectomy lymphedema syndrome I97.2
postmastoidectomy cholesteatoma — *see* Complications, postmastoidectomy, recurrent cholesteatoma
postvagotomy syndrome K91.1
postvalvulotomy syndrome I97.0
pulmonary insufficiency (acute) J95.2
chronic J95.3
following thoracic surgery J95.1
reattached body part — *see* Complications, reattached
respiratory — *see* Complications, respiratory system
shock (hypovolemic) T81.19 ☑
spleen (postoperative) D78.89
intraoperative D78.81
stitch abscess T81.4 ☑
subglottic stenosis (postsurgical) J95.5
testicular hypofunction E89.5
transplant — *see* Complications, organ or tissue transplant
urinary NEC N99.89
vaginal vault prolapse (posthysterectomy) N99.3
vascular (peripheral)
artery T81.719 ☑
mesenteric T81.710 ☑
renal T81.711 ☑
specified NEC T81.718 ☑
vein T81.72 ☑
wound infection T81.4 ☑
suture, permanent (wire) NEC T85.9 ☑
with repair of bone — *see* Complications, fixation device, internal
embolism T85.81 ☑
fibrosis T85.82 ☑
hemorrhage T85.83 ☑
infection and inflammation T85.79 ☑
mechanical
breakdown T85.612 ☑
displacement T85.622 ☑
malfunction T85.612 ☑
malposition T85.622 ☑
obstruction T85.692 ☑
perforation T85.692 ☑
protrusion T85.692 ☑
specified NEC T85.692 ☑
pain T85.84 ☑
specified type NEC T85.89 ☑
stenosis T85.85 ☑
thrombosis T85.86 ☑
tracheostomy J95.00
granuloma J95.09
hemorrhage J95.01
infection J95.02
malfunction J95.03
mechanical J95.03
obstruction J95.03
specified type NEC J95.09
tracheo-esophageal fistula J95.04
transfusion (blood) (lymphocytes) (plasma) T80.92 ☑
air emblism T80.0 ☑
circulatory overload E87.71
febrile nonhemolytic transfusion reaction R50.84
hemochromatosis E83.111
hemolysis T80.89 ☑
hemolytic reaction (antigen unspecified) T80.919 ☑
incompatibility reaction (antigen unspecified) T80.919 ☑
ABO T80.30 ☑
delayed serologic (DSTR) T80.39 ☑
hemolytic transfusion reaction (HTR) (unspecified time after transfusion) T80.319 ☑
acute (AHTR) (less than 24 hours after transfusion) T80.310 ☑

Complication(s) — *continued*
 transfusion — *continued*
  incompatibility reaction — *continued*
   ABO — *continued*
    hemolytic transfusion reaction — *contin-ued*
     delayed (DHTR) (24 hours or more after transfusion) T80.311 ☑
    specified NEC T80.39 ☑
   acute (antigen unspecified) T80.910 ☑
   delayed (antigen unspecified) T80.911 ☑
   delayed serologic (DSTR) T80.89 ☑
   non-ABO (minor antigens (Duffy) (Kell) (Kidd) (Lewis) (M) (N) (P) (S)) T80.A0 ☑ *(following* T80.4)
    delayed serologic (DSTR) T80.A9 ☑ *(following* T80.4)
    hemolytic transfusion reaction (HTR) (un-specified time after transfusion) T80.A19 ☑ *(following* T80.4)
     acute (AHTR) (less than 24 hours after transfusion) T80.A10 ☑ *(following* T80.4)
     delayed (DHTR) (24 hours or more after transfusion) T80.A11 ☑ *(following* T80.4)
    specified NEC T80.A9 ☑ *(following* T80.4)
   Rh (antigens (C) (c) (D) (E) (e)) (factor) T80.40 ☑
    delayed serologic (DSTR) T80.49 ☑
    hemolytic transfusion reaction (HTR) (un-specified time after transfusion) T80.419 ☑
     acute (AHTR) (less than 24 hours after transfusion) T80.410 ☑
     delayed (DHTR) (24 hours or more after transfusion) T80.411 ☑
    specified NEC T80.49 ☑
  infection T80.29 ☑
  reaction NEC T80.89 ☑
  sepsis T80.29 ☑
  shock T80.89 ☑
 transplant T86.90
  bone T86.839
   failure T86.831
   infection T86.832
   rejection T86.830
   specified type NEC T86.838
  bone marrow T86.00
   failure T86.02
   infection T86.03
   rejection T86.01
   specified type NEC T86.09
  cornea T86.849
   failure T86.841
   infection T86.842
   rejection T86.840
   specified type NEC T86.848
  failure T86.92
  heart T86.20
   with lung T86.30
   cardiac allograft vasculopathy T86.290
    failure T86.32
    infection T86.33
    rejection T86.31
    specified type NEC T86.39
   failure T86.22
   infection T86.23
   rejection T86.21
   specified type NEC T86.298
  infection T86.93
  intestine T86.859
   failure T86.851
   infection T86.852
   rejection T86.850
   specified type NEC T86.858
  kidney T86.10
   failure T86.12
   infection T86.13
   rejection T86.11
   specified type NEC T86.19
  liver T86.40
   failure T86.42
   infection T86.43
   rejection T86.41
   specified type NEC T86.49
  lung T86.819
   with heart T86.30
    failure T86.32

Complication(s) — *continued*
 transplant — *continued*
  lung — *continued*
   with heart — *continued*
    infection T86.33
    rejection T86.31
    specified type NEC T86.39
   failure T86.811
   infection T86.812
   rejection T86.810
   specified type NEC T86.818
  malignant neoplasm C80.2
  pancreas T86.899
   failure T86.891
   infection T86.892
   rejection T86.890
   specified type NEC T86.898
  peripheral blood stem cells T86.5
  post-transplant lymphoproliferative disorder (PTLD) D47.Z1 *(following* D47.4)
  rejection T86.91
  skin T86.829
   failure T86.821
   infection T86.822
   rejection T86.820
   specified type NEC T86.828
  specified
   tissue T86.899
    failure T86.891
    infection T86.892
    rejection T86.890
    specified type NEC T86.898
   type NEC T86.99
  stem cell (from peripheral blood) (from umbilical cord) T86.5
  umbilical cord stem cells T86.5
 trauma (early) T79.9
  specified NEC T79.8 ☑
 ultrasound therapy NEC T88.9 ☑
 umbilical cord NEC
  complicating delivery O69.9
  specified NEC O69.89 ☑
 umbrella device, vascular T82.9
  embolism T82.818 ☑
  fibrosis T82.828 ☑
  hemorrhage T82.838 ☑
  infection or inflammation T82.7 ☑
  mechanical
   breakdown T82.515 ☑
   displacement T82.525 ☑
   leakage T82.535 ☑
   malposition T82.525 ☑
   obstruction T82.595 ☑
   perforation T82.595 ☑
   protrusion T82.595 ☑
  pain T82.848 ☑
  specified type NEC T82.898 ☑
  stenosis T82.858 ☑
  thrombosis T82.868 ☑
 urethral catheter — *see* Complications, catheter, ure-thral, indwelling
 vaccination T88.1 ☑
  anaphylaxis NEC T80.52 ☑
  arthropathy — *see* Arthropathy, postimmunization
  cellulitis T88.0 ☑
  encephalitis or encephalomyelitis G04.02
  infection (general) (local) NEC T88.0 ☑
  meningitis G03.8
  myelitis G04.89
  protein sickness T80.62 ☑
  rash T88.1 ☑
  reaction (allergic) T88.1 ☑
   serum T80.62 ☑
  sepsis T88.0 ☑
  serum intoxication, sickness, rash, or other serum reaction NEC T80.62 ☑
   anaphylactic shock T80.52 ☑
  shock (allergic) (anaphylactic) T80.52 ☑
  vaccinia (generalized) (localized) T88.1 ☑
 vas deferens device or implant — *see* Complications, genitourinary, device or implant, genital tract
 vascular I99.9
  device or implant T82.9 ☑
   embolism T82.818 ☑
   fibrosis T82.828 ☑
   hemorrhage T82.838 ☑
   infection or inflammation T82.7 ☑

Complication(s) — *continued*
 vascular — *continued*
  device or implant — *continued*
   mechanical
    breakdown T82.519 ☑
     specified device NEC T82.518 ☑
    displacement T82.529 ☑
     specified device NEC T82.528 ☑
    leakage T82.539 ☑
     specified device NEC T82.538 ☑
    malposition T82.529 ☑
     specified device NEC T82.528 ☑
    obstruction T82.599 ☑
     specified device NEC T82.598 ☑
    perforation T82.599 ☑
     specified device NEC T82.598 ☑
    protrusion T82.599 ☑
     specified device NEC T82.598 ☑
   pain T82.848 ☑
   specified type NEC T82.898 ☑
   stenosis T82.858 ☑
   thrombosis T82.868 ☑
  dialysis catheter — *see* Complication, catheter, dialysis
  following infusion, therapeutic injection or transfu-sion T80.1 ☑
  graft T82.9
   embolism T82.818 ☑
   fibrosis T82.828 ☑
   hemorrhage T82.838 ☑
   mechanical
    breakdown T82.319 ☑
     aorta (bifurcation) T82.310 ☑
     carotid artery T82.311 ☑
     specified vessel NEC T82.318 ☑
    displacement T82.329 ☑
     aorta (bifurcation) T82.320 ☑
     carotid artery T82.321 ☑
     specified vessel NEC T82.328 ☑
    leakage T82.339 ☑
     aorta (bifurcation) T82.330 ☑
     carotid artery T82.331 ☑
     specified vessel NEC T82.338 ☑
    malposition T82.329 ☑
     aorta (bifurcation) T82.320 ☑
     carotid artery T82.321 ☑
     specified vessel NEC T82.328 ☑
    obstruction T82.399 ☑
     aorta (bifurcation) T82.390 ☑
     carotid artery T82.391 ☑
     specified vessel NEC T82.398 ☑
    perforation T82.399 ☑
     aorta (bifurcation) T82.390 ☑
     carotid artery T82.391 ☑
     specified vessel NEC T82.398 ☑
    protrusion T82.399 ☑
     aorta (bifurcation) T82.390 ☑
     carotid artery T82.391 ☑
     specified vessel NEC T82.398 ☑
   pain T82.848 ☑
   specified complication NEC T82.898 ☑
   stenosis T82.858 ☑
   thrombosis T82.868 ☑
  postoperative — *see* Complications, postoperative, circulatory
 vena cava device (filter) (sieve) (umbrella) — *see* Complications, umbrella device, vascular
 ventilation therapy NEC T81.81 ☑
 ventilator
  mechanical J95.850
   specified NEC J95.859
 ventricular (communicating) shunt (device) T85.9 ☑
  embolism T85.81 ☑
  fibrosis T85.82 ☑
  hemorrhage T85.83 ☑
  infection and inflammation T85.79 ☑
  mechanical
   breakdown T85.01 ☑
   displacement T85.02 ☑
   leakage T85.03 ☑
   malposition T85.02 ☑
   obstruction T85.09 ☑
   perforation T85.09 ☑
   protrusion T85.09 ☑
   specified NEC T85.09 ☑
  pain T85.84 ☑

Complication(s) — *continued*
  ventricular shunt — *continued*
    specified type NEC T85.89 ☑
    stenosis T85.85 ☑
    thrombosis T85.86 ☑
  wire suture, permanent (implanted) — *see* Complications, suture, permanent
Compressed air disease T70.3 ☑
Compression
  with injury — *code by* Nature of injury
  artery I77.1
    celiac, syndrome I77.4
  brachial plexus G54.0
  brain (stem) G93.5
    due to
      contusion (diffuse) — *see* Injury, intracranial, diffuse
        focal — *see* Injury, intracranial, focal
      injury NEC — *see* Injury, intracranial, diffuse
      traumatic — *see* Injury, intracranial, diffuse
  bronchus J98.09
  cauda equina G83.4
  celiac (artery) (axis) I77.4
  cerebral — *see* Compression, brain
  cervical plexus G54.2
  cord
    spinal — *see* Compression, spinal
    umbilical — *see* Compression, umbilical cord
  cranial nerve G52.9
    eighth H93.3 ☑
    eleventh G52.8
    fifth G50.8
    first G52.0
    fourth — *see* Strabismus, paralytic, fourth nerve
    ninth G52.1
    second — *see* Disorder, nerve, optic
    seventh G52.8
    sixth — *see* Strabismus, paralytic, sixth nerve
    tenth G52.2
    third — *see* Strabismus, paralytic, third nerve
    twelfth G52.3
  diver's squeeze T70.3 ☑
  during birth (newborn) P15.9
  esophagus K22.2
  eustachian tube — *see* Obstruction, eustachian tube, cartilaginous
  facies Q67.1
  fracture — *see* Fracture
  heart — *see* Disease, heart
  intestine — *see* Obstruction, intestine
  laryngeal nerve, recurrent G52.2
    with paralysis of vocal cords and larynx J38.00
      bilateral J38.02
      unilateral J38.01
  lumbosacral plexus G54.1
  lung J98.4
  lymphatic vessel I89.0
  medulla — *see* Compression, brain
  nerve (*see also* Disorder, nerve) G58.9
    arm NEC — *see* Mononeuropathy, upper limb
    axillary G54.0
    cranial — *see* Compression, cranial nerve
    leg NEC — *see* Mononeuropathy, lower limb
    median (in carpal tunnel) — *see* Syndrome, carpal tunnel
    optic — *see* Disorder, nerve, optic
    plantar — *see* Lesion, nerve, plantar
    posterior tibial (in tarsal tunnel) — *see* Syndrome, tarsal tunnel
    root or plexus NOS (in) G54.9
      intervertebral disc disorder NEC — *see* Disorder, disc, with, radiculopathy
        with myelopathy — *see* Disorder, disc, with, myelopathy
      neoplastic disease (*see also* Neoplasm) D49.9 [G55]
      spondylosis — *see* Spondylosis, with radiculopathy
    sciatic (acute) — *see* Lesion, nerve, sciatic
    sympathetic G90.8
    traumatic — *see* Injury, nerve
    ulnar — *see* Lesion, nerve, ulnar
    upper extremity NEC — *see* Mononeuropathy, upper limb
  spinal (cord) G95.20
    by displacement of intervertebral disc NEC (*see also* Disorder, disc, with, myelopathy)

Compression — *continued*
  spinal — *continued*
    nerve root NOS G54.9
      due to displacement of intervertebral disc NEC — *see* Disorder, disc, with, radiculopathy
        with myelopathy — *see* Disorder, disc, with, myelopathy
    specified NEC G95.29
    spondylogenic (cervical) (lumbar, lumbosacral) (thoracic) — *see* Spondylosis, with myelopathy NEC
    anterior — *see* Syndrome, anterior, spinal artery, compression
    traumatic — *see* Injury, spinal cord, by region
  subcostal nerve (syndrome) — *see* Mononeuropathy, upper limb, specified NEC
  sympathetic nerve NEC G90.8
  syndrome T79.5 ☑
  trachea J39.8
  ulnar nerve (by scar tissue) — *see* Lesion, nerve, ulnar
  umbilical cord
    complicating delivery O69.2 ☑
      cord around neck O69.1 ☑
      prolapse O69.0 ☑
      specified NEC O69.2 ☑
  ureter N13.5
  vein I87.1
  vena cava (inferior) (superior) I87.1
Compulsion, compulsive
  gambling F63.0
  neurosis F42
  personality F60.5
  states F42
  swearing F42
    in Gilles de la Tourette's syndrome F95.2
  tics and spasms F95.9
Concato's disease (pericardial polyserositis) A19.9
  nontubercular I31.1
  pleural — *see* Pleurisy, with effusion
Concavity chest wall M95.4
Concealed penis Q55.69
Concern (normal) **about sick person in family** Z63.6
Concrescence (teeth) K00.2
Concretio cordis I31.1
  rheumatic I09.2
Concretion (*see also* Calculus)
  appendicular K38.1
  canaliculus — *see* Dacryolith
  clitoris N90.89
  conjunctiva H11.12- ☑
  eyelid — *see* Disorder, eyelid, specified type NEC
  lacrimal passages — *see* Dacryolith
  prepuce (male) N47.8
  salivary gland (any) K11.5
  seminal vesicle N50.8
  tonsil J35.8
Concussion (brain) (cerebral) (current) S06.0X- ☑
  blast (air) (hydraulic) (immersion) (underwater)
    abdomen or thorax — *see* Injury, blast, by site
    ear with acoustic nerve injury — *see* Injury, nerve, acoustic, specified type NEC
  cauda equina S34.3 ☑
  conus medullaris S34.02 ☑
  ocular S05.8X- ☑
  spinal (cord)
    cervical S14.0 ☑
    lumbar S34.01 ☑
    sacral S34.02 ☑
    thoracic S24.0 ☑
  syndrome F07.81
Condition — *see* Disease
Conditions arising in the perinatal period — *see* Newborn, affected by
Conduct disorder — *see* Disorder, conduct
Condyloma A63.0
  acuminatum A63.0
  gonorrheal A54.09
  latum A51.31
  syphilitic A51.31
    congenital A50.07
  venereal, syphilitic A51.31
Conflagration (*see also* Burn)
  asphyxia (by inhalation of gases, fumes or vapors) (*see also* Table of Drugs and Chemicals) T59.9- ☑
Conflict (with) (*see also* Discord)
  family Z73.9
  marital Z63.0

Conflict — *continued*
  marital — *continued*
    involving divorce or estrangement Z63.5
  parent-child Z62.820
    parent-adopted child Z62.821
    parent-biological child Z62.820
    parent-foster child Z62.822
  social role NEC Z73.5
Confluent — *see* condition
Confusion, confused R41.0
  epileptic F05
  mental state (psychogenic) F44.89
  psychogenic F44.89
  reactive (from emotional stress, psychological trauma) F44.89
Confusional arousals G47.51
Congelation T69.9 ☑
Congenital (*see also* condition)
  aortic septum Q25.4
  intrinsic factor deficiency D51.0
  malformation — *see* Anomaly
Congestion, congestive
  bladder N32.89
  bowel K63.89
  brain G93.89
  breast N64.59
  bronchial J98.09
  catarrhal J31.0
  chest R09.89
  chill, malarial — *see* Malaria
  circulatory NEC I99.8
  duodenum K31.89
  eye — *see* Hyperemia, conjunctiva
  facial, due to birth injury P15.4
  general R68.89
  glottis J37.0
  heart — *see* Failure, heart, congestive
  hepatic K76.1
  hypostatic (lung) — *see* Edema, lung
  intestine K63.89
  kidney N28.89
  labyrinth H83.8 ☑
  larynx J37.0
  liver K76.1
  lung R09.89
    active or acute — *see* Pneumonia
  malaria, malarial — *see* Malaria
  nasal R09.81
  nose R09.81
  orbit, orbital (*see also* Exophthalmos)
    inflammatory (chronic) — *see* Inflammation, orbit
  ovary N83.8
  pancreas K86.8
  pelvic, female N94.89
  pleural J94.8
  prostate (active) N42.1
  pulmonary — *see* Congestion, lung
  renal N28.89
  retina H35.81
  seminal vesicle N50.1
  spinal cord G95.19
  spleen (chronic) D73.2
  stomach K31.89
  trachea — *see* Tracheitis
  urethra N36.8
  uterus N85.8
    with subinvolution N85.3
  venous (passive) I87.8
  viscera R68.89
Congestive — *see* Congestion
Conical
  cervix (hypertrophic elongation) N88.4
  cornea — *see* Keratoconus
  teeth K00.2
Conjoined twins Q89.4
Conjugal maladjustment Z63.0
  involving divorce or estrangement Z63.5
Conjunctiva — *see* condition
Conjunctivitis (staphylococcal) (streptococcal) NOS H10.9
  Acanthamoeba B60.12
  acute H10.3- ☑
    atopic H10.1- ☑
    chemical (*see also* Corrosion, cornea) H10.21- ☑
    mucopurulent H10.02- ☑
      follicular H10.01- ☑
    pseudomembranous H10.22- ☑

Index

Conjunctivitis — Constriction

Conjunctivitis — *continued*
acute — *continued*
  serous except viral H10.23- ☑
    viral — *see* Conjunctivitis, viral
  toxic H10.21- ☑
adenoviral (acute) (follicular) B30.1
allergic (acute) — *see* Conjunctivitis, acute, atopic
  chronic H10.45
    vernal H10.44
anaphylactic — *see* Conjunctivitis, acute, atopic
Apollo B30.3
atopic (acute) — *see* Conjunctivitis, acute, atopic
Béal's B30.2
blennorrhagic (gonococcal) (neonatorum) A54.31
chemical (acute) (*see also* Corrosion, cornea)
    H10.21- ☑
chlamydial A74.0
  due to trachoma A71.1
  neonatal P39.1
chronic (nodosa) (petrificans) (phlyctenular) H10.40- ☑
  allergic H10.45
    vernal H10.44
  follicular H10.43- ☑
  giant papillary H10.41- ☑
  simple H10.42- ☑
  vernal H10.44
coxsackievirus 24 B30.3
diphtheritic A36.86
due to
  dust — *see* Conjunctivitis, acute, atopic
  filariasis B74.9
  mucocutaneous leishmaniasis B55.2
enterovirus type 70 (hemorrhagic) B30.3
epidemic (viral) B30.9
  hemorrhagic B30.3
gonococcal (neonatorum) A54.31
granular (trachomatous) A71.1
  sequelae (late effect) B94.0
hemorrhagic (acute) (epidemic) B30.3
herpes zoster B02.31
in (due to)
  Acanthamoeba B60.12
  adenovirus (acute) (follicular) B30.1
  Chlamydia A74.0
  coxsackievirus 24 B30.3
  diphtheria A36.86
  enterovirus type 70 (hemorrhagic) B30.3
  filariasis B74.9
  gonococci A54.31
  herpes (simplex) virus B00.53
    zoster B02.31
  infectious disease NEC B99 ☑
  meningococci A39.89
  mucocutaneous leishmaniasis B55.2
  rosacea L71.9
  syphilis (late) A52.71
  zoster B02.31
inclusion A74.0
infantile P39.1
  gonococcal A54.31
Koch-Weeks' — *see* Conjunctivitis, acute, mucopuru-
    lent
light — *see* Conjunctivitis, acute, atopic
ligneous — *see* Blepharoconjunctivitis, ligneous
meningococcal A39.89
mucopurulent — *see* Conjunctivitis, acute, mucopuru-
    lent
neonatal P39.1
  gonococcal A54.31
Newcastle B30.8
of Béal B30.2
parasitic
  filariasis B74.9
  mucocutaneous leishmaniasis B55.2
Parinaud's H10.89
petrificans H10.89
rosacea L71.9
specified NEC H10.89
swimming-pool B30.1
trachomatous A71.1
  acute A71.0
  sequelae (late effect) B94.0
traumatic NEC H10.89
tuberculous A18.59
tularemic A21.1
tularensis A21.1
viral B30.9

Conjunctivitis — *continued*
viral — *continued*
  due to
    adenovirus B30.1
    enterovirus B30.3
  specified NEC B30.8
Conjunctivochalasis H11.82- ☑
Connective tissue — *see* condition
Conn's syndrome E26.01
Conradi (-Hunermann) **disease** Q77.3
Consanguinity Z84.3
  counseling Z71.89
Conscious simulation (of illness) Z76.5
Consecutive — *see* condition
Consolidation lung (base) — *see* Pneumonia, lobar
Constipation (atonic) (neurogenic) (simple) (spastic)
    K59.00
  drug-induced — *see* Table of Drugs and Chemicals
  outlet dysfunction K59.02
  psychogenic F45.8
  slow transit K59.01
  specified NEC K59.09
Constitutional (*see also* condition)
  substandard F60.7
Constitutionally substandard F60.7
Constriction (*see also* Stricture)
  auditory canal — *see* Stenosis, external ear canal
  bronchial J98.09
  duodenum K31.5
  esophagus K22.2
  external
    abdomen, abdominal (wall) S30.841 ☑
    alveolar process S00.542 ☑
    ankle S90.54- ☑
    antecubital space — *see* Constriction, external,
        forearm
    arm (upper) S40.84- ☑
    auricle — *see* Constriction, external, ear
    axilla — *see* Constriction, external, arm
    back, lower S30.840 ☑
    breast S20.14- ☑
    brow S00.84 ☑
    buttock S30.840 ☑
    calf — *see* Constriction, external, leg
    canthus — *see* Constriction, external, eyelid
    cheek S00.84 ☑
      internal S00.542 ☑
    chest wall — *see* Constriction, external, thorax
    chin S00.84 ☑
    clitoris S30.844 ☑
    costal region — *see* Constriction, external, thorax
    digit(s)
      foot — *see* Constriction, external, toe
      hand — *see* Constriction, external, finger
    ear S00.44- ☑
    elbow S50.34- ☑
    epididymis S30.843 ☑
    epigastric region S30.841 ☑
    esophagus, cervical S10.14 ☑
    eyebrow — *see* Constriction, external, eyelid
    eyelid S00.24- ☑
    face S00.84 ☑
    finger(s) S60.44- ☑
      index S60.44- ☑
      little S60.44- ☑
      middle S60.44- ☑
      ring S60.44- ☑
    flank S30.841 ☑
    foot (except toe(s) alone) S90.84- ☑
      toe — *see* Constriction, external, toe
    forearm S50.84- ☑
      elbow only — *see* Constriction, external, elbow
    forehead S00.84 ☑
    genital organs, external
      female S30.846 ☑
      male S30.845 ☑
    groin S30.841 ☑
    gum S00.542 ☑
    hand S60.54- ☑
    head S00.94 ☑
      ear — *see* Constriction, external, ear
      eyelid — *see* Constriction, external, eyelid
      lip S00.541 ☑
      nose S00.34 ☑
      oral cavity S00.542 ☑
      scalp S00.04 ☑

Constriction — *continued*
external — *continued*
  head — *continued*
    specified site NEC S00.84 ☑
  heel — *see* Constriction, external, foot
  hip S70.24- ☑
  inguinal region S30.841 ☑
  interscapular region S20.449 ☑
  jaw S00.84 ☑
  knee S80.24- ☑
  labium (majus) (minus) S30.844 ☑
  larynx S10.14 ☑
  leg (lower) S80.84- ☑
    knee — *see* Constriction, external, knee
    upper — *see* Constriction, external, thigh
  lip S00.541 ☑
  lower back S30.840 ☑
  lumbar region S30.840 ☑
  malar region S00.84 ☑
  mammary — *see* Constriction, external, breast
  mastoid region S00.84 ☑
  mouth S00.542 ☑
  nail
    finger — *see* Constriction, external, finger
    toe — *see* Constriction, external, toe
  nasal S00.34 ☑
  neck S10.94 ☑
    specified site NEC S10.84 ☑
    throat S10.14 ☑
  nose S00.34 ☑
  occipital region S00.04 ☑
  oral cavity S00.542 ☑
  orbital region — *see* Constriction, external, eyelid
  palate S00.542 ☑
  palm — *see* Constriction, external, hand
  parietal region S00.04 ☑
  pelvis S30.840 ☑
  penis S30.842 ☑
  perineum
    female S30.844 ☑
    male S30.840 ☑
  periocular area — *see* Constriction, external, eyelid
  phalanges
    finger — *see* Constriction, external, finger
    toe — *see* Constriction, external, toe
  pharynx S10.14 ☑
  pinna — *see* Constriction, external, ear
  popliteal space — *see* Constriction, external, knee
  prepuce S30.842 ☑
  pubic region S30.840 ☑
  pudendum
    female S30.846 ☑
    male S30.845 ☑
  sacral region S30.840 ☑
  scalp S00.04 ☑
  scapular region — *see* Constriction, external,
      shoulder
  scrotum S30.843 ☑
  shin — *see* Constriction, external, leg
  shoulder S40.24- ☑
  sternal region S20.349 ☑
  submaxillary region S00.84 ☑
  submental region S00.84 ☑
  subungual
    finger(s) — *see* Constriction, external, finger
    toe(s) — *see* Constriction, external, toe
  supraclavicular fossa S10.84 ☑
  supraorbital S00.84 ☑
  temple S00.84 ☑
  temporal region S00.84 ☑
  testis S30.843 ☑
  thigh S70.34- ☑
  thorax, thoracic (wall) S20.94 ☑
    back S20.44- ☑
    front S20.34- ☑
  throat S10.14 ☑
  thumb S60.34- ☑
  toe(s) (lesser) S90.44- ☑
    great S90.44- ☑
  tongue S00.542 ☑
  trachea S10.14 ☑
  tunica vaginalis S30.843 ☑
  uvula S00.542 ☑
  vagina S30.844 ☑
  vulva S30.844 ☑
  wrist S60.84- ☑

Constriction — *continued*
gallbladder — *see* Obstruction, gallbladder
intestine — *see* Obstruction, intestine
larynx J38.6
    congenital Q31.8
        specified NEC Q31.8
        subglottic Q31.1
organ or site, congenital NEC — *see* Atresia, by site
prepuce (acquired) (congenital) N47.1
pylorus (adult hypertrophic) K31.1
    congenital or infantile Q40.0
    newborn Q40.0
ring dystocia (uterus) O62.4
spastic (*see also* Spasm)
    ureter N13.5
ureter N13.5
    with infection N13.6
urethra — *see* Stricture, urethra
visual field (peripheral) (functional) — *see* Defect, visual field

Constrictive — *see* condition
Consultation
    without complaint or sickness Z71.9
        feared complaint unfounded Z71.1
        specified reason NEC Z71.89
    medical — *see* Counseling, medical
    religious Z71.81
    specified reason NEC Z71.89
    spiritual Z71.81
Consumption — *see* Tuberculosis
Contact (with) (*see also* Exposure (to))
    acariasis Z20.7
    AIDS virus Z20.6
    air pollution Z77.110
    algae and algae toxins Z77.121
    algae bloom Z77.121
    anthrax Z20.810
    aromatic amines Z77.020
    aromatic (hazardous) compounds NEC Z77.028
    aromatic dyes NOS Z77.028
    arsenic Z77.010
    asbestos Z77.090
    bacterial disease NEC Z20.818
    benzene Z77.021
    blue-green algae bloom Z77.121
    body fluids (potentially hazardous) Z77.21
    brown tide Z77.121
    chemicals (chiefly nonmedicinal) (hazardous) NEC Z77.098
    cholera Z20.09
    chromium compounds Z77.018
    communicable disease Z20.9
        bacterial NEC Z20.818
        specified NEC Z20.89
        viral NEC Z20.828
    cyanobacteria bloom Z77.121
    dyes Z77.098
    Escherichia coli (E. coli) Z20.01
    fiberglass — *see* Table of Drugs and Chemicals, fiberglass
    German measles Z20.4
    gonorrhea Z20.2
    hazardous metals NEC Z77.018
    hazardous substances NEC Z77.29
    hazards in the physical environment NEC Z77.128
    hazards to health NEC Z77.9
    HIV Z20.6
    HTLV-III/LAV Z20.6
    human immunodeficiency virus (HIV) Z20.6
    infection Z20.9
        specified NEC Z20.89
    infestation (parasitic) NEC Z20.7
    intestinal infectious disease NEC Z20.09
        Escherichia coli (E. coli) Z20.01
    lead Z77.011
    meningococcus Z20.811
    mold (toxic) Z77.120
    nickel dust Z77.018
    noise Z77.122
    parasitic disease Z20.7
    pediculosis Z20.7
    pfiesteria piscicida Z77.121
    poliomyelitis Z20.89
    pollution
        air Z77.110
        environmental NEC Z77.118
        soil Z77.112
        water Z77.111

Contact — *continued*
    polycyclic aromatic hydrocarbons Z77.028
    rabies Z20.3
    radiation, naturally occurring NEC Z77.123
    radon Z77.123
    red tide (Florida) Z77.121
    rubella Z20.4
    sexually-transmitted disease Z20.2
    smallpox (laboratory) Z20.89
    syphilis Z20.2
    tuberculosis Z20.1
    uranium Z77.012
    varicella Z20.820
    venereal disease Z20.2
    viral disease NEC Z20.828
    viral hepatitis Z20.5
    water pollution Z77.111
Contamination, food — *see* Intoxication, foodborne
Contraception, contraceptive
    advice Z30.09
    counseling Z30.09
    device (intrauterine) (in situ) Z97.5
        causing menorrhagia T83.83 ☑
        checking Z30.431
        complications — *see* Complications, intrauterine, contraceptive device
        in place Z97.5
        initial prescription Z30.014
        reinsertion Z30.433
        removal Z30.432
        replacement Z30.433
    emergency (postcoital) Z30.012
    initial prescription Z30.019
        injectable Z30.013
        intrauterine device Z30.014
        pills Z30.011
        postcoital (emergency) Z30.012
        specified type NEC Z30.018
        subdermal implantable Z30.019
    maintenance Z30.40
        examination Z30.8
        injectable Z30.42
        intrauterine device Z30.431
        pills Z30.41
        specified type NEC Z30.49
        subdermal implantable Z30.49
    management Z30.9
        specified NEC Z30.8
    postcoital (emergency) Z30.012
    prescription Z30.019
        repeat Z30.40
    sterilization Z30.2
    surveillance (drug) — *see* Contraception, maintenance
Contraction(s), contracture, contracted
    Achilles tendon (*see also* Short, tendon, Achilles)
        congenital Q66.89
    amputation stump (surgical) (flexion) (late) (next proximal joint) T87.89
    anus K59.8
    bile duct (common) (hepatic) K83.8
    bladder N32.89
        neck or sphincter N32.0
    bowel, cecum, colon or intestine, any part — *see* Obstruction, intestine
    Braxton Hicks — *see* False, labor
    breast implant, capsular T85.44 ☑
    bronchial J98.09
    burn (old) — *see* Cicatrix
    cervix — *see* Stricture, cervix
    cicatricial — *see* Cicatrix
    conjunctiva, trachomatous, active A71.1
        sequelae (late effect) B94.0
    Dupuytren's M72.0
    eyelid — *see* Disorder, eyelid function
    fascia (lata) (postural) M72.8
        Dupuytren's M72.0
        palmar M72.0
        plantar M72.2
    finger NEC (*see also* Deformity, finger)
        congenital Q68.1
        joint — *see* Contraction, joint, hand
    flaccid — *see* Contraction, paralytic
    gallbladder K82.0
    heart valve — *see* Endocarditis
    hip — *see* Contraction, joint, hip
    hourglass
        bladder N32.89
            congenital Q64.79

Contraction(s), contracture, contracted — *continued*
    hourglass — *continued*
        gallbladder K82.0
            congenital Q44.1
        stomach K31.89
            congenital Q40.2
            psychogenic F45.8
    uterus (complicating delivery) O62.4
    hysterical F44.4
    internal os — *see* Stricture, cervix
    joint (abduction) (acquired) (adduction) (flexion) (rotation) M24.50
        ankle M24.57- ☑
        congenital NEC Q68.8
            hip Q65.89
        elbow M24.52- ☑
        foot joint M24.57- ☑
        hand joint M24.54- ☑
        hip M24.55- ☑
            congenital Q65.89
        hysterical F44.4
        knee M24.56- ☑
        shoulder M24.51- ☑
        wrist M24.53- ☑
    kidney (granular) (secondary) N26.9
        congenital Q63.8
        hydronephritic — *see* Hydronephrosis
        Page N26.2
        pyelonephritic — *see* Pyelitis, chronic
        tuberculous A18.11
    ligament (*see also* Disorder, ligament)
        congenital Q79.8
    muscle (postinfective) (postural) NEC M62.40
        with contracture of joint — *see* Contraction, joint
        ankle M62.47- ☑
        congenital Q79.8
            sternocleidomastoid Q68.0
        extraocular — *see* Strabismus
        eye (extrinsic) — *see* Strabismus
        foot M62.47- ☑
        forearm M62.43- ☑
        hand M62.44- ☑
        hysterical F44.4
        ischemic (Volkmann's) T79.6 ☑
        lower leg M62.46- ☑
        multiple sites M62.49
        pelvic region M62.45- ☑
        posttraumatic — *see* Strabismus, paralytic
        psychogenic F45.8
            conversion reaction F44.4
        shoulder region M62.41- ☑
        specified site NEC M62.48
        thigh M62.45- ☑
        upper arm M62.42- ☑
    neck — *see* Torticollis
    ocular muscle — *see* Strabismus
    organ or site, congenital NEC — *see* Atresia, by site
    outlet (pelvis) — *see* Contraction, pelvis
    palmar fascia M72.0
    paralytic
        joint — *see* Contraction, joint
        muscle (*see also* Contraction, muscle NEC)
            ocular — *see* Strabismus, paralytic
    pelvis (acquired) (general) M95.5
        with disproportion (fetopelvic) O33.1
            causing obstructed labor O65.1
            inlet O33.2
            mid-cavity O33.3 ☑
            outlet O33.3 ☑
    plantar fascia M72.2
    premature
        atrium I49.1
        auriculoventricular I49.49
        heart I49.49
        junctional I49.2
        supraventricular I49.1
        ventricular I49.3
    prostate N42.89
    pylorus NEC (*see also* Pylorospasm)
        psychogenic F45.8
    rectum, rectal (sphincter) K59.8
    ring (Bandl's) (complicating delivery) O62.4
    scar — *see* Cicatrix
    spine — *see* Dorsopathy, deforming
    sternocleidomastoid (muscle), congenital Q68.0
    stomach K31.89
        hourglass K31.89

Contraction(s), contracture, contracted — continued
- stomach — continued
  - hourglass — continued
    - congenital Q40.2
    - psychogenic F45.8
  - psychogenic F45.8
- tendon (sheath) M62.40
  - with contracture of joint — see Contraction, joint
  - Achilles — see Short, tendon, Achilles
  - ankle M62.47-
    - Achilles — see Short, tendon, Achilles
  - foot M62.47- ☑
  - forearm M62.43- ☑
  - hand M62.44- ☑
  - lower leg M62.46- ☑
  - multiple sites M62.49
  - neck M62.48
  - pelvic region M62.45- ☑
  - shoulder region M62.41- ☑
  - specified site NEC M62.48
  - thigh M62.45- ☑
  - thorax M62.48
  - trunk M62.48
  - upper arm M62.42- ☑
- toe — see Deformity, toe, specified NEC
- ureterovesical orifice (postinfectional) N13.5
  - with infection N13.6
- urethra (see also Stricture, urethra)
  - orifice N32.0
- uterus N85.8
  - abnormal NEC O62.9
  - clonic (complicating delivery) O62.4
  - dyscoordinate (complicating delivery) O62.4
  - hourglass (complicating delivery) O62.4
  - hypertonic O62.4
  - hypotonic NEC O62.2
  - inadequate
    - primary O62.0
    - secondary O62.1
  - incoordinate (complicating delivery) O62.4
  - poor O62.2
  - tetanic (complicating delivery) O62.4
- vagina (outlet) N89.5
- vesical N32.89
  - neck or urethral orifice N32.0
- visual field — see Defect, visual field, generalized
- Volkmann's (ischemic) T79.6

Contusion (skin surface intact) T14.8
- abdomen, abdominal (muscle) (wall) S30.1 ☑
- adnexa, eye NEC S05.8X- ☑
- adrenal gland S37.812 ☑
- alveolar process S00.532 ☑
- ankle S90.0- ☑
- antecubital space — see Contusion, forearm
- anus S30.3 ☑
- arm (upper) S40.02- ☑
  - lower (with elbow) — see Contusion, forearm
- auditory canal — see Contusion, ear
- auricle — see Contusion, ear
- axilla — see Contusion, arm, upper
- back (see also Contusion, thorax, back)
  - lower S30.0 ☑
- bile duct S36.13 ☑
- bladder S37.22 ☑
- bone NEC T14.8
- brain (diffuse) — see Injury, intracranial, diffuse
  - focal — see Injury, intracranial, focal
- brainstem S06.38- ☑
- breast S20.0- ☑
- broad ligament S37.892 ☑
- brow S00.83 ☑
- buttock S30.0 ☑
- canthus, eye S00.1- ☑
- cauda equina S34.3 ☑
- cerebellar, traumatic S06.37- ☑
- cerebral S06.33- ☑
  - left side S06.32- ☑
  - right side S06.31- ☑
- cheek S00.83 ☑
  - internal S00.532 ☑
- chest (wall) — see Contusion, thorax
- chin S00.83 ☑
- clitoris S30.23 ☑
- colon — see Injury, intestine, large, contusion
- common bile duct S36.13 ☑
- conjunctiva S05.1- ☑

Contusion — continued
- conjunctiva — continued
  - with foreign body (in conjunctival sac) — see Foreign body, conjunctival sac
- conus medullaris (spine) S34.139
- cornea — see Contusion, eyeball
  - with foreign body — see Foreign body, cornea
- corpus cavernosum S30.21 ☑
- cortex (brain) (cerebral) — see Injury, intracranial, diffuse
  - focal — see Injury, intracranial, focal
- costal region — see Contusion, thorax
- cystic duct S36.13 ☑
- diaphragm S27.802 ☑
- duodenum S36.420 ☑
- ear S00.43- ☑
- elbow S50.0- ☑
  - with forearm — see Contusion, forearm
- epididymis S30.22 ☑
- epigastric region S30.1 ☑
- epiglottis S10.0 ☑
- esophagus (thoracic) S27.812 ☑
  - cervical S10.0 ☑
- eyeball S05.1- ☑
- eyebrow S00.1- ☑
- eyelid (and periocular area) S00.1- ☑
- face NEC S00.83 ☑
- fallopian tube S37.529 ☑
  - bilateral S37.522 ☑
  - unilateral S37.521 ☑
- femoral triangle S30.1 ☑
- finger(s) S60.00 ☑
  - with damage to nail (matrix) S60.10 ☑
  - index S60.02- ☑
    - with damage to nail S60.12- ☑
  - little S60.05- ☑
    - with damage to nail S60.15- ☑
  - middle S60.03- ☑
    - with damage to nail S60.13- ☑
  - ring S60.04- ☑
    - with damage to nail S60.14- ☑
  - thumb — see Contusion, thumb
- flank S30.1 ☑
- foot (except toe(s) alone) S90.3- ☑
  - toe — see Contusion, toe
- forearm S50.1- ☑
  - elbow only — see Contusion, elbow
- forehead S00.83 ☑
- gallbladder S36.122 ☑
- genital organs, external
  - female S30.202 ☑
  - male S30.201 ☑
- globe (eye) — see Contusion, eyeball
- groin S30.1 ☑
- gum S00.532 ☑
- hand S60.22- ☑
  - finger(s) — see Contusion, finger
  - wrist — see Contusion, wrist
- head S00.93 ☑
  - ear — see Contusion, ear
  - eyelid — see Contusion, eyelid
  - lip S00.531 ☑
  - nose S00.33 ☑
  - oral cavity S00.532 ☑
  - scalp S00.03 ☑
  - specified part NEC S00.83 ☑
- heel — see Contusion, foot
- hepatic duct S36.13 ☑
- hip S70.0- ☑
- ileum S36.428 ☑
- iliac region S30.1 ☑
- inguinal region S30.1 ☑
- interscapular region S20.229 ☑
- intra-abdominal organ S36.92 ☑
  - colon — see Injury, intestine, large, contusion
  - liver S36.112 ☑
  - pancreas — see Contusion, pancreas
  - rectum S36.62 ☑
  - small intestine — see Injury, intestine, small, contusion
  - specified organ NEC S36.892 ☑
  - spleen — see Contusion, spleen
  - stomach S36.32 ☑
- iris (eye) — see Contusion, eyeball
- jaw S00.83 ☑
- jejunum S36.428 ☑

Contusion — continued
- kidney S37.01- ☑
  - major (greater than 2 cm) S37.02- ☑
  - minor (less than 2 cm) S37.01- ☑
- knee S80.0- ☑
- labium (majus) (minus) S30.23 ☑
- lacrimal apparatus, gland or sac S05.8X- ☑
- larynx S10.0 ☑
- leg (lower) S80.1- ☑
  - knee — see Contusion, knee
- lens — see Contusion, eyeball
- lip S00.531 ☑
- liver S36.112 ☑
- lower back S30.0 ☑
- lumbar region S30.0 ☑
- lung S27.329 ☑
  - bilateral S27.322 ☑
  - unilateral S27.321 ☑
- malar region S00.83 ☑
- mastoid region S00.83 ☑
- membrane, brain — see Injury, intracranial, diffuse
  - focal — see Injury, intracranial, focal
- mesentery S36.892 ☑
- mesosalpinx S37.892 ☑
- mouth S00.532 ☑
- muscle — see Contusion, by site
- nail
  - finger — see Contusion, finger, with damage to nail
  - toe — see Contusion, toe, with damage to nail
- nasal S00.33 ☑
- neck S10.93 ☑
  - specified site NEC S10.83 ☑
  - throat S10.0 ☑
- nerve — see Injury, nerve
- newborn P54.5
- nose S00.33 ☑
- occipital
  - lobe (brain) — see Injury, intracranial, diffuse
    - focal — see Injury, intracranial, focal
  - region (scalp) S00.03 ☑
- orbit (region) (tissues) S05.1- ☑
- ovary S37.429 ☑
  - bilateral S37.422 ☑
  - unilateral S37.421 ☑
- palate S00.532 ☑
- pancreas S36.229 ☑
  - body S36.221 ☑
  - head S36.220 ☑
  - tail S36.222 ☑
- parietal
  - lobe (brain) — see Injury, intracranial, diffuse
    - focal — see Injury, intracranial, focal
  - region (scalp) S00.03 ☑
- pelvic organ S37.92 ☑
  - adrenal gland S37.812 ☑
  - bladder S37.22 ☑
  - fallopian tube — see Contusion, fallopian tube
  - kidney — see Contusion, kidney
  - ovary — see Contusion, ovary
  - prostate S37.822 ☑
  - specified organ NEC S37.892 ☑
  - ureter S37.12 ☑
  - urethra S37.32 ☑
  - uterus S37.62 ☑
- pelvis S30.0 ☑
- penis S30.21 ☑
- perineum
  - female S30.23 ☑
  - male S30.0 ☑
- periocular area S00.1- ☑
- peritoneum S36.81 ☑
- periurethral tissue — see Contusion, urethra
- pharynx S10.0 ☑
- pinna — see Contusion, ear
- popliteal space — see Contusion, knee
- prepuce S30.21 ☑
- prostate S37.822 ☑
- pubic region S30.1 ☑
- pudendum
  - female S30.202 ☑
  - male S30.201 ☑
- quadriceps femoris — see Contusion, thigh
- rectum S36.62 ☑
- retroperitoneum S36.892 ☑
- round ligament S37.892 ☑

70

☑ Additional Character Required — Refer to the Tabular List for Character Selection ▽ Subterms under main terms may continue to next column or page

Corrosion

Index

Contusion — *continued*
- sacral region S30.0 ☑
- scalp S00.03 ☑
  - due to birth injury P12.3
- scapular region — *see* Contusion, shoulder
- sclera — *see* Contusion, eyeball
- scrotum S30.22 ☑
- seminal vesicle S37.892 ☑
- shoulder S40.01- ☑
- skin NEC T14.8
- small intestine — *see* Injury, intestine, small, contusion
- spermatic cord S30.22 ☑
- spinal cord — *see* Injury, spinal cord, by region
  - cauda equina S34.3 ☑
  - conus medullaris S34.139 ☑
- spleen S36.029 ☑
  - major S36.021 ☑
  - minor S36.020 ☑
- sternal region S20.219 ☑
- stomach S36.32 ☑
- subconjunctival S05.1- ☑
- subcutaneous NEC T14.8
- submaxillary region S00.83 ☑
- submental region S00.83 ☑
- subperiosteal NEC T14.8
- subungual
  - finger — *see* Contusion, finger, with damage to nail
  - toe — *see* Contusion, toe, with damage to nail
- supraclavicular fossa S10.83 ☑
- supraorbital S00.83 ☑
- suprarenal gland S37.812 ☑
- temple (region) S00.83 ☑
- temporal
  - lobe (brain) — *see* Injury, intracranial, diffuse
    - focal — *see* Injury, intracranial, focal
  - region S00.83 ☑
- testis S30.22 ☑
- thigh S70.1- ☑
- thorax (wall) S20.20 ☑
  - back S20.22- ☑
  - front S20.21- ☑
- throat S10.0 ☑
- thumb S60.01- ☑
  - with damage to nail S60.11- ☑
- toe(s) (lesser) S90.12- ☑
  - with damage to nail S90.22- ☑
  - great S90.11- ☑
    - with damage to nail S90.21- ☑
    - specified type NEC S90.221 ☑
- tongue S00.532 ☑
- trachea (cervical) S10.0 ☑
  - thoracic S27.52 ☑
- tunica vaginalis S30.22 ☑
- tympanum, tympanic membrane — *see* Contusion, ear
- ureter S37.12 ☑
- urethra S37.32 ☑
- urinary organ NEC S37.892 ☑
- uterus S37.62 ☑
- uvula S00.532 ☑
- vagina S30.23 ☑
- vas deferens S37.892 ☑
- vesical S37.22 ☑
- vocal cord(s) S10.0 ☑
- vulva S30.23 ☑
- wrist S60.21- ☑

Conus (congenital) (any type) Q14.8
- cornea — *see* Keratoconus
- medullaris syndrome G95.81

Conversion hysteria, neurosis or reaction F44.9
Converter, tuberculosis (test reaction) R76.11
Conviction (legal), **anxiety concerning** Z65.0
- with imprisonment Z65.1
Convulsions (idiopathic) (*see also* Seizure(s)) R56.9
- apoplectiform (cerebral ischemia) I67.82
- benign neonatal (familial) — *see* Epilepsy, generalized, idiopathic
- dissociative F44.5
- epileptic — *see* Epilepsy
- epileptiform, epileptoid — *see* Seizure, epileptiform
- ether (anesthetic) — *see* Table of Drugs and Chemicals, by drug
- febrile R56.00
  - with status epilepticus G40.901
  - complex R56.01

Convulsions — *continued*
- febrile — *continued*
  - complex — *continued*
    - with status epilepticus G40.901
  - simple R56.00
- hysterical F44.5
- infantile P90
  - epilepsy — *see* Epilepsy
- jacksonian — *see* Epilepsy, localization-related, symptomatic, with simple partial seizures
- myoclonic G25.3
- neonatal, benign (familial) — *see* Epilepsy, generalized, idiopathic
- newborn P90
- obstetrical (nephritic) (uremic) — *see* Eclampsia
- paretic A52.17
- post traumatic R56.1
- psychomotor — *see* Epilepsy, localization-related, symptomatic, with complex partial seizures
- recurrent R56.9
- reflex R25.8
- scarlatinal A38.8
- tetanus, tetanic — *see* Tetanus
- thymic E32.8

Convulsive (*see also* Convulsions)
Cooley's anemia D56.1
Coolie itch B76.9
Cooper's
- disease — *see* Mastopathy, cystic
- hernia — *see* Hernia, abdomen, specified site NEC
Copra itch B88.0
Coprophagy F50.8
Coprophobia F40.298
Coproporphyria, hereditary E80.29
Cor
- biloculare Q20.8
- bovis, bovinum — *see* Hypertrophy, cardiac
- pulmonale (chronic) I27.81
  - acute I26.09
- triatriatum, triatrium Q24.2
- triloculare Q20.8
  - biatrium Q20.4
  - biventriculare Q21.1
Corbus' disease (gangrenous balanitis) N48.1
Cord (*see also* condition)
- around neck (tightly) (with compression)
  - complicating delivery O69.1 ☑
- bladder G95.89
  - tabetic A52.19
Cordis ectopia Q24.8
Corditis (spermatic) N49.1
Corectopia Q13.2
Cori's disease (glycogen storage) E74.03
Corkhandler's disease or lung J67.3
Corkscrew esophagus K22.4
Corkworker's disease or lung J67.3
Corn (infected) L84
Cornea (*see also* condition)
- donor Z52.5
- plana Q13.4
Cornelia de Lange syndrome Q87.1
Cornu cutaneum L85.8
Cornual gestation or pregnancy O00.8
Coronary (artery) — *see* condition
Coronavirus, as cause of disease classified elsewhere B97.29
- SARS-associated B97.21
Corpora (*see also* condition)
- amylacea, prostate N42.89
- cavernosa — *see* condition
Corpulence — *see* Obesity
Corpus — *see* condition
Corrected transposition Q20.5
Corrosion (injury) (acid) (caustic) (chemical) (lime) (external) (internal) T30.4
- abdomen, abdominal (muscle) (wall) T21.42 ☑
  - first degree T21.52 ☑
  - second degree T21.62 ☑
  - third degree T21.72 ☑
- above elbow T22.439 ☑
  - first degree T22.539 ☑
  - left T22.432 ☑
    - first degree T22.532 ☑
    - second degree T22.632 ☑
    - third degree T22.732 ☑
  - right T22.431 ☑
    - first degree T22.531 ☑

Corrosion — *continued*
- above elbow — *continued*
  - right — *continued*
    - second degree T22.631 ☑
    - third degree T22.731 ☑
  - second degree T22.639 ☑
  - third degree T22.739 ☑
- alimentary tract NEC T28.7 ☑
- ankle T25.419 ☑
  - first degree T25.519 ☑
  - left T25.412 ☑
    - first degree T25.512 ☑
    - second degree T25.612 ☑
    - third degree T25.712 ☑
  - multiple with foot — *see* Corrosion, lower, limb, multiple, ankle and foot
  - right T25.411 ☑
    - first degree T25.511 ☑
    - second degree T25.611 ☑
    - third degree T25.711 ☑
  - second degree T25.619 ☑
  - third degree T25.719 ☑
- anus — *see* Corrosion, buttock
- arm(s) (meaning upper limb(s)) — *see* Corrosion, upper limb
- axilla T22.449 ☑
  - first degree T22.549 ☑
  - left T22.442 ☑
    - first degree T22.542 ☑
    - second degree T22.642 ☑
    - third degree T22.742 ☑
  - right T22.441 ☑
    - first degree T22.541 ☑
    - second degree T22.641 ☑
    - third degree T22.741 ☑
  - second degree T22.649 ☑
  - third degree T22.749 ☑
- back (lower) T21.44 ☑
  - first degree T21.54 ☑
  - second degree T21.64 ☑
  - third degree T21.74 ☑
  - upper T21.43 ☑
    - first degree T21.53 ☑
    - second degree T21.63 ☑
    - third degree T21.73 ☑
- blisters — *code as* Corrosion, second degree, by site
- breast(s) — *see* Corrosion, chest wall
- buttock(s) T21.45 ☑
  - first degree T21.55 ☑
  - second degree T21.65 ☑
  - third degree T21.75 ☑
- calf T24.439 ☑
  - first degree T24.539 ☑
  - left T24.432 ☑
    - first degree T24.532 ☑
    - second degree T24.632 ☑
    - third degree T24.732 ☑
  - right T24.431 ☑
    - first degree T24.531 ☑
    - second degree T24.631 ☑
    - third degree T24.731 ☑
  - second degree T24.639 ☑
  - third degree T24.739 ☑
- canthus (eye) — *see* Corrosion, eyelid
- cervix T28.8 ☑
- cheek T20.46 ☑
  - first degree T20.56 ☑
  - second degree T20.66 ☑
  - third degree T20.76 ☑
- chest wall T21.41 ☑
  - first degree T21.51 ☑
  - second degree T21.61 ☑
  - third degree T21.71 ☑
- chin T20.43 ☑
  - first degree T20.53 ☑
  - second degree T20.63 ☑
  - third degree T20.73 ☑
- colon T28.7 ☑
- conjunctiva (and cornea) — *see* Corrosion, cornea
- cornea (and conjunctiva) T26.6- ☑
- deep necrosis of underlying tissue — *code as* Corrosion, third degree, by site
- dorsum of hand T23.469 ☑
  - first degree T23.569 ☑
  - left T23.462 ☑

Contusion — Corrosion

Corrosion — *continued*
  dorsum of hand — *continued*
    left — *continued*
      first degree T23.562 ☑
      second degree T23.662 ☑
      third degree T23.762 ☑
    right T23.461 ☑
      first degree T23.561 ☑
      second degree T23.661 ☑
      third degree T23.761 ☑
    second degree T23.669 ☑
    third degree T23.769 ☑
  ear (auricle) (external) (canal) T20.41 ☑
    drum T28.91
    first degree T20.51 ☑
    second degree T20.61 ☑
    third degree T20.71 ☑
  elbow T22.429 ☑
    first degree T22.529 ☑
    left T22.422 ☑
      first degree T22.522 ☑
      second degree T22.622 ☑
      third degree T22.722 ☑
    right T22.421 ☑
      first degree T22.521 ☑
      second degree T22.621 ☑
      third degree T22.721 ☑
    second degree T22.629 ☑
    third degree T22.729 ☑
  entire body — *see* Corrosion, multiple body regions
  epidermal loss — *code as* Corrosion, second degree, by site
  epiglottis T27.4 ☑
  erythema, erythematous — *code as* Corrosion, first degree, by site
  esophagus T28.6 ☑
  extent (percentage of body surface)
    less than 10 percent T32.0
    10-19 percent (0-9 percent third degree) T32.10
      with 10-19 percent third degree T32.11
    20-29 percent (0-9 percent third degree) T32.20
      with
        10-19 percent third degree T32.21
        20-29 percent third degree T32.22
    30-39 percent (0-9 percent third degree) T32.30
      with
        10-19 percent third degree T32.31
        20-29 percent third degree T32.32
        30-39 percent third degree T32.33
    40-49 percent (0-9 percent third degree) T32.40
      with
        10-19 percent third degree T32.41
        20-29 percent third degree T32.42
        30-39 percent third degree T32.43
        40-49 percent third degree T32.44
    50-59 percent (0-9 percent third degree) T32.50
      with
        10-19 percent third degree T32.51
        20-29 percent third degree T32.52
        30-39 percent third degree T32.53
        40-49 percent third degree T32.54
        50-59 percent third degree T32.55
    60-69 percent (0-9 percent third degree) T32.60
      with
        10-19 percent third degree T32.61
        20-29 percent third degree T32.62
        30-39 percent third degree T32.63
        40-49 percent third degree T32.64
        50-59 percent third degree T32.65
        60-69 percent third degree T32.66
    70-79 percent (0-9 percent third degree) T32.70
      with
        10-19 percent third degree T32.71
        20-29 percent third degree T32.72
        30-39 percent third degree T32.73
        40-49 percent third degree T32.74
        50-59 percent third degree T32.75
        60-69 percent third degree T32.76
        70-79 percent third degree T32.77
    80-89 percent (0-9 percent third degree) T32.80
      with
        10-19 percent third degree T32.81
        20-29 percent third degree T32.82
        30-39 percent third degree T32.83
        40-49 percent third degree T32.84
        50-59 percent third degree T32.85
        60-69 percent third degree T32.86

Corrosion — *continued*
  extent — *continued*
    80-89 percent — *continued*
      with — *continued*
        70-79 percent third degree T32.87
        80-89 percent third degree T32.88
    90 percent or more (0-9 percent third degree) T32.90
      with
        10-19 percent third degree T32.91
        20-29 percent third degree T32.92
        30-39 percent third degree T32.93
        40-49 percent third degree T32.94
        50-59 percent third degree T32.95
        60-69 percent third degree T32.96
        70-79 percent third degree T32.97
        80-89 percent third degree T32.98
        90-99 percent third degree T32.99
  extremity — *see* Corrosion, limb
  eye(s) and adnexa T26.9- ☑
    with resulting rupture and destruction of eyeball T26.7-
    conjunctival sac — *see* Corrosion, cornea
    cornea — *see* Corrosion, cornea
    lid — *see* Corrosion, eyelid
    periocular area — *see* Corrosion eyelid
    specified site NEC T26.8- ☑
  eyeball — *see* Corrosion, eye
  eyelid(s) T26.5- ☑
  face — *see* Corrosion, head
  finger T23.429 ☑
    first degree T23.529 ☑
    left T23.422 ☑
      first degree T23.522 ☑
      second degree T23.622 ☑
      third degree T23.722 ☑
    multiple sites (without thumb) T23.439 ☑
      with thumb T23.449 ☑
        first degree T23.549 ☑
        left T23.442 ☑
          first degree T23.542 ☑
          second degree T23.642 ☑
          third degree T23.742 ☑
        right T23.441 ☑
          first degree T23.541 ☑
          second degree T23.641 ☑
          third degree T23.741 ☑
      second degree T23.649 ☑
      third degree T23.749 ☑
    first degree T23.539 ☑
    left T23.432 ☑
      first degree T23.532 ☑
      second degree T23.632 ☑
      third degree T23.732 ☑
    right T23.431 ☑
      first degree T23.531 ☑
      second degree T23.631 ☑
      third degree T23.731 ☑
    second degree T23.639 ☑
    third degree T23.739 ☑
    right T23.421 ☑
      first degree T23.521 ☑
      second degree T23.621 ☑
      third degree T23.721 ☑
    second degree T23.629 ☑
    third degree T23.729 ☑
  flank — *see* Corrosion, abdomen
  foot T25.429 ☑
    first degree T25.529 ☑
    left T25.422 ☑
      first degree T25.522 ☑
      second degree T25.622 ☑
      third degree T25.722 ☑
    multiple with ankle — *see* Corrosion, lower, limb, multiple, ankle and foot
    right T25.421 ☑
      first degree T25.521 ☑
      second degree T25.621 ☑
      third degree T25.721 ☑
    second degree T25.629 ☑
    third degree T25.729 ☑
  forearm T22.419 ☑
    first degree T22.519 ☑
    left T22.412 ☑
      first degree T22.512 ☑
      second degree T22.612 ☑

Corrosion — *continued*
  forearm — *continued*
    left — *continued*
      third degree T22.712 ☑
    right T22.411 ☑
      first degree T22.511 ☑
      second degree T22.611 ☑
      third degree T22.711 ☑
    second degree T22.619 ☑
    third degree T22.719 ☑
  forehead T20.46 ☑
    first degree T20.56 ☑
    second degree T20.66 ☑
    third degree T20.76 ☑
  fourth degree — *code as* Corrosion, third degree, by site
  full thickness skin loss — *code as* Corrosion, third degree, by site
  gastrointestinal tract NEC T28.7 ☑
  genital organs
    external
      female T21.47 ☑
        first degree T21.57 ☑
        second degree T21.67 ☑
        third degree T21.77 ☑
      male T21.46 ☑
        first degree T21.56 ☑
        second degree T21.66 ☑
        third degree T21.76 ☑
    internal T28.8 ☑
  groin — *see* Corrosion, abdominal wall
  hand(s) T23.409 ☑
    back — *see* Corrosion, dorsum of hand
    finger — *see* Corrosion, finger
    first degree T23.509 ☑
    left T23.402 ☑
      first degree T23.502 ☑
      second degree T23.602 ☑
      third degree T23.702 ☑
    multiple sites with wrist T23.499 ☑
      first degree T23.599 ☑
      left T23.492 ☑
        first degree T23.592 ☑
        second degree T23.692 ☑
        third degree T23.792 ☑
      right T23.491 ☑
        first degree T23.591 ☑
        second degree T23.691 ☑
        third degree T23.791 ☑
      second degree T23.699 ☑
      third degree T23.799 ☑
    palm — *see* Corrosion, palm
    right T23.401 ☑
      first degree T23.501 ☑
      second degree T23.601 ☑
      third degree T23.701 ☑
    second degree T23.609 ☑
    third degree T23.709 ☑
    thumb — *see* Corrosion, thumb
  head (and face) (and neck) T20.40 ☑
    cheek — *see* Corrosion, cheek
    chin — *see* Corrosion, chin
    ear — *see* Corrosion, ear
    eye(s) only — *see* Corrosion, eye
    first degree T20.50 ☑
    forehead — *see* Corrosion, forehead
    lip — *see* Corrosion, lip
    multiple sites T20.49 ☑
      first degree T20.59 ☑
      second degree T20.69 ☑
      third degree T20.79 ☑
    neck — *see* Corrosion, neck
    nose — *see* Corrosion, nose
    scalp — *see* Corrosion, scalp
    second degree T20.60 ☑
    third degree T20.70 ☑
  hip(s) — *see* Corrosion, lower, limb
  inhalation — *see* Corrosion, respiratory tract
  internal organ(s) (*see also* Corrosion, by site) T28.90 ☑
    alimentary tract T28.7 ☑
      esophagus T28.6 ☑
    esophagus T28.6 ☑
    genitourinary T28.8 ☑
    mouth T28.5 ☑
    pharynx T28.5 ☑
    specified organ NEC T28.99 ☑

☑ **Additional Character Required** — Refer to the Tabular List for Character Selection   ▽ **Subterms under main terms may continue to next column or page**

Corrosion — *continued*
- interscapular region — *see* Corrosion, back, upper
- intestine (large) (small) T28.7 ☑
- knee T24.429 ☑
  - first degree T24.529 ☑
  - left T24.422 ☑
    - first degree T24.522 ☑
    - second degree T24.622 ☑
    - third degree T24.722 ☑
  - right T24.421 ☑
    - first degree T24.521 ☑
    - second degree T24.621 ☑
    - third degree T24.721 ☑
  - second degree T24.629 ☑
  - third degree T24.729 ☑
- labium (majus) (minus) — *see* Corrosion, genital organs, external, female
- lacrimal apparatus, duct, gland or sac — *see* Corrosion, eye, specified site NEC
- larynx T27.4 ☑
  - with lung T27.5 ☑
- leg(s) (meaning lower limb(s)) — *see* Corrosion, lower limb
- limb(s)
  - lower — *see* Corrosion, lower, limb
  - upper — *see* Corrosion, upper limb
- lip(s) T20.42 ☑
  - first degree T20.52 ☑
  - second degree T20.62 ☑
  - third degree T20.72 ☑
- lower
  - back — *see* Corrosion, back
  - limb T24.409 ☑
    - ankle — *see* Corrosion, ankle
    - calf — *see* Corrosion, calf
    - first degree T24.509 ☑
    - foot — *see* Corrosion, foot
    - knee — *see* Corrosion, knee
    - left T24.402 ☑
      - first degree T24.502 ☑
      - second degree T24.602 ☑
      - third degree T24.702 ☑
    - multiple sites, except ankle and foot T24.499 ☑
      - ankle and foot T25.499 ☑
        - first degree T25.599 ☑
        - left T25.492 ☑
          - first degree T25.592 ☑
          - second degree T25.692 ☑
          - third degree T25.792 ☑
        - right T25.491 ☑
          - first degree T25.591 ☑
          - second degree T25.691 ☑
          - third degree T25.791 ☑
        - second degree T25.699 ☑
        - third degree T25.799 ☑
      - first degree T24.599 ☑
      - left T24.492 ☑
        - first degree T24.592 ☑
        - second degree T24.692 ☑
        - third degree T24.792 ☑
      - right T24.491 ☑
        - first degree T24.591 ☑
        - second degree T24.691 ☑
        - third degree T24.791 ☑
      - second degree T24.699 ☑
      - third degree T24.799 ☑
    - right T24.401 ☑
      - first degree T24.501 ☑
      - second degree T24.601 ☑
      - third degree T24.701 ☑
    - second degree T24.609 ☑
    - thigh — *see* Corrosion, thigh
    - third degree T24.709 ☑
- lung (with larynx and trachea) T27.5 ☑
- mouth T28.5 ☑
- neck T20.47 ☑
  - first degree T20.57 ☑
  - second degree T20.67 ☑
  - third degree T20.77 ☑
- nose (septum) T20.44 ☑
  - first degree T20.54 ☑
  - second degree T20.64 ☑
  - third degree T20.74 ☑
- ocular adnexa — *see* Corrosion, eye
- orbit region — *see* Corrosion, eyelid

Corrosion — *continued*
- palm T23.459 ☑
  - first degree T23.559 ☑
  - left T23.452 ☑
    - first degree T23.552 ☑
    - second degree T23.652 ☑
    - third degree T23.752 ☑
  - right T23.451 ☑
    - first degree T23.551 ☑
    - second degree T23.651 ☑
    - third degree T23.751 ☑
  - second degree T23.659 ☑
  - third degree T23.759 ☑
- partial thickness — *code as* Corrosion, unspecified degree, by site
- pelvis — *see* Corrosion, trunk
- penis — *see* Corrosion, genital organs, external, male
- perineum
  - female — *see* Corrosion, genital organs, external, female
  - male — *see* Corrosion, genital organs, external, male
- periocular area — *see* Corrosion, eyelid
- pharynx T28.5 ☑
- rectum T28.7 ☑
- respiratory tract T27.7 ☑
  - larynx — *see* Corrosion, larynx
  - specified part NEC T27.6 ☑
  - trachea — *see* Corrosion, larynx
- sac, lacrimal — *see* Corrosion, eye, specified site NEC
- scalp T20.45 ☑
  - first degree T20.55 ☑
  - second degree T20.65 ☑
  - third degree T20.75 ☑
- scapular region T22.469 ☑
  - first degree T22.569 ☑
  - left T22.462 ☑
    - first degree T22.562 ☑
    - second degree T22.662 ☑
    - third degree T22.762 ☑
  - right T22.461 ☑
    - first degree T22.561 ☑
    - second degree T22.661 ☑
    - third degree T22.761 ☑
  - second degree T22.669 ☑
  - third degree T22.769 ☑
- sclera — *see* Corrosion, eye, specified site NEC
- scrotum — *see* Corrosion, genital organs, external, male
- shoulder T22.459 ☑
  - first degree T22.559 ☑
  - left T22.452 ☑
    - first degree T22.552 ☑
    - second degree T22.652 ☑
    - third degree T22.752 ☑
  - right T22.451 ☑
    - first degree T22.551 ☑
    - second degree T22.651 ☑
    - third degree T22.751 ☑
  - second degree T22.659 ☑
  - third degree T22.759 ☑
- stomach T28.7 ☑
- temple — *see* Corrosion, head
- testis — *see* Corrosion, genital organs, external, male
- thigh T24.419 ☑
  - first degree T24.519 ☑
  - left T24.412 ☑
    - first degree T24.512 ☑
    - second degree T24.612 ☑
    - third degree T24.712 ☑
  - right T24.411 ☑
    - first degree T24.511 ☑
    - second degree T24.611 ☑
    - third degree T24.711 ☑
  - second degree T24.619 ☑
  - third degree T24.719 ☑
- thorax (external) — *see* Corrosion, trunk
- throat (meaning pharynx) T28.5 ☑
- thumb(s) T23.419 ☑
  - first degree T23.519 ☑
  - left T23.412 ☑
    - first degree T23.512 ☑
    - second degree T23.612 ☑
    - third degree T23.712 ☑
  - multiple sites with fingers T23.449 ☑

Corrosion — *continued*
- thumb(s) — *continued*
  - multiple sites with fingers — *continued*
    - first degree T23.549 ☑
    - left T23.442 ☑
      - first degree T23.542 ☑
      - second degree T23.642 ☑
      - third degree T23.742 ☑
    - right T23.441 ☑
      - first degree T23.541 ☑
      - second degree T23.641 ☑
      - third degree T23.741 ☑
    - second degree T23.649 ☑
    - third degree T23.749 ☑
  - right T23.411 ☑
    - first degree T23.511 ☑
    - second degree T23.611 ☑
    - third degree T23.711 ☑
  - second degree T23.619 ☑
  - third degree T23.719 ☑
- toe T25.439 ☑
  - first degree T25.539 ☑
  - left T25.432 ☑
    - first degree T25.532 ☑
    - second degree T25.632 ☑
    - third degree T25.732 ☑
  - right T25.431 ☑
    - first degree T25.531 ☑
    - second degree T25.631 ☑
    - third degree T25.731 ☑
  - second degree T25.639 ☑
  - third degree T25.739 ☑
- tongue T28.5 ☑
- tonsil(s) T28.5 ☑
- total body — *see* Corrosion, multiple body regions
- trachea T27.4 ☑
  - with lung T27.5 ☑
- trunk T21.40 ☑
  - abdominal wall — *see* Corrosion, abdominal wall
  - anus — *see* Corrosion, buttock
  - axilla — *see* Corrosion, upper limb
  - back — *see* Corrosion, back
  - breast — *see* Corrosion, chest wall
  - buttock — *see* Corrosion, buttock
  - chest wall — *see* Corrosion, chest wall
  - first degree T21.50 ☑
  - flank — *see* Corrosion, abdominal wall
  - genital
    - female — *see* Corrosion, genital organs, external, female
    - male — *see* Corrosion, genital organs, external, male
  - groin — *see* Corrosion, abdominal wall
  - interscapular region — *see* Corrosion, back, upper
  - labia — *see* Corrosion, genital organs, external, female
  - lower back — *see* Corrosion, back
  - penis — *see* Corrosion, genital organs, external, male
  - perineum
    - female — *see* Corrosion, genital organs, external, female
    - male — *see* Corrosion, genital organs, external, male
  - scapular region — *see* Corrosion, upper limb
  - scrotum — *see* Corrosion, genital organs, external, male
  - second degree T21.60 ☑
  - shoulder — *see* Corrosion, upper limb
  - specified site NEC T21.49 ☑
    - first degree T21.59 ☑
    - second degree T21.69 ☑
    - third degree T21.79 ☑
  - testes — *see* Corrosion, genital organs, external, male
  - third degree T21.70 ☑
  - upper back — *see* Corrosion, back, upper
  - vagina T28.8 ☑
  - vulva — *see* Corrosion, genital organs, external, female
- unspecified site with extent of body surface involved specified
  - less than 10 percent T32.0
  - 10-19 percent (0-9 percent third degree) T32.10
    - with 10-19 percent third degree T32.11
  - 20-29 percent (0-9 percent third degree) T32.20

Corrosion — *continued*
  unspecified site with extent of body surface involved
    specified — *continued*
      20-29 percent — *continued*
        with
          10-19 percent third degree T32.21
          20-29 percent third degree T32.22
      30-39 percent (0-9 percent third degree) T32.30
        with
          10-19 percent third degree T32.31
          20-29 percent third degree T32.32
          30-39 percent third degree T32.33
      40-49 percent (0-9 percent third degree) T32.40
        with
          10-19 percent third degree T32.41
          20-29 percent third degree T32.42
          30-39 percent third degree T32.43
          40-49 percent third degree T32.44
      50-59 percent (0-9 percent third degree) T32.50
        with
          10-19 percent third degree T32.51
          20-29 percent third degree T32.52
          30-39 percent third degree T32.53
          40-49 percent third degree T32.54
          50-59 percent third degree T32.55
      60-69 percent (0-9 percent third degree) T32.60
        with
          10-19 percent third degree T32.61
          20-29 percent third degree T32.62
          30-39 percent third degree T32.63
          40-49 percent third degree T32.64
          50-59 percent third degree T32.65
          60-69 percent third degree T32.66
      70-79 percent (0-9 percent third degree) T32.70
        with
          10-19 percent third degree T32.71
          20-29 percent third degree T32.72
          30-39 percent third degree T32.73
          40-49 percent third degree T32.74
          50-59 percent third degree T32.75
          60-69 percent third degree T32.76
          70-79 percent third degree T32.77
      80-89 percent (0-9 percent third degree) T32.80
        with
          10-19 percent third degree T32.81
          20-29 percent third degree T32.82
          30-39 percent third degree T32.83
          40-49 percent third degree T32.84
          50-59 percent third degree T32.85
          60-69 percent third degree T32.86
          70-79 percent third degree T32.87
          80-89 percent third degree T32.88
      90 percent or more (0-9 percent third degree)
        T32.90
        with
          10-19 percent third degree T32.91
          20-29 percent third degree T32.92
          30-39 percent third degree T32.93
          40-49 percent third degree T32.94
          50-59 percent third degree T32.95
          60-69 percent third degree T32.96
          70-79 percent third degree T32.97
          80-89 percent third degree T32.98
          90-99 percent third degree T32.99
  upper limb (axilla) (scapular region) T22.40- ☑
    above elbow — *see* Corrosion, above elbow
    axilla — *see* Corrosion, axilla
    elbow — *see* Corrosion, elbow
    first degree T22.50- ☑
    forearm — *see* Corrosion, forearm
    hand — *see* Corrosion, hand
    interscapular region — *see* Corrosion, back, upper
    multiple sites T22.499 ☑
      first degree T22.599 ☑
      left T22.492 ☑
        first degree T22.592 ☑
        second degree T22.692 ☑
        third degree T22.792 ☑
      right T22.491 ☑
        first degree T22.591 ☑
        second degree T22.691 ☑
        third degree T22.791 ☑
      second degree T22.699 ☑
      third degree T22.799 ☑
    scapular region — *see* Corrosion, scapular region
    second degree T22.60- ☑
    shoulder — *see* Corrosion, shoulder
    third degree T22.70- ☑

Corrosion — *continued*
  upper limb — *continued*
    wrist –- *see* Corrosion, hand
  uterus T28.8 ☑
  vagina T28.8 ☑
  vulva — *see* Corrosion, genital organs, external, female
  wrist T23.479 ☑
    first degree T23.579 ☑
    left T23.472 ☑
      first degree T23.572 ☑
      second degree T23.672 ☑
      third degree T23.772 ☑
    multiple sites with hand T23.499 ☑
      first degree T23.599 ☑
      left T23.492 ☑
        first degree T23.592 ☑
        second degree T23.692 ☑
        third degree T23.792 ☑
      right T23.491 ☑
        first degree T23.591 ☑
        second degree T23.691 ☑
        third degree T23.791 ☑
      second degree T23.699 ☑
      third degree T23.799 ☑
    right T23.471 ☑
      first degree T23.571 ☑
      second degree T23.671 ☑
      third degree T23.771 ☑
    second degree T23.679 ☑
    third degree T23.779 ☑
Corrosive burn — *see* Corrosion
Corsican fever — *see* Malaria
Cortical — *see* condition
Cortico-adrenal — *see* condition
Coryza (acute) J00
  with grippe or influenza — *see* Influenza, with, respiratory manifestations NEC
  syphilitic
    congenital (chronic) A50.05
Costen's syndrome or complex M26.69
Costiveness — *see* Constipation
Costochondritis M94.0
Cot death R99
Cotard's syndrome F22
Cotia virus B08.8
Cotton wool spots (retinal) H35.81
Cotungo's disease — *see* Sciatica
Cough (affected) (chronic) (epidemic) (nervous) R05
  with hemorrhage — *see* Hemoptysis
  bronchial R05
    with grippe or influenza — *see* Influenza, with, respiratory manifestations NEC
  functional F45.8
  hysterical F45.8
  laryngeal, spasmodic R05
  psychogenic F45.8
  smokers' J41.0
  tea taster's B49
Counseling (for) Z71.9
  abuse NEC
    perpetrator Z69.82
    victim Z69.81
  alcohol abuser Z71.41
    family Z71.42
  child abuse
    nonparental
      perpetrator Z69.021
      victim Z69.020
    parental
      perpetrator Z69.011
      victim Z69.010
  consanguinity Z71.89
  contraceptive Z30.09
  dietary Z71.3
  drug abuser Z71.51
    family member Z71.52
  family Z71.89
  fertility preservation (prior to cancer therapy) (prior to removal of gonads) Z31.62
  for non-attending third party Z71.0
    related to sexual behavior or orientation Z70.2
  genetic NEC Z31.5
  health (advice) (education) (instruction) — *see* Counseling, medical
  human immunodeficiency virus (HIV) Z71.7
  impotence Z70.1
  insulin pump use Z46.81

Counseling — *continued*
  medical (for) Z71.9
    boarding school resident Z59.3
    consanguinity Z71.89
    feared complaint and no disease found Z71.1
    human immunodeficiency virus (HIV) Z71.7
    institutional resident Z59.3
    on behalf of another Z71.0
      related to sexual behavior or orientation Z70.2
    person living alone Z60.2
    specified reason NEC Z71.89
  natural family planning
    procreative Z31.61
    to avoid pregnancy Z30.02
  perpetrator (of)
    abuse NEC Z69.82
    child abuse
      non-parental Z69.021
      parental Z69.011
    rape NEC Z69.82
    spousal abuse Z69.12
  procreative NEC Z31.69
    fertility preservation (prior to cancer therapy) (prior to removal of gonads) Z31.62
    using natural family planning Z31.61
  promiscuity Z70.1
  rape victim Z69.81
  religious Z71.81
  sex, sexual (related to) Z70.9
    attitude(s) Z70.0
    behavior or orientation Z70.1
    combined concerns Z70.3
    non-responsiveness Z70.1
    on behalf of third party Z70.2
    specified reason NEC Z70.8
  specified reason NEC Z71.89
  spiritual Z71.81
  spousal abuse (perpetrator) Z69.12
    victim Z69.11
  substance abuse Z71.89
    alcohol Z71.41
    drug Z71.51
    tobacco Z71.6
  tobacco use Z71.6
  use (of)
    insulin pump Z46.81
  victim (of)
    abuse Z69.81
    child abuse
      by parent Z69.010
      non-parental Z69.020
    rape NEC Z69.81
Coupled rhythm R00.8
Couvelaire syndrome or uterus (complicating delivery) O45.8X- ☑
Cowperitis — *see* Urethritis
Cowper's gland — *see* condition
Cowpox B08.010
  due to vaccination T88.1 ☑
Coxa
  magna M91.4- ☑
  plana M91.2- ☑
  valga (acquired) (*see also* Deformity, limb, specified type NEC, thigh)
    congenital Q65.81
    sequelae (late effect) of rickets E64.3
  vara (acquired) (*see also* Deformity, limb, specified type NEC, thigh)
    congenital Q65.82
    sequelae (late effect) of rickets E64.3
Coxalgia, coxalgic (nontuberculous) (*see also* Pain, joint, hip)
  tuberculous A18.02
Coxitis — *see* Monoarthritis, hip
Coxsackie (virus) (infection) B34.1
  as cause of disease classified elsewhere B97.11
  carditis B33.20
  central nervous system NEC A88.8
  endocarditis B33.21
  enteritis A08.39
  meningitis (aseptic) A87.0
  myocarditis B33.22
  pericarditis B33.23
  pharyngitis B08.5
  pleurodynia B33.0
  specific disease NEC B33.8
Crabs, meaning pubic lice B85.3
Crack baby P04.41

Cracked nipple N64.0
  associated with
    lactation O92.13
      pregnancy O92.11- ☑
      puerperium O92.12
Cracked tooth K03.81
Cradle cap L21.0
Craft neurosis F48.8
Cramp(s) R25.2
  abdominal — *see* Pain, abdominal
  bathing T75.1 ☑
  colic R10.83
    psychogenic F45.8
  due to immersion T75.1 ☑
  fireman T67.2 ☑
  heat T67.2 ☑
  immersion T75.1 ☑
  intestinal — *see* Pain, abdominal
    psychogenic F45.8
  leg, sleep related G47.62
  limb (lower) (upper) NEC R25.2
    sleep related G47.62
  linotypist's F48.8
    organic G25.89
  muscle (limb) (general) R25.2
    due to immersion T75.1 ☑
    psychogenic F45.8
  occupational (hand) F48.8
    organic G25.89
  salt-depletion E87.1
  sleep related, leg G47.62
  stoker's T67.2 ☑
  swimmer's T75.1 ☑
  telegrapher's F48.8
    organic G25.89
  typist's F48.8
    organic G25.89
  uterus N94.89
    menstrual — *see* Dysmenorrhea
  writer's F48.8
    organic G25.89
Cranial — *see* condition
Craniocleidodysostosis Q74.0
Craniofenestria (skull) Q75.8
Craniolacunia (skull) Q75.8
Craniopagus Q89.4
Craniopathy, metabolic M85.2
Craniopharyngeal — *see* condition
Craniopharyngioma D44.4
Craniorachischisis (totalis) Q00.1
Cranioschisis Q75.8
Craniostenosis Q75.0
Craniosynostosis Q75.0
Craniotabes (cause unknown) M83.8
  neonatal P96.3
  rachitic E64.3
  syphilitic A50.56
Cranium — *see* condition
Craw-craw — *see* Onchocerciasis
Creaking joint — *see* Derangement, joint, specified type NEC
Creeping
  eruption B76.9
  palsy or paralysis G12.22
Crenated tongue K14.8
Creotoxism A05.9
Crepitus
  caput Q75.8
  joint — *see* Derangement, joint, specified type NEC
Crescent or conus choroid, congenital Q14.3
CREST syndrome M34.1
Cretin, cretinism (congenital) (endemic) (nongoitrous) (sporadic) E00.9
  pelvis
    with disproportion (fetopelvic) O33.0
      causing obstructed labor O65.0
  type
    hypothyroid E00.1
    mixed E00.2
    myxedematous E00.1
    neurological E00.0
Creutzfeldt-Jakob disease or syndrome (with dementia) A81.00
  familial A81.09
  iatrogenic A81.09
  specified NEC A81.09
  sporadic A81.09

Creutzfeldt-Jakob disease or syndrome — *continued*
  variant (vCJD) A81.01
Crib death R99
Cribriform hymen Q52.3
Cri-du-chat syndrome Q93.4
Crigler-Najjar disease or syndrome E80.5
Crime, victim of Z65.4
Crimean hemorrhagic fever A98.0
Criminalism F60.2
Crisis
  abdomen R10.0
  acute reaction F43.0
  addisonian E27.2
  adrenal (cortical) E27.2
  celiac K90.0
  Dietl's N13.8
  emotional (*see also* Disorder, adjustment)
    acute reaction to stress F43.0
    specific to childhood and adolescence F93.8
  glaucomatocyclitic — *see* Glaucoma, secondary, inflammation
  heart — *see* Failure, heart
  nitritoid I95.2
    correct substance properly administered — *see* Table of Drugs and Chemicals, by drug, adverse effect
    overdose or wrong substance given or taken — *see* Table of Drugs and Chemicals, by drug, poisoning
  oculogyric H51.8
    psychogenic F45.8
  Pel's (tabetic) A52.11
  psychosexual identity F64.2
  renal N28.0
  sickle-cell D57.00
    with
      acute chest syndrome D57.01
      splenic sequestration D57.02
  state (acute reaction) F43.0
  tabetic A52.11
  thyroid — *see* Thyrotoxicosis with thyroid storm
  thyrotoxic — *see* Thyrotoxicosis with thyroid storm
Crocq's disease (acrocyanosis) I73.89
Crohn's disease — *see* Enteritis, regional
Crooked septum, nasal J34.2
Cross syndrome E70.328
Crossbite (anterior) (posterior) M26.24
Cross-eye — *see* Strabismus, convergent concomitant
Croup, croupous (catarrhal) (infectious) (inflammatory) (nondiphtheritic) J05.0
  bronchial J20.9
  diphtheritic A36.2
  false J38.5
  spasmodic J38.5
    diphtheritic A36.2
  stridulous J38.5
    diphtheritic A36.2
Crouzon's disease Q75.1
Crowding, tooth, teeth, fully erupted M26.31
CRST syndrome M34.1
Cruchet's disease A85.8
Cruelty in children (*see also* Disorder, conduct)
Crural ulcer — *see* Ulcer, lower limb
Crush, crushed, crushing T14.8
  abdomen S38.1 ☑
  ankle S97.0- ☑
  arm (upper) (and shoulder) S47.- ☑
  axilla — *see* Crush, arm
  back, lower S38.1 ☑
  buttock S38.1 ☑
  cheek S07.0 ☑
  chest S28.0 ☑
  cranium S07.1 ☑
  ear S07.0 ☑
  elbow S57.0- ☑
  extremity
    lower
      ankle — *see* Crush, ankle
      below knee — *see* Crush, leg
      foot — *see* Crush, foot
      hip — *see* Crush, hip
      knee — *see* Crush, knee
      thigh — *see* Crush, thigh
      toe — *see* Crush, toe
    upper
      below elbow S67.9- ☑

Crush, crushed, crushing — *continued*
  extremity — *continued*
    upper — *continued*
      elbow — *see* Crush, elbow
      finger — *see* Crush, finger
      forearm — *see* Crush, forearm
      hand — *see* Crush, hand
      thumb — *see* Crush, thumb
      upper arm — *see* Crush, arm
      wrist — *see* Crush, wrist
  face S07.0 ☑
  finger(s) S67.1- ☑
    with hand (and wrist) — *see* Crush, hand, specified site NEC
    index S67.19- ☑
    little S67.19- ☑
    middle S67.19- ☑
    ring S67.19- ☑
    thumb — *see* Crush, thumb
  foot S97.8- ☑
    toe — *see* Crush, toe
  forearm S57.8- ☑
  genitalia, external
    female S38.002 ☑
      vagina S38.03 ☑
      vulva S38.03 ☑
    male S38.001 ☑
      penis S38.01 ☑
      scrotum S38.02 ☑
      testis S38.02 ☑
  hand (except fingers alone) S67.2- ☑
    with wrist S67.4- ☑
  head S07.9 ☑
    specified NEC S07.8 ☑
  heel — *see* Crush, foot
  hip S77.0- ☑
    with thigh S77.2- ☑
  internal organ (abdomen, chest, or pelvis) NEC T14.8
  knee S87.0- ☑
  labium (majus) (minus) S38.03 ☑
  larynx S17.0 ☑
  leg (lower) S87.8- ☑
    knee — *see* Crush, knee
  lip S07.0 ☑
  lower
    back S38.1 ☑
    leg — *see* Crush, leg
  neck S17.9 ☑
  nerve — *see* Injury, nerve
  nose S07.0 ☑
  pelvis S38.1 ☑
  penis S38.01 ☑
  scalp S07.8 ☑
  scapular region — *see* Crush, arm
  scrotum S38.02 ☑
  severe, unspecified site T14.8
  shoulder (and upper arm) — *see* Crush, arm
  skull S07.1 ☑
  syndrome (complication of trauma) T79.5 ☑
  testis S38.02 ☑
  thigh S77.1- ☑
    with hip S77.2- ☑
  throat S17.8 ☑
  thumb S67.0- ☑
    with hand (and wrist) — *see* Crush, hand, specified site NEC
  toe(s) S97.10- ☑
    great S97.11- ☑
    lesser S97.12- ☑
  trachea S17.0 ☑
  vagina S38.03 ☑
  vulva S38.03 ☑
  wrist S67.3- ☑
    with hand S67.4- ☑
Crusta lactea L21.0
Crusts R23.4
Crutch paralysis — *see* Injury, brachial plexus
Cruveilhier-Baumgarten cirrhosis, disease or syndrome K74.69
Cruveilhier's atrophy or disease G12.8
Crying (constant) (continuous) (excessive)
  child, adolescent, or adult R45.83
  infant (baby) (newborn) R68.11
Cryofibrinogenemia D89.2
Cryoglobulinemia (essential) (idiopathic) (mixed) (primary) (purpura) (secondary) (vasculitis) D89.1

Cryoglobulinemia — *continued*
  with lung involvement D89.1 [J99]
Cryptitis (anal) (rectal) K62.89
Cryptococcosis, cryptococcus (infection) (neoformans)
    B45.9
  bone B45.3
  cerebral B45.1
  cutaneous B45.2
  disseminated B45.7
  generalized B45.7
  meningitis B45.1
  meningocerebralis B45.1
  osseous B45.3
  pulmonary B45.0
  skin B45.2
  specified NEC B45.8
Cryptopapillitis (anus) K62.89
Cryptophthalmos Q11.2
  syndrome Q87.0
Cryptorchid, cryptorchism, cryptorchidism Q53.9
  bilateral Q53.20
    abdominal Q53.21
    perineal Q53.22
  unilateral Q53.10
    abdominal Q53.11
    perineal Q53.12
Cryptosporidiosis A07.2
  hepatobiliary B88.8
  respiratory B88.8
Cryptostromosis J67.6
Crystalluria R82.99
Cubitus
  congenital Q68.8
  valgus (acquired) M21.0- ☑
    congenital Q68.8
    sequelae (late effect) of rickets E64.3
  varus (acquired) M21.1- ☑
    congenital Q68.8
    sequelae (late effect) of rickets E64.3
Cultural deprivation or shock Z60.3
Curling esophagus K22.4
Curling's ulcer — *see* Ulcer, peptic, acute
Curschmann (-Batten) (-Steinert) **disease or syndrome**
    G71.11
Curse, Ondine's — *see* Apnea, sleep
Curvature
  organ or site, congenital NEC — *see* Distortion
  penis (lateral) Q55.61
  Pott's (spinal) A18.01
  radius, idiopathic, progressive (congenital) Q74.0
  spine (acquired) (angular) (idiopathic) (incorrect)
      (postural) — *see* Dorsopathy, deforming
    congenital Q67.5
    due to or associated with
      Charcot-Marie-Tooth disease (*see also* subcate-
          gory M49.8) G60.0
      osteitis
        deformans M88.88
        fibrosa cystica (*see also* subcategory M49.8)
            E21.0
      tuberculosis (Pott's curvature) A18.01
    sequelae (late effect) of rickets E64.3
    tuberculous A18.01
Cushingoid due to steroid therapy E24.2
  correct substance properly administered — *see* Table
      of Drugs and Chemicals, by drug, adverse effect
  overdose or wrong substance given or taken — *see*
      Table of Drugs and Chemicals, by drug, poison-
      ing
Cushing's
  syndrome or disease E24.9
    drug-induced E24.2
    iatrogenic E24.2
    pituitary-dependent E24.0
    specified NEC E24.8
  ulcer — *see* Ulcer, peptic, acute
Cusp, Carabelli — *omit code*
Cut (external) (*see also* Laceration)
  muscle — *see* Injury, muscle
Cutaneous (*see also* condition)
  hemorrhage R23.3
  larva migrans B76.9
Cutis (*see also* condition)
  hyperelastica Q82.8
    acquired L57.4
  laxa (hyperelastica) — *see* Dermatolysis
  marmorata R23.8

Cutis — *continued*
  osteosis L94.2
  pendula — *see* Dermatolysis
  rhomboidalis nuchae L57.2
  verticis gyrata Q82.8
    acquired L91.8
Cyanosis R23.0
  due to
    patent foramen botalli Q21.1
    persistent foramen ovale Q21.1
  enterogenous D74.8
  paroxysmal digital — *see* Raynaud's disease
    with gangrene I73.01
  retina, retinal H35.89
Cyanotic heart disease I24.9
  congenital Q24.9
Cycle
  anovulatory N97.0
  menstrual, irregular N92.6
Cyclencephaly Q04.9
Cyclical vomiting (*see also* Vomiting, cyclical) G43.A0
    (*following* G43.7)
  psychogenic F50.8
Cyclitis (*see also* Iridocyclitis) H20.9
  chronic — *see* Iridocyclitis, chronic
  Fuchs' heterochromic H20.81- ☑
  granulomatous — *see* Iridocyclitis, chronic
  lens-induced — *see* Iridocyclitis, lens-induced
  posterior H30.2- ☑
Cycloid personality F34.0
Cyclophoria H50.54
Cyclopia, cyclops Q87.0
Cyclopism Q87.0
Cyclosporiasis A07.4
Cyclothymia F34.0
Cyclothymic personality F34.0
Cyclotropia H50.41- ☑
Cylindroma (*see also* Neoplasm, malignant, by site)
  eccrine dermal — *see* Neoplasm, skin, benign
  skin — *see* Neoplasm, skin, benign
Cylindruria R82.99
Cynanche
  diphtheritic A36.2
  tonsillaris J36
Cynophobia F40.218
Cynorexia R63.2
Cyphosis — *see* Kyphosis
Cyprus fever — *see* Brucellosis
Cyst (colloid) (mucous) (simple) (retention)
  adenoid (infected) J35.8
  adrenal gland E27.8
    congenital Q89.1
  air, lung J98.4
  allantoic Q64.4
  alveolar process (jaw bone) M27.40
  amnion, amniotic O41.8X- ☑
  anterior
    chamber (eye) — *see* Cyst, iris
    nasopalatine K09.1
  antrum J34.1
  anus K62.89
  apical (tooth) (periodontal) K04.8
  appendix K38.8
  arachnoid, brain (acquired) G93.0
    congenital Q04.6
  arytenoid J38.7
  Baker's M71.2- ☑
    ruptured M66.0
    tuberculous A18.02
  Bartholin's gland N75.0
  bile duct (common) (hepatic) K83.5
  bladder (multiple) (trigone) N32.89
  blue dome (breast) — *see* Cyst, breast
  bone (local) NEC M85.60
    aneurysmal M85.50
      ankle M85.57- ☑
      foot M85.57- ☑
      forearm M85.53- ☑
      hand M85.54- ☑
      jaw M27.49
      lower leg M85.56- ☑
      multiple site M85.59
      neck M85.58
      rib M85.58
      shoulder M85.51- ☑
      skull M85.58
      specified site NEC M85.58

Cyst — *continued*
  bone — *continued*
    aneurysmal — *continued*
      thigh M85.55- ☑
      toe M85.57- ☑
      upper arm M85.52- ☑
      vertebra M85.58
    solitary M85.40
      ankle M85.47- ☑
      fibula M85.46- ☑
      foot M85.47- ☑
      hand M85.44- ☑
      humerus M85.42- ☑
      jaw M27.49
      neck M85.48
      pelvis M85.45- ☑
      radius M85.43- ☑
      rib M85.48
      shoulder M85.41- ☑
      skull M85.48
      specified site NEC M85.48
      tibia M85.46- ☑
      toe M85.47- ☑
      ulna M85.43- ☑
      vertebra M85.48
    specified type NEC M85.60
      ankle M85.67- ☑
      foot M85.67- ☑
      forearm M85.63- ☑
      hand M85.64- ☑
      jaw M27.40
        developmental (nonodontogenic) K09.1
        odontogenic K09.0
        latent M27.0
      lower leg M85.66- ☑
      multiple site M85.69
      neck M85.68
      rib M85.68
      shoulder M85.61- ☑
      skull M85.68
      specified site NEC M85.68
      thigh M85.65- ☑
      toe M85.67- ☑
      upper arm M85.62- ☑
      vertebra M85.68
  brain (acquired) G93.0
    congenital Q04.6
    hydatid B67.99 [G94]
    third ventricle (colloid), congenital Q04.6
  branchial (cleft) Q18.0
  branchiogenic Q18.0
  breast (benign) (blue dome) (pedunculated) (solitary)
      N60.0- ☑
    involution — *see* Dysplasia, mammary, specified
        type NEC
    sebaceous — *see* Dysplasia, mammary, specified
        type NEC
  broad ligament (benign) N83.8
  bronchogenic (mediastinal) (sequestration) J98.4
    congenital Q33.0
  buccal K09.8
  bulbourethral gland N36.8
  bursa, bursal NEC M71.30
    with rupture — *see* Rupture, synovium
    ankle M71.37- ☑
    elbow M71.32- ☑
    foot M71.37- ☑
    hand M71.34- ☑
    hip M71.35- ☑
    multiple sites M71.39
    pharyngeal J39.2
    popliteal space — *see* Cyst, Baker's
    shoulder M71.31- ☑
    specified site NEC M71.38
    wrist M71.33- ☑
  calcifying odontogenic D16.5
    upper jaw (bone) (maxilla) D16.4
  canal of Nuck (female) N94.89
    congenital Q52.4
  canthus — *see* Cyst, conjunctiva
  carcinomatous — *see* Neoplasm, malignant, by site
  cauda equina G95.89
  cavum septi pellucidi — *see* Cyst, brain
  celomic (pericardium) Q24.8
  cerebellopontine (angle) — *see* Cyst, brain
  cerebellum — *see* Cyst, brain
  cerebral — *see* Cyst, brain

☑ **Additional Character Required** — Refer to the Tabular List for Character Selection   ▽ **Subterms under main terms may continue to next column or page**

Cyst — *continued*
- cervical lateral Q18.1
- cervix NEC N88.8
  - embryonic Q51.6
  - nabothian N88.8
- chiasmal optic NEC — *see* Disorder, optic, chiasm
- chocolate (ovary) N80.1
- choledochus, congenital Q44.4
- chorion O41.8X- ☑
- choroid plexus G93.0
- ciliary body — *see* Cyst, iris
- clitoris N90.7
- colon K63.89
- common (bile) duct K83.5
- congenital NEC Q89.8
  - adrenal gland Q89.1
  - epiglottis Q31.8
  - esophagus Q39.8
  - fallopian tube Q50.4
  - kidney Q61.00
    - more than one (multiple) Q61.02
      - specified as polycystic Q61.3
        - adult type Q61.2
        - infantile type NEC Q61.19
          - collecting duct dilation Q61.11
    - solitary Q61.01
  - larynx Q31.8
  - liver Q44.6
  - lung Q33.0
  - mediastinum Q34.1
  - ovary Q50.1
  - oviduct Q50.4
  - periurethral (tissue) Q64.79
  - prepuce Q55.69
  - salivary gland (any) Q38.4
  - sublingual Q38.6
  - submaxillary gland Q38.6
  - thymus (gland) Q89.2
  - tongue Q38.3
  - ureterovesical orifice Q62.8
  - vulva Q52.79
- conjunctiva H11.44- ☑
- cornea H18.89- ☑
- corpora quadrigemina G93.0
- corpus
  - albicans N83.29
  - luteum (hemorrhagic) (ruptured) N83.1
- Cowper's gland (benign) (infected) N36.8
- cranial meninges G93.0
- craniobuccal pouch E23.6
- craniopharyngeal pouch E23.6
- cystic duct K82.8
- Cysticercus — *see* Cysticercosis
- Dandy-Walker Q03.1
  - with spina bifida — *see* Spina bifida
- dental (root) K04.8
  - developmental K09.0
  - eruption K09.0
  - primordial K09.0
- dentigerous (mandible) (maxilla) K09.0
- dermoid — *see* Neoplasm, benign, by site
  - with malignant transformation C56.- ☑
  - implantation
    - external area or site (skin) NEC L72.0
    - iris — *see* Cyst, iris, implantation
    - vagina N89.8
    - vulva N90.7
  - mouth K09.8
  - oral soft tissue K09.8
  - sacrococcygeal — *see* Cyst, pilonidal
- developmental K09.1
  - odontogenic K09.0
  - oral region (nonodontogenic) K09.1
  - ovary, ovarian Q50.1
- dura (cerebral) G93.0
  - spinal G96.19
- ear (external) Q18.1
- echinococcal — *see* Echinococcus
- embryonic
  - cervix uteri Q51.6
  - fallopian tube Q50.4
  - vagina Q51.6
- endometrium, endometrial (uterus) N85.8
  - ectopic — *see* Endometriosis
- enterogenous Q43.8
- epidermal, epidermoid (inclusion) (*see also* Cyst, skin) L72.0
  - mouth K09.8

Cyst — *continued*
- epidermal, epidermoid (*see also* Cyst, skin) — *continued*
  - oral soft tissue K09.8
- epididymis N50.3
- epiglottis J38.7
- epiphysis cerebri E34.8
- epithelial (inclusion) L72.0
- epoophoron Q50.5
- eruption K09.0
- esophagus K22.8
- ethmoid sinus J34.1
- external female genital organs NEC N90.7
- eyelid (sebaceous) H02.829
  - infected — *see* Hordeolum
  - left H02.826
    - lower H02.825
    - upper H02.824
  - right H02.823
    - lower H02.822
    - upper H02.821
- eye NEC H57.8
  - congenital Q15.8
- fallopian tube N83.8
  - congenital Q50.4
- fimbrial (twisted) Q50.4
- fissural (oral region) K09.1
- follicle (graafian) (hemorrhagic) N83.0
  - nabothian N88.8
- follicular (atretic) (hemorrhagic) (ovarian) N83.0
  - dentigerous K09.0
  - odontogenic K09.0
  - skin L72.9
    - specified NEC L72.8
- frontal sinus J34.1
- gallbladder K82.8
- ganglion — *see* Ganglion
- Gartner's duct Q52.4
- gingiva K09.0
- gland of Moll — *see* Cyst, eyelid
- globulomaxillary K09.1
- graafian follicle (hemorrhagic) N83.0
- granulosal lutein (hemorrhagic) N83.1
- hemangiomatous D18.00
  - intra-abdominal D18.03
  - intracranial D18.02
  - skin D18.01
  - specified site NEC D18.09
- hydatid (*see also* Echinococcus) B67.90
  - brain B67.99 [G94]
  - liver (*see also* Cyst, liver, hydatid) B67.8
  - lung NEC B67.99 [J99]
  - Morgagni
    - female Q50.5
    - male (epididymal) Q55.4
      - testicular Q55.29
  - specified site NEC B67.99
- hymen N89.8
  - embryonic Q52.4
- hypopharynx J39.2
- hypophysis, hypophyseal (duct) (recurrent) E23.6
  - cerebri E23.6
- implantation (dermoid)
  - external area or site (skin) NEC L72.0
  - iris — *see* Cyst, iris, implantation
  - vagina N89.8
  - vulva N90.7
- incisive canal K09.1
- inclusion (epidermal) (epithelial) (epidermoid) (squamous) L72.0
  - not of skin — *code under* Cyst, by site
- intestine (large) (small) K63.89
- intracranial — *see* Cyst, brain
- intraligamentous (*see also* Disorder, ligament)
  - knee — *see* Derangement, knee
- intrasellar E23.6
- iris H21.309
  - exudative H21.31- ☑
  - idiopathic H21.30- ☑
  - implantation H21.32- ☑
  - parasitic H21.33- ☑
  - pars plana (primary) H21.34- ☑
    - exudative H21.35- ☑
- jaw (bone) M27.40
  - aneurysmal M27.49
  - developmental (odontogenic) K09.0
  - fissural K09.1
  - hemorrhagic M27.49

Cyst — *continued*
- jaw — *continued*
  - traumatic M27.49
- joint NEC — *see* Disorder, joint, specified type NEC
- kidney (acquired) N28.1
  - calyceal — *see* Hydronephrosis
  - congenital Q61.00
    - more than one (multiple) Q61.02
      - specified as polycystic Q61.3
        - adult type (autosomal dominant) Q61.2
        - infantile type (autosomal recessive) NEC Q61.19
          - collecting duct dilation Q61.11
  - pyelogenic — *see* Hydronephrosis
  - simple N28.1
  - solitary (single) Q61.01
    - acquired N28.1
- labium (majus) (minus) N90.7
  - sebaceous N90.7
- lacrimal (*see also* Disorder, lacrimal system, specified NEC)
  - gland H04.13- ☑
  - passages or sac — *see* Disorder, lacrimal system, specified NEC
- larynx J38.7
- lateral periodontal K09.0
- lens H27.8
  - congenital Q12.8
- lip (gland) K13.0
- liver (idiopathic) (simple) K76.89
  - congenital Q44.6
  - hydatid B67.8
    - granulosus B67.0
    - multilocularis B67.5
- lung J98.4
  - congenital Q33.0
  - giant bullous J43.9
- lutein N83.1
- lymphangiomatous D18.1
- lymphoepithelial, oral soft tissue K09.8
- macula — *see* Degeneration, macula, hole
- malignant — *see* Neoplasm, malignant, by site
- mammary gland — *see* Cyst, breast
- mandible M27.40
  - dentigerous K09.0
  - radicular K04.8
- maxilla M27.40
  - dentigerous K09.0
  - radicular K04.8
- medial, face and neck Q18.8
- median
  - anterior maxillary K09.1
  - palatal K09.1
- mediastinum, congenital Q34.1
- meibomian (gland) — *see* Chalazion
  - infected — *see* Hordeolum
- membrane, brain G93.0
- meninges (cerebral) G93.0
  - spinal G96.19
- meniscus, knee — *see* Derangement, knee, meniscus, cystic
- mesentery, mesenteric K66.8
  - chyle I89.8
- mesonephric duct
  - female Q50.5
  - male Q55.4
- milk N64.89
- Morgagni (hydatid)
  - female Q50.5
  - male (epididymal) Q55.4
    - testicular Q55.29
- mouth K09.8
- Müllerian duct Q50.4
  - appendix testis Q55.29
  - cervix Q51.6
  - fallopian tube Q50.4
  - female Q50.4
  - male Q55.29
  - prostatic utricle Q55.4
  - vagina (embryonal) Q52.4
- multilocular (ovary) D39.10
  - benign — *see* Neoplasm, benign, by site
- myometrium N85.8
- nabothian (follicle) (ruptured) N88.8
- nasoalveolar K09.1
- nasolabial K09.1
- nasopalatine (anterior) (duct) K09.1
- nasopharynx J39.2

Cyst — *continued*
- neoplastic — *see* Neoplasm, uncertain behavior, by site
  - benign — *see* Neoplasm, benign, by site
- nervous system NEC G96.8
- neuroenteric (congenital) Q06.8
- nipple — *see* Cyst, breast
- nose (turbinates) J34.1
  - sinus J34.1
- odontogenic, developmental K09.0
- omentum (lesser) K66.8
  - congenital Q45.8
- ora serrata — *see* Cyst, retina, ora serrata
- oral
  - region K09.9
    - developmental (nonodontogenic) K09.1
    - specified NEC K09.8
  - soft tissue K09.9
    - specified NEC K09.8
- orbit H05.81- ☑
- ovary, ovarian (twisted) N83.20
  - adherent N83.20
  - chocolate N80.1
  - corpus
    - albicans N83.29
    - luteum (hemorrhagic) N83.1
  - dermoid D27.9
  - developmental Q50.1
  - due to failure of involution NEC N83.20
  - endometrial N80.1
  - follicular (graafian) (hemorrhagic) N83.0
  - hemorrhagic N83.20
  - in pregnancy or childbirth O34.8- ☑
    - with obstructed labor O65.5
  - multilocular D39.10
  - pseudomucinous D27.9
  - retention N83.29
  - serous N83.20
  - specified NEC N83.29
  - theca lutein (hemorrhagic) N83.1
  - tuberculous A18.18
- oviduct N83.8
- palate (median) (fissural) K09.1
- palatine papilla (jaw) K09.1
- pancreas, pancreatic (hemorrhagic) (true) K86.2
  - congenital Q45.2
  - false K86.3
- paralabral
  - hip M24.85- ☑
  - shoulder S43.43- ☑
- paramesonephric duct Q50.4
  - female Q50.4
  - male Q55.29
- paranephric N28.1
- paraphysis, cerebri, congenital Q04.6
- parasitic B89
- parathyroid (gland) E21.4
- paratubal N83.8
- paraurethral duct N36.8
- paroophoron Q50.5
- parotid gland K11.6
- parovarian Q50.5
- pelvis, female N94.89
  - in pregnancy or childbirth O34.8- ☑
    - causing obstructed labor O65.5
- penis (sebaceous) N48.89
- periapical K04.8
- pericardial (congenital) Q24.8
  - acquired (secondary) I31.8
- pericoronal K09.0
- periodontal K04.8
  - lateral K09.0
- peripelvic (lymphatic) N28.1
- peritoneum K66.8
  - chylous I89.8
- periventricular, acquired, newborn P91.1
- pharynx (wall) J39.2
- pilar L72.11
- pilonidal (infected) (rectum) L05.91
  - with abscess L05.01
  - malignant C44.59- ☑
- pituitary (duct) (gland) E23.6
- placenta O43.19- ☑
- pleura J94.8
- popliteal — *see* Cyst, Baker's
- porencephalic Q04.6
  - acquired G93.0
- postanal (infected) — *see* Cyst, pilonidal

Cyst — *continued*
- postmastoidectomy cavity (mucosal) — *see* Complications, postmastoidectomy, cyst
- preauricular Q18.1
- prepuce N47.4
  - congenital Q55.69
- primordial (jaw) K09.0
- prostate N42.83
- pseudomucinous (ovary) D27.9
- pupillary, miotic H21.27- ☑
- radicular (residual) K04.8
- radiculodental K04.8
- ranular K11.8
- Rathke's pouch E23.6
- rectum (epithelium) (mucous) K62.89
- renal — *see* Cyst, kidney
- residual (radicular) K04.8
- retention (ovary) N83.29
  - salivary gland K11.6
- retina H33.19- ☑
  - ora serrata H33.11- ☑
  - parasitic H33.12- ☑
- retroperitoneal K68.9
- sacrococcygeal (dermoid) — *see* Cyst, pilonidal
- salivary gland or duct (mucous extravasation or retention) K11.6
- Sampson's N80.1
- sclera H15.89
- scrotum L72.9
  - sebaceous L72.3
- sebaceous (duct) (gland) L72.3
  - breast — *see* Dysplasia, mammary, specified type NEC
  - eyelid — *see* Cyst, eyelid
  - genital organ NEC
    - female N94.89
    - male N50.8
  - scrotum L72.3
- semilunar cartilage (knee) (multiple) — *see* Derangement, knee, meniscus, cystic
- seminal vesicle N50.8
- serous (ovary) N83.20
- sinus (accessory) (nasal) J34.1
- Skene's gland N36.8
- skin L72.9
  - breast — *see* Dysplasia, mammary, specified type NEC
  - epidermal, epidermoid L72.0
  - epithelial L72.0
  - eyelid — *see* Cyst, eyelid
  - genital organ NEC
    - female N90.7
    - male N50.8
  - inclusion L72.0
  - scrotum L72.9
  - sebaceous L72.3
  - sweat gland or duct L74.8
- solitary
  - bone — *see* Cyst, bone, solitary
  - jaw M27.40
  - kidney N28.1
- spermatic cord N50.8
- sphenoid sinus J34.1
- spinal meninges G96.19
- spleen NEC D73.4
  - congenital Q89.09
  - hydatid (*see also* Echinococcus) B67.99 [D77]
- Stafne's M27.0
- subarachnoid intrasellar R93.0
- subcutaneous, pheomycotic (chromomycotic) B43.2
- subdural (cerebral) G93.0
  - spinal cord G96.19
- sublingual gland K11.6
- submandibular gland K11.6
- submaxillary gland K11.6
- suburethral N36.8
- suprarenal gland E27.8
- suprasellar — *see* Cyst, brain
- sweat gland or duct L74.8
- synovial (*see also* Cyst, bursa)
  - ruptured — *see* Rupture, synovium
- tarsal — *see* Chalazion
- tendon (sheath) — *see* Disorder, tendon, specified type NEC
- testis N44.2
  - tunica albuginea N44.1
- theca lutein (ovary) N83.1
- Thornwaldt's J39.2

Cyst — *continued*
- thymus (gland) E32.8
- thyroglossal duct (infected) (persistent) Q89.2
- thyroid (gland) E04.1
- thyrolingual duct (infected) (persistent) Q89.2
- tongue K14.8
- tonsil J35.8
- tooth — *see* Cyst, dental
- Tornwaldt's J39.2
- trichilemmal (proliferating) L72.12
- trichodermal L72.12
- tubal (fallopian) N83.8
  - inflammatory — *see* Salpingitis, chronic
- tubo-ovarian N83.8
  - inflammatory N70.13
- tunica
  - albuginea testis N44.1
  - vaginalis N50.8
- turbinate (nose) J34.1
- Tyson's gland N48.89
- urachus, congenital Q64.4
- ureter N28.89
- ureterovesical orifice N28.89
- urethra, urethral (gland) N36.8
- uterine ligament N83.8
- uterus (body) (corpus) (recurrent) N85.8
  - embryonic Q51.818
    - cervix Q51.6
- vagina, vaginal (implantation) (inclusion) (squamous cell) (wall) N89.8
  - embryonic Q52.4
- vallecula, vallecular (epiglottis) J38.7
- vesical (orifice) N32.89
- vitreous body H43.89
- vulva (implantation) (inclusion) N90.7
  - congenital Q52.79
  - sebaceous gland N90.7
- vulvovaginal gland N90.7
- wolffian
  - female Q50.5
  - male Q55.4

Cystadenocarcinoma — *see* Neoplasm, malignant, by site
- bile duct C22.1
- endometrioid — *see* Neoplasm, malignant, by site
  - specified site — *see* Neoplasm, malignant, by site
  - unspecified site
    - female C56.9
    - male C61
- mucinous
  - papillary
    - specified site — *see* Neoplasm, malignant, by site
    - unspecified site C56.9
  - specified site — *see* Neoplasm, malignant, by site
  - unspecified site C56.9
- papillary
  - mucinous
    - specified site — *see* Neoplasm, malignant, by site
    - unspecified site C56.9
  - pseudomucinous
    - specified site — *see* Neoplasm, malignant, by site
    - unspecified site C56.9
  - serous
    - specified site — *see* Neoplasm, malignant, by site
    - unspecified site C56.9
  - specified site — *see* Neoplasm, malignant, by site
  - unspecified site C56.9
- pseudomucinous
  - papillary
    - specified site — *see* Neoplasm, malignant, by site
    - unspecified site C56.9
  - specified site — *see* Neoplasm, malignant, by site
  - unspecified site C56.9
- serous
  - papillary
    - specified site — *see* Neoplasm, malignant, by site
    - unspecified site C56.9
  - specified site — *see* Neoplasm, malignant, by site
  - unspecified site C56.9

Cystadenofibroma
- clear cell — *see* Neoplasm, benign, by site
- endometrioid D27.9

Cystadenofibroma — *continued*
  endometrioid — *continued*
    borderline malignancy D39.1- ☑
    malignant C56.- ☑
  mucinous
    specified site — *see* Neoplasm, benign, by site
    unspecified site D27.9
  serous
    specified site — *see* Neoplasm, benign, by site
    unspecified site D27.9
  specified site — *see* Neoplasm, benign, by site
  unspecified site D27.9
Cystadenoma (*see also* Neoplasm, benign, by site)
  bile duct D13.4
  endometrioid — *see* Neoplasm, benign, by site
    borderline malignancy — *see* Neoplasm, uncertain
        behavior, by site
  malignant — *see* Neoplasm, malignant, by site
  mucinous
    borderline malignancy
      ovary C56.- ☑
      specified site NEC — *see* Neoplasm, uncertain
          behavior, by site
      unspecified site C56.9
    papillary
      borderline malignancy
        ovary C56.- ☑
        specified site NEC — *see* Neoplasm, uncer-
            tain behavior, by site
        unspecified site C56.9
      specified site — *see* Neoplasm, benign, by site
      unspecified site D27.9
    specified site — *see* Neoplasm, benign, by site
    unspecified site D27.9
  papillary
    borderline malignancy
      ovary C56.- ☑
      specified site NEC — *see* Neoplasm, uncertain
          behavior, by site
      unspecified site C56.9
    lymphomatosum
      specified site — *see* Neoplasm, benign, by site
      unspecified site D11.9
    mucinous
      borderline malignancy
        ovary C56.- ☑
        specified site NEC — *see* Neoplasm, uncer-
            tain behavior, by site
        unspecified site C56.9
      specified site — *see* Neoplasm, benign, by site
      unspecified site D27.9
    pseudomucinous
      borderline malignancy
        ovary C56.- ☑
        specified site NEC — *see* Neoplasm, uncer-
            tain behavior, by site
        unspecified site C56.9
      specified site — *see* Neoplasm, benign, by site
      unspecified site D27.9
    serous
      borderline malignancy
        ovary C56.- ☑
        specified site NEC — *see* Neoplasm, uncer-
            tain behavior, by site
        unspecified site C56.9
      specified site — *see* Neoplasm, benign, by site
      unspecified site D27.9
    specified site — *see* Neoplasm, benign, by site
    unspecified site D27.9
  pseudomucinous
    borderline malignancy
      ovary C56.- ☑
      specified site NEC — *see* Neoplasm, uncertain
          behavior, by site
      unspecified site C56.9
    papillary
      borderline malignancy
        ovary C56.- ☑
        specified site NEC — *see* Neoplasm, uncer-
            tain behavior, by site
        unspecified site C56.9
      specified site — *see* Neoplasm, benign, by site
      unspecified site D27.9
    specified site — *see* Neoplasm, benign, by site

Cystadenoma — *continued*
  pseudomucinous — *continued*
    unspecified site D27.9
    serous
      borderline malignancy
        ovary C56.- ☑
        specified site NEC — *see* Neoplasm, uncertain
            behavior, by site
        unspecified site C56.9
      papillary
        borderline malignancy
          ovary C56.- ☑
          specified site NEC — *see* Neoplasm, uncer-
              tain behavior, by site
          unspecified site C56.9
        specified site — *see* Neoplasm, benign, by site
        unspecified site D27.9
    specified site — *see* Neoplasm, benign, by site
    unspecified site D27.9
Cystathionine synthase deficiency E72.11
Cystathioninemia E72.19
Cystathioninuria E72.19
Cystic (*see also* condition)
  breast (chronic) — *see* Mastopathy, cystic
  corpora lutea (hemorrhagic) N83.1
  duct — *see* condition
  eyeball (congenital) Q11.0
  fibrosis — *see* Fibrosis, cystic
  kidney (congenital) Q61.9
    adult type Q61.2
    infantile type NEC Q61.19
      collecting duct dilatation Q61.11
    medullary Q61.5
  liver, congenital Q44.6
  lung disease J98.4
    congenital Q33.0
  mastitis, chronic — *see* Mastopathy, cystic
  medullary, kidney Q61.5
  meniscus — *see* Derangement, knee, meniscus, cystic
  ovary N83.20
Cysticercosis, cysticerciasis B69.9
  with
    epileptiform fits B69.0
    myositis B69.81
  brain B69.0
  central nervous system B69.0
  cerebral B69.0
  ocular B69.1
  specified NEC B69.89
Cysticercus cellulose infestation — *see* Cysticercosis
Cystinosis (malignant) E72.04
Cystinuria E72.01
Cystitis (exudative) (hemorrhagic) (septic) (suppurative)
    N30.90
  with
    fibrosis — *see* Cystitis, chronic, interstitial
    hematuria N30.91
    leukoplakia — *see* Cystitis, chronic, interstitial
    malakoplakia — *see* Cystitis, chronic, interstitial
    metaplasia — *see* Cystitis, chronic, interstitial
    prostatitis N41.3
  acute N30.00
    with hematuria N30.01
    of trigone N30.30
      with hematuria N30.31
  allergic — *see* Cystitis, specified type NEC
  amebic A06.81
  bilharzial B65.9 [N33]
  blennorrhagic (gonococcal) A54.01
  bullous — *see* Cystitis, specified type NEC
  calculous N21.0
  chlamydial A56.01
  chronic N30.20
    with hematuria N30.21
    interstitial N30.10
      with hematuria N30.11
    of trigone N30.30
      with hematuria N30.31
    specified NEC N30.20
      with hematuria N30.21
  cystic (a) — *see* Cystitis, specified type NEC
  diphtheritic A36.85
  echinococcal
    granulosus B67.39

Cystitis — *continued*
  echinococcal — *continued*
    multilocularis B67.69
  emphysematous — *see* Cystitis, specified type NEC
  encysted — *see* Cystitis, specified type NEC
  eosinophilic — *see* Cystitis, specified type NEC
  follicular — *see* Cystitis, of trigone
  gangrenous — *see* Cystitis, specified type NEC
  glandularis — *see* Cystitis, specified type NEC
  gonococcal A54.01
  incrusted — *see* Cystitis, specified type NEC
  interstitial (chronic) — *see* Cystitis, chronic, interstitial
  irradiation N30.40
    with hematuria N30.41
  irritation — *see* Cystitis, specified type NEC
  malignant — *see* Cystitis, specified type NEC
  of trigone N30.30
    with hematuria N30.31
  panmural — *see* Cystitis, chronic, interstitial
  polyposa — *see* Cystitis, specified type NEC
  prostatic N41.3
  puerperal (postpartum) O86.22
  radiation — *see* Cystitis, irradiation
  specified type NEC N30.80
    with hematuria N30.81
  subacute — *see* Cystitis, chronic
  submucous — *see* Cystitis, chronic, interstitial
  syphilitic (late) A52.76
  trichomonal A59.03
  tuberculous A18.12
  ulcerative — *see* Cystitis, chronic, interstitial
Cystocele (-urethrocele)
  female N81.10
    with prolapse of uterus — *see* Prolapse, uterus
    lateral N81.12
    midline N81.11
    paravaginal N81.12
  in pregnancy or childbirth O34.8- ☑
    causing obstructed labor O65.5
  male N32.89
Cystolithiasis N21.0
Cystoma (*see also* Neoplasm, benign, by site)
  endometrial, ovary N80.1
  mucinous
    specified site — *see* Neoplasm, benign, by site
    unspecified site D27.9
  serous
    specified site — *see* Neoplasm, benign, by site
    unspecified site D27.9
  simple (ovary) N83.29
Cystoplegia N31.2
Cystoptosis N32.89
Cystopyelitis — *see* Pyelonephritis
Cystorrhagia N32.89
Cystosarcoma phyllodes D48.6- ☑
  benign D24- ☑
  malignant — *see* Neoplasm, breast, malignant
Cystostomy
  attention to Z43.5
  complication — *see* Complications, cystostomy
  status Z93.50
    appendico-vesicostomy Z93.52
    cutaneous Z93.51
    specified NEC Z93.59
Cystourethritis — *see* Urethritis
Cystourethrocele (*see also* Cystocele)
  female N81.10
    with uterine prolapse — *see* Prolapse, uterus
    lateral N81.12
    midline N81.11
    paravaginal N81.12
  male N32.89
Cytomegalic inclusion disease
  congenital P35.1
Cytomegalovirus infection B25.9
Cytomycosis (reticuloendothelial) B39.4
Cytopenia D75.9
  refractory
    with multilineage dysplasia D46.A (*following* D46.2)
      and ring sideroblasts (RCMD RS) D46.B (*follow-*
          ing D46.2)
Czerny's disease (periodic hydrarthrosis of the knee) —
  see Effusion, joint, knee

D

Da Costa's syndrome F45.8
Daae (-Finsen) **disease** (epidemic pleurodynia) B33.0
Dabney's grip B33.0
Dacryoadenitis, dacryadenitis H04.00- ☑
  acute H04.01- ☑
  chronic H04.02- ☑
Dacryocystitis H04.30- ☑
  acute H04.32- ☑
  chronic H04.41- ☑
  neonatal P39.1
  phlegmonous H04.31- ☑
  syphilitic A52.71
    congenital (early) A50.01
  trachomatous, active A71.1
    sequelae (late effect) B94.0
Dacryocystoblenorrhea — see Inflammation, lacrimal, passages, chronic
Dacryocystocele — see Disorder, lacrimal system, changes
Dacryolith, dacryolithiasis H04.51- ☑
Dacryoma — see Disorder, lacrimal system, changes
Dacryopericystitis — see Dacryocystitis
Dacryops H04.11- ☑
Dacryostenosis (see also Stenosis, lacrimal)
  congenital Q10.5
Dactylitis
  bone — see Osteomyelitis
  sickle-cell D57.00
    Hb C D57.219
    Hb SS D57.00
    specified NEC D57.819
  skin L08.9
  syphilitic A52.77
  tuberculous A18.03
Dactylolysis spontanea (ainhum) L94.6
Dactylosymphysis Q70.9
  fingers — see Syndactylism, complex, fingers
  toes — see Syndactylism, complex, toes
Damage
  arteriosclerotic — see Arteriosclerosis
  brain (nontraumatic) G93.9
    anoxic, hypoxic G93.1
      resulting from a procedure G97.82
    child NEC G80.9
    due to birth injury P11.2
  cardiorenal (vascular) — see Hypertension, cardiorenal
  cerebral NEC — see Damage, brain
  coccyx, complicating delivery O71.6
  coronary — see Disease, heart, ischemic
  eye, birth injury P15.3
  liver (nontraumatic) K76.9
    alcoholic K70.9
    due to drugs — see Disease, liver, toxic
    toxic — see Disease, liver, toxic
  medication T88.7 ☑
  pelvic
    joint or ligament, during delivery O71.6
    organ NEC
      during delivery O71.5
      following ectopic or molar pregnancy O08.6
  renal — see Disease, renal
  subendocardium, subendocardial — see Degeneration, myocardial
  vascular I99.9
Dana-Putnam syndrome (subacute combined sclerosis with pernicious anemia) — see Degeneration, combined
Danbolt (-Cross) **syndrome** (acrodermatitis enteropathica) E83.2
Dandruff L21.0
Dandy-Walker syndrome Q03.1
  with spina bifida — see Spina bifida
Danlos' syndrome Q79.6
Darier (-White) **disease** (congenital) Q82.8
  meaning erythema annulare centrifugum L53.1
Darier-Roussy sarcoid D86.3
Darling's disease or histoplasmosis B39.4
Darwin's tubercle Q17.8

Dawson's (inclusion body) **encephalitis** A81.1
De Beurmann (-Gougerot) **disease** B42.1
De la Tourette's syndrome F95.2
De Lange's syndrome Q87.1
De Morgan's spots (senile angiomas) I78.1
De Quervain's
  disease (tendon sheath) M65.4
  syndrome E34.51
  thyroiditis (subacute granulomatous thyroiditis) E06.1
De Toni-Fanconi (-Debré) **syndrome** E72.09
  with cystinosis E72.04
Dead
  fetus, retained (mother) O36.4 ☑
    early pregnancy O02.1
  labyrinth H83.2 ☑
  ovum, retained O02.0
Deaf nonspeaking NEC H91.3
Deafmutism (acquired) (congenital) NEC H91.3
  hysterical F44.6
  syphilitic, congenital (see also subcategory) H94.8 A50.09
Deafness (acquired) (complete) (hereditary) (partial) H91.9- ☑
  with blue sclera and fragility of bone Q78.0
  auditory fatigue — see Deafness, specified type NEC
  aviation T70.0 ☑
    nerve injury — see Injury, nerve, acoustic, specified type NEC
  boilermaker's H83.3 ☑
  central — see Deafness, sensorineural
  conductive H90.2
    and sensorineural, mixed H90.8
      bilateral H90.6
    bilateral H90.0
    unilateral H90.1- ☑
  congenital H90.5
    with blue sclera and fragility of bone Q78.0
  due to toxic agents — see Deafness, ototoxic
  emotional (hysterical) F44.6
  functional (hysterical) F44.6
  high frequency H91.9- ☑
  hysterical F44.6
  low frequency H91.9- ☑
  mental R48.8
  mixed conductive and sensorineural H90.8
    bilateral H90.6
    unilateral H90.7- ☑
  nerve — see Deafness, sensorineural
  neural — see Deafness, sensorineural
  noise-induced (see also subcategory) H83.3 ☑
    nerve injury — see Injury, nerve, acoustic, specified type NEC
  nonspeaking H91.3
  ototoxic H91.0 ☑
  perceptive — see Deafness, sensorineural
  psychogenic (hysterical) F44.6
  sensorineural H90.5
    and conductive, mixed H90.8
      bilateral H90.6
    bilateral H90.3
    unilateral H90.4- ☑
  sensory — see Deafness, sensorineural
  specified type NEC H91.8 ☑
  sudden (idiopathic) H91.2- ☑
  syphilitic A52.15
  transient ischemic H93.01- ☑
  traumatic — see Injury, nerve, acoustic, specified type NEC
  word (developmental) H93.25
Death (cause unknown) (of) (unexplained) (unspecified cause) R99
  brain G93.82
  cardiac (sudden) (with successful resuscitation) — code to underlying disease
    family history of Z82.41
    personal history of Z86.74
  family member (assumed) Z63.4
Debility (chronic) (general) (nervous) R53.81
  congenital or neonatal NOS P96.9
  nervous R53.81
  old age R54
  senile R54

Débove's disease (splenomegaly) R16.1
Decalcification
  bone — see Osteoporosis
  teeth K03.89
Decapsulation, kidney N28.89
Decay
  dental — see Caries, dental
  senile R54
  tooth, teeth — see Caries, dental
Deciduitis (acute)
  following ectopic or molar pregnancy O08.0
Decline (general) — see Debility
  cognitive, age-associated R41.81
Decompensation
  cardiac (acute) (chronic) — see Disease, heart
  cardiovascular — see Disease, cardiovascular
  heart — see Disease, heart
  hepatic — see Failure, hepatic
  myocardial (acute) (chronic) — see Disease, heart
  respiratory J98.8
Decompression sickness T70.3 ☑
Decrease (d)
  absolute neutrophile count — see Neutropenia
  blood
    platelets — see Thrombocytopenia
    pressure R03.1
      due to shock following
        injury T79.4 ☑
        operation T81.19 ☑
  estrogen E28.39
    postablative E89.40
      asymptomatic E89.40
      symptomatic E89.41
  fragility of erythrocytes D58.8
  function
    lipase (pancreatic) K90.3
    ovary in hypopituitarism E23.0
    parenchyma of pancreas K86.8
    pituitary (gland) (anterior) (lobe) E23.0
      posterior (lobe) E23.0
  functional activity R68.89
  glucose R73.09
  hematocrit R71.0
  hemoglobin R71.0
  leukocytes D72.819
    specified NEC D72.818
  libido R68.82
  lymphocytes D72.810
  platelets D69.6
  respiration, due to shock following injury T79.4 ☑
  sexual desire R68.82
  tear secretion NEC — see Syndrome, dry eye
  tolerance
    fat K90.4
    glucose R73.09
    pancreatic K90.3
    salt and water E87.8
  vision NEC H54.7
  white blood cell count D72.819
    specified NEC D72.818
Decubitus (ulcer) — see Ulcer, pressure, by site
  cervix N86
Deepening acetabulum — see Derangement, joint, specified type NEC, hip
Defect, defective Q89.9
  3-beta-hydroxysteroid dehydrogenase E25.0
  11-hydroxylase E25.0
  21-hydroxylase E25.0
  abdominal wall, congenital Q79.59
  antibody immunodeficiency D80.9
  aorticopulmonary septum Q21.4
  atrial septal (ostium secundum type) Q21.1
    following acute myocardial infarction (current complication) I23.1
    ostium primum type Q21.2
  atrioventricular
    canal Q21.2
    septum Q21.2
  auricular septal Q21.1
  bilirubin excretion NEC E80.6
  biosynthesis, androgen (testicular) E29.1
  bulbar septum Q21.0

Defect, defective — *continued*
catalase E80.3
cell membrane receptor complex (CR3) D71
circulation I99.9
  congenital Q28.9
  newborn Q28.9
coagulation (factor) (*see also* Deficiency, factor) D68.9
  with
    ectopic pregnancy O08.1
    molar pregnancy O08.1
  acquired D68.4
  antepartum with hemorrhage — *see* Hemorrhage,
    antepartum, with coagulation defect
  due to
    liver disease D68.4
    vitamin K deficiency D68.4
  hereditary NEC D68.2
  intrapartum O67.0
  newborn, transient P61.6
  postpartum O72.3
  specified type NEC D68.8
complement system D84.1
conduction (heart) I45.9
  bone — *see* Deafness, conductive
congenital, organ or site not listed — *see* Anomaly,
  by site
coronary sinus Q21.1
cushion, endocardial Q21.2
degradation, glycoprotein E77.1
dental bridge, crown, fillings — *see* Defect, dental
  restoration
dental restoration K08.50
  specified NEC K08.59
dentin (hereditary) K00.5
Descemet's membrane, congenital Q13.89
developmental (*see also* Anomaly)
  cauda equina Q06.3
diaphragm
  with elevation, eventration or hernia — *see* Hernia,
    diaphragm
  congenital Q79.1
    with hernia Q79.0
    gross (with hernia) Q79.0
ectodermal, congenital Q82.9
Eisenmenger's Q21.8
enzyme
  catalase E80.3
  peroxidase E80.3
esophagus, congenital Q39.9
extensor retinaculum M62.89
fibrin polymerization D68.2
filling
  bladder R93.4
  kidney R93.4
  stomach R93.3
  ureter R93.4
Gerbode Q21.0
glycoprotein degradation E77.1
Hageman (factor) D68.2
hearing — *see* Deafness
high grade F70
interatrial septal Q21.1
interauricular septal Q21.1
interventricular septal Q21.0
  with dextroposition of aorta, pulmonary stenosis
    and hypertrophy of right ventricle Q21.3
  in tetralogy of Fallot Q21.3
learning (specific) — *see* Disorder, learning
lymphocyte function antigen-1 (LFA-1) D84.0
lysosomal enzyme, post-translational modification
  E77.0
major osseous M89.70
  ankle M89.77- ☑
  carpus M89.74- ☑
  clavicle M89.71- ☑
  femur M89.75- ☑
  fibula M89.76- ☑
  fingers M89.74- ☑
  foot M89.77- ☑
  forearm M89.73- ☑
  hand M89.74- ☑
  humerus M89.72- ☑
  lower leg M89.76- ☑
  metacarpus M89.74- ☑
  metatarsus M89.77- ☑
  multiple sites M89.79
  pelvic region M89.75- ☑
  pelvis M89.75- ☑

Defect, defective — *continued*
major osseous — *continued*
  radius M89.73- ☑
  scapula M89.71- ☑
  shoulder region M89.71- ☑ ·
  specified NEC M89.78
  tarsus M89.77- ☑
  thigh M89.75- ☑
  tibia M89.76- ☑
  toes M89.77- ☑
  ulna M89.73- ☑
mental — *see* Disability, intellectual
modification, lysosomal enzymes, post-translational
  E77.0
obstructive, congenital
  renal pelvis Q62.39
  ureter Q62.39
    atresia — *see* Atresia, ureter
    cecoureterocele Q62.32
    megaureter Q62.2
    orthotopic ureterocele Q62.31
osseous, major M89.70
  ankle M89.77- ☑
  carpus M89.74- ☑
  clavicle M89.71- ☑
  femur M89.75- ☑
  fibula M89.76- ☑
  fingers M89.74- ☑
  foot M89.77- ☑
  forearm M89.73- ☑
  hand M89.74- ☑
  humerus M89.72- ☑
  lower leg M89.76- ☑
  metacarpus M89.74- ☑
  metatarsus M89.77- ☑
  multiple sites M89.9
  pelvic region M89.75- ☑
  pelvis M89.75- ☑
  radius M89.73- ☑
  scapula M89.71- ☑
  shoulder region M89.71- ☑
  specified NEC M89.78
  tarsus M89.77- ☑
  thigh M89.75- ☑
  tibia M89.76- ☑
  toes M89.77- ☑
  ulna M89.73- ☑
osteochondral NEC (*see also* Deformity) M95.8
ostium
  primum Q21.2
  secundum Q21.1
peroxidase E80.3
placental blood supply — *see* Insufficiency, placental
platelets, qualitative D69.1
  constitutional D68.0
postural NEC, spine — *see* Dorsopathy, deforming
reduction
  limb Q73.8
    lower Q72.9- ☑
      absence — *see* Agenesis, leg
        foot — *see* Agenesis, foot
      longitudinal
        femur Q72.4- ☑
        fibula Q72.6- ☑
        tibia Q72.5- ☑
      specified type NEC Q72.89- ☑
      split foot Q72.7- ☑
    specified type NEC Q73.8
    upper Q71.9- ☑
      absence — *see* Agenesis, arm
        forearm — *see* Agenesis, forearm
        hand — *see* Agenesis, hand
      lobster-claw hand Q71.6- ☑
      longitudinal
        radius Q71.4- ☑
        ulna Q71.5- ☑
      specified type NEC Q71.89- ☑
renal pelvis Q63.8
  obstructive Q62.39
respiratory system, congenital Q34.9
restoration, dental K08.50
  specified NEC K08.59
retinal nerve bundle fibers H35.89
septal (heart) NOS Q21.9
  acquired (atrial) (auricular) (ventricular) (old) I51.0
  atrial Q21.1

Defect, defective — *continued*
septal — *continued*
  atrial — *continued*
    concurrent with acute myocardial infarction —
      see Infarct, myocardium
    following acute myocardial infarction (current
      complication) I23.1
    ventricular (*see also* Defect, ventricular septal)
      Q21.0
  sinus venosus Q21.1
speech R47.9
  developmental F80.9
  specified NEC R47.89
Taussig-Bing (aortic transposition and overriding pulmonary artery) Q20.1
teeth, wedge K03.1
vascular (local) I99.9
  congenital Q27.9
ventricular septal Q21.0
  concurrent with acute myocardial infarction — *see*
    Infarct, myocardium
  following acute myocardial infarction (current
    complication) I23.2
  in tetralogy of Fallot Q21.3
vision NEC H54.7
visual field H53.40
  bilateral
    heteronymous H53.47
    homonymous H53.46- ☑
  generalized contraction H53.48- ☑
  localized
    arcuate H53.43- ☑
    scotoma (central area) H53.41- ☑
      blind spot area H53.42- ☑
    sector H53.43- ☑
    specified type NEC H53.45- ☑
voice R49.9
  specified NEC R49.8
wedge, tooth, teeth (abrasion) K03.1
Deferentitis N49.1
  gonorrheal (acute) (chronic) A54.23
Defibrination (syndrome) D65
  antepartum — *see* Hemorrhage, antepartum, with
    coagulation defect, disseminated intravascular
    coagulation
  following ectopic or molar pregnancy O08.1
  intrapartum O67.0
  newborn P60
  postpartum O72.3
Deficiency, deficient
  3-beta hydroxysteroid dehydrogenase E25.0
  5-alpha reductase (with male pseudo-
    hermaphroditism) E29.1
  11-hydroxylase E25.0
  21-hydroxylase E25.0
  abdominal muscle syndrome Q79.4
  AC globulin (congenital) (hereditary) D68.2
    acquired D68.4
  accelerator globulin (Ac G) (blood) D68.2
  acid phosphatase E83.39
  activating factor (blood) D68.2
  adenosine deaminase (ADA) D81.3
  aldolase (hereditary) E74.19
  alpha-1-antitrypsin E88.01
  amino-acids E72.9
  anemia — *see* Anemia
  aneurin E51.9
  antibody with
    hyperimmunoglobulinemia D80.6
    near-normal immunoglobins D80.6
  antidiuretic hormone E23.2
  anti-hemophilic
    factor (A) D66
      B D67
      C D68.1
    globulin (AHG) NEC D66
  antithrombin (antithrombin III) D68.59
  ascorbic acid E54
  attention (disorder) (syndrome) F98.8
    with hyperactivity — *see* Disorder, attention-deficit
      hyperactivity
  autoprothrombin
    C D68.2
    I D68.2
    II D67
  beta-glucuronidase E76.29
  biotin E53.8
  biotin-dependent carboxylase D81.819

Index

Deficiency, deficient — Deficiency, deficient

Deficiency, deficient — continued
biotinidase D81.810
brancher enzyme (amylopectinosis) E74.03
C1 esterase inhibitor (C1-INH) D84.1
calciferol E55.9
  with
    adult osteomalacia M83.8
    rickets — see Rickets
calcium (dietary) E58
calorie, severe E43
  with marasmus E41
    and kwashiorkor E42
cardiac — see Insufficiency, myocardial
carnitine E71.40
  due to
    hemodialysis E71.43
    inborn errors of metabolism E71.42
    Valproic acid therapy E71.43
  iatrogenic E71.43
  muscle palmityltransferase E71.314
  primary E71.41
  secondary E71.448
carotene E50.9
central nervous system G96.8
ceruloplasmin (Wilson) E83.01
choline E53.8
Christmas factor D67
chromium E61.4
clotting (blood) (see also Deficiency, coagulation factor) D68.9
clotting factor NEC (hereditary) (see also Deficiency, factor) D68.2
coagulation NOS D68.9
  with
    ectopic pregnancy O08.1
    molar pregnancy O08.1
  acquired (any) D68.4
  antepartum hemorrhage — see Hemorrhage, antepartum, with coagulation defect
  clotting factor NEC (see also Deficiency, factor) D68.2
  due to
    hyperprothrombinemia D68.4
    liver disease D68.4
    vitamin K deficiency D68.4
  newborn, transient P61.6
  postpartum O72.3
  specified NEC D68.8
cognitive F09
color vision H53.50
  achromatopsia H53.51
  acquired H53.52
  deuteranomaly H53.53
  protanomaly H53.54
  specified type NEC H53.59
  tritanomaly H53.55
combined glucocorticoid and mineralocorticoid E27.49
contact factor D68.2
copper (nutritional) E61.0
corticoadrenal E27.40
  primary E27.1
craniofacial axis Q75.0
cyanocobalamin E53.8
debrancher enzyme (limit dextrinosis) E74.03
dehydrogenase
  long chain/very long chain acyl CoA E71.310
  medium chain acyl CoA E71.311
  short chain acyl CoA E71.312
diet E63.9
dihydropyrimidine dehydrogenase (DPD) E88.89
disaccharidase E73.9
edema — see Malnutrition, severe
endocrine E34.9
energy-supply — see Malnutrition
enzymes, circulating NEC E88.09
ergosterol E55.9
  with
    adult osteomalacia M83.8
    rickets — see Rickets
essential fatty acid (EFA) E63.0
factor (see also Deficiency, coagulation)
  Hageman D68.2
  I (congenital) (hereditary) D68.2
  II (congenital) (hereditary) D68.2
  IX (congenital) (functional) (hereditary) (with functional defect) D67
  multiple (congenital) D68.8
    acquired D68.4

Deficiency, deficient — continued
factor (see also Deficiency, coagulation) — continued
  V (congenital) (hereditary) D68.2
  VII (congenital) (hereditary) D68.2
  VIII (congenital) (functional) (hereditary) (with functional defect) D66
    with vascular defect D68.0
  X (congenital) (hereditary) D68.2
  XI (congenital) (hereditary) D68.1
  XII (congenital) (hereditary) D68.2
  XIII (congenital) (hereditary) D68.2
femoral, proximal focal (congenital) — see Defect, reduction, lower limb, longitudinal, femur
fibrinase D68.2
fibrinogen (congenital) (hereditary) D68.2
  acquired D65
fibrin-stabilizing factor (congenital) (hereditary) D68.2
  acquired D68.4
folate E53.8
folic acid E53.8
foreskin N47.3
fructokinase E74.11
fructose 1,6-diphosphatase E74.19
fructose-1-phosphate aldolase E74.19
galactokinase E74.29
galactose-1-phosphate uridyl transferase E74.29
gammaglobulin in blood D80.1
  hereditary D80.0
glass factor D68.2
glucocorticoid E27.49
  mineralocorticoid E27.49
glucose-6-phosphatase E74.01
glucose-6-phosphate dehydrogenase anemia D55.0
glucuronyl transferase E80.5
glycogen synthetase E74.09
gonadotropin (isolated) E23.0
growth hormone (idiopathic) (isolated) E23.0
Hageman factor D68.2
hemoglobin D64.9
hepatophosphorylase E74.09
homogentisate 1,2-dioxygenase E70.29
hormone
  anterior pituitary (partial) NEC E23.0
    growth E23.0
  growth (isolated) E23.0
  pituitary E23.0
  testicular E29.1
hypoxanthine- (guanine)-phosphoribosyltransferase (HG- PRT) (total H-PRT) E79.1
immunity D84.9
  cell-mediated D84.8
    with thrombocytopenia and eczema D82.0
  combined D81.9
  humoral D80.9
  IgA (secretory) D80.2
  IgG D80.3
  IgM D80.4
immuno — see Immunodeficiency
immunoglobulin, selective
  A (IgA) D80.2
  G (IgG) (subclasses) D80.3
  M (IgM) D80.4
inositol (B complex) E53.8
intrinsic
  factor (congenital) D51.0
  sphincter N36.42
    with urethral hypermobility N36.43
iodine E61.8
  congenital syndrome — see Syndrome, iodine-deficiency, congenital
iron E61.1
  anemia D50.9
kalium E87.6
kappa-light chain D80.8
labile factor (congenital) (hereditary) D68.2
  acquired D68.4
lacrimal fluid (acquired) (see also Syndrome, dry eye)
  congenital Q10.6
lactase
  congenital E73.0
  secondary E73.1
Laki-Lorand factor D68.2
lecithin cholesterol acyltransferase E78.6
lipocaic K86.8
lipoprotein (familial) (high density) E78.6
liver phosphorylase E74.09
lysosomal alpha-1, 4 glucosidase E74.02

Deficiency, deficient — continued
magnesium E61.2
major histocompatibility complex
  class I D81.6
  class II D81.7
manganese E61.3
menadione (vitamin K) E56.1
  newborn P53
mental (familial) (hereditary) — see Disability, intellectual
methylenetetrahydrofolate reductase (MTHFR) E72.12
mineralocorticoid E27.49
  with glucocorticoid E27.49
mineral NEC E61.8
molybdenum (nutritional) E61.5
moral F60.2
multiple nutrient elements E61.7
muscle
  carnitine (palmityltransferase) E71.314
  phosphofructokinase E74.09
myoadenylate deaminase E79.2
myocardial — see Insufficiency, myocardial
myophosphorylase E74.04
NADH diaphorase or reductase (congenital) D74.0
NADH-methemoglobin reductase (congenital) D74.0
natrium E87.1
niacin (amide) (-tryptophan) E52
nicotinamide E52
nicotinic acid E52
number of teeth — see Anodontia
nutrient element E61.9
  multiple E61.7
  specified NEC E61.8
nutrition, nutritional E63.9
  sequelae — see Sequelae, nutritional deficiency
  specified NEC E63.8
ornithine transcarbamylase E72.4
ovarian E28.39
oxygen — see Anoxia
pantothenic acid E53.8
parathyroid (gland) E20.9
perineum (female) N81.89
phenylalanine hydroxylase E70.1
phosphoenolpyruvate carboxykinase E74.4
phosphofructokinase E74.19
phosphomannomutase E74.8
phosphomannose isomerase E74.8
phosphomannosyl mutase E74.8
phosphorylase kinase, liver E74.09
pituitary hormone (isolated) E23.0
plasma thromboplastin
  antecedent (PTA) D68.1
  component (PTC) D67
platelet NEC D69.1
  constitutional D68.0
polyglandular E31.8
  autoimmune E31.0
potassium (K) E87.6
prepuce N47.3
proaccelerin (congenital) (hereditary) D68.2
  acquired D68.4
proconvertin factor (congenital) (hereditary) D68.2
  acquired D68.4
protein (see also Malnutrition) E46
  anemia D53.0
  C D68.59
  S D68.59
prothrombin (congenital) (hereditary) D68.2
  acquired D68.4
Prower factor D68.2
pseudocholinesterase E88.09
PTA (plasma thromboplastin antecedent) D68.1
PTC (plasma thromboplastin component) D67
purine nucleoside phosphorylase (PNP) D81.5
pyracin (alpha) (beta) E53.1
pyridoxal E53.1
pyridoxamine E53.1
pyridoxine (derivatives) E53.1
pyruvate
  carboxylase E74.4
  dehydrogenase E74.4
riboflavin (vitamin B2) E53.0
salt E87.1
secretion
  ovary E28.39
  salivary gland (any) K11.7
  urine R34
selenium (dietary) E59

Deficiency, deficient — *continued*
  serum antitrypsin, familial E88.01
  short stature homeobox gene (SHOX)
    with
      dyschondrosteosis Q78.8
      short stature (idiopathic) E34.3
      Turner's syndrome Q96.9
  sodium (Na) E87.1
  SPCA (factor VII) D68.2
  sphincter, intrinsic N36.42
    with urethral hypermobility N36.43
  stable factor (congenital) (hereditary) D68.2
    acquired D68.4
  Stuart-Prower (factor X) D68.2
  sucrase E74.39
  sulfatase E75.29
  sulfite oxidase E72.19
  thiamin, thiaminic (chloride) E51.9
    beriberi (dry) E51.11
      wet E51.12
  thrombokinase D68.2
    newborn P53
  thyroid (gland) — *see* Hypothyroidism
  tocopherol E56.0
  tooth bud K00.0
  transcobalamine II (anemia) D51.2
  vanadium E61.6
  vascular I99.9
  vasopressin E23.2
  viosterol — *see* Deficiency, calciferol
  vitamin (multiple) NOS E56.9
    A E50.9
      with
        Bitot's spot (corneal) E50.1
        follicular keratosis E50.8
        keratomalacia E50.4
        manifestations NEC E50.8
        night blindness E50.5
        scar of cornea, xerophthalmic E50.6
        xeroderma E50.8
        xerophthalmia E50.7
        xerosis
          conjunctival E50.0
            and Bitot's spot E50.1
          cornea E50.2
            and ulceration E50.3
      sequelae E64.1
    B (complex) NOS E53.9
      with
        beriberi (dry) E51.11
          wet E51.12
        pellagra E52
    B1 NOS E51.9
      beriberi (dry) E51.11
        with circulatory system manifestations
          E51.11
        wet E51.12
    B2 (riboflavin) E53.0
    B6 E53.1
    B12 E53.8
    C E54
      sequelae E64.2
    D E55.9
      with
        adult osteomalacia M83.8
        rickets — *see* Rickets
      25-hydroxylase E83.32
    E E56.0
    folic acid E53.8
    G E53.0
    group B E53.9
      specified NEC E53.8
    H (biotin) E53.8
    K E56.1
      of newborn P53
    nicotinic E52
    P E56.8
    PP (pellagra-preventing) E52
    specified NEC E56.8
    thiamin E51.9
      beriberi — *see* Beriberi
  zinc, dietary E60
Deficit (*see also* Deficiency)
  attention and concentration R41.840
    disorder — *see* Attention, deficit
  cognitive communication R41.841
  cognitive NEC R41.89

Deficit — *continued*
  cognitive — *continued*
    following
      cerebral infarction I69.31
      cerebrovascular disease I69.91
        specified disease NEC I69.81
      intracerebral hemorrhage I69.11
      nontraumatic intracranial hemorrhage NEC
        I69.21
      subarachnoid hemorrhage I69.01
  concentration R41.840
  executive function R41.844
  frontal lobe R41.844
  neurologic NEC R29.818
    ischemic
      reversible (RIND) I63.9
        prolonged (PRIND) I63.9
  oxygen R09.02
  prolonged reversible ischemic neurologic (PRIND) I63.9
  psychomotor R41.843
  visuospatial R41.842
Deflection
  radius — *see* Deformity, limb, specified type NEC,
    forearm
  septum (acquired) (nasal) (nose) J34.2
  spine — *see* Curvature, spine
  turbinate (nose) J34.2
Defluvium
  capillorum — *see* Alopecia
  ciliorum — *see* Madarosis
  unguium L60.8
Deformity Q89.9
  abdomen, congenital Q89.9
  abdominal wall
    acquired M95.8
    congenital Q79.59
  acquired (unspecified site) M95.9
  adrenal gland Q89.1
  alimentary tract, congenital Q45.9
    upper Q40.9
  ankle (joint) (acquired) (*see also* Deformity, lower
    leg)
    abduction — *see* Contraction, joint, ankle
    congenital Q68.8
    contraction — *see* Contraction, joint, ankle
    specified type NEC — *see* Deformity, limb, foot,
      specified NEC
  anus (acquired) K62.89
    congenital Q43.9
  aorta (arch) (congenital) Q25.4
    acquired I77.89
  aortic
    arch, acquired I77.89
    cusp or valve (congenital) Q23.8
      acquired (*see also* Endocarditis, aortic) I35.8
  arm (acquired) (upper) (*see also* Deformity, limb, upper
    arm)
    congenital Q68.8
    forearm — *see* Deformity, limb, forearm
  artery (congenital) (peripheral) NOS Q27.9
    acquired I77.89
    coronary (acquired) I25.9
      congenital Q24.5
    umbilical Q27.0
  atrial septal Q21.1
  auditory canal (external) (congenital) (*see also* Malfor-
    mation, ear, external)
    acquired — *see* Disorder, ear, external, specified
      type NEC
  auricle
    ear (congenital) (*see also* Malformation, ear, exter-
      nal)
      acquired — *see* Disorder, pinna, deformity
  back — *see* Dorsopathy, deforming
  bile duct (common) (congenital) (hepatic) Q44.5
    acquired K83.8
  biliary duct or passage (congenital) Q44.5
    acquired K83.8
  bladder (neck) (trigone) (sphincter) (acquired) N32.89
    congenital Q64.79
  bone (acquired) NOS M95.9
    congenital Q79.9
    turbinate M95.0
  brain (congenital) Q04.9
    acquired G93.89
    reduction Q04.3
  breast (acquired) N64.89
    congenital Q83.9

Deformity — *continued*
  breast — *continued*
    reconstructed N65.0
  bronchus (congenital) Q32.4
    acquired NEC J98.09
  bursa, congenital Q79.9
  canaliculi (lacrimalis) (acquired) (*see also* Disorder,
    lacrimal system, changes)
    congenital Q10.6
  canthus, acquired — *see* Disorder, eyelid, specified
    type NEC
  capillary (acquired) I78.8
  cardiovascular system, congenital Q28.9
  caruncle, lacrimal (acquired) (*see also* Disorder,
    lacrimal system, changes)
    congenital Q10.6
  cascade, stomach K31.2
  cecum (congenital) Q43.9
    acquired K63.89
  cerebral, acquired G93.89
    congenital Q04.9
  cervix (uterus) (acquired) NEC N88.8
    congenital Q51.9
  cheek (acquired) M95.2
    congenital Q18.9
  chest (acquired) (wall) M95.4
    congenital Q67.8
    sequelae (late effect) of rickets E64.3
  chin (acquired) M95.2
    congenital Q18.9
  choroid (congenital) Q14.3
    acquired H31.8
    plexus Q07.8
      acquired G96.19
  cicatricial — *see* Cicatrix
  cilia, acquired — *see* Disorder, eyelid, specified type
    NEC
  clavicle (acquired) M95.8
    congenital Q68.8
  clitoris (congenital) Q52.6
    acquired N90.89
  clubfoot — *see* Clubfoot
  coccyx (acquired) — *see* subcategory M43.8 ☑
  colon (congenital) Q43.9
    acquired K63.89
  concha (ear), congenital (*see also* Malformation, ear,
    external)
    acquired — *see* Disorder, pinna, deformity
  cornea (acquired) H18.70
    congenital Q13.4
    descemetocele — *see* Descemetocele
    ectasia — *see* Ectasia, cornea
    specified NEC H18.79- ☑
    staphyloma — *see* Staphyloma, cornea
  coronary artery (acquired) I25.9
    congenital Q24.5
  cranium (acquired) — *see* Deformity, skull
  cricoid cartilage (congenital) Q31.8
    acquired J38.7
  cystic duct (congenital) Q44.5
    acquired K82.8
  Dandy-Walker Q03.1
    with spina bifida — *see* Spina bifida
  diaphragm (congenital) Q79.1
    acquired J98.6
  digestive organ NOS Q45.9
  ductus arteriosus Q25.0
  duodenal bulb K31.89
  duodenum (congenital) Q43.9
    acquired K31.89
  dura — *see* Deformity, meninges
  ear (acquired) (*see also* Disorder, pinna, deformity)
    congenital (external) Q17.9
      internal Q16.5
      middle Q16.4
        ossicles Q16.3
      ossicles Q16.3
  ectodermal (congenital) NEC Q84.9
  ejaculatory duct (congenital) Q55.4
    acquired N50.8
  elbow (joint) (acquired) (*see also* Deformity, limb, up-
    per arm)
    congenital Q68.8
    contraction — *see* Contraction, joint, elbow
  endocrine gland NEC Q89.2
  epididymis (congenital) Q55.4
    acquired N50.8
  epiglottis (congenital) Q31.8

Deformity — *continued*
  epiglottis — *continued*
    acquired J38.7
  esophagus (congenital) Q39.9
    acquired K22.8
  eustachian tube (congenital) NEC Q17.8
  eye, congenital Q15.9
  eyebrow (congenital) Q18.8
  eyelid (acquired) (*see also* Disorder, eyelid, specified type NEC)
    congenital Q10.3
  face (acquired) M95.2
    congenital Q18.9
  fallopian tube, acquired N83.8
  femur (acquired) — *see* Deformity, limb, specified type NEC, thigh
  fetal
    with fetopelvic disproportion O33.7
    causing obstructed labor O66.3
  finger (acquired) M20.00- ☑
    boutonniere M20.02- ☑
    congenital Q68.1
    flexion contracture — *see* Contraction, joint, hand
    mallet finger M20.01- ☑
    specified NEC M20.09- ☑
    swan-neck M20.03- ☑
  flexion (joint) (acquired) (*see also* Deformity, limb, flexion) M21.20
    congenital NOS Q74.9
      hip Q65.89
  foot (acquired) (*see also* Deformity, limb, lower leg)
    cavovarus (congenital) Q66.1
    congenital NOS Q66.9
      specified type NEC Q66.89
    specified type NEC — *see* Deformity, limb, foot, specified NEC
    valgus (congenital) Q66.6
      acquired — *see* Deformity, valgus, ankle
    varus (congenital) NEC Q66.3
      acquired — *see* Deformity, varus, ankle
  forearm (acquired) (*see also* Deformity, limb, forearm)
    congenital Q68.8
  forehead (acquired) M95.2
    congenital Q75.8
  frontal bone (acquired) M95.2
    congenital Q75.8
  gallbladder (congenital) Q44.1
    acquired K82.8
  gastrointestinal tract (congenital) NOS Q45.9
    acquired K63.89
  genitalia, genital organ(s) or system NEC
    female (congenital) Q52.9
      acquired N94.89
      external Q52.70
    male (congenital) Q55.9
      acquired N50.8
  globe (eye) (congenital) Q15.8
    acquired H44.89
  gum, acquired NEC K06.8
  hand (acquired) — *see* Deformity, limb, hand
    congenital Q68.1
  head (acquired) M95.2
    congenital Q75.8
  heart (congenital) Q24.9
    septum Q21.9
      auricular Q21.1
      ventricular Q21.0
    valve (congenital) NEC Q24.8
      acquired — *see* Endocarditis
  heel (acquired) — *see* Deformity, foot
  hepatic duct (congenital) Q44.5
    acquired K83.8
  hip (joint) (acquired) (*see also* Deformity, limb, thigh)
    congenital Q65.9
    due to (previous) juvenile osteochondrosis — *see* Coxa, plana
    flexion — *see* Contraction, joint, hip
  hourglass — *see* Contraction, hourglass
  humerus (acquired) M21.82- ☑
    congenital Q74.0
  hypophyseal (congenital) Q89.2
  ileocecal (coil) (valve) (acquired) K63.89
    congenital Q43.9
  ileum (congenital) Q43.9
    acquired K63.89
  ilium (acquired) M95.5
    congenital Q74.2
  integument (congenital) Q84.9

Deformity — *continued*
  intervertebral cartilage or disc (acquired) — *see* Disorder, disc, specified NEC
  intestine (large) (small) (congenital) NOS Q43.9
    acquired K63.89
  intrinsic minus or plus (hand) — *see* Deformity, limb, specified type NEC, forearm
  iris (acquired) H21.89
    congenital Q13.2
  ischium (acquired) M95.5
    congenital Q74.3
  jaw (acquired) (congenital) M26.9
  joint (acquired) NEC M21.90
    congenital Q68.8
    elbow M21.92- ☑
    hand M21.94- ☑
    hip M21.95- ☑
    knee M21.96- ☑
    shoulder M21.92- ☑
    wrist M21.93- ☑
  kidney(s) (calyx) (pelvis) (congenital) Q63.9
    acquired N28.89
    artery (congenital) Q27.2
      acquired I77.89
  Klippel-Feil (brevicollis) Q76.1
  knee (acquired) NEC (*see also* Deformity, limb, lower leg)
    congenital Q68.2
  labium (majus) (minus) (congenital) Q52.79
    acquired N90.89
  lacrimal passages or duct (congenital) NEC Q10.6
    acquired — *see* Disorder, lacrimal system, changes
  larynx (muscle) (congenital) Q31.8
    acquired J38.7
    web (glottic) Q31.0
  leg (upper) (acquired) NEC (*see also* Deformity, limb, thigh)
    congenital Q68.8
    lower leg — *see* Deformity, limb, lower leg
  lens (acquired) H27.8
    congenital Q12.9
  lid (fold) (acquired) (*see also* Disorder, eyelid, specified type NEC)
    congenital Q10.3
  ligament (acquired) — *see* Disorder, ligament
    congenital Q79.9
  limb (acquired) M21.90
    clawfoot M21.53- ☑
    clawhand M21.51- ☑
    clubfoot M21.54- ☑
    clubhand M21.52- ☑
    congenital, except reduction deformity Q74.9
    flat foot M21.4- ☑
    flexion M21.20
      ankle M21.27- ☑
      elbow M21.22- ☑
      finger M21.24- ☑
      hip M21.25- ☑
      knee M21.26- ☑
      shoulder M21.21- ☑
      toe M21.27- ☑
      wrist M21.23- ☑
    foot
      claw — *see* Deformity, limb, clawfoot
      club — *see* Deformity, limb, clubfoot
      drop M21.37- ☑
      flat — *see* Deformity, limb, flat foot
      specified NEC M21.6X- ☑
    forearm M21.93- ☑
    hand M21.94- ☑
    lower leg M21.96- ☑
    specified type NEC M21.80
      forearm M21.83- ☑
      lower leg M21.86- ☑
      thigh M21.85- ☑
      upper arm M21.82- ☑
    thigh M21.95- ☑
    unequal length M21.70
      short site is
        femur M21.75- ☑
        fibula M21.76- ☑
        humerus M21.72- ☑
        radius M21.73- ☑
        tibia M21.76- ☑
        ulna M21.73- ☑
    upper arm M21.92- ☑
    valgus — *see* Deformity, valgus

Deformity — *continued*
  limb — *continued*
    varus — *see* Deformity, varus
    wrist drop M21.33- ☑
  lip (acquired) NEC K13.0
    congenital Q38.0
  liver (congenital) Q44.7
    acquired K76.89
  lumbosacral (congenital) (joint) (region) Q76.49
    acquired — *see* subcategory M43.8 ☑
    kyphosis — *see* Kyphosis, congenital
    lordosis — *see* Lordosis, congenital
  lung (congenital) Q33.9
    acquired J98.4
  lymphatic system, congenital Q89.9
  Madelung's (radius) Q74.0
  mandible (acquired) (congenital) M26.9
  maxilla (acquired) (congenital) M26.9
  meninges or membrane (congenital) Q07.9
    cerebral Q04.8
      acquired G96.19
    spinal cord (congenital) G96.19
      acquired G96.19
  metacarpus (acquired) — *see* Deformity, limb, forearm
    congenital Q74.0
  metatarsus (acquired) — *see* Deformity, foot
    congenital Q66.9
  middle ear (congenital) Q16.4
    ossicles Q16.3
  mitral (leaflets) (valve) I05.8
    parachute Q23.2
    stenosis, congenital Q23.2
  mouth (acquired) K13.79
    congenital Q38.6
  multiple, congenital NEC Q89.7
  muscle (acquired) M62.89
    congenital Q79.9
      sternocleidomastoid Q68.0
  musculoskeletal system (acquired) M95.9
    congenital Q79.9
    specified NEC M95.8
  nail (acquired) L60.8
    congenital Q84.6
  nasal — *see* Deformity, nose
  neck (acquired) M95.3
    congenital Q18.9
      sternocleidomastoid Q68.0
  nervous system (congenital) Q07.9
  nipple (congenital) Q83.9
    acquired N64.89
  nose (acquired) (cartilage) M95.0
    bone (turbinate) M95.0
    congenital Q30.9
      bent or squashed Q67.4
    saddle M95.0
      syphilitic A50.57
    septum (acquired) J34.2
      congenital Q30.8
    sinus (wall) (congenital) Q30.8
      acquired M95.0
    syphilitic (congenital) A50.57
      late A52.73
  ocular muscle (congenital) Q10.3
    acquired — *see* Strabismus, mechanical
  opticociliary vessels (congenital) Q13.2
  orbit (eye) (acquired) H05.30
    atrophy — *see* Atrophy, orbit
    congenital Q10.7
    due to
      bone disease NEC H05.32- ☑
      trauma or surgery H05.33- ☑
    enlargement — *see* Enlargement, orbit
    exostosis — *see* Exostosis, orbit
  organ of Corti (congenital) Q16.5
  ovary (congenital) Q50.39
    acquired N83.8
  oviduct, acquired N83.8
  palate (congenital) Q38.5
    acquired M27.8
    cleft (congenital) — *see* Cleft, palate
  pancreas (congenital) Q45.3
    acquired K86.8
  parathyroid (gland) Q89.2
  parotid (gland) (congenital) Q38.4
    acquired K11.8
  patella (acquired) — *see* Disorder, patella, specified NEC
  pelvis, pelvic (acquired) (bony) M95.5

Deformity — *continued*
　pelvis, pelvic — *continued*
　　with disproportion (fetopelvic) O33.0
　　　causing obstructed labor O65.0
　　congenital Q74.2
　　rachitic sequelae (late effect) E64.3
　penis (glans) (congenital) Q55.69
　　acquired N48.89
　pericardium (congenital) Q24.8
　　acquired — *see* Pericarditis
　pharynx (congenital) Q38.8
　　acquired J39.2
　pinna, acquired (*see also* Disorder, pinna, deformity)
　　congenital Q17.9
　pituitary (congenital) Q89.2
　posture — *see* Dorsopathy, deforming
　prepuce (congenital) Q55.69
　　acquired N47.8
　prostate (congenital) Q55.4
　　acquired N42.89
　pupil (congenital) Q13.2
　　acquired — *see* Abnormality, pupillary
　pylorus (congenital) Q40.3
　　acquired K31.89
　rachitic (acquired), old or healed E64.3
　radius (acquired) (*see also* Deformity, limb, forearm)
　　congenital Q68.8
　rectum (congenital) Q43.9
　　acquired K62.89
　reduction (extremity) (limb), congenital (*see also* condition and site) Q73.8
　　brain Q04.3
　　lower — *see* Defect, reduction, lower limb
　　upper — *see* Defect, reduction, upper limb
　renal — *see* Deformity, kidney
　respiratory system (congenital) Q34.9
　rib (acquired) M95.4
　　congenital Q76.6
　　cervical Q76.5
　rotation (joint) (acquired) — *see* Deformity, limb, specified site NEC
　　congenital Q74.9
　　hip — *see* Deformity, limb, specified type NEC, thigh
　　congenital Q65.89
　sacroiliac joint (congenital) — *see* subcategory Q74.2
　　acquired — *see* subcategory M43.8 ☑
　sacrum (acquired) — *see* subcategory M43.8 ☑
　saddle
　　back — *see* Lordosis
　　nose M95.0
　　　syphilitic A50.57
　salivary gland or duct (congenital) Q38.4
　　acquired K11.8
　scapula (acquired) M95.8
　　congenital Q68.8
　scrotum (congenital) (*see also* Malformation, testis and scrotum)
　　acquired N50.8
　seminal vesicles (congenital) Q55.4
　　acquired N50.8
　septum, nasal (acquired) J34.2
　shoulder (joint) (acquired) — *see* Deformity, limb, upper arm
　　congenital Q74.0
　　contraction — *see* Contraction, joint, shoulder
　sigmoid (flexure) (congenital) Q43.9
　　acquired K63.89
　skin (congenital) Q82.9
　skull (acquired) M95.2
　　congenital Q75.8
　　　with
　　　　anencephaly Q00.0
　　　　encephalocele — *see* Encephalocele
　　　　hydrocephalus Q03.9
　　　　　with spina bifida — *see* Spina bifida, by site, with hydrocephalus
　　　　microcephaly Q02
　soft parts, organs or tissues (of pelvis)
　　in pregnancy or childbirth NEC O34.8- ☑
　　　causing obstructed labor O65.5
　spermatic cord (congenital) Q55.4
　　acquired N50.8
　　torsion — *see* Torsion, spermatic cord
　spinal — *see* Dorsopathy, deforming
　　column (acquired) — *see* Dorsopathy, deforming
　　congenital Q67.5
　　cord (congenital) Q06.9

Deformity — *continued*
　spinal — *see* Dorsopathy, deforming — *continued*
　　cord — *continued*
　　　acquired G95.89
　　　nerve root (congenital) Q07.9
　spine (acquired) (*see also* Dorsopathy, deforming)
　　congenital Q67.5
　　rachitic E64.3
　　specified NEC — *see* Dorsopathy, deforming, specified NEC
　spleen
　　acquired D73.89
　　congenital Q89.09
　Sprengel's (congenital) Q74.0
　sternocleidomastoid (muscle), congenital Q68.0
　sternum (acquired) M95.4
　　congenital NEC Q76.7
　stomach (congenital) Q40.3
　　acquired K31.89
　submandibular gland (congenital) Q38.4
　submaxillary gland (congenital) Q38.4
　　acquired K11.8
　talipes — *see* Talipes
　testis (congenital) (*see also* Malformation, testis and scrotum)
　　acquired N44.8
　　　torsion — *see* Torsion, testis
　thigh (acquired) (*see also* Deformity, limb, thigh)
　　congenital NEC Q68.8
　thorax (acquired) (wall) M95.4
　　congenital Q67.8
　　sequelae of rickets E64.3
　thumb (acquired) (*see also* Deformity, finger)
　　congenital NEC Q68.1
　thymus (tissue) (congenital) Q89.2
　thyroid (gland) (congenital) Q89.2
　　cartilage Q31.8
　　acquired J38.7
　tibia (acquired) (*see also* Deformity, limb, specified type NEC, lower leg)
　　congenital NEC Q68.8
　　saber (syphilitic) A50.56
　toe (acquired) M20.6- ☑
　　congenital Q66.9
　　hallux rigidus M20.2- ☑
　　hallux valgus M20.1- ☑
　　hallux varus M20.3- ☑
　　hammer toe M20.4- ☑
　　specified NEC M20.5X- ☑
　tongue (congenital) Q38.3
　　acquired K14.8
　tooth, teeth K00.2
　trachea (rings) (congenital) Q32.1
　　acquired J39.8
　transverse aortic arch (congenital) Q25.4
　tricuspid (leaflets) (valve) I07.8
　　atresia or stenosis Q22.4
　　Ebstein's Q22.5
　trunk (acquired) M95.8
　　congenital Q89.9
　ulna (acquired) (*see also* Deformity, limb, forearm)
　　congenital NEC Q68.8
　urachus, congenital Q64.4
　ureter (opening) (congenital) Q62.8
　　acquired N28.89
　urethra (congenital) Q64.79
　　acquired N36.8
　urinary tract (congenital) Q64.9
　　urachus Q64.4
　uterus (congenital) Q51.9
　　acquired N85.8
　uvula (congenital) Q38.5
　vagina (acquired) N89.8
　　congenital Q52.4
　valgus NEC M21.00
　　ankle M21.07- ☑
　　elbow M21.02- ☑
　　hip M21.05- ☑
　　knee M21.06- ☑
　valve, valvular (congenital) (heart) Q24.8
　　acquired — *see* Endocarditis
　varus NEC M21.10
　　ankle M21.17- ☑
　　elbow M21.12- ☑
　　hip M21.15 ☑
　　knee M21.16- ☑
　　tibia — *see* Osteochondrosis, juvenile, tibia

Deformity — *continued*
　vas deferens (congenital) Q55.4
　　acquired N50.8
　vein (congenital) Q27.9
　　great Q26.9
　vertebra — *see* Dorsopathy, deforming
　vertical talus (congenital) Q66.80
　　left foot Q66.82
　　right foot Q66.81
　vesicourethral orifice (acquired) N32.89
　　congenital NEC Q64.79
　vessels of optic papilla (congenital) Q14.2
　visual field (contraction) — *see* Defect, visual field
　vitreous body, acquired H43.89
　vulva (congenital) Q52.79
　　acquired N90.89
　wrist (joint) (acquired) (*see also* Deformity, limb, forearm)
　　congenital Q68.8
　　contraction — *see* Contraction, joint, wrist

Degeneration, degenerative
　adrenal (capsule) (fatty) (gland) (hyaline) (infectional) E27.8
　amyloid (*see also* Amyloidosis) E85.9
　anterior cornua, spinal cord G12.29
　anterior labral S43.49- ☑
　aorta, aortic I70.0
　　fatty I77.89
　aortic valve (heart) — *see* Endocarditis, aortic
　arteriovascular — *see* Arteriosclerosis
　artery, arterial (atheromatous) (calcareous) (*see also* Arteriosclerosis)
　　cerebral, amyloid E85.4 [I68.0]
　　medial — *see* Arteriosclerosis, extremities
　articular cartilage NEC — *see* Derangement, joint, articular cartilage, by site
　atheromatous — *see* Arteriosclerosis
　basal nuclei or ganglia G23.9
　　specified NEC G23.8
　bone NEC — *see* Disorder, bone, specified type NEC
　brachial plexus G54.0
　brain (cortical) (progressive) G31.9
　　alcoholic G31.2
　　arteriosclerotic I67.2
　　childhood G31.9
　　　specified NEC G31.89
　　cystic G31.89
　　　congenital Q04.6
　　in
　　　alcoholism G31.2
　　　beriberi E51.2
　　　cerebrovascular disease I67.9
　　　congenital hydrocephalus Q03.9
　　　　with spina bifida (*see also* Spina bifida)
　　　Fabry-Anderson disease E75.21
　　　Gaucher's disease E75.22
　　　Hunter's syndrome E76.1
　　　lipidosis
　　　　cerebral E75.4
　　　　generalized E75.6
　　　mucopolysaccharidosis — *see* Mucopolysaccharidosis
　　　myxedema E03.9 [G32.89]
　　　neoplastic disease (*see also* Neoplasm) D49.6 [G32.89]
　　　Niemann-Pick disease E75.249 [G32.89]
　　　sphingolipidosis E75.3 [G32.89]
　　　vitamin B12 deficiency E53.8 [G32.89]
　　senile NEC G31.1
　breast N64.89
　Bruch's membrane — *see* Degeneration, choroid
　capillaries (fatty) I78.8
　　amyloid E85.8 [I79.8]
　cardiac (*see also* Degeneration, myocardial)
　　valve, valvular — *see* Endocarditis
　cardiorenal — *see* Hypertension, cardiorenal
　cardiovascular (*see also* Disease, cardiovascular)
　　renal — *see* Hypertension, cardiorenal
　cerebellar NOS G31.9
　　alcoholic G31.2
　　primary (hereditary) (sporadic) G11.9
　cerebral — *see* Degeneration, brain
　cerebrovascular I67.9
　　due to hypertension I67.4
　cervical plexus G54.2
　cervix N88.8
　　due to radiation (intended effect) N88.8
　　　adverse effect or misadventure N99.89

Degeneration, degenerative — *continued*
chamber angle H21.21- ☑
changes, spine or vertebra — *see* Spondylosis
chorioretinal (*see also* Degeneration, choroid)
   hereditary H31.20
choroid (colloid) (drusen) H31.10- ☑
   atrophy — *see* Atrophy, choroidal
   hereditary — *see* Dystrophy, choroidal, hereditary
ciliary body H21.22- ☑
cochlear — *see* subcategory H83.8 ☑
combined (spinal cord) (subacute) E53.8 [G32.0]
   with anemia (pernicious) D51.0 [G32.0]
      due to dietary vitamin B12 deficiency
         D51.3 [G32.0]
   in (due to)
      vitamin B12 deficiency E53.8 [G32.0]
         anemia D51.9 [G32.0]
conjunctiva H11.10
   concretions — *see* Concretion, conjunctiva
   deposits — *see* Deposit, conjunctiva
   pigmentations — *see* Pigmentation, conjunctiva
   pinguecula — *see* Pinguecula
   xerosis — *see* Xerosis, conjunctiva
cornea H18.40
   calcerous H18.43
      band keratopathy H18.42- ☑
   familial, hereditary — *see* Dystrophy, cornea
   hyaline (of old scars) H18.49
   keratomalacia — *see* Keratomalacia
   nodular H18.45- ☑
   peripheral H18.46- ☑
   senile H18.41- ☑
   specified type NEC H18.49
cortical (cerebellar) (parenchymatous) G31.89
   alcoholic G31.2
   diffuse, due to arteriopathy I67.2
corticobasal G31.85
cutis L98.8
   amyloid E85.4 [L99]
dental pulp K04.2
disc disease — *see* Degeneration, intervertebral disc
   NEC
dorsolateral (spinal cord) — *see* Degeneration, combined
extrapyramidal G25.9
eye, macular (*see also* Degeneration, macula)
   congenital or hereditary — *see* Dystrophy, retina
facet joints — *see* Spondylosis
fatty
   liver NEC K76.0
      alcoholic K70.0
grey matter (brain) (Alpers') G31.81
heart (*see also* Degeneration, myocardial)
   amyloid E85.4 [I43]
   atheromatous — *see* Disease, heart, ischemic, atherosclerotic
   ischemic — *see* Disease, heart, ischemic
hepatolenticular (Wilson's) E83.01
hepatorenal K76.7
hyaline (diffuse) (generalized)
   localized — *see* Degeneration, by site
infrapatellar fat pad M79.4
intervertebral disc NOS
   with
      myelopathy — *see* Disorder, disc, with, myelopathy
      radiculitis or radiculopathy — *see* Disorder, disc, with, radiculopathy
   cervical, cervicothoracic — *see* Disorder, disc, cervical, degeneration
      with
         myelopathy — *see* Disorder, disc, cervical, with myelopathy
         neuritis, radiculitis or radiculopathy — *see* Disorder, disc, cervical, with neuritis
   lumbar region M51.36
      with
         myelopathy M51.06
         neuritis, radiculitis, radiculopathy or sciatica M51.16
   lumbosacral region M51.37
      with
         neuritis, radiculitis, radiculopathy or sciatica M51.17
   sacrococcygeal region M53.3
   thoracic region M51.34

Degeneration, degenerative — *continued*
intervertebral disc — *continued*
   thoracic region — *continued*
      with
         myelopathy M51.04
         neuritis, radiculitis, radiculopathy M51.14
   thoracolumbar region M51.35
      with
         myelopathy M51.05
         neuritis, radiculitis, radiculopathy M51.15
intestine, amyloid E85.4
iris (pigmentary) H21.23- ☑
ischemic — *see* Ischemia
joint disease — *see* Osteoarthritis
kidney N28.89
   amyloid E85.4 [N29]
   cystic, congenital Q61.9
   fatty N28.89
   polycystic Q61.3
      adult type (autosomal dominant) Q61.2
      infantile type (autosomal recessive) NEC Q61.19
         collecting duct dilatation Q61.11
Kuhnt-Junius (*see also* Degeneration, macula) H35.32
lens — *see* Cataract
lenticular (familial) (progressive) (Wilson's) (with cirrhosis of liver) E83.01
liver (diffuse) NEC K76.89
   amyloid E85.4 [K77]
   cystic K76.89
      congenital Q44.6
   fatty NEC K76.0
      alcoholic K70.0
   hypertrophic K76.89
   parenchymatous, acute or subacute K72.00
      with coma K72.01
   pigmentary K76.89
   toxic (acute) K71.9
lung J98.4
lymph gland I89.8
   hyaline I89.8
macula, macular (acquired) (age-related) (senile) H35.30
   angioid streaks H35.33
   atrophic age-related H35.31
   congenital or hereditary — *see* Dystrophy, retina
   cystoid H35.35- ☑
   drusen H35.36- ☑
   exudative H35.32
   hole H35.34- ☑
   nonexudative H35.31
   puckering H35.37- ☑
   toxic H35.38- ☑
membranous labyrinth, congenital (causing impairment of hearing) Q16.5
meniscus — *see* Derangement, meniscus
mitral — *see* Insufficiency, mitral
Mönckeberg's — *see* Arteriosclerosis, extremities
motor centers, senile G31.1
multi-system G90.3
mural — *see* Degeneration, myocardial
muscle (fatty) (fibrous) (hyaline) (progressive) M62.89
   heart — *see* Degeneration, myocardial
myelin, central nervous system G37.9
myocardial, myocardium (fatty) (hyaline) (senile) I51.5
   with rheumatic fever (conditions in I00) I09.0
      active, acute or subacute I01.2
         with chorea I02.0
      inactive or quiescent (with chorea) I09.0
   hypertensive — *see* Hypertension, heart
   rheumatic — *see* Degeneration, myocardial, with rheumatic fever
   syphilitic A52.06
nasal sinus (mucosa) J32.9
   frontal J32.1
   maxillary J32.0
nerve — *see* Disorder, nerve
nervous system G31.9
   alcoholic G31.2
   amyloid E85.4 [G99.8]
   autonomic G90.9
   fatty G31.89
   specified NEC G31.89
nipple N64.89
olivopontocerebellar (hereditary) (familial) G23.8
osseous labyrinth — *see* subcategory H83.8 ☑
ovary N83.8
   cystic N83.20
   microcystic N83.20

Degeneration, degenerative — *continued*
pallidal pigmentary (progressive) G23.0
pancreas K86.8
   tuberculous A18.83
penis N48.89
pigmentary (diffuse) (general)
   localized — *see* Degeneration, by site
   pallidal (progressive) G23.0
pineal gland E34.8
pituitary (gland) E23.6
popliteal fat pad M79.4
posterolateral (spinal cord) — *see* Degeneration, combined
pulmonary valve (heart) I37.8
pulp (tooth) K04.2
pupillary margin H21.24- ☑
renal — *see* Degeneration, kidney
retina H35.9
   hereditary (cerebroretinal) (congenital) (juvenile) (macula) (peripheral) (pigmentary) — *see* Dystrophy, retina
   Kuhnt-Junius (*see also* Degeneration, macula) H35.32
   macula (cystic) (exudative) (hole) (nonexudative) (pseudohole) (senile) (toxic) — *see* Degeneration, macula
   peripheral H35.40
      lattice H35.41- ☑
      microcystoid H35.42- ☑
      paving stone H35.43- ☑
      secondary
         pigmentary H35.45- ☑
         vitreoretinal H35.46- ☑
      senile reticular H35.44- ☑
   pigmentary (primary) (*see also* Dystrophy, retina)
      secondary — *see* Degeneration, retina, peripheral, secondary
   posterior pole — *see* Degeneration, macula
saccule, congenital (causing impairment of hearing) Q16.5
senile R54
   brain G31.1
   cardiac, heart or myocardium — *see* Degeneration, myocardial
   motor centers G31.1
   vascular — *see* Arteriosclerosis
sinus (cystic) (*see also* Sinusitis)
   polypoid J33.1
skin L98.8
   amyloid E85.4 [L99]
   colloid L98.8
spinal (cord) G31.89
   amyloid E85.4 [G32.89]
   combined (subacute) — *see* Degeneration, combined
   dorsolateral — *see* Degeneration, combined
   familial NEC G31.89
   fatty G31.89
   funicular — *see* Degeneration, combined
   posterolateral — *see* Degeneration, combined
   subacute combined — *see* Degeneration, combined
   tuberculous A17.81
spleen D73.0
   amyloid E85.4 [D77]
stomach K31.89
striatonigral G23.2
suprarenal (capsule) (gland) E27.8
synovial membrane (pulpy) — *see* Disorder, synovium, specified type NEC
tapetoretinal — *see* Dystrophy, retina
thymus (gland) E32.8
   fatty E32.8
thyroid (gland) E07.89
tricuspid (heart) (valve) I07.9
tuberculous NEC — *see* Tuberculosis
turbinate J34.89
uterus (cystic) N85.8
vascular (senile) — *see* Arteriosclerosis
   hypertensive — *see* Hypertension
vitreoretinal, secondary — *see* Degeneration, retina, peripheral, secondary, vitreoretinal
vitreous (body) H43.81- ☑
Wallerian — *see* Disorder, nerve
Wilson's hepatolenticular E83.01

Deglutition
paralysis
hysterical F44.4
pneumonia J69.Ø
Degos' disease I77.89
Dehiscence (of)
amputation stump T87.81
cesarean wound O90.0
closure of
cornea T81.31 ☑
craniotomy T81.32 ☑
fascia (muscular) (superficial) T81.32 ☑
internal organ or tissue T81.32 ☑
laceration (external) (internal) T81.33 ☑
ligament T81.32 ☑
mucosa T81.31 ☑
muscle or muscle flap T81.32 ☑
ribs or rib cage T81.32 ☑
skin and subcutaneous tissue (full-thickness) (superficial) T81.31 ☑
skull T81.32 ☑
sternum (sternotomy) T81.32 ☑
tendon T81.32 ☑
traumatic laceration (external) (internal) T81.33 ☑
episiotomy O90.1
operation wound NEC T81.31 ☑
external operation wound (superficial) T81.31 ☑
internal operation wound (deep) T81.32 ☑
perineal wound (postpartum) O90.1
traumatic injury wound repair T81.33 ☑
wound T81.30 ☑
traumatic repair T81.33 ☑
Dehydration E86.Ø
hypertonic E87.Ø
hypotonic E87.1
newborn P74.1
Déjérine-Roussy syndrome G89.Ø
Déjérine-Sottas disease or neuropathy (hypertrophic)
G60.Ø
Déjérine-Thomas atrophy G23.8
Delay, delayed
any plane in pelvis
complicating delivery O66.9
birth or delivery NOS O63.9
closure, ductus arteriosus (Botalli) P29.3
coagulation — see Defect, coagulation
conduction (cardiac) (ventricular) I45.9
delivery, second twin, triplet, etc O63.2
development R62.50
global F88
intellectual (specific) F81.9
language F80.9
due to hearing loss F80.4
learning F81.9
pervasive F84.9
physiological R62.50
specified stage NEC R62.0
reading F81.0
sexual E30.0
speech F80.9
due to hearing loss F80.4
spelling F81.81
gastric emptying K30
menarche E30.0
menstruation (cause unknown) N91.0
milestone R62.0
passage of meconium (newborn) P76.0
primary respiration P28.9
puberty (constitutional) E30.0
separation of umbilical cord P96.82
sexual maturation, female E30.0
sleep phase syndrome G47.21
union, fracture — see Fracture, by site
vaccination Z28.9
Deletion(s)
autosome Q93.9
identified by fluorescence in situ hybridization
(FISH) Q93.89
identified by in situ hybridization (ISH) Q93.89
chromosome
with complex rearrangements NEC Q93.7
part of NEC Q93.5
seen only at prometaphase Q93.89
short arm
22q11.2 Q93.81
4 Q93.3
5p Q93.4

Deletion(s) — continued
chromosome — continued
specified NEC Q93.89
long arm chromosome 18 or 21 Q93.89
with complex rearrangements NEC Q93.7
microdeletions NEC Q93.88
Delhi boil or button B55.1
Delinquency (juvenile) (neurotic) F91.8
group Z72.81Ø
Delinquent immunization status Z28.3
Delirium, delirious (acute or subacute) (not alcohol- or
drug-induced) (with dementia) R41.Ø
alcoholic (acute) (tremens) (withdrawal) F10.921
with intoxication F10.921
in
abuse F10.121
dependence F10.221
due to (secondary to)
alcohol
intoxication F10.921
in
abuse F10.121
dependence F10.221
withdrawal F10.231
amphetamine intoxication F15.921
in
abuse F15.121
dependence F15.221
anxiolytic
intoxication F13.921
in
abuse F13.121
dependence F13.221
withdrawal F13.231
cannabis intoxication (acute) F12.921
in
abuse F12.121
dependence F12.221
cocaine intoxication (acute) F14.921
in
abuse F14.121
dependence F14.221
general medical condition F05
hallucinogen intoxication F16.921
in
abuse F16.121
dependence F16.221
hypnotic
intoxication F13.921
in
abuse F13.121
dependence F13.221
withdrawal F13.231
inhalant intoxication (acute) F18.921
in
abuse F18.121
dependence F18.221
multiple etiologies F05
opioid intoxication (acute) F11.921
in
abuse F11.121
dependence F11.221
phencyclidine intoxication (acute) F16.921
in
abuse F16.121
dependence F16.221
psychoactive substance NEC intoxication (acute)
F19.921
in
abuse F19.121
dependence F19.221
sedative
intoxication F13.921
in
abuse F13.121
dependence F13.221
withdrawal F13.231
unknown etiology F05
exhaustion F43.Ø
hysterical F44.89
postprocedural (postoperative) F05
puerperal F05
thyroid — see Thyrotoxicosis with thyroid storm
traumatic — see Injury, intracranial
tremens (alcohol-induced) F10.231
sedative-induced F13.231
Delivery (childbirth) (labor)
arrested active phase O62.1

Delivery — continued
cesarean (for)
without indication O82
abnormal
pelvis (bony) (deformity) (major) NEC with disproportion (fetopelvic) O33.0
with obstructed labor O65.0
presentation or position O32.9 ☑
abruptio placentae (see also Abruptio placentae)
O45.9-
acromion presentation O32.2 ☑
atony, uterus O62.2
breech presentation O32.1 ☑
incomplete O32.8 ☑
brow presentation O32.3 ☑
cephalopelvic disproportion O33.9
cerclage O34.3- ☑
chin presentation O32.3 ☑
cicatrix of cervix O34.4- ☑
contracted pelvis (general)
inlet O33.2
outlet O33.3 ☑
cord presentation or prolapse O69.0 ☑
cystocele O34.8- ☑
deformity (acquired) (congenital)
pelvic organs or tissues NEC O34.8- ☑
pelvis (bony) NEC O33.0
disproportion NOS O33.9
eclampsia — see Eclampsia
face presentation O32.3 ☑
failed
forceps O66.5
induction of labor O61.9
instrumental O61.1
mechanical O61.1
medical O61.0
specified NEC O61.8
surgical O61.1
trial of labor NOS O66.40
following previous cesarean delivery O66.41
vacuum extraction O66.5
ventouse O66.5
fetal-maternal hemorrhage O43.01- ☑
hemorrhage (intrapartum) O67.9
with coagulation defect O67.0
specified cause NEC O67.8
high head at term O32.4 ☑
hydrocephalic fetus O33.6
incarceration of uterus O34.51- ☑
incoordinate uterine action O62.4
increased size, fetus O33.5
inertia, uterus O62.2
primary O62.0
secondary O62.1
lateroversion, uterus O34.59- ☑
mal lie O32.9 ☑
malposition
fetus O32.9 ☑
pelvic organs or tissues NEC O34.8- ☑
uterus NEC O34.59- ☑
malpresentation NOS O32.9 ☑
oblique presentation O32.2 ☑
occurring after 37 completed weeks of gestation
but before 39 completed weeks gestation
due to (spontaneous) onset of labor O75.82
oversize fetus O33.5 ☑
pelvic tumor NEC O34.8- ☑
placenta previa O44.1- ☑
without hemorrhage O44.0- ☑
placental insufficiency O36.51- ☑
planned, occurring after 37 completed weeks of
gestation but before 39 completed weeks
gestation due to (spontaneous) onset of labor O75.82
polyp, cervix O34.4- ☑
causing obstructed labor O65.5
poor dilatation, cervix O62.0
pre-eclampsia O14.9- ☑
mild O14.0- ☑
moderate O14.0- ☑
severe
with hemolysis, elevated liver enzymes and
low platelet count (HELLP) O14.2- ☑
previous
cesarean delivery O34.21
surgery (to)
cervix O34.4- ☑

Delivery — *continued*
  cesarean — *continued*
    previous — *continued*
      surgery — *continued*
        gynecological NEC O34.8- ☑
        rectum O34.7- ☑
        uterus O34.29
        vagina O34.6- ☑
    prolapse
      arm or hand O32.2 ☑
      uterus O34.52- ☑
    prolonged labor NOS O63.9
    rectocele O34.8- ☑
    retroversion
      uterus O34.53- ☑
    rigid
      cervix O34.4- ☑
      pelvic floor O34.8- ☑
      perineum O34.7- ☑
      vagina O34.6- ☑
      vulva O34.7- ☑
    sacculation, pregnant uterus O34.59- ☑
    scar(s)
      cervix O34.4- ☑
      cesarean delivery O34.21
      uterus O34.29
    Shirodkar suture in situ O34.3- ☑
    shoulder presentation O32.2 ☑
    stenosis or stricture, cervix O34.4- ☑
    streptococcus B carrier state O99.824
    transverse presentation or lie O32.2 ☑
    tumor, pelvic organs or tissues NEC O34.8- ☑
      cervix O34.4- ☑
    umbilical cord presentation or prolapse O69.0 ☑
  completely normal case O80
  complicated O75.9
    by
      abnormal, abnormality (of)
        forces of labor O62.9
          specified type NEC O62.8
        glucose O99.814
        uterine contractions NOS O62.9
      abruptio placentae (*see also* Abruptio placentae) O45.9- ☑
      abuse
        physical O9A.32 (*following* O99)
        psychological O9A.52 (*following* O99)
        sexual O9A.42 (*following* O99)
      adherent placenta O72.0
        without hemorrhage O73.0
      alcohol use O99.314
      anemia (pre-existing) O99.02
      anesthetic death O74.8
      annular detachment of cervix O71.3
      atony, uterus O62.2
      attempted vacuum extraction and forceps O66.5
      Bandl's ring O62.4
      bariatric surgery status O99.844
      biliary tract disorder O26.62
      bleeding — *see* Delivery, complicated by, hemorrhage
      blood disorder NEC O99.12
      cervical dystocia (hypotonic) O62.2
        primary O62.0
        secondary O62.1
      circulatory system disorder O99.42
      compression of cord (umbilical) NEC O69.2 ☑
      condition NEC O99.89
      contraction, contracted ring O62.4
      cord (umbilical)
        around neck
          with compression O69.1 ☑
          without compression O69.81 ☑
        bruising O69.5 ☑
        complication O69.9 ☑
          specified NEC O69.89 ☑
        compression NEC O69.2 ☑
        entanglement O69.2 ☑
          without compression O69.82 ☑
        hematoma O69.5 ☑
        presentation O69.0 ☑
        prolapse O69.0 ☑
        short O69.3 ☑
        thrombosis (vessels) O69.5 ☑
        vascular lesion O69.5 ☑
      Couvelaire uterus O45.8X- ☑

Delivery — *continued*
  complicated — *continued*
    by — *continued*
      damage to (injury to) NEC
        perineum O71.82
        periurethral tissue O71.82
        vulva O71.82
      delay following rupture of membranes (spontaneous) — *see* Pregnancy, complicated by, premature rupture of membranes
      depressed fetal heart tones O76
      diabetes O24.92
        gestational O24.429
          diet controlled O24.420
          insulin controlled O24.424
        pre-existing O24.32
          specified NEC O24.82
          type 1 O24.02
          type 2 O24.12
      diastasis recti (abdominis) O71.89
      dilatation
        bladder O66.8
        cervix incomplete, poor or slow O62.0
      disease NEC O99.89
      disruptio uteri — *see* Delivery, complicated by, rupture, uterus
      drug use O99.324
      dysfunction, uterus NOS O62.9
        hypertonic O62.4
        hypotonic O62.2
          primary O62.0
          secondary O62.1
        incoordinate O62.4
      eclampsia O15.1
      embolism (pulmonary) — *see* Embolism, obstetric
      endocrine, nutritional or metabolic disease NEC O99.284
      failed
        attempted vaginal birth after previous cesarean delivery O66.41
        induction of labor O61.9
          instrumental O61.1
          mechanical O61.1
          medical O61.0
          specified NEC O61.8
          surgical O61.1
        trial of labor O66.40
      female genital mutilation O65.5
      fetal
        abnormal acid-base balance O68
        acidemia O68
        acidosis O68
        alkalosis O68
        death, early O02.1
        deformity O66.3
        heart rate or rhythm (abnormal) (non-reassuring) O76
        hypoxia O77.8
        stress O77.9
          due to drug administration O77.1
          electrocardiographic evidence of O77.8
          specified NEC O77.8
          ultrasound evidence of O77.8
      fever during labor O75.2
      gastric banding status O99.844
      gastric bypass status O99.844
      gastrointestinal disease NEC O99.62
      gestational diabetes O24.429
        diet controlled O24.420
        insulin (and diet) controlled O24.424
      gonorrhea O98.22
      hematoma O71.7
        ischial spine O71.7
        pelvic O71.7
        vagina O71.7
        vulva or perineum O71.7
      hemorrhage (uterine) O67.9
        associated with
          afibrinogenemia O67.0
          coagulation defect O67.0
          hyperfibrinolysis O67.0
          hypofibrinogenemia O67.0
        due to
          low-lying placenta O44.1- ☑
          placenta previa O44.1- ☑

Delivery — *continued*
  complicated — *continued*
    by — *continued*
      hemorrhage — *continued*
        due to — *continued*
          premature separation of placenta (normally implanted) (*see also* Abruptio placentae) O45.9- ☑
          retained placenta O72.0
          uterine leiomyoma O67.8
        placenta NEC O67.8
        postpartum NEC (atonic) (immediate) O72.1
          with retained or trapped placenta O72.0
          delayed O72.2
          secondary O72.2
          third stage O72.0
      hourglass contraction, uterus O62.4
      hypertension, hypertensive (pre-existing) — *see* Hypertension, complicated by, childbirth (labor)
      hypotension O26.5- ☑
      incomplete dilatation (cervix) O62.0
      incoordinate uterus contractions O62.4
      inertia, uterus O62.2
        during latent phase of labor O62.0
        primary O62.0
        secondary O62.1
      infection (maternal) O98.92
        carrier state NEC O99.834
        gonorrhea O98.22
        human immunodeficiency virus (HIV) O98.72
        sexually transmitted NEC O98.32
        specified NEC O98.82
        syphilis O98.12
        tuberculosis O98.02
        viral hepatitis O98.42
        viral NEC O98.52
      injury (to mother) (*see also* Delivery, complicated, by, damage to) O71.9
        nonobstetric O9A.22 (*following* O99)
          caused by abuse — *see* Delivery, complicated by, abuse
      intrauterine fetal death, early O02.1
      inversion, uterus O71.2
      laceration (perineal) O70.9
        anus (sphincter) O70.4
          with third degree laceration O70.2
            with mucosa O70.3
          without third degree laceration O70.4
        bladder (urinary) O71.5
        bowel O71.5
        cervix (uteri) O71.3
        fourchette O70.0
        hymen O70.0
        labia O70.0
        pelvic
          floor O70.1
          organ NEC O71.5
        perineum, perineal O70.9
          first degree O70.0
          fourth degree O70.3
          muscles O70.1
          second degree O70.1
          skin O70.0
          slight O70.0
          third degree O70.2
        peritoneum (pelvic) O71.5
        rectovaginal (septum) (without perineal laceration) O71.4
          with perineum O70.2
            with anal or rectal mucosa O70.3
        specified NEC O71.89
        sphincter ani — *see* Delivery, complicated, by, laceration, anus (sphincter)
        urethra O71.5
        uterus O71.81
          before labor O71.81
        vagina, vaginal (deep) (high) (without perineal laceration) O71.4
          with perineum O70.0
          muscles, with perineum O70.1
        vulva O70.0
      liver disorder O26.62
      malignancy O9A.12 (*following* O99)
      malnutrition O25.2

Delivery — *continued*
　complicated — *continued*
　　by — *continued*
　　　malposition, malpresentation
　　　　without obstruction (*see also* Delivery,
　　　　　complicated by, obstruction) O32.9 ☑
　　　　　breech O32.1 ☑
　　　　　compound O32.6 ☑
　　　　　face (brow) (chin) O32.3 ☑
　　　　　footling O32.8 ☑
　　　　　high head O32.4 ☑
　　　　　oblique O32.2 ☑
　　　　　specified NEC O32.8 ☑
　　　　　transverse O32.2 ☑
　　　　　unstable lie O32.0 ☑
　　　　placenta (with hemorrhage) O44.1- ☑
　　　　　without hemorrhage O44.0- ☑
　　　　uterus or cervix O65.5
　　　meconium in amniotic fluid O77.0
　　　mental disorder NEC O99.344
　　　metrorrhexis — *see* Delivery, complicated by,
　　　　rupture, uterus
　　　nervous system disorder O99.354
　　　obesity (pre-existing) O99.214
　　　obesity surgery status O99.844
　　　obstetric trauma O71.9
　　　　specified NEC O71.89
　　　obstructed labor
　　　　due to
　　　　　breech (complete) (frank) presentation
　　　　　　O64.1 ☑
　　　　　　incomplete O64.8 ☑
　　　　　brow presenation O64.3 ☑
　　　　　buttock presentation O64.1 ☑
　　　　　chin presentation O64.2 ☑
　　　　　compound presentation O64.5 ☑
　　　　　contracted pelvis O65.1
　　　　　deep transverse arrest O64.0 ☑
　　　　　deformed pelvis O65.0
　　　　　dystocia (fetal) O66.9
　　　　　　due to
　　　　　　　conjoined twins O66.3
　　　　　　　fetal
　　　　　　　　abnormality NEC O66.3
　　　　　　　　ascites O66.3
　　　　　　　　hydrops O66.3
　　　　　　　　meningomyelocele O66.3
　　　　　　　　sacral teratoma O66.3
　　　　　　　　tumor O66.3
　　　　　　　hydrocephalic fetus O66.3
　　　　　　　shoulder O66.0
　　　　　face presentation O64.2 ☑
　　　　　fetopelvic disproportion O65.4
　　　　　footling presentation O64.8 ☑
　　　　　impacted shoulders O66.0
　　　　　incomplete rotation of fetal head
　　　　　　O64.0 ☑
　　　　　large fetus O66.2
　　　　　locked twins O66.1
　　　　　malposition O64.9 ☑
　　　　　　specified NEC O64.8 ☑
　　　　　malpresentation O64.9 ☑
　　　　　　specified NEC O64.8 ☑
　　　　　multiple fetuses NEC O66.6
　　　　　pelvic
　　　　　　abnormality (maternal) O65.9
　　　　　　　organ O65.5
　　　　　　　specified NEC O65.8
　　　　　　contraction
　　　　　　　inlet O65.2
　　　　　　　mid-cavity O65.3
　　　　　　　outlet O65.3
　　　　　persistent (position)
　　　　　　occipitoiliac O64.0 ☑
　　　　　　occipitoposterior O64.0 ☑
　　　　　　occipitosacral O64.0 ☑
　　　　　　occipitotransverse O64.0 ☑
　　　　　prolapsed arm O64.4 ☑
　　　　　shoulder presentation O64.4 ☑
　　　　specified NEC O66.8
　　　pathological retraction ring, uterus O62.4
　　　penetration, pregnant uterus by instrument
　　　　O71.1
　　　perforation — *see* Delivery, complicated by,
　　　　laceration

Delivery — *continued*
　complicated — *continued*
　　by — *continued*
　　　placenta, placental
　　　　ablatio (*see also* Abruptio placentae)
　　　　　O45.9- ☑
　　　　abnormality O43.9- ☑
　　　　　specified NEC O43.89- ☑
　　　　abruptio (*see also* Abruptio placentae)
　　　　　O45.9- ☑
　　　　accreta O43.21- ☑
　　　　adherent (with hemorrhage) O72.0
　　　　　without hemorrhage O73.0
　　　　detachment (premature) (*see also* Abruptio
　　　　　placentae) O45.9- ☑
　　　　disorder O43.9- ☑
　　　　　specified NEC O43.89- ☑
　　　　hemorrhage NEC O67.8
　　　　increta O43.22- ☑
　　　　low (implantation) O44.1- ☑
　　　　　without hemorrhage O44.0- ☑
　　　　malformation O43.10- ☑
　　　　malposition O44.1- ☑
　　　　　without hemorrhage O44.0- ☑
　　　　percreta O43.23- ☑
　　　　previa (central) (lateral) (low) (marginal)
　　　　　(partial) (total) O44.1- ☑
　　　　　without hemorrhage O44.0- ☑
　　　　retained (with hemorrhage) O72.0
　　　　　without hemorrhage O73.0
　　　　separation (premature) O45.9- ☑
　　　　　specified NEC O45.8X- ☑
　　　　vicious insertion O44.1- ☑
　　　precipitate labor O62.3
　　　premature rupture, membranes (*see also* Preg-
　　　　nancy, complicated by, premature rup-
　　　　ture of membranes) O42.90
　　　prolapse
　　　　arm or hand O32.2 ☑
　　　　cord (umbilical) O69.0 ☑
　　　　foot or leg O32.8 ☑
　　　　uterus O34.52- ☑
　　　prolonged labor O63.9
　　　　first stage O63.0
　　　　second stage O63.1
　　　protozoal disease (maternal) O98.62
　　　respiratory disease NEC O99.52
　　　retained membranes or portions of placenta
　　　　O72.2
　　　　without hemorrhage O73.1
　　　retarded birth O63.9
　　　retention of secundines (with hemorrhage)
　　　　O72.0
　　　　without hemorrhage O73.0
　　　　partial O72.2
　　　　　without hemorrhage O73.1
　　　rupture
　　　　bladder (urinary) O71.5
　　　　cervix O71.3
　　　　pelvic organ NEC O71.5
　　　　urethra O71.5
　　　　uterus (during or after labor) O71.1
　　　　　before labor O71.0- ☑
　　　separation, pubic bone (symphysis pubis) O71.6
　　　shock O75.1
　　　shoulder presentation O64.4 ☑
　　　skin disorder NEC O99.72
　　　spasm, cervix O62.4
　　　stenosis or stricture, cervix O65.5
　　　streptococcus B carrier state O99.824
　　　subluxation of symphysis (pubis) O26.72
　　　syphilis (maternal) O98.12
　　　tear — *see* Delivery, complicated by, laceration
　　　tetanic uterus O62.4
　　　trauma (obstetrical) (*see also* Delivery, compli-
　　　　cated, by, damage to) O71.9
　　　　non-obstetric O9A.22 (*following* O99)
　　　　periurethral O71.82
　　　　specified NEC O71.89
　　　tuberculosis (maternal) O98.02
　　　tumor, pelvic organs or tissues NEC O65.5
　　　umbilical cord around neck
　　　　with compression O69.1 ☑
　　　　without compression O69.81 ☑
　　　uterine inertia O62.2
　　　　during latent phase of labor O62.0
　　　　primary O62.0

Delivery — *continued*
　complicated — *continued*
　　by — *continued*
　　　uterine inertia — *continued*
　　　　secondary O62.1
　　　vasa previa O69.4 ☑
　　　velamentous insertion of cord O43.12- ☑
　　　specified complication NEC O75.89
　delayed NOS O63.9
　　following rupture of membranes
　　　artificial O75.5
　　second twin, triplet, etc. O63.2
　forceps, low following failed vacuum extraction O66.5
　missed (at or near term) O36.4 ☑
　normal O80
　obstructed — *see* Delivery, complicated by, obstruc-
　　tion
　precipitate O62.3
　preterm (*see also* Pregnancy, complicated by, preterm
　　labor) O60.10 ☑
　spontaneous O80
　term pregnancy NOS O80
　uncomplicated O80
　vaginal, following previous cesarean delivery O34.21
Delusions (paranoid) — *see* Disorder, delusional
Dementia (degenerative (primary)) (old age) (persisting)
　F03.90
　with
　　aggressive behavior F03.91
　　behavioral disturbance F03.91
　　combative behavior F03.91
　　Lewy bodies G31.83 [F02.80]
　　　with behavioral disturbance G31.83 [F02.81]
　　Parkinsonism G31.83 [F02.80]
　　　with behavioral disturbance G31.83 [F02.81]
　　Parkinson's disease G20 [F02.80]
　　　with behavioral disturbance G20 [F02.81]
　　violent behavior F03.91
　alcoholic F10.97
　　with dependence F10.27
　Alzheimer's type — *see* Disease, Alzheimer's
　arteriosclerotic — *see* Dementia, vascular
　atypical, Alzheimer's type — *see* Disease, Alzheimer's,
　　specified NEC
　congenital — *see* Disability, intellectual
　frontal (lobe) G31.09 [F02.80]
　　with behavioral disturbance G31.09 [F02.81]
　frontotemporal G31.09 [F02.80]
　　with behavioral disturbance G31.09 [F02.81]
　　specified NEC G31.09 [F02.80]
　　　with behavioral disturbance G31.09 [F02.81]
　in (due to)
　　with behavioral disturbance G31.83 [F02.81]
　　alcohol F10.97
　　　with dependence F10.27
　　Alzheimer's disease — *see* Disease, Alzheimer's
　　arteriosclerotic brain disease — *see* Dementia,
　　　vascular
　　cerebral lipidoses E75.- ☑ [F02.80]
　　　with behavioral disturbance E75.- ☑ [F02.81]
　　Creutzfeldt-Jakob disease (*see also* Creutzfeldt-
　　　Jakob disease or syndrome (with dementia))
　　　A81.00
　　epilepsy G40.- ☑ [F02.80]
　　　with behavioral disturbance G40.- ☑ [F02.81]
　　hepatolenticular degeneration E83.01 [F02.80]
　　　with behavioral disturbance E83.01 [F02.81]
　　human immunodeficiency virus (HIV) disease
　　　B20 [F02.80]
　　　with behavioral disturbance B20 [F02.81]
　　Huntington's disease or chorea G10
　　hypercalcemia E83.52 [F02.80]
　　　with behavioral disturbance E83.52 [F02.81]
　　hypothyroidism, acquired E03.9 [F02.80]
　　　with behavioral disturbance E03.9 [F02.81]
　　　due to iodine deficiency E01.8 [F02.80]
　　　　with behavioral disturbance E01.8 [F02.81]
　　inhalants F18.97
　　　with dependence F18.27
　　multiple
　　　etiologies F03 ☑
　　　sclerosis G35 [F02.80]
　　　　with behavioral disturbance G35 [F02.81]
　　neurosyphilis A52.17 [F02.80]
　　　with behavioral disturbance A52.17 [F02.81]
　　　juvenile A50.49 [F02.80]
　　　　with behavioral disturbance A50.49 [F02.81]
　　niacin deficiency E52 [F02.80]

Index

Delivery — Dementia

Dementia — *continued*
  in — *continued*
    niacin deficiency — *continued*
      with behavioral disturbance E52 [F02.81]
    paralysis agitans G20 [F02.80]
      with behavioral disturbance G20 [F02.81]
    Parkinson's disease G20 [F02.80]
    pellagra E52 [F02.80]
      with behavioral disturbance E52 [F02.81]
    Pick's G31.01 [F02.80]
      with behavioral disturbance G31.01 [F02.81]
    polyarteritis nodosa M30.0 [F02.80]
      with behavioral disturbance M30.0 [F02.81]
    psychoactive drug F19.97
      with dependence F19.27
        inhalants F18.97
          with dependence F18.27
        sedatives, hypnotics or anxiolytics F13.97
          with dependence F13.27
    sedatives, hypnotics or anxiolytics F13.97
      with dependence F13.27
    systemic lupus erythematosus M32.- ☑ [F02.80]
      with behavioral disturbance M32.- ☑ [F02.81]
    trypanosomiasis
      African B56.9 [F02.80]
        with behavioral disturbance B56.9 [F02.81]
    unknown etiology F03 ☑
    vitamin B12 deficiency E53.8 [F02.80]
      with behavioral disturbance E53.8 [F02.81]
    volatile solvents F18.97
      with dependence F18.27
  infantile, infantilis F84.3
  Lewy body G31.83 [F02.80]
    with behavioral disturbance G31.83 [F02.81]
  multi-infarct — *see* Dementia, vascular
  paralytica, paralytic (syphilitic) A52.17 [F02.80]
    with behavioral disturbance A52.17 [F02.81]
    juvenilis A50.45
  paretic A52.17
  praecox — *see* Schizophrenia
  presenile F03 ☑
    Alzheimer's type — *see* Disease, Alzheimer's, early onset
  primary degenerative F03 ☑
  progressive, syphilitic A52.17
  senile F03 ☑
    with acute confusional state F05
    Alzheimer's type — *see* Disease, Alzheimer's, late onset
    depressed or paranoid type F03 ☑
  vascular (acute onset) (mixed) (multi-infarct) (subcortical) F01.50
    with behavioral disturbance F01.51
Demineralization, bone — *see* Osteoporosis
Demodex folliculorum (infestation) B88.0
Demophobia F40.248
Demoralization R45.3
Demyelination, demyelinization
  central nervous system G37.9
    specified NEC G37.8
  corpus callosum (central) G37.1
  disseminated, acute G36.9
    specified NEC G36.8
  global G35
  in optic neuritis G36.0
Dengue (classical) (fever) A90
  hemorrhagic A91
  sandfly A93.1
Dennie-Marfan syphilitic syndrome A50.45
Dens evaginatus, in dente or invaginatus K00.2
Dense breasts R92.2
Density
  increased, bone (disseminated) (generalized) (spotted) — *see* Disorder, bone, density and structure, specified type NEC
  lung (nodular) J98.4
Dental (*see also* condition)
  examination Z01.20
    with abnormal findings Z01.21
  restoration
    aesthetically inadequate or displeasing K08.56
    defective K08.50
      specified NEC K08.59
    failure of marginal integrity K08.51
    failure of periodontal anatomical integrity K08.54
Dentia praecox K00.6
Denticles (pulp) K04.2
Dentigerous cyst K09.0

Dentin
  irregular (in pulp) K04.3
  opalescent K00.5
  secondary (in pulp) K04.3
  sensitive K03.89
Dentinogenesis imperfecta K00.5
Dentinoma — *see* Cyst, calcifying odontogenic
Dentition (syndrome) K00.7
  delayed K00.6
  difficult K00.7
  precocious K00.6
  premature K00.6
  retarded K00.6
Dependence (on) (syndrome) F19.20
  with remission F19.21
  alcohol (ethyl) (methyl) (without remission) F10.20
    with
      amnestic disorder, persisting F10.26
      anxiety disorder F10.280
      dementia, persisting F10.27
      intoxication F10.229
        with delirium F10.221
        uncomplicated F10.220
      mood disorder F10.24
      psychotic disorder F10.259
        with
          delusions F10.250
          hallucinations F10.251
      remission F10.21
      sexual dysfunction F10.281
      sleep disorder F10.282
      specified disorder NEC F10.288
      withdrawal F10.239
        with
          delirium F10.231
          perceptual disturbance F10.232
        uncomplicated F10.230
    counseling and surveillance Z71.41
  amobarbital — *see* Dependence, drug, sedative
  amphetamine(s) (type) — *see* Dependence, drug, stimulant NEC
  amytal (sodium) — *see* Dependence, drug, sedative
  analgesic NEC F55.8
  anesthetic (agent) (gas) (general) (local) NEC — *see* Dependence, drug, psychoactive NEC
  anxiolytic NEC — *see* Dependence, drug, sedative
  barbital(s) — *see* Dependence, drug, sedative
  barbiturate(s) (compounds) (drugs classifiable to T42) — *see* Dependence, drug, sedative
  benzedrine — *see* Dependence, drug, stimulant NEC
  bhang — *see* Dependence, drug, cannabis
  bromide(s) NEC — *see* Dependence, drug, sedative
  caffeine — *see* Dependence, drug, stimulant NEC
  cannabis (sativa) (indica) (resin) (derivatives) (type) — *see* Dependence, drug, cannabis
  chloral (betaine) (hydrate) — *see* Dependence, drug, sedative
  chlordiazepoxide — *see* Dependence, drug, sedative
  coca (leaf) (derivatives) — *see* Dependence, drug, cocaine
  cocaine — *see* Dependence, drug, cocaine
  codeine — *see* Dependence, drug, opioid
  combinations of drugs F19.20
  dagga — *see* Dependence, drug, cannabis
  demerol — *see* Dependence, drug, opioid
  dexamphetamine — *see* Dependence, drug, stimulant NEC
  dexedrine — *see* Dependence, drug, stimulant NEC
  dextromethorphan — *see* Dependence, drug, opioid
  dextromoramide — *see* Dependence, drug, opioid
  dextro-nor-pseudo-ephedrine — *see* Dependence, drug, stimulant NEC
  dextrorphan — *see* Dependence, drug, opioid
  diazepam — *see* Dependence, drug, sedative
  dilaudid — *see* Dependence, drug, opioid
  D-lysergic acid diethylamide — *see* Dependence, drug, hallucinogen
  drug NEC F19.20
    with sleep disorder F19.282
    cannabis F12.20
      with
        anxiety disorder F12.280
        intoxication F12.229
          with
            delirium F12.221
            perceptual disturbance F12.222
          uncomplicated F12.220

Dependence — *continued*
  drug — *continued*
    cannabis — *continued*
      with — *continued*
        other specified disorder F12.288
        psychosis F12.259
          delusions F12.250
          hallucinations F12.251
        unspecified disorder F12.29
      in remission F12.21
    cocaine F14.20
      with
        anxiety disorder F14.280
        intoxication F14.229
          with
            delirium F14.221
            perceptual disturbance F14.222
          uncomplicated F14.220
        mood disorder F14.24
        other specified disorder F14.288
        psychosis F14.259
          delusions F14.250
          hallucinations F14.251
        sexual dysfunction F14.281
        sleep disorder F14.282
        unspecified disorder F14.29
        withdrawal F14.23
      in remission F14.21
    withdrawal symptoms in newborn P96.1
    counseling and surveillance Z71.51
    hallucinogen F16.20
      with
        anxiety disorder F16.280
        flashbacks F16.283
        intoxication F16.229
          with delirium F16.221
          uncomplicated F16.220
        mood disorder F16.24
        other specified disorder F16.288
        perception disorder, persisting F16.283
        psychosis F16.259
          delusions F16.250
          hallucinations F16.251
        unspecified disorder F16.29
      in remission F16.21
    in remission F19.21
    inhalant F18.20
      with
        anxiety disorder F18.280
        dementia, persisting F18.27
        intoxication F18.229
          with delirium F18.221
          uncomplicated F18.220
        mood disorder F18.24
        other specified disorder F18.288
        psychosis F18.259
          delusions F18.250
          hallucinations F18.251
        unspecified disorder F18.29
      in remission F18.21
    nicotine F17.200
      with disorder F17.209
        remission F17.201
        specified disorder NEC F17.208
        withdrawal F17.203
      chewing tobacco F17.220
        with disorder F17.229
          remission F17.221
          specified disorder NEC F17.228
          withdrawal F17.223
      cigarettes F17.210
        with disorder F17.219
          remission F17.211
          specified disorder NEC F17.218
          withdrawal F17.213
      specified product NEC F17.290
        with disorder F17.299
          remission F17.291
          specified disorder NEC F17.298
          withdrawal F17.293
    opioid F11.20
      with
        intoxication F11.229
          with
            delirium F11.221
            perceptual disturbance F11.222
          uncomplicated F11.220
        mood disorder F11.24

Dependence — *continued*
  drug — *continued*
    opioid — *continued*
      with — *continued*
        other specified disorder F11.288
        psychosis F11.259
          delusions F11.250
          hallucinations F11.251
        sexual dysfunction F11.281
        sleep disorder F11.282
        unspecified disorder F11.29
        withdrawal F11.23
      in remission F11.21
    psychoactive NEC F19.20
      with
        amnestic disorder F19.26
        anxiety disorder F19.280
        dementia F19.27
        intoxication F19.229
          with
            delirium F19.221
            perceptual disturbance F19.222
          uncomplicated F19.220
        mood disorder F19.24
        other specified disorder F19.288
        psychosis F19.259
          delusions F19.250
          hallucinations F19.251
        sexual dysfunction F19.281
        sleep disorder F19.282
        unspecified disorder F19.29
        withdrawal F19.239
          with
            delirium F19.231
            perceptual disturbance F19.232
          uncomplicated F19.230
    sedative, hypnotic or anxiolytic F13.20
      with
        amnestic disorder F13.26
        anxiety disorder F13.280
        dementia, persisting F13.27
        intoxication F13.229
          with delirium F13.221
          uncomplicated F13.220
        mood disorder F13.24
        other specified disorder F13.288
        psychosis F13.259
          delusions F13.250
          hallucinations F13.251
        sexual dysfunction F13.281
        sleep disorder F13.282
        unspecified disorder F13.29
        withdrawal F13.239
          with
            delirium F13.231
            perceptual disturbance F13.232
          uncomplicated F13.230
      in remission F13.21
    stimulant NEC F15.20
      with
        anxiety disorder F15.280
        intoxication F15.229
          with
            delirium F15.221
            perceptual disturbance F15.222
          uncomplicated F15.220
        mood disorder F15.24
        other specified disorder F15.288
        psychosis F15.259
          delusions F15.250
          hallucinations F15.251
        sexual dysfunction F15.281
        sleep disorder F15.282
        unspecified disorder F15.29
        withdrawal F15.23
      in remission F15.21
  ethyl
    alcohol (without remission) F10.20
      with remission F10.21
    bromide — *see* Dependence, drug, sedative
    carbamate F19.20
    chloride F19.20
    morphine — *see* Dependence, drug, opioid
  ganja — *see* Dependence, drug, cannabis
  glue (airplane) (sniffing) — *see* Dependence, drug, inhalant
  glutethimide — *see* Dependence, drug, sedative

Dependence — *continued*
  hallucinogenics — *see* Dependence, drug, hallucinogen
  hashish — *see* Dependence, drug, cannabis
  hemp — *see* Dependence, drug, cannabis
  heroin (salt) (any) — *see* Dependence, drug, opioid
  hypnotic NEC — *see* Dependence, drug, sedative
  Indian hemp — *see* Dependence, drug, cannabis
  inhalants — *see* Dependence, drug, inhalant
  khat — *see* Dependence, drug, stimulant NEC
  laudanum — *see* Dependence, drug, opioid
  LSD (-25) (derivatives) — *see* Dependence, drug, hallucinogen
  luminal — *see* Dependence, drug, sedative
  lysergic acid — *see* Dependence, drug, hallucinogen
  maconha — *see* Dependence, drug, cannabis
  marihuana — *see* Dependence, drug, cannabis
  meprobamate — *see* Dependence, drug, sedative
  mescaline — *see* Dependence, drug, hallucinogen
  methadone — *see* Dependence, drug, opioid
  methamphetamine(s) — *see* Dependence, drug, stimulant NEC
  methaqualone — *see* Dependence, drug, sedative
  methyl
    alcohol (without remission) F10.20
      with remission F10.21
    bromide — *see* Dependence, drug, sedative
    morphine — *see* Dependence, drug, opioid
    phenidate — *see* Dependence, drug, stimulant NEC
    sulfonal — *see* Dependence, drug, sedative
  morphine (sulfate) (sulfite) (type) — *see* Dependence, drug, opioid
  narcotic (drug) NEC — *see* Dependence, drug, opioid
  nembutal — *see* Dependence, drug, sedative
  neraval — *see* Dependence, drug, sedative
  neravan — *see* Dependence, drug, sedative
  neurobarb — *see* Dependence, drug, sedative
  nicotine — *see* Dependence, drug, nicotine
  nitrous oxide F19.20
  nonbarbiturate sedatives and tranquilizers with similar effect — *see* Dependence, drug, sedative
  on
    artificial heart (fully implantable) (mechanical) Z95.812
    aspirator Z99.0
    care provider (because of) Z74.9
      impaired mobility Z74.09
      need for
        assistance with personal care Z74.1
        continuous supervision Z74.3
      no other household member able to render care Z74.2
      specified reason NEC Z74.8
    machine Z99.89
      enabling NEC Z99.89
      specified type NEC Z99.89
    renal dialysis (hemodialysis) (peritoneal) Z99.2
    respirator Z99.11
    ventilator Z99.11
    wheelchair Z99.3
  opiate — *see* Dependence, drug, opioid
  opioids — *see* Dependence, drug, opioid
  opium (alkaloids) (derivatives) (tincture) — *see* Dependence, drug, opioid
  oxygen (long-term) (supplemental) Z99.81
  paraldehyde — *see* Dependence, drug, sedative
  paregoric — *see* Dependence, drug, opioid
  PCP (phencyclidine) (*see also* Abuse, drug, hallucinogen) F16.20
  pentobarbital — *see* Dependence, drug, sedative
  pentobarbitone (sodium) — *see* Dependence, drug, sedative
  pentothal — *see* Dependence, drug, sedative
  peyote — *see* Dependence, drug, hallucinogen
  phencyclidine (PCP) (and related substances) (*see also* Abuse, drug, hallucinogen) F16.20
  phenmetrazine — *see* Dependence, drug, stimulant NEC
  phenobarbital — *see* Dependence, drug, sedative
  polysubstance F19.20
  psilocibin, psilocin, psilocyn, psilocyline — *see* Dependence, drug, hallucinogen
  psychostimulant NEC — *see* Dependence, drug, stimulant NEC
  secobarbital — *see* Dependence, drug, sedative
  seconal — *see* Dependence, drug, sedative

Dependence — *continued*
  sedative NEC — *see* Dependence, drug, sedative
  specified drug NEC — *see* Dependence, drug
  stimulant NEC — *see* Dependence, drug, stimulant NEC
  substance NEC — *see* Dependence, drug
  supplemental oxygen Z99.81
  tobacco — *see* Dependence, drug, nicotine
    counseling and surveillance Z71.6
  tranquilizer NEC — *see* Dependence, drug, sedative
  vitamin B6 E53.1
  volatile solvents — *see* Dependence, drug, inhalant
Dependency
  care-provider Z74.9
  passive F60.7
  reactions (persistent) F60.7
Depersonalization (in neurotic state) (neurotic) (syndrome) F48.1
Depletion
  extracellular fluid E86.9
  plasma E86.1
  potassium E87.6
    nephropathy N25.89
  salt or sodium E87.1
    causing heat exhaustion or prostration T67.4 ☑
    nephropathy N28.9
  volume NOS E86.9
Deployment (current) (military) status Z56.82
  in theater or in support of military war, peacekeeping and humanitarian operations Z56.82
  personal history of Z91.82
    military war, peacekeeping and humanitarian deployment (current or past conflict) Z91.82
  returned from Z91.82
Depolarization, premature I49.40
  atrial I49.1
  junctional I49.2
  specified NEC I49.49
  ventricular I49.3
Deposit
  bone in Boeck's sarcoid D86.89
  calcareous, calcium — *see* Calcification
  cholesterol
    retina H35.89
    vitreous (body) (humor) — *see* Deposit, crystalline
  conjunctiva H11.11- ☑
  cornea H18.00- ☑
    argentous H18.02- ☑
    due to metabolic disorder H18.03- ☑
    Kayser-Fleischer ring H18.04- ☑
    pigmentation — *see* Pigmentation, cornea
  crystalline, vitreous (body) (humor) H43.2- ☑
  hemosiderin in old scars of cornea — *see* Pigmentation, cornea, stromal
  metallic in lens — *see* Cataract, specified NEC
  skin R23.8
  tooth, teeth (betel) (black) (green) (materia alba) (orange) (tobacco) K03.6
  urate, kidney — *see* Calculus, kidney
Depraved appetite — *see* Pica
Depressed
  HDL cholesterol E78.6
Depression (acute) (mental) F32.9
  agitated (single episode) F32.2
  anaclitic — *see* Disorder, adjustment
  anxiety F41.8
    persistent F34.1
  arches (*see also* Deformity, limb, flat foot)
  atypical (single episode) F32.8
  basal metabolic rate R94.8
  bone marrow D75.89
  central nervous system R09.2
  cerebral R29.818
    newborn P91.4
  cerebrovascular I67.9
  chest wall M95.4
  climacteric (single episode) F32.8
  endogenous (without psychotic symptoms) F33.2
    with psychotic symptoms F33.3
  functional activity R68.89
  hysterical F44.89
  involutional (single episode) F32.8
  major F32.9
    with psychotic symptoms F32.3
    recurrent — *see* Disorder, depressive, recurrent
  manic-depressive — *see* Disorder, depressive, recurrent

Depression — *continued*
- masked (single episode) F32.8
- medullary G93.89
- menopausal (single episode) F32.8
- metatarsus — *see* Depression, arches
- monopolar F33.9
- nervous F34.1
- neurotic F34.1
- nose M95.0
- postnatal F53
- postpartum F53
- post-psychotic of schizophrenia F32.8
- post-schizophrenic F32.8
- psychogenic (reactive) (single episode) F32.9
- psychoneurotic F34.1
- psychotic (single episode) F32.3
  - recurrent F33.3
- reactive (psychogenic) (single episode) F32.9
  - psychotic (single episode) F32.3
- recurrent — *see* Disorder, depressive, recurrent
- respiratory center G93.89
- seasonal — *see* Disorder, depressive, recurrent
- senile F03 ☑
- severe, single episode F32.2
- situational F43.21
- skull Q67.4
- specified NEC (single episode) F32.8
- sternum M95.4
- visual field — *see* Defect, visual field
- vital (recurrent) (without psychotic symptoms) F33.2
  - with psychotic symptoms F33.3
  - single episode F32.2

Deprivation
- cultural Z60.3
- effects NOS T73.9
  - specified NEC T73.8 ☑
- emotional NEC Z65.8
  - affecting infant or child — *see* Maltreatment, child, psychological
- food T73.0
- protein — *see* Malnutrition
- sleep Z72.820
- social Z60.4
  - affecting infant or child — *see* Maltreatment, child, psychological
- specified NEC T73.8 ☑
- vitamins — *see* Deficiency, vitamin
- water T73.1 ☑

Derangement
- ankle (internal) — *see* Derangement, joint, ankle
- cartilage (articular) NEC — *see* Derangement, joint, articular cartilage, by site
  - recurrent — *see* Dislocation, recurrent
- cruciate ligament, anterior, current injury — *see* Sprain, knee, cruciate, anterior
- elbow (internal) — *see* Derangement, joint, elbow
- hip (joint) (internal) (old) — *see* Derangement, joint, hip
- joint (internal) M24.9
  - ankylosis — *see* Ankylosis
  - articular cartilage M24.10
    - ankle M24.17- ☑
    - elbow M24.12- ☑
    - foot M24.17- ☑
    - hand M24.14- ☑
    - hip M24.15- ☑
    - knee NEC M23.9- ☑
    - loose body — *see* Loose, body
    - shoulder M24.11- ☑
    - wrist M24.13- ☑
  - contracture — *see* Contraction, joint
  - current injury (*see also* Dislocation)
    - knee, meniscus or cartilage — *see* Tear, meniscus
  - dislocation
    - pathological — *see* Dislocation, pathological
    - recurrent — *see* Dislocation, recurrent
  - knee — *see* Derangement, knee
  - ligament — *see* Disorder, ligament
  - loose body — *see* Loose, body
  - recurrent — *see* Dislocation, recurrent
  - specified type NEC M24.80
    - ankle M24.87- ☑
    - elbow M24.82- ☑
    - foot joint M24.87- ☑
    - hand joint M24.84- ☑
    - hip M24.85- ☑

Derangement — *continued*
- joint — *continued*
  - specified type — *continued*
    - shoulder M24.81- ☑
    - wrist M24.83- ☑
  - temporomandibular M26.69
- knee (recurrent) M23.9- ☑
  - ligament disruption, spontaneous M23.60- ☑
    - anterior cruciate M23.61- ☑
    - capsular M23.67- ☑
    - instability, chronic M23.5- ☑
    - lateral collateral M23.64- ☑
    - medial collateral M23.63- ☑
    - posterior cruciate M23.62- ☑
  - loose body M23.4- ☑
  - meniscus M23.30- ☑
    - cystic M23.00- ☑
      - lateral M23.002
        - anterior horn M23.04- ☑
        - posterior horn M23.05- ☑
        - specified NEC M23.06- ☑
      - medial M23.005
        - anterior horn M23.01- ☑
        - posterior horn M23.02- ☑
        - specified NEC M23.03- ☑
    - degenerate — *see* Derangement, knee, meniscus, specified NEC
    - detached — *see* Derangement, knee, meniscus, specified NEC
    - due to old tear or injury M23.20- ☑
      - lateral M23.20- ☑
        - anterior horn M23.24- ☑
        - posterior horn M23.25- ☑
        - specified NEC M23.26- ☑
      - medial M23.20- ☑
        - anterior horn M23.21- ☑
        - posterior horn M23.22- ☑
        - specified NEC M23.23- ☑
    - retained — *see* Derangement, knee, meniscus, specified NEC
    - specified NEC M23.30- ☑
      - lateral M23.30- ☑
        - anterior horn M23.34- ☑
        - posterior horn M23.35- ☑
        - specified NEC M23.36- ☑
      - medial M23.30- ☑
        - anterior horn M23.31- ☑
        - posterior horn M23.32- ☑
        - specified NEC M23.33- ☑
    - old M23.8X- ☑
    - specified NEC — *see* subcategory M23.8 ☑
  - low back NEC — *see* Dorsopathy, specified NEC
  - meniscus — *see* Derangement, knee, meniscus
- mental — *see* Psychosis
- patella, specified NEC — *see* Disorder, patella, derangement NEC
- semilunar cartilage (knee) — *see* Derangement, knee, meniscus, specified NEC
- shoulder (internal) — *see* Derangement, joint, shoulder

Dercum's disease E88.2
Derealization (neurotic) F48.1
Dermal — *see* condition
Dermaphytid — *see* Dermatophytosis
Dermatitis (eczematous) L30.9
- ab igne L59.0
- acarine B88.0
- actinic (due to sun) L57.8
  - other than from sun L59.8
- allergic — *see* Dermatitis, contact, allergic
- ambustionis, due to burn or scald — *see* Burn
- amebic A06.7
- ammonia L22
- arsenical (ingested) L27.8
- artefacta L98.1
  - psychogenic F54
- atopic L20.9
  - psychogenic F54
  - specified NEC L20.89
- autoimmune progesterone L30.8
- berlock, berloque L56.2
- blastomycotic B40.3
- blister beetle L24.89
- bullous, bullosa L13.9
  - mucosynechial, atrophic L12.1
  - seasonal L30.8

Dermatitis — *continued*
- bullous, bullosa — *continued*
  - specified NEC L13.8
- calorica L59.0
  - due to burn or scald — *see* Burn
- caterpillar L24.89
- cercarial B65.3
- combustionis L59.0
  - due to burn or scald — *see* Burn
- congelationis T69.1 ☑
- contact (occupational) L25.9
  - allergic L23.9
    - due to
      - adhesives L23.1
      - cement L23.5
      - chemical products NEC L23.5
      - chromium L23.0
      - cosmetics L23.2
      - dander (cat) (dog) L23.81
      - drugs in contact with skin L23.3
      - dyes L23.4
      - food in contact with skin L23.6
      - hair (cat) (dog) L23.81
      - insecticide L23.5
      - metals L23.0
      - nickel L23.0
      - plants, non-food L23.7
      - plastic L23.5
      - rubber L23.5
      - specified agent NEC L23.89
    - due to
      - cement L25.3
      - chemical products NEC L25.3
      - cosmetics L25.0
      - dander (cat) (dog) L23.81
      - drugs in contact with skin L25.1
      - dyes L25.2
      - food in contact with skin L25.4
      - hair (cat) (dog) L23.81
      - plants, non-food L25.5
      - specified agent NEC L25.8
    - irritant L24.9
      - due to
        - cement L25.3
        - chemical products NEC L24.5
        - cosmetics L24.3
        - detergents L24.0
        - drugs in contact with skin L24.4
        - food in contact with skin L24.6
        - oils and greases L24.1
        - plants, non-food L24.7
        - solvents L24.2
        - specified agent NEC L24.89
- contusiformis L52
- diabetic — *see* E08-E13 with .620
- diaper L22
- diphtheritica A36.3
- dry skin L85.3
- due to
  - acetone (contact) (irritant) L24.2
  - acids (contact) (irritant) L24.5
  - adhesive(s) (allergic) (contact) (plaster) L23.1
    - irritant L24.5
  - alcohol (irritant) (skin contact) (substances in category T51) L24.2
    - taken internally L27.8
  - alkalis (contact) (irritant) L24.5
  - arsenic (ingested) L27.8
  - carbon disulfide (contact) (irritant) L24.2
  - caustics (contact) (irritant) L24.5
  - cement (contact) L25.3
  - cereal (ingested) L27.2
  - chemical(s) NEC L25.3
    - taken internally L27.8
  - chlorocompounds L24.2
  - chromium (contact) (irritant) L24.81
  - coffee (ingested) L27.2
  - cold weather L30.8
  - cosmetics (contact) L25.0
    - allergic L23.2
    - irritant L24.3
  - cyclohexanes L24.2
  - dander (cat) (dog) L23.81
  - Demodex species B88.0
  - Dermanyssus gallinae B88.0
  - detergents (contact) (irritant) L24.0
  - dichromate L24.81

Dermatitis — *continued*
  due to — *continued*
    drugs and medicaments (generalized) (internal use) L27.0
      external — *see* Dermatitis, due to, drugs, in contact with skin
      in contact with skin L25.1
        allergic L23.3
        irritant L24.4
      localized skin eruption L27.1
      specified substance — *see* Table of Drugs and Chemicals
    dyes (contact) L25.2
      allergic L23.4
      irritant L24.89
    epidermophytosis — *see* Dermatophytosis
    esters L24.2
    external irritant NEC L24.9
    fish (ingested) L27.2
    flour (ingested) L27.2
    food (ingested) L27.2
      in contact with skin L25.4
    fruit (ingested) L27.2
    furs (allergic) (contact) L23.81
    glues — *see* Dermatitis, due to, adhesives
    glycols L24.2
    greases NEC (contact) (irritant) L24.1
    hair (cat) (dog) L23.81
    hot
      objects and materials — *see* Burn
      weather or places L59.0
    hydrocarbons L24.2
    infrared rays L59.8
    ingestion, ingested substance L27.9
      chemical NEC L27.8
      drugs and medicaments — *see* Dermatitis, due to, drugs
      food L27.2
      specified NEC L27.8
    insecticide in contact with skin L24.5
    internal agent L27.9
      drugs and medicaments (generalized) — *see* Dermatitis, due to, drugs
      food L27.2
    irradiation — *see* Dermatitis, due to, radioactive substance
    ketones L24.2
    lacquer tree (allergic) (contact) L23.7
    light (sun) NEC L57.8
      acute L56.8
      other L59.8
    Liponyssoides sanguineus B88.0
    low temperature L30.8
    meat (ingested) L27.2
    metals, metal salts (contact) (irritant) L24.81
    milk (ingested) L27.2
    nickel (contact) (irritant) L24.81
    nylon (contact) (irritant) L24.5
    oils NEC (contact) (irritant) L24.1
    paint solvent (contact) (irritant) L24.2
    petroleum products (contact) (irritant) (substances in T52.0) L24.2
    plants NEC (contact) L25.5
      allergic L23.7
      irritant L24.7
    plasters (adhesive) (any) (allergic) (contact) L23.1
      irritant L24.5
    plastic (contact) L25.3
    preservatives (contact) — *see* Dermatitis, due to, chemical, in contact with skin
    primrose (allergic) (contact) L23.7
    primula (allergic) (contact) L23.7
    radiation L59.8
      nonionizing (chronic exposure) L57.8
      sun NEC L57.8
        acute L56.8
    radioactive substance L58.9
      acute L58.0
      chronic L58.1
    radium L58.9
      acute L58.0
      chronic L58.1
    ragweed (allergic) (contact) L23.7
    Rhus (allergic) (contact) (diversiloba) (radicans) (toxicodendron) (venenata) (verniciflua) L23.7
    rubber (contact) L24.5
    Senecio jacobaea (allergic) (contact) L23.7

Dermatitis — *continued*
  due to — *continued*
    solvents (contact) (irritant) (substances in category T52) L24.2
    specified agent NEC (contact) L25.8
      allergic L23.89
      irritant L24.89
    sunshine NEC L57.8
      acute L56.8
    tetrachlorethylene (contact) (irritant) L24.2
    toluene (contact) (irritant) L24.2
    turpentine (contact) L24.2
    ultraviolet rays (sun NEC) (chronic exposure) L57.8
      acute L56.8
    vaccine or vaccination L27.0
      specified substance — *see* Table of Drugs and Chemicals
    varicose veins — *see* Varix, leg, with, inflammation
    X-rays L58.9
      acute L58.0
      chronic L58.1
  dyshydrotic L30.1
  dysmenorrheica N94.6
  escharotica — *see* Burn
  exfoliative, exfoliativa (generalized) L26
    neonatorum L00
  eyelid (*see also* Dermatosis, eyelid)
    allergic H01.119
      left H01.116
        lower H01.115
        upper H01.114
      right H01.113
        lower H01.112
        upper H01.111
    contact — *see* Dermatitis, eyelid, allergic
    due to
      Demodex species B88.0
      herpes (zoster) B02.39
        simplex B00.59
    eczematous H01.139
      left H01.136
        lower H01.135
        upper H01.134
      right H01.133
        lower H01.132
        upper H01.131
  facta, factitia, factitial L98.1
    psychogenic F54
  flexural NEC L20.82
  friction L30.4
  fungus B36.9
    specified type NEC B36.8
  gangrenosa, gangrenous infantum L08.0
  harvest mite B88.0
  heat L59.0
  herpesviral, vesicular (ear) (lip) B00.1
  herpetiformis (bullous) (erythematous) (pustular) (vesicular) L13.0
    juvenile L12.2
    senile L12.0
  hiemalis L30.8
  hypostatic, hypostatica — *see* Varix, leg, with, inflammation
  infectious eczematoid L30.3
  infective L30.3
  irritant — *see* Dermatitis, contact, irritant
  Jacquet's (diaper dermatitis) L22
  Leptus B88.0
  lichenified NEC L28.0
  medicamentosa (generalized) (internal use) — *see* Dermatitis, due to drugs
  mite B88.0
  multiformis L13.0
    juvenile L12.2
  napkin L22
  neurotica L13.0
  nummular L30.0
  papillaris capillitii L73.0
  pellagrous E52
  perioral L71.0
  photocontact L56.2
  polymorpha dolorosa L13.0
  pruriginosa L13.0
  pruritic NEC L30.8
  psychogenic F54
  purulent L08.0
  pustular
    contagious B08.02

Dermatitis — *continued*
  pustular — *continued*
    subcorneal L13.1
  pyococcal L08.0
  pyogenica L08.0
  repens L40.2
  Ritter's (exfoliativa) L00
  Schamberg's L81.7
  schistosome B65.3
  seasonal bullous L30.8
  seborrheic L21.9
    infantile L21.1
    specified NEC L21.8
  sensitization NOS L23.9
  septic L08.0
  solare L57.8
  specified NEC L30.8
  stasis I87.2
    with varicose ulcer — *see* Varix, leg, with ulcer, with inflammation
    due to postthrombotic syndrome — *see* Syndrome, postthrombotic
  suppurative L08.0
  traumatic NEC L30.4
  trophoneurotica L13.0
  ultraviolet (sun) (chronic exposure) L57.8
    acute L56.8
  varicose — *see* Varix, leg, with, inflammation
  vegetans L10.1
  verrucosa B43.0
  vesicular, herpesviral B00.1
Dermatoarthritis, lipoid E78.81
Dermatochalasis, eyelid H02.839
  left H02.836
    lower H02.835
    upper H02.834
  right H02.833
    lower H02.832
    upper H02.831
Dermatofibroma (lenticulare) — *see* Neoplasm, skin, benign
  protuberans — *see* Neoplasm, skin, uncertain behavior
Dermatofibrosarcoma (pigmented) (protuberans) — *see* Neoplasm, skin, malignant
Dermatographia L50.3
Dermatolysis (exfoliativa) (congenital) Q82.8
  acquired L57.4
  eyelids — *see* Blepharochalasis
  palpebrarum — *see* Blepharochalasis
  senile L57.4
Dermatomegaly NEC Q82.8
Dermatomucosomyositis M33.10
  with
    myopathy M33.12
    respiratory involvement M33.11
    specified organ involvement NEC M33.19
Dermatomycosis B36.9
  furfuracea B36.0
  specified type NEC B36.8
Dermatomyositis (acute) (chronic) (*see also* Dermatopolymyositis)
  in (due to) neoplastic disease (*see also* Neoplasm) D49.9 [M36.0]
Dermatoneuritis of children — *see* Poisoning, mercury
Dermatophilosis A48.8
Dermatophytid L30.2
Dermatophytide — *see* Dermatophytosis
Dermatophytosis (epidermophyton) (infection) (Microsporum) (tinea) (Trichophyton) B35.9
  beard B35.0
  body B35.4
  capitis B35.0
  corporis B35.4
  deep-seated B35.8
  disseminated B35.8
  foot B35.3
  granulomatous B35.8
  groin B35.6
  hand B35.2
  nail B35.1
  perianal (area) B35.6
  scalp B35.0
  specified NEC B35.8
Dermatopolymyositis M33.90
  with
    myopathy M33.92
    respiratory involvement M33.91
    specified organ involvement NEC M33.99

Dermatopolymyositis — continued
  in neoplastic disease (see also Neoplasm)
    D49.9 [M36.0]
  juvenile M33.00
    with
      myopathy M33.02
      respiratory involvement M33.01
      specified organ involvement NEC M33.09
  specified NEC M33.10
    myopathy M33.12
    respiratory involvement M33.11
    specified organ involvement NEC M33.19
Dermatopolyneuritis — see Poisoning, mercury
Dermatorrhexis Q79.6
  acquired L57.4
Dermatosclerosis (see also Scleroderma)
  localized L94.0
Dermatosis L98.9
  Andrews' L08.89
  Bowen's — see Neoplasm, skin, in situ
  bullous L13.9
    specified NEC L13.8
  exfoliativa L26
  eyelid (noninfectious)
    dermatitis — see Dermatitis, eyelid
    discoid lupus erythematosus — see Lupus, erythematosus, eyelid
    xeroderma — see Xeroderma, acquired, eyelid
  factitial L98.1
  febrile neutrophilic L98.2
  gonococcal A54.89
  herpetiformis L13.0
    juvenile L12.2
  linear IgA L13.8
  menstrual NEC L98.8
  neutrophilic, febrile L98.2
  occupational — see Dermatitis, contact
  papulosa nigra L82.1
  pigmentary L81.9
    progressive L81.7
    Schamberg's L81.7
  psychogenic F54
  purpuric, pigmented L81.7
  pustular, subcorneal L13.1
  transient acantholytic L11.1
Dermographia, dermographism L50.3
Dermoid (cyst) (see also Neoplasm, benign, by site)
  with malignant transformation C56- ☑
  due to radiation (nonionizing) L57.8
Dermopathy
  infiltrative with thyrotoxicosis — see Thyrotoxicosis
  nephrogenic fibrosing L90.8
Dermophytosis — see Dermatophytosis
Descemetocele H18.73- ☑
Descemet's membrane — see condition
Descending — see condition
Descensus uteri — see Prolapse, uterus
Desert
  rheumatism B38.0
  sore — see Ulcer, skin
Desertion (newborn) — see Maltreatment
Desmoid (extra-abdominal) (tumor) — see Neoplasm, connective tissue, uncertain behavior
  abdominal D48.1
Despondency F32.9
Desquamation, skin R23.4
Destruction, destructive (see also Damage)
  articular facet (see also Derangement, joint, specified type NEC)
    knee M23.8X- ☑
    vertebra — see Spondylosis
  bone (see also Disorder, bone, specified type NEC)
    syphilitic A52.77
  joint (see also Derangement, joint, specified type NEC)
    sacroiliac M53.3
  rectal sphincter K62.89
  septum (nasal) J34.89
  tuberculous NEC — see Tuberculosis
  tympanum, tympanic membrane (nontraumatic) — see Disorder, tympanic membrane, specified NEC
  vertebral disc — see Degeneration, intervertebral disc
Destructiveness (see also Disorder, conduct)
  adjustment reaction — see Disorder, adjustment
Desultory labor O62.2
Detachment
  cartilage — see Sprain

Detachment — continued
  cervix, annular N88.8
    complicating delivery O71.3
  choroid (old) (postinfectional) (simple) (spontaneous)
    H31.40- ☑
    hemorrhagic H31.41- ☑
    serous H31.42- ☑
  ligament — see Sprain
  meniscus (knee) (see also Derangement, knee, meniscus, specified NEC)
    current injury — see Tear, meniscus
    due to old tear or injury — see Derangement, knee, meniscus, due to old tear
  retina (without retinal break) (serous) H33.2- ☑
    with retinal:
      break H33.00- ☑
        giant H33.03- ☑
        multiple H33.02- ☑
        single H33.01- ☑
      dialysis H33.04- ☑
    pigment epithelium — see Degeneration, retina, separation of layers, pigment epithelium detachment
    rhegmatogenous — see Detachment, retina, with retinal, break
    specified NEC H33.8
    total H33.05- ☑
    traction H33.4- ☑
  vitreous (body) H43.81 ☑
Detergent asthma J69.8
Deterioration
  epileptic F06.8
  general physical R53.81
  heart, cardiac — see Degeneration, myocardial
  mental — see Psychosis
  myocardial, myocardium — see Degeneration, myocardial
  senile (simple) R54
Deuteranomaly (anomalous trichromat) H53.53
Deuteranopia (complete) (incomplete) H53.53
Development
  abnormal, bone Q79.9
  arrested R62.50
    bone — see Arrest, development or growth, bone
    child R62.50
    due to malnutrition E45
  defective, congenital (see also Anomaly, by site)
    cauda equina Q06.3
    left ventricle Q24.8
      in hypoplastic left heart syndrome Q23.4
    valve Q24.8
      pulmonary Q22.3
  delayed (see also Delay, development) R62.50
    arithmetical skills F81.2
    language (skills) (expressive) F80.1
    learning skill F81.9
    mixed skills F88
    motor coordination F82
    reading F81.0
    specified learning skill NEC F81.89
    speech F80.9
    spelling F81.81
    written expression F81.81
  imperfect, congenital (see also Anomaly, by site)
    heart Q24.9
    lungs Q33.6
  incomplete
    bronchial tree Q32.4
    organ or site not listed — see Hypoplasia, by site
    respiratory system Q34.9
  sexual, precocious NEC E30.1
  tardy, mental (see also Disability, intellectual) F79
Developmental — see condition
  testing, child — see Examination, child
Devergie's disease (pityriasis rubra pilaris) L44.0
Deviation (in)
  conjugate palsy (eye) (spastic) H51.0
  esophagus (acquired) K22.8
  eye, skew H51.8
  midline (jaw) (teeth) (dental arch) M26.29
    specified site NEC — see Malposition
  nasal septum J34.2
    congenital Q67.4
  opening and closing of the mandible M26.53
  organ or site, congenital NEC — see Malposition, congenital
  septum (nasal) (acquired) J34.2

Deviation — continued
  septum — continued
    congenital Q67.4
  sexual F65.9
    bestiality F65.89
    erotomania F52.8
    exhibitionism F65.2
    fetishism, fetishistic F65.0
      transvestism F65.1
    frotteurism F65.81
    masochism F65.51
    multiple F65.89
    necrophilia F65.89
    nymphomania F52.8
    pederosis F65.4
    pedophilia F65.4
    sadism, sadomasochism F65.52
    satyriasis F52.8
    specified type NEC F65.89
    transvestism F64.1
    voyeurism F65.3
  teeth, midline M26.29
  trachea J39.8
  ureter, congenital Q62.61
Device
  cerebral ventricle (communicating) in situ Z98.2
  contraceptive — see Contraceptive, device
  drainage, cerebrospinal fluid, in situ Z98.2
Devic's disease G36.0
Devil's
  grip B33.0
  pinches (purpura simplex) D69.2
Devitalized tooth K04.99
Devonshire colic — see Poisoning, lead
Dextraposition, aorta Q20.3
  in tetralogy of Fallot Q21.3
Dextrinosis, limit (debrancher enzyme deficiency) E74.03
Dextrocardia (true) Q24.0
  with
    complete transposition of viscera Q89.3
    situs inversus Q89.3
Dextrotransposition, aorta Q20.3
d-glycericacidemia E72.59
Dhat syndrome F48.8
Dhobi itch B35.6
Di George's syndrome D82.1
Di Guglielmo's disease C94.0- ☑
Diabetes, diabetic (mellitus) (sugar) E11.9
  with
    amyotrophy E11.44
    arthropathy NEC E11.618
    autonomic (poly)neuropathy E11.43
    cataract E11.36
    Charcot's joints E11.610
    chronic kidney disease E11.22
    circulatory complication NEC E11.59
    complication E11.8
      specified NEC E11.69
    dermatitis E11.620
    foot ulcer E11.621
    gangrene E11.52
    gastroparesis E11.43
    glomerulonephrosis, intracapillary E11.21
    glomerulosclerosis, intercapillary E11.21
    hyperglycemia E11.65
    hyperosmolarity E11.00
      with coma E11.01
    hypoglycemia E11.649
      with coma E11.641
    kidney complications NEC E11.29
    Kimmelstiel-Wilson disease E11.21
    loss of protective sensation (LOPS) — see Diabetes, by type, with neuropathy
    mononeuropathy E11.41
    myasthenia E11.44
    necrobiosis lipoidica E11.620
    nephropathy E11.21
    neuralgia E11.42
    neurologic complication NEC E11.49
    neuropathic arthropathy E11.610
    neuropathy E11.40
    ophthalmic complication NEC E11.39
    oral complication NEC E11.638
    periodontal disease E11.630
    peripheral angiopathy E11.51
      with gangrene E11.52
    polyneuropathy E11.42

Diabetes, diabetic — *continued*
  with — *continued*
    renal complication NEC E11.29
    renal tubular degeneration E11.29
    retinopathy E11.319
      with macular edema E11.311
      nonproliferative E11.329
        with macular edema E11.321
        mild E11.329
          with macular edema E11.321
        moderate E11.339
          with macular edema E11.331
        severe E11.349
          with macular edema E11.341
      proliferative E11.359
        with macular edema E11.351
    skin complication NEC E11.628
    skin ulcer NEC E11.622
  bronzed E83.110
  complicating pregnancy — *see* Pregnancy, complicated by, diabetes
  dietary counseling and surveillance Z71.3
  due to drug or chemical E09.9
    with
      amyotrophy E09.44
      arthropathy NEC E09.618
      autonomic (poly)neuropathy E09.43
      cataract E09.36
      Charcot's joints E09.610
      chronic kidney disease E09.22
      circulatory complication NEC E09.59
      complication E09.8
        specified NEC E09.69
      dermatitis E09.620
      foot ulcer E09.621
      gangrene E09.52
      gastroparesis E09.43
      glomerulonephrosis, intracapillary E09.21
      glomerulosclerosis, intercapillary E09.21
      hyperglycemia E09.65
      hyperosmolarity E09.00
        with coma E09.01
      hypoglycemia E09.649
        with coma E09.641
      ketoacidosis E09.10
        with coma E09.11
      kidney complications NEC E09.29
      Kimmelstiel-Wilson disease E09.21
      mononeuropathy E09.41
      myasthenia E09.44
      necrobiosis lipoidica E09.620
      nephropathy E09.21
      neuralgia E09.42
      neurologic complication NEC E09.49
      neuropathic arthropathy E09.610
      neuropathy E09.40
      ophthalmic complication NEC E09.39
      oral complication NEC E09.638
      periodontal disease E09.630
      peripheral angiopathy E09.51
        with gangrene E09.52
      polyneuropathy E09.42
      renal complication NEC E09.29
      renal tubular degeneration E09.29
      retinopathy E09.319
        with macular edema E09.311
        nonproliferative E09.329
          with macular edema E09.321
          mild E09.329
            with macular edema E09.321
          moderate E09.339
            with macular edema E09.331
          severe E09.349
            with macular edema E09.341
        proliferative E09.359
          with macular edema E09.351
      skin complication NEC E09.628
      skin ulcer NEC E09.622
  due to underlying condition E08.9
    with
      amyotrophy E08.44
      arthropathy NEC E08.618
      autonomic (poly)neuropathy E08.43
      cataract E08.36
      Charcot's joints E08.610
      chronic kidney disease E08.22
      circulatory complication NEC E08.59
      complication E08.8

Diabetes, diabetic — *continued*
  due to underlying condition — *continued*
    with — *continued*
      complication — *continued*
        specified NEC E08.69
      dermatitis E08.620
      foot ulcer E08.621
      gangrene E08.52
      gastroparesis E08.43
      glomerulonephrosis, intracapillary E08.21
      glomerulosclerosis, intercapillary E08.21
      hyperglycemia E08.65
      hyperosmolarity E08.00
        with coma E08.01
      hypoglycemia E08.649
        with coma E08.641
      ketoacidosis E08.10
        with coma E08.11
      kidney complications NEC E08.29
      Kimmelsteil-WIlson disease E08.21
      mononeuropathy E08.41
      myasthenia E08.44
      necrobiosis lipoidica E08.620
      nephropathy E08.21
      neuralgia E08.42
      neurologic complication NEC E08.49
      neuropathic arthropathy E08.610
      neuropathy E08.40
      ophthalmic complication NEC E08.39
      oral complication NEC E08.638
      periodontal disease E08.630
      peripheral angiopathy E08.51
        with gangrene E08.52
      polyneuropathy E08.42
      renal complication NEC E08.29
      renal tubular degeneration E08.29
      retinopathy E08.319
        with macular edema E08.311
        nonproliferative E08.329
          with macular edema E08.321
          mild E08.329
            with macular edema E08.321
          moderate E08.339
            with macular edema E08.331
          severe E08.349
            with macular edema E08.341
        proliferative E08.359
          with macular edema E08.351
      skin complication NEC E08.628
      skin ulcer NEC E08.622
  gestational (in pregnancy) O24.419
    affecting newborn P70.0
    diet controlled O24.410
    in childbirth O24.429
      diet controlled O24.420
      insulin (and diet) controlled O24.424
    insulin (and diet) controlled O24.414
    puerperal O24.439
      diet controlled O24.430
      insulin (and diet) controlled O24.434
  hepatogenous E13.9
  inadequately controlled — *code to* Diabetes, by type, with hyperglycemia
  insipidus E23.2
    nephrogenic N25.1
    pituitary E23.2
    vasopressin resistant N25.1
  insulin dependent — *code to* type of diabetes
  juvenile-onset — *see* Diabetes, type 1
  ketosis-prone — *see* Diabetes, type 1
  latent R73.09
  neonatal (transient) P70.2
  non-insulin dependent — *code to* type of diabetes
  out of control — *code to* Diabetes, by type, with hyperglycemia
  phosphate E83.39
  poorly controlled — *code to* Diabetes, by type, with hyperglycemia
  postpancreatectomy — *see* Diabetes, specified type NEC
  postprocedural — *see* Diabetes, specified type NEC
  secondary diabetes mellitus NEC — *see* Diabetes, specified type NEC
  specified type NEC E13.9
    with
      amyotrophy E13.44
      arthropathy NEC E13.618
      autonomic (poly)neuropathy E13.43

Diabetes, diabetic — *continued*
  specified type — *continued*
    with — *continued*
      cataract E13.36
      Charcot's joints E13.610
      chronic kidney disease E13.22
      circulatory complication NEC E13.59
      complication E13.8
        specified NEC E13.69
      dermatitis E13.620
      foot ulcer E13.621
      gangrene E13.52
      gastroparesis E13.43
      glomerulonephrosis, intracapillary E13.21
      glomerulosclerosis, intercapillary E13.21
      hyperglycemia E13.65
      hyperosmolarity E13.00
        with coma E13.01
      hypoglycemia E13.649
        with coma E13.641
      ketoacidosis E13.10
        with coma E13.11
      kidney complications NEC E13.29
      Kimmelstiel-Wilson disease E13.21
      mononeuropathy E13.41
      myasthenia E13.44
      necrobiosis lipoidica E13.620
      nephropathy E13.21
      neuralgia E13.42
      neurologic complication NEC E13.49
      neuropathic arthropathy E13.610
      neuropathy E13.40
      ophthalmic complication NEC E13.39
      oral complication NEC E13.638
      periodontal disease E13.630
      peripheral angiopathy E13.51
        with gangrene E13.52
      polyneuropathy E13.42
      renal complication NEC E13.29
      renal tubular degeneration E13.29
      retinopathy E13.319
        with macular edema E13.311
        nonproliferative E13.329
          with macular edema E13.321
          mild E13.329
            with macular edema E13.321
          moderate E13.339
            with macular edema E13.331
          severe E13.349
            with macular edema E13.341
        proliferative E13.359
          with macular edema E13.351
      skin complication NEC E13.628
      skin ulcer NEC E13.622
  steroid-induced — *see* Diabetes, due to, drug or chemical
  type 1 E10.9
    with
      amyotrophy E10.44
      arthropathy NEC E10.618
      autonomic (poly)neuropathy E10.43
      cataract E10.36
      Charcot's joints E10.610
      chronic kidney disease E10.22
      circulatory complication NEC E10.59
      complication E10.8
        specified NEC E10.69
      dermatitis E10.620
      foot ulcer E10.621
      gangrene E10.52
      gastroparesis E10.43
      glomerulonephrosis, intracapillary E10.21
      glomerulosclerosis, intercapillary E10.21
      hyperglycemia E10.65
      hypoglycemia E10.649
        with coma E10.641
      ketoacidosis E10.10
        with coma E10.11
      kidney complications NEC E10.29
      Kimmelstiel-Wilson disease E10.21
      mononeuropathy E10.41
      myasthenia E10.44
      necrobiosis lipoidica E10.620
      nephropathy E10.21
      neuralgia E10.42
      neurologic complication NEC E10.49
      neuropathic arthropathy E10.610
      neuropathy E10.40

Diabetes, diabetic — *continued*
  type 1 — *continued*
    with — *continued*
      ophthalmic complication NEC E10.39
      oral complication NEC E10.638
      periodontal disease E10.630
      peripheral angiopathy E10.51
        with gangrene E10.52
      polyneuropathy E10.42
      renal complication NEC E10.29
      renal tubular degeneration E10.29
      retinopathy E10.319
        with macular edema E10.311
        nonproliferative E10.329
          with macular edema E10.321
          mild E10.329
            with macular edema E10.321
          moderate E10.339
            with macular edema E10.331
          severe E10.349
            with macular edema E10.341
        proliferative E10.359
          with macular edema E10.351
      skin complication NEC E10.628
      skin ulcer NEC E10.622
  type 2 E11.9
    with
      amyotrophy E11.44
      arthropathy NEC E11.618
      autonomic (poly)neuropathy E11.43
      cataract E11.36
      Charcot's joints E11.610
      chronic kidney disease E11.22
      circulatory complication NEC E11.59
      complication E11.8
        specified NEC E11.69
      dermatitis E11.620
      foot ulcer E11.621
      gangrene E11.52
      gastroparesis E11.43
      glomerulonephrosis, intracapillary E11.21
      glomerulosclerosis, intercapillary E11.21
      hyperglycemia E11.65
      hyperosmolarity E11.00
        with coma E11.01
      hypoglycemia E11.649
        with coma E11.641
      kidney complications NEC E11.29
      Kimmelstiel-Wilson disease E11.21
      mononeuropathy E11.41
      myasthenia E11.44
      necrobiosis lipoidica E11.620
      nephropathy E11.21
      neuralgia E11.42
      neurologic complication NEC E11.49
      neuropathic arthropathy E11.610
      neuropathy E11.40
      ophthalmic complication NEC E11.39
      oral complication NEC E11.638
      periodontal disease E11.630
      peripheral angiopathy E11.51
        with gangrene E11.52
      polyneuropathy E11.42
      renal complication NEC E11.29
      renal tubular degeneration E11.29
      retinopathy E11.319
        with macular edema E11.311
        nonproliferative E11.329
          with macular edema E11.321
          mild E11.329
            with macular edema E11.321
          moderate E11.339
            with macular edema E11.331
          severe E11.349
            with macular edema E11.341
        proliferative E11.359
          with macular edema E11.351
      skin complication NEC E11.628
      skin ulcer NEC E11.622
Diacyclothrombopathia D69.1
Diagnosis deferred R69
Dialysis (intermittent) (treatment)
  noncompliance (with) Z91.15
  renal (hemodialysis) (peritoneal), status Z99.2
  retina, retinal — *see* Detachment, retina, with retinal, dialysis
Diamond-Blackfan anemia (congenital hypoplastic) D61.01

Diamond-Gardener syndrome (autoerythrocyte sensitization) D69.2
Diaper rash L22
Diaphoresis (excessive) R61
Diaphragm — *see* condition
Diaphragmalgia R07.1
Diaphragmatitis, diaphragmitis J98.6
Diaphysial aclasis Q78.6
Diaphysitis — *see* Osteomyelitis, specified type NEC
Diarrhea, diarrheal (disease) (infantile) (inflammatory) R19.7
  achlorhydric K31.83
  allergic K52.2
  amebic (*see also* Amebiasis) A06.0
    with abscess — *see* Abscess, amebic
    acute A06.0
    chronic A06.1
    nondysenteric A06.2
  bacillary — *see* Dysentery, bacillary
  balantidial A07.0
  cachectic NEC K52.89
  Chilomastix A07.8
  choleriformis A00.1
  chronic (noninfectious) K52.9
  coccidial A07.3
  Cochin-China K90.1
    strongyloidiasis B78.0
  Dientamoeba A07.8
  dietetic K52.2
  drug-induced K52.1
  due to
    bacteria A04.9
      specified NEC A04.8
    Campylobacter A04.5
    Capillaria philippinensis B81.1
    Clostridium difficile A04.7
    Clostridium perfringens (C) (F) A04.8
    Cryptosporidium A07.2
    drugs K52.1
    Escherichia coli A04.4
      enteroaggregative A04.4
      enterohemorrhagic A04.3
      enteroinvasive A04.2
      enteropathogenic A04.0
      enterotoxigenic A04.1
      specified NEC A04.4
    food hypersensitivity K52.2
    Necator americanus B76.1
    S. japonicum B65.2
    specified organism NEC A08.8
      bacterial A04.8
      viral A08.39
    Staphylococcus A04.8
    Trichuris trichiuria B79
    virus — *see* Enteritis, viral
    Yersinia enterocolitica A04.6
  dysenteric A09
  endemic A09
  epidemic A09
  flagellate A07.9
  Flexner's (ulcerative) A03.1
  functional K59.1
    following gastrointestinal surgery K91.89
    psychogenic F45.8
  Giardia lamblia A07.1
  giardial A07.1
  hill K90.1
  infectious A09
  malarial — *see* Malaria
  mite B88.0
  mycotic NEC B49
  neonatal (noninfectious) P78.3
  nervous F45.8
  neurogenic K59.1
  noninfectious K52.9
  postgastrectomy K91.1
  postvagotomy K91.1
  protozoal A07.9
    specified NEC A07.8
  psychogenic F45.8
  specified
    bacterium NEC A04.8
    virus NEC A08.39
  strongyloidiasis B78.0
  toxic K52.1
  trichomonal A07.8
  tropical K90.1
  tuberculous A18.32

Diarrhea, diarrheal — *continued*
  viral — *see* Enteritis, viral
Diastasis
  cranial bones M84.88
    congenital NEC Q75.8
  joint (traumatic) — *see* Dislocation
  muscle M62.00
    ankle M62.07- ☑
    congenital Q79.8
    foot M62.07- ☑
    forearm M62.03- ☑
    hand M62.04- ☑
    lower leg M62.06- ☑
    pelvic region M62.05- ☑
    shoulder region M62.01- ☑
    specified site NEC M62.08
    thigh M62.05- ☑
    upper arm M62.02- ☑
  recti (abdomen)
    complicating delivery O71.89
    congenital Q79.59
Diastema, tooth, teeth, fully erupted M26.32
Diastematomyelia Q06.2
Diataxia, cerebral G80.4
Diathesis
  allergic — *see* History, allergy
  bleeding (familial) D69.9
  cystine (familial) E72.00
  gouty — *see* Gout
  hemorrhagic (familial) D69.9
    newborn NEC P53
  spasmophilic R29.0
Diaz's disease or osteochondrosis (juvenile) (talus) — *see* Osteochondrosis, juvenile, tarsus
Dibothriocephalus, dibothriocephaliasis (latus) (infection) (infestation) B70.0
  larval B70.1
Dicephalus, dicephaly Q89.4
Dichotomy, teeth K00.2
Dichromat, dichromatopsia (congenital) — *see* Deficiency, color vision
Dichuchwa A65
Dicroceliasis B66.2
Didelphia, didelphys — *see* Double uterus
Didymytis N45.1
  with orchitis N45.3
Dietary
  inadequacy or deficiency E63.9
  surveillance and counseling Z71.3
Dietl's crisis N13.8
Dieulafoy lesion (hemorrhagic)
  duodenum K31.82
  esophagus K22.8
  intestine (colon) K63.81
  stomach K31.82
Difficult, difficulty (in)
  acculturation Z60.3
  feeding R63.3
    newborn P92.9
      breast P92.5
      specified NEC P92.8
    nonorganic (infant or child) F98.29
  intubation, in anesthesia T88.4 ☑
  mechanical, gastroduodenal stoma K91.89
    causing obstruction K91.3
  reading (developmental) F81.0
    secondary to emotional disorders F93.9
  spelling (specific) F81.81
    with reading disorder F81.89
    due to inadequate teaching Z55.8
  swallowing — *see* Dysphagia
  walking R26.2
  work
    conditions NEC Z56.5
    schedule Z56.3
Diffuse — *see* condition
Digestive — *see* condition
Dihydropyrimidine dehydrogenase disease (DPD) E88.89
Diktyoma — *see* Neoplasm, malignant, by site
Dilaceration, tooth K00.4
Dilatation
  anus K59.8
    venule — *see* Hemorrhoids
  aorta (focal) (general) — *see* Ectasia, aorta
    with aneurysm — *see* Aneurysm, aorta
  artery — *see* Aneurysm

Dilatation — *continued*
　bladder (sphincter) N32.89
　　congenital Q64.79
　blood vessel I99.8
　bronchial J47.9
　　with
　　　exacerbation (acute) J47.1
　　　lower respiratory infection J47.0
　calyx (due to obstruction) — *see* Hydronephrosis
　capillaries I78.8
　cardiac (acute) (chronic) (*see also* Hypertrophy, cardiac)
　　congenital Q24.8
　　　valve NEC Q24.8
　　　　pulmonary Q22.3
　　valve — *see* Endocarditis
　cavum septi pellucidi Q06.8
　cervix (uteri) (*see also* Incompetency, cervix)
　　incomplete, poor, slow complicating delivery O62.0
　colon K59.3
　　congenital Q43.1
　　psychogenic F45.8
　common duct (acquired) K83.8
　　congenital Q44.5
　cystic duct (acquired) K82.8
　　congenital Q44.5
　duct, mammary — *see* Ectasia, mammary duct
　duodenum K59.8
　esophagus K22.8
　　congenital Q39.5
　　due to achalasia K22.0
　eustachian tube, congenital Q17.8
　gallbladder K82.8
　gastric — *see* Dilatation, stomach
　heart (acute) (chronic) (*see also* Hypertrophy, cardiac)
　　congenital Q24.8
　　valve — *see* Endocarditis
　ileum K59.8
　　psychogenic F45.8
　jejunum K59.8
　　psychogenic F45.8
　kidney (calyx) (collecting structures) (cystic)
　　　(parenchyma) (pelvis) (idiopathic) N28.89
　lacrimal passages or duct — *see* Disorder, lacrimal
　　　system, changes
　lymphatic vessel I89.0
　mammary duct — *see* Ectasia, mammary duct
　Meckel's diverticulum (congenital) Q43.0
　　malignant — *see* Table of Neoplasms, small intes-
　　　tine, malignant
　myocardium (acute) (chronic) — *see* Hypertrophy,
　　　cardiac
　organ or site, congenital NEC — *see* Distortion
　pancreatic duct K86.8
　pericardium — *see* Pericarditis
　pharynx J39.2
　prostate N42.89
　pulmonary
　　artery (idiopathic) I28.8
　　valve, congenital Q22.3
　pupil H57.04
　rectum K59.3
　saccule, congenital Q16.5
　salivary gland (duct) K11.8
　sphincter ani K62.89
　stomach K31.89
　　acute K31.0
　　psychogenic F45.8
　submaxillary duct K11.8
　trachea, congenital Q32.1
　ureter (idiopathic) N28.82
　　congenital Q62.2
　　due to obstruction N13.4
　urethra (acquired) N36.8
　vasomotor I73.9
　vein I86.8
　ventricular, ventricle (acute) (chronic) (*see also* Hyper-
　　　trophy, cardiac)
　　cerebral, congenital Q04.8
　venule NEC I86.8
　vesical orifice N32.89
Dilated, dilation — *see* Dilatation
Diminished, diminution
　hearing (acuity) — *see* Deafness
　sense or sensation (cold) (heat) (tactile) (vibratory)
　　　R20.8
　vision NEC H54.7
　vital capacity R94.2
Diminuta taenia B71.0

Dimitri-Sturge-Weber disease Q85.8
Dimple
　parasacral, pilonidal or postanal — *see* Cyst, pilonidal
Dioctophyme renalis (infection) (infestation) B83.8
Dipetalonemiasis B74.4
Diphallus Q55.69
Diphtheria, diphtheritic (gangrenous) (hemorrhagic)
　　A36.9
　carrier (suspected) Z22.2
　cutaneous A36.3
　faucial A36.0
　infection of wound A36.3
　laryngeal A36.2
　myocarditis A36.81
　nasal, anterior A36.89
　nasopharyngeal A36.1
　neurological complication A36.89
　pharyngeal A36.0
　specified site NEC A36.89
　tonsillar A36.0
Diphyllobothriasis (intestine) B70.0
　larval B70.1
Diplacusis H93.22- ☑
Diplegia (upper limbs) G83.0
　congenital (cerebral) G80.8
　facial G51.0
　lower limbs G82.20
　spastic G80.1
Diplococcus, diplococcal — *see* condition
Diplopia H53.2
Dipsomania F10.20
　with
　　psychosis — *see* Psychosis, alcoholic
　　remission F10.21
Dipylidiasis B71.1
Direction, teeth, abnormal, fully erupted M26.30
Dirofilariasis B74.8
Dirt-eating child F98.3
Disability, disabilities
　heart — *see* Disease, heart
　intellectual F79
　　with
　　　autistic features F84.9
　　mild (I.Q. 50-69) F70
　　moderate (I.Q. 35-49) F71
　　profound (I.Q. under 20) F73
　　severe (I.Q. 20-34) F72
　　specified level NEC F78
　knowledge acquisition F81.9
　learning F81.9
　limiting activities Z73.6
　spelling, specific F81.81
Disappearance of family member Z63.4
Disarticulation — *see* Amputation
　meaning traumatic amputation — *see* Amputation,
　　　traumatic
Discharge (from)
　abnormal finding in — *see* Abnormal, specimen
　breast (female) (male) N64.52
　diencephalic autonomic idiopathic — *see* Epilepsy,
　　　specified NEC
　ear (*see also* Otorrhea)
　　blood — *see* Otorrhagia
　excessive urine R35.8
　nipple N64.52
　penile R36.9
　postnasal R09.82
　prison, anxiety concerning Z65.2
　urethral R36.9
　　without blood R36.0
　　hematospermia R36.1
　vaginal N89.8
Discitis, diskitis M46.40
　cervical region M46.42
　cervicothoracic region M46.43
　lumbar region M46.46
　lumbosacral region M46.47
　multiple sites M46.49
　occipito-atlanto-axial region M46.41
　pyogenic — *see* Infection, intervertebral disc, pyogenic
　sacrococcygeal region M46.48
　thoracic region M46.44
　thoracolumbar region M46.45
Discoid
　meniscus (congenital) Q68.6
　semilunar cartilage (congenital) — *see* Derangement,
　　　knee, meniscus, specified NEC

Discoloration
　nails L60.8
　teeth (posteruptive) K03.7
　　during formation K00.8
Discomfort
　chest R07.89
　visual H53.14- ☑
Discontinuity, ossicles, ear H74.2- ☑
Discord (with)
　boss Z56.4
　classmates Z55.4
　counselor Z64.4
　employer Z56.4
　family Z63.8
　fellow employees Z56.4
　in-laws Z63.1
　landlord Z59.2
　lodgers Z59.2
　neighbors Z59.2
　probation officer Z64.4
　social worker Z64.4
　teachers Z55.4
　workmates Z56.4
Discordant connection
　atrioventricular (congenital) Q20.5
　ventriculoarterial Q20.3
Discrepancy
　centric occlusion maximum intercuspation M26.55
　leg length (acquired) — *see* Deformity, limb, unequal
　　　length
　　congenital — *see* Defect, reduction, lower limb
　uterine size date O26.84- ☑
Discrimination
　ethnic Z60.5
　political Z60.5
　racial Z60.5
　religious Z60.5
　sex Z60.5
Disease, diseased (*see also* Syndrome)
　absorbent system I87.8
　acid-peptic K30
　Acosta's T70.29 ☑
　Adams-Stokes (-Morgagni) (syncope with heart block)
　　　I45.9
　Addison's anemia (pernicious) D51.0
　adenoids (and tonsils) J35.9
　adrenal (capsule) (cortex) (gland) (medullary) E27.9
　　hyperfunction E27.0
　　specified NEC E27.8
　ainhum L94.6
　airway
　　obstructive, chronic J44.9
　　　due to
　　　　cotton dust J66.0
　　　　specific organic dusts NEC J66.8
　　reactive — *see* Asthma
　akamushi (scrub typhus) A75.3
　Albers-Schönberg (marble bones) Q78.2
　Albert's — *see* Tendinitis, Achilles
　alimentary canal K63.9
　alligator-skin Q80.9
　　acquired L85.0
　alpha heavy chain C88.3
　alpine T70.29 ☑
　altitude T70.20 ☑
　alveolar ridge
　　edentulous K06.9
　　　specified NEC K06.8
　alveoli, teeth K08.9
　Alzheimer's G30.9 [F02.80]
　　with behavioral disturbance G30.9 [F02.81]
　　early onset G30.0 [F02.80]
　　　with behavioral disturbance G30.0 [F02.81]
　　late onset G30.1 [F02.80]
　　　with behavioral disturbance G30.1 [F02.81]
　　specified NEC G30.8 [F02.80]
　　　with behavioral disturbance G30.8 [F02.81]
　amyloid — *see* Amyloidosis
　Andersen's (glycogenosis IV) E74.09
　Andes T70.29 ☑
　Andrews' (bacterid) L08.89
　angiospastic I73.9
　　cerebral G45.9
　　vein I87.8
　anterior
　　chamber H21.9
　　horn cell G12.29

△ **Subterms under main terms may continue to next column or page**　　☑ **Additional Character Required** — Refer to the Tabular List for Character Selection　　**97**

Dilatation — Disease, diseased

Disease, diseased — continued

antiglomerular basement membrane (anti- GBM) anti-
    body M31.0
    tubulo-interstitial nephritis N12
antral — see Sinusitis, maxillary
anus K62.9
    specified NEC K62.89
aorta (nonsyphilitic) I77.9
    syphilitic NEC A52.02
aortic (heart) (valve) I35.9
    rheumatic I06.9
Apollo B30.3
aponeuroses — see Enthesopathy
appendix K38.9
    specified NEC K38.8
aqueous (chamber) H21.9
Arnold-Chiari — see Arnold-Chiari disease
arterial I77.9
    occlusive — see Occlusion, by site
        due to stricture or stenosis I77.1
arteriocardiorenal — see Hypertension, cardiorenal
arteriolar (generalized) (obliterative) I77.9
arteriorenal — see Hypertension, kidney
arteriosclerotic (see also Arteriosclerosis)
    cardiovascular — see Disease, heart, ischemic,
        atherosclerotic
    coronary (artery) — see Disease, heart, ischemic,
        atherosclerotic
    heart — see Disease, heart, ischemic, atherosclerot-
        ic
artery I77.9
    cerebral I67.9
    coronary I25.10
        with angina pectoris — see Arteriosclerosis,
            coronary (artery)
arthropod-borne NOS (viral) A94
    specified type NEC A93.8
atticoantral, chronic H66.20
    left H66.22
        with right H66.23
    right H66.21
        with left H66.23
auditory canal — see Disorder, ear, external
auricle, ear NEC — see Disorder, pinna
Australian X A83.4
autoimmune (systemic) NOS M35.9
    hemolytic (cold type) (warm type) D59.1
        drug-induced D59.0
    thyroid E06.3
aviator's — see Effect, adverse, high altitude
Ayala's Q78.5
Ayerza's (pulmonary artery sclerosis with pulmonary
    hypertension) I27.0
Babington's (familial hemorrhagic telangiectasia) I78.0
bacterial A49.9
    specified NEC A48.8
    zoonotic A28.9
        specified type NEC A28.8
Baelz's (cheilitis glandularis apostematosa) K13.0
bagasse J67.1
balloon — see Effect, adverse, high altitude
Bang's (brucella abortus) A23.1
Bannister's T78.3 ☑
barometer makers' — see Poisoning, mercury
Barraquer (-Simons') (progressive lipodystrophy) E88.1
Barrett's — see Barrett's, esophagus
Bartholin's gland N75.9
basal ganglia G25.9
    degenerative G23.9
        specified NEC G23.8
    specified NEC G25.89
Basedow's (exophthalmic goiter) — see Hyperthy-
    roidism, with, goiter (diffuse)
Bateman's B08.1
Batten-Steinert G71.11
Battey A31.0
Beard's (neurasthenia) F48.8
Becker
    idiopathic mural endomyocardial I42.3
    myotonia congenita G71.12
Begbie's (exophthalmic goiter) — see Hyperthy-
    roidism, with, goiter (diffuse)
behavioral, organic F07.9
Beigel's (white piedra) B36.2
Benson's — see Deposit, crystalline
Bernard-Soulier (thrombopathy) D69.1
Bernhardt (-Roth) — see Mononeuropathy, lower limb,
    meralgia paresthetica

Disease, diseased — continued

Biermer's (pernicious anemia) D51.0
bile duct (common) (hepatic) K83.9
    with calculus, stones — see Calculus, bile duct
    specified NEC K83.8
biliary (tract) K83.9
    specified NEC K83.8
Billroth's — see Spina bifida
bird fancier's J67.2
black lung J60
bladder N32.9
    in (due to)
        schistosomiasis (bilharziasis) B65.0 [N33]
    specified NEC N32.89
bleeder's D66
blood D75.9
    forming organs D75.9
    vessel I99.9
Bloodgood's — see Mastopathy, cystic
Bodechtel-Guttmann (subacute sclerosing panen-
    cephalitis) A81.1
bone (see also Disorder, bone)
    aluminum M83.4
    fibrocystic NEC
        jaw M27.49
bone-marrow D75.9
Borna A83.9
Bornholm (epidemic pleurodynia) B33.0
Bouchard's (myopathic dilatation of the stomach)
    K31.0
Bouillaud's (rheumatic heart disease) I01.9
Bourneville (-Brissaud) (tuberous sclerosis) Q85.1
Bouveret (-Hoffmann) (paroxysmal tachycardia) I47.9
bowel K63.9
    functional K59.9
        psychogenic F45.8
brain G93.9
    arterial, artery I67.9
    arteriosclerotic I67.2
    congenital Q04.9
    degenerative — see Degeneration, brain
    inflammatory — see Encephalitis
    organic G93.9
        arteriosclerotic I67.2
    parasitic NEC B71.9 [G94]
    senile NEC G31.1
    specified NEC G93.89
breast (see also Disorder, breast) N64.9
    cystic (chronic) — see Mastopathy, cystic
    fibrocystic — see Mastopathy, cystic
    Paget's
        female, unspecified side C50.91- ☑
        male, unspecified side C50.92- ☑
    specified NEC N64.89
Breda's — see Yaws
Bretonneau's (diphtheritic malignant angina) A36.0
Bright's — see Nephritis
    arteriosclerotic — see Hypertension, kidney
Brill's (recrudescent typhus) A75.1
Brill-Zinsser (recrudescent typhus) A75.1
Brion-Kayser — see Fever, paratyphoid
broad
    beta E78.2
    ligament (noninflammatory) N83.9
        inflammatory — see Disease, pelvis, inflamma-
            tory
        specified NEC N83.8
Brocq-Duhring (dermatitis herpetiformis) L13.0
Brocq's
    meaning
        dermatitis herpetiformis L13.0
        prurigo L28.2
bronchopulmonary J98.4
bronchus NEC J98.09
bronze Addison's E27.1
    tuberculous A18.7
budgerigar fancier's J67.2
Buerger's (thromboangiitis obliterans) I73.1
bullous L13.9
    chronic of childhood L12.2
    specified NEC L13.8
Bürger-Grütz (essential familial hyperlipemia) E78.3
bursa — see Bursopathy
caisson T70.3 ☑
California — see Coccidioidomycosis
capillaries I78.9
    specified NEC I78.8
Carapata A68.0

Disease, diseased — continued

cardiac — see Disease, heart
cardiopulmonary, chronic I27.9
cardiorenal (hepatic) (hypertensive) (vascular) — see
    Hypertension, cardiorenal
cardiovascular (atherosclerotic) I25.10
    with angina pectoris — see Arteriosclerosis, coro-
        nary (artery),
    congenital Q28.9
    hypertensive — see Hypertension, heart
    newborn P29.9
        specified NEC P29.89
    renal (hypertensive) — see Hypertension, cardiore-
        nal
    syphilitic (asymptomatic) A52.00
cartilage — see Disorder, cartilage
Castellani's A69.8
cat-scratch A28.1
Cavare's (familial periodic paralysis) G72.3
cecum K63.9
celiac (adult) (infantile) K90.0
cellular tissue L98.9
central core G71.2
cerebellar, cerebellum — see Disease, brain
cerebral (see also Disease, brain)
    degenerative — see Degeneration, brain
cerebrospinal G96.9
cerebrovascular I67.9
    acute I67.89
        embolic I63.4- ☑
        thrombotic I63.3- ☑
    arteriosclerotic I67.2
    specified NEC I67.89
cervix (uteri) (noninflammatory) N88.9
    inflammatory — see Cervicitis
    specified NEC N88.8
Chabert's A22.9
Chandler's (osteochondritis dissecans, hip) — see Os-
    teochondritis, dissecans, hip
Charlouis — see Yaws
Chédiak-Steinbrinck (-Higashi) (congenital gigantism
    of peroxidase granules) E70.330
chest J98.9
Chiari's (hepatic vein thrombosis) I82.0
Chicago B40.9
Chignon B36.8
chigo, chigoe B88.1
childhood granulomatous D71
Chinese liver fluke B66.1
chlamydial A74.9
    specified NEC A74.89
cholecystic K82.9
choroid H31.9
    specified NEC H31.8
Christmas D67
chronic bullous of childhood L12.2
chylomicron retention E78.3
ciliary body H21.9
    specified NEC H21.89
circulatory (system) NEC I99.8
    newborn P29.9
    syphilitic A52.00
        congenital A50.54
coagulation factor deficiency (congenital) — see De-
    fect, coagulation
coccidioidal — see Coccidioidomycosis
cold
    agglutinin or hemoglobinuria D59.1
        paroxysmal D59.6
    hemagglutinin (chronic) D59.1
collagen NOS (nonvascular) (vascular) M35.9
    specified NEC M35.8
colon K63.9
    functional K59.9
        congenital Q43.2
    ischemic K55.0
combined system — see Degeneration, combined
compressed air T70.3 ☑
Concato (pericardial polyserositis) A19.9
    nontubercular I31.1
    pleural — see Pleurisy, with effusion
conjunctiva H11.9
    chlamydial A74.0
    specified NEC H11.89
    viral B30.9
        specified NEC B30.8
connective tissue, systemic (diffuse) M35.9

Disease, diseased — *continued*
   connective tissue, systemic — *continued*
      in (due to)
         hypogammaglobulinemia D80.1 [M36.8]
         ochronosis E70.29 [M36.8]
      specified NEC M35.8
   Conor and Bruch's (boutonneuse fever) A77.1
   Cooper's — *see* Mastopathy, cystic
   Cori's (glycogenosis III) E74.03
   corkhandler's or corkworker's J67.3
   cornea H18.9
      specified NEC H18.89- ☑
   coronary (artery) — *see* Disease, heart, ischemic,
         atherosclerotic
      congenital Q24.5
      ostial, syphilitic (aortic) (mitral) (pulmonary) A52.03
   corpus cavernosum N48.9
      specified NEC N48.89
   Cotugno's — *see* Sciatica
   coxsackie (virus) NEC B34.1
   cranial nerve NOS G52.9
   Creutzfeldt-Jakob — *see* Creutzfeldt-Jakob disease or
         syndrome
   Crocq's (acrocyanosis) I73.89
   Crohn's — *see* Enteritis, regional
   Curschmann G71.11
   cystic
      breast (chronic) — *see* Mastopathy, cystic
      kidney, congenital Q61.9
      liver, congenital Q44.6
      lung J98.4
         congenital Q33.0
   cytomegalic inclusion (generalized) B25.9
      with pneumonia B25.0
      congenital P35.1
   cytomegaloviral B25.9
      specified NEC B25.8
   Czerny's (periodic hydrarthrosis of the knee) — *see*
         Effusion, joint, knee
   Daae (-Finsen) (epidemic pleurodynia) B33.0
   Darling's — *see* Histoplasmosis capsulati
   de Quervain's (tendon sheath) M65.4
      thyroid (subacute granulomatous thyroiditis) E06.1
   Débove's (splenomegaly) R16.1
   deer fly — *see* Tularemia
   Degos' I77.89
   demyelinating, demyelinizating (nervous system)
         G37.9
      multiple sclerosis G35
      specified NEC G37.8
   dense deposit (*see also* N00-N07 with fourth character
         .6) N05.6
   deposition, hydroxyapatite — *see* Disease, hydroxya-
         patite deposition
   Devergie's (pityriasis rubra pilaris) L44.0
   Devic's G36.0
   diaphorase deficiency D74.0
   diaphragm J98.6
   diarrheal, infectious NEC A09
   digestive system K92.9
      specified NEC K92.89
   disc, degenerative — *see* Degeneration, intervertebral
         disc
   discogenic (*see also* Displacement, intervertebral disc
         NEC)
      with myelopathy — *see* Disorder, disc, with,
            myelopathy
   diverticular — *see* Diverticula
   Dubois (thymus) A50.59 [E35]
   Duchenne-Griesinger G71.0
   Duchenne's
      muscular dystrophy G71.0
      pseudohypertrophy, muscles G71.0
   ductless glands E34.9
   Duhring's (dermatitis herpetiformis) L13.0
   duodenum K31.9
      specified NEC K31.89
   Dupré's (meningism) R29.1
   Dupuytren's (muscle contracture) M72.0
   Durand-Nicholas-Favre (climatic bubo) A55
   Duroziez's (congenital mitral stenosis) Q23.2
   ear — *see* Disorder, ear
   Eberth's — *see* Fever, typhoid
   Ebola (virus) A98.4
   Ebstein's heart Q22.5
   Echinococcus — *see* Echinococcus
   echovirus NEC B34.1
   Eddowes' (brittle bones and blue sclera) Q78.0

Disease, diseased — *continued*
   edentulous (alveolar) ridge K06.9
      specified NEC K06.8
   Edsall's T67.2 ☑
   Eichstedt's (pityriasis versicolor) B36.0
   Ellis-van Creveld (chondroectodermal dysplasia) Q77.6
   end stage renal (ESRD) N18.6
      due to hypertension I12.0
   endocrine glands or system NEC E34.9
   endomyocardial (eosinophilic) I42.3
   English (rickets) E55.0
   enteroviral, enterovirus NEC B34.1
      central nervous system NEC A88.8
   epidemic B99.9
      specified NEC B99.8
   epididymis N50.9
   Erb (-Landouzy) G71.0
   Erdheim-Chester (ECD) E88.89
   esophagus K22.9
      functional K22.4
      psychogenic F45.8
      specified NEC K22.8
   Eulenburg's (congenital paramyotonia) G71.19
   eustachian tube — *see* Disorder, eustachian tube
   external
      auditory canal — *see* Disorder, ear, external
      ear — *see* Disorder, ear, external
   extrapyramidal G25.9
      specified NEC G25.89
   eye H57.9
      anterior chamber H21.9
      inflammatory NEC H57.8
      muscle (external) — *see* Strabismus
      specified NEC H57.8
      syphilitic — *see* Oculopathy, syphilitic
   eyeball H44.9
      specified NEC H44.89
   eyelid — *see* Disorder, eyelid
      specified NEC — *see* Disorder, eyelid, specified type
            NEC
   eyeworm of Africa B74.3
   facial nerve (seventh) G51.9
      newborn (birth injury) P11.3
   Fahr (of brain) G23.8
   Fahr Volhard (of kidney) I12.- ☑
   fallopian tube (noninflammatory) N83.9
      inflammatory — *see* Salpingo-oophoritis
      specified NEC N83.8
   familial periodic paralysis G72.3
   Fanconi's (congenital pancytopenia) D61.09
   fascia NEC (*see also* Disorder, muscle)
      inflammatory — *see* Myositis
      specified NEC M62.89
   Fauchard's (periodontitis) — *see* Periodontitis
   Favre-Durand-Nicolas (climatic bubo) A55
   Fede's K14.0
   Feer's — *see* Poisoning, mercury
   female pelvic inflammatory (*see also* Disease, pelvis,
         inflammatory) N73.9
      syphilitic (secondary) A51.42
      tuberculous A18.17
   Fernels' (aortic aneurysm) I71.9
   fibrocaseous of lung — *see* Tuberculosis, pulmonary
   fibrocystic — *see* Fibrocystic disease
   Fiedler's (leptospiral jaundice) A27.0
   fifth B08.3
   file-cutter's — *see* Poisoning, lead
   fish-skin Q80.9
      acquired L85.0
   Flajani (-Basedow) (exophthalmic goiter) — *see* Hyper-
         thyroidism, with, goiter (diffuse)
   flax-dresser's J66.1
   fluke — *see* Infestation, fluke
   foot and mouth B08.8
   foot process N04.9
   Forbes' (glycogenosis III) E74.03
   Fordyce-Fox (apocrine miliaria) L75.2
   Fordyce's (ectopic sebaceous glands) (mouth) Q38.6
   Forestier's (rhizomelic pseudopolyarthritis) M35.3
      meaning ankylosing hyperostosis — *see* Hyperos-
            tosis, ankylosing
   Fothergill's
      neuralgia — *see* Neuralgia, trigeminal
      scarlatina anginosa A38.9
   Fournier (gangrene) N49.3
      female N76.89
   fourth B08.8
   Fox (-Fordyce) (apocrine miliaria) L75.2

Disease, diseased — *continued*
   Francis' — *see* Tularemia
   Franklin C88.2
   Frei's (climatic bubo) A55
   Friedreich's
      combined systemic or ataxia G11.1
      myoclonia G25.3
   frontal sinus — *see* Sinusitis, frontal
   fungus NEC B49
   Gaisböck's (polycythemia hypertonica) D75.1
   gallbladder K82.9
      calculus — *see* Calculus, gallbladder
      cholecystitis — *see* Cholecystitis
      cholesterolosis K82.4
      fistula — *see* Fistula, gallbladder
      hydrops K82.1
      obstruction — *see* Obstruction, gallbladder
      perforation K82.2
      specified NEC K82.8
   gamma heavy chain C88.2
   Gamna's (siderotic splenomegaly) D73.2
   Gamstorp's (adynamia episodica hereditaria) G72.3
   Gandy-Nanta (siderotic splenomegaly) D73.2
   ganister J62.8
   gastric — *see* Disease, stomach
   gastroesophageal reflux (GERD) K21.9
      with esophagitis K21.0
   gastrointestinal (tract) K92.9
      amyloid E85.4
      functional K59.9
         psychogenic F45.8
      specified NEC K92.89
   Gee (-Herter) (-Heubner) (-Thaysen) (nontropical sprue)
         K90.0
   genital organs
      female N94.9
      male N50.9
   Gerhardt's (erythromelalgia) I73.81
   Gibert's (pityriasis rosea) L42
   Gierke's (glycogenosis I) E74.01
   Gilles de la Tourette's (motor-verbal tic) F95.2
   gingiva K06.9
      specified NEC K06.8
   gland (lymph) I89.9
   Glanzmann's (hereditary hemorrhagic thrombasthenia)
         D69.1
   glass-blower's (cataract) — *see* Cataract, specified NEC
      salivary gland hypertrophy K11.1
   Glisson's — *see* Rickets
   globe H44.9
      specified NEC H44.89
   glomerular (*see also* Glomerulonephritis)
      with edema — *see* Nephrosis
      acute — *see* Nephritis, acute
      chronic — *see* Nephritis, chronic
      minimal change N05.0
      rapidly progressive N01.9
   glycogen storage E74.00
      Andersen's E74.09
      Cori's E74.03
      Forbes' E74.03
      generalized E74.00
      glucose-6-phosphatase deficiency E74.01
      heart E74.02 [I43]
      hepatorenal E74.09
      Hers' E74.09
      liver and kidney E74.09
      McArdle's E74.04
      muscle phosphofructokinase E74.09
      myocardium E74.02 [I43]
      Pompe's E74.02
      Tauri's E74.09
      type 0 E74.09
      type I E74.01
      type II E74.02
      type III E74.03
      type IV E74.09
      type V E74.04
      type VI-XI E74.09
      Von Gierke's E74.01
   Goldstein's (familial hemorrhagic telangiectasia) I78.0
   gonococcal NOS A54.9
   graft-versus-host (GVH) D89.813
      acute D89.810
      acute on chronic D89.812
      chronic D89.811
   grainhandler's J67.8
   granulomatous (childhood) (chronic) D71

Disease, diseased — *continued*
Graves' (exophthalmic goiter) — *see* Hyperthyroidism, with, goiter (diffuse)
Griesinger's — *see* Ancylostomiasis
Grisel's M43.6
Gruby's (tinea tonsurans) B35.0
Guillain-Barré G61.0
Guinon's (motor-verbal tic) F95.2
gum K06.9
gynecological N94.9
H (Hartnup's) E72.02
Haff — *see* Poisoning, mercury
Hageman (congenital factor XII deficiency) D68.2
hair (color) (shaft) L67.9
    follicles L73.9
        specified NEC L73.8
Hamman's (spontaneous mediastinal emphysema) J98.2
hand, foot and mouth B08.4
Hansen's — *see* Leprosy
Hantavirus, with pulmonary manifestations B33.4
    with renal manifestations A98.5
Harada's H30.81- ☑
Hartnup (pellagra-cerebellar ataxia-renal aminoaciduria) E72.02
Hart's (pellagra-cerebellar ataxia-renal aminoaciduria) E72.02
Hashimoto's (struma lymphomatosa) E06.3
Hb — *see* Disease, hemoglobin
heart (organic) I51.9
    with
        pulmonary edema (acute) (*see also* Failure, ventricular, left) I50.1
        rheumatic fever (conditions in I00)
            active I01.9
                with chorea I02.0
                    specified NEC I01.8
            inactive or quiescent (with chorea) I09.9
                specified NEC I09.89
    amyloid E85.4 [I43]
    aortic (valve) I35.9
    arteriosclerotic or sclerotic (senile) — *see* Disease, heart, ischemic, atherosclerotic
    artery, arterial — *see* Disease, heart, ischemic, atherosclerotic
    beer drinkers' I42.6
    beriberi (wet) E51.12
    black I27.0
    congenital Q24.9
        cyanotic Q24.9
        specified NEC Q24.8
    coronary — *see* Disease, heart, ischemic
    cryptogenic I51.9
    fibroid — *see* Myocarditis
    functional I51.89
        psychogenic F45.8
    glycogen storage E74.02 [I43]
    gonococcal A54.83
    hypertensive — *see* Hypertension, heart
    hyperthyroid (*see also* Hyperthyroidism) E05.90 [I43]
        with thyroid storm E05.91 [I43]
    ischemic (chronic or with a stated duration of over 4 weeks) I25.9
        atherosclerotic (of) I25.10
            with angina pectoris — *see* Arteriosclerosis, coronary (artery)
            coronary artery bypass graft — *see* Arteriosclerosis, coronary (artery), cardiomyopathy I25.5
            diagnosed on ECG or other special investigation, but currently presenting no symptoms I25.6
        silent I25.6
        specified form NEC I25.89
    kyphoscoliotic I27.1
    meningococcal A39.50
        endocarditis A39.51
        myocarditis A39.52
        pericarditis A39.53
    mitral I05.9
        specified NEC I05.8
    muscular — *see* Degeneration, myocardial
    psychogenic (functional) F45.8
    pulmonary (chronic) I27.9
        in schistosomiasis B65.9 [I52]
        specified NEC I27.89

Disease, diseased — *continued*
heart — *continued*
    rheumatic (chronic) (inactive) (old) (quiescent) (with chorea) I09.9
        active or acute I01.9
            with chorea (acute) (rheumatic) (Sydenham's) I02.0
        specified NEC I09.89
    senile — *see* Myocarditis
    syphilitic A52.06
        aortic A52.03
            aneurysm A52.01
        congenital A50.54 [I52]
    thyrotoxic (*see also* Thyrotoxicosis) E05.90 [I43]
        with thyroid storm E05.91 [I43]
    valve, valvular (obstructive) (regurgitant) (*see also* Endocarditis)
        congenital NEC Q24.8
            pulmonary Q22.3
    vascular — *see* Disease, cardiovascular
heavy chain NEC C88.2
    alpha C88.3
    gamma C88.2
    mu C88.2
Hebra's
    pityriasis
        maculata et circinata L42
        rubra pilaris L44.0
    prurigo L28.2
hematopoietic organs D75.9
hemoglobin or Hb
    abnormal (mixed) NEC D58.2
        with thalassemia D56.9
    AS genotype D57.3
    Bart's D56.0
    C (Hb-C) D58.2
        with other abnormal hemoglobin NEC D58.2
        elliptocytosis D58.1
        Hb-S D57.2- ☑
        sickle-cell D57.2- ☑
        thalassemia D56.8
    Constant Spring D58.2
    D (Hb-D) D58.2
    E (Hb-E) D58.2
    E-beta thalassemia D56.5
    elliptocytosis D58.1
    H (Hb-H) (thalassemia) D56.0
        with other abnormal hemoglobin NEC D56.9
        Constant Spring D56.0
    I thalassemia D56.9
    M D74.0
    S or SS D57.1
    SC D57.2- ☑
    SD D57.8- ☑
    SE D57.8- ☑
    spherocytosis D58.0
    unstable, hemolytic D58.2
hemolytic (newborn) P55.9
    autoimmune (cold type) (warm type) D59.1
    drug-induced D59.0
    due to or with
        incompatibility
            ABO (blood group) P55.1
            blood (group) (Duffy) (K(ell)) (Kidd) (Lewis) (M) (S) NEC P55.8
            Rh (blood group) (factor) P55.0
        Rh negative mother P55.0
    specified type NEC P55.8
    unstable hemoglobin D58.2
hemorrhagic D69.9
    newborn P53
Henoch (-Schönlein) (purpura nervosa) D69.0
hepatic — *see* Disease, liver
hepatolenticular E83.01
heredodegenerative NEC
    spinal cord G95.89
herpesviral, disseminated B00.7
Hers' (glycogenosis VI) E74.09
Herter (-Gee) (-Heubner) (nontropical sprue) K90.0
Heubner-Herter (nontropical sprue) K90.0
high fetal gene or hemoglobin thalassemia D56.9
Hildenbrand's — *see* Typhus
hip (joint) M25.9
    congenital Q65.89
    suppurative M00.9
    tuberculous A18.02
His (-Werner) (trench fever) A79.0
Hodgson's I71.2

Disease, diseased — *continued*
Hodgson's — *continued*
    ruptured I71.1
Holla — *see* Spherocytosis
hookworm B76.9
    specified NEC B76.8
host-versus-graft D89.813
    acute D89.810
    acute on chronic D89.812
    chronic D89.811
human immunodeficiency virus (HIV) B20
Huntington's G10
Hutchinson's (cheiropompholyx) — *see* Hutchinson's disease
hyaline (diffuse) (generalized)
    membrane (lung) (newborn) P22.0
        adult J80
hydatid — *see* Echinococcus
hydroxyapatite deposition M11.00
    ankle M11.07- ☑
    elbow M11.02- ☑
    foot joint M11.07- ☑
    hand joint M11.04- ☑
    hip M11.05- ☑
    knee M11.06- ☑
    multiple site M11.09
    shoulder M11.01- ☑
    vertebra M11.08
    wrist M11.03- ☑
hyperkinetic — *see* Hyperkinesia
hypertensive — *see* Hypertension
hypophysis E23.7
Iceland G93.3
I-cell E77.0
immune D89.9
immunoproliferative (malignant) C88.9
    small intestinal C88.3
    specified NEC C88.8
inclusion B25.9
    salivary gland B25.9
infectious, infective B99.9
    congenital P37.9
        specified NEC P37.8
        viral P35.9
            specified type NEC P35.8
    specified NEC B99.8
inflammatory
    penis N48.29
        abscess N48.21
        cellulitis N48.22
    prepuce N47.7
        balanoposthitis N47.6
    tubo-ovarian — *see* Salpingo-oophoritis
intervertebral disc (*see also* Disorder, disc)
    with myelopathy — *see* Disorder, disc, with, myelopathy
    cervical, cervicothoracic — *see* Disorder, disc, cervical
        with
            myelopathy — *see* Disorder, disc, cervical, with myelopathy
            neuritis, radiculitis or radiculopathy — *see* Disorder, disc, cervical, with neuritis
            specified NEC — *see* Disorder, disc, cervical, specified type NEC
    lumbar (with)
        myelopathy M51.06
        neuritis, radiculitis, radiculopathy or sciatica M51.16
        specified NEC M51.86
    lumbosacral (with)
        neuritis, radiculitis, radiculopathy or sciatica M51.17
        specified NEC M51.87
    specified NEC — *see* Disorder, disc, specified NEC
    thoracic (with)
        myelopathy M51.04
        neuritis, radiculitis or radiculopathy M51.14
        specified NEC M51.84
    thoracolumbar (with)
        myelopathy M51.05
        neuritis, radiculitis or radiculopathy M51.15
        specified NEC M51.85
intestine K63.9
    functional K59.9
        psychogenic F45.8
        specified NEC K59.8
    organic K63.9

☑ **Additional Character Required** — Refer to the Tabular List for Character Selection   ▧ Subterms under main terms may continue to next column or page

Disease, diseased — *continued*
- intestine — *continued*
  - protozoal A07.9
  - specified NEC K63.89
- iris H21.9
  - specified NEC H21.89
- iron metabolism or storage E83.10
- island (scrub typhus) A75.3
- itai-itai — *see* Poisoning, cadmium
- Jakob-Creutzfeldt — *see* Creutzfeldt-Jakob disease or syndrome
- jaw M27.9
  - fibrocystic M27.49
  - specified NEC M27.8
- jigger B88.1
- joint (*see also* Disorder, joint)
  - Charcot's — *see* Arthropathy, neuropathic (Charcot)
  - degenerative — *see* Osteoarthritis
    - multiple M15.9
    - spine — *see* Spondylosis
  - hypertrophic — *see* Osteoarthritis
  - sacroiliac M53.3
  - specified NEC — *see* Disorder, joint, specified type NEC
  - spine NEC — *see* Dorsopathy
  - suppurative — *see* Arthritis, pyogenic or pyemic
- Jourdain's (acute gingivitis) K05.00
  - nonplaque induced K05.01
  - plaque induced K05.00
- Kaschin-Beck (endemic polyarthritis) M12.10
  - ankle M12.17- ☑
  - elbow M12.12- ☑
  - foot joint M12.17- ☑
  - hand joint M12.14- ☑
  - hip M12.15- ☑
  - knee M12.16- ☑
  - multiple site M12.19
  - shoulder M12.11- ☑
  - vertebra M12.18
  - wrist M12.13- ☑
- Katayama B65.2
- Kedani (scrub typhus) A75.3
- Keshan E59
- kidney (functional) (pelvis) N28.9
  - chronic N18.9
    - hypertensive — *see* Hypertension, kidney
    - stage 1 N18.1
    - stage 2 (mild) N18.2
    - stage 3 (moderate) N18.3
    - stage 4 (severe) N18.4
    - stage 5 N18.5
  - complicating pregnancy — *see* Pregnancy, complicated by, renal disease
  - cystic (congenital) Q61.9
  - fibrocystic (congenital) Q61.8
  - hypertensive — *see* Hypertension, kidney
  - in (due to)
    - schistosomiasis (bilharziasis) B65.9 [N29]
  - multicystic Q61.4
  - polycystic Q61.3
    - adult type Q61.2
    - childhood type NEC Q61.19
      - collecting duct dilatation Q61.11
- Kimmelstiel (-Wilson) (intercapillary polycystic (congenital) glomerulosclerosis) — *see* E08-E13 with .21
- Kinnier Wilson's (hepatolenticular degeneration) E83.01
- kissing — *see* Mononucleosis, infectious
- Klebs' (*see also* Glomerulonephritis) N05- ☑
- Klippel-Feil (brevicollis) Q76.1
- Köhler-Pellegrini-Stieda (calcification, knee joint) — *see* Bursitis, tibial collateral
- Kok Q89.8
- König's (osteochondritis dissecans) — *see* Osteochondritis, dissecans
- Korsakoff's (nonalcoholic) F04
  - alcoholic F10.96
    - with dependence F10.26
- Kostmann's (infantile genetic agranulocytosis) D70.0
- kuru A81.81
- Kyasanur Forest A98.2
- labyrinth, ear — *see* Disorder, ear, inner
- lacrimal system — *see* Disorder, lacrimal system
- Lafora's — *see* Epilepsy, generalized, idiopathic
- Lancereaux-Mathieu (leptospiral jaundice) A27.0
- Landry's G61.0

Disease, diseased — *continued*
- Larrey-Weil (leptospiral jaundice) A27.0
- larynx J38.7
- legionnaires' A48.1
  - nonpneumonic A48.2
- Lenegre's I44.2
- lens H27.9
  - specified NEC H27.8
- Lev's (acquired complete heart block) I44.2
- Lewy body (dementia) G31.83 [F02.80]
  - with behavioral disturbance G31.83 [F02.81]
- Lichtheim's (subacute combined sclerosis with pernicious anemia) D51.0
- Lightwood's (renal tubular acidosis) N25.89
- Lignac's (cystinosis) E72.04
- lip K13.0
- lipid-storage E75.6
  - specified NEC E75.5
- Lipschütz's N76.6
- liver (chronic) (organic) K76.9
  - alcoholic (chronic) K70.9
    - acute — *see* Disease, liver, alcoholic, hepatitis
    - cirrhosis K70.30
      - with ascites K70.31
    - failure K70.40
      - with coma K70.41
    - fatty liver K70.0
    - fibrosis K70.2
    - hepatitis K70.10
      - with ascites K70.11
    - sclerosis K70.2
  - cystic, congenital Q44.6
  - drug-induced (idiosyncratic) (toxic) (predictable) (unpredictable) — *see* Disease, liver, toxic
  - end stage K72.90
    - due to hepatitis — *see* Hepatitis
  - fatty, nonalcoholic (NAFLD) K76.0
    - alcoholic K70.0
  - fibrocystic (congenital) Q44.6
  - fluke
    - Chinese B66.1
    - oriental B66.1
    - sheep B66.3
  - glycogen storage E74.09 [K77]
  - in (due to)
    - schistosomiasis (bilharziasis) B65.9 [K77]
  - inflammatory K75.9
    - alcoholic K70.1 ☑
    - specified NEC K75.89
  - polycystic (congenital) Q44.6
  - toxic K71.9
    - with
      - cholestasis K71.0
      - cirrhosis (liver) K71.7
      - fibrosis (liver) K71.7
      - focal nodular hyperplasia K71.8
      - hepatic granuloma K71.8
      - hepatic necrosis K71.10
        - with coma K71.11
      - hepatitis NEC K71.6
        - acute K71.2
        - chronic
          - active K71.50
            - with ascites K71.51
          - lobular K71.4
          - persistent K71.3
        - lupoid K71.50
          - with ascites K71.51
      - peliosis hepatis K71.8
      - veno-occlusive disease (VOD) of liver K71.8
  - veno-occlusive K76.5
- Lobo's (keloid blastomycosis) B48.0
- Lobstein's (brittle bones and blue sclera) Q78.0
- Ludwig's (submaxillary cellulitis) K12.2
- lumbosacral region M53.87
- lung J98.4
  - black J60
  - congenital Q33.9
  - cystic J98.4
    - congenital Q33.0
  - fibroid (chronic) — *see* Fibrosis, lung
  - fluke B66.4
    - oriental B66.4
  - in
    - amyloidosis E85.4 [J99]
    - sarcoidosis D86.0
    - Sjögren's syndrome M35.02

Disease, diseased — *continued*
- lung — *continued*
  - in — *continued*
    - systemic
      - lupus erythematosus M32.13
      - sclerosis M34.81
    - interstitial J84.9
      - of childhood, specified NEC J84.848
      - respiratory bronchiolitis J84.115
      - specified NEC J84.89
    - obstructive (chronic) J44.9
      - with
        - acute
          - bronchitis J44.0
          - exacerbation NEC J44.1
          - lower respiratory infection J44.0
        - alveolitis, allergic J67.9
        - asthma J44.9
        - bronchiectasis J47.9
          - with
            - exacerbation (acute) J47.1
            - lower respiratory infection J47.0
        - bronchitis J44.9
          - with
            - exacerbation (acute) J44.1
            - lower respiratory infection J44.0
        - emphysema J44.9
        - hypersensitivity pneumonitis J67.9
      - decompensated J44.1
        - with
          - exacerbation (acute) J44.1
    - polycystic J98.4
      - congenital Q33.0
    - rheumatoid (diffuse) (interstitial) — *see* Rheumatoid, lung
- Lutembacher's (atrial septal defect with mitral stenosis) Q21.1
- Lyme A69.20
- lymphatic (gland) (system) (channel) (vessel) I89.9
- lymphoproliferative D47.9
  - specified NEC D47.Z9 (*following* D47.4)
  - T-gamma D47.Z9 (*following* D47.4)
  - X-linked D82.3
- Magitot's M27.2
- malarial — *see* Malaria
- malignant (*see also* Neoplasm, malignant, by site)
- Manson's B65.1
- maple bark J67.6
- maple-syrup-urine E71.0
- Marburg (virus) A98.3
- Marion's (bladder neck obstruction) N32.0
- Marsh's (exophthalmic goiter) — *see* Hyperthyroidism, with, goiter (diffuse)
- mastoid (process) — *see* Disorder, ear, middle
- Mathieu's (leptospiral jaundice) A27.0
- Maxcy's A75.2
- McArdle (-Schmid-Pearson) (glycogenosis V) E74.04
- mediastinum J98.5
- medullary center (idiopathic) (respiratory) G93.89
- Meige's (chronic hereditary edema) Q82.0
- meningococcal — *see* Infection, meningococcal
- mental F99
  - organic F09
- mesenchymal M35.9
- mesenteric embolic K55.0
- metabolic, metabolism E88.9
  - bilirubin E80.7
- metal-polisher's J62.8
- metastatic (*see also* Neoplasm, secondary, by site) C79.9
- microvascular - code to condition
- microvillus
  - atrophy Q43.8
  - inclusion (MVD) Q43.8
- middle ear — *see* Disorder, ear, middle
- Mikulicz' (dryness of mouth, absent or decreased lacrimation) K11.8
- Milroy's (chronic hereditary edema) Q82.0
- Minamata — *see* Poisoning, mercury
- minicore G71.2
- Minor's G95.19
- Minot's (hemorrhagic disease, newborn) P53
- Minot-von Willebrand-Jürgens (angiohemophilia) D68.0
- Mitchell's (erythromelalgia) I73.81
- mitral (valve) I05.9
  - nonrheumatic I34.9
- mixed connective tissue M35.1

Disease, diseased — *continued*
moldy hay J67.0
Monge's T70.29 ☑
Morgagni-Adams-Stokes (syncope with heart block)
    I45.9
Morgagni's (syndrome) (hyperostosis frontalis interna)
    M85.2
Morton's (with metatarsalgia) — *see* Lesion, nerve,
    plantar
Morvan's G60.8
motor neuron (bulbar) (familial) (mixed type) (spinal)
    G12.20
    amyotrophic lateral sclerosis G12.21
    progressive bulbar palsy G12.22
    specified NEC G12.29
moyamoya I67.5
mu heavy chain disease C88.2
multicore G71.2
muscle (*see also* Disorder, muscle)
    inflammatory — *see* Myositis
    ocular (external) — *see* Strabismus
musculoskeletal system, soft tissue — *see also* Disor-
    der, soft tissue
    specified NEC — *see* Disorder, soft tissue, specified
        type NEC
mushroom workers' J67.5
mycotic B49
myelodysplastic, not classified C94.6
myeloproliferative, not classified C94.6
    chronic D47.1
myocardium, myocardial (*see also* Degeneration, my-
    ocardial) I51.5
    primary (idiopathic) I42.9
myoneural G70.9
Naegeli's D69.1
nails L60.9
    specified NEC L60.8
Nairobi (sheep virus) A93.8
nasal J34.9
nemaline body G71.2
nerve — *see* Disorder, nerve
nervous system G98.8
    autonomic G90.9
    central G96.9
        specified NEC G96.8
    congenital Q07.9
    parasympathetic G90.9
    specified NEC G98.8
    sympathetic G90.9
    vegetative G90.9
neuromuscular system G70.9
Newcastle B30.8
Nicolas (-Durand)-Favre (climatic bubo) A55
nipple N64.9
    Paget's C50.01- ☑
        female C50.01- ☑
        male C50.02- ☑
Nishimoto (-Takeuchi) I67.5
nonarthropod-borne NOS (viral) B34.9
    enterovirus NEC B34.1
nonautoimmune hemolytic D59.4
    drug-induced D59.2
Nonne-Milroy-Meige (chronic hereditary edema) Q82.0
nose J34.9
nucleus pulposus — *see* Disorder, disc
nutritional E63.9
oast-house-urine E72.19
ocular
    herpesviral B00.50
    zoster B02.30
obliterative vascular I77.1
Ohara's — *see* Tularemia
Opitz's (congestive splenomegaly) D73.2
Oppenheim-Urbach (necrobiosis lipoidica diabetico-
    rum) — *see* E08-E13 with .620
optic nerve NEC — *see* Disorder, nerve, optic
orbit — *see* Disorder, orbit
Oriental liver fluke B66.1
Oriental lung fluke B66.4
Ormond's N13.5
Oropouche virus A93.0
Osler-Rendu (familial hemorrhagic telangiectasia) I78.0
osteofibrocystic E21.0
Otto's M24.7
outer ear — *see* Disorder, ear, external
ovary (noninflammatory) N83.9
    cystic N83.20
    inflammatory — *see* Salpingo-oophoritis

Disease, diseased — *continued*
ovary — *continued*
    polycystic E28.2
    specified NEC N83.8
Owren's (congenital) — *see* Defect, coagulation
pancreas K86.9
    cystic K86.2
    fibrocystic E84.9
    specified NEC K86.8
panvalvular I08.9
    specified NEC I08.8
parametrium (noninflammatory) N83.9
parasitic B89
    cerebral NEC B71.9 [G94]
    intestinal NEC B82.9
    mouth B37.0
    skin NOS B88.9
    specified type — *see* Infestation
    tongue B37.0
parathyroid (gland) E21.5
    specified NEC E21.4
Parkinson's G20
parodontal K05.6
Parrot's (syphilitic osteochondritis) A50.02
Parry's (exophthalmic goiter) — *see* Hyperthyroidism,
    with, goiter (diffuse)
Parson's (exophthalmic goiter) — *see* Hyperthyroidism,
    with, goiter (diffuse)
Paxton's (white piedra) B36.2
pearl-worker's — *see* Osteomyelitis, specified type
    NEC
Pellegrini-Stieda (calcification, knee joint) — *see* Bur-
    sitis, tibial collateral
pelvis, pelvic
    female NOS N94.9
        specified NEC N94.89
    gonococcal (acute) (chronic) A54.24
    inflammatory (female) N73.9
        acute N73.0
        chronic N73.1
        specified NEC N73.8
        syphilitic (secondary) A51.42
            late A52.76
        tuberculous A18.17
    organ, female N94.9
    peritoneum, female NEC N94.89
penis N48.9
    inflammatory N48.29
        abscess N48.21
        cellulitis N48.22
    specified NEC N48.89
periapical tissues NOS K04.90
periodontal K05.6
    specified NEC K05.5
periosteum — *see* Disorder, bone, specified type NEC
peripheral
    arterial I73.9
    autonomic nervous system G90.9
    nerves — *see* Polyneuropathy
    vascular NOS I73.9
peritoneum K66.9
    pelvic, female NEC N94.89
    specified NEC K66.8
persistent mucosal (middle ear) H66.20
    left H66.22
        with right H66.23
    right H66.21
        with left H66.23
Petit's — *see* Hernia, abdomen, specified site NEC
pharynx J39.2
    specified NEC J39.2
Phocas' — *see* Mastopathy, cystic
photochromogenic (acid-fast bacilli) (pulmonary)
    A31.0
    nonpulmonary A31.9
Pick's G31.01 [F02.80]
    with behavioral disturbance G31.01 [F02.81]
pigeon fancier's J67.2
pineal gland E34.8
pink — *see* Poisoning, mercury
Pinkus' (lichen nitidus) L44.1
pinworm B80
Piry virus A93.8
pituitary (gland) E23.7
pituitary-snuff-taker's J67.8
pleura (cavity) J94.9
    specified NEC J94.8
pneumatic drill (hammer) T75.21 ☑

Disease, diseased — *continued*
Pollitzer's (hidradenitis suppurativa) L73.2
polycystic
    kidney or renal Q61.3
        adult type Q61.2
        childhood type NEC Q61.19
            collecting duct dilatation Q61.11
    liver or hepatic Q44.6
    lung or pulmonary J98.4
        congenital Q33.0
    ovary, ovaries E28.2
    spleen Q89.09
polyethylene T84.05- ☑
Pompe's (glycogenosis II) E74.02
Posadas-Wernicke B38.9
Potain's (pulmonary edema) — *see* Edema, lung
prepuce N47.8
    inflammatory N47.7
        balanoposthitis N47.6
Pringle's (tuberous sclerosis) Q85.1
prion, central nervous system A81.9
    specified NEC A81.89
prostate N42.9
    specified NEC N42.89
protozoal B64
    acanthamebiasis — *see* Acanthamebiasis
    African trypanosomiasis — *see* African trypanoso-
        miasis
    babesiosis B60.0
    Chagas disease — *see* Chagas disease
    intestine, intestinal A07.9
    leishmaniasis — *see* Leishmaniasis
    malaria — *see* Malaria
    naegleriasis B60.2
    pneumocystosis B59
    specified organism NEC B60.8
    toxoplasmosis — *see* Toxoplasmosis
pseudo-Hurler's E77.0
psychiatric F99
psychotic — *see* Psychosis
Puente's (simple glandular cheilitis) K13.0
puerperal (*see also* Puerperal) O90.89
pulmonary (*see also* Disease, lung)
    artery I28.9
    chronic obstructive J44.9
        with
            acute bronchitis J44.0
            exacerbation (acute) J44.1
            lower respiratory infection (acute) J44.0
        decompensated J44.1
            with
                exacerbation (acute) J44.1
    heart I27.9
        specified NEC I27.89
    hypertensive (vascular) I27.0
    valve I37.9
        rheumatic I09.89
pulp (dental) NOS K04.90
pulseless M31.4
Putnam's (subacute combined sclerosis with pernicious
    anemia) D51.0
Pyle (-Cohn) (craniometaphyseal dysplasia) Q78.5
ragpicker's or ragsorter's A22.1
Raynaud's — *see* Raynaud's disease
reactive airway — *see* Asthma
Reclus' (cystic) — *see* Mastopathy, cystic
rectum K62.9
    specified NEC K62.89
Refsum's (heredopathia atactica polyneuritiformis)
    G60.1
renal (functional) (pelvis) (*see also* Disease, kidney)
    N28.9
    with
        edema — *see* Nephrosis
        glomerular lesion — *see* Glomerulonephritis
            with edema — *see* Nephrosis
        interstitial nephritis N12
    acute N28.9
    chronic (*see also* Disease, kidney, chronic) N18.9
    cystic, congenital Q61.9
    diabetic — *see* E08-E13 with .22
    end-stage (failure) N18.6
        due to hypertension I12.0
    fibrocystic (congenital) Q61.8
    hypertensive — *see* Hypertension, kidney
    lupus M32.14
    phosphate-losing (tubular) N25.0
    polycystic (congenital) Q61.3

Disease, diseased — *continued*
  renal (*see also* Disease, kidney) — *continued*
    polycystic — *continued*
      adult type Q61.2
      childhood type NEC Q61.19
        collecting duct dilatation Q61.11
      rapidly progressive N01.9
      subacute N01.9
    Rendu-Osler-Weber (familial hemorrhagic telangiectasia) I78.0
    renovascular (arteriosclerotic) — *see* Hypertension, kidney
  respiratory (tract) J98.9
    acute or subacute NOS J06.9
      due to
        chemicals, gases, fumes or vapors (inhalation) J68.3
        external agent J70.9
          specified NEC J70.8
        radiation J70.0
        smoke inhalation J70.5
      noninfectious J39.8
    chronic NOS J98.9
      due to
        chemicals, gases, fumes or vapors J68.4
        external agent J70.9
          specified NEC J70.8
        radiation J70.1
      newborn P27.9
        specified NEC P27.8
    due to
      chemicals, gases, fumes or vapors J68.9
        acute or subacute NEC J68.3
        chronic J68.4
      external agent J70.9
        specified NEC J70.8
    newborn P28.9
      specified type NEC P28.89
    upper J39.9
      acute or subacute J06.9
      noninfectious NEC J39.8
      specified NEC J39.8
      streptococcal J06.9
  retina, retinal H35.9
    Batten's or Batten-Mayou E75.4 [H36]
    specified NEC H35.89
  rheumatoid — *see* Arthritis, rheumatoid
  rickettsial NOS A79.9
    specified type NEC A79.89
  Riga (-Fede) (cachectic aphthae) K14.0
  Riggs' (compound periodontitis) — *see* Periodontitis
  Ritter's L00
  Rivalta's (cervicofacial actinomycosis) A42.2
  Robles' (onchocerciasis) B73.01
  Roger's (congenital interventricular septal defect) Q21.0
  Rosenthal's (factor XI deficiency) D68.1
  Ross River B33.1
  Rossbach's (hyperchlorhydria) K30
  Rotes Quérol — *see* Hyperostosis, ankylosing
  Roth (-Bernhardt) — *see* Mononeuropathy, lower limb, meralgia paresthetica
  Runeberg's (progressive pernicious anemia) D51.0
  sacroiliac NEC M53.3
  salivary gland or duct K11.9
    inclusion B25.9
    specified NEC K11.8
    virus B25.9
  sandworm B76.9
  Schimmelbusch's — *see* Mastopathy, cystic
  Schmorl's — *see* Schmorl's disease or nodes
  Schönlein (-Henoch) (purpura rheumatica) D69.0
  Schottmüller's — *see* Fever, paratyphoid
  Schultz's (agranulocytosis) — *see* Agranulocytosis
  Schwalbe-Ziehen-Oppenheim G24.1
  Schwartz-Jampel G71.13
  sclera H15.9
    specified NEC H15.89
  scrofulous (tuberculous) A18.2
  scrotum N50.9
  sebaceous glands L73.9
  semilunar cartilage, cystic (*see also* Derangement, knee, meniscus, cystic)
  seminal vesicle N50.9
  serum NEC (*see also* Reaction, serum) T80.69 ☑
  sexually transmitted A64
    anogenital
      herpesviral infection — *see* Herpes, anogenital

Disease, diseased — *continued*
  sexually transmitted — *continued*
    anogenital — *continued*
      warts A63.0
    chancroid A57
    chlamydial infection — *see* Chlamydia
    gonorrhea — *see* Gonorrhea
    granuloma inguinale A58
    specified organism NEC A63.8
    syphilis — *see* Syphilis
    trichomoniasis — *see* Trichomoniasis
  Sézary C84.1- ☑
  shimamushi (scrub typhus) A75.3
  shipyard B30.0
  sickle-cell D57.1
    with crisis (vasoocclusive pain) D57.00
      with
        acute chest syndrome D57.01
        splenic sequestration D57.02
    elliptocytosis D57.8- ☑
    Hb-C D57.20
      with crisis (vasoocclusive pain) D57.219
        with
          acute chest syndrome D57.211
          splenic sequestration D57.212
      without crisis D57.20
    Hb-SD D57.80
      with crisis D57.819
        with
          acute chest syndrome D57.811
          splenic sequestration D57.812
    Hb-SE D57.80
      with crisis D57.819
        with
          acute chest syndrome D57.811
          splenic sequestration D57.812
    specified NEC D57.80
      with crisis D57.819
        with
          acute chest syndrome D57.811
          splenic sequestration D57.812
    spherocytosis D57.80
      with crisis D57.819
        with
          acute chest syndrome D57.811
          splenic sequestration D57.812
    thalassemia D57.40
      with crisis (vasoocclusive pain) D57.419
        with
          acute chest syndrome D57.411
          splenic sequestration D57.412
      without crisis D57.40
  silo-filler's J68.8
    bronchitis J68.0
    pneumonitis J68.0
    pulmonary edema J68.1
  simian B B00.4
  Simons' (progressive lipodystrophy) E88.1
  sin nombre virus B33.4
  sinus — *see* Sinusitis
  Sirkari's B55.0
  sixth B08.20
    due to human herpesvirus 6 B08.21
    due to human herpesvirus 7 B08.22
  skin L98.9
    due to metabolic disorder NEC E88.9 [L99]
    specified NEC L98.8
  slim (HIV) B20
  small vessel I73.9
  Sneddon-Wilkinson (subcorneal pustular dermatosis) L13.1
  South African creeping B88.0
  spinal (cord) G95.9
    congenital Q06.9
    specified NEC G95.89
  spine (*see also* Spondylopathy)
    joint — *see* Dorsopathy
    tuberculous A18.01
  spinocerebellar (hereditary) G11.9
    specified NEC G11.8
  spleen D73.9
    amyloid E85.4 [D77]
    organic D73.9
    polycystic Q89.09
    postinfectional D73.89
  sponge-diver's — *see* Toxicity, venom, marine animal, sea anemone
  Startle Q89.8

Disease, diseased — *continued*
  Steinert's G71.11
  Sticker's (erythema infectiosum) B08.3
  Stieda's (calcification, knee joint) — *see* Bursitis, tibial collateral
  Stokes' (exophthalmic goiter) — *see* Hyperthyroidism, with, goiter (diffuse)
  Stokes-Adams (syncope with heart block) I45.9
  stomach K31.9
    functional, psychogenic F45.8
    specified NEC K31.89
  stonemason's J62.8
  storage
    glycogen — *see* Disease, glycogen storage
    mucopolysaccharide — *see* Mucopolysaccharidosis
  striatopallidal system NEC G25.89
  Stuart-Prower (congenital factor X deficiency) D68.2
  Stuart's (congenital factor X deficiency) D68.2
  subcutaneous tissue — *see* Disease, skin
  supporting structures of teeth K08.9
    specified NEC K08.8
  suprarenal (capsule) (gland) E27.9
    hyperfunction E27.0
    specified NEC E27.8
  sweat glands L74.9
    specified NEC L74.8
  Sweeley-Klionsky E75.21
  Swift (-Feer) — *see* Poisoning, mercury
  swimming-pool granuloma A31.1
  Sylvest's (epidemic pleurodynia) B33.0
  sympathetic nervous system G90.9
  synovium — *see* Disorder, synovium
  syphilitic — *see* Syphilis
  systemic tissue mast cell C96.2
  tanapox (virus) B08.71
  Tangier E78.6
  Tarral-Besnier (pityriasis rubra pilaris) L44.0
  Tauri's E74.09
  tear duct — *see* Disorder, lacrimal system
  tendon, tendinous (*see also* Disorder, tendon)
    nodular — *see* Trigger finger
  terminal vessel I73.9
  testis N50.9
  thalassemia Hb-S — *see* Disease, sickle-cell, thalassemia
  Thaysen-Gee (nontropical sprue) K90.0
  Thomsen G71.12
  throat J39.2
    septic J02.9
  thromboembolic — *see* Embolism
  thymus (gland) E32.9
    specified NEC E32.8
  thyroid (gland) E07.9
    heart (*see also* Hyperthyroidism) E05.90 [I43]
      with thyroid storm E05.91 [I43]
    specified NEC E07.89
  Tietze's M94.0
  tongue K14.9
    specified NEC K14.8
  tonsils, tonsillar (and adenoids) J35.9
  tooth, teeth K08.9
    hard tissues K03.9
      specified NEC K03.89
    pulp NEC K04.99
    specified NEC K08.8
  Tourette's F95.2
  trachea NEC J39.8
  tricuspid I07.9
    nonrheumatic I36.9
  triglyceride-storage E75.5
  trophoblastic — *see* Mole, hydatidiform
  tsutsugamushi A75.3
  tube (fallopian) (noninflammatory) N83.9
    inflammatory — *see* Salpingitis
    specified NEC N83.8
  tuberculous NEC — *see* Tuberculosis
  tubo-ovarian (noninflammatory) N83.9
    inflammatory — *see* Salpingo-oophoritis
    specified NEC N83.8
  tubotympanic, chronic — *see* Otitis, media, suppurative, chronic, tubotympanic
  tubulo-interstitial N15.9
    specified NEC N15.8
  tympanum — *see* Disorder, tympanic membrane
  Uhl's Q24.8
  Underwood's (sclerema neonatorum) P83.0
  Unverricht (-Lundborg) — *see* Epilepsy, generalized, idiopathic

Disease, diseased — *continued*
Urbach-Oppenheim (necrobiosis lipoidica diabeticorum) — *see* E08-E13 with .620
ureter N28.9
   in (due to)
      schistosomiasis (bilharziasis) B65.0 [N29]
urethra N36.9
   specified NEC N36.8
urinary (tract) N39.9
   bladder N32.9
      specified NEC N32.89
   specified NEC N39.8
uterus (noninflammatory) N85.9
   infective — *see* Endometritis
   inflammatory — *see* Endometritis
   specified NEC N85.8
uveal tract (anterior) H21.9
   posterior H31.9
vagabond's B85.1
vagina, vaginal (noninflammatory) N89.9
   inflammatory NEC N76.89
   specified NEC N89.8
valve, valvular I38
   multiple I08.9
      specified NEC I08.8
van Creveld-von Gierke (glycogenosis I) E74.01
vas deferens N50.9
vascular I99.9
   arteriosclerotic — *see* Arteriosclerosis
   ciliary body NEC — *see* Disorder, iris, vascular
   hypertensive — *see* Hypertension
   iris NEC — *see* Disorder, iris, vascular
   obliterative I77.1
      peripheral I73.9
   occlusive I99.8
   peripheral (occlusive) I73.9
      in diabetes mellitus — *see* E08-E13 with .51
vasomotor I73.9
vasospastic I73.9
vein I87.9
venereal (*see also* Disease, sexually transmitted) A64
   chlamydial NEC A56.8
      anus A56.3
      genitourinary NOS A56.2
      pharynx A56.4
      rectum A56.3
   fifth A55
   sixth A55
   specified nature or type NEC A63.8
vertebra, vertebral (*see also* Spondylopathy)
   disc — *see* Disorder, disc
vibration — *see* Vibration, adverse effects
viral, virus (*see also* Disease, by type of virus) B34.9
   arbovirus NOS A94
   arthropod-borne NOS A94
   congenital P35.9
      specified NEC P35.8
   Hanta (with renal manifestations) (Dobrava) (Pu-
      umala) (Seoul) A98.5
      with pulmonary manifestations (Andes) (Bayou)
         (Bermejo) (Black Creek Canal) (Choclo)
         (Juquitiba) (Laguna negra) (Lechiguanas)
         (New York) (Oran) (Sin nombre) B33.4
   Hantaan (Korean hemorrhagic fever) A98.5
   human immunodeficiency (HIV) B20
   Kunjin A83.4
   nonarthropod-borne NOS B34.9
   Powassan A84.8
   Rocio (encephalitis) A83.6
   Sin nombre (Hantavirus) (cardio)-pulmonary syn-
      drome) B33.4
   Tahyna B33.8
   vesicular stomatitis A93.8
vitreous H43.9
   specified NEC H43.89
vocal cord J38.3
Volkmann's, acquired T79.6- ☑
von Eulenburg's (congenital paramyotonia) G71.19
von Gierke's (glycogenosis I) E74.01
von Graefe's — *see* Strabismus, paralytic, ophthalmoplegia, progressive
von Willebrand (-Jürgens) (angiohemophilia) D68.0
Vrolik's (osteogenesis imperfecta) Q78.0
vulva (noninflammatory) N90.9
   inflammatory NEC N76.89
   specified NEC N90.89
Wallgren's (obstruction of splenic vein with collateral
   circulation) I87.8

Disease, diseased — *continued*
Wassilieff's (leptospiral jaundice) A27.0
wasting NEC R64
   due to malnutrition E41
Waterhouse-Friderichsen A39.1
Wegner's (syphilitic osteochondritis) A50.02
Weil's (leptospiral jaundice of lung) A27.0
Weir Mitchell's (erythromelalgia) I73.81
Werdnig-Hoffmann G12.0
Wermer's E31.21
Werner-His (trench fever) A79.0
Werner-Schultz (neutropenic splenomegaly) D73.81
Wernicke-Posadas B38.9
whipworm B79
white blood cells D72.9
   specified NEC D72.89
white matter R90.82
white-spot, meaning lichen sclerosus et atrophicus
   L90.0
      penis N48.0
      vulva N90.4
Wilkie's K55.1
Wilkinson-Sneddon (subcorneal pustular dermatosis)
   L13.1
Willis' — *see* Diabetes
Wilson's (hepatolenticular degeneration) E83.01
woolsorter's A22.1
yaba monkey tumor B08.72
yaba pox (virus) B08.72
zoonotic, bacterial A28.9
   specified type NEC A28.8
Disfigurement (due to scar) L90.5
Disgerminoma — *see* Dysgerminoma
DISH (diffuse idiopathic skeletal hyperostosis) — *see*
   Hyperostosis, ankylosing
Disinsertion, retina — *see* Detachment, retina
Dislocatable hip, congenital Q65.6
Dislocation (articular)
   with fracture — *see* Fracture
   acromioclavicular (joint) S43.10- ☑
      with displacement
         100%-200% S43.12- ☑
         more than 200% S43.13- ☑
      inferior S43.14- ☑
      posterior S43.15- ☑
   ankle S93.0- ☑
   astragalus — *see* Dislocation, ankle
   atlantoaxial S13.121 ☑
   atlantooccipital S13.111 ☑
   atloidooccipital S13.111 ☑
   breast bone S23.29 ☑
   capsule, joint — *code by* site under Dislocation
   carpal (bone) — *see* Dislocation, wrist
   carpometacarpal (joint) NEC S63.05- ☑
      thumb S63.04- ☑
   cartilage (joint) — *code by* site under Dislocation
   cervical spine (vertebra) — *see* Dislocation, vertebra,
      cervical
   chronic — *see* Dislocation, recurrent
   clavicle — *see* Dislocation, acromioclavicular joint
   coccyx S33.2 ☑
   congenital NEC Q68.8
   coracoid — *see* Dislocation, shoulder
   costal cartilage S23.29 ☑
   costochondral S23.29 ☑
   cricoarytenoid articulation S13.29 ☑
   cricothyroid articulation S13.29 ☑
   dorsal vertebra — *see* Dislocation, vertebra, thoracic
   ear ossicle — *see* Discontinuity, ossicles, ear
   elbow S53.10- ☑
      congenital Q68.8
      pathological — *see* Dislocation, pathological NEC,
         elbow
      radial head alone — *see* Dislocation, radial head
      recurrent — *see* Dislocation, recurrent, elbow
      traumatic S53.10- ☑
         anterior S53.11- ☑
         lateral S53.14- ☑
         medial S53.13- ☑
         posterior S53.12- ☑
         specified type NEC S53.19- ☑
   eye, nontraumatic — *see* Luxation, globe
   eyeball, nontraumatic — *see* Luxation, globe
   femur
      distal end — *see* Dislocation, knee
      proximal end — *see* Dislocation, hip

Dislocation — *continued*
   fibula
      distal end — *see* Dislocation, ankle
      proximal end — *see* Dislocation, knee
   finger S63.25- ☑
      index S63.25- ☑
      interphalangeal S63.27- ☑
         distal S63.29- ☑
            index S63.29- ☑
            little S63.29- ☑
            middle S63.29- ☑
            ring S63.29- ☑
         index S63.27- ☑
         little S63.27- ☑
         middle S63.27- ☑
         proximal S63.28- ☑
            index S63.28- ☑
            little S63.28- ☑
            middle S63.28- ☑
            ring S63.28- ☑
         ring S63.27- ☑
      little S63.25- ☑
      metacarpophalangeal S63.26- ☑
         index S63.26- ☑
         little S63.26- ☑
         middle S63.26- ☑
         ring S63.26- ☑
      middle S63.25- ☑
      recurrent — *see* Dislocation, recurrent, finger
      ring S63.25- ☑
      thumb — *see* Dislocation, thumb
   foot S93.30- ☑
      recurrent — *see* Dislocation, recurrent, foot
      specified site NEC S93.33- ☑
      tarsal joint S93.31- ☑
      tarsometatarsal joint S93.32- ☑
      toe — *see* Dislocation, toe
   fracture — *see* Fracture
   glenohumeral (joint) — *see* Dislocation, shoulder
   glenoid — *see* Dislocation, shoulder
   habitual — *see* Dislocation, recurrent
   hip S73.00- ☑
      anterior S73.03- ☑
         obturator S73.02- ☑
      central S73.04- ☑
      congenital (total) Q65.2
         bilateral Q65.1
         partial Q65.5
            bilateral Q65.4
            unilateral Q65.3- ☑
         unilateral Q65.0- ☑
      developmental M24.85- ☑
      pathological — *see* Dislocation, pathological NEC,
         hip
      fibula
      posterior S73.01- ☑
      recurrent — *see* Dislocation, recurrent, hip
   humerus, proximal end — *see* Dislocation, shoulder
   incomplete — *see* Subluxation, by site
   incus — *see* Discontinuity, ossicles, ear
   infracoracoid — *see* Dislocation, shoulder
   innominate (pubic junction) (sacral junction) S33.39 ☑
      acetabulum — *see* Dislocation, hip
   interphalangeal (joint(s))
      finger S63.279 ☑
         distal S63.29- ☑
            index S63.29- ☑
            little S63.29- ☑
            middle S63.29- ☑
            ring S63.29- ☑
         index S63.27- ☑
         little S63.27- ☑
         middle S63.27- ☑
         proximal S63.28- ☑
            index S63.28- ☑
            little S63.28- ☑
            middle S63.28- ☑
            ring S63.28- ☑
         ring S63.27- ☑
      foot or toe — *see* Dislocation, toe
      thumb S63.12- ☑
         distal joint S63.14- ☑
         proximal joint S63.13- ☑
   jaw (cartilage) (meniscus) S03.0 ☑
   joint prosthesis — *see* Complications, joint prosthesis,
      mechanical, displacement, by site
   knee S83.106 ☑

Dislocation — *continued*
　knee — *continued*
　　cap — *see* Dislocation, patella
　　congenital Q68.2
　　old M23.8X-
　　patella — *see* Dislocation, patella
　　pathological — *see* Dislocation, pathological NEC, knee
　　proximal tibia
　　　anteriorly S83.11- ☑
　　　laterally S83.14- ☑
　　　medially S83.13- ☑
　　　posteriorly S83.12- ☑
　　recurrent (*see also* Derangement, knee, specified NEC)
　　specified type NEC S83.19- ☑
　lacrimal gland H04.16- ☑
　lens (complete) H27.10
　　anterior H27.12- ☑
　　congenital Q12.1
　　ocular implant — *see* Complications, intraocular lens
　　partial H27.11- ☑
　　posterior H27.13- ☑
　　traumatic S05.8X- ☑
　ligament — *code by* site under Dislocation
　lumbar (vertebra) — *see* Dislocation, vertebra, lumbar
　lumbosacral (vertebra) (*see also* Dislocation, vertebra, lumbar)
　　congenital Q76.49
　mandible S03.0
　meniscus (knee) — *see* Tear, meniscus
　　other sites - code by site under Dislocation
　metacarpal (bone)
　　distal end — *see* Dislocation, finger
　　proximal end S63.06- ☑
　metacarpophalangeal (joint)
　　finger S63.26- ☑
　　　index S63.26- ☑
　　　little S63.26- ☑
　　　middle S63.26- ☑
　　　ring S63.26- ☑
　　thumb S63.11- ☑
　metatarsal (bone) — *see* Dislocation, foot
　metatarsophalangeal (joint(s)) — *see* Dislocation, toe
　midcarpal (joint) S63.03- ☑
　midtarsal (joint) — *see* Dislocation, foot
　neck S13.20 ☑
　　specified site NEC S13.29 ☑
　　vertebra — *see* Dislocation, vertebra, cervical
　nose (septal cartilage) S03.1 ☑
　occipitoatloid S13.111 ☑
　old — *see* Derangement, joint, specified type NEC
　ossicles, ear — *see* Discontinuity, ossicles, ear
　partial — *see* Subluxation, by site
　patella S83.006 ☑
　　congenital Q74.1
　　lateral S83.01- ☑
　　recurrent (nontraumatic) M22.0- ☑
　　　incomplete M22.1- ☑
　　specified type NEC S83.09- ☑
　pathological NEC M24.30
　　ankle M24.37- ☑
　　elbow M24.32- ☑
　　foot joint M24.37- ☑
　　hand joint M24.34- ☑
　　hip M24.35- ☑
　　knee M24.36- ☑
　　lumbosacral joint — *see* subcategory M53.2 ☑
　　pelvic region — *see* Dislocation, pathological, hip
　　sacroiliac — *see* subcategory M53.2 ☑
　　shoulder M24.31- ☑
　　wrist M24.33- ☑
　pelvis NEC S33.30 ☑
　　specified NEC S33.39 ☑
　phalanx
　　finger or hand — *see* Dislocation, finger
　　foot or toe — *see* Dislocation, toe
　prosthesis, internal — *see* Complications, prosthetic device, by site, mechanical
　radial head S53.006 ☑
　　anterior S53.01- ☑
　　posterior S53.02- ☑
　　specified type NEC S53.09- ☑
　radiocarpal (joint) S63.02- ☑
　radiohumeral (joint) — *see* Dislocation, radial head

　radioulnar (joint)
　　distal S63.01- ☑
　　proximal — *see* Dislocation, elbow
　radius
　　distal end — *see* Dislocation, wrist
　　proximal end — *see* Dislocation, radial head
　recurrent M24.40
　　ankle M24.47- ☑
　　elbow M24.42- ☑
　　finger M24.44- ☑
　　foot joint M24.47- ☑
　　hand joint M24.44- ☑
　　hip M24.45- ☑
　　knee M24.46- ☑
　　　patella — *see* Dislocation, patella, recurrent
　　patella — *see* Dislocation, patella, recurrent
　　sacroiliac — *see* subcategory M53.2 ☑
　　shoulder M24.41- ☑
　　toe M24.47- ☑
　　vertebra (*see also* subcategory) M43.5 ☑
　　　atlantoaxial M43.4
　　　　with myelopathy M43.3
　　wrist M24.43- ☑
　rib (cartilage) S23.29 ☑
　sacrococcygeal S33.2 ☑
　sacroiliac (joint) (ligament) S33.2 ☑
　　congenital Q74.2
　　recurrent — *see* subcategory M53.2 ☑
　sacrum S33.2 ☑
　scaphoid (bone) (hand) (wrist) — *see* Dislocation, wrist
　　foot — *see* Dislocation, foot
　scapula — *see* Dislocation, shoulder, girdle, scapula
　semilunar cartilage, knee — *see* Tear, meniscus
　septal cartilage (nose) S03.1 ☑
　septum (nasal) (old) J34.2
　sesamoid bone — *code by* site under Dislocation
　shoulder (blade) (ligament) (joint) (traumatic) S43.006 ☑
　　acromioclavicular — *see* Dislocation, acromioclavicular
　　chronic — *see* Dislocation, recurrent, shoulder
　　congenital Q68.8
　　girdle S43.30- ☑
　　　scapula S43.31- ☑
　　　specified site NEC S43.39- ☑
　　humerus S43.00- ☑
　　　anterior S43.01- ☑
　　　inferior S43.03- ☑
　　　posterior S43.02- ☑
　　pathological — *see* Dislocation, pathological NEC, shoulder
　　recurrent — *see* Dislocation, recurrent, shoulder
　　specified type NEC S43.08- ☑
　spine
　　cervical — *see* Dislocation, vertebra, cervical
　　congenital Q76.49
　　due to birth trauma P11.5
　　lumbar — *see* Dislocation, vertebra, lumbar
　　thoracic — *see* Dislocation, vertebra, thoracic
　spontaneous — *see* Dislocation, pathological
　sternoclavicular (joint) S43.206 ☑
　　anterior S43.21- ☑
　　posterior S43.22- ☑
　sternum S23.29 ☑
　subglenoid — *see* Dislocation, shoulder
　symphysis pubis S33.4 ☑
　talus — *see* Dislocation, ankle
　tarsal (bone(s)) (joint(s)) — *see* Dislocation, foot
　tarsometatarsal (joint(s)) — *see* Dislocation, foot
　temporomandibular (joint) S03.0 ☑
　thigh, proximal end — *see* Dislocation, hip
　thorax S23.20 ☑
　　specified site NEC S23.29 ☑
　　vertebra — *see* Dislocation, vertebra
　thumb S63.10- ☑
　　interphalangeal joint — *see* Dislocation, interphalangeal (joint), thumb
　　metacarpophalangeal joint — *see* Dislocation, metacarpophalangeal (joint), thumb
　thyroid cartilage S13.29 ☑
　tibia
　　distal end — *see* Dislocation, ankle
　　proximal end — *see* Dislocation, knee
　tibiofibular (joint)
　　distal — *see* Dislocation, ankle

Dislocation — *continued*
　tibiofibular — *continued*
　　superior — *see* Dislocation, knee
　toe(s) S93.106 ☑
　　great S93.10- ☑
　　　interphalangeal joint S93.11- ☑
　　　metatarsophalangeal joint S93.12- ☑
　　interphalangeal joint S93.119 ☑
　　lesser S93.106 ☑
　　　interphalangeal joint S93.11- ☑
　　　metatarsophalangeal joint S93.12- ☑
　　metatarsophalangeal joint S93.12- ☑
　tooth S03.2 ☑
　trachea S23.29 ☑
　ulna
　　distal end S63.07- ☑
　　proximal end — *see* Dislocation, elbow
　ulnohumeral (joint) — *see* Dislocation, elbow
　vertebra (articular process) (body) (traumatic)
　　cervical S13.101 ☑
　　　atlantoaxial joint S13.121 ☑
　　　atlantooccipital joint S13.111 ☑
　　　atloidooccipital joint S13.111 ☑
　　　joint between
　　　　C0 and C1 S13.111 ☑
　　　　C1 and C2 S13.121 ☑
　　　　C2 and C3 S13.131 ☑
　　　　C3 and C4 S13.141 ☑
　　　　C4 and C5 S13.151 ☑
　　　　C5 and C6 S13.161 ☑
　　　　C6 and C7 S13.171 ☑
　　　　C7 and T1 S13.181 ☑
　　　occipitoatloid joint S13.111 ☑
　　congenital Q76.49
　　lumbar S33.101 ☑
　　　joint between
　　　　L1 and L2 S33.111 ☑
　　　　L2 and L3 S33.121 ☑
　　　　L3 and L4 S33.131 ☑
　　　　L4 and L5 S33.141 ☑
　　nontraumatic — *see* Displacement, intervertebral disc
　　partial — *see* Subluxation, by site
　　recurrent NEC — *see* subcategory M43.5 ☑
　　thoracic S23.101 ☑
　　　joint between
　　　　T1 and T2 S23.111 ☑
　　　　T2 and T3 S23.121 ☑
　　　　T3 and T4 S23.123 ☑
　　　　T4 and T5 S23.131 ☑
　　　　T5 and T6 S23.133 ☑
　　　　T6 and T7 S23.141 ☑
　　　　T7 and T8 S23.143 ☑
　　　　T8 and T9 S23.151 ☑
　　　　T9 and T10 S23.153 ☑
　　　　T10 and T11 S23.161 ☑
　　　　T11 and T12 S23.163 ☑
　　　　T12 and L1 S23.171 ☑
　wrist (carpal bone) S63.006 ☑
　　carpometacarpal joint — *see* Dislocation, carpometacarpal (joint)
　　distal radioulnar joint — *see* Dislocation, radioulnar (joint), distal
　　metacarpal bone, proximal — *see* Dislocation, metacarpal (bone), proximal end
　　midcarpal — *see* Dislocation, midcarpal (joint)
　　radiocarpal joint — *see* Dislocation, radiocarpal (joint)
　　recurrent — *see* Dislocation, recurrent, wrist
　　specified site NEC S63.09- ☑
　　ulna — *see* Dislocation, ulna, distal end
　xiphoid cartilage S23.29 ☑
Disorder (of) (*see also* Disease)
　acantholytic L11.9
　　specified NEC L11.8
　acute
　　psychotic — *see* Psychosis, acute
　　stress F43.0
　adjustment (grief) F43.20
　　with
　　　anxiety F43.22
　　　　with depressed mood F43.23
　　　conduct disturbance F43.24
　　　　with emotional disturbance F43.25
　　　depressed mood F43.21
　　　　with anxiety F43.23

Disorder — *continued*
  adjustment — *continued*
    with — *continued*
      other specified symptom F43.29
  adrenal (capsule) (gland) (medullary) E27.9
    specified NEC E27.8
  adrenogenital E25.9
    drug-induced E25.8
    iatrogenic E25.8
    idiopathic E25.8
  adult personality (and behavior) F69
    specified NEC F68.8
  affective (mood) — *see* Disorder, mood
  aggressive, unsocialized F91.1
  alcohol-related F10.99
    with
      amnestic disorder, persisting F10.96
      anxiety disorder F10.980
      dementia, persisting F10.97
      intoxication F10.929
        with delirium F10.921
        uncomplicated F10.920
      mood disorder F10.94
      other specified F10.988
      psychotic disorder F10.959
        with
          delusions F10.950
          hallucinations F10.951
      sexual dysfunction F10.981
      sleep disorder F10.982
  allergic — *see* Allergy
  alveolar NEC J84.09
  amino-acid
    cystathioninuria E72.19
    cystinosis E72.04
    cystinuria E72.01
    glycinuria E72.09
    homocystinuria E72.11
    metabolism — *see* Disturbance, metabolism,
      amino-acid
    specified NEC E72.8
    neonatal, transitory P74.8
    renal transport NEC E72.09
    transport NEC E72.09
  amnesic, amnestic
    alcohol-induced F10.96
      with dependence F10.26
    due to (secondary to) general medical condition
      F04
    psychoactive NEC-induced F19.96
      with
        abuse F19.16
        dependence F19.26
    sedative, hypnotic or anxiolytic-induced F13.96
      with dependence F13.26
  anaerobic glycolysis with anemia D55.2
  anxiety F41.9
    due to (secondary to)
      alcohol F10.980
      amphetamine F15.980
        in
          abuse F15.180
          dependence F15.280
      anxiolytic F13.980
        in
          abuse F13.180
          dependence F13.280
      caffeine F15.980
        in
          abuse F15.180
          dependence F15.280
      cannabis F12.980
        in
          abuse F12.180
          dependence F12.280
      cocaine F14.980
        in
          abuse F14.180
          dependence F14.180
      general medical condition F06.4
      hallucinogen F16.980
        in
          abuse F16.180
          dependence F16.280
      hypnotic F13.980
        in
          abuse F13.180
          dependence F13.280

Disorder — *continued*
  anxiety — *continued*
    due to — *continued*
      inhalant F18.980
        in
          abuse F18.180
          dependence F18.280
      phencyclidine F16.980
        in
          abuse F16.180
          dependence F16.280
      psychoactive substance NEC F19.980
        in
          abuse F19.180
          dependence F19.280
      sedative F13.980
        in
          abuse F13.180
          dependence F13.280
      volatile solvents F18.980
        in
          abuse F18.180
          dependence F18.280
    generalized F41.1
    mixed
      with depression (mild) F41.8
      specified NEC F41.3
    organic F06.4
    phobic F40.9
      of childhood F40.8
    specified NEC F41.8
  aortic valve — *see* Endocarditis, aortic
  aromatic amino-acid metabolism E70.9
    specified NEC E70.8
  arteriole NEC I77.89
  artery NEC I77.89
  articulation — *see* Disorder, joint
  attachment (childhood)
    disinhibited F94.2
    reactive F94.1
  attention-deficit hyperactivity (adolescent) (adult)
    (child) F90.9
    combined type F90.2
    hyperactive type F90.1
    inattentive type F90.0
    specified type NEC F90.8
  attention-deficit without hyperactivity (adolescent)
    (adult) (child) F90.0
  auditory processing (central) H93.25
  autistic F84.0
  autonomic nervous system G90.9
    specified NEC G90.8
  avoidant, child or adolescent F40.10
  balance
    acid-base E87.8
      mixed E87.4
    electrolyte E87.8
    fluid NEC E87.8
  behavioral (disruptive) — *see* Disorder, conduct
  beta-amino-acid metabolism E72.8
  bile acid and cholesterol metabolism E78.70
    Barth syndrome E78.71
    other specified E78.79
    Smith-Lemli-Opitz syndrome E78.72
  bilirubin excretion E80.6
  binocular
    movement H51.9
      convergence
        excess H51.12
        insufficiency H51.11
      internuclear ophthalmoplegia — *see* Ophthal-
        moplegia, internuclear
      palsy of conjugate gaze H51.0
      specified type NEC H51.8
    vision NEC — *see* Disorder, vision, binocular
  bipolar (I) F31.9
    current episode
      depressed F31.9
        with psychotic features F31.5
        without psychotic features F31.30
          mild F31.31
          moderate F31.32
          severe (without psychotic features) F31.4
            with psychotic features F31.5
      hypomanic F31.0
      manic F31.9
        with psychotic features F31.2
        without psychotic features F31.10

Disorder — *continued*
  bipolar — *continued*
    current episode — *continued*
      manic — *continued*
        without psychotic features — *continued*
          mild F31.11
          moderate F31.12
          severe (without psychotic features)
            F31.13
            with psychotic features F31.2
      mixed F31.60
        mild F31.61
        moderate F31.62
        severe (without psychotic features) F31.63
          with psychotic features F31.64
        severe depression (without psychotic features)
          F31.4
          with psychotic features F31.5
    in remission (currently) F31.70
      in full remission
        most recent episode
          depressed F31.76
          hypomanic F31.72
          manic F31.74
          mixed F31.78
      in partial remission
        most recent episode
          depressed F31.75
          hypomanic F31.71
          manic F31.73
          mixed F31.77
    organic F06.30
    single manic episode F30.9
      mild F30.11
      moderate F30.12
      severe (without psychotic symptoms) F30.13
        with psychotic symptoms F30.2
    specified NEC F31.89
  bipolar II F31.81
  bladder N32.9
    functional NEC N31.9
    in schistosomiasis B65.0 [N33]
    specified NEC N32.89
  bleeding D68.9
  blood D75.9
    in congenital early syphilis A50.09 [D77]
  body dysmorphic F45.22
  bone M89.9
    continuity M84.9
      specified type NEC M84.80
        ankle M84.87- ☑
        fibula M84.86- ☑
        foot M84.87- ☑
        hand M84.84- ☑
        humerus M84.82- ☑
        neck M84.88
        pelvis M84.859
        radius M84.83- ☑
        rib M84.88
        shoulder M84.81- ☑
        skull M84.88
        thigh M84.85- ☑
        tibia M84.86- ☑
        ulna M84.83- ☑
        vertebra M84.88
    density and structure M85.9
      cyst (*see also* Cyst, bone, specified type NEC)
        aneurysmal — *see* Cyst, bone, aneurysmal
        solitary — *see* Cyst, bone, solitary
      diffuse idiopathic skeletal hyperostosis — *see*
        Hyperostosis, ankylosing
      fibrous dysplasia (monostotic) — *see* Dysplasia,
        fibrous, bone
      fluorosis — *see* Fluorosis, skeletal
      hyperostosis of skull M85.2
      osteitis condensans — *see* Osteitis, condensans
      specified type NEC M85.8- ☑
        ankle M85.87- ☑
        foot M85.87- ☑
        forearm M85.83- ☑
        hand M85.84- ☑
        lower leg M85.86- ☑
        multiple sites M85.89
        neck M85.88
        rib M85.88
        shoulder M85.81- ☑
        skull M85.88
        thigh M85.85- ☑

Disorder — *continued*
 bone — *continued*
  density and structure — *continued*
   specified type — *continued*
    upper arm M85.82- ☑
    vertebra M85.88
  development and growth NEC M89.20
   carpus M89.24- ☑
   clavicle M89.21- ☑
   femur M89.25- ☑
   fibula M89.26- ☑
   finger M89.24- ☑
   humerus M89.22- ☑
   ilium M89.259
   ischium M89.259
   metacarpus M89.24- ☑
   metatarsus M89.27- ☑
   multiple sites M89.29
   neck M89.28
   radius M89.23- ☑
   rib M89.28
   scapula M89.21- ☑
   skull M89.28
   tarsus M89.27- ☑
   tibia M89.26- ☑
   toe M89.27- ☑
   ulna M89.23- ☑
   vertebra M89.28
  specified type NEC M89.8X- ☑
 brachial plexus G54.0
 branched-chain amino-acid metabolism E71.2
  specified NEC E71.19
 breast N64.9
  agalactia — *see* Agalactia
  associated with
   lactation O92.70
    specified NEC O92.79
   pregnancy O92.20
    specified NEC O92.29
   puerperium O92.20
    specified NEC O92.29
  cracked nipple — *see* Cracked nipple
  galactorrhea — *see* Galactorrhea
  hypogalactia O92.4
  lactation disorder NEC O92.79
  mastitis — *see* Mastitis
  nipple infection — *see* Infection, nipple
  retracted nipple — *see* Retraction, nipple
  specified type NEC N64.89
 Briquet's F45.0
 bullous, in diseases classified elsewhere L14
 cannabis use
  due to drug abuse — *see* Abuse, drug, cannabis
  due to drug dependence — *see* Dependence, drug, cannabis
 carbohydrate
  absorption, intestinal NEC E74.39
  metabolism (congenital) E74.9
   specified NEC E74.8
 cardiac, functional I51.89
 carnitine metabolism E71.40
 cartilage M94.9
  articular NEC — *see* Derangement, joint, articular cartilage
  chondrocalcinosis — *see* Chondrocalcinosis
  specified type NEC M94.8X- ☑
   articular — *see* Derangement, joint, articular cartilage
   multiple sites M94.8X0
 catatonic
  due to (secondary to) known physiological condition F06.1
  organic F06.1
 central auditory processing H93.25
 cervical
  region NEC M53.82
  root (nerve) NEC G54.2
 character NOS F60.9
 childhood disintegrative NEC F84.3
 cholesterol and bile acid metabolism E78.70
  Barth syndrome E78.71
  other specified E78.79
  Smith-Lemli-Opitz syndrome E78.72
 choroid H31.9
  atrophy — *see* Atrophy, choroid
  degeneration — *see* Degeneration, choroid
  detachment — *see* Detachment, choroid

Disorder — *continued*
 choroid — *continued*
  dystrophy — *see* Dystrophy, choroid
  hemorrhage — *see* Hemorrhage, choroid
  rupture — *see* Rupture, choroid
  scar — *see* Scar, chorioretinal
  solar retinopathy — *see* Retinopathy, solar
  specified type NEC H31.8
 ciliary body — *see* Disorder, iris
  degeneration — *see* Degeneration, ciliary body
 coagulation (factor) (*see also* Defect, coagulation) D68.9
  newborn, transient P61.6
 coccyx NEC M53.3
 cognitive F09
  due to (secondary to) general medical condition F09
  persisting R41.89
   due to
    alcohol F10.97
     with dependence F10.27
    anxiolytics F13.97
     with dependence F13.27
    hypnotics F13.97
     with dependence F13.27
    sedatives F13.97
     with dependence F13.27
    specified substance NEC F19.97
     with
      abuse F19.17
      dependence F19.27
 communication F80.9
 conduct (childhood) F91.9
  adjustment reaction — *see* Disorder, adjustment
  adolescent onset type F91.2
  childhood onset type F91.1
  compulsive F63.9
  confined to family context F91.0
  depressive F91.8
  group type F91.2
  hyperkinetic — *see* Disorder, attention-deficit hyperactivity
  oppositional defiance F91.3
  socialized F91.2
  solitary aggressive type F91.1
  specified NEC F91.8
  unsocialized (aggressive) F91.1
 conduction, heart I45.9
 congenital glycosylation (CDG) E74.8
 conjunctiva H11.9
  infection — *see* Conjunctivitis
 connective tissue, localized L94.9
  specified NEC L94.8
 conversion — *see* Disorder, dissociative
 convulsive (secondary) — *see* Convulsions
 cornea H18.9
  deformity — *see* Deformity, cornea
  degeneration — *see* Degeneration, cornea
  deposits — *see* Deposit, cornea
  due to contact lens H18.82- ☑
   specified as edema — *see* Edema, cornea
  edema — *see* Edema, cornea
  keratitis — *see* Keratitis
  keratoconjunctivitis — *see* Keratoconjunctivitis
  membrane change — *see* Change, corneal membrane
  neovascularization — *see* Neovascularization, cornea
  scar — *see* Opacity, cornea
  specified type NEC H18.89- ☑
  ulcer — *see* Ulcer, cornea
 corpus cavernosum N48.9
 cranial nerve — *see* Disorder, nerve, cranial
 cyclothymic F34.0
 defiant oppositional F91.3
 delusional (persistent) (systematized) F22
  induced F24
 depersonalization F48.1
 depressive F32.9
  major F32.9
   with psychotic symptoms F32.3
   in remission (full) F32.5
    partial F32.4
   recurrent F33.9
   single episode F32.9
    mild F32.0
    moderate F32.1
    severe (without psychotic symptoms) F32.2

Disorder — *continued*
 depressive — *continued*
  major — *continued*
   single episode — *continued*
    severe — *continued*
     with psychotic symptoms F32.3
   organic F06.31
   recurrent F33.9
    current episode
     mild F33.0
     moderate F33.1
     severe (without psychotic symptoms) F33.2
      with psychotic symptoms F33.3
    in remission F33.40
     full F33.42
     partial F33.41
    specified NEC F33.8
   single episode — *see* Episode, depressive
  developmental F89
   arithmetical skills F81.2
   coordination (motor) F82
   expressive writing F81.81
   language F80.9
    expressive F80.1
    mixed receptive and expressive F80.2
    receptive type F80.2
    specified NEC F80.89
   learning F81.9
    arithmetical F81.2
    reading F81.0
   mixed F88
   motor coordination or function F82
   pervasive F84.9
    specified NEC F84.8
   phonological F80.0
   reading F81.0
   scholastic skills (*see also* Disorder, learning)
    mixed F81.89
   specified NEC F88
   speech F80.9
    articulation F80.0
    specified NEC F80.89
   written expression F81.81
  diaphragm J98.6
  digestive (system) K92.9
   newborn P78.9
    specified NEC P78.89
   postprocedural — *see* Complication, gastrointestinal
   psychogenic F45.8
  disc (intervertebral) M51.9
   with
    myelopathy
     cervical region M50.00
     cervicothoracic region M50.03
     high cervical region M50.01
     lumbar region M51.06
     mid-cervical region M50.02
     sacrococcygeal region M53.3
     thoracic region M51.04
     thoracolumbar region M51.05
    radiculopathy
     cervical region M50.10
     cervicothoracic region M50.13
     high cervical region M50.11
     lumbar region M51.16
     lumbosacral region M51.17
     mid-cervical region M50.12
     sacrococcygeal region M53.3
     thoracic region M51.14
     thoracolumbar region M51.15
   cervical M50.90
    with
     myelopathy M50.00
      C2-C3 M50.01
      C3-C4 M50.01
      C4-C5 M50.02
      C5-C6 M50.02
      C6-C7 M50.02
      C7-T1 M50.03
      cervicothoracic region M50.03
      high cervical region M50.01
      mid-cervical region M50.02
     neuritis, radiculitis or radiculopathy M50.10
      C2-C3 M50.11
      C3-C4 M50.11
      C4-C5 M50.12
      C5-C6 M50.12

Disorder — continued
  disc — continued
    cervical — continued
      with — continued
        neuritis, radiculitis or radiculopathy — continued
          C6-C7 M50.12
          C7-T1 M50.13
          cervicothoracic region M50.13
          high cervical region M50.11
          mid-cervical region M50.12
      C2-C3 M50.91
      C3-C4 M50.91
      C4-C5 M50.92
      C5-C6 M50.92
      C6-C7 M50.92
      C7-T1 M50.93
      cervicothoracic region M50.93
      degeneration M50.30
        C2-C3 M50.31
        C3-C4 M50.31
        C4-C5 M50.32
        C5-C6 M50.32
        C6-C7 M50.32
        C7-T1 M50.33
        cervicothoracic region M50.33
        high cervical region M50.31
        mid-cervical region M50.32
      displacement M50.20
        C2-C3 M50.21
        C3-C4 M50.21
        C4-C5 M50.22
        C5-C6 M50.22
        C6-C7 M50.22
        C7-T1 M50.23
        cervicothoracic region M50.23
        high cervical region M50.21
        mid-cervical region M50.22
      high cervical region M50.91
      mid-cervical region M50.92
      specified type NEC M50.80
        C2-C3 M50.81
        C3-C4 M50.81
        C4-C5 M50.82
        C5-C6 M50.82
        C6-C7 M50.82
        C7-T1 M50.83
        cervicothoracic region M50.83
        high cervical region M50.81
        mid-cervical region M50.82
    specified NEC
      lumbar region M51.86
      lumbosacral region M51.87
      sacrococcygeal region M53.3
      thoracic region M51.84
      thoracolumbar region M51.85
  disinhibited attachment (childhood) F94.2
  disintegrative, childhood NEC F84.3
  disruptive behavior F98.9
  dissocial personality F60.2
  dissociative F44.9
    affecting
      motor function F44.4
        and sensation F44.7
      sensation F44.6
        and motor function F44.7
    brief reactive F43.0
    due to (secondary to) general medical condition F06.8
    mixed F44.7
    organic F06.8
    other specified NEC F44.89
  double heterozygous sickling — see Disease, sickle-cell
  dream anxiety F51.5
  drug induced hemorrhagic D68.32
  drug related F19.99
    abuse — see Abuse, drug
    dependence — see Dependence, drug
  dysmorphic body F45.1
  dysthymic F34.1
  ear H93.9- ☑
    bleeding — see Otorrhagia
    deafness — see Deafness
    degenerative H93.09- ☑
    discharge — see Otorrhea
    external H61.9- ☑

Disorder — continued
  ear — continued
    external — continued
      auditory canal stenosis — see Stenosis, external ear canal
      exostosis — see Exostosis, external ear canal
      impacted cerumen — see Impaction, cerumen
      otitis — see Otitis, externa
      perichondritis — see Perichondritis, ear
      pinna — see Disorder, pinna
      specified type NEC H61.89- ☑
    inner H83.9- ☑
      vestibular dysfunction — see Disorder, vestibular function
    middle H74.9- ☑
      adhesive H74.1- ☑
      ossicle — see Abnormal, ear ossicles
      polyp — see Polyp, ear (middle)
      specified NEC, in diseases classified elsewhere H75.8- ☑
    postprocedural — see Complications, ear, procedure
    specified NEC, in diseases classified elsewhere H94.8- ☑
  eating (adult) (psychogenic) F50.9
    anorexia — see Anorexia
    bulimia F50.2
    child F98.29
      pica F98.3
      rumination disorder F98.21
    pica F50.8
      childhood F98.3
  electrolyte (balance) NEC E87.8
    with
      abortion — see Abortion by type complicated by specified condition NEC
      ectopic pregnancy O08.5
      molar pregnancy O08.5
    acidosis (metabolic) (respiratory) E87.2
    alkalosis (metabolic) (respiratory) E87.3
  elimination, transepidermal L87.9
    specified NEC L87.8
  emotional (persistent) F34.9
    of childhood F93.9
      specified NEC F93.8
  endocrine E34.9
    postprocedural E89.89
    specified NEC E89.89
  erectile (male) (organic) (see also Dysfunction, sexual, male, erectile) N52.9
    nonorganic F52.21
  erythematous — see Erythema
  esophagus K22.9
    functional K22.4
    psychogenic F45.8
  eustachian tube H69.9- ☑
    infection — see Salpingitis, eustachian
    obstruction — see Obstruction, eustachian tube
    patulous — see Patulous, eustachian tube
    specified NEC H69.8- ☑
  extrapyramidal G25.9
    in deseases classified elsewhere — see category G26
    specified type NEC G25.89
  eye H57.9
    postprocedural — see Complication, postprocedural, eye
  eyelid H02.9
    cyst — see Cyst, eyelid
    degenerative H02.70
      chloasma — see Chloasma, eyelid
      madarosis — see Madarosis
      specified type NEC H02.79
      vitiligo — see Vitiligo, eyelid
      xanthelasma — see Xanthelasma
    dermatochalasis — see Dermatochalasis
    edema — see Edema, eyelid
    elephantiasis — see Elephantiasis, eyelid
    foreign body, retained — see Foreign body, retained, eyelid
    function H02.59
      abnormal innervation syndrome — see Syndrome, abnormal innervation
      blepharochalasis — see Blepharochalasis
      blepharoclonus — see Blepharoclonus
      blepharophimosis — see Blepharophimosis
      blepharoptosis — see Blepharoptosis

Disorder — continued
  eyelid — continued
    function — continued
      lagophthalmos — see Lagophthalmos
      lid retraction — see Retraction, lid
      hypertrichosis — see Hypertrichosis, eyelid
      specified type NEC H02.89
      vascular H02.879
        left H02.876
          lower H02.875
          upper H02.874
        right H02.873
          lower H02.872
          upper H02.871
  factitious F68.10
    with predominantly
      physical symptoms F68.12
        with psychological symptoms F68.13
      psychological symptoms F68.11
        with physical symptoms F68.13
  factor, coagulation — see Defect, coagulation
  fatty acid
    metabolism E71.30
      specified NEC E71.39
    oxidation
      LCAD E71.310
      MCAD E71.311
      SCAD E71.312
      specified deficiency NEC E71.318
  feeding (infant or child) (see also Disorder, eating) R63.3
  feigned (with obvious motivation) Z76.5
    without obvious motivation — see Disorder, factitious
  female
    hypoactive sexual desire F52.0
    orgasmic F52.31
    sexual arousal F52.22
  fibroblastic M72.9
    specified NEC M72.8
  fluency
    adult onset F98.5
    childhood onset F80.81
    following
      cerebral infarction I69.323
      cerebrovascular disease I69.923
        specified disease NEC I69.823
      intracerebral hemorrhage I69.123
      nontraumatic intracranial hemorrhage NEC I69.223
      subarachnoid hemorrhage I69.023
    in conditions classified elsewhere R47.82
  fluid balance E87.8
  follicular (skin) L73.9
    specified NEC L73.8
  fructose metabolism E74.10
    essential fructosuria E74.11
    fructokinase deficiency E74.11
    fructose-1, 6-diphosphatase deficiency E74.19
    hereditary fructose intolerance E74.12
    other specified E74.19
  functional polymorphonuclear neutrophils D71
  gallbladder, biliary tract and pancreas in diseases classified elsewhere K87
  gamma-glutamyl cycle E72.8
  gastric (functional) K31.9
    motility K30
    psychogenic F45.8
    secretion K30
  gastrointestinal (functional) NOS K92.9
    newborn P78.9
    psychogenic F45.8
  gender-identity or -role F64.9
    childhood F64.2
    effect on relationship F66
    of adolescence or adulthood (nontranssexual) F64.1
    specified NEC F64.8
    uncertainty F66
  genitourinary system
    female N94.9
    male N50.9
    psychogenic F45.8
  globe H44.9
    degenerated condition H44.50
      absolute glaucoma H44.51- ☑
      atrophy H44.52- ☑
      leucocoria H44.53- ☑
    degenerative H44.30

☑ Additional Character Required — Refer to the Tabular List for Character Selection   ▽ Subterms under main terms may continue to next column or page

Disorder — *continued*
　globe — *continued*
　　degenerative — *continued*
　　　chalcosis H44.31- ☑
　　　myopia H44.2- ☑
　　　siderosis H44.32- ☑
　　　specified type NEC H44.39- ☑
　　endophthalmitis — *see* Endophthalmitis
　　foreign body, retained — *see* Foreign body, intraocular, old, retained
　　hemophthalmos — *see* Hemophthalmos
　　hypotony H44.40
　　　due to
　　　　ocular fistula H44.42- ☑
　　　　specified disorder NEC H44.43- ☑
　　　flat anterior chamber H44.41- ☑
　　　primary H44.44- ☑
　　luxation — *see* Luxation, globe
　　specified type NEC H44.89
　glomerular (in) N05.9
　　amyloidosis E85.4 [N08]
　　cryoglobulinemia D89.1 [N08]
　　disseminated intravascular coagulation D65 [N08]
　　Fabry's disease E75.21 [N08]
　　familial lecithin cholesterol acyltransferase deficiency E78.6 [N08]
　　Goodpasture's syndrome M31.0
　　hemolytic-uremic syndrome D59.3
　　Henoch (-Schönlein) purpura D69.0 [N08]
　　malariae malaria B52.0
　　microscopic polyangiitis M31.7 [N08]
　　multiple myeloma C90.0- ☑ [N08]
　　mumps B26.83
　　schistosomiasis B65.9 [N08]
　　sepsis NEC A41.- ☑ [N08]
　　　streptococcal A40.- ☑ [N08]
　　sickle-cell disorders D57.- ☑ [N08]
　　strongyloidiasis B78.9 [N08]
　　subacute bacterial endocarditis I33.0 [N08]
　　syphilis A52.75
　　systemic lupus erythematosus M32.14
　　thrombotic thrombocytopenic purpura M31.1 [N08]
　　Waldenström macroglobulinemia C88.0 [N08]
　　Wegener's granulomatosis M31.31
　gluconeogenesis E74.4
　glucosaminoglycan metabolism — *see* Disorder, metabolism, glucosaminoglycan
　glycine metabolism E72.50
　　d-glycericacidemia E72.59
　　hyperhydroxyprolinemia E72.59
　　hyperoxaluria E72.53
　　hyperprolinemia E72.59
　　non-ketotic hyperglycinemia E72.51
　　oxalosis E72.53
　　oxaluria E72.53
　　sarcosinemia E72.59
　　trimethylaminuria E72.52
　glycoprotein metabolism E77.9
　　specified NEC E77.8
　habit (and impulse) F63.9
　　involving sexual behavior NEC F65.9
　　specified NEC F63.89
　heart action I49.9
　hematological D75.9
　　newborn (transient) P61.9
　　　specified NEC P61.8
　hematopoietic organs D75.9
　hemorrhagic NEC D69.9
　　drug-induced D68.32
　　due to
　　　extrinsic circulating anticoagulants D68.32
　　　increase in
　　　　anti-IIa D68.32
　　　　anti-Xa D68.32
　　　intrinsic
　　　　circulating anticoagulants D68.318
　　　　increase in
　　　　　anti-IXa D68.318
　　　　　antithrombin D68.318
　　　　　anti-VIIIa D68.318
　　　　　anti-XIa D68.318
　　following childbirth O72.3
　hemostasis — *see* Defect, coagulation
　histidine metabolism E70.40
　　histidinemia E70.41
　　other specified E70.49

Disorder — *continued*
　hyperkinetic — *see* Disorder, attention-deficit hyperactivity
　hyperleucine-isoleucinemia E71.19
　hypervalinemia E71.19
　hypoactive sexual desire F52.0
　hypochondriacal F45.20
　　body dysmorphic F45.22
　　neurosis F45.21
　　other specified F45.29
　identity
　　dissociative F44.81
　　of childhood F93.8
　immune mechanism (immunity) D89.9
　　specified type NEC D89.89
　impaired renal tubular function N25.9
　　specified NEC N25.89
　impulse (control) F63.9
　inflammatory
　　pelvic, in diseases classified elsewhere — *see* category N74
　　penis N48.29
　　　abscess N48.21
　　　cellulitis N48.22
　integument, newborn P83.9
　　specified NEC P83.8
　intermittent explosive F63.81
　internal secretion pancreas — *see* Increased, secretion, pancreas, endocrine
　intestine, intestinal
　　carbohydrate absorption NEC E74.39
　　　postoperative K91.2
　　functional NEC K59.9
　　　postoperative K91.89
　　psychogenic F45.8
　　vascular K55.9
　　　chronic K55.1
　　　specified NEC K55.8
　intraoperative (intraprocedural) — *see* Complications, intraoperative
　involuntary emotional expression (IEED) F07.89
　iris H21.9
　　adhesions — *see* Adhesions, iris
　　atrophy — *see* Atrophy, iris
　　chamber angle recession — *see* Recession, chamber angle
　　cyst — *see* Cyst, iris
　　degeneration — *see* Degeneration, iris
　　in diseases classified elsewhere H22
　　iridodialysis — *see* Iridodialysis
　　iridoschisis — *see* Iridoschisis
　　miotic pupillary cyst — *see* Cyst, pupillary
　　pupillary
　　　abnormality — *see* Abnormality, pupillary
　　　membrane — *see* Membrane, pupillary
　　specified type NEC H21.89
　　vascular NEC H21.1X- ☑
　iron metabolism E83.10
　　specified NEC E83.19
　isovaleric acidemia E71.110
　jaw, developmental M27.0
　　temporomandibular — *see* Anomaly, dentofacial, temporomandibular joint
　joint M25.9
　　derangement — *see* Derangement, joint
　　effusion — *see* Effusion, joint
　　fistula — *see* Fistula, joint
　　hemarthrosis — *see* Hemarthrosis
　　instability — *see* Instability, joint
　　osteophyte — *see* Osteophyte
　　pain — *see* Pain, joint
　　psychogenic F45.8
　　specified type NEC M25.80
　　　ankle M25.87- ☑
　　　elbow M25.82- ☑
　　　foot joint M25.87- ☑
　　　hand joint M25.84- ☑
　　　hip M25.85- ☑
　　　knee M25.86- ☑
　　　shoulder M25.81- ☑
　　　wrist M25.83- ☑
　　stiffness — *see* Stiffness, joint
　ketone metabolism E71.32
　kidney N28.9
　　functional (tubular) N25.9
　　in
　　　schistosomiasis B65.9 [N29]

Disorder — *continued*
　kidney — *continued*
　　tubular function N25.9
　　　specified NEC N25.89
　lacrimal system H04.9
　　changes H04.69
　　　fistula — *see* Fistula, lacrimal
　　gland H04.19
　　　atrophy — *see* Atrophy, lacrimal gland
　　　cyst — *see* Cyst, lacrimal, gland
　　　dacryops — *see* Dacryops
　　　dislocation — *see* Dislocation, lacrimal gland
　　　dry eye syndrome — *see* Syndrome, dry eye
　　　infection — *see* Dacryoadenitis
　　　granuloma — *see* Granuloma, lacrimal
　　　inflammation — *see* Inflammation, lacrimal
　　　obstruction — *see* Obstruction, lacrimal
　　　specified NEC H04.89
　lactation NEC O92.79
　language (developmental) F80.9
　　expressive F80.1
　　mixed receptive and expressive F80.2
　　receptive F80.2
　late luteal phase dysphoric N94.89
　learning (specific) F81.9
　　acalculia R48.8
　　alexia R48.0
　　mathematics F81.2
　　reading F81.0
　　specified NEC F81.89
　　spelling F81.81
　　written expression F81.81
　lens H27.9
　　aphakia — *see* Aphakia
　　cataract — *see* Cataract
　　dislocation — *see* Dislocation, lens
　　specified type NEC H27.8
　ligament M24.20
　　ankle M24.27- ☑
　　attachment, spine — *see* Enthesopathy, spinal
　　elbow M24.22- ☑
　　foot joint M24.27- ☑
　　hand joint M24.24- ☑
　　hip M24.25- ☑
　　knee — *see* Derangement, knee, specified NEC
　　shoulder M24.21- ☑
　　vertebra M24.28
　　wrist M24.23- ☑
　ligamentous attachments (*see also* Enthesopathy)
　　spine — *see* Enthesopathy, spinal
　lipid
　　metabolism, congenital E78.9
　　storage E75.6
　　　specified NEC E75.5
　lipoprotein
　　deficiency (familial) E78.6
　　metabolism E78.9
　　　specified NEC E78.89
　liver K76.9
　　malarial B54 [K77]
　low back (*see also* Dorsopathy, specified NEC)
　lumbosacral
　　plexus G54.1
　　root (nerve) NEC G54.4
　lung, interstitial, drug-induced J70.4
　　acute J70.2
　　chronic J70.3
　lymphoproliferative, post-transplant (PTLD) D47.Z1 (*following* D47.4)
　lysine and hydroxylysine metabolism E72.3
　male
　　erectile (organic) (*see also* Dysfunction, sexual, male, erectile) N52.9
　　　nonorganic F52.21
　　hypoactive sexual desire F52.0
　　orgasmic F52.32
　manic F30.9
　　organic F06.33
　mastoid (*see also* Disorder, ear, middle)
　　postprocedural — *see* Complications, ear, procedure
　meniscus — *see* Derangement, knee, meniscus
　menopausal N95.9
　　specified NEC N95.8
　menstrual N92.6
　　psychogenic F45.8
　　specified NEC N92.5
　mental (or behavioral) (nonpsychotic) F99

Disorder — continued
  mental — continued
    due to (secondary to)
      amphetamine
        due to drug abuse — see Abuse, drug, stimulant
        due to drug dependence — see Dependence, drug, stimulant
      brain disease, damage and dysfunction F09
      caffeine use
        due to drug abuse — see Abuse, drug, stimulant
        due to drug dependence — see Dependence, drug, stimulant
      cannabis use
        due to drug abuse — see Abuse, drug, cannabis
        due to drug dependence — see Dependence, drug, cannabis
      general medical condition F09
      sedative or hypnotic use
        due to drug abuse — see Abuse, drug, sedative
        due to drug dependence — see Dependence, drug, sedative
      tobacco (nicotine) use — see Dependence, drug, nicotine
    following organic brain damage F07.9
      frontal lobe syndrome F07.0
      personality change F07.0
      postconcussional syndrome F07.81
      specified NEC F07.89
    infancy, childhood or adolescence F98.9
    neurotic — see Neurosis
    organic or symptomatic F09
    presenile, psychotic F03 ☑
    problem NEC
    psychoneurotic — see Neurosis
    psychotic — see Psychosis
    puerperal F53
    senile, psychotic NEC F03 ☑
  metabolic, amino acid, transitory, newborn P74.8
  metabolism NOS E88.9
    amino-acid E72.9
      aromatic E70.9
        albinism — see Albinism
        histidine E70.40
          histidinemia E70.41
          other specified E70.49
        hyperphenylalaninemia E70.1
          classical phenylketonuria E70.0
        other specified E70.8
        tryptophan E70.5
        tyrosine E70.20
          hypertyrosinemia E70.21
          other specified E70.29
      branched chain E71.2
        3-methylglutaconic aciduria E71.111
        hyperleucine-isoleucinemia E71.19
        hypervalinemia E71.19
        isovaleric acidemia E71.110
        maple syrup urine disease E71.0
        methylmalonic acidemia E71.120
        organic aciduria NEC E71.118
        other specified E71.19
        proprionate NEC E71.128
        proprionic acidemia E71.121
      glycine E72.50
        d-glycericacidemia E72.59
        hyperhydroxyprolinemia E72.59
        hyperoxaluria E72.53
        hyperprolinemia E72.59
        non-ketotic hyperglycinemia E72.51
        other specified E72.59
        sarcosinemia E72.59
        trimethylaminuria E72.52
      hydroxylysine E72.3
      lysine E72.3
      ornithine E72.4
      other specified E72.8
        beta-amino acid E72.8
        gamma-glutamyl cycle E72.8
      straight-chain E72.8
      sulfur-bearing E72.10
        homocystinuria E72.11
        methylenetetrahydrofolate reductase deficiency E72.12
        other specified E72.19

Disorder — continued
  metabolism — continued
    bile acid and cholesterol metabolism E78.70
    bilirubin E80.7
      specified NEC E80.6
    calcium E83.50
      hypercalcemia E83.52
      hypocalcemia E83.51
      other specified E83.59
    carbohydrate E74.9
      specified NEC E74.8
    cholesterol and bile acid metabolism E78.70
    congenital E88.9
    copper E83.00
      specified type NEC E83.09
      Wilson's disease E83.01
    cystinuria E72.01
    fructose E74.10
    galactose E74.20
    glucosaminoglycan E76.9
      mucopolysaccharidosis — see Mucopolysaccharidosis
      specified NEC E76.8
    glutamine E72.8
    glycine E72.50
    glycogen storage (hepatorenal) E74.09
    glycoprotein E77.9
      specified NEC E77.8
    glycosaminoglycan E76.9
      specified NEC E76.8
    in labor and delivery O75.89
    iron E83.10
    isoleucine E71.19
    leucine E71.19
    lipoid E78.9
    lipoprotein E78.9
      specified NEC E78.89
    magnesium E83.40
      hypermagnesemia E83.41
      hypomagnesemia E83.42
      other specified E83.49
    mineral E83.9
      specified NEC E83.89
    mitochondrial E88.40
      MELAS syndrome E88.41
      MERRF syndrome (myoclonic epilepsy associated with ragged-red fibers) E88.42
      other specified E88.49
    ornithine E72.4
    phosphatases E83.30
    phosphorus E83.30
      acid phosphatase deficiency E83.39
      hypophosphatasia E83.39
      hypophosphatemia E83.39
        familial E83.31
      other specified E83.39
      pseudovitamin D deficiency E83.32
    plasma protein NEC E88.09
    porphyrin — see Porphyria
    postprocedural E89.89
      specified NEC E89.89
    purine E79.9
      specified NEC E79.8
    pyrimidine E79.9
      specified NEC E79.8
    pyruvate E74.4
    serine E72.8
    sodium E87.8
    specified NEC E88.89
    threonine E72.8
    valine E71.19
    zinc E83.2
  methylmalonic acidemia E71.120
  micturition NEC R39.19
    feeling of incomplete emptying R39.14
    hesitancy R39.11
    poor stream R39.12
    psychogenic F45.8
    split stream R39.13
    straining R39.16
    urgency R39.15
  mitochondrial metabolism E88.40
  mitral (valve) — see Endocarditis, mitral
  mixed
    anxiety and depressive F41.8
    of scholastic skills (developmental) F81.89
    receptive expressive language F80.2
  mood F39

Disorder — continued
  mood — continued
    bipolar — see Disorder, bipolar
    depressive — see Disorder, depressive
    due to (secondary to)
      alcohol F10.94
      amphetamine F15.94
        in
          abuse F15.14
          dependence F15.24
      anxiolytic F13.94
        in
          abuse F13.14
          dependence F13.24
      cocaine F14.94
        in
          abuse F14.14
          dependence F14.24
      general medical condition F06.30
      hallucinogen F16.94
        in
          abuse F16.14
          dependence F16.24
      hypnotic F13.94
        in
          abuse F13.14
          dependence F13.24
      inhalant F18.94
        in
          abuse F18.14
          dependence F18.24
      opioid F11.94
        in
          abuse F11.14
          dependence F11.24
      phencyclidine (PCP) F16.94
        in
          abuse F16.14
          dependence F16.24
      physiological condition F06.30
        with
          depressive features F06.31
          major depressive-like episode F06.32
          manic features F06.33
          mixed features F06.34
      psychoactive substance NEC F19.94
        in
          abuse F19.14
          dependence F19.24
      sedative F13.94
        in
          abuse F13.14
          dependence F13.24
      volatile solvents F18.94
        in
          abuse F18.14
          dependence F18.24
    manic episode F30.9
      with psychotic symptoms F30.2
      without psychotic symptoms F30.10
        mild F30.11
        moderate F30.12
        severe F30.13
      in remission (full) F30.4
        partial F30.3
      specified type NEC F30.8
    organic F06.30
      right hemisphere F07.89
    persistent F34.9
      cyclothymia F34.0
      dysthymia F34.1
      specified type NEC F34.8
    recurrent F39
    right hemisphere organic F07.89
  movement G25.9
    drug-induced G25.70
      akathisia G25.71
      specified NEC G25.79
    hysterical F44.4
    in diseases classified elsewhere — see category G26
    periodic limb G47.61
      sleep related G47.61
    sleep related NEC G47.69
    specified NEC G25.89
    stereotyped F98.4
    treatment-induced G25.9
  multiple personality F44.81

☑ **Additional Character Required** — Refer to the Tabular List for Character Selection   ▽ Subterms under main terms may continue to next column or page

Index

Disorder — Disorder

Disorder — *continued*
  muscle M62.9
    attachment, spine — *see* Enthesopathy, spinal
    in trichinellosis — *see* Trichinellosis, with muscle
        disorder
    psychogenic F45.8
    specified type NEC M62.89
    tone, newborn P94.9
      specified NEC P94.8
  muscular
    attachments (*see also* Enthesopathy)
      spine — *see* Enthesopathy, spinal
    urethra N36.44
  musculoskeletal system, soft tissue — *see* Disorder,
      soft tissue
    postprocedural M96.89
    psychogenic F45.8
  myoneural G70.9
    due to lead G70.1
    specified NEC G70.89
    toxic G70.1
  myotonic NEC G71.19
  nail, in diseases classified elsewhere L62
  neck region NEC — *see* Dorsopathy, specified NEC
  nerve G58.9
    abducent NEC — *see* Strabismus, paralytic, sixth
        nerve
    accessory G52.8
    acoustic — *see* subcategory H93.3 ☑
    auditory — *see* subcategory H93.3 ☑
    auriculotemporal G50.8
    axillary G54.0
    cerebral — *see* Disorder, nerve, cranial
    cranial G52.9
      eighth — *see* subcategory H93.3 ☑
      eleventh G52.8
      fifth G50.9
      first G52.0
      fourth NEC — *see* Strabismus, paralytic, fourth
          nerve
      multiple G52.7
      ninth G52.1
      second NEC — *see* Disorder, nerve, optic
      seventh NEC G51.8
      sixth NEC — *see* Strabismus, paralytic, sixth
          nerve
      specified NEC G52.8
      tenth G52.2
      third NEC — *see* Strabismus, paralytic, third
          nerve
      twelfth G52.3
    entrapment — *see* Neuropathy, entrapment
    facial G51.9
      specified NEC G51.8
    femoral — *see* Lesion, nerve, femoral
    glossopharyngeal NEC G52.1
    hypoglossal G52.3
    intercostal G58.0
    lateral
      cutaneous of thigh — *see* Mononeuropathy,
          lower limb, meralgia paresthetica
      popliteal — *see* Lesion, nerve, popliteal
    lower limb — *see* Mononeuropathy, lower limb
    medial popliteal — *see* Lesion, nerve, popliteal,
        medial
    median NEC — *see* Lesion, nerve, median
    multiple G58.7
    oculomotor NEC — *see* Strabismus, paralytic, third
        nerve
    olfactory G52.0
    optic NEC H47.09- ☑
      hemorrhage into sheath — *see* Hemorrhage,
          optic nerve
      ischemic H47.01- ☑
    peroneal — *see* Lesion, nerve, popliteal
    phrenic G58.8
    plantar — *see* Lesion, nerve, plantar
    pneumogastric G52.2
    posterior tibial — *see* Syndrome, tarsal tunnel
    radial — *see* Lesion, nerve, radial
    recurrent laryngeal G52.2
    root G54.9
      cervical G54.2
      lumbosacral G54.1
      specified NEC G54.8
      thoracic G54.3
    sciatic NEC — *see* Lesion, nerve, sciatic

Disorder — *continued*
  nerve — *continued*
    specified NEC G58.8
      lower limb — *see* Mononeuropathy, lower limb,
          specified NEC
      upper limb — *see* Mononeuropathy, upper
          limb, specified NEC
    sympathetic G90.9
    tibial — *see* Lesion, nerve, popliteal, medial
    trigeminal G50.9
      specified NEC G50.8
    trochlear NEC — *see* Strabismus, paralytic, fourth
        nerve
    ulnar — *see* Lesion, nerve, ulnar
    upper limb — *see* Mononeuropathy, upper limb
    vagus G52.2
  nervous system G98.8
    autonomic (peripheral) G90.9
      specified NEC G90.8
    central G96.9
      specified NEC G96.8
    parasympathetic G90.9
    specified NEC G98.8
    sympathetic G90.9
    vegetative G90.9
  neurohypophysis NEC E23.3
  neurological NEC R29.818
  neuromuscular G70.9
    hereditary NEC G71.9
    specified NEC G70.89
    toxic G70.1
  neurotic F48.9
    specified NEC F48.8
  neutrophil, polymorphonuclear D71
  nicotine use — *see* Dependence, drug, nicotine
  nightmare F51.5
  nose J34.9
    specified NEC J34.89
  obsessive-compulsive F42
  odontogenesis NOS K00.9
  opioid use
    with
      opioid-induced psychotic disorder F11.959
        with
          delusions F11.950
          hallucinations F11.951
    due to drug abuse — *see* Abuse, drug, opioid
    due to drug dependence — *see* Dependence, drug,
        opioid
  oppositional defiant F91.3
  optic
    chiasm H47.49
      due to
        inflammatory disorder H47.41
        neoplasm H47.42
        vascular disorder H47.43
    disc H47.39- ☑
      coloboma — *see* Coloboma, optic disc
      drusen — *see* Drusen, optic disc
      pseudopapilledema — *see* Pseudopapilledema
    radiations — *see* Disorder, visual, pathway
    tracts — *see* Disorder, visual, pathway
  orbit H05.9
    cyst — *see* Cyst, orbit
    deformity — *see* Deformity, orbit
    edema — *see* Edema, orbit
    enophthalmos — *see* Enophthalmos
    exophthalmos — *see* Exophthalmos
    hemorrhage — *see* Hemorrhage, orbit
    inflammation — *see* Inflammation, orbit
    myopathy — *see* Myopathy, extraocular muscles
    retained foreign body — *see* Foreign body, orbit,
        old
    specified type NEC H05.89
  organic
    anxiety F06.4
    catatonic F06.1
    delusional F06.2
    dissociative F06.8
    emotionally labile (asthenic) F06.8
    mood (affective) F06.30
    schizophrenia-like F06.2
  orgasmic (female) F52.31
    male F52.32
  ornithine metabolism E72.4
  overanxious F41.1
    of childhood F93.8

Disorder — *continued*
  pain
    with related psychological factors F45.42
    exclusively related to psychological factors F45.41
  pancreatic internal secretion E16.9
    specified NEC E16.8
  panic F41.0
    with agoraphobia F40.01
  papulosquamous L44.9
    in diseases classified elsewhere L45
    specified NEC L44.8
  paranoid F22
    induced F24
    shared F24
  parathyroid (gland) E21.5
    specified NEC E21.4
  parietoalveolar NEC J84.09
  paroxysmal, mixed R56.9
  patella M22.9- ☑
    chondromalacia — *see* Chondromalacia, patella
    derangement NEC M22.3X- ☑
    recurrent
      dislocation — *see* Dislocation, patella, recurrent
      subluxation — *see* Dislocation, patella, recur-
          rent, incomplete
    specified NEC M22.8X- ☑
  patellofemoral M22.2X- ☑
  pentose phosphate pathway with anemia D55.1
  perception, due to hallucinogens F16.983
    in
      abuse F16.183
      dependence F16.283
  peripheral nervous system NEC G64
  peroxisomal E71.50
    biogenesis
      neonatal adrenoleukodystrophy E71.511
      specified disorder NEC E71.518
      Zellweger syndrome E71.510
    rhizomelic chondrodysplasia punctata E71.540
    specified form NEC E71.548
      group 1 E71.518
      group 2 E71.53
      group 3 E71.542
    X-linked adrenoleukodystrophy E71.529
      adolescent E71.521
      adrenomyeloneuropathy E71.522
      childhood E71.520
      specified form NEC E71.528
    Zellweger-like syndrome E71.541
  persistent
    (somatoform) pain F45.41
    affective (mood) F34.9
  personality (*see also* Personality) F60.9
    affective F34.0
    aggressive F60.3
    amoral F60.2
    anankastic F60.5
    antisocial F60.2
    anxious F60.6
    asocial F60.2
    asthenic F60.7
    avoidant F60.6
    borderline F60.3
    change (secondary) due to general medical condi-
        tion F07.0
    compulsive F60.5
    cyclothymic F34.0
    dependent (passive) F60.7
    depressive F34.1
    dissocial F60.2
    emotional instability F60.3
    expansive paranoid F60.0
    explosive F60.3
    following organic brain damage F07.9
    histrionic F60.4
    hyperthymic F34.0
    hypothymic F34.1
    hysterical F60.4
    immature F60.89
    inadequate F60.7
    labile F60.3
    mixed (nonspecific) F60.89
    moral deficiency F60.2
    narcissistic F60.81
    negativistic F60.89
    obsessional F60.5
    obsessive (-compulsive) F60.5
    organic F07.9

Disorder — *continued*
  personality (*see also* Personality) — *continued*
    overconscientious F60.5
    paranoid F60.0
    passive (-dependent) F60.7
    passive-aggressive F60.89
    pathological NEC F60.9
    pseudosocial F60.2
    psychopathic F60.2
    schizoid F60.1
    schizotypal F21
    self-defeating F60.7
    specified NEC F60.89
    type A F60.5
    unstable (emotional) F60.3
  pervasive, developmental F84.9
  phobic anxiety, childhood F40.8
  phosphate-losing tubular N25.0
  pigmentation L81.9
    choroid, congenital Q14.3
    diminished melanin formation L81.6
    iron L81.8
    specified NEC L81.8
  pinna (noninfective) H61.10- ☑
    deformity, acquired H61.11- ☑
    hematoma H61.12- ☑
    perichondritis — *see* Perichondritis, ear
    specified type NEC H61.19- ☑
  pituitary gland E23.7
    iatrogenic (postprocedural) E89.3
    specified NEC E23.6
  platelets D69.1
  plexus G54.9
    specified NEC G54.8
  polymorphonuclear neutrophils D71
  porphyrin metabolism — *see* Porphyria
  postconcussional F07.81
  posthallucinogen perception F16.983
    in
      abuse F16.183
      dependence F16.283
  postmenopausal N95.9
    specified NEC N95.8
  postprocedural (postoperative) — *see* Complications, postprocedural
  post-transplant lymphoproliferative D47.Z1 (*following* D47.4)
  post-traumatic stress (PTSD) F43.10
    acute F43.11
    chronic F43.12
  premenstrual dysphoric (PMDD) N94.3
  prepuce N47.8
  propionic acidemia E71.121
  prostate N42.9
    specified NEC N42.89
  psychogenic NOS (*see also* condition) F45.9
    anxiety F41.8
    appetite F50.9
    asthenic F48.8
    cardiovascular (system) F45.8
    compulsive F42
    cutaneous F54
    depressive F32.9
    digestive (system) F45.8
    dysmenorrheic F45.8
    dyspneic F45.8
    endocrine (system) F54
    eye NEC F45.8
    feeding — *see* Disorder, eating
    functional NEC F45.8
    gastric F45.8
    gastrointestinal (system) F45.8
    genitourinary (system) F45.8
    heart (function) (rhythm) F45.8
    hyperventilatory F45.8
    hypochondriacal — *see* Disorder, hypochondriacal
    intestinal F45.8
    joint F45.8
    learning F81.9
    limb F45.8
    lymphatic (system) F45.8
    menstrual F45.8
    micturition F45.8
    monoplegic NEC F44.4
    motor F44.4
    muscle F45.8
    musculoskeletal F45.8
    neurocirculatory F45.8

Disorder — *continued*
  psychogenic (*see also* condition) — *continued*
    obsessive F42
    occupational F48.8
    organ or part of body NEC F45.8
    paralytic NEC F44.4
    phobic F40.9
    physical NEC F45.8
    rectal F45.8
    respiratory (system) F45.8
    rheumatic F45.8
    sexual (function) F52.9
    skin (allergic) (eczematous) F54
    sleep F51.9
    specified part of body NEC F45.8
    stomach F45.8
  psychological F99
    associated with
      disease classified elsewhere F54
      sexual
        development F66
        relationship F66
      uncertainty about gender identity F66
  psychomotor NEC F44.4
    hysterical F44.4
  psychoneurotic (*see also* Neurosis)
    mixed NEC F48.8
  psychophysiologic — *see* Disorder, somatoform
  psychosexual F65.9
    development F66
    identity of childhood F64.2
  psychosomatic NOS — *see* Disorder, somatoform
    multiple F45.0
    undifferentiated F45.1
  psychotic — *see* Psychosis
    transient (acute) F23
  puberty E30.9
    specified NEC E30.8
  pulmonary (valve) — *see* Endocarditis, pulmonary
  purine metabolism E79.9
  pyrimidine metabolism E79.9
  pyruvate metabolism E74.4
  reactive attachment (childhood) F94.1
  reading R48.0
    developmental (specific) F81.0
  receptive language F80.2
  receptor, hormonal, peripheral (*see also* Syndrome, androgen insensitivity) E34.50
  recurrent brief depressive F33.8
  reflex R29.2
  refraction H52.7
    aniseikonia H52.32
    anisometropia H52.31
    astigmatism — *see* Astigmatism
    hypermetropia — *see* Hypermetropia
    myopia — *see* Myopia
    presbyopia H52.4
    specified NEC H52.6
  relationship F68.8
    due to sexual orientation F66
  REM sleep behavior G47.52
  renal function, impaired (tubular) N25.9
  resonance R49.9
    specified NEC R49.8
  respiratory function, impaired (*see also* Failure, respiration)
    postprocedural — *see* Complication, postoperative, respiratory system
    psychogenic F45.8
  retina H35.9
    angioid streaks H35.33
    changes in vascular appearance H35.01- ☑
    degeneration — *see* Degeneration, retina
    dystrophy (hereditary) — *see* Dystrophy, retina
    edema H35.81
    hemorrhage — *see* Hemorrhage, retina
    ischemia H35.82
    macular degeneration — *see* Degeneration, macula
    microaneurysms H35.04- ☑
    microvascular abnormality NEC H35.09
    neovascularization — *see* Neovascularization, retina
    retinopathy — *see* Retinopathy
    separation of layers H35.70
      central serous chorioretinopathy H35.71- ☑
      pigment epithelium detachment (serous) H35.72- ☑
      hemorrhagic H35.73- ☑

Disorder — *continued*
  retina — *continued*
    specified type NEC H35.89
      telangiectasis — *see* Telangiectasis, retina
      vasculitis — *see* Vasculitis, retina
  retroperitoneal K68.9
  right hemisphere organic affective F07.89
  rumination (infant or child) F98.21
  sacrum, sacrococcygeal NEC M53.3
  schizoaffective F25.9
    bipolar type F25.0
    depressive type F25.1
    manic type F25.0
    mixed type F25.0
    specified NEC F25.8
  schizoid of childhood F84.5
  schizophreniform F20.81
    brief F23
  schizotypal (personality) F21
  secretion, thyrocalcitonin E07.0
  seizure (*see also* Epilepsy) G40.909
    intractable G40.919
      with status epilepticus G40.911
  semantic pragmatic F80.89
    with autism F84.0
  sense of smell R43.1
    psychogenic F45.8
  separation anxiety, of childhood F93.0
  sexual
    arousal, female F52.22
    aversion F52.1
    function, psychogenic F52.9
    maturation F66
    nonorganic F52.9
    preference (*see also* Deviation, sexual) F65.9
      fetishistic transvestism F65.1
    relationship F66
  shyness, of childhood and adolescence F40.10
  sibling rivalry F93.8
  sickle-cell (sickling) (homozygous) — *see* Disease, sickle-cell
    heterozygous D57.3
    specified type NEC D57.8- ☑
    trait D57.3
  sinus (nasal) J34.9
    specified NEC J34.89
  skin L98.9
    atrophic L90.9
      specified NEC L90.8
    granulomatous L92.9
      specified NEC L92.8
    hypertrophic L91.9
      specified NEC L91.8
    infiltrative NEC L98.6
    newborn P83.9
      specified NEC P83.8
    psychogenic (allergic) (eczematous) F54
  sleep G47.9
    breathing-related — *see* Apnea, sleep
    circadian rhythm G47.20
      advance sleep phase type G47.22
      delayed sleep phase type G47.21
      due to
        alcohol
          abuse F10.182
          dependence F10.282
          use F10.982
        amphetamines
          abuse F15.182
          dependence F15.282
          use F15.982
        caffeine
          abuse F15.182
          dependence F15.282
          use F15.982
        cocaine
          abuse F14.182
          dependence F14.282
          use F14.982
        drug NEC
          abuse F19.182
          dependence F19.282
          use F19.982
        opioid
          abuse F11.182
          dependence F11.282
          use F11.982

Disorder — *continued*
  sleep — *continued*
    circadian rhythm — *continued*
      due to — *continued*
        psychoactive substance
          abuse F19.182
          dependence F19.282
          use F19.982
        sedative, hypnotic, or anxiolytic
          abuse F13.182
          dependence F13.282
          use F13.982
        stimulant NEC
          abuse F15.182
          dependence F15.282
          use F15.982
      free running type G47.24
      in conditions classified elsewhere G47.27
      irregular sleep wake type G47.23
      jet lag type G47.25
      shift work type G47.26
      specified NEC G47.29
    due to
      alcohol
        abuse F10.182
        dependence F10.282
        use F10.982
      amphetamine
        abuse F15.182
        dependence F15.282
        use F15.982
      anxiolytic
        abuse F13.182
        dependence F13.282
        use F13.982
      caffeine
        abuse F15.182
        dependence F15.282
        use F15.982
      cocaine
        abuse F14.182
        dependence F14.282
        use F14.982
      drug NEC
        abuse F19.182
        dependence F19.282
        use F19.982
      hypnotic
        abuse F13.182
        dependence F13.282
        use F13.982
      opioid
        abuse F11.182
        dependence F11.282
        use F11.982
      psychoactive substance NEC
        abuse F19.182
        dependence F19.282
        use F19.982
      sedative
        abuse F13.182
        dependence F13.282
        use F13.982
      stimulant NEC
        abuse F15.182
        dependence F15.282
        use F15.982
    emotional F51.9
    excessive somnolence — *see* Hypersomnia
    hypersomnia type — *see* Hypersomnia
    initiating or maintaining — *see* Insomnia
    nightmares F51.5
    nonorganic F51.9
      specified NEC F51.8
    parasomnia type G47.50
    specified NEC G47.8
    terrors F51.4
    walking F51.3
  sleep-wake pattern or schedule — *see* Disorder, sleep,
    circadian rhythm
  social
    anxiety of childhood F40.10
    functioning in childhood F94.9
      specified NEC F94.8
  soft tissue M79.9
    ankle M79.9
    due to use, overuse and pressure M70.90
      ankle M70.97- ☑

Disorder — *continued*
  soft tissue — *continued*
    due to use, overuse and pressure — *continued*
      bursitis — *see* Bursitis
      foot M70.97- ☑
      forearm M70.93- ☑
      hand M70.94- ☑
      lower leg M70.96- ☑
      multiple sites M70.99
      pelvic region M70.95- ☑
      shoulder region M70.91- ☑
      specified site NEC M70.98
      specified type NEC M70.80
        ankle M70.87- ☑
        foot M70.87- ☑
        forearm M70.83- ☑
        hand M70.84- ☑
        lower leg M70.86- ☑
        multiple sites M70.89
        pelvic region M70.85- ☑
        shoulder region M70.81- ☑
        specified site NEC M70.88
        thigh M70.85- ☑
        upper arm M70.82- ☑
      thigh M70.95- ☑
      upper arm M70.92- ☑
    foot M79.9
    forearm M79.9
    hand M79.9
    lower leg M79.9
    multiple sites M79.9
    occupational — *see* Disorder, soft tissue, due to
      use, overuse and pressure
    pelvic region M79.9
    shoulder region M79.9
    specified type NEC M79.89
    thigh M79.9
    upper arm M79.9
  somatization F45.0
  somatoform F45.9
    pain (persistent) F45.41
    somatization (multiple) (long-lasting) F45.0
    specified NEC F45.8
    undifferentiated F45.1
  somnolence, excessive — *see* Hypersomnia
  specific
    arithmetical F81.2
    developmental, of motor F82
    reading F81.0
    speech and language F80.9
    spelling F81.81
    written expression F81.81
  speech R47.9
    articulation (functional) (specific) F80.0
    developmental F80.9
    specified NEC R47.89
  spelling (specific) F81.81
  spine (*see also* Dorsopathy)
    ligamentous or muscular attachments, peripheral
      — *see* Enthesopathy, spinal
    specified NEC — *see* Dorsopathy, specified NEC
  stereotyped, habit or movement F98.4
  stomach (functional) — *see* Disorder, gastric
  stress F43.9
    post-traumatic F43.10
      acute F43.11
      chronic F43.12
  sulfur-bearing amino-acid metabolism E72.10
  sweat gland (eccrine) L74.9
    apocrine L75.9
      specified NEC L75.8
    specified NEC L74.8
  synovium M67.90
    acromioclavicular M67.91- ☑
    ankle M67.97- ☑
    elbow M67.92- ☑
    foot M67.97- ☑
    forearm M67.93- ☑
    hand M67.94- ☑
    hip M67.95- ☑
    knee M67.96- ☑
    multiple sites M67.99
    rupture — *see* Rupture, synovium
    shoulder M67.91- ☑
    specified type NEC M67.80
      acromioclavicular M67.81- ☑
      ankle M67.87- ☑

Disorder — *continued*
  synovium — *continued*
    specified type — *continued*
      elbow M67.82- ☑
      foot M67.87- ☑
      hand M67.84- ☑
      hip M67.85- ☑
      knee M67.86- ☑
      multiple sites M67.89
      wrist M67.83- ☑
    synovitis — *see* Synovitis
    upper arm M67.92- ☑
    wrist M67.93- ☑
  temperature regulation, newborn P81.9
    specified NEC P81.8
  temporomandibular joint — *see* Anomaly, dentofacial,
    temporomandibular joint
  tendon M67.90
    acromioclavicular M67.91- ☑
    ankle M67.97- ☑
    contracture — *see* Contracture, tendon
    elbow M67.92- ☑
    foot M67.97- ☑
    forearm M67.93- ☑
    hand M67.94- ☑
    hip M67.95- ☑
    knee M67.96- ☑
    multiple sites M67.99
    rupture — *see* Rupture, tendon
    shoulder M67.91- ☑
    specified type NEC M67.80
      acromioclavicular M67.81- ☑
      ankle M67.87- ☑
      elbow M67.82- ☑
      foot M67.87- ☑
      hand M67.84- ☑
      hip M67.85- ☑
      knee M67.86- ☑
      multiple sites M67.89
      trunk M67.88
      wrist M67.83- ☑
    synovitis — *see* Synovitis
    tendinitis — *see* Tendinitis
    tenosynovitis — *see* Tenosynovitis
    trunk M67.98
    upper arm M67.92- ☑
    wrist M67.93- ☑
  thoracic root (nerve) NEC G54.3
  thyrocalcitonin hypersecretion E07.0
  thyroid (gland) E07.9
    function NEC, neonatal, transitory P72.2
    iodine-deficiency related E01.8
    specified NEC E07.89
  tic — *see* Tic
  tooth K08.9
    development K00.9
      specified NEC K00.8
    eruption K00.6
  Tourette's F95.2
  trance and possession F44.89
  tricuspid (valve) — *see* Endocarditis, tricuspid
  tryptophan metabolism E70.5
  tubular, phosphate-losing N25.0
  tubulo-interstitial (in)
    brucellosis A23.9 [N16]
    cystinosis E72.04
    diphtheria A36.84
    glycogen storage disease E74.00 [N16]
    leukemia NEC C95.9- ☑ [N16]
    lymphoma NEC C85.9- ☑ [N16]
    mixed cryoglobulinemia D89.1 [N16]
    multiple myeloma C90.0- ☑ [N16]
    Salmonella infection A02.25
    sarcoidosis D86.84
    sepsis A41.9 [N16]
      streptococcal A40.9 [N16]
    systemic lupus erythematosus M32.15
    toxoplasmosis B58.83
    transplant rejection T86.91 [N16]
    Wilson's disease E83.01 [N16]
  tubulo-renal function, impaired N25.9
    specified NEC N25.89
  tympanic membrane H73.9- ☑
    atrophy — *see* Atrophy, tympanic membrane
    infection — *see* Myringitis
    perforation — *see* Perforation, tympanum
    specified NEC H73.89- ☑

Disorder — *continued*
- unsocialized aggressive F91.1
- urea cycle metabolism E72.20
  - argininemia E72.21
  - arginosuccinic aciduria E72.22
  - citrullinemia E72.23
  - ornithine transcarbamylase deficiency E72.4
  - other specified E72.29
- ureter (in) N28.9
  - schistosomiasis B65.0 [N29]
  - tuberculosis A18.11
- urethra N36.9
  - specified NEC N36.8
- urinary system N39.9
  - specified NEC N39.8
- valve, heart
  - aortic — *see* Endocarditis, aortic
  - mitral — *see* Endocarditis, mitral
  - pulmonary — *see* Endocarditis, pulmonary
  - rheumatic
    - aortic — *see* Endocarditis, aortic, rheumatic
    - mitral — *see* Endocarditis, mitral
    - pulmonary — *see* Endocarditis, pulmonary, rheumatic
    - tricuspid — *see* Endocarditis, tricuspid
  - tricuspid — *see* Endocarditis, tricuspid
- vestibular function H81.9- ☑
  - specified NEC — *see* subcategory H81.8 ☑
    - in diseases classified elsewhere H82.- ☑
  - vertigo — *see* Vertigo
- vision, binocular H53.30
  - abnormal retinal correspondence H53.31
  - diplopia H53.2
  - fusion with defective stereopsis H53.32
  - simultaneous perception H53.33
  - suppression H53.34
- visual
  - cortex
    - blindness H47.619
      - left brain H47.612
      - right brain H47.611
    - due to
      - inflammatory disorder H47.629
        - left brain H47.622
        - right brain H47.621
      - neoplasm H47.639
        - left brain H47.632
        - right brain H47.631
      - vascular disorder H47.649
        - left brain H47.642
        - right brain H47.641
  - pathway H47.9
    - due to
      - inflammatory disorder H47.51- ☑
      - neoplasm H47.52- ☑
      - vascular disorder H47.53- ☑
    - optic chiasm — *see* Disorder, optic, chiasm
- vitreous body H43.9
  - crystalline deposits — *see* Deposit, crystalline
  - degeneration — *see* Degeneration, vitreous
  - hemorrhage — *see* Hemorrhage, vitreous
  - opacities — *see* Opacity, vitreous
  - prolapse — *see* Prolapse, vitreous
  - specified type NEC H43.89
- voice R49.9
  - specified type NEC R49.8
- volatile solvent use
  - due to drug abuse — *see* Abuse, drug, inhalant
  - due to drug dependence — *see* Dependence, drug, inhalant
- white blood cells D72.9
  - specified NEC D72.89
- withdrawing, child or adolescent F40.10

Disorientation R41.0
Displacement, displaced
- acquired traumatic of bone, cartilage, joint, tendon NEC — *see* Dislocation
- adrenal gland (congenital) Q89.1
- appendix, retrocecal (congenital) Q43.8
- auricle (congenital) Q17.4
- bladder (acquired) N32.89
  - congenital Q64.19
- brachial plexus (congenital) Q07.8
- brain stem, caudal (congenital) Q04.8
- canaliculus (lacrimalis), congenital Q10.6
- cardia through esophageal hiatus (congenital) Q40.1
- cerebellum, caudal (congenital) Q04.8
- cervix — *see* Malposition, uterus

Displacement, displaced — *continued*
- colon (congenital) Q43.3
- device, implant or graft (*see also* Complications, by site and type, mechanical) T85.628 ☑
  - arterial graft NEC — *see* Complication, cardiovascular device, mechanical, vascular
  - breast (implant) T85.42 ☑
  - catheter NEC T85.628 ☑
    - dialysis (renal) T82.42 ☑
      - intraperitoneal T85.621 ☑
    - infusion NEC T82.524 ☑
      - spinal (epidural) (subdural) T85.620 ☑
    - urinary (indwelling) T83.028 ☑
      - cystostomy T83.020 ☑
  - electronic (electrode) (pulse generator) (stimulator) — *see* Complication, electronic stimulator
  - fixation, internal (orthopedic) NEC — *see* Complication, fixation device, mechanical
  - gastrointestinal — *see* Complications, prosthetic device, mechanical, gastrointestinal device
  - genital NEC T83.428 ☑
    - intrauterine contraceptive device T83.32 ☑
    - penile prosthesis T83.420 ☑
  - heart NEC — *see* Complication, cardiovascular device, mechanical
  - joint prosthesis — *see* Complications, joint prosthesis, mechanical
  - ocular — *see* Complications, prosthetic device, mechanical, ocular device
  - orthopedic NEC — *see* Complication, orthopedic, device or graft, mechanical
  - specified NEC T85.628 ☑
  - urinary NEC (*see also* Complication, genitourinary, device, urinary, mechanical)
    - graft T83.22 ☑
  - vascular NEC — *see* Complication, cardiovascular device, mechanical
  - ventricular intracranial shunt T85.02 ☑
- electronic stimulator
  - bone T84.320 ☑
  - cardiac — *see* Complications, cardiac device, electronic
  - nervous system — *see* Complication, prosthetic device, mechanical, electronic nervous system stimulator
  - urinary — *see* Complications, electronic stimulator, urinary
- esophageal mucosa into cardia of stomach, congenital Q39.8
- esophagus (acquired) K22.8
  - congenital Q39.8
- eyeball (acquired) (lateral) (old) — *see* Displacement, globe
  - congenital Q15.8
  - current — *see* Avulsion, eye
- fallopian tube (acquired) N83.4
  - congenital Q50.6
  - opening (congenital) Q50.6
- gallbladder (congenital) Q44.1
- gastric mucosa (congenital) Q40.2
- globe (acquired) (old) (lateral) H05.21- ☑
  - current — *see* Avulsion, eye
- heart (congenital) Q24.8
  - acquired I51.89
- hymen (upward) (congenital) Q52.4
- intervertebral disc NEC
  - with myelopathy — *see* Disorder, disc, with, myelopathy
  - cervical, cervicothoracic (with) M50.20
    - myelopathy — *see* Disorder, disc, cervical, with myelopathy
    - neuritis, radiculitis or radiculopathy — *see* Disorder, disc, cervical, with neuritis
  - due to trauma — *see* Dislocation, vertebra
  - lumbar region M51.26
    - with
      - myelopathy M51.06
      - neuritis, radiculitis, radiculopathy or sciatica M51.16
  - lumbosacral region M51.27
    - with
      - neuritis, radiculitis, radiculopathy or sciatica M51.17
  - sacrococcygeal region M53.3
  - thoracic region M51.24
    - with
      - myelopathy M51.04

Displacement, displaced — *continued*
- intervertebral disc — *continued*
  - thoracic region — *continued*
    - with — *continued*
      - neuritis, radiculitis, radiculopathy M51.14
    - thoracolumbar region M51.25
      - with
        - myelopathy M51.05
        - neuritis, radiculitis, radiculopathy M51.15
- intrauterine device T83.32 ☑
- kidney (acquired) N28.83
  - congenital Q63.2
- lachrymal, lacrimal apparatus or duct (congenital) Q10.6
- lens, congenital Q12.1
- macula (congenital) Q14.1
- Meckel's diverticulum Q43.0
  - malignant — *see* Table of Neoplasms, small intestine, malignant
- nail (congenital) Q84.6
  - acquired L60.8
- opening of Wharton's duct in mouth Q38.4
- organ or site, congenital NEC — *see* Malposition, congenital
- ovary (acquired) N83.4
  - congenital Q50.39
  - free in peritoneal cavity (congenital) Q50.39
  - into hernial sac N83.4
- oviduct (acquired) N83.4
  - congenital Q50.6
- parathyroid (gland) E21.4
- parotid gland (congenital) Q38.4
- punctum lacrimale (congenital) Q10.6
- sacro-iliac (joint) (congenital) Q74.2
  - current injury S33.2 ☑
  - old — *see* subcategory M53.2 ☑
- salivary gland (any) (congenital) Q38.4
- spleen (congenital) Q89.09
- stomach, congenital Q40.2
- sublingual duct Q38.4
- tongue (downward) (congenital) Q38.3
- tooth, teeth, fully erupted M26.30
  - horizontal M26.33
  - vertical M26.34
- trachea (congenital) Q32.1
- ureter or ureteric opening or orifice (congenital) Q62.62
- uterine opening of oviducts or fallopian tubes Q50.6
- uterus, uterine — *see* Malposition, uterus
- ventricular septum Q21.0
  - with rudimentary ventricle Q20.4

Disproportion
- between native and reconstructed breast N65.1
- fiber-type G71.2

Disruptio uteri — *see* Rupture, uterus
Disruption (of)
- ciliary body NEC H21.89
- closure of
  - cornea T81.31 ☑
  - craniotomy T81.32 ☑
  - fascia (muscular) (superficial) T81.32 ☑
  - internal organ or tissue T81.32 ☑
  - laceration (external) (internal) T81.33 ☑
  - ligament T81.32 ☑
  - mucosa T81.31 ☑
  - muscle or muscle flap T81.32 ☑
  - ribs or rib cage T81.32 ☑
  - skin and subcutaneous tissue (full-thickness) (superficial) T81.31 ☑
  - skull T81.32 ☑
  - sternum (sternotomy) T81.32 ☑
  - tendon T81.32 ☑
  - traumatic laceration (external) (internal) T81.33 ☑
- family Z63.8
  - due to
    - absence of family member due to military deployment Z63.31
    - absence of family member NEC Z63.32
    - alcoholism and drug addiction in family Z63.72
    - bereavement Z63.4
    - death (assumed) or disappearance of family member Z63.4
    - divorce or separation Z63.5
    - drug addiction in family Z63.72
    - return of family member from military deployment (current or past conflict) Z63.71
    - stressful life events NEC Z63.79
- iris NEC H21.89

Disruption — continued
  ligament(s) (see also Sprain)
    knee
      current injury — see Dislocation, knee
      old (chronic) — see Derangement, knee, instability
      spontaneous NEC — see Derangement, knee, disruption ligament
    ossicular chain — see Discontinuity, ossicles, ear
  pelvic ring (stable) S32.810 ☑
    unstable S32.811 ☑
  traumatic injury wound repair T81.33 ☑
  wound T81.30 ☑
    episiotomy O90.1
    operation T81.31 ☑
      cesarean O90.0
      external operation wound (superficial) T81.31 ☑
      internal operation wound (deep) T81.32 ☑
    perineal (obstetric) O90.1
    traumatic injury repair T81.33 ☑
Dissatisfaction with
  employment Z56.9
  school environment Z55.4
Dissecting — see condition
Dissection
  aorta I71.00
    abdominal I71.02
    thoracic I71.01
    thoracoabdominal I71.03
  artery
    carotid I77.71
    cerebral (nonruptured) I67.0
      ruptured — see Hemorrhage, intracranial, subarachnoid
    coronary I25.42
    iliac I77.72
    renal I77.73
    specified NEC I77.79
    vertebral I77.74
  traumatic — see Wound, open, by site
  vascular I99.8
  wound — see Wound, open
Disseminated — see condition
Dissociation
  auriculoventricular or atrioventricular (AV) (any degree) (isorhythmic) I45.89
    with heart block I44.2
  interference I45.89
Dissociative reaction, state F44.9
Dissolution, vertebra — see Osteoporosis
Distension, distention
  abdomen R14.0
  bladder N32.89
  cecum K63.89
  colon K63.89
  gallbladder K82.8
  intestine K63.89
  kidney N28.89
  liver K76.89
  seminal vesicle N50.8
  stomach K31.89
    acute K31.0
    psychogenic F45.8
  ureter — see Dilatation, ureter
  uterus N85.8
Distoma hepaticum infestation B66.3
Distomiasis B66.9
  bile passages B66.3
  hemic B65.9
  hepatic B66.3
    due to Clonorchis sinensis B66.1
  intestinal B66.5
  liver B66.3
    due to Clonorchis sinensis B66.1
  lung B66.4
  pulmonary B66.4
Distomolar (fourth molar) K00.1
Disto-occlusion (Division I) (Division II) M26.212
Distortion(s) (congenital)
  adrenal (gland) Q89.1
  arm NEC Q68.8
  bile duct or passage Q44.5
  bladder Q64.79
  brain Q04.9
  cervix (uteri) Q51.9
  chest (wall) Q67.8

Distortion(s) — continued
  chest — continued
    bones Q76.8
  clavicle Q74.0
  clitoris Q52.6
  coccyx Q76.49
  common duct Q44.5
  coronary Q24.5
  cystic duct Q44.5
  ear (auricle) (external) Q17.3
    inner Q16.5
    middle Q16.4
      ossicles Q16.3
  endocrine NEC Q89.2
  eustachian tube Q17.8
  eye (adnexa) Q15.8
  face bone(s) NEC Q75.8
  fallopian tube Q50.6
  femur NEC Q68.8
  fibula NEC Q68.8
  finger(s) Q68.1
  foot Q66.9
  genitalia, genital organ(s)
    female Q52.8
      external Q52.79
      internal NEC Q52.8
  gyri Q04.8
  hand bone(s) Q68.1
  heart (auricle) (ventricle) Q24.8
    valve (cusp) Q24.8
  hepatic duct Q44.5
  humerus NEC Q68.8
  hymen Q52.4
  intrafamilial communications Z63.8
  jaw NEC M26.89
  labium (majus) (minus) Q52.79
  leg NEC Q68.8
  lens Q12.8
  liver Q44.7
  lumbar spine Q76.49
    with disproportion O33.8
      causing obstructed labor O65.0
  lumbosacral (joint) (region) Q76.49
    kyphosis — see Kyphosis, congenital
    lordosis — see Lordosis, congenital
  nerve Q07.8
  nose Q30.8
  organ
    of Corti Q16.5
    or site not listed — see Anomaly, by site
  ossicles, ear Q16.3
  oviduct Q50.6
  pancreas Q45.3
  parathyroid (gland) Q89.2
  pituitary (gland) Q89.2
  radius NEC Q68.8
  sacroiliac joint Q74.2
  sacrum Q76.49
  scapula Q74.0
  shoulder girdle Q74.0
  skull bone(s) NEC Q75.8
    with
      anencephalus Q00.0
      encephalocele — see Encephalocele
      hydrocephalus Q03.9
        with spina bifida — see Spina bifida, with hydrocephalus
      microcephaly Q02
  spinal cord Q06.8
  spine Q76.49
    kyphosis — see Kyphosis, congenital
    lordosis — see Lordosis, congenital
  spleen Q89.09
  sternum NEC Q76.7
  thorax (wall) Q67.8
    bony Q76.8
  thymus (gland) Q89.2
  thyroid (gland) Q89.2
  tibia NEC Q68.8
  toe(s) Q66.9
  tongue Q38.3
  trachea (cartilage) Q32.1
  ulna NEC Q68.8
  ureter Q62.8
  urethra Q64.79
    causing obstruction Q64.39
  uterus Q51.9
  vagina Q52.4

Distortion(s) — continued
  vertebra Q76.49
    kyphosis — see Kyphosis, congenital
    lordosis — see Lordosis, congenital
  visual (see also Disturbance, vision)
    shape and size H53.15
  vulva Q52.79
  wrist (bones) (joint) Q68.8
Distress
  abdomen — see Pain, abdominal
  acute respiratory (adult) (child) J80
  epigastric R10.13
  fetal P84
    complicating pregnancy — see Stress, fetal
  gastrointestinal (functional) K30
    psychogenic F45.8
  intestinal (functional) NOS K59.9
    psychogenic F45.8
  maternal, during labor and delivery O75.0
  respiratory R06.00
    adult J80
    child J80
    newborn P22.9
      specified NEC P22.8
    orthopnea R06.01
    psychogenic F45.8
    shortness of breath R06.02
    specified type NEC R06.09
Distribution vessel, atypical Q27.9
  coronary artery Q24.5
  precerebral Q28.1
Districhiasis L68.8
Disturbance(s) (see also Disease)
  absorption K90.9
    calcium E58
    carbohydrate K90.4
    fat K90.4
      pancreatic K90.3
    protein K90.4
    starch K90.4
    vitamin — see Deficiency, vitamin
  acid-base equilibrium E87.8
    mixed E87.4
  activity and attention (with hyperkinesis) — see Disorder, attention-deficit hyperactivity
  amino acid transport E72.00
  assimilation, food K90.9
  auditory nerve, except deafness — see subcategory H93.3 ☑
  behavior — see Disorder, conduct
  blood clotting (mechanism) (see also Defect, coagulation) D68.9
  cerebral
    nerve — see Disorder, nerve, cranial
    status, newborn P91.9
      specified NEC P91.8
  circulatory I99.9
  conduct (see also Disorder, conduct) F91.9
    adjustment reaction — see Disorder, adjustment
    compulsive F63.9
    disruptive F91.9
    hyperkinetic — see Disorder, attention-deficit hyperactivity
    socialized F91.2
    specified NEC F91.8
    unsocialized F91.1
  coordination R27.8
  cranial nerve — see Disorder, nerve, cranial
  deep sensibility — see Disturbance, sensation
  digestive K30
    psychogenic F45.8
  electrolyte (see also Imbalance, electrolyte)
    newborn, transitory P74.4
      hyperammonemia P74.6
      potassium balance P74.3
      sodium balance P74.2
      specified type NEC P74.4
  emotions specific to childhood and adolescence F93.9
    with
      anxiety and fearfulness NEC F93.8
      elective mutism F94.0
      oppositional disorder F91.3
      sensitivity (withdrawal) F40.10
      shyness F40.10
      social withdrawal F40.10
    involving relationship problems F93.8
    mixed F93.8
    specified NEC F93.8

Disturbance(s) — *continued*
  endocrine (gland) E34.9
    neonatal, transitory P72.9
      specified NEC P72.8
  equilibrium R42
  fructose metabolism E74.10
  gait — *see* Gait
    hysterical F44.4
    psychogenic F44.4
  gastrointestinal (functional) K30
    psychogenic F45.8
  habit, child F98.9
  hearing, except deafness and tinnitus — *see* Abnormal,
      auditory perception
  heart, functional (conditions in I44-I50)
    due to presence of (cardiac) prosthesis I97.19- ☑
      postoperative I97.89
        cardiac surgery I97.19- ☑
  hormones E34.9
  innervation uterus (parasympathetic) (sympathetic)
      N85.8
  keratinization NEC
    gingiva K05.10
      nonplaque induced K05.11
      plaque induced K05.10
    lip K13.0
    oral (mucosa) (soft tissue) K13.29
    tongue K13.29
  learning (specific) — *see* Disorder, learning
  memory — *see* Amnesia
    mild, following organic brain damage F06.8
  mental F99
    associated with diseases classified elsewhere F54
  metabolism E88.9
    with
      abortion — *see* Abortion, by type with other
          specified complication
      ectopic pregnancy O08.5
      molar pregnancy O08.5
    amino-acid E72.9
      aromatic E70.9
      branched-chain E71.2
      straight-chain E72.8
      sulfur-bearing E72.10
    ammonia E72.20
    arginine E72.21
    arginosuccinic acid E72.22
    carbohydrate E74.9
    cholesterol E78.9
    citrulline E72.23
    cystathionine E72.19
    general E88.9
    glutamine E72.8
    histidine E70.40
    homocystine E72.19
    hydroxylysine E72.3
    in labor or delivery O75.89
    iron E83.10
    lipoid E78.9
    lysine E72.3
    methionine E72.19
    neonatal, transitory P74.9
      calcium and magnesium P71.9
        specified type NEC P71.8
      carbohydrate metabolism P70.9
        specified type NEC P70.8
      specified NEC P74.8
    ornithine E72.4
    phosphate E83.39
    sodium NEC E87.8
    threonine E72.8
    tryptophan E70.5
    tyrosine E70.20
    urea cycle E72.20
  motor R29.2
  nervous, functional R45.0
  neuromuscular mechanism (eye), due to syphilis
      A52.15
  nutritional E63.9
    nail L60.3
  ocular motion H51.9
    psychogenic F45.8
  oculogyric H51.8
    psychogenic F45.8
  oculomotor H51.9
    psychogenic F45.8
  olfactory nerve R43.1
  optic nerve NEC — *see* Disorder, nerve, optic

Disturbance(s) — *continued*
  oral epithelium, including tongue NEC K13.29
  perceptual due to
    alcohol withdrawal F10.232
    amphetamine intoxication F15.922
      in
        abuse F15.122
        dependence F15.222
    anxiolytic withdrawal F13.232
    cannabis intoxication (acute) F12.922
      in
        abuse F12.122
        dependence F12.222
    cocaine intoxication (acute) F14.922
      in
        abuse F14.122
        dependence F14.222
    hypnotic withdrawal F13.232
    opioid intoxication (acute) F11.922
      in
        abuse F11.122
        dependence F11.222
    phencyclidine intoxication (acute) F19.922
      in
        abuse F19.122
        dependence F19.222
    sedative withdrawal F13.232
  personality (pattern) (trait) (*see also* Disorder, person-
      ality) F60.9
    following organic brain damage F07.9
  polyglandular E31.9
    specified NEC E31.8
  potassium balance, newborn P74.3
  psychogenic F45.9
  psychomotor F44.4
  psychophysical visual H53.16
  pupillary — *see* Anomaly, pupil, function
  reflex R29.2
  rhythm, heart I49.9
  salivary secretion K11.7
  sensation (cold) (heat) (localization) (tactile discrimi-
      nation) (texture) (vibratory) NEC R20.9
    hysterical F44.6
    skin R20.9
      anesthesia R20.0
      hyperesthesia R20.3
      hypoesthesia R20.1
      paresthesia R20.2
      specified type NEC R20.8
    smell R43.9
      and taste (mixed) R43.8
      anosmia R43.0
      parosmia R43.1
      specified NEC R43.8
    taste R43.9
      and smell (mixed) R43.8
      parageusia R43.2
      specified NEC R43.8
  sensory — *see* Disturbance, sensation
  situational (transient) (*see also* Disorder, adjustment)
    acute F43.0
  sleep G47.9
    nonorganic origin F51.9
  smell — *see* Disturbance, sensation, smell
  sociopathic F60.2
  sodium balance, newborn P74.2
  speech R47.9
    developmental F80.9
    specified NEC R47.89
  stomach (functional) K31.9
  sympathetic (nerve) G90.9
  taste — *see* Disturbance, sensation, taste
  temperature
    regulation, newborn P81.9
      specified NEC P81.8
    sense R20.8
      hysterical F44.6
  tooth
    eruption K00.6
    formation K00.4
    structure, hereditary NEC K00.5
  touch — *see* Disturbance, sensation
  vascular I99.9
    arteriosclerotic — *see* Arteriosclerosis
  vasomotor I73.9
  vasospastic I73.9
  vision, visual H53.9

Disturbance(s) — *continued*
  vision, visual — *continued*
    following
      cerebral infarction I69.398
      cerebrovascular disease I69.998
        specified NEC I69.898
      intracerebral hemorrhage I69.198
      nontraumatic intracranial hemorrhage NEC
          I69.298
      specified disease NEC I69.898
      subarachnoid hemorrhage I69.098
    psychophysical H53.16
    specified NEC H53.8
    subjective H53.10
      day blindness H53.11
      discomfort H53.14- ☑
      distortions of shape and size H53.15
      loss
        sudden H53.13- ☑
        transient H53.12- ☑
      specified type NEC H53.19
  voice R49.9
    psychogenic F44.4
    specified NEC R49.8
Diuresis R35.8
Diver's palsy, paralysis or squeeze T70.3 ☑
Diverticulitis (acute) K57.92
  bladder — *see* Cystitis
  ileum — *see* Diverticulitis, intestine, small
  intestine K57.92
    with
      abscess, perforation or peritonitis K57.80
        with bleeding K57.81
      bleeding K57.93
    congenital Q43.8
    large K57.32
      with
        abscess, perforation or peritonitis K57.20
          with bleeding K57.21
        bleeding K57.33
        small intestine K57.52
          with
            abscess, perforation or peritonitis
                K57.40
              with bleeding K57.41
            bleeding K57.53
    small K57.12
      with
        abscess, perforation or peritonitis K57.00
          with bleeding K57.01
        bleeding K57.13
        large intestine K57.52
          with
            abscess, perforation or peritonitis
                K57.40
              with bleeding K57.41
            bleeding K57.53
Diverticulosis K57.90
  with bleeding K57.91
  large intestine K57.30
    with
      bleeding K57.31
      small intestine K57.50
        with bleeding K57.51
  small intestine K57.10
    with
      bleeding K57.11
      large intestine K57.50
        with bleeding K57.51
Diverticulum, diverticula (multiple) K57.90
  appendix (noninflammatory) K38.2
  bladder (sphincter) N32.3
    congenital Q64.6
  bronchus (congenital) Q32.4
    acquired J98.09
  calyx, calyceal (kidney) N28.89
  cardia (stomach) K31.4
  cecum — *see* Diverticulosis, intestine, large
    congenital Q43.8
  colon — *see* Diverticulosis, intestine, large
    congenital Q43.8
  duodenum — *see* Diverticulosis, intestine, small
    congenital Q43.8
  epiphrenic (esophagus) K22.5
  esophagus (congenital) Q39.6
    acquired (epiphrenic) (pulsion) (traction) K22.5
  eustachian tube — *see* Disorder, eustachian tube,
      specified NEC

Diverticulum, diverticula — *continued*
  fallopian tube N83.8
  gastric K31.4
  heart (congenital) Q24.8
  ileum — *see* Diverticulosis, intestine, small
  jejunum — *see* Diverticulosis, intestine, small
  kidney (pelvis) (calyces) N28.89
    with calculus — *see* Calculus, kidney
  Meckel's (displaced) (hypertrophic) Q43.0
    malignant — *see* Table of Neoplasms, small intes-
        tine, malignant
  midthoracic K22.5
  organ or site, congenital NEC — *see* Distortion
  pericardium (congenital) (cyst) Q24.8
    acquired I31.8
  pharyngoesophageal (congenital) Q39.6
    acquired K22.5
  pharynx (congenital) Q38.7
  rectosigmoid — *see* Diverticulosis, intestine, large
    congenital Q43.8
  rectum — *see* Diverticulosis, intestine, large
  Rokitansky's K22.5
  seminal vesicle N50.8
  sigmoid — *see* Diverticulosis, intestine, large
    congenital Q43.8
  stomach (acquired) K31.4
    congenital Q40.2
  trachea (acquired) J39.8
    congenital Q32.8
  ureter (acquired) N28.89
    congenital Q62.8
  ureterovesical orifice N28.89
  urethra (acquired) N36.1
    congenital Q64.79
  ventricle, left (congenital) Q24.8
  vesical N32.3
    congenital Q64.6
  Zenker's (esophagus) K22.5
Division
  cervix uteri (acquired) N88.8
  glans penis Q55.69
  labia minora (congenital) Q52.79
  ligament (partial or complete) (current) (*see also*
      Sprain)
    with open wound — *see* Wound, open
  muscle (partial or complete) (current) (*see also* Injury,
      muscle)
    with open wound — *see* Wound, open
  nerve (traumatic) — *see* Injury, nerve
  spinal cord — *see* Injury, spinal cord, by region
  vein I87.8
Divorce, causing family disruption Z63.5
Dix-Hallpike neurolabyrinthitis — *see* Neuronitis,
    vestibular
Dizziness R42
  hysterical F44.89
  psychogenic F45.8
DMAC (disseminated mycobacterium avium- intracellu-
    lare complex) A31.2
DNR (do not resuscitate) Z66
Doan-Wiseman syndrome (primary splenic neutrope-
    nia) — *see* Agranulocytosis
Doehle-Heller aortitis A52.02
Dog bite — *see* Bite
Dohle body panmyelopathic syndrome D72.0
Dolichocephaly Q67.2
Dolichocolon Q43.8
Dolichostenomelia — *see* Syndrome, Marfan's
Donohue's syndrome E34.8
Donor (organ or tissue) Z52.9
  blood (whole) Z52.000
    autologous Z52.010
    specified component (lymphocytes) (platelets) NEC
        Z52.008
      autologous Z52.018
      specified donor NEC Z52.098
    specified donor NEC Z52.090
    stem cells Z52.001
      autologous Z52.011
      specified donor NEC Z52.091
  bone Z52.20
    autologous Z52.21
    marrow Z52.3
    specified type NEC Z52.29
  cornea Z52.5
  egg (Oocyte) Z52.819
    age 35 and over Z52.812
      anonymous recipient Z52.812
      designated recipient Z52.813

Donor — *continued*
  egg — *continued*
    under age 35 Z52.810
      anonymous recipient Z52.810
      designated recipient Z52.811
  kidney Z52.4
  liver Z52.6
  lung Z52.89
  lymphocyte — *see* Donor, blood, specified compo-
      nents NEC
  Oocyte — *see* Donor, egg
  platelets Z52.008
  potential, examination of Z00.5
  semen Z52.89
  skin Z52.10
    autologous Z52.11
    specified type NEC Z52.19
  specified organ or tissue NEC Z52.89
  sperm Z52.89
Donovanosis A58
Dorsalgia M54.9
  psychogenic F45.41
  specified NEC M54.89
Dorsopathy M53.9
  deforming M43.9
    specified NEC — *see* subcategory M43.8 ☑
  specified NEC M53.80
    cervical region M53.82
    cervicothoracic region M53.83
    lumbar region M53.86
    lumbosacral region M53.87
    occipito-atlanto-axial region M53.81
    sacrococcygeal region M53.88
    thoracic region M53.84
    thoracolumbar region M53.85
Double
  albumin E88.09
  aortic arch Q25.4
  auditory canal Q17.8
  auricle (heart) Q20.8
  bladder Q64.79
  cervix Q51.820
    with doubling of uterus (and vagina) Q51.10
      with obstruction Q51.11
  inlet ventricle Q20.4
  kidney with double pelvis (renal) Q63.0
  meatus urinarius Q64.75
  monster Q89.4
  outlet
    left ventricle Q20.2
    right ventricle Q20.1
  pelvis (renal) with double ureter Q62.5
  tongue Q38.3
  ureter (one or both sides) Q62.5
    with double pelvis (renal) Q62.5
  urethra Q64.74
  urinary meatus Q64.75
  uterus Q51.2
    with
      doubling of cervix (and vagina) Q51.10
        with obstruction Q51.11
      in pregnancy or childbirth O34.59- ☑
        causing obstructed labor O65.5
    vagina Q52.10
      with doubling of uterus (and cervix) Q51.10
        with obstruction Q51.11
  vision H53.2
  vulva Q52.79
Douglas' pouch, cul-de-sac — *see* condition
Down syndrome Q90.9
  meiotic nondisjunction Q90.0
  mitotic nondisjunction Q90.1
  mosaicism Q90.1
  translocation Q90.2
DPD (dihydropyrimidine dehydrogenase deficiency)
    E88.89
Dracontiasis B72
Dracunculiasis, dracunculosis B72
Dream state, hysterical F44.89
Drepanocytic anemia — *see* Disease, sickle-cell
Dresbach's syndrome (elliptocytosis) D58.1
Dreschlera (hawaiiensis) (infection) B43.8
Dressler's syndrome I24.1
Drift, ulnar — *see* Deformity, limb, specified type NEC,
    forearm
Drinking (alcohol)
  excessive, to excess NEC (without dependence) F10.10
    habitual (continual) (without remission) F10.20

Drinking — *continued*
  excessive, to excess — *continued*
    habitual — *continued*
      with remission F10.21
Drip, postnasal (chronic) R09.82
  due to
    allergic rhinitis — *see* Rhinitis, allergic
    common cold J00
    gastroesophageal reflux — *see* Reflux, gastroe-
        sophageal
    nasopharyngitis — *see* Nasopharyngitis
    other known condition — *code to* condition
    sinusitis — *see* Sinusitis
Droop
  facial R29.810
    cerebrovascular disease I69.992
      cerebral infarction I69.392
      intracerebral hemorrhage I69.192
      nontraumatic intracranial hemorrhage NEC
          I69.292
      specified disease NEC I69.892
      subarachnoid hemorrhage I69.092
Drop (in)
  attack NEC R55
  finger — *see* Deformity, finger
  foot — *see* Deformity, limb, foot, drop
  hematocrit (precipitous) R71.0
  hemoglobin R71.0
  toe — *see* Deformity, toe, specified NEC
  wrist — *see* Deformity, limb, wrist drop
Dropped heart beats I45.9
Dropsy, dropsical (*see also* Hydrops)
  abdomen R18.8
  brain — *see* Hydrocephalus
  cardiac, heart — *see* Failure, heart, congestive
  gangrenous — *see* Gangrene
  heart — *see* Failure, heart, congestive
  kidney — *see* Nephrosis
  lung — *see* Edema, lung
  newborn due to isoimmunization P56.0
  pericardium — *see* Pericarditis
Drowned, drowning (near) T75.1 ☑
Drowsiness R40.0
Drug
  abuse counseling and surveillance Z71.51
  addiction — *see* Dependence
  dependence — *see* Dependence
  habit — *see* Dependence
  harmful use — *see* Abuse, drug
  induced fever R50.2
  overdose — *see* Table of Drugs and Chemicals, by
      drug, poisoning
  poisoning — *see* Table of Drugs and Chemicals, by
      drug, poisoning
  resistant organism infection (*see also* Resistant, organ-
      ism, to, drug) Z16.30
  therapy
    long term (current) (prophylactic) — *see* Therapy,
        drug long-term (current) (prophylactic)
    short term — *omit code*
  wrong substance given or taken in error — *see* Table
      of Drugs and Chemicals, by drug, poisoning
Drunkenness (without dependence) F10.129
  acute in alcoholism F10.229
  chronic (without remission) F10.20
    with remission F10.21
  pathological (without dependence) F10.129
    with dependence F10.229
  sleep F51.9
Drusen
  macula (degenerative) (retina) — *see* Degeneration,
      macula, drusen
  optic disc H47.32- ☑
Dry, dryness (*see also* condition)
  larynx J38.7
  mouth R68.2
    due to dehydration E86.0
  nose J34.89
  socket (teeth) M27.3
  throat J39.2
DSAP L56.5
Duane's syndrome H50.81- ☑
Dubin-Johnson disease or syndrome E80.6
Dubois' disease (thymus gland) A50.59 [E35]
Dubowitz' syndrome Q87.1
Duchenne-Aran muscular atrophy G12.21
Duchenne-Griesinger disease G71.0

Index

Diverticulum, diverticula — Duchenne-Griesinger disease

Duchenne's
- disease or syndrome
  - motor neuron disease G12.22
  - muscular dystrophy G71.0
- locomotor ataxia (syphilitic) A52.11
- paralysis
  - birth injury P14.0
  - due to or associated with
    - motor neuron disease G12.22
    - muscular dystrophy G71.0

Ducrey's chancre A57
Duct, ductus — see condition
Duhring's disease (dermatitis herpetiformis) L13.0
Dullness, cardiac (decreased) (increased) R01.2
Dumb ague — see Malaria
Dumbness — see Aphasia
Dumdum fever B55.0
Dumping syndrome (postgastrectomy) K91.1
Duodenitis (nonspecific) (peptic) K29.80
- with bleeding K29.81

Duodenocholangitis — see Cholangitis
Duodenum, duodenal — see condition
Duplay's bursitis or periarthritis — see Tendinitis, calcific, shoulder
Duplication, duplex (see also Accessory)
- alimentary tract Q45.8
- anus Q43.4
- appendix (and cecum) Q43.4
- biliary duct (any) Q44.5
- bladder Q64.79
- cecum (and appendix) Q43.4
- cervix Q51.820
- chromosome NEC
  - with complex rearrangements NEC Q92.5
  - seen only at prometaphase Q92.8
- cystic duct Q44.5
- digestive organs Q45.8
- esophagus Q39.8
- frontonasal process Q75.8
- intestine (large) (small) Q43.4
- kidney Q63.0
- liver Q44.7
- pancreas Q45.3
- penis Q55.69
- respiratory organs NEC Q34.8
- salivary duct Q38.4
- spinal cord (incomplete) Q06.2
- stomach Q40.2

Dupré's disease (meningism) R29.1
Dupuytren's contraction or disease M72.0
Durand-Nicolas-Favre disease A55
Durotomy (inadvertent) (incidental) G97.41
Duroziez's disease (congenital mitral stenosis) Q23.2
Dutton's relapsing fever (West African) A68.1
Dwarfism E34.3
- achondroplastic Q77.4
- congenital E34.3
- constitutional E34.3
- hypochondroplastic Q77.4
- hypophyseal E23.0
- infantile E34.3
- Laron-type E34.3
- Lorain (-Levi) type E23.0
- metatropic Q77.8
- nephrotic-glycosuric (with hypophosphatemic rickets) E72.09
- nutritional E45
- pancreatic K86.8
- pituitary E23.0
- renal N25.0
- thanatophoric Q77.1

Dyke-Young anemia (secondary) (symptomatic) D59.1
Dysacusis — see Abnormal, auditory perception
Dysadrenocortism E27.9
- hyperfunction E27.0

Dysarthria R47.1
- following
  - cerebral infarction I69.322
  - cerebrovascular disease I69.922
    - specified disease NEC I69.822
  - intracerebral hemorrhage I69.122
  - nontraumatic intracranial hemorrhage NEC I69.222
  - subarachnoid hemorrhage I69.022

Dysautonomia (familial) G90.1
Dysbarism T70.3 ☑
Dysbasia R26.2
- angiosclerotica intermittens I73.9
- hysterical F44.4

Dysbasia — continued
- lordotica (progressiva) G24.1
- nonorganic origin F44.4
- psychogenic F44.4

Dysbetalipoproteinemia (familial) E78.2
Dyscalculia R48.8
- developmental F81.2

Dyschezia K59.00
Dyschondroplasia (with hemangiomata) Q78.4
Dyschromia (skin) L81.9
Dyscollagenosis M35.9
Dyscranio-pygo-phalangy Q87.0
Dyscrasia
- blood (with) D75.9
  - antepartum hemorrhage — see Hemorrhage, antepartum, with coagulation defect
  - intrapartum hemorrhage O67.0
  - newborn P61.9
    - specified type NEC P61.8
  - puerperal, postpartum O72.3
- polyglandular, pluriglandular E31.9

Dysendocrinism E34.9
Dysentery, dysenteric (catarrhal) (diarrhea) (epidemic) (hemorrhagic) (infectious) (sporadic) (tropical) A09
- abscess, liver A06.4
- amebic (see also Amebiasis) A06.0
  - with abscess — see Abscess, amebic
  - acute A06.0
  - chronic A06.1
- arthritis (see also category M01) A09
  - bacillary (see also category M01) A03.9
- bacillary A03.9
  - arthritis (see also category M01) A03.9
  - Boyd A03.2
  - Flexner A03.1
  - Schmitz (-Stutzer) A03.0
  - Shiga (-Kruse) A03.0
  - Shigella A03.9
    - boydii A03.2
    - dysenteriae A03.0
    - flexneri A03.1
    - group A A03.0
    - group B A03.1
    - group C A03.2
    - group D A03.3
    - sonnei A03.3
    - specified type NEC A03.8
  - Sonne A03.3
  - specified type NEC A03.8
- balantidial A07.0
- Balantidium coli A07.0
- Boyd's A03.2
- candidal B37.82
- Chilomastix A07.8
- Chinese A03.9
- coccidial A07.3
- Dientamoeba (fragilis) A07.8
- Embadomonas A07.8
- Entamoeba, entamebic — see Dysentery, amebic
- Flexner-Boyd A03.2
- Flexner's A03.1
- Giardia lamblia A07.1
- Hiss-Russell A03.1
- Lamblia A07.1
- leishmanial B55.0
- malarial — see Malaria
- metazoal B82.0
- monilial B37.82
- protozoal A07.9
- Salmonella A02.0
- schistosomal B65.1
- Schmitz (-Stutzer) A03.0
- Shiga (-Kruse) A03.0
- Shigella NOS — see Dysentery, bacillary
- Sonne A03.3
- strongyloidiasis B78.0
- trichomonal A07.8
- viral (see also Enteritis, viral) A08.4

Dysequilibrium R42
Dysesthesia R20.8
- hysterical F44.6

Dysfibrinogenemia (congenital) D68.2
Dysfunction
- adrenal E27.9
  - hyperfunction E27.0
- autonomic
  - due to alcohol G31.2
  - somatoform F45.8

Dysfunction — continued
- bladder N31.9
  - neurogenic NOS — see Dysfunction, bladder, neuromuscular
  - neuromuscular NOS N31.9
    - atonic (motor) (sensory) N31.2
    - autonomous N31.2
    - flaccid N31.2
    - nonreflex N31.2
    - reflex N31.1
    - specified NEC N31.8
    - uninhibited N31.0
- bleeding, uterus N93.8
- cerebral G93.89
- colon K59.9
  - psychogenic F45.8
- colostomy K94.03
- cystic duct K82.8
- cystostomy (stoma) — see Complications, cystostomy
- ejaculatory N53.19
  - anejaculatory orgasm N53.13
  - painful N53.12
  - premature F52.4
  - retarded N53.11
- endocrine NOS E34.9
- endometrium N85.8
- enterostomy K94.13
- gallbladder K82.8
- gastrostomy (stoma) K94.23
- gland, glandular NOS E34.9
- heart I51.89
- hemoglobin D75.89
- hepatic K76.89
- hypophysis E23.7
- hypothalamic NEC E23.3
- ileostomy (stoma) K94.13
- jejunostomy (stoma) K94.13
- kidney — see Disease, renal
- labyrinthine — see subcategory H83.2 ☑
- left ventricular, following sudden emotional stress I51.81
- liver K76.89
- male — see Dysfunction, sexual, male
- orgasmic (female) F52.31
  - male F52.32
- ovary E28.9
  - specified NEC E28.8
- papillary muscle I51.89
- parathyroid E21.4
- physiological NEC R68.89
  - psychogenic F59
- pineal gland E34.8
- pituitary (gland) E23.3
- platelets D69.1
- polyglandular E31.9
  - specified NEC E31.8
- psychophysiologic F59
- psychosexual F52.9
  - with
    - dyspareunia F52.6
    - premature ejaculation F52.4
    - vaginismus F52.5
- pylorus K31.9
- rectum K59.9
  - psychogenic F45.8
- reflex (sympathetic) — see Syndrome, pain, complex regional I
- segmental — see Dysfunction, somatic
- senile R54
- sexual (due to) R37
  - alcohol F10.981
  - amphetamine F15.981
    - in
      - abuse F15.181
      - dependence F15.281
  - anxiolytic F13.981
    - in
      - abuse F13.181
      - dependence F13.281
  - cocaine F14.981
    - in
      - abuse F14.181
      - dependence F14.281
  - excessive sexual drive F52.8
  - failure of genital response (male) F52.21
    - female F52.22
  - female N94.9
    - aversion F52.1

Dysfunction — *continued*
  sexual — *continued*
    female — *continued*
      dyspareunia N94.1
        psychogenic F52.6
      frigidity F52.22
      nymphomania F52.8
      orgasmic F52.31
      psychogenic F52.9
        aversion F52.1
        dyspareunia F52.6
        frigidity F52.22
        nymphomania F52.8
        orgasmic F52.31
        vaginismus F52.5
      vaginismus N94.2
        psychogenic F52.5
    hypnotic F13.981
      in
        abuse F13.181
        dependence F13.281
    inhibited orgasm (female) F52.31
      male F52.32
    lack
      of sexual enjoyment F52.1
      or loss of sexual desire F52.0
    male N53.9
      anejaculatory orgasm N53.13
      ejaculatory N53.19
        painful N53.12
        premature F52.4
        retarded N53.11
      erectile N52.9
        drug induced N52.2
        due to
          disease classified elsewhere N52.1
          drug N52.2
        postoperative (postprocedural) N52.39
          following
            prostatectomy N52.34
              radical N52.31
            radical cystectomy N52.32
            urethral surgery N52.33
        psychogenic F52.21
        specified cause NEC N52.8
        vasculogenic
          arterial insufficiency N52.01
            with corporo-venous occlusive N52.03
          corporo-venous occlusive N52.02
            with arterial insufficiency N52.03
      impotence — *see* Dysfunction, sexual, male, erectile
      psychogenic F52.9
        aversion F52.1
        erectile F52.21
        orgasmic F52.32
        premature ejaculation F52.4
        satyriasis F52.8
        specified type NEC F52.8
      specified type NEC N53.8
    nonorganic F52.9
      specified NEC F52.8
    opioid F11.981
      in
        abuse F11.181
        dependence F11.281
    orgasmic dysfunction (female) F52.31
      male F52.32
    premature ejaculation F52.4
    psychoactive substances NEC F19.981
      in
        abuse F19.181
        dependence F19.281
    psychogenic F52.9
    sedative F13.981
      in
        abuse F13.181
        dependence F13.281
    sexual aversion F52.1
    vaginismus (nonorganic) (psychogenic) F52.5
  sinoatrial node I49.5
  somatic M99.09
    abdomen M99.09
    acromioclavicular M99.07
    cervical region M99.01
    cervicothoracic M99.01
    costochondral M99.08

Dysfunction — *continued*
  somatic — *continued*
    costovertebral M99.08
    head region M99.00
    hip M99.05
    lower extremity M99.06
    lumbar region M99.03
    lumbosacral M99.03
    occipitocervical M99.00
    pelvic region M99.05
    pubic M99.05
    rib cage M99.08
    sacral region M99.04
    sacrococcygeal M99.04
    sacroiliac M99.04
    specified NEC M99.09
    sternochondral M99.08
    sternoclavicular M99.07
    thoracic region M99.02
    thoracolumbar M99.02
    upper extremity M99.07
  somatoform autonomic F45.8
  stomach K31.89
    psychogenic F45.8
  suprarenal E27.9
    hyperfunction E27.0
  symbolic R48.9
    specified type NEC R48.8
  temporomandibular (joint) M26.69
    joint-pain syndrome M26.62
  testicular (endocrine) E29.9
    specified NEC E29.8
  thymus E32.9
  thyroid E07.9
  ureterostomy (stoma) — *see* Complications, stoma, urinary tract
  urethrostomy (stoma) — *see* Complications, stoma, urinary tract
  uterus, complicating delivery O62.9
    hypertonic O62.4
    hypotonic O62.2
      primary O62.0
      secondary O62.1
  ventricular I51.9
    with congestive heart failure I50.9
    left, reversible, following sudden emotional stress I51.81

Dysgenesis
  gonadal (due to chromosomal anomaly) Q96.9
    pure Q99.1
  renal Q60.5
    bilateral Q60.4
    unilateral Q60.3
  reticular D72.0
  tidal platelet D69.3
Dysgerminoma
  specified site — *see* Neoplasm, malignant, by site
  unspecified site
    female C56.9
    male C62.90
Dysgeusia R43.2
Dysgraphia R27.8
Dyshidrosis, dysidrosis L30.1
Dyskaryotic cervical smear R87.619
Dyskeratosis L85.8
  cervix — *see* Dysplasia, cervix
  congenital Q82.8
  uterus NEC N85.8
Dyskinesia G24.9
  biliary (cystic duct or gallbladder) K82.8
  drug induced
    orofacial G24.01
  esophagus K22.4
  hysterical F44.4
  intestinal K59.8
  nonorganic origin F44.4
  orofacial (idiopathic) G24.4
    drug induced G24.01
  psychogenic F44.4
  subacute, drug induced G24.01
  tardive G24.01
    neuroleptic induced G24.01
  trachea J39.8
  tracheobronchial J98.09
Dyslalia (developmental) F80.0
Dyslexia R48.0
  developmental F81.0

Dyslipidemia E78.5
  depressed HDL cholesterol E78.6
  elevated fasting triglycerides E78.1
Dysmaturity (*see also* Light for dates)
  pulmonary (newborn) (Wilson-Mikity) P27.0
Dysmenorrhea (essential) (exfoliative) N94.6
  congestive (syndrome) N94.6
  primary N94.4
  psychogenic F45.8
  secondary N94.5
Dysmetabolic syndrome X E88.81
Dysmetria R27.8
Dysmorphism (due to)
  alcohol Q86.0
  exogenous cause NEC Q86.8
  hydantoin Q86.1
  warfarin Q86.2
Dysmorphophobia (nondelusional) F45.22
  delusional F22
Dysnomia R47.01
Dysorexia R63.0
  psychogenic F50.8
Dysostosis
  cleidocranial, cleidocranialis Q74.0
  craniofacial Q75.1
  Fairbank's (idiopathic familial generalized osteophytosis) Q78.9
  mandibulofacial (incomplete) Q75.4
  multiplex E76.01
  oculomandibular Q75.5
Dyspareunia (female) N94.1
  male N53.12
  nonorganic F52.6
  psychogenic F52.6
  secondary N94.1
Dyspepsia R10.13
  atonic K30
  functional (allergic) (congenital) (gastrointestinal) (occupational) (reflex) K30
  intestinal K59.8
  nervous F45.8
  neurotic F45.8
  psychogenic F45.8
Dysphagia R13.10
  cervical R13.19
  following
    cerebral infarction I69.391
    cerebrovascular disease I69.991
      specified NEC I69.891
    intracerebral hemorrhage I69.191
    nontraumatic intracranial hemorrhage NEC I69.291
    specified disease NEC I69.891
    subarachnoid hemorrhage I69.091
  functional (hysterical) F45.8
  hysterical F45.8
  nervous (hysterical) F45.8
  neurogenic R13.19
  oral phase R13.11
  oropharyngeal phase R13.12
  pharyneal phase R13.13
  pharyngoesophageal phase R13.14
  psychogenic F45.8
  sideropenic D50.1
  spastica K22.4
  specified NEC R13.19
Dysphagocytosis, congenital D71
Dysphasia R47.02
  developmental
    expressive type F80.1
    receptive type F80.2
  following
    cerebrovascular disease I69.921
    cerebral infarction I69.321
    intracerebral hemorrhage I69.121
    nontraumatic intracranial hemorrhage NEC I69.221
    specified disease NEC I69.821
    subarachnoid hemorrhage I69.021
Dysphonia R49.0
  functional F44.4
  hysterical F44.4
  psychogenic F44.4
  spastica J38.3
Dysphoria, postpartal O90.6
Dyspituitarism E23.3
Dysplasia (*see also* Anomaly)
  acetabular, congenital Q65.89
  alveolar capillary, with vein misalignment J84.843

Dysplasia — *continued*
- anus (histologically confirmed) (mild) (moderate) K62.82
  - severe D01.3
- arrhythmogenic right ventricular I42.8
- arterial, fibromuscular I77.3
- asphyxiating thoracic (congenital) Q77.2
- brain Q07.9
- bronchopulmonary, perinatal P27.1
- cervix (uteri) N87.9
  - mild N87.0
  - moderate N87.1
  - severe D06.9
- chondroectodermal Q77.6
- colon D12.6
- craniometaphyseal Q78.5
- dentinal K00.5
- diaphyseal, progressive Q78.3
- dystrophic Q77.5
- ectodermal (anhidrotic) (congenital) (hereditary) Q82.4
  - hidrotic Q82.8
- epithelial, uterine cervix — *see* Dysplasia, cervix
- eye (congenital) Q11.2
- fibrous
  - bone NEC (monostotic) M85.00
    - ankle M85.07- ☑
    - foot M85.07- ☑
    - forearm M85.03- ☑
    - hand M85.04- ☑
    - lower leg M85.06- ☑
    - multiple site M85.09
    - neck M85.08
    - rib M85.08
    - shoulder M85.01- ☑
    - skull M85.08
    - specified site NEC M85.08
    - thigh M85.05- ☑
    - toe M85.07- ☑
    - upper arm M85.02- ☑
    - vertebra M85.08
  - diaphyseal, progressive Q78.3
  - jaw M27.8
  - polyostotic Q78.1
- florid osseous (*see also* Cyst, calcifying odontogenic)
- high grade, focal D12.6
- hip, congenital Q65.89
- joint, congenital Q74.8
- kidney Q61.4
  - multicystic Q61.4
- leg Q74.2
- lung, congenital (not associated with short gestation) Q33.6
- mammary (gland) (benign) N60.9- ☑
  - cyst (solitary) — *see* Cyst, breast
  - cystic — *see* Mastopathy, cystic
  - duct ectasia — *see* Ectasia, mammary duct
  - fibroadenosis — *see* Fibroadenosis, breast
  - fibrosclerosis — *see* Fibrosclerosis, breast
  - specified type NEC N60.8- ☑
- metaphyseal (Jansen's) (McKusick's) (Schmid's) Q78.5
- muscle Q79.8
- oculodentodigital Q87.0
- periapical (cemental) (cemento-osseous) — *see* Cyst, calcifying odontogenic
- periosteum — *see* Disorder, bone, specified type NEC
- polyostotic fibrous Q78.1
- prostate (*see also* Neoplasia, intraepithelial, prostate) N42.3
  - severe D07.5
- renal Q61.4
  - multicystic Q61.4
- retinal, congenital Q14.1
- right ventricular, arrhythmogenic I42.8
- septo-optic Q04.4
- skin L98.8
- spinal cord Q06.1
- spondyloepiphyseal Q77.7
- thymic, with immunodeficiency D82.1
- vagina N89.3
  - mild N89.0
  - moderate N89.1
  - severe NEC D07.2
- vulva N90.3
  - mild N90.0
  - moderate N90.1
  - severe NEC D07.1

Dyspnea (nocturnal) (paroxysmal) R06.00
- asthmatic (bronchial) J45.909
  - with
    - bronchitis J45.909
      - with
        - exacerbation (acute) J45.901
        - status asthmaticus J45.902
      - chronic J44.9
    - exacerbation (acute) J45.901
    - status asthmaticus J45.902
  - cardiac — *see* Failure, ventricular, left
- cardiac — *see* Failure, ventricular, left
- functional F45.8
- hyperventilation R06.4
- hysterical F45.8
- newborn P28.89
- orthopnea R06.01
- psychogenic F45.8
- shortness of breath R06.02
- specified type NEC R06.09

Dyspraxia R27.8
- developmental (syndrome) F82

Dysproteinemia E88.09

Dysreflexia, autonomic G90.4

Dysrhythmia
- cardiac I49.9
  - newborn
    - bradycardia P29.12
      - occurring before birth P03.819
        - before onset of labor P03.810
        - during labor P03.811
    - tachycardia P29.11
  - postoperative I97.89
- cerebral or cortical — *see* Epilepsy

Dyssomnia — *see* Disorder, sleep

Dyssynergia
- biliary K83.8
- bladder sphincter N36.44
- cerebellaris myoclonica (Hunt's ataxia) G11.1

Dysthymia F34.1

Dysthyroidism E07.9

Dystocia O66.9
- affecting newborn P03.1
- cervical (hypotonic) O62.2
  - affecting newborn P03.6
  - primary O62.0
  - secondary O62.1
  - contraction ring O62.4
- fetal O66.9
  - abnormality NEC O66.3
  - conjoined twins O66.3
  - oversize O66.2
- maternal O66.9
- positional O64.9 ☑
- shoulder (girdle) O66.0
  - causing obstructed labor O66.0
- uterine NEC O62.4

Dystonia G24.9
- deformans progressiva G24.1
- drug induced NEC G24.09
  - acute G24.02
  - specified NEC G24.09
- familial G24.1
- idiopathic G24.1
  - familial G24.1
  - nonfamilial G24.2
  - orofacial G24.4
- lenticularis G24.8
- musculorum deformans G24.1
- neuroleptic induced (acute) G24.02
- orofacial (idiopathic) G24.4
- oromandibular G24.4
  - due to drug G24.01
- specified NEC G24.8
- torsion (familial) (idiopathic) G24.1
  - acquired G24.8
  - genetic G24.1
  - symptomatic (nonfamilial) G24.2

Dystonic movements R25.8

Dystrophy, dystrophia
- adiposogenital E23.6
- Becker's type G71.0
- cervical sympathetic G90.2
- choroid (hereditary) H31.20
  - central areolar H31.22
  - choroideremia H31.21
  - gyrate atrophy H31.23
  - specified type NEC H31.29

Dystrophy, dystrophia — *continued*
- cornea (hereditary) H18.50
  - endothelial H18.51
  - epithelial H18.52
  - granular H18.53
  - lattice H18.54
  - macular H18.55
  - specified type NEC H18.59
- Duchenne's type G71.0
- due to malnutrition E45
- Erb's G71.0
- Fuchs' H18.51
- Gower's muscular G71.0
- hair L67.8
- infantile neuraxonal G31.89
- Landouzy-Déjérine G71.0
- Leyden-Möbius G71.0
- muscular G71.0
  - benign (Becker type) G71.0
  - congenital (hereditary) (progressive) (with specific morphological abnormalities of the muscle fiber) G71.0
    - myotonic G71.11
  - distal G71.0
  - Duchenne type G71.0
  - Emery-Dreifuss G71.0
  - Erb type G71.0
  - facioscapulohumeral G71.0
  - Gower's G71.0
  - hereditary (progressive) G71.0
  - Landouzy-Déjérine type G71.0
  - limb-girdle G71.0
  - myotonic G71.11
  - progressive (hereditary) G71.0
    - Charcot-Marie (-Tooth) type G60.0
  - pseudohypertrophic (infantile) G71.0
  - severe (Duchenne type) G71.0
- myocardium, myocardial — *see* Degeneration, myocardial
- nail L60.3
  - congenital Q84.6
- nutritional E45
- ocular G71.0
- oculocerebrorenal E72.03
- oculopharyngeal G71.0
- ovarian N83.8
- polyglandular E31.8
- reflex (neuromuscular) (sympathetic) — *see* Syndrome, pain, complex regional I
- retinal (hereditary) H35.50
  - in
    - lipid storage disorders E75.6 [H36]
    - systemic lipidoses E75.6 [H36]
  - involving
    - pigment epithelium H35.54
    - sensory area H35.53
  - pigmentary H35.52
  - vitreoretinal H35.51
- Salzmann's nodular — *see* Degeneration, cornea, nodular
- scapuloperoneal G71.0
- skin NEC L98.8
- sympathetic (reflex) — *see* Syndrome, pain, complex regional I
  - cervical G90.2
- tapetoretinal H35.54
- thoracic, asphyxiating Q77.2
- unguium L60.3
  - congenital Q84.6
- vitreoretinal H35.51
- vulva N90.4
- yellow (liver) — *see* Failure, hepatic

Dysuria R30.0
- psychogenic F45.8

E

Eales' disease H35.06- ☑

Ear (*see also* condition)
- piercing Z41.3
- tropical B36.8
- wax (impacted) H61.20
  - left H61.22
    - with right H61.23
  - right H61.21
    - with left H61.23

Earache — *see* subcategory H92.0 ☑

Early satiety R68.81

Eaton-Lambert syndrome — see Syndrome, Lambert-Eaton
Eberth's disease (typhoid fever) A01.00
Ebola virus disease A98.4
Ebstein's anomaly or syndrome (heart) Q22.5
Eccentro-osteochondrodysplasia E76.29
Ecchondroma — see Neoplasm, bone, benign
Ecchondrosis D48.0
Ecchymosis R58
　conjunctiva — see Hemorrhage, conjunctiva
　eye (traumatic) — see Contusion, eyeball
　eyelid (traumatic) — see Contusion, eyelid
　newborn P54.5
　spontaneous R23.3
　traumatic — see Contusion
Echinococciasis — see Echinococcus
Echinococcosis — see Echinococcus
Echinococcus (infection) B67.90
　granulosus B67.4
　　bone B67.2
　　liver B67.0
　　lung B67.1
　　multiple sites B67.32
　　specified site NEC B67.39
　　thyroid B67.31 [E35]
　liver NOS B67.8
　　granulosus B67.0
　　multilocularis B67.5
　lung NEC B67.99
　　granulosus B67.1
　　multilocularis B67.69
　multilocularis B67.7
　　liver B67.5
　　multiple sites B67.61
　　specified site NEC B67.69
　specified site NEC B67.99
　　granulosus B67.39
　　multilocularis B67.69
　thyroid NEC B67.99
　　granulosus B67.31 [E35]
　　multilocularis B67.69 [E35]
Echinorhynchiasis B83.8
Echinostomiasis B66.8
Echolalia R48.8
Echovirus, as cause of disease classified elsewhere B97.12
Eclampsia, eclamptic (coma) (convulsions) (delirium) (with hypertension) NEC O15.9
　during labor and delivery O15.1
　postpartum O15.2
　pregnancy O15.0- ☑
　puerperal O15.2
Economic circumstances affecting care Z59.9
Economo's disease A85.8
Ectasia, ectasis
　annuloaortic I35.8
　aorta I77.819
　　with aneurysm — see Aneurysm, aorta
　　abdominal I77.811
　　thoracic I77.810
　　thoracoabdominal I77.812
　breast — see Ectasia, mammary duct
　capillary I78.8
　cornea H18.71- ☑
　gastric antral vascular (GAVE) K31.819
　　with hemorrhage K31.811
　　without hemorrhage K31.819
　mammary duct N60.4- ☑
　salivary gland (duct) K11.8
　sclera — see Sclerectasia
Ecthyma L08.0
　contagiosum B08.02
　gangrenosum L08.0
　infectiosum B08.02
Ectocardia Q24.8
Ectodermal dysplasia (anhidrotic) Q82.4
Ectodermosis erosiva pluriorificialis L51.1
Ectopic, ectopia (congenital)
　abdominal viscera Q45.8
　　due to defect in anterior abdominal wall Q79.59
　ACTH syndrome E24.3
　adrenal gland Q89.1
　anus Q43.5
　atrial beats I49.1
　beats I49.49
　　atrial I49.1
　　ventricular I49.3

Ectopic, ectopia — continued
　bladder Q64.10
　bone and cartilage in lung Q33.5
　brain Q04.8
　breast tissue Q83.8
　cardiac Q24.8
　cerebral Q04.8
　cordis Q24.8
　endometrium — see Endometriosis
　gastric mucosa Q40.2
　gestation — see Pregnancy, by site
　heart Q24.8
　hormone secretion NEC E34.2
　kidney (crossed) (pelvis) Q63.2
　lens, lentis Q12.1
　mole — see Pregnancy, by site
　organ or site NEC — see Malposition, congenital
　pancreas Q45.3
　pregnancy — see Pregnancy, ectopic
　pupil — see Abnormality, pupillary
　renal Q63.2
　sebaceous glands of mouth Q38.6
　spleen Q89.09
　testis Q53.00
　　bilateral Q53.02
　　unilateral Q53.01
　thyroid Q89.2
　tissue in lung Q33.5
　ureter Q62.63
　ventricular beats I49.3
　vesicae Q64.10
Ectromelia Q73.8
　lower limb — see Defect, reduction, limb, lower, specified type NEC
　upper limb — see Defect, reduction, limb, upper, specified type NEC
Ectropion H02.109
　cervix N86
　　with cervicitis N72
　congenital Q10.1
　eyelid (paralytic) H02.109
　　cicatricial H02.119
　　　left H02.116
　　　　lower H02.115
　　　　upper H02.114
　　　right H02.113
　　　　lower H02.112
　　　　upper H02.111
　　congenital Q10.1
　　left H02.106
　　　lower H02.105
　　　upper H02.104
　　mechanical H02.129
　　　left H02.126
　　　　lower H02.125
　　　　upper H02.124
　　　right H02.123
　　　　lower H02.122
　　　　upper H02.121
　　right H02.103
　　　lower H02.102
　　　upper H02.101
　　senile H02.139
　　　left H02.136
　　　　lower H02.135
　　　　upper H02.134
　　　right H02.133
　　　　lower H02.132
　　　　upper H02.131
　　spastic H02.149
　　　left H02.146
　　　　lower H02.145
　　　　upper H02.144
　　　right H02.143
　　　　lower H02.142
　　　　upper H02.141
　iris H21.89
　lip (acquired) K13.0
　　congenital Q38.0
　urethra N36.8
　uvea H21.89
Eczema (acute) (chronic) (erythematous) (fissum) (rubrum) (squamous) (see also Dermatitis) L30.9
　contact — see Dermatitis, contact
　dyshydrotic L30.1
　external ear — see Otitis, externa, acute, eczematoid
　flexural L20.82
　herpeticum B00.0

Eczema — continued
　hypertrophicum L28.0
　hypostatic — see Varix, leg, with, inflammation
　impetiginous L01.1
　infantile (due to any substance) L20.83
　　intertriginous L21.1
　　seborrheic L21.1
　intertriginous NEC L30.4
　　infantile L21.1
　intrinsic (allergic) L20.84
　lichenified NEC L28.0
　marginatum (hebrae) B35.6
　pustular L30.3
　stasis — see Varix, leg, with, inflammation
　vaccination, vaccinatum T88.1 ☑
　varicose — see Varix, leg, with, inflammation
Eczematid L30.2
Eddowes (-Spurway) **syndrome** Q78.0
Edema, edematous (infectious) (pitting) (toxic) R60.9
　with nephritis — see Nephrosis
　allergic T78.3 ☑
　amputation stump (surgical) (sequelae (late effect)) T87.89
　angioneurotic (allergic) (any site) (with urticaria) T78.3 ☑
　　hereditary D84.1
　angiospastic I73.9
　Berlin's (traumatic) S05.8X- ☑
　brain (cytotoxic) (vasogenic) G93.6
　　due to birth injury P11.0
　　newborn (anoxia or hypoxia) P52.4
　　　birth injury P11.0
　　traumatic — see Injury, intracranial, cerebral edema
　cardiac — see Failure, heart, congestive
　cardiovascular — see Failure, heart, congestive
　cerebral — see Edema, brain
　cerebrospinal — see Edema, brain
　cervix (uteri) (acute) N88.8
　　puerperal, postpartum O90.89
　chronic hereditary Q82.0
　circumscribed, acute T78.3 ☑
　　hereditary D84.1
　conjunctiva H11.42- ☑
　cornea H18.2- ☑
　　idiopathic H18.22- ☑
　　secondary H18.23- ☑
　　　due to contact lens H18.21- ☑
　due to
　　lymphatic obstruction I89.0
　　salt retention E87.0
　epiglottis — see Edema, glottis
　essential, acute T78.3 ☑
　　hereditary D84.1
　extremities, lower — see Edema, legs
　eyelid NEC H02.849
　　left H02.846
　　　lower H02.845
　　　upper H02.844
　　right H02.843
　　　lower H02.842
　　　upper H02.841
　familial, hereditary Q82.0
　famine — see Malnutrition, severe
　generalized R60.1
　glottis, glottic, glottidis (obstructive) (passive) J38.4
　　allergic T78.3 ☑
　　hereditary D84.1
　heart — see Failure, heart, congestive
　heat T67.7 ☑
　hereditary Q82.0
　inanition — see Malnutrition, severe
　intracranial G93.6
　iris H21.89
　joint — see Effusion, joint
　larynx — see Edema, glottis
　legs R60.0
　　due to venous obstruction I87.1
　　hereditary Q82.0
　localized R60.0
　　due to venous obstruction I87.1
　lower limbs — see Edema, legs
　lung J81.1
　　with heart condition or failure — see Failure, ventricular, left
　　acute J81.0
　　chemical (acute) J68.1
　　　chronic J68.1

Index

Edema, edematous — Elastic skin

Edema, edematous — *continued*
  lung — *continued*
    chronic J81.1
      due to
        chemicals, gases, fumes or vapors (inhalation) J68.1
        external agent J70.9
          specified NEC J70.8
        radiation J70.1
    due to
      chemicals, fumes or vapors (inhalation) J68.1
      external agent J70.9
        specified NEC J70.8
      high altitude T70.29 ☑
      near drowning T75.1 ☑
      radiation J70.0
    meaning failure, left ventricle I50.1
  lymphatic I89.0
    due to mastectomy I97.2
  macula H35.81
    cystoid, following cataract surgery — *see* Complications, postprocedural, following cataract surgery
    diabetic — *see* Diabetes, by type, with, retinopathy, with macular edema
  malignant — *see* Gangrene, gas
  Milroy's Q82.0
  nasopharynx J39.2
  newborn P83.30
    hydrops fetalis — *see* Hydrops, fetalis
    specified NEC P83.39
  nutritional (*see also* Malnutrition, severe)
    with dyspigmentation, skin and hair E40
  optic disc or nerve — *see* Papilledema
  orbit H05.22- ☑
  pancreas K86.8
  papilla, optic — *see* Papilledema
  penis N48.89
  periodic T78.3 ☑
    hereditary D84.1
  pharynx J39.2
  pulmonary — *see* Edema, lung
  Quincke's T78.3 ☑
    hereditary D84.1
  renal — *see* Nephrosis
  retina H35.81
    diabetic — *see* Diabetes, by type, with, retinopathy, with macular edema
  salt E87.0
  scrotum N50.8
  seminal vesicle N50.8
  spermatic cord N50.8
  spinal (cord) (vascular) (nontraumatic) G95.19
  starvation — *see* Malnutrition, severe
  stasis — *see* Hypertension, venous, (chronic)
  subglottic — *see* Edema, glottis
  supraglottic — *see* Edema, glottis
  testis N44.8
  tunica vaginalis N50.8
  vas deferens N50.8
  vulva (acute) N90.89
Edentulism — *see* Absence, teeth, acquired
Edsall's disease T67.2 ☑
Educational handicap Z55.9
  specified NEC Z55.8
Edward's syndrome — *see* Trisomy, 18
Effect(s) (of) (from) — *see* Effect, adverse NEC
Effect, adverse
  abnormal gravitational (G) forces or states T75.81 ☑
  abuse — *see* Maltreatment
  air pressure T70.9 ☑
    specified NEC T70.8 ☑
  altitude (high) — *see* Effect, adverse, high altitude
  anesthesia (*see also* Anesthesia) T88.59 ☑
    in labor and delivery O74.9
    in pregnancy NEC O29.3- ☑
    local, toxic
      in labor and delivery O74.4
      postpartum, puerperal O89.3
    postpartum, puerperal O89.9
    specified NEC T88.59 ☑
      in labor and delivery O74.8
      postpartum, puerperal O89.8
    spinal and epidural T88.59 ☑
      headache T88.59 ☑
        in labor and delivery O74.5
        postpartum, puerperal O89.4

Effect, adverse — *continued*
  anesthesia (*see also* Anesthesia) — *continued*
    spinal and epidural — *continued*
      specified NEC
        in labor and delivery O74.6
        postpartum, puerperal O89.5
  antitoxin — *see* Complications, vaccination
  atmospheric pressure T70.9 ☑
    due to explosion T70.8 ☑
    high T70.3 ☑
    low — *see* Effect, adverse, high altitude
    specified effect NEC T70.8 ☑
  biological, correct substance properly administered — *see* Effect, adverse, drug
  blood (derivatives) (serum) (transfusion) — *see* Complications, transfusion
  chemical substance — *see* Table of Drugs and Chemicals
  cold (temperature) (weather) T69.9 ☑
    chilblains T69.1 ☑
    frostbite — *see* Frostbite
    specified effect NEC T69.8 ☑
  drugs and medicaments T88.7 ☑
    specified drug — *see* Table of Drugs and Chemicals, by drug, adverse effect
    specified effect — *code to* condition
  electric current, electricity (shock) T75.4 ☑
    burn — *see* Burn
  exertion (excessive) T73.3 ☑
  exposure — *see* Exposure
  external cause NEC T75.89 ☑
  foodstuffs T78.1 ☑
    allergic reaction — *see* Allergy, food
      causing anaphylaxis — *see* Shock, anaphylactic, due to food
    noxious — *see* Poisoning, food, noxious
  gases, fumes, or vapors T59.9- ☑
    specified agent — *see* Table of Drugs and Chemicals
  glue (airplane) sniffing
    due to drug abuse — *see* Abuse, drug, inhalant
    due to drug dependence — *see* Dependence, drug, inhalant
  heat — *see* Heat
  high altitude NEC T70.29 ☑
    anoxia T70.29 ☑
    on
      ears T70.0 ☑
      sinuses T70.1 ☑
    polycythemia D75.1
  high pressure fluids T70.4 ☑
  hot weather — *see* Heat
  hunger T73.0 ☑
  immersion, foot — *see* Immersion
  immunization — *see* Complications, vaccination
  immunological agents — *see* Complications, vaccination
  infrared (radiation) (rays) NOS T66 ☑
    dermatitis or eczema L59.8
  infusion — *see* Complications, infusion
  lack of care of infants — *see* Maltreatment, child
  lightning — *see* Lightning
  medical care T88.9 ☑
    specified NEC T88.8 ☑
  medicinal substance, correct, properly administered — *see* Effect, adverse, drug
  motion T75.3 ☑
  noise, on inner ear — *see* subcategory H83.3 ☑
  overheated places — *see* Heat
  psychosocial, of work environment Z56.5
  radiation (diagnostic) (infrared) (natural source) (therapeutic) (ultraviolet) (X-ray) NOS T66 ☑
    dermatitis or eczema — *see* Dermatitis, due to, radiation
    fibrosis of lung J70.1
    pneumonitis J70.0
    pulmonary manifestations
      acute J70.0
      chronic J70.1
    skin L59.9
  radioactive substance NOS
    dermatitis or eczema — *see* Radiodermatitis
  reduced temperature T69.9 ☑
    immersion foot or hand — *see* Immersion
    specified effect NEC T69.8 ☑
  serum NEC (*see also* Reaction, serum) T80.69 ☑

Effect, adverse — *continued*
  specified NEC T78.8 ☑
    external cause NEC T75.89 ☑
  strangulation — *see* Asphyxia, traumatic
  submersion T75.1 ☑
  thirst T73.1 ☑
  toxic — *see* Toxicity
  transfusion — *see* Complications, transfusion
  ultraviolet (radiation) (rays) NOS T66 ☑
    burn — *see* Burn
    dermatitis or eczema — *see* Dermatitis, due to, ultraviolet rays
      acute L56.8
  vaccine (any) — *see* Complications, vaccination
  vibration — *see* Vibration, adverse effects
  water pressure NEC T70.9 ☑
    specified NEC T70.8 ☑
  weightlessness T75.82 ☑
  whole blood — *see* Complications, transfusion
  work environment Z56.5
Effects, late — *see* Sequelae
Effluvium
  anagen L65.1
  telogen L65.0
Effort syndrome (psychogenic) F45.8
Effusion
  amniotic fluid — *see* Pregnancy, complicated by, premature rupture of membranes
  brain (serous) G93.6
  bronchial — *see* Bronchitis
  cerebral G93.6
  cerebrospinal (*see also* Meningitis)
    vessel G93.6
  chest — *see* Effusion, pleura
  chylous, chyliform (pleura) J94.0
  intracranial G93.6
  joint M25.40
    ankle M25.47- ☑
    elbow M25.42- ☑
    foot joint M25.47- ☑
    hand joint M25.44- ☑
    hip M25.45- ☑
    knee M25.46- ☑
    shoulder M25.41- ☑
    specified joint NEC M25.48
    wrist M25.43- ☑
  malignant pleural J91.0
  meninges — *see* Meningitis
  pericardium, pericardial (noninflammatory) I31.3
    acute — *see* Pericarditis, acute
  peritoneal (chronic) R18.8
  pleura, pleurisy, pleuritic, pleuropericardial J90
    chylous, chyliform J94.0
    due to systemic lupus erythematosis M32.13
    influenzal — *see* Influenza, with, respiratory manifestations NEC
    malignant J91.0
    newborn P28.89
    tuberculous NEC A15.6
      primary (progressive) A15.7
  spinal — *see* Meningitis
  thorax, thoracic — *see* Effusion, pleura
Egg shell nails L60.3
  congenital Q84.6
Egyptian splenomegaly B65.1
Ehlers-Danlos syndrome Q79.6
Ehrlichiosis A77.40
  due to
    E. chafeensis A77.41
    E. sennetsu A79.81
    specified organism NEC A77.49
Eichstedt's disease B36.0
Eisenmenger's
  complex or syndrome I27.89
  defect Q21.8
Ejaculation
  painful N53.12
  premature F52.4
  retarded N53.11
  retrograde N53.14
  semen, painful N53.12
    psychogenic F52.6
Ekbom's syndrome (restless legs) G25.81
Ekman's syndrome (brittle bones and blue sclera) Q78.0
Elastic skin Q82.8
  acquired L57.4

Elastofibroma — *see* Neoplasm, connective tissue, benign

Elastoma (juvenile) Q82.8

    Miescher's L87.2

Elastomyofibrosis I42.4

Elastosis

    actinic, solar L57.8

    atrophicans (senile) L57.4

    perforans serpiginosa L87.2

    senilis L57.4

Elbow — *see* condition

Electric current, electricity, effects (concussion) (fatal) (nonfatal) (shock) T75.4 ☑

    burn — *see* Burn

Electric feet syndrome E53.8

Electrocution T75.4 ☑

    from electroshock gun (taser) T75.4 ☑

Electrolyte imbalance E87.8

    with

        abortion — *see* Abortion by type, complicated by, electrolyte imbalance

        ectopic pregnancy O08.5

        molar pregnancy O08.5

Elephantiasis (nonfilarial) I89.0

    arabicum — *see* Infestation, filarial

    bancroftian B74.0

    congenital (any site) (hereditary) Q82.0

    due to

        Brugia (malayi) B74.1

            timori B74.2

        mastectomy I97.2

        Wuchereria (bancrofti) B74.0

    eyelid H02.859

        left H02.856

            lower H02.855

            upper H02.854

        right H02.853

            lower H02.852

            upper H02.851

    filarial, filariensis — *see* Infestation, filarial

    glandular I89.0

    graecorum A30.9

    lymphangiectatic I89.0

    lymphatic vessel I89.0

        due to mastectomy I97.2

    scrotum (nonfilarial) I89.0

    streptococcal I89.0

    surgical I97.89

        postmastectomy I97.2

    telangiectodes I89.0

    vulva (nonfilarial) N90.89

Elevated, elevation

    antibody titer R76.0

    basal metabolic rate R94.8

    blood pressure (*see also* Hypertension)

        reading (incidental) (isolated) (nonspecific), no diagnosis of hypertension R03.0

    blood sugar R73.9

    body temperature (of unknown origin) R50.9

    cancer antigen 125 [CA 125] R97.1

    carcinoembryonic antigen [CEA] R97.0

    cholesterol E78.0

        with high triglycerides E78.2

    conjugate, eye H51.0

    C-reactive protein (CRP) R79.82

    diaphragm, congenital Q79.1

    erythrocyte sedimentation rate R70.0

    fasting glucose R73.01

    fasting triglycerides E78.1

    finding on laboratory examination — *see* Findings, abnormal, inconclusive, without diagnosis, by type of exam

    GFR (glomerular filtration rate) — *see* Findings, abnormal, inconclusive, without diagnosis, by type of exam

    glucose tolerance (oral) R73.02

    immunoglobulin level R76.8

    indoleacetic acid R82.5

    lactic acid dehydrogenase (LDH) level R74.0

    leukocytes D72.829

    lipoprotein a level E78.8 ☑

    liver function

        study R94.5

        test R79.89

            alkaline phosphatase R74.8

            aminotransferase R74.0

            bilirubin R17

            hepatic enzyme R74.8

Elevated, elevation — *continued*

    liver function — *continued*

        test — *continued*

            lactate dehydrogenase R74.0

    lymphocytes D72.820

    prostate specific antigen [PSA] R97.2

    Rh titer — *see* Complication(s), transfusion, incompatibility reaction, Rh (factor)

    scapula, congenital Q74.0

    sedimentation rate R70.0

    SGOT R74.0

    SGPT R74.0

    transaminase level R74.0

    triglycerides E78.1

        with high cholesterol E78.2

    tumor associated antigens [TAA] NEC R97.8

    tumor specific antigens [TSA] NEC R97.8

    urine level of

        17-ketosteroids R82.5

        catecholamine R82.5

        indoleacetic acid R82.5

        steroids R82.5

        vanillylmandelic acid (VMA) R82.5

    venous pressure I87.8

    white blood cell count D72.829

        specified NEC D72.828

Elliptocytosis (congenital) (hereditary) D58.1

    Hb C (disease) D58.1

    hemoglobin disease D58.1

    sickle-cell (disease) D57.8- ☑

        trait D57.3

Ellison-Zollinger syndrome E16.4

Ellis-van Creveld syndrome (chondroectodermal dysplasia) Q77.6

Elongated, elongation (congenital) (*see also* Distortion)

    bone Q79.9

    cervix (uteri) Q51.828

        acquired N88.4

        hypertrophic N88.4

    colon Q43.8

    common bile duct Q44.5

    cystic duct Q44.5

    frenulum, penis Q55.69

    labia minora (acquired) N90.6

    ligamentum patellae Q74.1

    petiolus (epiglottidis) Q31.8

    tooth, teeth K00.2

    uvula Q38.6

Eltor cholera A00.1

Emaciation (due to malnutrition) E41

Embadomoniasis A07.8

Embedded tooth, teeth K01.0

    root only K08.3

Embolic — *see* condition

Embolism (multiple) (paradoxical) I74.9

    air (any site) (traumatic) T79.0 ☑

        following

            abortion — *see* Abortion by type complicated by embolism

            ectopic pregnancy O08.2

            infusion, therapeutic injection or transfusion T80.0 ☑

            molar pregnancy O08.2

            procedure NEC

                artery T81.719 ☑

                    mesenteric T81.710 ☑

                    renal T81.711 ☑

                    specified NEC T81.718 ☑

                vein T81.72 ☑

        in pregnancy, childbirth or puerperium — *see* Embolism, obstetric

    amniotic fluid (pulmonary) (*see also* Embolism, obstetric)

        following

            abortion — *see* Abortion by type complicated by embolism

            ectopic pregnancy O08.2

            molar pregnancy O08.2

    aorta, aortic I74.10

        abdominal I74.09

            saddle I74.01

        bifurcation I74.09

        saddle I74.01

        thoracic I74.11

    artery I74.9

        auditory, internal I65.8

        basilar — *see* Occlusion, artery, basilar

Embolism — *continued*

    artery — *continued*

        carotid (common) (internal) — *see* Occlusion, artery, carotid

        cerebellar (anterior inferior) (posterior inferior) (superior) I66.3

        cerebral — *see* Occlusion, artery, cerebral

        choroidal (anterior) I66.8

        communicating posterior I66.8

        coronary (*see also* Infarct, myocardium)

            not resulting in infarction I24.0

        extremity I74.4

            lower I74.3

            upper I74.2

        hypophyseal I66.8

        iliac I74.5

        limb I74.4

            lower I74.3

            upper I74.2

        mesenteric (with gangrene) K55.0

        ophthalmic — *see* Occlusion, artery, retina

        peripheral I74.4

        pontine I66.8

        precerebral — *see* Occlusion, artery, precerebral

        pulmonary — *see* Embolism, pulmonary

        renal N28.0

        retinal — *see* Occlusion, artery, retina

        septic I76

        specified NEC I74.8

        vertebral — *see* Occlusion, artery, vertebral

    basilar (artery) I65.1

    blood clot

        following

            abortion — *see* Abortion by type complicated by embolism

            ectopic or molar pregnancy O08.2

        in pregnancy, childbirth or puerperium — *see* Embolism, obstetric

    brain (*see also* Occlusion, artery, cerebral)

        following

            abortion — *see* Abortion by type complicated by embolism

            ectopic or molar pregnancy O08.2

        puerperal, postpartum, childbirth — *see* Embolism, obstetric

    capillary I78.8

    cardiac (*see also* Infarct, myocardium)

        not resulting in infarction I24.0

    carotid (artery) (common) (internal) — *see* Occlusion, artery, carotid

    cavernous sinus (venous) — *see* Embolism, intracranial venous sinus

    cerebral — *see* Occlusion, artery, cerebral

    cholesterol — *see* Atheroembolism

    coronary (artery or vein) (systemic) — *see* Occlusion, coronary

    due to device, implant or graft (*see also* Complications, by site and type, specified NEC)

        arterial graft NEC T82.818 ☑

        breast (implant) T85.81 ☑

        catheter NEC T85.81 ☑

            dialysis (renal) T82.818 ☑

                intraperitoneal T85.81 ☑

            infusion NEC T82.818 ☑

                spinal (epidural) (subdural) T85.81 ☑

            urinary (indwelling) T83.81 ☑

        electronic (electrode) (pulse generator) (stimulator)

            bone T84.81 ☑

            cardiac T82.817 ☑

            nervous system (brain) (peripheral nerve) (spinal) T85.81 ☑

            urinary T83.81 ☑

        fixation, internal (orthopedic) NEC T84.81 ☑

        gastrointestinal (bile duct) (esophagus) T85.81 ☑

        genital NEC T83.81 ☑

        heart (graft) (valve) T82.817 ☑

        joint prosthesis T84.81 ☑

        ocular (corneal graft) (orbital implant) T85.81 ☑

        orthopedic (bone graft) NEC T86.838

        specified NEC T85.81 ☑

        urinary (graft) NEC T83.81 ☑

        vascular NEC T82.818 ☑

        ventricular intracranial shunt T85.81 ☑

    extremities

        lower — *see* Embolism, vein, lower extremity

            arterial I74.3

        upper I74.2

Embolism — continued
eye H34.9
fat (cerebral) (pulmonary) (systemic) T79.1 ☑
    complicating delivery — see Embolism, obstetric
    following
        abortion — see Abortion by type complicated
            by embolism
        ectopic or molar pregnancy O08.2
following
    abortion — see Abortion by type complicated by
        embolism
    ectopic or molar pregnancy O08.2
    infusion, therapeutic injection or transfusion
        air T80.0 ☑
heart (fatty) (see also Infarct, myocardium)
    not resulting in infarction I24.0
hepatic (vein) I82.0
in pregnancy, childbirth or puerperium — see Embolism, obstetric
intestine (artery) (vein) (with gangrene) K55.0
intracranial (see also Occlusion, artery, cerebral)
    venous sinus (any) G08
    nonpyogenic I67.6
intraspinal venous sinuses or veins G08
    nonpyogenic G95.19
kidney (artery) N28.0
lateral sinus (venous) — see Embolism, intracranial,
    venous sinus
leg — see Embolism, vein, lower extremity
    arterial I74.3
longitudinal sinus (venous) — see Embolism, intracranial, venous sinus
lung (massive) — see Embolism, pulmonary
meninges I66.8
mesenteric (artery) (vein) (with gangrene) K55.0
obstetric (in) (pulmonary)
    childbirth O88.82
        air O88.02
        amniotic fluid O88.12
        blood clot O88.22
        fat O88.82
        pyemic O88.32
        septic O88.32
        specified type NEC O88.82
    pregnancy O88.81- ☑
        air O88.01- ☑
        amniotic fluid O88.11- ☑
        blood clot O88.21- ☑
        fat O88.81- ☑
        pyemic O88.31- ☑
        septic O88.31- ☑
        specified type NEC O88.81- ☑
    puerperal O88.83
        air O88.03
        amniotic fluid O88.13
        blood clot O88.23
        fat O88.83
        pyemic O88.33
        septic O88.33
        specified type NEC O88.83
ophthalmic — see Occlusion, artery, retina
penis N48.81
peripheral artery NOS I74.4
pituitary E23.6
popliteal (artery) I74.3
portal (vein) I81
postoperative, postprocedural
    artery T81.719 ☑
        mesenteric T81.710 ☑
        renal T81.711 ☑
        specified NEC T81.718 ☑
    vein T81.72 ☑
precerebral artery — see Occlusion, artery, precerebral
puerperal — see Embolism, obstetric
pulmonary (acute) (artery) (vein) I26.99
    with acute cor pulmonale I26.09
    chronic I27.82
    following
        abortion — see Abortion by type complicated
            by embolism
        ectopic or molar pregnancy O08.2
    healed or old Z86.711
    in pregnancy, childbirth or puerperium — see
        Embolism, obstetric
    personal history of Z86.711
    saddle I26.92
        with acute cor pulmonale I26.02

Embolism — continued
pulmonary — continued
    septic I26.90
        with acute cor pulmonale I26.01
pyemic (multiple) I76
    following
        abortion — see Abortion by type complicated
            by embolism
        ectopic or molar pregnancy O08.2
    Hemophilus influenzae A41.3
    pneumococcal A40.3
        with pneumonia J13
    puerperal, postpartum, childbirth (any organism)
        — see Embolism, obstetric
    specified organism NEC A41.89
    staphylococcal A41.2
    streptococcal A40.9
renal (artery) N28.0
    vein I82.3
retina, retinal — see Occlusion, artery, retina
saddle
    abdominal aorta I74.01
    pulmonary artery I26.92
        with acute cor pulmonale I26.02
septic (arterial) I76
    complicating abortion — see Abortion, by type,
        complicated by, embolism
sinus — see Embolism, intracranial, venous sinus
soap complicating abortion — see Abortion, by type,
    complicated by, embolism
spinal cord G95.19
    pyogenic origin G06.1
spleen, splenic (artery) I74.8
upper extremity I74.2
vein (acute) I82.90
    antecubital I82.61- ☑
        chronic I82.71- ☑
    axillary I82.A1- ☑ (following I82.7)
        chronic I82.A2- ☑ (following I82.7)
    basilic I82.61- ☑
        chronic I82.71- ☑
    brachial I82.62- ☑
        chronic I82.72- ☑
    brachiocephalic (innominate) I82.290
        chronic I82.291
    cephalic I82.61- ☑
        chronic I82.71- ☑
    chronic I82.91
    deep (DVT) I82.40- ☑
        calf I82.4Z- ☑
            chronic I82.5Z- ☑
        lower leg I82.4Z- ☑
            chronic I82.5Z- ☑
        thigh I82.4Y- ☑
            chronic I82.5Y- ☑
        upper leg I82.4Y ☑
            chronic I82.5Y-
    femoral I82.41- ☑
        chronic I82.51- ☑
    iliac (iliofemoral) I82.42- ☑
        chronic I82.52- ☑
    innominate I82.290
        chronic I82.291
    internal jugular I82.C1- ☑ (following I82.7)
        chronic I82.C2- ☑ (following I82.7)
    lower extremity
        deep I82.40- ☑
            chronic I82.50- ☑
            specified NEC I82.49- ☑
                chronic NEC I82.59- ☑
        distal
            deep I82.4Z- ☑
        proximal
            deep I82.4Y- ☑
                chronic I82.5Y- ☑
        superficial I82.81- ☑
    popliteal I82.43- ☑
        chronic I82.53- ☑
    radial I82.62- ☑
        chronic I82.72- ☑
    renal I82.3
    saphenous (greater) (lesser) I82.81- ☑
    specified NEC I82.890
        chronic NEC I82.891
    subclavian I82.B1- ☑ (following I82.7)
        chronic I82.B2- ☑ (following I82.7)
    thoracic NEC I82.290

Embolism — continued
vein — continued
    thoracic — continued
        chronic I82.291
        tibial I82.44- ☑
            chronic I82.54- ☑
        ulnar I82.62- ☑
            chronic I82.72- ☑
        upper extremity I82.60- ☑
            chronic I82.70- ☑
            deep I82.62- ☑
                chronic I82.72- ☑
            superficial I82.61- ☑
                chronic I82.71- ☑
    vena cava
        inferior (acute) I82.220
            chronic I82.221
        superior (acute) I82.210
            chronic I82.211
    venous sinus G08
    vessels of brain — see Occlusion, artery, cerebral
Embolus — see Embolism
Embryoma (see also Neoplasm, uncertain behavior, by
    site)
    benign — see Neoplasm, benign, by site
    kidney C64.- ☑
    liver C22.0
    malignant (see also Neoplasm, malignant, by site)
        kidney C64.- ☑
        liver C22.0
        testis C62.9- ☑
            descended (scrotal) C62.1- ☑
            undescended C62.0- ☑
    testis C62.9- ☑
        descended (scrotal) C62.1- ☑
        undescended C62.0- ☑
Embryonic
    circulation Q28.9
    heart Q28.9
    vas deferens Q55.4
Embryopathia NOS Q89.9
Embryotoxon Q13.4
Emesis — see Vomiting
Emotional lability R45.86
Emotionality, pathological F60.3
Emotogenic disease — see Disorder, psychogenic
Emphysema (atrophic) (bullous) (chronic) (interlobular)
    (lung) (obstructive) (pulmonary) (senile) (vesicular)
    J43.9
    cellular tissue (traumatic) T79.7 ☑
        surgical T81.82 ☑
    centrilobular J43.2
    compensatory J98.3
    congenital (interstitial) P25.0
    conjunctiva H11.89
    connective tissue (traumatic) T79.7 ☑
        surgical T81.82 ☑
    due to chemicals, gases, fumes or vapors J68.4
    eyelid(s) — see Disorder, eyelid, specified type NEC
        surgical T81.82 ☑
        traumatic T79.7 ☑
    interstitial J98.2
        congenital P25.0
        perinatal period P25.0
    laminated tissue T79.7 ☑
        surgical T81.82 ☑
    mediastinal J98.2
        newborn P25.2
    orbit, orbital — see Disorder, orbit, specified type NEC
    panacinar J43.1
    panlobular J43.1
    specified NEC J43.8
    subcutaneous (traumatic) T79.7 ☑
        nontraumatic J98.2
        postprocedural T81.82 ☑
        surgical T81.82 ☑
    surgical T81.82 ☑
    thymus (gland) (congenital) E32.8
    traumatic (subcutaneous) T79.7 ☑
    unilateral J43.0
Empty nest syndrome Z60.0
Empyema (acute) (chest) (double) (pleura) (supradi-
    aphragmatic) (thorax) J86.9
    with fistula J86.0
    accessory sinus (chronic) — see Sinusitis
    antrum (chronic) — see Sinusitis, maxillary
    brain (any part) — see Abscess, brain

Empyema — *continued*
ethmoidal (chronic) (sinus) — *see* Sinusitis, ethmoidal
extradural — *see* Abscess, extradural
frontal (chronic) (sinus) — *see* Sinusitis, frontal
gallbladder K81.0
mastoid (process) (acute) — *see* Mastoiditis, acute
maxilla, maxillary M27.2
sinus (chronic) — *see* Sinusitis, maxillary
nasal sinus (chronic) — *see* Sinusitis
sinus (accessory) (chronic) (nasal) — *see* Sinusitis
sphenoidal (sinus) (chronic) — *see* Sinusitis, sphenoidal
subarachnoid — *see* Abscess, extradural
subdural — *see* Abscess, subdural
tuberculous A15.6
ureter — *see* Ureteritis
ventricular — *see* Abscess, brain
En coup de sabre lesion L94.1
Enamel pearls K00.2
Enameloma K00.2
Enanthema, viral B09
Encephalitis (chronic) (hemorrhagic) (idiopathic) (nonepidemic) (spurious) (subacute) G04.90
acute (*see also* Encephalitis, viral) A86
disseminated G04.00
infectious G04.01
noninfectious G04.81
postimmunization (postvaccination) G04.02
postinfectious G04.01
inclusion body A85.8
necrotizing hemorrhagic G04.30
postimmunization G04.32
postinfectious G04.31
specified NEC G04.39
arboviral, arbovirus NEC A85.2
arthropod-borne NEC (viral) A85.2
Australian A83.4
California (virus) A83.5
Central European (tick-borne) A84.1
Czechoslovakian A84.1
Dawson's (inclusion body) A81.1
diffuse sclerosing A81.1
disseminated, acute G04.00
due to
cat scratch disease A28.1
human immunodeficiency virus (HIV) disease B20 [G05.3]
malaria — *see* Malaria
rickettsiosis — *see* Rickettsiosis
smallpox inoculation G04.02
typhus — *see* Typhus
Eastern equine A83.2
endemic (viral) A86
epidemic NEC (viral) A86
equine (acute) (infectious) (viral) A83.9
Eastern A83.2
Venezuelan A92.2
Western A83.1
Far Eastern (tick-borne) A84.0
following vaccination or other immunization procedure G04.02
herpes zoster B02.0
herpesviral B00.4
due to herpesvirus 6 B10.01
due to herpesvirus 7 B10.09
specified NEC B10.09
Ilheus (virus) A83.8
in (due to)
actinomycosis A42.82
adenovirus A85.1
African trypanosomiasis B56.9 [G05.3]
Chagas' disease (chronic) B57.42
cytomegalovirus B25.8
enterovirus A85.0
herpes (simplex) virus B00.4
due to herpesvirus 6 B10.01
due to herpesvirus 7 B10.09
specified NEC B10.09
infectious disease NEC B99 ☑ [G05.3]
influenza — *see* Influenza, with, encephalopathy
listeriosis A32.12
measles B05.0
mumps B26.2
naegleriasis B60.2
parasitic disease NEC B89 [G05.3]
poliovirus A80.9 [G05.3]
rubella B06.01

Encephalitis — *continued*
in — *continued*
syphilis
congenital A50.42
late A52.14
systemic lupus erythematosus M32.19
toxoplasmosis (acquired) B58.2
congenital P37.1
tuberculosis A17.82
zoster B02.0
inclusion body A81.1
infectious (acute) (virus) NEC A86
Japanese (B type) A83.0
La Crosse A83.5
lead — *see* Poisoning, lead
lethargica (acute) (infectious) A85.8
louping ill A84.8
lupus erythematosus, systemic M32.19
lymphatica A87.2
Mengo A85.8
meningococcal A39.81
Murray Valley A83.4
otitic NEC H66.40 [G05.3]
parasitic NOS B71.9
periaxial G37.0
periaxialis (concentrica) (diffuse) G37.5
postchickenpox B01.11
postexanthematous NEC B09
postimmunization G04.02
postinfectious NEC G04.01
postmeasles B05.0
postvaccinal G04.02
postvaricella B01.11
postviral NEC A86
Powassan A84.8
Rasmussen G04.81
Rio Bravo A85.8
Russian
autumnal A83.0
spring-summer (taiga) A84.0
saturnine — *see* Poisoning, lead
specified NEC G04.81
St. Louis A83.3
subacute sclerosing A81.1
summer A83.0
suppurative G04.81
tick-borne A84.9
Torula, torular (cryptococcal) B45.1
toxic NEC G92
trichinosis B75 [G05.3]
type
B A83.0
C A83.3
van Bogaert's A81.1
Venezuelan equine A92.2
Vienna A85.8
viral, virus A86
arthropod-borne NEC A85.2
mosquito-borne A83.9
Australian X disease A83.4
California virus A83.5
Eastern equine A83.2
Japanese (B type) A83.0
Murray Valley A83.4
specified NEC A83.8
St. Louis A83.3
type B A83.0
type C A83.3
Western equine A83.1
tick-borne A84.9
biundulant A84.1
central European A84.1
Czechoslovakian A84.1
diphasic meningoencephalitis A84.1
Far Eastern A84.0
Russian spring-summer (taiga) A84.0
specified NEC A84.8
specified type NEC A85.8
Western equine A83.1
Encephalocele Q01.9
frontal Q01.0
nasofrontal Q01.1
occipital Q01.2
specified NEC Q01.8
Encephalocystocele — *see* Encephalocele
Encephaloduroarteriomyosynangiosis (EDAMS) I67.5
Encephalomalacia (brain) (cerebellar) (cerebral) — *see* Softening, brain

Encephalomeningitis — *see* Meningoencephalitis
Encephalomeningocele — *see* Encephalocele
Encephalomeningomyelitis — *see* Meningoencephalitis
Encephalomyelitis (*see also* Encephalitis) G04.90
acute disseminated G04.00
infectious G04.01
noninfectious G04.81
postimmunization G04.02
postinfectious G04.01
acute necrotizing hemorrhagic G04.30
postimmunization G04.32
postinfectious G04.31
specified NEC G04.39
benign myalgic G93.3
equine A83.9
Eastern A83.2
Venezuelan A92.2
Western A83.1
in diseases classified elsewhere G05.3
myalgic, benign G93.3
postchickenpox B01.11
postinfectious NEC G04.01
postmeasles B05.0
postvaccinal G04.02
postvaricella B01.11
rubella B06.01
specified NEC G04.81
Venezuelan equine A92.2
Encephalomyelocele — *see* Encephalocele
Encephalomyelomeningitis — *see* Meningoencephalitis
Encephalomyelopathy G96.9
Encephalomyeloradiculitis (acute) G61.0
Encephalomyeloradiculoneuritis (acute) (Guillain-Barré) G61.0
Encephalomyeloradiculopathy G96.9
Encephalopathia hyperbilirubinemica, newborn P57.9
due to isoimmunization (conditions in P55) P57.0
Encephalopathy (acute) G93.40
acute necrotizing hemorrhagic G04.30
postimmunization G04.32
postinfectious G04.31
specified NEC G04.39
alcoholic G31.2
anoxic — *see* Damage, brain, anoxic
arteriosclerotic I67.2
centrolobar progressive (Schilder) G37.0
congenital Q07.9
degenerative, in specified disease NEC G32.89
demyelinating callosal G37.1
due to
drugs (*see also* Table of Drugs and Chemicals) G92
hepatic — *see* Failure, hepatic
hyperbilirubinemic, newborn P57.9
due to isoimmunization (conditions in P55) P57.0
hypertensive I67.4
hypoglycemic E16.2
hypoxic — *see* Damage, brain, anoxic
hypoxic ischemic P91.60
mild P91.61
moderate P91.62
severe P91.63
in (due to) (with)
birth injury P11.1
hyperinsulinism E16.1 [G94]
influenza — *see* Influenza, with, encephalopathy
lack of vitamin (*see also* Deficiency, vitamin) E56.9 [G32.89]
neoplastic disease (*see also* Neoplasm) D49.9 [G13.1]
serum (*see also* Reaction, serum) T80.69 ☑
syphilis A52.17
trauma (postconcussional) F07.81
current injury — *see* Injury, intracranial
vaccination G04.02
lead — *see* Poisoning, lead
metabolic G93.41
drug induced G92
toxic G92
myoclonic, early, symptomatic — *see* Epilepsy, generalized, specified NEC
necrotizing, subacute (Leigh) G31.82
pellagrous E52 [G32.89]
portosystemic — *see* Failure, hepatic
postcontusional F07.81
current injury — *see* Injury, intracranial, diffuse

Encephalopathy — continued
  posthypoglycemic (coma) E16.1 [G94]
  postradiation G93.89
  saturnine — see Poisoning, lead
  septic G93.41
  specified NEC G93.49
  spongiform, subacute (viral) A81.09
  toxic G92
    metabolic G92
  traumatic (postconcussional) F07.81
    current injury — see Injury, intracranial
  vitamin B deficiency NEC E53.9 [G32.89]
    vitamin B1 E51.2
  Wernicke's E51.2
Encephalorrhagia — see Hemorrhage, intracranial, intracerebral
Encephalosis, posttraumatic F07.81
Enchondroma (see also Neoplasm, bone, benign)
Enchondromatosis (cartilaginous) (multiple) Q78.4
Encopresis R15.9
  functional F98.1
  nonorganic origin F98.1
  psychogenic F98.1
Encounter (with health service) (for) Z76.89
  adjustment and management (of)
    breast implant Z45.81 ☑
    implanted device NEC Z45.89
    myringotomy device (stent) (tube) Z45.82
  administrative purpose only Z02.9
    examination for
      adoption Z02.82
      armed forces Z02.3
      disability determination Z02.71
      driving license Z02.4
      employment Z02.1
      insurance Z02.6
      medical certificate NEC Z02.79
      paternity testing Z02.81
      residential institution admission Z02.2
      school admission Z02.0
      sports Z02.5
      specified reason NEC Z02.89
  aftercare — see Aftercare
  antenatal screening Z36
  assisted reproductive fertility procedure cycle Z31.83
  blood typing Z01.83
    Rh typing Z01.83
  breast augmentation or reduction Z41.1
  breast implant exchange (different material) (different size) Z45.81 ☑
  breast reconstruction following mastectomy Z42.1
  check-up — see Examination
  chemotherapy for neoplasm Z51.11
  colonoscopy, screening Z12.11
  counseling — see Counseling
  delivery, full-term, uncomplicated O80
    cesarean, without indication O82
  ear piercing Z41.3
  examination — see Examination
  expectant parent(s) (adoptive) pre-birth pediatrician visit Z76.81
  fertility preservation procedure (prior to cancer therapy) (prior to removal of gonads) Z31.84
  fitting (of) — see Fitting (and adjustment) (of)
  genetic
    counseling Z31.5
    testing — see Test, genetic
  hearing conservation and treatment Z01.12
  immunotherapy for neoplasm Z51.12
  in vitro fertilization cycle Z31.83
  instruction (in)
    child care (postpartal) (prenatal) Z32.3
    childbirth Z32.2
    natural family planning
      procreative Z31.61
      to avoid pregnancy Z30.02
  insulin pump titration Z46.81
  joint prosthesis insertion following prior explantation of joint prosthesis (staged procedure)
    hip Z47.32
    knee Z47.33
    shoulder Z47.31
  laboratory (as part of a general medical examination) Z00.00
    with abnormal findings Z00.01
  mental health services (for)
    abuse NEC
      perpetrator Z69.82

Encounter — continued
  mental health services — continued
    abuse — continued
      victim Z69.81
    child abuse
      nonparental
        perpetrator Z69.021
        victim Z69.020
      parental
        perpetrator Z69.011
        victim Z69.010
    spousal or partner abuse
      perpetrator Z69.12
      victim Z69.11
  observation (for) (ruled out)
    exposure to (suspected)
      anthrax Z03.810
      biological agent NEC Z03.818
  pediatrician visit, by expectant parent(s) (adoptive) Z76.81
  plastic and reconstructive surgery following medical procedure or healed injury NEC Z42.8
  pregnancy
    supervision of — see Pregnancy, supervision of
    test Z32.00
      result negative Z32.02
      result positive Z32.01
  radiation therapy (antineoplastic) Z51.0
  radiological (as part of a general medical examination) Z00.00
    with abnormal findings Z00.01
  reconstructive surgery following medical procedure or healed injury NEC Z42.8
  removal (of) (see also Removal)
    artificial
      arm Z44.00- ☑
        complete Z44.01- ☑
        partial Z44.02- ☑
      eye Z44.2- ☑
      leg Z44.10- ☑
        complete Z44.11- ☑
        partial Z44.12- ☑
    breast implant Z45.81 ☑
      tissue expander (without synchronous insertion of permanent implant) Z45.81 ☑
    device Z46.9
      specified NEC Z46.89
    external
      fixation device — code to fracture with seventh character D
      prosthesis, prosthetic device Z44.9
        breast Z44.3- ☑
        specified NEC Z44.8
    implanted device NEC Z45.89
    insulin pump Z46.81
    internal fixation device Z47.2
    myringotomy device (stent) (tube) Z45.82
    nervous system device NEC Z46.2
      brain neuropacemaker Z46.2
      visual substitution device Z46.2
        implanted Z45.31
    non-vascular catheter Z46.82
    orthodontic device Z46.4
    stent
      ureteral Z46.6
    urinary device Z46.6
  repeat cervical smear to confirm findings of recent normal smear following initial abnormal smear Z01.42
  respirator [ventilator] use during power failure Z99.12
  Rh typing Z01.83
  screening — see Screening
  specified NEC Z76.89
  sterilization Z30.2
  suspected condition, ruled out
    amniotic cavity and membrane Z03.71
    cervical shortening Z03.75
    fetal anomaly Z03.73
    fetal growth Z03.74
    maternal and fetal conditions NEC Z03.79
    oligohydramnios Z03.71
    placental problem Z03.72
    polyhydramnios Z03.71
  suspected exposure (to), ruled out
    anthrax Z03.810
    biological agents NEC Z03.818
  termination of pregnancy, elective Z33.2
  testing — see Test

Encounter — continued
  therapeutic drug level monitoring Z51.81
  titration, insulin pump Z46.81
  to determine fetal viability of pregnancy O36.80 ☑
  training
    insulin pump Z46.81
  X-ray of chest (as part of a general medical examination) Z00.00
    with abnormal findings Z00.01
Encystment — see Cyst
Endarteritis (bacterial, subacute) (infective) I77.6
  brain I67.7
  cerebral or cerebrospinal I67.7
  deformans — see Arteriosclerosis
  embolic — see Embolism
  obliterans (see also Arteriosclerosis)
    pulmonary I28.8
  pulmonary I28.8
  retina — see Vasculitis, retina
  senile — see Arteriosclerosis
  syphilitic A52.09
    brain or cerebral A52.04
    congenital A50.54 [I79.8]
  tuberculous A18.89
Endemic — see condition
Endocarditis (chronic) (marantic) (nonbacterial) (thrombotic) (valvular) I38
  with rheumatic fever (conditions in I00)
    active — see Endocarditis, acute, rheumatic
    inactive or quiescent (with chorea) I09.1
  acute or subacute I33.9
    infective I33.0
    rheumatic (aortic) (mitral) (pulmonary) (tricuspid) I01.1
      with chorea (acute) (rheumatic) (Sydenham's) I02.0
  aortic (heart) (nonrheumatic) (valve) I35.8
    with
      mitral disease I08.0
        with tricuspid (valve) disease I08.3
        active or acute I01.1
          with chorea (acute) (rheumatic) (Sydenham's) I02.0
      rheumatic fever (conditions in I00)
        active — see Endocarditis, acute, rheumatic
        inactive or quiescent (with chorea) I06.9
      tricuspid (valve) disease I08.2
        with mitral (valve) disease I08.3
    acute or subacute I33.9
    arteriosclerotic I35.8
    rheumatic I06.9
      with mitral disease I08.0
        with tricuspid (valve) disease I08.3
        active or acute I01.1
          with chorea (acute) (rheumatic) (Sydenham's) I02.0
      active or acute I01.1
        with chorea (acute) (rheumatic) (Sydenham's) I02.0
    specified NEC I06.8
    specified cause NEC I35.8
    syphilitic A52.03
  arteriosclerotic I38
  atypical verrucous (Libman-Sacks) M32.11
  bacterial (acute) (any valve) (subacute) I33.0
  candidal B37.6
  congenital Q24.8
  constrictive I33.0
  Coxiella burnetii A78 [I39]
  Coxsackie B33.21
  due to
    prosthetic cardiac valve T82.6 ☑
    Q fever A78 [I39]
    Serratia marcescens I33.0
    typhoid (fever) A01.02
  gonococcal A54.83
  infectious or infective (acute) (any valve) (subacute) I33.0
  lenta (acute) (any valve) (subacute) I33.0
  Libman-Sacks M32.11
  listerial A32.82
  Löffler's I42.3
  malignant (acute) (any valve) (subacute) I33.0
  meningococcal A39.51
  mitral (chronic) (double) (fibroid) (heart) (inactive) (valve) (with chorea) I05.9
    with
      aortic (valve) disease I08.0

Endocarditis — *continued*
 mitral — *continued*
  with — *continued*
   aortic disease — *continued*
    with tricuspid (valve) disease I08.3
     active or acute I01.1
      with chorea (acute) (rheumatic) (Sydenham's) I02.0
    rheumatic fever (conditions in I00)
     active — *see* Endocarditis, acute, rheumatic
     inactive or quiescent (with chorea) I05.9
    tricuspid (valve) disease I08.1
     with aortic (valve) disease I08.3
   active or acute I01.1
    with chorea (acute) (rheumatic) (Sydenham's) I02.0
   bacterial I33.0
  arteriosclerotic I34.8
  nonrheumatic I34.8
   acute or subacute I33.9
  specified NEC I05.8
 monilial B37.6
 multiple valves i08.9
  specified disorders I08.8
 mycotic (acute) (any valve) (subacute) I33.0
 pneumococcal (acute) (any valve) (subacute) I33.0
 pulmonary (chronic) (heart) (valve) I37.8
  with rheumatic fever (conditions in I00)
   active — *see* Endocarditis, acute, rheumatic
   inactive or quiescent (with chorea) I09.89
    with aortic, mitral or tricuspid disease I08.8
  acute or subacute I33.9
   rheumatic I01.1
    with chorea (acute) (rheumatic) (Sydenham's) I02.0
  arteriosclerotic I37.8
  congenital Q22.2
  rheumatic (chronic) (inactive) (with chorea) I09.89
   active or acute I01.1
    with chorea (acute) (rheumatic) (Sydenham's) I02.0
 syphilitic A52.03
 purulent (acute) (any valve) (subacute) I33.0
 Q fever A78 [I39]
 rheumatic (chronic) (inactive) (with chorea) I09.1
  active or acute (aortic) (mitral) (pulmonary) (tricuspid) I01.1
   with chorea (acute) (rheumatic) (Sydenham's) I02.0
 rheumatoid — *see* Rheumatoid, carditis
 septic (acute) (any valve) (subacute) I33.0
 streptococcal (acute) (any valve) (subacute) I33.0
 subacute — *see* Endocarditis, acute
 suppurative (acute) (any valve) (subacute) I33.0
 syphilitic A52.03
 toxic I33.9
 tricuspid (chronic) (heart) (inactive) (rheumatic) (valve) (with chorea) I07.9
  with
   aortic (valve) disease I08.2
    mitral (valve) disease I08.3
   mitral (valve) disease I08.1
    aortic (valve) disease I08.3
   rheumatic fever (conditions in I00)
    active — *see* Endocarditis, acute, rheumatic
    inactive or quiescent (with chorea) I07.8
  active or acute I01.1
   with chorea (acute) (rheumatic) (Sydenham's) I02.0
  arteriosclerotic I36.8
  nonrheumatic I36.8
   acute or subacute I33.9
  specified cause, except rheumatic I36.8
 tuberculous — *see* Tuberculosis, endocarditis
 typhoid A01.02
 ulcerative (acute) (any valve) (subacute) I33.0
 vegetative (acute) (any valve) (subacute) I33.0
 verrucous (atypical) (nonbacterial) (nonrheumatic) M32.11
Endocardium, endocardial (*see also* condition)
 cushion defect Q21.2
Endocervicitis (*see also* Cervicitis)
 due to intrauterine (contraceptive) device T83.6 ☑
 hyperplastic N72
Endocrine — *see* condition
Endocrinopathy, pluriglandular E31.9
Endodontic
 overfill M27.52

Endodontic — *continued*
 underfill M27.53
Endodontitis K04.0
Endomastoiditis — *see* Mastoiditis
Endometrioma N80.9
Endometriosis N80.9
 appendix N80.5
 bladder N80.8
 bowel N80.5
 broad ligament N80.3
 cervix N80.0
 colon N80.5
 cul-de-sac (Douglas') N80.3
 exocervix N80.0
 fallopian tube N80.2
 female genital organ NEC N80.8
 gallbladder N80.8
 in scar of skin N80.6
 internal N80.0
 intestine N80.5
 lung N80.8
 myometrium N80.0
 ovary N80.1
 parametrium N80.3
 pelvic peritoneum N80.3
 peritoneal (pelvic) N80.3
 rectovaginal septum N80.4
 rectum N80.5
 round ligament N80.3
 skin (scar) N80.6
 specified site NEC N80.8
 stromal D39.0
 umbilicus N80.8
 uterus (internal) N80.0
 vagina N80.4
 vulva N80.8
Endometritis (decidual) (nonspecific) (purulent) (senile) (atrophic) (suppurative) N71.9
 with ectopic pregnancy O08.0
 acute N71.0
 blenorrhagic (gonococcal) (acute) (chronic) A54.24
 cervix, cervical (with erosion or ectropion) (*see also* Cervicitis)
  hyperplastic N72
 chlamydial A56.11
 chronic N71.1
 following
  abortion — *see* Abortion by type complicated by genital infection
  ectopic or molar pregnancy O08.0
 gonococcal, gonorrheal (acute) (chronic) A54.24
 hyperplastic (*see also* Hyperplasia, endometrial) N85.00
  cervix N72
 puerperal, postpartum, childbirth O86.12
 subacute N71.0
 tuberculous A18.17
Endometrium — *see* condition
Endomyocardiopathy, South African I42.3
Endomyocarditis — *see* Endocarditis
Endomyofibrosis I42.3
Endomyometritis — *see* Endometritis
Endopericarditis — *see* Endocarditis
Endoperineuritis — *see* Disorder, nerve
Endophlebitis — *see* Phlebitis
Endophthalmia — *see* Endophthalmitis, purulent
Endophthalmitis (acute) (infective) (metastatic) (subacute) H44.009
 bleb associated (*see also* Bleb, inflammed (infected), postprocedural H59.4 ☑
 gonorrheal A54.39
 in (due to)
  cysticercosis B69.1
  onchocerciasis B73.01
  toxocariasis B83.0
 panuveitis — *see* Panuveitis
 parasitic H44.12- ☑
 purulent H44.00- ☑
  panophthalmitis — *see* Panophthalmitis
  vitreous abscess H44.02- ☑
 specified NEC H44.19
 sympathetic — *see* Uveitis, sympathetic
Endosalpingioma D28.2
Endosalpingiosis N94.89
Endosteitis — *see* Osteomyelitis
Endothelioma, bone — *see* Neoplasm, bone, malignant
Endotheliosis (hemorrhagic infectional) D69.8
Endotoxemia — code to condition

Endotrachelitis — *see* Cervicitis
Engelmann (-Camurati) **syndrome** Q78.3
English disease — *see* Rickets
Engman's disease L30.3
Engorgement
 breast N64.59
  newborn P83.4
  puerperal, postpartum O92.79
 lung (passive) — *see* Edema, lung
 pulmonary (passive) — *see* Edema, lung
 stomach K31.89
 venous, retina — *see* Occlusion, retina, vein, engorgement
Enlargement, enlarged (*see also* Hypertrophy)
 adenoids J35.2
  with tonsils J35.3
 alveolar ridge K08.8
  congenital — *see* Anomaly, alveolar
 apertures of diaphragm (congenital) Q79.1
 gingival K06.1
 heart, cardiac — *see* Hypertrophy, cardiac
 lacrimal gland, chronic H04.03- ☑
 liver — *see* Hypertrophy, liver
 lymph gland or node R59.9
  generalized R59.1
  localized R59.0
 orbit H05.34- ☑
 organ or site, congenital NEC — *see* Anomaly, by site
 parathyroid (gland) E21.0
 pituitary fossa R93.0
 prostate N40.0
  with lower urinary tract symptoms (LUTS) N40.1
  without lower urinary tract symtpoms (LUTS) N40.0
 sella turcica R93.0
 spleen — *see* Splenomegaly
 thymus (gland) (congenital) E32.0
 thyroid (gland) — *see* Goiter
 tongue K14.8
 tonsils J35.1
  with adenoids J35.3
 uterus N85.2
Enophthalmos H05.40- ☑
 due to
  orbital tissue atrophy H05.41- ☑
  trauma or surgery H05.42- ☑
Enostosis M27.8
Entamebic, entamebiasis — *see* Amebiasis
Entanglement
 umbilical cord(s) O69.2 ☑
  with compression O69.2 ☑
   without compression O69.82 ☑
  around neck (with compression) O69.1 ☑
   without compression O69.81 ☑
  of twins in monoamniotic sac O69.2 ☑
Enteralgia — *see* Pain, abdominal
Enteric — *see* condition
Enteritis (acute) (diarrheal) (hemorrhagic) (noninfective) (septic) K52.9
 adenovirus A08.2
 aertrycke infection A02.0
 allergic K52.2
 amebic (acute) A06.0
  with abscess — *see* Abscess, amebic
  chronic A06.1
   with abscess — *see* Abscess, amebic
   nondysenteric A06.2
  nondysenteric A06.2
 astrovirus A08.32
 bacillary NOS A03.9
 bacterial A04.9
  specified NEC A04.8
 calicivirus A08.31
 candidal B37.82
 Chilomastix A07.8
 choleriformis A00.1
 chronic (noninfectious) K52.9
  ulcerative — *see* Colitis, ulcerative
 cicatrizing (chronic) — *see* Enteritis, regional, small intestine
 Clostridium
  botulinum (food poisoning) A05.1
  difficile A04.7
 coccidial A07.3
 coxsackie virus A08.39
 dietetic K52.2
 drug-induced K52.1

Enteritis — *continued*
- due to
  - astrovirus A08.32
  - calicivirus A08.31
  - coxsackie virus A08.39
  - drugs K52.1
  - echovirus A08.39
  - enterovirus NEC A08.39
  - food hypersensitivity K52.2
  - infectious organism (bacterial) (viral) — *see* Enteritis, infectious
  - torovirus A08.39
  - Yersinia enterocolitica A04.6
- echovirus A08.39
- eltor A00.1
- enterovirus NEC A08.39
- eosinophilic K52.81
- epidemic (infectious) A09
- fulminant K55.0
- gangrenous — *see* Enteritis, infectious
- giardial A07.1
- infectious NOS A09
  - due to
    - adenovirus A08.2
    - Aerobacter aerogenes A04.8
    - Arizona (bacillus) A02.0
    - bacteria NOS A04.9
      - specified NEC A04.8
    - Campylobacter A04.5
    - Clostridium difficile A04.7
    - Clostridium perfringens A04.8
    - Enterobacter aerogenes A04.8
    - enterovirus A08.39
    - Escherichia coli A04.4
      - enteroaggregative A04.4
      - enterohemorrhagic A04.3
      - enteroinvasive A04.2
      - enteropathogenic A04.0
      - enterotoxigenic A04.1
      - specified NEC A04.4
    - specified
      - bacteria NEC A04.8
      - virus NEC A08.39
    - Staphylococcus A04.8
    - virus NEC A08.4
      - specified type NEC A08.39
    - Yersinia enterocolitica A04.6
  - specified organism NEC A08.8
- influenzal — *see* Influenza, with, digestive manifestations
- ischemic K55.9
  - acute K55.0
  - chronic K55.1
- microsporidial A07.8
- mucomembranous, myxomembranous — *see* Syndrome, irritable bowel
- mucous — *see* Syndrome, irritable bowel
- necroticans A05.2
- necrotizing of newborn — *see* Enterocolitis, necrotizing, in newborn
- neurogenic — *see* Syndrome, irritable bowel
- newborn necrotizing — *see* Enterocolitis, necrotizing, in newborn
- noninfectious K52.9
- norovirus A08.11
- parasitic NEC B82.9
- paratyphoid (fever) — *see* Fever, paratyphoid
- protozoal A07.9
  - specified NEC A07.8
- radiation K52.0
- regional (of) K50.90
  - with
    - complication K50.919
      - abscess K50.914
      - fistula K50.913
      - intestinal obstruction K50.912
      - rectal bleeding K50.911
      - specified complication NEC K50.918
  - colon — *see* Enteritis, regional, large intestine
  - duodenum — *see* Enteritis, regional, small intestine
  - ileum — *see* Enteritis, regional, small intestine
  - jejunum — *see* Enteritis, regional, small intestine
  - large bowel — *see* Enteritis, regional, large intestine
  - large intestine (colon) (rectum) K50.10
    - with
      - complication K50.119
        - abscess K50.114

Enteritis — *continued*
- regional — *continued*
  - large intestine — *continued*
    - with — *continued*
      - complication — *continued*
        - fistula K50.113
        - intestinal obstruction K50.112
        - rectal bleeding K50.111
        - small intestine (duodenum) (ileum) (jejunum) involvement K50.80
          - with
            - complication K50.819
              - abscess K50.814
              - fistula K50.813
              - intestinal obstruction K50.812
              - rectal bleeding K50.811
              - specified complication NEC K50.818
        - specified complication NEC K50.118
  - rectum — *see* Enteritis, regional, large intestine
  - small intestine (duodenum) (ileum) (jejunum) K50.00
    - with
      - complication K50.019
        - abscess K50.014
        - fistula K50.013
        - intestinal obstruction K50.012
        - large intestine (colon) (rectum) involvement K50.80
          - with
            - complication K50.819
              - abscess K50.814
              - fistula K50.813
              - intestinal obstruction K50.812
              - rectal bleeding K50.811
              - specified complication NEC K50.818
        - rectal bleeding K50.011
        - specified complication NEC K50.018
- rotaviral A08.0
- Salmonella, salmonellosis (arizonae) (cholerae-suis) (enteritidis) (typhimurium) A02.0
- segmental — *see* Enteritis, regional
- septic A09
- Shigella — *see* Infection, Shigella
- small round structured NEC A08.19
- spasmodic, spastic — *see* Syndrome, irritable bowel
- staphylococcal A04.8
  - due to food A05.0
- torovirus A08.39
- toxic NEC K52.1
  - due to Clostridium difficile A04.7
- trichomonal A07.8
- tuberculous A18.32
- typhosa A01.00
- ulcerative (chronic) — *see* Colitis, ulcerative
- viral A08.4
  - adenovirus A08.2
  - enterovirus A08.39
  - Rotavirus A08.0
  - small round structured NEC A08.19
  - specified NEC A08.39
  - virus specified NEC A08.39

Enterobiasis B80
Enterobius vermicularis (infection) (infestation) B80
Enterocele (*see also* Hernia, abdomen)
- pelvic, pelvis (acquired) (congenital) N81.5
- vagina, vaginal (acquired) (congenital) NEC N81.5
Enterocolitis (*see also* Enteritis) K52.9
- due to Clostridium difficile A04.7
- fulminant ischemic K55.0
- granulomatous — *see* Enteritis, regional
- hemorrhagic (acute) K55.0
  - chronic K55.1
- infectious NEC A09
- ischemic K55.9
- necrotizing
  - due to Clostridium difficile A04.7
  - in newborn P77.9
    - stage 1 (without pneumatosis, without perforation) P77.1
    - stage 2 (with pneumatosis, without perforation) P77.2
    - stage 3 (with pneumatosis, with perforation) P77.3
- noninfectious K52.9
  - newborn — *see* Enterocolitis, necrotizing, in newborn

Enterocolitis — *continued*
- pseudomembranous (newborn) A04.7
- radiation K52.0
  - newborn — *see* Enterocolitis, necrotizing, in newborn
- ulcerative (chronic) — *see* Pancolitis, ulcerative (chronic)
Enterogastritis — *see* Enteritis
Enteropathy K63.9
- gluten-sensitive K90.0
- hemorrhagic, terminal K55.0
- protein-losing K90.4
Enteroperitonitis — *see* Peritonitis
Enteroptosis K63.4
Enterorrhagia K92.2
Enterospasm (*see also* Syndrome, irritable, bowel)
- psychogenic F45.8
Enterostenosis (*see also* Obstruction, intestine) K56.69
Enterostomy
- complication — *see* Complication, enterostomy
- status Z93.4
Enterovirus, as cause of disease classified elsewhere B97.10
- coxsackievirus B97.11
- echovirus B97.12
- other specified B97.19
Enthesopathy (peripheral) M77.9
- Achilles tendinitis — *see* Tendinitis, Achilles
- ankle and tarsus M77.9
  - specified type NEC — *see* Enthesopathy, foot, specified type NEC
- anterior tibial syndrome M76.81- ☑
- calcaneal spur — *see* Spur, bone, calcaneal
- elbow region M77.8
  - lateral epicondylitis — *see* Epicondylitis, lateral
  - medial epicondylitis — *see* Epicondylitis, medial
- foot NEC M77.9
  - metatarsalgia — *see* Metatarsalgia
  - specified type NEC M77.5- ☑
- forearm M77.9
- gluteal tendinitis — *see* Tendinitis, gluteal
- hand M77.9
- hip — *see* Enthesopathy, lower limb, specified type NEC
- iliac crest spur — *see* Spur, bone, iliac crest
- iliotibial band syndrome — *see* Syndrome, iliotibial band
- knee — *see* Enthesopathy, lower limb, lower leg, specified type NEC
- lateral epicondylitis — *see* Epicondylitis, lateral
- lower limb (excluding foot) M76.9
  - Achilles tendinitis — *see* Tendinitis, Achilles
  - anterior tibial syndrome M76.81- ☑
  - gluteal tendinitis — *see* Tendinitis, gluteal
  - iliac crest spur — *see* Spur, bone, iliac crest
  - iliotibial band syndrome — *see* Syndrome, iliotibial band
  - patellar tendinitis — *see* Tendinitis, patellar
  - pelvic region — *see* Enthesopathy, lower limb, specified type NEC
  - peroneal tendinitis — *see* Tendinitis, peroneal
  - posterior tibial syndrome M76.82- ☑
  - psoas tendinitis — *see* Tendinitis, psoas
  - shoulder M77.9
  - specified type NEC M76.89- ☑
  - tibial collateral bursitis — *see* Bursitis, tibial collateral
- medial epicondylitis — *see* Epicondylitis, medial
- metatarsalgia — *see* Metatarsalgia
- multiple sites M77.9
- patellar tendinitis — *see* Tendinitis, patellar
- pelvis M77.9
- periarthritis of wrist — *see* Periarthritis, wrist
- peroneal tendinitis — *see* Tendinitis, peroneal
- posterior tibial syndrome M76.82- ☑
- psoas tendinitis — *see* Tendinitis, psoas
- shoulder region — *see* Lesion, shoulder
- specified site NEC M77.9
- specified type NEC M77.8
- spinal M46.00
  - cervical region M46.02
  - cervicothoracic region M46.03
  - lumbar region M46.06
  - lumbosacral region M46.07
  - multiple sites M46.09
  - occipito-atlanto-axial region M46.01
  - sacrococcygeal region M46.08

Enthesopathy — *continued*
  spinal — *continued*
    thoracic region M46.04
      thoracolumbar region M46.05
    tibial collateral bursitis — *see* Bursitis, tibial collateral
  upper arm M77.9
  wrist and carpus NEC M77.8
    calcaneal spur — *see* Spur, bone, calcaneal
    periarthritis of wrist — *see* Periarthritis, wrist
Entomophobia F40.218
Entomophthoromycosis B46.8
Entrance, air into vein — *see* Embolism, air
Entrapment, nerve — *see* Neuropathy, entrapment
Entropion (eyelid) (paralytic) H02.009
  cicatricial H02.019
    left H02.016
      lower H02.015
      upper H02.014
    right H02.013
      lower H02.012
      upper H02.011
  congenital Q10.2
  left H02.006
    lower H02.005
    upper H02.004
  mechanical H02.029
    left H02.026
      lower H02.025
      upper H02.024
    right H02.023
      lower H02.022
      upper H02.021
  right H02.003
    lower H02.002
    upper H02.001
  senile H02.039
    left H02.036
      lower H02.035
      upper H02.034
    right H02.033
      lower H02.032
      upper H02.031
  spastic H02.049
    left H02.046
      lower H02.045
      upper H02.044
    right H02.043
      lower H02.042
      upper H02.041
Enucleated eye (traumatic, current) S05.7- ☑
Enuresis R32
  functional F98.0
  habit disturbance F98.0
  nocturnal N39.44
    psychogenic F98.0
  nonorganic origin F98.0
  psychogenic F98.0
Eosinopenia — *see* Agranulocytosis
Eosinophilia (allergic) (hereditary) (idiopathic) (secondary) D72.1
  with
    angiolymphoid hyperplasia (ALHE) D18.01
  infiltrative J82
  Löffler's J82
  peritoneal — *see* Peritonitis, eosinophilic
  pulmonary NEC J82
  tropical (pulmonary) J82
Eosinophilia-myalgia syndrome M35.8
Ependymitis (acute) (cerebral) (chronic) (granular) — *see* Encephalomyelitis
Ependymoblastoma
  specified site — *see* Neoplasm, malignant, by site
  unspecified site C71.9
Ependymoma (epithelial) (malignant)
  anaplastic
    specified site — *see* Neoplasm, malignant, by site
    unspecified site C71.9
  benign
    specified site — *see* Neoplasm, benign, by site
    unspecified site D33.2
  myxopapillary D43.2
    specified site — *see* Neoplasm, uncertain behavior, by site
    unspecified site D43.2
  papillary D43.2
    specified site — *see* Neoplasm, uncertain behavior, by site
    unspecified site D43.2

Ependymoma — *continued*
  specified site — *see* Neoplasm, malignant, by site
  unspecified site C71.9
Ependymopathy G93.89
Ephelis, ephelides L81.2
Epiblepharon (congenital) Q10.3
Epicanthus, epicanthic fold (eyelid) (congenital) Q10.3
Epicondylitis (elbow)
  lateral M77.1- ☑
  medial M77.0- ☑
Epicystitis — *see* Cystitis
Epidemic — *see* condition
Epidermidalization, cervix — *see* Dysplasia, cervix
Epidermis, epidermal — *see* condition
Epidermodysplasia verruciformis B07.8
Epidermolysis
  bullosa (congenital) Q81.9
    acquired L12.30
      drug-induced L12.31
      specified cause NEC L12.35
    dystrophica Q81.2
    letalis Q81.1
    simplex Q81.0
    specified NEC Q81.8
  necroticans combustiformis L51.2
    due to drug — *see* Table of Drugs and Chemicals, by drug
Epidermophytid — *see* Dermatophytosis
Epidermophytosis (infected) — *see* Dermatophytosis
Epididymis — *see* condition
Epididymitis (acute) (nonvenereal) (recurrent) (residual) N45.1
  with orchitis N45.3
  blennorrhagic (gonococcal) A54.23
  caseous (tuberculous) A18.15
  chlamydial A56.19
  filarial (*see also* Infestation, filarial) B74.9 [N51]
  gonococcal A54.23
  syphilitic A52.76
  tuberculous A18.15
Epididymo-orchitis (*see also* Epididymitis) N45.3
Epidural — *see* condition
Epigastrium, epigastric — *see* condition
Epigastrocele — *see* Hernia, ventral
Epiglottis — *see* condition
Epiglottitis, epiglottiditis (acute) J05.10
  with obstruction J05.11
  chronic J37.0
Epignathus Q89.4
Epilepsia partialis continua (*see also* Kozhevnikof's epilepsy) G40.1- ☑
Epilepsy, epileptic, epilepsia (attack) (cerebral) (convulsion) (fit) (seizure) G40.909

> Note: the following terms are to be considered equivalent to intractable: pharmacoresistant (pharmacologically resistant), treatment resistant, refractory (medically) and poorly controlled

  with
    complex partial seizures — *see* Epilepsy, localization-related, symptomatic, with complex partial seizures
    grand mal seizures on awakening — *see* Epilepsy, generalized, specified NEC
    myoclonic absences — *see* Epilepsy, generalized, specified NEC
    myoclonic-astatic seizures — *see* Epilepsy, generalized, specified NEC
    simple partial seizures — *see* Epilepsy, localization-related, symptomatic, with simple partial seizures
  akinetic — *see* Epilepsy, generalized, specified NEC
  benign childhood with centrotemporal EEG spikes — *see* Epilepsy, localization-related, idiopathic
  benign myoclonic in infancy G40.80- ☑
  Bravais-jacksonian — *see* Epilepsy, localization-related, symptomatic, with simple partial seizures
  childhood
    with occipital EEG paroxysms — *see* Epilepsy, localization-related, idiopathic
    absence G40.A09 (*following* G40.3)
      intractable G40.A19 (*following* G40.3)
        with status epilepticus G40.A11 (*following* G40.3)
        without status epilepticus G40.A19 (*following* G40.3)
      not intractable G40.A09 (*following* G40.3)

Epilepsy, epileptic, epilepsia — *continued*
  childhood — *continued*
    absence — *continued*
      not intractable — *continued*
        with status epilepticus G40.A01 (*following* G40.3)
        without status epilepticus G40.A09 (*following* G40.3)
  climacteric — *see* Epilepsy, specified NEC
  cysticercosis B69.0
  deterioration (mental) F06.8
  due to syphilis A52.19
  focal — *see* Epilepsy, localization-related, symptomatic, with simple partial seizures
  generalized
    idiopathic G40.309
      intractable G40.319
        with status epilepticus G40.311
        without status epilepticus G40.319
      not intractable G40.309
        with status epilepticus G40.301
        without status epilepticus G40.309
    specified NEC G40.409
      intractable G40.419
        with status epilepticus G40.411
        without status epilepticus G40.419
      not intractable G40.409
        with status epilepticus G40.401
        without status epilepticus G40.409
  impulsive petit mal — *see* Epilepsy, juvenile myoclonic
  intractable G40.919
    with status epilepticus G40.911
    without status epilepticus G40.919
  juvenile absence G40.A09 (*following* G40.3)
    intractable G40.A19 (*following* G40.3)
      with status epilepticus G40.A11 (*following* G40.3)
      without status epilepticus G40.A19 (*following* G40.3)
    not intractable G40.A09 (*following* G40.3)
      with status epilepticus G40.A01 (*following* G40.3)
      without status epilepticus G40.A09 (*following* G40.3)
  juvenile myoclonic G40.B09 (*following* G40.3)
    intractable G40.B19 (*following* G40.3)
      with status epilepticus G40.B11 (*following* G40.3)
      without status epilepticus G40.B19 (*following* G40.3)
    not intractable G40.B09 (*following* G40.3)
      with status epilepticus G40.B01 (*following* G40.3)
      without status epilepticus G40.B09 (*following* G40.3)
  localization-related (focal) (partial)
    idiopathic G40.009
      with seizures of localized onset G40.009
        intractable G40.019
          with status epilepticus G40.011
          without status epilepticus G40.019
        not intractable G40.009
          with status epilepticus G40.001
          without status epilepticus G40.009
    symptomatic
      with complex partial seizures G40.209
        intractable G40.219
          with status epilepticus G40.211
          without status epilepticus G40.219
        not intractable G40.209
          with status epilepticus G40.201
          without status epilepticus G40.209
      with simple partial seizures G40.109
        intractable G40.119
          with status epilepticus G40.111
          without status epilepticus G40.119
        not intractable G40.109
          with status epilepticus G40.101
          without status epilepticus G40.109
  myoclonus, myoclonic (progressive) — *see* Epilepsy, generalized, specified NEC
  not intractable G40.909
    with status epilepticus G40.901
    without status epilepticus G40.909
  on awakening — *see* Epilepsy, generalized, specified NEC
  parasitic NOS B71.9 [G94]

Epilepsy, epileptic, epilepsia — *continued*
partialis continua (*see also* Kozhevnikof's epilepsy)
G40.1- ☑
peripheral — *see* Epilepsy, specified NEC
procursiva — *see* Epilepsy, localization-related,
symptomatic, with simple partial seizures
progressive (familial) myoclonic — *see* Epilepsy, generalized, idiopathic
reflex — *see* Epilepsy, specified NEC
related to
alcohol G40.509
not intractable G40.509
with status epilepticus G40.501
without status epilepticus G40.509
drugs G40.509
not intractable G40.509
with status epilepticus G40.501
without status epilepticus G40.509
external causes G40.509
not intractable G40.509
with status epilepticus G40.501
without status epilepticus G40.509
hormonal changes G40.509
not intractable G40.509
with status epilepticus G40.501
without status epilepticus G40.509
sleep deprivation G40.509
not intractable G40.509
with status epilepticus G40.501
without status epilepticus G40.509
stress G40.509
not intractable G40.509
with status epilepticus G40.501
without status epilepticus G40.509
somatomotor — *see* Epilepsy, localization-related,
symptomatic, with simple partial seizures
somatosensory — *see* Epilepsy, localization-related,
symptomatic, with simple partial seizures
spasms G40.822
intractable G40.824
with status epilepticus G40.823
without status epilepticus G40.824
not intractable G40.822
with status epilepticus G40.821
without status epilepticus G40.822
specified NEC G40.802
intractable G40.804
with status epilepticus G40.803
without status epilepticus G40.804
not intractable G40.802
with status epilepticus G40.801
without status epilepticus G40.802
syndromes
generalized
idiopathic G40.309
intractable G40.319
with status epilepticus G40.311
without status epilepticus G40.319
not intractable G40.309
with status epilepticus G40.301
without status epilepticus G40.309
specified NEC G40.409
intractable G40.419
with status epilepticus G40.411
without status epilepticus G40.419
not intractable G40.409
with status epilepticus G40.401
without status epilepticus G40.409
localization-related (focal) (partial)
idiopathic G40.009
with seizures of localized onset G40.009
intractable G40.019
with status epilepticus G40.011
without status epilepticus G40.019
not intractable G40.009
with status epilepticus G40.001
without status epilepticus G40.009
symptomatic
with complex partial seizures G40.209
intractable G40.219
with status epilepticus G40.211
without status epilepticus G40.219
not intractable G40.209
with status epilepticus G40.201
without status epilepticus G40.209
with simple partial seizures G40.109
intractable G40.119
with status epilepticus G40.111

Epilepsy, epileptic, epilepsia — *continued*
syndromes — *continued*
localization-related — *continued*
symptomatic — *continued*
with simple partial seizures — *continued*
intractable — *continued*
without status epilepticus G40.119
not intractable G40.109
with status epilepticus G40.101
without status epilepticus G40.109
specified NEC G40.802
intractable G40.804
with status epilepticus G40.803
without status epilepticus G40.804
not intractable G40.802
with status epilepticus G40.801
without status epilepticus G40.802
tonic (-clonic) — *see* Epilepsy, generalized, specified
NEC
twilight F05
uncinate (gyrus) — *see* Epilepsy, localization-related,
symptomatic, with complex partial seizures
Unverricht (-Lundborg) (familial myoclonic) — *see*
Epilepsy, generalized, idiopathic
visceral — *see* Epilepsy, specified NEC
visual — *see* Epilepsy, specified NEC
Epiloia Q85.1
Epimenorrhea N92.0
Epipharyngitis — *see* Nasopharyngitis
Epiphora H04.20- ☑
due to
excess lacrimation H04.21- ☑
insufficient drainage H04.22- ☑
Epiphyseal arrest — *see* Arrest, epiphyseal
Epiphyseolysis, epiphysiolysis — *see* Osteochondropathy
Epiphysitis (*see also* Osteochondropathy)
juvenile M92.9
syphilitic (congenital) A50.02
Epiplocele — *see* Hernia, abdomen
Epiploitis — *see* Peritonitis
Epiplosarcomphalocele — *see* Hernia, umbilicus
Episcleritis (suppurative) H15.10- ☑
in (due to)
syphilis A52.71
tuberculosis A18.51
nodular H15.12- ☑
periodica fugax H15.11- ☑
angioneurotic — *see* Edema, angioneurotic
syphilitic (late) A52.71
tuberculous A18.51
Episode
affective, mixed F39
depersonalization (in neurotic state) F48.1
depressive F32.9
major F32.9
mild F32.0
moderate F32.1
severe (without psychotic symptoms) F32.2
with psychotic symptoms F32.3
recurrent F33.9
brief F33.8
specified NEC F32.8
hypomanic F30.8
manic F30.9
with
psychotic symptoms F30.2
remission (full) F30.4
partial F30.3
without psychotic symptoms F30.10
mild F30.11
moderate F30.12
severe (without psychotic symptoms) F30.13
with psychotic symptoms F30.2
other specified F30.8
recurrent F31.89
psychotic F23
organic F06.8
schizophrenic (acute) NEC, brief F23
Epispadias (female) (male) Q64.0
Episplenitis D73.89
Epistaxis (multiple) R04.0
hereditary I78.0
vicarious menstruation N94.89
Epithelioma (malignant) (*see also* Neoplasm, malignant,
by site)
adenoides cysticum — *see* Neoplasm, skin, benign
basal cell — *see* Neoplasm, skin, malignant

Epithelioma — *continued*
benign — *see* Neoplasm, benign, by site
Bowen's — *see* Neoplasm, skin, in situ
calcifying, of Malherbe — *see* Neoplasm, skin, benign
external site — *see* Neoplasm, skin, malignant
intraepidermal, Jadassohn — *see* Neoplasm, skin, be-
nign
squamous cell — *see* Neoplasm, malignant, by site
Epitheliomatosis pigmented Q82.1
Epitheliopathy, multifocal placoid pigment
H30.14- ☑
Epithelium, epithelial — *see* condition
Epituberculosis (with atelectasis) (allergic) A15.7
Eponychia Q84.6
Epstein's
nephrosis or syndrome — *see* Nephrosis
pearl K09.8
Epulis (gingiva) (fibrous) (giant cell) K06.8
Equinia A24.0
Equinovarus (congenital) (talipes) Q66.0
acquired — *see* Deformity, limb, clubfoot
Equivalent
convulsive (abdominal) — *see* Epilepsy, specified NEC
epileptic (psychic) — *see* Epilepsy, localization-related,
symptomatic, with complex partial seizures
Erb (-Duchenne) **paralysis** (birth injury) (newborn) P14.0
Erb-Goldflam disease or syndrome G70.00
with exacerbation (acute) G70.01
in crisis G70.01
Erb's
disease G71.0
palsy, paralysis (brachial) (birth) (newborn) P14.0
spinal (spastic) syphilitic A52.17
pseudohypertrophic muscular dystrophy G71.0
Erdheim's syndrome (acromegalic macrospondylitis)
E22.0
Erection, painful (persistent) — *see* Priapism
Ergosterol deficiency (vitamin D) E55.9
with
adult osteomalacia M83.8
rickets — *see* Rickets
Ergotism (*see also* Poisoning, food, noxious, plant)
from ergot used as drug (migraine therapy) — *see*
Table of Drugs and Chemicals
Erosio interdigitalis blastomycetica B37.2
Erosion
artery I77.2
without rupture I77.89
bone — *see* Disorder, bone, density and structure,
specified NEC
bronchus J98.09
cartilage (joint) — *see* Disorder, cartilage, specified
type NEC
cervix (uteri) (acquired) (chronic) (congenital) N86
with cervicitis N72
cornea (nontraumatic) — *see* Ulcer, cornea
recurrent H18.83- ☑
traumatic — *see* Abrasion, cornea
dental (idiopathic) (occupational) (due to diet, drugs
or vomiting) K03.2
duodenum, postpyloric — *see* Ulcer, duodenum
esophagus K22.10
with bleeding K22.11
gastric — *see* Ulcer, stomach
gastrojejunal — *see* Ulcer, gastrojejunal
implanted mesh — *see* Complications, mesh
intestine K63.3
lymphatic vessel I89.8
pylorus, pyloric (ulcer) — *see* Ulcer, stomach
spine, aneurysmal A52.09
stomach — *see* Ulcer, stomach
teeth (idiopathic) (occupational) (due to diet, drugs
or vomiting) K03.2
urethra N36.8
uterus N85.8
Erotomania F52.8
Error
metabolism, inborn — *see* Disorder, metabolism
refractive — *see* Disorder, refraction
Eructation R14.2
nervous or psychogenic F45.8
Eruption
creeping B76.9
drug (generalized) (taken internally) L27.0
fixed L27.1
in contact with skin — *see* Dermatitis, due to drugs
localized L27.1

Eruption — *continued*
　Hutchinson, summer L56.4
　Kaposi's varicelliform B00.0
　napkin L22
　polymorphous light (sun) L56.4
　recalcitrant pustular L13.8
　ringed R23.8
　skin (nonspecific) R21
　　creeping (meaning hookworm) B76.9
　　due to inoculation/vaccination (generalized) (*see
　　　also* Dermatitis, due to, vaccine) L27.0
　　　localized L27.1
　　erysipeloid A26.0
　　feigned L98.1
　　Kaposi's varicelliform B00.0
　　lichenoid L28.0
　　meaning dermatitis — *see* Dermatitis
　　toxic NEC L53.0
　tooth, teeth, abnormal (incomplete) (late) (premature)
　　(sequence) K00.6
　vesicular R23.8
Erysipelas (gangrenous) (infantile) (newborn) (phleg-
　monous) (suppurative) A46
　external ear A46 [H62.40]
　puerperal, postpartum O86.89
Erysipeloid A26.9
　cutaneous (Rosenbach's) A26.0
　disseminated A26.8
　sepsis A26.7
　specified NEC A26.8
Erythema, erythematous (infectional) (inflammation)
　L53.9
　ab igne L59.0
　annulare (centrifugum) (rheumaticum) L53.1
　arthriticum epidemicum A25.1
　brucellum — *see* Brucellosis
　chronic figurate NEC L53.3
　chronicum migrans (Borrelia burgdorferi) A69.20
　diaper L22
　due to
　　chemical NEC L53.0
　　　in contact with skin L24.5
　　drug (internal use) — *see* Dermatitis, due to, drugs
　elevatum diutinum L95.1
　endemic E52
　epidemic, arthritic A25.1
　figuratum perstans L53.3
　gluteal L22
　heat — *code by site under* Burn, first degree
　ichthyosiforme congenitum bullous Q80.3
　in diseases classified elsewhere L54
　induratum (nontuberculous) L52
　　tuberculous A18.4
　infectiosum B08.3
　intertrigo L30.4
　iris L51.9
　marginatum L53.2
　　in (due to) acute rheumatic fever I00
　medicamentosum — *see* Dermatitis, due to, drugs
　migrans A26.0
　　chronicum A69.20
　　tongue K14.1
　multiforme (major) (minor) L51.9
　　bullous, bullosum L51.1
　　conjunctiva L51.1
　　nonbullous L51.0
　　pemphigoides L12.0
　　specified NEC L51.8
　napkin L22
　neonatorum P83.8
　　toxic P83.1
　nodosum L52
　　tuberculous A18.4
　palmar L53.8
　pernio T69.1 ☑
　rash, newborn P83.8
　scarlatiniform (recurrent) (exfoliative) L53.8
　solare L55.0
　specified NEC L53.8
　toxic, toxicum NEC L53.0
　　newborn P83.1
　tuberculous (primary) A18.4
Erythematous, erythematosus — *see* condition
Erythermalgia (primary) I73.81
Erythralgia I73.81
Erythrasma L08.1
Erythredema (polyneuropathy) — *see* Poisoning, mer-
　cury

Erythremia (acute) C94.0- ☑
　chronic D45
　secondary D75.1
Erythroblastopenia (*see also* Aplasia, red cell) D60.9
　congenital D61.01
Erythroblastophthisis D61.09
Erythroblastosis (fetalis) (newborn) P55.9
　due to
　　ABO (antibodies) (incompatibility) (isoimmuniza-
　　　tion) P55.1
　　Rh (antibodies) (incompatibility) (isoimmunization)
　　　P55.0
Erythrocyanosis (crurum) I73.89
Erythrocythemia — *see* Erythremia
Erythrocytosis (megalosplenic) (secondary) D75.1
　familial D75.0
　oval, hereditary — *see* Elliptocytosis
　secondary D75.1
　stress D75.1
Erythroderma (secondary) (*see also* Erythema) L53.9
　bullous ichthyosiform, congenital Q80.3
　desquamativum L21.1
　ichthyosiform, congenital (bullous) Q80.3
　neonatorum P83.8
　psoriaticum L40.8
Erythrodysesthesia, palmar plantar (PPE) L27.1
Erythrogenesis imperfecta D61.09
Erythroleukemia C94.0- ☑
Erythromelalgia I73.81
Erythrophagocytosis D75.89
Erythrophobia F40.298
Erythroplakia, oral epithelium, and tongue K13.29
Erythroplasia (Queyrat) D07.4
　specified site — *see* Neoplasm, skin, in situ
　unspecified site D07.4
Escherichia coli (E. coli), **as cause of disease classified
　elsewhere** B96.20
　non-O157 Shiga toxin-producing (with known O
　　group) B96.22
　non-Shiga toxin-producing B96.29
　O157 B96.21
　O157 with confirmation of Shiga toxin when H antigen
　　is unknown, or is not H7 B96.21
　O157:H- (nonmotile) with confirmation of Shiga toxin
　　B96.21
　O157:H7 with or without confirmation of Shiga toxin-
　　production B96.21
　　specified NEC B96.22
　Shiga toxin-producing (with unspecified O group)
　　(STEC) B96.23
　specified NEC B96.29
Esophagismus K22.4
Esophagitis (acute) (alkaline) (chemical) (chronic) (infec-
　tional) (necrotic) (peptic) (postoperative) K20.9
　candidal B37.81
　due to gastrointestinal reflux disease K21.0
　eosinophilic K20.0
　reflux K21.0
　specified NEC K20.8
　tuberculous A18.83
　ulcerative K22.10
　　with bleeding K22.11
Esophagocele K22.5
Esophagomalacia K22.8
Esophagospasm K22.4
Esophagostenosis K22.2
Esophagostomiasis B81.8
Esophagotracheal — *see* condition
Esophagus — *see* condition
Esophoria H50.51
　convergence, excess H51.12
　divergence, insufficiency H51.8
Esotropia — *see* Strabismus, convergent concomitant
Espundia B55.2
Essential — *see* condition
Esthesioneuroblastoma C30.0
Esthesioneurocytoma C30.0
Esthesioneuroepithelioma C30.0
Esthiomene A55
Estivo-autumnal malaria (fever) B50.9
Estrangement (marital) Z63.5
　parent-child NEC Z62.890
Estriasis — *see* Myiasis
Ethanolism — *see* Alcoholism
Etherism — *see* Dependence, drug, inhalant
Ethmoid, ethmoidal — *see* condition

Ethmoiditis (chronic) (nonpurulent) (purulent) (*see also*
　Sinusitis, ethmoidal)
　influenzal — *see* Influenza, with, respiratory manifes-
　　tations NEC
　Woakes' J33.1
Etinylism — *see* Alcoholism
Eulenburg's disease (congenital paramyotonia) G71.19
Eumycetoma B47.0
Eunuchoidism E29.1
　hypogonadotropic E23.0
European blastomycosis — *see* Cryptococcosis
Eustachian — *see* condition
Evaluation (for) (of)
　development state
　　adolescent Z00.3
　　period of
　　　delayed growth in childhood Z00.70
　　　　with abnormal findings Z00.71
　　　rapid growth in childhood Z00.2
　　puberty Z00.3
　growth and developmental state (period of rapid
　　growth) Z00.2
　　delayed growth Z00.70
　　　with abnormal findings Z00.71
　mental health (status) Z00.8
　　requested by authority Z04.6
　period of
　　delayed growth in childhood Z00.70
　　　with abnormal findings Z00.71
　　rapid growth in childhood Z00.2
　suspected condition — *see* Observation
Evans syndrome D69.41
**Event, apparent life threatening in newborn and
　infant** (ALTE) R68.13
Eventration (*see also* Hernia, ventral)
　colon into chest — *see* Hernia, diaphragm
　diaphragm (congenital) Q79.1
Eversion
　bladder N32.89
　cervix (uteri) N86
　　with cervicitis N72
　foot NEC (*see also* Deformity, valgus, ankle)
　　congenital Q66.6
　punctum lacrimale (postinfectional) (senile) H04.52- ☑
　ureter (meatus) N28.89
　urethra (meatus) N36.8
　uterus N81.4
Evidence
　cytologic
　　of malignancy on anal smear R85.614
　　of malignancy on cervical smear R87.614
　　of malignancy on vaginal smear R87.624
Evisceration
　birth injury P15.8
　traumatic NEC
　　eye — *see* Enucleated eye
Evulsion — *see* Avulsion
Ewing's sarcoma or tumor — *see* Neoplasm, bone,
　malignant
Examination (for) (following) (general) (of) (routine)
　Z00.00
　with abnormal findings Z00.01
　abuse, physical (alleged), ruled out
　　adult Z04.71
　　child Z04.72
　adolescent (development state) Z00.3
　alleged rape or sexual assault (victim), ruled out
　　adult Z04.41
　　child Z04.42
　allergy Z01.82
　annual (adult) (periodic) (physical) Z00.00
　　with abnormal findings Z00.01
　　gynecological Z01.419
　　　with abnormal findings Z01.411
　antibody response Z01.84
　blood — *see* Examination, laboratory
　blood pressure Z01.30
　　with abnormal findings Z01.31
　cancer staging — *see* Neoplasm, malignant, by site
　cervical Papanicolaou smear Z12.4
　　as part of routine gynecological examination
　　　Z01.419
　　　with abnormal findings Z01.411
　child (over 28 days old) Z00.129　*[handwritten: 6 month old]*
　　with abnormal findings Z00.121
　　under 28 days old — *see* Newborn, examination
　clinical research control or normal comparison (con-
　　trol) (participant) Z00.6

Index

Examination — Exhaustion, exhaustive

Examination — *continued*
  contraceptive (drug) maintenance (routine) Z30.8
    device (intrauterine) Z30.431
  dental Z01.20
    with abnormal findings Z01.21
  developmental — *see* Examination, child
  donor (potential) Z00.5
  ear Z01.10
    with abnormal findings NEC Z01.118
  eye Z01.00
    with abnormal findings Z01.01
  following
    accident NEC Z04.3
      transport Z04.1
      work Z04.2
    assault, alleged, ruled out
      adult Z04.71
      child Z04.72
    motor vehicle accident Z04.1
    treatment (for) Z09
      combined NEC Z09
        fracture Z09
          malignant neoplasm Z08
        malignant neoplasm Z08
        mental disorder Z09
        specified condition NEC Z09
  follow-up (routine) (following) Z09
    chemotherapy NEC Z09
      malignant neoplasm Z08
    fracture Z09
    malignant neoplasm Z08
    postpartum Z39.2
    psychotherapy Z09
    radiotherapy NEC Z09
      malignant neoplasm Z08
    surgery NEC Z09
      malignant neoplasm Z08
  gynecological Z01.419
    with abnormal findings Z01.411
    for contraceptive maintenance Z30.8
  health — *see* Examination, medical
  hearing Z01.10
    with abnormal findings NEC Z01.118
    following failed hearing screening Z01.110
  immunity status testing Z01.84
  laboratory (as part of a general medical examination)
    Z00.00
    with abnormal findings Z00.01
    preprocedural Z01.812
  lactating mother Z39.1
  medical (adult) (for) (of) Z00.00
    with abnormal findings Z00.01
    administrative purpose only Z02.9
      specified NEC Z02.89
    admission to
      armed forces Z02.3
      old age home Z02.2
      prison Z02.89
      residential institution Z02.2
      school Z02.0
        following illness or medical treatment Z02.0
      summer camp Z02.89
    adoption Z02.82
    blood alcohol or drug level Z02.83
    camp (summer) Z02.89
    clinical research, normal subject (control) (partici-
      pant) Z00.6
    control subject in clinical research (normal compar-
      ison) (participant) Z00.6
    donor (potential) Z00.5
    driving license Z02.4
    general (adult) Z00.00
      with abnormal findings Z00.01
    immigration Z02.89
    insurance purposes Z02.6
    marriage Z02.89
    medicolegal reasons NEC Z04.8
    naturalization Z02.89
    participation in sport Z02.5
    paternity testing Z02.81
    population survey Z00.8
    pre-employment Z02.1
    pre-operative — *see* Examination, pre-procedural
    pre-procedural
      cardiovascular Z01.810
      respiratory Z01.811
      specified NEC Z01.818

Examination — *continued*
  medical — *continued*
    preschool children
      for admission to school Z02.0
    prisoners
      for entrance into prison Z02.89
    recruitment for armed forces Z02.3
    specified NEC Z00.8
    sport competition Z02.5
  medicolegal reason NEC Z04.8
  newborn — *see* Newborn, examination
  pelvic (annual) (periodic) Z01.419
    with abnormal findings Z01.411
  period of rapid growth in childhood Z00.2
  periodic (adult) (annual) (routine) Z00.00
    with abnormal findings Z00.01
  physical (adult) (*see also* Examination, medical) Z00.00
    sports Z02.5
  postpartum
    immediately after delivery Z39.0
    routine follow-up Z39.2
  pre-chemotherapy (antineoplastic) Z01.818
  prenatal (normal pregnancy) (*see also* Pregnancy,
    normal) Z34.9- ☑
  pre-procedural (pre-operative)
    cardiovascular Z01.810
    laboratory Z01.812
    respiratory Z01.811
    specified NEC Z01.818
  prior to chemotherapy (antineoplastic) Z01.818
  psychiatric NEC Z00.8
    follow-up not needing further care Z09
    requested by authority Z04.6
  radiological (as part of a general medical examination)
    Z00.00
    with abnormal findings Z00.01
  repeat cervical smear to confirm findings of recent
    normal smear following initial abnormal smear
    Z01.42
  skin (hypersensitivity) Z01.82
  special (*see also* Examination, by type) Z01.89
    specified type NEC Z01.89
  specified type or reason NEC Z04.8
  teeth Z01.20
    with abnormal findings Z01.21
  urine — *see* Examination, laboratory
  vision Z01.00
    with abnormal findings Z01.01
Exanthem, exanthema (*see also* Rash)
  with enteroviral vesicular stomatitis B08.4
  Boston A88.0
  epidemic with meningitis A88.0 [G02]
  subitum B08.20
    due to human herpesvirus 6 B08.21
    due to human herpesvirus 7 B08.22
  viral, virus B09
    specified type NEC B08.8
Excess, excessive, excessively
  alcohol level in blood R78.0
  androgen (ovarian) E28.1
  attrition, tooth, teeth K03.0
  carotene, carotin (dietary) E67.1
  cold, effects of T69.9 ☑
    specified effect NEC T69.8 ☑
  convergence H51.12
  crying
    in child, adolescent, or adult R45.83
    in infant R68.11
  development, breast N62
  divergence H51.8
  drinking (alcohol) NEC (without dependence) F10.10
    habitual (continual) (without remission) F10.20
  eating R63.2
  estrogen E28.0
  fat (*see also* Obesity)
    in heart — *see* Degeneration, myocardial
    localized E65
  foreskin N47.8
  gas R14.0
  glucagon E16.3
  heat — *see* Heat
  intermaxillary vertical dimension of fully erupted teeth
    M26.37
  interocclusal distance of fully erupted teeth M26.37
  kalium E87.5
  large
    colon K59.3
      congenital Q43.8

Excess, excessive, excessively — *continued*
  large — *continued*
    infant P08.0
    organ or site, congenital NEC — *see* Anomaly, by
      site
  long
    organ or site, congenital NEC — *see* Anomaly, by
      site
  menstruation (with regular cycle) N92.0
    with irregular cycle N92.1
  napping Z72.821
  natrium E87.0
  number of teeth K00.1
  nutrient (dietary) NEC R63.2
  potassium (K) E87.5
  salivation K11.7
  secretion (*see also* Hypersecretion)
    milk O92.6
    sputum R09.3
    sweat R61
  sexual drive F52.8
  short
    organ or site, congenital NEC — *see* Anomaly, by
      site
    umbilical cord in labor or delivery O69.3 ☑
  skin, eyelid (acquired) — *see* Blepharochalasis
    congenital Q10.3
  sodium (Na) E87.0
  spacing of fully erupted teeth M26.32
  sputum R09.3
  sweating R61
  thirst R63.1
    due to deprivation of water T73.1 ☑
  tuberosity of jaw M26.07
  vitamin
    A (dietary) E67.0
      administered as drug (prolonged intake) — *see*
        Table of Drugs and Chemicals, vitamins,
        adverse effect
      overdose or wrong substance given or taken
        — *see* Table of Drugs and Chemicals, vi-
        tamins, poisoning
    D (dietary) E67.3
      administered as drug (prolonged intake) — *see*
        Table of Drugs and Chemicals, vitamins,
        adverse effect
      overdose or wrong substance given or taken
        — *see* Table of Drugs and Chemicals, vi-
        tamins, poisoning
  weight
    gain R63.5
    loss R63.4
Excitability, abnormal, under minor stress (personality disorder) F60.3
Excitation
  anomalous atrioventricular I45.6
  psychogenic F30.8
  reactive (from emotional stress, psychological trauma)
    F30.8
Excitement
  hypomanic F30.8
  manic F30.9
  mental, reactive (from emotional stress, psychological
    trauma) F30.8
  state, reactive (from emotional stress, psychological
    trauma) F30.8
Excoriation (traumatic) (*see also* Abrasion)
  neurotic L98.1
Exfoliation
  due to erythematous conditions according to extent
    of body surface involved L49.0
    less than 10 percent of body surface L49.0
    10-19 percent of body surface L49.1
    20-29 percent of body surface L49.2
    30-39 percent of body surface L49.3
    40-49 percent of body surface L49.4
    50-59 percent of body surface L49.5
    60-69 percent of body surface L49.6
    70-79 percent of body surface L49.7
    80-89 percent of body surface L49.8
    90-99 percent of body surface L49.9
  teeth, due to systemic causes K08.0
Exfoliative — *see* condition
Exhaustion, exhaustive (physical NEC) R53.83
  battle F43.0
  cardiac — *see* Failure, heart
  delirium F43.0

☑ **Additional Character Required — Refer to the Tabular List for Character Selection**   Subterms under main terms may continue to next column or page

Exhaustion, exhaustive — *continued*
- due to
  - cold T69.8 ☑
  - excessive exertion T73.3 ☑
  - exposure T73.2 ☑
  - neurasthenia F48.8
- heart — *see* Failure, heart
- heat (*see also* Heat, exhaustion) T67.5 ☑
  - due to
    - salt depletion T67.4 ☑
    - water depletion T67.3 ☑
- maternal, complicating delivery O75.81
- mental F48.8
- myocardium, myocardial — *see* Failure, heart
- nervous F48.8
- old age R54
- psychogenic F48.8
- psychosis F43.0
- senile R54
- vital NEC Z73.0

Exhibitionism F65.2
Exocervicitis — *see* Cervicitis
Exomphalos Q79.2
- meaning hernia — *see* Hernia, umbilicus

Exophoria H50.52
- convergence, insufficiency H51.11
- divergence, excess H51.8

Exophthalmos H05.2- ☑
- congenital Q15.8
- constant NEC H05.24- ☑
- displacement, globe — *see* Displacement, globe
- due to thyrotoxicosis (hyperthyroidism) — *see* Hyperthyroidism, with, goiter (diffuse)
- dysthyroid — *see* Hyperthyroidism, with, goiter (diffuse)
- goiter — *see* Hyperthyroidism, with, goiter (diffuse)
- intermittent NEC H05.25- ☑
- malignant — *see* Hyperthyroidism, with, goiter (diffuse)
- orbital
  - edema — *see* Edema, orbit
  - hemorrhage — *see* Hemorrhage, orbit
- pulsating NEC H05.26- ☑
- thyrotoxic, thyrotropic — *see* Hyperthyroidism, with, goiter (diffuse)

Exostosis (*see also* Disorder, bone)
- cartilaginous — *see* Neoplasm, bone, benign
- congenital (multiple) Q78.6
- external ear canal H61.81- ☑
- gonococcal A54.49
- jaw (bone) M27.8
- multiple, congenital Q78.6
- orbit H05.35- ☑
- osteocartilaginous — *see* Neoplasm, bone, benign
- syphilitic A52.77

Exotropia — *see* Strabismus, divergent concomitant
Explanation of
- investigation finding Z71.2
- medication Z71.89

Exposure (to) (*see also* Contact, with) T75.89 ☑
- acariasis Z20.7
- AIDS virus Z20.6
- air pollution Z77.110
- algae and algae toxins Z77.121
- algae bloom Z77.121
- anthrax Z20.810
- aromatic amines Z77.020
- aromatic (hazardous) compounds NEC Z77.028
- aromatic dyes NOS Z77.028
- arsenic Z77.010
- asbestos Z77.090
- bacterial disease NEC Z20.818
- benzene Z77.021
- blue-green algae bloom Z77.121
- body fluids (potentially hazardous) Z77.21
- brown tide Z77.121
- chemicals (chiefly nonmedicinal) (hazardous) NEC Z77.098
- cholera Z20.09
- chromium compounds Z77.018
- cold, effects of T69.9 ☑
  - specified effect NEC T69.8 ☑
- communicable disease Z20.9
  - bacterial NEC Z20.818
  - specified NEC Z20.89
  - viral NEC Z20.828
- cyanobacteria bloom Z77.121

Exposure — *continued*
- disaster Z65.5
- discrimination Z60.5
- dyes Z77.098
- effects of T73.9 ☑
- environmental tobacco smoke (acute) (chronic) Z77.22
- Escherichia coli (E. coli) Z20.01
- exhaustion due to T73.2 ☑
- fiberglass — *see* Table of Drugs and Chemicals, fiberglass
- German measles Z20.4
- gonorrhea Z20.2
- hazardous metals NEC Z77.018
- hazardous substances NEC Z77.29
- hazards in the physical environment NEC Z77.128
- hazards to health NEC Z77.9
- human immunodeficiency virus (HIV) Z20.6
- human T-lymphotropic virus type-1 (HTLV-1) Z20.89
- implanted
  - mesh — *see* Complications, mesh
  - prosthetic materials NEC — *see* Complications, prosthetic materials NEC
- infestation (parasitic) NEC Z20.7
- intestinal infectious disease NEC Z20.09
  - Escherichia coli (E. coli) Z20.01
- lead Z77.011
- meningococcus Z20.811
- mold (toxic) Z77.120
- nickel dust Z77.018
- noise Z77.122
- occupational
  - air contaminants NEC Z57.39
  - dust Z57.2
  - environmental tobacco smoke Z57.31
  - extreme temperature Z57.6
  - noise Z57.0
  - radiation Z57.1
  - risk factors Z57.9
    - specified NEC Z57.8
  - toxic agents (gases) (liquids) (solids) (vapors) in agriculture Z57.4
  - toxic agents (gases) (liquids) (solids) (vapors) in industry NEC Z57.5
  - vibration Z57.7
- parasitic disease NEC Z20.7
- pediculosis Z20.7
- persecution Z60.5
- pfiesteria piscicida Z77.121
- poliomyelitis Z20.89
- pollution
  - air Z77.110
  - environmental NEC Z77.118
  - soil Z77.112
  - water Z77.111
- polycyclic aromatic hydrocarbons Z77.028
- prenatal (drugs) (toxic chemicals) — *see* Newborn, affected by (suspected to be), noxious substances transmitted via placenta or breast milk
- rabies Z20.3
- radiation, naturally occurring NEC Z77.123
- radon Z77.123
- red tide (Florida) Z77.121
- rubella Z20.4
- second hand tobacco smoke (acute) (chronic) Z77.22
  - in the perinatal period P96.81
- sexually-transmitted disease Z20.2
- smallpox (laboratory) Z20.89
- syphilis Z20.2
- terrorism Z65.4
- torture Z65.4
- tuberculosis Z20.1
- uranium Z77.012
- varicella Z20.820
- venereal disease Z20.2
- viral disease NEC Z20.828
- war Z65.5
- water pollution Z77.111

Exsanguination — *see* Hemorrhage
Exstrophy
- abdominal contents Q45.8
- bladder Q64.10
  - cloacal Q64.12
  - specified type NEC Q64.19
  - supravesical fissure Q64.11

Extensive — *see* condition
Extra (*see also* Accessory)
- marker chromosomes (normal individual) Q92.61
  - in abnormal individual Q92.62

Extra — *continued*
- rib Q76.6
  - cervical Q76.5

Extrasystoles (supraventricular) I49.49
- atrial I49.1
- auricular I49.1
- junctional I49.2
- ventricular I49.3

Extrauterine gestation or pregnancy — *see* Pregnancy, by site
Extravasation
- blood R58
- chyle into mesentery I89.8
- pelvicalyceal N13.8
- pyelosinus N13.8
- urine (from ureter) R39.0
- vesicant agent
  - antineoplastic chemotherapy T80.810 ☑
  - other agent NEC T80.818 ☑

Extremity — *see* condition, limb
Extrophy — *see* Exstrophy
Extroversion
- bladder Q64.19
- uterus N81.4
  - complicating delivery O71.2
  - postpartal (old) N81.4

Extruded tooth (teeth) M26.34
Extrusion
- breast implant (prosthetic) T85.42 ☑
- eye implant (globe) (ball) T85.328 ☑
- intervertebral disc — *see* Displacement, intervertebral disc
- ocular lens implant (prosthetic) — *see* Complications, intraocular lens
- vitreous — *see* Prolapse, vitreous

Exudate
- pleural — *see* Effusion, pleura
- retina H35.89

Exudative — *see* condition
Eye, eyeball, eyelid — *see* condition
Eyestrain — *see* Disturbance, vision, subjective
Eyeworm disease of Africa B74.3

F

Faber's syndrome (achlorhydric anemia) D50.9
Fabry (-Anderson) **disease** E75.21
Faciocephalalgia, autonomic (*see also* Neuropathy, peripheral, autonomic) G90.09
Factor(s)
- psychic, associated with diseases classified elsewhere F54
- psychological
  - affecting physical conditions F54
  - or behavioral
    - affecting general medical condition F54
    - associated with disorders or diseases classified elsewhere F54

Fahr disease (of brain) G23.8
Fahr Volhard disease (of kidney) I12.- ☑
Failure, failed
- abortion — *see* Abortion, attempted
- aortic (valve) I35.8
  - rheumatic I06.8
- attempted abortion — *see* Abortion, attempted
- biventricular I50.9
- bone marrow — *see* Anemia, aplastic
- cardiac — *see* Failure, heart
- cardiorenal (chronic) I50.9
  - hypertensive I13.2
- cardiorespiratory (*see also* Failure, heart) R09.2
- cardiovascular (chronic) — *see* Failure, heart
- cerebrovascular I67.9
- cervical dilatation in labor O62.0
- circulation, circulatory (peripheral) R57.9
  - newborn P29.89
- compensation — *see* Disease, heart
- compliance with medical treatment or regimen — *see* Noncompliance
- congestive — *see* Failure, heart, congestive
- dental implant (endosseous) M27.69
  - due to
    - failure of dental prosthesis M27.63
    - lack of attached gingiva M27.62
    - occlusal trauma (poor prosthetic design) M27.62
    - parafunctional habits M27.62

Index

Failure, failed — Falling, falls

Failure, failed — *continued*
dental implant — *continued*
  due to — *continued*
    periodontal infection (peri-implantitis) M27.62
    poor oral hygiene M27.62
  osseointegration M27.61
    due to
      complications of systemic disease M27.61
      poor bone quality M27.61
    iatrogenic M27.61
  post-osseointegration
    biological M27.62
    due to complications of systemic disease M27.62
    iatrogenic M27.62
    mechanical M27.63
  pre-integration M27.61
  pre-osseointegration M27.61
  specified NEC M27.69
descent of head (at term) of pregnancy (mother) O32.4 ☑
endosseous dental implant — *see* Failure, dental implant
engagement of head (term of pregnancy) (mother) O32.4 ☑
erection (penile) (*see also* Dysfunction, sexual, male, erectile) N52.9
  nonorgqanic F52.21
examination(s), anxiety concerning Z55.2
expansion terminal respiratory units (newborn) (primary) P28.0
forceps NOS (with subsequent cesarean delivery) O66.5
gain weight (child over 28 days old) R62.51
  adult R62.7
  newborn P92.6
genital response (male) F52.21
  female F52.22
heart (acute) (senile) (sudden) I50.9
  with
    acute pulmonary edema — *see* Failure, ventricular, left
    decompensation — *see* Failure, heart, congestive
    dilatation — *see* Disease, heart
  arteriosclerotic I70.90
  biventricular I50.9
  combined left-right sided I50.9
  compensated I50.9
  complicating
    anesthesia (general) (local) or other sedation
      in labor and delivery O74.2
      in pregnancy O29.12- ☑
      postpartum, puerperal O89.1
    delivery (cesarean) (instrumental) O75.4
  congestive (compensated) (decompensated) I50.9
    with rheumatic fever (conditions in I00)
      active I01.8
      inactive or quiescent (with chorea) I09.81
    newborn P29.0
    rheumatic (chronic) (inactive) (with chorea) I09.81
      active or acute I01.8
        with chorea I02.0
  decompensated I50.9
  degenerative — *see* Degeneration, myocardial
  diastolic (congestive) I50.30
    acute (congestive) I50.31
      and (on) chronic (congestive) I50.33
    chronic (congestive) I50.32
      and (on) acute (congestive) I50.33
    combined with systolic (congestive) I50.40
      acute (congestive) I50.41
        and (on) chronic (congestive) I50.43
      chronic (congestive) I50.42
        and (on) acute (congestive) I50.43
  due to presence of cardiac prosthesis I97.13- ☑
  following cardiac surgery I97.13- ☑
  high output NOS I50.9
  hypertensive — *see* Hypertension, heart
  left (ventricular) — *see* Failure, ventricular, left
  low output (syndrome) NOS I50.9
  newborn P29.0
  organic — *see* Disease, heart
  peripartum O90.3
  postprocedural I97.13- ☑
  rheumatic (chronic) (inactive) I09.9
  right (ventricular) (secondary to left heart failure) — *see* Failure, heart, congestive

Failure, failed — *continued*
heart — *continued*
  systolic (congestive) I50.20
    acute (congestive) I50.21
      and (on) chronic (congestive) I50.23
    chronic (congestive) I50.22
      and (on) acute (congestive) I50.23
    combined with diastolic (congestive) I50.40
      acute (congestive) I50.41
        and (on) chronic (congestive) I50.43
      chronic (congestive) I50.42
        and (on) acute (congestive) I50.43
  thyrotoxic (*see also* Thyrotoxicosis) E05.90 [I43]
    with thyroid storm E05.91 [I43]
  valvular — *see* Endocarditis
hepatic K72.90
  with coma K72.91
  acute or subacute K72.00
    with coma K72.01
    due to drugs K71.10
      with coma K71.11
  alcoholic (acute) (chronic) (subacute) K70.40
    with coma K70.41
  chronic K72.10
    with coma K72.11
    due to drugs (acute) (subacute) (chronic) K71.10
      with coma K71.11
  due to drugs (acute) (subacute) (chronic) K71.10
    with coma K71.11
  postprocedural K91.82
hepatorenal K76.7
induction (of labor) O61.9
  abortion — *see* Abortion, attempted
  by
    oxytocic drugs O61.0
    prostaglandins O61.0
  instrumental O61.1
  mechanical O61.1
  medical O61.0
  specified NEC O61.8
  surgical O61.1
intubation during anesthesia T88.4 ☑
  in pregnancy O29.6- ☑
  labor and delivery O74.7
  postpartum, puerperal O89.6
involution, thymus (gland) E32.0
kidney (*see also* Disease, kidney, chronic) N19
  acute (*see also* Failure, renal, acute) N17.9
lactation (complete) O92.3
  partial O92.4
Leydig's cell, adult E29.1
liver — *see* Failure, hepatic
menstruation at puberty N91.0
mitral I05.8
myocardial, myocardium (*see also* Failure, heart) I50.9
  chronic (*see also* Failure, heart, congestive) I50.9
  congestive (*see also* Failure, heart, congestive) I50.9
orgasm (female) (psychogenic) F52.31
  male F52.32
ovarian (primary) E28.39
  iatrogenic E89.40
    asymptomatic E89.40
    symptomatic E89.41
  postprocedural (postablative) (postirradiation) (postsurgical) E89.40
    asymptomatic E89.40
    symptomatic E89.41
ovulation causing infertility N97.0
polyglandular, autoimmune E31.0
prosthetic joint implant — *see* Complications, joint prosthesis, mechanical, breakdown, by site
renal N19
  with
    tubular necrosis (acute) N17.0
  acute N17.9
    with
      cortical necrosis N17.1
      medullary necrosis N17.2
      tubular necrosis N17.0
    specified NEC N17.8
  chronic N18.9
    hypertensive — *see* Hypertension, kidney
  congenital P96.0
  end stage (chronic) N18.6
    due to hypertension I12.0
  following
    abortion — *see* Abortion by type complicated by specified condition NEC

Failure, failed — *continued*
renal — *continued*
  following — *continued*
    crushing T79.5 ☑
    ectopic or molar pregnancy O08.4
    labor and delivery (acute) O90.4
  hypertensive — *see* Hypertension, kidney
  postprocedural N99.0
respiration, respiratory J96.90
  with
    hypercapnia J96.92
    hypoxia J96.91
  acute J96.00
    with
      hypercapnia J96.02
      hypoxia J96.01
  acute and (on) chronic J96.20
    with
      hypercapnia J96.22
      hypoxia J96.21
  center G93.89
  chronic J96.10
    with
      hypercapnia J96.12
      hypoxia J96.11
  newborn P28.5
  postprocedural (acute) J95.821
    acute and chronic J95.822
rotation
  cecum Q43.3
  colon Q43.3
  intestine Q43.3
  kidney Q63.2
sedation (conscious) (moderate) during procedure T88.52 ☑
  history of Z92.83
segmentation (*see also* Fusion)
  fingers — *see* Syndactylism, complex, fingers
  vertebra Q76.49
    with scoliosis Q76.3
seminiferous tubule, adult E29.1
senile (general) R54
sexual arousal (male) F52.21
  female F52.22
testicular endocrine function E29.1
to thrive (child over 28 days old) R62.51
  adult R62.7
  newborn P92.6
transplant T86.92
  bone T86.831
    marrow T86.02
  cornea T86.841
  heart T86.22
    with lung(s) T86.32
  intestine T86.851
  kidney T86.12
  liver T86.42
  lung(s) T86.811
    with heart T86.32
  pancreas T86.891
  skin (allograft) (autograft) T86.821
  specified organ or tissue NEC T86.891
  stem cell (peripheral blood) (umbilical cord) T86.5
trial of labor (with subsequent cesarean delivery) O66.40
  following previous cesarean delivery O66.41
tubal ligation N99.89
urinary — *see* Disease, kidney, chronic
vacuum extraction NOS (with subsequent cesarean delivery) O66.5
vasectomy N99.89
ventouse NOS (with subsequent cesarean delivery) O66.5
ventricular (*see also* Failure, heart) I50.9
  left I50.1
    with rheumatic fever (conditions in I00)
      active I01.8
        with chorea I02.0
      inactive or quiescent (with chorea) I09.81
      rheumatic (chronic) (inactive) (with chorea) I09.81
        active or acute I01.8
          with chorea I02.0
  right (*see also* Failure, heart, congestive) I50.9
vital centers, newborn P91.8
Fainting (fit) R55
Fallen arches — *see* Deformity, limb, flat foot
Falling, falls (repeated) R29.6

Falling, falls — *continued*
  any organ or part — *see* Prolapse
Fallopian
  insufflation Z31.41
  tube — *see* condition
Fallot's
  pentalogy Q21.8
  tetrad or tetralogy Q21.3
  triad or trilogy Q22.3
False (*see also* condition)
  croup J38.5
  joint — *see* Nonunion, fracture
  labor (pains) O47.9
    at or after 37 completed weeks of gestation O47.1
    before 37 completed weeks of gestation O47.0-
  passage, urethra (prostatic) N36.5
  pregnancy F45.8
Family, familial (*see also* condition)
  disruption Z63.8
    involving divorce or separation Z63.5
  Li-Fraumeni (syndrome) Z15.01
  planning advice Z30.09
  problem Z63.9
    specified NEC Z63.8
  retinoblastoma C69.2- ☑
Famine (effects of) T73.0 ☑
  edema — *see* Malnutrition, severe
Fanconi (-de Toni)(-Debré) **syndrome** E72.09
  with cystinosis E72.04
Fanconi's anemia (congenital pancytopenia) D61.09
Farber's disease or syndrome E75.29
Farcy A24.0
Farmer's
  lung J67.0
  skin L57.8
Farsightedness — *see* Hypermetropia
Fascia — *see* condition
Fasciculation R25.3
Fasciitis M72.9
  diffuse (eosinophilic) M35.4
  infective M72.8
    necrotizing M72.6
  necrotizing M72.6
  nodular M72.4
  perirenal (with ureteral obstruction) N13.5
    with infection N13.6
  plantar M72.2
  specified NEC M72.8
  traumatic (old) M72.8
    current — *code by* site under Sprain
Fascioliasis B66.3
Fasciolopsis, fasciolopsiasis (intestinal) B66.5
Fascioscapulohumeral myopathy G71.0
Fast pulse R00.0
Fat
  embolism — *see* Embolism, fat
  excessive (*see also* Obesity)
    in heart — *see* Degeneration, myocardial
  in stool R19.5
  localized (pad) E65
    heart — *see* Degeneration, myocardial
    knee M79.4
    retropatellar M79.4
  necrosis
    breast N64.1
    mesentery K65.4
    omentum K65.4
  pad E65
    knee M79.4
Fatigue R53.83
  auditory deafness — *see* Deafness
  chronic R53.82
  combat F43.0
  general R53.83
    psychogenic F48.8
  heat (transient) T67.6 ☑
  muscle M62.89
  myocardium — *see* Failure, heart
  neoplasm-related R53.0
  nervous, neurosis F48.8
  operational F48.8
  psychogenic (general) F48.8
  senile R54
  voice R49.8
Fatness — *see* Obesity
Fatty (*see also* condition)
  apron E65

Fatty — *continued*
  degeneration — *see* Degeneration, fatty
  heart (enlarged) — *see* Degeneration, myocardial
  liver NEC K76.0
    alcoholic K70.0
    nonalcoholic K76.0
  necrosis — *see* Degeneration, fatty
Fauces — *see* condition
Fauchard's disease (periodontitis) — *see* Periodontitis
Faucitis J02.9
Favism (anemia) D55.0
Favus — *see* Dermatophytosis
Fazio-Londe disease or syndrome G12.1
Fear complex or reaction F40.9
Fear of — *see* Phobia
Feared complaint unfounded Z71.1
Febris, febrile (*see also* Fever)
  flava (*see also* Fever, yellow) A95.9
  melitensis A23.0
  pestis — *see* Plague
  recurrens — *see* Fever, relapsing
  rubra A38.9
Fecal
  incontinence R15.9
  smearing R15.1
  soiling R15.1
  urgency R15.2
Fecalith (impaction) K56.41
  appendix K38.1
  congenital P76.8
Fede's disease K14.0
Feeble rapid pulse due to shock following injury T79.4 ☑
Feeble-minded F70
Feeding
  difficulties R63.3
  problem R63.3
    newborn P92.9
      specified NEC P92.8
    nonorganic (adult) — *see* Disorder, eating
Feeling (of)
  foreign body in throat R09.89
Feer's disease — *see* Poisoning, mercury
Feet — *see* condition
Feigned illness Z76.5
Feil-Klippel syndrome (brevicollis) Q76.1
Feinmesser's (hidrotic) **ectodermal dysplasia** Q82.4
Felinophobia F40.218
Felon (*see also* Cellulitis, digit)
  with lymphangitis — *see* Lymphangitis, acute, digit
Felty's syndrome M05.00
  ankle M05.07- ☑
  elbow M05.02- ☑
  foot joint M05.07- ☑
  hand joint M05.04- ☑
  hip M05.05- ☑
  knee M05.06- ☑
  multiple site M05.09
  shoulder M05.01- ☑
  vertebra — *see* Spondylitis, ankylosing
  wrist M05.03- ☑
Female genital cutting status — *see* Female genital mutilation status (FGM)
Female genital mutilation status (FGM) N90.810
  specified NEC N90.818
  type I (clitorectomy status) N90.811
  type II (clitorectomy with excision of labia minora status) N90.812
  type III (infibulation status) N90.813
  type IV N90.818
Femur, femoral — *see* condition
Fenestration, fenestrated (*see also* Imperfect, closure)
  aortico-pulmonary Q21.4
  cusps, heart valve NEC Q24.8
    pulmonary Q22.3
  pulmonic cusps Q22.3
Fernell's disease (aortic aneurysm) I71.9
Fetid
  breath R19.6
  sweat L75.0
Fetishism F65.0
  transvestic F65.1
Fetus, fetal (*see also* condition)
  alcohol syndrome (dysmorphic) Q86.0
  compressus O31.0- ☑
  hydantoin syndrome Q86.1

Fetus, fetal — *continued*
  lung tissue P28.0
  papyraceous O31.0- ☑
Fever (inanition) (of unknown origin) (persistent) (with chills) (with rigor) R50.9
  abortus A23.1
  Aden (dengue) A90
  African tick-borne A68.1
  American
    mountain (tick) A93.2
    spotted A77.0
  aphthous B08.8
  arbovirus, arboviral A94
    hemorrhagic A94
    specified NEC A93.8
  Argentinian hemorrhagic A96.0
  Assam B55.0
  Australian Q A78
  Bangkok hemorrhagic A91
  Barmah forest A92.8
  Bartonella A44.0
  bilious, hemoglobinuric B50.8
  blackwater B50.8
  blister B00.1
  Bolivian hemorrhagic A96.1
  Bonvale dam T73.3 ☑
  boutonneuse A77.1
  brain — *see* Encephalitis
  Brazilian purpuric A48.4
  breakbone A90
  Bullis A77.0
  Bunyamwera A92.8
  Burdwan B55.0
  Bwamba A92.8
  Cameroon — *see* Malaria
  Canton A75.9
  catarrhal (acute) J00
    chronic J31.0
  cat-scratch A28.1
  Central Asian hemorrhagic A98.0
  cerebral — *see* Encephalitis
  cerebrospinal meningococcal A39.0
  Chagres B50.9
  Chandipura A92.8
  Changuinola A93.1
  Charcot's (biliary) (hepatic) (intermittent) — *see* Calculus, bile duct
  Chikungunya (viral) (hemorrhagic) A92.0
  Chitral A93.1
  Colombo — *see* Fever, paratyphoid
  Colorado tick (virus) A93.2
  congestive (remittent) — *see* Malaria
  Congo virus A98.0
  continued malarial B50.9
  Corsican — *see* Malaria
  Crimean-Congo hemorrhagic A98.0
  Cyprus — *see* Brucellosis
  dandy A90
  deer fly — *see* Tularemia
  dengue (virus) A90
    hemorrhagic A91
    sandfly A93.1
  desert B38.0
  drug induced R50.2
  due to
    conditions classified elsewhere R50.81
    heat T67.0 ☑
  enteric A01.00
  enteroviral exanthematous (Boston exanthem) A88.0
  ephemeral (of unknown origin) R50.9
  epidemic hemorrhagic A98.5
  erysipelatous — *see* Erysipelas
  estivo-autumnal (malarial) B50.9
  famine A75.0
  five day A79.0
  following delivery O86.4
  Fort Bragg A27.89
  gastroenteric A01.00
  gastromalarial — *see* Malaria
  Gibraltar — *see* Brucellosis
  glandular — *see* Mononucleosis, infectious
  Guama (viral) A92.8
  Haverhill A25.1
  hay (allergic) J30.1
    with asthma (bronchial) J45.909
      with
        exacerbation (acute) J45.901
        status asthmaticus J45.902

Fever — continued
  hay — continued
    due to
      allergen other than pollen J30.89
      pollen, any plant or tree J30.1
  heat (effects) T67.0 ☑
  hematuric, bilious B50.8
  hemoglobinuric (malarial) (bilious) B50.8
  hemorrhagic (arthropod-borne) NOS A94
    with renal syndrome A98.5
    arenaviral A96.9
      specified NEC A96.8
    Argentinian A96.0
    Bangkok A91
    Bolivian A96.1
    Central Asian A98.0
    Chikungunya A92.0
    Crimean-Congo A98.0
    dengue (virus) A91
    epidemic A98.5
    Junin (virus) A96.0
    Korean A98.5
    Kyasanur forest A98.2
    Machupo (virus) A96.1
    mite-borne A93.8
    mosquito-borne A92.8
    Omsk A98.1
    Philippine A91
    Russian A98.5
    Singapore A91
    Southeast Asia A91
    Thailand A91
    tick-borne NEC A93.8
    viral A99
      specified NEC A98.8
  hepatic — see Cholecystitis
  herpetic — see Herpes
  icterohemorrhagic A27.0
  Indiana A93.8
  infective B99.9
    specified NEC B99.8
  intermittent (bilious) (see also Malaria)
    of unknown origin R50.9
    pernicious B50.9
  iodide R50.2
  Japanese river A75.3
  jungle (see also Malaria)
    yellow A95.0
  Junin (virus) hemorrhagic A96.0
  Katayama B65.2
  kedani A75.3
  Kenya (tick) A77.1
  Kew Garden A79.1
  Korean hemorrhagic A98.5
  Lassa A96.2
  Lone Star A77.0
  Machupo (virus) hemorrhagic A96.1
  malaria, malarial — see Malaria
  Malta A23.9
  Marseilles A77.1
  marsh — see Malaria
  Mayaro (viral) A92.8
  Mediterranean (see also Brucellosis) A23.9
    familial E85.0
    tick A77.1
  meningeal — see Meningitis
  Meuse A79.0
  Mexican A75.2
  mianeh A68.1
  miasmatic — see Malaria
  mosquito-borne (viral) A92.9
    hemorrhagic A92.8
  mountain (see also Brucellosis)
    meaning Rocky Mountain spotted fever A77.0
    tick (American) (Colorado) (viral) A93.2
  Mucambo (viral) A92.8
  mud A27.9
  Neapolitan — see Brucellosis
  neutropenic D70.9
  newborn P81.9
    environmental P81.0
  Nine-Mile A78
  non-exanthematous tick A93.2
  North Asian tick-borne A77.2
  Omsk hemorrhagic A98.1
  O'nyong-nyong (viral) A92.1
  Oropouche (viral) A93.0
  Oroya A44.0

Fever — continued
  paludal — see Malaria
  Panama (malarial) B50.9
  Pappataci A93.1
  paratyphoid A01.4
    A A01.1
    B A01.2
    C A01.3
  parrot A70
  periodic (Mediterranean) E85.0
  persistent (of unknown origin) R50.9
  petechial A39.0
  pharyngoconjunctival B30.2
  Philippine hemorrhagic A91
  phlebotomus A93.1
  Piry (virus) A93.8
  Pixuna (viral) A92.8
  Plasmodium ovale B53.0
  polioviral (nonparalytic) A80.4
  Pontiac A48.2
  postimmunization R50.83
  postoperative R50.82
    due to infection T81.4 ☑
  posttransfusion R50.84
  postvaccination R50.83
  presenting with conditions classified elsewhere R50.81
  pretibial A27.89
  puerperal O86.4
  Q A78
  quadrilateral A78
  quartan (malaria) B52.9
  Queensland (coastal) (tick) A77.3
  quintan A79.0
  rabbit — see Tularemia
  rat-bite A25.9
    due to
      Spirillum A25.0
      Streptobacillus moniliformis A25.1
  recurrent — see Fever, relapsing
  relapsing (Borrelia) A68.9
    Carter's (Asiatic) A68.1
    Dutton's (West African) A68.1
    Koch's A68.9
    louse-borne A68.0
    Novy's
      louse-borne A68.0
      tick-borne A68.1
    Obermeyer's (European) A68.0
    tick-borne A68.1
  remittent (bilious) (congestive) (gastric) — see Malaria
  rheumatic (active) (acute) (chronic) (subacute) A38
    with central nervous system involvement I02.9
    active with heart involvement — see category I01 ☑
    inactive or quiescent with
      cardiac hypertrophy I09.89
      carditis I09.9
      endocarditis I09.1
        aortic (valve) I06.9
          with mitral (valve) disease I08.0
        mitral (valve) I05.9
          with aortic (valve) disease I08.0
        pulmonary (valve) I09.89
        tricuspid (valve) I07.8
      heart disease NEC I09.89
      heart failure (congestive) (conditions in I50.9) I09.81
      left ventricular failure (conditions in I50.1) I09.81
      myocarditis, myocardial degeneration (conditions in I51.4) I09.0
      pancarditis I09.9
      pericarditis I09.2
  Rift Valley (viral) A92.4
  Rocky Mountain spotted A77.0
  rose J30.1
  Ross River B33.1
  Russian hemorrhagic A98.5
  San Joaquin (Valley) B38.0
  sandfly A93.1
  Sao Paulo A77.0
  scarlet A38.9
  seven day (leptospirosis) (autumnal) (Japanese) A27.89
    dengue A90
  shin-bone A79.0
  Singapore hemorrhagic A91
  solar A90
  Songo A98.5

Fever — continued
  sore B00.1
  South African tick-bite A68.1
  Southeast Asia hemorrhagic A91
  spinal — see Meningitis
  spirillary A25.0
  splenic — see Anthrax
  spotted A77.9
    American A77.0
    Brazilian A77.0
    cerebrospinal meningitis A39.0
    Colombian A77.0
    due to Rickettsia
      australis A77.3
      conorii A77.1
      rickettsii A77.0
      sibirica A77.2
      specified type NEC A77.8
    Ehrlichiosis A77.40
      due to
        E. chafeensis A77.41
        specified organism NEC A77.49
    Rocky Mountain A77.0
  steroid R50.2
  streptobacillary A25.1
  subtertian B50.9
  Sumatran mite A75.3
  sun A90
  swamp A27.9
  swine A02.8
  sylvatic, yellow A95.0
  Tahyna B33.8
  tertian — see Malaria, tertian
  Thailand hemorrhagic A91
  thermic T67.0 ☑
  three-day A93.1
  tick
    American mountain A93.2
    Colorado A93.2
    Kemerovo A93.8
    Mediterranean A77.1
    mountain A93.2
    nonexanthematous A93.2
    Quaranfil A93.8
  tick-bite NEC A93.8
  tick-borne (hemorrhagic) NEC A93.8
  trench A79.0
  tsutsugamushi A75.3
  typhogastric A01.00
  typhoid (abortive) (hemorrhagic) (intermittent) (malignant) A01.00
    complicated by
      arthritis A01.04
      heart involvement A01.02
      meningitis A01.01
      osteomyelitis A01.05
      pneumonia A01.03
      specified NEC A01.09
  typhomalarial — see Malaria
  typhus — see Typhus (fever)
  undulant — see Brucellosis
  unknown origin R50.9
  uveoparotid D86.89
  valley B38.0
  Venezuelan equine A92.2
  vesicular stomatitis A93.8
  viral hemorrhagic — see Fever, hemorrhagic, by type of virus
  Volhynian A79.0
  Wesselsbron (viral) A92.8
  West
    African B50.8
    Nile (viral) A92.30
      with
        complications NEC A92.39
        cranial nerve disorders A92.32
        encephalitis A92.31
        encephalomyelitis A92.31
        neurologic manifestation NEC A92.32
        optic neuritis A92.32
        polyradiculitis A92.32
  Whitmore's — see Melioidosis
  Wolhynian A79.0
  worm B83.9
  yellow A95.9
    jungle A95.0
    sylvatic A95.0
    urban A95.1

Fever — *continued*
 Zika (viral) A92.8
Fibrillation
 atrial or auricular (established) I48.91
  chronic I48.2
  paroxysmal I48.0
  permanent I48.2
  persistent I48.1
 cardiac I49.8
 heart I49.8
 muscular M62.89
 ventricular I49.01
Fibrin
 ball or bodies, pleural (sac) J94.1
 chamber, anterior (eye) (gelatinous exudate) — *see*
   Iridocyclitis, acute
Fibrinogenolysis — *see* Fibrinolysis
Fibrinogenopenia D68.8
 acquired D65
 congenital D68.2
Fibrinolysis (hemorrhagic) (acquired) D65
 antepartum hemorrhage — *see* Hemorrhage, antepartum, with coagulation defect
 following
  abortion — *see* Abortion by type complicated by
    hemorrhage
  ectopic or molar pregnancy O08.1
 intrapartum O67.0
 newborn, transient P60
 postpartum O72.3
Fibrinopenia (hereditary) D68.2
 acquired D68.4
Fibrinopurulent — *see* condition
Fibrinous — *see* condition
Fibroadenoma
 cellular intracanalicular D24- ☑
 giant D24- ☑
 intracanalicular
  cellular D24- ☑
  giant D24- ☑
  specified site — *see* Neoplasm, benign, by site
  unspecified site D24- ☑
 juvenile D24- ☑
 pericanalicular
  specified site — *see* Neoplasm, benign, by site
  unspecified site D24- ☑
 phyllodes D24- ☑
 prostate D29.1
 specified site NEC — *see* Neoplasm, benign, by site
 unspecified site D24- ☑
Fibroadenosis, breast (chronic) (cystic) (diffuse) (periodic) (segmental) N60.2- ☑
Fibroangioma (*see also* Neoplasm, benign, by site)
 juvenile
  specified site — *see* Neoplasm, benign, by site
  unspecified site D10.6
Fibrochondrosarcoma — *see* Neoplasm, cartilage,
   malignant
Fibrocystic
 disease (*see also* Fibrosis, cystic)
  breast — *see* Mastopathy, cystic
  jaw M27.49
  kidney (congenital) Q61.8
  liver Q44.6
  pancreas E84.9
 kidney (congenital) Q61.8
Fibrodysplasia ossificans progressiva — *see* Myositis,
   ossificans, progressiva
Fibroelastosis (cordis) (endocardial) (endomyocardial)
   I42.4
Fibroid (tumor) (*see also* Neoplasm, connective tissue,
   benign)
 disease, lung (chronic) — *see* Fibrosis, lung
 heart (disease) — *see* Myocarditis
 in pregnancy or childbirth O34.1- ☑
  causing obstructed labor O65.5
 induration, lung (chronic) — *see* Fibrosis, lung
 lung — *see* Fibrosis, lung
 pneumonia (chronic) — *see* Fibrosis, lung
 uterus D25.9
Fibrolipoma — *see* Lipoma
Fibroliposarcoma — *see* Neoplasm, connective tissue,
   malignant
Fibroma (*see also* Neoplasm, connective tissue, benign)
 ameloblastic — *see* Cyst, calcifying odontogenic
 bone (nonossifying) — *see* Disorder, bone, specified
   type NEC

Fibroma — *continued*
 bone — *see* Disorder, bone, specified type — *continued*
  ossifying — *see* Neoplasm, bone, benign
 cementifying — *see* Neoplasm, bone, benign
 chondromyxoid — *see* Neoplasm, bone, benign
 desmoplastic — *see* Neoplasm, connective tissue,
   uncertain behavior
 durum — *see* Neoplasm, connective tissue, benign
 fascial — *see* Neoplasm, connective tissue, benign
 invasive — *see* Neoplasm, connective tissue, uncertain
   behavior
 molle — *see* Lipoma
 myxoid — *see* Neoplasm, connective tissue, benign
 nasopharynx, nasopharyngeal (juvenile) D10.6
 nonosteogenic (nonossifying) — *see* Dysplasia, fibrous
 odontogenic (central) — *see* Cyst, calcifying odontogenic
 ossifying — *see* Neoplasm, bone, benign
 periosteal — *see* Neoplasm, bone, benign
 soft — *see* Lipoma
Fibromatosis M72.9
 abdominal — *see* Neoplasm, connective tissue, uncertain behavior
 aggressive — *see* Neoplasm, connective tissue, uncertain behavior
 congenital generalized — *see* Neoplasm, connective
   tissue, uncertain behavior
 Dupuytren's M72.0
 gingival K06.1
 palmar (fascial) M72.0
 plantar (fascial) M72.2
 pseudosarcomatous (proliferative) (subcutaneous)
   M72.4
 retroperitoneal D48.3
 specified NEC M72.8
Fibromyalgia M79.7
Fibromyoma (*see also* Neoplasm, connective tissue, benign)
 uterus (corpus) (*see also* Leiomyoma, uterus)
  in pregnancy or childbirth — *see* Fibroid, in preg-
    nancy or childbirth
  causing obstructed labor O65.5
Fibromyositis M79.7
Fibromyxolipoma D17.9
Fibromyxoma — *see* Neoplasm, connective tissue, benign
Fibromyxosarcoma — *see* Neoplasm, connective tissue,
   malignant
Fibro-odontoma, ameloblastic — *see* Cyst, calcifying
   odontogenic
Fibro-osteoma — *see* Neoplasm, bone, benign
Fibroplasia, retrolental H35.17- ☑
Fibropurulent — *see* condition
Fibrosarcoma (*see also* Neoplasm, connective tissue,
   malignant)
 ameloblastic C41.1
  upper jaw (bone) C41.0
 congenital — *see* Neoplasm, connective tissue, malignant
 fascial — *see* Neoplasm, connective tissue, malignant
 infantile — *see* Neoplasm, connective tissue, malignant
 odontogenic C41.1
  upper jaw (bone) C41.0
 periosteal — *see* Neoplasm, bone, malignant
Fibrosclerosis
 breast N60.3- ☑
 multifocal M35.5
 penis (corpora cavernosa) N48.6
Fibrosis, fibrotic
 adrenal (gland) E27.8
 amnion O41.8X- ☑
 anal papillae K62.89
 arteriocapillary — *see* Arteriosclerosis
 bladder N32.89
  interstitial — *see* Cystitis, chronic, interstitial
  localized submucosal — *see* Cystitis, chronic, inter-
    stitial
  panmural — *see* Cystitis, chronic, interstitial
 breast — *see* Fibrosclerosis, breast
 capillary (*see also* Arteriosclerosis) I70.90
  lung (chronic) — *see* Fibrosis, lung
 cardiac — *see* Myocarditis
 cervix N88.8
 chorion O41.8X- ☑
 corpus cavernosum (sclerosing) N48.6

Fibrosis, fibrotic — *continued*
 cystic (of pancreas) E84.9
  with
   distal intestinal obstruction syndrome E84.19
   fecal impaction E84.19
   intestinal manifestations NEC E84.19
   pulmonary manifestations E84.0
   specified manifestations NEC E84.8
 due to device, implant or graft (*see also* Complications,
   by site and type, specified NEC) T85.82 ☑
  arterial graft NEC T82.828 ☑
  breast (implant) T85.82 ☑
  catheter NEC T85.82 ☑
   dialysis (renal) T82.828 ☑
    intraperitoneal T85.82 ☑
   infusion NEC T82.828 ☑
    spinal (epidural) (subdural) T85.82 ☑
   urinary (indwelling) T83.82 ☑
  electronic (electrode) (pulse generator) (stimulator)
   bone T84.82 ☑
   cardiac T82.827 ☑
   nervous system (brain) (peripheral nerve)
     (spinal) T85.82 ☑
   urinary T83.82 ☑
  fixation, internal (orthopedic) NEC T84.82 ☑
  gastrointestinal (bile duct) (esophagus) T85.82 ☑
  genital NEC T83.82 ☑
  heart NEC T82.827 ☑
  joint prosthesis T84.82 ☑
  ocular (corneal graft) (orbital implant) NEC
    T85.82 ☑
  orthopedic NEC T84.82 ☑
  specified NEC T85.82 ☑
  urinary NEC T83.82 ☑
  vascular NEC T82.828 ☑
  ventricular intracranial shunt T85.82 ☑
 ejaculatory duct N50.8
 endocardium — *see* Endocarditis
 endomyocardial (tropical) I42.3
 epididymis N50.8
 eye muscle — *see* Strabismus, mechanical
 heart — *see* Myocarditis
 hepatic — *see* Fibrosis, liver
 hepatolienal (portal hypertension) K76.6
 hepatosplenic (portal hypertension) K76.6
 infrapatellar fat pad M79.4
 intrascrotal N50.8
 kidney N26.9
 liver K74.0
  with sclerosis K74.2
  alcoholic K70.2
 lung (atrophic) (chronic) (confluent) (massive) (perialveolar) (peribronchial) J84.10
  with
   anthracosilicosis J60
   anthracosis J60
   asbestosis J61
   bagassosis J67.1
   bauxite J63.1
   berylliosis J63.2
   byssinosis J66.0
   calcicosis J62.8
   chalicosis J62.8
   dust reticulation J64
   farmer's lung J67.0
   ganister disease J62.8
   graphite J63.3
   pneumoconiosis NOS J64
   siderosis J63.4
   silicosis J62.8
  capillary J84.10
  congenital P27.8
  diffuse (idiopathic) J84.10
   chemicals, gases, fumes or vapors (inhalation)
     J68.4
   interstitial J84.10
    acute J84.114
   talc J62.0
  following radiation J70.1
  idiopathic J84.112
  postinflammatory J84.10
  silicotic J62.8
  tuberculous — *see* Tuberculosis, pulmonary
 lymphatic gland I89.8
 median bar — *see* Hyperplasia, prostate
 mediastinum (idiopathic) J98.5
 meninges G96.19

Fibrosis, fibrotic — *continued*
- myocardium, myocardial — *see* Myocarditis
- ovary N83.8
- oviduct N83.8
- pancreas K86.8
- penis NEC N48.6
- pericardium I31.0
- perineum, in pregnancy or childbirth O34.7- ☑
  - causing obstructed labor O65.5
- pleura J94.1
- popliteal fat pad M79.4
- prostate (chronic) — *see* Hyperplasia, prostate
- pulmonary (*see also* Fibrosis, lung) J84.10
  - congenital P27.8
  - idiopathic J84.112
- rectal sphincter K62.89
- retroperitoneal, idiopathic (with ureteral obstruction) N13.5
  - with infection N13.6
- sclerosing mesenteric (idiopathic) K65.4
- scrotum N50.8
- seminal vesicle N50.8
- senile R54
- skin L90.5
- spermatic cord N50.8
- spleen D73.89
  - in schistosomiasis (bilharziasis) B65.9 [D77]
- subepidermal nodular — *see* Neoplasm, skin, benign
- submucous (oral) (tongue) K13.5
- testis N44.8
  - chronic, due to syphilis A52.76
- thymus (gland) E32.8
- tongue, submucous K13.5
- tunica vaginalis N50.8
- uterus (non-neoplastic) N85.8
- vagina N89.8
- valve, heart — *see* Endocarditis
- vas deferens N50.8
- vein I87.8

Fibrositis (periarticular) M79.7
- nodular, chronic (Jaccoud's) (rheumatoid) — *see* Arthropathy, postrheumatic, chronic

Fibrothorax J94.1
Fibrotic — *see* Fibrosis
Fibrous — *see* condition
Fibroxanthoma (*see also* Neoplasm, connective tissue, benign)
- atypical — *see* Neoplasm, connective tissue, uncertain behavior
- malignant — *see* Neoplasm, connective tissue, malignant

Fibroxanthosarcoma — *see* Neoplasm, connective tissue, malignant
Fiedler's
- disease (icterohemorrhagic leptospirosis) A27.0
- myocarditis (acute) I40.1

Fifth disease B08.3
- venereal A55

Filaria, filarial, filariasis — *see* Infestation, filarial
Filatov's disease — *see* Mononucleosis, infectious
File-cutter's disease — *see* Poisoning, lead
Filling defect
- biliary tract R93.2
- bladder R93.4
- duodenum R93.3
- gallbladder R93.2
- gastrointestinal tract R93.3
- intestine R93.3
- kidney R93.4
- stomach R93.3
- ureter R93.4

Fimbrial cyst Q50.4
Financial problem affecting care NOS Z59.9
- bankruptcy Z59.8
- foreclosure on loan Z59.8

Findings, abnormal, inconclusive, without diagnosis (*see also* Abnormal)
- 17-ketosteroids, elevated R82.5
- acetonuria R82.4
- alcohol in blood R78.0
- anisocytosis R71.8
- antenatal screening of mother O28.9
  - biochemical O28.1
  - chromosomal O28.5
  - cytological O28.2
  - genetic O28.5
  - hematological O28.0
  - radiological O28.4

Findings, abnormal, inconclusive, without diagnosis — *continued*
- antenatal screening of mother — *continued*
  - specified NEC O28.8
  - ultrasonic O28.3
- antibody titer, elevated R76.0
- anticardiolipin antibody R76.0
- antiphosphatidylglycerol antibody R76.0
- antiphosphatidylinositol antibody R76.0
- antiphosphatidylserine antibody R76.0
- antiphospholipid antibody R76.0
- bacteriuria N39.0
- bicarbonate E87.8
- bile in urine R82.2
- blood sugar R73.09
  - high R73.9
  - low (transient) E16.2
- body fluid or substance, specified NEC R88.8
- casts, urine R82.99
- catecholamines R82.5
- cells, urine R82.99
- chloride E87.8
- cholesterol E78.9
  - high E78.0
    - with high triglycerides E78.2
- chyluria R82.0
- cloudy
  - dialysis effluent R88.0
  - urine R82.90
- creatinine clearance R94.4
- crystals, urine R82.99
- culture
  - blood R78.81
  - positive — *see* Positive, culture
- echocardiogram R93.1
- electrolyte level, urinary R82.99
- function study NEC R94.8
  - bladder R94.8
  - endocrine NEC R94.7
    - thyroid R94.6
  - kidney R94.4
  - liver R94.5
  - pancreas R94.8
  - placenta R94.8
  - pulmonary R94.2
  - spleen R94.8
- gallbladder, nonvisualization R93.2
- glucose (tolerance test) (non-fasting) R73.09
- glycosuria R81
- heart
  - shadow R93.1
  - sounds R01.2
- hematinuria R82.3
- hematocrit drop (precipitous) R71.0
- hemoglobinuria R82.3
- human papillomavirus (HPV) DNA test positive
  - cervix
    - high risk R87.810
    - low risk R87.820
  - vagina
    - high risk R87.811
    - low risk R87.821
- in blood (of substance not normally found in blood) R78.9
  - addictive drug NEC R78.4
  - alcohol (excessive level) R78.0
  - cocaine R78.2
  - hallucinogen R78.3
  - heavy metals (abnormal level) R78.79
  - lead R78.71
  - lithium (abnormal level) R78.89
  - opiate drug R78.1
  - psychotropic drug R78.5
  - specified substance NEC R78.89
  - steroid agent R78.6
- indoleacetic acid, elevated R82.5
- ketonuria R82.4
- lactic acid dehydrogenase (LDH) R74.0
- liver function test R79.89
- mammogram NEC R92.8
  - calcification (calculus) R92.1
  - inconclusive result (due to dense breasts) R92.2
  - microcalcification R92.0
- mediastinal shift R93.8
- melanin, urine R82.99
- myoglobinuria R82.1
- neonatal screening P09
- nonvisualization of gallbladder R93.2

Findings, abnormal, inconclusive, without diagnosis — *continued*
- odor of urine NOS R82.90
- Papanicolaou cervix R87.619
  - non-atypical endometrial cells R87.618
- pneumoencephalogram R93.0
- poikilocytosis R71.8
- potassium (deficiency) E87.6
  - excess E87.5
- PPD R76.11
- radiologic (X-ray) R93.8
  - abdomen R93.5
  - biliary tract R93.2
  - breast R92.8
  - gastrointestinal tract R93.3
  - genitourinary organs R93.8
  - head R93.0
  - inconclusive due to excess body fat of patient R93.9
  - intrathoracic organs NEC R93.1
  - placenta R93.8
  - retroperitoneum R93.5
  - skin R93.8
  - skull R93.0
  - subcutaneous tissue R93.8
- red blood cell (count) (morphology) (sickling) (volume) R71.8
- scan NEC R94.8
  - bladder R94.8
  - bone R94.8
  - kidney R94.4
  - liver R93.2
  - lung R94.2
  - pancreas R94.8
  - placental R94.8
  - spleen R94.8
  - thyroid R94.6
- sedimentation rate, elevated R70.0
- SGOT R74.0
- SGPT R74.0
- sodium (deficiency) E87.1
  - excess E87.0
- specified body fluid NEC R88.8
- stress test R94.39
- thyroid (function) (metabolic rate) (scan) (uptake) R94.6
- transaminase (level) R74.0
- triglycerides E78.9
  - high E78.1
    - with high cholesterol E78.2
- tuberculin skin test (without active tuberculosis) R76.11
- urine R82.90
  - acetone R82.4
  - bacteria N39.0
  - bile R82.2
  - casts or cells R82.99
  - chyle R82.0
  - culture positive R82.7
  - glucose R81
  - hemoglobin R82.3
  - ketone R82.4
  - sugar R81
- vanillylmandelic acid (VMA), elevated R82.5
- vectorcardiogram (VCG) R94.39
- ventriculogram R93.0
- white blood cell (count) (differential) (morphology) D72.9
- xerography R92.8

Finger — *see* condition
Fire, Saint Anthony's — *see* Erysipelas
Fire-setting
- pathological (compulsive) F63.1

Fish hook stomach K31.89
Fishmeal-worker's lung J67.8
Fissure, fissured
- anus, anal K60.2
  - acute K60.0
  - chronic K60.1
  - congenital Q43.8
- ear, lobule, congenital Q17.8
- epiglottis (congenital) Q31.8
- larynx J38.7
  - congenital Q31.8
- lip K13.0
  - congenital — *see* Cleft, lip
- nipple N64.0
  - associated with lactation O92.13

Fissure, fissured — *continued*
- nipple — *continued*
  - associated with — *continued*
    - pregnancy O92.11- ☑
    - puerperium O92.12
- nose Q30.2
- palate (congenital) — *see* Cleft, palate
- skin R23.4
- spine (congenital) (*see also* Spina bifida)
  - with hydrocephalus — *see* Spina bifida, by site, with hydrocephalus
- tongue (acquired) K14.5
  - congenital Q38.3

Fistula (cutaneous) L98.8
- abdomen (wall) K63.2
  - bladder N32.2
  - intestine NEC K63.2
  - ureter N28.89
  - uterus N82.5
- abdominorectal K63.2
- abdominosigmoidal K63.2
- abdominothoracic J86.0
- abdominouterine N82.5
  - congenital Q51.7
- abdominovesical N32.2
- accessory sinuses — *see* Sinusitis
- actinomycotic — *see* Actinomycosis
- alveolar antrum — *see* Sinusitis, maxillary
- alveolar process K04.6
- anorectal K60.5
- antrobuccal — *see* Sinusitis, maxillary
- antrum — *see* Sinusitis, maxillary
- anus, anal (recurrent) (infectional) K60.3
  - congenital Q43.6
    - with absence, atresia and stenosis Q42.2
  - tuberculous A18.32
- aorta-duodenal I77.2
- appendix, appendicular K38.3
- arteriovenous (acquired) (nonruptured) I77.0
  - brain I67.1
    - congenital Q28.2
      - ruptured I60.8
    - ruptured I60.8
  - cerebral — *see* Fistula, arteriovenous, brain
  - congenital (peripheral) (*see also* Malformation, arteriovenous)
    - brain Q28.2
      - ruptured I60.8
    - coronary Q24.5
    - pulmonary Q25.72
  - coronary I25.41
    - congenital Q24.5
  - pulmonary I28.0
    - congenital Q25.72
  - surgically created (for dialysis) Z99.2
    - complication — *see* Complication, arteriovenous, fistula, surgically created
  - traumatic — *see* Injury, blood vessel
- artery I77.2
- aural (mastoid) — *see* Mastoiditis, chronic
- auricle (*see also* Disorder, pinna, specified type NEC)
  - congenital Q18.1
- Bartholin's gland N82.8
- bile duct (common) (hepatic) K83.3
  - with calculus, stones — *see* Calculus, bile duct
- biliary (tract) — *see* Fistula, bile duct
- bladder (sphincter) NEC (*see also* Fistula, vesico-) N32.2
  - into seminal vesicle N32.2
- bone (*see also* Disorder, bone, specified type NEC)
  - with osteomyelitis, chronic — *see* Osteomyelitis, chronic, with draining sinus
- brain G93.89
  - arteriovenous (acquired) I67.1
    - congenital Q28.2
- branchial (cleft) Q18.0
- branchiogenous Q18.0
- breast N61
  - puerperal, postpartum or gestational, due to mastitis (purulent) — *see* Mastitis, obstetric, purulent
- bronchial J86.0
- bronchocutaneous, bronchomediastinal, bronchopleural, bronchopleuromediastinal (infective) J86.0
  - tuberculous NEC A15.5
- bronchoesophageal J86.0
  - congenital Q39.2
    - with atresia of esophagus Q39.1
- bronchovisceral J86.0

Fistula — *continued*
- buccal cavity (infective) K12.2
- cecosigmoidal K63.2
- cecum K63.2
- cerebrospinal (fluid) G96.0
- cervical, lateral Q18.1
- cervicoaural Q18.1
- cervicosigmoidal N82.4
- cervicovesical N82.1
- cervix N82.8
- chest (wall) J86.0
- cholecystenteric — *see* Fistula, gallbladder
- cholecystocolic — *see* Fistula, gallbladder
- cholecystocolonic — *see* Fistula, gallbladder
- cholecystoduodenal — *see* Fistula, gallbladder
- cholecystogastric — *see* Fistula, gallbladder
- cholecystointestinal — *see* Fistula, gallbladder
- choledochoduodenal — *see* Fistula, bile duct
- cholocolic K82.3
- coccyx — *see* Sinus, pilonidal
- colon K63.2
- colostomy K94.09
- common duct — *see* Fistula, bile duct
- congenital, site not listed — *see* Anomaly, by site
- coronary, arteriovenous I25.41
  - congenital Q24.5
- costal region J86.0
- cul-de-sac, Douglas' N82.8
- cystic duct (*see also* Fistula, gallbladder)
  - congenital Q44.5
- dental K04.6
- diaphragm J86.0
- duodenum K31.6
- ear (external) (canal) — *see* Disorder, ear, external, specified type NEC
- enterocolic K63.2
- enterocutaneous K63.2
- enterouterine N82.4
  - congenital Q51.7
- enterovaginal N82.4
  - congenital Q52.2
  - large intestine N82.3
  - small intestine N82.2
- enterovesical N32.1
- epididymis N50.8
  - tuberculous A18.15
- esophagobronchial J86.0
  - congenital Q39.2
    - with atresia of esophagus Q39.1
- esophagocutaneous K22.8
- esophagopleural-cutaneous J86.0
- esophagotracheal J86.0
  - congenital Q39.2
    - with atresia of esophagus Q39.1
- esophagus K22.8
  - congenital Q39.2
    - with atresia of esophagus Q39.1
- ethmoid — *see* Sinusitis, ethmoidal
- eyeball (cornea) (sclera) — *see* Disorder, globe, hypotony
- eyelid H01.8
- fallopian tube, external N82.5
- fecal K63.2
  - congenital Q43.6
  - from periapical abscess K04.6
- frontal sinus — *see* Sinusitis, frontal
- gallbladder K82.3
  - with calculus, cholelithiasis, stones — *see* Calculus, gallbladder
- gastric K31.6
- gastrocolic K31.6
  - congenital Q40.2
  - tuberculous A18.32
- gastroenterocolic K31.6
- gastroesophageal K31.6
- gastrojejunal K31.6
- gastrojejunocolic K31.6
- genital tract (female) N82.9
  - specified NEC N82.8
  - to intestine NEC N82.4
  - to skin N82.5
- hepatic artery-portal vein, congenital Q26.6
- hepatopleural J86.0
- hepatopulmonary J86.0
- ileorectal or ileosigmoidal K63.2
- ileovaginal N82.4
- ileovesical N32.1
- ileum K63.2

Fistula — *continued*
- in ano K60.3
  - tuberculous A18.32
- inner ear (labyrinth) — *see* subcategory H83.1 ☑
- intestine NEC K63.2
- intestinocolonic (abdominal) K63.2
- intestinoureteral N28.89
- intestinouterine N82.4
- intestinovaginal N82.4
  - large intestine N82.3
  - small intestine N82.2
- intestinovesical N32.1
- ischiorectal (fossa) K61.3
- jejunum K63.2
- joint M25.10
  - ankle M25.17- ☑
  - elbow M25.12- ☑
  - foot joint M25.17- ☑
  - hand joint M25.14- ☑
  - hip M25.15- ☑
  - knee M25.16- ☑
  - shoulder M25.11- ☑
  - specified joint NEC M25.18
  - tuberculous — *see* Tuberculosis, joint
  - vertebrae M25.18
  - wrist M25.13- ☑
- kidney N28.89
- labium (majus) (minus) N82.8
- labyrinth — *see* subcategory H83.1 ☑
- lacrimal (gland) (sac) H04.61- ☑
- lacrimonasal duct — *see* Fistula, lacrimal
- laryngotracheal, congenital Q34.8
- larynx J38.7
- lip K13.0
  - congenital Q38.0
- lumbar, tuberculous A18.01
- lung J86.0
- lymphatic I89.8
- mammary (gland) N61
- mastoid (process) (region) — *see* Mastoiditis, chronic
- maxillary J32.0
- medial, face and neck Q18.8
- mediastinal J86.0
- mediastinobronchial J86.0
- mediastinocutaneous J86.0
- middle ear — *see* subcategory H74.8 ☑
- mouth K12.2
- nasal J34.89
  - sinus — *see* Sinusitis
- nasopharynx J39.2
- nipple N64.0
- nose J34.89
- oral (cutaneous) K12.2
  - maxillary J32.0
  - nasal (with cleft palate) — *see* Cleft, palate
- orbit, orbital — *see* Disorder, orbit, specified type NEC
- oroantral J32.0
- oviduct, external N82.5
- palate (hard) M27.8
- pancreatic K86.8
- pancreaticoduodenal K86.8
- parotid (gland) K11.4
  - region K12.2
- penis N48.89
- perianal K60.3
- pericardium (pleura) (sac) — *see* Pericarditis
- pericecal K63.2
- perineorectal K60.4
- perineosigmoidal K63.2
- perineum, perineal (with urethral involvement) NEC N36.0
  - tuberculous A18.13
  - ureter N28.89
- perirectal K60.4
  - tuberculous A18.32
- peritoneum K65.9
- pharyngoesophageal J39.2
- pharynx J39.2
  - branchial cleft (congenital) Q18.0
- pilonidal (infected) (rectum) — *see* Sinus, pilonidal
- pleura, pleural, pleurocutaneous, pleuroperitoneal J86.0
  - tuberculous NEC A15.6
- pleuropericardial I31.8
- portal vein-hepatic artery, congenital Q26.6
- postauricular H70.81- ☑
- postoperative, persistent T81.83 ☑
  - specified site — *see* Fistula, by site

Fistula — *continued*
- preauricular (congenital) Q18.1
- prostate N42.89
- pulmonary J86.0
  - arteriovenous I28.0
    - congenital Q25.72
  - tuberculous — *see* Tuberculosis, pulmonary
- pulmonoperitoneal J86.0
- rectolabial N82.4
- rectosigmoid (intercommunicating) K63.2
- rectoureteral N28.89
- rectourethral N36.0
  - congenital Q64.73
- rectouterine N82.4
  - congenital Q51.7
- rectovaginal N82.3
  - congenital Q52.2
  - tuberculous A18.18
- rectovesical N32.1
  - congenital Q64.79
- rectovesicovaginal N82.3
- rectovulval N82.4
  - congenital Q52.79
- rectum (to skin) K60.4
  - congenital Q43.6
    - with absence, atresia and stenosis Q42.0
  - tuberculous A18.32
- renal N28.89
- retroauricular — *see* Fistula, postauricular
- salivary duct or gland (any) K11.4
  - congenital Q38.4
- scrotum (urinary) N50.8
  - tuberculous A18.15
- semicircular canals — *see* subcategory H83.1 ☑
- sigmoid K63.2
  - to bladder N32.1
- sinus — *see* Sinusitis
- skin L98.8
  - to genital tract (female) N82.5
- splenocolic D73.89
- stercoral K63.2
- stomach K31.6
- sublingual gland K11.4
- submandibular gland K11.4
- submaxillary (gland) K11.4
  - region K12.2
- thoracic J86.0
  - duct I89.8
- thoracoabdominal J86.0
- thoracogastric J86.0
- thoracointestinal J86.0
- thorax J86.0
- thyroglossal duct Q89.2
- thyroid E07.89
- trachea, congenital (external) (internal) Q32.1
- tracheoesophageal J86.0
  - congenital Q39.2
    - with atresia of esophagus Q39.1
  - following tracheostomy J95.04
- traumatic arteriovenous — *see* Injury, blood vessel, by site
- tuberculous — *code by* site under Tuberculosis
- typhoid A01.09
- umbilicourinary Q64.8
- urachus, congenital Q64.4
- ureter (persistent) N28.89
- ureteroabdominal N28.89
- ureterorectal N28.89
- ureterosigmoido-abdominal N28.89
- ureterovaginal N82.1
- ureterovesical N32.2
- urethra N36.0
  - congenital Q64.79
  - tuberculous A18.13
- urethroperineal N36.0
- urethroperineovesical N32.2
- urethrorectal N36.0
  - congenital Q64.73
- urethroscrotal N50.8
- urethrovaginal N82.1
- urethrovesical N32.2
- urinary (tract) (persistent) (recurrent) N36.0
- uteroabdominal N82.5
  - congenital Q51.7
- uteroenteric, uterointestinal N82.4
  - congenital Q51.7
- uterorectal N82.4
  - congenital Q51.7

Fistula — *continued*
- uteroureteric N82.1
- uterourethral Q51.7
- uterovaginal N82.8
- uterovesical N82.1
  - congenital Q51.7
- uterus N82.8
- vagina (postpartal) (wall) N82.8
- vaginocutaneous (postpartal) N82.5
- vaginointestinal NEC N82.4
  - large intestine N82.3
  - small intestine N82.2
- vaginoperineal N82.5
- vasocutaneous, congenital Q55.7
- vesical NEC N32.2
- vesicoabdominal N32.2
- vesicocervicovaginal N82.1
- vesicocolic N32.1
- vesicocutaneous N32.2
- vesicoenteric N32.1
- vesicointestinal N32.1
- vesicometrorectal N82.4
- vesicoperineal N32.2
- vesicorectal N32.1
  - congenital Q64.79
- vesicosigmoidal N32.1
- vesicosigmoidovaginal N82.3
- vesicoureteral N32.2
- vesicoureterovaginal N82.1
- vesicourethral N32.2
- vesicourethrorectal N32.1
- vesicouterine N82.1
  - congenital Q51.7
- vesicovaginal N82.0
- vulvorectal N82.4
  - congenital Q52.79

Fit R56.9
- epileptic — *see* Epilepsy
- fainting R55
- hysterical F44.5
- newborn P90

Fitting (and adjustment) (of)
- artificial
  - arm — *see* Admission, adjustment, artificial, arm
  - breast Z44.3 ☑
  - eye Z44.2 ☑
  - leg — *see* Admission, adjustment, artificial, leg
- automatic implantable cardiac defibrillator (with synchronous cardiac pacemaker) Z45.02
- brain neuropacemaker Z46.2
  - implanted Z45.42
- cardiac defibrillator — *see* Fitting (and adjustment) (of), automatic implantable cardiac defibrillator
- catheter, non-vascular Z46.82
- colostomy belt Z46.89
- contact lenses Z46.0
- cystostomy device Z46.6
- defibrillator, cardiac — *see* Fitting (and adjustment) (of), automatic implantable cardiac defibrillator
- dentures Z46.3
- device NOS Z46.9
  - abdominal Z46.89
  - gastrointestinal NEC Z46.59
  - implanted NEC Z45.89
  - nervous system Z46.2
    - implanted — *see* Admission, adjustment, device, implanted, nervous system
  - orthodontic Z46.4
  - orthoptic Z46.0
  - orthotic Z46.89
  - prosthetic (external) Z44.9
    - breast Z44.3 ☑
    - dental Z46.3
    - eye Z44.2 ☑
    - specified NEC Z44.8
  - specified NEC Z46.89
  - substitution
    - auditory Z46.2
      - implanted — *see* Admission, adjustment, device, implanted, hearing device
    - nervous system Z46.2
      - implanted — *see* Admission, adjustment, device, implanted, nervous system
    - visual Z46.2
      - implanted Z45.31
  - urinary Z46.6
- gastric lap band Z46.51
- gastrointestinal appliance NEC Z46.59

Fitting — *continued*
- glasses (reading) Z46.0
- hearing aid Z46.1
- ileostomy device Z46.89
- insulin pump Z46.81
- intestinal appliance NEC Z46.89
- myringotomy device (stent) (tube) Z45.82
- neuropacemaker Z46.2
  - implanted Z45.42
- non-vascular catheter Z46.82
- orthodontic device Z46.4
- orthopedic device (brace) (cast) (corset) (shoes) Z46.89
- pacemaker (cardiac) Z45.018
  - nervous system (brain) (peripheral nerve) (spinal cord) Z46.2
    - implanted Z45.42
  - pulse generator Z45.010
- portacath (port-a-cath) Z45.2
- prosthesis (external) Z44.9
  - arm — *see* Admission, adjustment, artificial, arm
  - breast Z44.3 ☑
  - dental Z46.3
  - eye Z44.2 ☑
  - leg — *see* Admission, adjustment, artificial, leg
  - specified NEC Z44.8
- spectacles Z46.0
- wheelchair Z46.89

Fitzhugh-Curtis syndrome
- due to
  - Chlamydia trachomatis A74.81
  - Neisseria gonorrhorea (gonococcal peritonitis) A54.85

Fitz's syndrome (acute hemorrhagic pancreatitis) K85.8

Fixation
- joint — *see* Ankylosis
- larynx J38.7
- stapes — *see* Ankylosis, ear ossicles
  - deafness — *see* Deafness, conductive
- uterus (acquired) — *see* Malposition, uterus
- vocal cord J38.3

Flabby ridge K06.8

Flaccid (*see also* condition)
- palate, congenital Q38.5

Flail
- chest S22.5 ☑
  - newborn (birth injury) P13.8
- joint (paralytic) M25.20
  - ankle M25.27- ☑
  - elbow M25.22- ☑
  - foot joint M25.27- ☑
  - hand joint M25.24- ☑
  - hip M25.25- ☑
  - knee M25.26- ☑
  - shoulder M25.21- ☑
  - specified joint NEC M25.28
  - wrist M25.23- ☑

Flajani's disease — *see* Hyperthyroidism, with, goiter (diffuse)

Flap, liver K71.3

Flashbacks (residual to hallucinogen use) F16.283

Flat
- chamber (eye) — *see* Disorder, globe, hypotony, flat anterior chamber
- chest, congenital Q67.8
- foot (acquired) (fixed type) (painful) (postural) (*see also* Deformity, limb, flat foot)
  - congenital (rigid) (spastic (everted)) Q66.5- ☑
  - rachitic sequelae (late effect) E64.3
- organ or site, congenital NEC — *see* Anomaly, by site
- pelvis M95.5
  - with disproportion (fetopelvic) O33.0
    - causing obstructed labor O65.0
  - congenital Q74.2

Flatau-Schilder disease G37.0

Flatback syndrome M40.30
- lumbar region M40.36
- lumbosacral region M40.37
- thoracolumbar region M40.35

Flattening
- head, femur M89.8X5
- hip — *see* Coxa, plana
- lip (congenital) Q18.8
- nose (congenital) Q67.4
  - acquired M95.0

Flatulence R14.3
- psychogenic F45.8

Flatus R14.3
  vaginalis N89.8
Flax-dresser's disease J66.1
Flea bite — *see* Injury, bite, by site, superficial, insect
Flecks, glaucomatous (subcapsular) — *see* Cataract, complicated
Fleischer (-Kayser) **ring** (cornea) H18.04- ☑
Fleshy mole O02.0
Flexibilitas cerea — *see* Catalepsy
Flexion
  amputation stump (surgical) T87.89
  cervix — *see* Malposition, uterus
  contracture, joint — *see* Contraction, joint
  deformity, joint (*see also* Deformity, limb, flexion) M21.20
    hip, congenital Q65.89
  uterus (*see also* Malposition, uterus)
    lateral — *see* Lateroversion, uterus
Flexner-Boyd dysentery A03.2
Flexner's dysentery A03.1
Flexure — *see* Flexion
Flint murmur (aortic insufficiency) I35.1
Floater, vitreous — *see* Opacity, vitreous
Floating
  cartilage (joint) (*see also* Loose, body, joint)
    knee — *see* Derangement, knee, loose body
  gallbladder, congenital Q44.1
  kidney N28.89
    congenital Q63.8
  spleen D73.89
Flooding N92.0
Floor — *see* condition
Floppy
  baby syndrome (nonspecific) P94.2
  iris syndrome (intraoperative) (IFIS) H21.81
  nonrheumatic mitral valve syndrome I34.1
Flu (*see also* Influenza)
  avian (*see also* Influenza, due to, identified novel influenza A virus) J09.X2
  bird (*see also* Influenza, due to, identified novel influenza A virus) J09.X2
  intestinal NEC A08.4
  swine (viruses that normally cause infections in pigs) (*see also* Influenza, due to, identified novel influenza A virus) J09.X2
Fluctuating blood pressure I99.8
Fluid
  abdomen R18.8
  chest J94.8
  heart — *see* Failure, heart, congestive
  joint — *see* Effusion, joint
  loss (acute) E86.9
    with
      hypernatremia E87.0
      hyponatremia E87.1
  lung — *see* Edema, lung
  overload E87.70
    specified NEC E87.79
  peritoneal cavity R18.8
  pleural cavity J94.8
  retention R60.9
Flukes NEC (*see also* Infestation, fluke)
  blood NEC — *see* Schistosomiasis
  liver B66.3
Fluor (vaginalis) N89.8
  trichomonal or due to Trichomonas (vaginalis) A59.00
Fluorosis
  dental K00.3
  skeletal M85.10
    ankle M85.17- ☑
    foot M85.17- ☑
    forearm M85.13- ☑
    hand M85.14- ☑
    lower leg M85.16- ☑
    multiple site M85.19
    neck M85.18
    rib M85.18
    shoulder M85.11- ☑
    skull M85.18
    specified site NEC M85.18
    thigh M85.15- ☑
    toe M85.17- ☑
    upper arm M85.12- ☑
    vertebra M85.18
Flush syndrome E34.0
Flushing R23.2
  menopausal N95.1

Flutter
  atrial or auricular I48.92
    atypical I48.4
    type I I48.3
    type II I48.4
    typical I48.3
  heart I49.8
    atrial or auricular I48.92
      atypical I48.4
      type I I48.3
      type II I48.4
      typical I48.3
    ventricular I49.02
  ventricular I49.02
FNHTR (febrile nonhemolytic transfusion reaction) R50.84
Fochier's abscess — *code by* site under Abscess
Focus, Assmann's — *see* Tuberculosis, pulmonary
Fogo selvagem L10.3
Foix-Alajouanine syndrome G95.19
Fold, folds (anomalous) (*see also* Anomaly, by site)
  Descemet's membrane — *see* Change, corneal membrane, Descemet's, fold
  epicanthic Q10.3
  heart Q24.8
Folie à deux F24
Follicle
  cervix (nabothian) (ruptured) N88.8
  graafian, ruptured, with hemorrhage N83.0
  nabothian N88.8
Follicular — *see* condition
Folliculitis (superficial) L73.9
  abscedens et suffodiens L66.3
  cyst N83.0
  decalvans L66.2
  deep — *see* Furuncle, by site
  gonococcal (acute) (chronic) A54.01
  keloid, keloidalis L73.0
  pustular L01.02
  ulerythematosa reticulata L66.4
Folliculome lipidique
  specified site — *see* Neoplasm, benign, by site
  unspecified site
    female D27.9
    male D29.20
Følling's disease E70.0
Follow-up — *see* Examination, follow-up
Fong's syndrome (hereditary osteo-onychodysplasia) Q78.5
Food
  allergy L27.2
  asphyxia (from aspiration or inhalation) — *see* Foreign body, by site
  choked on — *see* Foreign body, by site
  deprivation T73.0 ☑
    specified kind of food NEC E63.8
  intoxication — *see* Poisoning, food
  lack of T73.0 ☑
  poisoning — *see* Poisoning, food
  rejection NEC — *see* Disorder, eating
  strangulation or suffocation — *see* Foreign body, by site
  toxemia — *see* Poisoning, food
Foot — *see* condition
Foramen ovale (nonclosure) (patent) (persistent) Q21.1
Forbes' glycogen storage disease E74.03
Fordyce-Fox disease L75.2
Fordyce's disease (mouth) Q38.6
Forearm — *see* condition
Foreign body
  with
    laceration — *see* Laceration, by site, with foreign body
    puncture wound — *see* Puncture, by site, with foreign body
  accidentally left following a procedure T81.509 ☑
    aspiration T81.506 ☑
      resulting in
        adhesions T81.516 ☑
        obstruction T81.526 ☑
        perforation T81.536 ☑
        specified complication NEC T81.596 ☑
    cardiac catheterization T81.505 ☑
      resulting in
        acute reaction T81.60 ☑
          aseptic peritonitis T81.61 ☑
          specified NEC T81.69 ☑
        adhesions T81.515 ☑

Foreign body — *continued*
  accidentally left following a procedure — *continued*
    cardiac catheterization — *continued*
      resulting in — *continued*
        obstruction T81.525 ☑
        perforation T81.535 ☑
        specified complication NEC T81.595 ☑
    causing
      acute reaction T81.60 ☑
        aseptic peritonitis T81.61 ☑
        specified complication NEC T81.69 ☑
      adhesions T81.519 ☑
      aseptic peritonitis T81.61 ☑
      obstruction T81.529 ☑
      perforation T81.539 ☑
      specified complication NEC T81.599 ☑
    endoscopy T81.504 ☑
      resulting in
        adhesions T81.514 ☑
        obstruction T81.524 ☑
        perforation T81.534 ☑
        specified complication NEC T81.594 ☑
    immunization T81.503 ☑
      resulting in
        adhesions T81.513 ☑
        obstruction T81.523 ☑
        perforation T81.533 ☑
        specified complication NEC T81.593 ☑
    infusion T81.501 ☑
      resulting in
        adhesions T81.511 ☑
        obstruction T81.521 ☑
        perforation T81.531 ☑
        specified complication NEC T81.591 ☑
    injection T81.503 ☑
      resulting in
        adhesions T81.513 ☑
        obstruction T81.523 ☑
        perforation T81.533 ☑
        specified complication NEC T81.593 ☑
    kidney dialysis T81.502 ☑
      resulting in
        adhesions T81.512 ☑
        obstruction T81.522 ☑
        perforation T81.532 ☑
        specified complication NEC T81.592 ☑
    packing removal T81.507 ☑
      resulting in
        acute reaction T81.60 ☑
          aseptic peritonitis T81.61 ☑
          specified NEC T81.69 ☑
        adhesions T81.517 ☑
        obstruction T81.527 ☑
        perforation T81.537 ☑
        specified complication NEC T81.597 ☑
    puncture T81.506 ☑
      resulting in
        adhesions T81.516 ☑
        obstruction T81.526 ☑
        perforation T81.536 ☑
        specified complication NEC T81.596 ☑
    specified procedure NEC T81.508 ☑
      resulting in
        acute reaction T81.60 ☑
          aseptic peritonitis T81.61 ☑
          specified NEC T81.69 ☑
        adhesions T81.518 ☑
        obstruction T81.528 ☑
        perforation T81.538 ☑
        specified complication NEC T81.598 ☑
    surgical operation T81.500 ☑
      resulting in
        acute reaction T81.60 ☑
          aseptic peritonitis T81.61 ☑
          specified NEC T81.69 ☑
        adhesions T81.510 ☑
        obstruction T81.520 ☑
        perforation T81.530 ☑
        specified complication NEC T81.590 ☑
    transfusion T81.501 ☑
      resulting in
        adhesions T81.511 ☑
        obstruction T81.521 ☑
        perforation T81.531 ☑
        specified complication NEC T81.591 ☑

Index

Foreign body — *continued*
- alimentary tract T18.9 ☑
  - anus T18.5 ☑
  - colon T18.4 ☑
  - esophagus — *see* Foreign body, esophagus
  - mouth T18.0 ☑
  - multiple sites T18.8 ☑
  - rectosigmoid (junction) T18.5 ☑
  - rectum T18.5 ☑
  - small intestine T18.3 ☑
  - specified site NEC T18.8 ☑
  - stomach T18.2 ☑
- anterior chamber (eye) S05.5- ☑
- auditory canal — *see* Foreign body, entering through orifice, ear
- bronchus T17.508 ☑
  - causing
    - asphyxiation T17.500 ☑
      - food (bone) (seed) T17.520 ☑
      - gastric contents (vomitus) T17.510 ☑
      - specified type NEC T17.590 ☑
    - injury NEC T17.508 ☑
      - food (bone) (seed) T17.528 ☑
      - gastric contents (vomitus) T17.518 ☑
      - specified type NEC T17.598 ☑
- canthus — *see* Foreign body, conjunctival sac
- ciliary body (eye) S05.5- ☑
- conjunctival sac T15.1- ☑
- cornea T15.0- ☑
- entering through orifice
  - accessory sinus T17.0 ☑
  - alimentary canal T18.9 ☑
    - multiple parts T18.8 ☑
    - specified part NEC T18.8 ☑
  - alveolar process T18.0 ☑
  - antrum (Highmore's) T17.0 ☑
  - anus T18.5 ☑
  - appendix T18.4 ☑
  - auditory canal — *see* Foreign body, entering through orifice, ear
  - auricle — *see* Foreign body, entering through orifice, ear
  - bladder T19.8 ☑
  - bronchioles — *see* Foreign body, respiratory tract, specified site NEC
  - bronchus (main) — *see* Foreign body, bronchus
  - buccal cavity T18.0 ☑
  - canthus (inner) — *see* Foreign body, conjunctival sac
  - cecum T18.4 ☑
  - cervix (canal) (uteri) T19.3 ☑
  - colon T18.4 ☑
  - conjunctival sac — *see* Foreign body, conjunctival sac
  - cornea — *see* Foreign body, cornea
  - digestive organ or tract NOS T18.9 ☑
    - multiple parts T18.8 ☑
    - specified part NEC T18.8 ☑
  - duodenum T18.3 ☑
  - ear (external) T16.- ☑
  - esophagus — *see* Foreign body, esophagus
  - eye (external) NOS T15.9- ☑
    - conjunctival sac — *see* Foreign body, conjunctival sac
    - cornea — *see* Foreign body, cornea
    - specified part NEC T15.8- ☑
  - eyeball (*see also* Foreign body, entering through orifice, eye, specified part NEC)
    - with penetrating wound — *see* Puncture, eyeball
  - eyelid (*see also* Foreign body, conjunctival sac) with
    - laceration — *see* Laceration, eyelid, with foreign body
    - puncture — *see* Puncture, eyelid, with foreign body
    - superficial injury — *see* Foreign body, superficial, eyelid
  - gastrointestinal tract T18.9 ☑
    - multiple parts T18.8 ☑
    - specified part NEC T18.8 ☑
  - genitourinary tract T19.9 ☑
    - multiple parts T19.8 ☑
    - specified part NEC T19.8 ☑
  - globe — *see* Foreign body, entering through orifice, eyeball

Foreign body — *continued*
- entering through orifice — *continued*
  - gum T18.0 ☑
  - Highmore's antrum T17.0 ☑
  - hypopharynx — *see* Foreign body, pharynx
  - ileum T18.3 ☑
  - intestine (small) T18.3 ☑
    - large T18.4 ☑
  - lacrimal apparatus (punctum) — *see* Foreign body, entering through orifice, eye, specified part NEC
  - large intestine T18.4 ☑
  - larynx — *see* Foreign body, larynx
  - lung — *see* Foreign body, respiratory tract, specified site NEC
  - maxillary sinus T17.0 ☑
  - mouth T18.0 ☑
  - nasal sinus T17.0 ☑
  - nasopharynx — *see* Foreign body, pharynx
  - nose (passage) T17.1 ☑
  - nostril T17.1 ☑
  - oral cavity T18.0 ☑
  - palate T18.0 ☑
  - penis T19.4 ☑
  - pharynx — *see* Foreign body, pharynx
  - piriform sinus — *see* Foreign body, pharynx
  - rectosigmoid (junction) T18.5 ☑
  - rectum T18.5 ☑
  - respiratory tract — *see* Foreign body, respiratory tract
  - sinus (accessory) (frontal) (maxillary) (nasal) T17.0 ☑
    - piriform — *see* Foreign body, pharynx
  - small intestine T18.3 ☑
  - stomach T18.2 ☑
  - suffocation by — *see* Foreign body, by site
  - tear ducts or glands — *see* Foreign body, entering through orifice, eye, specified part NEC
  - throat — *see* Foreign body, pharynx
  - tongue T18.0 ☑
  - tonsil, tonsillar (fossa) — *see* Foreign body, pharynx
  - trachea — *see* Foreign body, trachea
  - ureter T19.8 ☑
  - urethra T19.0 ☑
  - uterus (any part) T19.3 ☑
  - vagina T19.2 ☑
  - vulva T19.2 ☑
- esophagus T18.108 ☑
  - causing
    - injury NEC T18.108 ☑
      - food (bone) (seed) T18.128 ☑
      - gastric contents (vomitus) T18.118 ☑
      - specified type NEC T18.198 ☑
    - tracheal compression T18.100 ☑
      - food (bone) (seed) T18.120 ☑
      - gastric contents (vomitus) T18.110 ☑
      - specified type NEC T18.190 ☑
- felling of, in throat R09.89
- fragment — *see* Retained, foreign body fragments (type of)
- genitourinary tract T19.9 ☑
  - bladder T19.1 ☑
  - multiple parts T19.8 ☑
  - penis T19.4 ☑
  - specified site NEC T19.8 ☑
  - urethra T19.0 ☑
  - uterus T19.3 ☑
    - IUD Z97.5
  - vagina T19.2 ☑
    - contraceptive device Z97.5
  - vulva T19.2 ☑
- granuloma (old) (soft tissue) (*see also* Granuloma, foreign body)
  - skin L92.3
- in
  - laceration — *see* Laceration, by site, with foreign body
  - puncture wound — *see* Puncture, by site, with foreign body
  - soft tissue (residual) M79.5
- inadvertently left in operation wound — *see* Foreign body, accidentally left during a procedure
- ingestion, ingested NOS T18.9 ☑
- inhalation or inspiration — *see* Foreign body, by site
- internal organ, not entering through a natural orifice — code as specific injury with foreign body

Foreign body — *continued*
- intraocular S05.5- ☑
  - old, retained (nonmagnetic) H44.70- ☑
    - anterior chamber H44.71- ☑
    - ciliary body H44.72- ☑
    - iris H44.72- ☑
    - lens H44.73- ☑
    - magnetic H44.60- ☑
      - anterior chamber H44.61- ☑
      - ciliary body H44.62- ☑
      - iris H44.62- ☑
      - lens H44.63- ☑
      - posterior wall H44.64- ☑
      - specified site NEC H44.69- ☑
      - vitreous body H44.65- ☑
    - posterior wall H44.74- ☑
    - specified site NEC H44.79- ☑
    - vitreous body H44.75- ☑
- iris — *see* Foreign body, intraocular
- lacrimal punctum — *see* Foreign body, entering through orifice, eye, specified part NEC
- larynx T17.308 ☑
  - causing
    - asphyxiation T17.300 ☑
      - food (bone) (seed) T17.320 ☑
      - gastric contents (vomitus) T17.310 ☑
      - specified type NEC T17.390 ☑
    - injury NEC T17.308 ☑
      - food (bone) (seed) T17.328 ☑
      - gastric contents (vomitus) T17.318 ☑
      - specified type NEC T17.398 ☑
- lens — *see* Foreign body, intraocular
- ocular muscle S05.4- ☑
  - old, retained — *see* Foreign body, orbit, old
- old or residual
  - soft tissue (residual) M79.5
- operation wound, left accidentally — *see* Foreign body, accidentally left during a procedure
- orbit S05.4- ☑
  - old, retained H05.5- ☑
- pharynx T17.208 ☑
  - causing
    - asphyxiation T17.200 ☑
      - food (bone) (seed) T17.220 ☑
      - gastric contents (vomitus) T17.210 ☑
      - specified type NEC T17.290 ☑
    - injury NEC T17.208 ☑
      - food (bone) (seed) T17.228 ☑
      - gastric contents (vomitus) T17.218 ☑
      - specified type NEC T17.298 ☑
- respiratory tract T17.908 ☑
  - bronchioles — *see* Foreign body, respiratory tract, specified site NEC
  - bronchus -— *see* Foreign body, bronchus
  - causing
    - asphyxiation T17.900 ☑
      - food (bone) (seed) T17.920 ☑
      - gastric contents (vomitus) T17.910 ☑
      - specified type NEC T17.990 ☑
    - injury NEC T17.908 ☑
      - food (bone) (seed) T17.928 ☑
      - gastric contents (vomitus) T17.918 ☑
      - specified type NEC T17.998 ☑
  - larynx — *see* Foreign body, larynx
  - lung — *see* Foreign body, respiratory tract, specified site NEC
  - multiple parts — *see* Foreign body, respiratory tract, specified site NEC
  - nasal sinus T17.0 ☑
  - nasopharynx — *see* Foreign body, pharynx
  - nose T17.1 ☑
  - nostril T17.1 ☑
  - pharynx — *see* Foreign body, pharynx
  - specified site NEC T17.808 ☑
    - causing
      - asphyxiation T17.800 ☑
        - food (bone) (seed) T17.820 ☑
        - gastric contents (vomitus) T17.810 ☑
        - specified type NEC T17.890 ☑
      - injury NEC T17.808 ☑
        - food (bone) (seed) T17.828 ☑
        - gastric contents (vomitus) T17.818 ☑
        - specified type NEC T17.898 ☑
  - throat — *see* Foreign body, pharynx
  - trachea — *see* Foreign body, trachea
- retained (old) (nonmagnetic) (in)

Foreign body — *continued*
  retained — *continued*
    anterior chamber (eye) — *see* Foreign body, intraocular, old, retained, anterior chamber
      magnetic — *see* Foreign body, intraocular, old, retained, magnetic, anterior chamber
    ciliary body — *see* Foreign body, intraocular, old, retained, ciliary body
      magnetic — *see* Foreign body, intraocular, old, retained, magnetic, ciliary body
    eyelid H02.819
      left H02.816
        lower H02.815
        upper H02.814
      right H02.813
        lower H02.812
        upper H02.811
    fragments — *see* Retained, foreign body fragments (type of)
    globe — *see* Foreign body, intraocular, old, retained
      magnetic — *see* Foreign body, intraocular, old, retained, magnetic
    intraocular — *see* Foreign body, intraocular, old, retained
      magnetic — *see* Foreign body, intraocular, old, retained, magnetic
    iris — *see* Foreign body, intraocular, old, retained, iris
      magnetic — *see* Foreign body, intraocular, old, retained, magnetic, iris
    lens — *see* Foreign body, intraocular, old, retained, lens
      magnetic — *see* Foreign body, intraocular, old, retained, magnetic, lens
    muscle — *see* Foreign body, retained, soft tissue
    orbit — *see* Foreign body, orbit, old
    posterior wall of globe — *see* Foreign body, intraocular, old, retained, posterior wall
      magnetic — *see* Foreign body, intraocular, old, retained, magnetic, posterior wall
    retrobulbar — *see* Foreign body, orbit, old, retrobulbar
    soft tissue M79.5
    vitreous — *see* Foreign body, intraocular, old, retained, vitreous body
      magnetic — *see* Foreign body, intraocular, old, retained, magnetic, vitreous body
  retina S05.5- ☑
  superficial, without open wound
    abdomen, abdominal (wall) S30.851 ☑
    alveolar process S00.552 ☑
    ankle S90.55- ☑
    antecubital space — *see* Foreign body, superficial, forearm
    anus S30.857 ☑
    arm (upper) S40.85- ☑
    auditory canal — *see* Foreign body, superficial, ear
    auricle — *see* Foreign body, superficial, ear
    axilla — *see* Foreign body, superficial, arm
    back, lower S30.850 ☑
    breast S20.15- ☑
    brow S00.85 ☑
    buttock S30.850 ☑
    calf — *see* Foreign body, superficial, leg
    canthus — *see* Foreign body, superficial, eyelid
    cheek S00.85 ☑
      internal S00.552 ☑
    chest wall — *see* Foreign body, superficial, thorax
    chin S00.85 ☑
    clitoris S30.854 ☑
    costal region — *see* Foreign body, superficial, thorax
    digit(s)
      foot — *see* Foreign body, superficial, toe
      hand — *see* Foreign body, superficial, finger
    ear S00.45 ·
    elbow S50.35- ☑
    epididymis S30.853 ☑
    epigastric region S30.851 ☑
    epiglottis S10.15 ☑
    esophagus, cervical S10.15 ☑
    eyebrow — *see* Foreign body, superficial, eyelid
    eyelid S00.25- ☑
    face S00.85 ☑
    finger(s) S60.459 ☑
      index S60.45- ☑

Foreign body — *continued*
  superficial, without open wound — *continued*
    finger(s) — *continued*
      little S60.45- ☑
      middle S60.45- ☑
      ring S60.45- ☑
    flank S30.851 ☑
    foot (except toe(s) alone) S90.85- ☑
      toe — *see* Foreign body, superficial, toe
    forearm S50.85- ☑
      elbow only — *see* Foreign body, superficial, elbow
    forehead S00.85 ☑
    genital organs, external
      female S30.856 ☑
      male S30.855 ☑
    groin S30.851 ☑
    gum S00.552 ☑
    hand S60.55- ☑
    head S00.95 ☑
      ear — *see* Foreign body, superficial, ear
      eyelid — *see* Foreign body, superficial, eyelid
      lip S00.551 ☑
      nose S00.35 ☑
      oral cavity S00.552 ☑
      scalp S00.05 ☑
      specified site NEC S00.85 ☑
    heel — *see* Foreign body, superficial, foot
    hip S70.25- ☑
    inguinal region S30.851 ☑
    interscapular region S20.459 ☑
    jaw S00.85 ☑
    knee S80.25- ☑
    labium (majus) (minus) S30.854 ☑
    larynx S10.15 ☑
    leg (lower) S80.85- ☑
      knee — *see* Foreign body, superficial, knee
      upper — *see* Foreign body, superficial, thigh
    lip S00.551 ☑
    lower back S30.850 ☑
    lumbar region S30.850 ☑
    malar region S00.85 ☑
    mammary — *see* Foreign body, superficial, breast
    mastoid region S00.85 ☑
    mouth S00.552 ☑
    nail
      finger — *see* Foreign body, superficial, finger
      toe — *see* Foreign body, superficial, toe
    nape S10.85 ☑
    nasal S00.35 ☑
    neck S10.95 ☑
      specified site NEC S10.85 ☑
      throat S10.15 ☑
    nose S00.35 ☑
    occipital region S00.05 ☑
    oral cavity S00.552 ☑
    orbital region — *see* Foreign body, superficial, eyelid
    palate S00.552 ☑
    palm — *see* Foreign body, superficial, hand
    parietal region S00.05 ☑
    pelvis S30.850 ☑
    penis S30.852 ☑
    perineum
      female S30.854 ☑
      male S30.850 ☑
    periocular area — *see* Foreign body, superficial, eyelid
    phalanges
      finger — *see* Foreign body, superficial, finger
      toe — *see* Foreign body, superficial, toe
    pharynx S10.15 ☑
    pinna — *see* Foreign body, superficial, ear
    popliteal space — *see* Foreign body, superficial, knee
    prepuce S30.852 ☑
    pubic region S30.850 ☑
    pudendum
      female S30.856 ☑
      male S30.855 ☑
    sacral region S30.850 ☑
    scalp S00.05 ☑
    scapular region — *see* Foreign body, superficial, shoulder
    scrotum S30.853 ☑
    shin — *see* Foreign body, superficial, leg

Foreign body — *continued*
  superficial, without open wound — *continued*
    shoulder S40.25- ☑
    sternal region S20.359 ☑
    submaxillary region S00.85 ☑
    submental region S00.85 ☑
    subungual
      finger(s) — *see* Foreign body, superficial, finger
      toe(s) — *see* Foreign body, superficial, toe
    supraclavicular fossa S10.85 ☑
    supraorbital S00.85 ☑
    temple S00.85 ☑
    temporal region S00.85 ☑
    testis S30.853 ☑
    thigh S70.35- ☑
    thorax, thoracic (wall) S20.95 ☑
      back S20.45- ☑
      front S20.35- ☑
    throat S10.15 ☑
    thumb S60.35- ☑
    toe(s) (lesser) S90.456 ☑
      great S90.45- ☑
    tongue S00.552 ☑
    trachea S10.15 ☑
    tunica vaginalis S30.853 ☑
    tympanum, tympanic membrane — *see* Foreign body, superficial, ear
    uvula S00.552 ☑
    vagina S30.854 ☑
    vocal cords S10.15 ☑
    vulva S30.854 ☑
    wrist S60.85- ☑
  swallowed T18.9 ☑
  trachea T17.408 ☑
    causing
      asphyxiation T17.400 ☑
        food (bone) (seed) T17.420 ☑
        gastric contents (vomitus) T17.410 ☑
        specified type NEC T17.490 ☑
      injury NEC T17.408 ☑
        food (bone) (seed) T17.428 ☑
        gastric contents (vomitus) T17.418 ☑
        specified type NEC T17.498 ☑
  type of fragment — *see* Retained, foreign body fragments (type of)
  vitreous (humor) S05.5- ☑
Forestier's disease (rhizomelic pseudopolyarthritis) M35.3
  meaning ankylosing hyperostosis — *see* Hyperostosis, ankylosing
Formation
  hyalin in cornea — *see* Degeneration, cornea
  sequestrum in bone (due to infection) — *see* Osteomyelitis, chronic
  valve
    colon, congenital Q43.8
    ureter (congenital) Q62.39
Formication R20.2
Fort Bragg fever A27.89
Fossa (*see also* condition)
  pyriform — *see* condition
Foster-Kennedy syndrome H47.14- ☑
Fothergill's
  disease (trigeminal neuralgia) (*see also* Neuralgia, trigeminal)
    scarlatina anginosa A38.9
Foul breath R19.6
Foundling Z76.1
Fournier disease or gangrene N49.3
  female N76.89
Fourth
  cranial nerve — *see* condition
  molar K00.1
Foville's (peduncular) **disease or syndrome** G46.3
Fox (-Fordyce) disease (apocrine miliaria) L75.2
Fracture, burst — *see* Fracture, traumatic, by site
Fracture, chronic — *see* Fracture, pathological
Fracture, insufficiency — *see* Fracture, pathologic, by site
Fracture, pathological (pathologic) (*see also* Fracture, traumatic) M84.40
  ankle M84.47- ☑
  carpus M84.44- ☑
  clavicle M84.41- ☑
  dental implant M27.63
  dental restorative material K08.539

Fracture, pathological — *continued*
  dental restorative material — *continued*
    with loss of material KØ8.531
    without loss of material KØ8.53Ø
  due to
    neoplastic disease NEC (*see also* Neoplasm)
      M84.5Ø ✓
      ankle M84.57- ✓
      carpus M84.54- ✓
      clavicle M84.51- ✓
      femur M84.55- ✓
      fibula M84.56- ✓
      finger M84.54- ✓
      hip M84.559 ✓
      humerus M84.52- ✓
      ilium M84.55Ø ✓
      ischium M84.55Ø ✓
      metacarpus M84.54- ✓
      metatarsus M84.57- ✓
      neck M84.58 ✓
      pelvis M84.55Ø ✓
      radius M84.53- ✓
      rib M84.58 ✓
      scapula M84.51- ✓
      skull M84.58 ✓
      specified site NEC M84.58 ✓
      tarsus M84.57- ✓
      tibia M84.56- ✓
      toe M84.57- ✓
      ulna M84.53- ✓
      vertebra M84.58 ✓
    osteoporosis M80.80 ✓
      disuse — *see* Osteoporosis, specified type NEC, with pathological fracture
      drug-induced — *see* Osteoporosis, drug-induced, with pathological fracture
      idiopathic — *see* Osteoporosis, specified type NEC, with pathological fracture
      postmenopausal — *see* Osteoporosis, postmenopausal, with pathological fracture
      postoophorectomy — *see* Osteoporosis, postoophorectomy, with pathological fracture
      postsurgical malabsorption — *see* Osteoporosis, specified type NEC, with pathological fracture
      specified cause NEC — *see* Osteoporosis, specified type NEC, with pathological fracture
    specified disease NEC M84.6Ø ✓
      ankle M84.67- ✓
      carpus M84.64- ✓
      clavicle M84.61- ✓
      femur M84.65- ✓
      fibula M84.66- ✓
      finger M84.64- ✓
      hip M84.65- ✓
      humerus M84.62- ✓
      ilium M84.65Ø ✓
      ischium M84.65Ø ✓
      metacarpus M84.64- ✓
      metatarsus M84.67- ✓
      neck M84.68 ✓
      radius M84.63- ✓
      rib M84.68 ✓
      scapula M84.61- ✓
      skull M84.68 ✓
      tarsus M84.67- ✓
      tibia M84.66- ✓
      toe M84.67- ✓
      ulna M84.63- ✓
      vertebra M84.68 ✓
  femur M84.45- ✓
  fibula M84.46- ✓
  finger M84.44- ✓
  hip M84.459 ✓
  humerus M84.42- ✓
  ilium M84.454 ✓
  ischium M84.454 ✓
  joint prosthesis — *see* Complications, joint prosthesis, mechanical, breakdown, by site
    periprosthetic — *see* Complications, joint prosthesis, mechanical, periprosthesis, fracture, by site
  metacarpus M84.44- ✓
  metatarsus M84.47- ✓
  neck M84.48 ✓

Fracture, pathological — *continued*
  pelvis M84.454 ✓
  radius M84.43- ✓
  restorative material (dental) KØ8.539
    with loss of material KØ8.531
    without loss of material KØ8.53Ø
  rib M84.48 ✓
  scapula M84.41- ✓
  skull M84.48 ✓
  tarsus M84.47- ✓
  tibia M84.46- ✓
  toe M84.47- ✓
  ulna M84.43- ✓
  vertebra M84.48 ✓
Fracture, traumatic (abduction) (adduction) (separation)
  (*see also* Fracture, pathological) T14.8
  acetabulum S32.4Ø- ✓
    column
      anterior (displaced) (iliopubic) S32.43- ✓
        nondisplaced S32.436
      posterior (displaced) (ilioischial) S32.443 ✓
        nondisplaced S32.44- ✓
    dome (displaced) S32.48- ✓
      nondisplaced S32.48 ✓
    specified NEC S32.49- ✓
    transverse (displaced) S32.45- ✓
      with associated posterior wall fracture (displaced) S32.46- ✓
        nondisplaced S32.46- ✓
      nondisplaced S32.45- ✓
    wall
      anterior (displaced) S32.41- ✓
        nondisplaced S32.41- ✓
      medial (displaced) S32.47- ✓
        nondisplaced S32.47- ✓
      posterior (displaced) S32.42- ✓
        with associated transverse fracture (displaced) S32.46- ✓
        nondisplaced S32.46- ✓
        nondisplaced S32.42- ✓
  acromion — *see* Fracture, scapula, acromial process
  ankle S82.899 ✓
    bimalleolar (displaced) S82.84- ✓
      nondisplaced S82.84- ✓
    lateral malleolus only (displaced) S82.6- ✓
      nondisplaced S82.6- ✓
    medial malleolus (displaced) S82.5- ✓
      associated with Maisonneuve's fracture — *see* Fracture, Maisonneuve's
      nondisplaced S82.5- ✓
    talus — *see* Fracture, tarsal, talus
    trimalleolar (displaced) S82.85- ✓
      nondisplaced S82.85- ✓
  arm (upper) (*see also* Fracture, humerus, shaft)
    humerus — *see* Fracture, humerus
    radius — *see* Fracture, radius
    ulna — *see* Fracture, ulna
  astragalus — *see* Fracture, tarsal, talus
  atlas — *see* Fracture, neck, cervical vertebra, first
  axis — *see* Fracture, neck, cervical vertebra, second
  back — *see* Fracture, vertebra
  Barton's — *see* Barton's fracture
  base of skull — *see* Fracture, skull, base
  basicervical (basal) (femoral) S72.Ø ✓
  Bennett's — *see* Bennett's fracture
  bimalleolar — *see* Fracture, ankle, bimalleolar
  blow-out SØ2.3
  bone NEC T14.8
    birth injury P13.9
    following insertion of orthopedic implant, joint prosthesis or bone plate — *see* Fracture, following insertion of orthopedic implant, joint prosthesis or bone plate
    in (due to) neoplastic disease NEC — *see* Fracture, pathological, due to, neoplastic disease
    pathological (cause unknown) — *see* Fracture, pathological
  breast bone — *see* Fracture, sternum
  bucket handle (semilunar cartilage) — *see* Tear, meniscus
  burst — *see* Fracture, traumatic, by site
  calcaneus — *see* Fracture, tarsal, calcaneus
  carpal bone(s) S62.1Ø- ✓
    capitate (displaced) S62.13- ✓
      nondisplaced S62.13- ✓
    cuneiform — *see* Fracture, carpal bone, triquetrum

Fracture, traumatic — *continued*
  carpal bone(s) — *continued*
    hamate (body) (displaced) S62.143 ✓
      hook process (displaced) S62.15- ✓
        nondisplaced S62.15- ✓
      nondisplaced S62.14- ✓
    larger multangular — *see* Fracture, carpal bones, trapezium
    lunate (displaced) S62.12- ✓
      nondisplaced S62.12- ✓
    navicular S62.ØØ- ✓
      distal pole (displaced) S62.Ø1- ✓
        nondisplaced S62.Ø1- ✓
      middle third (displaced) S62.Ø2- ✓
        nondisplaced S62.Ø2- ✓
      proximal third (displaced) S62.Ø3- ✓
        nondisplaced S62.Ø3- ✓
      volar tuberosity — *see* Fracture, carpal bones, navicular, distal pole
    os magnum — *see* Fracture, carpal bones, capitate
    pisiform (displaced) S62.16- ✓
      nondisplaced S62.16- ✓
    semilunar — *see* Fracture, carpal bones, lunate
    smaller multangular — *see* Fracture, carpal bones, trapezoid
    trapezium (displaced) S62.17- ✓
      nondisplaced S62.17- ✓
    trapezoid (displaced) S62.18- ✓
      nondisplaced S62.18- ✓
    triquetrum (displaced) S62.11- ✓
      nondisplaced S62.11- ✓
    unciform — *see* Fracture, carpal bones, hamate
  cervical — *see* Fracture, vertebra, cervical
  clavicle S42.ØØ- ✓
    acromial end (displaced) S42.Ø3- ✓
      nondisplaced S42.Ø3- ✓
    birth injury P13.4
    lateral end — *see* Fracture, clavicle, acromial end
    shaft (displaced) S42.Ø2- ✓
      nondisplaced S42.Ø2- ✓
    sternal end (anterior) (displaced) S42.Ø1- ✓
      nondisplaced S42.Ø1- ✓
      posterior S42.Ø1- ✓
  coccyx S32.2
  collapsed — *see* Collapse, vertebra
  collar bone — *see* Fracture, clavicle
  Colles' — *see* Colles' fracture
  compression, not due to trauma — *see* Collapse, vertebra
  coronoid process — *see* Fracture, ulna, upper end, coronoid process
  corpus cavernosum penis S39.84Ø ✓
  costochondral cartilage S23.41
  costochondral, costosternal junction — *see* Fracture, rib
  cranium — *see* Fracture, skull
  cricoid cartilage S12.8
  cuboid (ankle) — *see* Fracture, tarsal, cuboid
  cuneiform
    foot — *see* Fracture, tarsal, cuneiform
    wrist — *see* Fracture, carpal, triquetrum
  delayed union — *see* Delay, union, fracture
  dental restorative material KØ8.539
    with loss of material KØ8.531
    without loss of material KØ8.53Ø
  due to
    birth injury — *see* Birth, injury, fracture
    osteoporosis — *see* Osteoporosis, with fracture
  Dupuytren's — *see* Fracture, ankle, lateral malleolus
  elbow S42.4Ø- ✓
  ethmoid (bone) (sinus) — *see* Fracture, skull, base
  face bone SØ2.92 ✓
  fatigue (*see also* Fracture, stress)
    vertebra M48.4Ø ✓
      cervical region M48.42 ✓
      cervicothoracic region M48.43 ✓
      lumbar region M48.46 ✓
      lumbosacral region M48.47 ✓
      occipito-atlanto-axial region M48.41 ✓
      sacrococcygeal region M48.48 ✓
      thoracic region M48.44 ✓
      thoracolumbar region M48.45 ✓
  femur, femoral S72.9- ✓
    basicervical (basal) S72.Ø ✓
    birth injury P13.2
    capital epiphyseal S79.Ø1- ✓

✓ **Additional Character Required** — Refer to the Tabular List for Character Selection   ·   ▽ **Subterms under main terms may continue to next column or page**

Fracture, traumatic — *continued*
- femur, femoral — *continued*
  - condyles, epicondyles — *see* Fracture, femur, lower end
  - distal end — *see* Fracture, femur, lower end
  - epiphysis
    - head — *see* Fracture, femur, upper end, epiphysis
    - lower — *see* Fracture, femur, lower end, epiphysis
    - upper — *see* Fracture, femur, upper end, epiphysis
  - following insertion of implant, prosthesis or plate M96.66- ☑
  - head — *see* Fracture, femur, upper end, head
  - intertrochanteric — *see* Fracture, femur, trochanteric
  - intratrochanteric — *see* Fracture, femur, trochanteric
  - lower end S72.40- ☑
    - condyle (displaced) S72.41- ☑
      - lateral (displaced) S72.42- ☑
        - nondisplaced S72.42- ☑
      - medial (displaced) S72.43- ☑
        - nondisplaced S72.43- ☑
      - nondisplaced S72.41- ☑
    - epiphysis (displaced) S72.44- ☑
      - nondisplaced S72.44- ☑
    - physeal S79.10- ☑
      - Salter-Harris
        - Type I S79.11- ☑
        - Type II S79.12- ☑
        - Type III S79.13- ☑
        - Type IV S79.14- ☑
        - specified NEC S79.19- ☑
    - specified NEC S72.49- ☑
    - supracondylar (displaced) S72.45- ☑
      - with intracondylar extension (displaced) S72.46- ☑
        - nondisplaced S72.46- ☑
      - nondisplaced S72.45- ☑
    - torus S72.47- ☑
  - neck — *see* Fracture, femur, upper end, neck
  - pertrochanteric — *see* Fracture, femur, trochanteric
  - shaft (lower third) (middle third) (upper third) S72.30- ☑
    - comminuted (displaced) S72.35- ☑
      - nondisplaced S72.35- ☑
    - oblique (displaced) S72.33- ☑
      - nondisplaced S72.33- ☑
    - segmental (displaced) S72.36- ☑
      - nondisplaced S72.36- ☑
    - specified NEC S72.39- ☑
    - spiral (displaced) S72.34- ☑
      - nondisplaced S72.34- ☑
    - transverse (displaced) S72.32- ☑
      - nondisplaced S72.32- ☑
  - specified site NEC — *see* subcategory S72.8 ☑
  - subcapital (displaced) S72.01- ☑
  - subtrochanteric (region) (section) (displaced) S72.2- ☑
    - nondisplaced S72.2- ☑
  - transcervical — *see* Fracture, femur, upper end, neck
  - transtrochanteric — *see* Fracture, femur, trochanteric
  - trochanteric S72.10- ☑
    - apophyseal (displaced) S72.14- ☑
      - nondisplaced S72.14- ☑
    - greater trochanter (displaced) S72.11- ☑
      - nondisplaced S72.11- ☑
    - intertrochanteric (displaced) S72.13- ☑
      - nondisplaced S72.13- ☑
    - lesser trochanter (displaced) S72.12- ☑
      - nondisplaced S72.12- ☑
  - upper end S72.00- ☑
    - apophyseal (displaced) S72.13- ☑
      - nondisplaced S72.13- ☑
    - cervicotrochanteric — *see* Fracture, femur, upper end, neck, base
    - epiphysis (displaced) S72.02- ☑
      - nondisplaced S72.02- ☑
    - head S72.05- ☑
      - articular (displaced) S72.06- ☑
        - nondisplaced S72.06- ☑

Fracture, traumatic — *continued*
- femur, femoral — *continued*
  - upper end — *continued*
    - head — *continued*
      - specified NEC S72.09- ☑
      - intertrochanteric (displaced) S72.14- ☑
        - nondisplaced S72.14- ☑
      - intracapsular S72.01- ☑
      - midcervical (displaced) S72.03- ☑
        - nondisplaced S72.03- ☑
      - neck S72.00- ☑
        - base (displaced) S72.04- ☑
          - nondisplaced S72.04- ☑
        - specified NEC S72.09- ☑
      - pertrochanteric — *see* Fracture, femur, upper end, trochanteric
      - physeal S79.00- ☑
        - Salter-Harris type I S79.01- ☑
        - specified NEC S79.09- ☑
      - subcapital (displaced) S72.01- ☑
      - subtrochanteric (displaced) S72.2- ☑
        - nondisplaced S72.2- ☑
      - transcervical — *see* Fracture, femur, upper end, midcervical
      - trochanteric S72.10- ☑
        - greater (displaced) S72.11- ☑
          - nondisplaced S72.11- ☑
        - lesser (displaced) S72.12- ☑
          - nondisplaced S72.12- ☑
  - fibula (shaft) (styloid) S82.40- ☑
    - comminuted (displaced) S82.45- ☑
      - nondisplaced S82.45- ☑
    - following insertion of implant, prosthesis or plate M96.67- ☑
    - involving ankle or malleolus — *see* Fracture, fibula, lateral malleolus
    - lateral malleolus (displaced) S82.6- ☑
      - nondisplaced S82.6- ☑
    - lower end
      - physeal S89.30- ☑
        - Salter-Harris
          - Type I S89.31- ☑
          - Type II S89.32- ☑
          - specified NEC S89.39- ☑
      - specified NEC S82.83- ☑
      - torus S82.82- ☑
    - oblique (displaced) S82.43- ☑
      - nondisplaced S82.43- ☑
    - segmental (displaced) S82.46- ☑
      - nondisplaced S82.46- ☑
    - specified NEC S82.49- ☑
    - spiral (displaced) S82.44- ☑
      - nondisplaced S82.44- ☑
    - transverse (displaced) S82.42- ☑
      - nondisplaced S82.42- ☑
    - upper end
      - physeal S89.20- ☑
        - Salter-Harris
          - Type I S89.21- ☑
          - Type II S89.22- ☑
          - specified NEC S89.29- ☑
      - specified NEC S82.83- ☑
      - torus S82.81- ☑
  - finger (except thumb) S62.60- ☑
    - distal phalanx (displaced) S62.63- ☑
      - nondisplaced S62.66- ☑
    - index S62.60- ☑
      - distal phalanx (displaced) S62.63- ☑
        - nondisplaced S62.66- ☑
      - medial phalanx (displaced) S62.62- ☑
        - nondisplaced S62.65- ☑
      - proximal phalanx (displaced) S62.61- ☑
        - nondisplaced S62.64- ☑
    - little S62.60- ☑
      - distal phalanx (displaced) S62.63- ☑
        - nondisplaced S62.66- ☑
      - medial phalanx (displaced) S62.62- ☑
        - nondisplaced S62.65- ☑
      - proximal phalanx (displaced) S62.61- ☑
        - nondisplaced S62.64- ☑
    - medial phalanx (displaced) S62.62- ☑
      - nondisplaced S62.65- ☑
    - middle S62.60- ☑
      - distal phalanx (displaced) S62.63- ☑
        - nondisplaced S62.66- ☑
      - medial phalanx (displaced) S62.62-

Fracture, traumatic — *continued*
- finger — *continued*
  - middle — *continued*
    - medial phalanx — *continued*
      - nondisplaced S62.65- ☑
      - proximal phalanx (displaced) S62.61- ☑
        - nondisplaced S62.64- ☑
    - proximal phalanx (displaced) S62.61- ☑
      - nondisplaced S62.64- ☑
    - ring S62.60- ☑
      - distal phalanx (displaced) S62.63- ☑
        - nondisplaced S62.66- ☑
      - medial phalanx (displaced) S62.62- ☑
        - nondisplaced S62.65- ☑
      - proximal phalanx (displaced) S62.61- ☑
        - nondisplaced S62.64- ☑
    - thumb — *see* Fracture, thumb
  - following insertion (intraoperative) (postoperative) of orthopedic implant, joint prosthesis or bone plate M96.69
    - femur M96.66- ☑
    - fibula M96.67- ☑
    - humerus M96.62- ☑
    - pelvis M96.65
    - radius M96.63- ☑
    - specified bone NEC M96.69
    - tibia M96.67- ☑
    - ulna M96.63- ☑
  - foot S92.90- ☑
    - astragalus — *see* Fracture, tarsal, talus
    - calcaneus — *see* Fracture, tarsal, calcaneus
    - cuboid — *see* Fracture, tarsal, cuboid
    - cuneiform — *see* Fracture, tarsal, cuneiform
    - metatarsal — *see* Fracture, metatarsal
    - navicular — *see* Fracture, tarsal, navicular
    - talus — *see* Fracture, tarsal, talus
    - tarsal — *see* Fracture, tarsal
    - toe — *see* Fracture, toe
  - forearm S52.9- ☑
    - radius — *see* Fracture, radius
    - ulna — *see* Fracture, ulna
  - fossa (anterior) (middle) (posterior) S02.19 ☑
  - frontal (bone) (skull) S02.0 ☑
    - sinus S02.19 ☑
  - glenoid (cavity) (scapula) — *see* Fracture, scapula, glenoid cavity
  - greenstick — *see* Fracture, by site
  - hallux — *see* Fracture, toe, great
  - hand S62.9- ☑
    - carpal — *see* Fracture, carpal bone
    - finger (except thumb) — *see* Fracture, finger
    - metacarpal — *see* Fracture, metacarpal
    - navicular (scaphoid) (hand) — *see* Fracture, carpal bone, navicular
    - thumb — *see* Fracture, thumb
  - healed or old
    - with complications — *code by* Nature of the complication
  - heel bone — *see* Fracture, tarsal, calcaneus
  - Hill-Sachs S42.29- ☑
  - hip — *see* Fracture, femur, neck
  - humerus S42.30- ☑
    - anatomical neck — *see* Fracture, humerus, upper end
    - articular process — *see* Fracture, humerus, lower end
    - capitellum — *see* Fracture, humerus, lower end, condyle, lateral
    - distal end — *see* Fracture, humerus, lower end
    - epiphysis
      - lower — *see* Fracture, humerus, lower end, physeal
      - upper — *see* Fracture, humerus, upper end, physeal
    - external condyle — *see* Fracture, humerus, lower end, condyle, lateral
    - following insertion of implant, prosthesis or plate M96.62- ☑
    - great tuberosity — *see* Fracture, humerus, upper end, greater tuberosity
    - intercondylar — *see* Fracture, humerus, lower end
    - internal epicondyle — *see* Fracture, humerus, lower end, epicondyle, medial
    - lesser tuberosity — *see* Fracture, humerus, upper end, lesser tuberosity
    - lower end S42.40- ☑

Index

Fracture, traumatic — Fracture, traumatic

Fracture, traumatic — *continued*
  humerus — *continued*
    lower end — *continued*
      condyle
        lateral (displaced) S42.45- ✓
          nondisplaced S42.45- ✓
        medial (displaced) S42.46- ✓
          nondisplaced S42.46- ✓
      epicondyle
        lateral (displaced) S42.43- ✓
          nondisplaced S42.43- ✓
        medial (displaced) S42.44- ✓
          incarcerated S42.44- ✓
          nondisplaced S42.44- ✓
      physeal S49.10- ✓
        Salter-Harris
          Type I S49.11- ✓
          Type II S49.12- ✓
          Type III S49.13- ✓
          Type IV S49.14- ✓
        specified NEC S49.19- ✓
      specified NEC (displaced) S42.49- ✓
        nondisplaced S42.49- ✓
      supracondylar (simple) (displaced) S42.41- ✓
        comminuted (displaced) S42.42- ✓
          nondisplaced S42.42- ✓
        nondisplaced S42.41- ✓
      torus S42.48- ✓
      transcondylar (displaced) S42.47- ✓
        nondisplaced S42.47- ✓
    proximal end — *see* Fracture, humerus, upper end
    shaft S42.30- ✓
      comminuted (displaced) S42.35- ✓
        nondisplaced S42.35- ✓
      greenstick S42.31- ✓
      oblique (displaced) S42.33- ✓
        nondisplaced S42.33- ✓
      segmental (displaced) S42.36- ✓
        nondisplaced S42.36- ✓
      specified NEC S42.39- ✓
      spiral (displaced) S42.34- ✓
        nondisplaced S42.34- ✓
      transverse (displaced) S42.32- ✓
        nondisplaced S42.32- ✓
    supracondylar — *see* Fracture, humerus, lower end
    surgical neck — *see* Fracture, humerus, upper end, surgical neck
    trochlea — *see* Fracture, humerus, lower end, condyle, medial
    tuberosity — *see* Fracture, humerus, upper end
    upper end S42.20- ✓
      anatomical neck — *see* Fracture, humerus, upper end, specified NEC
      articular head — *see* Fracture, humerus, upper end, specified NEC
      epiphysis — *see* Fracture, humerus, upper end, physeal
      greater tuberosity (displaced) S42.25- ✓
        nondisplaced S42.25- ✓
      lesser tuberosity (displaced) S42.26- ✓
        nondisplaced S42.26- ✓
      physeal S49.00- ✓
        Salter-Harris
          Type I S49.01- ✓
          Type II S49.02- ✓
          Type III S49.03- ✓
          Type IV S49.04- ✓
        specified NEC S49.09- ✓
      specified NEC (displaced) S42.29- ✓
        nondisplaced S42.29- ✓
      surgical neck (displaced) S42.21- ✓
        four-part S42.24- ✓
        nondisplaced S42.21- ✓
        three-part S42.23- ✓
        two-part (displaced) S42.22- ✓
          nondisplaced S42.22- ✓
      torus S42.27- ✓
      transepiphyseal — *see* Fracture, humerus, upper end, physeal
  hyoid bone S12.8 ✓
  ilium S32.30- ✓
    with disruption of pelvic ring — *see* Disruption, pelvic ring
    avulsion (displaced) S32.31- ✓
      nondisplaced S32.31- ✓
    specified NEC S32.39- ✓

  impaction, impacted — *code as* Fracture, by site
  innominate bone — *see* Fracture, ilium
  instep — *see* Fracture, foot
  ischium S32.60- ✓
    with disruption of pelvic ring — *see* Disruption, pelvic ring
    avulsion (displaced) S32.61- ✓
      nondisplaced S32.61- ✓
    specified NEC S32.69- ✓
  jaw (bone) (lower) — *see* Fracture, mandible
    upper — *see* Fracture, maxilla
  joint prosthesis — *see* Complications, joint prosthesis, mechanical, breakdown, by site
    periprosthetic — *see* Complications, joint prosthesis, mechanical, periprosthesis, fracture, by site
  knee cap — *see* Fracture, patella
  larynx S12.8 ✓
  late effects — *see* Sequelae, fracture
  leg (lower) S82.9- ✓
    ankle — *see* Fracture, ankle
    femur — *see* Fracture, femur
    fibula — *see* Fracture, fibula
    malleolus — *see* Fracture, ankle
    patella — *see* Fracture, patella
    specified site NEC S82.89- ✓
    tibia — *see* Fracture, tibia
  lumbar spine — *see* Fracture, vertebra, lumbar
  lumbosacral spine S32.9 ✓
  Maisonneuve's (displaced) S82.86- ✓
    nondisplaced S82.86- ✓
  malar bone (*see also* Fracture, maxilla) S02.400 ✓
  malleolus — *see* Fracture, ankle
  malunion — *see* Fracture, by site
  mandible (lower jaw (bone)) S02.609 ✓
    alveolus S02.67 ✓
    angle (of jaw) S02.65 ✓
    body, unspecified S02.600 ✓
    condylar process S02.61 ✓
    coronoid process S02.63 ✓
    ramus, unspecified S02.64 ✓
    specified site NEC S02.69 ✓
    subcondylar process S02.62 ✓
    symphysis S02.66 ✓
  manubrium (sterni) S22.21 ✓
    dissociation from sternum S22.23 ✓
  march — *see* Fracture, traumatic, stress, by site
  maxilla, maxillary (bone) (sinus) (superior) (upper jaw) S02.401 ✓
    alveolus S02.42 ✓
    inferior — *see* Fracture, mandible
    LeFort I S02.411 ✓
    LeFort II S02.412 ✓
    LeFort III S02.413 ✓
  metacarpal S62.309 ✓
    base (displaced) S62.319 ✓
      nondisplaced S62.349 ✓
    fifth S62.30- ✓
      base (displaced) S62.31- ✓
        nondisplaced S62.34- ✓
      neck (displaced) S62.33- ✓
        nondisplaced S62.36- ✓
      shaft (displaced) S62.32- ✓
        nondisplaced S62.35- ✓
      specified NEC S62.398 ✓
    first S62.20- ✓
      base NEC (displaced) S62.23- ✓
        nondisplaced S62.23- ✓
      Bennett's — *see* Bennett's fracture
      neck (displaced) S62.25- ✓
        nondisplaced S62.25- ✓
      shaft (displaced) S62.24- ✓
        nondisplaced S62.24- ✓
      specified NEC S62.29- ✓
    fourth S62.30- ✓
      base (displaced) S62.31- ✓
        nondisplaced S62.34- ✓
      neck (displaced) S62.33- ✓
        nondisplaced S62.36- ✓
      shaft (displaced) S62.32- ✓
        nondisplaced S62.35- ✓
      specified NEC S62.39- ✓
    neck (displaced) S62.33- ✓
      nondisplaced S62.36- ✓
    Rolando's — *see* Rolando's fracture

  metacarpal — *continued*
    second S62.30- ✓
      base (displaced) S62.31- ✓
        nondisplaced S62.34- ✓
      neck (displaced) S62.33- ✓
        nondisplaced S62.36- ✓
      shaft (displaced) S62.32- ✓
        nondisplaced S62.35- ✓
      specified NEC S62.39- ✓
    shaft (displaced) S62.32- ✓
      nondisplaced S62.35- ✓
    specified NEC S62.399 ✓
    third S62.30- ✓
      base (displaced) S62.31- ✓
        nondisplaced S62.34- ✓
      neck (displaced) S62.33- ✓
        nondisplaced S62.36- ✓
      shaft (displaced) S62.32- ✓
        nondisplaced S62.35- ✓
      specified NEC S62.39- ✓
  metastatic — *see* Fracture, pathological, due to, neoplastic disease (*see also* Neoplasm)
  metatarsal bone S92.30- ✓
    fifth (displaced) S92.35- ✓
      nondisplaced S92.35- ✓
    first (displaced) S92.31- ✓
      nondisplaced S92.31- ✓
    fourth (displaced) S92.34- ✓
      nondisplaced S92.34- ✓
    second (displaced) S92.32- ✓
      nondisplaced S92.32- ✓
    third (displaced) S92.33- ✓
      nondisplaced S92.33- ✓
  Monteggia's — *see* Monteggia's fracture
  multiple
    hand (and wrist) NEC — *see* Fracture, by site
    ribs — *see* Fracture, rib, multiple
  nasal (bone(s)) S02.2 ✓
  navicular (scaphoid) (foot) (*see also* Fracture, tarsal, navicular)
    hand — *see* Fracture, carpal, navicular
  neck S12.9 ✓
    cervical vertebra S12.9 ✓
      fifth (displaced) S12.400 ✓
        nondisplaced S12.401 ✓
        specified type NEC (displaced) S12.490 ✓
          nondisplaced S12.491 ✓
      first (displaced) S12.000 ✓
        burst (stable) S12.01 ✓
          unstable S12.02 ✓
        lateral mass (displaced) S12.040 ✓
          nondisplaced S12.041 ✓
        nondisplaced S12.001 ✓
        posterior arch (displaced) S12.030 ✓
          nondisplaced S12.031 ✓
        specified type NEC (displaced) S12.090 ✓
          nondisplaced S12.091 ✓
      fourth (displaced) S12.300 ✓
        nondisplaced S12.301 ✓
        specified type NEC (displaced) S12.390 ✓
          nondisplaced S12.391 ✓
      second (displaced) S12.100 ✓
        dens (anterior) (displaced) (type II) S12.110 ✓
          nondisplaced S12.112 ✓
          posterior S12.111 ✓
        specified type NEC (displaced) S12.120 ✓
          nondisplaced S12.121 ✓
        nondisplaced S12.101 ✓
        specified type NEC (displaced) S12.190 ✓
          nondisplaced S12.191 ✓
      seventh (displaced) S12.600 ✓
        nondisplaced S12.601 ✓
        specified type NEC (displaced) S12.690 ✓
          displaced S12.691 ✓
      sixth (displaced) S12.500 ✓
        nondisplaced S12.501 ✓
        specified type NEC (displaced) S12.590 ✓
          displaced S12.591 ✓
      third (displaced) S12.200 ✓
        nondisplaced S12.201 ✓
        specified type NEC (displaced) S12.290 ✓
          displaced S12.291 ✓

Fracture, traumatic — *continued*
  neck — *continued*
    hyoid bone S12.8 ☑
    larynx S12.8 ☑
    specified site NEC S12.8 ☑
    thyroid cartilage S12.8 ☑
    trachea S12.8 ☑
  neoplastic NEC — *see* Fracture, pathological, due to, neoplastic disease
  neural arch — *see* Fracture, vertebra
  newborn — *see* Birth, injury, fracture
  nontraumatic — *see* Fracture, pathological
  nonunion — *see* Nonunion, fracture
  nose, nasal (bone) (septum) S02.2 ☑
  occiput — *see* Fracture, skull, base, occiput
  odontoid process — *see* Fracture, neck, cervical vertebra, second
  olecranon (process) (ulna) — *see* Fracture, ulna, upper end, olecranon process
  orbit, orbital (bone) (region) S02.8 ☑
    floor (blow-out) S02.3 ☑
    roof S02.19 ☑
  os
    calcis — *see* Fracture, tarsal, calcaneus
    magnum — *see* Fracture, carpal, capitate
    pubis — *see* Fracture, pubis
  palate S02.8 ☑
  parietal bone (skull) S02.0 ☑
  patella S82.00- ☑
    comminuted (displaced) S82.04- ☑
      nondisplaced S82.04- ☑
    longitudinal (displaced) S82.02- ☑
      nondisplaced S82.02- ☑
    osteochondral (displaced) S82.01- ☑
      nondisplaced S82.01- ☑
    specified NEC S82.09- ☑
    transverse (displaced) S82.03- ☑
      nondisplaced S82.03- ☑
  pedicle (of vertebral arch) — *see* Fracture, vertebra
  pelvis, pelvic (bone) S32.9 ☑
    acetabulum — *see* Fracture, acetabulum
    circle — *see* Disruption, pelvic ring
    following insertion of implant, prosthesis or plate M96.65
    ilium — *see* Fracture, ilium
    ischium — *see* Fracture, ischium
    multiple
      with disruption of pelvic ring (circle) — *see* Disruption, pelvic ring
      without disruption of pelvic ring (circle) S32.82 ☑
    pubis — *see* Fracture, pubis
    sacrum — *see* Fracture, sacrum
    specified site NEC S32.89 ☑
  phalanx
    foot — *see* Fracture, toe
    hand — *see* Fracture, finger
  pisiform — *see* Fracture, carpal, pisiform
  pond — *see* Fracture, skull
  prosthetic device, internal — *see* Complications, prosthetic device, by site, mechanical
  pubis S32.50- ☑
    with disruption of pelvic ring — *see* Disruption, pelvic ring
    specified site NEC S32.59- ☑
    superior rim S32.51- ☑
  radius S52.9- ☑
    distal end — *see* Fracture, radius, lower end
    following insertion of implant, prosthesis or plate M96.63- ☑
    head — *see* Fracture, radius, upper end, head
    lower end S52.50- ☑
      Barton's — *see* Barton's fracture
      Colles' — *see* Colles' fracture
      extraarticular NEC S52.55- ☑
      intraarticular NEC S52.57- ☑
      physeal S59.20- ☑
        Salter-Harris
          Type I S59.21- ☑
          Type II S59.22- ☑
          Type III S59.23- ☑
          Type IV S59.24- ☑
        specified NEC S59.29- ☑
      Smith's — *see* Smith's fracture
      specified NEC S52.59- ☑
      styloid process (displaced) S52.51- ☑

Fracture, traumatic — *continued*
  radius — *continued*
    lower end — *continued*
      styloid process — *continued*
        nondisplaced S52.51- ☑
      torus S52.52- ☑
    neck — *see* Fracture, radius, upper end
    proximal end — *see* Fracture, radius, upper end
    shaft S52.30- ☑
      bent bone S52.38- ☑
      comminuted (displaced) S52.35- ☑
        nondisplaced S52.35- ☑
      Galeazzi's — *see* Galeazzi's fracture
      greenstick S52.31- ☑
      oblique (displaced) S52.33- ☑
        nondisplaced S52.33- ☑
      segmental (displaced) S52.36- ☑
        nondisplaced S52.36- ☑
      specified NEC S52.39- ☑
      spiral (displaced) S52.34- ☑
        nondisplaced S52.34- ☑
      transverse (displaced) S52.32- ☑
        nondisplaced S52.32- ☑
    upper end S52.10- ☑
      head (displaced) S52.12- ☑
        nondisplaced S52.12- ☑
      neck (displaced) S52.13- ☑
        nondisplaced S52.13- ☑
      physeal S59.10- ☑
        Salter-Harris
          Type I S59.11- ☑
          Type II S59.12- ☑
          Type III S59.13- ☑
          Type IV S59.14- ☑
        specified NEC S59.19- ☑
      specified NEC S52.18- ☑
      torus S52.11- ☑
  ramus
    inferior or superior, pubis — *see* Fracture, pubis
    mandible — *see* Fracture, mandible
  restorative material (dental) K08.539
    with loss of material K08.531
    without loss of material K08.530
  rib S22.3- ☑
    with flail chest — *see* Flail, chest
    multiple S22.4- ☑
      with flail chest — *see* Flail, chest
  root, tooth — *see* Fracture, tooth
  sacrum S32.10 ☑
    specified NEC S32.19 ☑
    Type
      1 S32.14 ☑
      2 S32.15 ☑
      3 S32.16 ☑
      4 S32.17 ☑
    Zone
      I S32.119 ☑
        displaced (minimally) S32.111 ☑
          severely S32.112 ☑
        nondisplaced S32.110 ☑
      II S32.129 ☑
        displaced (minimally) S32.121 ☑
          severely S32.122 ☑
        nondisplaced S32.120 ☑
      III S32.139 ☑
        displaced (minimally) S32.131 ☑
          severely S32.132 ☑
        nondisplaced S32.130 ☑
  scaphoid (hand) (*see also* Fracture, carpal, navicular)
    foot — *see* Fracture, tarsal, navicular
  scapula S42.10- ☑
    acromial process (displaced) S42.12- ☑
      nondisplaced S42.12- ☑
    body (displaced) S42.11- ☑
      nondisplaced S42.11- ☑
    coracoid process (displaced) S42.13- ☑
      nondisplaced S42.13- ☑
    glenoid cavity (displaced) S42.14- ☑
      nondisplaced S42.14- ☑
    neck (displaced) S42.15- ☑
      nondisplaced S42.15- ☑
    specified NEC S42.19- ☑
  semilunar bone, wrist — *see* Fracture, carpal, lunate
  sequelae — *see* Sequelae, fracture
  sesamoid bone
    hand — *see* Fracture, carpal

Fracture, traumatic — *continued*
  sesamoid bone — *continued*
    other — *code by* site under Fracture
  shepherd's — *see* Fracture, tarsal, talus
  shoulder (girdle) S42.9- ☑
    blade — *see* Fracture, scapula
  sinus (ethmoid) (frontal) S02.19 ☑
  skull S02.91 ☑
    base S02.10 ☑
      occiput S02.119 ☑
        condyle S02.113 ☑
          type I S02.110 ☑
          type II S02.111 ☑
          type III S02.112 ☑
        specified NEC S02.118 ☑
      specified NEC S02.19 ☑
    birth injury P13.0
    frontal bone S02.0 ☑
    parietal bone S02.0 ☑
    specified site NEC S02.8 ☑
    temporal bone S02.19 ☑
    vault S02.0 ☑
  Smith's — *see* Smith's fracture
  sphenoid (bone) (sinus) S02.19 ☑
  spine — *see* Fracture, vertebra
  spinous process — *see* Fracture, vertebra
  spontaneous (cause unknown) — *see* Fracture, pathological
  stave (of thumb) — *see* Fracture, metacarpal, first
  sternum S22.20 ☑
    with flail chest — *see* Flail, chest
    body S22.22 ☑
    manubrium S22.21 ☑
    xiphoid (process) S22.24 ☑
  stress M84.30 ☑
    ankle M84.37- ☑
    carpus M84.34- ☑
    clavicle M84.31- ☑
    femoral neck M84.359 ☑
    femur M84.35- ☑
    fibula M84.36- ☑
    finger M84.34- ☑
    hip M84.359 ☑
    humerus M84.32- ☑
    ilium M84.350 ☑
    ischium M84.350 ☑
    metacarpus M84.34- ☑
    metatarsus M84.37- ☑
    neck — *see* Fracture, fatigue, vertebra
    pelvis M84.350 ☑
    radius M84.33- ☑
    rib M84.38 ☑
    scapula M84.31- ☑
    skull M84.38 ☑
    tarsus M84.37- ☑
    tibia M84.36- ☑
    toe M84.37- ☑
    ulna M84.33- ☑
    vertebra — *see* Fracture, fatigue, vertebra
  supracondylar, elbow — *see* Fracture, humerus, lower end, supracondylar
  symphysis pubis — *see* Fracture, pubis
  talus (ankle bone) — *see* Fracture, tarsal, talus
  tarsal bone(s) S92.20- ☑
    astragalus — *see* Fracture, tarsal, talus
    calcaneus S92.00- ☑
      anterior process (displaced) S92.02- ☑
        nondisplaced S92.02- ☑
      body (displaced) S92.01- ☑
        nondisplaced S92.01- ☑
      extraarticular NEC (displaced) S92.05- ☑
        nondisplaced S92.05- ☑
      intraarticular (displaced) S92.06- ☑
        nondisplaced S92.06- ☑
      tuberosity (displaced) S92.04- ☑
        avulsion (displaced) S92.03- ☑
          nondisplaced S92.03- ☑
        nondisplaced S92.04- ☑
    cuboid (displaced) S92.21- ☑
      nondisplaced S92.21- ☑
    cuneiform
      intermediate (displaced) S92.23- ☑
        nondisplaced S92.23- ☑
      lateral (displaced) S92.22- ☑
        nondisplaced S92.22- ☑
      medial (displaced) S92.24- ☑

Fracture, traumatic — *continued*
  tarsal bone(s) — *continued*
    cuneiform — *continued*
      medial — *continued*
        nondisplaced S92.24- ☑
      navicular (displaced) S92.25- ☑
        nondisplaced S92.25- ☑
    scaphoid — *see* Fracture, tarsal, navicular
    talus S92.10- ☑
      avulsion (displaced) S92.15- ☑
        nondisplaced S92.15- ☑
      body (displaced) S92.12- ☑
        nondisplaced S92.12- ☑
      dome (displaced) S92.14- ☑
        nondisplaced S92.14- ☑
      head (displaced) S92.12- ☑
        nondisplaced S92.12- ☑
      lateral process (displaced) S92.14- ☑
        nondisplaced S92.14- ☑
      neck (displaced) S92.11- ☑
        nondisplaced S92.11- ☑
      posterior process (displaced) S92.13- ☑
        nondisplaced S92.13- ☑
      specified NEC S92.19- ☑
  temporal bone (styloid) S02.19 ☑
  thorax (bony) S22.9 ☑
    with flail chest — *see* Flail, chest
    rib S22.3- ☑
      multiple S22.4- ☑
        with flail chest — *see* Flail, chest
    sternum S22.20 ☑
      body S22.22 ☑
      manubrium S22.21 ☑
      xiphoid process S22.24 ☑
    vertebra (displaced) S22.009 ☑
      burst (stable) S22.001 ☑
        unstable S22.002 ☑
      eighth S22.069 ☑
        burst (stable) S22.061 ☑
          unstable S22.062 ☑
        specified type NEC S22.068 ☑
        wedge compression S22.060 ☑
      eleventh S22.089 ☑
        burst (stable) S22.081 ☑
          unstable S22.082 ☑
        specified type NEC S22.088 ☑
        wedge compression S22.080 ☑
      fifth S22.059 ☑
        burst (stable) S22.051 ☑
          unstable S22.052 ☑
        specified type NEC S22.058 ☑
        wedge compression S22.050 ☑
      first S22.019 ☑
        burst (stable) S22.011 ☑
          unstable S22.012 ☑
        specified type NEC S22.018 ☑
        wedge compression S22.010 ☑
      fourth S22.049 ☑
        burst (stable) S22.041 ☑
          unstable S22.042 ☑
        specified type NEC S22.048 ☑
        wedge compression S22.040 ☑
      ninth S22.079 ☑
        burst (stable) S22.071 ☑
          unstable S22.072 ☑
        specified type NEC S22.078 ☑
        wedge compression S22.070 ☑
      nondisplaced S22.001 ☑
      second S22.029 ☑
        burst (stable) S22.021 ☑
          unstable S22.022 ☑
        specified type NEC S22.028 ☑
        wedge compression S22.020 ☑
      seventh S22.069 ☑
        burst (stable) S22.061 ☑
          unstable S22.062 ☑
        specified type NEC S22.068 ☑
        wedge compression S22.060 ☑
      sixth S22.059 ☑
        burst (stable) S22.051 ☑
          unstable S22.052 ☑
        specified type NEC S22.058 ☑
        wedge compression S22.050 ☑
      specified type NEC S22.008 ☑
      tenth S22.079 ☑

Fracture, traumatic — *continued*
  thorax — *continued*
    vertebra — *continued*
      tenth — *continued*
        burst (stable) S22.071 ☑
          unstable S22.072 ☑
        specified type NEC S22.078 ☑
        wedge compression S22.070 ☑
      third S22.039 ☑
        burst (stable) S22.031 ☑
          unstable S22.032 ☑
        specified type NEC S22.038 ☑
        wedge compression S22.030 ☑
      twelfth S22.089 ☑
        burst (stable) S22.081 ☑
          unstable S22.082 ☑
        specified type NEC S22.088 ☑
        wedge compression S22.080 ☑
      wedge compression S22.000 ☑
  thumb S62.50- ☑
    distal phalanx (displaced) S62.52- ☑
      nondisplaced S62.52- ☑
    proximal phalanx (displaced) S62.51- ☑
      nondisplaced S62.51- ☑
  thyroid cartilage S12.8 ☑
  tibia (shaft) S82.20- ☑
    comminuted (displaced) S82.25- ☑
      nondisplaced S82.25- ☑
    condyles — *see* Fracture, tibia, upper end
    distal end — *see* Fracture, tibia, lower end
    epiphysis
      lower — *see* Fracture, tibia, lower end
      upper — *see* Fracture, tibia, upper end
    following insertion of implant, prosthesis or plate
      M96.67- ☑
    head (involving knee joint) — *see* Fracture, tibia,
      upper end
    intercondyloid eminence — *see* Fracture, tibia,
      upper end
    involving ankle or malleolus — *see* Fracture, ankle,
      medial malleolus
    lower end S82.30- ☑
      physeal S89.10- ☑
        Salter-Harris
          Type I S89.11- ☑
          Type II S89.12- ☑
          Type III S89.13- ☑
          Type IV S89.14- ☑
        specified NEC S89.19- ☑
      pilon (displaced) S82.87- ☑
        nondisplaced S82.87- ☑
      specified NEC S82.39- ☑
      torus S82.31- ☑
    malleolus — *see* Fracture, ankle, medial malleolus
    oblique (displaced) S82.23- ☑
      nondisplaced S82.23- ☑
    pilon — *see* Fracture, tibia, lower end, pilon
    proximal end — *see* Fracture, tibia, upper end
    segmental (displaced) S82.26- ☑
      nondisplaced S82.26- ☑
    specified NEC S82.29- ☑
    spine — *see* Fracture, upper end, spine
    spiral (displaced) S82.24- ☑
      nondisplaced S82.24- ☑
    transverse (displaced) S82.22- ☑
      nondisplaced S82.22- ☑
    tuberosity — *see* Fracture, tibia, upper end,
      tuberosity
    upper end S82.10- ☑
      bicondylar (displaced) S82.14- ☑
        nondisplaced S82.14- ☑
      lateral condyle (displaced) S82.12- ☑
        nondisplaced S82.12- ☑
      medial condyle (displaced) S82.13- ☑
        nondisplaced S82.13- ☑
      physeal S89.00- ☑
        Salter-Harris
          Type I S89.01- ☑
          Type II S89.02- ☑
          Type III S89.03- ☑
          Type IV S89.04- ☑
        specified NEC S89.09- ☑
      plateau — *see* Fracture, tibia, upper end, bi-
        condylar
      specified NEC S82.19- ☑
      spine (displaced) S82.11- ☑

Fracture, traumatic — *continued*
  tibia — *continued*
    upper end — *continued*
      spine — *continued*
        nondisplaced S82.11- ☑
      torus S82.16- ☑
      tuberosity (displaced) S82.15- ☑
        nondisplaced S82.15- ☑
  toe S92.91- ☑
    great (displaced) S92.40- ☑
      distal phalanx (displaced) S92.42- ☑
        nondisplaced S92.42- ☑
      nondisplaced S92.40- ☑
      proximal phalanx (displaced) S92.41- ☑
        nondisplaced S92.41- ☑
      specified NEC S92.49- ☑
    lesser (displaced) S92.50- ☑
      distal phalanx (displaced) S92.53- ☑
        nondisplaced S92.53- ☑
      medial phalanx (displaced) S92.52- ☑
        nondisplaced S92.52- ☑
      nondisplaced S92.50- ☑
      proximal phalanx (displaced) S92.51- ☑
        nondisplaced S92.51- ☑
      specified NEC S92.59- ☑
  tooth (root) S02.5 ☑
  trachea (cartilage) S12.8 ☑
  transverse process — *see* Fracture, vertebra
  trapezium or trapezoid bone — *see* Fracture, carpal
  trimalleolar — *see* Fracture, ankle, trimalleolar
  triquetrum (cuneiform of carpus) — *see* Fracture,
    carpal, triquetrum
  trochanter — *see* Fracture, femur, trochanteric
  tuberosity (external) — *code by* site under Fracture
  ulna (shaft) S52.20- ☑
    bent bone S52.28- ☑
    coronoid process — *see* Fracture, ulna, upper end,
      coronoid process
    distal end — *see* Fracture, ulna, lower end
    following insertion of implant, prosthesis or plate
      M96.63- ☑
    head S52.00- ☑
    lower end S52.60- ☑
      physeal S59.00- ☑
        Salter-Harris
          Type I S59.01- ☑
          Type II S59.02- ☑
          Type III S59.03- ☑
          Type IV S59.04- ☑
        specified NEC S59.09- ☑
      specified NEC S52.69- ☑
      styloid process (displaced) S52.61- ☑
        nondisplaced S52.61- ☑
      torus S52.62- ☑
    proximal end — *see* Fracture, ulna, upper end
    shaft S52.20- ☑
      comminuted (displaced) S52.25- ☑
        nondisplaced S52.25- ☑
      greenstick S52.21- ☑
      Monteggia's — *see* Monteggia's fracture
      oblique (displaced) S52.23- ☑
        nondisplaced S52.23- ☑
      segmental (displaced) S52.26- ☑
        nondisplaced S52.26- ☑
      specified NEC S52.29- ☑
      spiral (displaced) S52.24- ☑
        nondisplaced S52.24- ☑
      transverse (displaced) S52.22- ☑
        nondisplaced S52.22- ☑
    upper end S52.00- ☑
      coronoid process (displaced) S52.04- ☑
        nondisplaced S52.04- ☑
      olecranon process (displaced) S52.02- ☑
        with intraarticular extension S52.03- ☑
        nondisplaced S52.02- ☑
          with intraarticular extension S52.03- ☑
      specified NEC S52.09- ☑
      torus S52.01- ☑
  unciform — *see* Fracture, carpal, hamate
  vault of skull S02.0 ☑
  vertebra, vertebral (arch) (body) (column) (neural arch)
    (pedicle) (spinous process) (transverse process)
    atlas — *see* Fracture, neck, cervical vertebra, first
    axis — *see* Fracture, neck, cervical vertebra, second
    cervical (teardrop) S12.9 ☑

☑ Additional Character Required — Refer to the Tabular List for Character Selection   ▽ Subterms under main terms may continue to next column or page

Fracture, traumatic — *continued*
  vertebra, vertebral — *continued*
    cervical —- *continued*
      axis — *see* Fracture, neck, cervical vertebra, second
      first (atlas) — *see* Fracture, neck, cervical vertebra, first
      second (axis) — *see* Fracture, neck, cervical vertebra, second
    chronic M84.48 ☑
    coccyx S32.2 ☑
    dorsal — *see* Fracture, thorax, vertebra
    lumbar S32.009 ☑
      burst (stable) S32.001 ☑
        unstable S32.002 ☑
      fifth S32.059 ☑
        burst (stable) S32.051 ☑
          unstable S32.052 ☑
        specified type NEC S32.058 ☑
        wedge compression S32.050 ☑
      first S32.019 ☑
        burst (stable) S32.011 ☑
          unstable S32.012 ☑
        specified type NEC S32.018 ☑
        wedge compression S32.010 ☑
      fourth S32.049 ☑
        burst (stable) S32.041 ☑
          unstable S32.042 ☑
        specified type NEC S32.048 ☑
        wedge compression S32.040 ☑
      second S32.029 ☑
        burst (stable) S32.021 ☑
          unstable S32.022 ☑
        specified type NEC S32.028 ☑
        wedge compression S32.020 ☑
      specified type NEC S32.008 ☑
      third S32.039 ☑
        burst (stable) S32.031 ☑
          unstable S32.032 ☑
        specified type NEC S32.038 ☑
        wedge compression S32.030 ☑
      wedge compression S32.000 ☑
    metastatic — *see* Collapse, vertebra, in, specified disease NEC (*see also* Neoplasm)
    newborn (birth injury) P11.5
    sacrum S32.10 ☑
      specified NEC S32.19 ☑
      Type
        1 S32.14 ☑
        2 S32.15 ☑
        3 S32.16 ☑
        4 S32.17 ☑
      Zone
        I S32.119 ☑
          displaced (minimally) S32.111 ☑
            severely S32.112 ☑
          nondisplaced S32.110 ☑
        II S32.129 ☑
          displaced (minimally) S32.121 ☑
            severely S32.122 ☑
          nondisplaced S32.120 ☑
        III S32.139 ☑
          displaced (minimally) S32.131 ☑
            severely S32.132 ☑
          nondisplaced S32.130 ☑
    thoracic — *see* Fracture, thorax, vertebra
  vertex S02.0 ☑
  vomer (bone) S02.2 ☑
  wrist S62.10- ☑
    carpal — *see* Fracture, carpal bone
    navicular (scaphoid) (hand) — *see* Fracture, carpal, navicular
  xiphisternum, xiphoid (process) S22.24 ☑
  zygoma S02.402 ☑
Fragile, fragility
  autosomal site Q95.5
  bone, congenital (with blue sclera) Q78.0
  capillary (hereditary) D69.8
  hair L67.8
  nails L60.3
  non-sex chromosome site Q95.5
  X chromosome Q99.2
Fragilitas
  crinium L67.8
  ossium (with blue sclerae) (hereditary) Q78.0
  unguium L60.3

Fragilitas — *continued*
  unguium — *continued*
    congenital Q84.6
Fragments, cataract (lens), **following cataract surgery** H59.02- ☑
  retained foreign body — *see* Retained, foreign body fragments (type of)
Frailty (frail) R54
  mental R41.81
Frambesia, frambesial (tropica) (*see also* Yaws)
  initial lesion or ulcer A66.0
  primary A66.0
Frambeside
  gummatous A66.4
  of early yaws A66.2
Frambesioma A66.1
Franceschetti-Klein (-Wildervanck) **disease or syndrome** Q75.4
Francis' disease — *see* Tularemia
Franklin disease C88.2
Frank's essential thrombocytopenia D69.3
Fraser's syndrome Q87.0
Freckle(s) L81.2
  malignant melanoma in — *see* Melanoma
  melanotic (Hutchinson's) — *see* Melanoma, in situ
  retinal D49.81
Frederickson's hyperlipoproteinemia, type
  I and V E78.3
  IIA E78.0
  IIB and III E78.2
  IV E78.1
Freeman Sheldon syndrome Q87.0
Freezing (*see also* Effect, adverse, cold) T69.9 ☑
Freiberg's disease (infraction of metatarsal head or osteochondrosis) — *see* Osteochondrosis, juvenile, metatarsus
Frei's disease A55
Fremitus, friction, cardiac R01.2
Frenum, frenulum
  external os Q51.828
  tongue (shortening) (congenital) Q38.1
Frequency micturition (nocturnal) R35.0
  psychogenic F45.8
Frey's syndrome
  auriculotemporal G50.8
  hyperhidrosis L74.52
Friction
  burn — *see* Burn, by site
  fremitus, cardiac R01.2
  precordial R01.2
  sounds, chest R09.89
Friderichsen-Waterhouse syndrome or disease A39.1
Friedländer's B (bacillus) **NEC** (*see also* condition) A49.8
Friedreich's
  ataxia G11.1
  combined systemic disease G11.1
  facial hemihypertrophy Q67.4
  sclerosis (cerebellum) (spinal cord) G11.1
Frigidity F52.22
Fröhlich's syndrome E23.6
Frontal (*see also* condition)
  lobe syndrome F07.0
Frostbite (superficial) T33.90 ☑
  with
    partial thickness skin loss — *see* Frostbite (superficial), by site
    tissue necrosis T34.90 ☑
  abdominal wall T33.3 ☑
    with tissue necrosis T34.3 ☑
  ankle T33.81- ☑
    with tissue necrosis T34.81- ☑
  arm T33.4- ☑
    with tissue necrosis T34.4- ☑
    finger(s) — *see* Frostbite, finger
    hand — *see* Frostbite, hand
    wrist — *see* Frostbite, wrist
  ear T33.01- ☑
    with tissue necrosis T34.01- ☑
  face T33.09 ☑
    with tissue necrosis T34.09 ☑
  finger T33.53- ☑
    with tissue necrosis T34.53- ☑
  foot T33.82- ☑
    with tissue necrosis T34.82- ☑
  hand T33.52- ☑
    with tissue necrosis T34.52- ☑
  head T33.09 ☑

Frostbite — *continued*
  head — *continued*
    with tissue necrosis T34.09 ☑
    ear — *see* Frostbite, ear
    nose — *see* Frostbite, nose
  hip (and thigh) T33.6- ☑
    with tissue necrosis T34.6- ☑
  knee T33.7- ☑
    with tissue necrosis T34.7- ☑
  leg T33.9- ☑
    with tissue necrosis T34.9- ☑
    ankle — *see* Frostbite, ankle
    foot — *see* Frostbite, foot
    knee — *see* Frostbite, knee
    lower T33.7- ☑
      with tissue necrosis T34.7- ☑
    thigh — *see* Frostbite, hip
    toe — *see* Frostbite, toe
  limb
    lower T33.99 ☑
      with tissue necrosis T34.99 ☑
    upper — *see* Frostbite, arm
  neck T33.1 ☑
    with tissue necrosis T34.1 ☑
  nose T33.02 ☑
    with tissue necrosis T34.02 ☑
  pelvis T33.3 ☑
    with tissue necrosis T34.3 ☑
  specified site NEC T33.99 ☑
    with tissue necrosis T34.99 ☑
  thigh — *see* Frostbite, hip
  thorax T33.2 ☑
    with tissue necrosis T34.2 ☑
  toes T33.83- ☑
    with tissue necrosis T34.83- ☑
  trunk T33.99 ☑
    with tissue necrosis T34.99 ☑
  wrist T33.51- ☑
    with tissue necrosis T34.51- ☑
Frotteurism F65.81
Frozen (*see also* Effect, adverse, cold) T69.9 ☑
  pelvis (female) N94.89
    male K66.8
  shoulder — *see* Capsulitis, adhesive
Fructokinase deficiency E74.11
Fructose 1,6 diphosphatase deficiency E74.19
Fructosemia (benign) (essential) E74.12
Fructosuria (benign) (essential) E74.11
Fuchs'
  black spot (myopic) H44.2- ☑
  dystrophy (corneal endothelium) H18.51
  heterochromic cyclitis — *see* Cyclitis, Fuchs' heterochromic
Fucosidosis E77.1
Fugue R68.89
  dissociative F44.1
  hysterical (dissociative) F44.1
  postictal in epilepsy — *see* Epilepsy
  reaction to exceptional stress (transient) F43.0
Fulminant, fulminating — *see* condition
Functional (*see also* condition)
  bleeding (uterus) N93.8
Functioning, intellectual, borderline R41.83
Fundus — *see* condition
Fungemia NOS B49
Fungus, fungous
  cerebral G93.89
  disease NOS B49
  infection — *see* Infection, fungus
Funiculitis (acute) (chronic) (endemic) N49.1
  gonococcal (acute) (chronic) A54.23
  tuberculous A18.15
Funnel
  breast (acquired) M95.4
    congenital Q67.6
    sequelae (late effect) of rickets E64.3
  chest (acquired) M95.4
    congenital Q67.6
    sequelae (late effect) of rickets E64.3
  pelvis (acquired) M95.5
    with disproportion (fetopelvic) O33.3 ☑
      causing obstructed labor O65.3
    congenital Q74.2
FUO (fever of unknown origin) R50.9
Furfur L21.0
  microsporon B36.0

Index

Fracture, traumatic — Furfur

Index

Furrier's lung — Fussy baby

Furrier's lung J67.8
Furrowed K14.5
  nail(s) (transverse) L60.4
    congenital Q84.6
  tongue K14.5
    congenital Q38.3
Furuncle L02.92
  abdominal wall L02.221
  ankle — see Furuncle, lower limb
  antecubital space — see Furuncle, upper limb
  anus K61.0
  arm — see Furuncle, upper limb
  auditory canal, external — see Abscess, ear, external
  auricle (ear) — see Abscess, ear, external
  axilla (region) L02.42- ☑
  back (any part) L02.222
  breast N61
  buttock L02.32
  cheek (external) L02.02
  chest wall L02.223
  chin L02.02
  corpus cavernosum N48.21
  ear, external — see Abscess, ear, external
  external auditory canal — see Abscess, ear, external
  eyelid — see Abscess, eyelid
  face L02.02
  femoral (region) — see Furuncle, lower limb
  finger — see Furuncle, hand
  flank L02.221
  foot L02.62- ☑
  forehead L02.02
  gluteal (region) L02.32
  groin L02.224
  hand L02.52- ☑
  head L02.821
    face L02.02
  hip — see Furuncle, lower limb
  kidney — see Abscess, kidney
  knee — see Furuncle, lower limb
  labium (majus) (minus) N76.4
  lacrimal
    gland — see Dacryoadenitis
    passages (duct) (sac) — see Inflammation, lacrimal, passages, acute
  leg (any part) — see Furuncle, lower limb
  lower limb L02.42- ☑
  malignant A22.0
  mouth K12.2
  navel L02.226

Furuncle — continued
  neck L02.12
  nose J34.0
  orbit, orbital — see Abscess, orbit
  palmar (space) — see Furuncle, hand
  partes posteriores L02.32
  pectoral region L02.223
  penis N48.21
  perineum L02.225
  pinna — see Abscess, ear, external
  popliteal — see Furuncle, lower limb
  prepatellar — see Furuncle, lower limb
  scalp L02.821
  seminal vesicle N49.0
  shoulder — see Furuncle, upper limb
  specified site NEC L02.828
  submandibular K12.2
  temple (region) L02.02
  thumb — see Furuncle, hand
  toe — see Furuncle, foot
  trunk L02.229
    abdominal wall L02.221
    back L02.222
    chest wall L02.223
    groin L02.224
    perineum L02.225
    umbilicus L02.226
  umbilicus L02.226
  upper limb L02.42- ☑
  vulva N76.4
Furunculosis — see Furuncle
Fused — see Fusion, fused
Fusion, fused (congenital)
  astragaloscaphoid Q74.2
  atria Q21.1
  auditory canal Q16.1
  auricles, heart Q21.1
  binocular with defective stereopsis H53.32
  bone Q79.8
  cervical spine M43.22
  choanal Q30.0
  commissure, mitral valve Q23.2
  cusps, heart valve NEC Q24.8
    mitral Q23.2
    pulmonary Q22.1
    tricuspid Q22.4
  ear ossicles Q16.3
  fingers Q70.0 ☑
  hymen Q52.3

Fusion, fused — continued
  joint (acquired) (see also Ankylosis)
    congenital Q74.8
  kidneys (incomplete) Q63.1
  labium (majus) (minus) Q52.5
  larynx and trachea Q34.8
  limb, congenital Q74.8
    lower Q74.2
    upper Q74.0
  lobes, lung Q33.8
  lumbosacral (acquired) M43.27
    arthrodesis status Z98.1
    congenital Q76.49
    postprocedural status Z98.1
  nares, nose, nasal, nostril(s) Q30.0
  organ or site not listed — see Anomaly, by site
  ossicles Q79.9
    auditory Q16.3
  pulmonic cusps Q22.1
  ribs Q76.6
  sacroiliac (joint) (acquired) M43.28
    arthrodesis status Z98.1
    congenital Q74.2
    postprocedural status Z98.1
  spine (acquired) NEC M43.20
    arthrodesis status Z98.1
    cervical region M43.22
    cervicothoracic region M43.23
    congenital Q76.49
    lumbar M43.26
    lumbosacral region M43.27
    occipito-atlanto-axial region M43.21
    postoperative status Z98.1
    sacrococcygeal region M43.28
    thoracic region M43.24
    thoracolumbar region M43.25
  sublingual duct with submaxillary duct at opening in mouth Q38.4
  testes Q55.1
  toes Q70.2- ☑
  tooth, teeth K00.2
  trachea and esophagus Q39.8
  twins Q89.4
  vagina Q52.4
  ventricles, heart Q21.0
  vertebra (arch) — see Fusion, spine
  vulva Q52.5
Fusospirillosis (mouth) (tongue) (tonsil) A69.1
Fussy baby R68.12

150

☑ **Additional Character Required** — Refer to the Tabular List for Character Selection   ▽ **Subterms under main terms may continue to next column or page**

G

Gain in weight (abnormal) (excessive) (see also Weight, gain)

Gaisböck's disease (polycythemia hypertonica) D75.1

Gait abnormality R26.9
- ataxic R26.0
- falling R29.6
- hysterical (ataxic) (staggering) F44.4
- paralytic R26.1
- spastic R26.1
- specified type NEC R26.89
- staggering R26.0
- unsteadiness R26.81
- walking difficulty NEC R26.2

Galactocele (breast) N64.89
- puerperal, postpartum O92.79

Galactokinase deficiency E74.29

Galactophoritis N61
- gestational, puerperal, postpartum O91.2- ☑

Galactorrhea O92.6
- not associated with childbirth N64.3

Galactosemia (classic) (congenital) E74.21

Galactosuria E74.29

Galacturia R82.0
- schistosomiasis (bilharziasis) B65.0

Galeazzi's fracture S52.37- ☑

Galen's vein — see condition

Galeophobia F40.218

Gall duct — see condition

Gallbladder (see also condition)
- acute K81.0

Gallop rhythm R00.8

Gallstone (colic) (cystic duct) (gallbladder) (impacted) (multiple) (see also Calculus, gallbladder)
- with
  - cholecystitis — see Calculus, gallbladder, with cholecystitis
- bile duct (common) (hepatic) — see Calculus, bile duct
- causing intestinal obstruction K56.3
- specified NEC K80.80
  - with obstruction K80.81

Gambling Z72.6
- pathological (compulsive) F63.0

Gammopathy (of undetermined significance [MGUS]) D47.2
- associated with lymphoplasmacytic dyscrasia D47.2
- monoclonal D47.2
- polyclonal D89.0

Gamna's disease (siderotic splenomegaly) D73.1

Gamophobia F40.298

Gampsodactylia (congenital) Q66.7

Gamstorp's disease (adynamia episodica hereditaria) G72.3

Gandy-Nanta disease (siderotic splenomegaly) D73.1

Gang
- membership offenses Z72.810

Gangliocytoma D36.10

Ganglioglioma — see Neoplasm, uncertain behavior, by site

Ganglion (compound) (diffuse) (joint) (tendon (sheath)) M67.40
- ankle M67.47- ☑
- foot M67.47- ☑
- forearm M67.43- ☑
- hand M67.44- ☑
- lower leg M67.46- ☑
- multiple sites M67.49
- of yaws (early) (late) A66.6
- pelvic region M67.45- ☑
- periosteal — see Periostitis
- shoulder region M67.41- ☑
- specified site NEC M67.48
- thigh region M67.45- ☑
- tuberculous A18.09
- upper arm M67.42- ☑
- wrist M67.43- ☑

Ganglioneuroblastoma — see Neoplasm, nerve, malignant

Ganglioneuroma D36.10

Ganglioneuroma — continued
- malignant — see Neoplasm, nerve, malignant

Ganglioneuromatosis D36.10

Ganglionitis
- fifth nerve — see Neuralgia, trigeminal
- gasserian (postherpetic) (postzoster) B02.21
- geniculate G51.1
  - newborn (birth injury) P11.3
  - postherpetic, postzoster B02.21
- herpes zoster B02.21
- postherpetic geniculate B02.21

Gangliosidosis E75.10
- GM1 E75.19
- GM2 E75.00
  - other specified E75.09
  - Sandhoff disease E75.01
  - Tay-Sachs disease E75.02
- GM3 E75.19
- mucolipidosis IV E75.11

Gangosa A66.5

Gangrene, gangrenous (connective tissue) (dropsical) (dry) (moist) (skin) (ulcer) (see also Necrosis) I96
- with diabetes (mellitus) — see Diabetes, gangrene
- abdomen (wall) I96
- alveolar M27.3
- appendix K35.80
  - with
    - perforation or rupture K35.2
    - peritoneal abscess K35.3
    - peritonitis NEC K35.3
      - generalized (with perforation or rupture) K35.2
      - localized (with perforation or rupture) K35.3
- arteriosclerotic (general) (senile) — see Arteriosclerosis, extremities, with, gangrene
- auricle I96
- Bacillus welchii A48.0
- bladder (infectious) — see Cystitis, specified type NEC
- bowel, cecum, or colon — see Gangrene, intestine
- Clostridium perfringens or welchii A48.0
- cornea H18.89- ☑
- corpora cavernosa N48.29
  - noninfective N48.89
- cutaneous, spreading I96
- decubital — see Ulcer, pressure, by site
- diabetic (any site) — see Diabetes, gangrene
- emphysematous — see Gangrene, gas
- epidemic — see Poisoning, food, noxious, plant
- epididymis (infectional) N45.1
- erysipelas — see Erysipelas
- extremity (lower) (upper) I96
- Fournier N49.3
  - female N76.89
- fusospirochetal A69.0
- gallbladder — see Cholecystitis, acute
- gas (bacillus) A48.0
  - following
    - abortion — see Abortion by type complicated by infection
    - ectopic or molar pregnancy O08.0
- glossitis K14.0
- hernia — see Hernia, by site, with gangrene
- intestine, intestinal (hemorrhagic) (massive) K55.0
  - with
    - mesenteric embolism K55.0
    - obstruction — see Obstruction, intestine
- laryngitis J04.0
- limb (lower) (upper) I96
- lung J85.0
  - spirochetal A69.8
- lymphangitis I89.1
- Meleney's (synergistic) — see Ulcer, skin
- mesentery K55.0
  - with
    - embolism K55.0
    - intestinal obstruction — see Obstruction, intestine
- mouth A69.0
- ovary — see Oophoritis
- pancreas K85.9
- penis N48.29
  - noninfective N48.89

Gangrene, gangrenous — continued
- perineum I96
- pharynx (see also Pharyngitis)
  - Vincent's A69.1
- presenile I73.1
- progressive synergistic — see Ulcer, skin
- pulmonary J85.0
- pulpal (dental) K04.1
- quinsy J36
- Raynaud's (symmetric gangrene) I73.01
- retropharyngeal J39.2
- scrotum N49.3
  - noninfective N50.8
- senile (atherosclerotic) — see Arteriosclerosis, extremities, with, gangrene
- spermatic cord N49.1
  - noninfective N50.8
- spine I96
- spirochetal NEC A69.8
- spreading cutaneous I96
- stomatitis A69.0
- symmetrical I73.01
- testis (infectional) N45.2
  - noninfective N44.8
- throat (see also Pharyngitis)
  - diphtheritic A36.0
  - Vincent's A69.1
- thyroid (gland) E07.89
- tooth (pulp) K04.1
- tuberculous NEC — see Tuberculosis
- tunica vaginalis N49.1
  - noninfective N50.8
- umbilicus I96
- uterus — see Endometritis
- uvulitis K12.2
- vas deferens N49.1
  - noninfective N50.8
- vulva N76.89

Ganister disease J62.8

Ganser's syndrome (hysterical) F44.89

Gardner-Diamond syndrome (autoerythrocyte sensitization) D69.2

Gargoylism E76.01

Garré's disease, osteitis (sclerosing), osteomyelitis — see Osteomyelitis, specified type NEC

Garrod's pad, knuckle M72.1

Gartner's duct
- cyst Q52.4
- persistent Q50.6

Gas R14.3
- asphyxiation, inhalation, poisoning, suffocation NEC — see Table of Drugs and Chemicals
- excessive R14.0
- gangrene A48.0
  - following
    - abortion — see Abortion by type complicated by infection
    - ectopic or molar pregnancy O08.0
- on stomach R14.0
- pains R14.1

Gastralgia (see also Pain, abdominal)

Gastrectasis K31.0
- psychogenic F45.8

Gastric — see condition

Gastrinoma
- malignant
  - pancreas C25.4
  - specified site NEC — see Neoplasm, malignant, by site
  - unspecified site C25.4
- specified site — see Neoplasm, uncertain behavior
- unspecified site D37.9

Gastritis (simple) K29.70
- with bleeding K29.71
- acute (erosive) K29.00
  - with bleeding K29.01
- alcoholic K29.20
  - with bleeding K29.21
- allergic K29.60
  - with bleeding K29.61
- atrophic (chronic) K29.40
  - with bleeding K29.41

Gastritis — *continued*
  chronic (antral) (fundal) K29.50
    with bleeding K29.51
    atrophic K29.40
      with bleeding K29.41
    superficial K29.30
      with bleeding K29.31
  dietary counseling and surveillance Z71.3
  due to diet deficiency E63.9
  eosinophilic K52.81
  giant hypertrophic K29.60
    with bleeding K29.61
  granulomatous K29.60
    with bleeding K29.61
  hypertrophic (mucosa) K29.60
    with bleeding K29.61
  nervous F54
  spastic K29.60
    with bleeding K29.61
  specified NEC K29.60
    with bleeding K29.61
  superficial chronic K29.30
    with bleeding K29.31
  tuberculous A18.83
  viral NEC A08.4
Gastrocarcinoma — *see* Neoplasm, malignant, stomach
Gastrocolic — *see* condition
Gastrodisciasis, gastrodiscoidiasis B66.8
Gastroduodenitis K29.90
  with bleeding K29.91
  virus, viral A08.4
    specified type NEC A08.39
Gastrodynia — *see* Pain, abdominal
Gastroenteritis (acute) (chronic) (noninfectious) (*see also* Enteritis) K52.9
  allergic K52.2
  dietetic K52.2
  drug-induced K52.1
  due to
    Cryptosporidium A07.2
    drugs K52.1
    food poisoning — *see* intoxication, foodborne
    radiation K52.0
  eosinophilic K52.81
  epidemic (infectious) A09
  food hypersensitivity K52.2
  infectious — *see* Enteritis, infectious
  influenzal — *see* Influenza, with gastroenteritis
  noninfectious K52.9
    specified NEC K52.89
  rotaviral A08.0
  Salmonella A02.0
  toxic K52.1
  viral NEC A08.4
    acute infectious A08.39
      type Norwalk A08.11
    infantile (acute) A08.39
    Norwalk agent A08.11
    rotaviral A08.0
    severe of infants A08.39
    specified type NEC A08.39
Gastroenteropathy (*see also* Gastroenteritis) K52.9
  acute, due to Norovirus A08.11
  acute, due to Norwalk agent A08.11
  infectious A09
Gastroenteroptosis K63.4
Gastroesophageal laceration- hemorrhage syndrome K22.6
Gastrointestinal — *see* condition
Gastrojejunal — *see* condition
Gastrojejunitis (*see also* Enteritis) K52.9
Gastrojejunocolic — *see* condition
Gastroliths K31.89
Gastromalacia K31.89
Gastroparalysis K31.84
  diabetic — *see* Diabetes, gastroparalysis
Gastroparesis K31.84
  diabetic — *see* Diabetes, by type, with gastroparesis
Gastropathy K31.9
  congestive portal K31.89
  erythematous K29.70
  exudative K90.89
  portal hypertensive K31.89
Gastroptosis K31.89
Gastrorrhagia K92.2
  psychogenic F45.8
Gastroschisis (congenital) Q79.3
Gastrospasm (neurogenic) (reflex) K31.89

Gastrospasm — *continued*
  neurotic F45.8
  psychogenic F45.8
Gastrostaxis — *see* Gastritis, with bleeding
Gastrostenosis K31.89
Gastrostomy
  attention to Z43.1
  status Z93.1
Gastrosuccorrhea (continuous) (intermittent) K31.89
  neurotic F45.8
  psychogenic F45.8
Gatophobia F40.218
Gaucher's disease or splenomegaly (adult) (infantile) E75.22
Gee (-Herter)(-Thaysen) **disease** (nontropical sprue) K90.0
Gélineau's syndrome G47.419
  with cataplexy G47.411
Gemination, tooth, teeth K00.2
Gemistocytoma
  specified site — *see* Neoplasm, malignant, by site
  unspecified site C71.9
General, generalized — *see* condition
Genetic
  carrier (status)
    cystic fibrosis Z14.1
    hemophilia A (asymptomatic) Z14.01
      symptomatic Z14.02
    specified NEC Z14.8
  susceptibility to disease NEC Z15.89
    malignant neoplasm Z15.09
      breast Z15.01
      endometrium Z15.04
      ovary Z15.02
      prostate Z15.03
      specified NEC Z15.09
    multiple endocrine neoplasia Z15.81
Genital — *see* condition
Genito-anorectal syndrome A55
Genitourinary system — *see* condition
Genu
  congenital Q74.1
  extrorsum (acquired) (*see also* Deformity, varus, knee)
    congenital Q74.1
    sequelae (late effect) of rickets E64.3
  introrsum (acquired) (*see also* Deformity, valgus, knee)
    congenital Q74.1
    sequelae (late effect) of rickets E64.3
  rachitic (old) E64.3
  recurvatum (acquired) (*see also* Deformity, limb, specified type NEC, lower leg)
    congenital Q68.2
    sequelae (late effect) of rickets E64.3
  valgum (acquired) (knock-knee) M21.06- ☑
    congenital Q74.1
    sequelae (late effect) of rickets E64.3
  varum (acquired) (bowleg) M21.16- ☑
    congenital Q74.1
    sequelae (late effect) of rickets E64.3
Geographic tongue K14.1
Geophagia — *see* Pica
Geotrichosis B48.3
  stomatitis B48.3
Gephyrophobia F40.242
Gerbode defect Q21.0
GERD (gastroesophageal reflux disease) K21.9
Gerhardt's
  disease (erythromelalgia) I73.81
  syndrome (vocal cord paralysis) J38.00
    bilateral J38.02
    unilateral J38.01
German measles (*see also* Rubella)
  exposure to Z20.4
Germinoblastoma (diffuse) C85.9- ☑
  follicular C82.9- ☑
Germinoma — *see* Neoplasm, malignant, by site
Gerontoxon — *see* Degeneration, cornea, senile
Gerstmann's syndrome R48.8
  developmental F81.2
Gerstmann-Sträussler-Scheinker syndrome (GSS) A81.82
Gestation (period) (*see also* Pregnancy)
  ectopic — *see* Pregnancy, by site
  multiple O30.9- ☑
    greater than quadruplets — *see* Pregnancy, multiple (gestation), specified NEC
    specified NEC — *see* Pregnancy, multiple (gestation), specified NEC

Gestational
  mammary abscess O91.11- ☑
  purulent mastitis O91.11- ☑
  subareolar abscess O91.11- ☑
Ghon tubercle, primary infection A15.7
Ghost
  teeth K00.4
  vessels (cornea) H16.41- ☑
Ghoul hand A66.3
Gianotti-Crosti disease L44.4
Giant
  cell
    epulis K06.8
      peripheral granuloma K06.8
  esophagus, congenital Q39.5
  kidney, congenital Q63.3
  urticaria T78.3 ☑
    hereditary D84.1
Giardiasis A07.1
Gibert's disease or pityriasis L42
Giddiness R42
  hysterical F44.89
  psychogenic F45.8
Gierke's disease (glycogenosis I) E74.01
Gigantism (cerebral) (hypophyseal) (pituitary) E22.0
  constitutional E34.4
Gilbert's disease or syndrome E80.4
Gilchrist's disease B40.9
Gilford-Hutchinson disease E34.8
Gilles de la Tourette's disease or syndrome (motor-verbal tic) F95.2
Gingivitis K05.10
  acute (catarrhal) K05.00
    necrotizing A69.1
    nonplaque induced K05.01
    plaque induced K05.00
  chronic (desquamative) (hyperplastic) (simple marginal) (ulcerative) K05.10
    nonplaque induced K05.11
    plaque induced K05.10
  expulsiva — *see* Periodontitis
  necrotizing ulcerative (acute) A69.1
  pellagrous E52
    acute necrotizing A69.1
  Vincent's A69.1
Gingivoglossitis K14.0
Gingivopericementitis — *see* Periodontitis
Gingivosis — *see* Gingivitis, chronic
Gingivostomatitis K05.10
  herpesviral B00.2
  necrotizing ulcerative (acute) A69.1
Gland, glandular — *see* condition
Glanders A24.0
Glanzmann (-Naegeli) **disease or thrombasthenia** D69.1
Glasgow coma scale
  total score
    3-8 R40.243
    9-12 R40.242
    13-15 R40.241
Glass-blower's disease (cataract) — *see* Cataract, specified NEC
Glaucoma H40.9
  with
    increased episcleral venous pressure H40.81- ☑
    pseudoexfoliation of lens — *see* Glaucoma, open angle, primary, capsular
  absolute H44.51- ☑
  angle-closure (primary) H40.20- ☑
    acute (attack) (crisis) H40.21- ☑
    chronic H40.22- ☑
    intermittent H40.23- ☑
    residual stage H40.24- ☑
  borderline H40.00- ☑
  capsular (with pseudoexfoliation of lens) — *see* Glaucoma, open angle, primary, capsular
  childhood Q15.0
  closed angle — *see* Glaucoma, angle-closure
  congenital Q15.0
  corticosteroid-induced — *see* Glaucoma, secondary, drugs
  hypersecretion H40.82- ☑
  in (due to)
    amyloidosis E85.4 [H42]
    aniridia Q13.1 [H42]
    concussion of globe — *see* Glaucoma, secondary, trauma

Glaucoma — continued
  in — continued
    dislocation of lens — see Glaucoma, secondary
    disorder of lens NEC — see Glaucoma, secondary
    drugs — see Glaucoma, secondary, drugs
    endocrine disease NOS E34.9 [H42]
    eye
      inflammation — see Glaucoma, secondary, inflammation
      trauma — see Glaucoma, secondary, trauma
    hypermature cataract — see Glaucoma, secondary
    iridocyclitis — see Glaucoma, secondary, inflammation
    lens disorder — see Glaucoma, secondary
    Lowe's syndrome E72.03 [H42]
    metabolic disease NOS E88.9 [H42]
    ocular disorders NEC — see Glaucoma, secondary
    onchocerciasis B73.02
    pupillary block — see Glaucoma, secondary
    retinal vein occlusion — see Glaucoma, secondary
    Rieger's anomaly Q13.81 [H42]
    rubeosis of iris — see Glaucoma, secondary
    tumor of globe — see Glaucoma, secondary
  infantile Q15.0
  low tension — see Glaucoma, open angle, primary, low-tension
  malignant H40.83- ☑
  narrow angle — see Glaucoma, angle-closure
  newborn Q15.0
  noncongestive (chronic) — see Glaucoma, open angle
  nonobstructive — see Glaucoma, open angle
  obstructive (see also Glaucoma, angle-closure)
    due to lens changes — see Glaucoma, secondary
  open angle H40.10- ☑
    primary H40.11- ☑
      capsular (with pseudoexfoliation of lens) H40.14- ☑
      low-tension H40.12- ☑
      pigmentary H40.13- ☑
      residual stage H40.15- ☑
  phacolytic — see Glaucoma, secondary
  pigmentary — see Glaucoma, open angle, primary, pigmentary
  postinfectious — see Glaucoma, secondary, inflammation
  secondary (to) H40.5- ☑
    drugs H40.6- ☑
    inflammation H40.4- ☑
    trauma H40.3- ☑
  simple (chronic) H40.11 ☑
  simplex H40.11 ☑
  specified type NEC H40.89
  suspect H40.00- ☑
  syphilitic A52.71
  traumatic (see also Glaucoma, secondary, trauma)
    newborn (birth injury) P15.3
  tuberculous A18.59
Glaucomatous flecks (subcapsular) — see Cataract, complicated
Glazed tongue K14.4
Gleet (gonococcal) A54.01
Glénard's disease K63.4
Glioblastoma (multiforme)
  with sarcomatous component
    specified site — see Neoplasm, malignant, by site
    unspecified site C71.9
  giant cell
    specified site — see Neoplasm, malignant, by site
    unspecified site C71.9
  specified site — see Neoplasm, malignant, by site
  unspecified site C71.9
Glioma (malignant)
  astrocytic
    specified site — see Neoplasm, malignant, by site
    unspecified site C71.9
  mixed
    specified site — see Neoplasm, malignant, by site
    unspecified site C71.9
  nose Q30.8
  specified site NEC — see Neoplasm, malignant, by site
  subependymal D43.2
    specified site — see Neoplasm, uncertain behavior, by site
    unspecified site D43.2
  unspecified site C71.9
Gliomatosis cerebri C71.0

Glioneuroma — see Neoplasm, uncertain behavior, by site
Gliosarcoma
  specified site — see Neoplasm, malignant, by site
  unspecified site C71.9
Gliosis (cerebral) G93.89
  spinal G95.89
Glisson's disease — see Rickets
Globinuria R82.3
Globus (hystericus) F45.8
Glomangioma D18.00
  intra-abdominal D18.03
  intracranial D18.02
  skin D18.01
  specified site NEC D18.09
Glomangiomyoma D18.00
  intra-abdominal D18.03
  intracranial D18.02
  skin D18.01
  specified site NEC D18.09
Glomangiosarcoma — see Neoplasm, connective tissue, malignant
Glomerular
  disease in syphilis A52.75
  nephritis — see Glomerulonephritis
Glomerulitis — see Glomerulonephritis
Glomerulonephritis (see also Nephritis) N05.9
  with
    edema — see Nephrosis
    minimal change N05.0
    minor glomerular abnormality N05.0
  acute N00.9
  chronic N03.9
  crescentic (diffuse) NEC (see also N00-N07 with fourth character .7) N05.7
  dense deposit (see also N00-N07 with fourth character .6) N05.6
  diffuse
    crescentic (see also N00-N07 with fourth character .7) N05.7
    endocapillary proliferative (see also N00-N07 with fourth character .4) N05.4
    membranous (see also N00-N07 with fourth character .2) N05.2
    mesangial proliferative (see also N00-N07 with fourth character .3) N05.3
    mesangiocapillary (see also N00-N07 with fourth character .5) N05.5
    sclerosing N05.8
  endocapillary proliferative (diffuse) NEC (see also N00-N07 with fourth character .4) N05.4
  extracapillary NEC (see also N00-N07 with fourth character .7) N05.7
  focal (and segmental) (see also N00-N07 with fourth character .1) N05.1
  hypocomplementemic — see Glomerulonephritis, membranoproliferative
  IgA — see Nephropathy, IgA
  immune complex (circulating) NEC N05.8
  in (due to)
    amyloidosis E85.4 [N08]
    bilharziasis B65.9 [N08]
    cryoglobulinemia D89.1 [N08]
    defibrination syndrome D65 [N08]
    diabetes mellitus — see Diabetes, glomerulosclerosis
    disseminated intravascular coagulation D65 [N08]
    Fabry (-Anderson) disease E75.21 [N08]
    Goodpasture's syndrome M31.0
    hemolytic-uremic syndrome D59.3
    Henoch (-Schönlein) purpura D69.0 [N08]
    lecithin cholesterol acyltransferase deficiency E78.6 [N08]
    microscopic polyangiitis M31.7 [N08]
    multiple myeloma C90.0- ☑ [N08]
    Plasmodium malariae B52.0
    schistosomiasis B65.9 [N08]
    sepsis A41.9 [N08]
      streptococcal A40- ☑ [N08]
    sickle-cell disorders D57.- ☑ [N08]
    strongyloidiasis B78.9 [N08]
    subacute bacterial endocarditis I33.0 [N08]
    syphilis (late) congenital A50.59 [N08]
    systemic lupus erythematosus M32.14
    thrombotic thrombocytopenic purpura M31.1 [N08]
    typhoid fever A01.09
    Waldenström macroglobulinemia C88.0 [N08]

Glomerulonephritis — continued
  in -- continued
    Wegener's granulomatosis M31.31
  latent or quiescent N03.9
  lobular, lobulonodular — see Glomerulonephritis, membranoproliferative
  membranoproliferative (diffuse)(type 1 or 3) (see also N00-N07 with fourth character .5) N05.5
    dense deposit (type 2) NEC (see also N00-N07 with fourth character .6) N05.6
  membranous (diffuse) NEC (see also N00-N07 with fourth character .2) N05.2
  mesangial
    IgA/IgG — see Nephropathy, IgA
    proliferative (diffuse) NEC (see also N00-N07 with fourth character .3) N05.3
  mesangiocapillary (diffuse) NEC (see also N00-N07 with fourth character .5) N05.5
  necrotic, necrotizing NEC (see also N00- N07 with fourth character .8) N05.8
  nodular — see Glomerulonephritis, membranoproliferative
  poststreptococcal NEC N05.9
    acute N00.9
    chronic N03.9
    rapidly progressive N01.9
  proliferative NEC (see also N00-N07 with fourth character .8) N05.8
    diffuse (lupus) M32.14
  rapidly progressive N01.9
  sclerosing, diffuse N05.8
  specified pathology NEC (see also N00- N07 with fourth character .8) N05.8
  subacute N01.9
Glomerulopathy — see Glomerulonephritis
Glomerulosclerosis (see also Sclerosis, renal)
  intercapillary (nodular) (with diabetes) — see Diabetes, glomerulosclerosis
  intracapillary — see Diabetes, glomerulosclerosis
Glossagra K14.6
Glossalgia K14.6
Glossitis (chronic superficial) (gangrenous) (Moeller's) K14.0
  areata exfoliativa K14.1
  atrophic K14.4
  benign migratory K14.1
  cortical superficial, sclerotic K14.0
  Hunter's D51.0
  interstitial, sclerous K14.0
  median rhomboid K14.2
  pellagrous E52
  superficial, chronic K14.0
Glossocele K14.8
Glossodynia K14.6
  exfoliativa K14.4
Glossoncus K14.8
Glossopathy K14.9
Glossophytia K14.3
Glossoplegia K14.8
Glossoptosis K14.8
Glossopyrosis K14.6
Glossotrichia K14.3
Glossy skin L90.8
Glottis — see condition
Glottitis (see also Laryngitis) J04.0
Glucagonoma
  pancreas
    benign D13.7
    malignant C25.4
    uncertain behavior D37.8
  specified site NEC
    benign — see Neoplasm, benign, by site
    malignant — see Neoplasm, malignant, by site
    uncertain behavior — see Neoplasm, uncertain behavior, by site
  unspecified site
    benign D13.7
    malignant C25.4
    uncertain behavior D37.8
Glucoglycinuria E72.51
Glucose-galactose malabsorption E74.39
Glue
  ear — see Otitis, media, nonsuppurative, chronic, mucoid
  sniffing (airplane) — see Abuse, drug, inhalant
    dependence — see Dependence, drug, inhalant
Glutaric aciduria E72.3

Glycinemia E72.51
Glycinuria (renal) (with ketosis) E72.09
Glycogen
  infiltration — *see* Disease, glycogen storage
  storage disease — *see* Disease, glycogen storage
Glycogenosis (diffuse) (generalized) (*see also* Disease, glycogen storage)
  cardiac E74.02 [I43]
  diabetic, secondary — *see* Diabetes, glycogenosis, secondary
  pulmonary interstitial J84.842
Glycopenia E16.2
Glycosuria R81
  renal E74.8
Gnathostoma spinigerum (infection) (infestation), **gnathostomiasis** (wandering swelling) B83.1
Goiter (plunging) (substernal) E04.9
  with
    hyperthyroidism (recurrent) — *see* Hyperthyroidism, with, goiter
    thyrotoxicosis — *see* Hyperthyroidism, with, goiter
  adenomatous — *see* Goiter, nodular
  cancerous C73
  congenital (nontoxic) E03.0
    diffuse E03.0
    parenchymatous E03.0
    transitory, with normal functioning P72.0
  cystic E04.2
    due to iodine-deficiency E01.1
  due to
    enzyme defect in synthesis of thyroid hormone E07.1
    iodine-deficiency (endemic) E01.2
  dyshormonogenetic (familial) E07.1
  endemic (iodine-deficiency) E01.2
    diffuse E01.0
    multinodular E01.1
  exophthalmic — *see* Hyperthyroidism, with, goiter
  iodine-deficiency (endemic) E01.2
    diffuse E01.0
    multinodular E01.1
    nodular E01.1
  lingual Q89.2
  lymphadenoid E06.3
  malignant C73
  multinodular (cystic) (nontoxic) E04.2
    toxic or with hyperthyroidism E05.20
      with thyroid storm E05.21
  neonatal NEC P72.0
  nodular (nontoxic) (due to) E04.9
    with
      hyperthyroidism E05.20
        with thyroid storm E05.21
      thyrotoxicosis E05.20
        with thyroid storm E05.21
    endemic E01.1
    iodine-deficiency E01.1
    sporadic E04.9
    toxic E05.20
      with thyroid storm E05.21
    nontoxic E04.9
      diffuse (colloid) E04.0
      multinodular E04.2
      simple E04.0
      specified NEC E04.8
      uninodular E04.1
    simple E04.0
    toxic — *see* Hyperthyroidism, with, goiter
    uninodular (nontoxic) E04.1
      toxic or with hyperthyroidism E05.10
        with thyroid storm E05.11
Goiter-deafness syndrome E07.1
Goldberg syndrome Q89.8
Goldberg-Maxwell syndrome E34.51
Goldblatt's hypertension or kidney I70.1
Goldenhar (-Gorlin) **syndrome** Q87.0
Goldflam-Erb disease or syndrome G70.00
  with exacerbation (acute) G70.01
  in crisis G70.01
Goldscheider's disease Q81.8
Goldstein's disease (familial hemorrhagic telangiectasia) I78.0
Golfer's elbow — *see* Epicondylitis, medial
Gonadoblastoma
  specified site — *see* Neoplasm, uncertain behavior, by site
  unspecified site
    female D39.10

Gonadoblastoma — *continued*
  unspecified site — *continued*
    male D40.10
Gonecystitis — *see* Vesiculitis
Gongylonemiasis B83.8
Goniosynechiae — *see* Adhesions, iris, goniosynechiae
Gonococcemia A54.86
Gonococcus, gonococcal (disease) (infection) (*see also* condition) A54.9
  anus A54.6
  bursa, bursitis A54.49
  conjunctiva, conjunctivitis (neonatorum) A54.31
  endocardium A54.83
  eye A54.30
    conjunctivitis A54.31
    iridocyclitis A54.32
    keratitis A54.33
    newborn A54.31
    other specified A54.39
  fallopian tubes (acute) (chronic) A54.24
  genitourinary (organ) (system) (tract) (acute)
    lower A54.00
      with abscess (accessory gland) (periurethral) A54.1
    upper (*see also* condition) A54.29
  heart A54.83
  iridocyclitis A54.32
  joint A54.42
  lymphatic (gland) (node) A54.89
  meninges, meningitis A54.81
  musculoskeletal A54.40
    arthritis A54.42
    osteomyelitis A54.43
    other specified A54.49
    spondylopathy A54.41
  pelviperitonitis A54.24
  pelvis (acute) (chronic) A54.24
  pharynx A54.5
  proctitis A54.6
  pyosalpinx (acute) (chronic) A54.24
  rectum A54.6
  skin A54.89
  specified site NEC A54.89
  tendon sheath A54.49
  throat A54.5
  urethra (acute) (chronic) A54.01
    with abscess (accessory gland) (periurethral) A54.1
  vulva (acute) (chronic) A54.02
Gonocytoma
  specified site — *see* Neoplasm, uncertain behavior, by site
  unspecified site
    female D39.10
    male D40.10
Gonorrhea (acute) (chronic) A54.9
  Bartholin's gland (acute) (chronic) (purulent) A54.02
    with abscess (accessory gland) (periurethral) A54.1
  bladder A54.01
  cervix A54.03
  conjunctiva, conjunctivitis (neonatorum) A54.31
  contact Z20.2
  Cowper's gland (with abscess) A54.1
  exposure to Z20.2
  fallopian tube (acute) (chronic) A54.24
  kidney (acute) (chronic) A54.21
  lower genitourinary tract A54.00
    with abscess (accessory gland) (periurethral) A54.1
  ovary (acute) (chronic) A54.24
  pelvis (acute) (chronic) A54.24
    female pelvic inflammatory disease A54.24
  penis A54.09
  prostate (acute) (chronic) A54.22
  seminal vesicle (acute) (chronic) A54.23
  specified site not listed (*see also* Gonococcus) A54.89
  spermatic cord (acute) (chronic) A54.23
  urethra A54.01
    with abscess (accessory gland) (periurethral) A54.1
  vagina A54.02
  vas deferens (acute) (chronic) A54.23
  vulva A54.02
Goodall's disease A08.19
Goodpasture's syndrome M31.0
Gopalan's syndrome (burning feet) E53.0
Gorlin-Chaudry-Moss syndrome Q87.0
Gottron's papules L94.4
Gougerot-Blum syndrome (pigmented purpuric lichenoid dermatitis) L81.7

Gougerot-Carteaud disease or syndrome (confluent reticulate papillomatosis) L83
Gougerot's syndrome (trisymptomatic) L81.7
Gouley's syndrome (constrictive pericarditis) I31.1
Goundou A66.6
Gout, chronic (*see also* Gout, gouty) M1A.9 ☑ (*following* M08)
  drug-induced M1A.20 ☑ (*following* M08)
    ankle M1A.27- ☑ (*following* M08)
    elbow M1A.22- ☑ (*following* M08)
    foot joint M1A.27- ☑ (*following* M08)
    hand joint M1A.24- ☑ (*following* M08)
    hip M1A.25- ☑ (*following* M08)
    knee M1A.26- ☑ (*following* M08)
    multiple site M1A.29- ☑ (*following* M08)
    shoulder M1A.21- ☑ (*following* M08)
    vertebrae M1A.28 ☑ (*following* M08)
    wrist M1A.23- ☑ (*following* M08)
  idiopathic M1A.00 ☑ (*following* M08)
    ankle M1A.07- ☑ (*following* M08)
    elbow M1A.02- ☑ (*following* M08)
    foot joint M1A.07- ☑ (*following* M08)
    hand joint M1A.04- ☑ (*following* M08)
    hip M1A.05- ☑ (*following* M08)
    knee M1A.06- ☑ (*following* M08)
    multiple site M1A.09 ☑ (*following* M08)
    shoulder M1A.01- ☑ (*following* M08)
    vertebrae M1A.08 ☑ (*following* M08)
    wrist M1A.03- ☑ (*following* M08)
  in (due to) renal impairment M1A.30 ☑ (*following* M08)
    ankle M1A.37- ☑ (*following* M08)
    elbow M1A.32- ☑ (*following* M08)
    foot joint M1A.37- ☑ (*following* M08)
    hand joint M1A.34- ☑ (*following* M08)
    hip M1A.35- ☑ (*following* M08)
    knee M1A.36- ☑ (*following* M08)
    multiple site M1A.39 ☑ (*following* M08)
    shoulder M1A.31- ☑ (*following* M08)
    vertebrae M1A.38 ☑ (*following* M08)
    wrist M1A.33- ☑ (*following* M08)
  lead-induced M1A.10 ☑ (*following* M08)
    ankle M1A.17- ☑ (*following* M08)
    elbow M1A.12- ☑ (*following* M08)
    foot joint M1A.17- ☑ (*following* M08)
    hand joint M1A.14- ☑ (*following* M08)
    hip M1A.15- ☑ (*following* M08)
    knee M1A.16- ☑ (*following* M08)
    multiple site M1A.19 ☑ (*following* M08)
    shoulder M1A.11- ☑ (*following* M08)
    vertebrae M1A.18 ☑ (*following* M08)
    wrist M1A.13- ☑ (*following* M08)
  primary — *see* Gout, chronic, idiopathic
  saturnine — *see* Gout, chronic, lead-induced
  secondary NEC M1A.40 ☑ (*following* M08)
    ankle M1A.47- ☑ (*following* M08)
    elbow M1A.42- ☑ (*following* M08)
    foot joint M1A.47- ☑ (*following* M08)
    hand joint M1A.44- ☑ (*following* M08)
    hip M1A.45- ☑ (*following* M08)
    knee M1A.46- ☑ (*following* M08)
    multiple site M1A.49 ☑ (*following* M08)
    shoulder M1A.41- ☑ (*following* M08)
    vertebrae M1A.48 ☑ (*following* M08)
    wrist M1A.43- ☑ (*following* M08)
  syphilitic (*see also* subcategory M14.8-) A52.77
  tophi M1A.9 ☑ (*following* M08)
Gout, gouty (acute) (attack) (flare) (*see also* Gout, chronic) M10.9
  drug-induced M10.20
    ankle M10.27- ☑
    elbow M10.22- ☑
    foot joint M10.27- ☑
    hand joint M10.24- ☑
    hip M10.25- ☑
    knee M10.26- ☑
    multiple site M10.29
    shoulder M10.21- ☑
    vertebrae M10.28
    wrist M10.23- ☑
  idiopathic M10.00
    ankle M10.07- ☑
    elbow M10.02- ☑
    foot joint M10.07- ☑
    hand joint M10.04- ☑
    hip M10.05- ☑

☑ Additional Character Required — Refer to the Tabular List for Character Selection   Subterms under main terms may continue to next column or page

Gout, gouty — *continued*
  idiopathic — *continued*
    knee M10.06- ☑
    multiple site M10.09
    shoulder M10.01- ☑
    vertebrae M10.08
    wrist M10.03- ☑
  in (due to) renal impairment M10.30
    ankle M10.37- ☑
    elbow M10.32- ☑
    foot joint M10.37- ☑
    hand joint M10.34- ☑
    hip M10.35- ☑
    knee M10.36- ☑
    multiple site M10.39
    shoulder M10.31- ☑
    vertebrae M10.38
    wrist M10.33- ☑
  lead-induced M10.10
    ankle M10.17- ☑
    elbow M10.12- ☑
    foot joint M10.17- ☑
    hand joint M10.14- ☑
    hip M10.15- ☑
    knee M10.16- ☑
    multiple site M10.19
    shoulder M10.11- ☑
    vertebrae M10.18
    wrist M10.13- ☑
  primary — *see* Gout, idiopathic
  saturnine — *see* Gout, lead-induced
  secondary NEC M10.40
    ankle M10.47- ☑
    elbow M10.42- ☑
    foot joint M10.47- ☑
    hand joint M10.44- ☑
    hip M10.45- ☑
    knee M10.46- ☑
    multiple site M10.49
    shoulder M10.41- ☑
    vertebrae M10.48
    wrist M10.43- ☑
  syphilitic (*see also* subcategory M14.8-) A52.77
  tophi — *see* Gout, chronic
Gower's
  muscular dystrophy G71.0
  syndrome (vasovagal attack) R55
Gradenigo's syndrome — *see* Otitis, media, suppurative, acute
Graefe's disease — *see* Strabismus, paralytic, ophthalmoplegia, progressive
Graft-versus-host disease D89.813
  acute D89.810
  acute on chronic D89.812
  chronic D89.811
Grain mite (itch) B88.0
Grainhandler's disease or lung J67.8
Grand mal — *see* Epilepsy, generalized, specified NEC
Grand multipara status only (not pregnant) Z64.1
  pregnant — *see* Pregnancy, complicated by, grand multiparity
Granite worker's lung J62.8
Granular (*see also* condition)
  inflammation, pharynx J31.2
  kidney (contracting) — *see* Sclerosis, renal
  liver K74.69
Granulation tissue (abnormal) (excessive) L92.9
  postmastoidectomy cavity — *see* Complications, postmastoidectomy, granulation
Granulocytopenia (primary) (malignant) — *see* Agranulocytosis
Granuloma L92.9
  abdomen K66.8
    from residual foreign body L92.3
    pyogenicum L98.0
  actinic L57.5
  annulare (perforating) L92.0
  apical K04.5
  aural — *see* Otitis, externa, specified NEC
  beryllium (skin) L92.3
  bone
    eosinophilic C96.6
    from residual foreign body — *see* Osteomyelitis, specified type NEC
    lung C96.6
  brain (any site) G06.0
    schistosomiasis B65.9 [G07]

Granuloma — *continued*
  canaliculus lacrimalis — *see* Granuloma, lacrimal
  candidal (cutaneous) B37.2
  cerebral (any site) G06.0
  coccidioidal (primary) (progressive) B38.7
    lung B38.1
    meninges B38.4
  colon K63.89
  conjunctiva H11.22- ☑
  dental K04.5
  ear, middle — *see* Cholesteatoma
  eosinophilic C96.6
    bone C96.6
    lung C96.6
    oral mucosa K13.4
    skin L92.2
  eyelid H01.8
  facial (e) L92.2
  foreign body (in soft tissue) NEC M60.20
    ankle M60.27- ☑
    foot M60.27- ☑
    forearm M60.23- ☑
    hand M60.24- ☑
    in operation wound — *see* Foreign body, accidentally left during a procedure
    lower leg M60.26- ☑
    pelvic region M60.25- ☑
    shoulder region M60.21- ☑
    skin L92.3
    specified site NEC M60.28
    subcutaneous tissue L92.3
    thigh M60.25- ☑
    upper arm M60.22- ☑
  gangraenescens M31.2
  genito-inguinale A58
  giant cell (central) (reparative) (jaw) M27.1
    gingiva (peripheral) K06.8
  gland (lymph) I88.8
  hepatic NEC K75.3
    in (due to)
      berylliosis J63.2 [K77]
      sarcoidosis D86.89
  Hodgkin C81.9 ☑
  ileum K63.89
  infectious B99.9
    specified NEC B99.8
  inguinale (Donovan) (venereal) A58
  intestine NEC K63.89
  intracranial (any site) G06.0
  intraspinal (any part) G06.1
  iridocyclitis — *see* Iridocyclitis, chronic
  jaw (bone) (central) M27.1
    reparative giant cell M27.1
  kidney (*see also* Infection, kidney) N15.8
  lacrimal H04.81- ☑
  larynx J38.7
  lethal midline (faciale(e)) M31.2
  liver NEC — *see* Granuloma, hepatic
  lung (infectious) — *see also* Fibrosis, lung)
    coccidioidal B38.1
    eosinophilic C96.6
  Majocchi's B35.8
  malignant (facial(e)) M31.2
  mandible (central) M27.1
  midline (lethal) M31.2
  monilial (cutaneous) B37.2
  nasal sinus — *see* Sinusitis
  operation wound T81.89 ☑
    foreign body — *see* Foreign body, accidentally left during a procedure
    stitch T81.89 ☑
    talc — *see* Foreign body, accidentally left during a procedure
  oral mucosa K13.4
  orbit, orbital H05.11- ☑
  paracoccidioidal B41.8
  penis, venereal A58
  periapical K04.5
  peritoneum K66.8
    due to ova of helminths NOS (*see also* Helminthiasis) B83.9 [K67]
  postmastoidectomy cavity — *see* Complications, postmastoidectomy, recurrent cholesteatoma
  prostate N42.89
  pudendi (ulcerating) A58
  pulp, internal (tooth) K03.3
  pyogenic, pyogenicum (of) (skin) L98.0
    gingiva K06.8

Granuloma — *continued*
  pyogenic, pyogenicum — *continued*
    maxillary alveolar ridge K04.5
      oral mucosa K13.4
  rectum K62.89
  reticulohistiocytic D76.3
  rubrum nasi L74.8
  Schistosoma — *see* Schistosomiasis
  septic (skin) L98.0
  silica (skin) L92.3
  sinus (accessory) (infective) (nasal) — *see* Sinusitis
  skin L92.9
    from residual foreign body L92.3
    pyogenicum L98.0
  spine
    syphilitic (epidural) A52.19
    tuberculous A18.01
  stitch (postoperative) T81.89 ☑
  suppurative (skin) L98.0
  swimming pool A31.1
  talc (*see also* Granuloma, foreign body)
    in operation wound — *see* Foreign body, accidentally left during a procedure
  telangiectaticum (skin) L98.0
  tracheostomy J95.09
  trichophyticum B35.8
  tropicum A66.4
  umbilicus L92.9
  urethra N36.8
  uveitis — *see* Iridocyclitis, chronic
  vagina A58
  venereum A58
  vocal cord J38.3
Granulomatosis L92.9
  lymphoid C83.8- ☑
  miliary (listerial) A32.89
  necrotizing, respiratory M31.30
  progressive septic D71
  specified NEC L92.8
  Wegener's M31.30
    with renal involvement M31.31
Granulomatous tissue (abnormal) (excessive) L92.9
Granulosis rubra nasi L74.8
Graphite fibrosis (of lung) J63.3
Graphospasm F48.8
  organic G25.89
Grating scapula M89.8X1
Gravel (urinary) — *see* Calculus, urinary
Graves' disease — *see* Hyperthyroidism, with, goiter
Gravis — *see* condition
Grawitz tumor C64.- ☑
Gray syndrome (newborn) P93.0
Grayness, hair (premature) L67.1
  congenital Q84.2
Green sickness D50.8
Greenfield's disease
  meaning
    concentric sclerosis (encephalitis periaxialis concentrica) G37.5
    metachromatic leukodystrophy E75.25
Greenstick fracture — *code as* Fracture, by site
Grey syndrome (newborn) P93.0
Grief F43.21
  prolonged F43.29
  reaction (*see also* Disorder, adjustment) F43.20
Griesinger's disease B76.9
Grinder's lung or pneumoconiosis J62.8
Grinding, teeth
  psychogenic F45.8
  sleep related G47.63
Grip
  Dabney's B33.0
  devil's B33.0
Grippe, grippal (*see also* Influenza)
  Balkan A78
  summer, of Italy A93.1
Grisel's disease M43.6
Groin — *see* condition
Grooved tongue K14.5
Ground itch B76.9
Grover's disease or syndrome L11.1
Growing pains, children R29.898
Growth (fungoid) (neoplastic) (new) (*see also* Neoplasm)
  adenoid (vegetative) J35.8
  benign — *see* Neoplasm, benign, by site
  malignant — *see* Neoplasm, malignant, by site
  rapid, childhood Z00.2

Growth — *continued*
secondary — *see* Neoplasm, secondary, by site
Gruby's disease B35.Ø
Gubler-Millard paralysis or syndrome G46.3
Guerin-Stern syndrome Q74.3
Guidance, insufficient anterior (occlusal) M26.54
Guillain-Barré disease or syndrome G61.Ø
sequelae G65.Ø
Guinea worms (infection) (infestation) B72
Guinon's disease (motor-verbal tic) F95.2
Gull's disease EØ3.4
Gum — *see* condition
Gumboil KØ4.7
with sinus KØ4.6
Gumma (syphilitic) A52.79
artery A52.Ø9
cerebral A52.Ø4
bone A52.77
of yaws (late) A66.6
brain A52.19
cauda equina A52.19
central nervous system A52.3
ciliary body A52.71
congenital A5Ø.59
eyelid A52.71
heart A52.Ø6
intracranial A52.19
iris A52.71
kidney A52.75
larynx A52.73
leptomeninges A52.19
liver A52.74
meninges A52.19
myocardium A52.Ø6
nasopharynx A52.73
neurosyphilitic A52.3
nose A52.73
orbit A52.71
palate (soft) A52.79
penis A52.76
pericardium A52.Ø6
pharynx A52.73
pituitary A52.79
scrofulous (tuberculous) A18.4
skin A52.79
specified site NEC A52.79
spinal cord A52.19
tongue A52.79
tonsil A52.73
trachea A52.73
tuberculous A18.4
ulcerative due to yaws A66.4
ureter A52.75
yaws A66.4
bone A66.6
Gunn's syndrome QØ7.8
Gunshot wound (*see also* Wound, open)
fracture — *code as* Fracture, by site
internal organs — *see* Injury, by site
Gynandrism Q56.Ø
Gynandroblastoma
specified site — *see* Neoplasm, uncertain behavior, by site
unspecified site
female D39.1Ø
male D4Ø.1Ø
Gynecological examination (periodic) (routine) ZØ1.419
with abnormal findings ZØ1.411
Gynecomastia N62
Gynephobia F4Ø.291
Gyrate scalp Q82.8

H

H (Hartnup's) **disease** E72.Ø2
Haas' disease or osteochondrosis (juvenile) (head of humerus) — *see* Osteochondrosis, juvenile, humerus
Habit, habituation
bad sleep Z72.821
chorea F95.8
disturbance, child F98.9
drug — *see* Dependence, drug
irregular sleep Z72.821
laxative F55.2
spasm — *see* Tic
tic — *see* Tic

Haemophilus (H.) influenzae, as cause of disease classified elsewhere B96.3
Haff disease — *see* Poisoning, mercury
Hageman's factor defect, deficiency or disease D68.2
Haglund's disease or osteochondrosis (juvenile) (os tibiale externum) –– *see* Osteochondrosis, juvenile, tarsus
Hailey-Hailey disease Q82.8
Hair (*see also* condition)
plucking F63.3
in stereotyped movement disorder F98.4
tourniquet syndrome (*see also* Constriction, external, by site)
finger S6Ø.44- ☑
penis S3Ø.842 ☑
thumb S6Ø.34- ☑
toe S9Ø.44- ☑
Hairball in stomach T18.2 ☑
Hair-pulling, pathological (compulsive) F63.3
Hairy black tongue K14.3
Half vertebra Q76.49
Halitosis R19.6
Hallerman-Streiff syndrome Q87.Ø
Hallervorden-Spatz disease G23.Ø
Hallopeau's acrodermatitis or disease L4Ø.2
Hallucination R44.3
auditory R44.Ø
gustatory R44.2
olfactory R44.2
specified NEC R44.2
tactile R44.2
visual R44.1
Hallucinosis (chronic) F28
alcoholic (acute) F1Ø.951
in
abuse F1Ø.151
dependence F1Ø.251
drug-induced F19.951
cannabis F12.951
cocaine F14.951
hallucinogen F16.151
in
abuse F19.151
cannabis F12.151
cocaine F14.151
hallucinogen F16.151
inhalant F18.151
opioid F11.151
sedative, anxiolytic or hypnotic F13.151
stimulant NEC F15.151
dependence F19.251
cannabis F12.251
cocaine F14.251
hallucinogen F16.251
inhalant F18.251
opioid F11.251
sedative, anxiolytic or hypnotic F13.251
stimulant NEC F15.251
inhalant F18.951
opioid F11.951
sedative, anxiolytic or hypnotic F13.951
stimulant NEC F15.951
organic FØ6.Ø
Hallux
deformity (acquired) NEC M2Ø.5X- ☑
limitus M2Ø.5X- ☑
malleus (acquired) NEC M2Ø.3- ☑
rigidus (acquired) M2Ø.2- ☑
congenital Q74.2
sequelae (late effect) of rickets E64.3
valgus (acquired) M2Ø.1- ☑
congenital Q66.6
varus (acquired) M2Ø.3- ☑
congenital Q66.3
Halo, visual H53.19
Hamartoma, hamartoblastoma Q85.9
epithelial (gingival), odontogenic, central or peripheral — *see* Cyst, calcifying odontogenic
Hamartosis Q85.9
Hamman-Rich syndrome J84.114
Hammer toe (acquired) NEC (*see also* Deformity, toe, hammer toe)
congenital Q66.89
sequelae (late effect) of rickets E64.3
Hand — *see* condition
Hand-foot syndrome L27.1

Handicap, handicapped
educational Z55.9
specified NEC Z55.8
Hand-Schüller-Christian disease or syndrome C96.5
Hanging (asphyxia) (strangulation) (suffocation) — *see* Asphyxia, traumatic, due to mechanical threat
Hangnail (*see also* Cellulitis, digit)
with lymphangitis — *see* Lymphangitis, acute, digit
Hangover (alcohol) F1Ø.129
Hanhart's syndrome Q87.Ø
Hanot-Chauffard (-Troisier) **syndrome** E83.19
Hanot's cirrhosis or disease K74.3
Hansen's disease — *see* Leprosy
Hantaan virus disease (Korean hemorrhagic fever) A98.5
Hantavirus disease (with renal manifestations) (Dobrava) (Puumala) (Seoul) A98.5
with pulmonary manifestations (Andes) (Bayou) (Bermejo) (Black Creek Canal) (Choclo) (Juquitiba) (Laguna negra) (Lechiguanas) (New York) (Oran) (Sin nombre) B33.4
Happy puppet syndrome Q93.5
Harada's disease or syndrome H3Ø.81- ☑
Hardening
artery — *see* Arteriosclerosis
brain G93.89
Harelip (complete) (incomplete) — *see* Cleft, lip
Harlequin (newborn) Q8Ø.4
Harley's disease D59.6
Harmful use (of)
alcohol F1Ø.1Ø
anxiolytics — *see* Abuse, drug, sedative
cannabinoids — *see* Abuse, drug, cannabis
cocaine — *see* Abuse, drug, cocaine
drug — *see* Abuse, drug
hallucinogens — *see* Abuse, drug, hallucinogen
hypnotics — *see* Abuse, drug, sedative
opioids — *see* Abuse, drug, opioid
PCP (phencyclidine) — *see* Abuse, drug, hallucinogen
sedatives — *see* Abuse, drug, sedative
stimulants NEC — *see* Abuse, drug, stimulant
Harris' lines — *see* Arrest, epiphyseal
Hartnup's disease E72.Ø2
Harvester's lung J67.Ø
Harvesting ovum for in vitro fertilization Z31.83
Hashimoto's disease or thyroiditis EØ6.3
Hashitoxicosis (transient) EØ6.3
Hassal-Henle bodies or warts (cornea) H18.49
Haut mal — *see* Epilepsy, generalized, specified NEC
Haverhill fever A25.1
Hay fever (*see also* Fever, hay) J3Ø.1
Hayem-Widal syndrome D59.8
Haygarth's nodes M15.8
Haymaker's lung J67.Ø
Hb (abnormal)
Bart's disease D56.Ø
disease — *see* Disease, hemoglobin
trait — *see* Trait
Head — *see* condition
Headache R51
allergic NEC G44.89
associated with sexual activity G44.82
chronic daily R51
cluster G44.ØØ9
chronic G44.Ø29
intractable G44.Ø21
not intractable G44.Ø29
episodic G44.Ø19
intractable G44.Ø11
not intractable G44.Ø19
intractable G44.ØØ1
not intractable G44.ØØ9
cough (primary) G44.83
daily chronic R51
drug-induced NEC G44.4Ø
intractable G44.41
not intractable G44.4Ø
exertional (primary) G44.84
histamine G44.ØØ9
intractable G44.ØØ1
not intractable G44.ØØ9
hypnic G44.81
lumbar puncture G97.1
medication overuse G44.4Ø
intractable G44.41
not intractable G44.4Ø
menstrual — *see* Migraine, menstrual
migraine (type) (*see also* Migraine) G43.9Ø9

☑ **Additional Character Required** — Refer to the Tabular List for Character Selection   ▽ Subterms under main terms may continue to next column or page

Headache — *continued*
  nasal septum R51
  neuralgiform, short lasting unilateral, with conjunctival injection and tearing (SUNCT) G44.Ø59
    intractable G44.Ø51
    not intractable G44.Ø59
  new daily persistent (NDPH) G44.52
  orgasmic G44.82
  periodic syndromes in adults and children G43.CØ (*following* G43.7)
    with refractory migraine G43.C1 (*following* G43.7)
    without refractory migraine G43.CØ (*following* G43.7)
    intractable G43.C1 (*following* G43.7)
    not intractable G43.CØ (*following* G43.7)
  postspinal puncture G97.1
  post-traumatic G44.3Ø9
    acute G44.319
      intractable G44.311
      not intractable G44.319
    chronic G44.329
      intractable G44.321
      not intractable G44.329
    intractable G44.3Ø1
    not intractable G44.3Ø9
  pre-menstrual — *see* Migraine, menstrual
  preorgasmic G44.82
  primary
    cough G44.83
    exertional G44.84
    stabbing G44.85
    thunderclap G44.53
  rebound G44.4Ø
    intractable G44.41
    not intractable G44.4Ø
  short lasting unilateral neuralgiform, with conjunctival injection and tearing (SUNCT) G44.Ø59
    intractable G44.Ø51
    not intractable G44.Ø59
  specified syndrome NEC G44.89
  spinal and epidural anesthesia - induced T88.59 ☑
    in labor and delivery O74.5
    in pregnancy O29.4- ☑
    postpartum, puerperal O89.4
  spinal fluid loss (from puncture) G97.1
  stabbing (primary) G44.85
  tension (-type) G44.2Ø9
    chronic G44.229
      intractable G44.221
      not intractable G44.229
    episodic G44.219
      intractable G44.211
      not intractable G44.219
    intractable G44.2Ø1
    not intractable G44.2Ø9
  thunderclap (primary) G44.53
  vascular NEC G44.1
Healthy
  infant
    accompanying sick mother Z76.3
    receiving care Z76.2
  person accompanying sick person Z76.3
Hearing examination Z01.10
  with abnormal findings NEC Z01.118
  following failed hearing screening Z01.11Ø
  for hearing conservation and treatment Z01.12
Heart — *see* condition
Heart beat
  abnormality RØØ.9
    specified NEC RØØ.8
  awareness RØØ.2
  rapid RØØ.Ø
  slow RØØ.1
Heartburn R12
  psychogenic F45.8
Heat (effects) T67.9 ☑
  apoplexy T67.Ø ☑
  burn (*see also* Burn) L55.9
  collapse T67.1 ☑
  cramps T67.2 ☑
  dermatitis or eczema L59.Ø
  edema T67.7 ☑
  erythema — *code by site under* Burn, first degree
  excessive T67.9 ☑
    specified effect NEC T67.8 ☑
  exhaustion T67.5 ☑
    anhydrotic T67.3 ☑

Heat — *continued*
  exhaustion — *continued*
    due to
      salt (and water) depletion T67.4 ☑
      water depletion T67.3 ☑
        with salt depletion T67.4 ☑
  fatigue (transient) T67.6 ☑
  fever T67.Ø ☑
  hyperpyrexia T67.Ø ☑
  prickly L74.Ø
  prostration — *see* Heat, exhaustion
  pyrexia T67.Ø ☑
  rash L74.Ø
  specified effect NEC T67.8 ☑
  stroke T67.Ø ☑
  sunburn — *see* Sunburn
  syncope T67.1 ☑
Heavy-for-dates NEC (infant) (4ØØØg to 4499g) PØ8.1
  exceptionally (45ØØg or more) PØ8.Ø
Hebephrenia, hebephrenic (schizophrenia) F2Ø.1
Heberden's disease or nodes (with arthropathy) M15.1
Hebra's
  pityriasis L26
  prurigo L28.2
Heel — *see* condition
Heerfordt's disease D86.89
Hegglin's anomaly or syndrome D72.Ø
Heilmeyer-Schoner disease D45
Heine-Medin disease A8Ø.9
Heinz body anemia, congenital D58.2
Heliophobia F4Ø.228
Heller's disease or syndrome F84.3
HELLP syndrome (hemolysis, elevated liver enzymes and low platelet count) O14.2-
Helminthiasis (*see also* Infestation, helminth)
  Ancylostoma B76.Ø
  intestinal B82.Ø
    mixed types (types classifiable to more than one of the titles B65.Ø-B81.3 and B81.8) B81.4
    specified type NEC B81.8
  mixed types (intestinal) (types classifiable to more than one of the titles B65.Ø-B81.3 and B81.8) B81.4
  Necator (americanus) B76.1
  specified type NEC B83.8
Heloma L84
Hemangioblastoma — *see* Neoplasm, connective tissue, uncertain behavior
  malignant — *see* Neoplasm, connective tissue, malignant
Hemangioendothelioma (*see also* Neoplasm, uncertain behavior, by site)
  benign D18.ØØ
    intra-abdominal D18.Ø3
    intracranial D18.Ø2
    skin D18.Ø1
    specified site NEC D18.Ø9
  bone (diffuse) — *see* Neoplasm, bone, malignant
  epithelioid (*see also* Neoplasm, uncertain behavior, by site)
    malignant — *see* Neoplasm, malignant, by site
  malignant — *see* Neoplasm, connective tissue, malignant
Hemangiofibroma — *see* Neoplasm, benign, by site
Hemangiolipoma — *see* Lipoma
Hemangioma D18.ØØ
  arteriovenous D18.ØØ
    intra-abdominal D18.Ø3
    intracranial D18.Ø2
    skin D18.Ø1
    specified site NEC D18.Ø9
  capillary D18.ØØ
    intra-abdominal D18.Ø3
    intracranial D18.Ø2
    skin D18.Ø1
    specified site NEC D18.Ø9
  cavernous D18.ØØ
    intra-abdominal D18.Ø3
    intracranial D18.Ø2
    skin D18.Ø1
    specified site NEC D18.Ø9
  epithelioid D18.ØØ
    intra-abdominal D18.Ø3
    intracranial D18.Ø2
    skin D18.Ø1
    specified site NEC D18.Ø9
  histiocytoid D18.ØØ

Hemangioma — *continued*
  histiocytoid — *continued*
    intra-abdominal D18.Ø3
    intracranial D18.Ø2
    skin D18.Ø1
    specified site NEC D18.Ø9
  infantile D18.ØØ
    intra-abdominal D18.Ø3
    intracranial D18.Ø2
    skin D18.Ø1
    specified site NEC D18.Ø9
  intra-abdominal D18.Ø3
  intracranial D18.Ø2
  intramuscular D18.ØØ
    intra-abdominal D18.Ø3
    intracranial D18.Ø2
    skin D18.Ø1
    specified site NEC D18.Ø9
  juvenile D18.ØØ
  malignant — *see* Neoplasm, connective tissue, malignant
  plexiform D18.ØØ
    intra-abdominal D18.Ø3
    intracranial D18.Ø2
    skin D18.Ø1
    specified site NEC D18.Ø9
  racemose D18.ØØ
    intra-abdominal D18.Ø3
    intracranial D18.Ø2
    skin D18.Ø1
    specified site NEC D18.Ø9
  sclerosing — *see* Neoplasm, skin, benign
  simplex D18.ØØ
    intra-abdominal D18.Ø3
    intracranial D18.Ø2
    skin D18.Ø1
    specified site NEC D18.Ø9
  skin D18.Ø1
  specified site NEC D18.Ø9
  venous D18.ØØ
    intra-abdominal D18.Ø3
    intracranial D18.Ø2
    skin D18.Ø1
    specified site NEC D18.Ø9
  verrucous keratotic D18.ØØ
    intra-abdominal D18.Ø3
    intracranial D18.Ø2
    skin D18.Ø1
    specified site NEC D18.Ø9
Hemangiomatosis (systemic) I78.8
  involving single site — *see* Hemangioma
Hemangiopericytoma (*see also* Neoplasm, connective tissue, uncertain behavior)
  benign — *see* Neoplasm, connective tissue, benign
  malignant — *see* Neoplasm, connective tissue, malignant
Hemangiosarcoma — *see* Neoplasm, connective tissue, malignant
Hemarthrosis (nontraumatic) M25.ØØ
  ankle M25.Ø7- ☑
  elbow M25.Ø2- ☑
  foot joint M25.Ø7- ☑
  hand joint M25.Ø4- ☑
  hip M25.Ø5- ☑
  in hemophilic arthropathy — *see* Arthropathy, hemophilic
  knee M25.Ø6- ☑
  shoulder M25.Ø1- ☑
  specified joint NEC M25.Ø8
  traumatic — *see* Sprain, by site
  vertebrae M25.Ø8
  wrist M25.Ø3- ☑
Hematemesis K92.Ø
  with ulcer — *code by site under* Ulcer, with hemorrhage K27.4
  newborn, neonatal P54.Ø
    due to swallowed maternal blood P78.2
Hematidrosis L74.8
Hematinuria (*see also* Hemoglobinuria)
  malarial B5Ø.8
Hematobilia K83.8
Hematocele
  female NEC N94.89
    with ectopic pregnancy OØØ.9
    ovary N83.8
  male N5Ø.1
Hematochezia (*see also* Melena) K92.1

Index

Headache — Hematochezia

Hematochyluria (*see also* Infestation, filarial)
  schistosomiasis (bilharziasis) B65.0
Hematocolpos (with hematometra or hematosalpinx)
  N89.7
Hematocornea — *see* Pigmentation, cornea, stromal
Hematogenous — *see* condition
Hematoma (traumatic) (skin surface intact) (*see also*
  Contusion)
  with
    injury of internal organs — *see* Injury, by site
    open wound — *see* Wound, open
  amputation stump (surgical) (late) T87.89
  aorta, dissecting I71.00
    abdominal I71.02
    thoracic I71.01
    thoracoabdominal I71.03
  aortic intramural — *see* Dissection, aorta
  arterial (complicating trauma) — *see* Injury, blood
    vessel, by site
  auricle — *see* Contusion, ear
    nontraumatic — *see* Disorder, pinna, hematoma
  birth injury NEC P15.8
  brain (traumatic)
    with
      cerebral laceration or contusion (diffuse) — *see*
        Injury, intracranial, diffuse
        focal — *see* Injury, intracranial, focal
    cerebellar, traumatic S06.37-
    intracerebral, traumatic — *see* Injury, intracranial,
      intracerebral hemorrhage
    newborn NEC P52.4
      birth injury P10.1
    nontraumatic -— *see* Hemorrhage, intracranial
    subarachnoid, arachnoid, traumatic — *see* Injury,
      intracranial, subarachnoid hemorrhage
    subdural, traumatic — *see* Injury, intracranial,
      subdural hemorrhage
  breast (nontraumatic) N64.89
  broad ligament (nontraumatic) N83.7
    traumatic S37.892 ☑
  cerebellar, traumatic S06.37- ☑
  cerebral — *see* Hematoma, brain
  cerebrum S06.36- ☑
    left S06.35- ☑
    right S06.34- ☑
  cesarean delivery wound O90.2
  complicating delivery (perineal) (pelvic) (vagina) (vul-
    va) O71.7
  corpus cavernosum (nontraumatic) N48.89
  epididymis (nontraumatic) N50.1
  epidural (traumatic) — *see* Injury, intracranial, epidural
    hemorrhage
    spinal — *see* Injury, spinal cord, by region
  episiotomy O90.2
  face, birth injury P15.4
  genital organ NEC (nontraumatic)
    female (nonobstetric) N94.89
      traumatic S30.202 ☑
    male N50.1
      traumatic S30.201 ☑
  internal organs — *see* Injury, by site
  intracerebral, traumatic — *see* Injury, intracranial, in-
    tracerebral hemorrhage
  intraoperative — *see* Complications, intraoperative,
    hemorrhage
  labia (nontraumatic) (nonobstetric) N90.89
  liver (subcapsular) (nontraumatic) K76.89
    birth injury P15.0
  mediastinum — *see* Injury, intrathoracic
  mesosalpinx (nontraumatic) N83.7
    traumatic S37.898 ☑
  muscle — code by site under Contusion
  nontraumatic
    muscle M79.81
    soft tissue M79.81
  obstetrical surgical wound O90.2
  orbit, orbital (nontraumatic) (*see also* Hemorrhage,
    orbit)
    traumatic — *see* Contusion, orbit
  pelvis (female) (nontraumatic) (nonobstetric) N94.89
    obstetric O71.7
    traumatic — *see* Injury, by site
  penis (nontraumatic) N48.89
    birth injury P15.5
  perianal (nontraumatic) K64.5
  perineal S30.23 ☑
    complicating delivery O71.7

Hematoma — *continued*
  perirenal — *see* Injury, kidney
  pinna — *see* Contusion, ear
    nontraumatic — *see* Disorder, pinna, hematoma
  placenta O43.89- ☑
  postoperative (postprocedural) — *see* Complication,
    postprocedural, hemorrhage
  retroperitoneal (nontraumatic) K66.1
    traumatic S36.892 ☑
  scrotum, superficial S30.22 ☑
    birth injury P15.5
  seminal vesicle (nontraumatic) N50.1
    traumatic S37.892 ☑
  spermatic cord (traumatic) S37.892 ☑
    nontraumatic N50.1
  spinal (cord) (meninges) (*see also* Injury, spinal cord,
    by region)
    newborn (birth injury) P11.5
  spleen D73.5
    intraoperative — *see* Complications, intraoperative,
      hemorrhage, spleen
    postprocedural (postoperative) — *see* Complica-
      tions, postprocedural, hemorrhage, spleen
  sternocleidomastoid, birth injury P15.2
  sternomastoid, birth injury P15.2
  subarachnoid (traumatic) — *see* Injury, intracranial,
    subarachnoid hemorrhage
    newborn (nontraumatic) P52.5
      due to birth injury P10.3
    nontraumatic — *see* Hemorrhage, intracranial,
      subarachnoid
  subdural (traumatic) — *see* Injury, intracranial, subdu-
    ral hemorrhage
    newborn (localized) P52.8
      birth injury P10.0
    nontraumatic — *see* Hemorrhage, intracranial,
      subdural
  superficial, newborn P54.5
  testis (nontraumatic) N50.1
    birth injury P15.5
  tunica vaginalis (nontraumatic) N50.1
  umbilical cord, complicating delivery O69.5 ☑
  uterine ligament (broad) (nontraumatic) N83.7
    traumatic S37.892 ☑
  vagina (ruptured) (nontraumatic) N89.8
    complicating delivery O71.7
  vas deferens (nontraumatic) N50.1
    traumatic S37.892 ☑
  vitreous — *see* Hemorrhage, vitreous
  vulva (nontraumatic) (nonobstetric) N90.89
    complicating delivery O71.7
    newborn (birth injury) P15.5
Hematometra N85.7
  with hematocolpos N89.7
Hematomyelia (central) G95.19
  newborn (birth injury) P11.5
  traumatic T14.8
Hematomyelitis G04.90
Hematoperitoneum — *see* Hemoperitoneum
Hematophobia F40.230
Hematopneumothorax (see Hemothorax)
Hematopoiesis, cyclic D70.4
Hematoporphyria — *see* Porphyria
Hematorachis, hematorrhachis G95.19
  newborn (birth injury) P11.5
Hematosalpinx N83.6
  with
    hematocolpos N89.7
    hematometra N85.7
      with hematocolpos N89.7
  infectional — *see* Salpingitis
Hematospermia R36.1
Hematothorax (see Hemothorax)
Hematuria R31.9
  benign (familial) (of childhood) (*see also* Hematuria,
    idiopathic)
    essential microscopic R31.1
  due to sulphonamide, sulfonamide — *see* Table of
    Drugs and Chemicals, by drug
  endemic (*see also* Schistosomiasis) B65.0
  gross R31.0
  idiopathic N02.9
    with glomerular lesion
      crescentic (diffuse) glomerulonephritis N02.7
      dense deposit disease N02.6
      endocapillary proliferative glomerulonephritis
        N02.4

Hematuria — *continued*
  idiopathic — *continued*
    with glomerular lesion — *continued*
      focal and segmental hyalinosis or sclerosis
        N02.1
      membranoproliferative (diffuse) N02.5
      membranous (diffuse) N02.2
      mesangial proliferative (diffuse) N02.3
      mesangiocapillary (diffuse) N02.5
      minor abnormality N02.0
      proliferative NEC N02.8
      specified pathology NEC N02.8
  intermittent — *see* Hematuria, idiopathic
  malarial B50.8
  microscopic NEC R31.2
    benign essential R31.1
  paroxysmal (*see also* Hematuria, idiopathic)
    nocturnal D59.5
  persistent — *see* Hematuria, idiopathic
  recurrent — *see* Hematuria, idiopathic
  tropical (*see also* Schistosomiasis) B65.0
  tuberculous A18.13
Hemeralopia (day blindness) H53.11
  vitamin A deficiency E50.5
Hemi-akinesia R41.4
Hemianalgesia R20.0
Hemianencephaly Q00.0
Hemianesthesia R20.0
Hemianopia, hemianopsia (heteronymous) H53.47
  homonymous H53.46- ☑
  syphilitic A52.71
Hemiathetosis R25.8
Hemiatrophy R68.89
  cerebellar G31.9
  face, facial, progressive (Romberg) G51.8
  tongue K14.8
Hemiballism (us) G25.5
Hemicardia Q24.8
Hemicephalus, hemicephaly Q00.0
Hemichorea G25.5
Hemicolitis, left — *see* Colitis, left sided
Hemicrania
  congenital malformation Q00.0
  continua G44.51
  meaning migraine (*see also* Migraine) G43.909
  paroxysmal G44.039
    chronic G44.049
      intractable G44.041
      not intractable G44.049
    episodic G44.039
      intractable G44.031
      not intractable G44.039
    intractable G44.031
    not intractable G44.039
Hemidystrophy — *see* Hemiatrophy
Hemiectromelia Q73.8
Hemihypalgesia R20.8
Hemihypesthesia R20.1
Hemi-inattention R41.4
Hemimelia Q73.8
  lower limb — *see* Defect, reduction, lower limb, spec-
    ified type NEC
  upper limb — *see* Defect, reduction, upper limb,
    specified type NEC
Hemiparalysis — *see* Hemiplegia
Hemiparesis — *see* Hemiplegia
Hemiparesthesia R20.2
Hemiparkinsonism G20
Hemiplegia G81.9- ☑
  alternans facialis G83.89
  ascending NEC G81.90
    spinal G95.89
  congenital (cerebral) G80.8
    spastic G80.2
  embolic (current episode) I63.4- ☑
  flaccid G81.0- ☑
  following
    cerebrovascular disease I69.959
      cerebral infarction I69.35- ☑
      intracerebral hemorrhage I69.15- ☑
      nontraumatic intracranial hemorrhage NEC
        I69.25- ☑
      specified disease NEC I69.85- ☑
      stroke NOS I69.35- ☑
      subarachnoid hemorrhage I69.05- ☑
  hysterical F44.4
  newborn NEC P91.8

Hemiplegia — *continued*
  newborn — *continued*
    birth injury P11.9
    spastic G81.1- ☑
      congenital G80.2
    thrombotic (current episode) I63.3 ☑
Hemisection, spinal cord — *see* Injury, spinal cord, by region
Hemispasm (facial) R25.2
Hemisporosis B48.8
Hemitremor R25.1
Hemivertebra Q76.49
  failure of segmentation with scoliosis Q76.3
  fusion with scoliosis Q76.3
Hemochromatosis E83.119
  with refractory anemia D46.1
  due to repeated red blood cell transfusion E83.111
  hereditary (primary) E83.110
  primary E83.110
  specified NEC E83.118
Hemoglobin (*see also* condition)
  abnormal (disease) — *see* Disease, hemoglobin
  AS genotype D57.3
  Constant Spring D58.2
  E-beta thalassemia D56.5
  fetal, hereditary persistence (HPFH) D56.4
  H Constant Spring D56.0
  low NOS D64.9
  S (Hb S), heterozygous D57.3
Hemoglobinemia D59.9
  due to blood transfusion T80.89 ☑
  paroxysmal D59.6
    nocturnal D59.5
Hemoglobinopathy (mixed) D58.2
  with thalassemia D56.8
  sickle-cell D57.1
    with thalassemia D57.40
      with crisis (vasoocclusive pain) D57.419
        with
          acute chest syndrome D57.411
          splenic sequestration D57.412
      without crisis D57.40
Hemoglobinuria R82.3
  with anemia, hemolytic, acquired (chronic) NEC D59.6
  cold (agglutinin) (paroxysmal) (with Raynaud's syndrome) D59.6
  due to exertion or hemolysis NEC D59.6
  intermittent D59.6
  malarial B50.9
  march D59.6
  nocturnal (paroxysmal) D59.5
  paroxysmal (cold) D59.6
    nocturnal D59.5
Hemolymphangioma D18.1
Hemolysis
  intravascular
    with
      abortion — *see* Abortion, by type, complicated by, hemorrhage
      ectopic or molar pregnancy O08.1
      hemorrhage
        antepartum — *see* Hemorrhage, antepartum, with coagulation defect
        intrapartum (*see also* Hemorrhage, complicating, delivery) O67.0
      postpartum O72.3
  neonatal (excessive) P58.9
    specified NEC P58.8
Hemolytic — *see* condition
Hemopericardium I31.2
  following acute myocardial infarction (current complication) I23.0
  newborn P54.8
  traumatic — *see* Injury, heart, with hemopericardium
Hemoperitoneum K66.1
  infectional K65.9
  traumatic S36.899 ☑
    with open wound — *see* Wound, open, with penetration into peritoneal cavity
Hemophilia (classical) (familial) (hereditary) D66
  A D66
  acquired D68.311
  autoimmune D68.311
  B D67
  C D68.1
  calcipriva (*see also* Defect, coagulation) D68.4
  nonfamilial (*see also* Defect, coagulation) D68.4
  secondary D68.311

Hemophilia — *continued*
  vascular D68.0
Hemophthalmos H44.81- ☑
Hemopneumothorax (*see also* Hemothorax)
  traumatic S27.2 ☑
Hemoptysis R04.2
  newborn P26.9
  tuberculous — *see* Tuberculosis, pulmonary
Hemorrhage, hemorrhagic (concealed) R58
  abdomen R58
  accidental antepartum — *see* Hemorrhage, antepartum
  acute idiopathic pulmonary, in infants R04.81
  adenoid (J35.8)
  adrenal (capsule) (gland) E27.49
    medulla E27.8
    newborn P54.4
  after delivery — *see* Hemorrhage, postpartum
  alveolar
    lung, newborn P26.8
    process K08.8
  alveolus K08.8
  amputation stump (surgical) T87.89
  anemia (chronic) D50.0
    acute D62
  antepartum (with) O46.90
    with coagulation defect O46.00- ☑
      afibrinogenemia O46.01- ☑
      disseminated intravascular coagulation O46.02- ☑
      hypofibrinogenemia O46.01- ☑
      specified defect NEC O46.09- ☑
    before 20 weeks gestation O20.9
      specified type NEC O20.8
      threatened abortion O20.0
    due to
      abruptio placenta (*see also* Abruptio placentae) O45.9- ☑
      leiomyoma, uterus — *see* Hemorrhage, antepartum, specified cause NEC
      placenta previa O44.1- ☑
    specified cause NEC — *see* subcategory O46.8X- ☑
  anus (sphincter) K62.5
  apoplexy (stroke) — *see* Hemorrhage, intracranial, intracerebral
  arachnoid — *see* Hemorrhage, intracranial, subarachnoid
  artery R58
    brain — *see* Hemorrhage, intracranial, intracerebral
  basilar (ganglion) I61.0
  bladder N32.89
  bowel K92.2
    newborn P54.3
  brain (miliary) (nontraumatic) — *see* Hemorrhage, intracranial, intracerebral
    due to
      birth injury P10.1
      syphilis A52.05
    epidural or extradural (traumatic) — *see* Injury, intracranial, epidural hemorrhage
    newborn P52.4
      birth injury P10.1
    subarachnoid — *see* Hemorrhage, intracranial, subarachnoid
    subdural — *see* Hemorrhage, intracranial, subdural
  brainstem (nontraumatic) I61.3
    traumatic S06.38- ☑
  breast N64.59
  bronchial tube — *see* Hemorrhage, lung
  bronchopulmonary — *see* Hemorrhage, lung
  bronchus — *see* Hemorrhage, lung
  bulbar I61.5
  capillary I78.8
    primary D69.8
  cecum K92.2
  cerebellar, cerebellum (nontraumatic) I61.4
    newborn P52.6
    traumatic S06.37- ☑
  cerebral, cerebrum (*see also* Hemorrhage, intracranial, intracerebral)
    lobe I61.1
    newborn (anoxic) P52.4
      birth injury P10.1
  cerebromeningeal I61.8
  cerebrospinal — *see* Hemorrhage, intracranial, intracerebral
  cervix (uteri) (stump) NEC N88.8

Hemorrhage, hemorrhagic — *continued*
  chamber, anterior (eye) — *see* Hyphema
  childbirth — *see* Hemorrhage, complicating, delivery
  choroid H31.30- ☑
    expulsive H31.31- ☑
  ciliary body — *see* Hyphema
  cochlea — *see* subcategory H83.8 ☑
  colon K92.2
  complicating
    abortion — *see* Abortion, by type, complicated by, hemorrhage
    delivery O67.9
      associated with coagulation defect (afibrinogenemia) (DIC) (hyperfibrinolysis) O67.0
      specified cause NEC O67.8
    surgical procedure — *see* Hemorrhage, intraoperative
  conjunctiva H11.3- ☑
    newborn P54.8
  cord, newborn (stump) P51.9
  corpus luteum (ruptured) cyst N83.1
  cortical (brain) I61.1
  cranial — *see* Hemorrhage, intracranial
  cutaneous R23.3
    due to autosensitivity, erythrocyte D69.2
    newborn P54.5
  delayed
    following ectopic or molar pregnancy O08.1
    postpartum O72.2
  diathesis (familial) D69.9
  disease D69.9
    newborn P53
    specified type NEC D69.8
  due to or associated with
    afibrinogenemia or other coagulation defect (conditions in categories D65- D69)
      antepartum — *see* Hemorrhage, antepartum, with coagulation defect
      intrapartum O67.0
    dental implant M27.61
    device, implant or graft (*see also* Complications, by site and type, specified NEC) T85.83 ☑
      arterial graft NEC T82.838 ☑
      breast T85.83 ☑
      catheter NEC T85.83 ☑
        dialysis (renal) T82.838 ☑
          intraperitoneal T85.83 ☑
        infusion NEC T82.838 ☑
          spinal (epidural) (subdural) T85.83 ☑
        urinary (indwelling) T83.83 ☑
      electronic (electrode) (pulse generator) (stimulator)
        bone T84.83 ☑
        cardiac T82.837 ☑
        nervous system (brain) (peripheral nerve) (spinal) T85.83 ☑
        urinary T83.83 ☑
      fixation, internal (orthopedic) NEC T84.83 ☑
      gastrointestinal (bile duct) (esophagus) T85.83 ☑
      genital NEC T83.83 ☑
      heart NEC T82.837 ☑
      joint prosthesis T84.83 ☑
      ocular (corneal graft) (orbital implant) NEC T85.83 ☑
      orthopedic NEC T84.83 ☑
        bone graft T86.838
      specified NEC T85.83 ☑
      urinary NEC T83.83 ☑
      vascular NEC T82.838 ☑
      ventricular intracranial shunt T85.83 ☑
  duodenum, duodenal K92.2
    ulcer — *see* Ulcer, duodenum, with hemorrhage
  dura mater — *see* Hemorrhage, intracranial, subdural
  endotracheal — *see* Hemorrhage, lung
  epicranial subaponeurotic (massive), birth injury P12.2
  epidural (traumatic) (*see also* Injury, intracranial, epidural hemorrhage)
    nontraumatic I62.1
  esophagus K22.8
    varix I85.01
      secondary I85.11
  excessive, following ectopic gestation (subsequent episode) O08.1
  extradural (traumatic) — *see* Injury, intracranial, epidural hemorrhage
    birth injury P10.8

Hemorrhage, hemorrhagic — *continued*
- extradural — *see* Injury, intracranial, epidural hemorrhage — *continued*
    - newborn (anoxic) (nontraumatic) P52.8
    - nontraumatic I62.1
- eye NEC H57.8
    - fundus — *see* Hemorrhage, retina
    - lid — *see* Disorder, eyelid, specified type NEC
- fallopian tube N83.6
- fibrinogenolysis — *see* Fibrinolysis
- fibrinolytic (acquired) — *see* Fibrinolysis
- from
    - ear (nontraumatic) — *see* Otorrhagia
    - tracheostomy stoma J95.01
- fundus, eye — *see* Hemorrhage, retina
- funis — *see* Hemorrhage, umbilicus, cord
- gastric — *see* Hemorrhage, stomach
- gastroenteric K92.2
    - newborn P54.3
- gastrointestinal (tract) K92.2
    - newborn P54.3
- genital organ, male N50.1
- genitourinary (tract) NOS R31.9
- gingiva K06.8
- globe (eye) — *see* Hemophthalmos
- graafian follicle cyst (ruptured) N83.0
- gum K06.8
- heart I51.89
- hypopharyngeal (throat) R04.1
- intermenstrual (regular) N92.3
    - irregular N92.1
- internal (organs) NEC R58
    - capsule I61.0
    - ear — *see* subcategory H83.8 ☑
        - newborn P54.8
- intestine K92.2
    - newborn P54.3
- intra-abdominal R58
- intra-alveolar (lung), newborn P26.8
- intracerebral (nontraumatic) — *see* Hemorrhage, intracranial, intracerebral
- intracranial (nontraumatic) I62.9
    - birth injury P10.9
    - epidural, nontraumatic I62.1
    - extradural, nontraumatic I62.1
    - intracerebral (nontraumatic) (in) I61.9
        - brain stem I61.3
        - cerebellum I61.4
        - hemisphere I61.2
            - cortical (superficial) I61.1
            - subcortical (deep) I61.0
        - intraoperative
            - during a nervous system procedure G97.31
            - during other procedure G97.32
        - intraventricular I61.5
        - multiple localized I61.6
        - newborn P52.4
            - birth injury P10.1
        - postprocedural
            - following a nervous system procedure G97.51
            - following other procedure G97.52
        - specified NEC I61.8
        - superficial I61.1
        - traumatic (diffuse) — *see* Injury, intracranial, diffuse
        - focal — *see* Injury, intracranial, focal
    - newborn P52.9
    - specified NEC P52.8
    - subarachnoid (nontraumatic) (from) I60.9
        - intracranial (cerebral) artery I60.7
            - anterior communicating I60.2- ☑
            - basilar I60.4
            - carotid siphon and bifurcation I60.0- ☑
            - communicating I60.7
                - anterior I60.2- ☑
                - posterior I60.3- ☑
            - middle cerebral I60.1- ☑
            - posterior communicating I60.3- ☑
            - specified artery NEC I60.6
            - vertebral I60.5- ☑
        - newborn P52.5
            - birth injury P10.3
        - specified NEC I60.8
        - traumatic S06.6X- ☑
    - subdural (nontraumatic) I62.00
        - acute I62.01
        - birth injury P10.0

Hemorrhage, hemorrhagic — *continued*
- intracranial — *continued*
    - subdural — *continued*
        - chronic I62.03
        - newborn (anoxic) (hypoxic) P52.8
            - birth injury P10.0
        - spinal G95.19
        - subacute I62.02
        - traumatic — *see* Injury, intracranial, subdural hemorrhage
    - traumatic — *see* Injury, intracranial, focal brain injury
- intramedullary NEC G95.19
- intraocular — *see* Hemophthalmos
- intraoperative, intraprocedural — *see* Complication, hemorrhage (hematoma), intraoperative (intraprocedural), by site
- intrapartum — *see* Hemorrhage, complicating, delivery
- intrapelvic
    - female N94.89
    - male K66.1
- intraperitoneal K66.1
- intrapontine I61.3
- intraprocedural — *see* Complication, hemorrhage (hematoma), intraoperative (intraprocedural), by site
- intrauterine N85.7
    - complicating delivery (*see also* Hemorrhage, complicating, delivery) O67.9
    - postpartum — *see* Hemorrhage, postpartum
- intraventricular I61.5
    - newborn (nontraumatic) (*see also* Newborn, affected by, hemorrhage) P52.3
        - due to birth injury P10.2
        - grade
            - 1 P52.0
            - 2 P52.1
            - 3 P52.21
            - 4 P52.22
- intravesical N32.89
- iris (postinfectional) (postinflammatory) (toxic) — *see* Hyphema
- joint (nontraumatic) — *see* Hemarthrosis
- kidney N28.89
- knee (joint) (nontraumatic) — *see* Hemarthrosis, knee
- labyrinth — *see* subcategory H83.8 ☑
- lenticular striate artery I61.0
- ligature, vessel — *see* Hemorrhage, postoperative
- liver K76.89
- lung R04.89
    - newborn P26.9
        - massive P26.1
        - specified NEC P26.8
    - tuberculous — *see* Tuberculosis, pulmonary
- massive umbilical, newborn P51.0
- mediastinum — *see* Hemorrhage, lung
- medulla I61.3
- membrane (brain) I60.8
    - spinal cord — *see* Hemorrhage, spinal cord
- meninges, meningeal (brain) (middle) I60.8
    - spinal cord — *see* Hemorrhage, spinal cord
- mesentery K66.1
- metritis — *see* Endometritis
- mouth K13.79
- mucous membrane NEC R58
    - newborn P54.8
- muscle M62.89
- nail (subungual) L60.8
- nasal turbinate R04.0
    - newborn P54.8
- navel, newborn P51.9
- newborn P54.9
    - specified NEC P54.8
- nipple N64.59
- nose R04.0
    - newborn P54.8
- omentum K66.1
- optic nerve (sheath) H47.02- ☑
- orbit, orbital H05.23- ☑
- ovary NEC N83.8
- oviduct N83.6
- pancreas K86.8
- parathyroid (gland) (spontaneous) E21.4
- parturition — *see* Hemorrhage, complicating, delivery
- penis N48.89
- pericardium, pericarditis I31.2
- peritoneum, peritoneal K66.1

Hemorrhage, hemorrhagic — *continued*
- peritonsillar tissue J35.8
    - due to infection J36
- petechial R23.3
    - due to autosensitivity, erythrocyte D69.2
- pituitary (gland) E23.6
- pleura — *see* Hemorrhage, lung
- polioencephalitis, superior E51.2
- polymyositis — *see* Polymyositis
- pons, pontine I61.3
- posterior fossa (nontraumatic) I61.8
    - newborn P52.6
- postmenopausal N95.0
- postnasal R04.0
- postoperative — *see* Complications, postprocedural, hemorrhage, by site
- postpartum NEC (following delivery of placenta) O72.1
    - delayed or secondary O72.2
    - retained placenta O72.0
    - third stage O72.0
- pregnancy — *see* Hemorrhage, antepartum
- preretinal — *see* Hemorrhage, retina
- prostate N42.1
- puerperal — *see* Hemorrhage, postpartum
    - delayed or secondary O72.2
- pulmonary R04.89
    - newborn P26.9
        - massive P26.1
        - specified NEC P26.8
    - tuberculous — *see* Tuberculosis, pulmonary
- purpura (primary) D69.3
- rectum (sphincter) K62.5
    - newborn P54.2
- recurring, following initial hemorrhage at time of injury T79.2 ☑
- renal N28.89
- respiratory passage or tract R04.9
    - specified NEC R04.89
- retina, retinal (vessels) H35.6- ☑
    - diabetic — *see* Diabetes, retinal, hemorrhage
- retroperitoneal R58
- scalp R58
- scrotum N50.1
- secondary (nontraumatic) R58
    - following initial hemorrhage at time of injury T79.2 ☑
- seminal vesicle N50.1
- skin R23.3
    - newborn P54.5
- slipped umbilical ligature P51.8
- spermatic cord N50.1
- spinal (cord) G95.19
    - newborn (birth injury) P11.5
- spleen D73.5
    - intraoperative — *see* Complications, intraoperative, hemorrhage, spleen
    - postprocedural — *see* Complications, postprocedural, hemorrhage, spleen
- stomach K92.2
    - newborn P54.3
    - ulcer — *see* Ulcer, stomach, with hemorrhage
- subarachnoid (nontraumatic) — *see* Hemorrhage, intracranial, subarachnoid
- subconjunctival (*see also* Hemorrhage, conjunctiva)
    - birth injury P15.3
- subcortical (brain) I61.0
- subcutaneous R23.3
- subdiaphragmatic R58
- subdural (acute) (nontraumatic) — *see* Hemorrhage, intracranial, subdural
- subependymal
    - newborn P52.0
        - with intraventricular extension P52.1
            - and intracerebral extension P52.22
- subgaleal P12.1
- subhyaloid — *see* Hemorrhage, retina
- subperiosteal — *see* Disorder, bone, specified type NEC
- subretinal — *see* Hemorrhage, retina
- subtentorial — *see* Hemorrhage, intracranial, subdural
- subungual L60.8
- suprarenal (capsule) (gland) E27.49
    - newborn P54.4
- tentorium (traumatic) NEC — *see* Hemorrhage, brain
    - newborn (birth injury) P10.4
- testis N50.1
- third stage (postpartum) O72.0
- thorax — *see* Hemorrhage, lung

Hemorrhage, hemorrhagic — *continued*
  throat R04.1
  thymus (gland) E32.8
  thyroid (cyst) (gland) E07.89
  tongue K14.8
  tonsil J35.8
  trachea — *see* Hemorrhage, lung
  tracheobronchial R04.89
    newborn P26.0
  traumatic — *code to specific injury*
    cerebellar — *see* Hemorrhage, brain
    intracranial — *see* Hemorrhage, brain
    recurring or secondary (following initial hemor-
      rhage at time of injury) T79.2 ☑
  tuberculous NEC (*see also* Tuberculosis, pulmonary)
    A15.0
  tunica vaginalis N50.1
  ulcer — *code by* site under Ulcer, with hemorrhage
    K27.4
  umbilicus, umbilical
    cord
      after birth, newborn P51.9
      complicating delivery O69.5 ☑
    newborn P51.9
      massive P51.0
      slipped ligature P51.8
    stump P51.9
  urethra (idiopathic) N36.8
  uterus, uterine (abnormal) N93.9
    climacteric N92.4
    complicating delivery — *see* Hemorrhage, compli-
      cating, delivery
    dysfunctional or functional N93.8
    intermenstrual (regular) N92.3
      irregular N92.1
    postmenopausal N95.0
    postpartum — *see* Hemorrhage, postpartum
    preclimacteric or premenopausal N92.4
    prepubertal N93.8
    pubertal N92.2
  vagina (abnormal) N93.9
    newborn P54.6
  vas deferens N50.1
  vasa previa O69.4 ☑
  ventricular I61.5
  vesical N32.89
  viscera NEC R58
    newborn P54.8
  vitreous (humor) (intraocular) H43.1- ☑
  vulva N90.89
Hemorrhoids (bleeding) (without mention of degree)
    K64.9
  1st degree (grade/stage I) (without prolapse outside
    of anal canal) K64.0
  2nd degree (grade/stage II) (that prolapse with
    straining but retract spontaneously) K64.1
  3rd degree (grade/stage III) (that prolapse with
    straining and require manual replacement back
    inside anal canal) K64.2
  4th degree (grade/stage IV) (with prolapsed tissue that
    cannot be manually replaced) K64.3
  complicating
    pregnancy O22.4 ☑
    puerperium O87.2
  external K64.4
    with
      thrombosis K64.5
  internal (without mention of degree) K64.8
  prolapsed K64.8
  skin tags
    anus K64.4
    residual K64.4
  specified NEC K64.8
  strangulated (*see also* Hemorrhoids, by degree) K64.8
  thrombosed (*see also* Hemorrhoids, by degree) K64.5
  ulcerated (*see also* Hemorrhoids, by degree) K64.8
Hemosalpinx N83.6
  with
    hematocolpos N89.7
    hematometra N85.7
      with hematocolpos N89.7
Hemosiderosis (dietary) E83.19
  pulmonary, idiopathic E83.1- ☑ [J84.03]
  transfusion T80.89 ☑
Hemothorax (bacterial) (nontuberculous) J94.2
  newborn P54.8
  traumatic S27.1 ☑
    with pneumothorax S27.2 ☑

Hemothorax — *continued*
  tuberculous NEC A15.6
Henoch (-Schönlein) **disease or syndrome** (purpura)
    D69.0
Henpue, henpuye A66.6
Hepar lobatum (syphilitic) A52.74
Hepatalgia K76.89
Hepatitis K75.9
  acute B17.9
    with coma K72.01
    with hepatic failure — *see* Failure, hepatic
    alcoholic — *see* Hepatitis, alcoholic
    infectious B15.9
      with hepatic coma B15.0
    viral B17.9
  alcoholic (acute) (chronic) K70.10
    with ascites K70.11
  amebic — *see* Abscess, liver, amebic
  anicteric, (viral) — *see* Hepatitis, viral
  antigen-associated (HAA) — *see* Hepatitis, B
  Australia-antigen (positive) — *see* Hepatitis, B
  autoimmune K75.4
  B B19.10
    with hepatic coma B19.11
    acute B16.9
      with
        delta-agent (coinfection) (without hepatic
          coma) B16.1
          with hepatic coma B16.0
        hepatic coma (without delta-agent coinfec-
          tion) B16.2
    chronic B18.1
      with delta-agent B18.0
  bacterial NEC K75.89
  C (viral) B19.20
    with hepatic coma B19.21
    acute B17.10
      with hepatic coma B17.11
    chronic B18.2
  catarrhal (acute) B15.9
    with hepatic coma B15.0
  cholangiolitic K75.89
  cholestatic K75.89
  chronic K73.9
    active NEC K73.2
    lobular NEC K73.1
    persistent NEC K73.0
    specified NEC K73.8
  cytomegaloviral B25.1
  due to ethanol (acute) (chronic) — *see* Hepatitis, alco-
    holic
  epidemic B15.9
    with hepatic coma B15.0
  fulminant NEC (viral) — *see* Hepatitis, viral
  granulomatous NEC K75.3
  herpesviral B00.81
  history of
    B Z86.19
    C Z86.19
  homologous serum — *see* Hepatitis, viral, type B
  in (due to)
    mumps B26.81
    toxoplasmosis (acquired) B58.1
      congenital (active) P37.1 [K77]
  infectious, infective (acute) (chronic) (subacute) B15.9
    with hepatic coma B15.0
  inoculation — *see* Hepatitis, viral, type B
  interstitial (chronic) K74.69
  lupoid NEC K75.4
  malignant NEC (with hepatic failure) K72.90
    with coma K72.91
  neonatal (idiopathic) (toxic) P59.29
  neonatal giant cell P59.29
  newborn P59.29
  postimmunization — *see* Hepatitis, viral, type B
  post-transfusion — *see* Hepatitis, viral, type B
  reactive, nonspecific K75.2
  serum — *see* Hepatitis, viral, type B
  specified type NEC
    with hepatic failure — *see* Failure, hepatic
  syphilitic (late) A52.74
    congenital (early) A50.08 [K77]
      late A50.59 [K77]
    secondary A51.45
  toxic (*see also* Disease, liver, toxic) K71.6
  tuberculous A18.83
  viral, virus B19.9
    with hepatic coma B19.0

Hepatitis — *continued*
  viral, virus — *continued*
    acute B17.9
    chronic B18.9
      specified NEC B18.8
      type
        B B18.1
          with delta-agent B18.0
        C B18.2
    congenital P35.3
    coxsackie B33.8 [K77]
    cytomegalic inclusion B25.1
    in remission, any type — *code to* Hepatitis, chronic,
      by type
    non-A, non-B B17.8
    specified type NEC (with or without coma) B17.8
    type
      A B15.9
        with hepatic coma B15.0
      B B19.10
        with hepatic coma B19.11
        acute B16.9
          with
            delta-agent (coinfection) (without
              hepatic coma) B16.1
              with hepatic coma B16.0
            hepatic coma (without delta-agent
              coinfection) B16.2
        chronic B18.1
          with delta-agent B18.0
      C B19.20
        with hepatic coma B19.21
        acute B17.10
          with hepatic coma B17.11
        chronic B18.2
      E B17.2
    non-A, non-B B17.8
Hepatization lung (acute) — *see* Pneumonia, lobar
Hepatoblastoma C22.2
Hepatocarcinoma C22.0
Hepatocholangiocarcinoma C22.0
Hepatocholangioma, benign D13.4
Hepatocholangitis K75.89
Hepatolenticular degeneration E83.01
Hepatoma (malignant) C22.0
  benign D13.4
  embryonal C22.0
Hepatomegaly (*see also* Hypertrophy, liver)
  with splenomegaly R16.2
  congenital Q44.7
  in mononucleosis
    gammaherpesviral B27.09
    infectious specified NEC B27.89
Hepatoptosis K76.89
Hepatorenal syndrome following labor and delivery
    O90.4
Hepatosis K76.89
Hepatosplenomegaly R16.2
  hyperlipemic (Bürger-Grütz type) E78.3 [K77]
Hereditary — *see* condition
Heredodegeneration, macular — *see* Dystrophy, retina
Heredopathia atactica polyneuritiformis G60.1
Heredosyphilis — *see* Syphilis, congenital
Herlitz' syndrome Q81.1
Hermansky-Pudlak syndrome E70.331
Hermaphrodite, hermaphroditism (true) Q56.0
  46,XX with streak gonads Q99.1
  46,XX/46,XY Q99.0
  46,XY with streak gonads Q99.1
  chimera 46,XX/46,XY Q99.0
Hernia, hernial (acquired) (recurrent) K46.9
  with
    gangrene — *see* Hernia, by site, with, gangrene
    incarceration — *see* Hernia, by site, with, obstruc-
      tion
    irreducible — *see* Hernia, by site, with, obstruction
    obstruction — *see* Hernia, by site, with, obstruction
    strangulation — *see* Hernia, by site, with, obstruc-
      tion
  abdomen, abdominal K46.9
    with
      gangrene (and obstruction) K46.1
      obstruction K46.0
    femoral — *see* Hernia, femoral
    incisional — *see* Hernia, incisional
    inguinal — *see* Hernia, inguinal
    specified site NEC K45.8

Hernia, hernial — *continued*
  abdomen, abdominal — *continued*
    specified site — *continued*
      with
        gangrene (and obstruction) K45.1
        obstruction K45.0
      umbilical — *see* Hernia, umbilical
      wall — *see* Hernia, ventral
  appendix — *see* Hernia, abdomen
  bladder (mucosa) (sphincter)
    congenital (female) (male) Q79.51
    female — *see* Cystocele
    male N32.89
  brain, congenital — *see* Encephalocele
  cartilage, vertebra — *see* Displacement, intervertebral disc
  cerebral, congenital (*see also* Encephalocele)
    endaural Q01.8
  ciliary body (traumatic) S05.2- ☑
  colon — *see* Hernia, abdomen
  Cooper's — *see* Hernia, abdomen, specified site NEC
  crural — *see* Hernia, femoral
  diaphragm, diaphragmatic K44.9
    with
      gangrene (and obstruction) K44.1
      obstruction K44.0
    congenital Q79.0
  direct (inguinal) — *see* Hernia, inguinal
  diverticulum, intestine — *see* Hernia, abdomen
  double (inguinal) — *see* Hernia, inguinal, bilateral
  due to adhesions (with obstruction) K56.5
  epigastric (*see also* Hernia, ventral) K43.9
  esophageal hiatus — *see* Hernia, hiatal
  external (inguinal) — *see* Hernia, inguinal
  fallopian tube N83.4
  fascia M62.89
  femoral K41.90
    with
      gangrene (and obstruction) K41.40
        not specified as recurrent K41.40
        recurrent K41.41
      obstruction K41.30
        not specified as recurrent K41.30
        recurrent K41.31
    bilateral K41.20
      with
        gangrene (and obstruction) K41.10
          not specified as recurrent K41.10
          recurrent K41.11
        obstruction K41.00
          not specified as recurrent K41.00
          recurrent K41.01
      not specified as recurrent K41.20
      recurrent K41.21
    not specified as recurrent K41.90
    recurrent K41.91
    unilateral K41.90
      with
        gangrene (and obstruction) K41.40
          not specified as recurrent K41.40
          recurrent K41.41
        obstruction K41.30
          not specified as recurrent K41.30
          recurrent K41.31
      not specified as recurrent K41.90
      recurrent K41.91
  foramen magnum G93.5
    congenital Q01.8
  funicular (umbilical) (*see also* Hernia, umbilicus)
    spermatic (cord) — *see* Hernia, inguinal
  gastrointestinal tract — *see* Hernia, abdomen
  Hesselbach's — *see* Hernia, femoral, specified site NEC
  hiatal (esophageal) (sliding) K44.9
    with
      gangrene (and obstruction) K44.1
      obstruction K44.0
    congenital Q40.1
  hypogastric — *see* Hernia, ventral
  incarcerated (*see also* Hernia, by site, with obstruction)
    with gangrene — *see* Hernia, by site, with gangrene
  incisional K43.2
    with
      gangrene (and obstruction) K43.1
      obstruction K43.0
  indirect (inguinal) — *see* Hernia, inguinal
  inguinal (direct) (external) (funicular) (indirect) (internal) (oblique) (scrotal) (sliding) K40.90

Hernia, hernial — *continued*
  inguinal — *continued*
    with
      gangrene (and obstruction) K40.40
        not specified as recurrent K40.40
        recurrent K40.41
      obstruction K40.30
        not specified as recurrent K40.30
        recurrent K40.31
    bilateral K40.20
      with
        gangrene (and obstruction) K40.10
          not specified as recurrent K40.10
          recurrent K40.11
        obstruction K40.00
          not specified as recurrent K40.00
          recurrent K40.01
      not specified as recurrent K40.20
      recurrent K40.21
    not specified as recurrent K40.90
    recurrent K40.91
    unilateral K40.90
      with
        gangrene (and obstruction) K40.40
          not specified as recurrent K40.40
          recurrent K40.41
        obstruction K40.30
          not specified as recurrent K40.30
          recurrent K40.31
      not specified as recurrent K40.90
      recurrent K40.91
  internal (*see also* Hernia, abdomen)
    inguinal — *see* Hernia, inguinal
  interstitial — *see* Hernia, abdomen
  intervertebral cartilage or disc — *see* Displacement, intervertebral disc
  intestine, intestinal — *see* Hernia, by site
  intra-abdominal — *see* Hernia, abdomen
  iris (traumatic) S05.2- ☑
  irreducible (*see also* Hernia, by site, with obstruction)
    with gangrene — *see* Hernia, by site, with gangrene
  ischiatic — *see* Hernia, abdomen, specified site NEC
  ischiorectal — *see* Hernia, abdomen, specified site NEC
  lens (traumatic) S05.2- ☑
  linea (alba) (semilunaris) — *see* Hernia, ventral
  Littre's — *see* Hernia, abdomen
  lumbar — *see* Hernia, abdomen, specified site NEC
  lung (subcutaneous) J98.4
  mediastinum J98.5
  mesenteric (internal) — *see* Hernia, abdomen
  midline — *see* Hernia, ventral
  muscle (sheath) M62.89
  nucleus pulposus — *see* Displacement, intervertebral disc
  oblique (inguinal) — *see* Hernia, inguinal
  obstructive (*see also* Hernia, by site, with obstruction)
    with gangrene — *see* Hernia, by site, with gangrene
  obturator — *see* Hernia, abdomen, specified site NEC
  omental — *see* Hernia, abdomen
  ovary N83.4
  oviduct N83.4
  paraesophageal (*see also* Hernia, diaphragm)
    congenital Q40.1
  parastomal K43.5
    with
      gangrene (and obstruction) K43.4
      obstruction K43.3
  paraumbilical — *see* Hernia, umbilicus
  perineal — *see* Hernia, abdomen, specified site NEC
  Petit's — *see* Hernia, abdomen, specified site NEC
  postoperative — *see* Hernia, incisional
  pregnant uterus — *see* Abnormal, uterus in pregnancy or childbirth
  prevesical N32.89
  properitoneal — *see* Hernia, abdomen, specified site NEC
  pudendal — *see* Hernia, abdomen, specified site NEC
  rectovaginal N81.6
  retroperitoneal — *see* Hernia, abdomen, specified site NEC
  Richter's — *see* Hernia, abdomen, with obstruction
  Rieux's, Riex's — *see* Hernia, abdomen, specified site NEC

Hernia, hernial — *continued*
  sac condition (adhesion) (dropsy) (inflammation) (laceration) (suppuration) — *code by site under* Hernia
  sciatic — *see* Hernia, abdomen, specified site NEC
  scrotum, scrotal — *see* Hernia, inguinal
  sliding (inguinal) (*see also* Hernia, inguinal)
    hiatus — *see* Hernia, hiatal
  spigelian — *see* Hernia, ventral
  spinal — *see* Spina bifida
  strangulated (*see also* Hernia, by site, with obstruction)
    with gangrene — *see* Hernia, by site, with gangrene
  subxiphoid — *see* Hernia, ventral
  supra-umbilicus — *see* Hernia, ventral
  tendon — *see* Disorder, tendon, specified type NEC
  Treitz's (fossa) — *see* Hernia, abdomen, specified site NEC
  tunica vaginalis Q55.29
  umbilicus, umbilical K42.9
    with
      gangrene (and obstruction) K42.1
      obstruction K42.0
  ureter N28.89
  urethra, congenital Q64.79
  urinary meatus, congenital Q64.79
  uterus N81.4
    pregnant — *see* Abnormal, uterus in pregnancy or childbirth
  vaginal (anterior) (wall) — *see* Cystocele
  Velpeau's — *see* Hernia, femoral
  ventral K43.9
    with
      gangrene (and obstruction) K43.7
      obstruction K43.6
    incisional K43.2
      with
        gangrene (and obstruction) K43.1
        obstruction K43.0
      recurrent — *see* Hernia, incisional
    specified NEC K43.9
      with
        gangrene (and obstruction) K43.7
        obstruction K43.6
  vesical
    congenital (female) (male) Q79.51
    female — *see* Cystocele
    male N32.89
  vitreous (into wound) S05.2- ☑
    into anterior chamber — *see* Prolapse, vitreous
Herniation (*see also* Hernia)
  brain (stem) G93.5
  cerebral G93.5
  mediastinum J98.5
  nucleus pulposus — *see* Displacement, intervertebral disc
Herpangina B08.5
Herpes, herpesvirus, herpetic B00.9
  anogenital A60.9
    perianal skin A60.1
    rectum A60.1
    urogenital tract A60.00
      cervix A60.03
      male genital organ NEC A60.02
      penis A60.01
      specified site NEC A60.09
      vagina A60.04
      vulva A60.04
  blepharitis (zoster) B02.39
    simplex B00.59
  circinatus B35.4
    bullosus L12.0
  conjunctivitis (simplex) B00.53
    zoster B02.31
  cornea B02.33
  encephalitis B00.4
    due to herpesvirus 6 B10.01
    due to herpesvirus 7 B10.09
    specified NEC B10.09
  eye (zoster) B02.30
    simplex B00.50
  eyelid (zoster) B02.39
    simplex B00.59
  facialis B00.1
  febrilis B00.1
  geniculate ganglionitis B02.21
  genital, genitalis A60.00
    female A60.09

Herpes, herpesvirus, herpetic — *continued*
genital, genitalis — *continued*
male A60.02
gestational, gestationis O26.4- ☑
gingivostomatitis B00.2
human B00.9
1 — *see* Herpes, simplex
2 — *see* Herpes, simplex
3 — *see* Varicella
4 — *see* Mononucleosis, Epstein-Barr (virus)
5 — *see* Disease, cytomegalic inclusion (generalized)
6
encephalitis B10.01
specified NEC B10.81
7
encephalitis B10.09
specified NEC B10.82
8 B10.89
infection NEC B10.89
Kaposi's sarcoma associated B10.89
iridocyclitis (simplex) B00.51
zoster B02.32
iris (vesicular erythema multiforme) L51.9
iritis (simplex) B00.51
Kaposi's sarcoma associated B10.89
keratitis (simplex) (dendritic) (disciform) (interstitial) B00.52
zoster (interstitial) B02.33
keratoconjunctivitis (simplex) B00.52
zoster B02.33
labialis B00.1
lip B00.1
meningitis (simplex) B00.3
zoster B02.1
ophthalmicus (zoster) NEC B02.30
simplex B00.50
penis A60.01
perianal skin A60.1
pharyngitis, pharyngotonsillitis B00.2
rectum A60.1
scrotum A60.02
sepsis B00.7
simplex B00.9
complicated NEC B00.89
congenital P35.2
conjunctivitis B00.53
external ear B00.1
eyelid B00.59
hepatitis B00.81
keratitis (interstitial) B00.52
myeitis B00.82
specified complication NEC B00.89
visceral B00.89
stomatitis B00.2
tonsurans B35.0
visceral B00.89
vulva A60.04
whitlow B00.89
zoster (*see also* condition) B02.9
auricularis B02.21
complicated NEC B02.8
conjunctivitis B02.31
disseminated B02.7
encephalitis B02.0
eye (lid) B02.39
geniculate ganglionitis B02.21
keratitis (interstitial) B02.33
meningitis B02.1
myelitis B02.24
neuritis, neuralgia B02.29
ophthalmicus NEC B02.30
oticus B02.21
polyneuropathy B02.23
specified complication NEC B02.8
trigeminal neuralgia B02.22
Herpesvirus (human) — *see* Herpes
Herpetophobia F40.218
Herrick's anemia — *see* Disease, sickle-cell
Hers' disease E74.09
Herter-Gee syndrome K90.0
Herxheimer's reaction R68.89
Hesitancy
of micturition R39.11
urinary R39.11
Hesselbach's hernia — *see* Hernia, femoral, specified site NEC
Heterochromia (congenital) Q13.2

Heterochromia — *continued*
cataract — *see* Cataract, complicated
cyclitis (Fuchs) — *see* Cyclitis, Fuchs' heterochromic
hair L67.1
iritis — *see* Cyclitis, Fuchs' heterochromic
retained metallic foreign body (nonmagnetic) — *see* Foreign body, intraocular, old, retained
magnetic — *see* Foreign body, intraocular, old, retained, magnetic
uveitis — *see* Cyclitis, Fuchs' heterochromic
Heterophoria — *see* Strabismus, heterophoria
Heterophyes, heterophyiasis (small intestine) B66.8
Heterotopia, heterotopic (*see also* Malposition, congenital)
cerebralis Q04.8
Heterotropia — *see* Strabismus
Heubner-Herter disease K90.0
Hexadactylism Q69.9
HGSIL (cytology finding) (high grade squamous intraepithelial lesion on cytologic smear) (Pap smear finding)
anus R85.613
cervix R87.613
biopsy (histology) finding — *code to* CIN II or CIN III
vagina R87.623
biopsy (histology) finding — *code to* VAIN II or VAIN III
Hibernoma — *see* Lipoma
Hiccup, hiccough R06.6
epidemic B33.0
psychogenic F45.8
Hidden penis (congenital) Q55.64
acquired N48.83
Hidradenitis (axillaris) (suppurative) L73.2
Hidradenoma (nodular) (*see also* Neoplasm, skin, benign)
clear cell — *see* Neoplasm, skin, benign
papillary — *see* Neoplasm, skin, benign
Hidrocystoma — *see* Neoplasm, skin, benign
High
altitude effects T70.20 ☑
anoxia T70.29 ☑
on
ears T70.0 ☑
sinuses T70.1 ☑
polycythemia D75.1
arch
foot Q66.7
palate, congenital Q38.5
arterial tension — *see* Hypertension
basal metabolic rate R94.8
blood pressure (*see also* Hypertension)
borderline R03.0
reading (incidental) (isolated) (nonspecific), without diagnosis of hypertension R03.0
cholesterol E78.0
with high triglycerides E78.2
diaphragm (congenital) Q79.1
expressed emotional level within family Z63.8
head at term O32.4 ☑
palate, congenital Q38.5
risk
infant NEC Z76.2
sexual behavior (heterosexual) Z72.51
bisexual Z72.53
homosexual Z72.52
temperature (of unknown origin) R50.9
thoracic rib Q76.6
triglycerides E78.1
with high cholesterol E78.2
Hildenbrand's disease A75.0
Hilum — *see* condition
Hip — *see* condition
Hippel's disease Q85.8
Hippophobia F40.218
Hippus H57.09
Hirschsprung's disease or megacolon Q43.1
Hirsutism, hirsuties L68.0
Hirudiniasis
external B88.3
internal B83.4
Hiss-Russell dysentery A03.1
Histidinemia, histidinuria E70.41
Histiocytoma (*see also* Neoplasm, skin, benign)
fibrous (*see also* Neoplasm, skin, benign)
atypical — *see* Neoplasm, connective tissue, uncertain behavior

Histiocytoma — *continued*
fibrous (*see also* Neoplasm, skin, benign) — *continued*
malignant — *see* Neoplasm, connective tissue, malignant
Histiocytosis D76.3
acute differentiated progressive C96.0
Langerhans' cell NEC C96.6
multifocal X
multisystemic (disseminated) C96.0
unisystemic C96.5
pulmonary, adult (adult PLCH) J84.82
unifocal (X) C96.6
lipid, lipoid D76.3
essential E75.29
malignant C96.A (following C96.6)
mononuclear phagocytes NEC D76.1
Langerhans' cells C96.6
non-Langerhans cell D76.3
polyostotic sclerosing D76.3
sinus, with massive lymphadenopathy D76.3
syndrome NEC D76.3
X NEC C96.6
acute (progressive) C96.0
chronic C96.6
multifocal C96.5
multisystemic C96.0
unifocal C96.6
Histoplasmosis B39.9
with pneumonia NEC B39.2
African B39.5
American — *see* Histoplasmosis, capsulati
capsulati B39.4
disseminated B39.3
generalized B39.3
pulmonary B39.2
acute B39.0
chronic B39.1
Darling's B39.4
duboisii B39.5
lung NEC B39.2
History
family (of) (*see also* History, personal (of))
alcohol abuse Z81.1
allergy NEC Z84.89
anemia Z83.2
arthritis Z82.61
asthma Z82.5
blindness Z82.1
cardiac death (sudden) Z82.41
carrier of genetic disease Z84.81
chromosomal anomaly Z82.79
chronic
disabling disease NEC Z82.8
lower respiratory disease Z82.5
colonic polyps Z83.71
congenital malformations and deformations Z82.79
polycystic kidney Z82.71
consanguinity Z84.3
deafness Z82.2
diabetes mellitus Z83.3
disability NEC Z82.8
disease or disorder (of)
allergic NEC Z84.89
behavioral NEC Z81.8
blood and blood-forming organs Z83.2
cardiovascular NEC Z82.49
chronic disabling NEC Z82.8
digestive Z83.79
ear NEC Z83.52
endocrine NEC Z83.49
eye NEC Z83.518
glaucoma Z83.511
genitourinary NEC Z84.2
glaucoma Z83.511
hematological Z83.2
immune mechanism Z83.2
infectious NEC Z83.1
ischemic heart Z82.49
kidney Z84.1
mental NEC Z81.8
metabolic NEC Z83.49
musculoskeletal NEC Z82.69
neurological NEC Z82.0
nutritional Z83.49
parasitic NEC Z83.1
psychiatric NEC Z81.8
respiratory NEC Z83.6

History — *continued*
- family (*see also* History, personal) — *continued*
  - disease or disorder — *continued*
    - skin and subcutaneous tissue NEC Z84.0
    - specified NEC Z84.89
    - drug abuse NEC Z81.3
    - epilepsy Z82.0
    - genetic disease carrier Z84.81
    - glaucoma Z83.511
    - hearing loss Z82.2
    - human immunodeficiency virus (HIV) infection Z83.0
    - Huntington's chorea Z82.0
    - intellectual disability Z81.0
    - leukemia Z80.6
    - malignant neoplasm (of) NOS Z80.9
      - bladder Z80.52
      - breast Z80.3
      - bronchus Z80.1
      - digestive organ Z80.0
      - gastrointestinal tract Z80.0
      - genital organ Z80.49
        - ovary Z80.41
        - prostate Z80.42
        - specified organ NEC Z80.49
        - testis Z80.43
      - hematopoietic NEC Z80.7
      - intrathoracic organ NEC Z80.2
      - kidney Z80.51
      - lung Z80.1
      - lymphatic NEC Z80.7
      - ovary Z80.41
      - prostate Z80.42
      - respiratory organ NEC Z80.2
      - specified site NEC Z80.8
      - testis Z80.43
      - trachea Z80.1
      - urinary organ or tract Z80.59
        - bladder Z80.52
        - kidney Z80.51
    - mental
      - disorder NEC Z81.8
    - multiple endocrine neoplasia (MEN) syndrome Z83.41
    - osteoporosis Z82.62
    - polycystic kidney Z82.71
    - polyps (colon) Z83.71
    - psychiatric disorder Z81.8
    - psychoactive substance abuse NEC Z81.3
    - respiratory condition NEC Z83.6
      - asthma and other lower respiratory conditions Z82.5
    - self-harmful behavior Z81.8
    - skin condition Z84.0
    - specified condition NEC Z84.89
    - stroke (cerebrovascular) Z82.3
    - substance abuse NEC Z81.4
      - alcohol Z81.1
      - drug NEC Z81.3
      - psychoactive NEC Z81.3
      - tobacco Z81.2
    - sudden cardiac death Z82.41
    - tobacco abuse Z81.2
    - violence, violent behavior Z81.8
    - visual loss Z82.1
  - personal (of) (*see also* History, family (of)))
    - abuse
      - adult Z91.419
        - physical and sexual Z91.410
        - psychological Z91.411
      - childhood Z62.819
        - physical Z62.810
        - psychological Z62.811
        - sexual Z62.810
    - alcohol dependence F10.21
    - allergy (to) Z88.9
      - analgesic agent NEC Z88.6
      - anesthetic Z88.4
      - antibiotic agent NEC Z88.1
      - anti-infective agent NEC Z88.3
      - contrast media Z91.041
      - drugs, medicaments and biological substances Z88.9
        - specified NEC Z88.8
      - food Z91.018
        - additives Z91.02
        - eggs Z91.012
        - milk products Z91.011

History — *continued*
- personal (*see also* History, family) — *continued*
  - allergy — *continued*
    - food — *continued*
      - peanuts Z91.010
      - seafood Z91.013
      - specified food NEC Z91.018
    - insect Z91.038
      - bee Z91.030
    - latex Z91.040
    - medicinal agents Z88.9
      - specified NEC Z88.8
    - narcotic agent NEC Z88.5
    - nonmedicinal agents Z91.048
    - penicillin Z88.0
    - serum Z88.7
    - specified NEC Z91.09
    - sulfonamides Z88.2
    - vaccine Z88.7
  - anaphylactic shock Z87.892
  - anaphylaxis Z87.892
  - behavioral disorders Z86.59
  - benign carcinoid tumor Z86.012
  - benign neoplasm Z86.018
    - brain Z86.011
    - carcinoid Z86.012
    - colonic polyps Z86.010
  - brain injury (traumatic) Z87.820
  - breast implant removal Z98.86
  - calculi, renal Z87.442
  - cancer — *see* History, personal (of), malignant neoplasm (of)
  - cardiac arrest (death), successfully resuscitated Z86.74
  - cerebral infarction without residual deficit Z86.73
  - cervical dysplasia Z87.410
  - chemotherapy for neoplastic condition Z92.21
  - childhood abuse — *see* History, personal (of), abuse
  - cleft lip (corrected) Z87.730
  - cleft palate (corrected) Z87.730
  - collapsed vertebra (healed) Z87.311
    - due to osteoporosis Z87.310
  - combat and operational stress reaction Z86.51
  - congenital malformation (corrected) Z87.798
    - circulatory system (corrected) Z87.74
    - digestive system (corrected) NEC Z87.738
    - ear (corrected) Z87.720
    - eye (corrected) Z87.721
    - face and neck (corrected) Z87.790
    - genitourinary system (corrected) NEC Z87.718
    - heart (corrected) Z87.74
    - integument (corrected) Z87.76
    - limb(s) (corrected) Z87.76
    - musculoskeletal system (corrected) Z87.76
    - neck (corrected) Z87.790
    - nervous system (corrected) NEC Z87.728
    - respiratory system (corrected) Z87.75
    - sense organs (corrected) NEC Z87.728
    - specified NEC Z87.798
  - contraception Z92.0
  - deployment (military) Z91.82
  - diabetic foot ulcer Z86.31
  - disease or disorder (of) Z87.898
    - anaphylaxis Z87.892
    - blood and blood-forming organs Z86.2
    - circulatory system Z86.79
      - specified condition NEC Z86.79
    - connective tissue Z87.39
    - digestive system Z87.19
      - colonic polyp Z86.010
      - peptic ulcer disease Z87.11
      - specified condition NEC Z87.19
    - ear Z86.69
    - endocrine Z86.39
      - diabetic foot ulcer Z86.31
      - gestational diabetes Z86.32
      - specified type NEC Z86.39
    - eye Z86.69
    - genital (track) system NEC
      - female Z87.42
      - male Z87.438
    - hematological Z86.2
    - Hodgkin Z85.71
    - immune mechanism Z86.2
    - infectious Z86.19
      - malaria Z86.13

History — *continued*
- personal (*see also* History, family) — *continued*
  - disease or disorder — *continued*
    - infectious — *continued*
      - Methicillin resistant Staphylococcus aureus (MRSA) Z86.14
      - poliomyelitis Z86.12
      - specified NEC Z86.19
      - tuberculosis Z86.11
    - mental NEC Z86.59
    - metabolic Z86.39
      - diabetic foot ulcer Z86.31
      - gestational diabetes Z86.32
      - specified type NEC Z86.39
    - musculoskeletal NEC Z87.39
    - nervous system Z86.69
    - nutritional Z86.39
    - parasitic Z86.19
    - respiratory system NEC Z87.09
    - sense organs Z86.69
    - skin Z87.2
    - specified site or type NEC Z87.898
    - subcutaneous tissue Z87.2
    - trophoblastic Z87.59
    - urinary system NEC Z87.448
  - drug dependence — *see* Dependence, drug, by type, in remission
  - drug therapy
    - antineoplastic chemotherapy Z92.21
    - estrogen Z92.23
    - immunosupression Z92.25
    - inhaled steroids Z92.240
    - monoclonal drug Z92.22
    - specified NEC Z92.29
    - steroid Z92.241
    - systemic steroids Z92.241
  - dysplasia
    - cervical Z87.410
    - prostatic Z87.430
    - vaginal Z87.411
    - vulvar Z87.412
  - embolism (venous) Z86.718
    - pulmonary Z86.711
  - encephalitis Z86.61
  - estrogen therapy Z92.23
  - extracorporeal membrane oxygenation (ECMO) Z92.81
  - failed conscious sedation Z92.83
  - failed moderate sedation Z92.83
  - fall, falling Z91.81
  - fracture (healed)
    - fatigue Z87.312
    - fragility Z87.310
    - osteoporosis Z87.310
    - pathological NEC Z87.311
    - stress Z87.312
    - traumatic Z87.81
  - gestational diabetes Z86.32
  - hepatitis
    - B Z86.19
    - C Z86.19
  - Hodgkin disease Z85.71
  - hyperthermia, malignant Z88.4
  - hypospadias (corrected) Z87.710
  - hysterectomy Z90.710
  - immunosupression therapy Z92.25
  - in situ neoplasm
    - breast Z86.000
    - cervix uteri Z86.001
    - specified NEC Z86.008
  - in utero procedure during pregnancy Z98.870
  - in utero procedure while a fetus Z98.871
  - infection NEC Z86.19
    - central nervous system Z86.61
    - Methicillin resistant Staphylococcus aureus (MRSA) Z86.14
    - urinary (recurrent) (tract) Z87.440
  - injury NEC Z87.828
  - irradiation Z92.3
  - kidney stones Z87.442
  - leukemia Z85.6
  - lymphoma (non-Hodgkin) Z85.72
  - malignant melanoma (skin) Z85.820
  - malignant neoplasm (of) Z85.9
    - accessory sinuses Z85.22
    - anus NEC Z85.048
      - carcinoid Z85.040
    - bladder Z85.51

☑ **Additional Character Required** — Refer to the Tabular List for Character Selection

⬇ **Subterms under main terms may continue to next column or page**

History — *continued*
  personal (*see also* History, family) — *continued*
    malignant neoplasm — *continued*
      bone Z85.830
      brain Z85.841
      breast Z85.3
      bronchus NEC Z85.118
        carcinoid Z85.110
      carcinoid — *see* History, personal (of), malignant neoplasm, by site, carcinioid
      cervix Z85.41
      colon NEC Z85.038
        carcinoid Z85.030
      digestive organ Z85.00
        specified NEC Z85.09
      endocrine gland NEC Z85.858
      epididymis Z85.48
      esophagus Z85.01
      eye Z85.840
      gastrointestinal tract — *see* History, malignant neoplasm, digestive organ
      genital organ
        female Z85.40
          specified NEC Z85.44
        male Z85.45
          specified NEC Z85.49
      hematopoietic NEC Z85.79
      intrathoracic organ Z85.20
      kidney NEC Z85.528
        carcinoid Z85.520
      large intestine NEC Z85.038
        carcinoid Z85.030
      larynx Z85.21
      liver Z85.05
      lung NEC Z85.118
        carcinoid Z85.110
      mediastinum Z85.29
      Merkel cell Z85.821
      middle ear Z85.22
      nasal cavities Z85.22
      nervous system NEC Z85.848
      oral cavity Z85.819
        specified site NEC Z85.818
      ovary Z85.43
      pancreas Z85.07
      pelvis Z85.53
      pharynx Z85.819
        specified site NEC Z85.818
      pleura Z85.29
      prostate Z85.46
      rectosigmoid junction NEC Z85.048
        carcinoid Z85.040
      rectum NEC Z85.048
        carcinoid Z85.040
      respiratory organ Z85.20
      sinuses, accessory Z85.22
      skin NEC Z85.828
        melanoma Z85.820
        Merkel cell Z85.821
      small intestine NEC Z85.068
        carcinoid Z85.060
      soft tissue Z85.831
      specified site NEC Z85.89
      stomach NEC Z85.028
        carcinoid Z85.020
      testis Z85.47
      thymus NEC Z85.238
        carcinoid Z85.230
      thyroid Z85.850
      tongue Z85.810
      trachea Z85.12
      urinary organ or tract Z85.50
        specified NEC Z85.59
      uterus Z85.42
    maltreatment Z91.89
    medical treatment NEC Z92.89
    melanoma (malignant) (skin) Z85.820
    meningitis Z86.61
    mental disorder Z86.59
    Merkel cell carcinoma (skin) Z85.821
    Methicillin resistant Staphylococcus aureus (MRSA) Z86.14
    military deployment Z91.82
    military war, peacekeeping and humanitarian deployment (current or past conflict) Z91.82
    myocardial infarction (old) I25.2
    neglect (in)
      adult Z91.412

History — *continued*
  personal (*see also* History, family) — *continued*
    neglect — *continued*
      childhood Z62.812
    neoplasm
      benign Z86.018
        brain Z86.011
        colon polyp Z86.010
      in situ
        breast Z86.000
        cervix uteri Z86.001
        specified NEC Z86.008
      malignant — *see* History of, malignant neoplasm
      uncertain behavior Z86.03
    nephrotic syndrome Z87.441
    nicotine dependence Z87.891
    noncompliance with medical treatment or regimen — *see* Noncompliance
    nutritional deficiency Z86.39
    obstetric complications Z87.59
      childbirth Z87.59
      pregnancy Z87.59
      pre-term labor Z87.51
      puerperium Z87.59
    osteoporosis fractures Z87.31 ☑
    parasuicide (attempt) Z91.5
    physical trauma NEC Z87.828
      self-harm or suicide attempt Z91.5
    pneumonia (recurrent) Z87.01
    poisoning NEC Z91.89
      self-harm or suicide attempt Z91.5
    poor personal hygiene Z91.89
    preterm labor Z87.51
    procedure during pregnancy Z98.870
    procedure while a fetus Z98.871
    prolonged reversible ischemic neurologic deficit (PRIND) Z86.73
    prostatic dysplasia Z87.430
    psychological
      abuse
        adult Z91.411
        child Z62.811
      trauma, specified NEC Z91.49
    radiation therapy Z92.3
    removal
      implant
        breast Z98.86
    renal calculi Z87.442
    respiratory condition NEC Z87.09
    retained foreign body fully removed Z87.821
    risk factors NEC Z91.89
    self-harm Z91.5
    self-poisoning attempt Z91.5
    sex reassignment Z87.890
    sleep-wake cycle problem Z72.821
    specified NEC Z87.898
    steroid therapy (systemic) Z92.241
      inhaled Z92.240
    stroke without residual deficits Z86.73
    substance abuse NEC F10-F19 with fifth character 1
    sudden cardiac arrest Z86.74
    sudden cardiac death successfully resuscitated Z86.74
    suicide attempt Z91.5
    surgery NEC Z98.89
      sex reassignment Z87.890
      transplant — *see* Transplant
    thrombophlebitis Z86.72
    thrombosis (venous) Z86.718
      pulmonary Z86.711
    tobacco dependence Z87.891
    transient ischemic attack (TIA) without residual deficits Z86.73
    trauma (physical) NEC Z87.828
      psychological NEC Z91.49
      self-harm Z91.5
    traumatic brain injury Z87.820
    unhealthy sleep-wake cycle Z72.821
    urinary calculi Z87.442
    urinary (recurrent) (tract) infection(s) Z87.440
    vaginal dysplasia Z87.411
    venous thrombosis or embolism Z86.718
      pulmonary Z86.711
    vulvar dysplasia Z87.412
His-Werner disease A79.0
HIV (*see also* Human, immunodeficiency virus) B20

HIV — *continued*
  laboratory evidence (nonconclusive) R75
  nonconclusive test (in infants) R75
  positive, seropositive Z21
Hives (bold) — *see* Urticaria
Hoarseness R49.0
Hobo Z59.0
Hodgkin disease — *see* Lymphoma, Hodgkin
Hodgson's disease I71.2
  ruptured I71.1
Hoffa-Kastert disease E88.89
Hoffa's disease E88.89
Hoffmann-Bouveret syndrome I47.9
Hoffmann's syndrome E03.9 [G73.7]
Hole (round)
  macula H35.34- ☑
  retina (without detachment) — *see* Break, retina, round hole
    with detachment — *see* Detachment, retina, with retinal, break
Holiday relief care Z75.5
Hollenhorst's plaque — *see* Occlusion, artery, retina
Hollow foot (congenital) Q66.7
  acquired — *see* Deformity, limb, foot, specified NEC
Holoprosencephaly Q04.2
Holt-Oram syndrome Q87.2
Homelessness Z59.0
Homesickness — *see* Disorder, adjustment
Homocystinemia, homocystinuria E72.11
Homogentisate 1,2-dioxygenase deficiency E70.29
Homologous serum hepatitis (prophylactic) (therapeutic) — *see* Hepatitis, viral, type B
Honeycomb lung J98.4
  congenital Q33.0
Hooded
  clitoris Q52.6
  penis Q55.69
Hookworm (anemia) (disease) (infection) (infestation) B76.9
  specified NEC B76.8
Hordeolum (eyelid) (externum) (recurrent) H00.019
  internum H00.029
    left H00.026
      lower H00.025
      upper H00.024
    right H00.023
      lower H00.022
      upper H00.021
  left H00.016
    lower H00.015
    upper H00.014
  right H00.013
    lower H00.012
    upper H00.011
Horn
  cutaneous L85.8
  nail L60.2
    congenital Q84.6
Horner (-Claude Bernard) **syndrome** G90.2
  traumatic — *see* Injury, nerve, cervical sympathetic
Horseshoe kidney (congenital) Q63.1
Horton's headache or neuralgia G44.099
  intractable G44.091
  not intractable G44.099
Hospital hopper syndrome — *see* Disorder, factitious
Hospitalism in children — *see* Disorder, adjustment
Hostility R45.5
  towards child Z62.3
Hot flashes
  menopausal N95.1
Hourglass (contracture) (*see also* Contraction, hourglass)
  stomach K31.89
    congenital Q40.2
    stricture K31.2
Household, housing circumstance affecting care Z59.9
  specified NEC Z59.8
Housemaid's knee — *see* Bursitis, prepatellar
Hudson (-Stähli) **line** (cornea) — *see* Pigmentation, cornea, anterior
Human
  bite (open wound) (*see also* Bite)
    intact skin surface — *see* Bite, superficial
  herpesvirus — *see* Herpes
  immunodeficiency virus (HIV) disease (infection) B20
    asymptomatic status Z21
    contact Z20.6

Human — *continued*
immunodeficiency virus disease — *continued*
counseling Z71.7
dementia B20 [F02.80]
with behavioral disturbance B20 [F02.81]
exposure to Z20.6
laboratory evidence R75
type-2 (HIV 2) as cause of disease classified elsewhere B97.35
papillomavirus (HPV)
DNA test positive
high risk
cervix R87.810
vagina R87.811
low risk
cervix R87.820
vagina R87.821
screening for Z11.51
T-cell lymphotropic virus
type-1 (HTLV-I) infection B33.3
as cause of disease classified elsewhere B97.33
carrier Z22.6
type-2 (HTLV-II) as cause of disease classified elsewhere B97.34
Humidifier lung or pneumonitis J67.7
Humiliation (experience) **in childhood** Z62.898
Humpback (acquired) — *see* Kyphosis
Hunchback (acquired) — *see* Kyphosis
Hunger T73.0 ☑
air, psychogenic F45.8
Hungry bone syndrome E83.81
Hunner's ulcer — *see* Cystitis, chronic, interstitial
Hunter's
glossitis D51.0
syndrome E76.1
Huntington's disease or chorea G10
with dementia G10 [F02.80]
with behavioral disturbance G10 [F02.81]
Hunt's
disease or syndrome (herpetic geniculate ganglionitis)
B02.21
dyssynergia cerebellaris myoclonica G11.1
neuralgia B02.21
Hurler (-Scheie) **disease or syndrome** E76.02
Hurst's disease G36.1
Hurthle cell
adenocarcinoma C73
adenoma D34
carcinoma C73
tumor D34
Hutchinson-Boeck disease or syndrome — *see* Sarcoidosis
Hutchinson-Gilford disease or syndrome E34.8
Hutchinson's
disease, meaning
angioma serpiginosum L81.7
pompholyx (cheiropompholyx) L30.1
prurigo estivalis L56.4
summer eruption or summer prurigo L56.4
melanotic freckle — *see* Melanoma, in situ
malignant melanoma in — *see* Melanoma
teeth or incisors (congenital syphilis) A50.52
triad (congenital syphilis) A50.53
Hyalin plaque, sclera, senile H15.89
Hyaline membrane (disease) (lung) (pulmonary) (newborn) P22.0
Hyalinosis
cutis (et mucosae) E78.89
focal and segmental (glomerular) (*see also* N00-N07
with fourth character .1) N05.1
Hyalitis, hyalosis, asteroid (*see also* Deposit, crystalline)
syphilitic (late) A52.71
Hydatid
cyst or tumor — *see* Echinococcus
mole — *see* Hydatidiform mole
Morgagni
female Q50.5
male (epididymal) Q55.4
testicular Q55.29
Hydatidiform mole (benign) (complicating pregnancy)
(delivered) (undelivered) O01.9
classical O01.0
complete O01.0
incomplete O01.1
invasive D39.2
malignant D39.2
partial O01.1
Hydatidosis — *see* Echinococcus

Hydradenitis (axillaris) (suppurative) L73.2
Hydradenoma — *see* Hidradenoma
Hydramnios O40.- ☑
Hydrancephaly, hydranencephaly Q04.3
with spina bifida — *see* Spina bifida, with hydrocephalus
Hydrargyrism NEC — *see* Poisoning, mercury
Hydrarthrosis (*see also* Effusion, joint)
gonococcal A54.42
intermittent M12.40
ankle M12.47- ☑
elbow M12.42- ☑
foot joint M12.47- ☑
hand joint M12.44- ☑
hip M12.45- ☑
knee M12.46- ☑
multiple site M12.49
shoulder M12.41- ☑
specified joint NEC M12.48
wrist M12.43- ☑
of yaws (early) (late) (*see also* subcategory M14.8-)
A66.6
syphilitic (late) A52.77
congenital A50.55 [M12.80]
Hydremia D64.89
Hydrencephalocele (congenital) — *see* Encephalocele
Hydrencephalomeningocele (congenital) — *see* Encephalocele
Hydroa R23.8
aestivale L56.4
vacciniforme L56.4
Hydroadenitis (axillaris) (suppurative) L73.2
Hydrocalycosis — *see* Hydronephrosis
Hydrocele (spermatic cord) (testis) (tunica vaginalis)
N43.3
canal of Nuck N94.89
communicating N43.2
congenital P83.5
congenital P83.5
encysted N43.0
female NEC N94.89
infected N43.1
newborn P83.5
round ligament N94.89
specified NEC N43.2
spinalis — *see* Spina bifida
vulva N90.89
Hydrocephalus (acquired) (external) (internal) (malignant) (recurrent) G91.9
aqueduct Sylvius stricture Q03.0
causing disproportion O33.6 ☑
with obstructed labor O66.3
communicating G91.0
congenital (external) (internal) Q03.9
with spina bifida Q05.4
cervical Q05.0
dorsal Q05.1
lumbar Q05.2
lumbosacral Q05.2
sacral Q05.3
thoracic Q05.1
thoracolumbar Q05.1
specified NEC Q03.8
due to toxoplasmosis (congenital) P37.1
foramen Magendie block (acquired) G91.1
congenital (*see also* Hydrocephalus, congenital)
Q03.1
in (due to)
infectious disease NEC B89 [G91.4]
neoplastic disease NEC (*see also* Neoplasm) G91.4
parasitic disease B89 [G91.4]
newborn Q03.9
with spina bifida — *see* Spina bifida, with hydrocephalus
noncommunicating G91.1
normal pressure G91.2
secondary G91.0
obstructive G91.1
otitic G93.2
post-traumatic NEC G91.3
secondary G91.4
post-traumatic G91.3
specified NEC G91.8
syphilitic, congenital A50.49
Hydrocolpos (congenital) N89.8
Hydrocystoma — *see* Neoplasm, skin, benign
Hydroencephalocele (congenital) — *see* Encephalocele

Hydroencephalomeningocele (congenital) — *see* En-
cephalocele
Hydrohematopneumothorax — *see* Hemothorax
Hydromeningitis — *see* Meningitis
Hydromeningocele (spinal) (*see also* Spina bifida)
cranial — *see* Encephalocele
Hydrometra N85.8
Hydrometrocolpos N89.8
Hydromicrocephaly Q02
Hydromphalos (since birth) Q45.8
Hydromyelia Q06.4
Hydromyelocele — *see* Spina bifida
Hydronephrosis (atrophic) (early) (functionless) (intermittent) (primary) (secondary) NEC N13.30
with
infection N13.6
obstruction (by) (of)
renal calculus N13.2
with infection N13.6
ureteral NEC N13.1
with infection N13.6
calculus N13.2
with infection N13.6
ureteropelvic junction (congenital) Q62.0
with infection N13.6
ureteral stricture NEC N13.1
with infection N13.6
congenital Q62.0
specified type NEC N13.39
tuberculous A18.11
Hydropericarditis — *see* Pericarditis
Hydropericardium — *see* Pericarditis
Hydroperitoneum R18.8
Hydrophobia — *see* Rabies
Hydrophthalmos Q15.0
Hydropneumohemothorax — *see* Hemothorax
Hydropneumopericarditis — *see* Pericarditis
Hydropneumopericardium — *see* Pericarditis
Hydropneumothorax J94.8
traumatic — *see* Injury, intrathoracic, lung
tuberculous NEC A15.6
Hydrops R60.9
abdominis R18.8
articulorum intermittens — *see* Hydrarthrosis, intermittent
cardiac — *see* Failure, heart, congestive
causing obstructed labor (mother) O66.3
endolymphatic H81.0- ☑
fetal — *see* Pregnancy, complicated by, hydrops, fetalis
fetalis P83.2
due to
ABO isoimmunization P56.0
alpha thalassemia D56.0
hemolytic disease P56.90
specified NEC P56.99
isoimmunization (ABO) (Rh) P56.0
other specified nonhemolytic disease NEC P83.2
Rh incompatibility P56.0
during pregnancy — *see* Pregnancy, complicated
by, hydrops, fetalis
gallbladder K82.1
joint — *see* Effusion, joint
labyrinth H81.0- ☑
newborn (idiopathic) P83.2
due to
ABO isoimmunization P56.0
alpha thalassemia D56.0
hemolytic disease P56.90
specified NEC P56.99
isoimmunization (ABO) (Rh) P56.0
Rh incompatibility P56.0
nutritional — *see* Malnutrition, severe
pericardium — *see* Pericarditis
pleura — *see* Hydrothorax
spermatic cord — *see* Hydrocele
Hydropyonephrosis N13.6
Hydrorachis Q06.4
Hydrorrhea (nasal) J34.89
pregnancy — *see* Rupture, membranes, premature
Hydrosadenitis (axillaris) (suppurative) L73.2
Hydrosalpinx (fallopian tube) (follicularis) N70.11
Hydrothorax (double) (pleura) J94.8
chylous (nonfilarial) I89.8
filarial (*see also* Infestation, filarial) B74.9 [J91.8]
traumatic — *see* Injury, intrathoracic
tuberculous NEC (non primary) A15.6
Hydroureter (*see also* Hydronephrosis) N13.4

Hydroureter — *continued*
　with infection N13.6
　congenital Q62.39
Hydroureteronephrosis — *see* Hydronephrosis
Hydrourethra N36.8
Hydroxykynureninuria E70.8
Hydroxylysinemia E72.3
Hydroxyprolinemia E72.59
Hygiene, sleep
　abuse Z72.821
　inadequate Z72.821
　poor Z72.821
Hygroma (congenital) (cystic) D18.1
　praepatellare, prepatellar — *see* Bursitis, prepatellar
Hymen — *see* condition
Hymenolepis, hymenolepiasis (diminuta) (infection)
　　(infestation) (nana) B71.0
Hypalgesia R20.8
Hyperacidity (gastric) K31.89
　psychogenic F45.8
Hyperactive, hyperactivity F90.9
　basal cell, uterine cervix — *see* Dysplasia, cervix
　bowel sounds R19.12
　cervix epithelial (basal) — *see* Dysplasia, cervix
　child F90.9
　　attention deficit — *see* Disorder, attention-deficit
　　　hyperactivity
　detrusor muscle N32.81
　gastrointestinal K31.89
　　psychogenic F45.8
　nasal mucous membrane J34.3
　stomach K31.89
　thyroid (gland) — *see* Hyperthyroidism
Hyperacusis H93.23- ☑
Hyperadrenalism E27.5
Hyperadrenocorticism E24.9
　congenital E25.0
　iatrogenic E24.2
　　correct substance properly administered — *see*
　　　Table of Drugs and Chemicals, by drug, ad-
　　　verse effect
　　overdose or wrong substance given or taken —
　　　see Table of Drugs and Chemicals, by drug,
　　　poisoning
　not associated with Cushing's syndrome E27.0
　pituitary-dependent E24.0
Hyperaldosteronism E26.9
　familial (type I) E26.02
　glucocorticoid-remediable E26.02
　primary (due to (bilateral) adrenal hyperplasia) E26.09
　primary NEC E26.09
　secondary E26.1
　specified NEC E26.89
Hyperalgesia R20.8
Hyperalimentation R63.2
　carotene, carotin E67.1
　specified NEC E67.8
　vitamin
　　A E67.0
　　D E67.3
Hyperaminoaciduria
　arginine E72.21
　cystine E72.01
　lysine E72.3
　ornithine E72.4
Hyperammonemia (congenital) E72.20
Hyperazotemia — *see* Uremia
Hyperbetalipoproteinemia (familial) E78.0
　with prebetalipoproteinemia E78.2
Hyperbilirubinemia
　constitutional E80.6
　familial conjugated E80.6
　neonatal (transient) — *see* Jaundice, newborn
Hypercalcemia, hypocalciuric, familial E83.52
Hypercalciuria, idiopathic E83.52
Hypercapnia R06.89
　newborn P84
Hypercarotenemia, hypercarotinemia (dietary) E67.1
Hypercementosis K03.4
Hyperchloremia E87.8
Hyperchlorhydria K31.89
　neurotic F45.8
　psychogenic F45.8
Hypercholesterinemia — *see* Hypercholesterolemia
Hypercholesterolemia (essential) (familial) (hereditary)
　　(primary) (pure) E78.0
　with hyperglyceridemia, endogenous E78.2

Hypercholesterolemia — *continued*
　dietary counseling and surveillance Z71.3
Hyperchylia gastrica, psychogenic F45.8
Hyperchylomicronemia (familial) (primary) E78.3
　with hyperbetalipoproteinemia E78.3
Hypercoagulable (state) D68.59
　activated protein C resistance D68.51
　antithrombin (III) deficiency D68.59
　factor V Leiden mutation D68.51
　primary NEC D68.59
　protein C deficiency D68.59
　protein S deficiency D68.59
　prothrombin gene mutation D68.52
　secondary D68.69
　specified NEC D68.69
Hypercoagulation (state) D68.59
Hypercorticalism, pituitary-dependent E24.0
Hypercorticosolism — *see* Cushing's, syndrome
Hypercorticosteronism E24.2
　correct substance properly administered — *see* Table
　　of Drugs and Chemicals, by drug, adverse effect
　overdose or wrong substance given or taken — *see*
　　Table of Drugs and Chemicals, by drug, poison-
　　ing
Hypercortisonism E24.2
　correct substance properly administered — *see* Table
　　of Drugs and Chemicals, by drug, adverse effect
　overdose or wrong substance given or taken — *see*
　　Table of Drugs and Chemicals, by drug, poison-
　　ing
Hyperekplexia Q89.8
Hyperelectrolytemia E87.8
Hyperemesis R11.10
　with nausea R11.2
　gravidarum (mild) O21.0
　　with
　　　carbohydrate depletion O21.1
　　　dehydration O21.1
　　　electrolyte imbalance O21.1
　　　metabolic disturbance O21.1
　　severe (with metabolic disturbance) O21.1
　projectile R11.12
　psychogenic F45.8
Hyperemia (acute) (passive) R68.89
　anal mucosa K62.89
　bladder N32.89
　cerebral I67.89
　conjunctiva H11.43- ☑
　ear internal, acute — *see* subcategory H83.0 ☑
　enteric K59.8
　eye — *see* Hyperemia, conjunctiva
　eyelid (active) (passive) — *see* Disorder, eyelid, speci-
　　fied type NEC
　intestine K59.8
　iris — *see* Disorder, iris, vascular
　kidney N28.89
　labyrinth — *see* subcategory H83.0 ☑
　liver (active) K76.89
　lung (passive) — *see* Edema, lung
　pulmonary (passive) — *see* Edema, lung
　renal N28.89
　retina H35.89
　stomach K31.89
Hyperesthesia (body surface) R20.3
　larynx (reflex) J38.7
　　hysterical F44.89
　pharynx (reflex) J39.2
　　hysterical F44.89
Hyperestrogenism (drug-induced) (iatrogenic) E28.0
Hyperexplexia Q89.8
Hyperfibrinolysis — *see* Fibrinolysis
Hyperfructosemia E74.19
Hyperfunction
　adrenal cortex, not associated with Cushing's syn-
　　drome E27.0
　　medulla E27.5
　　　adrenomedullary E27.5
　　virilism E25.9
　　　congenital E25.0
　ovarian E28.8
　pancreas K86.8
　parathyroid (gland) E21.3
　pituitary (gland) (anterior) E22.9
　　specified NEC E22.8
　polyglandular E31.1
　testicular E29.0

Hypergammaglobulinemia D89.2
　polyclonal D89.0
　Waldenström D89.0
Hypergastrinemia E16.4
Hyperglobulinemia R77.1
Hyperglycemia, hyperglycemic (transient) R73.9
　coma — *see* Diabetes, by type, with coma
　postpancreatectomy E89.1
Hyperglyceridemia (endogenous) (essential) (familial)
　　(hereditary) (pure) E78.1
　mixed E78.3
Hyperglycinemia (non-ketotic) E72.51
Hypergonadism
　ovarian E28.8
　testicular (primary) (infantile) E29.0
Hyperheparinemia D68.32
Hyperhidrosis, hyperidrosis R61
　focal
　　primary L74.519
　　　axilla L74.510
　　　face L74.511
　　　palms L74.512
　　　soles L74.513
　　secondary L74.52
　generalized R61
　localized
　　primary L74.519
　　　axilla L74.510
　　　face L74.511
　　　palms L74.512
　　　soles L74.513
　　secondary L74.52
　psychogenic F45.8
　secondary R61
　　focal L74.52
Hyperhistidinemia E70.41
Hyperhomocysteinemia E72.11
Hyperhydroxyprolinemia E72.59
Hyperinsulinism (functional) E16.1
　with
　　coma (hypoglycemic) E15
　　encephalopathy E16.1 [G94]
　ectopic E16.1
　therapeutic misadventure (from administration of in-
　　sulin) — *see* subcategory T38.3 ☑
Hyperkalemia E87.5
Hyperkeratosis (see also Keratosis) L85.9
　cervix N88.0
　due to yaws (early) (late) (palmar or plantar) A66.3
　follicularis Q82.8
　　penetrans (in cutem) L87.0
　palmoplantaris climacterica L85.1
　pinta A67.1
　senile (with pruritus) L57.0
　universalis congenita Q80.8
　vocal cord J38.3
　vulva N90.4
Hyperkinesia, hyperkinetic (disease) (reaction) (syn-
　　drome) (childhood) (adolescence) (see also Disorder,
　　attention-deficit hyperactivity)
　heart I51.89
Hyperleucine-isoleucinemia E71.19
Hyperlipemia, hyperlipidemia E78.5
　combined E78.2
　　familial E78.4
　group
　　A E78.0
　　B E78.1
　　C E78.2
　　D E78.3
　mixed E78.2
　specified NEC E78.4
Hyperlipidosis E75.6
　hereditary NEC E75.5
Hyperlipoproteinemia E78.5
　Fredrickson's type
　　I E78.3
　　IIa E78.0
　　IIb E78.2
　　III E78.2
　　IV E78.1
　　V E78.3
　low-density-lipoprotein-type (LDL) E78.0
　very-low-density-lipoprotein-type (VLDL) E78.1
Hyperlucent lung, unilateral J43.0
Hyperlysinemia E72.3
Hypermagnesemia E83.41
　neonatal P71.8

Hypermenorrhea N92.0
Hypermethioninemia E72.19
Hypermetropia (congenital) H52.0- ☑
Hypermobility, hypermotility
  cecum — see Syndrome, irritable bowel
  coccyx — see subcategory M53.2 ☑
  colon — see Syndrome, irritable bowel
    psychogenic F45.8
  ileum K58.9
  intestine (see also Syndrome, irritable bowel) K58.9
    psychogenic F45.8
  meniscus (knee) — see Derangement, knee, meniscus
  scapula — see Instability, joint, shoulder
  stomach K31.89
    psychogenic F45.8
  syndrome M35.7
  urethra N36.41
    with intrinsic sphincter deficiency N36.43
Hypernasality R49.21
Hypernatremia E87.0
Hypernephroma C64.- ☑
Hyperopia — see Hypermetropia
Hyperorexia nervosa F50.2
Hyperornithinemia E72.4
Hyperosmia R43.1
Hyperosmolality E87.0
Hyperostosis (monomelic) (see also Disorder, bone, density and structure, specified NEC)
  ankylosing (spine) M48.10
    cervical region M48.12
    cervicothoracic region M48.13
    lumbar region M48.16
    lumbosacral region M48.17
    multiple sites M48.19
    occipito-atlanto-axial region M48.11
    sacrococcygeal region M48.18
    thoracic region M48.14
    thoracolumbar region M48.15
  cortical (skull) M85.2 ☑
    infantile M89.8X- ☑
  frontal, internal of skull M85.2
  interna frontalis M85.2
  skeletal, diffuse idiopathic — see Hyperostosis, ankylosing
  skull M85.2
    congenital Q75.8
  vertebral, ankylosing — see Hyperostosis, ankylosing
Hyperovarism E28.8
Hyperoxaluria (primary) E72.53
Hyperparathyroidism E21.3
  primary E21.0
  secondary (renal) N25.81
    non-renal E21.1
  specified NEC E21.2
  tertiary E21.2
Hyperpathia R20.8
Hyperperistalsis R19.2
  psychogenic F45.8
Hyperpermeability, capillary I78.8
Hyperphagia R63.2
Hyperphenylalaninemia NEC E70.1
Hyperphoria (alternating) H50.53
Hyperphosphatemia E83.39
Hyperpiesis, hyperpiesia — see Hypertension
Hyperpigmentation (see also Pigmentation)
  melanin NEC L81.4
  postinflammatory L81.0
Hyperpinealism E34.8
Hyperpituitarism E22.9
Hyperplasia, hyperplastic
  adenoids J35.2
  adrenal (capsule) (cortex) (gland) E27.8
    with
      sexual precocity (male) E25.9
        congenital E25.0
      virilism, adrenal E25.9
        congenital E25.0
      virilization (female) E25.9
        congenital E25.0
    congenital E25.0
      salt-losing E25.0
  adrenomedullary E27.5
  angiolymphoid, eosinophilia (ALHE) D18.01
  appendix (lymphoid) K38.0
  artery, fibromuscular I77.3
  bone (see also Hypertrophy, bone)
    marrow D75.89

Hyperplasia, hyperplastic — continued
  breast (see also Hypertrophy, breast)
    ductal (atypical) N60.9- ☑
  C-cell, thyroid E07.0
  cementation (tooth) (teeth) K03.4
  cervical gland R59.0
  cervix (uteri) (basal cell) (endometrium) (polypoid) (see also Dysplasia, cervix)
    congenital Q51.828
  clitoris, congenital Q52.6
  denture K06.2
  endocervicitis N72
  endometrium, endometrial (adenomatous) (benign) (cystic) (glandular) (glandular-cystic) (polypoid) N85.00
    with atypia N85.02
    cervix — see Dysplasia, cervix
    complex (without atypia) N85.01
    simple (without atypia) N85.01
  epithelial L85.9
    focal, oral, including tongue K13.29
    nipple N62
    skin L85.9
    tongue K13.29
    vaginal wall N89.3
  erythroid D75.89
  fibromuscular of artery (carotid) (renal) I77.3
  genital
    female NEC N94.89
    male N50.8
  gingiva K06.1
  glandularis cystica uteri (interstitialis) (see also Hyperplasia, endometrial) N85.00
  gum K06.1
  hymen, congenital Q52.4
  irritative, edentulous (alveolar) K06.2
  jaw M26.09
    alveolar M26.79
    lower M26.03
      alveolar M26.72
    upper M26.01
      alveolar M26.71
  kidney (congenital) Q63.3
  labia N90.6
    epithelial N90.3
  liver (congenital) Q44.7
    nodular, focal K76.89
  lymph gland or node R59.9
  mandible, mandibular M26.03
    alveolar M26.72
    unilateral condylar M27.8
  maxilla, maxillary M26.01
    alveolar M26.71
  myometrium, myometrial N85.2
  neuroendocrine cell, of infancy J84.841
  nose
    lymphoid J34.89
    polypoid J33.9
  oral mucosa (irritative) K13.6
  organ or site, congenital NEC — see Anomaly, by site
  ovary N83.8
  palate, papillary (irritative) K13.6
  pancreatic islet cells E16.9
    alpha E16.8
      with excess
        gastrin E16.4
        glucagon E16.3
    beta E16.1
  parathyroid (gland) E21.0
  pharynx (lymphoid) J39.2
  prostate (adenofibromatous) (nodular) N40.0
    with lower urinary tract symptoms (LUTS) N40.1
    without lower urinary tract symtpoms (LUTS) N40.0
  renal artery I77.89
  reticulo-endothelial (cell) D75.89
  salivary gland (any) K11.1
  Schimmelbusch's — see Mastopathy, cystic
  suprarenal capsule (gland) E27.8
  thymus (gland) (persistent) E32.0
  thyroid (gland) — see Goiter
  tonsils (faucial) (infective) (lingual) (lymphoid) J35.1
    with adenoids J35.3
  unilateral condylar M27.8
  uterus, uterine N85.2
    endometrium (glandular) (see also Hyperplasia, endometrial) N85.00
  vulva N90.6
    epithelial N90.3

Hyperpnea — see Hyperventilation
Hyperpotassemia E87.5
Hyperprebetalipoproteinemia (familial) E78.1
Hyperprolactinemia E22.1
Hyperprolinemia (type I) (type II) E72.59
Hyperproteinemia E88.09
Hyperprothrombinemia, causing coagulation factor deficiency D68.4
Hyperpyrexia R50.9
  heat (effects) T67.0 ☑
  malignant, due to anesthetic T88.3 ☑
  rheumatic — see Fever, rheumatic
  unknown origin R50.9
Hyper-reflexia R29.2
Hypersalivation K11.7
Hypersecretion
  ACTH (not associated with Cushing's syndrome) E27.0
    pituitary E24.0
  adrenaline E27.5
  adrenomedullary E27.5
  androgen (testicular) E29.0
    ovarian (drug-induced) (iatrogenic) E28.1
  calcitonin E07.0
  catecholamine E27.5
  corticoadrenal E24.9
  cortisol E24.9
  epinephrine E27.5
  estrogen E28.0
  gastric K31.89
    psychogenic F45.8
  gastrin E16.4
  glucagon E16.3
  hormone(s)
    ACTH (not associated with Cushing's syndrome) E27.0
      pituitary E24.0
    antidiuretic E22.2
    growth E22.0
    intestinal NEC E34.1
    ovarian androgen E28.1
    pituitary E22.9
    testicular E29.0
    thyroid stimulating E05.80
      with thyroid storm E05.81
  insulin — see Hyperinsulinism
  lacrimal glands — see Epiphora
  medulloadrenal E27.5
  milk O92.6
  ovarian androgens E28.1
  salivary gland (any) K11.7
  thyrocalcitonin E07.0
  upper respiratory J38.8
Hypersegmentation, leukocytic, hereditary D72.0
Hypersensitive, hypersensitiveness, hypersensitivity (see also Allergy)
  carotid sinus G90.01
  colon — see Irritable, colon
  drug T88.7 ☑
  gastrointestinal K52.2
    psychogenic F45.8
  labyrinth — see subcategory H83.2 ☑
  pain R20.8
  pneumonitis — see Pneumonitis, allergic
  reaction T78.40 ☑
    upper respiratory tract NEC J39.3
Hypersomnia (organic) G47.10
  due to
    alcohol
      abuse F10.182
      dependence F10.282
      use F10.982
    amphetamines
      abuse F15.182
      dependence F15.282
      use F15.982
    caffeine
      abuse F15.182
      dependence F15.282
      use F15.982
    cocaine
      abuse F14.182
      dependence F14.282
      use F14.982
    drug NEC
      abuse F19.182
      dependence F19.282
      use F19.982
    medical condition G47.14

☑ **Additional Character Required** — Refer to the Tabular List for Character Selection   ▽ Subterms under main terms may continue to next column or page

Hypersomnia — *continued*
  due to — *continued*
    mental disorder F51.13
    opioid
      abuse F11.182
      dependence F11.282
      use F11.982
    psychoactive substance NEC
      abuse F19.182
      dependence F19.282
      use F19.982
    sedative, hypnotic, or anxiolytic
      abuse F13.182
      dependence F13.282
      use F13.982
    stimulant NEC
      abuse F15.182
      dependence F15.282
      use F15.982
  idiopathic G47.11
    with long sleep time G47.11
    without long sleep time G47.12
  menstrual related G47.13
  nonorganic origin F51.11
    specified NEC F51.19
  not due to a substance or known physiological condition F51.11
    specified NEC F51.19
  primary F51.11
  recurrent G47.13
  specified NEC G47.19
Hypersplenia, hypersplenism D73.1
Hyperstimulation, ovaries (associated with induced ovulation) N98.1
Hypersusceptibility — *see* Allergy
Hypertelorism (ocular) (orbital) Q75.2
Hypertension, hypertensive (accelerated) (benign) (essential) (idiopathic) (malignant) (systemic) I10
  with
    heart involvement (conditions in I51.4 - I51.9 due to hypertension) — *see* Hypertension, heart
    kidney involvement — *see* Hypertension, kidney
  benign, intracranial G93.2
  borderline R03.0
  cardiorenal (disease) I13.10
    with heart failure I13.0
      with stage 1 through stage 4 chronic kidney disease I13.0
      with stage 5 or end stage renal disease I13.2
    without heart failure I13.10
      with stage 1 through stage 4 chronic kidney disease I13.10
      with stage 5 or end stage renal disease I13.11
  cardiovascular
    disease (arteriosclerotic) (sclerotic) — *see* Hypertension, heart
    renal (disease) — *see* Hypertension, cardiorenal
  chronic venous — *see* Hypertension, venous (chronic)
  complicating
    childbirth (labor) O10.92
      with
        heart disease O10.12
          with renal disease O10.32
        renal disease O10.22
          with heart disease O10.32
      essential O10.02
      secondary O10.42
    pregnancy O16.- ☑
      with edema (*see also* Pre-eclampsia) O14.9- ☑
      gestational (pregnancy induced) (transient) (without proteinuria) O13.- ☑
        with proteinuria O14.9- ☑
          mild pre-eclampsia O14.0- ☑
          moderate pre-eclampsia O14.0- ☑
          severe pre-eclampsia O14.1- ☑
            with hemolysis, elevated liver enzymes and low platelet count (HELLP) O14.2- ☑
      pre-existing O10.91- ☑
        with
          heart disease O10.11- ☑
            with renal disease O10.31- ☑
          pre-eclampsia O11.- ☑
          renal disease O10.21- ☑
            with heart disease O10.31- ☑
        essential O10.01- ☑
        secondary O10.41- ☑
    puerperium, pre-existing O10.93

Hypertension, hypertensive — *continued*
  complicating — *continued*
    puerperium, pre-existing — *continued*
      with
        heart disease O10.13
          with renal disease O10.33
        renal disease O10.23
          with heart disease O10.33
      essential O10.03
    pregnancy-induced O13.9
    secondary O10.43
  due to
    endocrine disorders I15.2
    pheochromocytoma I15.2
    renal disorders NEC I15.1
      arterial I15.0
    renovascular disorders I15.0
    specified disease NEC I15.8
  encephalopathy I67.4
  gestational (without significant proteinuria) (pregnancy-induced) (transient) O13.- ☑
    with significant proteinuria — *see* Pre-eclampsia
  Goldblatt's I70.1
  heart (disease) (conditions in I51.4-I51.9 due to hypertension) I11.9
    with
      heart failure (congestive) I11.0
      kidney disease (chronic) — *see* Hypertension, cardiorenal
  intracranial (benign) G93.2
  kidney I12.9
    with
      heart disease — *see* Hypertension, cardiorenal
      stage 1 through stage 4 chronic kidney disease I12.9
      stage 5 chronic kidney disease (CKD) or end stage renal disease (ESRD) I12.0
  lesser circulation I27.0
  newborn P29.2
    pulmonary (persistent) P29.3
  ocular H40.05- ☑
  pancreatic duct — *code to* underlying condition
    with chronic pancreatitis K86.1
  portal (due to chronic liver disease) (idiopathic) K76.6
    gastropathy K31.89
    in (due to) schistosomiasis (bilharziasis) B65.9 [K77]
  postoperative I97.3
  psychogenic F45.8
  pulmonary (artery) (secondary) NEC I27.2
    with
      cor pulmonale (chronic) I27.2
        acute I26.09
      right heart ventricular strain/failure I27.2
        acute I26.09
    of newborn (persistent) P29.3
    primary (idiopathic) I27.0
  renal — *see* Hypertension, kidney
  renovascular I15.0
  secondary NEC I15.9
    due to
      endocrine disorders I15.2
      pheochromocytoma I15.2
      renal disorders NEC I15.1
        arterial I15.0
      renovascular disorders I15.0
    specified NEC I15.8
  venous (chronic)
    due to
      deep vein thrombosis — *see* Syndrome, post-thrombotic
    idiopathic I87.309
      with
        inflammation I87.32- ☑
          with ulcer I87.33- ☑
        specified complication NEC I87.39- ☑
        ulcer I87.31- ☑
          with inflammation I87.33- ☑
      asymptomatic I87.30- ☑
Hypertensive urgency — *see* Hypertension
Hyperthecosis ovary E28.8
Hyperthermia (of unknown origin) (*see also* Hyperpyrexia)
  malignant, due to anesthesia T88.3 ☑
  newborn P81.9
    environmental P81.0
Hyperthyroid (recurrent) — *see* Hyperthyroidism
Hyperthyroidism (latent) (pre-adult) (recurrent) E05.90

Hyperthyroidism — *continued*
  with
    goiter (diffuse) E05.00
      with thyroid storm E05.01
    nodular (multinodular) E05.20
      with thyroid storm E05.21
    uninodular E05.10
      with thyroid storm E05.11
    storm E05.91
  due to ectopic thyroid tissue E05.30
    with thyroid storm E05.31
  neonatal, transitory P72.1
  specified NEC E05.80
    with thyroid storm E05.81
Hypertony, hypertonia, hypertonicity
  bladder N31.8
  congenital P94.1
  stomach K31.89
    psychogenic F45.8
  uterus, uterine (contractions) (complicating delivery) O62.4
Hypertrichosis L68.9
  congenital Q84.2
  eyelid H02.869
    left H02.866
      lower H02.865
      upper H02.864
    right H02.863
      lower H02.862
      upper H02.861
  lanuginosa Q84.2
    acquired L68.1
  localized L68.2
  specified NEC L68.8
Hypertriglyceridemia, essential E78.1
Hypertrophy, hypertrophic
  adenofibromatous, prostate — *see* Enlargement, enlarged, prostate
  adenoids (infective) J35.2
    with tonsils J35.3
  adrenal cortex E27.8
  alveolar process or ridge — *see* Anomaly, alveolar
  anal papillae K62.89
  artery I77.89
    congenital NEC Q27.8
      digestive system Q27.8
      lower limb Q27.8
      specified site NEC Q27.8
      upper limb Q27.8
  auricular — *see* Hypertrophy, cardiac
  Bartholin's gland N75.8
  bile duct (common) (hepatic) K83.8
  bladder (sphincter) (trigone) N32.89
  bone M89.30
    carpus M89.34- ☑
    clavicle M89.31- ☑
    femur M89.35- ☑
    fibula M89.36- ☑
    finger M89.34- ☑
    humerus M89.32- ☑
    ilium M89.359
    ischium M89.359
    metacarpus M89.34- ☑
    metatarsus M89.37- ☑
    multiple sites M89.39
    neck M89.38
    radius M89.33- ☑
    rib M89.38
    scapula M89.31- ☑
    skull M89.38
    tarsus M89.37- ☑
    tibia M89.36- ☑
    toe M89.37- ☑
    ulna M89.33- ☑
    vertebra M89.38
  brain G93.89
  breast N62
    cystic — *see* Mastopathy, cystic
    newborn P83.4
    pubertal, massive N62
    puerperal, postpartum — *see* Disorder, breast, specified type NEC
    senile (parenchymatous) N62
  cardiac (chronic) (idiopathic) I51.7
    with rheumatic fever (conditions in I00)
      active I01.8
      inactive or quiescent (with chorea) I09.89
    congenital NEC Q24.8

Index

Hypertrophy, hypertrophic — Hypofunction

Hypertrophy, hypertrophic — *continued*
  cardiac — *continued*
    fatty — *see* Degeneration, myocardial
    hypertensive — *see* Hypertension, heart
    rheumatic (with chorea) I09.89
      active or acute I01.8
        with chorea I02.0
    valve — *see* Endocarditis
  cartilage — *see* Disorder, cartilage, specified type NEC
  cecum — *see* Megacolon
  cervix (uteri) N88.8
    congenital Q51.828
    elongation N88.4
  clitoris (cirrhotic) N90.89
    congenital Q52.6
  colon (*see also* Megacolon)
    congenital Q43.2
  conjunctiva, lymphoid H11.89
  corpora cavernosa N48.89
  cystic duct K82.8
  duodenum K31.89
  endometrium (glandular) (*see also* Hyperplasia, endometrial) N85.00
    cervix N88.8
  epididymis N50.8
  esophageal hiatus (congenital) Q79.1
    with hernia — *see* Hernia, hiatal
  eyelid — *see* Disorder, eyelid, specified type NEC
  fat pad E65
    knee (infrapatellar) (popliteal) (prepatellar) (retropatellar) M79.4
  foot (congenital) Q74.2
  frenulum, frenum (tongue) K14.8
    lip K13.0
  gallbladder K82.8
  gastric mucosa K29.60
    with bleeding K29.61
  gland, glandular R59.9
    generalized R59.1
    localized R59.0
  gum (mucous membrane) K06.1
  heart (idiopathic) (*see also* Hypertrophy, cardiac)
    valve (*see also* Endocarditis) I38
  hemifacial Q67.4
  hepatic — *see* Hypertrophy, liver
  hiatus (esophageal) Q79.1
  hilus gland R59.0
  hymen, congenital Q52.4
  ileum K63.89
  intestine NEC K63.89
  jejunum K63.89
  kidney (compensatory) N28.81
    congenital Q63.3
  labium (majus) (minus) N90.6
  ligament — *see* Disorder, ligament
  lingual tonsil (infective) J35.1
    with adenoids J35.3
  lip K13.0
    congenital Q18.6
  liver R16.0
    acute K76.89
    cirrhotic — *see* Cirrhosis, liver
    congenital Q44.7
    fatty — *see* Fatty, liver
  lymph, lymphatic gland R59.9
    generalized R59.1
    localized R59.0
    tuberculous — *see* Tuberculosis, lymph gland
  mammary gland — *see* Hypertrophy, breast
  Meckel's diverticulum (congenital) Q43.0
    malignant — *see* Table of Neoplasms, small intestine, malignant
  median bar — *see* Hyperplasia, prostate
  meibomian gland — *see* Chalazion
  meniscus, knee, congenital Q74.1
  metatarsal head — *see* Hypertrophy, bone, metatarsus
  metatarsus — *see* Hypertrophy, bone, metatarsus
  mucous membrane
    alveolar ridge K06.2
    gum K06.1
    nose (turbinate) J34.3
  muscle M62.89
  muscular coat, artery I77.89
  myocardium (*see also* Hypertrophy, cardiac)
    idiopathic I42.2
  myometrium N85.2
  nail L60.2
    congenital Q84.5

Hypertrophy, hypertrophic — *continued*
  nasal J34.89
    alae J34.89
    bone J34.89
    cartilage J34.89
    mucous membrane (septum) J34.3
    sinus J34.89
    turbinate J34.3
  nasopharynx, lymphoid (infectional) (tissue) (wall) J35.2
  nipple N62
  organ or site, congenital NEC — *see* Anomaly, by site
  ovary N83.8
  palate (hard) M27.8
    soft K13.79
  pancreas, congenital Q45.3
  parathyroid (gland) E21.0
  parotid gland K11.1
  penis N48.89
  pharyngeal tonsil J35.2
  pharynx J39.2
    lymphoid (infectional) (tissue) (wall) J35.2
  pituitary (anterior) (fossa) (gland) E23.6
  prepuce (congenital) N47.8
    female N90.89
  prostate — *see* Enlargement, enlarged, prostate
    congenital Q55.4
  pseudomuscular G71.0
  pylorus (adult) (muscle) (sphincter) K31.1
    congenital or infantile Q40.0
  rectal, rectum (sphincter) K62.89
  rhinitis (turbinate) J31.0
  salivary gland (any) K11.1
    congenital Q38.4
  scaphoid (tarsal) — *see* Hypertrophy, bone, tarsus
  scar L91.0
  scrotum N50.8
  seminal vesicle N50.8
  sigmoid — *see* Megacolon
  skin L91.9
    specified NEC L91.8
  spermatic cord N50.8
  spleen — *see* Splenomegaly
  spondylitis — *see* Spondylosis
  stomach K31.89
  sublingual gland K11.1
  submandibular gland K11.1
  suprarenal cortex (gland) E27.8
  synovial NEC M67.20
    acromioclavicular M67.21- ☑
    ankle M67.27- ☑
    elbow M67.22- ☑
    foot M67.27- ☑
    hand M67.24- ☑
    hip M67.25- ☑
    knee M67.26- ☑
    multiple sites M67.29
    specified site NEC M67.28
    wrist M67.23- ☑
  tendon — *see* Disorder, tendon, specified type NEC
  testis N44.8
    congenital Q55.29
  thymic, thymus (gland) (congenital) E32.0
  thyroid (gland) — *see* Goiter
  toe (congenital) Q74.2
    acquired (*see also* Deformity, toe, specified NEC)
  tongue K14.8
    congenital Q38.2
    papillae (foliate) K14.3
  tonsils (faucial) (infective) (lingual) (lymphoid) J35.1
    with adenoids J35.3
  tunica vaginalis N50.8
  ureter N28.89
  urethra N36.8
  uterus N85.2
    neck (with elongation) N88.4
    puerperal O90.89
  uvula K13.79
  vagina N89.8
  vas deferens N50.8
  vein I87.8
  ventricle, ventricular (heart) (*see also* Hypertrophy, cardiac)
    congenital Q24.8
    in tetralogy of Fallot Q21.3
  verumontanum N36.8
  vocal cord J38.3
  vulva N90.6

Hypertrophy, hypertrophic — *continued*
  vulva — *continued*
    stasis (nonfilarial) N90.6
Hypertropia H50.2- ☑
Hypertyrosinemia E70.21
Hyperuricemia (asymptomatic) E79.0
Hypervalinemia E71.19
Hyperventilation (tetany) R06.4
  hysterical F45.8
  psychogenic F45.8
  syndrome F45.8
Hypervitaminosis (dietary) NEC E67.8
  A E67.0
    administered as drug (prolonged intake) — *see* Table of Drugs and Chemicals, vitamins, adverse effect
    overdose or wrong substance given or taken — *see* Table of Drugs and Chemicals, vitamins, poisoning
  B6 E67.2
  D E67.3
    administered as drug (prolonged intake) — *see* Table of Drugs and Chemicals, vitamins, adverse effect
    overdose or wrong substance given or taken — *see* Table of Drugs and Chemicals, vitamins, poisoning
  K E67.8
    administered as drug (prolonged intake) — *see* Table of Drugs and Chemicals, vitamins, adverse effect
    overdose or wrong substance given or taken — *see* Table of Drugs and Chemicals, vitamins, poisoning
Hypervolemia E87.70
  specified NEC E87.79
Hypesthesia R20.1
  cornea — *see* Anesthesia, cornea
Hyphema H21.0- ☑
  traumatic S05.1- ☑
Hypoacidity, gastric K31.89
  psychogenic F45.8
Hypoadrenalism, hypoadrenia E27.40
  primary E27.1
  tuberculous A18.7
Hypoadrenocorticism E27.40
  pituitary E23.0
  primary E27.1
Hypoalbuminemia E88.09
Hypoaldosteronism E27.40
Hypoalphalipoproteinemia E78.6
Hypobarism T70.29 ☑
Hypobaropathy T70.29 ☑
Hypobetalipoproteinemia (familial) E78.6
Hypocalcemia E83.51
  dietary E58
  neonatal P71.1
    due to cow's milk P71.0
  phosphate-loading (newborn) P71.1
Hypochloremia E87.8
Hypochlorhydria K31.89
  neurotic F45.8
  psychogenic F45.8
Hypochondria, hypochondriac, hypochondriasis (reaction) F45.21
  sleep F51.03
Hypochondrogenesis Q77.0
Hypochondroplasia Q77.4
Hypochromasia, blood cells D50.8
Hypodontia — *see* Anodontia
Hypoeosinophilia D72.89
Hypoesthesia R20.1
Hypofibrinogenemia D68.8
  acquired D65
  congenital (hereditary) D68.2
Hypofunction
  adrenocortical E27.40
    drug-induced E27.3
    postprocedural E89.6
    primary E27.1
  adrenomedullary, postprocedural E89.6
  cerebral R29.818
  corticoadrenal NEC E27.40
  intestinal K59.8
  labyrinth — *see* subcategory H83.2 ☑
  ovary E28.39
  pituitary (gland) (anterior) E23.0

☑ **Additional Character Required** — Refer to the Tabular List for Character Selection   ▽ Subterms under main terms may continue to next column or page

Hypofunction — *continued*
testicular E29.1
postprocedural (postsurgical) (postirradiation) (iatrogenic) E89.5
Hypogalactia O92.4
Hypogammaglobulinemia (*see also* Agammaglobulinemia) D80.1
hereditary D80.0
nonfamilial D80.1
transient, of infancy D80.7
Hypogenitalism (congenital) — *see* Hypogonadism
Hypoglossia Q38.3
Hypoglycemia (spontaneous) E16.2
coma E15
diabetic — *see* Diabetes, coma
diabetic — *see* Diabetes, hypoglycemia
dietary counseling and surveillance Z71.3
drug-induced E16.0
with coma (nondiabetic) E15
due to insulin E16.0
with coma (nondiabetic) E15
therapeutic misadventure — *see* subcategory T38.3 ☑
functional, nonhyperinsulinemic E16.1
iatrogenic E16.0
with coma (nondiabetic) E15
in infant of diabetic mother P70.1
gestational diabetes P70.0
infantile E16.1
leucine-induced E71.19
neonatal (transitory) P70.4
iatrogenic P70.3
reactive (not drug-induced) E16.1
transitory neonatal P70.4
Hypogonadism
female E28.39
hypogonadotropic E23.0
male E29.1
ovarian (primary) E28.39
pituitary E23.0
testicular (primary) E29.1
Hypohidrosis, hypoidrosis L74.4
Hypoinsulinemia, postprocedural E89.1
Hypokalemia E87.6
Hypoleukocytosis — *see* Agranulocytosis
Hypolipoproteinemia (alpha) (beta) E78.6
Hypomagnesemia E83.42
neonatal P71.2
Hypomania, hypomanic reaction F30.8
Hypomenorrhea — *see* Oligomenorrhea
Hypometabolism R63.8
Hypomotility
gastrointestinal (tract) K31.89
psychogenic F45.8
intestine K59.8
psychogenic F45.8
stomach K31.89
psychogenic F45.8
Hyponasality R49.22
Hyponatremia E87.1
Hypo-osmolality E87.1
Hypo-ovarianism, hypo-ovarism E28.39
Hypoparathyroidism E20.9
familial E20.8
idiopathic E20.0
neonatal, transitory P71.4
postprocedural E89.2
specified NEC E20.8
Hypoperfusion (in)
newborn P96.89
Hypopharyngitis — *see* Laryngopharyngitis
Hypophoria H50.53
Hypophosphatemia, hypophosphatasia (acquired) (congenital) (renal) E83.39
familial E83.31
Hypophyseal, hypophysis (*see also* condition)
dwarfism E23.0
gigantism E22.0
Hypopiesis — *see* Hypotension
Hypopinealism E34.8
Hypopituitarism (juvenile) E23.0
drug-induced E23.1
due to
hypophysectomy E89.3
radiotherapy E89.3
iatrogenic NEC E23.1
postirradiation E89.3

Hypopituitarism — *continued*
postpartum E23.0
postprocedural E89.3
Hypoplasia, hypoplastic
adrenal (gland), congenital Q89.1
alimentary tract, congenital Q45.8
upper Q40.8
anus, anal (canal) Q42.3
with fistula Q42.2
aorta, aortic Q25.4
ascending, in hypoplastic left heart syndrome Q23.4
valve Q23.1
in hypoplastic left heart syndrome Q23.4
areola, congenital Q83.8
arm (congenital) — *see* Defect, reduction, upper limb
artery (peripheral) Q27.8
brain (congenital) Q28.3
coronary Q24.5
digestive system Q27.8
lower limb Q27.8
pulmonary Q25.79
functional, unilateral J43.0
retinal (congenital) Q14.1
specified site NEC Q27.8
umbilical Q27.0
upper limb Q27.8
auditory canal Q17.8
causing impairment of hearing Q16.9
biliary duct or passage Q44.5
bone NOS Q79.9
face Q75.8
marrow D61.9
megakaryocytic D69.49
skull — *see* Hypoplasia, skull
brain Q02
gyri Q04.3
part of Q04.3
breast (areola) N64.82
bronchus Q32.4
cardiac Q24.8
carpus — *see* Defect, reduction, upper limb, specified type NEC
cartilage hair Q78.5
cecum Q42.8
cementum K00.4
cephalic Q02
cerebellum Q04.3
cervix (uteri), congenital Q51.821
clavicle (congenital) Q74.0
coccyx Q76.49
colon Q42.9
specified NEC Q42.8
corpus callosum Q04.0
cricoid cartilage Q31.2
digestive organ(s) or tract NEC Q45.8
upper (congenital) Q40.8
ear (auricle) (lobe) Q17.2
middle Q16.4
enamel of teeth (neonatal) (postnatal) (prenatal) K00.4
endocrine (gland) NEC Q89.2
endometrium N85.8
epididymis (congenital) Q55.4
epiglottis Q31.2
erythroid, congenital D61.01
esophagus (congenital) Q39.8
eustachian tube Q17.8
eye Q11.2
eyelid (congenital) Q10.3
face Q18.8
bone(s) Q75.8
femur (congenital) — *see* Defect, reduction, lower limb, specified type NEC
fibula (congenital) — *see* Defect, reduction, lower limb, specified type NEC
finger (congenital) — *see* Defect, reduction, upper limb, specified type NEC
foot — *see* Defect, reduction, lower limb, specified type NEC
gallbladder Q44.1
genitalia, genital organ(s)
female, congenital Q52.8
external Q52.79
internal NEC Q52.8
in adiposogenital dystrophy E23.6
glottis Q31.2
hair Q84.2

Hypoplasia, hypoplastic — *continued*
hand (congenital) — *see* Defect, reduction, upper limb, specified type NEC
heart Q24.8
humerus (congenital) — *see* Defect, reduction, upper limb, specified type NEC
intestine (small) Q41.9
large Q42.9
specified NEC Q42.8
jaw M26.09
alveolar M26.79
lower M26.04
alveolar M26.74
upper M26.02
alveolar M26.73
kidney(s) Q60.5
bilateral Q60.4
unilateral Q60.3
labium (majus) (minus), congenital Q52.79
larynx Q31.2
left heart syndrome Q23.4
leg (congenital) — *see* Defect, reduction, lower limb
limb Q73.8
lower (congenital) — *see* Defect, reduction, lower limb
upper (congenital) — *see* Defect, reduction, upper limb
liver Q44.7
lung (lobe) (not associated with short gestation) Q33.6
associated with immaturity, low birth weight, prematurity, or short gestation P28.0
mammary (areola), congenital Q83.8
mandible, mandibular M26.04
alveolar M26.74
unilateral condylar M27.8
maxillary M26.02
alveolar M26.73
medullary D61.9
megakaryocytic D69.49
metacarpus — *see* Defect, reduction, upper limb, specified type NEC
metatarsus — *see* Defect, reduction, lower limb, specified type NEC
muscle Q79.8
nail(s) Q84.6
nose, nasal Q30.1
optic nerve H47.03- ☑
osseous meatus (ear) Q17.8
ovary, congenital Q50.39
pancreas Q45.0
parathyroid (gland) Q89.2
parotid gland Q38.4
patella Q74.1
pelvis, pelvic girdle Q74.2
penis (congenital) Q55.62
peripheral vascular system Q27.8
digestive system Q27.8
lower limb Q27.8
specified site NEC Q27.8
upper limb Q27.8
pituitary (gland) (congenital) Q89.2
pulmonary (not associated with short gestation) Q33.6
artery, functional J43.0
associated with short gestation P28.0
radioulnar — *see* Defect, reduction, upper limb, specified type NEC
radius — *see* Defect, reduction, upper limb
rectum Q42.1
with fistula Q42.0
respiratory system NEC Q34.8
rib Q76.6
right heart syndrome Q22.6
sacrum Q76.49
scapula Q74.0
scrotum Q55.1
shoulder girdle Q74.0
skin Q82.8
skull (bone) Q75.8
with
anencephaly Q00.0
encephalocele — *see* Encephalocele
hydrocephalus Q03.9
with spina bifida — *see* Spina bifida, by site, with hydrocephalus
microcephaly Q02
spinal (cord) (ventral horn cell) Q06.1
spine Q76.49
sternum Q76.7

Hypoplasia, hypoplastic — *continued*
 tarsus — *see* Defect, reduction, lower limb, specified
  type NEC
 testis Q55.1
 thymic, with immunodeficiency D82.1
 thymus (gland) Q89.2
  with immunodeficiency D82.1
 thyroid (gland) E03.1
  cartilage Q31.2
 tibiofibular (congenital) — *see* Defect, reduction,
  lower limb, specified type NEC
 toe — *see* Defect, reduction, lower limb, specified type
  NEC
 tongue Q38.3
 Turner's K00.4
 ulna (congenital) — *see* Defect, reduction, upper limb
 umbilical artery Q27.0
 unilateral condylar M27.8
 ureter Q62.8
 uterus, congenital Q51.811
 vagina Q52.4
 vascular NEC peripheral Q27.8
  brain Q28.3
  digestive system Q27.8
  lower limb Q27.8
  specified site NEC Q27.8
  upper limb Q27.8
 vein(s) (peripheral) Q27.8
  brain Q28.3
  digestive system Q27.8
  great Q26.8
  lower limb Q27.8
  specified site NEC Q27.8
  upper limb Q27.8
 vena cava (inferior) (superior) Q26.8
 vertebra Q76.49
 vulva, congenital Q52.79
 zonule (ciliary) Q12.8
Hypopotassemia E87.6
Hypoproconvertinemia, congenital (hereditary) D68.2
Hypoproteinemia E77.8
Hypoprothrombinemia (congenital) (hereditary) (idiopathic) D68.2
 acquired D68.4
 newborn, transient P61.6
Hypoptyalism K11.7
Hypopyon (eye) (anterior chamber) — *see* Iridocyclitis,
  acute, hypopyon
Hypopyrexia R68.0
Hyporeflexia R29.2
Hyposecretion
 ACTH E23.0
 antidiuretic hormone E23.2
 ovary E28.39
 salivary gland (any) K11.7
 vasopressin E23.2
Hyposegmentation, leukocytic, hereditary D72.0
Hyposiderinemia D50.9
Hypospadias Q54.9
 balanic Q54.0
 coronal Q54.0
 glandular Q54.0
 penile Q54.1
 penoscrotal Q54.2
 perineal Q54.3
 specified NEC Q54.8
Hypospermatogenesis — *see* Oligospermia
Hyposplenism D73.0
Hypostasis pulmonary, passive — *see* Edema, lung
Hypostatic — *see* condition
Hyposthenuria N28.89
Hypotension (arterial) (constitutional) I95.9
 chronic I95.89
 drug-induced I95.2
 due to (of) hemodialysis I95.3
 iatrogenic I95.89
 idiopathic (permanent) I95.0
 intracranial, following ventricular shunting (ventriculostomy) G97.2
 intra-dialytic I95.3
 maternal, syndrome (following labor and delivery)
  O26.5- ☑
 neurogenic, orthostatic G90.3
 orthostatic (chronic) I95.1
  due to drugs I95.2
  neurogenic G90.3
 postoperative I95.81
 postural I95.1

Hypotension — *continued*
 specified NEC I95.89
Hypothermia (accidental) T68 ☑
 due to anesthesia, anesthetic T88.51 ☑
 low environmental temperature T68 ☑
 neonatal P80.9
  environmental (mild) NEC P80.8
  mild P80.8
  severe (chronic) (cold injury syndrome) P80.0
  specified NEC P80.8
 not associated with low environmental temperature
  R68.0
Hypothyroidism (acquired) E03.9
 congenital (without goiter) E03.1
  with goiter (diffuse) E03.0
 due to
  exogenous substance NEC E03.2
  iodine-deficiency, acquired E01.8
   subclinical E02
  irradiation therapy E89.0
  medicament NEC E03.2
  P-aminosalicylic acid (PAS) E03.2
  phenylbutazone E03.2
  resorcinol E03.2
  sulfonamide E03.2
  surgery E89.0
  thiourea group drugs E03.2
 iatrogenic NEC E03.2
 iodine-deficiency (acquired) E01.8
  congenital — *see* Syndrome, iodine- deficiency,
   congenital
  subclinical E02
 neonatal, transitory P72.2
 postinfectious E03.3
 postirradiation E89.0
 postprocedural E89.0
 postsurgical E89.0
 specified NEC E03.8
 subclinical, iodine-deficiency related E02
Hypotonia, hypotonicity, hypotony
 bladder N31.2
 congenital (benign) P94.2
 eye — *see* Disorder, globe, hypotony
Hypotrichosis — *see* Alopecia
Hypotropia H50.2- ☑
Hypoventilation R06.89
 congenital central alveolar G47.35
 sleep related
  idiopathic nonobstructive alveolar G47.34
  in conditions classified elsewhere G47.36
Hypovitaminosis — *see* Deficiency, vitamin
Hypovolemia E86.1
 surgical shock T81.19 ☑
 traumatic (shock) T79.4 ☑
Hypoxemia R09.02
 newborn P84
 sleep related, in conditions classified elsewhere G47.36
Hypoxia (*see also* Anoxia) R09.02
 cerebral, during a procedure NEC G97.81
  postprocedural NEC G97.82
 intrauterine P84
 myocardial — *see* Insufficiency, coronary
 newborn P84
 sleep-related G47.34
Hypsarrhythmia — *see* Epilepsy, generalized, specified
  NEC
Hysteralgia, pregnant uterus O26.89- ☑
Hysteria, hysterical (conversion) (dissociative state)
  F44.9
 anxiety F41.8
 convulsions F44.5
 psychosis, acute F44.9
Hysteroepilepsy F44.5

I

Ichthyoparasitism due to Vandellia cirrhosa B88.8
Ichthyosis (congenital) Q80.9
 acquired L85.0
 fetalis Q80.4
 hystrix Q80.8
 lamellar Q80.2
 lingual K13.29
 palmaris and plantaris Q82.8
 simplex Q80.0
 vera Q80.8
 vulgaris Q80.0

Ichthyosis — *continued*
 X-linked Q80.1
Ichthyotoxism — *see* Poisoning, fish
 bacterial — *see* Intoxication, foodborne
Icteroanemia, hemolytic (acquired) D59.9
 congenital — *see* Spherocytosis
Icterus (*see also* Jaundice)
 conjunctiva R17
 gravis, newborn P55.0
 hematogenous (acquired) D59.9
 hemolytic (acquired) D59.9
  congenital — *see* Spherocytosis
 hemorrhagic (acute) (leptospiral) (spirochetal) A27.0
  newborn P53
 infectious B15.9
  with hepatic coma B15.0
  leptospiral A27.0
  spirochetal A27.0
 neonatorum — *see* Jaundice, newborn
 newborn P59.9
 spirochetal A27.0
Ictus solaris, solis T67.0 ☑
Id reaction (due to bacteria) L30.2
Ideation
 homicidal R45.850
 suicidal R45.851
Identity disorder (child) F64.9
 gender role F64.2
 psychosexual F64.2
Idioglossia F80.0
Idiopathic — *see* condition
Idiot, idiocy (congenital) F73
 amaurotic (Bielschowsky(-Jansky)) (family) (infantile
  (late)) (juvenile (late)) (Vogt-Spielmeyer) E75.4
 microcephalic Q02
IgE asthma J45.909
IIAC (idiopathic infantile arterial calcification) Q28.8
Ileitis (chronic) (noninfectious) (*see also* Enteritis) K52.9
 backwash — *see* Pancolitis, ulcerative (chronic)
 infectious A09
 regional (ulcerative) — *see* Enteritis, regional, small
  intestine
 segmental — *see* Enteritis, regional
 terminal (ulcerative) — *see* Enteritis, regional, small
  intestine
Ileocolitis (*see also* Enteritis) K52.9
 infectious A09
 regional — *see* Enteritis, regional
Ileostomy
 attention to Z43.2
 malfunctioning K94.13
 status Z93.2
  with complication — *see* Complications, enterostomy
Ileotyphus — *see* Typhoid
Ileum — *see* condition
Ileus (bowel) (colon) (inhibitory) (intestine) K56.7
 adynamic K56.0
 due to gallstone (in intestine) K56.3
 duodenal (chronic) K31.5
 gallstone K56.3
 mechanical NEC K56.69
 meconium P76.0
  in cystic fibrosis E84.11
  meaning meconium plug (without cystic fibrosis)
   P76.0
 myxedema K59.8
 neurogenic K56.0
  Hirschsprung's disease or megacolon Q43.1
 newborn
  due to meconium P76.0
   in cystic fibrosis E84.11
   meaning meconium plug (without cystic fibro-
    sis) P76.0
  transitory P76.1
 obstructive K56.69
 paralytic K56.0
Iliac — *see* condition
Iliotibial band syndrome M76.3- ☑
Illiteracy Z55.0
Illness (*see also* Disease) R69
 manic-depressive — *see* Disorder, bipolar
Imbalance R26.89
 autonomic G90.8
 constituents of food intake E63.1
 electrolyte E87.8

Imbalance — *continued*
　electrolyte — *continued*
　　with
　　　abortion — *see* Abortion by type, complicated by, electrolyte imbalance
　　　molar pregnancy O08.5
　　due to hyperemesis gravidarum O21.1
　　following ectopic or molar pregnancy O08.5
　　neonatal, transitory NEC P74.4
　　　potassium P74.3
　　　sodium P74.2
　endocrine E34.9
　eye muscle NOS H50.9
　hormone E34.9
　hysterical F44.4
　labyrinth — *see* subcategory H83.2 ☑
　posture R29.3
　protein-energy — *see* Malnutrition
　sympathetic G90.8
Imbecile, imbecility (I.Q. 35-49) F71
Imbedding, intrauterine device T83.39 ☑
Imbibition, cholesterol (gallbladder) K82.4
Imbrication, teeth,, fully erupted M26.30
Imerslund (-Gräsbeck) **syndrome** D51.1
Immature (*see also* Immaturity)
　birth (less than 37 completed weeks) — *see* Preterm, newborn
　extremely (less than 28 completed weeks) — *see* Immaturity, extreme
　personality F60.89
Immaturity (less than 37 completed weeks) (*see also* Preterm, newborn)
　extreme of newborn (less than 28 completed weeks of gestation) (less than 196 completed days of gestation) (unspecified weeks of gestation) P07.20
　　gestational age
　　　less than 23 completed weeks P07.21
　　　23 completed weeks (23 weeks, 0 days through 23 weeks, 6 days) P07.22
　　　24 completed weeks (24 weeks, 0 days through 24 weeks, 6 days) P07.23
　　　25 completed weeks (25 weeks, 0 days through 25 weeks, 6 days) P07.24
　　　26 completed weeks (26 weeks, 0 days through 26 weeks, 6 days) P07.25
　　　27 completed weeks (27 weeks, 0 days through 27 weeks, 6 days) P07.26
　fetus or infant light-for-dates — *see* Light-for-dates
　lung, newborn P28.0
　organ or site NEC — *see* Hypoplasia
　pulmonary, newborn P28.0
　reaction F60.89
　sexual (female) (male), after puberty E30.0
Immersion T75.1 ☑
　foot T69.02- ☑
　hand T69.01- ☑
Immobile, immobility
　complete, due to severe physical disability or frailty R53.2
　intestine K59.8
　syndrome (paraplegic) M62.3
Immune reconstitution (inflammatory) syndrome [IRIS] D89.3
Immunization (*see also* Vaccination)
　ABO — *see* Incompatibility, ABO
　　in newborn P55.1
　complication — *see* Complications, vaccination
　encounter for Z23
　not done (not carried out) Z28.9
　　because (of)
　　　acute illness of patient Z28.01
　　　allergy to vaccine (or component) Z28.04
　　　caregiver refusal Z28.82
　　　chronic illness of patient Z28.02
　　　contraindication NEC Z28.09
　　　group pressure Z28.1
　　　guardian refusal Z28.82
　　　immune compromised state of patient Z28.03
　　　parent refusal Z28.82
　　　patient had disease being vaccinated against Z28.81
　　　patient refusal Z28.21
　　　patient's belief Z28.1
　　　religious beliefs of patient Z28.1
　　　specified reason NEC Z28.89
　　　　of patient Z28.29
　　　unspecified patient reason Z28.20

Immunization — *continued*
　Rh factor
　　affecting management of pregnancy NEC O36.09- ☑
　　　anti-D antibody O36.01- ☑
　　from transfusion — *see* Complication(s), transfusion, incompatibility reaction, Rh (factor)
Immunocytoma C83.0- ☑
Immunodeficiency D84.9
　with
　　adenosine-deaminase deficiency D81.3
　　antibody defects D80.9
　　　specified type NEC D80.8
　　hyperimmunoglobulinemia D80.6
　　increased immunoglobulin M (IgM) D80.5
　　major defect D82.9
　　　specified type NEC D82.8
　　partial albinism D82.8
　　short-limbed stature D82.2
　　thrombocytopenia and eczema D82.0
　antibody with
　　hyperimmunoglobulinemia D80.6
　　near-normal immunoglobulins D80.6
　autosomal recessive, Swiss type D80.0
　combined D81.9
　　biotin-dependent carboxylase D81.819
　　　biotinidase D81.810
　　　holocarboxylase synthetase D81.818
　　　specified type NEC D81.818
　　severe (SCID) D81.9
　　　with
　　　　low or normal B-cell numbers D81.2
　　　　low T- and B-cell numbers D81.1
　　　　reticular dysgenesis D81.0
　　specified type NEC D81.89
　common variable D83.9
　　with
　　　abnormalities of B-cell numbers and function D83.0
　　　autoantibodies to B- or T-cells D83.2
　　　immunoregulatory T-cell disorders D83.1
　　specified type NEC D83.8
　following hereditary defective response to Epstein-Barr virus (EBV) D82.3
　selective, immunoglobulin
　　A (IgA) D80.2
　　G (IgG) (subclasses) D80.3
　　M (IgM) D80.4
　severe combined (SCID) D81.9
　specified type NEC D84.8
　X-linked, with increased IgM D80.5
Immunotherapy (encounter for)
　antineoplastic Z51.12
Impaction, impacted
　bowel, colon, rectum (*see also* Impaction, fecal) K56.49
　　by gallstone K56.3
　calculus — *see* Calculus
　cerumen (ear) (external) H61.2- ☑
　cuspid — *see* Impaction, tooth
　dental (same or adjacent tooth) K01.1
　fecal, feces K56.41
　fracture — *see* Fracture, by site
　gallbladder — *see* Calculus, gallbladder
　gallstone(s) — *see* Calculus, gallbladder
　　bile duct (common) (hepatic) — *see* Calculus, bile duct
　　cystic duct — *see* Calculus, gallbladder
　　in intestine, with obstruction (any part) K56.3
　intestine (calculous) NEC (*see also* Impaction, fecal) K56.49
　　gallstone, with ileus K56.3
　intrauterine device (IUD) T83.39 ☑
　molar — *see* Impaction, tooth
　shoulder, causing obstructed labor O66.0
　tooth, teeth K01.1
　turbinate J34.89
Impaired, impairment (function)
　auditory discrimination — *see* Abnormal, auditory perception
　cognitive, mild, so stated G31.84
　dual sensory Z73.82
　fasting glucose R73.01
　glucose tolerance (oral) R73.02
　hearing — *see* Deafness
　heart — *see* Disease, heart
　kidney N28.9
　　disorder resulting from N25.9
　　　specified NEC N25.89

Impaired, impairment — *continued*
　liver K72.90
　　with coma K72.91
　mastication K08.8
　mild cognitive, so stated G31.84
　mobility
　　ear ossicles — *see* Ankylosis, ear ossicles
　　requiring care provider Z74.09
　myocardium, myocardial — *see* Insufficiency, myocardial
　rectal sphincter R19.8
　renal (acute) (chronic) N28.9
　　disorder resulting from N25.9
　　　specified NEC N25.89
　vision H54.7
　　both eyes H54.3
Impediment, speech R47.9
　psychogenic (childhood) F98.8
　slurring R47.81
　specified NEC R47.89
Impending
　coronary syndrome I20.0
　delirium tremens F10.239
　myocardial infarction I20.0
Imperception auditory (acquired) (*see also* Deafness)
　congenital H93.25
Imperfect
　aeration, lung (newborn) NEC — *see* Atelectasis
　closure (congenital)
　　alimentary tract NEC Q45.8
　　　lower Q43.8
　　　upper Q40.8
　　atrioventricular ostium Q21.2
　　atrium (secundum) Q21.1
　　branchial cleft or sinus Q18.0
　　choroid Q14.3
　　cricoid cartilage Q31.8
　　cusps, heart valve NEC Q24.8
　　　pulmonary Q22.3
　　ductus
　　　arteriosus Q25.0
　　　Botalli Q25.0
　　ear drum (causing impairment of hearing) Q16.4
　　esophagus with communication to bronchus or trachea Q39.1
　　eyelid Q10.3
　　foramen
　　　botalli Q21.1
　　　ovale Q21.1
　　genitalia, genital organ(s) or system
　　　female Q52.8
　　　　external Q52.79
　　　　internal NEC Q52.8
　　　male Q55.8
　　glottis Q31.8
　　interatrial ostium or septum Q21.1
　　interauricular ostium or septum Q21.1
　　interventricular ostium or septum Q21.0
　　larynx Q31.8
　　lip — *see* Cleft, lip
　　nasal septum Q30.3
　　nose Q30.2
　　omphalomesenteric duct Q43.0
　　optic nerve entry Q14.2
　　organ or site not listed — *see* Anomaly, by site
　　ostium
　　　interatrial Q21.1
　　　interauricular Q21.1
　　　interventricular Q21.0
　　palate — *see* Cleft, palate
　　preauricular sinus Q18.1
　　retina Q14.1
　　roof of orbit Q75.8
　　sclera Q13.5
　　septum
　　　aorticopulmonary Q21.4
　　　atrial (secundum) Q21.1
　　　between aorta and pulmonary artery Q21.4
　　　heart Q21.9
　　　interatrial (secundum) Q21.1
　　　interauricular (secundum) Q21.1
　　　interventricular Q21.0
　　　　in tetralogy of Fallot Q21.3
　　　nasal Q30.3
　　　ventricular Q21.0
　　　　with pulmonary stenosis or atresia, dextra-position of aorta, and hypertrophy of right ventricle Q21.3

Imperfect — *continued*
  closure — *continued*
    septum — *continued*
      ventricular — *continued*
        in tetralogy of Fallot Q21.3
    skull Q75.Ø
      with
        anencephaly QØØ.Ø
        encephalocele — *see* Encephalocele
        hydrocephalus QØ3.9
          with spina bifida — *see* Spina bifida, by site, with hydrocephalus
        microcephaly QØ2
    spine (with meningocele) — *see* Spina bifida
    trachea Q32.1
    tympanic membrane (causing impairment of hearing) Q16.4
    uterus Q51.818
    vitelline duct Q43.Ø
  erection — *see* Dysfunction, sexual, male, erectile
  fusion — *see* Imperfect, closure
  inflation, lung (newborn) — *see* Atelectasis
  posture R29.3
  rotation, intestine Q43.3
  septum, ventricular Q21.Ø
Imperfectly descended testis — *see* Cryptorchid
Imperforate (congenital) (*see also* Atresia)
  anus Q42.3
    with fistula Q42.2
  cervix (uteri) Q51.828
  esophagus Q39.Ø
    with tracheoesophageal fistula Q39.1
  hymen Q52.3
  jejunum Q41.1
  pharynx Q38.8
  rectum Q42.1
    with fistula Q42.Ø
  urethra Q64.39
  vagina Q52.4
Impervious (congenital) (*see also* Atresia)
  anus Q42.3
    with fistula Q42.2
  bile duct Q44.2
  esophagus Q39.Ø
    with tracheoesophageal fistula Q39.1
  intestine (small) Q41.9
    large Q42.9
      specified NEC Q42.8
  rectum Q42.1
    with fistula Q42.Ø
  ureter — *see* Atresia, ureter
  urethra Q64.39
Impetiginization of dermatoses LØ1.1
Impetigo (any organism) (any site) (circinate) (contagiosa) (simplex) (vulgaris) LØ1.ØØ
  Bockhart's LØ1.Ø2
  bullous, bullosa LØ1.Ø3
  external ear LØ1.ØØ [H62.4Ø]
  follicularis LØ1.Ø2
  furfuracea L3Ø.5
  herpetiformis L4Ø.1
    nonobstetrical L4Ø.1
  neonatorum LØ1.Ø3
  nonbullous LØ1.Ø1
  specified type NEC LØ1.Ø9
  ulcerative LØ1.Ø9
Impingement (on teeth)
  soft tissue
    anterior M26.81
    posterior M26.82
Implant, endometrial N8Ø.9
Implantation
  anomalous — *see* Anomaly, by site
    ureter Q62.63
  cyst
    external area or site (skin) NEC L72.Ø
    iris — *see* Cyst, iris, implantation
    vagina N89.8
    vulva N9Ø.7
  dermoid (cyst) — *see* Implantation, cyst
Impotence (sexual) N52.9
  counseling Z7Ø.1
  organic origin (*see also* Dysfunction, sexual, male, erectile) N52.9
  psychogenic F52.21
Impression, basilar Q75.8
Imprisonment, anxiety concerning Z65.1
Improper care (child) (newborn) — *see* Maltreatment

Improperly tied umbilical cord (causing hemorrhage) P51.8
Impulsiveness (impulsive) R45.87
Inability to swallow — *see* Aphagia
Inaccessible, inaccessibility
  health care NEC Z75.3
    due to
      waiting period Z75.2
        for admission to facility elsewhere Z75.1
  other helping agencies Z75.4
Inactive — *see* condition
Inadequate, inadequacy
  aesthetics of dental restoration KØ8.56
  biologic, constitutional, functional, or social F6Ø.7
  development
    child R62.5Ø
    genitalia
      after puberty NEC E3Ø.Ø
      congenital
        female Q52.8
          external Q52.79
          internal Q52.8
        male Q55.8
    lungs Q33.6
      associated with short gestation P28.Ø
    organ or site not listed — *see* Anomaly, by site
  diet (causing nutritional deficiency) E63.9
  eating habits Z72.4
  environment, household Z59.1
  family support Z63.8
  food (supply) NEC Z59.4
    hunger effects T73.Ø ☑
  functional F6Ø.7
  household care, due to
    family member
      handicapped or ill Z74.2
      on vacation Z75.5
      temporarily away from home Z74.2
    technical defects in home Z59.1
    temporary absence from home of person rendering care Z74.2
  housing (heating) (space) Z59.1
  income (financial) Z59.6
  intrafamilial communication Z63.8
  material resources Z59.9
  mental — *see* Disability, intellectual
  parental supervision or control of child Z62.Ø
  personality F6Ø.7
  pulmonary
    function RØ6.89
      newborn P28.5
    ventilation, newborn P28.5
  sample of cytologic smear
    anus R85.615
    cervix R87.615
    vagina R87.625
  social F6Ø.7
    insurance Z59.7
    skills NEC Z73.4
  supervision of child by parent Z62.Ø
  teaching affecting education Z55.8
  welfare support Z59.7
Inanition R64
  with edema — *see* Malnutrition, severe
  due to
    deprivation of food T73.Ø ☑
    malnutrition — *see* Malnutrition
  fever R5Ø.9
Inappropriate
  change in quantitative human chorionic gonadotropin (hCG) in early pregnancy OØ2.81
  diet or eating habits Z72.4
  level of quantitative human chorionic gonadotropin (hCG) for gestational age in early pregnancy OØ2.81
  secretion
    antidiuretic hormone (ADH) (excessive) E22.2
      deficiency E23.2
    pituitary (posterior) E22.2
Inattention at or after birth — *see* Neglect
Incarceration, incarcerated
  enterocele K46.Ø
    gangrenous K46.1
  epiplocele K46.Ø
    gangrenous K46.1
  exophthalmos K42.Ø
    gangrenous K42.1
  hernia (*see also* Hernia, by site, with obstruction)

Incarceration, incarcerated — *continued*
  hernia (*see also* Hernia, by site, with obstruction) — *continued*
    with gangrene — *see* Hernia, by site, with gangrene
  iris, in wound — *see* Injury, eye, laceration, with prolapse
  lens, in wound — *see* Injury, eye, laceration, with prolapse
  omphalocele K42.Ø
  prison, anxiety concerning Z65.1
  rupture — *see* Hernia, by site
  sarcoepiplocele K46.Ø
    gangrenous K46.1
  sarcoepiplomphalocele K42.Ø
    with gangrene K42.1
  uterus N85.8
    gravid O34.51- ☑
      causing obstructed labor O65.5
Incised wound
  external — *see* Laceration
  internal organs — *see* Injury, by site
Incision, incisional
  hernia K43.2
    with
      gangrene (and obstruction) K43.1
      obstruction K43.Ø
  surgical, complication — *see* Complications, surgical procedure
  traumatic
    external — *see* Laceration
    internal organs — *see* Injury, by site
Inclusion
  azurophilic leukocytic D72.Ø
  blennorrhea (neonatal) (newborn) P39.1
  gallbladder in liver (congenital) Q44.1
Incompatibility
  ABO
    affecting management of pregnancy O36.11- ☑
      anti-A sensitization O36.11- ☑
      anti-B sensitization O36.19- ☑
      specified NEC O36.19- ☑
    infusion or transfusion reaction — *see* Complication(s), transfusion, incompatibility reaction, ABO
    newborn P55.1
  blood (group) (Duffy) (K(ell)) (Kidd) (Lewis) (M) (S) NEC
    affecting management of pregnancy O36.11- ☑
      anti-A sensitization O36.11- ☑
      anti-B sensitization O36.19- ☑
    infusion or transfusion reaction T8Ø.89 ☑
    newborn P55.8
  divorce or estrangement Z63.5
  Rh (blood group) (factor) Z31.82
    affecting management of pregnancy NEC O36.Ø9- ☑
      anti-D antibody O36.Ø1- ☑
    infusion or transfusion reaction — *see* Complication(s), transfusion, incompatibility reaction, Rh (factor)
    newborn P55.Ø
  rhesus — *see* Incompatibility, Rh
Incompetency, incompetent, incompetence
  annular
    aortic (valve) — *see* Insufficiency, aortic
    mitral (valve) I34.Ø
    pulmonary valve (heart) I37.1
  aortic (valve) — *see* Insufficiency, aortic
  cardiac valve — *see* Endocarditis
  cervix, cervical (os) N88.3
    in pregnancy O34.3- ☑
  chronotropic I45.89
    with
      autonomic dysfunction G9Ø.8
      ischemic heart disease I25.89
      left ventricular dysfunction I51.89
      sinus node dysfunction I49.8
  esophagogastric (junction) (sphincter) K22.Ø
  mitral (valve) — *see* Insufficiency, mitral
  pelvic fundus N81.89
  pubocervical tissue N81.82
  pulmonary valve (heart) I37.1
    congenital Q22.3
  rectovaginal tissue N81.83
  tricuspid (annular) (valve) — *see* Insufficiency, tricuspid
  valvular — *see* Endocarditis
    congenital Q24.8

Incompetency, incompetent, incompetence —
    continued
  vein, venous (saphenous) (varicose) — *see* Varix, leg
Incomplete (*see also* condition)
  bladder, emptying R33.9
  defecation R15.0
  expansion lungs (newborn) NEC — *see* Atelectasis
  rotation, intestine Q43.3
Inconclusive
  diagnostic imaging due to excess body fat of patient
      R93.9
  findings on diagnostic imaging of breast NEC R92.8
  mammogram (due to dense breasts) R92.2
Incontinence R32
  anal sphincter R15.9
  feces R15.9
    nonorganic origin F98.1
  overflow N39.490
  psychogenic F45.8
  rectal R15.9
  reflex N39.498
  stress (female) (male) N39.3
    and urge N39.46
  urethral sphincter R32
  urge N39.41
    and stress (female) (male) N39.46
  urine (urinary) R32
    continuous N39.45
    due to cognitive impairment, or severe physical
        disability or immobility R39.81
    functional R39.81
    mixed (stress and urge) N39.46
    nocturnal N39.44
    nonorganic origin F98.0
    overflow N39.490
    post dribbling N39.43
    reflex N39.498
    specified NEC N39.498
    stress (female) (male) N39.3
      and urge N39.46
    total N39.498
    unaware N39.42
    urge N39.41
      and stress (female) (male) N39.46
Incontinentia pigmenti Q82.3
Incoordinate, incoordination
  esophageal-pharyngeal (newborn) — *see* Dysphagia
  muscular R27.8
  uterus (action) (contractions) (complicating delivery)
      O62.4
Increase, increased
  abnormal, in development R63.8
  androgens (ovarian) E28.1
  anticoagulants (antithrombin) (anti-VIIIa) (anti-IXa)
      (anti-Xa) (anti-XIa) — *see* Circulating anticoagu-
      lants
  cold sense R20.8
  estrogen E28.0
  function
    adrenal
      cortex — *see* Cushing's, syndrome
      medulla E27.5
    pituitary (gland) (anterior) (lobe) E22.9
      posterior E22.2
  heat sense R20.8
  intracranial pressure (benign) G93.2
  permeability, capillaries I78.8
  pressure, intracranial G93.2
  secretion
    gastrin E16.4
    glucagon E16.3
    pancreas, endocrine E16.9
      growth hormone-releasing hormone E16.8
      pancreatic polypeptide E16.8
      somatostatin E16.8
      vasoactive-intestinal polypeptide E16.8
  sphericity, lens Q12.4
  splenic activity D73.1
  venous pressure I87.8
    portal K76.6
Increta placenta O43.22- ☑
Incrustation, cornea, foreign body (lead)(zinc) — *see*
    Foreign body, cornea
Incyclophoria H50.54
Incyclotropia — *see* Cyclotropia
Indeterminate sex Q56.4
India rubber skin Q82.8
Indigestion (acid) (bilious) (functional) K30

Indigestion — *continued*
  catarrhal K31.89
  due to decomposed food NOS A05.9
  nervous F45.8
  psychogenic F45.8
Indirect — *see* condition
Induratio penis plastica N48.6
Induration, indurated
  brain G93.89
  breast (fibrous) N64.51
    puerperal, postpartum O92.29
  broad ligament N83.8
  chancre
    anus A51.1
    congenital A50.07
    extragenital NEC A51.2
  corpora cavernosa (penis) (plastic) N48.6
  liver (chronic) K76.89
  lung (black) (chronic) (fibroid) (*see also* Fibrosis, lung)
      J84.10
    essential brown J84.03
  penile (plastic) N48.6
  phlebitic — *see* Phlebitis
  skin R23.4
Inebriety (without dependence) — *see* Alcohol, intoxica-
    tion
Inefficiency, kidney N28.9
Inelasticity, skin R23.4
Inequality, leg (length) (acquired) (*see also* Deformity,
    limb, unequal length)
  congenital — *see* Defect, reduction, lower limb
  lower leg — *see* Deformity, limb, unequal length
Inertia
  bladder (neurogenic) N31.2
  stomach K31.89
    psychogenic F45.8
  uterus, uterine during labor O62.2
    during latent phase of labor O62.0
    primary O62.0
    secondary O62.1
  vesical (neurogenic) N31.2
Infancy, infantile, infantilism (*see also* condition)
  celiac K90.0
  genitalia, genitals (after puberty) E30.0
  Herter's (nontropical sprue) K90.0
  intestinal K90.0
  Lorain E23.0
  pancreatic K86.8
  pelvis M95.5
    with disproportion (fetopelvic) O33.1
      causing obstructed labor O65.1
  pituitary E23.0
  renal N25.0
  uterus — *see* Infantile, genitalia
Infant(s) (*see also* Infancy)
  excessive crying R68.11
  irritable child R68.12
  lack of care — *see* Neglect
  liveborn (singleton) Z38.2
    born in hospital Z38.00
      by cesarean Z38.01
    born outside hospital Z38.1
    multiple NEC Z38.8
      born in hospital Z38.68
        by cesarean Z38.69
      born outside hospital Z38.7
    quadruplet Z38.8
      born in hospital Z38.63
        by cesarean Z38.64
      born outside hospital Z38.7
    quintuplet Z38.8
      born in hospital Z38.65
        by cesarean Z38.66
      born outside hospital Z38.7
    triplet Z38.8
      born in hospital Z38.61
        by cesarean Z38.62
      born outside hospital Z38.7
    twin Z38.5
      born in hospital Z38.30
        by cesarean Z38.31
      born outside hospital Z38.4
  of diabetic mother (syndrome of) P70.1
    gestational diabetes P70.0
Infantile (*see also* condition)
  genitalia, genitals E30.0
  os, uterine E30.0
  penis E30.0

Infantile — *continued*
  testis E29.1
  uterus E30.0
Infantilism — *see* Infancy
Infarct, infarction
  adrenal (capsule) (gland) E27.49
  appendices epiploicae K55.0
  bowel K55.0
  brain (stem) — *see* Infarct, cerebral
  breast N64.89
  brewer's (kidney) N28.0
  cardiac — *see* Infarct, myocardium
  cerebellar — *see* Infarct, cerebral
  cerebral (*see also* Occlusion, artery cerebral or precere-
      bral, with infarction) I63.9
    aborted I63.9
    cortical I63.9
    due to
      cerebral venous thrombosis, nonpyogenic I63.6
      embolism
        cerebral arteries I63.4- ☑
        precerebral arteries I63.1- ☑
      occlusion NEC
        cerebral arteries I63.5- ☑
        precerebral arteries I63.2- ☑
      stenosis NEC
        cerebral arteries I63.5- ☑
        precerebral arteries I63.2- ☑
      thrombosis
        cerebral artery I63.3- ☑
        precerebral artery I63.0- ☑
    intraoperative
      during cardiac surgery I97.810
      during other surgery I97.811
    postprocedural
      following cardiac surgery I97.820
      following other surgery I97.821
    specified NEC I63.8
  colon (acute) (agnogenic) (embolic) (hemorrhagic)
      (nonocclusive) (nonthrombotic) (occlusive)
      (segmental) (thrombotic) (with gangrene) K55.0
  coronary artery — *see* Infarct, myocardium
  embolic — *see* Embolism
  fallopian tube N83.8
  gallbladder K82.8
  heart — *see* Infarct, myocardium
  hepatic K76.3
  hypophysis (anterior lobe) E23.6
  impending (myocardium) I20.0
  intestine (acute) (agnogenic) (embolic) (hemorrhagic)
      (nonocclusive) (nonthrombotic) (occlusive)
      (thrombotic) (with gangrene) K55.0
  kidney N28.0
  liver K76.3
  lung (embolic) (thrombotic) — *see* Embolism, pul-
      monary
  lymph node I89.8
  mesentery, mesenteric (embolic) (thrombotic) (with
      gangrene) K55.0
  muscle (ischemic) M62.20
    ankle M62.27- ☑
    foot M62.27- ☑
    forearm M62.23- ☑
    hand M62.24- ☑
    lower leg M62.26- ☑
    pelvic region M62.25- ☑
    shoulder region M62.21- ☑
    specified site NEC M62.28
    thigh M62.25- ☑
    upper arm M62.22- ☑
  myocardium, myocardial (acute) (with stated duration
      of 4 weeks or less) I21.3
    diagnosed on ECG, but presenting no symptoms
        I25.2
    healed or old I25.2
    intraoperative
      during cardiac surgery I97.790
      during other surgery I97.791
    non-Q wave I21.4
    non-ST elevation (NSTEMI) I21.4
      subsequent I22.2
    nontransmural I21.4
    past (diagnosed on ECG or other investigation, but
        currently presenting no symptoms) I25.2
    postprocedural
      following cardiac surgery I97.190
      following other surgery I97.191
    Q wave (see also, Infarct, myocardium, by site) I21.3

Infarct, infarction — continued
  myocardium, myocardial — continued
    ST elevation (STEMI) I21.3
      anterior (anteroapical) (anterolateral) (anteroseptal) (Q wave) (wall) I21.09
        subsequent I22.0
      inferior (diaphragmatic) (inferolateral) (inferoposterior) (wall) NEC I21.19
        subsequent I22.1
      inferoposterior transmural (Q wave) I21.11
      involving
        coronary artery of anterior wall NEC I21.09
        coronary artery of inferior wall NEC I21.19
        diagonal coronary artery I21.02
        left anterior descending coronary artery I21.02
        left circumflex coronary artery I21.21
        left main coronary artery I21.01
        oblique marginal coronary artery I21.21
        right coronary artery I21.11
      lateral (apical-lateral) (basal-lateral) (high) I21.29
        subsequent I22.8
      posterior (posterobasal) (posterolateral) (posteroseptal) (true) I21.29
        subsequent I22.8
      septal I21.29
        subsequent I22.8
      specified NEC I21.29
        subsequent I22.8
      subsequent I22.9
    subsequent (recurrent) (reinfarction) I22.9
      anterior (anteroapical) (anterolateral) (anteroseptal) (wall) I22.0
      diaphragmatic (wall) I22.1
      inferior (diaphragmatic) (inferolateral) (inferoposterior) (wall) I22.1
      lateral (apical-lateral) (basal-lateral) (high) I22.8
      non-ST elevation (NSTEMI) I22.2
      posterior (posterobasal) (posterolateral) (posteroseptal) (true) I22.8
      septal I22.8
      specified NEC I22.8
      ST elevation I22.9
        anterior (anteroapical) (anterolateral) (anteroseptal) (wall) I22.0
        inferior (diaphragmatic) (inferolateral) (inferoposterior) (wall) I22.1
        specified NEC I22.8
      subendocardial I22.2
      transmural I22.9
        anterior (anteroapical) (anterolateral) (anteroseptal) (wall) I22.0
        diaphragmatic (wall) I22.1
        inferior (diaphragmatic) (inferolateral) (inferoposterior) (wall) I22.1
        lateral (apical-lateral) (basal-lateral) (high) I22.8
        posterior (posterobasal) (posterolateral) (posteroseptal) (true) I22.8
        specified NEC I22.8
    syphilitic A52.06
    transmural I21.3
      anterior (anteroapical) (anterolateral) (anteroseptal) (Q wave) (wall) NEC I21.09
      inferior (diaphragmatic) (inferolateral) (inferoposterior) (Q wave) (wall) NEC I21.19
      inferoposterior (Q wave) I21.11
      lateral (apical-lateral) (basal-lateral) (high) NEC I21.29
      posterior (posterobasal) (posterolateral) (posteroseptal) (true) NEC I21.29
      septal NEC I21.29
      specified NEC I21.29
  nontransmural I21.4
  omentum K55.0
  ovary N83.8
  pancreas K86.8
  papillary muscle — see Infarct, myocardium
  parathyroid gland E21.4
  pituitary (gland) E23.6
  placenta O43.81- ☑
  prostate N42.89
  pulmonary (artery) (vein) (hemorrhagic) — see Embolism, pulmonary
  renal (embolic) (thrombotic) N28.0
  retina, retinal (artery) — see Occlusion, artery, retina
  spinal (cord) (acute) (embolic) (nonembolic) G95.11

Infarct, infarction — continued
  spleen D73.5
    embolic or thrombotic I74.8
  subendocardial (acute) (nontransmural) I21.4
  suprarenal (capsule) (gland) E27.49
  testis N50.1
  thrombotic (see also Thrombosis)
    artery, arterial — see Embolism
  thyroid (gland) E07.89
  ventricle (heart) — see Infarct, myocardium
Infecting — see condition
Infection, infected, infective (opportunistic) B99.9
  with
    drug resistant organism — see Resistance (to), drug (see also specific organism)
    lymphangitis — see Lymphangitis
    organ dysfunction (acute) R65.20
      with septic shock R65.21
  abscess (skin) — code by site under Abscess
  Absidia — see Mucormycosis
  Acanthamoeba — see Acanthamebiasis
  Acanthocheilonema (perstans) (streptocerca) B74.4
  accessory sinus (chronic) — see Sinusitis
  achorion — see Dermatophytosis
  Acremonium falciforme B47.0
  acromioclavicular M00.9
  Actinobacillus (actinomycetem-comitans) A28.8
    mallei A24.0
    muris A25.1
  Actinomadura B47.1
  Actinomyces (israelii) (see also Actinomycosis) A42.9
  Actinomycetales — see Actinomycosis
  actinomycotic NOS — see Actinomycosis
  adenoid (and tonsil) J03.90
    chronic J35.02
  adenovirus NEC
    as cause of disease classified elsewhere B97.0
    unspecified nature or site B34.0
  aerogenes capsulatus A48.0
  aertrycke — see Infection, salmonella
  alimentary canal NOS — see Enteritis, infectious
  Allescheria boydii B48.2
  Alternaria B48.8
  alveolus, alveolar (process) K04.7
  Ameba, amebic (histolytica) — see Amebiasis
  amniotic fluid, sac or cavity O41.10- ☑
    chorioamnionitis O41.12- ☑
    placentitis O41.14- ☑
  amputation stump (surgical) — see Complication, amputation stump, infection
  Ancylostoma (duodenalis) B76.0
  Anisakiasis, Anisakis larvae B81.0
  anthrax — see Anthrax
  antrum (chronic) — see Sinusitis, maxillary
  anus, anal (papillae) (sphincter) K62.89
  arbovirus (arbor virus) A94
    specified type NEC A93.8
  artificial insemination N98.0
  Ascaris lumbricoides — see Ascariasis
  Ascomycetes B47.0
  Aspergillus (flavus) (fumigatus) (terreus) — see Aspergillosis
  atypical
    acid-fast (bacilli) — see Mycobacterium, atypical
    mycobacteria — see Mycobacterium, atypical
    virus A81.9
      specified type NEC A81.89
  auditory meatus (external) — see Otitis, externa, infective
  auricle (ear) — see Otitis, externa, infective
  axillary gland (lymph) L04.2
  Bacillus A49.9
    abortus A23.1
    anthracis — see Anthrax
    Ducrey's (any location) A57
    Flexner's A03.1
    Friedländer's NEC A49.8
    gas (gangrene) A48.0
    mallei A24.0
    melitensis A23.0
    paratyphoid, paratyphosus A01.4
      A A01.1
      B A01.2
      C A01.3
    Shiga (-Kruse) A03.0
    suipestifer — see Infection, salmonella
    swimming pool A31.1

Infection, infected, infective — continued
  Bacillus — continued
    typhosa A01.00
    welchii — see Gangrene, gas
  bacterial NOS A49.9
    as cause of disease classified elsewhere B96.89
      Bacteroides fragilis [B. fragilis] B96.6
      Clostridium perfringens [C. perfringens] B96.7
      Enterobacter sakazakii B96.89
      Enterococcus B95.2
      Escherichia coli [E. coli] (see also Escherichia coli) B96.20
      Helicobacter pylori [H.pylori] B96.81
      Hemophilus influenzae [H. influenzae] B96.3
      Klebsiella pneumoniae [K. pneumoniae] B96.1
      Mycoplasma pneumoniae [M. pneumoniae] B96.0
      Proteus (mirabilis) (morganii) B96.4
      Pseudomonas (aeruginosa) (mallei) (pseudomallei) B96.5
      Staphylococcus B95.8
        aureus (methicillin susceptible) (MSSA) B95.61
          methicillin resistant (MRSA) B95.62
        specified NEC B95.7
      Streptococcus B95.5
        group A B95.0
        group B B95.1
        pneumoniae B95.3
        specified NEC B95.4
      Vibrio vulnificus B96.82
    specified NEC A48.8
  Bacterium
    paratyphosum A01.4
      A A01.1
      B A01.2
      C A01.3
    typhosum A01.00
  Bacteroides NEC A49.8
    fragilis, as cause of disease classified elsewhere B96.6
  Balantidium coli A07.0
  Bartholin's gland N75.8
  Basidiobolus B46.8
  bile duct (common) (hepatic) — see Cholangitis
  bladder — see Cystitis
  Blastomyces, blastomycotic (see also Blastomycosis)
    brasiliensis — see Paracoccidioidomycosis
    dermatitidis — see Blastomycosis
    European — see Cryptococcosis
    Loboi B48.0
    North American B40.9
    South American — see Paracoccidioidomycosis
  bleb, postprocedure — see Blebitis
  bone — see Osteomyelitis
  Bordetella — see Whooping cough
  Borrelia bergdorfi A69.20
  brain (see also Encephalitis) G04.90
    membranes — see Meningitis
    septic G06.0
      meninges — see Meningitis, bacterial
  branchial cyst Q18.0
  breast — see Mastitis
  bronchus — see Bronchitis
  Brucella A23.9
    abortus A23.1
    canis A23.3
    melitensis A23.0
    mixed A23.8
    specified NEC A23.8
    suis A23.2
  Brugia (malayi) B74.1
    timori B74.2
  bursa — see Bursitis, infective
  buttocks (skin) L08.9
  Campylobacter, intestinal A04.5
    as cause of disease classified elsewhere B96.81
  Candida (albicans) (tropicalis) — see Candidiasis
  candiru B88.8
  Capillaria (intestinal) B81.1
    hepatica B83.8
    philippinensis B81.1
  cartilage — see Disorder, cartilage, specified type NEC
  cat liver fluke B66.0
  catheter-related bloodstream (CRBSI) T80.211 ☑
  cellulitis — code by site under Cellulitis
  central line-associated T80.219 ☑
    bloodstream (CLABSI) T80.211 ☑

Infection, infected, infective — *continued*
 central line-associated — *continued*
  specified NEC T80.218 ☑
 Cephalosporium falciforme B47.0
 cerebrospinal — *see* Meningitis
 cervical gland (lymph) L04.0
 cervix — *see* Cervicitis
 cesarean delivery wound (puerperal) O86.0
 cestodes — *see* Infestation, cestodes
 chest J22
 Chilomastix (intestinal) A07.8
 Chlamydia, chlamydial A74.9
  anus A56.3
  genitourinary tract A56.2
   lower A56.00
   specified NEC A56.19
  lymphogranuloma A55
  pharynx A56.4
  psittaci A70
  rectum A56.3
  sexually transmitted NEC A56.8
 cholera — *see* Cholera
 Cladosporium
  bantianum (brain abscess) B43.1
  carrionii B43.0
  castellanii B36.1
  trichoides (brain abscess) B43.1
  werneckii B36.1
 Clonorchis (sinensis) (liver) B66.1
 Clostridium NEC
  bifermentans A48.0
  botulinum (food poisoning) A05.1
   infant A48.51
   wound A48.52
  difficile
   as cause of disease classified elsewhere B96.89
   foodborne (disease) A04.7
   gas gangrene A48.0
   necrotizing enterocolitis A04.7
   sepsis A41.4
  gas-forming NEC A48.0
  histolyticum A48.0
  novyi, causing gas gangrene A48.0
  oedematiens A48.0
  perfringens
   as cause of disease classified elsewhere B96.7
   due to food A05.2
   foodborne (disease) A05.2
   gas gangrene A48.0
   sepsis A41.4
  septicum, causing gas gangrene A48.0
  sordellii, causing gas gangrene A48.0
  welchii
   as cause of disease classified elsewhere B96.7
   foodborne (disease) A05.2
   gas gangrene A48.0
   necrotizing enteritis A05.2
   sepsis A41.4
 Coccidioides (immitis) — *see* Coccidioidomycosis
 colon — *see* Enteritis, infectious
 colostomy K94.02
 common duct — *see* Cholangitis
 congenital P39.9
  Candida (albicans) P37.5
  cytomegalovirus P35.1
  hepatitis, viral P35.3
  herpes simplex P35.2
  infectious or parasitic disease P37.9
   specified NEC P37.8
  listeriosis (disseminated) P37.2
  malaria NEC P37.4
   falciparum P37.3
  Plasmodium falciparum P37.3
  poliomyelitis P35.8
  rubella P35.0
  skin P39.4
  toxoplasmosis (acute) (subacute) (chronic) P37.1
  tuberculosis P37.0
  urinary (tract) P39.3
  vaccinia P35.8
  virus P35.9
   specified type NEC P35.8
 Conidiobolus B46.8
 coronavirus NEC B34.2
  as cause of disease classified elsewhere B97.29
  severe acute respiratory syndrome (SARS associated) B97.21
 corpus luteum — *see* Salpingo-oophoritis

Infection, infected, infective — *continued*
 Corynebacterium diphtheriae — *see* Diphtheria
 cotia virus B08.8
 Coxiella burnetii A78
 coxsackie — *see* Coxsackie
 Cryptococcus neoformans — *see* Cryptococcosis
 Cryptosporidium A07.2
 Cunninghamella — *see* Mucormycosis
 cyst — *see* Cyst
 cystic duct (*see also* Cholecystitis) K81.9
 Cysticercus cellulosae — *see* Cysticercosis
 cytomegalovirus, cytomegaloviral B25.9
  congenital P35.1
  maternal, maternal care for (suspected) damage to fetus O35.3 ☑
  mononucleosis B27.10
   with
    complication NEC B27.19
    meningitis B27.12
    polyneuropathy B27.11
 delta-agent (acute), in hepatitis B carrier B17.0
 dental (pulpal origin) K04.7
 Deuteromycetes B47.0
 Dicrocoelium dendriticum B66.2
 Dipetalonema (perstans) (streptocerca) B74.4
 diphtherial — *see* Diphtheria
 Diphyllobothrium (adult) (latum) (pacificum) B70.0
  larval B70.1
 Diplogonoporus (grandis) B71.8
 Dipylidium caninum B67.4
 Dirofilaria B74.8
 Dracunculus medinensis B72
 Drechslera (hawaiiensis) B43.8
 Ducrey Haemophilus (any location) A57
 due to or resulting from
  artificial insemination N98.0
  central venous catheter T80.219 ☑
   bloodstream T80.211 ☑
   exit or insertion site T80.212 ☑
   localized T80.212 ☑
   port or reservoir T80.212 ☑
   specified NEC T80.218 ☑
   tunnel T80.212 ☑
  device, implant or graft (*see also* Complications, by site and type, infection or inflammation) T85.79 ☑
   arterial graft NEC T82.7 ☑
   breast (implant) T85.79 ☑
   catheter NEC T85.79 ☑
    dialysis (renal) T82.7 ☑
     intraperitoneal T85.71 ☑
    infusion NEC T82.7 ☑
     spinal (epidural) (subdural) T85.79 ☑
    urinary (indwelling) T83.51 ☑
   electronic (electrode) (pulse generator) (stimulator)
    bone T84.7 ☑
    cardiac T82.7 ☑
    nervous system (brain) (peripheral nerve) (spinal) T85.79 ☑
    urinary T83.59 ☑
   fixation, internal (orthopedic) NEC — *see* Complication, fixation device, infection
   gastrointestinal (bile duct) (esophagus) T85.79 ☑
   genital NEC T83.6 ☑
   heart NEC T82.7 ☑
    valve (prosthesis) T82.6 ☑
     graft T82.7 ☑
   joint prosthesis — *see* Complication, joint prosthesis, infection
   ocular (corneal graft) (orbital implant) NEC T85.79 ☑
   orthopedic NEC T84.7 ☑
   specified NEC T85.79 ☑
   urinary NEC T83.59 ☑
   vascular NEC T82.7 ☑
   ventricular intracranial shunt T85.79 ☑
  Hickman catheter T80.219 ☑
   bloodstream T80.211 ☑
   localized T80.212 ☑
   specified NEC T80.218 ☑
  immunization or vaccination T88.0 ☑
  infusion, injection or transfusion NEC T80.29 ☑
  injury NEC — *code by* site under Wound, open
  peripherally inserted central catheter (PICC) T80.219 ☑

Infection, infected, infective — *continued*
 due to or resulting from — *continued*
  peripherally inserted central catheter — *continued*
   bloodstream T80.211 ☑
   localized T80.212 ☑
   specified NEC T80.218 ☑
  portacath (port-a-cath) T80.219 ☑
   bloodstream T80.211 ☑
   localized T80.212 ☑
   specified NEC T80.218 ☑
  surgery T81.4 ☑
  triple lumen catheter T80.219 ☑
   bloodstream T80.211 ☑
   localized T80.212 ☑
   specified NEC T80.218 ☑
  umbilical venous catheter T80.219 ☑
   bloodstream T80.211 ☑
   localized T80.212 ☑
   specified NEC T80.218 ☑
 during labor NEC O75.3
 ear (middle) (*see also* Otitis media)
  external — *see* Otitis, externa, infective
  inner — *see* subcategory H83.0 ☑
 Eberthella typhosa A01.00
 Echinococcus — *see* Echinococcus
 echovirus
  as cause of disease classified elsewhere B97.12
  unspecified nature or site B34.1
 endocardium I33.0
 endocervix — *see* Cervicitis
 Entamoeba — *see* Amebiasis
 enteric — *see* Enteritis, infectious
 Enterobacter sakazakii B96.89
 Enterobius vermicularis B80
 enterostomy K94.12
 enterovirus B34.1
  as cause of disease classified elsewhere B97.10
   coxsackievirus B97.11
   echovirus B97.12
   specified NEC B97.19
 Entomophthora B46.8
 Epidermophyton — *see* Dermatophytosis
 epididymis — *see* Epididymitis
 episiotomy (puerperal) O86.0
 Erysipelothrix (insidiosa) (rhusiopathiae) — *see* Erysipeloid
 erythema infectiosum B08.3
 Escherichia (E.) coli NEC A49.8
  as cause of disease classified elsewhere (*see also* Escherichia coli) B96.20
  congenital P39.8
   sepsis P36.4
  generalized A41.51
  intestinal — *see* Enteritis, infectious, due to, Escherichia coli
 ethmoidal (chronic) (sinus) — *see* Sinusitis, ethmoidal
 eustachian tube (ear) — *see* Salpingitis, eustachian
 external auditory canal (meatus) NEC — *see* Otitis, externa, infective
 eye (purulent) — *see* Endophthalmitis, purulent
 eyelid — *see* Inflammation, eyelid
 fallopian tube — *see* Salpingo-oophoritis
 Fasciola (gigantica) (hepatica) (indica) B66.3
 Fasciolopsis (buski) B66.5
 filarial — *see* Infestation, filarial
 finger (skin) L08.9
  nail L03.01- ☑
   fungus B35.1
 fish tapeworm B70.0
  larval B70.1
 flagellate, intestinal A07.9
 fluke — *see* Infestation, fluke
 focal
  teeth (pulpal origin) K04.7
  tonsils J35.01
 Fonsecaea (compactum) (pedrosoi) B43.0
 food — *see* Intoxication, foodborne
 foot (skin) L08.9
  dermatophytic fungus B35.3
 Francisella tularensis — *see* Tularemia
 frontal (sinus) (chronic) — *see* Sinusitis, frontal
 fungus NOS B49
  beard B35.0
  dermatophytic — *see* Dermatophytosis
  foot B35.3
  groin B35.6

Infection, infected, infective — *continued*
- fungus — *continued*
  - hand B35.2
  - nail B35.1
  - pathogenic to compromised host only B48.8
  - perianal (area) B35.6
  - scalp B35.0
  - skin B36.9
    - foot B35.3
    - hand B35.2
    - toenails B35.1
- Fusarium B48.8
- gallbladder — *see* Cholecystitis
- gas bacillus — *see* Gangrene, gas
- gastrointestinal — *see* Enteritis, infectious
- generalized NEC — *see* Sepsis
- genital organ or tract
  - female — *see* Disease, pelvis, inflammatory
  - male N49.9
    - multiple sites N49.8
    - specified NEC N49.8
- Ghon tubercle, primary A15.7
- Giardia lamblia A07.1
- gingiva (chronic) K05.10
  - acute K05.00
    - nonplaque induced K05.01
    - plaque induced K05.00
  - nonplaque induced K05.11
  - plaque induced K05.10
- glanders A24.0
- glenosporopsis B48.0
- Gnathostoma (spinigerum) B83.1
- Gongylonema B83.8
- gonococcal — *see* Gonococcus
- gram-negative bacilli NOS A49.9
- guinea worm B72
- gum (chronic) K05.10
  - acute K05.00
    - nonplaque induced K05.01
    - plaque induced K05.00
  - nonplaque induced K05.11
  - plaque induced K05.10
- Haemophilus — *see* Infection, Hemophilus
- heart — *see* Carditis
- Helicobacter pylori A04.8
  - as cause of disease classified elsewhere B96.81
- helminths B83.9
  - intestinal B82.0
    - mixed (types classifiable to more than one of the titles B65.0-B81.3 and B81.8) B81.4
    - specified type NEC B81.8
  - specified type NEC B83.8
- Hemophilus
  - aegyptius, systemic A48.4
  - ducrey (any location) A57
  - generalized A41.3
  - influenzae NEC A49.2
    - as cause of disease classified elsewhere B96.3
- herpes (simplex) (*see also* Herpes)
  - congenital P35.2
  - disseminated B00.7
  - zoster B02.9
- herpesvirus, herpesviral — *see* Herpes
- Heterophyes (heterophyes) B66.8
- hip (joint) NEC M00.9
  - due to internal joint prosthesis
    - left T84.52 ☑
    - right T84.51 ☑
  - skin NEC L08.9
- Histoplasma — *see* Histoplasmosis
  - American B39.4
  - capsulatum B39.4
- hookworm B76.9
- human
  - papilloma virus A63.0
  - T-cell lymphotropic virus type-1 (HTLV-1) B33.3
- hydrocele N43.0
- Hymenolepis B71.0
- hypopharynx — *see* Pharyngitis
- inguinal (lymph) glands L04.1
  - due to soft chancre A57
- intervertebral disc, pyogenic M46.30
  - cervical region M46.32
  - cervicothoracic region M46.33
  - lumbar region M46.36
  - lumbosacral region M46.37
  - multiple sites M46.39
  - occipito-atlanto-axial region M46.31

Infection, infected, infective — *continued*
- intervertebral disc, pyogenic — *continued*
  - sacrococcygeal region M46.38
  - thoracic region M46.34
  - thoracolumbar region M46.35
- intestine, intestinal — *see* Enteritis, infectious
  - specified NEC A08.8
- intra-amniotic affecting newborn NEC P39.2
- Isospora belli or hominis A07.3
- Japanese B encephalitis A83.0
- jaw (bone) (lower) (upper) M27.2
- joint NEC M00.9
  - due to internal joint prosthesis T84.50 ☑
- kidney (cortex) (hematogenous) N15.9
  - with calculus N20.0
    - with hydronephrosis N13.6
  - following ectopic gestation O08.83
  - pelvis and ureter (cystic) N28.85
  - puerperal (postpartum) O86.21
  - specified NEC N15.8
- Klebsiella (K.) pneumoniae NEC A49.8
  - as cause of disease classified elsewhere B96.1
- knee (joint) NEC M00.9
  - due to internal joint prosthesis
    - left T84.54 ☑
    - right T84.53 ☑
  - joint M00.9
  - skin L08.9
- Koch's — *see* Tuberculosis
- labia (majora) (minora) (acute) — *see* Vulvitis
- lacrimal
  - gland — *see* Dacryoadenitis
  - passages (duct) (sac) — *see* Inflammation, lacrimal, passages
- lancet fluke B66.2
- larynx NEC J38.7
- leg (skin) NOS L08.9
- Legionella pneumophila A48.1
  - nonpneumonic A48.2
- Leishmania (*see also* Leishmaniasis)
  - aethiopica B55.1
  - braziliensis B55.2
  - chagasi B55.0
  - donovani B55.0
  - infantum B55.0
  - major B55.1
  - mexicana B55.1
  - tropica B55.1
- lentivirus, as cause of disease classified elsewhere B97.31
- Leptosphaeria senegalensis B47.0
- Leptospira interrogans A27.9
  - autumnalis A27.89
  - canicola A27.89
  - hebdomadis A27.89
  - icterohaemorrhagiae A27.0
  - pomona A27.89
  - specified type NEC A27.89
- leptospirochetal NEC — *see* Leptospirosis
- Listeria monocytogenes (*see also* Listeriosis)
  - congenital P37.2
- Loa loa B74.3
  - with conjunctival infestation B74.3
  - eyelid B74.3
- Loboa loboi B48.0
- local, skin (staphylococcal) (streptococcal) L08.9
  - abscess — *code by* site under Abscess
  - cellulitis — *code by* site under Cellulitis
  - specified NEC L08.89
  - ulcer — *see* Ulcer, skin
- Loefflerella mallei A24.0
- lung (*see also* Pneumonia) J18.9
  - atypical Mycobacterium A31.0
  - spirochetal A69.8
  - tuberculous — *see* Tuberculosis, pulmonary
  - virus — *see* Pneumonia, viral
- lymph gland (*see also* Lymphadenitis, acute)
  - mesenteric I88.0
- lymphoid tissue, base of tongue or posterior pharynx, NEC (chronic) J35.03
- Madurella (grisea) (mycetomii) B47.0
- major
  - following ectopic or molar pregnancy O08.0
  - puerperal, postpartum, childbirth O85
- Malassezia furfur B36.0
- Malleomyces
  - mallei A24.0
  - pseudomallei (whitmori) — *see* Melioidosis

Infection, infected, infective — *continued*
- mammary gland N61
- Mansonella (ozzardi) (perstans) (streptocerca) B74.4
- mastoid — *see* Mastoiditis
- maxilla, maxillary M27.2
  - sinus (chronic) — *see* Sinusitis, maxillary
- mediastinum J98.5
- Medina (worm) B72
- meibomian cyst or gland — *see* Hordeolum
- meninges — *see* Meningitis, bacterial
- meningococcal (*see also* condition) A39.9
  - adrenals A39.1
  - brain A39.81
  - cerebrospinal A39.0
  - conjunctiva A39.89
  - endocardium A39.51
  - heart A39.50
    - endocardium A39.51
    - myocardium A39.52
    - pericardium A39.53
  - joint A39.83
  - meninges A39.0
  - meningococcemia A39.4
    - acute A39.2
    - chronic A39.3
  - myocardium A39.52
  - pericardium A39.53
  - retrobulbar neuritis A39.82
  - specified site NEC A39.89
- mesenteric lymph nodes or glands NEC I88.0
- Metagonimus B66.8
- metatarsophalangeal M00.9
- methicillin
  - resistant Staphylococcus aureus (MRSA) A49.02
  - susceptible Staphylococcus aureus (MSSA) A49.01
- Microsporum, microsporic — *see* Dermatophytosis
- mixed flora (bacterial) NEC A49.8
- Monilia — *see* Candidiasis
- Monosporium apiospermum B48.2
- mouth, parasitic B37.0
- Mucor — *see* Mucormycosis
- muscle NEC — *see* Myositis, infective
- mycelium NOS B49
- mycetoma B47.9
  - actinomycotic NEC B47.1
  - mycotic NEC B47.0
- Mycobacterium, mycobacterial — *see* Mycobacterium
- Mycoplasma NEC A49.3
  - pneumoniae, as cause of disease classified elsewhere B96.0
- mycotic NOS B49
  - pathogenic to compromised host only B48.8
  - skin NOS B36.9
- myocardium NEC I40.0
- nail (chronic)
  - with lymphangitis — *see* Lymphangitis, acute, digit
  - finger L03.01- ☑
    - fungus B35.1
  - ingrowing L60.0
  - toe L03.03- ☑
    - fungus B35.1
- nasal sinus (chronic) — *see* Sinusitis
- nasopharynx — *see* Nasopharyngitis
- navel L08.82
- Necator americanus B76.1
- Neisseria — *see* Gonococcus
- Neotestudina rosatii B47.0
- newborn P39.9
  - intra-amniotic NEC P39.2
  - skin P39.4
  - specified type NEC P39.8
- nipple N61
  - associated with
    - lactation O91.03
    - pregnancy O91.01- ☑
    - puerperium O91.02
- Nocardia — *see* Nocardiosis
- obstetrical surgical wound (puerperal) O86.0
- Oesophagostomum (apiostomum) B81.8
- Oestrus ovis — *see* Myiasis
- Oidium albicans B37.9
- Onchocerca (volvulus) — *see* Onchocerciasis
- oncovirus, as cause of disease classified elsewhere B97.32
- operation wound T81.4 ☑
- Opisthorchis (felineus) (viverrini) B66.0
- orbit, orbital — *see* Inflammation, orbit

Infection, infected, infective — *continued*
  orthopoxvirus NEC B08.09
  ovary — *see* Salpingo-oophoritis
  Oxyuris vermicularis B80
  pancreas (acute) K85.9
    abscess — *see* Pancreatitis, acute
    specified NEC K85.8
  papillomavirus, as cause of disease classified elsewhere
      B97.7
  papovavirus NEC B34.4
  Paracoccidioides brasiliensis — *see* Paracoccidioidomy-
      cosis
  Paragonimus (westermani) B66.4
  parainfluenza virus B34.8
  parameningococcus NOS A39.9
  parapoxvirus B08.60
    specified NEC B08.69
  parasitic B89
  Parastrongylus
    cantonensis B83.2
    costaricensis B81.3
    paratyphoid A01.4
      Type A A01.1
      Type B A01.2
      Type C A01.3
  paraurethral ducts N34.2
  parotid gland — *see* Sialoadenitis
  parvovirus NEC B34.3
    as cause of disease classified elsewhere B97.6
  Pasteurella NEC A28.0
    multocida A28.0
    pestis — *see* Plague
    pseudotuberculosis A28.0
    septica (cat bite) (dog bite) A28.0
    tularensis — *see* Tularemia
  pelvic, female — *see* Disease, pelvis, inflammatory
  Penicillium (marneffei) B48.4
  penis (glans) (retention) NEC N48.29
  periapical K04.5
  peridental, periodontal K05.20
    generalized K05.22
    localized K05.21
  perinatal period P39.9
    specified type NEC P39.8
  perineal repair (puerperal) O86.0
  periorbital — *see* Inflammation, orbit
  perirectal K62.89
  perirenal — *see* Infection, kidney
  peritoneal — *see* Peritonitis
  periureteral N28.89
  Petriellidium boydii B48.2
  pharynx (*see also* Pharyngitis)
    coxsackievirus B08.5
    posterior, lymphoid (chronic) J35.03
  Phialophora
    gougerotii (subcutaneous abscess or cyst) B43.2
    jeanselmei (subcutaneous abscess or cyst) B43.2
    verrucosa (skin) B43.0
  Piedraia hortae B36.3
  pinta A67.9
    intermediate A67.1
    late A67.2
    mixed A67.3
    primary A67.0
  pinworm B80
  pityrosporum furfur B36.0
  pleuro-pneumonia-like organism (PPLO) NEC A49.3
    as cause of disease classified elsewhere B96.0
  pneumococcus, pneumococcal NEC A49.1
    as cause of disease classified elsewhere B95.3
    generalized (purulent) A40.3
      with pneumonia J13
  Pneumocystis carinii (pneumonia) B59
  Pneumocystis jiroveci (pneumonia) B59
  port or reservoir T80.212 ☑
  postoperative T81.4 ☑
  postoperative wound T81.4 ☑
  postprocedural T81.4 ☑
  postvaccinal T88.0 ☑
  prepuce NEC N47.7
    with penile inflammation N47.6
  prion — *see* Disease, prion, central nervous system
  prostate (capsule) — *see* Prostatitis
  Proteus (mirabilis) (morganii) (vulgaris) NEC A49.8
    as cause of disease classified elsewhere B96.4
  protozoal NEC B64
    intestinal A07.9
      specified NEC A07.8

Infection, infected, infective — *continued*
  protozoal — *continued*
    specified NEC B60.8
  Pseudoallescheria boydii B48.2
  Pseudomonas NEC A49.8
    as cause of disease classified elsewhere B96.5
    mallei A24.0
    pneumonia J15.1
    pseudomallei — *see* Melioidosis
  puerperal O86.4
    genitourinary tract NEC O86.89
    major or generalized O85
    minor O86.4
    specified NEC O86.89
  pulmonary — *see* Infection, lung
  purulent — *see* Abscess
  Pyrenochaeta romeroi B47.0
  Q fever A78
  rectum (sphincter) K62.89
  renal (*see also* Infection, kidney)
    pelvis and ureter (cystic) N28.85
  reovirus, as cause of disease classified elsewhere B97.5
  respiratory (tract) NEC J98.8
    acute J22
    chronic J98.8
    influenzal (upper) (acute) — *see* Influenza, with,
        respiratory manifestations NEC
    lower (acute) J22
      chronic — *see* Bronchitis, chronic
    rhinovirus J00
    syncytial virus, as cause of disease classified else-
        where B97.4
    upper (acute) NOS J06.9
      chronic J39.8
      streptococcal J06.9
      viral NOS J06.9
  resulting from
    presence of internal prosthesis, implant, graft —
        see Complications, by site and type, infection
  retortamoniasis A07.8
  retroperitoneal NEC K68.9
  retrovirus B33.3
    as cause of disease classified elsewhere B97.30
    human
      immunodeficiency, type 2 (HIV 2) B97.35
      T-cell lymphotropic
        type I (HTLV-I) B97.33
        type II (HTLV-II) B97.34
    lentivirus B97.31
    oncovirus B97.32
    specified NEC B97.39
  Rhinosporidium (seeberi) B48.1
  rhinovirus
    as cause of disease classified elsewhere B97.89
    unspecified nature or site B34.8
  Rhizopus — *see* Mucormycosis
  rickettsial NOS A79.9
  roundworm (large) NEC B82.0
    Ascariasis (*see also* Ascariasis) B77.9
  rubella — *see* Rubella
  Saccharomyces — *see* Candidiasis
  salivary duct or gland (any) — *see* Sialoadenitis
  Salmonella (aertrycke) (arizonae) (callinarum)
      (cholerae-suis) (enteritidis) (suipestifer) (ty-
      phimurium) A02.9
    with
      (gastro)enteritis A02.0
      sepsis A02.1
      specified manifestation NEC A02.8
    due to food (poisoning) A02.9
    hirschfeldii A01.3
    localized A02.20
      arthritis A02.23
      meningitis A02.21
      osteomyelitis A02.24
      pneumonia A02.22
      pyelonephritis A02.25
      specified NEC A02.29
    paratyphi A01.4
      A A01.1
      B A01.2
      C A01.3
    schottmuelleri A01.2
    typhi, typhosa — *see* Typhoid
  Sarcocystis A07.8
  scabies B86
  Schistosoma — *see* Infestation, Schistosoma
  scrotum (acute) NEC N49.2

Infection, infected, infective — *continued*
  seminal vesicle — *see* Vesiculitis
  septic
    localized, skin — *see* Abscess
  sheep liver fluke B66.3
  Shigella A03.9
    boydii A03.2
    dysenteriae A03.0
    flexneri A03.1
    group
      A A03.0
      B A03.1
      C A03.2
      D A03.3
    Schmitz (-Stutzer) A03.0
    schmitzii A03.0
    shigae A03.0
    sonnei A03.3
    specified NEC A03.8
  shoulder (joint) NEC M00.9
    due to internal joint prosthesis T84.59 ☑
    skin NEC L08.9
  sinus (accessory) (chronic) (nasal) (*see also* Sinusitis)
    pilonidal — *see* Sinus, pilonidal
    skin NEC L08.89
  Skene's duct or gland — *see* Urethritis
  skin (local) (staphylococcal) (streptococcal) L08.9
    abscess — *code by* site under Abscess
    cellulitis — *code by* site under Cellulitis
    due to fungus B36.9
      specified type NEC B36.8
    mycotic B36.9
      specified type NEC B36.8
    newborn P39.4
    ulcer — *see* Ulcer, skin
  slow virus A81.9
    specified NEC A81.89
  Sparganum (mansoni) (proliferum) (baxteri) B70.1
  specific (*see also* Syphilis)
    to perinatal period — *see* Infection, congenital
  specified NEC B99.8
  spermatic cord NEC N49.1
  sphenoidal (sinus) — *see* Sinusitis, sphenoidal
  spinal cord NOS (*see also* Myelitis) G04.91
    abscess G06.1
    meninges — *see* Meningitis
    streptococcal G04.89
  Spirillum A25.0
  spirochetal NOS A69.9
    lung A69.8
    specified NEC A69.8
  Spirometra larvae B70.1
  spleen D73.89
  Sporotrichum, Sporothrix (schenckii) — *see* Sporotri-
      chosis
  staphylococcal, unspecified site
    as cause of disease classified elsewhere B95.8
      aureus (methicillin susceptible) (MSSA) B95.61
        methicillin resistant (MRSA) B95.62
      specified NEC B95.7
    aureus (methicillin susceptible) (MSSA) A49.01
      methicillin resistant (MRSA) A49.02
    food poisoning A05.0
    generalized (purulent) A41.2
    pneumonia — *see* Pneumonia, staphylococcal
  Stellantchasmus falcatus B66.8
  streptobacillus moniliformis A25.1
  streptococcal NEC A49.1
    as cause of disease classified elsewhere B95.5
    B genitourinary complicating
      childbirth O98.82
      pregnancy O98.81- ☑
      puerperium O98.83
    congenital
      sepsis P36.10
        group B P36.0
        specified NEC P36.19
    generalized (purulent) A40.9
  Streptomyces B47.1
  Strongyloides (stercoralis) — *see* Strongyloidiasis
  stump (amputation) (surgical) — *see* Complication,
      amputation stump, infection
  subcutaneous tissue, local L08.9
  suipestifer — *see* Infection, salmonella
  swimming pool bacillus A31.1
  Taenia — *see* Infestation, Taenia
  Taeniarhynchus saginatus B68.1
  tapeworm — *see* Infestation, tapeworm

Index

Infection, infected, infective — Infestation

Infection, infected, infective — *continued*
tendon (sheath) — *see* Tenosynovitis, infective NEC
Ternidens diminutus B81.8
testis — *see* Orchitis
threadworm B80
throat — *see* Pharyngitis
thyroglossal duct K14.8
toe (skin) L08.9
  cellulitis L03.03- ☑
    fungus B35.1
  nail L03.03- ☑
    fungus B35.1
tongue NEC K14.0
  parasitic B37.0
tonsil (and adenoid) (faucial) (lingual) (pharyngeal) —
    see Tonsillitis
tooth, teeth K04.7
  periapical K04.7
  peridental, periodontal K05.20
    generalized K05.22
    localized K05.21
  pulp K04.0
  socket M27.3
TORCH — *see* Infection, congenital
  without active infection P00.2
Torula histolytica — *see* Cryptococcosis
Toxocara (canis) (cati) (felis) B83.0
Toxoplasma gondii — *see* Toxoplasma
trachea, chronic J42
trematode NEC — *see* Infestation, fluke
trench fever A79.0
Treponema pallidum — *see* Syphilis
Trichinella (spiralis) B75
Trichomonas A59.9
  cervix A59.09
  intestine A07.8
  prostate A59.02
  specified site NEC A59.8
  urethra A59.03
  urogenitalis A59.00
  vagina A59.01
  vulva A59.01
Trichophyton, trichophytic — *see* Dermatophytosis
Trichosporon (beigelii) cutaneum B36.2
Trichostrongylus B81.2
Trichuris (trichiura) B79
Trombicula (irritans) B88.0
Trypanosoma
  brucei
    gambiense B56.0
    rhodesiense B56.1
  cruzi — *see* Chagas' disease
tubal — *see* Salpingo-oophoritis
tuberculous NEC — *see* Tuberculosis
tubo-ovarian — *see* Salpingo-oophoritis
tunica vaginalis N49.1
tunnel T80.212 ☑
tympanic membrane NEC — *see* Myringitis
typhoid (abortive) (ambulant) (bacillus) — *see* Typhoid
typhus A75.9
  flea-borne A75.2
  mite-borne A75.3
  recrudescent A75.1
  tick-borne A77.9
    African A77.1
    North Asian A77.2
umbilicus L08.82
ureter N28.86
urethra — *see* Urethritis
urinary (tract) N39.0
  bladder — *see* Cystitis
  complicating
    pregnancy O23.4- ☑
      specified type NEC O23.3- ☑
  kidney — *see* Infection, kidney
  newborn P39.3
  puerperal (postpartum) O86.20
  tuberculous A18.13
  urethra — *see* Urethritis
uterus, uterine — *see* Endometritis
vaccination T88.0 ☑
vaccinia not from vaccination B08.011
vagina (acute) — *see* Vaginitis
varicella B01.9
varicose veins — *see* Varix
vas deferens NEC N49.1
vesical — *see* Cystitis

Infection, infected, infective — *continued*
Vibrio
  cholerae A00.0
    El Tor A00.1
  parahaemolyticus (food poisoning) A05.3
  vulnificus
    as cause of disease classified elsewhere B96.82
    foodborne intoxication A05.5
Vincent's (gum) (mouth) (tonsil) A69.1
virus, viral NOS B34.9
  adenovirus
    as cause of disease classified elsewhere B97.0
    unspecified nature or site B34.0
  arborvirus, arbovirus arthropod-borne A94
  as cause of disease classified elsewhere B97.89
    adenovirus B97.0
    coronavirus B97.29
      SARS-associated B97.21
    coxsackievirus B97.11
    echovirus B97.12
    enterovirus B97.10
      coxsackievirus B97.11
      echovirus B97.12
      specified NEC B97.19
    human
      immunodeficiency, type 2 (HIV 2) B97.35
      metapneumovirus B97.81
      T-cell lymphotropic,
        type I (HTLV-I) B97.33
        type II (HTLV-II) B97.34
    papillomavirus B97.7
    parvovirus B97.6
    reovirus B97.5
    respiratory syncytial B97.4
    retrovirus B97.30
      human
        immunodeficiency, type 2 (HIV 2) B97.35
        T-cell lymphotropic,
          type I (HTLV-I) B97.33
          type II (HTLV-II) B97.34
      lentivirus B97.31
      oncovirus B97.32
      specified NEC B97.39
    specified NEC B97.89
  central nervous system A89
    atypical A81.9
      specified NEC A81.89
    enterovirus NEC A88.8
      meningitis A87.0
    slow virus A81.9
      specified NEC A81.89
    specified NEC A88.8
  chest J98.8
  cotia B08.8
  coxsackie (*see also* Infection, coxsackie) B34.1
    as cause of disease classified elsewhere B97.11
  ECHO
    as cause of disease classified elsewhere B97.12
    unspecified nature or site B34.1
  encephalitis, tick-borne A84.9
  enterovirus, as cause of disease classified elsewhere
    B97.10
    coxsackievirus B97.11
    echovirus B97.12
    specified NEC B97.19
  exanthem NOS B09
  human metapneumovirus as cause of disease
    classified elsewhere B97.81
  human papilloma as cause of disease classified
    elsewhere B97.7
  intestine — *see* Enteritis, viral
  respiratory syncytial
    as cause of disease classified elsewhere B97.4
    bronchopneumonia J12.1
    common cold syndrome J00
    nasopharyngitis (acute) J00
  rhinovirus
    as cause of disease classified elsewhere B97.89
    unspecified nature or site B34.8
  slow A81.9
    specified NEC A81.89
  specified type NEC B33.8
    as cause of disease classified elsewhere B97.89
    unspecified nature or site B34.8
  unspecified nature or site B34.9
  West Nile — *see* Virus, West Nile
vulva (acute) — *see* Vulvitis
West Nile — *see* Virus, West Nile

Infection, infected, infective — *continued*
whipworm B79
worms B83.9
  specified type NEC B83.8
Wuchereria (bancrofti) B74.0
  malayi B74.1
yatapoxvirus B08.70
  specified NEC B08.79
yeast (*see also* Candidiasis) B37.9
yellow fever — *see* Fever, yellow
Yersinia
  enterocolitica (intestinal) A04.6
  pestis — *see* Plague
  pseudotuberculosis A28.2
Zeis' gland — *see* Hordeolum
zoonotic bacterial NOS A28.9
Zopfia senegalensis B47.0
Infective, infectious — *see* condition
Infertility
female N97.9
  age-related N97.8
  associated with
    anovulation N97.0
    cervical (mucus) disease or anomaly N88.3
    congenital anomaly
      cervix N88.3
      fallopian tube N97.1
      uterus N97.2
      vagina N97.8
    dysmucorrhea N88.3
    fallopian tube disease or anomaly N97.1
    pituitary-hypothalamic origin E23.0
    specified origin NEC N97.8
    Stein-Leventhal syndrome E28.2
    uterine disease or anomaly N97.2
    vaginal disease or anomaly N97.8
  due to
    cervical anomaly N88.3
    fallopian tube anomaly N97.1
    ovarian failure E28.39
    Stein-Leventhal syndrome E28.2
    uterine anomaly N97.2
    vaginal anomaly N97.8
  nonimplantation N97.2
  origin
    cervical N88.3
    tubal (block) (occlusion) (stenosis) N97.1
    uterine N97.2
    vaginal N97.8
male N46.9
  azoospermia N46.01
    extratesticular cause N46.029
      drug therapy N46.021
      efferent duct obstruction N46.023
      infection N46.022
      radiation N46.024
      specified cause NEC N46.029
      systemic disease N46.025
  oligospermia N46.11
    extratesticular cause N46.129
      drug therapy N46.121
      efferent duct obstruction N46.123
      infection N46.122
      radiation N46.124
      specified cause NEC N46.129
      systemic disease N46.125
  specified type NEC N46.8
Infestation B88.9
Acanthocheilonema (perstans) (streptocerca) B74.4
Acariasis B88.0
  demodex folliculorum B88.0
  sarcoptes scabiei B86
  trombiculae B88.0
Agamofilaria streptocerca B74.4
Ancylostoma, ankylostoma (braziliense) (caninum)
  (ceylanicum) (duodenale) B76.0
  americanum B76.1
  new world B76.1
Anisakis larvae, anisakiasis B81.0
arthropod NEC B88.2
Ascaris lumbricoides — *see* Ascariasis
Balantidium coli A07.0
beef tapeworm B68.1
Bothriocephalus (latus) B70.0
  larval B70.1
broad tapeworm B70.0
  larval B70.1
Brugia (malayi) B74.1

☑ **Additional Character Required** — Refer to the Tabular List for Character Selection   ▽ **Subterms under main terms may continue to next column or page**

Infestation — *continued*
  Brugia — *continued*
    timori B74.2
  candiru B88.8
  Capillaria
    hepatica B83.8
    philippinensis B81.1
  cat liver fluke B66.0
  cestodes B71.9
    diphyllobothrium — *see* Infestation, diphyllobothrium
    dipylidiasis B71.1
    hymenolepiasis B71.0
    specified type NEC B71.8
  chigger B88.0
  chigo, chigoe B88.1
  Clonorchis (sinensis) (liver) B66.1
  coccidial A07.3
  crab-lice B85.3
  Cysticercus cellulosae — *see* Cysticercosis
  Demodex (folliculorum) B88.0
  Dermanyssus gallinae B88.0
  Dermatobia (hominis) — *see* Myiasis
  Dibothriocephalus (latus) B70.0
    larval B70.1
  Dicrocoelium dendriticum B66.2
  Diphyllobothrium (adult) (latum) (intestinal) (pacificum) B70.0
    larval B70.1
  Diplogonoporus (grandis) B71.8
  Dipylidium caninum B67.4
  Distoma hepaticum B66.3
  dog tapeworm B67.4
  Dracunculus medinensis B72
  dragon worm B72
  dwarf tapeworm B71.0
  Echinococcus — *see* Echinococcus
  Echinostomum ilocanum B66.8
  Entamoeba (histolytica) — *see* Infection, Ameba
  Enterobius vermicularis B80
  eyelid
    in (due to)
      leishmaniasis B55.1
      loiasis B74.3
      onchocerciasis B73.09
      phthiriasis B85.3
      parasitic NOS B89
  eyeworm B74.3
  Fasciola (gigantica) (hepatica) (indica) B66.3
  Fasciolopsis (buski) (intestine) B66.5
  filarial B74.9
    bancroftian B74.0
    conjunctiva B74.9
    due to
      Acanthocheilonema (perstans) (streptocerca) B74.4
      Brugia (malayi) B74.1
        timori B74.2
      Dracunculus medinensis B72
      guinea worm B72
      loa loa B74.3
      Mansonella (ozzardi) (perstans) (streptocerca) B74.4
      Onchocerca volvulus B73.00
        eye B73.00
        eyelid B73.09
      Wuchereria (bancrofti) B74.0
    Malayan B74.1
    ozzardi B74.4
    specified type NEC B74.8
  fish tapeworm B70.0
    larval B70.1
  fluke B66.9
    blood NOS — *see* Schistosomiasis
    cat liver B66.0
    intestinal B66.5
    lancet B66.2
    liver (sheep) B66.3
      cat B66.0
      Chinese B66.1
      due to clonorchiasis B66.1
      oriental B66.1
    lung (oriental) B66.4
    sheep liver B66.3
    specified type NEC B66.8
  fly larvae — *see* Myiasis
  Gasterophilus (intestinalis) — *see* Myiasis
  Gastrodiscoides hominis B66.8

Infestation — *continued*
  Giardia lamblia A07.1
  Gnathostoma (spinigerum) B83.1
  Gongylonema B83.8
  guinea worm B72
  helminth B83.9
    angiostrongyliasis B83.2
      intestinal B81.3
    gnathostomiasis B83.1
    hirudiniasis, internal B83.4
    intestinal B82.0
      angiostrongyliasis B81.3
      anisakiasis B81.0
      ascariasis — *see* Ascariasis
      capillariasis B81.1
      cysticercosis — *see* Cysticercosis
      diphyllobothriasis — *see* Infestation, diphyllobothriasis
      dracunculiasis B72
      echinococcus — *see* Echinococcosis
      enterobiasis B80
      filariasis — *see* Infestation, filarial
      fluke — *see* Infestation, fluke
      hookworm — *see* Infestation, hookworm
      mixed (types classifiable to more than one of the titles B65.0-B81.3 and B81.8) B81.4
      onchocerciasis — *see* Onchocerciasis
      schistosomiasis — *see* Infestation, schistosoma
      specified
        cestode NEC — *see* Infestation, cestode
        type NEC B81.8
      strongyloidiasis — *see* Strongyloidiasis
      taenia — *see* Infestation, taenia
      trichinellosis B75
      trichostrongyliasis B81.2
      trichuriasis B79
    specified type NEC B83.8
    syngamiasis B83.3
    visceral larva migrans B83.0
  Heterophyes (heterophyes) B66.8
  hookworm B76.9
    ancylostomiasis B76.0
    necatoriasis B76.1
    specified type NEC B76.8
  Hymenolepis (diminuta) (nana) B71.0
  intestinal NEC B82.9
  leeches (aquatic) (land) — *see* Hirudiniasis
  Leishmania — *see* Leishmaniasis
  lice, louse — *see* Infestation, Pediculus
  Linguatula B88.8
  Liponyssoides sanguineus B88.0
  Loa loa B74.3
    conjunctival B74.3
    eyelid B74.3
  louse — *see* Infestation, Pediculus
  maggots — *see* Myiasis
  Mansonella (ozzardi) (perstans) (streptocerca) B74.4
  Medina (worm) B72
  Metagonimus (yokogawai) B66.8
  microfilaria streptocerca — *see* Onchocerciasis
    eye B73.00
    eyelid B73.09
  mites B88.9
    scabic B86
  Monilia (albicans) — *see* Candidiasis
  mouth B37.0
  Necator americanus B76.1
  nematode NEC (intestinal) B82.0
    Ancylostoma B76.0
    conjunctiva NEC B83.9
    Enterobius vermicularis B80
    Gnathostoma spinigerum B83.1
    physaloptera B80
    specified NEC B81.8
    trichostrongylus B81.2
    trichuris (trichuria) B79
  Oesophagostomum (apiostomum) B81.8
  Oestrus ovis (see also Myiasis) B87.9
  Onchocerca (volvulus) — *see* Onchocerciasis
  Opisthorchis (felineus) (viverrini) B66.0
  orbit, parasitic NOS B89
  Oxyuris vermicularis B80
  Paragonimus (westermani) B66.4
  parasite, parasitic B89
    eyelid B89
    intestinal NOS B82.9
    mouth B37.0
    skin B88.9

Infestation — *continued*
  parasite, parasitic — *continued*
    tongue B37.0
  Parastrongylus
    cantonensis B83.2
    costaricensis B81.3
  Pediculus B85.2
    body B85.1
    capitis (humanus) (any site) B85.0
    corporis (humanus) (any site) B85.1
    head B85.0
    mixed (classifiable to more than one of the titles B85.0 - B85.3) B85.4
    pubis (any site) B85.3
  Pentastoma B88.8
  Phthirus (pubis) (any site) B85.3
    with any infestation classifiable to B85.0 - B85.2 B85.4
  pinworm B80
  pork tapeworm (adult) B68.0
  protozoal NEC B64
    intestinal A07.9
      specified NEC A07.8
    specified NEC B60.8
  pubic, louse B85.3
  rat tapeworm B71.0
  red bug B88.0
  roundworm (large) NEC B82.0
    Ascariasis (see also Ascariasis) B77.9
  sandflea B88.1
  Sarcoptes scabiei B86
  scabies B86
  Schistosoma B65.9
    bovis B65.8
    cercariae B65.3
    haematobium B65.0
    intercalatum B65.8
    japonicum B65.2
    mansoni B65.1
    mattheei B65.8
    mekongi B65.8
    specified type NEC B65.8
    spindale B65.8
  screw worms — *see* Myiasis
  skin NOS B88.9
  Sparganum (mansoni) (proliferum) (baxteri) B70.1
    larval B70.1
  specified type NEC B88.8
  Spirometra larvae B70.1
  Stellantchasmus falcatus B66.8
  Strongyloides stercoralis — *see* Strongyloidiasis
  Taenia B68.9
    diminuta B71.0
    echinococcus — *see* Echinococcus
    mediocanellata B68.1
    nana B71.0
    saginata B68.1
    solium (intestinal form) B68.0
      larval form — *see* Cysticercosis
  Taeniarhynchus saginatus B68.1
  tapeworm B71.9
    beef B68.1
    broad B70.0
      larval B70.1
    dog B67.4
    dwarf B71.0
    fish B70.0
      larval B70.1
    pork B68.0
    rat B71.0
  Ternidens diminutus B81.8
  Tetranychus molestissimus B88.0
  threadworm B80
  tongue B37.0
  Toxocara (canis) (cati) (felis) B83.0
  trematode(s) NEC — *see* Infestation, fluke
  Trichinella (spiralis) B75
  Trichocephalus B79
  Trichomonas — *see* Trichomoniasis
  Trichostrongylus B81.2
  Trichuris (trichiura) B79
  Trombicula (irritans) B88.0
  Tunga penetrans B88.1
  Uncinaria americana B76.1
  Vandellia cirrhosa B88.8
  whipworm B79
  worms B83.9
    intestinal B82.0

Infestation — *continued*
  Wuchereria (bancrofti) B74.0
Infiltrate, infiltration
  amyloid (generalized) (localized) — *see* Amyloidosis
  calcareous NEC R89.7
    localized — *see* Degeneration, by site
  calcium salt R89.7
  cardiac
    fatty — *see* Degeneration, myocardial
    glycogenic E74.02 [I43]
  corneal — *see* Edema, cornea
  eyelid — *see* Inflammation, eyelid
  glycogen, glycogenic — *see* Disease, glycogen storage
  heart, cardiac
    fatty — *see* Degeneration, myocardial
    glycogenic E74.02 [I43]
  inflammatory in vitreous H43.89
  kidney N28.89
  leukemic — *see* Leukemia
  liver K76.89
    fatty — *see* Fatty, liver NEC
    glycogen (*see also* Disease, glycogen storage)
      E74.03 [K77]
  lung R91.8
    eosinophilic J82
  lymphatic (*see also* Leukemia, lymphatic) C91.9- ☑
    gland I88.9
  muscle, fatty M62.89
  myocardium, myocardial
    fatty — *see* Degeneration, myocardial
    glycogenic E74.02 [I43]
  on chest x-ray R91.8
  pulmonary R91.8
    with eosinophilia J82
  skin (lymphocytic) L98.6
  thymus (gland) (fatty) E32.8
  urine R39.0
  vesicant agent
    antineoplastic chemotherapy T80.810 ☑
    other agent NEC T80.818 ☑
  vitreous body H43.89
Infirmity R68.89
  senile R54
Inflammation, inflamed, inflammatory (with exudation)
  abducent (nerve) — *see* Strabismus, paralytic, sixth nerve
  accessory sinus (chronic) — *see* Sinusitis
  adrenal (gland) E27.8
  alveoli, teeth M27.3
    scorbutic E54
  anal canal, anus K62.89
  antrum (chronic) — *see* Sinusitis, maxillary
  appendix — *see* Appendicitis
  arachnoid — *see* Meningitis
  areola N61
    puerperal, postpartum or gestational — *see* Infection, nipple
  areolar tissue NOS L08.9
  artery — *see* Arteritis
  auditory meatus (external) — *see* Otitis, externa
  Bartholin's gland N75.8
  bile duct (common) (hepatic) or passage — *see* Cholangitis
  bladder — *see* Cystitis
  bone — *see* Osteomyelitis
  brain (*see also* Encephalitis)
    membrane — *see* Meningitis
  breast N61
    puerperal, postpartum, gestational — *see* Mastitis, obstetric
  broad ligament — *see* Disease, pelvis, inflammatory
  bronchi — *see* Bronchitis
  catarrhal J00
  cecum — *see* Appendicitis
  cerebral (*see also* Encephalitis)
    membrane — *see* Meningitis
  cerebrospinal
    meningococcal A39.0
  cervix (uteri) — *see* Cervicitis
  chest J98.8
  chorioretinal H30.9- ☑
    cyclitis — *see* Cyclitis
    disseminated H30.10- ☑
      generalized H30.13- ☑
      peripheral H30.12- ☑
      posterior pole H30.11- ☑

Inflammation, inflamed, inflammatory — *continued*
  chorioretinal — *continued*
    epitheliopathy — *see* Epitheliopathy
    focal H30.00- ☑
      juxtapapillary H30.01- ☑
      macular H30.04- ☑
      paramacular — *see* Inflammation, chorioretinal, focal, macular
      peripheral H30.03- ☑
      posterior pole H30.02- ☑
    specified type NEC H30.89- ☑
  choroid — *see* Inflammation, chorioretinal
  chronic, postmastoidectomy cavity — *see* Complications, postmastoidectomy, inflammation
  colon — *see* Enteritis
  connective tissue (diffuse) NEC — *see* Disorder, soft tissue, specified type NEC
  cornea — *see* Keratitis
  corpora cavernosa N48.29
  cranial nerve — *see* Disorder, nerve, cranial
  Douglas' cul-de-sac or pouch (chronic) N73.0
  due to device, implant or graft (*see also* Complications, by site and type, infection or inflammation)
    arterial graft T82.7 ☑
    breast (implant) T85.79 ☑
    catheter T85.79 ☑
      dialysis (renal) T82.7 ☑
        intraperitoneal T85.71 ☑
      infusion T82.7 ☑
        spinal (epidural) (subdural) T85.79 ☑
      urinary (indwelling) T83.51 ☑
    electronic (electrode) (pulse generator) (stimulator)
      bone T84.7 ☑
      cardiac T82.7 ☑
      nervous system (brain) (peripheral nerve) (spinal) T85.79 ☑
      urinary T83.59 ☑
    fixation, internal (orthopedic) NEC — *see* Complication, fixation device, infection
    gastrointestinal (bile duct) (esophagus) T85.79 ☑
    genital NEC T83.6 ☑
    heart NEC T82.7 ☑
      valve (prosthesis) T82.6 ☑
      graft T82.7 ☑
    joint prosthesis — *see* Complication, joint prosthesis, infection
    ocular (corneal graft) (orbital implant) NEC T85.79 ☑
    orthopedic NEC T84.7 ☑
    specified NEC T85.79 ☑
    urinary NEC T83.59 ☑
    vascular NEC T82.7 ☑
    ventricular intracranial shunt T85.79 ☑
  duodenum K29.80
    with bleeding K29.81
  dura mater — *see* Meningitis
  ear (middle) (*see also* Otitis, media)
    external — *see* Otitis, externa
    inner — *see* subcategory H83.0 ☑
  epididymis — *see* Epididymitis
  esophagus K20.9
  ethmoidal (sinus) (chronic) — *see* Sinusitis, ethmoidal
  eustachian tube (catarrhal) — *see* Salpingitis, eustachian
  eyelid H01.9
    abscess — *see* Abscess, eyelid
    blepharitis — *see* Blepharitis
    chalazion — *see* Chalazion
    dermatosis (noninfectious) — *see* Dermatosis, eyelid
    hordeolum — *see* Hordeolum
    specified NEC H01.8
  fallopian tube — *see* Salpingo-oophoritis
  fascia — *see* Myositis
  follicular, pharynx J31.2
  frontal (sinus) (chronic) — *see* Sinusitis, frontal
  gallbladder — *see* Cholecystitis
  gastric — *see* Gastritis
  gastrointestinal — *see* Enteritis
  genital organ (internal) (diffuse)
    female — *see* Disease, pelvis, inflammatory
    male N49.9
      multiple sites N49.8
      specified NEC N49.8
  gland (lymph) — *see* Lymphadenitis

Inflammation, inflamed, inflammatory — *continued*
  glottis — *see* Laryngitis
  granular, pharynx J31.2
  gum K05.10
    nonplaque induced K05.11
    plaque induced K05.10
  heart — *see* Carditis
  hepatic duct — *see* Cholangitis
  ileoanal (internal) pouch K91.850
  ileum (*see also* Enteritis)
    regional or terminal — *see* Enteritis, regional
  intestinal pouch K91.850
  intestine (any part) — *see* Enteritis
  jaw (acute) (bone) (chronic) (lower) (suppurative) (upper) M27.2
  joint NEC — *see* Arthritis
    sacroiliac M46.1
  kidney — *see* Nephritis
  knee (joint) M13.169
    tuberculous A18.02
  labium (majus) (minus) — *see* Vulvitis
  lacrimal
    gland — *see* Dacryoadenitis
    passages (duct) (sac) (*see also* Dacryocystitis)
      canaliculitis — *see* Canaliculitis, lacrimal
  larynx — *see* Laryngitis
  leg NOS L08.9
  lip K13.0
  liver (capsule) (*see also* Hepatitis)
    chronic K73.9
    suppurative K75.0
  lung (acute) (*see also* Pneumonia)
    chronic J98.4
  lymph gland or node — *see* Lymphadenitis
  lymphatic vessel — *see* Lymphangitis
  maxilla, maxillary M27.2
    sinus (chronic) — *see* Sinusitis, maxillary
  membranes of brain or spinal cord — *see* Meningitis
  meninges — *see* Meningitis
  mouth K12.1
  muscle — *see* Myositis
  myocardium — *see* Myocarditis
  nasal sinus (chronic) — *see* Sinusitis
  nasopharynx — *see* Nasopharyngitis
  navel L08.82
  nerve NEC — *see* Neuralgia
  nipple N61
    puerperal, postpartum or gestational — *see* Infection, nipple
  nose — *see* Rhinitis
  oculomotor (nerve) — *see* Strabismus, paralytic, third nerve
  optic nerve — *see* Neuritis, optic
  orbit (chronic) H05.10
    acute H05.00
      abscess — *see* Abscess, orbit
      cellulitis — *see* Cellulitis, orbit
      osteomyelitis — *see* Osteomyelitis, orbit
      periostitis — *see* Periostitis, orbital
      tenonitis — *see* Tenonitis, eye
    granuloma — *see* Granuloma, orbit
    myositis — *see* Myositis, orbital
  ovary — *see* Salpingo-oophoritis
  oviduct — *see* Salpingo-oophoritis
  pancreas (acute) — *see* Pancreatitis
  parametrium N73.0
  parotid region L08.9
  pelvis, female — *see* Disease, pelvis, inflammatory
  penis (corpora cavernosa) N48.29
  perianal K62.89
  pericardium — *see* Pericarditis
  perineum (female) (male) L08.9
  perirectal K62.89
  peritoneum — *see* Peritonitis
  periuterine — *see* Disease, pelvis, inflammatory
  perivesical — *see* Cystitis
  petrous bone (acute) (chronic) — *see* Petrositis
  pharynx (acute) — *see* Pharyngitis
  pia mater — *see* Meningitis
  pleura — *see* Pleurisy
  polyp, colon (*see also* Polyp, colon, inflammatory) K51.40
  prostate (*see also* Prostatitis)
    specified type NEC N41.8
  rectosigmoid — *see* Rectosigmoiditis
  rectum (*see also* Proctitis) K62.89

Inflammation, inflamed, inflammatory — *continued*
- respiratory, upper (*see also* Infection, respiratory, upper) J06.9
  - acute, due to radiation J70.0
  - chronic, due to external agent — *see* condition, respiratory, chronic, due to
  - due to
    - chemicals, gases, fumes or vapors (inhalation) J68.2
    - radiation J70.1
- retina — *see* Chorioretinitis
- retrocecal — *see* Appendicitis
- retroperitoneal — *see* Peritonitis
- salivary duct or gland (any) (suppurative) — *see* Sialoadenitis
- scorbutic, alveoli, teeth E54
- scrotum N49.2
- seminal vesicle — *see* Vesiculitis
- sigmoid — *see* Enteritis
- sinus — *see* Sinusitis
- Skene's duct or gland — *see* Urethritis
- skin L08.9
- spermatic cord N49.1
- sphenoidal (sinus) — *see* Sinusitis, sphenoidal
- spinal
  - cord — *see* Encephalitis
  - membrane — *see* Meningitis
  - nerve — *see* Disorder, nerve
- spine — *see* Spondylopathy, inflammatory
- spleen (capsule) D73.89
- stomach — *see* Gastritis
- subcutaneous tissue L08.9
- suprarenal (gland) E27.8
- synovial — *see* Tenosynovitis
- tendon (sheath) NEC — *see* Tenosynovitis
- testis — *see* Orchitis
- throat (acute) — *see* Pharyngitis
- thymus (gland) E32.8
- thyroid (gland) — *see* Thyroiditis
- tongue K14.0
- tonsil — *see* Tonsillitis
- trachea — *see* Tracheitis
- trochlear (nerve) — *see* Strabismus, paralytic, fourth nerve
- tubal — *see* Salpingo-oophoritis
- tuberculous NEC — *see* Tuberculosis
- tubo-ovarian — *see* Salpingo-oophoritis
- tunica vaginalis N49.1
- tympanic membrane — *see* Tympanitis
- umbilicus, umbilical L08.82
- uterine ligament — *see* Disease, pelvis, inflammatory
- uterus (catarrhal) — *see* Endometritis
- uveal tract (anterior) NOS (*see also* Iridocyclitis)
  - posterior — *see* Chorioretinitis
- vagina — *see* Vaginitis
- vas deferens N49.1
- vein (*see also* Phlebitis)
  - intracranial or intraspinal (septic) G08
  - thrombotic I80.9
    - leg — *see* Phlebitis, leg
    - lower extremity — *see* Phlebitis, leg
- vocal cord J38.3
- vulva — *see* Vulvitis
- Wharton's duct (suppurative) — *see* Sialoadenitis

Inflation, lung, imperfect (newborn) — *see* Atelectasis

Influenza (bronchial) (epidemic) (respiratory (upper)) (unidentified influenza virus) J11.1
- with
  - digestive manifestations J11.2
  - encephalopathy J11.81
  - enteritis J11.2
  - gastroenteritis J11.2
  - gastrointestinal manifestations J11.2
  - laryngitis J11.1
  - myocarditis J11.82
  - otitis media J11.83
  - pharyngitis J11.1
  - pneumonia J11.00
    - specified type J11.08
  - respiratory manifestations NEC J11.1
  - specified manifestation NEC J11.89
- A/H5N1 (*see also* Influenza, due to, identified novel influenza A virus) J09.X2
- avian (*see also* Influenza, due to, identified novel influenza A virus) J09.X2

Influenza — *continued*
- bird (*see also* Influenza, due to, identified novel influenza A virus) J09.X2
- due to
  - avian (*see also* Influenza, due to, identified novel influenza A virus) J09.X2
  - identified influenza virus NEC J10.1
    - with
      - digestive manifestations J10.2
      - encephalopathy J10.81
      - enteritis J10.2
      - gastroenteritis J10.2
      - gastrointestinal manifestations J10.2
      - laryngitis J10.1
      - myocarditis J10.82
      - otitis media J10.83
      - pharyngitis J10.1
      - pneumonia (unspecified type) J10.00
        - with same identified influenza virus J10.01
        - specified type NEC J10.08
      - respiratory manifestations NEC J10.1
      - specified manifestation NEC J10.89
  - identified novel influenza A virus J09.X2
    - with
      - digestive manifestations J09.X3
      - encephalopathy J09.X9
      - enteritis J09.X3
      - gastroenteritis J09.X3
      - gastrointestinal manifestations J09.X3
      - laryngitis J09.X2
      - myocarditis J09.X9
      - otitis media J09.X9
      - pharyngitis J09.X2
      - pneumonia J09.X1
      - respiratory manifestations NEC J09.X2
      - specified manifestation NEC J09.X9
      - upper respiratory symptoms J09.X2
- novel (2009) H1N1 influenza (*see also* Influenza, due to, identified influenza virus NEC) J10.1
- novel influenza A/H1N1 (*see also* Influenza, due to, identified influenza virus NEC) J10.1
- of other animal origin, not bird or swine (*see also* Influenza, due to, identified novel influenza A virus) J09.X2
- swine (viruses that normally cause infections in pigs) (*see also* Influenza, due to, identified novel influenza A virus) J09.X2

Influenzal — *see* Influenza

Influenza-like disease — *see* Influenza

Infraction, Freiberg's (metatarsal head) — *see* Osteochondrosis, juvenile, metatarsus

Infraeruption of tooth (teeth) M26.34

Infusion complication, misadventure, or reaction — *see* Complications, infusion

Ingestion
- chemical — *see* Table of Drugs and Chemicals, by substance, poisoning
- drug or medicament
  - correct substance properly administered — *see* Table of Drugs and Chemicals, by drug, adverse effect
  - overdose or wrong substance given or taken — *see* Table of Drugs and Chemicals, by drug, poisoning
- foreign body — *see* Foreign body, alimentary tract
- tularemia A21.3

Ingrowing
- hair (beard) L73.1
- nail (finger) (toe) L60.0

Inguinal (*see also* condition)
- testicle Q53.9
  - bilateral Q53.21
  - unilateral Q53.11

Inhalation
- anthrax A22.1
- flame T27.3 ☑
- food or foreign body — *see* Foreign body, by site
- gases, fumes, or vapors NEC T59.9- ☑
  - specified agent — *see* Table of Drugs and Chemicals, by substance
- liquid or vomitus — *see* Asphyxia
- meconium (newborn) P24.00
  - with
    - with respiratory symptoms P24.01
    - pneumonia (pneumonitis) P24.01
- mucus — *see* Asphyxia, mucus

Inhalation — *continued*
- oil or gasoline (causing suffocation) — *see* Foreign body, by site
- smoke J70.5
  - due to chemicals, gases, fumes and vapors J68.9
- steam — *see* Toxicity, vapors
- stomach contents or secretions — *see* Foreign body, by site
- due to anesthesia (general) (local) or other sedation T88.59 ☑
  - in labor and delivery O74.0
  - in pregnancy O29.01- ☑
  - postpartum, puerperal O89.01

Inhibition, orgasm
- female F52.31
- male F52.32

Inhibitor, systemic lupus erythematosus (presence of) D68.62

Iniencephalus, iniencephaly Q00.2

Injection, traumatic jet (air) (industrial) (water) (paint or dye) T70.4 ☑

Injury (*see also* specified injury type) T14.90
- abdomen, abdominal S39.91 ☑
  - blood vessel — *see* Injury, blood vessel, abdomen
  - cavity — *see* Injury, intra-abdominal
  - contusion S30.1 ☑
  - internal — *see* Injury, intra-abdominal
  - intra-abdominal organ — *see* Injury, intra-abdominal
  - nerve — *see* Injury, nerve, abdomen
  - open — *see* Wound, open, abdomen
  - specified NEC S39.81 ☑
  - superficial — *see* Injury, superficial, abdomen
- Achilles tendon S86.00- ☑
  - laceration S86.02- ☑
  - specified type NEC S86.09- ☑
  - strain S86.01- ☑
- acoustic, resulting in deafness — *see* Injury, nerve, acoustic
- adrenal (gland) S37.819 ☑
  - contusion S37.812 ☑
  - laceration S37.813 ☑
  - specified type NEC S37.818 ☑
- alveolar (process) S09.93 ☑
- ankle S99.91- ☑
  - contusion — *see* Contusion, ankle
  - dislocation — *see* Dislocation, ankle
  - fracture — *see* Fracture, ankle
  - nerve — *see* Injury, nerve, ankle
  - open — *see* Wound, open, ankle
  - specified type NEC S99.81- ☑
  - sprain — *see* Sprain, ankle
  - superficial — *see* Injury, superficial, ankle
- anterior chamber, eye — *see* Injury, eye, specified site NEC
- anus — *see* Injury, abdomen
- aorta (thoracic) S25.00 ☑
  - abdominal S35.00 ☑
    - laceration (minor) (superficial) S35.01 ☑
      - major S35.02 ☑
    - specified type NEC S35.09 ☑
  - laceration (minor) (superficial) S25.01 ☑
    - major S25.02 ☑
  - specified type NEC S25.09 ☑
- arm (upper) S49.9- ☑
  - blood vessel — *see* Injury, blood vessel, arm
  - contusion — *see* Contusion, arm, upper
  - fracture — *see* Fracture, humerus
  - lower — *see* Injury, forearm
  - muscle — *see* Injury, muscle, shoulder
  - nerve — *see* Injury, nerve, arm
  - open — *see* Wound, open, arm
  - specified type NEC S49.8- ☑
  - superficial — *see* Injury, superficial, arm
- artery (complicating trauma) (*see also* Injury, blood vessel, by site)
  - cerebral or meningeal — *see* Injury, intracranial
- auditory canal (external) (meatus) S09.91 ☑
- auricle, auris, ear S09.91 ☑
- axilla — *see* Injury, shoulder
- back — *see* Injury, back, lower
- bile duct S36.13 ☑
- birth (*see also* Birth, injury) P15.9
- bladder (sphincter) S37.20 ☑
  - at delivery O71.5
  - contusion S37.22 ☑

Injury — *continued*
 bladder — *continued*
  laceration S37.23 ☑
  obstetrical trauma O71.5
  specified type NEC S37.29 ☑
 blast (air) (hydraulic) (immersion) (underwater) NEC T14.8
  acoustic nerve trauma — *see* Injury, nerve, acoustic
  bladder — *see* Injury, bladder
  brain — *see* Concussion
  colon — *see* Injury, intestine, large
  ear (primary) S09.31- ☑
   secondary S09.39- ☑
  generalized T70.8 ☑
  lung — *see* Injury, intrathoracic, lung
  multiple body organs T70.8 ☑
  peritoneum S36.81 ☑
  rectum S36.61 ☑
  retroperitoneum S36.898 ☑
  small intestine S36.419 ☑
   duodenum S36.410 ☑
   specified site NEC S36.418 ☑
  specified
   intra-abdominal organ NEC S36.898 ☑
   pelvic organ NEC S37.899 ☑
 blood vessel NEC T14.8
  abdomen S35.9
   aorta — *see* Injury, aorta, abdominal
   celiac artery — *see* Injury, blood vessel, celiac artery
   iliac vessel — *see* Injury, blood vessel, iliac
   laceration S35.91 ☑
   mesenteric vessel — *see* Injury, mesenteric
   portal vein — *see* Injury, blood vessel, portal vein
   renal vessel — *see* Injury, blood vessel, renal
   specified vessel NEC S35.8X- ☑
   splenic vessel — *see* Injury, blood vessel, splenic
   vena cava — *see* Injury, vena cava, inferior
  ankle — *see* Injury, blood vessel, foot
  aorta (abdominal) (thoracic) — *see* Injury, aorta
  arm (upper) NEC S45.90- ☑
   forearm — *see* Injury, blood vessel, forearm
   laceration S45.91- ☑
   specified
    site NEC S45.80- ☑
     laceration S45.81- ☑
     specified type NEC S45.89- ☑
    type NEC S45.99- ☑
   superficial vein S45.30- ☑
    laceration S45.31- ☑
    specified type NEC S45.39- ☑
  axillary
   artery S45.00- ☑
    laceration S45.01- ☑
    specified type NEC S45.09- ☑
   vein S45.20- ☑
    laceration S45.21- ☑
    specified type NEC S45.29- ☑
  azygos vein — *see* Injury, blood vessel, thoracic, specified site NEC
  brachial
   artery S45.10- ☑
    laceration S45.11- ☑
    specified type NEC S45.19- ☑
   vein S45.20- ☑
    laceration S45.219 ☑
    specified type NEC S45.29- ☑
  carotid artery (common) (external) (internal, extracranial) S15.00- ☑
   internal, intracranial S06.8- ☑
   laceration (minor) (superficial) S15.01- ☑
    major S15.02- ☑
   specified type NEC S15.09- ☑
  celiac artery S35.219 ☑
   branch S35.299 ☑
    laceration (minor) (superficial) S35.291 ☑
     major S35.292 ☑
    specified NEC S35.298 ☑
   laceration (minor) (superficial) S35.211 ☑
    major S35.212 ☑
   specified type NEC S35.218 ☑
  cerebral — *see* Injury, intracranial
  deep plantar — *see* Injury, blood vessel, plantar artery

Injury — *continued*
 blood vessel — *continued*
  digital (hand) — *see* Injury, blood vessel, finger
  dorsal
   artery (foot) S95.00- ☑
    laceration S95.01- ☑
    specified type NEC S95.09- ☑
   vein (foot) S95.20- ☑
    laceration S95.21- ☑
    specified type NEC S95.29- ☑
  due to accidental laceration during procedure — *see* Laceration, accidental complicating surgery
  extremity — *see* Injury, blood vessel, limb
  femoral
   artery (common) (superficial) S75.00- ☑
    laceration (minor) (superficial) S75.01- ☑
     major S75.02- ☑
    specified type NEC S75.09- ☑
   vein (hip level) (thigh level) S75.10- ☑
    laceration (minor) (superficial) S75.11- ☑
     major S75.12- ☑
    specified type NEC S75.19- ☑
  finger S65.50- ☑
   index S65.50- ☑
    laceration S65.51- ☑
    specified type NEC S65.59- ☑
   laceration S65.51- ☑
   little S65.50- ☑
    laceration S65.51- ☑
    specified type NEC S65.59- ☑
   middle S65.50- ☑
    laceration S65.51- ☑
    specified type NEC S65.59- ☑
   specified type NEC S65.59- ☑
   thumb — *see* Injury, blood vessel, thumb
  foot S95.90- ☑
   dorsal
    artery — *see* Injury, blood vessel, dorsal, artery
    vein — *see* Injury, blood vessel, dorsal, vein
   laceration S95.91- ☑
   plantar artery — *see* Injury, blood vessel, plantar artery
   specified
    site NEC S95.80- ☑
     laceration S95.81- ☑
     specified type NEC S95.89- ☑
    specified type NEC S95.99- ☑
  forearm S55.90- ☑
   laceration S55.91- ☑
   radial artery — *see* Injury, blood vessel, radial artery
   specified
    site NEC S55.80- ☑
     laceration S55.81- ☑
     specified type NEC S55.89- ☑
    type NEC S55.99- ☑
   ulnar artery — *see* Injury, blood vessel, ulnar artery
   vein S55.20- ☑
    laceration S55.21- ☑
    specified type NEC S55.29- ☑
  gastric
   artery — *see* Injury, mesenteric, artery, branch
   vein — *see* Injury, blood vessel, abdomen
  gastroduodenal artery — *see* Injury, mesenteric, artery, branch
  greater saphenous vein (lower leg level) S85.30- ☑
   hip (and thigh) level S75.20- ☑
    laceration (minor) (superficial) S75.21- ☑
     major S75.22- ☑
    specified type NEC S75.29- ☑
   laceration S85.31- ☑
   specified type NEC S85.39- ☑
  hand (level) S65.90- ☑
   finger — *see* Injury, blood vessel, finger
   laceration S65.91- ☑
   palmar arch — *see* Injury, blood vessel, palmar arch
   radial artery — *see* Injury, blood vessel, radial artery, hand
   specified
    site NEC S65.80- ☑
     laceration S65.81- ☑
     specified type NEC S65.89- ☑

Injury — *continued*
 blood vessel — *continued*
  hand — *continued*
   specified — *continued*
    type NEC S65.99- ☑
   thumb — *see* Injury, blood vessel, thumb
   ulnar artery — *see* Injury, blood vessel, ulnar artery, hand
  head S09.0 ☑
   intracranial — *see* Injury, intracranial
   multiple S09.0 ☑
  hepatic
   artery — *see* Injury, mesenteric, artery
   vein — *see* Injury, vena cava, inferior
  hip S75.90- ☑
   femoral artery — *see* Injury, blood vessel, femoral, artery
   femoral vein — *see* Injury, blood vessel, femoral, vein
   greater saphenous vein — *see* Injury, blood vessel, greater saphenous, hip level
   laceration S75.91- ☑
   specified
    site NEC S75.80- ☑
     laceration S75.81- ☑
     specified type NEC S75.89- ☑
    type NEC S75.99- ☑
  hypogastric (artery) (vein) — *see* Injury, blood vessel, iliac
  iliac S35.5- ☑
   artery S35.51- ☑
   specified vessel NEC S35.5- ☑
   uterine vessel — *see* Injury, blood vessel, uterine
   vein S35.51- ☑
  innominate — *see* Injury, blood vessel, thoracic, innominate
  intercostal (artery) (vein) — *see* Injury, blood vessel, thoracic, intercostal
  jugular vein (external) S15.20- ☑
   internal S15.30- ☑
    laceration (minor) (superficial) S15.31- ☑
     major S15.32- ☑
    specified type NEC S15.39- ☑
   laceration (minor) (superficial) S15.21- ☑
    major S15.22- ☑
   specified type NEC S15.29- ☑
  leg (level) (lower) S85.90- ☑
   greater saphenous — *see* Injury, blood vessel, greater saphenous
   laceration S85.91- ☑
   lesser saphenous — *see* Injury, blood vessel, lesser saphenous
   peroneal artery — *see* Injury, blood vessel, peroneal artery
   popliteal
    artery — *see* Injury, blood vessel, popliteal, artery
    vein — *see* Injury, blood vessel, popliteal, vein
   specified
    site NEC S85.80- ☑
     laceration S85.81- ☑
     specified type NEC S85.89- ☑
    type NEC S85.99- ☑
   thigh — *see* Injury, blood vessel, hip
   tibial artery — *see* Injury, blood vessel, tibial artery
  lesser saphenous vein (lower leg level) S85.40- ☑
   laceration S85.41- ☑
   specified type NEC S85.49- ☑
  limb
   lower — *see* Injury, blood vessel, leg
   upper — *see* Injury, blood vessel, arm
  lower back — *see* Injury, blood vessel, abdomen
   specified NEC — *see* Injury, blood vessel, abdomen, specified, site NEC
  mammary (artery) (vein) — *see* Injury, blood vessel, thoracic, specified site NEC
  mesenteric (inferior) (superior)
   artery — *see* Injury, mesenteric, artery
   vein — *see* Injury, blood vessel, mesenteric, vein
  neck S15.9 ☑
   specified site NEC S15.8 ☑
  ovarian (artery) (vein) — *see* subcategory S35.8 ☑

Injury — *continued*
  blood vessel — *continued*
    palmar arch (superficial) S65.20- ☑
      deep S65.30- ☑
        laceration S65.31- ☑
        specified type NEC S65.39- ☑
      laceration S65.21- ☑
      specified type NEC S65.29- ☑
    pelvis — *see* Injury, blood vessel, abdomen
      specified NEC — *see* Injury, blood vessel, abdomen, specified, site NEC
    peroneal artery S85.20- ☑
      laceration S85.21- ☑
      specified type NEC S85.29- ☑
    plantar artery (deep) (foot) S95.10- ☑
      laceration S95.11- ☑
      specified type NEC S95.19- ☑
    popliteal
      artery S85.00- ☑
        laceration S85.01- ☑
        specified type NEC S85.09- ☑
      vein S85.50- ☑
        laceration S85.51- ☑
        specified type NEC S85.59- ☑
    portal vein S35.319 ☑
      laceration S35.311 ☑
      specified type NEC S35.318 ☑
    precerebral — *see* Injury, blood vessel, neck
    pulmonary (artery) (vein) — *see* Injury, blood vessel, thoracic, pulmonary
    radial artery (forearm level) S55.10- ☑
      hand and wrist (level) S65.10- ☑
        laceration S65.11- ☑
        specified type NEC S65.19- ☑
      laceration S55.11- ☑
      specified type NEC S55.19- ☑
    renal
      artery S35.40- ☑
        laceration S35.41- ☑
        specified NEC S35.49- ☑
      vein S35.40- ☑
        laceration S35.41- ☑
        specified NEC S35.49- ☑
    saphenous vein (greater) (lower leg level) — *see* Injury, blood vessel, greater saphenous
      hip and thigh level — *see* Injury, blood vessel, greater saphenous, hip level
      lesser — *see* Injury, blood vessel, lesser saphenous
    shoulder
      specified NEC — *see* Injury, blood vessel, arm, specified site NEC
      superficial vein — *see* Injury, blood vessel, arm, superficial vein
    specified NEC T14.8
    splenic
      artery — *see* Injury, blood vessel, celiac artery, branch
      vein S35.329 ☑
        laceration S35.321 ☑
        specified NEC S35.328 ☑
    subclavian — *see* Injury, blood vessel, thoracic, innominate
    thigh — *see* Injury, blood vessel, hip
    thoracic S25.90 ☑
      aorta S25.00 ☑
        laceration (minor) (superficial) S25.01 ☑
          major S25.02 ☑
        specified type NEC S25.09 ☑
      azygos vein — *see* Injury, blood vessel, thoracic, specified, site NEC
      innominate
        artery S25.10- ☑
          laceration (minor) (superficial) S25.11- ☑
            major S25.12- ☑
          specified type NEC S25.19- ☑
        vein S25.30- ☑
          laceration (minor) (superficial) S25.31- ☑
            major S25.32- ☑
          specified type NEC S25.39- ☑
      intercostal S25.50- ☑
        laceration S25.51- ☑
        specified type NEC S25.59- ☑
      laceration S25.91 ☑

  blood vessel — *continued*
    thoracic — *continued*
      mammary vessel — *see* Injury, blood vessel, thoracic, specified, site NEC
      pulmonary S25.40- ☑
        laceration (minor) (superficial) S25.41- ☑
          major S25.42- ☑
        specified type NEC S25.49- ☑
      specified
        site NEC S25.80- ☑
          laceration S25.81 ☑
          specified type NEC S25.89 ☑
        type NEC S25.99 ☑
      subclavian — *see* Injury, blood vessel, thoracic, innominate
      vena cava (superior) S25.20 ☑
        laceration (minor) (superficial) S25.21 ☑
          major S25.22 ☑
        specified type NEC S25.29 ☑
    thumb S65.40- ☑
      laceration S65.41- ☑
      specified type NEC S65.49- ☑
    tibial artery S85.10- ☑
      anterior S85.13- ☑
        laceration S85.14- ☑
        specified injury NEC S85.15- ☑
      laceration S85.11- ☑
      posterior S85.16- ☑
        laceration S85.17- ☑
        specified injury NEC S85.18- ☑
      specified injury NEC S85.12- ☑
    ulnar artery (forearm level) S55.00- ☑
      hand and wrist (level) S65.00- ☑
        laceration S65.01- ☑
        specified type NEC S65.09- ☑
      laceration S55.01- ☑
      specified type NEC S55.09- ☑
    upper arm (level) — *see* Injury, blood vessel, arm
    superficial vein — *see* Injury, blood vessel, arm, superficial vein
    uterine S35.5- ☑
      artery S35.53- ☑
      vein S35.53- ☑
    vena cava — *see* Injury, vena cava
    vertebral artery S15.10- ☑
      laceration (minor) (superficial) S15.11- ☑
        major S15.12- ☑
      specified type NEC S15.19- ☑
    wrist (level) — *see* Injury, blood vessel, hand
  brachial plexus S14.3 ☑
    newborn P14.3
  brain (traumatic) S06.9- ☑
    diffuse (axonal) S06.2X- ☑
    focal S06.30- ☑
    traumatic — *see* category S06 ☑
  brainstem S06.38- ☑
  breast NOS S29.9 ☑
  broad ligament — *see* Injury, pelvic organ, specified site NEC
  bronchus, bronchi — *see* Injury, intrathoracic, bronchus
  brow S09.90 ☑
  buttock S39.92 ☑
  canthus, eye S05.90 ☑
  cardiac plexus — *see* Injury, nerve, thorax, sympathetic
  cauda equina S34.3 ☑
  cavernous sinus — *see* Injury, intracranial
  cecum — *see* Injury, colon
  celiac ganglion or plexus — *see* Injury, nerve, lumbosacral, sympathetic
  cerebellum — *see* Injury, intracranial
  cerebral — *see* Injury, intracranial
  cervix (uteri) — *see* Injury, uterus
  cheek (wall) S09.93 ☑
  chest — *see* Injury, thorax
  childbirth (newborn) (*see also* Birth, injury)
    maternal NEC O71.9
  chin S09.93 ☑
  choroid (eye) — *see* Injury, eye, specified site NEC
  clitoris S39.94 ☑
  coccyx (*see also* Injury, back, lower)
    complicating delivery O71.6
  colon — *see* Injury, intestine, large
  common bile duct — *see* Injury, liver
  conjunctiva (superficial) — *see* Injury, eye, conjunctiva

  conus medullaris — *see* Injury, spinal, sacral cord
    spermatic (pelvic region) S37.898 ☑
      scrotal region S39.848 ☑
    spinal — *see* Injury, spinal cord, by region
  cornea — *see* Injury, eye, specified site NEC
    abrasion — *see* Injury, eye, cornea, abrasion
  cortex (cerebral) (*see also* Injury, intracranial)
    visual — *see* Injury, nerve, optic
  costal region NEC S29.9 ☑
  costochondral NEC S29.9 ☑
  cranial
    cavity — *see* Injury, intracranial
    nerve — *see* Injury, nerve, cranial
  crushing — *see* Crush
  cutaneous sensory nerve
  cystic duct — *see* Injury, liver
  deep tissue — *see* Contusion, by site
    meaning pressure ulcer — *see* Ulcer, pressure, unstageable, by site
  delivery (newborn) P15.9
    maternal NEC O71.9
  Descemet's membrane — *see* Injury, eyeball, penetrating
  diaphragm — *see* Injury, intrathoracic, diaphragm
  duodenum — *see* Injury, intestine, small, duodenum
  ear (auricle) (external) (canal) S09.91 ☑
    abrasion — *see* Abrasion, ear
    bite — *see* Bite, ear
    blister — *see* Blister, ear
    bruise — *see* Contusion, ear
    contusion — *see* Contusion, ear
    external constriction — *see* Constriction, external, ear
    hematoma — *see* Hematoma, ear
    inner — *see* Injury, ear, middle
    laceration — *see* Laceration, ear
    middle S09.30- ☑
      blast — *see* Injury, blast, ear
      specified NEC S09.39- ☑
    puncture — *see* Puncture, ear
    superficial — *see* Injury, superficial, ear
  eighth cranial nerve (acoustic or auditory) — *see* Injury, nerve, acoustic
  elbow S59.90- ☑
    contusion — *see* Contusion, elbow
    dislocation — *see* Dislocation, elbow
    fracture — *see* Fracture, ulna, upper end
    open — *see* Wound, open, elbow
    specified NEC S59.80- ☑
    sprain — *see* Sprain, elbow
    superficial — *see* Injury, superficial, elbow
  eleventh cranial nerve (accessory) — *see* Injury, nerve, accessory
  epididymis S39.94 ☑
  epigastric region S39.91 ☑
  epiglottis NEC S19.89 ☑
  esophageal plexus — *see* Injury, nerve, thorax, sympathetic
  esophagus (thoracic part) (*see also* Injury, intrathoracic, esophagus)
    cervical NEC S19.85 ☑
  eustachian tube S09.30 ☑
  eye S05.9- ☑
    avulsion S05.7- ☑
    ball — *see* Injury, eyeball
    conjunctiva S05.0- ☑
    cornea
      abrasion S05.0- ☑
      laceration S05.3- ☑
        with prolapse S05.2- ☑
    lacrimal apparatus S05.8X- ☑
    orbit penetration S05.4- ☑
    specified site NEC S05.8X- ☑
  eyeball S05.8X- ☑
    contusion S05.1- ☑
    penetrating S05.6- ☑
      with
        foreign body S05.5- ☑
        prolapse or loss of intraocular tissue S05.2- ☑
        without prolapse or loss of intraocular tissue S05.3- ☑
    specified type NEC S05.8- ☑
  eyebrow S09.93 ☑

Injury — *continued*

eyelid S09.93 ☑
  abrasion — *see* Abrasion, eyelid
  contusion — *see* Contusion, eyelid
  open — *see* Wound, open, eyelid
face S09.93 ☑
fallopian tube S37.509 ☑
  bilateral S37.502 ☑
    blast injury S37.512 ☑
    contusion S37.522 ☑
    laceration S37.532 ☑
    specified type NEC S37.592 ☑
  blast injury (primary) S37.519 ☑
    bilateral S37.512 ☑
    secondary — *see* Injury, fallopian tube, speci-
      fied type NEC
    unilateral S37.511 ☑
  contusion S37.529 ☑
    bilateral S37.522 ☑
    unilateral S37.521 ☑
  laceration S37.539 ☑
    bilateral S37.532 ☑
    unilateral S37.531 ☑
  specified type NEC S37.599 ☑
    bilateral S37.592 ☑
    unilateral S37.591 ☑
  unilateral S37.501 ☑
    blast injury S37.511 ☑
    contusion S37.521 ☑
    laceration S37.531 ☑
    specified type NEC S37.591 ☑
fascia — *see* Injury, muscle
fifth cranial nerve (trigeminal) — *see* Injury, nerve,
  trigeminal
finger (nail) S69.9- ☑
  blood vessel — *see* Injury, blood vessel, finger
  contusion — *see* Contusion, finger
  dislocation — *see* Dislocation, finger
  fracture — *see* Fracture, finger
  muscle — *see* Injury, muscle, finger
  nerve — *see* Injury, nerve, digital, finger
  open — *see* Wound, open, finger
  specified NEC S69.8- ☑
  sprain — *see* Sprain, finger
  superficial — *see* Injury, superficial, finger
first cranial nerve (olfactory) — *see* Injury, nerve, olfactory
flank — *see* Injury, abdomen
foot S99.92- ☑
  blood vessel — *see* Injury, blood vessel, foot
  contusion — *see* Contusion, foot
  dislocation — *see* Dislocation, foot
  fracture — *see* Fracture, foot
  muscle — *see* Injury, muscle, foot
  open — *see* Wound, open, foot
  specified type NEC S99.82- ☑
  sprain — *see* Sprain, foot
  superficial — *see* Injury, superficial, foot
forceps NOS P15.9
forearm S59.91- ☑
  blood vessel — *see* Injury, blood vessel, forearm
  contusion — *see* Contusion, forearm
  fracture — *see* Fracture, forearm
  muscle — *see* Injury, muscle, forearm
  nerve — *see* Injury, nerve, forearm
  open — *see* Wound, open, forearm
  specified NEC S59.81- ☑
  superficial — *see* Injury, superficial, forearm
forehead S09.90 ☑
fourth cranial nerve (trochlear) — *see* Injury, nerve,
  trochlear
gallbladder S36.129 ☑
  contusion S36.122 ☑
  laceration S36.123 ☑
  specified NEC S36.128 ☑
ganglion
  celiac, coeliac — *see* Injury, nerve, lumbosacral,
    sympathetic
  gasserian — *see* Injury, nerve, trigeminal
  stellate — *see* Injury, nerve, thorax, sympathetic
  thoracic sympathetic — *see* Injury, nerve, thorax,
    sympathetic
gasserian ganglion — *see* Injury, nerve, trigeminal
gastric artery — *see* Injury, blood vessel, celiac artery,
  branch

Injury — *continued*

gastroduodenal artery — *see* Injury, blood vessel,
  celiac artery, branch
gastrointestinal tract — *see* Injury, intra-abdominal
  with open wound into abdominal cavity — *see*
    Wound, open, with penetration into peri-
    toneal cavity
  colon — *see* Injury, intestine, large
  rectum — *see* Injury, intestine, large, rectum
    with open wound into abdominal cavity
    S36.61 ☑
  small intestine — *see* Injury, intestine, small
  specified site NEC — *see* Injury, intra-abdominal,
    specified, site NEC
  stomach — *see* Injury, stomach
genital organ(s)
  external S39.94 ☑
    specified NEC S39.848 ☑
  internal S37.90 ☑
    fallopian tube — *see* Injury, fallopian tube
    ovary — *see* Injury, ovary
    prostate — *see* Injury, prostate
    seminal vesicle — *see* Injury, pelvis, organ,
      specified site NEC
    uterus — *see* Injury, uterus
    vas deferens — *see* Injury, pelvis, organ, speci-
      fied site NEC
  obstetrical trauma O71.9
gland
  lacrimal laceration — *see* Injury, eye, specified site
    NEC
  salivary S09.90 ☑
  thyroid NEC S19.84 ☑
globe (eye) S05.90 ☑
  specified NEC S05.8X- ☑
groin — *see* Injury, abdomen
gum S09.90 ☑
hand S69.9- ☑
  blood vessel — *see* Injury, blood vessel, hand
  contusion — *see* Contusion, hand
  fracture — *see* Fracture, hand
  muscle — *see* Injury, muscle, hand
  nerve — *see* Injury, nerve, hand
  open — *see* Wound, open, hand
  specified NEC S69.8- ☑
  sprain — *see* Sprain, hand
  superficial — *see* Injury, superficial, hand
head S09.90 ☑
  with loss of consciousness S06.9- ☑
  specified NEC S09.8 ☑
heart S26.90 ☑
  with hemopericardium S26.00 ☑
    contusion S26.01 ☑
    laceration (mild) S26.020 ☑
      major S26.022 ☑
      moderate S26.021 ☑
    specified type NEC S26.09 ☑
  without hemopericardium S26.10 ☑
    contusion S26.11 ☑
    laceration S26.12 ☑
    specified type NEC S26.19 ☑
  contusion S26.91 ☑
  laceration S26.92 ☑
  specified type NEC S26.99 ☑
heel — *see* Injury, foot
hepatic
  artery — *see* Injury, blood vessel, celiac artery,
    branch
  duct — *see* Injury, liver
  vein — *see* Injury, vena cava, inferior
hip S79.91- ☑
  blood vessel — *see* Injury, blood vessel, hip
  contusion — *see* Contusion, hip
  dislocation — *see* Dislocation, hip
  fracture — *see* Fracture, femur, neck
  muscle — *see* Injury, muscle, hip
  nerve — *see* Injury, nerve, hip
  open — *see* Wound, open, hip
  specified NEC S79.81- ☑
  sprain — *see* Sprain, hip
  superficial — *see* Injury, superficial, hip
hymen S39.94 ☑
hypogastric
  blood vessel — *see* Injury, blood vessel, iliac
  plexus — *see* Injury, nerve, lumbosacral, sympa-
    thetic

Injury — *continued*

ileum — *see* Injury, intestine, small
iliac region S39.91 ☑
instrumental (during surgery) — *see* Laceration, accidental complicating surgery
birth injury — *see* Birth, injury
nonsurgical — *see* Injury, by site
obstetrical O71.9
  bladder O71.5
  cervix O71.3
  high vaginal O71.4
  perineal NOS O70.9
  urethra O71.5
  uterus O71.5
    with rupture or perforation O71.1
internal T14.8
  aorta — *see* Injury, aorta
  bladder (sphincter) — *see* Injury, bladder
  with
    ectopic or molar pregnancy O08.6
    following ectopic or molar pregnancy O08.6
    obstetrical trauma O71.5
  bronchus, bronchi — *see* Injury, intrathoracic,
    bronchus
  cecum — *see* Injury, intestine, large
  cervix (uteri) (*see also* Injury, uterus)
    with ectopic or molar pregnancy O08.6
    following ectopic or molar pregnancy O08.6
    obstetrical trauma O71.3
  chest — *see* Injury, intrathoracic
  gastrointestinal tract — *see* Injury, intra-abdominal
  heart — *see* Injury, heart
  intestine NEC — *see* Injury, intestine
  intrauterine — *see* Injury, uterus
  mesentery — *see* Injury, intra-abdominal, specified,
    site NEC
  pelvis, pelvic (organ) S37.90 ☑
    following ectopic or molar pregnancy (subse-
      quent episode) O08.6
    obstetrical trauma NEC O71.5
      rupture or perforation O71.1
    specified NEC S39.83 ☑
  rectum — *see* Injury, intestine, large, rectum
  stomach — *see* Injury, stomach
  ureter — *see* Injury, ureter
  urethra (sphincter) following ectopic or molar
    pregnancy O08.6
  uterus — *see* Injury, uterus
interscapular area — *see* Injury, thorax
intestine
  large S36.509 ☑
    ascending (right) S36.500 ☑
      blast injury (primary) S36.510 ☑
        secondary S36.590 ☑
      contusion S36.520 ☑
      laceration S36.530 ☑
      specified type NEC S36.590 ☑
    blast injury (primary) S36.519 ☑
      ascending (right) S36.510 ☑
      descending (left) S36.512 ☑
      rectum S36.61 ☑
      sigmoid S36.513 ☑
      specified site NEC S36.518 ☑
      transverse S36.511 ☑
    contusion S36.529 ☑
      ascending (right) S36.520 ☑
      descending (left) S36.522 ☑
      rectum S36.62 ☑
      sigmoid S36.523 ☑
      specified site NEC S36.528 ☑
      transverse S36.521 ☑
    descending (left) S36.502 ☑
      blast injury (primary) S36.512 ☑
        secondary S36.592 ☑
      contusion S36.522 ☑
      laceration S36.532 ☑
      specified type NEC S36.592 ☑
    laceration S36.539 ☑
      ascending (right) S36.530 ☑
      descending (left) S36.532 ☑
      rectum S36.63 ☑
      sigmoid S36.533 ☑
      specified site NEC S36.538 ☑
      transverse S36.531 ☑
    rectum S36.60 ☑
      blast injury (primary) S36.61 ☑

Injury — *continued*
  intestine — *continued*
    large — *continued*
      rectum — *continued*
        blast injury — *continued*
          secondary S36.69 ☑
        contusion S36.62 ☑
        laceration S36.63 ☑
        specified type NEC S36.69 ☑
      sigmoid S36.503 ☑
        blast injury (primary) S36.513 ☑
          secondary S36.593 ☑
        contusion S36.523 ☑
        laceration S36.533 ☑
        specified type NEC S36.593 ☑
      specified
        site NEC S36.508 ☑
          blast injury (primary) S36.518 ☑
            secondary S36.598 ☑
          contusion S36.528 ☑
          laceration S36.538 ☑
          specified type NEC S36.598 ☑
        type NEC S36.599 ☑
          ascending (right) S36.590 ☑
          descending (left) S36.592 ☑
          rectum S36.69 ☑
          sigmoid S36.593 ☑
          specified site NEC S36.598 ☑
          transverse S36.591 ☑
      transverse S36.501 ☑
        blast injury (primary) S36.511 ☑
          secondary S36.591 ☑
        contusion S36.521 ☑
        laceration S36.531 ☑
        specified type NEC S36.591 ☑
    small S36.409 ☑
      blast injury (primary) S36.419 ☑
        duodenum S36.410 ☑
        secondary S36.499 ☑
          duodenum S36.490 ☑
          specified site NEC S36.498 ☑
        specified site NEC S36.418 ☑
      contusion S36.429 ☑
        duodenum S36.420 ☑
        specified site NEC S36.428 ☑
      duodenum S36.400 ☑
        blast injury (primary) S36.410 ☑
          secondary S36.490 ☑
        contusion S36.420 ☑
        laceration S36.430 ☑
        specified NEC S36.490 ☑
      laceration S36.439 ☑
        duodenum S36.430 ☑
        specified site NEC S36.438 ☑
      specified
        site NEC S36.408 ☑
        type NEC S36.499 ☑
          duodenum S36.490 ☑
          specified site NEC S36.498 ☑
  intra-abdominal S36.90 ☑
    adrenal gland — *see* Injury, adrenal gland
    bladder — *see* Injury, bladder
    colon — *see* Injury, intestine, large
    contusion S36.92 ☑
    fallopian tube — *see* Injury, fallopian tube
    gallbladder — *see* Injury, gallbladder
    intestine — *see* Injury, intestine
    kidney — *see* Injury, kidney
    laceration S36.93 ☑
    liver — *see* Injury, liver
    ovary — *see* Injury, ovary
    pancreas — *see* Injury, pancreas
    pelvic NOS S37.90 ☑
    peritoneum — *see* Injury, intra-abdominal, speci-fied, site NEC
    prostate — *see* Injury, prostate
    rectum — *see* Injury, intestine, large, rectum
    retroperitoneum — *see* Injury, intra-abdominal, specified, site NEC
    seminal vesicle — *see* Injury, pelvis, organ, speci-fied site NEC
    small intestine — *see* Injury, intestine, small
    specified
      pelvic S37.90 ☑
      specified
        site NEC S37.899 ☑

Injury — *continued*
  intra-abdominal — *continued*
    specified — *continued*
      pelvic — *continued*
        specified — *continued*
          site — *continued*
            specified type NEC S37.898 ☑
          type NEC S37.99 ☑
      site NEC S36.899 ☑
        contusion S36.892 ☑
        laceration S36.893 ☑
        specified type NEC S36.898 ☑
      type NEC S36.99 ☑
    spleen — *see* Injury, spleen
    stomach — *see* Injury, stomach
    ureter — *see* Injury, ureter
    urethra — *see* Injury, urethra
    uterus — *see* Injury, uterus
    vas deferens — *see* Injury, pelvis, organ, specified site NEC
  intracranial (traumatic) S06.9- ☑
    cerebellar hemorrhage, traumatic — *see* Injury, intracranial, focal
    cerebral edema, traumatic S06.1X- ☑
      diffuse S06.1X- ☑
      focal S06.1X- ☑
    diffuse (axonal) S06.2X- ☑
    epidural hemorrhage (traumatic) S06.4X- ☑
    focal brain injury S06.30- ☑
      contusion — *see* Contusion, cerebral
      laceration — *see* Laceration, cerebral
    intracerebral hemorrhage, traumatic S06.36- ☑
      left side S06.35- ☑
      right side S06.34- ☑
    subarachnoid hemorrhage, traumatic S06.6X- ☑
    subdural hemorrhage, traumatic S06.5X- ☑
  intraocular — *see* Injury, eyeball, penetrating
  intrathoracic S27.9 ☑
    bronchus S27.409 ☑
      bilateral S27.402 ☑
      blast injury (primary) S27.419 ☑
        bilateral S27.412 ☑
        secondary — *see* Injury, intrathoracic, bronchus, specified type NEC
        unilateral S27.411 ☑
      contusion S27.429 ☑
        bilateral S27.422 ☑
        unilateral S27.421 ☑
      laceration S27.439 ☑
        bilateral S27.432 ☑
        unilateral S27.431 ☑
      specified type NEC S27.499 ☑
        bilateral S27.492 ☑
        unilateral S27.491 ☑
      unilateral S27.401 ☑
    diaphragm S27.809 ☑
      contusion S27.802 ☑
      laceration S27.803 ☑
      specified type NEC S27.808 ☑
    esophagus (thoracic) S27.819 ☑
      contusion S27.812 ☑
      laceration S27.813 ☑
      specified type NEC S27.818 ☑
    heart — *see* Injury, heart
    hemopneumothorax S27.2 ☑
    hemothorax S27.1 ☑
    lung S27.309 ☑
      aspiration J69.0
      bilateral S27.302 ☑
      blast injury (primary) S27.319 ☑
        bilateral S27.312 ☑
        secondary — *see* Injury, intrathoracic, lung, specified type NEC
        unilateral S27.311 ☑
      contusion S27.329 ☑
        bilateral S27.322 ☑
        unilateral S27.321 ☑
      laceration S27.339 ☑
        bilateral S27.332 ☑
        unilateral S27.331 ☑
      specified type NEC S27.399 ☑
        bilateral S27.392 ☑
        unilateral S27.391 ☑
      unilateral S27.301 ☑
    pleura S27.60 ☑
      laceration S27.63 ☑

Injury — *continued*
  intrathoracic — *continued*
    pleura — *continued*
      specified type NEC S27.69 ☑
    pneumothorax S27.0 ☑
    specified organ NEC S27.899 ☑
      contusion S27.892 ☑
      laceration S27.893 ☑
      specified type NEC S27.898 ☑
    thoracic duct — *see* Injury, intrathoracic, specified organ NEC
    thymus gland — *see* Injury, intrathoracic, specified organ NEC
    trachea, thoracic S27.50 ☑
      blast (primary) S27.51 ☑
      contusion S27.52 ☑
      laceration S27.53 ☑
      specified type NEC S27.59 ☑
  iris — *see* Injury, eye, specified site NEC
    penetrating — *see* Injury, eyeball, penetrating
  jaw S09.93 ☑
  jejunum — *see* Injury, intestine, small
  joint NOS T14.8
    old or residual — *see* Disorder, joint, specified type NEC
  kidney S37.00- ☑
    acute (nontraumatic) N17.9
    contusion — *see* Contusion, kidney
    laceration — *see* Laceration, kidney
    specified NEC S37.09- ☑
  knee S89.9- ☑
    contusion — *see* Contusion, knee
    dislocation — *see* Dislocation, knee
    meniscus (lateral) (medial) — *see* Sprain, knee, specified site NEC
      old injury or tear — *see* Derangement, knee, meniscus, due to old injury
    open — *see* Wound, open, knee
    specified NEC S89.8- ☑
    sprain — *see* Sprain, knee
    superficial — *see* Injury, superficial, knee
  labium (majus) (minus) S39.94 ☑
  labyrinth, ear S09.30- ☑
  lacrimal apparatus, duct, gland, or sac — *see* Injury, eye, specified site NEC
  larynx NEC S19.81 ☑
  leg (lower) S89.9- ☑
    blood vessel — *see* Injury, blood vessel, leg
    contusion — *see* Contusion, leg
    fracture — *see* Fracture, leg
    muscle — *see* Injury, muscle, leg
    nerve — *see* Injury, nerve, leg
    open — *see* Wound, open, leg
    specified NEC S89.8- ☑
    superficial — *see* Injury, superficial, leg
  lens, eye — *see* Injury, eye, specified site NEC
    penetrating — *see* Injury, eyeball, penetrating
  limb NEC T14.8
  lip S09.93 ☑
  liver S36.119 ☑
    contusion S36.112 ☑
    laceration S36.113 ☑
      major (stellate) S36.116 ☑
      minor S36.114 ☑
      moderate S36.115 ☑
    specified NEC S36.118 ☑
  lower back S39.92 ☑
    specified NEC S39.82 ☑
  lumbar, lumbosacral (region) S39.92 ☑
    plexus — *see* Injury, lumbosacral plexus
  lumbosacral plexus S34.4 ☑
  lung (*see also* Injury, intrathoracic, lung)
    aspiration J69.0
    transfusion-related (TRALI) J95.84
  lymphatic thoracic duct — *see* Injury, intrathoracic, specified organ NEC
  malar region S09.93 ☑
  mastoid region S09.90 ☑
  maxilla S09.93 ☑
  mediastinum — *see* Injury, intrathoracic, specified organ NEC
  membrane, brain — *see* Injury, intracranial
  meningeal artery — *see* Injury, intracranial, subdural hemorrhage
  meninges (cerebral) — *see* Injury, intracranial

Injury — continued
  mesenteric
    artery
      branch S35.299 ☑
        laceration (minor) (superficial) S35.291 ☑
          major S35.292 ☑
        specified NEC S35.298 ☑
      inferior S35.239 ☑
        laceration (minor) (superficial) S35.231 ☑
          major S35.232 ☑
        specified NEC S35.238 ☑
      superior S35.229 ☑
        laceration (minor) (superficial) S35.221 ☑
          major S35.222 ☑
        specified NEC S35.228 ☑
      plexus (inferior) (superior) — see Injury, nerve, lumbosacral, sympathetic
    vein
      inferior S35.349 ☑
        laceration S35.341 ☑
        specified NEC S35.348 ☑
      superior S35.339 ☑
        laceration S35.331 ☑
        specified NEC S35.338 ☑
  mesentery — see Injury, intra-abdominal, specified site NEC
  mesosalpinx — see Injury, pelvic organ, specified site NEC
  middle ear S09.30- ☑
  midthoracic region NOS S29.9 ☑
  mouth S09.93 ☑
  multiple NOS T07
  muscle (and fascia) (and tendon)
    abdomen S39.001 ☑
      laceration S39.021 ☑
      specified type NEC S39.091 ☑
      strain S39.011 ☑
    abductor
      thumb, forearm level — see Injury, muscle, thumb, abductor
    adductor
      thigh S76.20- ☑
        laceration S76.22- ☑
        specified type NEC S76.29- ☑
        strain S76.21- ☑
    ankle — see Injury, muscle, foot
    anterior muscle group, at leg level (lower) S86.20- ☑
      laceration S86.22- ☑
      specified type NEC S86.29- ☑
      strain S86.21- ☑
    arm (upper) — see Injury, muscle, shoulder
    biceps (parts NEC) S46.20- ☑
      laceration S46.22- ☑
      long head S46.10- ☑
        laceration S46.12- ☑
        specified type NEC S46.19- ☑
        strain S46.11- ☑
      specified type NEC S46.29- ☑
      strain S46.21- ☑
    extensor
      finger(s) (other than thumb) — see Injury, muscle, finger by site, extensor
      forearm level, specified NEC — see Injury, muscle, forearm, extensor
      thumb — see Injury, muscle, thumb, extensor
      toe (large) (ankle level) (foot level) — see Injury, muscle, toe, extensor
    finger
      extensor (forearm level) S56.40- ☑
        hand level S66.309 ☑
          laceration S66.329 ☑
          specified type NEC S66.399 ☑
          strain S66.319 ☑
        laceration S56.429 ☑
        specified type NEC S56.499 ☑
        strain S56.419 ☑
      flexor (forearm level) S56.10- ☑
        hand level S66.109 ☑
          laceration S66.129 ☑
          specified type NEC S66.199 ☑
          strain S66.119 ☑
        laceration S56.129 ☑
        specified type NEC S56.199 ☑
        strain S56.119 ☑
      index

Injury — continued
  muscle — continued
    finger — continued
      index — continued
        extensor (forearm level)
          hand level S66.308 ☑
            laceration S66.32- ☑
            specified type NEC S66.39- ☑
            strain S66.31- ☑
          specified type NEC S56.492- ☑
        flexor (forearm level)
          hand level S66.108 ☑
            laceration S66.12- ☑
            specified type NEC S66.19- ☑
            strain S66.11- ☑
          specified type NEC S56.19- ☑
          strain S56.11- ☑
        intrinsic S66.50- ☑
          laceration S66.52- ☑
          specified type NEC S66.59- ☑
          strain S66.51- ☑
      intrinsic S66.509 ☑
        laceration S66.529 ☑
        specified type NEC S66.599 ☑
        strain S66.519 ☑
      little
        extensor (forearm level)
          hand level S66.30- ☑
            laceration S66.32- ☑
            specified type NEC S66.39- ☑
            strain S66.31- ☑
          laceration S56.42- ☑
          specified type NEC S56.49- ☑
          strain S56.41- ☑
        flexor (forearm level)
          hand level S66.10- ☑
            laceration S66.12- ☑
            specified type NEC S66.19- ☑
            strain S66.11- ☑
          laceration S56.12- ☑
          specified type NEC S56.19- ☑
          strain S56.11- ☑
        intrinsic S66.50- ☑
          laceration S66.52- ☑
          specified type NEC S66.59- ☑
          strain S66.51- ☑
      middle
        extensor (forearm level)
          hand level S66.30- ☑
            laceration S66.32- ☑
            specified type NEC S66.39- ☑
            strain S66.31- ☑
          laceration S56.42- ☑
          specified type NEC S56.49- ☑
          strain S56.41- ☑
        flexor (forearm level)
          hand level S66.10- ☑
            laceration S66.12- ☑
            specified type NEC S66.19- ☑
            strain S66.11- ☑
          laceration S56.12- ☑
          specified type NEC S56.19- ☑
          strain S56.11- ☑
        intrinsic S66.50- ☑
          laceration S66.52- ☑
          specified type NEC S66.59- ☑
          strain S66.51- ☑
      ring
        extensor (forearm level)
          hand level S66.30- ☑
            laceration S66.32- ☑
            specified type NEC S66.39- ☑
            strain S66.31- ☑
          laceration S56.42- ☑
          specified type NEC S56.49- ☑
          strain S56.41- ☑
        flexor (forearm level)
          hand level S66.10- ☑
            laceration S66.12- ☑
            specified type NEC S66.19- ☑
            strain S66.11- ☑
          laceration S56.12- ☑
          specified type NEC S56.19- ☑
          strain S56.11- ☑
        intrinsic S66.50- ☑
          laceration S66.52- ☑

Injury — continued
  muscle — continued
    finger — continued
      ring — continued
        intrinsic — continued
          specified type NEC S66.59- ☑
          strain S66.51- ☑
    flexor
      finger(s) (other than thumb) — see Injury, muscle, finger
      forearm level, specified NEC — see Injury, muscle, forearm, flexor
      thumb — see Injury, muscle, thumb, flexor
      toe (long) (ankle level) (foot level) — see Injury, muscle, toe, flexor
    foot S96.90- ☑
      intrinsic S96.20- ☑
        laceration S96.22- ☑
        specified type NEC S96.29- ☑
        strain S96.21- ☑
      laceration S96.92- ☑
      long extensor, toe — see Injury, muscle, toe, extensor
      long flexor, toe — see Injury, muscle, toe, flexor
      specified
        site NEC S96.80- ☑
          laceration S96.82- ☑
          specified type NEC S96.89- ☑
          strain S96.81- ☑
        type S96.99- ☑
      strain S96.91- ☑
    forearm (level) S56.90- ☑
      extensor S56.50- ☑
        laceration S56.52- ☑
        specified type NEC S56.59- ☑
        strain S56.51- ☑
      flexor S56.20- ☑
        laceration S56.22- ☑
        specified type NEC S56.29- ☑
        strain S56.21- ☑
      laceration S56.92- ☑
      specified S56.99- ☑
        site NEC S56.80- ☑
          laceration S56.82- ☑
          strain S56.81- ☑
          type NEC S56.89- ☑
      strain S56.91- ☑
    hand (level) S66.90- ☑
      laceration S66.92- ☑
      specified
        site NEC S66.80- ☑
          laceration S66.82- ☑
          specified type NEC S66.89- ☑
          strain S66.81- ☑
          type NEC S66.99- ☑
      strain S66.91- ☑
    head S09.10 ☑
      laceration S09.12 ☑
      specified type NEC S09.19 ☑
      strain S09.11 ☑
    hip NEC S76.00- ☑
      laceration S76.02- ☑
      specified type NEC S76.09- ☑
      strain S76.01- ☑
    intrinsic
      ankle and foot level — see Injury, muscle, foot, intrinsic
      finger (other than thumb) — see Injury, muscle, finger by site, intrinsic
      foot (level) — see Injury, muscle, foot, intrinsic
      thumb — see Injury, muscle, thumb, intrinsic
    leg (level) (lower) S86.90- ☑
      Achilles tendon — see Injury, Achilles tendon
      anterior muscle group — see Injury, muscle, anterior muscle group
      laceration S86.92- ☑
      peroneal muscle group — see Injury, muscle, peroneal muscle group
      posterior muscle group — see Injury, muscle, posterior muscle group, leg level
      specified
        site NEC S86.80- ☑
          laceration S86.82- ☑
          specified type NEC S86.89- ☑
          strain S86.81- ☑
          type NEC S86.99- ☑

Injury — *continued*
- muscle — *continued*
  - leg — *continued*
    - strain S86.91- ☑
    - long
      - extensor toe, at ankle and foot level — *see* Injury, muscle, toe, extensor
      - flexor, toe, at ankle and foot level — *see* Injury, muscle, toe, flexor
      - head, biceps — *see* Injury, muscle, biceps, long head
    - lower back S39.002 ☑
      - laceration S39.022 ☑
      - specified type NEC S39.092 ☑
      - strain S39.012 ☑
    - neck (level) S16.9 ☑
      - laceration S16.2 ☑
      - specified type NEC S16.8 ☑
      - strain S16.1 ☑
    - pelvis S39.003 ☑
      - laceration S39.023 ☑
      - specified type NEC S39.093 ☑
      - strain S39.013 ☑
    - peroneal muscle group, at leg level (lower) S86.30- ☑
      - laceration S86.32- ☑
      - specified type NEC S86.39- ☑
      - strain S86.31- ☑
    - posterior muscle (group)
      - leg level (lower) S86.10- ☑
        - laceration S86.12- ☑
        - specified type NEC S86.19- ☑
        - strain S86.11- ☑
      - thigh level S76.30- ☑
        - laceration S76.32- ☑
        - specified type NEC S76.39- ☑
        - strain S76.31- ☑
    - quadriceps (thigh) S76.10- ☑
      - laceration S76.12- ☑
      - specified type NEC S76.19- ☑
      - strain S76.11- ☑
    - shoulder S46.90- ☑
      - laceration S46.92- ☑
      - rotator cuff — *see* Injury, rotator cuff
      - specified site NEC S46.80- ☑
        - laceration S46.82- ☑
        - specified type NEC S46.89- ☑
        - strain S46.81- ☑
      - specified type NEC S46.99- ☑
      - strain S46.91- ☑
    - thigh NEC (level) S76.90- ☑
      - adductor — *see* Injury, muscle, adductor, thigh
      - laceration S76.92- ☑
      - posterior muscle (group) — *see* Injury, muscle, posterior muscle, thigh level
      - quadriceps — *see* Injury, muscle, quadriceps
      - specified
        - site NEC S76.80- ☑
          - laceration S76.82- ☑
          - specified type NEC S76.89- ☑
          - strain S76.81- ☑
        - type NEC S76.99- ☑
      - strain S76.91- ☑
    - thorax (level) S29.009 ☑
      - back wall S29.002 ☑
      - front wall S29.001 ☑
      - laceration S29.029 ☑
        - back wall S29.022 ☑
        - front wall S29.021 ☑
      - specified type NEC S29.099 ☑
        - back wall S29.092 ☑
        - front wall S29.091 ☑
      - strain S29.019 ☑
        - back wall S29.012 ☑
        - front wall S29.011 ☑
    - thumb
      - abductor (forearm level) S56.30- ☑
        - laceration S56.32- ☑
        - specified type NEC S56.39- ☑
        - strain S56.31- ☑
      - extensor (forearm level) S56.30- ☑
        - hand level S66.20- ☑
          - laceration S66.22- ☑
          - specified type NEC S66.29- ☑
          - strain S66.21- ☑
        - laceration S56.32- ☑

Injury — *continued*
- muscle — *continued*
  - thumb — *continued*
    - extensor — *continued*
      - specified type NEC S56.39- ☑
      - strain S56.31- ☑
    - flexor (forearm level) S56.00- ☑
      - hand level S66.00- ☑
        - laceration S66.02- ☑
        - specified type NEC S66.09- ☑
        - strain S66.01- ☑
      - laceration S56.02- ☑
      - specified type NEC S56.09- ☑
      - strain S56.01- ☑
      - wrist level — *see* Injury, muscle, thumb, flexor, hand level
    - intrinsic S66.40- ☑
      - laceration S66.42- ☑
      - specified type NEC S66.49- ☑
      - strain S66.41- ☑
  - toe (*see also* Injury, muscle, foot)
    - extensor, long S96.10- ☑
      - laceration S96.12- ☑
      - specified type NEC S96.19- ☑
      - strain S96.11- ☑
    - flexor, long S96.00- ☑
      - laceration S96.02- ☑
      - specified type NEC S96.09- ☑
      - strain S96.01- ☑
  - triceps S46.30- ☑
    - laceration S46.32- ☑
    - specified type NEC S46.39- ☑
    - strain S46.31- ☑
  - wrist (and hand) level — *see* Injury, muscle, hand
- musculocutaneous nerve — *see* Injury, nerve, musculocutaneous
- myocardium — *see* Injury, heart
- nape — *see* Injury, neck
- nasal (septum) (sinus) S09.92 ☑
- nasopharynx S09.92 ☑
- neck S19.9 ☑
  - specified NEC S19.80 ☑
    - specified site NEC S19.89 ☑
- nerve NEC T14.8
  - abdomen S34.9 ☑
    - peripheral S34.6 ☑
    - specified site NEC S34.8 ☑
  - abducens S04.4- ☑
    - contusion S04.4- ☑
    - laceration S04.4- ☑
    - specified type NEC S04.4- ☑
  - abducent — *see* Injury, nerve, abducens
  - accessory S04.7- ☑
    - contusion S04.7- ☑
    - laceration S04.7- ☑
    - specified type NEC S04.7- ☑
  - acoustic S04.6- ☑
    - contusion S04.6- ☑
    - laceration S04.6- ☑
    - specified type NEC S04.6- ☑
  - ankle S94.9- ☑
    - cutaneous sensory S94.3- ☑
    - specified site NEC — *see* subcategory S94.8 ☑
  - anterior crural, femoral — *see* Injury, nerve, femoral
  - arm (upper) S44.9- ☑
    - axillary — *see* Injury, nerve, axillary
    - cutaneous — *see* Injury, nerve, cutaneous, arm
    - median — *see* Injury, nerve, median, upper arm
    - musculocutaneous — *see* Injury, nerve, musculocutaneous
    - radial — *see* Injury, nerve, radial, upper arm
    - specified site NEC — *see* subcategory S44.8 ☑
    - ulnar — *see* Injury, nerve, ulnar, arm
  - auditory — *see* Injury, nerve, acoustic
  - axillary S44.3- ☑
  - brachial plexus — *see* Injury, brachial plexus
  - cervical sympathetic S14.5 ☑
  - cranial S04.9 ☑
    - contusion S04.9 ☑
    - eighth (acoustic or auditory) — *see* Injury, nerve, acoustic
    - eleventh (accessory) — *see* Injury, nerve, accessory
    - fifth (trigeminal) — *see* Injury, nerve, trigeminal
    - first (olfactory) — *see* Injury, nerve, olfactory
    - fourth (trochlear) — *see* Injury, nerve, trochlear

Injury — *continued*
- nerve — *continued*
  - cranial — *continued*
    - laceration S04.9 ☑
    - ninth (glossopharyngeal) — *see* Injury, nerve, glossopharyngeal
    - second (optic) — *see* Injury, nerve, optic
    - seventh (facial) — *see* Injury, nerve, facial
    - sixth (abducent) — *see* Injury, nerve, abducens
    - specified
      - nerve NEC S04.89- ☑
        - contusion S04.89- ☑
        - laceration S04.89- ☑
        - specified type NEC S04.89- ☑
      - type NEC S04.9 ☑
    - tenth (pneumogastric or vagus) — *see* Injury, nerve, vagus
    - third (oculomotor) — *see* Injury, nerve, oculomotor
    - twelfth (hypoglossal) — *see* Injury, nerve, hypoglossal
  - cutaneous sensory
    - ankle (level) S94.3- ☑
    - arm (upper) (level) S44.5- ☑
    - foot (level) — *see* Injury, nerve, cutaneous sensory, ankle
    - forearm (level) S54.3- ☑
    - hip (level) S74.2- ☑
    - leg (lower level) S84.2- ☑
    - shoulder (level) — *see* Injury, nerve, cutaneous sensory, arm
    - thigh (level) — *see* Injury, nerve, cutaneous sensory, hip
  - deep peroneal — *see* Injury, nerve, peroneal, foot
  - digital
    - finger S64.4- ☑
      - index S64.49- ☑
      - little S64.49- ☑
      - middle S64.49- ☑
      - ring S64.49- ☑
    - thumb S64.3- ☑
    - toe — *see* Injury, nerve, ankle, specified site NEC
  - eighth cranial (acoustic or auditory) — *see* Injury, nerve, acoustic
  - eleventh cranial (accessory) — *see* Injury, nerve, accessory
  - facial S04.5- ☑
    - contusion S04.5- ☑
    - laceration S04.5- ☑
    - newborn P11.3
    - specified type NEC S04.5- ☑
  - femoral (hip level) (thigh level) S74.1- ☑
  - fifth cranial (trigeminal) — *see* Injury, nerve, trigeminal
  - finger (digital) — *see* Injury, nerve, digital, finger
  - first cranial (olfactory) — *see* Injury, nerve, olfactory
  - foot S94.9- ☑
    - cutaneous sensory S94.3- ☑
    - deep peroneal S94.2- ☑
    - lateral plantar S94.0- ☑
    - medial plantar S94.1- ☑
    - specified site NEC — *see* subcategory S94.8 ☑
  - forearm (level) S54.9- ☑
    - cutaneous sensory — *see* Injury, nerve, cutaneous sensory, forearm
    - median — *see* Injury, nerve, median
    - radial — *see* Injury, nerve, radial
    - specified site NEC — *see* subcategory S54.8 ☑
    - ulnar — *see* Injury, nerve, ulnar
  - fourth cranial (trochlear) — *see* Injury, nerve, trochlear
  - glossopharyngeal S04.89- ☑
    - specified type NEC S04.89- ☑
  - hand S64.9- ☑
    - median — *see* Injury, nerve, median, hand
    - radial — *see* Injury, nerve, radial, hand
    - specified NEC — *see* subcategory S64.8 ☑
    - ulnar — *see* Injury, nerve, ulnar, hand
  - hip (level) S74.9- ☑
    - cutaneous sensory — *see* Injury, nerve, cutaneous sensory, hip
    - femoral — *see* Injury, nerve, femoral
    - sciatic — *see* Injury, nerve, sciatic
    - specified site NEC — *see* subcategory S74.8 ☑
  - hypoglossal S04.89- ☑

Injury — *continued*
  nerve — *continued*
    hypoglossal — *continued*
      specified type NEC S04.89- ☑
    lateral plantar S94.0- ☑
    leg (lower) S84.9- ☑
      cutaneous sensory — *see* Injury, nerve, cutaneous sensory, leg
      peroneal — *see* Injury, nerve, peroneal
      specified site NEC — *see* subcategory S84.8 ☑
      tibial — *see* Injury, nerve, tibial
      upper — *see* Injury, nerve, thigh
    lower
      back — *see* Injury, nerve, abdomen, specified site NEC
        peripheral — *see* Injury, nerve, abdomen, peripheral
      limb — *see* Injury, nerve, leg
    lumbar plexus — *see* Injury, nerve, lumbosacral, sympathetic
    lumbar spinal — *see* Injury, nerve, spinal, lumbar
    lumbosacral
      plexus — *see* Injury, nerve, lumbosacral, sympathetic
      sympathetic S34.5 ☑
    medial plantar S94.1- ☑
    median (forearm level) S54.1- ☑
      hand (level) S64.1- ☑
      upper arm (level) S44.1- ☑
      wrist (level) — *see* Injury, nerve, median, hand
    musculocutaneous S44.4- ☑
    musculospiral (upper arm level) — *see* Injury, nerve, radial, upper arm
    neck S14.9 ☑
      peripheral S14.4 ☑
      specified site NEC S14.8 ☑
      sympathetic S14.5 ☑
    ninth cranial (glossopharyngeal) — *see* Injury, nerve, glossopharyngeal
    oculomotor S04.1- ☑
      contusion S04.1- ☑
      laceration S04.1- ☑
      specified type NEC S04.1- ☑
    olfactory S04.81- ☑
      specified type NEC S04.81- ☑
    optic S04.01- ☑
      contusion S04.01- ☑
      laceration S04.01- ☑
      specified type NEC S04.01- ☑
    pelvic girdle — *see* Injury, nerve, hip
    pelvis — *see* Injury, nerve, abdomen, specified site NEC
      peripheral — *see* Injury, nerve, abdomen, peripheral
    peripheral NEC T14.8
      abdomen — *see* Injury, nerve, abdomen, peripheral
      lower back — *see* Injury, nerve, abdomen, peripheral
      neck — *see* Injury, nerve, neck, peripheral
      pelvis — *see* Injury, nerve, abdomen, peripheral
      specified NEC T14.8
    peroneal (lower leg level) S84.1- ☑
      foot S94.2- ☑
    plexus
      brachial — *see* Injury, brachial plexus
      celiac, coeliac — *see* Injury, nerve, lumbosacral, sympathetic
      mesenteric, inferior — *see* Injury, nerve, lumbosacral, sympathetic
      sacral — *see* Injury, lumbosacral plexus
      spinal
        brachial — *see* Injury, brachial plexus
        lumbosacral — *see* Injury, lumbosacral plexus
    pneumogastric — *see* Injury, nerve, vagus
    radial (forearm level) S54.2- ☑
      hand (level) S64.2- ☑
      upper arm (level) S44.2- ☑
      wrist (level) — *see* Injury, nerve, radial, hand
    root — *see* Injury, nerve, spinal, root
    sacral plexus — *see* Injury, lumbosacral plexus
    sacral spinal — *see* Injury, nerve, spinal, sacral
    sciatic (hip level) (thigh level) S74.0- ☑
    second cranial (optic) — *see* Injury, nerve, optic
    seventh cranial (facial) — *see* Injury, nerve, facial

Injury — *continued*
  nerve — *continued*
    shoulder — *see* Injury, nerve, arm
    sixth cranial (abducent) — *see* Injury, nerve, abducens
    spinal
      plexus — *see* Injury, nerve, plexus, spinal
      root
        cervical S14.2 ☑
        dorsal S24.2 ☑
        lumbar S34.21 ☑
        sacral S34.22 ☑
        thoracic — *see* Injury, nerve, spinal, root, dorsal
    splanchnic — *see* Injury, nerve, lumbosacral, sympathetic
    sympathetic NEC — *see* Injury, nerve, lumbosacral, sympathetic
      cervical — *see* Injury, nerve, cervical sympathetic
    tenth cranial (pneumogastric or vagus) — *see* Injury, nerve, vagus
    thigh (level) — *see* Injury, nerve, hip
      cutaneous sensory — *see* Injury, nerve, cutaneous sensory, hip
      femoral — *see* Injury, nerve, femoral
      sciatic — *see* Injury, nerve, sciatic
      specified NEC — *see* Injury, nerve, hip
    third cranial (oculomotor) — *see* Injury, nerve, oculomotor
    thorax S24.9 ☑
      peripheral S24.3 ☑
      specified site NEC S24.8 ☑
      sympathetic S24.4 ☑
    thumb, digital — *see* Injury, nerve, digital, thumb
    tibial (lower leg level) (posterior) S84.0- ☑
    toe — *see* Injury, nerve, ankle
    trigeminal S04.3- ☑
      contusion S04.3- ☑
      laceration S04.3- ☑
      specified type NEC S04.3- ☑
    trochlear S04.2- ☑
      contusion S04.2- ☑
      laceration S04.2- ☑
      specified type NEC S04.2- ☑
    twelfth cranial (hypoglossal) — *see* Injury, nerve, hypoglossal
    ulnar (forearm level) S54.0- ☑
      arm (upper) (level) S44.0- ☑
      hand (level) S64.0- ☑
      wrist (level) — *see* Injury, nerve, ulnar, hand
    vagus S04.89- ☑
      specified type NEC S04.89- ☑
    wrist (level) — *see* Injury, nerve, hand
  ninth cranial nerve (glossopharyngeal) — *see* Injury, nerve, glossopharyngeal
  nose (septum) S09.92 ☑
  obstetrical O71.9
    specified NEC O71.89
  occipital (region) (scalp) S09.90 ☑
    lobe — *see* Injury, intracranial
  optic chiasm S04.02 ☑
  optic radiation S04.03- ☑
  optic tract and pathways S04.03- ☑
  orbit, orbital (region) — *see* Injury, eye
    penetrating (with foreign body) — *see* Injury, eye, orbit, penetrating
    specified NEC — *see* Injury, eye, specified site NEC
  ovary, ovarian S37.409 ☑
    bilateral S37.402 ☑
      contusion S37.422 ☑
      laceration S37.432 ☑
      specified type NEC S37.492 ☑
    blood vessel — *see* Injury, blood vessel, ovarian
    contusion S37.429 ☑
      bilateral S37.422 ☑
      unilateral S37.421 ☑
    laceration S37.439 ☑
      bilateral S37.432 ☑
      unilateral S37.431 ☑
    specified type NEC S37.499 ☑
      bilateral S37.492 ☑
      unilateral S37.491 ☑
    unilateral S37.401 ☑
      contusion S37.421 ☑
      laceration S37.431 ☑

Injury — *continued*
  ovary, ovarian — *continued*
    unilateral — *continued*
      specified type NEC S37.491 ☑
  palate (hard) (soft) S09.93 ☑
  pancreas S36.209 ☑
    body S36.201 ☑
      contusion S36.221 ☑
      laceration S36.231 ☑
        major S36.261 ☑
        minor S36.241 ☑
        moderate S36.251 ☑
      specified type NEC S36.291 ☑
    contusion S36.229 ☑
    head S36.200 ☑
      contusion S36.220 ☑
      laceration S36.230 ☑
        major S36.260 ☑
        minor S36.240 ☑
        moderate S36.250 ☑
      specified type NEC S36.290 ☑
    laceration S36.239 ☑
      major S36.269 ☑
      minor S36.249 ☑
      moderate S36.259 ☑
    specified type NEC S36.299 ☑
    tail S36.202 ☑
      contusion S36.222 ☑
      laceration S36.232 ☑
        major S36.262 ☑
        minor S36.242 ☑
        moderate S36.252 ☑
      specified type NEC S36.292 ☑
  parietal (region) (scalp) S09.90 ☑
    lobe — *see* Injury, intracranial
  patellar ligament (tendon) S76.10- ☑
    laceration S76.12- ☑
    specified NEC S76.19- ☑
    strain S76.11- ☑
  pelvis, pelvic (floor) S39.93 ☑
    complicating delivery O70.1
    joint or ligament, complicating delivery O71.6
    organ S37.90 ☑
      with ectopic or molar pregnancy O08.6
      complication of abortion — *see* Abortion
      contusion S37.92 ☑
      following ectopic or molar pregnancy O08.6
      laceration S37.93 ☑
      obstetrical trauma NEC O71.5
      specified
        site NEC S37.899 ☑
          contusion S37.892 ☑
          laceration S37.893 ☑
          specified type NEC S37.898 ☑
        type NEC S37.99 ☑
      specified NEC S39.83 ☑
  penis S39.94 ☑
  perineum S39.94 ☑
  peritoneum S36.81 ☑
    laceration S36.893 ☑
  periurethral tissue — *see* Injury, urethra
    complicating delivery O71.82
  phalanges
    foot — *see* Injury, foot
    hand — *see* Injury, hand
  pharynx NEC S19.85 ☑
  pleura — *see* Injury, intrathoracic, pleura
  plexus
    brachial — *see* Injury, brachial plexus
    cardiac — *see* Injury, nerve, thorax, sympathetic
    celiac, coeliac — *see* Injury, nerve, lumbosacral, sympathetic
    esophageal — *see* Injury, nerve, thorax, sympathetic
    hypogastric — *see* Injury, nerve, lumbosacral, sympathetic
    lumbar, lumbosacral — *see* Injury, lumbosacral plexus
    mesenteric — *see* Injury, nerve, lumbosacral, sympathetic
    pulmonary — *see* Injury, nerve, thorax, sympathetic
  postcardiac surgery (syndrome) I97.0
  prepuce S39.94 ☑
  prostate S37.829 ☑
    contusion S37.822 ☑

Injury — *continued*
  prostate — *continued*
    laceration S37.823 ☑
    specified type NEC S37.828 ☑
  pubic region S39.94 ☑
  pudendum S39.94 ☑
  pulmonary plexus — *see* Injury, nerve, thorax, sympathetic
  rectovaginal septum NEC S39.83 ☑
  rectum — *see* Injury, intestine, large, rectum
  retina — *see* Injury, eye, specified site NEC
    penetrating — *see* Injury, eyeball, penetrating
  retroperitoneal — *see* Injury, intra-abdominal, specified site NEC
  rotator cuff (muscle(s)) (tendon(s)) S46.00- ☑
    laceration S46.02- ☑
    specified type NEC S46.09- ☑
    strain S46.01- ☑
  round ligament — *see* Injury, pelvic organ, specified site NEC
  sacral plexus — *see* Injury, lumbosacral plexus
  salivary duct or gland S09.93 ☑
  scalp S09.90 ☑
    newborn (birth injury) P12.9
      due to monitoring (electrode) (sampling incision) P12.4
      specified NEC P12.89
        caput succedaneum P12.81
  scapular region — *see* Injury, shoulder
  sclera — *see* Injury, eye, specified site NEC
    penetrating — *see* Injury, eyeball, penetrating
  scrotum S39.94 ☑
  second cranial nerve (optic) — *see* Injury, nerve, optic
  seminal vesicle — *see* Injury, pelvic organ, specified site NEC
  seventh cranial nerve (facial) — *see* Injury, nerve, facial
  shoulder S49.9- ☑
    blood vessel — *see* Injury, blood vessel, arm
    contusion — *see* Contusion, shoulder
    dislocation — *see* Dislocation, shoulder
    fracture — *see* Fracture, shoulder
    muscle — *see* Injury, muscle, shoulder
    nerve — *see* Injury, nerve, shoulder
    open — *see* Wound, open, shoulder
    specified type NEC S49.8- ☑
    sprain — *see* Sprain, shoulder girdle
    superficial — *see* Injury, superficial, shoulder
  sinus
    cavernous — *see* Injury, intracranial
    nasal S09.92 ☑
  sixth cranial nerve (abducent) — *see* Injury, nerve, abducens
  skeleton, birth injury P13.9
    specified part NEC P13.8
  skin NEC T14.8
    surface intact — *see* Injury, superficial
  skull NEC S09.90 ☑
  specified NEC T14.8
  spermatic cord (pelvic region) S37.898 ☑
    scrotal region S39.848 ☑
  spinal (cord)
    cervical (neck) S14.109 ☑
      anterior cord syndrome S14.139 ☑
        C1 level S14.131 ☑
        C2 level S14.132 ☑
        C3 level S14.133 ☑
        C4 level S14.134 ☑
        C5 level S14.135 ☑
        C6 level S14.136 ☑
        C7 level S14.137 ☑
        C8 level S14.138 ☑
      Brown-Séquard syndrome S14.149 ☑
        C1 level S14.141 ☑
        C2 level S14.142 ☑
        C3 level S14.143 ☑
        C4 level S14.144 ☑
        C5 level S14.145 ☑
        C6 level S14.146 ☑
        C7 level S14.147 ☑
        C8 level S14.148 ☑
      C1 level S14.101 ☑
      C2 level S14.102 ☑
      C3 level S14.103 ☑
      C4 level S14.104 ☑
      C5 level S14.105 ☑
      C6 level S14.106 ☑

Injury — *continued*
  spinal — *continued*
    cervical — *continued*
      C7 level S14.107 ☑
      C8 level S14.108 ☑
      central cord syndrome S14.129 ☑
        C1 level S14.121 ☑
        C2 level S14.122 ☑
        C3 level S14.123 ☑
        C4 level S14.124 ☑
        C5 level S14.125 ☑
        C6 level S14.126 ☑
        C7 level S14.127 ☑
        C8 level S14.128 ☑
      complete lesion S14.119 ☑
        C1 level S14.111 ☑
        C2 level S14.112 ☑
        C3 level S14.113 ☑
        C4 level S14.114 ☑
        C5 level S14.115 ☑
        C6 level S14.116 ☑
        C7 level S14.117 ☑
        C8 level S14.118 ☑
      concussion S14.0 ☑
      edema S14.0 ☑
      incomplete lesion specified NEC S14.159 ☑
        C1 level S14.151 ☑
        C2 level S14.152 ☑
        C3 level S14.153 ☑
        C4 level S14.154 ☑
        C5 level S14.155 ☑
        C6 level S14.156 ☑
        C7 level S14.157 ☑
        C8 level S14.158 ☑
      posterior cord syndrome S14.159 ☑
        C1 level S14.151 ☑
        C2 level S14.152 ☑
        C3 level S14.153 ☑
        C4 level S14.154 ☑
        C5 level S14.155 ☑
        C6 level S14.156 ☑
        C7 level S14.157 ☑
        C8 level S14.158 ☑
    dorsal — *see* Injury, spinal, thoracic
    lumbar S34.109 ☑
      complete lesion S34.119 ☑
        L1 level S34.111 ☑
        L2 level S34.112 ☑
        L3 level S34.113 ☑
        L4 level S34.114 ☑
        L5 level S34.115 ☑
      concussion S34.01 ☑
      edema S34.01 ☑
      incomplete lesion S34.129 ☑
        L1 level S34.121 ☑
        L2 level S34.122 ☑
        L3 level S34.123 ☑
        L4 level S34.124 ☑
        L5 level S34.125 ☑
      L1 level S34.101 ☑
      L2 level S34.102 ☑
      L3 level S34.103 ☑
      L4 level S34.104 ☑
      L5 level S34.105 ☑
    nerve root NEC
      cervical — *see* Injury, nerve, spinal, root, cervical
      dorsal — *see* Injury, nerve, spinal, root, dorsal
      lumbar S34.21 ☑
      sacral S34.22 ☑
      thoracic — *see* Injury, nerve, spinal, root, dorsal
    plexus
      brachial — *see* Injury, brachial plexus
      lumbosacral — *see* Injury, lumbosacral plexus
    sacral S34.139 ☑
      complete lesion S34.131 ☑
      incomplete lesion S34.132 ☑
    thoracic S24.109 ☑
      anterior cord syndrome S24.139 ☑
        T1 level S24.131 ☑
        T2-T6 level S24.132 ☑
        T7-T10 level S24.133 ☑
        T11-T12 level S24.134 ☑
      Brown-Séquard syndrome S24.149 ☑
        T1 level S24.141 ☑

Injury — *continued*
  spinal — *continued*
    thoracic — *continued*
      Brown-Séquard syndrome — *continued*
        T2-T6 level S24.142 ☑
        T7-T10 level S24.143 ☑
        T11-T12 level S24.144 ☑
      complete lesion S24.119 ☑
        T1 level S24.111 ☑
        T2-T6 level S24.112 ☑
        T7-T10 level S24.113 ☑
        T11-T12 level S24.114 ☑
      concussion S24.0 ☑
      edema S24.0 ☑
      incomplete lesion specified NEC S24.159 ☑
        T1 level S24.151 ☑
        T2-T6 level S24.152 ☑
        T7-T10 level S24.153 ☑
        T11-T12 level S24.154 ☑
      posterior cord syndrome S24.159 ☑
        T1 level S24.151 ☑
        T2-T6 level S24.152 ☑
        T7-T10 level S24.153 ☑
        T11-T12 level S24.154 ☑
      T1 level S24.101 ☑
      T2-T6 level S24.102 ☑
      T7-T10 level S24.103 ☑
      T11-T12 level S24.104 ☑
  splanchnic nerve — *see* Injury, nerve, lumbosacral, sympathetic
  spleen S36.00 ☑
    contusion S36.029 ☑
      major S36.021 ☑
      minor S36.020 ☑
    laceration S36.039 ☑
      major (massive) (stellate) S36.032 ☑
      moderate S36.031 ☑
      superficial (capsular) (minor) S36.030 ☑
    specified type NEC S36.09 ☑
  splenic artery — *see* Injury, blood vessel, celiac artery, branch
  stellate ganglion — *see* Injury, nerve, thorax, sympathetic
  sternal region S29.9 ☑
  stomach S36.30 ☑
    contusion S36.32 ☑
    laceration S36.33 ☑
    specified type NEC S36.39 ☑
  subconjunctival — *see* Injury, eye, conjunctiva
  subcutaneous NEC T14.8
  submaxillary region S09.93 ☑
  submental region S09.93 ☑
  subungual
    fingers — *see* Injury, hand
    toes — *see* Injury, foot
  superficial NEC T14.8
    abdomen, abdominal (wall) S30.92 ☑
      abrasion S30.811 ☑
      bite S30.871 ☑
        insect S30.861 ☑
      contusion S30.1
      external constriction S30.841 ☑
      foreign body S30.851 ☑
    abrasion — *see* Abrasion, by site
    adnexa, eye NEC — *see* Injury, eye, specified site NEC
    alveolar process — *see* Injury, superficial, oral cavity
    ankle S90.91- ☑
      abrasion — *see* Abrasion, ankle
      bite — *see* Bite, ankle
      blister — *see* Blister, ankle
      contusion — *see* Contusion, ankle
      external constriction — *see* Constriction, external, ankle
      foreign body — *see* Foreign body, superficial, ankle
    anus S30.98 ☑
    arm (upper) S40.92- ☑
      abrasion — *see* Abrasion, arm
      bite — *see* Bite, superficial, arm
      blister — *see* Blister, arm (upper)
      contusion — *see* Contusion, arm
      external constriction — *see* Constriction, external, arm

Injury — continued
    superficial — continued
        arm — continued
            foreign body — see Foreign body, superficial, arm
            auditory canal (external) (meatus) — see Injury, superficial, ear
            auricle — see Injury, superficial, ear
            axilla — see Injury, superficial, arm
        back (see also Injury, superficial, thorax, back)
            lower S30.91 ☑
                abrasion S30.810 ☑
                contusion S30.0 ☑
                external constriction S30.840 ☑
                superficial
                    bite NEC S30.870 ☑
                    insect S30.860 ☑
                foreign body S30.850 ☑
        bite NEC — see Bite, superficial NEC, by site
        blister — see Blister, by site
        breast S20.10- ☑
            abrasion — see Abrasion, breast
            bite — see Bite, superficial, breast
            contusion — see Contusion, breast
            external constriction — see Constriction, external, breast
            foreign body — see Foreign body, superficial, breast
        brow — see Injury, superficial, head, specified NEC
        buttock S30.91 ☑
        calf — see Injury, superficial, leg
        canthus, eye — see Injury, superficial, periocular area
        cheek (external) — see Injury, superficial, head, specified NEC
            internal — see Injury, superficial, oral cavity
        chest wall — see Injury, superficial, thorax
        chin — see Injury, superficial, head NEC
        clitoris S30.95 ☑
        conjunctiva — see Injury, eye, conjunctiva
            with foreign body (in conjunctival sac) — see Foreign body, conjunctival sac
        contusion — see Contusion, by site
        costal region — see Injury, superficial, thorax
        digit(s)
            hand — see Injury, superficial, finger
        ear (auricle) (canal) (external) S00.40- ☑
            abrasion — see Abrasion, ear
            bite — see Bite, superficial, ear
            contusion — see Contusion, ear
            external constriction — see Constriction, external, ear
            foreign body — see Foreign body, superficial, ear
        elbow S50.90- ☑
            abrasion — see Abrasion, elbow
            bite — see Bite, superficial, elbow
            blister — see Blister, elbow
            contusion — see Contusion, elbow
            external constriction — see Constriction, external, elbow
            foreign body — see Foreign body, superficial, elbow
        epididymis S30.94 ☑
        epigastric region S30.92 ☑
        epiglottis — see Injury, superficial, throat
        esophagus
            cervical — see Injury, superficial, throat
        external constriction — see Constriction, external, by site
        extremity NEC T14.8
        eyeball NEC — see Injury, eye, specified site NEC
        eyebrow — see Injury, superficial, periocular area
        eyelid S00.20- ☑
            abrasion — see Abrasion, eyelid
            bite — see Bite, superficial, eyelid
            contusion — see Contusion, eyelid
            external constriction — see Constriction, external, eyelid
            foreign body — see Foreign body, superficial, eyelid
        face NEC — see Injury, superficial, head, specified NEC
        finger(s) S60.949 ☑
            abrasion — see Abrasion, finger
            bite — see Bite, superficial, finger

Injury — continued
    superficial — continued
        finger(s) — continued
            blister — see Blister, finger
            contusion — see Contusion, finger
            external constriction — see Constriction, external, finger
            foreign body — see Foreign body, superficial, finger
            index S60.94- ☑
            insect bite — see Bite, by site, superficial, insect
            little S60.94- ☑
            middle S60.94- ☑
            ring S60.94- ☑
        flank S30.92 ☑
        foot S90.92- ☑
            abrasion — see Abrasion, foot
            bite — see Bite, foot
            blister — see Blister, foot
            contusion — see Contusion, foot
            external constriction — see Constriction, external, foot
            foreign body — see Foreign body, superficial, foot
        forearm S50.91- ☑
            abrasion — see Abrasion, forearm
            bite — see Bite, forearm, superficial
            blister — see Blister, forearm
            contusion — see Contusion, forearm
            elbow only — see Injury, superficial, elbow
            external constriction — see Constriction, external, forearm
            foreign body — see Foreign body, superficial, forearm
        forehead — see Injury, superficial, head NEC
        foreign body — see Foreign body, superficial
        genital organs, external
            female S30.97 ☑
            male S30.96 ☑
        globe (eye) — see Injury, eye, specified site NEC
        groin S30.92 ☑
        gum — see Injury, superficial, oral cavity
        hand S60.92- ☑
            abrasion — see Abrasion, hand
            bite — see Bite, superficial, hand
            contusion — see Contusion, hand
            external constriction — see Constriction, external, hand
            foreign body — see Foreign body, superficial, hand
        head S00.90 ☑
            ear — see Injury, superficial, ear
            eyelid — see Injury, superficial, eyelid
            nose S00.30 ☑
            oral cavity S00.502 ☑
            scalp S00.00 ☑
            specified site NEC S00.80 ☑
        heel — see Injury, superficial, foot
        hip S70.91- ☑
            abrasion — see Abrasion, hip
            bite — see Bite, superficial, hip
            blister — see Blister, hip
            contusion — see Contusion, hip
            external constriction — see Constriction, external, hip
            foreign body — see Foreign body, superficial, hip
        iliac region — see Injury, superficial, abdomen
        inguinal region — see Injury, superficial, abdomen
        insect bite — see Bite, by site, superficial, insect
        interscapular region — see Injury, superficial, thorax, back
        jaw — see Injury, superficial, head, specified NEC
        knee S80.91- ☑
            abrasion — see Abrasion, knee
            bite — see Bite, superficial, knee
            blister — see Blister, knee
            contusion — see Contusion, knee
            external constriction — see Constriction, external, knee
            foreign body — see Foreign body, superficial, knee
        labium (majus) (minus) S30.95 ☑
        lacrimal (apparatus) (gland) (sac) — see Injury, eye, specified site NEC
        larynx — see Injury, superficial, throat

Injury — continued
    superficial — continued
        leg (lower) S80.92- ☑
            abrasion — see Abrasion, leg
            bite — see Bite, superficial, leg
            contusion — see Contusion, leg
            external constriction — see Constriction, external, leg
            foreign body — see Foreign body, superficial, leg
            knee — see Injury, superficial, knee
        limb NEC T14.8
        lip S00.501 ☑
        lower back S30.91 ☑
        lumbar region S30.91 ☑
        malar region — see Injury, superficial, head, specified NEC
        mammary — see Injury, superficial, breast
        mastoid region — see Injury, superficial, head, specified NEC
        mouth — see Injury, superficial, oral cavity
        muscle NEC T14.8
        nail NEC T14.8
            finger — see Injury, superficial, finger
            toe — see Injury, superficial, toe
        nasal (septum) — see Injury, superficial, nose
        neck S10.90 ☑
            specified site NEC S10.80 ☑
        nose (septum) S00.30 ☑
        occipital region — see Injury, superficial, scalp
        oral cavity S00.502 ☑
        orbital region — see Injury, superficial, periocular area
        palate — see Injury, superficial, oral cavity
        palm — see Injury, superficial, hand
        parietal region — see Injury, superficial, scalp
        pelvis S30.91 ☑
        penis S30.93 ☑
        perineum
            female S30.95 ☑
            male S30.91 ☑
        periocular area S00.20- ☑
            abrasion — see Abrasion, eyelid
            bite — see Bite, superficial, eyelid
            contusion — see Contusion, eyelid
            external constriction — see Constriction, external, eyelid
            foreign body — see Foreign body, superficial, eyelid
        phalanges
            finger — see Injury, superficial, finger
            toe — see Injury, superficial, toe
        pharynx — see Injury, superficial, throat
        pinna — see Injury, superficial, ear
        popliteal space — see Injury, superficial, knee
        prepuce S30.93 ☑
        pubic region S30.91 ☑
        pudendum
            female S30.97 ☑
            male S30.96 ☑
        sacral region S30.91 ☑
        scalp S00.00 ☑
        scapular region — see Injury, superficial, shoulder
        sclera — see Injury, eye, specified site NEC
        scrotum S30.94 ☑
        shin — see Injury, superficial, leg
        shoulder S40.91- ☑
            abrasion — see Abrasion, shoulder
            bite — see Bite, superficial, shoulder
            blister — see Blister, shoulder
            contusion — see Contusion, shoulder
            external constriction — see Constriction, external, shoulder
            foreign body — see Foreign body, superficial, shoulder
        skin NEC T14.8
        sternal region — see Injury, superficial, thorax, front
        subconjunctival — see Injury, eye, specified site NEC
        subcutaneous NEC T14.8
        submaxillary region — see Injury, superficial, head, specified NEC
        submental region — see Injury, superficial, head, specified NEC

☑ **Additional Character Required** — **Refer to the Tabular List for Character Selection**   ▽ **Subterms under main terms may continue to next column or page**

Injury — *continued*
  superficial — *continued*
    subungual
      finger(s) — *see* Injury, superficial, finger
      toe(s) — *see* Injury, superficial, toe
    supraclavicular fossa — *see* Injury, superficial, neck
    supraorbital — *see* Injury, superficial, head, specified NEC
    temple — *see* Injury, superficial, head, specified NEC
    temporal region — *see* Injury, superficial, head, specified NEC
    testis S30.94 ☑
    thigh S70.92- ☑
      abrasion — *see* Abrasion, thigh
      bite — *see* Bite, superficial, thigh
      blister — *see* Blister, thigh
      contusion — *see* Contusion, thigh
      external constriction — *see* Constriction, external, thigh
      foreign body — *see* Foreign body, superficial, thigh
    thorax, thoracic (wall) S20.90 ☑
      abrasion — *see* Abrasion, thorax
      back S20.40- ☑
      bite — *see* Bite, thorax, superficial
      blister — *see* Blister, thorax
      contusion — *see* Contusion, thorax
      external constriction — *see* Constriction, external, thorax
      foreign body — *see* Foreign body, superficial, thorax
      front S20.30- ☑
    throat S10.10 ☑
      abrasion S10.11 ☑
      bite S10.17 ☑
        insect S10.16 ☑
      blister S10.12 ☑
      contusion S10.0 ☑
      external constriction S10.14 ☑
      foreign body S10.15 ☑
    thumb S60.93- ☑
      abrasion — *see* Abrasion, thumb
      bite — *see* Bite, superficial, thumb
      blister — *see* Blister, thumb
      contusion — *see* Contusion, thumb
      external constriction — *see* Constriction, external, thumb
      foreign body — *see* Foreign body, superficial, thumb
      insect bite — *see* Bite, by site, superficial, insect
      specified type NEC S60.39 ☑
    toe(s) S90.93- ☑
      abrasion — *see* Abrasion, toe
      bite — *see* Bite, toe
      blister — *see* Blister, toe
      contusion — *see* Contusion, toe
      external constriction — *see* Constriction, external, toe
      foreign body — *see* Foreign body, superficial, toe
      great S90.93- ☑
    tongue — *see* Injury, superficial, oral cavity
    tooth, teeth — *see* Injury, superficial, oral cavity
    trachea S10.10 ☑
    tunica vaginalis S30.94 ☑
    tympanum, tympanic membrane — *see* Injury, superficial, ear
    uvula — *see* Injury, superficial, oral cavity
    vagina S30.95 ☑
    vocal cords — *see* Injury, superficial, throat
    vulva S30.95 ☑
    wrist S60.91- ☑
  supraclavicular region — *see* Injury, neck
  supraorbital S09.93 ☑
  suprarenal gland (multiple) — *see* Injury, adrenal
  surgical complication (external or internal site) — *see* Laceration, accidental complicating surgery
  temple S09.90 ☑
  temporal region S09.90 ☑
  tendon (*see also* Injury, muscle, by site)
    abdomen — *see* Injury, muscle, abdomen
    Achilles — *see* Injury, Achilles tendon
    lower back — *see* Injury, muscle, lower back
    pelvic organs — *see* Injury, muscle, pelvis

Injury — *continued*
  tenth cranial nerve (pneumogastric or vagus) — *see* Injury, nerve, vagus
  testis S39.94 ☑
  thigh S79.92-
    blood vessel — *see* Injury, blood vessel, hip
    contusion — *see* Contusion, thigh
    fracture — *see* Fracture, femur
    muscle — *see* Injury, muscle, thigh
    nerve — *see* Injury, nerve, thigh
    open — *see* Wound, open, thigh
    specified NEC S79.82- ☑
    superficial — *see* Injury, superficial, thigh
  third cranial nerve (oculomotor) — *see* Injury, nerve, oculomotor
  thorax, thoracic S29.9 ☑
    blood vessel — *see* Injury, blood vessel, thorax
    cavity — *see* Injury, intrathoracic
    dislocation — *see* Dislocation, thorax
    external (wall) S29.9 ☑
      contusion — *see* Contusion, thorax
      nerve — *see* Injury, nerve, thorax
      open — *see* Wound, open, thorax
      specified NEC S29.8 ☑
      sprain — *see* Sprain, thorax
      superficial — *see* Injury, superficial, thorax
    fracture — *see* Fracture, thorax
    internal — *see* Injury, intrathoracic
    intrathoracic organ — *see* Injury, intrathoracic
    sympathetic ganglion — *see* Injury, nerve, thorax, sympathetic
  throat (*see also* Injury, neck) S19.9 ☑
  thumb S69.9- ☑
    blood vessel — *see* Injury, blood vessel, thumb
    contusion — *see* Contusion, thumb
    dislocation — *see* Dislocation, thumb
    fracture — *see* Fracture, thumb
    muscle — *see* Injury, muscle, thumb
    nerve — *see* Injury, nerve, digital, thumb
    open — *see* Wound, open, thumb
    specified NEC S69.8- ☑
    sprain — *see* Sprain, thumb
    superficial — *see* Injury, superficial, thumb
  thymus (gland) — *see* Injury, intrathoracic, specified organ NEC
  thyroid (gland) NEC S19.84 ☑
  toe S99.92- ☑
    contusion — *see* Contusion, toe
    dislocation — *see* Dislocation, toe
    fracture — *see* Fracture, toe
    muscle — *see* Injury, muscle, toe
    open — *see* Wound, open, toe
    specified type NEC S99.82- ☑
    sprain — *see* Sprain, toe
    superficial — *see* Injury, superficial, toe
  tongue S09.93 ☑
  tonsil S09.93 ☑
  tooth S09.93 ☑
  trachea (cervical) NEC S19.82 ☑
    thoracic — *see* Injury, intrathoracic, trachea, thoracic
  transfusion-related acute lung (TRALI) J95.84
  tunica vaginalis S39.94 ☑
  twelfth cranial nerve (hypoglossal) — *see* Injury, nerve, hypoglossal
  ureter S37.10 ☑
    contusion S37.12 ☑
    laceration S37.13 ☑
    specified type NEC S37.19 ☑
  urethra (sphincter) S37.30 ☑
    at delivery O71.5
    contusion S37.32 ☑
    laceration S37.33 ☑
    specified type NEC S37.39 ☑
  urinary organ S37.90 ☑
    contusion S37.92 ☑
    laceration S37.93 ☑
    specified
      site NEC S37.899 ☑
        contusion S37.892 ☑
        laceration S37.893 ☑
        specified type NEC S37.898 ☑
      type NEC S37.99 ☑
  uterus, uterine S37.60 ☑
    with ectopic or molar pregnancy O08.6
    blood vessel — *see* Injury, blood vessel, iliac

Injury — *continued*
  uterus, uterine — *continued*
    contusion S37.62 ☑
    laceration S37.63 ☑
      cervix at delivery O71.3
    rupture associated with obstetrics — *see* Rupture, uterus
    specified type NEC S37.69 ☑
  uvula S09.93 ☑
  vagina S39.93 ☑
    abrasion S30.814 ☑
    bite S31.45 ☑
      insect S30.864 ☑
      superficial NEC S30.874 ☑
    contusion S30.23 ☑
    crush S38.03 ☑
    during delivery — *see* Laceration, vagina, during delivery
    external constriction S30.844 ☑
    insect bite S30.864 ☑
    laceration S31.41 ☑
      with foreign body S31.42 ☑
    open wound S31.40 ☑
    puncture S31.43 ☑
      with foreign body S31.44 ☑
    superficial S30.95 ☑
      foreign body S30.854 ☑
  vas deferens — *see* Injury, pelvic organ, specified site NEC
  vascular NEC T14.8
  vein — *see* Injury, blood vessel
  vena cava (superior) S25.20 ☑
    inferior S35.10 ☑
      laceration (minor) (superficial) S35.11 ☑
        major S35.12 ☑
      specified type NEC S35.19 ☑
    laceration (minor) (superficial) S25.21 ☑
      major S25.22 ☑
    specified type NEC S25.29 ☑
  vesical (sphincter) — *see* Injury, bladder
  visual cortex S04.04- ☑
  vitreous (humor) S05.90 ☑
    specified NEC S05.8X- ☑
  vocal cord NEC S19.83 ☑
  vulva S39.94 ☑
    abrasion S30.814 ☑
    bite S31.45 ☑
      insect S30.864 ☑
      superficial NEC S30.874 ☑
    contusion S30.23 ☑
    crush S38.03 ☑
    during delivery — *see* Laceration, perineum, female, during delivery
    external constriction S30.844 ☑
    insect bite S30.864 ☑
    laceration S31.41 ☑
      with foreign body S31.42 ☑
    open wound S31.40 ☑
    puncture S31.43 ☑
      with foreign body S31.44 ☑
    superficial S30.95 ☑
      foreign body S30.854 ☑
  whiplash (cervical spine) S13.4 ☑
  wrist S69.9- ☑
    blood vessel — *see* Injury, blood vessel, hand
    contusion — *see* Contusion, wrist
    dislocation — *see* Dislocation, wrist
    fracture — *see* Fracture, wrist
    muscle — *see* Injury, muscle, hand
    nerve — *see* Injury, nerve, hand
    open — *see* Wound, open, wrist
    specified NEC S69.8- ☑
    sprain — *see* Sprain, wrist
    superficial — *see* Injury, superficial, wrist

Inoculation (*see also* Vaccination)
  complication or reaction — *see* Complications, vaccination

Insanity, insane (*see also* Psychosis)
  adolescent — *see* Schizophrenia
  confusional F28
    acute or subacute F05
  delusional F22
  senile F03 ☑

Insect
  bite — *see* Bite, by site, superficial, insect

Insect — *continued*
  venomous, poisoning NEC (by) — *see* Venom, arthropod
Insensitivity
  adrenocorticotropin hormone (ACTH) E27.49
  androgen E34.50
    complete E34.51
    partial E34.52
Insertion
  cord (umbilical) lateral or velamentous O43.12- ☑
  intrauterine contraceptive device (encounter for) — *see* Intrauterine contraceptive device
Insolation (sunstroke) T67.0 ☑
Insomnia (organic) G47.00
  without objective findings F51.02
  adjustment F51.02
  adjustment disorder F51.02
  behavioral, of childhood Z73.819
    combined type Z73.812
    limit setting type Z73.811
    sleep-onset association type Z73.810
  childhood Z73.819
  chronic F51.04
    somatized tension F51.04
  conditioned F51.04
  due to
    alcohol
      abuse F10.182
      dependence F10.282
      use F10.982
    amphetamines
      abuse F15.182
      dependence F15.282
      use F15.982
    anxiety disorder F51.05
    caffeine
      abuse F15.182
      dependence F15.282
      use F15.982
    cocaine
      abuse F14.182
      dependence F14.282
      use F14.982
    depression F51.05
    drug NEC
      abuse F19.182
      dependence F19.282
      use F19.982
    medical condition G47.01
    mental disorder NEC F51.05
    opioid
      abuse F11.182
      dependence F11.282
      use F11.982
    psychoactive substance NEC
      abuse F19.182
      dependence F19.182
      use F19.982
    sedative, hypnotic, or anxiolytic
      abuse F13.182
      dependence F13.282
      use F13.982
    stimulant NEC
      abuse F15.182
      dependence F15.282
      use F15.982
  fatal familial (FFI) A81.83
  idiopathic F51.01
  learned F51.3
  nonorganic origin F51.01
  not due to a substance or known physiological condition F51.01
    specified NEC F51.09
  paradoxical F51.03
  primary F51.01
  psychiatric F51.05
  psychophysiologic F51.04
  related to psychopathology F51.05
  short-term F51.02
  specified NEC G47.09
  stress-related F51.02
  transient F51.02
Inspiration
  food or foreign body — *see* Foreign body, by site
  mucus — *see* Asphyxia, mucus
Inspissated bile syndrome (newborn) P59.1
Instability
  emotional (excessive) F60.3

Instability — *continued*
  joint (post-traumatic) M25.30
    ankle M25.37- ☑
    due to old ligament injury — *see* Disorder, ligament
    elbow M25.32- ☑
    flail — *see* Flail, joint
    foot M25.37- ☑
    hand M25.34- ☑
    hip M25.35- ☑
    knee M25.36- ☑
    lumbosacral — *see* subcategory M53.2 ☑
    prosthesis — *see* Complications, joint prosthesis, mechanical, displacement, by site
    sacroiliac — *see* subcategory M53.2 ☑
    secondary to
      old ligament injury — *see* Disorder, ligament
      removal of joint prosthesis M96.89
    shoulder (region) M25.31- ☑
    spine — *see* subcategory M53.2 ☑
    wrist M25.33- ☑
  knee (chronic) M23.5- ☑
  lumbosacral — *see* subcategory M53.2 ☑
  nervous F48.8
  personality (emotional) F60.3
  spine — *see* Instability, joint, spine
  vasomotor R55
Institutional syndrome (childhood) F94.2
Institutionalization, affecting child Z62.22
  disinhibited attachment F94.2
Insufficiency, insufficient
  accommodation, old age H52.4
  adrenal (gland) E27.40
    primary E27.1
  adrenocortical E27.40
    drug-induced E27.3
    iatrogenic E27.3
    primary E27.1
  anterior (occlusal) guidance M26.54
  anus K62.89
  aortic (valve) I35.1
    with
      mitral (valve) disease I08.0
        with tricuspid (valve) disease I08.3
      stenosis I35.2
      tricuspid (valve) disease I08.2
        with mitral (valve) disease I08.3
    congenital Q23.1
    rheumatic I06.1
      with
        mitral (valve) disease I08.0
          with tricuspid (valve) disease I08.3
        stenosis I06.2
          with mitral (valve) disease I08.0
            with tricuspid (valve) disease I08.3
        tricuspid (valve) disease I08.2
          with mitral (valve) disease I08.3
    specified cause NEC I35.1
    syphilitic A52.03
  arterial I77.1
    basilar G45.0
    carotid (hemispheric) G45.1
    cerebral I67.81
    coronary (acute or subacute) I24.8
    mesenteric K55.1
    peripheral I73.9
    precerebral (multiple) (bilateral) G45.2
    vertebral G45.0
  arteriovenous I99.8
  biliary K83.8
  cardiac (*see also* Insufficiency, myocardial)
    due to presence of (cardiac) prosthesis I97.11- ☑
    postprocedural I97.11- ☑
  cardiorenal, hypertensive I13.2
  cardiovascular — *see* Disease, cardiovascular
  cerebrovascular (acute) I67.81
    with transient focal neurological signs and symptoms G45.8
  circulatory NEC I99.8
    newborn P29.89
  convergence H51.11
  coronary (acute or subacute) I24.8
    chronic or with a stated duration of over 4 weeks I25.89
  corticoadrenal E27.40
    primary E27.1
  dietary E63.9
  divergence H51.8

Insufficiency, insufficient — *continued*
  food T73.0 ☑
  gastroesophageal K22.8
  gonadal
    ovary E28.39
    testis E29.1
  heart (*see also* Insufficiency, myocardial)
    newborn P29.0
    valve — *see* Endocarditis
  hepatic — *see* Failure, hepatic
  idiopathic autonomic G90.09
  interocclusal distance of fully erupted teeth (ridge) M26.36
  kidney N28.9
    acute N28.9
    chronic N18.9
  lacrimal (secretion) H04.12- ☑
    passages — *see* Stenosis, lacrimal
  liver — *see* Failure, hepatic
  lung — *see* Insufficiency, pulmonary
  mental (congenital) — *see* Disability, intellectual
  mesenteric K55.1
  mitral (valve) I34.0
    with
      aortic valve disease I08.0
        with tricuspid (valve) disease I08.3
      obstruction or stenosis I05.2
        with aortic valve disease I08.0
      tricuspid (valve) disease I08.1
        with aortic (valve) disease I08.3
    congenital Q23.3
    rheumatic I05.1
      with
        aortic valve disease I08.0
          with tricuspid (valve) disease I08.3
        obstruction or stenosis I05.2
          with aortic valve disease I08.0
            with tricuspid (valve) disease I08.3
        tricuspid (valve) disease I08.1
          with aortic (valve) disease I08.3
    active or acute I01.1
      with chorea, rheumatic (Sydenham's) I02.0
    specified cause, except rheumatic I34.0
  muscle (*see also* Disease, muscle)
    heart — *see* Insufficiency, myocardial
  ocular NEC H50.9
  myocardial, myocardium (with arteriosclerosis) I50.9
    with
      rheumatic fever (conditions in I00) I09.0
        active, acute or subacute I01.2
          with chorea I02.0
        inactive or quiescent (with chorea) I09.0
    congenital Q24.8
    hypertensive — *see* Hypertension, heart
    newborn P29.0
    rheumatic I09.0
      active, acute, or subacute I01.2
    syphilitic A52.06
  nourishment T73.0 ☑
  pancreatic K86.8
  parathyroid (gland) E20.9
  peripheral vascular (arterial) I73.9
  pituitary E23.0
  placental (mother) O36.51- ☑
  platelets D69.6
  prenatal care affecting management of pregnancy O09.3- ☑
  progressive pluriglandular E31.0
  pulmonary J98.4
    acute, following surgery (nonthoracic) J95.2
      thoracic J95.1
    chronic, following surgery J95.3
    following
      shock J98.4
      trauma J98.4
    newborn P28.5
    valve I37.1
      with stenosis I37.2
      congenital Q22.2
      rheumatic I09.89
        with aortic, mitral or tricuspid (valve) disease I08.8
  pyloric K31.89
  renal (acute) N28.9
    chronic N18.9
  respiratory R06.89
    newborn P28.5
  rotation — *see* Malrotation

Insufficiency, insufficient — continued
- sleep syndrome F51.12
- social insurance Z59.7
- suprarenal E27.40
  - primary E27.1
- tarso-orbital fascia, congenital Q10.3
- testis E29.1
- thyroid (gland) (acquired) E03.9
  - congenital E03.1
- tricuspid (valve) (rheumatic) I07.1
  - with
    - aortic (valve) disease I08.2
      - with mitral (valve) disease I08.3
    - mitral (valve) disease I08.1
      - with aortic (valve) disease I08.3
    - obstruction or stenosis I07.2
      - with aortic (valve) disease I08.2
        - with mitral (valve) disease I08.3
  - congenital Q22.8
  - nonrheumatic I36.1
    - with stenosis I36.2
- urethral sphincter R32
- valve, valvular (heart) — see Endocarditis
  - congenital Q24.8
- vascular I99.8
  - intestine K55.9
    - acute K55.0
  - mesenteric K55.1
  - peripheral I73.9
  - renal — see Hypertension, kidney
- velopharyngeal
  - acquired K13.79
  - congenital Q38.8
- venous (chronic) (peripheral) I87.2
- ventricular — see Insufficiency, myocardial
- welfare support Z59.7

Insufflation, fallopian Z31.41
Insular — see condition
Insulinoma
- pancreas
  - benign D13.7
  - malignant C25.4
  - uncertain behavior D37.8
- specified site
  - benign — see Neoplasm, by site, benign
  - malignant — see Neoplasm, by site, malignant
  - uncertain behavior — see Neoplasm, by site, uncertain behavior
- unspecified site
  - benign D13.7
  - malignant C25.4
  - uncertain behavior D37.8

Insuloma — see Insulinoma
Interference
- balancing side M26.56
- non-working side M26.56

Intermenstrual — see condition
Intermittent — see condition
Internal — see condition
Interrogation
- cardiac defibrillator (automatic) (implantable) Z45.02
- cardiac pacemaker Z45.018
- cardiac (event) (loop) recorder Z45.09
- infusion pump (implanted) (intrathecal) Z45.1
- neurostimulator Z46.2

Interruption
- bundle of His I44.30
- phase-shift, sleep cycle — see Disorder, sleep, circadian rhythm
- sleep phase-shift, or 24 hour sleep-wake cycle — see Disorder, sleep, circadian rhythm

Interstitial — see condition
Intertrigo L30.4
- labialis K13.0
Intervertebral disc — see condition
Intestine, intestinal — see condition
Intolerance
- carbohydrate K90.4
- disaccharide, hereditary E73.0
- fat NEC K90.4
  - pancreatic K90.3
- food K90.4
  - dietary counseling and surveillance Z71.3
- fructose E74.10
  - hereditary E74.12
- glucose (-galactose) E74.39
- gluten K90.0
- lactose E73.9

Intolerance — continued
- lactose — continued
  - specified NEC E73.8
- lysine E72.3
- milk NEC K90.4
  - lactose E73.9
- protein K90.4
- starch NEC K90.4
- sucrose (-isomaltose) E74.31

Intoxicated NEC (without dependence) — see Alcohol, intoxication
Intoxication
- acid E87.2
- alcoholic (acute) (without dependence) — see Alcohol, intoxication
- alimentary canal K52.1
- amphetamine (without dependence) — see Abuse, drug, stimulant, with intoxication
  - with dependence — see Dependence, drug, stimulant, with intoxication
- anxiolytic (acute) (without dependence) — see Abuse, drug, sedative, with intoxication
  - with dependence — see Dependence, drug, sedative, with intoxication
- caffeine (acute) (without dependence) — see Abuse, drug, stimulant, with intoxication
  - with dependence — see Dependence, drug, stimulant, with intoxication
- cannabinoids (acute) (without dependence) — see Abuse, drug, cannabis, with intoxication
  - with dependence — see Dependence, drug, cannabis, with intoxication
- chemical — see Table of Drugs and Chemicals
  - via placenta or breast milk — see - Absorption, chemical, through placenta
- cocaine (acute) (without dependence) — see Abuse, drug, cocaine, with intoxication
  - with dependence — see Dependence, drug, cocaine, with intoxication
- drug
  - acute (without dependence) — see Abuse, drug, by type with intoxication
    - with dependence — see Dependence, drug, by type with intoxication
  - addictive
    - via placenta or breast milk — see Absorption, drug, addictive, through placenta
  - newborn P93.8
    - gray baby syndrome P93.0
  - overdose or wrong substance given or taken — see Table of Drugs and Chemicals, by drug, poisoning
- enteric K52.1
- foodborne A05.9
  - bacterial A05.9
  - classical (Clostridium botulinum) A05.1
  - due to
    - Bacillus cereus A05.4
    - bacterium A05.9
      - specified NEC A05.8
    - Clostridium
      - botulinum A05.1
      - perfringens A05.2
      - welchii A05.2
    - Salmonella A02.9
      - with
        - (gastro)enteritis A02.0
        - localized infection(s) A02.20
          - arthritis A02.23
          - meningitis A02.21
          - osteomyelitis A02.24
          - pneumonia A02.22
          - pyelonephritis A02.25
          - specified NEC A02.29
        - sepsis A02.1
        - specified manifestation NEC A02.8
    - Staphylococcus A05.0
    - Vibrio
      - parahaemolyticus A05.3
      - vulnificus A05.5
  - enterotoxin, staphylococcal A05.0
  - noxious — see Poisoning, food, noxious
- gastrointestinal K52.1
- hallucinogenic (without dependence) — see Abuse, drug, hallucinogen, with intoxication
  - with dependence — see Dependence, drug, hallucinogen, with intoxication

Intoxication — continued
- hypnotic (acute) (without dependence) — see Abuse, drug, sedative, with intoxication
  - with dependence — see Dependence, drug, sedative, with intoxication
- inhalant (acute) (without dependence) — see Abuse, drug, inhalant, with intoxication
  - with dependence — see Dependence, drug, inhalant, with intoxication
- meaning
  - inebriation — see category F10 ☑
  - poisoning — see Table of Drugs and Chemicals
- methyl alcohol (acute) (without dependence) — see Alcohol, intoxication
- opioid (acute) (without dependence) — see Abuse, drug, opioid, with intoxication
  - with dependence — see Dependence, drug, opioid, with intoxication
- pathologic NEC (without dependence) — see Alcohol, intoxication
- phencyclidine (without dependence) — see Abuse, drug, psychoactive NEC, with intoxication
  - with dependence — see Dependence, drug, psychoactive NEC, with intoxication
- potassium (K) E87.5
- psychoactive substance NEC (without dependence) — see Abuse, drug, psychoactive NEC, with intoxication
  - with dependence — see Dependence, drug, psychoactive NEC, with intoxication
- sedative (acute) (without dependence) — see Abuse, drug, sedative, with intoxication
  - with dependence — see Dependence, drug, sedative, with intoxication
- serum (see also Reaction, serum) T80.69 ☑
- uremic — see Uremia
- volatile solvents (acute) (without dependence) — see Abuse, drug, inhalant, with intoxication
  - with dependence — see Dependence, drug, inhalant, with intoxication
- water E87.79

Intracranial — see condition
Intrahepatic gallbladder Q44.1
Intraligamentous — see condition
Intrathoracic (see also condition)
- kidney Q63.2
Intrauterine contraceptive device
- checking Z30.431
- in situ Z97.5
- insertion Z30.430
  - immediately following removal Z30.433
- management Z30.431
- reinsertion Z30.433
- removal Z30.432
- replacement Z30.433
- retention in pregnancy O26.3- ☑
Intraventricular — see condition
Intrinsic deformity — see Deformity
Intubation, difficult or failed T88.4 ☑
Intumescence, lens (eye) (cataract) — see Cataract
Intussusception (bowel) (colon) (enteric) (ileocecal) (ileocolic) (intestine) (rectum) K56.1
- appendix K38.8
- congenital Q43.8
- ureter (with obstruction) N13.5
Invagination (bowel, colon, intestine or rectum) K56.1
Inversion
- albumin-globulin (A-G) ratio E88.09
- bladder N32.89
- cecum — see Intussusception
- cervix N88.8
- chromosome in normal individual Q95.1
- circadian rhythm — see Disorder, sleep, circadian rhythm
- nipple N64.59
  - congenital Q83.8
  - gestational — see Retraction, nipple
  - puerperal, postpartum — see Retraction, nipple
- nyctohemeral rhythm — see Disorder, sleep, circadian rhythm
- optic papilla Q14.2
- organ or site, congenital NEC — see Anomaly, by site
- sleep rhythm — see Disorder, sleep, circadian rhythm
- testis (congenital) Q55.29
- uterus (chronic) (postinfectional) (postpartal, old) N85.5
  - postpartum O71.2

Inversion — *continued*
vagina (posthysterectomy) N99.3
ventricular Q20.5
Investigation (*see also* Examination) Z04.9
clinical research subject (control) (normal comparison) (participant) Z00.6
Involuntary movement, abnormal R25.9
Involution, involutional (*see also* condition)
breast, cystic — *see* Dysplasia, mammary, specified type NEC
depression (single episode) F32.8
recurrent episode F33.9
melancholia (recurrent episode) (single episode) F32.8
ovary, senile — *see* Atrophy, ovary
thymus failure E32.8
I.Q.
under 20 F73
20-34 F72
35-49 F71
50-69 F70
IRDS (type I) P22.0
type II P22.1
Irideremia Q13.1
Iridis rubeosis — *see* Disorder, iris, vascular
Iridochoroiditis (panuveitis) — *see* Panuveitis
Iridocyclitis H20.9
acute H20.0- ☑
hypopyon H20.05- ☑
primary H20.01- ☑
recurrent H20.02- ☑
secondary (noninfectious) H20.04- ☑
infectious H20.03- ☑
chronic H20.1- ☑
due to allergy — *see* Iridocyclitis, acute, secondary
endogenous — *see* Iridocyclitis, acute, primary
Fuchs' — *see* Cyclitis, Fuchs' heterochromic
gonococcal A54.32
granulomatous — *see* Iridocyclitis, chronic
herpes, herpetic (simplex) B00.51
zoster B02.32
hypopyon — *see* Iridocyclitis, acute, hypopyon
in (due to)
ankylosing spondylitis M45.9
gonococcal infection A54.32
herpes (simplex) virus B00.51
zoster B02.32
infectious disease NOS B99 ☑
parasitic disease NOS B89 [H22]
sarcoidosis D86.83
syphilis A51.43
tuberculosis A18.54
zoster B02.32
lens-induced H20.2- ☑
nongranulomatous — *see* Iridocyclitis, acute
recurrent — *see* Iridocyclitis, acute, recurrent
rheumatic — *see* Iridocyclitis, chronic
subacute — *see* Iridocyclitis, acute
sympathetic — *see* Uveitis, sympathetic
syphilitic (secondary) A51.43
tuberculous (chronic) A18.54
Vogt-Koyanagi H20.82- ☑
Iridocyclochoroiditis (panuveitis) — *see* Panuveitis
Iridodialysis H21.53- ☑
Iridodonesis H21.89
Iridoplegia (complete) (partial) (reflex) H57.09
Iridoschisis H21.25- ☑
Iris (*see also* condition)
bombé — *see* Membrane, pupillary
Iritis (*see also* Iridocyclitis)
chronic — *see* Iridocyclitis, chronic
diabetic — *see* E08-E13 with .39
due to
herpes simplex B00.51
leprosy A30.9 [H22]
gonococcal A54.32
gouty M10.9
granulomatous — *see* Iridocyclitis, chronic
lens induced — *see* Iridocyclitis, lens-induced
papulosa (syphilitic) A52.71
rheumatic — *see* Iridocyclitis, chronic
syphilitic (secondary) A51.43
congenital (early) A50.01
late A52.71
tuberculous A18.54
Iron — *see* condition
Iron-miner's lung J63.4
Irradiated enamel (tooth, teeth) K03.89

Irradiation effects, adverse T66 ☑
Irreducible, irreducibility — *see* condition
Irregular, irregularity
action, heart I49.9
alveolar process K08.8
bleeding N92.6
breathing R06.89
contour of cornea (acquired) — *see* Deformity, cornea
congenital Q13.4
contour, reconstructed breast N65.0
dentin (in pulp) K04.3
eye movements H55.89
nystagmus — *see* Nystagmus
saccadic H55.81
labor O62.2
menstruation (cause unknown) N92.6
periods N92.6
prostate N42.9
pupil — *see* Abnormality, pupillary
reconstructed breast N65.0
respiratory R06.89
septum (nasal) J34.2
shape, organ or site, congenital NEC — *see* Distortion
sleep-wake pattern (rhythm) G47.23
Irritable, irritability R45.4
bladder N32.89
bowel (syndrome) K58.9
with diarrhea K58.0
psychogenic F45.8
bronchial — *see* Bronchitis
cerebral, in newborn P91.3
colon K58.9
with diarrhea K58.0
psychogenic F45.8
duodenum K59.8
heart (psychogenic) F45.8
hip — *see* Derangement, joint, specified type NEC, hip
ileum K59.8
infant R68.12
jejunum K59.8
rectum K59.8
stomach K31.89
psychogenic F45.8
sympathetic G90.8
urethra N36.8
Irritation
anus K62.89
axillary nerve G54.0
bladder N32.89
brachial plexus G54.0
bronchial — *see* Bronchitis
cervical plexus G54.2
cervix — *see* Cervicitis
choroid, sympathetic — *see* Endophthalmitis
cranial nerve — *see* Disorder, nerve, cranial
gastric K31.89
psychogenic F45.8
globe, sympathetic — *see* Uveitis, sympathetic
labyrinth — *see* subcategory H83.2 ☑
lumbosacral plexus G54.1
meninges (traumatic) — *see* Injury, intracranial
nontraumatic — *see* Meningismus
nerve — *see* Disorder, nerve
nervous R45.0
penis N48.89
perineum NEC L29.3
peripheral autonomic nervous system G90.8
peritoneum — *see* Peritonitis
pharynx J39.2
plantar nerve — *see* Lesion, nerve, plantar
spinal (cord) (traumatic) (*see also* Injury, spinal cord, by region)
nerve G58.9
root NEC — *see* Radiculopathy
nontraumatic — *see* Myelopathy
stomach K31.89
psychogenic F45.8
sympathetic nerve NEC G90.8
ulnar nerve — *see* Lesion, nerve, ulnar
vagina N89.8
Ischemia, ischemic I99.8
bowel (transient)
acute K55.0
chronic K55.1
due to mesenteric artery insufficiency K55.1
brain — *see* Ischemia, cerebral
cardiac (see Disease, heart, ischemic)
cardiomyopathy I25.5

Ischemia, ischemic — *continued*
cerebral (chronic) (generalized) I67.82
arteriosclerotic I67.2
intermittent G45.9
newborn P91.0
recurrent focal G45.8
transient G45.9
colon chronic (due to mesenteric artery insufficiency) K55.1
coronary — *see* Disease, heart, ischemic
demand (coronary) (*see also* Angina) I24.8
heart (chronic or with a stated duration of over 4 weeks) I25.9
acute or with a stated duration of 4 weeks or less I24.9
subacute I24.9
infarction, muscle — *see* Infarct, muscle
intestine (large) (small) (transient) K55.9
acute K55.0
chronic K55.1
due to mesenteric artery insufficiency K55.1
kidney N28.0
mesenteric, acute K55.0
muscle, traumatic T79.6 ☑
myocardium, myocardial (chronic or with a stated duration of over 4 weeks) I25.9
acute, without myocardial infarction I24.0
silent (asymptomatic) I25.6
transient of newborn P29.4
renal N28.0
retina, retinal — *see* Occlusion, artery, retina
small bowel
acute K55.0
chronic K55.1
due to mesenteric artery insufficiency K55.1
spinal cord G95.11
subendocardial — *see* Insufficiency, coronary
supply (coronary) (*see also* Angina) I25.9
due to vasospasm I20.1
Ischial spine — *see* condition
Ischialgia — *see* Sciatica
Ischiopagus Q89.4
Ischium, ischial — *see* condition
Ischuria R34
Iselin's disease or osteochondrosis — *see* Osteochondrosis, juvenile, metatarsus
Islands of
parotid tissue in
lymph nodes Q38.6
neck structures Q38.6
submaxillary glands in
fascia Q38.6
lymph nodes Q38.6
neck muscles Q38.6
Islet cell tumor, pancreas D13.7
Isoimmunization NEC (*see also* Incompatibility)
affecting management of pregnancy (ABO) (with hydrops fetalis) O36.11-
anti-A sensitization O36.11- ☑
anti-B sensitization O36.19- ☑
anti-c sensitization O36.09- ☑
anti-C sensitization O36.09- ☑
anti-E sensitization O36.09- ☑
anti-e sensitization O36.09- ☑
Rh NEC O36.09- ☑
anti-D antibody O36.01- ☑
specified NEC O36.19- ☑
newborn P55.9
with
hydrops fetalis P56.0
kernicterus P57.0
ABO (blood groups) P55.1
Rhesus (Rh) factor P55.0
specified type NEC P55.8
Isolation, isolated
dwelling Z59.8
family Z63.79
social Z60.4
Isoleucinosis E71.19
Isomerism atrial appendages (with asplenia or polysplenia) Q20.6
Isosporiasis, isosporosis A07.3
Isovaleric acidemia E71.110
Issue of
medical certificate Z02.79
for disability determination Z02.71

Issue of — *continued*
  repeat prescription (appliance) (glasses) (medicinal substance, medicament, medicine) Z76.0
    contraception — *see* Contraception
Itch, itching (*see also* Pruritus)
  baker's L23.6
  barber's B35.0
  bricklayer's L24.5
  cheese B88.0
  clam digger's B65.3
  coolie B76.9
  copra B88.0
  dew B76.9
  dhobi B35.6
  filarial — *see* Infestation, filarial
  grain B88.0
  grocer's B88.0
  ground B76.9
  harvest B88.0
  jock B35.6
  Malabar B35.5
    beard B35.0
    foot B35.3
    scalp B35.0
  meaning scabies B86
  Norwegian B86
  perianal L29.0
  poultrymen's B88.0
  sarcoptic B86
  scabies B86
  scrub B88.0
  straw B88.0
  swimmer's B65.3
  water B76.9
  winter L29.8
Ivemark's syndrome (asplenia with congenital heart disease) Q89.01
Ivory bones Q78.2
Ixodiasis NEC B88.8

J

Jaccoud's syndrome — *see* Arthropathy, postrheumatic, chronic
Jackson's
  membrane Q43.3
  paralysis or syndrome G83.89
  veil Q43.3
Jacquet's dermatitis (diaper dermatitis) L22
Jadassohn-Pellizari's disease or anetoderma L90.2
Jadassohn's
  blue nevus — *see* Nevus
  intraepidermal epithelioma — *see* Neoplasm, skin, benign
Jaffe-Lichtenstein (-Uehlinger) syndrome — *see* Dysplasia, fibrous, bone NEC
Jakob-Creutzfeldt disease or syndrome — *see* Creutzfeldt-Jakob disease or syndrome
Jaksch-Luzet disease D64.89
Jamaican
  neuropathy G92
  paraplegic tropical ataxic-spastic syndrome G92
Janet's disease F48.8
Janiceps Q89.4
Jansky-Bielschowsky amaurotic idiocy E75.4
Japanese
  B-type encephalitis A83.0
  river fever A75.3
Jaundice (yellow) R17
  acholuric (familial) (splenomegalic) (*see also* Spherocytosis)
    acquired D59.8
  breast-milk (inhibitor) P59.3
  catarrhal (acute) B15.9
    with hepatic coma B15.0
  cholestatic (benign) R17
  due to or associated with
    delayed conjugation P59.8
      associated with (due to) preterm delivery P59.0
    preterm delivery P59.0
  epidemic (catarrhal) B15.9
    with hepatic coma B15.0
    leptospiral A27.0
    spirochetal A27.0
  familial nonhemolytic (congenital) (Gilbert) E80.4
    Crigler-Najjar E80.5
  febrile (acute) B15.9
    with hepatic coma B15.0

Jaundice — *continued*
  febrile — *continued*
    leptospiral A27.0
    spirochetal A27.0
  hematogenous D59.9
  hemolytic (acquired) D59.9
    congenital — *see* Spherocytosis
  hemorrhagic (acute) (leptospiral) (spirochetal) A27.0
  infectious (acute) (subacute) B15.9
    with hepatic coma B15.0
    leptospiral A27.0
    spirochetal A27.0
  leptospiral (hemorrhagic) A27.0
  malignant (without coma) K72.90
    with coma K72.91
  neonatal — *see* Jaundice, newborn
  newborn P59.9
    due to or associated with
      ABO
        antibodies P55.1
        incompatibility, maternal/fetal P55.1
        isoimmunization P55.1
      absence or deficiency of enzyme system for bilirubin conjugation (congenital) P59.8
      bleeding P58.1
      breast milk inhibitors to conjugation P59.3
        associated with preterm delivery P59.0
      bruising P58.0
      Crigler-Najjar syndrome E80.5
      delayed conjugation P59.8
        associated with preterm delivery P59.0
      drugs or toxins
        given to newborn P58.42
        transmitted from mother P58.41
      excessive hemolysis P58.9
        due to
          bleeding P58.1
          bruising P58.0
          drugs or toxins
            given to newborn P58.42
            transmitted from mother P58.41
          infection P58.2
          polycythemia P58.3
          swallowed maternal blood P58.5
      specified type NEC P58.8
      galactosemia E74.21
      Gilbert syndrome E80.4
      hemolytic disease P55.9
        ABO isoimmunization P55.1
        Rh isoimmunization P55.0
        specified NEC P55.8
      hepatocellular damage P59.20
        specified NEC P59.29
      hereditary hemolytic anemia P58.8
      hypothyroidism, congenital E03.1
      incompatibility, maternal/fetal NOS P55.9
      infection P58.2
      inspissated bile syndrome P59.1
      isoimmunization NOS P55.9
      mucoviscidosis E84.9
      polycythemia P58.3
      preterm delivery P59.0
      Rh
        antibodies P55.0
        incompatibility, maternal/fetal P55.0
        isoimmunization P55.0
      specified cause NEC P59.8
      swallowed maternal blood P58.5
      spherocytosis (congenital) D58.0
  nonhemolytic congenital familial (Gilbert) E80.4
  nuclear, newborn (*see also* Kernicterus of newborn) P57.9
  obstructive (*see also* Obstruction, bile duct) K83.1
  post-immunization — *see* Hepatitis, viral, type, B
  post-transfusion — *see* Hepatitis, viral, type, B
  regurgitation (*see also* Obstruction, bile duct) K83.1
  serum (homologous) (prophylactic) (therapeutic) — *see* Hepatitis, viral, type, B
  spirochetal (hemorrhagic) A27.0
  symptomatic R17
    newborn P59.9
Jaw — *see* condition
Jaw-winking phenomenon or syndrome Q07.8
Jealousy
  alcoholic F10.988
  childhood F93.8
  sibling F93.8
Jejunitis — *see* Enteritis

Jejunostomy status Z93.4
Jejunum, jejunal — *see* condition
Jensen's disease — *see* Inflammation, chorioretinal, focal, juxtapapillary
Jerks, myoclonic G25.3
Jervell-Lange-Nielsen syndrome I45.81
Jeune's disease Q77.2
Jigger disease B88.1
Job's syndrome (chronic granulomatous disease) D71
Joint (*see also* condition)
  mice — *see* Loose, body, joint
    knee M23.4- ☑
Jordan's anomaly or syndrome D72.0
Joseph-Diamond-Blackfan anemia (congenital hypoplastic) D61.01
Jungle yellow fever A95.0
Jüngling's disease — *see* Sarcoidosis
Juvenile — *see* condition

K

Kahler's disease C90.0- ☑
Kakke E51.11
Kala-azar B55.0
Kallmann's syndrome E23.0
Kanner's syndrome (autism) — *see* Psychosis, childhood
Kaposi's
  dermatosis (xeroderma pigmentosum) Q82.1
  lichen ruber L44.0
    acuminatus L44.0
  sarcoma
    colon C46.4
    connective tissue C46.1
    gastrointestinal organ C46.4
    lung C46.5- ☑
    lymph node (multiple) C46.3
    palate (hard) (soft) C46.2
    rectum C46.4
    skin (multiple sites) C46.0
    specified site NEC C46.7
    stomach C46.4
    unspecified site C46.9
  varicelliform eruption B00.0
    vaccinia T88.1 ☑
Kartagener's syndrome or triad (sinusitis, bronchiectasis, situs inversus) Q89.3
Karyotype
  with abnormality except iso (Xq) Q96.2
  45,X Q96.0
  46,X
    iso (Xq) Q96.1
  46,XX Q98.3
    with streak gonads Q50.32
    hermaphrodite (true) Q99.1
    male Q98.3
  46,XY
    with streak gonads Q56.1
    female Q97.3
    hermaphrodite (true) Q99.1
  47,XXX Q97.0
  47,XXY Q98.0
  47,XYY Q98.5
Kaschin-Beck disease — *see* Disease, Kaschin-Beck
Katayama's disease or fever B65.2
Kawasaki's syndrome M30.3
Kayser-Fleischer ring (cornea) (pseudosclerosis) H18.04- ☑
Kaznelson's syndrome (congenital hypoplastic anemia) D61.01
Kearns-Sayre syndrome H49.81- ☑
Kedani fever A75.3
Kelis L91.0
Kelly (-Patterson) **syndrome** (sideropenic dysphagia) D50.1
Keloid, cheloid L91.0
  acne L73.0
  Addison's L94.0
  cornea — *see* Opacity, cornea
  Hawkin's L91.0
  scar L91.0
Keloma L91.0
Kenya fever A77.1
Keratectasia (*see also* Ectasia, cornea)
  congenital Q13.4
Keratinization of alveolar ridge mucosa
  excessive K13.23
  minimal K13.22

Keratinized residual ridge mucosa
  excessive K13.23
  minimal K13.22
Keratitis (nodular) (nonulcerative) (simple) (zonular) H16.9
  with ulceration (central) (marginal) (perforated) (ring) — *see* Ulcer, cornea
  actinic — *see* Photokeratitis
  arborescens (herpes simplex) B00.52
  areolar H16.11- ☑
  bullosa H16.8
  deep H16.309
    specified type NEC H16.399
  dendritic (a) (herpes simplex) B00.52
  disciform (is) (herpes simplex) B00.52
    varicella B01.81
  filamentary H16.12- ☑
  gonococcal (congenital or prenatal) A54.33
  herpes, herpetic (simplex) B00.52
    zoster B02.33
  in (due to)
    acanthamebiasis B60.13
    adenovirus B30.0
    exanthema (*see also* Exanthem) B09
    herpes (simplex) virus B00.52
    measles B05.81
    syphilis A50.31
    tuberculosis A18.52
    zoster B02.33
  interstitial (nonsyphilitic) H16.30- ☑
    diffuse H16.32- ☑
    herpes, herpetic (simplex) B00.52
      zoster B02.33
    sclerosing H16.33- ☑
    specified type NEC H16.39- ☑
    syphilitic (congenital) (late) A50.31
    tuberculous A18.52
  macular H16.11- ☑
  nummular H16.11- ☑
  oyster shuckers' H16.8
  parenchymatous — *see* Keratitis, interstitial
  petrificans H16.8
  postmeasles B05.81
  punctata
    leprosa A30.9 [H16.14-] ☑
    syphilitic (profunda) A50.31
  punctate H16.14- ☑
  purulent H16.8
  rosacea L71.8
  sclerosing H16.33- ☑
  specified type NEC H16.8
  stellate H16.11- ☑
  striate H16.11- ☑
  superficial H16.10- ☑
    with conjunctivitis — *see* Keratoconjunctivitis
    due to light — *see* Photokeratitis
  suppurative H16.8
  syphilitic (congenital) (prenatal) A50.31
  trachomatous A71.1
    sequelae B94.0
  tuberculous A18.52
  vesicular H16.8
  xerotic (*see also* Keratomalacia) H16.8
    vitamin A deficiency E50.4
Keratoacanthoma L85.8
Keratocele — *see* Descemetocele
Keratoconjunctivitis H16.20- ☑
  Acanthamoeba B60.13
  adenoviral B30.0
  epidemic B30.0
  exposure H16.21- ☑
  herpes, herpetic (simplex) B00.52
    zoster B02.33
  in exanthema (*see also* Exanthem) B09
  infectious B30.0
  lagophthalmic — *see* Keratoconjunctivitis, specified type NEC
  neurotrophic H16.23- ☑
  phlyctenular H16.25- ☑
  postmeasles B05.81
  shipyard B30.0
  sicca (Sjogren's) M35.0- ☑
    not Sjogren's H16.22- ☑
  specified type NEC H16.29- ☑
  tuberculous (phlyctenular) A18.52
  vernal H16.26- ☑
Keratoconus H18.60- ☑

Keratoconus — *continued*
  congenital Q13.4
  stable H18.61- ☑
  unstable H18.62- ☑
Keratocyst (dental) (odontogenic) — *see* Cyst, calcifying odontogenic
Keratoderma, keratodermia (congenital) (palmaris et plantaris) (symmetrical) Q82.8
  acquired L85.1
    in diseases classified elsewhere L86
  climactericum L85.1
  gonococcal A54.89
  gonorrheal A54.89
  punctata L85.2
  Reiter's — *see* Reiter's disease
Keratodermatocele — *see* Descemetocele
Keratoglobus H18.79 ☑
  congenital Q15.8
    with glaucoma Q15.0
Keratohemia — *see* Pigmentation, cornea, stromal
Keratoiritis (*see also* Iridocyclitis)
  syphilitic A50.39
  tuberculous A18.54
Keratoma L57.0
  palmaris and plantaris hereditarium Q82.8
  senile L57.0
Keratomalacia H18.44- ☑
  vitamin A deficiency E50.4
Keratomegaly Q13.4
Keratomycosis B49
  nigrans, nigricans (palmaris) B36.1
Keratopathy H18.9
  band H18.42- ☑
  bullous (aphakic), following cataract surgery H59.01- ☑
  bullous H18.1- ☑
Keratoscleritis, tuberculous A18.52
Keratosis L57.0
  actinic L57.0
  arsenical L85.8
  congenital, specified NEC Q80.8
  female genital NEC N94.89
  follicularis Q82.8
    acquired L11.0
    congenita Q82.8
    et parafollicularis in cutem penetrans L87.0
    spinulosa (decalvans) Q82.8
    vitamin A deficiency E50.8
  gonococcal A54.89
  male genital (external) N50.8
  nigricans L83
  obturans, external ear (canal) — *see* Cholesteatoma, external ear
  palmaris et plantaris (inherited) (symmetrical) Q82.8
    acquired L85.1
  penile N48.89
  pharynx J39.2
  pilaris, acquired L85.8
  punctata (palmaris et plantaris) L85.2
  scrotal N50.8
  seborrheic L82.1
    inflamed L82.0
  senile L57.0
  solar L57.0
  tonsillaris J35.8
  vagina N89.4
  vegetans Q82.8
  vitamin A deficiency E50.8
  vocal cord J38.3
Kerato-uveitis — *see* Iridocyclitis
Kerion (celsi) B35.0
Kernicterus of newborn (not due to isoimmunization) P57.9
  due to isoimmunization (conditions in P55.0-P55.9) P57.0
  specified type NEC P57.8
Kerunoparalysis T75.09 ☑
Keshan disease E59
Ketoacidosis E87.2
  diabetic — *see* Diabetes, by type, with ketoacidosis
Ketonuria R82.4
Ketosis NEC E88.89
  diabetic — *see* Diabetes, by type, with with ketoacidosis
Kew Garden fever A79.1
Kidney — *see* condition

Kienböck's disease (*see also* Osteochondrosis, juvenile, hand, carpal lunate)
  adult M93.1
Kimmelstiel (-Wilson) **disease** — *see* Diabetes, Kimmelstiel (-Wilson) disease
Kink, kinking
  artery I77.1
  hair (acquired) L67.8
  ileum or intestine — *see* Obstruction, intestine
  Lane's — *see* Obstruction, intestine
  organ or site, congenital NEC — *see* Anomaly, by site
  ureter (pelvic junction) N13.5
    with
      hydronephrosis N13.1
        with infection N13.6
      pyelonephritis (chronic) N11.1
    congenital Q62.39
  vein(s) I87.8
    caval I87.1
    peripheral I87.1
Kinnier Wilson's disease (hepatolenticular degeneration) E83.01
Kissing spine M48.20
  cervical region M48.22
  cervicothoracic region M48.23
  lumbar region M48.26
  lumbosacral region M48.27
  occipito-atlanto-axial region M48.21
  thoracic region M48.24
  thoracolumbar region M48.25
Klatskin's tumor C22.1
Klauder's disease A26.8
Klebs' disease (*see also* Glomerulonephritis) N05- ☑
Klebsiella (K.) **pneumoniae, as cause of disease classified elsewhere** B96.1
Klein (e)-**Levin syndrome** G47.13
Kleptomania F63.2
Klinefelter's syndrome Q98.4
  karyotype 47,XXY Q98.0
  male with more than two X chromosomes Q98.1
Klippel-Feil deficiency, disease, or syndrome (brevicollis) Q76.1
Klippel's disease I67.2
Klippel-Trenaunay (-Weber) **syndrome** Q87.2
Klumpke (-Déjerine) **palsy, paralysis** (birth) (newborn) P14.1
Knee — *see* condition
Knock knee (acquired) M21.06- ☑
  congenital Q74.1
Knot(s)
  intestinal, syndrome (volvulus) K56.2
  surfer S89.8- ☑
  umbilical cord (true) O69.2 ☑
Knotting (of)
  hair L67.8
  intestine K56.2
Knuckle pad (Garrod's) M72.1
Koch's
  infection — *see* Tuberculosis
  relapsing fever A68.9
Koch-Weeks' conjunctivitis — *see* Conjunctivitis, acute, mucopurulent
Köebner's syndrome Q81.8
Köenig's disease (osteochondritis dissecans) — *see* Osteochondritis, dissecans
Köhler-Pellegrini-Steida disease or syndrome (calcification, knee joint) — *see* Bursitis, tibial collateral
Köhler's disease
  patellar — *see* Osteochondrosis, juvenile, patella
  tarsal navicular — *see* Osteochondrosis, juvenile, tarsus
Koilonychia L60.3
  congenital Q84.6
Kojevnikov's, epilepsy — *see* Kozhevnikof's epilepsy
Koplik's spots B05.9
Kopp's asthma E32.8
Korsakoff's (Wernicke) **disease, psychosis or syndrome** (alcoholic) F10.96
  with dependence F10.26
  drug-induced
    due to drug abuse — *see* Abuse, drug, by type, with amnestic disorder
    due to drug dependence — *see* Dependence, drug, by type, with amnestic disorder
  nonalcoholic F04
Korsakov's disease, psychosis or syndrome — *see* Korsakoff's disease

198

☑ **Additional Character Required** — Refer to the Tabular List for Character Selection   ☑ Subterms under main terms may continue to next column or page

Korsakow's disease, psychosis or syndrome — *see* Korsakoff's disease
Kostmann's disease or syndrome (infantile genetic agranulocytosis) — *see* Agranulocytosis
Kozhevnikof's epilepsy G40.109
  intractable G40.119
    with status epilepticus G40.111
    without status epilepticus G40.119
  not intractable G40.109
    with status epilepticus G40.101
    without status epilepticus G40.109
Krabbe's
  disease E75.23
  syndrome, congenital muscle hypoplasia Q79.8
Kraepelin-Morel disease — *see* Schizophrenia
Kraft-Weber-Dimitri disease Q85.8
Kraurosis
  ani K62.89
  penis N48.0
  vagina N89.8
  vulva N90.4
Kreotoxism A05.9
Krukenberg's
  spindle — *see* Pigmentation, cornea, posterior
  tumor C79.6- ☑
Kufs' disease E75.4
Kugelberg-Welander disease G12.1
Kuhnt-Junius degeneration (*see also* Degeneration, macula) H35.32
Kümmell's disease or spondylitis — *see* Spondylopathy, traumatic
Kupffer cell sarcoma C22.3
Kuru A81.81
Kussmaul's
  disease M30.0
  respiration E87.2
    in diabetic acidosis — *see* Diabetes, by type, with ketoacidosis
Kwashiorkor E40
  marasmic, marasmus type E42
Kyasanur Forest disease A98.2
Kyphoscoliosis, kyphoscoliotic (acquired) (*see also* Scoliosis) M41.9
  congenital Q67.5
  heart (disease) I27.1
  sequelae of rickets E64.3
  tuberculous A18.01
Kyphosis, kyphotic (acquired) M40.209
  cervical region M40.202
  cervicothoracic region M40.203
  congenital Q76.419
    cervical region Q76.412
    cervicothoracic region Q76.413
    occipito-atlanto-axial region Q76.411
    thoracic region Q76.414
    thoracolumbar region Q76.415
  Morquio-Brailsford type (spinal) (*see also* subcategory M49.8) E76.219
  postlaminectomy M96.3
  postradiation therapy M96.2
  postural (adolescent) M40.00
    cervicothoracic region M40.03
    thoracic region M40.04
    thoracolumbar region M40.05
  secondary NEC M40.10
    cervical region M40.12
    cervicothoracic region M40.13
    thoracic region M40.14
    thoracolumbar region M40.15
  sequelae of rickets E64.3
  specified type NEC M40.299
    cervical region M40.292
    cervicothoracic region M40.293
    thoracic region M40.294
    thoracolumbar region M40.295
  syphilitic, congenital A50.56
  thoracic region M40.204
  thoracolumbar region M40.205
  tuberculous A18.01
Kyrle disease L87.0

L

Labia, labium — *see* condition
Labile
  blood pressure R09.89
  vasomotor system I73.9

Labioglossal paralysis G12.29
Labium leporinum — *see* Cleft, lip
Labor — *see* Delivery
Labored breathing — *see* Hyperventilation
Labyrinthitis (circumscribed) (destructive) (diffuse) (inner ear) (latent) (purulent) (suppurative) (*see also* subcategory) H83.0 ☑
  syphilitic A52.79
Laceration
  with abortion — *see* Abortion, by type, complicated by laceration of pelvic organs
  abdomen, abdominal
    wall S31.119 ☑
      with
        foreign body S31.129 ☑
        penetration into peritoneal cavity S31.619 ☑
          with foreign body S31.629 ☑
      epigastric region S31.112 ☑
        with
          foreign body S31.122 ☑
          penetration into peritoneal cavity S31.612 ☑
            with foreign body S31.622 ☑
      left
        lower quadrant S31.114 ☑
          with
            foreign body S31.124 ☑
            penetration into peritoneal cavity S31.614 ☑
              with foreign body S31.624 ☑
        upper quadrant S31.111 ☑
          with
            foreign body S31.121 ☑
            penetration into peritoneal cavity S31.611 ☑
              with foreign body S31.621 ☑
      periumbilic region S31.115 ☑
        with
          foreign body S31.125 ☑
          penetration into peritoneal cavity S31.615 ☑
            with foreign body S31.625 ☑
      right
        lower quadrant S31.113 ☑
          with
            foreign body S31.123 ☑
            penetration into peritoneal cavity S31.613 ☑
              with foreign body S31.623 ☑
        upper quadrant S31.110 ☑
          with
            foreign body S31.120 ☑
            penetration into peritoneal cavity S31.610 ☑
              with foreign body S31.620 ☑
  accidental, complicating surgery — *see* Complications, surgical, accidental puncture or laceration
  Achilles tendon S86.02- ☑
  adrenal gland S37.813 ☑
  alveolar (process) — *see* Laceration, oral cavity
  ankle S91.01- ☑
    with
      foreign body S91.02- ☑
  antecubital space — *see* Laceration, elbow
  anus (sphincter) S31.831 ☑
    with
      ectopic or molar pregnancy O08.6
      foreign body S31.832 ☑
    complicating delivery — *see* Delivery, complicated, by, laceration, anus (sphincter)
    following ectopic or molar pregnancy O08.6
    nontraumatic, nonpuerperal — *see* Fissure, anus
  arm (upper) S41.11- ☑
    with foreign body S41.12- ☑
    lower — *see* Laceration, forearm
  auditory canal (external) (meatus) — *see* Laceration, ear
  auricle, ear — *see* Laceration, ear
  axilla — *see* Laceration, arm
  back (*see also* Laceration, thorax, back)
    lower S31.010 ☑
      with
        foreign body S31.020 ☑
        with penetration into retroperitoneal space S31.021 ☑

Laceration — *continued*
  back (*see also* Laceration, thorax, back) — *continued*
    lower — *continued*
      with — *continued*
        penetration into retroperitoneal space S31.011 ☑
  bile duct S36.13 ☑
  bladder S37.23 ☑
    with ectopic or molar pregnancy O08.6
    following ectopic or molar pregnancy O08.6
    obstetrical trauma O71.5
  blood vessel — *see* Injury, blood vessel
  bowel (*see also* Laceration, intestine)
    with ectopic or molar pregnancy O08.6
    complicating abortion — *see* Abortion, by type, complicated by, specified condition NEC
    following ectopic or molar pregnancy O08.6
    obstetrical trauma O71.5
  brain (any part) (cortex) (diffuse) (membrane) (*see also* Injury, intracranial, diffuse)
    during birth P10.8
      with hemorrhage P10.1
    focal — *see* Injury, intracranial, focal brain injury
  brainstem S06.38- ☑
  breast S21.01- ☑
    with foreign body S21.02- ☑
  broad ligament S37.893 ☑
    with ectopic or molar pregnancy O08.6
    following ectopic or molar pregnancy O08.6
    laceration syndrome N83.8
    obstetrical trauma O71.6
    syndrome (laceration) N83.8
  buttock S31.801 ☑
    with foreign body S31.802 ☑
    left S31.821 ☑
      with foreign body S31.822 ☑
    right S31.811 ☑
      with foreign body S31.812 ☑
  calf — *see* Laceration, leg
  canaliculus lacrimalis — *see* Laceration, eyelid
  canthus, eye — *see* Laceration, eyelid
  capsule, joint — *see* Sprain
  causing eversion of cervix uteri (old) N86
  central (perineal), complicating delivery O70.9
  cerebellum, traumatic S06.37- ☑
  cerebral S06.33- ☑
    during birth P10.8
      with hemorrhage P10.1
    left side S06.32- ☑
    right side S06.31- ☑
  cervix (uteri)
    with ectopic or molar pregnancy O08.6
    following ectopic or molar pregnancy O08.6
    nonpuerperal, nontraumatic N88.1
    obstetrical trauma (current) O71.3
    old (postpartal) N88.1
    traumatic S37.63 ☑
  cheek (external) S01.41- ☑
    with foreign body S01.42- ☑
    internal — *see* Laceration, oral cavity
  chest wall — *see* Laceration, thorax
  chin — *see* Laceration, head, specified site NEC
  chordae tendinae NEC I51.1
    concurrent with acute myocardial infarction — *see* Infarct, myocardium
    following acute myocardial infarction (current complication) I23.4
  clitoris — *see* Laceration, vulva
  colon — *see* Laceration, intestine, large, colon
  common bile duct S36.13 ☑
  cortex (cerebral) — *see* Injury, intracranial, diffuse
  costal region — *see* Laceration, thorax
  cystic duct S36.13 ☑
  diaphragm S27.803 ☑
  digit(s)
    foot — *see* Laceration, toe
    hand — *see* Laceration, finger
  duodenum S36.430 ☑
  ear (canal) (external) S01.31- ☑
    with foreign body S01.32- ☑
    drum S09.2- ☑
  elbow S51.01- ☑
    with
      foreign body S51.02- ☑
  epididymis — *see* Laceration, testis

Index

Korsakow's disease, psychosis or syndrome — Laceration

Subterms under main terms may continue to next column or page   ☑ Additional Character Required — Refer to the Tabular List for Character Selection   199

Index

Laceration — Laceration

Laceration — *continued*
  epigastric region — *see* Laceration, abdomen, wall, epigastric region
  esophagus K22.8
    traumatic
      cervical S11.21 ☑
        with foreign body S11.22 ☑
      thoracic S27.813 ☑
  eye (ball) S05.3- ☑
    with prolapse or loss of intraocular tissue S05.2- ☑
    penetrating S05.6- ☑
  eyebrow — *see* Laceration, eyelid
  eyelid S01.11- ☑
    with foreign body S01.12- ☑
  face NEC — *see* Laceration, head, specified site NEC
  fallopian tube S37.539 ☑
    bilateral S37.532 ☑
    unilateral S37.531 ☑
  finger(s) S61.219 ☑
    with
      damage to nail S61.319 ☑
        with
          foreign body S61.329 ☑
      foreign body S61.229 ☑
    index S61.218 ☑
      with
        damage to nail S61.318 ☑
          with
            foreign body S61.328 ☑
        foreign body S61.228 ☑
      left S61.211 ☑
        with
          damage to nail S61.311 ☑
            with
              foreign body S61.321 ☑
          foreign body S61.221 ☑
      right S61.210 ☑
        with
          damage to nail S61.310 ☑
            with
              foreign body S61.320 ☑
          foreign body S61.220 ☑
    little S61.218 ☑
      with
        damage to nail S61.318 ☑
          with
            foreign body S61.328 ☑
        foreign body S61.228 ☑
      left S61.217 ☑
        with
          damage to nail S61.317 ☑
            with
              foreign body S61.327 ☑
          foreign body S61.227 ☑
      right S61.216 ☑
        with
          damage to nail S61.316 ☑
            with
              foreign body S61.326 ☑
          foreign body S61.226 ☑
    middle S61.218 ☑
      with
        damage to nail S61.318 ☑
          with
            foreign body S61.328 ☑
        foreign body S61.228 ☑
      left S61.213 ☑
        with
          damage to nail S61.313 ☑
            with
              foreign body S61.323 ☑
          foreign body S61.223 ☑
      right S61.212 ☑
        with
          damage to nail S61.312 ☑
            with
              foreign body S61.322 ☑
          foreign body S61.222 ☑
    ring S61.218 ☑
      with
        damage to nail S61.318 ☑
          with
            foreign body S61.328 ☑
        foreign body S61.228 ☑
      left S61.215 ☑

Laceration — *continued*
  finger(s) — *continued*
    ring — *continued*
      left — *continued*
        with
          damage to nail S61.315 ☑
            with
              foreign body S61.325 ☑
          foreign body S61.225 ☑
      right S61.214 ☑
        with
          damage to nail S61.314 ☑
            with
              foreign body S61.324 ☑
          foreign body S61.224 ☑
  flank S31.119 ☑
    with foreign body S31.129 ☑
  foot (except toe(s) alone) S91.319 ☑
    with foreign body S91.329 ☑
    left S91.312 ☑
      with foreign body S91.322 ☑
    right S91.311 ☑
      with foreign body S91.321 ☑
    toe — *see* Laceration, toe
  forearm S51.819 ☑
    with
      foreign body S51.829 ☑
    elbow only — *see* Laceration, elbow
    left S51.812 ☑
      with
        foreign body S51.822 ☑
    right S51.811 ☑
      with
        foreign body S51.821 ☑
  forehead S01.81 ☑
    with foreign body S01.82 ☑
  fourchette O70.0
    with ectopic or molar pregnancy O08.6
    complicating delivery O70.0
    following ectopic or molar pregnancy O08.6
  gallbladder S36.123 ☑
  genital organs, external
    female S31.512 ☑
      with foreign body S31.522 ☑
      vagina — *see* Laceration, vagina
      vulva — *see* Laceration, vulva
    male S31.511 ☑
      with foreign body S31.521 ☑
      penis — *see* Laceration, penis
      scrotum — *see* Laceration, scrotum
      testis — *see* Laceration, testis
  groin — *see* Laceration, abdomen, wall
  gum — *see* Laceration, oral cavity
  hand S61.419 ☑
    with
      foreign body S61.429 ☑
    finger — *see* Laceration, finger
    left S61.412 ☑
      with
        foreign body S61.422 ☑
    right S61.411 ☑
      with
        foreign body S61.421 ☑
    thumb — *see* Laceration, thumb
  head S01.91 ☑
    with foreign body S01.92 ☑
    cheek — *see* Laceration, cheek
    ear — *see* Laceration, ear
    eyelid — *see* Laceration, eyelid
    lip — *see* Laceration, lip
    nose — *see* Laceration, nose
    oral cavity — *see* Laceration, oral cavity
    scalp S01.01 ☑
      with foreign body S01.02 ☑
    specified site NEC S01.81 ☑
      with foreign body S01.82 ☑
    temporomandibular area — *see* Laceration, cheek
  heart — *see* Injury, heart, laceration
  heel — *see* Laceration, foot
  hepatic duct S36.13 ☑
  hip S71.019 ☑
    with foreign body S71.029 ☑
    left S71.012 ☑
      with foreign body S71.022 ☑
    right S71.011 ☑
      with foreign body S71.021 ☑

Laceration — *continued*
  hymen — *see* Laceration, vagina
  hypochondrium — *see* Laceration, abdomen, wall
  hypogastric region — *see* Laceration, abdomen, wall
  ileum S36.438 ☑
  inguinal region — *see* Laceration, abdomen, wall
  instep — *see* Laceration, foot
  internal organ — *see* Injury, by site
  interscapular region — *see* Laceration, thorax, back
  intestine
    large
      colon S36.539 ☑
        ascending S36.530 ☑
        descending S36.532 ☑
        sigmoid S36.533 ☑
        specified site NEC S36.538 ☑
      rectum S36.63 ☑
      transverse S36.531 ☑
    small S36.439 ☑
      duodenum S36.430 ☑
      specified site NEC S36.438 ☑
  intra-abdominal organ S36.93 ☑
    intestine — *see* Laceration, intestine
    liver — *see* Laceration, liver
    pancreas — *see* Laceration, pancreas
    peritoneum S36.81 ☑
    specified site NEC S36.893 ☑
    spleen — *see* Laceration, spleen
    stomach — *see* Laceration, stomach
  intracranial NEC (*see also* Injury, intracranial, diffuse)
    birth injury P10.9
  jaw — *see* Laceration, head, specified site NEC
  jejunum S36.438 ☑
  joint capsule — *see* Sprain, by site
  kidney S37.03- ☑
    major (greater than 3 cm) (massive) (stellate) S37.06- ☑
    minor (less than 1 cm) S37.04- ☑
    moderate (1 to 3 cm) S37.05- ☑
      multiple S37.06- ☑
  knee S81.01- ☑
    with foreign body S81.02- ☑
  labium (majus) (minus) — *see* Laceration, vulva
  lacrimal duct — *see* Laceration, eyelid
  large intestine — *see* Laceration, intestine, large
  larynx S11.011 ☑
    with foreign body S11.012 ☑
  leg (lower) S81.819 ☑
    with foreign body S81.829 ☑
    foot — *see* Laceration, foot
    knee — *see* Laceration, knee
    left S81.812 ☑
      with foreign body S81.822 ☑
    right S81.811 ☑
      with foreign body S81.821 ☑
    upper — *see* Laceration, thigh
  ligament — *see* Sprain
  lip S01.511 ☑
    with foreign body S01.521 ☑
  liver S36.113 ☑
    major (stellate) S36.116 ☑
    minor S36.114 ☑
    moderate S36.115 ☑
  loin — *see* Laceration, abdomen, wall
  lower back — *see* Laceration, back, lower
  lumbar region — *see* Laceration, back, lower
  lung S27.339 ☑
    bilateral S27.332 ☑
    unilateral S27.331 ☑
  malar region — *see* Laceration, head, specified site NEC
  mammary — *see* Laceration, breast
  mastoid region — *see* Laceration, head, specified site NEC
  meninges — *see* Injury, intracranial, diffuse
  meniscus — *see* Tear, meniscus
  mesentery S36.893 ☑
  mesosalpinx S37.893 ☑
  mouth — *see* Laceration, oral cavity
  muscle — *see* Injury, muscle, by site, laceration
  nail
    finger — *see* Laceration, finger, with damage to nail
    toe — *see* Laceration, toe, with damage to nail
  nasal (septum) (sinus) — *see* Laceration, nose

☑ **Additional Character Required** — Refer to the Tabular List for Character Selection   Ⓥ Subterms under main terms may continue to next column or page

Laceration — *continued*
nasopharynx — *see* Laceration, head, specified site NEC ☑
neck S11.91 ☑
  with foreign body S11.92 ☑
  involving
    cervical esophagus S11.21 ☑
      with foreign body S11.22 ☑
    larynx — *see* Laceration, larynx
    pharynx — *see* Laceration, pharynx
    thyroid gland — *see* Laceration, thyroid gland
    trachea — *see* Laceration, trachea
  specified site NEC S11.81 ☑
    with foreign body S11.82 ☑
nerve — *see* Injury, nerve
nose (septum) (sinus) S01.21 ☑
  with foreign body S01.22 ☑
ocular NOS S05.3- ☑
  adnexa NOS S01.11- ☑
oral cavity S01.512 ☑
  with foreign body S01.522 ☑
orbit (eye) — *see* Wound, open, ocular, orbit
ovary S37.439 ☑
  bilateral S37.432 ☑
  unilateral S37.431 ☑
palate — *see* Laceration, oral cavity
palm — *see* Laceration, hand
pancreas S36.239 ☑
pelvic S31.010 ☑
  with
    foreign body S31.020 ☑
      penetration into retroperitoneal cavity S31.021 ☑
    penetration into retroperitoneal cavity S31.011 ☑
  floor (*see also* Laceration, back, lower)
    with ectopic or molar pregnancy O08.6
    complicating delivery O70.1
    following ectopic or molar pregnancy O08.6
    old (postpartal) N81.89
  organ S37.93 ☑
penis S31.21 ☑
  with foreign body S31.22 ☑
perineum
  female S31.41 ☑
    with
      ectopic or molar pregnancy O08.6
      foreign body S31.42 ☑
    during delivery O70.9
      first degree O70.0
      fourth degree O70.3
      second degree O70.1
      third degree O70.2
    old (postpartal) N81.89
    postpartal N81.89
    secondary (postpartal) O90.1
  male S31.119 ☑
    with foreign body S31.129 ☑
periocular area (with or without lacrimal passages) — *see* Laceration, eyelid
peritoneum S36.893 ☑
periumbilic region — *see* Laceration, abdomen, wall, periumbilic
periurethral tissue — *see* Laceration, urethra
phalanges
  finger — *see* Laceration, finger
  toe — *see* Laceration, toe
pharynx S11.21 ☑
  with foreign body S11.22 ☑
pinna — *see* Laceration, ear
popliteal space — *see* Laceration, knee
prepuce — *see* Laceration, penis
prostate S37.823 ☑
pubic region S31.119 ☑
  with foreign body S31.129 ☑
pudendum — *see* Laceration, genital organs, external
rectovaginal septum — *see* Laceration, vagina
rectum S36.63 ☑
retroperitoneum S36.893 ☑
round ligament S37.893 ☑
sacral region — *see* Laceration, back, lower
sacroiliac region — *see* Laceration, back, lower
salivary gland — *see* Laceration, oral cavity
scalp S01.01 ☑
  with foreign body S01.02 ☑
scapular region — *see* Laceration, shoulder

Laceration — *continued*
scrotum S31.31 ☑
  with foreign body S31.32 ☑
seminal vesicle S37.893 ☑
shin — *see* Laceration, leg
shoulder S41.019 ☑
  with foreign body S41.029 ☑
  left S41.012 ☑
    with foreign body S41.022 ☑
  right S41.011 ☑
    with foreign body S41.021 ☑
small intestine — *see* Laceration, intestine, small
spermatic cord — *see* Laceration, testis
spinal cord (meninges) (*see also* Injury, spinal cord, by region)
  due to injury at birth P11.5
  newborn (birth injury) P11.5
spleen S36.039 ☑
  major (massive) (stellate) S36.032 ☑
  moderate S36.031 ☑
  superficial (minor) S36.030 ☑
sternal region — *see* Laceration, thorax, front
stomach S36.33 ☑
submaxillary region — *see* Laceration, head, specified site NEC
submental region — *see* Laceration, head, specified site NEC
subungual
  finger(s) — *see* Laceration, finger, with damage to nail
  toe(s) — *see* Laceration, toe, with damage to nail
suprarenal gland — *see* Laceration, adrenal gland
temple, temporal region — *see* Laceration, head, specified site NEC
temporomandibular area — *see* Laceration, cheek
tendon — *see* Injury, muscle, by site, laceration
  Achilles S86.02- ☑
tentorium cerebelli — *see* Injury, intracranial, diffuse
testis S31.31 ☑
  with foreign body S31.32 ☑
thigh S71.11- ☑
  with foreign body S71.12- ☑
thorax, thoracic (wall) S21.91 ☑
  with foreign body S21.92 ☑
    back S21.22- ☑
      with penetration into thoracic cavity S21.42- ☑
    front S21.12- ☑
      with penetration into thoracic cavity S21.32- ☑
  back S21.21- ☑
    with
      foreign body S21.22- ☑
        with penetration into thoracic cavity S21.42- ☑
      penetration into thoracic cavity S21.41- ☑
  breast — *see* Laceration, breast
  front S21.11- ☑
    with
      foreign body S21.12- ☑
        with penetration into thoracic cavity S21.32- ☑
      penetration into thoracic cavity S21.31- ☑
thumb S61.019 ☑
  with
    damage to nail S61.119 ☑
      with
        foreign body S61.129 ☑
    foreign body S61.029 ☑
  left S61.012 ☑
    with
      damage to nail S61.112 ☑
        with
          foreign body S61.122 ☑
      foreign body S61.022 ☑
  right S61.011 ☑
    with
      damage to nail S61.111 ☑
        with
          foreign body S61.121 ☑
      foreign body S61.021 ☑
thyroid gland S11.11 ☑
  with foreign body S11.12 ☑
toe(s) S91.119 ☑
  with
    damage to nail S91.219 ☑

Laceration — *continued*
toe(s) — *continued*
  with — *continued*
    damage to nail — *continued*
      with
        foreign body S91.229 ☑
    foreign body S91.129 ☑
  great S91.113 ☑
    with
      damage to nail S91.213 ☑
        with
          foreign body S91.223 ☑
      foreign body S91.123 ☑
    left S91.112 ☑
      with
        damage to nail S91.212 ☑
          with
            foreign body S91.222 ☑
        foreign body S91.122 ☑
    right S91.111 ☑
      with
        damage to nail S91.211 ☑
          with
            foreign body S91.221 ☑
        foreign body S91.121 ☑
  lesser S91.116 ☑
    with
      damage to nail S91.216 ☑
        with
          foreign body S91.226 ☑
      foreign body S91.126 ☑
    left S91.115 ☑
      with
        damage to nail S91.215 ☑
          with
            foreign body S91.225 ☑
        foreign body S91.125 ☑
    right S91.114 ☑
      with
        damage to nail S91.214 ☑
          with
            foreign body S91.224 ☑
        foreign body S91.124 ☑
tongue — *see* Laceration, oral cavity
trachea S11.021 ☑
  with foreign body S11.022 ☑
tunica vaginalis — *see* Laceration, testis
tympanum, tympanic membrane — *see* Laceration, ear, drum
umbilical region S31.115 ☑
  with foreign body S31.125 ☑
ureter S37.13 ☑
urethra S37.33 ☑
  with or following ectopic or molar pregnancy O08.6
  obstetrical trauma O71.5
urinary organ NEC S37.893 ☑
uterus S37.63 ☑
  with ectopic or molar pregnancy O08.6
  following ectopic or molar pregnancy O08.6
  nonpuerperal, nontraumatic N85.8
  obstetrical trauma NEC O71.81
  old (postpartal) N85.8
uvula — *see* Laceration, oral cavity
vagina S31.41 ☑
  with
    ectopic or molar pregnancy O08.6
    foreign body S31.42 ☑
  during delivery O71.4
    with perineal laceration — *see* Laceration, perineum, female, during delivery
  following ectopic or molar pregnancy O08.6
  nonpuerperal, nontraumatic N89.8
  old (postpartal) N89.8
vas deferens S37.893 ☑
vesical — *see* Laceration, bladder
vocal cords S11.031 ☑
  with foreign body S11.032 ☑
vulva S31.41 ☑
  with
    ectopic or molar pregnancy O08.6
    foreign body S31.42 ☑
  complicating delivery O70.0
  following ectopic or molar pregnancy O08.6
  nonpuerperal, nontraumatic N90.89
  old (postpartal) N90.89
wrist S61.519 ☑

Laceration — *continued*
  wrist — *continued*
    with
      foreign body S61.529 ☑
    left S61.512 ☑
      with
        foreign body S61.522 ☑
    right S61.511 ☑
      with
        foreign body S61.521 ☑
Lack of
  achievement in school Z55.3
  adequate
    food Z59.4
    intermaxillary vertical dimension of fully erupted
      teeth M26.36
    sleep Z72.820
  appetite (see Anorexia) R63.0
  awareness R41.9
  care
    in home Z74.2
    of infant (at or after birth) T76.02 ☑
      confirmed T74.02 ☑
  cognitive functions R41.9
  coordination R27.9
    ataxia R27.0
    specified type NEC R27.8
  development (physiological) R62.50
    failure to thrive (child over 28 days old) R62.51
      adult R62.7
      newborn P92.6
    short stature R62.52
    specified type NEC R62.59
  energy R53.83
  financial resources Z59.6
  food T73.0 ☑
  growth R62.52
  heating Z59.1
  housing (permanent) (temporary) Z59.0
    adequate Z59.1
  learning experiences in childhood Z62.898
  leisure time (affecting life-style) Z73.2
  material resources Z59.9
  memory (see also Amnesia)
    mild, following organic brain damage F06.8
  ovulation N97.0
  parental supervision or control of child Z62.0
  person able to render necessary care Z74.2
  physical exercise Z72.3
  play experience in childhood Z62.898
  posterior occlusal support M26.57
  relaxation (affecting life-style) Z73.2
  sexual
    desire F52.0
    enjoyment F52.1
  shelter Z59.0
  sleep (adequate) Z72.820
  supervision of child by parent Z62.0
  support, posterior occlusal M26.57
  water T73.1 ☑
Lacrimal — *see* condition
Lacrimation, abnormal — *see* Epiphora
Lacrimonasal duct — *see* condition
Lactation, lactating (breast) (puerperal, postpartum)
  associated
    cracked nipple O92.13
    retracted nipple O92.03
  defective O92.4
  disorder NEC O92.79
  excessive O92.6
  failed (complete) O92.3
    partial O92.4
  mastitis NEC — *see* Mastitis, obstetric
  mother (care and/or examination) Z39.1
  nonpuerperal N64.3
Lacticemia, excessive E87.2
Lacunar skull Q75.8
Laennec's cirrhosis K74.69
  alcoholic K70.30
    with ascites K70.31
Lafora's disease — *see* Epilepsy, generalized, idiopathic
Lag, lid (nervous) — *see* Retraction, lid
Lagophthalmos (eyelid) (nervous) H02.209
  cicatricial H02.219
    left H02.216
      lower H02.215
      upper H02.214
    right H02.213

Lagophthalmos — *continued*
  cicatricial — *continued*
    right — *continued*
      lower H02.212
      upper H02.211
    keratoconjunctivitis — *see* Keratoconjunctivitis
    left H02.206
      lower H02.205
      upper H02.204
    mechanical H02.229
      left H02.226
        lower H02.225
        upper H02.224
      right H02.223
        lower H02.222
        upper H02.221
    paralytic H02.239
      left H02.236
        lower H02.235
        upper H02.234
      right H02.233
        lower H02.232
        upper H02.231
    right H02.203
      lower H02.202
      upper H02.201
Laki-Lorand factor deficiency — *see* Defect, coagulation, specified type NEC
Lalling F80.0
Lambert-Eaton syndrome — *see* Syndrome, Lambert-Eaton
Lambliasis, lambliosis A07.1
Landau-Kleffner syndrome — *see* Epilepsy, specified NEC
Landouzy-Déjérine dystrophy or facioscapulohumeral atrophy G71.0
Landouzy's disease (icterohemorrhagic leptospirosis) A27.0
Landry-Guillain-Barré, syndrome or paralysis G61.0
Landry's disease or paralysis G61.0
Lane's
  band Q43.3
  kink — *see* Obstruction, intestine
  syndrome K90.2
Langdon Down syndrome — *see* Trisomy, 21
Lapsed immunization schedule status Z28.3
Large
  baby (regardless of gestational age) (4000g to 4499g) P08.1
  ear, congenital Q17.1
  physiological cup Q14.2
  stature R68.89
Large-for-dates NEC (infant) (4000g to 4499g) P08.1
  affecting management of pregnancy O36.6- ☑
  exceptionally (4500g or more) P08.0
Larsen-Johansson disease orosteochondrosis — *see* Osteochondrosis, juvenile, patella
Larsen's syndrome (flattened facies and multiple congenital dislocations) Q74.8
Larva migrans
  cutaneous B76.9
    Ancylostoma B76.0
  visceral B83.0
Laryngeal — *see* condition
Laryngismus (stridulus) J38.5
  congenital P28.89
  diphtheritic A36.2
Laryngitis (acute) (edematous) (fibrinous) (infective) (infiltrative) (malignant) (membranous) (phlegmonous) (pneumococcal) (pseudomembranous) (septic) (subglottic) (suppurative) (ulcerative) J04.0
  with
    influenza, flu, or grippe — *see* Influenza, with, laryngitis
    tracheitis (acute) — *see* Laryngotracheitis
  atrophic J37.0
  catarrhal J37.0
  chronic J37.0
    with tracheitis (chronic) J37.1
  diphtheritic A36.2
  due to external agent — *see* Inflammation, respiratory, upper, due to
  H. influenzae J04.0
  Hemophilus influenzae J04.0
  hypertrophic J37.0
  influenzal — *see* Influenza, with, respiratory manifestations NEC
  obstructive J05.0

Laryngitis — *continued*
  sicca J37.0
  spasmodic J05.0
    acute J04.0
  streptococcal J04.0
  stridulous J05.0
  syphilitic (late) A52.73
    congenital A50.59 [J99]
      early A50.03 [J99]
  tuberculous A15.5
  Vincent's A69.1
Laryngocele (congenital) (ventricular) Q31.3
Laryngofissure J38.7
  congenital Q31.8
Laryngomalacia (congenital) Q31.5
Laryngopharyngitis (acute) J06.0
  chronic J37.0
  due to external agent — *see* Inflammation, respiratory, upper, due to
Laryngoplegia J38 00
  bilateral J38.02
  unilateral J38.01
Laryngoptosis J38.7
Laryngospasm J38.5
Laryngostenosis J38.6
Laryngotracheitis (acute) (Infectional) (infective) (viral) J04.2
  atrophic J37.1
  catarrhal J37.1
  chronic J37.1
  diphtheritic A36.2
  due to external agent — *see* Inflammation, respiratory, upper, due to
  Hemophilus influenzae J04.2
  hypertrophic J37.1
  influenzal — *see* Influenza, with, respiratory manifestations NEC
  pachydermic J38.7
  sicca J37.1
  spasmodic J38.5
    acute J05.0
  streptococcal J04.2
  stridulous J38.5
  syphilitic (late) A52.73
    congenital A50.59 [J99]
      early A50.03 [J99]
  tuberculous A15.5
  Vincent's A69.1
Laryngotracheobronchitis — *see* Bronchitis
Larynx, laryngeal — *see* condition
Lassa fever A96.2
Lassitude — *see* Weakness
Late
  talker R62.0
  walker R62.0
Late effect(s) — *see* Sequelae
Latent — *see* condition
Laterocession — *see* Lateroversion
Lateroflexion — *see* Lateroversion
Lateroversion
  cervix — *see* Lateroversion, uterus
  uterus, uterine (cervix) (postinfectional) (postpartal, old) N85.4
    congenital Q51.818
    in pregnancy or childbirth O34.59- ☑
Lathyrism — *see* Poisoning, food, noxious, plant
Launois' syndrome (pituitary gigantism) E22.0
Launois-Bensaude adenolipomatosis E88.89
Laurence-Moon (-Bardet)-**Biedl syndrome** Q87.89
Lax, laxity (see also Relaxation)
  ligament (ous) (see also Disorder, ligament)
    familial M35.7
    knee — *see* Derangement, knee
  skin (acquired) L57.4
    congenital Q82.8
Laxative habit F55.2
Lazy leukocyte syndrome D70.8
Lead miner's lung J63.6
Leak, leakage
  air NEC J93.82
    postprocedural J95.812
  amniotic fluid — *see* Rupture, membranes, premature
  blood (microscopic), fetal, into maternal circulation
    affecting management of pregnancy — *see* Pregnancy, complicated by
  cerebrospinal fluid G96.0
    from spinal (lumbar) puncture G97.0

☑ **Additional Character Required** — Refer to the Tabular List for Character Selection   ▽ Subterms under main terms may continue to next column or page

Leak, leakage — *continued*
 device, implant or graft (*see also* Complications, by site and type, mechanical)
  arterial graft NEC — *see* Complication, cardiovascular device, mechanical, vascular
  breast (implant) T85.43 ☑
  catheter NEC T85.638 ☑
   dialysis (renal) T82.43 ☑
    intraperitoneal T85.631 ☑
   infusion NEC T82.534 ☑
    spinal (epidural) (subdural) T85.630 ☑
   urinary, indwelling T83.038 ☑
    cystostomy T83.030 ☑
  gastrointestinal — *see* Complications, prosthetic device, mechanical, gastrointestinal device
  genital NEC T83.498 ☑
   penile prosthesis T83.490 ☑
  heart NEC — *see* Complication, cardiovascular device, mechanical
  joint prosthesis — *see* Complications, joint prosthesis, mechanical, specified NEC, by site
  ocular NEC — *see* Complications, prosthetic device, mechanical, ocular device
  orthopedic NEC — *see* Complication, orthopedic, device, mechanical
  persistent air J93.82
  specified NEC T85.638 ☑
  urinary NEC (*see also* Complication, genitourinary, device, urinary, mechanical)
   graft T83.23 ☑
  vascular NEC — *see* Complication, cardiovascular device, mechanical
  ventricular intracranial shunt T85.03 ☑
 urine — *see* Incontinence
Leaky heart — *see* Endocarditis
Learning defect (specific) F81.9
Leather bottle stomach C16.9
Leber's
 congenital amaurosis H35.50
 optic atrophy (hereditary) H47.22
Lederer's anemia D59.1
Leeches (external) — *see* Hirudiniasis
Leg — *see* condition
Legg (-Calvé)-**Perthes disease, syndrome or osteochondrosis** M91.1- ☑
Legionellosis A48.1
 nonpneumonic A48.2
Legionnaires'
 disease A48.1
  nonpneumonic A48.2
 pneumonia A48.1
Leigh's disease G31.82
Leiner's disease L21.1
Leiofibromyoma — *see* Leiomyoma
Leiomyoblastoma — *see* Neoplasm, connective tissue, benign
Leiomyofibroma (*see also* Neoplasm, connective tissue, benign)
 uterus (cervix) (corpus) D25.9
Leiomyoma (*see also* Neoplasm, connective tissue, benign)
 bizarre — *see* Neoplasm, connective tissue, benign
 cellular — *see* Neoplasm, connective tissue, benign
 epithelioid — *see* Neoplasm, connective tissue, benign
 uterus (cervix) (corpus) D25.9
  intramural D25.1
  submucous D25.0
  subserosal D25.2
 vascular — *see* Neoplasm, connective tissue, benign
Leiomyoma, leiomyomatosis (intravascular) — *see* Neoplasm, connective tissue, uncertain behavior
Leiomyosarcoma (*see also* Neoplasm, connective tissue, malignant)
 epithelioid — *see* Neoplasm, connective tissue, malignant
 myxoid — *see* Neoplasm, connective tissue, malignant
Leishmaniasis B55.9
 American (mucocutaneous) B55.2
  cutaneous B55.1
 Asian Desert B55.1
 Brazilian B55.2
 cutaneous (any type) B55.1
 dermal (*see also* Leishmaniasis, cutaneous)
  post-kala-azar B55.0
 eyelid B55.1
 infantile B55.0
 Mediterranean B55.0

Leishmaniasis — *continued*
 mucocutaneous (American) (New World) B55.2
 naso-oral B55.2
 nasopharyngeal B55.2
 old world B55.1
 tegumentaria diffusa B55.1
 visceral B55.0
Leishmanoid, dermal (*see also* Leishmaniasis, cutaneous)
 post-kala-azar B55.0
Lenegre's disease I44.2
Lengthening, leg — *see* Deformity, limb, unequal length
Lennert's lymphoma — *see* Lymphoma, Lennert's
Lennox-Gastaut syndrome G40.812
 intractable G40.814
  with status epilepticus G40.813
  without status epilepticus G40.814
 not intractable G40.812
  with status epilepticus G40.811
  without status epilepticus G40.812
Lens — *see* condition
Lenticonus (anterior) (posterior) (congenital) Q12.8
Lenticular degeneration, progressive E83.01
Lentiglobus (posterior) (congenital) Q12.8
Lentigo (congenital) L81.4
 maligna (*see also* Melanoma, in situ)
  melanoma — *see* Melanoma
Lentivirus, as cause of disease classified elsewhere B97.31
Leontiasis
 ossium M85.2
 syphilitic (late) A52.78
  congenital A50.59
Lepothrix A48.8
Lepra — *see* Leprosy
Leprechaunism E34.8
Leprosy A30.- ☑
 with muscle disorder A30.9 [M63.80]
  ankle A30.9 [M63.87-] ☑
  foot A30.9 [M63.87-] ☑
  forearm A30.9 [M63.83-] ☑
  hand A30.9 [M63.84-] ☑
  lower leg A30.9 [M63.86-] ☑
  multiple sites A30.9 [M63.89]
  pelvic region A30.9 [M63.85-] ☑
  shoulder region A30.9 [M63.81-] ☑
  specified site NEC A30.9 [M63.88]
  thigh A30.9 [M63.85-] ☑
  upper arm A30.9 [M63.82-] ☑
 anesthetic A30.9
 BB A30.3
 BL A30.4
 borderline (infiltrated) (neuritic) A30.3
  lepromatous A30.4
  tuberculoid A30.2
 BT A30.2
 dimorphous (infiltrated) (neuritic) A30.3
 I A30.0
 indeterminate (macular) (neuritic) A30.0
 lepromatous (diffuse) (infiltrated) (macular) (neuritic) (nodular) A30.5
 LL A30.5
 macular (early) (neuritic) (simple) A30.9
 maculoanesthetic A30.9
 mixed A30.3
 neural A30.9
 nodular A30.5
 primary neuritic A30.3
 specified type NEC A30.8
 TT A30.1
 tuberculoid (major) (minor) A30.1
Leptocytosis, hereditary D56.9
Leptomeningitis (chronic) (circumscribed) (hemorrhagic) (nonsuppurative) — *see* Meningitis
Leptomeningopathy G96.19
Leptospiral — *see* condition
Leptospirochetal — *see* condition
Leptospirosis A27.9
 canicola A27.89
 due to Leptospira interrogans serovar icterohaemorrhagiae A27.0
 icterohemorrhagica A27.0
 pomona A27.89
 Weil's disease A27.0
Leptus dermatitis B88.0
Leriche's syndrome (aortic bifurcation occlusion) I74.09
Leri's pleonosteosis Q78.8

Leri-Weill syndrome Q77.8
Lermoyez' syndrome — *see* Vertigo, peripheral NEC
Lesch-Nyhan syndrome E79.1
Leser-Trélat disease L82.1
 inflamed L82.0
Lesion(s) (nontraumatic)
 abducens nerve — *see* Strabismus, paralytic, sixth nerve
 alveolar process K08.9
 angiocentric immunoproliferative D47.Z9 (*following* D47.4)
 anorectal K62.9
 aortic (valve) I35.9
 auditory nerve — *see* subcategory H93.3 ☑
 basal ganglion G25.9
 bile duct — *see* Disease, bile duct
 biomechanical M99.9
  specified type NEC M99.89
   abdomen M99.89
   acromioclavicular M99.87
   cervical region M99.81
   cervicothoracic M99.81
   costochondral M99.88
   costovertebral M99.88
   head region M99.80
   hip M99.85
   lower extremity M99.86
   lumbar region M99.83
   lumbosacral M99.83
   occipitocervical M99.80
   pelvic region M99.85
   pubic M99.85
   rib cage M99.88
   sacral region M99.84
   sacrococcygeal M99.84
   sacroiliac M99.84
   specified NEC M99.89
   sternochondral M99.88
   sternoclavicular M99.87
   thoracic region M99.82
   thoracolumbar M99.82
   upper extremity M99.87
 bladder N32.9
 bone — *see* Disorder, bone
 brachial plexus G54.0
 brain G93.9
  congenital Q04.9
  vascular I67.9
   degenerative I67.9
   hypertensive I67.4
 buccal cavity K13.79
 calcified — *see* Calcification
 canthus — *see* Disorder, eyelid
 carate — *see* Pinta, lesions
 cardia K22.9
 cardiac (*see also* Disease, heart) I51.9
  congenital Q24.9
  valvular — *see* Endocarditis
 cauda equina G83.4
 cecum K63.9
 cerebral — *see* Lesion, brain
 cerebrovascular I67.9
  degenerative I67.9
  hypertensive I67.4
 cervical (nerve) root NEC G54.2
 chiasmal — *see* Disorder, optic, chiasm
 chorda tympani G51.8
 coin, lung R91.1
 colon K63.9
 congenital — *see* Anomaly, by site
 conjunctiva H11.9
 conus medullaris — *see* Injury, conus medullaris
 coronary artery — *see* Ischemia, heart
 cranial nerve G52.9
  eighth — *see* Disorder, ear
  eleventh G52.9
  fifth G50.9
  first G52.0
  fourth — *see* Strabismus, paralytic, fourth nerve
  seventh G51.9
  sixth — *see* Strabismus, paralytic, sixth nerve
  tenth G52.2
  twelfth G52.3
 cystic — *see* Cyst
 degenerative — *see* Degeneration
 duodenum K31.9
 edentulous (alveolar) ridge, associated with trauma, due to traumatic occlusion K06.2

Lesion(s) — *continued*
en coup de sabre L94.1
eyelid — *see* Disorder, eyelid
gasserian ganglion G50.8
gastric K31.9
gastroduodenal K31.9
gastrointestinal K63.9
gingiva, associated with trauma K06.2
glomerular
  focal and segmental (*see also* N00-N07 with fourth
    character .1) N05.1
  minimal change (*see also* N00-N07 with fourth
    character .0) N05.0
heart (organic) — *see* Disease, heart
hyperchromic, due to pinta (carate) A67.1
hyperkeratotic — *see* Hyperkeratosis
hypothalamic E23.7
ileocecal K63.9
ileum K63.9
iliohypogastric nerve G57.8- ☑
inflammatory — *see* Inflammation
intestine K63.9
intracerebral — *see* Lesion, brain
intrachiasmal (optic) — *see* Disorder, optic, chiasm
intracranial, space-occupying R90.0
joint — *see* Disorder, joint
  sacroiliac (old) M53.3
keratotic — *see* Keratosis
kidney — *see* Disease, renal
laryngeal nerve (recurrent) G52.2
lip K13.0
liver K76.9
lumbosacral
  plexus G54.1
  root (nerve) NEC G54.4
lung (coin) R91.1
maxillary sinus J32.0
mitral I05.9
Morel-Lavallée — *see* Hematoma, by site
motor cortex NEC G93.89
mouth K13.79
nerve G58.9
  femoral G57.2- ☑
  median G56.1- ☑
    carpal tunnel syndrome — *see* Syndrome,
      carpal tunnel
  plantar G57.6- ☑
  popliteal (lateral) G57.3- ☑
    medial G57.4- ☑
  radial G56.3- ☑
  sciatic G57.0- ☑
  spinal — *see* Injury, nerve, spinal
  ulnar G56.2- ☑
nervous system, congenital Q07.9
nonallopathic — *see* Lesion, biomechanical
nose (internal) J34.89
obstructive — *see* Obstruction
obturator nerve G57.8- ☑
oral mucosa K13.70
organ or site NEC — *see* Disease, by site
osteolytic — *see* Osteolysis
peptic K27.9
periodontal, due to traumatic occlusion K05.5
pharynx J39.2
pigment, pigmented (skin) L81.9
pinta — *see* Pinta, lesions
polypoid — *see* Polyp
prechiasmal (optic) — *see* Disorder, optic, chiasm
primary (*see also* Syphilis, primary) A51.0
  carate A67.0
  pinta A67.0
  yaws A66.0
pulmonary J98.4
  valve I37.9
pylorus K31.9
rectosigmoid K63.9
retina, retinal H35.9
sacroiliac (joint) (old) M53.3
salivary gland K11.9
  benign lymphoepithelial K11.8
saphenous nerve G57.8- ☑
sciatic nerve G57.0- ☑
secondary — *see* Syphilis, secondary
shoulder (region) M75.9- ☑
  specified NEC M75.8- ☑
sigmoid K63.9
sinus (accessory) (nasal) J34.89

Lesion(s) — *continued*
skin L98.9
  suppurative L08.0
SLAP S43.43- ☑
spinal cord G95.9
  congenital Q06.9
spleen D73.89
stomach K31.9
superior glenoid labrum S43.43- ☑
syphilitic — *see* Syphilis
tertiary — *see* Syphilis, tertiary
thoracic root (nerve) NEC G54.3
tonsillar fossa J35.9
tooth, teeth K08.9
  white spot
    chewing surface K02.51
    pit and fissure surface K02.51
    smooth surface K02.61
traumatic — *see* specific type of injury by site
tricuspid (valve) I07.9
  nonrheumatic I36.9
trigeminal nerve G50.9
ulcerated or ulcerative — *see* Ulcer, skin
uterus N85.9
vagus nerve G52.2
valvular — *see* Endocarditis
vascular I99.9
  affecting central nervous system I67.9
  following trauma NEC T14.8
  umbilical cord, complicating delivery O69.5 ☑
warty — *see* Verruca
white spot (tooth)
  chewing surface K02.51
  pit and fissure surface K02.51
  smooth surface K02.61
Lethargic — *see* condition
Lethargy R53.83
Letterer-Siwe's disease C96.0
Leukemia, leukemic C95.9- ☑
acute basophilic C94.8- ☑
acute bilineal C95.0- ☑
acute erythroid C94.0- ☑
acute lymphoblastic C91.0- ☑
acute megakaryoblastic C94.2- ☑
acute megakaryocytic C94.2- ☑
acute mixed lineage C95.0- ☑
acute monoblastic (monoblastic/monocytic) C93.0- ☑
acute monocytic (monoblastic/monocytic) C93.0- ☑
acute myeloblastic (minimal differentiation) (with
  maturation) C92.0- ☑
acute myeloid
  with
    11q23-abnormality C92.6- ☑
    dysplasia of remaining hematopoesis and/or
      myelodysplastic disease in its history
      C92.A- ☑ (*following* C92.6)
    multilineage dysplasia C92.A- ☑ (*following*
      C92.6)
    variation of MLL-gene C92.6- ☑
  M6 (a)(b) C94.0- ☑
  M7 C94.2- ☑
acute myelomonocytic C92.5- ☑
acute promyelocytic C92.4- ☑
adult T-cell (HTLV-1-associated) (acute variant)
  (chronic variant) (lymphomatoid variant)
  (smouldering variant) C91.5- ☑
aggressive NK-cell C94.8- ☑
AML (1/ETO) (M0) (M1) (M2) (without a FAB classification) C92.0- ☑
AML M3 C92.4- ☑
AML M4 (Eo with inv(16) or t(16;16)) C92.5- ☑
AML M5 C93.0- ☑
AML M5a C93.0- ☑
AML M5b C93.0- ☑
AML Me with t (15;17) and variants C92.4- ☑
atypical chronic myeloid, BCR/ABL-negative C92.2- ☑
biphenotypic acute C95.0- ☑
blast cell C95.0- ☑
Burkitt-type, mature B-cell C91.A- ☑ (*following* C91.6)
chronic lymphocytic, of B-cell type C91.1- ☑
chronic monocytic C93.1- ☑
chronic myelogenous (Philadelphia chromosome (Ph1)
  positive) (t(9;22)) (q34;q11) (with crisis of blast
  cells) C92.1- ☑
chronic myeloid, BCR/ABL-positive C92.1- ☑
  atypical, BCR/ABL-negative C92.2- ☑
chronic myelomonocytic C93.1- ☑

Leukemia, leukemic — *continued*
chronic neutrophilic D47.1
CMML (-1) (-2) (with eosinophilia) C93.1- ☑
granulocytic (*see also* Category C92) C92.9- ☑
hairy cell C91.4- ☑
juvenile myelomonocytic C93.3- ☑
lymphoid C91.9- ☑
  specified NEC C91.Z- ☑ (*following* C91.6)
mast cell C94.3- ☑
mature B-cell, Burkitt-type C91.A- ☑ (*following* C91.6)
monocytic (subacute) C93.9- ☑
  specified NEC C93.Z- ☑ (*following* C93.3)
myelogenous (*see also* Category C92) C92.9- ☑
myeloid C92.9- ☑
  specified NEC C92.Z- ☑ (*following* C92.6)
plasma cell C90.1- ☑
plasmacytic C90.1- ☑
prolymphocytic
  of B-cell type C91.3- ☑
  of T-cell type C91.6- ☑
specified NEC C94.8- ☑
stem cell, of unclear lineage C95.0- ☑
subacute lymphocytic C91.9- ☑
T-cell large granular lymphocytic C91.Z- ☑ (*following*
  C91.6)
unspecified cell type C95.9- ☑
  acute C95.0- ☑
  chronic C95.1- ☑
Leukemoid reaction (*see also* Reaction, leukemoid)
  D72.823
Leukoaraiosis (hypertensive) I67.81
Leukoariosis — *see* Leukoaraiosis
Leukocoria — *see* Disorder, globe, degenerated condition, leucocoria
Leukocytopenia D72.819
Leukocytosis D72.829
  eosinophilic D72.1
Leukoderma, leukodermia NEC L81.5
  syphilitic A51.39
    late A52.79
Leukodystrophy E75.29
Leukoedema, oral epithelium K13.29
Leukoencephalitis G04.81
  acute (subacute) hemorrhagic G36.1
    postimmunization or postvaccinal G04.02
  postinfectious G04.01
  subacute sclerosing A81.1
  van Bogaert's (sclerosing) A81.1
Leukoencephalopathy (*see also* Encephalopathy)
  G93.49
  Binswanger's I67.3
  heroin vapor G92
  metachromatic E75.25
  multifocal (progressive) A81.2
  postimmunization and postvaccinal G04.02
  progressive multifocal A81.2
  reversible, posterior G93.6
  van Bogaert's (sclerosing) A81.1
  vascular, progressive I67.3
Leukoerythroblastosis D75.9
Leukokeratosis (*see also* Leukoplakia)
  mouth K13.21
  nicotina palati K13.24
  oral mucosa K13.21
  tongue K13.21
  vocal cord J38.3
Leukokraurosis vulva (e) N90.4
Leukoma (cornea) (*see also* Opacity, cornea)
  adherent H17.0- ☑
  interfering with central vision — *see* Opacity, cornea,
    central
Leukomalacia, cerebral, newborn P91.2
  periventricular P91.2
Leukomelanopathy, hereditary D72.0
Leukonychia (punctata) (striata) L60.8
  congenital Q84.4
Leukopathia unguium L60.8
  congenital Q84.4
Leukopenia D72.819
  basophilic D72.818
  chemotherapy (cancer) induced D70.1
  congenital D70.0
  cyclic D70.0
  drug induced NEC D70.2
    due to cytoreductive cancer chemotherapy D70.1
  eosinophilic D72.818
  familial D70.0

Leukopenia — *continued*
  infantile genetic D70.0
  malignant D70.9
  periodic D70.0
  transitory neonatal P61.5
Leukopenic — *see* condition
Leukoplakia
  anus K62.89
  bladder (postinfectional) N32.89
  buccal K13.21
  cervix (uteri) N88.0
  esophagus K22.8
  gingiva K13.21
  hairy (oral mucosa) (tongue) K13.3
  kidney (pelvis) N28.89
  larynx J38.7
  lip K13.21
  mouth K13.21
  oral epithelium, including tongue (mucosa) K13.21
  palate K13.21
  pelvis (kidney) N28.89
  penis (infectional) N48.0
  rectum K62.89
  syphilitic (late) A52.79
  tongue K13.21
  ureter (postinfectional) N28.89
  urethra (postinfectional) N36.8
  uterus N85.8
  vagina N89.4
  vocal cord J38.3
  vulva N90.4
Leukorrhea N89.8
  due to Trichomonas (vaginalis) A59.00
  trichomonal A59.00
Leukosarcoma C85.9- ☑
Levocardia (isolated) Q24.1
  with situs inversus Q89.3
Levotransposition Q20.5
Lev's disease or syndrome (acquired complete heart block) I44.2
Levulosuria — *see* Fructosuria
Levurid L30.2
Lewy body (ies) (dementia) (disease) G31.83
Leyden-Moebius dystrophy G71.0
Leydig cell
  carcinoma
    specified site — *see* Neoplasm, malignant, by site
    unspecified site
      female C56.9
      male C62.9- ☑
  tumor
    benign
      specified site — *see* Neoplasm, benign, by site
      unspecified site
        female D27.- ☑
        male D29.2- ☑
    malignant
      specified site — *see* Neoplasm, malignant, by site
      unspecified site
        female C56.- ☑
        male C62.9- ☑
    specified site — *see* Neoplasm, uncertain behavior, by site
    unspecified site
      female D39.1- ☑
      male D40.1- ☑
Leydig-Sertoli cell tumor
  specified site — *see* Neoplasm, benign, by site
  unspecified site
    female D27.- ☑
    male D29.2- ☑
LGSIL (Low grade squamous intraepithelial lesion on cytologic smear of)
  anus R85.612
  cervix R87.612
  vagina R87.622
Liar, pathologic F60.2
Libido
  decreased R68.82
Libman-Sacks disease M32.11
Lice (infestation) B85.2
  body (Pediculus corporis) B85.1
  crab B85.3
  head (Pediculus capitis) B85.0
  mixed (classifiable to more than one of the titles B85.0-B85.3) B85.4

Lice — *continued*
  pubic (Phthirus pubis) B85.3
Lichen L28.0
  albus L90.0
    penis N48.0
    vulva N90.4
  amyloidosis E85.4 [L99]
  atrophicus L90.0
    penis N48.0
    vulva N90.4
  congenital Q82.8
  myxedematosus L98.5
  nitidus L44.1
  pilaris Q82.8
    acquired L85.8
  planopilaris L66.1
  planus (chronicus) L43.9
    annularis L43.8
    bullous L43.1
    follicular L66.1
    hypertrophic L43.0
    moniliformis L44.3
    of Wilson L43.9
    specified NEC L43.8
    subacute (active) L43.3
    tropicus L43.3
  ruber
    acuminatus L44.0
    moniliformis L44.3
    planus L43.9
  sclerosus (et atrophicus) L90.0
    penis N48.0
    vulva N90.4
  scrofulosus (primary) (tuberculous) A18.4
  simplex (chronicus) (circumscriptus) L28.0
  striatus L44.2
  urticatus L28.2
Lichenification L28.0
Lichenoides tuberculosis (primary) A18.4
Lichtheim's disease or syndrome — *see* Degeneration, combined
Lien migrans D73.89
Ligament — *see* condition
Light
  for gestational age — *see* Light for dates
  headedness R42
Light-for-dates (infant) P05.00
  with weight of
    1000-1249 grams P05.04
    1250-1499 grams P05.05
    1500-1749 grams P05.06
    1750-1999 grams P05.07
    2000-2499 grams P05.08
    499 grams or less P05.01
    500-749 grams P05.02
    750-999 grams P05.03
  affecting management of pregnancy O36.59- ☑
  and small-for-dates — *see* Small for dates
Lightning (effects) (stroke) (struck by) T75.00 ☑
  burn — *see* Burn
  foot E53.8
  shock T75.01 ☑
  specified effect NEC T75.09 ☑
Lightwood-Albright syndrome N25.89
Lightwood's disease or syndrome (renal tubular acidosis) N25.89
Lignac (-de Toni) (-Fanconi) (-Debré) disease or syndrome E72.09
  with cystinosis E72.04
Ligneous thyroiditis E06.5
Likoff's syndrome I20.8
Limb — *see* condition
Limbic epilepsy personality syndrome F07.0
Limitation, limited
  activities due to disability Z73.6
  cardiac reserve — *see* Disease, heart
  eye muscle duction, traumatic — *see* Strabismus, mechanical
  mandibular range of motion M26.52
Lindau (-von Hippel) disease Q85.8
Line(s)
  Beau's L60.4
  Harris' — *see* Arrest, epiphyseal
  Hudson's (cornea) — *see* Pigmentation, cornea, anterior
  Stähli's (cornea) — *see* Pigmentation, cornea, anterior
Linea corneae senilis — *see* Change, cornea, senile

Lingua
  geographica K14.1
  nigra (villosa) K14.3
  plicata K14.5
  tylosis K13.29
Lingual — *see* condition
Linguatulosis B88.8
Linitis (gastric) plastica C16.9
Lip — *see* condition
Lipedema — *see* Edema
Lipemia (*see also* Hyperlipidemia)
  retina, retinalis E78.3
Lipidosis E75.6
  cerebral (infantile) (juvenile) (late) E75.4
  cerebroretinal E75.4
  cerebroside E75.22
  cholesterol (cerebral) E75.5
  glycolipid E75.21
  hepatosplenomegalic E78.3
  sphingomyelin — *see* Niemann-Pick disease or syndrome
  sulfatide E75.29
Lipoadenoma — *see* Neoplasm, benign, by site
Lipoblastoma — *see* Lipoma
Lipoblastomatosis — *see* Lipoma
Lipochondrodystrophy E76.01
Lipochrome histiocytosis (familial) D71
Lipodermatosclerosis — *see* Varix, leg, with, inflammation
  ulcerated — *see* Varix, leg, with, ulcer, with inflammation by site
Lipodystrophia progressiva E88.1
Lipodystrophy (progressive) E88.1
  insulin E88.1
  intestinal K90.81
  mesenteric K65.4
Lipofibroma — *see* Lipoma
Lipofuscinosis, neuronal (with ceroidosis) E75.4
Lipogranuloma, sclerosing L92.8
Lipogranulomatosis E78.89
Lipoid (*see also* condition)
  histiocytosis D76.3
    essential E75.29
  nephrosis N04.9
  proteinosis of Urbach E78.89
Lipoidemia — *see* Hyperlipidemia
Lipoidosis — *see* Lipidosis
Lipoma D17.9
  fetal D17.9
    fat cell D17.9
  infiltrating D17.9
  intramuscular D17.9
  pleomorphic D17.9
  site classification
    arms (skin) (subcutaneous) D17.2- ☑
    connective tissue D17.30
      intra-abdominal D17.5
      intrathoracic D17.4
      peritoneum D17.79
      retroperitoneum D17.79
      specified site NEC D17.39
      spermatic cord D17.6
    face (skin) (subcutaneous) D17.0
    genitourinary organ NEC D17.72
    head (skin) (subcutaneous) D17.0
    intra-abdominal D17.5
    intrathoracic D17.4
    kidney D17.71
    legs (skin) (subcutaneous) D17.2- ☑
    neck (skin) (subcutaneous) D17.0
    peritoneum D17.79
    retroperitoneum D17.79
    skin D17.30
      specified site NEC D17.39
    specified site NEC D17.79
    spermatic cord D17.6
    subcutaneous D17.30
      specified site NEC D17.39
    trunk (skin) (subcutaneous) D17.1
    unspecified D17.9
  spindle cell D17.9
Lipomatosis E88.2
  dolorosa (Dercum) E88.2
  fetal — *see* Lipoma
  Launois-Bensaude E88.89
Lipomyoma — *see* Lipoma
Lipomyxoma — *see* Lipoma

Lipomyxosarcoma — see Neoplasm, connective tissue, malignant
Lipoprotein metabolism disorder E78.9
Lipoproteinemia E78.5
  broad-beta E78.2
  floating-beta E78.2
  hyper-pre-beta E78.1
Liposarcoma (see also Neoplasm, connective tissue, malignant)
  dedifferentiated — see Neoplasm, connective tissue, malignant
  differentiated type — see Neoplasm, connective tissue, malignant
  embryonal — see Neoplasm, connective tissue, malignant
  mixed type — see Neoplasm, connective tissue, malignant
  myxoid — see Neoplasm, connective tissue, malignant
  pleomorphic — see Neoplasm, connective tissue, malignant
  round cell — see Neoplasm, connective tissue, malignant
  well differentiated type — see Neoplasm, connective tissue, malignant
Liposynovitis prepatellaris E88.89
Lipping, cervix N86
Lipschütz disease or ulcer N76.6
Lipuria R82.0
  schistosomiasis (bilharziasis) B65.0
Lisping F80.0
Lissauer's paralysis A52.17
Lissencephalia, lissencephaly Q04.3
Listeriosis, listerellosis A32.9
  congenital (disseminated) P37.2
  cutaneous A32.0
  neonatal, newborn (disseminated) P37.2
  oculoglandular A32.81
  specified NEC A32.89
Lithemia E79.0
Lithiasis — see Calculus
Lithosis J62.8
Lithuria R82.99
Litigation, anxiety concerning Z65.3
Little leaguer's elbow — see Epicondylitis, medial
Little's disease G80.9
Littre's
  gland — see condition
  hernia — see Hernia, abdomen
Littritis — see Urethritis
Livedo (annularis) (racemosa) (reticularis) R23.1
Liver — see condition
Living alone (problems with) Z60.2
  with handicapped person Z74.2
Lloyd's syndrome — see Adenomatosis, endocrine
Loa loa, loaiasis, loasis B74.3
Lobar — see condition
Lobomycosis B48.0
Lobo's disease B48.0
Lobotomy syndrome F07.0
Lobstein (-Ekman) **disease or syndrome** Q78.0
Lobster-claw hand Q71.6- ☑
Lobulation (congenital) (see also Anomaly, by site)
  kidney, Q63.1
  liver, abnormal Q44.7
  spleen Q89.09
Lobule, lobular — see condition
Local, localized — see condition
Locked twins causing obstructed labor O66.1
Locked-in state G83.5
Locking
  joint — see Derangement, joint, specified type NEC
    knee — see Derangement, knee
Lockjaw — see Tetanus
Löffler's
  endocarditis I42.3
  eosinophilia J82
  pneumonia J82
  syndrome (eosinophilic pneumonitis) J82
Loiasis (with conjunctival infestation) (eyelid) B74.3
Lone Star fever A77.0
Long
  labor O63.9
    first stage O63.0
    second stage O63.1
  QT syndrome I45.81
Longitudinal stripes or grooves, nails L60.8
  congenital Q84.6

Long-term (current) (prophylactic) **drug therapy** (use of)
  agents affecting estrogen receptors and estrogen levels NEC Z79.818
  anastrozole (Arimidex) Z79.811
  antibiotics Z79.2
    short-term use — omit code
  anticoagulants Z79.01
  anti-inflammatory, non-steroidal (NSAID) Z79.1
  antiplatelet Z79.02
  antithrombotics Z79.02
  aromatase inhibitors Z79.811
  aspirin Z79.82
  birth control pill or patch Z79.3
  bisphosphonates Z79.83
  contraceptive, oral Z79.3
  drug, specified NEC Z79.899
  estrogen receptor downregulators Z79.818
  Evista Z79.810
  exemestane (Aromasin) Z79.811
  Fareston Z79.810
  fulvestrant (Faslodex) Z79.818
  gonadotropin-releasing hormone (GnRH) agonist Z79.818
  goserelin acetate (Zoladex) Z79.818
  hormone replacement (postmenopausal) Z79.890
  insulin Z79.4
  letrozole (Femara) Z79.811
  leuprolide acetate (leuprorelin) (Lupron) Z79.818
  megestrol acetate (Megace) Z79.818
  methadone for pain management Z79.891
  Nolvadex Z79.810
  non-steroidal anti-inflammatories (NSAID) Z79.1
  opiate analgesic Z79.891
  oral contraceptive Z79.3
  raloxifene (Evista) Z79.810
  selective estrogen receptor modulators (SERMs) Z79.810
  steroids
    inhaled Z79.51
    systemic Z79.52
  tamoxifen (Nolvadex) Z79.810
  toremifene (Fareston) Z79.810
Loop
  intestine — see Volvulus
  vascular on papilla (optic) Q14.2
Loose (see also condition)
  body
    joint M24.00
      ankle M24.07- ☑
      elbow M24.02- ☑
      hand M24.04- ☑
      hip M24.05- ☑
      knee M23.4- ☑
      shoulder (region) M24.01- ☑
      specified site NEC M24.08
      toe M24.07- ☑
      vertebra M24.08
      wrist M24.03- ☑
    knee M23.4- ☑
    sheath, tendon — see Disorder, tendon, specified type NEC
  cartilage — see Loose, body, joint
  tooth, teeth K08.8
Loosening
  aseptic
    joint prosthesis — see Complications, joint prosthesis, mechanical, loosening, by site
  epiphysis — see Osteochondropathy
  mechanical
    joint prosthesis — see Complications, joint prosthesis, mechanical, loosening, by site
Looser-Milkman (-Debray) **syndrome** M83.8
Lop ear (deformity) Q17.3
Lorain (-Levi) **short stature syndrome** E23.0
Lordosis M40.50
  acquired — see Lordosis, specified type NEC
  congenital Q76.429
    lumbar region Q76.426
    lumbosacral region Q76.427
    sacral region Q76.428
    sacrococcygeal region Q76.428
    thoracolumbar region Q76.425
  lumbar region M40.56
  lumbosacral region M40.57
  postsurgical M96.4
  postural — see Lordosis, specified type NEC
  rachitic (late effect) (sequelae) E64.3

Lordosis — continued
  sequelae of rickets E64.3
  specified type NEC M40.40
    lumbar region M40.46
    lumbosacral region M40.47
    thoracolumbar region M40.45
  thoracolumbar region M40.55
  tuberculous A18.01
Loss (of)
  appetite (see Anorexia) R63.0
    hysterical F50.8
    nonorganic origin F50.8
    psychogenic F50.8
  blood — see Hemorrhage
  consciousness, transient R55
    traumatic — see Injury, intracranial
  control, sphincter, rectum R15.9
    nonorganic origin F98.1
  elasticity, skin R23.4
  family (member) in childhood Z62.898
  fluid (acute) E86.9
    with
      hypernatremia E87.0
      hyponatremia E87.1
  function of labyrinth — see subcategory H83.2 ☑
  hair, nonscarring — see Alopecia
  hearing (see also Deafness)
    central NOS H90.5
    neural NOS H90.5
    perceptive NOS H90.5
    sensorineural NOS H90.5
    sensory NOS H90.5
  height R29.890
  limb or member, traumatic, current — see Amputation, traumatic
  love relationship in childhood Z62.898
  memory (see also Amnesia)
    mild, following organic brain damage F06.8
  mind — see Psychosis
  occlusal vertical dimension of fully erupted teeth M26.37
  organ or part — see Absence, by site, acquired
  ossicles, ear (partial) H74.32- ☑
  parent in childhood Z63.4
  pregnancy, recurrent N96
    without current pregnancy N96
    care in current pregnancy O26.2- ☑
  recurrent pregnancy — see Loss, pregnancy, recurrent
  self-esteem, in childhood Z62.898
  sense of
    smell — see Disturbance, sensation, smell
    taste — see Disturbance, sensation, taste
    touch R20.8
  sensory R44.9
    dissociative F44.6
  sexual desire F52.0
  sight (acquired) (complete) (congenital) — see Blindness
  substance of
    bone — see Disorder, bone, density and structure, specified NEC
    cartilage — see Disorder, cartilage, specified type NEC
      auricle (ear) — see Disorder, pinna, specified type NEC
    vitreous (humor) H15.89
  tooth, teeth — see Absence, teeth, acquired
  vision, visual H54.7
    both eyes H54.3
    one eye H54.60
      left (normal vision on right) H54.62
      right (normal vision on left) H54.61
    specified as blindness — see Blindness
    subjective
      sudden H53.13- ☑
      transient H53.12- ☑
  vitreous — see Prolapse, vitreous
  voice — see Aphonia
  weight (abnormal) (cause unknown) R63.4
Louis-Bar syndrome (ataxia-telangiectasia) G11.3
Louping ill (encephalitis) A84.8
Louse, lousiness — see Lice
Low
  achiever, school Z55.3
  back syndrome M54.5
  basal metabolic rate R94.8
  birthweight (2499 grams or less) P07.10

☑ **Additional Character Required** — Refer to the Tabular List for Character Selection   ▽ **Subterms under main terms may continue to next column or page**

Low — *continued*
  birthweight — *continued*
    with weight of
      1000-1249 grams P07.14
      1250-1499 grams P07.15
      1500-1749 grams P07.16
      1750-1999 grams P07.17
      2000-2499 grams P07.18
    extreme (999 grams or less) P07.00
      with weight of
        499 grams or less P07.01
        500-749 grams P07.02
        750-999 grams P07.03
    for gestational age — *see* Light for dates
  blood pressure (*see also* Hypotension)
    reading (incidental) (isolated) (nonspecific) R03.1
  cardiac reserve — *see* Disease, heart
  function (*see also* Hypofunction)
    kidney N28.9
  hematocrit D64.9
  hemoglobin D64.9
  income Z59.6
  level of literacy Z55.0
  lying
    kidney N28.89
    organ or site, congenital — *see* Malposition, congenital
  output syndrome (cardiac) — *see* Failure, heart
  platelets (blood) — *see* Thrombocytopenia
  reserve, kidney N28.89
  salt syndrome E87.1
  self esteem R45.81
  set ears Q17.4
  vision H54.2
    one eye (other eye normal) H54.50
      left (normal vision on right) H54.52
        other eye blind — *see* Blindness
      right (normal vision on left) H54.51
Low-density-lipoprotein-type (LDL) **hyperlipoproteinemia** E78.0
Lowe's syndrome E72.03
Lown-Ganong-Levine syndrome I45.6
LSD reaction (acute) (without dependence) F16.90
  with dependence F16.20
L-shaped kidney Q63.8
Ludwig's angina or disease K12.2
Lues (venerea), **luetic** — *see* Syphilis
Luetscher's syndrome (dehydration) E86.0
Lumbago, lumbalgia M54.5
  with sciatica M54.4- ☑
    due to intervertebral disc disorder M51.17
  due to displacement, intervertebral disc M51.27
    with sciatica M51.17
Lumbar — *see* condition
Lumbarization, vertebra, congenital Q76.49
Lumbermen's itch B88.0
Lump — *see* Mass
Lunacy — *see* Psychosis
Lung — *see* condition
Lupoid (miliary) **of Boeck** D86.3
Lupus
  anticoagulant D68.62
    with
      hemorrhagic disorder D68.312
      hypercoagulable state D68.62
      finding without diagnosis R76.0
  discoid (local) L93.0
  erythematosus (discoid) (local) L93.0
    disseminated — *see* Lupus, erythematosus, systemic
    eyelid H01.129
      left H01.126
        lower H01.125
        upper H01.124
      right H01.123
        lower H01.122
        upper H01.121
    profundus L93.2
    specified NEC L93.2
    subacute cutaneous L93.1
    systemic M32.9
      with organ or system involvement M32.10
        endocarditis M32.11
        lung M32.13
        pericarditis M32.12
        renal (glomerular) M32.14
          tubulo-interstitial M32.15
        specified organ or system NEC M32.19

Lupus — *continued*
  erythematosus — *continued*
    systemic — *continued*
      drug-induced M32.0
      inhibitor (presence of) D68.62
        with
          hemorrhagic disorder D68.312
          hypercoagulable state D68.62
        finding without diagnosis R76.0
      specified NEC M32.8
    exedens A18.4
    hydralazine M32.0
      correct substance properly administered — *see* Table of Drugs and Chemicals, by drug, adverse effect
      overdose or wrong substance given or taken — *see* Table of Drugs and Chemicals, by drug, poisoning
    nephritis (chronic) M32.14
    nontuberculous, not disseminated L93.0
    panniculitis L93.2
    pernio (Besnier) D86.3
    systemic — *see* Lupus, erythematosus, systemic
    tuberculous A18.4
      eyelid A18.4
    vulgaris A18.4
      eyelid A18.4
Luteinoma D27.- ☑
Lutembacher's disease or syndrome (atrial septal defect with mitral stenosis) Q21.1
Luteoma D27.- ☑
Lutz (-Splendore-de Almeida) **disease** — *see* Paracoccidioidomycosis
Luxation (*see also* Dislocation)
  eyeball (nontraumatic) — *see* Luxation, globe
    birth injury P15.3
  globe, nontraumatic H44.82- ☑
  lacrimal gland — *see* Dislocation, lacrimal gland
  lens (old) (partial) (spontaneous)
    congenital Q12.1
      syphilitic A50.39
Lycanthropy F22
Lyell's syndrome L51.2
  due to drug L51.2
    correct substance properly administered — *see* Table of Drugs and Chemicals, by drug, adverse effect
    overdose or wrong substance given or taken — *see* Table of Drugs and Chemicals, by drug, poisoning
Lyme disease A69.20
Lymph
  gland or node — *see* condition
  scrotum — *see* Infestation, filarial
Lymphadenitis I88.9
  with ectopic or molar pregnancy O08.0
  acute L04.9
    axilla L04.2
    face L04.0
    head L04.0
    hip L04.3
    limb
      lower L04.3
      upper L04.2
    neck L04.0
    shoulder L04.2
    specified site NEC L04.8
    trunk L04.1
  anthracosis (occupational) J60
  any site, except mesenteric I88.9
    chronic I88.1
    subacute I88.1
  breast
    gestational — *see* Mastitis, obstetric
    puerperal, postpartum (nonpurulent) O91.22
  chancroidal (congenital) A57
  chronic I88.1
    mesenteric I88.0
  due to
    Brugia (malayi) B74.1
      timori B74.2
    chlamydial lymphogranuloma A55
    diphtheria (toxin) A36.89
    lymphogranuloma venereum A55
    Wuchereria bancrofti B74.0
  following ectopic or molar pregnancy O08.0
  gonorrheal A54.89
  infective — *see* Lymphadenitis, acute

Lymphadenitis — *continued*
  mesenteric (acute) (chronic) (nonspecific) (subacute) I88.0
    due to Salmonella typhi A01.09
    tuberculous A18.39
  mycobacterial A31.8
  purulent — *see* Lymphadenitis, acute
  pyogenic — *see* Lymphadenitis, acute
  regional, nonbacterial I88.8
  septic — *see* Lymphadenitis, acute
  subacute, unspecified site I88.1
  suppurative — *see* Lymphadenitis, acute
  syphilitic (early) (secondary) A51.49
    late A52.79
  tuberculous — *see* Tuberculosis, lymph gland
  venereal (chlamydial) A55
Lymphadenoid goiter E06.3
Lymphadenopathy (generalized) R59.1
  angioimmunoblastic, with dysproteinemia (AILD) C86.5
  due to toxoplasmosis (acquired) B58.89
    congenital (acute) (subacute) (chronic) P37.1
  localized R59.0
  syphilitic (early) (secondary) A51.49
Lymphadenosis R59.1
Lymphangiectasis I89.0
  conjunctiva H11.89
  postinfectional I89.0
  scrotum I89.0
Lymphangiectatic elephantiasis, nonfilarial I89.0
Lymphangioendothelioma D18.1
  malignant — *see* Neoplasm, connective tissue, malignant
Lymphangioleiomyomatosis J84.81
Lymphangioma D18.1
  capillary D18.1
  cavernous D18.1
  cystic D18.1
  malignant — *see* Neoplasm, connective tissue, malignant
Lymphangiomyoma D18.1
Lymphangiomyomatosis J84.81
Lymphangiosarcoma — *see* Neoplasm, connective tissue, malignant
Lymphangitis I89.1
  with
    abscess — *code by* site under Abscess
    cellulitis — *code by* site under Cellulitis
    ectopic or molar pregnancy O08.0
  acute L03.91
    abdominal wall L03.321
    ankle — *see* Lymphangitis, acute, lower limb
    arm — *see* Lymphangitis, acute, upper limb
    auricle (ear) — *see* Lymphangitis, acute, ear
    axilla L03.12- ☑
    back (any part) L03.322
    buttock L03.327
    cervical (meaning neck) L03.222
    cheek (external) L03.212
    chest wall L03.323
    digit
      finger — *see* Lymphangitis, acute, finger
      toe — *see* Lymphangitis, acute, toe
    ear (external) H60.1- ☑
    external auditory canal — *see* Lymphangitis, acute, ear
    eyelid — *see* Abscess, eyelid
    face NEC L03.212
    finger (intrathecal) (periosteal) (subcutaneous) (subcuticular) L03.02- ☑
    foot — *see* Lymphangitis, acute, lower limb
    gluteal (region) L03.327
    groin L03.324
    hand — *see* Lymphangitis, acute, upper limb
    head NEC L03.891
      face (any part, except ear, eye and nose) L03.212
    heel — *see* Lymphangitis, acute, lower limb
    hip — *see* Lymphangitis, acute, lower limb
    jaw (region) L03.212
    knee — *see* Lymphangitis, acute, lower limb
    leg — *see* Lymphangitis, acute, lower limb
    lower limb L03.12- ☑
      toe — *see* Lymphangitis, acute, toe
    navel L03.326
    neck (region) L03.222
    orbit, orbital — *see* Cellulitis, orbit

Lymphangitis — continued
  acute — continued
    pectoral (region) L03.323
    perineal, perineum L03.325
    scalp (any part) L03.891
    shoulder — see Lymphangitis, acute, upper limb
    specified site NEC L03.898
    thigh — see Lymphangitis, acute, lower limb
    thumb (intrathecal) (periosteal) (subcutaneous) (subcuticular) — see Lymphangitis, acute, finger
    toe (intrathecal) (periosteal) (subcutaneous) (subcuticular) L03.04- ☑
    trunk L03.329
      abdominal wall L03.321
      back (any part) L03.322
      buttock L03.327
      chest wall L03.323
      groin L03.324
      perineal, perineum L03.325
      umbilicus L03.326
    umbilicus L03.326
    upper limb L03.12- ☑
      axilla — see Lymphangitis, acute, axilla
      finger — see Lymphangitis, acute, finger
      thumb — see Lymphangitis, acute, finger
      wrist — see Lymphangitis, acute, upper limb
  breast
    gestational — see Mastitis, obstetric
  chancroidal A57
  chronic (any site) I89.1
  due to
    Brugia (malayi) B74.1
      timori B74.2
    Wuchereria bancrofti B74.0
  following ectopic or molar pregnancy O08.89
  penis
    acute N48.29
    gonococcal (acute) (chronic) A54.09
  puerperal, postpartum, childbirth O86.89
  strumous, tuberculous A18.2
  subacute (any site) I89.1
  tuberculous — see Tuberculosis, lymph gland
Lymphatic (vessel) — see condition
Lymphatism E32.8
Lymphectasia I89.0
Lymphedema (acquired) (see also Elephantiasis)
  congenital Q82.0
  hereditary (chronic) (idiopathic) Q82.0
  postmastectomy I97.2
  praecox I89.0
  secondary I89.0
  surgical NEC I97.89
    postmastectomy (syndrome) I97.2
Lymphoblastic — see condition
Lymphoblastoma (diffuse) — see Lymphoma, lymphoblastic (diffuse)
  giant follicular — see Lymphoma, lymphoblastic (diffuse)
  macrofollicular — see Lymphoma, lymphoblastic (diffuse)
Lymphocele I89.8
Lymphocytic
  chorioencephalitis (acute) (serous) A87.2
  choriomeningitis (acute) (serous) A87.2
  meningoencephalitis A87.2
Lymphocytoma, benign cutis L98.8
Lymphocytopenia D72.810
Lymphocytosis (symptomatic) D72.820
  infectious B33.8
Lymphoepithelioma — see Neoplasm, malignant, by site
Lymphogranuloma (malignant) (see also Lymphoma, Hodgkin)
  chlamydial A55
  inguinale A55
  venereum (any site) (chlamydial) (with stricture of rectum) A55
Lymphogranulomatosis (malignant) (see also Lymphoma, Hodgkin)
  benign (Boeck's sarcoid) (Schaumann's) D86.1
Lymphohistiocytosis, hemophagocytic (familial) D76.1
Lymphoid — see condition
Lymphoma (of) (malignant) C85.90
  adult T-cell (HTLV-1-associated) (acute variant) (chronic variant) (lymphomatoid variant) (smouldering variant) C91.5- ☑

Lymphoma — continued
  anaplastic large cell
    ALK-negative C84.7- ☑
    ALK-positive C84.6- ☑
    CD30-positive C84.6- ☑
    primary cutaneous C86.6
  angioimmunoblastic T-cell C86.5
  BALT C88.4
  B-cell C85.1- ☑
  blastic NK-cell C86.4
  B-precursor C83.5- ☑
  bronchial-associated lymphoid tissue [BALT-lymphoma] C88.4
  Burkitt (atypical) C83.7- ☑
  Burkitt-like C83.7- ☑
  centrocytic C83.1- ☑
  cutaneous follicle center C82.6- ☑
  cutaneous T-cell C84.A- ☑ (following C84.7)
  diffuse follicle center C82.5- ☑
  diffuse large cell C83.3- ☑
    anaplastic C83.3- ☑
    B-cell C83.3- ☑
    CD30-positive C83.3- ☑
    centroblastic C83.3- ☑
    immunoblastic C83.3- ☑
    plasmablastic C83.3- ☑
    subtype not specified C83.3- ☑
    T-cell rich C83.3- ☑
  enteropathy-type (associated) (intestinal) T-cell C86.2
  extranodal marginal zone B-cell lymphoma of mucosa-associated lymphoid tissue [MALT-lymphoma] C88.4
  extranodal NK/T-cell, nasal type C86.0
  follicular C82.9- ☑
    grade
      I C82.0- ☑
      II C82.1- ☑
      III C82.2- ☑
      IIIa C82.3- ☑
      IIIb C82.4- ☑
    specified NEC C82.8- ☑
  hepatosplenic T-cell (alpha-beta) (gamma-delta) C86.1
  histiocytic C85.9- ☑
    true C96.A (following C96.6)
  Hodgkin C81.9 ☑
    classical C81.7- ☑
      lymphocyte depleted C81.3- ☑
      lymphocyte-rich C81.4- ☑
      mixed cellularity C81.2- ☑
      nodular sclerosis C81.1- ☑
      specified NEC C81.7- ☑
    lymphocyte depleted classical C81.3- ☑
    lymphocyte-rich classical C81.4- ☑
    mixed cellularity classical C81.2- ☑
    nodular
      lymphocyte predominant C81.0- ☑
      sclerosis classical C81.1- ☑
  intravascular large B-cell C83.8- ☑
  Lennert's C84.4- ☑
  lymphoblastic (diffuse) C83.5- ☑
  lymphoblastic B-cell C83.5- ☑
  lymphoblastic T-cell C83.5- ☑
  lymphoepithelioid C84.4- ☑
  lymphoplasmacytic C83.0- ☑
    with IgM-production C88.0
  MALT C88.4
  mantle cell C83.1- ☑
  mature T-cell NEC C84.4- ☑
  mature T/NK-cell C84.9- ☑
    specified NEC C84.Z- ☑ (following C84.7)
  mediastinal (thymic) large B-cell C85.2- ☑
  Mediterranean C88.3
  mucosa-associated lymphoid tissue [MALT-lymphoma] C88.4
  NK/T cell C84.9- ☑
  nodal marginal zone C83.0- ☑
  non-follicular (diffuse) C83.9- ☑
    specified NEC C83.8- ☑
  non-Hodgkin (see also Lymphoma, by type) C85.9- ☑
    specified NEC C85.8- ☑
  non-leukemic variant of B-CLL C83.0- ☑
  peripheral T-cell, not classified C84.4- ☑
  primary cutaneous
    anaplastic large cell C86.6
    CD30-positive large T-cell C86.6
  primary effusion B-cell C83.8- ☑

Lymphoma — continued
  SALT C88.4
  skin-associated lymphoid tissue [SALT-lymphoma] C88.4
  small cell B-cell C83.0- ☑
  splenic marginal zone C83.0- ☑
  subcutaneous panniculitis-like T-cell C86.3
  T-precursor C83.5- ☑
  true histiocytic C96.A (following C96.6)
Lymphomatosis — see Lymphoma
Lymphopathia venereum, veneris A55
Lymphopenia D72.810
Lymphoplasmacytic leukemia — see Leukemia, chronic lymphocytic, B-cell type
Lymphoproliferation, X-linked disease D82.3
Lymphoreticulosis, benign (of inoculation) A28.1
Lymphorrhea I89.8
Lymphosarcoma (diffuse) (see also Lymphoma) C85.9-
Lymphostasis I89.8
Lypemania — see Melancholia
Lysine and hydroxylysine metabolism disorder E72.3
Lyssa — see Rabies

M

Macacus ear Q17.3
Maceration, wet feet, tropical (syndrome) T69.02- ☑
MacLeod's syndrome J43.0
Macrocephalia, macrocephaly Q75.3
Macrocheilia, macrochilia (congenital) Q18.6
Macrocolon (see also Megacolon) Q43.1
Macrocornea Q15.8
  with glaucoma Q15.0
Macrocytic — see condition
Macrocytosis D75.89
Macrodactylia, macrodactylism (fingers) (thumbs) Q74.0
  toes Q74.2
Macrodontia K00.2
Macrogenia M26.05
Macrogenitosomia (adrenal) (male) (praecox) E25.9
  congenital E25.0
Macroglobulinemia (idiopathic) (primary) C88.0
  monoclonal (essential) D47.2
  Waldenström C88.0
Macroglossia (congenital) Q38.2
  acquired K14.8
Macrognathia, macrognathism (congenital) (mandibular) (maxillary) M26.09
Macrogyria (congenital) Q04.8
Macrohydrocephalus — see Hydrocephalus
Macromastia — see Hypertrophy, breast
Macrophthalmos Q11.3
  in congenital glaucoma Q15.0
Macropsia H53.15
Macrosigmoid K59.3
  congenital Q43.2
Macrospondylitis , acromegalic E22.0
Macrostomia (congenital) Q18.4
Macrotia (external ear) (congenital) Q17.1
Macula
  cornea, corneal — see Opacity, cornea
  degeneration (atrophic) (exudative) (senile) (see also Degeneration, macula)
    hereditary — see Dystrophy, retina
Maculae ceruleae B85.1
Maculopathy, toxic — see Degeneration, macula, toxic
Madarosis (eyelid) H02.729
  left H02.726
    lower H02.725
    upper H02.724
  right H02.723
    lower H02.722
    upper H02.721
Madelung's
  deformity (radius) Q74.0
  disease
    radial deformity Q74.0
    symmetrical lipomas, neck E88.89
Madness — see Psychosis
Madura
  foot B47.9
    actinomycotic B47.1
    mycotic B47.0
Maduromycosis B47.0
Maffucci's syndrome Q78.4

☑ Additional Character Required — Refer to the Tabular List for Character Selection   ▽ **Subterms under main terms may continue to next column or page**

Magnesium metabolism disorder — *see* Disorder, metabolism, magnesium
Main en griffe (acquired) (*see also* Deformity, limb, clawhand)
  congenital Q74.0
Maintenance (encounter for)
  antineoplastic chemotherapy Z51.11
  antineoplastic radiation therapy Z51.0
  methadone F11.20
Majocchi's
  disease L81.7
  granuloma B35.8
Major — *see* condition
Mal de los pintos — *see* Pinta
Mal de mer T75.3 ☑
Malabar itch (any site) B35.5
Malabsorption K90.9
  calcium K90.89
  carbohydrate K90.4
  disaccharide E73.9
  fat K90.4
  galactose E74.20
  glucose (-galactose) E74.39
  intestinal K90.9
    specified NEC K90.89
  isomaltose E74.31
  lactose E73.9
  methionine E72.19
  monosaccharide E74.39
  postgastrectomy K91.2
  postsurgical K91.2
  protein K90.4
  starch K90.4
  sucrose E74.39
  syndrome K90.9
    postsurgical K91.2
Malacia, bone (adult) M83.9
  juvenile — *see* Rickets
Malacoplakia
  bladder N32.89
  pelvis (kidney) N28.89
  ureter N28.89
  urethra N36.8
Malacosteon, juvenile — *see* Rickets
Maladaptation — *see* Maladjustment
Maladie de Roger Q21.0
Maladjustment
  conjugal Z63.0
    involving divorce or estrangement Z63.5
  educational Z55.4
  family Z63.9
  marital Z63.0
    involving divorce or estrangement Z63.5
  occupational NEC Z56.89
  simple, adult — *see* Disorder, adjustment
  situational — *see* Disorder, adjustment
  social Z60.9
    due to
      acculturation difficulty Z60.3
      discrimination and persecution (perceived) Z60.5
      exclusion and isolation Z60.4
      life-cycle (phase of life) transition Z60.0
      rejection Z60.4
      specified reason NEC Z60.8
Malaise R53.81
Malakoplakia — *see* Malacoplakia
Malaria, malarial (fever) B54
  with
    blackwater fever B50.8
      hemoglobinuric (bilious) B50.8
    hemoglobinuria B50.8
  accidentally induced (therapeutically) — *code by* type under Malaria
  algid B50.9
  cerebral B50.0 [G94]
  clinically diagnosed (without parasitological confirmation) B54
  congenital NEC P37.4
    falciparum P37.3
  congestion, congestive B54
  continued (fever) B50.9
  estivo-autumnal B50.9
  falciparum B50.9
    with complications NEC B50.8
      cerebral B50.0 [G94]
    severe B50.8
  hemorrhagic B54

Malaria, malarial — *continued*
  malariae B52.9
    with
      complications NEC B52.8
      glomerular disorder B52.0
  malignant (tertian) — *see* Malaria, falciparum
  mixed infections — *code to* first listed type in B50-B53
  ovale B53.0
  parasitologically confirmed NEC B53.8
  pernicious, acute — *see* Malaria, falciparum
  Plasmodium (P.)
    falciparum NEC — *see* Malaria, falciparum
    malariae NEC B52.9
      with Plasmodium
        falciparum (and or vivax) — *see* Malaria, falciparum
        vivax (*see also* Malaria, vivax)
          and falciparum — *see* Malaria, falciparum
    ovale B53.0
      with Plasmodium malariae (*see also* Malaria, malariae)
      and vivax (*see also* Malaria, vivax)
        and falciparum — *see* Malaria, falciparum
    simian B53.1
      with Plasmodium malariae (*see also* Malaria, malariae)
      and vivax (*see also* Malaria, vivax)
        and falciparum — *see* Malaria, falciparum
    vivax NEC B51.9
      with Plasmodium falciparum — *see* Malaria, falciparum
  quartan — *see* Malaria, malariae
  quotidian — *see* Malaria, falciparum
  recurrent B54
  remittent B54
  specified type NEC (parasitologically confirmed) B53.8
  spleen B54
  subtertian (fever) — *see* Malaria, falciparum
  tertian (benign) (*see also* Malaria, vivax)
    malignant B50.9
  tropical B50.9
  typhoid B54
  vivax B51.9
    with
      complications NEC B51.8
      ruptured spleen B51.0
Malassez's disease (cystic) N50.8
Malassimilation K90.9
Maldescent, testis Q53.9
  bilateral Q53.20
    abdominal Q53.21
    perineal Q53.22
  unilateral Q53.10
    abdominal Q53.11
    perineal Q53.12
Maldevelopment (*see also* Anomaly)
  brain Q07.9
  colon Q43.9
  hip Q74.2
    congenital dislocation Q65.2
      bilateral Q65.1
      unilateral Q65.0- ☑
  mastoid process Q75.8
  middle ear Q16.4
    except ossicles Q16.4
    ossicles Q16.3
  ossicles Q16.3
  spine Q76.49
  toe Q74.2
Male type pelvis Q74.2
  with disproportion (fetopelvic) O33.3 ☑
    causing obstructed labor O65.3
Malformation (congenital) (*see also* Anomaly)
  adrenal gland Q89.1
  affecting multiple systems with skeletal changes NEC Q87.5
  alimentary tract Q45.9
    specified type NEC Q45.8
    upper Q40.9
      specified type NEC Q40.8
  aorta Q25.9
    atresia Q25.2
    coarctation (preductal) (postductal) Q25.1
    patent ductus arteriosus Q25.0
    specified type NEC Q25.4

Malformation — *continued*
  aorta — *continued*
    stenosis (supravalvular) Q25.3
  aortic valve Q23.9
    specified NEC Q23.8
  arteriovenous, aneurysmatic (congenital) Q27.30
    brain Q28.2
    cerebral Q28.2
    peripheral Q27.30
      digestive system Q27.33
      lower limb Q27.32
      other specified site Q27.39
      renal vessel Q27.34
      upper limb Q27.31
    precerebral vessels (nonruptured) Q28.0
  auricle
    ear (congenital) Q17.3
      acquired H61.119
        left H61.112
          with right H61.113
        right H61.111
          with left H61.113
  bile duct Q44.5
  bladder Q64.79
    aplasia Q64.5
    diverticulum Q64.6
    exstrophy — *see* Exstrophy, bladder
    neck obstruction Q64.31
  bone Q79.9
    face Q75.9
      specified type NEC Q75.8
    skull Q75.9
      specified type NEC Q75.8
  brain (multiple) Q04.9
    arteriovenous Q28.2
    specified type NEC Q04.8
  branchial cleft Q18.2
  breast Q83.9
    specified type NEC Q83.8
  broad ligament Q50.6
  bronchus Q32.4
  bursa Q79.9
  cardiac
    chambers Q20.9
      specified type NEC Q20.8
    septum Q21.9
      specified type NEC Q21.8
  cerebral Q04.9
    vessels Q28.3
  cervix uteri Q51.9
    specified type NEC Q51.828
  Chiari
    Type I G93.5
    Type II Q07.01
  choroid (congenital) Q14.3
    plexus Q07.8
  circulatory system Q28.9
  cochlea Q16.5
  cornea Q13.4
  coronary vessels Q24.5
  corpus callosum (congenital) Q04.0
  diaphragm Q79.1
  digestive system NEC, specified type NEC Q45.8
  dura Q07.9
    brain Q04.9
    spinal Q06.9
  ear Q17.9
    causing impairment of hearing Q16.9
    external Q17.9
      accessory auricle Q17.0
      causing impairment of hearing Q16.9
        absence of
          auditory canal Q16.1
          auricle Q16.0
      macrotia Q17.1
      microtia Q17.2
      misplacement Q17.4
      misshapen NEC Q17.3
      prominence Q17.5
      specified type NEC Q17.8
    inner Q16.5
    middle Q16.4
      absence of eustachian tube Q16.2
      ossicles (fusion) Q16.3
    ossicles Q16.3
    specified type NEC Q17.8
  epididymis Q55.4
  esophagus Q39.9

Index

Magnesium metabolism disorder — Malformation

Malformation — *continued*
  esophagus — *continued*
    specified type NEC Q39.8
  eye Q15.9
    lid Q10.3
    specified NEC Q15.8
  fallopian tube Q50.6
  genital organ — *see* Anomaly, genitalia
  great
    artery Q25.9
      aorta — *see* Malformation, aorta
      pulmonary artery — *see* Malformation, pul-
        monary, artery
      specified type NEC Q25.8
    vein Q26.9
      anomalous
        portal venous connection Q26.5
        pulmonary venous connection Q26.4
          partial Q26.3
          total Q26.2
      persistent left superior vena cava Q26.1
      portal vein-hepatic artery fistula Q26.6
      specified type NEC Q26.8
      vena cava stenosis, congenital Q26.0
  gum Q38.6
  hair Q84.2
  heart Q24.9
    specified type NEC Q24.8
  integument Q84.9
    specified type NEC Q84.8
  internal ear Q16.5
  intestine Q43.9
    specified type NEC Q43.8
  iris Q13.2
  joint Q74.9
    ankle Q74.2
    lumbosacral Q76.49
    sacroiliac Q74.2
    specified type NEC Q74.8
  kidney Q63.9
    accessory Q63.0
    giant Q63.3
    horseshoe Q63.1
    hydronephrosis Q62.0
    malposition Q63.2
    specified type NEC Q63.8
  lacrimal apparatus Q10.6
  lingual Q38.3
  lip Q38.0
  liver Q44.7
  lung Q33.9
  meninges or membrane (congenital) Q07.9
    cerebral Q04.8
    spinal (cord) Q06.9
  middle ear Q16.4
    ossicles Q16.3
  mitral valve Q23.9
    specified NEC Q23.8
  Mondini's (congenital) (malformation, cochlea) Q16.5
  mouth (congenital) Q38.6
  multiple types NEC Q89.7
  musculoskeletal system Q79.9
  myocardium Q24.8
  nail Q84.6
  nervous system (central) Q07.9
  nose Q30.9
    specified type NEC Q30.8
  optic disc Q14.2
  orbit Q10.7
  ovary Q50.39
  palate Q38.5
  parathyroid gland Q89.2
  pelvic organs or tissues NEC
    in pregnancy or childbirth O34.8- ☑
      causing obstructed labor O65.5
  penis Q55.69
    aplasia Q55.5
    curvature (lateral) Q55.61
    hypoplasia Q55.62
  pericardium Q24.8
  peripheral vascular system Q27.9
    specified type NEC Q27.8
  pharynx Q38.8
  precerebral vessels Q28.1
  prostate Q55.4
  pulmonary
    arteriovenous Q25.72
    artery Q25.9

Malformation — *continued*
  pulmonary — *continued*
    artery — *continued*
      atresia Q25.5
      specified type NEC Q25.79
      stenosis Q25.6
    valve Q22.3
  renal artery Q27.2
  respiratory system Q34.9
  retina Q14.1
  scrotum — *see* Malformation, testis and scrotum
  seminal vesicles Q55.4
  sense organs NEC Q07.9
  skin Q82.9
  specified NEC Q89.8
  spinal
    cord Q06.9
    nerve root Q07.8
  spine Q76.49
    kyphosis — *see* Kyphosis, congenital
    lordosis — *see* Lordosis, congenital
  spleen Q89.09
  stomach Q40.3
    specified type NEC Q40.2
  teeth, tooth K00.9
  tendon Q79.9
  testis and scrotum Q55.20
    aplasia Q55.0
    hypoplasia Q55.1
    polyorchism Q55.21
    retractile testis Q55.22
    scrotal transposition Q55.23
    specified NEC Q55.29
  thorax, bony Q76.9
  throat Q38.8
  thyroid gland Q89.2
  tongue (congenital) Q38.3
    hypertrophy Q38.2
    tie Q38.1
  trachea Q32.1
  tricuspid valve Q22.9
    specified type NEC Q22.8
  umbilical cord NEC (complicating delivery) O69.89 ☑
  umbilicus Q89.9
  ureter Q62.8
    agenesis Q62.4
    duplication Q62.5
    malposition — *see* Malposition, congenital, ureter
    obstructive defect — *see* Defect, obstructive, ureter
    vesico-uretero-renal reflux Q62.7
  urethra Q64.79
    aplasia Q64.5
    duplication Q64.74
    posterior valves Q64.2
    prolapse Q64.71
    stricture Q64.32
  urinary system Q64.9
  uterus Q51.9
    specified type NEC Q51.818
  vagina Q52.4
  vas deferens Q55.4
    atresia Q55.3
  vascular system, peripheral Q27.9
  venous — *see* Anomaly, vein(s)
  vulva Q52.70

Malfunction (*see also* Dysfunction)
  cardiac electronic device T82.119 ☑
    electrode T82.110 ☑
    pulse generator T82.111 ☑
    specified type NEC T82.118 ☑
  catheter device NEC T85.618 ☑
    cystostomy T83.010 ☑
    dialysis (renal) (vascular) T82.41 ☑
      intraperitoneal T85.611 ☑
    infusion NEC T82.514 ☑
      spinal (epidural) (subdural) T85.610 ☑
    urinary, indwelling T83.018 ☑
  colostomy K94.03
    valve K94.03
  cystostomy (stoma) N99.512
    catheter T83.010 ☑
  enteric stoma K94.13
  enterostomy K94.13
  esophagostomy K94.33
  gastroenteric K31.89
  gastrostomy K94.23
  ileostomy K94.13
    valve K94.13

Malfunction — *continued*
  jejunostomy K94.13
  pacemaker — *see* Malfunction, cardiac electronic de-
    vice
  prosthetic device, internal — *see* Complications,
    prosthetic device, by site, mechanical
  tracheostomy J95.03
  urinary device NEC — *see* Complication, genitourinary,
    device, urinary, mechanical
  valve
    colostomy K94.03
    heart T82.09 ☑
    ileostomy K94.13
  vascular graft or shunt NEC — *see* Complication, car-
    diovascular device, mechanical, vascular
  ventricular (communicating shunt) T85.01 ☑
Malherbe's tumor — *see* Neoplasm, skin, benign
Malibu disease L98.8
Malignancy (*see also* Neoplasm, malignant, by site)
  unspecified site (primary) C80.1
Malignant — *see* condition
Malingerer, malingering Z76.5
Mallet finger (acquired) — *see* Deformity, finger, mallet
  finger
  congenital Q74.0
  sequelae of rickets E64.3
Malleus A24.0
Mallory's bodies R89.7
Mallory-Weiss syndrome K22.6
Malnutrition E46
  degree
    first E44.1
    mild (protein) E44.1
    moderate (protein) E44.0
    second E44.0
    severe (protein-energy) E43
      intermediate form E42
        with
          kwashiorkor (and marasmus) E42
          marasmus E41
    third E43
  following gastrointestinal surgery K91.2
  intrauterine
    light-for-dates — *see* Light for dates
    small-for-dates — *see* Small for dates
  lack of care, or neglect (child) (infant) T76.02 ☑
    confirmed T74.02 ☑
  malignant E40
  protein E46
    calorie E46
      mild E44.1
      moderate E44.0
      severe E43
        intermediate form E42
          with
            kwashiorkor (and marasmus) E42
            marasmus E41
    energy E46
      mild E44.1
      moderate E44.0
      severe E43
        intermediate form E42
          with
            kwashiorkor (and marasmus) E42
            marasmus E41
    severe (protein-energy) E43
      with
        kwashiorkor (and marasmus) E42
        marasmus E41
Malocclusion (teeth) M26.4
  Angle's M26.219
    class I M26.211
    class II M26.212
    class III M26.213
  due to
    abnormal swallowing M26.59
    mouth breathing M26.59
    tongue, lip or finger habits M26.59
  temporomandibular (joint) M26.69
Malposition
  cervix — *see* Malposition, uterus
  congenital
    adrenal (gland) Q89.1
    alimentary tract Q45.8
      lower Q43.8
      upper Q40.8
    aorta Q25.4
    appendix Q43.8

Malposition — continued
  congenital — continued
    arterial trunk Q20.0
    artery (peripheral) Q27.8
      coronary Q24.5
      digestive system Q27.8
      lower limb Q27.8
      pulmonary Q25.79
      specified site NEC Q27.8
      upper limb Q27.8
    auditory canal Q17.8
      causing impairment of hearing Q16.9
    auricle (ear) Q17.4
      causing impairment of hearing Q16.9
      cervical Q18.2
    biliary duct or passage Q44.5
    bladder (mucosa) — see Exstrophy, bladder
    brachial plexus Q07.8
    brain tissue Q04.8
    breast Q83.8
    bronchus Q32.4
    cecum Q43.8
    clavicle Q74.0
    colon Q43.8
    digestive organ or tract NEC Q45.8
      lower Q43.8
      upper Q40.8
    ear (auricle) (external) Q17.4
      ossicles Q16.3
    endocrine (gland) NEC Q89.2
    epiglottis Q31.8
    eustachian tube Q17.8
    eye Q15.8
    facial features Q18.8
    fallopian tube Q50.6
    finger(s) Q68.1
      supernumerary Q69.0
    foot Q66.9
    gallbladder Q44.1
    gastrointestinal tract Q45.8
    genitalia, genital organ(s) or tract
      female Q52.8
        external Q52.79
        internal NEC Q52.8
      male Q55.8
    glottis Q31.8
    hand Q68.1
    heart Q24.8
      dextrocardia Q24.0
        with complete transposition of viscera Q89.3
    hepatic duct Q44.5
    hip (joint) Q65.89
    intestine (large) (small) Q43.8
      with anomalous adhesions, fixation or malrotation Q43.3
    joint NEC Q68.8
    kidney Q63.2
    larynx Q31.8
    limb Q68.8
      lower Q68.8
      upper Q68.8
    liver Q44.7
    lung (lobe) Q33.8
    nail(s) Q84.6
    nerve Q07.8
    nervous system NEC Q07.8
    nose, nasal (septum) Q30.8
    organ or site not listed — see Anomaly, by site
    ovary Q50.39
    pancreas Q45.3
    parathyroid (gland) Q89.2
    patella Q74.1
    peripheral vascular system Q27.8
    pituitary (gland) Q89.2
    respiratory organ or system NEC Q34.8
    rib (cage) Q76.6
      supernumerary in cervical region Q76.5
    scapula Q74.0
    shoulder Q74.0
    spinal cord Q06.8
    spleen Q89.09
    sternum NEC Q76.7
    stomach Q40.2
    symphysis pubis Q74.2
    thymus (gland) Q89.2
    thyroid (gland) (tissue) Q89.2
      cartilage Q31.8
    toe(s) Q66.9

Malposition — continued
  congenital — continued
    toe(s) — continued
      supernumerary Q69.2
    tongue Q38.3
    trachea Q32.1
    ureter Q62.60
      deviation Q62.61
      displacement Q62.62
      ectopia Q62.63
      specified type NEC Q62.69
    uterus Q51.818
    vein(s) (peripheral) Q27.8
      great Q26.8
    vena cava (inferior) (superior) Q26.8
  device, implant or graft (see also Complications, by site and type, mechanical) T85.628 ☑
    arterial graft NEC — see Complication, cardiovascular device, mechanical, vascular
    breast (implant) T85.42 ☑
    catheter NEC T85.628 ☑
      cystostomy T83.020 ☑
      dialysis (renal) T82.42 ☑
        intraperitoneal T85.621 ☑
      infusion NEC T82.524 ☑
        spinal (epidural) (subdural) T85.620 ☑
      urinary, indwelling T83.028 ☑
    electronic (electrode) (pulse generator) (stimulator)
      bone T84.320 ☑
      cardiac T82.129 ☑
        electrode T82.120 ☑
        pulse generator T82.121 ☑
        specified type NEC T82.128 ☑
      nervous system — see Complication, prosthetic device, mechanical, electronic nervous system stimulator
      urinary — see Complication, genitourinary, device, urinary, mechanical
    fixation, internal (orthopedic) NEC — see Complication, fixation device, mechanical
    gastrointestinal — see Complications, prosthetic device, mechanical, gastrointestinal device
    genital NEC T83.428 ☑
      intrauterine contraceptive device T83.32 ☑
      penile prosthesis T83.420 ☑
    heart NEC — see Complication, cardiovascular device, mechanical
    joint prosthesis — see Complication, joint prosthesis, mechanical
    ocular NEC — see Complications, prosthetic device, mechanical, ocular device
    orthopedic NEC — see Complication, orthopedic, device, mechanical
    specified NEC T85.628 ☑
    urinary NEC (see also Complication, genitourinary, device, urinary, mechanical)
      graft T83.22 ☑
    vascular NEC — see Complication, cardiovascular device, mechanical
    ventricular intracranial shunt T85.02 ☑
  fetus — see Pregnancy, complicated by (management affected by), presentation, fetal
  gallbladder K82.8
  gastrointestinal tract, congenital Q45.8
  heart, congenital NEC Q24.8
  joint prosthesis — see Complications, joint prosthesis, mechanical, displacement, by site
  stomach K31.89
    congenital Q40.2
  tooth, teeth, fully erupted M26.30
  uterus (acute) (acquired) (adherent) (asymptomatic) (postinfectional) (postpartal, old) N85.4
    anteflexion or anteversion N85.4
      congenital Q51.818
    flexion N85.4
      lateral — see Lateroversion, uterus
    inversion N85.5
    lateral (flexion) (version) — see Lateroversion, uterus
    in pregnancy or childbirth — see subcategory O34.5 ☑
    retroflexion or retroversion — see Retroversion, uterus
Malposture R29.3
Malrotation
  cecum Q43.3
  colon Q43.3

Malrotation — continued
  intestine Q43.3
  kidney Q63.2
Malta fever — see Brucellosis
Maltreatment
  adult
    abandonment
      confirmed T74.01 ☑
      suspected T76.01 ☑
    confirmed T74.91 ☑
    history of Z91.419
    neglect
      confirmed T74.01 ☑
      suspected T76.01 ☑
    physical abuse
      confirmed T74.11 ☑
      suspected T76.11 ☑
    psychological abuse
      confirmed T74.31 ☑
      history of Z91.411
      suspected T76.31 ☑
    sexual abuse
      confirmed T74.21 ☑
      suspected T76.21 ☑
    suspected T76.91 ☑
  child
    abandonment
      confirmed T74.02 ☑
      suspected T76.02 ☑
    confirmed T74.92 ☑
    history of — see History, personal (of), abuse
    neglect
      confirmed T74.02 ☑
      history of — see History, personal (of), abuse
      suspected T76.02 ☑
    physical abuse
      confirmed T74.12 ☑
      history of — see History, personal (of), abuse
      suspected T76.12 ☑
    psychological abuse
      confirmed T74.32 ☑
      history of — see History, personal (of), abuse
      suspected T76.32 ☑
    sexual abuse
      confirmed T74.22 ☑
      history of — see History, personal (of), abuse
      suspected T76.22 ☑
    suspected T76.92 ☑
  personal history of Z91.89
Maltworker's lung J67.4
Malunion, fracture — see Fracture, by site
Mammillitis N61
  puerperal, postpartum O91.02
Mammitis — see Mastitis
Mammogram (examination) Z12.39
  routine Z12.31
Mammoplasia N62
Management (of)
  bone conduction hearing device (implanted) Z45.320
  cardiac pacemaker NEC Z45.018
  cerebrospinal fluid drainage device Z45.41
  cochlear device (implanted) Z45.321
  contraceptive Z30.9
    specified NEC Z30.8
  implanted device Z45.9
    specified NEC Z45.89
  infusion pump Z45.1
  procreative Z31.9
    male factor infertility in female Z31.81
    specified NEC Z31.89
  prosthesis (external) (see also Fitting) Z44.9
    implanted Z45.9
      specified NEC Z45.89
  renal dialysis catheter Z49.01
  vascular access device Z45.2
Mangled — see specified injury by site
Mania (monopolar) (see also Disorder, mood, manic episode)
  with psychotic symptoms F30.2
  without psychotic symptoms F30.10
    mild F30.11
    moderate F30.12
    severe F30.13
  Bell's F30.8
  chronic (recurrent) F31.89
  hysterical F44.89
  puerperal F30.8

Mania — continued
recurrent F31.89
Manic-depressive insanity, psychosis, or syndrome — see Disorder, bipolar
Mannosidosis E77.1
Mansonelliasis, mansonellosis B74.4
Manson's
disease B65.1
schistosomiasis B65.1
Manual — see condition
Maple-bark-stripper's lung (disease) J67.6
Maple-syrup-urine disease E71.0
Marable's syndrome (celiac artery compression) I77.4
Marasmus E41
due to malnutrition E41
intestinal E41
nutritional E41
senile R54
tuberculous NEC — see Tuberculosis
Marble
bones Q78.2
skin R23.8
Marburg virus disease A98.3
March
fracture — see Fracture, traumatic, stress, by site
hemoglobinuria D59.6
Marchesani (-Weill) **syndrome** Q87.0
Marchiafava (-Bignami) **syndrome or disease** G37.1
Marchiafava-Micheli syndrome D59.5
Marcus Gunn's syndrome Q07.8
Marfan's syndrome — see Syndrome, Marfan's
Marie-Bamberger disease — see Osteoarthropathy, hypertrophic, specified NEC
Marie-Charcot-Tooth neuropathic muscular atrophy G60.0
Marie's
cerebellar ataxia (late-onset) G11.2
disease or syndrome (acromegaly) E22.0
Marie-Strümpell arthritis, disease or spondylitis — see Spondylitis, ankylosing
Marion's disease (bladder neck obstruction) N32.0
Marital conflict Z63.0
Mark
port wine Q82.5
raspberry Q82.5
strawberry Q82.5
stretch L90.6
tattoo L81.8
Marker heterochromatin — see Extra, marker chromosomes
Maroteaux-Lamy syndrome (mild) (severe) E76.29
Marrow (bone)
arrest D61.9
poor function D75.89
Marseilles fever A77.1
Marsh fever — see Malaria
Marshall's (hidrotic) **ectodermal dysplasia** Q82.4
Marsh's disease (exophthalmic goiter) E05.00
with storm E05.01
Masculinization (female) **with adrenal hyperplasia** E25.9
congenital E25.0
Masculinovoblastoma D27.- ☑
Masochism (sexual) F65.51
Mason's lung J62.8
Mass
abdominal R19.00
epigastric R19.06
generalized R19.07
left lower quadrant R19.04
left upper quadrant R19.02
periumbilic R19.05
right lower quadrant R19.03
right upper quadrant R19.01
specified site NEC R19.09
breast N63
chest R22.2
cystic — see Cyst
ear H93.8- ☑
head R22.0
intra-abdominal (diffuse) (generalized) — see Mass, abdominal
kidney N28.89
liver R16.0
localized (skin) R22.9
chest R22.2
head R22.0

Mass — continued
localized — continued
limb
lower R22.4- ☑
upper R22.3- ☑
neck R22.1
trunk R22.2
lung R91.8
malignant — see Neoplasm, malignant, by site
neck R22.1
pelvic (diffuse) (generalized) — see Mass, abdominal
specified organ NEC — see Disease, by site
splenic R16.1
substernal thyroid — see Goiter
superficial (localized) R22.9
umbilical (diffuse) (generalized) R19.09
Massive — see condition
Mast cell
disease, systemic tissue D47.0
leukemia C94.3- ☑
sarcoma C96.2
tumor D47.0
malignant C96.2
Mastalgia N64.4
Masters-Allen syndrome N83.8
Mastitis (acute) (diffuse) (nonpuerperal) (subacute) N61
chronic (cystic) — see Mastopathy, cystic
cystic (Schimmelbusch's type) — see Mastopathy, cystic
fibrocystic — see Mastopathy, cystic
infective N61
newborn P39.0
interstitial, gestational or puerperal — see Mastitis, obstetric
neonatal (noninfective) P83.4
infective P39.0
obstetric (interstitial) (nonpurulent)
associated with
lactation O91.23
pregnancy O91.21- ☑
puerperium O91.22
purulent
associated with
lactation O91.13
pregnancy O91.11- ☑
puerperium O91.12
periductal — see Ectasia, mammary duct
phlegmonous — see Mastopathy, cystic
plasma cell — see Ectasia, mammary duct
Mastocytoma D47.0
malignant C96.2
Mastocytosis Q82.2
aggressive systemic C96.2
indolent systemic D47.0
malignant C96.2
systemic, associated with clonal hematopoetic non-mast-cell disease (SM-AHNMD) D47.0
Mastodynia N64.4
Mastoid — see condition
Mastoidalgia — see subcategory H92.0 ☑
Mastoiditis (coalescent) (hemorrhagic) (suppurative) H70.9- ☑
acute, subacute H70.00- ☑
complicated NEC H70.09- ☑
subperiosteal H70.01- ☑
chronic (necrotic) (recurrent) H70.1- ☑
in (due to)
infectious disease NEC B99 ☑ [H75.0-] ☑
parasitic disease NEC B89 [H75.0-] ☑
tuberculosis A18.03
petrositis — see Petrositis
postauricular fistula — see Fistula, postauricular
specified NEC H70.89- ☑
tuberculous A18.03
Mastopathy, mastopathia N64.9
chronica cystica — see Mastopathy, cystic
cystic (chronic) (diffuse) N60.1- ☑
with epithelial proliferation N60.3- ☑
diffuse cystic — see Mastopathy, cystic
estrogenic, oestrogenica N64.89
ovarian origin N64.89
Mastoplasia, mastoplastia N62
Masturbation (excessive) F98.8
Maternal care (for) — see Pregnancy (complicated by) (management affected by)
Matheiu's disease (leptospiral jaundice) A27.0

Mauclaire's disease or osteochondrosis — see Osteochondrosis, juvenile, hand, metacarpal
Maxcy's disease A75.2
Maxilla, maxillary — see condition
May (-Hegglin) **anomaly or syndrome** D72.0
McArdle (-Schmid)(-Pearson) **disease** (glycogen storage) E74.04
McCune-Albright syndrome Q78.1
McQuarrie's syndrome (idiopathic familial hypoglycemia) E16.2
Meadow's syndrome Q86.1
Measles (black) (hemorrhagic) (suppressed) B05.9
with
complications NEC B05.89
encephalitis B05.0
intestinal complications B05.4
keratitis (keratoconjunctivitis) B05.81
meningitis B05.1
otitis media B05.3
pneumonia B05.2
French — see Rubella
German — see Rubella
Liberty — see Rubella
Meatitis, urethral — see Urethritis
Meatus, meatal — see condition
Meat-wrappers' asthma J68.9
Meckel-Gruber syndrome Q61.9
Meckel's diverticulitis, diverticulum (displaced) (hypertrophic) Q43.0
malignant — see Table of Neoplasms, small intestine, malignant
Meconium
ileus, newborn P76.0
in cystic fibrosis E84.11
meaning meconium plug (without cystic fibrosis) P76.0
obstruction, newborn P76.0
due to fecaliths P76.0
in mucoviscidosis E84.11
peritonitis P78.0
plug syndrome (newborn) NEC P76.0
Median (see also condition)
arcuate ligament syndrome I77.4
bar (prostate) (vesical orifice) — see Hyperplasia, prostate
rhomboid glossitis K14.2
Mediastinal shift R93.8
Mediastinitis (acute) (chronic) J98.5
syphilitic A52.73
tuberculous A15.8
Mediastinopericarditis (see also Pericarditis)
acute I30.9
adhesive I31.0
chronic I31.8
rheumatic I09.2
Mediastinum, mediastinal — see condition
Medicine poisoning — see Table of Drugs and Chemicals, by drug, poisoning
Mediterranean
fever — see Brucellosis
familial E85.0
tick A77.1
kala-azar B55.0
leishmaniasis B55.0
tick fever A77.1
Medulla — see condition
Medullary cystic kidney Q61.5
Medullated fibers
optic (nerve) Q14.8
retina Q14.1
Medulloblastoma
desmoplastic C71.6
specified site — see Neoplasm, malignant, by site
unspecified site C71.6
Medulloepithelioma (see also Neoplasm, malignant, by site)
teratoid — see Neoplasm, malignant, by site
Medullomyoblastoma
specified site — see Neoplasm, malignant, by site
unspecified site C71.6
Meekeren-Ehlers-Danlos syndrome Q79.6
Megacolon (acquired) (functional) (not Hirschsprung's disease) (in) K59.3
Chagas' disease B57.32
congenital, congenitum (aganglionic) Q43.1
Hirschsprung's (disease) Q43.1
toxic NEC K59.3

☑ Additional Character Required -– Refer to the Tabular List for Character Selection   Subterms under main terms may continue to next column or page

Megacolon — *continued*
  toxic — *continued*
    due to Clostridium difficile A04.7
Megaesophagus (functional) K22.0
  congenital Q39.5
  in (due to) Chagas' disease B57.31
Megaiencephaly Q04.5
Megalerythema (epidemic) B08.3
Megaloappendix Q43.8
Megalocephalus, megalocephaly NEC Q75.3
Megalocornea Q15.8
  with glaucoma Q15.0
Megalocytic anemia D53.1
Megalodactylia (fingers) (thumbs) (congenital) Q74.0
  toes Q74.2
Megaloduodenum Q43.8
Megaloesophagus (functional) K22.0
  congenital Q39.5
Megalogastria (acquired) K31.89
  congenital Q40.2
Megalophthalmos Q11.3
Megalopsia H53.15
Megalosplenia — *see* Splenomegaly
Megaloureter N28.82
  congenital Q62.2
Megarectum K62.89
Megasigmoid K59.3
  congenital Q43.2
Megaureter N28.82
  congenital Q62.2
Megavitamin-B6 syndrome E67.2
Megrim — *see* Migraine
Meibomian
  cyst, infected — *see* Hordeolum
  gland — *see* condition
  sty, stye — *see* Hordeolum
Meibomitis — *see* Hordeolum
Meige-Milroy disease (chronic hereditary edema) Q82.0
Meige's syndrome Q82.0
Melalgia, nutritional E53.8
Melancholia F32.9
  climacteric (single episode) F32.8
    recurrent episode F33.9
  hypochondriac F45.29
  intermittent (single episode) F32.8
    recurrent episode F33.9
  involutional (single episode) F32.8
    recurrent episode F33.9
  menopausal (single episode) F32.8
    recurrent episode F33.9
  puerperal F32.8
  reactive (emotional stress or trauma) F32.3
  recurrent F33.9
  senile F03 ☑
  stuporous (single episode) F32.8
    recurrent episode F33.9
Melanemia R79.89
Melanoameloblastoma — *see* Neoplasm, bone, benign
Melanoblastoma — *see* Melanoma
Melanocarcinoma — *see* Melanoma
Melanocytoma, eyeball D31.4- ☑
Melanocytosis, neurocutaneous Q82.8
Melanoderma, melanodermia L81.4
Melanodontia, infantile K03.89
Melanodontoclasia K03.89
Melanoepithelioma — *see* Melanoma
Melanoma (malignant) C43.9
  acral lentiginous, malignant — *see* Melanoma, skin, by site
  amelanotic — *see* Melanoma, skin, by site
  balloon cell — *see* Melanoma, skin, by site
  benign — *see* Nevus
  desmoplastic, malignant — *see* Melanoma, skin, by site
  epithelioid cell — *see* Melanoma, skin, by site
    with spindle cell, mixed — *see* Melanoma, skin, by site
  in
    giant pigmented nevus — *see* Melanoma, skin, by site
    Hutchinson's melanotic freckle — *see* Melanoma, skin, by site
    junctional nevus — *see* Melanoma, skin, by site
    precancerous melanosis — *see* Melanoma, skin, by site
  in situ D03.9
    abdominal wall D03.59

Melanoma — *continued*
  in situ — *continued*
    ala nasi D03.39
    ankle D03.7- ☑
    anus, anal (margin) (skin) D03.51
    arm D03.6- ☑
    auditory canal D03.2- ☑
    auricle (ear) D03.2- ☑
    auricular canal (external) D03.2- ☑
    axilla, axillary fold D03.59
    back D03.59
    breast D03.52
    brow D03.39
    buttock D03.59
    canthus (eye) D03.1- ☑
    cheek (external) D03.39
    chest wall D03.59
    chin D03.39
    choroid D03.8
    conjunctiva D03.8
    ear (external) D03.2- ☑
    external meatus (ear) D03.2- ☑
    eye D03.8
    eyebrow D03.39
    eyelid (lower) (upper) D03.1- ☑
    face D03.30
      specified NEC D03.39
    female genital organ (external) NEC D03.8
    finger D03.6- ☑
    flank D03.59
    foot D03.7- ☑
    forearm D03.6- ☑
    forehead D03.39
    foreskin D03.8
    gluteal region D03.59
    groin D03.59
    hand D03.6- ☑
    heel D03.7- ☑
    helix D03.2- ☑
    hip D03.7- ☑
    interscapular region D03.59
    iris D03.8
    jaw D03.39
    knee D03.7- ☑
    labium (majus) (minus) D03.8
    lacrimal gland D03.8
    leg D03.7- ☑
    lip (lower) (upper) D03.0
    lower limb NEC D03.7- ☑
    male genital organ (external) NEC D03.8
    nail D03.9
      finger D03.6- ☑
      toe D03.7- ☑
    neck D03.4
    nose (external) D03.39
    orbit D03.8
    penis D03.8
    perianal skin D03.51
    perineum D03.51
    pinna D03.2- ☑
    popliteal fossa or space D03.7- ☑
    prepuce D03.8
    pudendum D03.8
    retina D03.8
    retrobulbar D03.8
    scalp D03.4
    scrotum D03.8
    shoulder D03.6- ☑
    specified site NEC D03.8
    submammary fold D03.52
    temple D03.39
    thigh D03.7- ☑
    toe D03.7- ☑
    trunk NEC D03.59
    umbilicus D03.59
    upper limb NEC D03.6- ☑
    vulva D03.8
  juvenile — *see* Nevus
  malignant, of soft parts except skin — *see* Neoplasm, connective tissue, malignant
  metastatic
    breast C79.81
    genital organ C79.82
    specified site NEC C79.89
  neurotropic, malignant — *see* Melanoma, skin, by site
  nodular — *see* Melanoma, skin, by site
  regressing, malignant — *see* Melanoma, skin, by site

Melanoma — *continued*
  skin C43.9
    abdominal wall C43.59
    ala nasi C43.31
    ankle C43.7- ☑
    anus, anal (skin) C43.51
    arm C43.6- ☑
    auditory canal (external) C43.2- ☑
    auricle (ear) C43.2- ☑
    auricular canal (external) C43.2- ☑
    axilla, axillary fold C43.59
    back C43.59
    breast (female) (male) C43.52
    brow C43.39
    buttock C43.59
    canthus (eye) C43.1- ☑
    cheek (external) C43.39
    chest wall C43.59
    chin C43.39
    ear (external) C43.2- ☑
    elbow C43.6- ☑
    external meatus (ear) C43.2- ☑
    eyebrow C43.39
    eyelid (lower) (upper) C43.1- ☑
    face C43.30
      specified NEC C43.39
    female genital organ (external) NEC C51.9
    finger C43.6- ☑
    flank C43.59
    foot C43.7- ☑
    forearm C43.6- ☑
    forehead C43.39
    foreskin C60.0
    glabella C43.39
    gluteal region C43.59
    groin C43.59
    hand C43.6- ☑
    heel C43.7- ☑
    helix C43.2- ☑
    hip C43.7- ☑
    interscapular region C43.59
    jaw (external) C43.39
    knee C43.7- ☑
    labium C51.9
      majus C51.0
      minus C51.1
    leg C43.7- ☑
    lip (lower) (upper) C43.0
    lower limb NEC C43.7- ☑
    male genital organ (external) NEC C63.9
    nail
      finger C43.6- ☑
      toe C43.7- ☑
    nasolabial groove C43.39
    nates C43.59
    neck C43.4
    nose (external) C43.31
    overlapping site C43.8
    palpebra C43.1- ☑
    penis C60.9
    perianal skin C43.51
    perineum C43.51
    pinna C43.2- ☑
    popliteal fossa or space C43.7- ☑
    prepuce C60.0
    pudendum C51.9
    scalp C43.4
    scrotum C63.2
    shoulder C43.6- ☑
    skin NEC C43.9
    submammary fold C43.52
    temple C43.39
    thigh C43.7- ☑
    toe C43.7- ☑
    trunk NEC C43.59
    umbilicus C43.59
    upper limb NEC C43.6- ☑
    vulva C51.9
      overlapping sites C51.8
  spindle cell
    with epithelioid, mixed — *see* Melanoma, skin, by site
    type A C69.4- ☑
    type B C69.4- ☑
  superficial spreading — *see* Melanoma, skin, by site
Melanosarcoma (*see also* Melanoma)
  epithelioid cell — *see* Melanoma

Melanosis L81.4
addisonian E27.1
tuberculous A18.7
adrenal E27.1
colon K63.89
conjunctiva — *see* Pigmentation, conjunctiva
congenital Q13.89
cornea (presenile) (senile) (*see also* Pigmentation, cornea)
congenital Q13.4
eye NEC H57.8
congenital Q15.8
lenticularis progressiva Q82.1
liver K76.89
precancerous (*see also* Melanoma, in situ)
malignant melanoma in — *see* Melanoma
Riehl's L81.4
sclera H15.89
congenital Q13.89
suprarenal E27.1
tar L81.4
toxic L81.4
Melanuria R82.99
MELAS syndrome E88.41
Melasma L81.1
adrenal (gland) E27.1
suprarenal (gland) E27.1
Melena K92.1
with ulcer — *code by* site under Ulcer, with hemorrhage K27.4
due to swallowed maternal blood P78.2
newborn, neonatal P54.1
due to swallowed maternal blood P78.2
Meleney's
gangrene (cutaneous) — *see* Ulcer, skin
ulcer (chronic undermining) — *see* Ulcer, skin
Melioidosis A24.9
acute A24.1
chronic A24.2
fulminating A24.1
pneumonia A24.1
pulmonary (chronic) A24.2
acute A24.1
subacute A24.2
sepsis A24.1
specified NEC A24.3
subacute A24.2
Melitensis, febris A23.0
Melkersson (-Rosenthal) **syndrome** G51.2
Mellitus, diabetes — *see* Diabetes
Melorheostosis (bone) — *see* Disorder, bone, density and structure, specified NEC
Meloschisis Q18.4
Melotia Q17.4
Membrana
capsularis lentis posterior Q13.89
epipapillaris Q14.2
Membranacea placenta O43.19- ☑
Membranaceous uterus N85.8
Membrane(s), membranous (*see also* condition)
cyclitic — *see* Membrane, pupillary
folds, congenital — *see* Web
Jackson's Q43.3
over face of newborn P28.9
premature rupture — *see* Rupture, membranes, premature
pupillary H21.4- ☑
persistent Q13.89
retained (with hemorrhage) (complicating delivery) O72.2
without hemorrhage O73.1
secondary cataract — *see* Cataract, secondary
unruptured (causing asphyxia) — *see* Asphyxia, newborn
vitreous — *see* Opacity, vitreous, membranes and strands
Membranitis — *see* Chorioamnionitis
Memory disturbance, lack or loss (*see also* Amnesia)
mild, following organic brain damage F06.8
Menadione deficiency E56.1
Menarche
delayed E30.0
precocious E30.1
Mendacity, pathologic F60.2
Mendelson's syndrome (due to anesthesia) J95.4
in labor and delivery O74.0
in pregnancy O29.01- ☑

Mendelson's syndrome — *continued*
obstetric O74.0
postpartum, puerperal O89.01
Ménétrier's disease or syndrome K29.60
with bleeding K29.61
Ménière's disease, syndrome or vertigo H81.0- ☑
Meninges, meningeal — *see* condition
Meningioma (*see also* Neoplasm, meninges, benign)
angioblastic — *see* Neoplasm, meninges, benign
angiomatous — *see* Neoplasm, meninges, benign
endotheliomatous — *see* Neoplasm, meninges, benign
fibroblastic — *see* Neoplasm, meninges, benign
fibrous — *see* Neoplasm, meninges, benign
hemangioblastic — *see* Neoplasm, meninges, benign
hemangiopericytic — *see* Neoplasm, meninges, benign
malignant — *see* Neoplasm, meninges, malignant
meningiothelial — *see* Neoplasm, meninges, benign
meningotheliomatous — *see* Neoplasm, meninges, benign
mixed — *see* Neoplasm, meninges, benign
multiple — *see* Neoplasm, meninges, uncertain behavior
papillary — *see* Neoplasm, meninges, uncertain behavior
psammomatous — *see* Neoplasm, meninges, benign
syncytial — *see* Neoplasm, meninges, benign
transitional — *see* Neoplasm, meninges, benign
Meningiomatosis (diffuse) — *see* Neoplasm, meninges, uncertain behavior
Meningism — *see* Meningismus
Meningismus (infectional) (pneumococcal) R29.1
due to serum or vaccine R29.1
influenzal — *see* Influenza, with, manifestations NEC
Meningitis (basal) (basic) (brain) (cerebral) (cervical) (congestive) (diffuse) (hemorrhagic) (infantile) (membranous) (metastatic) (nonspecific) (pontine) (progressive) (simple) (spinal) (subacute) (sympathetic) (toxic) G03.9
abacterial G03.0
actinomycotic A42.81
adenoviral A87.1
arbovirus A87.8
aseptic (acute) G03.0
bacterial G00.9
Escherichia coli (E. coli) G00.8
Friedländer (bacillus) G00.8
gram-negative G00.9
H. influenzae G00.0
Klebsiella G00.8
pneumococcal G00.1
specified organism NEC G00.8
staphylococcal G00.3
streptococcal (acute) G00.2
benign recurrent (Mollaret) G03.2
candidal B37.5
caseous (tuberculous) A17.0
cerebrospinal A39.0
chronic NEC G03.1
clear cerebrospinal fluid NEC G03.0
coxsackievirus A87.0
cryptococcal B45.1
diplococcal (gram positive) A39.0
echovirus A87.0
enteroviral A87.0
eosinophilic B83.2
epidemic NEC A39.0
Escherichia coli (E. coli) G00.8
fibrinopurulent G00.9
specified organism NEC G00.8
Friedländer (bacillus) G00.8
gonococcal A54.81
gram-negative cocci G00.9
gram-positive cocci G00.9
H. influenzae G00.0
Haemophilus (influenzae) G00.0
in (due to)
adenovirus A87.1
African trypanosomiasis B56.9 [G02]
anthrax A22.8
bacterial disease NEC A48.8 [G01]
Chagas' disease (chronic) B57.41
chickenpox B01.0
coccidioidomycosis B38.4
Diplococcus pneumoniae G00.1
enterovirus A87.0
herpes (simplex) virus B00.3
zoster B02.1

Meningitis — *continued*
in — *continued*
infectious mononucleosis B27.92
leptospirosis A27.81
Listeria monocytogenes A32.11
Lyme disease A69.21
measles B05.1
mumps (virus) B26.1
neurosyphilis (late) A52.13
parasitic disease NEC B89 [G02]
poliovirus A80.9 [G02]
preventive immunization, inoculation or vaccination G03.8
rubella B06.02
Salmonella infection A02.21
specified cause NEC G03.8
typhoid fever A01.01
varicella B01.0
viral disease NEC A87.8
whooping cough A37.90
zoster B02.1
infectious G00.9
influenzal (H. influenzae) G00.0
Klebsiella G00.8
leptospiral (aseptic) A27.81
lymphocytic (acute) (benign) (serous) A87.2
meningococcal A39.0
Mima polymorpha G00.8
Mollaret (benign recurrent) G03.2
monilial B37.5
mycotic NEC B49 [G02]
Neisseria A39.0
nonbacterial G03.0
nonpyogenic NEC G03.0
ossificans G96.19
pneumococcal G00.1
poliovirus A80.9 [G02]
postmeasles B05.1
purulent G00.9
specified organism NEC G00.8
pyogenic G00.9
specified organism NEC G00.8
Salmonella (arizonae) (Cholerae-Suis) (enteritidis) (typhimurium) A02.21
septic G00.9
specified organism NEC G00.8
serosa circumscripta NEC G03.0
serous NEC G93.2
specified organism NEC G00.8
sporotrichosis B42.81
staphylococcal G00.3
sterile G03.0
streptococcal (acute) G00.2
suppurative G00.9
specified organism NEC G00.8
syphilitic (late) (tertiary) A52.13
acute A51.41
congenital A50.41
secondary A51.41
Torula histolytica (cryptococcal) B45.1
traumatic (complication of injury) T79.8 ☑
tuberculous A17.0
typhoid A01.01
viral NEC A87.9
Yersinia pestis A20.3
Meningocele (spinal) (*see also* Spina bifida)
with hydrocephalus — *see* Spina bifida, by site, with hydrocephalus
acquired (traumatic) G96.19
cerebral — *see* Encephalocele
Meningocerebritis — *see* Meningoencephalitis
Meningococcemia A39.4
acute A39.2
chronic A39.3
Meningococcus, meningococcal (*see also* condition) A39.9
adrenalitis, hemorrhagic A39.1
carrier (suspected) of Z22.31
meningitis (cerebrospinal) A39.0
Meningoencephalitis (*see also* Encephalitis) G04.90
acute NEC (*see also* Encephalitis, viral) A86
bacterial NEC G04.2
California A83.5
diphasic A84.1
eosinophilic B83.2
epidemic A39.81
herpesviral, herpetic B00.4
due to herpesvirus 6 B10.01

☑ Additional Character Required — Refer to the Tabular List for Character Selection   ▽ Subterms under main terms may continue to next column or page

Meningoencephalitis — *continued*
　herpesviral, herpetic — *continued*
　　due to herpesvirus 7 B10.09
　　specified NEC B10.09
　in (due to)
　　blastomycosis NEC B40.81
　　diseases classified elsewhere G05.3
　　free-living amebae B60.2
　　H. influenzae G00.0
　　Hemophilus influenzae (H .influenzae) G04.2
　　herpes B00.4
　　　due to herpesvirus 6 B10.01
　　　due to herpesvirus 7 B10.09
　　　specified NEC B10.09
　　Lyme disease A69.22
　　mercury — *see* subcategory T56.1 ☑
　　mumps B26.2
　　Naegleria (amebae) (organisms) (fowleri) B60.2
　　Parastrongylus cantonensis B83.2
　　toxoplasmosis (acquired) B58.2
　　　congenital P37.1
　infectious (acute) (viral) A86
　influenzal (H. influenzae) G04.2
　Listeria monocytogenes A32.12
　lymphocytic (serous) A87.2
　mumps B26.2
　parasitic NEC B89 [G05.3]
　pneumococcal G00.1
　primary amebic B60.2
　specific (syphilitic) A52.14
　specified organism NEC G04.81
　staphylococcal G04.2
　streptococcal G04.2
　syphilitic A52.14
　toxic NEC G92
　　due to mercury — *see* subcategory T56.1 ☑
　tuberculous A17.82
　virus NEC A86
Meningoencephalocele (*see also* Encephalocele)
　syphilitic A52.19
　　congenital A50.49
Meningoencephalomyelitis (*see also* Meningoencephalitis)
　acute NEC (viral) A86
　　disseminated G04.00
　　　postimmunization or postvaccination G04.02
　　　postinfectious G04.01
　　due to
　　　actinomycosis A42.82
　　　Torula B45.1
　　　Toxoplasma or toxoplasmosis (acquired) B58.2
　　　　congenital P37.1
　　postimmunization or postvaccination G04.02
Meningoencephalomyelopathy G96.9
Meningoencephalopathy G96.9
Meningomyelitis (*see also* Meningoencephalitis)
　bacterial NEC G04.2
　blastomycotic NEC B40.81
　cryptococcal B45.1
　in diseases classified elsewhere G05.4
　meningococcal A39.81
　syphilitic A52.14
　tuberculous A17.82
Meningomyelocele (*see also* Spina bifida)
　syphilitic A52.19
Meningomyeloneuritis — *see* Meningoencephalitis
Meningoradiculitis — *see* Meningitis
Meningovascular — *see* condition
Menkes' disease or syndrome E83.09
　meaning maple-syrup-urine disease E71.0
Menometrorrhagia N92.1
Menopause, menopausal (asymptomatic) (state) Z78.0
　arthritis (any site) NEC — *see* Arthritis, specified form NEC
　bleeding N92.4
　depression (single episode) F32.8
　　agitated (single episode) F32.2
　　　recurrent episode F33.9
　　psychotic (single episode) F32.8
　　　recurrent episode F33.9
　　recurrent episode F33.9
　melancholia (single episode) F32.8
　　recurrent episode F33.9
　paranoid state F22
　premature E28.319
　　asymptomatic E28.319
　　　postirradiation E89.40
　　　postsurgical E89.40

Menopause, menopausal — *continued*
　premature — *continued*
　　symptomatic E28.310
　　　postirradiation E89.41
　　　postsurgical E89.41
　psychosis NEC F28
　symptomatic N95.1
　toxic polyarthritis NEC — *see* Arthritis, specified form
Menorrhagia (primary) N92.0
　climacteric N92.4
　　menopausal N92.4
　menopausal N92.4
　postclimacteric N95.0
　postmenopausal N95.0
　preclimacteric or premenopausal N92.4
　pubertal (menses retained) N92.2
Menostaxis N92.0
Menses, retention N94.89
Menstrual — *see* Menstruation
Menstruation
　absent — *see* Amenorrhea
　anovulatory N97.0
　cycle, irregular N92.6
　delayed N91.0
　disorder N93.9
　　psychogenic F45.8
　during pregnancy O20.8
　excessive (with regular cycle) N92.0
　　with irregular cycle N92.1
　　at puberty N92.2
　frequent N92.0
　infrequent — *see* Oligomenorrhea
　irregular N92.6
　　specified NEC N92.5
　latent N92.5
　membranous N92.5
　painful (*see also* Dysmenorrhea) N94.6
　　primary N94.4
　　psychogenic F45.8
　　secondary N94.5
　passage of clots N92.0
　precocious E30.1
　protracted N92.5
　rare — *see* Oligomenorrhea
　retained N94.89
　retrograde N92.5
　scanty — *see* Oligomenorrhea
　suppression N94.89
　vicarious (nasal) N94.89
Mental (*see also* condition)
　deficiency — *see* Disability, intellectual
　deterioration — *see* Psychosis
　disorder — *see* Disorder, mental
　exhaustion F48.8
　insufficiency (congenital) — *see* Disability, intellectual
　observation without need for further medical care Z03.89
　retardation — *see* Disability, intellectual
　subnormality — *see* Disability, intellectuall
　upset — *see* Disorder, mental
Meralgia paresthetica G57.1- ☑
Mercurial — *see* condition
Mercurialism — *see* subcategory T56.1 ☑
Merkel cell tumor — *see* Carcinoma, Merkel cell
Merocele — *see* Hernia, femoral
Meromelia
　lower limb — *see* Defect, reduction, lower limb
　　intercalary
　　　femur — *see* Defect, reduction, lower limb, specified type NEC
　　　　tibiofibular (complete) (incomplete) — *see* Defect, reduction, lower limb
　upper limb — *see* Defect, reduction, upper limb
　　intercalary, humeral, radioulnar — *see* Agenesis, arm, with hand present
MERRF syndrome (myoclonic epilepsy associated with ragged-red fiber) E88.42
Merzbacher-Pelizaeus disease E75.29
Mesaortitis — *see* Aortitis
Mesarteritis — *see* Arteritis
Mesencephalitis — *see* Encephalitis
Mesenchymoma (*see also* Neoplasm, connective tissue, uncertain behavior)
　benign — *see* Neoplasm, connective tissue, benign
　malignant — *see* Neoplasm, connective tissue, malignant

Mesenteritis
　retractile K65.4
　sclerosing K65.4
Mesentery, mesenteric — *see* condition
Mesiodens, mesiodentes K00.1
Mesio-occlusion M26.213
Mesocolon — *see* condition
Mesonephroma (malignant) — *see* Neoplasm, malignant, by site
　benign — *see* Neoplasm, benign, by site
Mesophlebitis — *see* Phlebitis
Mesostromal dysgenesia Q13.89
Mesothelioma (malignant) C45.9
　benign
　　mesentery D19.1
　　mesocolon D19.1
　　omentum D19.1
　　peritoneum D19.1
　　pleura D19.0
　　specified site NEC D19.7
　　unspecified site D19.9
　biphasic C45.9
　　benign
　　　mesentery D19.1
　　　mesocolon D19.1
　　　omentum D19.1
　　　peritoneum D19.1
　　　pleura D19.0
　　　specified site NEC D19.7
　　　unspecified site D19.9
　cystic D48.4
　epithelioid C45.9
　　benign
　　　mesentery D19.1
　　　mesocolon D19.1
　　　omentum D19.1
　　　peritoneum D19.1
　　　pleura D19.0
　　　specified site NEC D19.7
　　　unspecified site D19.9
　fibrous C45.9
　　benign
　　　mesentery D19.1
　　　mesocolon D19.1
　　　omentum D19.1
　　　peritoneum D19.1
　　　pleura D19.0
　　　specified site NEC D19.7
　　　unspecified site D19.9
　site classification
　　liver C45.7
　　lung C45.7
　　mediastinum C45.7
　　mesentery C45.1
　　mesocolon C45.1
　　omentum C45.1
　　pericardium C45.2
　　peritoneum C45.1
　　pleura C45.0
　　　parietal C45.0
　　retroperitoneum C45.7
　　specified site NEC C45.7
　　unspecified C45.9
Metabolic syndrome E88.81
Metagonimiasis B66.8
Metagonimus infestation (intestine) B66.8
Metal
　pigmentation L81.8
　polisher's disease J62.8
Metamorphopsia H53.15
Metaplasia
　apocrine (breast) — *see* Dysplasia, mammary, specified type NEC
　cervix (squamous) — *see* Dysplasia, cervix
　endometrium (squamous) (uterus) N85.8
　esophagus
　kidney (pelvis) (squamous) N28.89
　myelogenous D73.1
　myeloid (agnogenic) (megakaryocytic) D73.1
　spleen D73.1
　squamous cell, bladder N32.89
Metastasis, metastatic
　abscess — *see* Abscess
　calcification E83.59
　cancer
　　from specified site — *see* Neoplasm, malignant, by site

Index

Meningoencephalitis — Metastasis, metastatic

Metastasis, metastatic — *continued*
  cancer — *continued*
    to specified site — *see* Neoplasm, secondary, by site
    deposits (in) — *see* Neoplasm, secondary, by site
    disease (*see also* Neoplasm, secondary, by site) C79.9
    spread (to) — *see* Neoplasm, secondary, by site
Metastrongyliasis B83.8
Metatarsalgia M77.4- ☑
  anterior G57.6- ☑
  Morton's G57.6- ☑
Metatarsus, metatarsal (*see also* condition)
  valgus (abductus), congenital Q66.6
  varus (adductus) (congenital) Q66.2
Methadone use F11.20
Methemoglobinemia D74.9
  acquired (with sulfhemoglobinemia) D74.8
  congenital D74.0
  enzymatic (congenital) D74.0
  Hb M disease D74.0
  hereditary D74.0
  toxic D74.8
Methemoglobinuria — *see* Hemoglobinuria
Methioninemia E72.19
Methylmalonic acidemia E71.120
Metritis (catarrhal) (hemorrhagic) (septic) (suppurative) (*see also* Endometritis)
  cervical — *see* Cervicitis
Metropathia hemorrhagica N93.8
Metroperitonitis — *see* Peritonitis, pelvic, female
Metrorrhagia N92.1
  climacteric N92.4
  menopausal N92.4
  postpartum NEC (atonic) (following delivery of placenta) O72.1
    delayed or secondary O72.2
  preclimacteric or premenopausal N92.4
  psychogenic F45.8
Metrorrhexis — *see* Rupture, uterus
Metrosalpingitis N70.91
Metrostaxis N93.8
Metrovaginitis — *see* Endometritis
Meyer-Schwickerath and Weyers syndrome Q87.0
Meynert's amentia (nonalcoholic) F04
  alcoholic F10.96
    with dependence F10.26
Mibelli's disease (porokeratosis) Q82.8
Mice, joint — *see* Loose, body, joint
  knee M23.4- ☑
Micrencephalon, micrencephaly Q02
Microalbuminuria R80.9
Microaneurysm, retinal (*see also* Disorder, retina, microaneurysms)
  diabetic — *see* E08-E13 with .31
Microangiopathy (peripheral) I73.9
  thrombotic M31.1
Microcalcifications, breast R92.0
Microcephalus, microcephalic, microcephaly Q02
  due to toxoplasmosis (congenital) P37.1
Microcheilia Q18.7
Microcolon (congenital) Q43.8
Microcornea (congenital) Q13.4
Microcytic — *see* condition
Microdeletions NEC Q93.88
Microdontia K00.2
Microdrepanocytosis D57.40
  with crisis (vasoocclusive pain) D57.419
    with
      acute chest syndrome D57.411
      splenic sequestration D57.412
Microembolism
  atherothrombotic — *see* Atheroembolism
  retinal — *see* Occlusion, artery, retina
Microencephalon Q02
Microfilaria streptocerca infestation — *see* Onchocerciasis
Microgastria (congenital) Q40.2
Microgenia M26.06
Microgenitalia, congenital
  female Q52.8
  male Q55.8
Microglioma — *see* Lymphoma, non-Hodgkin, specified NEC
Microglossia (congenital) Q38.3
Micrognathia, micrognathism (congenital) (mandibular) (maxillary) M26.09
Microgyria (congenital) Q04.3

Microinfarct of heart — *see* Insufficiency, coronary
Microlentia (congenital) Q12.8
Microlithiasis, alveolar, pulmonary J84.02
Micromastia N64.82
Micromyelia (congenital) Q06.8
Micropenis Q55.62
Microphakia (congenital) Q12.8
Microphthalmos, microphthalmia (congenital) Q11.2
  due to toxoplasmosis P37.1
Micropsia H53.15
Microscopic polyangiitis (polyarteritis) M31.7
Microsporidiosis B60.8
  intestinal A07.8
Microsporon furfur infestation B36.0
Microsporosis (*see also* Dermatophytosis)
  nigra B36.1
Microstomia (congenital) Q18.5
Microtia (congenital) (external ear) Q17.2
Microtropia H50.40
Microvillus inclusion disease (MVD) (MVID) Q43.8
Micturition
  disorder NEC R39.19
    psychogenic F45.8
  frequency R35.0
    psychogenic F45.8
  hesitancy R39.11
  incomplete emptying R39.14
  nocturnal R35.1
  painful R30.9
    dysuria R30.0
    psychogenic F45.8
    tenesmus R30.1
  poor stream R39.12
  split stream R39.13
  straining R39.16
  urgency R39.15
Mid plane — *see* condition
Middle
  ear — *see* condition
  lobe (right) syndrome J98.19
Miescher's elastoma L87.2
Mietens' syndrome Q87.2
Migraine (idiopathic) G43.909
  with aura (acute-onset) (prolonged) (typical) (without headache) G43.109
    with refractory migraine G43.119
      with status migrainosus G43.111
      without status migrainosus G43.119
    without mention of refractory migraine G43.109
      with status migrainosus G43.101
      without status migrainosus G43.109
    intractable G43.119
      with status migrainosus G43.111
      without status migrainosus G43.119
    not intractable G43.109
      with status migrainosus G43.101
      without status migrainosus G43.109
    persistent G43.509
      with cerebral infarction G43.609
        with refractory migraine G43.619
          with status migrainosus G43.611
          without status migrainosus G43.619
        without refractory migraine G43.609
          with status migrainosus G43.601
          without status migrainosus G43.609
        intractable G43.619
          with status migrainosus G43.611
          without status migrainosus G43.619
        not intractable G43.609
          with status migrainosus G43.601
          without status migrainosus G43.609
      without cerebral infarction G43.509
        with refractory migraine G43.519
          with status migrainosus G43.511
          without status migrainosus G43.519
        without refractory migraine G43.509
          with status migrainosus G43.501
          without status migrainosus G43.509
        intractable G43.519
          with status migrainosus G43.511
          without status migrainosus G43.519
        not intractable G43.509
          with status migrainosus G43.501
          without status migrainosus G43.509
    with refractory migraine G43.919
      with status migrainosus G43.911
      without status migrainosus G43.919
  without aura G43.009

Migraine — *continued*
  without aura — *continued*
    with refractory migraine G43.019
      with status migrainosus G43.011
      without status migrainosus G43.019
    without mention of refractory migraine G43.009
      with status migrainosus G43.001
      without status migrainosus G43.009
  chronic G43.709
    with refractory migraine G43.719
      with status migrainosus G43.711
      without status migrainosus G43.719
    without refractory migraine G43.709
      with status migrainosus G43.701
      without status migrainosus G43.709
    intractable
      with status migrainosus G43.711
      without status migrainosus G43.719
    not intractable
      with status migrainosus G43.701
      without status migrainosus G43.709
  intractable
    with status migrainosus G43.011
    without status migrainosus G43.019
  not intractable
    with status migrainosus G43.001
    without status migrainosus G43.009
  without refractory migraine G43.909
    with status migrainosus G43.901
    without status migrainosus G43.919
  abdominal G43.D0 (*following* G43.7)
    with refractory migraine G43.D1 (*following* G43.7)
    without refractory migraine G43.D0 (*following* G43.7)
    intractable G43.D1 (*following* G43.7)
    not intractable G43.D0 (*following* G43.7)
  basilar — *see* Migraine, with aura
  classical — *see* Migraine, with aura
  common — *see* Migraine, without aura
  complicated G43.109
  equivalents — *see* Migraine, with aura
  familiar — *see* Migraine, hemiplegic
  hemiplegic G43.409
    with refractory migraine G43.419
      with status migrainosus G43.411
      without status migrainosus G43.419
    without refractory migraine G43.409
      with status migrainosus G43.401
      without status migrainosus G43.409
    intractable G43.419
      with status migrainosus G43.411
      without status migrainosus G43.419
    not intractable G43.409
      with status migrainosus G43.401
      without status migrainosus G43.409
  intractable G43.919
    with status migrainosus G43.911
    without status migrainosus G43.919
  menstrual G43.829
    with refractory migraine G43.839
      with status migrainosus G43.831
      without status migrainosus G43.839
    without refractory migraine G43.829
      with status migrainosus G43.821
      without status migrainosus G43.829
    intractable G43.839
      with status migrainosus G43.831
      without status migrainosus G43.839
    not intractable G43.829
      with status migrainosus G43.821
      without status migrainosus G43.829
  menstrually related — *see* Migraine, menstrual
  not intractable G43.909
    with status migrainosus G43.901
    without status migrainosus G43.919
  ophthalmoplegic G43.B0 (*following* G43.7)
    with refractory migraine G43.B1 (*following* G43.7)
    without refractory migraine G43.B0 (*following* G43.7)
    intractable G43.B1 (*following* G43.7)
    not intractable G43.B0 (*following* G43.7)
  persistent aura (with, without) cerebral infarction — *see* Migraine, with aura, persistent
  preceded or accompanied by transient focal neurological phenomena — *see* Migraine, with aura
  pre-menstrual — *see* Migraine, menstrual
  pure menstrual — *see* Migraine, menstrual
  retinal — *see* Migraine, with aura

☑ **Additional Character Required** — Refer to the Tabular List for Character Selection   ▽ Subterms under main terms may continue to next column or page

Migraine — *continued*
  specified NEC G43.809
    intractable G43.819
      with status migrainosus G43.811
      without status migrainosus G43.819
    not intractable G43.809
      with status migrainosus G43.801
      without status migrainosus G43.809
  sporadic — *see* Migraine, hemiplegic
  transformed — *see* Migraine, without aura, chronic
  triggered seizures — *see* Migraine, with aura
Migrant, social Z59.0
Migration, anxiety concerning Z60.3
Migratory, migrating (*see also* condition)
  person Z59.0
  testis Q55.29
Mikity-Wilson disease or syndrome P27.0
Mikulicz' disease or syndrome K11.8
Miliaria L74.3
  alba L74.1
  apocrine L75.2
  crystallina L74.1
  profunda L74.2
  rubra L74.0
  tropicalis L74.2
Miliary — *see* condition
Milium L72.0
  colloid L57.8
Milk
  crust L21.0
  excessive secretion O92.6
  poisoning — *see* Poisoning, food, noxious
  retention O92.79
  sickness — *see* Poisoning, food, noxious
  spots I31.0
Milk-alkali disease or syndrome E83.52
Milk-leg (deep vessels) (nonpuerperal) — *see* Embolism, vein, lower extremity
  complicating pregnancy O22.3- ☑
  puerperal, postpartum, childbirth O87.1
Milkman's disease or syndrome M83.8
Milky urine — *see* Chyluria
Millard-Gubler (-Foville) **paralysis or syndrome** G46.3
Millar's asthma J38.5
Miller Fisher syndrome G61.0
Mills' disease — *see* Hemiplegia
Millstone maker's pneumoconiosis J62.8
Milroy's disease (chronic hereditary edema) Q82.0
Minamata disease T26.1-
Miners' asthma or lung J60
Minkowski-Chauffard syndrome — *see* Spherocytosis
Minor — *see* condition
Minor's disease (hematomyelia) G95.19
Minot's disease (hemorrhagic disease), newborn P53
Minot-von Willebrand-Jurgens disease or syndrome (angiohemophilia) D68.0
Minus (and plus) **hand** (intrinsic) — *see* Deformity, limb, specified type NEC, forearm
Miosis (pupil) H57.03
Mirizzi's syndrome (hepatic duct stenosis) K83.1
Mirror writing F81.0
Misadventure (of) (prophylactic) (therapeutic) (*see also* Complications) T88.9 ☑
  administration of insulin (by accident) — *see* subcategory T38.3 ☑
  infusion — *see* Complications, infusion
  local applications (of fomentations, plasters, etc.) T88.9 ☑
    burn or scald — *see* Burn
    specified NEC T88.8 ☑
  medical care (early) (late) T88.9 ☑
    adverse effect of drugs or chemicals — *see* Table of Drugs and Chemicals
    burn or scald — *see* Burn
    specified NEC T88.8 ☑
  specified NEC T88.8 ☑
  surgical procedure (early) (late) — *see* Complications, surgical procedure
  transfusion — *see* Complications, transfusion
  vaccination or other immunological procedure — *see* Complications, vaccination
Miscarriage O03.9
Misdirection, aqueous H40.83- ☑
Misperception, sleep state F51.02
Misplaced, misplacement
  ear Q17.4
  kidney (acquired) N28.89

Misplaced, misplacement — *continued*
  kidney — *continued*
    congenital Q63.2
  organ or site, congenital NEC — *see* Malposition, congenital
Missed
  abortion O02.1
  delivery O36.4
Missing — *see* Absence
Misuse of drugs F19.99
Mitchell's disease (erythromelalgia) I73.81
Mite(s) (infestation) B88.9
  diarrhea B88.0
  grain (itch) B88.0
  hair follicle (itch) B88.0
  in sputum B88.0
Mitral — *see* condition
Mittelschmerz N94.0
Mixed — *see* condition
MNGIE (Mitochondrial Neurogastrointestinal Encephalopathy) **syndrome** E88.49
Mobile, mobility
  cecum Q43.3
  excessive — *see* Hypermobility
  gallbladder, congenital Q44.1
  kidney N28.89
  organ or site, congenital NEC — *see* Malposition, congenital
Mobitz heart block (atrioventricular) I44.1
Moebius, Möbius
  disease (ophthalmoplegic migraine) — *see* Migraine, ophthalmoplegic
  syndrome Q87.0
    congenital oculofacial paralysis (with other anomalies) Q87.0
    ophthalmoplegic migraine — *see* Migraine, ophthalmoplegic
Moeller's glossitis K14.0
Mohr's syndrome (Types I and II) Q87.0
Mola destruens D39.2
Molar pregnancy O02.0
Molarization of premolars K00.2
Molding, head (during birth) — *omit code*
Mole (pigmented) (*see also* Nevus)
  blood O02.0
  Breus' O02.0
  cancerous — *see* Melanoma
  carneous O02.0
  destructive D39.2
  fleshy O02.0
  hydatid, hydatidiform (benign) (complicating pregnancy) (delivered) (undelivered) O01.9
    classical O01.0
    complete O01.0
    incomplete O01.1
    invasive D39.2
    malignant D39.2
    partial O01.1
  intrauterine O02.0
  invasive (hydatidiform) D39.2
  malignant
    meaning
      malignant hydatidiform mole D39.2
      melanoma — *see* Melanoma
  nonhydatidiform O02.0
  nonpigmented — *see* Nevus
  pregnancy NEC O02.0
  skin — *see* Nevus
  tubal O00.1
  vesicular — *see* Mole, hydatidiform
Molimen, molimina (menstrual) N94.3
Molluscum contagiosum (epitheliale) B08.1
Mönckeberg's arteriosclerosis, disease, or sclerosis — *see* Arteriosclerosis, extremities
Mondini's malformation (cochlea) Q16.5
Mondor's disease I80.8
Monge's disease T70.29 ☑
Monilethrix (congenital) Q84.1
Moniliasis (*see also* Candidiasis) B37.9
  neonatal P37.5
Monitoring (encounter for)
  therapeutic drug level Z51.81
Monkey malaria B53.1
Monkeypox B04
Monoarthritis M13.10
  ankle M13.17- ☑
  elbow M13.12- ☑

Monoarthritis — *continued*
  foot joint M13.17- ☑
  hand joint M13.14- ☑
  hip M13.15- ☑
  knee M13.16- ☑
  shoulder M13.11- ☑
  wrist M13.13- ☑
Monoblastic — *see* condition
Monochromat (ism), monochromatopsia (acquired) (congenital) H53.51
Monocytic — *see* condition
Monocytopenia D72.818
Monocytosis (symptomatic) D72.821
Monomania — *see* Psychosis
Mononeuritis G58.9
  cranial nerve — *see* Disorder, nerve, cranial
  femoral nerve G57.2- ☑
  lateral
    cutaneous nerve of thigh G57.1- ☑
    popliteal nerve G57.3- ☑
  lower limb G57.9- ☑
    specified nerve NEC G57.8- ☑
  medial popliteal nerve G57.4- ☑
  median nerve G56.1- ☑
  multiplex G58.7
  plantar nerve G57.6- ☑
  posterior tibial nerve G57.5- ☑
  radial nerve G56.3- ☑
  sciatic nerve G57.0- ☑
  specified NEC G58.8
  tibial nerve G57.4- ☑
  ulnar nerve G56.2- ☑
  upper limb G56.9- ☑
    specified nerve NEC G56.8- ☑
  vestibular — *see* subcategory H93.3 ☑
Mononeuropathy G58.9
  carpal tunnel syndrome — *see* Syndrome, carpal tunnel
  diabetic NEC — *see* E08-E13 with .41
  femoral nerve — *see* Lesion, nerve, femoral
  ilioinguinal nerve G57.8- ☑
  in diseases classified elsewhere — *see* category G59
  intercostal G58.0
  lower limb G57.9- ☑
    causalgia — *see* Causalgia, lower limb
    femoral nerve — *see* Lesion, nerve, femoral
    meralgia paresthetica G57.1- ☑
    plantar nerve — *see* Lesion, nerve, plantar
    popliteal nerve — *see* Lesion, nerve, popliteal
    sciatic nerve — *see* Lesion, nerve, sciatic
    specified NEC G57.8- ☑
    tarsal tunnel syndrome — *see* Syndrome, tarsal tunnel
  median nerve — *see* Lesion, nerve, median
  multiplex G58.7
  obturator nerve G57.8- ☑
  popliteal nerve — *see* Lesion, nerve, popliteal
  radial nerve — *see* Lesion, nerve, radial
  saphenous nerve G57.8- ☑
  specified NEC G58.8
  tarsal tunnel syndrome — *see* Syndrome, tarsal tunnel
  tuberculous A17.83
  ulnar nerve — *see* Lesion, nerve, ulnar
  upper limb G56.9- ☑
    carpal tunnel syndrome — *see* Syndrome, carpal tunnel
    causalgia — *see* Causalgia
    median nerve — *see* Lesion, nerve, median
    radial nerve — *see* Lesion, nerve, radial
    specified site NEC G56.8- ☑
    ulnar nerve — *see* Lesion, nerve, ulnar
Mononucleosis, infectious B27.90
  with
    complication NEC B27.99
    meningitis B27.92
    polyneuropathy B27.91
  cytomegaloviral B27.10
    with
      complication NEC B27.19
      meningitis B27.12
      polyneuropathy B27.11
  Epstein-Barr (virus) B27.00
    with
      complication NEC B27.09
      meningitis B27.02
      polyneuropathy B27.01

Mononucleosis, infectious — *continued*
  gammaherpesviral B27.00
    with
      complication NEC B27.09
      meningitis B27.02
      polyneuropathy B27.01
  specified NEC B27.80
    with
      complication NEC B27.89
      meningitis B27.82
      polyneuropathy B27.81
Monoplegia G83.3- ☑
  congenital (cerebral) G80.8
    spastic G80.1
  embolic (current episode) I63.4 ☑
  following
    cerebrovascular disease
      cerebral infarction
        lower limb I69.34- ☑
        upper limb I69.33- ☑
      intracerebral hemorrhage
        lower limb I69.14- ☑
        upper limb I69.13- ☑
      lower limb I69.94- ☑
      nontraumatic intracranial hemorrhage NEC
        lower limb I69.24- ☑
        upper limb I69.23- ☑
      specified disease NEC
        lower limb I69.84- ☑
        upper limb I69.83- ☑
      stroke NOS
        lower limb I69.34- ☑
        upper limb I69.33- ☑
      subarachnoid hemorrhage
        lower limb I69.04- ☑
        upper limb I69.03- ☑
      upper limb I69.93- ☑
  hysterical (transient) F44.4
  lower limb G83.1- ☑
  psychogenic (conversion reaction) F44.4
  thrombotic (current episode) I63.3 ☑
  transient R29.818
  upper limb G83.2- ☑
Monorchism, monorchidism Q55.0
Monosomy (*see also* Deletion, chromosome) Q93.9
  specified NEC Q93.89
  whole chromosome
    meiotic nondisjunction Q93.0
    mitotic nondisjunction Q93.1
    mosaicism Q93.1
  X Q96.9
Monster, monstrosity (single) Q89.7
  acephalic Q00.0
  twin Q89.4
Monteggia's fracture (-dislocation) S52.27- ☑
Mooren's ulcer (cornea) — *see* Ulcer, cornea, Mooren's
Moore's syndrome — *see* Epilepsy, specified NEC
Mooser-Neill reaction A75.2
Mooser's bodies A75.2
Morbidity not stated or unknown R69
Morbilli — *see* Measles
Morbus (*see also* Disease)
  angelicus, anglorum E55.0
  Beigel B36.2
  caducus — *see* Epilepsy
  celiacus K90.0
  comitialis — *see* Epilepsy
  cordis (*see also* Disease, heart) I51.9
    valvulorum — *see* Endocarditis
  coxae senilis M16.9
    tuberculous A18.02
  hemorrhagicus neonatorum P53
  maculosus neonatorum P54.5
Morel (-Stewart)(-Morgagni) **syndrome** M85.2
Morel-Kraepelin disease — *see* Schizophrenia
Morel-Moore syndrome M85.2
Morgagni's
  cyst, organ, hydatid, or appendage
    female Q50.5
    male (epididymal) Q55.4
      testicular Q55.29
  syndrome M85.2
Morgagni-Stewart-Morel syndrome M85.2
Morgagni-Stokes-Adams syndrome I45.9
Morgagni-Turner (-Albright) **syndrome** Q96.9
Moria F07.0
Moron (I.Q. 50-69) F70

Morphea L94.0
Morphinism (without remission) F11.20
  with remission F11.21
Morphinomania (without remission) F11.20
  with remission F11.21
Morquio (-Ullrich)(-Brailsford) **disease or syndrome** —
  see Mucopolysaccharidosis
Mortification (dry) (moist) — *see* Gangrene
Morton's metatarsalgia (neuralgia)(neuroma) (syndrome) G57.6- ☑
Morvan's disease or syndrome G60.8
Mosaicism, mosaic (autosomal) (chromosomal)
  45,X/46,XX Q96.3
  45,X/other cell lines NEC with abnormal sex chromosome Q96.4
  sex chromosome
    female Q97.8
    lines with various numbers of X chromosomes Q97.2
    male Q98.7
  XY Q96.3
Moschowitz' disease M31.1
Mother yaw A66.0
Motion sickness (from travel, any vehicle) (from roundabouts or swings) T75.3 ☑
Mottled, mottling, teeth (enamel) (endemic) (nonendemic) K00.3
Mounier-Kuhn syndrome Q32.4
  with bronchiectasis J47.9
    exacerbation (acute) J47.1
    lower respiratory infection J47.0
  acquired J98.09
    with bronchiectasis J47.9
      with
        exacerbation (acute) J47.1
        lower respiratory infection J47.0
Mountain
  sickness T70.29 ☑
    with polycythemia , acquired (acute) D75.1
  tick fever A93.2
Mouse, joint — *see* Loose, body, joint
  knee M23.4- ☑
Mouth — *see* condition
Movable
  coccyx — *see* subcategory M53.2 ☑
  kidney N28.89
    congenital Q63.8
  spleen D73.89
Movements, dystonic R25.8
Moyamoya disease I67.5
MRSA (Methicillin resistant Staphylococcus aureus)
  infection A49.02
    as the cause of diseases classified elsewhere B95.62
    sepsis A41.02
MSSA (Methicillin susceptible Staphylococcus aureus)
  infection A49.01
    as the cause of diseases classified elsewhere B95.61
    sepsis A41.01
Mucha-Habermann disease L41.0
Mucinosis (cutaneous) (focal) (papular) (skin) L98.5
  oral K13.79
Mucocele
  appendix K38.8
  buccal cavity K13.79
  gallbladder K82.1
  lacrimal sac, chronic H04.43- ☑
  nasal sinus J34.1
  nose J34.1
  salivary gland (any) K11.6
  sinus (accessory) (nasal) J34.1
  turbinate (bone) (middle) (nasal) J34.1
  uterus N85.8
Mucolipidosis
  I E77.1
  II, III E77.0
  IV E75.11
Mucopolysaccharidosis E76.3
  beta-gluduronidase deficiency E76.29
  cardiopathy E76.3 [I52]
  Hunter's syndrome E76.1
  Hurler's syndrome E76.01
  Hurler-Scheie syndrome E76.02
  Maroteaux-Lamy syndrome E76.29
  Morquio syndrome E76.219
    A E76.210
    B E76.211
    classic E76.210

Mucopolysaccharidosis — *continued*
  Sanfilippo syndrome E76.22
  Scheie's syndrome E76.03
  specified NEC E76.29
  type
    I
      Hurler's syndrome E76.01
      Hurler-Scheie syndrome E76.02
      Scheie's syndrome E76.03
    II E76.1
    III E76.22
    IV E76.219
    IVA E76.210
    IVB E76.211
    VI E76.29
    VII E76.29
Mucormycosis B46.5
  cutaneous B46.3
  disseminated B46.4
  gastrointestinal B46.2
  generalized B46.4
  pulmonary B46.0
  rhinocerebral B46.1
  skin B46.3
  subcutaneous B46.3
Mucositis (ulcerative) K12.30   *Main Term*
  due to drugs NEC K12.32
  gastrointestinal K92.81
  mouth (oral) (oropharyngeal) K12.30
    due to antineoplastic therapy K12.31
    due to drugs NEC K12.32
    due to radiation K12.33
    specified NEC K12.39
    viral K12.39
  nasal J34.81
  oral cavity — *see* Mucositis, mouth
  oral soft tissues — *see* Mucositis, mouth
  vagina and vulva N76.81
Mucositis necroticans agranulocytica — *see* Agranulocytosis
Mucous (*see also* condition)
  patches (syphilitic) A51.39
    congenital A50.07
Mucoviscidosis E84.9
  with meconium obstruction E84.11
Mucus
  asphyxia or suffocation — *see* Asphyxia, mucus
  in stool R19.5
  plug — *see* Asphyxia, mucus
Muguet B37.0
Mulberry molars (congenital syphilis) A50.52
Müllerian mixed tumor
  specified site — *see* Neoplasm, malignant, by site
  unspecified site C54.9
Multicystic kidney (development) Q61.4
Multiparity (grand) Z64.1
  affecting management of pregnancy, labor and delivery (supervision only) O09.4- ☑
  requiring contraceptive management — *see* Contraception
Multipartita placenta O43.19- ☑
Multiple, multiplex (*see also* condition)
  digits (congenital) Q69.9
  endocrine neoplasia — *see* Neoplasia, endocrine, multiple (MEN)
  personality F44.81
Mumps B26.9
  arthritis B26.85
  complication NEC B26.89
  encephalitis B26.2
  hepatitis B26.81
  meningitis (aseptic) B26.1
  meningoencephalitis B26.2
  myocarditis B26.82
  oophoritis B26.89
  orchitis B26.0
  pancreatitis B26.3
  polyneuropathy B26.84
Mumu (*see also* Infestation, filarial) B74.9 [N51]
Münchhausen's syndrome — *see* Disorder, factitious
Münchmeyer's syndrome — *see* Myositis, ossificans, progressiva
Mural — *see* condition
Murmur (cardiac) (heart) (organic) R01.1
  abdominal R19.15
  aortic (valve) — *see* Endocarditis, aortic
  benign R01.0
  diastolic — *see* Endocarditis

Murmur — *continued*
Flint I35.1
functional R01.0
Graham Steell I37.1
innocent R01.0
mitral (valve) — *see* Insufficiency, mitral
nonorganic R01.0
presystolic, mitral — *see* Insufficiency, mitral
pulmonic (valve) I37.8
systolic (valvular) — *see* Endocarditis
tricuspid (valve) I07.9
valvular — *see* Endocarditis
Murri's disease (intermittent hemoglobinuria) D59.6
Muscle, muscular (*see also* condition)
carnitine (palmityltransferase) deficiency E71.314
Musculoneuralgia — *see* Neuralgia
Mushrooming hip — *see* Derangement, joint, specified NEC, hip
Mushroom-workers' (pickers') disease or lung J67.5
Mutation(s)
factor V Leiden D68.51
prothrombin gene D68.52
surfactant, of lung J84.83
Mutism (*see also* Aphasia)
deaf (acquired) (congenital) NEC H91.3
elective (adjustment reaction) (childhood) F94.0
hysterical F44.4
selective (childhood) F94.0
MVD (microvillus inclusion disease) Q43.8
MVID (microvillus inclusion disease) Q43.8
Myalgia M79.1
epidemic (cervical) B33.0
traumatic NEC T14.8
Myasthenia G70.9
congenital G70.2
cordis — *see* Failure, heart
developmental G70.2
gravis G70.00
with exacerbation (acute) G70.01
in crisis G70.01
neonatal, transient P94.0
pseudoparalytica G70.00
with exacerbation (acute) G70.01
in crisis G70.01
stomach, psychogenic F45.8
syndrome
in
diabetes mellitus — *see* E08-E13 with .44
neoplastic disease (*see also* Neoplasm) D49.9 [G73.3]
pernicious anemia D51.0 [G73.3]
thyrotoxicosis E05.90 [G73.3]
with thyroid storm E05.91 [G73.3]
Myasthenic M62.81
Mycelium infection B49
Mycetismus — *see* Poisoning, food, noxious, mushroom
Mycetoma B47.9
actinomycotic B47.1
bone (mycotic) B47.9 [M90.80]
eumycotic B47.0
foot B47.9
actinomycotic B47.1
mycotic B47.0
madurae NEC B47.9
mycotic B47.0
maduromycotic B47.0
mycotic B47.0
nocardial B47.1
Mycobacteriosis — *see* Mycobacterium
Mycobacterium, mycobacterial (infection) A31.9
anonymous A31.9
atypical A31.9
cutaneous A31.1
pulmonary A31.0
tuberculous — *see* Tuberculosis, pulmonary
specified site NEC A31.8
avium (intracellulare complex) A31.0
balnei A31.1
Battey A31.0
chelonei A31.8
cutaneous A31.1
extrapulmonary systemic A31.8
fortuitum A31.8
intracellulare (Battey bacillus) A31.0
kakaferifu A31.8
kansasii (yellow bacillus) A31.0
kasongo A31.8
leprae (*see also* Leprosy) A30.9

Mycobacterium, mycobacterial — *continued*
luciflavum A31.1
marinum (M. balnei) A31.1
nonspecific — *see* Mycobacterium, atypical
pulmonary (atypical) A31.0
tuberculous — *see* Tuberculosis, pulmonary
scrofulaceum A31.8
simiae A31.8
systemic, extrapulmonary A31.8
szulgai A31.8
terrae A31.8
triviale A31.8
tuberculosis (human, bovine) — *see* Tuberculosis
ulcerans A31.1
xenopi A31.8
Mycoplasma (M.) **pneumoniae, as cause of disease classified elsewhere** B96.0
Mycosis, mycotic B49
cutaneous NEC B36.9
ear B36.8
fungoides (extranodal) (solid organ) C84.0- ☑
mouth B37.0
nails B35.1
opportunistic B48.8
skin NEC B36.9
specified NEC B48.8
stomatitis B37.0
vagina, vaginitis (candidal) B37.3
Mydriasis (pupil) H57.04
Myelatelia Q06.1
Myelinolysis, pontine, central G37.2
Myelitis (acute) (ascending) (childhood) (chronic) (descending) (diffuse) (disseminated) (idiopathic) (pressure) (progressive) (spinal cord) (subacute) (*see also* Encephalitis) G04.91
herpes simplex B00.82
herpes zoster B02.24
in diseases classified elsewhere G05.4
necrotizing, subacute G37.4
optic neuritis in G36.0
postchickenpox B01.12
postherpetic B02.24
postimmunization G04.02
postinfectious NEC G04.89
postvaccinal G04.02
specified NEC G04.89
syphilitic (transverse) A52.14
toxic G92
transverse (in demyelinating diseases of central nervous system) G37.3
tuberculous A17.82
varicella B01.12
Myeloblastic — *see* condition
Myeloblastoma
granular cell (*see also* Neoplasm, connective tissue)
malignant — *see* Neoplasm, connective tissue, malignant
tongue D10.1
Myelocele — *see* Spina bifida
Myelocystocele — *see* Spina bifida
Myelocytic — *see* condition
Myelodysplasia D46.9
specified NEC D46.Z (*following* D46.4)
spinal cord (congenital) Q06.1
Myelodysplastic syndrome D46.9
with
5q deletion D46.C (*following* D46.2)
isolated del (5q) chromosomal abnormality D46.C (*following* D46.2)
specified NEC D46.Z (*following* D46.4)
Myeloencephalitis — *see* Encephalitis
Myelofibrosis D75.81
with myeloid metaplasia D47.4
acute C94.4- ☑
idiopathic (chronic) D47.4
primary D47.1
secondary D75.81
in myeloproliferative disease D47.4
Myelogenous — *see* condition
Myeloid — *see* condition
Myelokathexis D70.9
Myeloleukodystrophy E75.29
Myelolipoma — *see* Lipoma
Myeloma (multiple) C90.0- ☑
monostotic C90.3 ☑
plasma cell C90.0- ☑
plasma cell C90.0- ☑

Myeloma — *continued*
solitary (*see also* Plasmacytoma, solitary) C90.3- ☑
Myelomalacia G95.89
Myelomatosis C90.0- ☑
Myelomeningitis — *see* Meningoencephalitis
Myelomeningocele (spinal cord) — *see* Spina bifida
Myelo-osteo-musculodysplasia hereditaria Q79.8
Myelopathic
anemia D64.89
muscle atrophy — *see* Atrophy, muscle, spinal
pain syndrome G89.0
Myelopathy (spinal cord) G95.9
drug-induced G95.89
in (due to)
degeneration or displacement, intervertebral disc NEC — *see* Disorder, disc, with, myelopathy
infection — *see* Encephalitis
intervertebral disc disorder (*see also* Disorder, disc, with, myelopathy)
mercury — *see* subcategory T56.1 ☑
neoplastic disease (*see also* Neoplasm) D49.9 [G99.2]
pernicious anemia D51.0 [G99.2]
spondylosis — *see* Spondylosis, with myelopathy NEC
necrotic (subacute) (vascular) G95.19
radiation-induced G95.89
spondylogenic NEC — *see* Spondylosis, with myelopathy NEC
toxic G95.89
transverse, acute G37.3
vascular G95.19
vitamin B12 E53.8 [G32.0]
Myelophthisis D61.82
Myeloradiculitis G04.91
Myeloradiculodysplasia (spinal) Q06.1
Myelosarcoma C92.3- ☑
Myelosclerosis D75.89
with myeloid metaplasia D47.4
disseminated, of nervous system G35
megakaryocytic D47.4
with myeloid metaplasia D47.4
Myelosis
acute C92.0- ☑
aleukemic C92.9- ☑
chronic D47.1
erythremic (acute) C94.0- ☑
megakaryocytic C94.2- ☑
nonleukemic D72.828
subacute C92.9- ☑
Myiasis (cavernous) B87.9
aural B87.4
creeping B87.0
cutaneous B87.0
dermal B87.0
ear (external) (middle) B87.4
eye B87.2
genitourinary B87.81
intestinal B87.82
laryngeal B87.3
nasopharyngeal B87.3
ocular B87.2
orbit B87.2
skin B87.0
specified site NEC B87.89
traumatic B87.1
wound B87.1
Myoadenoma, prostate — *see* Hyperplasia, prostate
Myoblastoma
granular cell (*see also* Neoplasm, connective tissue, benign)
maiignant — *see* Neoplasm, connective tissue, malignant
tongue D10.1
Myocardial — *see* condition
Myocardiopathy (congestive) (constrictive) (familial) (hypertrophic nonobstructive) (idiopathic) (infiltrative) (obstructive) (primary) (restrictive) (sporadic) (*see also* Cardiomyopathy) I42.9
alcoholic I42.6
cobalt-beer I42.6
glycogen storage E74.02 [I43]
hypertrophic obstructive I42.1
in (due to)
beriberi E51.12
cardiac glycogenosis E74.02 [I43]
Friedreich's ataxia G11.1 [I43]

Myocardiopathy — continued
  in — continued
    myotonia atrophica G71.11 [I43]
    progressive muscular dystrophy G71.0 [I43]
  obscure (African) I42.8
  secondary I42.9
  thyrotoxic E05.90 [I43]
    with storm E05.91 [I43]
  toxic NEC I42.7
Myocarditis (with arteriosclerosis)(chronic)(fibroid) (interstitial) (old) (progressive) (senile) I51.4
  with
    rheumatic fever (conditions in I00) I09.0
      active — see Myocarditis, acute, rheumatic
      inactive or quiescent (with chorea) I09.0
  active I40.9
    rheumatic I01.2
      with chorea (acute) (rheumatic) (Sydenham's) I02.0
  acute or subacute (interstitial) I40.9
    due to
      streptococcus (beta-hemolytic) I01.2
    idiopathic I40.1
    rheumatic I01.2
      with chorea (acute) (rheumatic) (Sydenham's) I02.0
    specified NEC I40.8
  aseptic of newborn B33.22
  bacterial (acute) I40.0
  Coxsackie (virus) B33.22
  diphtheritic A36.81
  eosinophilic I40.1
  epidemic of newborn (Coxsackie) B33.22
  Fiedler's (acute) (isolated) I40.1
  giant cell (acute) (subacute) I40.1
  gonococcal A54.83
  granulomatous (idiopathic) (isolated) (nonspecific) I40.1
  hypertensive — see Hypertension, heart
  idiopathic (granulomatous) I40.1
  in (due to)
    diphtheria A36.81
    epidemic louse-borne typhus A75.0 [I41]
    Lyme disease A69.29
    sarcoidosis D86.85
    scarlet fever A38.1
    toxoplasmosis (acquired) B58.81
    typhoid A01.02
    typhus NEC A75.9 [I41]
  infective I40.0
  influenzal — see Influenza, with, myocarditis
  isolated (acute) I40.1
  meningococcal A39.52
  mumps B26.82
  nonrheumatic, active I40.9
  parenchymatous I40.9
  pneumococcal I40.0
  rheumatic (chronic) (inactive) (with chorea) I09.0
    active or acute I01.2
      with chorea (acute) (rheumatic) (Sydenham's) I02.0
  rheumatoid — see Rheumatoid, carditis
  septic I40.0
  staphylococcal I40.0
  suppurative I40.0
  syphilitic (chronic) A52.06
  toxic I40.8
    rheumatic — see Myocarditis, acute, rheumatic
  tuberculous A18.84
  typhoid A01.02
  valvular — see Endocarditis
  virus, viral I40.0
    of newborn (Coxsackie) B33.22
Myocardium, myocardial — see condition
Myocardosis — see Cardiomyopathy
Myoclonus, myoclonic, myoclonia (familial) (essential) (multifocal) (simplex) G25.3
  drug-induced G25.3
  epilepsy (see also Epilepsy, generalized, specified NEC) G40.4- ☑
    familial (progressive) G25.3
  epileptica G40.409
    with status epilepticus G40.401
  facial G51.3
  familial progressive G25.3
  Friedreich's G25.3
  jerks G25.3
  massive G25.3

Myoclonus, myoclonic, myoclonia — continued
  palatal G25.3
  pharyngeal G25.3
Myocytolysis I51.5
Myodiastasis — see Diastasis, muscle
Myoendocarditis — see Endocarditis
Myoepithelioma — see Neoplasm, benign, by site
Myofasciitis (acute) — see Myositis
Myofibroma (see also Neoplasm, connective tissue, benign)
  uterus (cervix) (corpus) — see Leiomyoma
Myofibromatosis D48.1
  infantile Q89.8
Myofibrosis M62.89
  heart — see Myocarditis
  scapulohumeral — see Lesion, shoulder, specified NEC
Myofibrositis M79.7
  scapulohumeral — see Lesion, shoulder, specified NEC
Myoglobulinuria, myoglobinuria (primary) R82.1
Myokymia, facial G51.4
Myolipoma — see Lipoma
Myoma (see also Neoplasm, connective tissue, benign)
  malignant — see Neoplasm, connective tissue, malignant
  prostate D29.1
  uterus (cervix) (corpus) — see Leiomyoma
Myomalacia M62.89
Myometritis — see Endometritis
Myometrium — see condition
Myonecrosis, clostridial A48.0
Myopathy G72.9
  acute
    necrotizing G72.81
      quadriplegic G72.81
  alcoholic G72.1
  benign congenital G71.2
  central core G71.2
  centronuclear G71.2
  congenital (benign) G71.2
  critical illness G72.81
  distal G71.0
  drug-induced G72.0
  endocrine NEC E34.9 [G73.7]
  extraocular muscles H05.82- ☑
  facioscapulohumeral G71.0
  hereditary G71.9
    specified NEC G71.8
  immune NEC G72.49
  in (due to)
    Addison's disease E27.1 [G73.7]
    alcohol G72.1
    amyloidosis E85.0 [G73.7]
    cretinism E00.9 [G73.7]
    Cushing's syndrome E24.9 [G73.7]
    drugs G72.0
    endocrine disease NEC E34.9 [G73.7]
    giant cell arteritis M31.6 [G73.7]
    glycogen storage disease E74.00 [G73.7]
    hyperadrenocorticism E24.9 [G73.7]
    hyperparathyroidism NEC E21.3 [G73.7]
    hypoparathyroidism E20.9 [G73.7]
    hypopituitarism E23.0 [G73.7]
    hypothyroidism E03.9 [G73.7]
    infectious disease NEC B99 ☑ [G73.7]
    lipid storage disease E75.6 [G73.7]
    metabolic disease NEC E88.9 [G73.7]
    myxedema E03.9 [G73.7]
    parasitic disease NEC B89 [G73.7]
    polyarteritis nodosa M30.0 [G73.7]
    rheumatoid arthritis — see Rheumatoid, myopathy
    sarcoidosis D86.87
    scleroderma M34.82
    sicca syndrome M35.03
    Sjögren's syndrome M35.03
    systemic lupus erythematosus M32.19
    thyrotoxicosis (hyperthyroidism) E05.90 [G73.7]
      with thyroid storm E05.91 [G73.7]
    toxic agent NEC G72.2
  inflammatory NEC G72.49
  intensive care (ICU) G72.81
  limb-girdle G71.0
  mitochondrial NEC G71.3
  myotubular G71.2
  mytonic, proximal (PROMM) G71.11
  nemaline G71.2
  ocular G71.0
  oculopharyngeal G71.0
  of critical illness G72.81

Myopathy — continued
  primary G71.9
    specified NEC G71.8
  progressive NEC G72.89
  proximal myotonic (PROMM) G71.11
  rod G71.2
  scapulohumeral G71.0
  specified NEC G72.89
  toxic G72.2
Myopericarditis (see also Pericarditis)
  chronic rheumatic I09.2
Myopia (axial) (congenital) H52.1- ☑
  degenerative (malignant) H44.2- ☑
  malignant H44.2- ☑
  pernicious H44.2- ☑
  progressive high (degenerative) H44.2- ☑
Myosarcoma — see Neoplasm, connective tissue, malignant
Myosis (pupil) H57.03
  stromal (endolymphatic) D39.0
Myositis M60.9
  clostridial A48.0
  due to posture — see Myositis, specified type NEC
  epidemic B33.0
  fibrosa or fibrous (chronic), Volkmann's T79.6 ☑
  foreign body granuloma — see Granuloma, foreign body
  in (due to)
    bilharziasis B65.9 [M63.8-] ☑
    cysticercosis B69.81
    leprosy A30.9 [M63.8-] ☑
    mycosis B49 [M63.8-] ☑
    sarcoidosis D86.87
    schistosomiasis B65.9 [M63.8-] ☑
    syphilis
      late A52.78
      secondary A51.49
    toxoplasmosis (acquired) B58.82
    trichinellosis B75 [M63.8-] ☑
    tuberculosis A18.09
  inclusion body [IBM] G72.41
  infective M60.009
    arm M60.002
      left M60.001
      right M60.000
    leg M60.005
      left M60.004
      right M60.003
    lower limb M60.005
      ankle M60.07- ☑
      foot M60.07- ☑
      lower leg M60.06- ☑
      thigh M60.05- ☑
      toe M60.07- ☑
    multiple sites M60.09
    specified site NEC M60.08
    upper limb M60.002
      finger M60.04- ☑
      forearm M60.03- ☑
      hand M60.04- ☑
      shoulder region M60.01- ☑
      upper arm M60.02- ☑
  interstitial M60.10
    ankle M60.17- ☑
    foot M60.17- ☑
    forearm M60.13- ☑
    hand M60.14- ☑
    lower leg M60.16- ☑
    multiple sites M60.19
    shoulder region M60.11- ☑
    specified site NEC M60.18
    thigh M60.15- ☑
    upper arm M60.12- ☑
  mycotic B49 [M63.8-] ☑
  orbital, chronic H05.12- ☑
  ossificans or ossifying (circumscripta) (see also Ossification, muscle, specified NEC)
    in (due to)
      burns M61.30
        ankle M61.37- ☑
        foot M61.37- ☑
        forearm M61.33- ☑
        hand M61.34- ☑
        lower leg M61.36- ☑
        multiple sites M61.39
        pelvic region M61.35- ☑
        shoulder region M61.31- ☑

Myositis — *continued*
   ossificans or ossifying (*see also* Ossification, muscle,
      specified) — *continued*
      in — *continued*
         burns — *continued*
            specified site NEC M61.38
            thigh M61.35- ☑
            upper arm M61.32- ☑
         quadriplegia or paraplegia M61.20
            ankle M61.27- ☑
            foot M61.27- ☑
            forearm M61.23- ☑
            hand M61.24- ☑
            lower leg M61.26- ☑
            multiple sites M61.29
            pelvic region M61.25- ☑
            shoulder region M61.21- ☑
            specified site NEC M61.28
            thigh M61.25- ☑
            upper arm M61.22- ☑
      progressiva M61.10
         ankle M61.17- ☑
         finger M61.14- ☑
         foot M61.17- ☑
         forearm M61.13- ☑
         hand M61.14- ☑
         lower leg M61.16- ☑
         multiple sites M61.19
         pelvic region M61.15- ☑
         shoulder region M61.11- ☑
         specified site NEC M61.18
         thigh M61.15- ☑
         toe M61.17- ☑
         upper arm M61.12- ☑
      traumatica M61.00
         ankle M61.07- ☑
         foot M61.07- ☑
         forearm M61.03- ☑
         hand M61.04- ☑

Myositis — *continued*
   ossificans or ossifying (*see also* Ossification, muscle,
      specified) — *continued*
      traumatica — *continued*
         lower leg M61.06- ☑
         multiple sites M61.09
         pelvic region M61.05- ☑
         shoulder region M61.01- ☑
         specified site NEC M61.08
         thigh M61.05- ☑
         upper arm M61.02- ☑
   purulent — *see* Myositis, infective
   specified type NEC M60.80
      ankle M60.87- ☑
      foot M60.87- ☑
      forearm M60.83- ☑
      hand M60.84- ☑
      lower leg M60.86- ☑
      multiple sites M60.89
      pelvic region M60.85- ☑
      shoulder region M60.81- ☑
      specified site NEC M60.88
      thigh M60.85- ☑
      upper arm M60.82- ☑
   suppurative — *see* Myositis, infective
   traumatic (old) — *see* Myositis, specified type NEC
Myospasia impulsiva F95.2
Myotonia (acquisita) (intermittens) M62.89
   atrophica G71.11
   chondrodystrophic G71.13
   congenita (acetazolamide responsive) (dominant)
      (recessive) G71.12
   drug-induced G71.14
   dystrophica G71.11
   fluctuans G71.19
   levior G71.12
   permanens G71.19
   symptomatic G71.19

Myotonic pupil — *see* Anomaly, pupil, function, tonic
   pupil
Myriapodiasis B88.2
Myringitis H73.2- ☑
   with otitis media — *see* Otitis, media
   acute H73.00- ☑
      bullous H73.01- ☑
      specified NEC H73.09- ☑
   bullous — *see* Myringitis, acute, bullous
   chronic H73.1- ☑
Mysophobia F40.228
Mytilotoxism — *see* Poisoning, fish
Myxadenitis labialis K13.0
Myxedema (adult) (idiocy) (infantile) (juvenile) (*see also*
   Hypothyroidism) E03.9
   circumscribed E05.90
      with storm E05.91
   coma E03.5
   congenital E00.1
   cutis L98.5
   localized (pretibial) E05.90
      with storm E05.91
   papular L98.5
Myxochondrosarcoma — *see* Neoplasm, cartilage,
   malignant
Myxofibroma — *see* Neoplasm, connective tissue, benign
   odontogenic — *see* Cyst, calcifying odontogenic
Myxofibrosarcoma — *see* Neoplasm, connective tissue,
   malignant
Myxolipoma D17.9
Myxoliposarcoma — *see* Neoplasm, connective tissue,
   malignant
Myxoma (*see also* Neoplasm, connective tissue, benign)
   nerve sheath — *see* Neoplasm, nerve, benign
   odontogenic — *see* Cyst, calcifying odontogenic
Myxosarcoma — *see* Neoplasm, connective tissue, malignant

N

Naegeli's
  disease Q82.8
  leukemia, monocytic C93.1- ☑
Naegleriasis (with meningoencephalitis) B60.2
Naffziger's syndrome G54.0
Naga sore — *see* Ulcer, skin
Nägele's pelvis M95.5
  with disproportion (fetopelvic) O33.0
    causing obstructed labor O65.0
Nail (*see also* condition)
  biting F98.8
  patella syndrome Q87.2
Nanism, nanosomia — *see* Dwarfism
Nanophyetiasis B66.8
Nanukayami A27.89
Napkin rash L22
Narcolepsy G47.419
  with cataplexy G47.411
  in conditions classified elsewhere G47.429
    with cataplexy G47.421
Narcosis R06.89
Narcotism — *see* Dependence
NARP (Neuropathy, Ataxia and Retinitis pigmentosa)
  syndrome E88.49
Narrow
  anterior chamber angle H40.03- ☑
  pelvis — *see* Contraction, pelvis
Narrowing (*see also* Stenosis)
  artery I77.1
    auditory, internal I65.8
    basilar — *see* Occlusion, artery, basilar
    carotid — *see* Occlusion, artery, carotid
    cerebellar — *see* Occlusion, artery, cerebellar
    cerebral — *see* Occlusion artery, cerebral
    choroidal — *see* Occlusion, artery, cerebral, specified NEC
    communicating posterior — *see* Occlusion, artery, cerebral, specified NEC
    coronary (*see also* Disease, heart, ischemic, atherosclerotic)
      congenital Q24.5
        syphilitic A50.54 [I52]
      due to syphilis NEC A52.06
    hypophyseal — *see* Occlusion, artery, cerebral, specified NEC
    pontine — *see* Occlusion, artery, cerebral, specified NEC
    precerebral — *see* Occlusion, artery, precerebral
    vertebral — *see* Occlusion, artery, vertebral
  auditory canal (external) — *see* Stenosis, external ear canal
  eustachian tube — *see* Obstruction, eustachian tube
  eyelid — *see* Disorder, eyelid function
  larynx J38.6
  mesenteric artery K55.0
  palate M26.89
  palpebral fissure — *see* Disorder, eyelid function
  ureter N13.5
    with infection N13.6
  urethra — *see* Stricture, urethra
Narrowness, abnormal, eyelid Q10.3
Nasal — *see* condition
Nasolachrymal, nasolacrimal — *see* condition
Nasopharyngeal (*see also* condition)
  pituitary gland Q89.2
  torticollis M43.6
Nasopharyngitis (acute) (infective) (streptococcal) (subacute) J00
  chronic (suppurative) (ulcerative) J31.1
Nasopharynx, nasopharyngeal — *see* condition
Natal tooth, teeth K00.6
Nausea (without vomiting) R11.0
  with vomiting R11.2
  gravidarum — *see* Hyperemesis, gravidarum
  marina T75.3 ☑
  navalis T75.3 ☑
Navel — *see* condition
Neapolitan fever — *see* Brucellosis

Near drowning T75.1 ☑
Nearsightedness — *see* Myopia
Near-syncope R55
Nebula, cornea — *see* Opacity, cornea
Necator americanus infestation B76.1
Necatoriasis B76.1
Neck — *see* condition
Necrobiosis R68.89
  lipoidica NEC L92.1
    with diabetes — *see* E08-E13 with .620
Necrolysis, toxic epidermal L51.2
  due to drug
    correct substance properly administered — *see* Table of Drugs and Chemicals, by drug, adverse effect
    overdose or wrong substance given or taken — *see* Table of Drugs and Chemicals, by drug, poisoning
Necrophilia F65.89
Necrosis, necrotic (ischemic) (*see also* Gangrene)
  adrenal (capsule) (gland) E27.49
  amputation stump (surgical) (late) T87.50
    arm T87.5- ☑
    leg T87.5- ☑
  antrum J32.0
  aorta (hyaline) (*see also* Aneurysm, aorta)
    cystic medial — *see* Dissection, aorta
  artery I77.5
  bladder (aseptic) (sphincter) N32.89
  bone (*see also* Osteonecrosis) M87.9
    aseptic or avascular — *see* Osteonecrosis
      idiopathic M87.00
    ethmoid J32.2
    jaw M27.2
    tuberculous — *see* Tuberculosis, bone
  brain I67.89
  breast (aseptic) (fat) (segmental) N64.1
  bronchus J98.09
  central nervous system NEC I67.89
  cerebellar I67.89
  cerebral I67.89
  colon K55.0
  cornea H18.40
  cortical (acute) (renal) N17.1
  cystic medial (aorta) — *see* Dissection, aorta
  dental pulp K04.1
  esophagus K22.8
  ethmoid (bone) J32.2
  eyelid — *see* Disorder, eyelid, degenerative
  fat, fatty (generalized) (*see also* Disorder, soft tissue, specified type NEC)
    abdominal wall K65.4
    breast (aseptic) (segmental) N64.1
    localized — *see* Degeneration, by site, fatty
    mesentery K65.4
    omentum K65.4
    pancreas K86.8
    peritoneum K65.4
    skin (subcutaneous), newborn P83.0
    subcutaneous, due to birth injury P15.6
  gallbladder — *see* Cholecystitis, acute
  heart — *see* Infarct, myocardium
  hip, aseptic or avascular — *see* Osteonecrosis, by type, femur
  intestine (acute) (hemorrhagic) (massive) K55.0
  jaw M27.2
  kidney (bilateral) N28.0
    acute N17.9
    cortical (acute) (bilateral) N17.1
      with ectopic or molar pregnancy O08.4
    medullary (bilateral) (in acute renal failure) (papillary) N17.2
    papillary (bilateral) (in acute renal failure) N17.2
    tubular N17.0
      with ectopic or molar pregnancy O08.4
      complicating
        abortion — *see* Abortion, by type, complicated by, tubular necrosis
        ectopic or molar pregnancy O08.4
        pregnancy — *see* Pregnancy, complicated by, diseases of, specified type or system NEC

Necrosis, necrotic — *continued*
  kidney — *continued*
    tubular — *continued*
      following ectopic or molar pregnancy O08.4
      traumatic T79.5 ☑
  larynx J38.7
  liver (with hepatic failure) (cell) — *see* Failure, hepatic
    hemorrhagic, central K76.2
  lung J85.0
  lymphatic gland — *see* Lymphadenitis, acute
  mammary gland (fat) (segmental) N64.1
  mastoid (chronic) — *see* Mastoiditis, chronic
  medullary (acute) (renal) N17.2
  mesentery K55.0
    fat K65.4
  mitral valve — *see* Insufficiency, mitral
  myocardium, myocardial — *see* Infarct, myocardium
  nose J34.89
  omentum (with mesenteric infarction) K55.0
    fat K65.4
  orbit, orbital — *see* Osteomyelitis, orbit
  ossicles, ear — *see* Abnormal, ear ossicles
  ovary N70.92
  pancreas (aseptic) (duct) (fat) K86.8
    acute (infective) — *see* Pancreatitis, acute
    infective — *see* Pancreatitis, acute
  papillary (acute) (renal) N17.2
  perineum N90.89
  peritoneum (with mesenteric infarction) K55.0
    fat K65.4
  pharynx J02.9
    in granulocytopenia — *see* Neutropenia
      Vincent's A69.1
  phosphorus — *see* subcategory T54.2 ☑
  pituitary (gland) (postpartum) (Sheehan) E23.0
  pressure — *see* Ulcer, pressure, by site
  pulmonary J85.0
  pulp (dental) K04.1
  radiation — *see* Necrosis, by site
  radium — *see* Necrosis, by site
  renal — *see* Necrosis, kidney
  sclera H15.89
  scrotum N50.8
  skin or subcutaneous tissue NEC I96
  spine, spinal (column) (*see also* Osteonecrosis, by type, vertebra)
    cord G95.19
  spleen D73.5
  stomach K31.89
  stomatitis (ulcerative) A69.0
  subcutaneous fat, newborn P83.8
  subendocardial (acute) I21.4
    chronic I25.89
  suprarenal (capsule) (gland) E27.49
  testis N50.8
  thymus (gland) E32.8
  tonsil J35.8
  trachea J39.8
  tuberculous NEC — *see* Tuberculosis
  tubular (acute) (anoxic) (renal) (toxic) N17.0
    postprocedural N99.0
  vagina N89.8
  vertebra (*see also* Osteonecrosis, by type, vertebra)
    tuberculous A18.01
  vulva N90.89
  X-ray — *see* Necrosis, by site
Necrospermia — *see* Infertility, male
Need (for)
  care provider because (of)
    assistance with personal care Z74.1
    continuous supervision required Z74.3
    impaired mobility Z74.09
    no other household member able to render care Z74.2
    specified reason NEC Z74.8
  immunization — *see* Vaccination
  vaccination — *see* Vaccination
Neglect
  adult
    confirmed T74.01 ☑
    history of Z91.412
    suspected T76.01 ☑

Neglect — *continued*
- child (childhood)
  - confirmed T74.02 ☑
  - history of Z62.812
  - suspected T76.02 ☑
- emotional, in childhood Z62.898
- hemispatial R41.4
- left-sided R41.4
- sensory R41.4
- visuospatial R41.4

Neisserian infection NEC — *see* Gonococcus
Nelaton's syndrome G60.8
Nelson's syndrome E24.1
Nematodiasis (intestinal) B82.0
- Ancylostoma B76.0
Neonatal (*see also* Newborn)
- acne L70.4
- bradycardia P29.12
- screening, abnormal findings on P09
- tachycardia P29.11
- tooth, teeth K00.6 ✓
Neonatorum — *see* condition
Neoplasia
- endocrine, multiple (MEN) E31.20
  - type I E31.21
  - type IIA E31.22
  - type IIB E31.23
- intraepithelial (histologically confirmed)
  - anal (AIN) (histologically confirmed) K62.82
    - grade I K62.82
    - grade II K62.82
    - severe D01.3
  - cervical glandular (histologically confirmed) D06.9
  - cervix (uteri) (CIN) (histologically confirmed) N87.9
    - glandular D06.9
    - grade I N87.0
    - grade II N87.1
    - grade III (severe dysplasia) (*see also* Carcinoma, cervix uteri, in situ) D06.9
  - prostate (histologically confirmed) (PIN I) (PIN II) N42.3
    - grade I N42.3
    - grade II N42.3
    - severe D07.5
  - vagina (histologically confirmed) (VAIN) N89.3
    - grade I N89.0
    - grade II N89.1
    - grade III (severe dysplasia) D07.2
  - vulva (histologically confirmed) (VIN) N90.3
    - grade I N90.0
    - grade II N90.1
    - grade III (severe dysplasia) D07.1
Neoplasm, neoplastic (*see also* Table of Neoplasms)
- lipomatous, benign — *see* Lipoma
Neovascularization
- ciliary body — *see* Disorder, iris, vascular
- cornea H16.40- ☑
  - deep H16.44- ☑
  - ghost vessels — *see* Ghost, vessels
  - localized H16.43- ☑
  - pannus — *see* Pannus
- iris — *see* Disorder, iris, vascular
- retina H35.05- ☑
Nephralgia N23
Nephritis, nephritic (albuminuric) (azotemic) (congenital) (disseminated) (epithelial) (familial) (focal) (granulomatous) (hemorrhagic) (infantile) (nonsuppurative, excretory) (uremic) N05.9
- with
  - dense deposit disease N05.6
  - diffuse
    - crescentic glomerulonephritis N05.7
    - endocapillary proliferative glomerulonephritis N05.4
    - membranous glomerulonephritis N05.2
    - mesangial proliferative glomerulonephritis N05.3
    - mesangiocapillary glomerulonephritis N05.5
  - edema — *see* Nephrosis
  - focal and segmental glomerular lesions N05.1
  - foot process disease N04.9
  - glomerular lesion
    - diffuse sclerosing N05.8
    - hypocomplementemic — *see* Nephritis, membranoproliferative
    - IgA — *see* Nephropathy, IgA
    - lobular, lobulonodular — *see* Nephritis, membranoproliferative

Nephritis, nephritic — *continued*
- with — *continued*
  - glomerular lesion — *continued*
    - nodular — *see* Nephritis, membranoproliferative
  - lesion of
    - glomerulonephritis, proliferative N05.8
    - renal necrosis N05.9
  - minor glomerular abnormality N05.0
  - specified morphological changes NEC N05.8
- acute N00.9
  - with
    - dense deposit disease N00.6
    - diffuse
      - crescentic glomerulonephritis N00.7
      - endocapillary proliferative glomerulonephritis N00.4
      - membranous glomerulonephritis N00.2
      - mesangial proliferative glomerulonephritis N00.3
      - mesangiocapillary glomerulonephritis N00.5
    - focal and segmental glomerular lesions N00.1
    - minor glomerular abnormality N00.0
    - specified morphological changes NEC N00.8
- amyloid E85.4 [N08]
- antiglomerular basement membrane (anti-GBM) antibody NEC
  - in Goodpasture's syndrome M31.0
- antitubular basement membrane (tubulo-interstitial) NEC N12
  - toxic — *see* Nephropathy, toxic
- arteriolar — *see* Hypertension, kidney
- arteriosclerotic — *see* Hypertension, kidney
- ascending — *see* Nephritis, tubulo-interstitial
- atrophic N03.9
- Balkan (endemic) N15.0
- calculous, calculus — *see* Calculus, kidney
- cardiac — *see* Hypertension, kidney
- cardiovascular — *see* Hypertension, kidney
- chronic N03.9
  - with
    - dense deposit disease N03.6
    - diffuse
      - crescentic glomerulonephritis N03.7
      - endocapillary proliferative glomerulonephritis N03.4
      - membranous glomerulonephritis N03.2
      - mesangial proliferative glomerulonephritis N03.3
      - mesangiocapillary glomerulonephritis N03.5
    - focal and segmental glomerular lesions N03.1
    - minor glomerular abnormality N03.0
    - specified morphological changes NEC N03.8
  - arteriosclerotic — *see* Hypertension, kidney
- cirrhotic N26.9
- complicating pregnancy O26.83- ☑
- croupous N00.9
- degenerative — *see* Nephrosis
- diffuse sclerosing N05.8
- due to
  - diabetes mellitus — *see* E08-E13 with .21
  - subacute bacterial endocarditis I33.0
  - systemic lupus erythematosus (chronic) M32.14
  - typhoid fever A01.09
- gonococcal (acute) (chronic) A54.21
- hypocomplementemic — *see* Nephritis, membranoproliferative
- IgA — *see* Nephropathy, IgA
- immune complex (circulating) NEC N05.8
- infective — *see* Nephritis, tubulo-interstitial
- interstitial — *see* Nephritis, tubulo-interstitial
- lead N14.3
- membranoproliferative (diffuse) (type 1 or 3) (*see also* N00-N07 with fourth character .5) N05.5
  - type 2 (*see also* N00-N07 with fourth character .6) N05.6
- minimal change N05.0
- necrotic, necrotizing NEC (*see also* N00-N07 with fourth character .8) N05.8
- nephrotic — *see* Nephrosis
- nodular — *see* Nephritis, membranoproliferative
- polycystic Q61.3
  - adult type Q61.2
  - autosomal
    - dominant Q61.2
    - recessive NEC Q61.19
  - childhood type NEC Q61.19
  - infantile type NEC Q61.19

Nephritis, nephritic — *continued*
- poststreptococcal N05.9
  - acute N00.9
  - chronic N03.9
  - rapidly progressive N01.9
- proliferative NEC (*see also* N00-N07 with fourth character .8) N05.8
- purulent — *see* Nephritis, tubulo-interstitial
- rapidly progressive N01.9
  - with
    - dense deposit disease N01.6
    - diffuse
      - crescentic glomerulonephritis N01.7
      - endocapillary proliferative glomerulonephritis N01.4
      - membranous glomerulonephritis N01.2
      - mesangial proliferative glomerulonephritis N01.3
      - mesangiocapillary glomerulonephritis N01.5
    - focal and segmental glomerular lesions N01.1
    - minor glomerular abnormality N01.0
    - specified morphological changes NEC N01.8
- salt losing or wasting NEC N28.89
- saturnine N14.3
- sclerosing, diffuse N05.8
- septic — *see* Nephritis, tubulo-interstitial
- specified pathology NEC (*see also* N00-N07 with fourth character .8) N05.8
- subacute N01.9
- suppurative — *see* Nephritis, tubulo-interstitial
- syphilitic (late) A52.75
  - congenital A50.59 [N08]
  - early (secondary) A51.44
- toxic — *see* Nephropathy, toxic
- tubal, tubular — *see* Nephritis, tubulo-interstitial
- tuberculous A18.11
- tubulo-interstitial (in) N12
  - acute (infectious) N10
  - chronic (infectious) N11.9
    - nonobstructive N11.8
      - reflux-associated N11.0
    - obstructive N11.1
    - specified NEC N11.8
  - due to
    - brucellosis A23.9 [N16]
    - cryoglobulinemia D89.1 [N16]
    - glycogen storage disease E74.00 [N16]
    - Sjögren's syndrome M35.04
- vascular — *see* Hypertension, kidney
- war N00.9
Nephroblastoma (epithelial) (mesenchymal) C64- ☑
Nephrocalcinosis E83.59 [N29]
Nephrocystitis, pustular — *see* Nephritis, tubulo-interstitial
Nephrolithiasis (congenital) (pelvis) (recurrent) (*see also* Calculus, kidney)
Nephroma C64- ☑
- mesoblastic D41.0- ☑
Nephronephritis — *see* Nephrosis
Nephronophthisis Q61.5
Nephropathia epidemica A98.5
Nephropathy (*see also* Nephritis) N28.9
- with
  - edema — *see* Nephrosis
  - glomerular lesion — *see* Glomerulonephritis
- amyloid, hereditary E85.0
- analgesic N14.0
  - with medullary necrosis, acute N17.2
- Balkan (endemic) N15.0
- chemical — *see* Nephropathy, toxic
- diabetic — *see* E08-E13 with .21
- drug-induced N14.2
  - specified NEC N14.1
- focal and segmental hyalinosis or sclerosis N02.1
- heavy metal-induced N14.3
- hereditary NEC N07.9
  - with
    - dense deposit disease N07.6
    - diffuse
      - crescentic glomerulonephritis N07.7
      - endocapillary proliferative glomerulonephritis N07.4
      - membranous glomerulonephritis N07.2
      - mesangial proliferative glomerulonephritis N07.3
      - mesangiocapillary glomerulonephritis N07.5
    - focal and segmental glomerular lesions N07.1
    - minor glomerular abnormality N07.0

Nephropathy — continued
  hereditary — continued
    with — continued
      specified morphological changes NEC N07.8
  hypercalcemic N25.89
  hypertensive — see Hypertension, kidney
  hypokalemic (vacuolar) N25.89
  IgA N02.8
    with glomerular lesion N02.9
      focal and segmental hyalinosis or sclerosis N02.1
      membranoproliferative (diffuse) N02.5
      membranous (diffuse) N02.2
      mesangial proliferative (diffuse) N02.3
      mesangiocapillary (diffuse) N02.5
      proliferative NEC N02.8
      specified pathology NEC N02.8
  lead N14.3
  membranoproliferative (diffuse) N02.5
  membranous (diffuse) N02.2
  mesangial (IgA/IgG) — see Nephropathy, IgA
    proliferative (diffuse) N02.3
  mesangiocapillary (diffuse) N02.5
  obstructive N13.8
  phenacetin N17.2
  phosphate-losing N25.0
  potassium depletion N25.89
  pregnancy-related O26.83- ☑
  proliferative NEC (see also N00-N07 with fourth character .8) N05.8
  protein-losing N25.89
  saturnine N14.3
  sickle-cell D57.- ☑ [N08]
  toxic NEC N14.4
    due to
      drugs N14.2
        analgesic N14.0
        specified NEC N14.1
      heavy metals N14.3
  vasomotor N17.0
  water-losing N25.89
Nephroptosis N28.83
Nephropyosis — see Abscess, kidney
Nephrorrhagia N28.89
Nephrosclerosis (arteriolar)(arteriosclerotic) (chronic) (hyaline) (see also Hypertension, kidney)
  hyperplastic — see Hypertension, kidney
  senile N26.9
Nephrosis, nephrotic (Epstein's) (syndrome) (congenital) N04.9
  with
    foot process disease N04.9
    glomerular lesion N04.1
    hypocomplementemic N04.5
  acute N04.9
  anoxic — see Nephrosis, tubular
  chemical — see Nephrosis, tubular
  cholemic K76.7
  diabetic — see E08-E13 with .21
  Finnish type (congenital) Q89.8
  hemoglobin N10
  hemoglobinuric — see Nephrosis, tubular
  in
    amyloidosis E85.4 [N08]
    diabetes mellitus — see E08-E13 with .21
    epidemic hemorrhagic fever A98.5
    malaria (malariae) B52.0
  ischemic — see Nephrosis, tubular
  lipoid N04.9
  lower nephron — see Nephrosis, tubular
  malarial (malariae) B52.0
  minimal change N04.0
  myoglobin N10
  necrotizing — see Nephrosis, tubular
  osmotic (sucrose) N25.89
  radiation N04.9
  syphilitic (late) A52.75
  toxic — see Nephrosis, tubular
  tubular (acute) N17.0
    postprocedural N99.0
    radiation N04.9
Nephrosonephritis, hemorrhagic (endemic) A98.5
Nephrostomy
  attention to Z43.6
  status Z93.6
Nerve (see also condition)
  injury — see Injury, nerve, by body site
Nerves R45.0

Nervous (see also condition) R45.0
  heart F45.8
  stomach F45.8
  tension R45.0
Nervousness R45.0
Nesidioblastoma
  pancreas D13.7
  specified site NEC — see Neoplasm, benign, by site
  unspecified site D13.7
Nettleship's syndrome Q82.2
Neumann's disease or syndrome L10.1
Neuralgia, neuralgic (acute) M79.2
  accessory (nerve) G52.8
  acoustic (nerve) — see subcategory H93.3 ☑
  auditory (nerve) — see subcategory H93.3 ☑
  ciliary G44.009
    intractable G44.001
    not intractable G44.009
  cranial
    nerve (see also Disorder, nerve, cranial)
      fifth or trigeminal — see Neuralgia, trigeminal
      postherpetic, postzoster B02.29
  ear — see subcategory H92.0 ☑
  facialis vera G51.1
  Fothergill's — see Neuralgia, trigeminal
  glossopharyngeal (nerve) G52.1
  Horton's G44.099
    intractable G44.091
    not intractable G44.099
  Hunt's B02.21
  hypoglossal (nerve) G52.3
  infraorbital — see Neuralgia, trigeminal
  malarial — see Malaria
  migrainous G44.009
    intractable G44.001
    not intractable G44.009
  Morton's G57.6- ☑
  nerve, cranial — see Disorder, nerve, cranial
  nose G52.0
  occipital M54.81
  olfactory G52.0
  penis N48.9
  perineum R10.2
  postherpetic NEC B02.29
    trigeminal B02.22
  pubic region R10.2
  scrotum R10.2
  Sluder's G44.89
  specified nerve NEC G58.8
  spermatic cord R10.2
  sphenopalatine (ganglion) G90.09
  trifacial — see Neuralgia, trigeminal
  trigeminal G50.0
    postherpetic, postzoster B02.22
  vagus (nerve) G52.2
  writer's F48.8
    organic G25.89
Neurapraxia — see Injury, nerve
Neurasthenia F48.8
  cardiac F45.8
  gastric F45.8
  heart F45.8
Neurilemmoma (see also Neoplasm, nerve, benign)
  acoustic (nerve) D33.3
  malignant (see also Neoplasm, nerve, malignant)
    acoustic (nerve) C72.4- ☑
Neurilemmosarcoma — see Neoplasm, nerve, malignant
Neurinoma — see Neoplasm, nerve, benign
Neurinomatosis — see Neoplasm, nerve, uncertain behavior
Neuritis (rheumatoid) M79.2
  abducens (nerve) — see Strabismus, paralytic, sixth nerve
  accessory (nerve) G52.8
  acoustic (nerve) (see also subcategory H93.3 ☑
    in (due to)
      infectious disease NEC B99 ☑ [H94.0-] ☑
      parasitic disease NEC B89 [H94.0-] ☑
      syphilitic A52.15
  alcoholic G62.1
    with psychosis — see Psychosis, alcoholic
  amyloid, any site E85.4 [G63]
  auditory (nerve) — see subcategory H93.3 ☑
  brachial — see Radiculopathy
    due to displacement, intervertebral disc — see Disorder, disc, cervical, with neuritis

Neuritis — continued
  cranial nerve
    due to Lyme disease A69.22
    eighth or acoustic or auditory — see subcategory H93.3 ☑
    eleventh or accessory G52.8
    fifth or trigeminal G51.0
    first or olfactory G52.0
    fourth or trochlear — see Strabismus, paralytic, fourth nerve
    second or optic — see Neuritis, optic
    seventh or facial G51.8
      newborn (birth injury) P11.3
    sixth or abducent — see Strabismus, paralytic, sixth nerve
    tenth or vagus G52.2
    third or oculomotor — see Strabismus, paralytic, third nerve
    twelfth or hypoglossal G52.3
  Déjérine-Sottas G60.0
  diabetic (mononeuropathy) — see E08-E13 with .41
    polyneuropathy — see E08-E13 with .42
  due to
    beriberi E51.11
    displacement, prolapse or rupture, intervertebral disc — see Disorder, disc, with, radiculopathy
    herniation, nucleus pulposus M51.9 [G55]
  endemic E51.11
  facial G51.8
    newborn (birth injury) P11.3
  general — see Polyneuropathy
  geniculate ganglion G51.1
    due to herpes (zoster) B02.21
  gouty M10.00 [G63]
  hypoglossal (nerve) G52.3
  ilioinguinal (nerve) G57.9- ☑
  infectious (multiple) NEC G61.0
  interstitial hypertrophic progressive G60.0
  lumbar M54.16
  lumbosacral M54.17
  multiple (see also Polyneuropathy)
    endemic E51.11
    infective, acute G61.0
  multiplex endemica E51.11
  nerve root — see Radiculopathy
  oculomotor (nerve) — see Strabismus, paralytic, third nerve
  olfactory nerve G52.0
  optic (nerve) (hereditary) (sympathetic) H46.9
    with demyelination G36.0
      in myelitis G36.0
    nutritional H46.2
    papillitis — see Papillitis, optic
    retrobulbar H46.1- ☑
    specified type NEC H46.8
    toxic H46.3
  peripheral (nerve) G62.9
    multiple — see Polyneuropathy
    single — see Mononeuritis
  pneumogastric (nerve) G52.2
  postherpetic, postzoster B02.29
  progressive hypertrophic interstitial G60.0
  retrobulbar (see also Neuritis, optic, retrobulbar)
    in (due to)
      late syphilis A52.15
      meningococcal infection A39.82
    meningococcal A39.82
    syphilitic A52.15
  sciatic (nerve) (see also Sciatica)
    due to displacement of intervertebral disc — see Disorder, disc, with, radiculopathy
  serum (see also Reaction, serum) T80.69 ☑
  shoulder-girdle G54.5
  specified nerve NEC G58.8
  spinal (nerve) root — see Radiculopathy
  syphilitic A52.15
  thenar (median) G56.1- ☑
  thoracic M54.14
  toxic NEC G62.2
  trochlear (nerve) — see Strabismus, paralytic, fourth nerve
  vagus (nerve) G52.2
Neuroastrocytoma — see Neoplasm, uncertain behavior, by site
Neuroavitaminosis E56.9 [G99.8]
Neuroblastoma
  olfactory C30.0
  specified site — see Neoplasm, malignant, by site

Neuroblastoma — *continued*
  unspecified site C74.90
Neurochorioretinitis — *see* Chorioretinitis
Neurocirculatory asthenia F45.8
Neurocysticercosis B69.0
Neurocytoma — *see* Neoplasm, benign, by site
Neurodermatitis (circumscribed) (circumscripta) (local) L28.0
  atopic L20.81
  diffuse (Brocq) L20.81
  disseminated L20.81
Neuroencephalomyelopathy, optic G36.0
Neuroepithelioma (*see also* Neoplasm, malignant, by site)
  olfactory C30.0
Neurofibroma (*see also* Neoplasm, nerve, benign)
  melanotic — *see* Neoplasm, nerve, benign
  multiple — *see* Neurofibromatosis
  plexiform — *see* Neoplasm, nerve, benign
Neurofibromatosis (multiple) (nonmalignant) Q85.00
  acoustic Q85.02
  malignant — *see* Neoplasm, nerve, malignant
  specified NEC Q85.09
  type 1 (von Recklinghausen) Q85.01
  type 2 Q85.02
Neurofibrosarcoma — *see* Neoplasm, nerve, malignant
Neurogenic (*see also* condition)
  bladder (*see also* Dysfunction, bladder, neuromuscular) N31.9
    cauda equina syndrome G83.4
  bowel NEC K59.2
  heart F45.8
Neuroglioma — *see* Neoplasm, uncertain behavior, by site
Neurolabyrinthitis (of Dix and Hallpike) — *see* Neuronitis, vestibular
Neurolathyrism — *see* Poisoning, food, noxious, plant
Neuroleprosy A30.9
Neuroma (*see also* Neoplasm, nerve, benign)
  acoustic (nerve) D33.3
  amputation (stump) (traumatic) (surgical complication) (late) T87.3- ☑
    arm T87.3- ☑
    leg T87.3- ☑
  digital (toe) G57.6- ☑
  interdigital (toe) G58.8
    lower limb G57.8- ☑
    upper limb G56.8- ☑
  intermetatarsal G57.8- ☑
  Morton's G57.6- ☑
  nonneoplastic
    arm G56.9- ☑
    leg G57.9- ☑
    lower extremity G57.9- ☑
    upper extremity G56.9- ☑
  optic (nerve) D33.3
  plantar G57.6- ☑
  plexiform — *see* Neoplasm, nerve, benign
  surgical (nonneoplastic)
    arm G56.9- ☑
    leg G57.9- ☑
    lower extremity G57.9- ☑
    upper extremity G56.9- ☑
Neuromyalgia — *see* Neuralgia
Neuromyasthenia (epidemic) (postinfectious) G93.3
Neuromyelitis G36.9
  ascending G61.0
  optica G36.0
Neuromyopathy G70.9
  paraneoplastic D49.9 [G13.0]
Neuromyotonia (Isaacs) G71.19
Neuronevus — *see* Nevus
Neuronitis G58.9
  ascending (acute) G57.2- ☑
  vestibular H81.2- ☑
Neuroparalytic — *see* condition
Neuropathy, neuropathic G62.9
  acute motor G62.81
  alcoholic G62.1
    with psychosis — *see* Psychosis, alcoholic
  arm G56.9- ☑
  autonomic, peripheral — *see* Neuropathy, peripheral, autonomic
  axillary G56.9- ☑
  bladder N31.9
    atonic (motor) (sensory) N31.2
    autonomous N31.2

Neuropathy, neuropathic — *continued*
  bladder — *continued*
    flaccid N31.2
    nonreflex N31.2
    reflex N31.1
    uninhibited N31.0
  brachial plexus G54.0
  cervical plexus G54.2
  chronic
    progressive segmentally demyelinating G62.89
    relapsing demyelinating G62.89
  Déjérine-Sottas G60.0
  diabetic — *see* E08-E13 with .40
    mononeuropathy — *see* E08-E13 with .41
    polyneuropathy — *see* E08-E13 with .42
  entrapment G58.9
    iliohypogastric nerve G57.8- ☑
    ilioinguinal nerve G57.8- ☑
    lateral cutaneous nerve of thigh G57.1- ☑
    median nerve G56.0- ☑
    obturator nerve G57.8- ☑
    peroneal nerve G57.3- ☑
    posterior tibial nerve G57.5- ☑
    saphenous nerve G57.8- ☑
    ulnar nerve G56.2- ☑
  facial nerve G51.9
  hereditary G60.9
    motor and sensory (types I-IV) G60.0
    sensory G60.8
    specified NEC G60.8
  hypertrophic G60.0
    Charcot-Marie-Tooth G60.0
    Déjérine-Sottas G60.0
    interstitial progressive G60.0
    of infancy G60.0
    Refsum G60.1
  idiopathic G60.9
    progressive G60.3
    specified NEC G60.8
  in association with hereditary ataxia G60.2
  intercostal G58.0
  ischemic — *see* Disorder, nerve
  Jamaica (ginger) G62.2
  leg NEC G57.9- ☑
  lower extremity G57.9- ☑
  lumbar plexus G54.1
  median nerve G56.1- ☑
  motor and sensory (*see also* Polyneuropathy)
    hereditary (types I-IV) G60.0
  multiple (acute) (chronic) — *see* Polyneuropathy
  optic (nerve) (*see also* Neuritis, optic)
    ischemic H47.01- ☑
  paraneoplastic (sensorial) (Denny Brown) D49.9 [G13.0]
  peripheral (nerve) (*see also* Polyneuropathy) G62.9
    autonomic G90.9
      idiopathic G90.09
      in (due to)
        amyloidosis E85.4 [G99.0]
        diabetes mellitus — *see* E08-E13 with .43
        endocrine disease NEC E34.9 [G99.0]
        gout M10.00 [G99.0]
        hyperthyroidism E05.90 [G99.0]
          with thyroid storm E05.91 [G99.0]
        metabolic disease NEC E88.9 [G99.0]
    idiopathic G60.9
      progressive G60.3
    in (due to)
      antitetanus serum G62.0
      arsenic G62.2
      drugs NEC G62.0
      lead G62.2
      organophosphate compounds G62.2
      toxic agent NEC G62.2
  plantar nerves G57.6- ☑
  progressive
    hypertrophic interstitial G60.0
    inflammatory G62.81
  radicular NEC — *see* Radiculopathy
  sacral plexus G54.1
  sciatic G57.0- ☑
  serum G61.1
  toxic NEC G62.2
  trigeminal sensory G50.8
  ulnar nerve G56.2- ☑
  uremic N18.9 [G63]
  vitamin B12 E53.8 [G63]
    with anemia (pernicious) D51.0 [G63]
      due to dietary deficiency D51.3 [G63]

Neurophthisis (*see also* Disorder, nerve)
  peripheral, diabetic — *see* E08-E13 with .42
Neuroretinitis — *see* Chorioretinitis
Neuroretinopathy, hereditary optic H47.22
Neurosarcoma — *see* Neoplasm, nerve, malignant
Neurosclerosis — *see* Disorder, nerve
Neurosis, neurotic F48.9
  anankastic F42
  anxiety (state) F41.1
    panic type F41.0
  asthenic F48.8
  bladder F45.8
  cardiac (reflex) F45.8
  cardiovascular F45.8
  character F60.9
  colon F45.8
  compensation F68.1 ☑
  compulsive, compulsion F42
  conversion F44.9
  craft F48.8
  cutaneous F45.8
  depersonalization F48.1
  depressive (reaction) (type) F34.1
  environmental F48.8
  excoriation L98.1
  fatigue F48.8
  functional — *see* Disorder, somatoform
  gastric F45.8
  gastrointestinal F45.8
  heart F45.8
  hypochondriacal F45.21
  hysterical F44.9
  incoordination F45.8
    larynx F45.8
    vocal cord F45.8
  intestine F45.8
  larynx (sensory) F45.8
    hysterical F44.4
  mixed NEC F48.8
  musculoskeletal F45.8
  obsessional F42
  obsessive-compulsive F42
  occupational F48.8
  ocular NEC F45.8
  organ — *see* Disorder, somatoform
  pharynx F45.8
  phobic F40.9
  posttraumatic (situational) F43.10
    acute F43.11
    chronic F43.12
  psychasthenic (type) F48.8
  railroad F48.8
  rectum F45.8
  respiratory F45.8
  rumination F45.8
  sexual F65.9
  situational F48.8
  social F40.10
    generalized F40.11
  specified type NEC F48.8
  state F48.9
    with depersonalization episode F48.1
  stomach F45.8
  traumatic F43.10
    acute F43.11
    chronic F43.12
  vasomotor F45.8
  visceral F45.8
  war F48.8

Neurospongioblastosis diffusa Q85.1
Neurosyphilis (arrested) (early) (gumma) (late) (latent) (recurrent) (relapse) A52.3
  with ataxia (cerebellar) (locomotor) (spastic) (spinal) A52.19
  aneurysm (cerebral) A52.05
  arachnoid (adhesive) A52.13
  arteritis (any artery) (cerebral) A52.04
  asymptomatic A52.2
  congenital A50.40
  dura (mater) A52.13
  general paresis A52.17
  hemorrhagic A52.05
  juvenile (asymptomatic) (meningeal) A50.40
  leptomeninges (aseptic) A52.13
  meningeal, meninges (adhesive) A52.13
  meningitis A52.13
  meningovascular (diffuse) A52.13
  optic atrophy A52.15

Neurosyphilis — *continued*
  parenchymatous (degenerative) A52.19
  paresis, paretic A52.17
    juvenile A50.45
  remission in (sustained) A52.3
  serological (without symptoms) A52.2
  specified nature or site NEC A52.19
  tabes, tabetic (dorsalis) A52.11
    juvenile A50.45
  taboparesis A52.17
    juvenile A50.45
  thrombosis (cerebral) A52.05
  vascular (cerebral) NEC A52.05
Neurothekeoma — *see* Neoplasm, nerve, benign
Neurotic — *see* Neurosis
Neurotoxemia — *see* Toxemia
Neutroclusion M26.211
Neutropenia, neutropenic (chronic) (genetic) (idiopathic) (immune) (infantile) (malignant) (pernicious) (splenic) D70.9
  congenital (primary) D70.0
  cyclic D70.4
  cytoreductive cancer chemotherapy sequela D70.1
  drug-induced D70.2
    due to cytoreductive cancer chemotherapy D70.1
  due to infection D70.3
  fever D70.9
  neonatal, transitory (isoimmune) (maternal transfer) P61.5
  periodic D70.4
  secondary (cyclic) (periodic) (splenic) D70.4
    drug-induced D70.2
      due to cytoreductive cancer chemotherapy D70.1
  toxic D70.8
Neutrophilia, hereditary giant D72.0
Nevocarcinoma — *see* Melanoma
Nevus D22.9
  achromic — *see* Neoplasm, skin, benign
  amelanotic — *see* Neoplasm, skin, benign
  angiomatous D18.00
    intra-abdominal D18.03
    intracranial D18.02
    skin D18.01
    specified site NEC D18.09
  araneus I78.1
  balloon cell — *see* Neoplasm, skin, benign
  bathing trunk D48.5
  blue — *see* Neoplasm, skin, benign
    cellular — *see* Neoplasm, skin, benign
    giant — *see* Neoplasm, skin, benign
    Jadassohn's — *see* Neoplasm, skin, benign
    malignant — *see* Melanoma
  capillary D18.00
    intra-abdominal D18.03
    intracranial D18.02
    skin D18.01
    specified site NEC D18.09
  cavernous D18.00
    intra-abdominal D18.03
    intracranial D18.02
    skin D18.01
    specified site NEC D18.09
  cellular — *see* Neoplasm, skin, benign
    blue — *see* Neoplasm, skin, benign
  choroid D31.3- ☑
  comedonicus Q82.5
  conjunctiva D31.0- ☑
  dermal — *see* Neoplasm, skin, benign
    with epidermal nevus — *see* Neoplasm, skin, benign
  dysplastic — *see* Neoplasm, skin, benign
  eye D31.9- ☑
  flammeus Q82.5
  hemangiomatous D18.00
    intra-abdominal D18.03
    intracranial D18.02
    skin D18.01
    specified site NEC D18.09
  iris D31.4- ☑
  lacrimal gland D31.5- ☑
  lymphatic D18.1
  magnocellular
    specified site — *see* Neoplasm, benign, by site
    unspecified site D31.40
  malignant — *see* Melanoma
  meaning hemangioma D18.00
    intra-abdominal D18.03

Nevus — *continued*
  meaning hemangioma — *continued*
    intracranial D18.02
    skin D18.01
    specified site NEC D18.09
  mouth (mucosa) D10.30
    specified site NEC D10.39
    white sponge Q38.6
  multiplex Q85.1
  non-neoplastic I78.1
  oral mucosa D10.30
    specified site NEC D10.39
    white sponge Q38.6
  orbit D31.6- ☑
  pigmented
    giant (*see also* Neoplasm, skin, uncertain behavior) D48.5
    malignant melanoma in — *see* Melanoma
  portwine Q82.5
  retina D31.2- ☑
  retrobulbar D31.6- ☑
  sanguineous Q82.5
  senile I78.1
  skin D22.9
    abdominal wall D22.5
    ala nasi D22.39
    ankle D22.7- ☑
    anus, anal D22.5
    arm D22.6- ☑
    auditory canal (external) D22.2- ☑
    auricle (ear) D22.2- ☑
    auricular canal (external) D22.2- ☑
    axilla, axillary fold D22.5
    back D22.5
    breast D22.5
    brow D22.39
    buttock D22.5
    canthus (eye) D22.1- ☑
    cheek (external) D22.39
    chest wall D22.5
    chin D22.39
    ear (external) D22.2- ☑
    external meatus (ear) D22.2- ☑
    eyebrow D22.39
    eyelid (lower) (upper) D22.1- ☑
    face D22.30
      specified NEC D22.39
    female genital organ (external) NEC D28.0
    finger D22.6- ☑
    flank D22.5
    foot D22.7- ☑
    forearm D22.6- ☑
    forehead D22.39
    foreskin D29.0
    genital organ (external) NEC
      female D28.0
      male D29.9
    gluteal region D22.5
    groin D22.5
    hand D22.6- ☑
    heel D22.7- ☑
    helix D22.2- ☑
    hip D22.7- ☑
    interscapular region D22.5
    jaw D22.39
    knee D22.7- ☑
    labium (majus) (minus) D28.0
    leg D22.7- ☑
    lip (lower) (upper) D22.0
    lower limb D22.7- ☑
    male genital organ (external) D29.9
    nail D22.9
      finger D22.6- ☑
      toe D22.7- ☑
    nasolabial groove D22.39
    nates D22.5
    neck D22.4
    nose (external) D22.39
    palpebra D22.1- ☑
    penis D29.0
    perianal skin D22.5
    perineum D22.5
    pinna D22.2- ☑
    popliteal fossa or space D22.7- ☑
    prepuce D29.0
    pudendum D28.0
    scalp D22.4

Nevus — *continued*
  skin — *continued*
    scrotum D29.4
    shoulder D22.6- ☑
    submammary fold D22.5
    temple D22.39
    thigh D22.7- ☑
    toe D22.7- ☑
    trunk NEC D22.5
    umbilicus D22.5
    upper limb D22.6- ☑
    vulva D28.0
  specified site NEC — *see* Neoplasm, by site, benign
  spider I78.1
  stellar I78.1
  strawberry Q82.5
  Sutton's — *see* Neoplasm, skin, benign
  unius lateris Q82.5
  Unna's Q82.5
  vascular Q82.5
  verrucous Q82.5
Newborn (infant) (liveborn) (singleton) Z38.2
  abstinence syndrome P96.1
  acne L70.4
  affected by (suspected to be)
    abnormalities of membranes P02.9
      specified NEC P02.8
    abruptio placenta P02.1
    amino-acid metabolic disorder, transitory P74.8
    amniocentesis (while in utero) P00.6
    amnionitis P02.7
    apparent life threatening event (ALTE) R68.13
    bleeding (into)
      cerebral cortex P52.22
      germinal matrix P52.0
      ventricles P52.1
    breech delivery P03.0
    cardiac arrest P29.81
    cardiomyopathy I42.8
      congenital I42.4
    cerebral ischemia P91.0
    Cesarean delivery P03.4
    chemotherapy agents P04.1
    chorioamnionitis P02.7
    cocaine (crack) P04.41
    complications of labor and delivery P03.9
      specified NEC P03.89
    compression of umbilical cord NEC P02.5
    contracted pelvis P03.1
    delivery P03.9
      Cesarean P03.4
      forceps P03.2
      vacuum extractor P03.3
    entanglement (knot) in umbilical cord P02.5
    environmental chemicals P04.6
    fetal (intrauterine)
      growth retardation P05.9
      malnutrition not light or small for gestational age P05.2
    forceps delivery P03.2
    heart rate abnormalities
      bradycardia P29.12
      intrauterine P03.819
        before onset of labor P03.810
        during labor P03.811
      tachycardia P29.11
    hemorrhage (antepartum) P02.1
      cerebellar (nontraumatic) P52.6
      intracerebral (nontraumatic) P52.4
      intracranial (nontraumatic) P52.9
        specified NEC P52.8
      intraventricular (nontraumatic) P52.3
        grade 1 P52.0
        grade 2 P52.1
        grade 3 P52.21
        grade 4 P52.22
      posterior fossa (nontraumatic) P52.6
      subarachnoid (nontraumatic) P52.5
      subependymal P52.0
        with intracerebral extension P52.22
        with intraventricular extension P52.21
          with enlargment of ventricles P52.21
        without intraventricular extension P52.0
    hypoxic ischemic encephalopathy [HIE] P91.60
      mild P91.61
      moderate P91.62
      severe P91.63
    induction of labor P03.89

226

☑ Additional Character Required — Refer to the Tabular List for Character Selection   ▽ Subterms under main terms may continue to next column or page

Newborn — *continued*
  affected by — *continued*
    intestinal perforation P78.0
    intrauterine (fetal) blood loss P50.9
      due to (from)
        cut end of co-twin cord P50.5
        hemorrhage into
          co-twin P50.3
          maternal circulation P50.4
        placenta P50.2
        ruptured cord blood P50.1
        vasa previa P50.0
      specified NEC P50.8
    intrauterine (fetal) hemorrhage P50.9
    intrauterine (in utero) procedure P96.5
    malpresentation (malposition) NEC P03.1
    maternal (complication of) (use of)
      alcohol P04.3
      analgesia (maternal) P04.0
      anesthesia (maternal) P04.0
      blood loss P02.1
      circulatory disease P00.3
      condition P00.9
        specified NEC P00.89
      delivery P03.9
        Cesarean P03.4
        forceps P03.2
        vacuum extractor P03.3
      diabetes mellitus (pre-existing) P70.1
      disorder P00.9
        specified NEC P00.89
      drugs (addictive) (illegal) NEC P04.49
      ectopic pregnancy P01.4
      gestational diabetes P70.0
      hemorrhage P02.1
      hypertensive disorder P00.0
      incompetent cervix P01.0
      infectious disease P00.2
      injury P00.5
      labor and delivery P03.9
      malpresentation before labor P01.7
      maternal death P01.6
      medical procedure P00.7
      medication P04.1
      multiple pregnancy P01.5
      nutritional disorder P00.4
      oligohydramnios P01.2
      parasitic disease P00.2
      periodontal disease P00.81
      placenta previa P02.0
      polyhydramnios P01.3
      precipitate delivery P03.5
      pregnancy P01.9
        specified P01.8
      premature rupture of membranes P01.1
      renal disease P00.1
      respiratory disease P00.3
      surgical procedure P00.6
      urinary tract disease P00.1
      uterine contraction (abnormal) P03.6
    meconium peritonitis P78.0
    medication (legal) (maternal use) (prescribed) P04.1
    membrane abnormalities P02.9
      specified NEC P02.8
    membranitis P02.7
    methamphetamine(s) P04.49
    mixed metabolic and respiratory acidosis P84
    neonatal abstinence syndrome P96.1
    noxious substances transmitted via placenta or
      breast milk P04.9
      specified NEC P04.8
    nutritional supplements P04.5
    placenta previa P02.0
    placental
      abnormality (functional) (morphological)
        P02.20
        specified NEC P02.29
      dysfunction P02.29
      infarction P02.29
      insufficiency P02.29
      separation NEC P02.1
      transfusion syndromes P02.3
    placentitis P02.7
    precipitate delivery P03.5
    prolapsed cord P02.4
    respiratory arrest P28.81
    slow intrauterine growth P05.9
    tobacco P04.2

Newborn — *continued*
  affected by — *continued*
    twin to twin transplacental transfusion P02.3
    umbilical cord (tightly) around neck P02.5
    umbilical cord condition P02.60
      short cord P02.69
      specified NEC P02.69
    uterine contractions (abnormal) P03.6
    vasa previa P02.69
      from intrauterine blood loss P50.0
  apnea P28.3
    obstructive P28.4
    primary P28.3
    specified P28.4
  born in hospital Z38.00
    by cesarean Z38.01
  born outside hospital Z38.1
  breast buds P96.89
  breast engorgement P83.4
  check-up — *see* Newborn, examination
  convulsion P90
  dehydration P74.1
  examination
    8 to 28 days old Z00.111
    under 8 days old Z00.110
  fever P81.9
    environmentally-induced P81.0
  hyperbilirubinemia P59.9
    of prematurity P59.0
  hypernatremia P74.2
  hyponatremia P74.2
  infection P39.9
    candidal P37.5
    specified NEC P39.8
    urinary tract P39.3
  jaundice P59.8
    due to
      breast milk inhibitor P59.3
      hepatocellular damage P59.20
        specified NEC P59.29
      preterm delivery P59.0
    of prematurity P59.0
    specified NEC P59.8
  late metabolic acidosis P74.0
  mastitis P39.0
    infective P39.0
    noninfective P83.4
  multiple born NEC Z38.8
    born in hospital Z38.68
      by cesarean Z38.69
    born outside hospital Z38.7
  omphalitis P38.9
    with mild hemorrhage P38.1
    without hemorrhage P38.9
  post-term P08.21
  prolonged gestation (over 42 completed weeks)
    P08.22
  quadruplet Z38.8
    born in hospital Z38.63
      by cesarean Z38.64
    born outside hospital Z38.7
  quintuplet Z38.8
    born in hospital Z38.65
      by cesarean Z38.66
    born outside hospital Z38.7
  seizure P90
  sepsis (congenital) P36.9
    due to
      anaerobes NEC P36.5
      Escherichia coli P36.4
      Staphylococcus P36.30
        aureus P36.2
        specified NEC P36.39
      Streptococcus P36.10
        group B P36.0
        specified NEC P36.19
      specified NEC P36.8
  triplet Z38.8
    born in hospital Z38.61
      by cesarean Z38.62
    born outside hospital Z38.7
  twin Z38.5
    born in hospital Z38.30
      by cesarean Z38.31
    born outside hospital Z38.4
  vomiting P92.09
    bilious P92.01
  weight check Z00.111

Newcastle conjunctivitis or disease B30.8
Nezelof's syndrome (pure alymphocytosis) D81.4
Niacin (amide) **deficiency** E52
Nicolas (-Durand)-**Favre disease** A55
Nicotine — *see* Tobacco
Nicotinic acid deficiency E52
Niemann-Pick disease or syndrome E75.249
  specified NEC E75.248
  type
    A E75.240
    B E75.241
    C E75.242
    D E75.243
Night
  blindness — *see* Blindness, night
  sweats R61
  terrors (child) F51.4
Nightmares (REM sleep type) F51.5
Nipple — *see* condition
Nisbet's chancre A57
Nishimoto (-Takeuchi) **disease** I67.5
Nitritoid crisis or reaction — *see* Crisis, nitritoid
Nitrosohemoglobinemia D74.8
Njovera A65
Nocardiosis, nocardiasis A43.9
  cutaneous A43.1
  lung A43.0
  pneumonia A43.0
  pulmonary A43.0
  specified site NEC A43.8
Nocturia R35.1
  psychogenic F45.8
Nocturnal — *see* condition
Nodal rhythm I49.8
Node(s) (*see also* Nodule)
  Bouchard's (with arthropathy) M15.2
  Haygarth's M15.8
  Heberden's (with arthropathy) M15.1
  larynx J38.7
  lymph — *see* condition
  milker's B08.03
  Osler's I33.0
  Schmorl's — *see* Schmorl's disease
  singer's J38.2
  teacher's J38.2
  tuberculous — *see* Tuberculosis, lymph gland
  vocal cord J38.2
Nodule(s), **nodular**
  actinomycotic — *see* Actinomycosis
  breast NEC N63
  colloid (cystic), thyroid E04.1
  cutaneous — *see* Swelling, localized
  endometrial (stromal) D26.1
  Haygarth's M15.8
  inflammatory — *see* Inflammation
  juxta-articular
    syphilitic A52.77
    yaws A66.7
  larynx J38.7
  lung, solitary (subsegmental branch of the bronchial
    tree) R91.1
    multiple R91.8
  milker's B08.03
  prostate N40.2
    with lower urinary tract symptoms (LUTS) N40.3
    without lower urinary tract symtpoms (LUTS) N40.2
  pulmonary, solitary (subsegmental branch of the
    bronchial tree) R91.1
  retrocardiac R09.89
  rheumatoid M06.30
    ankle M06.37- ☑
    elbow M06.32- ☑
    foot joint M06.37- ☑
    hand joint M06.34- ☑
    hip M06.35- ☑
    knee M06.36- ☑
    multiple site M06.39
    shoulder M06.31- ☑
    vertebra M06.38
    wrist M06.33- ☑
  scrotum (inflammatory) N49.2
  singer's J38.2
  solitary, lung (subsegmental branch of the bronchial
    tree) R91.1
    multiple R91.8
  subcutaneous — *see* Swelling, localized
  teacher's J38.2

Nodule(s), nodular — *continued*
thyroid (cold) (gland) (nontoxic) E04.1
with thyrotoxicosis E05.20
with thyroid storm E05.21
toxic or with hyperthyroidism E05.20
with thyroid storm E05.21
vocal cord J38.2
Noma (gangrenous) (hospital) (infective) A69.0
auricle I96
mouth A69.0
pudendi N76.89
vulvae N76.89
Nomad, nomadism Z59.0
Nonautoimmune hemolytic anemia D59.4
drug-induced D59.2
Nonclosure (*see also* Imperfect, closure)
ductus arteriosus (Botallo's) Q25.0
foramen
botalli Q21.1
ovale Q21.1
Noncompliance Z91.19
with
dialysis Z91.15
dietary regimen Z91.11
medical treatment Z91.19
medication regimen NEC Z91.14
underdosing (*see also* Table of Drugs and
Chemicals, categories T36-T50, with final
character 6) Z91.14
intentional NEC Z91.128
due to financial hardship of patient
Z91.120
unintentional NEC Z91.138
due to patient's age related debility
Z91.130
renal dialysis Z91.15
Nondescent (congenital) (*see also* Malposition, congenital)
cecum Q43.3
colon Q43.3
testicle Q53.9
bilateral Q53.20
abdominal Q53.21
perineal Q53.22
unilateral Q53.10
abdominal Q53.11
perineal Q53.12
Nondevelopment
brain Q02
part of Q04.3
heart Q24.8
organ or site, congenital NEC — *see* Hypoplasia
Nonengagement
head NEC O32.4 ☑
in labor, causing obstructed labor O64.8 ☑
Nonexanthematous tick fever A93.2
Nonexpansion, lung (newborn) P28.0
Nonfunctioning
cystic duct (*see also* Disease, gallbladder) K82.8
gallbladder (*see also* Disease, gallbladder) K82.8
kidney N28.9
labyrinth — *see* subcategory H83.2 ☑
Non-Hodgkin lymphoma NEC — *see* Lymphoma, non-Hodgkin
Nonimplantation, ovum N97.2
Noninsufflation, fallopian tube N97.1
Non-ketotic hyperglycemia E72.51
Nonne-Milroy syndrome Q82.0
Nonovulation N97.0
Nonpatent fallopian tube N97.1
Nonpneumatization, lung NEC P28.0
Nonrotation — *see* Malrotation
Nonsecretion, urine — *see* Anuria
Nonunion
fracture — *see* Fracture, by site
organ or site, congenital NEC — *see* Imperfect, closure
symphysis pubis, congenital Q74.2
Nonvisualization, gallbladder R93.2
Nonvital, nonvitalized tooth K04.99
Non-working side interference M26.56
Noonan's syndrome Q87.1
Normocytic anemia (infectional) due to blood loss
(chronic) D50.0
acute D62
Norrie's disease (congenital) Q15.8
North American blastomycosis B40.9
Norwegian itch B86

Nose, nasal — *see* condition
Nosebleed R04.0
Nose-picking F98.8
Nosomania F45.21
Nosophobia F45.22
Nostalgia F43.20
Notch of iris Q13.2
Notching nose, congenital (tip) Q30.2
Nothnagel's
syndrome — *see* Strabismus, paralytic, third nerve
vasomotor acroparesthesia I73.89
Novy's relapsing fever A68.9
louse-borne A68.0
tick-borne A68.1
Noxious
foodstuffs, poisoning by — *see* Poisoning, food, noxious, plant
substances transmitted through placenta or breast
milk P04.9
Nucleus pulposus — *see* condition
Numbness R20.0
Nuns' knee — *see* Bursitis, prepatellar
Nursemaid's elbow S53.03- ☑
Nutcracker esophagus K22.4
Nutmeg liver K76.1
Nutrient element deficiency E61.9
specified NEC E61.8
Nutrition deficient or insufficient (*see also* Malnutrition) E46
due to
insufficient food T73.0 ☑
lack of
care (child) T76.02 ☑
adult T76.01 ☑
food T73.0 ☑
Nutritional stunting E45
Nyctalopia (night blindness) — *see* Blindness, night
Nycturia R35.1
psychogenic F45.8
Nymphomania F52.8
Nystagmus H55.00
benign paroxysmal — *see* Vertigo, benign paroxysmal
central positional H81.4-
congenital H55.01
dissociated H55.04
latent H55.02
miners' H55.09
positional
benign paroxysmal H81.4- ☑
central H81.4- ☑
specified form NEC H55.09
visual deprivation H55.03

O

Obermeyer's relapsing fever (European) A68.0
Obesity E66.9
with alveolar hyperventilation E66.2
adrenal E27.8
complicating
childbirth O99.214
pregnancy O99.21- ☑
puerperium O99.215
constitutional E66.8
dietary counseling and surveillance Z71.3
drug-induced E66.1
due to
drug E66.1
excess calories E66.09
morbid E66.01
severe E66.01
endocrine E66.8
endogenous E66.8
familial E66.8
glandular E66.8
hypothyroid — *see* Hypothyroidism
morbid E66.01
with alveolar hypoventilation E66.2
due to excess calories E66.01
nutritional E66.09
pituitary E23.6
severe E66.01
specified type NEC E66.8
Oblique — *see* condition
Obliteration
appendix (lumen) K38.8
artery I77.1

Obliteration — *continued*
bile duct (noncalculous) K83.1
common duct (noncalculous) K83.1
cystic duct — *see* Obstruction, gallbladder
disease, arteriolar I77.1
endometrium N85.8
eye, anterior chamber — *see* Disorder, globe, hypotony
fallopian tube N97.1
lymphatic vessel I89.0
due to mastectomy I97.2
organ or site, congenital NEC — *see* Atresia, by site
ureter N13.5
with infection N13.6
urethra — *see* Stricture, urethra
vein I87.8
vestibule (oral) K08.8
Observation (following) (for) (without need for further
medical care) Z04.9
accident NEC Z04.3
at work Z04.2
transport Z04.1
adverse effect of drug Z03.6
alleged rape or sexual assault (victim), ruled out
adult Z04.41
child Z04.42
criminal assault Z04.8
development state
adolescent Z00.3
period of rapid growth in childhood Z00.2
puberty Z00.3
disease, specified NEC Z03.89
following work accident Z04.2
growth and development state — *see* Observation,
development state
injuries (accidental) NEC (*see also* Observation, accident)
newborn (for suspected condition, ruled out) — *see* -
Newborn, affected by (suspected to be), maternal (complication of) (use of)
postpartum
immediately after delivery Z39.0
routine follow-up Z39.2
pregnancy (normal) (without complication) Z34.9- ☑
high risk O09.9- ☑
suicide attempt, alleged NEC Z03.89
self-poisoning Z03.6
suspected, ruled out (*see also* Suspected condition,
ruled out)
abuse, physical
adult Z04.71
child Z04.72
accident at work Z04.2
adult battering victim Z04.71
child battering victim Z04.72
condition NEC Z03.89
newborn — *see* Newborn, affected by (suspected to be), maternal (complication of) (use of)
drug poisoning or adverse effect Z03.6
exposure (to)
anthrax Z03.810
biological agent NEC Z03.818
inflicted injury NEC Z04.8
suicide attempt, alleged Z03.89
self-poisoning Z03.6
toxic effects from ingested substance (drug) (poison) Z03.6
toxic effects from ingested substance (drug) (poison)
Z03.6
Obsession, obsessional state F42
Obsessive-compulsive neurosis or reaction F42
Obstetric embolism, septic — *see* Embolism, obstetric,
septic
Obstetrical trauma (complicating delivery) O71.9
with or following ectopic or molar pregnancy O08.6
specified type NEC O71.89
Obstipation — *see* Constipation
Obstruction, obstructed, obstructive
airway J98.8
with
allergic alveolitis J67.9
asthma J45.909
with
exacerbation (acute) J45.901
status asthmaticus J45.902
bronchiectasis J47.9

Obstruction, obstructed, obstructive — *continued*
airway — *continued*
  with — *continued*
    bronchiectasis — *continued*
      with
        exacerbation (acute) J47.1
        lower respiratory infection J47.0
      bronchitis (chronic) J44.9
      emphysema J43.9
    chronic J44.9
      with
        allergic alveolitis — *see* Pneumonitis, hypersensitivity
        bronchiectasis J47.9
          with
            exacerbation (acute) J47.1
            lower respiratory infection J47.0
    due to
      foreign body — *see* Foreign body, by site, causing asphyxia
      inhalation of fumes or vapors J68.9
      laryngospasm J38.5
  ampulla of Vater K83.1
  aortic (heart) (valve) — *see* Stenosis, aortic
  aortoiliac I74.09
  aqueduct of Sylvius G91.1
    congenital Q03.0
      with spina bifida — *see* Spina bifida, by site, with hydrocephalus
  Arnold-Chiari — *see* Arnold-Chiari disease
  artery (*see also* Embolism, artery) I74.9
    basilar (complete) (partial) — *see* Occlusion, artery, basilar
    carotid (complete) (partial) — *see* Occlusion, artery, carotid
    cerebellar — *see* Occlusion, artery, cerebellar
    cerebral (anterior) (middle) (posterior) — *see* Occlusion, artery, cerebral
    precerebral — *see* Occlusion, artery, precerebral
    renal N28.0
    retinal NEC — *see* Occlusion, artery, retina
    vertebral (complete) (partial) — *see* Occlusion, artery, vertebral
  band (intestinal) K56.69
  bile duct or passage (common) (hepatic) (noncalculous) K83.1
    with calculus K80.51
    congenital (causing jaundice) Q44.3
  biliary (duct) (tract) K83.1
    gallbladder K82.0
  bladder-neck (acquired) N32.0
    congenital Q64.31
    due to hyperplasia (hypertrophy) of prostate — *see* Hyperplasia, prostate
  bowel — *see* Obstruction, intestine
  bronchus J98.09
  canal, ear — *see* Stenosis, external ear canal
  cardia K22.2
  caval veins (inferior) (superior) I87.1
  cecum — *see* Obstruction, intestine
  circulatory I99.8
  colon — *see* Obstruction, intestine
  common duct (noncalculous) K83.1
  coronary (artery) — *see* Occlusion, coronary
  cystic duct (*see also* Obstruction, gallbladder)
    with calculus K80.21
  device, implant or graft (*see also* Complications, by site and type, mechanical) T85.698 ☑
    arterial graft NEC — *see* Complication, cardiovascular device, mechanical, vascular
    catheter NEC T85.628 ☑
      cystostomy T83.090 ☑
      dialysis (renal) T82.49 ☑
        intraperitoneal T85.691 ☑
      infusion NEC T82.594 ☑
        spinal (epidural) (subdural) T85.690 ☑
      urinary, indwelling T83.098 ☑
    due to infection T85.79 ☑
    gastrointestinal — *see* Complications, prosthetic device, mechanical, gastrointestinal device
    genital NEC T83.498 ☑
      intrauterine contraceptive device T83.39 ☑
      penile prosthesis T83.490 ☑
    heart NEC — *see* Complication, cardiovascular device, mechanical
    joint prosthesis — *see* Complications, joint prosthesis, mechanical, specified NEC, by site

Obstruction, obstructed, obstructive — *continued*
device, implant or graft (*see also* Complications, by site and type, mechanical) — *continued*
    orthopedic NEC — *see* Complication, orthopedic, device, mechanical
    specified NEC T85.628 ☑
    urinary NEC (*see also* Complication, genitourinary, device, urinary, mechanical)
      graft T83.29 ☑
    vascular NEC — *see* Complication, cardiovascular device, mechanical
    ventricular intracranial shunt T85.09 ☑
  due to foreign body accidentally left in operative wound T81.529 ☑
  duodenum K31.5
  ejaculatory duct N50.8
  esophagus K22.2
  eustachian tube (complete) (partial) H68.10- ☑
    cartilagenous (extrinsic) H68.13- ☑
      intrinsic H68.12- ☑
    osseous H68.11- ☑
  fallopian tube (bilateral) N97.1
  fecal K56.41
    with hernia — *see* Hernia, by site, with obstruction
  foramen of Monro (congenital) Q03.8
    with spina bifida — *see* Spina bifida, by site, with hydrocephalus
  foreign body — *see* Foreign body
  gallbladder K82.0
    with calculus, stones K80.21
    congenital Q44.1
  gastric outlet K31.1
  gastrointestinal — *see* Obstruction, intestine
  hepatic K76.89
    duct (noncalculous) K83.1
  ileum — *see* Obstruction, intestine
  iliofemoral (artery) I74.5
  intestine K56.60
    with
      adhesions (intestinal) (peritoneal) K56.5
    adynamic K56.0
    by gallstone K56.3
    congenital (small) Q41.9
      large Q42.9
        specified part NEC Q42.8
    neurogenic K56.0
      Hirschsprung's disease or megacolon Q43.1
    newborn P76.9
      due to
        fecaliths P76.8
        inspissated milk P76.2
        meconium (plug) P76.0
          in mucoviscidosis E84.11
      specified NEC P76.8
    postoperative K91.3
    reflex K56.0
    specified NEC K56.69
    volvulus K56.2
  intracardiac ball valve prosthesis T82.09 ☑
  jejunum — *see* Obstruction, intestine
  joint prosthesis — *see* Complications, joint prosthesis, mechanical, specified NEC, by site
  kidney (calices) N28.89
  labor — *see* Delivery
  lacrimal (passages) (duct)
    by
      dacryolith — *see* Dacryolith
      stenosis — *see* Stenosis, lacrimal
    congenital Q10.5
    neonatal H04.53- ☑
  lacrimonasal duct — *see* Obstruction, lacrimal
  lacteal, with steatorrhea K90.2
  laryngitis — *see* Laryngitis
  larynx NEC J38.6
    congenital Q31.8
  lung J98.4
    disease, chronic J44.9
  lymphatic I89.0
  meconium (plug)
    newborn P76.0
      due to fecaliths P76.0
      in mucoviscidosis E84.11
  mitral — *see* Stenosis, mitral
  nasal J34.89
  nasolacrimal duct (*see also* Obstruction, lacrimal)
    congenital Q10.5
  nasopharynx J39.2
  nose J34.89

Obstruction, obstructed, obstructive — *continued*
organ or site, congenital NEC — *see* Atresia, by site
pancreatic duct K86.8
parotid duct or gland K11.8
pelviureteral junction N13.5
  congenital Q62.39
pharynx J39.2
portal (circulation) (vein) I81
prostate (*see also* Hyperplasia, prostate)
  valve (urinary) N32.0
pulmonary valve (heart) I37.0
pyelonephritis (chronic) N11.1
pylorus
  adult K31.1
  congenital or infantile Q40.0
rectosigmoid — *see* Obstruction, intestine
rectum K62.4
renal N28.89
  outflow N13.8
  pelvis, congenital Q62.39
respiratory J98.8
  chronic J44.9
retinal (vessels) H34.9
salivary duct (any) K11.8
  with calculus K11.5
sigmoid — *see* Obstruction, intestine
sinus (accessory) (nasal) J34.89
Stensen's duct K11.8
stomach NEC K31.89
  acute K31.0
  congenital Q40.2
  due to pylorospasm K31.3
submandibular duct K11.8
submaxillary gland K11.8
  with calculus K11.5
thoracic duct I89.0
thrombotic — *see* Thrombosis
trachea J39.8
tracheostomy airway J95.03
tricuspid (valve) — *see* Stenosis, tricuspid
upper respiratory, congenital Q34.8
ureter (functional) (pelvic junction) NEC N13.5
  with
    hydronephrosis N13.1
      with infection N13.6
    pyelonephritis (chronic) N11.1
  congenital Q62.39
  due to calculus — *see* Calculus, ureter
urethra NEC N36.8
  congenital Q64.39
urinary (moderate) N13.9
  due to hyperplasia (hypertrophy) of prostate — *see* Hyperplasia, prostate
  organ or tract (lower) N13.9
  prostatic valve N32.0
  specified NEC N13.8
uropathy N13.9
uterus N85.8
vagina N89.5
valvular — *see* Endocarditis
vein, venous I87.1
  caval (inferior) (superior) I87.1
  thrombotic — *see* Thrombosis
vena cava (inferior) (superior) I87.1
vesical NEC N32.0
vesicourethral orifice N32.0
  congenital Q64.31
vessel NEC I99.8
Obturator — *see* condition
Occlusal wear, teeth K03.0
Occlusio pupillae — *see* Membrane, pupillary
Occlusion, occluded
anus K62.4
  congenital Q42.3
    with fistula Q42.2
aortoiliac (chronic) I74.09
aqueduct of Sylvius G91.1
  congenital Q03.0
    with spina bifida — *see* Spina bifida, by site, with hydrocephalus
artery (*see also* Embolism, artery) I74.9
  auditory, internal I65.8
  basilar I65.1
    with
      infarction I63.22
        due to
          embolism I63.12
          thrombosis I63.02

Occlusion, occluded — *continued*
artery (*see also* Embolism, artery) — *continued*
  brain or cerebral I66.9
    with infarction (due to) I63.5 ☑
      embolism I63.4 ☑
      thrombosis I63.3 ☑
  carotid I65.2- ☑
    with
      infarction I63.23- ☑
        due to
          embolism I63.13- ☑
          thrombosis I63.03- ☑
  cerebellar (anterior inferior) (posterior inferior)
      (superior) I66.3
    with infarction I63.54- ☑
      due to
        embolism I63.44- ☑
        thrombosis I63.34- ☑
  cerebral I66.9
    with infarction I63.50
      due to
        embolism I63.40
          specified NEC I63.49
        thrombosis I63.30
          specified NEC I63.39
  anterior I66.1- ☑
    with infarction I63.52- ☑
      due to
        embolism I63.42- ☑
        thrombosis I63.32- ☑
  middle I66.0- ☑
    with infarction I63.51- ☑
      due to
        embolism I63.41- ☑
        thrombosis I63.31- ☑
  posterior I66.2- ☑
    with infarction I63.53- ☑
      due to
        embolism I63.43- ☑
        thrombosis I63.33- ☑
  specified NEC I66.8
    with infarction I63.59
      due to
        embolism I63.4 ☑
        thrombosis I63.3 ☑
  choroidal (anterior) — *see* Occlusion, artery, pre-
      cerebral, specified NEC
  communicating posterior — *see* Occlusion, artery,
      cerebral, specified NEC
  complete
    coronary I25.82
    extremities I70.92
  coronary (acute) (thrombotic) (without myocardial
      infarction) I24.0
    with myocardial infarction — *see* Infarction,
        myocardium
    chronic total I25.82
    complete I25.82
    healed or old I25.2
    total (chronic) I25.82
  hypophyseal — *see* Occlusion, artery, precerebral,
      specified NEC
  iliac I74.5
  lower extremities due to stenosis or stricture I77.1
  mesenteric (embolic) (thrombotic) K55.0
  perforating — *see* Occlusion, artery, cerebral,
      specified NEC
  peripheral I77.9
    thrombotic or embolic I74.4
  pontine — *see* Occlusion, artery, cerebral, specified
      NEC
  precerebral I65.9
    with infarction I63.20
      due to
        embolism I63.10
          specified NEC I63.19
        thrombosis I63.00
          specified NEC I63.09
    specified NEC I63.29
  basilar — *see* Occlusion, artery, basilar
  carotid — *see* Occlusion, artery, carotid
  puerperal O88.23
  specified NEC I65.8
    with infarction I63.29
      due to
        embolism I63.19
        thrombosis I63.00

Occlusion, occluded — *continued*
artery (*see also* Embolism, artery) — *continued*
  precerebral — *continued*
    vertebral — *see* Occlusion, artery, vertebral
  renal N28.0
  retinal
    branch H34.23- ☑
    central H34.1- ☑
    partial H34.21- ☑
    transient H34.0- ☑
  spinal — *see* Occlusion, artery, precerebral, verte-
      bral
  total (chronic)
    coronary I25.82
    extremities I70.92
  vertebral I65.0- ☑
    with
      infarction I63.21- ☑
        due to
          embolism I63.11- ☑
          thrombosis I63.01- ☑
basilar artery — *see* Occlusion, artery, basilar
bile duct (common) (hepatic) (noncalculous) K83.1
bowel — *see* Obstruction, intestine
carotid (artery) (common) (internal) — *see* Occlusion,
    artery, carotid
centric (of teeth) M26.59
  maximum intercuspation discrepancy M26.55
cerebellar (artery) — *see* Occlusion, artery, cerebellar
cerebral (artery) — *see* Occlusion, artery, cerebral
cerebrovascular (*see also* Occlusion, artery, cerebral)
  with infarction I63.5
cervical canal — *see* Stricture, cervix
cervix (uteri) — *see* Stricture, cervix
choanal Q30.0
choroidal (artery) — *see* Occlusion, artery, precerebral,
    specified NEC
colon — *see* Obstruction, intestine
communicating posterior artery — *see* Occlusion,
    artery, precerebral, specified NEC
coronary (artery) (vein) (thrombotic) (*see also* Infarct,
    myocardium)
  chronic total I25.82
  healed or old I25.2
  not resulting in infarction I24.0
  total (chronic) I25.82
cystic duct — *see* Obstruction, gallbladder
embolic — *see* Embolism
fallopian tube N97.1
  congenital Q50.6
gallbladder (*see also* Obstruction, gallbladder)
  congenital (causing jaundice) Q44.1
gingiva, traumatic K06.2
hymen N89.6
  congenital Q52.3
hypophyseal (artery) — *see* Occlusion, artery, precere-
    bral, specified NEC
iliac artery I74.5
intestine — *see* Obstruction, intestine
lacrimal passages — *see* Obstruction, lacrimal
lung J98.4
lymph or lymphatic channel I89.0
mammary duct N64.89
mesenteric artery (embolic) (thrombotic) K55.0
nose J34.89
  congenital Q30.0
organ or site, congenital NEC — *see* Atresia, by site
oviduct N97.1
  congenital Q50.6
peripheral arteries
  due to stricture or stenosis I77.1
  upper extremity I74.4
pontine (artery) — *see* Occlusion, artery, precerebral,
    specified NEC
posterior lingual, of mandibular teeth M26.29
precerebral artery — *see* Occlusion, artery, precerebral
punctum lacrimale — *see* Obstruction, lacrimal
pupil — *see* Membrane, pupillary
pylorus, adult (*see also* Stricture, pylorus) K31.1
renal artery N28.0
retina, retinal
  artery — *see* Occlusion, artery, retinal
  vein (central) H34.81- ☑
    engorgement H34.82- ☑
    tributary H34.83- ☑
  vessels H34.9

Occlusion, occluded — *continued*
  spinal artery — *see* Occlusion, artery, precerebral,
      vertebral
  teeth (mandibular) (posterior lingual) M26.29
  thoracic duct I89.0
  thrombotic — *see* Thrombosis, artery
  traumatic
    edentulous (alveolar) ridge K06.2
    gingiva K06.2
    periodontal K05.5
  tubal N97.1
  ureter (complete) (partial) N13.5
    congenital Q62.10
  ureteropelvic junction N13.5
    congenital Q62.11
  ureterovesical orifice N13.5
    congenital Q62.12
  urethra — *see* Stricture, urethra
  uterus N85.8
  vagina N89.5
  vascular NEC I99.8
  vein — *see* Thrombosis
    retinal — *see* Occlusion, retinal, vein
  vena cava (inferior) (superior) — *see* Embolism, vena
      cava
  ventricle (brain) NEC G91.1
  vertebral (artery) — *see* Occlusion, artery, vertebral
  vessel (blood) I99.8
  vulva N90.5
Occult
  blood in feces (stools) R19.5
Occupational
  problems NEC Z56.89
Ochlophobia — *see* Agoraphobia
Ochronosis (endogenous) E70.29
Ocular muscle — *see* condition
Oculogyric crisis or disturbance H51.8
  psychogenic F45.8
Oculomotor syndrome H51.9
Oculopathy
  syphilitic NEC A52.71
    congenital
      early A50.01
      late A50.30
    early (secondary) A51.43
    late A52.71
Oddi's sphincter spasm K83.4
Odontalgia K08.8
Odontoameloblastoma — *see* Cyst, calcifying odonto-
    genic
Odontoclasia K03.89
Odontodysplasia, regional K00.4
Odontogenesis imperfecta K00.5
Odontoma (ameloblastic) (complex) (compound) (fi-
    broameloblastic) — *see* Cyst, calcifying odontogenic
Odontomyelitis (closed) (open) K04.0
Odontorrhagia K08.8
Odontosarcoma, ameloblastic C41.1
  upper jaw (bone) C41.0
Oestriasis — *see* Myiasis
Oguchi's disease H53.63
Ohara's disease — *see* Tularemia
Oidiomycosis — *see* Candidiasis
Oidium albicans infection — *see* Candidiasis
Old age (without mention of debility) R54
  dementia F03 ☑
Old (previous) **myocardial infarction** I25.2
Olfactory — *see* condition
Oligemia — *see* Anemia
Oligoastrocytoma
  specified site — *see* Neoplasm, malignant, by site
  unspecified site C71.9
Oligocythemia D64.9
Oligodendroblastoma
  specified site — *see* Neoplasm, malignant
  unspecified site C71.9
Oligodendroglioma
  anaplastic type
    specified site — *see* Neoplasm, malignant, by site
    unspecified site C71.9
  specified site — *see* Neoplasm, malignant, by site
  unspecified site C71.9
Oligodontia — *see* Anodontia
Oligoencephalon Q02
Oligohidrosis L74.4
Oligohydramnios O41.0- ☑
Oligohydrosis L74.4

Oligomenorrhea N91.5
  primary N91.3
  secondary N91.4
Oligophrenia (*see also* Disability, intellectual)
  phenylpyruvic E70.0
Oligospermia N46.11
  due to
    drug therapy N46.121
    efferent duct obstruction N46.123
    infection N46.122
    radiation N46.124
    specified cause NEC N46.129
    systemic disease N46.125
Oligotrichia — *see* Alopecia
Oliguria R34
  postprocedural N99.0
  with, complicating or following ectopic or molar
    pregnancy O08.4
Ollier's disease Q78.4
Omenotocele — *see* Hernia, abdomen, specified site
  NEC
Omentitis — *see* Peritonitis
Omentum, omental — *see* condition
Omphalitis (congenital) (newborn) P38.9
  with mild hemorrhage P38.1
  without hemorrhage P38.9
  not of newborn L08.82
  tetanus A33
Omphalocele Q79.2
Omphalomesenteric duct, persistent Q43.0
Omphalorrhagia, newborn P51.9
Omsk hemorrhagic fever A98.1
Onanism (excessive) F98.8
Onchocerciasis, onchocercosis B73.1
  with
    eye disease B73.00
      endophthalmitis B73.01
      eyelid B73.09
      glaucoma B73.02
      specified NEC B73.09
    eyelid B73.09
    eye NEC B73.00
Oncocytoma — *see* Neoplasm, benign, by site
Oncovirus, as cause of disease classified elsewhere
  B97.32
Ondine's curse — *see* Apnea, sleep
Oneirophrenia F23
Onychauxis L60.2
  congenital Q84.5
Onychia (*see also* Cellulitis, digit)
  with lymphangitis — *see* Lymphangitis, acute, digit
  candidal B37.2
  dermatophytic B35.1
Onychitis (*see also* Cellulitis, digit)
  with lymphangitis — *see* Lymphangitis, acute, digit
Onychocryptosis L60.0
Onychodystrophy L60.3
  congenital Q84.6
Onychogryphosis, onychogryposis L60.2
Onycholysis L60.1
Onychomadesis L60.8
Onychomalacia L60.3
Onychomycosis (finger) (toe) B35.1
Onycho-osteodysplasia Q79.8
Onychophagia F98.8
Onychophosis L60.8
Onychoptosis L60.8
Onychorrhexis L60.3
  congenital Q84.6
Onychoschizia L60.3
Onyxis (finger) (toe) L60.0
Onyxitis (*see also* Cellulitis, digit)
  with lymphangitis — *see* Lymphangitis, acute, digit
Oophoritis (cystic) (infectional) (interstitial) N70.92
  with salpingitis N70.93
  acute N70.02
    with salpingitis N70.03
  chronic N70.12
    with salpingitis N70.13
  complicating abortion — *see* Abortion, by type, com-
    plicated by, oophoritis
Oophorocele N83.4
Opacity, opacities
  cornea H17.- ☑
    central H17.1- ☑
    congenital Q13.3
    degenerative — *see* Degeneration, cornea

Opacity, opacities — *continued*
  cornea — *continued*
    hereditary — *see* Dystrophy, cornea
    inflammatory — *see* Keratitis
    minor H17.81- ☑
    peripheral H17.82- ☑
    sequelae of trachoma (healed) B94.0
    specified NEC H17.89
  enamel (teeth) (fluoride) (nonfluoride) K00.3
  lens — *see* Cataract
  snowball — *see* Deposit, crystalline
  vitreous (humor) NEC H43.39- ☑
    congenital Q14.0
    membranes and strands H43.31- ☑
Opalescent dentin (hereditary) K00.5
Open, opening
  abnormal, organ or site, congenital — *see* Imperfect,
    closure
  angle with
    borderline
      findings
        high risk H40.02- ☑
        low risk H40.01- ☑
      intraocular pressure H40.00- ☑
    cupping of discs H40.01- ☑
    glaucoma (primary) — *see* Glaucoma, open angle
  bite
    anterior M26.220
    posterior M26.221
  false — *see* Imperfect, closure
  margin on tooth restoration K08.51
  restoration margins of tooth K08.51
  wound — *see* Wound, open
Operational fatigue F48.8
Operative — *see* condition
Operculitis — *see* Periodontitis
Operculum — *see* Break, retina
Ophiasis L63.2
Ophthalmia (*see also* Conjunctivitis) H10.9
  actinic rays — *see* Photokeratitis
  allergic (acute) — *see* Conjunctivitis, acute, atopic
  blennorrhagic (gonococcal) (neonatorum) A54.31
  diphtheritic A36.86
  Egyptian A71.1
  electrica — *see* Photokeratitis
  gonococcal (neonatorum) A54.31
  metastatic — *see* Endophthalmitis, purulent
  migraine — *see* Migraine, ophthalmoplegic
  neonatorum, newborn P39.1
    gonococcal A54.31
  nodosa H16.24- ☑
  purulent — *see* Conjunctivitis, acute, mucopurulent
  spring — *see* Conjunctivitis, acute, atopic
  sympathetic — *see* Uveitis, sympathetic
Ophthalmitis — *see* Ophthalmia
Ophthalmocele (congenital) Q15.8
Ophthalmoneuromyelitis G36.0
Ophthalmoplegia (*see also* Strabismus, paralytic)
  anterior internuclear — *see* Ophthalmoplegia, inter-
    nuclear
  ataxia-areflexia G61.0
  diabetic — *see* E08-E13 with .39
  exophthalmic E05.00
    with thyroid storm E05.01
  external H49.88- ☑
    progressive H49.4- ☑
      with pigmentary retinopathy — *see* Kearns-
        Sayre syndrome
    total H49.3- ☑
  internal (complete) (total) H52.51- ☑
  internuclear H51.2- ☑
  migraine — *see* Migraine, ophthalmoplegic
  Parinaud's H49.88- ☑
  progressive external — *see* Ophthalmoplegia, external,
    progressive
  supranuclear, progressive G23.1
  total (external) — *see* Ophthalmoplegia, external, total
Opioid(s)
  abuse — *see* Abuse, drug, opioids
  dependence — *see* Dependence, drug, opioids
Opisthognathism M26.09
Opisthorchiasis (felineus) (viverrini) B66.0
Opitz' disease D73.2
Opiumism — *see* Dependence, drug, opioid
Oppenheim's disease G70.2
Oppenheim-Urbach disease (necrobiosis lipoidica dia-
  beticorum) — *see* E08-E13 with .620

Optic nerve — *see* condition
Orbit — *see* condition
Orchioblastoma C62.9- ☑
Orchitis (gangrenous) (nonspecific) (septic) (suppurative)
  N45.2
  blennorrhagic (gonococcal) (acute) (chronic) A54.23
  chlamydial A56.19
  filarial (*see also* Infestation, filarial) B74.9 [N51]
  gonococcal (acute) (chronic) A54.23
  mumps B26.0
  syphilitic A52.76
  tuberculous A18.15
Orf (virus disease) B08.02
Organic (*see also* condition)
  brain syndrome F09
  heart — *see* Disease, heart
  mental disorder F09
  psychosis F09
Orgasm
  anejaculatory N53.13
Oriental
  bilharziasis B65.2
  schistosomiasis B65.2
Orifice — *see* condition
Origin of both great vessels from right ventricle
  Q20.1
Ormond's disease (with ureteral obstruction) N13.5
  with infection N13.6
Ornithine metabolism disorder E72.4
Ornithinemia (Type I) (Type II) E72.4
Ornithosis A70
Orotaciduria, oroticaciduria (congenital) (hereditary)
  (pyrimidine deficiency) E79.8
  anemia D53.0
Orthodontics
  adjustment Z46.4
  fitting Z46.4
Orthopnea R06.01
Orthopoxvirus B08.09
  specified NEC B08.09
Os, uterus — *see* condition
Osgood-Schlatter disease or osteochondrosis — *see*
  Osteochondrosis, juvenile, tibia
Osler (-Weber)-**Rendu disease** I78.0
Osler's nodes I33.0
Osmidrosis L75.0
Osseous — *see* condition
Ossification
  artery — *see* Arteriosclerosis
  auricle (ear) — *see* Disorder, pinna, specified type NEC
  bronchial J98.09
  cardiac — *see* Degeneration, myocardial
  cartilage (senile) — *see* Disorder, cartilage, specified
    type NEC
  coronary (artery) — *see* Disease, heart, ischemic,
    atherosclerotic
  diaphragm J98.6
  ear, middle — *see* Otosclerosis
  falx cerebri G96.19
  fontanel, premature Q75.0
  heart (*see also* Degeneration, myocardial)
    valve — *see* Endocarditis
  larynx J38.7
  ligament — *see* Disorder, tendon, specified type NEC
    posterior longitudinal — *see* Spondylopathy,
      specified NEC
  meninges (cerebral) (spinal) G96.19
  multiple, eccentric centers — *see* Disorder, bone, de-
    velopment or growth
  muscle (*see also* Calcification, muscle)
    due to burns — *see* Myositis, ossificans, in, burns
    paralytic — *see* Myositis, ossificans, in, quadriplegia
    progressive — *see* Myositis, ossificans, progressiva
    specified NEC M61.50
      ankle M61.57- ☑
      foot M61.57- ☑
      forearm M61.53- ☑
      hand M61.54- ☑
      lower leg M61.56- ☑
      multiple sites M61.59
      pelvic region M61.55- ☑
      shoulder region M61.51- ☑
      specified site NEC M61.58
      thigh M61.55- ☑
      upper arm M61.52- ☑
    traumatic — *see* Myositis, ossificans, traumatica

Ossification — Osteochondropathy

Ossification — *continued*
  myocardium, myocardial — *see* Degeneration, myocardial
  penis N48.89
  periarticular — *see* Disorder, joint, specified type NEC
  pinna — *see* Disorder, pinna, specified type NEC
  rider's bone — *see* Ossification, muscle, specified NEC
  sclera H15.89
  subperiosteal, post-traumatic M89.8X- ☑
  tendon — *see* Disorder, tendon, specified type NEC
  trachea J39.8
  tympanic membrane — *see* Disorder, tympanic membrane, specified NEC
  vitreous (humor) — *see* Deposit, crystalline
Osteitis (*see also* Osteomyelitis)
  alveolar M27.3
  condensans M85.30
    ankle M85.37- ☑
    foot M85.37- ☑
    forearm M85.33- ☑
    hand M85.34- ☑
    lower leg M85.36- ☑
    multiple site M85.39
    neck M85.38
    rib M85.38
    shoulder M85.31- ☑
    skull M85.38
    specified site NEC M85.38
    thigh M85.35- ☑
    toe M85.37- ☑
    upper arm M85.32- ☑
    vertebra M85.38
  deformans M88.9
    in (due to)
      malignant neoplasm of bone C41.9 [M90.60]
      neoplastic disease (*see also* Neoplasm) D49.9 [M90.60]
        carpus D49.9 [M90.64-] ☑
        clavicle D49.9 [M90.61-] ☑
        femur D49.9 [M90.65-] ☑
        fibula D49.9 [M90.66-] ☑
        finger D49.9 [M90.64-] ☑
        humerus D49.9 [M90.62-] ☑
        ilium D49.9 [M90.65-] ☑
        ischium D49.9 [M90.65-] ☑
        metacarpus D49.9 [M90.64-] ☑
        metatarsus D49.9 [M90.67-] ☑
        multiple sites D49.9 [M90.69]
        neck D49.9 [M90.68]
        radius D49.9 [M90.63-] ☑
        rib D49.9 [M90.68]
        scapula D49.9 [M90.61-] ☑
        skull D49.9 [M90.68]
        tarsus D49.9 [M90.67-] ☑
        tibia D49.9 [M90.66-] ☑
        toe D49.9 [M90.67-] ☑
        ulna D49.9 [M90.63-] ☑
        vertebra D49.9 [M90.68]
    skull M88.0
    specified NEC — *see* Paget's disease, bone, by site
    vertebra M88.1
  due to yaws A66.6
  fibrosa NEC — *see* Cyst, bone, by site
    circumscripta — *see* Dysplasia, fibrous, bone NEC
    cystica (generalisata) E21.0
    disseminata Q78.1
    osteoplastica E21.0
  fragilitans Q78.0
  Garr's (sclerosing) — *see* Osteomyelitis, specified type NEC
  jaw (acute) (chronic) (lower) (suppurative) (upper) M27.2
  parathyroid E21.0
  petrous bone (acute) (chronic) — *see* Petrositis
  sclerotic, nonsuppurative — *see* Osteomyelitis, specified type NEC
  tuberculosa A18.09
    cystica D86.89
    multiplex cystoides D86.89
Osteoarthritis M19.90
  ankle M19.07- ☑
  elbow M19.02- ☑
  foot joint M19.07- ☑
  generalized M15.9
    erosive M15.4
    primary M15.0
    specified NEC M15.8

Osteoarthritis — *continued*
  hand joint M19.04- ☑
    first carpometacarpal joint M18.9
  hip M16.1- ☑
    bilateral M16.0
    due to hip dysplasia (unilateral) M16.3- ☑
      bilateral M16.2
  interphalangeal
    distal (Heberden) M15.1
    proximal (Bouchard) M15.2
  knee M17.9
    bilateral M17.0
  post-traumatic NEC M19.92
    ankle M19.17- ☑
    elbow M19.12- ☑
    foot joint M19.17- ☑
    hand joint M19.14- ☑
      first carpometacarpal joint M18.3- ☑
        bilateral M18.2
    hip M16.5- ☑
      bilateral M16.4
    knee M17.3- ☑
      bilateral M17.2
    shoulder M19.11- ☑
    wrist M19.13- ☑
  primary M19.91
    ankle M19.07- ☑
    elbow M19.02- ☑
    foot joint M19.07- ☑
    hand joint M19.04- ☑
      first carpometacarpal joint M18.1- ☑
        bilateral M18.0
    hip M16.1- ☑
      bilateral M16.0 ✓
    knee M17.1- ☑
      bilateral M17.0
    shoulder M19.01- ☑
    spine — *see* Spondylosis
    wrist M19.03- ☑
  secondary M19.93
    ankle M19.27- ☑
    elbow M19.22- ☑
    foot joint M19.27- ☑
    hand joint M19.24- ☑
      first carpometacarpal joint M18.5- ☑
        bilateral M18.4
    hip M16.7
      bilateral M16.6
    knee M17.5
      bilateral M17.4
    multiple M15.3
    shoulder M19.21- ☑
    spine — *see* Spondylosis
    wrist M19.23- ☑
  shoulder M19.01- ☑
  spine — *see* Spondylosis
  wrist M19.03- ☑
Osteoarthropathy (hypertrophic) M19.90
  ankle — *see* Osteoarthritis, primary, ankle
  elbow — *see* Osteoarthritis, primary, elbow
  foot joint — *see* Osteoarthritis, primary, foot
  hand joint — *see* Osteoarthritis, primary, hand joint
  knee joint — *see* Osteoarthritis, primary, knee
  multiple site — *see* Osteoarthritis, primary, multiple joint
  pulmonary (*see also* Osteoarthropathy, specified type NEC)
    hypertrophic — *see* Osteoarthropathy, hypertrophic, specified type NEC
  secondary — *see* Osteoarthropathy, specified type NEC
  secondary hypertrophic — *see* Osteoarthropathy, specified type NEC
  shoulder — *see* Osteoarthritis, primary, shoulder
  specified joint NEC — *see* Osteoarthritis, primary, specified joint NEC
  specified type NEC M89.40
    carpus M89.44- ☑
    clavicle M89.41- ☑
    femur M89.45- ☑
    fibula M89.46- ☑
    finger M89.44- ☑
    humerus M89.42- ☑
    ilium M89.459
    ischium M89.459
    metacarpus M89.44- ☑

Osteoarthropathy — *continued*
  specified type — *continued*
    metatarsus M89.47- ☑
    multiple sites M89.49
    neck M89.48
    radius M89.43- ☑
    rib M89.48
    scapula M89.41- ☑
    skull M89.48
    tarsus M89.47- ☑
    tibia M89.46- ☑
    toe M89.47- ☑
    ulna M89.43- ☑
    vertebra M89.48
  spine — *see* Spondylosis
  wrist — *see* Osteoarthritis, primary, wrist
Osteoarthrosis (degenerative) (hypertrophic) (joint) (*see also* Osteoarthritis)
  deformans alkaptonurica E70.29 [M36.8]
  erosive M15.4
  generalized M15.9
    primary M15.0
  polyarticular M15.9
  spine — *see* Spondylosis
Osteoblastoma — *see* Neoplasm, bone, benign
  aggressive — *see* Neoplasm, bone, uncertain behavior
Osteochondritis (*see also* Osteochondropathy, by site)
  Brailsford's — *see* Osteochondrosis, juvenile, radius
  dissecans M93.20
    ankle M93.27- ☑
    elbow M93.22- ☑
    foot M93.27- ☑
    hand M93.24- ☑
    hip M93.25- ☑
    knee M93.26- ☑
    multiple sites M93.29
    shoulder joint M93.21- ☑
    specified site NEC M93.28
    wrist M93.23- ☑
  juvenile M92.9
    patellar — *see* Osteochondrosis, juvenile, patella
  syphilitic (congenital) (early) A50.02 [M90.80]
    ankle A50.02 [M90.87-] ☑
    elbow A50.02 [M90.82-] ☑
    foot A50.02 [M90.87-] ☑
    forearm A50.02 [M90.83-] ☑
    hand A50.02 [M90.84-] ☑
    hip A50.02 [M90.85-] ☑
    knee A50.02 [M90.86-] ☑
    multiple sites A50.02 [M90.89]
    shoulder joint A50.02 [M90.81-] ☑
    specified site NEC A50.02 [M90.88]
Osteochondroarthrosis deformans endemica — *see* Disease, Kaschin-Beck
Osteochondrodysplasia Q78.9
  with defects of growth of tubular bones and spine Q77.9
    specified NEC Q77.8
  specified NEC Q78.8
Osteochondrodystrophy E78.9
Osteochondrolysis — *see* Osteochondritis, dissecans
Osteochondroma — *see* Neoplasm, bone, benign
Osteochondromatosis D48.0
  syndrome Q78.4
Osteochondromyxosarcoma — *see* Neoplasm, bone, malignant
Osteochondropathy M93.90
  ankle M93.97- ☑
  elbow M93.92- ☑
  foot M93.97- ☑
  hand M93.94- ☑
  hip M93.95- ☑
  Kienböck's disease of adults M93.1
  knee M93.96- ☑
  multiple joints M93.99
  osteochondritis dissecans — *see* Osteochondritis, dissecans
  osteochondrosis — *see* Osteochondrosis
  shoulder region M93.91- ☑
  slipped upper femoral epiphysis — *see* Slipped, epiphysis, upper femoral
  specified joint NEC M93.98
  specified type NEC M93.80
    ankle M93.87- ☑
    elbow M93.82- ☑
    foot M93.87- ☑

Osteochondropathy — continued
  specified type — continued
    hand M93.84- ☑
    hip M93.85- ☑
    knee M93.86- ☑
    multiple joints M93.89
    shoulder region M93.81- ☑
    specified joint NEC M93.88
    wrist M93.83- ☑
  syphilitic, congenital
    early A50.02 [M90.80]
    late A50.56 [M90.80]
  wrist M93.93- ☑
Osteochondrosarcoma — see Neoplasm, bone, malignant
Osteochondrosis (see also Osteochondropathy, by site)
  acetabulum (juvenile) M91.0
  adult — see Osteochondropathy, specified type NEC, by site
  astragalus (juvenile) — see Osteochondrosis, juvenile, tarsus
  Blount's — see Osteochondrosis, juvenile, tibia
  Buchanan's M91.0
  Burns' — see Osteochondrosis, juvenile, ulna
  calcaneus (juvenile) — see Osteochondrosis, juvenile, tarsus
  capitular epiphysis (femur) (juvenile) — see Legg-Calvé-Perthes disease
  carpal (juvenile) (lunate) (scaphoid) — see Osteochondrosis, juvenile, hand, carpal lunate
    adult M93.1
  coxae juvenilis — see Legg-Calvé-Perthes disease
  deformans juvenilis, coxae — see Legg-Calvé-Perthes disease
  Diaz's — see Osteochondrosis, juvenile, tarsus
  dissecans (knee) (shoulder) — see Osteochondritis, dissecans
  femoral capital epiphysis (juvenile) — see Legg-Calvé-Perthes disease
  femur (head), juvenile — see Legg-Calvé-Perthes disease
  fibula (juvenile) — see Osteochondrosis, juvenile, fibula
  foot NEC (juvenile) M92.8
  Freiberg's — see Osteochondrosis, juvenile, metatarsus
  Haas' (juvenile) — see Osteochondrosis, juvenile, humerus
  Haglund's — see Osteochondrosis, juvenile, tarsus
  hip (juvenile) — see Legg-Calvé-Perthes disease
  humerus (capitulum) (head) (juvenile) — see Osteochondrosis, juvenile, humerus
  ilium, iliac crest (juvenile) M91.0
  ischiopubic synchondrosis M91.0
  Iselin's — see Osteochondrosis, juvenile, metatarsus
  juvenile, juvenilis M92.9
    after congenital dislocation of hip reduction — see Osteochondrosis, juvenile, hip, specified NEC
    arm — see Osteochondrosis, juvenile, upper limb NEC
    capitular epiphysis (femur) — see Legg-Calvé-Perthes disease
    clavicle, sternal epiphysis — see Osteochondrosis, juvenile, upper limb NEC
    coxae — see Legg-Calvé-Perthes disease
    deformans M92.9
    fibula M92.5- ☑
    foot NEC M92.8
    hand M92.20- ☑
      carpal lunate M92.21- ☑
      metacarpal head M92.22- ☑
      specified site NEC M92.29- ☑
    head of femur — see Legg-Calvé-Perthes disease
    hip and pelvis M91.9- ☑
      coxa plana — see Coxa, plana
      femoral head — see Legg-Calvé-Perthes disease
      pelvis M91.0
      pseudocoxalgia — see Pseudocoxalgia
      specified NEC M91.8- ☑
    humerus M92.0- ☑
    limb
      lower NEC M92.8
      upper NEC — see Osteochondrosis, juvenile, upper limb NEC
    medial cuneiform bone — see Osteochondrosis, juvenile, tarsus
    metatarsus M92.7- ☑
    patella M92.4- ☑

Osteochondrosis — continued
  juvenile, juvenilis — continued
    radius M92.1- ☑
    specified site NEC M92.8
    spine M42.00
      cervical region M42.02
      cervicothoracic region M42.03
      lumbar region M42.06
      lumbosacral region M42.07
      multiple sites M42.09
      occipito-atlanto-axial region M42.01
      sacrococcygeal region M42.08
      thoracic region M42.04
      thoracolumbar region M42.05
    tarsus M92.6- ☑
    tibia M92.5- ☑
    ulna M92.1- ☑
    upper limb NEC M92.3- ☑
    vertebra (body) (epiphyseal plates) (Calvé's) (Scheuermann's) — see Osteochondrosis, juvenile, spine
  Kienböck's — see Osteochondrosis, juvenile, hand, carpal lunate
    adult M93.1
  Köhler's
    patellar — see Osteochondrosis, juvenile, patella
    tarsal navicular — see Osteochondrosis, juvenile, tarsus
  Legg-Perthes (-Calvé)(-Waldenström) — see Legg-Calvé-Perthes disease
  limb
    lower NEC (juvenile) M92.8
    upper NEC (juvenile) — see Osteochondrosis, juvenile, upper limb NEC
  lunate bone (carpal) (juvenile) (see also Osteochondrosis, juvenile, hand, carpal lunate)
    adult M93.1
  Mauclaire's — see Osteochondrosis, juvenile, hand, metacarpal
  metacarpal (head) (juvenile) — see Osteochondrosis, juvenile, hand, metacarpal
  metatarsus (fifth) (head) (juvenile) (second) — see Osteochondrosis, juvenile, metatarsus
  navicular (juvenile) — see Osteochondrosis, juvenile, tarsus
  os
    calcis (juvenile) — see Osteochondrosis, juvenile, tarsus
    tibiale externum (juvenile) — see Osteochondrosis, juvenile, tarsus
  Osgood-Schlatter — see Osteochondrosis, juvenile, tibia
  Panner's — see Osteochondrosis, juvenile, humerus
  patellar center (juvenile) (primary) (secondary) — see Osteochondrosis, juvenile, patella
  pelvis (juvenile) M91.0
  Pierson's M91.0
  radius (head) (juvenile) — see Osteochondrosis, juvenile, radius
  Scheuermann's — see Osteochondrosis, juvenile, spine
  Sever's — see Osteochondrosis, juvenile, tarsus
  Sinding-Larsen — see Osteochondrosis, juvenile, patella
  spine M42.9
    adult M42.10
      cervical region M42.12
      cervicothoracic region M42.13
      lumbar region M42.16
      lumbosacral region M42.17
      multiple sites M42.19
      occipito-atlanto-axial region M42.11
      sacrococcygeal region M42.18
      thoracic region M42.14
      thoracolumbar region M42.15
    juvenile — see Osteochondrosis, juvenile, spine
  symphysis pubis (juvenile) M91.0
  syphilitic (congenital) A50.02
  talus (juvenile) — see Osteochondrosis, juvenile, tarsus
  tarsus (navicular) (juvenile) — see Osteochondrosis, juvenile, tarsus
  tibia (proximal) (tubercle) (juvenile) — see Osteochondrosis, juvenile, tibia
  tuberculous — see Tuberculosis, bone
  ulna (lower) (juvenile) — see Osteochondrosis, juvenile, ulna
  van Neck's M91.0
  vertebral — see Osteochondrosis, spine

Osteoclastoma D48.0
  malignant — see Neoplasm, bone, malignant
Osteodynia — see Disorder, bone, specified type NEC
Osteodystrophy Q78.9
  azotemic N25.0
  congenital Q78.9
  parathyroid, secondary E21.1
  renal N25.0
Osteofibroma — see Neoplasm, bone, benign
Osteofibrosarcoma — see Neoplasm, bone, malignant
Osteogenesis imperfecta Q78.0
Osteogenic — see condition
Osteolysis M89.50
  carpus M89.54- ☑
  clavicle M89.51- ☑
  femur M89.55- ☑
  fibula M89.56- ☑
  finger M89.54- ☑
  humerus M89.52- ☑
  ilium M89.559
  ischium M89.559
  joint prosthesis (periprosthetic) — see Complications, joint prosthesis, mechanical, periprosthetic, osteolysis, by site
  metacarpus M89.54- ☑
  metatarsus M89.57- ☑
  multiple sites M89.59
  neck M89.58
  periprosthetic — see Complications, joint prosthesis, mechanical, periprosthetic, osteolysis, by site
  radius M89.53- ☑
  rib M89.58
  scapula M89.51- ☑
  skull M89.58
  tarsus M89.57- ☑
  tibia M89.56- ☑
  toe M89.57- ☑
  ulna M89.53- ☑
  vertebra M89.58
Osteoma (see also Neoplasm, bone, benign)
  osteoid (see also Neoplasm, bone, benign)
    giant — see Neoplasm, bone, benign
Osteomalacia M83.9
  adult M83.9
    drug-induced NEC M83.5
    due to
      malabsorption (postsurgical) M83.2
      malnutrition M83.3
    specified NEC M83.8
  aluminium-induced M83.4
  infantile — see Rickets
  juvenile — see Rickets
  oncogenic E83.89
  pelvis M83.8
  puerperal M83.0
  senile M83.1
  vitamin-D-resistant in adults E83.31 [M90.8-] ☑
    carpus E83.31 [M90.84-] ☑
    clavicle E83.31 [M90.81-] ☑
    femur E83.31 [M90.85-] ☑
    fibula E83.31 [M90.86-] ☑
    finger E83.31 [M90.84-] ☑
    humerus E83.31 [M90.82-] ☑
    ilium E83.31 [M90.859]
    ischium E83.31 [M90.859]
    metacarpus E83.31 [M90.84-] ☑
    metatarsus E83.31 [M90.87-] ☑
    multiple sites E83.31 [M90.89]
    neck E83.31 [M90.88]
    radius E83.31 [M90.83-] ☑
    rib E83.31 [M90.88]
    scapula E83.31 [M90.819]
    skull E83.31 [M90.88]
    tarsus E83.31 [M90.879]
    tibia E83.31 [M90.869]
    toe E83.31 [M90.879]
    ulna E83.31 [M90.839]
    vertebra E83.31 [M90.88]
Osteomyelitis (general) (infective) (localized) (neonatal) (purulent) (septic) (staphylococcal) (streptococcal) (suppurative) (with periostitis) M86.9
  acute M86.10
    carpus M86.14- ☑
    clavicle M86.11- ☑
    femur M86.15- ☑
    fibula M86.16- ☑
    finger M86.14- ☑

Index — Osteomyelitis — Osteonecrosis

Osteomyelitis — *continued*
acute — *continued*
  hematogenous M86.00
    carpus M86.04- ☑
    clavicle M86.01- ☑
    femur M86.05- ☑
    fibula M86.06- ☑
    finger M86.04- ☑
    humerus M86.02- ☑
    ilium M86.059
    ischium M86.059
    mandible M27.2
    metacarpus M86.04- ☑
    metatarsus M86.07- ☑
    multiple sites M86.09
    neck M86.08
    orbit H05.02- ☑
    petrous bone — *see* Petrositis
    radius M86.03- ☑
    rib M86.08
    scapula M86.01- ☑
    skull M86.08
    tarsus M86.07- ☑
    tibia M86.06- ☑
    toe M86.07- ☑
    ulna M86.03- ☑
    vertebra — *see* Osteomyelitis, vertebra
  humerus M86.12- ☑
  ilium M86.159
  ischium M86.159
  mandible M27.2
  metacarpus M86.14- ☑
  metatarsus M86.17- ☑
  multiple sites M86.19
  neck M86.18
  orbit H05.02- ☑
  petrous bone — *see* Petrositis
  radius M86.13- ☑
  rib M86.18
  scapula M86.11- ☑
  skull M86.18
  tarsus M86.17- ☑
  tibia M86.16- ☑
  toe M86.17- ☑
  ulna M86.13- ☑
  vertebra — *see* Osteomyelitis, vertebra
chronic (or old) M86.60
  with draining sinus M86.40
    carpus M86.44- ☑
    clavicle M86.41- ☑
    femur M86.45- ☑
    fibula M86.46- ☑
    finger M86.44- ☑
    humerus M86.42- ☑
    ilium M86.459
    ischium M86.459
    mandible M27.2
    metacarpus M86.44- ☑
    metatarsus M86.47- ☑
    multiple sites M86.49
    neck M86.48
    orbit H05.02- ☑
    petrous bone — *see* Petrositis
    radius M86.43- ☑
    rib M86.48
    scapula M86.41- ☑
    skull M86.48
    tarsus M86.47- ☑
    tibia M86.46- ☑
    toe M86.47- ☑
    ulna M86.43- ☑
    vertebra — *see* Osteomyelitis, vertebra
  carpus M86.64- ☑
  clavicle M86.61- ☑
  femur M86.65- ☑
  fibula M86.66- ☑
  finger M86.64- ☑
  hematogenous NEC M86.50
    carpus M86.54- ☑
    clavicle M86.51- ☑
    femur M86.55- ☑
    fibula M86.56- ☑
    finger M86.54- ☑
    humerus M86.52- ☑
    ilium M86.559
    ischium M86.559

Osteomyelitis — *continued*
chronic — *continued*
  hematogenous — *continued*
    mandible M27.2
    metacarpus M86.54- ☑
    metatarsus M86.57- ☑
    multifocal M86.30
      carpus M86.34- ☑
      clavicle M86.31- ☑
      femur M86.35- ☑
      fibula M86.36- ☑
      finger M86.34- ☑
      humerus M86.32- ☑
      ilium M86.359
      ischium M86.359
      metacarpus M86.34- ☑
      metatarsus M86.37- ☑
      multiple sites M86.39
      neck M86.38
      radius M86.33- ☑
      rib M86.38
      scapula M86.31- ☑
      skull M86.38
      tarsus M86.37- ☑
      tibia M86.36- ☑
      toe M86.37- ☑
      ulna M86.33- ☑
      vertebra — *see* Osteomyelitis, vertebra
    multiple sites M86.59
    neck M86.58
    orbit H05.02- ☑
    petrous bone — *see* Petrositis
    radius M86.53- ☑
    rib M86.58
    scapula M86.51- ☑
    skull M86.58
    tarsus M86.57- ☑
    tibia M86.56- ☑
    toe M86.57- ☑
    ulna M86.53- ☑
    vertebra — *see* Osteomyelitis, vertebra
  humerus M86.62- ☑
  ilium M86.659
  ischium M86.659
  mandible M27.2
  metacarpus M86.64- ☑
  metatarsus M86.67- ☑
  multifocal — *see* Osteomyelitis, chronic, hematogenous, multifocal
  multiple sites M86.69
  neck M86.68
  orbit H05.02- ☑
  petrous bone — *see* Petrositis
  radius M86.63- ☑
  rib M86.68
  scapula M86.61- ☑
  skull M86.68
  tarsus M86.67- ☑
  tibia M86.66- ☑
  toe M86.67- ☑
  ulna M86.63- ☑
  vertebra — *see* Osteomyelitis, vertebra
echinococcal B67.2
Garr's — *see* Osteomyelitis, specified type NEC
jaw (acute) (chronic) (lower) (neonatal) (suppurative) (upper) M27.2
nonsuppurating — *see* Osteomyelitis, specified type NEC
orbit H05.02- ☑
petrous bone — *see* Petrositis
Salmonella (arizonae) (cholerae-suis) (enteritidis) (typhimurium) A02.24
sclerosing, nonsuppurative — *see* Osteomyelitis, specified type NEC
specified type NEC (*see also* subcategory) M86.8X- ☑
  mandible M27.2
  orbit H05.02- ☑
  petrous bone — *see* Petrositis
  vertebra — *see* Osteomyelitis, vertebra
subacute M86.20
  carpus M86.24- ☑
  clavicle M86.21- ☑
  femur M86.25- ☑
  fibula M86.26- ☑
  finger M86.24- ☑
  humerus M86.22- ☑

Osteomyelitis — *continued*
subacute — *continued*
  mandible M27.2
  metacarpus M86.24- ☑
  metatarsus M86.27- ☑
  multiple sites M86.29
  neck M86.28
  orbit H05.02- ☑
  petrous bone — *see* Petrositis
  radius M86.23- ☑
  rib M86.28
  scapula M86.21- ☑
  skull M86.28
  tarsus M86.27- ☑
  tibia M86.26- ☑
  toe M86.27- ☑
  ulna M86.23- ☑
  vertebra — *see* Osteomyelitis, vertebra
syphilitic A52.77
  congenital (early) A50.02 [M90.80]
tuberculous — *see* Tuberculosis, bone
typhoid A01.05
vertebra M46.20
  cervical region M46.22
  cervicothoracic region M46.23
  lumbar region M46.26
  lumbosacral region M46.27
  occipito-atlanto-axial region M46.21
  sacrococcygeal region M46.28
  thoracic region M46.24
  thoracolumbar region M46.25
Osteomyelofibrosis D75.89
Osteomyelosclerosis D75.89
Osteonecrosis M87.9
due to
  drugs — *see* Osteonecrosis, secondary, due to, drugs
  trauma — *see* Osteonecrosis, secondary, due to, trauma
idiopathic aseptic M87.00
  ankle M87.07- ☑
  carpus M87.03- ☑
  clavicle M87.01- ☑
  femur M87.05- ☑
  fibula M87.06- ☑
  finger M87.04- ☑
  humerus M87.02- ☑
  ilium M87.050
  ischium M87.050
  metacarpus M87.04- ☑
  metatarsus M87.07- ☑
  multiple sites M87.09
  neck M87.08
  pelvis M87.050
  radius M87.03- ☑
  rib M87.08
  scapula M87.01- ☑
  skull M87.08
  tarsus M87.07- ☑
  tibia M87.06- ☑
  toe M87.07- ☑
  ulna M87.03- ☑
  vertebra M87.08
secondary NEC M87.30
  carpus M87.33- ☑
  clavicle M87.31- ☑
  due to
    drugs M87.10
      carpus M87.13- ☑
      clavicle M87.11- ☑
      femur M87.15- ☑
      fibula M87.16- ☑
      finger M87.14- ☑
      humerus M87.12- ☑
      ilium M87.159
      ischium M87.159
      jaw M87.180
      metacarpus M87.14- ☑
      metatarsus M87.17- ☑
      multiple sites M87.19
      neck M87.18
      radius M87.13- ☑
      rib M87.18 ☑
      scapula M87.11- ☑
      skull M87.18 ☑
      tarsus M87.17- ☑
      tibia M87.16- ☑

Osteonecrosis — *continued*
  secondary — *continued*
    due to — *continued*
      drugs — *continued*
        toe M87.17- ☑
        ulna M87.13- ☑
        vertebra M87.18 ☑
      hemoglobinopathy NEC D58.2 [M90.50]
        carpus D58.2 [M90.54-] ☑
        clavicle D58.2 [M90.51-] ☑
        femur D58.2 [M90.55-] ☑
        fibula D58.2 [M90.56-] ☑
        finger D58.2 [M90.54-] ☑
        humerus D58.2 [M90.52-] ☑
        ilium D58.2 [M90.55-] ☑
        ischium D58.2 [M90.55-] ☑
        metacarpus D58.2 [M90.54-] ☑
        metatarsus D58.2 [M90.57-] ☑
        multiple sites D58.2 [M90.58]
        neck D58.2 [M90.58]
        radius D58.2 [M90.53-] ☑
        rib D58.2 [M90.58]
        scapula D58.2 [M90.51-] ☑
        skull D58.2 [M90.58]
        tarsus D58.2 [M90.57-] ☑
        tibia D58.2 [M90.56-] ☑
        toe D58.2 [M90.57-] ☑
        ulna D58.2 [M90.53-] ☑
        vertebra D58.2 [M90.58]
      trauma (previous) M87.20
        carpus M87.23- ☑
        clavicle M87.21- ☑
        femur M87.25- ☑
        fibula M87.26- ☑
        finger M87.24- ☑
        humerus M87.22- ☑
        ilium M87.25- ☑
        ischium M87.25- ☑
        metacarpus M87.24- ☑
        metatarsus M87.27- ☑
        multiple sites M87.29
        neck M87.28
        radius M87.23- ☑
        rib M87.28
        scapula M87.21- ☑
        skull M87.28
        tarsus M87.27- ☑
        tibia M87.26- ☑
        toe M87.27- ☑
        ulna M87.23- ☑
        vertebra M87.28
  femur M87.35- ☑
  fibula M87.36- ☑
  finger M87.34- ☑
  humerus M87.32- ☑
  ilium M87.350
  in
    caisson disease T70.3 [M90.50]
      carpus T70.3 ☑ [M90.54-] ☑
      clavicle T70.3 ☑ [M90.51-] ☑
      femur T70.3 ☑ [M90.55-] ☑
      fibula T70.3 ☑ [M90.56-] ☑
      finger T70.3 ☑ [M90.54-] ☑
      humerus T70.3 ☑ [M90.52-] ☑
      ilium T70.3 ☑ [M90.55-] ☑
      ischium T70.3 ☑ [M90.55-] ☑
      metacarpus T70.3 ☑ [M90.54-] ☑
      metatarsus T70.3 ☑ [M90.57-] ☑
      multiple sites T70.3 ☑ [M90.59]
      neck T70.3 ☑ [M90.58]
      radius T70.3 ☑ [M90.53-] ☑
      rib T70.3 ☑ [M90.58]
      scapula T70.3 ☑ [M90.51-] ☑
      skull T70.3 ☑ [M90.58]
      tarsus T70.3 ☑ [M90.57-] ☑
      tibia T70.3 ☑ [M90.56-] ☑
      toe T70.3 ☑ [M90.57-] ☑
      ulna T70.3 ☑ [M90.53-] ☑
      vertebra T70.3 ☑ [M90.58]
  ischium M87.350
  metacarpus M87.34- ☑
  metatarsus M87.37- ☑
  multiple site M87 39
  neck M87.38
  radius M87.33- ☑
  rib M87.38

Osteonecrosis — *continued*
  secondary — *continued*
    scapula M87.319
    skull M87.38
    tarsus M87.379
    tibia M87.366
    toe M87.379
    ulna M87.33- ☑
    vertebra M87.38
  specified type NEC M87.80
    carpus M87.83- ☑
    clavicle M87.81- ☑
    femur M87.85- ☑
    fibula M87.86- ☑
    finger M87.84- ☑
    humerus M87.82- ☑
    ilium M87.85- ☑
    ischium M87.85- ☑
    metacarpus M87.84- ☑
    metatarsus M87.87- ☑
    multiple sites M87.89
    neck M87.88
    radius M87.83- ☑
    rib M87.88
    scapula M87.81- ☑
    skull M87.88
    tarsus M87.87- ☑
    tibia M87.86- ☑
    toe M87.87- ☑
    ulna M87.83- ☑
    vertebra M87.88

Osteo-onycho-arthro-dysplasia Q79.8
Osteo-onychodysplasia, hereditary Q79.8
Osteopathia condensans disseminata Q78.8
Osteopathy (*see also* Osteomyelitis, Osteonecrosis, Osteoporosis)
  after poliomyelitis M89.60
    carpus M89.64- ☑
    clavicle M89.61- ☑
    femur M89.65- ☑
    fibula M89.66- ☑
    finger M89.64- ☑
    humerus M89.62- ☑
    ilium M89.659
    ischium M89.659
    metacarpus M89.64- ☑
    metatarsus M89.67- ☑
    multiple sites M89.69
    neck M89.68
    radius M89.63- ☑
    rib M89.68
    scapula M89.61- ☑
    skull M89.68
    tarsus M89.67- ☑
    tibia M89.66- ☑
    toe M89.67- ☑
    ulna M89.63- ☑
    vertebra M89.68
  in (due to)
    renal osteodystrophy N25.0
    specified diseases classified elsewhere — *see* subcategory M90.8 ☑
Osteopenia M85.8- ☑
  borderline M85.8- ☑
Osteoperiostitis — *see* Osteomyelitis, specified type NEC
Osteopetrosis (familial) Q78.2
Osteophyte M25.70
  ankle M25.77- ☑
  elbow M25.72- ☑
  foot joint M25.77- ☑
  hand joint M25.74- ☑
  hip M25.75- ☑
  knee M25.76- ☑
  shoulder M25.71- ☑
  spine M25.78
  vertebrae M25.78
  wrist M25.73- ☑
Osteopoikilosis Q78.8
Osteoporosis (female) (male) M81.0
  with current pathological fracture M80.00 ☑
  age-related M81.0
    with current pathologic fracture M80.00 ☑
      carpus M80.04- ☑
      clavicle M80.01- ☑
      fibula M60.06- ☑

Osteoporosis — *continued*
  age-related — *continued*
    with current pathologic fracture — *continued*
      finger M80.04- ☑
      humerus M80.02- ☑
      ilium M80.05- ☑
      ischium M80.05- ☑
      metacarpus M80.04- ☑
      metatarsus M80.07- ☑
      pelvis M80.05- ☑
      radius M80.03- ☑
      scapula M80.01- ☑
      tarsus M80.07- ☑
      tibia M80.06- ☑
      toe M80.07- ☑
      ulna M80.03- ☑
      vertebra M80.08 ☑
  disuse M81.8
    with current pathological fracture M80.80 ☑
      carpus M80.84- ☑
      clavicle M80.81- ☑
      fibula M80.86- ☑
      finger M80.84- ☑
      humerus M80.82- ☑
      ilium M80.85- ☑
      ischium M80.85- ☑
      metacarpus M80.84- ☑
      metatarsus M80.87- ☑
      pelvis M80.85- ☑
      radius M80.83- ☑
      scapula M80.81- ☑
      tarsus M80.87- ☑
      tibia M80.86- ☑
      toe M80.87- ☑
      ulna M80.83- ☑
      vertebra M80.88 ☑
  drug-induced — *see* Osteoporosis, specified type NEC
  idiopathic — *see* Osteoporosis, specified type NEC
  involutional — *see* Osteoporosis, age-related
  Lequesne M81.6
  localized M81.6
  postmenopausal M81.0
    with pathological fracture M80.00 ☑
      carpus M80.04- ☑
      clavicle M80.01- ☑
      fibula M80.06- ☑
      finger M80.04- ☑
      humerus M80.02- ☑
      ilium M80.05- ☑
      ischium M80.05- ☑
      metacarpus M80.04- ☑
      metatarsus M80.07- ☑
      pelvis M80.05- ☑
      radius M80.03- ☑
      scapula M80.01- ☑
      tarsus M80.07- ☑
      tibia M80.06- ☑
      toe M80.07- ☑
      ulna M80.03- ☑
      vertebra M80.08 ☑
  postoophorectomy — *see* Osteoporosis, specified type NEC
  postsurgical malabsorption — *see* Osteoporosis, specified type NEC
  post-traumatic — *see* Osteoporosis, specified type NEC
  senile — *see* Osteoporosis, age-related
  specified type NEC M81.8
    with pathological fracture M80.80 ☑
      carpus M80.84- ☑
      clavicle M80.81- ☑
      fibula M80.86- ☑
      finger M80.84- ☑
      humerus M80.82- ☑
      ilium M80.85- ☑
      ischium M80.85- ☑
      metacarpus M80.84- ☑
      metatarsus M80.87- ☑
      pelvis M80.85- ☑
      radius M80.83- ☑
      scapula M80.81- ☑
      tarsus M80.87- ☑
      tibia M80.86- ☑
      toe M80.87- ☑
      ulna M80.83- ☑
      vertebra M80.88 ☑

Osteopsathyrosis (idiopathica) Q78.0
Osteoradionecrosis, jaw (acute) (chronic) (lower) (suppurative) (upper) M27.2
Osteosarcoma (any form) — *see* Neoplasm, bone, malignant
Osteosclerosis Q78.2
  acquired M85.8- ☑
  congenita Q77.4
  fragilitas (generalisata) Q78.2
  myelofibrosis D75.81
Osteosclerotic anemia D64.89
Osteosis
  cutis L94.2
  renal fibrocystic N25.0
Österreicher-Turner syndrome Q87.2
Ostium
  atrioventriculare commune Q21.2
  primum (arteriosum) (defect) (persistent) Q21.2
  secundum (arteriosum) (defect) (patent) (persistent) Q21.1
Ostrum-Furst syndrome Q75.8
Otalgia H92.0 ☑
Otitis (acute) H66.90
  with effusion (*see also* Otitis, media, nonsuppurative)
    purulent — *see* Otitis, media, suppurative
  adhesive — *see* subcategory H74.1 ☑
  chronic (*see also* Otitis, media, chronic)
    with effusion (*see also* Otitis, media, nonsuppurative, chronic)
  externa H60.9- ☑
    abscess — *see* Abscess, ear, external
    acute (noninfective) H60.50- ☑
      actinic H60.51- ☑
      chemical H60.52- ☑
      contact H60.53- ☑
      eczematoid H60.54- ☑
      infective — *see* Otitis, externa, infective
      reactive H60.55- ☑
      specified NEC H60.59- ☑
    cellulitis — *see* Cellulitis, ear
    chronic H60.6- ☑
    diffuse — *see* Otitis, externa, infective, diffuse
    hemorrhagic — *see* Otitis, externa, infective, hemorrhagic
    in (due to)
      aspergillosis B44.89
      candidiasis B37.84
      erysipelas A46 [H62.40]
      herpes (simplex) virus infection B00.1
        zoster B02.8
      impetigo L01.00 [H62.40]
      infectious disease NEC B99 ☑ [H62.4-]
      mycosis NEC B36.9 [H62.40]
      parasitic disease NEC B89 [H62.40]
      viral disease NEC B34.9 [H62.40]
      zoster B02.8
    infective NEC H60.39- ☑
      abscess — *see* Abscess, ear, external
      cellulitis — *see* Cellulitis, ear
      diffuse H60.31- ☑
      hemorrhagic H60.32- ☑
      swimmer's ear — *see* Swimmer's, ear
    malignant H60.2- ☑
    mycotic B36.9 [H62.40]
    necrotizing — *see* Otitis, externa, malignant
    Pseudomonas aeruginosa — *see* Otitis, externa, malignant
    reactive — *see* Otitis, externa, acute, reactive
    specified NEC — *see* subcategory H60.8 ☑
    tropical B36.8
  insidiosa — *see* Otosclerosis
  interna H83.0 ☑
  media (hemorrhagic) (staphylococcal) (streptococcal) H66.9- ☑
    with effusion (nonpurulent) — *see* Otitis, media, nonsuppurative
    acute, subacute H66.90
      allergic — *see* Otitis, media, nonsuppurative, acute, allergic
      exudative — *see* Otitis, media, nonsuppurative, acute
      mucoid — *see* Otitis, media, nonsuppurative, acute
      necrotizing (*see also* Otitis, media, suppurative, acute)
        in
          measles B05.3

Otitis — *continued*
  media — *continued*
    acute, subacute — *continued*
      necrotizing (*see also* Otitis, media, suppurative, acute) — *continued*
        in — *continued*
          scarlet fever A38.0
      nonsuppurative NEC — *see* Otitis, media, nonsuppurative, acute
      purulent — *see* Otitis, media, suppurative, acute
      sanguinous — *see* Otitis, media, nonsuppurative, acute
      secretory — *see* Otitis, media, nonsuppurative, acute, serous
      seromucinous — *see* Otitis, media, nonsuppurative, acute
      serous — *see* Otitis, media, nonsuppurative, acute, serous
      suppurative — *see* Otitis, media, suppurative, acute
    allergic — *see* Otitis, media, nonsuppurative
    catarrhal — *see* Otitis, media, nonsuppurative
    chronic H66.90
      with effusion (nonpurulent) — *see* Otitis, media, nonsuppurative, chronic
      allergic — *see* Otitis, media, nonsuppurative, chronic, allergic
      benign suppurative — *see* Otitis, media, suppurative, chronic, tubotympanic
      catarrhal — *see* Otitis, media, nonsuppurative, chronic, serous
      exudative — *see* Otitis, media, nonsuppurative, chronic
      mucinous — *see* Otitis, media, nonsuppurative, chronic, mucoid
      mucoid — *see* Otitis, media, nonsuppurative, chronic, mucoid
      nonsuppurative NEC — *see* Otitis, media, nonsuppurative, chronic
      purulent — *see* Otitis, media, suppurative, chronic
      secretory — *see* Otitis, media, nonsuppurative, chronic, mucoid
      seromucinous — *see* Otitis, media, nonsuppurative, chronic
      serous — *see* Otitis, media, nonsuppurative, chronic, serous
      suppurative — *see* Otitis, media, suppurative, chronic
      transudative — *see* Otitis, media, nonsuppurative, chronic, mucoid
    exudative — *see* Otitis, media, nonsuppurative
    in (due to) (with)
      influenza — *see* Influenza, with, otitis media
      measles B05.3
      scarlet fever A38.0
      tuberculosis A18.6
      viral disease NEC B34.- ☑ [H67.-] ☑
    mucoid — *see* Otitis, media, nonsuppurative
    nonsuppurative H65.9- ☑
      acute or subacute NEC H65.19- ☑
        allergic H65.11- ☑
          recurrent H65.11- ☑
        recurrent H65.19- ☑
        secretory — *see* Otitis, media, nonsuppurative, serous
        serous H65.0- ☑
          recurrent H65.0- ☑
      chronic H65.49- ☑
        allergic H65.41- ☑
        mucoid H65.3- ☑
        serous H65.2- ☑
      postmeasles B05.3
    purulent — *see* Otitis, media, suppurative
    secretory — *see* Otitis, media, nonsuppurative
    seromucinous — *see* Otitis, media, nonsuppurative
    serous — *see* Otitis, media, nonsuppurative
    suppurative H66.4- ☑
      acute H66.00- ☑
        with rupture of ear drum H66.01- ☑
        recurrent H66.00- ☑
          with rupture of ear drum H66.01- ☑
      chronic (*see also* subcategory) H66.3 ☑
        atticoantral H66.2- ☑
        benign — *see* Otitis, media, suppurative, chronic, tubotympanic

Otitis — *continued*
  media — *continued*
    suppurative — *continued*
      chronic (*see also* subcategory) — *continued*
        tubotympanic H66.1- ☑
      transudative — *see* Otitis, media, nonsuppurative
      tuberculous A18.6
Otocephaly Q18.2
Otolith syndrome — *see* subcategory H81.8 ☑
Otomycosis (diffuse) **NEC** B36.9 [H62.40]
  in
    aspergillosis B44.89
    candidiasis B37.84
    moniliasis B37.84
Otoporosis — *see* Otosclerosis
Otorrhagia (nontraumatic) H92.2- ☑
  traumatic — *code by* Type of injury
Otorrhea H92.1- ☑
  cerebrospinal G96.0
Otosclerosis (general) H80.9- ☑
  cochlear (endosteal) H80.2- ☑
  involving
    otic capsule — *see* Otosclerosis, cochlear
    oval window
      nonobliterative H80.0- ☑
      obliterative H80.1- ☑
    round window — *see* Otosclerosis, cochlear
  nonobliterative — *see* Otosclerosis, involving, oval window, nonobliterative
  obliterative — *see* Otosclerosis, involving, oval window, obliterative
  specified NEC H80.8- ☑
Otospongiosis — *see* Otosclerosis
Otto's disease or pelvis M24.7
Outcome of delivery Z37.9
  multiple births Z37.9
    all liveborn Z37.50
      quadruplets Z37.52
      quintuplets Z37.53
      sextuplets Z37.54
      specified number NEC Z37.59
      triplets Z37.51
    all stillborn Z37.7
    some liveborn Z37.60
      quadruplets Z37.62
      quintuplets Z37.63
      sextuplets Z37.64
      specified number NEC Z37.69
      triplets Z37.61
  single NEC Z37.9
    liveborn Z37.0
    stillborn Z37.1
  twins NEC Z37.9
    both liveborn Z37.2
    both stillborn Z37.4
    one liveborn, one stillborn Z37.3
Outlet — *see* condition
Ovalocytosis (congenital) (hereditary) — *see* Elliptocytosis
Ovarian — *See* Condition
Ovariocele N83.4
Ovaritis (cystic) — *see* Oophoritis
Ovary, ovarian (*see also* condition)
  resistant syndrome E28.39
  vein syndrome N13.8
Overactive (*see also* Hyperfunction)
  adrenal cortex NEC E27.0
  bladder N32.81
  hypothalamus E23.3
  thyroid — *see* Hyperthyroidism
Overactivity R46.3
  child — *see* Disorder, attention-deficit hyperactivity
Overbite (deep) (excessive) (horizontal) (vertical) M26.29
Overbreathing — *see* Hyperventilation
Overconscientious personality F60.5
Overdevelopment — *see* Hypertrophy
Overdistension — *see* Distension
Overdose, overdosage (drug) — *see* Table of Drugs and Chemicals, by drug, poisoning
Overeating R63.2
  nonorganic origin F50.8
  psychogenic F50.8
Overexertion (effects) (exhaustion) T73.3 ☑
Overexposure (effects) T73.9 ☑
  exhaustion T73.2 ☑
Overfeeding — *see* Overeating
  newborn P92.4

Overfill, endodontic M27.52

Overgrowth, bone — *see* Hypertrophy, bone

Overhanging of dental restorative material (unrepairable) K08.52

Overheated (places) (effects) — *see* Heat

Overjet (excessive horizontal) M26.23

Overlaid, overlying (suffocation) — *see* Asphyxia, traumatic, due to mechanical threat

Overlap, excessive horizontal (teeth) M26.23

Overlapping toe (acquired) (*see also* Deformity, toe, specified NEC)
　　congenital (fifth toe) Q66.89

Overload
　　circulatory, due to transfusion (blood) (blood components) (TACO) E87.71
　　fluid E87.70
　　　due to transfusion (blood) (blood components) E87.71
　　　specified NEC E87.79
　　iron, due to repeated red blood cell transfusions E83.111
　　potassium (K) E87.5
　　sodium (Na) E87.0

Overnutrition —- *see* Hyperalimentation

Overproduction (*see also* Hypersecretion)
　　ACTH E27.0
　　catecholamine E27.5
　　growth hormone E22.0

Overprotection, child by parent Z62.1

Overriding
　　aorta Q25.4
　　finger (acquired) — *see* Deformity, finger
　　　congenital Q68.1
　　toe (acquired) (*see also* Deformity, toe, specified NEC)
　　　congenital Q66.89

Overstrained R53.83
　　heart — *see* Hypertrophy, cardiac

Overuse, muscle NEC M70.8- ☑

Overweight E66.3

Overworked R53.83

Oviduct — *see* condition

Ovotestis Q56.0

Ovulation (cycle)
　　failure or lack of N97.0
　　pain N94.0

Ovum — *see* condition

Owren's disease or syndrome (parahemophilia) D68.2

Ox heart — *see* Hypertrophy, cardiac

Oxalosis E72.53

Oxaluria E72.53

Oxycephaly, oxycephalic Q75.0
　　syphilitic, congenital A50.02

Oxyuriasis B80

Oxyuris vermicularis (infestation) B80

Ozena J31.0

P

Pachyderma, pachydermia L85.9
　　larynx (verrucosa) J38.7

Pachydermatocele (congenital) Q82.8

Pachydermoperiostosis (*see also* Osteoarthropathy, hypertrophic, specified type NEC)
　　clubbed nail M89.40 [L62]

Pachygyria Q04.3

Pachymeningitis (adhesive) (basal) (brain) (cervical) (chronic)(circumscribed) (external) (fibrous) (hemorrhagic) (hypertrophic) (internal) (purulent) (spinal) (suppurative) — *see* Meningitis

Pachyonychia (congenital) Q84.5

Pacinian tumor — *see* Neoplasm, skin, benign

Pad, knuckle or Garrod's M72.1

Paget's disease
　　with infiltrating duct carcinoma — *see* Neoplasm, breast, malignant
　　bone M88.9
　　　carpus M88.84- ☑
　　　clavicle M88.81- ☑
　　　femur M88.85- ☑
　　　fibula M88.86- ☑
　　　finger M88.84- ☑
　　　humerus M88.82- ☑
　　　ilium M88.85- ☑
　　　in neoplastic disease — *see* Osteitis, deformans, in neoplastic disease
　　　ischium M88.85- ☑
　　　metacarpus M88.84- ☑

Paget's disease — *continued*
　　bone — *continued*
　　　metatarsus M88.87- ☑
　　　multiple sites M88.89
　　　neck M88.88
　　　radius M88.83- ☑
　　　rib M88.88
　　　scapula M88.81- ☑
　　　skull M88.0
　　　tarsus M88.87- ☑
　　　tibia M88.86- ☑
　　　toe M88.87- ☑
　　　ulna M88.83- ☑
　　　vertebra M88.88
　　breast (female) C50.01- ☑
　　　male C50.02- ☑
　　extramammary (*see also* Neoplasm, skin, malignant)
　　　anus C21.0
　　　　margin C44.590
　　　　skin C44.590
　　intraductal carcinoma — *see* Neoplasm, breast, malignant
　　malignant — *see* Neoplasm, skin, malignant
　　　breast (female) C50.01- ☑
　　　　male C50.02- ☑
　　　unspecified site (female) C50.01- ☑
　　　　male C50.02- ☑
　　mammary — *see* Paget's disease, breast
　　nipple — *see* Paget's disease, breast
　　osteitis deformans — *see* Paget's disease, bone

Paget-Schroetter syndrome I82.890

Pain(s) (*see also* Painful) R52
　　abdominal R10.9
　　　colic R10.83
　　　generalized R10.84
　　　　with acute abdomen R10.0
　　　lower R10.30
　　　　left quadrant R10.32
　　　　pelvic or perineal R10.2
　　　　periumbilical R10.33
　　　　right quadrant R10.31
　　　rebound — *see* Tenderness, abdominal, rebound
　　　severe with abdominal rigidity R10.0
　　　tenderness — *see* Tenderness, abdominal
　　　upper R10.10
　　　　epigastric R10.13
　　　　left quadrant R10.12
　　　　right quadrant R10.11
　　acute R52
　　　due to trauma G89.11
　　　neoplasm related G89.3
　　　postprocedural NEC G89.18
　　　post-thoracotomy G89.12
　　　specified by site — *code to* Pain, by site
　　adnexa (uteri) R10.2
　　anginoid — *see* Pain, precordial
　　anus K62.89
　　arm — *see* Pain, limb, upper
　　axillary (axilla) M79.62- ☑
　　back (postural) M54.9
　　bladder R39.89
　　　associated with micturition — *see* Micturition, painful
　　bone — *see* Disorder, bone, specified type NEC
　　breast N64.4
　　broad ligament R10.2
　　cancer associated (acute) (chronic) G89.3
　　cecum — *see* Pain, abdominal
　　cervicobrachial M53.1
　　chest (central) R07.9
　　　anterior wall R07.89
　　　atypical R07.89
　　　ischemic I20.9
　　　musculoskeletal R07.89
　　　non-cardiac R07.89
　　　on breathing R07.1
　　　pleurodynia R07.81
　　　precordial R07.2
　　　wall (anterior) R07.89
　　chronic G89.29
　　　associated with significant psychosocial dysfunction G89.4
　　　due to trauma G89.21
　　　neoplasm related G89.3
　　　postoperative NEC G89.28
　　　postprocedural NEC G89.28
　　　post-thoracotomy G89.22

Pain(s) — *continued*
　　chronic — *continued*
　　　specified NEC G89.29
　　coccyx M53.3
　　colon — *see* Pain, abdominal
　　coronary — *see* Angina
　　costochondral R07.1
　　diaphragm R07.1
　　due to cancer G89.3
　　due to device, implant or graft (*see also* Complications, by site and type, specified NEC) T85.84 ☑
　　　arterial graft NEC T82.848 ☑
　　　breast (implant) T85.84 ☑
　　　catheter NEC T85.84 ☑
　　　　dialysis (renal) T82.848 ☑
　　　　　intraperitoneal T85.84 ☑
　　　　infusion NEC T82.848 ☑
　　　　　spinal (epidural) (subdural) T85.84 ☑
　　　　urinary (indwelling) T83.84 ☑
　　　electronic (electrode) (pulse generator) (stimulator)
　　　　bone T84.84 ☑
　　　　cardiac T82.847 ☑
　　　　nervous system (brain) (peripheral nerve) (spinal) T85.84 ☑
　　　　urinary T83.84 ☑
　　　fixation, internal (orthopedic) NEC T84.84 ☑
　　　gastrointestinal (bile duct) (esophagus) T85.84 ☑
　　　genital NEC T83.84 ☑
　　　heart NEC T82.847 ☑
　　　infusion NEC T85.84 ☑
　　　joint prosthesis T84.84 ☑
　　　ocular (corneal graft) (orbital implant) NEC T85.84 ☑
　　　orthopedic NEC T84.84 ☑
　　　specified NEC T85.84 ☑
　　　urinary NEC T83.84 ☑
　　　vascular NEC T82.848 ☑
　　　ventricular intracranial shunt T85.84 ☑
　　due to malignancy (primary) (secondary) G89.3
　　ear — *see* subcategory H92.0 ☑
　　epigastric, epigastrium R10.13
　　eye — *see* Pain, ocular
　　face, facial R51
　　　atypical G50.1
　　female genital organs NEC N94.89
　　finger — *see* Pain, limb, upper
　　flank — *see* Pain, abdominal
　　foot — *see* Pain, limb, lower
　　gallbladder K82.9
　　gas (intestinal) R14.1
　　gastric — *see* Pain, abdominal
　　generalized NOS R52
　　genital organ
　　　female N94.89
　　　male N50.8
　　groin — *see* Pain, abdominal, lower
　　hand — *see* Pain, limb, upper
　　head — *see* Headache
　　heart — *see* Pain, precordial
　　infra-orbital — *see* Neuralgia, trigeminal
　　intercostal R07.82
　　intermenstrual N94.0
　　jaw R68.84
　　joint M25.50
　　　ankle M25.57- ☑
　　　elbow M25.52- ☑
　　　finger M79.64- ☑
　　　foot M25.57- ☑
　　　hand M79.64- ☑
　　　hip M25.55- ☑
　　　knee M25.56- ☑
　　　shoulder M25.51- ☑
　　　toe M25.57- ☑
　　　wrist M25.53- ☑
　　kidney N23
　　laryngeal R07.0
　　leg — *see* Pain, limb, lower
　　limb M79.609
　　　lower M79.60- ☑
　　　　foot M79.67- ☑
　　　　lower leg M79.66- ☑
　　　　thigh M79.65- ☑
　　　　toe M79.67- ☑
　　　upper M79.60- ☑
　　　　axilla M79.62- ☑
　　　　finger M79.64- ☑

Pain(s) — *continued*
  limb — *continued*
    upper — *continued*
      forearm M79.63- ☑
      hand M79.64- ☑
      upper arm M79.62- ☑
  loin M54.5
  low back M54.5
  lumbar region M54.5
  mandibular R68.84
  mastoid — *see* subcategory H92.0 ☑
  maxilla R68.84
  menstrual (*see also* Dysmenorrhea) N94.6
  metacarpophalangeal (joint) — *see* Pain, joint, hand
  metatarsophalangeal (joint) — *see* Pain, joint, foot
  mouth K13.79
  muscle — *see* Myalgia
  musculoskeletal (*see also* Pain, by site) M79.1
  myofascial M79.1
  nasal J34.89
  nasopharynx J39.2
  neck NEC M54.2
  nerve NEC — *see* Neuralgia
  neuromuscular — *see* Neuralgia
  nose J34.89
  ocular H57.1- ☑
  ophthalmic — *see* Pain, ocular
  orbital region — *see* Pain, ocular
  ovary N94.89
  over heart — *see* Pain, precordial
  ovulation N94.0
  pelvic (female) R10.2
  penis N48.89
  pericardial — *see* Pain, precordial
  perineal, perineum R10.2
  pharynx J39.2
  pleura, pleural, pleuritic R07.81
  postoperative NOS G89.18
  postprocedural NOS G89.18
  post-thoracotomy G89.12
  precordial (region) R07.2
  premenstrual N94.3
  psychogenic (persistent) (any site) F45.41
  radicular (spinal) — *see* Radiculopathy
  rectum K62.89
  respiration R07.1
  retrosternal R07.2
  rheumatoid, muscular — *see* Myalgia
  rib R07.81
  root (spinal) — *see* Radiculopathy
  round ligament (stretch) R10.2
  sacroiliac M53.3
  sciatic — *see* Sciatica
  scrotum N50.8
  seminal vesicle N50.8
  shoulder M25.51- ☑
  spermatic cord N50.8
  spinal root — *see* Radiculopathy
  spine M54.9
    cervical M54.2
    low back M54.5
      with sciatica M54.4- ☑
    thoracic M54.6
  stomach — *see* Pain, abdominal
  substernal R07.2
  temporomandibular (joint) M26.62
  testis N50.8
  thoracic spine M54.6
    with radicular and visceral pain M54.14
  throat R07.0
  tibia — *see* Pain, limb, lower
  toe — *see* Pain, limb, lower
  tongue K14.6
  tooth K08.8
  trigeminal — *see* Neuralgia, trigeminal
  tumor associated G89.3
  ureter N23
  urinary (organ) (system) N23
  uterus NEC N94.89
  vagina R10.2
  vertebrogenic (syndrome) M54.89
  vesical R39.89
    associated with micturition — *see* Micturition, painful
  vulva R10.2

Painful (*see also* Pain)
  coitus
    female N94.1

Painful — *continued*
  coitus — *continued*
    male N53.12
    psychogenic F52.6
  ejaculation (semen) N53.12
    psychogenic F52.6
  erection — *see* Priapism
  feet syndrome E53.8
  joint replacement (hip) (knee) T84.84 ☑
  menstruation — *see* Dysmenorrhea
    psychogenic F45.8
  micturition — *see* Micturition, painful
  respiration R07.1
  scar NEC L90.5
  wire sutures T81.89 ☑

Painter's colic — *see* subcategory T56.0 ☑
Palate — *see* condition
Palatoplegia K13.79
Palatoschisis — *see* Cleft, palate
Palilalia R48.8
Palliative care Z51.5
Pallor R23.1
  optic disc, temporal — *see* Atrophy, optic
Palmar (*see also* condition)
  fascia — *see* condition
Palpable
  cecum K63.89
  kidney N28.89
  ovary N83.8
  prostate N42.9
  spleen — *see* Splenomegaly
Palpitations (heart) R00.2
  psychogenic F45.8
Palsy (*see also* Paralysis) G83.9
  atrophic diffuse (progressive) G12.22
  Bell's (*see also* Palsy, facial)
    newborn P11.3
  brachial plexus NEC G54.0
    newborn (birth injury) P14.3
  brain — *see* Palsy, cerebral
  bulbar (progressive) (chronic) G12.22
    of childhood (Fazio-Londe) G12.1
    pseudo NEC G12.29
    supranuclear (progressive) G23.1
  cerebral (congenital) G80.9
    ataxic G80.4
    athetoid G80.3
    choreathetoid G80.3
    dipiegic G80.8
      spastic G80.1
    dyskinetic G80.3
      athetoid G80.3
      choreathetoid G80.3
      distonic G80.3
    dystonic G80.3
    hemiplegic G80.8
      spastic G80.2
    mixed G80.8
    monoplegic G80.8
      spastic G80.1
    paraplegic G80.8
      spastic G80.1
    quadriplegic G80.8
      spastic G80.0
    spastic G80.1
      diplegic G80.1
      hemiplegic G80.2
      monoplegic G80.1
      quadriplegic G80.0
      specified NEC G80.1
      tetrapelgic G80.0
    specified NEC G80.8
    syphilitic A52.12
      congenital A50.49
    tetraplegic G80.8
      spastic G80.0
  cranial nerve (*see also* Disorder, nerve, cranial)
    multiple G52.7
      in
        infectious disease B99 ☑ [G53]
        neoplastic disease (*see also* Neoplasm) D49.9 [G53]
        parasitic disease B89 [G53]
        sarcoidosis D86.82
  creeping G12.22
  diver's T70.3 ☑
  Erb's P14.0
  facial G51.0

Palsy — *continued*
  facial — *continued*
    newborn (birth injury) P11.3
  glossopharyngeal G52.1
  Klumpke (-Déjérine) P14.1
  lead — *see* subcategory T56.0 ☑
  median nerve (tardy) G56.1- ☑
  nerve G58.9
    specified NEC G58.8
  peroneal nerve (acute) (tardy) G57.3- ☑
  progressive supranuclear G23.1
  pseudobulbar NEC G12.29
  radial nerve (acute) G56.3- ☑
  seventh nerve (*see also* Palsy, facial)
    newborn P11.3
  shaking — *see* Parkinsonism
  spastic (cerebral) (spinal) G80.1
  ulnar nerve (tardy) G56.2- ☑
  wasting G12.29
Paludism — *see* Malaria
Panangiitis M30.0
Panaris, panaritium (*see also* Cellulitis, digit)
  with lymphangitis — *see* Lymphangitis, acute, digit
Panarteritis nodosa M30.0
  brain or cerebral I67.7
Pancake heart R93.1
  with cor pulmonale (chronic) I27.81
Pancarditis (acute) (chronic) I51.89
  rheumatic I09.89
    active or acute I01.8
Pancoast's syndrome or tumor C34.1- ☑
Pancolitis, ulcerative (chronic) K51.00
  with
    abscess K51.014
    complication K51.019
    fistula K51.013
    obstruction K51.012
    rectal bleeding K51.011
    specified complication NEC K51.018
Pancreas, pancreatic — *see* condition
Pancreatitis (annular) (apoplectic) (calcareous) (edematous) (hemorrhagic) (malignant) (recurrent) (subacute) (suppurative) K85.9
  acute K85.9
    alcohol induced K85.2
    biliary K85.1
    drug induced K85.3
    gallstone K85.1
    idiopathic K85.0
    specified NEC K85.8
  chronic (infectious) K86.1
    alcohol-induced K86.0
    recurrent K86.1
    relapsing K86.1
  cystic (chronic) K86.1
  cytomegaloviral B25.2
  fibrous (chronic) K86.1
  gallstone K85.1
  gangrenous K85.8
  interstitial (chronic) K86.1
    acute K85.8
  mumps B26.3
  recurrent (chronic) K86.1
  relapsing, chronic K86.1
  syphilitic A52.74
Pancreatoblastoma — *see* Neoplasm, pancreas, malignant
Pancreolithiasis K86.8
Pancytolysis D75.89
Pancytopenia (acquired) D61.818
  with
    malformations D61.09
    myelodysplastic syndrome — *see* Syndrome, myelodysplastic
  antineoplastic chemotherapy induced D61.810
  congenital D61.09
  drug-induced NEC D61.811
Panencephalitis, subacute, sclerosing A81.1
Panhematopenia D61.9
  congenital D61.09
  constitutional D61.09
  splenic, primary D73.1
Panhemocytopenia D61.9
  congenital D61.09
  constitutional D61.09
Panhypogonadism E29.1
Panhypopituitarism E23.0
  prepubertal E23.0

☑ Additional Character Required — Refer to the Tabular List for Character Selection   ▽ Subterms under main terms may continue to next column or page

Panic (attack) (state) F41.0
  reaction to exceptional stress (transient) F43.0
Panmyelopathy, familial, constitutional D61.09
Panmyelophthisis D61.82
  congenital D61.09
Panmyelosis (acute) (with myelofibrosis) C94.4- ☑
Panner's disease — *see* Osteochondrosis, juvenile, humerus
Panneuritis endemica E51.11
Panniculitis (nodular) (nonsuppurative) M79.3
  back M54.00
    cervical region M54.02
    cervicothoracic region M54.03
    lumbar region M54.06
    lumbosacral region M54.07
    multiple sites M54.09
    occipito-atlanto-axial region M54.01
    sacrococcygeal region M54.08
    thoracic region M54.04
    thoracolumbar region M54.05
  lupus L93.2
  mesenteric K65.4
  neck M54.02
    cervicothoracic region M54.03
    occipito-atlanto-axial region M54.01
  relapsing M35.6
Panniculus adiposus (abdominal) E65
Pannus (allergic) (cornea) (degenerativus) (keratic) H16.42- ☑
  abdominal (symptomatic) E65
  trachomatosus, trachomatous (active) A71.1
Panophthalmitis H44.01- ☑
Pansinusitis (chronic) (hyperplastic) (nonpurulent) (purulent) J32.4
  acute J01.40
    recurrent J01.41
  tuberculous A15.8
Panuveitis (sympathetic) H44.11- ☑
Panvalvular disease I08.9
  specified NEC I08.8
Papanicolaou smear, cervix Z12.4
  as part of routine gynecological examination Z01.419
    with abnormal findings Z01.411
  for suspected neoplasm Z12.4
  nonspecific abnormal finding R87.619
  routine Z01.419
    with abnormal findings Z01.411
Papilledema (choked disc) H47.10
  associated with
    decreased ocular pressure H47.12
    increased intracranial pressure H47.11
    retinal disorder H47.13
  Foster-Kennedy syndrome H47.14- ☑
Papillitis H46.00
  anus K62.89
  chronic lingual K14.4
  necrotizing, kidney N17.2
  optic H46.0- ☑
  rectum K62.89
  renal, necrotizing N17.2
  tongue K14.0
Papilloma (*see also* Neoplasm, benign, by site)
  acuminatum (female) (male) (anogenital) A63.0
  benign pinta (primary) A67.0
  bladder (urinary) (transitional cell) D41.4
  choroid plexus (lateral ventricle) (third ventricle) D33.0
    anaplastic C71.5
    fourth ventricle D33.1
    malignant C71.5
  renal pelvis (transitional cell) D41.1- ☑
    benign D30.1- ☑
  Schneiderian
    specified site — *see* Neoplasm, benign, by site
    unspecified site D14.0
  serous surface
    borderline malignancy
      specified site — *see* Neoplasm, uncertain behavior, by site
      unspecified site D39.10
    specified site — *see* Neoplasm, benign, by site
    unspecified site D27.9
  transitional (cell)
    bladder (urinary) D41.4
    inverted type — *see* Neoplasm, uncertain behavior, by site
    renal pelvis D41.1- ☑
    ureter D41.2- ☑

Papilloma —. *continued*
  ureter (transitional cell) D41.2- ☑
    benign D30.2- ☑
  urothelial — *see* Neoplasm, uncertain behavior, by site
  villous — *see* Neoplasm, uncertain behavior, by site
    adenocarcinoma in — *see* Neoplasm, malignant, by site
    in situ — *see* Neoplasm, in situ
  yaws, plantar or palmar A66.1
Papillomata, multiple, of yaws A66.1
Papillomatosis (*see also* Neoplasm, benign, by site)
  confluent and reticulated L83
  cystic, breast — *see* Mastopathy, cystic
  ductal, breast — *see* Mastopathy, cystic
  intraductal (diffuse) — *see* Neoplasm, benign, by site
  subareolar duct D24- ☑
Papillomavirus, as cause of disease classified elsewhere B97.7
Papillon-Léage and Psaume syndrome Q87.0
Papule(s) R23.8
  carate (primary) A67.0
  fibrous, of nose D22.39
  Gottron's L94.4
  pinta (primary) A67.0
Papulosis
  lymphomatoid C86.6
  malignant I77.89
Papyraceous fetus O31.0- ☑
Para-albuminemia E88.09
Paracephalus Q89.7
Parachute mitral valve Q23.2
Paracoccidioidomycosis B41.9
  disseminated B41.7
  generalized B41.7
  mucocutaneous-lymphangitic B41.8
  pulmonary B41.0
  specified NEC B41.8
  visceral B41.8
Paradentosis K05.4
Paraffinoma T88.8 ☑
Paraganglioma D44.7
  adrenal D35.0- ☑
    malignant C74.1- ☑
  aortic body D44.7
    malignant C75.5
  carotid body D44.6
    malignant C75.4
  chromaffin (*see also* Neoplasm, benign, by site)
    malignant — *see* Neoplasm, malignant, by site
  extra-adrenal D44.7
    malignant C75.5
      specified site — *see* Neoplasm, malignant, by site
      unspecified site C75.5
    specified site — *see* Neoplasm, uncertain behavior, by site
    unspecified site D44.7
  gangliocytic D13.2
    specified site — *see* Neoplasm, benign, by site
    unspecified site D13.2
  glomus jugulare D44.7
    malignant C75.5
  jugular D44.7
  malignant C75.5
    specified site — *see* Neoplasm, malignant, by site
    unspecified site C75.5
  nonchromaffin D44.7
    malignant C75.5
      specified site — *see* Neoplasm, malignant, by site
      unspecified site C75.5
    specified site -— *see* Neoplasm, uncertain behavior, by site
    unspecified site D44.7
  parasympathetic D44.7
    specified site — *see* Neoplasm, uncertain behavior, by site
    unspecified site D44.7
  specified site — *see* Neoplasm, uncertain behavior, by site
  sympathetic D44.7
    specified site — *see* Neoplasm, uncertain behavior, by site
    unspecified site D44.7
  unspecified site D44.7
Parageusia R43.2

Parageusia — *continued*
  psychogenic F45.8
Paragonimiasis B66.4
Paragranuloma, Hodgkin — *see* Lymphoma, Hodgkin, classical, specified NEC
Parahemophilia (*see also* Defect, coagulation) D68.2
Parakeratosis R23.4
  variegata L41.0
Paralysis, paralytic (complete) (incomplete) G83.9
  with
    syphilis A52.17
  abducens, abducent (nerve) — *see* Strabismus, paralytic, sixth nerve
  abductor, lower extremity G57.9- ☑
  accessory nerve G52.8
  accommodation (*see also* Paresis, of accommodation)
    hysterical F44.89
  acoustic nerve (except Deafness) H93.3 ☑
  agitans (*see also* Parkinsonism) G20
    arteriosclerotic G21.4
  alternating (oculomotor) G83.89
  amyotrophic G12.21
  ankle G57.9- ☑
  anus (sphincter) K62.89
  arm — *see* Monoplegia, upper limb
  ascending (spinal), acute G61.0
  association G12.29
  asthenic bulbar G70.00
    with exacerbation (acute) G70.01
    in crisis G70.01
  ataxic (hereditary) G11.9
    general (syphilitic) A52.17
  atrophic G58.9
    infantile, acute — *see* Poliomyelitis, paralytic
    progressive G12.22
    spinal (acute) — *see* Poliomyelitis, paralytic
  axillary G54.0
  Babinski-Nageotte's G83.89
  Bell's G51.0
    newborn P11.3
  Benedikt's G46.3
  birth injury P14.9
    spinal cord P11.5
  bladder (neurogenic) (sphincter) N31.2
  bowel, colon or intestine K56.0
  brachial plexus G54.0
    birth injury P14.3
    newborn (birth injury) P14.3
  brain G83.9
    diplegia G83.0
    triplegia G83.89
  bronchial J98.09
  Brown-Séquard G83.81
  bulbar (chronic) (progressive) G12.22
    infantile — *see* Poliomyelitis, paralytic
    poliomyelitic — *see* Poliomyelitis, paralytic
    pseudo G12.29
  bulbospinal G70.00
    with exacerbation (acute) G70.01
    in crisis G70.01
  cardiac (*see also* Failure, heart) I50.9
  cerebrocerebellar, diplegic G80.1
  cervical
    plexus G54.2
    sympathetic G90.09
  Céstan-Chenais G46.3
  Charcot-Marie-Tooth type G60.0
  Clark's G80.9
  colon K56.0
  compressed air T70.3 ☑
  compression
    arm G56.9- ☑
    leg G57.9- ☑
    lower extremity G57.9- ☑
    upper extremity G56.9- ☑
  congenital (cerebral) — *see* Palsy, cerebral
  conjugate movement (gaze) (of eye) H51.0
    cortical (nuclear) (supranuclear) H51.0
  cordis — *see* Failure, heart
  cranial or cerebral nerve G52.9
  creeping G12.22
  crossed leg G83.89
  crutch — *see* Injury, brachial plexus
  deglutition R13.0
    hysterical F44.4
  dementia A52.17
  descending (spinal) NEC G12.29
  diaphragm (flaccid) J98.6

Paralysis, paralytic — *continued*
  diaphragm — *continued*
    due to accidental dissection of phrenic nerve during procedure — *see* Puncture, accidental complicating surgery
  digestive organs NEC K59.8
  diplegic — *see* Diplegia
  divergence (nuclear) H51.8
  diver's T70.3 ☑
  Duchenne's
    birth injury P14.0
    due to or associated with
      motor neuron disease G12.22
      muscular dystrophy G71.0
    due to intracranial or spinal birth injury — *see* Palsy, cerebral
  embolic (current episode) I63.4 ☑
  Erb (-Duchenne) (birth) (newborn) P14.0
  Erb's syphilitic spastic spinal A52.17
  esophagus K22.8
  eye muscle (extrinsic) H49.9
    intrinsic (*see also* Paresis, of accommodation)
  facial (nerve) G51.0
    birth injury P11.3
    congenital P11.3
    following operation NEC — *see* Puncture, accidental complicating surgery
    newborn (birth injury) P11.3
  familial (recurrent) (periodic) G72.3
    spastic G11.4
  fauces J39.2
  finger G56.9- ☑
  gait R26.1
  gastric nerve (nondiabetic) G52.2
  gaze, conjugate H51.0
  general (progressive) (syphilitic) A52.17
    juvenile A50.45
  glottis J38.00
    bilateral J38.02
    unilateral J38.01
  gluteal G54.1
  Gubler (-Millard) G46.3
  hand — *see* Monoplegia, upper limb
  heart — *see* Arrest, cardiac
  hemiplegic — *see* Hemiplegia
  hyperkalemic periodic (familial) G72.3
  hypoglossal (nerve) G52.3
  hypokalemic periodic G72.3
  hysterical F44.4
  ileus K56.0
  infantile (*see also* Poliomyelitis, paralytic) A80.30
    bulbar — *see* Poliomyelitis, paralytic
    cerebral — *see* Palsy, cerebral
    spastic — *see* Palsy, cerebral, spastic
  infective — *see* Poliomyelitis, paralytic
  inferior nuclear G83.9
  internuclear — *see* Ophthalmoplegia, internuclear
  intestine K56.0
  iris H57.09
    due to diphtheria (toxin) A36.89
  ischemic, Volkmann's (complicating trauma) T79.6 ☑
  Jackson's G83.89
  jake — *see* Poisoning, food, noxious, plant
  Jamaica ginger (jake) G62.2
  juvenile general A50.45
  Klumpke (-Déjérine) (birth) (newborn) P14.1
  labioglossal (laryngeal) (pharyngeal) G12.29
  Landry's G61.0
  laryngeal nerve (recurrent) (superior) (unilateral) J38.00
    bilateral J38.02
    unilateral J38.01
  larynx J38.00
    bilateral J38.02
    due to diphtheria (toxin) A36.2
    unilateral J38.01
  lateral G12.21
  lead T56.0 ☑
  left side — *see* Hemiplegia
  leg G83.1- ☑
    both — *see* Paraplegia
    crossed G83.89
    hysterical F44.4
    psychogenic F44.4
    transient or transitory R29.818
      traumatic NEC — *see* Injury, nerve, leg
  levator palpebrae superioris — *see* Blepharoptosis, paralytic
  limb — *see* Monoplegia

Paralysis, paralytic — *continued*
  lip K13.0
  Lissauer's A52.17
  lower limb — *see* Monoplegia, lower limb
    both — *see* Paraplegia
  lung J98.4
  median nerve G56.1- ☑
  medullary (tegmental) G83.89
  mesencephalic NEC G83.89
    tegmental G83.89
  middle alternating G83.89
  Millard-Gubler-Foville G46.3
  monoplegic — *see* Monoplegia
  motor G83.9
  muscle, muscular NEC G72.89
    due to nerve lesion G58.9
    eye (extrinsic) H49.9
      intrinsic — *see* Paresis, of accommodation
      oblique — *see* Strabismus, paralytic, fourth nerve
    iris sphincter H21.9
    ischemic (Volkmann's) (complicating trauma) T79.6 ☑
    progressive G12.21
    pseudohypertrophic G71.0
  musculocutaneous nerve G56.9- ☑
  musculospiral G56.9- ☑
  nerve (*see also* Disorder, nerve)
    abducent — *see* Strabismus, paralytic, sixth nerve
    accessory G52.8
    auditory (except Deafness) H93.3 ☑
    birth injury P14.9
    cranial or cerebral G52.9
    facial G51.0
      birth injury P11.3
      congenital P11.3
      newborn (birth injury) P11.3
    fourth or trochlear — *see* Strabismus, paralytic, fourth nerve
    newborn (birth injury) P14.9
    oculomotor — *see* Strabismus, paralytic, third nerve
    phrenic (birth injury) P14.2
    radial G56.3- ☑
    seventh or facial G51.0
      newborn (birth injury) P11.3
    sixth or abducent — *see* Strabismus, paralytic, sixth nerve
    syphilitic A52.15
    third or oculomotor — *see* Strabismus, paralytic, third nerve
    trigeminal G50.9
    trochlear — *see* Strabismus, paralytic, fourth nerve
    ulnar G56.2- ☑
  normokalemic periodic G72.3
  ocular H49.9
    alternating G83.89
  oculofacial, congenital (Moebius) Q87.0
  oculomotor (external bilateral) (nerve) — *see* Strabismus, paralytic, third nerve
  palate (soft) K13.79
  paratrigeminal G50.9
  periodic (familial) (hyperkalemic) (hypokalemic) (myotonic) (normokalemic) (potassium sensitive) (secondary) G72.3
  peripheral autonomic nervous system — *see* Neuropathy, peripheral, autonomic
  peroneal (nerve) G57.3- ☑
  pharynx J39.2
  phrenic nerve G56.8- ☑
  plantar nerve(s) G57.6- ☑
  pneumogastric nerve G52.2
  poliomyelitis (current) — *see* Poliomyelitis, paralytic
  popliteal nerve G57.3- ☑
  postepileptic transitory G83.84
  progressive (atrophic) (bulbar) (spinal) G12.22
    general A52.17
    infantile acute — *see* Poliomyelitis, paralytic
    supranuclear G23.1
  pseudobulbar G12.29
  pseudohypertrophic (muscle) G71.0
  psychogenic F44.4
  quadriceps G57.9- ☑
  quadriplegic — *see* Tetraplegia
  radial nerve G56.3- ☑
  rectus muscle (eye) H49.9
  recurrent isolated sleep G47.53

Paralysis, paralytic — *continued*
  respiratory (muscle) (system) (tract) R06.81
    center NEC G93.89
    congenital P28.89
    newborn P28.89
  right side — *see* Hemiplegia
  saturnine T56.0 ☑
  sciatic nerve G57.0- ☑
  senile G83.9
  shaking — *see* Parkinsonism
  shoulder G56.9- ☑
  sleep, recurrent isolated G47.53
  spastic G83.9
    cerebral — *see* Palsy, cerebral, spastic
    congenital (cerebral) — *see* Palsy, cerebral, spastic
    familial G11.4
    hereditary G11.4
    quadriplegic G80.0
    syphilitic (spinal) A52.17
  sphincter, bladder — *see* Paralysis, bladder
  spinal (cord) G83.9
    accessory nerve G52.8
    acute — *see* Poliomyelitis, paralytic
    ascending acute G61.0
    atrophic (acute) (*see also* Poliomyelitis, paralytic)
      spastic, syphilitic A52.17
    congenital NEC — *see* Palsy, cerebral
    hereditary G95.89
    infantile — *see* Poliomyelitis, paralytic
    progressive G12.21
    sequelae NEC G83.89
  sternomastoid G52.8
  stomach K31.84
    diabetic — *see* Diabetes, by type, with gastroparesis
    nerve G52.2
      diabetic — *see* Diabetes, by type, with gastroparesis
  stroke — *see* Infarct, brain
  subcapsularis G56.8- ☑
  supranuclear (progressive) G23.1
  sympathetic G90.8
    cervical G90.09
    nervous system — *see* Neuropathy, peripheral, autonomic
  syndrome G83.9
    specified NEC G83.89
  syphilitic spastic spinal (Erb's) A52.17
  thigh G57.9- ☑
  throat J39.2
    diphtheritic A36.0
    muscle J39.2
  thrombotic (current episode) I63.3 ☑
  thumb G56.9- ☑
  tick — *see* Toxicity, venom, arthropod, specified NEC
  Todd's (postepileptic transitory paralysis) G83.84
  toe G57.6- ☑
  tongue K14.8
  transient R29.5
    arm or leg NEC R29.818
    traumatic NEC — *see* Injury, nerve
  trapezius G52.8
  traumatic, transient NEC — *see* Injury, nerve
  trembling — *see* Parkinsonism
  triceps brachii G56.9- ☑
  trigeminal nerve G50.9
  trochlear (nerve) — *see* Strabismus, paralytic, fourth nerve
  ulnar nerve G56.2- ☑
  upper limb — *see* Monoplegia, upper limb
  uremic N18.9 [G99.8]
  uveoparotitic D86.89
  uvula K13.79
    postdiphtheritic A36.0
  vagus nerve G52.2
  vasomotor NEC G90.8
  velum palati K13.79
  vesical — *see* Paralysis, bladder
  vestibular nerve (except Vertigo) H93.3 ☑
  vocal cords J38.00
    bilateral J38.02
    unilateral J38.01
  Volkmann's (complicating trauma) T79.6 ☑
  wasting G12.29
  Weber's G46.3
  wrist G56.9- ☑
Paramedial urethrovesical orifice Q64.79

☑ Additional Character Required — Refer to the Tabular List for Character Selection ▽ Subterms under main terms may continue to next column or page

Paramenia N92.6
Parametritis (see also Disease, pelvis, inflammatory)
   N73.2
  acute N73.0
  complicating abortion — see Abortion, by type, complicated by, parametritis
Parametrium, parametric — see condition
Paramnesia — see Amnesia
Paramolar K00.1
Paramyloidosis E85.8
Paramyoclonus multiplex G25.3
Paramyotonia (congenita) G71.19
Parangi — see Yaws
Paranoia (querulans) F22
  senile F03 ☑
Paranoid
  dementia (senile) F03 ☑
   praecox — see Schizophrenia
  personality F60.0
  psychosis (climacteric) (involutional) (menopausal)
   F22
   psychogenic (acute) F23
   senile F03 ☑
  reaction (acute) F23
   chronic F22
  schizophrenia F20.0
  state (climacteric) (involutional) (menopausal) (simple)
   F22
   senile F03 ☑
  tendencies F60.0
  traits F60.0
  trends F60.0
  type, psychopathic personality F60.0
Paraparesis — see Paraplegia
Paraphasia R47.02
Paraphilia F65.9
Paraphimosis (congenital) N47.2
  chancroidal A57
Paraphrenia, paraphrenic (late) F22
  schizophrenia F20.0
Paraplegia (lower) G82.20
  ataxic — see Degeneration, combined, spinal cord
  complete G82.21
  congenital (cerebral) G80.8
   spastic G80.1
  familial spastic G11.4
  functional (hysterical) F44.4
  hereditary, spastic G11.4
  hysterical F44.4
  incomplete G82.22
  Pott's A18.01
  psychogenic F44.4
  spastic
   Erb's spinal, syphilitic A52.17
   hereditary G11.4
   tropical G04.1
  syphilitic (spastic) A52.17
  tropical spastic G04.1
Parapoxvirus B08.60
  specified NEC B08.69
Paraproteinemia D89.2
  benign (familial) D89.2
  monoclonal D47.2
  secondary to malignant disease D47.2
Parapsoriasis L41.9
  en plaques L41.4
  guttata L41.1
  large plaque L41.4
  retiform, retiformis L41.5
  small plaque L41.3
  specified NEC L41.8
  varioliformis (acuta) L41.0
Parasitic (see also condition)
  disease NEC B89
  stomatitis B37.0
  sycosis (beard) (scalp) B35.0
  twin Q89.4
Parasitism B89
  intestinal B82.9
  skin B88.9
  specified — see Infestation
Parasitophobia F40.218
Parasomnia G47.50
  due to
   alcohol
    abuse F10.182
    dependence F10.282

Parasomnia — continued
  due to — continued
   alcohol — continued
    use F10.982
   amphetamines
    abuse F15.182
    dependence F15.282
    use F15.982
   caffeine
    abuse F15.182
    dependence F15.282
    use F15.982
   cocaine
    abuse F14.182
    dependence F14.282
    use F14.982
   drug NEC
    abuse F19.182
    dependence F19.282
    use F19.982
   opioid
    abuse F11.182
    dependence F11.282
    use F11.982
   psychoactive substance NEC
    abuse F19.182
    dependence F19.282
    use F19.982
   sedative, hypnotic, or anxiolytic
    abuse F13.182
    dependence F13.282
    use F13.982
   stimulant NEC
    abuse F15.182
    dependence F15.282
    use F15.982
  in conditions classified elsewhere G47.54
  nonorganic origin F51.8
  organic G47.50
  specified NEC G47.59
Paraspadias Q54.9
Paraspasmus facialis G51.8
Parasuicide (attempt)
  history of (personal) Z91.5
   in family Z81.8
Parathyroid gland — see condition
Parathyroid tetany E20.9
Paratrachoma A74.0
Paratyphilitis — see Appendicitis
Paratyphoid (fever) — see Fever, paratyphoid
Paratyphus — see Fever, paratyphoid
Paraurethral duct Q64.79
  nonorganic origin F51.5
Paraurethritis (see also Urethritis)
  gonococcal (acute) (chronic) (with abscess) A54.1
Paravaccinia NEC B08.04
Paravaginitis — see Vaginitis
Parencephalitis (see also Encephalitis)
  sequelae G09
Parent-child conflict — see Conflict, parent-child
  estrangement NEC Z62.890
Paresis (see also Paralysis)
  accommodation — see Paresis, of accommodation
  Bernhardt's G57.1- ☑
  bladder (sphincter) (see also Paralysis, bladder)
   tabetic A52.17
  bowel, colon or intestine K56.0
  extrinsic muscle, eye H49.9
  general (progressive) (syphilitic) A52.17
   juvenile A50.45
  heart — see Failure, heart
  insane (syphilitic) A52.17
  juvenile (general) A50.45
  of accommodation H52.52- ☑
  peripheral progressive (idiopathic) G60.3
  pseudohypertrophic G71.0
  senile G83.9
  syphilitic (general) A52.17
   congenital A50.45
  vesical NEC N31.2
Paresthesia (see also Disturbance, sensation)
  Bernhardt G57.1- ☑
Paretic — see condition
Parinaud's
  conjunctivitis H10.89
  oculoglandular syndrome H10.89
  ophthalmoplegia H49.88- ☑
Parkinsonism (idiopathic) (primary) G20

Parkinsonism — continued
  with neurogenic orthostatic hypotension (symptomatic) G90.3
  arteriosclerotic G21.4
  dementia G31.83 [F02.80]
   with behavioral disturbance G31.83 [F02.81]
  due to
   drugs NEC G21.19
    neuroleptic G21.11
  neuroleptic induced G21.11
  postencephalitic G21.3
  secondary G21.9
   due to
    arteriosclerosis G21.4
    drugs NEC G21.19
     neuroleptic G21.11
    encephalitis G21.3
    external agents NEC G21.2
    syphilis A52.19
   specified NEC G21.8
  syphilitic A52.19
  treatment-induced NEC G21.19
  vascular G21.4
Parkinson's disease, syndrome or tremor — see
  Parkinsonism
Parodontitis — see Periodontitis
Parodontosis K05.4
Paronychia (see also Cellulitis, digit)
  with lymphangitis -— see Lymphangitis, acute, digit
  candidal (chronic) B37.2
  tuberculous (primary) A18.4
Parorexia (psychogenic) F50.8
Parosmia R43.1
  psychogenic F45.8
Parotid gland — see condition
Parotitis, parotiditis (allergic)(nonspecific toxic) (purulent) (septic) (suppurative) (see also Sialoadenitis)
  epidemic — see Mumps
  infectious — see Mumps
  postoperative K91.89
  surgical K91.89
Parrot fever A70
Parrot's disease (early congenital syphilitic pseudoparalysis) A50.02
Parry-Romberg syndrome G51.8
Parry's disease or syndrome E05.00
  with thyroid storm E05.01
Pars planitis — see Cyclitis
Parsonage (-Aldren)-**Turner syndrome** G54.5
Parson's disease (exophthalmic goiter) E05.00
  with thyroid storm E05.01
Particolored infant Q82.8
Parturition — see Delivery
Parulis K04.7
  with sinus K04.6
Parvovirus, as cause of disease classified elsewhere
  B97.6
Pasini and Pierini's atrophoderma L90.3
Passage
  false, urethra N36.5
  meconium (newborn) during delivery P03.82
  of sounds or bougies — see Attention to, artificial,
   opening
Passive — see condition
  smoking Z77.22
Pasteurella septica A28.0
Pasteurellosis — see Infection, Pasteurella
PAT (paroxysmal atrial tachycardia) I47.1
Patau's syndrome — see Trisomy, 13
Patches
  mucous (syphilitic) A51.39
   congenital A50.07
  smokers' (mouth) K13.24
Patellar — see condition
Patent (see also Imperfect, closure)
  canal of Nuck Q52.4
  cervix N88.3
  ductus arteriosus or Botallo's Q25.0
  foramen
   botalli Q21.1
   ovale Q21.1
  interauricular septum Q21.1
  interventricular septum Q21.0
  omphalomesenteric duct Q43.0
  os (uteri) — see Patent, cervix
  ostium secundum Q21.1
  urachus Q64.4

▽ Subterms under main terms may continue to next column or page
☑ Additional Character Required — Refer to the Tabular List for Character Selection
241

Index

Patent — Perforation, perforated

Patent — *continued*
vitelline duct Q43.Ø
Paterson (-Brown)(-Kelly) **syndrome or web** D5Ø.1
Pathologic, pathological (*see also* condition)
asphyxia RØ9.Ø1
fire-setting F63.1
gambling F63.Ø
ovum OØ2.Ø
resorption, tooth KØ3.3
stealing F63.2
Pathology (of) — *see* Disease
periradicular, associated with previous endodontic
treatment NEC M27.59
Pattern, sleep-wake, irregular G47.23
Patulous (*see also* Imperfect, closure (congenital))
alimentary tract Q45.8
lower Q43.8
upper Q4Ø.8
eustachian tube H69.Ø- ☑
Pause, sinoatrial I49.5
Paxton's disease B36.2
Pearl(s)
enamel KØØ.2
Epstein's KØ9.8
Pearl-worker's disease — *see* Osteomyelitis, specified
type NEC
Pectenosis K62.4
Pectoral — *see* condition
Pectus
carinatum (congenital) Q67.7
acquired M95.4
rachitic sequelae (late effect) E64.3
excavatum (congenital) Q67.6
acquired M95.4
rachitic sequelae (late effect) E64.3
recurvatum (congenital) Q67.6
Pedatrophia E41
Pederosis F65.4
Pediculosis (infestation) B85.2
capitis (head-louse) (any site) B85.Ø
corporis (body-louse) (any site) B85.1
eyelid B85.Ø
mixed (classifiable to more than one of the titles B85.Ø-
B85.3) B85.4
pubis (pubic louse) (any site) B85.3
vestimenti B85.1
vulvae B85.3
Pediculus (infestation) — *see* Pediculosis
Pedophilia F65.4
Peg-shaped teeth KØØ.2
Pelade — *see* Alopecia, areata
Pelger-Huët anomaly or syndrome D72.Ø
Peliosis (rheumatica) D69.Ø
hepatis K76.4
with toxic liver disease K71.8
Pelizaeus-Merzbacher disease E75.29
Pellagra (alcoholic) (with polyneuropathy) E52
**Pellagra-cerebellar-ataxia-renal aminoaciduria
syndrome** E72.Ø2
Pellegrini (-Stieda) **disease or syndrome** — *see* Bursitis,
tibial collateral
Pellizzi's syndrome E34.8
Pel's crisis A52.11
Pelvic (*see also* condition)
examination (periodic) (routine) ZØ1.419
with abnormal findings ZØ1.411
kidney, congenital Q63.2
Pelviolithiasis — *see* Calculus, kidney
Pelviperitonitis (*see also* Peritonitis, pelvic)
gonococcal A54.24
puerperal O85
Pelvis — *see* condition or type
Pemphigoid L12.9
benign, mucous membrane L12.1
bullous L12.Ø
cicatricial L12.1
juvenile L12.2
ocular L12.1
specified NEC L12.8
Pemphigus L1Ø.9
benign familial (chronic) Q82.8
Brazilian L1Ø.3
circinatus L13.Ø
conjunctiva L12.1
drug-induced L1Ø.5
erythematosus L1Ø.4
foliaceus L1Ø.2

Pemphigus — *continued*
gangrenous — *see* Gangrene
neonatorum LØ1.Ø3
ocular L12.1
paraneoplastic L1Ø.81
specified NEC L1Ø.89
syphilitic (congenital) A5Ø.Ø6
vegetans L1Ø.1
vulgaris L1Ø.Ø
wildfire L1Ø.3
Pendred's syndrome EØ7.1
Pendulous
abdomen, in pregnancy — *see* Pregnancy, complicated by, abnormal, pelvic organs or tissues NEC
breast N64.89
Penetrating wound (*see also* Puncture)
with internal injury — *see* Injury, by site
eyeball — *see* Puncture, eyeball
orbit (with or without foreign body) — *see* Puncture,
orbit
uterus by instrument with or following ectopic or
molar pregnancy OØ8.6
Penicillosis B48.4
Penis — *see* condition
Penitis N48.29
Pentalogy of Fallot Q21.8
Pentasomy X syndrome Q97.1
Pentosuria (essential) E74.8
Percreta placenta - O43.23 ☑
Peregrinating patient — *see* Disorder, factitious
Perforation, perforated (nontraumatic) (of)
accidental during procedure (blood vessel) (nerve)
(organ) — *see* Complication, accidental puncture or laceration
antrum — *see* Sinusitis, maxillary
appendix K35.2
atrial septum, multiple Q21.1
attic, ear — *see* Perforation, tympanum, attic
bile duct (common) (hepatic) K83.2
cystic K82.2
bladder (urinary)
with or following ectopic or molar pregnancy OØ8.6
obstetrical trauma O71.5
traumatic S37.29 ☑
at delivery O71.5
bowel K63.1
with or following ectopic or molar pregnancy OØ8.6
newborn P78.Ø
obstetrical trauma O71.5
traumatic — *see* Laceration, intestine
broad ligament N83.8
with or following ectopic or molar pregnancy OØ8.6
obstetrical trauma O71.6
by
device, implant or graft (*see also* Complications,
by site and type, mechanical) T85.628 ☑
arterial graft NEC — *see* Complication, cardiovascular device, mechanical, vascular
breast (implant) T85.49 ☑
catheter NEC T85.698 ☑
cystostomy T83.Ø9Ø ☑
dialysis (renal) T82.49 ☑
intraperitoneal T85.691 ☑
infusion NEC T82.594 ☑
spinal (epidural) (subdural) T85.69Ø ☑
electronic (electrode) (pulse generator) (stimulator)
bone T84.39Ø ☑
cardiac T82.199 ☑
electrode T82.19Ø ☑
pulse generator T82.191 ☑
specified type NEC T82.198 ☑
nervous system — *see* Complication, prosthetic device, mechanical, electronic
nervous system stimulator
urinary — *see* Complication, genitourinary,
device, urinary, mechanical
fixation, internal (orthopedic) NEC — *see*
Complication, fixation device, mechanical
gastrointestinal — *see* Complications, prosthetic device, mechanical, gastrointestinal
device
genital NEC T83.498 ☑
intrauterine contraceptive device T83.39 ☑
penile prosthesis T83.49Ø ☑
heart NEC — *see* Complication, cardiovascular
device, mechanical

Perforation, perforated — *continued*
by — *continued*
device, implant or graft (*see also* Complications, by
site and type, mechanical) — *continued*
joint prosthesis — *see* Complications, joint
prosthesis, mechanical, specified NEC, by
site
ocular NEC — *see* Complications, prosthetic
device, mechanical, ocular device
orthopedic NEC — *see* Complication, orthopedic, device, mechanical
specified NEC T85.628 ☑
urinary, indwelling T83.Ø98 ☑
urinary NEC (*see also* Complication, genitourinary, device, urinary, mechanical)
graft T83.29 ☑
vascular NEC — *see* Complication, cardiovascular device, mechanical
ventricular intracranial shunt T85.Ø9 ☑
foreign body left accidentally in operative wound
T81.539 ☑
instrument (any) during a procedure, accidental
— *see* Puncture, accidental complicating
surgery
cecum K35.2
cervix (uteri) N88.8
with or following ectopic or molar pregnancy OØ8.6
obstetrical trauma O71.3
colon K63.1
newborn P78.Ø
obstetrical trauma O71.5
traumatic — *see* Laceration, intestine, large
common duct (bile) K83.2
cornea (due to ulceration) — *see* Ulcer, cornea, perforated
cystic duct K82.2
diverticulum (intestine) K57.8Ø
with bleeding K57.81
large intestine K57.2Ø
with
bleeding K57.21
small intestine K57.4Ø
with bleeding K57.41
small intestine K57.ØØ
with
bleeding K57.Ø1
large intestine K57.4Ø
with bleeding K57.41
ear drum — *see* Perforation, tympanum
esophagus K22.3
ethmoidal sinus — *see* Sinusitis, ethmoidal
frontal sinus — *see* Sinusitis, frontal
gallbladder K82.2
heart valve — *see* Endocarditis
ileum K63.1
newborn P78.Ø
obstetrical trauma O71.5
traumatic — *see* Laceration, intestine, small
instrumental, surgical (accidental) (blood vessel)
(nerve) (organ) — *see* Puncture, accidental
complicating surgery
intestine NEC K63.1
with ectopic or molar pregnancy OØ8.6
newborn P78.Ø
obstetrical trauma O71.5
traumatic — *see* Laceration, intestine
ulcerative NEC K63.1
newborn P78.Ø
jejunum, jejunal K63.1
obstetrical trauma O71.5
traumatic — *see* Laceration, intestine, small
ulcer — *see* Ulcer, gastrojejunal, with perforation
joint prosthesis — *see* Complications, joint prosthesis,
mechanical, specified NEC, by site
mastoid (antrum) (cell) — *see* Disorder, mastoid,
specified NEC
maxillary sinus — *see* Sinusitis, maxillary
membrana tympani — *see* Perforation, tympanum
nasal
septum J34.89
congenital Q3Ø.3
syphilitic A52.73
sinus J34.89
congenital Q3Ø.8
due to sinusitis — *see* Sinusitis
palate (*see also* Cleft, palate) Q35.9
syphilitic A52.79

Perforation, perforated — *continued*
  palatine vault (*see also* Cleft, palate, hard) Q35.1
    syphilitic A52.79
      congenital A50.59
  pars flaccida (ear drum) — *see* Perforation, tympanum, attic
  pelvic
    floor S31.030 ☑
      with
        ectopic or molar pregnancy O08.6
        penetration into retroperitoneal space S31.031 ☑
        retained foreign body S31.040 ☑
          with penetration into retroperitoneal space S31.041 ☑
      following ectopic or molar pregnancy O08.6
      obstetrical trauma O70.1
    organ S37.99 ☑
      adrenal gland S37.818 ☑
      bladder — *see* Perforation, bladder
      fallopian tube S37.599 ☑
        bilateral S37.592 ☑
        unilateral S37.591 ☑
      kidney S37.09- ☑
      obstetrical trauma O71.5
      ovary S37.499 ☑
        bilateral S37.492 ☑
        unilateral S37.491 ☑
      prostate S37.828 ☑
      specified organ NEC S37.898 ☑
      ureter — *see* Perforation, ureter
      urethra — *see* Perforation, urethra
      uterus — *see* Perforation, uterus
  perineum — *see* Laceration, perineum
  pharynx J39.2
  rectum K63.1
    newborn P78.0
    obstetrical trauma O71.5
    traumatic S36.63 ☑
  root canal space due to endodontic treatment M27.51
  sigmoid K63.1
    newborn P78.0
    obstetrical trauma O71.5
    traumatic S36.533 ☑
  sinus (accessory) (chronic) (nasal) J34.89
  sphenoidal sinus — *see* Sinusitis, sphenoidal
  surgical (accidental) (by instrument) (blood vessel) (nerve) (organ) — *see* Puncture, accidental complicating surgery
  traumatic
    external — *see* Puncture
    eye — *see* Puncture, eyeball
    internal organ — *see* Injury, by site
  tympanum, tympanic (membrane) (persistent post-traumatic) (postinflammatory) H72.9- ☑
    attic H72.1- ☑
      multiple — *see* Perforation, tympanum, multiple
      total — *see* Perforation, tympanum, total
    central H72.0- ☑
      multiple — *see* Perforation, tympanum, multiple
      total — *see* Perforation, tympanum, total
    marginal NEC — *see* subcategory H72.2 ☑
    multiple H72.81- ☑
    pars flaccida — *see* Perforation, tympanum, attic
    total H72.82- ☑
    traumatic, current episode S09.2- ☑
  typhoid, gastrointestinal — *see* Typhoid
  ulcer — *see* Ulcer, by site, with perforation
  ureter N28.89
    traumatic S37.19 ☑
  urethra N36.8
    with ectopic or molar pregnancy O08.6
    following ectopic or molar pregnancy O08.6
    obstetrical trauma O71.5
    traumatic S37.39 ☑
      at delivery O71.5
  uterus
    with ectopic or molar pregnancy O08.6
    by intrauterine contraceptive device T83.39 ☑
    following ectopic or molar pregnancy O08.6
    obstetrical trauma O71.1
    traumatic S37.69 ☑
      obstetric O71.1
  uvula K13.79
    syphilitic A52.79

Perforation, perforated — *continued*
  vagina O71.4
    obstetrical trauma O71.4
    other trauma — *see* Puncture, vagina
Periadenitis mucosa necrotica recurrens K12.0
Periappendicitis (acute) — *see* Appendicitis
Periarteritis nodosa (disseminated) (infectious) (necrotizing) M30.0
Periarthritis (joint) (*see also* Enthesopathy)
  Duplay's M75.0- ☑
  gonococcal A54.42
  humeroscapularis — *see* Capsulitis, adhesive
  scapulohumeral — *see* Capsulitis, adhesive
  shoulder — *see* Capsulitis, adhesive
  wrist M77.2- ☑
Periarthrosis (angioneural) — *see* Enthesopathy
Pericapsulitis, adhesive (shoulder) — *see* Capsulitis, adhesive
Pericarditis (with decompensation) (with effusion) I31.9
  with rheumatic fever (conditions in I00)
    active — *see* Pericarditis, rheumatic
    inactive or quiescent I09.2
  acute (hemorrhagic) (nonrheumatic) (Sicca) I30.9
    with chorea (acute) (rheumatic) (Sydenham's) I02.0
    benign I30.8
    nonspecific I30.0
    rheumatic I01.0
      with chorea (acute) (Sydenham's) I02.0
  adhesive or adherent (chronic) (external) (internal) I31.0
    acute — *see* Pericarditis, acute
    rheumatic I09.2
  bacterial (acute) (subacute) (with serous or seropurulent effusion) I30.1
  calcareous I31.1
  cholesterol (chronic) I31.8
    acute I30.9
  chronic (nonrheumatic) I31.9
    rheumatic I09.2
  constrictive (chronic) I31.1
  coxsackie B33.23
  fibrinocaseous (tuberculous) A18.84
  fibrinopurulent I30.1
  fibrinous I30.8
  fibrous I31.0
  gonococcal A54.83
  idiopathic I30.0
  in systemic lupus erythematosus M32.12
  infective I30.1
  meningococcal A39.53
  neoplastic (chronic) I31.8
    acute I30.9
  obliterans, obliterating I31.0
  plastic I31.0
  pneumococcal I30.1
  postinfarction I24.1
  purulent I30.1
  rheumatic (active) (acute) (with effusion) (with pneumonia) I01.0
    with chorea (acute) (rheumatic) (Sydenham's) I02.0
    chronic or inactive (with chorea) I09.2
  rheumatoid — *see* Rheumatoid, carditis
  septic I30.1
  serofibrinous I30.8
  staphylococcal I30.1
  streptococcal I30.1
  suppurative I30.1
  syphilitic A52.06
  tuberculous A18.84
  uremic N18.9 [I32]
  viral I30.1
Pericardium, pericardial — *see* condition
Pericellulitis — *see* Cellulitis
Pericementitis (chronic) (suppurative) (*see also* Periodontitis)
  acute K05.20
    generalized K05.22
    localized K05.21
Perichondritis
  auricle — *see* Perichondritis, ear
  bronchus J98.09
  ear (external) H61.00- ☑
    acute H61.01- ☑
    chronic H61.02- ☑
  external auditory canal — *see* Perichondritis, ear
  larynx J38.7
    syphilitic A52.73
    typhoid A01.09

Perichondritis — *continued*
  nose J34.89
  pinna — *see* Perichondritis, ear
  trachea J39.8
Periclasia K05.4
Pericoronitis — *see* Periodontitis
Pericystitis N30.90
  with hematuria N30.91
Peridiverticulitis (intestine) K57.92
  cecum — *see* Diverticulitis, intestine, large
  colon — *see* Diverticulitis, intestine, large
  duodenum — *see* Diverticulitis, intestine, small
  intestine — *see* Diverticulitis, intestine
  jejunum — *see* Diverticulitis, intestine, small
  rectosigmoid — *see* Diverticulitis, intestine, large
  rectum — *see* Diverticulitis, intestine, large
  sigmoid — *see* Diverticulitis, intestine, large
Periendocarditis — *see* Endocarditis
Periepididymitis N45.1
Perifolliculitis L01.02
  abscedens, caput, scalp L66.3
  capitis, abscedens (et suffodiens) L66.3
  superficial pustular L01.02
Perihepatitis K65.8
Perilabyrinthitis (acute) — *see* subcategory H83.0 ☑
Perimeningitis — *see* Meningitis
Perimetritis — *see* Endometritis
Perimetrosalpingitis — *see* Salpingo-oophoritis
Perineocele N81.81
Perinephric, perinephritic — *see* condition
Perinephritis (*see also* Infection, kidney)
  purulent — *see* Abscess, kidney
Perineum, perineal — *see* condition
Perineuritis NEC — *see* Neuralgia
Periodic — *see* condition
Periodontitis (chronic) (complex) (compound) (local) (simplex) K05.30
  acute K05.20
    generalized K05.22
    localized K05.21
  apical K04.5
    acute (pulpal origin) K04.4
  generalized K05.32
  localized K05.31
Periodontoclasia K05.4
Periodontosis (juvenile) K05.4
Periods (*see also* Menstruation)
  heavy N92.0
  irregular N92.6
  shortened intervals (irregular) N92.1
Perionychia (*see also* Cellulitis, digit)
  with lymphangitis — *see* Lymphangitis, acute, digit
Perioophoritis — *see* Salpingo-oophoritis
Periorchitis N45.2
Periosteum, periosteal — *see* condition
Periostitis (albuminosa) (circumscribed) (diffuse) (infective) (monomelic) (*see also* Osteomyelitis)
  alveolar M27.3
  alveolodental M27.3
  dental M27.3
  gonorrheal A54.43
  jaw (lower) (upper) M27.2
  orbit H05.03- ☑
  syphilitic A52.77
    congenital (early) A50.02 [M90.80]
    secondary A51.46
  tuberculous — *see* Tuberculosis, bone
  yaws (hypertrophic) (early) (late) A66.6 [M90.80]
Periostosis (hyperplastic) (*see also* Disorder, bone, specified type NEC)
  with osteomyelitis — *see* Osteomyelitis, specified type NEC
Peripartum
  cardiomyopathy O90.3
Periphlebitis — *see* Phlebitis
Periproctitis K62.89
Periprostatitis — *see* Prostatitis
Perirectal — *see* condition
Perirenal — *see* condition
Perisalpingitis — *see* Salpingo-oophoritis
Perisplenitis (infectional) D73.89
Peristalsis, visible or reversed R19.2
Peritendinitis — *see* Enthesopathy
Peritoneum, peritoneal — *see* condition
Peritonitis (adhesive) (bacterial) (fibrinous) (hemorrhagic) (idiopathic) (localized) (perforative) (primary) (with adhesions) (with effusion) K65.9

Index

Peritonitis — Perversion, perverted

Peritonitis — *continued*
  with or following
    abscess K65.1
    appendicitis K35.2
      with perforation or rupture K35.2
      generalized K35.2
      localized K35.3
    diverticular disease (intestine) K57.80
      with bleeding K57.81
      ectopic or molar pregnancy O08.0
      large intestine K57.20
        with
          bleeding K57.21
          small intestine K57.40
            with bleeding K57.41
      small intestine K57.00
        with
          bleeding K57.01
          large intestine K57.40
            with bleeding K57.41
  acute (generalized) K65.0
  aseptic T81.61 ☑
  bile, biliary K65.3
  chemical T81.61 ☑
  chlamydial A74.81
  chronic proliferative K65.8
  complicating abortion — *see* Abortion, by type, complicated by, pelvic peritonitis
  congenital P78.1
  diaphragmatic K65.0
  diffuse K65.0
  diphtheritic A36.89
  disseminated K65.0
  due to
    bile K65.3
    foreign
      body or object accidentally left during a procedure (instrument) (sponge) (swab) T81.599 ☑
      substance accidentally left during a procedure (chemical) (powder) (talc) T81.61 ☑
    talc T81.61 ☑
    urine K65.8
  eosinophilic K65.8
    acute K65.0
  fibrocaseous (tuberculous) A18.31
  fibropurulent K65.0
  following ectopic or molar pregnancy O08.0
  general (ized) K65.0
  gonococcal A54.85
  meconium (newborn) P78.0
  neonatal P78.1
    meconium P78.0
  pancreatic K65.0
  paroxysmal, familial E85.0
    benign E85.0
  pelvic
    female N73.5
      acute N73.3
      chronic N73.4
        with adhesions N73.6
    male K65.0
  periodic, familial E85.0
  proliferative, chronic K65.8
  puerperal, postpartum, childbirth O85
  purulent K65.0
  septic K65.0
  specified NEC K65.8
  spontaneous bacterial K65.2
  subdiaphragmatic K65.0
  subphrenic K65.0
  suppurative K65.0
  syphilitic A52.74
    congenital (early) A50.08 [K67]
  talc T81.61 ☑
  tuberculous A18.31
  urine K65.8
Peritonsillar — *see* condition
Peritonsillitis J36
Perityphlitis K37
Periureteritis N28.89
Periurethral — *see* condition
Periurethritis (gangrenous) — *see* Urethritis
Periuterine — *see* condition
Perivaginitis — *see* Vaginitis
Perivasculitis, retinal H35.06- ☑
Perivasitis (chronic) N49.1
Perivesiculitis (seminal) — *see* Vesiculitis

Perlèche NEC K13.0
  due to
    candidiasis B37.83
    moniliasis B37.83
    riboflavin deficiency E53.0
    vitamin B2 (riboflavin) deficiency E53.0
Pernicious — *see* condition
Pernio, perniosis T69.1 ☑
Perpetrator (of abuse) — *see* Index to External Causes of Injury, Perpetrator
Persecution
  delusion F22
  social Z60.5
Perseveration (tonic) R48.8
Persistence, persistent (congenital)
  anal membrane Q42.3
    with fistula Q42.2
  arteria stapedia Q16.3
  atrioventricular canal Q21.2
  branchial cleft Q18.0
  bulbus cordis in left ventricle Q21.8
  canal of Cloquet Q14.0
  capsule (opaque) Q12.8
  cilioretinal artery or vein Q14.8
  cloaca Q43.7
  communication — *see* Fistula, congenital
  convolutions
    aortic arch Q25.4
    fallopian tube Q50.6
    oviduct Q50.6
    uterine tube Q50.6
  double aortic arch Q25.4
  ductus arteriosus (Botalli) Q25.0
  fetal
    circulation P29.3
    form of cervix (uteri) Q51.828
    hemoglobin, hereditary (HPFH) D56.4
  foramen
    Botalli Q21.1
    ovale Q21.1
  Gartner's duct Q52.4
  hemoglobin, fetal (hereditary) (HPFH) D56.4
  hyaloid
    artery (generally incomplete) Q14.0
    system Q14.8
  hymen, in pregnancy or childbirth — *see* Pregnancy, complicated by, abnormal, vulva
  lanugo Q84.2
  left
    posterior cardinal vein Q26.8
    root with right arch of aorta Q25.4
    superior vena cava Q26.1
  Meckel's diverticulum Q43.0
    malignant — *see* Table of Neoplasms, small intestine, malignant
  mucosal disease (middle ear) — *see* Otitis, media, suppurative, chronic, tubotympanic
  nail(s), anomalous Q84.6
  omphalomesenteric duct Q43.0
  organ or site not listed — *see* Anomaly, by site
  ostium
    atrioventriculare commune Q21.2
    primum Q21.2
    secundum Q21.1
  ovarian rests in fallopian tube Q50.6
  pancreatic tissue in intestinal tract Q43.8
  primary (deciduous)
    teeth K00.6
    vitreous hyperplasia Q14.0
  pupillary membrane Q13.89
  rhesus (Rh) titer — *see* Complication(s), transfusion, incompatibility reaction, Rh (factor)
  right aortic arch Q25.4
  sinus
    urogenitalis
      female Q52.8
      male Q55.8
    venosus with imperfect incorporation in right auricle Q26.8
  thymus (gland) (hyperplasia) E32.0
  thyroglossal duct Q89.2
  thyrolingual duct Q89.2
  truncus arteriosus or communis Q20.0
  tunica vasculosa lentis Q12.2
  umbilical sinus Q64.4
  urachus Q64.4
  vitelline duct Q43.0

Person (with)
  admitted for clinical research, as a control subject (normal comparison) (participant) Z00.6
  awaiting admission to adequate facility elsewhere Z75.1
  concern (normal) about sick person in family Z63.6
  consulting on behalf of another Z71.0
  feigning illness Z76.5
  living (in)
    without
      adequate housing (heating) (space) Z59.1
      housing (permanent) (temporary) Z59.0
      person able to render necessary care Z74.2
      shelter Z59.0
    alone Z60.2
    boarding school Z59.3
    residential institution Z59.3
  on waiting list Z75.1
  sick or handicapped in family Z63.6
Personality (disorder) F60.9
  accentuation of traits (type A pattern) Z73.1
  affective F34.0
  aggressive F60.3
  amoral F60.2
  anacastic, anankastic F60.5
  antisocial F60.2
  anxious F60.6
  asocial F60.2
  asthenic F60.7
  avoidant F60.6
  borderline F60.3
  change due to organic condition (enduring) F07.0
  compulsive F60.5
  cycloid F34.0
  cyclothymic F34.0
  dependent F60.7
  depressive F34.1
  dissocial F60.2
  dual F44.81
  eccentric F60.89
  emotionally unstable F60.3
  expansive paranoid F60.0
  explosive F60.3
  fanatic F60.0
  haltose type F60.89
  histrionic F60.4
  hyperthymic F34.0
  hypothymic F34.1
  hysterical F60.4
  immature F60.89
  inadequate F60.7
  labile (emotional) F60.3
  mixed (nonspecific) F60.81
  morally defective F60.2
  multiple F44.81
  narcissistic F60.81
  obsessional F60.5
  obsessive (-compulsive) F60.5
  organic F07.0
  overconscientious F60.5
  paranoid F60.0
  passive (-dependent) F60.7
  passive-aggressive F60.89
  pathologic F60.9
  pattern defect or disturbance F60.9
  pseudopsychopathic (organic) F07.0
  pseudoretarded (organic) F07.0
  psychoinfantile F60.4
  psychoneurotic NEC F60.89
  psychopathic F60.2
  querulant F60.0
  sadistic F60.89
  schizoid F60.1
  self-defeating F60.7
  sensitive paranoid F60.0
  sociopathic (amoral) (antisocial) (asocial) (dissocial) F60.2
  specified NEC F60.89
  type A Z73.1
  unstable (emotional) F60.3
Perthes' disease — *see* Legg-Calvé-Perthes disease
Pertussis (*see also* Whooping cough) A37.90
Perversion, perverted
  appetite F50.8
    psychogenic F50.8
  function
    pituitary gland E23.2
      posterior lobe E22.2

☑ **Additional Character Required** — Refer to the Tabular List for Character Selection   ▽ **Subterms under main terms may continue to next column or page**

Perversion, perverted — *continued*
  sense of smell and taste R43.8
    psychogenic F45.8
  sexual — *see* Deviation, sexual
Pervious, congenital (*see also* Imperfect, closure)
  ductus arteriosus Q25.0
Pes (congenital) (*see also* Talipes)
  acquired (*see also* Deformity, limb, foot, specified NEC)
    planus — *see* Deformity, limb, flat foot
  adductus Q66.89
  cavus Q66.7
  deformity NEC, acquired — *see* Deformity, limb, foot, specified NEC
  planus (acquired) (any degree) (*see also* Deformity, limb, flat foot)
    rachitic sequelae (late effect) E64.3
  valgus Q66.6
Pest, pestis — *see* Plague
Petechia, petechiae R23.3
  newborn P54.5
Petechial typhus A75.9
Peter's anomaly Q13.4
Petit mal seizure — *see* Epilepsy, generalized, specified NEC
Petit's hernia — *see* Hernia, abdomen, specified site NEC
Petrellidosis B48.2
Petrositis H70.20- ☑
  acute H70.21- ☑
  chronic H70.22- ☑
Peutz-Jeghers disease or syndrome Q85.8
Peyronie's disease N48.6
Pfeiffer's disease — *see* Mononucleosis, infectious
Phagedena (dry) (moist) (sloughing) (*see also* Gangrene)
  geometric L88
  penis N48.29
  tropical — *see* Ulcer, skin
  vulva N76.6
Phagedenic — *see* condition
Phakoma H35.89
Phakomatosis (*see also* specific eponymous syndromes) Q85.9
  Bourneville's Q85.1
  specified NEC Q85.8
Phantom limb syndrome (without pain) G54.7
  with pain G54.6
Pharyngeal pouch syndrome D82.1
Pharyngitis (acute) (catarrhal)(gangrenous) (infective) (malignant) (membranous) (phlegmonous) (pseudomembranous) (simple) (subacute) (suppurative) (ulcerative) (viral) J02.9
  with influenza, flu, or grippe — *see* Influenza, with, pharyngitis
  aphthous B08.5
  atrophic J31.2
  chlamydial A56.4
  chronic (atrophic) (granular) (hypertrophic) J31.2
  coxsackievirus B08.5
  diphtheritic A36.0
  enteroviral vesicular B08.5
  follicular (chronic) J31.2
  fusospirochetal A69.1
  gonococcal A54.5
  granular (chronic) J31.2
  herpesviral B00.2
  hypertrophic J31.2
  infectional, chronic J31.2
  influenzal — *see* Influenza, with, respiratory manifestations NEC
  lymphonodular, acute (enteroviral) B08.8
  pneumococcal J02.8
  purulent J02.9
  putrid J02.9
  septic J02.0
  sicca J31.2
  specified organism NEC J02.8
  staphylococcal J02.8
  streptococcal J02.0
  syphilitic, congenital (early) A50.03
  tuberculous A15.8
  vesicular, enteroviral B08.5
  viral NEC J02.8
Pharyngoconjunctivitis, viral B30.2
Pharyngolaryngitis (acute) J06.0
  chronic J37.0
Pharyngoplegia J39.2
Pharyngotonsillitis, herpesviral B00.2

Pharyngotracheitis, chronic J42
Pharynx, pharyngeal — *see* condition
Phenomenon
  Arthus' — *see* Arthus' phenomenon
  jaw-winking Q07.8
  lupus erythematosus (LE) cell M32.9
  Raynaud's (secondary) I73.00
    with gangrene I73.01
  vasomotor R55
  vasospastic I73.9
  vasovagal R55
  Wenckebach's I44.1
Phenylketonuria E70.1
  classical E70.0
  maternal E70.1
Pheochromoblastoma
  specified site — *see* Neoplasm, malignant, by site
  unspecified site C74.10
Pheochromocytoma
  malignant
    specified site –– *see* Neoplasm, malignant, by site
    unspecified site C74.10
  specified site — *see* Neoplasm, benign, by site
  unspecified site D35.00
Pheohyphomycosis — *see* Chromomycosis
Pheomycosis — *see* Chromomycosis
Phimosis (congenital) (due to infection) N47.1
  chancroidal A57
Phlebectasia (*see also* Varix)
  congenital Q27.4
Phlebitis (infective) (pyemic) (septic) (suppurative) I80.9
  antepartum — *see* Thrombophlebitis, antepartum
  blue — *see* Phlebitis, leg, deep
  breast, superficial I80.8
  cavernous (venous) sinus — *see* Phlebitis, intracranial (venous) sinus
  cerebral (venous) sinus — *see* Phlebitis, intracranial (venous) sinus
  chest wall, superficial I80.8
  cranial (venous) sinus — *see* Phlebitis, intracranial (venous) sinus
  deep (vessels) — *see* Phlebitis, leg, deep
  due to implanted device — *see* Complications, by site and type, specified NEC
  during or resulting from a procedure T81.72 ☑
  femoral vein (superficial) I80.1- ☑
  femoropopliteal vein I80.0- ☑
  gestational — *see* Phlebopathy, gestational
  hepatic veins I80.8
  iliofemoral — *see* Phlebitis, femoral vein
  intracranial (venous) sinus (any) G08
    nonpyogenic I67.6
  intraspinal venous sinuses and veins G08
    nonpyogenic G95.19
  lateral (venous) sinus — *see* Phlebitis, intracranial (venous) sinus
  leg I80.3
    antepartum — *see* Thrombophlebitis, antepartum
    deep (vessels) NEC I80.20- ☑
      iliac I80.21- ☑
      popliteal vein I80.22- ☑
      specified vessel NEC I80.29- ☑
      tibial vein I80.23- ☑
    femoral vein (superficial) I80.1- ☑
    superficial (vessels) I80.0- ☑
  longitudinal sinus — *see* Phlebitis, intracranial (venous) sinus
  lower limb — *see* Phlebitis, leg
  migrans, migrating (superficial) I82.1
  pelvic
    with ectopic or molar pregnancy O08.0
    following ectopic or molar pregnancy O08.0
    puerperal, postpartum O87.1
  popliteal vein — *see* Phlebitis, leg, deep, popliteal
  portal (vein) K75.1
  postoperative T81.72 ☑
  pregnancy — *see* Thrombophlebitis, antepartum
  puerperal, postpartum, childbirth O87.0
    deep O87.1
    pelvic O87.1
    superficial O87.0
  retina — *see* Vasculitis, retina
  saphenous (accessory) (great) (long) (small) — *see* Phlebitis, leg, superficial
  sinus (meninges) — *see* Phlebitis, intracranial (venous) sinus
  specified site NEC I80.8

Phlebitis — *continued*
  syphilitic A52.09
  tibial vein — *see* Phlebitis, leg, deep, tibial
  ulcerative I80.9
    leg — *see* Phlebitis, leg
  umbilicus I80.8
  uterus (septic) — *see* Endometritis
  varicose (leg) (lower limb) — *see* Varix, leg, with, inflammation
Phlebofibrosis I87.8
Phleboliths I87.8
Phlebopathy,
  gestational O22.9- ☑
  puerperal O87.9
Phlebosclerosis I87.8
Phlebothrombosis (*see also* Thrombosis)
  antepartum — *see* Thrombophlebitis, antepartum
  pregnancy — *see* Thrombophlebitis, antepartum
  puerperal — *see* Thrombophlebitis, puerperal
Phlebotomus fever A93.1
Phlegmasia
  alba dolens O87.1
    nonpuerperal — *see* Phlebitis, femoral vein
  cerulea dolens — *see* Phlebitis, leg, deep
Phlegmon — *see* Abscess
Phlegmonous — *see* condition
Phlyctenulosis (allergic) (keratoconjunctivitis) (nontuberculous) (*see also* Keratoconjunctivitis)
  cornea — *see* Keratoconjunctivitis
  tuberculous A18.52
Phobia, phobic F40.9
  animal F40.218
    spiders F40.210
  examination F40.298
  reaction F40.9
  simple F40.298
  social F40.10
    generalized F40.11
  specific (isolated) F40.298
    animal F40.218
      spiders F40.210
    blood F40.230
    injection F40.231
    injury F40.233
    men F40.290
    natural environment F40.228
      thunderstorms F40.220
    situational F40.248
      bridges F40.242
      closed in spaces F40.240
      flying F40.243
      heights F40.241
    specified focus NEC F40.298
    transfusion F40.231
    women F40.291
  specified NEC F40.8
    medical care NEC F40.232
  state F40.9
Phocas' disease — *see* Mastopathy, cystic
Phocomelia Q73.1
  lower limb — *see* Agenesis, leg, with foot present
  upper limb — *see* Agenesis, arm, with hand present
Phoria H50.50
Phosphate-losing tubular disorder N25.0
Phosphatemia E83.39
Phosphaturia E83.39
Photodermatitis (sun) L56.8
  chronic L57.8
  due to drug L56.8
  light other than sun L59.8
Photokeratitis H16.13- ☑
Photophobia H53.14- ☑
Photophthalmia — *see* Photokeratitis
Photopsia H53.19
Photoretinitis — *see* Retinopathy, solar
Photosensitivity, photosensitization (sun) skin L56.8
  light other than sun L59.8
Phrenitis — *see* Encephalitis
Phrynoderma (vitamin A deficiency) E50.8
Phthiriasis (pubis) B85.3
  with any infestation classifiable to B85.0-B85.2 B85.4
Phthirus infestation — *see* Phthiriasis
Phthisis (*see also* Tuberculosis)
  bulbi (infectional) — *see* Disorder, globe, degenerated condition, atrophy
  eyeball (due to infection) — *see* Disorder, globe, degenerated condition, atrophy

Phycomycosis — see Zygomycosis
Physalopteriasis B81.8
Physical restraint status Z78.1
Phytobezoar T18.9 ☑
  intestine T18.3 ☑
  stomach T18.2 ☑
Pian — see Yaws
Pianoma A66.1
Pica F50.8
  in adults F50.8
  infant or child F98.3
Picking, nose F98.8
Pick-Niemann disease — see Niemann-Pick disease or
  syndrome
Pick's
  cerebral atrophy G31.01 [F02.80]
    with behavioral disturbance G31.01 [F02.81]
  disease or syndrome (brain) G31.01 [F02.80]
    with behavioral disturbance G31.01 [F02.81]
Pickwickian syndrome E66.2
Piebaldism E70.39
Piedra (beard) (scalp) B36.8
  black B36.3
  white B36.2
Pierre Robin deformity or syndrome Q87.0
Pierson's disease or osteochondrosis M91.0
Pig-bel A05.2
Pigeon
  breast or chest (acquired) M95.4
    congenital Q67.7
    rachitic sequelae (late effect) E64.3
  breeder's disease or lung J67.2
  fancier's disease or lung J67.2
  toe — see Deformity, toe, specified NEC
Pigmentation (abnormal) (anomaly) L81.9
  conjunctiva H11.13- ☑
  cornea (anterior) H18.01- ☑
    posterior H18.05- ☑
    stromal H18.06- ☑
  diminished melanin formation NEC L81.6
  iron L81.8
  lids, congenital Q82.8
  limbus corneae — see Pigmentation, cornea
  metals L81.8
  optic papilla, congenital Q14.2
  retina, congenital (grouped) (nevoid) Q14.1
  scrotum, congenital Q82.8
  tattoo L81.8
Piles (see also Hemorrhoids) K64.9
Pili
  annulati or torti (congenital) Q84.1
  incarnati L73.1
Pill roller hand (intrinsic) — see Parkinsonism
Pilomatrixoma — see Neoplasm, skin, benign
  malignant — see Neoplasm, skin, malignant
Pilonidal — see condition
Pimple R23.8
Pinched nerve — see Neuropathy, entrapment
Pindborg tumor — see Cyst, calcifying odontogenic
Pineal body or gland — see condition
Pinealoblastoma C75.3
Pinealoma D44.5
  malignant C75.3
Pineoblastoma C75.3
Pineocytoma D44.5
Pinguecula H11.15- ☑
Pingueculitis H10.81- ☑
Pinhole meatus (see also Stricture, urethra) N35.9
Pink
  disease — see subcategory T56.1 ☑
  eye — see Conjunctivitis, acute, mucopurulent
Pinkus' disease (lichen nitidus) L44.1
Pinpoint
  meatus — see Stricture, urethra
  os (uteri) — see Stricture, cervix
Pins and needles R20.2
Pinta A67.9
  cardiovascular lesions A67.2
  chancre (primary) A67.0
  erythematous plaques A67.1
  hyperchromic lesions A67.1
  hyperkeratosis A67.1
  lesions A67.9
    cardiovascular A67.2
    hyperchromic A67.1
    intermediate A67.1
    late A67.2

Pinta — continued
  lesions — continued
    mixed A67.3
    primary A67.0
    skin (achromic) (cicatricial) (dyschromic) A67.2
      hyperchromic A67.1
      mixed (achromic and hyperchromic) A67.3
  papule (primary) A67.0
  skin lesions (achromic) (cicatricial) (dyschromic) A67.2
    hyperchromic A67.1
    mixed (achromic and hyperchromic) A67.3
  vitiligo A67.2
Pintids A67.1
Pinworm (disease) (infection) (infestation) B80
Piroplasmosis B60.0
Pistol wound — see Gunshot wound
Pitchers' elbow — see Derangement, joint, specified
  type NEC, elbow
Pithecoid pelvis Q74.2
  with disproportion (fetopelvic) O33.0
    causing obstructed labor O65.0
Pithiatism F48.8
Pitted — see Pitting
Pitting (see also Edema) R60.9
  lip R60.0
  nail L60.8
  teeth K00.4
Pituitary gland — see condition
Pituitary-snuff-taker's disease J67.8
Pityriasis (capitis) L21.0
  alba L30.5
  circinata (et maculata) L42
  furfuracea L21.0
  Hebra's L26
  lichenoides L41.0
    chronica L41.1
    et varioliformis (acuta) L41.0
  maculata (et circinata) L30.5
  nigra B36.1
  pilaris, Hebra's L44.0
  rosea L42
  rotunda L44.8
  rubra (Hebra) pilaris L44.0
  simplex L30.5
  specified type NEC L30.5
  streptogenes L30.5
  versicolor (scrotal) B36.0
Placenta, placental — see Pregnancy, complicated by
  (care of) (management affected by), specified condition
Placentitis O41.14- ☑
Plagiocephaly Q67.3
Plague A20.9
  abortive A20.8
  ambulatory A20.8
  asymptomatic A20.8
  bubonic A20.0
  cellulocutaneous A20.1
  cutaneobubonic A20.1
  lymphatic gland A20.0
  meningitis A20.3
  pharyngeal A20.8
  pneumonic (primary) (secondary) A20.2
  pulmonary, pulmonic A20.2
  septicemic A20.7
  tonsillar A20.8
    septicemic A20.7
Planning, family
  contraception Z30.9
  procreation Z31.69
Plaque(s)
  artery, arterial — see Arteriosclerosis
  calcareous — see Calcification
  coronary, lipid rich I25.83
  epicardial I31.8
  erythematous, of pinta A67.1
  Hollenhorst's — see Occlusion, artery, retina
  lipid rich, coronary I25.83
  pleural (without asbestos) J92.9
    with asbestos J92.0
  tongue K13.29
Plasmacytoma C90.3- ☑
  extramedullary C90.2- ☑
  medullary C90.0- ☑
  solitary C90.3- ☑
Plasmacytopenia D72.818
Plasmacytosis D72.822
Plaster ulcer — see Ulcer, pressure, by site

Plateau iris syndrome (post-iridectomy) (postprocedu
  ral) (without glaucoma) H21.82
  with glaucoma H40.22- ☑
Platybasia Q75.8
Platyonychia (congenital) Q84.6
  acquired L60.8
Platypelloid pelvis M95.5
  with disproportion (fetopelvic) O33.0
    causing obstructed labor O65.0
  congenital Q74.2
Platyspondylisis Q76.49
Plaut (-Vincent) **disease** (see also Vincent's) A69.1
Plethora R23.2
  newborn P61.1
Pleura, pleural — see condition
Pleuralgia R07.81
Pleurisy (acute) (adhesive) (chronic) (costal) (diaphrag
  matic) (double) (dry) (fibrinous) (fibrous) (interlobar)
  (latent) (plastic) (primary) (residual) (sicca) (sterile)
  (subacute) (unresolved) R09.1
  with
    adherent pleura J86.0
    effusion J90
      chylous, chyliform J94.0
      tuberculous (non primary) A15.6
        primary (progressive) A15.7
    tuberculosis — see Pleurisy, tuberculous (non pri
      mary)
  encysted — see Pleurisy, with effusion
  exudative — see Pleurisy, with effusion
  fibrinopurulent, fibropurulent — see Pyothorax
  hemorrhagic — see Hemothorax
  pneumococcal J90
  purulent — see Pyothorax
  septic — see Pyothorax
  serofibrinous — see Pleurisy, with effusion
  seropurulent — see Pyothorax
  serous — see Pleurisy, with effusion
  staphylococcal J86.9
  streptococcal J90
  suppurative — see Pyothorax
  traumatic (post) (current) — see Injury, intrathoracic,
    pleura
  tuberculous (with effusion) (non primary) A15.6
    primary (progressive) A15.7
Pleuritis sicca — see Pleurisy
Pleurobronchopneumonia — see Pneumonia, broncho-
Pleurodynia R07.81
  epidemic B33.0
  viral B33.0
Pleuropericarditis (see also Pericarditis)
  acute I30.9
Pleuropneumonia (acute) (bilateral) (double) (septic)
  (see also Pneumonia) J18.8
  chronic — see Fibrosis, lung
Pleuro-pneumonia-like-organism (PPLO), as cause of
  disease classified elsewhere B96.0
Pleurorrhea — see Pleurisy, with effusion
Plexitis, brachial G54.0
Plica
  polonica B85.0
  syndrome, knee M67.5- ☑
  tonsil J35.8
Plicated tongue K14.5
Plug
  bronchus NEC J98.09
  meconium (newborn) NEC syndrome P76.0
  mucus — see Asphyxia, mucus
Plumbism — see subcategory T56.0 ☑
Plummer's disease E05.20
  with thyroid storm E05.21
Plummer-Vinson syndrome D50.1
Pluricarential syndrome of infancy E40
Plus (and minus) **hand** (intrinsic) — see Deformity, limb,
  specified type NEC, forearm
Pneumathemia — see Air, embolism
Pneumatic hammer (drill) syndrome T75.21 ☑
Pneumatocele (lung) J98.4
  intracranial G93.89
  tension J44.9
Pneumatosis
  cystoides intestinalis K63.89
  intestinalis K63.89
  peritonei K66.8
Pneumaturia R39.89
Pneumoblastoma — see Neoplasm, lung, malignant
Pneumocephalus G93.89

☑ **Additional Character Required** — Refer to the Tabular List for Character Selection   ▽ **Subterms under main terms may continue to next column or page**

Pneumococcemia A40.3
Pneumococcus, pneumococcal — *see* condition
Pneumoconiosis (due to) (inhalation of) J64
  with tuberculosis (any type in A15) J65
  aluminum J63.0
  asbestos J61
  bagasse, bagassosis J67.1
  bauxite J63.1
  beryllium J63.2
  coal miners' (simple) J60
  coalworkers' (simple) J60
  collier's J60
  cotton dust J66.0
  diatomite (diatomaceous earth) J62.8
  dust
    inorganic NEC J63.6
    lime J62.8
    marble J62.8
    organic NEC J66.8
  fumes or vapors (from silo) J68.9
  graphite J63.3
  grinder's J62.8
  kaolin J62.8
  mica J62.8
  millstone maker's J62.8
  mineral fibers NEC J61
  miner's J60
  moldy hay J67.0
  potter's J62.8
  rheumatoid — *see* Rheumatoid, lung
  sandblaster's J62.8
  silica, silicate NEC J62.8
    with carbon J60
  stonemason's J62.8
  talc (dust) J62.0
Pneumocystis carinii pneumonia B59
Pneumocystis jiroveci (pneumonia) B59
Pneumocystosis (with pneumonia) B59
Pneumohemopericardium I31.2
Pneumohemothorax J94.2
  traumatic S27.2 ☑
Pneumohydropericardium — *see* Pericarditis
Pneumohydrothorax — *see* Hydrothorax
Pneumomediastinum J98.2
  congenital or perinatal P25.2
Pneumomycosis B49 [J99]
Pneumonia (acute) (double) (migratory) (purulent)
  (septic) (unresolved) J18.9
  with
    influenza — *see* Influenza, with, pneumonia
    lung abscess J85.1
      due to specified organism — *see* Pneumonia,
        in (due to)
  adenoviral J12.0
  adynamic J18.2
  alba A50.04
  allergic (eosinophilic) J82
  alveolar — *see* Pneumonia, lobar
  anaerobes J15.8
  anthrax A22.1
  apex, apical — *see* Pneumonia, lobar
  Ascaris B77.81
  aspiration J69.0
    due to
      aspiration of microorganisms
        bacterial J15.9
        viral J12.9
      food (regurgitated) J69.0
      gastric secretions J69.0
      milk (regurgitated) J69.0
      oils, essences J69.1
      solids, liquids NEC J69.8
      vomitus J69.0
    newborn P24.81
      amniotic fluid (clear) P24.11
      blood P24.21
      food (regurgitated) P24.31
      liquor (amnii) P24.11
      meconium P24.01
      milk P24.31
      mucus P24.11
      specified NEC P24.81
      stomach contents P24.31
    postprocedural J95.4
  atypical NEC J18.9
  bacillus J15.9
    specified NEC J15.8
  bacterial J15.9

Pneumonia — *continued*
  bacterial — *continued*
    specified NEC J15.8
  Bacteroides (fragilis) (oralis) (melaninogenicus) J15.8
  basal, basic, basilar — *see* Pneumonia, by type
  bronchiolitis obliterans organized (BOOP) J84.89
  broncho-, bronchial (confluent) (croupous) (diffuse)
    (disseminated) (hemorrhagic) (involving lobes)
    (lobar) (terminal) J18.0
    allergic (eosinophilic) J82
    aspiration — *see* Pneumonia, aspiration
    bacterial J15.9
      specified NEC J15.8
    chronic — *see* Fibrosis, lung
    diplococcal J13
    Eaton's agent J15.7
    Escherichia coli (E. coli) J15.5
    Friedländer's bacillus J15.0
    Hemophilus influenzae J14
    hypostatic J18.2
    inhalation (*see also* Pneumonia, aspiration)
      due to fumes or vapors (chemical) J68.0
      of oils or essences J69.1
    Klebsiella (pneumoniae) J15.0
    lipid, lipoid J69.1
      endogenous J84.89
    Mycoplasma (pneumoniae) J15.7
    pleuro-pneumonia-like-organisms (PPLO) J15.7
    pneumococcal J13
    Proteus J15.6
    Pseudomonas J15.1
    Serratia marcescens J15.6
    specified organism NEC J16.8
    staphylococcal — *see* Pneumonia, staphylococcal
    streptococcal NEC J15.4
      group B J15.3
      pneumoniae J13
    viral, virus — *see* Pneumonia, viral
  Butyrivibrio (fibriosolvens) J15.8
  Candida B37.1
  caseous — *see* Tuberculosis, pulmonary
  catarrhal — *see* Pneumonia, broncho
  chlamydial J16.0
    congenital P23.1
  cholesterol J84.89
  cirrhotic (chronic) — *see* Fibrosis, lung
  Clostridium (haemolyticum) (novyi) J15.8
  confluent — *see* Pneumonia, broncho
  congenital (infective) P23.9
    due to
      bacterium NEC P23.6
      Chlamydia P23.1
      Escherichia coli P23.4
      Haemophilus influenzae P23.6
      infective organism NEC P23.8
      Klebsiella pneumoniae P23.6
      Mycoplasma P23.6
      Pseudomonas P23.5
      Staphylococcus P23.2
      Streptococcus (except group B) P23.6
        group B P23.3
      viral agent P23.0
    specified NEC P23.8
  croupous — *see* Pneumonia, lobar
  cryptogenic organizing J84.116
  cytomegalic inclusion B25.0
  cytomegaloviral B25.0
  deglutition — *see* Pneumonia, aspiration
  desquamative interstitial J84.117
  diffuse — *see* Pneumonia, broncho
  diplococcal, diplococcus (broncho-) (lobar) J13
  disseminated (focal) — *see* Pneumonia, broncho
  Eaton's agent J15.7
  embolic, embolism — *see* Embolism, pulmonary
  Enterobacter J15.6
  eosinophilic J82
  Escherichia coli (E. coli) J15.5
  Eubacterium J15.8
  fibrinous — *see* Pneumonia, lobar
  fibroid, fibrous (chronic) — *see* Fibrosis, lung
  Friedländer's bacillus J15.0
  Fusobacterium (nucleatum) J15.8
  gangrenous J85.0
  giant cell (measles) B05.2
  gonococcal A54.84
  gram-negative bacteria NEC J15.6
    anaerobic J15.8
  Hemophilus influenzae (broncho) (lobar) J14

Pneumonia — *continued*
  human metapneumovirus J12.3
  hypostatic (broncho) (lobar) J18.2
  in (due to)
    actinomycosis A42.0
    adenovirus J12.0
    anthrax A22.1
    ascariasis B77.81
    aspergillosis B44.9
    Bacillus anthracis A22.1
    Bacterium anitratum J15.6
    candidiasis B37.1
    chickenpox B01.2
    Chlamydia J16.0
      neonatal P23.1
    coccidioidomycosis B38.2
      acute B38.0
      chronic B38.1
    cytomegalovirus disease B25.0
    Diplococcus (pneumoniae) J13
    Eaton's agent J15.7
    Enterobacter J15.6
    Escherichia coli (E. coli) J15.5
    Friedländer's bacillus J15.0
    fumes and vapors (chemical) (inhalation) J68.0
    gonorrhea A54.84
    Hemophilus influenzae (H. influenzae) J14
    Herellea J15.6
    histoplasmosis B39.2
      acute B39.0
      chronic B39.1
    human metapneumovirus J12.3
    Klebsiella (pneumoniae) J15.0
    measles B05.2
    Mycoplasma (pneumoniae) J15.7
    nocardiosis, nocardiasis A43.0
    ornithosis A70
    parainfluenza virus J12.2
    pleuro-pneumonia-like-organism (PPLO) J15.7
    pneumococcus J13
    pneumocystosis (Pneumocystis carinii) (Pneumo-
      cystis jiroveci) B59
    Proteus J15.6
    Pseudomonas NEC J15.1
      pseudomallei A24.1
    psittacosis A70
    Q fever A78
    respiratory syncytial virus J12.1
    rheumatic fever I00 [J17]
    rubella B06.81
    Salmonella (infection) A02.22
      typhi A01.03
    schistosomiasis B65.9 [J17]
    Serratia marcescens J15.6
    specified
      bacterium NEC J15.8
      organism NEC J16.8
    spirochetal NEC A69.8
    Staphylococcus J15.20
      aureus (methicillin susceptible) (MSSA) J15.211
        methicillin resistant (MRSA) J15.212
      specified NEC J15.29
    Streptococcus J15.4
      group B J15.3
      pneumoniae J13
      specified NEC J15.4
    toxoplasmosis B58.3
    tularemia A21.2
    typhoid (fever) A01.03
    varicella B01.2
    virus — *see* Pneumonia, viral
    whooping cough A37.91
      due to
        Bordetella parapertussis A37.11
        Bordetella pertussis A37.01
        specified NEC A37.81
    Yersinia pestis A20.2
  inhalation of food or vomit — *see* Pneumonia, aspira-
    tion
  interstitial J84.9
    chronic J84.111
    desquamative J84.117
    due to
      collagen vascular disease J84.17
      known underlying cause J84.17
    idiopathic NOS J84.111
    in disease classified elsewhere J84.17

Index

Pneumonia — Poisoning

Pneumonia — continued
  interstitial — continued
    lymphocytic (due to collagen vascular disease) (in diseases classified elsewhere) J84.17
    lymphoid J84.2
    non-specific J84.89
      due to
        collagen vascular disease J84.17
        known underlying cause J84.17
      idiopathic J84.113
      in diseases classified elsewhere J84.17
    plasma cell B59
    pseudomonas J15.1
    usual J84.112
      due to collagen vascular disease J84.17
      idiopathic J84.112
      in diseases classified elsewhere J84.17
  Klebsiella (pneumoniae) J15.0
  lipid, lipoid (exogenous) J69.1
    endogenous J84.89
  lobar (disseminated) (double) (interstitial) J18.1
    bacterial J15.9
      specified NEC J15.8
    chronic — see Fibrosis, lung
    Escherichia coli (E. coli) J15.5
    Friedländer's bacillus J15.0
    Hemophilus influenzae J14
    hypostatic J18.2
    Klebsiella (pneumoniae) J15.0
    pneumococcal J13
    Proteus J15.6
    Pseudomonas J15.1
    specified organism NEC J16.8
    staphylococcal — see Pneumonia, staphylococcal
    streptococcal NEC J15.4
    Streptococcus pneumoniae J13
    viral, virus — see Pneumonia, viral
  lobular — see Pneumonia, broncho
  Löffler's J82
  lymphoid interstitial J84.2
  massive — see Pneumonia, lobar
  meconium P24.01
  MSSA (methicillin susceptible Staphylococcus aureus) J15.211
  multilobar — see Pneumonia, by type
  Mycoplasma (pneumoniae) J15.7
  necrotic J85.0
  neonatal P23.9
    aspiration — see Aspiration, by substance, with pneumonia
  nitrogen dioxide J68.9
  organizing J84.89
    due to
      collagen vascular disease J84.17
      known underlying cause J84.17
      in diseases classified elsewhere J84.17
  orthostatic J18.2
  parainfluenza virus J12.2
  parenchymatous — see Fibrosis, lung
  passive J18.2
  patchy — see Pneumonia, broncho
  Peptococcus J15.8
  Peptostreptococcus J15.8
  plasma cell (of infants) B59
  pleurolobar — see Pneumonia, lobar
  pleuro-pneumonia-like organism (PPLO) J15.7
  pneumococcal (broncho) (lobar) J13
  Pneumocystis (carinii) (jiroveci) B59
  postinfectional NEC B99 ☑ [J17]
  postmeasles B05.2
  Proteus J15.6
  Pseudomonas J15.1
  psittacosis A70
  radiation J70.0
  respiratory syncytial virus J12.1
  resulting from a procedure J95.89
  rheumatic I00 [J17]
  Salmonella (arizonae) (cholerae-suis) (enteritidis) (typhimurium) A02.22
    typhi A01.03
    typhoid fever A01.03
  SARS-associated coronavirus J12.81
  segmented, segmental — see Pneumonia, broncho-
  Serratia marcescens J15.6
  specified NEC J18.8
    bacterium NEC J15.8
    organism NEC J16.8
    virus NEC J12.89

Pneumonia — continued
  spirochetal NEC A69.8
  staphylococcal (broncho) (lobar) J15.20
    aureus (methicillin susceptible) (MSSA) J15.211
      methicillin resistant (MRSA) J15.212
    specified NEC J15.29
  static, stasis J18.2
  streptococcal NEC (broncho) (lobar) J15.4
    group
      A J15.4
      B J15.3
      specified NEC J15.4
  Streptococcus pneumoniae J13
  syphilitic, congenital (early) A50.04
  traumatic (complication) (early) (secondary) T79.8 ☑
  tuberculous (any) — see Tuberculosis, pulmonary
  tularemic A21.2
  varicella B01.2
  Veillonella J15.8
  ventilator associated J95.851
  viral, virus (broncho) (interstitial) (lobar) J12.9
    adenoviral J12.0
    congenital P23.0
    human metapneumovirus J12.3
    parainfluenza J12.2
    respiratory syncytial J12.1
    SARS-associated coronavirus J12.81
    specified NEC J12.89
  white (congenital) A50.04

Pneumonic — see condition

Pneumonitis (acute) (primary) (see also Pneumonia)
  air-conditioner J67.7
  allergic (due to) J67.9
    organic dust NEC J67.8
    red cedar dust J67.8
    sequoiosis J67.8
    wood dust J67.8
  aspiration J69.0
    due to
      anesthesia J95.4
        during
          labor and delivery O74.0
          pregnancy O29.01- ☑
          puerperium O89.01
      fumes or gases J68.0
    obstetric O74.0
  chemical (due to gases, fumes or vapors) (inhalation) J68.0
    due to anesthesia J95.4
  cholesterol J84.89
  chronic — see Fibrosis, lung
  congenital rubella P35.0
  crack (cocaine) J68.0
  due to
    beryllium J68.0
    cadmium J68.0
    crack (cocaine) J68.0
    detergent J69.8
    fluorocarbon-polymer J68.0
    food, vomit (aspiration) J69.0
    fumes or vapors J68.0
    gases, fumes or vapors (inhalation) J68.0
    inhalation
      blood J69.8
      essences J69.1
      food (regurgitated), milk, vomit J69.0
      oils, essences J69.1
      saliva J69.0
      solids, liquids NEC J69.8
    manganese J68.0
    nitrogen dioxide J68.0
    oils, essences J69.1
    solids, liquids NEC J69.8
    toxoplasmosis (acquired) B58.3
      congenital P37.1
    vanadium J68.0
    ventilator J95.851
  eosinophilic J82
  hypersensitivity J67.9
    air conditioner lung J67.7
    bagassosis J67.1
    bird fancier's lung J67.2
    farmer's lung J67.0
    maltworker's lung J67.4
    maple bark-stripper's lung J67.6
    mushroom worker's lung J67.5
    specified organic dust NEC J67.8
    suberosis J67.3

Pneumonitis — continued
  interstitial (chronic) J84.89
    acute J84.114
    lymphoid J84.2
    non-specific J84.89
      idiopathic J84.113
  lymphoid, interstitial J84.2
  meconium P24.01
  postanesthetic J95.4
    correct substance properly administered — see Table of Drugs and Chemicals, by drug, adverse effect
    in labor and delivery O74.0
    in pregnancy O29.01- ☑
      obstetric O74.0
    overdose or wrong substance given or taken (by accident) — see Table of Drugs and Chemicals, by drug, poisoning
    postpartum, puerperal O89.01
  postoperative J95.4
    obstetric O74.0
  radiation J70.0
  rubella, congenital P35.0
  ventilation (air-conditioning) J67.7
  ventilator associated J95.851
  wood-dust J67.8

Pneumonoconiosis — see Pneumoconiosis
Pneumoparotid K11.8
Pneumopathy NEC J98.4
  alveolar J84.09
  due to organic dust NEC J66.8
  parietoalveolar J84.09
Pneumopericarditis (see also Pericarditis)
  acute I30.9
Pneumopericardium (see also Pericarditis)
  congenital P25.3
  newborn P25.3
  traumatic (post) — see Injury, heart
Pneumophagia (psychogenic) F45.8
Pneumopleurisy, pneumopleuritis (see also Pneumonia) J18.8
Pneumopyopericardium I30.1
Pneumopyothorax — see Pyopneumothorax
  with fistula J86.0
Pneumorrhagia (see also Hemorrhage, lung)
  tuberculous — see Tuberculosis, pulmonary
Pneumothorax NOS J93.9
  acute J93.83
  chronic J93.81
  congenital P25.1
  perinatal period P25.1
  postprocedural J95.811
  specified NEC J93.83
  spontaneous NOS J93.83
    newborn P25.1
    primary J93.11
    secondary J93.12
    tension J93.0
  tense valvular, infectional J93.0
  tension (spontaneous) J93.0
  traumatic S27.0 ☑
    with hemothorax S27.2 ☑
  tuberculous — see Tuberculosis, pulmonary
Podagra (see also Gout) M10.9
Podencephalus Q01.9
Poikilocytosis R71.8
Poikiloderma L81.6
  Civatte's L57.3
  congenital Q82.8
  vasculare atrophicans L94.5
Poikilodermatomyositis M33.10
  with
    myopathy M33.12
    respiratory involvement M33.11
    specified organ involvement NEC M33.19
Pointed ear (congenital) Q17.3
Poison ivy, oak, sumac or other plant dermatitis (allergic) (contact) L23.7
Poisoning (acute) (see also Table of Drugs and Chemicals)
  algae and toxins T65.82- ☑
  Bacillus B (aertrycke) (cholerae (suis)) (paratyphosus) (suipestifer) A02.9
    botulinus A05.1
  bacterial toxins A05.9
  berries, noxious — see Poisoning, food, noxious, berries
  botulism A05.1
  ciguatera fish T61.0- ☑

☑ Additional Character Required — Refer to the Tabular List for Character Selection   ▽ Subterms under main terms may continue to next column or page

Poisoning — *continued*
Clostridium botulinum A05.1
death-cap (Amanita phalloides) (Amanita verna) —
see Poisoning, food, noxious, mushrooms
drug — *see* Table of Drugs and Chemicals, by drug,
poisoning
epidemic, fish (noxious) — *see* Poisoning, seafood
bacterial A05.9
fava bean D55.0
fish (noxious) T61.9- ☑
bacterial — *see* Intoxication, foodborne, by agent
ciguatera fish — *see* Poisoning, ciguatera fish
scombroid fish — *see* Poisoning, scombroid fish
specified type NEC T61.77- ☑
food (acute) (diseased) (infected) (noxious) NEC
T62.9- ☑
bacterial — *see* Intoxication, foodborne, by agent
due to
Bacillus (aertrycke) (choleraesuis) (paratyphosus) (suipestifer) A02.9
botulinus A05.1
Clostridium (perfringens) (Welchii) A05.2
salmonella (aertrycke) (callinarum) (choleraesuis) (enteritidis) (paratyphi) (suipestifer)
A02.9
with
gastroenteritis A02.0
sepsis A02.1
staphylococcus A05.0
Vibrio
parahaemolyticus A05.3
vulnificus A05.5
noxious or naturally toxic T62.9- ☑
berries — *see* subcategory T62.1 ☑
fish — *see* Poisoning, seafood
mushrooms — *see* subcategory T62.0X ☑
plants NEC — *see* subcategory T62.2X ☑
seafood — *see* Poisoning, seafood
specified NEC — *see* subcategory T62.8X ☑
ichthyotoxism — *see* Poisoning, seafood
kreotoxism, food A05.9
latex T65.81- ☑
lead T56.0- ☑
mushroom — *see* Poisoning, food, noxious, mushroom
mussels (*see also* Poisoning, shellfish)
bacterial — *see* Intoxication, foodborne, by agent
nicotine (tobacco) T65.2- ☑
noxious foodstuffs — *see* Poisoning, food, noxious
plants, noxious — *see* Poisoning, food, noxious, plants
NEC
ptomaine — *see* Poisoning, food
radiation J70.0
Salmonella (arizonae) (cholerae-suis) (enteritidis) (typhimurium) A02.9
scombroid fish T61.1- ☑
seafood (noxious) T61.9- ☑
bacterial — *see* Intoxication, foodborne, by agent
fish — *see* Poisoning, fish
shellfish — *see* Poisoning, shellfish
specified NEC — *see* subcategory T61.8X ☑
shellfish (amnesic) (azaspiracid) (diarrheic) (neurotoxic)
(noxious) (paralytic) T61.78- ☑
bacterial — *see* Intoxication, foodborne, by agent
ciguatera mollusk — *see* Poisoning, ciguatera fish
specified substance NEC T65.891 ☑
Staphylococcus, food A05.0
tobacco (nicotine) T65.2- ☑
water E87.79
Poker spine — *see* Spondylitis, ankylosing
Poland syndrome Q79.8
Polioencephalitis (acute) (bulbar) A80.9
inferior G12.22
influenzal — *see* Influenza, with, encephalopathy
superior hemorrhagic (acute) (Wernicke's) E51.2
Wernicke's E51.2
Polioencephalomyelitis (acute) (anterior) A80.9
with beriberi E51.2
Polioencephalopathy, superior hemorrhagic E51.2
with
beriberi E51.11
pellagra E52
Poliomeningoencephalitis — *see* Meningoencephalitis
Poliomyelitis (acute) (anterior) (epidemic) A80.9
with paralysis (bulbar) — *see* Poliomyelitis, paralytic
abortive A80.4
ascending (progressive) — *see* Poliomyelitis, paralytic
bulbar (paralytic) — *see* Poliomyelitis, paralytic

Poliomyelitis — *continued*
congenital P35.8
nonepidemic A80.9
nonparalytic A80.4
paralytic A80.30
specified NEC A80.39
vaccine-associated A80.0
wild virus
imported A80.1
indigenous A80.2
spinal, acute A80.9
Poliosis (eyebrow) (eyelashes) L67.1
circumscripta, acquired L67.1
Pollakiuria R35.0
psychogenic F45.8
Pollinosis J30.1
Pollitzer's disease L73.2
Polyadenitis (*see also* Lymphadenitis)
malignant A20.0
Polyalgia M79.89
Polyangiitis M30.0
microscopic M31.7
overlap syndrome M30.8
Polyarteritis
microscopic M31.7
nodosa M30.0
with lung involvement M30.1
juvenile M30.2
related condition NEC M30.8
Polyarthralgia — *see* Pain, joint
Polyarthritis, polyarthropathy (*see also* Arthritis) M13.0
due to or associated with other specified conditions
— *see* Arthritis
epidemic (Australian) (with exanthema) B33.1
infective — *see* Arthritis, pyogenic or pyemic
inflammatory M06.4
juvenile (chronic) (seronegative) M08.3
migratory — *see* Fever, rheumatic
rheumatic, acute — *see* Fever, rheumatic
Polyarthrosis M15.9
post-traumatic M15.3
primary M15.0
specified NEC M15.8
Polycarential syndrome of infancy E40
Polychondritis (atrophic) (chronic) (*see also* Disorder,
cartilage, specified type NEC)
relapsing M94.1
Polycoria Q13.2
Polycystic (disease)
degeneration, kidney Q61.3
autosomal dominant (adult type) Q61.2
autosomal recessive (infantile type) NEC Q61.19
kidney Q61.3
autosomal
dominant Q61.2
recessive NEC Q61.19
autosomal dominant (adult type) Q61.2
autosomal recessive (childhood type) NEC Q61.19
infantile type NEC Q61.19
liver Q44.6
lung J98.4
congenital Q33.0
ovary, ovaries E28.2
spleen Q89.09
Polycythemia (secondary) D75.1
acquired D75.1
benign (familial) D75.0
due to
donor twin P61.1
erythropoietin D75.1
fall in plasma volume D75.1
high altitude D75.1
maternal-fetal transfusion P61.1
stress D75.1
emotional D75.1
erythropoietin D75.1
familial (benign) D75.0
Gaisböck's (hypertonica) D75.1
high altitude D75.1
hypertonica D75.1
hypoxemic D75.1
neonatorum P61.1
nephrogenous D75.1
relative D75.1
secondary D75.1
spurious D75.1
stress D75.1
vera D45

Polycytosis cryptogenica D75.1
Polydactylism, polydactyly Q69.9
toes Q69.2
Polydipsia R63.1
Polydystrophy, pseudo-Hurler E77.0
Polyembryoma — *see* Neoplasm, malignant, by site
Polyglandular
deficiency E31.0
dyscrasia E31.9
dysfunction E31.9
syndrome E31.8
Polyhydramnios O40.- ☑
Polymastia Q83.1
Polymenorrhea N92.0
Polymyalgia M35.3
arteritica, giant cell M31.5
rheumatica M35.3
with giant cell arteritis M31.5
Polymyositis (acute) (chronic) (hemorrhagic) M33.20
with
myopathy M33.22
respiratory involvement M33.21
skin involvement — *see* Dermatopolymyositis
specified organ involvement NEC M33.29
ossificans (generalisata) (progressiva) — *see* Myositis,
ossificans, progressiva
Polyneuritis, polyneuritic (*see also* Polyneuropathy)
acute (post-)infective G61.0
alcoholic G62.1
cranialis G52.7
demyelinating, chronic inflammatory (CIDP) G61.81
diabetic — *see* Diabetes, polyneuropathy
diphtheritic A36.83
due to lack of vitamin NEC E56.9 [G63]
endemic E51.11
erythredema — *see* subcategory T56.1 ☑
febrile, acute G61.0
hereditary ataxic G60.1
idiopathic, acute G61.0
infective (acute) G61.0
inflammatory, chronic demyelinating (CIDP) G61.81
nutritional E63.9 [G63]
postinfective (acute) G61.0
specified NEC G62.89
Polyneuropathy (peripheral) G62.9
alcoholic G62.1
amyloid (Portuguese) E85.1 [G63]
arsenical G62.2
critical illness G62.81
demyelinating, chronic inflammatory (CIDP) G61.81
diabetic — *see* Diabetes, polyneuropathy
drug-induced G62.0
hereditary G60.9
specified NEC G60.8
idiopathic G60.9
progressive G60.3
in (due to)
alcohol G62.1
sequelae G65.2
amyloidosis, familial (Portuguese) E85.1 [G63]
antitetanus serum G61.1
arsenic G62.2
sequelae G65.2
avitaminosis NEC E56.9 [G63]
beriberi E51.11
collagen vascular disease NEC M35.9 [G63]
deficiency (of)
B (-complex) vitamins E53.9 [G63]
vitamin B6 E53.1 [G63]
diabetes — *see* Diabetes, polyneuropathy
diphtheria A36.83
drug or medicament G62.0
correct substance properly administered — *see*
Table of Drugs and Chemicals, by drug,
adverse effect
overdose or wrong substance given or taken
— *see* Table of Drugs and Chemicals, by
drug, poisoning
endocrine disease NEC E34.9 [G63]
herpes zoster B02.23
hypoglycemia E16.2 [G63]
infectious
disease NEC B99 ☑ [G63]
mononucleosis B27.91
lack of vitamin NEC E56.9 [G63]
lead G62.2
sequelae G65.2
leprosy A30.9 [G63]

Polyneuropathy — continued
in — continued
Lyme disease A69.22
metabolic disease NEC E88.9 [G63]
microscopic polyangiitis M31.7 [G63]
mumps B26.84
neoplastic disease (see also Neoplasm) D49.9 [G63]
nutritional deficiency NEC E63.9 [G63]
organophosphate compounds G62.2
sequelae G65.2
parasitic disease NEC B89 [G63]
pellagra E52 [G63]
polyarteritis nodosa M30.0
porphyria E80.20 [G63]
radiation G62.82
rheumatoid arthritis — see Rheumatoid, polyneuropathy
sarcoidosis D86.89
serum G61.1
syphilis (late) A52.15
congenital A50.43
systemic
connective tissue disorder M35.9 [G63]
lupus erythematosus M32.19
toxic agent NEC G62.2
sequelae G65.2
triorthocresyl phosphate G62.2
sequelae G65.2
tuberculosis A17.89
uremia N18.9 [G63]
vitamin B12 deficiency E53.8 [G63]
with anemia (pernicious) D51.0 [G63]
due to dietary deficiency D51.3 [G63]
zoster B02.23
inflammatory G61.9
chronic demyelinating (CIDP) G61.81
sequelae G65.1
specified NEC G61.89
lead G62.2
sequelae G65.2
nutritional NEC E63.9 [G63]
postherpetic (zoster) B02.23
progressive G60.3
radiation-induced G62.82
sensory (hereditary) (idiopathic) G60.8
specified NEC G62.89
syphilitic (late) A52.15
congenital A50.43
Polyopia H53.8
Polyorchism, polyorchidism Q55.21
Polyosteoarthritis (see also Osteoarthritis, generalized)
M15.9
post-traumatic M15.3
specified NEC M15.8
Polyostotic fibrous dysplasia Q78.1
Polyotia Q17.0
Polyp, polypus
accessory sinus J33.8
adenocarcinoma in — see Neoplasm, malignant, by
site
adenocarcinoma in situ in — see Neoplasm, in situ, by
site
adenoid tissue J33.0
adenomatous (see also Neoplasm, benign, by site)
adenocarcinoma in — see Neoplasm, malignant,
by site
adenocarcinoma in situ in — see Neoplasm, in situ,
by site
carcinoma in — see Neoplasm, malignant, by site
carcinoma in situ in — see Neoplasm, in situ, by
site
multiple — see Neoplasm, benign
adenocarcinoma in — see Neoplasm, malignant, by site
adenocarcinoma in situ in — see Neoplasm, in
situ, by site
antrum J33.8
anus, anal (canal) K62.0
Bartholin's gland N84.3
bladder D41.4
carcinoma in — see Neoplasm, malignant, by site
carcinoma in situ in — see Neoplasm, in situ, by site
cecum D12.0
cervix (uteri) N84.1
in pregnancy or childbirth — see Pregnancy,
complicated by, abnormal, cervix
mucous N84.1
nonneoplastic N84.1

Polyp, polypus — continued
choanal J33.0
cholesterol K82.4
clitoris N84.3
colon K63.5
adenomatous D12.6
ascending D12.2
cecum D12.0
descending D12.4
inflammatory K51.40
with
abscess K51.414
complication K51.419
specified NEC K51.418
fistula K51.413
intestinal obstruction K51.412
rectal bleeding K51.411
sigmoid D12.5
transverse D12.3
corpus uteri N84.0
dental K04.0
duodenum K31.7
ear (middle) H74.4- ☑
endometrium N84.0
ethmoidal (sinus) J33.8
fallopian tube N84.8
female genital tract N84.9
specified NEC N84.8
frontal (sinus) J33.8
gallbladder K82.4
gingiva, gum K06.8
labia, labium (majus) (minus) N84.3
larynx (mucous) J38.1
adenomatous D14.1
malignant — see Neoplasm, malignant, by site
maxillary (sinus) J33.8
middle ear — see Polyp, ear (middle)
myometrium N84.0
nares
anterior J33.9
posterior J33.0
nasal (mucous) J33.9
cavity J33.0
septum J33.0
nasopharyngeal J33.0
nose (mucous) J33.9
oviduct N84.8
pharynx J39.2
placenta O90.89
prostate — see Enlargement, enlarged, prostate
pudenda, pudendum N84.3
pulpal (dental) K04.0
rectum (nonadenomatous) K62.1
adenomatous — see Polyp, adenomatous
septum (nasal) J33.0
sinus (accessory) (ethmoidal) (frontal) (maxillary)
(sphenoidal) J33.8
sphenoidal (sinus) J33.8
stomach K31.7
adenomatous D13.1
tube, fallopian N84.8
turbinate, mucous membrane J33.8
umbilical, newborn P83.6
ureter N28.89
urethra N36.2
uterus (body) (corpus) (mucous) N84.0
cervix N84.1
in pregnancy or childbirth — see Pregnancy,
complicated by, tumor, uterus
vagina N84.2
vocal cord (mucous) J38.1
vulva N84.3
Polyphagia R63.2
Polyploidy Q92.7
Polypoid — see condition
Polyposis (see also Polyp)
coli (adenomatous) D12.6
adenocarcinoma in C18.9
adenocarcinoma in situ in — see Neoplasm, in situ,
by site
carcinoma in C18.9
colon (adenomatous) D12.6
familial D12.6
adenocarcinoma in situ in — see Neoplasm, in situ,
by site
intestinal (adenomatous) D12.6
malignant lymphomatous C83.1- ☑

Polyposis — continued
multiple, adenomatous (see also Neoplasm, benign)
D36.9
Polyradiculitis — see Polyneuropathy
Polyradiculoneuropathy (acute) (postinfective) (seg-
mentally demyelinating) G61.0
Polyserositis
due to pericarditis I31.1
pericardial I31.1
periodic, familial E85.0
tuberculous A19.9
acute A19.1
chronic A19.8
Polysplenia syndrome Q89.09
Polysyndactyly (see also Syndactylism, syndactyly) Q70.4
Polytrichia L68.3
Polyunguia Q84.6
Polyuria R35.8
nocturnal R35.1
psychogenic F45.8
Pompe's disease (glycogen storage) E74.02
Pompholyx L30.1
Poncet's disease (tuberculous rheumatism) A18.09
Pond fracture — see Fracture, skull
Ponos B55.0
Pons, pontine — see condition
Poor
aesthetic of existing restoration of tooth K08.56
contractions, labor O62.2
gingival margin to tooth restoration K08.51
personal hygiene R46.0
prenatal care, affecting management of pregnancy
— see Pregnancy, complicated by, insufficient,
prenatal care
sucking reflex (newborn) R29.2
urinary stream R39.12
vision NEC H54.7
Poradenitis, nostras inguinalis or venerea A55
Porencephaly (congenital) (developmental) (true) Q04.6
acquired G93.0
nondevelopmental G93.0
traumatic (post) F07.89
Porocephaliasis B88.8
Porokeratosis Q82.8
Poroma, eccrine — see Neoplasm, skin, benign
Porphyria (South African) E80.20
acquired E80.20
acute intermittent (hepatic) (Swedish) E80.21
cutanea tarda (hereditary) (symptomatic) E80.1
due to drugs E80.20
correct substance properly administered — see
Table of Drugs and Chemicals, by drug, adverse effect
overdose or wrong substance given or taken —
see Table of Drugs and Chemicals, by drug,
poisoning
erythropoietic (congenital) (hereditary) E80.0
hepatocutaneous type E80.1
secondary E80.20
toxic NEC E80.20
variegata E80.20
Porphyrinuria — see Porphyria
Porphyruria — see Porphyria
Port wine nevus, mark, or stain Q82.5
Portal — see condition
Posadas-Wernicke disease B38.9
Positive
culture (nonspecific)
blood R78.81
bronchial washings R84.5
cerebrospinal fluid R83.5
cervix uteri R87.5
nasal secretions R84.5
nipple discharge R89.5
nose R84.5
staphylococcus (Methicillin susceptible) Z22.321
Methicillin resistant Z22.322
peritoneal fluid R85.5
pleural fluid R84.5
prostatic secretions R86.5
saliva R85.5
seminal fluid R86.5
sputum R84.5
synovial fluid R89.5
throat scrapings R84.5
urine R82.7
vagina R87.5
vulva R87.5

☑ Additional Character Required — Refer to the Tabular List for Character Selection   ⬙ Subterms under main terms may continue to next column or page

Positive — continued
 culture — continued
  wound secretions R89.5
 PPD (skin test) R76.11
 serology for syphilis A53.0
  with signs or symptoms — code as Syphilis, by site and stage
  false R76.8
 skin test, tuberculin (without active tuberculosis) R76.11
 test, human immunodeficiency virus (HIV) R75
 VDRL A53.0
  with signs or symptoms — code by site and stage under Syphilis A53.9
 Wassermann reaction A53.0
Postcardiotomy syndrome I97.0
Postcaval ureter Q62.62
Postcholecystectomy syndrome K91.5
Postclimacteric bleeding N95.0
Postcommissurotomy syndrome I97.0
Postconcussional syndrome F07.81
Postcontusional syndrome F07.81
Postcricoid region — see condition
Post-dates (40-42 weeks) (pregnancy) (mother) O48.0
 more than 42 weeks gestation O48.1
Postencephalitic syndrome F07.89
Posterior — see condition
Posterolateral sclerosis (spinal cord) — see Degeneration, combined
Postexanthematous — see condition
Postfebrile — see condition
Postgastrectomy dumping syndrome K91.1
Posthemiplegic chorea — see Monoplegia
Posthemorrhagic anemia (chronic) D50.0
 acute D62
 newborn P61.3
Postherpetic neuralgia (zoster) B02.29
 trigeminal B02.22
Posthitis N47.7
Postimmunization complication or reaction — see Complications, vaccination
Postinfectious — see condition
Postlaminectomy syndrome NEC M96.1
Postleukotomy syndrome F07.0
Postmastectomy lymphedema (syndrome) I97.2
Postmaturity, postmature (over 42 weeks)
 maternal (over 42 weeks gestation) O48.1
 newborn P08.22
Postmeasles complication NEC (see also condition) B05.89
Postmenopausal
 endometrium (atrophic) N95.8
  suppurative (see also Endometritis) N71.9
 osteoporosis — see Osteoporosis, postmenopausal
Postnasal drip R09.82
 due to
  allergic rhinitis — see Rhinitis, allergic
  common cold J00
  gastroesophageal reflux — see Reflux, gastroesophageal
  nasopharyngitis — see Nasopharyngitis
  other known condition — code to condition
  sinusitis — see Sinusitis
Postnatal — see condition
Postoperative (postprocedural) — see Complication, postoperative
 pneumothorax, therapeutic Z98.3
 state NEC Z98.89
Postpancreatectomy hyperglycemia E89.1
Postpartum — see Puerperal
Postphlebitic syndrome — see Syndrome, postthrombotic
Postpolio (myelitic) **syndrome** G14
Postpoliomyelitic (see also condition)
 osteopathy — see Osteopathy, after poliomyelitis
Postprocedural (see also Postoperative)
 hypoinsulinemia E89.1
Postschizophrenic depression F32.8
Postsurgery status (see also Status (post))
 pneumothorax, therapeutic Z98.3
Post-term (40-42 weeks) (pregnancy) (mother) O48.0
 infant P08.21
 more than 42 weeks gestation (mother) O48.1
Post-traumatic brain syndrome, nonpsychotic F07.81
Post-typhoid abscess A01.09
Postures, hysterical F44.2

Postvaccinal reaction or complication — see Complications, vaccination
Postvalvulotomy syndrome I97.0
Potain's
 disease (pulmonary edema) — see Edema, lung
 syndrome (gastrectasis with dyspepsia) K31.0
Potter's
 asthma J62.8
 facies Q60.6
 lung J62.8
 syndrome (with renal agenesis) Q60.6
Pott's
 curvature (spinal) A18.01
 disease or paraplegia A18.01
 spinal curvature A18.01
 tumor, puffy — see Osteomyelitis, specified type NEC
Pouch
 bronchus Q32.4
 Douglas' — see condition
 esophagus, esophageal, congenital Q39.6
  acquired K22.5
 gastric K31.4
 Hartmann's K82.8
 pharynx, pharyngeal (congenital) Q38.7
Pouchitis K91.850
Poultrymen's itch B88.0
Poverty NEC Z59.6
 extreme Z59.5
Poxvirus NEC B08.8
Prader-Willi syndrome Q87.1
Preauricular appendage or tag Q17.0
Prebetalipoproteinemia (acquired) (essential) (familial) (hereditary) (primary) (secondary) E78.1
 with chylomicronemia E78.3
Precipitate labor or delivery O62.3
Preclimacteric bleeding (menorrhagia) N92.4
Precocious
 adrenarche E30.1
 menarche E30.1
 menstruation E30.1
 pubarche E30.1
 puberty E30.1
  central E22.8
 sexual development NEC E30.1
 thelarche E30.8
Precocity, sexual (constitutional) (cryptogenic) (female) (idiopathic) (male) E30.1
 with adrenal hyperplasia E25.9
  congenital E25.0
Precordial pain R07.2
Predeciduous teeth K00.2
Prediabetes, prediabetic R73.09
 complicating
  pregnancy — see Pregnancy, complicated by, diseases of, specified type or system NEC
  puerperium O99.89
Predislocation status of hip at birth Q65.6
Pre-eclampsia O14.9- ☑
 with pre-existing hypertension — see Hypertension, complicating pregnancy, pre-existing, with, pre-eclampsia
 mild O14.0- ☑
 moderate O14.0- ☑
 severe O14.1- ☑
  with hemolysis, elevated liver enzymes and low platelet count (HELLP) O14.2- ☑
Pre-eruptive color change, teeth, tooth K00.8
Pre-excitation atrioventricular conduction I45.6
Preglaucoma H40.00- ☑
Pregnancy (single) (uterine) (see also Delivery and Puerperal)

> Note: The Tabular must be reviewed for assignment of appropriate seventh character for multiple gestation codes in Chapter 15

> Note: The Tabular must be reviewed for assignment of the appropriate character indicating the trimester of the pregnancy

 abdominal (ectopic) O00.0
  with viable fetus O36.7- ☑
 ampullar O00.1
 biochemical O02.81
 broad ligament O00.8
 cervical O00.8
 chemical O02.81

Pregnancy — continued
 complicated by (care of) (management affected by)
  abnormal, abnormality
   cervix O34.4- ☑
    causing obstructed labor O65.5
   cord (umbilical) O69.9 ☑
   findings on antenatal screening of mother O28.9
    biochemical O28.1
    chromosomal O28.5
    cytological O28.2
    genetic O28.5
    hematological O28.0
    radiological O28.4
    specified NEC O28.8
    ultrasonic O28.3
   glucose (tolerance) NEC O99.810
   pelvic organs O34.9- ☑
    specified NEC O34.8- ☑
     causing obstructed labor O65.5
   pelvis (bony) (major) NEC O33.0
   perineum O34.7- ☑
   position
    placenta O44.1- ☑
     without hemorrhage O44.0- ☑
    uterus O34.59- ☑
   uterus O34.59- ☑
    causing obstructed labor O65.5
    congenital O34.0- ☑
   vagina O34.6- ☑
    causing obstructed labor O65.5
   vulva O34.7- ☑
    causing obstructed labor O65.5
  abruptio placentae — see Abruptio placentae
  abscess or cellulitis
   bladder O23.1- ☑
   breast O91.11- ☑
   genital organ or tract O23.9- ☑
  abuse
   physical O9A.31 ☑ (following O99)
   psychological O9A.51 ☑ (following O99)
   sexual O9A.41 ☑ (following O99)
  adverse effect anesthesia O29.9- ☑
   aspiration pneumonitis O29.01- ☑
   cardiac arrest O29.11- ☑
   cardiac complication NEC O29.19- ☑
   cardiac failure O29.12- ☑
   central nervous system complication NEC O29.29- ☑
   cerebral anoxia O29.21- ☑
   failed or difficult intubation O29.6- ☑
   inhalation of stomach contents or secretions NOS O29.01- ☑
   local, toxic reaction O29.3X ☑
   Mendelson's syndrome O29.01- ☑
   pressure collapse of lung O29.02- ☑
   pulmonary complications NEC O29.09- ☑
   specified NEC O29.8X- ☑
   spinal and epidural type NEC O29.5X ☑
    induced headache O29.4- ☑
  albuminuria O12.1- ☑
  alcohol use O99.31- ☑
  amnionitis O41.12- ☑
  anaphylactoid syndrome of pregnancy O88.01- ☑
  anemia (conditions in D50-D64) (pre-existing) O99.01- ☑
   complicating the puerperium O99.03
  antepartum hemorrhage O46.9- ☑
   with coagulation defect — see Hemorrhage, antepartum, with coagulation defect
   specified NEC O46.8X- ☑
  appendicitis O99.61- ☑
  atrophy (yellow) (acute) liver (subacute) O26.61- ☑
  bariatric surgery status O99.84- ☑
  bicornis or bicornuate uterus O34.59- ☑
  biliary tract problems O26.61- ☑
  breech presentation O32.1 ☑
  cardiovascular diseases (conditions in I00-I09, I20-I52, I70-I99) O99.41- ☑
  cerebrovascular disorders (conditions in I60-I69) O99.41- ☑
  cervical shortening O26.87- ☑
  cervicitis O23.51- ☑
  chloasma (gravidarum) O26.89- ☑
  cholecystitis O99.61- ☑
  cholestasis (intrahepatic) O26.61- ☑

Pregnancy — continued
complicated by — continued
  chorioamnionitis O41.12- ☑
  circulatory system disorder (conditions in I00-I09, I20-I99, O99.41-)
  compound presentation O32.6 ☑
  conjoined twins O30.02- ☑
  connective system disorders (conditions in M00-M99) O99.89
  contracted pelvis (general) O33.1
    inlet O33.2
    outlet O33.3 ☑
  convulsions (eclamptic) (uremic) (see also Eclampsia) O15.9
  cracked nipple O92.11- ☑
  cystitis O23.1- ☑
  cystocele O34.8- ☑
  death of fetus (near term) O36.4 ☑
    early pregnancy O02.1
    of one fetus or more in multiple gestation O31.2- ☑
  deciduitis O41.14- ☑
  decreased fetal movement O36.81- ☑
  dental problems O99.61- ☑
  diabetes (mellitus) O24.91- ☑
    gestational (pregnancy induced) — see Diabetes, gestational
    pre-existing O24.31- ☑
      specified NEC O24.81- ☑
      type 1 O24.01- ☑
      type 2 O24.11- ☑
  digestive system disorders (conditions in K00-K93) O99.61- ☑
  diseases of — see Pregnancy, complicated by, specified body system disease
    biliary tract O26.61- ☑
    blood NEC (conditions in D65-D77) O99.11- ☑
    liver O26.61- ☑
    specified NEC O99.89
  disorders of — see Pregnancy, complicated by, specified body system disorder
    amniotic fluid and membranes O41.9- ☑
      specified NEC O41.8X- ☑
    biliary tract O26.61- ☑
    ear and mastoid process (conditions in H60-H95) O99.89
    eye and adnexa (conditions in H00-H59) O99.89
    liver O26.61- ☑
    skin (conditions in L00-L99) O99.71- ☑
    specified NEC O99.89
  displacement, uterus NEC O34.59- ☑
    causing obstructed labor O65.5
  disproportion (due to) O33.9
    fetal deformities NEC O33.7
    generally contracted pelvis O33.1
    hydrocephalic fetus O33.6
    inlet contraction of pelvis O33.2
    mixed maternal and fetal origin O33.4
    specified NEC O33.8
  double uterus O34.59- ☑
    causing obstructed labor O65.5
  drug use (conditions in F11-F19) O99.32- ☑
  eclampsia, eclamptic (coma) (convulsions) (delirium) (nephritis) (uremia) (see also Eclampsia) O15.- ☑
  ectopic pregnancy — see Pregnancy, ectopic
  edema O12.0- ☑
    with
      gestational hypertension, mild (see also Preeclampsia) O14.0- ☑
      proteinuria O12.2- ☑
  effusion, amniotic fluid — see Pregnancy, complicated by, premature rupture of membranes
  elderly
    multigravida O09.52- ☑
    primigravida O09.51- ☑
  embolism (see also Embolism, obstetric, pregnancy) O88.- ☑
  endocrine diseases NEC O99.28- ☑
  endometritis O86.12
  excessive weight gain O26.0- ☑
  exhaustion O26.81- ☑
    during labor and delivery O75.81
  face presentation O32.3
  failed induction of labor O61.9
    instrumental O61.1
    mechanical O61.1

Pregnancy — continued
complicated by — continued
  failed induction of labor — continued
    medical O61.0
    specified NEC O61.8
    surgical O61.1
  failed or difficult intubation for anesthesia O29.6- ☑
  false labor (pains) O47.9
    at or after 37 completed weeks of pregnancy O47.1
    before 37 completed weeks of pregnancy O47.0- ☑
  fatigue O26.81- ☑
    during labor and delivery O75.81
  fatty metamorphosis of liver O26.61- ☑
  female genital mutilation O34.8- ☑ [N90.81-] ☑
  fetal (maternal care for)
    abnormality or damage O35.9 ☑
      acid-base balance O68
      specified type NEC O35.8 ☑
    acidemia O68
    acidosis O68
    alkalosis O68
    anemia and thrombocytopenia O36.82- ☑
    anencephaly O35.0 ☑
    chromosomal abnormality (conditions in Q90-Q99) O35.1 ☑
    conjoined twins O30.02- ☑
    damage from
      amniocentesis O35.7 ☑
      biopsy procedures O35.7 ☑
      drug addiction O35.5 ☑
      hematological investigation O35.7 ☑
      intrauterine contraceptive device O35.7 ☑
      maternal
        alcohol addiction O35.4 ☑
        cytomegalovirus infection O35.3 ☑
        disease NEC O35.8 ☑
        drug addiction O35.5 ☑
        listeriosis O35.8 ☑
        rubella O35.3 ☑
        toxoplasmosis O35.8 ☑
        viral infection O35.3 ☑
      medical procedure NEC O35.7 ☑
      radiation O35.6 ☑
    death (near term) O36.4 ☑
      early pregnancy O02.1
    decreased movement O36.81- ☑
    disproportion due to deformity (fetal) O33.7
    excessive growth (large for dates) O36.6- ☑
    growth retardation O36.59- ☑
      light for dates O36.59- ☑
      small for dates O36.59- ☑
    heart rate irregularity (bradycardia) (decelerations) (tachycardia) O76
    hereditary disease O35.2 ☑
    hydrocephalus O35.0 ☑
    intrauterine death O36.4 ☑
    poor growth O36.59- ☑
      light for dates O36.59- ☑
      small for dates O36.59- ☑
    problem O36.9- ☑
      specified NEC O36.89- ☑
    reduction (elective) O31.3- ☑
    selective termination O31.3- ☑
    spina bifida O35.0 ☑
    thrombocytopenia O36.82- ☑
  fibroid (tumor) (uterus) O34.1- ☑
  fissure of nipple O92.11- ☑
  gallstones O99.61- ☑
  gastric banding status O99.84- ☑
  gastric bypass status O99.84- ☑
  genital herpes (asymptomatic) (history of) (inactive) O98.51- ☑
  genital tract infection O23.9- ☑
  glomerular diseases (conditions in N00-N07) O26.83- ☑
    with hypertension, pre-existing — see Hypertension, complicating, pregnancy, pre-existing, with, renal disease
  gonorrhea O98.21- ☑
  grand multiparity O09.4 ☑
  habitual aborter — see Pregnancy, complicated by, recurrent pregnancy loss

Pregnancy — continued
complicated by — continued
  HELLP syndrome (hemolysis, elevated liver enzymes and low platelet count) O14.2- ☑
  hemorrhage
    antepartum — see Hemorrhage, antepartum
    before 20 completed weeks gestation O20.9
      specified NEC O20.8
    due to premature separation, placenta (see also Abruptio placentae) O45.9- ☑
    early O20.9
      specified NEC O20.8
    threatened abortion O20.0
  hemorrhoids O22.4- ☑
  hepatitis (viral) O98.41- ☑
  herniation of uterus O34.59- ☑
  high
    head at term O32.4 ☑
    risk — see Supervision (of) (for), high-risk
  history of in utero procedure during previous pregnancy O09.82- ☑
  HIV O98.71- ☑
  human immunodeficiency virus (HIV) disease O98.71- ☑
  hydatidiform mole (see also Mole, hydatidiform) O01.9
  hydramnios O40.- ☑
  hydrocephalic fetus (disproportion) O33.6 ☑
  hydrops
    amnii O40.- ☑
    fetalis O36.2- ☑
      associated with isoimmunization (see also Pregnancy, complicated by, isoimmunization) O36.11- ☑
  hydrorrhea O42.90
  hyperemesis (gravidarum) (mild) (see also Hyperemesis, gravidarum) O21.0
  hypertension — see Hypertension, complicating pregnancy
  hypertensive
    heart and renal disease, pre-existing — see Hypertension, complicating, pregnancy, pre-existing, with, heart disease, with renal disease
    heart disease, pre-existing — see Hypertension, complicating, pregnancy, pre-existing, with, heart disease
    renal disease, pre-existing — see Hypertension, complicating, pregnancy, pre-existing, with, renal disease
  hypotension O26.5- ☑
  immune disorders NEC (conditions in D80-D89) O99.11- ☑
  incarceration, uterus O34.51- ☑
  incompetent cervix O34.3- ☑
  inconclusive fetal viability O36.80 ☑
  infection(s) O98.91- ☑
    amniotic fluid or sac O41.10- ☑
    bladder O23.1- ☑
    carrier state NEC O99.830
      streptococcus B O99.820
    genital organ or tract O23.9- ☑
      specified NEC O23.59- ☑
    genitourinary tract O23.9- ☑
    gonorrhea O98.21- ☑
    hepatitis (viral) O98.41- ☑
    HIV O98.71- ☑
    human immunodeficiency virus (HIV) O98.71- ☑
    kidney O23.0- ☑
    nipple O91.01- ☑
    parasitic disease O98.91- ☑
      specified NEC O98.81- ☑
    protozoal disease O98.61- ☑
    sexually transmitted NEC O98.3ï- ☑
    specified type NEC O98.81- ☑
    syphilis O98.11- ☑
    tuberculosis O98.01- ☑
    urethra O23.2- ☑
    urinary (tract) O23.4- ☑
      specified NEC O23.3- ☑
    viral disease O98.51- ☑
  injury or poisoning (conditions in S00-T88) O9A.21- ☑ (following O99)
    due to abuse
      physical O9A.31- ☑ (following O99)

☑ Additional Character Required — Refer to the Tabular List for Character Selection   ▽ Subterms under main terms may continue to next column or page

Pregnancy — *continued*
  complicated by — *continued*
    injury or poisoning — *continued*
      due to abuse — *continued*
        psychological O9A.51- ☑ (*following* O99)
        sexual O9A.41- ☑ (*following* O99)
    insufficient
      prenatal care O09.3- ☑
      weight gain O26.1- ☑
    insulin resistance O26.89
    intrauterine fetal death (near term) O36.4 ☑
      early pregnancy O02.1
      multiple gestation (one fetus or more)
        O31.2- ☑
    isoimmunization O36.11- ☑
      anti-A sensitization O36.11- ☑
      anti-B sensitization O36.19- ☑
      Rh O36.09- ☑
        anti-D antibody O36.01- ☑
      specified NEC O36.19- ☑
    laceration of uterus NEC O71.81
    malformation
      placenta, placental (vessel) O43.10- ☑
        specified NEC O43.19- ☑
      uterus (congenital) O34.0- ☑
    malnutrition (conditions in E40-E46) O25.1- ☑
    maternal hypotension syndrome O26.5- ☑
    mental disorders (conditions in F01-F09, F20-F99)
      O99.34- ☑
      alcohol use O99.31- ☑
      drug use O99.32- ☑
      smoking O99.33- ☑
    mentum presentation O32.3 ☑
    metabolic disorders O99.28- ☑
    missed
      abortion O02.1
      delivery O36.4 ☑
    multiple gestations O30.9- ☑
      conjoined twins O30.02- ☑
      quadruplet — *see* Pregnancy, quadruplet
      specified complication NEC O31.8X- ☑
      specified number of multiples NEC — *see*
        Pregnancy, multiple (gestation), specified
        NEC
      triplet — *see* Pregnancy, triplet
      twin — *see* Pregnancy, twin
    musculoskeletal condition (conditions is M00-M99)
      O99.89
    necrosis, liver (conditions in K72) O26.61- ☑
    neoplasm
      benign
        cervix O34.4- ☑
        corpus uteri O34.1- ☑
        uterus O34.1- ☑
      malignant O9A.11- ☑ (*following* O99)
    nephropathy NEC O26.83- ☑
    nervous system condition (conditions in G00-G99)
      O99.35- ☑
    nutritional diseases NEC O99.28- ☑
    obesity (pre-existing) O99.21- ☑
    obesity surgery status O99.84- ☑
    oblique lie or presentation O32.2 ☑
    older mother — *see* Pregnancy, complicated by,
      elderly
    oligohydramnios O41.0- ☑
      with premature rupture of membranes (*see also*
        Pregnancy, complicated by, premature
        rupture of membranes) O42.- ☑
    onset (spontaneous) of labor after 37 completed
      weeks of gestation but before 39 completed
      weeks gestation, with delivery by (planned)
      cesarean section O75.82
    oophoritis O23.52- ☑
    overdose, drug (*see also* Table of Drugs and
      Chemicals, by drug, poisoning) O9A.21- ☑
      (*following* O99)
    oversize fetus O33.5 ☑
    papyraceous fetus O31.0- ☑
    pelvic inflammatory disease O99.89
    periodontal disease O99.61- ☑
    peripheral neuritis O26.82- ☑
    peritoneal (pelvic) adhesions O99.89
    phlebitis O22.9- ☑
    phlebopathy O22.9- ☑
    phlebothrombosis (superficial) O22.2- ☑
      deep O22.3- ☑

Pregnancy — *continued*
  complicated by — *continued*
    placenta accreta O43.21- ☑
    placenta increta O43.22- ☑
    placenta percreta O43.23- ☑
    placenta previa O44.1- ☑
      without hemorrhage O44.0- ☑
    placental disorder O43.9- ☑
      specified NEC O43.89- ☑
    placental dysfunction O43.89- ☑
    placental infarction O43.81- ☑
    placental insufficiency O36.51- ☑
    placental transfusion syndromes
      fetomaternal O43.01- ☑
      fetus to fetus O43.02- ☑
      maternofetal O43.01- ☑
    placentitis O41.14- ☑
    pneumonia O99.51- ☑
    poisoning (*see also* Table of Drugs and Chemicals)
      O9A.21 ☑ (*following* O99)
    polyhydramnios O40- ☑
    polymorphic eruption of pregnancy O26.86
    poor obstetric history NEC O09.29- ☑
    postmaturity (post-term) (40 to 42 weeks) O48.0
      more than 42 completed weeks gestation
        (prolonged) O48.1
    pre-eclampsia O14.9- ☑
      mild O14.0- ☑
      moderate O14.0- ☑
      severe O14.1- ☑
        with hemolysis, elevated liver enzymes and
          low platelet count (HELLP) O14.2- ☑
    premature labor — *see* Pregnancy, complicated
      by, preterm labor
    premature rupture of membranes O42.90
      with onset of labor
        after 24 hours O42.10
          after 37 weeks gestation O42.12
          pre-term (before 37 completed weeks
            of gestation) O42.11- ☑
        within 24 hours O42.00
          after 37 weeks gestation O42.02
          pre-term (before 37 completed weeks
            of gestation) O42.01- ☑
      after 37 weeks gestation O42.92
      full-term O42.92
      pre-term (before 37 completed weeks of gesta-
        tion) O42.91- ☑
    premature separation of placenta (*see also* Abrup-
      tio placentae) O45.9- ☑
    presentation, fetal — *see* Delivery, complicated
      by, malposition
    preterm delivery O60.10 ☑
    preterm labor
      with delivery O60.10 ☑
        preterm O60.10 ☑
        term O60.20 ☑
      without delivery O60.00
        second trimester O60.02
        third trimester O60.03
      second trimester
        with preterm delivery
          second trimester O60.12 ☑
          third trimester O60.13 ☑
        with term delivery O60.22 ☑
        without delivery O60.02
      third trimester
        with term delivery O60.23 ☑
        with third trimester preterm delivery
          O60.14 ☑
        without delivery O60.03
    previous history of — *see* Pregnancy, supervision
      of, high-risk
    prolapse, uterus O34.52- ☑
    proteinuria (gestational) O12.1- ☑
      with edema O12.2- ☑
    pruritic urticarial papules and plaques of pregnancy
      (PUPPP) O26.86
    pruritus (neurogenic) O26.89- ☑
    psychosis or psychoneurosis (puerperal) F53
    ptyalism O26.89- ☑
    PUPPP (pruritic urticarial papules and plaques of
      pregnancy) O26.86
    pyelitis O23.0- ☑
    recurrent pregnancy loss O26.2- ☑
    renal disease or failure NEC O26.83- ☑

Pregnancy — *continued*
  complicated by — *continued*
    renal disease or failure — *continued*
      with secondary hypertension, pre-existing —
        see Hypertension, complicating, pregnan-
        cy, pre-existing, secondary
      hypertensive, pre-existing — *see* Hypertension,
        complicating, pregnancy, pre-existing,
        with, renal disease
    respiratory condition (conditions in J00-J99)
      O99.51- ☑
    retained, retention
      dead ovum O02.0
      intrauterine contraceptive device O26.3- ☑
    retroversion, uterus O34.53- ☑
    Rh immunization, incompatibility or sensitization
      NEC O36.09- ☑
      anti-D antibody O36.01- ☑
    rupture
      amnion (premature) (*see also* Pregnancy, com-
        plicated by, premature rupture of mem-
        branes) O42- ☑
      membranes (premature) (*see also* Pregnancy,
        complicated by, premature rupture of
        membranes) O42- ☑
      uterus (during labor) O71.1
        before onset of labor O71.0- ☑
    salivation (excessive) O26.89- ☑
    salpingitis O23.52- ☑
    salpingo-oophoritis O23.52- ☑
    sepsis (conditions in A40, A41) O98.81- ☑
    size date discrepancy (uterine) O26.84- ☑
    skin condition (conditions in L00-L99) O99.71- ☑
    smoking (tobacco) O99.33- ☑
    social problem O09.7- ☑
    specified condition NEC O26.89- ☑
    spotting O26.85- ☑
    streptococcus B carrier state O99.820
    subluxation of symphysis (pubis) O26.71- ☑
    syphilis (conditions in A50-A53) O98.11- ☑
    threatened
      abortion O20.0
      labor O47.9
        at or after 37 completed weeks of gestation
          O47.1
        before 37 completed weeks of gestation
          O47.0- ☑
    thrombophlebitis (superficial) O22.2- ☑
    thrombosis O22.9- ☑
      cerebral venous O22.5- ☑
      cerebrovenous sinus O22.5- ☑
      deep O22.3- ☑
    torsion of uterus O34.59- ☑
    toxemia O14.9- ☑
    transverse lie or presentation O32.2 ☑
    tuberculosis (conditions in A15-A19) O98.01- ☑
    tumor (benign)
      cervix O34.4- ☑
      malignant O9A.11- ☑ (*following* O99)
      uterus O34.1- ☑
    unstable lie O32.0 ☑
    upper respiratory infection O99.51- ☑
    urethritis O23.2- ☑
    uterine size date discrepancy O26.84- ☑
    vaginitis or vulvitis O23.59- ☑
    varicose veins (lower extremities) O22.0- ☑
      genitals O22.1- ☑
      legs O22.0- ☑
      perineal O22.1- ☑
      vaginal or vulval O22.1- ☑
    venereal disease NEC (conditions in A63.8)
      O98.31- ☑
    venous disorders O22.9- ☑
      specified NEC O22.8X- ☑
    very young mother — *see* Pregnancy, complicated
      by, young mother
    viral diseases (conditions in A80-B09, B25-B34)
      O98.51- ☑
    vomiting O21.9
      due to diseases classified elsewhere O21.8
      hyperemesis gravidarum (mild) (*see also* Hyper-
        emesis, gravidarum) O21.0
      late (occurring after 20 weeks of gestation)
        O21.2
  young mother
    multigravida O09.62- ☑

Pregnancy — continued
  complicated by — continued
    young mother — continued
      primigravida O09.61- ☑
  complicated NOS O26.9- ☑
  concealed O09.3- ☑
  continuing following
    elective fetal reduction of one or more fetus
      O31.3- ☑
    intrauterine death of one or more fetus O31.2- ☑
    spontaneous abortion of one or more fetus
      O31.1- ☑
  cornual O00.8
  ectopic (ruptured) O00.9
    abdominal O00.0
      with viable fetus O36.7- ☑
    cervical O00.8
    complicated (by) O08.9
      afibrinogenemia O08.1
      cardiac arrest O08.81
      chemical damage of pelvic organ(s) O08.6
      circulatory collapse O08.3
      defibrination syndrome O08.1
      electrolyte imbalance O08.5
      embolism (amniotic fluid) (blood clot) (pul-
        monary) (septic) O08.2
      endometritis O08.0
      genital tract and pelvic infection O08.0
      hemorrhage (delayed) (excessive) O08.1
      infection
        genital tract or pelvic O08.0
        kidney O08.83
        urinary tract O08.3
      intravascular coagulation O08.1
      laceration of pelvic organ(s) O08.6
      metabolic disorder O08.5
      oliguria O08.4
      oophoritis O08.0
      parametritis O08.0
      pelvic peritonitis O08.0
      perforation of pelvic organ(s) O08.6
      renal failure or shutdown O08.4
      salpingitis or salpingo-oophoritis O08.0
      sepsis O08.82
      shock O08.83
        septic O08.82
      specified condition NEC O08.89
      tubular necrosis (renal) O08.4
      uremia O08.4
      urinary infection O08.83
      venous complication NEC O08.7
        embolism O08.2
    cornual O00.8
    intraligamentous O00.8
    mural O00.8
    ovarian O00.2
    specified site NEC O00.8
    tubal (ruptured) O00.1
  examination (normal) Z34.9- ☑
    first Z34.0- ☑
    high-risk — see Pregnancy, supervision of, high-
      risk
    specified Z34.8- ☑
  extrauterine — see Pregnancy, ectopic
  fallopian O00.1
  false F45.8
  hidden O09.3- ☑
  high-risk — see Pregnancy, supervision of, high-risk
  incidental finding Z33.1
  interstitial O00.8
  intraligamentous O00.8
  intramural O00.8
  intraperitoneal O00.0
  isthmian O00.1
  mesometric (mural) O00.8
  molar NEC O02.0
    complicated (by) O08.9
      afibrinogenemia O08.1
      cardiac arrest O08.81
      chemical damage of pelvic organ(s) O08.6
      circulatory collapse O08.3
      defibrination syndrome O08.1
      electrolyte imbalance O08.5
      embolism (amniotic fluid) (blood clot) (pul-
        monary) (septic) O08.2
      endometritis O08.0
      genital tract and pelvic infection O08.0
      hemorrhage (delayed) (excessive) O03.1

Pregnancy — continued
  molar — continued
    complicated — continued
      infection
        genital tract or pelvic O08.0
        kidney O08.83
        urinary tract O08.83
      intravascular coagulation O08.1
      laceration of pelvic organ(s) O08.6
      metabolic disorder O08.5
      oliguria O08.4
      oophoritis O08.0
      parametritis O08.0
      pelvic peritonitis O08.0
      perforation of pelvic organ(s) O08.6
      renal failure or shutdown O08.4
      salpingitis or salpingo-oophoritis O08.0
      sepsis O08.82
      shock O08.3
        septic O08.82
      specified condition NEC O08.89
      tubular necrosis (renal) O08.4
      uremia O08.4
      urinary infection O08.83
      venous complication NEC O08.7
        embolism O08.2
    hydatidiform (see also Mole, hydatidiform) O01.9
  multiple (gestation) O30.9- ☑
    greater than quadruplets — see Pregnancy, multi-
      ple (gestation), specified NEC
    specified NEC O30.80- ☑
      with
        two or more monoamniotic fetuses
          O30.82- ☑
        two or more monochorionic fetuses
          O30.81- ☑
      two or more monoamniotic fetuses O30.82- ☑
      two or more monochorionic fetuses O30.81- ☑
      unable to determine number of placenta and
        number of amniotic sacs O30.89- ☑
      unspecified number of placenta and unspeci-
        fied number of amniotic sacs O30.80- ☑
  mural O00.8
  normal (supervision of) Z34.9- ☑
    first Z34.0- ☑
    high-risk — see Pregnancy, supervision of, high-
      risk
    specified Z34.8- ☑
  ovarian O00.2
  postmature (40 to 42 weeks) O48.0
    more than 42 weeks gestation O48.1
  post-term (40 to 42 weeks) O48.0
  prenatal care only Z34.9- ☑
    first Z34.0- ☑
    high-risk — see Pregnancy, supervision of, high-
      risk
    specified Z34.8- ☑
  prolonged (more than 42 weeks gestation) O48.1
  quadruplet O30.20- ☑
    with
      two or more monoamniotic fetuses O30.22- ☑
      two or more monochorionic fetuses O30.21- ☑
    two or more monoamniotic fetuses O30.22- ☑
    two or more monochorionic fetuses O30.21- ☑
    unable to determine number of placenta and
      number of amniotic sacs O30.29- ☑
    unspecified number of placenta and unspecified
      number of amniotic sacs O30.20- ☑
  quintuplet — see Pregnancy, multiple (gestation),
    specified NEC
  sextuplet — see Pregnancy, multiple (gestation),
    specified NEC
  supervision of
    concealed pregnancy O09.3- ☑
    elderly mother
      multigravida O09.52- ☑
      primigravida O09.51- ☑
    hidden pregnancy O09.3- ☑
    high-risk O09.9- ☑
      due to (history of)
        ectopic pregnancy O09.1- ☑
        elderly — see Pregnancy, supervision, elder-
          ly mother
        grand multiparity O09.4
        in utero procedure during previous pregnan-
          cy O09.82- ☑
        in vitro fertilization O09.81- ☑

Pregnancy — continued
  supervision of — continued
    high-risk — continued
      due to — continued
        infertility O09.0- ☑
        insufficient prenatal care O09.3- ☑
        molar pregnancy O09.1- ☑
        multiple previous pregnancies O09.4- ☑
        older mother — see Pregnancy, supervision
          of, elderly mother
        poor reproductive or obstetric history NEC
          O09.29- ☑
        pre-term labor O09.21- ☑
        previous
          neonatal death O09.29- ☑
        social problems O09.7- ☑
        specified NEC O09.89- ☑
        very young mother — see Pregnancy, super-
          vision, young mother
      resulting from in vitro fertilization O09.81- ☑
    normal Z34.9- ☑
      first Z34.0- ☑
      specified NEC Z34.8- ☑
    young mother
      multigravida O09.62- ☑
      primigravida O09.61- ☑
  triplet O30.10- ☑
    with
      two or more monoamniotic fetuses O30.12- ☑
      two or more monochrorionic fetuses O30.11- ☑
    two or more monoamniotic fetuses O30.12- ☑
    two or more monochrorionic fetuses O30.11- ☑
    unable to determine number of placenta and
      number of amniotic sacs O30.19- ☑
    unspecified number of placenta and unspecified
      number of amniotic sacs O30.10- ☑
  tubal (with abortion) (with rupture) O00.1
  twin O30.00- ☑
    conjoined O30.02- ☑
    dichorionic/diamniotic (two placenta, two amniotic
      sacs) O30.04- ☑
    monochorionic/diamniotic (one placenta, two
      amniotic sacs) O30.03- ☑
    monochorionic/monoamniotic (one placenta, one
      amniotic sac) O30.01- ☑
    unable to determine number of placenta and
      number of amniotic sacs O30.09- ☑
    unspecified number of placenta and unspecified
      number of amniotic sacs O30.00- ☑
  unwanted Z64.0
  weeks of gestation
    less than 8 weeks Z3A.01 (following Z36)
    8 weeks Z3A.08 (following Z36)
    9 weeks Z3A.09 (following Z36)
    10 weeks Z3A.10 (following Z36)
    11 weeks Z3A.11 (following Z36)
    12 weeks Z3A.12 (following Z36)
    13 weeks Z3A.13 (following Z36)
    14 weeks Z3A.14 (following Z36)
    15 weeks Z3A.15 (following Z36)
    16 weeks Z3A.16 (following Z36)
    17 weeks Z3A.17 (following Z36)
    18 weeks Z3A.18 (following Z36)
    19 weeks Z3A.19 (following Z36)
    20 weeks Z3A.20 (following Z36)
    21 weeks Z3A.21 (following Z36)
    22 weeks Z3A.22 (following Z36)
    23 weeks Z3A.23 (following Z36)
    24 weeks Z3A.24 (following Z36)
    25 weeks Z3A.25 (following Z36)
    26 weeks Z3A.26 (following Z36)
    27 weeks Z3A.27 (following Z36)
    28 weeks Z3A.28 (following Z36)
    29 weeks Z3A.29 (following Z36)
    30 weeks Z3A.30 (following Z36)
    31 weeks Z3A.31 (following Z36)
    32 weeks Z3A.32 (following Z36)
    33 weeks Z3A.33 (following Z36)
    34 weeks Z3A.34 (following Z36)
    35 weeks Z3A.35 (following Z36)
    36 weeks Z3A.36 (following Z36)
    37 weeks Z3A.37 (following Z36)
    38 weeks Z3A.38 (following Z36)
    39 weeks Z3A.39 (following Z36)
    40 weeks Z3A.40 (following Z36)
    41 weeks Z3A.41 (following Z36)
    42 weeks Z3A.42 (following Z36)

254

☑ Additional Character Required — Refer to the Tabular List for Character Selection   ▽ Subterms under main terms may continue to next column or page

Pregnancy — *continued*
  weeks of gestation — *continued*
    greater than 42 weeks Z3A.49 *(following* Z36)
    not specified Z3A.00 *(following* Z36)
Preiser's disease — *see* Osteonecrosis, secondary, due to, trauma, metacarpus
Pre-kwashiorkor — *see* Malnutrition, severe
Preleukemia (syndrome) D46.9
Preluxation, hip, congenital Q65.6
Premature (*see also* condition)
  adrenarche E27.0
  aging E34.8
  beats I49.40
    atrial I49.1
    auricular I49.1
    supraventricular I49.1
  birth NEC — *see* Preterm, newborn
  closure, foramen ovale Q21.8
  contraction
    atrial I49.1
    atrioventricular I49.2
    auricular I49.1
    auriculoventricular I49.49
    heart (extrasystole) I49.49
    junctional I49.2
    ventricular I49.3
  delivery (*see also* Pregnancy, complicated by, preterm labor) O60.10 ☑
  ejaculation F52.4
  infant NEC — *see* Preterm, newborn
    light-for-dates — *see* Light for dates
  labor — *see* Pregnancy, complicated by, preterm labor
  lungs P28.0
  menopause E28.319
    asymptomatic E28.319
    symptomatic E28.310
  newborn
    less than 37 completed weeks — *see* Preterm, newborn
    extreme (less than 28 completed weeks) — *see* Immaturity, extreme
  puberty E30.1
  rupture membranes or amnion — *see* Pregnancy, complicated by, premature rupture of membranes
  senility E34.8
  thelarche E30.8
  ventricular systole I49.3
Prematurity NEC (less than 37 completed weeks) — *see* Preterm, newborn
  extreme (less than 28 completed weeks) — *see* Immaturity, extreme
Premenstrual
  dysphoric disorder (PMDD) N94.3
  tension (syndrome) N94.3
Premolarization, cuspids K00.2
Prenatal
  care, normal pregnancy — *see* Pregnancy, normal
  screening of mother Z36
  teeth K00.6
Preparatory care for subsequent treatment NEC
  for dialysis Z49.01
    peritoneal Z49.02
Prepartum — *see* condition
Preponderance, left or right ventricular I51.7
Prepuce — *see* condition
PRES (posterior reversible encephalopathy syndrome) I67.83
Presbycardia R54
Presbycusis, presbyacusia H91.1- ☑
Presbyesophagus K22.8
Presbyophrenia F03 ☑
Presbyopia H52.4
Prescription of contraceptives (initial) Z30.019
  emergency (postcoital) Z30.012
  implantable subdermal Z30.019
  injectable Z30.013
  intrauterine contraceptive device Z30.014
  pills Z30.011
  postcoital (emergency) Z30.012
  repeat Z30.40
    implantable subdermal Z30.49
    injectable Z30.42
    pills Z30.41
    specified type NEC Z30.49
  specified type NEC Z30.018

Presence (of)
  ankle-joint implant (functional) (prosthesis) Z96.66- ☑
  aortocoronary (bypass) graft Z95.1
  arterial-venous shunt (dialysis) Z99.2
  artificial
    eye (globe) Z97.0
    heart (fully implantable) (mechanical) Z95.812
      valve Z95.2
    larynx Z96.3
    lens (intraocular) Z96.1
    limb (complete) (partial) Z97.1- ☑
      arm Z97.1- ☑
        bilateral Z97.15
      leg Z97.1- ☑
        bilateral Z97.16
  audiological implant (functional) Z96.29
  bladder implant (functional) Z96.0
  bone
    conduction hearing device Z96.29
    implant (functional) NEC Z96.7
    joint (prosthesis) — *see* Presence, joint implant
  cardiac
    defibrillator (functional) (with synchronous cardiac pacemaker) Z95.810
    implant or graft Z95.9
      specified type NEC Z95.818
    pacemaker Z95.0
  cerebrospinal fluid drainage device Z98.2
  cochlear implant (functional) Z96.21
  contact lens (es) Z97.3
  coronary artery graft or prosthesis Z95.5
  CSF shunt Z98.2
  dental prosthesis device Z97.2
  dentures Z97.2
  device (external) NEC Z97.8
    cardiac NEC Z95.818
    heart assist Z95.811
    implanted (functional) Z96.9
      specified NEC Z96.89
    prosthetic Z97.8
  ear implant Z96.20
    cochlear implant Z96.21
    myringotomy tube Z96.22
    specified type NEC Z96.29
  elbow-joint implant (functional) (prosthesis) Z96.62- ☑
  endocrine implant (functional) NEC Z96.49
  eustachian tube stent or device (functional) Z96.29
  external hearing-aid or device Z97.4
  finger-joint implant (functional) (prosthetic) Z96.69- ☑
  functional implant Z96.9
    specified NEC Z96.89
  graft
    cardiac NEC Z95.818
    vascular NEC Z95.828
  hearing-aid or device (external) Z97.4
    implant (bone) (cochlear) (functional) Z96.21
  heart assist device Z95.811
  heart valve implant (functional) Z95.2
    prosthetic Z95.2
    specified type NEC Z95.4
    xenogenic Z95.3
  hip-joint implant (functional) (prosthesis) Z96.64- ☑
  implanted device (artificial) (functional) (prosthetic) Z96.9
    automatic cardiac defibrillator (with synchronous cardiac pacemaker) Z95.810
    cardiac pacemaker Z95.0
    cochlear Z96.21
    dental Z96.5
    heart Z95.812
    heart valve Z95.2
      prosthetic Z95.2
      specified NEC Z95.4
      xenogenic Z95.3
    insulin pump Z96.41
    intraocular lens Z96.1
    joint Z96.60
      ankle Z96.66- ☑
      elbow Z96.62- ☑
      finger Z96.69- ☑
      hip Z96.64- ☑
      knee Z96.65- ☑
      shoulder Z96.61- ☑
      specified NEC Z96.698
      wrist Z96.63- ☑
    larynx Z96.3
    myringotomy tube Z96.22

Presence — *continued*
  implanted device — *continued*
    otological Z96.20
      cochlear Z96.21
      eustachian stent Z96.29
      myringotomy Z96.22
      specified NEC Z96.29
      stapes Z96.29
    skin Z96.81
    skull plate Z96.7
    specified NEC Z96.89
    urogenital Z96.0
  insulin pump (functional) Z96.41
  intestinal bypass or anastomosis Z98.0
  intraocular lens (functional) Z96.1
  intrauterine contraceptive device (IUD) Z97.5
  intravascular implant (functional) (prosthetic) NEC Z95.9
    coronary artery Z95.5
    defibrillator (with synchronous cardiac pacemaker) Z95.810
    peripheral vessel (with angioplasty) Z95.820
  joint implant (prosthetic) (any) Z96.60
    ankle — *see* Presence, ankle joint implant
    elbow — *see* Presence, elbow joint implant
    finger — *see* Presence, finger joint implant
    hip — *see* Presence, hip joint implant
    knee — *see* Presence, knee joint implant
    shoulder — *see* Presence, shoulder joint implant
    specified joint NEC Z96.698
    wrist — *see* Presence, wrist joint implant
  knee-joint implant (functional) (prosthesis) Z96.65- ☑
  laryngeal implant (functional) Z96.3
  mandibular implant (dental) Z96.5
  myringotomy tube(s) Z96.22
  orthopedic-joint implant (prosthetic) (any) — *see* Presence, joint implant
  otological implant (functional) Z96.29
  shoulder-joint implant (functional) (prosthesis) Z96.61- ☑
  skull-plate implant Z96.7
  spectacles Z97.3
  stapes implant (functional) Z96.29
  systemic lupus erythematosus [SLE] inhibitor D68.62
  tendon implant (functional) (graft) Z96.7
  tooth root(s) implant Z96.5
  ureteral stent Z96.0
  urethral stent Z96.0
  urogenital implant (functional) Z96.0
  vascular implant or device Z95.9
    access port device Z95.828
    specified type NEC Z95.828
  wrist-joint implant (functional) (prosthesis) Z96.63- ☑
Presenile (*see also* condition)
  dementia F03 ☑
  premature aging E34.8
Presentation, fetal — *see* Delivery, complicated by, malposition
Prespondylolisthesis (congenital) Q76.2
Pressure
  area, skin — *see* Ulcer, pressure, by site
  brachial plexus G54.0
  brain G93.5
    injury at birth NEC P11.1
  cerebral — *see* Pressure, brain
  chest R07.89
  cone, tentorial G93.5
  hyposystolic (*see also* Hypotension)
    incidental reading, without diagnosis of hypotension R03.1
  increased
    intracranial (benign) G93.2
      injury at birth P11.0
    intraocular H40.05- ☑
  lumbosacral plexus G54.1
  mediastinum J98.5
  necrosis (chronic) — *see* Ulcer, pressure, by site
  parental, inappropriate (excessive) Z62.6
  sore (chronic) — *see* Ulcer, pressure, by site
  spinal cord G95.20
  ulcer (chronic) — *see* Ulcer, pressure, by site
  venous, increased I87.8
Pre-syncope R55
Preterm
  delivery (*see also* Pregnancy, complicated by, preterm labor) O60.10 ☑
  labor — *see* Pregnancy, complicated by, preterm labor
  newborn (infant) P07.30

Preterm — *continued*
  newborn — *continued*
    gestational age
      28 completed weeks (28 weeks, Ø days through 28 weeks, 6 days) PØ7.31
      29 completed weeks (29 weeks, Ø days through 29 weeks, 6 days) PØ7.32
      3Ø completed weeks (3Ø weeks, Ø days through 3Ø weeks, 6 days) PØ7.33
      31 completed weeks (31 weeks, Ø days through 31 weeks, 6 days) PØ7.34
      32 completed weeks (32 weeks, Ø days through 32 weeks, 6 days) PØ7.35
      33 completed weeks (33 weeks, Ø days through 33 weeks, 6 days) PØ7.36
      34 completed weeks (34 weeks, Ø days through 34 weeks, 6 days) PØ7.37
      35 completed weeks (35 weeks, Ø days through 35 weeks, 6 days) PØ7.38
      36 completed weeks (36 weeks, Ø days through 36 weeks, 6 days) PØ7.39

Previa
  placenta (low) (marginal) (partial) (total) (with hemorrhage) O44.1- ☑
    without hemorrhage O44.Ø- ☑
  vasa O69.4 ☑
Priapism N48.3Ø
  due to
    disease classified elsewhere N48.32
    drug N48.33
    specified cause NEC N48.39
    trauma N48.31
Prickling sensation (skin) R2Ø.2
Prickly heat L74.Ø
Primary — *see* condition
Primigravida
  elderly, affecting management of pregnancy, labor and delivery (supervision only) — *see* Pregnancy, complicated by, elderly, primigravida
  older, affecting management of pregnancy, labor and delivery (supervision only) — *see* Pregnancy, complicated by, elderly, primigravida
  very young, affecting management of pregnancy, labor and delivery (supervision only) — *see* Pregnancy, complicated by, young mother, primigravida
Primipara
  elderly, affecting management of pregnancy, labor and delivery (supervision only) — *see* Pregnancy, complicated by, elderly, primigravida
  older, affecting management of pregnancy, labor and delivery (supervision only) — *see* Pregnancy, complicated by, elderly, primigravida
  very young, affecting management of pregnancy, labor and delivery (supervision only) — *see* Pregnancy, complicated by, young mother, primigravida
Primus varus (bilateral) Q66.2
PRIND (Prolonged reversible ischemic neurologic deficit) I63.9
Pringle's disease (tuberous sclerosis) Q85.1
Prinzmetal angina I2Ø.1
Prizefighter ear — *see* Cauliflower ear
Problem (with) (related to)
  academic Z55.8
  acculturation Z6Ø.3
  adjustment (to)
    change of job Z56.1
    life-cycle transition Z6Ø.Ø
    pension Z6Ø.Ø
    retirement Z6Ø.Ø
  adopted child Z62.821
  alcoholism in family Z63.72
  atypical parenting situation Z62.9
  bankruptcy Z59.8
  behavioral (adult) F69
    drug seeking Z72.89
  birth of sibling affecting child Z62.898
  care (of)
    provider dependency Z74.9
      specified NEC Z74.8
    sick or handicapped person in family or household Z63.6
  child
    abuse (affecting the child) — *see* Maltreatment, child
    custody or support proceedings Z65.3
    in care of non-parental family member Z62.21
    in foster care Z62.21
    in welfare custody Z62.21

Problem — *continued*
  child — *continued*
    living in orphanage or group home Z62.22
  child-rearing Z62.9
    specified NEC Z62.898
  communication (developmental) F8Ø.9
  conflict or discord (with)
    boss Z56.4
    classmates Z55.4
    counselor Z64.4
    employer Z56.4
    family Z63.9
      specified NEC Z63.8
    probation officer Z64.4
    social worker Z64.4
    teachers Z55.4
    workmates Z56.4
  conviction in legal proceedings Z65.Ø
    with imprisonment Z65.1
  counselor Z64.4
  creditors Z59.8
  digestive K92.9
  drug addict in family Z63.72
  ear — *see* Disorder, ear
  economic Z59.9
    affecting care Z59.9
    specified NEC Z59.8
  education Z55.9
    specified NEC Z55.8
  employment Z56.9
    change of job Z56.1
    discord Z56.4
    environment Z56.5
    sexual harassment Z56.81
    specified NEC Z56.89
    stressful schedule Z56.3
    stress NEC Z56.6
    threat of job loss Z56.2
    unemployment Z56.Ø
  enuresis, child F98.Ø
  eye H57.9
  failed examinations (school) Z55.2
  falling Z91.81
  family (*see also* Disruption, family) Z63.9
    specified NEC Z63.8
  feeding (elderly) (infant) R63.3
    newborn P92.9
      breast P92.5
      overfeeding P92.4
      slow P92.2
      specified NEC P92.8
      underfeeding P92.3
    nonorganic F5Ø.8
  finance Z59.9
    specified NEC Z59.8
  foreclosure on loan Z59.8
  foster child Z62.822
  frightening experience(s) in childhood Z62.898
  genital NEC
    female N94.9
    male N5Ø.9
  health care Z75.9
    specified NEC Z75.8
  hearing — *see* Deafness
  homelessness Z59.Ø
  housing Z59.9
    inadequate Z59.1
    isolated Z59.8
    specified NEC Z59.8
  identity (of childhood) F93.8
  illegitimate pregnancy (unwanted) Z64.Ø
  illiteracy Z55.Ø
  impaired mobility Z74.Ø9
  imprisonment or incarceration Z65.1
  inadequate teaching affecting education Z55.8
  inappropriate (excessive) parental pressure Z62.6
  influencing health status NEC Z78.9
  in-law Z63.1
  institutionalization, affecting child Z62.22
  intrafamilial communication Z63.8
  jealousy, child F93.8
  landlord Z59.2
  language (developmental) F8Ø.9
  learning (developmental) F81.9
  legal Z65.3
    conviction without imprisonment Z65.Ø
    imprisonment Z65.1
    release from prison Z65.2

Problem — *continued*
  life-management Z73.9
    specified NEC Z73.89
  life-style Z72.9
    gambling Z72.6
    high-risk sexual behavior (heterosexual) Z72.51
      bisexual Z72.53
      homosexual Z72.52
    inappropriate eating habits Z72.4
    self-damaging behavior NEC Z72.89
    specified NEC Z72.89
    tobacco use Z72.Ø
  literacy Z55.9
    low level Z55.Ø
    specified NEC Z55.8
  living alone Z6Ø.2
  lodgers Z59.2
  loss of love relationship in childhood Z62.898
  marital Z63.Ø
    involving
      divorce Z63.5
      estrangement Z63.5
      gender identity F66
  mastication KØ8.8
  medical
    care, within family Z63.6
    facilities Z75.9
      specified NEC Z75.8
  mental F48.9
  multiparity Z64.1
  negative life events in childhood Z62.9
    altered pattern of family relationships Z62.898
    frightening experience Z62.898
    loss of
      love relationship Z62.898
      self-esteem Z62.898
    physical abuse (alleged) — *see* Maltreatment, child
    removal from home Z62.29
    specified event NEC Z62.898
  neighbor Z59.2
  neurological NEC R29.818
  new step-parent affecting child Z62.898
  none (feared complaint unfounded) Z71.1
  occupational NEC Z56.89
  parent-child — *see* Conflict, parent-child
  personal hygiene Z91.89
  personality F69
  phase-of-life transition, adjustment Z6Ø.Ø
  presence of sick or disabled person in family or household Z63.79
    needing care Z63.6
  primary support group (family) Z63.9
    specified NEC Z63.8
  probation officer Z64.4
  psychiatric F99
  psychosexual (development) F66
  psychosocial Z65.9
    specified NEC Z65.8
  relationship Z63.9
    childhood F93.8
  release from prison Z65.2
  removal from home affecting child Z62.29
  seeking and accepting known hazardous and harmful
    behavioral or psychological interventions Z65.8
    chemical, nutritional or physical interventions Z65.8
  sexual function (nonorganic) F52.9
  sight H54.7
  sleep disorder, child F51.9
  smell — *see* Disturbance, sensation, smell
  social
    environment Z6Ø.9
      specified NEC Z6Ø.8
    exclusion and rejection Z6Ø.4
    worker Z64.4
  speech R47.9
    developmental F8Ø.9
    specified NEC R47.89
  swallowing — *see* Dysphagia
  taste — *see* Disturbance, sensation, taste
  tic, child F95.Ø
  underachievement in school Z55.3
  unemployment Z56.Ø
    threatened Z56.2
  unwanted pregnancy Z64.Ø
  upbringing Z62.9
    specified NEC Z62.898
  urinary N39.9
  voice production R47.89

256

☑ Additional Character Required — Refer to the Tabular List for Character Selection   ▽ Subterms under main terms may continue to next column or page

Problem — continued
  work schedule (stressful) Z56.3
Procedure (surgical)
  for purpose other than remedying health state Z41.9
    specified NEC Z41.8
  not done Z53.9
    because of
      administrative reasons Z53.8
      contraindication Z53.09
        smoking Z53.01
      patient's decision Z53.20
        for reasons of belief or group pressure Z53.1
        left against medical advice (AMA) Z53.21
        specified reason NEC Z53.29
      specified reason NEC Z53.8
Procidentia (uteri) N81.3
Proctalgia K62.89
  fugax K59.4
  spasmodic K59.4
Proctitis K62.89
  amebic (acute) A06.0
  chlamydial A56.3
  gonococcal A54.6
  granulomatous — see Enteritis, regional, large intestine
  herpetic A60.1
  radiation K62.7
  tuberculous A18.32
  ulcerative (chronic) K51.20
    with
      complication K51.219
        abscess K51.214
        fistula K51.213
        obstruction K51.212
        rectal bleeding K51.211
        specified NEC K51.218
Proctocele
  female (without uterine prolapse) N81.6
    with uterine prolapse N81.2
      complete N81.3
  male K62.3
Proctocolitis, mucosal — see Rectosigmoiditis, ulcerative
Proctoptosis K62.3
Proctorrhagia K62.5
Proctosigmoiditis K63.89
  ulcerative (chronic) — see Rectosigmoiditis, ulcerative
Proctospasm K59.4
  psychogenic F45.8
Profichet's disease — see Disorder, soft tissue, specified type NEC
Progeria E34.8
Prognathism (mandibular) (maxillary) M26.19
Progonoma (melanotic) — see Neoplasm, benign, by site
Progressive — see condition
Prolactinoma
  specified site — see Neoplasm, benign, by site
  unspecified site D35.2
Prolapse, prolapsed
  anus, anal (canal) (sphincter) K62.2
  arm or hand O32.2 ☑
    causing obstructed labor O64.4 ☑
  bladder (mucosa) (sphincter) (acquired)
    congenital Q79.4
    female — see Cystocele
    male N32.89
  breast implant (prosthetic) T85.49 ☑
  cecostomy K94.09
  cecum K63.4
  cervix, cervical (hypertrophied) N81.2
    anterior lip, obstructing labor O65.5
    congenital Q51.828
    postpartal, old N81.2
    stump N81.85
  ciliary body (traumatic) — see Laceration, eye(ball), with prolapse or loss of interocular tissue
  colon (pedunculated) K63.4
  colostomy K94.09
  disc (intervertebral) — see Displacement, intervertebral disc
  eye implant (orbital) T85.398 ☑
    lens (ocular) — see Complications, intraocular lens
  fallopian tube N83.4
  gastric (mucosa) K31.89
  genital, female N81.9
    specified NEC N81.89
  globe, nontraumatic — see Luxation, globe

Prolapse, prolapsed — continued
  ileostomy bud K94.19
  intervertebral disc — see Displacement, intervertebral disc
  intestine (small) K63.4
  iris (traumatic) — see Laceration, eye(ball), with prolapse or loss of interocular tissue
    nontraumatic H21.89
  kidney N28.83
    congenital Q63.2
  laryngeal muscles or ventricle J38.7
  liver K76.89
  meatus urinarius N36.8
  mitral (valve) I34.1
  ocular lens implant — see Complications, intraocular lens
  organ or site, congenital NEC — see Malposition, congenital
  ovary N83.4
  pelvic floor, female N81.89
  perineum, female N81.89
  rectum (mucosa) (sphincter) K62.3
    due to trichuris trichuria B79
  spleen D73.89
  stomach K31.89
  umbilical cord
    complicating delivery O69.0 ☑
  urachus, congenital Q64.4
  ureter N28.89
    with obstruction N13.5
      with infection N13.6
  ureterovesical orifice N28.89
  urethra (acquired) (infected) (mucosa) N36.8
    congenital Q64.71
  urinary meatus N36.8
    congenital Q64.72
  uterovaginal N81.4
    complete N81.3
    incomplete N81.2
  uterus (with prolapse of vagina) N81.4
    complete N81.3
    congenital Q51.818
    first degree N81.2
    in pregnancy or childbirth — see Pregnancy, complicated by, abnormal, uterus
    incomplete N81.2
    postpartal (old) N81.4
    second degree N81.2
    third degree N81.3
  uveal (traumatic) — see Laceration, eye(ball), with prolapse or loss of interocular tissue
  vagina (anterior) (wall) — see Cystocele
    with prolapse of uterus N81.4
      complete N81.3
      incomplete N81.2
    posterior wall N81.6
    posthysterectomy N99.3
  vitreous (humor) H43.0- ☑
    in wound — see Laceration, eye(ball), with prolapse or loss of interocular tissue
  womb — see Prolapse, uterus
Prolapsus, female N81.9
  specified NEC N81.89
Proliferation(s)
  primary cutaneous CD30-positive large T-cell C86.6
Proliferative — see condition
Prolonged, prolongation (of)
  bleeding (time) (idiopathic) R79.1
  coagulation (time) R79.1
  gestation (over 42 completed weeks)
    mother O48.1
    newborn P08.22
  interval I44.0
  labor O63.9
    first stage O63.0
    second stage O63.1
  partial thromboplastin time (PTT) R79.1
  pregnancy (more than 42 weeks gestation) O48.1
  prothrombin time R79.1
  QT interval I45.81
  uterine contractions in labor O62.4
Prominence, prominent
  auricle (congenital) (ear) Q17.5
  ischial spine or sacral promontory
    with disproportion (fetopelvic) O33.0
      causing obstructed labor O65.0
  nose (congenital) acquired M95.0
Promiscuity — see High, risk, sexual behavior

Pronation
  ankle — see Deformity, limb, foot, specified NEC
  foot (see also Deformity, limb, foot, specified NEC)
    congenital Q74.2
Prophylactic
  administration of
    antibiotics, long-term Z79.2
      short-term use — omit code
    drug (see also Long-term (current) drug therapy (use of)) Z79.899
  medication Z79.899
  organ removal (for neoplasia management) Z40.00
    breast Z40.01
    ovary Z40.02
    specified site NEC Z40.09
  surgery Z40.9
    for risk factors related to malignant neoplasm — see Prophylactic, organ removal
    specified NEC Z40.8
  vaccination Z23
Propionic acidemia E71.121
Proptosis (ocular) (see also Exophthalmos)
  thyroid — see Hyperthyroidism, with goiter
Prosecution, anxiety concerning Z65.3
Prosopagnosia R48.3
Prostadynia N42.81
Prostate, prostatic — see condition
Prostatism — see Hyperplasia, prostate
Prostatitis (congestive) (suppurative) (with cystitis) N41.9
  acute N41.0
  cavitary N41.8
  chronic N41.1
  diverticular N41.8
  due to Trichomonas (vaginalis) A59.02
  fibrous N41.1
  gonococcal (acute) (chronic) A54.22
  granulomatous N41.4
  hypertrophic N41.1
  subacute N41.1
  trichomonal A59.02
  tuberculous A18.14
Prostatocystitis N41.3
Prostatorrhea N42.89
Prostatosis N42.82
Prostration R53.83
  heat (see also Heat, exhaustion)
    anhydrotic T67.3 ☑
    due to
      salt (and water) depletion T67.4 ☑
      water depletion T67.3 ☑
  nervous F48.8
  senile R54
Protanomaly (anomalous trichromat) H53.54
Protanopia (complete) (incomplete) H53.54
Protection (against) (from) — see Prophylactic
Protein
  deficiency NEC — see Malnutrition
  malnutrition — see Malnutrition
  sickness (see also Reaction, serum) T80.69 ☑
Proteinemia R77.9
Proteinosis
  alveolar (pulmonary) J84.01
  lipid or lipoid (of Urbach) E78.89
Proteinuria R80.9
  Bence Jones R80.3
  complicating pregnancy — see Proteinuria, gestational
  gestational O12.1- ☑
    with edema O12.2- ☑
  idiopathic R80.0
  isolated R80.0
    with glomerular lesion N06.9
      dense deposit disease N06.6
      diffuse
        crescentic glomerulonephritis N06.7
        endocapillary proliferative glomerulonephritis N06.4
        mesangiocapillary glomerulonephritis N06.5
      focal and segmental hyalinosis or sclerosis N06.1
      membranous (diffuse) N06.2
      mesangial proliferative (diffuse) N06.3
      minimal change N06.0
      specified pathology NEC N06.8
  orthostatic R80.2
    with glomerular lesion — see Proteinuria, isolated, with glomerular lesion
  persistent R80.1

Proteinuria — *continued*
  persistent — *continued*
    with glomerular lesion — *see* Proteinuria, isolated, with glomerular lesion
    postural R80.2
      with glomerular lesion — *see* Proteinuria, isolated, with glomerular lesion
    pre-eclamptic — *see* Pre-eclampsia
    specified type NEC R80.8
Proteolysis, pathologic D65
Proteus (mirabilis) (morganii), **as cause of disease classified elsewhere** B96.4
Prothrombin gene mutation D68.52
Protoporphyria, erythropoietic E80.0
Protozoal (*see also* condition)
  disease B64
    specified NEC B60.8
Protrusion, protrusio
  acetabuli M24.7
  acetabulum (into pelvis) M24.7
  device, implant or graft (*see also* Complications, by site and type, mechanical) T85.698 ☑
    arterial graft NEC — *see* Complication, cardiovascular device, mechanical, vascular
    breast (implant) T85.49 ☑
    catheter NEC T85.698 ☑
      cystostomy T83.090 ☑
      dialysis (renal) T82.49 ☑
        intraperitoneal T85.691 ☑
      infusion NEC T82.594 ☑
        spinal (epidural) (subdural) T85.690 ☑
      urinary, indwelling T83.098 ☑
    electronic (electrode) (pulse generator) (stimulator) bone T84.390 ☑
    nervous system — *see* Complication, prosthetic device, mechanical, electronic nervous system stimulator
    fixation, internal (orthopedic) NEC — *see* Complication, fixation device, mechanical
    gastrointestinal — *see* Complications, prosthetic device, mechanical, gastrointestinal device
    genital NEC T83.498 ☑
      intrauterine contraceptive device T83.39 ☑
      penile prosthesis T83.490 ☑
    heart NEC — *see* Complication, cardiovascular device, mechanical
    joint prosthesis — *see* Complications, joint prosthesis, mechanical, specified NEC, by site
    ocular NEC — *see* Complications, prosthetic device, mechanical, ocular device
    orthopedic NEC — *see* Complication, orthopedic, device, mechanical
    specified NEC T85.628 ☑
    urinary NEC (*see also* Complication, genitourinary, device, urinary, mechanical)
      graft T83.29 ☑
    vascular NEC — *see* Complication, cardiovascular device, mechanical
    ventricular intracranial shunt T85.09 ☑
  intervertebral disc — *see* Displacement, intervertebral disc
  joint prosthesis — *see* Complications, joint prosthesis, mechanical, specified NEC, by site
  nucleus pulposus — *see* Displacement, intervertebral disc
Prune belly (syndrome) Q79.4
Prurigo (ferox) (gravis) (Hebrae) (Hebra's) (mitis) (simplex) L28.2
  Besnier's L20.0
  estivalis L56.4
  nodularis L28.1
  psychogenic F45.8
Pruritus, pruritic (essential) L29.9
  ani, anus L29.0
    psychogenic F45.8
  anogenital L29.3
    psychogenic F45.8
  due to onchocerca volvulus B73.1
  gravidarum — *see* Pregnancy, complicated by, specified pregnancy-related condition NEC
  hiemalis L29.8
  neurogenic (any site) F45.8
  perianal L29.0
  psychogenic (any site) F45.8
  scroti, scrotum L29.1
    psychogenic F45.8
  senile, senilis L29.8

Pruritus, pruritic — *continued*
  specified NEC L29.8
    psychogenic F45.8
  Trichomonas A59.9
  vulva, vulvae L29.2
    psychogenic F45.8
Pseudarthrosis, pseudoarthrosis (bone) — *see* Nonunion, fracture
  clavicle, congenital Q74.0
  joint, following fusion or arthrodesis M96.0
Pseudoaneurysm — *see* Aneurysm
Pseudoangina (pectoris) — *see* Angina
Pseudoangioma I81
Pseudoarteriosus Q28.8
Pseudoarthrosis — *see* Pseudarthrosis
Pseudobulbar affect (PBA) F48.8
Pseudochromhidrosis L67.8
Pseudocirrhosis, liver, pericardial I31.1
Pseudocowpox B08.03
Pseudocoxalgia M91.3- ☑
Pseudocroup J38.5
Pseudo-Cushing's syndrome, alcohol-induced E24.4
Pseudocyesis F45.8
Pseudocyst
  lung J98.4
  pancreas K86.3
  retina — *see* Cyst, retina
Pseudoelephantiasis neuroarthritica Q82.0
Pseudoexfoliation, capsule (lens) — *see* Cataract, specified NEC
Pseudofolliculitis barbae L73.1
Pseudoglioma H44.89
Pseudohemophilia (Bernuth's) (hereditary) (type B) D68.0
  Type A D69.8
  vascular D69.8
Pseudohermaphroditism Q56.3
  adrenal E25.8
  female Q56.2
    with adrenocortical disorder E25.8
    without adrenocortical disorder Q56.2
    adrenal, congenital E25.0
  male Q56.1
    with
      5-alpha-reductase deficiency E29.1
      adrenocortical disorder E25.8
      androgen resistance E34.51
      cleft scrotum Q56.1
      feminizing testis E34.51
    without gonadal disorder Q56.1
    adrenal E25.8
Pseudo-Hurler's polydystrophy E77.0
Pseudohydrocephalus G93.2
Pseudohypertrophic muscular dystrophy (Erb's) G71.0
Pseudohypertrophy, muscle G71.0
Pseudohypoparathyroidism E20.1
Pseudoinsomnia F51.03
Pseudoleukemia, infantile D64.89
Pseudomembranous — *see* condition
Pseudomeningocele (cerebral) (infective) (post-traumatic) G96.19
  postprocedural (spinal) G97.82
Pseudomenses (newborn) P54.6
Pseudomenstruation (newborn) P54.6
Pseudomonas
  aeruginosa, as cause of disease classified elsewhere B96.5
  mallei infection A24.0
    as cause of disease classified elsewhere B96.5
  pseudomallei, as cause of disease classified elsewhere B96.5
Pseudomyotonia G71.19
Pseudomyxoma peritonei C78.6
Pseudoneuritis, optic (nerve) (disc) (papilla), **congenital** Q14.2
Pseudo-obstruction intestine (acute) (chronic) (idiopathic) (intermittent secondary) (primary) K59.8
Pseudopapilledema H47.33- ☑
  congenital Q14.2
Pseudoparalysis
  arm or leg R29.818
  atonic, congenital P94.2
Pseudopelade L66.0
Pseudophakia Z96.1
Pseudopolyarthritis, rhizomelic M35.3
Pseudopolycythemia D75.1
Pseudopseudohypoparathyroidism E20.1

Pseudopterygium H11.81- ☑
Pseudoptosis (eyelid) — *see* Blepharochalasis
Pseudopuberty, precocious
  female heterosexual E25.8
  male isosexual E25.8
Pseudorickets (renal) N25.0
Pseudorubella B08.20
Pseudosclerema, newborn P83.8
Pseudosclerosis (brain)
  Jakob's — *see* Creutzfeldt-Jakob disease or syndrome
  of Westphal (Strümpell) E83.01
  spastic — *see* Creutzfeldt-Jakob disease or syndrome
Pseudotetanus — *see* Convulsions
Pseudotetany R29.0
  hysterical F44.5
Pseudotruncus arteriosus Q25.4
Pseudotuberculosis A28.2
  enterocolitis A04.8
  pasteurella (infection) A28.0
Pseudotumor
  cerebri G93.2
  orbital H05.11 ☑
Pseudoxanthoma elasticum Q82.8
Psilosis (sprue) (tropical) K90.1
  nontropical K90.0
Psittacosis A70
Psoitis M60.88
Psoriasis L40.9
  arthropathic L40.50
    arthritis mutilans L40.52
    distal interphalangeal L40.51
    juvenile L40.54
    other specified L40.59
    spondylitis L40.53
  buccal K13.29
  flexural L40.8
  guttate L40.4
  mouth K13.29
  nummular L40.0
  plaque L40.0
  psychogenic F54
  pustular (generalized) L40.1
    palmaris et plantaris L40.3
  specified NEC L40.8
  vulgaris L40.0
Psychasthenia F48.8
Psychiatric disorder or problem F99
Psychogenic (*see also* condition)
  factors associated with physical conditions F54
Psychological and behavioral factors affecting medical condition F59
Psychoneurosis, psychoneurotic (*see also* Neurosis)
  anxiety (state) F41.1
  depersonalization F48.1
  hypochondriacal F45.21
  hysteria F44.9
  neurasthenic F48.8
  personality NEC F60.89
Psychopathy, psychopathic
  affectionless F94.2
  autistic F84.5
  constitution, post-traumatic F07.81
  personality — *see* Disorder, personality
  sexual — *see* Deviation, sexual
  state F60.2
Psychosexual identity disorder of childhood F64.2
Psychosis, psychotic F29
  acute (transient) F23
    hysterical F44.9
  affective — *see* Disorder, mood
  alcoholic F10.959
    with
      abuse F10.159
      anxiety disorder F10.980
        with
          abuse F10.180
          dependence F10.280
      delirium tremens F10.231
      delusions F10.950
        with
          abuse F10.150
          dependence F10.250
      dementia F10.97
        with dependence F10.27
      dependence F10.259
      hallucinosis F10.951

☑ **Additional Character Required — Refer to the Tabular List for Character Selection**   ▽ Subterms under main terms may continue to next column or page

Psychosis, psychotic — *continued*
  alcoholic — *continued*
    with
      hallucinosis — *continued*
        with
          abuse F10.151
          dependence F10.251
      mood disorder F10.94
        with
          abuse F10.14
          dependence F10.24
      paranoia F10.950
        with
          abuse F10.150
          dependence F10.250
      persisting amnesia F10.96
        with dependence F10.26
    amnestic confabulatory F10.96
      with dependence F10.26
    delirium tremens F10.231
    Korsakoff's, Korsakov's, Korsakow's F10.26
    paranoid type F10.950
      with
        abuse F10.150
        dependence F10.250
  anergastic — *see* Psychosis, organic
  arteriosclerotic (simple type) (uncomplicated) F01.50
    with behavioral disturbance F01.51
  childhood F84.0
    atypical F84.8
  climacteric — *see* Psychosis, involutional
  confusional F29
    acute or subacute F05
    reactive F23
  cycloid F23
  depressive — *see* Disorder, depressive
  disintegrative (childhood) F84.3
  drug-induced — *see* F11-F19 with .X59
    paranoid and hallucinatory states — *see* F11-F19
      with .X50 or .X51
  due to or associated with
    addiction, drug — *see* F11-F19 with .X59
    dependence
      alcohol F10.259
      drug — *see* F11-F19 with .X59
    epilepsy F06.8
    Huntington's chorea F06.8
    ischemia, cerebrovascular (generalized) F06.8
    multiple sclerosis F06.8
    physical disease F06.8
    presenile dementia F03 ☑
    senile dementia F03 ☑
    vascular disease (arteriosclerotic) (cerebral) F01.50
      with behavioral disturbance F01.51
  epileptic F06.8
  episode F23
    due to or associated with physical condition F06.8
  exhaustive F43.0
  hallucinatory, chronic F28
  hypomanic F30.8
  hysterical (acute) F44.9
  induced F24
  infantile F84.0
    atypical F84.8
  infective (acute) (subacute) F05
  involutional F28
    depressive — *see* Disorder, depressive
    melancholic — *see* Disorder, depressive
    paranoid (state) F22
  Korsakoff's, Korsakov's, Korsakow's (nonalcoholic) F04
    alcoholic F10.96
      in dependence F10.26
    induced by other psychoactive substance — *see*
      categories F11-F19 with .X5X
  mania, manic (single episode) F30.2
    recurrent type F31.89
  manic-depressive — *see* Disorder, mood
  menopausal — *see* Psychosis, involutional
  mixed schizophrenic and affective F25.8
  multi-infarct (cerebrovascular) F01.50
    with behavioral disturbance F01.51
  nonorganic F29
    specified NEC F28
  organic F09
    due to or associated with
      arteriosclerosis (cerebral) — *see* Psychosis, ar-
        teriosclerotic

Psychosis, psychotic — *continued*
  organic — *continued*
    due to or associated with — *continued*
      cerebrovascular disease, arteriosclerotic — *see*
        Psychosis, arteriosclerotic
      childbirth — *see* Psychosis, puerperal
      Creutzfeldt-Jakob disease or syndrome — *see*
        Creutzfeldt-Jakob disease or syndrome
      dependence, alcohol F10.259
      disease
        alcoholic liver F10.259
        brain, arteriosclerotic — *see* Psychosis, arte-
          riosclerotic
        cerebrovascular F01.50
          with behavioral disturbance F01.51
        Creutzfeldt-Jakob — *see* Creutzfeldt-Jakob
          disease or syndrome
        endocrine or metabolic F06.8
          acute or subacute F05
        liver, alcoholic F10.259
      epilepsy transient (acute) F05
      infection
        brain (intracranial) F06.8
          acute or subacute F05
      intoxication
        alcoholic (acute) F10.259
        drug F11-F19 with .X59
      ischemia, cerebrovascular (generalized) — *see*
        Psychosis, arteriosclerotic
      puerperium — *see* Psychosis, puerperal
      trauma, brain (birth) (from electric current)
        (surgical) F06.8
        acute or subacute F05
    infective F06.8
      acute or subacute F05
    post-traumatic F06.8
      acute or subacute F05
  paranoiac F22
  paranoid (climacteric) (involutional) (menopausal) F22
    psychogenic (acute) F23
    schizophrenic F20.0
    senile F03 ☑
  postpartum F53
  presbyophrenic (type) F03 ☑
  presenile F03 ☑
  psychogenic (paranoid) F23
    depressive F32.3
  puerperal F53
    specified type — *see* Psychosis, by type
  reactive (brief) (transient) (emotional stress) (psycho-
    logical trauma) F23
    depressive F32.3
      recurrent F33.3
    excitative type F30.8
  schizoaffective F25.9
    depressive type F25.1
    manic type F25.0
  schizophrenia, schizophrenic — *see* Schizophrenia
  schizophrenia-like, in epilepsy F06.2
  schizophreniform F20.81
    affective type F25.9
    brief F23
    confusional type F23
    depressive type F25.1
    manic type F25.0
    mixed type F25.0
  senile NEC F03 ☑
    depressed or paranoid type F03 ☑
    simple deterioration F03 ☑
    specified type — *code to* condition
  shared F24
  situational (reactive) F23
  symbiotic (childhood) F84.3
  symptomatic F09

Psychosomatic — *see* Disorder, psychosomatic
Psychosyndrome, organic F07.9
**Psychotic episode due to or associated with physical
  condition** F06.8
Pterygium (eye) H11.00- ☑
  amyloid H11.01- ☑
  central H11.02- ☑
  colli Q18.3
  double H11.03- ☑
  peripheral
    progressive H11.05- ☑
    stationary H11.04- ☑
  recurrent H11.06- ☑

Ptilosis (eyelid) — *see* Madarosis
Ptomaine (poisoning) — *see* Poisoning, food
Ptosis (*see also* Blepharoptosis)
  adiposa (false) — *see* Blepharoptosis
  breast N64.81
  cecum K63.4
  colon K63.4
  congenital (eyelid) Q10.0
    specified site NEC — *see* Anomaly, by site
  eyelid — *see* Blepharoptosis
    congenital Q10.0
  gastric K31.89
  intestine K63.4
  kidney N28.83
  liver K76.89
  renal N28.83
  splanchnic K63.4
  spleen D73.89
  stomach K31.89
  viscera K63.4
PTP D69.51
Ptyalism (periodic) K11.7
  hysterical F45.8
  pregnancy — *see* Pregnancy, complicated by, specified
    pregnancy-related condition NEC
  psychogenic F45.8
Ptyalolithiasis K11.5
Pubarche, precocious E30.1
Pubertas praecox E30.1
Puberty (development state) Z00.3
  bleeding (excessive) N92.2
  delayed E30.0
  precocious (constitutional) (cryptogenic) (idiopathic)
    E30.1
    central E22.8
    due to
      ovarian hyperfunction E28.1
        estrogen E28.0
      testicular hyperfunction E29.0
  premature E30.1
    due to
      adrenal cortical hyperfunction E25.8
      pineal tumor E34.8
      pituitary (anterior) hyperfunction E22.8
Puckering, macula — *see* Degeneration, macula, puckering
Pudenda, pudendum — *see* condition
Puente's disease (simple glandular cheilitis) K13.0
Puerperal, puerperium (complicated by, complications)
  abnormal glucose (tolerance test) O99.815
  abscess
    areola O91.02
      associated with lactation O91.03
    Bartholin's gland O86.19
    breast O91.12
      associated with lactation O91.13
    cervix (uteri) O86.11
    genital organ NEC O86.19
    kidney O86.21
    mammary O91.12
      associated with lactation O91.13
    nipple O91.02
      associated with lactation O91.03
    peritoneum O85
    subareolar O91.12
      associated with lactation O91.13
    urinary tract — *see* Puerperal, infection, urinary
    uterus O86.12
    vagina (wall) O86.13
    vaginorectal O86.13
    vulvovaginal gland O86.13
  adnexitis O86.19
  afibrinogenemia, or other coagulation defect O72.3
  albuminuria (acute) (subacute) — *see* Proteinuria,
    gestational
  alcohol use O99.315
  anemia O90.81
    pre-existing (pre-pregnancy) O99.03
  anesthetic death O89.8
  apoplexy O99.43
  bariatric surgery status O99.845
  blood disorder NEC O99.13
  blood dyscrasia O72.3
  cardiomyopathy O90.3
  cerebrovascular disorder (conditions in I60-I69) O99.43
  cervicitis O86.11
  circulatory system disorder O99.43
  coagulopathy (any) O72.3

Puerperal, puerperium — *continued*
- complications O90.9
  - specified NEC O90.89
- convulsions — *see* Eclampsia
- cystitis O86.22
- cystopyelitis O86.29
- delirium NEC F05
- diabetes O24.93
  - gestational — *see* Puerperal, gestational diabetes
  - pre-existing O24.33
    - specified NEC O24.83
    - type 1 O24.03
    - type 2 O24.13
- digestive system disorder O99.63
- disease O90.9
  - breast NEC O92.29
  - cerebrovascular (acute) O99.43
  - nonobstetric NEC O99.89
  - tubo-ovarian O86.19
  - Valsuani's O99.03
- disorder O90.9
  - biliary tract O26.63
  - lactation O92.70
  - liver O26.63
  - nonobstetric NEC O99.89
- disruption
  - cesarean wound O90.0
  - episiotomy wound O90.1
  - perineal laceration wound O90.1
- drug use O99.325
- eclampsia (with pre-existing hypertension) O15.2
- embolism (pulmonary) (blood clot) — *see* Embolism, obstetric, puerperal
- endocrine, nutritional or metabolic disease NEC O99.285
- endophlebitis — *see* Puerperal, phlebitis
- endotrachelitis O86.11
- failure
  - lactation (complete) O92.3
    - partial O92.4
  - renal, acute O90.4
- fever (of unknown origin) O86.4
  - septic O85
- fissure, nipple O92.12
  - associated with lactation O92.13
- fistula
  - breast (due to mastitis) O91.12
    - associated with lactation O91.13
  - nipple O91.02
    - associated with lactation O91.03
- galactophoritis O91.22
  - associated with lactation O91.23
- galactorrhea O92.6
- gastric banding status O99.845
- gastric bypass status O99.845
- gastrointestinal disease NEC O99.63
- gestational diabetes O24.439
  - diet controlled O24.430
  - insulin (and diet) controlled O24.434
- gonorrhea O98.23
- hematoma, subdural O99.43
- hemiplegia, cerebral O99.355
  - due to cerbrovascular disorder O99.43
- hemorrhage O72.1
  - brain O99.43
  - bulbar O99.43
  - cerebellar O99.43
  - cerebral O99.43
  - cortical O99.43
  - delayed or secondary O72.2
  - extradural O99.43
  - internal capsule O99.43
  - intracranial O99.43
  - intrapontine O99.43
  - meningeal O99.43
  - pontine O99.43
  - retained placenta O72.0
  - subarachnoid O99.43
  - subcortical O99.43
  - subdural O99.43
  - third stage O72.0
  - uterine, delayed O72.2
  - ventricular O99.43
- hemorrhoids O87.2
- hepatorenal syndrome O90.4
- hypertension — *see* Hypertension, complicating, puerperium
- hypertrophy, breast O92.29

Puerperal, puerperium — *continued*
- induration breast (fibrous) O92.29
- infection O86.4
  - cervix O86.11
  - generalized O85
  - genital tract NEC O86.19
    - obstetric surgical wound O86.0
  - kidney (bacillus coli) O86.21
  - maternal O98.93
    - carrier state NEC O99.835
    - gonorrhea O98.23
    - human immunodeficiency virus (HIV) O98.73
    - protozoal O98.63
    - sexually transmitted NEC O98.33
    - specified NEC O98.83
    - streptococcus B carrier state O99.825
    - syphilis O98.13
    - tuberculosis O98.03
    - viral hepatitis O98.43
    - viral NEC O98.53
  - nipple O91.02
    - associated with lactation O91.03
  - peritoneum O85
  - renal O86.21
  - specified NEC O86.89
  - urinary (asymptomatic) (tract) NEC O86.20
    - bladder O86.22
    - kidney O86.21
    - specified site NEC O86.29
    - urethra O86.22
  - vagina O86.13
  - vein — *see* Puerperal, phlebitis
- ischemia, cerebral O99.43
- lymphangitis O86.89
  - breast O91.22
    - associated with lactation O91.23
- malignancy O9A.13 (*following* O99)
- malnutrition O25.3
- mammillitis O91.02
  - associated with lactation O91.03
- mammitis O91.22
  - associated with lactation O91.23
- mania F30.8
- mastitis O91.22
  - associated with lactation O91.23
  - purulent O91.12
    - associated with lactation O91.13
- melancholia — *see* Disorder, depressive
- mental disorder NEC O99.345
- metroperitonitis O85
- metrorrhagia — *see* Hemorrhage, postpartum
- metrosalpingitis O86.19
- metrovaginitis O86.13
- milk leg O87.1
- monoplegia, cerebral O99.43
- mood disturbance O90.6
- necrosis, liver (acute) (subacute) (conditions in subcategory K72.0) O26.63
  - with renal failure O90.4
- nervous system disorder O99.355
- obesity (pre-existing prior to pregnancy) O99.215
- obesity surgery status O99.845
- occlusion, precerebral artery O99.43
- paralysis
  - bladder (sphincter) O90.89
  - cerebral O99.43
- paralytic stroke O99.43
- parametritis O85
- paravaginitis O86.13
- pelviperitonitis O85
- perimetritis O86.12
- perimetrosalpingitis O86.19
- perinephritis O86.21
- periphlebitis — *see* Puerperal phlebitis
- peritoneal infection O85
- peritonitis (pelvic) O85
- perivaginitis O86.13
- phlebitis O87.0
  - deep O87.1
  - pelvic O87.1
  - superficial O87.0
- phlebothrombosis, deep O87.1
- phlegmasia alba dolens O87.1
- placental polyp O90.89
- pneumonia, embolic — *see* Embolism, obstetric, puerperal
- pre-eclampsia — *see* Pre-eclampsia
- psychosis F53

Puerperal, puerperium — *continued*
- pyelitis O86.21
- pyelocystitis O86.29
- pyelonephritis O86.21
- pyelonephrosis O86.21
- pyemia O85
- pyocystitis O86.29
- pyohemia O85
- pyometra O86.12
- pyonephritis O86.21
- pyosalpingitis O86.19
- pyrexia (of unknown origin) O86.4
- renal
  - disease NEC O90.89
  - failure O90.4
- respiratory disease NEC O99.53
- retention
  - decidua — *see* Retention, decidua
  - placenta O72.0
  - secundines — *see* Retention, secundines
- retrated nipple O92.02
- salpingo-ovaritis O86.19
- salpingoperitonitis O85
- secondary perineal tear O90.1
- sepsis (pelvic) O85
- sepsis O85
- septic thrombophlebitis O86.81
- skin disorder NEC O99.73
- specified condition NEC O99.89
- stroke O99.43
- subinvolution (uterus) O90.89
- subluxation of symphysis (pubis) O26.73
- suppuration — *see* Puerperal, abscess
- tetanus A34
- thelitis O91.02
  - associated with lactation O91.03
- thrombocytopenia O72.3
- thrombophlebitis (superficial) O87.0
  - deep O87.1
  - pelvic O87.1
  - septic O86.81
- thrombosis (venous) — *see* Thrombosis, puerperal
- thyroiditis O90.5
- toxemia (eclamptic) (pre-eclamptic) (with convulsions) O15.2
- trauma, non-obstetric O9A.23 (*following* O99)
  - caused by abuse (physical) (suspected) O9A.33 (*following* O99)
    - confirmed O9A.33 (*following* O99)
    - psychological (suspected) O9A.53 (*following* O99)
      - confirmed O9A.53 (*following* O99)
    - sexual (suspected) O9A.43 (*following* O99)
      - confirmed O9A.43 (*following* O99)
- uremia (due to renal failure) O90.4
- urethritis O86.22
- vaginitis O86.13
- varicose veins (legs) O87.4
  - vulva or perineum O87.8
- venous O87.9
- vulvitis O86.19
- vulvovaginitis O86.13
- white leg O87.1

Puerperium — *see* Puerperal
Pulmolithiasis J98.4
Pulmonary — *see* condition
Pulpitis (acute) (anachoretic) (chronic) (hyperplastic) (irreversible) (putrescent) (reversible) (suppurative) (ulcerative) K04.0
Pulpless tooth K04.99
Pulse
- alternating R00.8
- bigeminal R00.8
- fast R00.0
- feeble, rapid due to shock following injury T79.4 ☑
- rapid R00.0
- weak R09.89

Pulsus alternans or trigeminus R00.8
Punch drunk F07.81
Punctum lacrimale occlusion — *see* Obstruction, lacrimal
Puncture
- abdomen, abdominal
  - wall S31.139 ☑
    - with
      - foreign body S31.149 ☑
      - penetration into peritoneal cavity S31.639 ☑

Puncture — *continued*
  abdomen, abdominal — *continued*
    wall — *continued*
      with — *continued*
        penetration into peritoneal cavity — *continued*
          with foreign body S31.649 ☑
      epigastric region S31.132 ☑
        with
          foreign body S31.142 ☑
          penetration into peritoneal cavity S31.632 ☑
            with foreign body S31.642 ☑
      left
        lower quadrant S31.134 ☑
          with
            foreign body S31.144 ☑
            penetration into peritoneal cavity S31.634 ☑
              with foreign body S31.644 ☑
        upper quadrant S31.131 ☑
          with
            foreign body S31.141 ☑
            penetration into peritoneal cavity S31.631 ☑
              with foreign body S31.641 ☑
      periumbilic region S31.135 ☑
        with
          foreign body S31.145 ☑
          penetration into peritoneal cavity S31.635 ☑
            with foreign body S31.645 ☑
      right
        lower quadrant S31.133 ☑
          with
            foreign body S31.143 ☑
            penetration into peritoneal cavity S31.633 ☑
              with foreign body S31.643 ☑
        upper quadrant S31.130 ☑
          with
            foreign body S31.140 ☑
            penetration into peritoneal cavity S31.630 ☑
              with foreign body S31.640 ☑
  accidental, complicating surgery — *see* Complication, accidental puncture or laceration
  alveolar (process) — *see* Puncture, oral cavity
  ankle S91.039 ☑
    with
      foreign body S91.049 ☑
    left S91.032 ☑
      with
        foreign body S91.042 ☑
    right S91.031 ☑
      with
        foreign body S91.041 ☑
  anus S31.833 ☑
    with foreign body S31.834 ☑
  arm (upper) S41.139 ☑
    with foreign body S41.149 ☑
    left S41.132 ☑
      with foreign body S41.142 ☑
    lower — *see* Puncture, forearm
    right S41.131 ☑
      with foreign body S41.141 ☑
  auditory canal (external) (meatus) — *see* Puncture, ear
  auricle, ear — *see* Puncture, ear
  axilla — *see* Puncture, arm
  back (*see also* Puncture, thorax, back)
    lower S31.030 ☑
      with
        foreign body S31.040 ☑
          with penetration into retroperitoneal space S31.041 ☑
        penetration into retroperitoneal space S31.031 ☑
  bladder (traumatic) S37.29 ☑
    nontraumatic N32.89
  breast S21.039 ☑
    with foreign body S21.049 ☑
    left S21.032 ☑
      with foreign body S21.042 ☑
    right S21.031 ☑
      with foreign body S21.041 ☑

Puncture — *continued*
  buttock S31.803 ☑
    with foreign body S31.804 ☑
    left S31.823 ☑
      with foreign body S31.824 ☑
    right S31.813 ☑
      with foreign body S31.814 ☑
  by
    device, implant or graft — *see* Complications, by site and type, mechanical
    foreign body left accidentally in operative wound T81.539 ☑
    instrument (any) during a procedure, accidental — *see* Puncture, accidental complicating surgery
  calf — *see* Puncture, leg
  canaliculus lacrimalis — *see* Puncture, eyelid
  canthus, eye — *see* Puncture, eyelid
  cervical esophagus S11.23 ☑
    with foreign body S11.24 ☑
  cheek (external) S01.439 ☑
    with foreign body S01.449 ☑
    internal — *see* Puncture, oral cavity
    left S01.432 ☑
      with foreign body S01.442 ☑
    right S01.431 ☑
      with foreign body S01.441 ☑
  chest wall — *see* Puncture, thorax
  chin — *see* Puncture, head, specified site NEC
  clitoris — *see* Puncture, vulva
  costal region — *see* Puncture, thorax
  digit(s)
    foot — *see* Puncture, toe
    hand — *see* Puncture, finger
  ear (canal) (external) S01.339 ☑
    with foreign body S01.349 ☑
    drum S09.2- ☑
    left S01.332 ☑
      with foreign body S01.342 ☑
    right S01.331 ☑
      with foreign body S01.341 ☑
  elbow S51.039 ☑
    with
      foreign body S51.049 ☑
    left S51.032 ☑
      with
        foreign body S51.042 ☑
    right S51.031 ☑
      with
        foreign body S51.041 ☑
  epididymis — *see* Puncture, testis
  epigastric region — *see* Puncture, abdomen, wall, epigastric
  epiglottis S11.83 ☑
    with foreign body S11.84 ☑
  esophagus
    cervical S11.23 ☑
      with foreign body S11.24 ☑
    thoracic S27.818 ☑
  eyeball S05.6- ☑
    with foreign body S05.5- ☑
  eyebrow — *see* Puncture, eyelid
  eyelid S01.13- ☑
    with foreign body S01.14- ☑
    left S01.132 ☑
      with foreign body S01.142 ☑
    right S01.131 ☑
      with foreign body S01.141 ☑
  face NEC — *see* Puncture, head, specified site NEC
  finger(s) S61.239 ☑
    with
      damage to nail S61.339 ☑
        with
          foreign body S61.349 ☑
      foreign body S61.249 ☑
    index S61.238 ☑
      with
        damage to nail S61.338 ☑
          with
            foreign body S61.348 ☑
        foreign body S61.248 ☑
      left S61.231 ☑
        with
          damage to nail S61.331 ☑
            with
              foreign body S61.341 ☑

Puncture –– *continued*
  finger(s) — *continued*
    index — *continued*
      left — *continued*
        with — *continued*
          foreign body S61.241 ☑
      right S61.230 ☑
        with
          damage to nail S61.330 ☑
            with
              foreign body S61.340 ☑
          foreign body S61.240 ☑
    little S61.238 ☑
      with
        damage to nail S61.338 ☑
          with
            foreign body S61.348 ☑
        foreign body S61.248 ☑
      left S61.237 ☑
        with
          damage to nail S61.337 ☑
            with
              foreign body S61.347 ☑
          foreign body S61.247 ☑
      right S61.236 ☑
        with
          damage to nail S61.336 ☑
            with
              foreign body S61.346 ☑
          foreign body S61.246 ☑
    middle S61.238 ☑
      with
        damage to nail S61.338 ☑
          with
            foreign body S61.348 ☑
        foreign body S61.248 ☑
      left S61.233 ☑
        with
          damage to nail S61.333 ☑
            with
              foreign body S61.343 ☑
          foreign body S61.243 ☑
      right S61.232 ☑
        with
          damage to nail S61.332 ☑
            with
              foreign body S61.342 ☑
          foreign body S61.242 ☑
    ring S61.238 ☑
      with
        damage to nail S61.338 ☑
          with
            foreign body S61.348 ☑
        foreign body S61.248 ☑
      left S61.235 ☑
        with
          damage to nail S61.335 ☑
            with
              foreign body S61.345 ☑
          foreign body S61.245 ☑
      right S61.234 ☑
        with
          damage to nail S61.334 ☑
            with
              foreign body S61.344 ☑
          foreign body S61.244 ☑
  flank S31.139 ☑
    with foreign body S31.149 ☑
  foot (except toe(s) alone) S91.339 ☑
    with foreign body S91.349 ☑
    left S91.332 ☑
      with foreign body S91.342 ☑
    right S91.331 ☑
      with foreign body S91.341 ☑
    toe — *see* Puncture, toe
  forearm S51.839 ☑
    with
      foreign body S51.849 ☑
    elbow only — *see* Puncture, elbow
    left S51.832 ☑
      with
        foreign body S51.842 ☑
    right S51.831 ☑
      with
        foreign body S51.841 ☑
  forehead — *see* Puncture, head, specified site NEC

Index · **Puncture — Puncture**

Puncture — *continued*
genital organs, external
female S31.532 ☑
with foreign body S31.542 ☑
vagina — *see* Puncture, vagina
vulva — *see* Puncture, vulva
male S31.531 ☑
with foreign body S31.541 ☑
penis — *see* Puncture, penis
scrotum — *see* Puncture, scrotum
testis — *see* Puncture, testis
groin — *see* Puncture, abdomen, wall
gum — *see* Puncture, oral cavity
hand S61.439 ☑
with
foreign body S61.449 ☑
finger — *see* Puncture, finger
left S61.432 ☑
with
foreign body S61.442 ☑
right S61.431 ☑
with
foreign body S61.441 ☑
thumb — *see* Puncture, thumb
head S01.93 ☑
with foreign body S01.94 ☑
cheek — *see* Puncture, cheek
ear — *see* Puncture, ear
eyelid — *see* Puncture, eyelid
lip — *see* Puncture, oral cavity
nose — *see* Puncture, nose
oral cavity — *see* Puncture, oral cavity
scalp S01.03 ☑
with foreign body S01.04 ☑
specified site NEC S01.83 ☑
with foreign body S01.84 ☑
temporomandibular area — *see* Puncture, cheek
heart S26.99 ☑
with hemopericardium S26.09 ☑
without hemopericardium S26.19 ☑
heel — *see* Puncture, foot
hip S71.039 ☑
with foreign body S71.049 ☑
left S71.032 ☑
with foreign body S71.042 ☑
right S71.031 ☑
with foreign body S71.041 ☑
hymen — *see* Puncture, vagina
hypochondrium — *see* Puncture, abdomen, wall
hypogastric region — *see* Puncture, abdomen, wall
inguinal region — *see* Puncture, abdomen, wall
instep — *see* Puncture, foot
internal organs — *see* Injury, by site
interscapular region — *see* Puncture, thorax, back
intestine
large
colon S36.599 ☑
ascending S36.590 ☑
descending S36.592 ☑
sigmoid S36.593 ☑
specified site NEC S36.598 ☑
transverse S36.591 ☑
rectum S36.69 ☑
small S36.499 ☑
duodenum S36.490 ☑
specified site NEC S36.498 ☑
intra-abdominal organ S36.99 ☑
gallbladder S36.128 ☑
intestine — *see* Puncture, intestine
liver S36.118 ☑
pancreas — *see* Puncture, pancreas
peritoneum S36.81 ☑
specified site NEC S36.898 ☑
spleen S36.09 ☑
stomach S36.39 ☑
jaw — *see* Puncture, head, specified site NEC
knee S81.039 ☑
with foreign body S81.049 ☑
left S81.032 ☑
with foreign body S81.042 ☑
right S81.031 ☑
with foreign body S81.041 ☑
labium (majus) (minus) — *see* Puncture, vulva
lacrimal duct — *see* Puncture, eyelid
larynx S11.013 ☑
with foreign body S11.014 ☑

Puncture — *continued*
leg (lower) S81.839 ☑
with foreign body S81.849 ☑
foot — *see* Puncture, foot
knee — *see* Puncture, knee
left S81.832 ☑
with foreign body S81.842 ☑
right S81.831 ☑
with foreign body S81.841 ☑
upper — *see* Puncture, thigh
lip S01.531 ☑
with foreign body S01.541 ☑
loin — *see* Puncture, abdomen, wall
lower back — *see* Puncture, back, lower
lumbar region — *see* Puncture, back, lower
malar region — *see* Puncture, head, specified site NEC
mammary — *see* Puncture, breast
mastoid region — *see* Puncture, head, specified site NEC
mouth — *see* Puncture, oral cavity
nail
finger — *see* Puncture, finger, with damage to nail
toe — *see* Puncture, toe, with damage to nail
nasal (septum) (sinus) — *see* Puncture, nose
nasopharynx — *see* Puncture, head, specified site NEC
neck S11.93 ☑
with foreign body S11.94 ☑
involving
cervical esophagus — *see* Puncture, cervical esophagus
larynx — *see* Puncture, larynx
pharynx — *see* Puncture, pharynx
thyroid gland — *see* Puncture, thyroid gland
trachea — *see* Puncture, trachea
specified site NEC S11.83 ☑
with foreign body S11.84 ☑
nose (septum) (sinus) S01.23 ☑
with foreign body S01.24 ☑
ocular — *see* Puncture, eyeball
oral cavity S01.532 ☑
with foreign body S01.542 ☑
orbit S05.4- ☑
palate — *see* Puncture, oral cavity
palm — *see* Puncture, hand
pancreas S36.299 ☑
body S36.291 ☑
head S36.290 ☑
tail S36.292 ☑
pelvis — *see* Puncture, back, lower
penis S31.23 ☑
with foreign body S31.24 ☑
perineum
female S31.43 ☑
with foreign body S31.44 ☑
male S31.139 ☑
with foreign body S31.149 ☑
periocular area (with or without lacrimal passages) — *see* Puncture, eyelid
phalanges
finger — *see* Puncture, finger
toe — *see* Puncture, toe
pharynx S11.23 ☑
with foreign body S11.24 ☑
pinna — *see* Puncture, ear
popliteal space — *see* Puncture, knee
prepuce — *see* Puncture, penis
pubic region S31.139 ☑
with foreign body S31.149 ☑
pudendum — *see* Puncture, genital organs, external
rectovaginal septum — *see* Puncture, vagina
sacral region — *see* Puncture, back, lower
sacroiliac region — *see* Puncture, back, lower
salivary gland — *see* Puncture, oral cavity
scalp S01.03 ☑
with foreign body S01.04 ☑
scapular region — *see* Puncture, shoulder
scrotum S31.33 ☑
with foreign body S31.34 ☑
shin — *see* Puncture, leg
shoulder S41.039 ☑
with foreign body S41.049 ☑
left S41.032 ☑
with foreign body S41.042 ☑
right S41.031 ☑
with foreign body S41.041 ☑
spermatic cord — *see* Puncture, testis

Puncture — *continued*
sternal region — *see* Puncture, thorax, front
submaxillary region — *see* Puncture, head, specified site NEC
submental region — *see* Puncture, head, specified site NEC
subungual
finger(s) — *see* Puncture, finger, with damage to nail
toe — *see* Puncture, toe, with damage to nail
supraclavicular fossa — *see* Puncture, neck, specified site NEC
temple, temporal region — *see* Puncture, head, specified site NEC
temporomandibular area — *see* Puncture, cheek
testis S31.33 ☑
with foreign body S31.34 ☑
thigh S71.139 ☑
with foreign body S71.149 ☑
left S71.132 ☑
with foreign body S71.142 ☑
right S71.131 ☑
with foreign body S71.141 ☑
thorax, thoracic (wall) S21.93 ☑
with foreign body S21.94 ☑
back S21.23- ☑
with
foreign body S21.24- ☑
with penetration S21.44 ☑
penetration S21.43 ☑
breast — *see* Puncture, breast
front S21.13- ☑
with
foreign body S21.14- ☑
with penetration S21.34 ☑
penetration S21.33 ☑
throat — *see* Puncture, neck
thumb S61.039 ☑
with
damage to nail S61.139 ☑
with
foreign body S61.149 ☑
foreign body S61.049 ☑
left S61.032 ☑
with
damage to nail S61.132 ☑
with
foreign body S61.142 ☑
foreign body S61.042 ☑
right S61.031 ☑
with
damage to nail S61.131 ☑
with
foreign body S61.141 ☑
foreign body S61.041 ☑
thyroid gland S11.13 ☑
with foreign body S11.14 ☑
toe(s) S91.139 ☑
with
damage to nail S91.239 ☑
with
foreign body S91.249 ☑
foreign body S91.149 ☑
great S91.133 ☑
with
damage to nail S91.233 ☑
with
foreign body S91.243 ☑
foreign body S91.143 ☑
left S91.132 ☑
with
damage to nail S91.232 ☑
with
foreign body S91.242 ☑
foreign body S91.142 ☑
right S91.131 ☑
with
damage to nail S91.231 ☑
with
foreign body S91.241 ☑
foreign body S91.141 ☑
lesser S91.136 ☑
with
damage to nail S91.236 ☑
with
foreign body S91.246 ☑

Puncture — *continued*
  toe(s) — *continued*
    lesser — *continued*
      with — *continued*
        foreign body S91.146 ☑
       left S91.135 ☑
        with
          damage to nail S91.235 ☑
            with
              foreign body S91.245 ☑
          foreign body S91.145 ☑
       right S91.134 ☑
        with
          damage to nail S91.234 ☑
            with
              foreign body S91.244 ☑
          foreign body S91.144 ☑
  tongue — *see* Puncture, oral cavity
  trachea S11.023 ☑
    with foreign body S11.024 ☑
  tunica vaginalis — *see* Puncture, testis
  tympanum, tympanic membrane S09.2- ☑
  umbilical region S31.135 ☑
    with foreign body S31.145 ☑
  uvula — *see* Puncture, oral cavity
  vagina S31.43 ☑
    with foreign body S31.44 ☑
  vocal cords S11.033 ☑
    with foreign body S11.034 ☑
  vulva S31.43 ☑
    with foreign body S31.44 ☑
  wrist S61.539 ☑
    with
      foreign body S61.549 ☑
    left S61.532 ☑
      with
        foreign body S61.542 ☑
    right S61.531 ☑
      with
        foreign body S61.541 ☑
PUO (pyrexia of unknown origin) R50.9
Pupillary membrane (persistent) Q13.89
Pupillotonia — *see* Anomaly, pupil, function, tonic pupil
Purpura D69.2
  abdominal D69.0
  allergic D69.0
  anaphylactoid D69.0
  annularis telangiectodes L81.7
  arthritic D69.0
  autoerythrocyte sensitization D69.2
  autoimmune D69.0
  bacterial D69.0
  Bateman's (senile) D69.2
  capillary fragility (hereditary) (idiopathic) D69.8
  cryoglobulinemic D89.1
  Devil's pinches D69.2
  fibrinolytic — *see* Fibrinolysis
  fulminans, fulminous D65
  gangrenous D65
  hemorrhagic, hemorrhagica D69.3
    not due to thrombocytopenia D69.0
  Henoch (-Schönlein) (allergic) D69.0
  hypergammaglobulinemic (benign) (Waldenström)
    D89.0
  idiopathic (thrombocytopenic) D69.3
    nonthrombocytopenic D69.0
  immune thrombocytopenic D69.3
  infectious D69.0
  malignant D69.0
  neonatorum P54.5
  nervosa D69.0
  newborn P54.5
  nonthrombocytopenic D69.2
    hemorrhagic D69.0
    idiopathic D69.0
  nonthrombopenic D69.2
  peliosis rheumatica D69.0
  posttransfusion (post-transfusion) (from fresh) whole
    blood or blood products) D69.51
  primary D69.49
  red cell membrane sensitivity D69.2
  rheumatica D69.0
  Schönlein (-Henoch) (allergic) D69.0
  scorbutic E54 [D77]
  senile D69.2
  simplex D69.2
  symptomatica D69.0

Purpura — *continued*
  telangiectasia annularis L81.7
  thrombocytopenic D69.49
    congenital D69.42
    hemorrhagic D69.3
    hereditary D69.42
    idiopathic D69.3
    immune D69.3
    neonatal, transitory P61.0
    thrombotic M31.1
  thrombohemolytic — *see* Fibrinolysis
  thrombolytic — *see* Fibrinolysis
  thrombopenic D69.49
  thrombotic, thrombocytopenic M31.1
  toxic D69.0
  vascular D69.0
  visceral symptoms D69.0
Purpuric spots R23.3
Purulent — *see* condition
Pus
  in
    stool R19.5
    urine N39.0
  tube (rupture) — *see* Salpingo-oophoritis
Pustular rash L08.0
Pustule (nonmalignant) L08.9
  malignant A22.0
Pustulosis palmaris et plantaris L40.3
Putnam (-Dana) **disease or syndrome** — *see* Degeneration, combined
Putrescent pulp (dental) K04.1
Pyarthritis, pyarthrosis — *see* Arthritis, pyogenic or pyemic
  tuberculous — *see* Tuberculosis, joint
Pyelectasis — *see* Hydronephrosis
Pyelitis (congenital) (uremic) (*see also* Pyelonephritis)
  with
    calculus — *see* category N20 ☑
      with hydronephrosis N13.2
    contracted kidney N11.9
  acute N10
  chronic N11.9
    with calculus — *see* category N20 ☑
      with hydronephrosis N13.2
  cystica N28.84
  puerperal (postpartum) O86.21
  tuberculous A18.11
Pyelocystitis — *see* Pyelonephritis
Pyelonephritis (*see also* Nephritis, tubulo-interstitial)
  with
    calculus — *see* category N20 ☑
      with hydronephrosis N13.2
    contracted kidney N11.9
  acute N10
  calculous — *see* category N20 ☑
    with hydronephrosis N13.2
  chronic N11.9
    with calculus — *see* category N20 ☑
      with hydronephrosis N13.2
    associated with ureteral obstruction or stricture
      N11.1
    nonobstructive N11.8
      with reflux (vesicoureteral) N11.0
    obstructive N11.1
    specified NEC N11.8
  in (due to)
    brucellosis A23.9 [N16]
    cryoglobulinemia (mixed) D89.1 [N16]
    cystinosis E72.04
    diphtheria A36.84
    glycogen storage disease E74.09 [N16]
    leukemia NEC C95.9- ☑ [N16]
    lymphoma NEC C85.90 [N16]
    multiple myeloma C90.0- ☑ [N16]
    obstruction N11.1
    Salmonella infection A02.25
    sarcoidosis D86.84
    sepsis A41.9 [N16]
    Sjögren's disease M35.04
    toxoplasmosis B58.83
    transplant rejection T86.91 [N16]
    Wilson's disease E83.01 [N16]
  nonobstructive N12
    with reflux (vesicoureteral) N11.0
    chronic N11.8
  syphilitic A52.75
Pyelonephrosis (obstructive) N11.1
  chronic N11.9

Pyelophlebitis I80.8
Pyeloureteritis cystica N28.85
Pyemia, pyemic (fever) (infection) (purulent) (*see also* Sepsis)
  joint — *see* Arthritis, pyogenic or pyemic
  liver K75.1
  pneumococcal A40.3
  portal K75.1
  postvaccinal T88.0 ☑
  puerperal, postpartum, childbirth O85
  specified organism NEC A41.89
  tuberculous — *see* Tuberculosis, miliary
Pygopagus Q89.4
Pyknoepilepsy (idiopathic) — *see* Pyknolepsy
Pyknolepsy G40.A09 (*following* G40.3)
  intractable G40.A19 (*following* G40.3)
    with status epilepticus G40.A11 (*following* G40.3)
    without status epilepticus G40.A19 (*following* G40.3)
  not intractable G40.A09 (*following* G40.3)
    with status epilepticus G40.A01 (*following* G40.3)
    without status epilepticus G40.A09 (*following* G40.3)
Pylephlebitis K75.1
Pyle's syndrome Q78.5
Pylethrombophlebitis K75.1
Pylethrombosis K75.1
Pyloritis K29.90
  with bleeding K29.91
Pylorospasm (reflex) **NEC** K31.3
  congenital or infantile Q40.0
  neurotic F45.8
  newborn Q40.0
  psychogenic F45.8
Pylorus, pyloric — *see* condition
Pyoarthrosis — *see* Arthritis, pyogenic or pyemic
Pyocele
  mastoid — *see* Mastoiditis, acute
  sinus (accessory) — *see* Sinusitis
  turbinate (bone) J32.9
  urethra (*see also* Urethritis) N34.0
Pyocolpos — *see* Vaginitis
Pyocystitis N30.80
  with hematuria N30.81
Pyoderma, pyodermia L08.0
  gangrenosum L88
  newborn P39.4
  phagedenic L88
  vegetans L08.81
Pyodermatitis L08.0
  vegetans L08.81
Pyogenic — *see* condition
Pyohydronephrosis N13.6
Pyometra, pyometrium, pyometritis — *see* Endometritis
Pyomyositis (tropical) — *see* Myositis, infective
Pyonephritis N12
Pyonephrosis N13.6
  tuberculous A18.11
Pyo-oophoritis — *see* Salpingo-oophoritis
Pyo-ovarium — *see* Salpingo-oophoritis
Pyopericarditis, pyopericardium I30.1
Pyophlebitis — *see* Phlebitis
Pyopneumopericardium I30.1
Pyopneumothorax (infective) J86.9
  with fistula J86.0
  tuberculous NEC A15.6
Pyosalpinx, pyosalpingitis (*see also* Salpingo-oophoritis)
Pyothorax J86.9
  with fistula J86.0
  tuberculous NEC A15.6
Pyoureter N28.89
  tuberculous A18.11
Pyramidopallidonigral syndrome G20
Pyrexia (of unknown origin) R50.9
  atmospheric T67.0 ☑
  during labor NEC O75.2
  heat T67.0 ☑
  newborn P81.9
    environmentally-induced P81.0
  persistent R50.9
  puerperal O86.4
Pyroglobulinemia NEC E88.09
Pyromania F63.1
Pyrosis R12
Pyuria (bacterial) N39.0

Q

Q fever A78
  with pneumonia A78
Quadricuspid aortic valve Q23.8
Quadrilateral fever A78
Quadriparesis — *see* Quadriplegia
  meaning muscle weakness M62.81
Quadriplegia G82.50
  complete
    C1-C4 level G82.51
    C5-C7 level G82.53
  congenital (cerebral) (spinal) G80.8
    spastic G80.0
  embolic (current episode) I63.4 ☑
  functional R53.2
  incomplete
    C1-C4 level G82.52
    C5-C7 level G82.54
  thrombotic (current episode) I63.3 ☑
  traumatic — *code to* injury with seventh character S
    current episode — *see* Injury, spinal (cord), cervical
Quadruplet, pregnancy — *see* Pregnancy, quadruplet
Quarrelsomeness F60.3
Queensland fever A77.3
Quervain's disease M65.4
  thyroid E06.1
Queyrat's erythroplasia D07.4
  penis D07.4
  specified site — *see* Neoplasm, skin, in situ
  unspecified site D07.4
Quincke's disease or edema T78.3 ☑
  hereditary D84.1
Quinsy (gangrenous) J36
Quintan fever A79.0
Quintuplet, pregnancy — *see* Pregnancy, quintuplet

R

Rabbit fever — *see* Tularemia
Rabies A82.9
  contact Z20.3
  exposure to Z20.3
  inoculation reaction — *see* Complications, vaccination
  sylvatic A82.0
  urban A82.1
Rachischisis — *see* Spina bifida
Rachitic (*see also* condition)
  deformities of spine (late effect) (sequelae) E64.3
  pelvis (late effect) (sequelae) E64.3
    with disproportion (fetopelvic) O33.0
      causing obstructed labor O65.0
Rachitis, rachitism (acute) (tarda) (*see also* Rickets)
  renalis N25.0
  sequelae E64.3
Radial nerve — *see* condition
Radiation
  burn — *see* Burn
  effects NOS T66 ☑
  sickness NOS T66 ☑
  therapy, encounter for Z51.0
Radiculitis (pressure) (vertebrogenic) — *see* Radiculopathy
Radiculomyelitis (*see also* Encephalitis)
  toxic, due to
    Clostridium tetani A35
    Corynebacterium diphtheriae A36.82
Radiculopathy M54.10
  cervical region M54.12
  cervicothoracic region M54.13
  due to
    disc disorder
      C3 M50.11
      C4 M50.11
      C5 M50.12
      C6 M50.12
      C7 M50.12
      C8 M50.13
    displacement of intervertebral disc — *see* Disorder,
      disc, with, radiculopathy
  leg M54.1- ☑
  lumbar region M54.16
  lumbosacral region M54.17
  occipito-atlanto-axial region M54.11
  postherpetic B02.29
  sacrococcygeal region M54.18

Radiculopathy — *continued*
  syphilitic A52.11
  thoracic region (with visceral pain) M54.14
  thoracolumbar region M54.15
Radiodermal burns (acute, chronic, or occupational) —
  see Burn
Radiodermatitis L58.9
  acute L58.0
  chronic L58.1
Radiotherapy session Z51.0
Rage, meaning rabies — *see* Rabies
Ragpicker's disease A22.1
Ragsorter's disease A22.1
Raillietiniasis B71.8
Railroad neurosis F48.8
Railway spine F48.8
Raised (*see also* Elevated)
  antibody titer R76.0
Rake teeth, tooth M26.39
Rales R09.89
Ramifying renal pelvis Q63.8
Ramsay-Hunt disease or syndrome (*see also* Hunt's
  disease) B02.21
  meaning dyssynergia cerebellaris myoclonica G11.1
Ranula K11.6
  congenital Q38.4
Rape
  adult
    confirmed T74.21 ☑
    suspected T76.21 ☑
  alleged, observation or examination, ruled out
    adult Z04.41
    child Z04.42
  child
    confirmed T74.22 ☑
    suspected T76.22 ☑
Rapid
  feeble pulse, due to shock, following injury T79.4 ☑
  heart (beat) R00.0
    psychogenic F45.8
  second stage (delivery) O62.3
  time-zone change syndrome — *see* Disorder, sleep,
    circadian rhythm, psychogenic
Rarefaction, bone — *see* Disorder, bone, density and
  structure, specified NEC
Rash (toxic) R21
  canker A38.9
  diaper L22
  drug (internal use) L27.0
    contact (*see also* Dermatitis, due to, drugs, external)
      L25.1
  following immunization T88.1 ☑
  food — *see* Dermatitis, due to, food
  heat L74.0
  napkin (psoriasiform) L22
  nettle — *see* Urticaria
  pustular L08.0
  rose R21
    epidemic B06.9
  scarlet A38.9
  serum (*see also* Reaction, serum) T80.69 ☑
  wandering tongue K14.1
Rasmussen aneurysm — *see* Tuberculosis, pulmonary
Rasmussen encephalitis G04.81
Rat-bite fever A25.9
  due to Streptobacillus moniliformis A25.1
  spirochetal (morsus muris) A25.0
Rathke's pouch tumor D44.3
Raymond (-Céstan) **syndrome** I65.8
Raynaud's disease, phenomenon or syndrome (secondary) I73.00
  with gangrene (symmetric) I73.01
RDS (newborn) (type I) P22.0
  type II P22.1
Reaction (*see also* Disorder)
  adaptation — *see* Disorder, adjustment
  adjustment (anxiety) (conduct disorder) (depressiveness) (distress) — *see* Disorder, adjustment
    with
      mutism, elective (child) (adolescent) F94.0
  adverse
    food (any) (ingested) NEC T78.1 ☑
      anaphylactic — *see* Shock, anaphylactic, due
        to food
  affective — *see* Disorder, mood
  allergic — *see* Allergy
  anaphylactic — *see* Shock, anaphylactic

Reaction — *continued*
  anaphylactoid — *see* Shock, anaphylactic
  anesthesia — *see* Anesthesia, complication
  antitoxin (prophylactic) (therapeutic) — *see* Complications, vaccination
  anxiety F41.1
  Arthus — *see* Arthus' phenomenon
  asthenic F48.8
  combat and operational stress F43.0
  compulsive F42
  conversion F44.9
  crisis, acute F43.0
  deoxyribonuclease (DNA) (DNase) hypersensitivity
    D69.2
  depressive (single episode) F32.9
    affective (single episode) F31.4
      recurrent episode F33.9
    neurotic F34.1
    psychoneurotic F34.1
    psychotic F32.3
    recurrent — *see* Disorder, depressive, recurrent
  dissociative F44.9
  drug NEC T88.7 ☑
    addictive — *see* Dependence, drug
      transmitted via placenta or breast milk — *see*
        Absorption, drug, addictive, through
        placenta
    allergic — *see* Allergy, drug
    lichenoid L43.2
    newborn P93.8
      gray baby syndrome P93.0
    overdose or poisoning (by accident) — *see* Table
      of Drugs and Chemicals, by drug, poisoning
    photoallergic L56.1
    phototoxic L56.0
    withdrawal — *see* Dependence, by drug, with,
      withdrawal
      infant of dependent mother P96.1
      newborn P96.1
    wrong substance given or taken (by accident) —
      see Table of Drugs and Chemicals, by drug,
      poisoning
  fear F40.9
    child (abnormal) F93.8
  febrile nonhemolytic transfusion (FNHTR) R50.84
  fluid loss, cerebrospinal G97.1
  foreign
    body NEC — *see* Granuloma, foreign body
      in operative wound (inadvertently left) — *see*
        Foreign body, accidentally left during a
        procedure
    substance accidentally left during a procedure
      (chemical) (powder) (talc) T81.60 ☑
      aseptic peritonitis T81.61 ☑
      body or object (instrument) (sponge) (swab)
        — *see* Foreign body, accidentally left
        during a procedure
      specified reaction NEC T81.69 ☑
  grief — *see* Disorder, adjustment
  Herxheimer's R68.89
  hyperkinetic — *see* Hyperkinesia
  hypochondriacal F45.20
  hypoglycemic, due to insulin E16.0
    with coma (diabetic) — *see* Diabetes, coma
      nondiabetic E15
    therapeutic misadventure — *see* subcategory
      T38.3 ☑
  hypomanic F30.8
  hysterical F44.9
  immunization — *see* Complications, vaccination
  incompatibility
    ABO blood group (infusion) (transfusion) — *see*
      Complication(s), transfusion, incompatibility
      reaction, ABO
    delayed serologic T80.39 ☑
    minor blood group (Duffy) (E) (K(ell)) (Kidd) (Lewis)
      (M) (N) (P) (S) T80.89 ☑
    Rh (factor) (infusion) (transfusion) — *see* Complication(s), transfusion, incompatibility reaction,
      Rh (factor)
  inflammatory — *see* Infection
  infusion — *see* Complications, infusion
  inoculation (immune serum) — *see* Complications,
    vaccination
  insulin T38.3- ☑
  involutional psychotic — *see* Disorder, depressive
  leukemoid D72.823

Reaction — *continued*
  leukemoid — *continued*
    basophilic D72.823
    lymphocytic D72.823
    monocytic D72.823
    myelocytic D72.823
    neutrophilic D72.823
  LSD (acute)
    due to drug abuse — *see* Abuse, drug, hallucinogen
    due to drug dependence — *see* Dependence, drug, hallucinogen
  lumbar puncture G97.1
  manic-depressive — *see* Disorder, bipolar
  neurasthenic F48.8
  neurogenic — *see* Neurosis
  neurotic F48.9
  neurotic-depressive F34.1
  nitritoid — *see* Crisis, nitritoid
  nonspecific
    to
      cell mediated immunity measurement of gamma interferon antigen response without active tuberculosis R76.12
      QuantiFERON-TB test (QFT) without active tuberculosis R76.12
      tuberculin test (*see also* Reaction, tuberculin skin test) R76.11
  obsessive-compulsive F42
  organic, acute or subacute — *see* Delirium
  paranoid (acute) F23
    chronic F22
    senile F03 ☑
  passive dependency F60.7
  phobic F40.9
  post-traumatic stress, uncomplicated Z73.3
  psychogenic F99
  psychoneurotic (*see also* Neurosis)
    compulsive F42
    depersonalization F48.1
    depressive F34.1
    hypochondriacal F45.20
    neurasthenic F48.8
    obsessive F42
  psychophysiologic — *see* Disorder, somatoform
  psychosomatic — *see* Disorder, somatoform
  psychotic — *see* Psychosis
  scarlet fever toxin — *see* Complications, vaccination
  schizophrenic F23
    acute (brief) (undifferentiated) F23
    latent F21
    undifferentiated (acute) (brief) F23
  serological for syphilis — *see* Serology for syphilis
  serum T80.69 ☑
    anaphylactic (immediate) (*see also* Shock, anaphylactic) T80.59 ☑
    specified reaction NEC
      due to
        administration of blood and blood products T80.61 ☑
        immunization T80.62 ☑
        serum specified NEC T80.69 ☑
        vaccination T80.62 ☑
  situational — *see* Disorder, adjustment
  somatization — *see* Disorder, somatoform
  spinal puncture G97.1
  stress (severe) F43.9
    acute (agitation) ("daze") (disorientation) (disturbance of consciousness) (flight reaction) (fugue) F43.0
    specified NEC F43.8
  surgical procedure — *see* Complications, surgical procedure
  tetanus antitoxin — *see* Complications, vaccination
  toxic, to local anesthesia T81.89 ☑
    in labor and delivery O74.4
    in pregnancy O29.3X- ☑
    postpartum, puerperal O89.3
  toxin-antitoxin — *see* Complications, vaccination
  transfusion (blood) (bone marrow) (lymphocytes) (allergic) — *see* Complications, transfusion
  tuberculin skin test, abnormal R76.11
  vaccination (any) — *see* Complications, vaccination
  withdrawing, child or adolescent F93.8
Reactive airway disease — *see* Asthma
Reactive depression — *see* Reaction, depressive

Rearrangement
  chromosomal
    balanced (in) Q95.9
      abnormal individual (autosomal) Q95.2
        non-sex (autosomal) chromosomes Q95.2
        sex/non-sex chromosomes Q95.3
      specified NEC Q95.8
Recalcitrant patient — *see* Noncompliance
Recanalization, thrombus — *see* Thrombosis
Recession, receding
  chamber angle (eye) H21.55- ☑
  chin M26.09
  gingival (generalized) (localized) (postinfective) (postoperative) K06.0
Recklinghausen disease Q85.01
  bones E21.0
Reclus' disease (cystic) — *see* Mastopathy, cystic
Recrudescent typhus (fever) A75.1
Recruitment, auditory H93.21- ☑
Rectalgia K62.89
Rectitis K62.89
Rectocele
  female (without uterine prolapse) N81.6
    with uterine prolapse N81.4
      incomplete N81.2
  in pregnancy — *see* Pregnancy, complicated by, abnormal, pelvic organs or tissues NEC
  male K62.3
Rectosigmoid junction — *see* condition
Rectosigmoiditis K63.89
  ulcerative (chronic) K51.30
    with
      complication K51.319
        abscess K51.314
        fistula K51.313
        obstruction K51.312
        rectal bleeding K51.311
        specified NEC K51.318
Rectourethral — *see* condition
Rectovaginal — *see* condition
Rectovesical — *see* condition
Rectum, rectal — *see* condition
Recurrent — *see* condition
  pregnancy loss — *see* Loss (of), pregnancy, recurrent
Red bugs B88.0
Red tide (*see also* Table of Drugs and Chemicals) T65.82- ☑
Red-cedar lung or pneumonitis J67.8
Reduced
  mobility Z74.09
  ventilatory or vital capacity R94.2
Redundant, redundancy
  anus (congenital) Q43.8
  clitoris N90.89
  colon (congenital) Q43.8
  foreskin (congenital) N47.8
  intestine (congenital) Q43.8
  labia N90.6
  organ or site, congenital NEC — *see* Accessory
  panniculus (abdominal) E65
  prepuce (congenital) N47.8
  pylorus K31.89
  rectum (congenital) Q43.8
  scrotum N50.8
  sigmoid (congenital) Q43.8
  skin (of face) L57.4
    eyelids — *see* Blepharochalasis
  stomach K31.89
Reduplication — *see* Duplication
Reflex R29.2
  hyperactive gag J39.2
  pupillary, abnormal — *see* Anomaly, pupil, function
  vasoconstriction I73.9
  vasovagal R55
Reflux K21.9
  acid K21.9
  esophageal K21.9
    with esophagitis K21.0
    newborn P78.83
  gastroesophageal K21.9
    with esophagitis K21.0
  mitral — *see* Insufficiency, mitral
  ureteral — *see* Reflux, vesicoureteral
  vesicoureteral (with scarring) N13.70
    with
      nephropathy N13.729
        with hydroureter N13.739

Reflux — *continued*
  vesicoureteral — *continued*
    with — *continued*
      nephropathy — *continued*
        with hydroureter — *continued*
          bilateral N13.732
          unilateral N13.731
        without hydroureter N13.729
          bilateral N13.722
          unilateral N13.721
        bilateral N13.722
        unilateral N13.721
      pyelonephritis (chronic) N11.0
    without nephropathy N13.71
    congenital Q62.7
Reforming, artificial openings — *see* Attention to, artificial, opening
Refractive error — *see* Disorder, refraction
Refsum's disease or syndrome G60.1
Refusal of
  food, psychogenic F50.8
  treatment (because of) Z53.20
    left against medical advice (AMA) Z53.21
    patient's decision NEC Z53.29
    reasons of belief or group pressure Z53.1
Regional — *see* condition
Regurgitation R11.10
  aortic (valve) — *see* Insufficiency, aortic
  food (*see also* Vomiting)
    with reswallowing — *see* Rumination
    newborn P92.1
  gastric contents — *see* Vomiting
  heart — *see* Endocarditis
  mitral (valve) — *see* Insufficiency, mitral
    congenital Q23.3
  myocardial — *see* Endocarditis
  pulmonary (valve) (heart) I37.1
    congenital Q22.2
    syphilitic A52.03
  tricuspid — *see* Insufficiency, tricuspid
  valve, valvular — *see* Endocarditis
    congenital Q24.8
  vesicoureteral — *see* Reflux, vesicoureteral
Reichmann's disease or syndrome K31.89
Reifenstein syndrome E34.52
Reinsertion, contraceptive device Z30.433
Reiter's disease, syndrome, or urethritis M02.30
  ankle M02.37- ☑
  elbow M02.32- ☑
  foot joint M02.37- ☑
  hand joint M02.34- ☑
  hip M02.35- ☑
  knee M02.36- ☑
  multiple site M02.39
  shoulder M02.31- ☑
  vertebra M02.38
  wrist M02.33- ☑
Rejection
  food, psychogenic F50.8
  transplant T86.91
    bone T86.830
      marrow T86.01
    cornea T86.840
    heart T86.21
      with lung(s) T86.31
    intestine T86.850
    kidney T86.11
    liver T86.41
    lung(s) T86.810
      with heart T86.31
    organ (immune or nonimmune cause) T86.91
    pancreas T86.890
    skin (allograft) (autograft) T86.820
    specified NEC T86.890
    stem cell (peripheral blood) (umbilical cord) T86.5
Relapsing fever A68.9
  Carter's (Asiatic) A68.1
  Dutton's (West African) A68.1
  Koch's A68.9
  louse-borne (epidemic) A68.0
  Novy's (American) A68.1
  Obermeyers's (European) A68.0
  Spirillum A68.9
  tick-borne (endemic) A68.1
Relationship
  occlusal
    open anterior M26.220

Relationship — *continued*
  occlusal — *continued*
    open posterior M26.221
Relaxation
  anus (sphincter) K62.89
    psychogenic F45.8
  arch (foot) (see also Deformity, limb, flat foot)
  back ligaments — *see* Instability, joint, spine
  bladder (sphincter) N31.2
  cardioesophageal K21.9
  cervix — *see* Incompetency, cervix
  diaphragm J98.6
  joint (capsule) (ligament) (paralytic) — *see* Flail, joint
    congenital NEC Q74.8
  lumbosacral (joint) — *see* subcategory M53.2 ☑
  pelvic floor N81.89
  perineum N81.89
  posture R29.3
  rectum (sphincter) K62.89
  sacroiliac (joint) — *see* subcategory M53.2 ☑
  scrotum N50.8
  urethra (sphincter) N36.44
  vesical N31.2
Release from prison, anxiety concerning Z65.2
Remains
  canal of Cloquet Q14.0
  capsule (opaque) Q14.8
Remittent fever (malarial) B54
Remnant
  canal of Cloquet Q14.0
  capsule (opaque) Q14.8
  cervix, cervical stump (acquired) (postoperative) N88.8
  cystic duct, postcholecystectomy K91.5
  fingernail L60.8
    congenital Q84.6
  meniscus, knee — *see* Derangement, knee, meniscus, specified NEC
  thyroglossal duct Q89.2
  tonsil J35.8
    infected (chronic) J35.01
  urachus Q64.4
Removal (from) (of)
  artificial
    arm Z44.00- ☑
      complete Z44.01- ☑
      partial Z44.02- ☑
    eye Z44.2- ☑
    leg Z44.10- ☑
      complete Z44.11- ☑
      partial Z44.12- ☑
  breast implant Z45.81 ☑
  cardiac pulse generator (battery) (end-of-life) Z45.010
  catheter (urinary) (indwelling) Z46.6
    from artificial opening — *see* Attention to, artificial, opening
    non-vascular Z46.82
    vascular NEC Z45.2
  device Z46.9
    contraceptive Z30.432
    implanted NEC Z45.89
    specified NEC Z46.89
  drains Z48.03
  dressing (nonsurgical) Z48.00
    surgical Z48.01
  external
    fixation device — *code to* fracture with seventh character D
    prosthesis, prosthetic device Z44.9
      breast Z44.3- ☑
      specified NEC Z44.8
  home in childhood (to foster home or institution) Z62.29
  ileostomy Z43.2
  insulin pump Z46.81
  myringotomy device (stent) (tube) Z45.82
  nervous system device NEC Z46.2
    brain neuropacemaker Z46.2
    visual substitution device Z46.2
      implanted Z45.31
  non-vascular catheter Z46.82
  organ, prophylactic (for neoplasia management) — *see* Prophylactic, organ removal
  orthodontic device Z46.4
  staples Z48.02
  stent
    ureteral Z46.6
  suture Z48.02
  urinary device Z46.6

Removal — *continued*
  vascular access device or catheter Z45.2
Ren
  arcuatus Q63.1
  mobile, mobilis N28.89
    congenital Q63.8
  unguliformis Q63.1
Renal — *see* condition
Rendu-Osler-Weber disease or syndrome I78.0
Reninoma D41.0- ☑
Renon-Delille syndrome E23.3
Reovirus, as cause of disease classified elsewhere B97.5
Repeated falls NEC R29.6
Replaced chromosome by dicentric ring Q93.2
Replacement by artificial or mechanical device or prosthesis of
  bladder Z96.0
  blood vessel NEC Z95.828
  bone NEC Z96.7
  cochlea Z96.21
  coronary artery Z95.5
  eustachian tube Z96.29
  eye globe Z97.0
  heart Z95.812
    valve Z95.2
      prosthetic Z95.2
      specified NEC Z95.4
      xenogenic Z95.3
  intestine Z96.89
  joint Z96.60
    hip — *see* Presence, hip joint implant
    knee — *see* Presence, knee joint implant
    specified site NEC Z96.698
  larynx Z96.3
  lens Z96.1
  limb(s) — *see* Presence, artificial, limb
  mandible NEC (for tooth root implant(s)) Z96.5
  organ NEC Z96.89
  peripheral vessel NEC Z95.828
  stapes Z96.29
  teeth Z97.2
  tendon Z96.7
  tissue NEC Z96.89
  tooth root(s) Z96.5
  vessel NEC Z95.828
    coronary (artery) Z95.5
Request for expert evidence Z04.8
Reserve, decreased or low
  cardiac — *see* Disease, heart
  kidney N28.89
Residual (see also condition)
  ovary syndrome N99.83
  state, schizophrenic F20.5
  urine R39.19
Resistance, resistant (to)
  activated protein C D68.51
  complicating pregnancy O26.89 ☑
  insulin E88.81
  organism(s)
    to
      drug
        aminoglycosides Z16.29
        amoxicillin Z16.11
        ampicillin Z16.11
        antibiotic(s) Z16.20
          multiple Z16.24
          specified NEC Z16.29
        antifungal Z16.32
        antimicrobial (single) Z16.30
          multiple Z16.35
          specified NEC Z16.39
        antimycbacterial (single) Z16.341
          multiple Z16.342
        antiparasitic Z16.31
        antiviral Z16.33
        beta lactam antibiotics Z16.10
          specified NEC Z16.19
        cephalosporins Z16.19
        extended beta lactamase (ESBL) Z16.12
        fluoroquinolones Z16.23
        macrolides Z16.29
        methicillin — *see* MRSA
        multiple drugs (MDRO)
          antibiotics Z16.24
        penicillins Z16.11
        quinine (and related compounds) Z16.31
        quinolones Z16.23

Resistance, resistant — *continued*
  organism(s) — *continued*
    to — *continued*
      drug — *continued*
        sulfonamides Z16.29
        tetracyclines Z16.29
        tuberculostatics (single) Z16.341
          multiple Z16.342
        vancomycin Z16.21
          related antibiotics Z16.22
  thyroid hormone E07.89
Resorption
  dental (roots) K03.3
    alveoli M26.79
  teeth (external) (internal) (pathological) (roots) K03.3
Respiration
  Cheyne-Stokes R06.3
  decreased due to shock, following injury T79.4 ☑
  disorder of, psychogenic F45.8
  insufficient, or poor R06.89
    newborn P28.5
  painful R07.1
  sighing, psychogenic F45.8
Respiratory (see also condition)
  distress syndrome (newborn) (type I) P22.0
    type II P22.1
  syncytial virus, as cause of disease classified elsewhere B97.4
Respite care Z75.5
Response (drug)
  photoallergic L56.1
  phototoxic L56.0
Restless legs (syndrome) G25.81
Restlessness R45.1
Restoration (of)
  dental
    aesthetically inadequate or displeasing K08.56
    defective K08.50
      specified NEC K08.59
    failure of marginal integrity K08.51
    failure of periodontal anatomical intergrity K08.54
  organ continuity from previous sterilization (tuboplasty) (vasoplasty) Z31.0
    aftercare Z31.42
  tooth (existing)
    contours biologically incompatible with oral health K08.54
    open margins K08.51
    overhanging K08.52
    poor aesthetic K08.56
    poor gingival margins K08.51
  unsatisfactory, of tooth K08.50
    specified NEC K08.59
Restorative material (dental)
  allergy to K08.55
  fractured K08.539
    with loss of material K08.531
    without loss of material K08.530
  unrepairable overhanging of K08.52
Restriction of housing space Z59.1
Rests, ovarian, in fallopian tube Q50.6
Restzustand (schizophrenic) F20.5
Retained (see also Retention)
  cholelithiasis following cholecystectomy K91.86
  foreign body fragments (type of) Z18.9
    acrylics Z18.2
    animal quill(s) or spines Z18.31
    cement Z18.83
    concrete Z18.83
    crystalline Z18.83
    depleted isotope Z18.09
    depleted uranium Z18.01
    diethylhexylphthalates Z18.2
    glass Z18.81
    isocyanate Z18.2
    magnetic metal Z18.11
    metal Z18.10
    nonmagnectic metal Z18.12
    nontherapeutic radioactive Z18.09
    organic NEC Z18.39
    plastic Z18.2
    quill(s) (animal) Z18.31
    radioactive (nontherapeutic) NEC Z18.09
    specified NEC Z18.89
    spine(s) (animal) Z18.31
    stone Z18.83
    tooth (teeth) Z18.32
    wood Z18.33

☑ Additional Character Required — Refer to the Tabular List for Character Selection   ▽ Subterms under main terms may continue to next column or page

Retained — *continued*
  fragments (type of) Z18.9
    acrylics Z18.2
    animal quill(s) or spines Z18.31
    cement Z18.83
    concrete Z18.83
    crystalline Z18.83
    depleted isotope Z18.09
    depleted uranium Z18.01
    diethylhexylphthalates Z18.2
    glass Z18.81
    isocyanate Z18.2
    magnetic metal Z18.11
    metal Z18.10
    nonmagnectic metal Z18.12
    nontherapeutic radioactive Z18.09
    organic NEC Z18.39
    plastic Z18.2
    quill(s) (animal) Z18.31
    radioactive (nontherapeutic) NEC Z18.09
    specified NEC Z18.89
    spine(s) (animal) Z18.31
    stone Z18.83
    tooth (teeth) Z18.32
    wood Z18.33
  gallstones, following cholecystectomy K91.86
Retardation
  development, developmental, specific — *see* Disorder, developmental
  endochondral bone growth — *see* Disorder, bone, development or growth
  growth R62.50
    due to malnutrition E45
  mental — *see* Disability, intellectual
  motor function, specific F82
  physical (child) R62.52
    due to malnutrition E45
  reading (specific) F81.0
  spelling (specific) (without reading disorder) F81.81
Retching — *see* Vomiting
Retention (*see also* Retained)
  bladder — *see* Retention, urine
  carbon dioxide E87.2
  cholelithiasis following cholecystectomy K91.86
  cyst — *see* Cyst
  dead
    fetus (at or near term) (mother) O36.4 ☑
      early fetal death O02.1
    ovum O02.0
  decidua (fragments) (following delivery) (with hemorrhage) O72.2
    without hemorrhage O73.1
  deciduous tooth K00.6
  dental root K08.3
  fecal — *see* Constipation
  fetus
    dead O36.4 ☑
      early O02.1
  fluid R60.9
  foreign body (*see also* Foreign body, retained)
    current trauma — *code as* Foreign body, by site or type
  gallstones, following cholecystectomy K91.86
  gastric K31.89
  intrauterine contraceptive device, in pregnancy — *see* Pregnancy, complicated by, retention, intrauterine device
  membranes (complicating delivery) (with hemorrhage) O72.2
    with abortion — *see* Abortion, by type
    without hemorrhage O73.1
  meniscus — *see* Derangement, meniscus
  menses N94.89
  milk (puerperal, postpartum) O92.79
  nitrogen, extrarenal R39.2
  ovary syndrome N99.83
  placenta (total) (with hemorrhage) O72.0
    without hemorrhage O73.0
    portions or fragments (with hemorrhage) O72.2
      without hemorrhage O73.1
  products of conception
    early pregnancy (dead fetus) O02.1
    following
      delivery (with hemorrhage) O72.2
        without hemorrhage O73.1
  secundines (following delivery) (with hemorrhage) O72.0
    without hemorrhage O73.0

Retention — *continued*
  secundines — *continued*
    complicating puerperium (delayed hemorrhage) O72.2
    partial O72.2
      without hemorrhage O73.1
  smegma, clitoris N90.89
  urine R33.9
    drug-induced R33.0
    due to hyperplasia (hypertrophy) of prostate — *see* Hyperplasia, prostate
    organic R33.8
      drug-induced R33.0
    psychogenic F45.8
    specified NEC R33.8
  water (in tissues) — *see* Edema
Reticulation, dust — *see* Pneumoconiosis
Reticulocytosis R70.1
Reticuloendotheliosis
  acute infantile C96.0
  leukemic C91.4- ☑
  malignant C96.9
  nonlipid C96.0
Reticulohistiocytoma (giant-cell) D76.3
Reticuloid, actinic L57.1
Reticulosis (skin)
  acute of infancy C96.0
  hemophagocytic, familial D76.1
  histiocytic medullary C96.9
  lipomelanotic I89.8
  malignant (midline) C86.0
  nonlipid C96.0
  polymorphic C83.8- ☑
  Sézary — *see* Sézary disease
Retina, retinal (*see also* condition)
  dark area D49.81
Retinitis (*see also* Inflammation, chorioretinal)
  albuminurica N18.9 [H32]
  diabetic — *see* Diabetes, retinitis
  disciformis — *see* Degeneration, macula
  focal — *see* Inflammation, chorioretinal, focal
  gravidarum — *see* Pregnancy, complicated by, specified pregnancy-related condition NEC
  juxtapapillaris — *see* Inflammation, chorioretinal, focal, juxtapapillary
  luetic — *see* Retinitis, syphilitic
  pigmentosa H35.52
  proliferans — *see* Disorder, globe, degenerative, specified type NEC
  proliferating — *see* Disorder, globe, degenerative, specified type NEC
  renal N18.9 [H32]
  syphilitic (early) (secondary) A51.43
    central, recurrent A52.71
    congenital (early) A50.01 [H32]
    late A52.71
  tuberculous A18.53
Retinoblastoma C69.2- ☑
  differentiated C69.2- ☑
  undifferentiated C69.2- ☑
Retinochoroiditis (*see also* Inflammation, chorioretinal)
  disseminated — *see* Inflammation, chorioretinal, disseminated
    syphilitic A52.71
  focal — *see* Inflammation, chorioretinal
  juxtapapillaris — *see* Inflammation, chorioretinal, focal, juxtapapillary
Retinopathy (background) H35.00
  arteriosclerotic I70.8 [H35.0-] ☑
  atherosclerotic I70.8 [H35.0-] ☑
  central serous — *see* Chorioretinopathy, central serous
  Coats H35.02- ☑
  diabetic — *see* Diabetes, retinopathy
  exudative H35.02- ☑
  hypertensive H35.03- ☑
  in (due to)
    diabetes — *see* Diabetes, retinopathy
    sickle-cell disorders D57.- ☑ [H36]
  of prematurity H35.10- ☑
    stage 0 H35.11- ☑
    stage 1 H35.12- ☑
    stage 2 H35.13- ☑
    stage 3 H35.14- ☑
    stage 4 H35.15- ☑
    stage 5 H35.16- ☑
  pigmentary, congenital — *see* Dystrophy, retina
  proliferative NEC H35.2- ☑

Retinopathy — *continued*
  proliferative — *continued*
    diabetic — *see* Diabetes, retinopathy, proliferative
    sickle-cell D57.- ☑ [H36]
  solar H31.02- ☑
Retinoschisis H33.10- ☑
  congenital Q14.1
  specified type NEC H33.19- ☑
Retortamoniasis A07.8
Retractile testis Q55.22
Retraction
  cervix — *see* Retroversion, uterus
  drum (membrane) — *see* Disorder, tympanic membrane, specified NEC
  finger — *see* Deformity, finger
  lid H02.539
    left H02.536
      lower H02.535
      upper H02.534
    right H02.533
      lower H02.532
      upper H02.531
  lung J98.4
  mediastinum J98.5
  nipple N64.53
    associated with
      lactation O92.03
      pregnancy O92.01- ☑
      puerperium O92.02
    congenital Q83.8
  palmar fascia M72.0
  pleura — *see* Pleurisy
  ring, uterus (Bandl's) (pathological) O62.4
  sternum (congenital) Q76.7
    acquired M95.4
  uterus — *see* Retroversion, uterus
  valve (heart) — *see* Endocarditis
Retrobulbar — *see* condition
Retrocecal — *see* condition
Retrocession — *see* Retroversion
Retrodisplacement — *see* Retroversion
Retroflection, retroflexion — *see* Retroversion
Retrognathia, retrognathism (mandibular) (maxillary) M26.19
Retrograde menstruation N92.5
Retroperineal — *see* condition
Retroperitoneal — *see* condition
Retroperitonitis K68.9
Retropharyngeal — *see* condition
Retroplacental — *see* condition
Retroposition — *see* Retroversion
Retroprosthetic membrane T85.398 ☑
Retrosternal thyroid (congenital) Q89.2
Retroversion, retroverted
  cervix — *see* Retroversion, uterus
  female NEC — *see* Retroversion, uterus
  iris H21.89
  testis (congenital) Q55.29
  uterus (acquired) (acute) (any degree) (asymptomatic) (cervix) (postinfectional) (postpartal, old) N85.4
    congenital Q51.818
    in pregnancy O34.53- ☑
Retrovirus, as cause of disease classified elsewhere B97.30
  human
    immunodeficiency, type 2 (HIV 2) B97.35
    T-cell lymphotropic
      type I (HTLV-I) B97.33
      type II (HTLV-II) B97.34
  lentivirus B97.31
  oncovirus B97.32
  specified NEC B97.39
Retrusion, premaxilla (developmental) M26.09
Rett's disease or syndrome F84.2
Reverse peristalsis R19.2
Reye's syndrome G93.7
Rh (factor)
  hemolytic disease (newborn) P55.0
  incompatibility, immunization or sensitization
    affecting management of pregnancy NEC O36.09- ☑
      anti-D antibody O36.01- ☑
    newborn P55.0
    transfusion reaction — *see* Complication(s), transfusion, incompatibility reaction, Rh (factor)
  negative mother affecting newborn P55.0

Index

Rh — RIND

Rh — *continued*
  titer elevated — *see* Complication(s), transfusion, incompatibility reaction, Rh (factor)
  transfusion reaction — *see* Complication(s), transfusion, incompatibility reaction, Rh (factor)
Rhabdomyolysis (idiopathic) NEC M62.82
  traumatic T79.6
Rhabdomyoma (*see also* Neoplasm, connective tissue, benign)
  adult — *see* Neoplasm, connective tissue, benign
  fetal — *see* Neoplasm, connective tissue, benign
  glycogenic — *see* Neoplasm, connective tissue, benign
Rhabdomyosarcoma (any type) — *see* Neoplasm, connective tissue, malignant
Rhabdosarcoma — *see* Rhabdomyosarcoma
Rhesus (factor) **incompatibility** — *see* Rh, incompatibility
Rheumatic (acute) (subacute) (chronic)
  adherent pericardium I09.2
  coronary arteritis I01.9
  degeneration, myocardium I09.0
  fever (acute) — *see* Fever, rheumatic
  heart — *see* Disease, heart, rheumatic
  myocardial degeneration — *see* Degeneration, myocardium
  myocarditis (chronic) (inactive) (with chorea) I09.0
    with chorea (acute) (rheumatic) (Sydenham's) I02.0
    active or acute I01.2
  pancarditis, acute I01.8
    with chorea (acute) (rheumatic) Sydenham's) I02.0
  pericarditis (active) (acute) (with effusion) (with pneumonia) I01.0
    with chorea (acute) (rheumatic) (Sydenham's) I02.0
    chronic or inactive I09.2
  pneumonia I00 [J17]
  torticollis M43.6
  typhoid fever A01.09
Rheumatism (articular) (neuralgic) (nonarticular) M79.0
  gout — *see* Arthritis, rheumatoid
  intercostal, meaning Tietze's disease M94.0
  palindromic (any site) M12.30
    ankle M12.37- ☑
    elbow M12.32- ☑
    foot joint M12.37- ☑
    hand joint M12.34- ☑
    hip M12.35- ☑
    knee M12.36- ☑
    multiple site M12.39
    shoulder M12.31- ☑
    specified joint NEC M12.38
    vertebrae M12.38
    wrist M12.33- ☑
  sciatic M54.4- ☑
Rheumatoid (*see also* condition)
  arthritis (*see also* Arthritis, rheumatoid)
    with involvement of organs NEC M05.60
      ankle M05.67- ☑
      elbow M05.62- ☑
      foot joint M05.67- ☑
      hand joint M05.64- ☑
      hip M05.65- ☑
      knee M05.66- ☑
      multiple site M05.69
      shoulder M05.61- ☑
      vertebra — *see* Spondylitis, ankylosing
      wrist M05.63- ☑
    seronegative — *see* Arthritis, rheumatoid, seronegative
    seropositive — *see* Arthritis, rheumatoid, seropositive
  carditis M05.30
    ankle M05.37- ☑
    elbow M05.32- ☑
    foot joint M05.37- ☑
    hand joint M05.34- ☑
    hip M05.35- ☑
    knee M05.36- ☑
    multiple site M05.39
    shoulder M05.31- ☑
    vertebra — *see* Spondylitis, ankylosing
    wrist M05.33- ☑
  endocarditis — *see* Rheumatoid, carditis
  lung (disease) M05.10
    ankle M05.17- ☑
    elbow M05.12- ☑
    foot joint M05.17- ☑
    hand joint M05.14- ☑

Rheumatoid — *continued*
  lung — *continued*
    hip M05.15- ☑
    knee M05.16- ☑
    multiple site M05.19
    shoulder M05.11- ☑
    vertebra — *see* Spondylitis, ankylosing
    wrist M05.13- ☑
  myocarditis — *see* Rheumatoid, carditis
  myopathy M05.40
    ankle M05.47- ☑
    elbow M05.42- ☑
    foot joint M05.47- ☑
    hand joint M05.44- ☑
    hip M05.45- ☑
    knee M05.46- ☑
    multiple site M05.49
    shoulder M05.41- ☑
    vertebra — *see* Spondylitis, ankylosing
    wrist M05.43- ☑
  pericarditis — *see* Rheumatoid, carditis
  polyarthritis — *see* Arthritis, rheumatoid
  polyneuropathy M05.50
    ankle M05.57- ☑
    elbow M05.52- ☑
    foot joint M05.57- ☑
    hand joint M05.54- ☑
    hip M05.55- ☑
    knee M05.56- ☑
    multiple site M05.59
    shoulder M05.51- ☑
    vertebra — *see* Spondylitis, ankylosing
    wrist M05.53- ☑
  vasculitis M05.20
    ankle M05.27- ☑
    elbow M05.22- ☑
    foot joint M05.27- ☑
    hand joint M05.24- ☑
    hip M05.25- ☑
    knee M05.26- ☑
    multiple site M05.29
    shoulder M05.21- ☑
    vertebra — *see* Spondylitis, ankylosing
    wrist M05.23- ☑
Rhinitis (atrophic) (catarrhal) (chronic) (croupous) (fibrinous) (granulomatous) (hyperplastic) (hypertrophic) (membranous) (obstructive) (purulent) (suppurative) (ulcerative) J31.0
  with
    sore throat — *see* Nasopharyngitis
  acute J00
  allergic J30.9
    with asthma J45.909
      with
        exacerbation (acute) J45.901
        status asthmaticus J45.902
    due to
      food J30.5
      pollen J30.1
    nonseasonal J30.89
    perennial J30.89
    seasonal NEC J30.2
    specified NEC J30.89
  infective J00
  pneumococcal J00
  syphilitic A52.73
    congenital A50.05 [J99]
  tuberculous A15.8
  vasomotor J30.0
Rhinoantritis (chronic) — *see* Sinusitis, maxillary
Rhinodacryolith — *see* Dacryolith
Rhinolith (nasal sinus) J34.89
Rhinomegaly J34.89
Rhinopharyngitis (acute) (subacute) (*see also* Nasopharyngitis)
  chronic J31.1
  destructive ulcerating A66.5
  mutilans A66.5
Rhinophyma L71.1
Rhinorrhea J34.89
  cerebrospinal (fluid) G96.0
  paroxysmal — *see* Rhinitis, allergic
  spasmodic — *see* Rhinitis, allergic
Rhinosalpingitis — *see* Salpingitis, eustachian
Rhinoscleroma A48.8
Rhinosporidiosis B48.1
Rhinovirus infection NEC B34.8

Rhizomelic chondrodysplasia punctata E71.540
Rhythm
  atrioventricular nodal I49.8
  disorder I49.9
    coronary sinus I49.8
    ectopic I49.8
    nodal I49.8
  escape I49.9
  heart, abnormal I49.9
  idioventricular I44.2
  nodal I49.8
  sleep, inversion G47.2- ☑
    nonorganic origin — *see* Disorder, sleep, circadian rhythm, psychogenic
Rhytidosis facialis L98.8
Rib (*see also* condition)
  cervical Q76.5
Riboflavin deficiency E53.0
Rice bodies (*see also* Loose, body, joint)
  knee M23.4- ☑
Richter syndrome — *see* Leukemia, chronic lymphocytic, B-cell type
Richter's hernia — *see* Hernia, abdomen, with obstruction
Ricinism — *see* Poisoning, food, noxious, plant
Rickets (active) (acute) (adolescent) (chest wall) (congenital) (current) (infantile) (intestinal) E55.0
  adult — *see* Osteomalacia
  celiac K90.0
  hypophosphatemic with nephrotic-glycosuric dwarfism E72.09
  inactive E64.3
  kidney N25.0
  renal N25.0
  sequelae, any E64.3
  vitamin-D-resistant E83.31 [M90.80]
Rickettsial disease A79.9
  specified type NEC A79.89
Rickettsialpox (Rickettsia akari) A79.1
Rickettsiosis A79.9
  due to
    Ehrlichia sennetsu A79.81
    Rickettsia akari (rickettsialpox) A79.1
  specified type NEC A79.89
  tick-borne A77.9
  vesicular A79.1
Rider's bone — *see* Ossification, muscle, specified NEC
Ridge, alveolus (*see also* condition)
  flabby K06.8
Ridged ear, congenital Q17.3
Riedel's
  lobe, liver Q44.7
  struma, thyroiditis or disease E06.5
Rieger's anomaly or syndrome Q13.81
Riehl's melanosis L81.4
Rietti-Greppi-Micheli anemia D56.9
Rieux's hernia — *see* Hernia, abdomen, specified site NEC
Riga (-Fede) **disease** K14.0
Riggs' disease — *see* Periodontitis
Right middle lobe syndrome J98.11
Rigid, rigidity (*see also* condition)
  abdominal R19.30
    with severe abdominal pain R10.0
    epigastric R19.36
    generalized R19.37
    left lower quadrant R19.34
    left upper quadrant R19.32
    periumbilic R19.35
    right lower quadrant R19.33
    right upper quadrant R19.31
  articular, multiple, congenital Q68.8
  cervix (uteri) in pregnancy — *see* Pregnancy, complicated by, abnormal, cervix
  hymen (acquired) (congenital) N89.6
  nuchal R29.1
  pelvic floor in pregnancy — *see* Pregnancy, complicated by, abnormal, pelvic organs or tissues NEC
  perineum or vulva in pregnancy — *see* Pregnancy, complicated by, abnormal, vulva
  spine — *see* Dorsopathy, specified NEC
  vagina in pregnancy — *see* Pregnancy, complicated by, abnormal, vagina
Rigors R68.89
  with fever R50.9
Riley-Day syndrome G90.1
RIND (reversible ischemic neurologic deficit) I63.9

Ring(s)
- aorta (vascular) Q25.4
- Bandl's O62.4
- contraction, complicating delivery O62.4
- esophageal, lower (muscular) K22.2
- Fleischer's (cornea) H18.04- ☑
- hymenal, tight (acquired) (congenital) N89.6
- Kayser-Fleischer (cornea) H18.04- ☑
- retraction, uterus, pathological O62.4
- Schatzki's (esophagus) (lower) K22.2
  - congenital Q39.3
- Soemmering's — see Cataract, secondary
- vascular (congenital) Q25.8
  - aorta Q25.4

Ringed hair (congenital) Q84.1

Ringworm B35.9
- beard B35.0
- black dot B35.0
- body B35.4
- Burmese B35.5
- corporeal B35.4
- foot B35.3
- groin B35.6
- hand B35.2
- honeycomb B35.0
- nails B35.1
- perianal (area) B35.6
- scalp B35.0
- specified NEC B35.8
- Tokelau B35.5

Rise, venous pressure I87.8

Risk, suicidal
- meaning personal history of attempted suicide Z91.5
- meaning suicidal ideation — see Ideation, suicidal

Ritter's disease L00

Rivalry, sibling Z62.891

Rivalta's disease A42.2

River blindness B73.01

Robert's pelvis Q74.2
- with disproportion (fetopelvic) O33.0
  - causing obstructed labor O65.0

Robin (-Pierre) **syndrome** Q87.0

Robinow-Silvermann-Smith syndrome Q87.1

Robinson's (hidrotic) **ectodermal dysplasia or syndrome** Q82.4

Robles' disease B73.01

Rocky Mountain (spotted) **fever** A77.0

Roetheln — see Rubella

Roger's disease Q21.0

Rokitansky-Aschoff sinuses (gallbladder) K82.8

Rolando's fracture (displaced) S62.22- ☑
- nondisplaced S62.22- ☑

Romano-Ward (prolonged QT interval) **syndrome** I45.81

Romberg's disease or syndrome G51.8

Roof, mouth — see condition

Rosacea L71.9
- acne L71.9
- keratitis L71.8
- specified NEC L71.8

Rosary, rachitic E55.0

Rose
- cold J30.1
- fever J30.1
- rash R21
  - epidemic B06.9

Rosenbach's erysipeloid A26.0

Rosenthal's disease or syndrome D68.1

Roseola B09
- infantum B08.20
  - due to human herpesvirus 6 B08.21
  - due to human herpesvirus 7 B08.22

Ross River disease or fever B33.1

Rossbach's disease K31.89
- psychogenic F45.8

Rostan's asthma (cardiac) — see Failure, ventricular, left

Rotation
- anomalous, incomplete or insufficient, intestine Q43.3
- cecum (congenital) Q43.3
- colon (congenital) Q43.3
- spine, incomplete or insufficient — see Dorsopathy, deforming, specified NEC
- tooth, teeth, fully erupted M26.35
- vertebra, incomplete or insufficient — see Dorsopathy, deforming, specified NEC

Rotes Quérol disease or syndrome — see Hyperostosis, ankylosing

Roth (-Bernhardt) **disease or syndrome** — see Meralgia paraesthetica

Rothmund (-Thomson) **syndrome** Q82.8

Rotor's disease or syndrome E80.6

Round
- back (with wedging of vertebrae) — see Kyphosis
  - sequelae (late effect) of rickets E64.3
- worms (large) (infestation) NEC B82.0
  - Ascariasis (see also Ascariasis) B77.9

Roussy-Lévy syndrome G60.0

Rubella (German measles) B06.9
- complication NEC B06.09
  - neurological B06.00
- congenital P35.0
- contact Z20.4
- exposure to Z20.4
- maternal
  - care for (suspected) damage to fetus O35.3 ☑
    - manifest rubella in infant P35.0
  - suspected damage to fetus affecting management of pregnancy O35.3 ☑
- specified complications NEC B06.89

Rubeola (meaning measles) — see Measles
- meaning rubella — see Rubella

Rubeosis, iris — see Disorder, iris, vascular

Rubinstein-Taybi syndrome Q87.2

Rudimentary (congenital) (see also Agenesis)
- arm — see Defect, reduction, upper limb
- bone Q79.9
- cervix uteri Q51.828
- eye Q11.2
- lobule of ear Q17.3
- patella Q74.1
- respiratory organs in thoracopagus Q89.4
- tracheal bronchus Q32.4
- uterus Q51.818
  - in male Q56.1
- vagina Q52.0

Ruled out condition — see Observation, suspected

Rumination R11.10
- with nausea R11.2
- disorder of infancy F98.21
- neurotic F42
- newborn P92.1
- obsessional F42
- psychogenic F42

Runeberg's disease D51.0

Runny nose R09.89

Rupia (syphilitic) A51.39
- congenital A50.06
- tertiary A52.79

Rupture, ruptured
- abscess (spontaneous) — code by site under Abscess
- aneurysm — see Aneurysm
- anus (sphincter) — see Laceration, anus
- aorta, aortic I71.8
  - abdominal I71.3
  - arch I71.1
  - ascending I71.1
  - descending I71.8
    - abdominal I71.3
    - thoracic I71.1
  - syphilitic A52.01
  - thoracoabdominal I71.5
  - thorax, thoracic I71.1
  - transverse I71.1
  - traumatic — see Injury, aorta, laceration, major
  - valve or cusp (see also Endocarditis, aortic) I35.8
- appendix (with peritonitis) K35.2
- arteriovenous fistula, brain I60.8
- artery I77.2
  - brain — see Hemorrhage, intracranial, intracerebral
  - coronary — see Infarct, myocardium
  - heart — see Infarct, myocardium
  - pulmonary I28.8
  - traumatic (complication) — see Injury, blood vessel
- bile duct (common) (hepatic) K83.2
  - cystic K82.2
- bladder (sphincter) (nontraumatic) (spontaneous) N32.89
  - following ectopic or molar pregnancy O08.6
  - obstetrical trauma O71.5
  - traumatic S37.29 ☑
- blood vessel (see also Hemorrhage)
  - brain — see Hemorrhage, intracranial, intracerebral
  - heart — see Infarct, myocardium

Rupture, ruptured — continued
- blood vessel (see also Hemorrhage) — continued
  - traumatic (complication) — see Injury, blood vessel, laceration, major, by site
- bone — see Fracture
- bowel (nontraumatic) K63.1
- brain
  - aneurysm (congenital) (see also Hemorrhage, intracranial, subarachnoid)
    - syphilitic A52.05
  - hemorrhagic — see Hemorrhage, intracranial, intracerebral
- capillaries I78.8
- cardiac (auricle) (ventricle) (wall) I23.3
  - with hemopericardium I23.0
  - infectional I40.9
  - traumatic — see Injury, heart
- cartilage (articular) (current) (see also Sprain)
  - knee S83.3- ☑
  - semilunar — see Tear, meniscus
- cecum (with peritonitis) K65.0
  - with peritoneal abscess K35.3
  - traumatic S36.598 ☑
- celiac artery, traumatic — see Injury, blood vessel, celiac artery, laceration, major
- cerebral aneurysm (congenital) (see Hemorrhage, intracranial, subarachnoid)
- cervix (uteri)
  - with ectopic or molar pregnancy O08.6
  - following ectopic or molar pregnancy O08.6
  - obstetrical trauma O71.3
  - traumatic S37.69 ☑
- chordae tendineae NEC I51.1
  - concurrent with acute myocardial infarction — see Infarct, myocardium
  - following acute myocardial infarction (current complication) I23.4
- choroid (direct) (indirect) (traumatic) H31.32- ☑
- circle of Willis I60.6
- colon (nontraumatic) K63.1
  - traumatic — see Injury, intestine, large
- cornea (traumatic) — see Injury, eye, laceration
- coronary (artery) (thrombotic) — see Infarct, myocardium
- corpus luteum (infected) (ovary) N83.1
- cyst — see Cyst
- cystic duct K82.2
- Descemet's membrane — see Change, corneal membrane, Descemet's, rupture
  - traumatic — see Injury, eye, laceration
- diaphragm, traumatic — see Injury, intrathoracic, diaphragm
- disc — see Rupture, intervertebral disc
- diverticulum (intestine) K57.80
  - with bleeding K57.81
  - bladder N32.3
  - large intestine K57.20
    - with
      - bleeding K57.21
      - small intestine K57.40
        - with bleeding K57.41
  - small intestine K57.00
    - with
      - bleeding K57.01
      - large intestine K57.40
        - with bleeding K57.41
- duodenal stump K31.89
- ear drum (nontraumatic) (see also Perforation, tympanum)
  - traumatic S09.2- ☑
  - due to blast injury — see Injury, blast, ear
- esophagus K22.3
- eye (without prolapse or loss of intraocular tissue) — see Injury, eye, laceration
- fallopian tube NEC (nonobstetric) (nontraumatic) N83.8
  - due to pregnancy O00.1
- fontanel P13.1
- gallbladder K82.2
  - traumatic S36.128 ☑
- gastric (see also Rupture, stomach)
  - vessel K92.2
- globe (eye) (traumatic) — see Injury, eye, laceration
- graafian follicle (hematoma) N83.0
- heart — see Rupture, cardiac
- hymen (nontraumatic) (nonintentional) N89.8
- internal organ, traumatic — see Injury, by site

Rupture, ruptured — *continued*
- intervertebral disc — *see* Displacement, intervertebral disc
  - traumatic — *see* Rupture, traumatic, intervertebral disc
- intestine NEC (nontraumatic) K63.1
  - traumatic — *see* Injury, intestine
- iris (*see also* Abnormality, pupillary)
  - traumatic — *see* Injury, eye, laceration
- joint capsule, traumatic — *see* Sprain
- kidney (traumatic) S37.06- ☑
  - birth injury P15.8
  - nontraumatic N28.89
- lacrimal duct (traumatic) — *see* Injury, eye, specified site NEC
- lens (cataract) (traumatic) — *see* Cataract, traumatic
- ligament, traumatic — *see* Rupture, traumatic, ligament, by site
- liver S36.116 ☑
  - birth injury P15.0
- lymphatic vessel I89.8
- marginal sinus (placental) (with hemorrhage) — *see* Hemorrhage, antepartum, specified cause NEC
- membrana tympani (nontraumatic) — *see* Perforation, tympanum
- membranes (spontaneous)
  - artificial
    - delayed delivery following O75.5
  - delayed delivery following — *see* Pregnancy, complicated by, premature rupture of membranes
- meningeal artery I60.8
- meniscus (knee) (*see also* Tear, meniscus)
  - old — *see* Derangement, meniscus
  - site other than knee — *code as* Sprain
- mesenteric artery, traumatic — *see* Injury, mesenteric, artery, laceration, major
- mesentery (nontraumatic) K66.8
  - traumatic — *see* Injury, intra-abdominal, specified, site NEC
- mitral (valve) I34.8
- muscle (traumatic) (*see also* Strain)
  - diastasis — *see* Diastasis, muscle
  - nontraumatic M62.10
    - ankle M62.17- ☑
    - foot M62.17- ☑
    - forearm M62.13- ☑
    - hand M62.14- ☑
    - lower leg M62.16- ☑
    - pelvic region M62.15- ☑
    - shoulder region M62.11- ☑
    - specified site NEC M62.18
    - thigh M62.15- ☑
    - upper arm M62.12- ☑
  - traumatic — *see* Strain, by site
- musculotendinous junction NEC, nontraumatic — *see* Rupture, tendon, spontaneous
- mycotic aneurysm causing cerebral hemorrhage — *see* Hemorrhage, intracranial, subarachnoid
- myocardium, myocardial — *see* Rupture, cardiac
  - traumatic — *see* Injury, heart
- nontraumatic, meaning hernia — *see* Hernia
- obstructed — *see* Hernia, by site, obstructed
- operation wound — *see* Disruption, wound, operation
- ovary, ovarian N83.8
  - corpus luteum cyst N83.1
  - follicle (graafian) N83.0
- oviduct (nonobstetric) (nontraumatic) N83.8
  - due to pregnancy O00.1
- pancreas (nontraumatic) K86.8
  - traumatic S36.299 ☑
- papillary muscle NEC I51.2
  - following acute myocardial infarction (current complication) I23.5
- pelvic
  - floor, complicating delivery O70.1
  - organ NEC, obstetrical trauma O71.5
- perineum (nonobstetric) (nontraumatic) N90.89
  - complicating delivery — *see* Delivery, complicated, by, laceration, anus (sphincter)
- postoperative wound — *see* Disruption, wound, operation
- prostate (traumatic) S37.828 ☑
- pulmonary
  - artery I28.8
  - valve (heart) I37.8
  - vein I28.8

Rupture, ruptured — *continued*
- pulmonary — *continued*
  - vessel I28.8
- pus tube — *see* Salpingitis
- pyosalpinx — *see* Salpingitis
- rectum (nontraumatic) K63.1
  - traumatic S36.69
- retina, retinal (traumatic) (without detachment) (*see also* Break, retina)
  - with detachment — *see* Detachment, retina, with retinal, break
- rotator cuff (nontraumatic) M75.10- ☑
  - complete M75.12- ☑
  - incomplete M75.11- ☑
- sclera — *see* Injury, eye, laceration
- sigmoid (nontraumatic) K63.1
  - traumatic S36.593
- spinal cord (*see also* Injury, spinal cord, by region)
  - due to injury at birth P11.5
  - newborn (birth injury) P11.5
- spleen (traumatic) S36.09
  - birth injury P15.1
  - congenital (birth injury) P15.1
  - due to P. vivax malaria B51.0
  - nontraumatic D73.5
  - spontaneous D73.5
- splenic vein R58
  - traumatic — *see* Injury, blood vessel, splenic vein
- stomach (nontraumatic) (spontaneous) K31.89
  - traumatic S36.39
- suprasinatus (complete) (incomplete) (nontraumatic) — *see* Tear, rotator cuff
- symphysis pubis
  - obstetric O71.6
  - traumatic S33.4 ☑
- synovium (cyst) M66.10
  - ankle M66.17- ☑
  - elbow M66.12- ☑
  - finger M66.14- ☑
  - foot M66.17- ☑
  - forearm M66.13- ☑
  - hand M66.14- ☑
  - pelvic region M66.15- ☑
  - shoulder region M66.11- ☑
  - specified site NEC M66.18
  - thigh M66.15- ☑
  - toe M66.17- ☑
  - upper arm M66.12- ☑
  - wrist M66.13- ☑
- tendon (traumatic) — *see* Strain
  - nontraumatic (spontaneous) M66.9
    - ankle M66.87- ☑
    - extensor M66.20
      - ankle M66.27- ☑
      - foot M66.27- ☑
      - forearm M66.23- ☑
      - hand M66.24- ☑
      - lower leg M66.26- ☑
      - multiple sites M66.29
      - pelvic region M66.25- ☑
      - shoulder region M66.21- ☑
      - specified site NEC M66.28
      - thigh M66.25- ☑
      - upper arm M66.22- ☑
    - flexor M66.30
      - ankle M66.37- ☑
      - foot M66.37- ☑
      - forearm M66.33- ☑
      - hand M66.34- ☑
      - lower leg M66.36- ☑
      - multiple sites M66.39
      - pelvic region M66.35- ☑
      - shoulder region M66.31- ☑
      - specified site NEC M66.38
      - thigh M66.35- ☑
      - upper arm M66.32- ☑
    - foot M66.87- ☑
    - forearm M66.83- ☑
    - hand M66.84- ☑
    - lower leg M66.86- ☑
    - multiple sites M66.89
    - pelvic region M66.85- ☑
    - shoulder region M66.81- ☑
    - specified
      - site NEC M66.88
      - tendon M66.80

Rupture, ruptured — *continued*
- tendon — *see* Strain — *continued*
  - nontraumatic — *continued*
    - thigh M66.85- ☑
    - upper arm M66.82- ☑
- thoracic duct I89.8
- tonsil J35.8
- traumatic
  - aorta — *see* Injury, aorta, laceration, major
  - diaphragm — *see* Injury, intrathoracic, diaphragm
  - external site — *see* Wound, open, by site
  - eye — *see* Injury, eye, laceration
  - internal organ — *see* Injury, by site
  - intervertebral disc
    - cervical S13.0 ☑
    - lumbar S33.0 ☑
    - thoracic S23.0 ☑
  - kidney S37.06- ☑
  - ligament (*see also* Sprain)
    - ankle — *see* Sprain, ankle
    - carpus — *see* Rupture, traumatic, ligament, wrist
    - collateral (hand) — *see* Rupture, traumatic, ligament, finger, collateral
    - finger (metacarpophalangeal) (interphalangeal) S63.40- ☑
      - collateral S63.41- ☑
        - index S63.41- ☑
        - little S63.41- ☑
        - middle S63.41- ☑
        - ring S63.41- ☑
      - index S63.40- ☑
      - little S63.40- ☑
      - middle S63.40- ☑
      - palmar S63.42- ☑
        - index S63.42- ☑
        - little S63.42- ☑
        - middle S63.42- ☑
        - ring S63.42- ☑
      - ring S63.40- ☑
      - specified site NEC S63.499 ☑
        - index S63.49- ☑
        - little S63.49- ☑
        - middle S63.49- ☑
        - ring S63.49- ☑
      - volar plate S63.43- ☑
        - index S63.43- ☑
        - little S63.43- ☑
        - middle S63.43- ☑
        - ring S63.43- ☑
    - foot — *see* Sprain, foot
    - radial collateral S53.2- ☑
    - radiocarpal — *see* Rupture, traumatic, ligament, wrist, radiocarpal
    - ulnar collateral S53.3- ☑
    - ulnocarpal — *see* Rupture, traumatic, ligament, wrist, ulnocarpal
    - wrist S63.30- ☑
      - collateral S63.31- ☑
      - radiocarpal S63.32- ☑
      - specified site NEC S63.39- ☑
      - ulnocarpal (palmar) S63.33- ☑
  - liver S36.116 ☑
  - membrana tympani — *see* Rupture, ear drum, traumatic
  - muscle or tendon — *see* Strain
  - myocardium — *see* Injury, heart
  - pancreas S36.299 ☑
  - rectum S36.69 ☑
  - sigmoid S36.593 ☑
  - spleen S36.09 ☑
  - stomach S36.39 ☑
  - symphysis pubis S33.4 ☑
  - tympanum, tympanic (membrane) — *see* Rupture, ear drum, traumatic
  - ureter S37.19 ☑
  - uterus S37.69 ☑
  - vagina — *see* Injury, vagina
  - vena cava — *see* Injury, vena cava, laceration, major
- tricuspid (heart) (valve) I07.8
- tube, tubal (nonobstetric) (nontraumatic) N83.8
  - abscess — *see* Salpingitis
  - due to pregnancy O00.1

Rupture, ruptured — *continued*
tympanum, tympanic (membrane) (nontraumatic)
(*see also* Perforation, tympanic membrane)
H72.9- ☑
traumatic — *see* Rupture, ear drum, traumatic
umbilical cord, complicating delivery O69.89 ☑
ureter (traumatic) S37.19 ☑
nontraumatic N28.89
urethra (nontraumatic) N36.8
with ectopic or molar pregnancy O08.6
following ectopic or molar pregnancy O08.6
obstetrical trauma O71.5
traumatic S37.39 ☑
uterosacral ligament (nonobstetric) (nontraumatic)
N83.8
uterus (traumatic) S37.69 ☑
before labor O71.0- ☑
during or after labor O71.1
nonpuerperal, nontraumatic N85.8
pregnant (during labor) O71.1
before labor O71.0- ☑
vagina — *see* Injury, vagina
valve, valvular (heart) — *see* Endocarditis
varicose vein — *see* Varix
varix — *see* Varix
vena cava R58
traumatic — *see* Injury, vena cava, laceration, major
vesical (urinary) N32.89
vessel (blood) R58
pulmonary I28.8
traumatic — *see* Injury, blood vessel
viscus R19.8
vulva complicating delivery O70.0
Russell-Silver syndrome Q87.1
Russian spring-summer type encephalitis A84.0
Rust's disease (tuberculous cervical spondylitis) A18.01
Ruvalcaba-Myhre-Smith syndrome E71.440
Rytand-Lipsitch syndrome I44.2

S

Saber, sabre shin or tibia (syphilitic) A50.56 [M90.8-] ☑
Sac lacrimal — *see* condition
Saccharomyces infection B37.9
Saccharopinuria E72.3
Saccular — *see* condition
Sacculation
aorta (nonsyphilitic) — *see* Aneurysm, aorta
bladder N32.3
intralaryngeal (congenital) (ventricular) Q31.3
larynx (congenital) (ventricular) Q31.3
organ or site, congenital — *see* Distortion
pregnant uterus — *see* Pregnancy, complicated by,
abnormal, uterus
ureter N28.89
urethra N36.1
vesical N32.3
Sachs' amaurotic familial idiocy or disease E75.02
Sachs-Tay disease E75.02
Sacks-Libman disease M32.11
Sacralgia M53.3
Sacralization Q76.49
Sacrodynia M53.3
Sacroiliac joint — *see* condition
Sacroiliitis NEC M46.1
Sacrum — *see* condition
Saddle
back — *see* Lordosis
embolus
abdominal aorta I74.01
pulmonary artery I26.92
with acute cor pulmonale I26.02
injury — *code to* condition
nose M95.0
due to syphilis A50.57
Sadism (sexual) F65.52
Sadness, postpartal O90.6
Sadomasochism F65.50
Saemisch's ulcer (cornea) — *see* Ulcer, cornea, central
Sahib disease B55.0
Sailors' skin L57.8
Saint
Anthony's fire — *see* Erysipelas
triad — *see* Hernia, diaphragm
Vitus' dance — *see* Chorea, Sydenham's
Salaam
attack(s) — *see* Epilepsy, spasms

Salaam — *continued*
tic R25.8
Salicylism
abuse F55.8
overdose or wrong substance given — *see* Table of
Drugs and Chemicals, by drug, poisoning
Salivary duct or gland — *see* condition
Salivation, excessive K11.7
Salmonella — *see* Infection, Salmonella
Salmonellosis A02.0
Salpingitis (catarrhal) (fallopian tube) (nodular) (pseud-
ofollicular) (purulent) (septic) N70.91
with oophoritis N70.93
acute N70.01
with oophoritis N70.03
chlamydial A56.11
chronic N70.11
with oophoritis N70.13
complicating abortion — *see* Abortion, by type, complicated by, salpingitis
ear — *see* Salpingitis, eustachian
eustachian (tube) H68.00- ☑
acute H68.01- ☑
chronic H68.02- ☑
follicularis N70.11
with oophoritis N70.13
gonococcal (acute) (chronic) A54.24
interstitial, chronic N70.11
with oophoritis N70.13
isthmica nodosa N70.11
with oophoritis N70.13
specific (gonococcal) (acute) (chronic) A54.24
tuberculous (acute) (chronic) A18.17
venereal (gonococcal) (acute) (chronic) A54.24
Salpingocele N83.4
Salpingo-oophoritis (catarrhal) (purulent) (ruptured)
(septic) (suppurative) N70.93
acute N70.03
with ectopic or molar pregnancy O08.0
following ectopic or molar pregnancy O08.0
gonococcal A54.24
chronic N70.13
following ectopic or molar pregnancy O08.0
gonococcal (acute) (chronic) A54.24
puerperal O86.19
specific (gonococcal) (acute) (chronic) A54.24
subacute N70.03
tuberculous (acute) (chronic) A18.17
venereal (gonococcal) (acute) (chronic) A54.24
Salpingo-ovaritis — *see* Salpingo-oophoritis
Salpingoperitonitis — *see* Salpingo-oophoritis
Salzmann's nodular dystrophy — *see* Degeneration,
cornea, nodular
Sampson's cyst or tumor N80.1
San Joaquin (Valley) **fever** B38.0
Sandblaster's asthma, lung or pneumoconiosis J62.8
Sander's disease (paranoia) F22
Sandfly fever A93.1
Sandhoff's disease E75.01
Sanfilippo (Type B) (Type C) (Type D) **syndrome** E76.22
Sanger-Brown ataxia G11.2
Sao Paulo fever or typhus A77.0
Saponification, mesenteric K65.8
Sarcocele (benign)
syphilitic A52.76
congenital A50.59
Sarcocystosis A07.8
Sarcoepiplocele — *see* Hernia
Sarcoepiplomphalocele Q79.2
Sarcoid (*see also* Sarcoidosis)
arthropathy D86.86
Boeck's D86.9
Darier-Roussy D86.3
iridocyclitis D86.83
meningitis D86.81
myocarditis D86.85
myositis D86.87
pyelonephritis D86.84
Spiegler-Fendt L08.89
Sarcoidosis D86.9
with
cranial nerve palsies D86.82
hepatic granuloma D86.89
polyarthritis D86.86
tubulo-interstitial nephropathy D86.84
combined sites NEC D86.89
lung D86.0

Sarcoidosis — *continued*
lung — *continued*
and lymph nodes D86.2
lymph nodes D86.1
and lung D86.2
meninges D86.81
skin D86.3
specified type NEC D86.89
Sarcoma (of) (*see also* Neoplasm, connective tissue, malignant)
alveolar soft part — *see* Neoplasm, connective tissue,
malignant
ameloblastic C41.1
upper jaw (bone) C41.0
botryoid — *see* Neoplasm, connective tissue, malignant
botryoides — *see* Neoplasm, connective tissue, malignant
cerebellar C71.6
circumscribed (arachnoidal) C71.6
circumscribed (arachnoidal) cerebellar C71.6
clear cell (*see also* Neoplasm, connective tissue, malignant)
kidney C64.- ☑
dendritic cells (accessory cells) C96.4
embryonal — *see* Neoplasm, connective tissue, malignant
endometrial (stromal) C54.1
isthmus C54.0
epithelioid (cell) — *see* Neoplasm, connective tissue,
malignant
Ewing's — *see* Neoplasm, bone, malignant
follicular dendritic cell C96.4
germinoblastic (diffuse) — *see* Lymphoma, diffuse
large cell
follicular — *see* Lymphoma, follicular, specified
NEC
giant cell (except of bone) (*see also* Neoplasm, connective tissue, malignant)
bone — *see* Neoplasm, bone, malignant
glomoid — *see* Neoplasm, connective tissue, malignant
granulocytic C92.3- ☑
hemangioendothelial — *see* Neoplasm, connective
tissue, malignant
hemorrhagic, multiple — *see* Sarcoma, Kaposi's
histiocytic C96.A (*following* C96.6)
Hodgkin — *see* Lymphoma, Hodgkin
immunoblastic (diffuse) — *see* Lymphoma, diffuse
large cell
interdigitating dendritic cell C96.4
Kaposi's
colon C46.4
connective tissue C46.1
gastrointestinal organ C46.4
lung C46.5- ☑
lymph node(s) C46.3
palate (hard) (soft) C46.2
rectum C46.4
skin C46.0
specified site NEC C46.7
stomach C46.4
unspecified site C46.9
Kupffer cell C22.3
Langerhans cell C96.4
leptomeningeal — *see* Neoplasm, meninges, malignant
liver NEC C22.4
lymphangioendothelial — *see* Neoplasm, connective
tissue, malignant
lymphoblastic — *see* Lymphoma, lymphoblastic (diffuse)
lymphocytic — *see* Lymphoma, small cell B-cell
mast cell C96.2
melanotic — *see* Melanoma
meningeal — *see* Neoplasm, meninges, malignant
meningothelial — *see* Neoplasm, meninges, malignant
mesenchymal (*see also* Neoplasm, connective tissue,
malignant)
mixed — *see* Neoplasm, connective tissue, malignant
mesothelial — *see* Mesothelioma
monstrocellular
specified site — *see* Neoplasm, malignant, by site
unspecified site C71.9
myeloid C92.3- ☑
neurogenic — *see* Neoplasm, nerve, malignant

Sarcoma — *continued*
  odontogenic C41.1
    upper jaw (bone) C41.0
  osteoblastic — *see* Neoplasm, bone, malignant
  osteogenic (*see also* Neoplasm, bone, malignant)
    juxtacortical — *see* Neoplasm, bone, malignant
    periosteal — *see* Neoplasm, bone, malignant
  periosteal (*see also* Neoplasm, bone, malignant)
    osteogenic — *see* Neoplasm, bone, malignant
  pleomorphic cell — *see* Neoplasm, connective tissue, malignant
  reticulum cell (diffuse) — *see* Lymphoma, diffuse large cell
    nodular — *see* Lymphoma, follicular
    pleomorphic cell type — *see* Lymphoma, diffuse large cell
  rhabdoid — *see* Neoplasm, malignant, by site
  round cell — *see* Neoplasm, connective tissue, malignant
  small cell — *see* Neoplasm, connective tissue, malignant
  soft tissue — *see* Neoplasm, connective tissue, malignant
  spindle cell — *see* Neoplasm, connective tissue, malignant
  stromal (endometrial) C54.1
    isthmus C54.0
  synovial (*see also* Neoplasm, connective tissue, malignant)
    biphasic — *see* Neoplasm, connective tissue, malignant
    epithelioid cell — *see* Neoplasm, connective tissue, malignant
    spindle cell — *see* Neoplasm, connective tissue, malignant
Sarcomatosis
  meningeal — *see* Neoplasm, meninges, malignant
  specified site NEC — *see* Neoplasm, connective tissue, malignant
  unspecified site C80.1
Sarcosinemia E72.59
Sarcosporidiosis (intestinal) A07.8
Satiety, early R68.81
Saturnine — *see* condition
Saturnism
  overdose or wrong substance given or taken — *see* Table of Drugs and Chemicals, by drug, poisoning
Satyriasis F52.8
Sauriasis — *see* Ichthyosis
SBE (subacute bacterial endocarditis) I33.0
Scabies (any site) B86
Scabs R23.4
Scaglietti-Dagnini syndrome E22.0
Scald — *see* Burn
Scalenus anticus (anterior) **syndrome** G54.0
Scales R23.4
Scaling, skin R23.4
Scalp — *see* condition
Scapegoating affecting child Z62.3
Scaphocephaly Q75.0
Scapulalgia M89.8X1
Scapulohumeral myopathy G71.0
Scar, scarring (*see also* Cicatrix) L90.5
  adherent L90.5
  atrophic L90.5
  cervix
    in pregnancy or childbirth — *see* Pregnancy, complicated by, abnormal cervix
  cheloid L91.0
  chorioretinal H31.00- ☑
    posterior pole macula H31.01- ☑
    postsurgical H59.81- ☑
    solar retinopathy H31.02- ☑
    specified type NEC H31.09- ☑
  choroid — *see* Scar, chorioretinal
  conjunctiva H11.24- ☑
  cornea H17.9
    xerophthalmic (*see also* Opacity, cornea)
      vitamin A deficiency E50.6
  duodenum, obstructive K31.5
  hypertrophic L91.0
  keloid L91.0
  labia N90.89
  lung (base) J98.4
  macula — *see* Scar, chorioretinal, posterior pole
  muscle M62.89

Scar, scarring — *continued*
  myocardium, myocardial I25.2
  painful L90.5
  posterior pole (eye) — *see* Scar, chorioretinal, posterior pole
  retina — *see* Scar, chorioretinal
  trachea J39.8
  uterus N85.8
    in pregnancy O34.29
  vagina N89.8
    postoperative N99.2
  vulva N90.89
Scarabiasis B88.2
Scarlatina (anginosa) (maligna) (ulcerosa) A38.9
  myocarditis (acute) A38.1
    old — *see* Myocarditis
  otitis media A38.0
Scarlet fever (albuminuria) (angina) A38.9
Schamberg's disease (progressive pigmentary dermatosis) L81.7
Schatzki's ring (acquired) (esophagus) (lower) K22.2
  congenital Q39.3
Schaufenster krankheit I20.8
Schaumann's
  benign lymphogranulomatosis D86.1
  disease or syndrome — *see* Sarcoidosis
Scheie's syndrome E76.03
Schenck's disease B42.1
Scheuermann's disease or osteochondrosis — *see* Osteochondrosis, juvenile, spine
Schilder (-Flatau) **disease** G37.0
Schilling-type monocytic leukemia C93.0- ☑
Schimmelbusch's disease, cystic mastitis, or hyperplasia — *see* Mastopathy, cystic
Schistosoma infestation — *see* Infestation, Schistosoma
Schistosomiasis B65.9
  with muscle disorder B65.9 [M63.80]
    ankle B65.9 [M63.87-] ☑
    foot B65.9 [M63.87-] ☑
    forearm B65.9 [M63.83-] ☑
    hand B65.9 [M63.84-] ☑
    lower leg B65.9 [M63.86-] ☑
    multiple sites B65.9 [M63.89]
    pelvic region B65.9 [M63.85-] ☑
    shoulder region B65.9 [M63.81-] ☑
    specified site NEC B65.9 [M63.88]
    thigh B65.9 [M63.85-] ☑
    upper arm B65.9 [M63.82-] ☑
  Asiatic B65.2
  bladder B65.0
  chestermani B65.8
  colon B65.1
  cutaneous B65.3
  due to
    S. haematobium B65.0
    S. japonicum B65.2
    S. mansoni B65.1
    S. mattheii B65.8
  Eastern B65.2
  genitourinary tract B65.0
  intestinal B65.1
  lung NEC B65.9 [J99]
    pneumonia B65.9 [J17]
  Manson's (intestinal) B65.1
  oriental B65.2
  pulmonary NEC B65.9 [J99]
    pneumonia B65.9
  Schistosoma
    haematobium B65.0
    japonicum B65.2
    mansoni B65.1
  specified type NEC B65.8
  urinary B65.0
  vesical B65.0
Schizencephaly Q04.6
Schizoaffective psychosis F25.9
Schizodontia K00.2
Schizoid personality F60.1
Schizophrenia, schizophrenic F20.9
  acute (brief) (undifferentiated) F23
  atypical (form) F20.3
  borderline F21
  catalepsy F20.2
  catatonic (type) (excited) (withdrawn) F20.2
  cenesthopathic, cenesthesiopathic F20.89
  childhood type F84.5
  chronic undifferentiated F20.5

Schizophrenia, schizophrenic — *continued*
  cyclic F25.0
  disorganized (type) F20.1
  flexibilitas cerea F20.2
  hebephrenic (type) F20.1
  incipient F21
  latent F21
  negative type F20.5
  paranoid (type) F20.0
  paraphrenic F20.0
  post-psychotic depression F32.8
  prepsychotic F21
  prodromal F21
  pseudoneurotic F21
  pseudopsychopathic F21
  reaction F23
  residual (state) (type) F20.5
  restzustand F20.5
  schizoaffective (type) — *see* Psychosis, schizoaffective
  simple (type) F20.89
  simplex F20.89
  specified type NEC F20.89
  stupor F20.2
  syndrome of childhood F84.5
  undifferentiated (type) F20.3
    chronic F20.5
Schizothymia (persistent) F60.1
Schlatter-Osgood disease or osteochondrosis — *see* Osteochondrosis, juvenile, tibia
Schlatter's tibia — *see* Osteochondrosis, juvenile, tibia
Schmidt's syndrome (polyglandular, autoimmune) E31.0
Schmincke's carcinoma or tumor — *see* Neoplasm, nasopharynx, malignant
Schmitz (-Stutzer) **dysentery** A03.0
Schmorl's disease or nodes
  lumbar region M51.46
  lumbosacral region M51.47
  sacrococcygeal region M53.3
  thoracic region M51.44
  thoracolumbar region M51.45
Schneiderian
  papilloma — *see* Neoplasm, nasopharynx, benign
    specified site — *see* Neoplasm, benign, by site
    unspecified site D14.0
  specified site — *see* Neoplasm, malignant, by site
    unspecified site C30.0
Scholte's syndrome (malignant carcinoid) E34.0
Scholz (-Bielchowsky-Henneberg) **disease or syndrome** E75.25
Schönlein (-Henoch) disease or purpura (primary) (rheumatic) D69.0
Schottmuller's disease A01.4
Schroeder's syndrome (endocrine hypertensive) E27.0
Schüller-Christian disease or syndrome C96.5
Schultze's type acroparesthesia, simple I73.89
Schultz's disease or syndrome — *see* Agranulocytosis
Schwalbe-Ziehen-Oppenheim disease G24.1
Schwannoma (*see also* Neoplasm, nerve, benign)
  malignant (*see also* Neoplasm, nerve, malignant)
    with rhabdomyoblastic differentiation — *see* Neoplasm, nerve, malignant
  melanocytic — *see* Neoplasm, nerve, benign
  pigmented — *see* Neoplasm, nerve, benign
Schwannomatosis Q85.03
Schwartz (-Jampel) **syndrome** G71.13
Schwartz-Bartter syndrome E22.2
Schweniger-Buzzi anetoderma L90.1
Sciatic — *see* condition
Sciatica (infective)
  with lumbago M54.4- ☑
    due to intervertebral disc disorder — *see* Disorder, disc, with, radiculopathy
  due to displacement of intervertebral disc (with lumbago) — *see* Disorder, disc, with, radiculopathy
  wallet M54.3- ☑
Scimitar syndrome Q26.8
Sclera — *see* condition
Sclerectasia H15.84- ☑
Scleredema
  adultorum — *see* Sclerosis, systemic
  Buschke's — *see* Sclerosis, systemic
  newborn P83.0
Sclerema (adiposum) (edematosum) (neonatorum) (newborn) P83.0
  adultorum — *see* Sclerosis, systemic
Scleriasis — *see* Scleroderma
Scleritis H15.00- ☑

Scleritis — *continued*
  with corneal involvement H15.04- ✔
    anterior H15.01- ✔
    brawny H15.02- ✔
    in (due to) zoster B02.34
    posterior H15.03- ✔
    specified type NEC H15.09- ✔
  syphilitic A52.71
  tuberculous (nodular) A18.51
Sclerochoroiditis H31.8
Scleroconjunctivitis — *see* Scleritis
Sclerocystic ovary syndrome E28.2
Sclerodactyly, sclerodactylia L94.3
Scleroderma, sclerodermia (acrosclerotic) (diffuse)
      (generalized) (progressive) (pulmonary) (*see also*
      Sclerosis, systemic) M34.9
  circumscribed L94.0
  linear L94.1
  localized L94.0
  newborn P83.8
  systemic M34.9
Sclerokeratitis H16.8
  tuberculous A18.52
Scleroma nasi A48.8
Scleromalacia (perforans) H15.05- ✔
Scleromyxedema L98.5
Sclérose en plaques G35
Sclerosis, sclerotic
  adrenal (gland) E27.8
  Alzheimer's — *see* Disease, Alzheimer's
  amyotrophic (lateral) G12.21
  aorta, aortic I70.0
    valve — *see* Endocarditis, aortic
  artery, arterial, arteriolar, arteriovascular — *see* Arteriosclerosis
  ascending multiple G35
  brain (generalized) (lobular) G37.9
    artery, arterial I67.2
    diffuse G37.0
    disseminated G35
    insular G35
    Krabbe's E75.23
    miliary G35
    multiple G35
    presenile (Alzheimer's) — *see* Disease, Alzheimer's, early onset
    senile (arteriosclerotic) I67.2
    stem, multiple G35
    tuberous Q85.1
  bulbar, multiple G35
  bundle of His I44.39
  cardiac — *see* Disease, heart, ischemic, atherosclerotic
  cardiorenal — *see* Hypertension, cardiorenal
  cardiovascular (*see also* Disease, cardiovascular)
    renal — *see* Hypertension, cardiorenal
  cerebellar — *see* Sclerosis, brain
  cerebral — *see* Sclerosis, brain
  cerebrospinal (disseminated) (multiple) G35
  cerebrovascular I67.2
  choroid — *see* Degeneration, choroid
  combined (spinal cord) (*see also* Degeneration, combined)
    multiple G35
  concentric (Balo) G37.5
  cornea — *see* Opacity, cornea
  coronary (artery) I25.10
    with angina pectoris — *see* Arteriosclerosis, coronary (artery),
  corpus cavernosum
    female N90.89
    male N48.6
  diffuse (brain) (spinal cord) G37.0
  disseminated G35
  dorsal G35
  dorsolateral (spinal cord) — *see* Degeneration, combined
  endometrium N85.5
  extrapyramidal G25.9
  eye, nuclear (senile) — *see* Cataract, senile, nuclear
  focal and segmental (glomerular) (*see also* N00-N07 with fourth character .1) N05.1
  Friedreich's (spinal cord) G11.1
  funicular (spermatic cord) N50.8
  general (vascular) — *see* Arteriosclerosis
  gland (lymphatic) I89.8
  hepatic K74.1
    alcoholic K70.2

Sclerosis, sclerotic — *continued*
  hereditary
    cerebellar G11.9
    spinal (Friedreich's ataxia) G11.1
  hippocampal G93.81
  insular G35
  kidney — *see* Sclerosis, renal
  larynx J38.7
  lateral (amyotrophic) (descending) (primary) (spinal) G12.21
  lens, senile nuclear — *see* Cataract, senile, nuclear
  liver K74.1
    with fibrosis K74.2
      alcoholic K70.2
    alcoholic K70.2
    cardiac K76.1
  lung — *see* Fibrosis, lung
  mastoid — *see* Mastoiditis, chronic
  mesial temporal G93.81
  mitral I05.8
  Mönckeberg's (medial) — *see* Arteriosclerosis, extremities
  multiple (brain stem) (cerebral) (generalized) (spinal cord) G35
  myocardium, myocardial — *see* Disease, heart, ischemic, atherosclerotic
  nuclear (senile), eye — *see* Cataract, senile, nuclear
  ovary N83.8
  pancreas K86.8
  penis N48.6
  peripheral arteries — *see* Arteriosclerosis, extremities
  plaques G35
  pluriglandular E31.8
  polyglandular E31.8
  posterolateral (spinal cord) — *see* Degeneration, combined
  presenile (Alzheimer's) — *see* Disease, Alzheimer's, early onset
  primary, lateral G12.29
  progressive, systemic M34.0
  pulmonary — *see* Fibrosis, lung
    artery I27.0
    valve (heart) — *see* Endocarditis, pulmonary
  renal N26.9
    with
      cystine storage disease E72.09
      hypertensive heart disease (conditions in I11) — *see* Hypertension, cardiorenal
      arteriolar (hyaline) (hyperplastic) — *see* Hypertension, kidney
  retina (senile) (vascular) H35.00
  senile (vascular) — *see* Arteriosclerosis
  spinal (cord) (progressive) G95.89
    ascending G61.0
    combined (*see also* Degeneration, combined)
      multiple G35
      syphilitic A52.11
    disseminated G35
    dorsolateral — *see* Degeneration, combined
    hereditary (Friedreich's) (mixed form) G11.1
    lateral (amyotrophic) G12.21
    multiple G35
    posterior (syphilitic) A52.11
  stomach K31.89
  subendocardial, congenital I42.4
  systemic M34.9
    with
      lung involvement M34.81
      myopathy M34.82
      polyneuropathy M34.83
    drug-induced M34.2
    due to chemicals NEC M34.2
    progressive M34.0
    specified NEC M34.89
  temporal (mesial) G93.81
  tricuspid (heart) (valve) I07.8
  tuberous (brain) Q85.1
  tympanic membrane — *see* Disorder, tympanic membrane, specified NEC
  valve, valvular (heart) — *see* Endocarditis
  vascular — *see* Arteriosclerosis
  vein I87.8
Scoliosis (acquired) (postural) M41.9
  adolescent (idiopathic) — *see* Scoliosis, idiopathic, juvenile
  congenital Q67.5
    due to bony malformation Q76.3
    failure of segmentation (hemivertebra) Q76.3

Scoliosis — *continued*
  congenital — *continued*
    hemivertebra fusion Q76.3
    postural Q67.5
  idiopathic M41.20
    adolescent M41.129
      cervical region M41.122
      cervicothoracic region M41.123
      lumbar region M41.126
      lumbosacral region M41.127
      thoracic region M41.124
      thoracolumbar region M41.125
    cervical region M41.22
    cervicothoracic region M41.23
    infantile M41.00
      cervical region M41.02
      cervicothoracic region M41.03
      lumbar region M41.06
      lumbosacral region M41.07
      sacrococcygeal region M41.08
      thoracic region M41.04
      thoracolumbar region M41.05
    juvenile M41.119
      cervical region M41.112
      cervicothoracic region M41.113
      lumbar region M41.116
      lumbosacral region M41.117
      thoracic region M41.114
      thoracolumbar region M41.115
    lumbar region M41.26
    lumbosacral region M41.27
    thoracic region M41.24
    thoracolumbar region M41.25
  neuromuscular M41.40
    cervical region M41.42
    cervicothoracic region M41.43
    lumbar region M41.46
    lumbosacral region M41.47
    occipito-atlanto-axial region M41.41
    thoracic region M41.44
    thoracolumbar region M41.45
  paralytic — *see* Scoliosis, neuromuscular
  postradiation therapy M96.5
  rachitic (late effect or sequelae) E64.3 [M49.80]
    cervical region E64.3 [M49.82]
    cervicothoracic region E64.3 [M49.83]
    lumbar region E64.3 [M49.86]
    lumbosacral region E64.3 [M49.87]
    multiple sites E64.3 [M49.89]
    occipito-atlanto-axial region E64.3 [M49.81]
    sacrococcygeal region E64.3 [M49.88]
    thoracic region E64.3 [M49.84]
    thoracolumbar region E64.3 [M49.85]
  sciatic M54.4- ✔
  secondary (to) NEC M41.50
    cerebral palsy, Friedreich's ataxia, poliomyelitis, neuromuscular disorders — *see* Scoliosis, neuromuscular
    cervical region M41.52
    cervicothoracic region M41.53
    lumbar region M41.56
    lumbosacral region M41.57
    thoracic region M41.54
    thoracolumbar region M41.55
  specified form NEC M41.80
    cervical region M41.82
    cervicothoracic region M41.83
    lumbar region M41.86
    lumbosacral region M41.87
    thoracic region M41.84
    thoracolumbar region M41.85
  thoracogenic M41.30
    thoracic region M41.34
    thoracolumbar region M41.35
  tuberculous A18.01
Scoliotic pelvis
  with disproportion (fetopelvic) O33.0
    causing obstructed labor O65.0
Scorbutus, scorbutic (*see also* Scurvy)
  anemia D53.2
Scotoma (arcuate) (Bjerrum) (central) (ring) (*see also* Defect, visual field, localized, scotoma)
  scintillating H53.19
Scratch — *see* Abrasion
Scratchy throat R09.89
Screening (for) Z13.9
  alcoholism Z13.89
  anemia Z13.0

Screening — continued
anomaly, congenital Z13.89
antenatal, of mother Z36
arterial hypertension Z13.6
arthropod-borne viral disease NEC Z11.59
bacteriuria, asymptomatic Z13.89
behavioral disorder Z13.89
brain injury, traumatic Z13.850
bronchitis, chronic Z13.83
brucellosis Z11.2
cardiovascular disorder Z13.6
cataract Z13.5
chlamydial diseases Z11.8
cholera Z11.0
chromosomal abnormalities (nonprocreative) NEC
    Z13.79
colonoscopy Z12.11
congenital
    dislocation of hip Z13.89
    eye disorder Z13.5
    malformation or deformation Z13.89
contamination NEC Z13.88
cystic fibrosis Z13.228
dengue fever Z11.59
dental disorder Z13.84
depression Z13.89
developmental handicap Z13.4
    in early childhood Z13.4
diabetes mellitus Z13.1
diphtheria Z11.2
disability, intellectual Z13.4
disease or disorder Z13.9
    bacterial NEC Z11.2
        intestinal infectious Z11.0
        respiratory tuberculosis Z11.1
    blood or blood-forming organ Z13.0
    cardiovascular Z13.6
    Chagas' Z11.6
    chlamydial Z11.8
    dental Z13.89
    developmental Z13.4
    digestive tract NEC Z13.818
        lower GI Z13.811
        upper GI Z13.810
    ear Z13.5
    endocrine Z13.29
    eye Z13.5
    genitourinary Z13.89
    heart Z13.6
    human immunodeficiency virus (HIV) infection
        Z11.4
    immunity Z13.0
    infection
        intestinal Z11.0
            specified NEC Z11.6
    infectious Z11.9
    mental Z13.89
    metabolic Z13.228
    neurological Z13.89
    nutritional Z13.21
        metabolic Z13.228
            lipoid disorders Z13.220
    protozoal Z11.6
        intestinal Z11.0
    respiratory Z13.83
    rheumatic Z13.828
    rickettsial Z11.8
    sexually-transmitted NEC Z11.3
        human immunodeficiency virus (HIV) Z11.4
    sickle-cell (trait) Z13.0
    skin Z13.89
    specified NEC Z13.89
    spirochetal Z11.8
    thyroid Z13.29
    vascular Z13.6
    venereal Z11.3
    viral NEC Z11.59
        human immunodeficiency virus (HIV) Z11.4
        intestinal Z11.0
elevated titer Z13.89
emphysema Z13.83
encephalitis, viral (mosquito- or tick-borne) Z11.59
exposure to contaminants (toxic) Z13.88
fever
    dengue Z11.59
    hemorrhagic Z11.59
    yellow Z11.59
filariasis Z11.6

Screening — continued
galactosemia Z13.228
gastrointestinal condition Z13.818
genetic (nonprocreative) - for procreative management — see Testing, genetic, for procreative management
    disease carrier status (nonprocreative) Z13.71
    specified NEC (nonprocreative) Z13.79
genitourinary condition Z13.89
glaucoma Z13.5
gonorrhea Z11.3
gout Z13.89
helminthiasis (intestinal) Z11.6
hematopoietic malignancy Z12.89
hemoglobinopathies NEC Z13.0
hemorrhagic fever Z11.59
Hodgkin disease Z12.89
human immunodeficiency virus (HIV) Z11.4
human papillomavirus Z11.51
hypertension Z13.6
immunity disorders Z13.0
infection
    mycotic Z11.8
    parasitic Z11.8
ingestion of radioactive substance Z13.88
intellectual disability Z13.4
intestinal
    helminthiasis Z11.6
    infectious disease Z11.0
leishmaniasis Z11.6
leprosy Z11.2
leptospirosis Z11.8
leukemia Z12.89
lymphoma Z12.89
malaria Z11.6
malnutrition Z13.29
    metabolic Z13.228
    nutritional Z13.21
measles Z11.59
mental disorder Z13.89
metabolic errors, inborn Z13.228
multiphasic Z13.89
musculoskeletal disorder Z13.828
    osteoporosis Z13.820
mycoses Z11.8
myocardial infarction (acute) Z13.6
neoplasm (malignant) (of) Z12.9
    bladder Z12.6
    blood Z12.89
    breast Z12.39
        routine mammogram Z12.31
    cervix Z12.4
    colon Z12.11
    genitourinary organs NEC Z12.79
        bladder Z12.6
        cervix Z12.4
        ovary Z12.73
        prostate Z12.5
        testis Z12.71
        vagina Z12.72
    hematopoietic system Z12.89
    intestinal tract Z12.10
        colon Z12.11
        rectum Z12.12
        small intestine Z12.13
    lung Z12.2
    lymph (glands) Z12.89
    nervous system Z12.82
    oral cavity Z12.81
    prostate Z12.5
    rectum Z12.12
    respiratory organs Z12.2
    skin Z12.83
    small intestine Z12.13
    specified site NEC Z12.89
    stomach Z12.0
nephropathy Z13.89
nervous system disorders NEC Z13.858
neurological condition Z13.89
osteoporosis Z13.820
parasitic infestation Z11.9
    specified NEC Z11.8
phenylketonuria Z13.228
plague Z11.8
poisoning (chemical) (heavy metal) Z13.88
poliomyelitis Z11.59
postnatal, chromosomal abnormalities Z13.89
prenatal, of mother Z36

Screening — continued
protozoal disease Z11.6
    intestinal Z11.0
pulmonary tuberculosis Z11.1
radiation exposure Z13.88
respiratory condition Z13.83
respiratory tuberculosis Z11.1
rheumatoid arthritis Z13.828
rubella Z11.59
schistosomiasis Z11.6
sexually-transmitted disease NEC Z11.3
    human immunodeficiency virus (HIV) Z11.4
sickle-cell disease or trait Z13.0
skin condition Z13.89
sleeping sickness Z11.6
special Z13.9
    specified NEC Z13.89
syphilis Z11.3
tetanus Z11.2
trachoma Z11.8
traumatic brain injury Z13.850
trypanosomiasis Z11.6
tuberculosis, respiratory Z11.1
venereal disease Z11.3
viral encephalitis (mosquito- or tick-borne) Z11.59
whooping cough Z11.2
worms, intestinal Z11.6
yaws Z11.8
yellow fever Z11.59
Scrofula, scrofulosis (tuberculosis of cervical lymph
    glands) A18.2
Scrofulide (primary) (tuberculous) A18.4
Scrofuloderma, scrofulodermia (any site) (primary)
    A18.4
Scrofulosus lichen (primary) (tuberculous) A18.4
Scrofulous — see condition
Scrotal tongue K14.5
Scrotum — see condition
Scurvy, scorbutic E54
    anemia D53.2
    gum E54
    infantile E54
    rickets E55.0 [M90.80]
Sealpox B08.62
Seasickness T75.3 ☑
Seatworm (infection) (infestation) B80
Sebaceous (see also condition)
    cyst — see Cyst, sebaceous
Seborrhea, seborrheic L21.9
    capillitii R23.8
    capitis L21.0
    dermatitis L21.9
        infantile L21.1
    eczema L21.9
        infantile L21.1
    sicca L21.0
Seckel's syndrome Q87.1
Seclusion, pupil — see Membrane, pupillary
Second hand tobacco smoke exposure (acute)
    (chronic) Z77.22
    in the perinatal period P96.81
Secondary
    dentin (in pulp) K04.3
    neoplasm, secondaries — see Table of Neoplasms,
        secondary
Secretion
    antidiuretic hormone, inappropriate E22.2
    catecholamine, by pheochromocytoma E27.5
    hormone
        antidiuretic, inappropriate (syndrome) E22.2
        by
            carcinoid tumor E34.0
            pheochromocytoma E27.5
        ectopic NEC E34.2
    urinary
        excessive R35.8
        suppression R34
Section
    nerve, traumatic — see Injury, nerve
Segmentation, incomplete (congenital) (see also Fusion)
    bone NEC Q78.8
    lumbosacral (joint) (vertebra) Q76.49
Seitelberger's syndrome (infantile neuraxonal dystrophy) G31.89
Seizure(s) (see also Convulsions) R56.9
    akinetic — see Epilepsy, generalized, specified NEC
    atonic — see Epilepsy, generalized, specified NEC

☑ Additional Character Required — Refer to the Tabular List for Character Selection   ▽ Subterms under main terms may continue to next column or page

Index

Seizure(s) — Septic

Seizure(s) — continued
autonomic (hysterical) F44.5
convulsive — see Convulsions
cortical (focal) (motor) — see Epilepsy, localization-
related, symptomatic, with simple partial
seizures
disorder (see also Epilepsy) G40.909
due to stroke — see Sequelae (of), disease, cerebrovascular, by type, specified NEC
epileptic — see Epilepsy
febrile (simple) R56.00
with status epilepticus G40.901
complex (atypical) (complicated) R56.01
with status epilepticus G40.901
grand mal G40.409
intractable G40.419
with status epilepticus G40.411
without status epilepticus G40.419
not intractable G40.409
with status epilepticus G40.401
without status epilepticus G40.409
heart — see Disease, heart
hysterical F44.5
intractable G40.919
with status epilepticus G40.911
Jacksonian (focal) (motor type) (sensory type) — see
Epilepsy, localization-related, symptomatic, with
simple partial seizures
newborn P90
nonspecific epileptic
atonic — see Epilepsy, generalized, specified NEC
clonic — see Epilepsy, generalized, specified NEC
myoclonic — see Epilepsy, generalized, specified
NEC
tonic — see Epilepsy, generalized, specified NEC
tonic-clonic — see Epilepsy, generalized, specified
NEC
partial, developing into secondarily generalized
seizures
complex — see Epilepsy, localization-related,
symptomatic, with complex partial seizures
simple — see Epilepsy, localization-related, symptomatic, with simple partial seizures
petit mal G40.409
intractable G40.419
with status epilepticus G40.411
without status epilepticus G40.419
not intractable G40.409
with status epilepticus G40.401
without status epilepticus G40.409
post traumatic R56.1
recurrent G40.909
specified NEC G40.89
uncinate — see Epilepsy, localization-related, symptomatic, with complex partial seizures
Selenium deficiency, dietary E59
Self-damaging behavior (life-style) Z72.89
Self-harm (attempted)
history (personal) Z91.5
in family Z81.8
Self-mutilation (attempted)
history (personal) Z91.5
in family Z81.8
Self-poisoning
history (personal) Z91.5
in family Z81.8
observation following (alleged) attempt Z03.6
Semicoma R40.1
Seminal vesiculitis N49.0
Seminoma C62.9- ☑
specified site — see Neoplasm, malignant, by site
Senear-Usher disease or syndrome L10.4
Senectus R54
Senescence (without mention of psychosis) R54
Senile, senility (see also condition) R41.81
with
acute confusional state F05
mental changes NOS F03 ☑
psychosis NEC — see Psychosis, senile
asthenia R54
cervix (atrophic) N88.8
debility R54
endometrium (atrophic) N85.8
fallopian tube (atrophic) — see Atrophy, fallopian tube
heart (failure) R54
ovary (atrophic) — see Atrophy, ovary
premature E34.8

Senile, senility — continued
vagina, vaginitis (atrophic) N95.2
wart L82.1
Sensation
burning (skin) R20.8
tongue K14.6
loss of R20.8
prickling (skin) R20.2
tingling (skin) R20.2
Sense loss
smell — see Disturbance, sensation, smell
taste — see Disturbance, sensation, taste
touch R20.8
Sensibility disturbance (cortical) (deep) (vibratory)
R20.9
Sensitive, sensitivity (see also Allergy)
carotid sinus G90.01
child (excessive) F93.8
cold, autoimmune D59.1
dentin K03.89
latex Z91.040
methemoglobin D74.8
tuberculin, without clinical or radiological symptoms
R76.11
visual
glare H53.71
impaired contrast H53.72
Sensitiver Beziehungswahn F22
Sensitization, auto-erythrocytic D69.2
Separation
anxiety, abnormal (of childhood) F93.0
apophysis, traumatic — code as Fracture, by site
choroid — see Detachment, choroid
epiphysis, epiphyseal
nontraumatic (see also Osteochondropathy, specified type NEC)
upper femoral — see Slipped, epiphysis, upper
femoral
traumatic — code as Fracture, by site
fracture — see Fracture
infundibulum cardiac from right ventricle by a partition
Q24.3
joint (traumatic) (current) — code by site under Dislocation
pubic bone, obstetrical trauma O71.6
retina, retinal — see Detachment, retina
symphysis pubis, obstetrical trauma O71.6
tracheal ring, incomplete, congenital Q32.1
Sepsis (generalized) (unspecified organism) A41.9
with
organ dysfunction (acute) (multiple) R65.20
with septic shock R65.21
actinomycotic A42.7
adrenal hemorrhage syndrome (meningococcal) A39.1
anaerobic A41.4
Bacillus anthracis A22.7
Brucella (see also Brucellosis) A23.9
candidal B37.7
cryptogenic A41.9
due to device, implant or graft T85.79 ☑
arterial graft NEC T82.7 ☑
breast (implant) T85.79 ☑
catheter NEC T85.79 ☑
dialysis (renal) T82.7 ☑
intraperitoneal T85.71 ☑
infusion NEC T82.7 ☑
spinal (epidural) (subdural) T85.79 ☑
urinary (indwelling) T83.51 ☑
ectopic or molar pregnancy O08.82
electronic (electrode) (pulse generator) (stimulator)
bone T84.7 ☑
cardiac T82.7 ☑
nervous system (brain) (peripheral nerve)
(spinal) T85.79 ☑
urinary T83.59 ☑
fixation, internal (orthopedic) — see Complication,
fixation device, infection
gastrointestinal (bile duct) (esophagus) T85.79 ☑
genital T83.6 ☑
heart NEC T82.7 ☑
valve (prosthesis) T82.6 ☑
graft T82.7 ☑
joint prosthesis — see Complication, joint prosthesis, infection
ocular (corneal graft) (orbital implant) T85.79 ☑
orthopedic NEC T84.7 ☑

Sepsis — continued
due to device, implant or graft — continued
orthopedic — continued
fixation device, internal — see Complication,
fixation device, infection
specified NEC T85.79 ☑
vascular T82.7 ☑
ventricular intracranial shunt T85.79 ☑
during labor O75.3
Enterococcus A41.81
Erysipelothrix (rhusiopathiae) (erysipeloid) A26.7
Escherichia coli (E. coli) A41.5 ☑
extraintestinal yersiniosis A28.2
following
abortion (subsequent episode) O08.0
current episode — see Abortion
ectopic or molar pregnancy O08.82
immunization T88.0 ☑
infusion, therapeutic injection or transfusion NEC
T80.29 ☑
gangrenous A41.9
gonococcal A54.86
Gram-negative (organism) A41.5 ☑
anaerobic A41.4
Haemophilus influenzae A41.3
herpesviral B00.7
intra-abdominal K65.1
intraocular — see Endophthalmitis, purulent
Listeria monocytogenes A32.7
localized — code to specific localized infection
in operation wound T81.4 ☑
skin — see Abscess
malleus A24.0
melioidosis A24.1
meningeal — see Meningitis
meningococcal A39.4
acute A39.2
chronic A39.3
MSSA (Methicillin susceptible Staphylococcus aureus)
A41.01
newborn P36.9
due to
anaerobes NEC P36.5
Escherichia coli P36.4
Staphylococcus P36.30
aureus P36.2
specified NEC P36.39
Streptococcus P36.10
group B P36.0
specified NEC P36.19
specified NEC P36.8
Pasteurella multocida A28.0
pelvic, puerperal, postpartum, childbirth O85
pneumococcal A40.3
postprocedural T81.4 ☑
puerperal, postpartum, childbirth (pelvic) O85
Salmonella (arizonae) (cholerae-suis) (enteritidis) (typhimurium) A02.1
severe R65.20
with septic shock R65.21
Shigella (see also Dysentery, bacillary) A03.9
skin, localized — see Abscess
specified organism NEC A41.89
Staphylococcus, staphylococcal A41.2
aureus (methicillin susceptible) (MSSA) A41.01
methicillin resistant (MRSA) A41.02
coagulase-negative A41.1
specified NEC A41.1
Streptococcus, streptococcal A40.9
agalactiae A40.1
group
A A40.0
B A40.1
D A41.81
neonatal P36.10
group B P36.0
specified NEC P36.19
pneumoniae A40.3
pyogenes A40.0
specified NEC A40.8
tracheostomy stoma J95.02
tularemic A21.7
umbilical, umbilical cord (newborn) — see Sepsis,
newborn
Yersinia pestis A20.7
Septate — see Septum
Septic — see condition
arm — see Cellulitis, upper limb

Septic — *continued*
  arm — *see* Cellulitis, upper limb — *continued*
    with lymphangitis — *see* Lymphangitis, acute, upper limb
  embolus — *see* Embolism
  finger — *see* Cellulitis, digit
    with lymphangitis — *see* Lymphangitis, acute, digit
  foot — *see* Cellulitis, lower limb
    with lymphangitis — *see* Lymphangitis, acute, lower limb
  gallbladder (acute) K81.0
  hand — *see* Cellulitis, upper limb
    with lymphangitis — *see* Lymphangitis, acute, upper limb
  joint — *see* Arthritis, pyogenic or pyemic
  leg — *see* Cellulitis, lower limb
    with lymphangitis — *see* Lymphangitis, acute, lower limb
  nail (*see also* Cellulitis, digit)
    with lymphangitis — *see* Lymphangitis, acute, digit
  sore (*see also* Abscess)
    throat J02.0
      streptococcal J02.0
  spleen (acute) D73.89
  teeth, tooth (pulpal origin) K04.4
  throat — *see* Pharyngitis
  thrombus — *see* Thrombosis
  toe — *see* Cellulitis, digit
    with lymphangitis — *see* Lymphangitis, acute, digit
  tonsils, chronic J35.01
    with adenoiditis J35.03
  uterus — *see* Endometritis
Septicemia A41.9
  meaning sepsis — *see* Sepsis
Septum, septate (congenital) (*see also* Anomaly, by site)
  anal Q42.3
    with fistula Q42.2
  aqueduct of Sylvius Q03.0
    with spina bifida — *see* Spina bifida, by site, with hydrocephalus
  uterus (complete) (partial) Q51.2
  vagina Q52.10
    in pregnancy — *see* Pregnancy, complicated by, abnormal vagina
      causing obstructed labor O65.5
    longitudinal (with or without obstruction) Q52.12
    transverse Q52.11
Sequelae (of) (*see also* condition)
  abscess, intracranial or intraspinal (conditions in G06) G09
  amputation — *code to* injury with seventh character S
  burn and corrosion — *code to* injury with seventh character S
  calcium deficiency E64.8
  cerebrovascular disease — *see* Sequelae, disease, cerebrovascular
  childbirth O94
  contusion — *code to* injury with seventh character S
  corrosion — *see* Sequelae, burn and corrosion
  crushing injury — *code to* injury with seventh character S
  disease
    cerebrovascular I69.90
      alteration of sensation I69.998
      aphasia I69.920
      apraxia I69.990
      ataxia I69.993
      cognitive deficits I69.91
      disturbance of vision I69.998
      dysarthria I69.922
      dysphagia I69.991
      dysphasia I69.921
      facial droop I69.992
      facial weakness I69.992
      fluency disorder I69.923
      hemiplegia I69.95- ☑
      hemorrhage
        intracerebral — *see* Sequelae, hemorrhage, intracerebral
        intracranial, nontraumatic NEC — *see* Sequelae, hemorrhage, intracranial, nontraumatic

Sequelae — *continued*
  disease — *continued*
    cerebrovascular — *continued*
      hemorrhage — *continued*
        subarachnoid — *see* Sequelae, hemorrhage, subarachnoid
      language deficit I69.928
      monoplegia
        lower limb I69.84- ☑
        upper limb I69.93- ☑
      paralytic syndrome I69.96- ☑
      specified effect NEC I69.998
      specified type NEC I69.80
        alteration of sensation I69.898
        aphasia I69.820
        apraxia I69.890
        ataxia I69.893
        cognitive deficits I69.81
        disturbance of vision I69.898
        dysarthria I69.822
        dysphagia I69.891
        dysphasia I69.821
        facial droop I69.892
        facial weakness I69.892
        fluency disorder I69.823
        hemiplegia I69.85- ☑
        language deficit I69.828
        monoplegia
          lower limb I69.84- ☑
          upper limb I69.83- ☑
        paralytic syndrome I69.86- ☑
        specified effect NEC I69.898
      speech deficit I69.928
        speech deficit I69.828
    stroke NOS — *see* Sequelae, stroke NOS
  dislocation — *code to* injury with seventh character S
  encephalitis or encephalomyelitis (conditions in G04) G09
    in infectious disease NEC B94.8
    viral B94.1
  external cause — *code to* injury with seventh character S
  foreign body entering natural orifice — *code to* injury with seventh character S
  fracture — *code to* injury with seventh character S
  frostbite — *code to* injury with seventh character S
  Hansen's disease B92
  hemorrhage
    intracerebral I69.10
      alteration of sensation I69.198
      aphasia I69.120
      apraxia I69.190
      ataxia I69.193
      cognitive deficits I69.11
      disturbance of vision I69.198
      dysarthria I69.122
      dysphagia I69.191
      dysphasia I69.121
      facial droop I69.192
      facial weakness I69.192
      fluency disorder I69.123
      hemiplegia I69.15- ☑
      language deficit NEC I69.128
      monoplegia
        lower limb I69.14- ☑
        upper limb I69.13- ☑
      paralytic syndrome I69.16- ☑
      specified effect NEC I69.198
      speech deficit NEC I69.128
    intracranial, nontraumatic NEC I69.20
      alteration of sensation I69.298
      aphasia I69.220
      apraxia I69.290
      ataxia I69.293
      cognitive deficits I69.21
      disturbance of vision I69.298
      dysarthria I69.222
      dysphagia I69.291
      dysphasia I69.221
      facial droop I69.292
      facial weakness I69.292
      fluency disorder I69.223
      hemiplegia I69.25- ☑
      language deficit NEC I69.228
      monoplegia
        lower limb I69.24- ☑
        upper limb I69.23- ☑
      paralytic syndrome I69.26- ☑

Sequelae — *continued*
  hemorrhage — *continued*
    intracranial, nontraumatic — *continued*
      specified effect NEC I69.298
      speech deficit NEC I69.228
    subarachnoid I69.00
      alteration of sensation I69.098
      aphasia I69.020
      apraxia I69.090
      ataxia I69.093
      cognitive deficits I69.01
      disturbance of vision I69.098
      dysarthria I69.022
      dysphagia I69.091
      dysphasia I69.021
      facial droop I69.092
      facial weakness I69.092
      fluency disorder I69.023
      hemiplegia I69.05- ☑
      language deficit NEC I69.028
      monoplegia
        lower limb I69.04- ☑
        upper limb I69.03- ☑
      paralytic syndrome I69.06- ☑
      specified effect NEC I69.098
      speech deficit NEC I69.028
  hepatitis, viral B94.2
  hyperalimentation E68
  infarction
    cerebral I69.30
      alteration of sensation I69.398
      aphasia I69.320
      apraxia I69.390
      ataxia I69.393
      cognitive deficits I69.31
      disturbance of vision I69.398
      dysarthria I69.322
      dysphagia I69.391
      dysphasia I69.321
      facial droop I69.392
      facial weakness I69.392
      fluency disorder I69.323
      hemiplegia I69.35- ☑
      language deficit NEC I69.328
      monoplegia
        lower limb I69.34- ☑
        upper limb I69.33- ☑
      paralytic syndrome I69.36- ☑
      specified effect NEC I69.398
      speech deficit NEC I69.328
  infection, pyogenic, intracranial or intraspinal G09
  infectious disease B94.9
    specified NEC B94.8
  injury — *code to* injury with seventh character S
  leprosy B92
  meningitis
    bacterial (conditions in G00) G09
    other or unspecified cause (conditions in G03) G09
  muscle (and tendon) injury — *code to* injury with seventh character S
  myelitis — *see* Sequelae, encephalitis
  niacin deficiency E64.8
  nutritional deficiency E64.9
    specified NEC E64.8
  obstetrical condition O94
  parasitic disease B94.9
  phlebitis or thrombophlebitis of intracranial or intraspinal venous sinuses and veins (conditions in G08) G09
  poisoning — *code to* poisoning with seventh character S
    nonmedicinal substance — *see* Sequelae, toxic effect, nonmedicinal substance
  poliomyelitis (acute) B91
  pregnancy O94
  protein-energy malnutrition E64.0
  puerperium O94
  rickets E64.3
  selenium deficiency E64.8
  sprain and strain — *code to* injury with seventh character S
  stroke NOS I69.30
    alteration in sensation I69.398
    aphasia I69.320
    apraxia I69.390
    ataxia I69.393
    cognitive deficits I69.31
    disturbance of vision I69.398

Sequelae — *continued*
  stroke — *continued*
    dysarthria I69.322
    dysphagia I69.391
    dysphasia I69.321
    facial droop I69.392
    facial weakness I69.392
    hemiplegia I69.35-
    language deficit NEC I69.328
    monoplegia
      lower limb I69.34- ☑
      upper limb I69.33- ☑
    paralytic syndrome I69.36- ☑
    specified effect NEC I69.398
    speech deficit NEC I69.328
  tendon and muscle injury — *code to* injury with seventh character S
  thiamine deficiency E64.8
  trachoma B94.0
  tuberculosis B90.9
    bones and joints B90.2
    central nervous system B90.0
    genitourinary B90.1
    pulmonary (respiratory) B90.9
    specified organs NEC B90.8
  viral
    encephalitis B94.1
    hepatitis B94.2
  vitamin deficiency NEC E64.8
    A E64.1
    B E64.8
    C E64.2
  wound, open — *code to* injury with seventh character S

Sequestration (*see also* Sequestrum)
  lung, congenital Q33.2

Sequestrum
  bone — *see* Osteomyelitis, chronic
  dental M27.2
  jaw bone M27.2
  orbit — *see* Osteomyelitis, orbit
  sinus (accessory) (nasal) — *see* Sinusitis

Sequoiosis lung or pneumonitis J67.8

Serology for syphilis
  doubtful
    with signs or symptoms — *code by* site and stage under Syphilis
    follow-up of latent syphilis — *see* Syphilis, latent
  negative, with signs or symptoms — *code by* site and stage under Syphilis
  positive A53.0
    with signs or symptoms — *code by* site and stage under Syphilis
  reactivated A53.0

Seroma (*see also* Hematoma)
  traumatic, secondary and recurrent T79.2 ☑

Seropurulent — *see* condition

Serositis, multiple K65.8
  pericardial I31.1
  peritoneal K65.8

Serous — *see* condition

Sertoli cell
  adenoma
    specified site — *see* Neoplasm, benign, by site
    unspecified site
      female D27.9
      male D29.20
  carcinoma
    specified site — *see* Neoplasm, malignant, by site
    unspecified site (male) C62.9- ☑
      female C56.9
  tumor
    with lipid storage
      specified site — *see* Neoplasm, benign, by site
      unspecified site
        female D27.9
        male D29.20
    specified site — *see* Neoplasm, benign, by site
    unspecified site
      female D27.9
      male D29.20

Sertoli-Leydig cell tumor — *see* Neoplasm, benign, by site
  specified site — *see* Neoplasm, benign, by site
  unspecified site
    female D27.9
    male D29.20

Serum
  allergy, allergic reaction (*see also* Reaction, serum) T80.69 ☑
    shock (*see also* Shock, anaphylactic) T80.59 ☑
  arthritis (*see also* Reaction, serum) T80.69 ☑
  complication or reaction NEC (*see also* Reaction, serum) T80.69 ☑
  disease NEC (*see also* Reaction, serum) T80.69 ☑
  hepatitis (*see also* Hepatitis, viral, type B)
    carrier (suspected) of Z22.51
  intoxication (*see also* Reaction, serum) T80.69 ☑
  neuritis (*see also* Reaction, serum) T80.69 ☑
  neuropathy G61.1
  poisoning NEC (*see also* Reaction, serum) T80.69 ☑
  rash NEC (*see also* Reaction, serum) T80.69 ☑
  reaction NEC (*see also* Reaction, serum) T80.69 ☑
  sickness NEC (*see also* Reaction, serum) T80.69 ☑
  urticaria (*see also* Reaction, serum) T80.69 ☑

Sesamoiditis M25.8- ☑

Severe sepsis R65.20
  with septic shock R65.21

Sever's disease or osteochondrosis — *see* Osteochondrosis, juvenile, tarsus

Sex
  chromosome mosaics Q97.8
    lines with various numbers of X chromosomes Q97.2
  education Z70.8
  reassignment surgery status Z87.890

Sextuplet pregnancy — *see* Pregnancy, sextuplet

Sexual
  function, disorder of (psychogenic) F52.9
  immaturity (female) (male) E30.0
  impotence (psychogenic) organic origin NEC — *see* Dysfunction, sexual, male
  precocity (constitutional) (cryptogenic)(female) (idiopathic) (male) E30.1

Sexuality, pathologic — *see* Deviation, sexual

Sézary disease C84.1- ☑

Shadow, lung R91.8

Shaking palsy or paralysis — *see* Parkinsonism

Shallowness, acetabulum — *see* Derangement, joint, specified type NEC, hip

Shaver's disease J63.1

Sheath (tendon) — *see* condition

Sheathing, retinal vessels H35.01- ☑

Shedding
  nail L60.8
  premature, primary (deciduous) teeth K00.6

Sheehan's disease or syndrome E23.0

Shelf, rectal K62.89

Shell teeth K00.5

Shellshock (current) F43.0
  lasting state — *see* Disorder, post-traumatic stress

Shield kidney Q63.1

Shift
  auditory threshold (temporary) H93.24- ☑
  mediastinal R93.8

Shifting sleep-work schedule (affecting sleep) G47.26

Shiga (-Kruse) **dysentery** A03.0

Shiga's bacillus A03.0

Shigella (dysentery) — *see* Dysentery, bacillary

Shigellosis A03.9
  Group A A03.0
  Group B A03.1
  Group C A03.2
  Group D A03.3

Shin splints S86.89- ☑

Shingles — *see* Herpes, zoster

Shipyard disease or eye B30.0

Shirodkar suture, in pregnancy — *see* Pregnancy, complicated by, incompetent cervix

Shock R57.9
  with ectopic or molar pregnancy O08.3
  adrenal (cortical) (Addisonian) E27.2
  adverse food reaction (anaphylactic) — *see* Shock, anaphylactic, due to food
  allergic — *see* Shock, anaphylactic
  anaphylactic T78.2 ☑
    chemical — *see* Table of Drugs and Chemicals
    due to drug or medicinal substance
      correct substance properly administered T88.6 ☑
      overdose or wrong substance given or taken (by accident) — *see* Table of Drugs and Chemicals, by drug, poisoning

Shock — *continued*
  anaphylactic — *continued*
    due to food (nonpoisonous) T78.00 ☑
      additives T78.06 ☑
      dairy products T78.07 ☑
      eggs T78.08 ☑
      fish T78.03 ☑
        shellfish T78.02 ☑
      fruit T78.04 ☑
      milk T78.07 ☑
      nuts T78.05 ☑
        peanuts T78.01 ☑
      peanuts T78.01 ☑
      seeds T78.05 ☑
      specified type NEC T78.09 ☑
      vegetable T78.04 ☑
    following sting(s) — *see* Venom
    immunization T80.52 ☑
    serum T80.59 ☑
      blood and blood products T80.51 ☑
      immunization T80.52 ☑
      specified NEC T80.59 ☑
      vaccination T80.52 ☑
  anaphylactoid — *see* Shock, anaphylactic
  anesthetic
    correct substance properly administered T88.2 ☑
    overdose or wrong substance given or taken — *see* Table of Drugs and Chemicals, by drug, poisoning
    specified anesthetic — *see* Table of Drugs and Chemicals, by drug, poisoning
  cardiogenic R57.0
  chemical substance — *see* Table of Drugs and Chemicals
  complicating ectopic or molar pregnancy O08.3
  culture — *see* Disorder, adjustment
  drug
    due to correct substance properly administered T88.6 ☑
    overdose or wrong substance given or taken (by accident) — *see* Table of Drugs and Chemicals, by drug, poisoning
  during or after labor and delivery O75.1
  electric T75.4 ☑
    (taser) T75.4 ☑
  endotoxic R65.21
    postprocedural (during or resulting from a procedure, not elsewhere classified) T81.12 ☑
  following
    ectopic or molar pregnancy O08.3
    injury (immediate) (delayed) T79.4 ☑
    labor and delivery O75.1
  food (anaphylactic) — *see* Shock, anaphylactic, due to food
  from electroshock gun (taser) T75.4 ☑
  gram-negative R65.21
    postprocedural (during or resulting from a procedure, not elsewhere classified) T81.12 ☑
  hematologic R57.8
  hemorrhagic
    surgery (intraoperative) (postoperative) T81.19 ☑
    trauma T79.4 ☑
  hypovolemic R57.1
    surgical T81.19 ☑
    traumatic T79.4 ☑
  insulin E15
    therapeutic misadventure — *see* subcategory T38.3 ☑
  kidney N17.0
    traumatic (following crushing) T79.5 ☑
  lightning T75.01 ☑
  lung J80
  obstetric O75.1
    with ectopic or molar pregnancy O08.3
    following ectopic or molar pregnancy O08.3
  pleural (surgical) T81.19 ☑
    due to trauma T79.4 ☑
  postprocedural (postoperative) T81.10 ☑
    with ectopic or molar pregnancy O08.3
    cardiogenic T81.11 ☑
    endotoxic T81.12 ☑
    following ectopic or molar pregnancy O08.3
    gram-negative T81.12 ☑
    hypovolemic T81.19 ☑
    septic T81.12 ☑
    specified type NEC T81.19 ☑

Shock — continued
  psychic F43.0
  septic (due to severe sepsis) R65.21
  specified NEC R57.8
  surgical T81.10 ☑
  taser gun (taser) T75.4 ☑
  therapeutic misadventure NEC T81.10 ☑
  thyroxin
    overdose or wrong substance given or taken —
      see Table of Drugs and Chemicals, by drug,
      poisoning
  toxic, syndrome A48.3
  transfusion — see Complications, transfusion
  traumatic (immediate) (delayed) T79.4 ☑
Shoemaker's chest M95.4
Short, shortening, shortness
  arm (acquired) (see also Deformity, limb, unequal
      length)
    congenital Q71.81- ☑
    forearm — see Deformity, limb, unequal length
  bowel syndrome K91.2
  breath R06.02
  cervical (complicating pregnancy) O26.87- ☑
    non-gravid uterus N88.3
  common bile duct, congenital Q44.5
  cord (umbilical), complicating delivery O69.3 ☑
  cystic duct, congenital Q44.5
  esophagus (congenital) Q39.8
  femur (acquired) — see Deformity, limb, unequal
      length, femur
    congenital — see Defect, reduction, lower limb,
      longitudinal, femur
  frenum, frenulum, linguae (congenital) Q38.1
  hip (acquired) (see also Deformity, limb, unequal
      length)
    congenital Q65.89
  leg (acquired) (see also Deformity, limb, unequal
      length)
    congenital Q72.81- ☑
    lower leg (see also Deformity, limb, unequal length)
  limbed stature, with immunodeficiency D82.2
  lower limb (acquired) (see also Deformity, limb, un-
      equal length)
    congenital Q72.81- ☑
  organ or site, congenital NEC — see Distortion
  palate, congenital Q38.5
  radius (acquired) (see also Deformity, limb, unequal
      length)
    congenital — see Defect, reduction, upper limb,
      longitudinal, radius
  rib syndrome Q77.2
  stature (child) (hereditary) (idiopathic) NEC R62.52
    constitutional E34.3
    due to endocrine disorder E34.3
    Laron-type E34.3
  tendon (see also Contraction, tendon)
    with contracture of joint — see Contraction, joint
    Achilles (acquired) M67.0- ☑
      congenital Q66.89
    congenital Q79.8
  thigh (acquired) (see also Deformity, limb, unequal
      length, femur)
    congenital — see Defect, reduction, lower limb,
      longitudinal, femur
  tibialis anterior (tendon) — see Contraction, tendon
  umbilical cord
    complicating delivery O69.3 ☑
  upper limb, congenital — see Defect, reduction, upper
      limb, specified type NEC
  urethra N36.8
  uvula, congenital Q38.5
  vagina (congenital) Q52.4
Shortsightedness — see Myopia
Shoshin (acute fulminating beriberi) E51.11
Shoulder — see condition
Shovel-shaped incisors K00.2
Shower, thromboembolic — see Embolism
Shunt
  arterial-venous (dialysis) Z99.2
  arteriovenous, pulmonary (acquired) I28.0
    congenital Q25.72
  cerebral ventricle (communicating) in situ Z98.2
  surgical, prosthetic, with complications — see Compli-
      cations, cardiovascular, device or implant
Shutdown, renal N28.9
Shy-Drager syndrome G90.3

Sialadenitis, sialadenosis (any gland) (chronic) (period-
    ic) (suppurative) — see Sialoadenitis
Sialectasia K11.8
Sialidosis E77.1
Sialitis, silitis (any gland) (chronic) (suppurative) — see
    Sialoadenitis
Sialoadenitis (any gland) (periodic) (suppurative) K11.20
  acute K11.21
    recurrent K11.22
  chronic K11.23
Sialoadenopathy K11.9
Sialoangitis — see Sialoadenitis
Sialodochitis (fibrinosa) — see Sialoadenitis
Sialodocholithiasis K11.5
Sialolithiasis K11.5
Sialometaplasia, necrotizing K11.8
Sialorrhea (see also Ptyalism)
  periodic — see Sialoadenitis
Sialosis K11.7
Siamese twin Q89.4
Sibling rivalry Z62.891
Sicard's syndrome G52.7
Sicca syndrome M35.00
  with
    keratoconjunctivitis M35.01
    lung involvement M35.02
    myopathy M35.03
    renal tubulo-interstitial disorders M35.04
    specified organ involvement NEC M35.09
Sick R69
  or handicapped person in family Z63.79
    needing care at home Z63.6
  sinus (syndrome) I49.5
Sick-euthyroid syndrome E07.81
Sickle-cell
  anemia — see Disease, sickle-cell
  trait D57.3
Sicklemia (see also Disease, sickle-cell)
  trait D57.3
Sickness
  air (travel) T75.3 ☑
  airplane T75.3 ☑
  alpine T70.29 ☑
  altitude T70.20 ☑
  Andes T70.29 ☑
  aviator's T70.29 ☑
  balloon T70.29 ☑
  car T75.3 ☑
  compressed air T70.3 ☑
  decompression T70.3 ☑
  green D50.8
  milk — see Poisoning, food, noxious
  motion T75.3 ☑
  mountain T70.29 ☑
    acute D75.1
  protein (see also Reaction, serum) T80.69 ☑
  radiation T66 ☑
  roundabout (motion) T75.3 ☑
  sea T75.3 ☑
  serum NEC (see also Reaction, serum) T80.69 ☑
  sleeping (African) B56.9
    by Trypanosoma B56.9
      brucei
        gambiense B56.0
        rhodesiense B56.1
    East African B56.1
    Gambian B56.0
    Rhodesian B56.1
    West African B56.0
  swing (motion) T75.3 ☑
  train (railway) (travel) T75.3 ☑
  travel (any vehicle) T75.3 ☑
Sideropenia — see Anemia, iron deficiency
Siderosilicosis J62.8
Siderosis (lung) J63.4
  eye (globe) — see Disorder, globe, degenerative,
      siderosis
Siemens' syndrome (ectodermal dysplasia) Q82.8
Sighing R06.89
  psychogenic F45.8
Sigmoid (see also condition)
  flexure — see condition
  kidney Q63.1
Sigmoiditis (see also Enteritis) K52.9
  infectious A09
  noninfectious K52.9
Silfversköld's syndrome Q78.9

Silicosiderosis J62.8
Silicosis, silicotic (simple) (complicated) J62.8
  with tuberculosis J65
Silicotuberculosis J65
Silo-fillers' disease J68.8
  bronchitis J68.0
  pneumonitis J68.0
  pulmonary edema J68.1
Silver's syndrome Q87.1
Simian malaria B53.1
Simmonds' cachexia or disease E23.0
Simons' disease or syndrome (progressive lipodystro-
    phy) E88.1
Simple, simplex — see condition
Simulation, conscious (of illness) Z76.5
Simultanagnosia (asimultagnosia) R48.3
Sin Nombre virus disease (Hantavirus) (cardio)-pul-
    monary syndrome) B33.4
Sinding-Larsen disease or osteochondrosis — see
    Osteochondrosis, juvenile, patella
Singapore hemorrhagic fever A91
Singer's node or nodule J38.2
Single
  atrium Q21.2
  coronary artery Q24.5
  umbilical artery Q27.0
  ventricle Q20.4
Singuitus R06.6
  epidemicus B33.0
Sinus (see also Fistula)
  abdominal K63.89
  arrest I45.5
  arrhythmia I49.8
  bradycardia R00.1
  branchial cleft (internal) (external) Q18.0
  coccygeal — see Sinus, pilonidal
  dental K04.6
  dermal (congenital) Q06.8
    with abscess Q06.8
    coccygeal, pilonidal — see Sinus, coccygeal
  infected, skin NEC L08.89
  marginal, ruptured or bleeding — see Hemorrhage,
      antepartum, specified cause NEC
  medial, face and neck Q18.8
  pause I45.5
  pericranii Q01.9
  pilonidal (infected) (rectum) L05.92
    with abscess L05.02
  preauricular Q18.1
  rectovaginal N82.3
  Rokitansky-Aschoff (gallbladder) K82.8
  sacrococcygeal (dermoid) (infected) — see Sinus, pi-
      lonidal
  tachycardia R00.0
    paroxysmal I47.1
  tarsi syndrome M25.57- ☑
  testis N50.8
  tract (postinfective) — see Fistula
  urachus Q64.4
Sinusitis (accessory) (chronic) (hyperplastic) (nasal)
    (nonpurulent) (purulent) J32.9
  acute J01.90
    ethmoidal J01.20
      recurrent J01.21
    frontal J01.10
      recurrent J01.11
    involving more than one sinus, other than pansi-
        nusitis J01.80
      recurrent J01.81
    maxillary J01.00
      recurrent J01.01
    pansinusitis J01.40
      recurrent J01.41
    recurrent J01.91
    specified NEC J01.80
      recurrent J01.81
    sphenoidal J01.30
      recurrent J01.31
  allergic — see Rhinitis, allergic
  due to high altitude T70.1 ☑
  ethmoidal J32.2
    acute J01.20
      recurrent J01.21
  frontal J32.1
    acute J01.10
      recurrent J01.11
  influenzal — see Influenza, with, respiratory manifes-
      tations NEC

☑ Additional Character Required — Refer to the Tabular List for Character Selection   ▽ Subterms under main terms may continue to next column or page

Sinusitis — *continued*
  involving more than one sinus but not pansinusitis J32.8
    acute J01.80
      recurrent J01.81
  maxillary J32.0
    acute J01.00
      recurrent J01.01
  sphenoidal J32.3
    acute J01.30
      recurrent J01.31
  tuberculous, any sinus A15.8
Sinusitis-bronchiectasis-situs inversus (syndrome) (triad) Q89.3
Sipple's syndrome E31.22
Sirenomelia (syndrome) Q87.2
Siriasis T67.0 ☑
Sirkari's disease B55.0
Siti A65
Situation, psychiatric F99
Situational
  disturbance (transient) — *see* Disorder, adjustment
    acute F43.0
  maladjustment — *see* Disorder, adjustment
  reaction — *see* Disorder, adjustment
    acute F43.0
Situs inversus or transversus (abdominalis) (thoracis) Q89.3
Sixth disease B08.20
  due to human herpesvirus 6 B08.21
  due to human herpesvirus 7 B08.22
Sjögren-Larsson syndrome Q87.1
Sjögren's syndrome or disease — *see* Sicca syndrome
Skeletal — *see* condition
Skene's gland — *see* condition
Skenitis — *see* Urethritis
Skerljevo A65
Skevas-Zerfus disease — *see* Toxicity, venom, marine animal, sea anemone
Skin (*see also* condition)
  clammy R23.1
  donor — *see* Donor, skin
  hidebound M35.9
Slate-dressers' or slate-miners' lung J62.8
Sleep
  apnea — *see* Apnea, sleep
  deprivation Z72.820
  disorder or disturbance G47.9
    child F51.9
    nonorganic origin F51.9
    specified NEC G47.8
  disturbance G47.9
    nonorganic origin F51.9
  drunkenness F51.9
  rhythm inversion G47.2- ☑
  terrors F51.4
  walking F51.3
    hysterical F44.89
Sleep hygiene
  abuse Z72.821
  inadequate Z72.821
  poor Z72.821
Sleeping sickness — *see* Sickness, sleeping
Sleeplessness — *see* Insomnia
  menopausal N95.1
Sleep-wake schedule disorder G47.20
Slim disease (in HIV infection) B20
Slipped, slipping
  epiphysis (traumatic) (*see also* Osteochondropathy, specified type NEC)
    capital femoral (traumatic)
      acute (on chronic) S79.01- ☑
    current traumatic — *code as* Fracture, by site
    upper femoral (nontraumatic) M93.00- ☑
      acute M93.01- ☑
        on chronic M93.03- ☑
      chronic M93.02- ☑
  intervertebral disc — *see* Displacement, intervertebral disc
  ligature, umbilical P51.8
  patella — *see* Disorder, patella, derangement NEC
  rib M89.8X8
  sacroiliac joint — *see* subcategory M53.2 ☑
  tendon — *see* Disorder, tendon
  ulnar nerve, nontraumatic — *see* Lesion, nerve, ulnar
  vertebra NEC — *see* Spondylolisthesis
Slocumb's syndrome E27.0

Sloughing (multiple) (phagedena) (skin) (*see also* Gangrene)
  abscess — *see* Abscess
  appendix K38.8
  fascia — *see* Disorder, soft tissue, specified type NEC
  scrotum N50.8
  tendon — *see* Disorder, tendon
  transplanted organ — *see* Rejection, transplant
  ulcer — *see* Ulcer, skin
Slow
  feeding, newborn P92.2
  flow syndrome, coronary I20.8
  heart (beat) R00.1
Slowing, urinary stream R39.19
Sluder's neuralgia (syndrome) G44.89
Slurred, slurring speech R47.81
Small (ness)
  for gestational age — *see* Small for dates
  introitus, vagina N89.6
  kidney (unknown cause) N27.9
    bilateral N27.1
    unilateral N27.0
  ovary (congenital) Q50.39
  pelvis
    with disproportion (fetopelvic) O33.1
      causing obstructed labor O65.1
  uterus N85.8
  white kidney N03.9
Small-and-light-for-dates — *see* Small for dates
Small-for-dates (infant) P05.10
  with weight of
    1000-1249 grams P05.14
    1250-1499 grams P05.15
    1500-1749 grams P05.16
    1750-1999 grams P05.17
    2000-2499 grams P05.18
    499 grams or less P05.11
    500-749 grams P05.12
    750-999 grams P05.13
Smallpox B03
Smearing, fecal R15.1
Smith-Lemli-Opitz syndrome E78.72
Smith's fracture S52.54- ☑
Smoker — *see* Dependence, drug, nicotine
Smoker's
  bronchitis J41.0
  cough J41.0
  palate K13.24
  throat J31.2
  tongue K13.24
Smoking
  passive Z77.22
Smothering spells R06.81
Snaggle teeth, tooth M26.39
Snapping
  finger — *see* Trigger finger
  hip — *see* Derangement, joint, specified type NEC, hip
    involving the iliotiblial band M76.3- ☑
  knee — *see* Derangement, knee
    involving the iliotiblial band M76.3- ☑
Sneddon-Wilkinson disease or syndrome (sub-corneal pustular dermatosis) L13.1
Sneezing (intractable) R06.7
Sniffing
  cocaine
    abuse — *see* Abuse, drug, cocaine
    dependence — *see* Dependence, drug, cocaine
  gasoline
    abuse — *see* Abuse, drug, inhalant
    dependence — *see* Dependence, drug, inhalant
  glue (airplane)
    abuse — *see* Abuse, drug, inhalant
    drug dependence — *see* Dependence, drug, inhalant
Sniffles
  newborn P28.89
Snoring R06.83
Snow blindness — *see* Photokeratitis
Snuffles (non-syphilitic) R06.5
  newborn P28.89
  syphilitic (infant) A50.05 [J99]
Social
  exclusion Z60.4
    due to discrimination or persecution (perceived) Z60.5
  migrant Z59.0
    acculturation difficulty Z60.3

Social — *continued*
  rejection Z60.4
    due to discrimination or persecution Z60.5
  role conflict NEC Z73.5
  skills inadequacy NEC Z73.4
  transplantation Z60.3
Sodoku A25.0
Soemmerring's ring — *see* Cataract, secondary
Soft (*see also* condition)
  nails L60.3
Softening
  bone — *see* Osteomalacia
  brain (necrotic) (progressive) G93.89
    congenital Q04.8
    embolic I63.4 ☑
    hemorrhagic — *see* Hemorrhage, intracranial, intracerebral
    occlusive I63.5 ☑
    thrombotic I63.3 ☑
  cartilage M94.2- ☑
    patella M22.4- ☑
  cerebellar — *see* Softening, brain
  cerebral — *see* Softening, brain
  cerebrospinal — *see* Softening, brain
  myocardial, heart — *see* Degeneration, myocardial
  spinal cord G95.89
  stomach K31.89
Soldier's
  heart F45.8
  patches I31.0
Solitary
  cyst, kidney N28.1
  kidney, congenital Q60.0
Solvent abuse — *see* Abuse, drug, inhalant
  dependence — *see* Dependence, drug, inhalant
Somatization reaction, somatic reaction — *see* Disorder, somatoform
Somnambulism F51.3
  hysterical F44.89
Somnolence R40.0
  nonorganic origin F51.11
Sonne dysentery A03.3
Soor B37.0
Sore
  bed — *see* Ulcer, pressure, by site
  chiclero B55.1
  Delhi B55.1
  desert — *see* Ulcer, skin
  eye H57.1- ☑
  Lahore B55.1
  mouth K13.79
    canker K12.0
  muscle M79.1
  Naga — *see* Ulcer, skin
  of skin — *see* Ulcer, skin
  oriental B55.1
  pressure — *see* Ulcer, pressure, by site
  skin L98.9
  soft A57
  throat (acute) (*see also* Pharyngitis)
    with influenza, flu, or grippe — *see* Influenza, with, respiratory manifestations NEC
    chronic J31.2
    coxsackie (virus) B08.5
    diphtheritic A36.0
    herpesviral B00.2
    influenzal — *see* Influenza, with, respiratory manifestations NEC
    septic J02.0
    streptococcal (ulcerative) J02.0
    viral NEC J02.8
      coxsackie B08.5
  tropical — *see* Ulcer, skin
  veldt — *see* Ulcer, skin
Soto's syndrome (cerebral gigantism) Q87.3
South African cardiomyopathy syndrome I42.8
Southeast Asian hemorrhagic fever A91
Spacing
  abnormal, tooth, teeth, fully erupted M26.30
  excessive, tooth, fully erupted M26.32
Spade-like hand (congenital) Q68.1
Spading nail L60.8
  congenital Q84.6
Spanish collar N47.1
Sparganosis B70.1
Spasm(s), spastic, spasticity (*see also* condition) R25.2
  accommodation — *see* Spasm, of accommodation

Spasm(s), spastic, spasticity — *continued*
- ampulla of Vater K83.4
- anus, ani (sphincter) (reflex) K59.4
  - psychogenic F45.8
- artery I73.9
  - cerebral G45.9
- Bell's G51.3
- bladder (sphincter, external or internal) N32.89
  - psychogenic F45.8
- bronchus, bronchiole J98.01
- cardia K22.0
- cardiac I20.1
- carpopedal — *see* Tetany
- cerebral (arteries) (vascular) G45.9
- cervix, complicating delivery O62.4
- ciliary body (of accommodation) -– *see* Spasm, of accommodation
- colon K58.9
  - with diarrhea K58.0
  - psychogenic F45.8
- common duct K83.8
- compulsive — *see* Tic
- conjugate H51.8
- coronary (artery) I20.1
- diaphragm (reflex) R06.6
  - epidemic B33.0
  - psychogenic F45.8
- duodenum K59.8
- epidemic diaphragmatic (transient) B33.0
- esophagus (diffuse) K22.4
  - psychogenic F45.8
- facial G51.3
- fallopian tube N83.8
- gastrointestinal (tract) K31.89
  - psychogenic F45.8
- glottis J38.5
  - hysterical F44.4
  - psychogenic F45.8
    - conversion reaction F44.4
  - reflex through recurrent laryngeal nerve J38.5
- habit — *see* Tic
- heart I20.1
- hemifacial (clonic) G51.3
- hourglass — *see* Contraction, hourglass
- hysterical F44.4
- infantile — *see* Epilepsy, spasms
- inferior oblique, eye H51.8
- intestinal (*see also* Syndrome, irritable bowel) K58.9
  - psychogenic F45.8
- larynx, laryngeal J38.5
  - hysterical F44.4
  - psychogenic F45.8
    - conversion reaction F44.4
- levator palpebrae superioris — *see* Disorder, eyelid function
- muscle NEC M62.838
  - back M62.830
- nerve, trigeminal G51.0
- nervous F45.8
- nodding F98.4
- occupational F48.8
- oculogyric H51.8
  - psychogenic F45.8
- of accommodation H52.53- ☑
- ophthalmic artery — *see* Occlusion, artery, retina
- perineal, female N94.89
- peroneo-extensor (*see also* Deformity, limb, flat foot)
- pharynx (reflex) J39.2
  - hysterical F45.8
  - psychogenic F45.8
- psychogenic F45.8
- pylorus NEC K31.3
  - adult hypertrophic K31.89
  - congenital or infantile Q40.0
  - psychogenic F45.8
- rectum (sphincter) K59.4
  - psychogenic F45.8
- retinal (artery) — *see* Occlusion, artery, retina
- sigmoid (*see also* Syndrome, irritable bowel) K58.9
  - psychogenic F45.8
- sphincter of Oddi K83.4
- stomach K31.89
  - neurotic F45.8
- throat J39.2
  - hysterical F45.8
  - psychogenic F45.8
- tic F95.9
  - chronic F95.1

Spasm(s), spastic, spasticity — *continued*
- tic — *continued*
  - transient of childhood F95.0
- tongue K14.8
- torsion (progressive) G24.1
- trigeminal nerve — *see* Neuralgia, trigeminal
- ureter N13.5
- urethra (sphincter) N35.9
- uterus N85.8
  - complicating labor O62.4
- vagina N94.2
  - psychogenic F52.5
- vascular I73.9
- vasomotor I73.9
- vein NEC I87.8
- viscera — *see* Pain, abdominal

Spasmodic — *see* condition

Spasmophilia — *see* Tetany

Spasmus nutans F98.4

Spastic, spasticity (*see also* Spasm)
- child (cerebral) (congenital) (paralysis) G80.1

Speaker's throat R49.8

Specific, specified — *see* condition

Speech
- defect, disorder, disturbance, impediment R47.9
  - psychogenic, in childhood and adolescence F98.8
  - slurring R47.81
  - specified NEC R47.89

Spencer's disease A08.19

Spens' syndrome (syncope with heart block) I45.9

Sperm counts (fertility testing) Z31.41
- postvasectomy Z30.8
- reversal Z31.42

Spermatic cord — *see* condition

Spermatocele N43.40
- congenital Q55.4
- multiple N43.42
- single N43.41

Spermatocystitis N49.0

Spermatocytoma C62.9- ☑
- specified site — *see* Neoplasm, malignant, by site

Spermatorrhea N50.8

Sphacelus — *see* Gangrene

Sphenoidal — *see* condition

Sphenoiditis (chronic) — *see* Sinusitis, sphenoidal

Sphenopalatine ganglion neuralgia G90.09

Sphericity, increased, lens (congenital) Q12.4

Spherocytosis (congenital) (familial) (hereditary) D58.0
- hemoglobin disease D58.0
- sickle-cell (disease) D57.8- ☑

Spherophakia Q12.4

Sphincter — *see* condition

Sphincteritis, sphincter of Oddi — *see* Cholangitis

Sphingolipidosis E75.3
- specified NEC E75.29

Sphingomyelinosis E75.3

Spicule tooth K00.2

Spider
- bite — *see* Toxicity, venom, spider
- fingers — *see* Syndrome, Marfan's
- nevus I78.1
- toes — *see* Syndrome, Marfan's
- vascular I78.1

Spiegler-Fendt
- benign lymphocytoma L98.8
- sarcoid L08.89

Spielmeyer-Vogt disease E75.4

Spina bifida (aperta) Q05.9
- with hydrocephalus NEC Q05.4
- cervical Q05.5
  - with hydrocephalus Q05.0
- dorsal Q05.6
  - with hydrocephalus Q05.1
- lumbar Q05.7
  - with hydrocephalus Q05.2
- lumbosacral Q05.7
  - with hydrocephalus Q05.2
- occulta Q76.0
- sacral Q05.8
  - with hydrocephalus Q05.3
- thoracic Q05.6
  - with hydrocephalus Q05.1
- thoracolumbar Q05.6
  - with hydrocephalus Q05.1

Spindle, Krukenberg's — *see* Pigmentation, cornea, posterior

Spine, spinal — *see* condition

Spiradenoma (eccrine) — *see* Neoplasm, skin, benign

Spirillosis A25.0

Spirillum
- minus A25.0
- obermeieri infection A68.0

Spirochetal — *see* condition

Spirochetosis A69.9
- arthritic, arthritica A69.9
- bronchopulmonary A69.8
- icterohemorrhagic A27.0
- lung A69.8

Spirometrosis B70.1

Spitting blood — *see* Hemoptysis

Splanchnoptosis K63.4

Spleen, splenic — *see* condition

Splenectasis — *see* Splenomegaly

Splenitis (interstitial) (malignant) (nonspecific) D73.89
- malarial (*see also* Malaria) B54 [D77]
- tuberculous A18.85

Splenocele D73.89

Splenomegaly, splenomegalia (Bengal) (cryptogenic) (idiopathic) (tropical) R16.1
- with hepatomegaly R16.2
- cirrhotic D73.2
- congenital Q89.09
- congestive, chronic D73.2
- Egyptian B65.1
- Gaucher's E75.22
- malarial (*see also* Malaria) B54 [D77]
- neutropenic D73.81
- Niemann-Pick — *see* Niemann-Pick disease or syndrome
- siderotic D73.2
- syphilitic A52.79
  - congenital (early) A50.08 [D77]

Splenopathy D73.9

Splenoptosis D73.89

Splenosis D73.89

Splinter — *see* Foreign body, superficial, by site

Split, splitting
- foot Q72.7- ☑
- heart sounds R01.2
- lip, congenital — *see* Cleft, lip
- nails L60.3
- urinary stream R39.13

Spondylarthrosis — *see* Spondylosis

Spondylitis (chronic) (*see also* Spondylopathy, inflammatory)
- ankylopoietica — *see* Spondylitis, ankylosing
- ankylosing (chronic) M45.9
  - with lung involvement M45.9 [J99]
  - cervical region M45.2
  - cervicothoracic region M45.3
  - juvenile M08.1
  - lumbar region M45.6
  - lumbosacral region M45.7
  - multiple sites M45.0
  - occipito-atlanto-axial region M45.1
  - sacrococcygeal region M45.8
  - thoracic region M45.4
  - thoracolumbar region M45.5
- atrophic (ligamentous) — *see* Spondylitis, ankylosing
- deformans (chronic) — *see* Spondylosis
- gonococcal A54.41
- gouty M10.08
- in (due to)
  - brucellosis A23.9 [M49.80]
    - cervical region A23.9 [M49.82]
    - cervicothoracic region A23.9 [M49.83]
    - lumbar region A23.9 [M49.86]
    - lumbosacral region A23.9 [M49.87]
    - multiple sites A23.9 [M49.89]
    - occipito-atlanto-axial region A23.9 [M49.81]
    - sacrococcygeal region A23.9 [M49.88]
    - thoracic region A23.9 [M49.84]
    - thoracolumbar region A23.9 [M49.85]
  - enterobacteria (*see also* subcategory M49.8) A04.9
  - tuberculosis A18.01
- infectious NEC — *see* Spondylopathy, infective
- juvenile ankylosing (chronic) M08.1
- Kümmell's — *see* Spondylopathy, traumatic
- Marie-Strümpell — *see* Spondylitis, ankylosing
- muscularis — *see* Spondylopathy, specified NEC
- psoriatic L40.53
- rheumatoid — *see* Spondylitis, ankylosing
- rhizomelica — *see* Spondylitis, ankylosing
- sacroiliac NEC M46.1

☑ **Additional Character Required** — Refer to the Tabular List for Character Selection   ▽ **Subterms under main terms may continue to next column or page**

Spondylitis — *continued*
　senescent, senile — *see* Spondylosis
　traumatic (chronic) or post-traumatic — *see* Spondylopathy, traumatic
　tuberculous A18.01
　typhosa A01.05
Spondylolisthesis (acquired) (degenerative) M43.10
　with disproportion (fetopelvic) O33.0
　　causing obstructed labor O65.0
　cervical region M43.12
　cervicothoracic region M43.13
　congenital Q76.2
　lumbar region M43.16
　lumbosacral region M43.17
　multiple sites M43.19
　occipito-atlanto-axial region M43.11
　sacrococcygeal region M43.18
　thoracic region M43.14
　thoracolumbar region M43.15
　traumatic (old) M43.10
　　acute
　　　fifth cervical (displaced) S12.430 ☑
　　　　nondisplaced S12.431 ☑
　　　　specified type NEC (displaced) S12.450 ☑
　　　　　nondisplaced S12.451 ☑
　　　　type III S12.44 ☑
　　　fourth cervical (displaced) S12.330 ☑
　　　　nondisplaced S12.331 ☑
　　　　specified type NEC (displaced) S12.350 ☑
　　　　　nondisplaced S12.351 ☑
　　　　type III S12.34 ☑
　　　second cervical (displaced) S12.130 ☑
　　　　nondisplaced S12.131 ☑
　　　　specified type NEC (displaced) S12.150 ☑
　　　　　nondisplaced S12.151 ☑
　　　　type III S12.14 ☑
　　　seventh cervical (displaced) S12.630 ☑
　　　　nondisplaced S12.631 ☑
　　　　specified type NEC (displaced) S12.650 ☑
　　　　　nondisplaced S12.651 ☑
　　　　type III S12.64 ☑
　　　sixth cervical (displaced) S12.530 ☑
　　　　nondisplaced S12.531 ☑
　　　　specified type NEC (displaced) S12.550 ☑
　　　　　nondisplaced S12.551 ☑
　　　　type III S12.54 ☑
　　　third cervical (displaced) S12.230 ☑
　　　　nondisplaced S12.231 ☑
　　　　specified type NEC (displaced) S12.250 ☑
　　　　　nondisplaced S12.251 ☑
　　　　type III S12.24 ☑
Spondylolysis (acquired) M43.00
　cervical region M43.02
　cervicothoracic region M43.03
　congenital Q76.2
　lumbar region M43.06
　lumbosacral region M43.07
　　with disproportion (fetopelvic) O33.0
　　　causing obstructed labor O65.8
　multiple sites M43.09
　occipito-atlanto-axial region M43.01
　sacrococcygeal region M43.08
　thoracic region M43.04
　thoracolumbar region M43.05
Spondylopathy M48.9
　infective NEC M46.50
　　cervical region M46.52
　　cervicothoracic region M46.53
　　lumbar region M46.56
　　lumbosacral region M46.57
　　multiple sites M46.59
　　occipito-atlanto-axial region M46.51
　　sacrococcygeal region M46.58
　　thoracic region M46.54
　　thoracolumbar region M46.55
　inflammatory M46.90
　　cervical region M46.92
　　cervicothoracic region M46.93
　　lumbar region M46.96
　　lumbosacral region M46.97
　　multiple sites M46.99
　　occipito-atlanto-axial region M46.91
　　sacrococcygeal region M46.98
　　specified type NEC M46.80
　　　cervical region M46.82
　　　cervicothoracic region M46.83
　　　lumbar region M46.86

Spondylopathy — *continued*
　inflammatory — *continued*
　　specified type — *continued*
　　　lumbosacral region M46.87
　　　multiple sites M46.89
　　　occipito-atlanto-axial region M46.81
　　　sacrococcygeal region M46.88
　　　thoracic region M46.84
　　　thoracolumbar region M46.85
　　thoracic region M46.94
　　thoracolumbar region M46.95
　neuropathic, in
　　syringomyelia and syringobulbia G95.0
　　tabes dorsalis A52.11
　specified NEC — *see* subcategory M48.8 ☑
　traumatic M48.30
　　cervical region M48.32
　　cervicothoracic region M48.33
　　lumbar region M48.36
　　lumbosacral region M48.37
　　occipito-atlanto-axial region M48.31
　　sacrococcygeal region M48.38
　　thoracic region M48.34
　　thoracolumbar region M48.35
Spondylosis M47.9
　with
　　disproportion (fetopelvic) O33.0
　　　causing obstructed labor O65.0
　　myelopathy NEC M47.10
　　　cervical region M47.12
　　　cervicothoracic region M47.13
　　　lumbar region M47.16
　　　occipito-atlanto-axial region M47.11
　　　thoracic region M47.14
　　　thoracolumbar region M47.15
　　radiculopathy M47.20
　　　cervical region M47.22
　　　cervicothoracic region M47.23
　　　lumbar region M47.26
　　　lumbosacral region M47.27
　　　occipito-atlanto-axial region M47.21
　　　sacrococcygeal region M47.28
　　　thoracic region M47.24
　　　thoracolumbar region M47.25
　without myelopathy or radiculopathy M47.819
　　cervical region M47.812
　　cervicothoracic region M47.813
　　lumbar region M47.816
　　lumbosacral region M47.817
　　occipito-atlanto-axial region M47.811
　　sacrococcygeal region M47.818
　　thoracic region M47.814
　　thoracolumbar region M47.815
　specified NEC M47.899
　　cervical region M47.892
　　cervicothoracic region M47.893
　　lumbar region M47.896
　　lumbosacral region M47.897
　　occipito-atlanto-axial region M47.891
　　sacrococcygeal region M47.898
　　thoracic region M47.894
　　thoracolumbar region M47.895
　traumatic — *see* Spondylopathy, traumatic
Sponge
　inadvertently left in operation wound — *see* Foreign body, accidentally left during a procedure
　kidney (medullary) Q61.5
Sponge-diver's disease — *see* Toxicity, venom, marine animal, sea anemone
Spongioblastoma (any type) — *see* Neoplasm, malignant, by site
　specified site — *see* Neoplasm, malignant, by site
　unspecified site C71.9
Spongioneuroblastoma — *see* Neoplasm, malignant, by site
Spontaneous (*see also* condition)
　fracture (cause unknown) — *see* Fracture, pathological
Spoon nail L60.3
　congenital Q84.6
Sporadic — *see* condition
Sporothrix schenckii infection — *see* Sporotrichosis
Sporotrichosis B42.9
　arthritis B42.82
　disseminated B42.7
　generalized B42.7
　lymphocutaneous (fixed) (progressive) B42.1
　pulmonary B42.0
　specified NEC B42.89

Spots, spotting (in) (of)
　Bitot's (*see also* Pigmentation, conjunctiva)
　　in the young child E50.1
　　vitamin A deficiency E50.1
　café, au lait L81.3
　Cayenne pepper I78.1
　cotton wool, retina — *see* Occlusion, artery, retina
　de Morgan's (senile angiomas) I78.1
　Fuchs' black (myopic) H44.2- ☑
　intermenstrual (regular) N92.0
　　irregular N92.1
　Koplik's B05.9
　liver L81.4
　pregnancy O26.85- ☑
　purpuric R23.3
　ruby I78.1
Spotted fever — *see* Fever, spotted N92.3
Sprain (joint) (ligament)
　acromioclavicular joint or ligament S43.5- ☑
　ankle S93.40- ☑
　　calcaneofibular ligament S93.41- ☑
　　deltoid ligament S93.42- ☑
　　internal collateral ligament — *see* Sprain, ankle, specified ligament NEC
　　specified ligament NEC S93.49- ☑
　　talofibular ligament — *see* Sprain, ankle, specified ligament NEC
　　tibiofibular ligament S93.43- ☑
　anterior longitudinal, cervical S13.4 ☑
　atlas, atlanto-axial, atlanto-occipital S13.4 ☑
　breast bone — *see* Sprain, sternum
　calcaneofibular — *see* Sprain, ankle
　carpal — *see* Sprain, wrist
　carpometacarpal — *see* Sprain, hand, specified site NEC
　cartilage
　　costal S23.41 ☑
　　semilunar (knee) — *see* Sprain, knee, specified site NEC
　　　with current tear — *see* Tear, meniscus
　　thyroid region S13.5 ☑
　　xiphoid — *see* Sprain, sternum
　cervical, cervicodorsal, cervicothoracic S13.4 ☑
　chondrosternal S23.421 ☑
　coracoclavicular S43.8- ☑
　coracohumeral S43.41- ☑
　coronary, knee — *see* Sprain, knee, specified site NEC
　costal cartilage S23.41 ☑
　cricoarytenoid articulation or ligament S13.5 ☑
　cricothyroid articulation S13.5 ☑
　cruciate, knee — *see* Sprain, knee, cruciate
　deltoid, ankle — *see* Sprain, ankle
　dorsal (spine) S23.3 ☑
　elbow S53.40- ☑
　　radial collateral ligament S53.43- ☑
　　radiohumeral S53.41- ☑
　　rupture
　　　radial collateral ligament — *see* Rupture, traumatic, ligament, radial collateral
　　　ulnar collateral ligament — *see* Rupture, traumatic, ligament, ulnar collateral
　　specified type NEC S53.49- ☑
　　ulnar collateral ligament S53.44- ☑
　　ulnohumeral S53.42- ☑
　femur, head — *see* Sprain, hip
　fibular collateral, knee — *see* Sprain, knee, collateral
　fibulocalcaneal — *see* Sprain, ankle
　finger(s) S63.61- ☑
　　index S63.61- ☑
　　interphalangeal (joint) S63.63- ☑
　　　index S63.63- ☑
　　　little S63.63- ☑
　　　middle S63.63- ☑
　　　ring S63.63- ☑
　　little S63.61- ☑
　　metacarpophalangeal (joint) S63.65- ☑
　　middle S63.61- ☑
　　ring S63.61- ☑
　　specified site NEC S63.69- ☑
　　　index S63.69- ☑
　　　little S63.69- ☑
　　　middle S63.69- ☑
　　　ring S63.69- ☑
　foot S93.60- ☑
　　specified ligament NEC S93.69- ☑
　　tarsal ligament S93.61- ☑

Sprain — *continued*
foot — *continued*
    tarsometatarsal ligament S93.62- ☑
    toe — *see* Sprain, toe
  hand S63.9- ☑
    finger — *see* Sprain, finger
    specified site NEC — *see* subcategory S63.8 ☑
    thumb — *see* Sprain, thumb
  head S03.9 ☑
  hip S73.10- ☑
    iliofemoral ligament S73.11- ☑
    ischiocapsular (ligament) S73.12- ☑
    specified NEC S73.19- ☑
  iliofemoral — *see* Sprain, hip
  innominate
    acetabulum — *see* Sprain, hip
    sacral junction S33.6 ☑
  internal
    collateral, ankle — *see* Sprain, ankle
    semilunar cartilage — *see* Sprain, knee, specified
      site NEC
  interphalangeal
    finger — *see* Sprain, finger, interphalangeal (joint)
    toe — *see* Sprain, toe, interphalangeal joint
  ischiocapsular — *see* Sprain, hip
  ischiofemoral — *see* Sprain, hip
  jaw (articular disc) (cartilage) (meniscus) S03.4 ☑
    old M26.69
  knee S83.9- ☑
    collateral ligament S83.40- ☑
      lateral (fibular) S83.42- ☑
      medial (tibial) S83.41- ☑
    cruciate ligament S83.50- ☑
      anterior S83.51- ☑
      posterior S83.52- ☑
    lateral (fibular) collateral ligament S83.42- ☑
    medial (tibial) collateral ligament S83.41- ☑
    patellar ligament S76.11- ☑
    specified site NEC S83.8X- ☑
    superior tibiofibular joint (ligament) S83.6- ☑
  lateral collateral, knee — *see* Sprain, knee, collateral
  lumbar (spine) S33.5 ☑
  lumbosacral S33.9 ☑
  mandible (articular disc) S03.4 ☑
    old M26.69
  medial collateral, knee — *see* Sprain, knee, collateral
  meniscus
    jaw S03.4 ☑
      old M26.69
    knee — *see* Sprain, knee, specified site NEC
      with current tear — *see* Tear, meniscus
        old — *see* Derangement, knee, meniscus,
          due to old tear
    mandible S03.4 ☑
      old M26.69
  metacarpal (distal) (proximal) — *see* Sprain, hand,
    specified site NEC
  metacarpophalangeal — *see* Sprain, finger, metacar-
    pophalangeal (joint)
  metatarsophalangeal — *see* Sprain, toe, metatarsopha-
    langeal joint
  midcarpal — *see* Sprain, hand, specified site NEC
  midtarsal — *see* Sprain, foot, specified site NEC
  neck S13.9 ☑
    anterior longitudinal cervical ligament S13.4 ☑
    atlanto-axial joint S13.4 ☑
    atlanto-occipital joint S13.4 ☑
    cervical spine S13.4 ☑
    cricoarytenoid ligament S13.5 ☑
    cricothyroid ligament S13.5 ☑
    specified site NEC S13.8 ☑
    thyroid region (cartilage) S13.5 ☑
  nose S03.8 ☑
  orbicular, hip — *see* Sprain, hip
  patella — *see* Sprain, knee, specified site NEC
  patellar ligament S76.11- ☑
  pelvis NEC S33.8 ☑
  phalanx
    finger — *see* Sprain, finger
    toe — *see* Sprain, toe
  pubofemoral — *see* Sprain, hip
  radiocarpal — *see* Sprain, wrist
  radiohumeral — *see* Sprain, elbow
  radius, collateral — *see* Rupture, traumatic, ligament,
    radial collateral
  rib (cage) S23.41 ☑

Sprain — *continued*
  rotator cuff (capsule) S43.42- ☑
  sacroiliac (region)
    chronic or old — *see* subcategory M53.2 ☑
    joint S33.6 ☑
  scaphoid (hand) — *see* Sprain, hand, specified site
    NEC
  scapula (r) — *see* Sprain, shoulder girdle, specified site
    NEC
  semilunar cartilage (knee) — *see* Sprain, knee, speci-
    fied site NEC
    with current tear — *see* Tear, meniscus
      old — *see* Derangement, knee, meniscus, due
        to old tear
  shoulder joint S43.40- ☑
    acromioclavicular joint (ligament) — *see* Sprain,
      acromioclavicular joint
    blade — *see* Sprain, shoulder, girdle, specified site
      NEC
    coracoclavicular joint (ligament) — *see* Sprain,
      coracoclavicular joint
    coracohumeral ligament — *see* Sprain, coraco-
      humeral joint
    girdle S43.9- ☑
      specified site NEC S43.8- ☑
    rotator cuff — *see* Sprain, rotator cuff
    specified site NEC S43.49- ☑
    sternoclavicular joint (ligament) — *see* Sprain,
      sternoclavicular joint
  spine
    cervical S13.4 ☑
    lumbar S33.5 ☑
    thoracic S23.3 ☑
  sternoclavicular joint S43.6- ☑
  sternum S23.429 ☑
    chondrosternal joint S23.421 ☑
    specified site NEC S23.428 ☑
    sternoclavicular (joint) (ligament) S23.420 ☑
  symphysis
    jaw S03.4 ☑
      old M26.69
    mandibular S03.4 ☑
      old M26.69
  talofibular — *see* Sprain, ankle
  tarsal — *see* Sprain, foot, specified site NEC
  tarsometatarsal — *see* Sprain, foot, specified site NEC
  temporomandibular S03.4 ☑
    old M26.69
  thorax S23.9 ☑
    ribs S23.41 ☑
    specified site NEC S23.8 ☑
    spine S23.3 ☑
    sternum — *see* Sprain, sternum
  thumb S63.60- ☑
    interphalangeal (joint) S63.62- ☑
    metacarpophalangeal (joint) S63.64- ☑
    specified site NEC S63.68- ☑
  thyroid cartilage or region S13.5 ☑
  tibia (proximal end) — *see* Sprain, knee, specified site
    NEC
  tibial collateral, knee — *see* Sprain, knee, collateral
  tibiofibular
    distal — *see* Sprain, ankle
    superior — *see* Sprain, knee, specified site NEC
  toe(s) S93.50- ☑
    great S93.50- ☑
    interphalangeal joint S93.51- ☑
      great S93.51- ☑
      lesser S93.51- ☑
    lesser S93.50- ☑
    metatarsophalangeal joint S93.52- ☑
      great S93.52- ☑
      lesser S93.52- ☑
  ulna, collateral — *see* Rupture, traumatic, ligament,
    ulnar collateral
  ulnohumeral — *see* Sprain, elbow
  wrist S63.50- ☑
    carpal S63.51- ☑
    radiocarpal S63.52- ☑
    specified site NEC S63.59- ☑
  xiphoid cartilage — *see* Sprain, sternum
Sprengel's deformity (congenital) Q74.0
Sprue (tropical) K90.1
  celiac K90.0
  idiopathic K90.0
  meaning thrush B37.0

Sprue — *continued*
  nontropical K90.0
Spur, bone (*see also* Enthesopathy)
  calcaneal M77.3- ☑
  iliac crest M76.2- ☑
  nose (septum) J34.89
Spurway's syndrome Q78.0
Sputum
  abnormal (amount) (color) (odor) (purulent) R09.3
  blood-stained R04.2
  excessive (cause unknown) R09.3
Squamous (*see also* condition)
  epithelium in
    cervical canal (congenital) Q51.828
    uterine mucosa (congenital) Q51.818
Squashed nose M95.0
  congenital Q67.4
Squeeze, diver's T70.3 ☑
Squint (*see also* Strabismus)
  accommodative — *see* Strabismus, convergent con-
    comitant
St. Hubert's disease A82.9
Stab (*see also* Laceration)
  internal organs — *see* Injury, by site
Stafne's cyst or cavity M27.0
Staggering gait R26.0
  hysterical F44.4
Staghorn calculus — *see* Calculus, kidney
Stähli's line (cornea) (pigment) — *see* Pigmentation,
  cornea, anterior
Stain, staining
  meconium (newborn) P96.83
  port wine Q82.5
  tooth, teeth (hard tissues) (extrinsic) K03.6
    due to
      accretions K03.6
      deposits (betel) (black) (green) (materia alba)
        (orange) (soft) (tobacco) K03.6
      metals (copper) (silver) K03.7
      nicotine K03.6
      pulpal bleeding K03.7
      tobacco K03.6
    intrinsic K00.8
Stammering (*see also* Disorder, fluency) F80.81
Standstill
  auricular I45.5
  cardiac — *see* Arrest, cardiac
  sinoatrial I45.5
  ventricular — *see* Arrest, cardiac
Stannosis J63.5
Stanton's disease — *see* Melioidosis
Staphylitis (acute) (catarrhal) (chronic) (gangrenous)
  (membranous) (suppurative) (ulcerative) K12.2
Staphylococcal scalded skin syndrome L00
Staphylococcemia A41.2
Staphylococcus, staphylococcal (*see also* condition)
  as cause of disease classified elsewhere B95.8
    aureus (methicillin susceptible) (MSSA) B95.61
      methicillin resistant (MRSA) B95.62
  specified NEC, as cause of disease classified elsewhere
    B95.7
Staphyloma (sclera)
  cornea H18.72- ☑
  equatorial H15.81- ☑
  localized (anterior) H15.82- ☑
  posticum H15.83- ☑
  ring H15.85- ☑
Stargardt's disease — *see* Dystrophy, retina
Starvation (inanition) (due to lack of food) T73.0 ☑
  edema — *see* Malnutrition, severe
Stasis
  bile (noncalculous) K83.1
  bronchus J98.09
    with infection — *see* Bronchitis
  cardiac — *see* Failure, heart, congestive
  cecum K59.8
  colon K59.8
  dermatitis — *see* Varix, leg, with, inflammation
  duodenal K31.5
  eczema — *see* Varix, leg, with, inflammation
  edema — *see* Hypertension, venous (chronic), idiopath-
    ic
  foot T69.0- ☑
  ileocecal coil K59.8
  ileum K59.8
  intestinal K59.8
  jejunum K59.8

282

☑ **Additional Character Required** — Refer to the Tabular List for Character Selection   ▽ **Subterms under main terms may continue to next column or page**

Stasis—continued
  kidney N19
  liver (cirrhotic) K76.1
  lymphatic I89.8
  pneumonia J18.2
  pulmonary — see Edema, lung
  rectal K59.8
  renal N19
    tubular N17.0
  ulcer — see Varix, leg, with, ulcer
    without varicose veins I87.2
  urine — see Retention, urine
  venous I87.8
State (of)
  affective and paranoid, mixed, organic psychotic F06.8
  agitated R45.1
    acute reaction to stress F43.0
  anxiety (neurotic) F41.1
  apprehension F41.1
  burn-out Z73.0
  climacteric, female Z78.0
    symptomatic N95.1
  compulsive F42
    mixed with obsessional thoughts F42
  confusional (psychogenic) F44.89
    acute (see also Delirium)
      with
        arteriosclerotic dementia F01.50
          with behavioral disturbance F01.51
        senility or dementia F05
      alcoholic F10.231
    epileptic F05
    reactive (from emotional stress, psychological
      trauma) F44.89
    subacute — see Delirium
  convulsive — see Convulsions
  crisis F43.0
  depressive F32.9
    neurotic F34.1
  dissociative F44.9
  emotional shock (stress) R45.7
  hypercoagulation — see Hypercoagulable
  locked-in G83.5
  menopausal Z78.0
    symptomatic N95.1
  neurotic F48.9
    with depersonalization F48.1
  obsessional F42
  oneiroid (schizophrenia-like) F23
  organic
    hallucinatory (nonalcoholic) F06.0
    paranoid (hallucinatory) F06.2
  panic F41.0
  paranoid F22
    climacteric F22
    involutional F22
    menopausal F22
    organic F06.2
    senile F03 ☑
    simple F22
  persistent vegetative R40.3
  phobic F40.9
  postleukotomy F07.0
  pregnant, incidental Z33.1
  psychogenic, twilight F44.89
  psychopathic (constitutional) F60.2
  psychotic, organic (see also Psychosis, organic)
    mixed paranoid and affective F06.8
    senile or presenile F03 ☑
    transient NEC F06.8
      with
        depression F06.31
        hallucinations F06.0
  residual schizophrenic F20.5
  restlessness R45.1
  stress (emotional) R45.7
  tension (mental) F48.9
    specified NEC F48.8
  transient organic psychotic NEC F06.8
    depressive type F06.31
    hallucinatory type F06.30
  twilight
    epileptic F05
    psychogenic F44.89
  vegetative, persistent R40.3
  vital exhaustion Z73.0
  withdrawal, — see Withdrawal, state

Status (post) (see also Presence (of))
  absence, epileptic — see Epilepsy, by type, with status
    epilepticus
  administration of tPA (rtPA) in a different facility
    within the last 24 hours prior to admission to
    current facility Z92.82
  adrenalectomy (unilateral) (bilateral) E89.6
  anastomosis Z98.0
  anginosus I20.9
  angioplasty (peripheral) Z98.62
    with implant Z95.820
    coronary artery Z98.61
      with implant Z95.5
  aortocoronary bypass Z95.1
  arthrodesis Z98.1
  artificial opening (of) Z93.9
    gastrointestinal tract Z93.4
    specified NEC Z93.8
    urinary tract Z93.6
    vagina Z93.8
  asthmaticus — see Asthma, by type, with status asth-
    maticus
  awaiting organ transplant Z76.82
  bariatric surgery Z98.84
  bed confinement Z74.01
  bleb, filtering (vitreous), after glaucoma surgery Z98.83
  breast implant Z98.82
    removal Z98.86
  cataract extraction Z98.4- ☑
  cholecystectomy Z90.49
  clitorectomy N90.811
    with excision of labia minora N90.812
  colectomy (complete) (partial) Z90.49
  colonization — see Carrier (suspected) of
  colostomy Z93.3
  convulsivus idiopathicus — see Epilepsy, by type, with
    status epilepticus
  coronary artery angioplasty — see Status, angioplasty,
    coronary artery
  cystectomy (urinary bladder) Z90.6
  cystostomy Z93.50
    appendico-vesicostomy Z93.52
    cutaneous Z93.51
    specified NEC Z93.59
  delinquent immunization Z28.3
  dental Z98.818
    crown Z98.811
    fillings Z98.811
    restoration Z98.811
    sealant Z98.810
    specified NEC Z98.818
  deployment (current) (military) Z56.82
  dialysis (hemodialysis) (peritoneal) Z99.2
  do not resuscitate (DNR) Z66
  donor — see Donor
  embedded fragments — see Retained, foreign body
    fragments (type of)
  embedded splinter — see Retained, foreign body
    fragments (type of)
  enterostomy Z93.4
  epileptic, epilepticus (see also Epilepsy, by type, with
    status epilepticus) G40.901
  estrogen receptor
    negative Z17.1
    positive Z17.0
  female genital cutting — see Female genital mutilation
    status
  female genital mutilation — see Female genital muti-
    lation status
  filtering (vitreous) bleb after glaucoma surgery Z98.83
  gastrectomy (complete) (partial) Z90.3
  gastric banding Z98.84
  gastric bypass for obesity Z98.84
  gastrostomy Z93.1
  human immunodeficiency virus (HIV) infection,
    asymptomatic Z21
  hysterectomy (complete) (total) Z90.710
    partial (with remaining cervial stump) Z90.711
  ileostomy Z93.2
  implant
    breast Z98.82
  infibulation N90.813
  intestinal bypass Z98.0
  jejunostomy Z93.4
  lapsed immunization schedule Z28.3
  laryngectomy Z90.02
  lymphaticus E32.8
  marmoratus G80.3

Status — continued
  mastectomy (unilateral) (bilateral) Z90.1- ☑
  military deployment status (current) Z56.82
    in theater or in support of military war, peacekeep-
      ing and humanitarian operations Z56.82
  nephrectomy (unilateral) (bilateral) Z90.5
  nephrostomy Z93.6
  obesity surgery Z98.84
  oophorectomy
    bilateral Z90.722
    unilateral Z90.721
  organ replacement
    by artificial or mechanical device or prosthesis of
      artery Z95.828
      bladder Z96.0
      blood vessel Z95.828
      breast Z97.8
      eye globe Z97.0
      heart Z95.812
        valve Z95.2
      intestine Z97.8
      joint Z96.60
        hip — see Presence, hip joint implant
        knee — see Presence, knee joint implant
        specified site NEC Z96.698
      kidney Z97.8
      larynx Z96.3
      lens Z96.1
      limbs — see Presence, artificial, limb
      liver Z97.8
      lung Z97.8
      pancreas Z97.8
    by organ transplant (heterologous)(homologous)
      — see Transplant
  pacemaker
    brain Z96.89
    cardiac Z95.0
    specified NEC Z96.89
  pancreatectomy Z90.410
    complete Z90.410
    partial Z90.411
    total Z90.410
  physical restraint Z78.1
  pneumonectomy (complete) (partial) Z90.2
  pneumothorax, therapeutic Z98.3
  postcommotio cerebri F07.81
  postoperative (postprocedural) NEC Z98.89
    breast implant Z98.82
    dental Z98.818
      crown Z98.811
      fillings Z98.811
      restoration Z98.811
      sealant Z98.810
      specified NEC Z98.818
    pneumothorax, therapeutic Z98.3
  postpartum (routine follow-up) Z39.2
    care immediately after delivery Z39.0
  postsurgical (postprocedural) NEC Z98.89
    pneumothorax, therapeutic Z98.3
  pregnancy, incidental Z33.1
  prosthesis coronary angioplasty Z95.5
  pseudophakia Z96.1
  renal dialysis (hemodialysis) (peritoneal) Z99.2
  retained foreign body — see Retained, foreign body
    fragments (type of)
  reversed jejunal transposition (for bypass) Z98.0
  salpingo-oophorectomy
    bilateral Z90.722
    unilateral Z90.721
  sex reassignment surgery status Z87.890
  shunt
    arteriovenous (for dialysis) Z99.2
    cerebrospinal fluid Z98.2
    ventricular (communicating) (for drainage) Z98.2
  splenectomy Z90.81
  thymicolymphaticus E32.8
  thymicus E32.8
  thymolymphaticus E32.8
  thyroidectomy (hypothyroidism) E89.0
  tooth (teeth) extraction (see also Absence, teeth, ac-
    quired) K08.409
  tPA (rtPA) administration in a different facility within
    the last 24 hours prior to admission to current
    facility Z92.82
  tracheostomy Z93.0
  transplant — see Transplant
    organ removed Z98.85
  tubal ligation Z98.51

Status — *continued*
  underimmunization Z28.3
  ureterostomy Z93.6
  urethrostomy Z93.6
  vagina, artificial Z93.8
  vasectomy Z98.52
  wheelchair confinement Z99.3
Stealing
  child problem F91.8
    in company with others Z72.810
  pathological (compulsive) F63.2
Steam burn — *see* Burn
Steatocystoma multiplex L72.2
Steatohepatitis (nonalcoholic) (NASH) K75.81
Steatoma L72.3
  eyelid (cystic) — *see* Dermatosis, eyelid
    infected — *see* Hordeolum
Steatorrhea (chronic) K90.4
  with lacteal obstruction K90.2
  idiopathic (adult) (infantile) K90.0
  pancreatic K90.3
  primary K90.0
  tropical K90.1
Steatosis E88.89
  heart — *see* Degeneration, myocardial
  kidney N28.89
  liver NEC K76.0
Steele-Richardson-Olszewski disease or syndrome
  G23.1
Steinbrocker's syndrome G90.8
Steinert's disease G71.11
Stein-Leventhal syndrome E28.2
Stein's syndrome E28.2
STEMI (*see also* Infarct, myocardium, ST elevation) I21.3
Stenocardia I20.8
Stenocephaly Q75.8
Stenosis, stenotic (cicatricial) (*see also* Stricture)
  ampulla of Vater K83.1
  anus, anal (canal) (sphincter) K62.4
    and rectum K62.4
    congenital Q42.3
      with fistula Q42.2
  aorta (ascending) (supraventricular) (congenital) Q25.3
    arteriosclerotic I70.0
    calcified I70.0
  aortic (valve) I35.0
    with insufficiency I35.2
    congenital Q23.0
    rheumatic I06.0
      with
        incompetency, insufficiency or regurgitation
          I06.2
          with mitral (valve) disease I08.0
            with tricuspid (valve) disease I08.3
        mitral (valve) disease I08.0
          with tricuspid (valve) disease I08.3
        tricuspid (valve) disease I08.2
          with mitral (valve) disease I08.3
    specified cause NEC I35.8
    syphilitic A52.03
  aqueduct of Sylvius (congenital) Q03.0
    with spina bifida — *see* Spina bifida, by site, with
      hydrocephalus
    acquired G91.1
  artery NEC (*see also* Arteriosclerosis) I77.1
    celiac I77.4
    cerebral — *see* Occlusion, artery, cerebral
    extremities — *see* Arteriosclerosis, extremities
    precerebral — *see* Occlusion, artery, precerebral
    pulmonary (congenital) Q25.6
      acquired I28.8
    renal I70.1
  bile duct (common) (hepatic) K83.1
    congenital Q44.3
  bladder-neck (acquired) N32.0
    congenital Q64.31
  brain G93.89
  bronchus J98.09
    congenital Q32.3
    syphilitic A52.72
  cardia (stomach) K22.2
    congenital Q39.3
  cardiovascular — *see* Disease, cardiovascular
  caudal M48.08
  cervix, cervical (canal) N88.2
    congenital Q51.828
    in pregnancy or childbirth — *see* Pregnancy,
      complicated by, abnormal cervix

Stenosis, stenotic — *continued*
  colon (*see also* Obstruction, intestine)
    congenital Q42.9
      specified NEC Q42.8
  colostomy K94.03
  common (bile) duct K83.1
    congenital Q44.3
  coronary (artery) — *see* Disease, heart, ischemic,
    atherosclerotic
  cystic duct — *see* Obstruction, gallbladder
  due to presence of device, implant or graft (*see also*
    Complications, by site and type, specified NEC)
    T85.85 ☑
    arterial graft NEC T82.858 ☑
    breast (implant) T85.85 ☑
    catheter T85.85 ☑
      dialysis (renal) T82.858 ☑
        intraperitoneal T85.85 ☑
      infusion NEC T82.858 ☑
        spinal (epidural) (subdural) T85.85 ☑
      urinary (indwelling) T83.85 ☑
    fixation, internal (orthopedic) NEC T84.85 ☑
    gastrointestinal (bile duct) (esophagus) T85.85 ☑
    genital NEC T83.85 ☑
    heart NEC T82.857 ☑
    joint prosthesis T84.85 ☑
    ocular (corneal graft) (orbital implant) NEC
      T85.85 ☑
    orthopedic NEC T84.85 ☑
    specified NEC T85.85 ☑
    urinary NEC T83.85 ☑
    vascular NEC T82.858 ☑
    ventricular intracranial shunt T85.85 ☑
  duodenum K31.5
    congenital Q41.0
  ejaculatory duct NEC N50.8
  endocervical os — *see* Stenosis, cervix
  enterostomy K94.13
  esophagus K22.2
    congenital Q39.3
    syphilitic A52.79
      congenital A50.59 [K23]
  eustachian tube — *see* Obstruction, eustachian tube
  external ear canal (acquired) H61.30- ☑
    congenital Q16.1
    due to
      inflammation H61.32- ☑
      trauma H61.31- ☑
    postprocedural H95.81- ☑
    specified cause NEC H61.39- ☑
  gallbladder — *see* Obstruction, gallbladder
  glottis J38.6
  heart valve (congenital) Q24.8
    aortic Q23.0
    mitral Q23.2
    pulmonary Q22.1
    tricuspid Q22.4
  hepatic duct K83.1
  hymen N89.6
  hypertrophic subaortic (idiopathic) I42.1
  ileum K56.69
    congenital Q41.2
  infundibulum cardia Q24.3
  intervertebral foramina (*see also* Lesion, biomechani-
    cal, specified NEC)
    connective tissue M99.79
      abdomen M99.79
      cervical region M99.71
      cervicothoracic M99.71
      head region M99.70
      lumbar region M99.73
      lumbosacral M99.73
      occipitocervical M99.70
      sacral region M99.74
      sacrococcygeal M99.74
      sacroiliac M99.74
      specified NEC M99.79
      thoracic region M99.72
      thoracolumbar M99.72
    disc M99.79
      abdomen M99.79
      cervical region M99.71
      cervicothoracic M99.71
      head region M99.70
      lower extremity M99.76
      lumbar region M99.73
      lumbosacral M99.73

Stenosis, stenotic — *continued*
  intervertebral foramina (*see also* Lesion, biomechanical,
    specified) — *continued*
    disc — *continued*
      occipitocervical M99.70
      pelvic M99.75
      rib cage M99.78
      sacral region M99.74
      sacrococcygeal M99.74
      sacroiliac M99.74
      specified NEC M99.79
      thoracic region M99.72
      thoracolumbar M99.72
      upper extremity M99.77
    osseous M99.69
      abdomen M99.69
      cervical region M99.61
      cervicothoracic M99.61
      head region M99.60
      lower extremity M99.66
      lumbar region M99.63
      lumbosacral M99.63
      occipitocervical M99.60
      pelvic M99.65
      rib cage M99.68
      sacral region M99.64
      sacrococcygeal M99.64
      sacroiliac M99.64
      specified NEC M99.69
      thoracic region M99.62
      thoracolumbar M99.62
      upper extremity M99.67
    subluxation — *see* Stenosis, intervertebral forami-
      na, osseous
  intestine (*see also* Obstruction, intestine)
    congenital (small) Q41.9
    large Q42.9
      specified NEC Q42.8
      specified NEC Q41.8
  jejunum K56.69
    congenital Q41.1
  lacrimal (passage)
    canaliculi H04.54- ☑
    congenital Q10.5
    duct H04.55- ☑
    punctum H04.56- ☑
    sac H04.57- ☑
  lacrimonasal duct — *see* Stenosis, lacrimal, duct
    congenital Q10.5
  larynx J38.6
    congenital NEC Q31.8
      subglottic Q31.1
    syphilitic A52.73
      congenital A50.59 [J99]
  mitral (chronic) (inactive) (valve) I05.0
    with
      aortic valve disease I08.0
      incompetency, insufficiency or regurgitation
        I05.2
    active or acute I01.1
      with rheumatic or Sydenham's chorea I02.0
    congenital Q23.2
    specified cause, except rheumatic I34.2
    syphilitic A52.03
  myocardium, myocardial (*see also* Degeneration, my-
    ocardial)
    hypertrophic subaortic (idiopathic) I42.1
  nares (anterior) (posterior) J34.89
    congenital Q30.0
  nasal duct (*see also* Stenosis, lacrimal, duct)
    congenital Q10.5
  nasolacrimal duct (*see also* Stenosis, lacrimal, duct)
    congenital Q10.5
  neural canal (*see also* Lesion, biomechanical, specified
    NEC)
    connective tissue M99.49
      abdomen M99.49
      cervical region M99.41
      cervicothoracic M99.41
      head region M99.40
      lower extremity M99.46
      lumbar region M99.43
      lumbosacral M99.43
      occipitocervical M99.40
      pelvic M99.45
      rib cage M99.48
      sacral region M99.44
      sacrococcygeal M99.44

☑ **Additional Character Required** — Refer to the Tabular List for Character Selection   ▽ **Subterms under main terms may continue to next column or page**

Stenosis, stenotic — *continued*
  neural canal (*see also* Lesion, biomechanical, specified) — *continued*
    connective tissue — *continued*
      sacroiliac M99.44
      specified NEC M99.49
      thoracic region M99.42
      thoracolumbar M99.42
      upper extremity M99.47
    intervertebral disc M99.59
      abdomen M99.59
      cervical region M99.51
      cervicothoracic M99.51
      head region M99.50
      lower extremity M99.56
      lumbar region M99.53
      lumbosacral M99.53
      occipitocervical M99.50
      pelvic M99.55
      rib cage M99.58
      sacral region M99.54
      sacrococcygeal M99.54
      sacroiliac M99.54
      specified NEC M99.59
      thoracic region M99.52
      thoracolumbar M99.52
      upper extremity M99.57
    osseous M99.39
      abdomen M99.39
      cervical region M99.31
      cervicothoracic M99.31
      head region M99.30
      lower extremity M99.36
      lumbar region M99.33
      lumbosacral M99.33
      occipitocervical M99.30
      pelvic M99.35
      rib cage M99.38
      sacral region M99.34
      sacrococcygeal M99.34
      sacroiliac M99.34
      specified NEC M99.39
      thoracic region M99.32
      thoracolumbar M99.32
      upper extremity M99.37
    subluxation M99.29
      cervical region M99.21
      cervicothoracic M99.21
      head region M99.20
      lower extremity M99.26
      lumbar region M99.23
      lumbosacral M99.23
      occipitocervical M99.20
      pelvic M99.25
      rib cage M99.28
      sacral region M99.24
      sacrococcygeal M99.24
      sacroiliac M99.24
      specified NEC M99.29
      thoracic region M99.22
      thoracolumbar M99.22
      upper extremity M99.27
  organ or site, congenital NEC — *see* Atresia, by site
  papilla of Vater K83.1
  pulmonary (artery) (congenital) Q25.6
    with ventricular septal defect, transposition of aorta, and hypertrophy of right ventricle Q21.3
    acquired I28.8
    in tetralogy of Fallot Q21.3
    infundibular Q24.3
    subvalvular Q24.3
    supravalvular Q25.6
    valve I37.0
      with insufficiency I37.2
      congenital Q22.1
      rheumatic I09.89
        with aortic, mitral or tricuspid (valve) disease I08.8
    vein, acquired I28.8
    vessel NEC I28.8
  pulmonic (congenital) Q22.1
    infundibular Q24.3
    subvalvular Q24.3
  pylorus (hypertrophic) (acquired) K31.1
    adult K31.1
    congenital Q40.0
    infantile Q40.0

Stenosis, stenotic — *continued*
  rectum (sphincter) — *see* Stricture, rectum
  renal artery I70.1
    congenital Q27.1
  salivary duct (any) K11.8
  sphincter of Oddi K83.1
  spinal M48.00
    cervical region M48.02
    cervicothoracic region M48.03
    lumbar region M48.06
    lumbosacral region M48.07
    occipito-atlanto-axial region M48.01
    sacrococcygeal region M48.08
    thoracic region M48.04
    thoracolumbar region M48.05
  stomach, hourglass K31.2
  subaortic (congenital) Q24.4
    hypertrophic (idiopathic) I42.1
  subglottic J38.6
    congenital Q31.1
    postprocedural J95.5
  trachea J39.8
    congenital Q32.1
    syphilitic A52.73
    tuberculous NEC A15.5
  tracheostomy J95.03
  tricuspid (valve) I07.0
    with
      aortic (valve) disease I08.2
      incompetency, insufficiency or regurgitation I07.2
        with aortic (valve) disease I08.2
          with mitral (valve) disease I08.3
        mitral (valve) disease I08.1
          with aortic (valve) disease I08.3
    congenital Q22.4
    nonrheumatic I36.0
      with insufficiency I36.2
  tubal N97.1
  ureter — *see* Atresia, ureter
  ureteropelvic junction, congenital Q62.11
  ureterovesical orifice, congenital Q62.12
  urethra (valve) (*see also* Stricture, urethra)
    congenital Q64.32
  urinary meatus, congenital Q64.33
  vagina N89.5
    congenital Q52.4
    in pregnancy — *see* Pregnancy, complicated by, abnormal vagina
      causing obstructed labor O65.5
  valve (cardiac) (heart) (*see also* Endocarditis) I38
    congenital Q24.8
      aortic Q23.0
      mitral Q23.2
      pulmonary Q22.1
      tricuspid Q22.4
  vena cava (inferior) (superior) I87.1
    congenital Q26.0
  vesicourethral orifice Q64.31
  vulva N90.5
Stent jail T82.897 ☑
Stercolith (impaction) K56.41
  appendix K38.1
Stercoraceous, stercoral ulcer K63.3
  anus or rectum K62.6
Stereotypies NEC F98.4
Sterility — *see* Infertility
Sterilization — *see* Encounter (for), sterilization
Sternalgia — *see* Angina
Sternopagus Q89.4
Sternum bifidum Q76.7
Steroid
  effects (adverse) (adrenocortical) (iatrogenic)
    cushingoid E24.2
      correct substance properly administered — *see* Table of Drugs and Chemicals, by drug, adverse effect
      overdose or wrong substance given or taken — *see* Table of Drugs and Chemicals, by drug, poisoning
    diabetes — *see* subcategory E09 ☑
      correct substance properly administered — *see* Table of Drugs and Chemicals, by drug, adverse effect
      overdose or wrong substance given or taken — *see* Table of Drugs and Chemicals, by drug, poisoning
    fever R50.2

Steroid — *continued*
  effects — *continued*
    insufficiency E27.3
      correct substance properly administered — *see* Table of Drugs and Chemicals, by drug, adverse effect
      overdose or wrong substance given or taken — *see* Table of Drugs and Chemicals, by drug, poisoning
  responder H40.04- ☑
Stevens-Johnson disease or syndrome L51.1
  toxic epidermal necrolysis overlap L51.3
Stewart-Morel syndrome M85.2
Sticker's disease B08.3
Sticky eye — *see* Conjunctivitis, acute, mucopurulent
Stieda's disease — *see* Bursitis, tibial collateral
Stiff neck — *see* Torticollis
Stiff-man syndrome G25.82
Stiffness, joint NEC M25.60
  ankle M25.67- ☑
  ankylosis — *see* Ankylosis, joint
  contracture — *see* Contraction, joint
  elbow M25.62- ☑
  foot M25.67- ☑
  hand M25.64- ☑
  hip M25.65- ☑
  knee M25.66- ☑
  shoulder M25.61- ☑
  wrist M25.63- ☑
Stigmata congenital syphilis A50.59
Stillbirth P95
Still-Felty syndrome — *see* Felty's syndrome
Still's disease or syndrome (juvenile) M08.20
  adult-onset M06.1
  ankle M08.27- ☑
  elbow M08.22- ☑
  foot joint M08.27- ☑
  hand joint M08.24- ☑
  hip M08.25- ☑
  knee M08.26- ☑
  multiple site M08.29
  shoulder M08.21- ☑
  vertebra M08.28
  wrist M08.23- ☑
Stimulation, ovary E28.1
Sting (venomous) (with allergic or anaphylactic shock) — *see* Table of Drugs and Chemicals, by animal or substance, poisoning
Stippled epiphyses Q78.8
Stitch
  abscess T81.4 ☑
  burst (in operation wound) — *see* Disruption, wound, operation
Stokes' disease E05.00
  with thyroid storm E05.01
Stokes-Adams disease or syndrome I45.9
Stokvis (-Talma) **disease** D74.8
Stoma malfunction
  colostomy K94.03
  enterostomy K94.13
  gastrostomy K94.23
  ileostomy K94.13
  tracheostomy J95.03
Stomach — *see* condition
Stomatitis (denture) (ulcerative) K12.1
  angular K13.0
    due to dietary or vitamin deficiency E53.0
  aphthous K12.0
  bovine B08.61
  candidal B37.0
  catarrhal K12.1
  diphtheritic A36.89
  due to
    dietary deficiency E53.0
    thrush B37.0
    vitamin deficiency
      B group NEC E53.9
      B2 (riboflavin) E53.0
  epidemic B08.8
  epizootic B08.8
  follicular K12.1
  gangrenous A69.0
  Geotrichum B48.3
  herpesviral, herpetic B00.2
  herpetiformis K12.0
  malignant K12.1
  membranous acute K12.1

Stomatitis — continued
    monilial B37.0
    mycotic B37.0
    necrotizing ulcerative A69.0
    parasitic B37.0
    septic K12.1
    spirochetal A69.1
    suppurative (acute) K12.2
    ulceromembranous A69.1
    vesicular K12.1
        with exanthem (enteroviral) B08.4
        virus disease A93.8
    Vincent's A69.1
Stomatocytosis D58.8
Stomatomycosis B37.0
Stomatorrhagia K13.79
Stone(s) (see also Calculus)
    bladder (diverticulum) N21.0
    cystine E72.09
    heart syndrome I50.1
    kidney N20.0
    prostate N42.0
    pulpal (dental) K04.2
    renal N20.0
    salivary gland or duct (any) K11.5
    urethra (impacted) N21.1
    urinary (duct) (impacted) (passage) N20.9
        bladder (diverticulum) N21.0
        lower tract N21.9
        specified NEC N21.8
        xanthine E79.8 [N22]
Stonecutter's lung J62.8
Stonemason's asthma, disease, lung or pneumoconiosis J62.8
Stoppage
    heart — see Arrest, cardiac
    urine — see Retention, urine
Storm, thyroid — see Thyrotoxicosis
Strabismus (congenital) (nonparalytic) H50.9
    concomitant H50.40
        convergent — see Strabismus, convergent concomitant
        divergent — see Strabismus, divergent concomitant
    convergent concomitant H50.00
        accommodative component H50.43
        alternating H50.05
            with
                A pattern H50.06
                specified nonconcomitances NEC H50.08
                V pattern H50.07
        monocular H50.01- ☑
            with
                A pattern H50.02- ☑
                specified nonconcomitances NEC H50.04- ☑
                V pattern H50.03- ☑
        intermittent H50.31- ☑
            alternating H50.32
    cyclotropia H50.1- ☑
    divergent concomitant H50.10
        alternating H50.15
            with
                A pattern H50.16
                specified nonconcomitances NEC H50.18
                V pattern H50.17
        monocular H50.11- ☑
            with
                A pattern H50.12- ☑
                specified nonconcomitances NEC H50.14- ☑
                V pattern H50.13- ☑
        intermittent H50.33 ☑
            alternating H50.34
    Duane's syndrome H50.81- ☑
    due to adhesions, scars H50.69
    heterophoria H50.50
        alternating H50.55
        cyclophoria H50.54
        esophoria H50.51
        exophoria H50.52
        vertical H50.53
    heterotropia H50.40
        intermittent H50.30
    hypertropia H50.2- ☑
    hypotropia — see Hypertropia
    latent H50.50
    mechanical H50.60
        Brown's sheath syndrome H50.61- ☑

Strabismus — continued
    mechanical — continued
        specified type NEC H50.69
    monofixation syndrome H50.42
    paralytic H49.9
        abducens nerve H49.2- ☑
        fourth nerve H49.1- ☑
        Kearns-Sayre syndrome H49.81- ☑
        ophthalmoplegia (external)
            progressive H49.4- ☑
                with pigmentary retinopathy H49.81- ☑
            total H49.3- ☑
        sixth nerve H49.2- ☑
        specified type NEC H49.88- ☑
        third nerve H49.0- ☑
        trochlear nerve H49.1- ☑
    specified type NEC H50.89
    vertical H50.2- ☑
Strain
    back S39.012 ☑
    cervical S16.1 ☑
    eye NEC — see Disturbance, vision, subjective
    heart — see Disease, heart
    low back S39.012 ☑
    mental NOS Z73.3
        work-related Z56.6
    muscle (tendon) — see Injury, muscle, by site, strain
    neck S16.1 ☑
    physical NOS Z73.3
        work-related Z56.6
    postural (see also Disorder, soft tissue, due to use)
    psychological NEC Z73.3
    tendon — see Injury, muscle, by site, strain
Straining, on urination R39.16
Strand, vitreous — see Opacity, vitreous, membranes and strands
Strangulation, strangulated (see also Asphyxia, traumatic)
    appendix K38.8
    bladder-neck N32.0
    bowel or colon K56.2
    food or foreign body — see Foreign body, by site
    hemorrhoids — see Hemorrhoids, with complication
    hernia (see also Hernia, by site, with obstruction)
        with gangrene — see Hernia, by site, with gangrene
    intestine (large) (small) K56.2
        with hernia (see also Hernia, by site, with obstruction)
            with gangrene — see Hernia, by site, with gangrene
    mesentery K56.2
    mucus — see Asphyxia, mucus
    omentum K56.2
    organ or site, congenital NEC — see Atresia, by site
    ovary — see Torsion, ovary
    penis N48.89
        foreign body T19.4 ☑
    rupture — see Hernia, by site, with obstruction
    stomach due to hernia (see also Hernia, by site, with obstruction)
        with gangrene — see Hernia, by site, with gangrene
    vesicourethral orifice N32.0
Strangury R30.0
Straw itch B88.0
Strawberry
    gallbladder K82.4
    mark Q82.5
    tongue (red) (white) K14.3
Streak(s)
    macula, angioid H35.33
    ovarian Q50.32
Strephosymbolia F81.0
    secondary to organic lesion R48.8
Streptobacillary fever A25.1
Streptobacillosis A25.1
Streptobacillus moniliformis A25.1
Streptococcus, streptococcal (see also condition)
    as cause of disease classified elsewhere B95.5
    group
        A, as cause of disease classified elsewhere B95.0
        B, as cause of disease classified elsewhere B95.1
        D, as cause of disease classified elsewhere B95.2
    pneumoniae, as cause of disease classified elsewhere B95.3

Streptococcus, streptococcal — continued
    specified NEC, as cause of disease classified elsewhere B95.4
Streptomycosis B47.1
Streptotrichosis A48.8
Stress F43.9
    family — see Disruption, family
    fetal P84
        complicating pregnancy O77.9
        due to drug administration O77.1
    mental NEC Z73.3
        work-related Z56.6
    physical NEC Z73.3
        work-related Z56.6
    polycythemia D75.1
    reaction (see also Reaction, stress) F43.9
    work schedule Z56.3
Stretching, nerve — see Injury, nerve
Striae albicantes, atrophicae or distensae (cutis) L90.6
Stricture (see also Stenosis)
    ampulla of Vater K83.1
    anus (sphincter) K62.4
        congenital Q42.3
            with fistula Q42.2
        infantile Q42.3
            with fistula Q42.2
    aorta (ascending) (congenital) Q25.3
        arteriosclerotic I70.0
        calcified I70.0
        supravalvular, congenital Q25.3
    aortic (valve) — see Stenosis, aortic
    aqueduct of Sylvius (congenital) Q03.0
        with spina bifida — see Spina bifida, by site, with hydrocephalus
        acquired G91.1
    artery I77.1
        basilar — see Occlusion, artery, basilar
        carotid — see Occlusion, artery, carotid
        celiac I77.4
        congenital (peripheral) Q27.8
            cerebral Q28.3
            coronary Q24.5
            digestive system Q27.8
            lower limb Q27.8
            retinal Q14.1
            specified site NEC Q27.8
            umbilical Q27.0
            upper limb Q27.8
        coronary — see Disease, heart, ischemic, atherosclerotic
            congenital Q24.5
        precerebral — see Occlusion, artery, precerebral
        pulmonary (congenital) Q25.6
            acquired I28.8
        renal I70.1
        vertebral — see Occlusion, artery, vertebral
    auditory canal (external) (congenital)
        acquired — see Stenosis, external ear canal
    bile duct (common) (hepatic) K83.1
        congenital Q44.3
        postoperative K91.89
    bladder N32.89
        neck N32.0
    bowel — see Obstruction, intestine
    brain G93.89
    bronchus J98.09
        congenital Q32.3
        syphilitic A52.72
    cardia (stomach) K22.2
        congenital Q39.3
    cardiac (see also Disease, heart)
        orifice (stomach) K22.2
    cecum — see Obstruction, intestine
    cervix, cervical (canal) N88.2
        congenital Q51.828
        in pregnancy — see Pregnancy, complicated by, abnormal cervix
            causing obstructed labor O65.5
    colon (see also Obstruction, intestine)
        congenital Q42.9
            specified NEC Q42.8
    colostomy K94.03
    common (bile) duct K83.1
    coronary (artery) — see Disease, heart, ischemic, atherosclerotic
    cystic duct — see Obstruction, gallbladder
    digestive organs NEC, congenital Q45.8
    duodenum K31.5

Stricture — *continued*
  duodenum — *continued*
    congenital Q41.0
  ear canal (external) (congenital) Q16.1
    acquired — *see* Stricture, auditory canal, acquired
  ejaculatory duct N50.8
  enterostomy K94.13
  esophagus K22.2
    congenital Q39.3
    syphilitic A52.79
      congenital A50.59 [K23]
  eustachian tube (*see also* Obstruction, eustachian tube)
    congenital Q17.8
  fallopian tube N97.1
    gonococcal A54.24
    tuberculous A18.17
  gallbladder — *see* Obstruction, gallbladder
  glottis J38.6
  heart (*see also* Disease, heart)
    valve (*see also* Endocarditis) I38
      aortic Q23.0
      mitral Q23.4
      pulmonary Q22.1
      tricuspid Q22.4
  hepatic duct K83.1
  hourglass, of stomach K31.2
  hymen N89.6
  hypopharynx J39.2
  ileum K56.69
    congenital Q41.2
  intestine (*see also* Obstruction, intestine)
    congenital (small) Q41.9
      large Q42.9
        specified NEC Q42.8
      specified NEC Q41.8
    ischemic K55.1
  jejunum K56.69
    congenital Q41.1
  lacrimal passages (*see also* Stenosis, lacrimal)
    congenital Q10.5
  larynx J38.6
    congenital NEC Q31.8
      subglottic Q31.1
    syphilitic A52.73
      congenital A50.59 [J99]
  meatus
    ear (congenital) Q16.1
      acquired — *see* Stricture, auditory canal, acquired
    osseous (ear) (congenital) Q16.1
      acquired — *see* Stricture, auditory canal, acquired
    urinarius (*see also* Stricture, urethra)
      congenital Q64.33
  mitral (valve) — *see* Stenosis, mitral
  myocardium, myocardial I51.5
    hypertrophic subaortic (idiopathic) I42.1
  nares (anterior) (posterior) J34.89
    congenital Q30.0
  nasal duct (*see also* Stenosis, lacrimal, duct)
    congenital Q10.5
  nasolacrimal duct (*see also* Stenosis, lacrimal, duct)
    congenital Q10.5
  nasopharynx J39.2
    syphilitic A52.73
  nose J34.89
    congenital Q30.0
  nostril (anterior) (posterior) J34.89
    congenital Q30.0
    syphilitic A52.73
      congenital A50.59 [J99]
  organ or site, congenital NEC — *see* Atresia, by site
  os uteri — *see* Stricture, cervix
  osseous meatus (ear) (congenital) Q16.1
    acquired — *see* Stricture, auditory canal, acquired
  oviduct — *see* Stricture, fallopian tube
  pelviureteric junction (congenital) Q62.11
  penis, by foreign body T19.4 ☑
  pharynx J39.2
  prostate N42.89
  pulmonary, pulmonic
    artery (congenital) Q25.6
      acquired I28.8
      noncongenital I28.8
    infundibulum (congenital) Q24.3
    valve I37.0
      congenital Q22.1
    vein, acquired I28.8

Stricture — *continued*
  pulmonary, pulmonic — *continued*
    vessel NEC I28.8
  punctum lacrimale (*see also* Stenosis, lacrimal, punctum)
    congenital Q10.5
  pylorus (hypertrophic) K31.1
    adult K31.1
    congenital Q40.0
    infantile Q40.0
  rectosigmoid K56.69
  rectum (sphincter) K62.4
    congenital Q42.1
      with fistula Q42.0
    due to
      chlamydial lymphogranuloma A55
      irradiation K91.89
      lymphogranuloma venereum A55
    gonococcal A54.6
    inflammatory (chlamydial) A55
    syphilitic A52.74
    tuberculous A18.32
  renal artery I70.1
    congenital Q27.1
  salivary duct or gland (any) K11.8
  sigmoid (flexure) — *see* Obstruction, intestine
  spermatic cord N50.8
  stoma (following) (of)
    colostomy K94.03
    enterostomy K94.13
    gastrostomy K94.23
    ileostomy K94.13
    tracheostomy J95.03
  stomach K31.89
    congenital Q40.2
    hourglass K31.2
  subaortic Q24.4
    hypertrophic (acquired) (idiopathic) I42.1
  subglottic J38.6
  syphilitic NEC A52.79
  trachea J39.8
    congenital Q32.1
    syphilitic A52.73
    tuberculous NEC A15.5
  tracheostomy J95.03
  tricuspid (valve) — *see* Stenosis, tricuspid
  tunica vaginalis N50.8
  ureter (postoperative) N13.5
    with
      hydronephrosis N13.1
        with infection N13.6
      pyelonephritis (chronic) N11.1
    congenital — *see* Atresia, ureter
    tuberculous A18.11
  ureteropelvic junction (congenital) Q62.11
  ureterovesical orifice N13.5
    with infection N13.6
  urethra (organic) (spasmodic) N35.9
    associated with schistosomiasis B65.0 [N37]
    congenital Q64.39
      valvular (posterior) Q64.2
    due to
      infection — *see* Stricture, urethra, postinfective
      trauma — *see* Stricture, urethra, post-traumatic
    gonococcal, gonorrheal A54.01
    infective NEC — *see* Stricture, urethra, postinfective
    late effect (sequelae) of injury — *see* Stricture, urethra, post-traumatic
    postcatheterization — *see* Stricture, urethra, postprocedural
    postinfective NEC
      female N35.12
      male N35.119
        anterior urethra N35.114
        bulbous urethra N35.112
        meatal N35.111
        membranous urethra N35.113
    postobstetric N35.021
    postoperative — *see* Stricture, urethra, postprocedural
    postprocedural
      female N99.12
      male N99.114
        anterior urethra N99.113
        bulbous urethra N99.111
        meatal N99.110
        membranous urethra N99.112

Stricture — *continued*
  urethra — *continued*
    post-traumatic
      female N35.028
        due to childbirth N35.021
      male N35.014
        anterior urethra N35.013
        bulbous urethra N35.011
        meatal N35.010
        membranous urethra N35.012
    sequela (late effect) of
      childbirth N35.021
      injury — *see* Stricture, urethra, post-traumatic
    specified cause NEC N35.8
    syphilitic A52.76
    traumatic — *see* Stricture, urethra, post-traumatic
    valvular (posterior), congenital Q64.2
  urinary meatus — *see* Stricture, urethra
  uterus, uterine (synechiae) N85.6
    os (external) (internal) — *see* Stricture, cervix
  vagina (outlet) — *see* Stenosis, vagina
  valve (cardiac) (heart) (*see also* Endocarditis)
    congenital
      aortic Q23.0
      mitral Q23.2
      pulmonary Q22.1
      tricuspid Q22.4
  vas deferens N50.8
    congenital Q55.4
  vein I87.1
  vena cava (inferior) (superior) NEC I87.1
    congenital Q26.0
  vesicourethral orifice N32.0
    congenital Q64.31
  vulva (acquired) N90.5
Stridor R06.1
  congenital (larynx) P28.89
Stridulous — *see* condition
Stroke (apoplectic) (brain) (embolic) (ischemic) (paralytic) (thrombotic) I63.9
  epileptic — *see* Epilepsy
  heat T67.0 ☑
  in evolution I63.9
  intraoperative
    during cardiac surgery I97.810
    during other surgery I97.811
  lightning — *see* Lightning
  meaning
    cerebral hemorrhage — *code to* Hemorrhage, intracranial
    cerebral infarction — *code to* Infarction, cerebral
  postprocedural
    following cardiac surgery I97.820
    following other surgery I97.821
  unspecified (NOS) I63.9
Stromatosis, endometrial D39.0
Strongyloidiasis, strongyloidosis B78.9
  cutaneous B78.1
  disseminated B78.7
  intestinal B78.0
Strophulus pruriginosus L28.2
Struck by lightning — *see* Lightning
Struma (*see also* Goiter)
  Hashimoto E06.3
  lymphomatosa E06.3
  nodosa (simplex) E04.9
    endemic E01.2
      multinodular E01.1
    multinodular E04.2
      iodine-deficiency related E01.1
    toxic or with hyperthyroidism E05.20
      with thyroid storm E05.21
      multinodular E05.20
        with thyroid storm E05.21
      uninodular E05.10
        with thyroid storm E05.11
    toxicosa E05.20
      with thyroid storm E05.21
      multinodular E05.20
        with thyroid storm E05.21
      uninodular E05.10
        with thyroid storm E05.11
    uninodular E04.1
  ovarii D27.- ☑
  Riedel's E06.5
Strumipriva cachexia E03.4
Strümpell-Marie spine — *see* Spondylitis, ankylosing
Strümpell-Westphal pseudosclerosis E83.01

Index

Stuart deficiency disease — Subnormal, subnormality

Stuart deficiency disease (factor X) D68.2
Stuart-Prower factor deficiency (factor X) D68.2
Student's elbow — see Bursitis, elbow, olecranon
Stump — see Amputation
Stunting, nutritional E45
Stupor (catatonic) R40.1
  depressive F32.8
  dissociative F44.2
  manic F30.2
  manic-depressive F31.89
  psychogenic (anergic) F44.2
  reaction to exceptional stress (transient) F43.0
Sturge (-Weber) (-Dimitri) (-Kalischer) **disease or syndrome** Q85.8
Stuttering F80.81
  adult onset F98.5
  childhood onset F80.81
  following cerebrovascular disease — see Disorder, fluency. following cerebrovascular disease
  in conditions classified elsewhere R47.82
Sty, stye (external) (internal) (meibomian) (zeisian) — see Hordeolum
Subacidity, gastric K31.89
  psychogenic F45.8
Subacute — see condition
Subarachnoid — see condition
Subcortical — see condition
Subcostal syndrome, nerve compression — see Mononeuropathy, upper limb, specified site NEC
Subcutaneous, subcuticular — see condition
Subdural — see condition
Subendocardium — see condition
Subependymoma
  specified site — see Neoplasm, uncertain behavior, by site
  unspecified site D43.2
Suberosis J67.3
Subglossitis — see Glossitis
Subhemophilia D66
Subinvolution
  breast (postlactational) (postpuerperal) N64.89
  puerperal O90.89
  uterus (chronic) (nonpuerperal) N85.3
    puerperal O90.89
Sublingual — see condition
Sublinguitis — see Sialoadenitis
Subluxatable hip Q65.6
Subluxation (see also Dislocation)
  acromioclavicular S43.11- ✓
  ankle S93.0- ✓
  atlantoaxial, recurrent M43.4
    with myelopathy M43.3
  carpometacarpal (joint) NEC S63.05- ✓
    thumb S63.04- ✓
  complex, vertebral — see Complex, subluxation
  congenital (see also Malposition, congenital)
    hip — see Dislocation, hip, congenital, partial
    joint (excluding hip)
      lower limb Q68.8
      shoulder Q68.8
      upper limb Q68.8
  elbow (traumatic) S53.10- ✓
    anterior S53.11- ✓
    lateral S53.14- ✓
    medial S53.13- ✓
    posterior S53.12- ✓
    specified type NEC S53.19- ✓
  finger S63.20- ✓
    index S63.20- ✓
    interphalangeal S63.22- ✓
      distal S63.24- ✓
        index S63.24- ✓
        little S63.24- ✓
        middle S63.24- ✓
        ring S63.24- ✓
      index S63.22- ✓
      little S63.22- ✓
      middle S63.22- ✓
      proximal S63.23- ✓
        index S63.23- ✓
        little S63.23- ✓
        middle S63.23- ✓
        ring S63.23- ✓
      ring S63.22- ✓
    little S63.20- ✓
    metacarpophalangeal S63.21- ✓

Subluxation — continued
  finger — continued
    metacarpophalangeal — continued
      index S63.21- ✓
      little S63.21- ✓
      middle S63.21- ✓
      ring S63.21- ✓
    middle S63.20- ✓
    ring S63.20- ✓
  foot S93.30- ✓
    specified site NEC S93.33- ✓
    tarsal joint S93.31- ✓
    tarsometatarsal joint S93.32- ✓
    toe — see Subluxation, toe
  hip S73.00- ✓
    anterior S73.03- ✓
      obturator S73.02- ✓
    central S73.04- ✓
    posterior S73.01- ✓
  interphalangeal (joint)
    finger S63.22- ✓
      distal joint S63.24- ✓
        index S63.24- ✓
        little S63.24- ✓
        middle S63.24- ✓
        ring S63.24- ✓
      index S63.22- ✓
      little S63.22- ✓
      middle S63.22- ✓
      proximal joint S63.23- ✓
        index S63.23- ✓
        little S63.23- ✓
        middle S63.23- ✓
        ring S63.23- ✓
      ring S63.22- ✓
    thumb S63.12- ✓
      distal joint S63.14- ✓
      proximal joint S63.13- ✓
    toe S93.13- ✓
      great S93.13- ✓
      lesser S93.13- ✓
  joint prosthesis — see Complications, joint prosthesis, mechanical, displacement, by site
  knee S83.10- ✓
    cap — see Subluxation, patella
    patella — see Subluxation, patella
    proximal tibia
      anteriorly S83.11- ✓
      laterally S83.14- ✓
      medially S83.13- ✓
      posteriorly S83.12- ✓
    specified type NEC S83.19- ✓
  lens — see Dislocation, lens, partial
  ligament, traumatic — see Sprain, by site
  metacarpal (bone)
    proximal end S63.06- ✓
  metacarpophalangeal (joint)
    finger S63.21- ✓
      index S63.21- ✓
      little S63.21- ✓
      middle S63.21- ✓
      ring S63.21- ✓
    thumb S63.11- ✓
  metatarsophalangeal joint S93.14- ✓
    great toe S93.14- ✓
    lesser toe S93.14- ✓
  midcarpal (joint) S63.03- ✓
  patella S83.00- ✓
    lateral S83.01- ✓
    recurrent (nontraumatic) — see Dislocation, patella, recurrent, incomplete
    specified type NEC S83.09- ✓
  pathological — see Dislocation, pathological
  radial head S53.00- ✓
    anterior S53.01- ✓
    nursemaid's elbow S53.03- ✓
    posterior S53.02- ✓
    specified type NEC S53.09- ✓
  radiocarpal (joint) S63.02- ✓
  radioulnar (joint)
    distal S63.01- ✓
    proximal — see Subluxation, elbow
  shoulder
    congenital Q68.8
    girdle S43.30- ✓
      scapula S43.31- ✓

Subluxation — continued
  shoulder — continued
    girdle — continued
      specified site NEC S43.39- ✓
    traumatic S43.00- ✓
      anterior S43.01- ✓
      inferior S43.03- ✓
      posterior S43.02- ✓
      specified type NEC S43.08- ✓
  sternoclavicular (joint) S43.20- ✓
    anterior S43.21- ✓
    posterior S43.22- ✓
  symphysis (pubis)
  thumb S63.103
    interphalangeal joint — see Subluxation, interphalangeal (joint), thumb
    metacarpophalangeal joint — see Subluxation, metacarpophalangeal (joint), thumb
  toe(s) S93.10- ✓
    great S93.10- ✓
      interphalangeal joint S93.13- ✓
      metatarsophalangeal joint S93.14- ✓
    interphalangeal joint S93.13- ✓
    lesser S93.10- ✓
      interphalangeal joint S93.13- ✓
      metatarsophalangeal joint S93.14- ✓
    metatarsophalangeal joint S93.149 ✓
  ulna
    distal end S63.07- ✓
    proximal end — see Subluxation, elbow
  ulnohumeral joint — see Subluxation, elbow
  vertebral
    recurrent NEC — see subcategory M43.5 ✓
    traumatic
      cervical S13.100 ✓
        atlantoaxial joint S13.120 ✓
        atlantooccipital joint S13.110 ✓
        atloidooccipital joint S13.110 ✓
        joint between
          C0 and C1 S13.110 ✓
          C1 and C2 S13.120 ✓
          C2 and C3 S13.130 ✓
          C3 and C4 S13.140 ✓
          C4 and C5 S13.150 ✓
          C5 and C6 S13.160 ✓
          C6 and C7 S13.170 ✓
          C7 and T1 S13.180 ✓
        occipitoatloid joint S13.110 ✓
      lumbar S33.100 ✓
        joint between
          L1 and L2 S33.110 ✓
          L2 and L3 S33.120 ✓
          L3 and L4 S33.130 ✓
          L4 and L5 S33.140 ✓
      thoracic S23.100 ✓
        joint between
          T1 and T2 S23.110 ✓
          T2 and T3 S23.120 ✓
          T3 and T4 S23.122 ✓
          T4 and T5 S23.130 ✓
          T5 and T6 S23.132 ✓
          T6 and T7 S23.140 ✓
          T7 and T8 S23.142 ✓
          T8 and T9 S23.150 ✓
          T9 and T10 S23.152 ✓
          T10 and T11 S23.160 ✓
          T11 and T12 S23.162 ✓
          T12 and L1 S23.170 ✓
  wrist (carpal bone) S63.00- ✓
    carpometacarpal joint — see Subluxation, carpometacarpal (joint)
    distal radioulnar joint — see Subluxation, radioulnar (joint), distal
    metacarpal bone, proximal — see Subluxation, metacarpal (bone), proximal end
    midcarpal — see Subluxation, midcarpal (joint)
    radiocarpal joint — see Subluxation, radiocarpal (joint)
    recurrent — see Dislocation, recurrent, wrist
    specified site NEC S63.09- ✓
    ulna — see Subluxation, ulna, distal end
Submaxillary — see condition
Submersion (fatal) (nonfatal) T75.1 ✓
Submucous — see condition
Subnormal, subnormality
  accommodation (old age) H52.4

Subnormal, subnormality — continued
  mental — see Disability, intellectual
  temperature (accidental) T68 ☑
Subphrenic — see condition
Subscapular nerve — see condition
Subseptus uterus Q51.2
Subsiding appendicitis K36
Substernal thyroid E04.9
  congenital Q89.2
Substitution disorder F44.9
Subtentorial — see condition
Subthyroidism (acquired) (see also Hypothyroidism)
  congenital E03.1
Succenturiate placenta O43.19- ☑
Sucking thumb, child (excessive) F98.8
Sudamen, sudamina L74.1
Sudanese kala-azar B55.0
Sudden
  hearing loss — see Deafness, sudden
  heart failure — see Failure, heart
Sudeck's atrophy, disease, or syndrome — see Algo-
    neurodystrophy
Suffocation — see Asphyxia, traumatic
Sugar
  blood
    high (transient) R73.9
    low (transient) E16.2
  in urine R81
Suicide, suicidal (attempted) T14.91
  by poisoning — see Table of Drugs and Chemicals
  history of (personal) Z91.5
    in family Z81.8
  ideation — see Ideation, suicidal
  risk
    meaning personal history of attempted suicide
        Z91.5
    meaning suicidal ideation — see Ideation, suicidal
  tendencies
    meaning personal history of attempted suicide
        Z91.5
    meaning suicidal ideation — see Ideation, suicidal
  trauma — see nature of injury by site
Suipestifer infection — see Infection, salmonella
Sulfhemoglobinemia, sulphemoglobinemia (ac-
    quired) (with methemoglobinemia) D74.8
Sumatran mite fever A75.3
Summer — see condition
Sunburn L55.9
  first degree L55.0
  second degree L55.1
  third degree L55.2
SUNCT (short lasting unilateral neuralgiform headache
    with conjunctival injection and tearing) G44.059
  intractable G44.051
  not intractable G44.059
Sunken acetabulum — see Derangement, joint, speci-
    fied type NEC, hip
Sunstroke T67.0 ☑
Superfecundation — see Pregnancy, multiple
Superfetation — see Pregnancy, multiple
Superinvolution (uterus) N85.8
Supernumerary (congenital)
  aortic cusps Q23.8
  auditory ossicles Q16.3
  bone Q79.8
  breast Q83.1
  carpal bones Q74.0
  cusps, heart valve NEC Q24.8
    aortic Q23.8
    mitral Q23.2
    pulmonary Q22.3
  digit(s) Q69.9
  ear (lobule) Q17.0
  fallopian tube Q50.6
  finger Q69.0
  hymen Q52.4
  kidney Q63.0
  lacrimonasal duct Q10.6
  lobule (ear) Q17.0
  mitral cusps Q23.2
  muscle Q79.8
  nipple(s) Q83.3
  organ or site not listed — see Accessory
  ossicles, auditory Q16.3
  ovary Q50.31
  oviduct Q50.6
  pulmonary, pulmonic cusps Q22.3

Supernumerary — continued
  rib Q76.6
    cervical or first (syndrome) Q76.5
  roots (of teeth) K00.2
  spleen Q89.09
  tarsal bones Q74.2
  teeth K00.1
  testis Q55.29
  thumb Q69.1
  toe Q69.2
  uterus Q51.2
  vagina Q52.1 ☑
  vertebra Q76.49
Supervision (of)
  contraceptive — see Prescription, contraceptives
  dietary (for) Z71.3
    allergy (food) Z71.3
    colitis Z71.3
    diabetes mellitus Z71.3
    food allergy or intolerance Z71.3
    gastritis Z71.3
    hypercholesterolemia Z71.3
    hypoglycemia Z71.3
    intolerance (food) Z71.3
    obesity Z71.3
    specified NEC Z71.3
  healthy infant or child Z76.2
    foundling Z76.1
  high-risk pregnancy — see Pregnancy, complicated
      by, high, risk
  lactation Z39.1
  pregnancy — see Pregnancy, supervision of
Supplemental teeth K00.1
Suppression
  binocular vision H53.34
  lactation O92.5
  menstruation N94.89
  ovarian secretion E28.39
  renal N28.9
  urine, urinary secretion R34
Suppuration, suppurative (see also condition)
  accessory sinus (chronic) — see Sinusitis
  adrenal gland
  antrum (chronic) — see Sinusitis, maxillary
  bladder — see Cystitis
  brain G06.0
    sequelae G09
  breast N61
    puerperal, postpartum or gestational — see Masti-
        tis, obstetric, purulent
  dental periosteum M27.3
  ear (middle) (see also Otitis, media)
    external NEC — see Otitis, externa, infective
    internal — see subcategory H83.0 ☑
  ethmoidal (chronic) (sinus) — see Sinusitis, ethmoidal
  fallopian tube — see Salpingo-oophoritis
  frontal (chronic) (sinus) — see Sinusitis, frontal
  gallbladder (acute) K81.0
  gum K05.20
    generalized K05.22
    localized K05.21
  intracranial G06.0
  joint — see Arthritis, pyogenic or pyemic
  labyrinthine — see subcategory H83.0 ☑
  lung — see Abscess, lung
  mammary gland N61
    puerperal, postpartum O91.12
      associated with lactation O91.13
  maxilla, maxillary M27.2
    sinus (chronic) — see Sinusitis, maxillary
  muscle — see Myositis, infective
  nasal sinus (chronic) — see Sinusitis
  pancreas, acute K85.8
  parotid gland — see Sialoadenitis
  pelvis, pelvic
    female — see Disease, pelvis, inflammatory
    male K65.0
  pericranial — see Osteomyelitis
  salivary duct or gland (any) — see Sialoadenitis
  sinus (accessory) (chronic) (nasal) — see Sinusitis
  sphenoidal sinus (chronic) — see Sinusitis, sphenoidal
  thymus (gland) E32.1
  thyroid (gland) E06.0
  tonsil — see Tonsillitis
  uterus — see Endometritis
Supraeruption of tooth (teeth) M26.34
Supraglottitis J04.30

Supraglottitis — continued
  with obstruction J04.31
Suprarenal (gland) — see condition
Suprascapular nerve — see condition
Suprasellar — see condition
Surfer's knots or nodules S89.8- ☑
Surgical
  emphysema T81.82 ☑
  procedures, complication or misadventure — see
      Complications, surgical procedures
  shock T81.10 ☑
Surveillance (of) (for) (see also Observation)
  alcohol abuse Z71.41
  contraceptive — see Prescription, contraceptives
  dietary Z71.3
  drug abuse Z71.51
Susceptibility to disease, genetic Z15.89
  malignant neoplasm Z15.09
    breast Z15.01
    endometrium Z15.04
    ovary Z15.02
    prostate Z15.03
    specified NEC Z15.09
  multiple endocrine neoplasia Z15.81
Suspected condition, ruled out (see also Observation,
    suspected)
  amniotic cavity and membrane Z03.71
  cervical shortening Z03.75
  fetal anomaly Z03.73
  fetal growth Z03.74
  maternal and fetal conditions NEC Z03.79
  oligohydramnios Z03.71
  placental problem Z03.72
  polyhydramnios Z03.71
Suspended uterus
  in pregnancy or childbirth — see Pregnancy, compli-
      cated by, abnormal uterus
Sutton's nevus D22.9
Suture
  burst (in operation wound) T81.31 ☑
    external operation wound T81.31 ☑
    internal operation wound T81.32 ☑
  inadvertently left in operation wound — see Foreign
      body, accidentally left during a procedure
  removal Z48.02
Swab inadvertently left in operation wound — see
    Foreign body, accidentally left during a procedure
Swallowed, swallowing
  difficulty — see Dysphagia
  foreign body — see Foreign body, alimentary tract
Swan-neck deformity (finger) — see Deformity, finger,
    swan-neck
Swearing, compulsive F42
  in Gilles de la Tourette's syndrome F95.2
Sweat, sweats
  fetid L75.0
  night R61
Sweating, excessive R61
Sweeley-Klionsky disease E75.21
Sweet's disease or dermatosis L98.2
Swelling (of) R60.9
  abdomen, abdominal (not referable to any particular
      organ) — see Mass, abdominal
  ankle — see Effusion, joint, ankle
  arm M79.89
    forearm M79.89
  breast N63
  Calabar B74.3
  cervical gland R59.0
  chest, localized R22.2
  ear H93.8- ☑
  extremity (lower) (upper) — see Disorder, soft tissue,
      specified type NEC
  finger M79.89
  foot M79.89
  glands R59.9
    generalized R59.1
    localized R59.0
  hand M79.89
  head (localized) R22.0
  inflammatory — see Inflammation
  intra-abdominal — see Mass, abdominal
  joint — see Effusion, joint
  leg M79.89
    lower M79.89
  limb — see Disorder, soft tissue, specified type NEC

Swelling — continued
  localized (skin) R22.9
    chest R22.2
    head R22.0
    limb
      lower — see Mass, localized, limb, lower
      upper — see Mass, localized, limb, upper
    neck R22.1
    trunk R22.2
  neck (localized) R22.1
  pelvic — see Mass, abdominal
  scrotum N50.8
  splenic — see Splenomegaly
  testis N50.8
  toe M79.89
  umbilical R19.09
  wandering, due to Gnathostoma (spinigerum) B83.1
  white — see Tuberculosis, arthritis
Swift (-Feer) disease
  overdose or wrong substance given or taken — see Table of Drugs and Chemicals, by drug, poisoning
Swimmer's
  cramp T75.1 ☑
  ear H60.33- ☑
  itch B65.3
Swimming in the head R42
Swollen — see Swelling
Swyer syndrome Q99.1
Sycosis L73.8
  barbae (not parasitic) L73.8
  contagiosa (mycotic) B35.0
  lupoides L73.8
  mycotic B35.0
  parasitic B35.0
  vulgaris L73.8
Sydenham's chorea — see Chorea, Sydenham's
Sylvatic yellow fever A95.0
Sylvest's disease B33.0
Symblepharon H11.23- ☑
  congenital Q10.3
Symond's syndrome G93.2
Sympathetic — see condition
Sympatheticotonia G90.8
Sympathicoblastoma
  specified site — see Neoplasm, malignant, by site
  unspecified site C74.90
Sympathogonioma — see Sympathicoblastoma
Symphalangy (fingers) (toes) Q70.9
Symptoms NEC R68.89
  breast NEC N64.59
  development NEC R63.8
  factitious, self-induced — see Disorder, factitious
  genital organs, female R10.2
  involving
    abdomen NEC R19.8
    appearance NEC R46.89
    awareness R41.9
      altered mental status R41.82
      amnesia — see Amnesia
      borderline intellectual functioning R41.83
      coma — see Coma
      disorientation R41.0
      neurologic neglect syndrome R41.4
      senile cognitive decline R41.81
      specified symptom NEC R41.89
    behavior NEC R46.89
    cardiovascular system NEC R09.89
    chest NEC R09.89
    circulatory system NEC R09.89
    cognitive functions R41.9
      altered mental status R41.82
      amnesia — see Amnesia
      borderline intellectual functioning R41.83
      coma — see Coma
      disorientation R41.0
      neurologic neglect syndrome R41.4
      senile cognitive decline R41.81
      specified symptom NEC R41.89
    development NEC R62.50
    digestive system NEC R19.8
    emotional state NEC R45.89
      emotional lability R45.86
    food and fluid intake R63.8
    general perceptions and sensations R44.9
      specified NEC R44.8
    musculoskeletal system R29.91

Symptoms — continued
  involving — continued
    musculoskeletal system — continued
      specified NEC R29.898
    nervous system R29.90
      specified NEC R29.818
    pelvis NEC R19.8
    respiratory system NEC R09.89
    skin and integument R23.9
    urinary system R39.9
  menopausal N95.1
  metabolism NEC R63.8
  neurotic F48.8
  of infancy R68.19
  pelvis NEC, female R10.2
  skin and integument NEC R23.9
  subcutaneous tissue NEC R23.9
Sympus Q74.2
Syncephalus Q89.4
Synchondrosis
  abnormal (congenital) Q78.8
  ischiopubic M91.0
Synchysis (scintillans) (senile) (vitreous body) H43.89
Syncope (near) (pre-) R55
  anginosa I20.8
  bradycardia R00.1
  cardiac R55
  carotid sinus G90.01
  due to spinal (lumbar) puncture G97.1
  heart R55
  heat T67.1 ☑
  laryngeal R05
  psychogenic F48.8
  tussive R05
  vasoconstriction R55
  vasodepressor R55
  vasomotor R55
  vasovagal R55
Syndactylism, syndactyly Q70.9
  complex (with synostosis)
    fingers Q70.0- ☑
    toes Q70.2- ☑
  simple (without synostosis)
    fingers Q70.1- ☑
    toes Q70.3- ☑
Syndrome (see also Disease)
  48,XXXX Q97.1
  49,XXXXX Q97.1
  5q minus NOS D46.C (following D46.2)
  abdominal
    acute R10.0
    muscle deficiency Q79.4
  abnormal innervation H02.519
    left H02.516
      lower H02.515
      upper H02.514
    right H02.513
      lower H02.512
      upper H02.511
  abstinence, neonatal P96.1
  acid pulmonary aspiration, obstetric O74.0
  acquired immunodeficiency — see Human, immunodeficiency virus (HIV) disease
  acute abdominal R10.0
  acute respiratory distress (adult) (child) J80
  Adair-Dighton Q78.0
  Adams-Stokes (-Morgagni) I45.9
  adiposogenital E23.6
  adrenal
    hemorrhage (meningococcal) A39.1
    meningococcic A39.1
  adrenocortical — see Cushing's, syndrome
  adrenogenital E25.9
    congenital, associated with enzyme deficiency E25.0
  afferent loop NEC K91.89
  Alagille's Q44.7
  alcohol withdrawal (without convulsions) — see Dependence, alcohol, with, withdrawal
  Alder's D72.0
  Aldrich (-Wiskott) D82.0
  alien hand R41.4
  Alport Q87.81
  alveolar hypoventilation E66.2
  alveolocapillary block J84.10
  amnesic, amnestic (confabulatory) (due to) — see Disorder, amnesic
  amyostatic (Wilson's disease) E83.01

Syndrome — continued
  androgen insensitivity E34.50
    complete E34.51
    partial E34.52
  androgen resistance (see also Syndrome, androgen insensitivity) E34.50
  Angelman Q93.5
  anginal — see Angina
  ankyloglossia superior Q38.1
  anterior
    chest wall R07.89
    cord G83.82
    spinal artery G95.19
      compression M47.019
        cervical region M47.012
        cervicothoracic region M47.013
        lumbar region M47.016
        occipito-atlanto-axial region M47.011
        thoracic region M47.014
        thoracolumbar region M47.015
    tibial M76.81- ☑
  antibody deficiency D80.9
    agammaglobulinemic D80.1
      hereditary D80.0
    congenital D80.0
    hypogammaglobulinemic D80.1
      hereditary D80.0
  anticardiolipin (-antibody) D68.61
  antiphospholipid (-antibody) D68.61
  aortic
    arch M31.4
    bifurcation I74.09
  aortomesenteric duodenum occlusion K31.5
  apical ballooning (transient left ventricular) I51.81
  arcuate ligament I77.4
  argentaffin, argintaffinoma E34.0
  Arnold-Chiari — see Arnold-Chiari disease
  Arrillaga-Ayerza I27.0
  Asherman's N85.6
  aspiration, of newborn — see Aspiration, by substance, with pneumonia
    meconium P24.01
  ataxia-telangiectasia G11.3
  auriculotemporal G50.8
  autoerythrocyte sensitization (Gardner-Diamond) D69.2
  autoimmune lymphoproliferative [ALPS] D89.82
  autoimmune polyglandular E31.0
  autosomal — see Abnormal, autosomes
  Avellis' G46.8
  Ayerza (-Arrillaga) I27.0
  Babinski-Nageotte G83.89
  Bakwin-Krida Q79.8
  bare lymphocyte D81.6
  Barré-Guillain G61.0
  Barré-Liéou M53.0
  Barrett's — see Barrett's, esophagus
  Barsony-Polgar K22.4
  Bársony-Teschendorf K22.4
  Barth E78.71
  Bartter's E26.81
  basal cell nevus Q87.89
  Basedow's E05.00
    with thyroid storm E05.01
  basilar artery G45.0
  Batten-Steinert G71.11
  battered
    baby or child — see Maltreatment, child, physical abuse
    spouse — see Maltreatment, adult, physical abuse
  Beals Q87.40
  Beau's I51.5
  Beck's I65.8
  Benedikt's G46.3
  Béquez César (-Steinbrinck-Chédiak-Higashi) E70.330
  Bernhardt-Roth — see Meralgia paresthetica
  Bernheim's I50.9
  big spleen D73.1
  bilateral polycystic ovarian E28.2
  Bing-Horton's — see Horton's headache
  Birt-Hogg-Dube syndrome Q87.89
  Björck (-Thorsen) E34.0
  black
    lung J60
    widow spider bite — see Toxicity, venom, spider, black widow
  Blackfan-Diamond D61.01

  ☑ **Additional Character Required** — Refer to the Tabular List for Character Selection   ⓦ **Subterms under main terms may continue to next column or page**

Syndrome — *continued*
- blind loop K90.2
  - congenital Q43.8
  - postsurgical K91.2
- blue sclera Q78.0
- blue toe I75.02- ☑
- Boder-Sedgewick G11.3
- Boerhaave's K22.3
- Borjeson Forssman Lehmann Q89.8
- Bouillaud's I01.9
- Bourneville (-Pringle) Q85.1
- Bouveret (-Hoffman) I47.9
- brachial plexus G54.0
- bradycardia-tachycardia I49.5
- brain (nonpsychotic) F09
  - with psychosis, psychotic reaction F09
  - acute or subacute — *see* Delirium
  - congenital — *see* Disability, intellectual
  - organic F09
    - post-traumatic (nonpsychotic) F07.81
      - psychotic F09
  - personality change F07.0
  - postcontusional F07.81
  - post-traumatic, nonpsychotic F07.81
  - psycho-organic F09
  - psychotic F06.8
- brain stem stroke G46.3
- Brandt's (acrodermatitis enteropathica) E83.2
- broad ligament laceration N83.8
- Brock's J98.11
- bronze baby P83.8
- Brown-Sequard G83.81
- bubbly lung P27.0
- Buchem's M85.2
- Budd-Chiari I82.0
- bulbar (progressive) G12.22
- Bürger-Grütz E78.3
- Burke's K86.8
- Burnett's (milk-alkali) E83.52
- burning feet E53.9
- Bywaters' T79.5 ☑
- Call-Fleming I67.841
- carbohydrate-deficient glycoprotein (CDGS) E77.8
- carcinogenic thrombophlebitis I82.1
- carcinoid E34.0
- cardiac asthma I50.1
- cardiacos negros I27.0
- cardiofaciocutaneous Q87.89
- cardiopulmonary-obesity E66.2
- cardiorenal — *see* Hypertension, cardiorenal
- cardiorespiratory distress (idiopathic), newborn P22.0
- cardiovascular renal — *see* Hypertension, cardiorenal
- carotid
  - artery (hemispheric) (internal) G45.1
  - body G90.01
  - sinus G90.01
- carpal tunnel G56.0- ☑
- Cassidy (-Scholte) E34.0
- cat cry Q93.4
- cat eye Q92.8
- cauda equina G83.4
- causalgia — *see* Causalgia
- celiac K90.0
  - artery compression I77.4
  - axis I77.4
- central pain G89.0
- cerebellar
  - hereditary G11.9
  - stroke G46.4
- cerebellomedullary malformation — *see* Spina bifida
- cerebral
  - artery
    - anterior G46.1
    - middle G46.0
    - posterior G46.2
  - gigantism E22.0
- cervical (root) M53.1
  - disc — *see* Disorder, disc, cervical, with neuritis
  - fusion Q76.1
  - posterior, sympathicus M53.0
  - rib Q76.5
  - sympathetic paralysis G90.2
- cervicobrachial (diffuse) M53.1
- cervicocranial M53.0
- cervicodorsal outlet G54.2
- cervicothoracic outlet G54.0
- Céstan (-Raymond) I65.8

Syndrome — *continued*
- Charcot's (angina cruris) (intermittent claudication) I73.9
- Charcot-Weiss-Baker G90.09
- CHARGE Q89.8
- Chédiak-Higashi (-Steinbrinck) E70.330
- chest wall R07.1
- Chiari's (hepatic vein thrombosis) I82.0
- Chilaiditi's Q43.3
- child maltreatment — *see* Maltreatment, child
- chondrocostal junction M94.0
- chondroectodermal dysplasia Q77.6
- chromosome 4 short arm deletion Q93.3
- chromosome 5 short arm deletion Q93.4
- chronic
  - pain G89.4
  - personality F68.8
- Clarke-Hadfield K86.8
- Clerambault's automatism G93.89
- Clouston's (hidrotic ectodermal dysplasia) Q82.4
- clumsiness, clumsy child F82
- cluster headache G44.009
  - intractable G44.001
  - not intractable G44.009
- Coffin-Lowry Q89.8
- cold injury (newborn) P80.0
- combined immunity deficiency D81.9
- compartment (deep) (posterior) (traumatic) T79.A0 ☑ (*following* T79.7)
  - abdomen T79.A3 ☑ (*following* T79.7)
  - lower extremity (hip, buttock, thigh, leg, foot, toes) T79.A2 ☑ (*following* T79.7)
  - nontraumatic
    - abdomen M79.A3 (*following* M79.7)
    - lower extremity (hip, buttock, thigh, leg, foot, toes) M79.A2- ☑ (*following* M79.7)
    - specified site NEC M79.A9 (*following* M79.7)
    - upper extremity (shoulder, arm, forearm, wrist, hand, fingers) M79.A1- ☑ (*following* M79.7)
  - postprocedural — *see* Syndrome, compartment, nontraumatic
  - specified site NEC T79.A9 ☑ (*following* T79.7)
  - upper extremity (shoulder, arm, forearm, wrist, hand, fingers) T79.A1 ☑ (*following* T79.7)
- complex regional pain — *see* Syndrome, pain, complex regional
- compression T79.5 ☑
  - anterior spinal — *see* Syndrome, anterior, spinal artery, compression
  - cauda equina G83.4
  - celiac artery I77.4
  - vertebral artery M47.029
    - cervical region M47.022
    - occipito-atlanto-axial region M47.021
- concussion F07.81
- congenital
  - affecting multiple systems NEC Q87.89
  - central alveolar hypoventilation G47.35
  - facial diplegia Q87.0
  - muscular hypertrophy-cerebral Q87.89
  - oculo-auriculovertebral Q87.0
  - oculofacial diplegia (Moebius) Q87.0
  - rubella (manifest) P35.0
- congestion-fibrosis (pelvic), female N94.89
- congestive dysmenorrhea N94.6
- connective tissue M35.9
  - overlap NEC M35.1
- Conn's E26.09
- conus medullaris G95.81
- cord
  - anterior G83.82
  - posterior G83.83
- coronary
  - acute NEC I24.9
  - insufficiency or intermediate I20.0
  - slow flow I20.8
- Costen's (complex) M26.69
- costochondral junction M94.0
- costoclavicular G54.0
- costovertebral E22.0
- Cowden Q85.8
- craniovertebral M53.0
- Creutzfeldt-Jakob — *see* Creutzfeldt-Jakob disease or syndrome
- crib death R99
- cricopharyngeal — *see* Dysphagia
- cri-du-chat Q93.4

Syndrome — *continued*
- croup J05.0
- CRPS I — *see* Syndrome, pain, complex regional I
- crush T79.5 ☑
- cryptophthalmos Q87.0
- cubital tunnel — *see* Lesion, nerve, ulnar
- Curschmann (-Batten) (-Steinert) G71.11
- Cushing's E24.9
  - alcohol-induced E24.4
  - drug-induced E24.2
  - due to
    - alcohol
    - drugs E24.2
    - ectopic ACTH E24.3
    - overproduction of pituitary ACTH E24.0
  - overdose or wrong substance given or taken — *see* Table of Drugs and Chemicals, by drug, poisoning
  - pituitary-dependent E24.0
  - specified type NEC E24.8
- cystic duct stump K91.5
- Dana-Putnam D51.0
- Danbolt (-Cross) (acrodermatitis enteropathica) E83.2
- Dandy-Walker Q03.1
  - with spina bifida Q07.01
- Danlos' Q79.8
- De Quervain E34.51
- de Toni-Fanconi (-Debré) E72.09
  - with cystinosis E72.04
- defibrination (*see also* Fibrinolysis)
  - with
    - antepartum hemorrhage — *see* Hemorrhage, antepartum, with coagulation defect
    - intrapartum hemorrhage — *see* Hemorrhage, complicating, delivery
  - newborn P60
  - postpartum O72.3
- Degos' I77.89
- Déjérine-Roussy G89.0
- delayed sleep phase G47.21
- demyelinating G37.9
- dependence — *see* F10-F19 with fourth character .2
- depersonalization (-derealization) F48.1
- di George's D82.1
- diabetes mellitus in newborn infant P70.2
- diabetes mellitus-hypertension-nephrosis — *see* Diabetes, nephrosis
- diabetes-nephrosis — *see* Diabetes, nephrosis
- diabetic amyotrophy — *see* Diabetes, amyotrophy
- Diamond-Blackfan D61.01
- Diamond-Gardener D69.2
- DIC (diffuse or disseminated intravascular coagulopathy) D65
- Dighton's Q78.0
- disequilibrium E87.8
- Döhle body-panmyelopathic D72.0
- dorsolateral medullary G46.4
- double athetosis G80.3
- Down (*see also* Down syndrome) Q90.9
- Dresbach's (elliptocytosis) D58.1
- Dressler's (postmyocardial infarction) I24.1
  - postcardiotomy I97.0
- drug withdrawal, infant of dependent mother P96.1
- dry eye H04.12- ☑
- due to abnormality
  - chromosomal Q99.9
  - sex
    - female phenotype Q97.9
    - male phenotype Q98.9
    - specified NEC Q99.8
- dumping (postgastrectomy) K91.1
  - nonsurgical K31.89
- Dupré's (meningism) R29.1
- dysmetabolic X E88.81
- dyspraxia, developmental F82
- Eagle-Barrett Q79.4
- Eaton-Lambert — *see* Syndrome, Lambert-Eaton
- Ebstein's Q22.5
- ectopic ACTH E24.3
- eczema-thrombocytopenia D82.0
- Eddowes' Q78.0
- effort (psychogenic) F45.8
- Ehlers-Danlos Q79.6
- Eisenmenger's I27.89
- Ekman's Q78.0
- electric feet E53.8
- Ellis-van Creveld Q77.6
- empty nest Z60.0

Syndrome — continued
endocrine-hypertensive E27.0
entrapment — see Neuropathy, entrapment
eosinophilia-myalgia M35.8
epileptic (see also Epilepsy, by type)
    absence G40.A09 (following G40.3)
        intractable G40.A19 (following G40.3)
            with status epilepticus G40.A11 (following G40.3)
            without status epilepticus G40.A19 (following G40.3)
        not intractable G40.A09 (following G40.3)
            with status epilepticus G40.A01 (following G40.3)
            without status epilepticus G40.A09 (following G40.3)
Erdheim-Chester (ECD) E88.89
Erdheim's E22.0
erythrocyte fragmentation D59.4
Evans D69.41
exhaustion F48.8
extrapyramidal G25.9
    specified NEC G25.89
eye retraction — see Strabismus
eyelid-malar-mandible Q87.0
Faber's D50.9
facial pain, paroxysmal G50.0
Fallot's Q21.3
familial eczema-thrombocytopenia (Wiskott-Aldrich) D82.0
Fanconi (-de Toni) (-Debré) E72.09
    with cystinosis E72.04
Fanconi's (anemia) (congenital pancytopenia) D61.09
fatigue
    chronic R53.82
    psychogenic F48.8
faulty bowel habit K59.3
Feil-Klippel (brevicollis) Q76.1
Felty's — see Felty's syndrome
fertile eunuch E23.0
fetal
    alcohol (dysmorphic) Q86.0
    hydantoin Q86.1
Fiedler's I40.1
first arch Q87.0
fish odor E72.8
Fisher's G61.0
Fitzhugh-Curtis
    due to
        Chlamydia trachomatis A74.81
        Neisseria gonorrhorea (gonococcal peritonitis) A54.85
Fitz's K85.0
Flajani (-Basedow) E05.00
    with thyroid storm E05.01
flatback — see Flatback syndrome
floppy
    baby P94.2
    iris (intraoeprative) (IFIS) H21.81
    mitral valve I34.1
flush E34.0
Foix-Alajouanine G95.19
Fong's Q79.8
foramen magnum G93.5
Foster-Kennedy H47.14- ☑
Foville's (peduncular) G46.3
fragile X Q99.2
Franceschetti Q75.4
Frey's
    auriculotemporal G50.8
    hyperhidrosis L74.52
Friderichsen-Waterhouse A39.1
Froin's G95.89
frontal lobe F07.0
Fukuhara E88.49
functional
    bowel K59.9
    prepubertal castrate E29.1
Gaisböck's D75.1
ganglion (basal ganglia brain) G25.9
    geniculi G51.1
Gardner-Diamond D69.2
gastroesophageal
    junction K22.0
    laceration-hemorrhage K22.6
gastrojejunal loop obstruction K91.89
Gee-Herter-Heubner K90.0
Gelineau's G47.419

Syndrome — continued
Gelineau's — continued
    with cataplexy G47.411
genito-anorectal A55
Gerstmann-Sträussler-Scheinker (GSS) A81.82
Gianotti-Crosti L44.4
giant platelet (Bernard-Soulier) D69.1
Gilles de la Tourette's F95.2
goiter-deafness E07.1
Goldberg Q89.8
Goldberg-Maxwell E34.51
Good's D83.8
Gopalan' (burning feet) E53.8
Gorlin's Q87.89
Gougerot-Blum L81.7
Gouley's I31.1
Gower's R55
gray or grey (newborn) P93.0
    platelet D69.1
Gubler-Millard G46.3
Guillain-Barré (-Strohl) G61.0
gustatory sweating G50.8
Hadfield-Clarke K86.8
hair tourniquet — see Constriction, external, by site
Hamman's J98.19
hand-foot L27.1
hand-shoulder G90.8
hantavirus (cardio)-pulmonary (HPS) (HCPS) B33.4
happy puppet Q93.5
Harada's H30.81- ☑
Hayem-Faber D50.9
headache NEC G44.89
    complicated NEC G44.59
Heberden's I20.8
Hedinger's E34.0
Hegglin's D72.0
HELLP (hemolysis, elevated liver enzymes and low platelet count) O14.2- ☑
hemolytic-uremic D59.3
hemophagocytic, infection-associated D76.2
Henoch-Schönlein D69.0
hepatic flexure K59.8
hepatopulmonary K76.81
hepatorenal K76.7
    following delivery O90.4
    postoperative or postprocedural K91.83
    postpartum, puerperal O90.4
hepatourologic K76.7
Herter (-Gee) (nontropical sprue) K90.0
Heubner-Herter K90.0
Heyd's K76.7
Hilger's G90.09
histamine-like (fish poisoning) — see Poisoning, fish
histiocytic D76.3
histiocytosis NEC D76.3
HIV infection, acute B20
Hoffmann-Werdnig G12.0
Hollander-Simons E88.1
Hoppe-Goldflam G70.00
    with exacerbation (acute) G70.01
    in crisis G70.01
Horner's G90.2
hungry bone E83.81
hunterian glossitis D51.0
Hutchinson's triad H30.53
hyperabduction G54.0
hyperammonemia-hyperornithinemia-homocitrullinemia E72.4
hypereosinophilic (idiopathic) D72.1
hyperimmunoglobulin E (IgE) D82.4
hyperkalemic E87.5
hyperkinetic — see Hyperkinesia
hypermobility M35.7
hypernatremia E87.0
hyperosmolarity E87.0
hyperperfusion G97.82
hypersplenic D73.1
hypertransfusion, newborn P61.1
hyperventilation F45.8
hyperviscosity (of serum)
    polycythemic D75.1
    sclerothymic D58.8
hypoglycemic (familial) (neonatal) E16.2
hypokalemic E87.6
hyponatremic E87.1
hypopituitarism E23.0
hypoplastic left-heart Q23.4
hypopotassemia E87.6

Syndrome — continued
hyposmolality E87.1
hypotension, maternal O26.5- ☑
hypothenar hammer I73.89
ICF (intravascular coagulation-fibrinolysis) D65
idiopathic
    cardiorespiratory distress, newborn P22.0
    nephrotic (infantile) N04.9
iliotibial band M76.3- ☑
immobility, immobilization (paraplegic) M62.3
immune reconstitution D89.3
immune reconstitution inflammatory [IRIS] D89.3
immunity deficiency, combined D81.9
immunodeficiency
    acquired — see Human, immunodeficiency virus (HIV) disease
    combined D81.9
impending coronary I20.0
impingement, shoulder M75.4- ☑
inappropriate secretion of antidiuretic hormone E22.2
infant
    gestational diabetes P70.0
    of diabetic mother P70.1
infantilism (pituitary) E23.0
inferior vena cava I87.1
inspissated bile (newborn) P59.1
institutional (childhood) F94.2
insufficient sleep F51.12
intermediate coronary (artery) I20.0
interspinous ligament — see Spondylopathy, specified NEC
intestinal
    carcinoid E34.0
    knot K56.2
intravascular coagulation-fibrinolysis (ICF) D65
iodine-deficiency, congenital E00.9
    type
        mixed E00.2
        myxedematous E00.1
        neurological E00.0
IRDS (idiopathic respiratory distress, newborn) P22.0
irritable
    bowel K58.9
        with diarrhea K58.0
        psychogenic F45.8
    heart (psychogenic) F45.8
    weakness F48.8
ischemic bowel (transient) K55.9
    chronic K55.1
    due to mesenteric artery insufficiency K55.1
IVC (intravascular coagulopathy) D65
Ivemark's Q89.01
Jaccoud's — see Arthropathy, postrheumatic, chronic
Jackson's G83.89
Jakob-Creutzfeldt — see Creutzfeldt-Jakob disease or syndrome
jaw-winking Q07.8
Jervell-Lange-Nielsen I45.81
jet lag G47.25
Job's D71
Joseph-Diamond-Blackfan D61.01
jugular foramen G52.7
Kabuki Q89.8
Kanner's (autism) F84.0
Kartagener's Q89.3
Kelly's D50.1
Kimmelstiel-Wilson — see Diabetes, specified type, with Kimmelstiel-Wilson disease
Klein (e)-Levine G47.13
Klippel-Feil (brevicollis) Q76.1
Köhler-Pellegrini-Steida — see Bursitis, tibial collateral
König's K59.8
Korsakoff (-Wernicke) (nonalcoholic) F04
    alcoholic F10.26
Kostmann's D70.0
Krabbe's congenital muscle hypoplasia Q79.8
labyrinthine — see subcategory H83.2 ☑
lacunar NEC G46.7
Lambert-Eaton G70.80
    in
        neoplastic disease G73.1
        specified disease NEC G70.81
Landau-Kleffner — see Epilepsy, specified NEC
Larsen's Q74.8
lateral
    cutaneous nerve of thigh G57.1- ☑
    medullary G46.4
Launois' E22.0

Syndrome — continued

lazy
  leukocyte D70.8
  posture M62.3
Lemiere I80.8
Lennox-Gastaut G40.812
  intractable G40.814
    with status epilepticus G40.813
    without status epilepticus G40.814
  not intractable G40.812
    with status epilepticus G40.811
    without status epilepticus G40.812
lenticular, progressive E83.01
Leopold-Levi's E05.90
Lev's I44.2
Lichtheim's D51.0
Li-Fraumeni Z15.01
Lightwood's N25.89
Lignac (de Toni) (-Fanconi) (-Debré) E72.09
  with cystinosis E72.04
Likoff's I20.8
limbic epilepsy personality F07.0
liver-kidney K76.7
lobotomy F07.0
Loffler's J82
long arm 18 or 21 deletion Q93.89
long QT I45.81
Louis-Barré G11.3
low
  atmospheric pressure T70.29 ☑
  back M54.5
  output (cardiac) I50.9
lower radicular, newborn (birth injury) P14.8
Luetscher's (dehydration) E86.0
Lupus anticoagulant D68.62
Lutembacher's Q21.1
macrophage activation D76.1
  due to infection D76.2
magnesium-deficiency R29.3
Mal de Debarquement R42
malabsorption K90.9
  postsurgical K91.2
malformation, congenital, due to
  alcohol Q86.0
  exogenous cause NEC Q86.8
  hydantoin Q86.1
  warfarin Q86.2
malignant
  carcinoid E34.0
  neuroleptic G21.0
Mallory-Weiss K22.6
mandibulofacial dysostosis Q75.4
manic-depressive — see Disorder, bipolar, affective
maple-syrup-urine E71.0
Marable's I77.4
Marfan's Q87.40
  with
    cardiovascular manifestations Q87.418
      aortic dilation Q87.410
    ocular manifestations Q87.42
    skeletal manifestations Q87.43
Marie's (acromegaly) E22.0
maternal hypotension — see Syndrome, hypotension, maternal
May (-Hegglin) D72.0
McArdle (-Schmidt) (-Pearson) E74.04
McQuarrie's E16.2
meconium plug (newborn) P76.0
median arcuate ligament I77.4
Meekeren-Ehlers-Danlos Q79.6
megavitamin-B6 E67.2
Meige G24.4
MELAS E88.41
Mendelson's O74.0
MERRF (myoclonic epilepsy associated with ragged-red fibers) E88.42
mesenteric
  artery (superior) K55.1
  vascular insufficiency K55.1
metabolic E88.81
metastatic carcinoid E34.0
micrognathia-glossoptosis Q87.0
midbrain NEC G93.89
middle lobe (lung) J98.19
middle radicular G54.0
migraine (see also Migraine) G43.909
Mikulicz' K11.8
milk-alkali E83.52

Syndrome — continued

Millard-Gubler G46.3
Miller-Dieker Q93.88
Miller-Fisher G61.0
Minkowski-Chauffard D58.0
Mirizzi's K83.1
MNGIE (Mitochondrial Neurogastrointestinal Encephalopathy) E88.49
Möbius, ophthalmoplegic migraine — see Migraine, ophthalmoplegic
monofixation H50.42
Morel-Moore M85.2
Morel-Morgagni M85.2
Morgagni (-Morel) (-Stewart) M85.2
Morgagni-Adams-Stokes I45.9
Mounier-Kuhn Q32.4
  with bronchiectasis J47.9
    with
      exacerbation (acute) J47.1
      lower respiratory infection J47.0
  acquired J98.09
    with bronchiectasis J47.9
      with
        exacerbation (acute) J47.1
        lower respiratory infection J47.0
mucocutaneous lymph node (acute febrile) (MCLS) M30.3
multiple endocrine neoplasia (MEN) — see Neoplasia, endocrine, multiple (MEN)
multiple operations — see Disorder, factitious
myasthenic G70.9
  in
    diabetes mellitus — see Diabetes, amyotrophy
    endocrine disease NEC E34.9 [G73.3]
    neoplastic disease (see also Neoplasm) D49.9 [G73.3]
    thyrotoxicosis (hyperthyroidism) E05.90 [G73.3]
      with thyroid storm E05.91 [G73.3]
myelodysplastic D46.9
  with
    5q deletion D46.C (following D46.2)
    isolated del (5q) chromosomal abnormality D46.C (following D46.2)
  lesions, low grade D46.20
  specified NEC D46.Z (following D46.4)
myelopathic pain G89.0
myeloproliferative (chronic) D47.1
myofascial pain M79.1
Naffziger's G54.0
nail patella Q87.2
NARP (Neuropathy, Ataxia and Retinitis pigmentosa) E88.49
neonatal abstinence P96.1
nephritic (see also Nephritis)
  with edema — see Nephrosis
  acute N00.9
  chronic N03.9
  rapidly progressive N01.9
nephrotic (congenital) (see also Nephrosis) N04.9
  with
    dense deposit disease N04.6
    diffuse
      crescentic glomerulonephritis N04.7
      endocapillary proliferative glomerulonephritis N04.4
      membranous glomerulonephritis N04.2
      mesangial proliferative glomerulonephritis N04.3
      mesangiocapillary glomerulonephritis N04.5
    focal and segmental glomerular lesions N04.1
    minor glomerular abnormality N04.0
    specified morphological changes NEC N04.8
  diabetic — see Diabetes, nephrosis
neurologic neglect R41.4
Nezelof's D81.4
Nonne-Milroy-Meige Q82.0
Nothnagel's vasomotor acroparesthesia I73.89
oculomotor H51.9
ophthalmoplegia-cerebellar ataxia — see Strabismus, paralytic, third nerve
oral-facial-digital Q87.0
organic
  affective F06.30
  amnesic (not alcohol- or drug-induced) F04
  brain F09
  depressive F06.31
  hallucinosis F06.0
  personality F07.0

Syndrome — continued

Ormond's N13.5
oro-facial-digital Q87.0
os trigonum Q68.8
Osler-Weber-Rendu I78.0
osteoporosis-osteomalacia M83.8
Osterreicher-Turner Q79.8
otolith — see subcategory H81.8 ☑
oto-palatal-digital Q87.0
outlet (thoracic) G54.0
ovary
  polycystic E28.2
  resistant E28.39
  sclerocystic E28.2
Owren's D68.2
Paget-Schroetter I82.890
pain (see also Pain)
  complex regional I G90.50
    lower limb G90.52- ☑
    specified site NEC G90.59
    upper limb G90.51- ☑
  complex regional II — see Causalgia
painful
  bruising D69.2
  feet E53.8
  prostate N42.81
paralysis agitans — see Parkinsonism
paralytic G83.9
  specified NEC G83.89
Parinaud's H51.0
parkinsonian — see Parkinsonism
Parkinson's — see Parkinsonism
paroxysmal facial pain G50.0
Parry's E05.00
  with thyroid storm E05.01
Parsonage (-Aldren)-Turner G54.5
patella clunk M25.86- ☑
Paterson (-Brown) (-Kelly) D50.1
pectoral girdle I77.89
pectoralis minor I77.89
Pelger-Huet D72.0
pellagra-cerebellar ataxia-renal aminoaciduria E72.02
pellagroid E52
Pellegrini-Stieda — see Bursitis, tibial collateral
pelvic congestion-fibrosis, female N94.89
penta X Q97.1
peptic ulcer — see Ulcer, peptic
perabduction I77.89
periodic headache, in adults and children — see Headache, periodic syndromes in adults and children
periurethral fibrosis N13.5
phantom limb (without pain) G54.7
  with pain G54.6
pharyngeal pouch D82.1
Pick's (heart) (liver) I31.1
Pickwickian E66.2
PIE (pulmonary infiltration with eosinophilia) J82
pigmentary pallidal degeneration (progressive) G23.0
pineal E34.8
pituitary E22.0
placental transfusion — see Pregnancy, complicated by, placental transfusion syndromes
plantar fascia M72.2
plateau iris (post-iridectomy) (postprocedural) H21.82
Plummer-Vinson D50.1
pluricarential of infancy E40
plurideficiency E40
pluriglandular (compensatory) E31.8
  autoimmune E31.0
pneumatic hammer T75.21 ☑
polyangiitis overlap M30.8
polycarential of infancy E40
polyglandular E31.8
  autoimmune E31.0
polysplenia Q89.09
pontine NEC G93.89
popliteal
  artery entrapment I77.89
  web Q87.89
post chemoembolization — code to associated conditions
postcardiac injury
  postcardiotomy I97.0
  postmyocardial infarction I24.1
postcardiotomy I97.0
postcholecystectomy K91.5
postcommissurotomy I97.0

Syndrome — *continued*
- postconcussional F07.81
- postcontusional F07.81
- postencephalitic F07.89
- posterior
  - cervical sympathetic M53.0
  - cord G83.83
  - fossa compression G93.5
  - reversible encephalopathy (PRES) I67.83
- postgastrectomy (dumping) K91.1
- postgastric surgery K91.1
- postinfarction I24.1
- postlaminectomy NEC M96.1
- postleukotomy F07.0
- postmastectomy lymphedema I97.2
- postmyocardial infarction I24.1
- postoperative NEC T81.9 ☑
  - blind loop K90.2
- postpartum panhypopituitary (Sheehan) E23.0
- postpolio (myelitic) G14
- postthrombotic I87.009
  - with
    - inflammation I87.02- ☑
      - with ulcer I87.03- ☑
    - specified complication NEC I87.09- ☑
    - ulcer I87.01- ☑
      - with inflammation I87.03- ☑
  - asymptomatic I87.00- ☑
- postvagotomy K91.1
- postvalvulotomy I97.0
- postviral NEC G93.3
  - fatigue G93.3
- Potain's K31.0
- potassium intoxication E87.5
- precerebral artery (multiple) (bilateral) G45.2
- preinfarction I20.0
- preleukemic D46.9
- premature senility E34.8
- premenstrual dysphoric N94.3
- premenstrual tension N94.3
- Prinzmetal-Massumi R07.1
- prune belly Q79.4
- pseudo -Turner's Q87.1
- pseudocarpal tunnel (sublimis) — *see* Syndrome, carpal tunnel
- pseudoparalytica G70.00
  - with exacerbation (acute) G70.01
  - in crisis G70.01
- psycho-organic (nonpsychotic severity) F07.9
  - acute or subacute F05
  - depressive type F06.31
  - hallucinatory type F06.0
  - nonpsychotic severity F07.0
  - specified NEC F07.89
- pulmonary
  - arteriosclerosis I27.0
  - dysmaturity (Wilson-Mikity) P27.0
  - hypoperfusion (idiopathic) P22.0
  - renal (hemorrhagic) (Goodpasture's) M31.0
- pure
  - motor lacunar G46.5
  - sensory lacunar G46.6
- Putnam-Dana D51.0
- pyramidopallidonigral G20
- pyriformis — *see* Lesion, nerve, sciatic
- QT interval prolongation I45.81
- radicular NEC — *see* Radiculopathy
  - upper limbs, newborn (birth injury) P14.3
- rapid time-zone change G47.25
- Rasmussen G04.81
- Raymond (-Céstan) I65.8
- Raynaud's I73.00
  - with gangrene I73.01
- RDS (respiratory distress syndrome, newborn) P22.0
- reactive airways dysfunction J68.3
- Refsum's G60.1
- Reifenstein E34.52
- renal glomerulohyalinosis-diabetic — *see* Diabetes, nephrosis
- Rendu-Osler-Weber I78.0
- residual ovary N99.83
- resistant ovary E28.39
- respiratory
  - distress
    - acute J80
      - adult J80
      - child J80
      - newborn (idiopathic) (type I) P22.0

Syndrome — *continued*
- respiratory — *continued*
  - distress — *continued*
    - newborn — *continued*
      - type II P22.1
- restless legs G25.81
- retinoblastoma (familial) C69.2 ☑
- retroperitoneal fibrosis N13.5
- retroviral seroconversion (acute) Z21
- Reye's G93.7
- Richter — *see* Leukemia, chronic lymphocytic, B-cell type
- Ridley's I50.1
- right
  - heart, hypoplastic Q22.6
  - ventricular obstruction — *see* Failure, heart, congestive
- Romano-Ward (prolonged QT interval) I45.81
- rotator cuff, shoulder (*see also* Tear, rotator cuff) M75.10- ☑
- Rotes Quérol — *see* Hyperostosis, ankylosing
- Roth — *see* Meralgia paresthetica
- rubella (congenital) P35.0
- Ruvalcaba-Myhre-Smith E71.440
- Rytand-Lipsitch I44.2
- salt
  - depletion E87.1
    - due to heat NEC T67.8 ☑
      - causing heat exhaustion or prostration T67.4 ☑
  - low E87.1
- salt-losing N28.89
- Scaglietti-Dagnini E22.0
- scalenus anticus (anterior) G54.0
- scapulocostal — *see* Mononeuropathy, upper limb, specified site NEC
- scapuloperoneal G71.0
- schizophrenic, of childhood NEC F84.5
- Schnitzler D47.2
- Scholte's E34.0
- Schroeder's E27.0
- Schüller-Christian C96.5
- Schwachman's — *see* Syndrome, Shwachman's
- Schwartz (-Jampel) G71.13
- Schwartz-Bartter E22.2
- scimitar Q26.8
- sclerocystic ovary E28.2
- Seitelberger's G31.89
- septicemic adrenal hemorrhage A39.1
- seroconversion, retroviral (acute) Z21
- serous meningitis G93.2
- severe acute respiratory (SARS) J12.81
- shaken infant T74.4
- shock (traumatic) T79.4 ☑
  - kidney N17.0
    - following crush injury T79.5 ☑
  - toxic A48.3
- shock-lung J80
- Shone's — *code to* specific anomalies
- short
  - bowel K91.2
  - rib Q77.2
- shoulder-hand — *see* Algoneurodystrophy
- Shwachman's D70.4
- sicca — *see* Sicca syndrome
- sick
  - cell E87.1
  - sinus I49.5
- sick-euthyroid E07.81
- sideropenic D50.1
- Siemens' ectodermal dysplasia Q82.4
- Silfversköld's Q78.9
- Simons' E88.1
- sinus tarsi M25.57- ☑
- sinusitis-bronchiectasis-situs inversus Q89.3
- Sipple's E31.22
- sirenomelia Q87.2
- Slocumb's E27.0
- slow flow, coronary I20.8
- Sluder's G44.89
- Smith-Magenis Q93.88
- Sneddon-Wilkinson L13.1
- Sotos' E22.0
- South African cardiomyopathy I42.8
- spasmodic
  - upward movement, eyes H51.8
  - winking F95.8
- Spen's I45.9

Syndrome — *continued*
- splenic
  - agenesis Q89.01
  - flexure K59.8
  - neutropenia D73.81
- Spurway's Q78.0
- staphylococcal scalded skin L00
- Stein-Leventhal E28.2
- Stein's E28.2
- Stevens-Johnson syndrome L51.1
  - toxic epidermal necrolysis overlap L51.3
- Stewart-Morel M85.2
- Stickler Q89.8
- stiff baby Q89.8
- stiff man G25.82
- Still-Felty — *see* Felty's syndrome
- Stokes (-Adams) I45.9
- stone heart I50.1
- straight back, congenital Q76.49
- subclavian steal G45.8
- subcoracoid-pectoralis minor G54.0
- subcostal nerve compression I77.89
- subphrenic interposition Q43.3
- superior
  - cerebellar artery I63.8
  - mesenteric artery K55.1
  - semi-circular canal dehiscence H83.8X- ☑
  - vena cava I87.1
- supine hypotensive (maternal) — *see* Syndrome, hypotension, maternal
- suprarenal cortical E27.0
- supraspinatus (*see also* Tear, rotator cuff) M75.10- ☑
- Susac G93.49
- swallowed blood P78.2
- sweat retention L74.0
- Swyer Q99.1
- Symond's G93.2
- sympathetic
  - cervical paralysis G90.2
  - pelvic, female N94.89
- systemic inflammatory response (SIRS), of non-infectious origin (without organ dysfunction) R65.10
  - with acute organ dysfunction R65.11
- tachycardia-bradycardia I49.5
- takotsubo I51.81
- TAR (thrombocytopenia with absent radius) Q87.2
- tarsal tunnel G57.5- ☑
- teething K00.7
- tegmental G93.89
- telangiectasic-pigmentation-cataract Q82.8
- temporal pyramidal apex — *see* Otitis, media, suppurative, acute
- temporomandibular joint-pain-dysfunction M26.62
- Terry's H44.2- ☑
- testicular feminization (*see also* Syndrome, androgen insensitivity) E34.51
- thalamic pain (hyperesthetic) G89.0
- thoracic outlet (compression) G54.0
- Thorson-Björck E34.0
- thrombocytopenia with absent radius (TAR) Q87.2
- thyroid-adrenocortical insufficiency E31.0
- tibial
  - anterior M76.81- ☑
  - posterior M76.82- ☑
- Tietze's M94.0
- time-zone (rapid) G47.25
- Toni-Fanconi E72.09
  - with cystinosis E72.04
- Touraine's Q79.8
- tourniquet — *see* Constriction, external, by site
- toxic shock A48.3
- transient left ventricular apical ballooning I51.81
- traumatic vasospastic T75.22 ☑
- Treacher Collins Q75.4
- triple X, female Q97.0
- trisomy Q92.9
  - 13 Q91.7
    - meiotic nondisjunction Q91.4
    - mitotic nondisjunction Q91.5
    - mosaicism Q91.5
    - translocation Q91.6
  - 18 Q91.3
    - meiotic nondisjunction Q91.0
    - mitotic nondisjunction Q91.1
    - mosaicism Q91.1
    - translocation Q91.2
  - 20 (q)(p) Q92.8
  - 21 Q90.9

Syndrome — continued
 trisomy — continued
  21 — continued
   meiotic nondisjunction Q90.0
   mitotic nondisjunction Q90.1
   mosaicism Q90.1
   translocation Q90.2
  22 Q92.8
 tropical wet feet T69.0- ☑
 Trousseau's I82.1
 tumor lysis (following antineoplastic chemotherapy) (spontaneous) NEC E88.3
 Twiddler's (due to)
  automatic implantable defibrillator T82.198 ☑
  cardiac pacemaker T82.198 ☑
 Unverricht (-Lundborg) — see Epilepsy, generalized, idiopathic
 upward gaze H51.8
 uremia, chronic (see also Disease, kidney, chronic) N18.9
 urethral N34.3
 urethro-oculo-articular — see Reiter's disease
 urohepatic K76.7
 vago-hypoglossal G52.7
 van Buchem's M85.2
 van der Hoeve's Q78.0
 vascular NEC in cerebrovascular disease G46.8
 vasoconstriction, reversible cerebrovascular I67.841
 vasomotor I73.9
 vasospastic (traumatic) T75.22 ☑
 vasovagal R55
 VATER Q87.2
 velo-cardio-facial Q93.81
 vena cava (inferior) (superior) (obstruction) I87.1
 vertebral
  artery G45.0
   compression — see Syndrome, anterior, spinal artery, compression
   steal G45.0
 vertebro-basilar artery G45.0
 vertebrogenic (pain) M54.89
 vertiginous — see Disorder, vestibular function
 Vinson-Plummer D50.1
 virus B34.9
 visceral larva migrans B83.0
 visual disorientation H53.8
 vitamin B6 deficiency E53.1
 vitreal corneal H59.01- ☑
 vitreous (touch) H59.01- ☑
 Vogt-Koyanagi H20.82- ☑
 Volkmann's T79.6 ☑
 von Schroetter's I82.890
 von Willebrand (-Jürgen) D68.0
 Waldenström-Kjellberg D50.1
 Wallenberg's G46.3
 water retention E87.79
 Waterhouse (-Friderichsen) A39.1
 Weber-Gubler G46.3
 Weber-Leyden G46.3
 Weber's G46.3
 Wegener's M31.30
  with
   kidney involvement M31.31
   lung involvement M31.30
    with kidney involvement M31.31
 Weingarten's (tropical eosinophilia) J82
 Weiss-Baker G90.09
 Werdnig-Hoffman G12.0
 Wermer's E31.21
 Werner's E34.8
 Wernicke-Korsakoff (nonalcoholic) F04
  alcoholic F10.26
 Westphal-Strümpell E83.01
 West's — see Epilepsy, spasms
 wet
  feet (maceration) (tropical) T69.0- ☑
  lung, newborn P22.1
 whiplash S13.4 ☑
 whistling face Q87.0
 Wilkie's K55.1
 Wilkinson-Sneddon L13.1
 Willebrand (-Jürgens) D68.0
 Wilson's (hepatolenticular degeneration) E83.01
 Wiskott-Aldrich D82.0
 withdrawal — see Withdrawal, state
  drug
   infant of dependent mother P96.1
   therapeutic use, newborn P96.2

Syndrome — continued
 Woakes' (ethmoiditis) J33.1
 Wright's (hyperabduction) I77.89
 X I20.9
 XXXX Q97.1
 XXXXX Q97.1
 XXXXY Q98.1
 XXY Q98.0
 yellow nail L60.5
 Zahorsky's B08.5
 Zellweger syndrome E71.510
 Zellweger-like syndrome E71.541
Synechia (anterior) (iris) (posterior) (pupil) (see also Adhesions, iris)
 intra-uterine (traumatic) N85.6
Synesthesia R20.8
Syngamiasis, syngamosis B83.3
Synodontia K00.2
Synorchidism, synorchism Q55.1
Synostosis (congenital) Q78.8
 astragalo-scaphoid Q74.2
 radioulnar Q74.0
Synovial sarcoma — see Neoplasm, connective tissue, malignant
Synovioma (malignant) (see also Neoplasm, connective tissue, malignant)
 benign — see Neoplasm, connective tissue, benign
Synoviosarcoma — see Neoplasm, connective tissue, malignant
Synovitis (see also Tenosynovitis)
 crepitant
  hand M70.0- ☑
  wrist M70.03- ☑
 gonococcal A54.49
 gouty — see Gout, idiopathic
 in (due to)
  crystals M65.8- ☑
  gonorrhea A54.49
  syphilis (late) A52.78
  use, overuse, pressure — see Disorder, soft tissue, due to use
 infective NEC — see Tenosynovitis, infective NEC
 specified NEC — see Tenosynovitis, specified type NEC
 syphilitic A52.78
  congenital (early) A50.02
 toxic — see Synovitis, transient
 transient M67.3- ☑
  ankle M67.37- ☑
  elbow M67.32- ☑
  foot joint M67.37- ☑
  hand joint M67.34- ☑
  hip M67.35- ☑
  knee M67.36- ☑
  multiple site M67.39
  pelvic region M67.35- ☑
  shoulder M67.31- ☑
  specified joint NEC M67.38
  wrist M67.33- ☑
 traumatic, current — see Sprain
 tuberculous — see Tuberculosis, synovitis
 villonodular (pigmented) M12.2- ☑
  ankle M12.27- ☑
  elbow M12.22- ☑
  foot joint M12.27- ☑
  hand joint M12.24- ☑
  hip M12.25- ☑
  knee M12.26- ☑
  multiple site M12.29
  pelvic region M12.25- ☑
  shoulder M12.21- ☑
  specified joint NEC M12.28
  vertebrae M12.28
  wrist M12.23- ☑
Syphilid A51.39
 congenital A50.06
 newborn A50.06
 tubercular (late) A52.79
Syphilis, syphilitic (acquired) A53.9
 abdomen (late) A52.79
 acoustic nerve A52.15
 adenopathy (secondary) A51.49
 adrenal (gland) (with cortical hypofunction) A52.79
 age under 2 years NOS (see also Syphilis, congenital, early)
  acquired A51.9
 alopecia (secondary) A51.32
 anemia (late) A52.79 [D63.8]

Syphilis, syphilitic — continued
 aneurysm (aorta) (ruptured) A52.01
  central nervous system A52.05
  congenital A50.54 [I79.0]
 anus (late) A52.74
  primary A51.1
  secondary A51.39
 aorta (arch) (abdominal) (thoracic) A52.02
  aneurysm A52.01
 aortic (insufficiency) (regurgitation) (stenosis) A52.03
  aneurysm A52.01
 arachnoid (adhesive) (cerebral) (spinal) A52.13
 asymptomatic — see Syphilis, latent
 ataxia (locomotor) A52.11
 atrophoderma maculatum A51.39
 auricular fibrillation A52.06
 bladder (late) A52.76
 bone A52.77
  secondary A51.46
 brain A52.17
 breast (late) A52.79
 bronchus (late) A52.72
 bubo (primary) A51.0
 bulbar palsy A52.19
 bursa (late) A52.78
 cardiac decompensation A52.06
 cardiovascular A52.00
 central nervous system (late) (recurrent) (relapse) (tertiary) A52.3
  with
   ataxia A52.11
   general paralysis A52.17
    juvenile A50.45
   paresis (general) A52.17
    juvenile A50.45
   tabes (dorsalis) A52.11
    juvenile A50.45
   taboparesis A52.17
    juvenile A50.45
  aneurysm A52.05
  congenital A50.40
  juvenile A50.40
  remission in (sustained) A52.3
  serology doubtful, negative, or positive A52.3
  specified nature or site NEC A52.19
  vascular A52.05
 cerebral A52.17
  meningovascular A52.13
  nerves (multiple palsies) A52.15
  sclerosis A52.17
  thrombosis A52.05
 cerebrospinal (tabetic type) A52.12
 cerebrovascular A52.05
 cervix (late) A52.76
 chancre (multiple) A51.0
  extragenital A51.2
  Rollet's A51.0
 Charcot's joint A52.16
 chorioretinitis A51.43
  congenital A50.01
  late A52.71
  prenatal A50.01
 choroiditis — see Syphilitic chorioretinitis
 choroidoretinitis — see Syphilitic chorioretinitis
 ciliary body (secondary) A51.43
  late A52.71
 colon (late) A52.74
 combined spinal sclerosis A52.11
 condyloma (latum) A51.31
 congenital A50.9
  with
   paresis (general) A50.45
   tabes (dorsalis) A50.45
   taboparesis A50.45
  early, or less than 2 years after birth NEC A50.2
   with manifestations — see Syphilis, congenital, early, symptomatic
   latent (without manifestations) A50.1
    negative spinal fluid test A50.1
    serology positive A50.1
   symptomatic A50.09
    cutaneous A50.06
    mucocutaneous A50.07
    oculopathy A50.01
    osteochondropathy A50.02
    pharyngitis A50.03
    pneumonia A50.04
    rhinitis A50.05

Syphilis, syphilitic — *continued*
congenital — *continued*
  early, or less than 2 years after birth — *continued*
    symptomatic — *continued*
      visceral A50.08
    chorioretinitis, choroiditis A50.01 [H32]
    interstitial keratitis A50.31
    juvenile neurosyphilis A50.45
    late, or 2 years or more after birth NEC A50.7
      chorioretinitis, choroiditis A50.32
      interstitial keratitis A50.31
      juvenile neurosyphilis A50.45
      latent (without manifestations) A50.6
        negative spinal fluid test A50.6
        serology positive A50.6
      symptomatic or with manifestations NEC A50.59
        arthropathy A50.55
        cardiovascular A50.54
        Clutton's joints A50.51
        Hutchinson's teeth A50.52
        Hutchinson's triad A50.53
        osteochondropathy A50.56
        saddle nose A50.57
  conjugal A53.9
    tabes A52.11
  conjunctiva (late) A52.71
  contact Z20.2
  cord bladder A52.19
  cornea, late A52.71
  coronary (artery) (sclerosis) A52.06
  coryza, congenital A50.05
  cranial nerve A52.15
    multiple palsies A52.15
  cutaneous — *see* Syphilis, skin
  dacryocystitis (late) A52.71
  degeneration, spinal cord A52.12
  dementia paralytica A52.17
    juvenilis A50.45
  destruction of bone A52.77
  dilatation, aorta A52.01
  due to blood transfusion A53.9
  dura mater A52.13
  ear A52.79
    inner A52.79
      nerve (eighth) A52.15
      neurorecurrence A52.15
  early A51.9
    cardiovascular A52.00
    central nervous system A52.3
    latent (without manifestations) (less than 2 years after infection) A51.5
      negative spinal fluid test A51.5
      serological relapse after treatment A51.5
      serology positive A51.5
    relapse (treated, untreated) A51.9
    skin A51.39
    symptomatic A51.9
      extragenital chancre A51.2
      primary, except extragenital chancre A51.0
      secondary (*see also* Syphilis, secondary) A51.39
        relapse (treated, untreated) A51.49
    ulcer A51.39
  eighth nerve (neuritis) A52.15
  endemic A65
  endocarditis A52.03
    aortic A52.03
    pulmonary A52.03
  epididymis (late) A52.76
  epiglottis (late) A52.73
  epiphysitis (congenital) (early) A50.02
  episcleritis (late) A52.71
  esophagus A52.79
  eustachian tube A52.73
  exposure to Z20.2
  eye A52.71
  eyelid (late) (with gumma) A52.71
  fallopian tube (late) A52.76
  fracture A52.77
  gallbladder (late) A52.74
  gastric (polyposis) (late) A52.74
  general A53.9
    paralysis A52.17
      juvenile A50.45
  genital (primary) A51.0
  glaucoma A52.71
  gumma NEC A52.79

Syphilis, syphilitic — *continued*
gumma — *continued*
  cardiovascular system A52.00
  central nervous system A52.3
  congenital A50.59
heart (block) (decompensation) (disease) (failure) A52.06 [I52]
  valve NEC A52.03
hemianesthesia A52.19
hemianopsia A52.71
hemiparesis A52.17
hemiplegia A52.17
hepatic artery A52.09
hepatis A52.74
hepatomegaly, congenital A50.08
hereditaria tarda — *see* Syphilis, congenital, late
hereditary — *see* Syphilis, congenital
Hutchinson's teeth A50.52
hyalitis A52.71
inactive — *see* Syphilis, latent
infantum — *see* Syphilis, congenital
inherited — *see* Syphilis, congenital
internal ear A52.79
intestine (late) A52.74
iris, iritis (secondary) A51.43
  late A52.71
joint (late) A52.77
keratitis (congenital) (interstitial) (late) A50.31
kidney (late) A52.75
lacrimal passages (late) A52.71
larynx (late) A52.73
late A52.9
  cardiovascular A52.00
  central nervous system A52.3
  kidney A52.75
  latent or 2 years or more after infection (without manifestations) A52.8
    negative spinal fluid test A52.8
    serology positive A52.8
  paresis A52.17
  specified site NEC A52.79
  symptomatic or with manifestations A52.79
  tabes A52.11
latent A53.0
  with signs or symptoms — *code by* site and stage under Syphilis
  early, or less than 2 years after infection A51.5
  central nervous system A52.2
  date of infection unspecified A53.0
  follow-up of latent syphilis A53.0
    date of infection unspecified A53.0
    late, or 2 years or more after infection A52.8
  late, or 2 years or more after infection A52.8
  positive serology (only finding) A53.0
    early, or less than 2 years after infection A51.5
    date of infection unspecified A53.0
    late, or 2 years or more after infection A52.8
lens (late) A52.71
leukoderma A51.39
  late A52.79
lienitis A52.79
lip A51.39
  chancre (primary) A51.2
  late A52.79
Lissauer's paralysis A52.17
liver A52.74
locomotor ataxia A52.11
lung A52.72
lymph gland (early) (secondary) A51.49
  late A52.79
lymphadenitis (secondary) A51.49
macular atrophy of skin A51.39
  striated A52.79
mediastinum (late) A52.73
meninges (adhesive) (brain) (spinal cord) A52.13
meningitis A52.13
  acute (secondary) A51.41
  congenital A50.41
meningoencephalitis A52.14
meningovascular A52.13
  congenital A50.41
mesarteritis A52.09
  brain A52.04
middle ear A52.77
mitral stenosis A52.03
monoplegia A52.17
mouth (secondary) A51.39
  late A52.79

Syphilis, syphilitic — *continued*
mucocutaneous (secondary) A51.39
  late A52.79
mucous
  membrane (secondary) A51.39
    late A52.79
  patches A51.39
    congenital A50.07
mulberry molars A50.52
muscle A52.78
myocardium A52.06
nasal sinus (late) A52.73
neonatorum — *see* Syphilis, congenital
nephrotic syndrome (secondary) A51.44
nerve palsy (any cranial nerve) A52.15
  multiple A52.15
nervous system, central A52.3
neuritis A52.15
  acoustic A52.15
neurorecidive of retina A52.19
neuroretinitis A52.19
newborn — *see* Syphilis, congenital
nodular superficial (late) A52.79
nonvenereal A65
nose (late) A52.73
  saddle back deformity A50.57
occlusive arterial disease A52.09
oculopathy A52.71
ophthalmic (late) A52.71
optic nerve (atrophy) (neuritis) (papilla) A52.15
orbit (late) A52.71
organic A53.9
osseous (late) A52.77
osteochondritis (congenital) (early) A50.02 [M90.80]
osteoporosis A52.77
ovary (late) A52.76
oviduct (late) A52.76
palate (late) A52.79
pancreas (late) A52.74
paralysis A52.17
  general A52.17
    juvenile A50.45
paresis (general) A52.17
  juvenile A50.45
paresthesia A52.19
Parkinson's disease or syndrome A52.19
paroxysmal tachycardia A52.06
pemphigus (congenital) A50.06
penis (chancre) A51.0
  late A52.76
pericardium A52.06
perichondritis, larynx (late) A52.73
periosteum (late) A52.77
  congenital (early) A50.02 [M90.80]
  early (secondary) A51.46
peripheral nerve A52.79
petrous bone (late) A52.77
pharynx (late) A52.73
  secondary A51.39
pituitary (gland) A52.79
pleura (late) A52.73
pneumonia, white A50.04
pontine lesion A52.17
portal vein A52.09
primary A51.0
  anal A51.1
  and secondary — *see* Syphilis, secondary
  central nervous system A52.3
  extragenital chancre NEC A51.2
    fingers A51.2
    genital A51.0
    lip A51.2
    specified site NEC A51.2
    tonsils A51.2
prostate (late) A52.76
ptosis (eyelid) A52.71
pulmonary (late) A52.72
  artery A52.09
pyelonephritis (late) A52.75
recently acquired, symptomatic A51.9
rectum (late) A52.74
respiratory tract (late) A52.73
retina, late A52.71
retrobulbar neuritis A52.15
salpingitis A52.76
sclera (late) A52.71
sclerosis
  cerebral A52.17

☑ Additional Character Required — Refer to the Tabular List for Character Selection   ▽ Subterms under main terms may continue to next column or page

Syphilis, syphilitic — continued
  sclerosis — continued
    coronary A52.06
    multiple A52.11
  scotoma (central) A52.71
  scrotum (late) A52.76
  secondary (and primary) A51.49
    adenopathy A51.49
    anus A51.39
    bone A51.46
    chorioretinitis, choroiditis A51.43
    hepatitis A51.45
    liver A51.45
    lymphadenitis A51.49
    meningitis (acute) A51.41
    mouth A51.39
    mucous membranes A51.39
    periosteum, periostitis A51.46
    pharynx A51.39
    relapse (treated, untreated) A51.49
    skin A51.39
    specified form NEC A51.49
    tonsil A51.39
    ulcer A51.39
    viscera NEC A51.49
    vulva A51.39
  seminal vesicle (late) A52.76
  seronegative with signs or symptoms — *code by* site
      and stage under Syphilis
  seropositive
    with signs or symptoms — *code by* site and stage
        under Syphilis
    follow-up of latent syphilis — *see* Syphilis, latent
    only finding — *see* Syphilis, latent
  seventh nerve (paralysis) A52.15
  sinus, sinusitis (late) A52.73
  skeletal system A52.77
  skin (with ulceration) (early) (secondary) A51.39
    late or tertiary A52.79
  small intestine A52.74
  spastic spinal paralysis A52.17
  spermatic cord (late) A52.76
  spinal (cord) A52.12

Syphilis, syphilitic — continued
  spleen A52.79
  splenomegaly A52.79
  spondylitis A52.77
  staphyloma A52.71
  stigmata (congenital) A50.59
  stomach A52.74
  synovium A52.78
  tabes dorsalis (late) A52.11
    juvenile A50.45
  tabetic type A52.11
    juvenile A50.45
  taboparesis A52.17
    juvenile A50.45
  tachycardia A52.06
  tendon (late) A52.78
  tertiary A52.9
    with symptoms NEC A52.79
    cardiovascular A52.00
    central nervous system A52.3
    multiple NEC A52.79
    specified site NEC A52.79
  testis A52.76
  thorax A52.73
  throat A52.73
  thymus (gland) (late) A52.79
  thyroid (late) A52.79
  tongue (late) A52.79
  tonsil (lingual) (late) A52.73
    primary A51.2
    secondary A51.39
  trachea (late) A52.73
  tunica vaginalis (late) A52.76
  ulcer (any site) (early) (secondary) A51.39
    late A52.79
    perforating A52.79
      foot A52.11
  urethra (late) A52.76
  urogenital (late) A52.76
  uterus (late) A52.76
  uveal tract (secondary) A51.43
    late A52.71
  uveitis (secondary) A51.43

Syphilis, syphilitic — continued
  uveitis — continued
    late A52.71
  uvula (late) (perforated) A52.79
  vagina A51.0
    late A52.76
  valvulitis NEC A52.03
  vascular A52.00
    brain (cerebral) A52.05
  ventriculi A52.74
  vesicae urinariae (late) A52.76
  viscera (abdominal) (late) A52.74
    secondary A51.49
  vitreous (opacities) (late) A52.71
    hemorrhage A52.71
  vulva A51.0
    late A52.76
    secondary A51.39
Syphiloma A52.79
  cardiovascular system A52.00
  central nervous system A52.3
  circulatory system A52.00
  congenital A50.59
Syphilophobia F45.29
Syringadenoma (*see also* Neoplasm, skin, benign)
  papillary — *see* Neoplasm, skin, benign
Syringobulbia G95.0
Syringocystadenoma — *see* Neoplasm, skin, benign
  papillary — *see* Neoplasm, skin, benign
Syringoma (*see also* Neoplasm, skin, benign)
  chondroid — *see* Neoplasm, skin, benign
Syringomyelia G95.0
Syringomyelitis — *see* Encephalitis
Syringomyelocele — *see* Spina bifida
Syringopontia G95.0
System, systemic (*see also* condition)
  disease, combined — *see* Degeneration, combined
  inflammatory response syndrome (SIRS) of non-infec-
      tious origin (without organ dysfunction) R65.10
    with acute organ dysfunction R65.11
  lupus erythematosus M32.9
    inhibitor present D68.62

Subterms under main terms may continue to next column or page   ☑ Additional Character Required — Refer to the Tabular List for Character Selection   297

Syphilis, syphilitic — System, systemic

T

Tabacism, tabacosis, tabagism (see also Poisoning, tobacco)
　meaning dependence (without remission) F17.200
　　with
　　　disorder F17.299
　　　　remission F17.211
　　　　specified disorder NEC F17.298
　　　　withdrawal F17.203
Tabardillo A75.9
　flea-borne A75.2
　louse-borne A75.0
Tabes, tabetic A52.10
　with
　　central nervous system syphilis A52.10
　　Charcot's joint A52.16
　　cord bladder A52.19
　　crisis, viscera (any) A52.19
　　paralysis, general A52.17
　　paresis (general) A52.17
　　perforating ulcer (foot) A52.19
　arthropathy (Charcot) A52.16
　bladder A52.19
　bone A52.11
　cerebrospinal A52.12
　congenital A50.45
　conjugal A52.10
　dorsalis A52.11
　　juvenile A50.49
　juvenile A50.49
　latent A52.19
　mesenterica A18.39
　paralysis, insane, general A52.17
　spasmodic A52.17
　syphilis (cerebrospinal) A52.12
Taboparalysis A52.17
Taboparesis (remission) A52.17
　juvenile A50.45
TAC (trigeminal autonomic cephalgia) **NEC** G44.099
　intractable G44.091
　not intractable G44.099
Tache noir S60.22- ☑
Tachyalimentation K91.2
Tachyarrhythmia, tachyrhythmia — see Tachycardia
Tachycardia R00.0
　atrial (paroxysmal) I47.1
　auricular I47.1
　AV nodal re-entry (re-entrant) I47.1
　junctional (paroxysmal) I47.1
　newborn P29.11
　nodal (paroxysmal) I47.1
　non-paroxysmal AV nodal I45.89
　paroxysmal (sustained) (nonsustained) I47.9
　　with sinus bradycardia I49.5
　　atrial (PAT) I47.1
　　atrioventricular (AV) (re-entrant) I47.1
　　　psychogenic F54
　　junctional I47.1
　　　ectopic I47.1
　　nodal I47.1
　　psychogenic (atrial) (supraventricular) (ventricular) F54
　　supraventricular (sustained) I47.1
　　　psychogenic F54
　　ventricular I47.2
　　　psychogenic F54
　psychogenic F45.8
　sick sinus I49.5
　sinoauricular NOS R00.0
　　paroxysmal I47.1
　sinus [sinusal] NOS R00.0
　　paroxysmal I47.1
　supraventricular I47.1
　ventricular (paroxysmal) (sustained) I47.2
　　psychogenic F54
Tachygastria K31.89
Tachypnea R06.82
　hysterical F45.8
　newborn (idiopathic) (transitory) P22.1
　psychogenic F45.8
　transitory, of newborn P22.1

TACO (transfusion associated circulatory overload) E87.71
Taenia (infection) (infestation) B68.9
　diminuta B71.0
　echinococcal infestation B67.90
　mediocanellata B68.1
　nana B71.0
　saginata B68.1
　solium (intestinal form) B68.0
　　larval form — see Cysticercosis
Taeniasis (intestine) — see Taenia
Tag (hypertrophied skin) (infected) L91.8
　adenoid J35.8
　anus K64.4
　hemorrhoidal K64.4
　hymen N89.8
　perineal N90.89
　preauricular Q17.0
　sentinel K64.4
　skin L91.8
　　accessory (congenital) Q82.8
　　anus K64.4
　　congenital Q82.8
　　preauricular Q17.0
　tonsil J35.8
　urethra, urethral N36.8
　vulva N90.89
Tahyna fever B33.8
Takahara's disease E80.3
Takayasu's disease or syndrome M31.4
Talcosis (pulmonary) J62.0
Talipes (congenital) Q66.89
　acquired, planus — see Deformity, limb, flat foot
　asymmetric Q66.89
　calcaneovalgus Q66.4
　calcaneovarus Q66.1
　calcaneus Q66.89
　cavus Q66.7
　equinovalgus Q66.6
　equinovarus Q66.0
　equinus Q66.89
　percavus Q66.7
　planovalgus Q66.6
　planus (acquired) (any degree) (see also Deformity, limb, flat foot)
　　congenital Q66.5- ☑
　　due to rickets (sequelae) E64.3
　valgus Q66.6
　varus Q66.3
Tall stature, constitutional E34.4
Talma's disease M62.89
Talon noir S90.3- ☑
　hand S60.22- ☑
　heel S90.3- ☑
　toe S90.1- ☑
Tamponade, heart I31.4
Tanapox (virus disease) B08.71
Tangier disease E78.6
Tantrum, child problem F91.8
Tapeworm (infection) (infestation) — see Infestation, tapeworm
Tapia's syndrome G52.7
TAR (thrombocytopenia with absent radius) **syndrome** Q87.2
Tarral-Besnier disease L44.0
Tarsal tunnel syndrome — see Syndrome, tarsal tunnel
Tarsalgia — see Pain, limb, lower
Tarsitis (eyelid) H01.8
　syphilitic A52.71
　tuberculous A18.4
Tartar (teeth) (dental calculus) K03.6
Tattoo (mark) L81.8
Tauri's disease E74.09
Taurodontism K00.2
Taussig-Bing syndrome Q20.1
Taybi's syndrome Q87.2
Tay-Sachs amaurotic familial idiocy or disease E75.02
TBI (traumatic brain injury) — see category S06 ☑
Teacher's node or nodule J38.2
Tear, torn (traumatic) (see also Laceration)
　with abortion — see Abortion
　annular fibrosis M51.35
　anus, anal (sphincter) S31.831 ☑

Tear, torn — continued
　anus, anal — continued
　　complicating delivery
　　　with third degree perineal laceration O70.2
　　　　with mucosa O70.3
　　　without third degree perineal laceration O70.4
　　nontraumatic (healed) (old) K62.81
　articular cartilage, old — see Derangement, joint, articular cartilage, by site
　bladder
　　with ectopic or molar pregnancy O08.6
　　following ectopic or molar pregnancy O08.6
　　obstetrical O71.5
　　traumatic — see Injury, bladder
　bowel
　　with ectopic or molar pregnancy O08.6
　　following ectopic or molar pregnancy O08.6
　　obstetrical trauma O71.5
　broad ligament
　　with ectopic or molar pregnancy O08.6
　　following ectopic or molar pregnancy O08.6
　　obstetrical trauma O71.6
　bucket handle (knee) (meniscus) — see Tear, meniscus
　capsule, joint — see Sprain
　cartilage (see also Sprain)
　　articular, old — see Derangement, joint, articular cartilage, by site
　cervix
　　with ectopic or molar pregnancy O08.6
　　following ectopic or molar pregnancy O08.6
　　obstetrical trauma (current) O71.3
　　old N88.1
　　traumatic — see Injury, uterus
　dural G97.41
　　nontraumatic G96.11
　internal organ — see Injury, by site
　knee cartilage
　　articular (current) S83.3- ☑
　　old — see Derangement, knee, meniscus, due to old tear
　ligament — see Sprain
　meniscus (knee) (current injury) S83.209 ☑
　　bucket-handle S83.20- ☑
　　lateral
　　　bucket-handle S83.25- ☑
　　　complex S83.27- ☑
　　　peripheral S83.26- ☑
　　　specified type NEC S83.28- ☑
　　medial
　　　bucket-handle S83.21- ☑
　　　complex S83.23- ☑
　　　peripheral S83.22- ☑
　　　specified type NEC S83.24- ☑
　　old — see Derangement, knee, meniscus, due to old tear
　　site other than knee — code as Sprain
　　specified type NEC S83.20- ☑
　muscle — see Strain
　pelvic
　　floor, complicating delivery O70.1
　　organ NEC, obstetrical trauma O71.5
　　　with ectopic or molar pregnancy O08.6
　　　following ectopic or molar pregnancy O08.6
　perineal, secondary O90.1
　periurethral tissue, obstetrical trauma O71.82
　　with ectopic or molar pregnancy O08.6
　　following ectopic or molar pregnancy O08.6
　rectovaginal septum — see Laceration, vagina
　retina, retinal (without detachment) (horseshoe) (see also Break, retina, horseshoe)
　　with detachment — see Detachment, retina, with retinal, break
　rotator cuff (nontraumatic) M75.10- ☑
　　complete M75.12- ☑
　　incomplete M75.11- ☑
　　traumatic S46.01- ☑
　　capsule S43.42- ☑
　semilunar cartilage, knee — see Tear, meniscus
　supraspinatus (complete) (incomplete) (nontraumatic) (see also Tear, rotator cuff) M75.10- ☑
　tendon — see Strain
　tentorial, at birth P10.4

Tear, torn — *continued*
  umbilical cord
    complicating delivery O69.89 ☑
  urethra
    with ectopic or molar pregnancy O08.6
    following ectopic or molar pregnancy O08.6
    obstetrical trauma O71.5
  uterus — *see* Injury, uterus
  vagina — *see* Laceration, vagina
  vessel, from catheter — *see* Puncture, accidental
    complicating surgery
  vulva, complicating delivery O70.0
Tear-stone — *see* Dacryolith
Teeth (*see also* condition)
  grinding
    psychogenic F45.8
    sleep related G47.63
Teething (syndrome) K00.7
Telangiectasia, telangiectasis (verrucous) I78.1
  ataxic (cerebellar) (Louis-Bar) G11.3
  familial I78.0
  hemorrhagic, hereditary (congenital) (senile) I78.0
  hereditary, hemorrhagic (congenital) (senile) I78.0
  juxtafoveal H35.07- ☑
  macular H35.07- ☑
  parafoveal H35.07- ☑
  retinal (idiopathic) (juxtafoveal) (macular) (parafoveal) H35.07- ☑
  spider I78.1
Telephone scatologia F65.89
Telescoped bowel or intestine K56.1
  congenital Q43.8
Temperature
  body, high (of unknown origin) R50.9
  cold, trauma from T69.9 ☑
    newborn P80.0
    specified effect NEC T69.8 ☑
Temple — *see* condition
Temporal — *see* condition
Temporomandibular joint pain-dysfunction syndrome M26.62
Temporosphenoidal — *see* condition
Tendency
  bleeding — *see* Defect, coagulation
  suicide
    meaning personal history of attempted suicide Z91.5
    meaning suicidal ideation — *see* Ideation, suicidal
  to fall R29.6
Tenderness, abdominal R10.819
  epigastric R10.816
  generalized R10.817
  left lower quadrant R10.814
  left upper quadrant R10.812
  periumbilic R10.815
  rebound R10.829
    epigastric R10.826
    generalized R10.827
    left lower quadrant R10.824
    left upper quadrant R10.822
    periumbilic R10.825
    right lower quadrant R10.823
    right upper quadrant R10.821
  right lower quadrant R10.813
  right upper quadrant R10.811
Tendinitis, tendonitis (*see also* Enthesopathy)
  Achilles M76.6- ☑
  adhesive — *see* Tenosynovitis, specified type NEC
    shoulder — *see* Capsulitis, adhesive
  bicipital M75.2- ☑
  calcific M65.2- ☑
    ankle M65.27- ☑
    foot M65.27- ☑
    forearm M65.23- ☑
    hand M65.24- ☑
    lower leg M65.26- ☑
    multiple sites M65.29
    pelvic region M65.25- ☑
    shoulder M75.3- ☑
    specified site NEC M65.28
    thigh M65.25- ☑
    upper arm M65.22- ☑
  due to use, overuse, pressure (*see also* Disorder, soft tissue, due to use)
    specified NEC — *see* Disorder, soft tissue, due to use, specified NEC
  gluteal M76.0- ☑

Tendinitis, tendonitis — *continued*
  patellar M76.5- ☑
  peroneal M76.7- ☑
  psoas M76.1- ☑
  tibial (posterior) M76.82- ☑
    anterior M76.81- ☑
  trochanteric — *see* Bursitis, hip, trochanteric
Tendon — *see* condition
Tendosynovitis — *see* Tenosynovitis
Tenesmus (rectal) R19.8
  vesical R30.1
Tennis elbow — *see* Epicondylitis, lateral
Tenonitis (*see also* Tenosynovitis)
  eye (capsule) H05.04- ☑
Tenontosynovitis — *see* Tenosynovitis
Tenontothecitis — *see* Tenosynovitis
Tenophyte — *see* Disorder, synovium, specified type NEC
Tenosynovitis (*see also* Synovitis) M65.9
  adhesive — *see* Tenosynovitis, specified type NEC
    shoulder — *see* Capsulitis, adhesive
  bicipital (calcifying) — *see* Tendinitis, bicipital
  gonococcal A54.49
  in (due to)
    crystals M65.8- ☑
    gonorrhea A54.49
    syphilis (late) A52.78
    use, overuse, pressure (*see also* Disorder, soft tissue, due to use)
      specified NEC — *see* Disorder, soft tissue, due to use, specified NEC
  infective NEC M65.1- ☑
    ankle M65.17- ☑
    foot M65.17- ☑
    forearm M65.13- ☑
    hand M65.14- ☑
    lower leg M65.16- ☑
    multiple sites M65.19
    pelvic region M65.15- ☑
    shoulder region M65.11- ☑
    specified site NEC M65.18
    thigh M65.15- ☑
    upper arm M65.12- ☑
  radial styloid M65.4
  shoulder region M65.81- ☑
    adhesive — *see* Capsulitis, adhesive
  specified type NEC M65.88
    ankle M65.87- ☑
    foot M65.87- ☑
    forearm M65.83- ☑
    hand M65.84- ☑
    lower leg M65.86- ☑
    multiple sites M65.89
    pelvic region M65.85- ☑
    shoulder region M65.81- ☑
    specified site NEC M65.88
    thigh M65.85- ☑
    upper arm M65.82- ☑
  tuberculous — *see* Tuberculosis, tenosynovitis
Tenovaginitis — *see* Tenosynovitis
Tension
  arterial, high (*see also* Hypertension)
    without diagnosis of hypertension R03.0
  headache G44.209
    intractable G44.201
    not intractable G44.209
  nervous R45.0
  pneumothorax J93.0
  premenstrual N94.3
  state (mental) F48.9
Tentorium — *see* condition
Teratencephalus Q89.8
Teratism Q89.7
Teratoblastoma (malignant) — *see* Neoplasm, malignant, by site
Teratocarcinoma (*see also* Neoplasm, malignant, by site)
  liver C22.7
Teratoma (solid) (*see also* Neoplasm, uncertain behavior, by site)
  with embryonal carcinoma, mixed — *see* Neoplasm, malignant, by site
  with malignant transformation — *see* Neoplasm, malignant, by site
  adult (cystic) — *see* Neoplasm, benign, by site
  benign — *see* Neoplasm, benign, by site

Teratoma — *continued*
  combined with choriocarcinoma — *see* Neoplasm, malignant, by site
  cystic (adult) — *see* Neoplasm, benign, by site
  differentiated — *see* Neoplasm, benign, by site
  embryonal (*see also* Neoplasm, malignant, by site)
    liver C22.7
  immature — *see* Neoplasm, malignant, by site
  liver C22.7
    adult, benign, cystic, differentiated type or mature D13.4
  malignant (*see also* Neoplasm, malignant, by site)
    anaplastic — *see* Neoplasm, malignant, by site
    intermediate — *see* Neoplasm, malignant, by site
    specified site — *see* Neoplasm, malignant, by site
    unspecified site C62.90
    undifferentiated — *see* Neoplasm, malignant, by site
  mature — *see* Neoplasm, uncertain behavior, by site
    malignant — *see* Neoplasm, by site, malignant, by site
  ovary D27.- ☑
    embryonal, immature or malignant C56- ☑
  solid — *see* Neoplasm, uncertain behavior, by site
  testis C62.9- ☑
    adult, benign, cystic, differentiated type or mature D29.2- ☑
    scrotal C62.1- ☑
    undescended C62.0- ☑
Termination
  anomalous (*see also* Malposition, congenital)
    right pulmonary vein Q26.3
  pregnancy, elective Z33.2
Ternidens diminutus infestation B81.8
Ternidensiasis B81.8
Terror(s) night (child) F51.4
Terrorism, victim of Z65.4
Terry's syndrome H44.2- ☑
Tertiary — *see* condition
Test, tests, testing (for)
  adequacy (for dialysis)
    hemodialysis Z49.31
    peritoneal Z49.32
  blood pressure Z01.30
    abnormal reading — *see* Blood, pressure
  blood typing Z01.83
    Rh typing Z01.83
  blood-alcohol Z04.8
    positive — *see* Findings, abnormal, in blood
  blood-drug Z04.8
    positive — *see* Findings, abnormal, in blood
  cardiac pulse generator (battery) Z45.010
  fertility Z31.41
  genetic
    disease carrier status for procreative management
      female Z31.430
      male Z31.440
    male partner of patient with recurrent pregnancy loss Z31.441
    procreative management NEC
      female Z31.438
      male Z31.448
  hearing Z01.10
    with abnormal findings NEC Z01.118
  HIV (human immunodeficiency virus)
    nonconclusive (in infants) R75
    positive Z21
    seropositive Z21
  immunity status Z01.84
  intelligence NEC Z01.89
  laboratory (as part of a general medical examination) Z00.00
    with abnormal finding Z00.01
    for medicolegal reason NEC Z04.8
  male partner of patient with recurrent pregnancy loss Z31.441
  Mantoux (for tuberculosis) Z11.1
    abnormal result R76.11
  pregnancy, positive first pregnancy — *see* Pregnancy, normal, first
  procreative Z31.49
    fertility Z31.41
  skin, diagnostic
    allergy Z01.82
    special screening examination — *see* Screening, by name of disease

Test, tests, testing — *continued*
skin, diagnostic — *continued*
Mantoux Z11.1
tuberculin Z11.1
specified NEC Z01.89
tuberculin Z11.1
abnormal result R76.11
vision Z01.00
with abnormal findings Z01.01
Wassermann Z11.3
positive — *see* Serology for syphilis, positive
Testicle, testicular, testis (*see also* condition)
feminization syndrome (*see also* Syndrome, androgen insensitivity) E34.51
migrans Q55.29
Tetanus, tetanic (cephalic) (convulsions) A35
with
abortion A34
ectopic or molar pregnancy O08.0
following ectopic or molar pregnancy O08.0
inoculation reaction (due to serum) — *see* Complications, vaccination
neonatorum A33
obstetrical A34
puerperal, postpartum, childbirth A34
Tetany (due to) R29.0
alkalosis E87.3
associated with rickets E55.0
convulsions R29.0
hysterical F44.5
functional (hysterical) F44.5
hyperkinetic R29.0
hysterical F44.5
hyperpnea R06.4
hysterical F44.5
psychogenic F45.8
hyperventilation (*see also* Hyperventilation) R06.4
hysterical F44.5
neonatal (without calcium or magnesium deficiency) P71.3
parathyroid (gland) E20.9
parathyroprival E89.2
post- (para)thyroidectomy E89.2
postoperative E89.2
pseudotetany R29.0
psychogenic (conversion reaction) F44.5
Tetralogy of Fallot Q21.3
Tetraplegia (chronic) (*see also* Quadriplegia) G82.50
Thailand hemorrhagic fever A91
Thalassanemia — *see* Thalassemia
Thalassemia (anemia) (disease) D56.9
with other hemoglobinopathy D56.8
alpha (major) (severe) (triple gene defect) D56.0
minor D56.3
silent carrier D56.3
trait D56.3
beta (severe) D56.1
homozygous D56.1
major D56.1
minor D56.3
trait D56.3
delta-beta (homozygous) D56.2
minor D56.3
trait D56.3
dominant D56.8
hemoglobin
C D56.8
E-beta D56.5
intermedia D56.1
major D56.1
minor D56.3
mixed D56.8
sickle-cell — *see* Disease, sickle-cell, thalassemia
specified type NEC D56.8
trait D56.3
variants D56.8
Thanatophoric dwarfism or short stature Q77.1
Thaysen-Gee disease (nontropical sprue) K90.0
Thaysen's disease K90.0
Thecoma D27- ☑
luteinized D27- ☑
malignant C56- ☑
Thelarche, premature E30.8
Thelaziasis B83.8
Thelitis N61
puerperal, postpartum or gestational — *see* Infection, nipple
Therapeutic — *see* condition

Therapy
drug, long-term (current) (prophylactic)
agents affecting estrogen receptors and estrogen levels NEC Z79.818
anastrozole (Arimidex) Z79.811
antibiotics Z79.2
short-term use — *omit code*
anticoagulants Z79.01
anti-inflammatory Z79.1
antiplatelet Z79.02
antithrombotics Z79.02
aromatase inhibitors Z79.811
aspirin Z79.82
birth control pill or patch Z79.3
bisphosphonates Z79.83
contraceptive, oral Z79.3
drug, specified NEC Z79.899
estrogen receptor downregulators Z79.818
Evista Z79.810
exemestane (Aromasin) Z79.811
Fareston Z79.810
fulvestrant (Faslodex) Z79.818
gonadotropin-releasing hormone (GnRH) agonist Z79.818
goserelin acetate (Zoladex) Z79.818
hormone replacement (postmenopausal) Z79.890
insulin Z79.4
letrozole (Femara) Z79.811
leuprolide acetate (leuprorelin) (Lupron) Z79.818
megestrol acetate (Megace) Z79.818
methadone
for pain management Z79.891
maintenance therapy F11.20
Nolvadex Z79.810
opiate analgesic Z79.891
oral contraceptive Z79.3
raloxifene (Evista) Z79.810
selective estrogen receptor modulators (SERMs) Z79.810
short term — *omit code*
steroids
inhaled Z79.51
systemic Z79.52
tamoxifen (Nolvadex) Z79.810
toremifene (Fareston) Z79.810
Thermic — *see* condition
Thermography (abnormal) (*see also* Abnormal, diagnostic imaging) R93.8
breast R92.8
Thermoplegia T67.0 ☑
Thesaurismosis, glycogen — *see* Disease, glycogen storage
Thiamin deficiency E51.9
specified NEC E51.8
Thiaminic deficiency with beriberi E51.11
Thibierge-Weissenbach syndrome — *see* Sclerosis, systemic
Thickening
bone — *see* Hypertrophy, bone
breast N64.59
endometrium R93.8
epidermal L85.9
specified NEC L85.8
hymen N89.6
larynx J38.7
nail L60.2
congenital Q84.5
periosteal — *see* Hypertrophy, bone
pleura J92.9
with asbestos J92.0
skin R23.4
subepiglottic J38.7
tongue K14.8
valve, heart — *see* Endocarditis
Thigh — *see* condition
Thinning vertebra — *see* Spondylopathy, specified NEC
Thirst, excessive R63.1
due to deprivation of water T73.1 ☑
Thomsen disease G71.12
Thoracic (*see also* condition)
kidney Q63.2
outlet syndrome G54.0
Thoracogastroschisis (congenital) Q79.8
Thoracopagus Q89.4
Thorax — *see* condition
Thorn's syndrome N28.89
Thorson-Björck syndrome E34.0
Threadworm (infection) (infestation) B80

Threatened
abortion O20.0
with subsequent abortion O03.9
job loss, anxiety concerning Z56.2
labor (without delivery) O47.9
after 37 completed weeks of gestation O47.1
before 37 completed weeks of gestation O47.0- ☑
loss of job, anxiety concerning Z56.2
miscarriage O20.0
unemployment, anxiety concerning Z56.2
Three-day fever A93.1
Threshers' lung J67.0
Thrix annulata (congenital) Q84.1
Throat — *see* condition
Thrombasthenia (Glanzmann) (hemorrhagic) (hereditary) D69.1
Thromboangiitis I73.1
obliterans (general) I73.1
cerebral I67.89
vessels
brain I67.89
spinal cord I67.89
Thromboarteritis — *see* Arteritis
Thromboasthenia (Glanzmann) (hemorrhagic) (hereditary) D69.1
Thrombocytasthenia (Glanzmann) D69.1
Thrombocythemia (essential) (hemorrhagic) (idiopathic) (primary) D47.3
Thrombocytopathy (dystrophic) (granulopenic) D69.1
Thrombocytopenia, thrombocytopenic D69.6
with absent radius (TAR) Q87.2
congenital D69.42
dilutional D69.59
due to
(massive) blood transfusion D69.59
drugs D69.59
extracorporeal circulation of blood D69.59
platelet alloimmunization D69.59
essential D69.3
heparin induced (HIT) D75.82
hereditary D69.42
idiopathic D69.3
neonatal, transitory P61.0
due to
exchange transfusion P61.0
idiopathic maternal thrombocytopenia P61.0
isoimmunization P61.0
primary NEC D69.49
idiopathic D69.3
puerperal, postpartum O72.3
secondary D69.59
transient neonatal P61.0
Thrombocytosis, essential D47.3
primary D47.3
Thromboembolism — *see* Embolism
Thrombopathy (Bernard-Soulier) D69.1
constitutional D68.0
Willebrand-Jurgens D68.0
Thrombopenia — *see* Thrombocytopenia
Thrombophilia D68.59
primary NEC D68.59
secondary NEC D68.69
specified NEC D68.69
Thrombophlebitis I80.9
antepartum O22.2- ☑
deep O22.3- ☑
superficial O22.2- ☑
cavernous (venous) sinus G08
complicating pregnancy O22.5- ☑
nonpyogenic I67.6
cerebral (sinus) (vein) G08
nonpyogenic I67.6
sequelae G09
due to implanted device — *see* Complications, by site and type, specified NEC
during or resulting from a procedure NEC T81.72 ☑
femoral vein (superficial) I80.1- ☑
femoropopliteal vein I80.0- ☑
hepatic (vein) I80.8
idiopathic, recurrent I82.1
iliofemoral I80.1- ☑
intracranial venous sinus (any) G08
nonpyogenic I67.6
sequelae G09
intraspinal venous sinuses and veins G08
nonpyogenic G95.19
lateral (venous) sinus G08
nonpyogenic I67.6

300
☑ **Additional Character Required** — Refer to the Tabular List for Character Selection
Ⓦ **Subterms under main terms may continue to next column or page**

Thrombophlebitis — *continued*
  leg I80.299
    superficial I80.0- ☑
  longitudinal (venous) sinus G08
    nonpyogenic I67.6
  lower extremity I80.299
  migrans, migrating I82.1
  pelvic
    with ectopic or molar pregnancy O08.0
    following ectopic or molar pregnancy O08.0
    puerperal O87.1
  popliteal vein — *see* Phlebitis, leg, deep, popliteal
  portal (vein) K75.1
  postoperative T81.72 ☑
  pregnancy — *see* Thrombophlebitis, antepartum
  puerperal, postpartum, childbirth O87.0
    deep O87.1
    pelvic O87.1
    septic O86.81
    superficial O87.0
  saphenous (greater) (lesser) I80.0- ☑
  sinus (intracranial) G08
    nonpyogenic I67.6
  specified site NEC I80.8
  tibial vein I80.23- ☑
Thrombosis, thrombotic (bland) (multiple) (progressive) (silent) (vessel) I82.90
  anal K64.5
  antepartum — *see* Thrombophlebitis, antepartum
  aorta, aortic I74.10
    abdominal I74.09
      saddle I74.01
    bifurcation I74.09
      saddle I74.01
    specified site NEC I74.19
    terminal I74.09
    thoracic I74.11
    valve — *see* Endocarditis, aortic
  apoplexy I63.3 ☑
  artery, arteries (postinfectional) I74.9
    auditory, internal — *see* Occlusion, artery, precerebral, specified NEC
    basilar — *see* Occlusion, artery, basilar
    carotid (common) (internal) — *see* Occlusion, artery, carotid
    cerebellar (anterior inferior) (posterior inferior) (superior) — *see* Occlusion, artery, cerebellar
    cerebral — *see* Occlusion, artery, cerebral
    choroidal (anterior) — *see* Occlusion, artery, cerebral, specified NEC
    communicating, posterior — *see* Occlusion, artery, cerebral, specified NEC
    coronary (*see also* Infarct, myocardium)
      not resulting in infarction I24.0
    hepatic I74.8
    hypophyseal — *see* Occlusion, artery, cerebral, specified NEC
    iliac I74.5
    limb I74.4
      lower I74.3
      upper I74.2
    meningeal, anterior or posterior — *see* Occlusion, artery, cerebral, specified NEC
    mesenteric (with gangrene) K55.0
    ophthalmic — *see* Occlusion, artery, retina
    pontine — *see* Occlusion, artery, cerebral, specified NEC
    precerebral — *see* Occlusion, artery, precerebral
    pulmonary (iatrogenic) — *see* Embolism, pulmonary
    renal N28.0
    retinal — *see* Occlusion, artery, retina
    spinal, anterior or posterior G95.11
    traumatic NEC T14.8
    vertebral — *see* Occlusion, artery, vertebral
  atrium, auricular (*see also* Infarct, myocardium)
    following acute myocardial infarction (current complication) I23.6
    not resulting in infarction I24.0
  basilar (artery) — *see* Occlusion, artery, basilar
  brain (artery) (stem) (*see also* Occlusion, artery, cerebral)
    due to syphilis A52.05
    puerperal O99.43
    sinus — *see* Thrombosis, intracranial venous sinus
  capillary I78.8

Thrombosis, thrombotic — *continued*
  cardiac (*see also* Infarct, myocardium)
    not resulting in infarction I24.0
    valve — *see* Endocarditis
  carotid (artery) (common) (internal) — *see* Occlusion, artery, carotid
  cavernous (venous) sinus — *see* Thrombosis, intracranial venous sinus
  cerebellar artery (anterior inferior) (posterior inferior) (superior) I66.3
  cerebral (artery) — *see* Occlusion, artery, cerebral
  cerebrovenous sinus (*see also* Thrombosis, intracranial venous sinus)
    puerperium O87.3
  chronic I82.91
  coronary (artery) (vein) (*see also* Infarct, myocardium)
    not resulting in infarction I24.0
  corpus cavernosum N48.89
  cortical I66.9
  deep — *see* Embolism, vein, lower extremity
  due to device, implant or graft (*see also* Complications, by site and type, specified NEC) T85.86 ☑
    arterial graft NEC T82.868 ☑
    breast (implant) T85.86 ☑
    catheter NEC T85.86 ☑
      dialysis (renal) T82.868 ☑
        intraperitoneal T85.86 ☑
      infusion NEC T82.868 ☑
        spinal (epidural) (subdural) T85.86 ☑
      urinary (indwelling) T83.86 ☑
    electronic (electrode) (pulse generator) (stimulator)
      bone T84.86 ☑
      cardiac T82.867 ☑
      nervous system (brain) (peripheral nerve) (spinal) T85.86 ☑
      urinary T83.86 ☑
    fixation, internal (orthopedic) NEC T84.86 ☑
    gastrointestinal (bile duct) (esophagus) T85.86 ☑
    genital NEC T83.86 ☑
    heart T82.867 ☑
    joint prosthesis T84.86 ☑
    ocular (corneal graft) (orbital implant) NEC T85.86 ☑
    orthopedic NEC T84.86 ☑
    specified NEC T85.86 ☑
    urinary NEC T83.86 ☑
    vascular NEC T82.868 ☑
    ventricular intracranial shunt T85.86 ☑
  during the puerperium — *see* Thrombosis, puerperal
  endocardial (*see also* Infarct, myocardium)
    not resulting in infarction I24.0
  eye — *see* Occlusion, retina
  genital organ
    female NEC N94.89
      pregnancy — *see* Thrombophlebitis, antepartum
    male N50.1
  gestational — *see* Phlebopathy, gestational
  heart (chamber) (*see also* Infarct, myocardium)
    not resulting in infarction I24.0
  hepatic (vein) I82.0
    artery I74.8
  history (of) Z86.718
  intestine (with gangrene) K55.0
  intracardiac NEC (apical) (atrial) (auricular) (ventricular) (old) I51.3
  intracranial (arterial) I66.9
    venous sinus (any) G08
      nonpyogenic origin I67.6
      puerperium O87.3
  intramural (*see also* Infarct, myocardium)
    not resulting in infarction I24.0
  intraspinal venous sinuses and veins G08
    nonpyogenic G95.19
  kidney (artery) N28.0
  lateral (venous) sinus — *see* Thrombosis, intracranial venous sinus
  leg — *see* Thrombosis, vein, lower extremity
    arterial I74.3
  liver (venous) I82.0
    artery I74.8
    portal vein I81
  longitudinal (venous) sinus — *see* Thrombosis, intracranial venous sinus
  lower limb — *see* Thrombosis, vein, lower extremity
  lung (iatrogenic) (postoperative) — *see* Embolism, pulmonary

Thrombosis, thrombotic — *continued*
  meninges (brain) (arterial) I66.8
  mesenteric (artery) (with gangrene) K55.0
    vein (inferior) (superior) I81
  mitral I34.8
  mural (*see also* Infarct, myocardium)
    due to syphilis A52.06
    not resulting in infarction I24.0
  omentum (with gangrene) K55.0
  ophthalmic — *see* Occlusion, retina
  pampiniform plexus (male) N50.1
  parietal (*see also* Infarct, myocardium)
    not resulting in infarction I24.0
  penis, superficial vein N48.81
  perianal venous K64.5
  peripheral arteries I74.4
    upper I74.2
  personal history (of) Z86.718
  portal I81
    due to syphilis A52.09
  precerebral artery — *see* Occlusion, artery, precerebral
  puerperal, postpartum O87.0
    brain (artery) O99.43
      venous (sinus) O87.3
    cardiac O99.43
    cerebral (artery) O99.43
      venous (sinus) O87.3
    superficial O87.0
  pulmonary (artery) (iatrogenic) (postoperative) (vein) — *see* Embolism, pulmonary
  renal (artery) N28.0
    vein I82.3
  resulting from presence of device, implant or graft — *see* Complications, by site and type, specified NEC
  retina, retinal — *see* Occlusion, retina
  scrotum N50.1
  seminal vesicle N50.1
  sigmoid (venous) sinus — *see* Thrombosis, intracranial venous sinus
  sinus, intracranial (any) — *see* Thrombosis, intracranial venous sinus
  specified site NEC I82.890
    chronic I82.891
  spermatic cord N50.1
  spinal cord (arterial) G95.11
    due to syphilis A52.09
    pyogenic origin G06.1
  spleen, splenic D73.5
    artery I74.8
  testis N50.1
  traumatic NEC T14.8
  tricuspid I07.8
  tumor — *see* Neoplasm, unspecified behavior, by site
  tunica vaginalis N50.1
  umbilical cord (vessels), complicating delivery O69.5 ☑
  vas deferens N50.1
  vein (acute) I82.90
    antecubital I82.61- ☑
      chronic I82.71- ☑
    axillary I82.A1- ☑ (*following* I82.7)
      chronic I82.A2- ☑ (*following* I82.7)
    basilic I82.61- ☑
      chronic I82.71- ☑
    brachial I82.62- ☑
      chronic I82.72- ☑
    brachiocephalic (innominate) I82.290
      chronic I82.291
    cephalic I82.61- ☑
      chronic I82.71- ☑
    cerebral, nonpyogenic I67.6
    chronic I82.91
    deep (DVT) I82.40- ☑
      calf I82.4Z- ☑
        chronic I82.5Z- ☑
      lower leg I82.4Z- ☑
        chronic I82.5Z- ☑
      thigh I82.4Y- ☑
        chronic I82.5Y- ☑
      upper leg I82.4Y ☑
        chronic I82.5y-
    femoral I82.41- ☑
      chronic I82.51- ☑
    iliac (iliofemoral) I82.42- ☑
      chronic I82.52- ☑
    innominate I82.290
      chronic I82.291

Thrombosis, thrombotic — *continued*
  vein — *continued*
    internal jugular I82.C1- ☑ (*following* I82.7)
      chronic I82.C2- ☑ (*following* I82.7)
    lower extremity
      deep I82.40- ☑
        chronic I82.50- ☑
        specified NEC I82.49- ☑
          chronic NEC I82.59- ☑
      distal
        deep I82.4Z- ☑
      proximal
        deep I82.4Y- ☑
          chronic I82.5Y- ☑
      superficial I82.81- ☑
    perianal K64.5
    popliteal I82.43- ☑
      chronic I82.53- ☑
    radial I82.62- ☑
      chronic I82.72- ☑
    renal I82.3
    saphenous (greater) (lesser) I82.81- ☑
    specified NEC I82.890
      chronic NEC I82.891
    subclavian I82.B1- ☑ (*following* I82.7)
      chronic I82.B2- ☑ (*following* I82.7)
    thoracic NEC I82.290
      chronic I82.291
    tibial I82.44- ☑
      chronic I82.54- ☑
    ulnar I82.62- ☑
      chronic I82.72- ☑
    upper extremity I82.60- ☑
      chronic I82.70- ☑
      deep I82.62- ☑
        chronic I82.72- ☑
      superficial I82.61- ☑
        chronic I82.71- ☑
  vena cava
    inferior I82.220
      chronic I82.221
    superior I82.210
      chronic I82.211
  venous, perianal K64.5
  ventricle (*see also* Infarct, myocardium)
    following acute myocardial infarction (current complication) I23.6
    not resulting in infarction I24.0
Thrombus — *see* Thrombosis
Thrush (*see also* Candidiasis)
  newborn P37.5
  oral B37.0
  vaginal B37.3
Thumb (*see also* condition)
  sucking (child problem) F98.8
Thymitis E32.8
Thymoma (benign) D15.0
  malignant C37
Thymus, thymic (gland) — *see* condition
Thyrocele — *see* Goiter
Thyroglossal (*see also* condition)
  cyst Q89.2
  duct, persistent Q89.2
Thyroid (gland) (body) (*see also* condition)
  hormone resistance E07.89
  lingual Q89.2
  nodule (cystic) (nontoxic) (single) E04.1
Thyroiditis E06.9
  acute (nonsuppurative) (pyogenic) (suppurative) E06.0
  autoimmune E06.3
  chronic (nonspecific) (sclerosing) E06.5
    with thyrotoxicosis, transient E06.2
    fibrous E06.5
    lymphadenoid E06.3
    lymphocytic E06.3
    lymphoid E06.3
  de Quervain's E06.1
  drug-induced E06.4
  fibrous (chronic) E06.5
  giant-cell (follicular) E06.1
  granulomatous (de Quervain) (subacute) E06.1
  Hashimoto's (struma lymphomatosa) E06.3
  iatrogenic E06.4
  ligneous E06.5
  lymphocytic (chronic) E06.3
  lymphoid E06.3
  lymphomatous E06.3

Thyroiditis — *continued*
  nonsuppurative E06.1
  postpartum, puerperal O90.5
  pseudotuberculous E06.1
  pyogenic E06.0
  radiation E06.4
  Riedel's E06.5
  subacute (granulomatous) E06.1
  suppurative E06.0
  tuberculous A18.81
  viral E06.1
  woody E06.5
Thyrolingual duct, persistent Q89.2
Thyromegaly E01.0
Thyrotoxic
  crisis — *see* Thyrotoxicosis
  heart disease or failure (*see also* Thyrotoxicosis) E05.90 [I43]
    with thyroid storm E05.91 [I43]
  storm — *see* Thyrotoxicosis
Thyrotoxicosis (recurrent) E05.90
  with
    goiter (diffuse) E05.00
      with thyroid storm E05.01
      adenomatous uninodular E05.10
        with thyroid storm E05.11
      multinodular E05.20
        with thyroid storm E05.21
      nodular E05.20
        with thyroid storm E05.21
      uninodular E05.10
        with thyroid storm E05.11
    infiltrative
      dermopathy E05.00
        with thyroid storm E05.01
      ophthalmopathy E05.00
        with thyroid storm E05.01
    single thyroid nodule E05.10
      with thyroid storm E05.11
    thyroid storm E05.91
  due to
    ectopic thyroid nodule or tissue E05.30
      with thyroid storm E05.31
    ingestion of (excessive) thyroid material E05.40
      with thyroid storm E05.41
    overproduction of thyroid-stimulating hormone E05.80
      with thyroid storm E05.81
    specified cause NEC E05.80
      with thyroid storm E05.81
  factitia E05.40
    with thyroid storm E05.41
  heart E05.90 [I43]
    with thyroid storm E05.91 [I43]
    failure E05.90 [I43]
  neonatal (transient) P72.1
  transient with chronic thyroiditis E06.2
Tibia vara — *see* Osteochondrosis, juvenile, tibia
Tic (disorder) F95.9
  breathing F95.8
  child problem F95.0
  compulsive F95.1
  de la Tourette F95.2
  degenerative (generalized) (localized) G25.69
    facial G25.69
  disorder
    chronic
      motor F95.1
      vocal F95.1
    combined vocal and multiple motor F95.2
    transient F95.0
  douloureux G50.0
    atypical G50.1
    postherpetic, postzoster B02.22
  drug-induced G25.61
  eyelid F95.8
  habit F95.9
    chronic F95.1
    transient of childhood F95.0
  lid, transient of childhood F95.0
  motor-verbal F95.2
  occupational F48.8
  orbicularis F95.8
    transient of childhood F95.0
  organic origin G25.69
  postchoreic G25.69
  psychogenic, compulsive F95.1
  salaam R25.8

Tic — *continued*
  spasm (motor or vocal) F95.9
    chronic F95.1
    transient of childhood F95.0
  specified NEC F95.8
Tick-borne — *see* condition
Tietze's disease or syndrome M94.0
Tight, tightness
  anus K62.89
  chest R07.89
  fascia (lata) M62.89
  foreskin (congenital) N47.1
  hymen, hymenal ring N89.6
  introitus (acquired) (congenital) N89.6
  rectal sphincter K62.89
  tendon — *see* Short, tendon
  urethral sphincter N35.9
Tilting vertebra — *see* Dorsopathy, deforming, specified NEC
Timidity, child F93.8
Tinea (intersecta) (tarsi) B35.9
  amiantacea L44.8
  asbestina B35.0
  barbae B35.0
  beard B35.0
  black dot B35.0
  blanca B36.2
  capitis B35.0
  corporis B35.4
  cruris B35.6
  flava B36.0
  foot B35.3
  furfuracea B36.0
  imbricata (Tokelau) B35.5
  kerion B35.0
  manuum B35.2
  microsporic — *see* Dermatophytosis
  nigra B36.1
  nodosa — *see* Piedra
  pedis B35.3
  scalp B35.0
  specified site NEC B35.8
  sycosis B35.0
  tonsurans B35.0
  trichophytic — *see* Dermatophytosis
  unguium B35.1
  versicolor B36.0
Tingling sensation (skin) R20.2
Tin-miner's lung J63.5
Tinnitus (audible) (aurium) (subjective) — *see* subcategory H93.1 ☑
Tipped tooth (teeth) M26.33
Tipping
  pelvis M95.5
    with disproportion (fetopelvic) O33.0
      causing obstructed labor O65.0
  tooth (teeth), fully erupted M26.33
Tiredness R53.83
Tissue — *see* condition
Tobacco (nicotine)
  dependence — *see* Dependence, drug, nicotine
  harmful use Z72.0
  heart — *see* Tobacco, toxic effect
  maternal use, affecting newborn P04.2
  toxic effect — *see* Table of Drugs and Chemicals, by substance, poisoning
    chewing tobacco — *see* Table of Drugs and Chemicals, by substance, poisoning
    cigarettes — *see* Table of Drugs and Chemicals, by substance, poisoning
  use Z72.0
    complicating
      childbirth O99.334
      pregnancy O99.33- ☑
      puerperium O99.335
    counseling and surveillance Z71.6
  withdrawal state — *see* Dependence, drug, nicotine
Tocopherol deficiency E56.0
Todd's
  cirrhosis K74.3
  paralysis (postepileptic) (transitory) G83.84
Toe — *see* condition
Toilet, artificial opening — *see* Attention to, artificial, opening
Tokelau (ringworm) B35.5
Tollwut — *see* Rabies

☑ **Additional Character Required** — Refer to the Tabular List for Character Selection   ▽ **Subterms under main terms may continue to next column or page**

Tommaselli's disease R31.9
    correct substance properly administered — see Table of Drugs and Chemicals, by drug, adverse effect
    overdose or wrong substance given or taken — see Table of Drugs and Chemicals, by drug, poisoning
Tongue (see also condition)
    tie Q38.1
Tonic pupil — see Anomaly, pupil, function, tonic pupil
Toni-Fanconi syndrome (cystinosis) E72.09
    with cystinosis E72.04
Tonsil — see condition
Tonsillitis (acute) (catarrhal) (croupous) (follicular) (gangrenous) (infective) (lacunar) (lingual) (malignant) (membranous) (parenchymatous) (phlegmonous) (pseudomembranous) (purulent) (septic) (subacute) (suppurative) (toxic) (ulcerative) (vesicular) (viral) J03.90
    chronic J35.01
      with adenoiditis J35.03
    diphtheritic A36.0
    hypertrophic J35.01
      with adenoiditis J35.03
    recurrent J03.91
    specified organism NEC J03.80
      recurrent J03.81
    staphylococcal J03.80
      recurrent J03.81
    streptococcal J03.00
      recurrent J03.01
    tuberculous A15.8
    Vincent's A69.1
Tooth, teeth — see condition
Toothache K08.8
Topagnosis R20.8
Tophi — see Gout, chronic
TORCH infection — see Infection, congenital
    without active infection P00.2
Torn — see Tear
Tornwaldt's cyst or disease J39.2
Torsion
    accessory tube — see Torsion, fallopian tube
    adnexa (female) — see Torsion, fallopian tube
    aorta, acquired I77.1
    appendix epididymis N44.04
    appendix testis N44.03
    bile duct (common) (hepatic) K83.8
      congenital Q44.5
    bowel, colon or intestine K56.2
    cervix — see Malposition, uterus
    cystic duct K82.8
    dystonia — see Dystonia, torsion
    epididymis (appendix) N44.04
    fallopian tube N83.52
      with ovary N83.53
    gallbladder K82.8
      congenital Q44.1
    hydatid of Morgagni
      female N83.52
      male N44.03
    kidney (pedicle) (leading to infarction) N28.0
    Meckel's diverticulum (congenital) Q43.0
      malignant — see Table of Neoplasms, small intestine, malignant
    mesentery K56.2
    omentum K56.2
    organ or site, congenital NEC — see Anomaly, by site
    ovary (pedicle) N83.51
      with fallopian tube N83.53
      congenital Q50.2
    oviduct — see Torsion, fallopian tube
    penis (acquired) N48.82
      congenital Q55.63
    spasm — see Dystonia, torsion
    spermatic cord N44.02
      extravaginal N44.01
      intravaginal N44.02
    spleen D73.5
    testis, testicle N44.00
      appendix N44.03
    tibia — see Deformity, limb, specified type NEC, lower leg
    uterus — see Malposition, uterus
Torticollis (intermittent) (spastic) M43.6
    congenital (sternomastoid) Q68.0
    due to birth injury P15.8
    hysterical F44.4
    ocular R29.891

Torticollis — continued
    psychogenic F45.8
      conversion reaction F44.4
    rheumatic M43.6
    rheumatoid M06.88
    spasmodic G24.3
    traumatic, current S13.4 ☑
Tortipelvis G24.1
Tortuous
    artery I77.1
    organ or site, congenital NEC — see Distortion
    retinal vessel, congenital Q14.1
    ureter N13.8
    urethra N36.8
    vein — see Varix
Torture, victim of Z65.4
Torula, torular (histolytica) (infection) — see Cryptococcosis
Torulosis — see Cryptococcosis
Torus (mandibularis) (palatinus) M27.0
    fracture — see Fracture, by site, torus
Touraine's syndrome Q79.8
Tourette's syndrome F95.2
Tourniquet syndrome — see Constriction, external, by site
Tower skull Q75.0
    with exophthalmos Q87.0
Toxemia R68.89
    bacterial — see Sepsis
    burn — see Burn
    eclamptic (with pre-existing hypertension) — see Eclampsia
    erysipelatous — see Erysipelas
    fatigue R68.89
    food — see Poisoning, food
    gastrointestinal K52.1
    intestinal K52.1
    kidney — see Uremia
    malarial — see Malaria
    myocardial — see Myocarditis, toxic
    of pregnancy — see Pre-eclampsia
    pre-eclamptic — see Pre-eclampsia
    small intestine K52.1
    staphylococcal, due to food A05.0
    stasis R68.89
    uremic — see Uremia
    urinary — see Uremia
Toxemica cerebropathia psychica (nonalcoholic) F04
    alcoholic — see Alcohol, amnestic disorder
Toxic (poisoning) (see also condition) T65.91 ☑
    effect — see Table of Drugs and Chemicals, by substance, poisoning
    shock syndrome A48.3
    thyroid (gland) — see Thyrotoxicosis
Toxicemia — see Toxemia
Toxicity — see Table of Drugs and Chemicals, by substance, poisoning
    fava bean D55.0
    food, noxious — see Poisoning, food
    from drug or nonmedicinal substance — see Table of Drugs and Chemicals, by drug
Toxicosis (see also Toxemia)
    capillary, hemorrhagic D69.0
Toxinfection, gastrointestinal K52.1
Toxocariasis B83.0
Toxoplasma, toxoplasmosis (acquired) B58.9
    with
      hepatitis B58.1
      meningoencephalitis B58.2
      ocular involvement B58.00
      other organ involvement B58.89
      pneumonia, pneumonitis B58.3
    congenital (acute) (subacute) (chronic) P37.1
    maternal, manifest toxoplasmosis in infant (acute) (subacute) (chronic) P37.1
tPA (rtPA) **administration in a different facility within the last 24 hours prior to admission to current facility** Z92.82
Trabeculation, bladder N32.89
Trachea — see condition
Tracheitis (catarrhal) (infantile) (membranous) (plastic) (septal) (suppurative) (viral) J04.10
    with
      bronchitis (15 years of age and above) J40
        acute or subacute — see Bronchitis, acute
        chronic J42
        tuberculous NEC A15.5

Tracheitis — continued
    with — continued
      bronchitis — continued
        under 15 years of age J20.9
      laryngitis (acute) J04.2
        chronic J37.1
        tuberculous NEC A15.5
    acute J04.10
      with obstruction J04.11
    chronic J42
      with
        bronchitis (chronic) J42
        laryngitis (chronic) J37.1
    diphtheritic (membranous) A36.89
    due to external agent — see Inflammation, respiratory, upper, due to
    syphilitic A52.73
    tuberculous A15.5
Trachelitis (nonvenereal) — see Cervicitis
Tracheobronchial — see condition
Tracheobronchitis (15 years of age and above) (see also Bronchitis)
    due to
      Bordetella bronchiseptica A37.80
        with pneumonia A37.81
      Francisella tularensis A21.8
Tracheobronchomegaly Q32.4
    with bronchiectasis J47.9
      with
        exacerbation (acute) J47.1
        lower respiratory infection J47.0
    acquired J98.09
      with bronchiectasis J47.9
        with
          exacerbation (acute) J47.1
          lower respiratory infection J47.0
Tracheobronchopneumonitis — see Pneumonia, broncho-
Tracheocele (external) (internal) J39.8
    congenital Q32.1
Tracheomalacia J39.8
    congenital Q32.0
Tracheopharyngitis (acute) J06.9
    chronic J42
    due to external agent — see Inflammation, respiratory, upper, due to
Tracheostenosis J39.8
Tracheostomy
    complication — see Complication, tracheostomy
    status Z93.0
      attention to Z43.0
      malfunctioning J95.03
Trachoma, trachomatous A71.9
    active (stage) A71.1
    contraction of conjunctiva A71.1
    dubium A71.0
    healed or sequelae B94.0
    initial (stage) A71.0
    pannus A71.1
    Türck's J37.0
Traction, vitreomacular H43.82- ☑
Train sickness T75.3 ☑
Trait(s)
    Hb-S D57.3
    hemoglobin
      abnormal NEC D58.2
        with thalassemia D56.3
      C — see Disease, hemoglobin C
      S (Hb-S) D57.3
    Lepore D56.3
    personality, accentuated Z73.1
    sickle-cell D57.3
      with elliptocytosis or spherocytosis D57.3
    type A personality Z73.1
Tramp Z59.0
Trance R41.89
    hysterical F44.89
Transaminasemia R74.0
Transection
    abdomen (partial) S38.3 ☑
    aorta (incomplete) (see also Injury, aorta)
      complete — see Injury, aorta, laceration, major
    carotid artery (incomplete) (see also Injury, blood vessel, carotid, laceration)
      complete — see Injury, blood vessel, carotid, laceration, major
    celiac artery (incomplete) S35.211 ☑
      branch (incomplete) S35.291 ☑

Transection — *continued*
celiac artery — *continued*
branch — *continued*
complete S35.292 ☑
complete S35.212 ☑
innominate
artery (incomplete) (*see also* Injury, blood vessel, thoracic, innominate, artery, laceration)
complete — *see* Injury, blood vessel, thoracic, innominate, artery, laceration, major
vein (incomplete) (*see also* Injury, blood vessel, thoracic, innominate, vein, laceration)
complete — *see* Injury, blood vessel, thoracic, innominate, vein, laceration, major
jugular vein (external) (incomplete) (*see also* Injury, blood vessel, jugular vein, laceration)
complete — *see* Injury, blood vessel, jugular vein, laceration, major
internal (incomplete) (*see also* Injury, blood vessel, jugular vein, internal, laceration)
complete — *see* Injury, blood vessel, jugular vein, internal, laceration, major
mesenteric artery (incomplete) (*see also* Injury, mesenteric, artery, laceration)
complete — *see* Injury, mesenteric artery, laceration, major
pulmonary vessel (incomplete) (*see also* Injury, blood vessel, thoracic, pulmonary, laceration)
complete — *see* Injury, blood vessel, thoracic, pulmonary, laceration, major
subclavian — *see* Transection, innominate
vena cava (incomplete) (*see also* Injury, vena cava)
complete — *see* Injury, vena cava, laceration, major
vertebral artery (incomplete) (*see also* Injury, blood vessel, vertebral, laceration)
complete — *see* Injury, blood vessel, vertebral, laceration, major
Transfusion
associated (red blood cell) hemochromatosis E83.111
blood
ABO incompatible — *see* Complication(s), transfusion, incompatibility reaction, ABO
minor blood group (Duffy) (E) (K(ell)) (Kidd) (Lewis) (M) (N) (P) (S) T80.89 ☑
reaction or complication — *see* Complications, transfusion
fetomaternal (mother) — *see* Pregnancy, complicated by, placenta, transfusion syndrome
maternofetal (mother) — *see* Pregnancy, complicated by, placenta, transfusion syndrome
placental (syndrome) (mother) — *see* Pregnancy, complicated by, placenta, transfusion syndrome
reaction (adverse) — *see* Complications, transfusion
related acute lung injury (TRALI) J95.84
twin-to-twin — *see* Pregnancy, complicated by, placenta, transfusion syndrome, fetus to fetus
Transient (meaning homeless) (*see also* condition) Z59.0
Translocation
balanced autosomal Q95.9
in normal individual Q95.0
chromosomes NEC Q99.8
balanced and insertion in normal individual Q95.0
Down syndrome Q90.2
trisomy
13 Q91.6
18 Q91.2
21 Q90.2
Translucency, iris — *see* Degeneration, iris
Transmission of chemical substances through the placenta — *see* Absorption, chemical, through placenta
Transparency, lung, unilateral J43.0
Transplant (ed) (status) Z94.9
awaiting organ Z76.82
bone Z94.6
marrow Z94.81
candidate Z76.82
complication — *see* Complication, transplant
cornea Z94.7
heart Z94.1
and lung(s) Z94.3
valve Z95.2
prosthetic Z95.2
specified NEC Z95.4
xenogenic Z95.3
intestine Z94.82
kidney Z94.0

Transplant — *continued*
liver Z94.4
lung(s) Z94.2
and heart Z94.3
organ (failure) (infection) (rejection) Z94.9
removal status Z98.85
pancreas Z94.83
skin Z94.5
social Z60.3
specified organ or tissue NEC Z94.89
stem cells Z94.84
tissue Z94.9
Transplants, ovarian, endometrial N80.1
Transposed — *see* Transposition
Transposition (congenital) (*see also* Malposition, congenital)
abdominal viscera Q89.3
aorta (dextra) Q20.3
appendix Q43.8
colon Q43.8
corrected Q20.5
great vessels (complete) (partial) Q20.3
heart Q24.0
with complete transposition of viscera Q89.3
intestine (large) (small) Q43.8
reversed jejunal (for bypass) (status) Z98.0
scrotum Q55.23
stomach Q40.2
with general transposition of viscera Q89.3
tooth, teeth, fully erupted M26.30
vessels, great (complete) (partial) Q20.3
viscera (abdominal) (thoracic) Q89.3
Transsexualism F64.1
Transverse (*see also* condition)
arrest (deep), in labor O64.0 ☑
lie (mother) O32.2 ☑
causing obstructed labor O64.8 ☑
Transvestism, transvestitism (dual-role) F64.1
fetishistic F65.1
Trapped placenta (with hemorrhage) O72.0
without hemorrhage O73.0
Trauma, traumatism (*see also* Injury)
acoustic — *see* subcategory H83.3 ☑
birth — *see* Birth, injury
complicating ectopic or molar pregnancy O08.6
during delivery O71.9
following ectopic or molar pregnancy O08.6
obstetric O71.9
specified NEC O71.89
Traumatic (*see also* condition)
brain injury — *see* category S06 ☑
Treacher Collins syndrome Q75.4
Treitz's hernia — *see* Hernia, abdomen, specified site NEC
Trematode infestation — *see* Infestation, fluke
Trematodiasis — *see* Infestation, fluke
Trembling paralysis — *see* Parkinsonism
Tremor(s) R25.1
drug induced G25.1
essential (benign) G25.0
familial G25.0
hereditary G25.0
hysterical F44.4
intention G25.2
medication induced postural G25.1
mercurial — *see* subcategory T56.1 ☑
Parkinson's — *see* Parkinsonism
psychogenic (conversion reaction) F44.4
senilis R54
specified type NEC G25.2
Trench
fever A79.0
foot — *see* Immersion, foot
mouth A69.1
Treponema pallidum infection — *see* Syphilis
Treponematosis
due to
T. pallidum — *see* Syphilis
T. pertenue — *see* Yaws
Triad
Hutchinson's (congenital syphilis) A50.53
Kartagener's Q89.3
Saint's — *see* Hernia, diaphragm
Trichiasis (eyelid) H02.059
with entropion — *see* Entropion
left H02.056
lower H02.055

Trichiasis — *continued*
left — *continued*
upper H02.054
right H02.053
lower H02.052
upper H02.051
Trichinella spiralis (infection) (infestation) B75
Trichinellosis, trichiniasis, trichinelliasis, trichinosis B75
with muscle disorder B75 [M63.80]
ankle B75 [M63.87-] ☑
foot B75 [M63.87-] ☑
forearm B75 [M63.83-] ☑
hand B75 [M63.84-] ☑
lower leg B75 [M63.86-] ☑
multiple sites B75 [M63.89]
pelvic region B75 [M63.85-] ☑
shoulder region B75 [M63.81-] ☑
specified site NEC B75 [M63.88]
thigh B75 [M63.85-] ☑
upper arm B75 [M63.82-] ☑
Trichobezoar T18.9 ☑
intestine T18.3 ☑
stomach T18.2 ☑
Trichocephaliasis, trichocephalosis B79
Trichocephalus infestation B79
Trichoclasis L67.8
Trichoepithelioma (*see also* Neoplasm, skin, benign)
malignant — *see* Neoplasm, skin, malignant
Trichofolliculoma — *see* Neoplasm, skin, benign
Tricholemmoma — *see* Neoplasm, skin, benign
Trichomoniasis A59.9
bladder A59.03
cervix A59.09
intestinal A07.8
prostate A59.02
seminal vesicles A59.09
specified site NEC A59.8
urethra A59.03
urogenitalis A59.00
vagina A59.01
vulva A59.01
Trichomycosis
axillaris A48.8
nodosa, nodularis B36.8
Trichonodosis L67.8
Trichophytid, trichophyton infection — *see* Dermatophytosis
Trichophytobezoar T18.9 ☑
intestine T18.3 ☑
stomach T18.2 ☑
Trichophytosis — *see* Dermatophytosis
Trichoptilosis L67.8
Trichorrhexis (nodosa) (invaginata) L67.0
Trichosis axillaris A48.8
Trichosporosis nodosa B36.2
Trichostasis spinulosa (congenital) Q84.1
Trichostrongyliasis, trichostrongylosis (small intestine) B81.2
Trichostrongylus infection B81.2
Trichotillomania F63.3
Trichromat, trichromatopsia, anomalous (congenital) H53.55
Trichuriasis B79
Trichuris trichiura (infection) (infestation) (any site) B79
Tricuspid (valve) — *see* condition
Trifid (*see also* Accessory)
kidney (pelvis) Q63.8
tongue Q38.3
Trigeminal neuralgia — *see* Neuralgia, trigeminal
Trigeminy R00.8
Trigger finger (acquired) M65.30
congenital Q74.0
index finger M65.32- ☑
little finger M65.35- ☑
middle finger M65.33- ☑
ring finger M65.34- ☑
thumb M65.31- ☑
Trigonitis (bladder) (chronic) (pseudomembranous) N30.30
with hematuria N30.31
Trigonocephaly Q75.0
Trilocular heart — *see* Cor triloculare
Trimethylaminuria E72.52
Tripartite placenta O43.19- ☑
Triphalangeal thumb Q74.0

Triple (*see also* Accessory)
kidneys Q63.0
uteri Q51.818
X, female Q97.0
Triplegia G83.89
congenital G80.8
Triplet (newborn) (*see also* Newborn, triplet)
complicating pregnancy — *see* Pregnancy, triplet
Triplication — *see* Accessory
Triploidy Q92.7
Trismus R25.2
neonatorum A33
newborn A33
Trisomy (syndrome) Q92.9
13 (partial) Q91.7
meiotic nondisjunction Q91.4
mitotic nondisjunction Q91.5
mosaicism Q91.5
translocation Q91.6
18 (partial) Q91.3
meiotic nondisjunction Q91.0
mitotic nondisjunction Q91.1
mosaicism Q91.1
translocation Q91.2
20 Q92.8
21 (partial) Q90.9
meiotic nondisjunction Q90.0
mitotic nondisjunction Q90.1
mosaicism Q90.1
translocation Q90.2
22 Q92.8
autosomes Q92.9
chromosome specified NEC Q92.8
partial Q92.2
due to unbalanced translocation Q92.5
specified NEC Q92.8
whole (nonsex chromosome)
meiotic nondisjunction Q92.0
mitotic nondisjunction Q92.1
mosaicism Q92.1
due to
dicentrics — *see* Extra, marker chromosomes
extra rings — *see* Extra, marker chromosomes
isochromosomes — *see* Extra, marker chromosomes
specified NEC Q92.8
whole chromosome Q92.9
meiotic nondisjunction Q92.0
mitotic nondisjunction Q92.1
mosaicism Q92.1
partial Q92.9
specified NEC Q92.8
Tritanomaly, tritanopia H53.55
Trombiculosis, trombiculiasis, trombidiosis B88.0
Trophedema (congenital) (hereditary) Q82.0
Trophoblastic disease (*see also* Mole, hydatidiform) O01.9
Tropholymphedema Q82.0
Trophoneurosis NEC G96.8
disseminated M34.9
Tropical — *see* condition
Trouble (*see also* Disease)
heart — *see* Disease, heart
kidney — *see* Disease, renal
nervous R45.0
sinus — *see* Sinusitis
Trousseau's syndrome (thrombophlebitis migrans) I82.1
Truancy, childhood
from school Z72.810
Truncus
arteriosus (persistent) Q20.0
communis Q20.0
Trunk — *see* condition
Trypanosomiasis
African B56.9
by Trypanosoma brucei
gambiense B56.0
rhodesiense B56.1
American — *see* Chagas' disease
Brazilian — *see* Chagas' disease
by Trypanosoma
brucei gambiense B56.0
brucei rhodesiense B56.1
cruzi — *see* Chagas' disease
gambiensis, Gambian B56.0
rhodesiensis, Rhodesian B56.1
South American — *see* Chagas' disease

Trypanosomiasis — *continued*
where
African trypanosomiasis is prevalent B56.9
Chagas' disease is prevalent B57.2
T-shaped incisors K00.2
Tsutsugamushi (disease) (fever) A75.3
Tube, tubal, tubular — *see* condition
Tubercle (*see also* Tuberculosis)
brain, solitary A17.81
Darwin's Q17.8
Ghon, primary infection A15.7
Tuberculid, tuberculide (indurating, subcutaneous) (lichenoid) (miliary) (papulonecrotic) (primary) (skin) A18.4
Tuberculoma (*see also* Tuberculosis)
brain A17.81
meninges (cerebral) (spinal) A17.1
spinal cord A17.81
Tuberculosis, tubercular, tuberculous (calcification) (calcified) (caseous) (chromogenic acid-fast bacilli) (degeneration) (fibrocaseous) (fistula) (interstitial) (isolated circumscribed lesions) (necrosis) (parenchymatous) (ulcerative) A15.9
with pneumoconiosis (any condition in J60-J64) J65
abdomen (lymph gland) A18.39
abscess (respiratory) A15.9
bone A18.03
hip A18.02
knee A18.02
sacrum A18.01
specified site NEC A18.03
spinal A18.01
vertebra A18.01
brain A17.81
breast A18.89
Cowper's gland A18.15
dura (mater) (cerebral) (spinal) A17.81
epidural (cerebral) (spinal) A17.81
female pelvis A18.17
frontal sinus A15.8
genital organs NEC A18.10
genitourinary A18.10
gland (lymphatic) — *see* Tuberculosis, lymph gland
hip A18.02
intestine A18.32
ischiorectal A18.32
joint NEC A18.02
hip A18.02
knee A18.02
specified NEC A18.02
vertebral A18.01
kidney A18.11
knee A18.02
latent R76.11
lumbar (spine) A18.01
lung — *see* Tuberculosis, pulmonary
meninges (cerebral) (spinal) A17.0
muscle A18.09
perianal (fistula) A18.32
perinephritic A18.11
perirectal A18.32
rectum A18.32
retropharyngeal A15.8
sacrum A18.01
scrofulous A18.2
scrotum A18.15
skin (primary) A18.4
spinal cord A17.81
spine or vertebra (column) A18.01
subdiaphragmatic A18.31
testis A18.15
urinary A18.13
uterus A18.17
accessory sinus — *see* Tuberculosis, sinus
Addison's disease A18.7
adenitis — *see* Tuberculosis, lymph gland
adenoids A15.8
adenopathy — *see* Tuberculosis, lymph gland
adherent pericardium A18.84
adnexa (uteri) A18.17
adrenal (capsule) (gland) A18.7
alimentary canal A18.32
anemia A18.89
ankle (joint) (bone) A18.02
anus A18.32
apex, apical — *see* Tuberculosis, pulmonary
appendicitis, appendix A18.32
arachnoid A17.0

Tuberculosis, tubercular, tuberculous — *continued*
artery, arteritis A18.89
cerebral A18.89
arthritis (chronic) (synovial) A18.02
spine or vertebra (column) A18.01
articular — *see* Tuberculosis, joint
ascites A18.31
asthma — *see* Tuberculosis, pulmonary
axilla, axillary (gland) A18.2
bladder A18.12
bone A18.03
hip A18.02
knee A18.02
limb NEC A18.03
sacrum A18.01
spine or vertebral column A18.01
bowel (miliary) A18.32
brain A17.81
breast A18.89
broad ligament A18.17
bronchi, bronchial, bronchus A15.5
ectasia, ectasis (bronchiectasis) — *see* Tuberculosis, pulmonary
fistula A15.5
primary (progressive) A15.7
gland or node A15.4
primary (progressive) A15.7
lymph gland or node A15.4
primary (progressive) A15.7
bronchiectasis — *see* Tuberculosis, pulmonary
bronchitis A15.5
bronchopleural A15.6
bronchopneumonia, bronchopneumonic — *see* Tuberculosis, pulmonary
bronchorrhagia A15.5
bronchotracheal A15.5
bronze disease A18.7
buccal cavity A18.83
bulbourethral gland A18.15
bursa A18.09
cachexia A15.9
cardiomyopathy A18.84
caries — *see* Tuberculosis, bone
cartilage A18.02
intervertebral A18.01
catarrhal — *see* Tuberculosis, respiratory
cecum A18.32
cellulitis (primary) A18.4
cerebellum A17.81
cerebral, cerebrum A17.81
cerebrospinal A17.81
meninges A17.0
cervical (lymph gland or node) A18.2
cervicitis, cervix (uteri) A18.16
chest — *see* Tuberculosis, respiratory
chorioretinitis A18.53
choroid, choroiditis A18.53
ciliary body A18.54
colitis A18.32
collier's J65
colliquativa (primary) A18.4
colon A18.32
complex, primary A15.7
congenital P37.0
conjunctiva A18.59
connective tissue (systemic) A18.89
contact Z20.1
cornea (ulcer) A18.52
Cowper's gland A18.15
coxae A18.02
coxalgia A18.02
cul-de-sac of Douglas A18.17
curvature, spine A18.01
cutis (colliquativa) (primary) A18.4
cyst, ovary A18.18
cystitis A18.12
dactylitis A18.03
diarrhea A18.32
diffuse — *see* Tuberculosis, miliary
digestive tract A18.32
disseminated — *see* Tuberculosis, miliary
duodenum A18.32
dura (mater) (cerebral) (spinal) A17.0
abscess (cerebral) (spinal) A17.81
dysentery A18.32
ear (inner) (middle) A18.6
bone A18.03
external (primary) A18.4

Index

Tuberculosis, tubercular, tuberculous — Tuberculosis, tubercular, tuberculous — Tuberculosis, tubercular, tuberculous

Tuberculosis, tubercular, tuberculous — *continued*

ear — *continued*
  skin (primary) A18.4
elbow A18.02
emphysema — *see* Tuberculosis, pulmonary
empyema A15.6
encephalitis A17.82
endarteritis A18.89
endocarditis A18.84
  aortic A18.84
  mitral A18.84
  pulmonary A18.84
  tricuspid A18.84
endocrine glands NEC A18.82
endometrium A18.17
enteric, enterica, enteritis A18.32
enterocolitis A18.32
epididymis, epididymitis A18.15
epidural abscess (cerebral) (spinal) A17.81
epiglottis A15.5
episcleritis A18.51
erythema (induratum) (nodosum) (primary) A18.4
esophagus A18.83
eustachian tube A18.6
exposure (to) Z20.1
exudative — *see* Tuberculosis, pulmonary
eye A18.50
eyelid (primary) (lupus) A18.4
fallopian tube (acute) (chronic) A18.17
fascia A18.09
fauces A15.8
female pelvic inflammatory disease A18.17
finger A18.03
first infection A15.7
gallbladder A18.83
ganglion A18.09
gastritis A18.83
gastrocolic fistula A18.32
gastroenteritis A18.32
gastrointestinal tract A18.32
general, generalized — *see* Tuberculosis, miliary
genital organs A18.10
genitourinary A18.10
genu A18.02
glandula suprarenalis A18.7
glandular, general A18.2
glottis A15.5
grinder's J65
gum A18.83
hand A18.03
heart A18.84
hematogenous — *see* Tuberculosis, miliary
hemoptysis — *see* Tuberculosis, pulmonary
hemorrhage NEC — *see* Tuberculosis, pulmonary
hemothorax A15.6
hepatitis A18.83
hilar lymph nodes A15.4
  primary (progressive) A15.7
hip (joint) (disease) (bone) A18.02
hydropneumothorax A15.6
hydrothorax A15.6
hypoadrenalism A18.7
hypopharynx A15.8
ileocecal (hyperplastic) A18.32
ileocolitis A18.32
ileum A18.32
iliac spine (superior) A18.03
immunological findings only A15.7
indurativa (primary) A18.4
infantile A15.7
infection A15.9
  without clinical manifestations A15.7
infraclavicular gland A18.2
inguinal gland A18.2
inguinalis A18.2
intestine (any part) A18.32
iridocyclitis A18.54
iris, iritis A18.54
ischiorectal A18.32
jaw A18.03
jejunum A18.32
joint A18.02
  vertebral A18.01
keratitis (interstitial) A18.52
keratoconjunctivitis A18.52
kidney A18.11
knee (joint) A18.02
kyphosis, kyphoscoliosis A18.01

Tuberculosis, tubercular, tuberculous — *continued*

laryngitis A15.5
larynx A15.5
leptomeninges, leptomeningitis (cerebral) (spinal) A17.0
lichenoides (primary) A18.4
linguae A18.83
lip A18.83
liver A18.83
lordosis A18.01
lung — *see* Tuberculosis, pulmonary
lupus vulgaris A18.4
lymph gland or node (peripheral) A18.2
  abdomen A18.39
  bronchial A15.4
    primary (progressive) A15.7
  cervical A18.2
  hilar A15.4
    primary (progressive) A15.7
  intrathoracic A15.4
    primary (progressive) A15.7
  mediastinal A15.4
    primary (progressive) A15.7
  mesenteric A18.39
  retroperitoneal A18.39
  tracheobronchial A15.4
    primary (progressive) A15.7
lymphadenitis — *see* Tuberculosis, lymph gland
lymphangitis — *see* Tuberculosis, lymph gland
lymphatic (gland) (vessel) — *see* Tuberculosis, lymph gland
mammary gland A18.89
marasmus A15.9
mastoiditis A18.03
mediastinal lymph gland or node A15.4
  primary (progressive) A15.7
mediastinitis A15.8
  primary (progressive) A15.7
mediastinum A15.8
  primary (progressive) A15.7
medulla A17.81
melanosis, Addisonian A18.7
meninges, meningitis (basilar) (cerebral) (cerebrospinal) (spinal) A17.0
meningoencephalitis A17.82
mesentery, mesenteric (gland or node) A18.39
miliary A19.9
  acute A19.2
    multiple sites A19.1
    single specified site A19.0
  chronic A19.8
  specified NEC A19.8
millstone makers' J65
miner's J65
molder's J65
mouth A18.83
multiple A19.9
  acute A19.1
  chronic A19.8
muscle A18.09
myelitis A17.82
myocardium, myocarditis A18.84
nasal (passage) (sinus) A15.8
nasopharynx A15.8
neck gland A18.2
nephritis A18.11
nerve (mononeuropathy) A17.83
nervous system A17.9
nose (septum) A15.8
ocular A18.50
omentum A18.31
oophoritis (acute) (chronic) A18.17
optic (nerve trunk) (papilla) A18.59
orbit A18.59
orchitis A18.15
organ, specified NEC A18.89
osseous — *see* Tuberculosis, bone
osteitis — *see* Tuberculosis, bone
osteomyelitis — *see* Tuberculosis, bone
otitis media A18.6
ovary, ovaritis (acute) (chronic) A18.17
oviduct (acute) (chronic) A18.17
pachymeningitis A17.0
palate (soft) A18.83
pancreas A18.83
papulonecrotic (a) (primary) A18.4
parathyroid glands A18.82
paronychia (primary) A18.4

Tuberculosis, tubercular, tuberculous — *continued*

parotid gland or region A18.83
pelvis (bony) A18.03
penis A18.15
peribronchitis A15.5
pericardium, pericarditis A18.84
perichondritis, larynx A15.5
periostitis — *see* Tuberculosis, bone
perirectal fistula A18.32
peritoneum NEC A18.31
peritonitis A18.31
pharynx, pharyngitis A15.8
phlyctenulosis (keratoconjunctivitis) A18.52
phthisis NEC — *see* Tuberculosis, pulmonary
pituitary gland A18.82
pleura, pleural, pleurisy, pleuritis (fibrinous) (obliterative) (purulent) (simple plastic) (with effusion) A15.6
  primary (progressive) A15.7
pneumonia, pneumonic — *see* Tuberculosis, pulmonary
pneumothorax (spontaneous) (tense valvular) — *see* Tuberculosis, pulmonary
polyneuropathy A17.89
polyserositis A19.9
  acute A19.1
  chronic A19.8
potter's J65
prepuce A18.15
primary (complex) A15.7
proctitis A18.32
prostate, prostatitis A18.14
pulmonalis — *see* Tuberculosis, pulmonary
pulmonary (cavitated) (fibrotic) (infiltrative) (nodular) A15.0
  childhood type or first infection A15.7
  primary (complex) A15.7
pyelitis A18.11
pyelonephritis A18.11
pyemia — *see* Tuberculosis, miliary
pyonephrosis A18.11
pyopneumothorax A15.6
pyothorax A15.6
rectum (fistula) (with abscess) A18.32
reinfection stage — *see* Tuberculosis, pulmonary
renal A18.11
renis A18.11
respiratory A15.9
  primary A15.7
  specified site NEC A15.8
retina, retinitis A18.53
retroperitoneal (lymph gland or node) A18.39
rheumatism NEC A18.09
rhinitis A15.8
sacroiliac (joint) A18.01
sacrum A18.01
salivary gland A18.83
salpingitis (acute) (chronic) A18.17
sandblaster's J65
sclera A18.51
scoliosis A18.01
scrofulous A18.2
scrotum A18.15
seminal tract or vesicle A18.15
senile A15.9
septic — *see* Tuberculosis, miliary
shoulder (joint) A18.02
  blade A18.03
sigmoid A18.32
sinus (any nasal) A15.8
  bone A18.03
  epididymis A18.15
skeletal NEC A18.03
skin (any site) (primary) A18.4
small intestine A18.32
soft palate A18.83
spermatic cord A18.15
spine, spinal (column) A18.01
  cord A17.81
  medulla A17.81
  membrane A17.0
  meninges A17.0
spleen, splenitis A18.85
spondylitis A18.01
sternoclavicular joint A18.02
stomach A18.83
stonemason's J65
subcutaneous tissue (cellular) (primary) A18.4

Tuberculosis, tubercular, tuberculous — *continued*
- subcutis (primary) A18.4
- subdeltoid bursa A18.83
- submaxillary (region) A18.83
- supraclavicular gland A18.2
- suprarenal (capsule) (gland) A18.7
- swelling, joint (*see also* category M01) (*see also* Tuberculosis, joint) A18.02
- symphysis pubis A18.02
- synovitis A18.09
  - articular A18.02
  - spine or vertebra A18.01
- systemic — *see* Tuberculosis, miliary
- tarsitis A18.4
- tendon (sheath) — *see* Tuberculosis, tenosynovitis
- tenosynovitis A18.09
  - spine or vertebra A18.01
- testis A18.15
- throat A15.8
- thymus gland A18.82
- thyroid gland A18.81
- tongue A18.83
- tonsil, tonsillitis A15.8
- trachea, tracheal A15.5
  - lymph gland or node A15.4
    - primary (progressive) A15.7
- tracheobronchial A15.5
  - lymph gland or node A15.4
    - primary (progressive) A15.7
- tubal (acute) (chronic) A18.17
- tunica vaginalis A18.15
- ulcer (skin) (primary) A18.4
  - bowel or intestine A18.32
  - specified NEC — *see* Tuberculosis, by site
- unspecified site A15.9
- ureter A18.11
- urethra, urethral (gland) A18.13
- urinary organ or tract A18.13
- uterus A18.17
- uveal tract A18.54
- uvula A18.83
- vagina A18.18
- vas deferens A18.15
- verruca, verrucosa (cutis) (primary) A18.4
- vertebra (column) A18.01
- vesiculitis A18.15
- vulva A18.18
- wrist (joint) A18.02

Tuberculum
- Carabelli — *see* Excludes Note at K00.2
- occlusal — *see* Excludes Note at K00.2
- paramolare K00.2

Tuberosity, enitre maxillary M26.07

Tuberous sclerosis (brain) Q85.1

Tubo-ovarian — *see* condition

Tuboplasty, after previous sterilization Z31.0
- aftercare Z31.42

Tubotympanitis, catarrhal (chronic) — *see* Otitis, media, nonsuppurative, chronic, serous

Tularemia A21.9
- with
  - conjunctivitis A21.1
  - pneumonia A21.2
- abdominal A21.3
- bronchopneumonic A21.2
- conjunctivitis A21.1
- cryptogenic A21.3
- enteric A21.3
- gastrointestinal A21.3
- generalized A21.7
- ingestion A21.3
- intestinal A21.3
- oculoglandular A21.1
- ophthalmic A21.1
- pneumonia (any), pneumonic A21.2
- pulmonary A21.2
- sepsis A21.7
- specified NEC A21.8
- typhoidal A21.7
- ulceroglandular A21.0

Tularensis conjunctivitis A21.1

Tumefaction (*see also* Swelling)
- liver — *see* Hypertrophy, liver

Tumor (*see also* Neoplasm, unspecified behavior, by site)
- acinar cell — *see* Neoplasm, uncertain behavior, by site
- acinic cell — *see* Neoplasm, uncertain behavior, by site

Tumor — *continued*
- adenocarcinoid — *see* Neoplasm, malignant, by site
- adenomatoid (*see also* Neoplasm, benign, by site)
  - odontogenic — *see* Cyst, calcifying odontogenic
- adnexal (skin) — *see* Neoplasm, skin, benign, by site
- adrenal
  - cortical (benign) D35.0- ☑
    - malignant C74.0- ☑
  - rest — *see* Neoplasm, benign, by site
- alpha-cell
  - malignant
    - pancreas C25.4
    - specified site NEC — *see* Neoplasm, malignant, by site
    - unspecified site C25.4
  - pancreas D13.7
  - specified site NEC — *see* Neoplasm, benign, by site
  - unspecified site D13.7
- aneurysmal — *see* Aneurysm
- aortic body D44.7
  - malignant C75.5
- Askin's — *see* Neoplasm, connective tissue, malignant
- basal cell (*see also* Neoplasm, skin, uncertain behavior) D48.5
- Bednar — *see* Neoplasm, skin, malignant
- benign (unclassified) — *see* Neoplasm, benign, by site
- beta-cell
  - malignant
    - pancreas C25.4
    - specified site NEC — *see* Neoplasm, malignant, by site
    - unspecified site C25.4
  - pancreas D13.7
  - specified site NEC — *see* Neoplasm, benign, by site
  - unspecified site D13.7
- Brenner D27.9
  - borderline malignancy D39.1- ☑
  - malignant C56- ☑
  - proliferating D39.1- ☑
- bronchial alveolar, intravascular D38.1
- Brooke's — *see* Neoplasm, skin, benign
- brown fat — *see* Lipoma
- Burkitt — *see* Lymphoma, Burkitt
- calcifying epithelial odontogenic — *see* Cyst, calcifying odontogenic
- carcinoid
  - benign D3A.00 (*following* D36)
    - appendix D3A.020 (*following* D36)
    - ascending colon D3A.022 (*following* D36)
    - bronchus (lung) D3A.090 (*following* D36)
    - cecum D3A.021 (*following* D36)
    - colon D3A.029 (*following* D36)
    - descending colon D3A.024 (*following* D36)
    - duodenum D3A.010 (*following* D36)
    - foregut NOS D3A.094 (*following* D36)
    - hindgut NOS D3A.096 (*following* D36)
    - ileum D3A.012 (*following* D36)
    - jejunum D3A.011 (*following* D36)
    - kidney D3A.093 (*following* D36)
    - large intestine D3A.029 (*following* D36)
    - lung (bronchus) D3A.090 (*following* D36)
    - midgut NOS D3A.095 (*following* D36)
    - rectum D3A.026 (*following* D36)
    - sigmoid colon D3A.025 (*following* D36)
    - small intestine D3A.019 (*following* D36)
    - specified NEC D3A.098 (*following* D36)
    - stomach D3A.092 (*following* D36)
    - thymus D3A.091 (*following* D36)
    - transverse colon D3A.023 (*following* D36)
  - malignant C7A.00 (*following* C75)
    - appendix C7A.020 (*following* C75)
    - ascending colon C7A.022 (*following* C75)
    - bronchus (lung) C7A.090 (*following* C75)
    - cecum C7A.021 (*following* C75)
    - colon C7A.029 (*following* C75)
    - descending colon C7A.024 (*following* C75)
    - duodenum C7A.010 (*following* C75)
    - foregut NOS C7A.094 (*following* C75)
    - hindgut NOS C7A.096 (*following* C75)
    - ileum C7A.012 (*following* C75)
    - jejunum C7A.011 (*following* C75)
    - kidney C7A.093 (*following* C75)
    - large intestine C7A.029 (*following* C75)
    - lung (bronchus) C7A.090 (*following* C75)
    - midgut NOS C7A.095 (*following* C75)
    - rectum C7A.026 (*following* C75)
    - sigmoid colon C7A.025 (*following* C75)
    - small intestine C7A.019 (*following* C75)

Tumor — *continued*
- carcinoid — *continued*
  - malignant — *continued*
    - specified NEC C7A.098 (*following* C75)
    - stomach C7A.092 (*following* C75)
    - thymus C7A.091 (*following* C75)
    - transverse colon C7A.023 (*following* C75)
  - mesentery metastasis C7B.04 (*following* C75)
  - secondary C7B.00 (*following* C75)
    - bone C7B.03 (*following* C75)
    - distant lymph nodes C7B.01 (*following* C75)
    - liver C7B.02 (*following* C75)
    - peritoneum C7B.04 (*following* C75)
    - specified NEC C7B.09 (*following* C75)
- carotid body D44.6
  - malignant C75.4
- cells (*see also* Neoplasm, unspecified behavior, by site)
  - benign — *see* Neoplasm, benign, by site
  - malignant — *see* Neoplasm, malignant, by site
  - uncertain whether benign or malignant — *see* Neoplasm, uncertain behavior, by site
- cervix, in pregnancy or childbirth — *see* Pregnancy, complicated by, tumor, cervix
- chondromatous giant cell — *see* Neoplasm, bone, benign
- chromaffin (*see also* Neoplasm, benign, by site)
  - malignant — *see* Neoplasm, malignant, by site
- Cock's peculiar L72.3
- Codman's — *see* Neoplasm, bone, benign
- dentigerous, mixed — *see* Cyst, calcifying odontogenic
- dermoid — *see* Neoplasm, benign, by site
  - with malignant transformation C56- ☑
- desmoid (extra-abdominal) (*see also* Neoplasm, connective tissue, uncertain behavior)
  - abdominal — *see* Neoplasm, connective tissue, uncertain behavior
- embolus — *see* Neoplasm, secondary, by site
- embryonal (mixed) (*see also* Neoplasm, uncertain behavior, by site)
  - liver C22.7
- endodermal sinus
  - specified site — *see* Neoplasm, malignant, by site
  - unspecified site
    - female C56.- ☑
    - male C62.90
- epithelial
  - benign — *see* Neoplasm, benign, by site
  - malignant — *see* Neoplasm, malignant, by site
- Ewing's — *see* Neoplasm, bone, malignant, by site
- fatty — *see* Lipoma
- fibroid — *see* Leiomyoma
- G cell
  - malignant
    - pancreas C25.4
    - specified site NEC — *see* Neoplasm, malignant, by site
    - unspecified site C25.4
  - specified site — *see* Neoplasm, uncertain behavior, by site
  - unspecified site D37.8
- germ cell (*see also* Neoplasm, malignant, by site)
  - mixed — *see* Neoplasm, malignant, by site
- ghost cell, odontogenic — *see* Cyst, calcifying odontogenic
- giant cell (*see also* Neoplasm, uncertain behavior, by site)
  - bone D48.0
    - malignant — *see* Neoplasm, bone, malignant
  - chondromatous — *see* Neoplasm, bone, benign
  - malignant — *see* Neoplasm, malignant, by site
  - soft parts — *see* Neoplasm, connective tissue, uncertain behavior
    - malignant — *see* Neoplasm, connective tissue, malignant
- glomus D18.00
  - intra-abdominal D18.03
  - intracranial D18.02
  - jugulare D44.7
    - malignant C75.5
  - skin D18.01
  - specified site NEC D18.09
- gonadal stromal — *see* Neoplasm, uncertain behavior, by site
- granular cell (*see also* Neoplasm, connective tissue, benign)
  - malignant — *see* Neoplasm, connective tissue, malignant

Index

Tumor — Turner's

Tumor — *continued*
granulosa cell D39.1- ☑
juvenile D39.1- ☑
malignant C56- ☑
granulosa cell-theca cell D39.1- ☑
malignant C56- ☑
Grawitz's C64- ☑
hemorrhoidal — *see* Hemorrhoids
hilar cell D27- ☑
hilus cell D27- ☑
Hurthle cell (benign) D34
malignant C73
hydatid — *see* Echinococcus
hypernephroid (*see also* Neoplasm, uncertain behavior, by site)
interstitial cell (*see also* Neoplasm, uncertain behavior, by site)
benign — *see* Neoplasm, benign, by site
malignant — *see* Neoplasm, malignant, by site
intravascular bronchial alveolar D38.1
islet cell — *see* Neoplasm, benign, by site
malignant — *see* Neoplasm, malignant, by site
pancreas C25.4
specified site NEC — *see* Neoplasm, malignant, by site
unspecified site C25.4
pancreas D13.7
specified site NEC — *see* Neoplasm, benign, by site
unspecified site D13.7
juxtaglomerular D41.0- ☑
Klatskin's C22.1
Krukenberg's C79.6- ☑
Leydig cell — *see* Neoplasm, uncertain behavior, by site
benign — *see* Neoplasm, benign, by site
specified site — *see* Neoplasm, benign, by site
unspecified site
female D27.9
male D29.20
malignant — *see* Neoplasm, malignant, by site
specified site — *see* Neoplasm, malignant, by site
unspecified site
female C56.9
male C62.90
specified site — *see* Neoplasm, uncertain behavior, by site
unspecified site
female D39.10
male D40.10
lipid cell, ovary D27- ☑
lipoid cell, ovary D27- ☑
malignant (*see also* Neoplasm, malignant, by site) C80.1
fusiform cell (type) C80.1
giant cell (type) C80.1
localized, plasma cell — *see* Plasmacytoma, solitary
mixed NEC C80.1
small cell (type) C80.1
spindle cell (type) C80.1
unclassified C80.1
mast cell D47.0
malignant C96.2
melanotic, neuroectodermal — *see* Neoplasm, benign, by site
Merkel cell — *see* Carcinoma, Merkel cell
mesenchymal
malignant — *see* Neoplasm, connective tissue, malignant
mixed — *see* Neoplasm, connective tissue, uncertain behavior
mesodermal, mixed (*see also* Neoplasm, malignant, by site)
liver C22.4
mesonephric (*see also* Neoplasm, uncertain behavior, by site)
malignant — *see* Neoplasm, malignant, by site
metastatic
from specified site — *see* Neoplasm, malignant, by site
of specified site — *see* Neoplasm, malignant, by site
to specified site — *see* Neoplasm, secondary, by site
mixed NEC (*see also* Neoplasm, benign, by site)
malignant — *see* Neoplasm, malignant, by site

Tumor — *continued*
mucinous of low malignant potential
specified site — *see* Neoplasm, malignant, by site
unspecified site C56.9
mucocarcinoid
specified site — *see* Neoplasm, malignant, by site
unspecified site C18.1
mucoepidermoid — *see* Neoplasm, uncertain behavior, by site
Müllerian, mixed
specified site — *see* Neoplasm, malignant, by site
unspecified site C54.9
myoepithelial — *see* Neoplasm, benign, by site
neuroectodermal (peripheral) — *see* Neoplasm, malignant, by site
primitive
specified site — *see* Neoplasm, malignant, by site
unspecified site C71.9
neuroendocrine D3A.8 (*following* D36)
malignant poorly differentiated C7A.1 (*following* C75)
secondary NEC C7B.8 (*following* C75)
specified NEC C7A.8 (*following* C75)
neurogenic olfactory C30.0
nonencapsulated sclerosing C73
odontogenic (adenomatoid) (benign) (calcifying epithelial) (keratocystic) (squamous) — *see* Cyst, calcifying odontogenic
malignant C41.1
upper jaw (bone) C41.0
ovarian stromal D39.1- ☑
ovary, in pregnancy — *see* Pregnancy, complicated by
pacinian — *see* Neoplasm, skin, benign
Pancoast's — *see* Pancoast's syndrome
papillary (*see also* Papilloma)
cystic D37.9
mucinous of low malignant potential C56- ☑
specified site — *see* Neoplasm, malignant, by site
unspecified site C56.9
serous of low malignant potential
specified site — *see* Neoplasm, malignant, by site
unspecified site C56.9
pelvic, in pregnancy or childbirth — *see* Pregnancy, complicated by
phantom F45.8
phyllodes D48.6- ☑
benign D24- ☑
malignant — *see* Neoplasm, breast, malignant
Pindborg — *see* Cyst, calcifying odontogenic
placental site trophoblastic D39.2
plasma cell (malignant) (localized) — *see* Plasmacytoma, solitary
polyvesicular vitelline
specified site — *see* Neoplasm, malignant, by site
unspecified site
female C56.9
male C62.90
Pott's puffy — *see* Osteomyelitis, specified NEC
Rathke's pouch D44.3
retinal anlage — *see* Neoplasm, benign, by site
salivary gland type, mixed — *see* Neoplasm, salivary gland, benign
malignant — *see* Neoplasm, salivary gland, malignant
Sampson's N80.1
Schmincke's — *see* Neoplasm, nasopharynx, malignant
sclerosing stromal D27- ☑
sebaceous — *see* Cyst, sebaceous
secondary — *see* Neoplasm, secondary, by site
carcinoid C7B.00 (*following* C75)
bone C7B.03 (*following* C75)
distant lymph nodes C7B.01 (*following* C75)
liver C7B.02 (*following* C75)
peritoneum C7B.04 (*following* C75)
specified NEC C7B.09 (*following* C75)
neuroendocrine NEC C7B.8 (*following* C75)
serous of low malignant potential
specified site — *see* Neoplasm, malignant, by site
unspecified site C56.9
Sertoli cell — *see* Neoplasm, benign, by site
with lipid storage
specified site — *see* Neoplasm, benign, by site
unspecified site

Tumor — *continued*
Sertoli cell — *see* Neoplasm, benign, by site — *continued*
with lipid storage — *continued*
unspecified site — *continued*
female D27.9
male D29.20
specified site — *see* Neoplasm, benign, by site
unspecified site
female D27.9
male D29.20
Sertoli-Leydig cell — *see* Neoplasm, benign, by site
specified site — *see* Neoplasm, benign, by site
unspecified site
female D27.9
male D29.20
sex cord (-stromal) — *see* Neoplasm, uncertain behavior, by site
with annular tubules D39.1- ☑
skin appendage — *see* Neoplasm, skin, benign
smooth muscle — *see* Neoplasm, connective tissue, uncertain behavior
soft tissue
benign — *see* Neoplasm, connective tissue, benign
malignant — *see* Neoplasm, connective tissue, malignant
sternomastoid (congenital) Q68.0
stromal
endometrial D39.0
gastric D48.1
benign D21.4
malignant C16.9
uncertain behavior D48.1
gastrointestinal
benign D21.4
malignant C49.4
uncertain behavior D48.1
intestine
benign D21.4
malignant C49.4
uncertain behavior D48.1
ovarian D39.1- ☑
stomach
benign D21.4
malignant C16.9
uncertain behavior D48.1
sweat gland (*see also* Neoplasm, skin, uncertain behavior)
benign — *see* Neoplasm, skin, benign
malignant — *see* Neoplasm, skin, malignant
syphilitic, brain A52.17
testicular D40.10
testicular stromal D40.1- ☑
theca cell D27.- ☑
theca cell-granulosa cell D39.1- ☑
Triton, malignant — *see* Neoplasm, nerve, malignant
trophoblastic, placental site D39.2
turban D23.4
uterus (body), in pregnancy or childbirth — *see* Pregnancy, complicated by, tumor, uterus
vagina, in pregnancy or childbirth — *see* Pregnancy, complicated by
varicose — *see* Varix
von Recklinghausen's — *see* Neurofibromatosis
vulva or perineum, in pregnancy or childbirth — *see* Pregnancy, complicated by
causing obstructed labor O65.5
Warthin's — *see* Neoplasm, salivary gland, benign
Wilms' C64- ☑
yolk sac — *see* Neoplasm, malignant, by site
specified site — *see* Neoplasm, malignant, by site
unspecified site
female C56.9
male C62.90
Tumor lysis syndrome (following antineoplastic chemotherapy) (spontaneous) NEC E88.3
Tumorlet — *see* Neoplasm, uncertain behavior, by site
Tungiasis B88.1
Tunica vasculosa lentis Q12.2
Turban tumor D23.4
Türck's trachoma J37.0
Turner-Kieser syndrome Q79.8
Turner-like syndrome Q87.1
Turner's
hypoplasia (tooth) K00.4
syndrome Q96.9
specified NEC Q96.8

Turner's — *continued*
tooth K00.4
Turner-Ullrich syndrome Q96.9
Tussis convulsiva — *see* Whooping cough
Twiddler's syndrome (due to)
automatic implantable defibrillatorT82.198
cardiac pacemaker T82.198 ☑
Twilight state
epileptic F05
psychogenic F44.89
Twin (newborn) (*see also* Newborn, twin)
conjoined Q89.4
pregnancy — *see* Pregnancy, twin, conjoined
Twinning, teeth K00.2
Twist, twisted
bowel, colon or intestine K56.2
hair (congenital) Q84.1
mesentery K56.2
omentum K56.2
organ or site, congenital NEC — *see* Anomaly, by site
ovarian pedicle — *see* Torsion, ovary
Twitching R25.3
Tylosis (acquired) L84
buccalis K13.29
linguae K13.29
palmaris et plantaris (congenital) (inherited) Q82.8
acquired L85.1
Tympanism R14.0
Tympanites (abdominal) (intestinal) R14.0
Tympanitis — *see* Myringitis
Tympanosclerosis H74.0 ☑
Tympanum — *see* condition
Tympany
abdomen R14.0
chest R09.89
Type A behavior pattern Z73.1
Typhlitis — *see* Appendicitis
Typhoenteritis — *see* Typhoid
Typhoid (abortive) (ambulant) (any site) (clinical) (fever) (hemorrhagic) (infection) (intermittent) (malignant) (rheumatic) (Widal negative) A01.00
with pneumonia A01.03
abdominal A01.09
arthritis A01.04
carrier (suspected) of Z22.0
cholecystitis (current) A01.09
endocarditis A01.02
heart involvement A01.02
inoculation reaction — *see* Complications, vaccination
meningitis A01.01
mesenteric lymph nodes A01.09
myocarditis A01.02
osteomyelitis A01.05
perichondritis, larynx A01.09
pneumonia A01.03
specified NEC A01.09
spine A01.05
ulcer (perforating) A01.09
Typhomalaria (fever) — *see* Malaria
Typhomania A01.00
Typhoperitonitis A01.09
Typhus (fever) A75.9
abdominal, abdominalis — *see* Typhoid
African tick A77.1
amarillic A95.9
brain A75.9 [G94]
cerebral A75.9 [G94]
classical A75.0
due to Rickettsia
prowazekii A75.0
recrudescent A75.1
tsutsugamushi A75.3
typhi A75.2
endemic (flea-borne) A75.2
epidemic (louse-borne) A75.0
exanthematicus SAI A75.0
brillii SAI A75.1
mexicanus SAI A75.2
typhus murinus A75.2
exanthematic NEC A75.0
flea-borne A75.2
India tick A77.1
Kenya (tick) A77.1
louse-borne A75.0
Mexican A75.2
mite-borne A75.3
murine A75.2
North Asian tick-borne A77.2

Typhus — *continued*
petechial A75.9
Queensland tick A77.3
rat A75.2
recrudescent A75.1
recurrens — *see* Fever, relapsing
Sao Paulo A77.0
scrub (China) (India) (Malaysia) (New Guinea) A75.3
shop (of Malaysia) A75.2
Siberian tick A77.2
tick-borne A77.9
tropical (mite-borne) A75.3
Tyrosinemia E70.21
newborn, transitory P74.5
Tyrosinosis E70.21
Tyrosinuria E70.29

U

Uhl's anomaly or disease Q24.8
Ulcer, ulcerated, ulcerating, ulceration, ulcerative
alveolar process M27.3
amebic (intestine) A06.1
skin A06.7
anastomotic — *see* Ulcer, gastrojejunal
anorectal K62.6
antral — *see* Ulcer, stomach
anus (sphincter) (solitary) K62.6
aorta — *see* Aneurysm
aphthous (oral) (recurrent) K12.0
genital organ(s)
female N76.6
male N50.8
artery I77.2
atrophic — *see* Ulcer, skin
decubitus — *see* Ulcer, pressure, by site
back L98.429
with
bone necrosis L98.424
exposed fat layer L98.422
muscle necrosis L98.423
skin breakdown only L98.421
Barrett's (esophagus) K22.10
with bleeding K22.11
bile duct (common) (hepatic) K83.8
bladder (solitary) (sphincter) NEC N32.89
bilharzial B65.9 [N33]
in schistosomiasis (bilharzial) B65.9 [N33]
submucosal — *see* Cystitis, interstitial
tuberculous A18.12
bleeding K27.4
bone — *see* Osteomyelitis, specified type NEC
bowel — *see* Ulcer, intestine
breast N61
bronchus J98.09
buccal (cavity) (traumatic) K12.1
Buruli A31.1
buttock L98.419
with
bone necrosis L98.414
exposed fat layer L98.412
muscle necrosis L98.413
skin breakdown only L98.411
cancerous — *see* Neoplasm, malignant, by site
cardia K22.10
with bleeding K22.11
cardioesophageal (peptic) K22.10
with bleeding K22.11
cecum — *see* Ulcer, intestine
cervix (uteri) (decubitus) (trophic) N86
with cervicitis N72
chancroidal A57
chiclero B55.1
chronic (cause unknown) — *see* Ulcer, skin
Cochin-China B55.1
colon — *see* Ulcer, intestine
conjunctiva H10.89
cornea H16.00- ☑
with hypopyon H16.03- ☑
central H16.01- ☑
dendritic (herpes simplex) B00.52
marginal H16.04- ☑
Mooren's H16.05- ☑
mycotic H16.06- ☑
perforated H16.07- ☑
ring H16.02- ☑
tuberculous (phlyctenular) A18.52

Ulcer, ulcerated, ulcerating, ulceration, ulcerative — *continued*
corpus cavernosum (chronic) N48.5
crural — *see* Ulcer, lower limb
Curling's — *see* Ulcer, peptic, acute
Cushing's — *see* Ulcer, peptic, acute
cystic duct K82.8
cystitis (interstitial) — *see* Cystitis, interstitial
decubitus — *see* Ulcer, pressure, by site
dendritic, cornea (herpes simplex) B00.52
diabetes, diabetic — *see* Diabetes, ulcer
Dieulafoy's K25.0
due to
infection NEC — *see* Ulcer, skin
radiation NEC L59.8
trophic disturbance (any region) — *see* Ulcer, skin
X-ray L58.1
duodenum, duodenal (eroded) (peptic) K26.9
with
hemorrhage K26.4
and perforation K26.6
perforation K26.5
acute K26.3
with
hemorrhage K26.0
and perforation K26.2
perforation K26.1
chronic K26.7
with
hemorrhage K26.4
and perforation K26.6
perforation K26.5
dysenteric A09
elusive — *see* Cystitis, interstitial
endocarditis (acute) (chronic) (subacute) I28.8
epiglottis J38.7
esophagus (peptic) K22.10
with bleeding K22.11
due to
aspirin K22.10
with bleeding K22.11
gastrointestinal reflux disease K21.0
ingestion of chemical or medicament K22.10
with bleeding K22.11
fungal K22.10
with bleeding K22.11
infective K22.10
with bleeding K22.11
varicose — *see* Varix, esophagus
eyelid (region) H01.8
fauces J39.2
Fenwick (-Hunner) (solitary) — *see* Cystitis, interstitial
fistulous — *see* Ulcer, skin
foot (indolent) (trophic) — *see* Ulcer, lower limb
frambesial, initial A66.0
frenum (tongue) K14.0
gallbladder or duct K82.8
gangrenous — *see* Gangrene
gastric — *see* Ulcer, stomach
gastrocolic — *see* Ulcer, gastrojejunal
gastroduodenal — *see* Ulcer, peptic
gastroesophageal — *see* Ulcer, stomach
gastrointestinal — *see* Ulcer, gastrojejunal
gastrojejunal (peptic) K28.9
with
hemorrhage K28.4
and perforation K28.6
perforation K28.5
acute K28.3
with
hemorrhage K28.0
and perforation K28.2
perforation K28.1
chronic K28.7
with
hemorrhage K28.4
and perforation K28.6
perforation K28.5
gastrojejunocolic — *see* Ulcer, gastrojejunal
gingiva K06.8
gingivitis K05.10
nonplaque induced K05.11
plaque induced K05.10
glottis J38.7
granuloma of pudenda A58
gum K06.8
gumma, due to yaws A66.4
heel — *see* Ulcer, lower limb

Ulcer, ulcerated, ulcerating, ulceration, ulcerative
— *continued*
- hemorrhoid (*see also* Hemorrhoids, by degree) K64.8
- Hunner's — *see* Cystitis, interstitial
- hypopharynx J39.2
- hypopyon (chronic) (subacute) — *see* Ulcer, cornea, with hypopyon
- hypostaticum — *see* Ulcer, varicose
- ileum — *see* Ulcer, intestine
- intestine, intestinal K63.3
  - with perforation K63.1
  - amebic A06.1
  - duodenal — *see* Ulcer, duodenum
  - granulocytopenic (with hemorrhage) — *see* Neutropenia
  - marginal — *see* Ulcer, gastrojejunal
  - perforating K63.1
    - newborn P78.0
  - primary, small intestine K63.3
  - rectum K62.6
  - stercoraceous, stercoral K63.3
  - tuberculous A18.32
  - typhoid (fever) — *see* Typhoid
  - varicose I86.8
- jejunum, jejunal — *see* Ulcer, gastrojejunal
- keratitis — *see* Ulcer, cornea
- knee — *see* Ulcer, lower limb
- labium (majus) (minus) N76.6
- laryngitis — *see* Laryngitis
- larynx (aphthous) (contact) J38.7
  - diphtheritic A36.2
- leg — *see* Ulcer, lower limb
- lip K13.0
- Lipschütz's N76.6
- lower limb (atrophic) (chronic) (neurogenic) (perforating) (pyogenic) (trophic) (tropical) L97.909
  - with
    - bone necrosis L97.904
    - exposed fat layer L97.902
    - muscle necrosis L97.903
    - skin breakdown only L97.901
  - ankle L97.309
    - with
      - bone necrosis L97.304
      - exposed fat layer L97.302
      - muscle necrosis L97.303
      - skin breakdown only L97.301
    - left L97.329
      - with
        - bone necrosis L97.324
        - exposed fat layer L97.322
        - muscle necrosis L97.323
        - skin breakdown only L97.321
    - right L97.319
      - with
        - bone necrosis L97.314
        - exposed fat layer L97.312
        - muscle necrosis L97.313
        - skin breakdown only L97.311
  - calf L97.209
    - with
      - bone necrosis L97.204
      - exposed fat layer L97.202
      - muscle necrosis L97.203
      - skin breakdown only L97.201
    - left L97.229
      - with
        - bone necrosis L97.224
        - exposed fat layer L97.222
        - muscle necrosis L97.223
        - skin breakdown only L97.221
    - right L97.219
      - with
        - bone necrosis L97.214
        - exposed fat layer L97.212
        - muscle necrosis L97.213
        - skin breakdown only L97.211
  - decubitus — *see* Ulcer, pressure, by site
  - foot specified NEC L97.509
    - with
      - bone necrosis L97.504
      - exposed fat layer L97.502
      - muscle necrosis L97.503
      - skin breakdown only L97.501
    - left L97.529
      - with
        - bone necrosis L97.524
        - exposed fat layer L97.522

Ulcer, ulcerated, ulcerating, ulceration, ulcerative
— *continued*
- lower limb — *continued*
  - foot specified — *continued*
    - left — *continued*
      - with — *continued*
        - muscle necrosis L97.523
        - skin breakdown only L97.521
    - right L97.519
      - with
        - bone necrosis L97.514
        - exposed fat layer L97.512
        - muscle necrosis L97.513
        - skin breakdown only L97.511
  - heel L97.409
    - with
      - bone necrosis L97.404
      - exposed fat layer L97.402
      - muscle necrosis L97.403
      - skin breakdown only L97.401
    - left L97.429
      - with
        - bone necrosis L97.424
        - exposed fat layer L97.422
        - muscle necrosis L97.423
        - skin breakdown only L97.421
    - right L97.419
      - with
        - bone necrosis L97.414
        - exposed fat layer L97.412
        - muscle necrosis L97.413
        - skin breakdown only L97.411
  - left L97.929
    - with
      - bone necrosis L97.924
      - exposed fat layer L97.922
      - muscle necrosis L97.923
      - skin breakdown only L97.921
  - leprous A30.1
  - lower leg NOS L97.909
    - with
      - bone necrosis L97.904
      - exposed fat layer L97.902
      - muscle necrosis L97.903
      - skin breakdown only L97.901
    - left L97.929
      - with
        - bone necrosis L97.924
        - exposed fat layer L97.922
        - muscle necrosis L97.923
        - skin breakdown only L97.921
    - right L97.919
      - with
        - bone necrosis L97.914
        - exposed fat layer L97.912
        - muscle necrosis L97.913
        - skin breakdown only L97.911
    - specified site NEC L97.809
      - with
        - bone necrosis L97.804
        - exposed fat layer L97.802
        - muscle necrosis L97.803
        - skin breakdown only L97.801
      - left L97.829
        - with
          - bone necrosis L97.824
          - exposed fat layer L97.822
          - muscle necrosis L97.823
          - skin breakdown only L97.821
      - right L97.819
        - with
          - bone necrosis L97.814
          - exposed fat layer L97.812
          - muscle necrosis L97.813
          - skin breakdown only L97.811
  - midfoot L97.409
    - with
      - bone necrosis L97.404
      - exposed fat layer L97.402
      - muscle necrosis L97.403
      - skin breakdown only L97.401
    - left L97.429
      - with
        - bone necrosis L97.424
        - exposed fat layer L97.422
        - muscle necrosis L97.423
        - skin breakdown only L97.421

Ulcer, ulcerated, ulcerating, ulceration, ulcerative
— *continued*
- lower limb — *continued*
  - midfoot — *continued*
    - right L97.419
      - with
        - bone necrosis L97.414
        - exposed fat layer L97.412
        - muscle necrosis L97.413
        - skin breakdown only L97.411
    - right L97.919
      - with
        - bone necrosis L97.914
        - exposed fat layer L97.912
        - muscle necrosis L97.913
        - skin breakdown only L97.911
  - syphilitic A52.19
  - thigh L97.109
    - with
      - bone necrosis L97.104
      - exposed fat layer L97.102
      - muscle necrosis L97.103
      - skin breakdown only L97.101
    - left L97.129
      - with
        - bone necrosis L97.124
        - exposed fat layer L97.122
        - muscle necrosis L97.123
        - skin breakdown only L97.121
    - right L97.119
      - with
        - bone necrosis L97.114
        - exposed fat layer L97.112
        - muscle necrosis L97.113
        - skin breakdown only L97.111
  - toe L97.509
    - with
      - bone necrosis L97.504
      - exposed fat layer L97.502
      - muscle necrosis L97.503
      - skin breakdown only L97.501
    - left L97.529
      - with
        - bone necrosis L97.524
        - exposed fat layer L97.522
        - muscle necrosis L97.523
        - skin breakdown only L97.521
    - right L97.519
      - with
        - bone necrosis L97.514
        - exposed fat layer L97.512
        - muscle necrosis L97.513
        - skin breakdown only L97.511
  - varicose — *see* Varix, leg, with, ulcer
- luetic — *see* Ulcer, syphilitic
- lung J98.4
  - tuberculous — *see* Tuberculosis, pulmonary
- malignant — *see* Neoplasm, malignant, by site
- marginal NEC — *see* Ulcer, gastrojejunal
- meatus (urinarius) N34.2
- Meckel's diverticulum Q43.0
  - malignant — *see* Table of Neoplasms, small intestine, malignant
- Meleney's (chronic undermining) — *see* Ulcer, skin
- Mooren's (cornea) — *see* Ulcer, cornea, Mooren's
- mycobacterial (skin) A31.1
- nasopharynx J39.2
- neck, uterus N86
- neurogenic NEC — *see* Ulcer, skin
- nose, nasal (passage) (infective) (septum) J34.0
  - skin — *see* Ulcer, skin
  - spirochetal A69.8
  - varicose (bleeding) I86.8
- oral mucosa (traumatic) K12.1
- palate (soft) K12.1
- penis (chronic) N48.5
- peptic (site unspecified) K27.9
  - with
    - hemorrhage K27.4
      - and perforation K27.6
    - perforation K27.5
  - acute K27.3
    - with
      - hemorrhage K27.0
        - and perforation K27.2
      - perforation K27.1
  - chronic K27.7

Ulcer, ulcerated, ulcerating, ulceration, ulcerative
— *continued*
- peptic — *continued*
  - chronic — *continued*
    - with
      - hemorrhage K27.4
        - and perforation K27.6
      - perforation K27.5
  - esophagus K22.10
    - with bleeding K22.11
  - newborn P78.82
- perforating K27.5
- skin — *see* Ulcer, skin
- peritonsillar J35.8
- phagedenic (tropical) — *see* Ulcer, skin
- pharynx J39.2
- phlebitis — *see* Phlebitis
- plaster — *see* Ulcer, pressure, by site
- popliteal space — *see* Ulcer, lower limb
- postpyloric — *see* Ulcer, duodenum
- prepuce N47.7
- prepyloric — *see* Ulcer, stomach
- pressure (pressure area) L89.9- ☑
  - ankle L89.5- ☑
  - back L89.1- ☑
  - buttock L89.3- ☑
  - coccyx L89.15- ☑
  - contiguous site of back, buttock, hip L89.4- ☑
  - elbow L89.0- ☑
  - face L89.81- ☑
  - head L89.81- ☑
  - heel L89.6- ☑
  - hip L89.2- ☑
  - sacral region (tailbone) L89.15- ☑
  - specified site NEC L89.89- ☑
  - stage 1 (healing) (pre-ulcer skin changes limited to persistent focal edema)
    - ankle L89.5- ☑
    - back L89.1- ☑
    - buttock L89.3- ☑
    - coccyx L89.15- ☑
    - contiguous site of back, buttock, hip L89.4- ☑
    - elbow L89.0- ☑
    - face L89.81- ☑
    - head L89.81- ☑
    - heel L89.6- ☑
    - hip L89.2- ☑
    - sacral region (tailbone) L89.15- ☑
    - specified site NEC L89.89- ☑
  - stage 2 (healing) (abrasion, blister, partial thickness skin loss involving epidermis and/or dermis)
    - ankle L89.5- ☑
    - back L89.1- ☑
    - buttock L89.3- ☑
    - coccyx L89.15- ☑
    - contiguous site of back, buttock, hip L89.4- ☑
    - elbow L89.0- ☑
    - face L89.81- ☑
    - head L89.81- ☑
    - heel L89.6- ☑
    - hip L89.2- ☑
    - sacral region (tailbone) L89.15- ☑
    - specified site NEC L89.89- ☑
  - stage 3 (healing) (full thickness skin loss involving damage or necrosis of subcutaneous tissue)
    - ankle L89.5- ☑
    - back L89.1- ☑
    - buttock L89.3- ☑
    - coccyx L89.15- ☑
    - contiguous site of back, buttock, hip L89.4- ☑
    - elbow L89.0- ☑
    - face L89.81- ☑
    - head L89.81- ☑
    - heel L89.6- ☑
    - hip L89.2- ☑
    - sacral region (tailbone) L89.15- ☑
    - specified site NEC L89.89- ☑
  - stage 4 (healing) (necrosis of soft tissues through to underlying muscle, tendon, or bone)
    - ankle L89.5- ☑
    - back L89.1- ☑
    - buttock L89.3- ☑
    - coccyx L89.15- ☑
    - contiguous site of back, buttock, hip L89.4- ☑
    - elbow L89.0- ☑
    - face L89.81- ☑

Ulcer, ulcerated, ulcerating, ulceration, ulcerative
— *continued*
- pressure — *continued*
  - stage 4 — *continued*
    - head L89.81- ☑
    - heel L89.6- ☑
    - hip L89.2- ☑
    - sacral region (tailbone) L89.15- ☑
    - specified site NEC L89.89- ☑
  - unspecified stage
    - ankle L89.5- ☑
    - back L89.1- ☑
    - buttock L89.3- ☑
    - coccyx L89.15- ☑
    - contiguous site of back, buttock, hip L89.4- ☑
    - elbow L89.0- ☑
    - face L89.81- ☑
    - head L89.81- ☑
    - heel L89.6- ☑
    - hip L89.2- ☑
    - sacral region (tailbone) L89.15- ☑
    - specified site NEC L89.89- ☑
  - unstageable
    - ankle L89.5- ☑
    - back L89.1- ☑
    - buttock L89.3- ☑
    - coccyx L89.15- ☑
    - contiguous site of back, buttock, hip L89.4- ☑
    - elbow L89.0- ☑
    - face L89.81- ☑
    - head L89.81- ☑
    - heel L89.6- ☑
    - hip L89.2- ☑
    - sacral region (tailbone) L89.15- ☑
    - specified site NEC L89.89- ☑
- primary of intestine K63.3
  - with perforation K63.1
- prostate N41.9
- pyloric — *see* Ulcer, stomach
- rectosigmoid K63.3
  - with perforation K63.1
- rectum (sphincter) (solitary) K62.6
  - stercoraceous, stercoral K62.6
- retina — *see* Inflammation, chorioretinal
- rodent (*see also* Neoplasm, skin, malignant)
- sclera — *see* Scleritis
- scrofulous (tuberculous) A18.2
- scrotum N50.8
  - tuberculous A18.15
  - varicose I86.1
- seminal vesicle N50.8
- sigmoid — *see* Ulcer, intestine
- skin (atrophic) (chronic) (neurogenic) (non-healing) (perforating) (pyogenic) (trophic) (tropical) L98.499
  - with gangrene — *see* Gangrene
  - amebic A06.7
  - back — *see* Ulcer, back
  - buttock — *see* Ulcer, buttock
  - decubitus — *see* Ulcer, pressure
  - lower limb — *see* Ulcer, lower limb
  - mycobacterial A31.1
  - specified site NEC L98.499
    - with
      - bone necrosis L98.494
      - exposed fat layer L98.492
      - muscle necrosis L98.493
      - skin breakdown only L98.491
  - tuberculous (primary) A18.4
  - varicose — *see* Ulcer, varicose
- sloughing — *see* Ulcer, skin
- solitary, anus or rectum (sphincter) K62.6
- sore throat J02.9
  - streptococcal J02.0
- spermatic cord N50.8
- spine (tuberculous) A18.01
- stasis (venous) — *see* Varix, leg, with, ulcer
  - without varicose veins I87.2
- stercoraceous, stercoral K63.3
  - with perforation K63.1
  - anus or rectum K62.6
- stoma, stomal — *see* Ulcer, gastrojejunal
- stomach (eroded) (peptic) (round) K25.9
  - with
    - hemorrhage K25.4
      - and perforation K25.6
    - perforation K25.5

Ulcer, ulcerated, ulcerating, ulceration, ulcerative
— *continued*
- stomach — *continued*
  - acute K25.3
    - with
      - hemorrhage K25.0
        - and perforation K25.2
      - perforation K25.1
    - chronic K25.7
      - with
        - hemorrhage K25.4
          - and perforation K25.6
        - perforation K25.5
  - stomal — *see* Ulcer, gastrojejunal
- stomatitis K12.1
- stress — *see* Ulcer, peptic
- strumous (tuberculous) A18.2
- submucosal, bladder — *see* Cystitis, interstitial
- syphilitic (any site) (early) (secondary) A51.39
  - late A52.79
    - perforating A52.79
      - foot A52.11
- testis N50.8
- thigh — *see* Ulcer, lower limb
- throat J39.2
  - diphtheritic A36.0
- toe — *see* Ulcer, lower limb
- tongue (traumatic) K14.0
- tonsil J35.8
  - diphtheritic A36.0
- trachea J39.8
- trophic — *see* Ulcer, skin
- tropical — *see* Ulcer, skin
- tuberculous — *see* Tuberculosis, ulcer
- tunica vaginalis N50.8
- turbinate J34.89
- typhoid (perforating) — *see* Typhoid
- unspecified site — *see* Ulcer, skin
- urethra (meatus) — *see* Urethritis
- uterus N85.8
  - cervix N86
    - with cervicitis N72
  - neck N86
    - with cervicitis N72
- vagina N76.5
  - in Behçet's disease M35.2 [N77.0]
  - pessary N89.8
- valve, heart I33.0
- varicose (lower limb, any part) (*see also* Varix, leg, with, ulcer)
  - broad ligament I86.2
  - esophagus — *see* Varix, esophagus
  - inflamed or infected — *see* Varix, leg, with ulcer, with inflammation
  - nasal septum I86.8
  - perineum I86.3
  - scrotum I86.1
  - specified site NEC I86.8
  - sublingual I86.0
  - vulva I86.3
- vas deferens N50.8
- vulva (acute) (infectional) N76.6
  - in (due to)
    - Behçet's disease M35.2 [N77.0]
    - herpesviral (herpes simplex) infection A60.04
    - tuberculosis A18.18
- vulvobuccal, recurring N76.6
- X-ray L58.1
- yaws A66.4

Ulcerosa scarlatina A38.8
Ulcus (*see also* Ulcer)
- cutis tuberculosum A18.4
- duodeni — *see* Ulcer, duodenum
- durum (syphilitic) A51.0
  - extragenital A51.2
- gastrojejunale — *see* Ulcer, gastrojejunal
- hypostaticum — *see* Ulcer, varicose
- molle (cutis) (skin) A57
- serpens corneae — *see* Ulcer, cornea, central
- ventriculi — *see* Ulcer, stomach
Ulegyria Q04.8
Ulerythema
- ophryogenes, congenital Q84.2
- sycosiforme L73.8
Ullrich (-Bonnevie)(-Turner) **syndrome** Q87.1
Ullrich-Feichtiger syndrome Q87.0
Ulnar — *see* condition
Ulorrhagia, ulorrhea K06.8

Umbilicus, umbilical — see condition
Unacceptable
  contours of tooth K08.54
  morphology of tooth K08.54
Unavailability (of)
  bed at medical facility Z75.1
  health service-related agencies Z75.4
  medical facilities (at) Z75.3
    due to
      investigation by social service agency Z75.2
      lack of services at home Z75.0
      remoteness from facility Z75.3
      waiting list Z75.1
    home Z75.0
    outpatient clinic Z75.3
  schooling Z55.1
  social service agencies Z75.4
Uncinaria americana infestation B76.1
Uncinariasis B76.9
Uncongenial work Z56.5
Unconscious (ness) — see Coma
Under observation — see Observation
Underachievement in school Z55.3
Underdevelopment (see also Undeveloped)
  nose Q30.1
  sexual E30.0
Underdosing (see also Table of Drugs and Chemicals, categories T36-T50, with final character 6) Z91.14
  intentional NEC Z91.128
    due to financial hardship of patient Z91.120
  unintentional NEC Z91.138
    due to patient's age related debility Z91.130
Underfeeding, newborn P92.3
Underfill, endodontic M27.53
Underimmunization status Z28.3
Undernourishment — see Malnutrition
Undernutrition — see Malnutrition
Underweight R63.6
  for gestational age — see Light for dates
Underwood's disease P83.0
Undescended (see also Malposition, congenital)
  cecum Q43.3
  colon Q43.3
  testicle — see Cryptorchid
Undeveloped, undevelopment (see also Hypoplasia)
  brain (congenital) Q02
  cerebral (congenital) Q02
  heart Q24.8
  lung Q33.6
  testis E29.1
  uterus E30.0
Undiagnosed (disease) R69
Undulant fever — see Brucellosis
Unemployment, anxiety concerning Z56.0
  threatened Z56.2
Unequal length (acquired) (limb) (see also Deformity, limb, unequal length)
  leg (see also Deformity, limb, unequal length)
    congenital Q72.9- ☑
Unextracted dental root K08.3
Unguis incarnatus L60.0
Unhappiness R45.2
Unicornate uterus Q51.4
Unilateral (see also condition)
  development, breast N64.89
  organ or site, congenital NEC — see Agenesis, by site
Unilocular heart Q20.8
Union, abnormal (see also Fusion)
  larynx and trachea Q34.8
Universal mesentery Q43.3
Unrepairable overhanging of dental restorative materials K08.52
Unsatisfactory
  restoration of tooth K08.50
    specified NEC K08.59
  sample of cytologic smear
    anus R85.615
    cervix R87.615
    vagina R87.625
  surroundings Z59.1
    work Z56.5
Unsoundness of mind — see Psychosis
Unstable
  back NEC — see Instability, joint, spine
  hip (congenital) Q65.6
    acquired — see Derangement, joint, specified type NEC, hip

Unstable — continued
  joint — see Instability, joint
    secondary to removal of joint prosthesis M96.89
  lie (mother) O32.0 ☑
  lumbosacral joint (congenital)
    acquired — see subcategory M53.2 ☑
  sacroiliac — see subcategory M53.2 ☑
  spine NEC — see Instability, joint, spine
Unsteadiness on feet R26.81
Untruthfulness, child problem F91.8
Unverricht (-Lundborg) disease or epilepsy — see Epilepsy, generalized, idiopathic
Unwanted pregnancy Z64.0
Upbringing, institutional Z62.22
  away from parents NEC Z62.29
  in care of non-parental family member Z62.21
  in foster care Z62.21
  in orphanage or group home Z62.22
  in welfare custody Z62.21
Upper respiratory — see condition
Upset
  gastric K30
  gastrointestinal K30
    psychogenic F45.8
  intestinal (large) (small) K59.9
    psychogenic F45.8
  menstruation N93.9
  mental F48.9
  stomach K30
    psychogenic F45.8
Urachus (see also condition)
  patent or persistent Q64.4
Urbach-Oppenheim disease (necrobiosis lipoidica diabeticorum) — see E08-E13 with .620
Urbach's lipoid proteinosis E78.89
Urbach-Wiethe disease E78.89
Urban yellow fever A95.1
Urea
  blood, high — see Uremia
  cycle metabolism disorder — see Disorder, urea cycle metabolism
Uremia, uremic N19
  with
    ectopic or molar pregnancy O08.4
    polyneuropathy N18.9 [G63]
  chronic (see also Disease, kidney, chronic) N18.9
    due to hypertension — see Hypertensive, kidney
  complicating
    ectopic or molar pregnancy O08.4
  congenital P96.0
  extrarenal R39.2
  following ectopic or molar pregnancy O08.4
  newborn P96.0
  prerenal R39.2
Ureter, ureteral — see condition
Ureteralgia N23
Ureterectasis — see Hydroureter
Ureteritis N28.89
  cystica N28.86
  due to calculus N20.1
    with calculus, kidney N20.2
      with hydronephrosis N13.2
  gonococcal (acute) (chronic) A54.21
  nonspecific N28.89
Ureterocele N28.89
  congenital (orthotopic) Q62.31
    ectopic Q62.32
Ureterolith, ureterolithiasis — see Calculus, ureter
Ureterostomy
  attention to Z43.6
  status Z93.6
Urethra, urethral — see condition
Urethralgia R39.89
Urethritis (anterior) (posterior) N34.2
  calculous N21.1
  candidal B37.41
  chlamydial A56.01
  diplococcal (gonococcal) A54.01
    with abscess (accessory gland) (periurethral) A54.1
  gonococcal A54.01
    with abscess (accessory gland) (periurethral) A54.1
  nongonococcal N34.1
    Reiter's — see Reiter's disease
  nonspecific N34.1
  nonvenereal N34.1
  postmenopausal N34.2
  puerperal O86.22

Urethritis — continued
  Reiter's — see Reiter's disease
  specified NEC N34.2
  trichomonal or due to Trichomonas (vaginalis) A59.03
Urethrocele N81.0
  with
    cystocele — see Cystocele
    prolapse of uterus — see Prolapse, uterus
Urethrolithiasis (with colic or infection) N21.1
Urethrorectal — see condition
Urethrorrhagia N36.8
Urethrorrhea R36.9
Urethrostomy
  attention to Z43.6
  status Z93.6
Urethrotrigonitis — see Trigonitis
Urethrovaginal — see condition
Urgency
  fecal R15.2
  hypertensive — see Hypertension
  urinary N39.41
Urhidrosis, uridrosis L74.8
Uric acid in blood (increased) E79.0
Uricacidemia (asymptomatic) E79.0
Uricemia (asymptomatic) E79.0
Uricosuria R82.99
Urinary — see condition
Urination
  frequent R35.0
  painful R30.9
Urine
  blood in — see Hematuria
  discharge, excessive R35.8
  enuresis, nonorganic origin F98.0
  extravasation R39.0
  frequency R35.0
  incontinence R32
    nonorganic origin F98.0
  intermittent stream R39.19
  pus in N39.0
  retention or stasis R33.9
    organic R33.8
      drug-induced R33.0
    psychogenic F45.8
  secretion
    deficient R34
    excessive R35.8
    frequency R35.0
  stream
    intermittent R39.19
    slowing R39.19
    splitting R39.13
    weak R39.12
Urinemia — see Uremia
Urinoma, urethra N36.8
Uroarthritis, infectious (Reiter's) — see Reiter's disease
Urodialysis R34
Urolithiasis — see Calculus, urinary
Uronephrosis — see Hydronephrosis
Uropathy N39.9
  obstructive N13.9
    specified NEC N13.8
  reflux N13.9
    specified NEC N13.8
  vesicoureteral reflux-associated — see Reflux, vesicoureteral
Urosepsis — code to condition
Urticaria L50.9
  with angioneurotic edema T78.3 ☑
    hereditary D84.1
  allergic L50.0
  cholinergic L50.5
  chronic L50.8
  cold, familial L50.2
  contact L50.6
  dermatographic L50.3
  due to
    cold or heat L50.2
    drugs L50.0
    food L50.0
    inhalants L50.0
    plants L50.6
    serum (see also Reaction, serum) T80.69 ☑
  factitial L50.3
  giant T78.3 ☑
    hereditary D84.1
  gigantea T78.3 ☑

☑ Additional Character Required — Refer to the Tabular List for Character Selection   ▽ Subterms under main terms may continue to next column or page

Urticaria — *continued*
  idiopathic L50.1
  larynx T78.3 ☑
    hereditary D84.1
  neonatorum P83.8
  nonallergic L50.1
  papulosa (Hebra) L28.2
  pigmentosa Q82.2
  recurrent periodic L50.8
  serum (*see also* Reaction, serum) T80.69 ☑
  solar L56.3
  specified type NEC L50.8
  thermal (cold) (heat) L50.2
  vibratory L50.4
  xanthelasmoidea Q82.2
Use (of)
  alcohol F10.99
    with sleep disorder F10.982
    harmful — *see* Abuse, alcohol
  amphetamines — *see* Use, stimulant NEC
  caffeine — *see* Use, stimulant NEC
  cannabis F12.90
    with
      anxiety disorder F12.980
      intoxication F12.929
        with
          delirium F12.921
          perceptual disturbance F12.922
        uncomplicated F12.920
      other specified disorder F12.988
      psychosis F12.959
        delusions F12.950
        hallucinations F12.951
      unspecified disorder F12.99
  cocaine F14.90
    with
      anxiety disorder F14.980
      intoxication F14.929
        with
          delirium F14.921
          perceptual disturbance F14.922
        uncomplicated F14.920
      other specified disorder F14.988
      psychosis F14.959
        delusions F14.950
        hallucinations F14.951
      sexual dysfunction F14.981
      sleep disorder F14.982
      unspecified disorder F14.99
    harmful — *see* Abuse, drug, cocaine
  drug(s) NEC F19.90
    with sleep disorder F19.982
    harmful — *see* Abuse, drug, by type
  hallucinogen NEC F16.90
    with
      anxiety disorder F16.980
      intoxication F16.929
        with
          delirium F16.921
        uncomplicated F16.920
      mood disorder F16.94
      other specified disorder F16.988
      perception disorder (flashbacks) F16.983
      psychosis F16.959
        delusions F16.950
        hallucinations F16.951
      unspecified disorder F16.99
    harmful — *see* Abuse, drug, hallucinogen NEC
  inhalants F18.90
    with
      anxiety disorder F18.980
      intoxication F18.929
        with delirium F18.921
        uncomplicated F18.920
      mood disorder F18.94
      other specified disorder F18.988
      persisting dementia F18.97
      psychosis F18.959
        delusions F18.950
        hallucinations F18.951
      unspecified disorder F18.99
    harmful — *see* Abuse, drug, inhalant
  methadone F11.20
  nonprescribed drugs F19.90
    harmful — *see* Abuse, non-psychoactive substance
  opioid F11.90

Use — *continued*
  opioid — *continued*
    with
      disorder F11.99
        mood F11.94
        sleep F11.982
        specified type NEC F11.988
      intoxication F11.929
        with
          delirium F11.921
          perceptual disturbance F11.922
        uncomplicated F11.920
      withdrawal F11.93
    harmful — *see* Abuse, drug, opioid
  patent medicines F19.90
    harmful — *see* Abuse, non-psychoactive substance
  psychoactive drug NEC F19.90
    with
      anxiety disorder F19.980
      intoxication F19.929
        with
          delirium F19.921
          perceptual disturbance F19.922
        uncomplicated F19.920
      mood disorder F19.94
      other specified disorder F19.988
      persisting
        amnestic disorder F19.96
        dementia F19.97
      psychosis F19.959
        delusions F19.950
        hallucinations F19.951
      sexual dysfunction F19.981
      sleep disorder F19.982
      unspecified disorder F19.99
      withdrawal F19.939
        with
          delirium F19.931
          perceptual disturbance F19.932
        uncomplicated F19.930
    harmful — *see* Abuse, drug NEC, psychoactive NEC
  sedative, hypnotic, or anxiolytic F13.90
    with
      anxiety disorder F13.980
      intoxication F13.929
        with
          delirium F13.921
        uncomplicated F13.920
      other specified disorder F13.988
      persisting
        amnestic disorder F13.96
        dementia F13.97
      psychosis F13.959
        delusions F13.950
        hallucinations F13.951
      sexual dysfunction F13.981
      sleep disorder F13.982
      unspecified disorder F13.99
    harmful — *see* Abuse, drug, sedative, hypnotic, or
      anxiolytic
  stimulant NEC F15.90
    with
      anxiety disorder F15.980
      intoxication F15.929
        with
          delirium F15.921
          perceptual disturbance F15.922
        uncomplicated F15.920
      mood disorder F15.94
      other specified disorder F15.988
      psychosis F15.959
        delusions F15.950
        hallucinations F15.951
      sexual dysfunction F15.981
      sleep disorder F15.982
      unspecified disorder F15.99
      withdrawal F15.93
    harmful — *see* Abuse, drug, stimulant NEC
  tobacco Z72.0
    with dependence — *see* Dependence, drug, nico-
      tine
  volatile solvents (*see also* Use, inhalant) F18.90
    harmful — *see* Abuse, drug, inhalant
Usher-Senear disease or syndrome L10.4
Uta B55.1
Uteromegaly N85.2
Uterovaginal — *see* condition
Uterovesical — *see* condition

Uveal — *see* condition
Uveitis (anterior) (*see also* Iridocyclitis)
  acute — *see* Iridocyclitis, acute
  chronic — *see* Iridocyclitis, chronic
  due to toxoplasmosis (acquired) B58.09
    congenital P37.1
  granulomatous — *see* Iridocyclitis, chronic
  heterochromic — *see* Cyclitis, Fuchs' heterochromic
  lens-induced — *see* Iridocyclitis, lens-induced
  posterior — *see* Chorioretinitis
  sympathetic H44.13- ☑
  syphilitic (secondary) A51.43
    congenital (early) A50.01
    late A52.71
  tuberculous A18.54
Uveoencephalitis — *see* Inflammation, chorioretinal
Uveokeratitis — *see* Iridocyclitis
Uveoparotitis D86.89
Uvula — *see* condition
Uvulitis (acute) (catarrhal) (chronic) (membranous)
  (suppurative) (ulcerative) K12.2

V

Vaccination (prophylactic)
  complication or reaction — *see* Complications, vacci-
    nation
  delayed Z28.9
  encounter for Z23
  not done — *see* Immunization, not done, because (of)
Vaccinia (generalized) (localized) T88.1 ☑
  without vaccination B08.011
  congenital P35.8
Vacuum, in sinus (accessory) (nasal) J34.89
Vagabond, vagabondage Z59.0
Vagabond's disease B85.1
Vagina, vaginal — *see* condition
Vaginalitis (tunica) (testis) N49.1
Vaginismus (reflex) N94.2
  functional F52.5
  nonorganic F52.5
  psychogenic F52.5
  secondary N94.2
Vaginitis (acute) (circumscribed) (diffuse) (emphysematous) (nonvenereal) (ulcerative) N76.0
  with ectopic or molar pregnancy O08.0
  amebic A06.82
  atrophic, postmenopausal N95.2
  bacterial N76.0
  blennorrhagic (gonococcal) A54.02
  candidal B37.3
  chlamydial A56.02
  chronic N76.1
  due to Trichomonas (vaginalis) A59.01
  following ectopic or molar pregnancy O08.0
  gonococcal A54.02
    with abscess (accessory gland) (periurethral) A54.1
  granuloma A58
  in (due to)
    candidiasis B37.3
    herpesviral (herpes simplex) infection A60.04
    pinworm infection B80 [N77.1]
  monilial B37.3
  mycotic (candidal) B37.3
  postmenopausal atrophic N95.2
  puerperal (postpartum) O86.13
  senile (atrophic) N95.2
  subacute or chronic N76.1
  syphilitic (early) A51.0
    late A52.76
  trichomonal A59.01
  tuberculous A18.18
Vaginosis — *see* Vaginitis
Vagotonia G52.2
Vagrancy Z59.0
VAIN — *see* Neoplasia, intraepithelial, vagina
Vallecula — *see* condition
Valley fever B38.0
Valsuani's disease — *see* Anemia, obstetric
Valve, valvular (formation) (*see also* condition)
  cerebral ventricle (communicating) in situ Z98.2
  cervix, internal os Q51.828
  congenital NEC — *see* Atresia, by site
  ureter (pelvic junction) (vesical orifice) Q62.39
  urethra (congenital) (posterior) Q64.2
Valvulitis (chronic) — *see* Endocarditis
Valvulopathy — *see* Endocarditis

Van Bogaert's leukoencephalopathy (sclerosing) (subacute) A81.1
Van Bogaert-Scherer-Epstein disease or syndrome E75.5
Van Buchem's syndrome M85.2
Van Creveld-von Gierke disease E74.01
Van der Hoeve (-de Kleyn) **syndrome** Q78.0
Van der Woude's syndrome Q38.0
Van Neck's disease or osteochondrosis M91.0
Vanishing lung J44.9
Vapor asphyxia or suffocation T59.9 ☑
  specified agent — *see* Table of Drugs and Chemicals
Variance, lethal ball, prosthetic heart valve T82.09 ☑
Variants, thalassemic D56.8
Variations in hair color L67.1
Varicella B01.9
  with
    complications NEC B01.89
    encephalitis B01.11
    encephalomyelitis B01.11
    meningitis B01.0
    myelitis B01.12
    pneumonia B01.2
  congenital P35.8
Varices — *see* Varix
Varicocele (scrotum) (thrombosed) I86.1
  ovary I86.2
  perineum I86.3
  spermatic cord (ulcerated) I86.1
Varicose
  aneurysm (ruptured) I77.0
  dermatitis — *see* Varix, leg, with, inflammation
  eczema — *see* Varix, leg, with, inflammation
  phlebitis — *see* Varix, with, inflammation
  tumor — *see* Varix
  ulcer (lower limb, any part) (*see also* Varix, leg, with, ulcer)
    anus (*see also* Hemorrhoids) K64.8
    esophagus — *see* Varix, esophagus
    inflamed or infected — *see* Varix, leg, with ulcer, with inflammation
    nasal septum I86.8
    perineum I86.3
    scrotum I86.1
    specified site NEC I86.8
  vein — *see* Varix
  vessel — *see* Varix, leg
Varicosis, varicosities, varicosity — *see* Varix
Variola (major) (minor) B03
Varioloid B03
Varix (lower limb) (ruptured) I83.90
  with
    edema I83.899
    inflammation I83.10
      with ulcer (venous) I83.209
    pain I83.819
    specified complication NEC I83.899
    stasis dermatitis I83.10
      with ulcer (venous) I83.209
    swelling I83.899
    ulcer I83.009
      with inflammation I83.209
  aneurysmal I77.0
  asymptomatic I83.9- ☑
  bladder I86.2
  broad ligament I86.2
  complicating
    childbirth (lower extremity) O87.4
      anus or rectum O87.2
      genital (vagina, vulva or perineum) O87.8
    pregnancy (lower extremity) O22.0- ☑
      anus or rectum O22.4- ☑
      genital (vagina, vulva or perineum) O22.1- ☑
    puerperium (lower extremity) O87.4
      anus or rectum O87.2
      genital (vagina, vulva, perineum) O87.8
  congenital (any site) Q27.8
  esophagus (idiopathic) (primary) (ulcerated) I85.00
    bleeding I85.01
    congenital Q27.8
    in (due to)
      alcoholic liver disease I85.10
        bleeding I85.11
      cirrhosis of liver I85.10
        bleeding I85.11
      portal hypertension I85.10
        bleeding I85.11

Varix — *continued*
  esophagus — *continued*
    in — *continued*
      schistosomiasis I85.10
        bleeding I85.11
      toxic liver disease I85.10
        bleeding I85.11
    secondary I85.10
      bleeding I85.11
  gastric I86.4
  inflamed or infected I83.10
    ulcerated I83.209
  labia (majora) I86.3
  leg (asymptomatic) I83.90
    with
      edema I83.899
      inflammation I83.10
        with ulcer — *see* Varix, leg, with, ulcer, with inflammation by site
      pain I83.819
      specified complication NEC I83.899
      swelling I83.899
      ulcer I83.009
        with inflammation I83.209
        ankle I83.003
          with inflammation I83.203
        calf I83.002
          with inflammation I83.202
        foot NEC I83.005
          with inflammation I83.205
        heel I83.004
          with inflammation I83.204
        lower leg NEC I83.008
          with inflammation I83.208
        midfoot I83.004
          with inflammation I83.204
        thigh I83.001
          with inflammation I83.201
    bilateral (asymptomatic) I83.93
      with
        edema I83.893
        pain I83.813
        specified complication NEC I83.893
        swelling I83.893
        ulcer I83.009
          with inflammation I83.209
    left (asymptomatic) I83.92
      with
        edema I83.892
        inflammation I83.12
          with ulcer — *see* Varix, leg, with, ulcer, with inflammation by site
        pain I83.812
        specified complication NEC I83.892
        swelling I83.892
        ulcer I83.029
          with inflammation I83.229
          ankle I83.023
            with inflammation I83.223
          calf I83.022
            with inflammation I83.222
          foot NEC I83.025
            with inflammation I83.225
          heel I83.024
            with inflammation I83.224
          lower leg NEC I83.028
            with inflammation I83.228
          midfoot I83.024
            with inflammation I83.224
          thigh I83.021
            with inflammation I83.221
    right (asymptomatic) I83.91
      with
        edema I83.891
        inflammation I83.11
          with ulcer — *see* Varix, leg, with, ulcer, with inflammation by site
        pain I83.811
        specified complication NEC I83.891
        swelling I83.891
        ulcer I83.019
          with inflammation I83.219
          ankle I83.013
            with inflammation I83.213
          calf I83.012
            with inflammation I83.212
          foot NEC I83.015
            with inflammation I83.215

Varix — *continued*
  leg — *continued*
    right — *continued*
      with — *continued*
        ulcer — *continued*
          heel I83.014
            with inflammation I83.214
          lower leg NEC I83.018
            with inflammation I83.218
          midfoot I83.014
            with inflammation I83.214
          thigh I83.011
            with inflammation I83.211
  nasal septum I86.8
  orbit I86.8
    congenital Q27.8
  ovary I86.2
  papillary I78.1
  pelvis I86.2
  perineum I86.3
  pharynx I86.8
  placenta O43.89- ☑
  renal papilla I86.8
  retina H35.09
  scrotum (ulcerated) I86.1
  sigmoid colon I86.8
  specified site NEC I86.8
  spinal (cord) (vessels) I86.8
  spleen, splenic (vein) (with phlebolith) I86.8
  stomach I86.4
  sublingual I86.0
  ulcerated I83.009
    inflamed or infected I83.209
  uterine ligament I86.2
  vagina I86.8
  vocal cord I86.8
  vulva I86.3
Vas deferens — *see* condition
Vas deferentitis N49.1
Vasa previa O69.4 ☑
  hemorrhage from, affecting newborn P50.0
Vascular (*see also* condition)
  loop on optic papilla Q14.2
  spasm I73.9
  spider I78.1
Vascularization, cornea — *see* Neovascularization, cornea
Vasculitis I77.6
  allergic D69.0
  cryoglobulinemic D89.1
  disseminated I77.6
  hypocomplementemic M31.8
  kidney I77.89
  livedoid L95.0
  nodular L95.8
  retina H35.06- ☑
  rheumatic — *see* Fever, rheumatic
  rheumatoid — *see* Rheumatoid, vasculitis
  skin (limited to) L95.9
    specified NEC L95.8
Vasculopathy, necrotizing M31.9
  cardiac allograft T86.290
  specified NEC M31.8
Vasitis (nodosa) N49.1
  tuberculous A18.15
Vasodilation I73.9
Vasomotor — *see* condition
Vasoplasty, after previous sterilization Z31.0
  aftercare Z31.42
Vasospasm (vasoconstriction) I73.9
  cerebral (cerebrovascular) (artery) I67.848
    reversible I67.841
  coronary I20.1
  nerve
    arm — *see* Mononeuropathy, upper limb
    brachial plexus G54.0
    cervical plexus G54.2
    leg — *see* Mononeuropathy, lower limb
  peripheral NOS I73.9
  retina (artery) — *see* Occlusion, artery, retina
Vasospastic — *see* condition
Vasovagal attack (paroxysmal) R55
  psychogenic F45.8
VATER syndrome Q87.2
Vater's ampulla — *see* condition
Vegetation, vegetative
  adenoid (nasal fossa) J35.8
  endocarditis (acute) (any valve) (subacute) I33.0

Vegetation, vegetative — *continued*
 heart (mycotic) (valve) I33.0
Veil
 Jackson's Q43.3
Vein, venous — *see* condition
Veldt sore — *see* Ulcer, skin
Velpeau's hernia — *see* Hernia, femoral
Venereal
 bubo A55
 disease A64
 granuloma inguinale A58
 lymphogranuloma (Durand-Nicolas-Favre) A55
Venofibrosis I87.8
Venom, venomous — *see* Table of Drugs and Chemicals,
  by animal or substance, poisoning
Venous — *see* condition
Ventilator lung, newborn P27.8
Ventral — *see* condition
Ventricle, ventricular (*see also* condition)
 escape I49.3
 inversion Q20.5
Ventriculitis (cerebral) (*see also* Encephalitis) G04.90
Ventriculostomy status Z98.2
Vernet's syndrome G52.7
Verneuil's disease (syphilitic bursitis) A52.78
Verruca (due to HPV) (filiformis) (simplex) (viral) (vulgaris)
  B07.9
 acuminata A63.0
 necrogenica (primary) (tuberculosa) A18.4
 plana B07.8
 plantaris B07.0
 seborrheica L82.1
  inflamed L82.0
 senile (seborrheic) L82.1
  inflamed L82.0
 tuberculosa (primary) A18.4
 venereal A63.0
Verrucosities — *see* Verruca
Verruga peruana, peruviana A44.1
Version
 with extraction
 cervix — *see* Malposition, uterus
 uterus (postinfectional) (postpartal, old) — *see* Malposition, uterus
Vertebra, vertebral — *see* condition
Vertical talus (congenital) Q66.80
 left foot Q66.82
 right foot Q66.81
Vertigo R42
 auditory — *see* Vertigo, aural
 aural H81.31- ☑
 benign paroxysmal (positional) H81.1- ☑
 central (origin) H81.4- ☑
 cerebral H81.4- ☑
 Dix and Hallpike (epidemic) — *see* Neuronitis,
   vestibular
 due to infrasound T75.23 ☑
 epidemic A88.1
  Dix and Hallpike — *see* Neuronitis, vestibular
  Pedersen's — *see* Neuronitis, vestibular
  vestibular neuronitis — *see* Neuronitis, vestibular
 hysterical F44.89
 infrasound T75.23 ☑
 labyrinthine — *see* subcategory H81.0 ☑
 laryngeal R05
 malignant positional H81.4- ☑
 Ménière's — *see* subcategory H81.0 ☑
 menopausal N95.1
 otogenic — *see* Vertigo, aural
 paroxysmal positional, benign — *see* Vertigo, benign
   paroxysmal
 Pedersen's (epidemic) — *see* Neuronitis, vestibular
 peripheral NEC H81.39- ☑
 positional
  benign paroxysmal — *see* Vertigo, benign parox-
    ysmal
  malignant H81.4- ☑
Very-low-density-lipoprotein-type (VLDL) **hyper-**
  lipoproteinemia E78.1
Vesania — *see* Psychosis
Vesical — *see* condition
Vesicle
 cutaneous R23.8
 seminal — *see* condition
 skin R23.8
Vesicocolic — *see* condition
Vesicoperineal — *see* condition

Vesicorectal — *see* condition
Vesicourethrorectal — *see* condition
Vesicovaginal — *see* condition
Vesicular — *see* condition
Vesiculitis (seminal) N49.0
 amebic A06.82
 gonorrheal (acute) (chronic) A54.23
 trichomonal A59.09
 tuberculous A18.15
Vestibulitis (ear) (*see also* subcategory) H83.0 ☑
 nose (external) J34.89
 vulvar N94.810
Vestibulopathy , acute peripheral (recurrent) — *see*
  Neuronitis, vestibular
Vestige, vestigial (*see also* Persistence)
 branchial Q18.0
 structures in vitreous Q14.0
Vibration
 adverse effects T75.20 ☑
  pneumatic hammer syndrome T75.21 ☑
  specified effect NEC T75.29 ☑
  vasospastic syndrome T75.22 ☑
  vertigo from infrasound T75.23 ☑
 exposure (occupational) Z57.7
 vertigo T75.23 ☑
Vibriosis A28.9
Victim (of)
 crime Z65.4
 disaster Z65.5
 terrorism Z65.4
 torture Z65.4
 war Z65.5
Vidal's disease L28.0
Villaret's syndrome G52.7
Villous — *see* condition
VIN — *see* Neoplasia, intraepithelial, vulva
Vincent's infection (angina) (gingivitis) A69.1
 stomatitis NEC A69.1
Vinson-Plummer syndrome D50.1
Violence, physical R45.6
Viosterol deficiency — *see* Deficiency, calciferol
Vipoma — *see* Neoplasm, malignant, by site
Viremia B34.9
Virilism (adrenal) E25.9
 congenital E25.0
Virilization (female) (suprarenal) E25.9
 congenital E25.0
 isosexual E28.2
Virulent bubo A57
Virus, viral (*see also* condition)
 as cause of disease classified elsewhere B97.89
 cytomegalovirus B25.9
 human immunodeficiency (HIV) — *see* Human, immunodeficiency virus (HIV) disease
 infection — *see* Infection, virus
 specified NEC B34.8
 swine influenza (viruses that normally cause infections
   in pigs) (*see also* Influenza, due to, identified
   novel influenza A virus) J09.X2
 West Nile (fever) A92.30
  with
   complications NEC A92.39
   cranial nerve disorders A92.32
   encephalitis A92.31
   encephalomyelitis A92.31
   neurologic manifestation NEC A92.32
   optic neuritis A92.32
   polyradiculitis A92.32
Viscera, visceral — *see* condition
Visceroptosis K63.4
Visible peristalsis R19.2
Vision, visual
 binocular, suppression H53.34
 blurred, blurring H53.8
  hysterical F44.6
 defect, defective NEC H54.7
 disorientation (syndrome) H53.8
 disturbance H53.9
  hysterical F44.6
 double H53.2
 examination Z01.00
  with abnormal findings Z01.01
 field, limitation (defect) — *see* Defect, visual field
 hallucinations R44.1
 halos H53.19
 loss — *see* Loss, vision

Vision, visual — *continued*
 loss — *see* Loss, vision — *continued*
  sudden — *see* Disturbance, vision, subjective, loss,
    sudden
 low (both eyes) — *see* Low, vision
 perception, simultaneous without fusion H53.33
Vitality, lack or want of R53.83
 newborn P96.89
Vitamin deficiency — *see* Deficiency, vitamin
Vitelline duct, persistent Q43.0
Vitiligo L80
 eyelid H02.739
  left H02.736
   lower H02.735
   upper H02.734
  right H02.733
   lower H02.732
   upper H02.731
 pinta A67.2
 vulva N90.89
Vitreal corneal syndrome H59.01- ☑
Vitreoretinopathy, proliferative (*see also* Retinopathy,
  proliferative)
 with retinal detachment — *see* Detachment, retina,
   traction
Vitreous (*see also* condition)
 touch syndrome — *see* Complication, postprocedural,
   following cataract surgery
Vocal cord — *see* condition
Vogt-Koyanagi syndrome H20.82- ☑
Vogt's disease or syndrome G80.3
Vogt-Spieimeyer amaurotic idiocy or disease E75.4
Voice
 change R49.9
  specified NEC R49.8
 loss — *see* Aphonia
Volhynian fever A79.0
Volkmann's ischemic contracture or paralysis (complicating trauma) T79.6 ☑
Volvulus (bowel) (colon) (duodenum) (intestine) K56.2
 with perforation K56.2
 congenital Q43.8
 fallopian tube — *see* Torsion, fallopian tube
 oviduct — *see* Torsion, fallopian tube
 stomach (due to absence of gastrocolic ligament)
   K31.89
Vomiting R11.10
 with nausea R11.2
 without nausea R11.11
 asphyxia — *see* Foreign body, by site, causing asphyxia, gastric contents
 bilious (cause unknown) R11.14
  following gastro-intestinal surgery K91.0
  in newborn P92.01
 blood — *see* Hematemesis
 causing asphyxia, choking, or suffocation — *see* Foreign body, by site
 cyclical G43.A0 (*following* G43.7)
  with refractory migraine G43.A1 (*following* G43.7)
  without refractory migraine G43.A0 (*following*
    G43.7)
  intractable G43.A1 (*following* G43.7)
  not intractable G43.A0 (*following* G43.7)
  psychogenic F50.8
 fecal mater R11.13
 following gastrointestinal surgery K91.0
  psychogenic F50.8
 functional K31.89
 hysterical F50.8
 nervous F50.8
 neurotic F50.8
 newborn NEC P92.09
  bilious P92.01
 periodic R11.10
  psychogenic F50.8
 projectile R11.12
 psychogenic F50.8
 uremic — *see* Uremia
Vomito negro — *see* Fever, yellow
Von Bezold's abscess — *see* Mastoiditis, acute
Von Economo-Cruchet disease A85.8
Von Eulenburg's disease G71.19
Von Gierke's disease E74.01
Von Hippel (-Lindau) **disease or syndrome** Q85.8
Von Jaksch's anemia or disease D64.89
Von Recklinghausen
 disease (neurofibromatosis) Q85.01

Von Recklinghausen — *continued*
  disease — *continued*
    bones E21.0
Von Schroetter's syndrome I82.890
Von Willebrand (-Jurgens)(-Minot) **disease or syndrome** D68.0
Von Zumbusch's disease L40.1
Voyeurism F65.3
Vrolik's disease Q78.0
Vulva — *see* condition
Vulvismus N94.2
Vulvitis (acute) (allergic) (atrophic) (hypertrophic) (intertriginous) (senile) N76.2
  with ectopic or molar pregnancy O08.0
  adhesive, congenital Q52.79
  blennorrhagic (gonococcal) A54.02
  candidal B37.3
  chlamydial A56.02
  due to Haemophilus ducreyi A57
  following ectopic or molar pregnancy O08.0
  gonococcal A54.02
    with abscess (accessory gland) (periurethral) A54.1
  herpesviral A60.04
  leukoplakic N90.4
  monilial B37.3
  puerperal (postpartum) O86.19
  subacute or chronic N76.3
  syphilitic (early) A51.0
    late A52.76
  trichomonal A59.01
  tuberculous A18.18
Vulvodynia N94.819
  specified NEC N94.818
Vulvorectal — *see* condition
Vulvovaginitis (acute) — *see* Vaginitis

W

Waiting list, person on Z75.1
  for organ transplant Z76.82
  undergoing social agency investigation Z75.2
Waldenström
  hypergammaglobulinemia D89.0
  syndrome or macroglobulinemia C88.0
Waldenström-Kjellberg syndrome D50.1
Walking
  difficulty R26.2
    psychogenic F44.4
  sleep F51.3
    hysterical F44.89
Wall, abdominal — *see* condition
Wallenberg's disease or syndrome G46.3
Wallgren's disease I87.8
Wandering
  gallbladder, congenital Q44.1
  in diseases classified elsewhere Z91.83
  kidney, congenital Q63.8
  organ or site, congenital NEC — *see* Malposition, congenital, by site
  pacemaker (heart) I49.8
  spleen D73.89
War neurosis F48.8
Wart (due to HPV) (filiform) (infectious) (viral) B07.9
  anogenital region (venereal) A63.0
  common B07.8
  external genital organs (venereal) A63.0
  flat B07.8
  Hassal-Henle's (of cornea) H18.49
  Peruvian A44.1
  plantar B07.0
  prosector (tuberculous) A18.4
  seborrheic L82.1
    inflamed L82.0
  senile (seborrheic) L82.1
    inflamed L82.0
  tuberculous A18.4
  venereal A63.0
Warthin's tumor — *see* Neoplasm, salivary gland, benign
Wassilieff's disease A27.0
Wasting
  disease R64
    due to malnutrition E41
  extreme (due to malnutrition) E41
  muscle NEC — *see* Atrophy, muscle
Water
  clefts (senile cataract) — *see* Cataract, senile, incipient
  deprivation of T73.1 ☑

Water — *continued*
  intoxication E87.79
  itch B76.9
  lack of T73.1 ☑
  loading E87.70
  on
    brain — *see* Hydrocephalus
    chest J94.8
    poisoning E87.79
Waterbrash R12
Waterhouse (-Friderichsen) **syndrome or disease** (meningococcal) A39.1
Water-losing nephritis N25.89
Watermelon stomach K31.819
  with hemorrhage K31.811
  without hemorrhage K31.819
Watsoniasis B66.8
Wax in ear — *see* Impaction, cerumen
Weak, weakening, weakness (generalized) R53.1
  arches (acquired) (*see also* Deformity, limb, flat foot)
  bladder (sphincter) R32
  facial R29.810
    following
      cerebrovascular disease I69.992
        cerebral infarction I69.392
        intracerebral hemorrhage I69.192
        nontraumatic intracranial hemorrhage NEC I69.292
        specified disease NEC I69.892
        stroke I69.392
        subarachnoid hemorrhage I69.092
  foot (double) — *see* Weak, arches
  heart, cardiac — *see* Failure, heart
  mind F70
  muscle M62.81
  myocardium — *see* Failure, heart
  newborn P96.89
  pelvic fundus N81.89
  pubocervical tissue N81.82
  rectovaginal tissue N81.83
  senile R54
  urinary stream R39.12
  valvular — *see* Endocarditis
Wear, worn (with normal or routine use)
  articular bearing surface of internal joint prosthesis — *see* Complications, joint prosthesis, mechanical, wear of articular bearing surfaces, by site
  device, implant or graft — *see* Complications, by site, mechanical complication
  tooth, teeth (approximal) (hard tissues) (interproximal) (occlusal) K03.0
Weather, weathered
  effects of
    cold T69.9 ☑
      specified effect NEC T69.8 ☑
    hot — *see* Heat
  skin L57.8
Weaver's syndrome Q87.3
Web, webbed (congenital)
  duodenal Q43.8
  esophagus Q39.4
  fingers Q70.1- ☑
  larynx (glottic) (subglottic) Q31.0
  neck (pterygium colli) Q18.3
  Paterson-Kelly D50.1
  popliteal syndrome Q87.89
  toes Q70.3- ☑
Weber-Christian disease M35.6
Weber-Cockayne syndrome (epidermolysis bullosa) Q81.8
Weber-Gubler syndrome G46.3
Weber-Leyden syndrome G46.3
Weber-Osler syndrome I78.0
Weber's paralysis or syndrome G46.3
Wedge-shaped or wedging vertebra — *see* Collapse, vertebra NEC
Wegener's granulomatosis or syndrome M31.30
  with
    kidney involvement M31.31
    lung involvement M31.30
      with kidney involvement M31.31
Wegner's disease A50.02
Weight
  1000-2499 grams at birth (low) — *see* Low, birthweight
  999 grams or less at birth (extremely low) — *see* Low, birthweight, extreme

Weight — *continued*
  gain (abnormal) (excessive) R63.5
    in pregnancy — *see* Pregnancy, complicated by, excessive weight gain
    low — *see* Pregnancy, complicated by, insufficient, weight gain
  loss (abnormal) (cause unknown) R63.4
Weightlessness (effect of) T75.82 ☑
Weil (I)-**Marchesani syndrome** Q87.1
Weil's disease A27.0
Weingarten's syndrome J82
Weir Mitchell's disease I73.81
Weiss-Baker syndrome G90.09
Wells' disease L98.3
Wen — *see* Cyst, sebaceous
Wenckebach's block or phenomenon I44.1
Werdnig-Hoffmann syndrome (muscular atrophy) G12.0
Werlhof's disease D69.3
Wermer's disease or syndrome E31.21
Werner-His disease A79.0
Werner's disease or syndrome E34.8
Wernicke-Korsakoff's syndrome or psychosis (alcoholic) F10.96
  with dependence F10.26
  drug-induced
    due to drug abuse — *see* Abuse, drug, by type, with amnestic disorder
    due to drug dependence — *see* Dependence, drug, by type, with amnestic disorder
  nonalcoholic F04
Wernicke-Posadas disease B38.9
Wernicke's
  developmental aphasia F80.2
  disease or syndrome E51.2
  encephalopathy E51.2
  polioencephalitis, superior E51.2
West African fever B50.8
Westphal-Strümpell syndrome E83.01
West's syndrome — *see* Epilepsy, spasms
Wet
  feet, tropical (maceration) (syndrome) — *see* Immersion, foot
  lung (syndrome), newborn P22.1
Wharton's duct — *see* condition
Wheal — *see* Urticaria
Wheezing R06.2
Whiplash injury S13.4 ☑
Whipple's disease (*see also* subcategory M14.8-) K90.81
Whipworm (disease) (infection) (infestation) B79
Whistling face Q87.0
White (*see also* condition)
  kidney, small N03.9
  leg, puerperal, postpartum, childbirth O87.1
  mouth B37.0
  patches of mouth K13.29
  spot lesions, teeth
    chewing surface K02.51
    pit and fissure surface K02.51
    smooth surface K02.61
Whitehead L70.0
Whitlow (*see also* Cellulitis, digit)
  with lymphangitis — *see* Lymphangitis, acute, digit
  herpesviral B00.89
Whitmore's disease or fever — *see* Melioidosis
Whooping cough A37.90
  with pneumonia A37.91
    due to Bordetella
      bronchiseptica A37.81
      parapertussis A37.11
      pertussis A37.01
    specified organism NEC A37.81
  due to
    Bordetella
      bronchiseptica A37.80
        with pneumonia A37.81
      parapertussis A37.10
        with pneumonia A37.11
      pertussis A37.00
        with pneumonia A37.01
    specified NEC A37.80
      with pneumonia A37.81
Wichman's asthma J38.5
Wide cranial sutures, newborn P96.3
Widening aorta — *see* Ectasia, aorta
  with aneurysm — *see* Aneurysm, aorta
Wilkie's disease or syndrome K55.1

Wilkinson-Sneddon disease or syndrome L13.1
Willebrand (-Jürgens) **thrombopathy** D68.0
Willige-Hunt disease or syndrome G23.1
Wilms' tumor C64- ☑
Wilson-Mikity syndrome P27.0
Wilson's
  disease or syndrome E83.01
  hepatolenticular degeneration E83.01
  lichen ruber L43.9
Window (*see also* Imperfect, closure)
  aorticopulmonary Q21.4
Winter — *see* condition
Wiskott-Aldrich syndrome D82.0
Withdrawal state (*see also* Dependence, drug by type,
  with withdrawal)
  newborn
    correct therapeutic substance properly adminis-
      tered P96.2
    infant of dependent mother P96.1
  therapeutic substance, neonatal P96.2
Witts' anemia D50.8
Witzelsucht F07.0
Woakes' ethmoiditis or syndrome J33.1
Wolff-Hirschorn syndrome Q93.3
Wolff-Parkinson-White syndrome I45.6
Wolhynian fever A79.0
Wolman's disease E75.5
Wood lung or pneumonitis J67.8
Woolly, wooly hair (congenital) (nevus) Q84.1
Woolsorter's disease A22.1
Word
  blindness (congenital) (developmental) F81.0
  deafness (congenital) (developmental) H93.25
Worm(s) (infection) (infestation) (*see also* Infestation,
  helminth)
  guinea B72
  in intestine NEC B82.0
Worm-eaten soles A66.3
Worn out — *see* Exhaustion
  cardiac
    defibrillator (with synchronous cardiace pacemak-
      er) Z45.02
    pacemaker
      battery Z45.010
      lead Z45.018
    device, implant or graft — *see* Complications, by site,
      mechanical
Worried well Z71.1
Worries R45.82
Wound, open
  abdomen, abdominal
    wall S31.109 ☑
      with penetration into peritoneal cavity
        S31.609 ☑
      bite — *see* Bite, abdomen, wall
      epigastric region S31.102 ☑
        with penetration into peritoneal cavity
          S31.602 ☑
        bite — *see* Bite, abdomen, wall, epigastric
          region
        laceration — *see* Laceration, abdomen, wall,
          epigastric region
        puncture — *see* Puncture, abdomen, wall,
          epigastric region
      laceration — *see* Laceration, abdomen, wall
      left
        lower quadrant S31.104 ☑
          with penetration into peritoneal cavity
            S31.604 ☑
          bite — *see* Bite, abdomen, wall, left,
            lower quadrant
          laceration — *see* Laceration, abdomen,
            wall, left, lower quadrant
          puncture — *see* Puncture, abdomen,
            wall, left, lower quadrant
        upper quadrant S31.101 ☑
          with penetration into peritoneal cavity
            S31.601 ☑
          bite — *see* Bite, abdomen, wall, left, up-
            per quadrant
          laceration — *see* Laceration, abdomen,
            wall, left, upper quadrant
          puncture — *see* Puncture, abdomen,
            wall, left, upper quadrant
      periumbilic region S31.105 ☑
        with penetration into peritoneal cavity
          S31.605 ☑

Wound, open — *continued*
  abdomen, abdominal — *continued*
    wall — *continued*
      periumbilic region — *continued*
        bite — *see* Bite, abdomen, wall, periumbilic
          region
        laceration — *see* Laceration, abdomen, wall,
          periumbilic region
        puncture — *see* Puncture, abdomen, wall,
          periumbilic region
      puncture — *see* Puncture, abdomen, wall
      right
        lower quadrant S31.103 ☑
          with penetration into peritoneal cavity
            S31.603 ☑
          bite — *see* Bite, abdomen, wall, right,
            lower quadrant
          laceration — *see* Laceration, abdomen,
            wall, right, lower quadrant
          puncture — *see* Puncture, abdomen,
            wall, right, lower quadrant
        upper quadrant S31.100 ☑
          with penetration into peritoneal cavity
            S31.600 ☑
          bite — *see* Bite, abdomen, wall, right,
            upper quadrant
          laceration — *see* Laceration, abdomen,
            wall, right, upper quadrant
          puncture — *see* Puncture, abdomen,
            wall, right, upper quadrant
    alveolar (process) — *see* Wound, open, oral cavity
    ankle S91.00- ☑
      bite — *see* Bite, ankle
      laceration — *see* Laceration, ankle
      puncture — *see* Puncture, ankle
    antecubital space — *see* Wound, open, elbow
    anterior chamber, eye — *see* Wound, open, ocular
    anus S31.839 ☑
      bite S31.835 ☑
      laceration — *see* Laceration, anus
      puncture — *see* Puncture, anus
    arm (upper) S41.10- ☑
      with amputation — *see* Amputation, traumatic,
        arm
      bite — *see* Bite, arm
      forearm — *see* Wound, open, forearm
      laceration — *see* Laceration, arm
      puncture — *see* Puncture, arm
    auditory canal (external) (meatus) — *see* Wound, open,
      ear
    auricle, ear — *see* Wound, open, ear
    axilla — *see* Wound, open, arm
    back (*see also* Wound, open, thorax, back)
      lower S31.000 ☑
        with penetration into retroperitoneal space
          S31.001 ☑
        bite — *see* Bite, back, lower
        laceration — *see* Laceration, back, lower
        puncture — *see* Puncture, back, lower
    bite — *see* Bite
    blood vessel — *see* Injury, blood vessel
    breast S21.00- ☑
      with amputation — *see* Amputation, traumatic,
        breast
      bite — *see* Bite, breast
      laceration — *see* Laceration, breast
      puncture — *see* Puncture, breast
    buttock S31.809 ☑
      bite — *see* Bite, buttock
      laceration — *see* Laceration, buttock
      left S31.829 ☑
      puncture — *see* Puncture, buttock
      right S31.819 ☑
    calf — *see* Wound, open, leg
    canaliculus lacrimalis — *see* Wound, open, eyelid
    canthus, eye — *see* Wound, open, eyelid
    cervical esophagus S11.20 ☑
      bite S11.25 ☑
      laceration — *see* Laceration, esophagus, traumatic,
        cervical
      puncture — *see* Puncture, cervical esophagus
    cheek (external) S01.40- ☑
      bite — *see* Bite, cheek
      internal — *see* Wound, open, oral cavity
      laceration — *see* Laceration, cheek
      puncture — *see* Puncture, cheek

Wound, open — *continued*
  chest wall — *see* Wound, open, thorax
  chin — *see* Wound, open, head, specified site NEC
  choroid — *see* Wound, open, ocular
  ciliary body (eye) — *see* Wound, open, ocular
  clitoris S31.40 ☑
    with amputation — *see* Amputation, traumatic,
      clitoris
    bite S31.45 ☑
    laceration — *see* Laceration, vulva
    puncture — *see* Puncture, vulva
  conjunctiva — *see* Wound, open, ocular
  cornea — *see* Wound, open, ocular
  costal region — *see* Wound, open, thorax
  Descemet's membrane — *see* Wound, open, ocular
  digit(s)
    foot — *see* Wound, open, toe
    hand — *see* Wound, open, finger
  ear (canal) (external) S01.30- ☑
    with amputation — *see* Amputation, traumatic,
      ear
    bite — *see* Bite, ear
    drum S09.2- ☑
    laceration — *see* Laceration, ear
    puncture — *see* Puncture, ear
  elbow S51.00- ☑
    bite — *see* Bite, elbow
    laceration — *see* Laceration, elbow
    puncture — *see* Puncture, elbow
  epididymis — *see* Wound, open, testis
  epigastric region S31.102 ☑
    with penetration into peritoneal cavity S31.602 ☑
    bite — *see* Bite, abdomen, wall, epigastric region
    laceration — *see* Laceration, abdomen, wall, epi-
      gastric region
    puncture — *see* Puncture, abdomen, wall, epigas-
      tric region
  epiglottis — *see* Wound, open, neck, specified site
    NEC
  esophagus (thoracic) S27.819 ☑
    cervical — *see* Wound, open, cervical esophagus
    laceration S27.813 ☑
    specified type NEC S27.818 ☑
  eye — *see* Wound, open, ocular
  eyeball — *see* Wound, open, ocular
  eyebrow — *see* Wound, open, eyelid
  eyelid S01.10- ☑
    bite — *see* Bite, eyelid
    laceration — *see* Laceration, eyelid
    puncture — *see* Puncture, eyelid
  face NEC — *see* Wound, open, head, specified site NEC
  finger(s) S61.209 ☑
    with
      amputation — *see* Amputation, traumatic, fin-
        ger
      damage to nail S61.309 ☑
    bite — *see* Bite, finger
    index S61.208 ☑
      with
        damage to nail S61.308 ☑
      left S61.201 ☑
        with
          damage to nail S61.301 ☑
      right S61.200 ☑
        with
          damage to nail S61.300 ☑
    laceration — *see* Laceration, finger
    little S61.208 ☑
      with
        damage to nail S61.308 ☑
      left S61.207 ☑
        with damage to nail S61.307 ☑
      right S61.206 ☑
        with damage to nail S61.306 ☑
    middle S61.208 ☑
      with
        damage to nail S61.308 ☑
      left S61.203 ☑
        with damage to nail S61.303 ☑
      right S61.202 ☑
        with damage to nail S61.302 ☑
    puncture — *see* Puncture, finger
    ring S61.208 ☑
      with
        damage to nail S61.308 ☑
      left S61.205 ☑

Wound, open — *continued*
  finger(s) — *continued*
    ring — *continued*
      left — *continued*
        with damage to nail S61.305 ☑
      right S61.204 ☑
        with damage to nail S61.304 ☑
  flank — *see* Wound, open, abdomen, wall
  foot (except toe(s) alone) S91.30- ☑
    with amputation — *see* Amputation, traumatic, foot
    bite — *see* Bite, foot
    laceration — *see* Laceration, foot
    puncture — *see* Puncture, foot
    toe — *see* Wound, open, toe
  forearm S51.80- ☑
    with
      amputation — *see* Amputation, traumatic, forearm
    bite — *see* Bite, forearm
    elbow only — *see* Wound, open, elbow
    laceration — *see* Laceration, forearm
    puncture — *see* Puncture, forearm
  forehead — *see* Wound, open, head, specified site NEC
  genital organs, external
    with amputation — *see* Amputation, traumatic, genital organs
    bite — *see* Bite, genital organ
    female S31.502 ☑
      vagina S31.40 ☑
      vulva S31.40 ☑
    laceration — *see* Laceration, genital organ
    male S31.501 ☑
      penis S31.20 ☑
      scrotum S31.30 ☑
      testes S31.30 ☑
    puncture — *see* Puncture, genital organ
  globe (eye) — *see* Wound, open, ocular
  groin — *see* Wound, open, abdomen, wall
  gum — *see* Wound, open, oral cavity
  hand S61.40- ☑
    with
      amputation — *see* Amputation, traumatic, hand
    bite — *see* Bite, hand
    finger(s) — *see* Wound, open, finger
    laceration — *see* Laceration, hand
    puncture — *see* Puncture, hand
    thumb — *see* Wound, open, thumb
  head S01.90 ☑
    bite — *see* Bite, head
    cheek — *see* Wound, open, cheek
    ear — *see* Wound, open, ear
    eyelid — *see* Wound, open, eyelid
    laceration — *see* Laceration, head
    lip — *see* Wound, open, lip
    nose S01.20 ☑
    oral cavity — *see* Wound, open, oral cavity
    puncture — *see* Puncture, head
    scalp — *see* Wound, open, scalp
    specified site NEC S01.80 ☑
    temporomandibular area — *see* Wound, open, cheek
  heel — *see* Wound, open, foot
  hip S71.00- ☑
    with amputation — *see* Amputation, traumatic, hip
    bite — *see* Bite, hip
    laceration — *see* Laceration, hip
    puncture — *see* Puncture, hip
  hymen S31.40 ☑
    bite — *see* Bite, vulva
    laceration — *see* Laceration, vagina
    puncture — *see* Puncture, vagina
  hypochondrium S31.109 ☑
    bite — *see* Bite, hypochondrium
    laceration — *see* Laceration, hypochondrium
    puncture — *see* Puncture, hypochondrium
  hypogastric region S31.109 ☑
    bite — *see* Bite, hypogastric region
    laceration — *see* Laceration, hypogastric region
    puncture — *see* Puncture, hypogastric region
  iliac (region) — *see* Wound, open, inguinal region
  inguinal region S31.109 ☑
    bite — *see* Bite, abdomen, wall, lower quadrant
    laceration — *see* Laceration, inguinal region

Wound, open — *continued*
  inguinal region — *continued*
    puncture — *see* Puncture, inguinal region
  instep — *see* Wound, open, foot
  interscapular region — *see* Wound, open, thorax, back
  intraocular — *see* Wound, open, ocular
  iris — *see* Wound, open, ocular
  jaw — *see* Wound, open, head, specified site NEC
  knee S81.00- ☑
    bite — *see* Bite, knee
    laceration — *see* Laceration, knee
    puncture — *see* Puncture, knee
  labium (majus) (minus) — *see* Wound, open, vulva
  laceration — *see* Laceration, by site
  lacrimal duct — *see* Wound, open, eyelid
  larynx S11.019 ☑
    bite — *see* Bite, larynx
    laceration — *see* Laceration, larynx
    puncture — *see* Puncture, larynx
  left
    lower quadrant S31.104 ☑
      with penetration into peritoneal cavity S31.604 ☑
      bite — *see* Bite, abdomen, wall, left, lower quadrant
      laceration — *see* Laceration, abdomen, wall, left, lower quadrant
      puncture — *see* Puncture, abdomen, wall, left, lower quadrant
    upper quadrant S31.101 ☑
      with penetration into peritoneal cavity S31.601 ☑
      bite — *see* Bite, abdomen, wall, left, upper quadrant
      laceration — *see* Laceration, abdomen, wall, left, upper quadrant
      puncture — *see* Puncture, abdomen, wall, left, upper quadrant
  leg (lower) S81.80- ☑
    with amputation — *see* Amputation, traumatic, leg
    ankle — *see* Wound, open, ankle
    bite — *see* Bite, leg
    foot — *see* Wound, open, foot
    knee — *see* Wound, open, knee
    laceration — *see* Laceration, leg
    puncture — *see* Puncture, leg
    toe — *see* Wound, open, toe
    upper — *see* Wound, open, thigh
  lip S01.501 ☑
    bite — *see* Bite, lip
    laceration — *see* Laceration, lip
    puncture — *see* Puncture, lip
  loin S31.109 ☑
    bite — *see* Bite, abdomen, wall
    laceration — *see* Laceration, loin
    puncture — *see* Puncture, loin
  lower back — *see* Wound, open, back, lower
  lumbar region — *see* Wound, open, back, lower
  malar region — *see* Wound, open, head, specified site NEC
  mammary — *see* Wound, open, breast
  mastoid region — *see* Wound, open, head, specified site NEC
  mouth — *see* Wound, open, oral cavity
  nail
    finger — *see* Wound, open, finger, with damage to nail
    toe — *see* Wound, open, toe, with damage to nail
  nape (neck) — *see* Wound, open, neck
  nasal (septum) (sinus) — *see* Wound, open, nose
  nasopharynx — *see* Wound, open, head, specified site NEC
  neck S11.90 ☑
    bite — *see* Bite, neck
    involving
      cervical esophagus S11.20 ☑
      larynx — *see* Wound, open, larynx
      pharynx S11.20 ☑
      thyroid S11.10 ☑
      trachea (cervical) S11.029 ☑
        bite — *see* Bite, trachea
        laceration S11.021 ☑
          with foreign body S11.022 ☑
        puncture S11.023 ☑
          with foreign body S11.024 ☑

Wound, open — *continued*
  neck — *continued*
    laceration — *see* Laceration, neck
    puncture — *see* Puncture, neck
    specified site NEC S11.80 ☑
      specified type NEC S11.89 ☑
  nose (septum) (sinus) S01.20 ☑
    with amputation — *see* Amputation, traumatic, nose
    bite — *see* Bite, nose
    laceration — *see* Laceration, nose
    puncture — *see* Puncture, nose
  ocular S05.90 ☑
    avulsion (traumatic enucleation) S05.7- ☑
    eyeball S05.6- ☑
      with foreign body S05.5- ☑
    eyelid — *see* Wound, open, eyelid
    laceration and rupture S05.3- ☑
      with prolapse or loss of intraocular tissue S05.2- ☑
    orbit (penetrating) (with or without foreign body) S05.4- ☑
    periocular area — *see* Wound, open, eyelid
    specified NEC S05.8X- ☑
  oral cavity S01.502 ☑
    bite S01.552 ☑
    laceration — *see* Laceration, oral cavity
    puncture — *see* Puncture, oral cavity
  orbit — *see* Wound, open, ocular, orbit
  palate — *see* Wound, open, oral cavity
  palm — *see* Wound, open, hand
  pelvis, pelvic (*see also* Wound, open, back, lower)
    girdle — *see* Wound, open, hip
  penetrating — *see* Puncture, by site
  penis S31.20 ☑
    with amputation — *see* Amputation, traumatic, penis
    bite S31.25 ☑
    laceration — *see* Laceration, penis
    puncture — *see* Puncture, penis
  perineum
    bite — *see* Bite, perineum
    female S31.502 ☑
    laceration — *see* Laceration, perineum
    male S31.501 ☑
    puncture — *see* Puncture, perineum
  periocular area (with or without lacrimal passages) — *see* Wound, open, eyelid
  periumbilic region S31.105 ☑
    with penetration into peritoneal cavity S31.605 ☑
    bite — *see* Bite, abdomen, wall, periumbilic region
    laceration — *see* Laceration, abdomen, wall, periumbilic region
    puncture — *see* Puncture, abdomen, wall, periumbilic region
  phalanges
    finger — *see* Wound, open, finger
    toe — *see* Wound, open, toe
  pharynx S11.20 ☑
  pinna — *see* Wound, open, ear
  popliteal space — *see* Wound, open, knee
  prepuce — *see* Wound, open, penis
  pubic region — *see* Wound, open, back, lower
  pudendum — *see* Wound, open, genital organs, external
  puncture wound — *see* Puncture
  rectovaginal septum — *see* Wound, open, vagina
  right
    lower quadrant S31.103 ☑
      with penetration into peritoneal cavity S31.603 ☑
      bite — *see* Bite, abdomen, wall, right, lower quadrant
      laceration — *see* Laceration, abdomen, wall, right, lower quadrant
      puncture — *see* Puncture, abdomen, wall, right, lower quadrant
    upper quadrant S31.100 ☑
      with penetration into peritoneal cavity S31.600 ☑
      bite — *see* Bite, abdomen, wall, right, upper quadrant
      laceration — *see* Laceration, abdomen, wall, right, upper quadrant
      puncture — *see* Puncture, abdomen, wall, right, upper quadrant

☑ **Additional Character Required** — **Refer to the Tabular List for Character Selection**   ▽ **Subterms under main terms may continue to next column or page**

Wound, open — *continued*
  sacral region — *see* Wound, open, back, lower
  sacroiliac region — *see* Wound, open, back, lower
  salivary gland — *see* Wound, open, oral cavity
  scalp S01.00 ☑
    bite S01.05 ☑
    laceration — *see* Laceration, scalp
    puncture — *see* Puncture, scalp
  scalpel, newborn (birth injury) P15.8
  scapular region — *see* Wound, open, shoulder
  sclera — *see* Wound, open, ocular
  scrotum S31.30 ☑
    with amputation — *see* Amputation, traumatic, scrotum
    bite S31.35 ☑
    laceration — *see* Laceration, scrotum
    puncture — *see* Puncture, scrotum
  shin — *see* Wound, open, leg
  shoulder S41.00- ☑
    with amputation — *see* Amputation, traumatic, arm
    bite — *see* Bite, shoulder
    laceration — *see* Laceration, shoulder
    puncture — *see* Puncture, shoulder
  skin NOS T14.8
  spermatic cord — *see* Wound, open, testis
  sternal region — *see* Wound, open, thorax, front wall
  submaxillary region — *see* Wound, open, head, specified site NEC
  submental region — *see* Wound, open, head, specified site NEC
  subungual
    finger(s) — *see* Wound, open, finger
    toe(s) — *see* Wound, open, toe
  supraclavicular region — *see* Wound, open, neck, specified site NEC
  temple, temporal region — *see* Wound, open, head, specified site NEC
  temporomandibular area — *see* Wound, open, cheek
  testis S31.30 ☑
    with amputation — *see* Amputation, traumatic, testes
    bite S31.35 ☑
    laceration — *see* Laceration, testis
    puncture — *see* Puncture, testis
  thigh S71.10- ☑
    with amputation — *see* Amputation, traumatic, hip
    bite — *see* Bite, thigh
    laceration — *see* Laceration, thigh
    puncture — *see* Puncture, thigh
  thorax, thoracic (wall) S21.90 ☑
    back S21.20- ☑
      with penetration S21.40 ☑
    bite — *see* Bite, thorax
    breast — *see* Wound, open, breast
    front S21.10- ☑
      with penetration S21.30 ☑
    laceration — *see* Laceration, thorax
    puncture — *see* Puncture, thorax
  throat — *see* Wound, open, neck
  thumb S61.009 ☑
    with
      amputation — *see* Amputation, traumatic, thumb
      damage to nail S61.109 ☑
    bite — *see* Bite, thumb
    laceration — *see* Laceration, thumb
    left S61.002 ☑
      with
        damage to nail S61.102 ☑
    puncture — *see* Puncture, thumb
    right S61.001 ☑
      with
        damage to nail S61.101 ☑
  thyroid (gland) — *see* Wound, open, neck, thyroid
  toe(s) S91.109 ☑
    with
      amputation — *see* Amputation, traumatic, toe
      damage to nail S91.209 ☑
    bite — *see* Bite, toe
    great S91.103 ☑
      with
        damage to nail S91.203 ☑
      left S91.102 ☑

Wound, open — *continued*
  toe(s) — *continued*
    great — *continued*
      left — *continued*
        with
          damage to nail S91.202 ☑
      right S91.101 ☑
        with
          damage to nail S91.201 ☑
    laceration — *see* Laceration, toe
    lesser S91.106 ☑
      with
        damage to nail S91.206 ☑
      left S91.105 ☑
        with
          damage to nail S91.205 ☑
      right S91.104 ☑
        with
          damage to nail S91.204 ☑
    puncture — *see* Puncture, toe
  tongue — *see* Wound, open, oral cavity
  trachea (cervical region) — *see* Wound, open, neck, trachea
  tunica vaginalis — *see* Wound, open, testis
  tympanum, tympanic membrane S09.2- ☑
    laceration — *see* Laceration, ear, drum
    puncture — *see* Puncture, tympanum
  umbilical region — *see* Wound, open, abdomen, wall, periumbilic region
  uvula — *see* Wound, open, oral cavity
  vagina S31.40 ☑
    bite S31.45 ☑
    laceration — *see* Laceration, vagina
    puncture — *see* Puncture, vagina
  vitreous (humor) — *see* Wound, open, ocular
  vocal cord S11.039 ☑
    bite — *see* Bite, vocal cord
    laceration S11.031 ☑
      with foreign body S11.032 ☑
    puncture S11.033 ☑
      with foreign body S11.034 ☑
  vulva S31.40 ☑
    with amputation — *see* Amputation, traumatic, vulva
    bite S31.45 ☑
    laceration — *see* Laceration, vulva
    puncture — *see* Puncture, vulva
  wrist S61.50- ☑
    bite — *see* Bite, wrist
    laceration — *see* Laceration, wrist
    puncture — *see* Puncture, wrist
Wound, superficial — *see* Injury (*see also* specified injury type)
Wright's syndrome G54.0
Wrist — *see* condition
Wrong drug (by accident) (given in error) — *see* Table of Drugs and Chemicals, by drug, poisoning
Wry neck — *see* Torticollis
Wuchereria (bancrofti) **infestation** B74.0
Wuchereriasis B74.0
Wuchernde Struma Langhans C73

X

Xanthelasma (eyelid) (palpebrarum) H02.60
  left H02.66
    lower H02.65
    upper H02.64
  right H02.63
    lower H02.62
    upper H02.61
Xanthelasmatosis (essential) E78.2
Xanthinuria, hereditary E79.8
Xanthoastrocytoma
  specified site — *see* Neoplasm, malignant, by site
  unspecified site C71.9
Xanthofibroma — *see* Neoplasm, connective tissue, benign
Xanthogranuloma D76.3
Xanthoma(s), xanthomatosis (primary) (familial) (hereditary) E75.5
  with
    hyperlipoproteinemia
      Type I E78.3
      Type III E78.2
      Type IV E78.1

Xanthoma(s), xanthomatosis — *continued*
  with — *continued*
    hyperlipoproteinemia — *continued*
      Type V E78.3
    cerebrotendinous E75.5
    cutaneotendinous E75.5
    disseminatum (skin) E78.2
    eruptive E78.2
    hypercholesterinemic E78.0
    hypercholesterolemic E78.0
    hyperlipidemic E78.5
    joint E75.5
    multiple (skin) E78.2
    tendon (sheath) E75.5
    tuberosum E78.2
    tuberous E78.2
    tubo-eruptive E78.2
    verrucous, oral mucosa K13.4
Xanthosis R23.8
Xenophobia F40.10
Xeroderma (*see also* Ichthyosis)
  acquired L85.0
    eyelid H01.149
      left H01.146
        lower H01.145
        upper H01.144
      right H01.143
        lower H01.142
        upper H01.141
  pigmentosum Q82.1
  vitamin A deficiency E50.8
Xerophthalmia (vitamin A deficiency) E50.7
  unrelated to vitamin A deficiency — *see* Keratoconjunctivitis
Xerosis
  conjunctiva H11.14- ☑
    with Bitot's spots (*see also* Pigmentation, conjunctiva)
      vitamin A deficiency E50.1
    vitamin A deficiency E50.0
  cornea H18.89- ☑
    with ulceration — *see* Ulcer, cornea
      vitamin A deficiency E50.3
    vitamin A deficiency E50.2
  cutis L85.3
  skin L85.3
Xerostomia K11.7
Xiphopagus Q89.4
XO syndrome Q96.9
X-ray (of)
  abnormal findings — *see* Abnormal, diagnostic imaging
  breast (mammogram) (routine) Z12.31
  chest
    routine (as part of a general medical examination) Z00.00
      with abnormal findings Z00.01
  routine (as part of a general medical examination) Z00.00
    with abnormal findings Z00.01
XXXXY syndrome Q98.1
XXY syndrome Q98.0

Y

Yaba pox (virus disease) B08.72
Yatapoxvirus B08.70
  specified NEC B08.79
Yawning R06.89
  psychogenic F45.8
Yaws A66.9
  cutaneous, less than five years after infection A66.2
  bone lesions A66.6
  butter A66.1
  chancre A66.0
  early (cutaneous) (macular) (maculopapular) (micropapular) (papular) A66.2
    frambeside A66.2
    skin lesions NEC A66.2
  eyelid A66.2
  ganglion A66.6
  gangosis, gangosa A66.5
  gumma, gummata A66.4
    bone A66.6
  gummatous
    frambeside A66.4
    osteitis A66.6
    periostitis A66.6

Yaws — *continued*
hydrarthrosis (*see also* subcategory M14.8-) A66.6
hyperkeratosis (early) (late) A66.3
initial lesions A66.0
joint lesions (*see also* subcategory M14.8-) A66.6
juxta-articular nodules A66.7
late nodular (ulcerated) A66.4
latent (without clinical manifestations) (with positive
serology) A66.8
mother A66.0
mucosal A66.7
multiple papillomata A66.1
nodular, late (ulcerated) A66.4
osteitis A66.6
papilloma, plantar or palmar A66.1
periostitis (hypertrophic) A66.6
specified NEC A66.7

Yaws — *continued*
ulcers A66.4
wet crab A66.1
Yeast infection (*see also* Candidiasis) B37.9
Yellow
atrophy (liver) — *see* Failure, hepatic
fever — *see* Fever, yellow
jack — *see* Fever, yellow
jaundice — *see* Jaundice
nail syndrome L60.5
Yersiniosis (*see also* Infection, Yersinia)
extraintestinal A28.2
intestinal A04.6

Z

Zahorsky's syndrome (herpangina) B08.5

Zellweger's syndrome Q87.89
Zenker's diverticulum (esophagus) K22.5
Ziehen-Oppenheim disease G24.1
Zieve's syndrome K70.0
Zinc
deficiency, dietary E60
metabolism disorder E83.2
Zollinger-Ellison syndrome E16.4
Zona — *see* Herpes, zoster
Zoophobia F40.218
Zoster (herpes) — *see* Herpes, zoster
Zygomycosis B46.9
specified NEC B46.8
Zymotic — *see* condition

ICD-10-CM Neoplasm Table

Note: The list below gives the code number for neoplasms by anatomical site. For each site there are six possible code numbers according to whether the neoplasm in question is malignant, benign, in situ, of uncertain behavior, or of unspecified nature. The description of the neoplasm will often indicate which of the six columns is appropriate; e.g., malignant melanoma of skin, benign fibroadenoma of breast, carcinoma in situ of cervix uteri. Where such descriptors are not present, the remainder of the Index should be consulted where guidance is given to the appropriate column for each morphological (histological) variety listed; e.g., Mesonephroma – see Neoplasm, malignant; Embryoma (see also Neoplasm, uncertain behavior); Disease, Bowen's – see Neoplasm, skin, in situ. However, the guidance in the Index can be overridden if one of the descriptors mentioned above is present; e.g., malignant adenoma of colon is coded to C18.9 and not to D12.6 as the adjective "malignant" overrides the Index entry "Adenoma (see also Neoplasm, benign)." Codes listed with a dash -, following the code have a required 5th character for laterality. The tabular list must be reviewed for the complete code.

	Malignant Primary	Malignant Secondary	Ca in situ	Benign	Uncertain	Unspecified Behavior
Neoplasm, neoplastic	C80.1	C79.9	D09.9	D36.9	D48.9	D49.9
abdomen, abdominal	C76.2	C79.8-☑	D09.8	D36.7	D48.7	D49.89
cavity	C76.2	C79.8-☑	D09.8	D36.7	D48.7	D49.89
organ	C76.2	C79.8-☑	D09.8	D36.7	D48.7	D49.89
viscera	C76.2	C79.8-☑	D09.8	D36.7	D48.7	D49.89
wall — *see also* Neoplasm, abdomen, wall, skin	C44.509	C79.2	D04.5	D23.5	D48.5	D49.2
connective tissue	C49.4	C79.8-☑	—	D21.4	D48.1	D49.2
skin	C44.509	—	—	—	—	—
basal cell carcinoma	C44.519	—	—	—	—	—
specified type NEC	C44.599	—	—	—	—	—
squamous cell carcinoma	C44.529	—	—	—	—	—
abdominopelvic	C76.8	C79.8-☑	—	D36.7	D48.7	D49.89
accessory sinus — *see* Neoplasm, sinus						
acoustic nerve	C72.4-☑	C79.49	—	D33.3	D43.3	D49.7
adenoid (pharynx) (tissue)	C11.1	C79.89	D00.08	D10.6	D37.05	D49.0
adipose tissue — *see also* Neoplasm, connective, tissue	C49.4	C79.89	—	D21.9	D48.1	D49.2
adnexa (uterine)	C57.4	C79.89	D07.39	D28.7	D39.8	D49.5
adrenal	C74.9-☑	C79.7-☑	D09.3	D35.0-☑	D44.1-☑	D49.7
capsule	C74.9-☑	C79.7-☑	D09.3	D35.0-☑	D44.1-☑	D49.7
cortex	C74.0-☑	C79.7-☑	D09.3	D35.0-☑	D44.1-☑	D49.7
gland	C74.9-☑	C79.7-☑	D09.3	D35.0-☑	D44.1-☑	D49.7
medulla	C74.1-☑	C79.7-☑	D09.3	D35.0-☑	D44.1-☑	D49.7
ala nasi (external) — *see also* Neoplasm, skin, nose	C44.301	C79.2	D04.39	D23.39	D48.5	D49.2
alimentary canal or tract NEC	C26.9	C78.80	D01.9	D13.9	D37.9	D49.0
alveolar	C03.9	C79.89	D00.03	D10.39	D37.09	D49.0
mucosa	C03.9	C79.89	D00.03	D10.39	D37.09	D49.0
lower	C03.1	C79.89	D00.03	D10.39	D37.09	D49.0
upper	C03.0	C79.89	D00.03	D10.39	D37.09	D49.0
ridge or process	C41.1	C79.51	—	D16.5	D48.0	D49.2
carcinoma	C03.9	C79.8-☑	—	—	—	—
lower	C03.1	C79.8-☑	—	—	—	—
upper	C03.0	C79.8-☑	—	—	—	—
lower	C41.1	C79.51	—	D16.5	D48.0	D49.2
mucosa	C03.9	C79.89	D00.03	D10.39	D37.09	D49.0
lower	C03.1	C79.89	D00.03	D10.39	D37.09	D49.0
upper	C03.0	C79.89	D00.03	D10.39	D37.09	D49.0
upper	C41.0	C79.51	—	D16.4	D48.0	D49.2
sulcus	C06.1	C79.89	D00.02	D10.39	D37.09	D49.0
alveolus	C03.9	C79.89	D00.03	D10.39	D37.09	D49.0
lower	C03.1	C79.89	D00.03	D10.39	D37.09	D49.0
upper	C03.0	C79.89	D00.03	D10.39	D37.09	D49.0
ampulla of Vater	C24.1	C78.89	D01.5	D13.5	D37.6	D49.0
ankle NEC	C76.5-☑	C79.89	D04.7-☑	D36.7	D48.7	D49.89

	Malignant Primary	Malignant Secondary	Ca in situ	Benign	Uncertain	Unspecified Behavior
Neoplasm, neoplastic — *continued*						
anorectum, anorectal (junction)	C21.8	C78.5	D01.3	D12.9	D37.8	D49.0
antecubital fossa or space	C76.4-☑	C79.89	D04.6-☑	D36.7	D48.7	D49.89
antrum (Highmore) (maxillary)	C31.0	C78.39	D02.3	D14.0	D38.5	D49.1
pyloric	C16.3	C78.89	D00.2	D13.1	D37.1	D49.0
tympanicum	C30.1	C78.39	D02.3	D14.0	D38.5	D49.1
anus, anal	C21.0	C78.5	D01.3	D12.9	D37.8	D49.0
canal	C21.1	C78.5	D01.3	D12.9	D37.8	D49.0
cloacogenic zone	C21.2	C78.5	D01.3	D12.9	D37.8	D49.0
margin — *see also* Neoplasm, anus, skin	C44.500	C79.2	D04.5	D23.5	D48.5	D49.2
overlapping lesion with rectosigmoid junction or rectum	C21.8	—	—	—	—	—
skin	C44.500	C79.2	D04.5	D23.5	D48.5	D49.2
basal cell carcinoma	C44.510	—	—	—	—	—
specified type NEC	C44.590	—	—	—	—	—
squamous cell carcinoma	C44.520	—	—	—	—	—
sphincter	C21.1	C78.5	D01.3	D12.9	D37.8	D49.0
aorta (thoracic)	C49.3	C79.89	—	D21.3	D48.1	D49.2
abdominal	C49.4	C79.89	—	D21.4	D48.1	D49.2
aortic body	C75.5	C79.89	—	D35.6	D44.7	D49.7
aponeurosis	C49.9	C79.89	—	D21.9	D48.1	D49.2
palmar	C49.1-☑	C79.89	—	D21.1-☑	D48.1	D49.2
plantar	C49.2-☑	C79.89	—	D21.2-☑	D48.1	D49.2
appendix	C18.1	C78.5	D01.0	D12.1	D37.3	D49.0
arachnoid	C70.9	C79.49	—	D32.9	D42.9	D49.7
cerebral	C70.0	C79.32	—	D32.0	D42.0	D49.7
spinal	C70.1	C79.49	—	D32.1	D42.1	D49.7
areola	C50.0-☑	C79.81	D05-☑	D24-☑	D48.6-☑	D49.3
arm NEC	C76.4-☑	C79.89	D04.6-☑	D36.7	D48.7	D49.89
artery — *see* Neoplasm, connective tissue						
aryepiglottic fold	C13.1	C79.89	D00.08	D10.7	D37.05	D49.0
hypopharyngeal aspect	C13.1	C79.89	D00.08	D10.7	D37.05	D49.0
laryngeal aspect	C32.1	C78.39	D02.0	D14.1	D38.0	D49.1
marginal zone	C13.1	C79.89	D00.08	D10.7	D37.05	D49.0
arytenoid (cartilage)	C32.3	C78.39	D02.0	D14.1	D38.0	D49.1
fold — *see* Neoplasm, aryepiglottic						
associated with transplanted organ	C80.2	—	—	—	—	—
atlas	C41.2	C79.51	—	D16.6	D48.0	D49.2
atrium, cardiac	C38.0	C79.89	—	D15.1	D48.7	D49.89
auditory						
canal (external) (skin) A81	C44.20-☑	C79.2	D04.2-☑	D23.2-☑	D48.5	D49.2
internal	C30.1	C78.39	D02.3	D14.0	D38.5	D49.1
nerve	C72.4-☑	C79.49	—	D33.3	D43.3	D49.7
tube	C30.1	C78.39	D02.3	D14.0	D38.5	D49.1
opening	C11.2	C79.89	D00.08	D10.6	D37.05	D49.0
auricle, ear — *see also* Neoplasm, skin, ear	C44.20-☑	C79.2	D04.2-☑	D23.2-☑	D48.5	D49.2
auricular canal (external) — *see also* Neoplasm, skin, ear	C44.20-☑	C79.2	D04.2-☑	D23.2-☑	D48.5	D49.2
internal	C30.1	C78.39	D02.3	D14.0	D38.5	D49.2
autonomic nerve or nervous system NEC (see Neoplasm, nerve, peripheral)						
axilla, axillary	C76.1	C79.89	D09.8	D36.7	D48.7	D49.89
fold — *see also* Neoplasm, skin, trunk	C44.509	C79.2	D04.5	D23.5	D48.5	D49.2
back NEC	C76.8	C79.89	D04.5	D36.7	D48.7	D49.89

Neoplasm Table

Neoplasm, Bartholin's gland — Neoplasm, brain NEC

	Malignant Primary	Malignant Secondary	Ca in situ	Benign	Uncertain	Unspecified Behavior
Neoplasm, neoplastic — *continued*						
Bartholin's gland	C51.0	C79.82	D07.1	D28.0	D39.8	D49.5
basal ganglia	C71.0	C79.31	—	D33.0	D43.0	D49.6
basis pedunculi	C71.7	C79.31	—	D33.1	D43.1	D49.6
bile or biliary (tract)	C24.9	C78.89	D01.5	D13.5	D37.6	D49.0
canaliculi (biliferi) (intrahepatic)	C22.1	C78.7	D01.5	D13.4	D37.6	D49.0
canals, interlobular	C22.1	C78.89	D01.5	D13.4	D37.6	D49.0
duct or passage (common) (cystic) (extrahepatic)	C24.0	C78.89	D01.5	D13.5	D37.6	D49.0
interlobular	C22.1	C78.89	D01.5	D13.4	D37.6	D49.0
intrahepatic	C22.1	C78.7	D01.5	D13.4	D37.6	D49.0
and extrahepatic	C24.8	C78.89	D01.5	D13.5	D37.6	D49.0
bladder (urinary)	C67.9	C79.11	D09.0	D30.3	D41.4	D49.4
dome	C67.1	C79.11	D09.0	D30.3	D41.4	D49.4
neck	C67.5	C79.11	D09.0	D30.3	D41.4	D49.4
orifice	C67.9	C79.11	D09.0	D30.3	D41.4	D49.4
ureteric	C67.6	C79.11	D09.0	D30.3	D41.4	D49.4
urethral	C67.5	C79.11	D09.0	D30.3	D41.4	D49.4
overlapping lesion	C67.8	—	—	—	—	—
sphincter	C67.8	C79.11	D09.0	D30.3	D41.4	D49.4
trigone	C67.0	C79.11	D09.0	D30.3	D41.4	D49.4
urachus	C67.7	C79.11	D09.0	D30.3	D41.4	D49.4
wall	C67.9	C79.11	D09.0	D30.3	D41.4	D49.4
anterior	C67.3	C79.11	D09.0	D30.3	D41.4	D49.4
lateral	C67.2	C79.11	D09.0	D30.3	D41.4	D49.4
posterior	C67.4	C79.11	D09.0	D30.3	D41.4	D49.4
blood vessel — *see* Neoplasm, connective tissue						
bone (periosteum)	C41.9	C79.51	—	D16.9	D48.0	D49.2
acetabulum	C41.4	C79.51	—	D16.8	D48.0	D49.2
ankle	C40.3-✓	C79.51	—	D16.3-✓	—	—
arm NEC	C40.0-✓	C79.51	—	D16.0-✓	—	—
astragalus	C40.3-✓	C79.51	—	D16.3-✓	—	—
atlas	C41.2	C79.51	—	D16.6	D48.0	D49.2
axis	C41.2	C79.51	—	D16.6	D48.0	D49.2
back NEC	C41.2	C79.51	—	D16.6	D48.0	D49.2
calcaneus	C40.3-✓	C79.51	—	D16.3-✓	—	—
calvarium	C41.0	C79.51	—	D16.4	D48.0	D49.2
carpus (any)	C40.1-✓	C79.51	—	D16.1-✓	—	—
cartilage NEC	C41.9	C79.51	—	D16.9	D48.0	D49.2
clavicle	C41.3	C79.51	—	D16.7	D48.0	D49.2
clivus	C41.0	C79.51	—	D16.4	D48.0	D49.2
coccygeal vertebra	C41.4	C79.51	—	D16.8	D48.0	D49.2
coccyx	C41.4	C79.51	—	D16.8	D48.0	D49.2
costal cartilage	C41.3	C79.51	—	D16.7	D48.0	D49.2
costovertebral joint	C41.3	C79.51	—	D16.7	D48.0	D49.2
cranial	C41.0	C79.51	—	D16.4	D48.0	D49.2
cuboid	C40.3-✓	C79.51	—	D16.3-✓	—	—
cuneiform	C41.9	C79.51	—	D16.9	D48.0	D49.2
elbow	C40.0-✓	C79.51	—	D16.0-✓	—	—
ethmoid (labyrinth)	C41.0	C79.51	—	D16.4	D48.0	D49.2
face	C41.0	C79.51	—	D16.4	D48.0	D49.2
femur (any part)	C40.2-✓	C79.51	—	D16.2-✓	—	—
fibula (any part)	C40.2-✓	C79.51	—	D16.2-✓	—	—
finger (any)	C40.1-✓	C79.51	—	D16.1-✓	—	—
foot	C40.3-✓	C79.51	—	D16.3-✓	—	—
forearm	C40.0-✓	C79.51	—	D16.0-✓	—	—
frontal	C41.0	C79.51	—	D16.4	D48.0	D49.2
hand	C40.1-✓	C79.51	—	D16.1-✓	—	—
heel	C40.3-✓	C79.51	—	D16.3-✓	—	—
hip	C41.4	C79.51	—	D16.8	D48.0	D49.2
humerus (any part)	C40.0-✓	C79.51	—	D16.0-✓	—	—
hyoid	C41.0	C79.51	—	D16.4	D48.0	D49.2
ilium	C41.4	C79.51	—	D16.8	D48.0	D49.2
innominate	C41.4	C79.51	—	D16.8	D48.0	D49.2
intervertebral cartilage or disc	C41.2	C79.51	—	D16.6	D48.0	D49.2
ischium	C41.4	C79.51	—	D16.8	D48.0	D49.2
jaw (lower)	C41.1	C79.51	—	D16.5	D48.0	D49.2
knee	C40.2-✓	C79.51	—	D16.2-✓	—	—
leg NEC	C40.2-✓	C79.51	—	D16.2-✓	—	—
limb NEC	C40.9-✓	C79.51	—	D16.9	—	—

	Malignant Primary	Malignant Secondary	Ca in situ	Benign	Uncertain	Unspecified Behavior
Neoplasm, neoplastic — *continued*						
bone — *continued*						
limb — *continued*						
lower (long bones)	C40.2-✓	C79.51	—	D16.2-✓	—	—
short bones	C40.3-✓	C79.51	—	D16.3-✓	—	—
upper (long bones)	C40.0-✓	C79.51	—	D16.0-✓	—	—
short bones	C40.1-✓	C79.51	—	D16.1-✓	—	—
malar	C41.0	C79.51	—	D16.4	D48.0	D49.2
mandible	C41.1	C79.51	—	D16.5	D48.0	D49.2
marrow NEC (any bone)	C96.9	C79.52	—	—	D47.9	D49.89
mastoid	C41.0	C79.51	—	D16.4	D48.0	D49.2
maxilla, maxillary (superior)	C41.0	C79.51	—	D16.4	D48.0	D49.2
inferior	C41.1	C79.51	—	D16.5	D48.0	D49.2
metacarpus (any)	C40.1-✓	C79.51	—	D16.1-✓	—	—
metatarsus (any)	C40.3-✓	C79.51	—	D16.3-✓	—	—
navicular						
ankle	C40.3-✓	C79.51	—	—	—	—
hand	C40.1-✓	C79.51	—	—	—	—
nose, nasal	C41.0	C79.51	—	D16.4	D48.0	D49.2
occipital	C41.0	C79.51	—	D16.4	D48.0	D49.2
orbit	C41.0	C79.51	—	D16.4	D48.0	D49.2
overlapping sites	C40.8-✓	—	—	—	—	—
parietal	C41.0	C79.51	—	D16.4	D48.0	D49.2
patella	C40.2-✓	C79.51	—	—	—	—
pelvic	C41.4	C79.51	—	D16.8	D48.0	D49.2
phalanges						
foot	C40.3-✓	C79.51	—	—	—	—
hand	C40.1-✓	C79.51	—	—	—	—
pubic	C41.4	C79.51	—	D16.8	D48.0	D49.2
radius (any part)	C40.0-✓	C79.51	—	D16.0-✓	—	—
rib	C41.3	C79.51	—	D16.7	D48.0	D49.2
sacral vertebra	C41.4	C79.51	—	D16.8	D48.0	D49.2
sacrum	C41.4	C79.51	—	D16.8	D48.0	D49.2
scaphoid						
of ankle	C40.3-✓	C79.51	—	—	—	—
of hand	C40.1-✓	C79.51	—	—	—	—
scapula (any part)	C40.0-✓	C79.51	—	D16.0-✓	—	—
sella turcica	C41.0	C79.51	—	D16.4	D48.0	D49.2
shoulder	C40.0-✓	C79.51	—	D16.0-✓	—	—
skull	C41.0	C79.51	—	D16.4	D48.0	D49.2
sphenoid	C41.0	C79.51	—	D16.4	D48.0	D49.2
spine, spinal (column)	C41.2	C79.51	—	D16.6	D48.0	D49.2
coccyx	C41.4	C79.51	—	D16.8	D48.0	D49.2
sacrum	C41.4	C79.51	—	D16.8	D48.0	D49.2
sternum	C41.3	C79.51	—	D16.7	D48.0	D49.2
tarsus (any)	C40.3-✓	C79.51	—	—	—	—
temporal	C41.0	C79.51	—	D16.4	D48.0	D49.2
thumb	C40.1-✓	C79.51	—	—	—	—
tibia (any part)	C40.2-✓	C79.51	—	—	—	—
toe (any)	C40.3-✓	C79.51	—	—	—	—
trapezium	C40.1-✓	C79.51	—	—	—	—
trapezoid	C40.1-✓	C79.51	—	—	—	—
turbinate	C41.0	C79.51	—	D16.4	D48.0	D49.2
ulna (any part)	C40.0-✓	C79.51	—	D16.0-✓	—	—
unciform	C40.1-✓	C79.51	—	—	—	—
vertebra (column)	C41.2	C79.51	—	D16.6	D48.0	D49.2
coccyx	C41.4	C79.51	—	D16.8	D48.0	D49.2
sacrum	C41.4	C79.51	—	D16.8	D48.0	D49.2
vomer	C41.0	C79.51	—	D16.4	D48.0	D49.2
wrist	C40.1-✓	C79.51	—	—	—	—
xiphoid process	C41.3	C79.51	—	D16.7	D48.0	D49.2
zygomatic	C41.0	C79.51	—	D16.4	D48.0	D49.2
book-leaf (mouth) — ventral surface of tongue and floor of mouth	C06.89	C79.89	D00.00	D10.39	D37.09	D49.0
bowel — *see* Neoplasm, intestine						
brachial plexus	C47.1-✓	C79.89	—	D36.12	D48.2	D49.2
brain NEC	C71.9	C79.31	—	D33.2	D43.2	D49.6
basal ganglia	C71.0	C79.31	—	D33.0	D43.0	D49.6
cerebellopontine angle	C71.6	C79.31	—	D33.1	D43.1	D49.6
cerebellum NOS	C71.6	C79.31	—	D33.1	D43.1	D49.6
cerebrum	C71.0	C79.31	—	D33.0	D43.0	D49.6

☑ Additional Character Required — Refer to the Tabular List for Character Selection   Subterms under main terms may continue to next column or page

(handwritten note over Benign column: adenoma; handwritten note over Malignant Primary column, right side: melanoma)

Neoplasm, neoplastic — continued	Malignant Primary	Malignant Secondary	Ca in situ	Benign	Uncertain	Unspecified Behavior
brain — continued						
choroid plexus	C71.7	C79.31	—	D33.1	D43.1	D49.6
corpus callosum	C71.8	C79.31	—	D33.2	D43.2	D49.6
corpus striatum	C71.0	C79.31	—	D33.0	D43.0	D49.6
cortex (cerebral)	C71.0	C79.31	—	D33.0	D43.0	D49.6
frontal lobe	C71.1	C79.31	—	D33.0	D43.0	D49.6
globus pallidus	C71.0	C79.31	—	D33.0	D43.0	D49.6
hippocampus	C71.2	C79.31	—	D33.0	D43.0	D49.6
hypothalamus	C71.0	C79.31	—	D33.0	D43.0	D49.6
internal capsule	C71.0	C79.31	—	D33.0	D43.0	D49.6
medulla oblongata	C71.7	C79.31	—	D33.1	D43.1	D49.6
meninges	C70.0	C79.32	—	D32.0	D42.0	D49.7
midbrain	C71.7	C79.31	—	D33.1	D43.1	D49.6
occipital lobe	C71.4	C79.31	—	D33.0	D43.0	D49.6
overlapping lesion	C71.8	C79.31	—	—	—	—
parietal lobe	C71.3	C79.31	—	D33.0	D43.0	D49.6
peduncle	C71.7	C79.31	—	D33.1	D43.1	D49.6
pons	C71.7	C79.31	—	D33.1	D43.1	D49.6
stem	C71.7	C79.31	—	D33.1	D43.1	D49.6
tapetum	C71.8	C79.31	—	D33.2	D43.2	D49.6
temporal lobe	C71.2	C79.31	—	D33.0	D43.0	D49.6
thalamus	C71.0	C79.31	—	D33.0	D43.0	D49.6
uncus	C71.2	C79.31	—	D33.0	D43.0	D49.6
ventricle (floor)	C71.5	C79.31	—	D33.0	D43.0	D49.6
fourth	C71.7	C79.31	—	D33.1	D43.1	D49.6
branchial (cleft) (cyst) (vestiges)	C10.4	C79.89	D00.08	D10.5	D37.05	D49.0
breast (connective tissue) (glandular tissue) (soft parts)	C50.9-✓	C79.81	D05.-✓	D24.-✓	D48.6-✓	D49.3
areola	C50.0-✓	C79.81	D05.-✓	D24.-✓	D48.6-✓	D49.3
axillary tail	C50.6-✓	C79.81	D05.-✓	D24.-✓	D48.6-✓	D49.3
central portion	C50.1-✓	C79.81	D05.-✓	D24.-✓	D48.6-✓	D49.3
inner	C50.8-✓	C79.81	D05.-✓	D24.-✓	D48.6-✓	D49.3
lower	C50.8-✓	C79.81	D05.-✓	D24.-✓	D48.6-✓	D49.3
lower-inner quadrant	C50.3-✓	C79.81	D05.-✓	D24.-✓	D48.6-✓	D49.3
lower-outer quadrant	C50.5-✓	C79.81	D05.-✓	D24.-✓	D48.6-✓	D49.3
mastectomy site (skin) — see also Neoplasm, breast, skin	C44.501	C79.2	—	—	—	—
specified as breast tissue	C50.8-✓	C79.81	—	—	—	—
midline	C50.8-✓	C79.81	D05.-✓	D24.-✓	D48.6-✓	D49.3
nipple	C50.0-✓	C79.81	D05.-✓	D24.-✓	D48.6-✓	D49.3
outer	C50.8-✓	C79.81	D05.-✓	D24.-✓	D48.6-✓	D49.3
overlapping lesion	C50.8-✓	—	—	—	—	—
skin	C44.501	C79.2	D04.5	D23.5	D48.5	D49.2
basal cell carcinoma	C44.511	—	—	—	—	—
specified type NEC	C44.591	—	—	—	—	—
squamous cell carcinoma	C44.521	—	—	—	—	—
tail (axillary)	C50.6-✓	C79.81	D05.-✓	D24.-✓	D48.6-✓	D49.3
upper	C50.8-✓	C79.81	D05.-✓	D24.-✓	D48.6-✓	D49.3
upper-inner quadrant	C50.2-✓	C79.81	D05.-✓	D24.-✓	D48.6-✓	D49.3
upper-outer quadrant	C50.4-✓	C79.81	D05.-✓	D24.-✓	D48.6-✓	D49.3
broad ligament	C57.1-✓	C79.82	D07.39	D28.2	D39.8	D49.5
bronchiogenic, bronchogenic (lung)	C34.9-✓	C78.0-✓	D02.2-✓	D14.3-✓	D38.1	D49.1
bronchiole	C34.9-✓	C78.0-✓	D02.2-✓	D14.3-✓	D38.1	D49.1
bronchus	C34.9-✓	C78.0-✓	D02.2-✓	D14.3-✓	D38.1	D49.1
carina	C34.0-✓	C78.0-✓	D02.2-✓	D14.3-✓	D38.1	D49.1
lower lobe of lung	C34.3-✓	C78.0-✓	D02.2-✓	D14.3-✓	D38.1	D49.1
main	C34.0-✓	C78.0-✓	D02.2-✓	D14.3-✓	D38.1	D49.1
middle lobe of lung	C34.2	C78.0-✓	D02.21	D14.31	D38.1	D49.1
overlapping lesion	C34.8-✓	—	—	—	—	—
upper lobe of lung	C34.1-✓	C78.0-✓	D02.2-✓	D14.3-✓	D38.1	D49.1
brow	C44.309	C79.2	D04.39	D23.39	D48.5	D49.2
basal cell carcinoma	C44.319	—	—	—	—	—
specified type NEC	C44.399	—	—	—	—	—

Neoplasm, neoplastic — continued	Malignant Primary	Malignant Secondary	Ca in situ	Benign	Uncertain	Unspecified Behavior
brow — continued						
squamous cell carcinoma	C44.329	—	—	—	—	—
buccal (cavity)	C06.9	C79.89	D00.00	D10.39	D37.09	D49.0
commissure	C06.0	C79.89	D00.02	D10.39	D37.09	D49.0
groove (lower) (upper)	C06.1	C79.89	D00.02	D10.39	D37.09	D49.0
mucosa	C06.0	C79.89	D00.02	D10.39	D37.09	D49.0
sulcus (lower) (upper)	C06.1	C79.89	D00.02	D10.39	D37.09	D49.0
bulbourethral gland	C68.0	C79.19	D09.19	D30.4	D41.3	D49.5
bursa — see Neoplasm, connective tissue						
buttock NEC	C76.3	C79.89	D04.5	D36.7	D48.7	D49.89
calf	C76.5-✓	C79.89	D04.7-✓	D36.7	D48.7	D49.89
calvarium	C41.0	C79.51	—	D16.4	D48.0	D49.2
calyx, renal	C65.-✓	C79.0-✓	D09.19	D30.1-✓	D41.1-✓	D49.5
canal						
anal	C21.1	C78.5	D01.3	D12.9	D37.8	D49.0
auditory (external) — see also Neoplasm, skin, ear	C44.20-✓	C79.2	D04.2-✓	D23.2-✓	D48.5	D49.2
auricular (external) — see also Neoplasm, skin, ear	C44.20-✓	C79.2	D04.2-✓	D23.2-✓	D48.5	D49.2
canaliculi, biliary (biliferi) (intrahepatic)	C22.1	C78.7	D01.5	D13.4	D37.6	D49.0
canthus (eye) (inner) (outer)	C44.10-✓	C79.2	D04.1-✓	D23.1-✓	D48.5	D49.2
basal cell carcinoma	C44.11-✓	—	—	—	—	—
specified type NEC	C44.19-✓	—	—	—	—	—
squamous cell carcinoma	C44.12-✓	—	—	—	—	—
capillary — see Neoplasm, connective tissue						
caput coli	C18.0	C78.5	D01.0	D12.0	D37.4	D49.0
carcinoid — see Tumor, carcinoid						
cardia (gastric)	C16.0	C78.89	D00.2	D13.1	D37.1	D49.0
cardiac orifice (stomach)	C16.0	C78.89	D00.2	D13.1	D37.1	D49.0
cardio-esophageal junction	C16.0	C78.89	D00.2	D13.1	D37.1	D49.0
cardio-esophagus	C16.0	C78.89	D00.2	D13.1	D37.1	D49.0
carina (bronchus)	C34.0-✓	C78.0-✓	D02.2-✓	D14.3-✓	D38.1	D49.1
carotid (artery)	C49.0	C79.89	—	D21.0	D48.1	D49.2
body	C75.4	C79.89	—	D35.5	D44.6	D49.7
carpus (any bone)	C40.1-✓	C79.51	—	D16.1-✓	—	—
cartilage (articular) (joint) NEC — see also Neoplasm, bone	C41.9	C79.51	—	D16.9	D48.0	D49.2
arytenoid	C32.3	C78.39	D02.0	D14.1	D38.0	D49.1
auricular	C49.0	C79.89	—	D21.0	D48.1	D49.2
bronchi	C34.0-✓	C78.39	—	D14.3-✓	D38.1	D49.1
costal	C41.3	C79.51	—	D16.7	D48.0	D49.2
cricoid	C32.3	C78.39	D02.0	D14.1	D38.0	D49.1
cuneiform	C32.3	C78.39	D02.0	D14.1	D38.0	D49.1
ear (external)	C49.0	C79.89	—	D21.0	D48.1	D49.2
ensiform	C41.3	C79.51	—	D16.7	D48.0	D49.2
epiglottis	C32.1	C78.39	D02.0	D14.1	D38.0	D49.1
anterior surface	C10.1	C79.89	D00.08	D10.5	D37.05	D49.0
eyelid	C49.0	C79.89	—	D21.0	D48.1	D49.2
intervertebral	C41.2	C79.51	—	D16.6	D48.0	D49.2
larynx, laryngeal	C32.3	C78.39	D02.0	D14.1	D38.0	D49.1
nose, nasal	C30.0	C78.39	D02.3	D14.0	D38.5	D49.1
pinna	C49.0	C79.89	—	D21.0	D48.1	D49.2
rib	C41.3	C79.51	—	D16.7	D48.0	D49.2
semilunar (knee)	C40.2-✓	C79.51	—	D16.2-✓	D48.0	D49.2
thyroid	C32.3	C78.39	D02.0	D14.1	D38.0	D49.1
trachea	C33	C78.39	D02.1	D14.2	D38.1	D49.1
cauda equina	C72.1	C79.49	—	D33.4	D43.4	D49.7
cavity						
buccal	C06.9	C79.89	D00.00	D10.30	D37.09	D49.0
nasal	C30.0	C78.39	D02.3	D14.0	D38.5	D49.1
oral	C06.9	C79.89	D00.00	D10.30	D37.09	D49.0
peritoneal	C48.2	C78.6	—	D20.1	D48.4	D49.0
tympanic	C30.1	C78.39	D02.3	D14.0	D38.5	D49.1
cecum	C18.0	C78.5	D01.0	D12.0	D37.4	D49.0

Neoplasm, neoplastic — continued	Malignant Primary	Malignant Secondary	Ca in situ	Benign	Uncertain	Unspecified Behavior
central nervous system	C72.9	C79.40	—	—	—	—
cerebellopontine (angle)	C71.6	C79.31	—	D33.1	D43.1	D49.6
cerebellum, cerebellar	C71.6	C79.31	—	D33.1	D43.1	D49.6
cerebrum, cerebral (cortex) (hemisphere) (white matter)	C71.0	C79.31	—	D33.0	D43.0	D49.6
meninges	C70.0	C79.32	—	D32.0	D42.0	D49.7
peduncle	C71.7	C79.31	—	D33.1	D43.1	D49.6
ventricle	C71.5	C79.31	—	D33.0	D43.0	D49.6
fourth	C71.7	C79.31	—	D33.1	D43.1	D49.6
cervical region	C76.0	C79.89	D09.8	D36.7	D48.7	D49.89
cervix (cervical) (uteri) (uterus)	C53.9	C79.82	D06.9	D26.0	D39.0	D49.5
canal	C53.0	C79.82	D06.0	D26.0	D39.0	D49.5
endocervix (canal) (gland)	C53.0	C79.82	D06.0	D26.0	D39.0	D49.5
exocervix	C53.1	C79.82	D06.1	D26.0	D39.0	D49.5
external os	C53.1	C79.82	D06.1	D26.0	D39.0	D49.5
internal os	C53.0	C79.82	D06.0	D26.0	D39.0	D49.5
nabothian gland	C53.0	C79.82	D06.0	D26.0	D39.0	D49.5
overlapping lesion	C53.8	—	—	—	—	—
squamocolumnar junction	C53.8	C79.82	D06.7	D26.0	D39.0	D49.5
stump	C53.8	C79.82	D06.7	D26.0	D39.0	D49.5
cheek	C76.0	C79.89	D09.8	D36.7	D48.7	D49.89
external	C44.309	C79.2	D04.39	D23.39	D48.5	D49.2
basal cell carcinoma	C44.319					
specified type NEC	C44.399	—	—	—	—	—
squamous cell carcinoma	C44.329		—	—	—	—
inner aspect	C06.0	C79.89	D00.02	D10.39	D37.09	D49.0
internal	C06.0	C79.89	D00.02	D10.39	D37.09	D49.0
mucosa	C06.0	C79.89	D00.02	D10.39	D37.09	D49.0
chest (wall) NEC	C76.1	C79.89	D09.8	D36.7	D48.7	D49.89
chiasma opticum	C72.3-☑	C79.49	—	D33.3	D43.3	D49.7
chin	C44.309	C79.2	D04.39	D23.39	D48.5	D49.2
basal cell carcinoma	C44.319	—	—	—	—	—
specified type NEC	C44.399	—	—	—	—	—
squamous cell carcinoma	C44.329	—	—	—	—	—
choana	C11.3	C79.89	D00.08	D10.6	D37.05	D49.0
cholangiole	C22.1	C78.89	D01.5	D13.4	D37.6	D49.0
choledochal duct	C24.0	C78.89	D01.5	D13.5	D37.6	D49.0
choroid	C69.3-☑	C79.49	D09.2-☑	D31.3-☑	D48.7	D49.81
plexus	C71.5	C79.31	—	D33.0	D43.0	D49.6
ciliary body	C69.4-☑	C79.49	D09.2-☑	D31.4-☑	D48.7	D49.89
clavicle	C41.3	C79.51	—	D16.7	D48.0	D49.2
clitoris	C51.2	C79.82	D07.1	D28.0	D39.8	D49.5
clivus	C41.0	C79.51	—	D16.4	D48.0	D49.2
cloacogenic zone	C21.2	C78.5	D01.3	D12.9	D37.8	D49.0
coccygeal body or glomus	C49.5	C79.89	—	D21.5	D48.1	D49.2
vertebra	C41.4	C79.51	—	D16.8	D48.0	D49.2
coccyx	C41.4	C79.51	—	D16.8	D48.0	D49.2
colon — see also Neoplasm, intestine, large	C18.9	C78.5	—	—	—	—
with rectum	C19	C78.5	D01.1	D12.7	D37.5	D49.0
columnella — see also Neoplasm, skin, face	C44.390	C79.2	D04.39	D23.39	D48.5	D49.2
column, spinal — see Neoplasm, spine						
commissure labial, lip	C00.6	C79.89	D00.01	D10.39	D37.01	D49.0
laryngeal	C32.0	C78.39	D02.0	D14.1	D38.0	D49.1
common (bile) duct	C24.0	C78.89	D01.5	D13.5	D37.6	D49.0
concha — see also Neoplasm, skin, ear	C44.20-☑	C79.2	D04.2-☑	D23.2-☑	D48.5	D49.2
nose	C30.0	C78.39	D02.3	D14.0	D38.5	D49.1
conjunctiva	C69.0-☑	C79.49	D09.2-☑	D31.0-☑	D48.7	D49.89

Neoplasm, neoplastic — continued	Malignant Primary	Malignant Secondary	Ca in situ	Benign	Uncertain	Unspecified Behavior
connective tissue NEC	C49.9	C79.89	—	D21.9	D48.1	D49.2

Note: For neoplasms of connective tissue (blood vessel, bursa, fascia, ligament, muscle, peripheral nerves, sympathetic and parasympathetic nerves and ganglia, synovia, tendon, etc.) or of morphological types that indicate connective tissue, code according to the list under "Neoplasm, connective tissue". For sites that do not appear in this list, code to neoplasm of that site; e.g., fibrosarcoma, pancreas (C25.9)

Note: Morphological types that indicate connective tissue appear in their proper place in the alphabetic index with the instruction "see Neoplasm, connective tissue ...."

	Malignant Primary	Malignant Secondary	Ca in situ	Benign	Uncertain	Unspecified Behavior
abdomen	C49.4	C79.89	—	D21.4	D48.1	D49.2
abdominal wall	C49.4	C79.89	—	D21.4	D48.1	D49.2
ankle	C49.2-☑	C79.89	—	D21.2-☑	D48.1	D49.2
antecubital fossa or space	C49.1-☑	C79.89	—	D21.1-☑	D48.1	D49.2
arm	C49.1-☑	C79.89	—	D21.1-☑	D48.1	D49.2
auricle (ear)	C49.0	C79.89	—	D21.0	D48.1	D49.2
axilla	C49.3	C79.89	—	D21.3	D48.1	D49.2
back	C49.6	C79.89	—	D21.6	D48.1	D49.2
breast — see Neoplasm, breast						
buttock	C49.5	C79.89	—	D21.5	D48.1	D49.2
calf	C49.2-☑	C79.89	—	D21.2-☑	D48.1	D49.2
cervical region	C49.0	C79.89	—	D21.0	D48.1	D49.2
cheek	C49.0	C79.89	—	D21.0	D48.1	D49.2
chest (wall)	C49.3	C79.89	—	D21.3	D48.1	D49.2
chin	C49.0	C79.89	—	D21.0	D48.1	D49.2
diaphragm	C49.3	C79.89	—	D21.3	D48.1	D49.2
ear (external)	C49.0	C79.89	—	D21.0	D48.1	D49.2
elbow	C49.1-☑	C79.89	—	D21.1-☑	D48.1	D49.2
extrarectal	C49.5	C79.89	—	D21.5	D48.1	D49.2
extremity	C49.9	C79.89	—	D21.9	D48.1	D49.2
lower	C49.2-☑	C79.89	—	D21.2-☑	D48.1	D49.2
upper	C49.1-☑	C79.89	—	D21.1-☑	D48.1	D49.2
eyelid	C49.0	C79.89	—	D21.0	D48.1	D49.2
face	C49.0	C79.89	—	D21.0	D48.1	D49.2
finger	C49.1-☑	C79.89	—	D21.1-☑	D48.1	D49.2
flank	C49.6	C79.89	—	D21.6	D48.1	D49.2
foot	C49.2-☑	C79.89	—	D21.2-☑	D48.1	D49.2
forearm	C49.1-☑	C79.89	—	D21.1-☑	D48.1	D49.2
forehead	C49.0	C79.89	—	D21.0	D48.1	D49.2
gastric	C49.4	C79.89	—	D21.4	D48.1	D49.2
gastrointestinal	C49.4	C79.89	—	D21.4	D48.1	D49.2
gluteal region	C49.5	C79.89	—	D21.5	D48.1	D49.2
great vessels NEC	C49.3	C79.89	—	D21.3	D48.1	D49.2
groin	C49.5	C79.89	—	D21.5	D48.1	D49.2
hand	C49.1-☑	C79.89	—	D21.1-☑	D48.1	D49.2
head	C49.0	C79.89	—	D21.0	D48.1	D49.2
heel	C49.2-☑	C79.89	—	D21.2-☑	D48.1	D49.2
hip	C49.2-☑	C79.89	—	D21.2-☑	D48.1	D49.2
hypochondrium	C49.4	C79.89	—	D21.4	D48.1	D49.2
iliopsoas muscle	C49.5	C79.89	—	D21.5	D48.1	D49.2
infraclavicular region	C49.3	C79.89	—	D21.3	D48.1	D49.2
inguinal (canal) (region)	C49.5	C79.89	—	D21.5	D48.1	D49.2
intestinal	C49.4	C79.89	—	D21.4	D48.1	D49.2
intrathoracic	C49.3	C79.89	—	D21.3	D48.1	D49.2
ischiorectal fossa	C49.5	C79.89	—	D21.5	D48.1	D49.2
jaw	C03.9	C79.89	D00.03	D10.39	D48.1	D49.0
knee	C49.2-☑	C79.89	—	D21.2-☑	D48.1	D49.2
leg	C49.2-☑	C79.89	—	D21.2-☑	D48.1	D49.2
limb NEC	C49.9	C79.89	—	D21.9	D48.1	D49.2
lower	C49.2-☑	C79.89	—	D21.2-☑	D48.1	D49.2
upper	C49.1-☑	C79.89	—	D21.1-☑	D48.1	D49.2
nates	C49.5	C79.89	—	D21.5	D48.1	D49.2
neck	C49.0	C79.89	—	D21.0	D48.1	D49.2
orbit	C69.6-☑	C79.49	D09.2-☑	D31.6-☑	D48.1	D49.89
overlapping lesion	C49.8	—	—	—	—	—
pararectal	C49.5	C79.89	—	D21.5	D48.1	D49.2
para-urethral	C49.5	C79.89	—	D21.5	D48.1	D49.2
paravaginal	C49.5	C79.89	—	D21.5	D48.1	D49.2
pelvis (floor)	C49.5	C79.89	—	D21.5	D48.1	D49.2
pelvo-abdominal	C49.8	C79.89	—	D21.6	D48.1	D49.2
perineum	C49.5	C79.89	—	D21.5	D48.1	D49.2
perirectal (tissue)	C49.5	C79.89	—	D21.5	D48.1	D49.2

☑ Additional Character Required — Refer to the Tabular List for Character Selection ⬇ Subterms under main terms may continue to next column or page

Neoplasm, neoplastic — continued	Malignant Primary	Malignant Secondary	Ca in situ	Benign	Uncertain	Unspecified Behavior
connective tissue — continued						
periurethral (tissue)	C49.5	C79.89	—	D21.5	D48.1	D49.2
popliteal fossa or space	C49.2-✓	C79.89	—	D21.2-✓	D48.1	D49.2
presacral	C49.5	C79.89	—	D21.5	D48.1	D49.2
psoas muscle	C49.4	C79.89	—	D21.4	D48.1	D49.2
pterygoid fossa	C49.0	C79.89	—	D21.0	D48.1	D49.2
rectovaginal septum or wall	C49.5	C79.89	—	D21.5	D48.1	D49.2
rectovesical	C49.5	C79.89	—	D21.5	D48.1	D49.2
retroperitoneum	C48.0	C78.6	—	D20.0	D48.3	D49.0
sacrococcygeal region	C49.5	C79.89	—	D21.5	D48.1	D49.2
scalp	C49.0	C79.89	—	D21.0	D48.1	D49.2
scapular region	C49.3	C79.89	—	D21.3	D48.1	D49.2
shoulder	C49.1-✓	C79.89	—	D21.1-✓	D48.1	D49.2
skin (dermis) NEC — see also Neoplasm, skin, by site	C44.90	C79.2	D04.9	D23.9	D48.5	D49.2
stomach	C49.4	C79.89	—	D21.4	D48.1	D49.2
submental	C49.0	C79.89	—	D21.0	D48.1	D49.2
supraclavicular region	C49.0	C79.89	—	D21.0	D48.1	D49.2
temple	C49.0	C79.89	—	D21.0	D48.1	D49.2
temporal region	C49.0	C79.89	—	D21.0	D48.1	D49.2
thigh	C49.2-✓	C79.89	—	D21.2-✓	D48.1	D49.2
thoracic (duct) (wall)	C49.3	C79.89	—	D21.3	D48.1	D49.2
thorax	C49.3	C79.89	—	D21.3	D48.1	D49.2
thumb	C49.1-✓	C79.89	—	D21.1-✓	D48.1	D49.2
toe	C49.2-✓	C79.89	—	D21.2-✓	D48.1	D49.2
trunk	C49.6	C79.89	—	D21.6	D48.1	D49.2
umbilicus	C49.4	C79.89	—	D21.4	D48.1	D49.2
vesicorectal	C49.5	C79.89	—	D21.5	D48.1	D49.2
wrist	C49.1-✓	C79.89	—	D21.1-✓	D48.1	D49.2
conus medullaris	C72.0	C79.49	—	D33.4	D43.4	D49.7
cord (true) (vocal)	C32.0	C78.39	D02.0	D14.1	D38.0	D49.1
false	C32.1	C78.39	D02.0	D14.1	D38.0	D49.1
spermatic	C63.1-✓	C79.82	D07.69	D29.8	D40.8	D49.5
spinal (cervical) (lumbar) (thoracic)	C72.0	C79.49	—	D33.4	D43.4	D49.7
cornea (limbus)	C69.1-✓	C79.49	D09.2-✓	D31.1-✓	D48.7	D49.89
corpus						
albicans	C56.-✓	C79.6-✓	D07.39	D27.-✓	D39.1-✓	D49.5
callosum, brain	C71.0	C79.31	—	D33.2	D43.2	D49.6
cavernosum	C60.2	C79.82	D07.4	D29.0	D40.8	D49.5
gastric	C16.2	C78.89	D00.2	D13.1	D37.1	D49.0
overlapping sites	C54.8	—	—	—	—	—
penis	C60.2	C79.82	D07.4	D29.0	D40.8	D49.5
striatum, cerebrum	C71.0	C79.31	—	D33.0	D43.0	D49.6
uteri	C54.9	C79.82	D07.0	D26.1	D39.0	D49.5
isthmus	C54.0	C79.82	D07.0	D26.1	D39.0	D49.5
cortex						
adrenal	C74.0-✓	C79.7-✓	D09.3	D35.0-✓	D44.1-✓	D49.7
cerebral	C71.0	C79.31	—	D33.0	D43.0	D49.6
costal cartilage	C41.3	C79.51	—	D16.7	D48.0	D49.2
costovertebral joint	C41.3	C79.51	—	D16.7	D48.0	D49.2
Cowper's gland	C68.0	C79.19	D09.19	D30.4	D41.3	D49.5
cranial (fossa, any)	C71.9	C79.31	—	D33.2	D43.2	D49.6
meninges	C70.0	C79.32	—	D32.0	D42.0	D49.7
nerve	C72.50	C79.49	—	D33.3	D43.3	D49.7
specified NEC	C72.59	C79.49	—	D33.3	D43.3	D49.7
craniobuccal pouch	C75.2	C79.89	D09.3	D35.2	D44.3	D49.7
craniopharyngeal (duct) (pouch)	C75.2	C79.89	D09.3	D35.3	D44.4	D49.7
cricoid	C13.0	C79.89	D00.08	D10.7	D37.05	D49.0
cartilage	C32.3	C78.39	D02.0	D14.1	D38.0	D49.1
cricopharynx	C13.0	C79.89	D00.08	D10.7	D37.05	D49.0
crypt of Morgagni	C21.8	C78.5	D01.3	D12.9	D37.8	D49.0
crystalline lens	C69.4-✓	C79.49	D09.2-✓	D31.4-✓	D48.7	D49.89
cul-de-sac (Douglas')	C48.1	C78.6	—	D20.1	D48.4	D49.0
cuneiform cartilage	C32.3	C78.39	D02.0	D14.1	D38.0	D49.1
cutaneous — see Neoplasm, skin						
cutis — see Neoplasm, skin						

Neoplasm, neoplastic — continued	Malignant Primary	Malignant Secondary	Ca in situ	Benign	Uncertain	Unspecified Behavior
cystic (bile) duct (common)	C24.0	C78.89	D01.5	D13.5	D37.6	D49.0
dermis — see Neoplasm, skin						
diaphragm	C49.3	C79.89	—	D21.3	D48.1	D49.2
digestive organs, system, tube, or tract NEC	C26.9	C78.89	D01.9	D13.9	D37.9	D49.0
disc, intervertebral	C41.2	C79.51	—	D16.6	D48.0	D49.2
disease, generalized	C80.0	—	—	—	—	—
disseminated	C80.0	—	—	—	—	—
Douglas' cul-de-sac or pouch	C48.1	C78.6	—	D20.1	D48.4	D49.0
duodenojejunal junction	C17.8	C78.4	D01.49	D13.39	D37.2	D49.0
duodenum	C17.0	C78.4	D01.49	D13.2	D37.2	D49.0
dura (cranial) (mater)	C70.9	C79.49	—	D32.9	D42.9	D49.7
cerebral	C70.0	C79.32	—	D32.0	D42.0	D49.7
spinal	C70.1	C79.49	—	D32.1	D42.1	D49.7
ear (external) — see also Neoplasm, skin, ear						
auricle or auris — see also Neoplasm, skin, ear	C44.20-✓	C79.2	D04.2-✓	D23.2-✓	D48.5	D49.2
canal, external — see also Neoplasm, skin, ear	C44.20-✓	C79.2	D04.2-✓	D23.2-✓	D48.5	D49.2
cartilage	C49.0	C79.89	—	D21.0	D48.1	D49.2
external meatus — see also Neoplasm, skin, ear	C44.20-✓	C79.2	D04.2-✓	D23.2-✓	D48.5	D49.2
inner	C30.1	C78.39	D02.3	D14.0	D38.5	D49.1
lobule — see also Neoplasm, skin, ear	C44.20-✓	C79.2	D04.2-✓	D23.2-✓	D48.5	D49.2
middle	C30.1	C78.39	D02.3	D14.0	D38.5	D49.1
overlapping lesion with accessory sinuses	C31.8	—	—	—	—	—
skin	C44.20-✓	C79.2	D04.2-✓	D23.2-✓	D48.5	D49.2
basal cell carcinoma	C44.21-✓	—	—	—	—	—
specified type NEC	C44.29-✓	—	—	—	—	—
squamous cell carcinoma	C44.22-✓	—	—	—	—	—
earlobe	C44.20-✓	C79.2	D04.2-✓	D23.2-✓	D48.5	D49.2
basal cell carcinoma	C44.21-✓	—	—	—	—	—
specified type NEC	C44.29-✓	—	—	—	—	—
squamous cell carcinoma	C44.22-✓	—	—	—	—	—
ejaculatory duct	C63.7	C79.82	D07.69	D29.8	D40.8	D49.5
elbow NEC	C76.4-✓	C79.89	D04.6-✓	D36.7	D48.7	D49.89
endocardium	C38.0	C79.89	—	D15.1	D48.7	D49.89
endocervix (canal) (gland)	C53.0	C79.82	D06.0	D26.0	D39.0	D49.5
endocrine gland NEC	C75.9	C79.89	D09.3	D35.9	D44.9	D49.7
pluriglandular	C75.8	C79.89	D09.3	D35.7	D44.9	D49.7
endometrium (gland) (stroma)	C54.1	C79.82	D07.0	D26.1	D39.0	D49.5
ensiform cartilage	C41.3	C79.51	—	D16.7	D48.0	D49.2
enteric — see Neoplasm, intestine						
ependyma (brain)	C71.5	C79.31	—	D33.0	D43.0	D49.6
fourth ventricle	C71.7	C79.31	—	D33.1	D43.1	D49.6
epicardium	C38.0	C79.89	—	D15.1	D48.7	D49.89
epididymis	C63.0-✓	C79.82	D07.69	D29.3-✓	D40.8	D49.5
epidural	C72.9	C79.49	—	D33.9	D43.9	D49.7
epiglottis	C32.1	C78.39	D02.0	D14.1	D38.0	D49.1
anterior aspect or surface	C10.1	C79.89	D00.08	D10.5	D37.05	D49.0
cartilage	C32.3	C78.39	D02.0	D14.1	D38.0	D49.1
free border (margin)	C10.1	C79.89	D00.08	D10.5	D37.05	D49.0
junctional region	C10.8	C79.89	D00.08	D10.5	D37.05	D49.0
posterior (laryngeal) surface	C32.1	C78.39	D02.0	D14.1	D38.0	D49.1

Neoplasm Table

Neoplasm, connective tissue NEC — Neoplasm, epiglottis

Neoplasm Table

Neoplasm, epiglottis — Neoplasm, gland, glandular

Neoplasm, neoplastic — continued	Malignant Primary	Malignant Secondary	Ca in situ	Benign	Uncertain	Unspecified Behavior
epiglottis — continued						
suprahyoid portion	C32.1	C78.39	D02.0	D14.1	D38.0	D49.1
esophagogastric junction	C16.0	C78.89	D00.2	D13.1	D37.1	D49.0
esophagus	C15.9	C78.89	D00.1	D13.0	D37.8	D49.0
abdominal	C15.5	C78.89	D00.1	D13.0	D37.8	D49.0
cervical	C15.3	C78.89	D00.1	D13.0	D37.8	D49.0
distal (third)	C15.5	C78.89	D00.1	D13.0	D37.8	D49.0
lower (third)	C15.5	C78.89	D00.1	D13.0	D37.8	D49.0
middle (third)	C15.4	C78.89	D00.1	D13.0	D37.8	D49.0
overlapping lesion	C15.8	—	—	—	—	—
proximal (third)	C15.3	C78.89	D00.1	D13.0	D37.8	D49.0
thoracic	C15.4	C78.89	D00.1	D13.0	D37.8	D49.0
upper (third)	C15.3	C78.89	D00.1	D13.0	D37.8	D49.0
ethmoid (sinus)	C31.1	C78.39	D02.3	D14.0	D38.5	D49.1
bone or labyrinth	C41.0	C79.51	—	D16.4	D48.0	D49.2
eustachian tube	C30.1	C78.39	D02.3	D14.0	D38.5	D49.1
exocervix	C53.1	C79.82	D06.1	D26.0	D39.0	D49.5
external						
meatus (ear) — see also Neoplasm, skin, ear	C44.20-☑	C79.2	D04.2-☑	D23.2-☑	D48.5	D49.2
os, cervix uteri	C53.1	C79.82	D06.1	D26.0	D39.0	D49.5
extradural	C72.9	C79.49	—	D33.9	D43.9	D49.7
extrahepatic (bile) duct	C24.0	C78.89	D01.5	D13.5	D37.6	D49.0
overlapping lesion with gallbladder	C24.8	—	—	—	—	—
extraocular muscle	C69.6-☑	C79.49	D09.2-☑	D31.6-☑	D48.7	D49.89
extrarectal	C76.3	C79.89	D09.8	D36.7	D48.7	D49.89
extremity	C76.8	C79.89	D04.8	D36.7	D48.7	D49.89
lower	C76.5-☑	C79.89	D04.7-☑	D36.7	D48.7	D49.89
upper	C76.4-☑	C79.89	D04.6-☑	D36.7	D48.7	D49.89
eyeball	C69.9-☑	C79.49	D09.2-☑	D31.9-☑	D48.7	D49.89
eyebrow	C44.309	C79.2	D04.39	D23.39	D48.5	D49.2
basal cell carcinoma	C44.319	—	—	—	—	—
specified type NEC	C44.399	—	—	—	—	—
squamous cell carcinoma	C44.329	—	—	—	—	—
eyelid (lower) (skin) (upper)	C44.10-☑					
basal cell carcinoma	C44.11-☑					
cartilage	C49.0	C79.89		D21.0	D48.1	D49.2
specified type NEC	C44.19-☑					
squamous cell carcinoma	C44.12-☑					
eye NEC	C69.9-☑	C79.49	D09.2-☑	D31.9-☑	D48.7	D49.89
overlapping sites	C69.8-☑					
face NEC	C76.0	C79.89	D04.39	D36.7	D48.7	D49.89
fallopian tube (accessory)	C57.0-☑	C79.82	D07.39	D28.2	D39.8	D49.5
falx (cerebella) (cerebri)	C70.0	C79.32	—	D32.0	D42.0	D49.7
fascia — see also Neoplasm, connective tissue						
palmar	C49.1-☑	C79.89		D21.1-☑	D48.1	D49.2
plantar	C49.2-☑	C79.89		D21.2-☑	D48.1	D49.2
fatty tissue — see Neoplasm, connective tissue						
fauces, faucial NEC	C10.9	C79.89	D00.08	D10.5	D37.05	D49.0
pillars	C09.1	C79.89	D00.08	D10.5	D37.05	D49.0
tonsil	C09.9	C79.89	D00.08	D10.4	D37.05	D49.0
femur (any part)	C40.2-☑	—	—	D16.2-☑	—	—
fetal membrane	C58	C79.82	D07.0	D26.7	D39.2	D49.5
fibrous tissue — see Neoplasm, connective tissue						
fibula (any part)	C40.2-☑	C79.51	—	D16.2-☑	—	—
filum terminale	C72.0	C79.49	—	D33.4	D43.4	D49.7
finger NEC	C76.4-☑	C79.89	D04.6-☑	D36.7	D48.7	D49.89
flank NEC	C76.8	C79.89	D04.5	D36.7	D48.7	D49.89
follicle, nabothian	C53.0	C79.82	D06.0	D26.0	D39.0	D49.5
foot NEC	C76.5-☑	C79.89	D04.7-☑	D36.7	D48.7	D49.89
forearm NEC	C76.4-☑	C79.89	D04.6-☑	D36.7	D48.7	D49.89
forehead (skin)	C44.309	C79.2	D04.39	D23.39	D48.5	D49.2

Neoplasm, neoplastic — continued	Malignant Primary	Malignant Secondary	Ca in situ	Benign	Uncertain	Unspecified Behavior
forehead — continued						
basal cell carcinoma	C44.319	—	—	—	—	—
specified type NEC	C44.399	—	—	—	—	—
squamous cell carcinoma	C44.329	—	—	—	—	—
foreskin	C60.0	C79.82	D07.4	D29.0	D40.8	D49.5
fornix						
pharyngeal	C11.3	C79.89	D00.08	D10.6	D37.05	D49.0
vagina	C52	C79.82	D07.2	D28.1	D39.8	D49.5
fossa (of)						
anterior (cranial)	C71.9	C79.31	—	D33.2	D43.2	D49.6
cranial	C71.9	C79.31	—	D33.2	D43.2	D49.6
ischiorectal	C76.3	C79.89	D09.8	D36.7	D48.7	D49.89
middle (cranial)	C71.9	C79.31	—	D33.2	D43.2	D49.6
piriform	C12	C79.89	D00.08	D10.7	D37.05	D49.0
pituitary	C75.1	C79.89	D09.3	D35.2	D44.3	D49.7
posterior (cranial)	C71.9	C79.31	—	D33.2	D43.2	D49.6
pterygoid	C49.0	C79.89	—	D21.0	D48.1	D49.2
pyriform	C12	C79.89	D00.08	D10.7	D37.05	D49.0
Rosenmuller	C11.2	C79.89	D00.08	D10.6	D37.05	D49.0
tonsillar	C09.0	C79.89	D00.08	D10.5	D37.05	D49.0
fourchette	C51.9	C79.82	D07.1	D28.0	D39.8	D49.5
frenulum						
labii — see Neoplasm, lip, internal						
linguae	C02.2	C79.89	D00.07	D10.1	D37.02	D49.0
frontal						
bone	C41.0	C79.51	—	D16.4	D48.0	D49.2
lobe, brain	C71.1	C79.31	—	D33.0	D43.0	D49.6
pole	C71.1	C79.31	—	D33.0	D43.0	D49.6
sinus	C31.2	C78.39	D02.3	D14.0	D38.5	D49.1
fundus						
stomach	C16.1	C78.89	D00.2	D13.1	D37.1	D49.0
uterus	C54.3	C79.82	D07.0	D26.1	D39.0	D49.5
gallbladder	C23	C78.89	D01.5	D13.5	D37.6	D49.0
overlapping lesion with extrahepatic bile ducts	C24.8	—	—	—	—	—
gall duct (extrahepatic)	C24.0	C78.89	D01.5	D13.5	D37.6	D49.0
intrahepatic	C22.1	C78.7	D01.5	D13.4	D37.6	D49.0
ganglia — see also Neoplasm, nerve, peripheral	C47.9	C79.89		D36.10	D48.2	D49.2
basal	C71.0	C79.31	—	D33.0	D43.0	D49.6
cranial nerve	C72.50	C79.49	—	D33.3	D43.3	D49.7
Gartner's duct	C52	C79.82	D07.2	D28.1	D39.8	D49.5
gastric — see Neoplasm, stomach						
gastrocolic	C26.9	C78.89	D01.9	D13.9	D37.9	D49.0
gastroesophageal junction	C16.0	C78.89	D00.2	D13.1	D37.1	D49.0
gastrointestinal (tract) NEC	C26.9	C78.89	D01.9	D13.9	D37.9	D49.0
generalized	C80.0	—	—	—	—	—
genital organ or tract						
female NEC	C57.9	C79.82	D07.30	D28.9	D39.9	D49.5
overlapping lesion	C57.8	—	—	—	—	—
specified site NEC	C57.7	C79.82	D07.39	D28.7	D39.8	D49.5
male NEC	C63.9	C79.82	D07.60	D29.9	D40.9	D49.5
overlapping lesion	C63.8	—	—	—	—	—
specified site NEC	C63.7	C79.82	D07.69	D29.8	D40.8	D49.5
genitourinary tract						
female	C57.9	C79.82	D07.30	D28.9	D39.9	D49.5
male	C63.9	C79.82	D07.60	D29.9	D40.9	D49.5
gingiva (alveolar) (marginal)	C03.9	C79.89	D00.03	D10.39	D37.09	D49.0
lower	C03.1	C79.89	D00.03	D10.39	D37.09	D49.0
mandibular	C03.1	C79.89	D00.03	D10.39	D37.09	D49.0
maxillary	C03.0	C79.89	D00.03	D10.39	D37.09	D49.0
upper	C03.0	C79.89	D00.03	D10.39	D37.09	D49.0
gland, glandular (lymphatic) (system) — see also Neoplasm, lymph gland						
endocrine NEC	C75.9	C79.89	D09.3	D35.9	D44.9	D49.7

☑ Additional Character Required — Refer to the Tabular List for Character Selection   ▽ Subterms under main terms may continue to next column or page

Neoplasm, neoplastic — continued	Malignant Primary	Malignant Secondary	Ca in situ	Benign	Uncertain	Unspecified Behavior
gland, glandular — see also Neoplasm, lymph gland — continued						
salivary — see Neoplasm, salivary gland						
glans penis	C60.1	C79.82	D07.4	D29.0	D40.8	D49.5
globus pallidus	C71.0	C79.31	—	D33.0	D43.0	D49.6
glomus						
coccygeal	C49.5	C79.89	—	D21.5	D48.1	D49.2
jugularis	C75.5	C79.89	—	D35.6	D44.7	D49.7
glosso-epiglottic fold(s)	C10.1	C79.89	D00.08	D10.5	D37.05	D49.0
glossopalatine fold	C09.1	C79.89	D00.08	D10.5	D37.05	D49.0
glossopharyngeal sulcus	C09.0	C79.89	D00.08	D10.5	D37.05	D49.0
glottis	C32.0	C78.39	D02.0	D14.1	D38.0	D49.1
gluteal region	C76.3	C79.89	D04.5	D36.7	D48.7	D49.89
great vessels NEC	C49.3	C79.89	—	D21.3	D48.1	D49.2
groin NEC	C76.3	C79.89	D04.5	D36.7	D48.7	D49.89
gum	C03.9	C79.89	D00.03	D10.39	D37.09	D49.0
lower	C03.1	C79.89	D00.03	D10.39	D37.09	D49.0
upper	C03.0	C79.89	D00.03	D10.39	D37.09	D49.0
hand NEC	C76.4-☑	C79.89	D04.6-☑	D36.7	D48.7	D49.89
head NEC	C76.0	C79.89	D04.4	D36.7	D48.7	D49.89
heart	C38.0	C79.89	—	D15.1	D48.7	D49.89
heel NEC	C76.5-☑	C79.89	D04.7-☑	D36.7	D48.7	D49.89
helix — see also Neoplasm, skin, ear	C44.20-☑	C79.2	D04.2-☑	D23.2-☑	D48.5	D49.2
hematopoietic, hemopoietic tissue NEC	C96.9	—	—	—	—	—
specified NEC	C96.Z	—	—	—	—	—
hemisphere, cerebral	C71.0	C79.31	—	D33.0	D43.0	D49.6
hemorrhoidal zone	C21.1	C78.5	D01.3	D12.9	D37.8	D49.0
hepatic — see also Index to disease, by histology	C22.9	C78.7	D01.5	D13.4	D37.6	D49.0
duct (bile)	C24.0	C78.89	D01.5	D13.5	D37.6	D49.0
flexure (colon)	C18.3	C78.5	D01.0	D12.3	D37.4	D49.0
primary	C22.8	C78.7	D01.5	D13.4	D37.6	D49.0
hepatobiliary	C24.9	C78.89	D01.5	D13.5	D37.6	D49.0
hepatoblastoma	C22.2	C78.7	D01.5	D13.4	D37.6	D49.0
hepatoma	C22.0	C78.7	D01.5	D13.4	D37.6	D49.0
hilus of lung	C34.0-☑	C78.0-☑	D02.2-☑	D14.3-☑	D38.1	D49.1
hippocampus, brain	C71.2	C79.31	—	D33.0	D43.0	D49.6
hip NEC	C76.5-☑	C79.89	D04.7-☑	D36.7	D48.7	D49.89
humerus (any part)	C40.0-☑	C79.51	—	D16.0-☑	—	—
hymen	C52	C79.82	D07.2	D28.1	D39.8	D49.5
hypopharynx, hypopharyngeal NEC	C13.9	C79.89	D00.08	D10.7	D37.05	D49.0
overlapping lesion	C13.8	—	—	—	—	—
postcricoid region	C13.0	C79.89	D00.08	D10.7	D37.05	D49.0
posterior wall	C13.2	C79.89	D00.08	D10.7	D37.05	D49.0
pyriform fossa (sinus)	C12	C79.89	D00.08	D10.7	D37.05	D49.0
hypophysis	C75.1	C79.89	D09.3	D35.2	D44.3	D49.7
hypothalamus	C71.0	C79.31	—	D33.0	D43.0	D49.6
ileocecum, ileocecal (coil) (junction) (valve)	C18.0	C78.5	D01.0	D12.0	D37.4	D49.0
ileum	C17.2	C78.4	D01.49	D13.39	D37.2	D49.0
ilium	C41.4	C79.51	—	D16.8	D48.0	D49.2
immunoproliferative NEC	C88.9	—	—	—	—	—
infraclavicular (region)	C76.1	C79.89	D04.5	D36.7	D48.7	D49.89
inguinal (region)	C76.3	C79.89	D04.5	D36.7	D48.7	D49.89
insula	C71.0	C79.31	—	D33.0	D43.0	D49.6
insular tissue (pancreas)	C25.4	C78.89	D01.7	D13.7	D37.8	D49.0
brain	C71.0	C79.31	—	D33.0	D43.0	D49.6
interarytenoid fold	C13.1	C78.39	D00.08	D10.7	D37.05	D49.0
hypopharyngeal aspect	C13.1	C79.89	D00.08	D10.7	D37.05	D49.0
laryngeal aspect	C32.1	C78.39	D02.0	D14.1	D38.0	D49.1
marginal zone	C13.1	C79.89	D00.08	D10.7	D37.05	D49.0
interdental papillae	C03.9	C79.89	D00.03	D10.39	D37.09	D49.0

Neoplasm, neoplastic — continued	Malignant Primary	Malignant Secondary	Ca in situ	Benign	Uncertain	Unspecified Behavior
interdental papillae — continued						
lower	C03.1	C79.89	D00.03	D10.39	D37.09	D49.0
upper	C03.0	C79.89	D00.03	D10.39	D37.09	D49.0
internal						
capsule	C71.0	C79.31	—	D33.0	D43.0	D49.6
os (cervix)	C53.0	C79.82	D06.0	D26.0	D39.0	D49.5
intervertebral cartilage or disc	C41.2	C79.51	—	D16.6	D48.0	D49.2
intestine, intestinal	C26.0	C78.80	D01.40	D13.9	D37.8	D49.0
large	C18.9	C78.5	D01.0	D12.6	D37.4	D49.0
appendix	C18.1	C78.5	D01.0	D12.1	D37.3	D49.0
caput coli	C18.0	C78.5	D01.0	D12.0	D37.4	D49.0
cecum	C18.0	C78.5	D01.0	D12.0	D37.4	D49.0
colon	C18.9	C78.5	D01.0	D12.6	D37.4	D49.0
and rectum	C19	C78.5	D01.1	D12.7	D37.5	D49.0
ascending	C18.2	C78.5	D01.0	D12.2	D37.4	D49.0
caput	C18.0	C78.5	D01.0	D12.0	D37.4	D49.0
descending	C18.6	C78.5	D01.0	D12.4	D37.4	D49.0
distal	C18.6	C78.5	D01.0	D12.4	D37.4	D49.0
left	C18.6	C78.5	D01.0	D12.4	D37.4	D49.0
overlapping lesion	C18.8	—	—	—	—	—
pelvic	C18.7	C78.5	D01.0	D12.5	D37.4	D49.0
right	C18.2	C78.5	D01.0	D12.2	D37.4	D49.0
sigmoid (flexure)	C18.7	C78.5	D01.0	D12.5	D37.4	D49.0
transverse	C18.4	C78.5	D01.0	D12.3	D37.4	D49.0
hepatic flexure	C18.3	C78.5	D01.0	D12.3	D37.4	D49.0
ileocecum, ileocecal (coil) (valve)	C18.0	C78.5	D01.0	D12.0	D37.4	D49.0
overlapping lesion	C18.8	—	—	—	—	—
sigmoid flexure (lower) (upper)	C18.7	C78.5	D01.0	D12.5	D37.4	D49.0
splenic flexure	C18.5	C78.5	D01.0	D12.3	D37.4	D49.0
small	C17.9	C78.4	D01.40	D13.30	D37.2	D49.0
duodenum	C17.0	C78.4	D01.49	D13.2	D37.2	D49.0
ileum	C17.2	C78.4	D01.49	D13.39	D37.2	D49.0
jejunum	C17.1	C78.4	D01.49	D13.39	D37.2	D49.0
overlapping lesion	C17.8	—	—	—	—	—
tract NEC	C26.0	C78.89	D01.40	D13.9	D37.8	D49.0
intra-abdominal	C76.2	C79.89	D09.8	D36.7	D48.7	D49.89
intracranial NEC	C71.9	C79.31	—	D33.2	D43.2	D49.6
intrahepatic (bile) duct	C22.1	C78.7	D01.5	D13.4	D37.6	D49.0
intraocular	C69.9-☑	C79.49	D09.2-☑	D31.9-☑	D48.7	D49.89
intraorbital	C69.6-☑	C79.49	D09.2-☑	D31.6-☑	D48.7	D49.89
intrasellar	C75.1	C79.89	D09.3	D35.2	D44.3	D49.7
intrathoracic (cavity) (organs)	C76.1	C79.89	D09.8	D15.9	D48.7	D49.89
specified NEC	C76.1	C79.89	D09.8	D15.7	—	—
iris	C69.4-☑	C79.49	D09.2-☑	D31.4-☑	D48.7	D49.89
ischiorectal (fossa)	C76.3	C79.89	D09.8	D36.7	D48.7	D49.89
ischium	C41.4	C79.51	—	D16.8	D48.0	D49.2
island of Reil	C71.0	C79.31	—	D33.0	D43.0	D49.6
islands or islets of Langerhans	C25.4	C78.89	D01.7	D13.7	D37.8	D49.0
isthmus uteri	C54.0	C79.82	D07.0	D26.1	D39.0	D49.5
jaw	C76.0	C79.89	D09.8	D36.7	D48.7	D49.89
bone	C41.1	C79.51	—	D16.5	D48.0	D49.2
lower	C41.1	C79.51	—	D16.5	—	—
upper	C41.0	C79.51	—	D16.4	—	—
carcinoma (any type) (lower) (upper)	C76.0	C79.89	—	—	—	—
skin — see also Neoplasm, skin, face	C44.309	C79.2	D04.39	D23.39	D48.5	D49.2
soft tissues	C03.9	C79.89	D00.03	D10.39	D37.09	D49.0
lower	C03.1	C79.89	D00.03	D10.39	D37.09	D49.0
upper	C03.0	C79.89	D00.03	D10.39	D37.09	D49.0
jejunum	C17.1	C78.4	D01.49	D13.39	D37.2	D49.0
joint NEC — see also Neoplasm, bone	C41.9	C79.51	—	D16.9	D48.0	D49.2
acromioclavicular	C40.0-☑	C79.51	—	D16.0-☑	—	—
bursa or synovial membrane — see						

Neoplasm Table

Neoplasm, joint NEC — Neoplasm, lung

Neoplasm, neoplastic — continued	Malignant Primary	Malignant Secondary	Ca in situ	Benign	Uncertain	Unspecified Behavior
joint — see also Neoplasm, bone — continued						
bursa or synovial membrane — see Neoplasm, connective tissue — continued						
Neoplasm, connective tissue						
costovertebral	C41.3	C79.51	—	D16.7	D48.0	D49.2
sternocostal	C41.3	C79.51	—	D16.7	D48.0	D49.2
temporomandibular	C41.1	C79.51	—	D16.5	D48.0	D49.2
junction						
anorectal	C21.8	C78.5	D01.3	D12.9	D37.8	D49.0
cardioesophageal	C16.0	C78.89	D00.2	D13.1	D37.1	D49.0
esophagogastric	C16.0	C78.89	D00.2	D13.1	D37.1	D49.0
gastroesophageal	C16.0	C78.89	D00.2	D13.1	D37.1	D49.0
hard and soft palate	C05.9	C79.89	D00.00	D10.39	D37.09	D49.0
ileocecal	C18.0	C78.5	D01.0	D12.0	D37.4	D49.0
pelvirectal	C19	C78.5	D01.1	D12.7	D37.5	D49.0
pelviureteric	C65.-✓	C79.0-✓	D09.19	D30.1-✓	D41.1-✓	D49.5
rectosigmoid	C19	C78.5	D01.1	D12.7	D37.5	D49.0
squamocolumnar, of cervix	C53.8	C79.82	D06.7	D26.0	D39.0	D49.5
Kaposi's sarcoma — see Kaposi's, sarcoma						
kidney (parenchymal)	C64.-✓	C79.0-✓	D09.19	D30.0-✓	D41.0-✓	D49.5
calyx	C65.-✓	C79.0-✓	D09.19	D30.1-✓	D41.1-✓	D49.5
hilus	C65.-✓	C79.0-✓	D09.19	D30.1-✓	D41.1-✓	D49.5
pelvis	C65.-✓	C79.0-✓	D09.19	D30.1-✓	D41.1-✓	D49.5
knee NEC	C76.5-✓	C79.89	D04.7-✓	D36.7	D48.7	D49.89
labia (skin)	C51.9	C79.82	D07.1	D28.0	D39.8	D49.5
majora	C51.0	C79.82	D07.1	D28.0	D39.8	D49.5
minora	C51.1	C79.82	D07.1	D28.0	D39.8	D49.5
labial — see also Neoplasm, lip	C00.9	C79.89	D00.01	D10.0	D37.01	D49.0
sulcus (lower) (upper)	C06.1	C79.89	D00.02	D10.39	D37.09	D49.0
labium (skin)	C51.9	C79.82	D07.1	D28.0	D39.8	D49.5
majus	C51.0	C79.82	D07.1	D28.0	D39.8	D49.5
minus	C51.1	C79.82	D07.1	D28.0	D39.8	D49.5
lacrimal						
canaliculi	C69.5-✓	C79.49	D09.2-✓	D31.5-✓	D48.7	D49.89
duct (nasal)	C69.5-✓	C79.49	D09.2-✓	D31.5-✓	D48.7	D49.89
gland	C69.5-✓	C79.49	D09.2-✓	D31.5-✓	D48.7	D49.89
punctum	C69.5-✓	C79.49	D09.2-✓	D31.5-✓	D48.7	D49.89
sac	C69.5-✓	C79.49	D09.2-✓	D31.5-✓	D48.7	D49.89
Langerhans, islands or islets	C25.4	C78.89	D01.7	D13.7	D37.8	D49.0
laryngopharynx	C13.9	C79.89	D00.08	D10.7	D37.05	D49.0
larynx, laryngeal NEC	C32.9	C78.39	D02.0	D14.1	D38.0	D49.1
aryepiglottic fold	C32.1	C78.39	D02.0	D14.1	D38.0	D49.1
cartilage (arytenoid) (cricoid) (cuneiform) (thyroid)	C32.3	C78.39	D02.0	D14.1	D38.0	D49.1
commissure (anterior) (posterior)	C32.0	C78.39	D02.0	D14.1	D38.0	D49.1
extrinsic NEC	C32.1	C78.39	D02.0	D14.1	D38.0	D49.1
meaning hypopharynx	C13.9	C79.89	D00.08	D10.7	D37.05	D49.0
interarytenoid fold	C32.1	C78.39	D02.0	D14.1	D38.0	D49.1
intrinsic	C32.0	C78.39	D02.0	D14.1	D38.0	D49.1
overlapping lesion	C32.8	—	—	—	—	—
ventricular band	C32.1	C78.39	D02.0	D14.1	D38.0	D49.1
leg NEC	C76.5-✓	C79.89	D04.7-✓	D36.7	D48.7	D49.89
lens, crystalline	C69.4-✓	C79.49	D09.2-✓	D31.4-✓	D48.7	D49.89
lid (lower) (upper)	C44.10-✓	C79.2	D04.1-✓	D23.1-✓	D48.5	D49.2
basal cell carcinoma	C44.11-✓	—	—	—	—	—
specified type NEC	C44.19-✓	—	—	—	—	—
squamous cell carcinoma	C44.12-✓	—	—	—	—	—
ligament — see also Neoplasm, connective tissue						

Neoplasm, neoplastic — continued	Malignant Primary	Malignant Secondary	Ca in situ	Benign	Uncertain	Unspecified Behavior
ligament — see also Neoplasm, connective tissue — continued						
broad	C57.1-✓	C79.82	D07.39	D28.2	D39.8	D49.5
Mackenrodt's	C57.7	C79.82	D07.39	D28.7	D39.8	D49.5
non-uterine — see Neoplasm, connective tissue						
round	C57.2-✓	C79.82	—	D28.2	D39.8	D49.5
sacro-uterine	C57.3	C79.82	—	D28.2	D39.8	D49.5
uterine	C57.3	C79.82	—	D28.2	D39.8	D49.5
utero-ovarian	C57.7	C79.82	D07.39	D28.2	D39.8	D49.5
uterosacral	C57.3	C79.82	—	D28.2	D39.8	D49.5
limb	C76.8	C79.89	D04.8	D36.7	D48.7	D49.89
lower	C76.5-✓	C79.89	D04.7-✓	D36.7	D48.7	D49.89
upper	C76.4-✓	C79.89	D04.6-✓	D36.7	D48.7	D49.89
limbus of cornea	C69.1-✓	C79.49	D09.2-✓	D31.1-✓	D48.7	D49.89
lingual NEC — see also Neoplasm, tongue	C02.9	C79.89	D00.07	D10.1	D37.02	D49.0
lingula, lung	C34.1-✓	C78.0-✓	D02.2-✓	D14.3-✓	D38.1	D49.1
lip	C00.9	C79.89	D00.01	D10.0	D37.01	D49.0
buccal aspect — see Neoplasm, lip, internal						
commissure	C00.6	C79.89	D00.01	D10.0	D37.01	D49.0
external	C00.2	C79.89	D00.01	D10.0	D37.01	D49.0
lower	C00.1	C79.89	D00.01	D10.0	D37.01	D49.0
upper	C00.0	C79.89	D00.01	D10.0	D37.01	D49.0
frenulum — see Neoplasm, lip, internal						
inner aspect — see Neoplasm, lip, internal						
internal	C00.5	C79.89	D00.01	D10.0	D37.01	D49.0
lower	C00.4	C79.89	D00.01	D10.0	D37.01	D49.0
upper	C00.3	C79.89	D00.01	D10.0	D37.01	D49.0
lipstick area	C00.2	C79.89	D00.01	D10.0	D37.01	D49.0
lower	C00.1	C79.89	D00.01	D10.0	D37.01	D49.0
upper	C00.0	C79.89	D00.01	D10.0	D37.01	D49.0
lower	C00.1	C79.89	D00.01	D10.0	D37.01	D49.0
internal	C00.4	C79.89	D00.01	D10.0	D37.01	D49.0
mucosa — see Neoplasm, lip, internal						
oral aspect — see Neoplasm, lip, internal						
overlapping lesion	C00.8	—	—	—	—	—
with oral cavity or pharynx	C14.8	—	—	—	—	—
skin (commissure) (lower) (upper)	C44.00	C79.2	D04.0	D23.0	D48.5	D49.2
basal cell carcinoma	C44.01	—	—	—	—	—
specified type NEC	C44.09	—	—	—	—	—
squamous cell carcinoma	C44.02	—	—	—	—	—
upper	C00.0	C79.89	D00.01	D10.0	D37.01	D49.0
internal	C00.3	C79.89	D00.01	D10.0	D37.01	D49.0
vermilion border	C00.2	C79.89	D00.01	D10.0	D37.01	D49.0
lower	C00.1	C79.89	D00.01	D10.0	D37.01	D49.0
upper	C00.0	C79.89	D00.01	D10.0	D37.01	D49.0
lipomatous — see Lipoma, by site						
liver — see also Index to disease, by histology	C22.9	C78.7	D01.5	D13.4	D37.6	D49.0
primary	C22.8	C78.7	D01.5	D13.4	D37.6	D49.0
lumbosacral plexus	C47.5	C79.89	—	D36.16	D48.2	D49.2
lung	C34.9-✓	C78.0-✓	D02.2-✓	D14.3-✓	D38.1	D49.1
azygos lobe	C34.1-✓	C78.0-✓	D02.2-✓	D14.3-✓	D38.1	D49.1
carina	C34.0-✓	C78.0-✓	D02.2-✓	D14.3-✓	D38.1	D49.1
hilus	C34.0-✓	C78.0-✓	D02.2-✓	D14.3-✓	D38.1	D49.1
lingula	C34.1-✓	C78.0-✓	D02.2-✓	D14.3-✓	D38.1	D49.1
lobe NEC	C34.9-✓	C78.0-✓	D02.2-✓	D14.3-✓	D38.1	D49.1
lower lobe	C34.3-✓	C78.0-✓	D02.2-✓	D14.3-✓	D38.1	D49.1

✓ Additional Character Required — Refer to the Tabular List for Character Selection   Subterms under main terms may continue to next column or page

Neoplasm, neoplastic —	Malignant Primary	Malignant Secondary	Ca in situ	Benign	Uncertain	Unspecified Behavior
continued						
lung — *continued*						
main bronchus	C34.0-☑	C78.0-☑	D02.2-☑	D14.3-☑	D38.1	D49.1
mesothelioma — *see*						
Mesothelioma						
middle lobe	C34.2	C78.0-☑	D02.21	D14.31	D38.1	D49.1
overlapping lesion	C34.8-☑	—	—	—	—	
upper lobe	C34.1-☑	C78.0-☑	D02.2-☑	D14.3-☑	D38.1	D49.1
lymph, lymphatic channel						
NEC	C49.9	C79.89	—	D21.9	D48.1	D49.2
gland (secondary)	—	C77.9	—	D36.0	D48.7	D49.89
abdominal	—	C77.2	—	D36.0	D48.7	D49.89
aortic	—	C77.2	—	D36.0	D48.7	D49.89
arm	—	C77.3	—	D36.0	D48.7	D49.89
auricular (anterior)						
(posterior)	—	C77.0	—	D36.0	D48.7	D49.89
axilla, axillary	—	C77.3	—	D36.0	D48.7	D49.89
brachial	—	C77.3	—	D36.0	D48.7	D49.89
bronchial	—	C77.1	—	D36.0	D48.7	D49.89
bronchopulmonary	—	C77.1	—	D36.0	D48.7	D49.89
celiac	—	C77.2	—	D36.0	D48.7	D49.89
cervical	—	C77.0	—	D36.0	D48.7	D49.89
cervicofacial	—	C77.0	—	D36.0	D48.7	D49.89
Cloquet	—	C77.4	—	D36.0	D48.7	D49.89
colic	—	C77.2	—	D36.0	D48.7	D49.89
common duct	—	C77.2	—	D36.0	D48.7	D49.89
cubital	—	C77.3	—	D36.0	D48.7	D49.89
diaphragmatic	—	C77.1	—	D36.0	D48.7	D49.89
epigastric,						
inferior	—	C77.1	—	D36.0	D48.7	D49.89
epitrochlear	—	C77.3	—	D36.0	D48.7	D49.89
esophageal	—	C77.1	—	D36.0	D48.7	D49.89
face	—	C77.0	—	D36.0	D48.7	D49.89
femoral	—	C77.4	—	D36.0	D48.7	D49.89
gastric	—	C77.2	—	D36.0	D48.7	D49.89
groin	—	C77.4	—	D36.0	D48.7	D49.89
head	—	C77.0	—	D36.0	D48.7	D49.89
hepatic	—	C77.2	—	D36.0	D48.7	D49.89
hilar						
(pulmonary)	—	C77.1	—	D36.0	D48.7	D49.89
splenic	—	C77.2	—	D36.0	D48.7	D49.89
hypogastric	—	C77.5	—	D36.0	D48.7	D49.89
ileocolic	—	C77.2	—	D36.0	D48.7	D49.89
iliac	—	C77.5	—	D36.0	D48.7	D49.89
infraclavicular	—	C77.3	—	D36.0	D48.7	D49.89
inguina, inguinal	—	C77.4	—	D36.0	D48.7	D49.89
innominate	—	C77.1	—	D36.0	D48.7	D49.89
intercostal	—	C77.1	—	D36.0	D48.7	D49.89
intestinal	—	C77.2	—	D36.0	D48.7	D49.89
intrabdominal	—	C77.2	—	D36.0	D48.7	D49.89
intrapelvic	—	C77.5	—	D36.0	D48.7	D49.89
intrathoracic	—	C77.1	—	D36.0	D48.7	D49.89
jugular	—	C77.0	—	D36.0	D48.7	D49.89
leg	—	C77.4	—	D36.0	D48.7	D49.89
limb						
lower	—	C77.4	—	D36.0	D48.7	D49.89
upper	—	C77.3	—	D36.0	D48.7	D49.89
lower limb	—	C77.4	—	D36.0	D48.7	D49.89
lumbar	—	C77.2	—	D36.0	D48.7	D49.89
mandibular	—	C77.0	—	D36.0	D48.7	D49.89
mediastinal	—	C77.1	—	D36.0	D48.7	D49.89
mesenteric (inferior)						
(superior)	—	C77.2	—	D36.0	D48.7	D49.89
midcolic	—	C77.2	—	D36.0	D48.7	D49.89
multiple sites in						
categories C77.0-						
C77.5	—	C77.8	—	D36.0	D48.7	D49.89
neck	—	C77.0	—	D36.0	D48.7	D49.89
obturator	—	C77.5	—	D36.0	D48.7	D49.89
occipital	—	C77.0	—	D36.0	D48.7	D49.89
pancreatic	—	C77.2	—	D36.0	D48.7	D49.89
para-aortic	—	C77.2	—	D36.0	D48.7	D49.89
paracervical	—	C77.5	—	D36.0	D48.7	D49.89
parametrial	—	C77.5	—	D36.0	D48.7	D49.89
parasternal	—	C77.1	—	D36.0	D48.7	D49.89
parotid	—	C77.0	—	D36.0	D48.7	D49.89
pectoral	—	C77.3	—	D36.0	D48.7	D49.89
pelvic	—	C77.5	—	D36.0	D48.7	D49.89
peri-aortic	—	C77.2	—	D36.0	D48.7	D49.89
peripancreatic	—	C77.2	—	D36.0	D48.7	D49.89
popliteal	—	C77.4	—	D36.0	D48.7	D49.89
porta hepatis	—	C77.2	—	D36.0	D48.7	D49.89

Neoplasm, neoplastic —	Malignant Primary	Malignant Secondary	Ca in situ	Benign	Uncertain	Unspecified Behavior
continued						
lymph, lymphatic channel						
— *continued*						
gland — *continued*						
portal	—	C77.2	—	D36.0	D48.7	D49.89
preauricular	—	C77.0	—	D36.0	D48.7	D49.89
prelaryngeal	—	C77.0	—	D36.0	D48.7	D49.89
presymphysial	—	C77.5	—	D36.0	D48.7	D49.89
pretracheal	—	C77.0	—	D36.0	D48.7	D49.89
primary (any site)						
NEC	C96.9	—	—	—	—	—
pulmonary						
(hiler)	—	C77.1	—	D36.0	D48.7	D49.89
pyloric	—	C77.2	—	D36.0	D48.7	D49.89
retroperitoneal	—	C77.2	—	D36.0	D48.7	D49.89
retropharyngeal	—	C77.0	—	D36.0	D48.7	D49.89
Rosenmuller's	—	C77.4	—	D36.0	D48.7	D49.89
sacral	—	C77.5	—	D36.0	D48.7	D49.89
scalene	—	C77.0	—	D36.0	D48.7	D49.89
site NEC	—	C77.9	—	D36.0	D48.7	D49.89
splenic (hilar)	—	C77.2	—	D36.0	D48.7	D49.89
subclavicular	—	C77.3	—	D36.0	D48.7	D49.89
subinguinal	—	C77.4	—	D36.0	D48.7	D49.89
sublingual	—	C77.0	—	D36.0	D48.7	D49.89
submandibular	—	C77.0	—	D36.0	D48.7	D49.89
submaxillary	—	C77.0	—	D36.0	D48.7	D49.89
submental	—	C77.0	—	D36.0	D48.7	D49.89
subscapular	—	C77.3	—	D36.0	D48.7	D49.89
supraclavicular	—	C77.0	—	D36.0	D48.7	D49.89
thoracic	—	C77.1	—	D36.0	D48.7	D49.89
tibial	—	C77.4	—	D36.0	D48.7	D49.89
tracheal	—	C77.1	—	D36.0	D48.7	D49.89
tracheobronchial	—	C77.1	—	D36.0	D48.7	D49.89
upper limb	—	C77.3	—	D36.0	D48.7	D49.89
Virchow's	—	C77.0	—	D36.0	D48.7	D49.89
node — *see also*						
Neoplasm, lymph						
gland						
primary NEC	C96.9	—	—	—	—	—
vessel — *see also*						
Neoplasm,						
connective						
tissue	C49.9	C79.89	—	D21.9	D48.1	D49.2
Mackenrodt's						
ligament	C57.7	C79.82	D07.39	D28.7	D39.8	D49.5
malar	C41.0	C79.51	—	D16.4	D48.0	D49.2
region — *see*						
Neoplasm, cheek						
mammary gland — *see*						
Neoplasm, breast						
mandible	C41.1	C79.51	—	D16.5	D48.0	D49.2
alveolar						
mucosa						
(carcinoma)	C03.1	C79.89	D00.03	D10.39	D37.09	D49.0
ridge or process	C41.1	C79.51	—	D16.5	D48.0	D49.2
marrow (bone) NEC	C96.9	C79.52	—	—	D47.9	D49.89
mastectomy site (skin) —						
see also Neoplasm,						
breast, skin	C44.501	C79.2	—	—	—	—
specified as breast						
tissue	C50.8-☑	C79.81	—	—	—	—
mastoid (air cells)						
(antrum) (cavity)	C30.1	C78.39	D02.3	D14.0	D38.5	D49.1
bone or process	C41.0	C79.51	—	D16.4	D48.0	D49.2
maxilla, maxillary						
(superior)	C41.0	C79.51	—	D16.4	D48.0	D49.2
alveolar						
mucosa	C03.0	C79.89	D00.03	D10.39	D37.09	D49.0
ridge or process						
(carcinoma)	C41.0	C79.51	—	D16.4	D48.0	D49.2
antrum	C31.0	C78.39	D02.3	D14.0	D38.5	D49.1
carcinoma	C03.0	C79.51	—			
inferior — *see*						
Neoplasm,						
mandible						
sinus	C31.0	C78.39	D02.3	D14.0	D38.5	D49.1
meatus external (ear) —						
see also Neoplasm,						
skin, ear	C44.20-☑	C79.2	D04.2-☑	D23.2-☑	D48.5	D49.2
Meckel diverticulum,						
malignant	C17.3	C78.4	D01.49	D13.39	D37.2	D49.0

Neoplasm, neoplastic — continued

	Malignant Primary	Malignant Secondary	Ca in situ	Benign	Uncertain	Unspecified Behavior
mediastinum, mediastinal	C38.3	C78.1	—	D15.2	D38.3	D49.89
anterior	C38.1	C78.1	—	D15.2	D38.3	D49.89
posterior	C38.2	C78.1	—	D15.2	D38.3	D49.89
medulla adrenal	C74.1-✓	C79.7-✓	D09.3	D35.0-✓	D44.1-✓	D49.7
oblongata	C71.7	C79.31	—	D33.1	D43.1	D49.6
meibomian gland	C44.10-✓	C79.2	D04.1-✓	D23.1-✓	D48.5	D49.2
basal cell carcinoma	C44.11-✓	—	—	—	—	—
specified type NEC	C44.19-✓	—	—	—	—	—
squamous cell carcinoma	C44.12-✓	—	—	—	—	—
melanoma — see Melanoma						
meninges	C70.9	C79.49	—	D32.9	D42.9	D49.7
brain	C70.0	C79.32	—	D32.0	D42.0	D49.7
cerebral	C70.0	C79.32	—	D32.0	D42.0	D49.7
crainial	C70.0	C79.32	—	D32.0	D42.0	D49.7
intracranial	C70.0	C79.32	—	D32.0	D42.0	D49.7
spinal (cord)	C70.1	C79.49	—	D32.1	D42.1	D49.7
meniscus, knee joint (lateral) (medial)	C40.2-✓	C79.51	—	D16.2-✓	D48.0	D49.2
Merkel cell — see Carcinoma, Merkel cell						
mesentery, mesenteric	C48.1	C78.6	—	D20.1	D48.4	D49.0
mesoappendix	C48.1	C78.6	—	D20.1	D48.4	D49.0
mesocolon	C48.1	C78.6	—	D20.1	D48.4	D49.0
mesopharynx — see Neoplasm, oropharynx						
mesosalpinx	C57.1-✓	C79.82	D07.39	D28.2	D39.8	D49.5
mesothelial tissue — see Mesothelioma						
mesothelioma — see Mesothelioma						
mesovarium	C57.1-✓	C79.82	D07.39	D28.2	D39.8	D49.5
metacarpus (any bone)	C40.1-✓	C79.51	—	D16.1-✓	—	—
metastatic NEC — see also Neoplasm, by site, secondary	—	C79.9	—	—	—	—
metatarsus (any bone)	C40.3-✓	C79.51	—	D16.3-✓	—	—
midbrain	C71.7	C79.31	—	D33.1	D43.1	D49.6
milk duct — see Neoplasm, breast						
mons pubis	C51.9	C79.82	D07.1	D28.0	D39.8	D49.5
veneris	C51.9	C79.82	D07.1	D28.0	D39.8	D49.5
motor tract	C72.9	C79.49	—	D33.9	D43.9	D49.7
brain	C71.9	C79.31	—	D33.2	D43.2	D49.6
cauda equina	C72.1	C79.49	—	D33.4	D43.4	D49.7
spinal	C72.0	C79.49	—	D33.4	D43.4	D49.7
mouth	C06.9	C79.89	D00.00	D10.30	D37.09	D49.0
book-leaf	C06.89	C79.89	—	—	—	—
floor	C04.9	C79.89	D00.06	D10.2	D37.09	D49.0
anterior portion	C04.0	C79.89	D00.06	D10.2	D37.09	D49.0
lateral portion	C04.1	C79.89	D00.06	D10.2	D37.09	D49.0
overlapping lesion	C04.8	—	—	—	—	—
overlapping NEC	C06.80	—	—	—	—	—
roof	C05.9	C79.89	D00.00	D10.39	D37.09	D49.0
specified part NEC	C06.89	C79.89	D00.00	D10.39	D37.09	D49.0
vestibule	C06.1	C79.89	D00.00	D10.39	D37.09	D49.0
mucosa alveolar (ridge or process)	C03.9	C79.89	D00.03	D10.39	D37.09	D49.0
lower	C03.1	C79.89	D00.03	D10.39	D37.09	D49.0
upper	C03.0	C79.89	D00.03	D10.39	D37.09	D49.0
buccal	C06.0	C79.89	D00.02	D10.39	D37.09	D49.0
cheek	C06.0	C79.89	D00.02	D10.39	D37.09	D49.0
lip — see Neoplasm, lip, internal						
nasal	C30.0	C78.39	D02.3	D14.0	D38.5	D49.1
oral	C06.0	C79.89	D00.02	D10.39	D37.09	D49.0
Mullerian duct female	C57.7	C79.82	D07.39	D28.7	D39.8	D49.5
male	C63.7	C79.82	D07.69	D29.8	D40.8	D49.5

Neoplasm, neoplastic — continued

	Malignant Primary	Malignant Secondary	Ca in situ	Benign	Uncertain	Unspecified Behavior
muscle — see also Neoplasm, connective tissue extraocular	C69.6-✓	C79.49	D09.2-✓	D31.6-✓	D48.7	D49.89
myocardium	C38.0	C79.89	—	D15.1	D48.7	D49.89
myometrium	C54.2	C79.82	D07.0	D26.1	D39.0	D49.5
myopericardium	C38.0	C79.89	—	D15.1	D48.7	D49.89
nabothian gland (follicle)	C53.0	C79.82	D06.0	D26.0	D39.0	D49.5
nail — see also Neoplasm, skin, limb	C44.90	C79.2	D04.9	D23.9	D48.5	D49.2
finger — see also Neoplasm, skin, limb, upper	C44.60-✓	C79.2	D04.6-✓	D23.6-✓	D48.5	D49.2
toe — see also Neoplasm, skin, limb, lower	C44.70-✓	C79.2	D04.7-✓	D23.7-✓	D48.5	D49.2
nares, naris (anterior) (posterior)	C30.0	C78.39	D02.3	D14.0	D38.5	D49.1
nasal — see Neoplasm, nose						
nasolabial groove — see also Neoplasm, skin, face	C44.309	C79.2	D04.39	D23.39	D48.5	D49.2
nasolacrimal duct	C69.5-✓	C79.49	D09.2-✓	D31.5-✓	D48.7	D49.89
nasopharynx, nasopharyngeal	C11.9	C79.89	D00.08	D10.6	D37.05	D49.0
floor	C11.3	C79.89	D00.08	D10.6	D37.05	D49.0
overlapping lesion	C11.8	—	—	—	—	—
roof	C11.0	C79.89	D00.08	D10.6	D37.05	D49.0
wall	C11.9	C79.89	D00.08	D10.6	D37.05	D49.0
anterior	C11.3	C79.89	D00.08	D10.6	D37.05	D49.0
lateral	C11.2	C79.89	D00.08	D10.6	D37.05	D49.0
posterior	C11.1	C79.89	D00.08	D10.6	D37.05	D49.0
superior	C11.0	C79.89	D00.08	D10.6	D37.05	D49.0
nates — see also Neoplasm, skin, trunk	C44.509	C79.2	D04.5	D23.5	D48.5	D49.2
neck NEC	C76.0	C79.89	D09.8	D36.7	D48.7	D49.89
skin	C44.40	—	—	—	—	—
basal cell carcinoma	C44.41					
specified type NEC	C44.49					
squamous cell carcinoma	C44.42					
nerve (ganglion)	C47.9	C79.89	—	D36.10	D48.2	D49.2
abducens	C72.59	C79.49	—	D33.3	D43.3	D49.7
accessory (spinal)	C72.59	C79.49	—	D33.3	D43.3	D49.7
acoustic	C72.4-✓	C79.49	—	D33.3	D43.3	D49.7
auditory	C72.4-✓	C79.49	—	D33.3	D43.3	D49.7
autonomic NEC — see also Neoplasm, nerve, peripheral	C47.9	C79.89	—	D36.10	D48.2	D49.2
brachial	C47.1-✓	C79.89	—	D36.12	D48.2	D49.2
cranial	C72.50	C79.49	—	D33.3	D43.3	D49.7
specified NEC	C72.59	C79.49	—	D33.3	D43.3	D49.7
facial	C72.59	C79.49	—	D33.3	D43.3	D49.7
femoral	C47.2-✓	C79.89	—	D36.13	D48.2	D49.2
ganglion NEC — see also Neoplasm, nerve, peripheral	C47.9	C79.89	—	D36.10	D48.2	D49.2
glossopharyngeal	C72.59	C79.49	—	D33.3	D43.3	D49.7
hypoglossal	C72.59	C79.49	—	D33.3	D43.3	D49.7
intercostal	C47.3	C79.89	—	D36.14	D48.2	D49.2
lumbar	C47.6	C79.89	—	D36.17	D48.2	D49.2
median	C47.1-✓	C79.89	—	D36.12	D48.2	D49.2
obturator	C47.2-✓	C79.89	—	D36.13	D48.2	D49.2
oculomotor	C72.59	C79.49	—	D33.3	D43.3	D49.7
olfactory	C47.2-✓	C79.49	—	D33.3	D43.3	D49.7
optic	C72.3-✓	C79.49	—	D33.3	D43.3	D49.7
parasympathetic NEC	C47.9	C79.89	—	D36.10	D48.2	D49.2
peripheral NEC	C47.9	C79.89	—	D36.10	D48.2	D49.2
abdomen	C47.4	C79.89	—	D36.15	D48.2	D49.2
abdominal wall	C47.4	C79.89	—	D36.15	D48.2	D49.2
ankle	C47.2-✓	C79.89	—	D36.13	D48.2	D49.2

✓ Additional Character Required — Refer to the Tabular List for Character Selection   ▽ Subterms under main terms may continue to next column or page

Neoplasm, neoplastic — continued	Malignant Primary	Malignant Secondary	Ca in situ	Benign	Uncertain	Unspecified Behavior
nerve — continued						
peripheral — continued						
antecubital fossa or space	C47.1-☑	C79.89	—	D36.12	D48.2	D49.2
arm	C47.1-☑	C79.89	—	D36.12	D48.2	D49.2
auricle (ear)	C47.0	C79.89	—	D36.11	D48.2	D49.2
axilla	C47.3	C79.89	—	D36.12	D48.2	D49.2
back	C47.6	C79.89	—	D36.17	D48.2	D49.2
buttock	C47.5	C79.89	—	D36.16	D48.2	D49.2
calf	C47.2-☑	C79.89	—	D36.13	D48.2	D49.2
cervical region	C47.0	C79.89	—	D36.11	D48.2	D49.2
cheek	C47.0	C79.89	—	D36.11	D48.2	D49.2
chest (wall)	C47.3	C79.89	—	D36.14	D48.2	D49.2
chin	C47.0	C79.89	—	D36.11	D48.2	D49.2
ear (external)	C47.0	C79.89	—	D36.11	D48.2	D49.2
elbow	C47.1-☑	C79.89	—	D36.12	D48.2	D49.2
extrarectal	C47.5	C79.89	—	D36.16	D48.2	D49.2
extremity	C47.9	C79.89	—	D36.10	D48.2	D49.2
lower	C47.2-☑	C79.89	—	D36.13	D48.2	D49.2
upper	C47.1-☑	C79.89	—	D36.12	D48.2	D49.2
eyelid	C47.0	C79.89	—	D36.11	D48.2	D49.2
face	C47.0	C79.89	—	D36.11	D48.2	D49.2
finger	C47.1-☑	C79.89	—	D36.12	D48.2	D49.2
flank	C47.6	C79.89	—	D36.17	D48.2	D49.2
foot	C47.2-☑	C79.89	—	D36.13	D48.2	D49.2
forearm	C47.1-☑	C79.89	—	D36.12	D48.2	D49.2
forehead	C47.0	C79.89	—	D36.11	D48.2	D49.2
gluteal region	C47.5	C79.89	—	D36.16	D48.2	D49.2
groin	C47.5	C79.89	—	D36.16	D48.2	D49.2
hand	C47.1-☑	C79.89	—	D36.12	D48.2	D49.2
head	C47.0	C79.89	—	D36.11	D48.2	D49.2
heel	C47.2-☑	C79.89	—	D36.13	D48.2	D49.2
hip	C47.2-☑	C79.89	—	D36.13	D48.2	D49.2
infraclavicular region	C47.3	C79.89	—	D36.14	D48.2	D49.2
inguinal (canal) (region)	C47.5	C79.89	—	D36.16	D48.2	D49.2
intrathoracic	C47.3	C79.89	—	D36.14	D48.2	D49.2
ischiorectal fossa	C47.5	C79.89	—	D36.16	D48.2	D49.2
knee	C47.2-☑	C79.89	—	D36.13	D48.2	D49.2
leg	C47.2-☑	C79.89	—	D36.13	D48.2	D49.2
limb NEC	C47.9	C79.89	—	D36.10	D48.2	D49.2
lower	C47.2-☑	C79.89	—	D36.13	D48.2	D49.2
upper	C47.1-☑	C79.89	—	D36.12	D48.2	D49.2
nates	C47.5	C79.89	—	D36.16	D48.2	D49.2
neck	C47.0	C79.89	—	D36.11	D48.2	D49.2
orbit	C69.6-☑	C79.49	—	D31.6-☑	D48.7	D49.2
pararectal	C47.5	C79.89	—	D36.16	D48.2	D49.2
paraurethral	C47.5	C79.89	—	D36.16	D48.2	D49.2
paravaginal	C47.5	C79.89	—	D36.16	D48.2	D49.2
pelvis (floor)	C47.5	C79.89	—	D36.16	D48.2	D49.2
pelvoabdominal	C47.8	C79.89	—	D36.17	D48.2	D49.2
perineum	C47.5	C79.89	—	D36.16	D48.2	D49.2
perirectal (tissue)	C47.5	C79.89	—	D36.16	D48.2	D49.2
periurethral (tissue)	C47.5	C79.89	—	D36.16	D48.2	D49.2
popliteal fossa or space	C47.2-☑	C79.89	—	D36.13	D48.2	D49.2
presacral	C47.5	C79.89	—	D36.16	D48.2	D49.2
pterygoid fossa	C47.0	C79.89	—	D36.11	D48.2	D49.2
rectovaginal septum or wall	C47.5	C79.89	—	D36.16	D48.2	D49.2
rectovesical	C47.5	C79.89	—	D36.16	D48.2	D49.2
sacrococcygeal region	C47.5	C79.89	—	D36.16	D48.2	D49.2
scalp	C47.0	C79.89	—	D36.11	D48.2	D49.2
scapular region	C47.3	C79.89	—	D36.14	D48.2	D49.2
shoulder	C47.1-☑	C79.89	—	D36.12	D48.2	D49.2
submental	C47.0	C79.89	—	D36.11	D48.2	D49.2
supraclavicular region	C47.0	C79.89	—	D36.11	D48.2	D49.2
temple	C47.0	C79.89	—	D36.11	D48.2	D49.2
temporal region	C47.0	C79.89	—	D36.11	D48.2	D49.2
thigh	C47.2-☑	C79.89	—	D36.13	D48.2	D49.2
thoracic (duct) (wall)	C47.3	C79.89	—	D36.14	D48.2	D49.2
thorax	C47.3	C79.89	—	D36.14	D48.2	D49.2
thumb	C47.1-☑	C79.89	—	D36.12	D48.2	D49.2

Neoplasm, neoplastic — continued	Malignant Primary	Malignant Secondary	Ca in situ	Benign	Uncertain	Unspecified Behavior
nerve — continued						
peripheral — continued						
toe	C47.2-☑	C79.89	—	D36.13	D48.2	D49.2
trunk	C47.6	C79.89	—	D36.17	D48.2	D49.2
umbilicus	C47.4	C79.89	—	D36.15	D48.2	D49.2
vesicorectal	C47.5	C79.89	—	D36.16	D48.2	D49.2
wrist	C47.1-☑	C79.89	—	D36.12	D48.2	D49.2
radial	C47.1-☑	C79.89	—	D36.12	D48.2	D49.2
sacral	C47.5	C79.89	—	D36.16	D48.2	D49.2
sciatic	C47.2-☑	C79.89	—	D36.13	D48.2	D49.2
spinal NEC	C47.9	C79.89	—	D36.10	D48.2	D49.2
accessory	C72.59	C79.49	—	D33.3	D43.3	D49.7
sympathetic NEC — see also Neoplasm, nerve, peripheral	C47.9	C79.89	—	D36.10	D48.2	D49.2
trigeminal	C72.59	C79.49	—	D33.3	D43.3	D49.7
trochlear	C72.59	C79.49	—	D33.3	D43.3	D49.7
ulnar	C47.1-☑	C79.89	—	D36.12	D48.2	D49.2
vagus	C72.59	C79.49	—	D33.3	D43.3	D49.7
nervous system (central)	C72.9	C79.40	—	D33.9	D43.9	D49.7
autonomic — see Neoplasm, nerve, peripheral						
parasympathetic — see Neoplasm, nerve, peripheral						
specified site NEC	—	C79.49	—	D33.7	D43.8	
sympathetic — see Neoplasm, nerve, peripheral						
nevus — see Nevus						
nipple	C50.0-☑	C79.81	D05.-☑	D24.-☑	—	—
nose, nasal	C76.0	C79.89	D09.8	D36.7	D48.7	D49.89
ala (external) (nasi) — see also Neoplasm, nose, skin	C44.301	C79.2	D04.39	D23.39	D48.5	D49.2
bone	C41.0	C79.51	—	D16.4	D48.0	D49.2
cartilage	C30.0	C78.39	D02.3	D14.0	D38.5	D49.1
cavity	C30.0	C78.39	D02.3	D14.0	D38.5	D49.1
choana	C11.3	C79.89	D00.08	D10.6	D37.05	D49.0
external (skin) — see also Neoplasm, nose, skin	C44.301	C79.2	D04.39	D23.39	D48.5	D49.2
fossa	C30.0	C78.39	D02.3	D14.0	D38.5	D49.1
internal	C30.0	C78.39	D02.3	D14.0	D38.5	D49.1
mucosa	C30.0	C78.39	D02.3	D14.0	D38.5	D49.1
septum	C30.0	C78.39	D02.3	D14.0	D38.5	D49.1
posterior margin	C11.3	C79.89	D00.08	D10.6	D37.05	D49.0
sinus — see Neoplasm, sinus						
skin	C44.301	C79.2	D04.39	D23.39	D48.5	D49.2
basal cell carcinoma	C44.311	—	—	—	—	—
specified type NEC	C44.391	—	—	—	—	—
squamous cell carcinoma	C44.321	—	—	—	—	—
turbinate (mucosa)	C30.0	C78.39	D02.3	D14.0	D38.5	D49.1
bone	C41.0	C79.51	—	D16.4	D48.0	D49.2
vestibule	C30.0	C78.39	D02.3	D14.0	D38.5	D49.1
nostril	C30.0	C78.39	D02.3	D14.0	D38.5	D49.1
nucleus pulposus	C41.2	C79.51	—	D16.6	D48.0	D49.2
occipital						
bone	C41.0	C79.51	—	D16.4	D48.0	D49.2
lobe or pole, brain	C71.4	C79.31	—	D33.0	D43.0	D49.6
odontogenic — see Neoplasm, jaw bone						
olfactory nerve or bulb	C72.2-☑	C79.49	—	D33.3	D43.3	D49.7
olive (brain)	C71.7	C79.31	—	D33.1	D43.1	D49.6
omentum	C48.1	C78.6	—	D20.1	D48.4	D49.0
operculum (brain)	C71.0	C79.31	—	D33.0	D43.0	D49.6
optic nerve, chiasm, or tract	C72.3-☑	C79.49	—	D33.3	D43.3	D49.7
oral (cavity)	C06.9	C79.89	D00.00	D10.30	D37.09	D49.0
ill-defined	C14.8	C79.89	D00.00	D10.30	D37.09	D49.0
mucosa	C06.0	C79.89	D00.02	D10.39	D37.09	D49.0
orbit	C69.6-☑	C79.49	D09.2-☑	D31.6-☑	D48.7	D49.89

Neoplasm, neoplastic — continued	Malignant Primary	Malignant Secondary	Ca in situ	Benign	Uncertain	Unspecified Behavior
orbit — continued						
autonomic nerve	C69.6-☑	C79.49	—	D31.6-☑	D48.7	D49.2
bone	C41.0	C79.51	—	D16.4	D48.0	D49.2
eye	C69.6-☑	C79.49	D09.2-☑	D31.6-☑	D48.7	D49.89
peripheral nerves	C69.6-☑	C79.49	—	D31.6-☑	D48.7	D49.2
soft parts	C69.6-☑	C79.49	D09.2-☑	D31.6-☑	D48.7	D49.89
organ of Zuckerkandl	C75.5	C79.89	—	D35.6	D44.7	D49.7
oropharynx	C10.9	C79.89	D00.08	D10.5	D37.05	D49.0
branchial cleft (vestige)	C10.4	C79.89	D00.08	D10.5	D37.05	D49.0
junctional region	C10.8	C79.89	D00.08	D10.5	D37.05	D49.0
lateral wall	C10.2	C79.89	D00.08	D10.5	D37.05	D49.0
overlapping lesion	C10.8	—	—	—	—	—
pillars or fauces	C09.1	C79.89	D00.08	D10.5	D37.05	D49.0
posterior wall	C10.3	C79.89	D00.08	D10.5	D37.05	D49.0
vallecula	C10.0	C79.89	D00.08	D10.5	D37.05	D49.0
os						
external	C53.1	C79.82	D06.1	D26.0	D39.0	D49.5
internal	C53.0	C79.82	D06.0	D26.0	D39.0	D49.5
ovary	C56.-☑	C79.6-☑	D07.39	D27.-☑	D39.1-☑	D49.5
oviduct	C57.0-☑	C79.82	D07.39	D28.2	D39.8	D49.5
palate	C05.9	C79.89	D00.00	D10.39	D37.09	D49.5
hard	C05.0	C79.89	D00.05	D10.39	D37.09	D49.0
junction of hard and soft palate	C05.9	C79.89	D00.00	D10.39	D37.09	D49.0
overlapping lesions	C05.8	—	—	—	—	—
soft	C05.1	C79.89	D00.04	D10.39	D37.09	D49.0
nasopharyngeal surface	C11.3	C79.89	D00.08	D10.6	D37.05	D49.0
posterior surface	C11.3	C79.89	D00.08	D10.6	D37.05	D49.0
superior surface	C11.3	C79.89	D00.08	D10.6	D37.05	D49.0
palatoglossal arch	C09.1	C79.89	D00.00	D10.5	D37.09	D49.0
palatopharyngeal arch	C09.1	C79.89	D00.00	D10.5	D37.09	D49.0
pallium	C71.0	C79.31	—	D33.0	D43.0	D49.6
palpebra	C44.10-☑	C79.2	D04.1-☑	D23.1-☑	D48.5	D49.2
basal cell carcinoma	C44.11-☑	—	—	—	—	—
specified type NEC	C44.19-☑	—	—	—	—	—
squamous cell carcinoma	C44.12-☑	—	—	—	—	—
pancreas	C25.9	C78.89	D01.7	D13.6	D37.8	D49.0
body	C25.1	C78.89	D01.7	D13.6	D37.8	D49.0
duct (of Santorini) (of Wirsung)	C25.3	C78.89	D01.7	D13.6	D37.8	D49.0
ectopic tissue	C25.7	C78.89	—	D13.6	D37.8	D49.0
head	C25.0	C78.89	D01.7	D13.6	D37.8	D49.0
islet cells	C25.4	C78.89	D01.7	D13.7	D37.8	D49.0
neck	C25.7	C78.89	D01.7	D13.6	D37.8	D49.0
overlapping lesion	C25.8	—	—	—	—	—
tail	C25.2	C78.89	D01.7	D13.6	D37.8	D49.0
para-aortic body	C75.5	C79.89	—	D35.6	D44.7	D49.7
paraganglion NEC	C75.5	C79.89	—	D35.6	D44.7	D49.7
parametrium	C57.3	C79.82	—	D28.2	D39.8	D49.5
paranephric	C48.0	C78.6	—	D20.0	D48.3	D49.0
pararectal	C76.3	C79.89	—	D36.7	D48.7	D49.89
parasagittal (region)	C76.0	C79.89	D09.8	D36.7	D48.7	D49.89
parasellar	C72.9	C79.49	—	D33.9	D43.8	D49.7
parathyroid (gland)	C75.0	C79.89	D09.3	D35.1	D44.2	D49.7
paraurethral	C76.3	C79.89	—	D36.7	D48.7	D49.89
gland	C68.1	C79.19	D09.19	D30.8	D41.8	D49.5
paravaginal	C76.3	C79.89	—	D36.7	D48.7	D49.89
parenchyma, kidney	C64.-☑	C79.0-☑	D09.19	D30.0-☑	D41.0-☑	D49.5
parietal						
bone	C41.0	C79.51	—	D16.4	D48.0	D49.2
lobe, brain	C71.3	C79.31	—	D33.0	D43.0	D49.6
paroophoron	C57.1-☑	C79.82	D07.39	D28.2	D39.8	D49.5
parotid (duct) (gland)	C07	C79.89	D00.00	D11.0	D37.030	D49.0
parovarium	C57.1-☑	C79.82	D07.39	D28.2	D39.8	D49.5
patella	C40.20	C79.51	—	—	—	—
peduncle, cerebral	C71.7	C79.31	—	D33.1	D43.1	D49.6
pelvirectal junction	C19	C78.5	D01.1	D12.7	D37.5	D49.0
pelvis, pelvic	C76.3	C79.89	D09.8	D36.7	D48.7	D49.89
bone	C41.4	C79.51	—	D16.8	D48.0	D49.2
floor	C76.3	C79.89	D09.8	D36.7	D48.7	D49.89
renal	C65.-☑	C79.0-☑	D09.19	D30.1-☑	D41.1-☑	D49.5
viscera	C76.3	C79.89	D09.8	D36.7	D48.7	D49.89

Neoplasm, neoplastic — continued	Malignant Primary	Malignant Secondary	Ca in situ	Benign	Uncertain	Unspecified Behavior
pelvis, pelvic — continued						
wall	C76.3	C79.89	D09.8	D36.7	D48.7	D49.89
pelvo-abdominal	C76.8	C79.89	D09.8	D36.7	D48.7	D49.89
penis	C60.9	C79.82	D07.4	D29.0	D40.8	D49.5
body	C60.2	C79.82	D07.4	D29.0	D40.8	D49.5
corpus (cavernosum)	C60.2	C79.82	D07.4	D29.0	D40.8	D49.5
glans	C60.1	C79.82	D07.4	D29.0	D40.8	D49.5
overlapping sites	C60.8	—	—	—	—	—
skin NEC	C60.9	C79.82	D07.4	D29.0	D40.8	D49.5
periadrenal (tissue)	C48.0	C78.6	—	D20.0	D48.3	D49.0
perianal (skin) — see also Neoplasm, anus, skin	C44.500	C79.2	D04.5	D23.5	D48.5	D49.2
pericardium	C38.0	C79.89	—	D15.1	D48.7	D49.89
perinephric	C48.0	C78.6	—	D20.0	D48.3	D49.0
perineum	C76.3	C79.89	D09.8	D36.7	D48.7	D49.89
periodontal tissue NEC	C03.9	C79.89	D00.03	D10.39	D37.09	D49.0
periosteum — see Neoplasm, bone						
peripancreatic	C48.0	C78.6	—	D20.0	D48.3	D49.0
peripheral nerve NEC	C47.9	C79.89	—	D36.10	D48.2	D49.2
perirectal (tissue)	C76.3	C79.89	—	D36.7	D48.7	D49.89
perirenal (tissue)	C48.0	C78.6	—	D20.0	D48.3	D49.0
peritoneum, peritoneal (cavity)	C48.2	C78.6	—	D20.1	D48.4	D49.0
benign mesothelial tissue — see Mesothelioma, benign						
overlapping lesion	C48.8	—	—	—	—	—
with digestive organs	C26.9	—	—	—	—	—
parietal	C48.1	C78.6	—	D20.1	D48.4	D49.0
pelvic	C48.1	C78.6	—	D20.1	D48.4	D49.0
specified part NEC	C48.1	C78.6	—	D20.1	D48.4	D49.0
peritonsillar (tissue)	C76.0	C79.89	D09.8	D36.7	D48.7	D49.89
periurethral tissue	C76.3	C79.89	—	D36.7	D48.7	D49.89
phalanges						
foot	C40.3-☑	C79.51	—	D16.3-☑	—	—
hand	C40.1-☑	C79.51	—	D16.1-☑	—	—
pharynx, pharyngeal	C14.0	C79.89	D00.08	D10.9	D37.05	D49.0
bursa	C11.1	C79.89	D00.08	D10.6	D37.05	D49.0
fornix	C11.3	C79.89	D00.08	D10.6	D37.05	D49.0
recess	C11.2	C79.89	D00.08	D10.6	D37.05	D49.0
region	C14.0	C79.89	D00.08	D10.9	D37.05	D49.0
tonsil	C11.1	C79.89	D00.08	D10.6	D37.05	D49.0
wall (lateral) (posterior)	C14.0	C79.89	D00.08	D10.9	D37.05	D49.0
pia mater	C70.9	C79.40	—	D32.9	D42.9	D49.7
cerebral	C70.0	C79.32	—	D32.0	D42.0	D49.7
cranial	C70.0	C79.32	—	D32.0	D42.0	D49.7
spinal	C70.1	C79.49	—	D32.1	D42.1	D49.7
pillars of fauces	C09.1	C79.89	D00.08	D10.5	D37.05	D49.0
pineal (body) (gland)	C75.3	C79.89	D09.3	D35.4	D44.5	D49.7
pinna (ear) NEC — see also Neoplasm, skin, ear	C44.20-☑	C79.2	D04.2-☑	D23.2-☑	D48.5	D49.2
piriform fossa or sinus	C12	C79.89	D00.08	D10.7	D37.05	D49.0
pituitary (body) (fossa) (gland) (lobe)	C75.1	C79.89	D09.3	D35.2	D44.3	D49.7
placenta	C58	C79.82	D07.0	D26.7	D39.2	D49.5
pleura, pleural (cavity)	C38.4	C78.2	—	D19.0	D38.2	D49.1
overlapping lesion with heart or mediastinum	C38.8	—	—	—	—	—
parietal	C38.4	C78.2	—	D19.0	D38.2	D49.1
visceral	C38.4	C78.2	—	D19.0	D38.2	D49.1
plexus						
brachial	C47.1-☑	C79.89	—	D36.12	D48.2	D49.2
cervical	C47.0	C79.89	—	D36.11	D48.2	D49.2
choroid	C71.5	C79.31	—	D33.0	D43.0	D49.6
lumbosacral	C47.5	C79.89	—	D36.16	D48.2	D49.2
sacral	C47.5	C79.89	—	D36.16	D48.2	D49.2
pluriendocrine	C75.8	C79.89	D09.3	D35.7	D44.9	D49.7
pole						

☑ Additional Character Required — Refer to the Tabular List for Character Selection   ▽ Subterms under main terms may continue to next column or page

Neoplasm, neoplastic — continued	Malignant Primary	Malignant Secondary	Ca in situ	Benign	Uncertain	Unspecified Behavior
pole — continued						
frontal	C71.1	C79.31	—	D33.0	D43.0	D49.6
occipital	C71.4	C79.31	—	D33.0	D43.0	D49.6
pons (varolii)	C71.7	C79.31	—	D33.1	D43.1	D49.6
popliteal fossa or space	C76.5-✓	C79.89	D04.7-✓	D36.7	D48.7	D49.89
postcricoid (region)	C13.0	C79.89	D00.08	D10.7	D37.05	D49.0
posterior fossa (cranial)	C71.9	C79.31	—	D33.2	D43.2	D49.6
postnasal space	C11.9	C79.89	D00.08	D10.6	D37.05	D49.0
prepuce	C60.0	C79.82	D07.4	D29.0	D40.8	D49.5
prepylorus	C16.4	C78.89	D00.2	D13.1	D37.1	D49.0
presacral (region)	C76.3	C79.89	—	D36.7	D48.7	D49.89
prostate (gland)	C61	C79.82	D07.5	D29.1	D40.0	D49.5
utricle	C68.0	C79.19	D09.19	D30.4	D41.3	D49.5
pterygoid fossa	C49.0	C79.89	—	D21.0	D48.1	D49.2
pubic bone	C41.4	C79.51	—	D16.8	D48.0	D49.2
pudenda, pudendum (femae)	C51.9	C79.82	D07.1	D28.0	D39.8	D49.5
pulmonary — see also Neoplasm, lung	C34.9-✓	C78.0-✓	D02.2-✓	D14.3-✓	D38.1	D49.1
putamen	C71.0	C79.31	—	D33.0	D43.0	D49.6
pyloric						
antrum	C16.3	C78.89	D00.2	D13.1	D37.1	D49.0
canal	C16.4	C78.89	D00.2	D13.1	D37.1	D49.0
pylorus	C16.4	C78.89	D00.2	D13.1	D37.1	D49.0
pyramid (brain)	C71.7	C79.31	—	D33.1	D43.1	D49.6
pyriform fossa or sinus	C12	C79.89	D00.08	D10.7	D37.05	D49.0
radius (any part)	C40.0-✓	C79.51	—	D16.0-✓	—	—
Rathke's pouch	C75.1	C79.89	D09.3	D35.2	D44.3	D49.7
rectosigmoid (junction)	C19	C78.5	D01.1	D12.7	D37.5	D49.0
overlapping lesion with anus or rectum	C21.8	—	—	—	—	—
rectouterine pouch	C48.1	C78.6	—	D20.1	D48.4	D49.0
rectovaginal septum or wall	C76.3	C79.89	D09.8	D36.7	D48.7	D49.89
rectovesical septum	C76.3	C79.89	D09.8	D36.7	D48.7	D49.89
rectum (ampulla)	C20	C78.5	D01.2	D12.8	D37.5	D49.0
and colon	C19	C78.5	D01.1	D12.7	D37.5	D49.0
overlapping lesion with anus or rectosigmoid junction	C21.8	—	—	—	—	—
renal	C64.-✓	C79.0-✓	D09.19	D30.0-✓	D41.0-✓	D49.5
calyx	C65.-✓	C79.0-✓	D09.19	D30.1-✓	D41.1-✓	D49.5
hilus	C65.-✓	C79.0-✓	D09.19	D30.1-✓	D41.1-✓	D49.5
parenchyma	C64.-✓	C79.0-✓	D09.19	D30.0-✓	D41.0-✓	D49.5
pelvis	C65.-✓	C79.0-✓	D09.19	D30.1-✓	D41.1-✓	D49.5
respiratory						
organs or system NEC	C39.9	C78.30	D02.4	D14.4	D38.6	D49.1
tract NEC	C39.9	C78.30	D02.4	D14.4	D38.5	D49.1
upper	C39.0	C78.30	D02.4	D14.4	D38.5	D49.1
retina	C69.2-✓	C79.49	D09.2-✓	D31.2-✓	D48.7	D49.81
retrobulbar	C69.6-✓	C79.49	—	D31.6-✓	D48.7	D49.89
retrocecal	C48.0	C78.6	—	D20.0	D48.3	D49.0
retromolar (area) (triangle) (trigone)	C06.2	C79.89	D00.00	D10.39	D37.09	D49.0
retro-orbital	C76.0	C79.89	D09.8	D36.7	D48.7	D49.89
retroperitoneal (space) (tissue)	C48.0	C78.6	—	D20.0	D48.3	D49.0
retroperitoneum	C48.0	C78.6	—	D20.0	D48.3	D49.0
retropharyngeal	C14.0	C79.89	D00.08	D10.9	D37.05	D49.0
retrovesical (septum)	C76.3	C79.89	D09.8	D36.7	D48.7	D49.89
rhinencephalon	C71.0	C79.31	—	D33.0	D43.0	D49.6
rib	C41.3	C79.51	—	D16.7	D48.0	D49.2
Rosenmuller's fossa	C11.2	C79.89	D00.08	D10.6	D37.05	D49.0
round ligament	C57.2✓	C79.82	—	D28.2	D39.8	D49.5
sacrococcyx, sacrococcygeal	C41.4	C79.51	—	D16.8	D48.0	D49.2
region	C76.3	C79.89	D09.8	D36.7	D48.7	D49.89
sacrouterine ligament	C57.3	C79.82	—	D28.2	D39.8	D49.5
sacrum, sacral (vertebra)	C41.4	C79.51	—	D16.8	D48.0	D49.2

Neoplasm, neoplastic — continued	Malignant Primary	Malignant Secondary	Ca in situ	Benign	Uncertain	Unspecified Behavior
salivary gland or duct (major)	C08.9	C79.89	D00.00	D11.9	D37.039	D49.0
minor NEC	C06.9	C79.89	D00.00	D10.39	D37.04	D49.0
overlapping lesion	C08.9	—	—	—	—	—
parotid	C07	C79.89	D00.00	D11.0	D37.030	D49.0
pluriglandular	C08.9	C79.89	D00.00	D11.9	D37.039	D49.0
sublingual	C08.1	C79.89	D00.00	D11.7	D37.031	D49.0
submandibular	C08.0	C79.89	D00.00	D11.7	D37.032	D49.0
submaxillary	C08.0	C79.89	D00.00	D11.7	D37.032	D49.0
salpinx (uterine)	C57.0-✓	C79.82	D07.39	D28.2	D39.8	D49.5
Santorini's duct	C25.3	C78.89	D01.7	D13.6	D37.8	D49.0
scalp	C44.40	C79.2	D04.4	D23.4	D48.5	D49.2
basal cell carcinoma	C44.41	—	—	—	—	—
specified type NEC	C44.49	—	—	—	—	—
squamous cell carcinoma	C44.42	—	—	—	—	—
scapula (any part)	C40.0-✓	C79.51	—	D16.0-✓	—	—
scapular region	C76.1	C79.89	D09.8	D36.7	D48.7	D49.89
scar NEC — see also Neoplasm, skin, by site	C44.90	C79.2	D04.9	D23.9	D48.5	D49.2
sciatic nerve	C47.2-✓	C79.89	—	D36.13	D48.2	D49.2
sclera	C69.4-✓	C79.49	D09.2-✓	D31.4-✓	D48.7	D49.89
scrotum (skin)	C63.2	C79.82	D07.61	D29.4	D40.8	D49.5
sebaceous gland — see Neoplasm, skin						
sella turcica	C75.1	C79.89	D09.3	D35.2	D44.3	D49.7
bone	C41.0	C79.51	—	D16.4	D48.0	D49.2
semilunar cartilage (knee)	C40.2-✓	C79.51	—	D16.2-✓	D48.0	D49.2
seminal vesicle	C63.7	C79.82	D07.69	D29.8	D40.8	D49.5
septum						
nasal	C30.0	C78.39	D02.3	D14.0	D38.5	D49.1
posterior margin	C11.3	C79.89	D00.08	D10.6	D37.05	D49.0
rectovaginal	C76.3	C79.89	D09.8	D36.7	D48.7	D49.89
rectovesical	C76.3	C79.89	D09.8	D36.7	D48.7	D49.89
urethrovaginal	C57.9	C79.82	D07.30	D28.9	D39.9	D49.5
vesicovaginal	C57.9	C79.82	D07.30	D28.9	D39.9	D49.5
shoulder NEC	C76.4-✓	C79.89	D04.6-✓	D36.7	D48.7	D49.89
sigmoid flexure (lower) (upper)	C18.7	C78.5	D01.0	D12.5	D37.4	D49.0
sinus (accessory)	C31.9	C78.39	D02.3	D14.0	D38.5	D49.1
bone (any)	C41.0	C79.51	—	D16.4	D48.0	D49.2
ethmoidal	C31.1	C78.39	D02.3	D14.0	D38.5	D49.1
frontal	C31.2	C78.39	D02.3	D14.0	D38.5	D49.1
maxillary	C31.0	C78.39	D02.3	D14.0	D38.5	D49.1
nasal, paranasal NEC	C31.9	C78.39	D02.3	D14.0	D38.5	D49.1
overlapping lesion	C31.8	—	—	—	—	—
pyriform	C12	C79.89	D00.08	D10.7	D37.05	D49.0
sphenoid	C31.3	C78.39	D02.3	D14.0	D38.5	D49.1
skeleton, skeletal NEC	C41.9	C79.51	—	D16.9	D48.0	D49.2
Skene's gland	C68.1	C79.19	D09.19	D30.8	D41.8	D49.5
skin NOS	C44.90	C79.2	D04.9	D23.9	D48.5	D49.2
abdominal wall	C44.509	C79.2	D04.5	D23.5	D48.5	D49.2
basal cell carcinoma	C44.519	—	—	—	—	—
specified type NEC	C44.599	—	—	—	—	—
squamous cell carcinoma	C44.529	—	—	—	—	—
ala nasi — see also Neoplasm, nose, skin	C44.301	C79.2	D04.39	D23.39	D48.5	D49.2
ankle — see also Neoplasm, skin, limb, lower	C44.70-✓	C79.2	D04.7-✓	D23.7-✓	D48.5	D49.2
antecubital space — see also Neoplasm, skin, limb, upper	C44.60-✓	C79.2	D04.6-✓	D23.6-✓	D48.5	D49.2
anus	C44.500	C79.2	D04.5	D23.5	D48.5	D49.2
basal cell carcinoma	C44.510	—	—	—	—	—
specified type NEC	C44.590	—	—	—	—	—
squamous cell carcinoma	C44.520	—	—	—	—	—

Neoplasm Table

Neoplasm, skin NOS — Neoplasm, skin NOS

Neoplasm, neoplastic — continued skin — continued	Malignant Primary	Malignant Secondary	Ca in situ	Benign	Uncertain	Unspecified Behavior
arm — see also Neoplasm, skin, limb, upper	C44.60-☑	C79.2	D04.6-☑	D23.6-☑	D48.5	D49.2
auditory canal (external) — see also Neoplasm, skin, ear	C44.20-☑	C79.2	D04.2-☑	D23.2-☑	D48.5	D49.2
auricle (ear) — see also Neoplasm, skin, ear	C44.20-☑	C79.2	D04.2-☑	D23.2-☑	D48.5	D49.2
auricular canal (external) — see also Neoplasm, skin, ear	C44.20-☑	C79.2	D04.2-☑	D23.2-☑	D48.5	D49.2
axilla, axillary fold — see also Neoplasm, skin, trunk	C44.509	C79.2	D04.5	D23.5	D48.5	D49.2
back — see also Neoplasm, skin, trunk	C44.509	C79.2	D04.5	D23.5	D48.5	D49.2
basal cell carcinoma	C44.91	—	—	—	—	—
breast	C44.501	C79.2	D04.5	D23.5	D48.5	D49.2
basal cell carcinoma	C44.511	—	—	—	—	—
specified type NEC	C44.591	—	—	—	—	—
squamous cell carcinoma	C44.521	—	—	—	—	—
brow — see also Neoplasm, skin, face	C44.309	C79.2	D04.39	D23.39	D48.5	D49.2
buttock — see also Neoplasm, skin, trunk	C44.509	C79.2	D04.5	D23.5	D48.5	D49.2
calf — see also Neoplasm, skin, limb, lower	C44.70-☑	C79.2	D04.7-☑	D23.7-☑	D48.5	D49.2
canthus (eye) (inner) (outer)	C44.10-☑	C79.2	D04.1-☑	D23.1-☑	D48.5	D49.2
basal cell carcinoma	C44.11-☑	—	—	—	—	—
specified type NEC	C44.19-☑	—	—	—	—	—
squamous cell carcinoma	C44.12-☑	—	—	—	—	—
cervical region — see also Neoplasm, skin, neck	C44.40	C79.2	D04.4	D23.4	D48.5	D49.2
cheek (external) — see also Neoplasm, skin, face	C44.309	C79.2	D04.39	D23.39	D48.5	D49.2
chest (wall) — see also Neoplasm, skin, trunk	C44.509	C79.2	D04.5	D23.5	D48.5	D49.2
chin — see also Neoplasm, skin, face	C44.309	C79.2	D04.39	D23.39	D48.5	D49.2
clavicular area — see also Neoplasm, skin, trunk	C44.509	C79.2	D04.5	D23.5	D48.5	D49.2
clitoris	C51.2	C79.82	D07.1	D28.0	D39.8	D49.5
columnella — see also Neoplasm, skin, face	C44.309	C79.2	D04.39	D23.39	D48.5	D49.2
concha — see also Neoplasm, skin, ear	C44.20-☑	C79.2	D04.2-☑	D23.2-☑	D48.5	D49.2
ear (external)	C44.20-☑	C79.2	D04.2-☑	D23.2-☑	D48.5	D49.2
basal cell carcinoma	C44.21-☑	—	—	—	—	—
specified type NEC	C44.29-☑	—	—	—	—	—
squamous cell carcinoma	C44.22-☑	—	—	—	—	—
elbow — see also Neoplasm, skin, limb, upper	C44.60-☑	C79.2	D04.6-☑	D23.6-☑	D48.5	D49.2

Neoplasm, neoplastic — continued skin — continued	Malignant Primary	Malignant Secondary	Ca in situ	Benign	Uncertain	Unspecified Behavior
eyebrow — see also Neoplasm, skin, face	C44.309	C79.2	D04.39	D23.39	D48.5	D49.2
eyelid	C44.10-☑	C79.2	D04.1-☑	D23.1-☑	D48.5	D49.2
basal cell carcinoma	C44.11-☑	—	—	—	—	—
specified type NEC	C44.19-☑	—	—	—	—	—
squamous cell carcinoma	C44.12-☑	—	—	—	—	—
face NOS	C44.300	C79.2	D04.30	D23.30	D48.5	D49.2
basal cell carcinoma	C44.310	—	—	—	—	—
specified type NEC	C44.390	—	—	—	—	—
squamous cell carcinoma	C44.320	—	—	—	—	—
female genital organs (external)	C51.9	C79.82	D07.1	D28.0	D39.8	D49.5
clitoris	C51.2	C79.82	D07.1	D28.0	D39.8	D49.5
labium NEC	C51.9	C79.82	D07.1	D28.0	D39.8	D49.5
majus	C51.0	C79.82	D07.1	D28.0	D39.8	D49.5
minus	C51.1	C79.82	D07.1	D28.0	D39.8	D49.5
pudendum	C51.9	C79.82	D07.1	D28.0	D39.8	D49.5
vulva	C51.9	C79.82	D07.1	D28.0	D39.8	D49.5
finger — see also Neoplasm, skin, limb, upper	C44.60-☑	C79.2	D04.6-☑	D23.6-☑	D48.5	D49.2
flank — see also Neoplasm, skin, trunk	C44.509	C79.2	D04.5	D23.5	D48.5	D49.2
foot — see also Neoplasm, skin, limb, lower	C44.70-☑	C79.2	D04.7-☑	D23.7-☑	D48.5	D49.2
forearm — see also Neoplasm, skin, limb, upper	C44.60-☑	C79.2	D04.6-☑	D23.6-☑	D48.5	D49.2
forehead — see also Neoplasm, skin, face	C44.309	C79.2	D04.39	D23.39	D48.5	D49.2
glabella — see also Neoplasm, skin, face	C44.309	C79.2	D04.39	D23.39	D48.5	D49.2
gluteal region — see also Neoplasm, skin, trunk	C44.509	C79.2	D04.5	D23.5	D48.5	D49.2
groin — see also Neoplasm, skin, trunk	C44.509	C79.2	D04.5	D23.5	D48.5	D49.2
hand — see also Neoplasm, skin, limb, upper	C44.60-☑	C79.2	D04.6-☑	D23.6-☑	D48.5	D49.2
head NEC — see also Neoplasm, skin, scalp	C44.40	C79.2	D04.4	D23.4	D48.5	D49.2
heel — see also Neoplasm, skin, limb, lower	C44.70-☑	C79.2	D04.7-☑	D23.7-☑	D48.5	D49.2
helix — see also Neoplasm, skin, ear	C44.20-☑	C79.2	D04.2-☑	D23.2-☑	D48.5	D49.2
hip — see also Neoplasm, skin, limb, lower	C44.70-☑	C79.2	D04.7-☑	D23.7-☑	D48.5	D49.2
infraclavicular region — see also Neoplasm, skin, trunk	C44.509	C79.2	D04.5	D23.5	D48.5	D49.2
inguinal region — see also Neoplasm, skin, trunk	C44.509	C79.2	D04.5	D23.5	D48.5	D49.2
jaw — see also Neoplasm, skin, face	C44.309	C79.2	D04.39	D23.39	D48.5	D49.2
Kaposi's sarcoma — see Kaposi's, sarcoma, skin						
knee — see also Neoplasm, skin, limb, lower	C44.70-☑	C79.2	D04.7-☑	D23.7-☑	D48.5	D49.2
labia						

☑ Additional Character Required — Refer to the Tabular List for Character Selection   Subterms under main terms may continue to next column or page

Neoplasm, neoplastic — continued	Malignant Primary	Malignant Secondary	Ca in situ	Benign	Uncertain	Unspecified Behavior
skin — continued						
labia — continued						
majora	C51.0	C79.82	D07.1	D28.0	D39.8	D49.5
minora	C51.1	C79.82	D07.1	D28.0	D39.8	D49.5
leg — see also						
Neoplasm, skin, limb, lower	C44.70-☑	C79.2	D04.7-☑	D23.7-☑	D48.5	D49.2
lid (lower) (upper)	C44.10-☑	C79.2	D04.1-☑	D23.1-☑	D48.5	D49.2
basal cell						
carcinoma	C44.11-☑	—	—	—	—	—
specified type NEC	C44.19-☑	—	—	—	—	—
squamous cell						
carcinoma	C44.12-☑	—	—	—	—	—
limb NEC	C44.90	C79.2	D04.9	D23.9	D48.5	D49.2
basal cell						
carcinoma	C44.91					
lower	C44.70-☑	C79.2	D04.7-☑	D23.7-☑	D48.5	D49.2
basal cell						
carcinoma	C44.71-☑					
specified type NEC	C44.79-☑					
squamous cell						
carcinoma	C44.72-☑					
upper	C44.60-☑	C79.2	D04.6-☑	D23.6-☑	D48.5	D49.2
basal cell						
carcinoma	C44.61-☑					
specified type NEC	C44.69-☑					
squamous cell						
carcinoma	C44.62-☑	—				
lip (lower) (upper)	C44.00	C79.2	D04.0	D23.0	D48.5	D49.2
basal cell						
carcinoma	C44.01					
specified type NEC	C44.09					
squamous cell						
carcinoma	C44.02					
male genital organs	C63.9	C79.82	D07.60	D29.9	D40.8	D49.5
penis	C60.9	C79.82	D07.4	D29.0	D40.8	D49.5
prepuce	C60.0	C79.82	D07.4	D29.0	D40.8	D49.5
scrotum	C63.2	C79.82	D07.61	D29.4	D40.8	D49.5
mastectomy site (skin) — see also						
Neoplasm, skin, breast	C44.501	C79.2				
specified as breast tissue	C50.8-☑	C79.81	—			
meatus, acoustic (external) — see also Neoplasm, skin, ear	C44.20-☑	C79.2	D04.2-☑	D23.2-☑	D48.5	D49.2
melanotic — see Melanoma						
Merkel cell — see Carcinoma, Merkel cell						
nates — see also Neoplasm, skin, trunk	C44.509	C79.2	D04.5	D23.5	D48.5	D49.2
neck	C44.40	C79.2	D04.4	D23.4	D48.5	D49.2
basal cell						
carcinoma	C44.41	—	—	—	—	—
specified type NEC	C44.49	—	—	—	—	—
squamous cell						
carcinoma	C44.42	—	—	—	—	—
nevus — see Nevus, skin						
nose (external) — see also Neoplasm, nose, skin	C44.301	C79.2	D04.39	D23.39	D48.5	D49.2
overlapping lesion	C44.80					
basal cell						
carcinoma	C44.81	—				
specified type NEC	C44.89	—				
squamous cell						
carcinoma	C44.82	—				

Neoplasm, neoplastic — continued	Malignant Primary	Malignant Secondary	Ca in situ	Benign	Uncertain	Unspecified Behavior
skin — continued						
palm — see also Neoplasm, skin, limb, upper	C44.60-☑	C79.2	D04.6-☑	D23.6-☑	D48.5	D49.2
palpebra	C44.10-☑	C79.2	D04.1-☑	D23.1-☑	D48.5	D49.2
basal cell						
carcinoma	C44.11-☑	—	—	—	—	—
specified type NEC	C44.19-☑	—	—	—	—	—
squamous cell						
carcinoma	C44.12-☑	—	—	—	—	—
penis NEC	C60.9	C79.82	D07.4	D29.0	D40.8	D49.5
perianal — see also Neoplasm, skin, anus	C44.500	C79.2	D04.5	D23.5	D48.5	D49.2
perineum — see also Neoplasm, skin, anus	C44.500	C79.2	D04.5	D23.5	D48.5	D49.2
pinna — see also Neoplasm, skin, ear	C44.20-☑	C79.2	D04.2-☑	D23.2-☑	D48.5	D49.2
plantar — see also Neoplasm, skin, limb, lower	C44.70-☑	C79.2	D04.7-☑	D23.7-☑	D48.5	D49.2
popliteal fossa or space — see also Neoplasm, skin, limb, lower	C44.70-☑	C79.2	D04.7-☑	D23.7-☑	D48.5	D49.2
prepuce	C60.0	C79.82	D07.4	D29.0	D40.8	D49.5
pubes — see also Neoplasm, skin, trunk	C44.509	C79.2	D04.5	D23.5	D48.5	D49.2
sacrococcygeal region — see also Neoplasm, skin, trunk	C44.509	C79.2	D04.5	D23.5	D48.5	D49.2
scalp	C44.40	C79.2	D04.4	D23.4	D48.5	D49.2
basal cell						
carcinoma	C44.41	—	—	—	—	—
specified type NEC	C44.49	—	—	—	—	—
squamous cell						
carcinoma	C44.42	—	—	—	—	—
scapular region — see also Neoplasm, skin, trunk	C44.509	C79.2	D04.5	D23.5	D48.5	D49.2
scrotum	C63.2	C79.82	D07.61	D29.4	D40.8	D49.5
shoulder — see also Neoplasm, skin, limb, upper	C44.60-☑	C79.2	D04.6-☑	D23.6-☑	D48.5	D49.2
sole (foot) — see also Neoplasm, skin, limb, lower	C44.70-☑	C79.2	D04.7-☑	D23.7-☑	D48.5	D49.2
specified sites NEC	C44.80	C79.2	D04.8	D23.9	D48.5	D49.2
basal cell						
carcinoma	C44.81	—	—	—	—	—
specified type NEC	C44.89	—	—	—	—	—
squamous cell						
carcinoma	C44.82	—	—	—	—	—
specified type NEC	C44.99	—	—	—	—	—
squamous cell						
carcinoma	C44.92	—	—	—	—	—
submammary fold — see also Neoplasm, skin, trunk	C44.509	C79.2	D04.5	D23.5	D48.5	D49.2
supraclavicular region — see also Neoplasm, skin, neck	C44.40	C79.2	D04.4	D23.4	D48.5	D49.2
temple — see also Neoplasm, skin, face	C44.309	C79.2	D04.39	D23.39	D48.5	D49.2
thigh — see also Neoplasm, skin, limb, lower	C44.70-☑	C79.2	D04.7-☑	D23.7-☑	D48.5	D49.2
thoracic wall — see also Neoplasm, skin, trunk	C44.509	C79.2	D04.5	D23.5	D48.5	D49.2

Neoplasm Table

Neoplasm, skin NOS — Neoplasm, thyroglossal duct

Neoplasm, neoplastic —	Malignant Primary	Malignant Secondary	Ca in situ	Benign	Uncertain	Unspecified Behavior
continued						
skin — continued						
thumb — see also						
Neoplasm, skin, limb, upper	C44.60-☑	C79.2	D04.6-☑	D23.6-☑	D48.5	D49.2
toe — see also						
Neoplasm, skin, limb, lower	C44.70-☑	C79.2	D04.7-☑	D23.7-☑	D48.5	D49.2
tragus — see also						
Neoplasm, skin, ear	C44.20-☑	C79.2	D04.2-☑	D23.2-☑	D48.5	D49.2
trunk	C44.509	C79.2	D04.5	D23.5	D48.5	D49.2
basal cell carcinoma	C44.519	—	—	—	—	—
specified type NEC	C44.599	—	—	—	—	—
squamous cell carcinoma	C44.529	—	—	—	—	—
umbilicus — see also						
Neoplasm, skin, trunk	C44.509	C79.2	D04.5	D23.5	D48.5	D49.2
vulva	C51.9	C79.82	D07.1	D28.0	D39.8	D49.5
overlapping lesion	C51.8	—	—	—	—	—
wrist — see also						
Neoplasm, skin, limb, upper	C44.60-☑	C79.2	D04.6-☑	D23.6-☑	D48.5	D49.2
skull	C41.0	C79.51	—	D16.4	D48.0	D49.2
soft parts or tissues — see Neoplasm, connective tissue						
specified site NEC	C76.8	C79.89	D09.8	D36.7	D48.7	D49.89
spermatic cord	C63.1-☑	C79.82	D07.69	D29.8	D40.8	D49.5
sphenoid	C31.3	C78.39	D02.3	D14.0	D38.5	D49.1
bone	C41.0	C79.51	—	D16.4	D48.0	D49.2
sinus	C31.3	C78.39	D02.3	D14.0	D38.5	D49.1
sphincter						
anal	C21.1	C78.5	D01.3	D12.9	D37.8	D49.0
of Oddi	C24.0	C78.89	D01.5	D13.5	D37.6	D49.0
spine, spinal (column)	C41.2	C79.51	—	D16.6	D48.0	D49.2
bulb	C71.7	C79.31	—	D33.1	D43.1	D49.6
coccyx	C41.4	C79.51	—	D16.8	D48.0	D49.2
cord (cervical) (lumbar) (sacral)						
(thoracic)	C72.0	C79.49	—	D33.4	D43.4	D49.7
dura mater	C70.1	C79.49	—	D32.1	D42.1	D49.7
lumbosacral	C41.2	C79.51	—	D16.6	D48.0	D49.2
marrow NEC	C96.9	C79.52	—	—	D47.9	D49.89
membrane	C70.1	C79.49	—	D32.1	D42.1	D49.7
meninges	C70.1	C79.49	—	D32.1	D42.1	D49.7
nerve (root)	C47.9	C79.89	—	D36.10	D48.2	D49.2
pia mater	C70.1	C79.49	—	D32.1	D42.1	D49.7
root	C47.9	C79.89	—	D36.10	D48.2	D49.2
sacrum	C41.4	C79.51	—	D16.8	D48.0	D49.2
spleen, splenic NEC	C26.1	C78.89	D01.7	D13.9	D37.8	D49.0
flexure (colon)	C18.5	C78.5	D01.0	D12.3	D37.4	D49.0
stem, brain	C71.7	C79.31	—	D33.1	D43.1	D49.6
Stensen's duct	C07	C79.89	D00.00	D11.0	D37.030	D49.0
sternum	C41.3	C79.51	—	D16.7	D48.0	D49.2
stomach	C16.9	C78.89	D00.2	D13.1	D37.1	D49.0
antrum (pyloric)	C16.3	C78.89	D00.2	D13.1	D37.1	D49.0
body	C16.2	C78.89	D00.2	D13.1	D37.1	D49.0
cardia	C16.0	C78.89	D00.2	D13.1	D37.1	D49.0
cardiac orifice	C16.0	C78.89	D00.2	D13.1	D37.1	D49.0
corpus	C16.2	C78.89	D00.2	D13.1	D37.1	D49.0
fundus	C16.1	C78.89	D00.2	D13.1	D37.1	D49.0
greater curvature NEC	C16.6	C78.89	D00.2	D13.1	D37.1	D49.0
lesser curvature NEC	C16.5	C78.89	D00.2	D13.1	D37.1	D49.0
overlapping lesion	C16.8	—	—	—	—	—
prepylorus	C16.4	C78.89	D00.2	D13.1	D37.1	D49.0
pylorus	C16.4	C78.89	D00.2	D13.1	D37.1	D49.0
wall NEC	C16.9	C78.89	D00.2	D13.1	D37.1	D49.0
anterior NEC	C16.8	C78.89	D00.2	D13.1	D37.1	D49.0
posterior NEC	C16.8	C78.89	D00.2	D13.1	D37.1	D49.0
stroma, endometrial	C54.1	C79.82	D07.0	D26.1	D39.0	D49.5
stump, cervical	C53.8	C79.82	D06.7	D26.0	D39.0	D49.5
subcutaneous (nodule) (tissue) NEC — see						

Neoplasm, neoplastic —	Malignant Primary	Malignant Secondary	Ca in situ	Benign	Uncertain	Unspecified Behavior
continued						
subcutaneous — see Neoplasm, connective tissue — continued						
Neoplasm, connective tissue						
subdural	C70.9	C79.32	—	D32.9	D42.9	D49.7
subglottis, subglottic	C32.2	C78.39	D02.0	D14.1	D38.0	D49.1
sublingual	C04.9	C79.89	D00.06	D10.2	D37.09	D49.0
gland or duct	C08.1	C79.89	D00.00	D11.7	D37.031	D49.0
submandibular gland	C08.0	C79.89	D00.00	D11.7	D37.032	D49.0
submaxillary gland or duct	C08.0	C79.89	D00.00	D11.7	D37.032	D49.0
submental	C76.0	C79.89	D09.8	D36.7	D48.7	D49.89
subpleural	C34.9-☑	C78.0-☑	D02.2-☑	D14.3-☑	D38.1	D49.1
substernal	C38.1	C78.1	—	D15.2	D38.3	D49.89
sudoriferous, sudoriparous gland, site unspecified	C44.90	C79.2	D04.9	D23.9	D48.5	D49.2
specified site — see Neoplasm, skin						
supraclavicular region	C76.0	C79.89	D09.8	D36.7	D48.7	D49.89
supraglottis	C32.1	C78.39	D02.0	D14.1	D38.0	D49.1
suprarenal	C74.9-☑	C79.7-☑	D09.3	D35.0-☑	D44.1-☑	D49.7
capsule	C74.9-☑	C79.7-☑	D09.3	D35.0-☑	D44.1-☑	D49.7
cortex	C74.0-☑	C79.7-☑	D09.3	D35.0-☑	D44.1-☑	D49.7
gland	C74.9-☑	C79.7-☑	D09.3	D35.0-☑	D44.1-☑	D49.7
medulla	C74.1-☑	C79.7-☑	D09.3	D35.0-☑	D44.1-☑	D49.7
suprasellar (region)	C71.9	C79.31	—	D33.2	D43.2	D49.6
supratentorial (brain)						
NEC	C71.0	C79.31	—	D33.0	D43.0	D49.6
sweat gland (apocrine) (eccrine), site unspecified	C44.90	C79.2	D04.9	D23.9	D48.5	D49.2
specified site — see Neoplasm, skin						
sympathetic nerve or nervous system						
NEC	C47.9	C79.89	—	D36.10	D48.2	D49.2
symphysis pubis	C41.4	C79.51	—	D16.8	D48.0	D49.2
synovial membrane — see Neoplasm, connective tissue						
tapetum, brain	C71.8	C79.31	—	D33.2	D43.2	D49.6
tarsus (any bone)	C40.3-☑	C79.51	—	D16.3-☑	—	—
temple (skin) — see also Neoplasm, skin, face	C44.309	C79.2	D04.39	D23.39	D48.5	D49.2
temporal						
bone	C41.0	C79.51	—	D16.4	D48.0	D49.2
lobe or pole	C71.2	C79.31	—	D33.0	D43.0	D49.6
region	C76.0	C79.89	D09.8	D36.7	D48.7	D49.89
skin — see also Neoplasm, skin, face	C44.309	C79.2	D04.39	D23.39	D48.5	D49.2
tendon (sheath) — see Neoplasm, connective tissue						
tentorium (cerebelli)	C70.0	C79.32	—	D32.0	D42.0	D49.7
testis, testes	C62.9-☑	C79.82	D07.69	D29.2-☑	D40.1-☑	D49.5
descended	C62.1-☑	C79.82	D07.69	D29.2-☑	D40.1-☑	D49.5
ectopic	C62.0-☑	C79.82	D07.69	D29.2-☑	D40.1-☑	D49.5
retained	C62.0-☑	C79.82	D07.69	D29.2-☑	D40.1-☑	D49.5
scrotal	C62.1-☑	C79.82	D07.69	D29.2-☑	D40.1-☑	D49.5
undescended	C62.0-☑	C79.82	D07.69	D29.2-☑	D40.1-☑	D49.5
unspecified whether descended or undescended	C62.9-☑	C79.82	D07.69	D29.2-☑	D40.1-☑	D49.5
thalamus	C71.0	C79.31	—	D33.0	D43.0	D49.6
thigh NEC	C76.5-☑	C79.89	D04.7-☑	D36.7	D48.7	D49.89
thorax, thoracic (cavity) (organs NEC)	C76.1	C79.89	D09.8	D36.7	D48.7	D49.89
duct	C49.3	C79.89	—	D21.3	D48.1	D49.2
wall NEC	C76.1	C79.89	D09.8	D36.7	D48.7	D49.89
throat	C14.0	C79.89	D00.08	D10.9	D37.05	D49.0
thumb NEC	C76.4-☑	C79.89	D04.6-☑	D36.7	D48.7	D49.89
thymus (gland)	C37	C79.89	D09.3	D15.0	D38.4	D49.89
thyroglossal duct	C73	C79.89	D09.3	D34	D44.0	D49.7

☑ Additional Character Required — Refer to the Tabular List for Character Selection   🔻 Subterms under main terms may continue to next column or page

Neoplasm, neoplastic — continued	Malignant Primary	Malignant Secondary	Ca in situ	Benign	Uncertain	Unspecified Behavior
thyroid (gland)	C73	C79.89	D09.3	D34	D44.0	D49.7
cartilage	C32.3	C78.39	D02.0	D14.1	D38.0	D49.1
tibia (any part)	C40.2-☑	C79.51	—	D16.2-☑	—	—
toe NEC	C76.5-☑	C79.89	D04.7-☑	D36.7	D48.7	D49.89
tongue	C02.9	C79.89	D00.07	D10.1	D37.02	D49.0
anterior (two-thirds) NEC	C02.3	C79.89	D00.07	D10.1	D37.02	D49.0
dorsal surface	C02.0	C79.89	D00.07	D10.1	D37.02	D49.0
ventral surface	C02.2	C79.89	D00.07	D10.1	D37.02	D49.0
base (dorsal surface)	C01	C79.89	D00.07	D10.1	D37.02	D49.0
border (lateral)	C02.1	C79.89	D00.07	D10.1	D37.02	D49.0
dorsal surface NEC	C02.0	C79.89	D00.07	D10.1	D37.02	D49.0
fixed part NEC	C01	C79.89	D00.07	D10.1	D37.02	D49.0
foreamen cecum	C02.0	C79.89	D00.07	D10.1	D37.02	D49.0
frenulum linguae	C02.2	C79.89	D00.07	D10.1	D37.02	D49.0
junctional zone	C02.8	C79.89	D00.07	D10.1	D37.02	D49.0
margin (lateral)	C02.1	C79.89	D00.07	D10.1	D37.02	D49.0
midline NEC	C02.0	C79.89	D00.07	D10.1	D37.02	D49.0
mobile part NEC	C02.3	C79.89	D00.07	D10.1	D37.02	D49.0
overlapping lesion	C02.8	—	—	—	—	—
posterior (third)	C01	C79.89	D00.07	D10.1	D37.02	D49.0
root	C01	C79.89	D00.07	D10.1	D37.02	D49.0
surface (dorsal)	C02.0	C79.89	D00.07	D10.1	D37.02	D49.0
base	C01	C79.89	D00.07	D10.1	D37.02	D49.0
ventral	C02.2	C79.89	D00.07	D10.1	D37.02	D49.0
tip	C02.1	C79.89	D00.07	D10.1	D37.02	D49.0
tonsil	C02.4	C79.89	D00.07	D10.1	D37.02	D49.0
tonsil	C09.9	C79.89	D00.08	D10.4	D37.05	D49.0
fauces, faucial	C09.9	C79.89	D00.08	D10.4	D37.05	D49.0
lingual	C02.4	C79.89	D00.07	D10.1	D37.02	D49.0
overlapping sites	C09.8	—	—	—	—	—
palatine	C09.9	C79.89	D00.08	D10.4	D37.05	D49.0
pharyngeal	C11.1	C79.89	D00.08	D10.6	D37.05	D49.0
pillar (anterior) (posterior)	C09.1	C79.89	D00.08	D10.5	D37.05	D49.0
tonsillar fossa	C09.0	C79.89	D00.08	D10.5	D37.05	D49.0
tooth socket NEC	C03.9	C79.89	D00.03	D10.39	D37.09	D49.0
trachea (cartilage) (mucosa)	C33	C78.39	D02.1	D14.2	D38.1	D49.1
overlapping lesion with bronchus or lung	C34.8-☑	—	—	—	—	—
tracheobronchial	C34.8-☑	C78.39	D02.1	D14.2	D38.1	D49.1
overlapping lesion with lung	C34.8-☑	—	—	—	—	—
tragus — see also Neoplasm, skin, ear	C44.20-☑	C79.2	D04.2-☑	D23.2-☑	D48.5	D49.2
trunk NEC	C76.8	C79.89	D04.5	D36.7	D48.7	D49.89
tubo-ovarian	C57.8	C79.82	D07.39	D28.7	D39.8	D49.5
tunica vaginalis	C63.7	C79.82	D07.69	D29.8	D40.8	D49.5
turbinate (bone)	C41.0	C79.51	—	D16.4	D48.0	D49.2
nasal	C30.0	C78.39	D02.3	D14.0	D38.5	D49.1
tympanic cavity	C30.1	C78.39	D02.3	D14.0	D38.5	D49.1
ulna (any part)	C40.0-☑	C79.51	—	D16.0-☑	—	—
umbilicus, umbilical — see also Neoplasm, skin, trunk	C44.509	C79.2	D04.5	D23.5	D48.5	D49.2
uncus, brain	C71.2	C79.31	—	D33.0	D43.0	D49.6
unknown site or unspecified	C80.1	C79.9	D09.9	D36.9	D48.9	D49.9
urachus	C67.7	C79.11	D09.0	D30.3	D41.4	D49.4
ureter-bladder (junction)	C67.6	C79.11	D09.0	D30.3	D41.4	D49.4
ureter, ureteral	C66.-☑	C79.19	D09.19	D30.2-☑	D41.2-☑	D49.5
orifice (bladder)	C67.6	C79.11	D09.0	D30.3	D41.4	D49.4
urethra, urethral (gland)	C68.0	C79.19	D09.19	D30.4	D41.3	D49.5
orifice, internal	C67.5	C79.11	D09.0	D30.3	D41.4	D49.4
urethrovaginal (septum)	C57.9	C79.82	D07.30	D28.9	D39.8	D49.5
urinary organ or system	C68.9	C79.10	D09.10	D30.9	D41.9	D49.5
bladder — see Neoplasm, bladder						
overlapping lesion	C68.8	—	—	—	—	—
specified sites NEC	C68.8	C79.19	D09.19	D30.8	D41.8	D49.5
utero-ovarian	C57.8	C79.82	D07.39	D28.7	D39.8	D49.5
ligament	C57.1-☑	C79.82	D07.39	D28.2	D39.8	D49.5
uterosacral ligament	C57.3	C79.82	—	D28.2	D39.8	D49.5
uterus, uteri, uterine	C55	C79.82	D07.0	D26.9	D39.0	D49.5
adnexa NEC	C57.4	C79.82	D07.39	D28.7	D39.8	D49.5
body	C54.9	C79.82	D07.0	D26.1	D39.0	D49.5
cervix	C53.9	C79.82	D06.9	D26.0	D39.0	D49.5
cornu	C54.9	C79.82	D07.0	D26.1	D39.0	D49.5
corpus	C54.9	C79.82	D07.0	D26.1	D39.0	D49.5
endocervix (canal) (gland)	C53.0	C79.82	D06.0	D26.0	D39.0	D49.5
endometrium	C54.1	C79.82	D07.0	D26.1	D39.0	D49.5
exocervix	C53.1	C79.82	D06.1	D26.0	D39.0	D49.5
external os	C53.1	C79.82	D06.1	D26.0	D39.0	D49.5
fundus	C54.3	C79.82	D07.0	D26.1	D39.0	D49.5
internal os	C53.0	C79.82	D06.0	D26.0	D39.0	D49.5
isthmus	C54.0	C79.82	D07.0	D26.1	D39.0	D49.5
ligament	C57.3	C79.82	—	D28.2	D39.8	D49.5
broad	C57.1-☑	C79.82	D07.39	D28.2	D39.8	D49.5
round	C57.2-☑	C79.82	—	D28.2	D39.8	D49.5
lower segment	C54.0	C79.82	D07.0	D26.1	D39.0	D49.5
myometrium	C54.2	C79.82	D07.0	D26.1	D39.0	D49.5
overlapping sites	C54.8	—	—	—	—	—
squamocolumnar junction	C53.8	C79.82	D06.7	D26.0	D39.0	D49.5
tube	C57.0-☑	C79.82	D07.39	D28.2	D39.8	D49.5
utricle, prostatic	C68.0	C79.19	D09.19	D30.4	D41.3	D49.5
uveal tract	C69.4-☑	C79.49	D09.2-☑	D31.4-☑	D48.7	D49.89
uvula	C05.2	C79.89	D00.04	D10.39	D37.09	D49.0
vagina, vaginal (fornix) (vault) (wall)	C52	C79.82	D07.2	D28.1	D39.8	D49.5
vaginovesical	C57.9	C79.82	D07.30	D28.9	D39.9	D49.5
septum	C57.9	C79.82	D07.30	D28.9	D39.9	D49.5
vallecula (epigiottis)	C10.0	C79.89	D00.08	D10.5	D37.05	D49.0
vascular — see Neoplasm, connective tissue						
vas deferens	C63.1-☑	C79.82	D07.69	D29.8	D40.8	D49.5
Vater's ampulla	C24.1	C78.89	D01.5	D13.5	D37.6	D49.0
vein, venous — see Neoplasm, connective tissue						
vena cava (abdominal) (inferior)	C49.4	C79.89	—	D21.4	D48.1	D49.2
superior	C49.3	C79.89	—	D21.3	D48.1	D49.2
ventricle (cerebral) (floor) (lateral) (third)	C71.5	C79.31	—	D33.0	D43.0	D49.6
cardiac (left) (right)	C38.0	C79.89	—	D15.1	D48.7	D49.89
fourth	C71.7	C79.31	—	D33.1	D43.1	D49.6
ventricular band of larynx	C32.1	C78.39	D02.0	D14.1	D38.0	D49.1
ventriculus — see Neoplasm, stomach						
vermillion border — see Neoplasm, lip						
vermis, cerebellum	C71.6	C79.31	—	D33.1	D43.1	D49.6
vertebra (column)	C41.2	C79.51	—	D16.6	D48.0	D49.2
coccyx	C41.4	C79.51	—	D16.8	D48.0	D49.2
marrow NEC	C96.9	C79.52	—	—	D47.9	D49.89
sacrum	C41.4	C79.51	—	D16.8	D48.0	D49.2
vesical — see Neoplasm, bladder						
vesicle, seminal	C63.7	C79.82	D07.69	D29.8	D40.8	D49.5
vesicocervical tissue	C57.9	C79.82	D07.30	D28.9	D39.9	D49.5
vesicorectal	C76.3	C79.82	D09.8	D36.7	D48.7	D49.89
vesicovaginal	C57.9	C79.82	D07.30	D28.9	D39.9	D49.5
septum	C57.9	C79.82	D07.30	D28.9	D39.8	D49.5
vessel (blood) — see Neoplasm, connective tissue						
vestibular gland, greater	C51.0	C79.82	D07.1	D28.0	D39.8	D49.5
vestibule						
mouth	C06.1	C79.89	D00.00	D10.39	D37.09	D49.0
nose	C30.0	C78.39	D02.3	D14.0	D38.5	D49.1
Virchow's gland	C77.0	C77.0	—	D36.0	D48.7	D49.89
viscera NEC	C76.8	C79.89	D09.8	D36.7	D48.7	D49.89
vocal cords (true)	C32.0	C78.39	D02.0	D14.1	D38.0	D49.1
false	C32.1	C78.39	D02.0	D14.1	D38.0	D49.1
vomer	C41.0	C79.51	—	D16.4	D48.0	D49.2
vulva	C51.9	C79.82	D07.1	D28.0	D39.8	D49.5
vulvovaginal gland	C51.0	C79.82	D07.1	D28.0	D39.8	D49.5
Waldeyer's ring	C14.2	C79.89	D00.08	D10.9	D37.05	D49.0
Wharton's duct	C08.0	C79.89	D00.00	D11.7	D37.032	D49.0

	Malignant Primary	Malignant Secondary	Ca in situ	Benign	Uncertain	Unspecified Behavior
Neoplasm, neoplastic —						
continued						
white matter (central)						
(cerebral)	C71.Ø	C79.31	—	D33.Ø	D43.Ø	D49.6
windpipe	C33	C78.39	DØ2.1	D14.2	D38.1	D49.1
Wirsung's duct	C25.3	C78.89	DØ1.7	D13.6	D37.8	D49.Ø
wolffian (body) (duct)						
female	C57.7	C79.82	DØ7.39	D28.7	D39.8	D49.5
male	C63.7	C79.82	DØ7.69	D29.8	D4Ø.8	D49.5
womb — *see* Neoplasm,						
uterus						
wrist NEC	C76.4-☑	C79.89	DØ4.6-☑	D36.7	D48.7	D49.89
xiphoid process	C41.3	C79.51	—	D16.7	D48.Ø	D49.2
Zuckerkandl organ	C75.5	C79.89	—	D35.6	D44.7	D49.7

☑ Additional Character Required — Refer to the Tabular List for Character Selection   ▽ Subterms under main terms may continue to next column or page

ICD-10-CM Table of Drugs and Chemicals

Anesthesia (handwritten)

Poisoning (watermark)

Substance	Poisoning, Accidental (unintentional)	Poisoning, Intentional Self-harm	Poisoning, Assault	Poisoning, Undetermined	Adverse Effect	Under-dosing
14-Hydroxydihydromorphinone	T40.2X1	T40.2X2	T40.2X3	T40.2X4	T40.2X5	T40.2X6
1-Propanol	T51.3X1	T51.3X2	T51.3X3	T51.3X4	—	—
2,3,7,8-Tetrachlorodibenzo-p-dioxin	T53.7X1	T53.7X2	T53.7X3	T53.7X4	—	—
2,4,5-T (trichlorophenoxyacetic acid)	T60.1X1	T60.1X2	T60.1X3	T60.1X4	—	—
2,4,5-Trichlorophenoxyacetic acid	T60.3X1	T60.3X2	T60.3X3	T60.3X4	—	—
2,4-D (dichlorophenoxyacetic acid)	T60.3X1	T60.3X2	T60.3X3	T60.3X4	—	—
2,4-Toluene diisocyanate	T65.0X1	T65.0X2	T65.0X3	T65.0X4	—	—
2-Deoxy-5-fluorouridine	T45.1X1	T45.1X2	T45.1X3	T45.1X4	T45.1X5	T45.1X6
2-Ethoxyethanol	T52.3X1	T52.3X2	T52.3X3	T52.3X4	—	—
2-Methoxyethanol	T52.3X1	T52.3X2	T52.3X3	T52.3X4	—	—
2-Propanol	T51.2X1	T51.2X2	T51.2X3	T51.2X4	—	—
4-Aminobutyric acid	T43.8X1	T43.8X2	T43.8X3	T43.8X4	T43.8X5	T43.8X6
4-Aminophenol derivatives	T39.1X1	T39.1X2	T39.1X3	T39.1X4	T39.1X5	T39.1X6
5-Deoxy-5-fluorouridine	T45.1X1	T45.1X2	T45.1X3	T45.1X4	T45.1X5	T45.1X6
5-Methoxypsoralen (5-MOP)	T50.991	T50.992	T50.993	T50.994	T50.995	T50.996
8-Aminoquinoline drugs	T37.2X1	T37.2X2	T37.2X3	T37.2X4	T37.2X5	T37.2X6
8-Methoxypsoralen (8-MOP)	T50.991	T50.992	T50.993	T50.994	T50.995	T50.996
ABOB	T37.5X1	T37.5X2	T37.5X3	T37.5X4	T37.5X5	T37.5X6
Abrine	T62.2X1	T62.2X2	T62.2X3	T62.2X4	—	—
Abrus (seed)	T62.2X1	T62.2X2	T62.2X3	T62.2X4	—	—
Absinthe	T51.0X1	T51.0X2	T51.0X3	T51.0X4	—	—
beverage	T51.0X1	T51.0X2	T51.0X3	T51.0X4	—	—
Acaricide	T60.8X1	T60.8X2	T60.8X3	T60.8X4	—	—
Acebutolol	T44.7X1	T44.7X2	T44.7X3	T44.7X4	T44.7X5	T44.7X6
Acecarbromal	T42.6X1	T42.6X2	T42.6X3	T42.6X4	T42.6X5	T42.6X6
Aceclidine	T44.1X1	T44.1X2	T44.1X3	T44.1X4	T44.1X5	T44.1X6
Acedapsone	T37.0X1	T37.0X2	T37.0X3	T37.0X4	T37.0X5	T37.0X6
Acefylline piperazine	T48.6X1	T48.6X2	T48.6X3	T48.6X4	T48.6X5	T48.6X6
Acemorphan	T40.2X1	T40.2X2	T40.2X3	T40.2X4	T40.2X5	T40.2X6
Acenocoumarin	T45.511	T45.512	T45.513	T45.514	T45.515	T45.516
Acenocoumarol	T45.511	T45.512	T45.513	T45.514	T45.515	T45.516
Acepifylline	T48.6X1	T48.6X2	T48.6X3	T48.6X4	T48.6X5	T48.6X6
Acepromazine	T43.3X1	T43.3X2	T43.3X3	T43.3X4	T43.3X5	T43.3X6
Acesulfamethoxypyridazine	T37.0X1	T37.0X2	T37.0X3	T37.0X4	T37.0X5	T37.0X6
Acetal	T52.8X1	T52.8X2	T52.8X3	T52.8X4	—	—
Acetaldehyde (vapor)	T52.8X1	T52.8X2	T52.8X3	T52.8X4	—	—
liquid	T65.891	T65.892	T65.893	T65.894	—	—
Acetaminophen	T39.1X1	T39.1X2	T39.1X3	T39.1X4	T39.1X5	T39.1X6
Acetaminosalol	T39.1X1	T39.1X2	T39.1X3	T39.1X4	T39.1X5	T39.1X6
Acetanilide	T39.1X1	T39.1X2	T39.1X3	T39.1X4	T39.1X5	T39.1X6
Acetarsol	T37.3X1	T37.3X2	T37.3X3	T37.3X4	T37.3X5	T37.3X6
Acetazolamide	T50.2X1	T50.2X2	T50.2X3	T50.2X4	T50.2X5	T50.2X6
Acetiamine	T45.2X1	T45.2X2	T45.2X3	T45.2X4	T45.2X5	T45.2X6
Acetic						
acid	T54.2X1	T54.2X2	T54.2X3	T54.2X4	—	—
with sodium acetate (ointment)	T49.3X1	T49.3X2	T49.3X3	T49.3X4	T49.3X5	T49.3X6
ester (solvent)(vapor)	T52.8X1	T52.8X2	T52.8X3	T52.8X4	—	—
irrigating solution	T50.3X1	T50.3X2	T50.3X3	T50.3X4	T50.3X5	T50.3X6
medicinal (lotion)	T49.2X1	T49.2X2	T49.2X3	T49.2X4	T49.2X5	T49.2X6
anhydride	T65.891	T65.892	T65.893	T65.894	—	—
ether (vapor)	T52.8X1	T52.8X2	T52.8X3	T52.8X4	—	—
Acetohexamide	T38.3X1	T38.3X2	T38.3X3	T38.3X4	T38.3X5	T38.3X6
Acetohydroxamic acid	T50.991	T50.992	T50.993	T50.994	T50.995	T50.996
Acetomenaphthone	T45.7X1	T45.7X2	T45.7X3	T45.7X4	T45.7X5	T45.7X6
Acetomorphine	T40.1X1	T40.1X2	T40.1X3	T40.1X4	—	—
Acetone (oils)	T52.4X1	T52.4X2	T52.4X3	T52.4X4	—	—
chlorinated	T52.4X1	T52.4X2	T52.4X3	T52.4X4	—	—
vapor	T52.4X1	T52.4X2	T52.4X3	T52.4X4	—	—
Acetonitrile	T52.8X1	T52.8X2	T52.8X3	T52.8X4	—	—
Acetophenazine	T43.3X1	T43.3X2	T43.3X3	T43.3X4	T43.3X5	T43.3X6
Acetophenetedin	T39.1X1	T39.1X2	T39.1X3	T39.1X4	T39.1X5	T39.1X6
Acetophenone	T52.4X1	T52.4X2	T52.4X3	T52.4X4	—	—
Acetorphine	T40.2X1	T40.2X2	T40.2X3	T40.2X4	—	—
Acetosulfone (sodium)	T37.1X1	T37.1X2	T37.1X3	T37.1X4	T37.1X5	T37.1X6
Acetrizoate (sodium)	T50.8X1	T50.8X2	T50.8X3	T50.8X4	T50.8X5	T50.8X6
Acetrizoic acid	T50.8X1	T50.8X2	T50.8X3	T50.8X4	T50.8X5	T50.8X6
Acetyl						
bromide	T53.6X1	T53.6X2	T53.6X3	T53.6X4	—	—
chloride	T53.6X1	T53.6X2	T53.6X3	T53.6X4	—	—
Acetylcarbromal	T42.6X1	T42.6X2	T42.6X3	T42.6X4	T42.6X5	T42.6X6

Substance	Poisoning, Accidental (unintentional)	Poisoning, Intentional Self-harm	Poisoning, Assault	Poisoning, Undetermined	Adverse Effect	Under-dosing
Acetylcholine						
chloride	T44.1X1	T44.1X2	T44.1X3	T44.1X4	T44.1X5	T44.1X6
derivative	T44.1X1	T44.1X2	T44.1X3	T44.1X4	T44.1X5	T44.1X6
Acetylcysteine	T48.4X1	T48.4X2	T48.4X3	T48.4X4	T48.4X5	T48.4X6
Acetyldigitoxin	T46.0X1	T46.0X2	T46.0X3	T46.0X4	T46.0X5	T46.0X6
Acetyldigoxin	T46.0X1	T46.0X2	T46.0X3	T46.0X4	T46.0X5	T46.0X6
Acetyldihydrocodeine	T40.2X1	T40.2X2	T40.2X3	T40.2X4	—	—
Acetyldihydrocodeinone	T40.2X1	T40.2X2	T40.2X3	T40.2X4	—	—
Acetylene (gas)	T59.891	T59.892	T59.893	T59.894	—	—
dichloride	T53.6X1	T53.6X2	T53.6X3	T53.6X4	—	—
incomplete combustion of	T58.11	T58.12	T58.13	T58.14	—	—
industrial	T59.891	T59.892	T59.893	T59.894	—	—
tetrachloride	T53.6X1	T53.6X2	T53.6X3	T53.6X4	—	—
vapor	T53.6X1	T53.6X2	T53.6X3	T53.6X4	—	—
Acetylpheneturide	T42.6X1	T42.6X2	T42.6X3	T42.6X4	T42.6X5	T42.6X6
Acetylphenylhydrazine	T39.8X1	T39.8X2	T39.8X3	T39.8X4	T39.8X5	T39.8X6
Acetylsalicylic acid (salts)	T39.011	T39.012	T39.013	T39.014	T39.015	T39.016
enteric coated	T39.011	T39.012	T39.013	T39.014	T39.015	T39.016
Acetylsulfamethoxypyridazine	T37.0X1	T37.0X2	T37.0X3	T37.0X4	T37.0X5	T37.0X6
Achromycin	T36.4X1	T36.4X2	T36.4X3	T36.4X4	T36.4X5	T36.4X6
ophthalmic preparation	T49.5X1	T49.5X2	T49.5X3	T49.5X4	T49.5X5	T49.5X6
topical NEC	T49.0X1	T49.0X2	T49.0X3	T49.0X4	T49.0X5	T49.0X6
Aciclovir	T37.5X1	T37.5X2	T37.5X3	T37.5X4	T37.5X5	T37.5X6
Acidifying agent NEC	T50.901	T50.902	T50.903	T50.904	T50.905	T50.906
Acid (corrosive) NEC	T54.2X1	T54.2X2	T54.2X3	T54.2X4	—	—
Acipimox	T46.6X1	T46.6X2	T46.6X3	T46.6X4	T46.6X5	T46.6X6
Acitretin	T50.991	T50.992	T50.993	T50.994	T50.995	T50.996
Aclarubicin	T45.1X1	T45.1X2	T45.1X3	T45.1X4	T45.1X5	T45.1X6
Aclatonium napadisilate	T48.1X1	T48.1X2	T48.1X3	T48.1X4	T48.1X5	T48.1X6
Aconite (wild)	T46.991	T46.992	T46.993	T46.994	T46.995	T46.996
Aconitine	T46.991	T46.992	T46.993	T46.994	T46.995	T46.996
Aconitum ferox	T46.991	T46.992	T46.993	T46.994	T46.995	T46.996
Acridine	T65.6X1	T65.6X2	T65.6X3	T65.6X4	—	—
vapor	T59.891	T59.892	T59.893	T59.894	—	—
Acriflavine	T37.91	T37.92	T37.93	T37.94	T37.95	T37.96
Acriflavinium chloride	T49.0X1	T49.0X2	T49.0X3	T49.0X4	T49.0X5	T49.0X6
Acrinol	T49.0X1	T49.0X2	T49.0X3	T49.0X4	T49.0X5	T49.0X6
Acrisorcin	T49.0X1	T49.0X2	T49.0X3	T49.0X4	T49.0X5	T49.0X6
Acrivastine	T45.0X1	T45.0X2	T45.0X3	T45.0X4	T45.0X5	T45.0X6
Acrolein (gas)	T59.891	T59.892	T59.893	T59.894	—	—
liquid	T54.1X1	T54.1X2	T54.1X3	T54.1X4	—	—
Acrylamide	T65.891	T65.892	T65.893	T65.894	—	—
Acrylic resin	T49.3X1	T49.3X2	T49.3X3	T49.3X4	T49.3X5	T49.3X6
Acrylonitrile	T65.891	T65.892	T65.893	T65.894	—	—
Actaea spicata	T62.2X1	T62.2X2	T62.2X3	T62.2X4	—	—
berry	T62.1X1	T62.1X2	T62.1X3	T62.1X4	—	—
Acterol	T37.3X1	T37.3X2	T37.3X3	T37.3X4	T37.3X5	T37.3X6
ACTH	T38.811	T38.812	T38.813	T38.814	T38.815	T38.816
Actinomycin C	T45.1X1	T45.1X2	T45.1X3	T45.1X4	T45.1X5	T45.1X6
Actinomycin D	T45.1X1	T45.1X2	T45.1X3	T45.1X4	T45.1X5	T45.1X6
Activated charcoal — see also Charcoal, medicinal	T47.6X1	T47.6X2	T47.6X3	T47.6X4	T47.6X5	T47.6X6
Acyclovir	T37.5X1	T37.5X2	T37.5X3	T37.5X4	T37.5X5	T37.5X6
Adenine	T45.2X1	T45.2X2	T45.2X3	T45.2X4	T45.2X5	T45.2X6
arabinoside	T37.5X1	T37.5X2	T37.5X3	T37.5X4	T37.5X5	T37.5X6
Adenosine (phosphate)	T46.2X1	T46.2X2	T46.2X3	T46.2X4	T46.2X5	T46.2X6
ADH	T38.891	T38.892	T38.893	T38.894	T38.895	T38.896
Adhesive NEC	T65.891	T65.892	T65.893	T65.894	—	—
Adicillin	T36.0X1	T36.0X2	T36.0X3	T36.0X4	T36.0X5	T36.0X6
Adiphenine	T44.3X1	T44.3X2	T44.3X3	T44.3X4	T44.3X5	T44.3X6
Adipiodone	T50.8X1	T50.8X2	T50.8X3	T50.8X4	T50.8X5	T50.8X6
Adjunct, pharmaceutical	T50.901	T50.902	T50.903	T50.904	T50.905	T50.906
Adrenal (extract, cortex or medulla) (glucocorticoids) (hormones) (mineralocorticoids)	T38.0X1	T38.0X2	T38.0X3	T38.0X4	T38.0X5	T38.0X6
ENT agent	T49.6X1	T49.6X2	T49.6X3	T49.6X4	T49.6X5	T49.6X6
ophthalmic preparation	T49.5X1	T49.5X2	T49.5X3	T49.5X4	T49.5X5	T49.5X6
topical NEC	T49.0X1	T49.0X2	T49.0X3	T49.0X4	T49.0X5	T49.0X6
Adrenalin — see Adrenaline						
Adrenaline	T44.5X1	T44.5X2	T44.5X3	T44.5X4	T44.5X5	T44.5X6
Adrenergic NEC	T44.901	T44.902	T44.903	T44.904	T44.905	T44.906
blocking agent NEC	T44.8X1	T44.8X2	T44.8X3	T44.8X4	T44.8X5	T44.8X6
beta, heart	T44.7X1	T44.7X2	T44.7X3	T44.7X4	T44.7X5	T44.7X6
specified NEC	T44.991	T44.992	T44.993	T44.994	T44.995	T44.996
Adrenochrome						
derivative	T46.991	T46.992	T46.993	T46.994	T46.995	T46.996

Substance	Poisoning, Accidental (unintentional)	Poisoning, Intentional Self-harm	Poisoning, Assault	Poisoning, Undetermined	Adverse Effect	Under-dosing
Adrenochrome — *continued*						
(mono) semicarbazone	T46.991	T46.992	T46.993	T46.994	T46.995	T46.996
Adrenocorticotrophic hormone	T38.811	T38.812	T38.813	T38.814	T38.815	T38.816
Adrenocorticotrophin	T38.811	T38.812	T38.813	T38.814	T38.815	T38.816
Adriamycin	T45.1X1	T45.1X2	T45.1X3	T45.1X4	T45.1X5	T45.1X6
Aerosol spray NEC	T65.91	T65.92	T65.93	T65.94	—	—
Aerosporin	T36.8X1	T36.8X2	T36.8X3	T36.8X4	T36.8X5	T36.8X6
ENT agent	T49.6X1	T49.6X2	T49.6X3	T49.6X4	T49.6X5	T49.6X6
ophthalmic preparation	T49.5X1	T49.5X2	T49.5X3	T49.5X4	T49.5X5	T49.5X6
topical NEC	T49.0X1	T49.0X2	T49.0X3	T49.0X4	T49.0X5	T49.0X6
Aethusa cynapium	T62.2X1	T62.2X2	T62.2X3	T62.2X4	—	—
Afghanistan black	T40.7X1	T40.7X2	T40.7X3	T40.7X4	T40.7X5	T40.7X6
Aflatoxin	T64.01	T64.02	T64.03	T64.04	—	—
Afloqualone	T42.8X1	T42.8X2	T42.8X3	T42.8X4	T42.8X5	T42.8X6
African boxwood	T62.2X1	T62.2X2	T62.2X3	T62.2X4	—	—
Agar	T47.4X1	T47.4X2	T47.4X3	T47.4X4	T47.4X5	T47.4X6
Agonist						
predominantly						
alpha-adrenoreceptor	T44.4X1	T44.4X2	T44.4X3	T44.4X4	T44.4X5	T44.4X6
beta-adrenoreceptor	T44.5X1	T44.5X2	T44.5X3	T44.5X4	T44.5X5	T44.5X6
Agricultural agent NEC	T65.91	T65.92	T65.93	T65.94	—	—
Agrypnal	T42.3X1	T42.3X2	T42.3X3	T42.3X4	T42.3X5	T42.3X6
AHLG	T50.Z11	T50.Z12	T50.Z13	T50.Z14	T50.Z15	T50.Z16
Air contaminant(s), **source/type NOS**	T65.91	T65.92	T65.93	T65.94	—	—
Ajmaline	T46.2X1	T46.2X2	T46.2X3	T46.2X4	T46.2X5	T46.2X6
Akee	T62.1X1	T62.1X2	T62.1X3	T62.1X4	—	—
Akrinol	T49.0X1	T49.0X2	T49.0X3	T49.0X4	T49.0X5	T49.0X6
Akritoin	T37.8X1	T37.8X2	T37.8X3	T37.8X4	T37.8X5	T37.8X6
Alacepril	T46.4X1	T46.4X2	T46.4X3	T46.4X4	T46.4X5	T46.4X6
Alantolactone	T37.4X1	T37.4X2	T37.4X3	T37.4X4	T37.4X5	T37.4X6
Albamycin	T36.8X1	T36.8X2	T36.8X3	T36.8X4	T36.8X5	T36.8X6
Albendazole	T37.4X1	T37.4X2	T37.4X3	T37.4X4	T37.4X5	T37.4X6
Albumin						
bovine	T45.8X1	T45.8X2	T45.8X3	T45.8X4	T45.8X5	T45.8X6
human serum	T45.8X1	T45.8X2	T45.8X3	T45.8X4	T45.8X5	T45.8X6
salt-poor	T45.8X1	T45.8X2	T45.8X3	T45.8X4	T45.8X5	T45.8X6
normal human serum	T45.8X1	T45.8X2	T45.8X3	T45.8X4	T45.8X5	T45.8X6
Albuterol	T48.6X1	T48.6X2	T48.6X3	T48.6X4	T48.6X5	T48.6X6
Albutoin	T42.0X1	T42.0X2	T42.0X3	T42.0X4	T42.0X5	T42.0X6
Alclometasone	T49.0X1	T49.0X2	T49.0X3	T49.0X4	T49.0X5	T49.0X6
Alcohol	T51.91	T51.92	T51.93	T51.94	—	—
absolute	T51.0X1	T51.0X2	T51.0X3	T51.0X4	—	—
beverage	T51.0X1	T51.0X2	T51.0X3	T51.0X4	—	—
allyl	T51.8X1	T51.8X2	T51.8X3	T51.8X4	—	—
amyl	T51.3X1	T51.3X2	T51.3X3	T51.3X4	—	—
antifreeze	T51.1X1	T51.1X2	T51.1X3	T51.1X4	—	—
beverage	T51.0X1	T51.0X2	T51.0X3	T51.0X4	—	—
butyl	T51.3X1	T51.3X2	T51.3X3	T51.3X4	—	—
dehydrated	T51.0X1	T51.0X2	T51.0X3	T51.0X4	—	—
beverage	T51.0X1	T51.0X2	T51.0X3	T51.0X4	—	—
denatured	T51.0X1	T51.0X2	T51.0X3	T51.0X4	—	—
deterrent NEC	T50.6X1	T50.6X2	T50.6X3	T50.6X4	T50.6X5	T50.6X6
diagnostic (gastric function)	T50.8X1	T50.8X2	T50.8X3	T50.8X4	T50.8X5	T50.8X6
ethyl	T51.0X1	T51.0X2	T51.0X3	T51.0X4	—	—
beverage	T51.0X1	T51.0X2	T51.0X3	T51.0X4	—	—
grain	T51.0X1	T51.0X2	T51.0X3	T51.0X4	—	—
beverage	T51.0X1	T51.0X2	T51.0X3	T51.0X4	—	—
industrial	T51.0X1	T51.0X2	T51.0X3	T51.0X4	—	—
isopropyl	T51.2X1	T51.2X2	T51.2X3	T51.2X4	—	—
methyl	T51.1X1	T51.1X2	T51.1X3	T51.1X4	—	—
preparation for consumption	T51.0X1	T51.0X2	T51.0X3	T51.0X4	—	—
propyl	T51.3X1	T51.3X2	T51.3X3	T51.3X4	—	—
secondary	T51.2X1	T51.2X2	T51.2X3	T51.2X4	—	—
radiator	T51.1X1	T51.1X2	T51.1X3	T51.1X4	—	—
rubbing	T51.2X1	T51.2X2	T51.2X3	T51.2X4	—	—
specified type NEC	T51.8X1	T51.8X2	T51.8X3	T51.8X4	—	—
surgical	T51.0X1	T51.0X2	T51.0X3	T51.0X4	—	—
vapor (from any type of Alcohol)	T59.891	T59.892	T59.893	T59.894	—	—
wood	T51.1X1	T51.1X2	T51.1X3	T51.1X4	—	—
Alcuronium (chloride)	T48.1X1	T48.1X2	T48.1X3	T48.1X4	T48.1X5	T48.1X6
Aldactone	T50.0X1	T50.0X2	T50.0X3	T50.0X4	T50.0X5	T50.0X6
Aldesulfone sodium	T37.1X1	T37.1X2	T37.1X3	T37.1X4	T37.1X5	T37.1X6
Aldicarb	T60.0X1	T60.0X2	T60.0X3	T60.0X4	—	—
Aldomet	T46.5X1	T46.5X2	T46.5X3	T46.5X4	T46.5X5	T46.5X6
Aldosterone	T50.0X1	T50.0X2	T50.0X3	T50.0X4	T50.0X5	T50.0X6
Aldrin (dust)	T60.1X1	T60.1X2	T60.1X3	T60.1X4	—	—
Aleve — *see* Naproxen						
Alexitol sodium	T47.1X1	T47.1X2	T47.1X3	T47.1X4	T47.1X5	T47.1X6

Substance	Poisoning, Accidental (unintentional)	Poisoning, Intentional Self-harm	Poisoning, Assault	Poisoning, Undetermined	Adverse Effect	Under-dosing
Alfacalcidol	T45.2X1	T45.2X2	T45.2X3	T45.2X4	T45.2X5	T45.2X6
Alfadolone	T41.1X1	T41.1X2	T41.1X3	T41.1X4	T41.1X5	T41.1X6
Alfaxalone	T41.1X1	T41.1X2	T41.1X3	T41.1X4	T41.1X5	T41.1X6
Alfentanil	T40.4X1	T40.4X2	T40.4X3	T40.4X4	T40.4X5	T40.4X6
Alfuzosin (hydrochloride)	T44.8X1	T44.8X2	T44.8X3	T44.8X4	T44.8X5	T44.8X6
Algae (harmful) (toxin)	T65.821	T65.822	T65.823	T65.824	—	—
Algeldrate	T47.1X1	T47.1X2	T47.1X3	T47.1X4	T47.1X5	T47.1X6
Algin	T47.8X1	T47.8X2	T47.8X3	T47.8X4	T47.8X5	T47.8X6
Alglucerase	T45.3X1	T45.3X2	T45.3X3	T45.3X4	T45.3X5	T45.3X6
Alidase	T45.3X1	T45.3X2	T45.3X3	T45.3X4	T45.3X5	T45.3X6
Alimemazine	T43.3X1	T43.3X2	T43.3X3	T43.3X4	T43.3X5	T43.3X6
Aliphatic thiocyanates	T65.0X1	T65.0X2	T65.0X3	T65.0X4	—	—
Alizapride	T45.0X1	T45.0X2	T45.0X3	T45.0X4	T45.0X5	T45.0X6
Alkali (caustic)	T54.3X1	T54.3X2	T54.3X3	T54.3X4	—	—
Alkaline antiseptic solution (aromatic)	T49.6X1	T49.6X2	T49.6X3	T49.6X4	T49.6X5	T49.6X6
Alkalinizing agents (medicinal)	T50.901	T50.902	T50.903	T50.904	T50.905	T50.906
Alkalizing agent NEC	T50.901	T50.902	T50.903	T50.904	T50.905	T50.906
Alka-seltzer	T39.011	T39.012	T39.013	T39.014	T39.015	T39.016
Alkavervir	T46.5X1	T46.5X2	T46.5X3	T46.5X4	T46.5X5	T46.5X6
Alkonium (bromide)	T49.0X1	T49.0X2	T49.0X3	T49.0X4	T49.0X5	T49.0X6
Alkylating drug NEC	T45.1X1	T45.1X2	T45.1X3	T45.1X4	T45.1X5	T45.1X6
antimyeloproliferative	T45.1X1	T45.1X2	T45.1X3	T45.1X4	T45.1X5	T45.1X6
lymphatic	T45.1X1	T45.1X2	T45.1X3	T45.1X4	T45.1X5	T45.1X6
Alkylisocyanate	T65.0X1	T65.0X2	T65.0X3	T65.0X4	—	—
Allantoin	T49.4X1	T49.4X2	T49.4X3	T49.4X4	T49.4X5	T49.4X6
Allegron	T43.011	T43.012	T43.013	T43.014	T43.015	T43.016
Allethrin	T49.0X1	T49.0X2	T49.0X3	T49.0X4	T49.0X5	T49.0X6
Allobarbital	T42.3X1	T42.3X2	T42.3X3	T42.3X4	T42.3X5	T42.3X6
Allopurinol	T50.4X1	T50.4X2	T50.4X3	T50.4X4	T50.4X5	T50.4X6
Allyl						
alcohol	T51.8X1	T51.8X2	T51.8X3	T51.8X4	—	—
disulfide	T46.6X1	T46.6X2	T46.6X3	T46.6X4	T46.6X5	T46.6X6
Allylestrenol	T38.5X1	T38.5X2	T38.5X3	T38.5X4	T38.5X5	T38.5X6
Allylisopropylacetylurea	T42.6X1	T42.6X2	T42.6X3	T42.6X4	T42.6X5	T42.6X6
Allylisopropylmalonylurea	T42.3X1	T42.3X2	T42.3X3	T42.3X4	T42.3X5	T42.3X6
Allylthiourea	T49.3X1	T49.3X2	T49.3X3	T49.3X4	T49.3X5	T49.3X6
Allyltribromide	T42.6X1	T42.6X2	T42.6X3	T42.6X4	T42.6X5	T42.6X6
Allypropymal	T42.3X1	T42.3X2	T42.3X3	T42.3X4	T42.3X5	T42.3X6
Almagate	T47.1X1	T47.1X2	T47.1X3	T47.1X4	T47.1X5	T47.1X6
Almasilate	T47.1X1	T47.1X2	T47.1X3	T47.1X4	T47.1X5	T47.1X6
Almitrine	T50.7X1	T50.7X2	T50.7X3	T50.7X4	T50.7X5	T50.7X6
Aloes	T47.2X1	T47.2X2	T47.2X3	T47.2X4	T47.2X5	T47.2X6
Aloglutamol	T47.1X1	T47.1X2	T47.1X3	T47.1X4	T47.1X5	T47.1X6
Aloin	T47.2X1	T47.2X2	T47.2X3	T47.2X4	T47.2X5	T47.2X6
Aloxidone	T42.2X1	T42.2X2	T42.2X3	T42.2X4	T42.2X5	T42.2X6
Alpha						
acetyldigoxin	T46.0X1	T46.0X2	T46.0X3	T46.0X4	T46.0X5	T46.0X6
adrenergic blocking drug	T44.6X1	T44.6X2	T44.6X3	T44.6X4	T44.6X5	T44.6X6
amylase	T45.3X1	T45.3X2	T45.3X3	T45.3X4	T45.3X5	T45.3X6
tocoferol (acetate)	T45.2X1	T45.2X2	T45.2X3	T45.2X4	T45.2X5	T45.2X6
tocopherol	T45.2X1	T45.2X2	T45.2X3	T45.2X4	T45.2X5	T45.2X6
Alphadolone	T41.1X1	T41.1X2	T41.1X3	T41.1X4	T41.1X5	T41.1X6
Alphaprodine	T40.4X1	T40.4X2	T40.4X3	T40.4X4	T40.4X5	T40.4X6
Alphaxalone	T41.1X1	T41.1X2	T41.1X3	T41.1X4	T41.1X5	T41.1X6
Alprazolam	T42.4X1	T42.4X2	T42.4X3	T42.4X4	T42.4X5	T42.4X6
Alprenolol	T44.7X1	T44.7X2	T44.7X3	T44.7X4	T44.7X5	T44.7X6
Alprostadil	T46.7X1	T46.7X2	T46.7X3	T46.7X4	T46.7X5	T46.7X6
Alsactide	T38.811	T38.812	T38.813	T38.814	T38.815	T38.816
Alseroxylon	T46.5X1	T46.5X2	T46.5X3	T46.5X4	T46.5X5	T46.5X6
Alteplase	T45.611	T45.612	T45.613	T45.614	T45.615	T45.616
Altizide	T50.2X1	T50.2X2	T50.2X3	T50.2X4	T50.2X5	T50.2X6
Altretamine	T45.1X1	T45.1X2	T45.1X3	T45.1X4	T45.1X5	T45.1X6
Alum (medicinal)	T49.4X1	T49.4X2	T49.4X3	T49.4X4	T49.4X5	T49.4X6
nonmedicinal (ammonium) (potassium)	T56.891	T56.892	T56.893	T56.894	—	—
Aluminium, aluminum						
acetate	T49.2X1	T49.2X2	T49.2X3	T49.2X4	T49.2X5	T49.2X6
solution	T49.0X1	T49.0X2	T49.0X3	T49.0X4	T49.0X5	T49.0X6
aspirin	T39.011	T39.012	T39.013	T39.014	T39.015	T39.016
bis (acetylsalicylate)	T39.011	T39.012	T39.013	T39.014	T39.015	T39.016
carbonate (gel, basic)	T47.1X1	T47.1X2	T47.1X3	T47.1X4	T47.1X5	T47.1X6
chlorhydroxide-complex	T47.1X1	T47.1X2	T47.1X3	T47.1X4	T47.1X5	T47.1X6
chloride	T49.2X1	T49.2X2	T49.2X3	T49.2X4	T49.2X5	T49.2X6
clofibrate	T46.6X1	T46.6X2	T46.6X3	T46.6X4	T46.6X5	T46.6X6
diacetate	T49.2X1	T49.2X2	T49.2X3	T49.2X4	T49.2X5	T49.2X6
glycinate	T47.1X1	T47.1X2	T47.1X3	T47.1X4	T47.1X5	T47.1X6
hydroxide (gel)	T47.1X1	T47.1X2	T47.1X3	T47.1X4	T47.1X5	T47.1X6
hydroxide-magnesium carb. gel	T47.1X1	T47.1X2	T47.1X3	T47.1X4	T47.1X5	T47.1X6
magnesium silicate	T47.1X1	T47.1X2	T47.1X3	T47.1X4	T47.1X5	T47.1X6
nicotinate	T46.7X1	T46.7X2	T46.7X3	T46.7X4	T46.7X5	T46.7X6

Substance	Poisoning, Accidental (unintentional)	Poisoning, Intentional Self-harm	Poisoning, Assault	Poisoning, Undetermined	Adverse Effect	Under-dosing
Aluminium, aluminum — *continued*						
ointment (surgical) (topical)	T49.3X1	T49.3X2	T49.3X3	T49.3X4	T49.3X5	T49.3X6
phosphate	T47.1X1	T47.1X2	T47.1X3	T47.1X4	T47.1X5	T47.1X6
salicylate	T39.091	T39.092	T39.093	T39.094	T39.095	T39.096
silicate	T47.1X1	T47.1X2	T47.1X3	T47.1X4	T47.1X5	T47.1X6
sodium silicate	T47.1X1	T47.1X2	T47.1X3	T47.1X4	T47.1X5	T47.1X6
subacetate	T49.2X1	T49.2X2	T49.2X3	T49.2X4	T49.2X5	T49.2X6
sulfate	T49.0X1	T49.0X2	T49.0X3	T49.0X4	T49.0X5	T49.0X6
tannate	T47.6X1	T47.6X2	T47.6X3	T47.6X4	T47.6X5	T47.6X6
topical NEC	T49.3X1	T49.3X2	T49.3X3	T49.3X4	T49.3X5	T49.3X6
Alurate	T42.3X1	T42.3X2	T42.3X3	T42.3X4	T42.3X5	T42.3X6
Alverine	T44.3X1	T44.3X2	T44.3X3	T44.3X4	T44.3X5	T44.3X6
Alvodine	T40.2X1	T40.2X2	T40.2X3	T40.2X4	T40.2X5	T40.2X6
Amanita phalloides	T62.0X1	T62.0X2	T62.0X3	T62.0X4	—	—
Amanitine	T62.0X1	T62.0X2	T62.0X3	T62.0X4	—	—
Amantadine	T42.8X1	T42.8X2	T42.8X3	T42.8X4	T42.8X5	T42.8X6
Ambazone	T49.6X1	T49.6X2	T49.6X3	T49.6X4	T49.6X5	T49.6X6
Ambenonium (chloride)	T44.0X1	T44.0X2	T44.0X3	T44.0X4	T44.0X5	T44.0X6
Ambroxol	T48.4X1	T48.4X2	T48.4X3	T48.4X4	T48.4X5	T48.4X6
Ambuphylline	T48.6X1	T48.6X2	T48.6X3	T48.6X4	T48.6X5	T48.6X6
Ambutonium bromide	T44.3X1	T44.3X2	T44.3X3	T44.3X4	T44.3X5	T44.3X6
Amcinonide	T49.0X1	T49.0X2	T49.0X3	T49.0X4	T49.0X5	T49.0X6
Amdinocilline	T36.0X1	T36.0X2	T36.0X3	T36.0X4	T36.0X5	T36.0X6
Ametazole	T50.8X1	T50.8X2	T50.8X3	T50.8X4	T50.8X5	T50.8X6
Amethocaine	T41.3X1	T41.3X2	T41.3X3	T41.3X4	T41.3X5	T41.3X6
regional	T41.3X1	T41.3X2	T41.3X3	T41.3X4	T41.3X5	T41.3X6
spinal	T41.3X1	T41.3X2	T41.3X3	T41.3X4	T41.3X5	T41.3X6
Amethopterin	T45.1X1	T45.1X2	T45.1X3	T45.1X4	T45.1X5	T45.1X6
Amezinium metilsulfate	T44.991	T44.992	T44.993	T44.994	T44.995	T44.996
Amfebutamone	T43.291	T43.292	T43.293	T43.294	T43.295	T43.296
Amfepramone	T50.5X1	T50.5X2	T50.5X3	T50.5X4	T50.5X5	T50.5X6
Amfetamine	T43.621	T43.622	T43.623	T43.624	T43.625	T43.626
Amfetaminil	T43.621	T43.622	T43.623	T43.624	T43.625	T43.626
Amfomycin	T36.8X1	T36.8X2	T36.8X3	T36.8X4	T36.8X5	T36.8X6
Amidefrine mesilate	T48.5X1	T48.5X2	T48.5X3	T48.5X4	T48.5X5	T48.5X6
Amidone	T40.3X1	T40.3X2	T40.3X3	T40.3X4	T40.3X5	T40.3X6
Amidopyrine	T39.2X1	T39.2X2	T39.2X3	T39.2X4	T39.2X5	T39.2X6
Amidotrizoate	T50.8X1	T50.8X2	T50.8X3	T50.8X4	T50.8X5	T50.8X6
Amiflamine	T43.1X1	T43.1X2	T43.1X3	T43.1X4	T43.1X5	T43.1X6
Amikacin	T36.5X1	T36.5X2	T36.5X3	T36.5X4	T36.5X5	T36.5X6
Amikhelline	T46.3X1	T46.3X2	T46.3X3	T46.3X4	T46.3X5	T46.3X6
Amiloride	T50.2X1	T50.2X2	T50.2X3	T50.2X4	T50.2X5	T50.2X6
Aminacrine	T49.0X1	T49.0X2	T49.0X3	T49.0X4	T49.0X5	T49.0X6
Amineptine	T43.011	T43.012	T43.013	T43.014	T43.015	T43.016
Aminitrozole	T37.3X1	T37.3X2	T37.3X3	T37.3X4	T37.3X5	T37.3X6
Aminoacetic acid (derivatives)	T50.3X1	T50.3X2	T50.3X3	T50.3X4	T50.3X5	T50.3X6
Amino acids	T50.3X1	T50.3X2	T50.3X3	T50.3X4	T50.3X5	T50.3X6
Aminoacridine	T49.0X1	T49.0X2	T49.0X3	T49.0X4	T49.0X5	T49.0X6
Aminobenzoic acid (-p)	T49.3X1	T49.3X2	T49.3X3	T49.3X4	T49.3X5	T49.3X6
Aminocaproic acid	T45.621	T45.622	T45.623	T45.624	T45.625	T45.626
Aminoethylisothiourium	T45.8X1	T45.8X2	T45.8X3	T45.8X4	T45.8X5	T45.8X6
Aminofenazone	T39.2X1	T39.2X2	T39.2X3	T39.2X4	T39.2X5	T39.2X6
Aminoglutethimide	T45.1X1	T45.1X2	T45.1X3	T45.1X4	T45.1X5	T45.1X6
Aminohippuric acid	T50.8X1	T50.8X2	T50.8X3	T50.8X4	T50.8X5	T50.8X6
Aminomethylbenzoic acid	T45.691	T45.692	T45.693	T45.694	T45.695	T45.696
Aminometradine	T50.2X1	T50.2X2	T50.2X3	T50.2X4	T50.2X5	T50.2X6
Aminopentamide	T44.3X1	T44.3X2	T44.3X3	T44.3X4	T44.3X5	T44.3X6
Aminophenazone	T39.2X1	T39.2X2	T39.2X3	T39.2X4	T39.2X5	T39.2X6
Aminophenol	T54.0X1	T54.0X2	T54.0X3	T54.0X4	—	—
Aminophenylpyridone	T43.591	T43.592	T43.593	T43.594	T43.595	T43.596
Aminophylline	T48.6X1	T48.6X2	T48.6X3	T48.6X4	T48.6X5	T48.6X6
Aminopterin sodium	T45.1X1	T45.1X2	T45.1X3	T45.1X4	T45.1X5	T45.1X6
Aminopyrine	T39.2X1	T39.2X2	T39.2X3	T39.2X4	T39.2X5	T39.2X6
Aminorex	T50.5X1	T50.5X2	T50.5X3	T50.5X4	T50.5X5	T50.5X6
Aminosalicylic acid	T37.1X1	T37.1X2	T37.1X3	T37.1X4	T37.1X5	T37.1X6
Aminosalylum	T37.1X1	T37.1X2	T37.1X3	T37.1X4	T37.1X5	T37.1X6
Amiodarone	T46.2X1	T46.2X2	T46.2X3	T46.2X4	T46.2X5	T46.2X6
Amiphenazole	T50.7X1	T50.7X2	T50.7X3	T50.7X4	T50.7X5	T50.7X6
Amiquinsin	T46.5X1	T46.5X2	T46.5X3	T46.5X4	T46.5X5	T46.5X6
Amisometradine	T50.2X1	T50.2X2	T50.2X3	T50.2X4	T50.2X5	T50.2X6
Amisulpride	T43.591	T43.592	T43.593	T43.594	T43.595	T43.596
Amitriptyline	T43.011	T43.012	T43.013	T43.014	T43.015	T43.016
Amitriptylinoxide	T43.011	T43.012	T43.013	T43.014	T43.015	T43.016
Amlexanox	T48.6X1	T48.6X2	T48.6X3	T48.6X4	T48.6X5	T48.6X6
Ammonia (fumes) (gas) (vapor)	T59.891	T59.892	T59.893	T59.894	—	—
aromatic spirit	T48.991	T48.992	T48.993	T48.994	T48.995	T48.996
liquid (household)	T54.3X1	T54.3X2	T54.3X3	T54.3X4	—	—
Ammoniated mercury	T49.0X1	T49.0X2	T49.0X3	T49.0X4	T49.0X5	T49.0X6
Ammonium						
acid tartrate	T49.5X1	T49.5X2	T49.5X3	T49.5X4	T49.5X5	T49.5X6

Substance	Poisoning, Accidental (unintentional)	Poisoning, Intentional Self-harm	Poisoning, Assault	Poisoning, Undetermined	Adverse Effect	Under-dosing
Ammonium — *continued*						
bromide	T42.6X1	T42.6X2	T42.6X3	T42.6X4	T42.6X5	T42.6X6
carbonate	T54.3X1	T54.3X2	T54.3X3	T54.3X4	—	—
chloride	T50.991	T50.992	T50.993	T50.994	T50.995	T50.996
expectorant	T48.4X1	T48.4X2	T48.4X3	T48.4X4	T48.4X5	T48.4X6
compounds (household) NEC	T54.3X1	T54.3X2	T54.3X3	T54.3X4	—	—
fumes (any usage)	T59.891	T59.892	T59.893	T59.894	—	—
industrial	T54.3X1	T54.3X2	T54.3X3	T54.3X4	—	—
ichthyosulronate	T49.4X1	T49.4X2	T49.4X3	T49.4X4	T49.4X5	T49.4X6
mandelate	T37.91	T37.92	T37.93	T37.94	T37.95	T37.96
sulfamate	T60.3X1	T60.3X2	T60.3X3	T60.3X4	—	—
sulfonate resin	T47.8X1	T47.8X2	T47.8X3	T47.8X4	T47.8X5	T47.8X6
Amobarbital (sodium)	T42.3X1	T42.3X2	T42.3X3	T42.3X4	T42.3X5	T42.3X6
Amodiaquine	T37.2X1	T37.2X2	T37.2X3	T37.2X4	T37.2X5	T37.2X6
Amopyroquin (e)	T37.2X1	T37.2X2	T37.2X3	T37.2X4	T37.2X5	T37.2X6
Amoxapine	T43.011	T43.012	T43.013	T43.014	T43.015	T43.016
Amoxicillin	T36.0X1	T36.0X2	T36.0X3	T36.0X4	T36.0X5	T36.0X6
Amperozide	T43.591	T43.592	T43.593	T43.594	T43.595	T43.596
Amphenidone	T43.591	T43.592	T43.593	T43.594	T43.595	T43.596
Amphetamine NEC	T43.621	T43.622	T43.623	T43.624	T43.625	T43.626
Amphomycin	T36.8X1	T36.8X2	T36.8X3	T36.8X4	T36.8X5	T36.8X6
Amphotalide	T37.4X1	T37.4X2	T37.4X3	T37.4X4	T37.4X5	T37.4X6
Amphotericin B	T36.7X1	T36.7X2	T36.7X3	T36.7X4	T36.7X5	T36.7X6
topical	T49.0X1	T49.0X2	T49.0X3	T49.0X4	T49.0X5	T49.0X6
Ampicillin	T36.0X1	T36.0X2	T36.0X3	T36.0X4	T36.0X5	T36.0X6
Amprotropine	T44.3X1	T44.3X2	T44.3X3	T44.3X4	T44.3X5	T44.3X6
Amsacrine	T45.1X1	T45.1X2	T45.1X3	T45.1X4	T45.1X5	T45.1X6
Amygdaline	T62.2X1	T62.2X2	T62.2X3	T62.2X4	—	—
Amyl						
acetate	T52.8X1	T52.8X2	T52.8X3	T52.8X4	—	—
vapor	T59.891	T59.892	T59.893	T59.894	—	—
alcohol	T51.3X1	T51.3X2	T51.3X3	T51.3X4	—	—
chloride	T53.6X1	T53.6X2	T53.6X3	T53.6X4	—	—
formate	T52.8X1	T52.8X2	T52.8X3	T52.8X4	—	—
nitrite	T46.3X1	T46.3X2	T46.3X3	T46.3X4	T46.3X5	T46.3X6
propionate	T65.891	T65.892	T65.893	T65.894	—	—
Amylase	T47.5X1	T47.5X2	T47.5X3	T47.5X4	T47.5X5	T47.5X6
Amyleine, regional	T41.3X1	T41.3X2	T41.3X3	T41.3X4	T41.3X5	T41.3X6
Amylene						
dichloride	T53.6X1	T53.6X2	T53.6X3	T53.6X4	—	—
hydrate	T51.3X1	T51.3X2	T51.3X3	T51.3X4	—	—
Amylmetacresol	T49.6X1	T49.6X2	T49.6X3	T49.6X4	T49.6X5	T49.6X6
Amylobarbitone	T42.3X1	T42.3X2	T42.3X3	T42.3X4	T42.3X5	T42.3X6
Amylocaine, regional	T41.3X1	T41.3X2	T41.3X3	T41.3X4	T41.3X5	T41.3X6
infiltration (subcutaneous)	T41.3X1	T41.3X2	T41.3X3	T41.3X4	T41.3X5	T41.3X6
nerve block (peripheral) (plexus)	T41.3X1	T41.3X2	T41.3X3	T41.3X4	T41.3X5	T41.3X6
spinal	T41.3X1	T41.3X2	T41.3X3	T41.3X4	T41.3X5	T41.3X6
topical (surface)	T41.3X1	T41.3X2	T41.3X3	T41.3X4	T41.3X5	T41.3X6
Amylopectin	T47.6X1	T47.6X2	T47.6X3	T47.6X4	T47.6X5	T47.6X6
Amytal (sodium)	T42.3X1	T42.3X2	T42.3X3	T42.3X4	T42.3X5	T42.3X6
Anabolic steroid	T38.7X1	T38.7X2	T38.7X3	T38.7X4	T38.7X5	T38.7X6
Analeptic NEC	T50.7X1	T50.7X2	T50.7X3	T50.7X4	T50.7X5	T50.7X6
Analgesic	T39.91	T39.92	T39.93	T39.94	T39.95	T39.96
anti-inflammatory NEC	T39.91	T39.92	T39.93	T39.94	T39.95	T39.96
propionic acid derivative	T39.311	T39.312	T39.313	T39.314	T39.315	T39.316
antirheumatic NEC	T39.4X1	T39.4X2	T39.4X3	T39.4X4	T39.4X5	T39.4X6
aromatic NEC	T39.1X1	T39.1X2	T39.1X3	T39.1X4	T39.1X5	T39.1X6
narcotic NEC	T40.601	T40.602	T40.603	T40.604	T40.605	T40.606
combination	T40.601	T40.602	T40.603	T40.604	T40.605	T40.606
obstetric	T40.601	T40.602	T40.603	T40.604	T40.605	T40.606
non-narcotic NEC	T39.91	T39.92	T39.93	T39.94	T39.95	T39.96
combination	T39.91	T39.92	T39.93	T39.94	T39.95	T39.96
pyrazole	T39.2X1	T39.2X2	T39.2X3	T39.2X4	T39.2X5	T39.2X6
specified NEC	T39.8X1	T39.8X2	T39.8X3	T39.8X4	T39.8X5	T39.8X6
Analgin	T39.2X1	T39.2X2	T39.2X3	T39.2X4	T39.2X5	T39.2X6
Anamirta cocculus	T62.1X1	T62.1X2	T62.1X3	T62.1X4	—	—
Ancillin	T36.0X1	T36.0X2	T36.0X3	T36.0X4	T36.0X5	T36.0X6
Ancrod	T45.691	T45.692	T45.693	T45.694	T45.695	T45.696
Androgen	T38.7X1	T38.7X2	T38.7X3	T38.7X4	T38.7X5	T38.7X6
Androgen-estrogen mixture	T38.7X1	T38.7X2	T38.7X3	T38.7X4	T38.7X5	T38.7X6
Androstalone	T38.7X1	T38.7X2	T38.7X3	T38.7X4	T38.7X5	T38.7X6
Androstanolone	T38.7X1	T38.7X2	T38.7X3	T38.7X4	T38.7X5	T38.7X6
Androsterone	T38.7X1	T38.7X2	T38.7X3	T38.7X4	T38.7X5	T38.7X6
Anemone pulsatilla	T62.2X1	T62.2X2	T62.2X3	T62.2X4	—	—
Anesthesia						
caudal	T41.3X1	T41.3X2	T41.3X3	T41.3X4	T41.3X5	T41.3X6
endotracheal	T41.0X1	T41.0X2	T41.0X3	T41.0X4	T41.0X5	T41.0X6
epidural	T41.3X1	T41.3X2	T41.3X3	T41.3X4	T41.3X5	T41.3X6
inhalation	T41.0X1	T41.0X2	T41.0X3	T41.0X4	T41.0X5	T41.0X6
local	T41.3X1	T41.3X2	T41.3X3	T41.3X4	T41.3X5	T41.3X6

Substance	Poisoning, Accidental (unintentional)	Poisoning, Intentional Self-harm	Poisoning, Assault	Poisoning, Undetermined	Adverse Effect	Under-dosing
Anesthesia — continued						
mucosal	T41.3X1	T41.3X2	T41.3X3	T41.3X4	T41.3X5	T41.3X6
muscle relaxation	T48.1X1	T48.1X2	T48.1X3	T48.1X4	T48.1X5	T48.1X6
nerve blocking	T41.3X1	T41.3X2	T41.3X3	T41.3X4	T41.3X5	T41.3X6
plexus blocking	T41.3X1	T41.3X2	T41.3X3	T41.3X4	T41.3X5	T41.3X6
potentiated	T41.201	T41.202	T41.203	T41.204	T41.205	T41.206
rectal	T41.201	T41.202	T41.203	T41.204	T41.205	T41.206
general	T41.201	T41.202	T41.203	T41.204	T41.205	T41.206
local	T41.3X1	T41.3X2	T41.3X3	T41.3X4	T41.3X5	T41.3X6
regional	T41.3X1	T41.3X2	T41.3X3	T41.3X4	T41.3X5	T41.3X6
surface	T41.3X1	T41.3X2	T41.3X3	T41.3X4	T41.3X5	T41.3X6
Anesthetic NEC — see also	T41.41	T41.42	T41.43	T41.44	T41.45	T41.46
Anesthesia						
with muscle relaxant	T41.201	T41.202	T41.203	T41.204	T41.205	T41.206
general	T41.201	T41.202	T41.203	T41.204	T41.205	T41.206
local	T41.3X1	T41.3X2	T41.3X3	T41.3X4	T41.3X5	T41.3X6
gaseous NEC	T41.0X1	T41.0X2	T41.0X3	T41.0X4	T41.0X5	T41.0X6
general NEC	T41.201	T41.202	T41.203	T41.204	T41.205	T41.206
halogenated hydrocarbon derivatives NEC	T41.0X1	T41.0X2	T41.0X3	T41.0X4	T41.0X5	T41.0X6
infiltration NEC	T41.3X1	T41.3X2	T41.3X3	T41.3X4	T41.3X5	T41.3X6
intravenous NEC	T41.1X1	T41.1X2	T41.1X3	T41.1X4	T41.1X5	T41.1X6
local NEC	T41.3X1	T41.3X2	T41.3X3	T41.3X4	T41.3X5	T41.3X6
rectal	T41.201	T41.202	T41.203	T41.204	T41.205	T41.206
general	T41.201	T41.202	T41.203	T41.204	T41.205	T41.206
local	T41.3X1	T41.3X2	T41.3X3	T41.3X4	T41.3X5	T41.3X6
regional NEC	T41.3X1	T41.3X2	T41.3X3	T41.3X4	T41.3X5	T41.3X6
spinal NEC	T41.3X1	T41.3X2	T41.3X3	T41.3X4	T41.3X5	T41.3X6
thiobarbiturate	T41.1X1	T41.1X2	T41.1X3	T41.1X4	T41.1X5	T41.1X6
topical	T41.3X1	T41.3X2	T41.3X3	T41.3X4	T41.3X5	T41.3X6
Aneurine	T45.2X1	T45.2X2	T45.2X3	T45.2X4	T45.2X5	T45.2X6
Angio-Conray	T50.8X1	T50.8X2	T50.8X3	T50.8X4	T50.8X5	T50.8X6
Angiotensin	T44.5X1	T44.5X2	T44.5X3	T44.5X4	T44.5X5	T44.5X6
Angiotensinamide	T44.991	T44.992	T44.993	T44.994	T44.995	T44.996
Anhydrohydroxy-progesterone	T38.5X1	T38.5X2	T38.5X3	T38.5X4	T38.5X5	T38.5X6
Anhydron	T50.2X1	T50.2X2	T50.2X3	T50.2X4	T50.2X5	T50.2X6
Anileridine	T40.4X1	T40.4X2	T40.4X3	T40.4X4	T40.4X5	T40.4X6
Aniline (dye) (liquid)	T65.3X1	T65.3X2	T65.3X3	T65.3X4	—	—
analgesic	T39.1X1	T39.1X2	T39.1X3	T39.1X4	T39.1X5	T39.1X6
derivatives, therapeutic NEC	T39.1X1	T39.1X2	T39.1X3	T39.1X4	T39.1X5	T39.1X6
vapor	T65.3X1	T65.3X2	T65.3X3	T65.3X4	—	—
Aniscoropine	T44.3X1	T44.3X2	T44.3X3	T44.3X4	T44.3X5	T44.3X6
Anise oil	T47.5X1	T47.5X2	T47.5X3	T47.5X4	T47.5X5	T47.5X6
Anisidine	T65.3X1	T65.3X2	T65.3X3	T65.3X4	—	—
Anisindione	T45.511	T45.512	T45.513	T45.514	T45.515	T45.516
Anisotropine	T44.3X1	T44.3X2	T44.3X3	T44.3X4	T44.3X5	T44.3X6
methyl-bromide	T45.611	T45.612	T45.613	T45.614	T45.615	T45.616
Anistreplase	T45.611	T45.612	T45.613	T45.614	T45.615	T45.616
Anorexiant (central)	T50.5X1	T50.5X2	T50.5X3	T50.5X4	T50.5X5	T50.5X6
Anorexic agents	T50.5X1	T50.5X2	T50.5X3	T50.5X4	T50.5X5	T50.5X6
Ansamycin	T36.6X1	T36.6X2	T36.6X3	T36.6X4	T36.6X5	T36.6X6
Ant (bite) (sting)	T63.421	T63.422	T63.423	T63.424		
Antabuse	T50.6X1	T50.6X2	T50.6X3	T50.6X4	T50.6X5	T50.6X6
Antacid NEC	T47.1X1	T47.1X2	T47.1X3	T47.1X4	T47.1X5	T47.1X6
Antagonist						
Aldosterone	T50.0X1	T50.0X2	T50.0X3	T50.0X4	T50.0X5	T50.0X6
alpha-adrenoreceptor	T44.6X1	T44.6X2	T44.6X3	T44.6X4	T44.6X5	T44.6X6
anticoagulant	T45.7X1	T45.7X2	T45.7X3	T45.7X4	T45.7X5	T45.7X6
beta-adrenoreceptor	T44.7X1	T44.7X2	T44.7X3	T44.7X4	T44.7X5	T44.7X6
extrapyramidal NEC	T44.3X1	T44.3X2	T44.3X3	T44.3X4	T44.3X5	T44.3X6
folic acid	T45.1X1	T45.1X2	T45.1X3	T45.1X4	T45.1X5	T45.1X6
H2 receptor	T47.0X1	T47.0X2	T47.0X3	T47.0X4	T47.0X5	T47.0X6
heavy metal	T45.8X1	T45.8X2	T45.8X3	T45.8X4	T45.8X5	T45.8X6
narcotic analgesic	T50.7X1	T50.7X2	T50.7X3	T50.7X4	T50.7X5	T50.7X6
opiate	T50.7X1	T50.7X2	T50.7X3	T50.7X4	T50.7X5	T50.7X6
pyrimidine	T45.1X1	T45.1X2	T45.1X3	T45.1X4	T45.1X5	T45.1X6
serotonin	T46.5X1	T46.5X2	T46.5X3	T46.5X4	T46.5X5	T46.5X6
Antazolin (e)	T45.0X1	T45.0X2	T45.0X3	T45.0X4	T45.0X5	T45.0X6
Anterior pituitary hormone NEC	T38.811	T38.812	T38.813	T38.814	T38.815	T38.816
Anthelmintic NEC	T37.4X1	T37.4X2	T37.4X3	T37.4X4	T37.4X5	T37.4X6
Anthiolimine	T37.4X1	T37.4X2	T37.4X3	T37.4X4	T37.4X5	T37.4X6
Anthralin	T49.4X1	T49.4X2	T49.4X3	T49.4X4	T49.4X5	T49.4X6
Anthramycin	T45.1X1	T45.1X2	T45.1X3	T45.1X4	T45.1X5	T45.1X6
Antiadrenergic NEC	T44.8X1	T44.8X2	T44.8X3	T44.8X4	T44.8X5	T44.8X6
Antiallergic NEC	T45.0X1	T45.0X2	T45.0X3	T45.0X4	T45.0X5	T45.0X6
Antiandrogen NEC	T38.6X1	T38.6X2	T38.6X3	T38.6X4	T38.6X5	T38.6X6
Anti-anemic (drug) (preparation)	T45.8X1	T45.8X2	T45.8X3	T45.8X4	T45.8X5	T45.8X6
Antianxiety drug NEC	T43.501	T43.502	T43.503	T43.504	T43.505	T43.506
Antiaris toxicaria	T65.891	T65.892	T65.893	T65.894	—	—
Antiarteriosclerotic drug	T46.6X1	T46.6X2	T46.6X3	T46.6X4	T46.6X5	T46.6X6

Substance	Poisoning, Accidental (unintentional)	Poisoning, Intentional Self-harm	Poisoning, Assault	Poisoning, Undetermined	Adverse Effect	Under-dosing
Antiasthmatic drug NEC	T48.6X1	T48.6X2	T48.6X3	T48.6X4	T48.6X5	T48.6X6
Antibiotic NEC	T36.91	T36.92	T36.93	T36.94	T36.95	T36.96
aminoglycoside	T36.5X1	T36.5X2	T36.5X3	T36.5X4	T36.5X5	T36.5X6
anticancer	T45.1X1	T45.1X2	T45.1X3	T45.1X4	T45.1X5	T45.1X6
antifungal	T36.7X1	T36.7X2	T36.7X3	T36.7X4	T36.7X5	T36.7X6
antimycobacterial	T36.5X1	T36.5X2	T36.5X3	T36.5X4	T36.5X5	T36.5X6
antineoplastic	T45.1X1	T45.1X2	T45.1X3	T45.1X4	T45.1X5	T45.1X6
b-lactam NEC	T36.1X1	T36.1X2	T36.1X3	T36.1X4	T36.1X5	T36.1X6
cephalosporin (group)	T36.1X1	T36.1X2	T36.1X3	T36.1X4	T36.1X5	T36.1X6
chloramphenicol (group)	T36.2X1	T36.2X2	T36.2X3	T36.2X4	T36.2X5	T36.2X6
ENT	T49.6X1	T49.6X2	T49.6X3	T49.6X4	T49.6X5	T49.6X6
eye	T49.5X1	T49.5X2	T49.5X3	T49.5X4	T49.5X5	T49.5X6
fungicidal (local)	T49.0X1	T49.0X2	T49.0X3	T49.0X4	T49.0X5	T49.0X6
intestinal	T36.8X1	T36.8X2	T36.8X3	T36.8X4	T36.8X5	T36.8X6
local	T49.0X1	T49.0X2	T49.0X3	T49.0X4	T49.0X5	T49.0X6
macrolides	T36.3X1	T36.3X2	T36.3X3	T36.3X4	T36.3X5	T36.3X6
polypeptide	T36.8X1	T36.8X2	T36.8X3	T36.8X4	T36.8X5	T36.8X6
specified NEC	T36.8X1	T36.8X2	T36.8X3	T36.8X4	T36.8X5	T36.8X6
tetracycline (group)	T36.4X1	T36.4X2	T36.4X3	T36.4X4	T36.4X5	T36.4X6
throat	T49.6X1	T49.6X2	T49.6X3	T49.6X4	T49.6X5	T49.6X6
Anticancer agents NEC	T45.1X1	T45.1X2	T45.1X3	T45.1X4	T45.1X5	T45.1X6
Anticholesterolemic drug NEC	T46.6X1	T46.6X2	T46.6X3	T46.6X4	T46.6X5	T46.6X6
Anticholinergic NEC	T44.3X1	T44.3X2	T44.3X3	T44.3X4	T44.3X5	T44.3X6
Anticholinesterase	T44.0X1	T44.0X2	T44.0X3	T44.0X4	T44.0X5	T44.0X6
organophosphorus	T44.0X1	T44.0X2	T44.0X3	T44.0X4	T44.0X5	T44.0X6
insecticide	T60.0X1	T60.0X2	T60.0X3	T60.0X4	—	—
nerve gas	T59.891	T59.892	T59.893	T59.894		
reversible	T44.0X1	T44.0X2	T44.0X3	T44.0X4	T44.0X5	T44.0X6
ophthalmological	T49.5X1	T49.5X2	T49.5X3	T49.5X4	T49.5X5	T49.5X6
Anticoagulant NEC	T45.511	T45.512	T45.513	T45.514	T45.515	T45.516
Antagonist	T45.7X1	T45.7X2	T45.7X3	T45.7X4	T45.7X5	T45.7X6
Anti-common-cold drug NEC	T48.5X1	T48.5X2	T48.5X3	T48.5X4	T48.5X5	T48.5X6
Anticonvulsant	T42.71	T42.72	T42.73	T42.74	T42.75	T42.76
barbiturate	T42.3X1	T42.3X2	T42.3X3	T42.3X4	T42.3X5	T42.3X6
combination (with barbiturate)	T42.3X1	T42.3X2	T42.3X3	T42.3X4	T42.3X5	T42.3X6
hydantoin	T42.0X1	T42.0X2	T42.0X3	T42.0X4	T42.0X5	T42.0X6
hypnotic NEC	T42.6X1	T42.6X2	T42.6X3	T42.6X4	T42.6X5	T42.6X6
oxazolidinedione	T42.2X1	T42.2X2	T42.2X3	T42.2X4	T42.2X5	T42.2X6
pyrimidinedione	T42.6X1	T42.6X2	T42.6X3	T42.6X4	T42.6X5	T42.6X6
specified NEC	T42.6X1	T42.6X2	T42.6X3	T42.6X4	T42.6X5	T42.6X6
succinimide	T42.2X1	T42.2X2	T42.2X3	T42.2X4	T42.2X5	T42.2X6
Antidepressant	T43.201	T43.202	T43.203	T43.204	T43.205	T43.206
monoamine oxidase inhibitor	T43.1X1	T43.1X2	T43.1X3	T43.1X4	T43.1X5	T43.1X6
selective serotonin norepinephrine reuptake inhibitor	T43.211	T43.212	T43.213	T43.214	T43.215	T43.216
selective serotonin reuptake inhibitor	T43.221	T43.222	T43.223	T43.224	T43.225	T43.226
specified NEC	T43.291	T43.292	T43.293	T43.294	T43.295	T43.296
tetracyclic	T43.021	T43.022	T43.023	T43.024	T43.025	T43.026
triazolopyridine	T43.211	T43.212	T43.213	T43.214	T43.215	T43.216
tricyclic	T43.011	T43.012	T43.013	T43.014	T43.015	T43.016
Antidiabetic NEC	T38.3X1	T38.3X2	T38.3X3	T38.3X4	T38.3X5	T38.3X6
biguanide	T38.3X1	T38.3X2	T38.3X3	T38.3X4	T38.3X5	T38.3X6
and sulfonyl combined	T38.3X1	T38.3X2	T38.3X3	T38.3X4	T38.3X5	T38.3X6
combined	T38.3X1	T38.3X2	T38.3X3	T38.3X4	T38.3X5	T38.3X6
sulfonylurea	T38.3X1	T38.3X2	T38.3X3	T38.3X4	T38.3X5	T38.3X6
Antidiarrheal drug NEC	T47.6X1	T47.6X2	T47.6X3	T47.6X4	T47.6X5	T47.6X6
absorbent	T47.6X1	T47.6X2	T47.6X3	T47.6X4	T47.6X5	T47.6X6
Anti-D immunoglobulin (human)	T50.Z11	T50.Z12	T50.Z13	T50.Z14	T50.Z15	T50.Z16
Antidiphtheria serum	T50.Z11	T50.Z12	T50.Z13	T50.Z14	T50.Z15	T50.Z16
Antidiuretic hormone	T38.891	T38.892	T38.893	T38.894	T38.895	T38.896
Antidote NEC	T50.6X1	T50.6X2	T50.6X3	T50.6X4	T50.6X5	T50.6X6
heavy metal	T45.8X1	T45.8X2	T45.8X3	T45.8X4	T45.8X5	T45.8X6
Antidysrhythmic NEC	T46.2X1	T46.2X2	T46.2X3	T46.2X4	T46.2X5	T46.2X6
Antiemetic drug	T45.0X1	T45.0X2	T45.0X3	T45.0X4	T45.0X5	T45.0X6
Antiepilepsy agent	T42.71	T42.72	T42.73	T42.74	T42.75	T42.76
combination	T42.5X1	T42.5X2	T42.5X3	T42.5X4	T42.5X5	T42.5X6
mixed	T42.5X1	T42.5X2	T42.5X3	T42.5X4	T42.5X5	T42.5X6
specified, NEC	T42.6X1	T42.6X2	T42.6X3	T42.6X4	T42.6X5	T42.6X6
Antiestrogen NEC	T38.6X1	T38.6X2	T38.6X3	T38.6X4	T38.6X5	T38.6X6
Antifertility pill	T38.4X1	T38.4X2	T38.4X3	T38.4X4	T38.4X5	T38.4X6
Antifibrinolytic drug	T45.621	T45.622	T45.623	T45.624	T45.625	T45.626
Antifilarial drug	T37.4X1	T37.4X2	T37.4X3	T37.4X4	T37.4X5	T37.4X6
Antiflatulent	T47.5X1	T47.5X2	T47.5X3	T47.5X4	T47.5X5	T47.5X6
Antifreeze	T65.91	T65.92	T65.93	T65.94	—	—
alcohol	T51.1X1	T51.1X2	T51.1X3	T51.1X4	—	—
ethylene glycol	T51.8X1	T51.8X2	T51.8X3	T51.8X4	—	—

Table of Drugs and Chemicals

Substance	Poisoning, Accidental (unintentional)	Poisoning, Intentional Self-harm	Poisoning, Assault	Poisoning, Undetermined	Adverse Effect	Under-dosing
Antifungal						
antibiotic (systemic)	T36.7X1	T36.7X2	T36.7X3	T36.7X4	T36.7X5	T36.7X6
anti-infective NEC	T37.91	T37.92	T37.93	T37.94	T37.95	T37.96
disinfectant, local	T49.0X1	T49.0X2	T49.0X3	T49.0X4	T49.0X5	T49.0X6
nonmedicinal (spray)	T60.3X1	T60.3X2	T60.3X3	T60.3X4	—	—
topical	T49.0X1	T49.0X2	T49.0X3	T49.0X4	T49.0X5	T49.0X6
Anti-gastric-secretion drug NEC	T47.1X1	T47.1X2	T47.1X3	T47.1X4	T47.1X5	T47.1X6
Antigonadotrophin NEC	T38.6X1	T38.6X2	T38.6X3	T38.6X4	T38.6X5	T38.6X6
Antihallucinogen	T43.501	T43.502	T43.503	T43.504	T43.505	T43.506
Antihelmintics	T37.4X1	T37.4X2	T37.4X3	T37.4X4	T37.4X5	T37.4X6
Antihemophilic						
factor	T45.8X1	T45.8X2	T45.8X3	T45.8X4	T45.8X5	T45.8X6
fraction	T45.8X1	T45.8X2	T45.8X3	T45.8X4	T45.8X5	T45.8X6
globulin concentrate	T45.7X1	T45.7X2	T45.7X3	T45.7X4	T45.7X5	T45.7X6
human plasma	T45.8X1	T45.8X2	T45.8X3	T45.8X4	T45.8X5	T45.8X6
plasma, dried	T45.7X1	T45.7X2	T45.7X3	T45.7X4	T45.7X5	T45.7X6
Antihemorrhoidal preparation	T49.2X1	T49.2X2	T49.2X3	T49.2X4	T49.2X5	T49.2X6
Antiheparin drug	T45.7X1	T45.7X2	T45.7X3	T45.7X4	T45.7X5	T45.7X6
Antihistamine	T45.0X1	T45.0X2	T45.0X3	T45.0X4	T45.0X5	T45.0X6
Antihookworm drug	T37.4X1	T37.4X2	T37.4X3	T37.4X4	T37.4X5	T37.4X6
Anti-human lymphocytic globulin	T50.Z11	T50.Z12	T50.Z13	T50.Z14	T50.Z15	T50.Z16
Antihyperlipidemic drug	T46.6X1	T46.6X2	T46.6X3	T46.6X4	T46.6X5	T46.6X6
Antihypertensive drug NEC	T46.5X1	T46.5X2	T46.5X3	T46.5X4	T46.5X5	T46.5X6
Anti-infective NEC	T37.91	T37.92	T37.93	T37.94	T37.95	T37.96
anthelmintic	T37.4X1	T37.4X2	T37.4X3	T37.4X4	T37.4X5	T37.4X6
antibiotics	T36.91	T36.92	T36.93	T36.94	T36.95	T36.96
specified NEC	T36.8X1	T36.8X2	T36.8X3	T36.8X4	T36.8X5	T36.8X6
antimalarial	T37.2X1	T37.2X2	T37.2X3	T37.2X4	T37.2X5	T37.2X6
antimycobacterial NEC	T37.1X1	T37.1X2	T37.1X3	T37.1X4	T37.1X5	T37.1X6
antibiotics	T36.5X1	T36.5X2	T36.5X3	T36.5X4	T36.5X5	T36.5X6
antiprotozoal NEC	T37.3X1	T37.3X2	T37.3X3	T37.3X4	T37.3X5	T37.3X6
blood	T37.2X1	T37.2X2	T37.2X3	T37.2X4	T37.2X5	T37.2X6
antiviral	T37.5X1	T37.5X2	T37.5X3	T37.5X4	T37.5X5	T37.5X6
arsenical	T37.8X1	T37.8X2	T37.8X3	T37.8X4	T37.8X5	T37.8X6
bismuth, local	T49.0X1	T49.0X2	T49.0X3	T49.0X4	T49.0X5	T49.0X6
ENT	T49.6X1	T49.6X2	T49.6X3	T49.6X4	T49.6X5	T49.6X6
eye NEC	T49.5X1	T49.5X2	T49.5X3	T49.5X4	T49.5X5	T49.5X6
heavy metals NEC	T37.8X1	T37.8X2	T37.8X3	T37.8X4	T37.8X5	T37.8X6
local NEC	T49.0X1	T49.0X2	T49.0X3	T49.0X4	T49.0X5	T49.0X6
specified NEC	T49.0X1	T49.0X2	T49.0X3	T49.0X4	T49.0X5	T49.0X6
mixed	T37.91	T37.92	T37.93	T37.94	T37.95	T37.96
ophthalmic preparation	T49.5X1	T49.5X2	T49.5X3	T49.5X4	T49.5X5	T49.5X6
topical NEC	T49.0X1	T49.0X2	T49.0X3	T49.0X4	T49.0X5	T49.0X6
Anti-inflammatory drug NEC	T39.391	T39.392	T39.393	T39.394	T39.395	T39.396
local	T49.0X1	T49.0X2	T49.0X3	T49.0X4	T49.0X5	T49.0X6
nonsteroidal NEC	T39.391	T39.392	T39.393	T39.394	T39.395	T39.396
propionic acid derivative	T39.311	T39.312	T39.313	T39.314	T39.315	T39.316
specified NEC	T39.391	T39.392	T39.393	T39.394	T39.395	T39.396
Antikaluretic	T50.3X1	T50.3X2	T50.3X3	T50.3X4	T50.3X5	T50.3X6
Antiknock (tetraethyl lead)	T56.0X1	T56.0X2	T56.0X3	T56.0X4	—	—
Antilipemic drug NEC	T46.6X1	T46.6X2	T46.6X3	T46.6X4	T46.6X5	T46.6X6
Antimalarial	T37.2X1	T37.2X2	T37.2X3	T37.2X4	T37.2X5	T37.2X6
prophylactic NEC	T37.2X1	T37.2X2	T37.2X3	T37.2X4	T37.2X5	T37.2X6
pyrimidine derivative	T37.2X1	T37.2X2	T37.2X3	T37.2X4	T37.2X5	T37.2X6
Antimetabolite	T45.1X1	T45.1X2	T45.1X3	T45.1X4	T45.1X5	T45.1X6
Antimitotic agent	T45.1X1	T45.1X2	T45.1X3	T45.1X4	T45.1X5	T45.1X6
Antimony (compounds) (vapor) NEC	T56.891	T56.892	T56.893	T56.894	—	—
anti-infectives	T37.8X1	T37.8X2	T37.8X3	T37.8X4	T37.8X5	T37.8X6
dimercaptosuccinate	T37.3X1	T37.3X2	T37.3X3	T37.3X4	T37.3X5	T37.3X6
hydride	T56.891	T56.892	T56.893	T56.894	—	—
pesticide (vapor)	T60.8X1	T60.8X2	T60.8X3	T60.8X4	—	—
potassium (sodium)	T37.8X1	T37.8X2	T37.8X3	T37.8X4	T37.8X5	T37.8X6
tartrate						
sodium	T37.3X1	T37.3X2	T37.3X3	T37.3X4	T37.3X5	T37.3X6
dimercaptosuccinate						
tartrated	T37.8X1	T37.8X2	T37.8X3	T37.8X4	T37.8X5	T37.8X6
Antimuscarinic NEC	T44.3X1	T44.3X2	T44.3X3	T44.3X4	T44.3X5	T44.3X6
Antimycobacterial drug NEC	T37.1X1	T37.1X2	T37.1X3	T37.1X4	T37.1X5	T37.1X6
antibiotics	T36.5X1	T36.5X2	T36.5X3	T36.5X4	T36.5X5	T36.5X6
combination	T37.1X1	T37.1X2	T37.1X3	T37.1X4	T37.1X5	T37.1X6
Antinausea drug	T45.0X1	T45.0X2	T45.0X3	T45.0X4	T45.0X5	T45.0X6
Antinematode drug	T37.4X1	T37.4X2	T37.4X3	T37.4X4	T37.4X5	T37.4X6
Antineoplastic NEC	T45.1X1	T45.1X2	T45.1X3	T45.1X4	T45.1X5	T45.1X6
alkaloidal	T45.1X1	T45.1X2	T45.1X3	T45.1X4	T45.1X5	T45.1X6
antibiotics	T45.1X1	T45.1X2	T45.1X3	T45.1X4	T45.1X5	T45.1X6
combination	T45.1X1	T45.1X2	T45.1X3	T45.1X4	T45.1X5	T45.1X6
estrogen	T38.5X1	T38.5X2	T38.5X3	T38.5X4	T38.5X5	T38.5X6

Substance	Poisoning, Accidental (unintentional)	Poisoning, Intentional Self-harm	Poisoning, Assault	Poisoning, Undetermined	Adverse Effect	Under-dosing
Antineoplastic — *continued*						
steroid	T38.7X1	T38.7X2	T38.7X3	T38.7X4	T38.7X5	T38.7X6
Antiparasitic drug (systemic)	T37.91	T37.92	T37.93	T37.94	T37.95	T37.96
local	T49.0X1	T49.0X2	T49.0X3	T49.0X4	T49.0X5	T49.0X6
specified NEC	T37.8X1	T37.8X2	T37.8X3	T37.8X4	T37.8X5	T37.8X6
Antiparkinsonism drug	T42.8X1	T42.8X2	T42.8X3	T42.8X4	T42.8X5	T42.8X6
Antiperspirant NEC	T49.2X1	T49.2X2	T49.2X3	T49.2X4	T49.2X5	T49.2X6
Antiphlogistic NEC	T39.4X1	T39.4X2	T39.4X3	T39.4X4	T39.4X5	T39.4X6
Antiplatyhelmintic drug	T37.4X1	T37.4X2	T37.4X3	T37.4X4	T37.4X5	T37.4X6
Antiprotozoal drug NEC	T37.3X1	T37.3X2	T37.3X3	T37.3X4	T37.3X5	T37.3X6
blood	T37.2X1	T37.2X2	T37.2X3	T37.2X4	T37.2X5	T37.2X6
local	T49.0X1	T49.0X2	T49.0X3	T49.0X4	T49.0X5	T49.0X6
Antipruritic drug NEC	T49.1X1	T49.1X2	T49.1X3	T49.1X4	T49.1X5	T49.1X6
Antipsychotic drug	T43.501	T43.502	T43.503	T43.504	T43.505	T43.506
specified NEC	T43.591	T43.592	T43.593	T43.594	T43.595	T43.596
Antipyretic	T39.91	T39.92	T39.93	T39.94	T39.95	T39.96
specified NEC	T39.8X1	T39.8X2	T39.8X3	T39.8X4	T39.8X5	T39.8X6
Antipyrine	T39.2X1	T39.2X2	T39.2X3	T39.2X4	T39.2X5	T39.2X6
Antirabies hyperimmune serum	T50.Z11	T50.Z12	T50.Z13	T50.Z14	T50.Z15	T50.Z16
Antirheumatic NEC	T39.4X1	T39.4X2	T39.4X3	T39.4X4	T39.4X5	T39.4X6
Antirigidity drug NEC	T42.8X1	T42.8X2	T42.8X3	T42.8X4	T42.8X5	T42.8X6
Antischistosomal drug	T37.4X1	T37.4X2	T37.4X3	T37.4X4	T37.4X5	T37.4X6
Antiscorpion sera	T50.Z11	T50.Z12	T50.Z13	T50.Z14	T50.Z15	T50.Z16
Antiseborrheics	T49.4X1	T49.4X2	T49.4X3	T49.4X4	T49.4X5	T49.4X6
Antiseptics (external) (medicinal)	T49.0X1	T49.0X2	T49.0X3	T49.0X4	T49.0X5	T49.0X6
Antistine	T45.0X1	T45.0X2	T45.0X3	T45.0X4	T45.0X5	T45.0X6
Antitapeworm drug	T37.4X1	T37.4X2	T37.4X3	T37.4X4	T37.4X5	T37.4X6
Antitetanus immunoglobulin	T50.Z11	T50.Z12	T50.Z13	T50.Z14	T50.Z15	T50.Z16
Antithyroid drug NEC	T38.2X1	T38.2X2	T38.2X3	T38.2X4	T38.2X5	T38.2X6
Antitoxin	T50.Z11	T50.Z12	T50.Z13	T50.Z14	T50.Z15	T50.Z16
diphtheria	T50.Z11	T50.Z12	T50.Z13	T50.Z14	T50.Z15	T50.Z16
gas gangrene	T50.Z11	T50.Z12	T50.Z13	T50.Z14	T50.Z15	T50.Z16
tetanus	T50.Z11	T50.Z12	T50.Z13	T50.Z14	T50.Z15	T50.Z16
Antitrichomonal drug	T37.3X1	T37.3X2	T37.3X3	T37.3X4	T37.3X5	T37.3X6
Antituberculars	T37.1X1	T37.1X2	T37.1X3	T37.1X4	T37.1X5	T37.1X6
antibiotics	T36.5X1	T36.5X2	T36.5X3	T36.5X4	T36.5X5	T36.5X6
Antitussive NEC	T48.3X1	T48.3X2	T48.3X3	T48.3X4	T48.3X5	T48.3X6
codeine mixture	T40.2X1	T40.2X2	T40.2X3	T40.2X4	T40.2X5	T40.2X6
opiate	T40.2X1	T40.2X2	T40.2X3	T40.2X4	T40.2X5	T40.2X6
Antivaricose drug	T46.8X1	T46.8X2	T46.8X3	T46.8X4	T46.8X5	T46.8X6
Antivenin, antivenom (sera)	T50.Z11	T50.Z12	T50.Z13	T50.Z14	T50.Z15	T50.Z16
crotaline	T50.Z11	T50.Z12	T50.Z13	T50.Z14	T50.Z15	T50.Z16
spider bite	T50.Z11	T50.Z12	T50.Z13	T50.Z14	T50.Z15	T50.Z16
Antivertigo drug	T45.0X1	T45.0X2	T45.0X3	T45.0X4	T45.0X5	T45.0X6
Antiviral drug NEC	T37.5X1	T37.5X2	T37.5X3	T37.5X4	T37.5X5	T37.5X6
eye	T49.5X1	T49.5X2	T49.5X3	T49.5X4	T49.5X5	T49.5X6
Antiwhipworm drug	T37.4X1	T37.4X2	T37.4X3	T37.4X4	T37.4X5	T37.4X6
Ant poison — *see* Insecticide						
Antrol — *see also* by specific chemical substance	T60.91	T60.92	T60.93	T60.94		
fungicide	T60.91	T60.92	T60.93	T60.94	—	—
ANTU (alpha naphthylthiourea)	T60.4X1	T60.4X2	T60.4X3	T60.4X4	—	—
Apalcillin	T36.0X1	T36.0X2	T36.0X3	T36.0X4	T36.0X5	T36.0X6
APC	T48.5X1	T48.5X2	T48.5X3	T48.5X4	T48.5X5	T48.5X6
Aplonidine	T44.4X1	T44.4X2	T44.4X3	T44.4X4	T44.4X5	T44.4X6
Apomorphine	T47.7X1	T47.7X2	T47.7X3	T47.7X4	T47.7X5	T47.7X6
Appetite depressants, central	T50.5X1	T50.5X2	T50.5X3	T50.5X4	T50.5X5	T50.5X6
Apraclonidine (hydrochloride)	T44.4X1	T44.4X2	T44.4X3	T44.4X4	T44.4X5	T44.4X6
Apresoline	T46.5X1	T46.5X2	T46.5X3	T46.5X4	T46.5X5	T46.5X6
Aprindine	T46.2X1	T46.2X2	T46.2X3	T46.2X4	T46.2X5	T46.2X6
Aprobarbital	T42.3X1	T42.3X2	T42.3X3	T42.3X4	T42.3X5	T42.3X6
Apronalide	T42.6X1	T42.6X2	T42.6X3	T42.6X4	T42.6X5	T42.6X6
Aprotinin	T45.621	T45.622	T45.623	T45.624	T45.625	T45.626
Aptocaine	T41.3X1	T41.3X2	T41.3X3	T41.3X4	T41.3X5	T41.3X6
Aqua fortis	T54.2X1	T54.2X2	T54.2X3	T54.2X4	—	—
Ara-A	T37.5X1	T37.5X2	T37.5X3	T37.5X4	T37.5X5	T37.5X6
Ara-C	T45.1X1	T45.1X2	T45.1X3	T45.1X4	T45.1X5	T45.1X6
Arachis oil	T49.3X1	T49.3X2	T49.3X3	T49.3X4	T49.3X5	T49.3X6
cathartic	T47.4X1	T47.4X2	T47.4X3	T47.4X4	T47.4X5	T47.4X6
Aralen	T37.2X1	T37.2X2	T37.2X3	T37.2X4	T37.2X5	T37.2X6
Arecoline	T44.1X1	T44.1X2	T44.1X3	T44.1X4	T44.1X5	T44.1X6
Arginine	T50.991	T50.992	T50.993	T50.994	T50.995	T50.996
glutamate	T50.991	T50.992	T50.993	T50.994	T50.995	T50.996
Argyrol	T49.0X1	T49.0X2	T49.0X3	T49.0X4	T49.0X5	T49.0X6
ENT agent	T49.6X1	T49.6X2	T49.6X3	T49.6X4	T49.6X5	T49.6X6

Table of Drugs and Chemicals

Antifungal — Argyrol

Table of Drugs and Chemicals

Argyrol — Benzalkonium

Substance	Poisoning, Accidental (unintentional)	Poisoning, Intentional Self-harm	Poisoning, Assault	Poisoning, Undetermined	Adverse Effect	Under-dosing
Argyrol — *continued*						
ophthalmic preparation	T49.5X1	T49.5X2	T49.5X3	T49.5X4	T49.5X5	T49.5X6
Aristocort	T38.0X1	T38.0X2	T38.0X3	T38.0X4	T38.0X5	T38.0X6
ENT agent	T49.6X1	T49.6X2	T49.6X3	T49.6X4	T49.6X5	T49.6X6
ophthalmic preparation	T49.5X1	T49.5X2	T49.5X3	T49.5X4	T49.5X5	T49.5X6
topical NEC	T49.0X1	T49.0X2	T49.0X3	T49.0X4	T49.0X5	T49.0X6
Aromatics, corrosive	T54.1X1	T54.1X2	T54.1X3	T54.1X4	—	—
disinfectants	T54.1X1	T54.1X2	T54.1X3	T54.1X4	—	—
Arsenate of lead	T57.0X1	T57.0X2	T57.0X3	T57.0X4	—	—
herbicide	T57.0X1	T57.0X2	T57.0X3	T57.0X4	—	—
Arsenic, arsenicals (compounds) (dust) (vapor) **NEC**	T57.0X1	T57.0X2	T57.0X3	T57.0X4	—	—
anti-infectives	T37.8X1	T37.8X2	T37.8X3	T37.8X4	T37.8X5	T37.8X6
pesticide (dust) (fumes)	T57.0X1	T57.0X2	T57.0X3	T57.0X4	—	—
Arsine (gas)	T57.0X1	T57.0X2	T57.0X3	T57.0X4	—	—
Arsphenamine (silver)	T37.8X1	T37.8X2	T37.8X3	T37.8X4	T37.8X5	T37.8X6
Arsthinol	T37.3X1	T37.3X2	T37.3X3	T37.3X4	T37.3X5	T37.3X6
Artane	T44.3X1	T44.3X2	T44.3X3	T44.3X4	T44.3X5	T44.3X6
Arthropod (venomous) **NEC**	T63.481	T63.482	T63.483	T63.484	—	—
Articaine	T41.3X1	T41.3X2	T41.3X3	T41.3X4	T41.3X5	T41.3X6
Asbestos	T57.8X1	T57.8X2	T57.8X3	T57.8X4	—	—
Ascaridole	T37.4X1	T37.4X2	T37.4X3	T37.4X4	T37.4X5	T37.4X6
Ascorbic acid	T45.2X1	T45.2X2	T45.2X3	T45.2X4	T45.2X5	T45.2X6
Asiaticoside	T49.0X1	T49.0X2	T49.0X3	T49.0X4	T49.0X5	T49.0X6
Asparaginase	T45.1X1	T45.1X2	T45.1X3	T45.1X4	T45.1X5	T45.1X6
Aspidium (oleoresin)	T37.4X1	T37.4X2	T37.4X3	T37.4X4	T37.4X5	T37.4X6
Aspirin (aluminum) (soluble)	T39.011	T39.012	T39.013	T39.014	T39.015	T39.016
Aspoxicillin	T36.0X1	T36.0X2	T36.0X3	T36.0X4	T36.0X5	T36.0X6
Astemizole	T45.0X1	T45.0X2	T45.0X3	T45.0X4	T45.0X5	T45.0X6
Astringent (local)	T49.2X1	T49.2X2	T49.2X3	T49.2X4	T49.2X5	T49.2X6
specified NEC	T49.2X1	T49.2X2	T49.2X3	T49.2X4	T49.2X5	T49.2X6
Astromicin	T36.5X1	T36.5X2	T36.5X3	T36.5X4	T36.5X5	T36.5X6
Ataractic drug NEC	T43.501	T43.502	T43.503	T43.504	T43.505	T43.506
Atenolol	T44.7X1	T44.7X2	T44.7X3	T44.7X4	T44.7X5	T44.7X6
Atonia drug, intestinal	T47.4X1	T47.4X2	T47.4X3	T47.4X4	T47.4X5	T47.4X6
Atophan	T50.4X1	T50.4X2	T50.4X3	T50.4X4	T50.4X5	T50.4X6
Atracurium besilate	T48.1X1	T48.1X2	T48.1X3	T48.1X4	T48.1X5	T48.1X6
Atropine	T44.3X1	T44.3X2	T44.3X3	T44.3X4	T44.3X5	T44.3X6
derivative	T44.3X1	T44.3X2	T44.3X3	T44.3X4	T44.3X5	T44.3X6
methonitrate	T44.3X1	T44.3X2	T44.3X3	T44.3X4	T44.3X5	T44.3X6
Attapulgite	T47.6X1	T47.6X2	T47.6X3	T47.6X4	T47.6X5	T47.6X6
Auramine	T65.891	T65.892	T65.893	T65.894	—	—
dye	T65.6X1	T65.6X2	T65.6X3	T65.6X4	—	—
fungicide	T60.3X1	T60.3X2	T60.3X3	T60.3X4	—	—
Auranofin	T39.4X1	T39.4X2	T39.4X3	T39.4X4	T39.4X5	T39.4X6
Aurantiin	T46.991	T46.992	T46.993	T46.994	T46.995	T46.996
Aureomycin	T36.4X1	T36.4X2	T36.4X3	T36.4X4	T36.4X5	T36.4X6
ophthalmic preparation	T49.5X1	T49.5X2	T49.5X3	T49.5X4	T49.5X5	T49.5X6
topical NEC	T49.0X1	T49.0X2	T49.0X3	T49.0X4	T49.0X5	T49.0X6
Aurothioglucose	T39.4X1	T39.4X2	T39.4X3	T39.4X4	T39.4X5	T39.4X6
Aurothioglycanide	T39.4X1	T39.4X2	T39.4X3	T39.4X4	T39.4X5	T39.4X6
Aurothiomalate sodium	T39.4X1	T39.4X2	T39.4X3	T39.4X4	T39.4X5	T39.4X6
Aurotioprol	T39.4X1	T39.4X2	T39.4X3	T39.4X4	T39.4X5	T39.4X6
Automobile fuel	T52.0X1	T52.0X2	T52.0X3	T52.0X4	—	—
Autonomic nervous system agent NEC	T44.901	T44.902	T44.903	T44.904	T44.905	T44.906
Avlosulfon	T37.1X1	T37.1X2	T37.1X3	T37.1X4	T37.1X5	T37.1X6
Avomine	T42.6X1	T42.6X2	T42.6X3	T42.6X4	T42.6X5	T42.6X6
Axerophthol	T45.2X1	T45.2X2	T45.2X3	T45.2X4	T45.2X5	T45.2X6
Azacitidine	T45.1X1	T45.1X2	T45.1X3	T45.1X4	T45.1X5	T45.1X6
Azacyclonol	T43.591	T43.592	T43.593	T43.594	T43.595	T43.596
Azadirachta	T60.2X1	T60.2X2	T60.2X3	T60.2X4	—	—
Azanidazole	T37.3X1	T37.3X2	T37.3X3	T37.3X4	T37.3X5	T37.3X6
Azapetine	T46.7X1	T46.7X2	T46.7X3	T46.7X4	T46.7X5	T46.7X6
Azapropazone	T39.2X1	T39.2X2	T39.2X3	T39.2X4	T39.2X5	T39.2X6
Azaribine	T45.1X1	T45.1X2	T45.1X3	T45.1X4	T45.1X5	T45.1X6
Azaserine	T45.1X1	T45.1X2	T45.1X3	T45.1X4	T45.1X5	T45.1X6
Azatadine	T45.0X1	T45.0X2	T45.0X3	T45.0X4	T45.0X5	T45.0X6
Azatepa	T45.1X1	T45.1X2	T45.1X3	T45.1X4	T45.1X5	T45.1X6
Azathioprine	T45.1X1	T45.1X2	T45.1X3	T45.1X4	T45.1X5	T45.1X6
Azelaic acid	T49.0X1	T49.0X2	T49.0X3	T49.0X4	T49.0X5	T49.0X6
Azelastine	T45.0X1	T45.0X2	T45.0X3	T45.0X4	T45.0X5	T45.0X6
Azidocillin	T36.0X1	T36.0X2	T36.0X3	T36.0X4	T36.0X5	T36.0X6
Azidothymidine	T37.5X1	T37.5X2	T37.5X3	T37.5X4	T37.5X5	T37.5X6
Azinphos (ethyl) (methyl)	T60.0X1	T60.0X2	T60.0X3	T60.0X4	—	—
Aziridine (chelating)	T54.1X1	T54.1X2	T54.1X3	T54.1X4	—	—
Azithromycin	T36.3X1	T36.3X2	T36.3X3	T36.3X4	T36.3X5	T36.3X6
Azlocillin	T36.0X1	T36.0X2	T36.0X3	T36.0X4	T36.0X5	T36.0X6
Azobenzene smoke	T65.3X1	T65.3X2	T65.3X3	T65.3X4	—	—
acaricide	T60.8X1	T60.8X2	T60.8X3	T60.8X4	—	—
Azosulfamide	T37.0X1	T37.0X2	T37.0X3	T37.0X4	T37.0X5	T37.0X6
AZT	T37.5X1	T37.5X2	T37.5X3	T37.5X4	T37.5X5	T37.5X6
Aztreonam	T36.1X1	T36.1X2	T36.1X3	T36.1X4	T36.1X5	T36.1X6

Substance	Poisoning, Accidental (unintentional)	Poisoning, Intentional Self-harm	Poisoning, Assault	Poisoning, Undetermined	Adverse Effect	Under-dosing
Azulfidine	T37.0X1	T37.0X2	T37.0X3	T37.0X4	T37.0X5	T37.0X6
Azuresin	T50.8X1	T50.8X2	T50.8X3	T50.8X4	T50.8X5	T50.8X6
b-acetyldigoxin	T46.0X1	T46.0X2	T46.0X3	T46.0X4	T46.0X5	T46.0X6
P-Acetamidophenol	T39.1X1	T39.1X2	T39.1X3	T39.1X4	T39.1X5	T39.1X6
Bacampicillin	T36.0X1	T36.0X2	T36.0X3	T36.0X4	T36.0X5	T36.0X6
Bacillus						
lactobacillus	T47.8X1	T47.8X2	T47.8X3	T47.8X4	T47.8X5	T47.8X6
subtilis	T47.6X1	T47.6X2	T47.6X3	T47.6X4	T47.6X5	T47.6X6
Bacimycin	T49.0X1	T49.0X2	T49.0X3	T49.0X4	T49.0X5	T49.0X6
ophthalmic preparation	T49.5X1	T49.5X2	T49.5X3	T49.5X4	T49.5X5	T49.5X6
Bacitracin zinc	T49.0X1	T49.0X2	T49.0X3	T49.0X4	T49.0X5	T49.0X6
with neomycin	T49.0X1	T49.0X2	T49.0X3	T49.0X4	T49.0X5	T49.0X6
ENT agent	T49.6X1	T49.6X2	T49.6X3	T49.6X4	T49.6X5	T49.6X6
ophthalmic preparation	T49.5X1	T49.5X2	T49.5X3	T49.5X4	T49.5X5	T49.5X6
topical NEC	T49.0X1	T49.0X2	T49.0X3	T49.0X4	T49.0X5	T49.0X6
Baclofen	T42.8X1	T42.8X2	T42.8X3	T42.8X4	T42.8X5	T42.8X6
Baking soda	T50.991	T50.992	T50.993	T50.994	T50.995	T50.996
BAL	T45.8X1	T45.8X2	T45.8X3	T45.8X4	T45.8X5	T45.8X6
Bambuterol	T48.6X1	T48.6X2	T48.6X3	T48.6X4	T48.6X5	T48.6X6
Bamethan (sulfate)	T46.7X1	T46.7X2	T46.7X3	T46.7X4	T46.7X5	T46.7X6
Bamifylline	T48.6X1	T48.6X2	T48.6X3	T48.6X4	T48.6X5	T48.6X6
Bamipine	T45.0X1	T45.0X2	T45.0X3	T45.0X4	T45.0X5	T45.0X6
Baneberry — *see* Actaea spicata						
Banewort — *see* Belladonna						
Barbenyl	T42.3X1	T42.3X2	T42.3X3	T42.3X4	T42.3X5	T42.3X6
Barbexaclone	T42.6X1	T42.6X2	T42.6X3	T42.6X4	T42.6X5	T42.6X6
Barbital	T42.3X1	T42.3X2	T42.3X3	T42.3X4	T42.3X5	T42.3X6
sodium	T42.3X1	T42.3X2	T42.3X3	T42.3X4	T42.3X5	T42.3X6
Barbitone	T42.3X1	T42.3X2	T42.3X3	T42.3X4	T42.3X5	T42.3X6
Barbiturate NEC	T42.3X1	T42.3X2	T42.3X3	T42.3X4	T42.3X5	T42.3X6
with tranquilizer	T42.3X1	T42.3X2	T42.3X3	T42.3X4	T42.3X5	T42.3X6
anesthetic (intravenous)	T41.1X1	T41.1X2	T41.1X3	T41.1X4	T41.1X5	T41.1X6
Barium (carbonate) (chloride) (sulfite)	T57.8X1	T57.8X2	T57.8X3	T57.8X4	—	—
diagnostic agent	T50.8X1	T50.8X2	T50.8X3	T50.8X4	T50.8X5	T50.8X6
pesticide	T60.4X1	T60.4X2	T60.4X3	T60.4X4	—	—
rodenticide	T60.4X1	T60.4X2	T60.4X3	T60.4X4	—	—
sulfate (medicinal)	T50.8X1	T50.8X2	T50.8X3	T50.8X4	T50.8X5	T50.8X6
Barrier cream	T49.3X1	T49.3X2	T49.3X3	T49.3X4	T49.3X5	T49.3X6
Basic fuchsin	T49.0X1	T49.0X2	T49.0X3	T49.0X4	T49.0X5	T49.0X6
Battery acid or fluid	T54.2X1	T54.2X2	T54.2X3	T54.2X4	—	—
Bay rum	T51.8X1	T51.8X2	T51.8X3	T51.8X4	—	—
b-benzalbutyramide	T46.6X1	T46.6X2	T46.6X3	T46.6X4	T46.6X5	T46.6X6
BCG (vaccine)	T50.A91	T50.A92	T50.A93	T50.A94	T50.A95	T50.A96
BCNU	T45.1X1	T45.1X2	T45.1X3	T45.1X4	T45.1X5	T45.1X6
Bearsfoot	T62.2X1	T62.2X2	T62.2X3	T62.2X4	—	—
Beclamide	T42.6X1	T42.6X2	T42.6X3	T42.6X4	T42.6X5	T42.6X6
Beclomethasone	T44.5X1	T44.5X2	T44.5X3	T44.5X4	T44.5X5	T44.5X6
Bee (sting) (venom)	T63.441	T63.442	T63.443	T63.444	—	—
Befunolol	T49.5X1	T49.5X2	T49.5X3	T49.5X4	T49.5X5	T49.5X6
Bekanamycin	T36.5X1	T36.5X2	T36.5X3	T36.5X4	T36.5X5	T36.5X6
Belladonna — *see also* Nightshade						
alkaloids	T44.3X1	T44.3X2	T44.3X3	T44.3X4	T44.3X5	T44.3X6
extract	T44.3X1	T44.3X2	T44.3X3	T44.3X4	T44.3X5	T44.3X6
herb	T44.3X1	T44.3X2	T44.3X3	T44.3X4	T44.3X5	T44.3X6
Bemegride	T50.7X1	T50.7X2	T50.7X3	T50.7X4	T50.7X5	T50.7X6
Benactyzine	T44.3X1	T44.3X2	T44.3X3	T44.3X4	T44.3X5	T44.3X6
Benadryl	T45.0X1	T45.0X2	T45.0X3	T45.0X4	T45.0X5	T45.0X6
Benaprizine	T44.3X1	T44.3X2	T44.3X3	T44.3X4	T44.3X5	T44.3X6
Benazepril	T46.4X1	T46.4X2	T46.4X3	T46.4X4	T46.4X5	T46.4X6
Bencyclane	T46.7X1	T46.7X2	T46.7X3	T46.7X4	T46.7X5	T46.7X6
Bendazol	T46.3X1	T46.3X2	T46.3X3	T46.3X4	T46.3X5	T46.3X6
Bendrofluazide	T50.2X1	T50.2X2	T50.2X3	T50.2X4	T50.2X5	T50.2X6
Bendroflumethiazide	T50.2X1	T50.2X2	T50.2X3	T50.2X4	T50.2X5	T50.2X6
Benemid	T50.4X1	T50.4X2	T50.4X3	T50.4X4	T50.4X5	T50.4X6
Benethamine penicillin	T36.0X1	T36.0X2	T36.0X3	T36.0X4	T36.0X5	T36.0X6
Benexate	T47.1X1	T47.1X2	T47.1X3	T47.1X4	T47.1X5	T47.1X6
Benfluorex	T46.6X1	T46.6X2	T46.6X3	T46.6X4	T46.6X5	T46.6X6
Benfotiamine	T45.2X1	T45.2X2	T45.2X3	T45.2X4	T45.2X5	T45.2X6
Benisone	T49.0X1	T49.0X2	T49.0X3	T49.0X4	T49.0X5	T49.0X6
Benomyl	T60.0X1	T60.0X2	T60.0X3	T60.0X4	—	—
Benoquin	T49.8X1	T49.8X2	T49.8X3	T49.8X4	T49.8X5	T49.8X6
Benoxinate	T41.3X1	T41.3X2	T41.3X3	T41.3X4	T41.3X5	T41.3X6
Benperidol	T43.4X1	T43.4X2	T43.4X3	T43.4X4	T43.4X5	T43.4X6
Benproperine	T48.3X1	T48.3X2	T48.3X3	T48.3X4	T48.3X5	T48.3X6
Benserazide	T42.8X1	T42.8X2	T42.8X3	T42.8X4	T42.8X5	T42.8X6
Bentazepam	T42.4X1	T42.4X2	T42.4X3	T42.4X4	T42.4X5	T42.4X6
Bentiromide	T50.8X1	T50.8X2	T50.8X3	T50.8X4	T50.8X5	T50.8X6
Bentonite	T49.3X1	T49.3X2	T49.3X3	T49.3X4	T49.3X5	T49.3X6
Benzalbutyramide	T46.6X1	T46.6X2	T46.6X3	T46.6X4	T46.6X5	T46.6X6
Benzalkonium (chloride)	T49.0X1	T49.0X2	T49.0X3	T49.0X4	T49.0X5	T49.0X6
ophthalmic preparation	T49.5X1	T49.5X2	T49.5X3	T49.5X4	T49.5X5	T49.5X6

Additional Character May Be Required — Refer to the Tabular List for Character Selection ▽ Subterms under main terms may continue to next column or page

Substance	Poisoning, Accidental (unintentional)	Poisoning, Intentional Self-harm	Poisoning, Assault	Poisoning, Undetermined	Adverse Effect	Under-dosing
Benzamidosalicylate (calcium)	T37.1X1	T37.1X2	T37.1X3	T37.1X4	T37.1X5	T37.1X6
Benzamine	T41.3X1	T41.3X2	T41.3X3	T41.3X4	T41.3X5	T41.3X6
lactate	T49.1X1	T49.1X2	T49.1X3	T49.1X4	T49.1X5	T49.1X6
Benzamphetamine	T50.5X1	T50.5X2	T50.5X3	T50.5X4	T50.5X5	T50.5X6
Benzapril hydrochloride	T46.5X1	T46.5X2	T46.5X3	T46.5X4	T46.5X5	T46.5X6
Benzathine benzylpenicillin	T36.0X1	T36.0X2	T36.0X3	T36.0X4	T36.0X5	T36.0X6
Benzathine penicillin	T36.0X1	T36.0X2	T36.0X3	T36.0X4	T36.0X5	T36.0X6
Benzatropine	T42.8X1	T42.8X2	T42.8X3	T42.8X4	T42.8X5	T42.8X6
Benzbromarone	T50.4X1	T50.4X2	T50.4X3	T50.4X4	T50.4X5	T50.4X6
Benzcarbimine	T45.1X1	T45.1X2	T45.1X3	T45.1X4	T45.1X5	T45.1X6
Benzedrex	T44.991	T44.992	T44.993	T44.994	T44.995	T44.996
Benzedrine (amphetamine)	T43.621	T43.622	T43.623	T43.624	T43.625	T43.626
Benzenamine	T65.3X1	T65.3X2	T65.3X3	T65.3X4	—	—
Benzene	T52.1X1	T52.1X2	T52.1X3	T52.1X4	—	—
homologues (acetyl) (dimethyl) (methyl) (solvent)	T52.2X1	T52.2X2	T52.2X3	T52.2X4	—	—
Benzethonium (chloride)	T49.0X1	T49.0X2	T49.0X3	T49.0X4	T49.0X5	T49.0X6
Benzfetamine	T50.5X1	T50.5X2	T50.5X3	T50.5X4	T50.5X5	T50.5X6
Benzhexol	T44.3X1	T44.3X2	T44.3X3	T44.3X4	T44.3X5	T44.3X6
Benzhydramine (chloride)	T45.0X1	T45.0X2	T45.0X3	T45.0X4	T45.0X5	T45.0X6
Benzidine	T65.891	T65.892	T65.893	T65.894	—	—
Benziionium bromide	T44.3X1	T44.3X2	T44.3X3	T44.3X4	T44.3X5	—
Benzimidazole	T60.3X1	T60.3X2	T60.3X3	T60.3X4	—	—
Benzin (e) — see Ligroin						
Benziodarone	T46.3X1	T46.3X2	T46.3X3	T46.3X4	T46.3X5	T46.3X6
Benznidazole	T37.3X1	T37.3X2	T37.3X3	T37.3X4	T37.3X5	T37.3X6
Benzocaine	T41.3X1	T41.3X2	T41.3X3	T41.3X4	T41.3X5	T41.3X6
Benzodiapin	T42.4X1	T42.4X2	T42.4X3	T42.4X4	T42.4X5	T42.4X6
Benzodiazepine NEC	T42.4X1	T42.4X2	T42.4X3	T42.4X4	T42.4X5	T42.4X6
Benzoic acid	T49.0X1	T49.0X2	T49.0X3	T49.0X4	T49.0X5	T49.0X6
with salicylic acid	T49.0X1	T49.0X2	T49.0X3	T49.0X4	T49.0X5	T49.0X6
Benzoin (tincture)	T48.5X1	T48.5X2	T48.5X3	T48.5X4	T48.5X5	T48.5X6
Benzol (benzene)	T52.1X1	T52.1X2	T52.1X3	T52.1X4	—	—
vapor	T52.0X1	T52.0X2	T52.0X3	T52.0X4	—	—
Benzomorphan	T40.2X1	T40.2X2	T40.2X3	T40.2X4	T40.2X5	T40.2X6
Benzonatate	T48.3X1	T48.3X2	T48.3X3	T48.3X4	T48.3X5	T48.3X6
Benzophenones	T49.3X1	T49.3X2	T49.3X3	T49.3X4	T49.3X5	T49.3X6
Benzopyrone	T46.991	T46.992	T46.993	T46.994	T46.995	T46.996
Benzothiadiazides	T50.2X1	T50.2X2	T50.2X3	T50.2X4	T50.2X5	T50.2X6
Benzoxonium chloride	T49.0X1	T49.0X2	T49.0X3	T49.0X4	T49.0X5	T49.0X6
Benzoylpas calcium	T37.1X1	T37.1X2	T37.1X3	T37.1X4	T37.1X5	T37.1X6
Benzoyl peroxide	T49.0X1	T49.0X2	T49.0X3	T49.0X4	T49.0X5	T49.0X6
Benzperidin	T43.591	T43.592	T43.593	T43.594	T43.595	T43.596
Benzperidol	T43.591	T43.592	T43.593	T43.594	T43.595	T43.596
Benzphetamine	T50.5X1	T50.5X2	T50.5X3	T50.5X4	T50.5X5	T50.5X6
Benzpyrinium bromide	T44.1X1	T44.1X2	T44.1X3	T44.1X4	T44.1X5	T44.1X6
Benzquinamide	T45.0X1	T45.0X2	T45.0X3	T45.0X4	T45.0X5	T45.0X6
Benzthiazide	T50.2X1	T50.2X2	T50.2X3	T50.2X4	T50.2X5	T50.2X6
Benztropine						
anticholinergic	T44.3X1	T44.3X2	T44.3X3	T44.3X4	T44.3X5	T44.3X6
antiparkinson	T42.8X1	T42.8X2	T42.8X3	T42.8X4	T42.8X5	T42.8X6
Benzydamine	T49.0X1	T49.0X2	T49.0X3	T49.0X4	T49.0X5	T49.0X6
Benzyl						
acetate	T52.8X1	T52.8X2	T52.8X3	T52.8X4	—	—
alcohol	T49.0X1	T49.0X2	T49.0X3	T49.0X4	T49.0X5	T49.0X6
benzoate	T49.0X1	T49.0X2	T49.0X3	T49.0X4	T49.0X5	T49.0X6
Benzoic acid	T49.0X1	T49.0X2	T49.0X3	T49.0X4	T49.0X5	T49.0X6
morphine	T40.2X1	T40.2X2	T40.2X3	T40.2X4	—	—
nicotinate	T46.6X1	T46.6X2	T46.6X3	T46.6X4	T46.6X5	T46.6X6
penicillin	T36.0X1	T36.0X2	T36.0X3	T36.0X4	T36.0X5	T36.0X6
Benzylhydrochlorthiazide	T50.2X1	T50.2X2	T50.2X3	T50.2X4	T50.2X5	T50.2X6
Benzylpenicillin	T36.0X1	T36.0X2	T36.0X3	T36.0X4	T36.0X5	T36.0X6
Benzylthiouracil	T38.2X1	T38.2X2	T38.2X3	T38.2X4	T38.2X5	T38.2X6
Bephenium	T37.4X1	T37.4X2	T37.4X3	T37.4X4	T37.4X5	T37.4X6
hydroxynaphthoate						
Bepridil	T46.1X1	T46.1X2	T46.1X3	T46.1X4	T46.1X5	T46.1X6
Bergamot oil	T65.891	T65.892	T65.893	T65.894	—	—
Bergapten	T50.991	T50.992	T50.993	T50.994	T50.995	T50.996
Berries, poisonous	T62.1X1	T62.1X2	T62.1X3	T62.1X4	—	—
Beryllium (compounds)	T56.7X1	T56.7X2	T56.7X3	T56.7X4	—	—
beta adrenergic blocking agent, heart	T44.7X1	T44.7X2	T44.7X3	T44.7X4	T44.7X5	T44.7X6
Betacarotene	T45.2X1	T45.2X2	T45.2X3	T45.2X4	T45.2X5	T45.2X6
Beta-Chlor	T42.6X1	T42.6X2	T42.6X3	T42.6X4	T42.6X5	T42.6X6
Betahistine	T46.7X1	T46.7X2	T46.7X3	T46.7X4	T46.7X5	T46.7X6
Betaine	T47.5X1	T47.5X2	T47.5X3	T47.5X4	T47.5X5	T47.5X6
Betamethasone	T49.0X1	T49.0X2	T49.0X3	T49.0X4	T49.0X5	T49.0X6
topical	T49.0X1	T49.0X2	T49.0X3	T49.0X4	T49.0X5	T49.0X6
Betamicin	T36.8X1	T36.8X2	T36.8X3	T36.8X4	T36.8X5	T36.8X6
Betanidine	T46.5X1	T46.5X2	T46.5X3	T46.5X4	T46.5X5	T46.5X6
Betaxolol	T44.7X1	T44.7X2	T44.7X3	T44.7X4	T44.7X5	T44.7X6

Substance	Poisoning, Accidental (unintentional)	Poisoning, Intentional Self-harm	Poisoning, Assault	Poisoning, Undetermined	Adverse Effect	Under-dosing
Betazole	T50.8X1	T50.8X2	T50.8X3	T50.8X4	T50.8X5	T50.8X6
Bethanechol	T44.1X1	T44.1X2	T44.1X3	T44.1X4	T44.1X5	T44.1X6
chloride	T44.1X1	T44.1X2	T44.1X3	T44.1X4	T44.1X5	T44.1X6
Bethanidine	T46.5X1	T46.5X2	T46.5X3	T46.5X4	T46.5X5	T46.5X6
Betoxycaine	T41.3X1	T41.3X2	T41.3X3	T41.3X4	T41.3X5	T41.3X6
Betula oil	T49.3X1	T49.3X2	T49.3X3	T49.3X4	T49.3X5	T49.3X6
Bevantolol	T44.7X1	T44.7X2	T44.7X3	T44.7X4	T44.7X5	T44.7X6
Bevonium metilsulfate	T44.3X1	T44.3X2	T44.3X3	T44.3X4	T44.3X5	T44.3X6
Bezafibrate	T46.6X1	T46.6X2	T46.6X3	T46.6X4	T46.6X5	T46.6X6
Bezitramide	T40.4X1	T40.4X2	T40.4X3	T40.4X4	T40.4X5	T40.4X6
BHA	T50.991	T50.992	T50.993	T50.994	T50.995	T50.996
Bhang	T40.7X1	T40.7X2	T40.7X3	T40.7X4	T40.7X5	T40.7X6
BHC (medicinal)	T49.0X1	T49.0X2	T49.0X3	T49.0X4	T49.0X5	T49.0X6
nonmedicinal (vapor)	T53.6X1	T53.6X2	T53.6X3	T53.6X4	—	—
Bialamicol	T37.3X1	T37.3X2	T37.3X3	T37.3X4	T37.3X5	T37.3X6
Bibenzonium bromide	T48.3X1	T48.3X2	T48.3X3	T48.3X4	T48.3X5	T48.3X6
Bibrocathol	T49.5X1	T49.5X2	T49.5X3	T49.5X4	T49.5X5	T49.5X6
Bichloride of mercury — see Mercury, chloride						
Bichromates (calcium) (potassium)(sodium) (crystals)	T57.8X1	T57.8X2	T57.8X3	T57.8X4		
fumes	T56.2X1	T56.2X2	T56.2X3	T56.2X4	—	
Biclotymol	T49.6X1	T49.6X2	T49.6X3	T49.6X4	T49.6X5	T49.6X6
Bicucculine	T50.7X1	T50.7X2	T50.7X3	T50.7X4	T50.7X5	T50.7X6
Bifemelane	T43.291	T43.292	T43.293	T43.294	T43.295	T43.296
Biguanide derivatives, oral	T38.3X1	T38.3X2	T38.3X3	T38.3X4	T38.3X5	T38.3X6
Bile salts	T47.5X1	T47.5X2	T47.5X3	T47.5X4	T47.5X5	T47.5X6
Biligrafin	T50.8X1	T50.8X2	T50.8X3	T50.8X4	T50.8X5	T50.8X6
Bilopaque	T50.8X1	T50.8X2	T50.8X3	T50.8X4	T50.8X5	T50.8X6
Binifibrate	T46.6X1	T46.6X2	T46.6X3	T46.6X4	T46.6X5	T46.6X6
Binitrobenzol	T65.3X1	T65.3X2	T65.3X3	T65.3X4	—	—
Bioflavonoid(s)	T46.991	T46.992	T46.993	T46.994	T46.995	T46.996
Biological substance NEC	T50.901	T50.902	T50.903	T50.904	T50.905	T50.906
Biotin	T45.2X1	T45.2X2	T45.2X3	T45.2X4	T45.2X5	T45.2X6
Biperiden	T44.3X1	T44.3X2	T44.3X3	T44.3X4	T44.3X5	T44.3X6
Bisacodyl	T47.2X1	T47.2X2	T47.2X3	T47.2X4	T47.2X5	T47.2X6
Bisbentiamine	T45.2X1	T45.2X2	T45.2X3	T45.2X4	T45.2X5	T45.2X6
Bisbutiamine	T45.2X1	T45.2X2	T45.2X3	T45.2X4	T45.2X5	T45.2X6
Bisdequalinium (salts) (diacetate)	T49.6X1	T49.6X2	T49.6X3	T49.6X4	T49.6X5	T49.6X6
Bishydroxycoumarin	T45.511	T45.512	T45.513	T45.514	T45.515	T45.516
Bismarsen	T37.8X1	T37.8X2	T37.8X3	T37.8X4	T37.8X5	T37.8X6
Bismuth salts	T47.6X1	T47.6X2	T47.6X3	T47.6X4	T47.6X5	T47.6X6
aluminate	T47.1X1	T47.1X2	T47.1X3	T47.1X4	T47.1X5	T47.1X6
anti-infectives	T37.8X1	T37.8X2	T37.8X3	T37.8X4	T37.8X5	T37.8X6
formic iodide	T49.0X1	T49.0X2	T49.0X3	T49.0X4	T49.0X5	T49.0X6
glycolylarsenate	T49.0X1	T49.0X2	T49.0X3	T49.0X4	T49.0X5	T49.0X6
nonmedicinal (compounds) NEC	T65 91	T65.92	T65.93	T65.94	—	—
subcarbonate	T47.6X1	T47.6X2	T47.6X3	T47.6X4	T47.6X5	T47.6X6
subsalicylate	T37.8X1	T37.8X2	T37.8X3	T37.8X4	T37.8X5	T37.8X6
sulfarsphenamine	T37.8X1	T37.8X2	T37.8X3	T37.8X4	T37.8X5	T37.8X6
Bisoprolol	T44.7X1	T44.7X2	T44.7X3	T44.7X4	T44.7X5	T44.7X6
Bisoxatin	T47.2X1	T47.2X2	T47.2X3	T47.2X4	T47.2X5	T47.2X6
Bisulepin (hydrochloride)	T45.0X1	T45.0X2	T45.0X3	T45.0X4	T45.0X5	T45.0X6
Bithionol	T37.8X1	T37.8X2	T37.8X3	T37.8X4	T37.8X5	T37.8X6
anthelminthic	T37.4X1	T37.4X2	T37.4X3	T37.4X4	T37.4X5	T37.4X6
Bitolterol	T48.6X1	T48.6X2	T48.6X3	T48.6X4	T48.6X5	T48.6X6
Bitoscanate	T37.4X1	T37.4X2	T37.4X3	T37.4X4	T37.4X5	T37.4X6
Bitter almond oil	T62.8X1	T62.8X2	T62.8X3	T62.8X4	—	—
Bittersweet	T62.2X1	T62.2X2	T62.2X3	T62.2X4	—	—
Black						
flag	T60.91	T60.92	T60.93	T60.94	—	—
henbane	T62.2X1	T62.2X2	T62.2X3	T62.2X4	—	—
leaf (40)	T60.91	T60.92	T60.93	T60.94	—	—
widow spider (bite)	T63.311	T63.312	T63.313	T63.314	—	—
antivenin	T50.Z11	T50.Z12	T50.Z13	T50.Z14	T50.Z15	T50.Z16
Blast furnace gas (carbon monoxide from)	T58.8X1	T58.8X2	T58.8X3	T58.8X4	—	—
Bleach	T54.91	T54.92	T54.93	T54.94	—	—
Bleaching agent (medicinal)	T49.4X1	T49.4X2	T49.4X3	T49.4X4	T49.4X5	T49.4X6
Bleomycin	T45.1X1	T45.1X2	T45.1X3	T45.1X4	T45.1X5	T45.1X6
Blockain	T41.3X1	T41.3X2	T41.3X3	T41.3X4	T41.3X5	T41.3X6
infiltration (subcutaneous)	T41.3X1	T41.3X2	T41.3X3	T41.3X4	T41.3X5	T41.3X6
nerve block (peripheral) (plexus)	T41.3X1	T41.3X2	T41.3X3	T41.3X4	T41.3X5	T41.3X6
topical (surface)	T41.3X1	T41.3X2	T41.3X3	T41.3X4	T41.3X5	T41.3X6
Blockers, calcium channel	T46.1X1	T46.1X2	T46.1X3	T46.1X4	T46.1X5	T46.1X6
Blood (derivatives) (natural) (plasma) (whole)	T45.8X1	T45.8X2	T45.8X3	T45.8X4	T45.8X5	T45.8X6
dried	T45.8X1	T45.8X2	T45.8X3	T45.8X4	T45.8X5	T45.8X6
drug affecting NEC	T45.91	T45.92	T45.93	T45.94	T45.95	T45.96

Substance	Poisoning, Accidental (unintentional)	Poisoning, Intentional Self-harm	Poisoning, Assault	Poisoning, Undetermined	Adverse Effect	Under-dosing
Blood — continued						
expander NEC	T45.8X1	T45.8X2	T45.8X3	T45.8X4	T45.8X5	T45.8X6
fraction NEC	T45.8X1	T45.8X2	T45.8X3	T45.8X4	T45.8X5	T45.8X6
substitute (macromolecular)	T45.8X1	T45.8X2	T45.8X3	T45.8X4	T45.8X5	T45.8X6
Blue velvet	T40.2X1	T40.2X2	T40.2X3	T40.2X4	—	—
Bone meal	T62.8X1	T62.8X2	T62.8X3	T62.8X4	—	—
Bonine	T45.0X1	T45.0X2	T45.0X3	T45.0X4	T45.0X5	T45.0X6
Bopindolol	T44.7X1	T44.7X2	T44.7X3	T44.7X4	T44.7X5	T44.7X6
Boracic acid	T49.0X1	T49.0X2	T49.0X3	T49.0X4	T49.0X5	T49.0X6
ENT agent	T49.6X1	T49.6X2	T49.6X3	T49.6X4	T49.6X5	T49.6X6
ophthalmic preparation	T49.5X1	T49.5X2	T49.5X3	T49.5X4	T49.5X5	T49.5X6
Borane complex	T57.8X1	T57.8X2	T57.8X3	T57.8X4	—	—
Borate(s)	T57.8X1	T57.8X2	T57.8X3	T57.8X4	—	—
buffer	T50.991	T50.992	T50.993	T50.994	T50.995	T50.996
cleanser	T54.91	T54.92	T54.93	T54.94	—	—
sodium	T57.8X1	T57.8X2	T57.8X3	T57.8X4	—	—
Borax (cleanser)	T54.91	T54.92	T54.93	T54.94	—	—
Bordeaux mixture	T60.3X1	T60.3X2	T60.3X3	T60.3X4	—	—
Boric acid	T49.0X1	T49.0X2	T49.0X3	T49.0X4	T49.0X5	T49.0X6
ENT agent	T49.6X1	T49.6X2	T49.6X3	T49.6X4	T49.6X5	T49.6X6
ophthalmic preparation	T49.5X1	T49.5X2	T49.5X3	T49.5X4	T49.5X5	T49.5X6
Bornaprine	T44.3X1	T44.3X2	T44.3X3	T44.3X4	T44.3X5	T44.3X6
Boron	T57.8X1	T57.8X2	T57.8X3	T57.8X4	—	—
hydride NEC	T57.8X1	T57.8X2	T57.8X3	T57.8X4	—	—
fumes or gas	T57.8X1	T57.8X2	T57.8X3	T57.8X4	—	—
trifluoride	T59.891	T59.892	T59.893	T59.894	—	—
Botox	T48.291	T48.292	T48.293	T48.294	T48.295	T48.296
Botulinus anti-toxin (type A, B)	T50.Z11	T50.Z12	T50.Z13	T50.Z14	T50.Z15	T50.Z16
Brake fluid vapor	T59.891	T59.892	T59.893	T59.894	—	—
Brallobarbital	T42.3X1	T42.3X2	T42.3X3	T42.3X4	T42.3X5	T42.3X6
Bran (wheat)	T47.4X1	T47.4X2	T47.4X3	T47.4X4	T47.4X5	T47.4X6
Brass (fumes)	T56.891	T56.892	T56.893	T56.894	—	—
Brasso	T52.0X1	T52.0X2	T52.0X3	T52.0X4	—	—
Bretylium tosilate	T46.2X1	T46.2X2	T46.2X3	T46.2X4	T46.2X5	T46.2X6
Brevital (sodium)	T41.1X1	T41.1X2	T41.1X3	T41.1X4	T41.1X5	T41.1X6
Brinase	T45.3X1	T45.3X2	T45.3X3	T45.3X4	T45.3X5	T45.3X6
British antilewisite	T45.8X1	T45.8X2	T45.8X3	T45.8X4	T45.8X5	T45.8X6
Brodifacoum	T60.4X1	T60.4X2	T60.4X3	T60.4X4	—	—
Bromal (hydrate)	T42.6X1	T42.6X2	T42.6X3	T42.6X4	T42.6X5	T42.6X6
Bromazepam	T42.4X1	T42.4X2	T42.4X3	T42.4X4	T42.4X5	T42.4X6
Bromazine	T45.0X1	T45.0X2	T45.0X3	T45.0X4	T45.0X5	T45.0X6
Brombenzylcyanide	T59.3X1	T59.3X2	T59.3X3	T59.3X4	—	—
Bromelains	T45.3X1	T45.3X2	T45.3X3	T45.3X4	T45.3X5	T45.3X6
Bromethalin	T60.4X1	T60.4X2	T60.4X3	T60.4X4	—	—
Bromhexine	T48.4X1	T48.4X2	T48.4X3	T48.4X4	T48.4X5	T48.4X6
Bromide salts	T42.6X1	T42.6X2	T42.6X3	T42.6X4	T42.6X5	T42.6X6
Bromindione	T45.511	T45.512	T45.513	T45.514	T45.515	T45.516
Bromine						
compounds (medicinal)	T42.6X1	T42.6X2	T42.6X3	T42.6X4	T42.6X5	T42.6X6
sedative	T42.6X1	T42.6X2	T42.6X3	T42.6X4	T42.6X5	T42.6X6
vapor	T59.891	T59.892	T59.893	T59.894	—	—
Bromisoval	T42.6X1	T42.6X2	T42.6X3	T42.6X4	T42.6X5	T42.6X6
Bromisovalum	T42.6X1	T42.6X2	T42.6X3	T42.6X4	T42.6X5	T42.6X6
Bromobenzylcyanide	T59.3X1	T59.3X2	T59.3X3	T59.3X4	—	—
Bromochlorosalicylani-lide	T49.0X1	T49.0X2	T49.0X3	T49.0X4	T49.0X5	T49.0X6
Bromocriptine	T42.8X1	T42.8X2	T42.8X3	T42.8X4	T42.8X5	T42.8X6
Bromodiphenhydramine	T45.0X1	T45.0X2	T45.0X3	T45.0X4	T45.0X5	T45.0X6
Bromoform	T42.6X1	T42.6X2	T42.6X3	T42.6X4	T42.6X5	T42.6X6
Bromophenol blue reagent	T50.991	T50.992	T50.993	T50.994	T50.995	T50.996
Bromopride	T47.8X1	T47.8X2	T47.8X3	T47.8X4	T47.8X5	T47.8X6
Bromosalicylchloranitide	T49.0X1	T49.0X2	T49.0X3	T49.0X4	T49.0X5	T49.0X6
Bromosalicylhydroxamic acid	T37.1X1	T37.1X2	T37.1X3	T37.1X4	T37.1X5	T37.1X6
Bromo-seltzer	T39.1X1	T39.1X2	T39.1X3	T39.1X4	T39.1X5	T39.1X6
Bromoxynil	T60.3X1	T60.3X2	T60.3X3	T60.3X4	—	—
Bromperidol	T43.4X1	T43.4X2	T43.4X3	T43.4X4	T43.4X5	T43.4X6
Brompheniramine	T45.0X1	T45.0X2	T45.0X3	T45.0X4	T45.0X5	T45.0X6
Bromsulfophthalein	T50.8X1	T50.8X2	T50.8X3	T50.8X4	T50.8X5	T50.8X6
Bromural	T42.6X1	T42.6X2	T42.6X3	T42.6X4	T42.6X5	T42.6X6
Bromvaletone	T42.6X1	T42.6X2	T42.6X3	T42.6X4	T42.6X5	T42.6X6
Bronchodilator NEC	T48.6X1	T48.6X2	T48.6X3	T48.6X4	T48.6X5	T48.6X6
Brotizolam	T42.4X1	T42.4X2	T42.4X3	T42.4X4	T42.4X5	T42.4X6
Brovincamine	T46.7X1	T46.7X2	T46.7X3	T46.7X4	T46.7X5	T46.7X6
Brown recluse spider (bite) (venom)	T63.331	T63.332	T63.333	T63.334	—	—
Brown spider (bite) (venom)	T63.391	T63.392	T63.393	T63.394	—	—
Broxaterol	T48.6X1	T48.6X2	T48.6X3	T48.6X4	T48.6X5	T48.6X6
Broxuridine	T45.1X1	T45.1X2	T45.1X3	T45.1X4	T45.1X5	T45.1X6
Broxyquinoline	T37.8X1	T37.8X2	T37.8X3	T37.8X4	T37.8X5	T37.8X6
Bruceine	T48.291	T48.292	T48.293	T48.294	T48.295	T48.296
Brucia	T62.2X1	T62.2X2	T62.2X3	T62.2X4	—	—
Brucine	T65.1X1	T65.1X2	T65.1X3	T65.1X4	—	—
Brunswick green — see Copper						
Bruten — see Ibuprofen						
Bryonia	T47.2X1	T47.2X2	T47.2X3	T47.2X4	T47.2X5	T47.2X6
Buclizine	T45.0X1	T45.0X2	T45.0X3	T45.0X4	T45.0X5	T45.0X6
Buclosamide	T49.0X1	T49.0X2	T49.0X3	T49.0X4	T49.0X5	T49.0X6
Budesonide	T44.5X1	T44.5X2	T44.5X3	T44.5X4	T44.5X5	T44.5X6
Budralazine	T46.5X1	T46.5X2	T46.5X3	T46.5X4	T46.5X5	T46.5X6
Bufferin	T39.011	T39.012	T39.013	T39.014	T39.015	T39.016
Buflomedil	T46.7X1	T46.7X2	T46.7X3	T46.7X4	T46.7X5	T46.7X6
Buformin	T38.3X1	T38.3X2	T38.3X3	T38.3X4	T38.3X5	T38.3X6
Bufotenine	T40.991	T40.992	T40.993	T40.994	—	—
Bufrolin	T48.6X1	T48.6X2	T48.6X3	T48.6X4	T48.6X5	T48.6X6
Bufylline	T48.6X1	T48.6X2	T48.6X3	T48.6X4	T48.6X5	T48.6X6
Bulk filler	T50.5X1	T50.5X2	T50.5X3	T50.5X4	T50.5X5	T50.5X6
cathartic	T47.4X1	T47.4X2	T47.4X3	T47.4X4	T47.4X5	T47.4X6
Bumetanide	T50.1X1	T50.1X2	T50.1X3	T50.1X4	T50.1X5	T50.1X6
Bunaftine	T46.2X1	T46.2X2	T46.2X3	T46.2X4	T46.2X5	T46.2X6
Bunamiodyl	T50.8X1	T50.8X2	T50.8X3	T50.8X4	T50.8X5	T50.8X6
Bunazosin	T44.6X1	T44.6X2	T44.6X3	T44.6X4	T44.6X5	T44.6X6
Bunitrolol	T44.7X1	T44.7X2	T44.7X3	T44.7X4	T44.7X5	T44.7X6
Buphenine	T46.7X1	T46.7X2	T46.7X3	T46.7X4	T46.7X5	T46.7X6
Bupivacaine	T41.3X1	T41.3X2	T41.3X3	T41.3X4	T41.3X5	T41.3X6
infiltration (subcutaneous)	T41.3X1	T41.3X2	T41.3X3	T41.3X4	T41.3X5	T41.3X6
nerve block (peripheral) (plexus)	T41.3X1	T41.3X2	T41.3X3	T41.3X4	T41.3X5	T41.3X6
spinal	T41.3X1	T41.3X2	T41.3X3	T41.3X4	T41.3X5	T41.3X6
Bupranolol	T44.7X1	T44.7X2	T44.7X3	T44.7X4	T44.7X5	T44.7X6
Buprenorphine	T40.4X1	T40.4X2	T40.4X3	T40.4X4	T40.4X5	T40.4X6
Bupropion	T43.291	T43.292	T43.293	T43.294	T43.295	T43.296
Burimamide	T47.1X1	T47.1X2	T47.1X3	T47.1X4	T47.1X5	T47.1X6
Buserelin	T38.891	T38.892	T38.893	T38.894	T38.895	T38.896
Buspirone	T43.591	T43.592	T43.593	T43.594	T43.595	T43.596
Busulfan, busulphan	T45.1X1	T45.1X2	T45.1X3	T45.1X4	T45.1X5	T45.1X6
Butabarbital (sodium)	T42.3X1	T42.3X2	T42.3X3	T42.3X4	T42.3X5	T42.3X6
Butabarbitone	T42.3X1	T42.3X2	T42.3X3	T42.3X4	T42.3X5	T42.3X6
Butabarpal	T42.3X1	T42.3X2	T42.3X3	T42.3X4	T42.3X5	T42.3X6
Butacaine	T41.3X1	T41.3X2	T41.3X3	T41.3X4	T41.3X5	T41.3X6
Butalamine	T46.7X1	T46.7X2	T46.7X3	T46.7X4	T46.7X5	T46.7X6
Butalbital	T42.3X1	T42.3X2	T42.3X3	T42.3X4	T42.3X5	T42.3X6
Butallylonal	T42.3X1	T42.3X2	T42.3X3	T42.3X4	T42.3X5	T42.3X6
Butamben	T41.3X1	T41.3X2	T41.3X3	T41.3X4	T41.3X5	T41.3X6
Butamirate	T48.3X1	T48.3X2	T48.3X3	T48.3X4	T48.3X5	T48.3X6
Butane (distributed in mobile container)	T59.891	T59.892	T59.893	T59.894	—	—
distributed through pipes	T59.891	T59.892	T59.893	T59.894	—	—
incomplete combustion	T58.11	T58.12	T58.13	T58.14	—	—
Butanilicaine	T41.3X1	T41.3X2	T41.3X3	T41.3X4	T41.3X5	T41.3X6
Butanol	T51.3X1	T51.3X2	T51.3X3	T51.3X4	—	—
Butanone, 2-butanone	T52.4X1	T52.4X2	T52.4X3	T52.4X4	—	—
Butantrone	T49.4X1	T49.4X2	T49.4X3	T49.4X4	T49.4X5	T49.4X6
Butaperazine	T43.3X1	T43.3X2	T43.3X3	T43.3X4	T43.3X5	T43.3X6
Butazolidin	T39.2X1	T39.2X2	T39.2X3	T39.2X4	T39.2X5	T39.2X6
Butetamate	T48.6X1	T48.6X2	T48.6X3	T48.6X4	T48.6X5	T48.6X6
Butethal	T42.3X1	T42.3X2	T42.3X3	T42.3X4	T42.3X5	T42.3X6
Butethamate	T44.3X1	T44.3X2	T44.3X3	T44.3X4	T44.3X5	T44.3X6
Buthalitone (sodium)	T41.1X1	T41.1X2	T41.1X3	T41.1X4	T41.1X5	T41.1X6
Butisol (sodium)	T42.3X1	T42.3X2	T42.3X3	T42.3X4	T42.3X5	T42.3X6
Butizide	T50.2X1	T50.2X2	T50.2X3	T50.2X4	T50.2X5	T50.2X6
Butobarbital	T42.3X1	T42.3X2	T42.3X3	T42.3X4	T42.3X5	T42.3X6
sodium	T42.3X1	T42.3X2	T42.3X3	T42.3X4	T42.3X5	T42.3X6
Butobarbitone	T42.3X1	T42.3X2	T42.3X3	T42.3X4	T42.3X5	T42.3X6
Butoconazole (nitrate)	T49.0X1	T49.0X2	T49.0X3	T49.0X4	T49.0X5	T49.0X6
Butorphanol	T40.4X1	T40.4X2	T40.4X3	T40.4X4	T40.4X5	T40.4X6
Butriptyline	T43.011	T43.012	T43.013	T43.014	T43.015	T43.016
Butropium bromide	T44.3X1	T44.3X2	T44.3X3	T44.3X4	T44.3X5	T44.3X6
Buttercups	T62.2X1	T62.2X2	T62.2X3	T62.2X4	—	—
Butter of antimony — see Antimony						
Butyl						
acetate (secondary)	T52.8X1	T52.8X2	T52.8X3	T52.8X4	—	—
alcohol	T51.3X1	T51.3X2	T51.3X3	T51.3X4	—	—
aminobenzoate	T41.3X1	T41.3X2	T41.3X3	T41.3X4	T41.3X5	T41.3X6
butyrate	T52.8X1	T52.8X2	T52.8X3	T52.8X4	—	—
carbinol	T51.3X1	T51.3X2	T51.3X3	T51.3X4	—	—
carbitol	T52.3X1	T52.3X2	T52.3X3	T52.3X4	—	—
cellosolve	T52.3X1	T52.3X2	T52.3X3	T52.3X4	—	—
chloral (hydrate)	T42.6X1	T42.6X2	T42.6X3	T42.6X4	T42.6X5	T42.6X6
formate	T52.8X1	T52.8X2	T52.8X3	T52.8X4	—	—
lactate	T52.8X1	T52.8X2	T52.8X3	T52.8X4	—	—
propionate	T52.8X1	T52.8X2	T52.8X3	T52.8X4	—	—
scopolamine bromide	T44.3X1	T44.3X2	T44.3X3	T44.3X4	T44.3X5	T44.3X6
thiobarbital sodium	T41.1X1	T41.1X2	T41.1X3	T41.1X4	T41.1X5	T41.1X6

Additional Character May Be Required — Refer to the Tabular List for Character Selection   ▽ Subterms under main terms may continue to next column or page

Substance	Poisoning, Accidental (unintentional)	Poisoning, Intentional Self-harm	Poisoning, Assault	Poisoning, Undetermined	Adverse Effect	Under-dosing
Butylated hydroxyanisole	T50.991	T50.992	T50.993	T50.994	T50.995	T50.996
Butylchloral hydrate	T42.6X1	T42.6X2	T42.6X3	T42.6X4	T42.6X5	T42.6X6
Butyltoluene	T52.2X1	T52.2X2	T52.2X3	T52.2X4	—	—
Butyn	T41.3X1	T41.3X2	T41.3X3	T41.3X4	T41.3X5	T41.3X6
Butyrophenone (-based tranquilizers)	T43.4X1	T43.4X2	T43.4X3	T43.4X4	T43.4X5	T43.4X6
Cabergoline	T42.8X1	T42.8X2	T42.8X3	T42.8X4	T42.8X5	T42.8X6
Cacodyl, cacodylic acid	T57.0X1	T57.0X2	T57.0X3	T57.0X4	—	—
Cactinomycin	T45.1X1	T45.1X2	T45.1X3	T45.1X4	T45.1X5	T45.1X6
Cade oil	T49.4X1	T49.4X2	T49.4X3	T49.4X4	T49.4X5	T49.4X6
Cadexomer iodine	T49.0X1	T49.0X2	T49.0X3	T49.0X4	T49.0X5	T49.0X6
Cadmium (chloride) (fumes) (oxide)	T56.3X1	T56.3X2	T56.3X3	T56.3X4	—	—
sulfide (medicinal) NEC	T49.4X1	T49.4X2	T49.4X3	T49.4X4	T49.4X5	T49.4X6
Cadralazine	T46.5X1	T46.5X2	T46.5X3	T46.5X4	T46.5X5	T46.5X6
Caffeine	T43.611	T43.612	T43.613	T43.614	T43.615	T43.616
Calabar bean	T62.2X1	T62.2X2	T62.2X3	T62.2X4	—	—
Caladium seguinum	T62.2X1	T62.2X2	T62.2X3	T62.2X4	—	—
Calamine (lotion)	T49.3X1	T49.3X2	T49.3X3	T49.3X4	T49.3X5	T49.3X6
Calcifediol	T45.2X1	T45.2X2	T45.2X3	T45.2X4	T45.2X5	T45.2X6
Calciferol	T45.2X1	T45.2X2	T45.2X3	T45.2X4	T45.2X5	T45.2X6
Calcitonin	T50.991	T50.992	T50.993	T50.994	T50.995	T50.996
Calcitriol	T45.2X1	T45.2X2	T45.2X3	T45.2X4	T45.2X5	T45.2X6
Calcium	T50.3X1	T50.3X2	T50.3X3	T50.3X4	T50.3X5	T50.3X6
actylsalicylate	T39.011	T39.012	T39.013	T39.014	T39.015	T39.016
benzamidosalicylate	T37.1X1	T37.1X2	T37.1X3	T37.1X4	T37.1X5	T37.1X6
bromide	T42.6X1	T42.6X2	T42.6X3	T42.6X4	T42.6X5	T42.6X6
bromolactobionate	T42.6X1	T42.6X2	T42.6X3	T42.6X4	T42.6X5	T42.6X6
carbaspirin	T39.011	T39.012	T39.013	T39.014	T39.015	T39.016
carbimide	T50.6X1	T50.6X2	T50.6X3	T50.6X4	T50.6X5	T50.6X6
carbonate	T47.1X1	T47.1X2	T47.1X3	T47.1X4	T47.1X5	T47.1X6
chloride	T50.991	T50.992	T50.993	T50.994	T50.995	T50.996
anhydrous	T50.991	T50.992	T50.993	T50.994	T50.995	T50.996
cyanide	T57.8X1	T57.8X2	T57.8X3	T57.8X4	—	—
dioctyl sulfosuccinate	T47.4X1	T47.4X2	T47.4X3	T47.4X4	T47.4X5	T47.4X6
disodium edathamil	T45.8X1	T45.8X2	T45.8X3	T45.8X4	T45.8X5	T45.8X6
disodium edetate	T45.8X1	T45.8X2	T45.8X3	T45.8X4	T45.8X5	T45.8X6
dobesilate	T46.991	T46.992	T46.993	T46.994	T46.995	T46.996
EDTA	T45.8X1	T45.8X2	T45.8X3	T45.8X4	T45.8X5	T45.8X6
ferrous citrate	T45.4X1	T45.4X2	T45.4X3	T45.4X4	T45.4X5	T45.4X6
folinate	T45.8X1	T45.8X2	T45.8X3	T45.8X4	T45.8X5	T45.8X6
glubionate	T50.3X1	T50.3X2	T50.3X3	T50.3X4	T50.3X5	T50.3X6
gluconate	T50.3X1	T50.3X2	T50.3X3	T50.3X4	T50.3X5	T50.3X6
gluconogalactogluconate	T50.3X1	T50.3X2	T50.3X3	T50.3X4	T50.3X5	T50.3X6
hydrate, hydroxide	T54.3X1	T54.3X2	T54.3X3	T54.3X4	—	—
hypochlorite	T54.3X1	T54.3X2	T54.3X3	T54.3X4	—	—
iodide	T48.4X1	T48.4X2	T48.4X3	T48.4X4	T48.4X5	T48.4X6
ipodate	T50.8X1	T50.8X2	T50.8X3	T50.8X4	T50.8X5	T50.8X6
lactate	T50.3X1	T50.3X2	T50.3X3	T50.3X4	T50.3X5	T50.3X6
leucovorin	T45.8X1	T45.8X2	T45.8X3	T45.8X4	T45.8X5	T45.8X6
mandelate	T37.91	T37.92	T37.93	T37.94	T37.95	T37.96
oxide	T54.3X1	T54.3X2	T54.3X3	T54.3X4	—	—
pantothenate	T45.2X1	T45.2X2	T45.2X3	T45.2X4	T45.2X5	T45.2X6
phosphate	T50.3X1	T50.3X2	T50.3X3	T50.3X4	T50.3X5	T50.3X6
salicylate	T39.091	T39.092	T39.093	T39.094	T39.095	T39.096
salts	T50.3X1	T50.3X2	T50.3X3	T50.3X4	T50.3X5	T50.3X6
Calculus-dissolving drug	T50.991	T50.992	T50.993	T50.994	T50.995	T50.996
Calomel	T49.0X1	T49.0X2	T49.0X3	T49.0X4	T49.0X5	T49.0X6
Caloric agent	T50.3X1	T50.3X2	T50.3X3	T50.3X4	T50.3X5	T50.3X6
Calusterone	T38.7X1	T38.7X2	T38.7X3	T38.7X4	T38.7X5	T38.7X6
Camazepam	T42.4X1	T42.4X2	T42.4X3	T42.4X4	T42.4X5	T42.4X6
Camomile	T49.0X1	T49.0X2	T49.0X3	T49.0X4	T49.0X5	T49.0X6
Camoquin	T37.2X1	T37.2X2	T37.2X3	T37.2X4	T37.2X5	T37.2X6
Camphor						
insecticide	T60.2X1	T60.2X2	T60.2X3	T60.2X4	—	—
medicinal	T49.8X1	T49.8X2	T49.8X3	T49.8X4	T49.8X5	T49.8X6
Camylofin	T44.3X1	T44.3X2	T44.3X3	T44.3X4	T44.3X5	T44.3X6
Cancer chemotherapy drug regimen	T45.1X1	T45.1X2	T45.1X3	T45.1X4	T45.1X5	T45.1X6
Candeptin	T49.0X1	T49.0X2	T49.0X3	T49.0X4	T49.0X5	T49.0X6
Candicidin	T49.0X1	T49.0X2	T49.0X3	T49.0X4	T49.0X5	T49.0X6
Cannabinol	T40.7X1	T40.7X2	T40.7X3	T40.7X4	T40.7X5	T40.7X6
Cannabis (derivatives)	T40.7X1	T40.7X2	T40.7X3	T40.7X4	T40.7X5	T40.7X6
Canned heat	T51.1X1	T51.1X2	T51.1X3	T51.1X4	—	—
Canrenoic acid	T50.0X1	T50.0X2	T50.0X3	T50.0X4	T50.0X5	T50.0X6
Canrenone	T50.0X1	T50.0X2	T50.0X3	T50.0X4	T50.0X5	T50.0X6
Cantharides, cantharidin, cantharis	T49.8X1	T49.8X2	T49.8X3	T49.8X4	T49.8X5	T49.8X6
Canthaxanthin	T50.991	T50.992	T50.993	T50.994	T50.995	T50.996
Capillary-active drug NEC	T46.901	T46.902	T46.903	T46.904	T46.905	T46.906
Capreomycin	T36.8X1	T36.8X2	T36.8X3	T36.8X4	T36.8X5	T36.8X6
Capsicum	T49.4X1	T49.4X2	T49.4X3	T49.4X4	T49.4X5	T49.4X6
Captafol	T60.3X1	T60.3X2	T60.3X3	T60.3X4	—	—

Substance	Poisoning, Accidental (unintentional)	Poisoning, Intentional Self-harm	Poisoning, Assault	Poisoning, Undetermined	Adverse Effect	Under-dosing
Captan	T60.3X1	T60.3X2	T60.3X3	T60.3X4	—	—
Captodiame, captodiamine	T43.591	T43.592	T43.593	T43.594	T43.595	T43.596
Captopril	T46.4X1	T46.4X2	T46.4X3	T46.4X4	T46.4X5	T46.4X6
Caramiphen	T44.3X1	T44.3X2	T44.3X3	T44.3X4	T44.3X5	T44.3X6
Carazolol	T44.7X1	T44.7X2	T44.7X3	T44.7X4	T44.7X5	T44.7X6
Carbachol	T44.1X1	T44.1X2	T44.1X3	T44.1X4	T44.1X5	T44.1X6
Carbacrylamine (resin)	T50.3X1	T50.3X2	T50.3X3	T50.3X4	T50.3X5	T50.3X6
Carbamate (insecticide)	T60.0X1	T60.0X2	T60.0X3	T60.0X4	—	—
Carbamate (sedative)	T42.6X1	T42.6X2	T42.6X3	T42.6X4	T42.6X5	T42.6X6
herbicide	T60.0X1	T60.0X2	T60.0X3	T60.0X4	—	—
insecticide	T60.0X1	T60.0X2	T60.0X3	T60.0X4	—	—
Carbamazepine	T42.1X1	T42.1X2	T42.1X3	T42.1X4	T42.1X5	T42.1X6
Carbamide	T47.3X1	T47.3X2	T47.3X3	T47.3X4	T47.3X5	T47.3X6
peroxide	T49.0X1	T49.0X2	T49.0X3	T49.0X4	T49.0X5	T49.0X6
topical	T49.8X1	T49.8X2	T49.8X3	T49.8X4	T49.8X5	T49.8X6
Carbamylcholine chloride	T44.1X1	T44.1X2	T44.1X3	T44.1X4	T44.1X5	T44.1X6
Carbaril	T60.0X1	T60.0X2	T60.0X3	T60.0X4	—	—
Carbarsone	T37.3X1	T37.3X2	T37.3X3	T37.3X4	T37.3X5	T37.3X6
Carbaryl	T60.0X1	T60.0X2	T60.0X3	T60.0X4	—	—
Carbaspirin	T39.011	T39.012	T39.013	T39.014	T39.015	T39.016
Carbazochrome (salicylate) (sodium sulfonate)	T49.4X1	T49.4X2	T49.4X3	T49.4X4	T49.4X5	T49.4X6
Carbenicillin	T36.0X1	T36.0X2	T36.0X3	T36.0X4	T36.0X5	T36.0X6
Carbenoxolone	T47.1X1	T47.1X2	T47.1X3	T47.1X4	T47.1X5	T47.1X6
Carbetapentane	T48.3X1	T48.3X2	T48.3X3	T48.3X4	T48.3X5	T48.3X6
Carbethyl salicylate	T39.091	T39.092	T39.093	T39.094	T39.095	T39.096
Carbidopa (with levodopa)	T42.8X1	T42.8X2	T42.8X3	T42.8X4	T42.8X5	T42.8X6
Carbimazole	T38.2X1	T38.2X2	T38.2X3	T38.2X4	T38.2X5	T38.2X6
Carbinol	T51.1X1	T51.1X2	T51.1X3	T51.1X4	—	—
Carbinoxamine	T45.0X1	T45.0X2	T45.0X3	T45.0X4	T45.0X5	T45.0X6
Carbiphene	T39.8X1	T39.8X2	T39.8X3	T39.8X4	T39.8X5	T39.8X6
Carbitol	T52.3X1	T52.3X2	T52.3X3	T52.3X4	—	—
Carbocaine	T41.3X1	T41.3X2	T41.3X3	T41.3X4	T41.3X5	T41.3X6
infiltration (subcutaneous)	T41.3X1	T41.3X2	T41.3X3	T41.3X4	T41.3X5	T41.3X6
nerve block (peripheral) (plexus)	T41.3X1	T41.3X2	T41.3X3	T41.3X4	T41.3X5	T41.3X6
topical (surface)	T41.3X1	T41.3X2	T41.3X3	T41.3X4	T41.3X5	T41.3X6
Carbocisteine	T48.4X1	T48.4X2	T48.4X3	T48.4X4	T48.4X5	T48.4X6
Carbocromen	T46.3X1	T46.3X2	T46.3X3	T46.3X4	T46.3X5	T46.3X6
Carbol fuchsin	T49.0X1	T49.0X2	T49.0X3	T49.0X4	T49.0X5	T49.0X6
Carbolic acid — see also Phenol	T54.0X1	T54.0X2	T54.0X3	T54.0X4	—	—
Carbolonium (bromide)	T48.1X1	T48.1X2	T48.1X3	T48.1X4	T48.1X5	T48.1X6
Carbo medicinalis	T47.6X1	T47.6X2	T47.6X3	T47.6X4	T47.6X5	T47.6X6
Carbomycin	T36.8X1	T36.8X2	T36.8X3	T36.8X4	T36.8X5	T36.8X6
Carbon						
bisulfide (liquid)	T65.4X1	T65.4X2	T65.4X3	T65.4X4	—	—
vapor	T65.4X1	T65.4X2	T65.4X3	T65.4X4	—	—
dioxide (gas)	T59.7X1	T59.7X2	T59.7X3	T59.7X4	—	—
medicinal	T41.5X1	T41.5X2	T41.5X3	T41.5X4	T41.5X5	T41.5X6
nonmedicinal	T59.7X1	T59.7X2	T59.7X3	T59.7X4	—	—
snow	T49.4X1	T49.4X2	T49.4X3	T49.4X4	T49.4X5	T49.4X6
disulfide (liquid)	T65.4X1	T65.4X2	T65.4X3	T65.4X4	—	—
vapor	T65.4X1	T65.4X2	T65.4X3	T65.4X4	—	—
monoxide (from incomplete combustion)	T58.91	T58.92	T58.93	T58.94	—	—
blast furnace gas	T58.8X1	T58.8X2	T58.8X3	T58.8X4	—	—
butane (distributed in mobile container)	T58.11	T58.12	T58.13	T58.14	—	—
distributed through pipes	T58.11	T58.12	T58.13	T58.14	—	—
charcoal fumes	T58.2X1	T58.2X2	T58.2X3	T58.2X4	—	—
coal	T58.2X1	T58.2X2	T58.2X3	T58.2X4	—	—
coke (in domestic stoves, fireplaces)	T58.2X1	T58.2X2	T58.2X3	T58.2X4	—	—
exhaust gas (motor) not in transit	T58.01	T58.02	T58.03	T58.04	—	—
combustion engine, any not in watercraft	T58.01	T58.02	T58.03	T58.04	—	—
farm tractor, not in transit	T58.01	T58.02	T58.03	T58.04	—	—
gas engine	T58.01	T58.02	T58.03	T58.04	—	—
motor pump	T58.01	T58.02	T58.03	T58.04	—	—
motor vehicle, not in transit	T58.01	T58.02	T58.03	T58.04	—	—
fuel (in domestic use)	T58.2X1	T58.2X2	T58.2X3	T58.2X4	—	—
gas (piped)	T58.11	T58.12	T58.13	T58.14	—	—
in mobile container	T58.11	T58.12	T58.13	T58.14	—	—
piped (natural)	T58.11	T58.12	T58.13	T58.14	—	—
utility	T58.11	T58.12	T58.13	T58.14	—	—
in mobile container	T58.11	T58.12	T58.13	T58.14	—	—
gas (piped)	T58.11	T58.12	T58.13	T58.14	—	—
illuminating gas	T58.11	T58.12	T58.13	T58.14	—	—

Substance	Poisoning, Accidental (unintentional)	Poisoning, Intentional Self-harm	Poisoning, Assault	Poisoning, Undetermined	Adverse Effect	Under-dosing
Carbon — continued						
monoxide — continued						
industrial fuels or gases, any	T58.8X1	T58.8X2	T58.8X3	T58.8X4	—	—
kerosene (in domestic stoves, fireplaces)	T58.2X1	T58.2X2	T58.2X3	T58.2X4	—	—
kiln gas or vapor	T58.8X1	T58.8X2	T58.8X3	T58.8X4	—	—
motor exhaust gas, not in transit	T58.01	T58.02	T58.03	T58.04	—	—
piped gas (manufactured) (natural)	T58.11	T58.12	T58.13	T58.14	—	—
producer gas	T58.8X1	T58.8X2	T58.8X3	T58.8X4	—	—
propane (distributed in mobile container)	T58.11	T58.12	T58.13	T58.14	—	—
distributed through pipes	T58.11	T58.12	T58.13	T58.14	—	—
solid (in domestic stoves, fireplaces)	T58.2X1	T58.2X2	T58.2X3	T58.2X4	—	—
specified source NEC	T58.8X1	T58.8X2	T58.8X3	T58.8X4	—	—
stove gas	T58.11	T58.12	T58.13	T58.14	—	—
piped	T58.11	T58.12	T58.13	T58.14	—	—
utility gas	T58.11	T58.12	T58.13	T58.14	—	—
piped	T58.11	T58.12	T58.13	T58.14	—	—
water gas	T58.11	T58.12	T58.13	T58.14	—	—
wood (in domestic stoves, fireplaces)	T58.2X1	T58.2X2	T58.2X3	T58.2X4	—	—
tetrachloride (vapor) NEC	T53.0X1	T53.0X2	T53.0X3	T53.0X4	—	—
liquid (cleansing agent) NEC	T53.0X1	T53.0X2	T53.0X3	T53.0X4	—	—
solvent	T53.0X1	T53.0X2	T53.0X3	T53.0X4	—	—
Carbonic acid gas	T59.7X1	T59.7X2	T59.7X3	T59.7X4	—	—
anhydrase inhibitor NEC	T50.2X1	T50.2X2	T50.2X3	T50.2X4	T50.2X5	T50.2X6
Carbophenothion	T60.0X1	T60.0X2	T60.0X3	T60.0X4	—	—
Carboplatin	T45.1X1	T45.1X2	T45.1X3	T45.1X4	T45.1X5	T45.1X6
Carboprost	T48.0X1	T48.0X2	T48.0X3	T48.0X4	T48.0X5	T48.0X6
Carboquone	T45.1X1	T45.1X2	T45.1X3	T45.1X4	T45.1X5	T45.1X6
Carbowax	T49.3X1	T49.3X2	T49.3X3	T49.3X4	T49.3X5	T49.3X6
Carboxymethylcellulose	T47.4X1	T47.4X2	T47.4X3	T47.4X4	T47.4X5	T47.4X6
Carbrital	T42.3X1	T42.3X2	T42.3X3	T42.3X4	T42.3X5	T42.3X6
Carbromal	T42.6X1	T42.6X2	T42.6X3	T42.6X4	T42.6X5	T42.6X6
Carbutamide	T38.3X1	T38.3X2	T38.3X3	T38.3X4	T38.3X5	T38.3X6
Carbuterol	T48.6X1	T48.6X2	T48.6X3	T48.6X4	T48.6X5	T48.6X6
Cardiac						
depressants	T46.2X1	T46.2X2	T46.2X3	T46.2X4	T46.2X5	T46.2X6
rhythm regulator	T46.2X1	T46.2X2	T46.2X3	T46.2X4	T46.2X5	T46.2X6
specified NEC	T46.2X1	T46.2X2	T46.2X3	T46.2X4	T46.2X5	T46.2X6
Cardiografin	T50.8X1	T50.8X2	T50.8X3	T50.8X4	T50.8X5	T50.8X6
Cardiogreen	T50.8X1	T50.8X2	T50.8X3	T50.8X4	T50.8X5	T50.8X6
Cardiotonic (glycoside) **NEC**	T46.0X1	T46.0X2	T46.0X3	T46.0X4	T46.0X5	T46.0X6
Cardiovascular drug NEC	T46.901	T46.902	T46.903	T46.904	T46.905	T46.906
Cardrase	T50.2X1	T50.2X2	T50.2X3	T50.2X4	T50.2X5	T50.2X6
Carfecillin	T36.0X1	T36.0X2	T36.0X3	T36.0X4	T36.0X5	T36.0X6
Carfenazine	T43.3X1	T43.3X2	T43.3X3	T43.3X4	T43.3X5	T43.3X6
Carfusin	T49.0X1	T49.0X2	T49.0X3	T49.0X4	T49.0X5	T49.0X6
Carindacillin	T36.0X1	T36.0X2	T36.0X3	T36.0X4	T36.0X5	T36.0X6
Carisoprodol	T42.8X1	T42.8X2	T42.8X3	T42.8X4	T42.8X5	T42.8X6
Carmellose	T47.4X1	T47.4X2	T47.4X3	T47.4X4	T47.4X5	T47.4X6
Carminative	T47.5X1	T47.5X2	T47.5X3	T47.5X4	T47.5X5	T47.5X6
Carmofur	T45.1X1	T45.1X2	T45.1X3	T45.1X4	T45.1X5	T45.1X6
Carmustine	T45.1X1	T45.1X2	T45.1X3	T45.1X4	T45.1X5	T45.1X6
Carotene	T45.2X1	T45.2X2	T45.2X3	T45.2X4	T45.2X5	T45.2X6
Carphenazine	T43.3X1	T43.3X2	T43.3X3	T43.3X4	T43.3X5	T43.3X6
Carpipramine	T42.4X1	T42.4X2	T42.4X3	T42.4X4	T42.4X5	T42.4X6
Carprofen	T39.311	T39.312	T39.313	T39.314	T39.315	T39.316
Carpronium chloride	T44.3X1	T44.3X2	T44.3X3	T44.3X4	T44.3X5	T44.3X6
Carrageenan	T47.8X1	T47.8X2	T47.8X3	T47.8X4	T47.8X5	T47.8X6
Carteolol	T44.7X1	T44.7X2	T44.7X3	T44.7X4	T44.7X5	T44.7X6
Carter's Little Pills	T47.2X1	T47.2X2	T47.2X3	T47.2X4	T47.2X5	T47.2X6
Cascara (sagrada)	T47.2X1	T47.2X2	T47.2X3	T47.2X4	T47.2X5	T47.2X6
Cassava	T62.2X1	T62.2X2	T62.2X3	T62.2X4	—	—
Castellani's paint	T49.0X1	T49.0X2	T49.0X3	T49.0X4	T49.0X5	T49.0X6
Castor						
bean	T62.2X1	T62.2X2	T62.2X3	T62.2X4	—	—
oil	T47.2X1	T47.2X2	T47.2X3	T47.2X4	T47.2X5	T47.2X6
Catalase	T45.3X1	T45.3X2	T45.3X3	T45.3X4	T45.3X5	T45.3X6
Caterpillar (sting)	T63.431	T63.432	T63.433	T63.434	—	—
Catha (edulis) (tea)	T43.691	T43.692	T43.693	T43.694	—	—
Cathartic NEC	T47.4X1	T47.4X2	T47.4X3	T47.4X4	T47.4X5	T47.4X6
anthracene derivative	T47.2X1	T47.2X2	T47.2X3	T47.2X4	T47.2X5	T47.2X6
bulk	T47.4X1	T47.4X2	T47.4X3	T47.4X4	T47.4X5	T47.4X6
contact	T47.2X1	T47.2X2	T47.2X3	T47.2X4	T47.2X5	T47.2X6
emollient NEC	T47.4X1	T47.4X2	T47.4X3	T47.4X4	T47.4X5	T47.4X6
irritant NEC	T47.2X1	T47.2X2	T47.2X3	T47.2X4	T47.2X5	T47.2X6

Substance	Poisoning, Accidental (unintentional)	Poisoning, Intentional Self-harm	Poisoning, Assault	Poisoning, Undetermined	Adverse Effect	Under-dosing
Cathartic — continued						
mucilage	T47.4X1	T47.4X2	T47.4X3	T47.4X4	T47.4X5	T47.4X6
saline	T47.3X1	T47.3X2	T47.3X3	T47.3X4	T47.3X5	T47.3X6
vegetable	T47.2X1	T47.2X2	T47.2X3	T47.2X4	T47.2X5	T47.2X6
Cathine	T50.5X1	T50.5X2	T50.5X3	T50.5X4	T50.5X5	T50.5X6
Cathomycin	T36.8X1	T36.8X2	T36.8X3	T36.8X4	T36.8X5	T36.8X6
Cation exchange resin	T50.3X1	T50.3X2	T50.3X3	T50.3X4	T50.3X5	T50.3X6
Caustic(s) NEC	T54.91	T54.92	T54.93	T54.94	—	—
alkali	T54.3X1	T54.3X2	T54.3X3	T54.3X4	—	—
hydroxide	T54.3X1	T54.3X2	T54.3X3	T54.3X4	—	—
potash	T54.3X1	T54.3X2	T54.3X3	T54.3X4	—	—
soda	T54.3X1	T54.3X2	T54.3X3	T54.3X4	—	—
specified NEC	T54.91	T54.92	T54.93	T54.94	—	—
Ceepryn	T49.0X1	T49.0X2	T49.0X3	T49.0X4	T49.0X5	T49.0X6
ENT agent	T49.6X1	T49.6X2	T49.6X3	T49.6X4	T49.6X5	T49.6X6
lozenges	T49.6X1	T49.6X2	T49.6X3	T49.6X4	T49.6X5	T49.6X6
Cefacetrile	T36.1X1	T36.1X2	T36.1X3	T36.1X4	T36.1X5	T36.1X6
Cefaclor	T36.1X1	T36.1X2	T36.1X3	T36.1X4	T36.1X5	T36.1X6
Cefadroxil	T36.1X1	T36.1X2	T36.1X3	T36.1X4	T36.1X5	T36.1X6
Cefalexin	T36.1X1	T36.1X2	T36.1X3	T36.1X4	T36.1X5	T36.1X6
Cefaloglycin	T36.1X1	T36.1X2	T36.1X3	T36.1X4	T36.1X5	T36.1X6
Cefaloridine	T36.1X1	T36.1X2	T36.1X3	T36.1X4	T36.1X5	T36.1X6
Cefalosporins	T36.1X1	T36.1X2	T36.1X3	T36.1X4	T36.1X5	T36.1X6
Cefalotin	T36.1X1	T36.1X2	T36.1X3	T36.1X4	T36.1X5	T36.1X6
Cefamandole	T36.1X1	T36.1X2	T36.1X3	T36.1X4	T36.1X5	T36.1X6
Cefamycin antibiotic	T36.1X1	T36.1X2	T36.1X3	T36.1X4	T36.1X5	T36.1X6
Cefapirin	T36.1X1	T36.1X2	T36.1X3	T36.1X4	T36.1X5	T36.1X6
Cefatrizine	T36.1X1	T36.1X2	T36.1X3	T36.1X4	T36.1X5	T36.1X6
Cefazedone	T36.1X1	T36.1X2	T36.1X3	T36.1X4	T36.1X5	T36.1X6
Cefazolin	T36.1X1	T36.1X2	T36.1X3	T36.1X4	T36.1X5	T36.1X6
Cefbuperazone	T36.1X1	T36.1X2	T36.1X3	T36.1X4	T36.1X5	T36.1X6
Cefetamet	T36.1X1	T36.1X2	T36.1X3	T36.1X4	T36.1X5	T36.1X6
Cefixime	T36.1X1	T36.1X2	T36.1X3	T36.1X4	T36.1X5	T36.1X6
Cefmenoxime	T36.1X1	T36.1X2	T36.1X3	T36.1X4	T36.1X5	T36.1X6
Cefmetazole	T36.1X1	T36.1X2	T36.1X3	T36.1X4	T36.1X5	T36.1X6
Cefminox	T36.1X1	T36.1X2	T36.1X3	T36.1X4	T36.1X5	T36.1X6
Cefonicid	T36.1X1	T36.1X2	T36.1X3	T36.1X4	T36.1X5	T36.1X6
Cefoperazone	T36.1X1	T36.1X2	T36.1X3	T36.1X4	T36.1X5	T36.1X6
Ceforanide	T36.1X1	T36.1X2	T36.1X3	T36.1X4	T36.1X5	T36.1X6
Cefotaxime	T36.1X1	T36.1X2	T36.1X3	T36.1X4	T36.1X5	T36.1X6
Cefotetan	T36.1X1	T36.1X2	T36.1X3	T36.1X4	T36.1X5	T36.1X6
Cefotiam	T36.1X1	T36.1X2	T36.1X3	T36.1X4	T36.1X5	T36.1X6
Cefoxitin	T36.1X1	T36.1X2	T36.1X3	T36.1X4	T36.1X5	T36.1X6
Cefpimizole	T36.1X1	T36.1X2	T36.1X3	T36.1X4	T36.1X5	T36.1X6
Cefpiramide	T36.1X1	T36.1X2	T36.1X3	T36.1X4	T36.1X5	T36.1X6
Cefradine	T36.1X1	T36.1X2	T36.1X3	T36.1X4	T36.1X5	T36.1X6
Cefroxadine	T36.1X1	T36.1X2	T36.1X3	T36.1X4	T36.1X5	T36.1X6
Cefsulodin	T36.1X1	T36.1X2	T36.1X3	T36.1X4	T36.1X5	T36.1X6
Ceftazidime	T36.1X1	T36.1X2	T36.1X3	T36.1X4	T36.1X5	T36.1X6
Cefteram	T36.1X1	T36.1X2	T36.1X3	T36.1X4	T36.1X5	T36.1X6
Ceftezole	T36.1X1	T36.1X2	T36.1X3	T36.1X4	T36.1X5	T36.1X6
Ceftizoxime	T36.1X1	T36.1X2	T36.1X3	T36.1X4	T36.1X5	T36.1X6
Ceftriaxone	T36.1X1	T36.1X2	T36.1X3	T36.1X4	T36.1X5	T36.1X6
Cefuroxime	T36.1X1	T36.1X2	T36.1X3	T36.1X4	T36.1X5	T36.1X6
Cefuzonam	T38.0X1	T38.0X2	T38.0X3	T38.0X4	T38.0X5	T38.0X6
Celestone	T49.0X1	T49.0X2	T49.0X3	T49.0X4	T49.0X5	T49.0X6
topical	T49.0X1	T49.0X2	T49.0X3	T49.0X4	T49.0X5	T49.0X6
Celiprolol	T44.7X1	T44.7X2	T44.7X3	T44.7X4	T44.7X5	T44.7X6
Cell stimulants and proliferants	T49.8X1	T49.8X2	T49.8X3	T49.8X4	T49.8X5	T49.8X6
Cellosolve	T52.91	T52.92	T52.93	T52.94	—	—
Cellulose						
cathartic	T47.4X1	T47.4X2	T47.4X3	T47.4X4	T47.4X5	T47.4X6
hydroxyethyl	T47.4X1	T47.4X2	T47.4X3	T47.4X4	T47.4X5	T47.4X6
nitrates (topical)	T49.3X1	T49.3X2	T49.3X3	T49.3X4	T49.3X5	T49.3X6
oxidized	T49.4X1	T49.4X2	T49.4X3	T49.4X4	T49.4X5	T49.4X6
Centipede (bite)	T63.411	T63.412	T63.413	T63.414	—	—
Central nervous system						
depressants	T42.71	T42.72	T42.73	T42.74	T42.75	T42.76
anesthetic (general) NEC	T41.201	T41.202	T41.203	T41.204	T41.205	T41.206
gases NEC	T41.0X1	T41.0X2	T41.0X3	T41.0X4	T41.0X5	T41.0X6
intravenous	T41.1X1	T41.1X2	T41.1X3	T41.1X4	T41.1X5	T41.1X6
barbiturates	T42.3X1	T42.3X2	T42.3X3	T42.3X4	T42.3X5	T42.3X6
benzodiazepines	T42.4X1	T42.4X2	T42.4X3	T42.4X4	T42.4X5	T42.4X6
bromides	T42.6X1	T42.6X2	T42.6X3	T42.6X4	T42.6X5	T42.6X6
cannabis sativa	T40.7X1	T40.7X2	T40.7X3	T40.7X4	T40.7X5	T40.7X6
chloral hydrate	T42.6X1	T42.6X2	T42.6X3	T42.6X4	T42.6X5	T42.6X6
ethanol	T51.0X1	T51.0X2	T51.0X3	T51.0X4	—	—
hallucinogenics	T40.901	T40.902	T40.903	T40.904	T40.905	T40.906
hypnotics	T42.71	T42.72	T42.73	T42.74	T42.75	T42.76
specified NEC	T42.6X1	T42.6X2	T42.6X3	T42.6X4	T42.6X5	T42.6X6
muscle relaxants	T42.8X1	T42.8X2	T42.8X3	T42.8X4	T42.8X5	T42.8X6
paraldehyde	T42.6X1	T42.6X2	T42.6X3	T42.6X4	T42.6X5	T42.6X6

Additional Character May Be Required — Refer to the Tabular List for Character Selection ▽ Subterms under main terms may continue to next column or page

Substance	Poisoning, Accidental (unintentional)	Poisoning, Intentional Self-harm	Poisoning, Assault	Poisoning, Undetermined	Adverse Effect	Under-dosing
Central nervous system — *continued*						
depressants — *continued*						
sedatives;	T42.71	T42.72	T42.73	T42.74	T42.75	T42.76
sedative-hypnotics						
mixed NEC	T42.6X1	T42.6X2	T42.6X3	T42.6X4	T42.6X5	T42.6X6
specified NEC	T42.6X1	T42.6X2	T42.6X3	T42.6X4	T42.6X5	T42.6X6
muscle-tone depressants	T42.8X1	T42.8X2	T42.8X3	T42.8X4	T42.8X5	T42.8X6
stimulants	T43.601	T43.602	T43.603	T43.604	T43.605	T43.606
amphetamines	T43.621	T43.622	T43.623	T43.624	T43.625	T43.626
analeptics	T50.7X1	T50.7X2	T50.7X3	T50.7X4	T50.7X5	T50.7X6
antidepressants	T43.201	T43.202	T43.203	T43.204	T43.205	T43.206
opiate antagonists	T50.7X1	T50.7X2	T50.7X3	T50.7X4	T50.7X5	T50.7X6
specified NEC	T43.691	T43.692	T43.693	T43.694	T43.695	T43.696
Cephalexin	T36.1X1	T36.1X2	T36.1X3	T36.1X4	T36.1X5	T36.1X6
Cephaloglycin	T36.1X1	T36.1X2	T36.1X3	T36.1X4	T36.1X5	T36.1X6
Cephaloridine	T36.1X1	T36.1X2	T36.1X3	T36.1X4	T36.1X5	T36.1X6
Cephalosporins	T36.1X1	T36.1X2	T36.1X3	T36.1X4	T36.1X5	T36.1X6
N (adicillin)	T36.0X1	T36.0X2	T36.0X3	T36.0X4	T36.0X5	T36.0X6
Cephalothin	T36.1X1	T36.1X2	T36.1X3	T36.1X4	T36.1X5	T36.1X6
Cephalotin	T36.1X1	T36.1X2	T36.1X3	T36.1X4	T36.1X5	T36.1X6
Cephradine	T36.1X1	T36.1X2	T36.1X3	T36.1X4	T36.1X5	T36.1X6
Cerbera (odallam)	T62.2X1	T62.2X2	T62.2X3	T62.2X4	—	—
Cerberin	T46.0X1	T46.0X2	T46.0X3	T46.0X4	T46.0X5	T46.0X6
Cerebral stimulants	T43.601	T43.602	T43.603	T43.604	T43.605	T43.606
psychotherapeutic	T43.601	T43.602	T43.603	T43.604	T43.605	T43.606
specified NEC	T43.691	T43.692	T43.693	T43.694	T43.695	T43.696
Cerium oxalate	T45.0X1	T45.0X2	T45.0X3	T45.0X4	T45.0X5	T45.0X6
Cerous oxalate	T45.0X1	T45.0X2	T45.0X3	T45.0X4	T45.0X5	T45.0X6
Ceruletide	T50.8X1	T50.8X2	T50.8X3	T50.8X4	T50.8X5	T50.8X6
Cetalkonium (chloride)	T49.0X1	T49.0X2	T49.0X3	T49.0X4	T49.0X5	T49.0X6
Cethexonium chloride	T49.0X1	T49.0X2	T49.0X3	T49.0X4	T49.0X5	T49.0X6
Cetiedil	T46.7X1	T46.7X2	T46.7X3	T46.7X4	T46.7X5	T46.7X6
Cetirizine	T45.0X1	T45.0X2	T45.0X3	T45.0X4	T45.0X5	T45.0X6
Cetomacrogol	T50.991	T50.992	T50.993	T50.994	T50.995	T50.996
Cetotiamine	T45.2X1	T45.2X2	T45.2X3	T45.2X4	T45.2X5	T45.2X6
Cetoxime	T45.0X1	T45.0X2	T45.0X3	T45.0X4	T45.0X5	T45.0X6
Cetraxate	T47.1X1	T47.1X2	T47.1X3	T47.1X4	T47.1X5	T47.1X6
Cetrimide	T49.0X1	T49.0X2	T49.0X3	T49.0X4	T49.0X5	T49.0X6
Cetrimonium (bromide)	T49.0X1	T49.0X2	T49.0X3	T49.0X4	T49.0X5	T49.0X6
Cetylpyridinium chloride	T49.0X1	T49.0X2	T49.0X3	T49.0X4	T49.0X5	T49.0X6
ENT agent	T49.6X1	T49.6X2	T49.6X3	T49.6X4	T49.6X5	T49.6X6
lozenges	T49.6X1	T49.6X2	T49.6X3	T49.6X4	T49.6X5	T49.6X6
Cevadilla — *see* Sabadilla						
Cevitamic acid	T45.2X1	T45.2X2	T45.2X3	T45.2X4	T45.2X5	T45.2X6
Chalk, precipitated	T47.1X1	T47.1X2	T47.1X3	T47.1X4	T47.1X5	T47.1X6
Chamomile	T49.0X1	T49.0X2	T49.0X3	T49.0X4	T49.0X5	T49.0X6
Ch'an su	T46.0X1	T46.0X2	T46.0X3	T46.0X4	T46.0X5	T46.0X6
Charcoal	T47.6X1	T47.6X2	T47.6X3	T47.6X4	T47.6X5	T47.6X6
activated — *see also* Charcoal, medicinal	T47.6X1	T47.6X2	T47.6X3	T47.6X4	T47.6X5	T47.6X6
fumes (Carbon monoxide)	T58.2X1	T58.2X2	T58.2X3	T58.2X4	—	—
industrial	T58.8X1	T58.8X2	T58.8X3	T58.8X4	—	—
medicinal (activated)	T47.6X1	T47.6X2	T47.6X3	T47.6X4	T47.6X5	T47.6X6
antidiarrheal	T47.6X1	T47.6X2	T47.6X3	T47.6X4	T47.6X5	T47.6X6
poison control	T47.8X1	T47.8X2	T47.8X3	T47.8X4	T47.8X5	T47.8X6
specified use other than for diarrhea	T47.8X1	T47.8X2	T47.8X3	T47.8X4	T47.8X5	T47.8X6
topical	T49.8X1	T49.8X2	T49.8X3	T49.8X4	T49.8X5	T49.8X6
Chaulmosulfone	T37.1X1	T37.1X2	T37.1X3	T37.1X4	T37.1X5	T37.1X6
Chelating agent NEC	T50.6X1	T50.6X2	T50.6X3	T50.6X4	T50.6X5	T50.6X6
Chelidonium majus	T62.2X1	T62.2X2	T62.2X3	T62.2X4	—	—
Chemical substance NEC	T65.91	T65.92	T65.93	T65.94	—	—
Chenodeoxycholic acid	T47.5X1	T47.5X2	T47.5X3	T47.5X4	T47.5X5	T47.5X6
Chenodiol	T47.5X1	T47.5X2	T47.5X3	T47.5X4	T47.5X5	T47.5X6
Chenopodium	T37.4X1	T37.4X2	T37.4X3	T37.4X4	T37.4X5	T37.4X6
Cherry laurel	T62.2X1	T62.2X2	T62.2X3	T62.2X4	—	—
Chinidin (e)	T46.2X1	T46.2X2	T46.2X3	T46.2X4	T46.2X5	T46.2X6
Chiniofon	T37.8X1	T37.8X2	T37.8X3	T37.8X4	T37.8X5	T37.8X6
Chlophedianol	T48.3X1	T48.3X2	T48.3X3	T48.3X4	T48.3X5	T48.3X6
Chloral	T42.6X1	T42.6X2	T42.6X3	T42.6X4	T42.6X5	T42.6X6
derivative	T42.6X1	T42.6X2	T42.6X3	T42.6X4	T42.6X5	T42.6X6
hydrate	T42.6X1	T42.6X2	T42.6X3	T42.6X4	T42.6X5	T42.6X6
Chloralamide	T42.6X1	T42.6X2	T42.6X3	T42.6X4	T42.6X5	T42.6X6
Chloralodol	T42.6X1	T42.6X2	T42.6X3	T42.6X4	T42.6X5	T42.6X6
Chloralose	T60.4X1	T60.4X2	T60.4X3	T60.4X4	—	—
Chlorambucil	T45.1X1	T45.1X2	T45.1X3	T45.1X4	T45.1X5	T45.1X6
Chloramine	T57.8X1	T57.8X2	T57.8X3	T57.8X4	—	—
T	T49.0X1	T49.0X2	T49.0X3	T49.0X4	T49.0X5	T49.0X6
topical	T49.0X1	T49.0X2	T49.0X3	T49.0X4	T49.0X5	T49.0X6
Chloramphenicol	T36.2X1	T36.2X2	T36.2X3	T36.2X4	T36.2X5	T36.2X6
ENT agent	T49.6X1	T49.6X2	T49.6X3	T49.6X4	T49.6X5	T49.6X6
ophthalmic preparation	T49.5X1	T49.5X2	T49.5X3	T49.5X4	T49.5X5	T49.5X6
Chloramphenicol — *continued*						
topical NEC	T49.0X1	T49.0X2	T49.0X3	T49.0X4	T49.0X5	T49.0X6
Chlorate (potassium) (sodium)	T60.3X1	T60.3X2	T60.3X3	T60.3X4	—	—
NEC						
herbicide	T60.3X1	T60.3X2	T60.3X3	T60.3X4	—	—
Chlorazanil	T50.2X1	T50.2X2	T50.2X3	T50.2X4	T50.2X5	T50.2X6
Chlorbenzene, chlorbenzol	T53.7X1	T53.7X2	T53.7X3	T53.7X4	—	—
Chlorbenzoxamine	T44.3X1	T44.3X2	T44.3X3	T44.3X4	T44.3X5	T44.3X6
Chlorbutol	T42.6X1	T42.6X2	T42.6X3	T42.6X4	T42.6X5	T42.6X6
Chlorcyclizine	T45.0X1	T45.0X2	T45.0X3	T45.0X4	T45.0X5	T45.0X6
Chlordan (e) (dust)	T60.1X1	T60.1X2	T60.1X3	T60.1X4	—	—
Chlordantoin	T49.0X1	T49.0X2	T49.0X3	T49.0X4	T49.0X5	T49.0X6
Chlordiazepoxide	T42.4X1	T42.4X2	T42.4X3	T42.4X4	T42.4X5	T42.4X6
Chlordiethyl benzamide	T49.3X1	T49.3X2	T49.3X3	T49.3X4	T49.3X5	T49.3X6
Chloresium	T49.8X1	T49.8X2	T49.8X3	T49.8X4	T49.8X5	T49.8X6
Chlorethiazol	T42.6X1	T42.6X2	T42.6X3	T42.6X4	T42.6X5	T42.6X6
Chlorethyl — *see* Ethyl chloride						
Chloretone	T42.6X1	T42.6X2	T42.6X3	T42.6X4	T42.6X5	T42.6X6
Chlorex	T53.6X1	T53.6X2	T53.6X3	T53.6X4	—	—
insecticide	T60.1X1	T60.1X2	T60.1X3	T60.1X4	—	—
Chlorfenvinphos	T60.0X1	T60.0X2	T60.0X3	T60.0X4	—	—
Chlorhexadol	T42.6X1	T42.6X2	T42.6X3	T42.6X4	T42.6X5	T42.6X6
Chlorhexamide	T45.1X1	T45.1X2	T45.1X3	T45.1X4	T45.1X5	T45.1X6
Chlorhexidine	T49.0X1	T49.0X2	T49.0X3	T49.0X4	T49.0X5	T49.0X6
Chlorhydroxyquinolin	T49.0X1	T49.0X2	T49.0X3	T49.0X4	T49.0X5	T49.0X6
Chloride of lime (bleach)	T54.3X1	T54.3X2	T54.3X3	T54.3X4	—	—
Chlorimipramine	T43.011	T43.012	T43.013	T43.014	T43.015	T43.016
Chlorinated						
camphene	T53.6X1	T53.6X2	T53.6X3	T53.6X4	—	—
diphenyl	T53.7X1	T53.7X2	T53.7X3	T53.7X4	—	—
hydrocarbons NEC	T53.91	T53.92	T53.93	T53.94	—	—
solvents	T53.91	T53.92	T53.93	T53.94	—	—
lime (bleach)	T54.3X1	T54.3X2	T54.3X3	T54.3X4	—	—
and boric acid solution	T49.0X1	T49.0X2	T49.0X3	T49.0X4	T49.0X5	T49.0X6
naphthalene (insecticide)	T60.1X1	T60.1X2	T60.1X3	T60.1X4	—	—
industrial (non-pesticide)	T53.7X1	T53.7X2	T53.7X3	T53.7X4	—	—
pesticide NEC	T60.8X1	T60.8X2	T60.8X3	T60.8X4	—	—
soda — *see also* sodium hypochlorite						
solution	T49.0X1	T49.0X2	T49.0X3	T49.0X4	T49.0X5	T49.0X6
Chlorine (fumes) (gas)	T59.4X1	T59.4X2	T59.4X3	T59.4X4	—	—
bleach	T54.3X1	T54.3X2	T54.3X3	T54.3X4	—	—
compound gas NEC	T59.4X1	T59.4X2	T59.4X3	T59.4X4	—	—
disinfectant	T59.4X1	T59.4X2	T59.4X3	T59.4X4	—	—
releasing agents NEC	T59.4X1	T59.4X2	T59.4X3	T59.4X4	—	—
Chlorisondamine chloride	T46.991	T46.992	T46.993	T46.994	T46.995	T46.996
Chlormadinone	T38.5X1	T38.5X2	T38.5X3	T38.5X4	T38.5X5	T38.5X6
Chlormephos	T60.0X1	T60.0X2	T60.0X3	T60.0X4	—	—
Chlormerodrin	T50.2X1	T50.2X2	T50.2X3	T50.2X4	T50.2X5	T50.2X6
Chlormethiazole	T42.6X1	T42.6X2	T42.6X3	T42.6X4	T42.6X5	T42.6X6
Chlormethine	T45.1X1	T45.1X2	T45.1X3	T45.1X4	T45.1X5	T45.1X6
Chlormethylenecycline	T36.4X1	T36.4X2	T36.4X3	T36.4X4	T36.4X5	T36.4X6
Chlormezanone	T42.6X1	T42.6X2	T42.6X3	T42.6X4	T42.6X5	T42.6X6
Chloroacetic acid	T60.3X1	T60.3X2	T60.3X3	T60.3X4	—	—
Chloroacetone	T59.3X1	T59.3X2	T59.3X3	T59.3X4	—	—
Chloroacetophenone	T59.3X1	T59.3X2	T59.3X3	T59.3X4	—	—
Chloroaniline	T53.7X1	T53.7X2	T53.7X3	T53.7X4	—	—
Chlorobenzene, chlorobenzol	T53.7X1	T53.7X2	T53.7X3	T53.7X4	—	—
Chlorobromomethane (fire extinguisher)	T53.6X1	T53.6X2	T53.6X3	T53.6X4	—	—
Chlorobutanol	T49.0X1	T49.0X2	T49.0X3	T49.0X4	T49.0X5	T49.0X6
Chlorocresol	T49.0X1	T49.0X2	T49.0X3	T49.0X4	T49.0X5	T49.0X6
Chlorodehydromethyltestosterone	T38.7X1	T38.7X2	T38.7X3	T38.7X4	T38.7X5	T38.7X6
Chlorodinitrobenzene	T53.7X1	T53.7X2	T53.7X3	T53.7X4	—	—
dust or vapor	T53.7X1	T53.7X2	T53.7X3	T53.7X4	—	—
Chlorodiphenyl	T53.7X1	T53.7X2	T53.7X3	T53.7X4	—	—
Chloroethane — *see* Ethyl chloride						
Chloroethylene	T53.6X1	T53.6X2	T53.6X3	T53.6X4	—	—
Chlorofluorocarbons	T53.5X1	T53.5X2	T53.5X3	T53.5X4	—	—
Chloroform (fumes) (vapor)	T53.1X1	T53.1X2	T53.1X3	T53.1X4	—	—
anesthetic	T41.0X1	T41.0X2	T41.0X3	T41.0X4	T41.0X5	T41.0X6
solvent	T53.1X1	T53.1X2	T53.1X3	T53.1X4	—	—
water, concentrated	T41.0X1	T41.0X2	T41.0X3	T41.0X4	T41.0X5	T41.0X6
Chloroguanide	T37.2X1	T37.2X2	T37.2X3	T37.2X4	T37.2X5	T37.2X6
Chloromycetin	T36.2X1	T36.2X2	T36.2X3	T36.2X4	T36.2X5	T36.2X6
ENT agent	T49.6X1	T49.6X2	T49.6X3	T49.6X4	T49.6X5	T49.6X6
ophthalmic preparation	T49.5X1	T49.5X2	T49.5X3	T49.5X4	T49.5X5	T49.5X6
otic solution	T49.6X1	T49.6X2	T49.6X3	T49.6X4	T49.6X5	T49.6X6
topical NEC	T49.0X1	T49.0X2	T49.0X3	T49.0X4	T49.0X5	T49.0X6
Chloronitrobenzene	T53.7X1	T53.7X2	T53.7X3	T53.7X4	—	—
dust or vapor	T53.7X1	T53.7X2	T53.7X3	T53.7X4	—	—

Table of Drugs and Chemicals

Chlorophacinone — Clofibrate

Substance	Poisoning, Accidental (unintentional)	Poisoning, Intentional Self-harm	Poisoning, Assault	Poisoning, Undetermined	Adverse Effect	Under-dosing
Chlorophacinone	T60.4X1	T60.4X2	T60.4X3	T60.4X4	—	—
Chlorophenol	T53.7X1	T53.7X2	T53.7X3	T53.7X4	—	—
Chlorophenothane	T60.1X1	T60.1X2	T60.1X3	T60.1X4	—	—
Chlorophyll	T50.991	T50.992	T50.993	T50.994	T50.995	T50.996
Chloropicrin (fumes)	T53.6X1	T53.6X2	T53.6X3	T53.6X4	—	—
fumigant	T60.8X1	T60.8X2	T60.8X3	T60.8X4	—	—
fungicide	T60.3X1	T60.3X2	T60.3X3	T60.3X4	—	—
pesticide	T60.8X1	T60.8X2	T60.8X3	T60.8X4	—	—
Chloroprocaine	T41.3X1	T41.3X2	T41.3X3	T41.3X4	T41.3X5	T41.3X6
infiltration (subcutaneous)	T41.3X1	T41.3X2	T41.3X3	T41.3X4	T41.3X5	T41.3X6
nerve block (peripheral) (plexus)	T41.3X1	T41.3X2	T41.3X3	T41.3X4	T41.3X5	T41.3X6
spinal	T41.3X1	T41.3X2	T41.3X3	T41.3X4	T41.3X5	T41.3X6
Chloroptic	T49.5X1	T49.5X2	T49.5X3	T49.5X4	T49.5X5	T49.5X6
Chloropurine	T45.1X1	T45.1X2	T45.1X3	T45.1X4	T45.1X5	T45.1X6
Chloropyramine	T45.0X1	T45.0X2	T45.0X3	T45.0X4	T45.0X5	T45.0X6
Chloropyrifos	T60.0X1	T60.0X2	T60.0X3	T60.0X4	—	—
Chloropyrilene	T45.0X1	T45.0X2	T45.0X3	T45.0X4	T45.0X5	T45.0X6
Chloroquine	T37.2X1	T37.2X2	T37.2X3	T37.2X4	T37.2X5	T37.2X6
Chlorothalonil	T60.3X1	T60.3X2	T60.3X3	T60.3X4	—	—
Chlorothen	T45.0X1	T45.0X2	T45.0X3	T45.0X4	T45.0X5	T45.0X6
Chlorothiazide	T50.2X1	T50.2X2	T50.2X3	T50.2X4	T50.2X5	T50.2X6
Chlorothymol	T49.4X1	T49.4X2	T49.4X3	T49.4X4	T49.4X5	T49.4X6
Chlorotrianisene	T38.5X1	T38.5X2	T38.5X3	T38.5X4	T38.5X5	T38.5X6
Chlorovinyldichloroarsine, not in war	T57.0X1	T57.0X2	T57.0X3	T57.0X4	—	—
Chloroxine	T49.4X1	T49.4X2	T49.4X3	T49.4X4	T49.4X5	T49.4X6
Chloroxylenol	T49.0X1	T49.0X2	T49.0X3	T49.0X4	T49.0X5	T49.0X6
Chlorphenamine	T45.0X1	T45.0X2	T45.0X3	T45.0X4	T45.0X5	T45.0X6
Chlorphenesin	T42.8X1	T42.8X2	T42.8X3	T42.8X4	T42.8X5	T42.8X6
topical (antifungal)	T49.0X1	T49.0X2	T49.0X3	T49.0X4	T49.0X5	T49.0X6
Chlorpheniramine	T45.0X1	T45.0X2	T45.0X3	T45.0X4	T45.0X5	T45.0X6
Chlorphenoxamine	T45.0X1	T45.0X2	T45.0X3	T45.0X4	T45.0X5	T45.0X6
Chlorphentermine	T50.5X1	T50.5X2	T50.5X3	T50.5X4	T50.5X5	T50.5X6
Chlorprocaine — see Chloroprocaine						
Chlorproguanil	T37.2X1	T37.2X2	T37.2X3	T37.2X4	T37.2X5	T37.2X6
Chlorpromazine	T43.3X1	T43.3X2	T43.3X3	T43.3X4	T43.3X5	T43.3X6
Chlorpropamide	T38.3X1	T38.3X2	T38.3X3	T38.3X4	T38.3X5	T38.3X6
Chlorprothixene	T43.4X1	T43.4X2	T43.4X3	T43.4X4	T43.4X5	T43.4X6
Chlorquinaldol	T49.0X1	T49.0X2	T49.0X3	T49.0X4	T49.0X5	T49.0X6
Chlorquinol	T49.0X1	T49.0X2	T49.0X3	T49.0X4	T49.0X5	T49.0X6
Chlortalidone	T50.2X1	T50.2X2	T50.2X3	T50.2X4	T50.2X5	T50.2X6
Chlortetracycline	T36.4X1	T36.4X2	T36.4X3	T36.4X4	T36.4X5	T36.4X6
Chlorthalidone	T50.2X1	T50.2X2	T50.2X3	T50.2X4	T50.2X5	T50.2X6
Chlorthion	T60.0X1	T60.0X2	T60.0X3	T60.0X4	—	—
Chlorthiophos	T60.0X1	T60.0X2	T60.0X3	T60.0X4	—	—
Chlortrianisene	T38.5X1	T38.5X2	T38.5X3	T38.5X4	T38.5X5	T38.5X6
Chlor-Trimeton	T45.0X1	T45.0X2	T45.0X3	T45.0X4	T45.0X5	T45.0X6
Chlorzoxazone	T42.8X1	T42.8X2	T42.8X3	T42.8X4	T42.8X5	T42.8X6
Choke damp	T59.7X1	T59.7X2	T59.7X3	T59.7X4	—	—
Cholagogues	T47.5X1	T47.5X2	T47.5X3	T47.5X4	T47.5X5	T47.5X6
Cholebrine	T50.8X1	T50.8X2	T50.8X3	T50.8X4	T50.8X5	T50.8X6
Cholecalciferol	T45.2X1	T45.2X2	T45.2X3	T45.2X4	T45.2X5	T45.2X6
Cholecystokinin	T50.8X1	T50.8X2	T50.8X3	T50.8X4	T50.8X5	T50.8X6
Cholera vaccine	T50.A91	T50.A92	T50.A93	T50.A94	T50.A95	T50.A96
Choleretic	T47.5X1	T47.5X2	T47.5X3	T47.5X4	T47.5X5	T47.5X6
Cholesterol-lowering agents	T46.6X1	T46.6X2	T46.6X3	T46.6X4	T46.6X5	T46.6X6
Cholestyramine (resin)	T46.6X1	T46.6X2	T46.6X3	T46.6X4	T46.6X5	T46.6X6
Cholic acid	T47.5X1	T47.5X2	T47.5X3	T47.5X4	T47.5X5	T47.5X6
Choline	T48.6X1	T48.6X2	T48.6X3	T48.6X4	T48.6X5	T48.6X6
chloride	T50.991	T50.992	T50.993	T50.994	T50.995	T50.996
dihydrogen citrate	T50.991	T50.992	T50.993	T50.994	T50.995	T50.996
salicylate	T39.091	T39.092	T39.093	T39.094	T39.095	T39.096
theophyllinate	T48.6X1	T48.6X2	T48.6X3	T48.6X4	T48.6X5	T48.6X6
Cholinergic (drug) NEC	T44.1X1	T44.1X2	T44.1X3	T44.1X4	T44.1X5	T44.1X6
muscle tone enhancer	T44.1X1	T44.1X2	T44.1X3	T44.1X4	T44.1X5	T44.1X6
organophosphorus	T44.0X1	T44.0X2	T44.0X3	T44.0X4	T44.0X5	T44.0X6
insecticide	T60.0X1	T60.0X2	T60.0X3	T60.0X4	—	—
nerve gas	T59.891	T59.892	T59.893	T59.894	—	—
trimethyl ammonium propanediol	T44.1X1	T44.1X2	T44.1X3	T44.1X4	T44.1X5	T44.1X6
Cholinesterase reactivator	T50.6X1	T50.6X2	T50.6X3	T50.6X4	T50.6X5	T50.6X6
Cholografin	T50.8X1	T50.8X2	T50.8X3	T50.8X4	T50.8X5	T50.8X6
Chorionic gonadotropin	T38.891	T38.892	T38.893	T38.894	T38.895	T38.896
Chromate	T56.2X1	T56.2X2	T56.2X3	T56.2X4	—	—
dust or mist	T56.2X1	T56.2X2	T56.2X3	T56.2X4	—	—
lead — see also lead	T56.0X1	T56.0X2	T56.0X3	T56.0X4	—	—
paint	T56.0X1	T56.0X2	T56.0X3	T56.0X4	—	—
Chromic						
acid	T56.2X1	T56.2X2	T56.2X3	T56.2X4	—	—
dust or mist	T56.2X1	T56.2X2	T56.2X3	T56.2X4	—	—
Chromic — continued						
phosphate 32P	T45.1X1	T45.1X2	T45.1X3	T45.1X4	T45.1X5	T45.1X6
Chromium	T56.2X1	T56.2X2	T56.2X3	T56.2X4	—	—
compounds — see Chromate						
sesquioxide	T50.8X1	T50.8X2	T50.8X3	T50.8X4	T50.8X5	T50.8X6
Chromomycin A3	T45.1X1	T45.1X2	T45.1X3	T45.1X4	T45.1X5	T45.1X6
Chromonar	T46.3X1	T46.3X2	T46.3X3	T46.3X4	T46.3X5	T46.3X6
Chromyl chloride	T56.2X1	T56.2X2	T56.2X3	T56.2X4	—	—
Chrysarobin	T49.4X1	T49.4X2	T49.4X3	T49.4X4	T49.4X5	T49.4X6
Chrysazin	T47.2X1	T47.2X2	T47.2X3	T47.2X4	T47.2X5	T47.2X6
Chymar	T45.3X1	T45.3X2	T45.3X3	T45.3X4	T45.3X5	T45.3X6
ophthalmic preparation	T49.5X1	T49.5X2	T49.5X3	T49.5X4	T49.5X5	T49.5X6
Chymopapain	T45.3X1	T45.3X2	T45.3X3	T45.3X4	T45.3X5	T45.3X6
Chymotrypsin	T45.3X1	T45.3X2	T45.3X3	T45.3X4	T45.3X5	T45.3X6
ophthalmic preparation	T49.5X1	T49.5X2	T49.5X3	T49.5X4	T49.5X5	T49.5X6
Cianidanol	T50.991	T50.992	T50.993	T50.994	T50.995	T50.996
Cianopramine	T43.011	T43.012	T43.013	T43.014	T43.015	T43.016
Cibenzoline	T46.2X1	T46.2X2	T46.2X3	T46.2X4	T46.2X5	T46.2X6
Ciclacillin	T36.0X1	T36.0X2	T36.0X3	T36.0X4	T36.0X5	T36.0X6
Ciclobarbital — see Hexobarbital						
Ciclonicate	T46.7X1	T46.7X2	T46.7X3	T46.7X4	T46.7X5	T46.7X6
Ciclopirox (olamine)	T49.0X1	T49.0X2	T49.0X3	T49.0X4	T49.0X5	T49.0X6
Ciclosporin	T45.1X1	T45.1X2	T45.1X3	T45.1X4	T45.1X5	T45.1X6
Cicuta maculata or virosa	T62.2X1	T62.2X2	T62.2X3	T62.2X4	—	—
Cicutoxin	T62.2X1	T62.2X2	T62.2X3	T62.2X4	—	—
Cigarette lighter fluid	T52.0X1	T52.0X2	T52.0X3	T52.0X4	—	—
Cigarettes (tobacco)	T65.221	T65.222	T65.223	T65.224	—	—
Ciguatoxin	T61.01	T61.02	T61.03	T61.04	—	—
Cilazapril	T46.4X1	T46.4X2	T46.4X3	T46.4X4	T46.4X5	T46.4X6
Cimetidine	T47.0X1	T47.0X2	T47.0X3	T47.0X4	T47.0X5	T47.0X6
Cimetropium bromide	T44.3X1	T44.3X2	T44.3X3	T44.3X4	T44.3X5	T44.3X6
Cinchocaine	T41.3X1	T41.3X2	T41.3X3	T41.3X4	T41.3X5	T41.3X6
topical (surface)	T41.3X1	T41.3X2	T41.3X3	T41.3X4	T41.3X5	T41.3X6
Cinchona	T37.2X1	T37.2X2	T37.2X3	T37.2X4	T37.2X5	T37.2X6
Cinchonine alkaloids	T37.2X1	T37.2X2	T37.2X3	T37.2X4	T37.2X5	T37.2X6
Cinchophen	T50.4X1	T50.4X2	T50.4X3	T50.4X4	T50.4X5	T50.4X6
Cinepazide	T46.7X1	T46.7X2	T46.7X3	T46.7X4	T46.7X5	T46.7X6
Cinnamedrine	T48.5X1	T48.5X2	T48.5X3	T48.5X4	T48.5X5	T48.5X6
Cinnarizine	T45.0X1	T45.0X2	T45.0X3	T45.0X4	T45.0X5	T45.0X6
Cinoxacin	T37.8X1	T37.8X2	T37.8X3	T37.8X4	T37.8X5	T37.8X6
Ciprofibrate	T46.6X1	T46.6X2	T46.6X3	T46.6X4	T46.6X5	T46.6X6
Ciprofloxacin	T36.8X1	T36.8X2	T36.8X3	T36.8X4	T36.8X5	T36.8X6
Cisapride	T47.8X1	T47.8X2	T47.8X3	T47.8X4	T47.8X5	T47.8X6
Cisplatin	T45.1X1	T45.1X2	T45.1X3	T45.1X4	T45.1X5	T45.1X6
Citalopram	T43.221	T43.222	T43.223	T43.224	T43.225	T43.226
Citanest	T41.3X1	T41.3X2	T41.3X3	T41.3X4	T41.3X5	T41.3X6
infiltration (subcutaneous)	T41.3X1	T41.3X2	T41.3X3	T41.3X4	T41.3X5	T41.3X6
nerve block (peripheral) (plexus)	T41.3X1	T41.3X2	T41.3X3	T41.3X4	T41.3X5	T41.3X6
Citric acid	T47.5X1	T47.5X2	T47.5X3	T47.5X4	T47.5X5	T47.5X6
Citrovorum (factor)	T45.8X1	T45.8X2	T45.8X3	T45.8X4	T45.8X5	T45.8X6
Claviceps purpurea	T62.2X1	T62.2X2	T62.2X3	T62.2X4	—	—
Clavulanic acid	T36.1X1	T36.1X2	T36.1X3	T36.1X4	T36.1X5	T36.1X6
Cleaner, cleansing agent, type not specified	T65.891	T65.892	T65.893	T65.894	—	—
of paint or varnish	T52.91	T52.92	T52.93	T52.94	—	—
specified type NEC	T65.891	T65.892	T65.893	T65.894	—	—
Clebopride	T47.8X1	T47.8X2	T47.8X3	T47.8X4	T47.8X5	T47.8X6
Clefamide	T37.3X1	T37.3X2	T37.3X3	T37.3X4	T37.3X5	T37.3X6
Clemastine	T45.0X1	T45.0X2	T45.0X3	T45.0X4	T45.0X5	T45.0X6
Clematis vitalba	T62.2X1	T62.2X2	T62.2X3	T62.2X4	—	—
Clemizole	T45.0X1	T45.0X2	T45.0X3	T45.0X4	T45.0X5	T45.0X6
penicillin	T36.0X1	T36.0X2	T36.0X3	T36.0X4	T36.0X5	T36.0X6
Clenbuterol	T48.6X1	T48.6X2	T48.6X3	T48.6X4	T48.6X5	T48.6X6
Clidinium bromide	T44.3X1	T44.3X2	T44.3X3	T44.3X4	T44.3X5	T44.3X6
Clindamycin	T36.8X1	T36.8X2	T36.8X3	T36.8X4	T36.8X5	T36.8X6
Clinofibrate	T46.6X1	T46.6X2	T46.6X3	T46.6X4	T46.6X5	T46.6X6
Clioquinol	T37.8X1	T37.8X2	T37.8X3	T37.8X4	T37.8X5	T37.8X6
Cliradon	T40.2X1	T40.2X2	T40.2X3	T40.2X4	—	—
Clobazam	T42.4X1	T42.4X2	T42.4X3	T42.4X4	T42.4X5	T42.4X6
Clobenzorex	T50.5X1	T50.5X2	T50.5X3	T50.5X4	T50.5X5	T50.5X6
Clobetasol	T49.0X1	T49.0X2	T49.0X3	T49.0X4	T49.0X5	T49.0X6
Clobetasone	T49.0X1	T49.0X2	T49.0X3	T49.0X4	T49.0X5	T49.0X6
Clobutinol	T48.3X1	T48.3X2	T48.3X3	T48.3X4	T48.3X5	T48.3X6
Clocortolone	T38.0X1	T38.0X2	T38.0X3	T38.0X4	T38.0X5	T38.0X6
Clodantoin	T49.0X1	T49.0X2	T49.0X3	T49.0X4	T49.0X5	T49.0X6
Clodronic acid	T50.991	T50.992	T50.993	T50.994	T50.995	T50.996
Clofazimine	T37.1X1	T37.1X2	T37.1X3	T37.1X4	T37.1X5	T37.1X6
Clofedanol	T48.3X1	T48.3X2	T48.3X3	T48.3X4	T48.3X5	T48.3X6
Clofenamide	T50.2X1	T50.2X2	T50.2X3	T50.2X4	T50.2X5	T50.2X6
Clofenotane	T49.0X1	T49.0X2	T49.0X3	T49.0X4	T49.0X5	T49.0X6
Clofezone	T39.2X1	T39.2X2	T39.2X3	T39.2X4	T39.2X5	T39.2X6
Clofibrate	T46.6X1	T46.6X2	T46.6X3	T46.6X4	T46.6X5	T46.6X6

Substance	Poisoning, Accidental (unintentional)	Poisoning, Intentional Self-harm	Poisoning, Assault	Poisoning, Undetermined	Adverse Effect	Under-dosing
Clofibride	T46.6X1	T46.6X2	T46.6X3	T46.6X4	T46.6X5	T46.6X6
Cloforex	T50.5X1	T50.5X2	T50.5X3	T50.5X4	T50.5X5	T50.5X6
Clomethiazole	T42.6X1	T42.6X2	T42.6X3	T42.6X4	T42.6X5	T42.6X6
Clometocillin	T36.0X1	T36.0X2	T36.0X3	T36.0X4	T36.0X5	T36.0X6
Clomifene	T38.5X1	T38.5X2	T38.5X3	T38.5X4	T38.5X5	T38.5X6
Clomiphene	T38.5X1	T38.5X2	T38.5X3	T38.5X4	T38.5X5	T38.5X6
Clomipramine	T43.011	T43.012	T43.013	T43.014	T43.015	T43.016
Clomocycline	T36.4X1	T36.4X2	T36.4X3	T36.4X4	T36.4X5	T36.4X6
Clonazepam	T42.4X1	T42.4X2	T42.4X3	T42.4X4	T42.4X5	T42.4X6
Clonidine	T46.5X1	T46.5X2	T46.5X3	T46.5X4	T46.5X5	T46.5X6
Clonixin	T39.8X1	T39.8X2	T39.8X3	T39.8X4	T39.8X5	T39.8X6
Clopamide	T50.2X1	T50.2X2	T50.2X3	T50.2X4	T50.2X5	T50.2X6
Clopenthixol	T43.4X1	T43.4X2	T43.4X3	T43.4X4	T43.4X5	T43.4X6
Cloperastine	T48.3X1	T48.3X2	T48.3X3	T48.3X4	T48.3X5	T48.3X6
Clophedianol	T48.3X1	T48.3X2	T48.3X3	T48.3X4	T48.3X5	T48.3X6
Cloponone	T36.2X1	T36.2X2	T36.2X3	T36.2X4	T36.2X5	T36.2X6
Cloprednol	T38.0X1	T38.0X2	T38.0X3	T38.0X4	T38.0X5	T38.0X6
Cloral betaine	T42.6X1	T42.6X2	T42.6X3	T42.6X4	T42.6X5	T42.6X6
Cloramfenicol	T36.2X1	T36.2X2	T36.2X3	T36.2X4	T36.2X5	T36.2X6
Clorazepate (dipotassium)	T42.4X1	T42.4X2	T42.4X3	T42.4X4	T42.4X5	T42.4X6
Clorexolone	T50.2X1	T50.2X2	T50.2X3	T50.2X4	T50.2X5	T50.2X6
Clorfenamine	T45.0X1	T45.0X2	T45.0X3	T45.0X4	T45.0X5	T45.0X6
Clorgiline	T43.1X1	T43.1X2	T43.1X3	T43.1X4	T43.1X5	T43.1X6
Clorotepine	T44.3X1	T44.3X2	T44.3X3	T44.3X4	T44.3X5	T44.3X6
Clorox (bleach)	T54.91	T54.92	T54.93	T54.94	—	—
Clorprenaline	T48.6X1	T48.6X2	T48.6X3	T48.6X4	T48.6X5	T48.6X6
Clortermine	T50.5X1	T50.5X2	T50.5X3	T50.5X4	T50.5X5	T50.5X6
Clotiapine	T43.591	T43.592	T43.593	T43.594	T43.595	T43.596
Clotiazepam	T42.4X1	T42.4X2	T42.4X3	T42.4X4	T42.4X5	T42.4X6
Clotibric acid	T46.6X1	T46.6X2	T46.6X3	T46.6X4	T46.6X5	T46.6X6
Clotrimazole	T49.0X1	T49.0X2	T49.0X3	T49.0X4	T49.0X5	T49.0X6
Cloxacillin	T36.0X1	T36.0X2	T36.0X3	T36.0X4	T36.0X5	T36.0X6
Cloxazolam	T42.4X1	T42.4X2	T42.4X3	T42.4X4	T42.4X5	T42.4X6
Cloxiquine	T49.0X1	T49.0X2	T49.0X3	T49.0X4	T49.0X5	T49.0X6
Clozapine	T42.4X1	T42.4X2	T42.4X3	T42.4X4	T42.4X5	T42.4X6
Coagulant NEC	T45.7X1	T45.7X2	T45.7X3	T45.7X4	T45.7X5	T45.7X6
Coal (carbon monoxide from) — see also Carbon, monoxide, coal	T58.2X1	T58.2X2	T58.2X3	T58.2X4	—	—
oil — see Kerosene						
tar	T49.1X1	T49.1X2	T49.1X3	T49.1X4	T49.1X5	T49.1X6
fumes	T59.891	T59.892	T59.893	T59.894	—	—
medicinal (ointment)	T49.4X1	T49.4X2	T49.4X3	T49.4X4	T49.4X5	T49.4X6
analgesics NEC	T39.2X1	T39.2X2	T39.2X3	T39.2X4	T39.2X5	T39.2X6
naphtha (solvent)	T52.0X1	T52.0X2	T52.0X3	T52.0X4	—	—
Cobalamine	T45.2X1	T45.2X2	T45.2X3	T45.2X4	T45.2X5	T45.2X6
Cobalt (nonmedicinal) (fumes) (industrial)	T56.891	T56.892	T56.893	T56.894	—	—
medicinal (trace) (chloride)	T45.8X1	T45.8X2	T45.8X3	T45.8X4	T45.8X5	T45.8X6
Cobra (venom)	T63.041	T63.042	T63.043	T63.044	—	—
Coca (leaf)	T40.5X1	T40.5X2	T40.5X3	T40.5X4	T40.5X5	T40.5X6
Cocaine	T40.5X1	T40.5X2	T40.5X3	T40.5X4	T40.5X5	T40.5X6
topical anesthetic	T41.3X1	T41.3X2	T41.3X3	T41.3X4	T41.3X5	T41.3X6
Cocarboxylase	T45.3X1	T45.3X2	T45.3X3	T45.3X4	T45.3X5	T45.3X6
Coccidioidin	T50.8X1	T50.8X2	T50.8X3	T50.8X4	T50.8X5	T50.8X6
Cocculus indicus	T62.1X1	T62.1X2	T62.1X3	T62.1X4	—	—
Cochineal	T65.6X1	T65.6X2	T65.6X3	T65.6X4	—	—
medicinal products	T50.991	T50.992	T50.993	T50.994	T50.995	T50.996
Codeine	T40.2X1	T40.2X2	T40.2X3	T40.2X4	T40.2X5	T40.2X6
Cod-liver oil	T45.2X1	T45.2X2	T45.2X3	T45.2X4	T45.2X5	T45.2X6
Coenzyme A	T50.991	T50.992	T50.993	T50.994	T50.995	T50.996
Coffee	T62.8X1	T62.8X2	T62.8X3	T62.8X4	—	—
Cogalactoisomerase	T50.991	T50.992	T50.993	T50.994	T50.995	T50.996
Cogentin	T44.3X1	T44.3X2	T44.3X3	T44.3X4	T44.3X5	T44.3X6
Coke fumes or gas (carbon monoxide)	T58.2X1	T58.2X2	T58.2X3	T58.2X4	—	—
industrial use	T58.8X1	T58.8X2	T58.8X3	T58.8X4	—	—
Colace	T47.4X1	T47.4X2	T47.4X3	T47.4X4	T47.4X5	T47.4X6
Colaspase	T45.1X1	T45.1X2	T45.1X3	T45.1X4	T45.1X5	T45.1X6
Colchicine	T50.4X1	T50.4X2	T50.4X3	T50.4X4	T50.4X5	T50.4X6
Colchicum	T62.2X1	T62.2X2	T62.2X3	T62.2X4	—	—
Cold cream	T49.3X1	T49.3X2	T49.3X3	T49.3X4	T49.3X5	T49.3X6
Colecalciferol	T45.2X1	T45.2X2	T45.2X3	T45.2X4	T45.2X5	T45.2X6
Colestipol	T46.6X1	T46.6X2	T46.6X3	T46.6X4	T46.6X5	T46.6X6
Colestyramine	T46.6X1	T46.6X2	T46.6X3	T46.6X4	T46.6X5	T46.6X6
Colimycin	T36.8X1	T36.8X2	T36.8X3	T36.8X4	T36.8X5	T36.8X6
Colistimethate	T36.8X1	T36.8X2	T36.8X3	T36.8X4	T36.8X5	T36.8X6
Colistin	T36.8X1	T36.8X2	T36.8X3	T36.8X4	T36.8X5	T36.8X6
sulfate (eye preparation)	T49.5X1	T49.5X2	T49.5X3	T49.5X4	T49.5X5	T49.5X6
Collagen	T50.991	T50.992	T50.993	T50.994	T50.995	T50.996
Collagenase	T49.4X1	T49.4X2	T49.4X3	T49.4X4	T49.4X5	T49.4X6
Collodion	T49.3X1	T49.3X2	T49.3X3	T49.3X4	T49.3X5	T49.3X6
Colocynth	T47.2X1	T47.2X2	T47.2X3	T47.2X4	T47.2X5	T47.2X6

Substance	Poisoning, Accidental (unintentional)	Poisoning, Intentional Self-harm	Poisoning, Assault	Poisoning, Undetermined	Adverse Effect	Under-dosing
Colophony adhesive	T49.3X1	T49.3X2	T49.3X3	T49.3X4	T49.3X5	T49.3X6
Colorant — see also Dye	T50.991	T50.992	T50.993	T50.994	T50.995	T50.996
Coloring matter — see Dye(s)						
Combustion gas (after combustion) — see Carbon, monoxide						
prior to combustion	T59.891	T59.892	T59.893	T59.894	—	—
Compazine	T43.3X1	T43.3X2	T43.3X3	T43.3X4	T43.3X5	T43.3X6
Compound						
42 (warfarin)	T60.4X1	T60.4X2	T60.4X3	T60.4X4	—	—
269 (endrin)	T60.1X1	T60.1X2	T60.1X3	T60.1X4	—	—
497 (dieldrin)	T60.1X1	T60.1X2	T60.1X3	T60.1X4	—	—
1080 (sodium fluoroacetate)	T60.4X1	T60.4X2	T60.4X3	T60.4X4	—	—
3422 (parathion)	T60.0X1	T60.0X2	T60.0X3	T60.0X4	—	—
3911 (phorate)	T60.0X1	T60.0X2	T60.0X3	T60.0X4	—	—
3956 (toxaphene)	T60.1X1	T60.1X2	T60.1X3	T60.1X4	—	—
4049 (malathion)	T60.0X1	T60.0X2	T60.0X3	T60.0X4	—	—
4069 (malathion)	T60.0X1	T60.0X2	T60.0X3	T60.0X4	—	—
4124 (dicapthon)	T60.0X1	T60.0X2	T60.0X3	T60.0X4	—	—
E (cortisone)	T38.0X1	T38.0X2	T38.0X3	T38.0X4	T38.0X5	T38.0X6
F (hydrocortisone)	T38.0X1	T38.0X2	T38.0X3	T38.0X4	T38.0X5	T38.0X6
Congener, anabolic	T38.7X1	T38.7X2	T38.7X3	T38.7X4	T38.7X5	T38.7X6
Congo red	T50.8X1	T50.8X2	T50.8X3	T50.8X4	T50.8X5	T50.8X6
Coniine, conine	T62.2X1	T62.2X2	T62.2X3	T62.2X4	—	—
Conium (maculatum)	T62.2X1	T62.2X2	T62.2X3	T62.2X4	—	—
Conjugated estrogenic substances	T38.5X1	T38.5X2	T38.5X3	T38.5X4	T38.5X5	T38.5X6
Contac	T48.5X1	T48.5X2	T48.5X3	T48.5X4	T48.5X5	T48.5X6
Contact lens solution	T49.5X1	T49.5X2	T49.5X3	T49.5X4	T49.5X5	T49.5X6
Contraceptive (oral)	T38.4X1	T38.4X2	T38.4X3	T38.4X4	T38.4X5	T38.4X6
vaginal	T49.8X1	T49.8X2	T49.8X3	T49.8X4	T49.8X5	T49.8X6
Contrast medium, radiography	T50.8X1	T50.8X2	T50.8X3	T50.8X4	T50.8X5	T50.8X6
Convallaria glycosides	T46.0X1	T46.0X2	T46.0X3	T46.0X4	T46.0X5	T46.0X6
Convallaria majalis	T62.2X1	T62.2X2	T62.2X3	T62.2X4	—	—
berry	T62.1X1	T62.1X2	T62.1X3	T62.1X4	—	—
Copperhead snake (bite) (venom)	T63.061	T63.062	T63.063	T63.064	—	—
Copper (dust) (fumes) (nonmedicinal) NEC	T56.4X1	T56.4X2	T56.4X3	T56.4X4	—	—
arsenate, arsenite	T57.0X1	T57.0X2	T57.0X3	T57.0X4	—	—
insecticide	T60.2X1	T60.2X2	T60.2X3	T60.2X4	—	—
emetic	T47.7X1	T47.7X2	T47.7X3	T47.7X4	T47.7X5	T47.7X6
fungicide	T60.3X1	T60.3X2	T60.3X3	T60.3X4	—	—
gluconate	T49.0X1	T49.0X2	T49.0X3	T49.0X4	T49.0X5	T49.0X6
insecticide	T60.2X1	T60.2X2	T60.2X3	T60.2X4	—	—
medicinal (trace)	T45.8X1	T45.8X2	T45.8X3	T45.8X4	T45.8X5	T45.8X6
oleate	T49.0X1	T49.0X2	T49.0X3	T49.0X4	T49.0X5	T49.0X6
sulfate	T56.4X1	T56.4X2	T56.4X3	T56.4X4	—	—
cupric	T56.4X1	T56.4X2	T56.4X3	T56.4X4	—	—
fungicide	T60.3X1	T60.3X2	T60.3X3	T60.3X4	—	—
medicinal						
ear	T49.6X1	T49.6X2	T49.6X3	T49.6X4	T49.6X5	T49.6X6
emetic	T47.7X1	T47.7X2	T47.7X3	T47.7X4	T47.7X5	T47.7X6
eye	T49.5X1	T49.5X2	T49.5X3	T49.5X4	T49.5X5	T49.5X6
cuprous	T56.4X1	T56.4X2	T56.4X3	T56.4X4	—	—
fungicide	T60.3X1	T60.3X2	T60.3X3	T60.3X4	—	—
medicinal						
ear	T49.6X1	T49.6X2	T49.6X3	T49.6X4	T49.6X5	T49.6X6
emetic	T47.7X1	T47.7X2	T47.7X3	T47.7X4	T47.7X5	T47.7X6
eye	T49.5X1	T49.5X2	T49.5X3	T49.5X4	T49.5X5	T49.5X6
Coral (sting)	T63.691	T63.692	T63.693	T63.694		
snake (bite) (venom)	T63.021	T63.022	T63.023	T63.024		
Corbadrine	T49.6X1	T49.6X2	T49.6X3	T49.6X4	T49.6X5	T49.6X6
Cordite	T65.891	T65.892	T65.893	T65.894		
vapor	T59.891	T59.892	T59.893	T59.894		
Cordran	T49.0X1	T49.0X2	T49.0X3	T49.0X4	T49.0X5	T49.0X6
Corn cures	T49.4X1	T49.4X2	T49.4X3	T49.4X4	T49.4X5	T49.4X6
Cornhusker's lotion	T49.3X1	T49.3X2	T49.3X3	T49.3X4	T49.3X5	T49.3X6
Corn starch	T49.3X1	T49.3X2	T49.3X3	T49.3X4	T49.3X5	T49.3X6
Coronary vasodilator NEC	T46.3X1	T46.3X2	T46.3X3	T46.3X4	T46.3X5	T46.3X6
Corrosive NEC	T54.91	T54.92	T54.93	T54.94		
acid NEC	T54.2X1	T54.2X2	T54.2X3	T54.2X4		
aromatics	T54.1X1	T54.1X2	T54.1X3	T54.1X4		
disinfectant	T54.1X1	T54.1X2	T54.1X3	T54.1X4		
fumes NEC	T54.91	T54.92	T54.93	T54.94		
specified NEC	T54.91	T54.92	T54.93	T54.94		
sublimate	T56.1X1	T56.1X2	T56.1X3	T56.1X4		
Cortate	T38.0X1	T38.0X2	T38.0X3	T38.0X4	T38.0X5	T38.0X6
Cort-Dome	T38.0X1	T38.0X2	T38.0X3	T38.0X4	T38.0X5	T38.0X6
ENT agent	T49.6X1	T49.6X2	T49.6X3	T49.6X4	T49.6X5	T49.6X6
ophthalmic preparation	T49.5X1	T49.5X2	T49.5X3	T49.5X4	T49.5X5	T49.5X6

Substance	Poisoning, Accidental (unintentional)	Poisoning, Intentional Self-harm	Poisoning, Assault	Poisoning, Undetermined	Adverse Effect	Under-dosing
Cort-Dome — *continued*						
topical NEC	T49.0X1	T49.0X2	T49.0X3	T49.0X4	T49.0X5	T49.0X6
Cortef	T38.0X1	T38.0X2	T38.0X3	T38.0X5	T38.0X6
ENT agent	T49.6X1	T49.6X2	T49.6X3	T49.6X4	T49.6X5	T49.6X6
ophthalmic preparation	T49.5X1	T49.5X2	T49.5X3	T49.5X4	T49.5X5	T49.5X6
topical NEC	T49.0X1	T49.0X2	T49.0X3	T49.0X4	T49.0X5	T49.0X6
Corticosteroid	T38.0X1	T38.0X2	T38.0X3	T38.0X4	T38.0X5	T38.0X6
ENT agent	T49.6X1	T49.6X2	T49.6X3	T49.6X4	T49.6X5	T49.6X6
mineral	T50.0X1	T50.0X2	T50.0X3	T50.0X4	T50.0X5	T50.0X6
ophthalmic	T49.5X1	T49.5X2	T49.5X3	T49.5X4	T49.5X5	T49.5X6
topical NEC	T49.0X1	T49.0X2	T49.0X3	T49.0X4	T49.0X5	T49.0X6
Corticotropin	T38.811	T38.812	T38.813	T38.814	T38.815	T38.816
Cortisol	T49.0X1	T49.0X2	T49.0X3	T49.0X4	T49.0X5	T49.0X6
ENT agent	T49.6X1	T49.6X2	T49.6X3	T49.6X4	T49.6X5	T49.6X6
ophthalmic preparation	T49.5X1	T49.5X2	T49.5X3	T49.5X4	T49.5X5	T49.5X6
topical NEC	T49.0X1	T49.0X2	T49.0X3	T49.0X4	T49.0X5	T49.0X6
Cortisone (acetate)	T38.0X1	T38.0X2	T38.0X3	T38.0X4	T38.0X5	T38.0X6
ENT agent	T49.6X1	T49.6X2	T49.6X3	T49.6X4	T49.6X5	T49.6X6
ophthalmic preparation	T49.5X1	T49.5X2	T49.5X3	T49.5X4	T49.5X5	T49.5X6
topical NEC	T49.0X1	T49.0X2	T49.0X3	T49.0X4	T49.0X5	T49.0X6
Cortivazol	T38.0X1	T38.0X2	T38.0X3	T38.0X4	T38.0X5	T38.0X6
Cortogen	T38.0X1	T38.0X2	T38.0X3	T38.0X4	T38.0X5	T38.0X6
ENT agent	T49.6X1	T49.6X2	T49.6X3	T49.6X4	T49.6X5	T49.6X6
ophthalmic preparation	T49.5X1	T49.5X2	T49.5X3	T49.5X4	T49.5X5	T49.5X6
Cortone	T38.0X1	T38.0X2	T38.0X3	T38.0X4	T38.0X5	T38.0X6
ENT agent	T49.6X1	T49.6X2	T49.6X3	T49.6X4	T49.6X5	T49.6X6
ophthalmic preparation	T49.5X1	T49.5X2	T49.5X3	T49.5X4	T49.5X5	T49.5X6
Cortril	T38.0X1	T38.0X2	T38.0X3	T38.0X4	T38.0X5	T38.0X6
ENT agent	T49.6X1	T49.6X2	T49.6X3	T49.6X4	T49.6X5	T49.6X6
ophthalmic preparation	T49.5X1	T49.5X2	T49.5X3	T49.5X4	T49.5X5	T49.5X6
topical NEC	T49.0X1	T49.0X2	T49.0X3	T49.0X4	T49.0X5	T49.0X6
Corynebacterium parvum	T45.1X1	T45.1X2	T45.1X3	T45.1X4	T45.1X5	T45.1X6
Cosmetic preparation	T49.8X1	T49.8X2	T49.8X3	T49.8X4	T49.8X5	T49.8X6
Cosmetics	T49.8X1	T49.8X2	T49.8X3	T49.8X4	T49.8X5	T49.8X6
Cosyntropin	T38.811	T38.812	T38.813	T38.814	T38.815	T38.816
Cotarnine	T45.7X1	T45.7X2	T45.7X3	T45.7X4	T45.7X5	T45.7X6
Co-trimoxazole	T36.8X1	T36.8X2	T36.8X3	T36.8X4	T36.8X5	T36.8X6
Cottonseed oil	T49.3X1	T49.3X2	T49.3X3	T49.3X4	T49.3X5	T49.3X6
Cough mixture (syrup)	T48.4X1	T48.4X2	T48.4X3	T48.4X4	T48.4X5	T48.4X6
containing opiates	T40.2X1	T40.2X2	T40.2X3	T40.2X4	T40.2X5	T40.2X6
expectorants	T48.4X1	T48.4X2	T48.4X3	T48.4X4	T48.4X5	T48.4X6
Coumadin	T45.511	T45.512	T45.513	T45.514	T45.515	T45.516
rodenticide	T60.4X1	T60.4X2	T60.4X3	T60.4X4	—	—
Coumaphos	T60.0X1	T60.0X2	T60.0X3	T60.0X4	—	—
Coumarin	T45.511	T45.512	T45.513	T45.514	T45.515	T45.516
Coumetarol	T45.511	T45.512	T45.513	T45.514	T45.515	T45.516
Cowbane	T62.2X1	T62.2X2	T62.2X3	T62.2X4	—	—
Cozyme	T45.2X1	T45.2X2	T45.2X3	T45.2X4	T45.2X5	T45.2X6
Crack	T40.5X1	T40.5X2	T40.5X3	T40.5X4	—	—
Crataegus extract	T46.0X1	T46.0X2	T46.0X3	T46.0X4	T46.0X5	T46.0X6
Creolin	T54.1X1	T54.1X2	T54.1X3	T54.1X4	—	—
disinfectant	T54.1X1	T54.1X2	T54.1X3	T54.1X4	—	—
Creosol (compound)	T49.0X1	T49.0X2	T49.0X3	T49.0X4	—	—
Creosote (coal tar)	T49.0X1	T49.0X2	T49.0X3	T49.0X4	T49.0X5	T49.0X6
(beechwood)						
medicinal (expectorant)	T48.4X1	T48.4X2	T48.4X3	T48.4X4	T48.4X5	T48.4X6
syrup	T48.4X1	T48.4X2	T48.4X3	T48.4X4	T48.4X5	T48.4X6
Cresol(s)	T49.0X1	T49.0X2	T49.0X3	T49.0X4	T49.0X5	T49.0X6
and soap solution	T49.0X1	T49.0X2	T49.0X3	T49.0X4	T49.0X5	T49.0X6
Cresyl acetate	T49.0X1	T49.0X2	T49.0X3	T49.0X4	T49.0X5	T49.0X6
Cresylic acid	T49.0X1	T49.0X2	T49.0X3	T49.0X4	T49.0X5	T49.0X6
Crimidine	T60.4X1	T60.4X2	T60.4X3	T60.4X4	—	—
Croconazole	T37.8X1	T37.8X2	T37.8X3	T37.8X4	T37.8X5	T37.8X6
Cromoglicic acid	T48.6X1	T48.6X2	T48.6X3	T48.6X4	T48.6X5	T48.6X6
Cromolyn	T48.6X1	T48.6X2	T48.6X3	T48.6X4	T48.6X5	T48.6X6
Cromonar	T46.3X1	T46.3X2	T46.3X3	T46.3X4	T46.3X5	T46.3X6
Cropropamide	T39.8X1	T39.8X2	T39.8X3	T39.8X4	T39.8X5	T39.8X6
with crotethamide	T50.7X1	T50.7X2	T50.7X3	T50.7X4	T50.7X5	T50.7X6
Crotamiton	T49.0X1	T49.0X2	T49.0X3	T49.0X4	T49.0X5	T49.0X6
Crotethamide	T39.8X1	T39.8X2	T39.8X3	T39.8X4	T39.8X5	T39.8X6
with cropropamide	T50.7X1	T50.7X2	T50.7X3	T50.7X4	T50.7X5	T50.7X6
Croton (oil)	T47.2X1	T47.2X2	T47.2X3	T47.2X4	T47.2X5	T47.2X6
chloral	T42.6X1	T42.6X2	T42.6X3	T42.6X4	T42.6X5	T42.6X6
Crude oil	T52.0X1	T52.0X2	T52.0X3	T52.0X4	—	—
Cryogenine	T39.8X1	T39.8X2	T39.8X3	T39.8X4	T39.8X5	T39.8X6
Cryolite (vapor)	T60.1X1	T60.1X2	T60.1X3	T60.1X4	—	—
insecticide	T60.1X1	T60.1X2	T60.1X3	T60.1X4	—	—
Cryptenamine (tannates)	T46.5X1	T46.5X2	T46.5X3	T46.5X4	T46.5X5	T46.5X6
Crystal violet	T49.0X1	T49.0X2	T49.0X3	T49.0X4	T49.0X5	T49.0X6
Cuckoopint	T62.2X1	T62.2X2	T62.2X3	T62.2X4	—	—
Cumetharol	T45.511	T45.512	T45.513	T45.514	T45.515	T45.516
Cupric						
acetate	T60.3X1	T60.3X2	T60.3X3	T60.3X4	—	—

Substance	Poisoning, Accidental (unintentional)	Poisoning, Intentional Self-harm	Poisoning, Assault	Poisoning, Undetermined	Adverse Effect	Under-dosing
Cupric — *continued*						
acetoarsenite	T57.0X1	T57.0X2	T57.0X3	T57.0X4	—	—
arsenate	T57.0X1	T57.0X2	T57.0X3	T57.0X4	—	—
gluconate	T49.0X1	T49.0X2	T49.0X3	T49.0X4	T49.0X5	T49.0X6
oleate	T49.0X1	T49.0X2	T49.0X3	T49.0X4	T49.0X5	T49.0X6
sulfate	T56.4X1	T56.4X2	T56.4X3	T56.4X4	—	—
Cuprous sulfate — *see also*	T56.4X1	T56.4X2	T56.4X3	T56.4X4	—	—
Copper sulfate						
Curare, curarine	T48.1X1	T48.1X2	T48.1X3	T48.1X4	T48.1X5	T48.1X6
Cyamemazine	T43.3X1	T43.3X2	T43.3X3	T43.3X4	T43.3X5	T43.3X6
Cyamopsis tetragonoloba	T46.6X1	T46.6X2	T46.6X3	T46.6X4	T46.6X5	T46.6X6
Cyanacetyl hydrazide	T37.1X1	T37.1X2	T37.1X3	T37.1X4	T37.1X5	T37.1X6
Cyanic acid (gas)	T59.891	T59.892	T59.893	T59.894		
Cyanide(s) (compounds)	T65.0X1	T65.0X2	T65.0X3	T65.0X4	—	—
(potassium) (sodium)						
NEC						
dust or gas (inhalation) NEC	T57.3X1	T57.3X2	T57.3X3	T57.3X4	—	—
fumigant	T65.0X1	T65.0X2	T65.0X3	T65.0X4	—	—
hydrogen	T57.3X1	T57.3X2	T57.3X3	T57.3X4	—	—
mercuric — *see* Mercury						
pesticide (dust) (fumes)	T65.0X1	T65.0X2	T65.0X3	T65.0X4	—	—
Cyanoacrylate adhesive	T49.3X1	T49.3X2	T49.3X3	T49.3X4	T49.3X5	T49.3X6
Cyanocobalamin	T45.8X1	T45.8X2	T45.8X3	T45.8X4	T45.8X5	T45.8X6
Cyanogen (chloride) (gas)	T59.891	T59.892	T59.893	T59.894		
NEC						
Cyclacillin	T36.0X1	T36.0X2	T36.0X3	T36.0X4	T36.0X5	T36.0X6
Cyclaine	T41.3X1	T41.3X2	T41.3X3	T41.3X4	T41.3X5	T41.3X6
Cyclamate	T50.991	T50.992	T50.993	T50.994	T50.995	T50.996
Cyclamen europaeum	T62.2X1	T62.2X2	T62.2X3	T62.2X4	—	—
Cyclandelate	T46.7X1	T46.7X2	T46.7X3	T46.7X4	T46.7X5	T46.7X6
Cyclazocine	T50.7X1	T50.7X2	T50.7X3	T50.7X4	T50.7X5	T50.7X6
Cyclizine	T45.0X1	T45.0X2	T45.0X3	T45.0X4	T45.0X5	T45.0X6
Cyclobarbital	T42.3X1	T42.3X2	T42.3X3	T42.3X4	T42.3X5	T42.3X6
Cyclobarbitone	T42.3X1	T42.3X2	T42.3X3	T42.3X4	T42.3X5	T42.3X6
Cyclobenzaprine	T48.1X1	T48.1X2	T48.1X3	T48.1X4	T48.1X5	T48.1X6
Cyclodrine	T44.3X1	T44.3X2	T44.3X3	T44.3X4	T44.3X5	T44.3X6
Cycloguanil embonate	T37.2X1	T37.2X2	T37.2X3	T37.2X4	T37.2X5	T37.2X6
Cyclohexane	T52.8X1	T52.8X2	T52.8X3	T52.8X4	—	—
Cyclohexanol	T51.8X1	T51.8X2	T51.8X3	T51.8X4	—	—
Cyclohexanone	T52.4X1	T52.4X2	T52.4X3	T52.4X4	—	—
Cycloheximide	T60.3X1	T60.3X2	T60.3X3	T60.3X4	—	—
Cyclohexyl acetate	T52.8X1	T52.8X2	T52.8X3	T52.8X4	—	—
Cycloleucin	T45.1X1	T45.1X2	T45.1X3	T45.1X4	T45.1X5	T45.1X6
Cyclomethycaine	T41.3X1	T41.3X2	T41.3X3	T41.3X4	T41.3X5	T41.3X6
Cyclopentamine	T44.4X1	T44.4X2	T44.4X3	T44.4X4	T44.4X5	T44.4X6
Cyclopenthiazide	T50.2X1	T50.2X2	T50.2X3	T50.2X4	T50.2X5	T50.2X6
Cyclopentolate	T44.3X1	T44.3X2	T44.3X3	T44.3X4	T44.3X5	T44.3X6
Cyclophosphamide	T45.1X1	T45.1X2	T45.1X3	T45.1X4	T45.1X5	T45.1X6
Cycloplegic drug	T49.5X1	T49.5X2	T49.5X3	T49.5X4	T49.5X5	T49.5X6
Cyclopropane	T41.291	T41.292	T41.293	T41.294	T41.295	T41.296
Cyclopyrabital	T39.8X1	T39.8X2	T39.8X3	T39.8X4	T39.8X5	T39.8X6
Cycloserine	T37.1X1	T37.1X2	T37.1X3	T37.1X4	T37.1X5	T37.1X6
Cyclosporin	T45.1X1	T45.1X2	T45.1X3	T45.1X4	T45.1X5	T45.1X6
Cyclothiazide	T50.2X1	T50.2X2	T50.2X3	T50.2X4	T50.2X5	T50.2X6
Cycrimine	T44.3X1	T44.3X2	T44.3X3	T44.3X4	T44.3X5	T44.3X6
Cyhalothrin	T60.1X1	T60.1X2	T60.1X3	T60.1X4	—	—
Cymarin	T46.0X1	T46.0X2	T46.0X3	T46.0X4	T46.0X5	T46.0X6
Cypermethrin	T60.1X1	T60.1X2	T60.1X3	T60.1X4	—	—
Cyphenothrin	T60.2X1	T60.2X2	T60.2X3	T60.2X4	—	—
Cyproheptadine	T45.0X1	T45.0X2	T45.0X3	T45.0X4	T45.0X5	T45.0X6
Cyproterone	T38.6X1	T38.6X2	T38.6X3	T38.6X4	T38.6X5	T38.6X6
Cysteamine	T50.6X1	T50.6X2	T50.6X3	T50.6X4	T50.6X5	T50.6X6
Cytarabine	T45.1X1	T45.1X2	T45.1X3	T45.1X4	T45.1X5	T45.1X6
Cytisus						
laburnum	T62.2X1	T62.2X2	T62.2X3	T62.2X4	—	—
scoparius	T62.2X1	T62.2X2	T62.2X3	T62.2X4	—	—
Cytochrome C	T47.5X1	T47.5X2	T47.5X3	T47.5X4	T47.5X5	T47.5X6
Cytomel	T38.1X1	T38.1X2	T38.1X3	T38.1X4	T38.1X5	T38.1X6
Cytosine arabinoside	T45.1X1	T45.1X2	T45.1X3	T45.1X4	T45.1X5	T45.1X6
Cytoxan	T45.1X1	T45.1X2	T45.1X3	T45.1X4	T45.1X5	T45.1X6
Cytozyme	T45.7X1	T45.7X2	T45.7X3	T45.7X4	T45.7X5	T45.7X6
S-Carboxymethylcysteine	T48.4X1	T48.4X2	T48.4X3	T48.4X4	T48.4X5	T48.4X6
Dacarbazine	T45.1X1	T45.1X2	T45.1X3	T45.1X4	T45.1X5	T45.1X6
Dactinomycin	T45.1X1	T45.1X2	T45.1X3	T45.1X4	T45.1X5	T45.1X6
DADPS	T37.1X1	T37.1X2	T37.1X3	T37.1X4	T37.1X5	T37.1X6
Dakin's solution	T49.0X1	T49.0X2	T49.0X3	T49.0X4	T49.0X5	T49.0X6
Dalapon (sodium)	T60.3X1	T60.3X2	T60.3X3	T60.3X4	—	—
Dalmane	T42.4X1	T42.4X2	T42.4X3	T42.4X4	T42.4X5	T42.4X6
Danazol	T38.6X1	T38.6X2	T38.6X3	T38.6X4	T38.6X5	T38.6X6
Danilone	T45.511	T45.512	T45.513	T45.514	T45.515	T45.516
Danthron	T47.2X1	T47.2X2	T47.2X3	T47.2X4	T47.2X5	T47.2X6
Dantrolene	T42.8X1	T42.8X2	T42.8X3	T42.8X4	T42.8X5	T42.8X6
Dantron	T47.2X1	T47.2X2	T47.2X3	T47.2X4	T47.2X5	T47.2X6

Additional Character May Be Required — Refer to the Tabular List for Character Selection   ▽ Subterms under main terms may continue to next column or page

Substance	Poisoning, Accidental (unintentional)	Poisoning, Intentional Self-harm	Poisoning, Assault	Poisoning, Undetermined	Adverse Effect	Under-dosing
Daphne (gnidium) (mezereum)	T62.2X1	T62.2X2	T62.2X3	T62.2X4	—	—
berry	T62.1X1	T62.1X2	T62.1X3	T62.1X4	—	—
Dapsone	T37.1X1	T37.1X2	T37.1X3	T37.1X4	T37.1X5	T37.1X6
Daraprim	T37.2X1	T37.2X2	T37.2X3	T37.2X4	T37.2X5	T37.2X6
Darnel	T62.2X1	T62.2X2	T62.2X3	T62.2X4	—	—
Darvon	T39.8X1	T39.8X2	T39.8X3	T39.8X4	T39.8X5	T39.8X6
Daunomycin	T45.1X1	T45.1X2	T45.1X3	T45.1X4	T45.1X5	T45.1X6
Daunorubicin	T45.1X1	T45.1X2	T45.1X3	T45.1X4	T45.1X5	T45.1X6
DBI	T38.3X1	T38.3X2	T38.3X3	T38.3X4	T38.3X5	T38.3X6
D-Con	T60.91	T60.92	T60.93	T60.94	—	—
insecticide	T60.2X1	T60.2X2	T60.2X3	T60.2X4	—	—
rodenticide	T60.4X1	T60.4X2	T60.4X3	T60.4X4	—	—
DDAVP	T38.891	T38.892	T38.893	T38.894	T38.895	T38.896
DDE (bis(chlorophenyl)-dichloroethylene)	T60.2X1	T60.2X2	T60.2X3	T60.2X4	—	—
DDS	T37.1X1	T37.1X2	T37.1X3	T37.1X4	T37.1X5	T37.1X6
DDT (dust)	T60.1X1	T60.1X2	T60.1X3	T60.1X4	—	—
Deadly nightshade — see also Belladonna						
berry	T62.1X1	T62.1X2	T62.1X3	T62.1X4	—	—
Deamino-D-arginine vasopressin	T38.891	T38.892	T38.893	T38.894	T38.895	T38.896
Deanol (aceglumate)	T50.991	T50.992	T50.993	T50.994	T50.995	T50.996
Debrisoquine	T46.5X1	T46.5X2	T46.5X3	T46.5X4	T46.5X5	T46.5X6
Decaborane	T57.8X1	T57.8X2	T57.8X3	T57.8X4	—	—
fumes	T59.891	T59.892	T59.893	T59.894	—	—
Decadron	T38.0X1	T38.0X2	T38.0X3	T38.0X4	T38.0X5	T38.0X6
ENT agent	T49.6X1	T49.6X2	T49.6X3	T49.6X4	T49.6X5	T49.6X6
ophthalmic preparation	T49.5X1	T49.5X2	T49.5X3	T49.5X4	T49.5X5	T49.5X6
topical NEC	T49.0X1	T49.0X2	T49.0X3	T49.0X4	T49.0X5	T49.0X6
Decahydronaphthalene	T52.8X1	T52.8X2	T52.8X3	T52.8X4	—	—
Decalin	T52.8X1	T52.8X2	T52.8X3	T52.8X4	—	—
Decamethonium (bromide)	T48.1X1	T48.1X2	T48.1X3	T48.1X4	T48.1X5	T48.1X6
Decholin	T47.5X1	T47.5X2	T47.5X3	T47.5X4	T47.5X5	T47.5X6
Declomycin	T36.4X1	T36.4X2	T36.4X3	T36.4X4	T36.4X5	T36.4X6
Decongestant, nasal (mucosa)	T48.5X1	T48.5X2	T48.5X3	T48.5X4	T48.5X5	T48.5X6
combination	T48.5X1	T48.5X2	T48.5X3	T48.5X4	T48.5X5	T48.5X6
Deet	T60.8X1	T60.8X2	T60.8X3	T60.8X4	—	—
Deferoxamine	T45.8X1	T45.8X2	T45.8X3	T45.8X4	T45.8X5	T45.8X6
Deflazacort	T38.0X1	T38.0X2	T38.0X3	T38.0X4	T38.0X5	T38.0X6
Deglycyrrhizinized extract of licorice	T48.4X1	T48.4X2	T48.4X3	T48.4X4	T48.4X5	T48.4X6
Dehydrocholic acid	T47.5X1	T47.5X2	T47.5X3	T47.5X4	T47.5X5	T47.5X6
Dehydroemetine	T37.3X1	T37.3X2	T37.3X3	T37.3X4	T37.3X5	T37.3X6
Dekalin	T52.8X1	T52.8X2	T52.8X3	T52.8X4	—	—
Delalutin	T38.5X1	T38.5X2	T38.5X3	T38.5X4	T38.5X5	T38.5X6
Delorazepam	T42.4X1	T42.4X2	T42.4X3	T42.4X4	T42.4X5	T42.4X6
Delphinium	T62.2X1	T62.2X2	T62.2X3	T62.2X4	—	—
Deltamethrin	T60.1X1	T60.1X2	T60.1X3	T60.1X4	—	—
Deltasone	T38.0X1	T38.0X2	T38.0X3	T38.0X4	T38.0X5	T38.0X6
Deltra	T38.0X1	T38.0X2	T38.0X3	T38.0X4	T38.0X5	T38.0X6
Delvinal	T42.3X1	T42.3X2	T42.3X3	T42.3X4	T42.3X5	T42.3X6
Demecarium (bromide)	T49.5X1	T49.5X2	T49.5X3	T49.5X4	T49.5X5	T49.5X6
Demeclocycline	T36.4X1	T36.4X2	T36.4X3	T36.4X4	T36.4X5	T36.4X6
Demecolcine	T45.1X1	T45.1X2	T45.1X3	T45.1X4	T45.1X5	T45.1X6
Demegestone	T38.5X1	T38.5X2	T38.5X3	T38.5X4	T38.5X5	T38.5X6
Demelanizing agents	T49.8X1	T49.8X2	T49.8X3	T49.8X4	T49.8X5	T49.8X6
Demephion -O and -S	T60.0X1	T60.0X2	T60.0X3	T60.0X4	—	—
Demerol	T40.2X1	T40.2X2	T40.2X3	T40.2X4	T40.2X5	T40.2X6
Demethylchlortetracycline	T36.4X1	T36.4X2	T36.4X3	T36.4X4	T36.4X5	T36.4X6
Demethyltetracycline	T36.4X1	T36.4X2	T36.4X3	T36.4X4	T36.4X5	T36.4X6
Demeton -O and -S	T60.0X1	T60.0X2	T60.0X3	T60.0X4	—	—
Demulcent (external)	T49.3X1	T49.3X2	T49.3X3	T49.3X4	T49.3X5	T49.3X6
specified NEC	T49.3X1	T49.3X2	T49.3X3	T49.3X4	T49.3X5	T49.3X6
Demulen	T38.4X1	T38.4X2	T38.4X3	T38.4X4	T38.4X5	T38.4X6
Denatured alcohol	T51.0X1	T51.0X2	T51.0X3	T51.0X4	—	—
Dendrid	T49.5X1	T49.5X2	T49.5X3	T49.5X4	T49.5X5	T49.5X6
Dental drug, topical application NEC	T49.7X1	T49.7X2	T49.7X3	T49.7X4	T49.7X5	T49.7X6
Dentifrice	T49.7X1	T49.7X2	T49.7X3	T49.7X4	T49.7X5	T49.7X6
Deodorant spray (feminine hygiene)	T49.8X1	T49.8X2	T49.8X3	T49.8X4	T49.8X5	T49.8X6
Deoxycortone	T50.0X1	T50.0X2	T50.0X3	T50.0X4	T50.0X5	T50.0X6
Deoxyribonuclease (pancreatic)	T45.3X1	T45.3X2	T45.3X3	T45.3X4	T45.3X5	T45.3X6
Depilatory	T49.4X1	T49.4X2	T49.4X3	T49.4X4	T49.4X5	T49.4X6
Deprenalin	T42.8X1	T42.8X2	T42.8X3	T42.8X4	T42.8X5	T42.8X6
Deprenyl	T42.8X1	T42.8X2	T42.8X3	T42.8X4	T42.8X5	T42.8X6
Depressant						
appetite (central)	T50.5X1	T50.5X2	T50.5X3	T50.5X4	T50.5X5	T50.5X6
cardiac	T46.2X1	T46.2X2	T46.2X3	T46.2X4	T46.2X5	T46.2X6
Depressant — continued						
central nervous system (anesthetic) — see also Central nervous system, depressants	T42.71	T42.72	T42.73	T42.74	T42.75	T42.76
general anesthetic	T41.201	T41.202	T41.203	T41.204	T41.205	T41.206
muscle tone	T42.8X1	T42.8X2	T42.8X3	T42.8X4	T42.8X5	T42.8X6
muscle tone, central	T42.8X1	T42.8X2	T42.8X3	T42.8X4	T42.8X5	T42.8X6
psychotherapeutic	T43.501	T43.502	T43.503	T43.504	T43.505	T43.506
Depressant, appetite	T50.5X1	T50.5X2	T50.5X3	T50.5X4	T50.5X5	T50.5X6
Deptropine	T45.0X1	T45.0X2	T45.0X3	T45.0X4	T45.0X5	T45.0X6
Dequalinium (chloride)	T49.0X1	T49.0X2	T49.0X3	T49.0X4	T49.0X5	T49.0X6
Derris root	T60.2X1	T60.2X2	T60.2X3	T60.2X4	—	—
Deserpidine	T46.5X1	T46.5X2	T46.5X3	T46.5X4	T46.5X5	T46.5X6
Desferrioxamine	T45.8X1	T45.8X2	T45.8X3	T45.8X4	T45.8X5	T45.8X6
Desipramine	T43.011	T43.012	T43.013	T43.014	T43.015	T43.016
Deslanoside	T46.0X1	T46.0X2	T46.0X3	T46.0X4	T46.0X5	T46.0X6
Desloughing agent	T49.4X1	T49.4X2	T49.4X3	T49.4X4	T49.4X5	T49.4X6
Desmethylimipramine	T43.011	T43.012	T43.013	T43.014	T43.015	T43.016
Desmopressin	T38.891	T38.892	T38.893	T38.894	T38.895	T38.896
Desocodeine	T40.2X1	T40.2X2	T40.2X3	T40.2X4	T40.2X5	T40.2X6
Desogestrel	T38.5X1	T38.5X2	T38.5X3	T38.5X4	T38.5X5	T38.5X6
Desomorphine	T40.2X1	T40.2X2	T40.2X3	T40.2X4	—	—
Desonide	T49.0X1	T49.0X2	T49.0X3	T49.0X4	T49.0X5	T49.0X6
Desoximetasone	T49.0X1	T49.0X2	T49.0X3	T49.0X4	T49.0X5	T49.0X6
Desoxycorticosteroid	T50.0X1	T50.0X2	T50.0X3	T50.0X4	T50.0X5	T50.0X6
Desoxycortone	T50.0X1	T50.0X2	T50.0X3	T50.0X4	T50.0X5	T50.0X6
Desoxyephedrine	T43.621	T43.622	T43.623	T43.624	T43.625	T43.626
Detaxtran	T46.6X1	T46.6X2	T46.6X3	T46.6X4	T46.6X5	T46.6X6
Detergent	T49.2X1	T49.2X2	T49.2X3	T49.2X4	T49.2X5	T49.2X6
external medication	T49.2X1	T49.2X2	T49.2X3	T49.2X4	T49.2X5	T49.2X6
local	T49.2X1	T49.2X2	T49.2X3	T49.2X4	T49.2X5	T49.2X6
medicinal	T49.2X1	T49.2X2	T49.2X3	T49.2X4	T49.2X5	T49.2X6
nonmedicinal	T55.1X1	T55.1X2	T55.1X3	T55.1X4	—	—
specified NEC	T55.1X1	T55.1X2	T55.1X3	T55.1X4	—	—
Deterrent, alcohol	T50.6X1	T50.6X2	T50.6X3	T50.6X4	T50.6X5	T50.6X6
Detoxifying agent	T50.6X1	T50.6X2	T50.6X3	T50.6X4	T50.6X5	T50.6X6
Detrothyronine	T38.1X1	T38.1X2	T38.1X3	T38.1X4	T38.1X5	T38.1X6
Dettol (external medication)	T49.0X1	T49.0X2	T49.0X3	T49.0X4	T49.0X5	T49.0X6
Dexamethasone	T38.0X1	T38.0X2	T38.0X3	T38.0X4	T38.0X5	T38.0X6
ENT agent	T49.6X1	T49.6X2	T49.6X3	T49.6X4	T49.6X5	T49.6X6
ophthalmic preparation	T49.5X1	T49.5X2	T49.5X3	T49.5X4	T49.5X5	T49.5X6
topical NEC	T49.0X1	T49.0X2	T49.0X3	T49.0X4	T49.0X5	T49.0X6
Dexamfetamine	T43.621	T43.622	T43.623	T43.624	T43.625	T43.626
Dexamphetamine	T43.621	T43.622	T43.623	T43.624	T43.625	T43.626
Dexbrompheniramine	T45.0X1	T45.0X2	T45.0X3	T45.0X4	T45.0X5	T45.0X6
Dexchlorpheniramine	T45.0X1	T45.0X2	T45.0X3	T45.0X4	T45.0X5	T45.0X6
Dexedrine	T43.621	T43.622	T43.623	T43.624	T43.625	T43.626
Dexetimide	T44.3X1	T44.3X2	T44.3X3	T44.3X4	T44.3X5	T44.3X6
Dexfenfluramine	T50.5X1	T50.5X2	T50.5X3	T50.5X4	T50.5X5	T50.5X6
Dexpanthenol	T45.2X1	T45.2X2	T45.2X3	T45.2X4	T45.2X5	T45.2X6
Dextran (40) (70) (150)	T45.8X1	T45.8X2	T45.8X3	T45.8X4	T45.8X5	T45.8X6
Dextriferron	T45.4X1	T45.4X2	T45.4X3	T45.4X4	T45.4X5	T45.4X6
Dextroamphetamine	T43.621	T43.622	T43.623	T43.624	T43.625	T43.626
Dextro calcium pantothenate	T45.2X1	T45.2X2	T45.2X3	T45.2X4	T45.2X5	T45.2X6
Dextromethorphan	T48.3X1	T48.3X2	T48.3X3	T48.3X4	T48.3X5	T48.3X6
Dextromoramide	T40.4X1	T40.4X2	T40.4X3	T40.4X4	—	—
topical	T49.8X1	T49.8X2	T49.8X3	T49.8X4	T49.8X5	T49.8X6
Dextro pantothenyl alcohol	T45.2X1	T45.2X2	T45.2X3	T45.2X4	T45.2X5	T45.2X6
Dextropropoxyphene	T40.4X1	T40.4X2	T40.4X3	T40.4X4	—	—
Dextrorphan	T40.2X1	T40.2X2	T40.2X3	T40.2X4	T40.2X5	T40.2X6
Dextrose	T50.3X1	T50.3X2	T50.3X3	T50.3X4	T50.3X5	T50.3X6
concentrated solution, intravenous	T46.8X1	T46.8X2	T46.8X3	T46.8X4	T46.8X5	T46.8X6
Dextrothyroxin	T38.1X1	T38.1X2	T38.1X3	T38.1X4	T38.1X5	T38.1X6
Dextrothyroxine sodium	T38.1X1	T38.1X2	T38.1X3	T38.1X4	T38.1X5	T38.1X6
DFP	T44.0X1	T44.0X2	T44.0X3	T44.0X4	T44.0X5	T44.0X6
DHE	T37.3X1	T37.3X2	T37.3X3	T37.3X4	T37.3X5	T37.3X6
45	T46.5X1	T46.5X2	T46.5X3	T46.5X4	T46.5X5	T46.5X6
Diabinese	T38.3X1	T38.3X2	T38.3X3	T38.3X4	T38.3X5	T38.3X6
Diacetone alcohol	T52.4X1	T52.4X2	T52.4X3	T52.4X4	—	—
Diacetyl monoxime	T50.991	T50.992	T50.993	T50.994	—	—
Diacetylmorphine	T40.1X1	T40.1X2	T40.1X3	T40.1X4	—	—
Diachylon plaster	T49.4X1	T49.4X2	T49.4X3	T49.4X4	T49.4X5	T49.4X6
Diaethylstilboestrolum	T38.5X1	T38.5X2	T38.5X3	T38.5X4	T38.5X5	T38.5X6
Diagnostic agent NEC	T50.8X1	T50.8X2	T50.8X3	T50.8X4	T50.8X5	T50.8X6
Dial (soap)	T49.2X1	T49.2X2	T49.2X3	T49.2X4	T49.2X5	T49.2X6
sedative	T42.3X1	T42.3X2	T42.3X3	T42.3X4	T42.3X5	T42.3X6
Dialkyl carbonate	T52.91	T52.92	T52.93	T52.94	—	—
Diallylbarbituric acid	T42.3X1	T42.3X2	T42.3X3	T42.3X4	T42.3X5	T42.3X6
Diallymal	T42.3X1	T42.3X2	T42.3X3	T42.3X4	T42.3X5	T42.3X6

Substance	Poisoning, Accidental (unintentional)	Poisoning, Intentional Self-harm	Poisoning, Assault	Poisoning, Undetermined	Adverse Effect	Under-dosing
Dialysis solution (intraperitoneal)	T50.3X1	T50.3X2	T50.3X3	T50.3X4	T50.3X5	T50.3X6
Diaminodiphenylsulfone	T37.1X1	T37.1X2	T37.1X3	T37.1X4	T37.1X5	T37.1X6
Diamorphine	T40.1X1	T40.1X2	T40.1X3	T40.1X4	—	—
Diamox	T50.2X1	T50.2X2	T50.2X3	T50.2X4	T50.2X5	T50.2X6
Diamthazole	T49.0X1	T49.0X2	T49.0X3	T49.0X4	T49.0X5	T49.0X6
Dianthone	T47.2X1	T47.2X2	T47.2X3	T47.2X4	T47.2X5	T47.2X6
Diaphenylsulfone	T37.0X1	T37.0X2	T37.0X3	T37.0X4	T37.0X5	T37.0X6
Diasone (sodium)	T37.1X1	T37.1X2	T37.1X3	T37.1X4	T37.1X5	T37.1X6
Diastase	T47.5X1	T47.5X2	T47.5X3	T47.5X4	T47.5X5	T47.5X6
Diatrizoate	T50.8X1	T50.8X2	T50.8X3	T50.8X4	T50.8X5	T50.8X6
Diazepam	T42.4X1	T42.4X2	T42.4X3	T42.4X4	T42.4X5	T42.4X6
Diazinon	T60.0X1	T60.0X2	T60.0X3	T60.0X4	—	—
Diazomethane (gas)	T59.891	T59.892	T59.893	T59.894	—	—
Diazoxide	T46.5X1	T46.5X2	T46.5X3	T46.5X4	T46.5X5	T46.5X6
Dibekacin	T36.5X1	T36.5X2	T36.5X3	T36.5X4	T36.5X5	T36.5X6
Dibenamine	T44.6X1	T44.6X2	T44.6X3	T44.6X4	T44.6X5	T44.6X6
Dibenzepin	T43.011	T43.012	T43.013	T43.014	T43.015	T43.016
Dibenzheptropine	T45.0X1	T45.0X2	T45.0X3	T45.0X4	T45.0X5	T45.0X6
Dibenzyline	T44.6X1	T44.6X2	T44.6X3	T44.6X4	T44.6X5	T44.6X6
Diborane (gas)	T59.891	T59.892	T59.893	T59.894	—	—
Dibromochloropropane	T60.8X1	T60.8X2	T60.8X3	T60.8X4	—	—
Dibromodulcitol	T45.1X1	T45.1X2	T45.1X3	T45.1X4	T45.1X5	T45.1X6
Dibromoethane	T53.6X1	T53.6X2	T53.6X3	T53.6X4	—	—
Dibromomannitol	T45.1X1	T45.1X2	T45.1X3	T45.1X4	T45.1X5	T45.1X6
Dibromopropamidine isethionate	T49.0X1	T49.0X2	T49.0X3	T49.0X4	T49.0X5	T49.0X6
Dibrompropamidine	T49.0X1	T49.0X2	T49.0X3	T49.0X4	T49.0X5	T49.0X6
Dibucaine	T41.3X1	T41.3X2	T41.3X3	T41.3X4	T41.3X5	T41.3X6
topical (surface)	T41.3X1	T41.3X2	T41.3X3	T41.3X4	T41.3X5	T41.3X6
Dibunate sodium	T48.3X1	T48.3X2	T48.3X3	T48.3X4	T48.3X5	T48.3X6
Dibutoline sulfate	T44.3X1	T44.3X2	T44.3X3	T44.3X4	T44.3X5	T44.3X6
Dicamba	T60.3X1	T60.3X2	T60.3X3	T60.3X4	—	—
Dicapthon	T60.0X1	T60.0X2	T60.0X3	T60.0X4	—	—
Dichlobenil	T60.3X1	T60.3X2	T60.3X3	T60.3X4	—	—
Dichlone	T60.3X1	T60.3X2	T60.3X3	T60.3X4	—	—
Dichloralphenazone	T42.6X1	T42.6X2	T42.6X3	T42.6X4	T42.6X5	T42.6X6
Dichlorbenzidine	T65.3X1	T65.3X2	T65.3X3	T65.3X4	—	—
Dichlorhydrin	T52.8X1	T52.8X2	T52.8X3	T52.8X4	—	—
Dichlorhydroxyquinoline	T37.8X1	T37.8X2	T37.8X3	T37.8X4	T37.8X5	T37.8X6
Dichlorobenzene	T53.7X1	T53.7X2	T53.7X3	T53.7X4	—	—
Dichlorobenzyl alcohol	T49.6X1	T49.6X2	T49.6X3	T49.6X4	T49.6X5	T49.6X6
Dichlorodifluoromethane	T53.5X1	T53.5X2	T53.5X3	T53.5X4	—	—
Dichloroethane	T52.8X1	T52.8X2	T52.8X3	T52.8X4	—	—
Dichloroethylene	T53.6X1	T53.6X2	T53.6X3	T53.6X4	—	—
Dichloroethyl sulfide, not in war	T59.891	T59.892	T59.893	T59.894	—	—
Dichloroformoxine, not in war	T59.891	T59.892	T59.893	T59.894	—	—
Dichlorohydrin, alpha-dichlorohydrin	T52.8X1	T52.8X2	T52.8X3	T52.8X4	—	—
Dichloromethane (solvent)	T53.4X1	T53.4X2	T53.4X3	T53.4X4	—	—
vapor	T53.4X1	T53.4X2	T53.4X3	T53.4X4	—	—
Dichloronaphthoquinone	T60.3X1	T60.3X2	T60.3X3	T60.3X4	—	—
Dichlorophen	T37.4X1	T37.4X2	T37.4X3	T37.4X4	T37.4X5	T37.4X6
Dichloropropene	T60.3X1	T60.3X2	T60.3X3	T60.3X4	—	—
Dichloropropionic acid	T60.3X1	T60.3X2	T60.3X3	T60.3X4	—	—
Dichlorphenamide	T50.2X1	T50.2X2	T50.2X3	T50.2X4	T50.2X5	T50.2X6
Dichlorvos	T60.0X1	T60.0X2	T60.0X3	T60.0X4	—	—
Diclofenac	T39.391	T39.392	T39.393	T39.394	T39.395	T39.396
Diclofenamide	T50.2X1	T50.2X2	T50.2X3	T50.2X4	T50.2X5	T50.2X6
Diclofensine	T43.291	T43.292	T43.293	T43.294	T43.295	T43.296
Diclonixine	T39.8X1	T39.8X2	T39.8X3	T39.8X4	T39.8X5	T39.8X6
Dicloxacillin	T36.0X1	T36.0X2	T36.0X3	T36.0X4	T36.0X5	T36.0X6
Dicophane	T49.0X1	T49.0X2	T49.0X3	T49.0X4	T49.0X5	T49.0X6
Dicoumarol, dicoumarin, dicumarol	T45.511	T45.512	T45.513	T45.514	T45.515	T45.516
Dicrotophos	T60.0X1	T60.0X2	T60.0X3	T60.0X4	—	—
Dicyanogen (gas)	T65.0X1	T65.0X2	T65.0X3	T65.0X4	—	—
Dicyclomine	T44.3X1	T44.3X2	T44.3X3	T44.3X4	T44.3X5	T44.3X6
Dicycloverine	T44.3X1	T44.3X2	T44.3X3	T44.3X4	T44.3X5	T44.3X6
Dideoxycytidine	T37.5X1	T37.5X2	T37.5X3	T37.5X4	T37.5X5	T37.5X6
Dideoxyinosine	T37.5X1	T37.5X2	T37.5X3	T37.5X4	T37.5X5	T37.5X6
Dieldrin (vapor)	T60.1X1	T60.1X2	T60.1X3	T60.1X4	—	—
Diemal	T42.3X1	T42.3X2	T42.3X3	T42.3X4	T42.3X5	T42.3X6
Dienestrol	T38.5X1	T38.5X2	T38.5X3	T38.5X4	T38.5X5	T38.5X6
Dienoestrol	T38.5X1	T38.5X2	T38.5X3	T38.5X4	T38.5X5	T38.5X6
Dietetic drug NEC	T50.901	T50.902	T50.903	T50.904	T50.905	T50.906
Diethazine	T42.8X1	T42.8X2	T42.8X3	T42.8X4	T42.8X5	T42.8X6
Diethyl						
barbituric acid	T42.3X1	T42.3X2	T42.3X3	T42.3X4	T42.3X5	T42.3X6
carbamazine	T37.4X1	T37.4X2	T37.4X3	T37.4X4	T37.4X5	T37.4X6
carbinol	T51.3X1	T51.3X2	T51.3X3	T51.3X4	—	—

Substance	Poisoning, Accidental (unintentional)	Poisoning, Intentional Self-harm	Poisoning, Assault	Poisoning, Undetermined	Adverse Effect	Under-dosing
Diethyl — continued						
carbonate	T52.8X1	T52.8X2	T52.8X3	T52.8X4	—	—
ether (vapor) — see also ether	T41.0X1	T41.0X2	T41.0X3	T41.0X4	T41.0X5	T41.0X6
oxide	T52.8X1	T52.8X2	T52.8X3	T52.8X4	—	—
propion	T50.5X1	T50.5X2	T50.5X3	T50.5X4	T50.5X5	T50.5X6
stilbestrol	T38.5X1	T38.5X2	T38.5X3	T38.5X4	T38.5X5	T38.5X6
toluamide (nonmedicinal)	T60.8X1	T60.8X2	T60.8X3	T60.8X4	—	—
medicinal	T49.3X1	T49.3X2	T49.3X3	T49.3X4	T49.3X5	T49.3X6
Diethylcarbamazine	T37.4X1	T37.4X2	T37.4X3	T37.4X4	T37.4X5	T37.4X6
Diethylene						
dioxide	T52.8X1	T52.8X2	T52.8X3	T52.8X4	—	—
glycol (monoacetate) (monobutyl ether) (monoethyl ether)	T52.3X1	T52.3X2	T52.3X3	T52.3X4	—	—
Diethylhexylphthalate	T65.891	T65.892	T65.893	T65.894	—	—
Diethylpropion	T50.5X1	T50.5X2	T50.5X3	T50.5X4	T50.5X5	T50.5X6
Diethylstilbestrol	T38.5X1	T38.5X2	T38.5X3	T38.5X4	T38.5X5	T38.5X6
Diethylstilboestrol	T38.5X1	T38.5X2	T38.5X3	T38.5X4	T38.5X5	T38.5X6
Diethylsulfone-diethylmethane	T42.6X1	T42.6X2	T42.6X3	T42.6X4	T42.6X5	T42.6X6
Diethyltoluamide	T49.0X1	T49.0X2	T49.0X3	T49.0X4	T49.0X5	T49.0X6
Diethyltryptamine (DET)	T40.991	T40.992	T40.993	T40.994	—	—
Difebarbamate	T42.3X1	T42.3X2	T42.3X3	T42.3X4	T42.3X5	T42.3X6
Difencloxazine	T40.2X1	T40.2X2	T40.2X3	T40.2X4	T40.2X5	T40.2X6
Difenidol	T45.0X1	T45.0X2	T45.0X3	T45.0X4	T45.0X5	T45.0X6
Difenoxin	T47.6X1	T47.6X2	T47.6X3	T47.6X4	T47.6X5	T47.6X6
Difetarsone	T37.3X1	T37.3X2	T37.3X3	T37.3X4	T37.3X5	T37.3X6
Diffusin	T45.3X1	T45.3X2	T45.3X3	T45.3X4	T45.3X5	T45.3X6
Diflorasone	T49.0X1	T49.0X2	T49.0X3	T49.0X4	T49.0X5	T49.0X6
Diflos	T44.0X1	T44.0X2	T44.0X3	T44.0X4	T44.0X5	T44.0X6
Diflubenzuron	T60.1X1	T60.1X2	T60.1X3	T60.1X4	—	—
Diflucortolone	T49.0X1	T49.0X2	T49.0X3	T49.0X4	T49.0X5	T49.0X6
Diflunisal	T39.091	T39.092	T39.093	T39.094	T39.095	T39.096
Difluoromethyldopa	T42.8X1	T42.8X2	T42.8X3	T42.8X4	T42.8X5	T42.8X6
Difluorophate	T44.0X1	T44.0X2	T44.0X3	T44.0X4	T44.0X5	T44.0X6
Digestant NEC	T47.5X1	T47.5X2	T47.5X3	T47.5X4	T47.5X5	T47.5X6
Digitalin (e)	T46.0X1	T46.0X2	T46.0X3	T46.0X4	T46.0X5	T46.0X6
Digitalis (leaf)(glycoside)	T46.0X1	T46.0X2	T46.0X3	T46.0X4	T46.0X5	T46.0X6
lanata	T46.0X1	T46.0X2	T46.0X3	T46.0X4	T46.0X5	T46.0X6
purpurea	T46.0X1	T46.0X2	T46.0X3	T46.0X4	T46.0X5	T46.0X6
Digitoxin	T46.0X1	T46.0X2	T46.0X3	T46.0X4	T46.0X5	T46.0X6
Digitoxose	T46.0X1	T46.0X2	T46.0X3	T46.0X4	T46.0X5	T46.0X6
Digoxin	T46.0X1	T46.0X2	T46.0X3	T46.0X4	T46.0X5	T46.0X6
Digoxine	T46.0X1	T46.0X2	T46.0X3	T46.0X4	T46.0X5	T46.0X6
Dihydralazine	T46.5X1	T46.5X2	T46.5X3	T46.5X4	T46.5X5	T46.5X6
Dihydrazine	T46.5X1	T46.5X2	T46.5X3	T46.5X4	T46.5X5	T46.5X6
Dihydrocodeine	T40.2X1	T40.2X2	T40.2X3	T40.2X4	T40.2X5	T40.2X6
Dihydrocodeinone	T40.2X1	T40.2X2	T40.2X3	T40.2X4	T40.2X5	T40.2X6
Dihydroergocornine	T46.7X1	T46.7X2	T46.7X3	T46.7X4	T46.7X5	T46.7X6
Dihydroergocristine (mesilate)	T46.7X1	T46.7X2	T46.7X3	T46.7X4	T46.7X5	T46.7X6
Dihydroergokryptine	T46.7X1	T46.7X2	T46.7X3	T46.7X4	T46.7X5	T46.7X6
Dihydroergotamine	T46.5X1	T46.5X2	T46.5X3	T46.5X4	T46.5X5	T46.5X6
Dihydroergotoxine	T46.7X1	T46.7X2	T46.7X3	T46.7X4	T46.7X5	T46.7X6
mesilate	T46.7X1	T46.7X2	T46.7X3	T46.7X4	T46.7X5	T46.7X6
Dihydrohydroxycodeinone	T40.2X1	T40.2X2	T40.2X3	T40.2X4	T40.2X5	T40.2X6
Dihydrohydroxymorphinone	T40.2X1	T40.2X2	T40.2X3	T40.2X4	T40.2X5	T40.2X6
Dihydroisocodeine	T40.2X1	T40.2X2	T40.2X3	T40.2X4	T40.2X5	T40.2X6
Dihydromorphine	T40.2X1	T40.2X2	T40.2X3	T40.2X4	—	—
Dihydromorphinone	T40.2X1	T40.2X2	T40.2X3	T40.2X4	T40.2X5	T40.2X6
Dihydrostreptomycin	T36.5X1	T36.5X2	T36.5X3	T36.5X4	T36.5X5	T36.5X6
Dihydrotachysterol	T45.2X1	T45.2X2	T45.2X3	T45.2X4	T45.2X5	T45.2X6
Dihydroxyaluminum aminoacetate	T47.1X1	T47.1X2	T47.1X3	T47.1X4	T47.1X5	T47.1X6
Dihydroxyaluminum sodium carbonate	T47.1X1	T47.1X2	T47.1X3	T47.1X4	T47.1X5	T47.1X6
Dihydroxyanthraquinone	T47.2X1	T47.2X2	T47.2X3	T47.2X4	T47.2X5	T47.2X6
Dihydroxycodeinone	T40.2X1	T40.2X2	T40.2X3	T40.2X4	T40.2X5	T40.2X6
Dihydroxypropyl theophylline	T50.2X1	T50.2X2	T50.2X3	T50.2X4	T50.2X5	T50.2X6
Diiodohydroxyquin	T37.8X1	T37.8X2	T37.8X3	T37.8X4	T37.8X5	T37.8X6
topical	T49.0X1	T49.0X2	T49.0X3	T49.0X4	T49.0X5	T49.0X6
Diiodohydroxyquinoline	T37.8X1	T37.8X2	T37.8X3	T37.8X4	T37.8X5	T37.8X6
Diiodotyrosine	T38.2X1	T38.2X2	T38.2X3	T38.2X4	T38.2X5	T38.2X6
Diisopromine	T44.3X1	T44.3X2	T44.3X3	T44.3X4	T44.3X5	T44.3X6
Diisopropylamine	T46.3X1	T46.3X2	T46.3X3	T46.3X4	T46.3X5	T46.3X6
Diisopropylfluorophosphonate	T44.0X1	T44.0X2	T44.0X3	T44.0X4	T44.0X5	T44.0X6
Dilantin	T42.0X1	T42.0X2	T42.0X3	T42.0X4	T42.0X5	T42.0X6
Dilaudid	T40.2X1	T40.2X2	T40.2X3	T40.2X4	T40.2X5	T40.2X6
Dilazep	T46.3X1	T46.3X2	T46.3X3	T46.3X4	T46.3X5	T46.3X6
Dill	T47.5X1	T47.5X2	T47.5X3	T47.5X4	T47.5X5	T47.5X6
Diloxanide	T37.3X1	T37.3X2	T37.3X3	T37.3X4	T37.3X5	T37.3X6
Diltiazem	T46.1X1	T46.1X2	T46.1X3	T46.1X4	T46.1X5	T46.1X6

Substance	Poisoning, Accidental (unintentional)	Poisoning, Intentional Self-harm	Poisoning, Assault	Poisoning, Undetermined	Adverse Effect	Under-dosing
Dimazole	T49.0X1	T49.0X2	T49.0X3	T49.0X4	T49.0X5	T49.0X6
Dimefline	T50.7X1	T50.7X2	T50.7X3	T50.7X4	T50.7X5	T50.7X6
Dimefox	T60.0X1	T60.0X2	T60.0X3	T60.0X4	—	—
Dimemorfan	T48.3X1	T48.3X2	T48.3X3	T48.3X4	T48.3X5	T48.3X6
Dimenhydrinate	T45.0X1	T45.0X2	T45.0X3	T45.0X4	T45.0X5	T45.0X6
Dimercaprol (British anti-lewisite)	T45.8X1	T45.8X2	T45.8X3	T45.8X4	T45.8X5	T45.8X6
Dimercaptopropanol	T45.8X1	T45.8X2	T45.8X3	T45.8X4	T45.8X5	T45.8X6
Dimestrol	T38.5X1	T38.5X2	T38.5X3	T38.5X4	T38.5X5	T38.5X6
Dimetane	T45.0X1	T45.0X2	T45.0X3	T45.0X4	T45.0X5	T45.0X6
Dimethicone	T47.1X1	T47.1X2	T47.1X3	T47.1X4	T47.1X5	T47.1X6
Dimethindene	T45.0X1	T45.0X2	T45.0X3	T45.0X4	T45.0X5	T45.0X6
Dimethisoquin	T49.1X1	T49.1X2	T49.1X3	T49.1X4	T49.1X5	T49.1X6
Dimethisterone	T38.5X1	T38.5X2	T38.5X3	T38.5X4	T38.5X5	T38.5X6
Dimethoate	T60.0X1	T60.0X2	T60.0X3	T60.0X4	—	—
Dimethocaine	T41.3X1	T41.3X2	T41.3X3	T41.3X4	T41.3X5	T41.3X6
Dimethoxanate	T48.3X1	T48.3X2	T48.3X3	T48.3X4	T48.3X5	T48.3X6
Dimethyl						
arsine, arsinic acid	T57.0X1	T57.0X2	T57.0X3	T57.0X4	—	—
carbinol	T51.2X1	T51.2X2	T51.2X3	T51.2X4	—	—
carbonate	T52.8X1	T52.8X2	T52.8X3	T52.8X4	—	—
diguanide	T38.3X1	T38.3X2	T38.3X3	T38.3X4	T38.3X5	T38.3X6
ketone	T52.4X1	T52.4X2	T52.4X3	T52.4X4	—	—
vapor	T52.4X1	T52.4X2	T52.4X3	T52.4X4	—	—
meperidine	T40.2X1	T40.2X2	T40.2X3	T40.2X4	T40.2X5	T40.2X6
parathion	T60.0X1	T60.0X2	T60.0X3	T60.0X4	—	—
phthlate	T49.3X1	T49.3X2	T49.3X3	T49.3X4	T49.3X5	T49.3X6
polysiloxane	T47.8X1	T47.8X2	T47.8X3	T47.8X4	T47.8X5	T47.8X6
sulfate (fumes)	T59.891	T59.892	T59.893	T59.894	—	—
liquid	T65.891	T65.892	T65.893	T65.894	—	—
sulfoxide (nonmedicinal)	T52.8X1	T52.8X2	T52.8X3	T52.8X4	—	—
medicinal	T49.4X1	T49.4X2	T49.4X3	T49.4X4	T49.4X5	T49.4X6
tryptamine	T40.991	T40.992	T40.993	T40.994	—	—
tubocurarine	T48.1X1	T48.1X2	T48.1X3	T48.1X4	T48.1X5	T48.1X6
Dimethylamine sulfate	T49.4X1	T49.4X2	T49.4X3	T49.4X4	T49.4X5	T49.4X6
Dimethylformamide	T52.8X1	T52.8X2	T52.8X3	T52.8X4	—	—
Dimethyltubocurarinium chloride	T48.1X1	T48.1X2	T48.1X3	T48.1X4	T48.1X5	T48.1X6
Dimeticone	T47.1X1	T47.1X2	T47.1X3	T47.1X4	T47.1X5	T47.1X6
Dimetilan	T60.0X1	T60.0X2	T60.0X3	T60.0X4	—	—
Dimetindene	T45.0X1	T45.0X2	T45.0X3	T45.0X4	T45.0X5	T45.0X6
Dimetotiazine	T43.3X1	T43.3X2	T43.3X3	T43.3X4	T43.3X5	T43.3X6
Dimorpholamine	T50.7X1	T50.7X2	T50.7X3	T50.7X4	T50.7X5	T50.7X6
Dimoxyline	T46.3X1	T46.3X2	T46.3X3	T46.3X4	T46.3X5	T46.3X6
Dinitrobenzene	T65.3X1	T65.3X2	T65.3X3	T65.3X4	—	—
vapor	T59.891	T59.892	T59.893	T59.894	—	—
Dinitrobenzol	T65.3X1	T65.3X2	T65.3X3	T65.3X4	—	—
vapor	T59.891	T59.892	T59.893	T59.894	—	—
Dinitrobutylphenol	T65.3X1	T65.3X2	T65.3X3	T65.3X4	—	—
Dinitro (-ortho-)cresol (pesticide) (spray)	T65.3X1	T65.3X2	T65.3X3	T65.3X4	—	—
Dinitrocyclohexylphenol	T65.3X1	T65.3X2	T65.3X3	T65.3X4	—	—
Dinitrophenol	T65.3X1	T65.3X2	T65.3X3	T65.3X4	—	—
Dinoprost	T48.0X1	T48.0X2	T48.0X3	T48.0X4	T48.0X5	T48.0X6
Dinoprostone	T48.0X1	T48.0X2	T48.0X3	T48.0X4	T48.0X5	T48.0X6
Dinoseb	T60.3X1	T60.3X2	T60.3X3	T60.3X4	—	—
Dioctyl sulfosuccinate (calcium) (sodium)	T47.4X1	T47.4X2	T47.4X3	T47.4X4	T47.4X5	T47.4X6
Diodone	T50.8X1	T50.8X2	T50.8X3	T50.8X4	T50.8X5	T50.8X6
Diodoquin	T37.8X1	T37.8X2	T37.8X3	T37.8X4	T37.8X5	T37.8X6
Dionin	T40.2X1	T40.2X2	T40.2X3	T40.2X4	T40.2X5	T40.2X6
Diosmin	T46.991	T46.992	T46.993	T46.994	T46.995	T46.996
Dioxane	T52.8X1	T52.8X2	T52.8X3	T52.8X4	—	—
Dioxathion	T60.0X1	T60.0X2	T60.0X3	T60.0X4	—	—
Dioxin	T53.7X1	T53.7X2	T53.7X3	T53.7X4	—	—
Dioxopromethazine	T43.3X1	T43.3X2	T43.3X3	T43.3X4	T43.3X5	T43.3X6
Dioxyline	T46.3X1	T46.3X2	T46.3X3	T46.3X4	T46.3X5	T46.3X6
Dipentene	T52.8X1	T52.8X2	T52.8X3	T52.8X4	—	—
Diperodon	T41.3X1	T41.3X2	T41.3X3	T41.3X4	T41.3X5	T41.3X6
Diphacinone	T60.4X1	T60.4X2	T60.4X3	T60.4X4	—	—
Diphemanil	T44.3X1	T44.3X2	T44.3X3	T44.3X4	T44.3X5	T44.3X6
metilsulfate	T44.3X1	T44.3X2	T44.3X3	T44.3X4	T44.3X5	T44.3X6
Diphenadione	T45.511	T45.512	T45.513	T45.514	T45.515	T45.516
rodenticide	T60.4X1	T60.4X2	T60.4X3	T60.4X4	—	—
Diphenhydramine	T45.0X1	T45.0X2	T45.0X3	T45.0X4	T45.0X5	T45.0X6
Diphenidol	T45.0X1	T45.0X2	T45.0X3	T45.0X4	T45.0X5	T45.0X6
Diphenoxylate	T47.6X1	T47.6X2	T47.6X3	T47.6X4	T47.6X5	T47.6X6
Diphenylamine	T65.3X1	T65.3X2	T65.3X3	T65.3X4	—	—
Diphenylbutazone	T39.2X1	T39.2X2	T39.2X3	T39.2X4	T39.2X5	T39.2X6
Diphenylchlorarsine, not in war	T57.0X1	T57.0X2	T57.0X3	T57.0X4	—	—
Diphenylhydantoin	T42.0X1	T42.0X2	T42.0X3	T42.0X4	T42.0X5	T42.0X6
Diphenylmethane dye	T52.1X1	T52.1X2	T52.1X3	T52.1X4	—	—

Substance	Poisoning, Accidental (unintentional)	Poisoning, Intentional Self-harm	Poisoning, Assault	Poisoning, Undetermined	Adverse Effect	Under-dosing
Diphenylpyraline	T45.0X1	T45.0X2	T45.0X3	T45.0X4	T45.0X5	T45.0X6
Diphtheria						
antitoxin	T50.Z11	T50.Z12	T50.Z13	T50.Z14	T50.Z15	T50.Z16
toxoid	T50.A91	T50.A92	T50.A93	T50.A94	T50.A95	T50.A96
with tetanus toxoid	T50.A21	T50.A22	T50.A23	T50.A24	T50.A25	T50.A26
with pertussis component	T50.A11	T50.A12	T50.A13	T50.A14	T50.A15	T50.A16
vaccine	T50.A91	T50.A92	T50.A93	T50.A94	T50.A95	T50.A96
combination						
without pertussis	T50.A21	T50.A22	T50.A23	T50.A24	T50.A25	T50.A26
including pertussis	T50.A11	T50.A12	T50.A13	T50.A14	T50.A15	T50.A16
Diphylline	T50.2X1	T50.2X2	T50.2X3	T50.2X4	T50.2X5	T50.2X6
Dipipanone	T40.4X1	T40.4X2	T40.4X3	T40.4X4	—	—
Dipivefrine	T49.5X1	T49.5X2	T49.5X3	T49.5X4	T49.5X5	T49.5X6
Diplovax	T50.B91	T50.B92	T50.B93	T50.B94	T50.B95	T50.B96
Diprophylline	T50.2X1	T50.2X2	T50.2X3	T50.2X4	T50.2X5	T50.2X6
Dipropyline	T48.291	T48.292	T48.293	T48.294	T48.295	T48.296
Dipyridamole	T46.3X1	T46.3X2	T46.3X3	T46.3X4	T46.3X5	T46.3X6
Dipyrone	T39.2X1	T39.2X2	T39.2X3	T39.2X4	T39.2X5	T39.2X6
Diquat (dibromide)	T60.3X1	T60.3X2	T60.3X3	T60.3X4	—	—
Disinfectant	T65.891	T65.892	T65.893	T65.894	—	—
alkaline	T54.3X1	T54.3X2	T54.3X3	T54.3X4	—	—
aromatic	T54.1X1	T54.1X2	T54.1X3	T54.1X4	—	—
intestinal	T37.8X1	T37.8X2	T37.8X3	T37.8X4	T37.8X5	T37.8X6
Disipal	T42.8X1	T42.8X2	T42.8X3	T42.8X4	T42.8X5	T42.8X6
Disodium edetate	T50.6X1	T50.6X2	T50.6X3	T50.6X4	T50.6X5	T50.6X6
Disoprofol	T41.291	T41.292	T41.293	T41.294	T41.295	T41.296
Disopyramide	T46.2X1	T46.2X2	T46.2X3	T46.2X4	T46.2X5	T46.2X6
Distigmine (bromide)	T44.0X1	T44.0X2	T44.0X3	T44.0X4	T44.0X5	T44.0X6
Disulfamide	T50.2X1	T50.2X2	T50.2X3	T50.2X4	T50.2X5	T50.2X6
Disulfanilamide	T37.0X1	T37.0X2	T37.0X3	T37.0X4	T37.0X5	T37.0X6
Disulfiram	T50.6X1	T50.6X2	T50.6X3	T50.6X4	T50.6X5	T50.6X6
Disulfoton	T60.0X1	T60.0X2	T60.0X3	T60.0X4	—	—
Dithiazanine iodide	T37.4X1	T37.4X2	T37.4X3	T37.4X4	T37.4X5	T37.4X6
Dithiocarbamate	T60.0X1	T60.0X2	T60.0X3	T60.0X4	—	—
Dithranol	T49.4X1	T49.4X2	T49.4X3	T49.4X4	T49.4X5	T49.4X6
Diucardin	T50.2X1	T50.2X2	T50.2X3	T50.2X4	T50.2X5	T50.2X6
Diupres	T50.2X1	T50.2X2	T50.2X3	T50.2X4	T50.2X5	T50.2X6
Diuretic NEC	T50.2X1	T50.2X2	T50.2X3	T50.2X4	T50.2X5	T50.2X6
benzothiadiazine	T50.2X1	T50.2X2	T50.2X3	T50.2X4	T50.2X5	T50.2X6
carbonic acid anhydrase inhibitors	T50.2X1	T50.2X2	T50.2X3	T50.2X4	T50.2X5	T50.2X6
furfuryl NEC	T50.2X1	T50.2X2	T50.2X3	T50.2X4	T50.2X5	T50.2X6
loop (high-ceiling)	T50.1X1	T50.1X2	T50.1X3	T50.1X4	T50.1X5	T50.1X6
mercurial NEC	T50.2X1	T50.2X2	T50.2X3	T50.2X4	T50.2X5	T50.2X6
osmotic	T50.2X1	T50.2X2	T50.2X3	T50.2X4	T50.2X5	T50.2X6
purine NEC	T50.2X1	T50.2X2	T50.2X3	T50.2X4	T50.2X5	T50.2X6
saluretic NEC	T50.2X1	T50.2X2	T50.2X3	T50.2X4	T50.2X5	T50.2X6
sulfonamide	T50.2X1	T50.2X2	T50.2X3	T50.2X4	T50.2X5	T50.2X6
thiazide NEC	T50.2X1	T50.2X2	T50.2X3	T50.2X4	T50.2X5	T50.2X6
xanthine	T50.2X1	T50.2X2	T50.2X3	T50.2X4	T50.2X5	T50.2X6
Diurgin	T50.2X1	T50.2X2	T50.2X3	T50.2X4	T50.2X5	T50.2X6
Diuril	T50.2X1	T50.2X2	T50.2X3	T50.2X4	T50.2X5	T50.2X6
Diuron	T60.3X1	T60.3X2	T60.3X3	T60.3X4	—	—
Divalproex	T42.6X1	T42.6X2	T42.6X3	T42.6X4	T42.6X5	T42.6X6
Divinyl ether	T41.0X1	T41.0X2	T41.0X3	T41.0X4	T41.0X5	T41.0X6
Dixanthogen	T49.0X1	T49.0X2	T49.0X3	T49.0X4	T49.0X5	T49.0X6
Dixyrazine	T43.3X1	T43.3X2	T43.3X3	T43.3X4	T43.3X5	T43.3X6
D-lysergic acid diethylamide	T40.8X1	T40.8X2	T40.8X3	T40.8X4	—	—
DMCT	T36.4X1	T36.4X2	T36.4X3	T36.4X4	T36.4X5	T36.4X6
DMSO — see Dimethyl sulfoxide						
DNBP	T60.3X1	T60.3X2	T60.3X3	T60.3X4	—	—
DNOC	T65.3X1	T65.3X2	T65.3X3	T65.3X4	—	—
Dobutamine	T44.5X1	T44.5X2	T44.5X3	T44.5X4	T44.5X5	T44.5X6
DOCA	T38.0X1	T38.0X2	T38.0X3	T38.0X4	T38.0X5	T38.0X6
Docusate sodium	T47.4X1	T47.4X2	T47.4X3	T47.4X4	T47.4X5	T47.4X6
Dodicin	T49.0X1	T49.0X2	T49.0X3	T49.0X4	T49.0X5	T49.0X6
Dofamium chloride	T49.0X1	T49.0X2	T49.0X3	T49.0X4	T49.0X5	T49.0X6
Dolophine	T40.3X1	T40.3X2	T40.3X3	T40.3X4	T40.3X5	T40.3X6
Doloxene	T39.8X1	T39.8X2	T39.8X3	T39.8X4	T39.8X5	T39.8X6
Domestic gas (after combustion) — see Gas, utility						
prior to combustion	T59.891	T59.892	T59.893	T59.894	—	—
Domiodol	T48.4X1	T48.4X2	T48.4X3	T48.4X4	T48.4X5	T48.4X6
Domiphen (bromide)	T49.0X1	T49.0X2	T49.0X3	T49.0X4	T49.0X5	T49.0X6
Domperidone	T45.0X1	T45.0X2	T45.0X3	T45.0X4	T45.0X5	T45.0X6
Dopa	T42.8X1	T42.8X2	T42.8X3	T42.8X4	T42.8X5	T42.8X6
Dopamine	T44.991	T44.992	T44.993	T44.994	T44.995	T44.996
Doriden	T42.6X1	T42.6X2	T42.6X3	T42.6X4	T42.6X5	T42.6X6
Dormiral	T42.3X1	T42.3X2	T42.3X3	T42.3X4	T42.3X5	T42.3X6
Dormison	T42.6X1	T42.6X2	T42.6X3	T42.6X4	T42.6X5	T42.6X6
Dornase	T48.4X1	T48.4X2	T48.4X3	T48.4X4	T48.4X5	T48.4X6

Table of Drugs and Chemicals

Dorsacaine — Esmolol

Substance	Poisoning, Accidental (unintentional)	Poisoning, Intentional Self-harm	Poisoning, Assault	Poisoning, Undetermined	Adverse Effect	Under-dosing
Dorsacaine	T41.3X1	T41.3X2	T41.3X3	T41.3X4	T41.3X5	T41.3X6
Dosulepin	T43.011	T43.012	T43.013	T43.014	T43.015	T43.016
Dothiepin	T43.011	T43.012	T43.013	T43.014	T43.015	T43.016
Doxantrazole	T48.6X1	T48.6X2	T48.6X3	T48.6X4	T48.6X5	T48.6X6
Doxapram	T50.7X1	T50.7X2	T50.7X3	T50.7X4	T50.7X5	T50.7X6
Doxazosin	T44.6X1	T44.6X2	T44.6X3	T44.6X4	T44.6X5	T44.6X6
Doxepin	T43.011	T43.012	T43.013	T43.014	T43.015	T43.016
Doxifluridine	T45.1X1	T45.1X2	T45.1X3	T45.1X4	T45.1X5	T45.1X6
Doxorubicin	T45.1X1	T45.1X2	T45.1X3	T45.1X4	T45.1X5	T45.1X6
Doxycycline	T36.4X1	T36.4X2	T36.4X3	T36.4X4	T36.4X5	T36.4X6
Doxylamine	T45.0X1	T45.0X2	T45.0X3	T45.0X4	T45.0X5	T45.0X6
Dramamine	T45.0X1	T45.0X2	T45.0X3	T45.0X4	T45.0X5	T45.0X6
Drano (drain cleaner)	T54.3X1	T54.3X2	T54.3X3	T54.3X4	—	—
Dressing, live pulp	T49.7X1	T49.7X2	T49.7X3	T49.7X4	T49.7X5	T49.7X6
Drocode	T40.2X1	T40.2X2	T40.2X3	T40.2X4	T40.2X5	T40.2X6
Dromoran	T40.2X1	T40.2X2	T40.2X3	T40.2X4	T40.2X5	T40.2X6
Dromostanolone	T38.7X1	T38.7X2	T38.7X3	T38.7X4	T38.7X5	T38.7X6
Dronabinol	T40.7X1	T40.7X2	T40.7X3	T40.7X4	T40.7X5	T40.7X6
Droperidol	T43.591	T43.592	T43.593	T43.594	T43.595	T43.596
Dropropizine	T48.3X1	T48.3X2	T48.3X3	T48.3X4	T48.3X5	T48.3X6
Drostanolone	T38.7X1	T38.7X2	T38.7X3	T38.7X4	T38.7X5	T38.7X6
Drotaverine	T44.3X1	T44.3X2	T44.3X3	T44.3X4	T44.3X5	T44.3X6
Drotrecogin alfa	T45.511	T45.512	T45.513	T45.514	T45.515	T45.516
Drug NEC	T50.901	T50.902	T50.903	T50.904	T50.905	T50.906
specified NEC	T50.991	T50.992	T50.993	T50.994	T50.995	T50.996
DTIC	T45.1X1	T45.1X2	T45.1X3	T45.1X4	T45.1X5	T45.1X6
Duboisine	T44.3X1	T44.3X2	T44.3X3	T44.3X4	T44.3X5	T44.3X6
Dulcolax	T47.2X1	T47.2X2	T47.2X3	T47.2X4	T47.2X5	T47.2X6
Duponol (C) (EP)	T49.2X1	T49.2X2	T49.2X3	T49.2X4	T49.2X5	T49.2X6
Durabolin	T38.7X1	T38.7X2	T38.7X3	T38.7X4	T38.7X5	T38.7X6
Dyclone	T41.3X1	T41.3X2	T41.3X3	T41.3X4	T41.3X5	T41.3X6
Dyclonine	T41.3X1	T41.3X2	T41.3X3	T41.3X4	T41.3X5	T41.3X6
Dydrogesterone	T38.5X1	T38.5X2	T38.5X3	T38.5X4	T38.5X5	T38.5X6
Dye NEC	T65.6X1	T65.6X2	T65.6X3	T65.6X4	—	—
antiseptic	T49.0X1	T49.0X2	T49.0X3	T49.0X4	T49.0X5	T49.0X6
diagnostic agents	T50.8X1	T50.8X2	T50.8X3	T50.8X4	T50.8X5	T50.8X6
pharmaceutical NEC	T50.901	T50.902	T50.903	T50.904	T50.905	T50.906
Dyflos	T44.0X1	T44.0X2	T44.0X3	T44.0X4	T44.0X5	T44.0X6
Dymelor	T38.3X1	T38.3X2	T38.3X3	T38.3X4	T38.3X5	T38.3X6
Dynamite	T65.3X1	T65.3X2	T65.3X3	T65.3X4	—	—
fumes	T59.891	T59.892	T59.893	T59.894	—	—
Dyphylline	T44.3X1	T44.3X2	T44.3X3	T44.3X4	T44.3X5	T44.3X6
b-eucaine	T49.1X1	T49.1X2	T49.1X3	T49.1X4	T49.1X5	T49.1X6
Ear drug NEC	T49.6X1	T49.6X2	T49.6X3	T49.6X4	T49.6X5	T49.6X6
Ear preparations	T49.6X1	T49.6X2	T49.6X3	T49.6X4	T49.6X5	T49.6X6
Echothiophate, echothiopate, ecothiopate	T49.5X1	T49.5X2	T49.5X3	T49.5X4	T49.5X5	T49.5X6
Econazole	T49.0X1	T49.0X2	T49.0X3	T49.0X4	T49.0X5	T49.0X6
Ecothiopate iodide	T49.5X1	T49.5X2	T49.5X3	T49.5X4	T49.5X5	T49.5X6
Ecstasy	T43.621	T43.622	T43.623	T43.624	T43.625	T43.626
Ectylurea	T42.6X1	T42.6X2	T42.6X3	T42.6X4	T42.6X5	T42.6X6
Edathamil disodium	T45.8X1	T45.8X2	T45.8X3	T45.8X4	T45.8X5	T45.8X6
Edecrin	T50.1X1	T50.1X2	T50.1X3	T50.1X4	T50.1X5	T50.1X6
Edetate, disodium (calcium)	T45.8X1	T45.8X2	T45.8X3	T45.8X4	T45.8X5	T45.8X6
Edoxudine	T49.5X1	T49.5X2	T49.5X3	T49.5X4	T49.5X5	T49.5X6
Edrophonium	T44.0X1	T44.0X2	T44.0X3	T44.0X4	T44.0X5	T44.0X6
chloride	T44.0X1	T44.0X2	T44.0X3	T44.0X4	T44.0X5	T44.0X6
EDTA	T50.6X1	T50.6X2	T50.6X3	T50.6X4	T50.6X5	T50.6X6
Eflornithine	T37.2X1	T37.2X2	T37.2X3	T37.2X4	T37.2X5	T37.2X6
Efloxate	T46.3X1	T46.3X2	T46.3X3	T46.3X4	T46.3X5	T46.3X6
Elase	T49.8X1	T49.8X2	T49.8X3	T49.8X4	T49.8X5	T49.8X6
Elastase	T47.5X1	T47.5X2	T47.5X3	T47.5X4	T47.5X5	T47.5X6
Elaterium	T47.2X1	T47.2X2	T47.2X3	T47.2X4	T47.2X5	T47.2X6
Elcatonin	T50.991	T50.992	T50.993	T50.994	T50.995	T50.996
Elder	T62.2X1	T62.2X2	T62.2X3	T62.2X4	—	—
berry, (unripe)	T62.1X1	T62.1X2	T62.1X3	T62.1X4	—	—
Electrolyte balance drug	T50.3X1	T50.3X2	T50.3X3	T50.3X4	T50.3X5	T50.3X6
Electrolytes NEC	T50.3X1	T50.3X2	T50.3X3	T50.3X4	T50.3X5	T50.3X6
Electrolytic agent NEC	T50.3X1	T50.3X2	T50.3X3	T50.3X4	T50.3X5	T50.3X6
Elemental diet	T50.901	T50.902	T50.903	T50.904	T50.905	T50.906
Elliptinium acetate	T45.1X1	T45.1X2	T45.1X3	T45.1X4	T45.1X5	T45.1X6
Embramine	T45.0X1	T45.0X2	T45.0X3	T45.0X4	T45.0X5	T45.0X6
Emepronium (salts)	T44.3X1	T44.3X2	T44.3X3	T44.3X4	T44.3X5	T44.3X6
bromide	T44.3X1	T44.3X2	T44.3X3	T44.3X4	T44.3X5	T44.3X6
Emetic NEC	T47.7X1	T47.7X2	T47.7X3	T47.7X4	T47.7X5	T47.7X6
Emetine	T37.3X1	T37.3X2	T37.3X3	T37.3X4	T37.3X5	T37.3X6
Emollient NEC	T49.3X1	T49.3X2	T49.3X3	T49.3X4	T49.3X5	T49.3X6
Emorfazone	T39.8X1	T39.8X2	T39.8X3	T39.8X4	T39.8X5	T39.8X6
Emylcamate	T43.591	T43.592	T43.593	T43.594	T43.595	T43.596
Enalapril	T46.4X1	T46.4X2	T46.4X3	T46.4X4	T46.4X5	T46.4X6
Enalaprilat	T46.4X1	T46.4X2	T46.4X3	T46.4X4	T46.4X5	T46.4X6
Encainide	T46.2X1	T46.2X2	T46.2X3	T46.2X4	T46.2X5	T46.2X6
Endocaine	T41.3X1	T41.3X2	T41.3X3	T41.3X4	T41.3X5	T41.3X6
Endosulfan	T60.2X1	T60.2X2	T60.2X3	T60.2X4	—	—
Endothall	T60.3X1	T60.3X2	T60.3X3	T60.3X4	—	—
Endralazine	T46.5X1	T46.5X2	T46.5X3	T46.5X4	T46.5X5	T46.5X6
Endrin	T60.1X1	T60.1X2	T60.1X3	T60.1X4	—	—
Enflurane	T41.0X1	T41.0X2	T41.0X3	T41.0X4	T41.0X5	T41.0X6
Enhexymal	T42.3X1	T42.3X2	T42.3X3	T42.3X4	T42.3X5	T42.3X6
Enocitabine	T45.1X1	T45.1X2	T45.1X3	T45.1X4	T45.1X5	T45.1X6
Enovid	T38.4X1	T38.4X2	T38.4X3	T38.4X4	T38.4X5	T38.4X6
Enoxacin	T36.8X1	T36.8X2	T36.8X3	T36.8X4	T36.8X5	T36.8X6
Enoxaparin (sodium)	T45.511	T45.512	T45.513	T45.514	T45.515	T45.516
Enpiprazole	T43.591	T43.592	T43.593	T43.594	T43.595	T43.596
Enprofylline	T48.6X1	T48.6X2	T48.6X3	T48.6X4	T48.6X5	T48.6X6
Enprostil	T47.1X1	T47.1X2	T47.1X3	T47.1X4	T47.1X5	T47.1X6
Enterogastrone	T38.891	T38.892	T38.893	T38.894	T38.895	T38.896
ENT preparations (anti-infectives)	T49.6X1	T49.6X2	T49.6X3	T49.6X4	T49.6X5	T49.6X6
Enviomycin	T36.8X1	T36.8X2	T36.8X3	T36.8X4	T36.8X5	T36.8X6
Enzodase	T45.3X1	T45.3X2	T45.3X3	T45.3X4	T45.3X5	T45.3X6
Enzyme NEC	T45.3X1	T45.3X2	T45.3X3	T45.3X4	T45.3X5	T45.3X6
depolymerizing	T49.8X1	T49.8X2	T49.8X3	T49.8X4	T49.8X5	T49.8X6
fibrolytic	T45.3X1	T45.3X2	T45.3X3	T45.3X4	T45.3X5	T45.3X6
gastric	T47.5X1	T47.5X2	T47.5X3	T47.5X4	T47.5X5	T47.5X6
intestinal	T47.5X1	T47.5X2	T47.5X3	T47.5X4	T47.5X5	T47.5X6
local action	T49.4X1	T49.4X2	T49.4X3	T49.4X4	T49.4X5	T49.4X6
proteolytic	T49.4X1	T49.4X2	T49.4X3	T49.4X4	T49.4X5	T49.4X6
thrombolytic	T45.3X1	T45.3X2	T45.3X3	T45.3X4	T45.3X5	T45.3X6
EPAB	T41.3X1	T41.3X2	T41.3X3	T41.3X4	T41.3X5	T41.3X6
Epanutin	T42.0X1	T42.0X2	T42.0X3	T42.0X4	T42.0X5	T42.0X6
Ephedra	T44.991	T44.992	T44.993	T44.994	T44.995	T44.996
Ephedrine	T44.991	T44.992	T44.993	T44.994	T44.995	T44.996
Epichlorhydrin, epichlorohydrin	T52.8X1	T52.8X2	T52.8X3	T52.8X4	—	—
Epicillin	T36.0X1	T36.0X2	T36.0X3	T36.0X4	T36.0X5	T36.0X6
Epiestriol	T38.5X1	T38.5X2	T38.5X3	T38.5X4	T38.5X5	T38.5X6
Epilim — see Sodium valproate						
Epimestrol	T38.5X1	T38.5X2	T38.5X3	T38.5X4	T38.5X5	T38.5X6
Epinephrine	T44.5X1	T44.5X2	T44.5X3	T44.5X4	T44.5X5	T44.5X6
Epirubicin	T45.1X1	T45.1X2	T45.1X3	T45.1X4	T45.1X5	T45.1X6
Epitiostanol	T38.7X1	T38.7X2	T38.7X3	T38.7X4	T38.7X5	T38.7X6
Epitizide	T50.2X1	T50.2X2	T50.2X3	T50.2X4	T50.2X5	T50.2X6
EPN	T60.0X1	T60.0X2	T60.0X3	T60.0X4	—	—
EPO	T45.8X1	T45.8X2	T45.8X3	T45.8X4	T45.8X5	T45.8X6
Epoetin alpha	T45.8X1	T45.8X2	T45.8X3	T45.8X4	T45.8X5	T45.8X6
Epomediol	T50.991	T50.992	T50.993	T50.994	T50.995	T50.996
Epoprostenol	T45.521	T45.522	T45.523	T45.524	T45.525	T45.526
Epoxy resin	T65.891	T65.892	T65.893	T65.894	—	—
Eprazinone	T48.4X1	T48.4X2	T48.4X3	T48.4X4	T48.4X5	T48.4X6
Epsilon aminocaproic acid	T45.621	T45.622	T45.623	T45.624	T45.625	T45.626
Epsom salt	T47.3X1	T47.3X2	T47.3X3	T47.3X4	T47.3X5	T47.3X6
Eptazocine	T40.4X1	T40.4X2	T40.4X3	T40.4X4	T40.4X5	T40.4X6
Equanil	T43.591	T43.592	T43.593	T43.594	T43.595	T43.596
Equisetum	T62.2X1	T62.2X2	T62.2X3	T62.2X4	—	—
diuretic	T50.2X1	T50.2X2	T50.2X3	T50.2X4	T50.2X5	T50.2X6
Ergobasine	T48.0X1	T48.0X2	T48.0X3	T48.0X4	T48.0X5	T48.0X6
Ergocalciferol	T45.2X1	T45.2X2	T45.2X3	T45.2X4	T45.2X5	T45.2X6
Ergoloid mesylates	T46.7X1	T46.7X2	T46.7X3	T46.7X4	T46.7X5	T46.7X6
Ergometrine	T48.0X1	T48.0X2	T48.0X3	T48.0X4	T48.0X5	T48.0X6
Ergonovine	T48.0X1	T48.0X2	T48.0X3	T48.0X4	T48.0X5	T48.0X6
Ergotamine	T46.5X1	T46.5X2	T46.5X3	T46.5X4	T46.5X5	T46.5X6
Ergotocine	T48.0X1	T48.0X2	T48.0X3	T48.0X4	T48.0X5	T48.0X6
Ergotrate	T48.0X1	T48.0X2	T48.0X3	T48.0X4	T48.0X5	T48.0X6
Ergot NEC	T64.81	T64.82	T64.83	T64.84	—	—
derivative	T48.0X1	T48.0X2	T48.0X3	T48.0X4	T48.0X5	T48.0X6
medicinal (alkaloids)	T48.0X1	T48.0X2	T48.0X3	T48.0X4	T48.0X5	T48.0X6
prepared	T48.0X1	T48.0X2	T48.0X3	T48.0X4	T48.0X5	T48.0X6
Eritrityl tetranitrate	T46.3X1	T46.3X2	T46.3X3	T46.3X4	T46.3X5	T46.3X6
Erythrityl tetranitrate	T46.3X1	T46.3X2	T46.3X3	T46.3X4	T46.3X5	T46.3X6
Erythrol tetranitrate	T46.3X1	T46.3X2	T46.3X3	T46.3X4	T46.3X5	T46.3X6
Erythromycin (salts)	T36.3X1	T36.3X2	T36.3X3	T36.3X4	T36.3X5	T36.3X6
ophthalmic preparation	T49.5X1	T49.5X2	T49.5X3	T49.5X4	T49.5X5	T49.5X6
topical NEC	T49.0X1	T49.0X2	T49.0X3	T49.0X4	T49.0X5	T49.0X6
Erythropoietin	T45.8X1	T45.8X2	T45.8X3	T45.8X4	T45.8X5	T45.8X6
human	T45.8X1	T45.8X2	T45.8X3	T45.8X4	T45.8X5	T45.8X6
Escin	T46.991	T46.992	T46.993	T46.994	T46.995	T46.996
Esculin	T45.2X1	T45.2X2	T45.2X3	T45.2X4	T45.2X5	T45.2X6
Esculoside	T45.2X1	T45.2X2	T45.2X3	T45.2X4	T45.2X5	T45.2X6
ESDT (ether-soluble tar distillate)	T49.1X1	T49.1X2	T49.1X3	T49.1X4	T49.1X5	T49.1X6
Eserine	T49.5X1	T49.5X2	T49.5X3	T49.5X4	T49.5X5	T49.5X6
Esflurbiprofen	T39.311	T39.312	T39.313	T39.314	T39.315	T39.316
Eskabarb	T42.3X1	T42.3X2	T42.3X3	T42.3X4	T42.3X5	T42.3X6
Eskalith	T43.8X1	T43.8X2	T43.8X3	T43.8X4	T43.8X5	T43.8X6
Esmolol	T44.7X1	T44.7X2	T44.7X3	T44.7X4	T44.7X5	T44.7X6

Substance	Poisoning, Accidental (unintentional)	Poisoning, Intentional Self-harm	Poisoning, Assault	Poisoning, Undetermined	Adverse Effect	Underdosing
Estanozolol	T38.7X1	T38.7X2	T38.7X3	T38.7X4	T38.7X5	T38.7X6
Estazolam	T42.4X1	T42.4X2	T42.4X3	T42.4X4	T42.4X5	T42.4X6
Estradiol	T38.5X1	T38.5X2	T38.5X3	T38.5X4	T38.5X5	T38.5X6
with testosterone	T38.7X1	T38.7X2	T38.7X3	T38.7X4	T38.7X5	T38.7X6
benzoate	T38.5X1	T38.5X2	T38.5X3	T38.5X4	T38.5X5	T38.5X6
Estramustine	T45.1X1	T45.1X2	T45.1X3	T45.1X4	T45.1X5	T45.1X6
Estriol	T38.5X1	T38.5X2	T38.5X3	T38.5X4	T38.5X5	T38.5X6
Estrogen	T38.5X1	T38.5X2	T38.5X3	T38.5X4	T38.5X5	T38.5X6
with progesterone	T38.5X1	T38.5X2	T38.5X3	T38.5X4	T38.5X5	T38.5X6
conjugated	T38.5X1	T38.5X2	T38.5X3	T38.5X4	T38.5X5	T38.5X6
Estrone	T38.5X1	T38.5X2	T38.5X3	T38.5X4	T38.5X5	T38.5X6
Estropipate	T38.5X1	T38.5X2	T38.5X3	T38.5X4	T38.5X5	T38.5X6
Etacrynate sodium	T50.1X1	T50.1X2	T50.1X3	T50.1X4	T50.1X5	T50.1X6
Etacrynic acid	T50.1X1	T50.1X2	T50.1X3	T50.1X4	T50.1X5	T50.1X6
Etafedrine	T48.6X1	T48.6X2	T48.6X3	T48.6X4	T48.6X5	T48.6X6
Etafenone	T46.3X1	T46.3X2	T46.3X3	T46.3X4	T46.3X5	T46.3X6
Etambutol	T37.1X1	T37.1X2	T37.1X3	T37.1X4	T37.1X5	T37.1X6
Etamiphyllin	T48.6X1	T48.6X2	T48.6X3	T48.6X4	T48.6X5	T48.6X6
Etamivan	T50.7X1	T50.7X2	T50.7X3	T50.7X4	T50.7X5	T50.7X6
Etamsylate	T45.7X1	T45.7X2	T45.7X3	T45.7X4	T45.7X5	T45.7X6
Etebenecid	T50.4X1	T50.4X2	T50.4X3	T50.4X4	T50.4X5	T50.4X6
Ethacridine	T49.0X1	T49.0X2	T49.0X3	T49.0X4	T49.0X5	T49.0X6
Ethacrynic acid	T50.1X1	T50.1X2	T50.1X3	T50.1X4	T50.1X5	T50.1X6
Ethadione	T42.2X1	T42.2X2	T42.2X3	T42.2X4	T42.2X5	T42.2X6
Ethambutol	T37.1X1	T37.1X2	T37.1X3	T37.1X4	T37.1X5	T37.1X6
Ethamide	T50.2X1	T50.2X2	T50.2X3	T50.2X4	T50.2X5	T50.2X6
Ethamivan	T50.7X1	T50.7X2	T50.7X3	T50.7X4	T50.7X5	T50.7X6
Ethamsylate	T45.7X1	T45.7X2	T45.7X3	T45.7X4	T45.7X5	T45.7X6
Ethanol	T51.0X1	T51.0X2	T51.0X3	T51.0X4	—	—
beverage	T51.0X1	T51.0X2	T51.0X3	T51.0X4	—	—
Ethanolamine oleate	T46.8X1	T46.8X2	T46.8X3	T46.8X4	T46.8X5	T46.8X6
Ethaverine	T44.3X1	T44.3X2	T44.3X3	T44.3X4	T44.3X5	T44.3X6
Ethchlorvynol	T42.6X1	T42.6X2	T42.6X3	T42.6X4	T42.6X5	T42.6X6
Ethebenecid	T50.4X1	T50.4X2	T50.4X3	T50.4X4	T50.4X5	T50.4X6
Ether (vapor)	T41.0X1	T41.0X2	T41.0X3	T41.0X4	T41.0X5	T41.0X6
anesthetic	T41.0X1	T41.0X2	T41.0X3	T41.0X4	T41.0X5	T41.0X6
divinyl	T41.0X1	T41.0X2	T41.0X3	T41.0X4	T41.0X5	T41.0X6
ethyl (medicinal)	T41.0X1	T41.0X2	T41.0X3	T41.0X4	T41.0X5	T41.0X6
nonmedicinal	T52.8X1	T52.8X2	T52.8X3	T52.8X4	—	—
petroleum — see Ligroin						
solvent	T52.8X1	T52.8X2	T52.8X3	T52.8X4	—	—
Ethiazide	T50.2X1	T50.2X2	T50.2X3	T50.2X4	T50.2X5	T50.2X6
Ethidium chloride (vapor)	T59.891	T59.892	T59.893	T59.894	—	—
Ethinamate	T42.6X1	T42.6X2	T42.6X3	T42.6X4	T42.6X5	T42.6X6
Ethinylestradiol, ethinyloestradiol	T38.5X1	T38.5X2	T38.5X3	T38.5X4	T38.5X5	T38.5X6
with						
levonorgestrel	T38.4X1	T38.4X2	T38.4X3	T38.4X4	T38.4X5	T38.4X6
norethisterone	T38.4X1	T38.4X2	T38.4X3	T38.4X4	T38.4X5	T38.4X6
Ethiodized oil (131 I)	T50.8X1	T50.8X2	T50.8X3	T50.8X4	T50.8X5	T50.8X6
Ethion	T60.0X1	T60.0X2	T60.0X3	T60.0X4	—	—
Ethionamide	T37.1X1	T37.1X2	T37.1X3	T37.1X4	T37.1X5	T37.1X6
Ethioniamide	T37.1X1	T37.1X2	T37.1X3	T37.1X4	T37.1X5	T37.1X6
Ethisterone	T38.5X1	T38.5X2	T38.5X3	T38.5X4	T38.5X5	T38.5X6
Ethobral	T42.3X1	T42.3X2	T42.3X3	T42.3X4	T42.3X5	T42.3X6
Ethocaine (infiltration) (topical)	T41.3X1	T41.3X2	T41.3X3	T41.3X4	T41.3X5	T41.3X6
nerve block (peripheral) (plexus)	T41.3X1	T41.3X2	T41.3X3	T41.3X4	T41.3X5	T41.3X6
spinal	T41.3X1	T41.3X2	T41.3X3	T41.3X4	T41.3X5	T41.3X6
Ethoheptazine	T40.4X1	T40.4X2	T40.4X3	T40.4X4	T40.4X5	T40.4X6
Ethopropazine	T44.3X1	T44.3X2	T44.3X3	T44.3X4	T44.3X5	T44.3X6
Ethosuximide	T42.2X1	T42.2X2	T42.2X3	T42.2X4	T42.2X5	T42.2X6
Ethotoin	T42.0X1	T42.0X2	T42.0X3	T42.0X4	T42.0X5	T42.0X6
Ethoxazene	T37.91	T37.92	T37.93	T37.94	T37.95	T37.96
Ethoxazorutoside	T46.991	T46.992	T46.993	T46.994	T46.995	T46.996
Ethoxzolamide	T50.2X1	T50.2X2	T50.2X3	T50.2X4	T50.2X5	T50.2X6
Ethyl						
acetate	T52.8X1	T52.8X2	T52.8X3	T52.8X4	—	—
alcohol	T51.0X1	T51.0X2	T51.0X3	T51.0X4	—	—
beverage	T51.0X1	T51.0X2	T51.0X3	T51.0X4	—	—
aldehyde (vapor)	T59.891	T59.892	T59.893	T59.894	—	—
liquid	T52.8X1	T52.8X2	T52.8X3	T52.8X4	—	—
aminobenzoate	T41.3X1	T41.3X2	T41.3X3	T41.3X4	T41.3X5	T41.3X6
aminophenothiazine	T43.3X1	T43.3X2	T43.3X3	T43.3X4	T43.3X5	T43.3X6
benzoate	T52.8X1	T52.8X2	T52.8X3	T52.8X4	—	—
biscoumacetate	T45.511	T45.512	T45.513	T45.514	T45.515	T45.516
bromide (anesthetic)	T41.0X1	T41.0X2	T41.0X3	T41.0X4	T41.0X5	T41.0X6
carbamate	T45.1X1	T45.1X2	T45.1X3	T45.1X4	T45.1X5	T45.1X6
carbinol	T51.3X1	T51.3X2	T51.3X3	T51.3X4	—	—
carbonate	T52.8X1	T52.8X2	T52.8X3	T52.8X4	—	—
chaulmoograte	T37.1X1	T37.1X2	T37.1X3	T37.1X4	T37.1X5	T37.1X6
chloride (anesthetic)	T41.0X1	T41.0X2	T41.0X3	T41.0X4	T41.0X5	T41.0X6

Substance	Poisoning, Accidental (unintentional)	Poisoning, Intentional Self-harm	Poisoning, Assault	Poisoning, Undetermined	Adverse Effect	Underdosing
Ethyl — continued						
chloride — continued						
anesthetic (local)	T41.3X1	T41.3X2	T41.3X3	T41.3X4	T41.3X5	T41.3X6
inhaled	T41.0X1	T41.0X2	T41.0X3	T41.0X4	T41.0X5	T41.0X6
local	T49.4X1	T49.4X2	T49.4X3	T49.4X4	T49.4X5	T49.4X6
solvent	T53.6X1	T53.6X2	T53.6X3	T53.6X4	—	—
dibunate	T48.3X1	T48.3X2	T48.3X3	T48.3X4	T48.3X5	T48.3X6
dichloroarsine (vapor)	T57.0X1	T57.0X2	T57.0X3	T57.0X4	—	—
estranol	T38.7X1	T38.7X2	T38.7X3	T38.7X4	T38.7X5	T38.7X6
ether — see also ether	T52.8X1	T52.8X2	T52.8X3	T52.8X4		
formate NEC (solvent)	T52.0X1	T52.0X2	T52.0X3	T52.0X4		
fumarate	T49.4X1	T49.4X2	T49.4X3	T49.4X4	T49.4X5	T49.4X6
hydroxyisobutyrate NEC (solvent)	T52.8X1	T52.8X2	T52.8X3	T52.8X4		
iodoacetate	T59.3X1	T59.3X2	T59.3X3	T59.3X4		
lactate NEC (solvent)	T52.8X1	T52.8X2	T52.8X3	T52.8X4		
loflazepate	T42.4X1	T42.4X2	T42.4X3	T42.4X4	T42.4X5	T42.4X6
mercuric chloride	T56.1X1	T56.1X2	T56.1X3	T56.1X4	—	—
methylcarbinol	T51.8X1	T51.8X2	T51.8X3	T51.8X4	—	—
morphine	T40.2X1	T40.2X2	T40.2X3	T40.2X4	T40.2X5	T40.2X6
noradrenaline	T48.6X1	T48.6X2	T48.6X3	T48.6X4	T48.6X5	T48.6X6
oxybutyrate NEC (solvent)	T52.8X1	T52.8X2	T52.8X3	T52.8X4	—	—
Ethylene (gas)	T59.891	T59.892	T59.893	T59.894		
anesthetic (general)	T41.0X1	T41.0X2	T41.0X3	T41.0X4	T41.0X5	T41.0X6
chlorohydrin	T52.8X1	T52.8X2	T52.8X3	T52.8X4	—	—
vapor	T53.6X1	T53.6X2	T53.6X3	T53.6X4	—	—
dichloride	T52.8X1	T52.8X2	T52.8X3	T52.8X4	—	—
vapor	T53.6X1	T53.6X2	T53.6X3	T53.6X4	—	—
dinitrate	T52.3X1	T52.3X2	T52.3X3	T52.3X4	—	—
glycol(s)	T52.8X1	T52.8X2	T52.8X3	T52.8X4	—	—
dinitrate	T52.3X1	T52.3X2	T52.3X3	T52.3X4	—	—
monobutyl ether	T52.3X1	T52.3X2	T52.3X3	T52.3X4	—	—
imine	T54.1X1	T54.1X2	T54.1X3	T54.1X4	—	—
oxide (fumigant) (nonmedicinal)	T59.891	T59.892	T59.893	T59.894	—	—
medicinal	T49.0X1	T49.0X2	T49.0X3	T49.0X4	T49.0X5	T49.0X6
Ethylenediaminetetra-acetic acid	T50.6X1	T50.6X2	T50.6X3	T50.6X4	T50.6X5	T50.6X6
Ethylenediamine theophylline	T48.6X1	T48.6X2	T48.6X3	T48.6X4	T48.6X5	T48.6X6
Ethylenedinitrilotetra-acetate	T50.6X1	T50.6X2	T50.6X3	T50.6X4	T50.6X5	T50.6X6
Ethylestrenol	T38.7X1	T38.7X2	T38.7X3	T38.7X4	T38.7X5	T38.7X6
Ethylhydroxycellulose	T47.4X1	T47.4X2	T47.4X3	T47.4X4	T47.4X5	T47.4X6
Ethylidene						
chloride NEC	T53.6X1	T53.6X2	T53.6X3	T53.6X4	—	—
diacetate	T60.3X1	T60.3X2	T60.3X3	T60.3X4	—	—
dicoumarin	T45.511	T45.512	T45.513	T45.514	T45.515	T45.516
dicoumarol	T45.511	T45.512	T45.513	T45.514	T45.515	T45.516
diethyl ether	T52.0X1	T52.0X2	T52.0X3	T52.0X4	—	—
Ethylmorphine	T40.2X1	T40.2X2	T40.2X3	T40.2X4	T40.2X5	T40.2X6
Ethylnorepinephrine	T48.6X1	T48.6X2	T48.6X3	T48.6X4	T48.6X5	T48.6X6
Ethylparachlorophen-oxyisobutyrate	T46.6X1	T46.6X2	T46.6X3	T46.6X4	T46.6X5	T46.6X6
Ethynodiol	T38.4X1	T38.4X2	T38.4X3	T38.4X4	T38.4X5	T38.4X6
with mestranol diacetate	T38.4X1	T38.4X2	T38.4X3	T38.4X4	T38.4X5	T38.4X6
Etidocaine	T41.3X1	T41.3X2	T41.3X3	T41.3X4	T41.3X5	T41.3X6
infiltration (subcutaneous)	T41.3X1	T41.3X2	T41.3X3	T41.3X4	T41.3X5	T41.3X6
nerve (peripheral) (plexus)	T41.3X1	T41.3X2	T41.3X3	T41.3X4	T41.3X5	T41.3X6
Etidronate	T50.991	T50.992	T50.993	T50.994	T50.995	T50.996
Etidronic acid (disodium salt)	T50.991	T50.992	T50.993	T50.994	T50.995	T50.996
Etifoxine	T42.6X1	T42.6X2	T42.6X3	T42.6X4	T42.6X5	T42.6X6
Etilefrine	T44.4X1	T44.4X2	T44.4X3	T44.4X4	T44.4X5	T44.4X6
Etilfen	T42.3X1	T42.3X2	T42.3X3	T42.3X4	T42.3X5	T42.3X6
Etinodiol	T38.4X1	T38.4X2	T38.4X3	T38.4X4	T38.4X5	T38.4X6
Etiroxate	T46.6X1	T46.6X2	T46.6X3	T46.6X4	T46.6X5	T46.6X6
Etizolam	T42.4X1	T42.4X2	T42.4X3	T42.4X4	T42.4X5	T42.4X6
Etodolac	T39.391	T39.392	T39.393	T39.394	T39.395	T39.396
Etofamide	T37.3X1	T37.3X2	T37.3X3	T37.3X4	T37.3X5	T37.3X6
Etofibrate	T46.6X1	T46.6X2	T46.6X3	T46.6X4	T46.6X5	T46.6X6
Etofylline	T46.7X1	T46.7X2	T46.7X3	T46.7X4	T46.7X5	T46.7X6
clofibrate	T46.6X1	T46.6X2	T46.6X3	T46.6X4	T46.6X5	T46.6X6
Etoglucid	T45.1X1	T45.1X2	T45.1X3	T45.1X4	T45.1X5	T45.1X6
Etomidate	T41.1X1	T41.1X2	T41.1X3	T41.1X4	T41.1X5	T41.1X6
Etomide	T39.8X1	T39.8X2	T39.8X3	T39.8X4	T39.8X5	T39.8X6
Etomidoline	T44.3X1	T44.3X2	T44.3X3	T44.3X4	T44.3X5	T44.3X6
Etoposide	T45.1X1	T45.1X2	T45.1X3	T45.1X4	T45.1X5	T45.1X6
Etorphine	T40.2X1	T40.2X2	T40.2X3	T40.2X4	T40.2X5	T40.2X6
Etoval	T42.3X1	T42.3X2	T42.3X3	T42.3X4	T42.3X5	T42.3X6
Etozolin	T50.1X1	T50.1X2	T50.1X3	T50.1X4	T50.1X5	T50.1X6
Etretinate	T50.991	T50.992	T50.993	T50.994	T50.995	T50.996
Etryptamine	T43.691	T43.692	T43.693	T43.694	T43.695	T43.696
Etybenzatropine	T44.3X1	T44.3X2	T44.3X3	T44.3X4	T44.3X5	T44.3X6

Table of Drugs and Chemicals

Etynodiol — Fluocinonide

Substance	Poisoning, Accidental (unintentional)	Poisoning, Intentional Self-harm	Poisoning, Assault	Poisoning, Undetermined	Adverse Effect	Under-dosing
Etynodiol	T38.4X1	T38.4X2	T38.4X3	T38.4X4	T38.4X5	T38.4X6
Eucaine	T41.3X1	T41.3X2	T41.3X3	T41.3X4	T41.3X5	T41.3X6
Eucalyptus oil	T49.7X1	T49.7X2	T49.7X3	T49.7X4	T49.7X5	T49.7X6
Eucatropine	T49.5X1	T49.5X2	T49.5X3	T49.5X4	T49.5X5	T49.5X6
Eucodal	T40.2X1	T40.2X2	T40.2X3	T40.2X4	T40.2X5	T40.2X6
Euneryl	T42.3X1	T42.3X2	T42.3X3	T42.3X4	T42.3X5	T42.3X6
Euphthalmine	T44.3X1	T44.3X2	T44.3X3	T44.3X4	T44.3X5	T44.3X6
Eurax	T49.0X1	T49.0X2	T49.0X3	T49.0X4	T49.0X5	T49.0X6
Euresol	T49.4X1	T49.4X2	T49.4X3	T49.4X4	T49.4X5	T49.4X6
Euthroid	T38.1X1	T38.1X2	T38.1X3	T38.1X4	T38.1X5	T38.1X6
Evans blue	T50.8X1	T50.8X2	T50.8X3	T50.8X4	T50.8X5	T50.8X6
Evipal	T42.3X1	T42.3X2	T42.3X3	T42.3X4	T42.3X5	T42.3X6
sodium	T41.1X1	T41.1X2	T41.1X3	T41.1X4	T41.1X5	T41.1X6
Evipan	T42.3X1	T42.3X2	T42.3X3	T42.3X4	T42.3X5	T42.3X6
sodium	T41.1X1	T41.1X2	T41.1X3	T41.1X4	T41.1X5	T41.1X6
Exalamide	T49.0X1	T49.0X2	T49.0X3	T49.0X4	T49.0X5	T49.0X6
Exalgin	T39.1X1	T39.1X2	T39.1X3	T39.1X4	T39.1X5	T39.1X6
Excipients, pharmaceutical	T50.901	T50.902	T50.903	T50.904	T50.905	T50.906
Exhaust gas (engine) (motor vehicle)	T58.01	T58.02	T58.03	T58.04	—	—
Ex-Lax (phenolphthalein)	T47.2X1	T47.2X2	T47.2X3	T47.2X4	T47.2X5	T47.2X6
Expectorant NEC	T48.4X1	T48.4X2	T48.4X3	T48.4X4	T48.4X5	T48.4X6
Extended insulin zinc suspension	T38.3X1	T38.3X2	T38.3X3	T38.3X4	T38.3X5	T38.3X6
External medications (skin) (mucous membrane)	T49.91	T49.92	T49.93	T49.94	T49.95	T49.96
dental agent	T49.7X1	T49.7X2	T49.7X3	T49.7X4	T49.7X5	T49.7X6
ENT agent	T49.6X1	T49.6X2	T49.6X3	T49.6X4	T49.6X5	T49.6X6
ophthalmic preparation	T49.5X1	T49.5X2	T49.5X3	T49.5X4	T49.5X5	T49.5X6
specified NEC	T49.8X1	T49.8X2	T49.8X3	T49.8X4	T49.8X5	T49.8X6
Extrapyramidal antagonist NEC	T44.3X1	T44.3X2	T44.3X3	T44.3X4	T44.3X5	T44.3X6
Eye agents (anti-infective)	T49.5X1	T49.5X2	T49.5X3	T49.5X4	T49.5X5	T49.5X6
Eye drug NEC	T49.5X1	T49.5X2	T49.5X3	T49.5X4	T49.5X5	T49.5X6
FAC (fluorouracil + doxorubicin + cyclophosphamide)	T45.1X1	T45.1X2	T45.1X3	T45.1X4	T45.1X5	T45.1X6
Factor						
I (fibrinogen)	T45.8X1	T45.8X2	T45.8X3	T45.8X4	T45.8X5	T45.8X6
III (thromboplastin)	T45.8X1	T45.8X2	T45.8X3	T45.8X4	T45.8X5	T45.8X6
IX complex	T45.7X1	T45.7X2	T45.7X3	T45.7X4	T45.7X5	T45.7X6
human	T45.8X1	T45.8X2	T45.8X3	T45.8X4	T45.8X5	T45.8X6
VIII (antihemophilic Factor) (concentrate)	T45.8X1	T45.8X2	T45.8X3	T45.8X4	T45.8X5	T45.8X6
Famotidine	T47.0X1	T47.0X2	T47.0X3	T47.0X4	T47.0X5	T47.0X6
Fat suspension, intravenous	T50.991	T50.992	T50.993	T50.994	T50.995	T50.996
Fazadinium bromide	T48.1X1	T48.1X2	T48.1X3	T48.1X4	T48.1X5	T48.1X6
Febarbamate	T42.3X1	T42.3X2	T42.3X3	T42.3X4	T42.3X5	T42.3X6
Fecal softener	T47.4X1	T47.4X2	T47.4X3	T47.4X4	T47.4X5	T47.4X6
Fedrilate	T48.3X1	T48.3X2	T48.3X3	T48.3X4	T48.3X5	T48.3X6
Felodipine	T46.1X1	T46.1X2	T46.1X3	T46.1X4	T46.1X5	T46.1X6
Felypressin	T38.891	T38.892	T38.893	T38.894	T38.895	T38.896
Femoxetine	T43.221	T43.222	T43.223	T43.224	T43.225	T43.226
Fenalcomine	T46.3X1	T46.3X2	T46.3X3	T46.3X4	T46.3X5	T46.3X6
Fenamisal	T37.1X1	T37.1X2	T37.1X3	T37.1X4	T37.1X5	T37.1X6
Fenazone	T39.2X1	T39.2X2	T39.2X3	T39.2X4	T39.2X5	T39.2X6
Fenbendazole	T37.4X1	T37.4X2	T37.4X3	T37.4X4	T37.4X5	T37.4X6
Fenbutrazate	T50.5X1	T50.5X2	T50.5X3	T50.5X4	T50.5X5	T50.5X6
Fencamfamine	T43.691	T43.692	T43.693	T43.694	T43.695	T43.696
Fendiline	T46.1X1	T46.1X2	T46.1X3	T46.1X4	T46.1X5	T46.1X6
Fenetylline	T43.691	T43.692	T43.693	T43.694	T43.695	T43.696
Fenflumizole	T39.391	T39.392	T39.393	T39.394	T39.395	T39.396
Fenfluramine	T50.5X1	T50.5X2	T50.5X3	T50.5X4	T50.5X5	T50.5X6
Fenobarbital	T42.3X1	T42.3X2	T42.3X3	T42.3X4	T42.3X5	T42.3X6
Fenofibrate	T46.6X1	T46.6X2	T46.6X3	T46.6X4	T46.6X5	T46.6X6
Fenoprofen	T39.311	T39.312	T39.313	T39.314	T39.315	T39.316
Fenoterol	T48.6X1	T48.6X2	T48.6X3	T48.6X4	T48.6X5	T48.6X6
Fenoverine	T44.3X1	T44.3X2	T44.3X3	T44.3X4	T44.3X5	T44.3X6
Fenoxazoline	T48.5X1	T48.5X2	T48.5X3	T48.5X4	T48.5X5	T48.5X6
Fenproporex	T50.5X1	T50.5X2	T50.5X3	T50.5X4	T50.5X5	T50.5X6
Fenquizone	T50.2X1	T50.2X2	T50.2X3	T50.2X4	T50.2X5	T50.2X6
Fentanyl	T40.4X1	T40.4X2	T40.4X3	T40.4X4	T40.4X5	T40.4X6
Fentazin	T43.3X1	T43.3X2	T43.3X3	T43.3X4	T43.3X5	T43.3X6
Fenthion	T60.0X1	T60.0X2	T60.0X3	T60.0X4	—	—
Fenticlor	T49.0X1	T49.0X2	T49.0X3	T49.0X4	T49.0X5	T49.0X6
Fenylbutazone	T39.2X1	T39.2X2	T39.2X3	T39.2X4	T39.2X5	T39.2X6
Feprazone	T39.2X1	T39.2X2	T39.2X3	T39.2X4	T39.2X5	T39.2X6
Fer de lance (bite) (venom)	T63.061	T63.062	T63.063	T63.064	—	—
Ferric — see also Iron						
chloride	T45.4X1	T45.4X2	T45.4X3	T45.4X4	T45.4X5	T45.4X6
citrate	T45.4X1	T45.4X2	T45.4X3	T45.4X4	T45.4X5	T45.4X6
hydroxide						
colloidal	T45.4X1	T45.4X2	T45.4X3	T45.4X4	T45.4X5	T45.4X6

Substance	Poisoning, Accidental (unintentional)	Poisoning, Intentional Self-harm	Poisoning, Assault	Poisoning, Undetermined	Adverse Effect	Under-dosing
Ferric — see also Iron — continued						
hydroxide — continued						
polymaltose	T45.4X1	T45.4X2	T45.4X3	T45.4X4	T45.4X5	T45.4X6
pyrophosphate	T45.4X1	T45.4X2	T45.4X3	T45.4X4	T45.4X5	T45.4X6
Ferritin	T45.4X1	T45.4X2	T45.4X3	T45.4X4	T45.4X5	T45.4X6
Ferrocholinate	T45.4X1	T45.4X2	T45.4X3	T45.4X4	T45.4X5	T45.4X6
Ferrodextrane	T45.4X1	T45.4X2	T45.4X3	T45.4X4	T45.4X5	T45.4X6
Ferropolimaler	T45.4X1	T45.4X2	T45.4X3	T45.4X4	T45.4X5	T45.4X6
Ferrous — see also Iron						
phosphate	T45.4X1	T45.4X2	T45.4X3	T45.4X4	T45.4X5	T45.4X6
salt	T45.4X1	T45.4X2	T45.4X3	T45.4X4	T45.4X5	T45.4X6
with folic acid	T45.4X1	T45.4X2	T45.4X3	T45.4X4	T45.4X5	T45.4X6
Ferrous fumerate, gluconate, lactate, salt NEC, sulfate (medicinal)	T45.4X1	T45.4X2	T45.4X3	T45.4X4	T45.4X5	T45.4X6
Ferrovanadium (fumes)	T59.891	T59.892	T59.893	T59.894	—	—
Ferrum — see Iron						
Fertilizers NEC	T65.891	T65.892	T65.893	T65.894	—	—
with herbicide mixture	T60.3X1	T60.3X2	T60.3X3	T60.3X4	—	—
Fetoxilate	T47.6X1	T47.6X2	T47.6X3	T47.6X4	T47.6X5	T47.6X6
Fiber, dietary	T47.4X1	T47.4X2	T47.4X3	T47.4X4	T47.4X5	T47.4X6
Fiberglass	T65.831	T65.832	T65.833	T65.834	—	—
Fibrinogen (human)	T45.8X1	T45.8X2	T45.8X3	T45.8X4	T45.8X5	T45.8X6
Fibrinolysin (human)	T45.691	T45.692	T45.693	T45.694	T45.695	T45.696
Fibrinolysis						
affecting drug	T45.601	T45.602	T45.603	T45.604	T45.605	T45.606
inhibitor NEC	T45.621	T45.622	T45.623	T45.624	T45.625	T45.626
Fibrinolytic drug	T45.611	T45.612	T45.613	T45.614	T45.615	T45.616
Filix mas	T37.4X1	T37.4X2	T37.4X3	T37.4X4	T37.4X5	T37.4X6
Filtering cream	T49.3X1	T49.3X2	T49.3X3	T49.3X4	T49.3X5	T49.3X6
Fiorinal	T39.011	T39.012	T39.013	T39.014	T39.015	T39.016
Firedamp	T59.891	T59.892	T59.893	T59.894	—	—
Fish, noxious, nonbacterial	T61.91	T61.92	T61.93	T61.94	—	—
ciguatera	T61.01	T61.02	T61.03	T61.04	—	—
scombroid	T61.11	T61.12	T61.13	T61.14	—	—
shell	T61.781	T61.782	T61.783	T61.784	—	—
specified NEC	T61.771	T61.772	T61.773	T61.774	—	—
Flagyl	T37.3X1	T37.3X2	T37.3X3	T37.3X4	T37.3X5	T37.3X6
Flavine adenine dinucleotide	T45.2X1	T45.2X2	T45.2X3	T45.2X4	T45.2X5	T45.2X6
Flavodic acid	T46.991	T46.992	T46.993	T46.994	T46.995	T46.996
Flavoxate	T44.3X1	T44.3X2	T44.3X3	T44.3X4	T44.3X5	T44.3X6
Flaxedil	T48.1X1	T48.1X2	T48.1X3	T48.1X4	T48.1X5	T48.1X6
Flaxseed (medicinal)	T49.3X1	T49.3X2	T49.3X3	T49.3X4	T49.3X5	T49.3X6
Flecainide	T46.2X1	T46.2X2	T46.2X3	T46.2X4	T46.2X5	T46.2X6
Fleroxacin	T36.8X1	T36.8X2	T36.8X3	T36.8X4	T36.8X5	T36.8X6
Floctafenine	T39.8X1	T39.8X2	T39.8X3	T39.8X4	T39.8X5	T39.8X6
Flomax	T44.6X1	T44.6X2	T44.6X3	T44.6X4	T44.6X5	T44.6X6
Flomoxef	T36.1X1	T36.1X2	T36.1X3	T36.1X4	T36.1X5	T36.1X6
Flopropione	T44.3X1	T44.3X2	T44.3X3	T44.3X4	T44.3X5	T44.3X6
Florantyrone	T47.5X1	T47.5X2	T47.5X3	T47.5X4	T47.5X5	T47.5X6
Floraquin	T37.8X1	T37.8X2	T37.8X3	T37.8X4	T37.8X5	T37.8X6
Florinef	T38.0X1	T38.0X2	T38.0X3	T38.0X4	T38.0X5	T38.0X6
ENT agent	T49.6X1	T49.6X2	T49.6X3	T49.6X4	T49.6X5	T49.6X6
ophthalmic preparation	T49.5X1	T49.5X2	T49.5X3	T49.5X4	T49.5X5	T49.5X6
topical NEC	T49.0X1	T49.0X2	T49.0X3	T49.0X4	T49.0X5	T49.0X6
Flowers of sulfur	T49.4X1	T49.4X2	T49.4X3	T49.4X4	T49.4X5	T49.4X6
Floxuridine	T45.1X1	T45.1X2	T45.1X3	T45.1X4	T45.1X5	T45.1X6
Fluanisone	T43.4X1	T43.4X2	T43.4X3	T43.4X4	T43.4X5	T43.4X6
Flubendazole	T37.4X1	T37.4X2	T37.4X3	T37.4X4	T37.4X5	T37.4X6
Fluclorolone acetonide	T49.0X1	T49.0X2	T49.0X3	T49.0X4	T49.0X5	T49.0X6
Flucloxacillin	T36.0X1	T36.0X2	T36.0X3	T36.0X4	T36.0X5	T36.0X6
Fluconazole	T37.8X1	T37.8X2	T37.8X3	T37.8X4	T37.8X5	T37.8X6
Flucytosine	T37.8X1	T37.8X2	T37.8X3	T37.8X4	T37.8X5	T37.8X6
Fludeoxyglucose (18F)	T50.8X1	T50.8X2	T50.8X3	T50.8X4	T50.8X5	T50.8X6
Fludiazepam	T42.4X1	T42.4X2	T42.4X3	T42.4X4	T42.4X5	T42.4X6
Fludrocortisone	T50.0X1	T50.0X2	T50.0X3	T50.0X4	T50.0X5	T50.0X6
ENT agent	T49.6X1	T49.6X2	T49.6X3	T49.6X4	T49.6X5	T49.6X6
ophthalmic preparation	T49.5X1	T49.5X2	T49.5X3	T49.5X4	T49.5X5	T49.5X6
topical NEC	T49.0X1	T49.0X2	T49.0X3	T49.0X4	T49.0X5	T49.0X6
Fludroxycortide	T49.0X1	T49.0X2	T49.0X3	T49.0X4	T49.0X5	T49.0X6
Flufenamic acid	T39.391	T39.392	T39.393	T39.394	T39.395	T39.396
Fluindione	T45.511	T45.512	T45.513	T45.514	T45.515	T45.516
Flumequine	T37.8X1	T37.8X2	T37.8X3	T37.8X4	T37.8X5	T37.8X6
Flumethasone	T49.0X1	T49.0X2	T49.0X3	T49.0X4	T49.0X5	T49.0X6
Flumethiazide	T50.2X1	T50.2X2	T50.2X3	T50.2X4	T50.2X5	T50.2X6
Flumidin	T37.5X1	T37.5X2	T37.5X3	T37.5X4	T37.5X5	T37.5X6
Flunarizine	T46.7X1	T46.7X2	T46.7X3	T46.7X4	T46.7X5	T46.7X6
Flunidazole	T37.8X1	T37.8X2	T37.8X3	T37.8X4	T37.8X5	T37.8X6
Flunisolide	T48.6X1	T48.6X2	T48.6X3	T48.6X4	T48.6X5	T48.6X6
Flunitrazepam	T42.4X1	T42.4X2	T42.4X3	T42.4X4	T42.4X5	T42.4X6
Fluocinolone (acetonide)	T49.0X1	T49.0X2	T49.0X3	T49.0X4	T49.0X5	T49.0X6
Fluocinonide	T49.0X1	T49.0X2	T49.0X3	T49.0X4	T49.0X5	T49.0X6

Additional Character May Be Required — Refer to the Tabular List for Character Selection   ▽ **Subterms under main terms may continue to next column or page**

Substance	Poisoning, Accidental (unintentional)	Poisoning, Intentional Self-harm	Poisoning, Assault	Poisoning, Undetermined	Adverse Effect	Under-dosing
Fluocortin (butyl)	T49.0X1	T49.0X2	T49.0X3	T49.0X4	T49.0X5	T49.0X6
Fluocortolone	T49.0X1	T49.0X2	T49.0X3	T49.0X4	T49.0X5	T49.0X6
Fluohydrocortisone	T38.0X1	T38.0X2	T38.0X3	T38.0X4	T38.0X5	T38.0X6
ENT agent	T49.6X1	T49.6X2	T49.6X3	T49.6X4	T49.6X5	T49.6X6
ophthalmic preparation	T49.5X1	T49.5X2	T49.5X3	T49.5X4	T49.5X5	T49.5X6
topical NEC	T49.0X1	T49.0X2	T49.0X3	T49.0X4	T49.0X5	T49.0X6
Fluonid	T49.0X1	T49.0X2	T49.0X3	T49.0X4	T49.0X5	T49.0X6
Fluopromazine	T43.3X1	T43.3X2	T43.3X3	T43.3X4	T43.3X5	T43.3X6
Fluoracetate	T60.8X1	T60.8X2	T60.8X3	T60.8X4	—	—
Fluorescein	T50.8X1	T50.8X2	T50.8X3	T50.8X4	T50.8X5	T50.8X6
Fluorhydrocortisone	T50.0X1	T50.0X2	T50.0X3	T50.0X4	T50.0X5	T50.0X6
Fluoride (nonmedicinal) (pesticide) (sodium) NEC	T60.8X1	T60.8X2	T60.8X3	T60.8X4	—	—
hydrogen — see Hydrofluoric acid						
medicinal NEC	T50.991	T50.992	T50.993	T50.994	T50.995	T50.996
dental use	T49.7X1	T49.7X2	T49.7X3	T49.7X4	T49.7X5	T49.7X6
not pesticide NEC	T54.91	T54.92	T54.93	T54.94	—	—
stannous	T49.7X1	T49.7X2	T49.7X3	T49.7X4	T49.7X5	T49.7X6
Fluorinated corticosteroids	T38.0X1	T38.0X2	T38.0X3	T38.0X4	T38.0X5	T38.0X6
Fluorine (gas)	T59.5X1	T59.5X2	T59.5X3	T59.5X4	—	—
salt — see Fluoride(s)						
Fluoristan	T49.7X1	T49.7X2	T49.7X3	T49.7X4	T49.7X5	T49.7X6
Fluormetholone	T49.0X1	T49.0X2	T49.0X3	T49.0X4	T49.0X5	T49.0X6
Fluoroacetate	T60.8X1	T60.8X2	T60.8X3	T60.8X4	—	—
Fluorocarbon monomer	T53.6X1	T53.6X2	T53.6X3	T53.6X4	—	—
Fluorocytosine	T37.8X1	T37.8X2	T37.8X3	T37.8X4	T37.8X5	T37.8X6
Fluorodeoxyuridine	T45.1X1	T45.1X2	T45.1X3	T45.1X4	T45.1X5	T45.1X6
Fluorometholone	T49.0X1	T49.0X2	T49.0X3	T49.0X4	T49.0X5	T49.0X6
ophthalmic preparation	T49.5X1	T49.5X2	T49.5X3	T49.5X4	T49.5X5	T49.5X6
Fluorophosphate insecticide	T60.0X1	T60.0X2	T60.0X3	T60.0X4	—	—
Fluorosol	T46.3X1	T46.3X2	T46.3X3	T46.3X4	T46.3X5	T46.3X6
Fluorouracil	T45.1X1	T45.1X2	T45.1X3	T45.1X4	T45.1X5	T45.1X6
Fluorphenylalanine	T49.5X1	T49.5X2	T49.5X3	T49.5X4	T49.5X5	T49.5X6
Fluothane	T41.0X1	T41.0X2	T41.0X3	T41.0X4	T41.0X5	T41.0X6
Fluoxetine	T43.221	T43.222	T43.223	T43.224	T43.225	T43.226
Fluoxymesterone	T38.7X1	T38.7X2	T38.7X3	T38.7X4	T38.7X5	T38.7X6
Flupenthixol	T43.4X1	T43.4X2	T43.4X3	T43.4X4	T43.4X5	T43.4X6
Flupentixol	T43.4X1	T43.4X2	T43.4X3	T43.4X4	T43.4X5	T43.4X6
Fluphenazine	T43.3X1	T43.3X2	T43.3X3	T43.3X4	T43.3X5	T43.3X6
Fluprednidene	T49.0X1	T49.0X2	T49.0X3	T49.0X4	T49.0X5	T49.0X6
Fluprednisolone	T38.0X1	T38.0X2	T38.0X3	T38.0X4	T38.0X5	T38.0X6
Fluradoline	T39.8X1	T39.8X2	T39.8X3	T39.8X4	T39.8X5	T39.8X6
Flurandrenolide	T49.0X1	T49.0X2	T49.0X3	T49.0X4	T49.0X5	T49.0X6
Flurandrenolone	T49.0X1	T49.0X2	T49.0X3	T49.0X4	T49.0X5	T49.0X6
Flurazepam	T42.4X1	T42.4X2	T42.4X3	T42.4X4	T42.4X5	T42.4X6
Flurbiprofen	T39.311	T39.312	T39.313	T39.314	T39.315	T39.316
Flurobate	T49.0X1	T49.0X2	T49.0X3	T49.0X4	T49.0X5	T49.0X6
Fluroxene	T41.0X1	T41.0X2	T41.0X3	T41.0X4	T41.0X5	T41.0X6
Fluspirilene	T43.591	T43.592	T43.593	T43.594	T43.595	T43.596
Flutamide	T38.6X1	T38.6X2	T38.6X3	T38.6X4	T38.6X5	T38.6X6
Flutazolam	T42.4X1	T42.4X2	T42.4X3	T42.4X4	T42.4X5	T42.4X6
Fluticasone propionate	T49.1X1	T49.1X2	T49.1X3	T49.1X4	T49.1X5	T49.1X6
Flutoprazepam	T42.4X1	T42.4X2	T42.4X3	T42.4X4	T42.4X5	T42.4X6
Flutropium bromide	T48.6X1	T48.6X2	T48.6X3	T48.6X4	T48.6X5	T48.6X6
Fluvoxamine	T43.221	T43.222	T43.223	T43.224	T43.225	T43.226
Folacin	T45.8X1	T45.8X2	T45.8X3	T45.8X4	T45.8X5	T45.8X6
Folic acid	T45.8X1	T45.8X2	T45.8X3	T45.8X4	T45.8X5	T45.8X6
with ferrous salt	T45.2X1	T45.2X2	T45.2X3	T45.2X4	T45.2X5	T45.2X6
antagonist	T45.1X1	T45.1X2	T45.1X3	T45.1X4	T45.1X5	T45.1X6
Folinic acid	T45.8X1	T45.8X2	T45.8X3	T45.8X4	T45.8X5	T45.8X6
Folium stramoniae	T48.6X1	T48.6X2	T48.6X3	T48.6X4	T48.6X5	T48.6X6
Follicle-stimulating hormone, human	T38.811	T38.812	T38.813	T38.814	T38.815	T38.816
Folpet	T60.3X1	T60.3X2	T60.3X3	T60.3X4	—	—
Fominoben	T48.3X1	T48.3X2	T48.3X3	T48.3X4	T48.3X5	T48.3X6
Food, foodstuffs, noxious, nonbacterial, NEC	T62.91	T62.92	T62.93	T62.94	—	—
berries	T62.1X1	T62.1X2	T62.1X3	T62.1X4	—	—
fish — see also Fish	T61.91	T61.92	T61.93	T61.94	—	—
mushrooms	T62.0X1	T62.0X2	T62.0X3	T62.0X4	—	—
plants	T62.2X1	T62.2X2	T62.2X3	T62.2X4	—	—
seafood	T61.91	T61.92	T61.93	T61.94	—	—
specified NEC	T61.8X1	T61.8X2	T61.8X3	T61.8X4	—	—
seeds	T62.2X1	T62.2X2	T62.2X3	T62.2X4	—	—
shellfish	T61.781	T61.782	T61.783	T61.784	—	—
specified NEC	T62.8X1	T62.8X2	T62.8X3	T62.8X4	—	—
Fool's parsley	T62.2X1	T62.2X2	T62.2X3	T62.2X4	—	—
Formaldehyde (solution), gas or vapor	T59.2X1	T59.2X2	T59.2X3	T59.2X4	—	—
fungicide	T60.3X1	T60.3X2	T60.3X3	T60.3X4	—	—
Formalin	T59.2X1	T59.2X2	T59.2X3	T59.2X4	—	—
Formalin — continued						
fungicide	T60.3X1	T60.3X2	T60.3X3	T60.3X4	—	—
vapor	T59.2X1	T59.2X2	T59.2X3	T59.2X4	—	—
Formic acid	T54.2X1	T54.2X2	T54.2X3	T54.2X4	—	—
vapor	T59.891	T59.892	T59.893	T59.894	—	—
Foscarnet sodium	T37.5X1	T37.5X2	T37.5X3	T37.5X4	T37.5X5	T37.5X6
Fosfestrol	T38.5X1	T38.5X2	T38.5X3	T38.5X4	T38.5X5	T38.5X6
Fosfomycin	T36.8X1	T36.8X2	T36.8X3	T36.8X4	T36.8X5	T36.8X6
Fosfonet sodium	T37.5X1	T37.5X2	T37.5X3	T37.5X4	T37.5X5	T37.5X6
Fosinopril	T46.4X1	T46.4X2	T46.4X3	T46.4X4	T46.4X5	T46.4X6
sodium	T46.4X1	T46.4X2	T46.4X3	T46.4X4	T46.4X5	T46.4X6
Fowler's solution	T57.0X1	T57.0X2	T57.0X3	T57.0X4	—	—
Foxglove	T62.2X1	T62.2X2	T62.2X3	T62.2X4	—	—
Framycetin	T36.5X1	T36.5X2	T36.5X3	T36.5X4	T36.5X5	T36.5X6
Frangula	T47.2X1	T47.2X2	T47.2X3	T47.2X4	T47.2X5	T47.2X6
extract	T47.2X1	T47.2X2	T47.2X3	T47.2X4	T47.2X5	T47.2X6
Frei antigen	T50.8X1	T50.8X2	T50.8X3	T50.8X4	T50.8X5	T50.8X6
Freon	T53.5X1	T53.5X2	T53.5X3	T53.5X4	—	—
Fructose	T50.3X1	T50.3X2	T50.3X3	T50.3X4	T50.3X5	T50.3X6
Frusemide	T50.1X1	T50.1X2	T50.1X3	T50.1X4	T50.1X5	T50.1X6
FSH	T38.811	T38.812	T38.813	T38.814	T38.815	T38.816
Ftorafur	T45.1X1	T45.1X2	T45.1X3	T45.1X4	T45.1X5	T45.1X6
Fuel						
automobile	T52.0X1	T52.0X2	T52.0X3	T52.0X4	—	—
exhaust gas, not in transit	T58.01	T58.02	T58.03	T58.04	—	—
vapor NEC	T52.0X1	T52.0X2	T52.0X3	T52.0X4	—	—
gas (domestic use) — see also Carbon, monoxide, fuel, utility	T59.891	T59.892	T59.893	T59.894	—	—
utility	T59.891	T59.892	T59.893	T59.894	—	—
incomplete combustion of — see Carbon, monoxide, fuel, utility						
in mobile container	T59.891	T59.892	T59.893	T59.894	—	—
piped (natural)	T59.891	T59.892	T59.893	T59.894	—	—
industrial, incomplete combustion	T58.8X1	T58.8X2	T58.8X3	T58.8X4	—	—
Fugillin	T36.8X1	T36.8X2	T36.8X3	T36.8X4	T36.8X5	T36.8X6
Fulminate of mercury	T56.1X1	T56.1X2	T56.1X3	T56.1X4	—	—
Fulvicin	T36.7X1	T36.7X2	T36.7X3	T36.7X4	T36.7X5	T36.7X6
Fumadil	T36.8X1	T36.8X2	T36.8X3	T36.8X4	T36.8X5	T36.8X6
Fumagillin	T36.8X1	T36.8X2	T36.8X3	T36.8X4	T36.8X5	T36.8X6
Fumaric acid	T49.4X1	T49.4X2	T49.4X3	T49.4X4	T49.4X5	T49.4X6
Fumes (from)	T59.91	T59.92	T59.93	T59.94	—	—
carbon monoxide — see Carbon, monoxide						
charcoal (domestic use) — see Charcoal, fumes						
chloroform — see Chloroform						
coke (in domestic stoves, fireplaces) — see Coke fumes						
corrosive NEC	T54.91	T54.92	T54.93	T54.94	—	—
ether — see ether						
freons	T53.5X1	T53.5X2	T53.5X3	T53.5X4	—	—
hydrocarbons	T59.891	T59.892	T59.893	T59.894	—	—
petroleum (liquefied)	T59.891	T59.892	T59.893	T59.894	—	—
distributed through pipes (pure or mixed with air)	T59.891	T59.892	T59.893	T59.894	—	—
lead — see lead						
metal — see Metals, or the specified metal						
nitrogen dioxide	T59.0X1	T59.0X2	T59.0X3	T59.0X4	—	—
pesticides — see Pesticides						
petroleum (liquefied)	T59.891	T59.892	T59.893	T59.894	—	—
distributed through pipes (pure or mixed with air)	T59.891	T59.892	T59.893	T59.894	—	—
polyester	T59.891	T59.892	T59.893	T59.894	—	—
specified source NEC — see also substance specified	T59.891	T59.892	T59.893	T59.894	—	—
sulfur dioxide	T59.1X1	T59.1X2	T59.1X3	T59.1X4	—	—
Fumigant NEC	T60.91	T60.92	T60.93	T60.94	—	—
Fungicide NEC (nonmedicinal)	T60.3X1	T60.3X2	T60.3X3	T60.3X4	—	—
Fungi, noxious, used as food	T62.0X1	T62.0X2	T62.0X3	T62.0X4	—	—
Fungizone	T36.7X1	T36.7X2	T36.7X3	T36.7X4	T36.7X5	T36.7X6
topical	T49.0X1	T49.0X2	T49.0X3	T49.0X4	T49.0X5	T49.0X6
Furacin	T49.0X1	T49.0X2	T49.0X3	T49.0X4	T49.0X5	T49.0X6
Furadantin	T37.91	T37.92	T37.93	T37.94	T37.95	T37.96
Furazolidone	T37.8X1	T37.8X2	T37.8X3	T37.8X4	T37.8X5	T37.8X6

Substance	Poisoning, Accidental (unintentional)	Poisoning, Intentional Self-harm	Poisoning, Assault	Poisoning, Undetermined	Adverse Effect	Under-dosing
Furazolium chloride	T49.0X1	T49.0X2	T49.0X3	T49.0X4	T49.0X5	T49.0X6
Furfural	T52.8X1	T52.8X2	T52.8X3	T52.8X4	—	—
Furnace (coal burning) (domestic),	T58.2X1	T58.2X2	T58.2X3	T58.2X4	—	—
gas from						
industrial	T58.8X1	T58.8X2	T58.8X3	T58.8X4	—	—
Furniture polish	T65.891	T65.892	T65.893	T65.894	—	—
Furosemide	T50.1X1	T50.1X2	T50.1X3	T50.1X4	T50.1X5	T50.1X6
Furoxone	T37.91	T37.92	T37.93	T37.94	T37.95	T37.96
Fursultiamine	T45.2X1	T45.2X2	T45.2X3	T45.2X4	T45.2X5	T45.2X6
Fusafungine	T36.8X1	T36.8X2	T36.8X3	T36.8X4	T36.8X5	T36.8X6
Fusel oil (any) (amyl) (butyl)	T51.3X1	T51.3X2	T51.3X3	T51.3X4	—	—
(propyl), vapor						
Fusidate (ethanolamine)	T36.8X1	T36.8X2	T36.8X3	T36.8X4	T36.8X5	T36.8X6
(sodium)						
Fusidic acid	T36.8X1	T36.8X2	T36.8X3	T36.8X4	T36.8X5	T36.8X6
Fytic acid, nonasodium	T50.6X1	T50.6X2	T50.6X3	T50.6X4	T50.6X5	T50.6X6
b-Galactosidase	T47.5X1	T47.5X2	T47.5X3	T47.5X4	T47.5X5	T47.5X6
GABA	T43.8X1	T43.8X2	T43.8X3	T43.8X4	T43.8X5	T43.8X6
Gadopentetic acid	T50.8X1	T50.8X2	T50.8X3	T50.8X4	T50.8X5	T50.8X6
Galactose	T50.3X1	T50.3X2	T50.3X3	T50.3X4	T50.3X5	T50.3X6
Galantamine	T44.0X1	T44.0X2	T44.0X3	T44.0X4	T44.0X5	T44.0X6
Gallamine (triethiodide)	T48.1X1	T48.1X2	T48.1X3	T48.1X4	T48.1X5	T48.1X6
Gallium citrate	T50.991	T50.992	T50.993	T50.994	T50.995	T50.996
Gallopamil	T46.1X1	T46.1X2	T46.1X3	T46.1X4	T46.1X5	T46.1X6
Gamboge	T47.2X1	T47.2X2	T47.2X3	T47.2X4	T47.2X5	T47.2X6
Gamimune	T50.Z11	T50.Z12	T50.Z13	T50.Z14	T50.Z15	T50.Z16
Gamma-aminobutyric acid	T43.8X1	T43.8X2	T43.8X3	T43.8X4	T43.8X5	T43.8X6
Gamma-benzene hexachloride	T49.0X1	T49.0X2	T49.0X3	T49.0X4	T49.0X5	T49.0X6
(medicinal)						
nonmedicinal, vapor	T53.6X1	T53.6X2	T53.6X3	T53.6X4	—	—
Gamma-BHC (medicinal) — see	T49.0X1	T49.0X2	T49.0X3	T49.0X4	T49.0X5	T49.0X6
also Gamma-benzene						
hexachloride						
Gamma globulin	T50.Z11	T50.Z12	T50.Z13	T50.Z14	T50.Z15	T50.Z16
Gamulin	T50.Z11	T50.Z12	T50.Z13	T50.Z14	T50.Z15	T50.Z16
Ganciclovir (sodium)	T37.5X1	T37.5X2	T37.5X3	T37.5X4	T37.5X5	T37.5X6
Ganglionic blocking drug NEC	T44.2X1	T44.2X2	T44.2X3	T44.2X4	T44.2X5	T44.2X6
specified NEC	T44.2X1	T44.2X2	T44.2X3	T44.2X4	T44.2X5	T44.2X6
Ganja	T40.7X1	T40.7X2	T40.7X3	T40.7X4	T40.7X5	T40.7X6
Garamycin	T36.5X1	T36.5X2	T36.5X3	T36.5X4	T36.5X5	T36.5X6
ophthalmic preparation	T49.5X1	T49.5X2	T49.5X3	T49.5X4	T49.5X5	T49.5X6
topical NEC	T49.0X1	T49.0X2	T49.0X3	T49.0X4	T49.0X5	T49.0X6
Gardenal	T42.3X1	T42.3X2	T42.3X3	T42.3X4	T42.3X5	T42.3X6
Gardepanyl	T42.3X1	T42.3X2	T42.3X3	T42.3X4	T42.3X5	T42.3X6
Gas	T59.91	T59.92	T59.93	T59.94	—	—
acetylene	T59.891	T59.892	T59.893	T59.894	—	—
incomplete combustion of	T58.11	T58.12	T58.13	T58.14	—	—
air contaminants, source or type	T59.91	T59.92	T59.93	T59.94	—	—
not specified						
anesthetic	T41.0X1	T41.0X2	T41.0X3	T41.0X4	T41.0X5	T41.0X6
blast furnace	T58.8X1	T58.8X2	T58.8X3	T58.8X4	—	—
butane — see butane						
carbon monoxide — see Carbon,						
monoxide						
chlorine	T59.4X1	T59.4X2	T59.4X3	T59.4X4	—	—
coal	T58.2X1	T58.2X2	T58.2X3	T58.2X4	—	—
cyanide	T57.3X1	T57.3X2	T57.3X3	T57.3X4	—	—
dicyanogen	T65.0X1	T65.0X2	T65.0X3	T65.0X4	—	—
domestic — see Domestic gas						
exhaust	T58.01	T58.02	T58.03	T58.04	—	—
from utility (for cooking, heating,						
or lighting) (after						
combustion) — see Carbon,						
monoxide, fuel, utility						
prior to combustion	T59.891	T59.892	T59.893	T59.894	—	—
from wood- or coal-burning	T58.2X1	T58.2X2	T58.2X3	T58.2X4	—	—
stove or fireplace						
fuel (domestic use) (after						
combustion) — see also						
Carbon, monoxide, fuel						
industrial use	T58.8X1	T58.8X2	T58.8X3	T58.8X4	—	—
prior to combustion	T59.891	T59.892	T59.893	T59.894	—	—
utility	T59.891	T59.892	T59.893	T59.894	—	—
incomplete combustion of						
— see Carbon,						
monoxide, fuel, utility						
in mobile container	T59.891	T59.892	T59.893	T59.894	—	—
piped (natural)	T59.891	T59.892	T59.893	T59.894	—	—
garage	T58.01	T58.02	T58.03	T58.04	—	—
hydrocarbon NEC	T59.891	T59.892	T59.893	T59.894	—	—

Substance	Poisoning, Accidental (unintentional)	Poisoning, Intentional Self-harm	Poisoning, Assault	Poisoning, Undetermined	Adverse Effect	Under-dosing
Gas — continued						
hydrocarbon — continued						
incomplete combustion of —						
see Carbon, monoxide,						
fuel, utility						
liquefied — see butane						
piped	T59.891	T59.892	T59.893	T59.894	—	—
hydrocyanic acid	T65.0X1	T65.0X2	T65.0X3	T65.0X4	—	—
illuminating (after	T58.11	T58.12	T58.13	T58.14	—	—
combustion)						
prior to combustion	T59.891	T59.892	T59.893	T59.894	—	—
incomplete combustion, any —						
see Carbon, monoxide						
kiln	T58.8X1	T58.8X2	T58.8X3	T58.8X4	—	—
lacrimogenic	T59.3X1	T59.3X2	T59.3X3	T59.3X4	—	—
liquefied petroleum — see						
butane						
marsh	T59.891	T59.892	T59.893	T59.894	—	—
motor exhaust, not in	T58.01	T58.02	T58.03	T58.04	—	—
transit						
mustard, not in war	T59.891	T59.892	T59.893	T59.894	—	—
natural	T59.891	T59.892	T59.893	T59.894	—	—
nerve, not in war	T59.91	T59.92	T59.93	T59.94	—	—
oil	T52.0X1	T52.0X2	T52.0X3	T52.0X4	—	—
petroleum (liquefied)	T59.891	T59.892	T59.893	T59.894	—	—
(distributed in mobile						
containers)						
piped (pure or mixed with	T59.891	T59.892	T59.893	T59.894	—	—
air)						
piped (manufactured) (natural)	T59.891	T59.892	T59.893	T59.894	—	—
NEC						
producer	T58.8X1	T58.8X2	T58.8X3	T58.8X4	—	—
propane — see propane						
refrigerant	T53.5X1	T53.5X2	T53.5X3	T53.5X4	—	—
(chlorofluoro-carbon)						
not chlorofluoro-carbon	T59.891	T59.892	T59.893	T59.894	—	—
sewer	T59.91	T59.92	T59.93	T59.94	—	—
specified source NEC	T59.91	T59.92	T59.93	T59.94	—	—
stove (after combustion)	T58.11	T58.12	T58.13	T58.14	—	—
prior to combustion	T59.891	T59.892	T59.893	T59.894	—	—
tear	T59.3X1	T59.3X2	T59.3X3	T59.3X4	—	—
therapeutic	T41.5X1	T41.5X2	T41.5X3	T41.5X4	T41.5X5	T41.5X6
utility (for cooking, heating, or	T59.891	T59.892	T59.893	T59.894	—	—
lighting) (piped) NEC						
incomplete combustion of —						
see Carbon, monoxide,						
fuel, utilty						
in mobile container	T59.891	T59.892	T59.893	T59.894	—	—
piped (natural)	T59.891	T59.892	T59.893	T59.894	—	—
water	T58.11	T58.12	T58.13	T58.14	—	—
incomplete combustion of —						
see Carbon, monoxide,						
fuel, utility						
Gaseous substance — see Gas						
Gasoline	T52.0X1	T52.0X2	T52.0X3	T52.0X4	—	—
vapor	T52.0X1	T52.0X2	T52.0X3	T52.0X4	—	—
Gastric enzymes	T47.5X1	T47.5X2	T47.5X3	T47.5X4	T47.5X5	T47.5X6
Gastrografin	T50.8X1	T50.8X2	T50.8X3	T50.8X4	T50.8X5	T50.8X6
Gastrointestinal drug	T47.91	T47.92	T47.93	T47.94	T47.95	T47.96
biological	T47.8X1	T47.8X2	T47.8X3	T47.8X4	T47.8X5	T47.8X6
specified NEC	T47.8X1	T47.8X2	T47.8X3	T47.8X4	T47.8X5	T47.8X6
Gaultheria procumbens	T62.2X1	T62.2X2	T62.2X3	T62.2X4	—	—
Gefarnate	T44.3X1	T44.3X2	T44.3X3	T44.3X4	T44.3X5	T44.3X6
Gelatin (intravenous)	T45.8X1	T45.8X2	T45.8X3	T45.8X4	T45.8X5	T45.8X6
absorbable (sponge)	T45.7X1	T45.7X2	T45.7X3	T45.7X4	T45.7X5	T45.7X6
Gelfilm	T49.8X1	T49.8X2	T49.8X3	T49.8X4	T49.8X5	T49.8X6
Gelfoam	T45.7X1	T45.7X2	T45.7X3	T45.7X4	T45.7X5	T45.7X6
Gelsemine	T50.991	T50.992	T50.993	T50.994	T50.995	T50.996
Gelsemium (sempervirens)	T62.2X1	T62.2X2	T62.2X3	T62.2X4	—	—
Gemeprost	T48.0X1	T48.0X2	T48.0X3	T48.0X4	T48.0X5	T48.0X6
Gemfibrozil	T46.6X1	T46.6X2	T46.6X3	T46.6X4	T46.6X5	T46.6X6
Gemonil	T42.3X1	T42.3X2	T42.3X3	T42.3X4	T42.3X5	T42.3X6
Gentamicin	T36.5X1	T36.5X2	T36.5X3	T36.5X4	T36.5X5	T36.5X6
ophthalmic preparation	T49.5X1	T49.5X2	T49.5X3	T49.5X4	T49.5X5	T49.5X6
topical NEC	T49.0X1	T49.0X2	T49.0X3	T49.0X4	T49.0X5	T49.0X6
Gentian	T47.5X1	T47.5X2	T47.5X3	T47.5X4	T47.5X5	T47.5X6
violet	T49.0X1	T49.0X2	T49.0X3	T49.0X4	T49.0X5	T49.0X6
Gepefrine	T44.4X1	T44.4X2	T44.4X3	T44.4X4	T44.4X5	T44.4X6
Gestonorone caproate	T38.5X1	T38.5X2	T38.5X3	T38.5X4	T38.5X5	T38.5X6
Gexane	T49.0X1	T49.0X2	T49.0X4	T49.0X5	T49.0X6	
Gila monster (venom)	T63.111	T63.112	T63.113	T63.114	—	—
Ginger	T47.5X1	T47.5X2	T47.5X3	T47.5X4	T47.5X5	T47.5X6
Jamaica — see Jamaica, ginger						

360

Additional Character May Be Required — Refer to the Tabular List for Character Selection   ▽ Subterms under main terms may continue to next column or page

Substance	Poisoning, Accidental (unintentional)	Poisoning, Intentional Self-harm	Poisoning, Assault	Poisoning, Undetermined	Adverse Effect	Underdosing
Gitalin	T46.0X1	T46.0X2	T46.0X3	T46.0X4	T46.0X5	T46.0X6
amorphous	T46.0X1	T46.0X2	T46.0X3	T46.0X4	T46.0X5	T46.0X6
Gitaloxin	T46.0X1	T46.0X2	T46.0X3	T46.0X4	T46.0X5	T46.0X6
Gitoxin	T46.0X1	T46.0X2	T46.0X3	T46.0X4	T46.0X5	T46.0X6
Glafenine	T39.8X1	T39.8X2	T39.8X3	T39.8X4	T39.8X5	T39.8X6
Glandular extract (medicinal) NEC	T50.Z91	T50.Z92	T50.Z93	T50.Z94	T50.Z95	T50.Z96
Glaucarubin	T37.3X1	T37.3X2	T37.3X3	T37.3X4	T37.3X5	T37.3X6
Glibenclamide	T38.3X1	T38.3X2	T38.3X3	T38.3X4	T38.3X5	T38.3X6
Glibornuride	T38.3X1	T38.3X2	T38.3X3	T38.3X4	T38.3X5	T38.3X6
Gliclazide	T38.3X1	T38.3X2	T38.3X3	T38.3X4	T38.3X5	T38.3X6
Glimidine	T38.3X1	T38.3X2	T38.3X3	T38.3X4	T38.3X5	T38.3X6
Glipizide	T38.3X1	T38.3X2	T38.3X3	T38.3X4	T38.3X5	T38.3X6
Gliquidone	T38.3X1	T38.3X2	T38.3X3	T38.3X4	T38.3X5	T38.3X6
Glisolamide	T38.3X1	T38.3X2	T38.3X3	T38.3X4	T38.3X5	T38.3X6
Glisoxepide	T38.3X1	T38.3X2	T38.3X3	T38.3X4	T38.3X5	T38.3X6
Globin zinc insulin	T38.3X1	T38.3X2	T38.3X3	T38.3X4	T38.3X5	T38.3X6
Globulin						
antilymphocytic	T50.Z11	T50.Z12	T50.Z13	T50.Z14	T50.Z15	T50.Z16
antirhesus	T50.Z11	T50.Z12	T50.Z13	T50.Z14	T50.Z15	T50.Z16
antivenin	T50.Z11	T50.Z12	T50.Z13	T50.Z14	T50.Z15	T50.Z16
antiviral	T50.Z11	T50.Z12	T50.Z13	T50.Z14	T50.Z15	T50.Z16
Glucagon	T38.3X1	T38.3X2	T38.3X3	T38.3X4	T38.3X5	T38.3X6
Glucocorticoids	T38.0X1	T38.0X2	T38.0X3	T38.0X4	T38.0X5	T38.0X6
Glucocorticosteroid	T38.0X1	T38.0X2	T38.0X3	T38.0X4	T38.0X5	T38.0X6
Gluconic acid	T50.991	T50.992	T50.993	T50.994	T50.995	T50.996
Glucosamine sulfate	T39.4X1	T39.4X2	T39.4X3	T39.4X4	T39.4X5	T39.4X6
Glucose	T50.3X1	T50.3X2	T50.3X3	T50.3X4	T50.3X5	T50.3X6
with sodium chloride	T50.3X1	T50.3X2	T50.3X3	T50.3X4	T50.3X5	T50.3X6
Glucosulfone sodium	T37.1X1	T37.1X2	T37.1X3	T37.1X4	T37.1X5	T37.1X6
Glucurolactone	T47.8X1	T47.8X2	T47.8X3	T47.8X4	T47.8X5	T47.8X6
Glue NEC	T52.8X1	T52.8X2	T52.8X3	T52.8X4	—	—
Glutamic acid	T47.5X1	T47.5X2	T47.5X3	T47.5X4	T47.5X5	T47.5X6
Glutaral (medicinal)	T49.0X1	T49.0X2	T49.0X3	T49.0X4	T49.0X5	T49.0X6
nonmedicinal	T65.891	T65.892	T65.893	T65.894	—	—
Glutaraldehyde (nonmedicinal)	T65.891	T65.892	T65.893	T65.894	—	—
medicinal	T49.0X1	T49.0X2	T49.0X3	T49.0X4	T49.0X5	T49.0X6
Glutathione	T50.6X1	T50.6X2	T50.6X3	T50.6X4	T50.6X5	T50.6X6
Glutethimide	T42.6X1	T42.6X2	T42.6X3	T42.6X4	T42.6X5	T42.6X6
Glyburide	T38.3X1	T38.3X2	T38.3X3	T38.3X4	T38.3X5	T38.3X6
Glycerin	T47.4X1	T47.4X2	T47.4X3	T47.4X4	T47.4X5	T47.4X6
Glycerol	T47.4X1	T47.4X2	T47.4X3	T47.4X4	T47.4X5	T47.4X6
borax	T49.6X1	T49.6X2	T49.6X3	T49.6X4	T49.6X5	T49.6X6
intravenous	T50.3X1	T50.3X2	T50.3X3	T50.3X4	T50.3X5	T50.3X6
iodinated	T48.4X1	T48.4X2	T48.4X3	T48.4X4	T48.4X5	T48.4X6
Glycerophosphate	T50.991	T50.992	T50.993	T50.994	T50.995	T50.996
Glyceryl						
gualacolate	T48.4X1	T48.4X2	T48.4X3	T48.4X4	T48.4X5	T48.4X6
nitrate	T46.3X1	T46.3X2	T46.3X3	T46.3X4	T46.3X5	T46.3X6
triacetate (topical)	T49.0X1	T49.0X2	T49.0X3	T49.0X4	T49.0X5	T49.0X6
trinitrate	T46.3X1	T46.3X2	T46.3X3	T46.3X4	T46.3X5	T46.3X6
Glycine	T50.3X1	T50.3X2	T50.3X3	T50.3X4	T50.3X5	T50.3X6
Glyclopyramide	T38.3X1	T38.3X2	T38.3X3	T38.3X4	T38.3X5	T38.3X6
Glycobiarsol	T37.3X1	T37.3X2	T37.3X3	T37.3X4	T37.3X5	T37.3X6
Glycols (ether)	T52.3X1	T52.3X2	T52.3X3	T52.3X4	—	—
Glyconiazide	T37.1X1	T37.1X2	T37.1X3	T37.1X4	T37.1X5	T37.1X6
Glycopyrrolate	T44.3X1	T44.3X2	T44.3X3	T44.3X4	T44.3X5	T44.3X6
Glycopyrronium	T44.3X1	T44.3X2	T44.3X3	T44.3X4	T44.3X5	T44.3X6
bromide	T44.3X1	T44.3X2	T44.3X3	T44.3X4	T44.3X5	T44.3X6
Glycoside, cardiac (stimulant)	T46.0X1	T46.0X2	T46.0X3	T46.0X4	T46.0X5	T46.0X6
Glycyclamide	T38.3X1	T38.3X2	T38.3X3	T38.3X4	T38.3X5	T38.3X6
Glycyrrhiza extract	T48.4X1	T48.4X2	T48.4X3	T48.4X4	T48.4X5	T48.4X6
Glycyrrhizic acid	T48.4X1	T48.4X2	T48.4X3	T48.4X4	T48.4X5	T48.4X6
Glycyrrhizinate potassium	T48.4X1	T48.4X2	T48.4X3	T48.4X4	T48.4X5	T48.4X6
Glymidine sodium	T38.3X1	T38.3X2	T38.3X3	T38.3X4	T38.3X5	T38.3X6
Glyphosate	T60.3X1	T60.3X2	T60.3X3	T60.3X4	—	—
Glyphylline	T48.6X1	T48.6X2	T48.6X3	T48.6X4	T48.6X5	T48.6X6
Gold						
colloidal (l98Au)	T45.1X1	T45.1X2	T45.1X3	T45.1X4	T45.1X5	T45.1X6
salts	T39.4X1	T39.4X2	T39.4X3	T39.4X4	T39.4X5	T39.4X6
Golden sulfide of antimony	T56.891	T56.892	T56.893	T56.894	—	—
Goldylocks	T62.2X1	T62.2X2	T62.2X3	T62.2X4	—	—
Gonadal tissue extract	T38.901	T38.902	T38.903	T38.904	T38.905	T38.906
female	T38.5X1	T38.5X2	T38.5X3	T38.5X4	T38.5X5	T38.5X6
male	T38.7X1	T38.7X2	T38.7X3	T38.7X4	T38.7X5	T38.7X6
Gonadorelin	T38.891	T38.892	T38.893	T38.894	T38.895	T38.896
Gonadotropin	T38.891	T38.892	T38.893	T38.894	T38.895	T38.896
chorionic	T38.891	T38.892	T38.893	T38.894	T38.895	T38.896
pituitary	T38.811	T38.812	T38.813	T38.814	T38.815	T38.816
Goserelin	T45.1X1	T45.1X2	T45.1X3	T45.1X4	T45.1X5	T45.1X6
Grain alcohol	T51.0X1	T51.0X2	T51.0X3	T51.0X4	—	—

Substance	Poisoning, Accidental (unintentional)	Poisoning, Intentional Self-harm	Poisoning, Assault	Poisoning, Undetermined	Adverse Effect	Underdosing
Gramicidin	T49.0X1	T49.0X2	T49.0X3	T49.0X4	T49.0X5	T49.0X6
Granisetron	T45.0X1	T45.0X2	T45.0X3	T45.0X4	T45.0X5	T45.0X6
Gratiola officinalis	T62.2X1	T62.2X2	T62.2X3	T62.2X4	—	—
Grease	T65.891	T65.892	T65.893	T65.894	—	—
Green hellebore	T62.2X1	T62.2X2	T62.2X3	T62.2X4	—	—
Green soap	T49.2X1	T49.2X2	T49.2X3	T49.2X4	T49.2X5	T49.2X6
Grifulvin	T36.7X1	T36.7X2	T36.7X3	T36.7X4	T36.7X5	T36.7X6
Griseofulvin	T36.7X1	T36.7X2	T36.7X3	T36.7X4	T36.7X5	T36.7X6
Growth hormone	T38.811	T38.812	T38.813	T38.814	T38.815	T38.816
Guaiacol derivatives	T48.4X1	T48.4X2	T48.4X3	T48.4X4	T48.4X5	T48.4X6
Guaiac reagent	T50.991	T50.992	T50.993	T50.994	T50.995	T50.996
Guaifenesin	T48.4X1	T48.4X2	T48.4X3	T48.4X4	T48.4X5	T48.4X6
Guaimesal	T48.4X1	T48.4X2	T48.4X3	T48.4X4	T48.4X5	T48.4X6
Guaiphenesin	T48.4X1	T48.4X2	T48.4X3	T48.4X4	T48.4X5	T48.4X6
Guamecycline	T36.4X1	T36.4X2	T36.4X3	T36.4X4	T36.4X5	T36.4X6
Guanabenz	T46.5X1	T46.5X2	T46.5X3	T46.5X4	T46.5X5	T46.5X6
Guanacline	T46.5X1	T46.5X2	T46.5X3	T46.5X4	T46.5X5	T46.5X6
Guanadrel	T46.5X1	T46.5X2	T46.5X3	T46.5X4	T46.5X5	T46.5X6
Guanatol	T37.2X1	T37.2X2	T37.2X3	T37.2X4	T37.2X5	T37.2X6
Guanethidine	T46.5X1	T46.5X2	T46.5X3	T46.5X4	T46.5X5	T46.5X6
Guanfacine	T46.5X1	T46.5X2	T46.5X3	T46.5X4	T46.5X5	T46.5X6
Guano	T65.891	T65.892	T65.893	T65.894	—	—
Guanochlor	T46.5X1	T46.5X2	T46.5X3	T46.5X4	T46.5X5	T46.5X6
Guanoclor	T46.5X1	T46.5X2	T46.5X3	T46.5X4	T46.5X5	T46.5X6
Guanoctine	T46.5X1	T46.5X2	T46.5X3	T46.5X4	T46.5X5	T46.5X6
Guanoxabenz	T46.5X1	T46.5X2	T46.5X3	T46.5X4	T46.5X5	T46.5X6
Guanoxan	T46.5X1	T46.5X2	T46.5X3	T46.5X4	T46.5X5	T46.5X6
Guar gum (medicinal)	T46.6X1	T46.6X2	T46.6X3	T46.6X4	T46.6X5	T46.6X6
Hachimycin	T36.7X1	T36.7X2	T36.7X3	T36.7X4	T36.7X5	T36.7X6
Hair						
dye	T49.4X1	T49.4X2	T49.4X3	T49.4X4	T49.4X5	T49.4X6
preparation NEC	T49.4X1	T49.4X2	T49.4X3	T49.4X4	T49.4X5	T49.4X6
Halazepam	T42.4X1	T42.4X2	T42.4X3	T42.4X4	T42.4X5	T42.4X6
Halcinolone	T49.0X1	T49.0X2	T49.0X3	T49.0X4	T49.0X5	T49.0X6
Halcinonide	T49.0X1	T49.0X2	T49.0X3	T49.0X4	T49.0X5	T49.0X6
Halethazole	T49.0X1	T49.0X2	T49.0X3	T49.0X4	T49.0X5	T49.0X6
Hallucinogen NEC	T40.901	T40.902	T40.903	T40.904	T40.905	T40.906
Halofantrine	T37.2X1	T37.2X2	T37.2X3	T37.2X4	T37.2X5	T37.2X6
Halofenate	T46.6X1	T46.6X2	T46.6X3	T46.6X4	T46.6X5	T46.6X6
Halometasone	T49.0X1	T49.0X2	T49.0X3	T49.0X4	T49.0X5	T49.0X6
Haloperidol	T43.4X1	T43.4X2	T43.4X3	T43.4X4	T43.4X5	T43.4X6
Haloprogin	T49.0X1	T49.0X2	T49.0X3	T49.0X4	T49.0X5	T49.0X6
Halotex	T49.0X1	T49.0X2	T49.0X3	T49.0X4	T49.0X5	T49.0X6
Halothane	T41.0X1	T41.0X2	T41.0X3	T41.0X4	T41.0X5	T41.0X6
Haloxazolam	T42.4X1	T42.4X2	T42.4X3	T42.4X4	T42.4X5	T42.4X6
Halquinols	T49.0X1	T49.0X2	T49.0X3	T49.0X4	T49.0X5	T49.0X6
Hamamelis	T49.2X1	T49.2X2	T49.2X3	T49.2X4	T49.2X5	T49.2X6
Haptendextran	T45.8X1	T45.8X2	T45.8X3	T45.8X4	T45.8X5	T45.8X6
Harmonyl	T46.5X1	T46.5X2	T46.5X3	T46.5X4	T46.5X5	T46.5X6
Hartmann's solution	T50.3X1	T50.3X2	T50.3X3	T50.3X4	T50.3X5	T50.3X6
Hashish	T40.7X1	T40.7X2	T40.7X3	T40.7X4	T40.7X5	T40.7X6
Hawaiian Woodrose seeds	T40.991	T40.992	T40.993	T40.994	—	—
HCB	T60.3X1	T60.3X2	T60.3X3	T60.3X4	—	—
HCH	T53.6X1	T53.6X2	T53.6X3	T53.6X4	—	—
medicinal	T49.0X1	T49.0X2	T49.0X3	T49.0X4	T49.0X5	T49.0X6
HCN	T57.3X1	T57.3X2	T57.3X3	T57.3X4	—	—
Headache cures, drugs, powders NEC	T50.901	T50.902	T50.903	T50.904	T50.905	T50.906
Heavenly Blue (morning glory)	T40.991	T40.992	T40.993	T40.994	—	—
Heavy metal antidote	T45.8X1	T45.8X2	T45.8X3	T45.8X4	T45.8X5	T45.8X6
Hedaquinium	T49.0X1	T49.0X2	T49.0X3	T49.0X4	T49.0X5	T49.0X6
Hedge hyssop	T62.2X1	T62.2X2	T62.2X3	T62.2X4	—	—
Heet	T49.8X1	T49.8X2	T49.8X3	T49.8X4	T49.8X5	T49.8X6
Helenin	T37.4X1	T37.4X2	T37.4X3	T37.4X4	T37.4X5	T37.4X6
Helium (nonmedicinal) NEC	T59.891	T59.892	T59.893	T59.894	—	—
medicinal	T48.991	T48.992	T48.993	T48.994	T48.995	T48.996
Hellebore (black) (green) (white)	T62.2X1	T62.2X2	T62.2X3	T62.2X4	—	—
Hematin	T45.8X1	T45.8X2	T45.8X3	T45.8X4	T45.8X5	T45.8X6
Hematinic preparation	T45.8X1	T45.8X2	T45.8X3	T45.8X4	T45.8X5	T45.8X6
Hematological agent	T45.91	T45.92	T45.93	T45.94	T45.95	T45.96
specified NEC	T45.8X1	T45.8X2	T45.8X3	T45.8X4	T45.8X5	T45.8X6
Hemlock	T62.2X1	T62.2X2	T62.2X3	T62.2X4	—	—
Hemostatic	T45.621	T45.622	T45.623	T45.624	T45.625	T45.626
drug, systemic	T45.621	T45.622	T45.623	T45.624	T45.625	T45.626
Hemostyptic	T49.4X1	T49.4X2	T49.4X3	T49.4X4	T49.4X5	T49.4X6
Henbane	T62.2X1	T62.2X2	T62.2X3	T62.2X4	—	—
Heparin (sodium)	T45.511	T45.512	T45.513	T45.514	T45.515	T45.516
action reverser	T45.7X1	T45.7X2	T45.7X3	T45.7X4	T45.7X5	T45.7X6
Heparin-fraction	T45.511	T45.512	T45.513	T45.514	T45.515	T45.516
Heparinoid (systemic)	T45.511	T45.512	T45.513	T45.514	T45.515	T45.516

Substance	Poisoning, Accidental (unintentional)	Poisoning, Intentional Self-harm	Poisoning, Assault	Poisoning, Undetermined	Adverse Effect	Under-dosing
Hepatic secretion stimulant	T47.8X1	T47.8X2	T47.8X3	T47.8X4	T47.8X5	T47.8X6
Hepatitis B						
immune globulin	T50.Z11	T50.Z12	T50.Z13	T50.Z14	T50.Z15	T50.Z16
vaccine	T50.B91	T50.B92	T50.B93	T50.B94	T50.B95	T50.B96
Hepronicate	T46.7X1	T46.7X2	T46.7X3	T46.7X4	T46.7X5	T46.7X6
Heptabarb	T42.3X1	T42.3X2	T42.3X3	T42.3X4	T42.3X5	T42.3X6
Heptabarbital	T42.3X1	T42.3X2	T42.3X3	T42.3X4	T42.3X5	T42.3X6
Heptabarbitone	T42.3X1	T42.3X2	T42.3X3	T42.3X4	T42.3X5	T42.3X6
Heptachlor	T60.1X1	T60.1X2	T60.1X3	T60.1X4	—	—
Heptalgin	T40.2X1	T40.2X2	T40.2X3	T40.2X4	T40.2X5	T40.2X6
Heptaminol	T46.3X1	T46.3X2	T46.3X3	T46.3X4	T46.3X5	T46.3X6
Herbicide NEC	T60.3X1	T60.3X2	T60.3X3	T60.3X4	—	—
Heroin	T40.1X1	T40.1X2	T40.1X3	T40.1X4	—	—
Herplex	T49.5X1	T49.5X2	T49.5X3	T49.5X4	T49.5X5	T49.5X6
HES	T45.8X1	T45.8X2	T45.8X3	T45.8X4	T45.8X5	T45.8X6
Hesperidin	T46.991	T46.992	T46.993	T46.994	T46.995	T46.996
Hetacillin	T36.0X1	T36.0X2	T36.0X3	T36.0X4	T36.0X5	T36.0X6
Hetastarch	T45.8X1	T45.8X2	T45.8X3	T45.8X4	T45.8X5	T45.8X6
HETP	T60.0X1	T60.0X2	T60.0X3	T60.0X4	—	—
Hexachlorobenzene (vapor)	T60.3X1	T60.3X2	T60.3X3	T60.3X4	—	—
Hexachlorocyclohexane	T53.6X1	T53.6X2	T53.6X3	T53.6X4	—	—
Hexachlorophene	T49.0X1	T49.0X2	T49.0X3	T49.0X4	T49.0X5	T49.0X6
Hexadiline	T46.3X1	T46.3X2	T46.3X3	T46.3X4	T46.3X5	T46.3X6
Hexadimethrine (bromide)	T45.7X1	T45.7X2	T45.7X3	T45.7X4	T45.7X5	T45.7X6
Hexadylamine	T46.3X1	T46.3X2	T46.3X3	T46.3X4	T46.3X5	T46.3X6
Hexaethyl tetraphosphate	T60.0X1	T60.0X2	T60.0X3	T60.0X4	—	—
Hexafluorenium bromide	T48.1X1	T48.1X2	T48.1X3	T48.1X4	T48.1X5	T48.1X6
Hexafluronium (bromide)	T48.1X1	T48.1X2	T48.1X3	T48.1X4	T48.1X5	T48.1X6
Hexa-germ	T49.2X1	T49.2X2	T49.2X3	T49.2X4	T49.2X5	T49.2X6
Hexahydrobenzol	T52.8X1	T52.8X2	T52.8X3	T52.8X4	—	—
Hexahydrocresol(s)	T51.8X1	T51.8X2	T51.8X3	T51.8X4	—	—
arsenide	T57.0X1	T57.0X2	T57.0X3	T57.0X4	—	—
arseniurated	T57.0X1	T57.0X2	T57.0X3	T57.0X4	—	—
cyanide	T57.3X1	T57.3X2	T57.3X3	T57.3X4	—	—
gas	T59.891	T59.892	T59.893	T59.894	—	—
Fluoride (liquid)	T57.8X1	T57.8X2	T57.8X3	T57.8X4	—	—
vapor	T59.891	T59.892	T59.893	T59.894	—	—
phophorated	T60.0X1	T60.0X2	T60.0X3	T60.0X4	—	—
sulfate	T57.8X1	T57.8X2	T57.8X3	T57.8X4	—	—
sulfide (gas)	T59.6X1	T59.6X2	T59.6X3	T59.6X4	—	—
arseniurated	T57.0X1	T57.0X2	T57.0X3	T57.0X4	—	—
sulfurated	T57.8X1	T57.8X2	T57.8X3	T57.8X4	—	—
Hexahydrophenol	T51.8X1	T51.8X2	T51.8X3	T51.8X4	—	—
Hexalen	T51.8X1	T51.8X2	T51.8X3	T51.8X4	—	—
Hexamethonium bromide	T44.2X1	T44.2X2	T44.2X3	T44.2X4	T44.2X5	T44.2X6
Hexamethylene	T52.8X1	T52.8X2	T52.8X3	T52.8X4	—	—
Hexamethylmelamine	T45.1X1	T45.1X2	T45.1X3	T45.1X4	T45.1X5	T45.1X6
Hexamidine	T49.0X1	T49.0X2	T49.0X3	T49.0X4	T49.0X5	T49.0X6
Hexamine (mandelate)	T37.8X1	T37.8X2	T37.8X3	T37.8X4	T37.8X5	T37.8X6
Hexanone, 2-hexanone	T52.4X1	T52.4X2	T52.4X3	T52.4X4	—	—
Hexanuorenium	T48.1X1	T48.1X2	T48.1X3	T48.1X4	T48.1X5	T48.1X6
Hexapropymate	T42.6X1	T42.6X2	T42.6X3	T42.6X4	T42.6X5	T42.6X6
Hexasonium iodide	T44.3X1	T44.3X2	T44.3X3	T44.3X4	T44.3X5	T44.3X6
Hexcarbacholine bromide	T48.1X1	T48.1X2	T48.1X3	T48.1X4	T48.1X5	T48.1X6
Hexemal	T42.3X1	T42.3X2	T42.3X3	T42.3X4	T42.3X5	T42.3X6
Hexestrol	T38.5X1	T38.5X2	T38.5X3	T38.5X4	T38.5X5	T38.5X6
Hexethal (sodium)	T42.3X1	T42.3X2	T42.3X3	T42.3X4	T42.3X5	T42.3X6
Hexetidine	T37.8X1	T37.8X2	T37.8X3	T37.8X4	T37.8X5	T37.8X6
Hexobarbital	T42.3X1	T42.3X2	T42.3X3	T42.3X4	T42.3X5	T42.3X6
rectal	T41.291	T41.292	T41.293	T41.294	T41.295	T41.296
sodium	T41.1X1	T41.1X2	T41.1X3	T41.1X4	T41.1X5	T41.1X6
Hexobendine	T46.3X1	T46.3X2	T46.3X3	T46.3X4	T46.3X5	T46.3X6
Hexocyclium	T44.3X1	T44.3X2	T44.3X3	T44.3X4	T44.3X5	T44.3X6
metilsulfate	T44.3X1	T44.3X2	T44.3X3	T44.3X4	T44.3X5	T44.3X6
Hexoestrol	T38.5X1	T38.5X2	T38.5X3	T38.5X4	T38.5X5	T38.5X6
Hexone	T52.4X1	T52.4X2	T52.4X3	T52.4X4	—	—
Hexoprenaline	T48.6X1	T48.6X2	T48.6X3	T48.6X4	T48.6X5	T48.6X6
Hexylcaine	T41.3X1	T41.3X2	T41.3X3	T41.3X4	T41.3X5	T41.3X6
Hexylresorcinol	T52.2X1	T52.2X2	T52.2X3	T52.2X4	—	—
HGH (human growth hormone)	T38.811	T38.812	T38.813	T38.814	T38.815	T38.816
Hinkle's pills	T47.2X1	T47.2X2	T47.2X3	T47.2X4	T47.2X5	T47.2X6
Histalog	T50.8X1	T50.8X2	T50.8X3	T50.8X4	T50.8X5	T50.8X6
Histamine (phosphate)	T50.8X1	T50.8X2	T50.8X3	T50.8X4	T50.8X5	T50.8X6
Histoplasmin	T50.8X1	T50.8X2	T50.8X3	T50.8X4	T50.8X5	T50.8X6
Holly berries	T62.2X1	T62.2X2	T62.2X3	T62.2X4	—	—
Homatropine	T44.3X1	T44.3X2	T44.3X3	T44.3X4	T44.3X5	T44.3X6
methylbromide	T44.3X1	T44.3X2	T44.3X3	T44.3X4	T44.3X5	T44.3X6
Homochlorcyclizine	T45.0X1	T45.0X2	T45.0X3	T45.0X4	T45.0X5	T45.0X6
Homosalate	T49.3X1	T49.3X2	T49.3X3	T49.3X4	T49.3X5	T49.3X6
Homo-tet	T50.Z11	T50.Z12	T50.Z13	T50.Z14	T50.Z15	T50.Z16
Hormone	T38.801	T38.802	T38.803	T38.804	T38.805	T38.806

Substance	Poisoning, Accidental (unintentional)	Poisoning, Intentional Self-harm	Poisoning, Assault	Poisoning, Undetermined	Adverse Effect	Under-dosing
Hormone — continued						
adrenal cortical steroids	T38.0X1	T38.0X2	T38.0X3	T38.0X4	T38.0X5	T38.0X6
androgenic	T38.7X1	T38.7X2	T38.7X3	T38.7X4	T38.7X5	T38.7X6
anterior pituitary NEC	T38.811	T38.812	T38.813	T38.814	T38.815	T38.816
antidiabetic agents	T38.3X1	T38.3X2	T38.3X3	T38.3X4	T38.3X5	T38.3X6
antidiuretic	T38.891	T38.892	T38.893	T38.894	T38.895	T38.896
cancer therapy	T45.1X1	T45.1X2	T45.1X3	T45.1X4	T45.1X5	T45.1X6
follicle stimulating	T38.811	T38.812	T38.813	T38.814	T38.815	T38.816
gonadotropic	T38.891	T38.892	T38.893	T38.894	T38.895	T38.896
pituitary	T38.811	T38.812	T38.813	T38.814	T38.815	T38.816
growth	T38.811	T38.812	T38.813	T38.814	T38.815	T38.816
luteinizing	T38.811	T38.812	T38.813	T38.814	T38.815	T38.816
ovarian	T38.5X1	T38.5X2	T38.5X3	T38.5X4	T38.5X5	T38.5X6
oxytocic	T48.0X1	T48.0X2	T48.0X3	T48.0X4	T48.0X5	T48.0X6
parathyroid (derivatives)	T50.991	T50.992	T50.993	T50.994	T50.995	T50.996
pituitary (posterior) NEC	T38.891	T38.892	T38.893	T38.894	T38.895	T38.896
anterior	T38.811	T38.812	T38.813	T38.814	T38.815	T38.816
specified, NEC	T38.891	T38.892	T38.893	T38.894	T38.895	T38.896
thyroid	T38.1X1	T38.1X2	T38.1X3	T38.1X4	T38.1X5	T38.1X6
Hornet (sting)	T63.451	T63.452	T63.453	T63.454	—	—
Horse anti-human lymphocytic serum	T50.Z11	T50.Z12	T50.Z13	T50.Z14	T50.Z15	T50.Z16
Horticulture agent NEC	T65.91	T65.92	T65.93	T65.94	—	—
with pesticide	T60.91	T60.92	T60.93	T60.94	—	—
Human						
albumin	T45.8X1	T45.8X2	T45.8X3	T45.8X4	T45.8X5	T45.8X6
growth hormone (HGH)	T38.811	T38.812	T38.813	T38.814	T38.815	T38.816
immune serum	T50.Z11	T50.Z12	T50.Z13	T50.Z14	T50.Z15	T50.Z16
Hyaluronidase	T45.3X1	T45.3X2	T45.3X3	T45.3X4	T45.3X5	T45.3X6
Hyazyme	T45.3X1	T45.3X2	T45.3X3	T45.3X4	T45.3X5	T45.3X6
Hycodan	T40.2X1	T40.2X2	T40.2X3	T40.2X4	T40.2X5	T40.2X6
Hydantoin derivative NEC	T42.0X1	T42.0X2	T42.0X3	T42.0X4	T42.0X5	T42.0X6
Hydeltra	T38.0X1	T38.0X2	T38.0X3	T38.0X4	T38.0X5	T38.0X6
Hydergine	T44.6X1	T44.6X2	T44.6X3	T44.6X4	T44.6X5	T44.6X6
Hydrabamine penicillin	T36.0X1	T36.0X2	T36.0X3	T36.0X4	T36.0X5	T36.0X6
Hydralazine	T46.5X1	T46.5X2	T46.5X3	T46.5X4	T46.5X5	T46.5X6
Hydrargaphen	T49.0X1	T49.0X2	T49.0X3	T49.0X4	T49.0X5	T49.0X6
Hydrargyri aminochloridum	T49.0X1	T49.0X2	T49.0X3	T49.0X4	T49.0X5	T49.0X6
Hydrastine	T48.291	T48.292	T48.293	T48.294	T48.295	T48.296
Hydrazine	T54.1X1	T54.1X2	T54.1X3	T54.1X4	—	—
monoamine oxidase inhibitors	T43.1X1	T43.1X2	T43.1X3	T43.1X4	T43.1X5	T43.1X6
Hydrazoic acid, azides	T54.2X1	T54.2X2	T54.2X3	T54.2X4	—	—
Hydriodic acid	T48.4X1	T48.4X2	T48.4X3	T48.4X4	T48.4X5	T48.4X6
Hydrocarbon gas	T59.891	T59.892	T59.893	T59.894	—	—
incomplete combustion of — see Carbon, monoxide, fuel, utility						
liquefied (mobile container)	T59.891	T59.892	T59.893	T59.894	—	—
piped (natural)	T59.891	T59.892	T59.893	T59.894	—	—
Hydrochloric acid (liquid)	T54.2X1	T54.2X2	T54.2X3	T54.2X4	—	—
medicinal (digestant)	T47.5X1	T47.5X2	T47.5X3	T47.5X4	T47.5X5	T47.5X6
vapor	T59.891	T59.892	T59.893	T59.894	—	—
Hydrochlorothiazide	T50.2X1	T50.2X2	T50.2X3	T50.2X4	T50.2X5	T50.2X6
Hydrocodone	T40.2X1	T40.2X2	T40.2X3	T40.2X4	T40.2X5	T40.2X6
Hydrocortisone (derivatives)	T49.0X1	T49.0X2	T49.0X3	T49.0X4	T49.0X5	T49.0X6
aceponate	T49.0X1	T49.0X2	T49.0X3	T49.0X4	T49.0X5	T49.0X6
ENT agent	T49.6X1	T49.6X2	T49.6X3	T49.6X4	T49.6X5	T49.6X6
ophthalmic preparation	T49.5X1	T49.5X2	T49.5X3	T49.5X4	T49.5X5	T49.5X6
topical NEC	T49.0X1	T49.0X2	T49.0X3	T49.0X4	T49.0X5	T49.0X6
Hydrocortone	T38.0X1	T38.0X2	T38.0X3	T38.0X4	T38.0X5	T38.0X6
ENT agent	T49.6X1	T49.6X2	T49.6X3	T49.6X4	T49.6X5	T49.6X6
ophthalmic preparation	T49.5X1	T49.5X2	T49.5X3	T49.5X4	T49.5X5	T49.5X6
topical NEC	T49.0X1	T49.0X2	T49.0X3	T49.0X4	T49.0X5	T49.0X6
Hydrocyanic acid (liquid)	T57.3X1	T57.3X2	T57.3X3	T57.3X4	—	—
gas	T65.0X1	T65.0X2	T65.0X3	T65.0X4	—	—
Hydroflumethiazide	T50.2X1	T50.2X2	T50.2X3	T50.2X4	T50.2X5	T50.2X6
Hydrofluoric acid (liquid)	T54.2X1	T54.2X2	T54.2X3	T54.2X4	—	—
vapor	T59.891	T59.892	T59.893	T59.894	—	—
Hydrogen	T59.891	T59.892	T59.893	T59.894	—	—
arsenide	T57.0X1	T57.0X2	T57.0X3	T57.0X4	—	—
arseniureted	T57.0X1	T57.0X2	T57.0X3	T57.0X4	—	—
chloride	T57.8X1	T57.8X2	T57.8X3	T57.8X4	—	—
cyanide (salts)	T57.3X1	T57.3X2	T57.3X3	T57.3X4	—	—
gas	T57.3X1	T57.3X2	T57.3X3	T57.3X4	—	—
Fluoride	T59.5X1	T59.5X2	T59.5X3	T59.5X4	—	—
vapor	T59.5X1	T59.5X2	T59.5X3	T59.5X4	—	—
peroxide	T49.0X1	T49.0X2	T49.0X3	T49.0X4	T49.0X5	T49.0X6
phosphureted	T57.1X1	T57.1X2	T57.1X3	T57.1X4	—	—
sulfide	T59.6X1	T59.6X2	T59.6X3	T59.6X4	—	—
arseniureted	T57.0X1	T57.0X2	T57.0X3	T57.0X4	—	—
sulfureted	T59.6X1	T59.6X2	T59.6X3	T59.6X4	—	—

Additional Character May Be Required — Refer to the Tabular List for Character Selection ▽ Subterms under main terms may continue to next column or page

Substance	Poisoning, Accidental (unintentional)	Poisoning, Intentional Self-harm	Poisoning, Assault	Poisoning, Undetermined	Adverse Effect	Under-dosing
Hydromethylpyridine	T46.7X1	T46.7X2	T46.7X3	T46.7X4	T46.7X5	T46.7X6
Hydromorphinol	T40.2X1	T40.2X2	T40.2X3	T40.2X4	—	—
Hydromorphinone	T40.2X1	T40.2X2	T40.2X3	T40.2X4	T40.2X5	T40.2X6
Hydromorphone	T40.2X1	T40.2X2	T40.2X3	T40.2X4	T40.2X5	T40.2X6
Hydromox	T50.2X1	T50.2X2	T50.2X3	T50.2X4	T50.2X5	T50.2X6
Hydrophilic lotion	T49.3X1	T49.3X2	T49.3X3	T49.3X4	T49.3X5	T49.3X6
Hydroquinidine	T46.2X1	T46.2X2	T46.2X3	T46.2X4	T46.2X5	T46.2X6
Hydroquinone	T52.2X1	T52.2X2	T52.2X3	T52.2X4	—	—
vapor	T59.891	T59.892	T59.893	T59.894	—	—
Hydrosulfuric acid (gas)	T59.6X1	T59.6X2	T59.6X3	T59.6X4	—	—
Hydrotalcite	T47.1X1	T47.1X2	T47.1X3	T47.1X4	T47.1X5	T47.1X6
Hydrous wool fat	T49.3X1	T49.3X2	T49.3X3	T49.3X4	T49.3X5	T49.3X6
Hydroxide, caustic	T54.3X1	T54.3X2	T54.3X3	T54.3X4	—	—
Hydroxocobalamin	T45.8X1	T45.8X2	T45.8X3	T45.8X4	T45.8X5	T45.8X6
Hydroxyamphetamine	T49.5X1	T49.5X2	T49.5X3	T49.5X4	T49.5X5	T49.5X6
Hydroxycarbamide	T45.1X1	T45.1X2	T45.1X3	T45.1X4	T45.1X5	T45.1X6
Hydroxychloroquine	T37.8X1	T37.8X2	T37.8X3	T37.8X4	T37.8X5	T37.8X6
Hydroxydihydrocodeinone	T40.2X1	T40.2X2	T40.2X3	T40.2X4	T40.2X5	T40.2X6
Hydroxyestrone	T38.5X1	T38.5X2	T38.5X3	T38.5X4	T38.5X5	T38.5X6
Hydroxyethyl starch	T45.8X1	T45.8X2	T45.8X3	T45.8X4	T45.8X5	T45.8X6
Hydroxymethylpentanone	T52.4X1	T52.4X2	T52.4X3	T52.4X4	—	—
Hydroxyphenamate	T43.591	T43.592	T43.593	T43.594	T43.595	T43.596
Hydroxyphenylbutazone	T39.2X1	T39.2X2	T39.2X3	T39.2X4	T39.2X5	T39.2X6
Hydroxyprogesterone	T38.5X1	T38.5X2	T38.5X3	T38.5X4	T38.5X5	T38.5X6
caproate	T38.5X1	T38.5X2	T38.5X3	T38.5X4	T38.5X5	T38.5X6
Hydroxyquinoline (derivatives) NEC	T37.8X1	T37.8X2	T37.8X3	T37.8X4	T37.8X5	T37.8X6
Hydroxystilbamidine	T37.3X1	T37.3X2	T37.3X3	T37.3X4	T37.3X5	T37.3X6
Hydroxytoluene (nonmedicinal)	T54.0X1	T54.0X2	T54.0X3	T54.0X4	—	—
medicinal	T49.0X1	T49.0X2	T49.0X3	T49.0X4	T49.0X5	T49.0X6
Hydroxyurea	T45.1X1	T45.1X2	T45.1X3	T45.1X4	T45.1X5	T45.1X6
Hydroxyzine	T43.591	T43.592	T43.593	T43.594	T43.595	T43.596
Hyoscine	T44.3X1	T44.3X2	T44.3X3	T44.3X4	T44.3X5	T44.3X6
Hyoscyamine	T44.3X1	T44.3X2	T44.3X3	T44.3X4	T44.3X5	T44.3X6
Hyoscyamus	T44.3X1	T44.3X2	T44.3X3	T44.3X4	T44.3X5	T44.3X6
dry extract	T44.3X1	T44.3X2	T44.3X3	T44.3X4	T44.3X5	T44.3X6
Hypaque	T50.8X1	T50.8X2	T50.8X3	T50.8X4	T50.8X5	T50.8X6
Hypertussis	T50.Z11	T50.Z12	T50.Z13	T50.Z14	T50.Z15	T50.Z16
Hypnotic	T42.71	T42.72	T42.73	T42.74	T42.75	T42.76
anticonvulsant	T42.71	T42.72	T42.73	T42.74	T42.75	T42.76
specified NEC	T42.6X1	T42.6X2	T42.6X3	T42.6X4	T42.6X5	T42.6X6
Hypochlorite	T49.0X1	T49.0X2	T49.0X3	T49.0X4	T49.0X5	T49.0X6
Hypophysis, posterior	T38.891	T38.892	T38.893	T38.894	T38.895	T38.896
Hypotensive NEC	T46.5X1	T46.5X2	T46.5X3	T46.5X4	T46.5X5	T46.5X6
Hypromellose	T49.5X1	T49.5X2	T49.5X3	T49.5X4	T49.5X5	T49.5X6
Ibacitabine	T37.5X1	T37.5X2	T37.5X3	T37.5X4	T37.5X5	T37.5X6
Ibopamine	T44.991	T44.992	T44.993	T44.994	T44.995	T44.996
Ibufenac	T39.311	T39.312	T39.313	T39.314	T39.315	T39.316
Ibuprofen	T39.311	T39.312	T39.313	T39.314	T39.315	T39.316
Ibuproxam	T39.311	T39.312	T39.313	T39.314	T39.315	T39.316
Ibuterol	T48.6X1	T48.6X2	T48.6X3	T48.6X4	T48.6X5	T48.6X6
Ichthammol	T49.0X1	T49.0X2	T49.0X3	T49.0X4	T49.0X5	T49.0X6
Ichthyol	T49.4X1	T49.4X2	T49.4X3	T49.4X4	T49.4X5	T49.4X6
Idarubicin	T45.1X1	T45.1X2	T45.1X3	T45.1X4	T45.1X5	T45.1X6
Idrocilamide	T42.8X1	T42.8X2	T42.8X3	T42.8X4	T42.8X5	T42.8X6
Ifenprodil	T46.7X1	T46.7X2	T46.7X3	T46.7X4	T46.7X5	T46.7X6
Ifosfamide	T45.1X1	T45.1X2	T45.1X3	T45.1X4	T45.1X5	T45.1X6
Iletin	T38.3X1	T38.3X2	T38.3X3	T38.3X4	T38.3X5	T38.3X6
Ilex	T62.2X1	T62.2X2	T62.2X3	T62.2X4	—	—
Illuminating gas (after combustion)	T58.11	T58.12	T58.13	T58.14	—	—
prior to combustion	T59.891	T59.892	T59.893	T59.894	—	—
Ilopan	T45.2X1	T45.2X2	T45.2X3	T45.2X4	T45.2X5	T45.2X6
Iloprost	T46.7X1	T46.7X2	T46.7X3	T46.7X4	T46.7X5	T46.7X6
Ilotycin	T36.3X1	T36.3X2	T36.3X3	T36.3X4	T36.3X5	T36.3X6
ophthalmic preparation	T49.5X1	T49.5X2	T49.5X3	T49.5X4	T49.5X5	T49.5X6
topical NEC	T49.0X1	T49.0X2	T49.0X3	T49.0X4	T49.0X5	T49.0X6
Imidazole-4-carboxamide	T45.1X1	T45.1X2	T45.1X3	T45.1X4	T45.1X5	T45.1X6
Iminostilbene	T42.1X1	T42.1X2	T42.1X3	T42.1X4	T42.1X5	T42.1X6
Imipenem	T36.0X1	T36.0X2	T36.0X3	T36.0X4	T36.0X5	T36.0X6
Imipramine	T43.011	T43.012	T43.013	T43.014	T43.015	T43.016
Immu-G	T50.Z11	T50.Z12	T50.Z13	T50.Z14	T50.Z15	T50.Z16
Immuglobin	T50.Z11	T50.Z12	T50.Z13	T50.Z14	T50.Z15	T50.Z16
Immune						
globulin	T50.Z11	T50.Z12	T50.Z13	T50.Z14	T50.Z15	T50.Z16
serum globulin	T50.Z11	T50.Z12	T50.Z13	T50.Z14	T50.Z15	T50.Z16
Immunoglobin human (intravenous) (normal)	T50.Z11	T50.Z12	T50.Z13	T50.Z14	T50.Z15	T50.Z16
unmodified	T50.Z11	T50.Z12	T50.Z13	T50.Z14	T50.Z15	T50.Z16
Immunosuppressive drug	T45.1X1	T45.1X2	T45.1X3	T45.1X4	T45.1X5	T45.1X6
Immu-tetanus	T50.Z11	T50.Z12	T50.Z13	T50.Z14	T50.Z15	T50.Z16
Indalpine	T43.221	T43.222	T43.223	T43.224	T43.225	T43.226
Indanazoline	T48.5X1	T48.5X2	T48.5X3	T48.5X4	T48.5X5	T48.5X6
Indandione (derivatives)	T45.511	T45.512	T45.513	T45.514	T45.515	T45.516
Indapamide	T46.5X1	T46.5X2	T46.5X3	T46.5X4	T46.5X5	T46.5X6
Indendione (derivatives)	T45.511	T45.512	T45.513	T45.514	T45.515	T45.516
Indenolol	T44.7X1	T44.7X2	T44.7X3	T44.7X4	T44.7X5	T44.7X6
Inderal	T44.7X1	T44.7X2	T44.7X3	T44.7X4	T44.7X5	T44.7X6
Indian						
hemp	T40.7X1	T40.7X2	T40.7X3	T40.7X4	T40.7X5	T40.7X6
tobacco	T62.2X1	T62.2X2	T62.2X3	T62.2X4	—	—
Indigo carmine	T50.8X1	T50.8X2	T50.8X3	T50.8X4	T50.8X5	T50.8X6
Indobufen	T45.521	T45.522	T45.523	T45.524	T45.525	T45.526
Indocin	T39.2X1	T39.2X2	T39.2X3	T39.2X4	T39.2X5	T39.2X6
Indocyanine green	T50.8X1	T50.8X2	T50.8X3	T50.8X4	T50.8X5	T50.8X6
Indometacin	T39.391	T39.392	T39.393	T39.394	T39.395	T39.396
Indomethacin	T39.391	T39.392	T39.393	T39.394	T39.395	T39.396
farnesil	T39.4X1	T39.4X2	T39.4X3	T39.4X4	T39.4X5	T39.4X6
Indoramin	T44.6X1	T44.6X2	T44.6X3	T44.6X4	T44.6X5	T44.6X6
Industrial						
alcohol	T51.0X1	T51.0X2	T51.0X3	T51.0X4	—	—
fumes	T59.891	T59.892	T59.893	T59.894	—	—
solvents (fumes) (vapors)	T52.91	T52.92	T52.93	T52.94	—	—
Influenza vaccine	T50.B91	T50.B92	T50.B93	T50.B94	T50.B95	T50.B96
Ingested substance NEC	T65.91	T65.92	T65.93	T65.94	—	—
INH	T37.1X1	T37.1X2	T37.1X3	T37.1X4	T37.1X5	T37.1X6
Inhalation, gas (noxious) — see Gas						
Inhibitor						
angiotensin-converting enzyme	T46.4X1	T46.4X2	T46.4X3	T46.4X4	T46.4X5	T46.4X6
carbonic anhydrase	T50.2X1	T50.2X2	T50.2X3	T50.2X4	T50.2X5	T50.2X6
fibrinolysis	T45.621	T45.622	T45.623	T45.624	T45.625	T45.626
monoamine oxidase NEC	T43.1X1	T43.1X2	T43.1X3	T43.1X4	T43.1X5	T43.1X6
hydrazine	T43.1X1	T43.1X2	T43.1X3	T43.1X4	T43.1X5	T43.1X6
postsynaptic	T43.8X1	T43.8X2	T43.8X3	T43.8X4	T43.8X5	T43.8X6
prothrombin synthesis	T45.511	T45.512	T45.513	T45.514	T45.515	T45.516
Ink	T65.891	T65.892	T65.893	T65.894	—	—
Inorganic substance NEC	T57.91	T57.92	T57.93	T57.94	—	—
Inosine pranobex	T37.5X1	T37.5X2	T37.5X3	T37.5X4	T37.5X5	T37.5X6
Inositol	T50.991	T50.992	T50.993	T50.994	T50.995	T50.996
nicotinate	T46.7X1	T46.7X2	T46.7X3	T46.7X4	T46.7X5	T46.7X6
Inproquone	T45.1X1	T45.1X2	T45.1X3	T45.1X4	T45.1X5	T45.1X6
Insecticide NEC	T60.91	T60.92	T60.93	T60.94		
carbamate	T60.0X1	T60.0X2	T60.0X3	T60.0X4		
chlorinated	T60.1X1	T60.1X2	T60.1X3	T60.1X4		
mixed	T60.91	T60.92	T60.93	T60.94		
organochlorine	T60.1X1	T60.1X2	T60.1X3	T60.1X4		
organophosphorus	T60.0X1	T60.0X2	T60.0X3	T60.0X4		
Insect (sting), venomous	T63.481	T63.482	T63.483	T63.484		
ant	T63.421	T63.422	T63.423	T63.424		
bee	T63.441	T63.442	T63.443	T63.444		
caterpillar	T63.431	T63.432	T63.433	T63.434		
hornet	T63.451	T63.452	T63.453	T63.454		
wasp	T63.461	T63.462	T63.463	T63.464		
Insular tissue extract	T38.3X1	T38.3X2	T38.3X3	T38.3X4	T38.3X5	T38.3X6
Insulin (amorphous) (globin) (isophane) (Lente) (NPH) (Semilente) (Ultralente)	T38.3X1	T38.3X2	T38.3X3	T38.3X4	T38.3X5	T38.3X6
defalan	T38.3X1	T38.3X2	T38.3X3	T38.3X4	T38.3X5	T38.3X6
human	T38.3X1	T38.3X2	T38.3X3	T38.3X4	T38.3X5	T38.3X6
injection, soluble	T38.3X1	T38.3X2	T38.3X3	T38.3X4	T38.3X5	T38.3X6
biphasic	T38.3X1	T38.3X2	T38.3X3	T38.3X4	T38.3X5	T38.3X6
intermediate acting	T38.3X1	T38.3X2	T38.3X3	T38.3X4	T38.3X5	T38.3X6
protamine zinc	T38.3X1	T38.3X2	T38.3X3	T38.3X4	T38.3X5	T38.3X6
slow acting	T38.3X1	T38.3X2	T38.3X3	T38.3X4	T38.3X5	T38.3X6
zinc						
protamine injection	T38.3X1	T38.3X2	T38.3X3	T38.3X4	T38.3X5	T38.3X6
suspension (amorphous) (crystalline)	T38.3X1	T38.3X2	T38.3X3	T38.3X4	T38.3X5	T38.3X6
Interferon (alpha) (beta) (gamma)	T37.5X1	T37.5X2	T37.5X3	T37.5X4	T37.5X5	T37.5X6
Intestinal motility control drug	T47.6X1	T47.6X2	T47.6X3	T47.6X4	T47.6X5	T47.6X6
biological	T47.8X1	T47.8X2	T47.8X3	T47.8X4	T47.8X5	T47.8X6
Intranarcon	T41.1X1	T41.1X2	T41.1X3	T41.1X4	T41.1X5	T41.1X6
Intravenous						
amino acids	T50.991	T50.992	T50.993	T50.994	T50.995	T50.996
fat suspension	T50.991	T50.992	T50.993	T50.994	T50.995	T50.996
Inulin	T50.8X1	T50.8X2	T50.8X3	T50.8X4	T50.8X5	T50.8X6
Invert sugar	T50.3X1	T50.3X2	T50.3X3	T50.3X4	T50.3X5	T50.3X6
Inza — see Naproxen						
Iobenzamic acid	T50.8X1	T50.8X2	T50.8X3	T50.8X4	T50.8X5	T50.8X6
Iocarmic acid	T50.8X1	T50.8X2	T50.8X3	T50.8X4	T50.8X5	T50.8X6
Iocetamic acid	T50.8X1	T50.8X2	T50.8X3	T50.8X4	T50.8X5	T50.8X6

Table of Drugs and Chemicals

Iodamide — Karaya

Substance	Poisoning, Accidental (unintentional)	Poisoning, Intentional Self-harm	Poisoning, Assault	Poisoning, Undetermined	Adverse Effect	Under-dosing
Iodamide	T50.8X1	T50.8X2	T50.8X3	T50.8X4	T50.8X5	T50.8X6
Iodide NEC — *see also* Iodine	T49.0X1	T49.0X2	T49.0X3	T49.0X4	T49.0X5	T49.0X6
mercury (ointment)	T49.0X1	T49.0X2	T49.0X3	T49.0X4	T49.0X5	T49.0X6
methylate	T49.0X1	T49.0X2	T49.0X3	T49.0X4	T49.0X5	T49.0X6
potassium (expectorant) NEC	T48.4X1	T48.4X2	T48.4X3	T48.4X4	T48.4X5	T48.4X6
Iodinated						
contrast medium	T50.8X1	T50.8X2	T50.8X3	T50.8X4	T50.8X5	T50.8X6
glycerol	T48.4X1	T48.4X2	T48.4X3	T48.4X4	T48.4X5	T48.4X6
human serum albumin (131I)	T50.8X1	T50.8X2	T50.8X3	T50.8X4	T50.8X5	T50.8X6
Iodine (antiseptic, external) (tincture) **NEC**	T49.0X1	T49.0X2	T49.0X3	T49.0X4	T49.0X5	T49.0X6
125 — *see also* Radiation sickness, and Exposure to radioactivce isotopes	T50.8X1	T50.8X2	T50.8X3	T50.8X4	T50.8X5	T50.8X6
therapeutic	T50.991	T50.992	T50.993	T50.994	T50.995	T50.996
131 — *see also* Radiation sickness, and Exposure to radioactivce isotopes	T50.8X1	T50.8X2	T50.8X3	T50.8X4	T50.8X5	T50.8X6
therapeutic	T38.2X1	T38.2X2	T38.2X3	T38.2X4	T38.2X5	T38.2X6
diagnostic	T50.8X1	T50.8X2	T50.8X3	T50.8X4	T50.8X5	T50.8X6
for thyroid conditions (antithyroid)	T38.2X1	T38.2X2	T38.2X3	T38.2X4	T38.2X5	T38.2X6
solution	T49.0X1	T49.0X2	T49.0X3	T49.0X4	T49.0X5	T49.0X6
vapor	T59.891	T59.892	T59.893	T59.894	—	—
Iodipamide	T50.8X1	T50.8X2	T50.8X3	T50.8X4	T50.8X5	T50.8X6
Iodized (poppy seed) oil	T50.8X1	T50.8X2	T50.8X3	T50.8X4	T50.8X5	T50.8X6
Iodobismitol	T37.8X1	T37.8X2	T37.8X3	T37.8X4	T37.8X5	T37.8X6
Iodochlorhydroxyquin	T37.8X1	T37.8X2	T37.8X3	T37.8X4	T37.8X5	T37.8X6
topical	T49.0X1	T49.0X2	T49.0X3	T49.0X4	T49.0X5	T49.0X6
Iodochlorhydroxyquinoline	T37.8X1	T37.8X2	T37.8X3	T37.8X4	T37.8X5	T37.8X6
Iodocholesterol (131I)	T50.8X1	T50.8X2	T50.8X3	T50.8X4	T50.8X5	T50.8X6
Iodoform	T49.0X1	T49.0X2	T49.0X3	T49.0X4	T49.0X5	T49.0X6
Iodohippuric acid	T50.8X1	T50.8X2	T50.8X3	T50.8X4	T50.8X5	T50.8X6
Iodopanoic acid	T50.8X1	T50.8X2	T50.8X3	T50.8X4	T50.8X5	T50.8X6
Iodophthalein (sodium)	T50.8X1	T50.8X2	T50.8X3	T50.8X4	T50.8X5	T50.8X6
Iodopyracet	T50.8X1	T50.8X2	T50.8X3	T50.8X4	T50.8X5	T50.8X6
Iodoquinol	T37.8X1	T37.8X2	T37.8X3	T37.8X4	T37.8X5	T37.8X6
Iodoxamic acid	T50.8X1	T50.8X2	T50.8X3	T50.8X4	T50.8X5	T50.8X6
Iofendylate	T50.8X1	T50.8X2	T50.8X3	T50.8X4	T50.8X5	T50.8X6
Ioglycamic acid	T50.8X1	T50.8X2	T50.8X3	T50.8X4	T50.8X5	T50.8X6
Iohexol	T50.8X1	T50.8X2	T50.8X3	T50.8X4	T50.8X5	T50.8X6
Ion exchange resin						
anion	T47.8X1	T47.8X2	T47.8X3	T47.8X4	T47.8X5	T47.8X6
cation	T50.3X1	T50.3X2	T50.3X3	T50.3X4	T50.3X5	T50.3X6
cholestyramine	T46.6X1	T46.6X2	T46.6X3	T46.6X4	T46.6X5	T46.6X6
intestinal	T47.8X1	T47.8X2	T47.8X3	T47.8X4	T47.8X5	T47.8X6
Iopamidol	T50.8X1	T50.8X2	T50.8X3	T50.8X4	T50.8X5	T50.8X6
Iopanoic acid	T50.8X1	T50.8X2	T50.8X3	T50.8X4	T50.8X5	T50.8X6
Iophenoic acid	T50.8X1	T50.8X2	T50.8X3	T50.8X4	T50.8X5	T50.8X6
Iopodate, sodium	T50.8X1	T50.8X2	T50.8X3	T50.8X4	T50.8X5	T50.8X6
Iopodic acid	T50.8X1	T50.8X2	T50.8X3	T50.8X4	T50.8X5	T50.8X6
Iopromide	T50.8X1	T50.8X2	T50.8X3	T50.8X4	T50.8X5	T50.8X6
Iopydol	T50.8X1	T50.8X2	T50.8X3	T50.8X4	T50.8X5	T50.8X6
Iotalamic acid	T50.8X1	T50.8X2	T50.8X3	T50.8X4	T50.8X5	T50.8X6
Iothalamate	T50.8X1	T50.8X2	T50.8X3	T50.8X4	T50.8X5	T50.8X6
Iothiouracil	T38.2X1	T38.2X2	T38.2X3	T38.2X4	T38.2X5	T38.2X6
Iotrol	T50.8X1	T50.8X2	T50.8X3	T50.8X4	T50.8X5	T50.8X6
Iotrolan	T50.8X1	T50.8X2	T50.8X3	T50.8X4	T50.8X5	T50.8X6
Iotroxate	T50.8X1	T50.8X2	T50.8X3	T50.8X4	T50.8X5	T50.8X6
Iotroxic acid	T50.8X1	T50.8X2	T50.8X3	T50.8X4	T50.8X5	T50.8X6
Ioversol	T50.8X1	T50.8X2	T50.8X3	T50.8X4	T50.8X5	T50.8X6
Ioxaglate	T50.8X1	T50.8X2	T50.8X3	T50.8X4	T50.8X5	T50.8X6
Ioxaglic acid	T50.8X1	T50.8X2	T50.8X3	T50.8X4	T50.8X5	T50.8X6
Ioxitalamic acid	T50.8X1	T50.8X2	T50.8X3	T50.8X4	T50.8X5	T50.8X6
Ipecac	T47.7X1	T47.7X2	T47.7X3	T47.7X4	T47.7X5	T47.7X6
Ipecacuanha	T48.4X1	T48.4X2	T48.4X3	T48.4X4	T48.4X5	T48.4X6
Ipodate, calcium	T50.8X1	T50.8X2	T50.8X3	T50.8X4	T50.8X5	T50.8X6
Ipral	T42.3X1	T42.3X2	T42.3X3	T42.3X4	T42.3X5	T42.3X6
Ipratropium (bromide)	T48.6X1	T48.6X2	T48.6X3	T48.6X4	T48.6X5	T48.6X6
Ipriflavone	T46.3X1	T46.3X2	T46.3X3	T46.3X4	T46.3X5	T46.3X6
Iprindole	T43.011	T43.012	T43.013	T43.014	T43.015	T43.016
Iproclozide	T43.1X1	T43.1X2	T43.1X3	T43.1X4	T43.1X5	T43.1X6
Iprofenin	T50.8X1	T50.8X2	T50.8X3	T50.8X4	T50.8X5	T50.8X6
Iproheptine	T49.2X1	T49.2X2	T49.2X3	T49.2X4	T49.2X5	T49.2X6
Iproniazid	T43.1X1	T43.1X2	T43.1X3	T43.1X4	T43.1X5	T43.1X6
Iproplatin	T45.1X1	T45.1X2	T45.1X3	T45.1X4	T45.1X5	T45.1X6
Iproveratril	T46.1X1	T46.1X2	T46.1X3	T46.1X4	T46.1X5	T46.1X6
Iron (compounds) (medicinal) NEC	T45.4X1	T45.4X2	T45.4X3	T45.4X4	T45.4X5	T45.4X6
ammonium	T45.4X1	T45.4X2	T45.4X3	T45.4X4	T45.4X5	T45.4X6
dextran injection	T45.4X1	T45.4X2	T45.4X3	T45.4X4	T45.4X5	T45.4X6

Substance	Poisoning, Accidental (unintentional)	Poisoning, Intentional Self-harm	Poisoning, Assault	Poisoning, Undetermined	Adverse Effect	Under-dosing
Iron (compounds) (medicinal) **NEC**						
— *continued*						
nonmedicinal	T56.891	T56.892	T56.893	T56.894	—	—
salts	T45.4X1	T45.4X2	T45.4X3	T45.4X4	T45.4X5	T45.4X6
sorbitex	T45.4X1	T45.4X2	T45.4X3	T45.4X4	T45.4X5	T45.4X6
sorbitol citric acid complex	T45.4X1	T45.4X2	T45.4X3	T45.4X4	T45.4X5	T45.4X6
Irrigating fluid (vaginal)	T49.8X1	T49.8X2	T49.8X3	T49.8X4	T49.8X5	T49.8X6
eye	T49.5X1	T49.5X2	T49.5X3	T49.5X4	T49.5X5	T49.5X6
Isepamicin	T36.5X1	T36.5X2	T36.5X3	T36.5X4	T36.5X5	T36.5X6
Isoaminile (citrate)	T48.3X1	T48.3X2	T48.3X3	T48.3X4	T48.3X5	T48.3X6
Isoamyl nitrite	T46.3X1	T46.3X2	T46.3X3	T46.3X4	T46.3X5	T46.3X6
Isobenzan	T60.1X1	T60.1X2	T60.1X3	T60.1X4		
Isobutyl acetate	T52.8X1	T52.8X2	T52.8X3	T52.8X4		
Isocarboxazid	T43.1X1	T43.1X2	T43.1X3	T43.1X4	T43.1X5	T43.1X6
Isoconazole	T49.0X1	T49.0X2	T49.0X3	T49.0X4	T49.0X5	T49.0X6
Isocyanate	T65.0X1	T65.0X2	T65.0X3	T65.0X4		
Isoephedrine	T44.991	T44.992	T44.993	T44.994	T44.995	T44.996
Isoetarine	T48.6X1	T48.6X2	T48.6X3	T48.6X4	T48.6X5	T48.6X6
Isoethadione	T42.2X1	T42.2X2	T42.2X3	T42.2X4	T42.2X5	T42.2X6
Isoetharine	T44.5X1	T44.5X2	T44.5X3	T44.5X4	T44.5X5	T44.5X6
Isoflurane	T41.0X1	T41.0X2	T41.0X3	T41.0X4	T41.0X5	T41.0X6
Isoflurophate	T44.0X1	T44.0X2	T44.0X3	T44.0X4	T44.0X5	T44.0X6
Isomaltose, ferric complex	T45.4X1	T45.4X2	T45.4X3	T45.4X4	T45.4X5	T45.4X6
Isometheptene	T44.3X1	T44.3X2	T44.3X3	T44.3X4	T44.3X5	T44.3X6
Isoniazid	T37.1X1	T37.1X2	T37.1X3	T37.1X4	T37.1X5	T37.1X6
with						
rifampicin	T36.6X1	T36.6X2	T36.6X3	T36.6X4	T36.6X5	T36.6X6
thioacetazone	T37.1X1	T37.1X2	T37.1X3	T37.1X4	T37.1X5	T37.1X6
Isonicotinic acid hydrazide	T37.1X1	T37.1X2	T37.1X3	T37.1X4	T37.1X5	T37.1X6
Isonipecaine	T40.4X1	T40.4X2	T40.4X3	T40.4X4	T40.4X5	T40.4X6
Isopentaquine	T37.2X1	T37.2X2	T37.2X3	T37.2X4	T37.2X5	T37.2X6
Isophane insulin	T38.3X1	T38.3X2	T38.3X3	T38.3X4	T38.3X5	T38.3X6
Isophorone	T65.891	T65.892	T65.893	T65.894	—	—
Isophosphamide	T45.1X1	T45.1X2	T45.1X3	T45.1X4	T45.1X5	T45.1X6
Isopregnenone	T38.5X1	T38.5X2	T38.5X3	T38.5X4	T38.5X5	T38.5X6
Isoprenaline	T48.6X1	T48.6X2	T48.6X3	T48.6X4	T48.6X5	T48.6X6
Isopromethazine	T43.3X1	T43.3X2	T43.3X3	T43.3X4	T43.3X5	T43.3X6
Isopropamide	T44.3X1	T44.3X2	T44.3X3	T44.3X4	T44.3X5	T44.3X6
iodide	T44.3X1	T44.3X2	T44.3X3	T44.3X4	T44.3X5	T44.3X6
Isopropanol	T51.2X1	T51.2X2	T51.2X3	T51.2X4	—	—
Isopropyl						
acetate	T52.8X1	T52.8X2	T52.8X3	T52.8X4	—	—
alcohol	T51.2X1	T51.2X2	T51.2X3	T51.2X4	—	—
medicinal	T49.4X1	T49.4X2	T49.4X3	T49.4X4	T49.4X5	T49.4X6
ether	T52.8X1	T52.8X2	T52.8X3	T52.8X4	—	—
Isopropylaminophenazone	T39.2X1	T39.2X2	T39.2X3	T39.2X4	T39.2X5	T39.2X6
Isoproterenol	T48.6X1	T48.6X2	T48.6X3	T48.6X4	T48.6X5	T48.6X6
Isosorbide dinitrate	T46.3X1	T46.3X2	T46.3X3	T46.3X4	T46.3X5	T46.3X6
Isothipendyl	T45.0X1	T45.0X2	T45.0X3	T45.0X4	T45.0X5	T45.0X6
Isotretinoin	T50.991	T50.992	T50.993	T50.994	T50.995	T50.996
Isoxazolyl penicillin	T36.0X1	T36.0X2	T36.0X3	T36.0X4	T36.0X5	T36.0X6
Isoxicam	T39.391	T39.392	T39.393	T39.394	T39.395	T39.396
Isoxsuprine	T46.7X1	T46.7X2	T46.7X3	T46.7X4	T46.7X5	T46.7X6
Ispagula	T47.4X1	T47.4X2	T47.4X3	T47.4X4	T47.4X5	T47.4X6
husk	T47.4X1	T47.4X2	T47.4X3	T47.4X4	T47.4X5	T47.4X6
Isradipine	T46.1X1	T46.1X2	T46.1X3	T46.1X4	T46.1X5	T46.1X6
I-thyroxine sodium	T38.1X1	T38.1X2	T38.1X3	T38.1X4	T38.1X5	T38.1X6
Itraconazole	T37.8X1	T37.8X2	T37.8X3	T37.8X4	T37.8X5	T37.8X6
Itramin tosilate	T46.3X1	T46.3X2	T46.3X3	T46.3X4	T46.3X5	T46.3X6
Ivermectin	T37.4X1	T37.4X2	T37.4X3	T37.4X4	T37.4X5	T37.4X6
Izoniazid	T37.1X1	T37.1X2	T37.1X3	T37.1X4	T37.1X5	T37.1X6
with thioacetazone	T37.1X1	T37.1X2	T37.1X3	T37.1X4	T37.1X5	T37.1X6
Jalap	T47.2X1	T47.2X2	T47.2X3	T47.2X4	T47.2X5	T47.2X6
Jamaica						
dogwood (bark)	T39.8X1	T39.8X2	T39.8X3	T39.8X4	T39.8X5	T39.8X6
ginger	T65.891	T65.892	T65.893	T65.894	—	—
root	T62.2X1	T62.2X2	T62.2X3	T62.2X4	—	—
Jatropha	T62.2X1	T62.2X2	T62.2X3	T62.2X4	—	—
curcas	T62.2X1	T62.2X2	T62.2X3	T62.2X4	—	—
Jectofer	T45.4X1	T45.4X2	T45.4X3	T45.4X4	T45.4X5	T45.4X6
Jellyfish (sting)	T63.621	T63.622	T63.623	T63.624		
Jequirity (bean)	T62.2X1	T62.2X2	T62.2X3	T62.2X4	—	—
Jimson weed (stramonium)	T62.2X1	T62.2X2	T62.2X3	T62.2X4	—	—
seeds	T62.2X1	T62.2X2	T62.2X3	T62.2X4	—	—
Josamycin	T36.3X1	T36.3X2	T36.3X3	T36.3X4	T36.3X5	T36.3X6
Juniper tar	T49.1X1	T49.1X2	T49.1X3	T49.1X4	T49.1X5	T49.1X6
Kallidinogenase	T46.7X1	T46.7X2	T46.7X3	T46.7X4	T46.7X5	T46.7X6
Kallikrein	T46.7X1	T46.7X2	T46.7X3	T46.7X4	T46.7X5	T46.7X6
Kanamycin	T36.5X1	T36.5X2	T36.5X3	T36.5X4	T36.5X5	T36.5X6
Kantrex	T36.5X1	T36.5X2	T36.5X3	T36.5X4	T36.5X5	T36.5X6
Kaolin	T47.6X1	T47.6X2	T47.6X3	T47.6X4	T47.6X5	T47.6X6
light	T47.6X1	T47.6X2	T47.6X3	T47.6X4	T47.6X5	T47.6X6
Karaya (gum)	T47.4X1	T47.4X2	T47.4X3	T47.4X4	T47.4X5	T47.4X6

Additional Character May Be Required — Refer to the Tabular List for Character Selection   ▽ **Subterms under main terms may continue to next column or page**

Substance	Poisoning, Accidental (unintentional)	Poisoning, Intentional Self-harm	Poisoning, Assault	Poisoning, Undetermined	Adverse Effect	Under-dosing
Kebuzone	T39.2X1	T39.2X2	T39.2X3	T39.2X4	T39.2X5	T39.2X6
Kelevan	T60.1X1	T60.1X2	T60.1X3	T60.1X4	—	—
Kemithal	T41.1X1	T41.1X2	T41.1X3	T41.1X4	T41.1X5	T41.1X6
Kenacort	T38.0X1	T38.0X2	T38.0X3	T38.0X4	T38.0X5	T38.0X6
Keratolytic drug NEC	T49.4X1	T49.4X2	T49.4X3	T49.4X4	T49.4X5	T49.4X6
anthracene	T49.4X1	T49.4X2	T49.4X3	T49.4X4	T49.4X5	T49.4X6
Keratoplastic NEC	T49.4X1	T49.4X2	T49.4X3	T49.4X4	T49.4X5	T49.4X6
Kerosene, kerosine (fuel) (solvent) NEC	T52.0X1	T52.0X2	T52.0X3	T52.0X4	—	—
insecticide	T52.0X1	T52.0X2	T52.0X3	T52.0X4	—	—
vapor	T52.0X1	T52.0X2	T52.0X3	T52.0X4	—	—
Ketamine	T41.291	T41.292	T41.293	T41.294	T41.295	T41.296
Ketazolam	T42.4X1	T42.4X2	T42.4X3	T42.4X4	T42.4X5	T42.4X6
Ketazon	T39.2X1	T39.2X2	T39.2X3	T39.2X4	T39.2X5	T39.2X6
Ketobemidone	T40.4X1	T40.4X2	T40.4X3	T40.4X4	—	—
Ketoconazole	T49.0X1	T49.0X2	T49.0X3	T49.0X4	T49.0X5	T49.0X6
Ketols	T52.4X1	T52.4X2	T52.4X3	T52.4X4	—	—
Ketone oils	T52.4X1	T52.4X2	T52.4X3	T52.4X4	—	—
Ketoprofen	T39.311	T39.312	T39.313	T39.314	T39.315	T39.316
Ketorolac	T39.8X1	T39.8X2	T39.8X3	T39.8X4	T39.8X5	T39.8X6
Ketotifen	T45.0X1	T45.0X2	T45.0X3	T45.0X4	T45.0X5	T45.0X6
Khat	T43.691	T43.692	T43.693	T43.694	—	—
Khellin	T46.3X1	T46.3X2	T46.3X3	T46.3X4	T46.3X5	T46.3X6
Khelloside	T46.3X1	T46.3X2	T46.3X3	T46.3X4	T46.3X5	T46.3X6
Kiln gas or vapor (carbon monoxide)	T58.8X1	T58.8X2	T58.8X3	T58.8X4	—	—
Kitasamycin	T36.3X1	T36.3X2	T36.3X3	T36.3X4	T36.3X5	T36.3X6
Konsyl	T47.4X1	T47.4X2	T47.4X3	T47.4X4	T47.4X5	T47.4X6
Kosam seed	T62.2X1	T62.2X2	T62.2X3	T62.2X4	—	—
Krait (venom)	T63.091	T63.092	T63.093	T63.094	—	—
Kwell (insecticide)	T60.1X1	T60.1X2	T60.1X3	T60.1X4	—	—
anti-infective (topical)	T49.0X1	T49.0X2	T49.0X3	T49.0X4	T49.0X5	T49.0X6
Labetalol	T44.8X1	T44.8X2	T44.8X3	T44.8X4	T44.8X5	T44.8X6
Laburnum (seeds)	T62.2X1	T62.2X2	T62.2X3	T62.2X4	—	—
leaves	T62.2X1	T62.2X2	T62.2X3	T62.2X4	—	—
Lachesine	T49.5X1	T49.5X2	T49.5X3	T49.5X4	T49.5X5	T49.5X6
Lacidipine	T46.5X1	T46.5X2	T46.5X3	T46.5X4	T46.5X5	T46.5X6
Lacquer	T65.6X1	T65.6X2	T65.6X3	T65.6X4	—	—
Lacrimogenic gas	T59.3X1	T59.3X2	T59.3X3	T59.3X4	—	—
Lactated potassic saline	T50.3X1	T50.3X2	T50.3X3	T50.3X4	T50.3X5	T50.3X6
Lactic acid	T49.8X1	T49.8X2	T49.8X3	T49.8X4	T49.8X5	T49.8X6
Lactobacillus						
acidophilus	T47.6X1	T47.6X2	T47.6X3	T47.6X4	T47.6X5	T47.6X6
compound	T47.6X1	T47.6X2	T47.6X3	T47.6X4	T47.6X5	T47.6X6
bifidus, lyophilized	T47.6X1	T47.6X2	T47.6X3	T47.6X4	T47.6X5	T47.6X6
bulgaricus	T47.6X1	T47.6X2	T47.6X3	T47.6X4	T47.6X5	T47.6X6
sporogenes	T47.6X1	T47.6X2	T47.6X3	T47.6X4	T47.6X5	T47.6X6
Lactoflavin	T45.2X1	T45.2X2	T45.2X3	T45.2X4	T45.2X5	T45.2X6
Lactose (as excipient)	T50.901	T50.902	T50.903	T50.904	T50.905	T50.906
Lactuca (virosa) (extract)	T42.6X1	T42.6X2	T42.6X3	T42.6X4	T42.6X5	T42.6X6
Lactucarium	T42.6X1	T42.6X2	T42.6X3	T42.6X4	T42.6X5	T42.6X6
Lactulose	T47.3X1	T47.3X2	T47.3X3	T47.3X4	T47.3X5	T47.3X6
Laevo — see Levo-						
Lanatosides	T46.0X1	T46.0X2	T46.0X3	T46.0X4	T46.0X5	T46.0X6
Lanolin	T49.3X1	T49.3X2	T49.3X3	T49.3X4	T49.3X5	T49.3X6
Largactil	T43.3X1	T43.3X2	T43.3X3	T43.3X4	T43.3X5	T43.3X6
Larkspur	T62.2X1	T62.2X2	T62.2X3	T62.2X4	—	—
Laroxyl	T43.011	T43.012	T43.013	T43.014	T43.015	T43.016
Lasix	T50.1X1	T50.1X2	T50.1X3	T50.1X4	T50.1X5	T50.1X6
Lassar's paste	T49.4X1	T49.4X2	T49.4X3	T49.4X4	T49.4X5	T49.4X6
Latamoxef	T36.1X1	T36.1X2	T36.1X3	T36.1X4	T36.1X5	T36.1X6
Latex	T65.811	T65.812	T65.813	T65.814	—	—
Lathyrus (seed)	T62.2X1	T62.2X2	T62.2X3	T62.2X4	—	—
Laudanum	T40.0X1	T40.0X2	T40.0X3	T40.0X4	—	—
Laudexium	T48.1X1	T48.1X2	T48.1X3	T48.1X4	T48.1X5	T48.1X6
Laughing gas	T41.0X1	T41.0X2	T41.0X3	T41.0X4	T41.0X5	T41.0X6
Laurel, black or cherry	T62.2X1	T62.2X2	T62.2X3	T62.2X4	—	—
Laurolinium	T49.0X1	T49.0X2	T49.0X3	T49.0X4	T49.0X5	T49.0X6
Lauryl sulfoacetate	T49.2X1	T49.2X2	T49.2X3	T49.2X4	T49.2X5	T49.2X6
Laxative NEC	T47.4X1	T47.4X2	T47.4X3	T47.4X4	T47.4X5	T47.4X6
osmotic	T47.3X1	T47.3X2	T47.3X3	T47.3X4	T47.3X5	T47.3X6
saline	T47.3X1	T47.3X2	T47.3X3	T47.3X4	T47.3X5	T47.3X6
stimulant	T47.2X1	T47.2X2	T47.2X3	T47.2X4	T47.2X5	T47.2X6
L-dopa	T42.8X1	T42.8X2	T42.8X3	T42.8X4	T42.8X5	T42.8X6
Lead (dust) (fumes) (vapor) NEC	T56.0X1	T56.0X2	T56.0X3	T56.0X4	—	—
acetate	T49.2X1	T49.2X2	T49.2X3	T49.2X4	T49.2X5	T49.2X6
alkyl (fuel additive)	T56.0X1	T56.0X2	T56.0X3	T56.0X4	—	—
anti-infectives	T37.8X1	T37.8X2	T37.8X3	T37.8X4	T37.8X5	T37.8X6
antiknock compound (tetraethyl)	T56.0X1	T56.0X2	T56.0X3	T56.0X4	—	—

Substance	Poisoning, Accidental (unintentional)	Poisoning, Intentional Self-harm	Poisoning, Assault	Poisoning, Undetermined	Adverse Effect	Under-dosing
Lead (dust) (fumes) (vapor) NEC						
— continued						
arsenate, arsenite (dust)(herbicide) (insecticide) (vapor)	T57.0X1	T57.0X2	T57.0X3	T57.0X4	—	—
carbonate	T56.0X1	T56.0X2	T56.0X3	T56.0X4	—	—
paint	T56.0X1	T56.0X2	T56.0X3	T56.0X4	—	—
chromate	T56.0X1	T56.0X2	T56.0X3	T56.0X4	—	—
paint	T56.0X1	T56.0X2	T56.0X3	T56.0X4	—	—
dioxide	T56.0X1	T56.0X2	T56.0X3	T56.0X4	—	—
inorganic	T56.0X1	T56.0X2	T56.0X3	T56.0X4	—	—
iodide	T56.0X1	T56.0X2	T56.0X3	T56.0X4	—	—
pigment (paint)	T56.0X1	T56.0X2	T56.0X3	T56.0X4	—	—
monoxide (dust)	T56.0X1	T56.0X2	T56.0X3	T56.0X4	—	—
paint	T56.0X1	T56.0X2	T56.0X3	T56.0X4	—	—
organic	T56.0X1	T56.0X2	T56.0X3	T56.0X4	—	—
oxide	T56.0X1	T56.0X2	T56.0X3	T56.0X4	—	—
paint	T56.0X1	T56.0X2	T56.0X3	T56.0X4	—	—
paint	T56.0X1	T56.0X2	T56.0X3	T56.0X4	—	—
salts	T56.0X1	T56.0X2	T56.0X3	T56.0X4	—	—
specified compound NEC	T56.0X1	T56.0X2	T56.0X3	T56.0X4	—	—
tetra-ethyl	T56.0X1	T56.0X2	T56.0X3	T56.0X4	—	—
Lebanese red	T40.7X1	T40.7X2	T40.7X3	T40.7X4	T40.7X5	T40.7X6
Lefetamine	T39.8X1	T39.8X2	T39.8X3	T39.8X4	T39.8X5	T39.8X6
Lenperone	T43.4X1	T43.4X2	T43.4X3	T43.4X4	T43.4X5	T43.4X6
Lente lietin (insulin)	T38.3X1	T38.3X2	T38.3X3	T38.3X4	T38.3X5	T38.3X6
Leptazol	T50.7X1	T50.7X2	T50.7X3	T50.7X4	T50.7X5	T50.7X6
Leptophos	T60.0X1	T60.0X2	T60.0X3	T60.0X4	—	—
Leritine	T40.2X1	T40.2X2	T40.2X3	T40.2X4	T40.2X5	T40.2X6
Letosteine	T48.4X1	T48.4X2	T48.4X3	T48.4X4	T48.4X5	T48.4X6
Letter	T38.1X1	T38.1X2	T38.1X3	T38.1X4	T38.1X5	T38.1X6
Lettuce opium	T42.6X1	T42.6X2	T42.6X3	T42.6X4	T42.6X5	T42.6X6
Leucinocaine	T41.3X1	T41.3X2	T41.3X3	T41.3X4	T41.3X5	T41.3X6
Leucocianidol	T46.991	T46.992	T46.993	T46.994	T46.995	T46.996
Leucovorin (factor)	T45.8X1	T45.8X2	T45.8X3	T45.8X4	T45.8X5	T45.8X6
Leukeran	T45.1X1	T45.1X2	T45.1X3	T45.1X4	T45.1X5	T45.1X6
Leuprolide	T38.891	T38.892	T38.893	T38.894	T38.895	T38.896
Levalbuterol	T48.6X1	T48.6X2	T48.6X3	T48.6X4	T48.6X5	T48.6X6
Levallorphan	T50.7X1	T50.7X2	T50.7X3	T50.7X4	T50.7X5	T50.7X6
Levamisole	T37.4X1	T37.4X2	T37.4X3	T37.4X4	T37.4X5	T37.4X6
Levanil	T42.6X1	T42.6X2	T42.6X3	T42.6X4	T42.6X5	T42.6X6
Levarterenol	T44.4X1	T44.4X2	T44.4X3	T44.4X4	T44.4X5	T44.4X6
Levdropropizine	T48.3X1	T48.3X2	T48.3X3	T48.3X4	T48.3X5	T48.3X6
Levobunolol	T49.5X1	T49.5X2	T49.5X3	T49.5X4	T49.5X5	T49.5X6
Levocabastine (hydrochloride)	T45.0X1	T45.0X2	T45.0X3	T45.0X4	T45.0X5	T45.0X6
Levocarnitine	T50.991	T50.992	T50.993	T50.994	T50.995	T50.996
Levodopa	T42.8X1	T42.8X2	T42.8X3	T42.8X4	T42.8X5	T42.8X6
with carbidopa	T42.8X1	T42.8X2	T42.8X3	T42.8X4	T42.8X5	T42.8X6
Levo-dromoran	T40.2X1	T40.2X2	T40.2X3	T40.2X4	T40.2X5	T40.2X6
Levoglutamide	T50.991	T50.992	T50.993	T50.994	T50.995	T50.996
Levoid	T38.1X1	T38.1X2	T38.1X3	T38.1X4	T38.1X5	T38.1X6
Levo-isomethadone	T40.3X1	T40.3X2	T40.3X3	T40.3X4	—	—
Levomepromazine	T43.3X1	T43.3X2	T43.3X3	T43.3X4	T43.3X5	T43.3X6
Levonordefrin	T49.6X1	T49.6X2	T49.6X3	T49.6X4	T49.6X5	T49.6X6
Levonorgestrel	T38.4X1	T38.4X2	T38.4X3	T38.4X4	T38.4X5	T38.4X6
with ethinylestradiol	T38.5X1	T38.5X2	T38.5X3	T38.5X4	T38.5X5	T38.5X6
Levopromazine	T43.3X1	T43.3X2	T43.3X3	T43.3X4	T43.3X5	T43.3X6
Levoprome	T42.6X1	T42.6X2	T42.6X3	T42.6X4	T42.6X5	T42.6X6
Levopropoxyphene	T40.4X1	T40.4X2	T40.4X3	T40.4X4	T40.4X5	T40.4X6
Levopropylhexedrine	T50.5X1	T50.5X2	T50.5X3	T50.5X4	T50.5X5	T50.5X6
Levoproxyphylline	T48.6X1	T48.6X2	T48.6X3	T48.6X4	T48.6X5	T48.6X6
Levorphanol	T40.4X1	T40.4X2	T40.4X3	T40.4X4	T40.4X5	T40.4X6
Levothyroxine	T38.1X1	T38.1X2	T38.1X3	T38.1X4	T38.1X5	T38.1X6
sodium	T38.1X1	T38.1X2	T38.1X3	T38.1X4	T38.1X5	T38.1X6
Levsin	T44.3X1	T44.3X2	T44.3X3	T44.3X4	T44.3X5	T44.3X6
Levulose	T50.3X1	T50.3X2	T50.3X3	T50.3X4	T50.3X5	T50.3X6
Lewisite (gas), not in war	T57.0X1	T57.0X2	T57.0X3	T57.0X4	—	—
Librium	T42.4X1	T42.4X2	T42.4X3	T42.4X4	T42.4X5	T42.4X6
Lidex	T49.0X1	T49.0X2	T49.0X3	T49.0X4	T49.0X5	T49.0X6
Lidocaine	T41.3X1	T41.3X2	T41.3X3	T41.3X4	T41.3X5	T41.3X6
regional	T41.3X1	T41.3X2	T41.3X3	T41.3X4	T41.3X5	T41.3X6
spinal	T41.3X1	T41.3X2	T41.3X3	T41.3X4	T41.3X5	T41.3X6
Lidofenin	T50.8X1	T50.8X2	T50.8X3	T50.8X4	T50.8X5	T50.8X6
Lidoflazine	T46.1X1	T46.1X2	T46.1X3	T46.1X4	T46.1X5	T46.1X6
Lighter fluid	T52.0X1	T52.0X2	T52.0X3	T52.0X4	—	—
Lignin hemicellulose	T47.6X1	T47.6X2	T47.6X3	T47.6X4	T47.6X5	T47.6X6
Lignocaine	T41.3X1	T41.3X2	T41.3X3	T41.3X4	T41.3X5	T41.3X6
regional	T41.3X1	T41.3X2	T41.3X3	T41.3X4	T41.3X5	T41.3X6
spinal	T41.3X1	T41.3X2	T41.3X3	T41.3X4	T41.3X5	T41.3X6
Ligroin (e) (solvent)	T52.0X1	T52.0X2	T52.0X3	T52.0X4	—	—
vapor	T59.891	T59.892	T59.893	T59.894	—	—
Ligustrum vulgare	T62.2X1	T62.2X2	T62.2X3	T62.2X4	—	—

Substance	Poisoning, Accidental (unintentional)	Poisoning, Intentional Self-harm	Poisoning, Assault	Poisoning, Undetermined	Adverse Effect	Under-dosing
Lily of the valley	T62.2X1	T62.2X2	T62.2X3	T62.2X4	—	—
Lime (chloride)	T54.3X1	T54.3X2	T54.3X3	T54.3X4	—	—
Limonene	T52.8X1	T52.8X2	T52.8X3	T52.8X4	—	—
Lincomycin	T36.8X1	T36.8X2	T36.8X3	T36.8X4	T36.8X5	T36.8X6
Lindane (insecticide) (nonmedicinal) (vapor)	T53.6X1	T53.6X2	T53.6X3	T53.6X4	—	—
medicinal	T49.0X1	T49.0X2	T49.0X3	T49.0X4	T49.0X5	T49.0X6
Liniments NEC	T49.91	T49.92	T49.93	T49.94	T49.95	T49.96
Linoleic acid	T46.6X1	T46.6X2	T46.6X3	T46.6X4	T46.6X5	T46.6X6
Linolenic acid	T46.6X1	T46.6X2	T46.6X3	T46.6X4	T46.6X5	T46.6X6
Linseed	T47.4X1	T47.4X2	T47.4X3	T47.4X4	T47.4X5	T47.4X6
Liothyronine	T38.1X1	T38.1X2	T38.1X3	T38.1X4	T38.1X5	T38.1X6
Liotrix	T38.1X1	T38.1X2	T38.1X3	T38.1X4	T38.1X5	T38.1X6
Lipancreatin	T47.5X1	T47.5X2	T47.5X3	T47.5X4	T47.5X5	T47.5X6
Lipo-alprostadil	T46.7X1	T46.7X2	T46.7X3	T46.7X4	T46.7X5	T46.7X6
Lipo-Lutin	T38.5X1	T38.5X2	T38.5X3	T38.5X4	T38.5X5	T38.5X6
Lipotropic drug NEC	T50.901	T50.902	T50.903	T50.904	T50.905	T50.906
Liquefied petroleum gases	T59.891	T59.892	T59.893	T59.894	—	—
piped (pure or mixed with air)	T59.891	T59.892	T59.893	T59.894	—	—
Liquid						
paraffin	T47.4X1	T47.4X2	T47.4X3	T47.4X4	T47.4X5	T47.4X6
petrolatum	T47.4X1	T47.4X2	T47.4X3	T47.4X4	T47.4X5	T47.4X6
topical	T49.3X1	T49.3X2	T49.3X3	T49.3X4	T49.3X5	T49.3X6
specified NEC	T65.891	T65.892	T65.893	T65.894	—	—
substance	T65.91	T65.92	T65.93	T65.94	—	—
Liquor creosolis compositus	T65.891	T65.892	T65.893	T65.894	—	—
Liquorice	T48.4X1	T48.4X2	T48.4X3	T48.4X4	T48.4X5	T48.4X6
extract	T47.8X1	T47.8X2	T47.8X3	T47.8X4	T47.8X5	T47.8X6
Lisinopril	T46.4X1	T46.4X2	T46.4X3	T46.4X4	T46.4X5	T46.4X6
Lisuride	T42.8X1	T42.8X2	T42.8X3	T42.8X4	T42.8X5	T42.8X6
Lithane	T43.8X1	T43.8X2	T43.8X3	T43.8X4	T43.8X5	T43.8X6
Lithium	T56.891	T56.892	T56.893	T56.894	—	—
gluconate	T43.591	T43.592	T43.593	T43.594	T43.595	T43.596
salts (carbonate)	T43.591	T43.592	T43.593	T43.594	T43.595	T43.596
Lithonate	T43.8X1	T43.8X2	T43.8X3	T43.8X4	T43.8X5	T43.8X6
Liver						
extract	T45.8X1	T45.8X2	T45.8X3	T45.8X4	T45.8X5	T45.8X6
for parenteral use	T45.8X1	T45.8X2	T45.8X3	T45.8X4	T45.8X5	T45.8X6
fraction 1	T45.8X1	T45.8X2	T45.8X3	T45.8X4	T45.8X5	T45.8X6
hydrolysate	T45.8X1	T45.8X2	T45.8X3	T45.8X4	T45.8X5	T45.8X6
Lizard (bite) (venom)	T63.121	T63.122	T63.123	T63.124	—	—
LMD	T45.8X1	T45.8X2	T45.8X3	T45.8X4	T45.8X5	T45.8X6
Lobelia	T62.2X1	T62.2X2	T62.2X3	T62.2X4	—	—
Lobeline	T50.7X1	T50.7X2	T50.7X3	T50.7X4	T50.7X5	T50.7X6
Local action drug NEC	T49.8X1	T49.8X2	T49.8X3	T49.8X4	T49.8X5	T49.8X6
Locorten	T49.0X1	T49.0X2	T49.0X3	T49.0X4	T49.0X5	T49.0X6
Lofepramine	T43.011	T43.012	T43.013	T43.014	T43.015	T43.016
Lolium temulentum	T62.2X1	T62.2X2	T62.2X3	T62.2X4	—	—
Lomotil	T47.6X1	T47.6X2	T47.6X3	T47.6X4	T47.6X5	T47.6X6
Lomustine	T45.1X1	T45.1X2	T45.1X3	T45.1X4	T45.1X5	T45.1X6
Lonidamine	T45.1X1	T45.1X2	T45.1X3	T45.1X4	T45.1X5	T45.1X6
Loperamide	T47.6X1	T47.6X2	T47.6X3	T47.6X4	T47.6X5	T47.6X6
Loprazolam	T42.4X1	T42.4X2	T42.4X3	T42.4X4	T42.4X5	T42.4X6
Lorajmine	T46.2X1	T46.2X2	T46.2X3	T46.2X4	T46.2X5	T46.2X6
Loratidine	T45.0X1	T45.0X2	T45.0X3	T45.0X4	T45.0X5	T45.0X6
Lorazepam	T42.4X1	T42.4X2	T42.4X3	T42.4X4	T42.4X5	T42.4X6
Lorcainide	T46.2X1	T46.2X2	T46.2X3	T46.2X4	T46.2X5	T46.2X6
Lormetazepam	T42.4X1	T42.4X2	T42.4X3	T42.4X4	T42.4X5	T42.4X6
Lotions NEC	T49.91	T49.92	T49.93	T49.94	—	T49.96
Lotusate	T42.3X1	T42.3X2	T42.3X3	T42.3X4	T42.3X5	T42.3X6
Lovastatin	T46.6X1	T46.6X2	T46.6X3	T46.6X4	T46.6X5	T46.6X6
Lowila	T49.2X1	T49.2X2	T49.2X3	T49.2X4	T49.2X5	T49.2X6
Loxapine	T43.591	T43.592	T43.593	T43.594	T43.595	T43.596
Lozenges (throat)	T49.6X1	T49.6X2	T49.6X3	T49.6X4	T49.6X5	T49.6X6
LSD	T40.8X1	T40.8X2	T40.8X3	T40.8X4	—	—
L-Tryptophan — see amino acid						
Lubricant, eye	T49.5X1	T49.5X2	T49.5X3	T49.5X4	T49.5X5	T49.5X6
Lubricating oil NEC	T52.0X1	T52.0X2	T52.0X3	T52.0X4	—	—
Lucanthone	T37.4X1	T37.4X2	T37.4X3	T37.4X4	T37.4X5	T37.4X6
Luminal	T42.3X1	T42.3X2	T42.3X3	T42.3X4	T42.3X5	T42.3X6
Lung irritant (gas) NEC	T59.91	T59.92	T59.93	T59.94	—	—
Luteinizing hormone	T38.811	T38.812	T38.813	T38.814	T38.815	T38.816
Lutocylol	T38.5X1	T38.5X2	T38.5X3	T38.5X4	T38.5X5	T38.5X6
Lutromone	T38.5X1	T38.5X2	T38.5X3	T38.5X4	T38.5X5	T38.5X6
Lututrin	T48.291	T48.292	T48.293	T48.294	T48.295	T48.296
Lye (concentrated)	T54.3X1	T54.3X2	T54.3X3	T54.3X4	—	—
Lygranum (skin test)	T50.8X1	T50.8X2	T50.8X3	T50.8X4	T50.8X5	T50.8X6
Lymecycline	T36.4X1	T36.4X2	T36.4X3	T36.4X4	T36.4X5	T36.4X6
Lymphogranuloma venereum antigen	T50.8X1	T50.8X2	T50.8X3	T50.8X4	T50.8X5	T50.8X6
Lynestrenol	T38.4X1	T38.4X2	T38.4X3	T38.4X4	T38.4X5	T38.4X6

Substance	Poisoning, Accidental (unintentional)	Poisoning, Intentional Self-harm	Poisoning, Assault	Poisoning, Undetermined	Adverse Effect	Under-dosing
Lyovac Sodium Edecrin	T50.1X1	T50.1X2	T50.1X3	T50.1X4	T50.1X5	T50.1X6
Lypressin	T38.891	T38.892	T38.893	T38.894	T38.895	T38.896
Lysergic acid diethylamide	T40.8X1	T40.8X2	T40.8X3	T40.8X4	—	—
Lysergide	T40.8X1	T40.8X2	T40.8X3	T40.8X4	—	—
Lysine vasopressin	T38.891	T38.892	T38.893	T38.894	T38.895	T38.896
Lysol	T54.1X1	T54.1X2	T54.1X3	T54.1X4	—	—
Lysozyme	T49.0X1	T49.0X2	T49.0X3	T49.0X4	T49.0X5	T49.0X6
Lytta (vitatta)	T49.8X1	T49.8X2	T49.8X3	T49.8X4	T49.8X5	T49.8X6
Mace	T59.3X1	T59.3X2	T59.3X3	T59.3X4	—	—
Macrogol	T50.991	T50.992	T50.993	T50.994	T50.995	T50.996
Macrolide						
anabolic drug	T38.7X1	T38.7X2	T38.7X3	T38.7X4	T38.7X5	T38.7X6
antibiotic	T36.3X1	T36.3X2	T36.3X3	T36.3X4	T36.3X5	T36.3X6
Mafenide	T49.0X1	T49.0X2	T49.0X3	T49.0X4	T49.0X5	T49.0X6
Magaldrate	T47.1X1	T47.1X2	T47.1X3	T47.1X4	T47.1X5	T47.1X6
Magic mushroom	T40.991	T40.992	T40.993	T40.994	—	—
Magnamycin	T36.8X1	T36.8X2	T36.8X3	T36.8X4	T36.8X5	T36.8X6
Magnesia magma	T47.1X1	T47.1X2	T47.1X3	T47.1X4	T47.1X5	T47.1X6
Magnesium NEC	T56.891	T56.892	T56.893	T56.894	—	—
carbonate	T47.1X1	T47.1X2	T47.1X3	T47.1X4	T47.1X5	T47.1X6
citrate	T47.4X1	T47.4X2	T47.4X3	T47.4X4	T47.4X5	T47.4X6
hydroxide	T47.1X1	T47.1X2	T47.1X3	T47.1X4	T47.1X5	T47.1X6
oxide	T47.1X1	T47.1X2	T47.1X3	T47.1X4	T47.1X5	T47.1X6
peroxide	T49.0X1	T49.0X2	T49.0X3	T49.0X4	T49.0X5	T49.0X6
salicylate	T39.091	T39.092	T39.093	T39.094	T39.095	T39.096
silicofluoride	T50.3X1	T50.3X2	T50.3X3	T50.3X4	T50.3X5	T50.3X6
sulfate	T47.4X1	T47.4X2	T47.4X3	T47.4X4	T47.4X5	T47.4X6
thiosulfate	T45.0X1	T45.0X2	T45.0X3	T45.0X4	T45.0X5	T45.0X6
trisilicate	T47.1X1	T47.1X2	T47.1X3	T47.1X4	T47.1X5	T47.1X6
Malathion (medicinal)	T49.0X1	T49.0X2	T49.0X3	T49.0X4	T49.0X5	T49.0X6
insecticide	T60.0X1	T60.0X2	T60.0X3	T60.0X4	—	—
Male fern extract	T37.4X1	T37.4X2	T37.4X3	T37.4X4	T37.4X5	T37.4X6
M-AMSA	T45.1X1	T45.1X2	T45.1X3	T45.1X4	T45.1X5	T45.1X6
Mandelic acid	T37.8X1	T37.8X2	T37.8X3	T37.8X4	T37.8X5	T37.8X6
Manganese (dioxide) (salts)	T57.2X1	T57.2X2	T57.2X3	T57.2X4	—	—
medicinal	T50.991	T50.992	T50.993	T50.994	T50.995	T50.996
Mannitol	T47.3X1	T47.3X2	T47.3X3	T47.3X4	T47.3X5	T47.3X6
hexanitrate	T46.3X1	T46.3X2	T46.3X3	T46.3X4	T46.3X5	T46.3X6
Mannomustine	T45.1X1	T45.1X2	T45.1X3	T45.1X4	T45.1X5	T45.1X6
MAO inhibitors	T43.1X1	T43.1X2	T43.1X3	T43.1X4	T43.1X5	T43.1X6
Mapharsen	T37.8X1	T37.8X2	T37.8X3	T37.8X4	T37.8X5	T37.8X6
Maphenide	T49.0X1	T49.0X2	T49.0X3	T49.0X4	T49.0X5	T49.0X6
Maprotiline	T43.021	T43.022	T43.023	T43.024	T43.025	T43.026
Marcaine	T41.3X1	T41.3X2	T41.3X3	T41.3X4	T41.3X5	T41.3X6
infiltration (subcutaneous)	T41.3X1	T41.3X2	T41.3X3	T41.3X4	T41.3X5	T41.3X6
nerve block (peripheral) (plexus)	T41.3X1	T41.3X2	T41.3X3	T41.3X4	T41.3X5	T41.3X6
Marezine	T45.0X1	T45.0X2	T45.0X3	T45.0X4	T45.0X5	T45.0X6
Marihuana	T40.7X1	T40.7X2	T40.7X3	T40.7X4	T40.7X5	T40.7X6
Marijuana	T40.7X1	T40.7X2	T40.7X3	T40.7X4	T40.7X5	T40.7X6
Marine (sting)	T63.691	T63.692	T63.693	T63.694	—	—
animals (sting)	T63.691	T63.692	T63.693	T63.694	—	—
plants (sting)	T63.711	T63.712	T63.713	T63.714	—	—
Marplan	T43.1X1	T43.1X2	T43.1X3	T43.1X4	T43.1X5	T43.1X6
Marsh gas	T59.891	T59.892	T59.893	T59.894	—	—
Marsilid	T43.1X1	T43.1X2	T43.1X3	T43.1X4	T43.1X5	T43.1X6
Matulane	T45.1X1	T45.1X2	T45.1X3	T45.1X4	T45.1X5	T45.1X6
Mazindol	T50.5X1	T50.5X2	T50.5X3	T50.5X4	T50.5X5	T50.5X6
MCPA	T60.3X1	T60.3X2	T60.3X3	T60.3X4	—	—
MDMA	T43.621	T43.622	T43.623	T43.624	T43.625	T43.626
Meadow saffron	T62.2X1	T62.2X2	T62.2X3	T62.2X4	—	—
Measles virus vaccine (attenuated)	T50.B91	T50.B92	T50.B93	T50.B94	T50.B95	T50.B96
Meat, noxious	T62.8X1	T62.8X2	T62.8X3	T62.8X4	—	—
Meballymal	T42.3X1	T42.3X2	T42.3X3	T42.3X4	T42.3X5	T42.3X6
Mebanazine	T43.1X1	T43.1X2	T43.1X3	T43.1X4	T43.1X5	T43.1X6
Mebaral	T42.3X1	T42.3X2	T42.3X3	T42.3X4	T42.3X5	T42.3X6
Mebendazole	T37.4X1	T37.4X2	T37.4X3	T37.4X4	T37.4X5	T37.4X6
Mebeverine	T44.3X1	T44.3X2	T44.3X3	T44.3X4	T44.3X5	T44.3X6
Mebhydrolin	T45.0X1	T45.0X2	T45.0X3	T45.0X4	T45.0X5	T45.0X6
Mebumal	T42.3X1	T42.3X2	T42.3X3	T42.3X4	T42.3X5	T42.3X6
Mebutamate	T43.591	T43.592	T43.593	T43.594	T43.595	T43.596
Mecamylamine	T44.2X1	T44.2X2	T44.2X3	T44.2X4	T44.2X5	T44.2X6
Mechlorethamine	T45.1X1	T45.1X2	T45.1X3	T45.1X4	T45.1X5	T45.1X6
Mecillinam	T36.0X1	T36.0X2	T36.0X3	T36.0X4	T36.0X5	T36.0X6
Meclizine (hydrochloride)	T45.0X1	T45.0X2	T45.0X3	T45.0X4	T45.0X5	T45.0X6
Meclocycline	T36.4X1	T36.4X2	T36.4X3	T36.4X4	T36.4X5	T36.4X6
Meclofenamate	T39.391	T39.392	T39.393	T39.394	T39.395	T39.396
Meclofenamic acid	T39.391	T39.392	T39.393	T39.394	T39.395	T39.396
Meclofenoxate	T43.691	T43.692	T43.693	T43.694	T43.695	T43.696
Meclozine	T45.0X1	T45.0X2	T45.0X3	T45.0X4	T45.0X5	T45.0X6
Mecobalamin	T45.8X1	T45.8X2	T45.8X3	T45.8X4	T45.8X5	T45.8X6
Mecoprop	T60.3X1	T60.3X2	T60.3X3	T60.3X4	—	—

Table of Drugs and Chemicals

Substance	Poisoning, Accidental (unintentional)	Poisoning, Intentional Self-harm	Poisoning, Assault	Poisoning, Undetermined	Adverse Effect	Under-dosing
Mecrilate	T49.3X1	T49.3X2	T49.3X3	T49.3X4	T49.3X5	T49.3X6
Mecysteine	T48.4X1	T48.4X2	T48.4X3	T48.4X4	T48.4X5	T48.4X6
Medazepam	T42.4X1	T42.4X2	T42.4X3	T42.4X4	T42.4X5	T42.4X6
Medicament NEC	T50.901	T50.902	T50.903	T50.904	T50.905	T50.906
Medinal	T42.3X1	T42.3X2	T42.3X3	T42.3X4	T42.3X5	T42.3X6
Medomin	T42.3X1	T42.3X2	T42.3X3	T42.3X4	T42.3X5	T42.3X6
Medrogestone	T38.5X1	T38.5X2	T38.5X3	T38.5X4	T38.5X5	T38.5X6
Medroxalol	T44.8X1	T44.8X2	T44.8X3	T44.8X4	T44.8X5	T44.8X6
Medroxyprogesterone acetate (depot)	T38.5X1	T38.5X2	T38.5X3	T38.5X4	T38.5X5	T38.5X6
Medrysone	T49.0X1	T49.0X2	T49.0X3	T49.0X4	T49.0X5	T49.0X6
Mefenamic acid	T39.391	T39.392	T39.393	T39.394	T39.395	T39.396
Mefenorex	T50.5X1	T50.5X2	T50.5X3	T50.5X4	T50.5X5	T50.5X6
Mefloquine	T37.2X1	T37.2X2	T37.2X3	T37.2X4	T37.2X5	T37.2X6
Mefruside	T50.2X1	T50.2X2	T50.2X3	T50.2X4	T50.2X5	T50.2X6
Megahallucinogen	T40.901	T40.902	T40.903	T40.904	T40.905	T40.906
Megestrol	T38.5X1	T38.5X2	T38.5X3	T38.5X4	T38.5X5	T38.5X6
Meglumine						
antimoniate	T37.8X1	T37.8X2	T37.8X3	T37.8X4	T37.8X5	T37.8X6
diatrizoate	T50.8X1	T50.8X2	T50.8X3	T50.8X4	T50.8X5	T50.8X6
iodipamide	T50.8X1	T50.8X2	T50.8X3	T50.8X4	T50.8X5	T50.8X6
iotroxate	T50.8X1	T50.8X2	T50.8X3	T50.8X4	T50.8X5	T50.8X6
MEK (methyl ethyl ketone)	T52.4X1	T52.4X2	T52.4X3	T52.4X4	—	—
Meladinin	T49.3X1	T49.3X2	T49.3X3	T49.3X4	T49.3X5	T49.3X6
Meladrazine	T44.3X1	T44.3X2	T44.3X3	T44.3X4	T44.3X5	T44.3X6
Melaleuca alternifolia oil	T49.0X1	T49.0X2	T49.0X3	T49.0X4	T49.0X5	T49.0X6
Melanizing agents	T49.3X1	T49.3X2	T49.3X3	T49.3X4	T49.3X5	T49.3X6
Melanocyte-stimulating hormone	T38.891	T38.892	T38.893	T38.894	T38.895	T38.896
Melarsonyl potassium	T37.3X1	T37.3X2	T37.3X3	T37.3X4	T37.3X5	T37.3X6
Melarsoprol	T37.3X1	T37.3X2	T37.3X3	T37.3X4	T37.3X5	T37.3X6
Melia azedarach	T62.2X1	T62.2X2	T62.2X3	T62.2X4	—	—
Melitracen	T43.011	T43.012	T43.013	T43.014	T43.015	T43.016
Mellaril	T43.3X1	T43.3X2	T43.3X3	T43.3X4	T43.3X5	T43.3X6
Meloxine	T49.3X1	T49.3X2	T49.3X3	T49.3X4	T49.3X5	T49.3X6
Melperone	T43.4X1	T43.4X2	T43.4X3	T43.4X4	T43.4X5	T43.4X6
Melphalan	T45.1X1	T45.1X2	T45.1X3	T45.1X4	T45.1X5	T45.1X6
Memantine	T43.8X1	T43.8X2	T43.8X3	T43.8X4	T43.8X5	T43.8X6
Menadiol	T45.7X1	T45.7X2	T45.7X3	T45.7X4	T45.7X5	T45.7X6
sodium sulfate	T45.7X1	T45.7X2	T45.7X3	T45.7X4	T45.7X5	T45.7X6
Menadione	T45.7X1	T45.7X2	T45.7X3	T45.7X4	T45.7X5	T45.7X6
sodium bisulfite	T45.7X1	T45.7X2	T45.7X3	T45.7X4	T45.7X5	T45.7X6
Menaphthone	T45.7X1	T45.7X2	T45.7X3	T45.7X4	T45.7X5	T45.7X6
Menaquinone	T45.7X1	T45.7X2	T45.7X3	T45.7X4	T45.7X5	T45.7X6
Menatetrenone	T45.7X1	T45.7X2	T45.7X3	T45.7X4	T45.7X5	T45.7X6
Meningococcal vaccine	T50.A91	T50.A92	T50.A93	T50.A94	T50.A95	T50.A96
Menningovax (-AC) (-C)	T50.A91	T50.A92	T50.A93	T50.A94	T50.A95	T50.A96
Menotropins	T38.811	T38.812	T38.813	T38.814	T38.815	T38.816
Menthol	T48.5X1	T48.5X2	T48.5X3	T48.5X4	T48.5X5	T48.5X6
Mepacrine	T37.2X1	T37.2X2	T37.2X3	T37.2X4	T37.2X5	T37.2X6
Meparfynol	T42.6X1	T42.6X2	T42.6X3	T42.6X4	T42.6X5	T42.6X6
Mepartricin	T36.7X1	T36.7X2	T36.7X3	T36.7X4	T36.7X5	T36.7X6
Mepazine	T43.3X1	T43.3X2	T43.3X3	T43.3X4	T43.3X5	T43.3X6
Mepenzolate	T44.3X1	T44.3X2	T44.3X3	T44.3X4	T44.3X5	T44.3X6
bromide	T44.3X1	T44.3X2	T44.3X3	T44.3X4	T44.3X5	T44.3X6
Meperidine	T40.4X1	T40.4X2	T40.4X3	T40.4X4	T40.4X5	T40.4X6
Mephebarbital	T42.3X1	T42.3X2	T42.3X3	T42.3X4	T42.3X5	T42.3X6
Mephenamin (e)	T42.8X1	T42.8X2	T42.8X3	T42.8X4	T42.8X5	T42.8X6
Mephenesin	T42.8X1	T42.8X2	T42.8X3	T42.8X4	T42.8X5	T42.8X6
Mephenhydramine	T45.0X1	T45.0X2	T45.0X3	T45.0X4	T45.0X5	T45.0X6
Mephenoxalone	T42.8X1	T42.8X2	T42.8X3	T42.8X4	T42.8X5	T42.8X6
Mephentermine	T44.991	T44.992	T44.993	T44.994	T44.995	T44.996
Mephenytoin	T42.0X1	T42.0X2	T42.0X3	T42.0X4	T42.0X5	T42.0X6
with phenobarbital	T42.3X1	T42.3X2	T42.3X3	T42.3X4	T42.3X5	T42.3X6
Mephobarbital	T42.3X1	T42.3X2	T42.3X3	T42.3X4	T42.3X5	T42.3X6
Mephosfolan	T60.0X1	T60.0X2	T60.0X3	T60.0X4	—	—
Mepindolol	T44.7X1	T44.7X2	T44.7X3	T44.7X4	T44.7X5	T44.7X6
Mepiperphenidol	T44.3X1	T44.3X2	T44.3X3	T44.3X4	T44.3X5	T44.3X6
Mepitiostane	T38.7X1	T38.7X2	T38.7X3	T38.7X4	T38.7X5	T38.7X6
Mepivacaine	T41.3X1	T41.3X2	T41.3X3	T41.3X4	T41.3X5	T41.3X6
epidural	T41.3X1	T41.3X2	T41.3X3	T41.3X4	T41.3X5	T41.3X6
Meprednisone	T38.0X1	T38.0X2	T38.0X3	T38.0X4	T38.0X5	T38.0X6
Meprobam	T43.591	T43.592	T43.593	T43.594	T43.595	T43.596
Meprobamate	T43.591	T43.592	T43.593	T43.594	T43.595	T43.596
Meproscillarin	T46.0X1	T46.0X2	T46.0X3	T46.0X4	T46.0X5	T46.0X6
Meprylcaine	T41.3X1	T41.3X2	T41.3X3	T41.3X4	T41.3X5	T41.3X6
Meptazinol	T39.8X1	T39.8X2	T39.8X3	T39.8X4	T39.8X5	T39.8X6
Mepyramine	T45.0X1	T45.0X2	T45.0X3	T45.0X4	T45.0X5	T45.0X6
Mequitazine	T43.3X1	T43.3X2	T43.3X3	T43.3X4	T43.3X5	T43.3X6
Meralluride	T50.2X1	T50.2X2	T50.2X3	T50.2X4	T50.2X5	T50.2X6
Merbaphen	T50.2X1	T50.2X2	T50.2X3	T50.2X4	T50.2X5	T50.2X6
Merbromin	T49.0X1	T49.0X2	T49.0X3	T49.0X4	T49.0X5	T49.0X6

Substance	Poisoning, Accidental (unintentional)	Poisoning, Intentional Self-harm	Poisoning, Assault	Poisoning, Undetermined	Adverse Effect	Under-dosing
Mercaptobenzothiazole salts	T49.0X1	T49.0X2	T49.0X3	T49.0X4	T49.0X5	T49.0X6
Mercaptomerin	T50.2X1	T50.2X2	T50.2X3	T50.2X4	T50.2X5	T50.2X6
Mercaptopurine	T45.1X1	T45.1X2	T45.1X3	T45.1X4	T45.1X5	T45.1X6
Mercumatilin	T50.2X1	T50.2X2	T50.2X3	T50.2X4	T50.2X5	T50.2X6
Mercuramide	T50.2X1	T50.2X2	T50.2X3	T50.2X4	T50.2X5	T50.2X6
Mercurochrome	T49.0X1	T49.0X2	T49.0X3	T49.0X4	T49.0X5	T49.0X6
Mercurophylline	T50.2X1	T50.2X2	T50.2X3	T50.2X4	T50.2X5	T50.2X6
Mercury, mercurial, mercuric, mercurous (compounds) (cyanide) (fumes) (nonmedicinal) (vapor) NEC	T56.1X1	T56.1X2	T56.1X3	T56.1X4	—	—
ammoniated	T49.0X1	T49.0X2	T49.0X3	T49.0X4	T49.0X5	T49.0X6
anti-infective						
local	T49.0X1	T49.0X2	T49.0X3	T49.0X4	T49.0X5	T49.0X6
systemic	T37.8X1	T37.8X2	T37.8X3	T37.8X4	T37.8X5	T37.8X6
topical	T49.0X1	T49.0X2	T49.0X3	T49.0X4	T49.0X5	T49.0X6
chloride (ammoniated)	T49.0X1	T49.0X2	T49.0X3	T49.0X4	T49.0X5	T49.0X6
fungicide	T56.1X1	T56.1X2	T56.1X3	T56.1X4	—	—
diuretic NEC	T50.2X1	T50.2X2	T50.2X3	T50.2X4	T50.2X5	T50.2X6
fungicide	T56.1X1	T56.1X2	T56.1X3	T56.1X4	—	—
organic (fungicide)	T56.1X1	T56.1X2	T56.1X3	T56.1X4	—	—
oxide, yellow	T49.0X1	T49.0X2	T49.0X3	T49.0X4	T49.0X5	T49.0X6
Mersalyl	T50.2X1	T50.2X2	T50.2X3	T50.2X4	T50.2X5	T50.2X6
Merthiolate	T49.0X1	T49.0X2	T49.0X3	T49.0X4	T49.0X5	T49.0X6
ophthalmic preparation	T49.5X1	T49.5X2	T49.5X3	T49.5X4	T49.5X5	T49.5X6
Meruvax	T50.B91	T50.B92	T50.B93	T50.B94	T50.B95	T50.B96
Mesalazine	T47.8X1	T47.8X2	T47.8X3	T47.8X4	T47.8X5	T47.8X6
Mescal buttons	T40.991	T40.992	T40.993	T40.994	—	—
Mescaline	T40.991	T40.992	T40.993	T40.994	—	—
Mesna	T48.4X1	T48.4X2	T48.4X3	T48.4X4	T48.4X5	T48.4X6
Mesoglycan	T46.6X1	T46.6X2	T46.6X3	T46.6X4	T46.6X5	T46.6X6
Mesoridazine	T43.3X1	T43.3X2	T43.3X3	T43.3X4	T43.3X5	T43.3X6
Mestanolone	T38.7X1	T38.7X2	T38.7X3	T38.7X4	T38.7X5	T38.7X6
Mesterolone	T38.7X1	T38.7X2	T38.7X3	T38.7X4	T38.7X5	T38.7X6
Mestranol	T38.5X1	T38.5X2	T38.5X3	T38.5X4	T38.5X5	T38.5X6
Mesulergine	T42.8X1	T42.8X2	T42.8X3	T42.8X4	T42.8X5	T42.8X6
Mesulfen	T49.0X1	T49.0X2	T49.0X3	T49.0X4	T49.0X5	T49.0X6
Mesuximide	T42.2X1	T42.2X2	T42.2X3	T42.2X4	T42.2X5	T42.2X6
Metabutethamine	T41.3X1	T41.3X2	T41.3X3	T41.3X4	T41.3X5	T41.3X6
Metactesylacetate	T49.0X1	T49.0X2	T49.0X3	T49.0X4	T49.0X5	T49.0X6
Metacycline	T36.4X1	T36.4X2	T36.4X3	T36.4X4	T36.4X5	T36.4X6
Metaldehyde (snail killer) NEC	T60.8X1	T60.8X2	T60.8X3	T60.8X4	—	—
Metals (heavy) (nonmedicinal)	T56.91	T56.92	T56.93	T56.94	—	—
dust, fumes, or vapor NEC	T56.91	T56.92	T56.93	T56.94	—	—
light NEC	T56.91	T56.92	T56.93	T56.94	—	—
dust, fumes, or vapor NEC	T56.91	T56.92	T56.93	T56.94	—	—
specified NEC	T56.891	T56.892	T56.893	T56.894	—	—
thallium	T56.811	T56.812	T56.813	T56.814	—	—
Metamfetamine	T43.621	T43.622	T43.623	T43.624	T43.625	T43.626
Metamizole sodium	T39.2X1	T39.2X2	T39.2X3	T39.2X4	T39.2X5	T39.2X6
Metampicillin	T36.0X1	T36.0X2	T36.0X3	T36.0X4	T36.0X5	T36.0X6
Metamucil	T47.4X1	T47.4X2	T47.4X3	T47.4X4	T47.4X5	T47.4X6
Metandienone	T38.7X1	T38.7X2	T38.7X3	T38.7X4	T38.7X5	T38.7X6
Metandrostenolone	T38.7X1	T38.7X2	T38.7X3	T38.7X4	T38.7X5	T38.7X6
Metaphen	T49.0X1	T49.0X2	T49.0X3	T49.0X4	T49.0X5	T49.0X6
Metaphos	T60.0X1	T60.0X2	T60.0X3	T60.0X4	—	—
Metapramine	T43.011	T43.012	T43.013	T43.014	T43.015	T43.016
Metaproterenol	T48.291	T48.292	T48.293	T48.294	T48.295	T48.296
Metaraminol	T44.4X1	T44.4X2	T44.4X3	T44.4X4	T44.4X5	T44.4X6
Metaxalone	T42.8X1	T42.8X2	T42.8X3	T42.8X4	T42.8X5	T42.8X6
Metenolone	T38.7X1	T38.7X2	T38.7X3	T38.7X4	T38.7X5	T38.7X6
Metergoline	T42.8X1	T42.8X2	T42.8X3	T42.8X4	T42.8X5	T42.8X6
Metescufylline	T46.991	T46.992	T46.993	T46.994	T46.995	T46.996
Metetoin	T42.0X1	T42.0X2	T42.0X3	T42.0X4	T42.0X5	T42.0X6
Metformin	T38.3X1	T38.3X2	T38.3X3	T38.3X4	T38.3X5	T38.3X6
Methacholine	T44.1X1	T44.1X2	T44.1X3	T44.1X4	T44.1X5	T44.1X6
Methacycline	T36.4X1	T36.4X2	T36.4X3	T36.4X4	T36.4X5	T36.4X6
Methadone	T40.3X1	T40.3X2	T40.3X3	T40.3X4	T40.3X5	T40.3X6
Methallenestril	T38.5X1	T38.5X2	T38.5X3	T38.5X4	T38.5X5	T38.5X6
Methallenoestril	T38.5X1	T38.5X2	T38.5X3	T38.5X4	T38.5X5	T38.5X6
Methamphetamine	T43.621	T43.622	T43.623	T43.624	T43.625	T43.626
Methampyrone	T39.2X1	T39.2X2	T39.2X3	T39.2X4	T39.2X5	T39.2X6
Methandienone	T38.7X1	T38.7X2	T38.7X3	T38.7X4	T38.7X5	T38.7X6
Methandiol	T38.7X1	T38.7X2	T38.7X3	T38.7X4	T38.7X5	T38.7X6
Methandrostenolone	T38.7X1	T38.7X2	T38.7X3	T38.7X4	T38.7X5	T38.7X6
Methane	T59.891	T59.892	T59.893	T59.894	—	—
Methanethiol	T59.891	T59.892	T59.893	T59.894	—	—
Methaniazide	T37.1X1	T37.1X2	T37.1X3	T37.1X4	T37.1X5	T37.1X6
Methanol (vapor)	T51.1X1	T51.1X2	T51.1X3	T51.1X4	—	—

Table of Drugs and Chemicals

Mecrilate — Methanol

Substance	Poisoning, Accidental (unintentional)	Poisoning, Intentional Self-harm	Poisoning, Assault	Poisoning, Undetermined	Adverse Effect	Under-dosing
Methantheline	T44.3X1	T44.3X2	T44.3X3	T44.3X4	T44.3X5	T44.3X6
Methanthelinium bromide	T44.3X1	T44.3X2	T44.3X3	T44.3X4	T44.3X5	T44.3X6
Methaphenilene	T45.0X1	T45.0X2	T45.0X3	T45.0X4	T45.0X5	T45.0X6
Methapyrilene	T45.0X1	T45.0X2	T45.0X3	T45.0X4	T45.0X5	T45.0X6
Methaqualone (compound)	T42.6X1	T42.6X2	T42.6X3	T42.6X4	T42.6X5	T42.6X6
Metharbital	T42.3X1	T42.3X2	T42.3X3	T42.3X4	T42.3X5	T42.3X6
Methazolamide	T50.2X1	T50.2X2	T50.2X3	T50.2X4	T50.2X5	T50.2X6
Methdilazine	T43.3X1	T43.3X2	T43.3X3	T43.3X4	T43.3X5	T43.3X6
Methedrine	T43.621	T43.622	T43.623	T43.624	T43.625	T43.626
Methenamine (mandelate)	T37.8X1	T37.8X2	T37.8X3	T37.8X4	T37.8X5	T37.8X6
Methenolone	T38.7X1	T38.7X2	T38.7X3	T38.7X4	T38.7X5	T38.7X6
Methergine	T48.0X1	T48.0X2	T48.0X3	T48.0X4	T48.0X5	T48.0X6
Methetoin	T42.0X1	T42.0X2	T42.0X3	T42.0X4	T42.0X5	T42.0X6
Methiacil	T38.2X1	T38.2X2	T38.2X3	T38.2X4	T38.2X5	T38.2X6
Methicillin	T36.0X1	T36.0X2	T36.0X3	T36.0X4	T36.0X5	T36.0X6
Methimazole	T38.2X1	T38.2X2	T38.2X3	T38.2X4	T38.2X5	T38.2X6
Methiodal sodium	T50.8X1	T50.8X2	T50.8X3	T50.8X4	T50.8X5	T50.8X6
Methionine	T50.991	T50.992	T50.993	T50.994	T50.995	T50.996
Methisazone	T37.5X1	T37.5X2	T37.5X3	T37.5X4	T37.5X5	T37.5X6
Methisoprinol	T37.5X1	T37.5X2	T37.5X3	T37.5X4	T37.5X5	T37.5X6
Methitural	T42.3X1	T42.3X2	T42.3X3	T42.3X4	T42.3X5	T42.3X6
Methixene	T44.3X1	T44.3X2	T44.3X3	T44.3X4	T44.3X5	T44.3X6
Methobarbital, methobarbitone	T42.3X1	T42.3X2	T42.3X3	T42.3X4	T42.3X5	T42.3X6
Methocarbamol	T42.8X1	T42.8X2	T42.8X3	T42.8X4	T42.8X5	T42.8X6
skeletal muscle relaxant	T48.1X1	T48.1X2	T48.1X3	T48.1X4	T48.1X5	T48.1X6
Methohexital	T41.1X1	T41.1X2	T41.1X3	T41.1X4	T41.1X5	T41.1X6
Methohexitone	T41.1X1	T41.1X2	T41.1X3	T41.1X4	T41.1X5	T41.1X6
Methoin	T42.0X1	T42.0X2	T42.0X3	T42.0X4	T42.0X5	T42.0X6
Methopholine	T39.8X1	T39.8X2	T39.8X3	T39.8X4	T39.8X5	T39.8X6
Methopromazine	T43.3X1	T43.3X2	T43.3X3	T43.3X4	T43.3X5	T43.3X6
Methorate	T48.3X1	T48.3X2	T48.3X3	T48.3X4	T48.3X5	T48.3X6
Methoserpidine	T46.5X1	T46.5X2	T46.5X3	T46.5X4	T46.5X5	T46.5X6
Methotrexate	T45.1X1	T45.1X2	T45.1X3	T45.1X4	T45.1X5	T45.1X6
Methotrimeprazine	T43.3X1	T43.3X2	T43.3X3	T43.3X4	T43.3X5	T43.3X6
Methoxa-Dome	T49.3X1	T49.3X2	T49.3X3	T49.3X4	T49.3X5	T49.3X6
Methoxamine	T44.4X1	T44.4X2	T44.4X3	T44.4X4	T44.4X5	T44.4X6
Methoxsalen	T50.991	T50.992	T50.993	T50.994	T50.995	T50.996
Methoxyaniline	T65.3X1	T65.3X2	T65.3X3	T65.3X4	—	—
Methoxybenzyl penicillin	T36.0X1	T36.0X2	T36.0X3	T36.0X4	T36.0X5	T36.0X6
Methoxychlor	T53.7X1	T53.7X2	T53.7X3	T53.7X4	—	—
Methoxy-DDT	T53.7X1	T53.7X2	T53.7X3	T53.7X4	—	—
Methoxyflurane	T41.0X1	T41.0X2	T41.0X3	T41.0X4	T41.0X5	T41.0X6
Methoxyphenamine	T48.6X1	T48.6X2	T48.6X3	T48.6X4	T48.6X5	T48.6X6
Methoxypromazine	T43.3X1	T43.3X2	T43.3X3	T43.3X4	T43.3X5	T43.3X6
Methscopolamine bromide	T44.3X1	T44.3X2	T44.3X3	T44.3X4	T44.3X5	T44.3X6
Methsuximide	T42.2X1	T42.2X2	T42.2X3	T42.2X4	T42.2X5	T42.2X6
Methyclothiazide	T50.2X1	T50.2X2	T50.2X3	T50.2X4	T50.2X5	T50.2X6
Methyl						
acetate	T52.4X1	T52.4X2	T52.4X3	T52.4X4	—	—
acetone	T52.4X1	T52.4X2	T52.4X3	T52.4X4	—	—
acrylate	T65.891	T65.892	T65.893	T65.894	—	—
alcohol	T51.1X1	T51.1X2	T51.1X3	T51.1X4	—	—
aminophenol	T65.3X1	T65.3X2	T65.3X3	T65.3X4	—	—
amphetamine	T43.621	T43.622	T43.623	T43.624	T43.625	T43.626
androstanolone	T38.7X1	T38.7X2	T38.7X3	T38.7X4	T38.7X5	T38.7X6
atropine	T44.3X1	T44.3X2	T44.3X3	T44.3X4	T44.3X5	T44.3X6
benzene	T52.2X1	T52.2X2	T52.2X3	T52.2X4	—	—
benzoate	T52.8X1	T52.8X2	T52.8X3	T52.8X4	—	—
benzol	T52.2X1	T52.2X2	T52.2X3	T52.2X4	—	—
bromide (gas)	T59.891	T59.892	T59.893	T59.894	—	—
fumigant	T60.8X1	T60.8X2	T60.8X3	T60.8X4	—	—
butanol	T51.3X1	T51.3X2	T51.3X3	T51.3X4	—	—
carbinol	T51.1X1	T51.1X2	T51.1X3	T51.1X4	—	—
carbonate	T52.8X1	T52.8X2	T52.8X3	T52.8X4	—	—
CCNU	T45.1X1	T45.1X2	T45.1X3	T45.1X4	T45.1X5	T45.1X6
cellosolve	T52.91	T52.92	T52.93	T52.94	—	—
cellulose	T47.4X1	T47.4X2	T47.4X3	T47.4X4	T47.4X5	T47.4X6
chloride (gas)	T59.891	T59.892	T59.893	T59.894	—	—
chloroformate	T59.3X1	T59.3X2	T59.3X3	T59.3X4	—	—
cyclohexane	T52.8X1	T52.8X2	T52.8X3	T52.8X4	—	—
cyclohexanol	T51.8X1	T51.8X2	T51.8X3	T51.8X4	—	—
cyclohexanone	T52.8X1	T52.8X2	T52.8X3	T52.8X4	—	—
cyclohexyl acetate	T52.8X1	T52.8X2	T52.8X3	T52.8X4	—	—
demeton	T60.0X1	T60.0X2	T60.0X3	T60.0X4	—	—
dihydromorphinone	T40.2X1	T40.2X2	T40.2X3	T40.2X4	T40.2X5	T40.2X6
ergometrine	T48.0X1	T48.0X2	T48.0X3	T48.0X4	T48.0X5	T48.0X6
ergonovine	T48.0X1	T48.0X2	T48.0X3	T48.0X4	T48.0X5	T48.0X6
ethyl ketone	T52.4X1	T52.4X2	T52.4X3	T52.4X4	—	—
glucamine antimonate	T37.8X1	T37.8X2	T37.8X3	T37.8X4	T37.8X5	T37.8X6
hydrazine	T65.891	T65.892	T65.893	T65.894	—	—
iodide	T65.891	T65.892	T65.893	T65.894	—	—
isobutyl ketone	T52.4X1	T52.4X2	T52.4X3	T52.4X4	—	—

Substance	Poisoning, Accidental (unintentional)	Poisoning, Intentional Self-harm	Poisoning, Assault	Poisoning, Undetermined	Adverse Effect	Under-dosing
Methyl — continued						
isothiocyanate	T60.3X1	T60.3X2	T60.3X3	T60.3X4	—	—
mercaptan	T59.891	T59.892	T59.893	T59.894	—	—
morphine NEC	T40.2X1	T40.2X2	T40.2X3	T40.2X4	T40.2X5	T40.2X6
nicotinate	T49.4X1	T49.4X2	T49.4X3	T49.4X4	T49.4X5	T49.4X6
paraben	T49.0X1	T49.0X2	T49.0X3	T49.0X4	T49.0X5	T49.0X6
parafynol	T42.6X1	T42.6X2	T42.6X3	T42.6X4	T42.6X5	T42.6X6
parathion	T60.0X1	T60.0X2	T60.0X3	T60.0X4	—	—
peridol	T43.4X1	T43.4X2	T43.4X3	T43.4X4	T43.4X5	T43.4X6
phenidate	T43.631	T43.632	T43.633	T43.634	T43.635	T43.636
prednisolone	T38.0X1	T38.0X2	T38.0X3	T38.0X4	T38.0X5	T38.0X6
ENT agent	T49.6X1	T49.6X2	T49.6X3	T49.6X4	T49.6X5	T49.6X6
ophthalmic preparation	T49.5X1	T49.5X2	T49.5X3	T49.5X4	T49.5X5	T49.5X6
topical NEC	T49.0X1	T49.0X2	T49.0X3	T49.0X4	T49.0X5	T49.0X6
propylcarbinol	T51.3X1	T51.3X2	T51.3X3	T51.3X4	—	—
rosaniline NEC	T49.0X1	T49.0X2	T49.0X3	T49.0X4	T49.0X5	T49.0X6
salicylate	T49.2X1	T49.2X2	T49.2X3	T49.2X4	T49.2X5	T49.2X6
sulfate (fumes)	T59.891	T59.892	T59.893	T59.894	—	—
liquid	T52.8X1	T52.8X2	T52.8X3	T52.8X4	—	—
sulfonal	T42.6X1	T42.6X2	T42.6X3	T42.6X4	T42.6X5	T42.6X6
testosterone	T38.7X1	T38.7X2	T38.7X3	T38.7X4	T38.7X5	T38.7X6
thiouracil	T38.2X1	T38.2X2	T38.2X3	T38.2X4	T38.2X5	T38.2X6
Methylamphetamine	T43.621	T43.622	T43.623	T43.624	T43.625	T43.626
Methylated spirit	T51.1X1	T51.1X2	T51.1X3	T51.1X4	—	—
Methylatropine nitrate	T44.3X1	T44.3X2	T44.3X3	T44.3X4	T44.3X5	T44.3X6
Methylbenactyzium bromide	T44.3X1	T44.3X2	T44.3X3	T44.3X4	T44.3X5	T44.3X6
Methylbenzethonium chloride	T49.0X1	T49.0X2	T49.0X3	T49.0X4	T49.0X5	T49.0X6
Methylcellulose	T47.4X1	T47.4X2	T47.4X3	T47.4X4	T47.4X5	T47.4X6
laxative	T47.4X1	T47.4X2	T47.4X3	T47.4X4	T47.4X5	T47.4X6
Methylchlorophenoxyacetic acid	T60.3X1	T60.3X2	T60.3X3	T60.3X4	—	—
Methyldopa	T46.5X1	T46.5X2	T46.5X3	T46.5X4	T46.5X5	T46.5X6
Methyldopate	T46.5X1	T46.5X2	T46.5X3	T46.5X4	T46.5X5	T46.5X6
Methylene						
blue	T50.6X1	T50.6X2	T50.6X3	T50.6X4	T50.6X5	T50.6X6
chloride or dichloride (solvent) NEC	T53.4X1	T53.4X2	T53.4X3	T53.4X4	—	—
Methylenedioxyamphetamine	T43.621	T43.622	T43.623	T43.624	T43.625	T43.626
Methylenedioxymethamphetamine	T43.621	T43.622	T43.623	T43.624	T43.625	T43.626
Methylergometrine	T48.0X1	T48.0X2	T48.0X3	T48.0X4	T48.0X5	T48.0X6
Methylergonovine	T48.0X1	T48.0X2	T48.0X3	T48.0X4	T48.0X5	T48.0X6
Methylestrenolone	T38.5X1	T38.5X2	T38.5X3	T38.5X4	T38.5X5	T38.5X6
Methylethyl cellulose	T50.991	T50.992	T50.993	T50.994	T50.995	T50.996
Methylhexabital	T42.3X1	T42.3X2	T42.3X3	T42.3X4	T42.3X5	T42.3X6
Methylmorphine	T40.2X1	T40.2X2	T40.2X3	T40.2X4	T40.2X5	T40.2X6
Methylparaben (ophthalmic)	T49.5X1	T49.5X2	T49.5X3	T49.5X4	T49.5X5	T49.5X6
Methylparafynol	T42.6X1	T42.6X2	T42.6X3	T42.6X4	T42.6X5	T42.6X6
Methylpentynol, methylpenthynol	T42.6X1	T42.6X2	T42.6X3	T42.6X4	T42.6X5	T42.6X6
Methylphenidate	T43.631	T43.632	T43.633	T43.634	T43.635	T43.636
Methylphenobarbital	T42.3X1	T42.3X2	T42.3X3	T42.3X4	T42.3X5	T42.3X6
Methylpolysiloxane	T47.1X1	T47.1X2	T47.1X3	T47.1X4	T47.1X5	T47.1X6
Methylprednisolone — see Methyl, prednisolone						
Methylrosaniline	T49.0X1	T49.0X2	T49.0X3	T49.0X4	T49.0X5	T49.0X6
Methylrosanilinium chloride	T49.0X1	T49.0X2	T49.0X3	T49.0X4	T49.0X5	T49.0X6
Methyltestosterone	T38.7X1	T38.7X2	T38.7X3	T38.7X4	T38.7X5	T38.7X6
Methylthionine chloride	T50.6X1	T50.6X2	T50.6X3	T50.6X4	T50.6X5	T50.6X6
Methylthioninium chloride	T50.6X1	T50.6X2	T50.6X3	T50.6X4	T50.6X5	T50.6X6
Methylthiouracil	T38.2X1	T38.2X2	T38.2X3	T38.2X4	T38.2X5	T38.2X6
Methyprylon	T42.6X1	T42.6X2	T42.6X3	T42.6X4	T42.6X5	T42.6X6
Methysergide	T46.5X1	T46.5X2	T46.5X3	T46.5X4	T46.5X5	T46.5X6
Metiamide	T47.1X1	T47.1X2	T47.1X3	T47.1X4	T47.1X5	T47.1X6
Meticillin	T36.0X1	T36.0X2	T36.0X3	T36.0X4	T36.0X5	T36.0X6
Meticrane	T50.2X1	T50.2X2	T50.2X3	T50.2X4	T50.2X5	T50.2X6
Metildigoxin	T46.0X1	T46.0X2	T46.0X3	T46.0X4	T46.0X5	T46.0X6
Metipranolol	T49.5X1	T49.5X2	T49.5X3	T49.5X4	T49.5X5	T49.5X6
Metirosine	T46.5X1	T46.5X2	T46.5X3	T46.5X4	T46.5X5	T46.5X6
Metisazone	T37.5X1	T37.5X2	T37.5X3	T37.5X4	T37.5X5	T37.5X6
Metixene	T44.3X1	T44.3X2	T44.3X3	T44.3X4	T44.3X5	T44.3X6
Metizoline	T48.5X1	T48.5X2	T48.5X3	T48.5X4	T48.5X5	T48.5X6
Metoclopramide	T45.0X1	T45.0X2	T45.0X3	T45.0X4	T45.0X5	T45.0X6
Metofenazate	T43.3X1	T43.3X2	T43.3X3	T43.3X4	T43.3X5	T43.3X6
Metofoline	T39.8X1	T39.8X2	T39.8X3	T39.8X4	T39.8X5	T39.8X6
Metolazone	T50.2X1	T50.2X2	T50.2X3	T50.2X4	T50.2X5	T50.2X6
Metopon	T40.2X1	T40.2X2	T40.2X3	T40.2X4	T40.2X5	T40.2X6
Metoprine	T45.1X1	T45.1X2	T45.1X3	T45.1X4	T45.1X5	T45.1X6
Metoprolol	T44.7X1	T44.7X2	T44.7X3	T44.7X4	T44.7X5	T44.7X6
Metrifonate	T60.0X1	T60.0X2	T60.0X3	T60.0X4	—	—

Substance	Poisoning, Accidental (unintentional)	Poisoning, Intentional Self-harm	Poisoning, Assault	Poisoning, Undetermined	Adverse Effect	Under-dosing
Metrizamide	T50.8X1	T50.8X2	T50.8X3	T50.8X4	T50.8X5	T50.8X6
Metrizoic acid	T50.8X1	T50.8X2	T50.8X3	T50.8X4	T50.8X5	T50.8X6
Metronidazole	T37.8X1	T37.8X2	T37.8X3	T37.8X4	T37.8X5	T37.8X6
Metycaine						
infiltration (subcutaneous)	T41.3X1	T41.3X2	T41.3X3	T41.3X4	T41.3X5	T41.3X6
nerve block (peripheral)	T41.3X1	T41.3X2	T41.3X3	T41.3X4	T41.3X5	T41.3X6
(plexus)						
topical (surface)	T41.3X1	T41.3X2	T41.3X3	T41.3X4	T41.3X5	T41.3X6
Metyrapone	T50.8X1	T50.8X2	T50.8X3	T50.8X4	T50.8X5	T50.8X6
Mevinphos	T60.0X1	T60.0X2	T60.0X3	T60.0X4	—	—
Mexazolam	T42.4X1	T42.4X2	T42.4X3	T42.4X4	T42.4X5	T42.4X6
Mexenone	T49.3X1	T49.3X2	T49.3X3	T49.3X4	T49.3X5	T49.3X6
Mexiletine	T46.2X1	T46.2X2	T46.2X3	T46.2X4	T46.2X5	T46.2X6
Mezereon	T62.2X1	T62.2X2	T62.2X3	T62.2X4	—	—
berries	T62.1X1	T62.1X2	T62.1X3	T62.1X4	—	—
Mezlocillin	T36.0X1	T36.0X2	T36.0X3	T36.0X4	T36.0X5	T36.0X6
Mianserin	T43.021	T43.022	T43.023	T43.024	T43.025	T43.026
Micatin	T49.0X1	T49.0X2	T49.0X3	T49.0X4	T49.0X5	T49.0X6
Miconazole	T49.0X1	T49.0X2	T49.0X3	T49.0X4	T49.0X5	T49.0X6
Micronomicin	T36.5X1	T36.5X2	T36.5X3	T36.5X4	T36.5X5	T36.5X6
Midazolam	T42.4X1	T42.4X2	T42.4X3	T42.4X4	T42.4X5	T42.4X6
Midecamycin	T36.3X1	T36.3X2	T36.3X3	T36.3X4	T36.3X5	T36.3X6
Mifepristone	T38.6X1	T38.6X2	T38.6X3	T38.6X4	T38.6X5	T38.6X6
Milk of magnesia	T47.1X1	T47.1X2	T47.1X3	T47.1X4	T47.1X5	T47.1X6
Millipede (tropical)	T63.411	T63.412	T63.413	T63.414	—	—
(venomous)						
Miltown	T43.591	T43.592	T43.593	T43.594	T43.595	T43.596
Milverine	T44.3X1	T44.3X2	T44.3X3	T44.3X4	T44.3X5	T44.3X6
Minaprine	T43.291	T43.292	T43.293	T43.294	T43.295	T43.296
Minaxolone	T41.291	T41.292	T41.293	T41.294	T41.295	T41.296
Mineral						
acids	T54.2X1	T54.2X2	T54.2X3	T54.2X4	—	—
oil (laxative)(medicinal)	T47.4X1	T47.4X2	T47.4X3	T47.4X4	T47.4X5	T47.4X6
emulsion	T47.2X1	T47.2X2	T47.2X3	T47.2X4	T47.2X5	T47.2X6
nonmedicinal	T52.0X1	T52.0X2	T52.0X3	T52.0X4	—	—
topical	T49.3X1	T49.3X2	T49.3X3	T49.3X4	T49.3X5	T49.3X6
salt NEC	T50.3X1	T50.3X2	T50.3X3	T50.3X4	T50.3X5	T50.3X6
spirits	T52.0X1	T52.0X2	T52.0X3	T52.0X4	—	—
Mineralocorticosteroid	T50.0X1	T50.0X2	T50.0X3	T50.0X4	T50.0X5	T50.0X6
Minocycline	T36.4X1	T36.4X2	T36.4X3	T36.4X4	T36.4X5	T36.4X6
Minoxidil	T46.7X1	T46.7X2	T46.7X3	T46.7X4	T46.7X5	T46.7X6
Miokamycin	T36.3X1	T36.3X2	T36.3X3	T36.3X4	T36.3X5	T36.3X6
Miotic drug	T49.5X1	T49.5X2	T49.5X3	T49.5X4	T49.5X5	T49.5X6
Mipafox	T60.0X1	T60.0X2	T60.0X3	T60.0X4	—	—
Mirex	T60.1X1	T60.1X2	T60.1X3	T60.1X4	—	—
Mirtazapine	T43.021	T43.022	T43.023	T43.024	T43.025	T43.026
Misonidazole	T37.3X1	T37.3X2	T37.3X3	T37.3X4	T37.3X5	T37.3X6
Misoprostol	T47.1X1	T47.1X2	T47.1X3	T47.1X4	T47.1X5	T47.1X6
Mithramycin	T45.1X1	T45.1X2	T45.1X3	T45.1X4	T45.1X5	T45.1X6
Mitobronitol	T45.1X1	T45.1X2	T45.1X3	T45.1X4	T45.1X5	T45.1X6
Mitoguazone	T45.1X1	T45.1X2	T45.1X3	T45.1X4	T45.1X5	T45.1X6
Mitolactol	T45.1X1	T45.1X2	T45.1X3	T45.1X4	T45.1X5	T45.1X6
Mitomycin	T45.1X1	T45.1X2	T45.1X3	T45.1X4	T45.1X5	T45.1X6
Mitopodozide	T45.1X1	T45.1X2	T45.1X3	T45.1X4	T45.1X5	T45.1X6
Mitotane	T45.1X1	T45.1X2	T45.1X3	T45.1X4	T45.1X5	T45.1X6
Mitoxantrone	T45.1X1	T45.1X2	T45.1X3	T45.1X4	T45.1X5	T45.1X6
Mivacurium chloride	T48.1X1	T48.1X2	T48.1X3	T48.1X4	T48.1X5	T48.1X6
Miyari bacteria	T47.6X1	T47.6X2	T47.6X3	T47.6X4	T47.6X5	T47.6X6
Moclobemide	T43.1X1	T43.1X2	T43.1X3	T43.1X4	T43.1X5	T43.1X6
Moderil	T46.5X1	T46.5X2	T46.5X3	T46.5X4	T46.5X5	T46.5X6
Mofebutazone	T39.2X1	T39.2X2	T39.2X3	T39.2X4	T39.2X5	T39.2X6
Mogadon — see Nitrazepam						
Molindone	T43.591	T43.592	T43.593	T43.594	T43.595	T43.596
Molsidomine	T46.3X1	T46.3X2	T46.3X3	T46.3X4	T46.3X5	T46.3X6
Mometasone	T49.0X1	T49.0X2	T49.0X3	T49.0X4	T49.0X5	T49.0X6
Monistat	T49.0X1	T49.0X2	T49.0X3	T49.0X4	T49.0X5	T49.0X6
Monkshood	T62.2X1	T62.2X2	T62.2X3	T62.2X4	—	—
Monoamine oxidase inhibitor NEC	T43.1X1	T43.1X2	T43.1X3	T43.1X4	T43.1X5	T43.1X6
hydrazine	T43.1X1	T43.1X2	T43.1X3	T43.1X4	T43.1X5	T43.1X6
Monobenzone	T49.4X1	T49.4X2	T49.4X3	T49.4X4	T49.4X5	T49.4X6
Monochloroacetic acid	T60.3X1	T60.3X2	T60.3X3	T60.3X4	—	—
Monochlorobenzene	T53.7X1	T53.7X2	T53.7X3	T53.7X4	—	—
Monoethanolamine	T46.8X1	T46.8X2	T46.8X3	T46.8X4	T46.8X5	T46.8X6
oleate	T46.8X1	T46.8X2	T46.8X3	T46.8X4	T46.8X5	T46.8X6
Monooctanoin	T50.991	T50.992	T50.993	T50.994	T50.995	T50.996
Monophenylbutazone	T39.2X1	T39.2X2	T39.2X3	T39.2X4	T39.2X5	T39.2X6
Monosodium glutamate	T65.891	T65.892	T65.893	T65.894	—	—
Monosulfiram	T49.0X1	T49.0X2	T49.0X3	T49.0X4	T49.0X5	T49.0X6
Monoxide, carbon — see Carbon, monoxide						
Monoxidine hydrochloride	T46.1X1	T46.1X2	T46.1X3	T46.1X4	T46.1X5	T46.1X6
Monuron	T60.3X1	T60.3X2	T60.3X3	T60.3X4	—	—
Moperone	T43.4X1	T43.4X2	T43.4X3	T43.4X4	T43.4X5	T43.4X6
Mopidamol	T45.1X1	T45.1X2	T45.1X3	T45.1X4	T45.1X5	T45.1X6
MOPP (mechloreth-amine + vincristine + prednisone + procarba-zine)	T45.1X1	T45.1X2	T45.1X3	T45.1X4	T45.1X5	T45.1X6
Morfin	T40.2X1	T40.2X2	T40.2X3	T40.2X4	T40.2X5	T40.2X6
Morinamide	T37.1X1	T37.1X2	T37.1X3	T37.1X4	T37.1X5	T37.1X6
Morning glory seeds	T40.991	T40.992	T40.993	T40.994	—	—
Moroxydine	T37.5X1	T37.5X2	T37.5X3	T37.5X4	T37.5X5	T37.5X6
Morphazinamide	T37.1X1	T37.1X2	T37.1X3	T37.1X4	T37.1X5	T37.1X6
Morphine	T40.2X1	T40.2X2	T40.2X3	T40.2X4	T40.2X5	T40.2X6
antagonist	T50.7X1	T50.7X2	T50.7X3	T50.7X4	T50.7X5	T50.7X6
Morpholinylethylmorphine	T40.2X1	T40.2X2	T40.2X3	T40.2X4	—	—
Morsuximide	T42.2X1	T42.2X2	T42.2X3	T42.2X4	T42.2X5	T42.2X6
Mosapramine	T43.591	T43.592	T43.593	T43.594	T43.595	T43.596
Moth balls — see also Pesticides	T60.2X1	T60.2X2	T60.2X3	T60.2X4		
naphthalene	T60.2X1	T60.2X2	T60.2X3	T60.2X4		
paradichlorobenzene	T60.1X1	T60.1X2	T60.1X3	T60.1X4		
Motor exhaust gas	T58.01	T58.02	T58.03	T58.04	—	—
Mouthwash (antiseptic) (zinc chloride)	T49.6X1	T49.6X2	T49.6X3	T49.6X4	T49.6X5	T49.6X6
Moxastine	T45.0X1	T45.0X2	T45.0X3	T45.0X4	T45.0X5	T45.0X6
Moxaverine	T44.3X1	T44.3X2	T44.3X3	T44.3X4	T44.3X5	T44.3X6
Moxisylyte	T46.7X1	T46.7X2	T46.7X3	T46.7X4	T46.7X5	T46.7X6
Mucilage, plant	T47.4X1	T47.4X2	T47.4X3	T47.4X4	T47.4X5	T47.4X6
Mucolytic drug	T48.4X1	T48.4X2	T48.4X3	T48.4X4	T48.4X5	T48.4X6
Mucomyst	T48.4X1	T48.4X2	T48.4X3	T48.4X4	T48.4X5	T48.4X6
Mucous membrane agents (external)	T49.91	T49.92	T49.93	T49.94	T49.95	T49.96
specified NEC	T49.8X1	T49.8X2	T49.8X3	T49.8X4	T49.8X5	T49.8X6
Mumps						
immune globulin (human)	T50.Z11	T50.Z12	T50.Z13	T50.Z14	T50.Z15	T50.Z16
skin test antigen	T50.8X1	T50.8X2	T50.8X3	T50.8X4	T50.8X5	T50.8X6
vaccine	T50.B91	T50.B92	T50.B93	T50.B94	T50.B95	T50.B96
Mumpsvax	T50.B91	T50.B92	T50.B93	T50.B94	T50.B95	T50.B96
Mupirocin	T49.0X1	T49.0X2	T49.0X3	T49.0X4	T49.0X5	T49.0X6
Muriatic acid — see Hydrochloric acid						
Muromonab-CD3	T45.1X1	T45.1X2	T45.1X3	T45.1X4	T45.1X5	T45.1X6
Muscle-action drug NEC	T48.201	T48.202	T48.203	T48.204	T48.205	T48.206
Muscle affecting agents NEC	T48.201	T48.202	T48.203	T48.204	T48.205	T48.206
oxytocic	T48.0X1	T48.0X2	T48.0X3	T48.0X4	T48.0X5	T48.0X6
relaxants	T48.201	T48.202	T48.203	T48.204	T48.205	T48.206
central nervous system	T42.8X1	T42.8X2	T42.8X3	T42.8X4	T42.8X5	T42.8X6
skeletal	T48.1X1	T48.1X2	T48.1X3	T48.1X4	T48.1X5	T48.1X6
smooth	T44.3X1	T44.3X2	T44.3X3	T44.3X4	T44.3X5	T44.3X6
Muscle relaxant — see Relaxant, muscle						
Muscle-tone depressant, central NEC	T42.8X1	T42.8X2	T42.8X3	T42.8X4	T42.8X5	T42.8X6
specified NEC	T42.8X1	T42.8X2	T42.8X3	T42.8X4	T42.8X5	T42.8X6
Mushroom, noxious	T62.0X1	T62.0X2	T62.0X3	T62.0X4	—	—
Mussel, noxious	T61.781	T61.782	T61.783	T61.784	—	—
Mustard (emetic)	T47.7X1	T47.7X2	T47.7X3	T47.7X4	T47.7X5	T47.7X6
black	T47.7X1	T47.7X2	T47.7X3	T47.7X4	T47.7X5	T47.7X6
gas, not in war	T59.91	T59.92	T59.93	T59.94	—	—
nitrogen	T45.1X1	T45.1X2	T45.1X3	T45.1X4	T45.1X5	T45.1X6
Mustine	T45.1X1	T45.1X2	T45.1X3	T45.1X4	T45.1X5	T45.1X6
M-vac	T45.1X1	T45.1X2	T45.1X3	T45.1X4	T45.1X5	T45.1X6
Mycifradin	T36.5X1	T36.5X2	T36.5X3	T36.5X4	T36.5X5	T36.5X6
topical	T49.0X1	T49.0X2	T49.0X3	T49.0X4	T49.0X5	T49.0X6
Mycitracin	T36.8X1	T36.8X2	T36.8X3	T36.8X4	T36.8X5	T36.8X6
ophthalmic preparation	T49.5X1	T49.5X2	T49.5X3	T49.5X4	T49.5X5	T49.5X6
Mycostatin	T36.7X1	T36.7X2	T36.7X3	T36.7X4	T36.7X5	T36.7X6
topical	T49.0X1	T49.0X2	T49.0X3	T49.0X4	T49.0X5	T49.0X6
Mycotoxins	T64.81	T64.82	T64.83	T64.84	—	—
aflatoxin	T64.01	T64.02	T64.03	T64.04	—	—
specified NEC	T64.81	T64.82	T64.83	T64.84	—	—
Mydriacyl	T44.3X1	T44.3X2	T44.3X3	T44.3X4	T44.3X5	T44.3X6
Mydriatic drug	T49.5X1	T49.5X2	T49.5X3	T49.5X4	T49.5X5	T49.5X6
Myelobromal	T45.1X1	T45.1X2	T45.1X3	T45.1X4	T45.1X5	T45.1X6
Myleran	T45.1X1	T45.1X2	T45.1X3	T45.1X4	T45.1X5	T45.1X6
Myochrysin (e)	T39.2X1	T39.2X2	T39.2X3	T39.2X4	T39.2X5	T39.2X6
Myoneural blocking agents	T48.1X1	T48.1X2	T48.1X3	T48.1X4	T48.1X5	T48.1X6
Myralact	T49.0X1	T49.0X2	T49.0X3	T49.0X4	T49.0X5	T49.0X6
Myristica fragrans	T62.2X1	T62.2X2	T62.2X3	T62.2X4	—	—
Myristicin	T65.891	T65.892	T65.893	T65.894	—	—
Mysoline	T42.3X1	T42.3X2	T42.3X3	T42.3X4	T42.3X5	T42.3X6
Nabilone	T40.7X1	T40.7X2	T40.7X3	T40.7X4	T40.7X5	T40.7X6
Nabumetone	T39.391	T39.392	T39.393	T39.394	T39.395	T39.396
Nadolol	T44.7X1	T44.7X2	T44.7X3	T44.7X4	T44.7X5	T44.7X6

Table of Drugs and Chemicals

Nafcillin — Nitromersol

Substance	Poisoning, Accidental (unintentional)	Poisoning, Intentional Self-harm	Poisoning, Assault	Poisoning, Undetermined	Adverse Effect	Under-dosing
Nafcillin	T36.0X1	T36.0X2	T36.0X3	T36.0X4	T36.0X5	T36.0X6
Nafoxidine	T38.6X1	T38.6X2	T38.6X3	T38.6X4	T38.6X5	T38.6X6
Naftazone	T46.991	T46.992	T46.993	T46.994	T46.995	T46.996
Naftidrofuryl (oxalate)	T46.7X1	T46.7X2	T46.7X3	T46.7X4	T46.7X5	T46.7X6
Naftifine	T49.0X1	T49.0X2	T49.0X3	T49.0X4	T49.0X5	T49.0X6
Nail polish remover	T52.91	T52.92	T52.93	T52.94	—	—
Nalbuphine	T40.4X1	T40.4X2	T40.4X3	T40.4X4	T40.4X5	T40.4X6
Naled	T60.0X1	T60.0X2	T60.0X3	T60.0X4	—	—
Nalidixic acid	T37.8X1	T37.8X2	T37.8X3	T37.8X4	T37.8X5	T37.8X6
Nalorphine	T50.7X1	T50.7X2	T50.7X3	T50.7X4	T50.7X5	T50.7X6
Naloxone	T50.7X1	T50.7X2	T50.7X3	T50.7X4	T50.7X5	T50.7X6
Naltrexone	T50.7X1	T50.7X2	T50.7X3	T50.7X4	T50.7X5	T50.7X6
Namenda	T43.8X1	T43.8X2	T43.8X3	T43.8X4	T43.8X5	T43.8X6
Nandrolone	T38.7X1	T38.7X2	T38.7X3	T38.7X4	T38.7X5	T38.7X6
Naphazoline	T48.5X1	T48.5X2	T48.5X3	T48.5X4	T48.5X5	T48.5X6
Naphtha (painters') (petroleum)	T52.0X1	T52.0X2	T52.0X3	T52.0X4	—	—
solvent	T52.0X1	T52.0X2	T52.0X3	T52.0X4	—	—
vapor	T52.0X1	T52.0X2	T52.0X3	T52.0X4	—	—
Naphthalene (non-chlorinated)	T60.2X1	T60.2X2	T60.2X3	T60.2X4	—	—
chlorinated	T60.1X1	T60.1X2	T60.1X3	T60.1X4	—	—
vapor	T60.1X1	T60.1X2	T60.1X3	T60.1X4	—	—
insecticide or moth repellent	T60.2X1	T60.2X2	T60.2X3	T60.2X4	—	—
chlorinated	T60.1X1	T60.1X2	T60.1X3	T60.1X4	—	—
vapor	T60.2X1	T60.2X2	T60.2X3	T60.2X4	—	—
chlorinated	T60.1X1	T60.1X2	T60.1X3	T60.1X4	—	—
Naphthol	T65.891	T65.892	T65.893	T65.894	—	—
Naphthylamine	T65.891	T65.892	T65.893	T65.894	—	—
Naphthylthiourea (ANTU)	T60.4X1	T60.4X2	T60.4X3	T60.4X4	—	—
Naprosyn — see Naproxen						
Naproxen	T39.311	T39.312	T39.313	T39.314	T39.315	T39.316
Narcotic (drug)	T40.601	T40.602	T40.603	T40.604	T40.605	T40.606
analgesic NEC	T40.601	T40.602	T40.603	T40.604	T40.605	T40.606
antagonist	T50.7X1	T50.7X2	T50.7X3	T50.7X4	T50.7X5	T50.7X6
specified NEC	T40.691	T40.692	T40.693	T40.694	T40.695	T40.696
synthetic	T40.4X1	T40.4X2	T40.4X3	T40.4X4	T40.4X5	T40.4X6
Narcotine	T48.3X1	T48.3X2	T48.3X3	T48.3X4	T48.3X5	T48.3X6
Nardil	T43.1X1	T43.1X2	T43.1X3	T43.1X4	T43.1X5	T43.1X6
Nasal drug NEC	T49.6X1	T49.6X2	T49.6X3	T49.6X4	T49.6X5	T49.6X6
Natamycin	T49.0X1	T49.0X2	T49.0X3	T49.0X4	T49.0X5	T49.0X6
Natrium cyanide — see Cyanide(s)						
Natural						
blood (product)	T45.8X1	T45.8X2	T45.8X3	T45.8X4	T45.8X5	T45.8X6
gas (piped)	T59.891	T59.892	T59.893	T59.894	—	—
incomplete combustion	T58.11	T58.12	T58.13	T58.14	—	—
Nealbarbital	T42.3X1	T42.3X2	T42.3X3	T42.3X4	T42.3X5	T42.3X6
Nectadon	T48.3X1	T48.3X2	T48.3X3	T48.3X4	T48.3X5	T48.3X6
Nedocromil	T48.6X1	T48.6X2	T48.6X3	T48.6X4	T48.6X5	T48.6X6
Nefopam	T39.8X1	T39.8X2	T39.8X3	T39.8X4	T39.8X5	T39.8X6
Nematocyst (sting)	T63.691	T63.692	T63.693	T63.694	—	—
Nembutal	T42.3X1	T42.3X2	T42.3X3	T42.3X4	T42.3X5	T42.3X6
Nemonapride	T43.591	T43.592	T43.593	T43.594	T43.595	T43.596
Neoarsphenamine	T37.8X1	T37.8X2	T37.8X3	T37.8X4	T37.8X5	T37.8X6
Neocinchophen	T50.4X1	T50.4X2	T50.4X3	T50.4X4	T50.4X5	T50.4X6
Neomycin (derivatives)	T36.5X1	T36.5X2	T36.5X3	T36.5X4	T36.5X5	T36.5X6
with bacitracin	T49.0X1	T49.0X2	T49.0X3	T49.0X4	T49.0X5	T49.0X6
neostigmine	T44.0X1	T44.0X2	T44.0X3	T44.0X4	T44.0X5	T44.0X6
ENT agent	T49.6X1	T49.6X2	T49.6X3	T49.6X4	T49.6X5	T49.6X6
ophthalmic preparation	T49.5X1	T49.5X2	T49.5X3	T49.5X4	T49.5X5	T49.5X6
topical NEC	T49.0X1	T49.0X2	T49.0X3	T49.0X4	T49.0X5	T49.0X6
Neonal	T42.3X1	T42.3X2	T42.3X3	T42.3X4	T42.3X5	T42.3X6
Neoprontosil	T37.0X1	T37.0X2	T37.0X3	T37.0X4	T37.0X5	T37.0X6
Neosalvarsan	T37.8X1	T37.8X2	T37.8X3	T37.8X4	T37.8X5	T37.8X6
Neosilversalvarsan	T37.8X1	T37.8X2	T37.8X3	T37.8X4	T37.8X5	T37.8X6
Neosporin	T36.8X1	T36.8X2	T36.8X3	T36.8X4	T36.8X5	T36.8X6
ENT agent	T49.6X1	T49.6X2	T49.6X3	T49.6X4	T49.6X5	T49.6X6
opthalmic preparation	T49.5X1	T49.5X2	T49.5X3	T49.5X4	T49.5X5	T49.5X6
topical NEC	T49.0X1	T49.0X2	T49.0X3	T49.0X4	T49.0X5	T49.0X6
Neostigmine bromide	T44.0X1	T44.0X2	T44.0X3	T44.0X4	T44.0X5	T44.0X6
Neraval	T42.3X1	T42.3X2	T42.3X3	T42.3X4	T42.3X5	T42.3X6
Neravan	T42.3X1	T42.3X2	T42.3X3	T42.3X4	T42.3X5	T42.3X6
Nerium oleander	T62.2X1	T62.2X2	T62.2X3	T62.2X4	—	—
Nerve gas, not in war	T59.91	T59.92	T59.93	T59.94	—	—
Nesacaine	T41.3X1	T41.3X2	T41.3X3	T41.3X4	T41.3X5	T41.3X6
infiltration (subcutaneous)	T41.3X1	T41.3X2	T41.3X3	T41.3X4	T41.3X5	T41.3X6
nerve block (peripheral) (plexus)	T41.3X1	T41.3X2	T41.3X3	T41.3X4	T41.3X5	T41.3X6
Netilmicin	T36.5X1	T36.5X2	T36.5X3	T36.5X4	T36.5X5	T36.5X6
Neurobarb	T42.3X1	T42.3X2	T42.3X3	T42.3X4	T42.3X5	T42.3X6

Substance	Poisoning, Accidental (unintentional)	Poisoning, Intentional Self-harm	Poisoning, Assault	Poisoning, Undetermined	Adverse Effect	Under-dosing
Neuroleptic drug NEC	T43.501	T43.502	T43.503	T43.504	T43.505	T43.506
Neuromuscular blocking drug	T48.1X1	T48.1X2	T48.1X3	T48.1X4	T48.1X5	T48.1X6
Neutral insulin injection	T38.3X1	T38.3X2	T38.3X3	T38.3X4	T38.3X5	T38.3X6
Neutral spirits	T51.0X1	T51.0X2	T51.0X3	T51.0X4	—	—
beverage	T51.0X1	T51.0X2	T51.0X3	T51.0X4	—	—
Niacin	T46.7X1	T46.7X2	T46.7X3	T46.7X4	T46.7X5	T46.7X6
Niacinamide	T45.2X1	T45.2X2	T45.2X3	T45.2X4	T45.2X5	T45.2X6
Nialamide	T43.1X1	T43.1X2	T43.1X3	T43.1X4	T43.1X5	T43.1X6
Niaprazine	T42.6X1	T42.6X2	T42.6X3	T42.6X4	T42.6X5	T42.6X6
Nicametate	T46.7X1	T46.7X2	T46.7X3	T46.7X4	T46.7X5	T46.7X6
Nicardipine	T46.1X1	T46.1X2	T46.1X3	T46.1X4	T46.1X5	T46.1X6
Nicergoline	T46.7X1	T46.7X2	T46.7X3	T46.7X4	T46.7X5	T46.7X6
Nickel (carbonyl) (tetra-carbonyl)(fumes) (vapor)	T56.891	T56.892	T56.893	T56.894	—	—
Nickelocene	T56.891	T56.892	T56.893	T56.894	—	—
Niclosamide	T37.4X1	T37.4X2	T37.4X3	T37.4X4	T37.4X5	T37.4X6
Nicofuranose	T46.7X1	T46.7X2	T46.7X3	T46.7X4	T46.7X5	T46.7X6
Nicomorphine	T40.2X1	T40.2X2	T40.2X3	T40.2X4	—	—
Nicorandil	T46.3X1	T46.3X2	T46.3X3	T46.3X4	T46.3X5	T46.3X6
Nicotiana (plant)	T62.2X1	T62.2X2	T62.2X3	T62.2X4	—	—
Nicotinamide	T45.2X1	T45.2X2	T45.2X3	T45.2X4	T45.2X5	T45.2X6
Nicotine (insecticide) (spray) (sulfate) NEC	T60.2X1	T60.2X2	T60.2X3	T60.2X4	—	—
from tobacco	T65.291	T65.292	T65.293	T65.294	—	—
cigarettes	T65.221	T65.222	T65.223	T65.224	—	—
not insecticide	T65.291	T65.292	T65.293	T65.294	—	—
Nicotinic acid	T46.7X1	T46.7X2	T46.7X3	T46.7X4	T46.7X5	T46.7X6
Nicotinyl alcohol	T46.7X1	T46.7X2	T46.7X3	T46.7X4	T46.7X5	T46.7X6
Nicoumalone	T45.511	T45.512	T45.513	T45.514	T45.515	T45.516
Nifedipine	T46.1X1	T46.1X2	T46.1X3	T46.1X4	T46.1X5	T46.1X6
Nifenazone	T39.2X1	T39.2X2	T39.2X3	T39.2X4	T39.2X5	T39.2X6
Nifuraldezone	T37.91	T37.92	T37.93	T37.94	T37.95	T37.96
Nifuratel	T37.8X1	T37.8X2	T37.8X3	T37.8X4	T37.8X5	T37.8X6
Nifurtimox	T37.3X1	T37.3X2	T37.3X3	T37.3X4	T37.3X5	T37.3X6
Nifurtoinol	T37.8X1	T37.8X2	T37.8X3	T37.8X4	T37.8X5	T37.8X6
Nightshade, deadly (solanum) — see also Belladonna	T62.2X1	T62.2X2	T62.2X3	T62.2X4	—	—
berry	T62.1X1	T62.1X2	T62.1X3	T62.1X4	—	—
Nikethamide	T50.7X1	T50.7X2	T50.7X3	T50.7X4	T50.7X5	T50.7X6
Nilstat	T36.7X1	T36.7X2	T36.7X3	T36.7X4	T36.7X5	T36.7X6
topical	T49.0X1	T49.0X2	T49.0X3	T49.0X4	T49.0X5	T49.0X6
Nilutamide	T38.6X1	T38.6X2	T38.6X3	T38.6X4	T38.6X5	T38.6X6
Nimesulide	T39.391	T39.392	T39.393	T39.394	T39.395	T39.396
Nimetazepam	T42.4X1	T42.4X2	T42.4X3	T42.4X4	T42.4X5	T42.4X6
Nimodipine	T46.1X1	T46.1X2	T46.1X3	T46.1X4	T46.1X5	T46.1X6
Nimorazole	T37.3X1	T37.3X2	T37.3X3	T37.3X4	T37.3X5	T37.3X6
Nimustine	T45.1X1	T45.1X2	T45.1X3	T45.1X4	T45.1X5	T45.1X6
Niridazole	T37.4X1	T37.4X2	T37.4X3	T37.4X4	T37.4X5	T37.4X6
Nisentil	T40.2X1	T40.2X2	T40.2X3	T40.2X4	T40.2X5	T40.2X6
Nisoldipine	T46.1X1	T46.1X2	T46.1X3	T46.1X4	T46.1X5	T46.1X6
Nitramine	T65.3X1	T65.3X2	T65.3X3	T65.3X4	—	—
Nitrate, organic	T46.3X1	T46.3X2	T46.3X3	T46.3X4	T46.3X5	T46.3X6
Nitrazepam	T42.4X1	T42.4X2	T42.4X3	T42.4X4	T42.4X5	T42.4X6
Nitrefazole	T50.6X1	T50.6X2	T50.6X3	T50.6X4	T50.6X5	T50.6X6
Nitrendipine	T46.1X1	T46.1X2	T46.1X3	T46.1X4	T46.1X5	T46.1X6
Nitric						
acid (liquid)	T54.2X1	T54.2X2	T54.2X3	T54.2X4	—	—
vapor	T59.891	T59.892	T59.893	T59.894	—	—
oxide (gas)	T59.0X1	T59.0X2	T59.0X3	T59.0X4	—	—
Nitrimidazine	T37.3X1	T37.3X2	T37.3X3	T37.3X4	T37.3X5	T37.3X6
Nitrite, amyl (medicinal) (vapor)	T46.3X1	T46.3X2	T46.3X3	T46.3X4	T46.3X5	T46.3X6
Nitroaniline	T65.3X1	T65.3X2	T65.3X3	T65.3X4	—	—
vapor	T59.891	T59.892	T59.893	T59.894	—	—
Nitrobenzene, nitrobenzol	T65.3X1	T65.3X2	T65.3X3	T65.3X4	—	—
vapor	T65.3X1	T65.3X2	T65.3X3	T65.3X4	—	—
Nitrocellulose	T65.891	T65.892	T65.893	T65.894	—	—
lacquer	T65.891	T65.892	T65.893	T65.894	—	—
Nitrodiphenyl	T65.3X1	T65.3X2	T65.3X3	T65.3X4	—	—
Nitrofural	T49.0X1	T49.0X2	T49.0X3	T49.0X4	T49.0X5	T49.0X6
Nitrofurantoin	T37.8X1	T37.8X2	T37.8X3	T37.8X4	T37.8X5	T37.8X6
Nitrofurazone	T49.0X1	T49.0X2	T49.0X3	T49.0X4	T49.0X5	T49.0X6
Nitrogen	T59.0X1	T59.0X2	T59.0X3	T59.0X4	—	—
mustard	T45.1X1	T45.1X2	T45.1X3	T45.1X4	T45.1X5	T45.1X6
Nitroglycerin, nitroglycerol (medicinal)	T46.3X1	T46.3X2	T46.3X3	T46.3X4	T46.3X5	T46.3X6
nonmedicinal	T65.5X1	T65.5X2	T65.5X3	T65.5X4	—	—
fumes	T65.5X1	T65.5X2	T65.5X3	T65.5X4	—	—
Nitroglycol	T52.3X1	T52.3X2	T52.3X3	T52.3X4	—	—
Nitrohydrochloric acid	T54.2X1	T54.2X2	T54.2X3	T54.2X4	—	—
Nitromersol	T49.0X1	T49.0X2	T49.0X3	T49.0X4	T49.0X5	T49.0X6

Substance	Poisoning, Accidental (unintentional)	Poisoning, Intentional Self-harm	Poisoning, Assault	Poisoning, Undetermined	Adverse Effect	Under-dosing
Nitronaphthalene	T65.891	T65.892	T65.893	T65.894	—	—
Nitrophenol	T54.0X1	T54.0X2	T54.0X3	T54.0X4	—	—
Nitropropane	T52.8X1	T52.8X2	T52.8X3	T52.8X4	—	—
Nitroprusside	T46.5X1	T46.5X2	T46.5X3	T46.5X4	T46.5X5	T46.5X6
Nitrosodimethylamine	T65.3X1	T65.3X2	T65.3X3	T65.3X4	—	—
Nitrothiazol	T37.4X1	T37.4X2	T37.4X3	T37.4X4	T37.4X5	T37.4X6
Nitrotoluene, nitrotoluol	T65.3X1	T65.3X2	T65.3X3	T65.3X4	—	—
vapor	T65.3X1	T65.3X2	T65.3X3	T65.3X4	—	—
Nitrous						
acid (liquid)	T54.2X1	T54.2X2	T54.2X3	T54.2X4	—	—
fumes	T59.891	T59.892	T59.893	T59.894	—	—
ether spirit	T46.3X1	T46.3X2	T46.3X3	T46.3X4	T46.3X5	T46.3X6
oxide	T41.0X1	T41.0X2	T41.0X3	T41.0X4	T41.0X5	T41.0X6
Nitroxoline	T37.8X1	T37.8X2	T37.8X3	T37.8X4	T37.8X5	T37.8X6
Nitrozone	T49.0X1	T49.0X2	T49.0X3	T49.0X4	T49.0X5	T49.0X6
Nizatidine	T47.0X1	T47.0X2	T47.0X3	T47.0X4	T47.0X5	T47.0X6
Nizofenone	T43.8X1	T43.8X2	T43.8X3	T43.8X4	T43.8X5	T43.8X6
Noctec	T42.6X1	T42.6X2	T42.6X3	T42.6X4	T42.6X5	T42.6X6
Noludar	T42.6X1	T42.6X2	T42.6X3	T42.6X4	T42.6X5	T42.6X6
Nomegestrol	T38.5X1	T38.5X2	T38.5X3	T38.5X4	T38.5X5	T38.5X6
Nomifensine	T43.291	T43.292	T43.293	T43.294	T43.295	T43.296
Nonoxinol	T49.8X1	T49.8X2	T49.8X3	T49.8X4	T49.8X5	T49.8X6
Nonylphenoxy	T49.8X1	T49.8X2	T49.8X3	T49.8X4	T49.8X5	T49.8X6
(polyethoxyethanol)						
Noptil	T42.3X1	T42.3X2	T42.3X3	T42.3X4	T42.3X5	T42.3X6
Noradrenaline	T44.4X1	T44.4X2	T44.4X3	T44.4X4	T44.4X5	T44.4X6
Noramidopyrine	T39.2X1	T39.2X2	T39.2X3	T39.2X4	T39.2X5	T39.2X6
methanesulfonate sodium	T39.2X1	T39.2X2	T39.2X3	T39.2X4	T39.2X5	T39.2X6
Norbormide	T60.4X1	T60.4X2	T60.4X3	T60.4X4	—	—
Nordazepam	T42.4X1	T42.4X2	T42.4X3	T42.4X4	T42.4X5	T42.4X6
Norepinephrine	T44.4X1	T44.4X2	T44.4X3	T44.4X4	T44.4X5	T44.4X6
Norethandrolone	T38.7X1	T38.7X2	T38.7X3	T38.7X4	T38.7X5	T38.7X6
Norethindrone	T38.4X1	T38.4X2	T38.4X3	T38.4X4	T38.4X5	T38.4X6
Norethisterone (acetate)	T38.4X1	T38.4X2	T38.4X3	T38.4X4	T38.4X5	T38.4X6
(enantate)						
with ethinylestradiol	T38.5X1	T38.5X2	T38.5X3	T38.5X4	T38.5X5	T38.5X6
Noretynodrel	T38.5X1	T38.5X2	T38.5X3	T38.5X4	T38.5X5	T38.5X6
Norfenefrine	T44.4X1	T44.4X2	T44.4X3	T44.4X4	T44.4X5	T44.4X6
Norfloxacin	T36.8X1	T36.8X2	T36.8X3	T36.8X4	T36.8X5	T36.8X6
Norgestrel	T38.4X1	T38.4X2	T38.4X3	T38.4X4	T38.4X5	T38.4X6
Norgestrienone	T38.4X1	T38.4X2	T38.4X3	T38.4X4	T38.4X5	T38.4X6
Norlestrin	T38.4X1	T38.4X2	T38.4X3	T38.4X4	T38.4X5	T38.4X6
Norlutin	T38.4X1	T38.4X2	T38.4X3	T38.4X4	T38.4X5	T38.4X6
Normal serum albumin (human),	T45.8X1	T45.8X2	T45.8X3	T45.8X4	T45.8X5	T45.8X6
salt-poor						
Normethandrone	T38.5X1	T38.5X2	T38.5X3	T38.5X4	T38.5X5	T38.5X6
Normison — see Benzodiazepines						
Normorphine	T40.2X1	T40.2X2	T40.2X3	T40.2X4	—	—
Norpseudoephedrine	T50.5X1	T50.5X2	T50.5X3	T50.5X4	T50.5X5	T50.5X6
Nortestosterone	T38.7X1	T38.7X2	T38.7X3	T38.7X4	T38.7X5	T38.7X6
(furanpropionate)						
Nortriptyline	T43.011	T43.012	T43.013	T43.014	T43.015	T43.016
Noscapine	T48.3X1	T48.3X2	T48.3X3	T48.3X4	T48.3X5	T48.3X6
Nose preparations	T49.6X1	T49.6X2	T49.6X3	T49.6X4	T49.6X5	T49.6X6
Novobiocin	T36.5X1	T36.5X2	T36.5X3	T36.5X4	T36.5X5	T36.5X6
Novocain (infiltration)	T41.3X1	T41.3X2	T41.3X3	T41.3X4	T41.3X5	T41.3X6
(topical)						
nerve block (peripheral)	T41.3X1	T41.3X2	T41.3X3	T41.3X4	T41.3X5	T41.3X6
(plexus)						
spinal	T41.3X1	T41.3X2	T41.3X3	T41.3X4	T41.3X5	T41.3X6
Noxious foodstuff	T62.91	T62.92	T62.93	T62.94	—	—
specified NEC	T62.8X1	T62.8X2	T62.8X3	T62.8X4	—	—
Noxiptiline	T43.011	T43.012	T43.013	T43.014	T43.015	T43.016
Noxytiolin	T49.0X1	T49.0X2	T49.0X3	T49.0X4	T49.0X5	T49.0X6
NPH Iletin (insulin)	T38.3X1	T38.3X2	T38.3X3	T38.3X4	T38.3X5	T38.3X6
Numorphan	T40.2X1	T40.2X2	T40.2X3	T40.2X4	T40.2X5	T40.2X6
Nunol	T42.3X1	T42.3X2	T42.3X3	T42.3X4	T42.3X5	T42.3X6
Nupercaine (spinal	T41.3X1	T41.3X2	T41.3X3	T41.3X4	T41.3X5	T41.3X6
anesthetic)						
topical (surface)	T41.3X1	T41.3X2	T41.3X3	T41.3X4	T41.3X5	T41.3X6
Nutmeg oil (liniment)	T49.3X1	T49.3X2	T49.3X3	T49.3X4	T49.3X5	T49.3X6
Nutritional supplement	T50.901	T50.902	T50.903	T50.904	T50.905	T50.906
Nux vomica	T65.1X1	T65.1X2	T65.1X3	T65.1X4	—	—
Nydrazid	T37.1X1	T37.1X2	T37.1X3	T37.1X4	T37.1X5	T37.1X6
Nylidrin	T46.7X1	T46.7X2	T46.7X3	T46.7X4	T46.7X5	T46.7X6
Nystatin	T36.7X1	T36.7X2	T36.7X3	T36.7X4	T36.7X5	T36.7X6
topical	T49.0X1	T49.0X2	T49.0X3	T49.0X4	T49.0X5	T49.0X6
Nytol	T45.0X1	T45.0X2	T45.0X3	T45.0X4	T45.0X5	T45.0X6
Obidoxime chloride	T50.6X1	T50.6X2	T50.6X3	T50.6X4	T50.6X5	T50.6X6
Octafonium (chloride)	T49.3X1	T49.3X2	T49.3X3	T49.3X4	T49.3X5	T49.3X6
Octamethyl pyrophosphoramide	T60.0X1	T60.0X2	T60.0X3	T60.0X4	—	—

Substance	Poisoning, Accidental (unintentional)	Poisoning, Intentional Self-harm	Poisoning, Assault	Poisoning, Undetermined	Adverse Effect	Under-dosing
Octanoin	T50.991	T50.992	T50.993	T50.994	T50.995	T50.996
Octatropine methylbromide	T44.3X1	T44.3X2	T44.3X3	T44.3X4	T44.3X5	T44.3X6
Octotiamine	T45.2X1	T45.2X2	T45.2X3	T45.2X4	T45.2X5	T45.2X6
Octoxinol (9)	T49.8X1	T49.8X2	T49.8X3	T49.8X4	T49.8X5	T49.8X6
Octreotide	T38.991	T38.992	T38.993	T38.994	T38.995	T38.996
Octyl nitrite	T46.3X1	T46.3X2	T46.3X3	T46.3X4	T46.3X5	T46.3X6
Oestradiol	T38.5X1	T38.5X2	T38.5X3	T38.5X4	T38.5X5	T38.5X6
Oestriol	T38.5X1	T38.5X2	T38.5X3	T38.5X4	T38.5X5	T38.5X6
Oestrogen	T38.5X1	T38.5X2	T38.5X3	T38.5X4	T38.5X5	T38.5X6
Oestrone	T38.5X1	T38.5X2	T38.5X3	T38.5X4	T38.5X5	T38.5X6
Ofloxacin	T36.8X1	T36.8X2	T36.8X3	T36.8X4	T36.8X5	T36.8X6
Oil (of)	T65.891	T65.892	T65.893	T65.894	—	—
bitter almond	T62.8X1	T62.8X2	T62.8X3	T62.8X4	—	—
cloves	T49.7X1	T49.7X2	T49.7X3	T49.7X4	T49.7X5	T49.7X6
colors	T65.6X1	T65.6X2	T65.6X3	T65.6X4	—	—
fumes	T59.891	T59.892	T59.893	T59.894	—	—
lubricating	T52.0X1	T52.0X2	T52.0X3	T52.0X4	—	—
Niobe	T52.8X1	T52.8X2	T52.8X3	T52.8X4	—	—
vitriol (liquid)	T54.2X1	T54.2X2	T54.2X3	T54.2X4	—	—
fumes	T54.2X1	T54.2X2	T54.2X3	T54.2X4	—	—
wintergreen (bitter) NEC	T49.3X1	T49.3X2	T49.3X3	T49.3X4	T49.3X5	T49.3X6
Oily preparation (for skin)	T49.3X1	T49.3X2	T49.3X3	T49.3X4	T49.3X5	T49.3X6
Ointment NEC	T49.3X1	T49.3X2	T49.3X3	T49.3X4	T49.3X5	T49.3X6
Olanzapine	T43.591	T43.592	T43.593	T43.594	T43.595	T43.596
Oleander	T62.2X1	T62.2X2	T62.2X3	T62.2X4	—	—
Oleandomycin	T36.3X1	T36.3X2	T36.3X3	T36.3X4	T36.3X5	T36.3X6
Oleandrin	T46.0X1	T46.0X2	T46.0X3	T46.0X4	T46.0X5	T46.0X6
Oleic acid	T46.6X1	T46.6X2	T46.6X3	T46.6X4	T46.6X5	T46.6X6
Oleovitamin A	T45.2X1	T45.2X2	T45.2X3	T45.2X4	T45.2X5	T45.2X6
Oleum ricini	T47.2X1	T47.2X2	T47.2X3	T47.2X4	T47.2X5	T47.2X6
Olive oil (medicinal) NEC	T47.4X1	T47.4X2	T47.4X3	T47.4X4	T47.4X5	T47.4X6
Olivomycin	T45.1X1	T45.1X2	T45.1X3	T45.1X4	T45.1X5	T45.1X6
Olsalazine	T47.8X1	T47.8X2	T47.8X3	T47.8X4	T47.8X5	T47.8X6
Omeprazole	T47.1X1	T47.1X2	T47.1X3	T47.1X4	T47.1X5	T47.1X6
OMPA	T60.0X1	T60.0X2	T60.0X3	T60.0X4	—	—
Oncovin	T45.1X1	T45.1X2	T45.1X3	T45.1X4	T45.1X5	T45.1X6
Ondansetron	T45.0X1	T45.0X2	T45.0X3	T45.0X4	T45.0X5	T45.0X6
Ophthaine	T41.3X1	T41.3X2	T41.3X3	T41.3X4	T41.3X5	T41.3X6
Ophthetic	T41.3X1	T41.3X2	T41.3X3	T41.3X4	T41.3X5	T41.3X6
Opiate NEC	T40.601	T40.602	T40.603	T40.604	T40.605	T40.606
antagonists	T50.7X1	T50.7X2	T50.7X3	T50.7X4	T50.7X5	T50.7X6
Opioid NEC	T40.2X1	T40.2X2	T40.2X3	T40.2X4	T40.2X5	T40.2X6
Opipramol	T43.011	T43.012	T43.013	T43.014	T43.015	T43.016
Opium alkaloids (total)	T40.0X1	T40.0X2	T40.0X3	T40.0X4	T40.0X5	T40.0X6
standardized powdered	T40.0X1	T40.0X2	T40.0X3	T40.0X4	T40.0X5	T40.0X6
tincture (camphorated)	T40.0X1	T40.0X2	T40.0X3	T40.0X4	T40.0X5	T40.0X6
Oracon	T38.4X1	T38.4X2	T38.4X3	T38.4X4	T38.4X5	T38.4X6
Oragrafin	T50.8X1	T50.8X2	T50.8X3	T50.8X4	T50.8X5	T50.8X6
Oral contraceptives	T38.4X1	T38.4X2	T38.4X3	T38.4X4	T38.4X5	T38.4X6
Oral rehydration salts	T50.3X1	T50.3X2	T50.3X3	T50.3X4	T50.3X5	T50.3X6
Orazamide	T50.991	T50.992	T50.993	T50.994	T50.995	T50.996
Orciprenaline	T48.291	T48.292	T48.293	T48.294	T48.295	T48.296
Organidin	T48.4X1	T48.4X2	T48.4X3	T48.4X4	T48.4X5	T48.4X6
Organonitrate NEC	T46.3X1	T46.3X2	T46.3X3	T46.3X4	T46.3X5	T46.3X6
Organophosphates	T60.0X1	T60.0X2	T60.0X3	T60.0X4	—	—
Orimune	T50.B91	T50.B92	T50.B93	T50.B94	T50.B95	T50.B96
Orinase	T38.3X1	T38.3X2	T38.3X3	T38.3X4	T38.3X5	T38.3X6
Ormeloxifene	T38.6X1	T38.6X2	T38.6X3	T38.6X4	T38.6X5	T38.6X6
Ornidazole	T37.3X1	T37.3X2	T37.3X3	T37.3X4	T37.3X5	T37.3X6
Ornithine aspartate	T50.991	T50.992	T50.993	T50.994	T50.995	T50.996
Ornoprostil	T47.1X1	T47.1X2	T47.1X3	T47.1X4	T47.1X5	T47.1X6
Orphenadrine	T42.8X1	T42.8X2	T42.8X3	T42.8X4	T42.8X5	T42.8X6
(hydrochloride)						
Ortal (sodium)	T42.3X1	T42.3X2	T42.3X3	T42.3X4	T42.3X5	T42.3X6
Orthoboric acid	T49.0X1	T49.0X2	T49.0X3	T49.0X4	T49.0X5	T49.0X6
ENT agent	T49.6X1	T49.6X2	T49.6X3	T49.6X4	T49.6X5	T49.6X6
ophthalmic preparation	T49.5X1	T49.5X2	T49.5X3	T49.5X4	T49.5X5	T49.5X6
Orthocaine	T41.3X1	T41.3X2	T41.3X3	T41.3X4	T41.3X5	T41.3X6
Orthodichlorobenzene	T53.7X1	T53.7X2	T53.7X3	T53.7X4	—	—
Ortho-Novum	T38.4X1	T38.4X2	T38.4X3	T38.4X4	T38.4X5	T38.4X6
Orthotolidine (reagent)	T54.2X1	T54.2X2	T54.2X3	T54.2X4	—	—
Osmic acid (liquid)	T54.2X1	T54.2X2	T54.2X3	T54.2X4	—	—
fumes	T54.2X1	T54.2X2	T54.2X3	T54.2X4	—	—
Osmotic diuretics	T50.2X1	T50.2X2	T50.2X3	T50.2X4	T50.2X5	T50.2X6
Otilonium bromide	T44.3X1	T44.3X2	T44.3X3	T44.3X4	T44.3X5	T44.3X6
Otorhinolaryngological drug NEC	T49.6X1	T49.6X2	T49.6X3	T49.6X4	T49.6X5	T49.6X6
Ouabain (e)	T46.0X1	T46.0X2	T46.0X3	T46.0X4	T46.0X5	T46.0X6
Ovarian						
hormone	T38.5X1	T38.5X2	T38.5X3	T38.5X4	T38.5X5	T38.5X6
stimulant	T38.5X1	T38.5X2	T38.5X3	T38.5X4	T38.5X5	T38.5X6
Ovral	T38.4X1	T38.4X2	T38.4X3	T38.4X4	T38.4X5	T38.4X6

Substance	Poisoning, Accidental (unintentional)	Poisoning, Intentional Self-harm	Poisoning, Assault	Poisoning, Undetermined	Adverse Effect	Under-dosing
Ovulen	T38.4X1	T38.4X2	T38.4X3	T38.4X4	T38.4X5	T38.4X6
Oxacillin	T36.0X1	T36.0X2	T36.0X3	T36.0X4	T36.0X5	T36.0X6
Oxalic acid	T54.2X1	T54.2X2	T54.2X3	T54.2X4	—	—
ammonium salt	T50.991	T50.992	T50.993	T50.994	T50.995	T50.996
Oxamniquine	T37.4X1	T37.4X2	T37.4X3	T37.4X4	T37.4X5	T37.4X6
Oxanamide	T43.591	T43.592	T43.593	T43.594	T43.595	T43.596
Oxandrolone	T38.7X1	T38.7X2	T38.7X3	T38.7X4	T38.7X5	T38.7X6
Oxantel	T37.4X1	T37.4X2	T37.4X3	T37.4X4	T37.4X5	T37.4X6
Oxapium iodide	T44.3X1	T44.3X2	T44.3X3	T44.3X4	T44.3X5	T44.3X6
Oxaprotiline	T43.021	T43.022	T43.023	T43.024	T43.025	T43.026
Oxaprozin	T39.311	T39.312	T39.313	T39.314	T39.315	T39.316
Oxatomide	T45.0X1	T45.0X2	T45.0X3	T45.0X4	T45.0X5	T45.0X6
Oxazepam	T42.4X1	T42.4X2	T42.4X3	T42.4X4	T42.4X5	T42.4X6
Oxazimedrine	T50.5X1	T50.5X2	T50.5X3	T50.5X4	T50.5X5	T50.5X6
Oxazolam	T42.4X1	T42.4X2	T42.4X3	T42.4X4	T42.4X5	T42.4X6
Oxazolidine derivatives	T42.2X1	T42.2X2	T42.2X3	T42.2X4	T42.2X5	T42.2X6
Oxazolidinedione (derivative)	T42.2X1	T42.2X2	T42.2X3	T42.2X4	T42.2X5	T42.2X6
Ox bile extract	T47.5X1	T47.5X2	T47.5X3	T47.5X4	T47.5X5	T47.5X6
Oxcarbazepine	T42.1X1	T42.1X2	T42.1X3	T42.1X4	T42.1X5	T42.1X6
Oxedrine	T44.4X1	T44.4X2	T44.4X3	T44.4X4	T44.4X5	T44.4X6
Oxeladin (citrate)	T48.3X1	T48.3X2	T48.3X3	T48.3X4	T48.3X5	T48.3X6
Oxendolone	T38.5X1	T38.5X2	T38.5X3	T38.5X4	T38.5X5	T38.5X6
Oxetacaine	T41.3X1	T41.3X2	T41.3X3	T41.3X4	T41.3X5	T41.3X6
Oxethazine	T41.3X1	T41.3X2	T41.3X3	T41.3X4	T41.3X5	T41.3X6
Oxetorone	T39.8X1	T39.8X2	T39.8X3	T39.8X4	T39.8X5	T39.8X6
Oxiconazole	T49.0X1	T49.0X2	T49.0X3	T49.0X4	T49.0X5	T49.0X6
Oxidizing agent NEC	T54.91	T54.92	T54.93	T54.94	—	—
Oxipurinol	T50.4X1	T50.4X2	T50.4X3	T50.4X4	T50.4X5	T50.4X6
Oxitriptan	T43.291	T43.292	T43.293	T43.294	T43.295	T43.296
Oxitropium bromide	T48.6X1	T48.6X2	T48.6X3	T48.6X4	T48.6X5	T48.6X6
Oxodipine	T46.1X1	T46.1X2	T46.1X3	T46.1X4	T46.1X5	T46.1X6
Oxolamine	T48.3X1	T48.3X2	T48.3X3	T48.3X4	T48.3X5	T48.3X6
Oxolinic acid	T37.8X1	T37.8X2	T37.8X3	T37.8X4	T37.8X5	T37.8X6
Oxomemazine	T43.3X1	T43.3X2	T43.3X3	T43.3X4	T43.3X5	T43.3X6
Oxophenarsine	T37.3X1	T37.3X2	T37.3X3	T37.3X4	T37.3X5	T37.3X6
Oxprenolol	T44.7X1	T44.7X2	T44.7X3	T44.7X4	T44.7X5	T44.7X6
Oxsoralen	T49.3X1	T49.3X2	T49.3X3	T49.3X4	T49.3X5	T49.3X6
Oxtriphylline	T48.6X1	T48.6X2	T48.6X3	T48.6X4	T48.6X5	T48.6X6
Oxybate sodium	T41.291	T41.292	T41.293	T41.294	T41.295	T41.296
Oxybuprocaine	T41.3X1	T41.3X2	T41.3X3	T41.3X4	T41.3X5	T41.3X6
Oxybutynin	T44.3X1	T44.3X2	T44.3X3	T44.3X4	T44.3X5	T44.3X6
Oxychlorosene	T49.0X1	T49.0X2	T49.0X3	T49.0X4	T49.0X5	T49.0X6
Oxycodone	T40.2X1	T40.2X2	T40.2X3	T40.2X4	T40.2X5	T40.2X6
Oxyfedrine	T46.3X1	T46.3X2	T46.3X3	T46.3X4	T46.3X5	T46.3X6
Oxygen	T41.5X1	T41.5X2	T41.5X3	T41.5X4	T41.5X5	T41.5X6
Oxylone	T49.0X1	T49.0X2	T49.0X3	T49.0X4	T49.0X5	T49.0X6
ophthalmic preparation	T49.5X1	T49.5X2	T49.5X3	T49.5X4	T49.5X5	T49.5X6
Oxymesterone	T38.7X1	T38.7X2	T38.7X3	T38.7X4	T38.7X5	T38.7X6
Oxymetazoline	T48.5X1	T48.5X2	T48.5X3	T48.5X4	T48.5X5	T48.5X6
Oxymetholone	T38.7X1	T38.7X2	T38.7X3	T38.7X4	T38.7X5	T38.7X6
Oxymorphone	T40.2X1	T40.2X2	T40.2X3	T40.2X4	T40.2X5	T40.2X6
Oxypertine	T43.591	T43.592	T43.593	T43.594	T43.595	T43.596
Oxyphenbutazone	T39.2X1	T39.2X2	T39.2X3	T39.2X4	T39.2X5	T39.2X6
Oxyphencyclimine	T44.3X1	T44.3X2	T44.3X3	T44.3X4	T44.3X5	T44.3X6
Oxyphenisatine	T47.2X1	T47.2X2	T47.2X3	T47.2X4	T47.2X5	T47.2X6
Oxyphenonium bromide	T44.3X1	T44.3X2	T44.3X3	T44.3X4	T44.3X5	T44.3X6
Oxypolygelatin	T45.8X1	T45.8X2	T45.8X3	T45.8X4	T45.8X5	T45.8X6
Oxyquinoline (derivatives)	T37.8X1	T37.8X2	T37.8X3	T37.8X4	T37.8X5	T37.8X6
Oxytetracycline	T36.4X1	T36.4X2	T36.4X3	T36.4X4	T36.4X5	T36.4X6
Oxytocic drug NEC	T48.0X1	T48.0X2	T48.0X3	T48.0X4	T48.0X5	T48.0X6
Oxytocin (synthetic)	T48.0X1	T48.0X2	T48.0X3	T48.0X4	T48.0X5	T48.0X6
Ozone	T59.891	T59.892	T59.893	T59.894	—	—
PABA	T49.3X1	T49.3X2	T49.3X3	T49.3X4	T49.3X5	T49.3X6
Packed red cells	T45.8X1	T45.8X2	T45.8X3	T45.8X4	T45.8X5	T45.8X6
Padimate	T49.3X1	T49.3X2	T49.3X3	T49.3X4	T49.3X5	T49.3X6
Paint NEC	T65.6X1	T65.6X2	T65.6X3	T65.6X4	—	—
cleaner	T52.91	T52.92	T52.93	T52.94	—	—
fumes NEC	T59.891	T59.892	T59.893	T59.894	—	—
lead (fumes)	T56.0X1	T56.0X2	T56.0X3	T56.0X4	—	—
solvent NEC	T52.8X1	T52.8X2	T52.8X3	T52.8X4	—	—
stripper	T52.8X1	T52.8X2	T52.8X3	T52.8X4	—	—
Palfium	T40.2X1	T40.2X2	T40.2X3	T40.2X4	—	—
Palm kernel oil	T50.991	T50.992	T50.993	T50.994	T50.995	T50.996
Paludrine	T37.2X1	T37.2X2	T37.2X3	T37.2X4	T37.2X5	T37.2X6
PAM (pralidoxime)	T50.6X1	T50.6X2	T50.6X3	T50.6X4	T50.6X5	T50.6X6
Pamaquine (naphthoute)	T37.2X1	T37.2X2	T37.2X3	T37.2X4	T37.2X5	T37.2X6
Panadol	T39.1X1	T39.1X2	T39.1X3	T39.1X4	T39.1X5	T39.1X6
Pancreatic						
digestive secretion stimulant	T47.8X1	T47.8X2	T47.8X3	T47.8X4	T47.8X5	T47.8X6
dornase	T45.3X1	T45.3X2	T45.3X3	T45.3X4	T45.3X5	T45.3X6
Pancreatin	T47.5X1	T47.5X2	T47.5X3	T47.5X4	T47.5X5	T47.5X6

Substance	Poisoning, Accidental (unintentional)	Poisoning, Intentional Self-harm	Poisoning, Assault	Poisoning, Undetermined	Adverse Effect	Under-dosing
Pancrelipase	T47.5X1	T47.5X2	T47.5X3	T47.5X4	T47.5X5	T47.5X6
Pancuronium (bromide)	T48.1X1	T48.1X2	T48.1X3	T48.1X4	T48.1X5	T48.1X6
Pangamic acid	T45.2X1	T45.2X2	T45.2X3	T45.2X4	T45.2X5	T45.2X6
Panthenol	T45.2X1	T45.2X2	T45.2X3	T45.2X4	T45.2X5	T45.2X6
topical	T49.8X1	T49.8X2	T49.8X3	T49.8X4	T49.8X5	T49.8X6
Pantopon	T40.0X1	T40.0X2	T40.0X3	T40.0X4	T40.0X5	T40.0X6
Pantothenic acid	T45.2X1	T45.2X2	T45.2X3	T45.2X4	T45.2X5	T45.2X6
Panwarfin	T45.511	T45.512	T45.513	T45.514	T45.515	T45.516
Papain	T47.5X1	T47.5X2	T47.5X3	T47.5X4	T47.5X5	T47.5X6
digestant	T47.5X1	T47.5X2	T47.5X3	T47.5X4	T47.5X5	T47.5X6
Papaveretum	T40.0X1	T40.0X2	T40.0X3	T40.0X4	T40.0X5	T40.0X6
Papaverine	T44.3X1	T44.3X2	T44.3X3	T44.3X4	T44.3X5	T44.3X6
Para-acetamidophenol	T39.1X1	T39.1X2	T39.1X3	T39.1X4	T39.1X5	T39.1X6
Para-aminobenzoic acid	T49.3X1	T49.3X2	T49.3X3	T49.3X4	T49.3X5	T49.3X6
Para-aminophenol derivatives	T39.1X1	T39.1X2	T39.1X3	T39.1X4	T39.1X5	T39.1X6
Para-aminosalicylic acid	T37.1X1	T37.1X2	T37.1X3	T37.1X4	T37.1X5	T37.1X6
Paracetaldehyde	T42.6X1	T42.6X2	T42.6X3	T42.6X4	T42.6X5	T42.6X6
Paracetamol	T39.1X1	T39.1X2	T39.1X3	T39.1X4	T39.1X5	T39.1X6
Parachlorophenol (camphorated)	T49.0X1	T49.0X2	T49.0X3	T49.0X4	T49.0X5	T49.0X6
Paracodin	T40.2X1	T40.2X2	T40.2X3	T40.2X4	T40.2X5	T40.2X6
Paradione	T42.2X1	T42.2X2	T42.2X3	T42.2X4	T42.2X5	T42.2X6
Paraffin(s) (wax)	T52.0X1	T52.0X2	T52.0X3	T52.0X4	—	—
liquid (medicinal)	T47.4X1	T47.4X2	T47.4X3	T47.4X4	T47.4X5	T47.4X6
nonmedicinal	T52.0X1	T52.0X2	T52.0X3	T52.0X4	—	—
Paraformaldehyde	T60.3X1	T60.3X2	T60.3X3	T60.3X4	—	—
Paraldehyde	T42.6X1	T42.6X2	T42.6X3	T42.6X4	T42.6X5	T42.6X6
Paramethadione	T42.2X1	T42.2X2	T42.2X3	T42.2X4	T42.2X5	T42.2X6
Paramethasone	T38.0X1	T38.0X2	T38.0X3	T38.0X4	T38.0X5	T38.0X6
acetate	T49.0X1	T49.0X2	T49.0X3	T49.0X4	T49.0X5	T49.0X6
Paraoxon	T60.0X1	T60.0X2	T60.0X3	T60.0X4	—	—
Paraquat	T60.3X1	T60.3X2	T60.3X3	T60.3X4	—	—
Parasympatholytic NEC	T44.3X1	T44.3X2	T44.3X3	T44.3X4	T44.3X5	T44.3X6
Parasympathomimetic drug NEC	T44.1X1	T44.1X2	T44.1X3	T44.1X4	T44.1X5	T44.1X6
Parathion	T60.0X1	T60.0X2	T60.0X3	T60.0X4	—	—
Parathormone	T50.991	T50.992	T50.993	T50.994	T50.995	T50.996
Parathyroid extract	T50.991	T50.992	T50.993	T50.994	T50.995	T50.996
Paratyphoid vaccine	T50.A91	T50.A92	T50.A93	T50.A94	T50.A95	T50.A96
Paredrine	T44.4X1	T44.4X2	T44.4X3	T44.4X4	T44.4X5	T44.4X6
Paregoric	T40.0X1	T40.0X2	T40.0X3	T40.0X4	T40.0X5	T40.0X6
Pargyline	T46.5X1	T46.5X2	T46.5X3	T46.5X4	T46.5X5	T46.5X6
Paris green	T57.0X1	T57.0X2	T57.0X3	T57.0X4	—	—
insecticide	T57.0X1	T57.0X2	T57.0X3	T57.0X4	—	—
Parnate	T43.1X1	T43.1X2	T43.1X3	T43.1X4	T43.1X5	T43.1X6
Paromomycin	T36.5X1	T36.5X2	T36.5X3	T36.5X4	T36.5X5	T36.5X6
Paroxypropione	T45.1X1	T45.1X2	T45.1X3	T45.1X4	T45.1X5	T45.1X6
Parzone	T40.2X1	T40.2X2	T40.2X3	T40.2X4	T40.2X5	T40.2X6
PAS	T37.1X1	T37.1X2	T37.1X3	T37.1X4	T37.1X5	T37.1X6
Pasiniazid	T37.1X1	T37.1X2	T37.1X3	T37.1X4	T37.1X5	T37.1X6
PBB (polybrominated biphenyls)	T65.891	T65.892	T65.893	T65.894	—	—
PCB	T65.891	T65.892	T65.893	T65.894	—	—
PCP						
meaning pentachlorophenol	T60.1X1	T60.1X2	T60.1X3	T60.1X4	—	—
fungicide	T60.3X1	T60.3X2	T60.3X3	T60.3X4	—	—
herbicide	T60.3X1	T60.3X2	T60.3X3	T60.3X4	—	—
insecticide	T60.1X1	T60.1X2	T60.1X3	T60.1X4	—	—
meaning phencyclidine	T40.991	T40.992	T40.993	T40.994	—	—
Peach kernel oil (emulsion)	T47.4X1	T47.4X2	T47.4X3	T47.4X4	T47.4X5	T47.4X6
Peanut oil (emulsion) NEC	T47.4X1	T47.4X2	T47.4X3	T47.4X4	T47.4X5	T47.4X6
topical	T49.3X1	T49.3X2	T49.3X3	T49.3X4	T49.3X5	T49.3X6
Pearly Gates (morning glory seeds)	T40.991	T40.992	T40.993	T40.994	—	—
Pecazine	T43.3X1	T43.3X2	T43.3X3	T43.3X4	T43.3X5	T43.3X6
Pectin	T47.6X1	T47.6X2	T47.6X3	T47.6X4	T47.6X5	T47.6X6
Pefloxacin	T37.8X1	T37.8X2	T37.8X3	T37.8X4	T37.8X5	T37.8X6
Pegademase, bovine	T50.Z91	T50.Z92	T50.Z93	T50.Z94	T50.Z95	T50.Z96
Pelletierine tannate	T37.4X1	T37.4X2	T37.4X3	T37.4X4	T37.4X5	T37.4X6
Pemirolast (potassium)	T48.6X1	T48.6X2	T48.6X3	T48.6X4	T48.6X5	T48.6X6
Pemoline	T50.7X1	T50.7X2	T50.7X3	T50.7X4	T50.7X5	T50.7X6
Pempidine	T44.2X1	T44.2X2	T44.2X3	T44.2X4	T44.2X5	T44.2X6
Penamecillin	T36.0X1	T36.0X2	T36.0X3	T36.0X4	T36.0X5	T36.0X6
Penbutolol	T44.7X1	T44.7X2	T44.7X3	T44.7X4	T44.7X5	T44.7X6
Penethamate	T36.0X1	T36.0X2	T36.0X3	T36.0X4	T36.0X5	T36.0X6
Penfluridol	T43.591	T43.592	T43.593	T43.594	T43.595	T43.596
Penflutizide	T50.2X1	T50.2X2	T50.2X3	T50.2X4	T50.2X5	T50.2X6
Pengitoxin	T46.0X1	T46.0X2	T46.0X3	T46.0X4	T46.0X5	T46.0X6
Penicillamine	T50.6X1	T50.6X2	T50.6X3	T50.6X4	T50.6X5	T50.6X6
Penicillin (any)	T36.0X1	T36.0X2	T36.0X3	T36.0X4	T36.0X5	T36.0X6
Penicillinase	T45.3X1	T45.3X2	T45.3X3	T45.3X4	T45.3X5	T45.3X6

Substance	Poisoning, Accidental (unintentional)	Poisoning, Intentional Self-harm	Poisoning, Assault	Poisoning, Undetermined	Adverse Effect	Under-dosing
Penicilloyl polylysine	T50.8X1	T50.8X2	T50.8X3	T50.8X4	T50.8X5	T50.8X6
Penimepicycline	T36.4X1	T36.4X2	T36.4X3	T36.4X4	T36.4X5	T36.4X6
Pentachloroethane	T53.6X1	T53.6X2	T53.6X3	T53.6X4	—	—
Pentachloronaphthalene	T53.7X1	T53.7X2	T53.7X3	T53.7X4	—	—
Pentachlorophenol	T60.1X1	T60.1X2	T60.1X3	T60.1X4	—	—
(pesticide)						
fungicide	T60.3X1	T60.3X2	T60.3X3	T60.3X4	—	—
herbicide	T60.3X1	T60.3X2	T60.3X3	T60.3X4	—	—
insecticide	T60.1X1	T60.1X2	T60.1X3	T60.1X4	—	—
Pentaerythritol	T46.3X1	T46.3X2	T46.3X3	T46.3X4	T46.3X5	T46.3X6
chloral	T42.6X1	T42.6X2	T42.6X3	T42.6X4	T42.6X5	T42.6X6
tetranitrate NEC	T46.3X1	T46.3X2	T46.3X3	T46.3X4	T46.3X5	T46.3X6
Pentaerythrityl tetranitrate	T46.3X1	T46.3X2	T46.3X3	T46.3X4	T46.3X5	T46.3X6
Pentagastrin	T50.8X1	T50.8X2	T50.8X3	T50.8X4	T50.8X5	T50.8X6
Pentalin	T53.6X1	T53.6X2	T53.6X3	T53.6X4	—	—
Pentamethonium bromide	T44.2X1	T44.2X2	T44.2X3	T44.2X4	T44.2X5	T44.2X6
Pentamidine	T37.3X1	T37.3X2	T37.3X3	T37.3X4	T37.3X5	T37.3X6
Pentanol	T51.3X1	T51.3X2	T51.3X3	T51.3X4	—	—
Pentapyrrolinium (bitartrate)	T44.2X1	T44.2X2	T44.2X3	T44.2X4	T44.2X5	T44.2X6
Pentaquine	T37.2X1	T37.2X2	T37.2X3	T37.2X4	T37.2X5	T37.2X6
Pentazocine	T40.4X1	T40.4X2	T40.4X3	T40.4X4	T40.4X5	T40.4X6
Pentetrazole	T50.7X1	T50.7X2	T50.7X3	T50.7X4	T50.7X5	T50.7X6
Penthienate bromide	T44.3X1	T44.3X2	T44.3X3	T44.3X4	T44.3X5	T44.3X6
Pentifylline	T46.7X1	T46.7X2	T46.7X3	T46.7X4	T46.7X5	T46.7X6
Pentobarbital	T42.3X1	T42.3X2	T42.3X3	T42.3X4	T42.3X5	T42.3X6
sodium	T42.3X1	T42.3X2	T42.3X3	T42.3X4	T42.3X5	T42.3X6
Pentobarbitone	T42.3X1	T42.3X2	T42.3X3	T42.3X4	T42.3X5	T42.3X6
Pentolonium tartrate	T44.2X1	T44.2X2	T44.2X3	T44.2X4	T44.2X5	T44.2X6
Pentosan polysulfate (sodium)	T39.8X1	T39.8X2	T39.8X3	T39.8X4	T39.8X5	T39.8X6
Pentostatin	T45.1X1	T45.1X2	T45.1X3	T45.1X4	T45.1X5	T45.1X6
Pentothal	T41.1X1	T41.1X2	T41.1X3	T41.1X4	T41.1X5	T41.1X6
Pentoxifylline	T46.7X1	T46.7X2	T46.7X3	T46.7X4	T46.7X5	T46.7X6
Pentoxyverine	T48.3X1	T48.3X2	T48.3X3	T48.3X4	T48.3X5	T48.3X6
Pentrinat	T46.3X1	T46.3X2	T46.3X3	T46.3X4	T46.3X5	T46.3X6
Pentylenetetrazole	T50.7X1	T50.7X2	T50.7X3	T50.7X4	T50.7X5	T50.7X6
Pentylsalicylamide	T37.1X1	T37.1X2	T37.1X3	T37.1X4	T37.1X5	T37.1X6
Pentymal	T42.3X1	T42.3X2	T42.3X3	T42.3X4	T42.3X5	T42.3X6
Peplomycin	T45.1X1	T45.1X2	T45.1X3	T45.1X4	T45.1X5	T45.1X6
Peppermint (oil)	T47.5X1	T47.5X2	T47.5X3	T47.5X4	T47.5X5	T47.5X6
Pepsin	T47.5X1	T47.5X2	T47.5X3	T47.5X4	T47.5X5	T47.5X6
digestant	T47.5X1	T47.5X2	T47.5X3	T47.5X4	T47.5X5	T47.5X6
Pepstatin	T47.1X1	T47.1X2	T47.1X3	T47.1X4	T47.1X5	T47.1X6
Peptavlon	T50.8X1	T50.8X2	T50.8X3	T50.8X4	T50.8X5	T50.8X6
Perazine	T43.3X1	T43.3X2	T43.3X3	T43.3X4	T43.3X5	T43.3X6
Percaine (spinal)	T41.3X1	T41.3X2	T41.3X3	T41.3X4	T41.3X5	T41.3X6
topical (surface)	T41.3X1	T41.3X2	T41.3X3	T41.3X4	T41.3X5	T41.3X6
Perchloroethylene	T53.3X1	T53.3X2	T53.3X3	T53.3X4	—	—
medicinal	T37.4X1	T37.4X2	T37.4X3	T37.4X4	T37.4X5	T37.4X6
vapor	T53.3X1	T53.3X2	T53.3X3	T53.3X4	—	—
Percodan	T40.2X1	T40.2X2	T40.2X3	T40.2X4	T40.2X5	T40.2X6
Percogesic — see also acetaminophen	T45.0X1	T45.0X2	T45.0X3	T45.0X4	T45.0X5	T45.0X6
Percorten	T38.0X1	T38.0X2	T38.0X3	T38.0X4	T38.0X5	T38.0X6
Pergolide	T42.8X1	T42.8X2	T42.8X3	T42.8X4	T42.8X5	T42.8X6
Pergonal	T38.811	T38.812	T38.813	T38.814	T38.815	T38.816
Perhexilene	T46.3X1	T46.3X2	T46.3X3	T46.3X4	T46.3X5	T46.3X6
Perhexiline (maleate)	T46.3X1	T46.3X2	T46.3X3	T46.3X4	T46.3X5	T46.3X6
Periactin	T45.0X1	T45.0X2	T45.0X3	T45.0X4	T45.0X5	T45.0X6
Periciazine	T43.3X1	T43.3X2	T43.3X3	T43.3X4	T43.3X5	T43.3X6
Periclor	T42.6X1	T42.6X2	T42.6X3	T42.6X4	T42.6X5	T42.6X6
Perindopril	T46.4X1	T46.4X2	T46.4X3	T46.4X4	T46.4X5	T46.4X6
Perisoxal	T39.8X1	T39.8X2	T39.8X3	T39.8X4	T39.8X5	T39.8X6
Peritoneal dialysis solution	T50.3X1	T50.3X2	T50.3X3	T50.3X4	T50.3X5	T50.3X6
Peritrate	T46.3X1	T46.3X2	T46.3X3	T46.3X4	T46.3X5	T46.3X6
Perlapine	T42.4X1	T42.4X2	T42.4X3	T42.4X4	T42.4X5	T42.4X6
Permanganate	T65.891	T65.892	T65.893	T65.894	—	—
Permethrin	T60.1X1	T60.1X2	T60.1X3	T60.1X4	—	—
Pernocton	T42.3X1	T42.3X2	T42.3X3	T42.3X4	T42.3X5	T42.3X6
Pernoston	T42.3X1	T42.3X2	T42.3X3	T42.3X4	T42.3X5	T42.3X6
Peronine	T40.2X1	T40.2X2	T40.2X3	T40.2X4	—	—
Perphenazine	T43.3X1	T43.3X2	T43.3X3	T43.3X4	T43.3X5	T43.3X6
Pertofrane	T43.011	T43.012	T43.013	T43.014	T43.015	T43.016
Pertussis						
immune serum (human)	T50.Z11	T50.Z12	T50.Z13	T50.Z14	T50.Z15	T50.Z16
vaccine (with diphtheria toxoid)	T50.A11	T50.A12	T50.A13	T50.A14	T50.A15	T50.A16
(with tetanus toxoid)						
Peruvian balsam	T49.0X1	T49.0X2	T49.0X3	T49.0X4	T49.0X5	T49.0X6
Peruvoside	T46.0X1	T46.0X2	T46.0X3	T46.0X4	T46.0X5	T46.0X6
Pesticide (dust) (fumes) (vapor)	T60.91	T60.92	T60.93	T60.94	—	—
NEC						

Substance	Poisoning, Accidental (unintentional)	Poisoning, Intentional Self-harm	Poisoning, Assault	Poisoning, Undetermined	Adverse Effect	Under-dosing
Pesticide (dust) (fumes) (vapor) NEC — continued						
arsenic	T57.0X1	T57.0X2	T57.0X3	T57.0X4	—	—
chlorinated	T60.1X1	T60.1X2	T60.1X3	T60.1X4	—	—
cyanide	T65.0X1	T65.0X2	T65.0X3	T65.0X4	—	—
kerosene	T52.0X1	T52.0X2	T52.0X3	T52.0X4	—	—
mixture (of compounds)	T60.91	T60.92	T60.93	T60.94	—	—
naphthalene	T60.2X1	T60.2X2	T60.2X3	T60.2X4	—	—
organochlorine (compounds)	T60.1X1	T60.1X2	T60.1X3	T60.1X4	—	—
petroleum (distillate) (products) NEC	T60.8X1	T60.8X2	T60.8X3	T60.8X4	—	—
specified ingredient NEC	T60.8X1	T60.8X2	T60.8X3	T60.8X4	—	—
strychnine	T65.1X1	T65.1X2	T65.1X3	T65.1X4	—	—
thallium	T60.4X1	T60.4X2	T60.4X3	T60.4X4	—	—
Pethidine	T40.4X1	T40.4X2	T40.4X3	T40.4X4	T40.4X5	T40.4X6
Petrichloral	T42.6X1	T42.6X2	T42.6X3	T42.6X4	T42.6X5	T42.6X6
Petrol	T52.0X1	T52.0X2	T52.0X3	T52.0X4	—	—
vapor	T52.0X1	T52.0X2	T52.0X3	T52.0X4	—	—
Petrolatum	T49.3X1	T49.3X2	T49.3X3	T49.3X4	T49.3X5	T49.3X6
hydrophilic	T49.3X1	T49.3X2	T49.3X3	T49.3X4	T49.3X5	T49.3X6
liquid	T47.4X1	T47.4X2	T47.4X3	T47.4X4	T47.4X5	T47.4X6
topical	T49.3X1	T49.3X2	T49.3X3	T49.3X4	T49.3X5	T49.3X6
nonmedicinal	T52.0X1	T52.0X2	T52.0X3	T52.0X4	—	—
red veterinary	T49.3X1	T49.3X2	T49.3X3	T49.3X4	T49.3X5	T49.3X6
white	T49.3X1	T49.3X2	T49.3X3	T49.3X4	T49.3X5	T49.3X6
Petroleum (products) NEC	T52.0X1	T52.0X2	T52.0X3	T52.0X4	—	—
benzine(s) — see Ligroin						
ether — see Ligroin						
jelly — see Petrolatum						
naphtha — see Ligroin						
pesticide	T60.8X1	T60.8X2	T60.8X3	T60.8X4	—	—
solids	T52.0X1	T52.0X2	T52.0X3	T52.0X4	—	—
solvents	T52.0X1	T52.0X2	T52.0X3	T52.0X4	—	—
vapor	T52.0X1	T52.0X2	T52.0X3	T52.0X4	—	—
Peyote	T40.991	T40.992	T40.993	T40.994	—	—
Phanodorm, phanodorn	T42.3X1	T42.3X2	T42.3X3	T42.3X4	T42.3X5	T42.3X6
Phanquinone	T37.3X1	T37.3X2	T37.3X3	T37.3X4	T37.3X5	T37.3X6
Phanquone	T37.3X1	T37.3X2	T37.3X3	T37.3X4	T37.3X5	T37.3X6
Pharmaceutical						
adjunct NEC	T50.901	T50.902	T50.903	T50.904	T50.905	T50.906
excipient NEC	T50.901	T50.902	T50.903	T50.904	T50.905	T50.906
sweetener	T50.901	T50.902	T50.903	T50.904	T50.905	T50.906
viscous agent	T50.901	T50.902	T50.903	T50.904	T50.905	T50.906
Phemitone	T42.3X1	T42.3X2	T42.3X3	T42.3X4	T42.3X5	T42.3X6
Phenacaine	T41.3X1	T41.3X2	T41.3X3	T41.3X4	T41.3X5	T41.3X6
Phenacemide	T42.6X1	T42.6X2	T42.6X3	T42.6X4	T42.6X5	T42.6X6
Phenacetin	T39.1X1	T39.1X2	T39.1X3	T39.1X4	T39.1X5	T39.1X6
Phenadoxone	T40.2X1	T40.2X2	T40.2X3	T40.2X4	—	—
Phenaglycodol	T43.591	T43.592	T43.593	T43.594	T43.595	T43.596
Phenantoin	T42.0X1	T42.0X2	T42.0X3	T42.0X4	T42.0X5	T42.0X6
Phenaphthazine reagent	T50.991	T50.992	T50.993	T50.994	T50.995	T50.996
Phenazocine	T40.4X1	T40.4X2	T40.4X3	T40.4X4	T40.4X5	T40.4X6
Phenazone	T39.2X1	T39.2X2	T39.2X3	T39.2X4	T39.2X5	T39.2X6
Phenazopyridine	T39.8X1	T39.8X2	T39.8X3	T39.8X4	T39.8X5	T39.8X6
Phenbenicillin	T36.0X1	T36.0X2	T36.0X3	T36.0X4	T36.0X5	T36.0X6
Phenbutrazate	T50.5X1	T50.5X2	T50.5X3	T50.5X4	T50.5X5	T50.5X6
Phencyclidine	T40.991	T40.992	T40.993	T40.994	T40.995	T40.996
Phendimetrazine	T50.5X1	T50.5X2	T50.5X3	T50.5X4	T50.5X5	T50.5X6
Phenelzine	T43.1X1	T43.1X2	T43.1X3	T43.1X4	T43.1X5	T43.1X6
Phenemal	T42.3X1	T42.3X2	T42.3X3	T42.3X4	T42.3X5	T42.3X6
Phenergan	T42.6X1	T42.6X2	T42.6X3	T42.6X4	T42.6X5	T42.6X6
Pheneticillin	T36.0X1	T36.0X2	T36.0X3	T36.0X4	T36.0X5	T36.0X6
Pheneturide	T42.6X1	T42.6X2	T42.6X3	T42.6X4	T42.6X5	T42.6X6
Phenformin	T38.3X1	T38.3X2	T38.3X3	T38.3X4	T38.3X5	T38.3X6
Phenglutarimide	T44.3X1	T44.3X2	T44.3X3	T44.3X4	T44.3X5	T44.3X6
Phenicarbazide	T39.8X1	T39.8X2	T39.8X3	T39.8X4	T39.8X5	T39.8X6
Phenindamine	T45.0X1	T45.0X2	T45.0X3	T45.0X4	T45.0X5	T45.0X6
Phenindione	T45.511	T45.512	T45.513	T45.514	T45.515	T45.516
Pheniprazine	T43.1X1	T43.1X2	T43.1X3	T43.1X4	T43.1X5	T43.1X6
Pheniramine	T45.0X1	T45.0X2	T45.0X3	T45.0X4	T45.0X5	T45.0X6
Phenisatin	T47.2X1	T47.2X2	T47.2X3	T47.2X4	T47.2X5	T47.2X6
Phenmetrazine	T50.5X1	T50.5X2	T50.5X3	T50.5X4	T50.5X5	T50.5X6
Phenobal	T42.3X1	T42.3X2	T42.3X3	T42.3X4	T42.3X5	T42.3X6
Phenobarbital	T42.3X1	T42.3X2	T42.3X3	T42.3X4	T42.3X5	T42.3X6
with						
mephenytoin	T42.3X1	T42.3X2	T42.3X3	T42.3X4	T42.3X5	T42.3X6
phenytoin	T42.3X1	T42.3X2	T42.3X3	T42.3X4	T42.3X5	T42.3X6
sodium	T42.3X1	T42.3X2	T42.3X3	T42.3X4	T42.3X5	T42.3X6
Phenobarbitone	T42.3X1	T42.3X2	T42.3X3	T42.3X4	T42.3X5	T42.3X6
Phenobutiodil	T50.8X1	T50.8X2	T50.8X3	T50.8X4	T50.8X5	T50.8X6
Phenoctide	T49.0X1	T49.0X2	T49.0X3	T49.0X4	T49.0X5	T49.0X6
Phenol	T49.0X1	T49.0X2	T49.0X3	T49.0X4	T49.0X5	T49.0X6

Table of Drugs and Chemicals — Phenol — Plant

Substance	Poisoning, Accidental (unintentional)	Poisoning, Intentional Self-harm	Poisoning, Assault	Poisoning, Undetermined	Adverse Effect	Under-dosing
Phenol — continued						
disinfectant	T54.0X1	T54.0X2	T54.0X3	T54.0X4	—	—
in oil injection	T46.8X1	T46.8X2	T46.8X3	T46.8X4	T46.8X5	T46.8X6
medicinal	T49.1X1	T49.1X2	T49.1X3	T49.1X4	T49.1X5	T49.1X6
nonmedicinal NEC	T54.0X1	T54.0X2	T54.0X3	T54.0X4	—	—
pesticide	T60.8X1	T60.8X2	T60.8X3	T60.8X4	—	—
red	T50.8X1	T50.8X2	T50.8X3	T50.8X4	T50.8X5	T50.8X6
Phenolic preparation	T49.1X1	T49.1X2	T49.1X3	T49.1X4	T49.1X5	T49.1X6
Phenolphthalein	T47.2X1	T47.2X2	T47.2X3	T47.2X4	T47.2X5	T47.2X6
Phenolsulfonphthalein	T50.8X1	T50.8X2	T50.8X3	T50.8X4	T50.8X5	T50.8X6
Phenomorphan	T40.2X1	T40.2X2	T40.2X3	T40.2X4		
Phenonyl	T42.3X1	T42.3X2	T42.3X3	T42.3X4	T42.3X5	T42.3X6
Phenoperidine	T40.4X1	T40.4X2	T40.4X3	T40.4X4		
Phenopyrazone	T46.991	T46.992	T46.993	T46.994	T46.995	T46.996
Phenoquin	T50.4X1	T50.4X2	T50.4X3	T50.4X4	T50.4X5	T50.4X6
Phenothiazine (psychotropic) NEC	T43.3X1	T43.3X2	T43.3X3	T43.3X4	T43.3X5	T43.3X6
insecticide	T60.2X1	T60.2X2	T60.2X3	T60.2X4		
Phenothrin	T49.0X1	T49.0X2	T49.0X3	T49.0X4	T49.0X5	T49.0X6
Phenoxybenzamine	T46.7X1	T46.7X2	T46.7X3	T46.7X4	T46.7X5	T46.7X6
Phenoxyethanol	T49.0X1	T49.0X2	T49.0X3	T49.0X4	T49.0X5	T49.0X6
Phenoxymethyl penicillin	T36.0X1	T36.0X2	T36.0X3	T36.0X4	T36.0X5	T36.0X6
Phenprobamate	T42.8X1	T42.8X2	T42.8X3	T42.8X4	T42.8X5	T42.8X6
Phenprocoumon	T45.511	T45.512	T45.513	T45.514	T45.515	T45.516
Phensuximide	T42.2X1	T42.2X2	T42.2X3	T42.2X4	T42.2X5	T42.2X6
Phentermine	T50.5X1	T50.5X2	T50.5X3	T50.5X4	T50.5X5	T50.5X6
Phenthicillin	T36.0X1	T36.0X2	T36.0X3	T36.0X4	T36.0X5	T36.0X6
Phentolamine	T46.7X1	T46.7X2	T46.7X3	T46.7X4	T46.7X5	T46.7X6
Phenyl						
butazone	T39.2X1	T39.2X2	T39.2X3	T39.2X4	T39.2X5	T39.2X6
enediamine	T65.3X1	T65.3X2	T65.3X3	T65.3X4	—	—
hydrazine	T65.3X1	T65.3X2	T65.3X3	T65.3X4	—	—
antineoplastic	T45.1X1	T45.1X2	T45.1X3	T45.1X4	T45.1X5	T45.1X6
mercuric compounds — see Mercury						
salicylate	T49.3X1	T49.3X2	T49.3X3	T49.3X4	T49.3X5	T49.3X6
Phenylalanine mustard	T45.1X1	T45.1X2	T45.1X3	T45.1X4	T45.1X5	T45.1X6
Phenylbutazone	T39.2X1	T39.2X2	T39.2X3	T39.2X4	T39.2X5	T39.2X6
Phenylenediamine	T65.3X1	T65.3X2	T65.3X3	T65.3X4	—	—
Phenylephrine	T44.4X1	T44.4X2	T44.4X3	T44.4X4	T44.4X5	T44.4X6
Phenylethylbiguanide	T38.3X1	T38.3X2	T38.3X3	T38.3X4	T38.3X5	T38.3X6
Phenylmercuric						
acetate	T49.0X1	T49.0X2	T49.0X3	T49.0X4	T49.0X5	T49.0X6
borate	T49.0X1	T49.0X2	T49.0X3	T49.0X4	T49.0X5	T49.0X6
nitrate	T49.0X1	T49.0X2	T49.0X3	T49.0X4	T49.0X5	T49.0X6
Phenylmethylbarbitone	T42.3X1	T42.3X2	T42.3X3	T42.3X4	T42.3X5	T42.3X6
Phenylpropanol	T47.5X1	T47.5X2	T47.5X3	T47.5X4	T47.5X5	T47.5X6
Phenylpropanolamine	T44.991	T44.992	T44.993	T44.994	T44.995	T44.996
Phenylsulfthion	T60.0X1	T60.0X2	T60.0X3	T60.0X4	—	—
Phenyltoloxamine	T45.0X1	T45.0X2	T45.0X3	T45.0X4	T45.0X5	T45.0X6
Phenyramidol, phenyramidon	T39.8X1	T39.8X2	T39.8X3	T39.8X4	T39.8X5	T39.8X6
Phenytoin	T42.0X1	T42.0X2	T42.0X3	T42.0X4	T42.0X5	T42.0X6
with Phenobarbital	T42.3X1	T42.3X2	T42.3X3	T42.3X4	T42.3X5	T42.3X6
pHisoHex	T49.2X1	T49.2X2	T49.2X3	T49.2X4	T49.2X5	T49.2X6
Pholcodine	T48.3X1	T48.3X2	T48.3X3	T48.3X4	T48.3X5	T48.3X6
Pholedrine	T46.991	T46.992	T46.993	T46.994	T46.995	T46.996
Phorate	T60.0X1	T60.0X2	T60.0X3	T60.0X4	—	—
Phosdrin	T60.0X1	T60.0X2	T60.0X3	T60.0X4	—	—
Phosfolan	T60.0X1	T60.0X2	T60.0X3	T60.0X4	—	—
Phosgene (gas)	T59.891	T59.892	T59.893	T59.894	—	—
Phosphamidon	T60.0X1	T60.0X2	T60.0X3	T60.0X4	—	—
Phosphate	T65.891	T65.892	T65.893	T65.894	—	—
laxative	T47.4X1	T47.4X2	T47.4X3	T47.4X4	T47.4X5	T47.4X6
organic	T60.0X1	T60.0X2	T60.0X3	T60.0X4	—	—
solvent	T52.91	T52.92	T52.93	T52.94	—	—
tricresyl	T65.891	T65.892	T65.893	T65.894	—	—
Phosphine	T57.1X1	T57.1X2	T57.1X3	T57.1X4	—	—
fumigant	T57.1X1	T57.1X2	T57.1X3	T57.1X4	—	—
Phospholine	T49.5X1	T49.5X2	T49.5X3	T49.5X4	T49.5X5	T49.5X6
Phosphoric acid	T54.2X1	T54.2X2	T54.2X3	T54.2X4	—	—
Phosphorus (compound)	T57.1X1	T57.1X2	T57.1X3	T57.1X4	—	—
NEC						
pesticide	T60.0X1	T60.0X2	T60.0X3	T60.0X4	—	—
Phthalates	T65.891	T65.892	T65.893	T65.894	—	—
Phthalic anhydride	T65.891	T65.892	T65.893	T65.894	—	—
Phthalimidoglutarimide	T42.6X1	T42.6X2	T42.6X3	T42.6X4	T42.6X5	T42.6X6
Phthalylsulfathiazole	T37.0X1	T37.0X2	T37.0X3	T37.0X4	T37.0X5	T37.0X6
Phylloquinone	T45.7X1	T45.7X2	T45.7X3	T45.7X4	T45.7X5	T45.7X6
Physeptone	T40.3X1	T40.3X2	T40.3X3	T40.3X4	T40.3X5	T40.3X6
Physostigma venenosum	T62.2X1	T62.2X2	T62.2X3	T62.2X4	—	—
Physostigmine	T49.5X1	T49.5X2	T49.5X3	T49.5X4	T49.5X5	T49.5X6
Phytolacca decandra	T62.2X1	T62.2X2	T62.2X3	T62.2X4		

Substance	Poisoning, Accidental (unintentional)	Poisoning, Intentional Self-harm	Poisoning, Assault	Poisoning, Undetermined	Adverse Effect	Under-dosing
Phytolacca decandra — continued						
berries	T62.1X1	T62.1X2	T62.1X3	T62.1X4	—	—
Phytomenadione	T45.7X1	T45.7X2	T45.7X3	T45.7X4	T45.7X5	T45.7X6
Phytonadione	T45.7X1	T45.7X2	T45.7X3	T45.7X4	T45.7X5	T45.7X6
Picoperine	T48.3X1	T48.3X2	T48.3X3	T48.3X4	T48.3X5	T48.3X6
Picosulfate (sodium)	T47.2X1	T47.2X2	T47.2X3	T47.2X4	T47.2X5	T47.2X6
Picric (acid)	T54.2X1	T54.2X2	T54.2X3	T54.2X4	—	—
Picrotoxin	T50.7X1	T50.7X2	T50.7X3	T50.7X4	T50.7X5	T50.7X6
Piketoprofen	T49.0X1	T49.0X2	T49.0X3	T49.0X4	T49.0X5	T49.0X6
Pilocarpine	T44.1X1	T44.1X2	T44.1X3	T44.1X4	T44.1X5	T44.1X6
Pilocarpus (jaborandi) extract	T44.1X1	T44.1X2	T44.1X3	T44.1X4	T44.1X5	T44.1X6
Pilsicainide (hydrochloride)	T46.2X1	T46.2X2	T46.2X3	T46.2X4	T46.2X5	T46.2X6
Pimaricin	T36.7X1	T36.7X2	T36.7X3	T36.7X4	T36.7X5	T36.7X6
Pimeclone	T50.7X1	T50.7X2	T50.7X3	T50.7X4	T50.7X5	T50.7X6
Pimelic ketone	T52.8X1	T52.8X2	T52.8X3	T52.8X4	—	—
Pimethixene	T45.0X1	T45.0X2	T45.0X3	T45.0X4	T45.0X5	T45.0X6
Piminodine	T40.2X1	T40.2X2	T40.2X3	T40.2X4	T40.2X5	T40.2X6
Pimozide	T43.591	T43.592	T43.593	T43.594	T43.595	T43.596
Pinacidil	T46.5X1	T46.5X2	T46.5X3	T46.5X4	T46.5X5	T46.5X6
Pinaverium bromide	T44.3X1	T44.3X2	T44.3X3	T44.3X4	T44.3X5	T44.3X6
Pinazepam	T42.4X1	T42.4X2	T42.4X3	T42.4X4	T42.4X5	T42.4X6
Pindolol	T44.7X1	T44.7X2	T44.7X3	T44.7X4	T44.7X5	T44.7X6
Pindone	T60.4X1	T60.4X2	T60.4X3	T60.4X4	—	—
Pine oil (disinfectant)	T65.891	T65.892	T65.893	T65.894	—	—
Pinkroot	T37.4X1	T37.4X2	T37.4X3	T37.4X4	T37.4X5	T37.4X6
Pipadone	T40.2X1	T40.2X2	T40.2X3	T40.2X4	—	—
Pipamazine	T45.0X1	T45.0X2	T45.0X3	T45.0X4	T45.0X5	T45.0X6
Pipamperone	T43.4X1	T43.4X2	T43.4X3	T43.4X4	T43.4X5	T43.4X6
Pipazetate	T48.3X1	T48.3X2	T48.3X3	T48.3X4	T48.3X5	T48.3X6
Pipemidic acid	T37.8X1	T37.8X2	T37.8X3	T37.8X4	T37.8X5	T37.8X6
Pipenzolate bromide	T44.3X1	T44.3X2	T44.3X3	T44.3X4	T44.3X5	T44.3X6
Piperacetazine	T43.3X1	T43.3X2	T43.3X3	T43.3X4	T43.3X5	T43.3X6
Piperacillin	T36.0X1	T36.0X2	T36.0X3	T36.0X4	T36.0X5	T36.0X6
Piperazine	T37.4X1	T37.4X2	T37.4X3	T37.4X4	T37.4X5	T37.4X6
estrone sulfate	T38.5X1	T38.5X2	T38.5X3	T38.5X4	T38.5X5	T38.5X6
Piper cubeba	T62.2X1	T62.2X2	T62.2X3	T62.2X4	—	—
Piperidione	T48.3X1	T48.3X2	T48.3X3	T48.3X4	T48.3X5	T48.3X6
Piperidolate	T44.3X1	T44.3X2	T44.3X3	T44.3X4	T44.3X5	T44.3X6
Piperocaine	T41.3X1	T41.3X2	T41.3X3	T41.3X4	T41.3X5	T41.3X6
infiltration (subcutaneous)	T41.3X1	T41.3X2	T41.3X3	T41.3X4	T41.3X5	T41.3X6
nerve block (peripheral) (plexus)	T41.3X1	T41.3X2	T41.3X3	T41.3X4	T41.3X5	T41.3X6
topical (surface)	T41.3X1	T41.3X2	T41.3X3	T41.3X4	T41.3X5	T41.3X6
Piperonyl butoxide	T60.8X1	T60.8X2	T60.8X3	T60.8X4	—	—
Pipethanate	T44.3X1	T44.3X2	T44.3X3	T44.3X4	T44.3X5	T44.3X6
Pipobroman	T45.1X1	T45.1X2	T45.1X3	T45.1X4	T45.1X5	T45.1X6
Pipotiazine	T43.3X1	T43.3X2	T43.3X3	T43.3X4	T43.3X5	T43.3X6
Pipoxizine	T45.0X1	T45.0X2	T45.0X3	T45.0X4	T45.0X5	T45.0X6
Pipradrol	T43.691	T43.692	T43.693	T43.694	T43.695	T43.696
Piprinhydrinate	T45.0X1	T45.0X2	T45.0X3	T45.0X4	T45.0X5	T45.0X6
Pirarubicin	T45.1X1	T45.1X2	T45.1X3	T45.1X4	T45.1X5	T45.1X6
Pirazinamide	T37.1X1	T37.1X2	T37.1X3	T37.1X4	T37.1X5	T37.1X6
Pirbuterol	T48.6X1	T48.6X2	T48.6X3	T48.6X4	T48.6X5	T48.6X6
Pirenzepine	T47.1X1	T47.1X2	T47.1X3	T47.1X4	T47.1X5	T47.1X6
Piretanide	T50.1X1	T50.1X2	T50.1X3	T50.1X4	T50.1X5	T50.1X6
Piribedil	T42.8X1	T42.8X2	T42.8X3	T42.8X4	T42.8X5	T42.8X6
Piridoxilate	T46.3X1	T46.3X2	T46.3X3	T46.3X4	T46.3X5	T46.3X6
Piritramide	T40.4X1	T40.4X2	T40.4X3	T40.4X4	—	—
Piromidic acid	T37.8X1	T37.8X2	T37.8X3	T37.8X4	T37.8X5	T37.8X6
Piroxicam	T39.391	T39.392	T39.393	T39.394	T39.395	T39.396
beta-cyclodextrin complex	T39.8X1	T39.8X2	T39.8X3	T39.8X4	T39.8X5	T39.8X6
Pirozadil	T46.6X1	T46.6X2	T46.6X3	T46.6X4	T46.6X5	T46.6X6
Piscidia (bark) (erythrina)	T39.8X1	T39.8X2	T39.8X3	T39.8X4	T39.8X5	T39.8X6
Pitch	T65.891	T65.892	T65.893	T65.894	—	—
Pitkin's solution	T41.3X1	T41.3X2	T41.3X3	T41.3X4	T41.3X5	T41.3X6
Pitocin	T48.0X1	T48.0X2	T48.0X3	T48.0X4	T48.0X5	T48.0X6
Pitressin (tannate)	T38.891	T38.892	T38.893	T38.894	T38.895	T38.896
Pituitary extracts (posterior)	T38.891	T38.892	T38.893	T38.894	T38.895	T38.896
anterior	T38.811	T38.812	T38.813	T38.814	T38.815	T38.816
Pituitrin	T38.891	T38.892	T38.893	T38.894	T38.895	T38.896
Pivampicillin	T36.0X1	T36.0X2	T36.0X3	T36.0X4	T36.0X5	T36.0X6
Pivmecillinam	T36.0X1	T36.0X2	T36.0X3	T36.0X4	T36.0X5	T36.0X6
Placental hormone	T38.891	T38.892	T38.893	T38.894	T38.895	T38.896
Placidyl	T42.6X1	T42.6X2	T42.6X3	T42.6X4	T42.6X5	T42.6X6
Plague vaccine	T50.A91	T50.A92	T50.A93	T50.A94	T50.A95	T50.A96
Plant						
food or fertilizer NEC	T65.891	T65.892	T65.893	T65.894	—	—
containing herbicide	T60.3X1	T60.3X2	T60.3X3	T60.3X4	—	—
noxious, used as food	T62.2X1	T62.2X2	T62.2X3	T62.2X4	—	—
berries	T62.1X1	T62.1X2	T62.1X3	T62.1X4	—	—
seeds	T62.2X1	T62.2X2	T62.2X3	T62.2X4	—	—

Table of Drugs and Chemicals

Substance	Poisoning, Accidental (unintentional)	Poisoning, Intentional Self-harm	Poisoning, Assault	Poisoning, Undetermined	Adverse Effect	Under-dosing
Plant — *continued*						
noxious, used as food — *continued*						
specified type NEC	T62.2X1	T62.2X2	T62.2X3	T62.2X4	—	—
Plasma	T45.8X1	T45.8X2	T45.8X3	T45.8X4	T45.8X5	T45.8X6
expander NEC	T45.8X1	T45.8X2	T45.8X3	T45.8X4	T45.8X5	T45.8X6
protein fraction (human)	T45.8X1	T45.8X2	T45.8X3	T45.8X4	T45.8X5	T45.8X6
Plasmanate	T45.8X1	T45.8X2	T45.8X3	T45.8X4	T45.8X5	T45.8X6
Plasminogen (tissue) activator	T45.611	T45.612	T45.613	T45.614	T45.615	T45.616
Plaster dressing	T49.3X1	T49.3X2	T49.3X3	T49.3X4	T49.3X5	T49.3X6
Plastic dressing	T49.3X1	T49.3X2	T49.3X3	T49.3X4	T49.3X5	T49.3X6
Plegicil	T43.3X1	T43.3X2	T43.3X3	T43.3X4	T43.3X5	T43.3X6
Plicamycin	T45.1X1	T45.1X2	T45.1X3	T45.1X4	T45.1X5	T45.1X6
Podophyllotoxin	T49.8X1	T49.8X2	T49.8X3	T49.8X4	T49.8X5	T49.8X6
Podophyllum (resin)	T49.4X1	T49.4X2	T49.4X3	T49.4X4	T49.4X5	T49.4X6
Poisonous berries	T62.1X1	T62.1X2	T62.1X3	T62.1X4	—	—
Poison NEC	T65.91	T65.92	T65.93	T65.94	—	—
Pokeweed (any part)	T62.2X1	T62.2X2	T62.2X3	T62.2X4	—	—
Poldine metilsulfate	T44.3X1	T44.3X2	T44.3X3	T44.3X4	T44.3X5	T44.3X6
Polidexide (sulfate)	T46.6X1	T46.6X2	T46.6X3	T46.6X4	T46.6X5	T46.6X6
Polidocanol	T46.8X1	T46.8X2	T46.8X3	T46.8X4	T46.8X5	T46.8X6
Poliomyelitis vaccine	T50.B91	T50.B92	T50.B93	T50.B94	T50.B95	T50.B96
Polish (car) (floor) (furni-ture) (metal) (porcelain) (silver)	T65.891	T65.892	T65.893	T65.894	—	—
abrasive	T65.891	T65.892	T65.893	T65.894	—	—
porcelain	T65.891	T65.892	T65.893	T65.894	—	—
Poloxalkol	T47.4X1	T47.4X2	T47.4X3	T47.4X4	T47.4X5	T47.4X6
Poloxamer	T47.4X1	T47.4X2	T47.4X3	T47.4X4	T47.4X5	T47.4X6
Polyaminostyrene resins	T50.3X1	T50.3X2	T50.3X3	T50.3X4	T50.3X5	T50.3X6
Polycarbophil	T47.4X1	T47.4X2	T47.4X3	T47.4X4	T47.4X5	T47.4X6
Polychlorinated biphenyl	T65.891	T65.892	T65.893	T65.894	—	—
Polycycline	T36.4X1	T36.4X2	T36.4X3	T36.4X4	T36.4X5	T36.4X6
Polyester fumes	T59.891	T59.892	T59.893	T59.894	—	—
Polyester resin hardener	T52.91	T52.92	T52.93	T52.94	—	—
fumes	T59.891	T59.892	T59.893	T59.894	—	—
Polyestradiol phosphate	T38.5X1	T38.5X2	T38.5X3	T38.5X4	T38.5X5	T38.5X6
Polyethanolamine alkyl sulfate	T49.2X1	T49.2X2	T49.2X3	T49.2X4	T49.2X5	T49.2X6
Polyethylene adhesive	T49.3X1	T49.3X2	T49.3X3	T49.3X4	T49.3X5	T49.3X6
Polyferose	T45.4X1	T45.4X2	T45.4X3	T45.4X4	T45.4X5	T45.4X6
Polygeline	T45.8X1	T45.8X2	T45.8X3	T45.8X4	T45.8X5	T45.8X6
Polymyxin	T36.8X1	T36.8X2	T36.8X3	T36.8X4	T36.8X5	T36.8X6
B	T36.8X1	T36.8X2	T36.8X3	T36.8X4	T36.8X5	T36.8X6
ENT agent	T49.6X1	T49.6X2	T49.6X3	T49.6X4	T49.6X5	T49.6X6
ophthalmic preparation	T49.5X1	T49.5X2	T49.5X3	T49.5X4	T49.5X5	T49.5X6
topical NEC	T49.0X1	T49.0X2	T49.0X3	T49.0X4	T49.0X5	T49.0X6
E sulfate (eye preparation)	T49.5X1	T49.5X2	T49.5X3	T49.5X4	T49.5X5	T49.5X6
Polynoxylin	T49.0X1	T49.0X2	T49.0X3	T49.0X4	T49.0X5	T49.0X6
Polyoestradiol phosphate	T38.5X1	T38.5X2	T38.5X3	T38.5X4	T38.5X5	T38.5X6
Polyoxymethyleneurea	T49.0X1	T49.0X2	T49.0X3	T49.0X4	T49.0X5	T49.0X6
Polysilane	T47.8X1	T47.8X2	T47.8X3	T47.8X4	T47.8X5	T47.8X6
Polytetrafluoroethylene (inhaled)	T59.891	T59.892	T59.893	T59.894	—	—
Polythiazide	T50.2X1	T50.2X2	T50.2X3	T50.2X4	T50.2X5	T50.2X6
Polyvidone	T45.8X1	T45.8X2	T45.8X3	T45.8X4	T45.8X5	T45.8X6
Polyvinylpyrrolidone	T45.8X1	T45.8X2	T45.8X3	T45.8X4	T45.8X5	T45.8X6
Pontocaine (hydrochloride) (infiltration) (topical)	T41.3X1	T41.3X2	T41.3X3	T41.3X4	T41.3X5	T41.3X6
nerve block (peripheral) (plexus)	T41.3X1	T41.3X2	T41.3X3	T41.3X4	T41.3X5	T41.3X6
spinal	T41.3X1	T41.3X2	T41.3X3	T41.3X4	T41.3X5	T41.3X6
Porfiromycin	T45.1X1	T45.1X2	T45.1X3	T45.1X4	T45.1X5	T45.1X6
Posterior pituitary hormone NEC	T38.891	T38.892	T38.893	T38.894	T38.895	T38.896
Pot	T40.7X1	T40.7X2	T40.7X3	T40.7X4	T40.7X5	T40.7X6
Potash (caustic)	T54.3X1	T54.3X2	T54.3X3	T54.3X4	—	—
Potassic saline injection (lactated)	T50.3X1	T50.3X2	T50.3X3	T50.3X4	T50.3X5	T50.3X6
Potassium-removing resin	T50.3X1	T50.3X2	T50.3X3	T50.3X4	T50.3X5	T50.3X6
Potassium-retaining drug	T50.3X1	T50.3X2	T50.3X3	T50.3X4	T50.3X5	T50.3X6
Potassium (salts) **NEC**	T50.3X1	T50.3X2	T50.3X3	T50.3X4	T50.3X5	T50.3X6
aminobenzoate	T45.8X1	T45.8X2	T45.8X3	T45.8X4	T45.8X5	T45.8X6
aminosalicylate	T37.1X1	T37.1X2	T37.1X3	T37.1X4	T37.1X5	T37.1X6
antimony ' tartrate'	T37.8X1	T37.8X2	T37.8X3	T37.8X4	T37.8X5	T37.8X6
arsenite (solution)	T57.0X1	T57.0X2	T57.0X3	T57.0X4	—	—
bichromate	T56.2X1	T56.2X2	T56.2X3	T56.2X4	—	—
bisulfate	T47.3X1	T47.3X2	T47.3X3	T47.3X4	T47.3X5	T47.3X6
bromide	T42.6X1	T42.6X2	T42.6X3	T42.6X4	T42.6X5	T42.6X6
canrenoate	T50.0X1	T50.0X2	T50.0X3	T50.0X4	T50.0X5	T50.0X6
carbonate	T54.3X1	T54.3X2	T54.3X3	T54.3X4	—	—
chlorate NEC	T65.891	T65.892	T65.893	T65.894	—	—
chloride	T50.3X1	T50.3X2	T50.3X3	T50.3X4	T50.3X5	T50.3X6
Potassium (salts) **NEC** — *continued*						
citrate	T50.991	T50.992	T50.993	T50.994	T50.995	T50.996
cyanide	T65.0X1	T65.0X2	T65.0X3	T65.0X4	—	—
ferric hexacyanoferrate (medicinal)	T50.6X1	T50.6X2	T50.6X3	T50.6X4	T50.6X5	T50.6X6
nonmedicinal	T65.891	T65.892	T65.893	T65.894	—	—
Fluoride	T57.8X1	T57.8X2	T57.8X3	T57.8X4	—	—
glucaldrate	T47.1X1	T47.1X2	T47.1X3	T47.1X4	T47.1X5	T47.1X6
hydroxide	T54.3X1	T54.3X2	T54.3X3	T54.3X4	—	—
iodate	T49.0X1	T49.0X2	T49.0X3	T49.0X4	T49.0X5	T49.0X6
iodide	T48.4X1	T48.4X2	T48.4X3	T48.4X4	T48.4X5	T48.4X6
nitrate	T57.8X1	T57.8X2	T57.8X3	T57.8X4	—	—
oxalate	T65.891	T65.892	T65.893	T65.894	—	—
perchlorate (nonmedicinal) NEC	T65.891	T65.892	T65.893	T65.894	—	—
antithyroid	T38.2X1	T38.2X2	T38.2X3	T38.2X4	T38.2X5	T38.2X6
medicinal	T38.2X1	T38.2X2	T38.2X3	T38.2X4	T38.2X5	T38.2X6
Permanganate (nonmedicinal)	T65.891	T65.892	T65.893	T65.894	—	—
medicinal	T49.0X1	T49.0X2	T49.0X3	T49.0X4	T49.0X5	T49.0X6
sulfate	T47.2X1	T47.2X2	T47.2X3	T47.2X4	T47.2X5	T47.2X6
Povidone	T45.8X1	T45.8X2	T45.8X3	T45.8X4	T45.8X5	T45.8X6
iodine	T49.0X1	T49.0X2	T49.0X3	T49.0X4	T49.0X5	T49.0X6
Practolol	T44.7X1	T44.7X2	T44.7X3	T44.7X4	T44.7X5	T44.7X6
Prajmalium bitartrate	T46.2X1	T46.2X2	T46.2X3	T46.2X4	T46.2X5	T46.2X6
Pralidoxime (iodide)	T50.6X1	T50.6X2	T50.6X3	T50.6X4	T50.6X5	T50.6X6
chloride	T50.6X1	T50.6X2	T50.6X3	T50.6X4	T50.6X5	T50.6X6
Pramiverine	T44.3X1	T44.3X2	T44.3X3	T44.3X4	T44.3X5	T44.3X6
Pramocaine	T49.1X1	T49.1X2	T49.1X3	T49.1X4	T49.1X5	T49.1X6
Pramoxine	T49.1X1	T49.1X2	T49.1X3	T49.1X4	T49.1X5	T49.1X6
Prasterone	T38.7X1	T38.7X2	T38.7X3	T38.7X4	T38.7X5	T38.7X6
Pravastatin	T46.6X1	T46.6X2	T46.6X3	T46.6X4	T46.6X5	T46.6X6
Prazepam	T42.4X1	T42.4X2	T42.4X3	T42.4X4	T42.4X5	T42.4X6
Praziquantel	T37.4X1	T37.4X2	T37.4X3	T37.4X4	T37.4X5	T37.4X6
Prazitone	T43.291	T43.292	T43.293	T43.294	T43.295	T43.296
Prazosin	T44.6X1	T44.6X2	T44.6X3	T44.6X4	T44.6X5	T44.6X6
Prednicarbate	T49.0X1	T49.0X2	T49.0X3	T49.0X4	T49.0X5	T49.0X6
Prednimustine	T45.1X1	T45.1X2	T45.1X3	T45.1X4	T45.1X5	T45.1X6
Prednisolone	T38.0X1	T38.0X2	T38.0X3	T38.0X4	T38.0X5	T38.0X6
ENT agent	T49.6X1	T49.6X2	T49.6X3	T49.6X4	T49.6X5	T49.6X6
ophthalmic preparation	T49.5X1	T49.5X2	T49.5X3	T49.5X4	T49.5X5	T49.5X6
steaglate	T49.0X1	T49.0X2	T49.0X3	T49.0X4	T49.0X5	T49.0X6
topical NEC	T49.0X1	T49.0X2	T49.0X3	T49.0X4	T49.0X5	T49.0X6
Prednisone	T38.0X1	T38.0X2	T38.0X3	T38.0X4	T38.0X5	T38.0X6
Prednylidene	T38.0X1	T38.0X2	T38.0X3	T38.0X4	T38.0X5	T38.0X6
Pregnandiol	T38.5X1	T38.5X2	T38.5X3	T38.5X4	T38.5X5	T38.5X6
Pregneninolone	T38.5X1	T38.5X2	T38.5X3	T38.5X4	T38.5X5	T38.5X6
Preludin	T43.691	T43.692	T43.693	T43.694	T43.695	T43.696
Premarin	T38.5X1	T38.5X2	T38.5X3	T38.5X4	T38.5X5	T38.5X6
Premedication anesthetic	T41.201	T41.202	T41.203	T41.204	T41.205	T41.206
Prenalterol	T44.5X1	T44.5X2	T44.5X3	T44.5X4	T44.5X5	T44.5X6
Prenoxdiazine	T48.3X1	T48.3X2	T48.3X3	T48.3X4	T48.3X5	T48.3X6
Prenylamine	T46.3X1	T46.3X2	T46.3X3	T46.3X4	T46.3X5	T46.3X6
Preparation H	T49.8X1	T49.8X2	T49.8X3	T49.8X4	T49.8X5	T49.8X6
Preparation, local	T49.4X1	T49.4X2	T49.4X3	T49.4X4	T49.4X5	T49.4X6
Preservative (nonmedicinal)	T65.891	T65.892	T65.893	T65.894	—	—
medicinal	T50.901	T50.902	T50.903	T50.904	T50.905	T50.906
wood	T60.91	T60.92	T60.93	T60.94	—	—
Prethcamide	T50.7X1	T50.7X2	T50.7X3	T50.7X4	T50.7X5	T50.7X6
Pride of China	T62.2X1	T62.2X2	T62.2X3	T62.2X4	—	—
Pridinol	T44.3X1	T44.3X2	T44.3X3	T44.3X4	T44.3X5	T44.3X6
Prifinium bromide	T44.3X1	T44.3X2	T44.3X3	T44.3X4	T44.3X5	T44.3X6
Prilocaine	T41.3X1	T41.3X2	T41.3X3	T41.3X4	T41.3X5	T41.3X6
infiltration (subcutaneous)	T41.3X1	T41.3X2	T41.3X3	T41.3X4	T41.3X5	T41.3X6
nerve block (peripheral) (plexus)	T41.3X1	T41.3X2	T41.3X3	T41.3X4	T41.3X5	T41.3X6
regional	T41.3X1	T41.3X2	T41.3X3	T41.3X4	T41.3X5	T41.3X6
Primaquine	T37.2X1	T37.2X2	T37.2X3	T37.2X4	T37.2X5	T37.2X6
Primidone	T42.6X1	T42.6X2	T42.6X3	T42.6X4	T42.6X5	T42.6X6
Primula (veris)	T62.2X1	T62.2X2	T62.2X3	T62.2X4	—	—
Prinadol	T40.2X1	T40.2X2	T40.2X3	T40.2X4	T40.2X5	T40.2X6
Priscol, Priscoline	T44.6X1	T44.6X2	T44.6X3	T44.6X4	T44.6X5	T44.6X6
Pristinamycin	T36.3X1	T36.3X2	T36.3X3	T36.3X4	T36.3X5	T36.3X6
Privet	T62.2X1	T62.2X2	T62.2X3	T62.2X4	—	—
berries	T62.1X1	T62.1X2	T62.1X3	T62.1X4	—	—
Privine	T44.4X1	T44.4X2	T44.4X3	T44.4X4	T44.4X5	T44.4X6
Pro-Banthine	T44.3X1	T44.3X2	T44.3X3	T44.3X4	T44.3X5	T44.3X6
Probarbital	T42.3X1	T42.3X2	T42.3X3	T42.3X4	T42.3X5	T42.3X6
Probenecid	T50.4X1	T50.4X2	T50.4X3	T50.4X4	T50.4X5	T50.4X6
Probucol	T46.6X1	T46.6X2	T46.6X3	T46.6X4	T46.6X5	T46.6X6
Procainamide	T46.2X1	T46.2X2	T46.2X3	T46.2X4	T46.2X5	T46.2X6
Procaine	T41.3X1	T41.3X2	T41.3X3	T41.3X4	T41.3X5	T41.3X6

Plant — Procaine

Substance	Poisoning, Accidental (unintentional)	Poisoning, Intentional Self-harm	Poisoning, Assault	Poisoning, Undetermined	Adverse Effect	Under-dosing
Procaine — continued						
benzylpenicillin	T36.0X1	T36.0X2	T36.0X3	T36.0X4	T36.0X5	T36.0X6
nerve block (periphreal) (plexus)	T41.3X1	T41.3X2	T41.3X3	T41.3X4	T41.3X5	T41.3X6
penicillin G	T36.0X1	T36.0X2	T36.0X3	T36.0X4	T36.0X5	T36.0X6
regional	T41.3X1	T41.3X2	T41.3X3	T41.3X4	T41.3X5	T41.3X6
spinal	T41.3X1	T41.3X2	T41.3X3	T41.3X4	T41.3X5	T41.3X6
Procalmidol	T43.591	T43.592	T43.593	T43.594	T43.595	T43.596
Procarbazine	T45.1X1	T45.1X2	T45.1X3	T45.1X4	T45.1X5	T45.1X6
Procaterol	T44.5X1	T44.5X2	T44.5X3	T44.5X4	T44.5X5	T44.5X6
Prochlorperazine	T43.3X1	T43.3X2	T43.3X3	T43.3X4	T43.3X5	T43.3X6
Procyclidine	T44.3X1	T44.3X2	T44.3X3	T44.3X4	T44.3X5	T44.3X6
Producer gas	T58.8X1	T58.8X2	T58.8X3	T58.8X4	—	—
Profadol	T40.4X1	T40.4X2	T40.4X3	T40.4X4	T40.4X5	T40.4X6
Profenamine	T44.3X1	T44.3X2	T44.3X3	T44.3X4	T44.3X5	T44.3X6
Profenil	T44.3X1	T44.3X2	T44.3X3	T44.3X4	T44.3X5	T44.3X6
Proflavine	T49.0X1	T49.0X2	T49.0X3	T49.0X4	T49.0X5	T49.0X6
Progabide	T42.6X1	T42.6X2	T42.6X3	T42.6X4	T42.6X5	T42.6X6
Progesterone	T38.5X1	T38.5X2	T38.5X3	T38.5X4	T38.5X5	T38.5X6
Progestin	T38.5X1	T38.5X2	T38.5X3	T38.5X4	T38.5X5	T38.5X6
oral contraceptive	T38.4X1	T38.4X2	T38.4X3	T38.4X4	T38.4X5	T38.4X6
Progestogen NEC	T38.5X1	T38.5X2	T38.5X3	T38.5X4	T38.5X5	T38.5X6
Progestone	T38.5X1	T38.5X2	T38.5X3	T38.5X4	T38.5X5	T38.5X6
Proglumide	T47.1X1	T47.1X2	T47.1X3	T47.1X4	T47.1X5	T47.1X6
Proguanil	T37.2X1	T37.2X2	T37.2X3	T37.2X4	T37.2X5	T37.2X6
Prolactin	T38.811	T38.812	T38.813	T38.814	T38.815	T38.816
Prolintane	T43.691	T43.692	T43.693	T43.694	T43.695	T43.696
Proloid	T38.1X1	T38.1X2	T38.1X3	T38.1X4	T38.1X5	T38.1X6
Proluton	T38.5X1	T38.5X2	T38.5X3	T38.5X4	T38.5X5	T38.5X6
Promacetin	T37.1X1	T37.1X2	T37.1X3	T37.1X4	T37.1X5	T37.1X6
Promazine	T43.3X1	T43.3X2	T43.3X3	T43.3X4	T43.3X5	T43.3X6
Promedol	T40.2X1	T40.2X2	T40.2X3	T40.2X4	—	—
Promegestone	T38.5X1	T38.5X2	T38.5X3	T38.5X4	T38.5X5	T38.5X6
Promethazine (teoclate)	T43.3X1	T43.3X2	T43.3X3	T43.3X4	T43.3X5	T43.3X6
Promin	T37.1X1	T37.1X2	T37.1X3	T37.1X4	T37.1X5	T37.1X6
Pronase	T45.3X1	T45.3X2	T45.3X3	T45.3X4	T45.3X5	T45.3X6
Pronestyl (hydrochloride)	T46.2X1	T46.2X2	T46.2X3	T46.2X4	T46.2X5	T46.2X6
Pronetalol	T44.7X1	T44.7X2	T44.7X3	T44.7X4	T44.7X5	T44.7X6
Prontosil	T37.0X1	T37.0X2	T37.0X3	T37.0X4	T37.0X5	T37.0X6
Propachlor	T60.3X1	T60.3X2	T60.3X3	T60.3X4	—	—
Propafenone	T46.2X1	T46.2X2	T46.2X3	T46.2X4	T46.2X5	T46.2X6
Propallylonal	T42.3X1	T42.3X2	T42.3X3	T42.3X4	T42.3X5	T42.3X6
Propamidine	T49.0X1	T49.0X2	T49.0X3	T49.0X4	T49.0X5	T49.0X6
Propane (distributed in mobile container)	T59.891	T59.892	T59.893	T59.894	—	—
distributed through pipes	T59.891	T59.892	T59.893	T59.894	—	—
incomplete combustion	T58.11	T58.12	T58.13	T58.14	—	—
Propanidid	T41.291	T41.292	T41.293	T41.294	T41.295	T41.296
Propanil	T60.3X1	T60.3X2	T60.3X3	T60.3X4	—	—
Propantheline	T44.3X1	T44.3X2	T44.3X3	T44.3X4	T44.3X5	T44.3X6
bromide	T44.3X1	T44.3X2	T44.3X3	T44.3X4	T44.3X5	T44.3X6
Proparacaine	T41.3X1	T41.3X2	T41.3X3	T41.3X4	T41.3X5	T41.3X6
Propatylnitrate	T46.3X1	T46.3X2	T46.3X3	T46.3X4	T46.3X5	T46.3X6
Propicillin	T36.0X1	T36.0X2	T36.0X3	T36.0X4	T36.0X5	T36.0X6
Propiolactone	T49.0X1	T49.0X2	T49.0X3	T49.0X4	T49.0X5	T49.0X6
Propiomazine	T45.0X1	T45.0X2	T45.0X3	T45.0X4	T45.0X5	T45.0X6
Propionaidehyde (medicinal)	T42.6X1	T42.6X2	T42.6X3	T42.6X4	T42.6X5	T42.6X6
Propionate (calcium) (sodium)	T49.0X1	T49.0X2	T49.0X3	T49.0X4	T49.0X5	T49.0X6
Propion gel	T49.0X1	T49.0X2	T49.0X3	T49.0X4	T49.0X5	T49.0X6
Propitocaine	T41.3X1	T41.3X2	T41.3X3	T41.3X4	T41.3X5	T41.3X6
infiltration (subcutaneous)	T41.3X1	T41.3X2	T41.3X3	T41.3X4	T41.3X5	T41.3X6
nerve block (peripheral) (plexus)	T41.3X1	T41.3X2	T41.3X3	T41.3X4	T41.3X5	T41.3X6
Propofol	T41.291	T41.292	T41.293	T41.294	T41.295	T41.296
Propoxur	T60.0X1	T60.0X2	T60.0X3	T60.0X4	—	—
Propoxycaine	T41.3X1	T41.3X2	T41.3X3	T41.3X4	T41.3X5	T41.3X6
infiltration (subcutaneous)	T41.3X1	T41.3X2	T41.3X3	T41.3X4	T41.3X5	T41.3X6
nerve block (peripheral) (plexus)	T41.3X1	T41.3X2	T41.3X3	T41.3X4	T41.3X5	T41.3X6
topical (surface)	T41.3X1	T41.3X2	T41.3X3	T41.3X4	T41.3X5	T41.3X6
Propoxyphene	T40.4X1	T40.4X2	T40.4X3	T40.4X4	T40.4X5	T40.4X6
Propranolol	T44.7X1	T44.7X2	T44.7X3	T44.7X4	T44.7X5	T44.7X6
Propyl						
alcohol	T51.3X1	T51.3X2	T51.3X3	T51.3X4	—	—
carbinol	T51.3X1	T51.3X2	T51.3X3	T51.3X4	—	—
hexadrine	T44.4X1	T44.4X2	T44.4X3	T44.4X4	T44.4X5	T44.4X6
iodone	T50.8X1	T50.8X2	T50.8X3	T50.8X4	T50.8X5	T50.8X6
thiouracil	T38.2X1	T38.2X2	T38.2X3	T38.2X4	T38.2X5	T38.2X6
Propylaminophenothiazine	T43.3X1	T43.3X2	T43.3X3	T43.3X4	T43.3X5	T43.3X6
Propylene	T59.891	T59.892	T59.893	T59.894	—	—
Propylhexedrine	T48.5X1	T48.5X2	T48.5X3	T48.5X4	T48.5X5	T48.5X6

Substance	Poisoning, Accidental (unintentional)	Poisoning, Intentional Self-harm	Poisoning, Assault	Poisoning, Undetermined	Adverse Effect	Under-dosing
Propyliodone	T50.8X1	T50.8X2	T50.8X3	T50.8X4	T50.8X5	T50.8X6
Propylparaben (ophthalmic)	T49.5X1	T49.5X2	T49.5X3	T49.5X4	T49.5X5	T49.5X6
Propylthiouracil	T38.2X1	T38.2X2	T38.2X3	T38.2X4	T38.2X5	T38.2X6
Propyphenazone	T39.2X1	T39.2X2	T39.2X3	T39.2X4	T39.2X5	T39.2X6
Proquazone	T39.391	T39.392	T39.392	T39.394	T39.395	T39.396
Proscillaridin	T46.0X1	T46.0X2	T46.0X3	T46.0X4	T46.0X5	T46.0X6
Prostacyclin	T45.521	T45.522	T45.523	T45.524	T45.525	T45.526
Prostaglandin (I2)	T45.521	T45.522	T45.523	T45.524	T45.525	T45.526
E1	T46.7X1	T46.7X2	T46.7X3	T46.7X4	T46.7X5	T46.7X6
E2	T48.0X1	T48.0X2	T48.0X3	T48.0X4	T48.0X5	T48.0X6
F2 alpha	T48.0X1	T48.0X2	T48.0X3	T48.0X4	T48.0X5	T48.0X6
Prostigmin	T44.0X1	T44.0X2	T44.0X3	T44.0X4	T44.0X5	T44.0X6
Prosultiamine	T45.2X1	T45.2X2	T45.2X3	T45.2X4	T45.2X5	T45.2X6
Protamine sulfate	T45.7X1	T45.7X2	T45.7X3	T45.7X4	T45.7X5	T45.7X6
zinc insulin	T38.3X1	T38.3X2	T38.3X3	T38.3X4	T38.3X5	T38.3X6
Protease	T47.5X1	T47.5X2	T47.5X3	T47.5X4	T47.5X5	T47.5X6
Protectant, skin NEC	T49.3X1	T49.3X2	T49.3X3	T49.3X4	T49.3X5	T49.3X6
Protein hydrolysate	T50.991	T50.992	T50.993	T50.994	T50.995	T50.996
Prothiaden — see Dothiepin hydrochloride						
Prothionamide	T37.1X1	T37.1X2	T37.1X3	T37.1X4	T37.1X5	T37.1X6
Prothipendyl	T43.591	T43.592	T43.593	T43.594	T43.595	T43.596
Prothoate	T60.0X1	T60.0X2	T60.0X3	T60.0X4	—	—
Prothrombin						
activator	T45.7X1	T45.7X2	T45.7X3	T45.7X4	T45.7X5	T45.7X6
synthesis inhibitor	T45.511	T45.512	T45.513	T45.514	T45.515	T45.516
Protionamide	T37.1X1	T37.1X2	T37.1X3	T37.1X4	T37.1X5	T37.1X6
Protirelin	T38.891	T38.892	T38.893	T38.894	T38.895	T38.896
Protokylol	T48.6X1	T48.6X2	T48.6X3	T48.6X4	T48.6X5	T48.6X6
Protopam	T50.6X1	T50.6X2	T50.6X3	T50.6X4	T50.6X5	T50.6X6
Protoveratrine(s) (A) (B)	T46.5X1	T46.5X2	T46.5X3	T46.5X4	T46.5X5	T46.5X6
Protriptyline	T43.011	T43.012	T43.013	T43.014	T43.015	T43.016
Provera	T38.5X1	T38.5X2	T38.5X3	T38.5X4	T38.5X5	T38.5X6
Provitamin A	T45.2X1	T45.2X2	T45.2X3	T45.2X4	T45.2X5	T45.2X6
Proxibarbal	T42.3X1	T42.3X2	T42.3X3	T42.3X4	T42.3X5	T42.3X6
Proxymetacaine	T41.3X1	T41.3X2	T41.3X3	T41.3X4	T41.3X5	T41.3X6
Proxyphylline	T48.6X1	T48.6X2	T48.6X3	T48.6X4	T48.6X5	T48.6X6
Prozac — see Fluoxetine hydrochloride						
Prunus						
laurocerasus	T62.2X1	T62.2X2	T62.2X3	T62.2X4	—	—
virginiana	T62.2X1	T62.2X2	T62.2X3	T62.2X4	—	—
Prussian blue						
commercial	T65.891	T65.892	T65.893	T65.894	—	—
therapeutic	T50.6X1	T50.6X2	T50.6X3	T50.6X4	T50.6X5	T50.6X6
Prussic acid	T65.0X1	T65.0X2	T65.0X3	T65.0X4	—	—
vapor	T57.3X1	T57.3X2	T57.3X3	T57.3X4	—	—
Pseudoephedrine	T44.991	T44.992	T44.993	T44.994	T44.995	T44.996
Psilocin	T40.991	T40.992	T40.993	T40.994	—	—
Psilocybin	T40.991	T40.992	T40.993	T40.994	—	—
Psilocybine	T40.991	T40.992	T40.993	T40.994	—	—
Psoralene (nonmedicinal)	T65.891	T65.892	T65.893	T65.894	—	—
Psoralens (medicinal)	T50.991	T50.992	T50.993	T50.994	T50.995	T50.996
PSP (phenolsulfonphthalein)	T50.8X1	T50.8X2	T50.8X3	T50.8X4	T50.8X5	T50.8X6
Psychodysleptic drug NEC	T40.901	T40.902	T40.903	T40.904	T40.905	T40.906
Psychostimulant	T43.601	T43.602	T43.603	T43.604	T43.605	T43.606
amphetamine	T43.621	T43.622	T43.623	T43.624	T43.625	T43.626
caffeine	T43.611	T43.612	T43.613	T43.614	T43.615	T43.616
methylphenidate	T43.631	T43.632	T43.633	T43.634	T43.635	T43.636
specified NEC	T43.691	T43.692	T43.693	T43.694	T43.695	T43.696
Psychotherapeutic drug NEC	T43.91	T43.92	T43.93	T43.94	T43.95	T43.96
antidepressants — see also Antidepressant	T43.201	T43.202	T43.203	T43.204	T43.205	T43.206
specified NEC	T43.8X1	T43.8X2	T43.8X3	T43.8X4	T43.8X5	T43.8X6
tranquilizers NEC	T43.501	T43.502	T43.503	T43.504	T43.505	T43.506
Psychotomimetic agents	T40.901	T40.902	T40.903	T40.904	T40.905	T40.906
Psychotropic drug NEC	T43.91	T43.92	T43.93	T43.94	T43.95	T43.96
specified NEC	T43.8X1	T43.8X2	T43.8X3	T43.8X4	T43.8X5	T43.8X6
Psyllium hydrophilic mucilloid	T47.4X1	T47.4X2	T47.4X3	T47.4X4	T47.4X5	T47.4X6
Pteroylglutamic acid	T45.8X1	T45.8X2	T45.8X3	T45.8X4	T45.8X5	T45.8X6
Pteroyltriglutamate	T45.1X1	T45.1X2	T45.1X3	T45.1X4	T45.1X5	T45.1X6
PTFE — see Polytetrafluoroethylene						
Pulp						
devitalizing paste	T49.7X1	T49.7X2	T49.7X3	T49.7X4	T49.7X5	T49.7X6
dressing	T49.7X1	T49.7X2	T49.7X3	T49.7X4	T49.7X5	T49.7X6
Pulsatilla	T62.2X1	T62.2X2	T62.2X3	T62.2X4	—	—
Pumpkin seed extract	T37.4X1	T37.4X2	T37.4X3	T37.4X4	T37.4X5	T37.4X6
Purex (bleach)	T54.91	T54.92	T54.93	T54.94	—	—
Purgative NEC — see also Cathartic	T47.4X1	T47.4X2	T47.4X3	T47.4X4	T47.4X5	T47.4X6

Additional Character May Be Required — Refer to the Tabular List for Character Selection ▽ **Subterms under main terms may continue to next column or page**

Substance	Poisoning, Accidental (unintentional)	Poisoning, Intentional Self-harm	Poisoning, Assault	Poisoning, Undetermined	Adverse Effect	Under-dosing
Purine analogue (antineoplastic)	T45.1X1	T45.1X2	T45.1X3	T45.1X4	T45.1X5	T45.1X6
Purine diuretics	T50.2X1	T50.2X2	T50.2X3	T50.2X4	T50.2X5	T50.2X6
Purinethol	T45.1X1	T45.1X2	T45.1X3	T45.1X4	T45.1X5	T45.1X6
PVP	T45.8X1	T45.8X2	T45.8X3	T45.8X4	T45.8X5	T45.8X6
Pyrabital	T39.8X1	T39.8X2	T39.8X3	T39.8X4	T39.8X5	T39.8X6
Pyramidon	T39.2X1	T39.2X2	T39.2X3	T39.2X4	T39.2X5	T39.2X6
Pyrantel	T37.4X1	T37.4X2	T37.4X3	T37.4X4	T37.4X5	T37.4X6
Pyrathiazine	T45.0X1	T45.0X2	T45.0X3	T45.0X4	T45.0X5	T45.0X6
Pyrazinamide	T37.1X1	T37.1X2	T37.1X3	T37.1X4	T37.1X5	T37.1X6
Pyrazinoic acid (amide)	T37.1X1	T37.1X2	T37.1X3	T37.1X4	T37.1X5	T37.1X6
Pyrazole (derivatives)	T39.2X1	T39.2X2	T39.2X3	T39.2X4	T39.2X5	T39.2X6
Pyrazolone analgesic NEC	T39.2X1	T39.2X2	T39.2X3	T39.2X4	T39.2X5	T39.2X6
Pyrethrin, pyrethrum (nonmedicinal)	T60.2X1	T60.2X2	T60.2X3	T60.2X4	—	—
Pyrethrum extract	T49.0X1	T49.0X2	T49.0X3	T49.0X4	T49.0X5	T49.0X6
Pyribenzamine	T45.0X1	T45.0X2	T45.0X3	T45.0X4	T45.0X5	T45.0X6
Pyridine	T52.8X1	T52.8X2	T52.8X3	T52.8X4	—	—
aldoxime methiodide	T50.6X1	T50.6X2	T50.6X3	T50.6X4	T50.6X5	T50.6X6
aldoxime methyl chloride	T50.6X1	T50.6X2	T50.6X3	T50.6X4	T50.6X5	T50.6X6
vapor	T59.891	T59.892	T59.893	T59.894	—	—
Pyridium	T39.8X1	T39.8X2	T39.8X3	T39.8X4	T39.8X5	T39.8X6
Pyridostigmine bromide	T44.0X1	T44.0X2	T44.0X3	T44.0X4	T44.0X5	T44.0X6
Pyridoxal phosphate	T45.2X1	T45.2X2	T45.2X3	T45.2X4	T45.2X5	T45.2X6
Pyridoxine	T45.2X1	T45.2X2	T45.2X3	T45.2X4	T45.2X5	T45.2X6
Pyrilamine	T45.0X1	T45.0X2	T45.0X3	T45.0X4	T45.0X5	T45.0X6
Pyrimethamine	T37.2X1	T37.2X2	T37.2X3	T37.2X4	T37.2X5	T37.2X6
with sulfadoxine	T37.2X1	T37.2X2	T37.2X3	T37.2X4	T37.2X5	T37.2X6
Pyrimidine antagonist	T45.1X1	T45.1X2	T45.1X3	T45.1X4	T45.1X5	T45.1X6
Pyriminil	T60.4X1	T60.4X2	T60.4X3	T60.4X4	—	—
Pyrithione zinc	T49.4X1	T49.4X2	T49.4X3	T49.4X4	T49.4X5	T49.4X6
Pyrithyldione	T42.6X1	T42.6X2	T42.6X3	T42.6X4	T42.6X5	T42.6X6
Pyrogallic acid	T49.0X1	T49.0X2	T49.0X3	T49.0X4	T49.0X5	T49.0X6
Pyrogallol	T49.0X1	T49.0X2	T49.0X3	T49.0X4	T49.0X5	T49.0X6
Pyroxylin	T49.3X1	T49.3X2	T49.3X3	T49.3X4	T49.3X5	T49.3X6
Pyrrobutamine	T45.0X1	T45.0X2	T45.0X3	T45.0X4	T45.0X5	T45.0X6
Pyrrolizidine alkaloids	T62.8X1	T62.8X2	T62.8X3	T62.8X4	—	—
Pyrvinium chloride	T37.4X1	T37.4X2	T37.4X3	T37.4X4	T37.4X5	T37.4X6
PZI	T38.3X1	T38.3X2	T38.3X3	T38.3X4	T38.3X5	T38.3X6
Quaalude	T42.6X1	T42.6X2	T42.6X3	T42.6X4	T42.6X5	T42.6X6
Quarternary ammonium						
anti-infective	T49.0X1	T49.0X2	T49.0X3	T49.0X4	T49.0X5	T49.0X6
ganglion blocking	T44.2X1	T44.2X2	T44.2X3	T44.2X4	T44.2X5	T44.2X6
parasympatholytic	T44.3X1	T44.3X2	T44.3X3	T44.3X4	T44.3X5	T44.3X6
Quazepam	T42.4X1	T42.4X2	T42.4X3	T42.4X4	T42.4X5	T42.4X6
Quicklime	T54.3X1	T54.3X2	T54.3X3	T54.3X4	—	—
Quillaja extract	T48.4X1	T48.4X2	T48.4X3	T48.4X4	T48.4X5	T48.4X6
Quinacrine	T37.2X1	T37.2X2	T37.2X3	T37.2X4	T37.2X5	T37.2X6
Quinaglute	T46.2X1	T46.2X2	T46.2X3	T46.2X4	T46.2X5	T46.2X6
Quinalbarbital	T42.3X1	T42.3X2	T42.3X3	T42.3X4	T42.3X5	T42.3X6
Quinalbarbitone sodium	T42.3X1	T42.3X2	T42.3X3	T42.3X4	T42.3X5	T42.3X6
Quinalphos	T60.0X1	T60.0X2	T60.0X3	T60.0X4	—	—
Quinapril	T46.4X1	T46.4X2	T46.4X3	T46.4X4	T46.4X5	T46.4X6
Quinestradiol	T38.5X1	T38.5X2	T38.5X3	T38.5X4	T38.5X5	T38.5X6
Quinestradol	T38.5X1	T38.5X2	T38.5X3	T38.5X4	T38.5X5	T38.5X6
Quinestrol	T38.5X1	T38.5X2	T38.5X3	T38.5X4	T38.5X5	T38.5X6
Quinethazone	T50.2X1	T50.2X2	T50.2X3	T50.2X4	T50.2X5	T50.2X6
Quingestanol	T38.4X1	T38.4X2	T38.4X3	T38.4X4	T38.4X5	T38.4X6
Quinidine	T46.2X1	T46.2X2	T46.2X3	T46.2X4	T46.2X5	T46.2X6
Quinine	T37.2X1	T37.2X2	T37.2X3	T37.2X4	T37.2X5	T37.2X6
Quiniobine	T37.8X1	T37.8X2	T37.8X3	T37.8X4	T37.8X5	T37.8X6
Quinisocaine	T49.1X1	T49.1X2	T49.1X3	T49.1X4	T49.1X5	T49.1X6
Quinocide	T37.2X1	T37.2X2	T37.2X3	T37.2X4	T37.2X5	T37.2X6
Quinoline (derivatives) NEC	T37.8X1	T37.8X2	T37.8X3	T37.8X4	T37.8X5	T37.8X6
Quinupramine	T43.011	T43.012	T43.013	T43.014	T43.015	T43.016
Quotane	T41.3X1	T41.3X2	T41.3X3	T41.3X4	T41.3X5	T41.3X6
Rabies						
immune globulin (human)	T50.Z11	T50.Z12	T50.Z13	T50.Z14	T50.Z15	T50.Z16
vaccine	T50.B91	T50.B92	T50.B93	T50.B94	T50.B95	T50.B96
Racemoramide	T40.2X1	T40.2X2	T40.2X3	T40.2X4	—	—
Racemorphan	T40.2X1	T40.2X2	T40.2X3	T40.2X4	T40.2X5	T40.2X6
Racepinefrin	T44.5X1	T44.5X2	T44.5X3	T44.5X4	T44.5X5	T44.5X6
Raclopride	T43.591	T43.592	T43.593	T43.594	T43.595	T43.596
Radiator alcohol	T51.1X1	T51.1X2	T51.1X3	T51.1X4	—	—
Radioactive drug NEC	T50.8X1	T50.8X2	T50.8X3	T50.8X4	T50.8X5	T50.8X6
Radio-opaque (drugs) (materials)	T50.8X1	T50.8X2	T50.8X3	T50.8X4	T50.8X5	T50.8X6
Ramifenazone	T39.2X1	T39.2X2	T39.2X3	T39.2X4	T39.2X5	T39.2X6
Ramipril	T46.4X1	T46.4X2	T46.4X3	T46.4X4	T46.4X5	T46.4X6
Ranitidine	T47.0X1	T47.0X2	T47.0X3	T47.0X4	T47.0X5	T47.0X6
Ranunculus	T62.2X1	T62.2X2	T62.2X3	T62.2X4	—	—
Rat poison NEC	T60.4X1	T60.4X2	T60.4X3	T60.4X4	—	—
Rattlesnake (venom)	T63.011	T63.012	T63.013	T63.014		

Substance	Poisoning, Accidental (unintentional)	Poisoning, Intentional Self-harm	Poisoning, Assault	Poisoning, Undetermined	Adverse Effect	Under-dosing
Raubasine	T46.7X1	T46.7X2	T46.7X3	T46.7X4	T46.7X5	T46.7X6
Raudixin	T46.5X1	T46.5X2	T46.5X3	T46.5X4	T46.5X5	T46.5X6
Rautensin	T46.5X1	T46.5X2	T46.5X3	T46.5X4	T46.5X5	T46.5X6
Rautina	T46.5X1	T46.5X2	T46.5X3	T46.5X4	T46.5X5	T46.5X6
Rautotal	T46.5X1	T46.5X2	T46.5X3	T46.5X4	T46.5X5	T46.5X6
Rauwiloid	T46.5X1	T46.5X2	T46.5X3	T46.5X4	T46.5X5	T46.5X6
Rauwoldin	T46.5X1	T46.5X2	T46.5X3	T46.5X4	T46.5X5	T46.5X6
Rauwolfia (alkaloids)	T46.5X1	T46.5X2	T46.5X3	T46.5X4	T46.5X5	T46.5X6
Razoxane	T45.1X1	T45.1X2	T45.1X3	T45.1X4	T45.1X5	T45.1X6
Realgar	T57.0X1	T57.0X2	T57.0X3	T57.0X4	—	—
Recombinant (R) — see specific protein						
Red blood cells, packed	T45.8X1	T45.8X2	T45.8X3	T45.8X4	T45.8X5	T45.8X6
Red squill (scilliroside)	T60.4X1	T60.4X2	T60.4X3	T60.4X4	—	—
Reducing agent, industrial NEC	T65.891	T65.892	T65.893	T65.894	—	—
Refrigerant gas (chlorofluorocarbon)	T53.5X1	T53.5X2	T53.5X3	T53.5X4	—	—
not chlorofluorocarbon	T59.891	T59.892	T59.893	T59.894	—	—
Regroton	T50.2X1	T50.2X2	T50.2X3	T50.2X4	T50.2X5	T50.2X6
Rehydration salts (oral)	T50.3X1	T50.3X2	T50.3X3	T50.3X4	T50.3X5	T50.3X6
Rela	T42.8X1	T42.8X2	T42.8X3	T42.8X4	T42.8X5	T42.8X6
Relaxant, muscle						
anesthetic	T48.1X1	T48.1X2	T48.1X3	T48.1X4	T48.1X5	T48.1X6
central nervous system	T42.8X1	T42.8X2	T42.8X3	T42.8X4	T42.8X5	T42.8X6
skeletal NEC	T48.1X1	T48.1X2	T48.1X3	T48.1X4	T48.1X5	T48.1X6
smooth NEC	T44.3X1	T44.3X2	T44.3X3	T44.3X4	T44.3X5	T44.3X6
Remoxipride	T43.591	T43.592	T43.593	T43.594	T43.595	T43.596
Renese	T50.2X1	T50.2X2	T50.2X3	T50.2X4	T50.2X5	T50.2X6
Renografin	T50.8X1	T50.8X2	T50.8X3	T50.8X4	T50.8X5	T50.8X6
Replacement solution	T50.3X1	T50.3X2	T50.3X3	T50.3X4	T50.3X5	T50.3X6
Reproterol	T48.6X1	T48.6X2	T48.6X3	T48.6X4	T48.6X5	T48.6X6
Rescinnamine	T46.5X1	T46.5X2	T46.5X3	T46.5X4	T46.5X5	T46.5X6
Reserpin (e)	T46.5X1	T46.5X2	T46.5X3	T46.5X4	T46.5X5	T46.5X6
Resorcin, resorcinol (nonmedicinal)	T65.891	T65.892	T65.893	T65.894	—	—
medicinal	T49.4X1	T49.4X2	T49.4X3	T49.4X4	T49.4X5	T49.4X6
Respaire	T48.4X1	T48.4X2	T48.4X3	T48.4X4	T48.4X5	T48.4X6
Respiratory drug NEC	T48.901	T48.902	T48.903	T48.904	T48.905	T48.906
antiasthmatic NEC	T48.6X1	T48.6X2	T48.6X3	T48.6X4	T48.6X5	T48.6X6
anti-common-cold NEC	T48.5X1	T48.5X2	T48.5X3	T48.5X4	T48.5X5	T48.5X6
expectorant NEC	T48.4X1	T48.4X2	T48.4X3	T48.4X4	T48.4X5	T48.4X6
stimulant	T48.901	T48.902	T48.903	T48.904	T48.905	T48.906
Retinoic acid	T49.0X1	T49.0X2	T49.0X3	T49.0X4	T49.0X5	T49.0X6
Retinol	T45.2X1	T45.2X2	T45.2X3	T45.2X4	T45.2X5	T45.2X6
Rh (D) immune globulin (human)	T50.Z11	T50.Z12	T50.Z13	T50.Z14	T50.Z15	T50.Z16
Rhodine	T39.011	T39.012	T39.013	T39.014	T39.015	T39.016
RhoGAM	T50.Z11	T50.Z12	T50.Z13	T50.Z14	T50.Z15	T50.Z16
Rhubarb						
dry extract	T47.2X1	T47.2X2	T47.2X3	T47.2X4	T47.2X5	T47.2X6
tincture, compound	T47.2X1	T47.2X2	T47.2X3	T47.2X4	T47.2X5	T47.2X6
Ribavirin	T37.5X1	T37.5X2	T37.5X3	T37.5X4	T37.5X5	T37.5X6
Riboflavin	T45.2X1	T45.2X2	T45.2X3	T45.2X4	T45.2X5	T45.2X6
Ribostamycin	T36.5X1	T36.5X2	T36.5X3	T36.5X4	T36.5X5	T36.5X6
Ricin	T62.2X1	T62.2X2	T62.2X3	T62.2X4	—	—
Ricinus communis	T62.2X1	T62.2X2	T62.2X3	T62.2X4	—	—
Rickettsial vaccine NEC	T50.A91	T50.A92	T50.A93	T50.A94	T50.A95	T50.A96
Rifabutin	T36.6X1	T36.6X2	T36.6X3	T36.6X4	T36.6X5	T36.6X6
Rifamide	T36.6X1	T36.6X2	T36.6X3	T36.6X4	T36.6X5	T36.6X6
Rifampicin	T36.6X1	T36.6X2	T36.6X3	T36.6X4	T36.6X5	T36.6X6
with isoniazid	T37.1X1	T37.1X2	T37.1X3	T37.1X4	T37.1X5	T37.1X6
Rifampin	T36.6X1	T36.6X2	T36.6X3	T36.6X4	T36.6X5	T36.6X6
Rifamycin	T36.6X1	T36.6X2	T36.6X3	T36.6X4	T36.6X5	T36.6X6
Rifaximin	T36.6X1	T36.6X2	T36.6X3	T36.6X4	T36.6X5	T36.6X6
Rimantadine	T37.5X1	T37.5X2	T37.5X3	T37.5X4	T37.5X5	T37.5X6
Rimazolium metilsulfate	T39.8X1	T39.8X2	T39.8X3	T39.8X4	T39.8X5	T39.8X6
Rimifon	T37.1X1	T37.1X2	T37.1X3	T37.1X4	T37.1X5	T37.1X6
Rimiterol	T48.6X1	T48.6X2	T48.6X3	T48.6X4	T48.6X5	T48.6X6
Ringer (lactate) solution	T50.3X1	T50.3X2	T50.3X3	T50.3X4	T50.3X5	T50.3X6
Ristocetin	T36.8X1	T36.8X2	T36.8X3	T36.8X4	T36.8X5	T36.8X6
Ritalin	T43.631	T43.632	T43.633	T43.634	T43.635	T43.636
Ritodrine	T44.5X1	T44.5X2	T44.5X3	T44.5X4	T44.5X5	T44.5X6
Roach killer — see Insecticide						
Rociverine	T44.3X1	T44.3X2	T44.3X3	T44.3X4		T44.3X6
Rocky Mountain spotted fever vaccine	T50.A91	T50.A92	T50.A93	T50.A94	T50.A95	T50.A96
Rodenticide NEC	T60.4X1	T60.4X2	T60.4X3	T60.4X4	—	—
Rohypnol	T42.4X1	T42.4X2	T42.4X3	T42.4X4	T42.4X5	T42.4X6
Rokitamycin	T36.3X1	T36.3X2	T36.3X3	T36.3X4	T36.3X5	T36.3X6
Rolaids	T47.1X1	T47.1X2	T47.1X3	T47.1X4	T47.1X5	T47.1X6
Rolitetracycline	T36.4X1	T36.4X2	T36.4X3	T36.4X4	T36.4X5	T36.4X6
Romilar	T48.3X1	T48.3X2	T48.3X3	T48.3X4	T48.3X5	T48.3X6

Substance	Poisoning, Accidental (unintentional)	Poisoning, Intentional Self-harm	Poisoning, Assault	Poisoning, Undetermined	Adverse Effect	Under-dosing
Ronifibrate	T46.6X1	T46.6X2	T46.6X3	T46.6X4	T46.6X5	T46.6X6
Rosaprostol	T47.1X1	T47.1X2	T47.1X3	T47.1X4	T47.1X5	T47.1X6
Rose bengal sodium (131I)	T50.8X1	T50.8X2	T50.8X3	T50.8X4	T50.8X5	T50.8X6
Rose water ointment	T49.3X1	T49.3X2	T49.3X3	T49.3X4	T49.3X5	T49.3X6
Rosoxacin	T37.8X1	T37.8X2	T37.8X3	T37.8X4	T37.8X5	T37.8X6
Rotenone	T60.2X1	T60.2X2	T60.2X3	T60.2X4	—	—
Rotoxamine	T45.0X1	T45.0X2	T45.0X3	T45.0X4	T45.0X5	T45.0X6
Rough-on-rats	T60.4X1	T60.4X2	T60.4X3	T60.4X4	—	—
Roxatidine	T47.0X1	T47.0X2	T47.0X3	T47.0X4	T47.0X5	T47.0X6
Roxithromycin	T36.3X1	T36.3X2	T36.3X3	T36.3X4	T36.3X5	T36.3X6
Rt-PA	T45.611	T45.612	T45.613	T45.614	T45.615	T45.616
Rubbing alcohol	T51.2X1	T51.2X2	T51.2X3	T51.2X4	—	—
Rubefacient	T49.4X1	T49.4X2	T49.4X3	T49.4X4	T49.4X5	T49.4X6
Rubella vaccine	T50.B91	T50.B92	T50.B93	T50.B94	T50.B95	T50.B96
Rubeola vaccine	T50.B91	T50.B92	T50.B93	T50.B94	T50.B95	T50.B96
Rubidium chloride Rb82	T50.8X1	T50.8X2	T50.8X3	T50.8X4	T50.8X5	T50.8X6
Rubidomycin	T45.1X1	T45.1X2	T45.1X3	T45.1X4	T45.1X5	T45.1X6
Rue	T62.2X1	T62.2X2	T62.2X3	T62.2X4	—	—
Rufocromomycin	T45.1X1	T45.1X2	T45.1X3	T45.1X4	T45.1X5	T45.1X6
Russel's viper venin	T45.7X1	T45.7X2	T45.7X3	T45.7X4	T45.7X5	T45.7X6
Ruta (graveolens)	T62.2X1	T62.2X2	T62.2X3	T62.2X4	—	—
Rutinum	T46.991	T46.992	T46.993	T46.994	T46.995	T46.996
Rutoside	T46.991	T46.992	T46.993	T46.994	T46.995	T46.996
b-sitosterol(s)	T46.6X1	T46.6X2	T46.6X3	T46.6X4	T46.6X5	T46.6X6
Sabadilla (plant)	T62.2X1	T62.2X2	T62.2X3	T62.2X4	—	—
pesticide	T60.2X1	T60.2X2	T60.2X3	T60.2X4	—	—
Saccharated iron oxide	T45.8X1	T45.8X2	T45.8X3	T45.8X4	T45.8X5	T45.8X6
Saccharin	T50.901	T50.902	T50.903	T50.904	T50.905	T50.906
Saccharomyces boulardii	T47.6X1	T47.6X2	T47.6X3	T47.6X4	T47.6X5	T47.6X6
Safflower oil	T46.6X1	T46.6X2	T46.6X3	T46.6X4	T46.6X5	T46.6X6
Safrazine	T43.1X1	T43.1X2	T43.1X3	T43.1X4	T43.1X5	T43.1X6
Salazosulfapyridine	T37.0X1	T37.0X2	T37.0X3	T37.0X4	T37.0X5	T37.0X6
Salbutamol	T48.6X1	T48.6X2	T48.6X3	T48.6X4	T48.6X5	T48.6X6
Salicylamide	T39.091	T39.092	T39.093	T39.094	T39.095	T39.096
Salicylate NEC	T39.091	T39.092	T39.093	T39.094	T39.095	T39.096
methyl	T49.3X1	T49.3X2	T49.3X3	T49.3X4	T49.3X5	T49.3X6
theobromine calcium	T50.2X1	T50.2X2	T50.2X3	T50.2X4	T50.2X5	T50.2X6
Salicylazosulfapyridine	T37.0X1	T37.0X2	T37.0X3	T37.0X4	T37.0X5	T37.0X6
Salicylhydroxamic acid	T49.0X1	T49.0X2	T49.0X3	T49.0X4	T49.0X5	T49.0X6
Salicylic acid	T49.4X1	T49.4X2	T49.4X3	T49.4X4	T49.4X5	T49.4X6
with benzoic acid	T49.4X1	T49.4X2	T49.4X3	T49.4X4	T49.4X5	T49.4X6
congeners	T39.091	T39.092	T39.093	T39.094	T39.095	T39.096
derivative	T39.091	T39.092	T39.093	T39.094	T39.095	T39.096
salts	T39.091	T39.092	T39.093	T39.094	T39.095	T39.096
Salinazid	T37.1X1	T37.1X2	T37.1X3	T37.1X4	T37.1X5	T37.1X6
Salmeterol	T48.6X1	T48.6X2	T48.6X3	T48.6X4	T48.6X5	T48.6X6
Salol	T49.3X1	T49.3X2	T49.3X3	T49.3X4	T49.3X5	T49.3X6
Salsalate	T39.091	T39.092	T39.093	T39.094	T39.095	T39.096
Salt-replacing drug	T50.901	T50.902	T50.903	T50.904	T50.905	T50.906
Salt-retaining mineralocorticoid	T50.0X1	T50.0X2	T50.0X3	T50.0X4	T50.0X5	T50.0X6
Salt substitute	T50.901	T50.902	T50.903	T50.904	T50.905	T50.906
Saluretic NEC	T50.2X1	T50.2X2	T50.2X3	T50.2X4	T50.2X5	T50.2X6
Saluron	T50.2X1	T50.2X2	T50.2X3	T50.2X4	T50.2X5	T50.2X6
Salvarsan 606 (neosilver) (silver)	T37.8X1	T37.8X2	T37.8X3	T37.8X4	T37.8X5	T37.8X6
Sambucus canadensis	T62.2X1	T62.2X2	T62.2X3	T62.2X4	—	—
berry	T62.1X1	T62.1X2	T62.1X3	T62.1X4	—	—
Sandril	T46.5X1	T46.5X2	T46.5X3	T46.5X4	T46.5X5	T46.5X6
Sanguinaria canadensis	T62.2X1	T62.2X2	T62.2X3	T62.2X4	—	—
Saniflush (cleaner)	T54.2X1	T54.2X2	T54.2X3	T54.2X4	—	—
Santonin	T37.4X1	T37.4X2	T37.4X3	T37.4X4	T37.4X5	T37.4X6
Santyl	T49.8X1	T49.8X2	T49.8X3	T49.8X4	T49.8X5	T49.8X6
Saralasin	T46.5X1	T46.5X2	T46.5X3	T46.5X4	T46.5X5	T46.5X6
Sarcolysin	T45.1X1	T45.1X2	T45.1X3	T45.1X4	T45.1X5	T45.1X6
Sarkomycin	T45.1X1	T45.1X2	T45.1X3	T45.1X4	T45.1X5	T45.1X6
Saroten	T43.011	T43.012	T43.013	T43.014	T43.015	T43.016
Saturnine — see Lead						
Savin (oil)	T49.4X1	T49.4X2	T49.4X3	T49.4X4	T49.4X5	T49.4X6
Scammony	T47.2X1	T47.2X2	T47.2X3	T47.2X4	T47.2X5	T47.2X6
Scarlet red	T49.8X1	T49.8X2	T49.8X3	T49.8X4	T49.8X5	T49.8X6
Scheele's green	T57.0X1	T57.0X2	T57.0X3	T57.0X4	—	—
insecticide	T57.0X1	T57.0X2	T57.0X3	T57.0X4	—	—
Schizontozide (blood) (tissue)	T37.2X1	T37.2X2	T37.2X3	T37.2X4	T37.2X5	T37.2X6
Schradan	T60.0X1	T60.0X2	T60.0X3	T60.0X4	—	—
Schweinfurth green	T57.0X1	T57.0X2	T57.0X3	T57.0X4	—	—
insecticide	T57.0X1	T57.0X2	T57.0X3	T57.0X4	—	—
Scilla, rat poison	T60.4X1	T60.4X2	T60.4X3	T60.4X4	—	—
Scillaren	T60.4X1	T60.4X2	T60.4X3	T60.4X4	—	—
Sclerosing agent	T46.8X1	T46.8X2	T46.8X3	T46.8X4	T46.8X5	T46.8X6
Scombrotoxin	T61.11	T61.12	T61.13	T61.14	—	—
Scopolamine	T44.3X1	T44.3X2	T44.3X3	T44.3X4	T44.3X5	T44.3X6
Scopolia extract	T44.3X1	T44.3X2	T44.3X3	T44.3X4	T44.3X5	T44.3X6
Scouring powder	T65.891	T65.892	T65.893	T65.894	—	—
Sea						
anemone (sting)	T63.631	T63.632	T63.633	T63.634	—	—
cucumber (sting)	T63.691	T63.692	T63.693	T63.694	—	—
snake (bite) (venom)	T63.091	T63.092	T63.093	T63.094	—	—
urchin spine (puncture)	T63.691	T63.692	T63.693	T63.694	—	—
Seafood	T61.91	T61.92	T61.93	T61.94	—	—
specified NEC	T61.8X1	T61.8X2	T61.8X3	T61.8X4	—	—
Secbutabarbital	T42.3X1	T42.3X2	T42.3X3	T42.3X4	T42.3X5	T42.3X6
Secbutabarbitone	T42.3X1	T42.3X2	T42.3X3	T42.3X4	T42.3X5	T42.3X6
Secnidazole	T37.3X1	T37.3X2	T37.3X3	T37.3X4	T37.3X5	T37.3X6
Secobarbital	T42.3X1	T42.3X2	T42.3X3	T42.3X4	T42.3X5	T42.3X6
Seconal	T42.3X1	T42.3X2	T42.3X3	T42.3X4	T42.3X5	T42.3X6
Secretin	T50.8X1	T50.8X2	T50.8X3	T50.8X4	T50.8X5	T50.8X6
Sedative NEC	T42.71	T42.72	T42.73	T42.74	T42.75	T42.76
mixed NEC	T42.6X1	T42.6X2	T42.6X3	T42.6X4	T42.6X5	T42.6X6
Sedormid	T42.6X1	T42.6X2	T42.6X3	T42.6X4	T42.6X5	T42.6X6
Seed disinfectant or dressing	T60.8X1	T60.8X2	T60.8X3	T60.8X4	—	—
Seeds (poisonous)	T62.2X1	T62.2X2	T62.2X3	T62.2X4	—	—
Selegiline	T42.8X1	T42.8X2	T42.8X3	T42.8X4	T42.8X5	T42.8X6
Selenium NEC	T56.891	T56.892	T56.893	T56.894	—	—
disulfide or sulfide	T49.4X1	T49.4X2	T49.4X3	T49.4X4	T49.4X5	T49.4X6
fumes	T59.891	T59.892	T59.893	T59.894	—	—
sulfide	T49.4X1	T49.4X2	T49.4X3	T49.4X4	T49.4X5	T49.4X6
Selenomethionine (75Se)	T50.8X1	T50.8X2	T50.8X3	T50.8X4	T50.8X5	T50.8X6
Selsun	T49.4X1	T49.4X2	T49.4X3	T49.4X4	T49.4X5	T49.4X6
Semustine	T45.1X1	T45.1X2	T45.1X3	T45.1X4	T45.1X5	T45.1X6
Senega syrup	T48.4X1	T48.4X2	T48.4X3	T48.4X4	T48.4X5	T48.4X6
Senna	T47.2X1	T47.2X2	T47.2X3	T47.2X4	T47.2X5	T47.2X6
Sennoside A+B	T47.2X1	T47.2X2	T47.2X3	T47.2X4	T47.2X5	T47.2X6
Septisol	T49.2X1	T49.2X2	T49.2X3	T49.2X4	T49.2X5	T49.2X6
Seractide	T38.811	T38.812	T38.813	T38.814	T38.815	T38.816
Serax	T42.4X1	T42.4X2	T42.4X3	T42.4X4	T42.4X5	T42.4X6
Serenesil	T42.6X1	T42.6X2	T42.6X3	T42.6X4	T42.6X5	T42.6X6
Serenium (hydrochloride)	T37.91	T37.92	T37.93	T37.94	T37.95	T37.96
Serepax — see Oxazepam						
Sermorelin	T38.891	T38.892	T38.893	T38.894	T38.895	T38.896
Sernyl	T41.1X1	T41.1X2	T41.1X3	T41.1X4	T41.1X5	T41.1X6
Serotonin	T50.991	T50.992	T50.993	T50.994	T50.995	T50.996
Serpasil	T46.5X1	T46.5X2	T46.5X3	T46.5X4	T46.5X5	T46.5X6
Serrapeptase	T45.3X1	T45.3X2	T45.3X3	T45.3X4	T45.3X5	T45.3X6
Serum						
antibotulinus	T50.Z11	T50.Z12	T50.Z13	T50.Z14	T50.Z15	T50.Z16
anticytotoxic	T50.Z11	T50.Z12	T50.Z13	T50.Z14	T50.Z15	T50.Z16
antidiphtheria	T50.Z11	T50.Z12	T50.Z13	T50.Z14	T50.Z15	T50.Z16
antimeningococcus	T50.Z11	T50.Z12	T50.Z13	T50.Z14	T50.Z15	T50.Z16
anti-Rh	T50.Z11	T50.Z12	T50.Z13	T50.Z14	T50.Z15	T50.Z16
anti-snake-bite	T50.Z11	T50.Z12	T50.Z13	T50.Z14	T50.Z15	T50.Z16
antitetanic	T50.Z11	T50.Z12	T50.Z13	T50.Z14	T50.Z15	T50.Z16
antitoxic	T50.Z11	T50.Z12	T50.Z13	T50.Z14	T50.Z15	T50.Z16
complement (inhibitor)	T45.8X1	T45.8X2	T45.8X3	T45.8X4	T45.8X5	T45.8X6
convalescent	T50.Z11	T50.Z12	T50.Z13	T50.Z14	T50.Z15	T50.Z16
hemolytic complement	T45.8X1	T45.8X2	T45.8X3	T45.8X4	T45.8X5	T45.8X6
immune (human)	T50.Z11	T50.Z12	T50.Z13	T50.Z14	T50.Z15	T50.Z16
protective NEC	T50.Z11	T50.Z12	T50.Z13	T50.Z14	T50.Z15	T50.Z16
Setastine	T45.0X1	T45.0X2	T45.0X3	T45.0X4	T45.0X5	T45.0X6
Setoperone	T43.591	T43.592	T43.593	T43.594	T43.595	T43.596
Sewer gas	T59.91	T59.92	T59.93	T59.94	—	—
Shampoo	T55.0X1	T55.0X2	T55.0X3	T55.0X4	—	—
Shellfish, noxious, nonbacterial	T61.781	T61.782	T61.783	T61.784	—	—
Sildenafil	T46.7X1	T46.7X2	T46.7X3	T46.7X4	T46.7X5	T46.7X6
Silibinin	T50.991	T50.992	T50.993	T50.994	T50.995	T50.996
Silicone NEC	T65.891	T65.892	T65.893	T65.894	—	—
medicinal	T49.3X1	T49.3X2	T49.3X3	T49.3X4	T49.3X5	T49.3X6
Silvadene	T49.0X1	T49.0X2	T49.0X3	T49.0X4	T49.0X5	T49.0X6
Silver	T49.0X1	T49.0X2	T49.0X3	T49.0X4	T49.0X5	T49.0X6
anti-infectives	T49.0X1	T49.0X2	T49.0X3	T49.0X4	T49.0X5	T49.0X6
arsphenamine	T37.8X1	T37.8X2	T37.8X3	T37.8X4	T37.8X5	T37.8X6
colloidal	T49.0X1	T49.0X2	T49.0X3	T49.0X4	T49.0X5	T49.0X6
nitrate	T49.0X1	T49.0X2	T49.0X3	T49.0X4	T49.0X5	T49.0X6
ophthalmic preparation	T49.5X1	T49.5X2	T49.5X3	T49.5X4	T49.5X5	T49.5X6
toughened (keratolytic)	T49.4X1	T49.4X2	T49.4X3	T49.4X4	T49.4X5	T49.4X6
nonmedicinal (dust)	T56.891	T56.892	T56.893	T56.894	—	—
protein	T49.5X1	T49.5X2	T49.5X3	T49.5X4	T49.5X5	T49.5X6
salvarsan	T37.8X1	T37.8X2	T37.8X3	T37.8X4	T37.8X5	T37.8X6
sulfadiazine	T49.4X1	T49.4X2	T49.4X3	T49.4X4	T49.4X5	T49.4X6
Silymarin	T50.991	T50.992	T50.993	T50.994	T50.995	T50.996
Simaldrate	T47.1X1	T47.1X2	T47.1X3	T47.1X4	T47.1X5	T47.1X6
Simazine	T60.3X1	T60.3X2	T60.3X3	T60.3X4	—	—
Simethicone	T47.1X1	T47.1X2	T47.1X3	T47.1X4	T47.1X5	T47.1X6

Additional Character May Be Required — Refer to the Tabular List for Character Selection   ▽ **Subterms under main terms may continue to next column or page**

Substance	Poisoning, Accidental (unintentional)	Poisoning, Intentional Self-harm	Poisoning, Assault	Poisoning, Undetermined	Adverse Effect	Under-dosing
Simfibrate	T46.6X1	T46.6X2	T46.6X3	T46.6X4	T46.6X5	T46.6X6
Simvastatin	T46.6X1	T46.6X2	T46.6X3	T46.6X4	T46.6X5	T46.6X6
Sincalide	T50.8X1	T50.8X2	T50.8X3	T50.8X4	T50.8X5	T50.8X6
Sinequan	T43.011	T43.012	T43.013	T43.014	T43.015	T43.016
Singoserp	T46.5X1	T46.5X2	T46.5X3	T46.5X4	T46.5X5	T46.5X6
Sintrom	T45.511	T45.512	T45.513	T45.514	T45.515	T45.516
Sisomicin	T36.5X1	T36.5X2	T36.5X3	T36.5X4	T36.5X5	T36.5X6
Sitosterols	T46.6X1	T46.6X2	T46.6X3	T46.6X4	T46.6X5	T46.6X6
Skeletal muscle relaxants	T48.1X1	T48.1X2	T48.1X3	T48.1X4	T48.1X5	T48.1X6
Skin						
agents (external)	T49.91	T49.92	T49.93	T49.94	T49.95	T49.96
specified NEC	T49.8X1	T49.8X2	T49.8X3	T49.8X4	T49.8X5	T49.8X6
test antigen	T50.8X1	T50.8X2	T50.8X3	T50.8X4	T50.8X5	T50.8X6
Sleep-eze	T45.0X1	T45.0X2	T45.0X3	T45.0X4	T45.0X5	T45.0X6
Sleeping draught, pill	T42.71	T42.72	T42.73	T42.74	T42.75	T42.76
Smallpox vaccine	T50.B11	T50.B12	T50.B13	T50.B14	T50.B15	T50.B16
Smelter fumes NEC	T56.91	T56.92	T56.93	T56.94	—	—
Smog	T59.1X1	T59.1X2	T59.1X3	T59.1X4	—	—
Smoke NEC	T59.811	T59.812	T59.813	T59.814	—	—
Smooth muscle relaxant	T44.3X1	T44.3X2	T44.3X3	T44.3X4	T44.3X5	T44.3X6
Snail killer NEC	T60.8X1	T60.8X2	T60.8X3	T60.8X4	—	—
Snake venom or bite	T63.001	T63.002	T63.003	T63.004	—	—
hemocoagulase	T45.7X1	T45.7X2	T45.7X3	T45.7X4	T45.7X5	T45.7X6
Snuff	T65.211	T65.212	T65.213	T65.214	—	—
Soap (powder) (product)	T55.0X1	T55.0X2	T55.0X3	T55.0X4	—	—
enema	T47.4X1	T47.4X2	T47.4X3	T47.4X4	T47.4X5	T47.4X6
medicinal, soft	T49.2X1	T49.2X2	T49.2X3	T49.2X4	T49.2X5	T49.2X6
superfatted	T49.2X1	T49.2X2	T49.2X3	T49.2X4	T49.2X5	T49.2X6
Sobrerol	T48.4X1	T48.4X2	T48.4X3	T48.4X4	T48.4X5	T48.4X6
Soda (caustic)	T54.3X1	T54.3X2	T54.3X3	T54.3X4	—	—
bicarb	T47.1X1	T47.1X2	T47.1X3	T47.1X4	T47.1X5	T47.1X6
chlorinated — see Sodium, hypochlorite						
Sodium						
acetosulfone	T37.1X1	T37.1X2	T37.1X3	T37.1X4	T37.1X5	T37.1X6
acetrizoate	T50.8X1	T50.8X2	T50.8X3	T50.8X4	T50.8X5	T50.8X6
acid phosphate	T50.3X1	T50.3X2	T50.3X3	T50.3X4	T50.3X5	T50.3X6
alginate	T47.8X1	T47.8X2	T47.8X3	T47.8X4	T47.8X5	T47.8X6
amidotrizoate	T50.8X1	T50.8X2	T50.8X3	T50.8X4	T50.8X5	T50.8X6
aminopterin	T45.1X1	T45.1X2	T45.1X3	T45.1X4	T45.1X5	T45.1X6
amylosulfate	T47.8X1	T47.8X2	T47.8X3	T47.8X4	T47.8X5	T47.8X6
amytal	T42.3X1	T42.3X2	T42.3X3	T42.3X4	T42.3X5	T42.3X6
antimony gluconate	T37.3X1	T37.3X2	T37.3X3	T37.3X4	T37.3X5	T37.3X6
arsenate	T57.0X1	T57.0X2	T57.0X3	T57.0X4	—	—
aurothiomalate	T39.4X1	T39.4X2	T39.4X3	T39.4X4	T39.4X5	T39.4X6
aurothiosulfate	T39.4X1	T39.4X2	T39.4X3	T39.4X4	T39.4X5	T39.4X6
barbiturate	T42.3X1	T42.3X2	T42.3X3	T42.3X4	T42.3X5	T42.3X6
basic phosphate	T47.4X1	T47.4X2	T47.4X3	T47.4X4	T47.4X5	T47.4X6
bicarbonate	T47.1X1	T47.1X2	T47.1X3	T47.1X4	T47.1X5	T47.1X6
bichromate	T57.8X1	T57.8X2	T57.8X3	T57.8X4	—	—
biphosphate	T50.3X1	T50.3X2	T50.3X3	T50.3X4	T50.3X5	T50.3X6
bisulfate	T65.891	T65.892	T65.893	T65.894	—	—
borate						
cleanser	T57.8X1	T57.8X2	T57.8X3	T57.8X4	—	—
eye	T49.5X1	T49.5X2	T49.5X3	T49.5X4	T49.5X5	T49.5X6
therapeutic	T49.8X1	T49.8X2	T49.8X3	T49.8X4	T49.8X5	T49.8X6
bromide	T42.6X1	T42.6X2	T42.6X3	T42.6X4	T42.6X5	T42.6X6
cacodylate (nonmedicinal) NEC	T50.8X1	T50.8X2	T50.8X3	T50.8X4	T50.8X5	T50.8X6
anti-infective	T37.8X1	T37.8X2	T37.8X3	T37.8X4	T37.8X5	T37.8X6
herbicide	T60.3X1	T60.3X2	T60.3X3	T60.3X4	—	—
calcium edetate	T45.8X1	T45.8X2	T45.8X3	T45.8X4	T45.8X5	T45.8X6
carbonate NEC	T54.3X1	T54.3X2	T54.3X3	T54.3X4	—	—
chlorate NEC	T65.891	T65.892	T65.893	T65.894	—	—
herbicide	T54.91	T54.92	T54.93	T54.94	—	—
chloride	T50.3X1	T50.3X2	T50.3X3	T50.3X4	T50.3X5	T50.3X6
with glucose	T50.3X1	T50.3X2	T50.3X3	T50.3X4	T50.3X5	T50.3X6
chromate	T65.891	T65.892	T65.893	T65.894	—	—
citrate	T50.991	T50.992	T50.993	T50.994	T50.995	T50.996
cromoglicate	T48.6X1	T48.6X2	T48.6X3	T48.6X4	T48.6X5	T48.6X6
cyanide	T65.0X1	T65.0X2	T65.0X3	T65.0X4	—	—
cyclamate	T50.3X1	T50.3X2	T50.3X3	T50.3X4	T50.3X5	T50.3X6
dehydrocholate	T45.8X1	T45.8X2	T45.8X3	T45.8X4	T45.8X5	T45.8X6
diatrizoate	T50.8X1	T50.8X2	T50.8X3	T50.8X4	T50.8X5	T50.8X6
dibunate	T48.4X1	T48.4X2	T48.4X3	T48.4X4	T48.4X5	T48.4X6
dioctyl sulfosuccinate	T47.4X1	T47.4X2	T47.4X3	T47.4X4	T47.4X5	T47.4X6
dipantoyl ferrate	T45.8X1	T45.8X2	T45.8X3	T45.8X4	T45.8X5	T45.8X6
edetate	T45.8X1	T45.8X2	T45.8X3	T45.8X4	T45.8X5	T45.8X6
ethacrynate	T50.1X1	T50.1X2	T50.1X3	T50.1X4	T50.1X5	T50.1X6
feredetate	T45.8X1	T45.8X2	T45.8X3	T45.8X4	T45.8X5	T45.8X6
Fluoride — see Fluoride						
fluoroacetate (dust) (pesticide)	T60.4X1	T60.4X2	T60.4X3	T60.4X4	—	—

Substance	Poisoning, Accidental (unintentional)	Poisoning, Intentional Self-harm	Poisoning, Assault	Poisoning, Undetermined	Adverse Effect	Under-dosing
Sodium — continued						
free salt	T50.3X1	T50.3X2	T50.3X3	T50.3X4	T50.3X5	T50.3X6
fusidate	T36.8X1	T36.8X2	T36.8X3	T36.8X4	T36.8X5	T36.8X6
glucaldrate	T47.1X1	T47.1X2	T47.1X3	T47.1X4	T47.1X5	T47.1X6
glucosulfone	T37.1X1	T37.1X2	T37.1X3	T37.1X4	T37.1X5	T37.1X6
glutamate	T45.8X1	T45.8X2	T45.8X3	T45.8X4	T45.8X5	T45.8X6
hydrogen carbonate	T50.3X1	T50.3X2	T50.3X3	T50.3X4	T50.3X5	T50.3X6
hydroxide	T54.3X1	T54.3X2	T54.3X3	T54.3X4	—	—
hypochlorite (bleach) NEC	T54.3X1	T54.3X2	T54.3X3	T54.3X4	—	—
disinfectant	T54.3X1	T54.3X2	T54.3X3	T54.3X4	—	—
medicinal (anti-infective) (external)	T49.0X1	T49.0X2	T49.0X3	T49.0X4	T49.0X5	T49.0X6
vapor	T54.3X1	T54.3X2	T54.3X3	T54.3X4	—	—
hyposulfite	T49.0X1	T49.0X2	T49.0X3	T49.0X4	T49.0X5	T49.0X6
indigotin disulfonate	T50.8X1	T50.8X2	T50.8X3	T50.8X4	T50.8X5	T50.8X6
iodide	T50.991	T50.992	T50.993	T50.994	T50.995	T50.996
I-131	T50.8X1	T50.8X2	T50.8X3	T50.8X4	T50.8X5	T50.8X6
therapeutic	T38.2X1	T38.2X2	T38.2X3	T38.2X4	T38.2X5	T38.2X6
iodohippurate (131I)	T50.8X1	T50.8X2	T50.8X3	T50.8X4	T50.8X5	T50.8X6
iopodate	T50.8X1	T50.8X2	T50.8X3	T50.8X4	T50.8X5	T50.8X6
iothalamate	T50.8X1	T50.8X2	T50.8X3	T50.8X4	T50.8X5	T50.8X6
iron edetate	T45.4X1	T45.4X2	T45.4X3	T45.4X4	T45.4X5	T45.4X6
lactate (compound solution)	T45.8X1	T45.8X2	T45.8X3	T45.8X4	T45.8X5	T45.8X6
lauryl (sulfate)	T49.2X1	T49.2X2	T49.2X3	T49.2X4	T49.2X5	T49.2X6
L-triiodothyronine	T38.1X1	T38.1X2	T38.1X3	T38.1X4	T38.1X5	T38.1X6
magnesium citrate	T50.991	T50.992	T50.993	T50.994	T50.995	T50.996
mersalate	T50.2X1	T50.2X2	T50.2X3	T50.2X4	T50.2X5	T50.2X6
metasilicate	T65.891	T65.892	T65.893	T65.894	—	—
metrizoate	T50.8X1	T50.8X2	T50.8X3	T50.8X4	T50.8X5	T50.8X6
monofluoroacetate (pesticide)	T60.1X1	T60.1X2	T60.1X3	T60.1X4	—	—
morrhuate	T46.8X1	T46.8X2	T46.8X3	T46.8X4	T46.8X5	T46.8X6
nafcillin	T36.0X1	T36.0X2	T36.0X3	T36.0X4	T36.0X5	T36.0X6
nitrate (oxidizing agent)	T65.891	T65.892	T65.893	T65.894	—	—
nitrite	T50.6X1	T50.6X2	T50.6X3	T50.6X4	T50.6X5	T50.6X6
nitroferricyanide	T46.5X1	T46.5X2	T46.5X3	T46.5X4	T46.5X5	T46.5X6
nitroprusside	T46.5X1	T46.5X2	T46.5X3	T46.5X4	T46.5X5	T46.5X6
oxalate	T65.891	T65.892	T65.893	T65.894	—	—
oxide/peroxide	T65.891	T65.892	T65.893	T65.894	—	—
oxybate	T41.291	T41.292	T41.293	T41.294	T41.295	T41.296
para-aminohippurate	T50.8X1	T50.8X2	T50.8X3	T50.8X4	T50.8X5	T50.8X6
perborate (nonmedicinal) NEC	T65.891	T65.892	T65.893	T65.894	—	—
medicinal	T49.0X1	T49.0X2	T49.0X3	T49.0X4	T49.0X5	T49.0X6
soap	T55.0X1	T55.0X2	T55.0X3	T55.0X4	—	—
percarbonate — see Sodium, perborate						
pertechnetate Tc99m	T50.8X1	T50.8X2	T50.8X3	T50.8X4	T50.8X5	T50.8X6
phosphate						
cellulose	T45.8X1	T45.8X2	T45.8X3	T45.8X4	T45.8X5	T45.8X6
dibasic	T47.2X1	T47.2X2	T47.2X3	T47.2X4	T47.2X5	T47.2X6
monobasic	T47.2X1	T47.2X2	T47.2X3	T47.2X4	T47.2X5	T47.2X6
phytate	T50.6X1	T50.6X2	T50.6X3	T50.6X4	T50.6X5	T50.6X6
picosulfate	T47.2X1	T47.2X2	T47.2X3	T47.2X4	T47.2X5	T47.2X6
polyhydroxyaluminium monocarbonate	T47.1X1	T47.1X2	T47.1X3	T47.1X4	T47.1X5	T47.1X6
polystyrene sulfonate	T50.3X1	T50.3X2	T50.3X3	T50.3X4	T50.3X5	T50.3X6
propionate	T49.0X1	T49.0X2	T49.0X3	T49.0X4	T49.0X5	T49.0X6
propyl hydroxybenzoate	T50.991	T50.992	T50.993	T50.994	T50.995	T50.996
psylliate	T46.8X1	T46.8X2	T46.8X3	T46.8X4	T46.8X5	T46.8X6
removing resins	T50.3X1	T50.3X2	T50.3X3	T50.3X4	T50.3X5	T50.3X6
salicylate	T39.091	T39.092	T39.093	T39.094	T39.095	T39.096
salt NEC	T50.3X1	T50.3X2	T50.3X3	T50.3X4	T50.3X5	T50.3X6
selenate	T60.2X1	T60.2X2	T60.2X3	T60.2X4	—	—
stibogluconate	T37.3X1	T37.3X2	T37.3X3	T37.3X4	T37.3X5	T37.3X6
sulfate	T47.4X1	T47.4X2	T47.4X3	T47.4X4	T47.4X5	T47.4X6
sulfoxone	T37.1X1	T37.1X2	T37.1X3	T37.1X4	T37.1X5	T37.1X6
tetradecyl sulfate	T46.8X1	T46.8X2	T46.8X3	T46.8X4	T46.8X5	T46.8X6
thiopental	T41.1X1	T41.1X2	T41.1X3	T41.1X4	T41.1X5	T41.1X6
thiosalicylate	T39.091	T39.092	T39.093	T39.094	T39.095	T39.096
thiosulfate	T50.6X1	T50.6X2	T50.6X3	T50.6X4	T50.6X5	T50.6X6
tolbutamide	T38.3X1	T38.3X2	T38.3X3	T38.3X4	T38.3X5	T38.3X6
(L)-triiodothyronine	T38.1X1	T38.1X2	T38.1X3	T38.1X4	T38.1X5	T38.1X6
tyropanoate	T50.8X1	T50.8X2	T50.8X3	T50.8X4	T50.8X5	T50.8X6
valproate	T42.6X1	T42.6X2	T42.6X3	T42.6X4	T42.6X5	T42.6X6
versenate	T50.6X1	T50.6X2	T50.6X3	T50.6X4	T50.6X5	T50.6X6
Sodium-free salt	T50.901	T50.902	T50.903	T50.904	T50.905	T50.906
Sodium-removing resin	T50.3X1	T50.3X2	T50.3X3	T50.3X4	T50.3X5	T50.3X6
Soft soap	T55.0X1	T55.0X2	T55.0X3	T55.0X4	—	—
Solanine	T62.2X1	T62.2X2	T62.2X3	T62.2X4	—	—
berries	T62.1X1	T62.1X2	T62.1X3	T62.1X4	—	—
Solanum dulcamara	T62.2X1	T62.2X2	T62.2X3	T62.2X4	—	—

Substance	Poisoning, Accidental (unintentional)	Poisoning, Intentional Self-harm	Poisoning, Assault	Poisoning, Undetermined	Adverse Effect	Under-dosing
Solanum dulcamara — continued						
berries	T62.1X1	T62.1X2	T62.1X3	T62.1X4	—	—
Solapsone	T37.1X1	T37.1X2	T37.1X3	T37.1X4	T37.1X5	T37.1X6
Solar lotion	T49.3X1	T49.3X2	T49.3X3	T49.3X4	T49.3X5	T49.3X6
Solasulfone	T37.1X1	T37.1X2	T37.1X3	T37.1X4	T37.1X5	T37.1X6
Soldering fluid	T65.891	T65.892	T65.893	T65.894	—	—
Solid substance	T65.91	T65.92	T65.93	T65.94	—	—
specified NEC	T65.891	T65.892	T65.893	T65.894	—	—
Solvent, industrial NEC	T52.91	T52.92	T52.93	T52.94	—	—
naphtha	T52.0X1	T52.0X2	T52.0X3	T52.0X4	—	—
petroleum	T52.0X1	T52.0X2	T52.0X3	T52.0X4	—	—
specified NEC	T52.8X1	T52.8X2	T52.8X3	T52.8X4	—	—
Soma	T42.8X1	T42.8X2	T42.8X3	T42.8X4	T42.8X5	T42.8X6
Somatorelin	T38.891	T38.892	T38.893	T38.894	T38.895	T38.896
Somatostatin	T38.991	T38.992	T38.993	T38.994	T38.995	T38.996
Somatotropin	T38.811	T38.812	T38.813	T38.814	T38.815	T38.816
Somatrem	T38.811	T38.812	T38.813	T38.814	T38.815	T38.816
Somatropin	T38.811	T38.812	T38.813	T38.814	T38.815	T38.816
Sominex	T45.0X1	T45.0X2	T45.0X3	T45.0X4	T45.0X5	T45.0X6
Somnos	T42.6X1	T42.6X2	T42.6X3	T42.6X4	T42.6X5	T42.6X6
Somonal	T42.3X1	T42.3X2	T42.3X3	T42.3X4	T42.3X5	T42.3X6
Soneryl	T42.3X1	T42.3X2	T42.3X3	T42.3X4	T42.3X5	T42.3X6
Soothing syrup	T50.901	T50.902	T50.903	T50.904	T50.905	T50.906
Sopor	T42.6X1	T42.6X2	T42.6X3	T42.6X4	T42.6X5	T42.6X6
Soporific	T42.71	T42.72	T42.73	T42.74	T42.75	T42.76
Soporific drug	T42.71	T42.72	T42.73	T42.74	T42.75	T42.76
specified type NEC	T42.6X1	T42.6X2	T42.6X3	T42.6X4	T42.6X5	T42.6X6
Sorbide nitrate	T46.3X1	T46.3X2	T46.3X3	T46.3X4	T46.3X5	T46.3X6
Sorbitol	T47.4X1	T47.4X2	T47.4X3	T47.4X4	T47.4X5	T47.4X6
Sotalol	T44.7X1	T44.7X2	T44.7X3	T44.7X4	T44.7X5	T44.7X6
Sotradecol	T46.8X1	T46.8X2	T46.8X3	T46.8X4	T46.8X5	T46.8X6
Soysterol	T46.6X1	T46.6X2	T46.6X3	T46.6X4	T46.6X5	T46.6X6
Spacoline	T44.3X1	T44.3X2	T44.3X3	T44.3X4	T44.3X5	T44.3X6
Spanish fly	T49.8X1	T49.8X2	T49.8X3	T49.8X4	T49.8X5	T49.8X6
Sparine	T43.3X1	T43.3X2	T43.3X3	T43.3X4	T43.3X5	T43.3X6
Sparteine	T48.0X1	T48.0X2	T48.0X3	T48.0X4	T48.0X5	T48.0X6
Spasmolytic						
anticholinergics	T44.3X1	T44.3X2	T44.3X3	T44.3X4	T44.3X5	T44.3X6
autonomic	T44.3X1	T44.3X2	T44.3X3	T44.3X4	T44.3X5	T44.3X6
bronchial NEC	T48.6X1	T48.6X2	T48.6X3	T48.6X4	T48.6X5	T48.6X6
quaternary ammonium	T44.3X1	T44.3X2	T44.3X3	T44.3X4	T44.3X5	T44.3X6
skeletal muscle NEC	T48.1X1	T48.1X2	T48.1X3	T48.1X4	T48.1X5	T48.1X6
Spectinomycin	T36.5X1	T36.5X2	T36.5X3	T36.5X4	T36.5X5	T36.5X6
Speed	T43.621	T43.622	T43.623	T43.624	T43.625	T43.626
Spermicide	T49.8X1	T49.8X2	T49.8X3	T49.8X4	T49.8X5	T49.8X6
Spider (bite) (venom)	T63.391	T63.392	T63.393	T63.394	—	—
antivenin	T50.Z11	T50.Z12	T50.Z13	T50.Z14	T50.Z15	T50.Z16
Spigelia (root)	T37.4X1	T37.4X2	T37.4X3	T37.4X4	T37.4X5	T37.4X6
Spindle inactivator	T50.4X1	T50.4X2	T50.4X3	T50.4X4	T50.4X5	T50.4X6
Spiperone	T43.4X1	T43.4X2	T43.4X3	T43.4X4	T43.4X5	T43.4X6
Spiramycin	T36.3X1	T36.3X2	T36.3X3	T36.3X4	T36.3X5	T36.3X6
Spirapril	T46.4X1	T46.4X2	T46.4X3	T46.4X4	T46.4X5	T46.4X6
Spirilene	T43.591	T43.592	T43.593	T43.594	T43.595	T43.596
Spirit(s) (neutral) NEC	T51.0X1	T51.0X2	T51.0X3	T51.0X4	—	—
beverage	T51.0X1	T51.0X2	T51.0X3	T51.0X4	—	—
industrial	T51.0X1	T51.0X2	T51.0X3	T51.0X4	—	—
mineral	T52.0X1	T52.0X2	T52.0X3	T52.0X4	—	—
of salt — see Hydrochloric acid						
surgical	T51.0X1	T51.0X2	T51.0X3	T51.0X4	—	—
Spironolactone	T50.0X1	T50.0X2	T50.0X3	T50.0X4	T50.0X5	T50.0X6
Spiroperidol	T43.4X1	T43.4X2	T43.4X3	T43.4X4	T43.4X5	T43.4X6
Sponge, absorbable (gelatin)	T45.7X1	T45.7X2	T45.7X3	T45.7X4	T45.7X5	T45.7X6
Sporostacin	T49.0X1	T49.0X2	T49.0X3	T49.0X4	T49.0X5	T49.0X6
Spray (aerosol)	T65.91	T65.92	T65.93	T65.94	—	—
cosmetic	T65.891	T65.892	T65.893	T65.894	—	—
medicinal NEC	T50.901	T50.902	T50.903	T50.904	T50.905	T50.906
pesticides — see Pesticides						
specified content — see specific substance						
Spurge flax	T62.2X1	T62.2X2	T62.2X3	T62.2X4	—	—
Spurges	T62.2X1	T62.2X2	T62.2X3	T62.2X4	—	—
Sputum viscosity-lowering drug	T48.4X1	T48.4X2	T48.4X3	T48.4X4	T48.4X5	T48.4X6
Squill	T46.0X1	T46.0X2	T46.0X3	T46.0X4	T46.0X5	T46.0X6
rat poison	T60.4X1	T60.4X2	T60.4X3	T60.4X4	—	—
Squirting cucumber (cathartic)	T47.2X1	T47.2X2	T47.2X3	T47.2X4	T47.2X5	T47.2X6
Stains	T65.6X1	T65.6X2	T65.6X3	T65.6X4	—	—
Stannous fluoride	T49.7X1	T49.7X2	T49.7X3	T49.7X4	T49.7X5	T49.7X6
Stanolone	T38.7X1	T38.7X2	T38.7X3	T38.7X4	T38.7X5	T38.7X6
Stanozolol	T38.7X1	T38.7X2	T38.7X3	T38.7X4	T38.7X5	T38.7X6

Substance	Poisoning, Accidental (unintentional)	Poisoning, Intentional Self-harm	Poisoning, Assault	Poisoning, Undetermined	Adverse Effect	Under-dosing
Staphisagria or stavesacre (pediculicide)	T49.0X1	T49.0X2	T49.0X3	T49.0X4	T49.0X5	T49.0X6
Starch	T50.901	T50.902	T50.903	T50.904	T50.905	T50.906
Stelazine	T43.3X1	T43.3X2	T43.3X3	T43.3X4	T43.3X5	T43.3X6
Stemetil	T43.3X1	T43.3X2	T43.3X3	T43.3X4	T43.3X5	T43.3X6
Stepronin	T48.4X1	T48.4X2	T48.4X3	T48.4X4	T48.4X5	T48.4X6
Sterculia	T47.4X1	T47.4X2	T47.4X3	T47.4X4	T47.4X5	T47.4X6
Sternutator gas	T59.891	T59.892	T59.893	T59.894	—	—
Steroid	T38.0X1	T38.0X2	T38.0X3	T38.0X4	T38.0X5	T38.0X6
anabolic	T38.7X1	T38.7X2	T38.7X3	T38.7X4	T38.7X5	T38.7X6
androgenic	T38.7X1	T38.7X2	T38.7X3	T38.7X4	T38.7X5	T38.7X6
antineoplastic, hormone	T38.7X1	T38.7X2	T38.7X3	T38.7X4	T38.7X5	T38.7X6
estrogen	T38.5X1	T38.5X2	T38.5X3	T38.5X4	T38.5X5	T38.5X6
ENT agent	T49.6X1	T49.6X2	T49.6X3	T49.6X4	T49.6X5	T49.6X6
ophthalmic preparation	T49.5X1	T49.5X2	T49.5X3	T49.5X4	T49.5X5	T49.5X6
topical NEC	T49.0X1	T49.0X2	T49.0X3	T49.0X4	T49.0X5	T49.0X6
Stibine	T56.891	T56.892	T56.893	T56.894	—	—
Stibogluconate	T37.3X1	T37.3X2	T37.3X3	T37.3X4	T37.3X5	T37.3X6
Stibophen	T37.4X1	T37.4X2	T37.4X3	T37.4X4	T37.4X5	T37.4X6
Stilbamidine (isetionate)	T37.3X1	T37.3X2	T37.3X3	T37.3X4	T37.3X5	T37.3X6
Stilbestrol	T38.5X1	T38.5X2	T38.5X3	T38.5X4	T38.5X5	T38.5X6
Stilboestrol	T38.5X1	T38.5X2	T38.5X3	T38.5X4	T38.5X5	T38.5X6
Stimulant						
central nervous system — see also Psychostimulant	T43.601	T43.602	T43.603	T43.604	T43.605	T43.606
analeptics	T50.7X1	T50.7X2	T50.7X3	T50.7X4	T50.7X5	T50.7X6
opiate antagonist	T50.7X1	T50.7X2	T50.7X3	T50.7X4	T50.7X5	T50.7X6
psychotherapeutic NEC — see also Psychotherapeutic drug	T43.601	T43.602	T43.603	T43.604	T43.605	T43.606
specified NEC	T43.691	T43.692	T43.693	T43.694	T43.695	T43.696
respiratory	T48.901	T48.902	T48.903	T48.904	T48.905	T48.906
Stone-dissolving drug	T50.901	T50.902	T50.903	T50.904	T50.905	T50.906
Storage battery (cells) (acid)	T54.2X1	T54.2X2	T54.2X3	T54.2X4	—	—
Stovaine	T41.3X1	T41.3X2	T41.3X3	T41.3X4	T41.3X5	T41.3X6
infiltration (subcutaneous)	T41.3X1	T41.3X2	T41.3X3	T41.3X4	T41.3X5	T41.3X6
nerve block (peripheral) (plexus)	T41.3X1	T41.3X2	T41.3X3	T41.3X4	T41.3X5	T41.3X6
spinal	T41.3X1	T41.3X2	T41.3X3	T41.3X4	T41.3X5	T41.3X6
topical (surface)	T41.3X1	T41.3X2	T41.3X3	T41.3X4	T41.3X5	T41.3X6
Stovarsal	T37.8X1	T37.8X2	T37.8X3	T37.8X4	T37.8X5	T37.8X6
Stove gas — see Gas, stove						
Stoxil	T49.5X1	T49.5X2	T49.5X3	T49.5X4	T49.5X5	T49.5X6
Stramonium	T48.6X1	T48.6X2	T48.6X3	T48.6X4	T48.6X5	T48.6X6
natural state	T62.2X1	T62.2X2	T62.2X3	T62.2X4	—	—
Streptodornase	T45.3X1	T45.3X2	T45.3X3	T45.3X4	T45.3X5	T45.3X6
Streptoduocin	T36.5X1	T36.5X2	T36.5X3	T36.5X4	T36.5X5	T36.5X6
Streptokinase	T45.611	T45.612	T45.613	T45.614	T45.615	T45.616
Streptomycin (derivative)	T36.5X1	T36.5X2	T36.5X3	T36.5X4	T36.5X5	T36.5X6
Streptonivicin	T36.5X1	T36.5X2	T36.5X3	T36.5X4	T36.5X5	T36.5X6
Streptovarycin	T36.5X1	T36.5X2	T36.5X3	T36.5X4	T36.5X5	T36.5X6
Streptozocin	T45.1X1	T45.1X2	T45.1X3	T45.1X4	T45.1X5	T45.1X6
Streptozotocin	T45.1X1	T45.1X2	T45.1X3	T45.1X4	T45.1X5	T45.1X6
Stripper (paint) (solvent)	T52.8X1	T52.8X2	T52.8X3	T52.8X4	—	—
Strobane	T60.1X1	T60.1X2	T60.1X3	T60.1X4	—	—
Strofantina	T46.0X1	T46.0X2	T46.0X3	T46.0X4	T46.0X5	T46.0X6
Strophanthin (g) (k)	T46.0X1	T46.0X2	T46.0X3	T46.0X4	T46.0X5	T46.0X6
Strophanthus	T46.0X1	T46.0X2	T46.0X3	T46.0X4	T46.0X5	T46.0X6
Strophantin	T46.0X1	T46.0X2	T46.0X3	T46.0X4	T46.0X5	T46.0X6
Strophantin-g	T46.0X1	T46.0X2	T46.0X3	T46.0X4	T46.0X5	T46.0X6
Strychnine (nonmedicinal) (pesticide) (salts)	T65.1X1	T65.1X2	T65.1X3	T65.1X4	—	—
medicinal	T48.291	T48.292	T48.293	T48.294	T48.295	T48.296
Strychnos (ignatii) — see Strychnine						
Styramate	T42.8X1	T42.8X2	T42.8X3	T42.8X4	T42.8X5	T42.8X6
Styrene	T65.891	T65.892	T65.893	T65.894	—	—
Succinimide, antiepileptic or anticonvulsant	T42.2X1	T42.2X2	T42.2X3	T42.2X4	T42.2X5	T42.2X6
mercuric — see Mercury						
Succinylcholine	T48.1X1	T48.1X2	T48.1X3	T48.1X4	T48.1X5	T48.1X6
Succinylsulfathiazole	T37.0X1	T37.0X2	T37.0X3	T37.0X4	T37.0X5	T37.0X6
Sucralfate	T47.1X1	T47.1X2	T47.1X3	T47.1X4	T47.1X5	T47.1X6
Sucrose	T50.3X1	T50.3X2	T50.3X3	T50.3X4	T50.3X5	T50.3X6
Sufentanil	T40.4X1	T40.4X2	T40.4X3	T40.4X4	T40.4X5	T40.4X6
Sulbactam	T36.0X1	T36.0X2	T36.0X3	T36.0X4	T36.0X5	T36.0X6
Sulbenicillin	T36.0X1	T36.0X2	T36.0X3	T36.0X4	T36.0X5	T36.0X6
Sulbentine	T49.0X1	T49.0X2	T49.0X3	T49.0X4	T49.0X5	T49.0X6
Sulfacetamide	T49.0X1	T49.0X2	T49.0X3	T49.0X4	T49.0X5	T49.0X6
ophthalmic preparation	T49.5X1	T49.5X2	T49.5X3	T49.5X4	T49.5X5	T49.5X6
Sulfachlorpyridazine	T37.0X1	T37.0X2	T37.0X3	T37.0X4	T37.0X5	T37.0X6
Sulfacitine	T37.0X1	T37.0X2	T37.0X3	T37.0X4	T37.0X5	T37.0X6
Sulfadiasulfone sodium	T37.0X1	T37.0X2	T37.0X3	T37.0X4	T37.0X5	T37.0X6

Substance	Poisoning, Accidental (unintentional)	Poisoning, Intentional Self-harm	Poisoning, Assault	Poisoning, Undetermined	Adverse Effect	Underdosing
Sulfadiazine	T37.0X1	T37.0X2	T37.0X3	T37.0X4	T37.0X5	T37.0X6
silver (topical)	T49.0X1	T49.0X2	T49.0X3	T49.0X4	T49.0X5	T49.0X6
Sulfadimethoxine	T37.0X1	T37.0X2	T37.0X3	T37.0X4	T37.0X5	T37.0X6
Sulfadimidine	T37.0X1	T37.0X2	T37.0X3	T37.0X4	T37.0X5	T37.0X6
Sulfadoxine	T37.0X1	T37.0X2	T37.0X3	T37.0X4	T37.0X5	T37.0X6
with pyrimethamine	T37.2X1	T37.2X2	T37.2X3	T37.2X4	T37.2X5	T37.2X6
Sulfaethidole	T37.0X1	T37.0X2	T37.0X3	T37.0X4	T37.0X5	T37.0X6
Sulfafurazole	T37.0X1	T37.0X2	T37.0X3	T37.0X4	T37.0X5	T37.0X6
Sulfaguanidine	T37.0X1	T37.0X2	T37.0X3	T37.0X4	T37.0X5	T37.0X6
Sulfalene	T37.0X1	T37.0X2	T37.0X3	T37.0X4	T37.0X5	T37.0X6
Sulfaloxate	T37.0X1	T37.0X2	T37.0X3	T37.0X4	T37.0X5	T37.0X6
Sulfaloxic acid	T37.0X1	T37.0X2	T37.0X3	T37.0X4	T37.0X5	T37.0X6
Sulfamazone	T39.2X1	T39.2X2	T39.2X3	T39.2X4	T39.2X5	T39.2X6
Sulfamerazine	T37.0X1	T37.0X2	T37.0X3	T37.0X4	T37.0X5	T37.0X6
Sulfameter	T37.0X1	T37.0X2	T37.0X3	T37.0X4	T37.0X5	T37.0X6
Sulfamethazine	T37.0X1	T37.0X2	T37.0X3	T37.0X4	T37.0X5	T37.0X6
Sulfamethizole	T37.0X1	T37.0X2	T37.0X3	T37.0X4	T37.0X5	T37.0X6
Sulfamethoxazole	T37.0X1	T37.0X2	T37.0X3	T37.0X4	T37.0X5	T37.0X6
with trimethoprim	T36.8X1	T36.8X2	T36.8X3	T36.8X4	T36.8X5	T36.8X6
Sulfamethoxydiazine	T37.0X1	T37.0X2	T37.0X3	T37.0X4	T37.0X5	T37.0X6
Sulfamethoxypyridazine	T37.0X1	T37.0X2	T37.0X3	T37.0X4	T37.0X5	T37.0X6
Sulfamethylthiazole	T37.0X1	T37.0X2	T37.0X3	T37.0X4	T37.0X5	T37.0X6
Sulfametoxydiazine	T37.0X1	T37.0X2	T37.0X3	T37.0X4	T37.0X5	T37.0X6
Sulfamidopyrine	T39.2X1	T39.2X2	T39.2X3	T39.2X4	T39.2X5	T39.2X6
Sulfamonomethoxine	T37.0X1	T37.0X2	T37.0X3	T37.0X4	T37.0X5	T37.0X6
Sulfamoxole	T37.0X1	T37.0X2	T37.0X3	T37.0X4	T37.0X5	T37.0X6
Sulfamylon	T49.0X1	T49.0X2	T49.0X3	T49.0X4	T49.0X5	T49.0X6
Sulfan blue (diagnostic dye)	T50.8X1	T50.8X2	T50.8X3	T50.8X4	T50.8X5	T50.8X6
Sulfanilamide	T37.0X1	T37.0X2	T37.0X3	T37.0X4	T37.0X5	T37.0X6
Sulfanilylguanidine	T37.0X1	T37.0X2	T37.0X3	T37.0X4	T37.0X5	T37.0X6
Sulfaperin	T37.0X1	T37.0X2	T37.0X3	T37.0X4	T37.0X5	T37.0X6
Sulfaphenazole	T37.0X1	T37.0X2	T37.0X3	T37.0X4	T37.0X5	T37.0X6
Sulfaphenylthiazole	T37.0X1	T37.0X2	T37.0X3	T37.0X4	T37.0X5	T37.0X6
Sulfaproxyline	T37.0X1	T37.0X2	T37.0X3	T37.0X4	T37.0X5	T37.0X6
Sulfapyridine	T37.0X1	T37.0X2	T37.0X3	T37.0X4	T37.0X5	T37.0X6
Sulfapyrimidine	T37.0X1	T37.0X2	T37.0X3	T37.0X4	T37.0X5	T37.0X6
Sulfarsphenamine	T37.8X1	T37.8X2	T37.8X3	T37.8X4	T37.8X5	T37.8X6
Sulfasalazine	T37.0X1	T37.0X2	T37.0X3	T37.0X4	T37.0X5	T37.0X6
Sulfasuxidine	T37.0X1	T37.0X2	T37.0X3	T37.0X4	T37.0X5	T37.0X6
Sulfasymazine	T37.0X1	T37.0X2	T37.0X3	T37.0X4	T37.0X5	T37.0X6
Sulfated amylopectin	T47.8X1	T47.8X2	T47.8X3	T47.8X4	T47.8X5	T47.8X6
Sulfathiazole	T37.0X1	T37.0X2	T37.0X3	T37.0X4	T37.0X5	T37.0X6
Sulfatostearate	T49.2X1	T49.2X2	T49.2X3	T49.2X4	T49.2X5	T49.2X6
Sulfinpyrazone	T50.4X1	T50.4X2	T50.4X3	T50.4X4	T50.4X5	T50.4X6
Sulfiram	T49.0X1	T49.0X2	T49.0X3	T49.0X4	T49.0X5	T49.0X6
Sulfisomidine	T37.0X1	T37.0X2	T37.0X3	T37.0X4	T37.0X5	T37.0X6
Sulfisoxazole	T37.0X1	T37.0X2	T37.0X3	T37.0X4	T37.0X5	T37.0X6
ophthalmic preparation	T49.5X1	T49.5X2	T49.5X3	T49.5X4	T49.5X5	T49.5X6
Sulfobromophthalein (sodium)	T50.8X1	T50.8X2	T50.8X3	T50.8X4	T50.8X5	T50.8X6
Sulfobromphthalein	T50.8X1	T50.8X2	T50.8X3	T50.8X4	T50.8X5	T50.8X6
Sulfogaiacol	T48.4X1	T48.4X2	T48.4X3	T48.4X4	T48.4X5	T48.4X6
Sulfomyxin	T36.8X1	T36.8X2	T36.8X3	T36.8X4	T36.8X5	T36.8X6
Sulfonal	T42.6X1	T42.6X2	T42.6X3	T42.6X4	T42.6X5	T42.6X6
Sulfonamide NEC	T37.0X1	T37.0X2	T37.0X3	T37.0X4	T37.0X5	T37.0X6
eye	T49.5X1	T49.5X2	T49.5X3	T49.5X4	T49.5X5	T49.5X6
Sulfonazide	T37.1X1	T37.1X2	T37.1X3	T37.1X4	T37.1X5	T37.1X6
Sulfones	T37.1X1	T37.1X2	T37.1X3	T37.1X4	T37.1X5	T37.1X6
Sulfonethylmethane	T42.6X1	T42.6X2	T42.6X3	T42.6X4	T42.6X5	T42.6X6
Sulfonmethane	T42.6X1	T42.6X2	T42.6X3	T42.6X4	T42.6X5	T42.6X6
Sulfonphthal, sulfonphthol	T50.8X1	T50.8X2	T50.8X3	T50.8X4	T50.8X5	T50.8X6
Sulfonylurea derivatives, oral	T38.3X1	T38.3X2	T38.3X3	T38.3X4	T38.3X5	T38.3X6
Sulforidazine	T43.3X1	T43.3X2	T43.3X3	T43.3X4	T43.3X5	T43.3X6
Sulfoxone	T37.1X1	T37.1X2	T37.1X3	T37.1X4	T37.1X5	T37.1X6
Sulfuric acid	T54.2X1	T54.2X2	T54.2X3	T54.2X4	—	—
Sulfur, sulfurated, sulfuric, sulfurous, sulfuryl (compounds NEC) (medicinal)	T49.4X1	T49.4X2	T49.4X3	T49.4X4	T49.4X5	T49.4X6
acid	T54.2X1	T54.2X2	T54.2X3	T54.2X4	—	—
dioxide (gas)	T59.1X1	T59.1X2	T59.1X3	T59.1X4	—	—
ether — see Ether(s)						
hydrogen	T59.6X1	T59.6X2	T59.6X3	T59.6X4	—	—
medicinal (keratolytic) (ointment) NEC	T49.4X1	T49.4X2	T49.4X3	T49.4X4	T49.4X5	T49.4X6
ointment	T49.0X1	T49.0X2	T49.0X3	T49.0X4	T49.0X5	T49.0X6
pesticide (vapor)	T60.91	T60.92	T60.93	T60.94	—	—
vapor NEC	T59.891	T59.892	T59.893	T59.894	—	—
Sulglicotide	T47.1X1	T47.1X2	T47.1X3	T47.1X4	T47.1X5	T47.1X6
Sulindac	T39.391	T39.392	T39.393	T39.394	T39.395	T39.396
Sulisatin	T47.2X1	T47.2X2	T47.2X3	T47.2X4	T47.2X5	T47.2X6
Sulisobenzone	T49.3X1	T49.3X2	T49.3X3	T49.3X4	T49.3X5	T49.3X6
Sulkowitch's reagent	T50.8X1	T50.8X2	T50.8X3	T50.8X4	T50.8X5	T50.8X6
Sulmetozine	T44.3X1	T44.3X2	T44.3X3	T44.3X4	T44.3X5	T44.3X6
Suloctidil	T46.7X1	T46.7X2	T46.7X3	T46.7X4	T46.7X5	T46.7X6
Sulph- — see also Sulf-						
Sulphadiazine	T37.0X1	T37.0X2	T37.0X3	T37.0X4	T37.0X5	T37.0X6
Sulphadimethoxine	T37.0X1	T37.0X2	T37.0X3	T37.0X4	T37.0X5	T37.0X6
Sulphadimidine	T37.0X1	T37.0X2	T37.0X3	T37.0X4	T37.0X5	T37.0X6
Sulphadione	T37.1X1	T37.1X2	T37.1X3	T37.1X4	T37.1X5	T37.1X6
Sulphafurazole	T37.0X1	T37.0X2	T37.0X3	T37.0X4	T37.0X5	T37.0X6
Sulphamethizole	T37.0X1	T37.0X2	T37.0X3	T37.0X4	T37.0X5	T37.0X6
Sulphamethoxazole	T37.0X1	T37.0X2	T37.0X3	T37.0X4	T37.0X5	T37.0X6
Sulphan blue	T50.8X1	T50.8X2	T50.8X3	T50.8X4	T50.8X5	T50.8X6
Sulphaphenazole	T37.0X1	T37.0X2	T37.0X3	T37.0X4	T37.0X5	T37.0X6
Sulphapyridine	T37.0X1	T37.0X2	T37.0X3	T37.0X4	T37.0X5	T37.0X6
Sulphasalazine	T37.0X1	T37.0X2	T37.0X3	T37.0X4	T37.0X5	T37.0X6
Sulphinpyrazone	T50.4X1	T50.4X2	T50.4X3	T50.4X4	T50.4X5	T50.4X6
Sulpiride	T43.591	T43.592	T43.593	T43.594	T43.595	T43.596
Sulprostone	T48.0X1	T48.0X2	T48.0X3	T48.0X4	T48.0X5	T48.0X6
Sulpyrine	T39.2X1	T39.2X2	T39.2X3	T39.2X4	T39.2X5	T39.2X6
Sultamicillin	T36.0X1	T36.0X2	T36.0X3	T36.0X4	T36.0X5	T36.0X6
Sulthiame	T42.6X1	T42.6X2	T42.6X3	T42.6X4	T42.6X5	T42.6X6
Sultiame	T42.6X1	T42.6X2	T42.6X3	T42.6X4	T42.6X5	T42.6X6
Sultopride	T43.591	T43.592	T43.593	T43.594	T43.595	T43.596
Sumatriptan	T39.8X1	T39.8X2	T39.8X3	T39.8X4	T39.8X5	T39.8X6
Sunflower seed oil	T46.6X1	T46.6X2	T46.6X3	T46.6X4	T46.6X5	T46.6X6
Superinone	T48.4X1	T48.4X2	T48.4X3	T48.4X4	T48.4X5	T48.4X6
Suprofen	T39.311	T39.312	T39.313	T39.314	T39.315	T39.316
Suramin (sodium)	T37.4X1	T37.4X2	T37.4X3	T37.4X4	T37.4X5	T37.4X6
Surfacaine	T41.3X1	T41.3X2	T41.3X3	T41.3X4	T41.3X5	T41.3X6
Surital	T41.1X1	T41.1X2	T41.1X3	T41.1X4	T41.1X5	T41.1X6
Sutilains	T45.3X1	T45.3X2	T45.3X3	T45.3X4	T45.3X5	T45.3X6
Suxamethonium (chloride)	T48.1X1	T48.1X2	T48.1X3	T48.1X4	T48.1X5	T48.1X6
Suxethonium (chloride)	T48.1X1	T48.1X2	T48.1X3	T48.1X4	T48.1X5	T48.1X6
Suxibuzone	T39.2X1	T39.2X2	T39.2X3	T39.2X4	T39.2X5	T39.2X6
Sweetener	T50.901	T50.902	T50.903	T50.904	T50.905	T50.906
Sweet niter spirit	T46.3X1	T46.3X2	T46.3X3	T46.3X4	T46.3X5	T46.3X6
Sweet oil (birch)	T49.3X1	T49.3X2	T49.3X3	T49.3X4	T49.3X5	T49.3X6
Sym-dichloroethyl ether	T53.6X1	T53.6X2	T53.6X3	T53.6X4	—	—
Sympatholytic NEC	T44.8X1	T44.8X2	T44.8X3	T44.8X4	T44.8X5	T44.8X6
haloalkylamine	T44.8X1	T44.8X2	T44.8X3	T44.8X4	T44.8X5	T44.8X6
Sympathomimetic NEC	T44.901	T44.902	T44.903	T44.904	T44.905	T44.906
anti-common-cold	T48.5X1	T48.5X2	T48.5X3	T48.5X4	T48.5X5	T48.5X6
bronchodilator	T48.6X1	T48.6X2	T48.6X3	T48.6X4	T48.6X5	T48.6X6
specified NEC	T44.991	T44.992	T44.993	T44.994	T44.995	T44.996
Synagis	T50.B91	T50.B92	T50.B93	T50.B94	T50.B95	T50.B96
Synalar	T49.0X1	T49.0X2	T49.0X3	T49.0X4	T49.0X5	T49.0X6
Synthroid	T38.1X1	T38.1X2	T38.1X3	T38.1X4	T38.1X5	T38.1X6
Syntocinon	T48.0X1	T48.0X2	T48.0X3	T48.0X4	T48.0X5	T48.0X6
Syrosingopine	T46.5X1	T46.5X2	T46.5X3	T46.5X4	T46.5X5	T46.5X6
Systemic drug	T45.91	T45.92	T45.93	T45.94	T45.95	T45.96
specified NEC	T45.8X1	T45.8X2	T45.8X3	T45.8X4	T45.8X5	T45.8X6
Tablets — see also specified substance	T50.901	T50.902	T50.903	T50.904	T50.905	T50.906
Tace	T38.5X1	T38.5X2	T38.5X3	T38.5X4	T38.5X5	T38.5X6
Tacrine	T44.0X1	T44.0X2	T44.0X3	T44.0X4	T44.0X5	T44.0X6
Tadalafil	T46.7X1	T46.7X2	T46.7X3	T46.7X4	T46.7X5	T46.7X6
Talampicillin	T36.0X1	T36.0X2	T36.0X3	T36.0X4	T36.0X5	T36.0X6
Talbutal	T42.3X1	T42.3X2	T42.3X3	T42.3X4	T42.3X5	T42.3X6
Talc powder	T49.3X1	T49.3X2	T49.3X3	T49.3X4	T49.3X5	T49.3X6
Talcum	T49.3X1	T49.3X2	T49.3X3	T49.3X4	T49.3X5	T49.3X6
Taleranol	T38.6X1	T38.6X2	T38.6X3	T38.6X4	T38.6X5	T38.6X6
Tamoxifen	T38.6X1	T38.6X2	T38.6X3	T38.6X4	T38.6X5	T38.6X6
Tamsulosin	T44.6X1	T44.6X2	T44.6X3	T44.6X4	T44.6X5	T44.6X6
Tandearil, tanderil	T39.2X1	T39.2X2	T39.2X3	T39.2X4	T39.2X5	T39.2X6
Tannic acid	T49.2X1	T49.2X2	T49.2X3	T49.2X4	T49.2X5	T49.2X6
medicinal (astringent)	T49.2X1	T49.2X2	T49.2X3	T49.2X4	T49.2X5	T49.2X6
Tannin — see Tannic acid						
Tansy	T62.2X1	T62.2X2	T62.2X3	T62.2X4	—	—
TAO	T36.3X1	T36.3X2	T36.3X3	T36.3X4	T36.3X5	T36.3X6
Tapazole	T38.2X1	T38.2X2	T38.2X3	T38.2X4	T38.2X5	T38.2X6
Taractan	T43.591	T43.592	T43.593	T43.594	T43.595	T43.596
Tarantula (venomous)	T63.321	T63.322	T63.323	T63.324	—	—
Tartar emetic	T37.8X1	T37.8X2	T37.8X3	T37.8X4	T37.8X5	T37.8X6
Tartaric acid	T65.891	T65.892	T65.893	T65.894	—	—
Tartrated antimony (anti-infective)	T37.8X1	T37.8X2	T37.8X3	T37.8X4	T37.8X5	T37.8X6
Tartrate, laxative	T47.4X1	T47.4X2	T47.4X3	T47.4X4	T47.4X5	T47.4X6
Tar NEC	T52.0X1	T52.0X2	T52.0X3	T52.0X4	—	—
camphor	T60.1X1	T60.1X2	T60.1X3	T60.1X4	—	—
distillate	T49.1X1	T49.1X2	T49.1X3	T49.1X4	T49.1X5	T49.1X6
fumes	T59.891	T59.892	T59.893	T59.894	—	—
medicinal	T49.1X1	T49.1X2	T49.1X3	T49.1X4	T49.1X5	T49.1X6
ointment	T49.1X1	T49.1X2	T49.1X3	T49.1X4	T49.1X5	T49.1X6

Substance	Poisoning, Accidental (unintentional)	Poisoning, Intentional Self-harm	Poisoning, Assault	Poisoning, Undetermined	Adverse Effect	Under-dosing
Tauromustine	T45.1X1	T45.1X2	T45.1X3	T45.1X4	T45.1X5	T45.1X6
TCA — see Trichloroacetic acid						
TCDD	T53.7X1	T53.7X2	T53.7X3	T53.7X4	—	—
TDI (vapor)	T65.0X1	T65.0X2	T65.0X3	T65.0X4	—	—
Tear						
gas	T59.3X1	T59.3X2	T59.3X3	T59.3X4	—	—
solution	T49.5X1	T49.5X2	T49.5X3	T49.5X4	T49.5X5	T49.5X6
Teclothiazide	T50.2X1	T50.2X2	T50.2X3	T50.2X4	T50.2X5	T50.2X6
Teclozan	T37.3X1	T37.3X2	T37.3X3	T37.3X4	T37.3X5	T37.3X6
Tegafur	T45.1X1	T45.1X2	T45.1X3	T45.1X4	T45.1X5	T45.1X6
Tegretol	T42.1X1	T42.1X2	T42.1X3	T42.1X4	T42.1X5	T42.1X6
Teicoplanin	T36.8X1	T36.8X2	T36.8X3	T36.8X4	T36.8X5	T36.8X6
Telepaque	T50.8X1	T50.8X2	T50.8X3	T50.8X4	T50.8X5	T50.8X6
Tellurium	T56.891	T56.892	T56.893	T56.894	—	—
fumes	T56.891	T56.892	T56.893	T56.894	—	—
TEM	T45.1X1	T45.1X2	T45.1X3	T45.1X4	T45.1X5	T45.1X6
Temazepam	T42.4X1	T42.4X2	T42.4X3	T42.4X4	T42.4X5	T42.4X6
Temocillin	T36.0X1	T36.0X2	T36.0X3	T36.0X4	T36.0X5	T36.0X6
Tenamfetamine	T43.621	T43.622	T43.623	T43.624	T43.625	T43.626
Teniposide	T45.1X1	T45.1X2	T45.1X3	T45.1X4	T45.1X5	T45.1X6
Tenitramine	T46.3X1	T46.3X2	T46.3X3	T46.3X4	T46.3X5	T46.3X6
Tenoglicin	T48.4X1	T48.4X2	T48.4X3	T48.4X4	T48.4X5	T48.4X6
Tenonitrozole	T37.3X1	T37.3X2	T37.3X3	T37.3X4	T37.3X5	T37.3X6
Tenoxicam	T39.391	T39.392	T39.393	T39.394	T39.395	T39.396
TEPA	T45.1X1	T45.1X2	T45.1X3	T45.1X4	T45.1X5	T45.1X6
TEPP	T60.0X1	T60.0X2	T60.0X3	T60.0X4	—	—
Teprotide	T46.5X1	T46.5X2	T46.5X3	T46.5X4	T46.5X5	T46.5X6
Terazosin	T44.6X1	T44.6X2	T44.6X3	T44.6X4	T44.6X5	T44.6X6
Terbufos	T60.0X1	T60.0X2	T60.0X3	T60.0X4	—	—
Terbutaline	T48.6X1	T48.6X2	T48.6X3	T48.6X4	T48.6X5	T48.6X6
Terconazole	T49.0X1	T49.0X2	T49.0X3	T49.0X4	T49.0X5	T49.0X6
Terfenadine	T45.0X1	T45.0X2	T45.0X3	T45.0X4	T45.0X5	T45.0X6
Teriparatide (acetate)	T50.991	T50.992	T50.993	T50.994	T50.995	T50.996
Terizidone	T37.1X1	T37.1X2	T37.1X3	T37.1X4	T37.1X5	T37.1X6
Terlipressin	T38.891	T38.892	T38.893	T38.894	T38.895	T38.896
Terodiline	T46.3X1	T46.3X2	T46.3X3	T46.3X4	T46.3X5	T46.3X6
Teroxalene	T37.4X1	T37.4X2	T37.4X3	T37.4X4	T37.4X5	T37.4X6
Terpin (cis) hydrate	T48.4X1	T48.4X2	T48.4X3	T48.4X4	T48.4X5	T48.4X6
Terramycin	T36.4X1	T36.4X2	T36.4X3	T36.4X4	T36.4X5	T36.4X6
Tertatolol	T44.7X1	T44.7X2	T44.7X3	T44.7X4	T44.7X5	T44.7X6
Tessalon	T48.3X1	T48.3X2	T48.3X3	T48.3X4	T48.3X5	T48.3X6
Testolactone	T38.7X1	T38.7X2	T38.7X3	T38.7X4	T38.7X5	T38.7X6
Testosterone	T38.7X1	T38.7X2	T38.7X3	T38.7X4	T38.7X5	T38.7X6
Tetanus toxoid or vaccine	T50.A91	T50.A92	T50.A93	T50.A94	T50.A95	T50.A96
antitoxin	T50.Z11	T50.Z12	T50.Z13	T50.Z14	T50.Z15	T50.Z16
immune globulin (human)	T50.Z11	T50.Z12	T50.Z13	T50.Z14	T50.Z15	T50.Z16
toxoid	T50.A91	T50.A92	T50.A93	T50.A94	T50.A95	T50.A96
with diphtheria toxoid	T50.A21	T50.A22	T50.A23	T50.A24	T50.A25	T50.A26
with pertussis	T50.A11	T50.A12	T50.A13	T50.A14	T50.A15	T50.A16
Tetrabenazine	T43.591	T43.592	T43.593	T43.594	T43.595	T43.596
Tetracaine	T41.3X1	T41.3X2	T41.3X3	T41.3X4	T41.3X5	T41.3X6
nerve block (peripheral) (plexus)	T41.3X1	T41.3X2	T41.3X3	T41.3X4	T41.3X5	T41.3X6
regional	T41.3X1	T41.3X2	T41.3X3	T41.3X4	T41.3X5	T41.3X6
spinal	T41.3X1	T41.3X2	T41.3X3	T41.3X4	T41.3X5	T41.3X6
Tetrachlorethylene — see Tetrachloroethylene						
Tetrachlormethiazide	T50.2X1	T50.2X2	T50.2X3	T50.2X4	T50.2X5	T50.2X6
Tetrachloroethane	T53.6X1	T53.6X2	T53.6X3	T53.6X4	—	—
vapor	T53.6X1	T53.6X2	T53.6X3	T53.6X4	—	—
paint or varnish	T53.6X1	T53.6X2	T53.6X3	T53.6X4	—	—
Tetrachloroethylene (liquid)	T53.3X1	T53.3X2	T53.3X3	T53.3X4	—	—
medicinal	T37.4X1	T37.4X2	T37.4X3	T37.4X4	T37.4X5	T37.4X6
vapor	T53.3X1	T53.3X2	T53.3X3	T53.3X4	—	—
Tetrachloromethane — see Carbon tetrachloride						
Tetracosactide	T38.811	T38.812	T38.813	T38.814	T38.815	T38.816
Tetracosactrin	T38.811	T38.812	T38.813	T38.814	T38.815	T38.816
Tetracycline	T36.4X1	T36.4X2	T36.4X3	T36.4X4	T36.4X5	T36.4X6
ophthalmic preparation	T49.5X1	T49.5X2	T49.5X3	T49.5X4	T49.5X5	T49.5X6
topical NEC	T49.0X1	T49.0X2	T49.0X3	T49.0X4	T49.0X5	T49.0X6
Tetradifon	T60.8X1	T60.8X2	T60.8X3	T60.8X4	—	—
Tetradotoxin	T61.771	T61.772	T61.773	T61.774		
Tetraethyl						
lead	T56.0X1	T56.0X2	T56.0X3	T56.0X4	—	—
pyrophosphate	T60.0X1	T60.0X2	T60.0X3	T60.0X4	—	—
Tetraethylammonium chloride	T44.2X1	T44.2X2	T44.2X3	T44.2X4	T44.2X5	T44.2X6
Tetraethylthiuram disulfide	T50.6X1	T50.6X2	T50.6X3	T50.6X4	T50.6X5	T50.6X6
Tetrahydroaminoacridine	T44.0X1	T44.0X2	T44.0X3	T44.0X4	T44.0X5	T44.0X6
Tetrahydrocannabinol	T40.7X1	T40.7X2	T40.7X3	T40.7X4	T40.7X5	T40.7X6
Tetrahydrofuran	T52.8X1	T52.8X2	T52.8X3	T52.8X4	—	—
Tetrahydronaphthalene	T52.8X1	T52.8X2	T52.8X3	T52.8X4	—	—
Tetrahydrozoline	T49.5X1	T49.5X2	T49.5X3	T49.5X4	T49.5X5	T49.5X6
Tetralin	T52.8X1	T52.8X2	T52.8X3	T52.8X4	—	—
Tetramethrin	T60.2X1	T60.2X2	T60.2X3	T60.2X4	—	—
Tetramethylthiuram (disulfide) NEC	T60.3X1	T60.3X2	T60.3X3	T60.3X4	—	—
medicinal	T49.0X1	T49.0X2	T49.0X3	T49.0X4	T49.0X5	T49.0X6
Tetramisole	T37.4X1	T37.4X2	T37.4X3	T37.4X4	T37.4X5	T37.4X6
Tetranicotinoyl fructose	T46.7X1	T46.7X2	T46.7X3	T46.7X4	T46.7X5	T46.7X6
Tetrazepam	T42.4X1	T42.4X2	T42.4X3	T42.4X4	T42.4X5	T42.4X6
Tetronal	T42.6X1	T42.6X2	T42.6X3	T42.6X4	T42.6X5	T42.6X6
Tetryl	T65.3X1	T65.3X2	T65.3X3	T65.3X4	—	—
Tetrylammonium chloride	T44.2X1	T44.2X2	T44.2X3	T44.2X4	T44.2X5	T44.2X6
Tetryzoline	T49.5X1	T49.5X2	T49.5X3	T49.5X4	T49.5X5	T49.5X6
Thalidomide	T45.1X1	T45.1X2	T45.1X3	T45.1X4	T45.1X5	T45.1X6
Thallium (compounds) (dust)	T56.811	T56.812	T56.813	T56.814	—	—
NEC						
pesticide	T60.4X1	T60.4X2	T60.4X3	T60.4X4	—	—
THC	T40.7X1	T40.7X2	T40.7X3	T40.7X4	T40.7X5	T40.7X6
Thebacon	T48.3X1	T48.3X2	T48.3X3	T48.3X4	T48.3X5	T48.3X6
Thebaine	T40.2X1	T40.2X2	T40.2X3	T40.2X4	T40.2X5	T40.2X6
Thenoic acid	T49.6X1	T49.6X2	T49.6X3	T49.6X4	T49.6X5	T49.6X6
Thenyldiamine	T45.0X1	T45.0X2	T45.0X3	T45.0X4	T45.0X5	T45.0X6
Theobromine (calcium salicylate)	T48.6X1	T48.6X2	T48.6X3	T48.6X4	T48.6X5	T48.6X6
sodium salicylate	T48.6X1	T48.6X2	T48.6X3	T48.6X4	T48.6X5	T48.6X6
Theophyllamine	T48.6X1	T48.6X2	T48.6X3	T48.6X4	T48.6X5	T48.6X6
Theophylline	T48.6X1	T48.6X2	T48.6X3	T48.6X4	T48.6X5	T48.6X6
aminobenzoic acid	T48.6X1	T48.6X2	T48.6X3	T48.6X4	T48.6X5	T48.6X6
ethylenediamine	T48.6X1	T48.6X2	T48.6X3	T48.6X4	T48.6X5	T48.6X6
piperazine	T48.6X1	T48.6X2	T48.6X3	T48.6X4	T48.6X5	T48.6X6
p-amino-benzoate						
Thiabendazole	T37.4X1	T37.4X2	T37.4X3	T37.4X4	T37.4X5	T37.4X6
Thialbarbital	T41.1X1	T41.1X2	T41.1X3	T41.1X4	T41.1X5	T41.1X6
Thiamazole	T38.2X1	T38.2X2	T38.2X3	T38.2X4	T38.2X5	T38.2X6
Thiambutosine	T37.1X1	T37.1X2	T37.1X3	T37.1X4	T37.1X5	T37.1X6
Thiamine	T45.2X1	T45.2X2	T45.2X3	T45.2X4	T45.2X5	T45.2X6
Thiamphenicol	T36.2X1	T36.2X2	T36.2X3	T36.2X4	T36.2X5	T36.2X6
Thiamylal	T41.1X1	T41.1X2	T41.1X3	T41.1X4	T41.1X5	T41.1X6
sodium	T41.1X1	T41.1X2	T41.1X3	T41.1X4	T41.1X5	T41.1X6
Thiazesim	T43.291	T43.292	T43.293	T43.294	T43.295	T43.296
Thiazides (diuretics)	T50.2X1	T50.2X2	T50.2X3	T50.2X4	T50.2X5	T50.2X6
Thiazinamium metilsulfate	T43.3X1	T43.3X2	T43.3X3	T43.3X4	T43.3X5	T43.3X6
Thiethylperazine	T43.3X1	T43.3X2	T43.3X3	T43.3X4	T43.3X5	T43.3X6
Thimerosal	T49.0X1	T49.0X2	T49.0X3	T49.0X4	T49.0X5	T49.0X6
ophthalmic preparation	T49.5X1	T49.5X2	T49.5X3	T49.5X4	T49.5X5	T49.5X6
Thioacetazone	T37.1X1	T37.1X2	T37.1X3	T37.1X4	T37.1X5	T37.1X6
with isoniazid	T37.1X1	T37.1X2	T37.1X3	T37.1X4	T37.1X5	T37.1X6
Thiobarbital sodium	T41.1X1	T41.1X2	T41.1X3	T41.1X4	T41.1X5	T41.1X6
Thiobarbiturate anesthetic	T41.1X1	T41.1X2	T41.1X3	T41.1X4	T41.1X5	T41.1X6
Thiobismol	T37.8X1	T37.8X2	T37.8X3	T37.8X4	T37.8X5	T37.8X6
Thiobutabarbital sodium	T41.1X1	T41.1X2	T41.1X3	T41.1X4	T41.1X5	T41.1X6
Thiocarbamate (insecticide)	T60.0X1	T60.0X2	T60.0X3	T60.0X4	—	—
Thiocarbamide	T38.2X1	T38.2X2	T38.2X3	T38.2X4	T38.2X5	T38.2X6
Thiocarbarsone	T37.8X1	T37.8X2	T37.8X3	T37.8X4	T37.8X5	T37.8X6
Thiocarlide	T37.1X1	T37.1X2	T37.1X3	T37.1X4	T37.1X5	T37.1X6
Thioctamide	T50.991	T50.992	T50.993	T50.994	T50.995	T50.996
Thioctic acid	T50.991	T50.992	T50.993	T50.994	T50.995	T50.996
Thiofos	T60.0X1	T60.0X2	T60.0X3	T60.0X4	—	—
Thioglycolate	T49.4X1	T49.4X2	T49.4X3	T49.4X4	T49.4X5	T49.4X6
Thioglycolic acid	T65.891	T65.892	T65.893	T65.894	—	—
Thioguanine	T45.1X1	T45.1X2	T45.1X3	T45.1X4	T45.1X5	T45.1X6
Thiomercaptomerin	T50.2X1	T50.2X2	T50.2X3	T50.2X4	T50.2X5	T50.2X6
Thiomerin	T50.2X1	T50.2X2	T50.2X3	T50.2X4	T50.2X5	T50.2X6
Thiomersal	T49.0X1	T49.0X2	T49.0X3	T49.0X4	T49.0X5	T49.0X6
Thionazin	T60.0X1	T60.0X2	T60.0X3	T60.0X4	—	—
Thiopental (sodium)	T41.1X1	T41.1X2	T41.1X3	T41.1X4	T41.1X5	T41.1X6
Thiopentone (sodium)	T41.1X1	T41.1X2	T41.1X3	T41.1X4	T41.1X5	T41.1X6
Thiopropazate	T43.3X1	T43.3X2	T43.3X3	T43.3X4	T43.3X5	T43.3X6
Thioproperazine	T43.3X1	T43.3X2	T43.3X3	T43.3X4	T43.3X5	T43.3X6
Thioridazine	T43.3X1	T43.3X2	T43.3X3	T43.3X4	T43.3X5	T43.3X6
Thiosinamine	T49.3X1	T49.3X2	T49.3X3	T49.3X4	T49.3X5	T49.3X6
Thiotepa	T45.1X1	T45.1X2	T45.1X3	T45.1X4	T45.1X5	T45.1X6
Thiothixene	T43.4X1	T43.4X2	T43.4X3	T43.4X4	T43.4X5	T43.4X6
Thiouracil (benzyl) (methyl) (propyl)	T38.2X1	T38.2X2	T38.2X3	T38.2X4	T38.2X5	T38.2X6
Thiourea	T38.2X1	T38.2X2	T38.2X3	T38.2X4	T38.2X5	T38.2X6
Thiphenamil	T44.3X1	T44.3X2	T44.3X3	T44.3X4	T44.3X5	T44.3X6
Thiram	T60.3X1	T60.3X2	T60.3X3	T60.3X4	—	—
medicinal	T49.2X1	T49.2X2	T49.2X3	T49.2X4	T49.2X5	T49.2X6
Thonzylamine (systemic)	T45.0X1	T45.0X2	T45.0X3	T45.0X4	T45.0X5	T45.0X6
mucosal decongestant	T48.5X1	T48.5X2	T48.5X3	T48.5X4	T48.5X5	T48.5X6

Substance	Poisoning, Accidental (unintentional)	Poisoning, Intentional Self-harm	Poisoning, Assault	Poisoning, Undetermined	Adverse Effect	Under-dosing
Thorazine	T43.3X1	T43.3X2	T43.3X3	T43.3X4	T43.3X5	T43.3X6
Thorium dioxide suspension	T50.8X1	T50.8X2	T50.8X3	T50.8X4	T50.8X5	T50.8X6
Thornapple	T62.2X1	T62.2X2	T62.2X3	T62.2X4	—	—
Throat drug NEC	T49.6X1	T49.6X2	T49.6X3	T49.6X4	T49.6X5	T49.6X6
Thrombin	T45.7X1	T45.7X2	T45.7X3	T45.7X4	T45.7X5	T45.7X6
Thrombolysin	T45.611	T45.612	T45.613	T45.614	T45.615	T45.616
Thromboplastin	T45.7X1	T45.7X2	T45.7X3	T45.7X4	T45.7X5	T45.7X6
Thurfyl nicotinate	T46.7X1	T46.7X2	T46.7X3	T46.7X4	T46.7X5	T46.7X6
Thymol	T49.0X1	T49.0X2	T49.0X3	T49.0X4	T49.0X5	T49.0X6
Thymopentin	T37.5X1	T37.5X2	T37.5X3	T37.5X4	T37.5X5	T37.5X6
Thymoxamine	T46.7X1	T46.7X2	T46.7X3	T46.7X4	T46.7X5	T46.7X6
Thymus extract	T38.891	T38.892	T38.893	T38.894	T38.895	T38.896
Thyreotrophic hormone	T38.811	T38.812	T38.813	T38.814	T38.815	T38.816
Thyroglobulin	T38.1X1	T38.1X2	T38.1X3	T38.1X4	T38.1X5	T38.1X6
Thyroid (hormone)	T38.1X1	T38.1X2	T38.1X3	T38.1X4	T38.1X5	T38.1X6
Thyrolar	T38.1X1	T38.1X2	T38.1X3	T38.1X4	T38.1X5	T38.1X6
Thyrotrophin	T38.811	T38.812	T38.813	T38.814	T38.815	T38.816
Thyrotropic hormone	T38.811	T38.812	T38.813	T38.814	T38.815	T38.816
Thyroxine	T38.1X1	T38.1X2	T38.1X3	T38.1X4	T38.1X5	T38.1X6
Tiabendazole	T37.4X1	T37.4X2	T37.4X3	T37.4X4	T37.4X5	T37.4X6
Tiamizide	T50.2X1	T50.2X2	T50.2X3	T50.2X4	T50.2X5	T50.2X6
Tianeptine	T43.291	T43.292	T43.293	T43.294	T43.295	T43.296
Tiapamil	T46.1X1	T46.1X2	T46.1X3	T46.1X4	T46.1X5	T46.1X6
Tiapride	T43.591	T43.592	T43.593	T43.594	T43.595	T43.596
Tiaprofenic acid	T39.311	T39.312	T39.313	T39.314	T39.315	T39.316
Tiaramide	T39.8X1	T39.8X2	T39.8X3	T39.8X4	T39.8X5	T39.8X6
Ticarcillin	T36.0X1	T36.0X2	T36.0X3	T36.0X4	T36.0X5	T36.0X6
Ticlatone	T49.0X1	T49.0X2	T49.0X3	T49.0X4	T49.0X5	T49.0X6
Ticlopidine	T45.521	T45.522	T45.523	T45.524	T45.525	T45.526
Ticrynafen	T50.1X1	T50.1X2	T50.1X3	T50.1X4	T50.1X5	T50.1X6
Tidiacic	T50.991	T50.992	T50.993	T50.994	T50.995	T50.996
Tiemonium	T44.3X1	T44.3X2	T44.3X3	T44.3X4	T44.3X5	T44.3X6
iodide	T44.3X1	T44.3X2	T44.3X3	T44.3X4	T44.3X5	T44.3X6
Tienilic acid	T50.1X1	T50.1X2	T50.1X3	T50.1X4	T50.1X5	T50.1X6
Tifenamil	T44.3X1	T44.3X2	T44.3X3	T44.3X4	T44.3X5	T44.3X6
Tigan	T45.0X1	T45.0X2	T45.0X3	T45.0X4	T45.0X5	T45.0X6
Tigloidine	T44.3X1	T44.3X2	T44.3X3	T44.3X4	T44.3X5	T44.3X6
Tilactase	T47.5X1	T47.5X2	T47.5X3	T47.5X4	T47.5X5	T47.5X6
Tiletamine	T41.291	T41.292	T41.293	T41.294	T41.295	T41.296
Tilidine	T40.4X1	T40.4X2	T40.4X3	T40.4X4	—	—
Timepidium bromide	T44.3X1	T44.3X2	T44.3X3	T44.3X4	T44.3X5	T44.3X6
Timiperone	T43.4X1	T43.4X2	T43.4X3	T43.4X4	T43.4X5	T43.4X6
Timolol	T44.7X1	T44.7X2	T44.7X3	T44.7X4	T44.7X5	T44.7X6
Tincture, iodine — see Iodine						
Tindal	T43.3X1	T43.3X2	T43.3X3	T43.3X4	T43.3X5	T43.3X6
Tinidazole	T37.3X1	T37.3X2	T37.3X3	T37.3X4	T37.3X5	T37.3X6
Tinoridine	T39.8X1	T39.8X2	T39.8X3	T39.8X4	T39.8X5	T39.8X6
Tin (chloride) (dust) (oxide)	T56.6X1	T56.6X2	T56.6X3	T56.6X4	—	—
NEC						
anti-infectives	T37.8X1	T37.8X2	T37.8X3	T37.8X4	T37.8X5	T37.8X6
Tiocarlide	T37.1X1	T37.1X2	T37.1X3	T37.1X4	T37.1X5	T37.1X6
Tioclomarol	T45.511	T45.512	T45.513	T45.514	T45.515	T45.516
Tioconazole	T49.0X1	T49.0X2	T49.0X3	T49.0X4	T49.0X5	T49.0X6
Tioguanine	T45.1X1	T45.1X2	T45.1X3	T45.1X4	T45.1X5	T45.1X6
Tiopronin	T50.991	T50.992	T50.993	T50.994	T50.995	T50.996
Tiotixene	T43.4X1	T43.4X2	T43.4X3	T43.4X4	T43.4X5	T43.4X6
Tioxolone	T49.4X1	T49.4X2	T49.4X3	T49.4X4	T49.4X5	T49.4X6
Tipepidine	T48.3X1	T48.3X2	T48.3X3	T48.3X4	T48.3X5	T48.3X6
Tiquizium bromide	T44.3X1	T44.3X2	T44.3X3	T44.3X4	T44.3X5	T44.3X6
Tiratricol	T38.1X1	T38.1X2	T38.1X3	T38.1X4	T38.1X5	T38.1X6
Tisopurine	T50.4X1	T50.4X2	T50.4X3	T50.4X4	T50.4X5	T50.4X6
Titanium (compounds)	T56.891	T56.892	T56.893	T56.894	—	—
(vapor)	T49.3X1	T49.3X2	T49.3X3	T49.3X4	T49.3X5	T49.3X6
dioxide	T49.3X1	T49.3X2	T49.3X3	T49.3X4	T49.3X5	T49.3X6
ointment	T49.3X1	T49.3X2	T49.3X3	T49.3X4	T49.3X5	T49.3X6
oxide	T49.3X1	T49.3X2	T49.3X3	T49.3X4	T49.3X5	T49.3X6
tetrachloride	T56.891	T56.892	T56.893	T56.894	—	—
Titanocene	T56.891	T56.892	T56.893	T56.894	—	—
Titroid	T38.1X1	T38.1X2	T38.1X3	T38.1X4	T38.1X5	T38.1X6
Tizanidine	T42.8X1	T42.8X2	T42.8X3	T42.8X4	T42.8X5	T42.8X6
TMTD	T60.3X1	T60.3X2	T60.3X3	T60.3X4	—	—
TNT (fumes)	T65.3X1	T65.3X2	T65.3X3	T65.3X4	—	—
Toadstool	T62.0X1	T62.0X2	T62.0X3	T62.0X4	—	—
Tobacco NEC	T65.291	T65.292	T65.293	T65.294	—	—
cigarettes	T65.221	T65.222	T65.223	T65.224	—	—
Indian	T62.2X1	T62.2X2	T62.2X3	T62.2X4	—	—
smoke, second-hand	T65.221	T65.222	T65.223	T65.224	—	—
Tobramycin	T36.5X1	T36.5X2	T36.5X3	T36.5X4	T36.5X5	T36.5X6
Tocainide	T46.2X1	T46.2X2	T46.2X3	T46.2X4	T46.2X5	T46.2X6
Tocoferol	T45.2X1	T45.2X2	T45.2X3	T45.2X4	T45.2X5	T45.2X6
Tocopherol	T45.2X1	T45.2X2	T45.2X3	T45.2X4	T45.2X5	T45.2X6
acetate	T45.2X1	T45.2X2	T45.2X3	T45.2X4	T45.2X5	T45.2X6

Substance	Poisoning, Accidental (unintentional)	Poisoning, Intentional Self-harm	Poisoning, Assault	Poisoning, Undetermined	Adverse Effect	Under-dosing
Tocosamine	T48.0X1	T48.0X2	T48.0X3	T48.0X4	T48.0X5	T48.0X6
Todralazine	T46.5X1	T46.5X2	T46.5X3	T46.5X4	T46.5X5	T46.5X6
Tofisopam	T42.4X1	T42.4X2	T42.4X3	T42.4X4	T42.4X5	T42.4X6
Tofranil	T43.011	T43.012	T43.013	T43.014	T43.015	T43.016
Toilet deodorizer	T65.891	T65.892	T65.893	T65.894	—	—
Tolamolol	T44.7X1	T44.7X2	T44.7X3	T44.7X4	T44.7X5	T44.7X6
Tolazamide	T38.3X1	T38.3X2	T38.3X3	T38.3X4	T38.3X5	T38.3X6
Tolazoline	T46.7X1	T46.7X2	T46.7X3	T46.7X4	T46.7X5	T46.7X6
Tolbutamide (sodium)	T38.3X1	T38.3X2	T38.3X3	T38.3X4	T38.3X5	T38.3X6
Tolciclate	T49.0X1	T49.0X2	T49.0X3	T49.0X4	T49.0X5	T49.0X6
Tolmetin	T39.391	T39.392	T39.393	T39.394	T39.395	T39.396
Tolnaftate	T49.0X1	T49.0X2	T49.0X3	T49.0X4	T49.0X5	T49.0X6
Tolonidine	T46.5X1	T46.5X2	T46.5X3	T46.5X4	T46.5X5	T46.5X6
Toloxatone	T42.6X1	T42.6X2	T42.6X3	T42.6X4	T42.6X5	T42.6X6
Tolperisone	T44.3X1	T44.3X2	T44.3X3	T44.3X4	T44.3X5	T44.3X6
Tolserol	T42.8X1	T42.8X2	T42.8X3	T42.8X4	T42.8X5	T42.8X6
Toluene (liquid)	T52.2X1	T52.2X2	T52.2X3	T52.2X4	—	—
diisocyanate	T65.0X1	T65.0X2	T65.0X3	T65.0X4	—	—
Toluidine	T65.891	T65.892	T65.893	T65.894	—	—
vapor	T59.891	T59.892	T59.893	T59.894	—	—
Toluol (liquid)	T52.2X1	T52.2X2	T52.2X3	T52.2X4	—	—
vapor	T52.2X1	T52.2X2	T52.2X3	T52.2X4	—	—
Toluylenediamine	T65.3X1	T65.3X2	T65.3X3	T65.3X4	—	—
Tolylene-2,4-diisocyanate	T65.0X1	T65.0X2	T65.0X3	T65.0X4	—	—
Tonic NEC	T50.901	T50.902	T50.903	T50.904	T50.905	T50.906
Topical action drug NEC	T49.91	T49.92	T49.93	T49.94	T49.95	T49.96
ear, nose or throat	T49.6X1	T49.6X2	T49.6X3	T49.6X4	T49.6X5	T49.6X6
eye	T49.5X1	T49.5X2	T49.5X3	T49.5X4	T49.5X5	T49.5X6
skin	T49.91	T49.92	T49.93	T49.94	T49.95	T49.96
specified NEC	T49.8X1	T49.8X2	T49.8X3	T49.8X4	T49.8X5	T49.8X6
Toquizine	T44.3X1	T44.3X2	T44.3X3	T44.3X4	T44.3X5	T44.3X6
Toremifene	T38.6X1	T38.6X2	T38.6X3	T38.6X4	T38.6X5	T38.6X6
Tosylchloramide sodium	T49.8X1	T49.8X2	T49.8X3	T49.8X4	T49.8X5	T49.8X6
Toxaphene (dust) (spray)	T60.1X1	T60.1X2	T60.1X3	T60.1X4	—	—
Toxin, diphtheria (Schick Test)	T50.8X1	T50.8X2	T50.8X3	T50.8X4	T50.8X5	T50.8X6
Toxoid						
combined	T50.A21	T50.A22	T50.A23	T50.A24	T50.A25	T50.A26
diphtheria	T50.A91	T50.A92	T50.A93	T50.A94	T50.A95	T50.A96
tetanus	T50.A91	T50.A92	T50.A93	T50.A94	T50.A95	T50.A96
Trace element NEC	T45.8X1	T45.8X2	T45.8X3	T45.8X4	T45.8X5	T45.8X6
Tractor fuel NEC	T52.0X1	T52.0X2	T52.0X3	T52.0X4	—	—
Tragacanth	T50.991	T50.992	T50.993	T50.994	T50.995	T50.996
Tramadol	T40.4X1	T40.4X2	T40.4X3	T40.4X4	T40.4X5	T40.4X6
Tramazoline	T48.5X1	T48.5X2	T48.5X3	T48.5X4	T48.5X5	T48.5X6
Tranexamic acid	T45.621	T45.622	T45.623	T45.624	T45.625	T45.626
Tranilast	T45.0X1	T45.0X2	T45.0X3	T45.0X4	T45.0X5	T45.0X6
Tranquilizer NEC	T43.501	T43.502	T43.503	T43.504	T43.505	T43.506
with hypnotic or sedative	T42.6X1	T42.6X2	T42.6X3	T42.6X4	T42.6X5	T42.6X6
benzodiazepine NEC	T42.4X1	T42.4X2	T42.4X3	T42.4X4	T42.4X5	T42.4X6
butyrophenone NEC	T43.4X1	T43.4X2	T43.4X3	T43.4X4	T43.4X5	T43.4X6
carbamate	T43.591	T43.592	T43.593	T43.594	T43.595	T43.596
dimethylamine	T43.3X1	T43.3X2	T43.3X3	T43.3X4	T43.3X5	T43.3X6
ethylamine	T43.3X1	T43.3X2	T43.3X3	T43.3X4	T43.3X5	T43.3X6
hydroxyzine	T43.591	T43.592	T43.593	T43.594	T43.595	T43.596
major NEC	T43.501	T43.502	T43.503	T43.504	T43.505	T43.506
penothiazine NEC	T43.3X1	T43.3X2	T43.3X3	T43.3X4	T43.3X5	T43.3X6
phenothiazine-based	T43.3X1	T43.3X2	T43.3X3	T43.3X4	T43.3X5	T43.3X6
piperazine NEC	T43.3X1	T43.3X2	T43.3X3	T43.3X4	T43.3X5	T43.3X6
piperidine	T43.3X1	T43.3X2	T43.3X3	T43.3X4	T43.3X5	T43.3X6
propylamine	T43.3X1	T43.3X2	T43.3X3	T43.3X4	T43.3X5	T43.3X6
specified NEC	T43.591	T43.592	T43.593	T43.594	T43.595	T43.596
thioxanthene NEC	T43.591	T43.592	T43.593	T43.594	T43.595	T43.596
Tranxene	T42.4X1	T42.4X2	T42.4X3	T42.4X4	T42.4X5	T42.4X6
Tranylcypromine	T43.1X1	T43.1X2	T43.1X3	T43.1X4	T43.1X5	T43.1X6
Trapidil	T46.3X1	T46.3X2	T46.3X3	T46.3X4	T46.3X5	T46.3X6
Trasentine	T44.3X1	T44.3X2	T44.3X3	T44.3X4	T44.3X5	T44.3X6
Travert	T50.3X1	T50.3X2	T50.3X3	T50.3X4	T50.3X5	T50.3X6
Trazodone	T43.211	T43.212	T43.213	T43.214	T43.215	T43.216
Trecator	T37.1X1	T37.1X2	T37.1X3	T37.1X4	T37.1X5	T37.1X6
Treosulfan	T45.1X1	T45.1X2	T45.1X3	T45.1X4	T45.1X5	T45.1X6
Tretamine	T45.1X1	T45.1X2	T45.1X3	T45.1X4	T45.1X5	T45.1X6
Tretinoin	T49.0X1	T49.0X2	T49.0X3	T49.0X4	T49.0X5	T49.0X6
Tretoquinol	T48.6X1	T48.6X2	T48.6X3	T48.6X4	T48.6X5	T48.6X6
Triacetin	T49.0X1	T49.0X2	T49.0X3	T49.0X4	T49.0X5	T49.0X6
Triacetoxyanthracene	T49.4X1	T49.4X2	T49.4X3	T49.4X4	T49.4X5	T49.4X6
Triacetyloleandomycin	T36.3X1	T36.3X2	T36.3X3	T36.3X4	T36.3X5	T36.3X6
Triamcinolone	T49.0X1	T49.0X2	T49.0X3	T49.0X4	T49.0X5	T49.0X6
ENT agent	T49.6X1	T49.6X2	T49.6X3	T49.6X4	T49.6X5	T49.6X6
hexacetonide	T49.0X1	T49.0X2	T49.0X3	T49.0X4	T49.0X5	T49.0X6
ophthalmic preparation	T49.5X1	T49.5X2	T49.5X3	T49.5X4	T49.5X5	T49.5X6
topical NEC	T49.0X1	T49.0X2	T49.0X3	T49.0X4	T49.0X5	T49.0X6
Triampyzine	T44.3X1	T44.3X2	T44.3X3	T44.3X4	T44.3X5	T44.3X6

Substance	Poisoning, Accidental (unintentional)	Poisoning, Intentional Self-harm	Poisoning, Assault	Poisoning, Undetermined	Adverse Effect	Underdosing
Triamterene	T50.2X1	T50.2X2	T50.2X3	T50.2X4	T50.2X5	T50.2X6
Triazine (herbicide)	T60.3X1	T60.3X2	T60.3X3	T60.3X4	—	—
Triaziquone	T45.1X1	T45.1X2	T45.1X3	T45.1X4	T45.1X5	T45.1X6
Triazolam	T42.4X1	T42.4X2	T42.4X3	T42.4X4	T42.4X5	T42.4X6
Triazole (herbicide)	T60.3X1	T60.3X2	T60.3X3	T60.3X4	—	—
Tribenoside	T46.991	T46.992	T46.993	T46.994	T46.995	T46.996
Tribromacetaldehyde	T42.6X1	T42.6X2	T42.6X3	T42.6X4	T42.6X5	T42.6X6
Tribromoethanol, rectal	T41.291	T41.292	T41.293	T41.294	T41.295	T41.296
Tribromomethane	T42.6X1	T42.6X2	T42.6X3	T42.6X4	T42.6X5	T42.6X6
Trichlorethane	T53.2X1	T53.2X2	T53.2X3	T53.2X4	—	—
Trichlorethylene	T53.2X1	T53.2X2	T53.2X3	T53.2X4	—	—
Trichlorfon	T60.0X1	T60.0X2	T60.0X3	T60.0X4	—	—
Trichlormethiazide	T50.2X1	T50.2X2	T50.2X3	T50.2X4	T50.2X5	T50.2X6
Trichlormethine	T45.1X1	T45.1X2	T45.1X3	T45.1X4	T45.1X5	T45.1X6
Trichloroacetic acid, Trichloracetic acid	T54.2X1	T54.2X2	T54.2X3	T54.2X4	—	—
medicinal	T49.4X1	T49.4X2	T49.4X3	T49.4X4	T49.4X5	T49.4X6
Trichloroethane	T53.2X1	T53.2X2	T53.2X3	T53.2X4	—	—
Trichloroethanol	T42.6X1	T42.6X2	T42.6X3	T42.6X4	T42.6X5	T42.6X6
Trichloroethylene (liquid)	T53.2X1	T53.2X2	T53.2X3	T53.2X4	—	—
(vapor)						
anesthetic (gas)	T41.0X1	T41.0X2	T41.0X3	T41.0X4	T41.0X5	T41.0X6
vapor NEC	T53.2X1	T53.2X2	T53.2X3	T53.2X4	—	—
Trichloroethyl phosphate	T42.6X1	T42.6X2	T42.6X3	T42.6X4	T42.6X5	T42.6X6
Trichlorofluoromethane NEC	T53.5X1	T53.5X2	T53.5X3	T53.5X4	—	—
Trichloronate	T60.0X1	T60.0X2	T60.0X3	T60.0X4	—	—
Trichloropropane	T53.6X1	T53.6X2	T53.6X3	T53.6X4	—	—
Trichlorotriethylamine	T45.1X1	T45.1X2	T45.1X3	T45.1X4	T45.1X5	T45.1X6
Trichomonacides NEC	T37.3X1	T37.3X2	T37.3X3	T37.3X4	T37.3X5	T37.3X6
Trichomycin	T36.7X1	T36.7X2	T36.7X3	T36.7X4	T36.7X5	T36.7X6
Triclobisonium chloride	T49.0X1	T49.0X2	T49.0X3	T49.0X4	T49.0X5	T49.0X6
Triclocarban	T49.0X1	T49.0X2	T49.0X3	T49.0X4	T49.0X5	T49.0X6
Triclofos	T42.6X1	T42.6X2	T42.6X3	T42.6X4	T42.6X5	T42.6X6
Triclosan	T49.0X1	T49.0X2	T49.0X3	T49.0X4	T49.0X5	T49.0X6
Tricresyl phosphate	T65.891	T65.892	T65.893	T65.894	—	—
solvent	T52.91	T52.92	T52.93	T52.94	—	—
Tricyclamol chloride	T44.3X1	T44.3X2	T44.3X3	T44.3X4	T44.3X5	T44.3X6
Tridesilon	T49.0X1	T49.0X2	T49.0X3	T49.0X4	T49.0X5	T49.0X6
Tridihexethyl iodide	T44.3X1	T44.3X2	T44.3X3	T44.3X4	T44.3X5	T44.3X6
Tridione	T42.2X1	T42.2X2	T42.2X3	T42.2X4	T42.2X5	T42.2X6
Trientine	T45.8X1	T45.8X2	T45.8X3	T45.8X4	T45.8X5	T45.8X6
Triethanolamine NEC	T54.3X1	T54.3X2	T54.3X3	T54.3X4	—	—
detergent	T54.3X1	T54.3X2	T54.3X3	T54.3X4	—	—
trinitrate (biphosphate)	T46.3X1	T46.3X2	T46.3X3	T46.3X4	T46.3X5	T46.3X6
Triethanomelamine	T45.1X1	T45.1X2	T45.1X3	T45.1X4	T45.1X5	T45.1X6
Triethylenemelamine	T45.1X1	T45.1X2	T45.1X3	T45.1X4	T45.1X5	T45.1X6
Triethylenephosphoramide	T45.1X1	T45.1X2	T45.1X3	T45.1X4	T45.1X5	T45.1X6
Triethylenethiophosphoramide	T45.1X1	T45.1X2	T45.1X3	T45.1X4	T45.1X5	T45.1X6
Trifluoperazine	T43.3X1	T43.3X2	T43.3X3	T43.3X4	T43.3X5	T43.3X6
Trifluoroethyl vinyl ether	T41.0X1	T41.0X2	T41.0X3	T41.0X4	T41.0X5	T41.0X6
Trifluperidol	T43.4X1	T43.4X2	T43.4X3	T43.4X4	T43.4X5	T43.4X6
Triflupromazine	T43.3X1	T43.3X2	T43.3X3	T43.3X4	T43.3X5	T43.3X6
Trifluridine	T37.5X1	T37.5X2	T37.5X3	T37.5X4	T37.5X5	T37.5X6
Triflusal	T45.521	T45.522	T45.523	T45.524	T45.525	T45.526
Trihexyphenidyl	T44.3X1	T44.3X2	T44.3X3	T44.3X4	T44.3X5	T44.3X6
Triiodothyronine	T38.1X1	T38.1X2	T38.1X3	T38.1X4	T38.1X5	T38.1X6
Trilene	T41.0X1	T41.0X2	T41.0X3	T41.0X4	T41.0X5	T41.0X6
Trilostane	T38.991	T38.992	T38.993	T38.994	T38.995	T38.996
Trimebutine	T44.3X1	T44.3X2	T44.3X3	T44.3X4	T44.3X5	T44.3X6
Trimecaine	T41.3X1	T41.3X2	T41.3X3	T41.3X4	T41.3X5	T41.3X6
Trimeprazine (tartrate)	T44.3X1	T44.3X2	T44.3X3	T44.3X4	T44.3X5	T44.3X6
Trimetaphan camsilate	T44.2X1	T44.2X2	T44.2X3	T44.2X4	T44.2X5	T44.2X6
Trimetazidine	T46.7X1	T46.7X2	T46.7X3	T46.7X4	T46.7X5	T46.7X6
Trimethadione	T42.2X1	T42.2X2	T42.2X3	T42.2X4	T42.2X5	T42.2X6
Trimethaphan	T44.2X1	T44.2X2	T44.2X3	T44.2X4	T44.2X5	T44.2X6
Trimethidinium	T44.2X1	T44.2X2	T44.2X3	T44.2X4	T44.2X5	T44.2X6
Trimethobenzamide	T45.0X1	T45.0X2	T45.0X3	T45.0X4	T45.0X5	T45.0X6
Trimethoprim	T37.8X1	T37.8X2	T37.8X3	T37.8X4	T37.8X5	T37.8X6
with sulfamethoxazole	T36.8X1	T36.8X2	T36.8X3	T36.8X4	T36.8X5	T36.8X6
Trimethylcarbinol	T51.3X1	T51.3X2	T51.3X3	T51.3X4	—	—
Trimethylpsoralen	T49.3X1	T49.3X2	T49.3X3	T49.3X4	T49.3X5	T49.3X6
Trimeton	T45.0X1	T45.0X2	T45.0X3	T45.0X4	T45.0X5	T45.0X6
Trimetrexate	T45.1X1	T45.1X2	T45.1X3	T45.1X4	T45.1X5	T45.1X6
Trimipramine	T43.011	T43.012	T43.013	T43.014	T43.015	T43.016
Trimustine	T45.1X1	T45.1X2	T45.1X3	T45.1X4	T45.1X5	T45.1X6
Trinitrine	T46.3X1	T46.3X2	T46.3X3	T46.3X4	T46.3X5	T46.3X6
Trinitrobenzol	T65.3X1	T65.3X2	T65.3X3	T65.3X4	—	—
Trinitrophenol	T65.3X1	T65.3X2	T65.3X3	T65.3X4	—	—
Trinitrotoluene (fumes)	T65.3X1	T65.3X2	T65.3X3	T65.3X4	—	—
Trional	T42.6X1	T42.6X2	T42.6X3	T42.6X4	T42.6X5	T42.6X6
Triorthocresyl phosphate	T65.891	T65.892	T65.893	T65.894	—	—
Trioxide of arsenic	T57.0X1	T57.0X2	T57.0X3	T57.0X4	—	—

Substance	Poisoning, Accidental (unintentional)	Poisoning, Intentional Self-harm	Poisoning, Assault	Poisoning, Undetermined	Adverse Effect	Underdosing
Trioxysalen	T49.4X1	T49.4X2	T49.4X3	T49.4X4	T49.4X5	T49.4X6
Tripamide	T50.2X1	T50.2X2	T50.2X3	T50.2X4	T50.2X5	T50.2X6
Triparanol	T46.6X1	T46.6X2	T46.6X3	T46.6X4	T46.6X5	T46.6X6
Tripelennamine	T45.0X1	T45.0X2	T45.0X3	T45.0X4	T45.0X5	T45.0X6
Triperiden	T44.3X1	T44.3X2	T44.3X3	T44.3X4	T44.3X5	T44.3X6
Triperidol	T43.4X1	T43.4X2	T43.4X3	T43.4X4	T43.4X5	T43.4X6
Triphenylphosphate	T65.891	T65.892	T65.893	T65.894	—	—
Triple						
bromides	T42.6X1	T42.6X2	T42.6X3	T42.6X4	T42.6X5	T42.6X6
carbonate	T47.1X1	T47.1X2	T47.1X3	T47.1X4	T47.1X5	T47.1X6
vaccine						
DPT	T50.A11	T50.A12	T50.A13	T50.A14	T50.A15	T50.A16
including pertussis	T50.A11	T50.A12	T50.A13	T50.A14	T50.A15	T50.A16
MMR	T50.B91	T50.B92	T50.B93	T50.B94	T50.B95	T50.B96
Triprolidine	T45.0X1	T45.0X2	T45.0X3	T45.0X4	T45.0X5	T45.0X6
Trisodium hydrogen edetate	T50.6X1	T50.6X2	T50.6X3	T50.6X4	T50.6X5	T50.6X6
Trisoralen	T49.3X1	T49.3X2	T49.3X3	T49.3X4	T49.3X5	T49.3X6
Trisulfapyrimidines	T37.0X1	T37.0X2	T37.0X3	T37.0X4	T37.0X5	T37.0X6
Trithiozine	T44.3X1	T44.3X2	T44.3X3	T44.3X4	T44.3X5	T44.3X6
Tritiozine	T44.3X1	T44.3X2	T44.3X3	T44.3X4	T44.3X5	T44.3X6
Tritoqualine	T45.0X1	T45.0X2	T45.0X3	T45.0X4	T45.0X5	T45.0X6
Trofosfamide	T45.1X1	T45.1X2	T45.1X3	T45.1X4	T45.1X5	T45.1X6
Troleandomycin	T36.3X1	T36.3X2	T36.3X3	T36.3X4	T36.3X5	T36.3X6
Trolnitrate (phosphate)	T46.3X1	T46.3X2	T46.3X3	T46.3X4	T46.3X5	T46.3X6
Tromantadine	T37.5X1	T37.5X2	T37.5X3	T37.5X4	T37.5X5	T37.5X6
Trometamol	T50.2X1	T50.2X2	T50.2X3	T50.2X4	T50.2X5	T50.2X6
Tromethamine	T50.2X1	T50.2X2	T50.2X3	T50.2X4	T50.2X5	T50.2X6
Tronothane	T41.3X1	T41.3X2	T41.3X3	T41.3X4	T41.3X5	T41.3X6
Tropacine	T44.3X1	T44.3X2	T44.3X3	T44.3X4	T44.3X5	T44.3X6
Tropatepine	T44.3X1	T44.3X2	T44.3X3	T44.3X4	T44.3X5	T44.3X6
Tropicamide	T44.3X1	T44.3X2	T44.3X3	T44.3X4	T44.3X5	T44.3X6
Trospium chloride	T44.3X1	T44.3X2	T44.3X3	T44.3X4	T44.3X5	T44.3X6
Troxerutin	T46.991	T46.992	T46.993	T46.994	T46.995	T46.996
Troxidone	T42.2X1	T42.2X2	T42.2X3	T42.2X4	T42.2X5	T42.2X6
Tryparsamide	T37.3X1	T37.3X2	T37.3X3	T37.3X4	T37.3X5	T37.3X6
Trypsin	T45.3X1	T45.3X2	T45.3X3	T45.3X4	T45.3X5	T45.3X6
Tryptizol	T43.011	T43.012	T43.013	T43.014	T43.015	T43.016
TSH	T38.811	T38.812	T38.813	T38.814	T38.815	T38.816
Tuaminoheptane	T48.5X1	T48.5X2	T48.5X3	T48.5X4	T48.5X5	T48.5X6
Tuberculin, purified protein derivative (PPD)	T50.8X1	T50.8X2	T50.8X3	T50.8X4	T50.8X5	T50.8X6
Tubocurare	T48.1X1	T48.1X2	T48.1X3	T48.1X4	T48.1X5	T48.1X6
Tubocurarine (chloride)	T48.1X1	T48.1X2	T48.1X3	T48.1X4	T48.1X5	T48.1X6
Tulobuterol	T48.6X1	T48.6X2	T48.6X3	T48.6X4	T48.6X5	T48.6X6
Turpentine (spirits of)	T52.8X1	T52.8X2	T52.8X3	T52.8X4	—	—
vapor	T52.8X1	T52.8X2	T52.8X3	T52.8X4	—	—
Tybamate	T43.591	T43.592	T43.593	T43.594	T43.595	T43.596
Tyloxapol	T48.4X1	T48.4X2	T48.4X3	T48.4X4	T48.4X5	T48.4X6
Tymazoline	T48.5X1	T48.5X2	T48.5X3	T48.5X4	T48.5X5	T48.5X6
Typhoid-paratyphoid vaccine	T50.A91	T50.A92	T50.A93	T50.A94	T50.A95	T50.A96
Typhus vaccine	T50.A91	T50.A92	T50.A93	T50.A94	T50.A95	T50.A96
Tyropanoate	T50.8X1	T50.8X2	T50.8X3	T50.8X4	T50.8X5	T50.8X6
Tyrothricin	T49.6X1	T49.6X2	T49.6X3	T49.6X4	T49.6X5	T49.6X6
ENT agent	T49.6X1	T49.6X2	T49.6X3	T49.6X4	T49.6X5	T49.6X6
ophthalmic preparation	T49.5X1	T49.5X2	T49.5X3	T49.5X4	T49.5X5	T49.5X6
Ufenamate	T39.391	T39.392	T39.393	T39.394	T39.395	T39.396
Ultraviolet light protectant	T49.3X1	T49.3X2	T49.3X3	T49.3X4	T49.3X5	T49.3X6
Undecenoic acid	T49.0X1	T49.0X2	T49.0X3	T49.0X4	T49.0X5	T49.0X6
Undecoylium	T49.0X1	T49.0X2	T49.0X3	T49.0X4	T49.0X5	T49.0X6
Undecylenic acid (derivatives)	T49.0X1	T49.0X2	T49.0X3	T49.0X4	T49.0X5	T49.0X6
Unna's boot	T49.3X1	T49.3X2	T49.3X3	T49.3X4	T49.3X5	T49.3X6
Unsaturated fatty acid	T46.6X1	T46.6X2	T46.6X3	T46.6X4	T46.6X5	T46.6X6
Uracil mustard	T45.1X1	T45.1X2	T45.1X3	T45.1X4	T45.1X5	T45.1X6
Uramustine	T45.1X1	T45.1X2	T45.1X3	T45.1X4	T45.1X5	T45.1X6
Urapidil	T46.5X1	T46.5X2	T46.5X3	T46.5X4	T46.5X5	T46.5X6
Urari	T48.1X1	T48.1X2	T48.1X3	T48.1X4	T48.1X5	T48.1X6
Urate oxidase	T50.4X1	T50.4X2	T50.4X3	T50.4X4	T50.4X5	T50.4X6
Urea	T47.3X1	T47.3X2	T47.3X3	T47.3X4	T47.3X5	T47.3X6
peroxide	T49.0X1	T49.0X2	T49.0X3	T49.0X4	T49.0X5	T49.0X6
stibamine	T37.4X1	T37.4X2	T37.4X3	T37.4X4	T37.4X5	T37.4X6
topical	T49.8X1	T49.8X2	T49.8X3	T49.8X4	T49.8X5	T49.8X6
Urethane	T45.1X1	T45.1X2	T45.1X3	T45.1X4	T45.1X5	T45.1X6
Urginea (maritima) (scilla) — see Squill						
Uric acid metabolism drug NEC	T50.4X1	T50.4X2	T50.4X3	T50.4X4	T50.4X5	T50.4X6
Uricosuric agent	T50.4X1	T50.4X2	T50.4X3	T50.4X4	T50.4X5	T50.4X6
Urinary anti-infective	T37.8X1	T37.8X2	T37.8X3	T37.8X4	T37.8X5	T37.8X6
Urofollitropin	T38.811	T38.812	T38.813	T38.814	T38.815	T38.816
Urokinase	T45.611	T45.612	T45.613	T45.614	T45.615	T45.616

Substance	Poisoning, Accidental (unintentional)	Poisoning, Intentional Self-harm	Poisoning, Assault	Poisoning, Undetermined	Adverse Effect	Under-dosing
Urokon	T50.8X1	T50.8X2	T50.8X3	T50.8X4	T50.8X5	T50.8X6
Ursodeoxycholic acid	T50.991	T50.992	T50.993	T50.994	T50.995	T50.996
Ursodiol	T50.991	T50.992	T50.993	T50.994	T50.995	T50.996
Urtica	T62.2X1	T62.2X2	T62.2X3	T62.2X4	—	—
Utility gas — see Gas, utility						
Vaccine NEC	T50.Z91	T50.Z92	T50.Z93	T50.Z94	T50.Z95	T50.Z96
antineoplastic	T50.Z91	T50.Z92	T50.Z93	T50.Z94	T50.Z95	T50.Z96
bacterial NEC	T50.A91	T50.A92	T50.A93	T50.A94	T50.A95	T50.A96
with						
other bacterial	T50.A21	T50.A22	T50.A23	T50.A24	T50.A25	T50.A26
component						
pertussis component	T50.A11	T50.A12	T50.A13	T50.A14	T50.A15	T50.A16
viral-rickettsial	T50.A21	T50.A22	T50.A23	T50.A24	T50.A25	T50.A26
component						
mixed NEC	T50.A21	T50.A22	T50.A23	T50.A24	T50.A25	T50.A26
BCG	T50.A91	T50.A92	T50.A93	T50.A94	T50.A95	T50.A96
cholera	T50.A91	T50.A92	T50.A93	T50.A94	T50.A95	T50.A96
diphtheria	T50.A91	T50.A92	T50.A93	T50.A94	T50.A95	T50.A96
with tetanus	T50.A21	T50.A22	T50.A23	T50.A24	T50.A25	T50.A26
and pertussis	T50.A11	T50.A12	T50.A13	T50.A14	T50.A15	T50.A16
influenza	T50.B91	T50.B92	T50.B93	T50.B94	T50.B95	T50.B96
measles	T50.B91	T50.B92	T50.B93	T50.B94	T50.B95	T50.B96
with mumps and rubella	T50.B91	T50.B92	T50.B93	T50.B94	T50.B95	T50.B96
meningococcal	T50.A91	T50.A92	T50.A93	T50.A94	T50.A95	T50.A96
mumps	T50.B91	T50.B92	T50.B93	T50.B94	T50.B95	T50.B96
paratyphoid	T50.A91	T50.A92	T50.A93	T50.A94	T50.A95	T50.A96
pertussis	T50.A11	T50.A12	T50.A13	T50.A14	T50.A15	T50.A16
with diphtheria	T50.A11	T50.A12	T50.A13	T50.A14	T50.A15	T50.A16
and tetanus	T50.A11	T50.A12	T50.A13	T50.A14	T50.A15	T50.A16
with other component	T50.A11	T50.A12	T50.A13	T50.A14	T50.A15	T50.A16
plague	T50.A91	T50.A92	T50.A93	T50.A94	T50.A95	T50.A96
poliomyelitis	T50.B91	T50.B92	T50.B93	T50.B94	T50.B95	T50.B96
poliovirus	T50.B91	T50.B92	T50.B93	T50.B94	T50.B95	T50.B96
rabies	T50.B91	T50.B92	T50.B93	T50.B94	T50.B95	T50.B96
respiratory syncytial virus	T50.B91	T50.B92	T50.B93	T50.B94	T50.B95	T50.B96
rickettsial NEC	T50.A91	T50.A92	T50.A93	T50.A94	T50.A95	T50.A96
with						
bacterial component	T50.A21	T50.A22	T50.A23	T50.A24	T50.A25	T50.A26
Rocky Mountain spotted fever	T50.A91	T50.A92	T50.A93	T50.A94	T50.A95	T50.A96
rubella	T50.B91	T50.B92	T50.B93	T50.B94	T50.B95	T50.B96
sabin oral	T50.B91	T50.B92	T50.B93	T50.B94	T50.B95	T50.B96
smallpox	T50.B11	T50.B12	T50.B13	T50.B14	T50.B15	T50.B16
TAB	T50.A91	T50.A92	T50.A93	T50.A94	T50.A95	T50.A96
tetanus	T50.A91	T50.A92	T50.A93	T50.A94	T50.A95	T50.A96
typhoid	T50.A91	T50.A92	T50.A93	T50.A94	T50.A95	T50.A96
typhus	T50.A91	T50.A92	T50.A93	T50.A94	T50.A95	T50.A96
viral NEC	T50.B91	T50.B92	T50.B93	T50.B94	T50.B95	T50.B96
yellow fever	T50.B91	T50.B92	T50.B93	T50.B94	T50.B95	T50.B96
Vaccinia immune globulin	T50.Z11	T50.Z12	T50.Z13	T50.Z14	T50.Z15	T50.Z16
Vaginal contraceptives	T49.8X1	T49.8X2	T49.8X3	T49.8X4	T49.8X5	T49.8X6
Valerian						
root	T42.6X1	T42.6X2	T42.6X3	T42.6X4	T42.6X5	T42.6X6
tincture	T42.6X1	T42.6X2	T42.6X3	T42.6X4	T42.6X5	T42.6X6
Valethamate bromide	T44.3X1	T44.3X2	T44.3X3	T44.3X4	T44.3X5	T44.3X6
Valisone	T49.0X1	T49.0X2	T49.0X3	T49.0X4	T49.0X5	T49.0X6
Valium	T42.4X1	T42.4X2	T42.4X3	T42.4X4	T42.4X5	T42.4X6
Valmid	T42.6X1	T42.6X2	T42.6X3	T42.6X4	T42.6X5	T42.6X6
Valnoctamide	T42.6X1	T42.6X2	T42.6X3	T42.6X4	T42.6X5	T42.6X6
Valproate (sodium)	T42.6X1	T42.6X2	T42.6X3	T42.6X4	T42.6X5	T42.6X6
Valproic acid	T42.6X1	T42.6X2	T42.6X3	T42.6X4	T42.6X5	T42.6X6
Valpromide	T42.6X1	T42.6X2	T42.6X3	T42.6X4	T42.6X5	T42.6X6
Vanadium	T56.891	T56.892	T56.893	T56.894	—	—
Vancomycin	T36.8X1	T36.8X2	T36.8X3	T36.8X4	T36.8X5	T36.8X6
Vapor — see also Gas	T59.91	T59.92	T59.93	T59.94	—	—
kiln (carbon monoxide)	T58.8X1	T58.8X2	T58.8X3	T58.8X4	—	—
lead — see lead						
specified source NEC	T59.891	T59.892	T59.893	T59.894	—	—
Vardenafil	T46.7X1	T46.7X2	T46.7X3	T46.7X4	T46.7X5	T46.7X6
Varicose reduction drug	T46.8X1	T46.8X2	T46.8X3	T46.8X4	T46.8X5	T46.8X6
Varnish	T65.4X1	T65.4X2	T65.4X3	T65.4X4	—	—
cleaner	T52.91	T52.92	T52.93	T52.94	—	—
Vaseline	T49.3X1	T49.3X2	T49.3X3	T49.3X4	T49.3X5	T49.3X6
Vasodilan	T46.7X1	T46.7X2	T46.7X3	T46.7X4	T46.7X5	T46.7X6
Vasodilator						
coronary NEC	T46.3X1	T46.3X2	T46.3X3	T46.3X4	T46.3X5	T46.3X6
peripheral NEC	T46.7X1	T46.7X2	T46.7X3	T46.7X4	T46.7X5	T46.7X6
Vasopressin	T38.891	T38.892	T38.893	T38.894	T38.895	T38.896
Vasopressor drugs	T38.891	T38.892	T38.893	T38.894	T38.895	T38.896
Vecuronium bromide	T48.1X1	T48.1X2	T48.1X3	T48.1X4	T48.1X5	T48.1X6
Vegetable extract, astringent	T49.2X1	T49.2X2	T49.2X3	T49.2X4	T49.2X5	T49.2X6
Venlafaxine	T43.211	T43.212	T43.213	T43.214	T43.215	T43.216

Substance	Poisoning, Accidental (unintentional)	Poisoning, Intentional Self-harm	Poisoning, Assault	Poisoning, Undetermined	Adverse Effect	Under-dosing
Venom, venomous (bite) (sting)	T63.91	T63.92	T63.93	T63.94	—	—
amphibian NEC	T63.831	T63.832	T63.833	T63.834	—	—
animal NEC	T63.891	T63.892	T63.893	T63.894	—	—
ant	T63.421	T63.422	T63.423	T63.424	—	—
arthropod NEC	T63.481	T63.482	T63.483	T63.484	—	—
bee	T63.441	T63.442	T63.443	T63.444	—	—
centipede	T63.411	T63.412	T63.413	T63.414	—	—
fish	T63.591	T63.592	T63.593	T63.594	—	—
frog	T63.811	T63.812	T63.813	T63.814	—	—
hornet	T63.451	T63.452	T63.453	T63.454	—	—
insect NEC	T63.481	T63.482	T63.483	T63.484	—	—
lizard	T63.121	T63.122	T63.123	T63.124	—	—
marine						
animals	T63.691	T63.692	T63.693	T63.694	—	—
bluebottle	T63.611	T63.612	T63.613	T63.614	—	—
jellyfish NEC	T63.621	T63.622	T63.623	T63.624	—	—
Portugese Man-o-war	T63.611	T63.612	T63.613	T63.614	—	—
sea anemone	T63.631	T63.632	T63.633	T63.634	—	—
specified NEC	T63.691	T63.692	T63.693	T63.694	—	—
fish	T63.591	T63.592	T63.593	T63.594	—	—
plants	T63.711	T63.712	T63.713	T63.714	—	—
sting ray	T63.511	T63.512	T63.513	T63.514	—	—
millipede (tropical)	T63.411	T63.412	T63.413	T63.414	—	—
plant NEC	T63.791	T63.792	T63.793	T63.794	—	—
marine	T63.711	T63.712	T63.713	T63.714	—	—
reptile	T63.191	T63.192	T63.193	T63.194	—	—
gila monster	T63.111	T63.112	T63.113	T63.114	—	—
lizard NEC	T63.121	T63.122	T63.123	T63.124	—	—
scorpion	T63.2X1	T63.2X2	T63.2X3	T63.2X4	—	—
snake	T63.001	T63.002	T63.003	T63.004	—	—
African NEC	T63.081	T63.082	T63.083	T63.084	—	—
American (North) (South) NEC	T63.061	T63.062	T63.063	T63.064	—	—
Asian	T63.081	T63.082	T63.083	T63.084	—	—
Australian	T63.071	T63.072	T63.073	T63.074	—	—
cobra	T63.041	T63.042	T63.043	T63.044	—	—
coral snake	T63.021	T63.022	T63.023	T63.024	—	—
rattlesnake	T63.011	T63.012	T63.013	T63.014	—	—
specified NEC	T63.091	T63.092	T63.093	T63.094	—	—
taipan	T63.031	T63.032	T63.033	T63.034	—	—
specified NEC	T63.891	T63.892	T63.893	T63.894	—	—
spider	T63.301	T63.302	T63.303	T63.304	—	—
black widow	T63.311	T63.312	T63.313	T63.314	—	—
brown recluse	T63.331	T63.332	T63.333	T63.334	—	—
specified NEC	T63.391	T63.392	T63.393	T63.394	—	—
tarantula	T63.321	T63.322	T63.323	T63.324	—	—
sting ray	T63.511	T63.512	T63.513	T63.514	—	—
toad	T63.821	T63.822	T63.823	T63.824	—	—
wasp	T63.461	T63.462	T63.463	T63.464	—	—
Venous sclerosing drug NEC	T46.8X1	T46.8X2	T46.8X3	T46.8X4	T46.8X5	T46.8X6
Ventolin — see Albuterol						
Veramon	T42.3X1	T42.3X2	T42.3X3	T42.3X4	T42.3X5	T42.3X6
Verapamil	T46.1X1	T46.1X2	T46.1X3	T46.1X4	T46.1X5	T46.1X6
Veratrine	T46.5X1	T46.5X2	T46.5X3	T46.5X4	T46.5X5	T46.5X6
Veratrum						
album	T62.2X1	T62.2X2	T62.2X3	T62.2X4	—	—
alkaloids	T46.5X1	T46.5X2	T46.5X3	T46.5X4	T46.5X5	T46.5X6
viride	T62.2X1	T62.2X2	T62.2X3	T62.2X4	—	—
Verdigris	T60.3X1	T60.3X2	T60.3X3	T60.3X4	—	—
Veronal	T42.3X1	T42.3X2	T42.3X3	T42.3X4	T42.3X5	T42.3X6
Veroxil	T37.4X1	T37.4X2	T37.4X3	T37.4X4	T37.4X5	T37.4X6
Versenate	T50.6X1	T50.6X2	T50.6X3	T50.6X4	T50.6X5	T50.6X6
Versidyne	T39.8X1	T39.8X2	T39.8X3	T39.8X4	T39.8X5	T39.8X6
Vetrabutine	T48.0X1	T48.0X2	T48.0X3	T48.0X4	T48.0X5	T48.0X6
Vidarabine	T37.5X1	T37.5X2	T37.5X3	T37.5X4	T37.5X5	T37.5X6
Vienna						
green	T57.0X1	T57.0X2	T57.0X3	T57.0X4	—	—
insecticide	T60.2X1	T60.2X2	T60.2X3	T60.2X4	—	—
red	T57.0X1	T57.0X2	T57.0X3	T57.0X4	—	—
pharmaceutical dye	T50.991	T50.992	T50.993	T50.994	T50.995	T50.996
Vigabatrin	T42.6X1	T42.6X2	T42.6X3	T42.6X4	T42.6X5	T42.6X6
Viloxazine	T43.291	T43.292	T43.293	T43.294	T43.295	T43.296
Viminol	T39.8X1	T39.8X2	T39.8X3	T39.8X4	T39.8X5	T39.8X6
Vinbarbital, vinbarbitone	T42.3X1	T42.3X2	T42.3X3	T42.3X4	T42.3X5	T42.3X6
Vinblastine	T45.1X1	T45.1X2	T45.1X3	T45.1X4	T45.1X5	T45.1X6
Vinburnine	T46.7X1	T46.7X2	T46.7X3	T46.7X4	T46.7X5	T46.7X6
Vincamine	T45.1X1	T45.1X2	T45.1X3	T45.1X4	T45.1X5	T45.1X6
Vincristine	T45.1X1	T45.1X2	T45.1X3	T45.1X4	T45.1X5	T45.1X6
Vindesine	T45.1X1	T45.1X2	T45.1X3	T45.1X4	T45.1X5	T45.1X6
Vinesthene, vinethene	T41.0X1	T41.0X2	T41.0X3	T41.0X4	T41.0X5	T41.0X6
Vinorelbine tartrate	T45.1X1	T45.1X2	T45.1X3	T45.1X4	T45.1X5	T45.1X6

Table of Drugs and Chemicals

Vinpocetine — Zyprexa

Substance	Poisoning, Accidental (unintentional)	Poisoning, Intentional Self-harm	Poisoning, Assault	Poisoning, Undetermined	Adverse Effect	Under-dosing
Vinpocetine	T46.7X1	T46.7X2	T46.7X3	T46.7X4	T46.7X5	T46.7X6
Vinyl						
acetate	T65.891	T65.892	T65.893	T65.894	—	—
bital	T42.3X1	T42.3X2	T42.3X3	T42.3X4	T42.3X5	T42.3X6
bromide	T65.891	T65.892	T65.893	T65.894	—	—
chloride	T59.891	T59.892	T59.893	T59.894	—	—
ether	T41.0X1	T41.0X2	T41.0X3	T41.0X4	T41.0X5	T41.0X6
Vinylbital	T42.3X1	T42.3X2	T42.3X3	T42.3X4	T42.3X5	T42.3X6
Vinylidene chloride	T65.891	T65.892	T65.893	T65.894	—	—
Vioform	T37.8X1	T37.8X2	T37.8X3	T37.8X4	T37.8X5	T37.8X6
topical	T49.0X1	T49.0X2	T49.0X3	T49.0X4	T49.0X5	T49.0X6
Viomycin	T36.8X1	T36.8X2	T36.8X3	T36.8X4	T36.8X5	T36.8X6
Viosterol	T45.2X1	T45.2X2	T45.2X3	T45.2X4	T45.2X5	T45.2X6
Viper (venom)	T63.091	T63.092	T63.093	T63.094	—	—
Viprynium	T37.4X1	T37.4X2	T37.4X3	T37.4X4	T37.4X5	T37.4X6
Viquidil	T46.7X1	T46.7X2	T46.7X3	T46.7X4	T46.7X5	T46.7X6
Viral vaccine NEC	T50.B91	T50.B92	T50.B93	T50.B94	T50.B95	T50.B96
Virginiamycin	T36.8X1	T36.8X2	T36.8X3	T36.8X4	T36.8X5	T36.8X6
Virugon	T37.5X1	T37.5X2	T37.5X3	T37.5X4	T37.5X5	T37.5X6
Viscous agent	T50.901	T50.902	T50.903	T50.904	T50.905	T50.906
Visine	T49.5X1	T49.5X2	T49.5X3	T49.5X4	T49.5X5	T49.5X6
Visnadine	T46.3X1	T46.3X2	T46.3X3	T46.3X4	T46.3X5	T46.3X6
Vitamin NEC	T45.2X1	T45.2X2	T45.2X3	T45.2X4	T45.2X5	T45.2X6
A	T45.2X1	T45.2X2	T45.2X3	T45.2X4	T45.2X5	T45.2X6
B1	T45.2X1	T45.2X2	T45.2X3	T45.2X4	T45.2X5	T45.2X6
B2	T45.2X1	T45.2X2	T45.2X3	T45.2X4	T45.2X5	T45.2X6
B6	T45.2X1	T45.2X2	T45.2X3	T45.2X4	T45.2X5	T45.2X6
B12	T45.2X1	T45.2X2	T45.2X3	T45.2X4	T45.2X5	T45.2X6
B15	T45.2X1	T45.2X2	T45.2X3	T45.2X4	T45.2X5	T45.2X6
B NEC	T45.2X1	T45.2X2	T45.2X3	T45.2X4	T45.2X5	T45.2X6
nicotinic acid	T46.7X1	T46.7X2	T46.7X3	T46.7X4	T46.7X5	T46.7X6
C	T45.2X1	T45.2X2	T45.2X3	T45.2X4	T45.2X5	T45.2X6
D	T45.2X1	T45.2X2	T45.2X3	T45.2X4	T45.2X5	T45.2X6
D2	T45.2X1	T45.2X2	T45.2X3	T45.2X4	T45.2X5	T45.2X6
D3	T45.2X1	T45.2X2	T45.2X3	T45.2X4	T45.2X5	T45.2X6
E	T45.2X1	T45.2X2	T45.2X3	T45.2X4	T45.2X5	T45.2X6
E acetate	T45.2X1	T45.2X2	T45.2X3	T45.2X4	T45.2X5	T45.2X6
hematopoietic	T45.8X1	T45.8X2	T45.8X3	T45.8X4	T45.8X5	T45.8X6
K1	T45.7X1	T45.7X2	T45.7X3	T45.7X4	T45.7X5	T45.7X6
K2	T45.7X1	T45.7X2	T45.7X3	T45.7X4	T45.7X5	T45.7X6
K NEC	T45.7X1	T45.7X2	T45.7X3	T45.7X4	T45.7X5	T45.7X6
PP	T45.2X1	T45.2X2	T45.2X3	T45.2X4	T45.2X5	T45.2X6
ulceroprotectant	T47.1X1	T47.1X2	T47.1X3	T47.1X4	T47.1X5	T47.1X6
Vleminckx's solution	T49.4X1	T49.4X2	T49.4X3	T49.4X4	T49.4X5	T49.4X6
Voltaren — see Diclofenac						
sodium						
Warfarin	T45.511	T45.512	T45.513	T45.514	T45.515	T45.516
rodenticide	T60.4X1	T60.4X2	T60.4X3	T60.4X4	—	—
sodium	T60.4X1	T60.4X2	T60.4X3	T60.4X4	—	—
Wasp (sting)	T63.461	T63.462	T63.463	T63.464	—	—
Water						
balance drug	T50.3X1	T50.3X2	T50.3X3	T50.3X4	T50.3X5	T50.3X6
distilled	T50.3X1	T50.3X2	T50.3X3	T50.3X4	T50.3X5	T50.3X6
gas — see Gas, water						
incomplete combustion of — see Carbon, monoxide, fuel, utility						
hemlock	T62.2X1	T62.2X2	T62.2X3	T62.2X4	—	—
moccasin (venom)	T63.061	T63.062	T63.063	T63.064	—	—
purified	T50.3X1	T50.3X2	T50.3X3	T50.3X4	T50.3X5	T50.3X6
Wax (paraffin) (petroleum)	T52.0X1	T52.0X2	T52.0X3	T52.0X4	—	—
automobile	T65.891	T65.892	T65.893	T65.894	—	—
floor	T52.0X1	T52.0X2	T52.0X3	T52.0X4	—	—
Weed killers NEC	T60.3X1	T60.3X2	T60.3X3	T60.3X4	—	—
Welldorm	T42.6X1	T42.6X2	T42.6X3	T42.6X4	T42.6X5	T42.6X6
White						
arsenic	T57.0X1	T57.0X2	T57.0X3	T57.0X4	—	—
hellebore	T62.2X1	T62.2X2	T62.2X3	T62.2X4	—	—
lotion (keratolytic)	T49.4X1	T49.4X2	T49.4X3	T49.4X4	T49.4X5	T49.4X6
spirit	T52.0X1	T52.0X2	T52.0X3	T52.0X4	—	—
Whitewash	T65.891	T65.892	T65.893	T65.894	—	—
Whole blood (human)	T45.8X1	T45.8X2	T45.8X3	T45.8X4	T45.8X5	T45.8X6
Wild						
black cherry	T62.2X1	T62.2X2	T62.2X3	T62.2X4	—	—
poisonous plants NEC	T62.2X1	T62.2X2	T62.2X3	T62.2X4	—	—
Window cleaning fluid	T65.891	T65.892	T65.893	T65.894	—	—
Wintergreen (oil)	T49.3X1	T49.3X2	T49.3X3	T49.3X4	T49.3X5	T49.3X6
Wisterine	T62.2X1	T62.2X2	T62.2X3	T62.2X4	—	—
Witch hazel	T49.2X1	T49.2X2	T49.2X3	T49.2X4	T49.2X5	T49.2X6
Wood alcohol or spirit	T51.1X1	T51.1X2	T51.1X3	T51.1X4	—	—
Wool fat (hydrous)	T49.3X1	T49.3X2	T49.3X3	T49.3X4	T49.3X5	T49.3X6
Woorali	T48.1X1	T48.1X2	T48.1X3	T48.1X4	T48.1X5	T48.1X6
Wormseed, American	T37.4X1	T37.4X2	T37.4X3	T37.4X4	T37.4X5	T37.4X6

Substance	Poisoning, Accidental (unintentional)	Poisoning, Intentional Self-harm	Poisoning, Assault	Poisoning, Undetermined	Adverse Effect	Under-dosing
Xamoterol	T44.5X1	T44.5X2	T44.5X3	T44.5X4	T44.5X5	T44.5X6
Xanthine diuretics	T50.2X1	T50.2X2	T50.2X3	T50.2X4	T50.2X5	T50.2X6
Xanthinol nicotinate	T46.7X1	T46.7X2	T46.7X3	T46.7X4	T46.7X5	T46.7X6
Xanthotoxin	T49.3X1	T49.3X2	T49.3X3	T49.3X4	T49.3X5	T49.3X6
Xantinol nicotinate	T46.7X1	T46.7X2	T46.7X3	T46.7X4	T46.7X5	T46.7X6
Xantocillin	T36.0X1	T36.0X2	T36.0X3	T36.0X4	T36.0X5	T36.0X6
Xenon (127Xe) (133Xe)	T50.8X1	T50.8X2	T50.8X3	T50.8X4	T50.8X5	T50.8X6
Xenysalate	T49.4X1	T49.4X2	T49.4X3	T49.4X4	T49.4X5	T49.4X6
Xibornol	T37.8X1	T37.8X2	T37.8X3	T37.8X4	T37.8X5	T37.8X6
Xigris	T45.511	T45.512	T45.513	T45.514	T45.515	T45.516
Xipamide	T50.2X1	T50.2X2	T50.2X3	T50.2X4	T50.2X5	T50.2X6
Xylene (vapor)	T52.2X1	T52.2X2	T52.2X3	T52.2X4	—	—
Xylocaine (infiltration) (topical)	T41.3X1	T41.3X2	T41.3X3	T41.3X4	T41.3X5	T41.3X6
nerve block (peripheral) (plexus)	T41.3X1	T41.3X2	T41.3X3	T41.3X4	T41.3X5	T41.3X6
spinal	T41.3X1	T41.3X2	T41.3X3	T41.3X4	T41.3X5	T41.3X6
Xylol (vapor)	T52.2X1	T52.2X2	T52.2X3	T52.2X4	—	—
Xylometazoline	T48.5X1	T48.5X2	T48.5X3	T48.5X4	T48.5X5	T48.5X6
Yeast	T45.2X1	T45.2X2	T45.2X3	T45.2X4	T45.2X5	T45.2X6
dried	T45.2X1	T45.2X2	T45.2X3	T45.2X4	T45.2X5	T45.2X6
Yellow						
fever vaccine	T50.B91	T50.B92	T50.B93	T50.B94	T50.B95	T50.B96
jasmine	T62.2X1	T62.2X2	T62.2X3	T62.2X4	—	—
phenolphthalein	T47.2X1	T47.2X2	T47.2X3	T47.2X4	T47.2X5	T47.2X6
Yew	T62.2X1	T62.2X2	T62.2X3	T62.2X4	—	—
Yohimbic acid	T40.991	T40.992	T40.993	T40.994	T40.995	T40.996
Zactane	T39.8X1	T39.8X2	T39.8X3	T39.8X4	T39.8X5	T39.8X6
Zalcitabine	T37.5X1	T37.5X2	T37.5X3	T37.5X4	T37.5X5	T37.5X6
Zaroxolyn	T50.2X1	T50.2X2	T50.2X3	T50.2X4	T50.2X5	T50.2X6
Zephiran (topical)	T49.0X1	T49.0X2	T49.0X3	T49.0X4	T49.0X5	T49.0X6
ophthalmic preparation	T49.5X1	T49.5X2	T49.5X3	T49.5X4	T49.5X5	T49.5X6
Zeranol	T38.7X1	T38.7X2	T38.7X3	T38.7X4	T38.7X5	T38.7X6
Zerone	T51.1X1	T51.1X2	T51.1X3	T51.1X4	—	—
Zidovudine	T37.5X1	T37.5X2	T37.5X3	T37.5X4	T37.5X5	T37.5X6
Zimeldine	T43.221	T43.222	T43.223	T43.224	T43.225	T43.226
Zinc (compounds) (fumes) (vapor) NEC	T56.5X1	T56.5X2	T56.5X3	T56.5X4	—	—
anti-infectives	T49.0X1	T49.0X2	T49.0X3	T49.0X4	T49.0X5	T49.0X6
antivaricose	T46.8X1	T46.8X2	T46.8X3	T46.8X4	T46.8X5	T46.8X6
bacitracin	T49.0X1	T49.0X2	T49.0X3	T49.0X4	T49.0X5	T49.0X6
chloride (mouthwash)	T49.6X1	T49.6X2	T49.6X3	T49.6X4	T49.6X5	T49.6X6
chromate	T56.5X1	T56.5X2	T56.5X3	T56.5X4	—	—
gelatin	T49.3X1	T49.3X2	T49.3X3	T49.3X4	T49.3X5	T49.3X6
oxide	T49.3X1	T49.3X2	T49.3X3	T49.3X4	T49.3X5	T49.3X6
plaster	T49.3X1	T49.3X2	T49.3X3	T49.3X4	T49.3X5	T49.3X6
peroxide	T49.0X1	T49.0X2	T49.0X3	T49.0X4	T49.0X5	T49.0X6
pesticides	T56.5X1	T56.5X2	T56.5X3	T56.5X4	—	—
phosphide	T60.4X1	T60.4X2	T60.4X3	T60.4X4	—	—
pyrithionate	T49.4X1	T49.4X2	T49.4X3	T49.4X4	T49.4X5	T49.4X6
stearate	T49.3X1	T49.3X2	T49.3X3	T49.3X4	T49.3X5	T49.3X6
sulfate	T49.5X1	T49.5X2	T49.5X3	T49.5X4	T49.5X5	T49.5X6
ENT agent	T49.6X1	T49.6X2	T49.6X3	T49.6X4	T49.6X5	T49.6X6
ophthalmic solution	T49.5X1	T49.5X2	T49.5X3	T49.5X4	T49.5X5	T49.5X6
topical NEC	T49.0X1	T49.0X2	T49.0X3	T49.0X4	T49.0X5	T49.0X6
undecylenate	T49.0X1	T49.0X2	T49.0X3	T49.0X4	T49.0X5	T49.0X6
Zineb	T60.0X1	T60.0X2	T60.0X3	T60.0X4	—	—
Zinostatin	T45.1X1	T45.1X2	T45.1X3	T45.1X4	T45.1X5	T45.1X6
Zipeprol	T48.3X1	T48.3X2	T48.3X3	T48.3X4	T48.3X5	T48.3X6
Zofenopril	T46.4X1	T46.4X2	T46.4X3	T46.4X4	T46.4X5	T46.4X6
Zolpidem	T42.6X1	T42.6X2	T42.6X3	T42.6X4	T42.6X5	T42.6X6
Zomepirac	T39.391	T39.392	T39.393	T39.394	T39.395	T39.396
Zopiclone	T42.6X1	T42.6X2	T42.6X3	T42.6X4	T42.6X5	T42.6X6
Zorubicin	T45.1X1	T45.1X2	T45.1X3	T45.1X4	T45.1X5	T45.1X6
Zotepine	T43.591	T43.592	T43.593	T43.594	T43.595	T43.596
Zovant	T45.511	T45.512	T45.513	T45.514	T45.515	T45.516
Zoxazolamine	T42.8X1	T42.8X2	T42.8X3	T42.8X4	T42.8X5	T42.8X6
Zuclopenthixol	T43.4X1	T43.4X2	T43.4X3	T43.4X4	T43.4X5	T43.4X6
Zygadenus (venenosus)	T62.2X1	T62.2X2	T62.2X3	T62.2X4	—	—
Zyprexa	T43.591	T43.592	T43.593	T43.594	T43.595	T43.596

A

Abandonment (causing exposure to weather conditions) (with intent to injure or kill) NEC X58 ☑
Abuse (adult) (child) (mental) (physical) (sexual) X58 ☑
Accident (to) X58 ☑
  aircraft (in transit) (powered) (*see also* Accident, transport, aircraft)
    due to, caused by cataclysm — *see* Forces of nature, by type
  animal-drawn vehicle — *see* Accident, transport, animal-drawn vehicle occupant
  animal-rider — *see* Accident, transport, animal-rider
  automobile — *see* Accident, transport, car occupant
  bare foot water skier V94.4 ☑
  boat, boating (*see also* Accident, watercraft)
    striking swimmer
      powered V94.11 ☑
      unpowered V94.12 ☑
  bus — *see* Accident, transport, bus occupant
  <Insert new term here>
  cable car, not on rails V98.Ø ☑
    on rails — *see* Accident, transport, streetcar occupant
  car — *see* Accident, transport, car occupant
  caused by, due to
    animal NEC W64 ☑
    chain hoist W24.Ø ☑
    cold (excessive) — *see* Exposure, cold
    corrosive liquid, substance — *see* Table of Drugs and Chemicals
    cutting or piercing instrument — *see* Contact, with, by type of instrument
    drive belt W24.Ø ☑
    electric
      current — *see* Exposure, electric current
      motor (*see also* Contact, with, by type of machine) W31.3 ☑
      current (of) W86.8 ☑
    environmental factor NEC X58 ☑
    explosive material — *see* Explosion
    fire, flames — *see* Exposure, fire
    firearm missile — *see* Discharge, firearm by type
    heat (excessive) — *see* Heat
    hot — *see* Contact, with, hot
    ignition — *see* Ignition
    lifting device W24.Ø ☑
    lightning — *see* subcategory T75.Ø ☑
      causing fire — *see* Exposure, fire
    machine, machinery — *see* Contact, with, by type of machine
    natural factor NEC X58 ☑
    pulley (block) W24.Ø ☑
    radiation — *see* Radiation
    steam X13.1 ☑
      inhalation X13.Ø ☑
      pipe X16 ☑
    thunderbolt — *see* subcategory T75.Ø ☑
      causing fire — *see* Exposure, fire
    transmission device W24.1 ☑
  coach — *see* Accident, transport, bus occupant
  coal car — *see* Accident, transport, industrial vehicle occupant
  diving (*see also* Fall, into, water)
    with
      drowning or submersion — *see* Drowning
  forklift — *see* Accident, transport, industrial vehicle occupant
  heavy transport vehicle NOS — *see* Accident, transport, truck occupant
  ice yacht V98.2 ☑
  in
    medical, surgical procedure
      as, or due to misadventure — *see* Misadventure
      causing an abnormal reaction or later complication without mention of misadventure (*see also* Complication of or following, by type of procedure) Y84.9
  land yacht V98.1 ☑
  late effect of — *see* WØØ-X58 with 7th character S

Accident — *continued*
  logging car — *see* Accident, transport, industrial vehicle occupant
  machine, machinery (*see also* Contact, with, by type of machine)
    on board watercraft V93.69 ☑
      explosion — *see* Explosion, in, watercraft
      fire — *see* Burn, on board watercraft
      powered craft V93.63 ☑
        ferry boat V93.61 ☑
        fishing boat V93.62 ☑
        jetskis V93.63 ☑
        liner V93.61 ☑
        merchant ship V93.6Ø ☑
        passenger ship V93.61 ☑
        sailboat V93.63 ☑
  mine tram — *see* Accident, transport, industrial vehicle occupant
  mobility scooter (motorized) — *see* Accident, transport, pedestrian, conveyance, specified type NEC
  motor scooter — *see* Accident, transport, motorcyclist
  motor vehicle NOS (traffic) (*see also* Accident, transport) V89.2 ☑
    nontraffic V89.Ø ☑
    three-wheeled NOS — *see* Accident, transport, three-wheeled motor vehicle occupant
  motorcycle NOS — *see* Accident, transport, motorcyclist
  nonmotor vehicle NOS (nontraffic) (*see also* Accident, transport) V89.1 ☑
    traffic NOS V89.3 ☑
  nontraffic (victim's mode of transport NOS) V88.9 ☑
    collision (between) V88.7 ☑
      bus and truck V88.5 ☑
      car and:
        bus V88.3 ☑
        pickup V88.2 ☑
        three-wheeled motor vehicle V88.Ø ☑
        train V88.6 ☑
        truck V88.4 ☑
        two-wheeled motor vehicle V88.Ø ☑
        van V88.2 ☑
      specified vehicle NEC and:
        three-wheeled motor vehicle V88.1 ☑
        two-wheeled motor vehicle V88.1 ☑
      known mode of transport — *see* Accident, transport, by type of vehicle
    noncollision V88.8 ☑
  on board watercraft V93.89 ☑
    powered craft V93.83 ☑
      ferry boat V93.81 ☑
      fishing boat V93.82 ☑
      jetskis V93.83 ☑
      liner V93.81 ☑
      merchant ship V93.8Ø ☑
      passenger ship V93.81 ☑
    unpowered craft V93.88 ☑
      canoe V93.85 ☑
      inflatable V93.86 ☑
        in tow
          recreational V94.31 ☑
          specified NEC V94.32 ☑
      kayak V93.85 ☑
      sailboat V93.84 ☑
      surf-board V93.88 ☑
      water skis V93.87 ☑
      windsurfer V93.88 ☑
  parachutist V97.29 ☑
    entangled in object V97.21 ☑
    injured on landing V97.22 ☑
  pedal cycle — *see* Accident, transport, pedal cyclist
  pedestrian (on foot)
    with
      another pedestrian W51 ☑
        with fall WØ3 ☑
          due to ice or snow WØØ.Ø ☑
      on pedestrian conveyance NEC VØØ.Ø9 ☑
      roller skater (in-line) VØØ.Ø1 ☑
      skate boarder VØØ.Ø2 ☑
      transport vehicle — *see* Accident, transport

Accident — *continued*
  pedestrian — *continued*
    on pedestrian conveyance — *see* Accident, transport, pedestrian, conveyance
  pick-up truck or van — *see* Accident, transport, pickup truck occupant
  quarry truck — *see* Accident, transport, industrial vehicle occupant
  railway vehicle (any) (in motion) — *see* Accident, transport, railway vehicle occupant
    due to cataclysm — *see* Forces of nature, by type
  scooter (non-motorized) — *see* Accident, transport, pedestrian, conveyance, scooter
  sequelae of — *see* categories WØØ-X58 with 7th character S
  skateboard — *see* Accident, transport, pedestrian, conveyance, skateboard
  ski(ing) — *see* Accident, transport, pedestrian, conveyance
    lift V98.3 ☑
  specified cause NEC X58 ☑
  streetcar — *see* Accident, transport, streetcar occupant
  traffic (victim's mode of transport NOS) V87.9 ☑
    collision (between) V87.7 ☑
      bus and truck V87.5 ☑
      car and:
        bus V87.3 ☑
        pickup V87.2 ☑
        three-wheeled motor vehicle V87.Ø ☑
        train V87.6 ☑
        truck V87.4 ☑
        two-wheeled motor vehicle V87.Ø ☑
        van V87.2 ☑
      specified vehicle NEC and:
        three-wheeled motor vehicle V87.1 ☑
        two-wheeled motor vehicle V87.1 ☑
      known mode of transport — *see* Accident, transport, by type of vehicle
    noncollision V87.8 ☑
  transport (involving injury to) V99 ☑
    18 wheeler — *see* Accident, transport, truck occupant
    agricultural vehicle occupant (nontraffic) V84.9 ☑
      driver V84.5 ☑
      hanger-on V84.7 ☑
      passenger V84.6 ☑
      traffic V84.3 ☑
        driver V84.Ø ☑
        hanger-on V84.2 ☑
        passenger V84.1 ☑
      while boarding or alighting V84.4 ☑
    aircraft NEC V97.89 ☑
      military NEC V97.818 ☑
        with civlian aircraft V97.81Ø ☑
        civilian injured by V97.811 ☑
      occupant injured (in)
        nonpowered craft accident V96.9 ☑
          balloon V96.ØØ ☑
            collision V96.Ø3 ☑
            crash V96.Ø1 ☑
            explosion V96.Ø5 ☑
            fire V96.Ø4 ☑
            forced landing V96.Ø2 ☑
            specified type NEC V96.Ø9 ☑
          glider V96.2Ø ☑
            collision V96.23 ☑
            crash V96.21 ☑
            explosion V96.25 ☑
            fire V96.24 ☑
            forced landing V96.22 ☑
            specified type NEC V96.29 ☑
          hang glider V96.1Ø ☑
            collision V96.13 ☑
            crash V96.11 ☑
            explosion V96.15 ☑
            fire V96.14 ☑
            forced landing V96.12 ☑
            specified type NEC V96.19 ☑
          specified craft NEC V96.8 ☑
        powered craft accident V95.9 ☑

Accident — *continued*
transport — *continued*
aircraft — *continued*
occupant injured — *continued*
powered craft accident — *continued*
fixed wing
commercial V95.30 ☑
collision V95.33 ☑
crash V95.31 ☑
explosion V95.35 ☑
fire V95.34 ☑
forced landing V95.32 ☑
specified type NEC V95.39 ☑
private V95.20 ☑
collision V95.23 ☑
crash V95.21 ☑
explosion V95.25 ☑
fire V95.24 ☑
forced landing V95.22 ☑
specified type NEC V95.29 ☑
glider V95.10 ☑
collision V95.13 ☑
crash V95.11 ☑
explosion V95.15 ☑
fire V95.14 ☑
forced landing V95.12 ☑
specified type NEC V95.19 ☑
helicopter V95.00 ☑
collision V95.03 ☑
crash V95.01 ☑
explosion V95.05 ☑
fire V95.04 ☑
forced landing V95.02 ☑
specified type NEC V95.09 ☑
spacecraft V95.40 ☑
collision V95.43 ☑
crash V95.41 ☑
explosion V95.45 ☑
fire V95.44 ☑
forced landing V95.42 ☑
specified type NEC V95.49 ☑
specified craft NEC V95.8 ☑
ultralight V95.10 ☑
collision V95.13 ☑
crash V95.11 ☑
explosion V95.15 ☑
fire V95.14 ☑
forced landing V95.12 ☑
specified type NEC V95.19 ☑
specified accident NEC V97.0 ☑
while boarding or alighting V97.1 ☑
person (injured by)
falling from, in or on aircraft V97.0 ☑
machinery on aircraft V97.89 ☑
on ground with aircraft involvement V97.39 ☑
rotating propeller V97.32 ☑
struck by object falling from aircraft V97.31 ☑
sucked into aircraft jet V97.33 ☑
while boarding or alighting aircraft V97.1 ☑
airport (battery-powered) passenger vehicle — *see* Accident, transport, industrial vehicle occupant
all-terrain vehicle occupant (nontraffic) V86.99 ☑
driver V86.59 ☑
dune buggy — *see* Accident, transport, dune buggy occupant
hanger-on V86.79 ☑
passenger V86.69 ☑
snowmobile — *see* Accident, transport, snowmobile occupant
traffic V86.39 ☑
driver V86.09 ☑
hanger-on V86.29 ☑
passenger V86.19 ☑
while boarding or alighting V86.49 ☑
ambulance occupant (traffic) V86.31 ☑
driver V86.01 ☑
hanger-on V86.21 ☑
nontraffic V86.91 ☑
driver V86.51 ☑
hanger-on V86.71 ☑
passenger V86.61 ☑
passenger V86.11 ☑
while boarding or alighting V86.41 ☑

Accident — *continued*
transport — *continued*
animal-drawn vehicle occupant (in) V80.929 ☑
collision (with)
animal V80.12 ☑
being ridden V80.711 ☑
animal-drawn vehicle V80.721 ☑
bus V80.42 ☑
car V80.42 ☑
fixed or stationary object V80.82 ☑
military vehicle V80.920 ☑
nonmotor vehicle V80.791 ☑
pedal cycle V80.22 ☑
pedestrian V80.12 ☑
pickup V80.42 ☑
railway train or vehicle V80.62 ☑
specified motor vehicle NEC V80.52 ☑
streetcar V80.731 ☑
truck V80.42 ☑
two- or three-wheeled motor vehicle V80.32 ☑
van V80.42 ☑
noncollision V80.02 ☑
specified circumstance NEC V80.928 ☑
animal-rider V80.919 ☑
collision (with)
animal V80.11 ☑
being ridden V80.710 ☑
animal-drawn vehicle V80.720 ☑
bus V80.41 ☑
car V80.41 ☑
fixed or stationary object V80.81 ☑
military vehicle V80.910 ☑
nonmotor vehicle V80.790 ☑
pedal cycle V80.21 ☑
pedestrian V80.11 ☑
pickup V80.41 ☑
railway train or vehicle V80.61 ☑
specified motor vehicle NEC V80.51 ☑
streetcar V80.730 ☑
truck V80.41 ☑
two- or three-wheeled motor vehicle V80.31 ☑
van V80.41 ☑
noncollision V80.018 ☑
specified as horse rider V80.010 ☑
specified circumstance NEC V80.918 ☑
armored car — *see* Accident, transport, truck occupant
battery-powered truck (baggage) (mail) — *see* Accident, transport, industrial vehicle occupant
bus occupant V79.9 ☑
collision (with)
animal (traffic) V70.9 ☑
being ridden (traffic) V76.9 ☑
nontraffic V76.3 ☑
while boarding or alighting V76.4 ☑
nontraffic V70.3 ☑
while boarding or alighting V70.4 ☑
animal-drawn vehicle (traffic) V76.9 ☑
nontraffic V76.3 ☑
while boarding or alighting V76.4 ☑
bus (traffic) V74.9 ☑
nontraffic V74.3 ☑
while boarding or alighting V74.4 ☑
car (traffic) V73.9 ☑
nontraffic V73.3 ☑
while boarding or alighting V73.4 ☑
motor vehicle NOS (traffic) V79.60 ☑
nontraffic V79.20 ☑
specified type NEC (traffic) V79.69 ☑
nontraffic V79.29 ☑
pedal cycle (traffic) V71.9 ☑
nontraffic V71.3 ☑
while boarding or alighting V71.4 ☑
pickup truck (traffic) V73.9 ☑
nontraffic V73.3 ☑
while boarding or alighting V73.4 ☑
railway vehicle (traffic) V75.9 ☑
nontraffic V75.3 ☑
while boarding or alighting V75.4 ☑
specified vehicle NEC (traffic) V76.9 ☑
nontraffic V76.3 ☑
while boarding or alighting V76.4 ☑
stationary object (traffic) V77.9 ☑

Accident — *continued*
transport — *continued*
bus occupant — *continued*
collision — *continued*
stationary object — *continued*
nontraffic V77.3 ☑
while boarding or alighting V77.4 ☑
streetcar (traffic) V76.9 ☑
nontraffic V76.3 ☑
while boarding or alighting V76.4 ☑
three wheeled motor vehicle (traffic) V72.9 ☑
nontraffic V72.3 ☑
while boarding or alighting V72.4 ☑
truck (traffic) V74.9 ☑
nontraffic V74.3 ☑
while boarding or alighting V74.4 ☑
two wheeled motor vehicle (traffic) V72.9 ☑
nontraffic V72.3 ☑
while boarding or alighting V72.4 ☑
van (traffic) V73.9 ☑
nontraffic V73.3 ☑
while boarding or alighting V73.4 ☑
driver
collision (with)
animal (traffic) V70.5 ☑
being ridden (traffic) V76.5 ☑
nontraffic V76.0 ☑
nontraffic V70.0 ☑
animal-drawn vehicle (traffic) V76.5 ☑
nontraffic V76.0 ☑
bus (traffic) V74.5 ☑
nontraffic V74.0 ☑
car (traffic) V73.5 ☑
nontraffic V73.0 ☑
motor vehicle NOS (traffic) V79.40 ☑
nontraffic V79.00 ☑
specified type NEC (traffic) V79.49 ☑
nontraffic V79.09 ☑
pedal cycle (traffic) V71.5 ☑
nontraffic V71.0 ☑
pickup truck (traffic) V73.5 ☑
nontraffic V73.0 ☑
railway vehicle (traffic) V75.5 ☑
nontraffic V75.0 ☑
specified vehicle NEC (traffic) V76.5 ☑
nontraffic V76.0 ☑
stationary object (traffic) V77.5 ☑
nontraffic V77.0 ☑
streetcar (traffic) V76.5 ☑
nontraffic V76.0 ☑
three wheeled motor vehicle (traffic) V72.5 ☑
nontraffic V72.0 ☑
truck (traffic) V74.5 ☑
nontraffic V74.0 ☑
two wheeled motor vehicle (traffic) V72.5 ☑
nontraffic V72.0 ☑
van (traffic) V73.5 ☑
nontraffic V73.0 ☑
noncollision accident (traffic) V78.5 ☑
nontraffic V78.0 ☑
hanger-on
collision (with)
animal (traffic) V70.7 ☑
being ridden (traffic) V76.7 ☑
nontraffic V76.2 ☑
nontraffic V70.2 ☑
animal-drawn vehicle (traffic) V76.7 ☑
nontraffic V76.2 ☑
bus (traffic) V74.7 ☑
nontraffic V74.2 ☑
car (traffic) V73.7 ☑
nontraffic V73.2 ☑
pedal cycle (traffic) V71.7 ☑
nontraffic V71.2 ☑
pickup truck (traffic) V73.7 ☑
nontraffic V73.2 ☑
railway vehicle (traffic) V75.7 ☑
nontraffic V75.2 ☑
specified vehicle NEC (traffic) V76.7 ☑
nontraffic V76.2 ☑
stationary object (traffic) V77.7 ☑
nontraffic V77.2 ☑
streetcar (traffic) V76.7 ☑

☑ **Additional Character Required** — Refer to the Tabular List for Character Selection   ▽ **Subterms under main terms may continue to next column or page**

Accident — *continued*
　transport — *continued*
　　bus occupant — *continued*
　　　hanger-on — *continued*
　　　　collision — *continued*
　　　　　streetcar — *continued*
　　　　　　nontraffic V76.2 ☑
　　　　　three wheeled motor vehicle (traffic)
　　　　　　V72.7 ☑
　　　　　　nontraffic V72.2 ☑
　　　　　truck (traffic) V74.7 ☑
　　　　　　nontraffic V74.2 ☑
　　　　　two wheeled motor vehicle (traffic)
　　　　　　V72.7 ☑
　　　　　　nontraffic V72.2 ☑
　　　　　van (traffic) V73.7 ☑
　　　　　　nontraffic V73.2 ☑
　　　　noncollision accident (traffic) V78.7 ☑
　　　　　nontraffic V78.2 ☑
　　　　noncollision accident (traffic) V78.9 ☑
　　　　　nontraffic V78.3 ☑
　　　　　while boarding or alighting V78.4 ☑
　　　　nontraffic V79.3 ☑
　　　passenger
　　　　collision (with)
　　　　　animal (traffic) V70.6 ☑
　　　　　　being ridden (traffic) V76.6 ☑
　　　　　　　nontraffic V76.1 ☑
　　　　　　nontraffic V70.1 ☑
　　　　　animal-drawn vehicle (traffic) V76.6 ☑
　　　　　　nontraffic V76.1 ☑
　　　　　bus (traffic) V74.6 ☑
　　　　　　nontraffic V74.1 ☑
　　　　　car (traffic) V73.6 ☑
　　　　　　nontraffic V73.1 ☑
　　　　　motor vehicle NOS (traffic) V79.50 ☑
　　　　　　nontraffic V79.10 ☑
　　　　　　specified type NEC (traffic) V79.59 ☑
　　　　　　　nontraffic V79.19 ☑
　　　　　pedal cycle (traffic) V71.6 ☑
　　　　　　nontraffic V71.1 ☑
　　　　　pickup truck (traffic) V73.6 ☑
　　　　　　nontraffic V73.1 ☑
　　　　　railway vehicle (traffic) V75.6 ☑
　　　　　　nontraffic V75.1 ☑
　　　　　specified vehicle NEC (traffic) V76.6 ☑
　　　　　　nontraffic V76.1 ☑
　　　　　stationary object (traffic) V77.6 ☑
　　　　　　nontraffic V77.1 ☑
　　　　　streetcar (traffic) V76.6 ☑
　　　　　　nontraffic V76.1 ☑
　　　　　three wheeled motor vehicle (traffic)
　　　　　　V72.6 ☑
　　　　　　nontraffic V72.1 ☑
　　　　　truck (traffic) V74.6 ☑
　　　　　　nontraffic V74.1 ☑
　　　　　two wheeled motor vehicle (traffic)
　　　　　　V72.6 ☑
　　　　　　nontraffic V72.1 ☑
　　　　　van (traffic) V73.6 ☑
　　　　　　nontraffic V73.1 ☑
　　　　noncollision accident (traffic) V78.6 ☑
　　　　　nontraffic V78.1 ☑
　　　specified type NEC V79.88 ☑
　　　military vehicle V79.81 ☑
　　cable car, not on rails V98.0 ☑
　　　on rails — *see* Accident, transport, streetcar
　　　　occupant
　　car occupant V49.9 ☑
　　　ambulance occupant — *see* Accident, transport,
　　　　ambulance occupant
　　　collision (with)
　　　　animal (traffic) V40.9 ☑
　　　　　being ridden (traffic) V46.9 ☑
　　　　　　nontraffic V46.3 ☑
　　　　　　while boarding or alighting V46.4 ☑
　　　　　nontraffic V40.3 ☑
　　　　　while boarding or alighting V40.4 ☑
　　　　animal-drawn vehicle (traffic) V46.9 ☑
　　　　　nontraffic V46.3 ☑
　　　　　while boarding or alighting V46.4 ☑
　　　　bus (traffic) V44.9 ☑
　　　　　nontraffic V44.3 ☑
　　　　　while boarding or alighting V44.4 ☑
　　　　car (traffic) V43.92 ☑
　　　　　nontraffic V43.32 ☑

Accident — *continued*
　transport — *continued*
　　car occupant — *continued*
　　　collision — *continued*
　　　　car — *continued*
　　　　　while boarding or alighting V43.42 ☑
　　　　motor vehicle NOS (traffic) V49.60 ☑
　　　　　nontraffic V49.20 ☑
　　　　　specified type NEC (traffic) V49.69 ☑
　　　　　　nontraffic V49.29 ☑
　　　　pedal cycle (traffic) V41.9 ☑
　　　　　nontraffic V41.3 ☑
　　　　　while boarding or alighting V41.4 ☑
　　　　pickup truck (traffic) V43.93 ☑
　　　　　nontraffic V43.33 ☑
　　　　　while boarding or alighting V43.43 ☑
　　　　railway vehicle (traffic) V45.9 ☑
　　　　　nontraffic V45.3 ☑
　　　　　while boarding or alighting V45.4 ☑
　　　　specified vehicle NEC (traffic) V46.9 ☑
　　　　　nontraffic V46.3 ☑
　　　　　while boarding or alighting V46.4 ☑
　　　　sport utility vehicle (traffic) V43.91 ☑
　　　　　nontraffic V43.31 ☑
　　　　　while boarding or alighting V43.41 ☑
　　　　stationary object (traffic) V47.92 ☑
　　　　　nontraffic V47.32 ☑
　　　　　while boarding or alighting V47.4 ☑
　　　　streetcar (traffic) V46.9 ☑
　　　　　nontraffic V46.3 ☑
　　　　　while boarding or alighting V46.4 ☑
　　　　three wheeled motor vehicle (traffic)
　　　　　V42.9 ☑
　　　　　nontraffic V42.3 ☑
　　　　　while boarding or alighting V42.4 ☑
　　　　truck (traffic) V44.9 ☑
　　　　　nontraffic V44.3 ☑
　　　　　while boarding or alighting V44.4 ☑
　　　　two wheeled motor vehicle (traffic) V42.9 ☑
　　　　　nontraffic V42.3 ☑
　　　　　while boarding or alighting V42.4 ☑
　　　　van (traffic) V43.94 ☑
　　　　　nontraffic V43.34 ☑
　　　　　while boarding or alighting V43.44 ☑
　　　driver
　　　　collision (with)
　　　　　animal (traffic) V40.5 ☑
　　　　　　being ridden (traffic) V46.5 ☑
　　　　　　　nontraffic V46.0 ☑
　　　　　　nontraffic V40.0 ☑
　　　　　animal-drawn vehicle (traffic) V46.5 ☑
　　　　　　nontraffic V46.0 ☑
　　　　　bus (traffic) V44.5 ☑
　　　　　　nontraffic V44.0 ☑
　　　　　car (traffic) V43.52 ☑
　　　　　　nontraffic V43.02 ☑
　　　　　motor vehicle NOS (traffic) V49.40 ☑
　　　　　　nontraffic V49.00 ☑
　　　　　　specified type NEC (traffic) V49.49 ☑
　　　　　　　nontraffic V49.09 ☑
　　　　　pedal cycle (traffic) V41.5 ☑
　　　　　　nontraffic V41.0 ☑
　　　　　pickup truck (traffic) V43.53 ☑
　　　　　　nontraffic V43.03 ☑
　　　　　railway vehicle (traffic) V45.5 ☑
　　　　　　nontraffic V45.0 ☑
　　　　　specified vehicle NEC (traffic) V46.5 ☑
　　　　　　nontraffic V46.0 ☑
　　　　　sport utility vehicle (traffic) V43.51 ☑
　　　　　　nontraffic V43.01 ☑
　　　　　stationary object (traffic) V47.52 ☑
　　　　　　nontraffic V47.02 ☑
　　　　　streetcar (traffic) V46.5 ☑
　　　　　　nontraffic V46.0 ☑
　　　　　three wheeled motor vehicle (traffic)
　　　　　　V42.5 ☑
　　　　　　nontraffic V42.0 ☑
　　　　　truck (traffic) V44.5 ☑
　　　　　　nontraffic V44.0 ☑
　　　　　two wheeled motor vehicle (traffic)
　　　　　　V42.5 ☑
　　　　　　nontraffic V42.0 ☑
　　　　　van (traffic) V43.54 ☑
　　　　　　nontraffic V43.04 ☑
　　　　noncollision accident (traffic) V48.5 ☑
　　　　　nontraffic V48.0 ☑

Accident — *continued*
　transport — *continued*
　　car occupant — *continued*
　　　hanger-on
　　　　collision (with)
　　　　　animal (traffic) V40.7 ☑
　　　　　　being ridden (traffic) V46.7 ☑
　　　　　　　nontraffic V46.2 ☑
　　　　　　nontraffic V40.2 ☑
　　　　　animal-drawn vehicle (traffic) V46.7 ☑
　　　　　　nontraffic V46.2 ☑
　　　　　bus (traffic) V44.7 ☑
　　　　　　nontraffic V44.2 ☑
　　　　　car (traffic) V43.72 ☑
　　　　　　nontraffic V43.22 ☑
　　　　　pedal cycle (traffic) V41.7 ☑
　　　　　　nontraffic V41.2 ☑
　　　　　pickup truck (traffic) V43.73 ☑
　　　　　　nontraffic V43.23 ☑
　　　　　railway vehicle (traffic) V45.7 ☑
　　　　　　nontraffic V45.2 ☑
　　　　　specified vehicle NEC (traffic) V46.7 ☑
　　　　　　nontraffic V46.2 ☑
　　　　　sport utility vehicle (traffic) V43.71 ☑
　　　　　　nontraffic V43.21 ☑
　　　　　stationary object (traffic) V47.7 ☑
　　　　　　nontraffic V47.2 ☑
　　　　　streetcar (traffic) V46.7 ☑
　　　　　　nontraffic V46.2 ☑
　　　　　three wheeled motor vehicle (traffic)
　　　　　　V42.7 ☑
　　　　　　nontraffic V42.2 ☑
　　　　　truck (traffic) V44.7 ☑
　　　　　　nontraffic V44.2 ☑
　　　　　two wheeled motor vehicle (traffic)
　　　　　　V42.7 ☑
　　　　　　nontraffic V42.2 ☑
　　　　　van (traffic) V43.74 ☑
　　　　　　nontraffic V43.24 ☑
　　　　noncollision accident (traffic) V48.7 ☑
　　　　　nontraffic V48.2 ☑
　　　noncollision accident (traffic) V48.9 ☑
　　　　nontraffic V48.3 ☑
　　　　while boarding or alighting V48.4 ☑
　　　nontraffic V49.3 ☑
　　　passenger
　　　　collision (with)
　　　　　animal (traffic) V40.6 ☑
　　　　　　being ridden (traffic) V46.6 ☑
　　　　　　　nontraffic V46.1 ☑
　　　　　　nontraffic V40.1 ☑
　　　　　animal-drawn vehicle (traffic) V46.6 ☑
　　　　　　nontraffic V46.1 ☑
　　　　　bus (traffic) V44.6 ☑
　　　　　　nontraffic V44.1 ☑
　　　　　car (traffic) V43.62 ☑
　　　　　　nontraffic V43.12 ☑
　　　　　motor vehicle NOS (traffic) V49.50 ☑
　　　　　　nontraffic V49.10 ☑
　　　　　　specified type NEC (traffic) V49.59 ☑
　　　　　　　nontraffic V49.19 ☑
　　　　　pedal cycle (traffic) V41.6 ☑
　　　　　　nontraffic V41.1 ☑
　　　　　pickup truck (traffic) V43.63 ☑
　　　　　　nontraffic V43.13 ☑
　　　　　railway vehicle (traffic) V45.6 ☑
　　　　　　nontraffic V45.1 ☑
　　　　　specified vehicle NEC (traffic) V46.6 ☑
　　　　　　nontraffic V46.1 ☑
　　　　　sport utility vehicle (traffic) V43.61 ☑
　　　　　　nontraffic V43.11 ☑
　　　　　stationary object (traffic) V47.62 ☑
　　　　　　nontraffic V47.12 ☑
　　　　　streetcar (traffic) V46.6 ☑
　　　　　　nontraffic V46.1 ☑
　　　　　three wheeled motor vehicle (traffic)
　　　　　　V42.6 ☑
　　　　　　nontraffic V42.1 ☑
　　　　　truck (traffic) V44.6 ☑
　　　　　　nontraffic V44.1 ☑
　　　　　two wheeled motor vehicle (traffic)
　　　　　　V42.6 ☑
　　　　　　nontraffic V42.1 ☑
　　　　　van (traffic) V43.64 ☑
　　　　　　nontraffic V43.14 ☑
　　　　noncollision accident (traffic) V48.6 ☑

Accident — *continued*
  transport — *continued*
    car occupant — *continued*
      passenger — *continued*
        noncollision accident — *continued*
          nontraffic V48.1 ☑
        specified type NEC V49.88 ☑
        military vehicle V49.81 ☑
      coal car — *see* Accident, transport, industrial vehicle occupant
      construction vehicle occupant (nontraffic) V85.9 ☑
        driver V85.5 ☑
        hanger-on V85.7 ☑
        passenger V85.6 ☑
        traffic V85.3 ☑
          driver V85.0 ☑
          hanger-on V85.2 ☑
          passenger V85.1 ☑
        while boarding or alighting V85.4 ☑
      dirt bike rider — *see* Accident, transport, all-terrain vehicle occupant
      due to cataclysm — *see* Forces of nature, by type
      dune buggy occupant (nontraffic) V86.93 ☑
        driver V86.53 ☑
        hanger-on V86.73 ☑
        passenger V86.63 ☑
        traffic V86.33 ☑
          driver V86.03 ☑
          hanger-on V86.23 ☑
          passenger V86.13 ☑
        while boarding or alighting V86.43 ☑
      forklift — *see* Accident, transport, industrial vehicle occupant
      go cart — *see* Accident, transport, all-terrain vehicle occupant
      golf cart — *see* Accident, transport, all-terrain vehicle occupant
      heavy transport vehicle occupant — *see* Accident, transport, truck occupant
      ice yacht V98.2 ☑
      industrial vehicle occupant (nontraffic) V83.9 ☑
        driver V83.5 ☑
        hanger-on V83.7 ☑
        passenger V83.6 ☑
        traffic V83.3 ☑
          driver V83.0 ☑
          hanger-on V83.2 ☑
          passenger V83.1 ☑
        while boarding or alighting V83.4 ☑
      interurban electric car — *see* Accident, transport, streetcar
      land yacht V98.1 ☑
      logging car — *see* Accident, transport, industrial vehicle occupant
      military vehicle occupant (traffic) V86.34 ☑
        driver V86.04 ☑
        hanger-on V86.24 ☑
        nontraffic V86.94 ☑
          driver V86.54 ☑
          hanger-on V86.74 ☑
          passenger V86.64 ☑
        passenger V86.14 ☑
        while boarding or alighting V86.44 ☑
      mine tram — *see* Accident, transport, industrial vehicle occupant
      motor vehicle NEC occupant (traffic) V86.39 ☑
        driver V86.09 ☑
        hanger-on V86.29 ☑
        nontraffic V86.99 ☑
          driver V86.59 ☑
          hanger-on V86.79 ☑
          passenger V86.69 ☑
        passenger V86.19 ☑
        while boarding or alighting V86.49 ☑
      motorcoach — *see* Accident, transport, bus occupant
      motorcyclist V29.9 ☑
        collision (with)
          animal (traffic) V20.9 ☑
            being ridden (traffic) V26.9 ☑
              nontraffic V26.2 ☑
              while boarding or alighting V26.3 ☑
            nontraffic V20.2 ☑
              while boarding or alighting V20.3 ☑
          animal-drawn vehicle (traffic) V26.9 ☑
            nontraffic V26.2 ☑

Accident — *continued*
  transport — *continued*
    motorcyclist — *continued*
      collision — *continued*
        animal-drawn vehicle — *continued*
          while boarding or alighting V26.3 ☑
        bus (traffic) V24.9 ☑
          nontraffic V24.2 ☑
          while boarding or alighting V24.3 ☑
        car (traffic) V23.9 ☑
          nontraffic V23.2 ☑
          while boarding or alighting V23.3 ☑
        motor vehicle NOS (traffic) V29.60 ☑
          nontraffic V29.20 ☑
          specified type NEC (traffic) V29.69 ☑
            nontraffic V29.29 ☑
        pedal cycle (traffic) V21.9 ☑
          nontraffic V21.2 ☑
          while boarding or alighting V21.3 ☑
        pickup truck (traffic) V23.9 ☑
          nontraffic V23.2 ☑
          while boarding or alighting V23.3 ☑
        railway vehicle (traffic) V25.9 ☑
          nontraffic V25.2 ☑
          while boarding or alighting V25.3 ☑
        specified vehicle NEC (traffic) V26.9 ☑
          nontraffic V26.2 ☑
          while boarding or alighting V26.3 ☑
        stationary object (traffic) V27.9 ☑
          nontraffic V27.2 ☑
          while boarding or alighting V27.3 ☑
        streetcar (traffic) V26.9 ☑
          nontraffic V26.2 ☑
          while boarding or alighting V26.3 ☑
        three wheeled motor vehicle (traffic) V22.9 ☑
          nontraffic V22.2 ☑
          while boarding or alighting V22.3 ☑
        truck (traffic) V24.9 ☑
          nontraffic V24.2 ☑
          while boarding or alighting V24.3 ☑
        two wheeled motor vehicle (traffic) V22.9 ☑
          nontraffic V22.2 ☑
          while boarding or alighting V22.3 ☑
        van (traffic) V23.9 ☑
          nontraffic V23.2 ☑
          while boarding or alighting V23.3 ☑
      driver
        collision (with)
          animal (traffic) V20.4 ☑
            being ridden (traffic) V26.4 ☑
              nontraffic V26.0 ☑
            nontraffic V20.0 ☑
          animal-drawn vehicle (traffic) V26.4 ☑
            nontraffic V26.0 ☑
          bus (traffic) V24.4 ☑
            nontraffic V24.0 ☑
          car (traffic) V23.4 ☑
            nontraffic V23.0 ☑
          motor vehicle NOS (traffic) V29.40 ☑
            nontraffic V29.00 ☑
            specified type NEC (traffic) V29.49 ☑
              nontraffic V29.09 ☑
          pedal cycle (traffic) V21.4 ☑
            nontraffic V21.0 ☑
          pickup truck (traffic) V23.4 ☑
            nontraffic V23.0 ☑
          railway vehicle (traffic) V25.4 ☑
            nontraffic V25.0 ☑
          specified vehicle NEC (traffic) V26.4 ☑
            nontraffic V26.0 ☑
          stationary object (traffic) V27.4 ☑
            nontraffic V27.0 ☑
          streetcar (traffic) V26.4 ☑
            nontraffic V26.0 ☑
          three wheeled motor vehicle (traffic) V22.4 ☑
            nontraffic V22.0 ☑
          truck (traffic) V24.4 ☑
            nontraffic V24.0 ☑
          two wheeled motor vehicle (traffic) V22.4 ☑
            nontraffic V22.0 ☑
          van (traffic) V23.4 ☑
            nontraffic V23.0 ☑
        noncollision accident (traffic) V28.4 ☑

Accident — *continued*
  transport — *continued*
    motorcyclist — *continued*
      driver — *continued*
        noncollision accident — *continued*
          nontraffic V28.0 ☑
      noncollision accident (traffic) V28.9 ☑
        nontraffic V28.2 ☑
        while boarding or alighting V28.3 ☑
      nontraffic V29.3 ☑
      passenger
        collision (with)
          animal (traffic) V20.5 ☑
            being ridden (traffic) V26.5 ☑
              nontraffic V26.1 ☑
            nontraffic V20.1 ☑
          animal-drawn vehicle (traffic) V26.5 ☑
            nontraffic V26.1 ☑
          bus (traffic) V24.5 ☑
            nontraffic V24.1 ☑
          car (traffic) V23.5 ☑
            nontraffic V23.1 ☑
          motor vehicle NOS (traffic) V29.50 ☑
            nontraffic V29.10 ☑
            specified type NEC (traffic) V29.59 ☑
              nontraffic V29.19 ☑
          pedal cycle (traffic) V21.5 ☑
            nontraffic V21.1 ☑
          pickup truck (traffic) V23.5 ☑
            nontraffic V23.1 ☑
          railway vehicle (traffic) V25.5 ☑
            nontraffic V25.1 ☑
          specified vehicle NEC (traffic) V26.5 ☑
            nontraffic V26.1 ☑
          stationary object (traffic) V27.5 ☑
            nontraffic V27.1 ☑
          streetcar (traffic) V26.5 ☑
            nontraffic V26.1 ☑
          three wheeled motor vehicle (traffic) V22.5 ☑
            nontraffic V22.1 ☑
          truck (traffic) V24.5 ☑
            nontraffic V24.1 ☑
          two wheeled motor vehicle (traffic) V22.5 ☑
            nontraffic V22.1 ☑
          van (traffic) V23.5 ☑
            nontraffic V23.1 ☑
        noncollision accident (traffic) V28.5 ☑
          nontraffic V28.1 ☑
      specified type NEC V29.88 ☑
        military vehicle V29.81 ☑
    occupant (of)
      aircraft (powered) V95.9 ☑
        fixed wing
          commercial — *see* Accident, transport, aircraft, occupant, powered, fixed wing, commercial
          private — *see* Accident, transport, aircraft, occupant, powered, fixed wing, private
        nonpowered V96.9 ☑
        specified NEC V95.8 ☑
      airport battery-powered vehicle — *see* Accident, transport, industrial vehicle occupant
      all-terrain vehicle (ATV) — *see* Accident, transport, all-terrain vehicle occupant
      animal-drawn vehicle — *see* Accident, transport, animal-drawn vehicle occupant
      automobile — *see* Accident, transport, car occupant
      balloon V96.00 ☑
      battery-powered vehicle — *see* Accident, transport, industrial vehicle occupant
      bicycle — *see* Accident, transport, pedal cyclist
        motorized — *see* Accident, transport, motorcycle rider
      boat NEC — *see* Accident, watercraft
      bulldozer — *see* Accident, transport, construction vehicle occupant
      bus — *see* Accident, transport, bus occupant
      cable car (on rails) (*see also* Accident, transport, streetcar occupant)
        not on rails V98.0 ☑
      car (*see also* Accident, transport, car occupant)

Accident — *continued*
  transport — *continued*
    occupant — *continued*
      car (*see also* Accident, transport, car occupant) — *continued*
        cable (on rails) (*see also* Accident, transport, streetcar occupant)
          not on rails V98.0 ☑
      coach — *see* Accident, transport, bus occupant
      coal-car — *see* Accident, transport, industrial vehicle occupant
      digger — *see* Accident, transport, construction vehicle occupant
      dump truck — *see* Accident, transport, construction vehicle occupant
      earth-leveler — *see* Accident, transport, construction vehicle occupant
      farm machinery (self-propelled) — *see* Accident, transport, agricultural vehicle occupant
      forklift — *see* Accident, transport, industrial vehicle occupant
      glider (unpowered) V96.20 ☑
        hang V96.10 ☑
        powered (microlight) (ultralight) — *see* Accident, transport, aircraft, occupant, powered, glider
      glider (unpowered) NEC V96.20 ☑
      hang-glider V96.10 ☑
      harvester — *see* Accident, transport, agricultural vehicle occupant
      heavy (transport) vehicle — *see* Accident, transport, truck occupant
      helicopter — *see* Accident, transport, aircraft, occupant, helicopter
      ice-yacht V98.2 ☑
      kite (carrying person) V96.8 ☑
      land-yacht V98.1 ☑
      logging car — *see* Accident, transport, industrial vehicle occupant
      mechanical shovel — *see* Accident, transport, construction vehicle occupant
      microlight — *see* Accident, transport, aircraft, occupant, powered, glider
      minibus — *see* Accident, transport, car occupant
      minivan — *see* Accident, transport, car occupant
      moped — *see* Accident, transport, motorcycle
      motor scooter — *see* Accident, transport, motorcycle
      motorcycle (with sidecar) — *see* Accident, transport, motorcycle
      pedal cycle (*see also* Accident, transport, pedal cyclist)
      pick-up (truck) — *see* Accident, transport, pickup truck occupant
      railway (train) (vehicle) (subterranean) (elevated) — *see* Accident, transport, railway vehicle occupant
      rickshaw — *see* Accident, transport, pedal cycle
        motorized — *see* Accident, transport, three-wheeled motor vehicle
        pedal driven — *see* Accident, transport, pedal cyclist
      road-roller — *see* Accident, transport, construction vehicle occupant
      ship NOS V94.9 ☑
      ski-lift (chair) (gondola) V98.3 ☑
      snowmobile — *see* Accident, transport, snowmobile occupant
      spacecraft, spaceship — *see* Accident, transport, aircraft, occupant, spacecraft
      sport utility vehicle — *see* Accident, transport, car occupant
      streetcar (interurban) (operating on public street or highway) — *see* Accident, transport, streetcar occupant
      SUV — *see* Accident, transport, car occupant
      téléférique V98.0 ☑
      three-wheeled vehicle (motorized) (*see also* Accident, transport, three-wheeled motor vehicle occupant)
        nonmotorized — *see* Accident, transport, pedal cycle
      tractor (farm) (and trailer) — *see* Accident, transport, agricultural vehicle occupant

Accident — *continued*
  transport — *continued*
    occupant — *continued*
      train — *see* Accident, transport, railway vehicle occupant
      tram — *see* Accident, transport, streetcar occupant
        in mine or quarry — *see* Accident, transport, industrial vehicle occupant
      tricycle — *see* Accident, transport, pedal cycle
        motorized — *see* Accident, transport, three-wheeled motor vehicle
      trolley — *see* Accident, transport, streetcar occupant
        in mine or quarry — *see* Accident, transport, industrial vehicle occupant
      tub, in mine or quarry — *see* Accident, transport, industrial vehicle occupant
      ultralight — *see* Accident, transport, aircraft, occupant, powered, glider
      van — *see* Accident, transport, van occupant
      vehicle NEC V89.9 ☑
        heavy transport — *see* Accident, transport, truck occupant
        motor (traffic) NEC V89.2 ☑
          nontraffic NEC V89.0 ☑
      watercraft NOS V94.9 ☑
        causing drowning B — *see* Drowning, resulting from accident to boat
  parachutist V97.29 ☑
    after accident to aircraft — *see* Accident, transport, aircraft
    entangled in object V97.21 ☑
    injured on landing V97.22 ☑
  pedal cyclist V19.9 ☑
    collision (with)
      animal (traffic) V10.9 ☑
        being ridden (traffic) V16.9 ☑
          nontraffic V16.2 ☑
          while boarding or alighting V16.3 ☑
        nontraffic V10.2 ☑
        while boarding or alighting V10.3 ☑
      animal-drawn vehicle (traffic) V16.9 ☑
        nontraffic V16.2 ☑
        while boarding or alighting V16.3 ☑
      bus (traffic) V14.9 ☑
        nontraffic V14.2 ☑
        while boarding or alighting V14.3 ☑
      car (traffic) V13.9 ☑
        nontraffic V13.2 ☑
        while boarding or alighting V13.3 ☑
      motor vehicle NOS (traffic) V19.60 ☑
        nontraffic V19.20 ☑
        specified type NEC (traffic) V19.69 ☑
          nontraffic V19.29 ☑
      pedal cycle (traffic) V11.9 ☑
        nontraffic V11.2 ☑
        while boarding or alighting V11.3 ☑
      pickup truck (traffic) V13.9 ☑
        nontraffic V13.2 ☑
        while boarding or alighting V13.3 ☑
      railway vehicle (traffic) V15.9 ☑
        nontraffic V15.2 ☑
        while boarding or alighting V15.3 ☑
      specified vehicle NEC (traffic) V16.9 ☑
        nontraffic V16.2 ☑
        while boarding or alighting V16.3 ☑
      stationary object (traffic) V17.9 ☑
        nontraffic V17.2 ☑
        while boarding or alighting V17.3 ☑
      streetcar (traffic) V16.9 ☑
        nontraffic V16.2 ☑
        while boarding or alighting V16.3 ☑
      three wheeled motor vehicle (traffic) V12.9 ☑
        nontraffic V12.2 ☑
        while boarding or alighting V12.3 ☑
      truck (traffic) V14.9 ☑
        nontraffic V14.2 ☑
        while boarding or alighting V14.3 ☑
      two wheeled motor vehicle (traffic) V12.9 ☑
        nontraffic V12.2 ☑
        while boarding or alighting V12.3 ☑
      van (traffic) V13.9 ☑
        nontraffic V13.2 ☑
        while boarding or alighting V13.3 ☑

Accident — *continued*
  transport — *continued*
    pedal cyclist — *continued*
      driver
        collision (with)
          animal (traffic) V10.4 ☑
            being ridden (traffic) V16.4 ☑
              nontraffic V16.0 ☑
            nontraffic V10.0 ☑
          animal-drawn vehicle (traffic) V16.4 ☑
            nontraffic V16.0 ☑
          bus (traffic) V14.4 ☑
            nontraffic V14.0 ☑
          car (traffic) V13.4 ☑
            nontraffic V13.0 ☑
          motor vehicle NOS (traffic) V19.40 ☑
            nontraffic V19.00 ☑
            specified type NEC (traffic) V19.49 ☑
              nontraffic V19.09 ☑
          pedal cycle (traffic) V11.4 ☑
            nontraffic V11.0 ☑
          pickup truck (traffic) V13.4 ☑
            nontraffic V13.0 ☑
          railway vehicle (traffic) V15.4 ☑
            nontraffic V15.0 ☑
          specified vehicle NEC (traffic) V16.4 ☑
            nontraffic V16.0 ☑
          stationary object (traffic) V17.4 ☑
            nontraffic V17.0 ☑
          streetcar (traffic) V16.4 ☑
            nontraffic V16.0 ☑
          three wheeled motor vehicle (traffic) V12.4 ☑
            nontraffic V12.0 ☑
          truck (traffic) V14.4 ☑
            nontraffic V14.0 ☑
          two wheeled motor vehicle (traffic) V12.4 ☑
            nontraffic V12.0 ☑
          van (traffic) V13.4 ☑
            nontraffic V13.0 ☑
        noncollision accident (traffic) V18.4 ☑
          nontraffic V18.0 ☑
        noncollision accident (traffic) V18.9 ☑
          nontraffic V18.2 ☑
          while boarding or alighting V18.3 ☑
        nontraffic V19.3 ☑
      passenger
        collision (with)
          animal (traffic) V10.5 ☑
            being ridden (traffic) V16.5 ☑
              nontraffic V16.1 ☑
            nontraffic V10.1 ☑
          animal-drawn vehicle (traffic) V16.5 ☑
            nontraffic V16.1 ☑
          bus (traffic) V14.5 ☑
            nontraffic V14.1 ☑
          car (traffic) V13.5 ☑
            nontraffic V13.1 ☑
          motor vehicle NOS (traffic) V19.50 ☑
            nontraffic V19.10 ☑
            specified type NEC (traffic) V19.59 ☑
              nontraffic V19.19 ☑
          pedal cycle (traffic) V11.5 ☑
            nontraffic V11.1 ☑
          pickup truck (traffic) V13.5 ☑
            nontraffic V13.1 ☑
          railway vehicle (traffic) V15.5 ☑
            nontraffic V15.1 ☑
          specified vehicle NEC (traffic) V16.5 ☑
            nontraffic V16.1 ☑
          stationary object (traffic) V17.5 ☑
            nontraffic V17.1 ☑
          streetcar (traffic) V16.5 ☑
            nontraffic V16.1 ☑
          three wheeled motor vehicle (traffic) V12.5 ☑
            nontraffic V12.1 ☑
          truck (traffic) V14.5 ☑
            nontraffic V14.1 ☑
          two wheeled motor vehicle (traffic) V12.5 ☑
            nontraffic V12.1 ☑
          van (traffic) V13.5 ☑
            nontraffic V13.1 ☑
        noncollision accident (traffic) V18.5 ☑

Accident — *continued*
  transport — *continued*
    pedal cyclist — *continued*
      passenger — *continued*
        noncollision accident — *continued*
          nontraffic V18.1 ☑
        specified type NEC V19.88 ☑
        military vehicle V19.81 ☑
    pedestrian
      conveyance (occupant) V09.9 ☑
        babystroller V00.828 ☑
          collision (with) V09.9 ☑
            animal being ridden or animal drawn
              vehicle V06.99 ☑
              nontraffic V06.09 ☑
              traffic V06.19 ☑
            bus or heavy transport V04.99 ☑
              nontraffic V04.09 ☑
              traffic V04.19 ☑
            car V03.99 ☑
              nontraffic V03.09 ☑
              traffic V03.19 ☑
            pedal cycle V01.99 ☑
              nontraffic V01.09 ☑
              traffic V01.19 ☑
            pick-up truck or van V03.99 ☑
              nontraffic V03.09 ☑
              traffic V03.19 ☑
            railway (train) (vehicle) V05.99 ☑
              nontraffic V05.09 ☑
              traffic V05.19 ☑
            stationary object V00.822 ☑
            streetcar V06.99 ☑
              nontraffic V06.09 ☑
              traffic V06.19 ☑
            two- or three-wheeled motor vehicle V02.99 ☑
              nontraffic V02.09 ☑
              traffic V02.19 ☑
            vehicle V09.9 ☑
              animal-drawn V06.99 ☑
                nontraffic V06.09 ☑
                traffic V06.19 ☑
              motor
                nontraffic V09.00 ☑
                traffic V09.20 ☑
          fall V00.821 ☑
          nontraffic V09.1 ☑
            involving motor vehicle NEC V09.00 ☑
          traffic V09.3 ☑
            involving motor vehicle NEC V09.20 ☑
        flat-bottomed NEC V00.388 ☑
          collision (with) V09.9 ☑
            animal being ridden or animal drawn
              vehicle V06.99 ☑
              nontraffic V06.09 ☑
              traffic V06.19 ☑
            bus or heavy transport V04.99 ☑
              nontraffic V04.09 ☑
              traffic V04.19 ☑
            car V03.99 ☑
              nontraffic V03.09 ☑
              traffic V03.19 ☑
            pedal cycle V01.99 ☑
              nontraffic V01.09 ☑
              traffic V01.19 ☑
            pick-up truck or van V03.99 ☑
              nontraffic V03.09 ☑
              traffic V03.19 ☑
            railway (train) (vehicle) V05.99 ☑
              nontraffic V05.09 ☑
              traffic V05.19 ☑
            stationary object V00.382 ☑
            streetcar V06.99 ☑
              nontraffic V06.09 ☑
              traffic V06.19 ☑
            two- or three-wheeled motor vehicle V02.99 ☑
              nontraffic V02.09 ☑
              traffic V02.19 ☑
            vehicle V09.9 ☑
              animal-drawn V06.99 ☑
                nontraffic V06.09 ☑
                traffic V06.19 ☑

Accident — *continued*
  transport — *continued*
    pedestrian — *continued*
      conveyance — *continued*
        flat-bottomed — *continued*
          collision — *continued*
            vehicle — *continued*
              motor
                nontraffic V09.00 ☑
                traffic V09.20 ☑
          fall V00.381 ☑
          nontraffic V09.1 ☑
            involving motor vehicle NEC V09.00 ☑
          snow
            board — *see* Accident, transport, pedestrian, conveyance, snow board
            ski — *see* Accident, transport, pedestrian, conveyance, skis (snow)
          traffic V09.3 ☑
            involving motor vehicle NEC V09.20 ☑
        gliding type NEC V00.288 ☑
          collision (with) V09.9 ☑
            animal being ridden or animal drawn
              vehicle V06.99 ☑
              nontraffic V06.09 ☑
              traffic V06.19 ☑
            bus or heavy transport V04.99 ☑
              nontraffic V04.09 ☑
              traffic V04.19 ☑
            car V03.99 ☑
              nontraffic V03.09 ☑
              traffic V03.19 ☑
            pedal cycle V01.99 ☑
              nontraffic V01.09 ☑
              traffic V01.19 ☑
            pick-up truck or van V03.99 ☑
              nontraffic V03.09 ☑
              traffic V03.19 ☑
            railway (train) (vehicle) V05.99 ☑
              nontraffic V05.09 ☑
              traffic V05.19 ☑
            stationary object V00.282 ☑
            streetcar V06.99 ☑
              nontraffic V06.09 ☑
              traffic V06.19- ☑
            two- or three-wheeled motor vehicle V02.99 ☑
              nontraffic V02.09 ☑
              traffic V02.19 ☑
            vehicle V09.9 ☑
              animal-drawn V06.99 ☑
                nontraffic V06.09 ☑
                traffic V06.19 ☑
              motor
                nontraffic V09.00 ☑
                traffic V09.20 ☑
         fall V00.281 ☑
        heelies — *see* Accident, transport, pedestrian, conveyance, heelies
        ice skate — *see* Accident, transport, pedestrian, conveyance, ice skate
        nontraffic V09.1 ☑
          involving motor vehicle NEC V09.00 ☑
        sled — *see* Accident, transport, pedestrian, conveyance, sled
        traffic V09.3 ☑
          involving motor vehicle NEC V09.20 ☑
          wheelies — *see* Accident, transport, pedestrian, conveyance, heelies
        heelies V00.158 ☑
          colliding with stationary object V00.152 ☑
          fall V00.151 ☑
        ice skates V00.218 ☑
          collision (with) V09.9 ☑
            animal being ridden or animal drawn
              vehicle V06.99 ☑
              nontraffic V06.09 ☑
              traffic V06.19 ☑

Accident — *continued*
  transport — *continued*
    pedestrian — *continued*
      conveyance — *continued*
        ice skates — *continued*
          collision — *continued*
            bus or heavy transport V04.99 ☑
              nontraffic V04.09 ☑
              traffic V04.19 ☑
            car V03.99 ☑
              nontraffic V03.09 ☑
              traffic V03.19 ☑
            pedal cycle V01.99 ☑
              nontraffic V01.09 ☑
              traffic V01.19 ☑
            pick-up truck or van V03.99 ☑
              nontraffic V03.09 ☑
              traffic V03.19 ☑
            railway (train) (vehicle) V05.99 ☑
              nontraffic V05.09 ☑
              traffic V05.19 ☑
            stationary object V00.212 ☑
            streetcar V06.99 ☑
              nontraffic V06.09 ☑
              traffic V06.19 ☑
            two- or three-wheeled motor vehicle V02.99 ☑
              nontraffic V02.09 ☑
              traffic V02.19 ☑
            vehicle V09.9 ☑
              animal-drawn V06.99 ☑
                nontraffic V06.09 ☑
                traffic V06.19 ☑
              motor
                nontraffic V09.00 ☑
                traffic V09.20 ☑
         fall V00.211 ☑
        nontraffic V09.1 ☑
          involving motor vehicle NEC V09.00 ☑
        traffic V09.3 ☑
          involving motor vehicle NEC V09.20 ☑
        motorized mobility scooter V00.838 ☑
          collision with stationary object V00.832 ☑
          fall from V00.831 ☑
        nontraffic V09.1 ☑
          involving motor vehicle V09.00 ☑
            military V09.01 ☑
            specified type NEC V09.09 ☑
        roller skates (non in-line) V00.128 ☑
          collision (with) V09.9 ☑
            animal being ridden or animal drawn
              vehicle V06.91 ☑
              nontraffic V06.01 ☑
              traffic V06.11 ☑
            bus or heavy transport V04.91 ☑
              nontraffic V04.01 ☑
              traffic V04.11 ☑
            car V03.91 ☑
              nontraffic V03.01 ☑
              traffic V03.11 ☑
            pedal cycle V01.91 ☑
              nontraffic V01.01 ☑
              traffic V01.11 ☑
            pick-up truck or van V03.91 ☑
              nontraffic V03.01 ☑
              traffic V03.11 ☑
            railway (train) (vehicle) V05.91 ☑
              nontraffic V05.01 ☑
              traffic V05.11 ☑
            stationary object V00.122 ☑
            streetcar V06.91 ☑
              nontraffic V06.01 ☑
              traffic V06.11 ☑
            two- or three-wheeled motor vehicle V02.91 ☑
              nontraffic V02.01 ☑
              traffic V02.11 ☑
            vehicle V09.9 ☑
              animal-drawn V06.91 ☑
                nontraffic V06.01 ☑
                traffic V06.11 ☑
              motor
                nontraffic V09.00 ☑

☑ Additional Character Required — Refer to the Tabular List for Character Selection   ▽ Subterms under main terms may continue to next column or page

Accident — *continued*
 transport — *continued*
  pedestrian — *continued*
   conveyance — *continued*
    roller skates — *continued*
     collision — *continued*
      vehicle — *continued*
       motor — *continued*
        traffic V09.20 ☑
     fall V00.121 ☑
     in-line V00.118 ☑
      collision — *see also* Accident, transport, pedestrian, conveyance occupant, roller skates, collision
       with stationary object V00.112 ☑
      fall V00.111 ☑
      nontraffic V09.1 ☑
       involving motor vehicle NEC V09.00 ☑
      traffic V09.3 ☑
       involving motor vehicle NEC V09.20 ☑
    rolling shoes V00.158 ☑
     colliding with stationary object V00.152 ☑
     fall V00.151 ☑
    rolling type NEC V00.188 ☑
     collision (with) V09.9 ☑
      animal being ridden or animal drawn vehicle V06.99 ☑
       nontraffic V06.09 ☑
       traffic V06.19 ☑
      bus or heavy transport V04.99 ☑
       nontraffic V04.09 ☑
       traffic V04.19 ☑
      car V03.99 ☑
       nontraffic V03.09 ☑
       traffic V03.19 ☑
      pedal cycle V01.99 ☑
       nontraffic V01.09 ☑
       traffic V01.19 ☑
      pick-up truck or van V03.99 ☑
       nontraffic V03.09 ☑
       traffic V03.19 ☑
      railway (train) (vehicle) V05.99 ☑
       nontraffic V05.09 ☑
       traffic V05.19 ☑
      stationary object V00.182 ☑
      streetcar V06.99 ☑
       nontraffic V06.09 ☑
       traffic V06.19 ☑
      two- or three-wheeled motor vehicle V02.99 ☑
       nontraffic V02.09 ☑
       traffic V02.19 ☑
      vehicle V09.9 ☑
       animal-drawn V06.99 ☑
        nontraffic V06.09 ☑
        traffic V06.19 ☑
       motor
        nontraffic V09.00 ☑
        traffic V09.20 ☑
     fall V00.181 ☑
    in-line roller skate — *see* Accident, transport, pedestrian, conveyance, roller skate, in-line
    nontraffic V09.1 ☑
     involving motor vehicle NEC V09.00 ☑
    roller skate — *see* Accident, transport, pedestrian, conveyance, roller skate
    scooter (non-motorized) — *see* Accident, transport, pedestrian, conveyance, scooter
    skateboard — *see* Accident, transport, pedestrian, conveyance, skateboard
    traffic V09.3 ☑
     involving motor vehicle NEC V09.20 ☑
    scooter (non-motorized) V00.148 ☑
     collision (with) V09.9 ☑
      animal being ridden or animal drawn vehicle V06.99 ☑

Accident — *continued*
 transport — *continued*
  pedestrian — *continued*
   conveyance — *continued*
    scooter — *continued*
     collision — *continued*
      animal being ridden or animal drawn vehicle — *continued*
       nontraffic V06.09 ☑
       traffic V06.19 ☑
      bus or heavy transport V04.99 ☑
       nontraffic V04.09 ☑
       traffic V04.19 ☑
      car V03.99 ☑
       nontraffic V03.09 ☑
       traffic V03.19 ☑
      pedal cycle V01.99 ☑
       nontraffic V01.09 ☑
       traffic V01.19 ☑
      pick-up truck or van V03.99 ☑
       nontraffic V03.09 ☑
       traffic V03.19 ☑
      railway (train) (vehicle) V05.99 ☑
       nontraffic V05.09 ☑
       traffic V05.19 ☑
      stationary object V00.142 ☑
      streetcar V06.99 ☑
       nontraffic V06.09 ☑
       traffic V06.19 ☑
      two- or three-wheeled motor vehicle V02.99 ☑
       nontraffic V02.09 ☑
       traffic V02.19 ☑
      vehicle V09.9 ☑
       animal-drawn V06.99 ☑
        nontraffic V06.09 ☑
        traffic V06.19 ☑
       motor
        nontraffic V09.00 ☑
        traffic V09.20 ☑
     fall V00.141 ☑
     nontraffic V09.1 ☑
      involving motor vehicle NEC V09.00 ☑
     traffic V09.3 ☑
      involving motor vehicle NEC V09.20 ☑
    skate board V00.138 ☑
     collision (with) V09.9 ☑
      animal being ridden or animal drawn vehicle V06.92 ☑
       nontraffic V06.02 ☑
       traffic V06.12 ☑
      bus or heavy transport V04.92 ☑
       nontraffic V04.02 ☑
       traffic V04.12 ☑
      car V03.92 ☑
       nontraffic V03.02 ☑
       traffic V03.12 ☑
      pedal cycle V01.92 ☑
       nontraffic V01.02 ☑
       traffic V01.12 ☑
      pick-up truck or van V03.92 ☑
       nontraffic V03.02 ☑
       traffic V03.12 ☑
      railway (train) (vehicle) V05.92 ☑
       nontraffic V05.02 ☑
       traffic V05.12 ☑
      stationary object V00.132 ☑
      streetcar V06.92 ☑
       nontraffic V06.02 ☑
       traffic V06.12 ☑
      two- or three-wheeled motor vehicle V02.92 ☑
       nontraffic V02.02 ☑
       traffic V02.12 ☑
      vehicle V09.9 ☑
       animal-drawn V06.92 ☑
        nontraffic V06.02 ☑
        traffic V06.12 ☑
       motor
        nontraffic V09.00 ☑
        traffic V09.20 ☑
     fall V00.131 ☑
     nontraffic V09.1 ☑

Accident — *continued*
 transport — *continued*
  pedestrian — *continued*
   conveyance — *continued*
    skate board — *continued*
     nontraffic — *continued*
      involving motor vehicle NEC V09.00 ☑
     traffic V09.3 ☑
      involving motor vehicle NEC V09.20 ☑
    skis (snow) V00.328 ☑
     collision (with) V09.9 ☑
      animal being ridden or animal drawn vehicle V06.99 ☑
       nontraffic V06.09 ☑
       traffic V06.19 ☑
      bus or heavy transport V04.99 ☑
       nontraffic V04.09 ☑
       traffic V04.19 ☑
      car V03.99 ☑
       nontraffic V03.09 ☑
       traffic V03.19 ☑
      pedal cycle V01.99 ☑
       nontraffic V01.09 ☑
       traffic V01.19 ☑
      pick-up truck or van V03.99 ☑
       nontraffic V03.09 ☑
       traffic V03.19 ☑
      railway (train) (vehicle) V05.99 ☑
       nontraffic V05.09 ☑
       traffic V05.19 ☑
      stationary object V00.322 ☑
      streetcar V06.99 ☑
       nontraffic V06.09 ☑
       traffic V06.19 ☑
      two- or three-wheeled motor vehicle V02.99 ☑
       nontraffic V02.09 ☑
       traffic V02.19 ☑
      vehicle V09.9 ☑
       animal-drawn V06.99 ☑
        nontraffic V06.09 ☑
        traffic V06.19 ☑
       motor
        nontraffic V09.00 ☑
        traffic V09.20 ☑
     fall V00.321 ☑
     nontraffic V09.1 ☑
      involving motor vehicle NEC V09.00 ☑
     traffic V09.3 ☑
      involving motor vehicle NEC V09.20 ☑
    sled V00.228 ☑
     collision (with) V09.9 ☑
      animal being ridden or animal drawn vehicle V06.99 ☑
       nontraffic V06.09 ☑
       traffic V06.19 ☑
      bus or heavy transport V04.99 ☑
       nontraffic V04.09 ☑
       traffic V04.19 ☑
      car V03.99 ☑
       nontraffic V03.09 ☑
       traffic V03.19 ☑
      pedal cycle V01.99 ☑
       nontraffic V01.09 ☑
       traffic V01.19 ☑
      pick-up truck or van V03.99 ☑
       nontraffic V03.09 ☑
       traffic V03.19 ☑
      railway (train) (vehicle) V05.99 ☑
       nontraffic V05.09 ☑
       traffic V05.19 ☑
      stationary object V00.222 ☑
      streetcar V06.99 ☑
       nontraffic V06.09 ☑
       traffic V06.19 ☑
      two- or three-wheeled motor vehicle V02.99 ☑
       nontraffic V02.09 ☑
       traffic V02.19 ☑
      vehicle V09.9 ☑
       animal-drawn V06.99 ☑
        nontraffic V06.09 ☑

Accident — *continued*
 transport — *continued*
  pedestrian — *continued*
   conveyance — *continued*
    sled — *continued*
     collision — *continued*
      vehicle — *continued*
       animal-drawn — *continued*
        traffic V06.19 ☑
       motor
        nontraffic V09.00 ☑
        traffic V09.20 ☑
     fall V00.221 ☑
     nontraffic V09.1 ☑
      involving motor vehicle NEC
        V09.00 ☑
     traffic V09.3 ☑
      involving motor vehicle NEC
        V09.20 ☑
    snow board V00.318 ☑
     collision (with) V09.9 ☑
      animal being ridden or animal drawn
        vehicle V06.99 ☑
        nontraffic V06.09 ☑
        traffic V06.19 ☑
      bus or heavy transport V04.99 ☑
        nontraffic V04.09 ☑
        traffic V04.19 ☑
      car V03.99 ☑
        nontraffic V03.09 ☑
        traffic V03.19 ☑
      pedal cycle V01.99 ☑
        nontraffic V01.09 ☑
        traffic V01.19 ☑
      pick-up truck or van V03.99 ☑
        nontraffic V03.09 ☑
        traffic V03.19 ☑
      railway (train) (vehicle) V05.99 ☑
        nontraffic V05.09 ☑
        traffic V05.19 ☑
      stationary object V00.312 ☑
      streetcar V06.99 ☑
        nontraffic V06.09 ☑
        traffic V06.19 ☑
      two- or three-wheeled motor vehicle
        V02.99 ☑
        nontraffic V02.09 ☑
        traffic V02.19 ☑
      vehicle V09.9 ☑
        animal-drawn V06.99 ☑
         nontraffic V06.09 ☑
         traffic V06.19 ☑
        motor
         nontraffic V09.00 ☑
         traffic V09.20 ☑
     fall V00.311 ☑
     nontraffic V09.1 ☑
      involving motor vehicle NEC
        V09.00 ☑
     traffic V09.3 ☑
      involving motor vehicle NEC
        V09.20 ☑
    specified type NEC V00.898 ☑
     collision (with) V09.9 ☑
      animal being ridden or animal drawn
        vehicle V06.99 ☑
        nontraffic V06.09 ☑
        traffic V06.19 ☑
      bus or heavy transport V04.99 ☑
        nontraffic V04.09 ☑
        traffic V04.19 ☑
      car V03.99 ☑
        nontraffic V03.09 ☑
        traffic V03.19 ☑
      pedal cycle V01.99 ☑
        nontraffic V01.09 ☑
        traffic V01.19 ☑
      pick-up truck or van V03.99 ☑
        nontraffic V03.09 ☑
        traffic V03.19 ☑
      railway (train) (vehicle) V05.99 ☑
        nontraffic V05.09 ☑
        traffic V05.19 ☑
      stationary object V00.892 ☑
      streetcar V06.99 ☑
        nontraffic V06.09 ☑

Accident — *continued*
 transport — *continued*
  pedestrian — *continued*
   conveyance — *continued*
    specified type — *continued*
     collision — *continued*
      streetcar — *continued*
       traffic V06.19 ☑
      two- or three-wheeled motor vehicle
        V02.99 ☑
        nontraffic V02.09 ☑
        traffic V02.19 ☑
      vehicle V09.9 ☑
        animal-drawn V06.99 ☑
         nontraffic V06.09 ☑
         traffic V06.19 ☑
        motor
         nontraffic V09.00 ☑
         traffic V09.20 ☑
     fall V00.891 ☑
     nontraffic V09.1 ☑
      involving motor vehicle NEC
        V09.00 ☑
     traffic V09.3 ☑
      involving motor vehicle NEC
        V09.20 ☑
   traffic V09.3 ☑
    involving motor vehicle V09.20 ☑
     military V09.21 ☑
     specified type NEC V09.29 ☑
   wheelchair (powered) V00.818 ☑
    collision (with) V09.9 ☑
     animal being ridden or animal drawn
        vehicle V06.99 ☑
        nontraffic V06.09 ☑
        traffic V06.19 ☑
     bus or heavy transport V04.99 ☑
        nontraffic V04.09 ☑
        traffic V04.19 ☑
     car V03.99 ☑
        nontraffic V03.09 ☑
        traffic V03.19 ☑
     pedal cycle V01.99 ☑
        nontraffic V01.09 ☑
        traffic V01.19 ☑
     pick-up truck or van V03.99 ☑
        nontraffic V03.09 ☑
        traffic V03.19 ☑
     railway (train) (vehicle) V05.99 ☑
        nontraffic V05.09 ☑
        traffic V05.19 ☑
     stationary object V00.812 ☑
     streetcar V06.99 ☑
        nontraffic V06.09 ☑
        traffic V06.19 ☑
     two- or three-wheeled motor vehicle
        V02.99 ☑
        nontraffic V02.09 ☑
        traffic V02.19 ☑
     vehicle V09.9 ☑
        animal-drawn V06.99 ☑
         nontraffic V06.09 ☑
         traffic V06.19 ☑
        motor
         nontraffic V09.00 ☑
         traffic V09.20 ☑
    fall V00.811 ☑
    nontraffic V09.1 ☑
     involving motor vehicle NEC
        V09.00 ☑
    traffic V09.3 ☑
     involving motor vehicle NEC
        V09.20 ☑
   wheeled shoe V00.158 ☑
    colliding with stationary object
        V00.152 ☑
    fall V00.151 ☑
  on foot (*see also* Accident, pedestrian)
   collision (with)
    animal being ridden or animal drawn
        vehicle V06.90 ☑
        nontraffic V06.00 ☑
        traffic V06.10 ☑
    bus or heavy transport V04.90 ☑
        nontraffic V04.00 ☑
        traffic V04.10 ☑

Accident — *continued*
 transport — *continued*
  pedestrian — *continued*
   on foot (*see also* Accident, pedestrian) — *continued*
    collision — *continued*
     car V03.90 ☑
        nontraffic V03.00 ☑
        traffic V03.10 ☑
     pedal cycle V01.90 ☑
        nontraffic V01.00 ☑
        traffic V01.10 ☑
     pick-up truck or van V03.90 ☑
        nontraffic V03.00 ☑
        traffic V03.10 ☑
     railway (train) (vehicle) V05.90 ☑
        nontraffic V05.00 ☑
        traffic V05.10 ☑
     streetcar V06.90 ☑
        nontraffic V06.00 ☑
        traffic V06.10 ☑
     two- or three-wheeled motor vehicle
        V02.90 ☑
        nontraffic V02.00 ☑
        traffic V02.10 ☑
     vehicle V09.9 ☑
        animal-drawn V06.90 ☑
         nontraffic V06.00 ☑
         traffic V06.10 ☑
        motor
   nontraffic V09.1 ☑
    involving motor vehicle V09.00 ☑
     military V09.01 ☑
     specified type NEC V09.09 ☑
   traffic V09.3 ☑
    involving motor vehicle V09.20 ☑
     military V09.21 ☑
     specified type NEC V09.29 ☑
  person NEC (unknown way or transportation)
   V99
  collision (between)
   bus (with)
    heavy transport vehicle (traffic) V87.5 ☑
     nontraffic V88.5 ☑
   car (with)
    bus (traffic) V87.3 ☑
     nontraffic V88.3 ☑
    heavy transport vehicle (traffic) V87.4 ☑
     nontraffic V88.4 ☑
    nontraffic V88.5 ☑
    pick-up truck or van (traffic) V87.2 ☑
     nontraffic V88.2 ☑
    train or railway vehicle (traffic) V87.6 ☑
     nontraffic V88.6 ☑
    two-or three-wheeled motor vehicle
        (traffic) V87.0 ☑
     nontraffic V88.0 ☑
   motor vehicle (traffic) NEC V87.7 ☑
    nontraffic V88.7 ☑
   two-or three-wheeled vehicle (with) (traffic)
    motor vehicle NEC V87.1 ☑
     nontraffic V88.1 ☑
   nonmotor vehicle (collision) (noncollision)
        (traffic) V87.9 ☑
    nontraffic V88.9 ☑
  pickup truck occupant V59.9 ☑
   collision (with)
    animal (traffic) V50.9 ☑
     being ridden (traffic) V56.9 ☑
      nontraffic V56.3 ☑
       while boarding or alighting V56.4 ☑
     nontraffic V50.3 ☑
      while boarding or alighting V50.4 ☑
    animal-drawn vehicle (traffic) V56.9 ☑
     nontraffic V56.3 ☑
      while boarding or alighting V56.4 ☑
    bus (traffic) V54.9 ☑
     nontraffic V54.3 ☑
      while boarding or alighting V54.4 ☑
    car (traffic) V53.9 ☑
     nontraffic V53.3 ☑
      while boarding or alighting V53.4 ☑
    motor vehicle NOS (traffic) V59.60 ☑
     nontraffic V59.20 ☑
      specified type NEC (traffic) V59.69 ☑
       nontraffic V59.29 ☑

Accident — *continued*
  transport — *continued*
    pickup truck occupant — *continued*
      collision — *continued*
        pedal cycle (traffic) V51.9 ☑
          nontraffic V51.3 ☑
          while boarding or alighting V51.4 ☑
        pickup truck (traffic) V53.9 ☑
          nontraffic V53.3 ☑
          while boarding or alighting V53.4 ☑
        railway vehicle (traffic) V55.9 ☑
          nontraffic V55.3 ☑
          while boarding or alighting V55.4 ☑
        specified vehicle NEC (traffic) V56.9 ☑
          nontraffic V56.3 ☑
          while boarding or alighting V56.4 ☑
        stationary object (traffic) V57.9 ☑
          nontraffic V57.3 ☑
          while boarding or alighting V57.4 ☑
        streetcar (traffic) V56.9 ☑
          nontraffic V56.3 ☑
          while boarding or alighting V56.4 ☑
        three wheeled motor vehicle (traffic) V52.9 ☑
          nontraffic V52.3 ☑
          while boarding or alighting V52.4 ☑
        truck (traffic) V54.9 ☑
          nontraffic V54.3 ☑
          while boarding or alighting V54.4 ☑
        two wheeled motor vehicle (traffic) V52.9 ☑
          nontraffic V52.3 ☑
          while boarding or alighting V52.4 ☑
        van (traffic) V53.9 ☑
          nontraffic V53.3 ☑
          while boarding or alighting V53.4 ☑
      driver
        collision (with)
          animal (traffic) V50.5 ☑
            being ridden (traffic) V56.5 ☑
              nontraffic V56.0 ☑
            nontraffic V50.0 ☑
          animal-drawn vehicle (traffic) V56.5 ☑
            nontraffic V56.0 ☑
          bus (traffic) V54.5 ☑
            nontraffic V54.0 ☑
          car (traffic) V53.5 ☑
            nontraffic V53.0 ☑
          motor vehicle NOS (traffic) V59.40 ☑
            nontraffic V59.00 ☑
            specified type NEC (traffic) V59.49 ☑
              nontraffic V59.09 ☑
          pedal cycle (traffic) V51.5 ☑
            nontraffic V51.0 ☑
          pickup truck (traffic) V53.5 ☑
            nontraffic V53.0 ☑
          railway vehicle (traffic) V55.5 ☑
            nontraffic V55.0 ☑
          specified vehicle NEC (traffic) V56.5 ☑
            nontraffic V56.0 ☑
          stationary object (traffic) V57.5 ☑
            nontraffic V57.0 ☑
          streetcar (traffic) V56.5 ☑
            nontraffic V56.0 ☑
          three wheeled motor vehicle (traffic) V52.5 ☑
            nontraffic V52.0 ☑
          truck (traffic) V54.5 ☑
            nontraffic V54.0 ☑
          two wheeled motor vehicle (traffic) V52.5 ☑
            nontraffic V52.0 ☑
          van (traffic) V53.5 ☑
            nontraffic V53.0 ☑
        noncollision accident (traffic) V58.5 ☑
          nontraffic V58.0 ☑
      hanger-on
        collision (with)
          animal (traffic) V50.7 ☑
            being ridden (traffic) V56.7 ☑
              nontraffic V56.2 ☑
            nontraffic V50.2 ☑
          animal-drawn vehicle (traffic) V56.7 ☑
            nontraffic V56.2 ☑
          bus (traffic) V54.7 ☑
            nontraffic V54.2 ☑
          car (traffic) V53.7 ☑

Accident — *continued*
  transport — *continued*
    pickup truck occupant — *continued*
      hanger-on — *continued*
        collision — *continued*
          car — *continued*
            nontraffic V53.2 ☑
          pedal cycle (traffic) V51.7 ☑
            nontraffic V51.2 ☑
          pickup truck (traffic) V53.7 ☑
            nontraffic V53.2 ☑
          railway vehicle (traffic) V55.7 ☑
            nontraffic V55.2 ☑
          specified vehicle NEC (traffic) V56.7 ☑
            nontraffic V56.2 ☑
          stationary object (traffic) V57.7 ☑
            nontraffic V57.2 ☑
          streetcar (traffic) V56.7 ☑
            nontraffic V56.2 ☑
          three wheeled motor vehicle (traffic) V52.7 ☑
            nontraffic V52.2 ☑
          truck (traffic) V54.7 ☑
            nontraffic V54.2 ☑
          two wheeled motor vehicle (traffic) V52.7 ☑
            nontraffic V52.2 ☑
          van (traffic) V53.7 ☑
            nontraffic V53.2 ☑
        noncollision accident (traffic) V58.7 ☑
          nontraffic V58.2 ☑
      noncollision accident (traffic) V58.9 ☑
        nontraffic V58.3 ☑
        while boarding or alighting V58.4 ☑
      nontraffic V59.3 ☑
      passenger
        collision (with)
          animal (traffic) V50.6 ☑
            being ridden (traffic) V56.6 ☑
              nontraffic V56.1 ☑
            nontraffic V50.1 ☑
          animal-drawn vehicle (traffic) V56.6 ☑
            nontraffic V56.1 ☑
          bus (traffic) V54.6 ☑
            nontraffic V54.1 ☑
          car (traffic) V53.6 ☑
            nontraffic V53.1 ☑
          motor vehicle NOS (traffic) V59.50 ☑
            nontraffic V59.10 ☑
            specified type NEC (traffic) V59.59 ☑
              nontraffic V59.19 ☑
          pedal cycle (traffic) V51.6 ☑
            nontraffic V51.1 ☑
          pickup truck (traffic) V53.6 ☑
            nontraffic V53.1 ☑
          railway vehicle (traffic) V55.6 ☑
            nontraffic V55.1 ☑
          specified vehicle NEC (traffic) V56.6 ☑
            nontraffic V56.1 ☑
          stationary object (traffic) V57.6 ☑
            nontraffic V57.1 ☑
          streetcar (traffic) V56.6 ☑
            nontraffic V56.1 ☑
          three wheeled motor vehicle (traffic) V52.6 ☑
            nontraffic V52.1 ☑
          truck (traffic) V54.6 ☑
            nontraffic V54.1 ☑
          two wheeled motor vehicle (traffic) V52.6 ☑
            nontraffic V52.1 ☑
          van (traffic) V53.6 ☑
            nontraffic V53.1 ☑
        noncollision accident (traffic) V58.6 ☑
          nontraffic V58.1 ☑
      specified type NEC V59.88 ☑
      military vehicle V59.81 ☑
    quarry truck — *see* Accident, transport, industrial vehicle occupant
    race car — *see* Accident, transport, motor vehicle NEC occupant
    railway vehicle occupant V81.9 ☑
      collision (with) V81.3 ☑
        motor vehicle (non-military) (traffic) V81.1 ☑
          military V81.83 ☑

Accident — *continued*
  transport — *continued*
    railway vehicle occupant — *continued*
      collision — *continued*
        motor vehicle — *continued*
          nontraffic V81.0 ☑
        rolling stock V81.2 ☑
        specified object NEC V81.3 ☑
      during derailment V81.7 ☑
        with antecedent collision B — *see* Accident, transport, railway vehicle occupant, collision
      explosion V81.81 ☑
      fall (in railway vehicle) V81.5 ☑
        during derailment V81.7 ☑
          with antecedent collision B — *see* Accident, transport, railway vehicle occupant, collision
        from railway vehicle V81.6 ☑
          during derailment V81.7 ☑
            with antecedent collision B — *see* Accident, transport, railway vehicle occupant, collision
        while boarding or alighting V81.4 ☑
      fire V81.81 ☑
      object falling onto train V81.82 ☑
      specified type NEC V81.89 ☑
      while boarding or alighting V81.4 ☑
    ski lift V98.3 ☑
    snowmobile occupant (nontraffic) V86.92 ☑
      driver V86.52 ☑
      hanger-on V86.72 ☑
      passenger V86.62 ☑
      traffic V86.32 ☑
        driver V86.02 ☑
        hanger-on V86.22 ☑
        passenger V86.12 ☑
      while boarding or alighting V86.42 ☑
    specified NEC V98.8 ☑
    sport utility vehicle occupant (*see also* Accident, transport, car occupant)
      collision (with)
        stationary object (traffic) V47.91 ☑
          nontraffic V47.31 ☑
      driver
        collision (with)
          stationary object (traffic) V47.51 ☑
            nontraffic V47.01 ☑
      passenger
        collision (with)
          stationary object (traffic) V47.61 ☑
            nontraffic V47.11 ☑
    streetcar occupant V82.9 ☑
      collision (with) V82.3 ☑
        motor vehicle (traffic) V82.1 ☑
          nontraffic V82.0 ☑
        rolling stock V82.2 ☑
      during derailment V82.7 ☑
        with antecedent collision B — *see* Accident, transport, streetcar occupant, collision
      fall (in streetcar) V82.5 ☑
        during derailment V82.7 ☑
          with antecedent collision B — *see* Accident, transport, streetcar occupant, collision
        from streetcar V82.6 ☑
          during derailment V82.7 ☑
            with antecedent collision B — *see* Accident, transport, streetcar occupant, collision
        while boarding or alighting V82.4 ☑
      while boarding or alighting V82.4 ☑
      specified type NEC V82.8 ☑
      while boarding or alighting V82.4 ☑
    three-wheeled motor vehicle occupant V39.9 ☑
      collision (with)
        animal (traffic) V30.9 ☑
          being ridden (traffic) V36.9 ☑
            nontraffic V36.3 ☑
            while boarding or alighting V36.4 ☑
          nontraffic V30.3 ☑
          while boarding or alighting V30.4 ☑
        animal-drawn vehicle (traffic) V36.9 ☑
          nontraffic V36.3 ☑
          while boarding or alighting V36.4 ☑
        bus (traffic) V34.9 ☑

Accident — *continued*
transport — *continued*
  three-wheeled motor vehicle occupant — *continued*
    collision — *continued*
      bus — *continued*
        nontraffic V34.3 ☑
        while boarding or alighting V34.4 ☑
      car (traffic) V33.9 ☑
        nontraffic V33.3 ☑
        while boarding or alighting V33.4 ☑
      motor vehicle NOS (traffic) V39.60 ☑
        nontraffic V39.20 ☑
        specified type NEC (traffic) V39.69 ☑
          nontraffic V39.29 ☑
      pedal cycle (traffic) V31.9 ☑
        nontraffic V31.3 ☑
        while boarding or alighting V31.4 ☑
      pickup truck (traffic) V33.9 ☑
        nontraffic V33.3 ☑
        while boarding or alighting V33.4 ☑
      railway vehicle (traffic) V35.9 ☑
        nontraffic V35.3 ☑
        while boarding or alighting V35.4 ☑
      specified vehicle NEC (traffic) V36.9 ☑
        nontraffic V36.3 ☑
        while boarding or alighting V36.4 ☑
      stationary object (traffic) V37.9 ☑
        nontraffic V37.3 ☑
        while boarding or alighting V37.4 ☑
      streetcar (traffic) V36.9 ☑
        nontraffic V36.3 ☑
        while boarding or alighting V36.4 ☑
      three wheeled motor vehicle (traffic) V32.9 ☑
        nontraffic V32.3 ☑
        while boarding or alighting V32.4 ☑
      truck (traffic) V34.9 ☑
        nontraffic V34.3 ☑
        while boarding or alighting V34.4 ☑
      two wheeled motor vehicle (traffic) V32.9 ☑
        nontraffic V32.3 ☑
        while boarding or alighting V32.4 ☑
      van (traffic) V33.9 ☑
        nontraffic V33.3 ☑
        while boarding or alighting V33.4 ☑
    driver
      collision (with)
        animal (traffic) V30.5 ☑
          being ridden (traffic) V36.5 ☑
            nontraffic V36.0 ☑
          nontraffic V30.0 ☑
        animal-drawn vehicle (traffic) V36.5 ☑
          nontraffic V36.0 ☑
        bus (traffic) V34.5 ☑
          nontraffic V34.0 ☑
        car (traffic) V33.5 ☑
          nontraffic V33.0 ☑
        motor vehicle NOS (traffic) V39.40 ☑
          nontraffic V39.00 ☑
          specified type NEC (traffic) V39.49 ☑
            nontraffic V39.09 ☑
        pedal cycle (traffic) V31.5 ☑
          nontraffic V31.0 ☑
        pickup truck (traffic) V33.5 ☑
          nontraffic V33.0 ☑
        railway vehicle (traffic) V35.5 ☑
          nontraffic V35.0 ☑
        specified vehicle NEC (traffic) V36.5 ☑
          nontraffic V36.0 ☑
        stationary object (traffic) V37.5 ☑
          nontraffic V37.0 ☑
        streetcar (traffic) V36.5 ☑
          nontraffic V36.0 ☑
        three wheeled motor vehicle (traffic) V32.5 ☑
          nontraffic V32.0 ☑
        truck (traffic) V34.5 ☑
          nontraffic V34.0 ☑
        two wheeled motor vehicle (traffic) V32.5 ☑
          nontraffic V32.0 ☑
        van (traffic) V33.5 ☑
          nontraffic V33.0 ☑
      noncollision accident (traffic) V38.5 ☑
        nontraffic V38.0 ☑

Accident — *continued*
transport — *continued*
  three-wheeled motor vehicle occupant — *continued*
    hanger-on
      collision (with)
        animal (traffic) V30.7 ☑
          being ridden (traffic) V36.7 ☑
            nontraffic V36.2 ☑
          nontraffic V30.2 ☑
        animal-drawn vehicle (traffic) V36.7 ☑
          nontraffic V36.2 ☑
        bus (traffic) V34.7 ☑
          nontraffic V34.2 ☑
        car (traffic) V33.7 ☑
          nontraffic V33.2 ☑
        pedal cycle (traffic) V31.7 ☑
          nontraffic V31.2 ☑
        pickup truck (traffic) V33.7 ☑
          nontraffic V33.2 ☑
        railway vehicle (traffic) V35.7 ☑
          nontraffic V35.2 ☑
        specified vehicle NEC (traffic) V36.7 ☑
          nontraffic V36.2 ☑
        stationary object (traffic) V37.7 ☑
          nontraffic V37.2 ☑
        streetcar (traffic) V36.7 ☑
          nontraffic V36.2 ☑
        three wheeled motor vehicle (traffic) V32.7 ☑
          nontraffic V32.2 ☑
        truck (traffic) V34.7 ☑
          nontraffic V34.2 ☑
        two wheeled motor vehicle (traffic) V32.7 ☑
          nontraffic V32.2 ☑
        van (traffic) V33.7 ☑
          nontraffic V33.2 ☑
      noncollision accident (traffic) V38.7 ☑
        nontraffic V38.2 ☑
    noncollision accident (traffic) V38.9 ☑
      nontraffic V38.3 ☑
      while boarding or alighting V38.4 ☑
    nontraffic V39.3 ☑
    passenger
      collision (with)
        animal (traffic) V30.6 ☑
          being ridden (traffic) V36.6 ☑
            nontraffic V36.1 ☑
          nontraffic V30.1 ☑
        animal-drawn vehicle (traffic) V36.6 ☑
          nontraffic V36.1 ☑
        bus (traffic) V34.6 ☑
          nontraffic V34.1 ☑
        car (traffic) V33.6 ☑
          nontraffic V33.1 ☑
        motor vehicle NOS (traffic) V39.50 ☑
          nontraffic V39.10 ☑
          specified type NEC (traffic) V39.59 ☑
            nontraffic V39.19 ☑
        pedal cycle (traffic) V31.6 ☑
          nontraffic V31.1 ☑
        pickup truck (traffic) V33.6 ☑
          nontraffic V33.1 ☑
        railway vehicle (traffic) V35.6 ☑
          nontraffic V35.1 ☑
        specified vehicle NEC (traffic) V36.6 ☑
          nontraffic V36.1 ☑
        stationary object (traffic) V37.6 ☑
          nontraffic V37.1 ☑
        streetcar (traffic) V36.6 ☑
          nontraffic V36.1 ☑
        three wheeled motor vehicle (traffic) V32.6 ☑
          nontraffic V32.1 ☑
        truck (traffic) V34.6 ☑
          nontraffic V34.1 ☑
        two wheeled motor vehicle (traffic) V32.6 ☑
          nontraffic V32.1 ☑
        van (traffic) V33.6 ☑
          nontraffic V33.1 ☑
      noncollision accident (traffic) V38.6 ☑
        nontraffic V38.1 ☑
    specified type NEC V39.89 ☑
    military vehicle V39.81 ☑

Accident — *continued*
transport — *continued*
  tractor (farm) (and trailer) — *see* Accident, transport, agricultural vehicle occupant
  tram — *see* Accident, transport, streetcar
    in mine or quarry — *see* Accident, transport, industrial vehicle occupant
  trolley — *see* Accident, transport, streetcar
    in mine or quarry — *see* Accident, transport, industrial vehicle occupant
  truck (heavy) occupant V69.9 ☑
    collision (with)
      animal (traffic) V60.9 ☑
        being ridden (traffic) V66.9 ☑
          nontraffic V66.3 ☑
          while boarding or alighting V66.4 ☑
        nontraffic V60.3 ☑
        while boarding or alighting V60.4 ☑
      animal-drawn vehicle (traffic) V66.9 ☑
        nontraffic V66.3 ☑
        while boarding or alighting V66.4 ☑
      bus (traffic) V64.9 ☑
        nontraffic V64.3 ☑
        while boarding or alighting V64.4 ☑
      car (traffic) V63.9 ☑
        nontraffic V63.3 ☑
        while boarding or alighting V63.4 ☑
      motor vehicle NOS (traffic) V69.60 ☑
        nontraffic V69.20 ☑
        specified type NEC (traffic) V69.69 ☑
          nontraffic V69.29 ☑
      pedal cycle (traffic) V61.9 ☑
        nontraffic V61.3 ☑
        while boarding or alighting V61.4 ☑
      pickup truck (traffic) V63.9 ☑
        nontraffic V63.3 ☑
        while boarding or alighting V63.4 ☑
      railway vehicle (traffic) V65.9 ☑
        nontraffic V65.3 ☑
        while boarding or alighting V65.4 ☑
      specified vehicle NEC (traffic) V66.9 ☑
        nontraffic V66.3 ☑
        while boarding or alighting V66.4 ☑
      stationary object (traffic) V67.9 ☑
        nontraffic V67.3 ☑
        while boarding or alighting V67.4 ☑
      streetcar (traffic) V66.9 ☑
        nontraffic V66.3 ☑
        while boarding or alighting V66.4 ☑
      three wheeled motor vehicle (traffic) V62.9 ☑
        nontraffic V62.3 ☑
        while boarding or alighting V62.4 ☑
      truck (traffic) V64.9 ☑
        nontraffic V64.3 ☑
        while boarding or alighting V64.4 ☑
      two wheeled motor vehicle (traffic) V62.9 ☑
        nontraffic V62.3 ☑
        while boarding or alighting V62.4 ☑
      van (traffic) V63.9 ☑
        nontraffic V63.3 ☑
        while boarding or alighting V63.4 ☑
    driver
      collision (with)
        animal (traffic) V60.5 ☑
          being ridden (traffic) V66.5 ☑
            nontraffic V66.0 ☑
          nontraffic V60.0 ☑
        animal-drawn vehicle (traffic) V66.5 ☑
          nontraffic V66.0 ☑
        bus (traffic) V64.5 ☑
          nontraffic V64.0 ☑
        car (traffic) V63.5 ☑
          nontraffic V63.0 ☑
        motor vehicle NOS (traffic) V69.40 ☑
          nontraffic V69.00 ☑
          specified type NEC (traffic) V69.49 ☑
            nontraffic V69.09 ☑
        pedal cycle (traffic) V61.5 ☑
          nontraffic V61.0 ☑
        pickup truck (traffic) V63.5 ☑
          nontraffic V63.0 ☑
        railway vehicle (traffic) V65.5 ☑
          nontraffic V65.0 ☑
        specified vehicle NEC (traffic) V66.5 ☑
          nontraffic V66.0 ☑

☑ Additional Character Required — Refer to the Tabular List for Character Selection   ▽ Subterms under main terms may continue to next column or page

Accident — *continued*
  transport — *continued*
    truck occupant — *continued*
      driver — *continued*
        collision — *continued*
          stationary object (traffic) V67.5 ☑
            nontraffic V67.0 ☑
          streetcar (traffic) V66.5 ☑
            nontraffic V66.0 ☑
          three wheeled motor vehicle (traffic) V62.5 ☑
            nontraffic V62.0 ☑
          truck (traffic) V64.5 ☑
            nontraffic V64.0 ☑
          two wheeled motor vehicle (traffic) V62.5 ☑
            nontraffic V62.0 ☑
          van (traffic) V63.5 ☑
            nontraffic V63.0 ☑
        noncollision accident (traffic) V68.5 ☑
          nontraffic V68.0 ☑
      dump — *see* Accident, transport, construction vehicle occupant
      hanger-on
        collision (with)
          animal (traffic) V60.7 ☑
            being ridden (traffic) V66.7 ☑
              nontraffic V66.2 ☑
            nontraffic V60.2 ☑
          animal-drawn vehicle (traffic) V66.7 ☑
            nontraffic V66.2 ☑
          bus (traffic) V64.7 ☑
            nontraffic V64.2 ☑
          car (traffic) V63.7 ☑
            nontraffic V63.2 ☑
          pedal cycle (traffic) V61.7 ☑
            nontraffic V61.2 ☑
          pickup truck (traffic) V63.7 ☑
            nontraffic V63.2 ☑
          railway vehicle (traffic) V65.7 ☑
            nontraffic V65.2 ☑
          specified vehicle NEC (traffic) V66.7 ☑
            nontraffic V66.2 ☑
          stationary object (traffic) V67.7 ☑
            nontraffic V67.2 ☑
          streetcar (traffic) V66.7 ☑
            nontraffic V66.2 ☑
          three wheeled motor vehicle (traffic) V62.7 ☑
            nontraffic V62.2 ☑
          truck (traffic) V64.7 ☑
            nontraffic V64.2 ☑
          two wheeled motor vehicle (traffic) V62.7 ☑
            nontraffic V62.2 ☑
          van (traffic) V63.7 ☑
            nontraffic V63.2 ☑
        noncollision accident (traffic) V68.7 ☑
          nontraffic V68.2 ☑
      noncollision accident (traffic) V68.9 ☑
        nontraffic V68.3 ☑
        while boarding or alighting V68.4 ☑
      nontraffic V69.3 ☑
      passenger
        collision (with)
          animal (traffic) V60.6 ☑
            being ridden (traffic) V66.6 ☑
              nontraffic V66.1- ☑
            nontraffic V60.1 ☑
          animal-drawn vehicle (traffic) V66.6 ☑
            nontraffic V66.1 ☑
          bus (traffic) V64.6 ☑
            nontraffic V64.1 ☑
          car (traffic) V63.6 ☑
            nontraffic V63.1 ☑
          motor vehicle NOS (traffic) V69.50 ☑
            nontraffic V69.10 ☑
            specified type NEC (traffic) V69.59 ☑
              nontraffic V69.19 ☑
          pedal cycle (traffic) V61.6 ☑
            nontraffic V61.1 ☑
          pickup truck (traffic) V63.6 ☑
            nontraffic V63.1 ☑
          railway vehicle (traffic) V65.6 ☑
            nontraffic V65.1 ☑
          specified vehicle NEC (traffic) V66.6 ☑

Accident — *continued*
  transport — *continued*
    truck occupant — *continued*
      passenger — *continued*
        collision — *continued*
          specified vehicle — *continued*
            nontraffic V66.1 ☑
          stationary object (traffic) V67.6 ☑
            nontraffic V67.1 ☑
          streetcar (traffic) V66.6 ☑
            nontraffic V66.1 ☑
          three wheeled motor vehicle (traffic) V62.6 ☑
            nontraffic V62.1 ☑
          truck (traffic) V64.6 ☑
            nontraffic V64.1 ☑
          two wheeled motor vehicle (traffic) V62.6 ☑
            nontraffic V62.1 ☑
          van (traffic) V63.6 ☑
            nontraffic V63.1 ☑
        noncollision accident (traffic) V68.6 ☑
          nontraffic V68.1 ☑
      pickup — *see* Accident, transport, pickup truck occupant
      specified type NEC V69.88 ☑
      military vehicle V69.81 ☑
    van occupant V59.9 ☑
      collision (with)
        animal (traffic) V50.9 ☑
          being ridden (traffic) V56.9 ☑
            nontraffic V56.3 ☑
            while boarding or alighting V56.4 ☑
          nontraffic V50.3 ☑
          while boarding or alighting V50.4 ☑
        animal-drawn vehicle (traffic) V56.9 ☑
          nontraffic V56.3 ☑
          while boarding or alighting V56.4 ☑
        bus (traffic) V54.9 ☑
          nontraffic V54.3 ☑
          while boarding or alighting V54.4 ☑
        car (traffic) V53.9 ☑
          nontraffic V53.3 ☑
          while boarding or alighting V53.4 ☑
        motor vehicle NOS (traffic) V59.60 ☑
          nontraffic V59.20 ☑
          specified type NEC (traffic) V59.69 ☑
            nontraffic V59.29 ☑
        pedal cycle (traffic) V51.9 ☑
          nontraffic V51.3 ☑
          while boarding or alighting V51.4 ☑
        pickup truck (traffic) V53.9 ☑
          nontraffic V53.3 ☑
          while boarding or alighting V53.4 ☑
        railway vehicle (traffic) V55.9 ☑
          nontraffic V55.3 ☑
          while boarding or alighting V55.4 ☑
        specified vehicle NEC (traffic) V56.9 ☑
          nontraffic V56.3 ☑
          while boarding or alighting V56.4 ☑
        stationary object (traffic) V57.9 ☑
          nontraffic V57.3 ☑
          while boarding or alighting V57.4 ☑
        streetcar (traffic) V56.9 ☑
          nontraffic V56.3 ☑
          while boarding or alighting V56.4 ☑
        three wheeled motor vehicle (traffic) V52.9 ☑
          nontraffic V52.3 ☑
          while boarding or alighting V52.4 ☑
        truck (traffic) V54.9 ☑
          nontraffic V54.3 ☑
          while boarding or alighting V54.4 ☑
        two wheeled motor vehicle (traffic) V52.9 ☑
          nontraffic V52.3 ☑
          while boarding or alighting V52.4 ☑
        van (traffic) V53.9 ☑
          nontraffic V53.3 ☑
          while boarding or alighting V53.4 ☑
      driver
        collision (with)
          animal (traffic) V50.5 ☑
            being ridden (traffic) V56.5 ☑
              nontraffic V56.0 ☑
            nontraffic V50.0 ☑
          animal-drawn vehicle (traffic) V56.5 ☑

Accident — *continued*
  transport — *continued*
    van occupant — *continued*
      driver — *continued*
        collision — *continued*
          animal-drawn vehicle — *continued*
            nontraffic V56.0 ☑
          bus (traffic) V54.5 ☑
            nontraffic V54.0 ☑
          car (traffic) V53.5 ☑
            nontraffic V53.0 ☑
          motor vehicle NOS (traffic) V59.40 ☑
            nontraffic V59.00 ☑
            specified type NEC (traffic) V59.49 ☑
              nontraffic V59.09 ☑
          pedal cycle (traffic) V51.5 ☑
            nontraffic V51.0 ☑
          pickup truck (traffic) V53.5 ☑
            nontraffic V53.0 ☑
          railway vehicle (traffic) V55.5 ☑
            nontraffic V55.0 ☑
          specified vehicle NEC (traffic) V56.5 ☑
            nontraffic V56.0 ☑
          stationary object (traffic) V57.5 ☑
            nontraffic V57.0 ☑
          streetcar (traffic) V56.5 ☑
            nontraffic V56.0 ☑
          three wheeled motor vehicle (traffic) V52.5 ☑
            nontraffic V52.0 ☑
          truck (traffic) V54.5 ☑
            nontraffic V54.0 ☑
          two wheeled motor vehicle (traffic) V52.5 ☑
            nontraffic V52.0 ☑
          van (traffic) V53.5 ☑
            nontraffic V53.0 ☑
        noncollision accident (traffic) V58.5 ☑
          nontraffic V58.0 ☑
      hanger-on
        collision (with)
          animal (traffic) V50.7 ☑
            being ridden (traffic) V56.7 ☑
              nontraffic V56.2 ☑
            nontraffic V50.2 ☑
          animal-drawn vehicle (traffic) V56.7 ☑
            nontraffic V56.2 ☑
          bus (traffic) V54.7 ☑
            nontraffic V54.2 ☑
          car (traffic) V53.7 ☑
            nontraffic V53.2 ☑
          pedal cycle (traffic) V51.7 ☑
            nontraffic V51.2 ☑
          pickup truck (traffic) V53.7 ☑
            nontraffic V53.2 ☑
          railway vehicle (traffic) V55.7 ☑
            nontraffic V55.2 ☑
          specified vehicle NEC (traffic) V56.7 ☑
            nontraffic V56.2 ☑
          stationary object (traffic) V57.7 ☑
            nontraffic V57.2 ☑
          streetcar (traffic) V56.7 ☑
            nontraffic V56.2 ☑
          three wheeled motor vehicle (traffic) V52.7 ☑
            nontraffic V52.2 ☑
          truck (traffic) V54.7 ☑
            nontraffic V54.2 ☑
          two wheeled motor vehicle (traffic) V52.7 ☑
            nontraffic V52.2 ☑
          van (traffic) V53.7 ☑
            nontraffic V53.2 ☑
        noncollision accident (traffic) V58.7 ☑
          nontraffic V58.2 ☑
      noncollision accident (traffic) V58.9 ☑
        nontraffic V58.3 ☑
        while boarding or alighting V58.4 ☑
      nontraffic V59.3 ☑
      passenger
        collision (with)
          animal (traffic) V50.6 ☑
            being ridden (traffic) V56.6 ☑
              nontraffic V56.1 ☑
            nontraffic V50.1 ☑
          animal-drawn vehicle (traffic) V56.6 ☑

Accident — *continued*
  transport — *continued*
    van occupant — *continued*
      passenger — *continued*
        collision — *continued*
          animal-drawn vehicle — *continued*
            nontraffic V56.1 ☑
          bus (traffic) V54.6 ☑
            nontraffic V54.1 ☑
          car (traffic) V53.6 ☑
            nontraffic V53.1 ☑
          motor vehicle NOS (traffic) V59.50 ☑
            nontraffic V59.10 ☑
            specified type NEC (traffic) V59.59 ☑
              nontraffic V59.19 ☑
          pedal cycle (traffic) V51.6 ☑
            nontraffic V51.1 ☑
          pickup truck (traffic) V53.6 ☑
            nontraffic V53.1 ☑
          railway vehicle (traffic) V55.6 ☑
            nontraffic V55.1 ☑
          specified vehicle NEC (traffic) V56.6 ☑
            nontraffic V56.1 ☑
          stationary object (traffic) V57.6 ☑
            nontraffic V57.1 ☑
          streetcar (traffic) V56.6 ☑
            nontraffic V56.1 ☑
          three wheeled motor vehicle (traffic) V52.6 ☑
            nontraffic V52.1 ☑
          truck (traffic) V54.6 ☑
            nontraffic V54.1 ☑
          two wheeled motor vehicle (traffic) V52.6 ☑
            nontraffic V52.1 ☑
          van (traffic) V53.6 ☑
            nontraffic V53.1 ☑
         noncollision accident (traffic) V58.6 ☑
           nontraffic V58.1 ☑
        specified type NEC V59.88 ☑
        military vehicle V59.81 ☑
      watercraft occupant — *see* Accident, watercraft
    vehicle NEC V89.9 ☑
    animal-drawn NEC — *see* Accident, transport, animal-drawn vehicle occupant
    special
      agricultural — *see* Accident, transport, agricultural vehicle occupant
      construction — *see* Accident, transport, construction vehicle occupant
      industrial — *see* Accident, transport, industrial vehicle occupant
    three-wheeled NEC (motorized) — *see* Accident, transport, three-wheeled motor vehicle occupant
  watercraft V94.9 ☑
    causing
      drowning B — *see* Drowning, due to, accident to, watercraft
      injury NEC V91.89 ☑
        crushed between craft and object V91.19 ☑
          powered craft V91.13 ☑
            ferry boat V91.11 ☑
            fishing boat V91.12 ☑
            jetskis V91.13 ☑
            liner V91.11 ☑
            merchant ship V91.10 ☑
            passenger ship V91.11 ☑
          unpowered craft V91.18 ☑
            canoe V91.15 ☑
            inflatable V91.16 ☑
            kayak V91.15 ☑
            sailboat V91.14 ☑
            surf-board V91.18 ☑
            windsurfer V91.18 ☑
        fall on board V91.29 ☑
          powered craft V91.23 ☑
            ferry boat V91.21 ☑
            fishing boat V91.22 ☑
            jetskis V91.23 ☑
            liner V91.21 ☑
            merchant ship V91.20 ☑
            passenger ship V91.21 ☑
          unpowered craft
            canoe V91.25 ☑
            inflatable V91.26 ☑

Accident — *continued*
  watercraft — *continued*
    causing — *continued*
      injury — *continued*
        fall on board — *continued*
          unpowered craft — *continued*
            kayak V91.25 ☑
            sailboat V91.24 ☑
        fire on board causing burn V91.09 ☑
          powered craft V91.03 ☑
            ferry boat V91.01 ☑
            fishing boat V91.02 ☑
            jetskis V91.03 ☑
            liner V91.01 ☑
            merchant ship V91.00 ☑
            passenger ship V91.01 ☑
          unpowered craft V91.08 ☑
            canoe V91.05 ☑
            inflatable V91.06 ☑
            kayak V91.05 ☑
            sailboat V91.04 ☑
            surf-board V91.08 ☑
            water skis V91.07 ☑
            windsurfer V91.08 ☑
        hit by falling object V91.39 ☑
          powered craft V91.33 ☑
            ferry boat V91.31 ☑
            fishing boat V91.32 ☑
            jetskis V91.33 ☑
            liner V91.31 ☑
            merchant ship V91.30 ☑
            passenger ship V91.31 ☑
          unpowered craft V91.38 ☑
            canoe V91.35 ☑
            inflatable V91.36 ☑
            kayak V91.35 ☑
            sailboat V91.34 ☑
            surf-board V91.38 ☑
            water skis V91.37 ☑
            windsurfer V91.38 ☑
        specified type NEC V91.89 ☑
          powered craft V91.83 ☑
            ferry boat V91.81 ☑
            fishing boat V91.82 ☑
            jetskis V91.83 ☑
            liner V91.81 ☑
            merchant ship V91.80 ☑
            passenger ship V91.81 ☑
          unpowered craft V91.88 ☑
            canoe V91.85 ☑
            inflatable V91.86 ☑
            kayak V91.85 ☑
            sailboat V91.84 ☑
            surf-board V91.88 ☑
            water skis V91.87 ☑
            windsurfer V91.88 ☑
      due to, caused by cataclysm — *see* Forces of nature, by type
      military V94.818 ☑
        with civilian watercraft V94.810 ☑
        civilian in water injured by V94.811 ☑
      nonpowered, struck by
        nonpowered vessel V94.22 ☑
        powered vessel V94.21 ☑
      specified type NEC V94.89 ☑
      striking swimmer
        powered V94.11 ☑
        unpowered V94.12 ☑
Acid throwing (assault) Y08.89 ☑
Activity (involving) (of victim at time of event) Y93.9
  aerobic and step exercise (class) Y93.A3 (*following* Y93.7)
  alpine skiing Y93.23
  animal care NEC Y93.K9 (*following* Y93.7)
  arts and handcrafts NEC Y93.D9 (*following* Y93.7)
  athletics played as a team or group NEC Y93.69
  athletics played individually NEC Y93.59
  athletics NEC Y93.79
  baking Y93.G3 (*following* Y93.7)
  ballet Y93.41
  barbells Y93.B3 (*following* Y93.7)
  BASE (Building, Antenna, Span, Earth) jumping Y93.33
  baseball Y93.64
  basketball Y93.67
  bathing (personal) Y93.E1 (*following* Y93.7)
  beach volleyball Y93.68

Activity — *continued*
  bike riding Y93.55
  boogie boarding Y93.18
  bowling Y93.54
  boxing Y93.71
  brass instrument playing Y93.J4 (*following* Y93.7)
  building construction Y93.H3 (*following* Y93.7)
  bungee jumping Y93.34
  calisthenics Y93.A2 (*following* Y93.7)
  canoeing (in calm and turbulent water) Y93.16
  capture the flag Y93.6A
  cardiorespiratory exercise NEC Y93.A9 (*following* Y93.7)
  caregiving (providing) NEC Y93.F9 (*following* Y93.7)
    bathing Y93.F1 (*following* Y93.7)
    lifting Y93.F2 (*following* Y93.7)
  cellular
    communication device Y93.C2 (*following* Y93.7)
    telephone Y93.C2 (*following* Y93.7)
  challenge course Y93.A5 (*following* Y93.7)
  cheerleading Y93.45
  circuit training Y93.A4 (*following* Y93.7)
  cleaning
    floor Y93.E5 (*following* Y93.7)
  climbing NEC Y93.39
    mountain Y93.31
    rock Y93.31
    wall Y93.31
  clothing care and maintenance NEC Y93.E9 (*following* Y93.7)
  combatives Y93.75
  computer
    keyboarding Y93.C1 (*following* Y93.7)
    technology NEC Y93.C9 (*following* Y93.7)
  confidence course Y93.A5 (*following* Y93.7)
  construction (building) Y93.H3 (*following* Y93.7)
  cooking and baking Y93.G3 (*following* Y93.7)
  cool down exercises Y93.A2 (*following* Y93.7)
  cricket Y93.69
  crocheting Y93.D1 (*following* Y93.7)
  cross country skiing Y93.24
  dancing (all types) Y93.41
  digging
    dirt Y93.H1 (*following* Y93.7)
  dirt digging Y93.H1 (*following* Y93.7)
  dishwashing Y93.G1 (*following* Y93.7)
  diving (platform) (springboard) Y93.12
    underwater Y93.15
  dodge ball Y93.6A
  downhill skiing Y93.23
  drum playing Y93.J2 (*following* Y93.7)
  dumbbells Y93.B3 (*following* Y93.7)
  electronic
    devices NEC Y93.C9 (*following* Y93.7)
      hand held interactive Y93.C2 (*following* Y93.7)
    game playing (using) (with)
      interactive device Y93.C2 (*following* Y93.7)
      keyboard or other stationary device Y93.C1 (*following* Y93.7)
  elliptical machine Y93.A1 (*following* Y93.7)
  exercise(s)
    machines ((primarily) for)
      cardiorespiratory conditioning Y93.A1 (*following* Y93.7)
      muscle strengthening Y93.B1 (*following* Y93.7)
    muscle strengthening (non-machine) NEC Y93.B9 (*following* Y93.7)
  external motion NEC Y93.I9 (*following* Y93.7)
    rollercoaster Y93.I1 (*following* Y93.7)
  field hockey Y93.65
  figure skating (pairs) (singles) Y93.21
  flag football Y93.62
  floor mopping and cleaning Y93.E5 (*following* Y93.7)
  food preparation and clean up Y93.G1 (*following* Y93.7)
  football (American) NOS Y93.61
    flag Y93.62
    tackle Y93.61
    touch Y93.62
  four square Y93.6A
  free weights Y93.B3 (*following* Y93.7)
  frisbee (ultimate) Y93.74
  furniture
    building Y93.D3 (*following* Y93.7)
    finishing Y93.D3 (*following* Y93.7)
    repair Y93.D3 (*following* Y93.7)
  game playing (electronic)
    using interactive device Y93.C2 (*following* Y93.7)
    using keyboard or other stationary device Y93.C1 (*following* Y93.7)

Activity — *continued*
gardening Y93.H2 (*following* Y93.7)
golf Y93.53
grass drills Y93.A6 (*following* Y93.7)
grilling and smoking food Y93.G2 (*following* Y93.7)
grooming and shearing an animal Y93.K3 (*following* Y93.7)
guerilla drills Y93.A6 (*following* Y93.7)
gymnastics (rhythmic) Y93.43
hand held interactive electronic device Y93.C2 (*following* Y93.7)
handball Y93.73
handcrafts NEC Y93.D9 (*following* Y93.7)
hang gliding Y93.35
hiking (on level or elevated terrain) Y93.01
hockey (ice) Y93.22
 field Y93.65
horseback riding Y93.52
household (interior) maintenance NEC Y93.E9 (*following* Y93.7)
ice NEC Y93.29
 dancing Y93.21
 hockey Y93.22
 skating Y93.21
inline roller skating Y93.51
ironing Y93.E4 (*following* Y93.7)
judo Y93.75
jumping jacks Y93.A2 (*following* Y93.7)
jumping rope Y93.56
jumping (off) NEC Y93.39
 BASE (Building, Antenna, Span, Earth) Y93.33
 bungee Y93.34
 jacks Y93.A2 (*following* Y93.7)
 rope Y93.56
karate Y93.75
kayaking (in calm and turbulent water) Y93.16
keyboarding (computer) Y93.C1 (*following* Y93.7)
kickball Y93.6A
knitting Y93.D1 (*following* Y93.7)
lacrosse Y93.65
land maintenance NEC Y93.H9 (*following* Y93.7)
landscaping Y93.H2 (*following* Y93.7)
laundry Y93.E2 (*following* Y93.7)
machines (exercise)
 primarily for cardiorespiratory conditioning Y93.A1 (*following* Y93.7)
 primarily for muscle strengthening Y93.B1 (*following* Y93.7)
maintenance
 exterior building NEC Y93.H9 (*following* Y93.7)
 household (interior) NEC Y93.E9 (*following* Y93.7)
 land Y93.H9 (*following* Y93.7)
 property Y93.H9 (*following* Y93.7)
marching (on level or elevated terrain) Y93.01
martial arts Y93.75
microwave oven Y93.G3 (*following* Y93.7)
milking an animal Y93.K2 (*following* Y93.7)
mopping (floor) Y93.E5 (*following* Y93.7)
mountain climbing Y93.31
muscle strengthening
 exercises (non-machine) NEC Y93.B9 (*following* Y93.7)
 machines Y93.B1 (*following* Y93.7)
musical keyboard (electronic) playing Y93.J1 (*following* Y93.7)
nordic skiing Y93.24
obstacle course Y93.A5 (*following* Y93.7)
oven (microwave) Y93.G3 (*following* Y93.7)
packing up and unpacking in moving to a new residence Y93.E6 (*following* Y93.7)
parasailing Y93.19
percussion instrument playing NEC Y93.J2 (*following* Y93.7)
personal
 bathing and showering Y93.E1 (*following* Y93.7)
 hygiene NEC Y93.E8 (*following* Y93.7)
 showering Y93.E1 (*following* Y93.7)
physical games generally associated with school recess, summer camp and children Y93.6A
physical training NEC Y93.A9 (*following* Y93.7)
piano playing Y93.J1 (*following* Y93.7)
pilates Y93.B4 (*following* Y93.7)
platform diving Y93.12
playing musical instrument
 brass instrument Y93.J4 (*following* Y93.7)
 drum Y93.J2 (*following* Y93.7)
 musical keyboard (electronic) Y93.J1 (*following* Y93.7)

Activity — *continued*
playing musical instrument — *continued*
 percussion instrument NEC Y93.J2 (*following* Y93.7)
 piano Y93.J1 (*following* Y93.7)
 string instrument Y93.J3 (*following* Y93.7)
 winds instrument Y93.J4 (*following* Y93.7)
property maintenance
 exterior NEC Y93.H9 (*following* Y93.7)
 interior NEC Y93.E9 (*following* Y93.7)
pruning (garden and lawn) Y93.H2 (*following* Y93.7)
pull-ups Y93.B2 (*following* Y93.7)
push-ups Y93.B2 (*following* Y93.7)
racquetball Y93.73
rafting (in calm and turbulent water) Y93.16
raking (leaves) Y93.H1 (*following* Y93.7)
rappelling Y93.32
refereeing a sports activity Y93.81
residential relocation Y93.E6 (*following* Y93.7)
rhythmic gymnastics Y93.43
rhythmic movement NEC Y93.49
riding
 horseback Y93.52
 rollercoaster Y93.I1 (*following* Y93.7)
rock climbing Y93.31
roller skating (inline) Y93.51
rollercoaster riding Y93.I1 (*following* Y93.7)
rough housing and horseplay Y93.83
rowing (in calm and turbulent water) Y93.16
rugby Y93.63
running Y93.02
SCUBA diving Y93.15
sewing Y93.D2 (*following* Y93.7)
shoveling Y93.H1 (*following* Y93.7)
 dirt Y93.H1 (*following* Y93.7)
 snow Y93.H1 (*following* Y93.7)
showering (personal) Y93.E1 (*following* Y93.7)
sit-ups Y93.B2 (*following* Y93.7)
skateboarding Y93.51
skating (ice) Y93.21
 roller Y93.51
skiing (alpine) (downhill) Y93.23
 cross country Y93.24
 nordic Y93.24
 water Y93.17
sledding (snow) Y93.23
sleeping (sleep) Y93.84
smoking and grilling food Y93.G2 (*following* Y93.7)
snorkeling Y93.15
snow NEC Y93.29
 boarding Y93.23
 shoveling Y93.H1 (*following* Y93.7)
 sledding Y93.23
 tubing Y93.23
soccer Y93.66
softball Y93.64
specified NEC Y93.89
spectator at an event Y93.82
sports NEC Y93.79
 sports played as a team or group NEC Y93.69
 sports played individually NEC Y93.59
springboard diving Y93.12
squash Y93.73
stationary bike Y93.A1 (*following* Y93.7)
step (stepping) exercise (class) Y93.A3 (*following* Y93.7)
stepper machine Y93.A1 (*following* Y93.7)
stove Y93.G3 (*following* Y93.7)
string instrument playing Y93.J3 (*following* Y93.7)
surfing Y93.18
 wind Y93.18
swimming Y93.11
tackle football Y93.61
tap dancing Y93.41
tennis Y93.73
tobogganing Y93.23
touch football Y93.62
track and field events (non-running) Y93.57
 running Y93.02
trampoline Y93.44
treadmill Y93.A1 (*following* Y93.7)
trimming shrubs Y93.H2 (*following* Y93.7)
tubing (in calm and turbulent water) Y93.16
 snow Y93.23
ultimate frisbee Y93.74
underwater diving Y93.15
unpacking in moving to a new residence Y93.E6 (*following* Y93.7)
use of stove, oven and microwave oven Y93.G3 (*following* Y93.7)

Activity — *continued*
vacuuming Y93.E3 (*following* Y93.7)
volleyball (beach) (court) Y93.68
wake boarding Y93.17
walking (on level or elevated terrain) Y93.01
 an animal Y93.K1 (*following* Y93.7)
walking an animal Y93.K1 (*following* Y93.7)
wall climbing Y93.31
warm up and cool down exercises Y93.A2 (*following* Y93.7)
water NEC Y93.19
 aerobics Y93.14
 craft NEC Y93.19
 exercise Y93.14
 polo Y93.13
 skiing Y93.17
 sliding Y93.18
 survival training and testing Y93.19
weeding (garden and lawn) Y93.H2 (*following* Y93.7)
wind instrument playing Y93.J4 (*following* Y93.7)
windsurfing Y93.18
wrestling Y93.72
yoga Y93.42
Adverse effect of drugs — *see* Table of Drugs and Chemicals
Aerosinusitis — *see* Air, pressure
After-effect, late — *see* Sequelae
Air
blast in war operations — *see* War operations, air blast
pressure
 change, rapid
 during
 ascent W94.29 ☑
 while (in) (surfacing from)
 aircraft W94.23 ☑
 deep water diving W94.21 ☑
 underground W94.22 ☑
 descent W94.39 ☑
 in
 aircraft W94.31 ☑
 water W94.32 ☑
 high, prolonged W94.0 ☑
 low, prolonged W94.12 ☑
 due to residence or long visit at high altitude W94.11 ☑
Alpine sickness W94.11 ☑
Altitude sickness W94.11 ☑
Anaphylactic shock, anaphylaxis — *see* Table of Drugs and Chemicals
Andes disease W94.11 ☑
Arachnidism, arachnoidism X58 ☑
Arson (with intent to injure or kill) X97 ☑
Asphyxia, asphyxiation
by
 food (bone) (seed) — *see* categories T17 and T18 ☑
 gas (*see also* Table of Drugs and Chemicals)
 legal
 execution — *see* Legal, intervention, gas
 intervention — *see* Legal, intervention, gas
from
 fire (*see also* Exposure, fire)
 in war operations — *see* War operations, fire
 ignition — *see* Ignition
 vomitus T17.81 ☑
in war operations — *see* War operations, restriction of airway
Aspiration
food (any type) (into respiratory tract) (with asphyxia, obstruction respiratory tract, suffocation) — *see* categories T17 and T18 ☑
foreign body — *see* Foreign body, aspiration
vomitus (with asphyxia, obstruction respiratory tract, suffocation) T17.81 ☑
Assassination (attempt) — *see* Assault
Assault (homicidal) (by) (in) Y09
arson X97 ☑
bite (of human being) Y04.1 ☑
bodily force Y04.8 ☑
 bite Y04.1 ☑
 bumping into Y04.2 ☑
 sexual — *see* subcategories T74.0, T76.0 ☑
 unarmed fight Y04.0 ☑
bomb X96.9 ☑
 antipersonnel X96.0 ☑
 fertilizer X96.3 ☑
 gasoline X96.1 ☑

Assault — *continued*
- bomb — *continued*
  - letter X96.2 ☑
  - petrol X96.1 ☑
  - pipe X96.3 ☑
  - specified NEC X96.8 ☑
- brawl (hand) (fists) (foot) (unarmed) Y04.0 ☑
- burning, burns (by fire) NEC X97 ☑
  - acid Y08.89 ☑
  - caustic, corrosive substance Y08.89 ☑
  - chemical from swallowing caustic, corrosive substance — *see* Table of Drugs and Chemicals
  - cigarette(s) X97 ☑
  - hot object X98.9 ☑
    - fluid NEC X98.2 ☑
    - household appliance X98.3 ☑
    - specified NEC X98.8 ☑
    - steam X98.0 ☑
    - tap water X98.1 ☑
    - vapors X98.0 ☑
  - scalding — *see* Assault, burning
  - steam X98.0 ☑
  - vitriol Y08.89 ☑
- caustic, corrosive substance (gas) Y08.89 ☑
- crashing of
  - aircraft Y08.81 ☑
  - motor vehicle Y03.8 ☑
    - pushed in front of Y02.0 ☑
    - run over Y03.0 ☑
    - specified NEC Y03.8 ☑
- cutting or piercing instrument X99.9 ☑
  - dagger X99.2 ☑
  - glass X99.0 ☑
  - knife X99.1 ☑
  - specified NEC X99.8 ☑
  - sword X99.2 ☑
- dagger X99.2 ☑
- drowning (in) X92.9 ☑
  - bathtub X92.0 ☑
  - natural water X92.3 ☑
  - specified NEC X92.8 ☑
  - swimming pool X92.1 ☑
    - following fall X92.2 ☑
- dynamite X96.8 ☑
- explosive(s) (material) X96.9 ☑
- fight (hand) (fists) (foot) (unarmed) Y04.0 ☑
  - with weapon — *see* Assault, by type of weapon
- fire X97 ☑
- firearm X95.9 ☑
  - airgun X95.01 ☑
  - handgun X93 ☑
  - hunting rifle X94.1 ☑
  - larger X94.9 ☑
    - specified NEC X94.8 ☑
  - machine gun X94.2 ☑
  - shotgun X94.0 ☑
  - specified NEC X95.8 ☑
- from high place Y01 ☑
- gunshot (wound) NEC — *see* Assault, firearm, by type
- incendiary device X97 ☑
- injury Y09 ☑
  - to child due to criminal abortion attempt NEC Y08.89 ☑
- knife X99.1 ☑
- late effect of — *see* categories X92-Y08 with 7th character S
- placing before moving object NEC Y02.8 ☑
  - motor vehicle Y02.0 ☑
- poisoning — *see* categories T36-T65 with 7th character S
- puncture, any part of body — *see* Assault, cutting or piercing instrument
- pushing
  - before moving object NEC Y02.8 ☑
    - motor vehicle Y02.0 ☑
    - subway train Y02.1 ☑
    - train Y02.1 ☑
  - from high place Y01 ☑
- rape T74.2- ☑
- scalding — *see* Assault, burning
- sequelae of — *see* categories X92-Y08 with 7th character S
- sexual (by bodily force) T74.2- ☑
- shooting — *see* Assault, firearm
- specified means NEC Y08.89 ☑

Assault — *continued*
- stab, any part of body — *see* Assault, cutting or piercing instrument
- steam X98.0 ☑
- striking against
  - other person Y04.2 ☑
  - sports equipment Y08.09 ☑
    - baseball bat Y08.02 ☑
    - hockey stick Y08.01 ☑
- struck by
  - sports equipment Y08.09 ☑
    - baseball bat Y08.02 ☑
    - hockey stick Y08.01 ☑
- submersion — *see* Assault, drowning
- violence Y09 ☑
- weapon Y09 ☑
  - blunt Y00 ☑
  - cutting or piercing — *see* Assault, cutting or piercing instrument
  - firearm — *see* Assault, firearm
- wound Y09 ☑
  - cutting — *see* Assault, cutting or piercing instrument
  - gunshot — *see* Assault, firearm
  - knife X99.1 ☑
  - piercing — *see* Assault, cutting or piercing instrument
  - puncture — *see* Assault, cutting or piercing instrument
  - stab — *see* Assault, cutting or piercing instrument
- **Attack by mammals NEC** W55.89 ☑
- **Avalanche** — *see* Landslide
- **Aviator's disease** — *see* Air, pressure

B

Barotitis, barodontalgia, barosinusitis, barotrauma (otitic) (sinus) — *see* Air, pressure
Battered (baby) (child) (person) (syndrome) X58 ☑
Bayonet wound W26.1 ☑
- in
  - legal intervention — *see* Legal, intervention, sharp object, bayonet
  - war operations — *see* War operations, combat
  - stated as undetermined whether accidental or intentional Y28.8 ☑
  - suicide (attempt) X78.2 ☑
Bean in nose — *see* categories T17 and T18 ☑
Bed set on fire NEC — *see* Exposure, fire, uncontrolled, building, bed
Beheading (by guillotine)
- homicide X99.9 ☑
- legal execution — *see* Legal, intervention
Bending, injury in — *see* category Y93 ☑
Bends — *see* Air, pressure, change
Bite, bitten by
- alligator W58.01 ☑
- arthropod (nonvenomous) NEC W57 ☑
- bull W55.21 ☑
- cat W55.01 ☑
- cow W55.21 ☑
- crocodile W58.11 ☑
- dog W54.0 ☑
- goat W55.31 ☑
- hoof stock NEC W55.31 ☑
- horse W55.11 ☑
- human being (accidentally) W50.3 ☑
  - with intent to injure or kill Y04.1 ☑
  - as, or caused by, a crowd or human stampede (with fall) W52 ☑
  - assault Y04.1 ☑
  - homicide (attempt) Y04.1 ☑
  - in
    - fight Y04.1 ☑
- insect (nonvenomous) W57 ☑
- lizard (nonvenomous) W59.01 ☑
- mammal NEC W55.81 ☑
- mammal NEC W55.81 ☑
  - marine W56.31 ☑
- marine animal (nonvenomous) W56.81 ☑
- millipede W57 ☑
- moray eel W56.51 ☑
- mouse W53.01 ☑
- person(s) (accidentally) W50.3 ☑
  - with intent to injure or kill Y04.1 ☑

Bite, bitten by — *continued*
- person(s) — *continued*
  - as, or caused by, a crowd or human stampede (with fall) W52 ☑
  - assault Y04.1 ☑
  - homicide (attempt) Y04.1 ☑
  - in
    - fight Y04.1 ☑
- pig W55.41 ☑
- raccoon W55.51 ☑
- rat W53.11 ☑
- reptile W59.81 ☑
  - lizard W59.01 ☑
  - snake W59.11 ☑
  - turtle W59.21 ☑
    - terrestrial W59.81 ☑
- rodent W53.81 ☑
  - mouse W53.01 ☑
  - rat W53.11 ☑
  - specified NEC W53.81 ☑
  - squirrel W53.21 ☑
- shark W56.41 ☑
- sheep W55.31 ☑
- snake (nonvenomous) W59.11 ☑
- spider (nonvenomous) W57 ☑
- squirrel W53.21 ☑
Blast (air) in war operations — *see* War operations, blast
Blizzard X37.2 ☑
Blood alcohol level Y90.9
- less than 20mg/100ml Y90.0
- 20-39mg/100ml Y90.1
- 40-59mg/100ml Y90.2
- 60-79mg/100ml Y90.3
- 80-99mg/100ml Y90.4
- 100-119mg/100ml Y90.5
- 120-199mg/100ml Y90.6
- 200-239mg/100ml Y90.7
- presence in blood, level not specified Y90.9
Blow X58 ☑
- by law-enforcing agent, police (on duty) — *see* Legal, intervention, manhandling
- blunt object — *see* Legal, intervention, blunt object
Blowing up — *see* Explosion
Brawl (hand) (fists) (foot) Y04.0 ☑
Breakage (accidental) (part of)
- ladder (causing fall) W11 ☑
- scaffolding (causing fall) W12 ☑
Broken
- glass, contact with — *see* Contact, with, glass
- power line (causing electric shock) W85 ☑
Bumping against, into (accidentally)
- object NEC W22.8 ☑
  - with fall — *see* Fall, due to, bumping against, object
  - caused by crowd or human stampede (with fall) W52 ☑
  - sports equipment W21.9 ☑
- person(s) W51 ☑
  - with fall W03 ☑
    - due to ice or snow W00.0 ☑
  - assault Y04.2 ☑
  - caused by, a crowd or human stampede (with fall) W52 ☑
  - homicide (attempt) Y04.2 ☑
- sports equipment W21.9 ☑
Burn, burned, burning (accidental) (by) (from) (on)
- acid NEC — *see* Table of Drugs and Chemicals
- bed linen — *see* Exposure, fire, uncontrolled, in building, bed
- blowtorch X08.8 ☑
  - with ignition of clothing NEC X06.2 ☑
    - nightwear X05 ☑
- bonfire, campfire (controlled) (*see also* Exposure, fire, controlled, not in building)
  - uncontrolled — *see* Exposure, fire, uncontrolled, not in building
- candle X08.8 ☑
  - with ignition of clothing NEC X06.2 ☑
    - nightwear X05 ☑
- caustic liquid, substance (external) (internal) NEC — *see* Table of Drugs and Chemicals
- chemical (external) (internal) (*see also* Table of Drugs and Chemicals)
  - in war operations — *see* War operations. fire
- cigar(s) or cigarette(s) X08.8 ☑
  - with ignition of clothing NEC X06.2 ☑

Burn, burned, burning — *continued*
- cigar(s) or cigarette(s) — *continued*
  - with ignition of clothing — *continued*
    - nightwear X05 ☑
- clothes, clothing NEC (from controlled fire) X06.2 ☑
  - with conflagration — *see* Exposure, fire, uncontrolled, building
    - not in building or structure — *see* Exposure, fire, uncontrolled, not in building
- cooker (hot) X15.8 ☑
  - stated as undetermined whether accidental or intentional Y27.3 ☑
  - suicide (attempt) X77.3 ☑
- electric blanket X16 ☑
- engine (hot) X17 ☑
- fire, flames — *see* Exposure, fire
- flare, Very pistol — *see* Discharge, firearm NEC
- heat
  - from appliance (electrical) (household) X15.8 ☑
    - cooker X15.8 ☑
    - hotplate X15.2 ☑
    - kettle X15.8 ☑
    - light bulb X15.8 ☑
    - saucepan X15.3 ☑
    - skillet X15.3 ☑
    - stated as undetermined whether accidental or intentional Y27.3 ☑
    - stove X15.0 ☑
    - suicide (attempt) X77.3 ☑
    - toaster X15.1 ☑
  - in local application or packing during medical or surgical procedure Y63.5
- heating
  - appliance, radiator or pipe X16 ☑
- homicide (attempt) — *see* Assault, burning
- hot
  - air X14.1 ☑
  - cooker X15.8 ☑
  - drink X10.0 ☑
  - engine X17 ☑
  - fat X10.2 ☑
  - fluid NEC X12 ☑
  - food X10.1 ☑
  - gases X14.1 ☑
  - heating appliance X16 ☑
  - household appliance NEC X15.8 ☑
  - kettle X15.8 ☑
  - liquid NEC X12 ☑
  - machinery X17 ☑
  - metal (molten) (liquid) NEC X18 ☑
  - object (not producing fire or flames) NEC X19 ☑
  - oil (cooking) X10.2 ☑
  - pipe(s) X16 ☑
  - radiator X16 ☑
  - saucepan (glass) (metal) X15.3 ☑
  - stove (kitchen) X15.0 ☑
  - substance NEC X19 ☑
    - caustic or corrosive NEC — *see* Table of Drugs and Chemicals
  - toaster X15.1 ☑
  - tool X17 ☑
  - vapor X13.1 ☑
  - water (tap) — *see* Contact, with, hot, tap water
- hotplate X15.2 ☑
  - suicide (attempt) X77.3 ☑
- ignition — *see* Ignition
- in war operations — *see* War operations, fire
- inflicted by other person X97 ☑
  - by hot objects, hot vapor, and steam — *see* Assault, burning, hot object
- internal, from swallowed caustic, corrosive liquid, substance — *see* Table of Drugs and Chemicals
- iron (hot) X15.8 ☑
  - stated as undetermined whether accidental or intentional Y27.3 ☑
  - suicide (attempt) X77.3 ☑
- kettle (hot) X15.8 ☑
  - stated as undetermined whether accidental or intentional Y27.3 ☑
  - suicide (attempt) X77.3 ☑
- lamp (flame) X08.8 ☑
  - with ignition of clothing NEC X06.2 ☑
    - nightwear X05 ☑
- lighter (cigar) (cigarette) X08.8 ☑
  - with ignition of clothing NEC X06.2 ☑
    - nightwear X05 ☑

Burn, burned, burning — *continued*
- lightning — *see* subcategory T75.0 ☑
  - causing fire — *see* Exposure, fire
- liquid (boiling) (hot) NEC X12 ☑
  - stated as undetermined whether accidental or intentional Y27.2 ☑
  - suicide (attempt) X77.2 ☑
- local application of externally applied substance in medical or surgical care Y63.5
- machinery (hot) X17 ☑
- matches X08.8 ☑
  - with ignition of clothing NEC X06.2 ☑
    - nightwear X05 ☑
- mattress — *see* Exposure, fire, uncontrolled, building, bed
- medicament, externally applied Y63.5
- metal (hot) (liquid) (molten) NEC X18 ☑
- nightwear (nightclothes, nightdress, gown, pajamas, robe) X05 ☑
- object (hot) NEC X19 ☑
- on board watercraft
  - due to
    - accident to watercraft V91.09 ☑
      - powered craft V91.03 ☑
        - ferry boat V91.01 ☑
        - fishing boat V91.02 ☑
        - jetskis V91.03 ☑
        - liner V91.01 ☑
        - merchant ship V91.00 ☑
        - passenger ship V91.01 ☑
      - unpowered craft V91.08 ☑
        - canoe V91.05 ☑
        - inflatable V91.06 ☑
        - kayak V91.05 ☑
        - sailboat V91.04 ☑
        - surf-board V91.08 ☑
        - water skis V91.07 ☑
        - windsurfer V91.08 ☑
    - fire on board V93.09 ☑
      - ferry boat V93.01 ☑
      - fishing boat V93.02 ☑
      - jetskis V93.03 ☑
      - liner V93.01 ☑
      - merchant ship V93.00 ☑
      - passenger ship V93.01 ☑
      - powered craft NEC V93.03 ☑
      - sailboat V93.04 ☑
    - specified heat source NEC on board V93.19 ☑
      - ferry boat V93.11 ☑
      - fishing boat V93.12 ☑
      - jetskis V93.13 ☑
      - liner V93.11 ☑
      - merchant ship V93.10 ☑
      - passenger ship V93.11 ☑
      - powered craft NEC V93.13 ☑
      - sailboat V93.14 ☑
- pipe (hot) X16 ☑
- smoking X08.8 ☑
  - with ignition of clothing NEC X06.2 ☑
    - nightwear X05 ☑
- powder — *see* Powder burn
- radiator (hot) X16 ☑
- saucepan (hot) (glass) (metal) X15.3 ☑
  - stated as undetermined whether accidental or intentional Y27.3 ☑
  - suicide (attempt) X77.3 ☑
- self-inflicted X76 ☑
  - stated as undetermined whether accidental or intentional Y26 ☑
- stated as undetermined whether accidental or intentional Y27.0 ☑
- steam X13.1 ☑
  - pipe X16 ☑
    - stated as undetermined whether accidental or intentional Y27.8 ☑
  - stated as undetermined whether accidental or intentional Y27.0 ☑
  - suicide (attempt) X77.0 ☑
- stove (hot) (kitchen) X15.0 ☑
  - stated as undetermined whether accidental or intentional Y27.3 ☑
  - suicide (attempt) X77.3 ☑
- substance (hot) NEC X19 ☑
  - boiling X12 ☑
    - stated as undetermined whether accidental or intentional Y27.2 ☑

Burn, burned, burning — *continued*
- substance — *continued*
  - boiling — *continued*
    - suicide (attempt) X77.2 ☑
  - molten (metal) X18 ☑
  - suicide (attempt) NEC X76 ☑
  - hot
    - household appliance X77.3 ☑
    - object X77.9 ☑
- therapeutic misadventure
  - heat in local application or packing during medical or surgical procedure Y63.5
  - overdose of radiation Y63.2
- toaster (hot) X15.1 ☑
  - stated as undetermined whether accidental or intentional Y27.3 ☑
  - suicide (attempt) X77.3 ☑
- tool (hot) X17 ☑
- torch, welding X08.8 ☑
  - with ignition of clothing NEC X06.2 ☑
    - nightwear X05 ☑
- trash fire (controlled) — *see* Exposure, fire, controlled, not in building
  - uncontrolled — *see* Exposure, fire, uncontrolled, not in building
- vapor (hot) X13.1 ☑
  - stated as undetermined whether accidental or intentional Y27.0 ☑
  - suicide (attempt) X77.0 ☑
- Very pistol — *see* Discharge, firearm NEC

Butted by animal W55.82 ☑
- bull W55.22 ☑
- cow W55.22 ☑
- goat W55.32 ☑
- horse W55.12 ☑
- pig W55.42 ☑
- sheep W55.32 ☑

C

Caisson disease — *see* Air, pressure, change
Campfire (exposure to) (controlled) (*see also* Exposure, fire, controlled, not in building)
- uncontrolled — *see* Exposure, fire, uncontrolled, not in building
Capital punishment (any means) — *see* Legal, intervention
Car sickness T75.3 ☑
Casualty (not due to war) NEC X58 ☑
- war — *see* War operations
Cat
- bite W55.01 ☑
- scratch W55.03 ☑
Cataclysm, cataclysmic (any injury) NEC — *see* Forces of nature
Catching fire — *see* Exposure, fire
Caught
- between
  - folding object W23.0 ☑
  - objects (moving) (stationary and moving) W23.0 ☑
    - and machinery — *see* Contact, with, by type of machine
  - stationary W23.1 ☑
  - sliding door and door frame W23.0 ☑
- by, in
  - machinery (moving parts of) — *see* Contact, with, by type of machine
  - washing-machine wringer W23.0 ☑
- under packing crate (due to losing grip) W23.1 ☑
Cave-in caused by cataclysmic earth surface movement or eruption — *see* Landslide
Change(s) in air pressure — *see* Air, pressure, change
Choked, choking (on) (any object except food or vomitus)
- food (bone) (seed) — *see* categories T17 and T18 ☑
- vomitus T17.81- ☑
Civil insurrection — *see* War operations
Cloudburst (any injury) X37.8 ☑
Cold, exposure to (accidental) (excessive) (extreme) (natural) (place) NEC — *see* Exposure, cold
Collapse
- building W20.1 ☑
  - burning (uncontrolled fire) X00.2 ☑
- dam or man-made structure (causing earth movement) X36.0 ☑
- machinery — *see* Contact, with, by type of machine

Collapse — *continued*
structure W20.1 ✓
burning (uncontrolled fire) X00.2 ✓
Collision (accidental) NEC (*see also* Accident, transport) V89.9 ✓
pedestrian W51 ✓
with fall W03 ✓
due to ice or snow W00.0 ✓
involving pedestrian conveyance — *see* Accident, transport, pedestrian, conveyance
and
crowd or human stampede (with fall) W52 ✓
object W22.8 ✓
with fall — *see* Fall, due to, bumping against, object
person(s) — *see* Collision, pedestrian
transport vehicle NEC V89.9 ✓
and
avalanche, fallen or not moving — *see* Accident, transport
falling or moving — *see* Landslide
landslide, fallen or not moving — *see* Accident, transport
falling or moving — *see* Landslide
due to cataclysm — *see* Forces of nature, by type
intentional, purposeful suicide (attempt) — *see* Suicide, collision
Combustion, spontaneous — *see* Ignition
Complication (delayed) **of or following** (medical or surgical procedure) Y84.9
with misadventure — *see* Misadventure
amputation of limb(s) Y83.5
anastomosis (arteriovenous) (blood vessel) (gastrojejunal) (tendon) (natural or artificial material) Y83.2
aspiration (of fluid) Y84.4
tissue Y84.8
biopsy Y84.8
blood
sampling Y84.7
transfusion
procedure Y84.8
bypass Y83.2
catheterization (urinary) Y84.6
cardiac Y84.0
colostomy Y83.3
cystostomy Y83.3
dialysis (kidney) Y84.1
drug — *see* Table of Drugs and Chemicals
due to misadventure — *see* Misadventure
duodenostomy Y83.3
electroshock therapy Y84.3
external stoma, creation of Y83.3
formation of external stoma Y83.3
gastrostomy Y83.3
graft Y83.2
hypothermia (medically-induced) Y84.8
implant, implantation (of)
artificial
internal device (cardiac pacemaker) (electrodes in brain) (heart valve prosthesis) (orthopedic) Y83.1
material or tissue (for anastomosis or bypass) Y83.2
with creation of external stoma Y83.3
natural tissues (for anastomosis or bypass) Y83.2
with creation of external stoma Y83.3
infusion
procedure Y84.8
injection — *see* Table of Drugs and Chemicals
procedure Y84.8
insertion of gastric or duodenal sound Y84.5
insulin-shock therapy Y84.3
paracentesis (abdominal) (thoracic) (aspirative) Y84.4
procedures other than surgical operation — *see* Complication of or following, by type of procedure
radiological procedure or therapy Y84.2
removal of organ (partial) (total) NEC Y83.6
sampling
blood Y84.7
fluid NEC Y84.4
tissue Y84.8
shock therapy Y84.3
surgical operation NEC (*see also* Complication of or following, by type of operation) Y83.9
reconstructive NEC Y83.4

Complication (delayed) **of or following** — *continued*
surgical operation (*see also* Complication of or following, by type of operation) — *continued*
reconstructive — *continued*
with
anastomosis, bypass or graft Y83.2
formation of external stoma Y83.3
specified NEC Y83.8
transfusion (*see also* Table of Drugs and Chemicals)
procedure Y84.8
transplant, transplantation (heart) (kidney) (liver) (whole organ, any) Y83.0
partial organ Y83.4
ureterostomy Y83.3
vaccination (*see also* Table of Drugs and Chemicals)
procedure Y84.8
Compression
divers' squeeze — *see* Air, pressure, change
trachea by
food (lodged in esophagus) — *see* categories T17 and T18 ✓
vomitus (lodged in esophagus) T17.81- ✓
Conflagration — *see* Exposure, fire, uncontrolled
Constriction (external)
hair W49.01 ✓
jewelry W49.04 ✓
ring W49.04 ✓
rubber band W49.03 ✓
specified item NEC W49.09 ✓
string W49.02 ✓
thread W49.02 ✓
Contact (accidental)
with
abrasive wheel (metalworking) W31.1 ✓
alligator W58.09 ✓
bite W58.01 ✓
crushing W58.03 ✓
strike W58.02 ✓
amphibian W62.9 ✓
frog W62.0 ✓
toad W62.1 ✓
animal (nonvenomous) NEC W64 ✓
marine W56.89 ✓
bite W56.81 ✓
dolphin — *see* Contact, with, dolphin
fish NEC — *see* Contact, with, fish
mammal — *see* Contact, with, mammal, marine
orca — *see* Contact, with, orca
sea lion — *see* Contact, with, sea lion
shark — *see* Contact, with, shark
strike W56.82 ✓
animate mechanical force NEC W64 ✓
arrow W21.89 ✓
not thrown, projected or falling W45.8 ✓
arthropods (nonvenomous) W57
axe W27.0 ✓
band-saw (industrial) W31.2 ✓
bayonet — *see* Bayonet wound
bee(s) X58 ✓
bench-saw (industrial) W31.2 ✓
bird W61.99 ✓
bite W61.91 ✓
chicken — *see* Contact, with, chicken
duck — *see* Contact, with, duck
goose — *see* Contact, with, goose
macaw — *see* Contact, with, macaw
parrot — *see* Contact, with, parrot
psittacine — *see* Contact, with, psittacine
strike W61.92 ✓
turkey — *see* Contact, with, turkey
blender W29.0 ✓
boiling water X12 ✓
stated as undetermined whether accidental or intentional Y27.2 ✓
suicide (attempt) X77.2 ✓
bore, earth-drilling or mining (land) (seabed) W31.0 ✓
buffalo — *see* Contact, with, hoof stock NEC
bull W55.29 ✓
bite W55.21 ✓
gored W55.22 ✓
strike W55.22 ✓
bumper cars W31.81 ✓
camel — *see* Contact, with, hoof stock NEC

Contact — *continued*
with — *continued*
can
lid W45.2 ✓
opener W27.4 ✓
powered W29.0 ✓
cat W55.09 ✓
bite W55.01 ✓
scratch W55.03 ✓
caterpillar (venomous) X58 ✓
centipede (venomous) X58 ✓
chain
hoist W24.0 ✓
agricultural operations W30.89 ✓
saw W29.3 ✓
chicken W61.39 ✓
peck W61.33 ✓
strike W61.32 ✓
chisel W27.0 ✓
circular saw W31.2 ✓
cobra X58 ✓
combine (harvester) W30.0 ✓
conveyer belt W24.1 ✓
cooker (hot) X15.8 ✓
stated as undetermined whether accidental or intentional Y27.3 ✓
suicide (attempt) X77.3 ✓
coral X58 ✓
cotton gin W31.82 ✓
cow W55.29 ✓
bite W55.21 ✓
strike W55.22 ✓
crane W24.0 ✓
agricultural operations W30.89 ✓
crocodile W58.19 ✓
bite W58.11 ✓
crushing W58.13 ✓
strike W58.12 ✓
dagger W26.1 ✓
stated as undetermined whether accidental or intentional Y28.2 ✓
suicide (attempt) X78.2 ✓
dairy equipment W31.82 ✓
dart W21.89 ✓
not thrown, projected or falling W45.8 ✓
deer — *see* Contact, with, hoof stock NEC
derrick W24.0 ✓
agricultural operations W30.89 ✓
hay W30.2 ✓
dog W54.8 ✓
bite W54.0 ✓
strike W54.1 ✓
dolphin W56.09 ✓
bite W56.01 ✓
strike W56.02 ✓
donkey — *see* Contact, with, hoof stock NEC
drill (powered) W29.8 ✓
earth (land) (seabed) W31.0 ✓
nonpowered W27.8 ✓
drive belt W24.0 ✓
agricultural operations W30.89 ✓
dry ice — *see* Exposure, cold, man-made
dryer (clothes) (powered) (spin) W29.2 ✓
duck W61.69 ✓
bite W61.61 ✓
strike W61.62 ✓
earth (-)
drilling machine (industrial) W31.0 ✓
scraping machine in stationary use W31.83 ✓
edge of stiff paper W45.1 ✓
electric
beater W29.0 ✓
blanket X16 ✓
fan W29.2 ✓
commercial W31.82 ✓
knife W29.1 ✓
mixer W29.0 ✓
elevator (building) W24.0 ✓
agricultural operations W30.89 ✓
grain W30.3 ✓
engine(s), hot NEC X17 ✓
excavating machine W31.0 ✓
farm machine W30.9 ✓
feces — *see* Contact, with, by type of animal
fer de lance X58 ✓

✓ Additional Character Required — Refer to the Tabular List for Character Selection   ▼ Subterms under main terms may continue to next column or page

Contact — *continued*
　with — *continued*
　　fish W56.59 ☑
　　　bite W56.51 ☑
　　　shark — *see* Contact, with, shark
　　　strike W56.52 ☑
　　flying horses W31.81 ☑
　　forging (metalworking) machine W31.1 ☑
　　fork W27.4 ☑
　　forklift (truck) W24.0 ☑
　　　agricultural operations W30.89 ☑
　　frog W62.0 ☑
　　garden
　　　cultivator (powered) W29.3 ☑
　　　　riding W30.89 ☑
　　　fork W27.1 ☑
　　gas turbine W31.3 ☑
　　Gila monster X58 ☑
　　giraffe — *see* Contact, with, hoof stock NEC
　　glass (sharp) (broken) W25 ☑
　　　with subsequent fall W18.02 ☑
　　　assault X99.0 ☑
　　　due to fall — *see* Fall, by type
　　　stated as undetermined whether accidental or
　　　　intentional Y28.0 ☑
　　　suicide (attempt) X78.0 ☑
　　goat W55.39 ☑
　　　bite W55.31 ☑
　　　strike W55.32 ☑
　　goose W61.59 ☑
　　　bite W61.51 ☑
　　　strike W61.52 ☑
　　hand
　　　saw W27.0 ☑
　　　tool (not powered) NEC W27.8 ☑
　　　　powered W29.8 ☑
　　harvester W30.0 ☑
　　hay-derrick W30.2 ☑
　　heating
　　　appliance (hot) X16 ☑
　　　pad (electric) X16 ☑
　　heat NEC X19 ☑
　　　from appliance (electrical) (household) — *see*
　　　　Contact, with, hot, household appliance
　　　heating appliance X16 ☑
　　hedge-trimmer (powered) W29.3 ☑
　　hoe W27.1 ☑
　　hoist (chain) (shaft) NEC W24.0 ☑
　　　agricultural W30.89 ☑
　　hoof stock NEC W55.39 ☑
　　　bite W55.31 ☑
　　　strike W55.32 ☑
　　hornet(s) X58 ☑
　　horse W55.19 ☑
　　　bite W55.11 ☑
　　　strike W55.12 ☑
　　hot
　　　air X14.1 ☑
　　　　inhalation X14.0 ☑
　　　cooker X15.8 ☑
　　　drinks X10.0 ☑
　　　engine X17 ☑
　　　fats X10.2 ☑
　　　fluids NEC X12 ☑
　　　　assault X98.2 ☑
　　　　suicide (attempt) X77.2 ☑
　　　　undetermined whether accidental or inten-
　　　　　tional Y27.2 ☑
　　　food X10.1 ☑
　　　gases X14.1 ☑
　　　　inhalation X14.0 ☑
　　　heating appliance X16 ☑
　　　household appliance X15.8 ☑
　　　　assault X98.3 ☑
　　　　cooker X15.8 ☑
　　　　hotplate X15.2 ☑
　　　　kettle X15.8 ☑
　　　　light bulb X15.8 ☑
　　　　object NEC X19 ☑
　　　　　assault X98.8 ☑
　　　　　stated as undetermined whether acciden-
　　　　　　tal or intentional Y27.9 ☑
　　　　　suicide (attempt) X77.8 ☑
　　　　saucepan X15.3 ☑
　　　　skillet X15.3 ☑

Contact — *continued*
　with — *continued*
　　hot — *continued*
　　　household appliance — *continued*
　　　　stated as undetermined whether accidental
　　　　　or intentional Y27.3 ☑
　　　　stove X15.0 ☑
　　　　suicide (attempt) X77.3 ☑
　　　　toaster X15.1 ☑
　　　kettle X15.8 ☑
　　　light bulb X15.8 ☑
　　　liquid NEC (*see also* Burn) X12 ☑
　　　　drinks X10.0 ☑
　　　　stated as undetermined whether accidental
　　　　　or intentional Y27.2 ☑
　　　　suicide (attempt) X77.2 ☑
　　　　tap water X11.8 ☑
　　　　　stated as undetermined whether acciden-
　　　　　　tal or intentional Y27.1 ☑
　　　　　suicide (attempt) X77.1 ☑
　　　machinery X17 ☑
　　　metal (molten) (liquid) NEC X18 ☑
　　　object (not producing fire or flames) NEC X19 ☑
　　　oil (cooking) X10.2 ☑
　　　pipe X16 ☑
　　　plate X15.2 ☑
　　　radiator X16 ☑
　　　saucepan (glass) (metal) X15.3 ☑
　　　skillet X15.3 ☑
　　　stove (kitchen) X15.0 ☑
　　　substance NEC X19 ☑
　　　tap-water X11.8 ☑
　　　　assault X98.1 ☑
　　　　heated on stove X12 ☑
　　　　　stated as undetermined whether acciden-
　　　　　　tal or intentional Y27.2 ☑
　　　　　suicide (attempt) X77.2 ☑
　　　　in bathtub X11.0 ☑
　　　　running X11.1 ☑
　　　　stated as undetermined whether accidental
　　　　　or intentional Y27.1 ☑
　　　　suicide (attempt) X77.1 ☑
　　　toaster X15.1 ☑
　　　tool X17 ☑
　　　vapors X13.1 ☑
　　　　inhalation X13.0 ☑
　　　water (tap) X11.8 ☑
　　　　boiling X12 ☑
　　　　　stated as undetermined whether acciden-
　　　　　　tal or intentional Y27.2 ☑
　　　　　suicide (attempt) X77.2 ☑
　　　　heated on stove X12 ☑
　　　　　stated as undetermined whether acciden-
　　　　　　tal or intentional Y27.2 ☑
　　　　　suicide (attempt) X77.2 ☑
　　　　in bathtub X11.0 ☑
　　　　running X11.1 ☑
　　　　stated as undetermined whether accidental
　　　　　or intentional Y27.1 ☑
　　　　suicide (attempt) X77.1 ☑
　　hotplate X15.2 ☑
　　ice-pick W27.4 ☑
　　insect (nonvenomous) NEC W57 ☑
　　kettle (hot) X15.8 ☑
　　knife W26.0 ☑
　　　assault X99.1 ☑
　　　electric W29.1 ☑
　　　stated as undetermined whether accidental or
　　　　intentional Y28.1 ☑
　　　suicide (attempt) X78.1 ☑
　　lathe (metalworking) W31.1 ☑
　　　turnings W45.8 ☑
　　　woodworking W31.2 ☑
　　lawnmower (powered) (ridden) W28 ☑
　　　causing electrocution W86.8 ☑
　　　suicide (attempt) X83.1 ☑
　　　unpowered W27.1 ☑
　　lift, lifting (devices) W24.0 ☑
　　　agricultural operations W30.89 ☑
　　　shaft W24.0 ☑
　　liquefied gas — *see* Exposure, cold, man-made
　　liquid air, hydrogen, nitrogen — *see* Exposure, cold,
　　　man-made
　　lizard (nonvenomous) W59.09 ☑
　　　bite W59.01 ☑
　　　strike W59.02 ☑

Contact — *continued*
　with — *continued*
　　llama — *see* Contact, with, hoof stock NEC
　　macaw W61.19 ☑
　　　bite W61.11 ☑
　　　strike W61.12 ☑
　　machine, machinery W31.9 ☑
　　　abrasive wheel W31.1 ☑
　　　agricultural including animal-powered
　　　　W30.9 ☑
　　　　combine harvester W30.0 ☑
　　　　grain storage elevator W30.3 ☑
　　　　hay derrick W30.2 ☑
　　　　power take-off device W30.1 ☑
　　　　reaper W30.0 ☑
　　　　specified NEC W30.89 ☑
　　　　thresher W30.0 ☑
　　　　transport vehicle, stationary W30.81 ☑
　　　band saw W31.2 ☑
　　　bench saw W31.2 ☑
　　　circular saw W31.2 ☑
　　　commercial NEC W31.82 ☑
　　　drilling, metal (industrial) W31.1 ☑
　　　earth-drilling W31.0 ☑
　　　earthmoving or scraping W31.89 ☑
　　　excavating W31.89 ☑
　　　forging machine W31.1 ☑
　　　gas turbine W31.3 ☑
　　　hot X17 ☑
　　　internal combustion engine W31.3 ☑
　　　land drill W31.0 ☑
　　　lathe W31.1 ☑
　　　lifting (devices) W24.0 ☑
　　　metal drill W31.1 ☑
　　　metalworking (industrial) W31.1 ☑
　　　milling, metal W31.1 ☑
　　　mining W31.0 ☑
　　　molding W31.2 ☑
　　　overhead plane W31.2 ☑
　　　power press, metal W31.1 ☑
　　　prime mover W31.3 ☑
　　　printing W31.89 ☑
　　　radial saw W31.2 ☑
　　　recreational W31.81 ☑
　　　roller-coaster W31.81 ☑
　　　rolling mill, metal W31.1 ☑
　　　sander W31.2 ☑
　　　seabed drill W31.0 ☑
　　　shaft
　　　　hoist W31.0 ☑
　　　　lift W31.0 ☑
　　　specified NEC W31.89 ☑
　　　spinning W31.89 ☑
　　　steam engine W31.3 ☑
　　　transmission W24.1 ☑
　　　undercutter W31.0 ☑
　　　water driven turbine W31.3 ☑
　　　weaving W31.89 ☑
　　　woodworking or forming (industrial) W31.2 ☑
　　mammal (feces) (urine) W55.89 ☑
　　　bull — *see* Contact, with, bull
　　　cat — *see* Contact, with, cat
　　　cow — *see* Contact, with, cow
　　　goat — *see* Contact, with, goat
　　　hoof stock — *see* Contact, with, hoof stock
　　　horse — *see* Contact, with, horse
　　　marine W56.39 ☑
　　　　dolphin — *see* Contact, with, dolphin
　　　　orca — *see* Contact, with, orca
　　　　sea lion — *see* Contact, with, sea lion
　　　　specified NEC W56.39 ☑
　　　　　bite W56.31 ☑
　　　　　strike W56.32 ☑
　　　pig — *see* Contact, with, pig
　　　raccoon — *see* Contact, with, raccoon
　　　rodent — *see* Contact, with, rodent
　　　sheep — *see* Contact, with, sheep
　　　specified NEC W55.89 ☑
　　　　bite W55.81 ☑
　　　　strike W55.82 ☑
　　marine
　　　animal W56.89 ☑
　　　　bite W56.81 ☑
　　　　dolphin — *see* Contact, with, dolphin
　　　　fish NEC — *see* Contact, with, fish

Contact — *continued*
  with — *continued*
    marine — *continued*
      animal — *continued*
        mammal — *see* Contact, with, mammal, marine
        orca — *see* Contact, with, orca
        sea lion — *see* Contact, with, sea lion
        shark — *see* Contact, with, shark
        strike W56.82 ☑
    meat
      grinder (domestic) W29.0 ☑
        industrial W31.82 ☑
        nonpowered W27.4 ☑
      slicer (domestic) W29.0 ☑
        industrial W31.82 ☑
    merry go round W31.81 ☑
    metal, hot (liquid) (molten) NEC X18 ☑
    millipede W57 ☑
    nail W45.0 ☑
      gun W29.4 ☑
    needle (sewing) W27.3 ☑
      hypodermic W46.0 ☑
        contaminated W46.1 ☑
    object (blunt) NEC
      hot NEC X19
      legal intervention — *see* Legal, intervention, blunt object
      sharp NEC W45.8 ☑
        inflicted by other person NEC W45.8 ☑
          stated as
            intentional homicide (attempt) — *see* Assault, cutting or piercing instrument
        legal intervention — *see* Legal, intervention, sharp object
        self-inflicted X78.9 ☑
    orca W56.29 ☑
      bite W56.21 ☑
      strike W56.22 ☑
    overhead plane W31.2 ☑
    paper (as sharp object) W45.1 ☑
    paper-cutter W27.5 ☑
    parrot W61.09 ☑
      bite W61.01 ☑
      strike W61.02 ☑
    pig W55.49 ☑
      bite W55.41 ☑
      strike W55.42 ☑
    pipe, hot X16 ☑
    pitchfork W27.1 ☑
    plane (metal) (wood) W27.0 ☑
      overhead W31.2 ☑
    plant thorns, spines, sharp leaves or other mechanisms W60 ☑
    powered
      garden cultivator W29.3 ☑
      household appliance, implement, or machine W29.8 ☑
      saw (industrial) W31.2 ☑
        hand W29.8 ☑
    printing machine W31.89 ☑
    psittacine bird W61.29 ☑
      bite W61.21 ☑
      macaw — *see* Contact, with, macaw
      parrot — *see* Contact, with, parrot
      strike W61.22 ☑
    pulley (block) (transmission) W24.0 ☑
      agricultural operations W30.89 ☑
    raccoon W55.59 ☑
      bite W55.51 ☑
      strike W55.52 ☑
    radial-saw (industrial) W31.2 ☑
    radiator (hot) X16 ☑
    rake W27.1 ☑
    rattlesnake X58 ☑
    reaper W30.0 ☑
    reptile W59.89 ☑
      lizard — *see* Contact, with, lizard
      snake — *see* Contact, with, snake
      specified NEC W59.89 ☑
        bite W59.81 ☑
        crushing W59.83 ☑
        strike W59.82 ☑
      turtle — *see* Contact, with, turtle
    rivet gun (powered) W29.4 ☑

Contact — *continued*
  with — *continued*
    road scraper — *see* Accident, transport, construction vehicle
    rodent (feces) (urine) W53.89 ☑
      bite W53.81 ☑
      mouse W53.09 ☑
        bite W53.01 ☑
      rat W53.19 ☑
        bite W53.11 ☑
      specified NEC W53.89 ☑
        bite W53.81 ☑
      squirrel W53.29 ☑
        bite W53.21 ☑
    roller coaster W31.81 ☑
    rope NEC W24.0 ☑
      agricultural operations W30.89 ☑
    saliva — *see* Contact, with, by type of animal
    sander W29.8 ☑
      industrial W31.2 ☑
    saucepan (hot) (glass) (metal) X15.3 ☑
    saw W27.0 ☑
      band (industrial) W31.2 ☑
      bench (industrial) W31.2 ☑
      chain W29.3 ☑
      hand W27.0 ☑
    sawing machine, metal W31.1 ☑
    scissors W27.2 ☑
    scorpion X58 ☑
    screwdriver W27.0 ☑
      powered W29.8 ☑
    sea
      anemone, cucumber or urchin (spine) X58 ☑
      lion W56.19 ☑
        bite W56.11 ☑
        strike W56.12 ☑
    serpent — *see* Contact, with, snake, by type
    sewing-machine (electric) (powered) W29.2 ☑
      not powered W27.8 ☑
    shaft (hoist) (lift) (transmission) NEC W24.0 ☑
      agricultural W30.89 ☑
    shark W56.49 ☑
      bite W56.41 ☑
      strike W56.42 ☑
    shears (hand) W27.2 ☑
      powered (industrial) W31.1 ☑
        domestic W29.2 ☑
    sheep W55.39 ☑
      bite W55.31 ☑
      strike W55.32 ☑
    shovel W27.8 ☑
      steam — *see* Accident, transport, construction vehicle
    snake (nonvenomous) W59.19 ☑
      bite W59.11 ☑
      crushing W59.13 ☑
      strike W59.12 ☑
    spade W27.1 ☑
    spider (venomous) X58 ☑
    spin-drier W29.2 ☑
    spinning machine W31.89 ☑
    splinter W45.8 ☑
    sports equipment W21.9 ☑
    staple gun (powered) W29.8 ☑
    steam X13.1 ☑
      engine W31.3 ☑
      inhalation X13.0 ☑
      pipe X16 ☑
      shovel W31.89 ☑
    stove (hot) (kitchen) X15.0 ☑
    substance, hot NEC X19 ☑
      molten (metal) X18 ☑
    sword W26.1 ☑
      assault X99.2 ☑
      stated as undetermined whether accidental or intentional Y28.2 ☑
      suicide (attempt) X78.2 ☑
    tarantula X58 ☑
    thresher W30.0 ☑
    tin can lid W45.2 ☑
    toad W62.1 ☑
    toaster (hot) X15.1 ☑
    tool W27.8 ☑
      hand (not powered) W27.8 ☑
        auger W27.0 ☑

Contact — *continued*
  with — *continued*
    tool — *continued*
      hand — *continued*
        axe W27.0 ☑
        can opener W27.4 ☑
        chisel W27.0 ☑
        fork W27.4 ☑
        garden W27.1 ☑
        handsaw W27.0 ☑
        hoe W27.1 ☑
        ice-pick W27.4 ☑
        kitchen utensil W27.4 ☑
        manual
          lawn mower W27.1 ☑
          sewing machine W27.8 ☑
        meat grinder W27.4 ☑
        needle (sewing) W27.3 ☑
          hypodermic W46.0 ☑
            contaminated W46.1 ☑
        paper cutter W27.5 ☑
        pitchfork W27.1 ☑
        rake W27.1 ☑
        scissors W27.2 ☑
        screwdriver W27.0 ☑
        specified NEC W27.8 ☑
        workbench W27.0 ☑
      hot X17 ☑
      powered W29.8 ☑
        blender W29.0 ☑
          commercial W31.82 ☑
        can opener W29.0 ☑
          commercial W31.82 ☑
        chainsaw W29.3 ☑
        clothes dryer W29.2 ☑
          commercial W31.82 ☑
        dishwasher W29.2 ☑
          commercial W31.82 ☑
        edger W29.3 ☑
        electric fan W29.2 ☑
          commercial W31.82 ☑
        electric knife W29.1 ☑
        food processor W29.0 ☑
          commercial W31.82 ☑
        garbage disposal W29.0 ☑
          commercial W31.82 ☑
        garden tool W29.3 ☑
        hedge trimmer W29.3 ☑
        ice maker W29.0 ☑
          commercial W31.82 ☑
        kitchen appliance W29.0 ☑
          commercial W31.82 ☑
        lawn mower W28 ☑
        meat grinder W29.0 ☑
          commercial W31.82 ☑
        mixer W29.0 ☑
          commercial W31.82 ☑
        rototiller W29.3 ☑
        sewing machine W29.2 ☑
          commercial W31.82 ☑
        washing machine W29.2 ☑
          commercial W31.82 ☑
      transmission device (belt, cable, chain, gear, pinion, shaft) W24.1 ☑
        agricultural operations W30.89 ☑
      turbine (gas) (water-driven) W31.3 ☑
      turkey W61.49 ☑
        peck W61.43 ☑
        strike W61.42 ☑
      turtle (nonvenomous) W59.29 ☑
        bite W59.21 ☑
        strike W59.22 ☑
        terrestrial W59.89 ☑
          bite W59.81 ☑
          crushing W59.83 ☑
          strike W59.82 ☑
      under-cutter W31.0 ☑
    urine — *see* Contact, with, by type of animal
    vehicle
      agricultural use (transport) — *see* Accident, transport, agricultural vehicle
        not on public highway W30.81 ☑
      industrial use (transport) — *see* Accident, transport, industrial vehicle
        not on public highway W31.83 ☑

☑ Additional Character Required — Refer to the Tabular List for Character Selection   ▽ Subterms under main terms may continue to next column or page

Contact — *continued*
  with — *continued*
    vehicle — *continued*
      off-road use (transport) — *see* Accident, transport, all-terrain or off-road vehicle
        not on public highway W31.83 ☑
      special construction use (transport) — *see* Accident, transport, construction vehicle
        not on public highway W31.83 ☑
    venomous
      animal X58 ☑
      arthropods X58 ☑
      lizard X58 ☑
      marine animal NEC X58 ☑
      marine plant NEC X58 ☑
      millipedes (tropical) X58 ☑
      plant(s) X58 ☑
      snake X58 ☑
      spider X58 ☑
      viper X58 ☑
    washing-machine (powered) W29.2 ☑
    wasp X58 ☑
    weaving-machine W31.89 ☑
    winch W24.0 ☑
      agricultural operations W30.89 ☑
    wire NEC W24.0 ☑
      agricultural operations W30.89 ☑
    wood slivers W45.8 ☑
    yellow jacket X58 ☑
    zebra — *see* Contact, with, hoof stock NEC
Coup de soleil X32 ☑
Crash
  aircraft (in transit) (powered) V95.9 ☑
    balloon V96.01 ☑
    fixed wing NEC (private) V95.21 ☑
      commercial V95.31 ☑
    glider V96.21 ☑
      hang V96.11 ☑
      powered V95.11 ☑
    helicopter V95.01 ☑
    in war operations — *see* War operations, destruction of aircraft
    microlight V95.11 ☑
    nonpowered V96.9 ☑
      specified NEC V96.8 ☑
    powered NEC V95.8 ☑
    stated as
      homicide (attempt) Y08.81 ☑
      suicide (attempt) X83.0 ☑
    ultralight V95.11 ☑
  spacecraft V95.41 ☑
  transport vehicle NEC (*see also* Accident, transport) V89.9 ☑
    homicide (attempt) Y03.8 ☑
    motor NEC (traffic) V89.2 ☑
      homicide (attempt) Y03.8 ☑
    suicide (attempt) — *see* Suicide, collision
Cruelty (mental) (physical) (sexual) X58 ☑
Crushed (accidentally) X58 ☑
  between objects (moving) (stationary and moving) W23.0 ☑
    stationary W23.1 ☑
  by
    alligator W58.03 ☑
    avalanche NEC — *see* Landslide
    cave-in W20.0 ☑
      caused by cataclysmic earth surface movement — *see* Landslide
    crocodile W58.13 ☑
    crowd or human stampede W52 ☑
    falling
      aircraft V97.39 ☑
        in war operations — *see* War operations, destruction of aircraft
      earth, material W20.0 ☑
        caused by cataclysmic earth surface movement — *see* Landslide
      object NEC W20.8 ☑
    landslide NEC — *see* Landslide
    lizard (nonvenomous) W59.09 ☑
    machinery — *see* Contact, with, by type of machine
    reptile NEC W59.89 ☑
    snake (nonvenomous) W59.13 ☑
  in
    machinery — *see* Contact, with, by type of machine

Cut, cutting (any part of body) (accidental) (*see also* Contact, with, by object or machine)
  during medical or surgical treatment as misadventure — *see* Index to Diseases and Injuries, Complications
  homicide (attempt) — *see* Assault, cutting or piercing instrument
  inflicted by other person — *see* Assault, cutting or piercing instrument
  legal
    execution — *see* Legal, intervention
    intervention — *see* Legal, intervention, sharp object
  machine NEC (*see also* Contact, with, by type of machine) W31.9 ☑
  self-inflicted — *see* Suicide, cutting or piercing instrument
  suicide (attempt) — *see* Suicide, cutting or piercing instrument
Cyclone (any injury) X37.1 ☑

D

Decapitation (accidental circumstances) NEC X58 ☑
  homicide X99.9 ☑
  legal execution — *see* Legal, intervention
Dehydration from lack of water X58 ☑
Deprivation X58 ☑
Derailment (accidental)
  railway (rolling stock) (train) (vehicle) (without antecedent collision) V81.7 ☑
    with antecedent collision — *see* Accident, transport, railway vehicle occupant
  streetcar (without antecedent collision) V82.7 ☑
    with antecedent collision — *see* Accident, transport, streetcar occupant
Descent
  parachute (voluntary) (without accident to aircraft) V97.29 ☑
    due to accident to aircraft — *see* Accident, transport, aircraft
Desertion X58 ☑
Destitution X58 ☑
Disability, late effect or sequela of injury — *see* Sequelae
Discharge (accidental)
  airgun W34.010 ☑
    assault X95.01 ☑
    homicide (attempt) X95.01 ☑
    stated as undetermined whether accidental or intentional Y24.0 ☑
    suicide (attempt) X74.01 ☑
  BB gun — *see* Discharge, airgun
  firearm (accidental) W34.00 ☑
    assault X95.9 ☑
    handgun (pistol) (revolver) W32.0 ☑
      assault X93 ☑
      homicide (attempt) X93 ☑
      legal intervention — *see* Legal, intervention, firearm, handgun
      stated as undetermined whether accidental or intentional Y22 ☑
      suicide (attempt) X72 ☑
    homicide (attempt) X95.9 ☑
    hunting rifle W33.02 ☑
      assault X94.1 ☑
      homicide (attempt) X94.1 ☑
      legal intervention
        injuring
          bystander Y35.032 ☑
          law enforcement personnel Y35.031 ☑
          suspect Y35.033 ☑
      stated as undetermined whether accidental or intentional Y23.1 ☑
      suicide (attempt) X73.1 ☑
    larger W33.00 ☑
      assault X94.9 ☑
      homicide (attempt) X94.9 ☑
      hunting rifle — *see* Discharge, firearm, hunting rifle
      legal intervention — *see* Legal, intervention, firearm by type of firearm
      machine gun — *see* Discharge, firearm, machine gun
      shotgun — *see* Discharge, firearm, shotgun
      specified NEC W33.09 ☑

Discharge — *continued*
  firearm — *continued*
    larger — *continued*
      specified — *continued*
        assault X94.8 ☑
        homicide (attempt) X94.8 ☑
        legal intervention
          injuring
            bystander Y35.092 ☑
            law enforcement personnel Y35.091 ☑
            suspect Y35.093 ☑
        stated as undetermined whether accidental or intentional Y23.8 ☑
        suicide (attempt) X73.8 ☑
      stated as undetermined whether accidental or intentional Y23.9 ☑
      suicide (attempt) X73.9 ☑
    legal intervention
      injuring
        bystander Y35.002 ☑
        law enforcement personnel Y35.001 ☑
        suspect Y35.03 ☑
      using rubber bullet
        injuring
          bystander Y35.042 ☑
          law enforcement personnel Y35.041 ☑
          suspect Y35.043 ☑
    machine gun W33.03 ☑
      assault X94.2 ☑
      homicide (attempt) X94.2 ☑
      legal intervention — *see* Legal, intervention, firearm, machine gun
      stated as undetermined whether accidental or intentional Y23.3 ☑
      suicide (attempt) X73.2 ☑
    pellet gun — *see* Discharge, airgun
    shotgun W33.01 ☑
      assault X94.0 ☑
      homicide (attempt) X94.0 ☑
      legal intervention — *see* Legal, intervention, firearm, specified NEC
      stated as undetermined whether accidental or intentional Y23.0 ☑
      suicide (attempt) X73.0 ☑
    specified NEC W34.09 ☑
      assault X95.8 ☑
      homicide (attempt) X95.8 ☑
      legal intervention — *see* Legal, intervention, firearm, specified NEC
      stated as undetermined whether accidental or intentional Y24.8 ☑
      suicide (attempt) X74.8 ☑
    stated as undetermined whether accidental or intentional Y24.9 ☑
    suicide (attempt) X74.9 ☑
    Very pistol W34.09 ☑
      assault X95.8 ☑
      homicide (attempt) X95.8 ☑
      stated as undetermined whether accidental or intentional Y24.8 ☑
      suicide (attempt) X74.8 ☑
  firework(s) W39 ☑
    stated as undetermined whether accidental or intentional Y25 ☑
  gas-operated gun NEC W34.018 ☑
    airgun — *see* Discharge, airgun
    assault X95.09 ☑
    homicide (attempt) X95.09 ☑
    paintball gun — *see* Discharge, paintball gun
    stated as undetermined whether accidental or intentional Y24.8 ☑
    suicide (attempt) X74.09 ☑
  gun NEC (*see also* Discharge, firearm NEC)
    air — *see* Discharge, airgun
    BB — *see* Discharge, airgun
    for single hand use — *see* Discharge, firearm, handgun
    hand — *see* Discharge, firearm, handgun
    machine — *see* Discharge, firearm, machine gun
    other specified — *see* Discharge, firearm NEC
    paintball — *see* Discharge, paintball gun
    pellet — *see* Discharge, airgun
  handgun — *see* Discharge, firearm, handgun
  machine gun — *see* Discharge, firearm, machine gun
  paintball gun W34.011 ☑

Discharge — continued
  paintball gun — continued
    assault X95.02 ☑
    homicide (attempt) X95.02 ☑
    stated as undetermined whether accidental or intentional Y24.8 ☑
    suicide (attempt) X74.02 ☑
  pistol — see Discharge, firearm, handgun
    flare — see Discharge, firearm, Very pistol
    pellet — see Discharge, firearm, airgun
    Very — see Discharge, firearm, Very pistol
  revolver — see Discharge, firearm, handgun
  rifle (hunting) — see Discharge, firearm, hunting rifle
  shotgun — see Discharge, firearm, shotgun
  spring-operated gun NEC W34.018 ☑
    assault X95.09 ☑
    homicide (attempt) X95.09 ☑
    stated as undetermined whether accidental or intentional Y24.8 ☑
    suicide (attempt) X74.09 ☑
Disease
  Andes W94.11 ☑
  aviator's — see Air, pressure
  range W94.11 ☑
Diver's disease, palsy, paralysis, squeeze — see Air, pressure
Diving (into water) — see Accident, diving
Dog bite W54.0 ☑
Dragged by transport vehicle NEC (see also Accident, transport) V09.9 ☑
Drinking poison (accidental) — see Table of Drugs and Chemicals
Dropped (accidentally) **while being carried or supported by other person** W04 ☑
Drowning (accidental) W74 ☑
  assault X92.9 ☑
  due to
    accident (to)
      machinery — see Contact, with, by type of machine
      watercraft V90.89 ☑
        burning V90.29 ☑
          powered V90.23 ☑
            fishing boat V90.22 ☑
            jetskis V90.23 ☑
            merchant ship V90.20 ☑
            passenger ship V90.21 ☑
          unpowered V90.28 ☑
            canoe V90.25 ☑
            inflatable V90.26 ☑
            kayak V90.25 ☑
            sailboat V90.24 ☑
            water skis V90.27 ☑
        crushed V90.39 ☑
          powered V90.33 ☑
            fishing boat V90.32 ☑
            jetskis V90.33 ☑
            merchant ship V90.30 ☑
            passenger ship V90.31 ☑
          unpowered V90.38 ☑
            canoe V90.35 ☑
            inflatable V90.36 ☑
            kayak V90.35 ☑
            sailboat V90.34 ☑
            water skis V90.37 ☑
        overturning V90.09 ☑
          powered V90.03 ☑
            fishing boat V90.02 ☑
            jetskis V90.03 ☑
            merchant ship V90.00 ☑
            passenger ship V90.01 ☑
          unpowered V90.08 ☑
            canoe V90.05 ☑
            inflatable V90.06 ☑
            kayak V90.05 ☑
            sailboat V90.04 ☑
        sinking V90.19 ☑
          powered V90.13 ☑
            fishing boat V90.12 ☑
            jetskis V90.13 ☑
            merchant ship V90.10 ☑
            passenger ship V90.11 ☑
          unpowered V90.18 ☑
            canoe V90.15 ☑
            inflatable V90.16 ☑
            kayak V90.15 ☑

Drowning — continued
  due to — continued
    accident — continued
      watercraft — continued
        sinking — continued
          unpowered — continued
            sailboat V90.14 ☑
        specified type NEC V90.89 ☑
          powered V90.83 ☑
            fishing boat V90.82 ☑
            jetskis V90.83 ☑
            merchant ship V90.80 ☑
            passenger ship V90.81 ☑
          unpowered V90.88 ☑
            canoe V90.85 ☑
            inflatable V90.86 ☑
            kayak V90.85 ☑
            sailboat V90.84 ☑
            water skis V90.87 ☑
    avalanche — see Landslide
    cataclysmic
      earth surface movement NEC — see Forces of nature, earth movement
      storm — see Forces of nature, cataclysmic storm
    cloudburst X37.8 ☑
    cyclone X37.1 ☑
    fall overboard (from) V92.09 ☑
      powered craft V92.03 ☑
        ferry boat V92.01 ☑
        fishing boat V92.02 ☑
        jetskis V92.03 ☑
        liner V92.01 ☑
        merchant ship V92.00 ☑
        passenger ship V92.01 ☑
      resulting from
        accident to watercraft — see Drowning, due to, accident to, watercraft
        being washed overboard (from) V92.29 ☑
          powered craft V92.23 ☑
            ferry boat V92.21 ☑
            fishing boat V92.22 ☑
            jetskis V92.23 ☑
            liner V92.21 ☑
            merchant ship V92.20 ☑
            passenger ship V92.21 ☑
          unpowered craft V92.28 ☑
            canoe V92.25 ☑
            inflatable V92.26 ☑
            kayak V92.25 ☑
            sailboat V92.24 ☑
            surf-board V92.28 ☑
            water skis V92.27 ☑
            windsurfer V92.28 ☑
        motion of watercraft V92.19 ☑
          powered craft V92.13 ☑
            ferry boat V92.11 ☑
            fishing boat V92.12 ☑
            jetskis V92.13 ☑
            liner V92.11 ☑
            merchant ship V92.10 ☑
            passenger ship V92.11 ☑
          unpowered craft
            canoe V92.15 ☑
            inflatable V92.16 ☑
            kayak V92.15 ☑
            sailboat V92.14 ☑
      unpowered craft V92.08 ☑
        canoe V92.05 ☑
        inflatable V92.06 ☑
        kayak V92.05 ☑
        sailboat V92.04 ☑
        surf-board V92.08 ☑
        water skis V92.07 ☑
        windsurfer V92.08 ☑
    hurricane X37.0 ☑
    jumping into water from watercraft (involved in accident) (see also Drowning, due to, accident to, watercraft)
      without accident to or on watercraft W16.711 ☑
    tidal wave NEC — see Forces of nature, tidal wave
    torrential rain X37.8 ☑

Drowning — continued
  following
    fall
      into
        bathtub W16.211 ☑
        bucket W16.221 ☑
        fountain — see Drowning, following, fall, into, water, specified NEC
        quarry — see Drowning, following, fall, into, water, specified NEC
        reservoir — see Drowning, following, fall, into, water, specified NEC
        swimming-pool W16.011 ☑
          stated as undetermined whether accidental or intentional Y21.3 ☑
          striking
            bottom W16.021 ☑
            wall W16.031 ☑
          suicide (attempt) X71.2 ☑
        water NOS W16.41 ☑
          natural (lake) (open sea) (river) (stream) (pond) W16.111 ☑
            striking
              bottom W16.121 ☑
              side W16.131 ☑
          specified NEC W16.311 ☑
            striking
              bottom W16.321 ☑
              wall W16.331 ☑
      overboard NEC — see Drowning, due to, fall overboard
    jump or dive
      from boat W16.711 ☑
        striking bottom W16.721 ☑
      into
        fountain — see Drowning, following, jump or dive, into, water, specified NEC
        quarry — see Drowning, following, jump or dive, into, water, specified NEC
        reservoir — see Drowning, following, jump or dive, into, water, specified NEC
        swimming-pool W16.511 ☑
          striking
            bottom W16.521 ☑
            wall W16.531 ☑
          suicide (attempt) X71.2 ☑
        water NOS W16.91 ☑
          natural (lake) (open sea) (river) (stream) (pond) W16.611 ☑
          specified NEC W16.811 ☑
            bottom W16.821 ☑
            striking
              bottom W16.821 ☑
              wall W16.831 ☑
          striking
            bottom W16.821 ☑
            wal! W16.831 ☑
          striking bottom W16.621 ☑
  homicide (attempt) X92.9 ☑
  in
    bathtub (accidental) W65 ☑
      assault X92.0 ☑
      following fall W16.211 ☑
      stated as undetermined whether accidental or intentional Y21.1 ☑
      stated as undetermined whether accidental or intentional Y21.0 ☑
      suicide (attempt) X71.0 ☑
    lake — see Drowning, in, natural water
    natural water (lake) (open sea) (river) (stream) (pond) W69 ☑
      assault X92.3 ☑
      following
        dive or jump W16.611 ☑
          striking bottom W16.621 ☑
        fall W16.111 ☑
          striking
            bottom W16.121 ☑
            side W16.131 ☑
      stated as undetermined whether accidental or intentional Y21.4 ☑
      suicide (attempt) X71.3 ☑
    quarry — see Drowning, in, specified place NEC
    quenching tank — see Drowning, in, specified place NEC
    reservoir — see Drowning, in, specified place NEC

Drowning — *continued*
  in — *continued*
    river — *see* Drowning, in, natural water
    sea — *see* Drowning, in, natural water
    specified place NEC W73 ☑
      assault X92.8 ☑
      following
        dive or jump W16.811 ☑
          striking
            bottom W16.821 ☑
            wall W16.831 ☑
        fall W16.311 ☑
          striking
            bottom W16.321 ☑
            wall W16.331 ☑
      stated as undetermined whether accidental or
        intentional Y21.8 ☑
      suicide (attempt) X71.8 ☑
    stream — *see* Drowning, in, natural water
    swimming-pool W67 ☑
      assault X92.1 ☑
      following fall X92.2 ☑
      following
        dive or jump W16.511 ☑
          striking
            bottom W16.521 ☑
            wall W16.531 ☑
        fall W16.011 ☑
          striking
            bottom W16.021 ☑
            wall W16.031 ☑
      stated as undetermined whether accidental or
        intentional Y21.2 ☑
      following fall Y21.3 ☑
      suicide (attempt) X71.1 ☑
      following fall X71.2 ☑
    war operations — *see* War operations, restriction
      of airway
  resulting from accident to watercraft — *see* Drowning,
    due to, accident, watercraft
  self-inflicted X71.9 ☑
  stated as undetermined whether accidental or inten-
    tional Y21.9 ☑
  suicide (attempt) X71.9 ☑

E

Earth falling (on) W20.0 ☑
  caused by cataclysmic earth surface movement or
    eruption — *see* Landslide
Earth (surface) movement NEC — *see* Forces of nature,
  earth movement
Earthquake (any injury) X34 ☑
Effect(s) (adverse) **of**
  air pressure (any) — *see* Air, pressure
  cold, excessive (exposure to) — *see* Exposure, cold
  heat (excessive) — *see* Heat
  hot place (weather) B — *see* Heat
  insolation X30 ☑
  late — *see* Sequelae
  motion — *see* Motion
  nuclear explosion or weapon in war operations — *see*
    War operations, nuclear weapon
  radiation — *see* Radiation
  travel — *see* Travel
Electric shock (accidental) (by) (in) — *see* Exposure,
  electric current
Electrocution (accidental) — *see* Exposure, electric current
Endotracheal tube wrongly placed during anesthetic
  procedure
Entanglement
  in
    bed linen, causing suffocation T71 ☑
    wheel of pedal cycle V19.88 ☑
Entry of foreign body or material — *see* Foreign body
Environmental pollution related condition — *see*
  category Z57 ☑
Execution, legal (any method) — *see* Legal, intervention
Exhaustion
  cold — *see* Exposure, cold
  due to excessive exertion — *see* category Y93 ☑
  heat — *see* Heat
Explosion (accidental) (of) (with secondary fire) W40.9 ☑
  acetylene W40.1 ☑
  aerosol can W36.1 ☑

Explosion — *continued*
  air tank (compressed) (in machinery) W36.2 ☑
  aircraft (in transit) (powered) NEC V95.9 ☑
    balloon V96.05 ☑
    fixed wing NEC (private) V95.25 ☑
      commercial V95.35 ☑
    glider V96.25 ☑
      hang V96.15 ☑
      powered V95.15 ☑
    helicopter V95.05 ☑
    in war operations — *see* War operations, destruc-
      tion of aircraft
    microlight V95.15 ☑
    nonpowered V96.9 ☑
      specified NEC V96.8 ☑
    powered NEC V95.8 ☑
    stated as
      homicide (attempt) Y03.8 ☑
      suicide (attempt) X83.0 ☑
    ultralight V95.15 ☑
  anesthetic gas in operating room W40.1 ☑
  antipersonnel bomb W40.8 ☑
    assault X96.0 ☑
    homicide (attempt) X96.0 ☑
    suicide (attempt) X75 ☑
  assault X96.9 ☑
  bicycle tire W37.0 ☑
  blasting (cap) (materials) W40.0 ☑
  boiler (machinery), not on transport vehicle W35 ☑
    on watercraft — *see* Explosion, in, watercraft
  butane W40.1 ☑
  caused by other person X96.9 ☑
  coal gas W40.1 ☑
  detonator W40.0 ☑
  dump (munitions) W40.8 ☑
  dynamite W40.0 ☑
    in
      assault X96.8 ☑
      homicide (attempt) X96.8 ☑
      legal intervention
        injuring
          bystander Y35.112 ☑
          law enforcement personnel Y35.111 ☑
          suspect Y35.113 ☑
      suicide (attempt) X75 ☑
  explosive (material) W40.9 ☑
    gas W40.1 ☑
    in blasting operation W40.0 ☑
    specified NEC W40.8 ☑
      in
        assault X96.8 ☑
        homicide (attempt) X96.8 ☑
        legal intervention
          injuring
            bystander Y35.192 ☑
            law enforcement personnel
              Y35.191 ☑
            suspect Y35.193 ☑
        suicide (attempt) X75 ☑
  factory (munitions) W40.8 ☑
  fertilizer bomb W40.8 ☑
    assault X96.3 ☑
    homicide (attempt) X96.3 ☑
    suicide (attempt) X75 ☑
  firearm (parts) NEC W34.19 ☑
    airgun W34.110 ☑
    BB gun W34.110 ☑
    gas, air or spring-operated gun NEC W34.118 ☑
    hangun W32.1 ☑
    hunting rifle W33.12 ☑
    larger firearm W33.10 ☑
      specified NEC W33.19 ☑
    machine gun W33.13 ☑
    paintball gun W34.111 ☑
    pellet gun W34.110 ☑
    shotgun W33.11 ☑
    Very pistol [flare] W34.19 ☑
  fire-damp W40.1 ☑
  fireworks W39 ☑
  gas (coal) (explosive) W40.1 ☑
    cylinder W36.9 ☑
      aerosol can W36.1 ☑
      air tank W36.2 ☑
      pressurized W36.3 ☑
      specified NEC W36.8 ☑

Explosion — *continued*
  gasoline (fumes) (tank) not in moving motor vehicle
    W40.1 ☑
    bomb W40.8 ☑
      assault X96.1 ☑
      homicide (attempt) X96.1 ☑
      suicide (attempt) X75 ☑
    in motor vehicle — *see* Accident, transport, by type
      of vehicle
  grain store W40.8 ☑
  grenade W40.8 ☑
    in
      assault X96.8 ☑
      homicide (attempt) X96.8 ☑
      legal intervention
        injuring
          bystander Y35.192 ☑
          law enforcement personnel Y35.191 ☑
          suspect Y35.193 ☑
      suicide (attempt) X75 ☑
  handgun (parts) — *see* Explosion, firearm, hangun
    (parts)
  homicide (attempt) X96.9 ☑
    antipersonnel bomb — *see* Explosion, antiperson-
      nel bomb
    fertilizer bomb — *see* Explosion, fertilizer bomb
    gasoline bomb — *see* Explosion, gasoline bomb
    letter bomb — *see* Explosion, letter bomb
    pipe bomb — *see* Explosion, pipe bomb
    specified NEC X96.8 ☑
  hose, pressurized W37.8 ☑
  hot water heater, tank (in machinery) W35 ☑
    on watercraft — *see* Explosion, in, watercraft
  in, on
    dump W40.8 ☑
    factory W40.8 ☑
    mine (of explosive gases) NEC W40.1 ☑
    watercraft V93.59 ☑
      powered craft V93.53 ☑
        ferry boat V93.51 ☑
        fishing boat V93.52 ☑
        jetskis V93.53 ☑
        liner V93.51 ☑
        merchant ship V93.50 ☑
        passenger ship V93.51 ☑
        sailboat V93.54 ☑
  letter bomb W40.8 ☑
    assault X96.2 ☑
    homicide (attempt) X96.2 ☑
    suicide (attempt) X75 ☑
  machinery (*see also* Contact, with, by type of machine)
    on board watercraft — *see* Explosion, in, watercraft
    pressure vessel — *see* Explosion, by type of vessel
  methane W40.1 ☑
  mine W40.1 ☑
  missile NEC W40.8 ☑
  mortar bomb W40.8 ☑
    in
      assault X96.8 ☑
      homicide (attempt) X96.8 ☑
      legal intervention
        injuring
          bystander Y35.192 ☑
          law enforcement personnel Y35.191 ☑
          suspect Y35.193 ☑
      suicide (attempt) X75 ☑
  munitions (dump) (factory) W40.8 ☑
  pipe, pressurized W37.8 ☑
    bomb W40.8 ☑
      assault X96.4 ☑
      homicide (attempt) X96.4 ☑
      suicide (attempt) X75 ☑
  pressure, pressurized
    cooker W38 ☑
    gas tank (in machinery) W36.3 ☑
    hose W37.8 ☑
    pipe W37.8 ☑
    specified device NEC W38 ☑
    tire W37.8 ☑
      bicycle W37.0 ☑
    vessel (in machinery) W38 ☑
  propane W40.1 ☑
  self-inflicted X75 ☑
  shell (artillery) NEC W40.8 ☑
    during war operations — *see* War operations, ex-
      plosion

Explosion — *continued*
- shell — *continued*
  - in
    - legal intervention
      - injuring
        - bystander Y35.122 ☑
        - law enforcement personnel Y35.121 ☑
        - suspect Y35.123 ☑
    - war — *see* War operations, explosion
  - spacecraft V95.45 ☑
  - stated as undetermined whether accidental or intentional Y25 ☑
  - steam or water lines (in machinery) W37.8 ☑
  - stove W40.9 ☑
  - suicide (attempt) X75 ☑
  - tire, pressurized W37.8 ☑
    - bicycle W37.0 ☑
  - undetermined whether accidental or intentional Y25 ☑
  - vehicle tire NEC W37.8 ☑
    - bicycle W37.0 ☑
  - war operations — *see* War operations, explosion
- **Exposure** (to) X58 ☑
  - air pressure change — *see* Air, pressure
  - cold (accidental) (excessive) (extreme) (natural) (place) X31 ☑
    - assault Y08.89 ☑
    - due to
      - man-made conditions W93.8 ☑
        - dry ice (contact) W93.01 ☑
          - inhalation W93.02 ☑
        - liquid air (contact) (hydrogen) (nitrogen) W93.11 ☑
          - inhalation W93.12 ☑
        - refrigeration unit (deep freeze) W93.2 ☑
        - suicide (attempt) X83.2 ☑
      - weather (conditions) X31 ☑
    - homicide (attempt) Y08.89 ☑
    - self-inflicted X83.2 ☑
  - due to abandonment or neglect X58 ☑
  - electric current W86.8 ☑
    - appliance (faulty) W86.8 ☑
      - domestic W86.0 ☑
    - caused by other person Y08.89 ☑
    - conductor (faulty) W86.1 ☑
    - control apparatus (faulty) W86.1 ☑
    - electric power generating plant, distribution station W86.1 ☑
    - electroshock gun — *see* Exposure, electric current, taser
    - high-voltage cable W85 ☑
    - homicide (attempt) Y08.89 ☑
    - legal execution — *see* Legal, intervention, specified means NEC
    - lightning — *see* subcategory T75.0 ☑
    - live rail W86.8 ☑
    - misadventure in medical or surgical procedure in electroshock therapy Y63.4
    - motor (electric) (faulty) W86.8 ☑
      - domestic W86.0 ☑
    - self-inflicted X83.1 ☑
    - specified NEC W86.8 ☑
      - domestic W86.0 ☑
    - stun gun — *see* Exposure, electric current, taser
    - suicide (attempt) X83.1 ☑
    - taser W86.8 ☑
      - assault Y08.89 ☑
      - legal intervention — *see* category Y35 ☑
      - self-harm (intentional) X83.8 ☑
      - undetermined intent Y33 ☑
    - third rail W86.8 ☑
    - transformer (faulty) W86.1 ☑
    - transmission lines W85 ☑
  - environmental tobacco smoke X58 ☑
  - excessive
    - cold — *see* Exposure, cold
    - heat (natural) NEC X30 ☑
      - man-made W92 ☑
  - factor(s) NOS X58 ☑
    - environmental NEC X58 ☑
    - man-made NEC W99 ☑
    - natural NEC — *see* Forces of nature
    - specified NEC X58 ☑
  - fire, flames (accidental) X08.8 ☑
    - assault X97 ☑

Exposure — *continued*
- fire, flames — *continued*
  - campfire — *see* Exposure, fire, controlled, not in building
  - controlled (in)
    - with ignition (cf) clothing (*see also* Ignition, clothes) X06.2 ☑
      - nightwear X05 ☑
    - bonfire — *see* Exposure, fire, controlled, not in building
    - brazier (in building or structure) (*see also* Exposure, fire, controlled, building)
      - not in building or structure — *see* Exposure, fire, controlled, not in building
    - building or structure X02.0 ☑
      - with
        - fall from building X02.3 ☑
        - from building X02.5 ☑
        - injury due to building collapse X02.2 ☑
        - smoke inhalation X02.1 ☑
      - hit by object from building X02.4 ☑
      - specified mode of injury NEC X02.8 ☑
    - fireplace, furnace or stove — *see* Exposure, fire, controlled, building
    - not in building or structure X03.0 ☑
      - with
        - fall X03.3 ☑
        - smoke inhalation X03.1 ☑
      - hit by object X03.4 ☑
      - specified mode of injury NEC X03.8 ☑
    - trash — *see* Exposure, fire, controlled, not in building
  - fireplace — *see* Exposure, fire, controlled, building
  - fittings or furniture (in building or structure) (uncontrolled) — *see* Exposure, fire, uncontrolled, building
  - forest (uncontrolled) — *see* Exposure, fire, uncontrolled, not in building
  - grass (uncontrolled) — *see* Exposure, fire, uncontrolled, not in building
  - hay (uncontrolled) — *see* Exposure, fire, uncontrolled, not in building
  - homicide (attempt) X97 ☑
  - ignition of highly flammable material X04 ☑
  - in, of, on, starting in
    - machinery — *see* Contact, with, by type of machine
    - motor vehicle (in motion) (*see also* Accident, transport, occupant by type of vehicle) V87.8 ☑
      - with collision — *see* Collision
    - railway rolling stock, train, vehicle V81.81 ☑
      - with collision — *see* Accident, transport, railway vehicle occupant
    - street car (in motion) V82.8 ☑
      - with collision — *see* Accident, transport, streetcar occupant
    - transport vehicle NEC (*see also* Accident, transport)
      - with collision — *see* Collision
    - war operations (*see also* War operations, fire)
      - from nuclear explosion — *see* War operations, nuclear weapons
    - watercraft (in transit) (not in transit) V91.09 ☑
      - localized — *see* Burn, on board watercraft, due to, fire on board
      - powered craft V91.03 ☑
        - ferry boat V91.01 ☑
        - fishing boat V91.02 ☑
        - jet skis V91.03 ☑
        - liner V91.01 ☑
        - merchant ship V91.00 ☑
        - passenger ship V91.01 ☑
      - unpowered craft V91.08 ☑
        - canoe V91.05 ☑
        - inflatable V91.06 ☑
        - kayak V91.05 ☑
        - sailboat V91.04 ☑
        - surf-board V91.08 ☑
        - waterskis V91.07 ☑
        - windsurfer V91.08 ☑
  - lumber (uncontrolled) — *see* Exposure, fire, uncontrolled, not in building
  - mine (uncontrolled) — *see* Exposure, fire, uncontrolled, not in building

Exposure — *continued*
- fire, flames — *continued*
  - prairie (uncontrolled) — *see* Exposure, fire, uncontrolled, not in building
  - resulting from
    - explosion — *see* Explosion
    - lightning X08.8 ☑
  - self-inflicted X76 ☑
  - specified NEC X08.8 ☑
  - started by other person X97 ☑
  - stated as undetermined whether accidental or intentional Y26 ☑
  - stove — *see* Exposure, fire, controlled, building
  - suicide (attempt) X76 ☑
  - tunnel (uncontrolled) — *see* Exposure, fire, uncontrolled, not in building
  - uncontrolled
    - in building or structure X00.0 ☑
      - with
        - fall from building X00.3 ☑
        - injury due to building collapse X00.2 ☑
        - jump from building X00.5 ☑
        - smoke inhalation X00.1 ☑
      - bed X08.00 ☑
        - due to
          - cigarette X08.01 ☑
          - specified material NEC X08.09 ☑
      - furniture NEC X08.20 ☑
        - due to
          - cigarette X08.21 ☑
          - specified material NEC X08.29 ☑
      - hit by object from building X00.4 ☑
      - sofa X08.10 ☑
        - due to
          - cigarette X08.11 ☑
          - specified material NEC X08.19 ☑
      - specified mode of injury NEC X00.8 ☑
    - not in building or structure (any) X01.0 ☑
      - with
        - fall X01.3 ☑
        - smoke inhalation X01.1 ☑
      - hit by object X01.4 ☑
      - specified mode of injury NEC X01.8 ☑
  - undetermined whether accidental or intentional Y26 ☑
  - forces of nature NEC — *see* Forces of nature
  - G-forces (abnormal) W49.9 ☑
  - gravitational forces (abnormal) W49.9 ☑
  - heat (natural) NEC — *see* Heat
  - high-pressure jet (hydraulic) (pneumatic) W49.9 ☑
  - hydraulic jet W49.9 ☑
  - inanimate mechanical force W49.9 ☑
  - jet, high-pressure (hydraulic) (pneumatic) W49.9 ☑
  - lightning — *see* subcategory T75.0 ☑
    - causing fire — *see* Exposure, fire
  - mechanical forces NEC W49.9 ☑
    - animate NEC W64 ☑
    - inanimate NEC W49.9 ☑
  - noise W42.9 ☑
    - supersonic W42.0 ☑
  - noxious substance — *see* Table of Drugs and Chemicals
  - pneumatic jet W49.9 ☑
  - prolonged in deep-freeze unit or refrigerator W93.2 ☑
  - radiation — *see* Radiation
  - smoke (*see also* Exposure, fire)
    - tobacco, second hand Z77.22
  - specified factors NEC X58 ☑
  - sunlight X32 ☑
    - man-made (sun lamp) W89.8 ☑
    - tanning bed W89.1 ☑
  - supersonic waves W42.0 ☑
  - transmission line(s), electric W85 ☑
  - vibration W49.9 ☑
  - waves
    - infrasound W49.9 ☑
    - sound W42.9 ☑
    - supersonic W42.0 ☑
  - weather NEC — *see* Forces of nature
- **External cause status** Y99.9
  - child assisting in compensated work for family Y99.8
  - civilian activity done for financial or other compensation Y99.0
  - civilian activity done for income or pay Y99.0
  - family member assisting in compensated work for other family member Y99.8

External Causes Index

External cause status — Fall, falling

External cause status — *continued*
hobby not done for income Y99.8
leisure activity Y99.8
military activity Y99.1
off-duty activity of military personnel Y99.8
recreation or sport not for income or while a student
    Y99.8
specified NEC Y99.8
student activity Y99.8
volunteer activity Y99.2

F

Factors, supplemental
alcohol
    blood level
        less than 20mg/100ml Y90.0
        20-39mg/100ml Y90.1
        40-59mg/100ml Y90.2
        60-79mg/100ml Y90.3
        80-99mg/100ml Y90.4
        100-119mg/100ml Y90.5
        120-199mg/100ml Y90.6
        200-239mg/100ml Y90.7
        240mg/100ml or more Y90.8
        presence in blood, level not specified Y90.9
    presence in blood, but level not specified Y90.9
environmental-pollution-related condition- see Z57 ☑
nosocomial condition Y95
work-related condition Y99.0
Failure
in suture or ligature during surgical procedure Y65.2
mechanical, of instrument or apparatus (any) (during
    any medical or surgical procedure) Y65.8
sterile precautions (during medical and surgical care)
    — *see* Misadventure, failure, sterile precautions,
    by type of procedure
to
    introduce tube or instrument Y65.4
        endotracheal tube during anesthesia Y65.3
    make curve (transport vehicle) NEC — *see* Accident,
        transport
    remove tube or instrument Y65.4
Fall, falling (accidental) W19 ☑
building W20.1
    burning (uncontrolled fire) X00.3 ☑
down
    embankment W17.81 ☑
    escalator W10.0 ☑
    hill W17.81 ☑
    ladder W11 ☑
    ramp W10.2 ☑
    stairs, steps W10.9 ☑
due to
    bumping against
        object W18.00 ☑
            sharp glass W18.02 ☑
            specified NEC W18.09 ☑
            sports equipment W18.01 ☑
        person W03 ☑
            due to ice or snow W00.0 ☑
            on pedestrian conveyance — *see* Accident,
                transport, pedestrian, conveyance
    collision with another person W03 ☑
        due to ice or snow W00.0 ☑
        involving pedestrian conveyance — *see* Acci-
            dent, transport, pedestrian, conveyance
    grocery cart tipping over W17.82 ☑
    ice or snow W00.9 ☑
        from one level to another W00.2 ☑
        on stairs or steps W00.1 ☑
        involving pedestrian conveyance — *see* Acci-
            dent, transport, pedestrian, conveyance
        on same level W00.0 ☑
    slipping (on moving sidewalk) W01.0 ☑
        with subsequent striking against object
            W01.10 ☑
            furniture W01.190 ☑
            sharp object W01.119 ☑
                glass W01.110 ☑
                power tool or machine W01.111 ☑
                specified NEC W01.118 ☑
            specified NEC W01.198 ☑
    striking against
        object W18.00 ☑
            sharp glass W18.02 ☑
            specified NEC W18.09 ☑

Fall, falling — *continued*
due to — *continued*
    striking against — *continued*
        object — *continued*
            sports equipment W18.01 ☑
        person W03 ☑
            due to ice or snow W00.0 ☑
            on pedestrian conveyance — *see*
                transport, pedestrian, conveyance
earth (with asphyxia or suffocation (by pressure)) —
    see Earth, falling
from, off, out of
    aircraft NEC (with accident to aircraft NEC) V97.0 ☑
        while boarding or alighting V97.1 ☑
    balcony W13.0 ☑
    bed W06 ☑
    boat, ship, watercraft NEC (with drowning or sub-
        mersion) — *see* Drowning, due to, fall over-
        board
        with hitting bottom or object V94.0 ☑
    bridge W13.1 ☑
    building W13.9 ☑
        burning (uncontrolled fire) X00.3 ☑
    cavity W17.2 ☑
    chair W07 ☑
    cherry picker W17.89 ☑
    cliff W15 ☑
    dock W17.4 ☑
    embankment W17.81 ☑
    escalator W10.0 ☑
    flagpole W13.8 ☑
    furniture NEC W08 ☑
    grocery cart W17.82 ☑
    haystack W17.89 ☑
    high place NEC W17.89 ☑
        stated as undetermined whether accidental or
            intentional Y30 ☑
    hole W17.2 ☑
    incline W10.2 ☑
    ladder W11 ☑
    lifting device W17.89 ☑
    machine, machinery (*see also* Contact, with, by
        type of machine)
        not in operation W17.89 ☑
    manhole W17.1 ☑
    mobile elevated work platform [MEWP] W17.89 ☑
    motorized mobility scooter W05.2 ☑
    one level to another NEC W17.89 ☑
        intentional, purposeful, suicide (attempt)
            X80 ☑
        stated as undetermined whether accidental or
            intentional Y30 ☑
    pit W17.2 ☑
    playground equipment W09.8 ☑
        jungle gym W09.2 ☑
        slide W09.0 ☑
        swing W09.1 ☑
    quarry W17.89 ☑
    railing W13.9 ☑
    ramp W10.2 ☑
    roof W13.2 ☑
    scaffolding W12 ☑
    scooter (nonmotorized) W05.1 ☑
        motorized mobility W05.2 ☑
    sky lift W17.89 ☑
    stairs, steps W10.9 ☑
        curb W10.1 ☑
        due to ice or snow W00.1 ☑
        escalator W10.0 ☑
        incline W10.2 ☑
        ramp W10.2 ☑
        sidewalk curb W10.1 ☑
        specified NEC W10.8 ☑
    stepladder W11 ☑
    storm drain W17.1 ☑
    streetcar NEC V82.6 ☑
        with antecedent collision — *see* Accident,
            transport, streetcar occupant
        while boarding or alighting V82.4 ☑
    structure NEC W13.8 ☑
        burning (uncontrolled fire) X00.3 ☑
    table W08 ☑
    toilet W18.11 ☑
        with subsequent striking against object
            W18.12 ☑
    train NEC V81.6 ☑

Fall, falling — *continued*
from, off, out of — *continued*
    train — *continued*
        during derailment (without antecedent colli-
            sion) V81.7 ☑
            with antecedent collision — *see* Accident,
                transport, railway vehicle occupant
        while boarding or alighting V81.4 ☑
        transport vehicle after collision — *see* Accident,
            transport, by type of vehicle, collision
    tree W14 ☑
    vehicle (in motion) NEC (*see also* Accident, trans-
        port) V89.9 ☑
        motor NEC (*see also* Accident, transport, occu-
            pant, by type of vehicle) V87.8 ☑
        stationary W17.89 ☑
            while boarding or alighting B — *see* Acci-
                dent, transport, by type of vehicle,
                while boarding or alighting
    viaduct W13.8 ☑
    wall W13.8 ☑
    watercraft (*see also* Drowning, due to, fall over-
        board)
        with hitting bottom or object V94.0 ☑
    well W17.0 ☑
    wheelchair, non-moving W05.0 ☑
        powered — *see* Accident, transport, pedestrian,
            conveyance occupant, specified type NEC
    window W13.4 ☑
in, on
    aircraft NEC V97.0 ☑
        with accident to aircraft V97.0 ☑
        while boarding or alighting V97.1 ☑
    bathtub (empty) W18.2 ☑
        filled W16.212 ☑
            causing drowning W16.211 ☑
    escalator W10.0 ☑
    incline W10.2 ☑
    ladder W11 ☑
    machine, machinery — *see* Contact, with, by type
        of machine
    object, edged, pointed or sharp (with cut) — *see*
        Fall, by type
    playground equipment W09.8 ☑
        jungle gym W09.2 ☑
        slide W09.0 ☑
        swing W09.1 ☑
    ramp W10.2 ☑
    scaffolding W12 ☑
    shower W18.2 ☑
        causing drowning W16.211 ☑
    staircase, stairs, steps W10.9 ☑
        curb W10.1 ☑
        due to ice or snow W00.1 ☑
        escalator W10.0 ☑
        incline W10.2 ☑
        specified NEC W10.8 ☑
    streetcar (without antecedent collision) V82.5 ☑
        with antecedent collision — *see* Accident,
            transport, streetcar occupant
        while boarding or alighting V82.4 ☑
    train (without antecedent collision) V81.5 ☑
        with antecedent collision — *see* Accident,
            transport, railway vehicle occupant
        during derailment (without antecedent colli-
            sion) V81.7 ☑
            with antecedent collision — *see* Accident,
                transport, railway vehicle occupant
        while boarding or alighting V81.4 ☑
    transport vehicle after collision — *see* Accident,
        transport, by type of vehicle, collision
    watercraft V93.39 ☑
        due to
            accident to craft V91.29 ☑
                powered craft V91.23 ☑
                    ferry boat V91.21 ☑
                    fishing boat V91.22 ☑
                    jetskis V91.23 ☑
                    liner V91.21 ☑
                    merchant ship V91.20 ☑
                    passenger ship V91.21 ☑
                unpowered craft
                    canoe V91.25 ☑
                    inflatable V91.26 ☑
                    kayak V91.25 ☑
                    sailboat V91.24 ☑

Fall, falling — *continued*
  in, on — *continued*
    watercraft — *continued*
      powered craft V93.33 ☑
        ferry boat V93.31 ☑
        fishing boat V93.32 ☑
        jetskis V93.33 ☑
        liner V93.31 ☑
        merchant ship V93.30 ☑
        passenger ship V93.31 ☑
      unpowered craft V93.38 ☑
        canoe V93.35 ☑
        inflatable V93.36 ☑
        kayak V93.35 ☑
        sailboat V93.34 ☑
        surf-board V93.38 ☑
        windsurfer V93.38 ☑
  into
    cavity W17.2 ☑
    dock W17.4 ☑
    fire — *see* Exposure, fire, by type
    haystack W17.89 ☑
    hole W17.2 ☑
    lake — *see* Fall, into, water
    lake — *see* Fall, into, water
    manhole W17.1 ☑
    moving part of machinery — *see* Contact, with, by
      type of machine
    ocean — *see* Fall, into, water
    opening in surface NEC W17.89 ☑
    pit W17.2 ☑
    pond — *see* Fall, into, water
    quarry W17.89 ☑
    river — *see* Fall, into, water
    shaft W17.89 ☑
    storm drain W17.1 ☑
    stream — *see* Fall, into, water
    swimming pool (*see also* Fall, into, water, in,
      swimming pool)
      empty W17.3 ☑
    tank W17.89 ☑
    water W16.42 ☑
      causing drowning W16.41 ☑
      from watercraft — *see* Drowning, due to, fall
        overboard
      hitting diving board W21.4 ☑
      in
        bathtub W16.212 ☑
          causing drowning W16.211 ☑
        bucket W16.222 ☑
          causing drowning W16.221 ☑
        natural body of water W16.112 ☑
          causing drowning W16.111 ☑
          striking
            bottom W16.122 ☑
              causing drowning W16.121 ☑
            side W16.132 ☑
              causing drowning W16.131 ☑
        specified water NEC W16.312 ☑
          causing drowning W16.311 ☑
          striking
            bottom W16.322 ☑
              causing drowning W16.321 ☑
            wall W16.332 ☑
              causing drowning W16.331 ☑
        swimming pool W16.012 ☑
          causing drowning W16.011 ☑
          striking
            bottom W16.022 ☑
              causing drowning W16.031 ☑
            wall W16.032 ☑
              causing drowning W16.021 ☑
        utility bucket W16.222 ☑
          causing drowning W16.221 ☑
    well W17.0 ☑
  involving
    bed W06 ☑
    chair W07 ☑
    furniture NEC W08 ☑
    glass — *see* Fall, by type
    playground equipment W09.8 ☑
      jungle gym W09.2 ☑
      slide W09.0 ☑
      swing W09.1 ☑
    roller blades — *see* Accident, transport, pedestrian,
      conveyance

Fall, falling — *continued*
  involving — *continued*
    skateboard(s) — *see* Accident, transport, pedestri-
      an, conveyance
    skates (ice) (in line) (roller) — *see* Accident, trans-
      port, pedestrian, conveyance
    skis — *see* Accident, transport, pedestrian, con-
      veyance
    table W08 ☑
    wheelchair, non-moving W05.0 ☑
      powered — *see* Accident, transport, pedestrian,
        conveyance, specified type NEC
  object — *see* Struck by, object, falling
  off
    toilet W18.11 ☑
      with subsequent striking against object
        W18.12 ☑
  on same level W18.30 ☑
    due to
      specified NEC W18.39 ☑
      stepping on an object W18.31 ☑
  out of
    bed W06 ☑
    building NEC W13.8 ☑
    chair W07 ☑
    furniture NEC W08 ☑
    wheelchair, non-moving W05.0 ☑
      powered — *see* Accident, transport, pedestrian,
        conveyance, specified type NEC
    window W13.4 ☑
  over
    animal W01.0 ☑
    cliff W15 ☑
    embankment W17.81 ☑
    small object W01.0 ☑
  rock W20.8 ☑
  same level W18.30 ☑
    from
      being crushed, pushed, or stepped on by a
        crowd or human stampede W52 ☑
      collision, pushing, shoving, by or with other
        person W03 ☑
      slipping, stumbling, tripping W01.0 ☑
    involving ice or snow W00.0 ☑
      involving skates (ice) (roller), skateboard, skis
        — *see* Accident, transport, pedestrian,
        conveyance
  snowslide (avalanche) — *see* Landslide
  stone W20.8 ☑
  structure W20.1 ☑
    burning (uncontrolled fire) X00.3 ☑
  through
    bridge W13.1 ☑
    floor W13.3 ☑
    roof W13.2 ☑
    wall W13.8 ☑
    window W13.4 ☑
  timber W20.8 ☑
  tree (caused by lightning) W20.8 ☑
  while being carried or supported by other person(s)
    W04 ☑

Fallen on by
  animal (not being ridden) NEC W55.89 ☑
Felo-de-se — *see* Suicide
Fight (hand) (fists) (foot) — *see* Assault, fight
Fire (accidental) — *see* Exposure, fire
Firearm discharge — *see* Discharge, firearm
Fireball effects from nuclear explosion in war oper-
    ations — *see* War operations, nuclear weapons
Fireworks (explosion) W39 ☑
Flash burns from explosion — *see* Explosion
Flood (any injury) (caused by) X38 ☑
  collapse of man-made structure causing earth move-
    ment X36.0 ☑
  tidal wave — *see* Forces of nature, tidal wave
Food (any type) **in**
  air passages (with asphyxia, obstruction, or suffoca-
    tion) — *see* categories T17 and T18 ☑
  alimentary tract causing asphyxia (due to compression
    of trachea) — *see* categories T17 and T18 ☑
Forces of nature X39.8 ☑
  avalanche X36.1 ☑
    causing transport accident — *see* Accident, trans-
      port, by type of vehicle
  blizzard X37.2 ☑
  cataclysmic storm X37.9 ☑

Forces of nature — *continued*
  cataclysmic storm — *continued*
    with flood X38 ☑
    blizzard X37.2 ☑
    cloudburst X37.8 ☑
    cyclone X37.1 ☑
    dust storm X37.3 ☑
    hurricane X37.0 ☑
    specified storm NEC X37.8 ☑
    storm surge X37.0 ☑
    tornado X37.1 ☑
    twister X37.1 ☑
    typhoon X37.0 ☑
  cloudburst X37.8 ☑
  cold (natural) X31 ☑
  cyclone X37.1 ☑
  dam collapse causing earth movement X36.0 ☑
  dust storm X37.3 ☑
  earth movement X36.1 ☑
    caused by dam or structure collapse X36.0 ☑
    earthquake X34 ☑
  earthquake X34 ☑
  flood (caused by) X38 ☑
    dam collapse X36.0 ☑
    tidal wave B — *see* Forces of nature, tidal wave
  heat (natural) X30 ☑
  hurricane X37.0 ☑
  landslide X36.1 ☑
    causing transport accident — *see* Accident, trans-
      port, by type of vehicle
  lightning — *see* subcategory T75.0 ☑
    causing fire — *see* Exposure, fire
  mudslide X36.1 ☑
    causing transport accident — *see* Accident, trans-
      port, by type of vehicle
  radiation (natural) X39.08 ☑
    radon X39.01 ☑
  radon X39.01 ☑
  specified force NEC X39.8 ☑
  storm surge X37.0 ☑
  structure collapse causing earth movement X36.0 ☑
  sunlight X32 ☑
  tidal wave X37.41 ☑
    due to
      earthquake X37.41 ☑
      landslide X37.43 ☑
      storm X37.42 ☑
      volcanic eruption X37.41 ☑
  tornado X37.1 ☑
  tsunami X37.41 ☑
  twister X37.1 ☑
  typhoon X37.0 ☑
  volcanic eruption X35 ☑
Foreign body
  aspiration — *see* Index to Diseases and Injuries, For-
    eign body, respiratory tract
  entering through skin W45.8 ☑
    can lid W45.2 ☑
    nail W45.0 ☑
    paper W45.1 ☑
    specified NEC W45.8 ☑
    splinter W45.8 ☑
Forest fire (exposure to) — *see* Exposure, fire, uncon-
    trolled, not in building
Found injured X58 ☑
  from exposure (to) — *see* Exposure
  on
    highway, road(way), street V89.9 ☑
    railway right of way V81.9 ☑
Fracture (circumstances unknown or unspecified) X58 ☑
  due to specified cause NEC X58 ☑
Freezing — *see* Exposure, cold
Frostbite X31 ☑
  due to man-made conditions — *see* Exposure, cold,
    man-made
Frozen — *see* Exposure, cold

G

Gored by bull W55.22 ☑
Gunshot wound W34.00 ☑

H

Hailstones, injured by X39.8 ☑

Hanged herself or himself — *see* Hanging, self-inflicted
Hanging (accidental) (*see also* category) T71 ☑
  legal execution — *see* Legal, intervention, specified
    means NEC
Heat (effects of) (excessive) X30 ☑
  due to
    man-made conditions W92 ☑
      on board watercraft V93.29 ☑
        fishing boat V93.22 ☑
        merchant ship V93.20 ☑
        passenger ship V93.21 ☑
        sailboat V93.24 ☑
        specified powered craft NEC V93.23 ☑
    weather (conditions) X30 ☑
  from
    electric heating apparatus causing burning X16 ☑
    nuclear explosion in war operations — *see* War
      operations, nuclear weapons
  inappropriate in local application or packing in medical
    or surgical procedure Y63.5
Hemorrhage
  delayed following medical or surgical treatment
    without mention of misadventure — *see* Index
    to Diseases and Injuries, Complication(s)
  during medical or surgical treatment as misadventure
    — *see* Index to Diseases and Injuries, Complica-
    tion(s)
High
  altitude (effects) — *see* Air, pressure, low
  level of radioactivity, effects — *see* Radiation
  pressure (effects) — *see* Air, pressure, high
  temperature, effects — *see* Heat
Hit, hitting (accidental) by — *see* Struck by
Hitting against — *see* Striking against
Homicide (attempt) (justifiable) — *see* Assault
Hot
  place, effects (*see also* Heat)
  weather, effects X30 ☑
House fire (uncontrolled) — *see* Exposure, fire, uncon-
  trolled, building
Humidity, causing problem X39.8 ☑
Hunger X58 ☑
Hurricane (any injury) X37.0 ☑
Hypobarism, hypobaropathy — *see* Air, pressure, low

Ictus
  caloris (*see also* Heat)
  solaris X30 ☑
Ignition (accidental) (*see also* Exposure, fire) X08.8 ☑
  anesthetic gas in operating room W40.1 ☑
  apparel X06.2 ☑
    from highly flammable material X04 ☑
    nightwear X05 ☑
  bed linen (sheets) (spreads) (pillows) (mattress) — *see*
    Exposure, fire, uncontrolled, building, bed
  benzine X04 ☑
  clothes, clothing NEC (from controlled fire) X06.2 ☑
    from
      highly flammable material X04 ☑
  ether X04 ☑
    in operating room W40.1 ☑
  explosive material — *see* Explosion
  gasoline X04 ☑
  jewelry (plastic) (any) X06.0 ☑
  kerosene X04 ☑
  material
    explosive — *see* Explosion
    highly flammable with secondary explosion X04 ☑
  nightwear X05 ☑
  paraffin X04 ☑
  petrol X04 ☑
Immersion (accidental) (*see also* Drowning)
  hand or foot due to cold (excessive) X31 ☑
Implantation of quills of porcupine W55.89 ☑
Inanition (from) (hunger) X58 ☑
  thirst X58 ☑
Inappropriate operation performed
  correct operation on wrong side or body part (wrong
    side) (wrong site) Y65.53
  operation intended for another patient done on wrong
    patient Y65.52
  wrong operation performed on correct patient Y65.51
Inattention after, at birth (homicidal intent) (infantici-
  dal intent) X58 ☑

Incident, adverse
  device
    anesthesiology Y70.8
      accessory Y70.2
      diagnostic Y70.0
      miscellaneous Y70.8
      monitoring Y70.0
      prosthetic Y70.2
      rehabilitative Y70.1
      surgical Y70.3
      therapeutic Y70.1
    cardiovascular Y71.8
      accessory Y71.2
      diagnostic Y71.0
      miscellaneous Y71.8
      monitoring Y71.0
      prosthetic Y71.2
      rehabilitative Y71.1
      surgical Y71.3
      therapeutic Y71.1
    gastroenterology Y73.8
      accessory Y73.2
      diagnostic Y73.0
      miscellaneous Y73.8
      monitoring Y73.0
      prosthetic Y73.2
      rehabilitative Y73.1
      surgical Y73.3
      therapeutic Y73.1
    general
      hospital Y74.8
        accessory Y74.2
        diagnostic Y74.0
        miscellaneous Y74.8
        monitoring Y74.0
        prosthetic Y74.2
        rehabilitative Y74.1
        surgical Y74.3
        therapeutic Y74.1
      surgical Y81.8
        accessory Y81.2
        diagnostic Y81.0
        miscellaneous Y81.8
        monitoring Y81.0
        prosthetic Y81.2
        rehabilitative Y81.1
        surgical Y81.3
        therapeutic Y81.1
    gynecological Y76.8
      accessory Y76.2
      diagnostic Y76.0
      miscellaneous Y76.8
      monitoring Y76.0
      prosthetic Y76.2
      rehabilitative Y76.1
      surgical Y76.3
      therapeutic Y76.1
    medical Y82.9
      specified type NEC Y82.8
    neurological Y75.8
      accessory Y75.2
      diagnostic Y75.0
      miscellaneous Y75.8
      monitoring Y75.0
      prosthetic Y75.2
      rehabilitative Y75.1
      surgical Y75.3
      therapeutic Y75.1
    obstetrical Y76.8
      accessory Y76.2
      diagnostic Y76.0
      miscellaneous Y76.8
      monitoring Y76.0
      prosthetic Y76.2
      rehabilitative Y76.1
      surgical Y76.3
      therapeutic Y76.1
    ophthalmic Y77.8
      accessory Y77.2
      diagnostic Y77.0
      miscellaneous Y77.8
      monitoring Y77.0
      prosthetic Y77.2
      rehabilitative Y77.1
      surgical Y77.3
      therapeutic Y77.1
    orthopedic Y79.8
      accessory Y79.2

Incident, adverse — *continued*
  device — *continued*
    orthopedic — *continued*
      diagnostic Y79.0
      miscellaneous Y79.8
      monitoring Y79.0
      prosthetic Y79.2
      rehabilitative Y79.1
      surgical Y79.3
      therapeutic Y79.1
    otorhinolaryngological Y72.8
      accessory Y72.2
      diagnostic Y72.0
      miscellaneous Y72.8
      monitoring Y72.0
      prosthetic Y72.2
      rehabilitative Y72.1
      surgical Y72.3
      therapeutic Y72.1
    personal use Y74.8
      accessory Y74.2
      diagnostic Y74.0
      miscellaneous Y74.8
      monitoring Y74.0
      prosthetic Y74.2
      rehabilitative Y74.1
      surgical Y74.3
      therapeutic Y74.1
    physical medicine Y80.8
      accessory Y80.2
      diagnostic Y80.0
      miscellaneous Y80.8
      monitoring Y80.0
      prosthetic Y80.2
      rehabilitative Y80.1
      surgical Y80.3
      therapeutic Y80.1
    plastic surgical Y81.8
      accessory Y81.2
      diagnostic Y81.0
      miscellaneous Y81.8
      monitoring Y81.0
      prosthetic Y81.2
      rehabilitative Y81.1
      surgical Y81.3
      therapeutic Y81.1
    radiological Y78.8
      accessory Y78.2
      diagnostic Y78.0
      miscellaneous Y78.8
      monitoring Y78.0
      prosthetic Y78.2
      rehabilitative Y78.1
      surgical Y78.3
      therapeutic Y78.1
    urology Y73.8
      accessory Y73.2
      diagnostic Y73.0
      miscellaneous Y73.8
      monitoring Y73.0
      prosthetic Y73.2
      rehabilitative Y73.1
      surgical Y73.3
      therapeutic Y73.1
Incineration (accidental) — *see* Exposure, fire
Infanticide — *see* Assault
Infrasound waves (causing injury) W49.9 ☑
Ingestion
  foreign body (causing injury) (with obstruction) — *see*
    Foreign body, alimentary canal
  poisonous
    plant(s) X58 ☑
    substance NEC — *see* Table of Drugs and Chemicals
Inhalation
  excessively cold substance, man-made — *see* Expo-
    sure, cold, man-made
  food (any type) (into respiratory tract) (with asphyxia,
    obstruction respiratory tract, suffocation) — *see*
    categories T17 and T18 ☑
  foreign body -– *see* Foreign body, aspiration
  gastric contents (with asphyxia, obstruction respiratory
    passage, suffocation) T17.81- ☑
  hot air or gases X14.0 ☑
  liquid air, hydrogen, nitrogen W93.12 ☑
    suicide (attempt) X83.2 ☑
  steam X13.0 ☑
    assault X98.0 ☑

Inhalation — *continued*
  steam — *continued*
    stated as undetermined whether accidental or intentional Y27.0 ☑
    suicide (attempt) X77.0 ☑
  toxic gas — *see* Table of Drugs and Chemicals
  vomitus (with asphyxia, obstruction respiratory passage, suffocation) T17.81- ☑
Injury, injured (accidental(ly)) NOS X58 ☑
  by, caused by, from
    assault — *see* Assault
    law-enforcing agent, police, in course of legal intervention — *see* Legal intervention
  suicide (attempt) X83.8 ☑
  due to, in
    civil insurrection — *see* War operations
    fight (*see also* Assault, fight) Y04.0 ☑
    war operations — *see* War operations
  homicide (*see also* Assault) Y09
  inflicted (by)
    in course of arrest (attempted), suppression of disturbance, maintenance of order, by law-enforcing agents — *see* Legal intervention
    other person
      stated as
        accidental X58 ☑
        intentional, homicide (attempt) — *see* Assault
        undetermined whether accidental or intentional Y33 ☑
  purposely (inflicted) by other person(s) — *see* Assault
  self-inflicted X83.8 ☑
    stated as accidental X58 ☑
  specified cause NEC X58 ☑
  undetermined whether accidental or intentional Y33 ☑
Insolation, effects X30 ☑
Insufficient nourishment X58 ☑
Interruption of respiration (by)
  food (lodged in esophagus) — *see* categories T17 and T18 ☑
  vomitus (lodged in esophagus) T17.81- ☑
Intervention, legal — *see* Legal intervention
Intoxication
  drug — *see* Table of Drugs and Chemicals
  poison — *see* Table of Drugs and Chemicals

J

Jammed (accidentally)
  between objects (moving) (stationary and moving) W23.0 ☑
    stationary W23.1 ☑
Jumped, jumping
  before moving object NEC X81.8 ☑
    motor vehicle X81.0 ☑
    subway train X81.1 ☑
    train X81.1 ☑
    undetermined whether accidental or intentional Y31 ☑
  from
    boat (into water) voluntarily, without accident (to or on boat) W16.712 ☑
      with
        accident to or on boat — *see* Accident, watercraft
        drowning or submersion W16.711 ☑
          suicide (attempt) X71.3 ☑
      striking bottom W16.722 ☑
        causing drowning W16.721 ☑
    building (*see also* Jumped, from, high place) W13.9 ☑
      burning (uncontrolled fire) X00.5 ☑
    high place NEC W17.89 ☑
      suicide (attempt) X80 ☑
      undetermined whether accidental or intentional Y30 ☑
    structure (*see also* Jumped, from, high place) W13.9 ☑
      burning (uncontrolled fire) X00.5 ☑
  into water W16.92 ☑
    causing drowning W16.91 ☑
    from, off watercraft — *see* Jumped, from, boat
    in
      natural body W16.612 ☑
        causing drowning W16.611 ☑

Jumped, jumping — *continued*
  into water — *continued*
    in — *continued*
      natural body — *continued*
        striking bottom W16.622 ☑
          causing drowning W16.621 ☑
      specified place NEC W16.812 ☑
        causing drowning W16.811 ☑
        striking
          bottom W16.822 ☑
            causing drowning W16.821 ☑
          wall W16.832 ☑
            causing drowning W16.831 ☑
      swimming pool W16.512 ☑
        causing drowning W16.511 ☑
        striking
          bottom W16.522 ☑
            causing drowning W16.521 ☑
          wall W16.532 ☑
            causing drowning W16.531 ☑
  suicide (attempt) X71.3 ☑

K

Kicked by
  animal NEC W55.82 ☑
  person(s) (accidentally) W50.1 ☑
    with intent to injure or kill Y04.0 ☑
    as, or caused by, a crowd or human stampede (with fall) W52 ☑
    assault Y04.0 ☑
    homicide (attempt) Y04.0 ☑
    in
      fight Y04.0 ☑
      legal intervention
        injuring
          bystander Y35.812 ☑
          law enforcement personnel Y35.811 ☑
          suspect Y35.813 ☑
Kicking against
  object W22.8 ☑
    sports equipment W21.9 ☑
    stationary wW22.09
      sports equipment W21.89 ☑
  person — *see* Striking against, person
  sports equipment W21.9 ☑
Killed, killing (accidentally) NOS (*see also* Injury) X58 ☑
  in
    action — *see* War operations
    brawl, fight (hand) (fists) (foot) Y04.0 ☑
      by weapon (*see also* Assault)
        cutting, piercing — *see* Assault, cutting or piercing instrument
        firearm — *see* Discharge, firearm, by type, homicide
  self
    stated as
      accident NOS X58 ☑
      suicide — *see* Suicide
      undetermined whether accidental or intentional Y33 ☑
Knocked down (accidentally) (by) NOS X58 ☑
  animal (not being ridden) NEC (*see also* Struck by, by type of animal)
  crowd or human stampede W52 ☑
  person W51 ☑
    in brawl, fight Y04.0 ☑
  transport vehicle NEC (*see also* Accident, transport) V09.9 ☑

L

Laceration NEC — *see* Injury
Lack of
  care (helpless person) (infant) (newborn) X58 ☑
  food except as result of abandonment or neglect X58 ☑
    due to abandonment or neglect X58 ☑
  water except as result of transport accident X58 ☑
    due to transport accident B — *see* Accident, transport, by type
    helpless person, infant, newborn X58 ☑
Landslide (falling on transport vehicle) X36.1 ☑
  caused by collapse of man-made structure X36.0 ☑
Late effect — *see* Sequelae

Legal
  execution (any method) — *see* Legal, intervention
  intervention (by)
    baton — *see* Legal, intervention, blunt object, baton
    bayonet — *see* Legal, intervention, sharp object, bayonet
    blow — *see* Legal, intervention, manhandling
    blunt object
      baton
        injuring
          bystander Y35.312 ☑
          law enforcement personnel Y35.311 ☑
          suspect Y35.313 ☑
      injuring
        bystander Y35.302 ☑
        law enforcement personnel Y35.301 ☑
        suspect Y35.303 ☑
      specified NEC
        injuring
          bystander Y35.392 ☑
          law enforcement personnel Y35.391 ☑
          suspect Y35.393 ☑
      stave
        injuring
          bystander Y35.392 ☑
          law enforcement personnel Y35.391 ☑
          suspect Y35.393 ☑
    bomb — *see* Legal, intervention, explosive
    cutting or piercing instrument — *see* Legal, intervention, sharp object
    dynamite — *see* Legal, intervention, explosive, dynamite
    explosive(s)
      dynamite
        injuring
          bystander Y35.112 ☑
          law enforcement personnel Y35.111 ☑
          suspect Y35.113 ☑
      grenade
        injuring
          bystander Y35.192 ☑
          law enforcement personnel Y35.191 ☑
          suspect Y35.193 ☑
      injuring
        bystander Y35.102 ☑
        law enforcement personnel Y35.101 ☑
        suspect Y35.103 ☑
      mortar bomb
        injuring
          bystander Y35.192 ☑
          law enforcement personnel Y35.191 ☑
          suspect Y35.193 ☑
      shell
        injuring
          bystander Y35.122 ☑
          law enforcement personnel Y35.121 ☑
          suspect Y35.123 ☑
      specified NEC
        injuring
          bystander Y35.192 ☑
          law enforcement personnel Y35.191 ☑
          suspect Y35.193 ☑
    firearm(s) (discharge)
      handgun
        injuring
          bystander Y35.022 ☑
          law enforcement personnel Y35.021 ☑
          suspect Y35.023 ☑
      injuring
        bystander Y35.002 ☑
        law enforcement personnel Y35.001 ☑
        suspect Y35.003 ☑
      machine gun
        injuring
          bystander Y35.012 ☑
          law enforcement personnel Y35.011 ☑
          suspect Y35.013 ☑
      rifle pellet
        injuring
          bystander Y35.032 ☑
          law enforcement personnel Y35.031 ☑
          suspect Y35.033 ☑
      rubber bullet
        injuring
          bystander Y35.042 ☑
          law enforcement personnel Y35.041 ☑

Legal — *continued*
 intervention — *continued*
  firearm(s) — *continued*
   rubber bullet — *continued*
    injuring
     suspect Y35.043 ☑
   shotgun — *see* Legal, intervention, firearm, specified NEC
   specified NEC
    injuring
     bystander Y35.092 ☑
     law enforcement personnel Y35.091 ☑
     suspect Y35.093 ☑
  gas (asphyxiation) (poisoning)
   injuring
    bystander Y35.202 ☑
    law enforcement personnel Y35.201 ☑
    suspect Y35.203 ☑
   specified NEC
    injuring
     bystander Y35.292 ☑
     law enforcement personnel Y35.291 ☑
     suspect Y35.293 ☑
   tear gas
    injuring
     bystander Y35.212 ☑
     law enforcement personnel Y35.211 ☑
     suspect Y35.213 ☑
  grenade — *see* Legal, intervention, explosive, grenade
  injuring
   bystander Y35.92 ☑
   law enforcement personnel Y35.91 ☑
   suspect Y35.93 ☑
  late effect (of) — *see* with 7th character S Y35 ☑
  manhandling
   injuring
    bystander Y35.812 ☑
    law enforcement personnel Y35.811 ☑
    suspect Y35.813 ☑
  sequelae (of) — *see* with 7th character S Y35 ☑
  sharp objects
   bayonet
    injuring
     bystander Y35.412 ☑
     law enforcement personnel Y35.411 ☑
     suspect Y35.413 ☑
   injuring
    bystander Y35.402 ☑
    law enforcement personnel Y35.401 ☑
    suspect Y35.403 ☑
   specified NEC
    injuring
     bystander Y35.492 ☑
     law enforcement personnel Y35.491 ☑
     suspect Y35.493 ☑
  specified means NEC
   injuring
    bystander Y35.892 ☑
    law enforcement personnel Y35.891 ☑
    suspect Y35.893 ☑
  stabbing — *see* Legal, intervention, sharp object
  stave — *see* Legal, intervention, blunt object, stave
  tear gas — *see* Legal, intervention, gas, tear gas
  truncheon — *see* Legal, intervention, blunt object, stave
Lightning (shock) (stroke) (struck by) — *see* subcategory T75.0 ☑
 causing fire — *see* Exposure, fire
Loss of control (transport vehicle) NEC — *see* Accident, transport
Lost at sea NOS — *see* Drowning, due to, fall overboard
Low
 pressure (effects) — *see* Air, pressure, low
 temperature (effects) — *see* Exposure, cold
Lying before train, vehicle or other moving object X81.8 ☑
 subway train X81.1 ☑
 train X81.1 ☑
 undetermined whether accidental or intentional Y31 ☑
Lynching — *see* Assault

M

Malfunction (mechanism or component) (of)

Malfunction — *continued*
 firearm W34.10 ☑
  airgun W34.110 ☑
  BB gun W34.110 ☑
  gas, air or spring-operated gun NEC W34.118 ☑
  handgun W32.1 ☑
  hunting rifle W33.12 ☑
  larger firearm W33.10 ☑
   specified NEC W33.19 ☑
  machine gun W33.13 ☑
  paintball gun W34.111 ☑
  pellet gun W34.110 ☑
  shotgun W33.11 ☑
  specified NEC W34.19 ☑
  Very pistol [flare] W34.19 ☑
 handgun — *see* Malfunction, firearm, handgun
Maltreatment — *see* Perpetrator
Mangled (accidentally) NOS X58 ☑
Manhandling (in brawl, fight) Y04.0 ☑
 legal intervention — *see* Legal, intervention, manhandling
Manslaughter (nonaccidental) — *see* Assault
Mauled by animal NEC W55.89 ☑
Medical procedure, complication of (delayed or as an abnormal reaction without mention of misadventure) — *see* Complication of or following, by specified type of procedure
 due to or as a result of misadventure — *see* Misadventure
Melting (due to fire) (*see also* Exposure, fire)
 apparel NEC X06.3 ☑
 clothes, clothing NEC X06.3 ☑
  nightwear X05 ☑
 fittings or furniture (burning building) (uncontrolled fire) X00.8 ☑
 nightwear X05 ☑
 plastic jewelry X06.1 ☑
Mental cruelty X58 ☑
Military operations (injuries to military and civilians occuring during peacetime on military property and during routine military exercises and operations) (by) (from) (involving) Y37.90- ☑
 air blast Y37.20- ☑
 aircraft
  destruction — *see* Military operations, destruction of aircraft
  airway restriction — *see* Military operations, restriction of airways
 asphyxiation — *see* Military operations, restriction of airways
 biological weapons Y37.6X- ☑
 blast Y37.20- ☑
 blast fragments Y37.20- ☑
 blast wave Y37.20- ☑
 blast wind Y37.20- ☑
 bomb Y37.20- ☑
  dirty Y37.50- ☑
  gasoline Y37.31- ☑
  incendiary Y37.31- ☑
  petrol Y37.31- ☑
 bullet Y37.43- ☑
  incendiary Y37.32- ☑
  rubber Y37.41- ☑
 chemical weapons Y37.7X- ☑
 combat
  hand to hand (unarmed) combat Y37.44- ☑
  using blunt or piercing object Y37.45- ☑
 conflagration — *see* Military operations, fire
 conventional warfare NEC Y37.49- ☑
 depth-charge Y37.01- ☑
 destruction of aircraft Y37.10- ☑
  due to
   air to air missile Y37.11- ☑
   collision with other aircraft Y37.12- ☑
   detonation (accidental) of onboard munitions and explosives Y37.14- ☑
   enemy fire or explosives Y37.11- ☑
   explosive placed on aircraft Y37.11- ☑
   onboard fire Y37.13- ☑
   rocket propelled grenade [RPG] Y37.11- ☑
   small arms fire Y37.11- ☑
   surface to air missile Y37.11- ☑
  specified NEC Y37.19- ☑
 detonation (accidental) of
  onboard marine weapons Y37.05- ☑

Military operations — *continued*
 detonation of — *continued*
  own munitions or munitions launch device Y37.24- ☑
 dirty bomb Y37.50- ☑
 explosion (of) Y37.20- ☑
  aerial bomb Y37.21- ☑
  bomb NOS (*see also* Military operations, bomb(s)) Y37.20- ☑
  fragments Y37.20- ☑
  grenade Y37.29- ☑
  guided missile Y37.22- ☑
  improvised explosive device [IED] (person-borne) (roadside) (vehicle-borne) Y37.23- ☑
  land mine Y37.29- ☑
  marine mine (at sea) (in harbor) Y37.02- ☑
  marine weapon Y37.00- ☑
   specified NEC Y37.09- ☑
  own munitions or munitions launch device (accidental) Y37.24- ☑
  sea-based artillery shell Y37.03- ☑
  specified NEC Y37.29- ☑
  torpedo Y37.04- ☑
 fire Y37.30- ☑
  specified NEC Y37.39- ☑
 firearms
  discharge Y37.43- ☑
  pellets Y37.42- ☑
 flamethrower Y37.33- ☑
 fragments (from) (of)
  improvised explosive device [IED] (person-borne) (roadside) (vehicle-borne) Y37.26- ☑
  munitions Y37.25- ☑
  specified NEC Y37.29- ☑
  weapons Y37.27- ☑
 friendly fire Y37.92- ☑
 hand to hand (unarmed) combat Y37.44- ☑
 hot substances — *see* Military operations, fire
 incendiary bullet Y37.32- ☑
 nuclear weapon (effects of) Y37.50- ☑
  acute radiation exposure Y37.54- ☑
  blast pressure Y37.51- ☑
  direct blast Y37.51- ☑
  direct heat Y37.53- ☑
  fallout exposure Y37.54- ☑
  fireball Y37.53- ☑
  indirect blast (struck or crushed by blast debris) (being thrown by blast) Y37.52- ☑
  ionizing radiation (immediate exposure) Y37.54- ☑
  nuclear radiation Y37.54- ☑
  radiation
   ionizing (immediate exposure) Y37.54- ☑
   nuclear Y37.54- ☑
   thermal Y37.53- ☑
  secondary effects Y37.54- ☑
  specified NEC Y37.59- ☑
  thermal radiation Y37.53- ☑
 restriction of air (airway)
  intentional Y37.46- ☑
  unintentional Y37.47- ☑
 rubber bullets Y37.41- ☑
 shrapnel NOS Y37.29- ☑
 suffocation — *see* Military operations, restriction of airways
 unconventional warfare NEC Y37.7X- ☑
 underwater blast NOS Y37.00- ☑
 warfare
  conventional NEC Y37.49- ☑
  unconventional NEC Y37.7X- ☑
 weapon of mass destruction [WMD] Y37.91- ☑
 weapons
  biological weapons Y37.6X- ☑
  chemical Y37.7X- ☑
  nuclear (effects of) Y37.50- ☑
   acute radiation exposure Y37.54- ☑
   blast pressure Y37.51- ☑
   direct blast Y37.51- ☑
   direct heat Y37.53- ☑
   fallout exposure Y37.54- ☑
   fireball Y37.53- ☑
   indirect blast (struck or crushed by blast debris) (being thrown by blast) Y37.52- ☑
   radiation
    ionizing (immediate exposure) Y37.54- ☑
    nuclear Y37.54- ☑
    thermal Y37.53- ☑

Military operations — *continued*
  weapons — *continued*
    nuclear — *continued*
      secondary effects Y37.54- ☑
      specified NEC Y37.59- ☑
    of mass destruction [WMD] Y37.91- ☑
Misadventure(s) **to patient**(s) **during surgical or medical care** Y69
  contaminated medical or biological substance (blood, drug, fluid) Y64.9
    administered (by) NEC Y64.9
      immunization Y64.1
      infusion Y64.0
      injection Y64.1
      specified means NEC Y64.8
      transfusion Y64.0
      vaccination Y64.1
  excessive amount of blood or other fluid during transfusion or infusion Y63.0
  failure
    in dosage Y63.9
      electroshock therapy Y63.4
      inappropriate temperature (too hot or too cold) in local application and packing Y63.5
      infusion
        excessive amount of fluid Y63.0
        incorrect dilution of fluid Y63.1
      insulin-shock therapy Y63.4
      nonadministration of necessary drug or biological substance Y63.6
      overdose — *see* Table of Drugs and Chemicals
      radiation, in therapy Y63.2
      radiation
        overdose Y63.2
      specified procedure NEC Y63.8
      transfusion
        excessive amount of blood Y63.0
    mechanical, of instrument or apparatus (any) (during any procedure) Y65.8
    sterile precautions (during procedure) Y62.9
      aspiration of fluid or tissue (by puncture or catheterization, except heart) Y62.6
      biopsy (except needle aspiration) Y62.8
        needle (aspirating) Y62.6
      blood sampling Y62.6
      catheterization Y62.6
        heart Y62.5
      dialysis (kidney) Y62.2
      endoscopic examination Y62.4
      enema Y62.8
      immunization Y62.3
      infusion Y62.1
      injection Y62.3
      needle biopsy Y62.6
      paracentesis (abdominal) (thoracic) Y62.6
      perfusion Y62.2
      puncture (lumbar) Y62.6
      removal of catheter or packing Y62.8
      specified procedure NEC Y62.8
      surgical operation Y62.0
      transfusion Y62.1
      vaccination Y62.3
    suture or ligature during surgical procedure Y65.2
    to introduce or to remove tube or instrument B — *see* Failure, to
  hemorrhage — *see* Index to Diseases and Injuries, Complication(s)
  inadvertent exposure of patient to radiation Y63.3
  inappropriate
    operation performed — *see* Inappropriate operation performed
    temperature (too hot or too cold) in local application or packing Y63.5
  infusion (*see also* Misadventure, by type, infusion) Y69
    excessive amount of fluid Y63.0
    incorrect dilution of fluid Y63.1
    wrong fluid Y65.1
  mismatched blood in transfusion Y65.0
  nonadministration of necessary drug or biological substance
    overdose — *see* Table of Drugs and Chemicals
    radiation (in therapy) Y63.2
  perforation — *see* Index to Diseases and Injuries, Complication(s)
  performance of inappropriate operation — *see* !Inappropriate operation performed
  puncture — *see* Index to Diseases and Injuries, Complication(s)

Misadventure(s) **to patient**(s) **during surgical or medical care** — *continued*
  specified type NEC Y65.8
    failure
      suture or ligature during surgical operation Y65.2
      to introduce or to remove tube or instrument B — *see* Failure, to
    infusion of wrong fluid Y65.1
    performance of inappropriate operation — *see* Inappropriate operation performed
    transfusion of mismatched blood Y65.0
    wrong
      fluid in infusion Y65.1
      placement of endotracheal tube during anesthetic procedure Y65.3
  transfusion — *see* Misadventure, by type, transfusion
    excessive amount of blood Y63.0
    mismatched blood Y65.0
  wrong
    drug given in error — *see* Table of Drugs and Chemicals
    fluid in infusion Y65.1
    placement of endotracheal tube during anesthetic procedure Y65.3
Mismatched blood in transfusion Y65.0
Motion sickness T75.3 ☑
Mountain sickness W94.11 ☑
Mudslide (of cataclysmic nature) — *see* Landslide
Murder (attempt) — *see* Assault

N

Nail, contact with W45.0 ☑
  gun W29.4 ☑
Neglect (criminal) (homicidal intent) X58 ☑
Noise (causing injury) (pollution) W42.9 ☑
  supersonic W42.0 ☑
Nonadministration (of)
  drug or biological substance (necessary) Y63.6
  surgical and medical care Y66
Nosocomial condition Y95

O

Object
  falling
    from, in, on, hitting
      machinery — *see* Contact, with, by type of machine
  set in motion by
    accidental explosion or rupture of pressure vessel W38 ☑
    firearm — *see* Discharge, firearm, by type
    machine(ry) — *see* Contact, with, by type of machine
Overdose (drug) — *see* Table of Drugs and Chemicals
  radiation Y63.2
Overexertion — *see* category Y93 ☑
Overexposure (accidental) (to)
  cold (*see also* Exposure, cold) X31 ☑
    due to man-made conditions — *see* Exposure, cold, man-made
  heat (*see also* Heat) X30 ☑
  radiation — *see* Radiation
  radioactivity W88.0 ☑
  sun (sunburn) X32 ☑
  weather NEC — *see* Forces of nature
  wind NEC — *see* Forces of nature
Overheated — *see* Heat
Overturning (accidental)
  machinery — *see* Contact, with, by type of machine
  transport vehicle NEC (*see also* Accident, transport) V89.9 ☑
  watercraft (causing drowning, submersion) (*see also* Drowning, due to, accident to, watercraft, overturning)
    causing injury except drowning or submersion B — *see* Accident, watercraft, causing, injury NEC

P

Parachute descent (voluntary) (without accident to aircraft) V97.29 ☑

Parachute descent — *continued*
  due to accident to aircraft — *see* Accident, transport, aircraft
Pecked by bird W61.99 ☑
Perforation during medical or surgical treatment as misadventure — *see* Index to Diseases and Injuries, Complication(s)
Perpetrator, perpetration, of assault, maltreatment and neglect (by) Y07.9
  boyfriend Y07.03
  brother Y07.410
    stepbrother Y07.435
  coach Y07.53
  cousin
    female Y07.491
    male Y07.490
  daycare provider Y07.519
    at-home
      adult care Y07.512
      childcare Y07.510
    care center
      adult care Y07.513
      childcare Y07.511
  family member NEC Y07.499
  father Y07.11
    adoptive Y07.13
    foster Y07.420
    stepfather Y07.430
  foster father Y07.420
  foster mother Y07.421
  girl friend Y07.04
  healthcare provider Y07.529
    mental health Y07.521
    specified NEC Y07.528
  husband Y07.01
  instructor Y07.53
  mother Y07.12
    adoptive Y07.14
    foster Y07.421
    stepmother Y07.433
  nonfamily member Y07.50
    specified NEC Y07.59
  nurse Y07.528
  occupational therapist Y07.528
  partner of parent
    female Y07.434
    male Y07.432
  physical therapist Y07.528
  sister Y07.411
  speech therapist Y07.528
  stepbrother Y07.435
  stepfather Y07.430
  stepmother Y07.433
  stepsister Y07.436
  teacher Y07.53
  wife Y07.02
Piercing — *see* Contact, with, by type of object or machine
Pinched
  between objects (moving) (stationary and moving) W23.0 ☑
    stationary W23.1 ☑
Pinned under machine(ry) — *see* Contact, with, by type of machine
Place of occurrence Y92.9
  abandoned house Y92.89
  airplane Y92.813
  airport Y92.520
  ambulatory health services establishment NEC Y92.538
  ambulatory surgery center Y92.530
  amusement park Y92.831
  apartment (co-op) — *see* Place of occurrence, residence, apartment
  assembly hall Y92.29
  bank Y92.510
  barn Y92.71
  baseball field Y92.320
  basketball court Y92.310
  beach Y92.832
  boarding house — *see* Place of occurrence, residence, boarding house
  boat Y92.814
  bowling alley Y92.39
  bridge Y92.89
  building under construction Y92.61
  bus Y92.811
    station Y92.521
  cafe Y92.511

Place of occurrence — *continued*

campsite Y92.833
campus — *see* Place of occurrence, school
canal Y92.89
car Y92.810
casino Y92.59
children's home — *see* Place of occurrence, residence, institutional, orphanage
church Y92.22
cinema Y92.26
clubhouse Y92.29
coal pit Y92.64
college (community) Y92.214
condominium — *see* Place of occurrence, residence, apartment
construction area — *see* Place of occurrence, industrial and construction area
convalescent home — *see* Place of occurrence, residence, institutional, nursing home
court-house Y92.240
cricket ground Y92.328
cultural building Y92.258
    art gallery Y92.250
    museum Y92.251
    music hall Y92.252
    opera house Y92.253
    specified NEC Y92.258
    theater Y92.254
dancehall Y92.252
day nursery Y92.210
dentist office Y92.531
derelict house Y92.89
desert Y92.820
dockyard Y92.62
dock NOS Y92.89
doctor's office Y92.531
dormitory — *see* Place of occurrence, residence, institutional, school dormitory
dry dock Y92.62
factory (building) (premises) Y92.63
farm (land under cultivation) (outbuildings) Y92.79
    barn Y92.71
    chicken coop Y92.72
    field Y92.73
    hen house Y92.72
    house — *see* Place of occurrence, residence, house
    orchard Y92.74
    specified NEC Y92.79
football field Y92.321
forest Y92.821
freeway Y92.411
gallery Y92.250
garage (commercial) Y92.59
    boarding house Y92.044
    military base Y92.135
    mobile home Y92.025
    nursing home Y92.124
    orphanage Y92.114
    private house Y92.015
    reform school Y92.155
gas station Y92.524
gasworks Y92.69
golf course Y92.39
gravel pit Y92.64
grocery Y92.512
gymnasium Y92.39
handball court Y92.318
harbor Y92.89
harness racing course Y92.39
healthcare provider office Y92.531
highway (interstate) Y92.411
hill Y92.828
hockey rink Y92.330
home — *see* Place of occurrence, residence
hospice — *see* Place of occurrence, residence, institutional, nursing home
hospital Y92.239
    cafeteria Y92.233
    corridor Y92.232
    operating room Y92.234
    patient
        bathroom Y92.231
        room Y92.230
    specified NEC Y92.238
hotel Y92.59
house (*see also* Place of occurrence, residence)
    abandoned Y92.89
    under construction Y92.61

Place of occurrence — *continued*

industrial and construction area (yard) Y92.69
    building under construction Y92.61
    dock Y92.62
    dry dock Y92.62
    factory Y92.63
    gasworks Y92.69
    mine Y92.64
    oil rig Y92.65
    pit Y92.64
    power station Y92.69
    shipyard Y92.62
    specified NEC Y92.69
    tunnel under construction Y92.69
    workshop Y92.69
kindergarten Y92.211
lacrosse field Y92.328
lake Y92.828
library Y92.241
mall Y92.59
market Y92.512
marsh Y92.828
military
    base — *see* Place of occurrence, residence, institutional, military base
    training ground Y92.84
mine Y92.64
mosque Y92.22
motel Y92.59
motorway (interstate) Y92.411
mountain Y92.828
movie-house Y92.26
museum Y92.251
music-hall Y92.252
not applicable Y92.9
nuclear power station Y92.69
nursing home — *see* Place of occurrence, residence, institutional, nursing home
office building Y92.59
offshore installation Y92.65
oil rig Y92.65
old people's home — *see* Place of occurrence, residence, institutional, specified NEC
opera-house Y92.253
orphanage — *see* Place of occurrence, residence, institutional, orphanage
outpatient surgery center Y92.530
park (public) Y92.830
    amusement Y92.831
parking garage Y92.89
    lot Y92.481
pavement Y92.480
physician office Y92.531
polo field Y92.328
pond Y92.828
post office Y92.242
power station Y92.69
prairie Y92.828
prison — *see* Place of occurrence, residence, institutional, prison
public
    administration building Y92.248
        city hall Y92.243
        courthouse Y92.240
        library Y92.241
        post office Y92.242
        specified NEC Y92.248
    building NEC Y92.29
    hall Y92.29
    place NOS Y92.89
race course Y92.39
radio station Y92.59
railway line (bridge) Y92.85
ranch (outbuildings) — *see* Place of occurrence, farm
recreation area Y92.838
    amusement park Y92.831
    beach Y92.832
    campsite Y92.833
    park (public) Y92.830
    seashore Y92.832
    specified NEC Y92.838
reform school - — *see* Place of occurrence, residence, institutional, reform school
religious institution Y92.22
residence (non-institutional) (private) Y92.009
    apartment Y92.039
        bathroom Y92.031
        bedroom Y92.032

Place of occurrence — *continued*

residence — *continued*
    apartment — *continued*
        kitchen Y92.030
        specified NEC Y92.038
    bathroom Y92.002
    bedroom Y92.003
    boarding house Y92.049
        bathroom Y92.041
        bedroom Y92.042
        driveway Y92.043
        garage Y92.044
        garden Y92.046
        kitchen Y92.040
        specified NEC Y92.048
        swimming pool Y92.045
        yard Y92.046
    dining room Y92.001
    garden Y92.007
    home Y92.009
    house, single family Y92.019
        bathroom Y92.012
        bedroom Y92.013
        dining room Y92.011
        driveway Y92.014
        garage Y92.015
        garden Y92.017
        kitchen Y92.010
        specified NEC Y92.018
        swimming pool Y92.016
        yard Y92.017
    institutional Y92.10
        children's home — *see* Place of occurrence, residence, institutional, orphanage
        hospice — *see* Place of occurrence, residence, institutional, nursing home
        military base Y92.139
            barracks Y92.133
            garage Y92.135
            garden Y92.137
            kitchen Y92.130
            mess hall Y92.131
            specified NEC Y92.138
            swimming pool Y92.136
            yard Y92.137
        nursing home Y92.129
            bathroom Y92.121
            bedroom Y92.122
            driveway Y92.123
            garage Y92.124
            garden Y92.126
            kitchen Y92.120
            specified NEC Y92.128
            swimming pool Y92.125
            yard Y92.126
        orphanage Y92.119
            bathroom Y92.111
            bedroom Y92.112
            driveway Y92.113
            garage Y92.114
            garden Y92.116
            kitchen Y92.110
            specified NEC Y92.118
            swimming pool Y92.115
            yard Y92.116
        prison Y92.149
            bathroom Y92.142
            cell Y92.143
            courtyard Y92.147
            dining room Y92.141
            kitchen Y92.140
            specified NEC Y92.148
            swimming pool Y92.146
        reform school Y92.159
            bathroom Y92.152
            bedroom Y92.153
            dining room Y92.151
            driveway Y92.154
            garage Y92.155
            garden Y92.157
            kitchen Y92.150
            specified NEC Y92.158
            swimming pool Y92.156
            yard Y92.157
        school dormitory Y92.169
            bathroom Y92.162
            bedroom Y92.163
            dining room Y92.161

Place of occurrence — *continued*
　residence — *continued*
　　institutional — *continued*
　　　school dormitory — *continued*
　　　　kitchen Y92.160
　　　　specified NEC Y92.168
　　　specified NEC Y92.199
　　　　bathroom Y92.192
　　　　bedroom Y92.193
　　　　dining room Y92.191
　　　　driveway Y92.194
　　　　garage Y92.195
　　　　garden Y92.197
　　　　kitchen Y92.190
　　　　specified NEC Y92.198
　　　　swimming pool Y92.196
　　　　yard Y92.197
　　kitchen Y92.000
　　mobile home Y92.029
　　　bathroom Y92.022
　　　bedroom Y92.023
　　　dining room Y92.021
　　　driveway Y92.024
　　　garage Y92.025
　　　garden Y92.027
　　　kitchen Y92.020
　　　specified NEC Y92.028
　　　swimming pool Y92.026
　　　yard Y92.027
　　specified place in residence NEC Y92.009
　　specified residence type NEC Y92.099
　　　bathroom Y92.091
　　　bedroom Y92.092
　　　driveway Y92.093
　　　garage Y92.094
　　　garden Y92.096
　　　kitchen Y92.090
　　　specified NEC Y92.098
　　　swimming pool Y92.095
　　　yard Y92.096
　restaurant Y92.511
　riding school Y92.39
　river Y92.828
　road Y92.488
　rodeo ring Y92.39
　rugby field Y92.328
　same day surgery center Y92.530
　sand pit Y92.64
　school (private) (public) (state) Y92.219
　　college Y92.214
　　daycare center Y92.210
　　elementary school Y92.211
　　high school Y92.213
　　kindergarten Y92.211
　　middle school Y92.212
　　specified NEC Y92.218
　　trace school Y92.215
　　university Y92.214
　　vocational school Y92.215
　sea (shore) Y92.832
　senior citizen center Y92.29
　service area
　　airport Y92.520
　　bus station Y92.521
　　gas station Y92.524
　　highway rest stop Y92.523
　　railway station Y92.522
　shipyard Y92.62
　shop (commercial) Y92.513
　sidewalk Y92.480
　silo Y92.79
　skating rink (roller) Y92.331
　　ice Y92.330
　slaughter house Y92.86
　soccer field Y92.322
　specified place NEC Y92.89
　sports area Y92.39
　　athletic
　　　court Y92.318
　　　　basketball Y92.310
　　　　specified NEC Y92.318
　　　　squash Y92.311
　　　　tennis Y92.312
　　　field Y92.328
　　　　baseball Y92.320
　　　　cricket ground Y92.328
　　　　football Y92.321
　　　　hockey Y92.328

Place of occurrence — *continued*
　sports area — *continued*
　　athletic — *continued*
　　　field — *continued*
　　　　soccer Y92.322
　　　　specified NEC Y92.328
　　golf course Y92.39
　　gymnasium Y92.39
　　riding school Y92.39
　　skating rink (roller) Y92.331
　　　ice Y92.330
　　stadium Y92.39
　　swimming pool Y92.34
　squash court Y92.311
　stadium Y92.39
　steeplechasing course Y92.39
　store Y92.512
　stream Y92.828
　street and highway Y92.410
　　bike path Y92.482
　　freeway Y92.411
　　highway ramp Y92.415
　　interstate highway Y92.411
　　local residential or business street Y92.414
　　motorway Y92.411
　　parking lot Y92.481
　　parkway Y92.412
　　sidewalk Y92.480
　　specified NEC Y92.488
　　state road Y92.413
　subway car Y92.816
　supermarket Y92.512
　swamp Y92.828
　swimming pool (public) Y92.34
　　private (at) Y92.095
　　　boarding house Y92.045
　　　military base Y92.136
　　　mobile home Y92.026
　　　nursing home Y92.125
　　　orphanage Y92.115
　　　prison Y92.146
　　　reform school Y92.156
　　　single family residence Y92.016
　synagogue Y92.22
　television station Y92.59
　tennis court Y92.312
　theater Y92.254
　trade area Y92.59
　　bank Y92.510
　　cafe Y92.511
　　casino Y92.59
　　garage Y92.59
　　hotel Y92.59
　　market Y92.512
　　office building Y92.59
　　radio station Y92.59
　　restaurant Y92.511
　　shop Y92.513
　　shopping mall Y92.59
　　store Y92.512
　　supermarket Y92.512
　　television station Y92.59
　　warehouse Y92.59
　trailer park, residential — *see* Place of occurrence,
　　　residence, mobile home
　trailer site NOS Y92.89
　train Y92.815
　　station Y92.522
　truck Y92.812
　tunnel under construction Y92.69
　university Y92.214
　urgent (health) care center Y92.532
　vehicle (transport) Y92.818
　　airplane Y92.813
　　boat Y92.814
　　bus Y92.811
　　car Y92.810
　　specified NEC Y92.818
　　subway car Y92.816
　　train Y92.815
　　truck Y92.812
　warehouse Y92.59
　water reservoir Y92.89
　wilderness area Y92.828
　　desert Y92.820
　　forest Y92.821
　　marsh Y92.828
　　mountain Y92.828

Place of occurrence — *continued*
　wilderness area — *continued*
　　prairie Y92.828
　　specified NEC Y92.828
　　swamp Y92.828
　workshop Y92.69
　yard, private Y92.096
　　boarding house Y92.046
　　mobile home Y92.027
　　single family house Y92.017
　youth center Y92.29
　zoo (zoological garden) Y92.834
Plumbism — *see* Table of Drugs and Chemicals, lead
Poisoning (accidental) (by) (*see also* Table of Drugs and
　　Chemicals)
　by plant, thorns, spines, sharp leaves or other mecha-
　　　nisms NEC X58 ☑
　carbon monoxide
　　generated by
　　　motor vehicle — *see* Accident, transport
　　　watercraft (in transit) (not in transit) V93.89 ☑
　　　　ferry boat V93.81 ☑
　　　　fishing boat V93.82 ☑
　　　　jet skis V93.83 ☑
　　　　liner V93.81 ☑
　　　　merchant ship V93.80 ☑
　　　　passenger ship V93.81 ☑
　　　　powered craft NEC V93.83 ☑
　caused by injection of poisons into skin by plant
　　　thorns, spines, sharp leaves X58 ☑
　　marine or sea plants (venomous) X58 ☑
　execution — *see* Legal, intervention, gas
　　intervention
　　　by gas — *see* Legal, intervention, gas
　　　other specified means — *see* Legal, interven-
　　　　tion, specified means NEC
　exhaust gas
　　generated by
　　　motor vehicle — *see* Accident, transport
　　　watercraft (in transit) (not in transit) V93.89 ☑
　　　　ferry boat V93.81 ☑
　　　　fishing boat V93.82 ☑
　　　　jet skis V93.83 ☑
　　　　liner V93.81 ☑
　　　　merchant ship V93.80 ☑
　　　　passenger ship V93.81 ☑
　　　　powered craft NEC V93.83 ☑
　fumes or smoke due to
　　explosion (*see also* Explosion) W40.9 ☑
　　fire — *see* Exposure, fire
　　ignition — *see* Ignition
　gas
　　in legal intervention — *see* Legal, intervention, gas
　　legal execution — *see* Legal, intervention, gas
　in war operations — *see* War operations
　legal
Powder burn (by) (from)
　airgun W34.110 ☑
　BB gun W34.110 ☑
　firearm NEC W34.19 ☑
　gas, air or spring-operated gun NEC W34.118 ☑
　handgun W32.1 ☑
　hunting rifle W33.12 ☑
　larger firearm W33.10 ☑
　　specified NEC W33.19 ☑
　machine gun W33.13 ☑
　paintball gun W34.111 ☑
　pellet gun W34.110 ☑
　shotgun W33.11 ☑
　Very pistol [flare] W34.19 ☑
Premature cessation (of) **surgical and medical care**
　　Y66
Privation (food) (water) X58 ☑
Procedure (operation)
　correct, on wrong side or body part (wrong side)
　　　(wrong site) Y65.53
　intended for another patient done on wrong patient
　　　Y65.52
　performed on patient not scheduled for surgery Y65.52
　performed on wrong patient Y65.52
　wrong, performed on correct patient Y65.51
Prolonged
　sitting in transport vehicle — *see* Travel, by type of
　　　vehicle
　stay in
　　high altitude as cause of anoxia, barodontalgia,
　　　barotitis or hypoxia W94.11 ☑

Prolonged — *continued*
  stay in — *continued*
    weightless environment X52 ☑
Pulling, excessive — *see* category Y93 ☑
Puncture, puncturing (*see also* Contact, with, by type
  of object or machine)
  by
    plant thorns, spines, sharp leaves or other mecha-
      nisms NEC W60 ☑
    during medical or surgical treatment as misadventure
      — *see* Index to Diseases and Injuries, Complica-
      tion(s)
Pushed, pushing (accidental) (injury in) (overexertion)
  see category Y93 ☑
  by other person(s) (accidental) W51 ☑
    with fall W03 ☑
      due to ice or snow W00.0 ☑
    as, or caused by, a crowd or human stampede (with
      fall) W52 ☑
    before moving object NEC Y02.8 ☑
      motor vehicle Y02.0 ☑
      subway train Y02.1 ☑
      train Y02.1 ☑
    from
      high place NEC
        in accidental circumstances W17.89 ☑
        stated as
          intentional, homicide (attempt) Y01 ☑
          undetermined whether accidental or
            intentional Y30 ☑
      transport vehicle NEC (*see also* Accident, trans-
        port) V89.9 ☑
        stated as
          intentional, homicide (attempt)
            Y08.89 ☑

R

Radiation (exposure to)
  arc lamps W89.0 ☑
  atomic power plant (malfunction) NEC W88.1 ☑
  complication of or abnormal reaction to medical radio-
    therapy Y84.2
  electromagnetic, ionizing W88.0 ☑
  gamma rays W88.1 ☑
  in
    war operations (from or following nuclear explo-
      sion) — *see* War operations
  inadvertent exposure of patient (receiving test or
    therapy) Y63.3
  infrared (heaters and lamps) W90.1 ☑
    excessive heat from W92 ☑
  ionized, ionizing (particles, artificially accelerated)
    radioisotopes W88.1 ☑
    specified NEC W88.8 ☑
    x-rays W88.0 ☑
  isotopes, radioactive — *see* Radiation, radioactive
    isotopes
  laser(s) W90.2 ☑
    in war operations — *see* War operations
    misadventure in medical care Y63.2
  light sources (man-made visible and ultraviolet)
    W89.9 ☑
    natural X32 ☑
    specified NEC W89.8 ☑
    tanning bed W89.1 ☑
    welding light W89.0 ☑
  man-made visible light W89.9 ☑
    specified NEC W89.8 ☑
    tanning bed W89.1 ☑
    welding light W89.0 ☑
  microwave W90.8 ☑
  misadventure in medical or surgical procedure Y63.2
  natural NEC X39.08 ☑
    radon X39.01 ☑
  overdose (in medical or surgical procedure) Y63.2
  radar W90.0 ☑
  radioactive isotopes (any) W88.1 ☑
    atomic power plant malfunction W88.1 ☑
    misadventure in medical or surgical treatment
      Y63.2
  radiofrequency W90.0 ☑
  radium NEC W88.1 ☑
  sun X32 ☑
  ultraviolet (light) (man-made) W89.9 ☑
    natural X32 ☑

Radiation — *continued*
  ultraviolet — *continued*
    specified NEC W89.8 ☑
    tanning bed W89.1 ☑
    welding light W89.0 ☑
  welding arc, torch, or light W89.0 ☑
    excessive heat from W92 ☑
  x-rays (hard) (soft) W88.0 ☑
Range disease W94.11 ☑
Rape (attempted) T74.2- ☑
Rat bite W53.11 ☑
Reaction, abnormal to medical procedure (*see also*
  Complication of or following, by type of procedure)
  Y84.9
  with misadventure — *see* Misadventure
  biologicals — *see* Table of Drugs and Chemicals
  drugs — *see* Table of Drugs and Chemicals
  vaccine — *see* Table of Drugs and Chemicals
Recoil
  airgun W34.110 ☑
  BB gun W34.110 ☑
  firearm NEC W34.19 ☑
  gas, air or spring-operated gun NEC W34.118 ☑
  handgun W32.1 ☑
  hunting rifle W33.12 ☑
  larger firearm W33.10 ☑
    specified NEC W33.19 ☑
  machine gun W33.13 ☑
  paintball gun W34.111 ☑
  pellet W34.110 ☑
  shotgun W33.11 ☑
  Very pistol [flare] W34.19 ☑
Reduction in
  atmospheric pressure — *see* Air, pressure, change
Rock falling on or hitting (accidentally) (person)
  W20.8 ☑
  in cave-in W20.0 ☑
Run over (accidentally) (by)
  animal (not being ridden) NEC W55.89 ☑
  machinery — *see* Contact, with, by specified type of
    machine
  transport vehicle NEC (*see also* Accident, transport)
    V09.9 ☑
    intentional homicide (attempt) Y03.0 ☑
    motor NEC V09.20 ☑
      intentional homicide (attempt) Y03.0 ☑
Running
  before moving object X81.8 ☑
    motor vehicle X81.0 ☑
Running off, away
  animal (being ridden) (*see also* Accident, transport)
    V80.918 ☑
    not being ridden W55.89 ☑
  animal-drawn vehicle NEC (*see also* Accident, trans-
    port) V80.928 ☑
  highway, road(way), street
    transport vehicle NEC (*see also* Accident, transport)
      V89.9 ☑
Rupture pressurized devices — *see* Explosion, by type
  of device

S

Saturnism — *see* Table of Drugs and Chemicals, lead
Scald, scalding (accidental) (by) (from) (in) X19 ☑
  air (hot) X14.1 ☑
  gases (hot) X14.1 ☑
  homicide (attempt) — *see* Assault, burning, hot object
  inflicted by other person
    stated as intentional, homicide (attempt) — *see*
      Assault, burning, hot object
  liquid (boiling) (hot) NEC X12 ☑
    stated as undetermined whether accidental or in-
      tentional Y27.2 ☑
    suicide (attempt) X77.2 ☑
  local application of externally applied substance in
    medical or surgical care Y63.5
  metal (molten) (liquid) (hot) NEC X18 ☑
  self-inflicted X77.9 ☑
  stated as undetermined whether accidental or inten-
    tional Y27.8 ☑
  steam X13.1 ☑
    assault X98.0 ☑
    stated as undetermined whether accidental or in-
      tentional Y27.0 ☑
    suicide (attempt) X77.0 ☑

Scald, scalding — *continued*
  suicide (attempt) X77.9 ☑
  vapor (hot) X13.1 ☑
    assault X98.0 ☑
    stated as undetermined whether accidental or in-
      tentional Y27.0 ☑
    suicide (attempt) X77.0 ☑
Scratched by
  cat W55.03 ☑
  person(s) (accidentally) W50.4 ☑
    with intent to injure or kill Y04.0 ☑
    as, or caused by, a crowd or human stampede (with
      fall) W52 ☑
    assault Y04.0 ☑
    homicide (attempt) Y04.0 ☑
    in
      fight Y04.0 ☑
      legal intervention
        injuring
          bystander Y35.892 ☑
          law enforcement personnel Y35.891 ☑
          suspect Y35.893 ☑
Seasickness T75.3 ☑
Self-harm NEC (*see also* External cause by type, undetermined whether accidental or intentional)
  intentional — *see* Suicide
  poisoning NEC — *see* Table of Drugs and Chemicals,
    poisoning, accidental
Self-inflicted (injury) **NEC** (*see also* External cause by
  type, undetermined whether accidental or intentional)
  intentional — *see* Suicide
  poisoning NEC — *see* Table of Drugs and Chemicals,
    poisoning, accidental
Sequelae (of)
  accident NEC — *see* W00-X58 with 7th character S
  assault (homicidal) (any means) — *see* X92-Y08 with
    7th character S
  homicide, attempt (any means) — *see* X92-Y08 with
    7th character S
  injury undetermined whether accidentally or purposely
    inflicted — *see* Y21-Y33 with 7th character S
  intentional self-harm (classifiable to X71-X83) — *see*
    X71-X83 with 7th character S
  legal intervention — *see* with 7th character S Y35 ☑
  motor vehicle accident — *see* V00-V99 with 7th char-
    acter S
  suicide, attempt (any means) — *see* X71-X83 with 7th
    character S
  transport accident — *see* V00-V99 with 7th character
    S
  war operations — *see* War operations
Shock
  electric — *see* Exposure, electric current
  from electric appliance (any) (faulty) W86.8 ☑
    domestic W86.0 ☑
    suicide (attempt) X83.1 ☑
Shooting, shot (accidental(ly)) (*see also* Discharge,
  firearm, by type)
  herself or himself — *see* Discharge, firearm by type,
    self-inflicted
  homicide (attempt) — *see* Discharge, firearm by type,
    homicide
  in war operations — *see* War operations
  inflicted by other person — *see* Discharge, firearm by
    type, homicide
    accidental — *see* Discharge, firearm, by type of
      firearm
  legal
    execution — *see* Legal, intervention, firearm
    intervention — *see* Legal, intervention, firearm
  self-inflicted — *see* Discharge, firearm by type, suicide
    accidental — *see* Discharge, firearm, by type of
      firearm
  suicide (attempt) — *see* Discharge, firearm by type,
    suicide
Shoving (accidentally) **by other person** — *see* Pushed,
  by other person
Sickness
  alpine W94.11 ☑
  motion — *see* Motion
  mountain W94.11 ☑
Sinking (accidental)
  watercraft (causing drowning, submersion) (*see also*
    Drowning, due to, accident to, watercraft, sink-
    ing)

Sinking — *continued*
  watercraft (*see also* Drowning, due to, accident to, watercraft, sinking) — *continued*
    causing injury except drowning or submersion B — *see* Accident, watercraft, causing, injury NEC
Siriasis X32 ☑
Slashed wrists — *see* Cut, self-inflicted
Slipping (accidental) (on same level) (with fall) W01.0 ☑
  without fall W18.40 ☑
    due to
      specified NEC W18.49 ☑
      stepping from one level to another W18.43 ☑
      stepping into hole or opening W18.42 ☑
      stepping on object W18.41 ☑
    on
      ice W00.0 ☑
        with skates — *see* Accident, transport, pedestrian, conveyance
      mud W01.0 ☑
      oil W01.0 ☑
      snow W00.0 ☑
        with skis — *see* Accident, transport, pedestrian, conveyance
      surface (slippery) (wet) NEC W01.0 ☑
Sliver, wood, contact with W45.8 ☑
Smoldering (due to fire) — *see* Exposure, fire
Sodomy (attempted) **by force** T74.2 ☑
Sound waves (causing injury) W42.9 ☑
  supersonic W42.0 ☑
Splinter, contact with W45.8 ☑
Stab, stabbing B — *see* Cut
Starvation X58 ☑
Status of external cause Y99.9
  child assisting in compensated work for family Y99.8
  civilian activity done for financial or other compensation Y99.0
  civilian activity done for income or pay Y99.0
  family member assisting in compensated work for other family member Y99.8
  hobby not done for income Y99.8
  leisure activity Y99.8
  military activity Y99.1
  off-duty activity of military personnel Y99.8
  recreation or sport not for income or while a student Y99.8
  specified NEC Y99.8
  student activity Y99.8
  volunteer activity Y99.2
Stepped on
  by
    animal (not being ridden) NEC W55.89 ☑
    crowd or human stampede W52 ☑
    person W50.0 ☑
Stepping on
  object W22.8 ☑
    with fall W18.31 ☑
    sports equipment W21.9 ☑
    stationary W22.09 ☑
      sports equipment W21.89 ☑
  person W51 ☑
    by crowd or human stampede W52 ☑
    sports equipment W21.9 ☑
Sting
  arthropod, nonvenomous W57 ☑
  insect, nonvenomous W57 ☑
Storm (cataclysmic) — *see* Forces of nature, cataclysmic storm
Straining, excessive — *see* category Y93 ☑
Strangling — *see* Strangulation
Strangulation (accidental) T71 ☑
Strenuous movements — *see* category Y93 ☑
Striking against
  airbag (automobile) W22.10 ☑
    driver side W22.11 ☑
    front passenger side W22.12 ☑
    specified NEC W22.19 ☑
  bottom when
    diving or jumping into water (in) W16.822 ☑
      causing drowning W16.821 ☑
      from boat W16.722 ☑
        causing drowning W16.721 ☑
      natural body W16.622 ☑
        causing drowning W16.621 ☑
      swimming pool W16.522 ☑
        causing drowning W16.521 ☑

Striking against — *continued*
  bottom when — *continued*
    falling into water (in) W16.322 ☑
      causing drowning W16.321 ☑
      fountain — *see* Striking against, bottom when, falling into water, specified NEC
      natural body W16.122 ☑
        causing drowning W16.121 ☑
      reservoir — *see* Striking against, bottom when, falling into water, specified NEC
      specified NEC W16.322 ☑
        causing drowning W16.321 ☑
      swimming pool W16.022 ☑
        causing drowning W16.021 ☑
  diving board (swimming-pool) W21.4 ☑
  object W22.8 ☑
    with
      drowning or submersion — *see* Drowning
      fall — *see* Fall, due to, bumping against, object
    caused by crowd or human stampede (with fall) W52
    furniture W22.03 ☑
    lamppost W22.02 ☑
    sports equipment W21.9 ☑
    stationary W22.09 ☑
      sports equipment W21.89 ☑
    wall W22.01 ☑
  person(s) W51 ☑
    with fall W03 ☑
      due to ice or snow W00.0 ☑
    as, or caused by, a crowd or human stampede (with fall) W52 ☑
    assault Y04.2 ☑
    homicide (attempt) Y04.2 ☑
  sports equipment W21.9 ☑
  wall (when) W22.01 ☑
    diving or jumping into water (in) W16.832 ☑
      causing drowning W16.831 ☑
      swimming pool W16.532 ☑
        causing drowning W16.531 ☑
    falling into water (in) W16.332 ☑
      causing drowning W16.331 ☑
      fountain — *see* Striking against, wall when, falling into water, specified NEC
      natural body W16.132 ☑
        causing drowning W16.131 ☑
      reservoir — *see* Striking against, wall when, falling into water, specified NEC
      specified NEC W16.332 ☑
        causing drowning W16.331 ☑
      swimming pool W16.032 ☑
        causing drowning W16.031 ☑
    swimming pool (when) W22.042 ☑
      causing drowning W22.041 ☑
      diving or jumping into water W16.532 ☑
        causing drowning W16.531 ☑
      falling into water W16.032 ☑
        causing drowning W16.031 ☑
Struck (accidentally) **by**
  airbag (automobile) W22.10 ☑
    driver side W22.11 ☑
    front passenger side W22.12 ☑
    specified NEC W22.19 ☑
  alligator W58.02 ☑
  animal (not being ridden) NEC W55.89 ☑
  avalanche — *see* Landslide
  ball (hit) (thrown) W21.00 ☑
    assault Y08.09 ☑
    baseball W21.03 ☑
    basketball W21.05 ☑
    football W21.01 ☑
    golf ball W21.04 ☑
    soccer W21.02 ☑
    softball W21.07 ☑
    specified NEC W21.09 ☑
    volleyball W21.06 ☑
  bat or racquet
    baseball bat W21.11 ☑
      assault Y08.02 ☑
    golf club W21.13 ☑
      assault Y08.09 ☑
    specified NEC W21.19 ☑
      assault Y08.09 ☑
    tennis racquet W21.12 ☑
      assault Y08.09 ☑
  bullet (*see also* Discharge, firearm by type)

Struck (accidentally) **by** — *continued*
  bullet (*see also* Discharge, firearm by type) — *continued*
    in war operations — *see* War operations
  crocodile W58.12 ☑
  dog W54.1 ☑
  flare, Very pistol — *see* Discharge, firearm NEC
  hailstones X39.8 ☑
  hockey (ice)
    field
      puck W21.221 ☑
      stick W21.211 ☑
    puck W21.220 ☑
    stick W21.210 ☑
      assault Y08.01 ☑
  landslide — *see* Landslide
  law-enforcement agent (on duty) — *see* Legal, intervention, manhandling
    with blunt object — *see* Legal, intervention, blunt object
  lightning T75.0 ☑
    causing fire — *see* Exposure, fire
  machine — *see* Contact, with, by type of machine
  mammal NEC W55.89 ☑
    marine W56.32 ☑
  marine animal W56.82 ☑
  missile
    firearm — *see* Discharge, firearm by type
    in war operations — *see* War operations, missile
  object W22.8 ☑
    blunt W22.8 ☑
      assault Y00 ☑
      suicide (attempt) X79 ☑
      undetermined whether accidental or intentional Y29 ☑
    falling W20.8 ☑
      from, in, on
        building W20.1 ☑
          burning (uncontrolled fire) X00.4 ☑
        cataclysmic
          earth surface movement NEC — *see* Landslide
          storm — *see* Forces of nature, cataclysmic storm
        cave-in W20.0 ☑
        earthquake X34 ☑
        machine (in operation) — *see* Contact, with, by type of machine
        structure W20.1 ☑
          burning X00.4 ☑
        transport vehicle (in motion) — *see* Accident, transport, by type of vehicle
        watercraft V93.49 ☑
          due to
            accident to craft V91.39 ☑
              powered craft V91.33 ☑
                ferry boat V91.31 ☑
                fishing boat V91.32 ☑
                jetskis V91.33 ☑
                liner V91.31 ☑
                merchant ship V91.30 ☑
                passenger ship V91.31 ☑
              unpowered craft V91.38 ☑
                canoe V91.35 ☑
                inflatable V91.36 ☑
                kayak V91.35 ☑
                sailboat V91.34 ☑
                surf-board V91.38 ☑
                windsurfer V91.38 ☑
            powered craft V93.43 ☑
              ferry boat V93.41 ☑
              fishing boat V93.42 ☑
              jetskis V93.43 ☑
              liner V93.41 ☑
              merchant ship V93.40 ☑
              passenger ship V93.41 ☑
            unpowered craft V93.48 ☑
              sailboat V93.44 ☑
              surf-board V93.48 ☑
              windsurfer V93.48 ☑
    moving NEC W20.8 ☑
    projected W20.8 ☑
      assault Y00 ☑
      in sports W21.9 ☑
        assault Y08.09 ☑
        ball W21.00 ☑

☑ **Additional Character Required** — Refer to the Tabular List for Character Selection   ▽ **Subterms under main terms may continue to next column or page**

Struck (accidentally) **by** — *continued*
  object — *continued*
    projected — *continued*
      in sports — *continued*
        ball — *continued*
          baseball W21.03 ☑
          basketball W21.05 ☑
          football W21.01 ☑
          golf ball W21.04 ☑
          soccer W21.02 ☑
          softball W21.07 ☑
          specified NEC W21.09 ☑
          volleyball W21.06 ☑
        bat or racquet
          baseball bat W21.11 ☑
            assault Y08.02 ☑
          golf club W21.13 ☑
            assault Y08.09 ☑
          specified NEC W21.19 ☑
            assault Y08.09 ☑
          tennis racquet W21.12 ☑
            assault Y08.09 ☑
        hockey (ice)
          field
            puck W21.221 ☑
            stick W21.211 ☑
          puck W21.220 ☑
          stick W21.210 ☑
            assault Y08.01 ☑
        specified NEC W21.89 ☑
    set in motion by explosion — *see* Explosion
    thrown W20.8 ☑
      assault Y00 ☑
      in sports W21.9 ☑
        assault Y08.09 ☑
        ball W21.00 ☑
          baseball W21.03 ☑
          basketball W21.05 ☑
          football W21.01 ☑
          golf ball W21.04 ☑
          soccer W21.02 ☑
          soft ball W21.07 ☑
          specified NEC W21.09 ☑
          volleyball W21.06 ☑
        bat or racquet
          baseball bat W21.11 ☑
            assault Y08.02 ☑
          golf club W21.13 ☑
            assault Y08.09 ☑
          specified NEC W21.19 ☑
            assault Y08.09 ☑
          tennis racquet W21.12 ☑
            assault Y08.09 ☑
        hockey (ice)
          field
            puck W21.221 ☑
            stick W21.211 ☑
          puck W21.220 ☑
          stick W21.210 ☑
            assault Y08.01 ☑
        specified NEC W21.89 ☑
  other person(s) W50.0 ☑
    with
      blunt object W22.8 ☑
        intentional, homicide (attempt) Y00 ☑
        sports equipment W21.9 ☑
        undetermined whether accidental or intentional Y29 ☑
      fall W03 ☑
        due to ice or snow W00.0 ☑
    as, or caused by, a crowd or human stampede (with fall) W52 ☑
    assault Y04.2 ☑
    homicide (attempt) Y04.2 ☑
    in legal intervention
      injuring
        bystander Y35.812 ☑
        law enforcement personnel Y35.811 ☑
        suspect Y35.813 ☑
      sports equipment W21.9 ☑
    police (on duty) — *see* Legal, intervention, manhandling
      with blunt object — *see* Legal, intervention, blunt object
  sports equipment W21.9 ☑
    assault Y08.09 ☑

Struck (accidentally) **by** — *continued*
  sports equipment — *continued*
    ball W21.00 ☑
      baseball W21.03 ☑
      basketball W21.05 ☑
      football W21.01 ☑
      golf ball W21.04 ☑
      soccer W21.02 ☑
      soft ball W21.07 ☑
      specified NEC W21.09 ☑
      volleyball W21.06 ☑
    bat or racquet
      baseball bat W21.11 ☑
        assault Y08.02 ☑
      golf club W21.13 ☑
        assault Y08.09 ☑
      specified NEC W21.19 ☑
      tennis racquet W21.12 ☑
        assault Y08.09 ☑
    cleats (shoe) W21.31 ☑
    foot wear NEC W21.39 ☑
    football helmet W21.81 ☑
    hockey (ice)
      field
        puck W21.221 ☑
        stick W21.211 ☑
      puck W21.220 ☑
      stick W21.210 ☑
        assault Y08.01 ☑
    skate blades W21.32 ☑
    specified NEC W21.89 ☑
      assault Y08.09 ☑
  thunderbolt — *see* subcategory T75.0 ☑
    causing fire — *see* Exposure, fire
  transport vehicle NEC (*see also* Accident, transport)
    V09.9 ☑
    intentional, homicide (attempt) Y03.0 ☑
    motor NEC (*see also* Accident, transport) V09.20
      homicide Y03.0 ☑
  vehicle (transport) NEC — *see* Accident, transport, by type of vehicle
    stationary (falling from jack, hydraulic lift, ramp)
      W20.8 ☑
Stumbling
  without fall W18.40 ☑
    due to
      specified NEC W18.49 ☑
      stepping from one level to another W18.43 ☑
      stepping into hole or opening W18.42 ☑
      stepping on object W18.41 ☑
    over
      animal NEC W01.0 ☑
        with fall W18.09 ☑
      carpet, rug or (small) object W22.8 ☑
        with fall W18.09 ☑
      person W51 ☑
        with fall W03 ☑
          due to ice or snow W00.0 ☑
Submersion (accidental) — *see* Drowning
Suffocation (accidental) (by external means) (by pressure) (mechanical) (*see also* category) T71 ☑
  due to, by
    avalanche — *see* Landslide
    explosion — *see* Explosion
    fire — *see* Exposure, fire
    food, any type (aspiration) (ingestion) (inhalation) — *see* categories T17 and T18 ☑
    ignition — *see* Ignition
    landslide — *see* Landslide
    machine(ry) — *see* Contact, with, by type of machine
    vomitus (aspiration) (inhalation) T17.81- ☑
  in
    burning building X00.8 ☑
Suicide, suicidal (attempted) (by) X83.8 ☑
  blunt object X79 ☑
  burning, burns X76 ☑
    hot object X77.9 ☑
      fluid NEC X77.2 ☑
      household appliance X77.3 ☑
      specified NEC X77.8 ☑
      steam X77.0 ☑
      tap water X77.1 ☑
      vapors X77.0 ☑
  caustic substance — *see* Table of Drugs and Chemicals
  cold, extreme X83.2 ☑

Suicide, suicidal — *continued*
  collision of motor vehicle with
    motor vehicle X82.0 ☑
    specified NEC X82.8 ☑
    train X82.1 ☑
    tree X82.2 ☑
  crashing of aircraft X83.0 ☑
  cut (any part of body) X78.9 ☑
  cutting or piercing instrument X78.9 ☑
    dagger X78.2 ☑
    glass X78.0 ☑
    knife X78.1 ☑
    specified NEC X78.8 ☑
    sword X78.2 ☑
  drowning (in) X71.9 ☑
    bathtub X71.0 ☑
    natural water X71.3 ☑
    specified NEC X71.8 ☑
    swimming pool X71.1 ☑
      following fall X71.2 ☑
  electrocution X83.1 ☑
  explosive(s) (material) X75 ☑
  fire, flames X76 ☑
  firearm X74.9 ☑
    airgun X74.01 ☑
    handgun X72 ☑
    hunting rifle X73.1 ☑
    larger X73.9 ☑
      specified NEC X73.8 ☑
    machine gun X73.2 ☑
    shotgun X73.0 ☑
    specified NEC X74.8 ☑
  hanging X83.8 ☑
  hot object — *see* Suicide, burning, hot object
  jumping
    before moving object X81.8 ☑
      motor vehicle X81.0 ☑
      subway train X81.1 ☑
      train X81.1 ☑
    from high place X80 ☑
  late effect of attempt — *see* X71-X83 with 7th character S
  lying before moving object, train, vehicle X81.8 ☑
  poisoning — *see* Table of Drugs and Chemicals
  puncture (any part of body) — *see* Suicide, cutting or piercing instrument
  scald — *see* Suicide, burning, hot object
  sequelae of attempt — *see* X71-X83 with 7th character S
  sharp object (any) — *see* Suicide, cutting or piercing instrument
  shooting — *see* Suicide, firearm
  specified means NEC X83.8 ☑
  stab (any part of body) — *see* Suicide, cutting or piercing instrument
  steam, hot vapors X77.0 ☑
  strangulation X83.8 ☑
  submersion — *see* Suicide, drowning
  suffocation X83.8 ☑
  wound NEC X83.8 ☑
Sunstroke X32 ☑
Supersonic waves (causing injury) W42.0 ☑
Surgical procedure, complication of (delayed or as an abnormal reaction without mention of misadventure) (*see also* Complication of or following, by type of procedure)
  due to or as a result of misadventure — *see* Misadventure
Swallowed, swallowing
  foreign body — *see* Foreign body, alimentary canal
  poison — *see* Table of Drugs and Chemicals
  substance
    caustic or corrosive — *see* Table of Drugs and Chemicals
    poisonous — *see* Table of Drugs and Chemicals

T

Tackle in sport W03 ☑
Terrorism (involving) Y38.80 ☑
  biological weapons Y38.6X- ☑
  chemical weapons Y38.7X- ☑
  conflagration Y38.3X- ☑
  explosion Y38.2X- ☑
    destruction of aircraft Y38.1X- ☑
    marine weapons Y38.0X- ☑

Terrorism — *continued*
  fire Y38.3X- ☑
  firearms Y38.4X- ☑
  hot substances Y38.5X- ☑
  nuclear weapons Y38.5X- ☑
  specified method NEC Y38.89- ☑
Thirst X58 ☑
Threat to breathing
  aspiration — *see* Aspiration
  due to cave-in, falling earth or substance NEC T71 ☑
Thrown (accidentally)
  against part (any) of or object in transport vehicle (in motion) NEC (*see also* Accident, transport)
  from
    high place, homicide (attempt) Y01 ☑
    machinery — *see* Contact, with, by type of machine
    transport vehicle NEC (*see also* Accident, transport) V89.9 ☑
  off — *see* Thrown, from
Thunderbolt — *see* subcategory T75.0 ☑
  causing fire — *see* Exposure, fire
Tidal wave (any injury) NEC — *see* Forces of nature, tidal wave
Took
  overdose (drug) — *see* Table of Drugs and Chemicals
  poison — *see* Table of Drugs and Chemicals
Tornado (any injury) X37.1 ☑
Torrential rain (any injury) X37.8 ☑
Torture X58 ☑
Trampled by animal NEC W55.89 ☑
Trapped (accidentally)
  between objects (moving) (stationary and moving) — *see* Caught
  by part (any) of
    motorcycle V29.88 ☑
    pedal cycle V19.88 ☑
    transport vehicle NEC (*see also* Accident, transport) V89.9 ☑
Travel (effects) (sickness) T75.3 ☑
Tree falling on or hitting (accidentally) (person) W20.8 ☑
Tripping
  without fall W18.40 ☑
    due to
      specified NEC W18.49 ☑
      stepping from one level to another W18.43 ☑
      stepping into hole or opening W18.42 ☑
      stepping on object W18.41 ☑
    over
      animal W01.0 ☑
        with fall W01.0 ☑
      carpet, rug or (small) object W22.8 ☑
        with fall W18.09 ☑
      person W51 ☑
        with fall W03 ☑
          due to ice or snow W00.0 ☑
Twisted by person(s) (accidentally) W50.2 ☑
  with intent to injure or kill Y04.0 ☑
  as, or caused by, a crowd or human stampede (with fall) W52 ☑
  assault Y04.0 ☑
  homicide (attempt) Y04.0 ☑
  in
    fight Y04.0 ☑
    legal intervention — *see* Legal, intervention, manhandling
Twisting, excessive — *see* category Y93 ☑

U

Underdosing of necessary drugs, medicaments or biological substances Y63.6
Undetermined intent (contact) (exposure)
  automobile collision Y32 ☑
  blunt object Y29 ☑
  drowning (submersion) (in) Y21.9 ☑
    bathtub Y21.0 ☑
      after fall Y21.1 ☑
    natural water (lake) (ocean) (pond) (river) (stream) Y21.4 ☑
    specified place NEC Y21.8 ☑
    swimming pool Y21.2 ☑
      after fall Y21.3 ☑
  explosive material Y25 ☑
  fall, jump or push from high place Y30 ☑
  falling, lying or running before moving object Y31 ☑

Undetermined intent — *continued*
  fire Y26 ☑
  firearm discharge Y24.9 ☑
    airgun (BB) (pellet) Y24.0 ☑
    handgun (pistol) (revolver) Y22 ☑
    hunting rifle Y23.1 ☑
    larger Y23.9 ☑
      hunting rifle Y23.1 ☑
      machine gun Y23.3 ☑
      military Y23.2 ☑
      shotgun Y23.0 ☑
      specified type NEC Y23.8 ☑
    machine gun Y23.3 ☑
    military Y23.2 ☑
    shotgun Y23.0 ☑
    specified type NEC Y24.8 ☑
    Very pistol Y24.8 ☑
  hot object Y27.9 ☑
    fluid NEC Y27.2 ☑
    household appliance Y27.3 ☑
    specified object NEC Y27.8 ☑
    steam Y27.0 ☑
    tap water Y27.1 ☑
    vapor Y27.0 ☑
  jump, fall or push from high place Y30 ☑
  lying, falling or running before moving object Y31 ☑
  motor vehicle crash Y32 ☑
  push, fall or jump from high place Y30 ☑
  running, falling or lying before moving object Y31 ☑
  sharp object Y28.9 ☑
    dagger Y28.2 ☑
    glass Y28.0 ☑
    knife Y28.1 ☑
    specified object NEC Y28.8 ☑
    sword Y28.2 ☑
  smoke Y26 ☑
  specified event NEC Y33 ☑

V

Vibration (causing injury) W49.9 ☑
Victim (of)
  avalanche — *see* Landslide
  earth movements NEC — *see* Forces of nature, earth movement
  earthquake X34 ☑
  flood — *see* Flood
  landslide — *see* Landslide
  lightning — *see* subcategory T75.0 ☑
    causing fire — *see* Exposure, fire
  storm (cataclysmic) NEC — *see* Forces of nature, cataclysmic storm
  volcanic eruption X35 ☑
Volcanic eruption (any injury) X35 ☑
Vomitus, gastric contents in air passages (with asphyxia, obstruction or suffocation) T17.81- ☑

W

Walked into stationary object (any) W22.09 ☑
  furniture W22.03 ☑
  lamppost W22.02 ☑
  wall W22.01 ☑
War operations (injuries to military personnel and civilians during war, civil insurrection and peacekeeping missions) (by) (from) (involving) Y36.90 ☑
  after cessation of hostilities Y36.89- ☑
    explosion (of)
      bomb placed during war operations Y36.82- ☑
      mine placed during war operations Y36.81- ☑
      specified NEC Y36.88- ☑
  air blast Y36.20- ☑
  aircraft
    destruction — *see* War operations, destruction of aircraft
  airway restriction — *see* War operations, restriction of airways
  asphyxiation — *see* War operations, restriction of airways
  biological weapons Y36.6X- ☑
  blast Y36.20- ☑
  blast fragments Y36.20- ☑
  blast wave Y36.20- ☑
  blast wind Y36.20- ☑
  bomb Y36.20- ☑

War operations — *continued*
  bomb — *continued*
    dirty Y36.50- ☑
    gasoline Y36.31- ☑
    incendiary Y36.31- ☑
    petrol Y36.31- ☑
  bullet Y36.43- ☑
    incendiary Y36.32- ☑
    rubber Y36.41- ☑
  chemical weapons Y36.7X- ☑
  combat
    hand to hand (unarmed) combat Y36.44- ☑
    using blunt or piercing object Y36.45- ☑
  conflagration — *see* War operations, fire
  conventional warfare NEC Y36.49- ☑
  depth-charge Y36.01- ☑
  destruction of aircraft Y36.10- ☑
    due to
      air to air missile Y36.11- ☑
      collision with other aircraft Y36.12- ☑
      detonation (accidental) of onboard munitions and explosives Y36.14- ☑
      enemy fire or explosives Y36.11- ☑
      explosive placed on aircraft Y36.11- ☑
      onboard fire Y36.13- ☑
      rocket propelled grenade [RPG] Y36.11- ☑
      small arms fire Y36.11- ☑
      surface to air missile Y36.11- ☑
    specified NEC Y36.19- ☑
  detonation (accidental) of
    onboard marine weapons Y36.05- ☑
    own munitions or munitions launch device Y36.24- ☑
  dirty bomb Y36.50- ☑
  explosion (of) Y36.20- ☑
    aerial bomb Y36.21- ☑
    after cessation of hostilities
      bomb placed during war operations Y36.82- ☑
      mine placed during war operations Y36.81- ☑
    bomb NOS (*see also* War operations, bomb(s)) Y36.20- ☑
    fragments Y36.20- ☑
    grenade Y36.29- ☑
    guided missile Y36.22- ☑
    improvised explosive device [IED] (person-borne) (roadside) (vehicle-borne) Y36.23- ☑
    land mine Y36.29- ☑
    marine mine (at sea) (in harbor) Y36.02- ☑
    marine weapon Y36.00- ☑
      specified NEC Y36.09- ☑
    own munitions or munitions launch device (accidental) Y36.24- ☑
    sea-based artillery shell Y36.03- ☑
    specified NEC Y36.29- ☑
    torpedo Y36.04- ☑
  fire Y36.30- ☑
    specified NEC Y36.39- ☑
  firearms
    discharge Y36.43- ☑
    pellets Y36.42- ☑
  flamethrower Y36.33- ☑
  fragments (from) (of)
    improvised explosive device [IED] (person-borne) (roadside) (vehicle-borne) Y36.26- ☑
    munitions Y36.25- ☑
    specified NEC Y36.29- ☑
    weapons Y36.27- ☑
  friendly fire Y36.92 ☑
  hand to hand (unarmed) combat Y36.44- ☑
  hot substances — *see* War operations, fire
  incendiary bullet Y36.32- ☑
  nuclear weapon (effects of) Y36.50- ☑
    acute radiation exposure Y36.54- ☑
    blast pressure Y36.51- ☑
    direct blast Y36.51- ☑
    direct heat Y36.53- ☑
    fallout exposure Y36.54- ☑
    fireball Y36.53- ☑
    indirect blast (struck or crushed by blast debris) (being thrown by blast) Y36.52- ☑
    ionizing radiation (immediate exposure) Y36.54- ☑
    nuclear radiation Y36.54- ☑
    radiation
      ionizing (immediate exposure) Y36.54- ☑
      nuclear Y36.54- ☑
      thermal Y36.53- ☑

War operations — *continued*
  nuclear weapon — *continued*
    secondary effects Y36.54- ☑
    specified NEC Y36.59- ☑
    thermal radiation Y36.53- ☑
  restriction of air (airway)
    intentional Y36.46- ☑
    unintentional Y36.47- ☑
  rubber bullets Y36.41- ☑
  shrapnel NOS Y36.29- ☑
  suffocation — *see* War operations, restriction of airways
  unconventional warfare NEC Y36.7X- ☑
  underwater blast NOS Y36.00- ☑
  warfare
    conventional NEC Y36.49- ☑
    unconventional NEC Y36.7X- ☑
  weapon of mass destruction [WMD] Y36.91 ☑
  weapons
    biological weapons Y36.6X- ☑

War operations — *continued*
  weapons — *continued*
    chemical Y36.7X- ☑
    nuclear (effects of) Y36.50- ☑
      acute radiation exposure Y36.54- ☑
      blast pressure Y36.51- ☑
      direct blast Y36.51- ☑
      direct heat Y36.53- ☑
      fallout exposure Y36.54- ☑
      fireball Y36.53- ☑
      indirect blast (struck or crushed by blast debris) (being thrown by blast) Y36.52- ☑
      radiation
        ionizing (immediate exposure) Y36.54- ☑
        nuclear Y36.54- ☑
        thermal Y36.53- ☑
      secondary effects Y36.54- ☑
      specified NEC Y36.59- ☑
    of mass destruction [WMD] Y36.91 ☑

Washed
  away by flood — *see* Flood
  off road by storm (transport vehicle) — *see* Forces of nature, cataclysmic storm
Weather exposure NEC — *see* Forces of nature
Weightlessness (causing injury) (effects of) (in spacecraft, real or simulated) X52 ☑
Work related condition Y99.0
Wound (accidental) NEC (*see also* Injury) X58 ☑
  battle (*see also* War operations) Y36.90 ☑
  gunshot — *see* Discharge, firearm by type
Wreck transport vehicle NEC (*see also* Accident, transport) V89.9 ☑
Wrong
  device implanted into correct surgical site Y65.51
  fluid in infusion Y65.1
  patient, procedure performed on Y65.52
  procedure (operation) on correct patient Y65.51

Check the index with Main Term

Confirm the specific codes here.

ICD-10-CM Tabular List of Diseases and Injuries

Chapter 1. Certain Infectious and Parasitic Diseases (A00-B99)

> **INCLUDES** diseases generally recognized as communicable or transmissible
> Use additional code to identify resistance to antimicrobial drugs (Z16.-)
> **EXCLUDES 1** certain localized infections—see body system-related chapters
> **EXCLUDES 2** carrier or suspected carrier of infectious disease (Z22.-)
> infectious and parasitic diseases complicating pregnancy, childbirth and the puerperium (O98.-)
> infectious and parasitic diseases specific to the perinatal period (P35-P39)
> influenza and other acute respiratory infections (J00-J22)

This chapter contains the following blocks:

A00-A09	Intestinal infectious diseases
A15-A19	Tuberculosis
A20-A28	Certain zoonotic bacterial diseases
A30-A49	Other bacterial diseases
A50-A64	Infections with a predominantly sexual mode of transmission
A65-A69	Other spirochetal diseases
A70-A74	Other diseases caused by chlamydiae
A75-A79	Rickettsioses
A80-A89	Viral infections of the central nervous system
A90-A99	Arthropod-borne viral fevers and viral hemorrhagic fevers
B00-B09	Viral infections characterized by skin and mucous membrane lesions
B10	Other human herpesviruses
B15-B19	Viral hepatitis
B20	Human immunodeficiency virus [HIV] disease
B25-B34	Other viral diseases
B35-B49	Mycoses
B50-B64	Protozoal diseases
B65-B83	Helminthiases
B85-B89	Pediculosis, acariasis and other infestations
B90-B94	Sequelae of infectious and parasitic diseases
B95-B97	Bacterial and viral infectious agents
B99	Other infectious diseases

Intestinal Infectious Diseases (A00-A09)

☑4ᵗʰ A00 Cholera

> **CC Excl:** For CC codes in category A00, unless otherwise noted: A00.0-A00.9

A00.0 Cholera due to Vibrio cholerae 01, biovar cholerae `CC`
Classical cholera

A00.1 Cholera due to Vibrio cholerae 01, biovar eltor `CC`
Cholera eltor

A00.9 Cholera, unspecified `CC`

☑4ᵗʰ A01 Typhoid and paratyphoid fevers

> **CC Excl:** For CC codes in category A01, unless otherwise noted: A01.00-A01.4

☑5ᵗʰ A01.0 Typhoid fever
Infection due to Salmonella typhi

A01.00 Typhoid fever, unspecified `CC`

A01.01 Typhoid meningitis `CC`

A01.02 Typhoid fever with heart involvement `CC`
Typhoid endocarditis Typhoid myocarditis

A01.03 Typhoid pneumonia `CC`

A01.04 Typhoid arthritis `CC`

A01.05 Typhoid osteomyelitis `CC`

A01.09 Typhoid fever with other complications `CC`

A01.1 Paratyphoid fever A `CC`

A01.2 Paratyphoid fever B `CC`

A01.3 Paratyphoid fever C `CC`

A01.4 Paratyphoid fever, unspecified `CC`
Infection due to Salmonella paratyphi NOS

☑4ᵗʰ A02 Other salmonella infections
> **INCLUDES** infection or foodborne intoxication due to any Salmonella species other than S. typhi and S. paratyphi

A02.0 Salmonella enteritis `CC`
Salmonellosis
> **CC Excl:** A01.00-A01.09, A01.4-A02.0, A03.9-A05.2, A07.4, A08.0-A09, A48.51-A48.52, K30, K52.1-K52.2, K52.82-K52.9, K58.0-K58.9, K65.0, K65.2, K65.8, K68.12-K68.9, P76.8-P77.9, P78.1, P78.3-P78.89

A02.1 Salmonella sepsis `HIV` `MCC`
> **CC Excl:** A02.1, A20.7, A22.7, A26.7, A32.7, A39.2-A39.4, A40.0-A40.1, A40.8-A41.9, A42.7, A48.2-A48.4, A48.8-A49.9, A54.86, B00.7, B37.7, B92, B94.2-B96.89, M00.011-M00.012, M00.021-M00.022, M00.031- M00.032, M00.041-M00.042, M00.051-M00.052, M00.061-M00.062, M00.071-M00.072, P36.0-P36.9, P39.2, P39.4-P39.9, R65.10-R65.20, Z16.10-Z16.39

☑5ᵗʰ A02.2 Localized salmonella infections

A02.20 Localized salmonella infection, unspecified `HIV`

A02.21 Salmonella meningitis `HIV` `MCC`
> **CC Excl:** A02.21, A17.0-A17.1, A27.81, A39.0, A50.41, A51.41, A52.13, A54.82, A54.84, A54.89-A54.9, A74.81-A74.9, A87.0-A87.9, A96.2, A98.3-A98.4, B26.1, B33.24, B33.4-B33.8, B34.1-B34.2, B34.4-B34.8, B37.5, B38.4, B45.1, B58.2, B92, B94.2-B94.9, B97.10, B97.19, B97.29, B97.5-B97.6, B97.81-B97.89, G00.0-G03.9, G04.2, G32.89, G96.8-G96.9, G98.0-G98.8, G99.8

A02.22 Salmonella pneumonia `HIV` `MCC`
> **CC Excl:** A02.22, A15.0-A15.6, A15.8-A15.9, A17.9, A18.82, A18.84, A18.89, A20.2, A21.1, A22.1, A31.0, A37.01, A37.11, A37.81, A37.91, A42.0, A43.0, A48.1, B25.0, B39.0-B39.2, B44.0, B58.3, B59, B67.1, J09.X1-J09.X2, J10.00-J10.1, J11.00-J11.1, J12.0-J12.3, J12.89-J18.1, J18.8-J18.9, J22, J60, J62.0-J67.7, J68.0-J70.4, J70.8-J70.9, J98.4, J98.8-J99, R91.1

A02.23 Salmonella arthritis `HIV` `CC`
> **CC Excl:** A02.23, A18.02, A18.09, A39.83-A39.84, A54.40, A54.42-A54.43, A54.82, A54.84, A54.89-A54.9, B06.82, M00.00, M00.19, M00.29, M00.39, M00.49, M00.59, M00.69, M00.79, M00.08-M02.9, M05.40-M05.59, M05.70-M06.09, M06.20-M06.39, M06.80-M07.69, M11.00-M11.9, M12.10-M15.0, M15.3-M15.9, M16.2-M16.9, M17.2-M17.9, M18.2-M18.9, M19.111-M19.93, M24.10-M24.176, M25.00, M25.08-M25.18, M25.40-M25.676, M25.80-M25.9, M35.2, M36.1-M36.4, R29.4

A02.24 Salmonella osteomyelitis `HIV` `CC`
> **CC Excl:** A02.24, A18.03-A18.09, M46.20-M46.39, M86.00-M86.9

A02.25 Salmonella pyelonephritis `HIV` `CC`
Salmonella tubulo-interstitial nephropathy
> **CC Excl:** A02.25-A02.29

A02.29 Salmonella with other localized infection `HIV` `CC`
> **CC Excl:** See code: A02.25

A02.8 Other specified salmonella infections `HIV` `CC`
> **CC Excl:** A02.8

A02.9 Salmonella infection, unspecified `HIV` `CC`
> **CC Excl:** A02.9

☑4ᵗʰ A03 Shigellosis

A03.0 Shigellosis due to Shigella dysenteriae `CC`
Group A shigellosis [Shiga-Kruse dysentery]
> **CC Excl:** A00.1, A01.00-A01.09, A01.4-A02.0, A03.0, A03.9, A04.9-A05.2, A06.0-A06.2, A06.9, A07.1-A07.9, A08.4-A09, A18.32-A18.39, A18.83, A48.51-A48.52, B37.82, B82.9, J09.X3-J09.X9, J10.2-J10.89, J11.2-J11.89, K30, K31.84, K50.00-K51.919, K52.1-K52.2, K52.82-K55.1, K55.8-K55.9, K58.0-K58.9, P70.0-P70.4, P70.9-P71.9, P72.1, P72.9-P74.4, P74.9, P76.8-P77.9, P78.1, P78.3-P78.89, P94.0

A03.1 Shigellosis due to Shigela flexneri
Group B shigellosis

A03.2 Shigellosis due to Shigella boydii
Group C shigellosis

A03.3 Shigellosis due to Shigella sonnei
Group D shigellosis

A03.8 Other shigellosis

A03.9 Shigellosis, unspecified
Bacillary dysentery NOS

☑4ᵗʰ A04 Other bacterial intestinal infections
> **EXCLUDES 1** bacterial foodborne intoxications, NEC (A05.-)
> tuberculous enteritis (A18.32)

> **CC Excl:** For CC codes in category A04, unless otherwise noted:
> For codes A04.0-A04.4: A02.0, A03.9-A05.0, A05.2, A07.4, A08.0-A09, J09.X3-J09.X9, J10.2-J10.89, J11.2-J11.89, K30, K31.84, K52.1-K52.2, K52.82-K52.9, K58.0-K58.9, K65.0, K65.2, K65.8, K68.12-K68.9, P76.8-P77.9, P78.1, P78.3-P78.89 For codes A04.5-A04.8: A00.1, A01.00-A01.09, A01.4-A02.0, A03.9-A05.2, A06.0-A06.2, A06.9, A07.1-A09, A18.32-A18.39, A18.83, A48.51-A48.52, B37.82, B82.9, J09.X3-J09.X9, J10.2-J10.89, J11.2-J11.89, K30, K31.84, K50.00-K51.919, K52.1-K52.2, K52.82-K55.1, K55.8-K55.9, K58.0-K58.9, P70.0-P70.4, P70.9-P71.9, P72.1, P72.9-P74.4, P74.9, P76.8-P77.9, P78.1, P78.3-P78.89, P94.0

A04.0 Enteropathogenic Escherichia coli infection `CC`

☑ Additional Character Required   ✓x7ᵗʰ Xtension Alert   Unacceptable PDx   Manifestation   Hospital Acquired Condition   **EXCLUDES 1** Not Coded Here   **EXCLUDES 2** Not Included Here

Certain Infectious and Parasitic Diseases

A04.1–A09

A04.1   **Enterotoxigenic** Escherichia coli infection   `CC`

A04.2   **Enteroinvasive** Escherichia coli infection   `CC`

A04.3   **Enterohemorrhagic** Escherichia coli infection   `CC`

A04.4   **Other** intestinal Escherichia coli infections   `CC`
Escherichia coli enteritis NOS

A04.5   **Campylobacter** enteritis   `CC`

A04.6   **Enteritis** due to **Yersinia enterocolitica**   `CC`
EXCLUDES 1   *extraintestinal yersiniosis (A28.2)*

A04.7   **Enterocolitis** due to **Clostridium difficile**   `CC`
Foodborne intoxication by Clostridium difficile
Pseudomembraneous colitis

A04.8   **Other** specified bacterial intestinal infections   `CC`

A04.9   **Bacterial** intestinal infection, **unspecified**   `CC`
Bacterial enteritis NOS
CC Excl: A00.1, A01.00-A01.09, A01.4-A02.0, A03.9-A05.0, A05.2, A06.0-A06.2, A06.9, A07.1-A09, A18.32-A18.39, A18.83, B37.82, B82.9, J09.X3-J09.X9, J10.2-J10.89, J11.2-J11.89, K30, K31.84, K52.1-K52.2, K52.82-K52.9, K58.0-K58.9, K65.0, K65.2, K65.8, K68.12-K68.9, P76.8-P77.9, P78.1, P78.3-P78.89

✓4ᵗʰ **A05**   **Other bacterial foodborne intoxications, not elsewhere classified**
EXCLUDES 1   *Clostridium difficile foodborne intoxication and infection (A04.7)*
Escherichia coli infection (A04.0-A04.4)
listeriosis (A32.-)
salmonella foodborne intoxication and infection (A02.-)
toxic effect of noxious foodstuffs (T61-T62)

A05.0   **Foodborne** staphylococcal intoxication   `CC`
CC Excl: A00.0-A09, A48.51-A48.52

A05.1   **Botulism** food poisoning   `CC`
Botulism NOS
Classical foodborne intoxication due to Clostridium botulinum
EXCLUDES 1   *infant botulism (A48.51)*
wound botulism (A48.52)
CC Excl: A04.7-A05.2, A48.51-A48.52

A05.2   **Foodborne** Clostridium perfringens [Clostridium welchii] intoxication   `CC`
Enteritis necroticans
Pig-bel
CC Excl: A02.0, A03.9-A05.2, A07.4, A08.0-A09, A48.51-A48.52, J09.X3-J09.X9, J10.2-J10.89, J11.2-J11.89, K30, K31.84, K52.1-K52.2, K52.82-K52.9, K58.0-K58.9, K65.0, K65.2, K65.8, K68.12-K68.9, P76.8-P77.9, P78.1, P78.3-P78.89

A05.3   **Foodborne** Vibrio parahaemolyticus intoxication   `CC`
CC Excl: See code: A05.0

A05.4   **Foodborne** Bacillus cereus intoxication   `CC`
CC Excl: See code: A05.0

A05.5   **Foodborne** Vibrio vulnificus intoxication   `CC`
CC Excl: See code: A05.0

A05.8   **Other** specified bacterial foodborne intoxications   `CC`
CC Excl: See code: A05.0

A05.9   **Bacterial** foodborne intoxication, **unspecified**

✓4ᵗʰ **A06**   **Amebiasis**
INCLUDES   infection due to Entamoeba histolytica
EXCLUDES 1   *other protozoal intestinal diseases (A07.-)*
EXCLUDES 2   *acanthamebiasis (B60.1-)*
Naegleriasis (B60.2)

A06.0   **Acute amebic** dysentery   `CC`
Acute amebiasis
Intestinal amebiasis NOS
CC Excl: A06.0-A06.1, A07.4

A06.1   **Chronic** intestinal **amebiasis**   `CC`
CC Excl: See code: A06.0

A06.2   **Amebic** nondysenteric colitis   `CC`
CC Excl: A02.0, A03.9-A05.0, A05.2, A06.0-A06.2, A06.9, A07.1-A09, B82.9, J09.X3-J09.X9, J10.2-J10.89, J11.2-J11.89, K30, K31.84, K50.00-K51.919, K52.1-K52.2, K52.82-K55.1, K55.8-K55.9, K58.0-K58.9, P76.8-P77.9, P78.1, P78.3-P78.89

A06.3   **Ameboma** of intestine   `CC`
Ameboma NOS
CC Excl: A06.0-A06.6, A06.81-A06.89

A06.4   **Amebic** liver abscess   `MCC`
Hepatic amebiasis
CC Excl: A06.4, K75.0

A06.5   **Amebic** lung abscess   `MCC`
Amebic abscess of lung (and liver)
CC Excl: A06.5, J85.0-J85.2

A06.6   **Amebic** brain abscess   `MCC`
Amebic abscess of brain (and liver) (and lung)
CC Excl: A06.6, G06.0

A06.7   **Cutaneous** ameboma

✓5ᵗʰ **A06.8**   **Amebic** infection of other sites

     A06.81   **Amebic** cystitis   `CC`
       CC Excl: A06.0-A06.6, A06.81-A06.89

     A06.82   **Other** amebic genitourinary infections   `CC`
       Amebic balanitis   Amebic vulvovaginitis
       Amebic vesiculitis
       CC Excl: See code: A06.3

     A06.89   **Other** amebic infections   `CC`
       Amebic appendicitis   Amebic splenic abscess
       CC Excl: See code: A06.3

A06.9   **Amebiasis, unspecified**

✓4ᵗʰ **A07**   **Other protozoal intestinal diseases**

CC Excl: For CC codes in category A07, unless otherwise noted:
A02.0, A03.9-A05.0, A05.2, A06.0-A06.2, A06.9, A07.1-A09, B82.9, J09.X3-J09.X9, J10.2-J10.89, J11.2-J11.89, K30, K31.84, K52.1-K52.2, K52.82-K52.9, K58.0-K58.9

A07.0   **Balantidiasis**
Balantidial dysentery

A07.1   **Giardiasis [lambliasis]**   `CC`

A07.2   **Cryptosporidiosis**   `CC`

A07.3   **Isosporiasis**   `HIV` `CC`
Infection due to Isospora belli and Isospora hominis
Intestinal coccidiosis
Isosporosis

A07.4   **Cyclosporiasis**   `CC`
CC Excl: A02.0, A03.9-A05.0, A05.2, A06.0-A06.2, A06.9, A07.1-A09, B82.9, J09.X3-J09.X9, J10.2-J10.89, J11.2-J11.89, K30, K31.84, K52.1-K52.2, K52.82-K52.9, K58.0-K58.9, K65.0, K65.2, K65.8, K68.12-K68.9

A07.8   **Other** specified protozoal intestinal diseases   `CC`
Intestinal microsporidiosis   Sarcocystosis
Intestinal trichomoniasis   Sarcosporidiosis

A07.9   **Protozoal** intestinal disease, **unspecified**   `CC`
Flagellate diarrhea   Protozoal diarrhea
Protozoal colitis   Protozoal dysentery

✓4ᵗʰ **A08**   **Viral and other specified intestinal infections**
EXCLUDES 1   *influenza with involvement of gastrointestinal tract (J09.X3, J10.2, J11.2)*

CC Excl: For CC codes in category A08, unless otherwise noted:
A02.0, A03.9-A05.0, A05.2, A06.0-A06.2, A06.9, A07.1-A09, A18.32-A18.39, A18.83, B37.82, B82.9, J09.X3-J09.X9, J10.2-J10.89, J11.2-J11.89, K30, K31.84, K52.1-K52.2, K52.82-K52.9, K58.0-K58.9, K65.0, K65.2, K65.8, K68.12-K68.9, P76.8-P77.9, P78.1, P78.3-P78.89

A08.0   **Rotaviral** enteritis   `CC`

✓5ᵗʰ **A08.1**   **Acute** gastroenteropathy due to Norwalk agent and other small round viruses

     A08.11   **Acute** gastroenteropathy due to Norwalk agent   `CC`
       Acute gastroenteropathy due to Norovirus
       Acute gastroenteropathy due to Norwalk-like agent

     A08.19   **Acute** gastroenteropathy due to other small round viruses   `CC`
       Acute gastroenteropathy due to small round virus [SRV] NOS

A08.2   **Adenoviral** enteritis   `CC`

✓5ᵗʰ **A08.3**   **Other** viral enteritis

     A08.31   **Calicivirus** enteritis   `CC`

     A08.32   **Astrovirus** enteritis   `CC`

     A08.39   **Other** viral enteritis   `CC`
       Coxsackie virus enteritis   Enterovirus enteritis NEC
       Echovirus enteritis   Torovirus enteritis

A08.4   **Viral** intestinal infection, **unspecified**
Viral enteritis NOS   Viral gastroenteropathy NOS
Viral gastroenteritis NOS

A08.8   **Other** specified intestinal infections

A09   **Infectious** gastroenteritis and colitis, **unspecified**   `CC`
Infectious colitis NOS
Infectious enteritis NOS
Infectious gastroenteritis NOS
EXCLUDES 1   *colitis NOS (K52.9)*
diarrhea NOS (R19.7)
enteritis NOS (K52.9)
gastroenteritis NOS (K52.9)
noninfective gastroenteritis and colitis, unspecified (K52.9)
CC Excl: A00.0-A09, A48.51-A48.52

N Newborn: 0   **P** Pediatric: 0-17   **M** Maternity: 12-55   **A** Adult: 15-124   `MCC` Major CC Condition   `PDx MCC` PDx acts as own MCC   `CC` CC Condition   `PDx CC` PDx acts as own CC

424   ICD-10-CM Draft (2015)

Tuberculosis (A15-A19)

INCLUDES infections due to Mycobacterium tuberculosis and Mycobacterium bovis

EXCLUDES 1 congenital tuberculosis (P37.0)
nonspecific reaction to test for tuberculosis without active tuberculosis (R76.1-)
pneumoconiosis associated with tuberculosis, any type in A15 (J65)
positive PPD (R76.11)
positive tuberculin skin test without active tuberculosis (R76.11)
sequelae of tuberculosis (B90.-)
silicotuberculosis (J65)

✓4ᵗʰ A15 Respiratory tuberculosis

A15.0 Tuberculosis of lung   HIV CC
Tuberculous bronchiectasis
Tuberculous fibrosis of lung
Tuberculous pneumonia
Tuberculous pneumothorax
CC Excl: A15.0-A15.6, A15.8-A15.9, A17.9, A18.82, A18.84, A18.89-A19.9, A22.1, A31.0, A31.2-A31.9, A37.01, A37.11, A37.81, A37.91, A48.1, A49.3-A49.9, B25.0, B44.0, B90.9, B92, B94.2-B94.9, B96.0, B96.6-B96.89, J09.X1-J09.X2, J10.00-J10.1, J11.00-J11.1, J12.0-J12.3, J12.89-J18.1, J18.8-J18.9, J44.9, J47.0-J70.4, J70.8-J70.9, J98.4, R91.1

A15.4 Tuberculosis of intrathoracic lymph nodes   HIV CC
Tuberculosis of hilar lymph nodes
Tuberculosis of mediastinal lymph nodes
Tuberculosis of tracheobronchial lymph nodes
EXCLUDES 1 tuberculosis specified as primary (A15.7)
CC Excl: See code: A15.0

A15.5 Tuberculosis of larynx, trachea and bronchus   HIV CC
Tuberculosis of bronchus
Tuberculosis of glottis
Tuberculosis of larynx
Tuberculosis of trachea
CC Excl: See code: A15.0

A15.6 Tuberculous pleurisy   HIV CC
Tuberculosis of pleura Tuberculous empyema
EXCLUDES 1 primary respiratory tuberculosis (A15.7)
CC Excl: See code: A15.0

A15.7 Primary respiratory tuberculosis   HIV CC
CC Excl: A15.0-A17.82, A17.89-A19.9

A15.8 Other respiratory tuberculosis   HIV CC
Mediastinal tuberculosis
Nasopharyngeal tuberculosis
Tuberculosis of nose
Tuberculosis of sinus [any nasal]
CC Excl: A15.0-A17.82, A17.89, A18.31-A18.39, A18.83, A19.0-A19.9

A15.9 Respiratory tuberculosis unspecified   HIV CC
CC Excl: See code: A15.8

✓4ᵗʰ A17 Tuberculosis of nervous system

A17.0 Tuberculous meningitis   HIV MCC
Tuberculosis of meninges (cerebral)(spinal)
Tuberculous leptomeningitis
EXCLUDES 1 tuberculous meningoencephalitis (A17.82)
CC Excl: A02.21, A17.0-A17.1, A17.89-A17.9, A18.82, A18.84, A18.89, A27.81, A31.2-A31.9, A39.0, A49.3-A49.9, A50.41, A51.41, A52.13, A54.82, A54.84, A54.89-A54.9, A87.0-A87.9, B00.3, B02.1, B26.1, B37.5, B38.4, B45.1, B58.2, B90.0, B92, B94.2-B94.9, B96.0, B96.6-B96.89, G00.0-G03.9, G04.2, G32.89, G61.0, G96.8-G96.9, G98.0-G98.8, G99.8

A17.1 Meningeal tuberculoma   HIV MCC
Tuberculoma of meninges (cerebral) (spinal)
EXCLUDES 2 tuberculoma of brain and spinal cord (A17.81)
CC Excl: See code: A17.0

✓5ᵗʰ A17.8 Other tuberculosis of nervous system

A17.81 Tuberculoma of brain and spinal cord   HIV MCC
Tuberculous abscess of brain and spinal cord
CC Excl: A17.81-A17.82, A17.89-A17.9, A18.82, A18.84, A18.89, A31.2-A31.9, A49.3-A49.9, B90.0, B92, B94.2-B94.9, B96.0, B96.6-B96.89

A17.82 Tuberculous meningoencephalitis   HIV MCC
Tuberculous myelitis
CC Excl: See code: A17.81

A17.83 Tuberculous neuritis   HIV MCC
Tuberculous mononeuropathy
CC Excl: No Excl

A17.89 Other tuberculosis of nervous system   HIV MCC
Tuberculous polyneuropathy
CC Excl: A17.89-A17.9, A18.82, A18.84, A18.89, A31.2-A31.9, A49.3-A49.9, B90.0, B92, B94.2-B94.9, B96.0, B96.6-B96.89

A17.9 Tuberculosis of nervous system, unspecified   HIV CC
CC Excl: A17.9, A18.82, A18.84, A18.89, A31.2-A31.9, A49.3-A49.9, B92, B94.2-B94.9, B96.0, B96.6-B96.89

✓4ᵗʰ A18 Tuberculosis of other organs

✓5ᵗʰ A18.0 Tuberculosis of bones and joints

A18.01 Tuberculosis of spine   HIV CC
Pott's disease or curvature of spine
Tuberculous arthritis
Tuberculous osteomyelitis of spine
Tuberculous spondylitis
CC Excl: A18.01

A18.02 Tuberculous arthritis of other joints   HIV CC
Tuberculosis of hip (joint)
Tuberculosis of knee (joint)
CC Excl: A18.02

A18.03 Tuberculosis of other bones   HIV CC
Tuberculous mastoiditis
Tuberculous osteomyelitis
CC Excl: A18.01-A18.03

A18.09 Other musculoskeletal tuberculosis   HIV CC
Tuberculous myositis
Tuberculous synovitis
Tuberculous tenosynovitis
CC Excl: A18.01-A18.02, A18.09

✓5ᵗʰ A18.1 Tuberculosis of genitourinary system

A18.10 Tuberculosis of genitourinary system, unspecified   HIV CC
CC Excl: A17.9, A18.10, A18.82, A18.84, A18.89, A31.2-A31.9, A49.3-A49.9, B90.1, B92, B94.2-B94.9, B96.0, B96.6-B96.89

A18.11 Tuberculosis of kidney and ureter   HIV CC
CC Excl: A17.9-A18.13, A18.82, A18.84, A18.89, A31.2-A31.9, A49.3-A49.9, B90.1, B92, B94.2-B94.9, B96.0, B96.6-B96.89

A18.12 Tuberculosis of bladder   HIV CC
CC Excl: See code: A18.11

A18.13 Tuberculosis of other urinary organs   HIV CC
Tuberculous urethritis
CC Excl: See code: A18.11

A18.14 Tuberculosis of prostate   HIV CC A♂
CC Excl: A17.9, A18.10, A18.14-A18.15, A18.82, A18.84, A18.89, A31.2-A31.9, A49.3-A49.9, B90.1, B92, B94.2-B94.9, B96.0, B96.6-B96.89

A18.15 Tuberculosis of other male genital organs   HIV CC ♂
CC Excl: See code: A18.14

A18.16 Tuberculosis of cervix   HIV CC ♀
CC Excl: A17.9, A18.10, A18.16-A18.18, A18.82, A18.84, A18.89, A31.2-A31.9, A49.3-A49.9, B90.1, B92, B94.2-B94.9, B96.0, B96.6-B96.89

A18.17 Tuberculous female pelvic inflammatory disease   HIV CC ♀
Tuberculous endometritis
Tuberculous oophoritis and salpingitis
CC Excl: See code: A18.16

A18.18 Tuberculosis of other female genital organs   HIV CC ♀
Tuberculous ulceration of vulva
CC Excl: See code: A18.16

A18.2 Tuberculous peripheral lymphadenopathy   HIV CC
Tuberculous adenitis
EXCLUDES 2 tuberculosis of bronchial and mediastinal lymph nodes (A15.4)
tuberculosis of mesenteric and retroperitoneal lymph nodes (A18.39)
tuberculous tracheobronchial adenopathy (A15.4)
CC Excl: A17.9, A18.2, A18.82, A18.84, A18.89, A31.2-A31.9, A49.3-A49.9, B92, B94.2-B94.9, B96.0, B96.6-B96.89

✓5ᵗʰ A18.3 Tuberculosis of intestines, peritoneum and mesenteric glands

CC Excl: For CC/MCC codes in subcategory A18.3, unless otherwise noted: A17.9, A18.31-A18.39, A18.82-A18.84, A18.89, A31.2-A31.9, A49.3-A49.9, B92, B94.2-B94.9, B96.0, B96.6-B96.89

A18.31 Tuberculous peritonitis   HIV MCC
Tuberculous ascites

A18.32 Tuberculous enteritis   HIV CC
Tuberculosis of anus and rectum
Tuberculosis of intestine (large) (small)

A18.39 Retroperitoneal tuberculosis   HIV CC
Tuberculosis of mesenteric glands
Tuberculosis of retroperitoneal (lymph glands)

Certain Infectious and Parasitic Diseases

A18.4 Tuberculosis of skin and subcutaneous tissue `HIV` `CC`
Erythema induratum, tuberculous
Lupus excedens
Lupus vulgaris NOS
Lupus vulgaris of eyelid
Scrofuloderma
Tuberculosis of external ear
EXCLUDES 2   *lupus erythematosus (L93.-)*
lupus NOS (M32.9)
systemic (M32.-)
CC Excl: A15.0-A17.82, A17.89-A19.9

√5ᵗʰ **A18.5 Tuberculosis of eye**
EXCLUDES 2   *lupus vulgaris of eyelid (A18.4)*

CC Excl: For CC codes in subcategory A18.5, unless otherwise noted: A17.9, A18.50-A18.59, A18.82, A18.84, A18.89, A31.2-A31.9, A49.3-A49.9, B92, B94.2-B94.9, B96.0, B96.6-B96.89

A18.50 Tuberculosis of eye, unspecified `HIV` `CC`
A18.51 Tuberculous episcleritis `HIV` `CC`
A18.52 Tuberculous keratitis `HIV` `CC`
Tuberculous interstitial keratitis
Tuberculous keratoconjunctivitis (interstitial) (phlyctenular)
A18.53 Tuberculous chorioretinitis `HIV` `CC`
A18.54 Tuberculous iridocyclitis `HIV` `CC`
A18.59 Other tuberculosis of eye `HIV` `CC`
Tuberculous conjunctivitis

A18.6 Tuberculosis of (inner) (middle) ear `HIV` `CC`
Tuberculous otitis media
EXCLUDES 2   *tuberculosis of external ear (A18.4)*
tuberculous mastoiditis (A18.03)
CC Excl: A17.9, A18.6, A18.82, A18.84, A18.89, A31.2-A31.9, A49.3-A49.9, B92, B94.2-B94.9, B96.0, B96.6-B96.89

A18.7 Tuberculosis of adrenal glands `HIV` `CC`
Tuberculous Addison's disease
CC Excl: A17.9, A18.7, A18.82, A18.84, A18.89, A31.2-A31.9, A49.3-A49.9, B92, B94.2-B94.9, B96.0, B96.6-B96.89

√5ᵗʰ **A18.8 Tuberculosis of other specified organs**
A18.81 Tuberculosis of thyroid gland `HIV` `CC`
CC Excl: A17.9, A18.81-A18.82, A18.84, A18.89, A31.2-A31.9, A49.3-A49.9, B92, B94.2-B94.9, B96.0, B96.6-B96.89
A18.82 Tuberculosis of other endocrine glands `HIV` `CC`
Tuberculosis of pituitary gland
Tuberculosis of thymus gland
CC Excl: A17.9, A18.82, A18.84, A18.89, A31.2-A31.9, A49.3-A49.9, B92, B94.2-B94.9, B96.0, B96.6-B96.89
A18.83 Tuberculosis of digestive tract organs, not elsewhere classified `HIV` `CC`
EXCLUDES 1   *tuberculosis of intestine (A18.32)*
CC Excl: A17.9, A18.31-A18.39, A18.82-A18.84, A18.89, A31.2-A31.9, A49.3-A49.9, B92, B94.2-B94.9, B96.0, B96.6-B96.89
A18.84 Tuberculosis of heart `HIV` `CC`
Tuberculous cardiomyopathy
Tuberculous endocarditis
Tuberculous myocarditis
Tuberculous pericarditis
CC Excl: See code: A18.82
A18.85 Tuberculosis of spleen `HIV` `CC`
CC Excl: A17.9-A18.82, A18.84-A18.89, A31.2-A31.9, A49.3-A49.9, B92, B94.2-B94.9, B96.0, B96.6-B96.89
A18.89 Tuberculosis of other sites `HIV` `CC`
Tuberculosis of muscle
Tuberculous cerebral arteritis
CC Excl: See code: A18.82

√4ᵗʰ **A19 Miliary tuberculosis**
INCLUDES   disseminated tuberculosis
generalized tuberculosis
tuberculous polyserositis

CC Excl: For MCC codes in category A19, unless otherwise noted: A17.9, A18.82, A18.84, A18.89-A19.9, A31.2-A31.9, A49.3-A49.9, B92, B94.2-B94.9, B96.0, B96.6-B96.89

A19.0 Acute miliary tuberculosis of a single specified site `HIV` `MCC`
A19.1 Acute miliary tuberculosis of multiple sites `HIV` `MCC`
A19.2 Acute miliary tuberculosis, unspecified `HIV` `MCC`
A19.8 Other miliary tuberculosis `HIV` `MCC`
A19.9 Miliary tuberculosis, unspecified `HIV` `MCC`

Certain zoonotic bacterial diseases (A20-A28)

√4ᵗʰ **A20 Plague**
INCLUDES   infection due to Yersinia pestis

A20.0 Bubonic plague `MCC`
CC Excl: A20.0-A20.9
A20.1 Cellulocutaneous plague `MCC`
CC Excl: See code: A20.0
A20.2 Pneumonic plague `MCC`
CC Excl: A20.2-J12.81
A20.3 Plague meningitis `MCC`
CC Excl: A20.3-A20.8
A20.7 Septicemic plague `MCC`
CC Excl: A02.1, A20.0-A20.9, A22.7, A26.7, A32.7, A40.0-A40.1, A40.8-A41.9, A42.7, A54.86, B37.7, P36.0-P36.9, P39.2, P39.4-P39.9, R65.10-R65.20
A20.8 Other forms of plague `MCC`
Abortive plague
Asymptomatic plague
Pestis minor
CC Excl: See code: A20.3
A20.9 Plague, unspecified `MCC`
CC Excl: A20.9

√4ᵗʰ **A21 Tularemia**
INCLUDES   deer-fly fever
infection due to Francisella tularensis
rabbit fever

A21.0 Ulceroglandular tularemia `CC`
CC Excl: A21.0
A21.1 Oculoglandular tularemia `CC`
Ophthalmic tularemia
CC Excl: A21.1-J12.81
A21.2 Pulmonary tularemia `CC`
CC Excl: A22.1-A37.01, A37.11, A37.81, A37.91, A48.1, B25.0, B44.0, J09.X1-J09.X2, J10.00-J10.1, J11.00-J11.1, J15.29, J15.5-J18.0, J18.8-J18.9, J22, J60-J70.4, J70.8-J70.9, J98.4, J98.8-J99, R91.1
A21.3 Gastrointestinal tularemia `CC`
Abdominal tularemia
CC Excl: A21.3
A21.7 Generalized tularemia `CC`
CC Excl: A21.0-A21.9
A21.8 Other forms of tularemia `CC`
CC Excl: See code: A21.7
A21.9 Tulamirea, unspecified `CC`
CC Excl: See code: A21.7

√4ᵗʰ **A22 Anthrax**
INCLUDES   infection due to Bacillus anthracis

A22.0 Cutaneous anthrax `CC`
Malignant carbuncle   Malignant pustule
CC Excl: A22.0
A22.1 Pulmonary anthrax `MCC`
Inhalation anthrax   Woolsorter's disease
Ragpicker's disease
CC Excl: A15.0-A15.6, A15.8-A15.9, A17.9, A18.82, A18.84, A18.89, A20.2, A21.1-A21.2, A22.1, A31.0, A37.01, A37.11, A37.81,A37.91, A42.0, A43.0, A48.1, B25.0, B39.0-B39.2, B44.0, B58.3, B59, B67.1, J09.X1-J09.X2, J10.00-J10.1, J11.00-J11.1, J12.0-J18.1, J18.8-J18.9, J22, J44.9, J47.0-J70.4, J70.8-J70.9, J98.4, J98.8-J99, Q33.4, R91.1
A22.2 Gastrointestinal anthrax `CC`
CC Excl: A22.2
A22.7 Anthrax sepsis `PDx MCC` `MCC`
CC Excl: A02.1-A20.7, A22.7, A26.7, A32.7, A39.2-A39.4, A40.0-A40.1, A40.8-A41.9, A42.7, A48.2-A48.4, A48.8-A49.9, A54.86, B00.7, B37.7, B92, B94.2-B96.89, M00.011-M00.012, M00.021-M00.022, M00.031- M00.032, M00.041-M00.042, M00.051-M00.052, M00.061-M00.062, M00.071-M00.072, P36.0-P36.9, P39.2, P39.4-P39.9, R65.10-R65.20, Z16.10-Z16.39
A22.8 Other forms of anthrax `CC`
Anthrax meningitis
CC Excl: A22.8
A22.9 Anthrax, unspecified `CC`
CC Excl: A22.0-A22.9

√4ᵗʰ **A23 Brucellosis**
Malta fever   Undulant fever
Mediterranean fever
A23.0 Brucellosis due to Brucella melitensis
A23.1 Brucellosis due to Brucella abortus
A23.2 Brucellosis due to Brucella suis
A23.3 Brucellosis due to Brucella canis

Ⓝ Newborn: 0   Ⓟ Pediatric: 0-17   Ⓜ Maternity: 12-55   Ⓐ Adult: 15-124   `MCC` Major CC Condition   `PDx MCC` PDx acts as own MCC   `CC` CC Condition   `PDx CC` PDx acts as own CC

426   ICD-10-CM Draft (2015)

A23.8 Other brucellosis `CC`
CC Excl: A23.0-A23.9

A23.9 Brucellosis, unspecified `CC`
CC Excl: See code: A23.8

✓4ᵗʰ A24 Glanders and melioidosis

A24.0 Glanders `CC`
Infection due to Pseudomonas mallei   Malleus
CC Excl: A24.0

A24.1 Acute and fulminating melioidosis `CC`
Melioidosis pneumonia   Melioidosis sepsis
CC Excl: A24.1-A24.9

A24.2 Subacute and chronic melioidosis `CC`
CC Excl: See code: A24.1

A24.3 Other melioidosis `CC`
CC Excl: See code: A24.1

A24.9 Melioidosis, unspecified `CC`
Infection due to Pseudomonas pseudomallei NOS
Whitmore's disease
CC Excl: See code: A24.1

✓4ᵗʰ A25 Rat-bite fevers

CC Excl: For CC codes in category A25, unless otherwise noted:
A25.0-A25.9

A25.0 Spirillosis `CC`
Sodoku

A25.1 Streptobacillosis `CC`
Epidemic arthritic erythema   Streptobacillary rat-bite fever
Haverhill fever

A25.9 Rat-bite fever, unspecified `CC`

✓4ᵗʰ A26 Erysipeloid

A26.0 Cutaneous erysipeloid
Erythema migrans

A26.7 Erysipelothrix sepsis `PDx MCC` `MCC`
CC Excl: A02.1, A20.7, A22.7, A26.7, A32.7, A39.2-A39.4, A40.0-
A40.1, A40.8-A41.9, A42.7, A48.2-A48.4, A48.8-A49.9, A54.86,
B00.7, B37.7, B92, B94.2-B96.89, M00.011-M00.012, M00.021-
M00.022, M00.031- M00.032, M00.041-M00.042, M00.051-
M00.052, M00.061-M00.062, M00.071-M00.072, R65.10-R65.20,
Z16.10-Z16.39

A26.8 Other forms of erysipeloid

A26.9 Erysipeloid, unspecified

✓4ᵗʰ A27 Leptospirosis

CC Excl: For CC/MCC codes in category A27, unless otherwise
noted: A27.0-A27.9

A27.0 Leptospirosis icterohemorrhagica `CC`
Leptospiral or spirochetal jaundice (hemorrhagic)
Weil's disease

✓5ᵗʰ A27.8 Other forms of leptospirosis

A27.81 Aseptic meningitis in leptospirosis `MCC`
CC Excl: A02.21, A17.0-A17.1, A27.0-A27.9, A39.0,
A50.41, A51.41, A52.13, A54.82, A54.84, A54.89-A54.9,
A74.81-A74.9, A87.0-A87.9, A96.2, A98.3-A98.4, B26.1,
B33.24, B33.4-B33.8, B34.1-B34.2, B34.4-B34.8, B37.5,
B38.4, B45.1, B58.2, B92, B94.2-B94.9, B97.10, B97.19,
B97.29, B97.5-B97.6, B97.81-B97.89, G00.0-G03.9, G04.2,
G32.89, G61.0, G96.8-G96.9, G98.0-G98.8, G99.8

A27.89 Other forms of leptospirosis `CC`

A27.9 Leptospirosis, unspecified `CC`

✓4ᵗʰ A28 Other zoonotic bacterial diseases, not elsewhere classified

CC Excl: For CC codes in category A28, unless otherwise noted:
:A26.0, A26.8-A26.9, A28.0, A28.2-A28.9, A32.0-A32.12, A32.81-A32.9

A28.0 Pasteurellosis `CC`

A28.1 Cat-scratch disease `CC`
Cat-scratch fever
CC Excl: A28.1-B97.21

A28.2 Extraintestinal yersiniosis `CC`
EXCLUDES1 enteritis due to Yersinia enterocolitica (A04.6)
plague (A20.-)

A28.8 Other specified zoonotic bacterial diseases, not elsewhere classified `CC`

A28.9 Zoonotic bacterial disease, unspecified `CC`

Other bacterial diseases (A30-A49)

✓4ᵗʰ A30 Leprosy [Hansen's disease]
INCLUDES infection due to Mycobacterium leprae
EXCLUDES1 sequelae of leprosy (B92)

A30.0 Indeterminate leprosy `CC`
I leprosy
CC Excl: A30.0

A30.1 Tuberculoid leprosy `CC`
TT leprosy
CC Excl: A30.1

A30.2 Borderline tuberculoid leprosy `CC`
BT leprosy
CC Excl: A30.2-A30.4

A30.3 Borderline leprosy `CC`
BB leprosy
CC Excl: See code: A30.2

A30.4 Borderline lepromatous leprosy `CC`
BL leprosy
CC Excl: See code: A30.2

A30.5 Lepromatous leprosy `CC`
LL leprosy
CC Excl: A30.5

A30.8 Other forms of leprosy `CC`
CC Excl: A30.8

A30.9 Leprosy, unspecified `CC`
CC Excl: A30.9

✓4ᵗʰ A31 Infection due to other mycobacteria

CC Excl: For CC codes in category A31, unless otherwise noted:
A31.0-A31.9

EXCLUDES2 leprosy (A30.-)
tuberculosis (A15-A19)

A31.0 Pulmonary mycobacterial infection `CC`
Infection due to Mycobacterium avium
Infection due to Mycobacterium intracellulare [Battey bacillus]
Infection due to Mycobacterium kansasii
CC Excl: A15.0-A15.6, A15.8-A15.9, A17.9, A18.82, A18.84, A18.89,
A22.1, A31.0, A31.2-A31.9, A37.01, A37.11, A37.81, A37.91, A48.1,
A49.3-A49.9, B25.0, B44.0-B44.9, B90.9, B92, B94.2-B94.9, B96.0, B96.6-
B96.89, J09.X1-J09.X2, J10.00-J10.1, J11.00-J11.1, J12.0-J12.3,
J12.89-J18.1, J18.8-J18.9, J44.9, J47.0-J70.4, J70.8-J70.9, J98.4,
R91.1

A31.1 Cutaneous mycobacterial infection `CC`
Buruli ulcer
Infection due to Mycobacterium marinum
Infection due to Mycobacterium ulcerans

A31.2 Disseminated mycobacterium avium-intracellulare complex (DMAC) `HIV` `CC`
MAC sepsis

A31.8 Other mycobacterial infections `HIV` `CC`

A31.9 Mycobacterial infection, unspecified `HIV` `CC`
Atypical mycobacterial infection NOS
Mycobacteriosis NOS

✓4ᵗʰ A32 Listeriosis
INCLUDES listerial foodborne infection
EXCLUDES1 neonatal (disseminated) listeriosis (P37.2)

CC Excl: For CC/MCC codes in category A32, unless otherwise
noted: A26.0, A26.8-A26.9, A28.0, A28.2-A28.9, A32.0-A32.12,
A32.81-A32.9

A32.0 Cutaneous listeriosis `CC`

✓5ᵗʰ A32.1 Listerial meningitis and meningoencephalitis

A32.11 Listerial meningitis `CC`
A32.12 Listerial meningoencephalitis `CC`

A32.7 Listerial sepsis `PDx MCC` `MCC`
CC Excl: A02.1, A20.7, A22.7, A26.7, A32.7, A39.2-A39.4, A40.0-
A40.1, A40.8-A41.9, A42.7, A48.2-A48.4, A48.8-A49.9, A54.86,
B00.7, B37.7, B92, B94.2-B96.89, M00.011-M00.012, M00.021-
M00.022, M00.031- M00.032, M00.041-M00.042, M00.051-
M00.052, M00.061-M00.062, M00.071-M00.072, R65.10-R65.20,
Z16.10-Z16.39

✓5ᵗʰ A32.8 Other forms of listeriosis

A32.81 Oculoglandular listeriosis `CC`
A32.82 Listerial endocarditis `CC`
A32.89 Other forms of listeriosis `CC`
Listerial cerebral arteritis

A32.9 Listeriosis, unspecified `CC`

A33 Tetanus neonatorum `MCC` `N`
CC Excl: A33-P29.2, P29.4, P29.89-P29.9, P94.1-P94.9, P96.0, P96.3-P96.5, P96.82-P96.89

A34 Obstetrical tetanus `CC` `M` ♀
CC Excl: A34, O08.0, O08.2-O08.9, O20.0-O20.9, O25.10-O25.3, O26.10-O26.13, O26.30-O26.43, O26.63-O26.819, O26.841-O26.86, O26.891-O26.93, O29.011-O29.93, O35.7X-O35.7X, O44.00-O44.13, O45.8X1-O45.93, O75.4, O75.81, O75.89-O75.9, O80, O90.89, O99.111-O99.285, O99.330-O99.335, O99.350-O99.355, O99.511-O99.73, O99.820-O99.825, O99.840-O9A.53

A35 Other tetanus `MCC`
Tetanus NOS
 EXCLUDES 1 obstetrical tetanus (A34)
tetanus neonatorum (A33)
CC Excl: A35, B92, B94.2-B94.9

☑4ᵗʰ **A36 Diphtheria**

> CC Excl: For CC codes in category A36, unless otherwise noted: A36.0-A36.9

A36.0 Pharyngeal diphtheria `CC`
Diphtheritic membranous angina
Tonsillar diphtheria

A36.1 Nasopharyngeal diphtheria `CC`

A36.2 Laryngeal diphtheria `CC`
Diphtheritic laryngotracheitis

A36.3 Cutaneous diphtheria `CC`
 EXCLUDES 2 erythrasma (L08.1)

☑5ᵗʰ **A36.8 Other diphtheria**

A36.81 Diphtheritic cardiomyopathy `CC`
Diphtheritic myocarditis
CC Excl: A36.81, A52.06, B33.20-B33.22, I00, I01.2-I01.9, I09.0, I09.9, I23.6-I23.3, I23.6-I23.8, I40.0-I41, I51.0, I51.4, I87.8, I99.8-I99.9

A36.82 Diphtheritic radiculomyelitis `CC`
A36.83 Diphtheritic polyneuritis `CC`
A36.84 Diphtheritic tubulo-interstitial nephropathy `CC`
A36.85 Diphtheritic cystitis `CC`
A36.86 Diphtheritic conjunctivitis `CC`
A36.89 Other diphtheritic complications `CC`
Diphtheritic peritonitis

A36.9 Diphtheria, unspecified `CC`

☑4ᵗʰ **A37 Whooping cough**

> CC Excl: For CC/MCC codes in category A37, unless otherwise noted: For codes A37.00, A37.10, A37.80 and A37.90: A37.00-A37.91 For codes A37.01, A37.11, A37.81 and A37.91: A15.0-A15.6, A15.8-A15.9, A17.9, A18.82, A18.84, A18.89, A21.2, A22.1, A31.0, A37.00-A37.91, A42.0, A43.0, A48.1, B25.0, B39.0-B39.2, B44.0, B58.3, B59, B67.1, J09.X1-J09.X2, J10.00-J10.1, J11.00-J11.1, J12.0-J12.3, J12.89-J18.1, J18.8-J18.9, J22, J44.9, J47.0-J70.4, J70.8-J70.9, J98.4, J98.8-J99, Q33.4, R91.1

☑5ᵗʰ **A37.0 Whooping cough due to Bordetella pertussis**

A37.00 Whooping cough due to Bordetella pertussis without pneumonia `CC`
A37.01 Whooping cough due to Bordetella pertussis with pneumonia `PDx MCC` `MCC`

☑5ᵗʰ **A37.1 Whooping cough due to Bordetella parapertussis**

A37.10 Whooping cough due to Bordetella parapertussis without pneumonia `CC`
A37.11 Whooping cough due to Bordetella with parapertussis pneumonia `PDx MCC` `MCC`

☑5ᵗʰ **A37.8 Whooping cough due to other Bordetella species**

A37.80 Whooping cough due to other Bordetella species without pneumonia `CC`
A37.81 Whooping cough due to other Bordetella species with pneumonia `PDx MCC` `MCC`

☑5ᵗʰ **A37.9 Whooping cough, unspecified species**

A37.90 Whooping cough, unspecified species without pneumonia `CC`
A37.91 Whooping cough, unspecified species with pneumonia `PDx MCC` `MCC`

☑4ᵗʰ **A38 Scarlet fever**
 INCLUDES scarlatina
 EXCLUDES 2 streptococcal sore throat (J02.0)

> CC Excl: For MCC codes in category A38, unless otherwise noted: A38.0-A38.9, A46, J02.0, J03.00-J03.01

A38.0 Scarlet fever with otitis media `CC`

A38.1 Scarlet fever with myocarditis `CC`
A38.8 Scarlet fever with other complications `CC`
A38.9 Scarlet fever, uncomplicated `CC`
Scarlet fever, NOS

☑4ᵗʰ **A39 Meningococcal infection**

A39.0 Meningococcal meningitis `MCC`
CC Excl: A02.1, A17.0-A17.1, A27.81, A39.0, A39.89-A39.9, A39.3-A49.9, A50.41, A51.41, A52.13, A54.82, A54.84, A54.89-A54.9, A87.0-A87.9, B00.3, B02.1, B26.1, B37.5, B38.4, B45.1, B58.2, B92, B94.2-B94.9, B96.0, B96.6-B96.89, G00.0-G03.9, G04.2, G32.89, G61.0, G96.8-G96.9, G98.0-G98.8, G99.8

A39.1 Waterhouse-Friderichsen syndrome `MCC`
Meningococcal hemorrhagic adrenalitis
Meningococcic adrenal syndrome
CC Excl: A39.1, A39.89-A39.9, A49.3-A49.9, B92, B94.2-B94.9, B96.0, B96.6-B96.89

A39.2 Acute meningococcemia `MCC`
CC Excl: A02.1, A20.7, A22.7, A26.7, A32.7, A39.2-A39.4, A39.89-A40.1, A40.8-A41.9, A42.7, A49.3-A49.9, A54.86, B00.7, B37.7, B92, B94.2-B94.9, B96.0, B96.6-B96.89, R65.10-R65.20

A39.3 Chronic meningococcemia `MCC`
CC Excl: See code: A39.2

A39.4 Meningococcemia, unspecified `MCC`
CC Excl: See code: A39.2

☑5ᵗʰ **A39.5 Meningococcal heart disease**

A39.50 Meningococcal carditis, unspecified `MCC`
CC Excl: A39.50, A39.89-A39.9, A49.3-A49.9, B92, B94.2-B94.9, B96.0, B96.6-B96.89

A39.51 Meningococcal endocarditis `MCC`
CC Excl: A39.51, A39.89-A39.9, A49.3-A49.9, B92, B94.2-B94.9, B96.0, B96.6-B96.89

A39.52 Meningococcal myocarditis `MCC`
CC Excl: A39.52, A49.3-A49.9, B92, B94.2-B94.9, B96.0, B96.6-B96.89

A39.53 Meningococcal pericarditis `MCC`
CC Excl: A39.53, A39.89-A39.9, A49.3-A49.9, B92, B94.2-B94.9, B96.0, B96.6-B96.89

☑5ᵗʰ **A39.8 Other meningococcal infections**

A39.81 Meningococcal encephalitis `MCC`
CC Excl: A39.81, A39.89-A39.9, A49.3-A49.9, B92, B94.2-B94.9, B96.0, B96.6-B96.89

A39.82 Meningococcal retrobulbar neuritis `CC`
CC Excl: A39.82, A39.89-A39.9, A49.3-A49.9, B92, B94.2-B94.9, B96.0, B96.6-B96.89

A39.83 Meningococcal arthritis `CC`
CC Excl: A39.83-A39.9, A49.3-A49.9, B92, B94.2-B94.9, B96.0, B96.6-B96.89

A39.84 Postmeningococcal arthritis `CC`
CC Excl: See code: A39.83

A39.89 Other meningococcal infections `CC`
Meningococcal conjunctivitis
CC Excl: A39.89-A39.9, A49.3-A49.9, B92, B94.2-B94.9, B96.0, B96.6-B96.89

A39.9 Meningococcal infection, unspecified `CC`
Meningococcal disease NOS
CC Excl: See code: A39.89

☑4ᵗʰ **A40 Streptococcal sepsis**
Code first: postprocedural streptococcal sepsis (T81.4)
streptococcal sepsis during labor (O75.3)
streptococcal sepsis following abortion or ectopic or molar pregnancy (O03-O07, O08.0)
streptococcal sepsis following immunization (T88.0)
streptococcal sepsis following infusion, transfusion or therapeutic injection (T80.2-)
 EXCLUDES 1 neonatal (P36.0-P36.1)
puerperal sepsis (O85)
sepsis due to Streptococcus, group D (A41.81)

> CC Excl: For MCC codes in category A40, unless otherwise noted: A02.1, A20.7, A22.7, A26.7, A32.7, A39.2-A39.4, A40.0-A40.1, A40.8-A41.9, A42.7, A48.2-A48.4, A48.8-A49.9, A54.86, B00.7, B37.7, B92, B94.2-B96.89, M00.011-M00.012, M00.021-M00.022, M00.031-M00.032, M00.041-M00.042, M00.051-M00.052, M00.061-M00.062, M00.071-M00.072, R65.10-R65.20, Z16.10-Z16.39

A40.0 Sepsis due to streptococcus, group A `MCC`
A40.1 Sepsis due to streptococcus, group B `MCC`
A40.3 Sepsis due to Streptococcus pneumoniae `MCC`
Pneumococcal sepsis
CC Excl: No Excl
A40.8 Other streptococcal sepsis `MCC`
A40.9 Streptococcal sepsis, unspecified `HIV` `MCC`

A41 Other sepsis

Code first: postprocedural sepsis (T81.4)
sepsis during labor (O75.3)
sepsis following abortion, ectopic or molar pregnancy (O03-O07, O08.0)
sepsis following immunization (T88.0)
sepsis following infusion, transfusion or therapeutic injection (T80.2-)

EXCLUDES 1 bacteremia NOS (R78.81)
neonatal (P36.-)
puerperal sepsis (O85)
sepsis NOS (A41.9)
streptococcal sepsis (A40.-)

EXCLUDES 2 sepsis (due to) (in) actinomycotic (A42.7)
sepsis (due to) (in) anthrax (A22.7)
sepsis (due to) (in) candidal (B37.7)
sepsis (due to) (in) Erysipelothrix (A26.7)
sepsis (due to) (in) extraintestinal yersiniosis (A28.2)
sepsis (due to) (in) gonococcal (A54.86)
sepsis (due to) (in) herpesviral (B00.7)
sepsis (due to) (in) listerial (A32.7)
sepsis (due to) (in) melioidosis (A24.1)
sepsis (due to) (in) meningococcal (A39.2-A39.4)
sepsis (due to) (in) plague (A20.7)
sepsis (due to) (in) tularemia (A21.7)
toxic shock syndrome (A48.3)

AHA: 2014, 2Q, 13

CC Excl: For MCC codes in category A41, unless otherwise noted:
A02.1, A20.7, A22.7, A26.7, A32.7, A39.2-A39.4, A40.0-A40.1, A40.8-A41.9, A42.7, A48.2-A48.4, A48.8-A49.9, A54.86, B00.7, B37.7, B92, B94.2-B96.89, M00.011-M00.012, M00.021-M00.022, M00.031-M00.032, M00.041-M00.042, M00.051- M00.052, M00.061-M00.062, M00.071-M00.072, R65.10-R65.20, Z16.10-Z16.39

A41.0 Sepsis due to Staphylococcus aureus ✓

A41.01 Sepsis due to methicillin susceptible Staphylococcus aureus　　HIV MCC
MSSA sepsis
Staphylococcus aureus sepsis NOS

A41.02 Sepsis due to methicillin resistant Staphylococcus aureus　　HIV MCC
[handwritten: MRSA]

A41.1 Sepsis due to other specified staphylococcus　　HIV MCC
Coagulase negative staphylococcus sepsis

A41.2 Sepsis due to unspecified staphylococcus　　HIV MCC

A41.3 Sepsis due to Hemophilus influenzae　　HIV MCC

A41.4 Sepsis due to anaerobes　　HIV MCC
EXCLUDES 1 gas gangrene (A48.0)

A41.5 Sepsis due to other Gram-negative organisms

A41.50 Gram-negative sepsis, unspecified　　HIV MCC
Gram-negative sepsis NOS

A41.51 Sepsis due to Escherichia coli [E. coli]　　HIV MCC

A41.52 Sepsis due to Pseudomonas　　HIV MCC
Pseudomonas aeroginosa

A41.53 Sepsis due to Serratia　　HIV MCC

A41.59 Other Gram-negative sepsis　　HIV MCC

A41.8 Other specified sepsis

A41.81 Sepsis due to Enterococcus　　HIV MCC

A41.89 Other specified sepsis　　HIV MCC

A41.9 Sepsis, unspecified organism　　HIV MCC
Septicemia NOS

A42 Actinomycosis
EXCLUDES 1 actinomycetoma (B47.1)

A42.0 Pulmonary actinomycosis　　HIV CC
CC Excl: A42.0, A42.81-A43.0, A43.8-A43.9, B47.1, J12.81

A42.1 Abdominal actinomycosis　　HIV CC
CC Excl: A42.1, A42.81-A42.9, A43.8-A43.9, B47.1

A42.2 Cervicofacial actinomycosis　　HIV CC
CC Excl: A42.2, A42.81-A42.9, A43.8-A43.9, B47.1

A42.7 Actinomycotic sepsis　　HIV MCC
CC Excl: A02.1, A20.7, A22.7, A26.7, A32.7, A39.2-A39.4, A40.0-A40.1, A40.8-A41.9, A42.7, A48.2-A48.4, A48.8-A49.9, A54.86, B00.7, B37.7, B92, B94.2-B96.89, M00.011-M00.012, M00.021-M00.022, M00.031- M00.032, M00.041-M00.042, M00.051-M00.052, M00.061-M00.062, M00.071-M00.072, R65.10-R65.20, Z16.10-Z16.39

A42.8 Other forms of actinomycosis

CC Excl: For CC codes in subcategory A42.8, unless otherwise noted: A42.0-A42.2, A42.81-A43.9, B47.1-B47.9, L08.1

A42.81 Actinomycotic meningitis　　HIV CC

A42.82 Actinomycotic encephalitis　　HIV CC

A42.89 Other forms of actinomycosis　　HIV CC

A42.9 Actinomycosis, unspecified　　HIV CC
CC Excl: See code: A42.8

A43 Nocardiosis

A43.0 Pulmonary nocardiosis　　HIV CC
CC Excl: A42.0, A42.81-A43.0, A43.8-A43.9, B47.1, J12.81

A43.1 Cutaneous nocardiosis　　HIV CC
CC Excl: A42.81-A42.9, A43.1-A43.9, B47.1, L08.1

A43.8 Other forms of nocardiosis　　HIV CC
CC Excl: A42.0-A42.2, A42.81-A43.9, B47.1-B47.9, L08.1

A43.9 Nocardiosis, unspecified　　HIV CC
CC Excl: See code: A43.8

A44 Bartonellosis

CC Excl: For CC codes in category A44, unless otherwise noted:
A44.0-A44.9, A68.0-A68.9, A69.20-A69.29, A75.0-A79.9, B55.0-B57.5, B60.0

A44.0 Systemic bartonellosis　　CC
Oroya fever

A44.1 Cutaneous and mucocutaneous bartonellosis　　CC
Verruga peruana

A44.8 Other forms of bartonellosis　　CC

A44.9 Bartonellosis, unspecified　　CC

A46 Erysipelas
EXCLUDES 1 postpartum or puerperal erysipelas (O86.89)

A48 Other bacterial diseases, not elsewhere classified
EXCLUDES 1 actinomycetoma (B47.1)

A48.0 Gas gangrene　　MCC
Clostridial cellulitis
Clostridial myonecrosis
CC Excl: A48.0, B92, B94.2-B94.9

A48.1 Legionnaires' disease　　HIV MCC
CC Excl: A15.0-A15.6, A15.8-A15.9, A17.9, A18.82, A18.84, A18.89, A21.2, A22.1, A31.0, A37.01, A37.11, A37.81, A37.91, A42.0, A43.0, A48.1, B25.0, B39.0-B39.2, B44.0, B58.3, B59, B67.1, J09.X1-J09.X2, J10.00-J10.1, J11.00-J11.1, J12.0-J12.3, J12.89-J18.1, J18.8-J18.9, J22, J44.9, J47.0-J70.4, J70.8-J70.9, J98.4, J98.8-J99, Q33.4, R91.1

A48.2 Nonpneumonic Legionnaires' disease [Pontiac fever]

A48.3 Toxic shock syndrome　　MCC
Use additional code to identify the organism (B95, B96)
EXCLUDES 1 endotoxic shock NOS (R57.8)
sepsis NOS (A41.9)
CC Excl: A48.3, G89.0-G89.4, R09.89, R41.0-R41.3, R41.82, R41.9, R44.8-R44.9, R45.83-R45.84, R46.0-R46.89, R52, R57.0-R57.9, R65.21-R68.19, R68.81-R68.83, R68.89-R69

A48.4 Brazilian purpuric fever
Systemic Hemophilus aegyptius infection

A48.5 Other specified botulism
Non-foodborne intoxication due to toxins of Clostridium botulinum [C. botulinum]
EXCLUDES 1 food poisoning due to toxins of Clostridium botulinum (A05.1)

CC Excl: For CC codes in subcategory A48.5, unless otherwise noted: A04.7, A05.0-A05.2, A48.51-A48.52

A48.51 Infant botulism　　CC P

A48.52 Wound botulism　　CC
Non-foodborne botulism NOS
Use additional code for associated wound

A48.8 Other specified bacterial diseases

A49 Bacterial infection of unspecified site
EXCLUDES 1 bacterial agents as the cause of diseases classified elsewhere (B95-B96)
chlamydial infection NOS (A74.9)
meningococcal infection NOS (A39.9)
rickettsial infection NOS (A79.9)
spirochetal infection NOS (A69.9)

A49.0 Staphylococcal infection, unspecified site

A49.01 Methicillin susceptible Staphylococcus aureus infection, unspecified site
Methicillin susceptible Staphylococcus aureus (MSSA) infection
Staphylococcus aureus infection NOS

✓ Additional Character Required　　✓x7ᵗʰ Xtension Alert　　Unacceptable PDx　　Manifestation　　Hospital Acquired Condition　　**EXCLUDES 1** Not Coded Here　　**EXCLUDES 2** Not Included Here

ICD-10-CM Draft (2015)　　　　　　　　　　　　　　　　　　　　429

A49.02   **Methicillin resistant Staphylococcus aureus infection, unspecified site**
Methicillin resistant Staphylococcus aureus (MRSA) infection

A49.1   **Streptococcal infection, unspecified site**

A49.2   **Hemophilus influenzae infection, unspecified site**

A49.3   **Mycoplasma infection, unspecified site**

A49.8   **Other bacterial infections of unspecified site**

A49.9   **Bacterial infection, unspecified**
EXCLUDES 1   bacteremia NOS (R78.81)

Infections with a predominantly sexual mode of transmission (A50-A64)

EXCLUDES 1   human immunodeficiency virus [HIV] disease (B20)
nonspecific and nongonococcal urethritis (N34.1)
Reiter's disease (M02.3-)

✓4th A50   Congenital syphilis

✓5th A50.0   **Early congenital syphilis, symptomatic**
Any congenital syphilitic condition specified as early or manifest less than two years after birth.)

CC Excl: For CC codes in subcategory A50.0, unless otherwise noted: A50.01-A51.46, A51.5-A53.9

A50.01   **Early congenital syphilitic oculopathy**   CC

A50.02   **Early congenital syphilitic osteochondropathy**   CC

A50.03   **Early congenital syphilitic pharyngitis**   CC
Early congenital syphilitic laryngitis

A50.04   **Early congenital syphilitic pneumonia**   CC

A50.05   **Early congenital syphilitic rhinitis**   CC

A50.06   **Early cutaneous congenital syphilis**   CC

A50.07   **Early mucocutaneous congenital syphilis**   CC

A50.08   **Early visceral congenital syphilis**   CC

A50.09   **Other early congenital syphilis, symptomatic**   CC

A50.1   **Early congenital syphilis, latent**
Congenital syphilis without clinical manifestations, with positive serological reaction and negative spinal fluid test, less than two years after birth.

A50.2   **Early congenital syphilis, unspecified**   CC
Congenital syphilis NOS less than two years after birth.
CC Excl: A50.01-A51.46, A51.5-A54.85, A54.89-A58, A63.8-A64, B92, B94.2-B94.9, M02.30-M02.342

✓5th A50.3   **Late congenital syphilitic oculopathy**
EXCLUDES 1   Hutchinson's triad (A50.53)

CC Excl: For CC/MCC codes in subcategory A50.3, unless otherwise noted: A50.01-A51.46, A51.5-A53.9

A50.30   **Late congenital syphilitic oculopathy, unspecified**   CC

A50.31   **Late congenital syphilitic interstitial keratitis**   CC

A50.32   **Late congenital syphilitic chorioretinitis**   CC

A50.39   **Other late congenital syphilitic oculopathy**   CC

✓5th A50.4   **Late congenital neurosyphilis [juvenile neurosyphilis]**
Use additional code to identify any associated mental disorder
EXCLUDES 1   Hutchinson's triad (A50.53)

A50.40   **Late congenital neurosyphilis, unspecified**   CC
Juvenile neurosyphilis NOS
CC Excl: A50.01-A51.46, A51.5-A53.9, A56.00-A56.8, A63.8-A64, B92, B94.2-B94.9, N34.1

A50.41   **Late congenital syphilitic meningitis**   MCC
CC Excl: A02.21, A17.0-A17.1, A27.81, A39.0, A50.01-A51.46, A51.5-A53.9, A54.82, A54.84, A54.89-A54.9, A56.00-A56.8, A63.8-A64, A87.0-A87.9, B00.3, B02.1, B26.1, B37.5, B38.4, B45.1, B58.2, B92, B94.2-B94.9, G00.0-G03.9, G04.2, G32.89, G61.0, G96.8-G96.9, G98.0-G98.8, G99.8, N34.1

A50.42   **Late congenital syphilitic encephalitis**   MCC
CC Excl: A50.01-A51.46, A51.5-A53.9, A56.00-A56.8, A63.8-A64, B92, B94.2-B94.9, N34.1

A50.43   **Late congenital syphilitic polyneuropathy**   CC
CC Excl: See code: A50.42

A50.44   **Late congenital syphilitic optic nerve atrophy**   CC
CC Excl: A50.01-A51.46, A51.5-A53.9

A50.45   **Juvenile general paresis**   CC
Dementia paralytica juvenilis
Juvenile tabetoparetic neurosyphilis
CC Excl: See code: A50.40

A50.49   **Other late congenital neurosyphilis**   CC
Juvenile tabes dorsalis
CC Excl: See code: A50.40

✓5th A50.5   **Other late congenital syphilis, symptomatic**
Any congenital syphilitic condition specified as late or manifest two years or more after birth.

CC Excl: For CC codes in subcategory A50.5, unless otherwise noted: A50.01-A51.46, A51.5-A53.9

A50.51   **Clutton's joints**   CC

A50.52   **Hutchinson's teeth**   CC

A50.53   **Hutchinson's triad**   CC

A50.54   **Late congenital cardiovascular syphilis**   CC

A50.55   **Late congenital syphilitic arthropathy**   CC

A50.56   **Late congenital syphilitic osteochondropathy**   CC

A50.57   **Syphilitic saddle nose**   CC

A50.59   **Other late congenital syphilis, symptomatic**   CC

A50.6   **Late congenital syphilis, latent**
Congenital syphilis without clinical manifestations, with positive serological reaction and negative spinal fluid test, two years or more after birth.

A50.7   **Late congenital syphilis, unspecified**
Congenital syphilis NOS two years or more after birth.

A50.9   **Congenital syphilis, unspecified**

✓4th A51   Early syphilis

A51.0   **Primary genital syphilis**
Syphilitic chancre NOS

A51.1   **Primary anal syphilis**

A51.2   **Primary syphilis of other sites**

✓5th A51.3   **Secondary syphilis of skin and mucous membranes**

A51.31   **Condyloma latum**   CC
CC Excl: A50.01-A51.46, A51.5-A53.9

A51.32   **Syphilitic alopecia**   CC
CC Excl: A50.01-A51.46, A51.5-A54.85, A54.89-A58, A63.8-A64, M02.30-M02.39, N34.1

A51.39   **Other secondary syphilis of skin**   CC
Syphilitic leukoderma   Syphilitic mucous patch
EXCLUDES 1   late syphilitic leukoderma (A52.79)
CC Excl: See code: A51.31

✓5th A51.4   **Other secondary syphilis**

A51.41   **Secondary syphilitic meningitis**   MCC
CC Excl: A02.21, A17.0-A17.1, A27.81, A39.0, A50.01-A51.46, A51.5-A54.85, A54.89-A58, A63.8-A64, A74.81-A74.9, A87.0-A87.9, A96.2, A98.3-A98.4, B26.1, B33.24, B33.4-B33.8, B34.1-B34.2, B34.4-B34.8, B37.5, B38.4, B45.1, B58.2, B92, B94.2-B94.9, B97.10, B97.19, B97.29, B97.5-B97.6, B97.81-B97.89, G00.0-G03.9, G04.2, G32.89, G61.0, G96.8-G96.9, G98.0-G98.8, G99.8, M02.30-M02.39, N34.1

A51.42   **Secondary syphilitic female pelvic disease**   CC ♀
CC Excl: A50.01-A51.46, A51.5-A54.85, A54.89-A58, A63.8-A64, B92, B94.2-B94.9, M02.30-M02.39, N34.1

A51.43   **Secondary syphilitic oculopathy**   CC
Secondary syphilitic chorioretinitis
Secondary syphilitic iridocyclitis, iritis
Secondary syphilitic uveitis
CC Excl: A50.01-A51.46, A51.5-A53.9

A51.44   **Secondary syphilitic nephritis**   CC
CC Excl: A50.01-A51.46, A51.5-A54.85, A54.89-A58, A63.8-A64, B92, B94.2-B94.9, M02.30-M02.39, N34.1

A51.45   **Secondary syphilitic hepatitis**   CC
CC Excl: A50.01-A51.46, A51.5-A54.85, A54.89-A58, A63.8-A64, K71.0-K71.9, K73.1-K73.8, K74.0-K74.69, K75.2-K76.0, K76.4-K76.5, K76.89-K76.9, M02.30-M02.39, N34.1

A51.46   **Secondary syphilitic osteopathy**   CC
CC Excl: A18.09, A50.01-A51.46, A51.5-A54.85, A54.89-A58, A63.8-A64, A66.6, M02.30-M02.39, M84.80-M84.9, M85.10-M85.19, M85.80-M85.89, M86.30-M86.8X9, M89.20-M89.39, M89.50-M89.59, M89.8X0-M89.8X9, M94.1, M94.351-M94.8X9, N34.1

A51.49   **Other secondary syphilitic conditions**   CC
Secondary syphilitic lymphadenopathy
Secondary syphilitic myositis
CC Excl: No Excl

A51.5   **Early syphilis, latent**
Syphilis (acquired) without clinical manifestations, with positive serological reaction and negative spinal fluid test, less than two years after infection.

A51.9   **Early syphilis, unspecified**

Certain Infectious and Parasitic Diseases

A52–A54.39

✓4ᵗʰ **A52 Late syphilis**

✓5ᵗʰ **A52.0 Cardiovascular and cerebrovascular syphilis**

> **CC Excl:** For CC codes in subcategory A52.0, unless otherwise noted: A50.01-A51.46, A51.5-A53.9, A56.00-A56.8, A63.8-A64, B92, B94.2-B94.9, N34.1

A52.00 Cardiovascular syphilis, unspecified cc

A52.01 Syphilitic aneurysm of aorta cc

A52.02 Syphilitic aortitis cc

A52.03 Syphilitic endocarditis cc
Syphilitic aortic valve incompetence or stenosis
Syphilitic mitral valve stenosis
Syphilitic pulmonary valve regurgitation

A52.04 Syphilitic cerebral arteritis cc

A52.05 Other cerebrovascular syphilis cc
Syphilitic cerebral aneurysm (ruptured) (non-ruptured)
Syphilitic cerebral thrombosis

A52.06 Other syphilitic heart involvement cc
Syphilitic coronary artery disease
Syphilitic myocarditis
Syphilitic pericarditis

A52.09 Other cardiovascular syphilis cc

✓5ᵗʰ **A52.1 Symptomatic neurosyphilis**

> **CC Excl:** For CC/MCC codes in subcategory A52.1, unless otherwise noted: A50.01-A51.46, A51.5-A53.9, A56.00-A56.8, A63.8-A64, B92, B94.2-B94.9, N34.1

A52.10 Symptomatic neurosyphilis, unspecified cc

A52.11 Tabes dorsalis cc
Locomotor ataxia (progressive)
Tabetic neurosyphilis

A52.12 Other cerebrospinal syphilis cc

A52.13 Late syphilitic meningitis MCC
CC Excl: A02.21, A17.0-A17.1, A27.81, A39.0, A50.01-A51.46, A51.5-A53.9, A54.82, A54.84, A54.89-A54.9, A56.00-A56.8, A63.8-A64, A87.0-A87.9, B00.3, B02.1, B26.1, B37.5, B38.4, B45.1, B58.2, B92, B94.2-B94.9, G00.0-G03.9, G04.2, G32.89, G61.0, G96.8-G96.9, G98.0-G98.8, G99.8, N34.1

A52.14 Late syphilitic encephalitis MCC

A52.15 Late syphilitic neuropathy cc
Late syphilitic acoustic neuritis
Late syphilitic optic (nerve) atrophy
Late syphilitic polyneuropathy
Late syphilitic retrobulbar neuritis

A52.16 Charcôt's arthropathy (tabetic) cc

A52.17 General paresis cc
Dementia paralytica

A52.19 Other symptomatic neurosyphilis cc
Syphilitic parkinsonism

A52.2 Asymptomatic neurosyphilis cc
CC Excl: See code: A52.1

A52.3 Neurosyphilis, unspecified cc
Gumma (syphilitic)   Syphiloma
Syphilis (late)
CC Excl: See code: A52.1

✓5ᵗʰ **A52.7 Other symptomatic late syphilis**

> **CC Excl:** For CC codes in subcategory A52.7, unless otherwise noted: A50.01-A51.46, A51.5-A54.85, A54.89-A58, A63.8-A64, M02.30-M02.39, N34.1

A52.71 Late syphilitic oculopathy cc
Late syphilitic chorioretinitis
Late syphilitic episcleritis
CC Excl: A18.50-A18.59, A50.01-A51.46, A51.5-A54.85, A54.89-A58, A63.8-A64, H15.001-H15.009, H15.091-H15.129, M02.30-M02.39, N34.1

A52.72 Syphilis of lung and bronchus cc

A52.73 Symptomatic late syphilis of other respiratory organs cc

A52.74 Syphilis of liver and other viscera cc
Late syphilitic peritonitis

A52.75 Syphilis of kidney and ureter cc
Syphilitic glomerular disease

A52.76 Other genitourinary symptomatic late syphilis cc
Late syphilitic female pelvic inflammatory disease

A52.77 Syphilis of bone and joint cc

A52.78 Syphilis of other musculoskeletal tissue cc
Late syphilitic bursitis
Syphilis [stage unspecified] of bursa
Syphilis [stage unspecified] of muscle
Syphilis [stage unspecified] of synovium
Syphilis [stage unspecified] of tendon

A52.79 Other symptomatic late syphilis cc
Late syphilitic leukoderma   Syphilis of thyroid gland
Syphilis of adrenal gland   Syphilitic splenomegaly
Syphilis of pituitary gland
EXCLUDES 1 syphilitic leukoderma (secondary) (A51.39)

A52.8 Late syphilis, latent
Syphilis (acquired) without clinical manifestations, with positive serological reaction and negative spinal fluid test, two years or more after infection

A52.9 Late syphilis, unspecified

✓4ᵗʰ **A53 Other and unspecified syphilis**

A53.0 Latent syphilis, unspecified as early or late
Latent syphilis NOS   Positive serological reaction for syphilis

A53.9 Syphilis, unspecified
Infection due to Treponema pallidum NOS
Syphilis (acquired) NOS
EXCLUDES 1 syphilis NOS under two years of age (A50.2)

✓4ᵗʰ **A54 Gonococcal infection**

✓5ᵗʰ **A54.0 Gonococcal infection of lower genitourinary tract without periurethral or accessory gland abscess**

> **CC Excl:** For CC codes in subcategory A54.0, unless otherwise noted: A54.00-A54.29, A54.82, A54.84, A54.89-A54.9, A56.00-A56.8, A63.8-A64, B92, B94.2-B94.9, N34.1

> *EXCLUDES 1* gonococcal infection with genitourinary gland abscess (A54.1)
> gonococcal infection with periurethral abscess (A54.1)

A54.00 Gonococcal infection of lower genitourinary tract, unspecified cc

A54.01 Gonococcal cystitis and urethritis, unspecified cc

A54.02 Gonococcal vulvovaginitis, unspecified cc ♀

A54.03 Gonococcal cervicitis, unspecified cc ♀

A54.09 Other gonococcal infection of lower genitourinary tract cc

A54.1 Gonococcal infection of lower genitourinary tract with periurethral and accessory gland abscess cc
Gonococcal Bartholin's gland abscess
CC Excl: See code: A54.0

✓5ᵗʰ **A54.2 Gonococcal pelviperitonitis and other gonococcal genitourinary infection**

> **CC Excl:** For CC codes in subcategory A54.2, unless otherwise noted: A54.00-A54.29, A54.82, A54.84, A54.89-A54.9, A56.00-A56.8, A63.8-A64, B92, B94.2-B94.9, N34.1

A54.21 Gonococcal infection of kidney and ureter cc

A54.22 Gonococcal prostatitis cc ♂

A54.23 Gonococcal infection of other male genital organs cc ♂
Gonococcal epididymitis   Gonococcal orchitis

A54.24 Gonococcal female pelvic inflammatory disease cc ♀
Gonococcal pelviperitonitis
EXCLUDES 1 gonococcal peritonitis (A54.85)

A54.29 Other gonococcal genitourinary infections cc

✓5ᵗʰ **A54.3 Gonococcal infection of eye**

> **CC Excl:** For CC codes in subcategory A54.3, unless otherwise noted: A50.01-A51.46, A51.5-A54.85, A54.89-A58, A63.8-A64, M02.30-M02.39, N34.1

A54.30 Gonococcal infection of eye, unspecified cc

A54.31 Gonococcal conjunctivitis cc
Ophthalmia neonatorum due to gonococcus

A54.32 Gonococcal iridocyclitis cc

A54.33 Gonococcal keratitis cc

A54.39 Other gonococcal eye infection cc
Gonococcal endophthalmia

✓ Additional Character Required   ✓x7ᵗʰ Xtension Alert   Unacceptable PDx   Manifestation   Hospital Acquired Condition   *EXCLUDES 1* Not Coded Here   *EXCLUDES 2* Not Included Here

ICD-10-CM Draft (2015)   431

Certain Infectious and Parasitic Diseases

A54.4–A64

✓5ᵗʰ A54.4 Gonococcal infection of musculoskeletal system

> **CC Excl:** For CC codes in subcategory A54.4, unless
> otherwise noted: A02.23, A17.9, A18.02, A18.09, A18.82,
> A18.84, A18.89, A39.83-A39.84, A50.01-A51.46, A51.5-
> A54.85, A54.89-A58, A63.8-A64, B06.82, M00.00, M00.19,
> M00.29, M00.39, M00.49, M00.59, M00.69, M00.79, M00.08-
> M02.9, M05.40-M05.59, M05.70-M06.09, M06.20-M06.39,
> M06.80-M07.69, M11.00-M11.9, M12.10-M15.0, M15.3-
> M15.9, M16.2-M16.9, M17.2-M17.9, M18.2-M18.9, M19.111-
> M19.93, M24.10-M24.176, M25.00, M25.08-M25.18, M25.40-
> M25.676, M25.80-M25.9, M35.2, M36.1-M36.4, N34.1, R29.4

A54.40 Gonococcal infection of musculoskeletal system, `CC`
     unspecified

A54.41 Gonococcal spondylopathy `CC`

A54.42 Gonococcal arthritis `CC`
     EXCLUDES 2   gonococcal infection of spine (A54.41)

A54.43 Gonococcal osteomyelitis `CC`
     EXCLUDES 2   gonococcal infection of spine (A54.41)

A54.49 Gonococcal infection of other musculoskeletal `CC`
     tissue
     Gonococcal bursitis
     Gonococcal myositis
     Gonococcal synovitis
     Gonococcal tenosynovitis

A54.5 Gonococcal pharyngitis

A54.6 Gonococcal infection of anus and rectum

✓5ᵗʰ A54.8 Other gonococcal infections

A54.81 Gonococcal meningitis `MCC`
     CC Excl: A02.21, A17.0-A17.1, A27.81, A39.0, A50.01-
     A51.46, A51.5-A54.85, A54.89-A58, A63.8-A64, A74.81-
     A74.9, A87.0-A87.9, A96.2, A98.3-A98.4, B26.1, B33.24,
     B33.4-B33.8, B34.1-B34.2, B34.4-B34.8, B37.5, B38.4,
     B45.1, B58.2, B92, B94.2-B94.9, B97.10, B97.19, B97.29,
     B97.5-B97.6, B97.81-B97.89, G00.0-G03.9, G04.2, G32.89,
     G61.0, G96.8-G96.9, G98.0-G98.8, G99.8, M02.30-
     M02.39, N34.1

A54.82 Gonococcal brain abscess `CC`
     CC Excl: A50.01-A51.46, A51.5-A54.85, A54.89-A58,
     A63.8-A64, M02.30-M02.39, N25.81-N25.89, N34.1

A54.83 Gonococcal heart infection `CC`
     Gonococcal endocarditis
     Gonococcal myocarditis
     Gonococcal pericarditis
     CC Excl: A01.00-A01.09, A39.51, A50.01-A51.46, A51.5-
     A54.85, A54.89-A58, A63.8-A64, A78, B33.20-B33.22,
     B37.6, B40.0-B40.9, I00, I01.1-I02.0, I05.0-I07.9, I08.1-
     I08.3, I08.9-I09.1, I09.89-I09.9, I23.0-I23.3, I23.6-I23.8,
     I33.0-I41, I42.4, I51.0, I51.4, I87.8, I99.8-I99.9, M00.00,
     M00.08-M00.10, M00.18-M00.20, M00.28-M00.80,
     M00.88-M00.9, M02.30-M02.39, N34.1, Q22.2, Q23.8-
     Q23.9, Q24.8, T82.6XXA

A54.84 Gonococcal pneumonia `CC`
     CC Excl: See code: A54.82

A54.85 Gonococcal peritonitis `CC`
     EXCLUDES 1   gonococcal pelviperitonitis (A54.24)
     CC Excl: A18.31-A34, A50.01-A51.46, A51.5-A54.85,
     A54.89-A58, A63.8-A64, K35.2-K35.3, K63.4, K63.89-
     K63.9, K65.1, K65.3, K65.9, K67, K86.8, K92.89-K92.9,
     M02.30-M02.39, N34.1, N73.3-N73.4, N73.6, O08.0,
     O08.82, O85, O86.12, O86.81-O86.89, P78.0, R11.13,
     T81.60XA, T81.61XA, T81.69XA

A54.86 Gonococcal sepsis `PDx MCC` `MCC`
     CC Excl: A02.1, A20.7, A22.7, A26.7, A32.7, A39.2-A39.4,
     A40.0-A40.1, A40.8-A41.9, A42.7, A48.2-A48.4, A48.8-
     A49.9, A54.86, B00.7, B37.7, B92, B94.2-B96.89, M00.011-
     M00.012, M00.021-M00.022, M00.031- M00.032,
     M00.041-M00.042, M00.051- M00.052, M00.061-
     M00.062, M00.071-M00.072, R65.10-R65.20, Z16.10-
     Z16.39

A54.89 Other gonococcal infections `CC`
     Gonococcal keratoderma
     Gonococcal lymphadenitis
     CC Excl: See code: A54.82

A54.9 Gonococcal infection, unspecified `CC`
     CC Excl: See code: A54.82

A55 Chlamydial lymphogranuloma (venereum)
     Climatic or tropical bubo
     Durand-Nicolas-Favre disease
     Esthiomene
     Lymphogranuloma inguinale

✓4ᵗʰ A56 Other sexually transmitted chlamydial diseases
     INCLUDES   sexually transmitted diseases due to Chlamydia
          trachomatis
     EXCLUDES 1   neonatal chlamydial conjunctivitis (P39.1)
          neonatal chlamydial pneumonia (P23.1)
     EXCLUDES 2   chlamydial lymphogranuloma (A55)
          conditions classified to A74-

✓5ᵗʰ A56.0 Chlamydial infection of lower genitourinary tract

A56.00 Chlamydial infection of lower genitourinary tract,
     unspecified

A56.01 Chlamydial cystitis and urethritis

A56.02 Chlamydial vulvovaginitis ♀

A56.09 Other chlamydial infection of lower genitourinary
     tract
     Chlamydial cervicitis

✓5ᵗʰ A56.1 Chlamydial infection of pelviperitoneum and other
genitourinary organs

A56.11 Chlamydial female pelvic inflammatory disease ♀

A56.19 Other chlamydial genitourinary infection
     Chlamydial epididymitis
     Chlamydial orchitis

A56.2 Chlamydial infection of genitourinary tract, unspecified

A56.3 Chlamydial infection of anus and rectum

A56.4 Chlamydial infection of pharynx

A56.8 Sexually transmitted chlamydial infection of other sites

A57 Chancroid
     Ulcus molle

A58 Granuloma inguinale
     Donovanosis

✓4ᵗʰ A59 Trichomoniasis
     EXCLUDES 2   intestinal trichomoniasis (A07.8)

✓5ᵗʰ A59.0 Urogenital trichomoniasis

A59.00 Urogenital trichomoniasis, unspecified
     Fluor (vaginalis) due to Trichomonas
     Leukorrhea (vaginalis) due to Trichomonas

A59.01 Trichomonal vulvovaginitis ♀

A59.02 Trichomonal prostatitis ♂

A59.03 Trichomonal cystitis and urethritis

A59.09 Other urogenital trichomoniasis
     Trichomonas cervicitis

A59.8 Trichomoniasis of other sites

A59.9 Trichomoniasis, unspecified

✓4ᵗʰ A60 Anogenital herpesviral [herpes simplex] infections

✓5ᵗʰ A60.0 Herpesviral infection of genitalia and urogenital tract

A60.00 Herpesviral infection of urogenital system, `HIV`
     unspecified

A60.01 Herpesviral infection of penis `HIV` ♂

A60.02 Herpesviral infection of other male genital ♂
     organs

A60.03 Herpesviral cervicitis ♀

A60.04 Herpesviral vulvovaginitis `HIV` ♀
     Herpesviral [herpes simplex] ulceration
     Herpesviral [herpes simplex] vaginitis
     Herpesviral [herpes simplex] vulvitis

A60.09 Herpesviral infection of other urogenital tract `HIV`

A60.1 Herpesviral infection of perianal skin and rectum `HIV`

A60.9 Anogenital herpesviral infection, unspecified `HIV`

✓4ᵗʰ A63 Other predominantly sexually transmitted diseases, not
elsewhere classified
     EXCLUDES 2   molluscum contagiosum (B08.1)
          papilloma of cervix (D26.0)

A63.0 Anogenital (venereal) warts
     Anogenital warts due to (human) papillomavirus [HPV]
     Condyloma acuminatum

A63.8 Other specified predominantly sexually transmitted diseases

A64 Unspecified sexually transmitted disease

N Newborn: 0   **P** Pediatric: 0-17   **M** Maternity: 12-55   **A** Adult: 15-124   `MCC` Major CC Condition   `PDx MCC` PDx acts as own MCC   `CC` CC Condition   `PDx CC` PDx acts as own CC

432   ICD-10-CM Draft (2015)

Other spirochetal diseases (A65-A69)

EXCLUDES 2   leptospirosis (A27.-)
          syphilis (A50-A53)

A65   Nonvenereal syphilis
     Bejel
     Endemic syphilis
     Njovera

✓4ᵗʰ A66   Yaws
     INCLUDES   bouba
              frambesia (tropica)
              pian

A66.0   Initial lesions of yaws
     Chancre of yaws
     Frambesia, initial or primary
     Initial frambesial ulcer
     Mother yaw

A66.1   Multiple papillomata and wet crab yaws
     Frambesioma
     Pianoma
     Plantar or palmar papilloma of yaws

A66.2   Other early skin lesions of yaws
     Cutaneous yaws, less than five years after infection
     Early yaws (cutaneous) (macular) (maculopapular)
          (micropapular) (papular)
     Frambeside of early yaws

A66.3   Hyperkeratosis of yaws
     Ghoul hand
     Hyperkeratosis, palmar or plantar (early) (late) due to yaws
     Worm-eaten soles

A66.4   Gummata and ulcers of yaws
     Gummatous frambeside
     Nodular late yaws (ulcerated)

A66.5   Gangosa
     Rhinopharyngitis mutilans

A66.6   Bone and joint lesions of yaws
     Yaws ganglion
     Yaws goundou
     Yaws gumma, bone
     Yaws gummatous osteitis or periostitis
     Yaws hydrarthrosis
     Yaws osteitis
     Yaws periostitis (hypertrophic)

A66.7   Other manifestations of yaws
     Juxta-articular nodules of yaws
     Mucosal yaws

A66.8   Latent yaws
     Yaws without clinical manifestations, with positive serology

A66.9   Yaws, unspecified

✓4ᵗʰ A67   Pinta [carate]

A67.0   Primary lesions of pinta
     Chancre (primary) of pinta
     Papule (primary) of pinta

A67.1   Intermediate lesions of pinta
     Erythematous plaques of pinta
     Hyperchromic lesions of pinta
     Hyperkeratosis of pinta
     Pintids

A67.2   Late lesions of pinta
     Achromic skin lesions of pinta
     Cicatricial skin lesions of pinta
     Dyschromic skin lesions of pinta

A67.3   Mixed lesions of pinta
     Achromic with hyperchromic skin lesions of pinta [carate]

A67.9   Pinta, unspecified

✓4ᵗʰ A68   Relapsing fevers
     INCLUDES   recurrent fever
     EXCLUDES 2   Lyme disease (A69.2-)

     CC Excl: For CC codes in category A68, unless otherwise noted:
     A44.0-A44.9, A68.0-A68.9, A69.20-A69.29, A75.0-A79.9, B55.0-B57.5, B60.0

A68.0   Louse-borne relapsing fever   cc
     Relapsing fever due to Borrelia recurrentis

A68.1   Tick-borne relapsing fever   cc
     Relapsing fever due to any Borrelia species other than Borrelia recurrentis

A68.9   Relapsing fever, unspecified   cc

✓4ᵗʰ A69   Other spirochetal infections

A69.0   Necrotizing ulcerative stomatitis
     Cancrum oris   Noma
     Fusospirochetal gangrene   Stomatitis gangrenosa

A69.1   Other Vincent's infections   cc
     Fusospirochetal pharyngitis
     Necrotizing ulcerative (acute) gingivitis
     Necrotizing ulcerative (acute) gingivostomatitis
     Spirochetal stomatitis
     Trench mouth
     Vincent's angina
     Vincent's gingivitis
     CC Excl: A69.1

✓5ᵗʰ A69.2   Lyme disease
     Erythema chronicum migrans due to Borrelia burgdorferi

     CC Excl: For CC codes in subcategory A69.2, unless otherwise noted: A44.0-A44.9, A68.0-A68.9, A69.20-A69.29, A75.0-A79.9, B55.0-B57.5, B60.0

A69.20   Lyme disease, unspecified   cc
A69.21   Meningitis due to Lyme disease   cc
A69.22   Other neurologic disorders in Lyme disease   cc
     Cranial neuritis
     Meningoencephalitis
     Polyneuropathy
A69.23   Arthritis due to Lyme disease   cc
A69.29   Other conditions associated with Lyme disease   cc
     Myopericarditis due to Lyme disease

A69.8   Other specified spirochetal infections

A69.9   Spirochetal infection, unspecified

Other diseases caused by chlamydiae (A70-A74)

EXCLUDES 1   sexually transmitted chlamydial diseases (A55-A56)

A70   Chlamydia psittaci infections   cc
     Ornithosis
     Parrot fever
     Psittacosis
     CC Excl: A70

✓4ᵗʰ A71   Trachoma
     EXCLUDES 1   sequelae of trachoma (B94.0)

A71.0   Initial stage of trachoma
     Trachoma dubium

A71.1   Active stage of trachoma
     Granular conjunctivitis (trachomatous)
     Trachomatous follicular conjunctivitis
     Trachomatous pannus

A71.9   Trachoma, unspecified

✓4ᵗʰ A74   Other diseases caused by chlamydiae
     EXCLUDES 1   neonatal chlamydial conjunctivitis (P39.1)
                neonatal chlamydial pneumonia (P23.1)
                Reiter's disease (M02.3-)
                sexually transmitted chlamydial diseases (A55-A56)
     EXCLUDES 2   chlamydial pneumonia (J16.0)

A74.0   Chlamydial conjunctivitis
     Paratrachoma

✓5ᵗʰ A74.8   Other chlamydial diseases
A74.81   Chlamydial peritonitis
A74.89   Other chlamydial diseases

A74.9   Chlamydial infection, unspecified
     Chlamydiosis NOS

Rickettsioses (A75-A79)

✓4ᵗʰ A75   Typhus fever
     EXCLUDES 1   rickettsiosis due to Ehrlichia sennetsu (A79.81)

     CC Excl: For CC codes in category A75, unless otherwise noted:
     A44.0-A44.9, A68.0-A68.9, A69.20-A69.29, A75.0-A79.9, B55.0-B57.5, B60.0

A75.0   Epidemic louse-borne typhus fever due to Rickettsia prowazekii   cc
     Classical typhus (fever)
     Epidemic (louse-borne) typhus

A75.1   Recrudescent typhus [Brill's disease]   cc
     Brill-Zinsser disease

A75.2   Typhus fever due to Rickettsia typhi   cc
     Murine (flea-borne) typhus

Certain Infectious and Parasitic Diseases

A75.3–A83.1

A75.3 **Typhus fever due to** Rickettsia tsutsugamushi   CC
Scrub (mite-borne) typhus
Tsutsugamushi fever

A75.9 **Typhus fever,** unspecified   CC
Typhus (fever) NOS
CC Excl: A17.82, A44.0-A44.9, A50.42, A52.14, A68.0-A68.9,
A69.20-A69.29, A75.0-A79.9, A81.1, A81.82-A81.89, A83.0-A85.8,
A87.2, A88.0, A88.8, A92.1-A92.8, A93.0, B00.4, B00.82, B01.11-
B01.12, B04, B06.01, B08.09, B08.20-B08.22, B08.60-B08.79, B09-
B10.09, B26.2, B33.1, B45.0, B45.2-B45.9, B50.9, B55.0-B57.5, B58.2,
B60.0, B75, B97.10, B97.21, G04.00-G04.01, G04.31, G04.81-G05.4,
G37.0, G37.4-G37.5, J09.X3-J09.X9, J10.2-J10.89, J11.2-J11.89,
L44.4, M1A.10-M1A.19, P35.2-P35.9, P37.0-P37.4, P37.8-P37.9,
T56.0X1-T56.0X4 with 7th character A

✓4ᵗʰ **A77** **Spotted fever [tick-borne rickettsioses]**

CC Excl: For CC codes in category A77, unless otherwise noted:
A44.0-A44.9, A68.0-A68.9, A69.20-A69.29, A75.0-A79.9, B55.0-B57.5,
B60.0

A77.0 **Spotted fever due to** Rickettsia rickettsii   CC
Rocky Mountain spotted fever
Sao Paulo fever

A77.1 **Spotted fever due to** Rickettsia conorii   CC
African tick typhus
Boutonneuse fever
India tick typhus
Kenya tick typhus
Marseilles fever
Mediterranean tick fever

A77.2 **Spotted fever due to** Rickettsia siberica   CC
North Asian tick fever
Siberian tick typhus

A77.3 **Spotted fever due to** Rickettsia australis   CC
Queensland tick typhus

✓5ᵗʰ **A77.4** **Ehrlichiosis**
EXCLUDES 1 Rickettsiosis due to Ehrlichia sennetsu (A79.81)

A77.40 **Ehrlichiosis,** unspecified   CC

A77.41 **Ehrlichiosis chafeensis [E. chafeensis]**   CC

A77.49 **Other ehrlichiosis**   CC

A77.8 **Other spotted fevers**   CC

A77.9 **Spotted fever,** unspecified   CC
Tick-borne typhus NOS

A78 **Q fever**   CC
Infection due to Coxiella burnetii
Nine Mile fever
Quadrilateral fever
CC Excl: See code: A77

✓4ᵗʰ **A79** **Other rickettsioses**

A79.0 **Trench fever**   CC
Quintan fever   Wolhynian fever
CC Excl: See code: A77

A79.1 **Rickettsialpox due to** Rickettsia akari   CC
Kew Garden fever   Vesicular rickettsiosis
CC Excl: A77.0-A79.9

✓5ᵗʰ **A79.8** **Other specified rickettsioses**

A79.81 **Rickettsiosis due to** Ehrlichia sennetsu   CC
CC Excl: See code: A79.1

A79.89 **Other specified rickettsioses**   CC
CC Excl: See code: A79.1

A79.9 **Rickettsiosis,** unspecified   CC
Rickettsial infection NOS
CC Excl: See code: A79.1

Viral and prion infections of the central nervous system (A80-A89)

EXCLUDES 1 postpolio syndrome (G14)
sequelae of poliomyelitis (B91)
sequelae of viral encephalitis (B94.1)

✓4ᵗʰ **A80** **Acute poliomyelitis**

CC Excl: For MCC codes in category A80, unless otherwise noted:
A80.0-A80.39

A80.0 **Acute paralytic poliomyelitis,** vaccine-associated   MCC

A80.1 **Acute paralytic poliomyelitis,** wild virus, imported   MCC

A80.2 **Acute paralytic poliomyelitis,** wild virus, indigenous   MCC

✓5ᵗʰ **A80.3** **Acute paralytic poliomyelitis,** other and unspecified

A80.30 **Acute paralytic poliomyelitis,** unspecified   MCC

A80.39 **Other acute paralytic poliomyelitis**   MCC

A80.4 **Acute nonparalytic poliomyelitis**

A80.9 **Acute poliomyelitis,** unspecified

✓4ᵗʰ **A81** **Atypical virus infections of central nervous system**
INCLUDES diseases of the central nervous system caused by prions
Use additional code to identify:
dementia with behavioral disturbance (F02.81)
dementia without behavioral disturbance (F02.80)

✓5ᵗʰ **A81.0** **Creutzfeldt-Jakob disease**

A81.00 **Creutzfeldt-Jakob disease,** unspecified   CC
Jakob-Creutzfeldt disease, unspecified
CC Excl: A17.82, A50.42, A52.14, A75.9, A79.9, A81.00-
A81.9, A83.0-A85.8, A87.2, A88.0, A88.8, A92.1-A92.2,
A92.4-A92.8, A93.0, B00.4, B00.82, B01.11-B01.12, B04,
B06.01, B08.09, B08.20-B08.22, B08.60-B08.79, B09-
B10.09, B26.2, B33.1, B45.0, B45.2-B45.9, B58.2, B75,
B97.10, G04.00-G04.01, G04.31, G04.81-G05.4, G37.0,
G37.4-G37.5, I67.3, J09.X3-J09.X9, J10.2-J10.89, J11.2-
J11.89, L44.4, M1A.10-M1A.19, P35.2-P35.9, P37.0-P37.4,
P37.8-P37.9, T56.0X1-T56.0X4A

A81.01 **Variant Creutzfeldt-Jakob disease**   CC
vCJD
CC Excl: See code: A81.00

A81.09 **Other Creutzfeldt-Jakob disease**   CC
CJD
Familial Creutzfeldt-Jakob disease
Iatrogenic Creutzfeldt-Jakob disease
Sporadic Creutzfeldt-Jakob disease
Subacute spongiform encephalopathy (with
dementia)
CC Excl: See code: A81.00

A81.1 **Subacute sclerosing panencephalitis**   CC
Dawson's inclusion body encephalitis
Van Bogaert's sclerosing leukoencephalopathy
CC Excl: A81.1, B92, B94.2-B94.9

A81.2 **Progressive multifocal leukoencephalopathy**   HIV CC
Multifocal leukoencephalopathy NOS
CC Excl: A17.82, A50.42, A52.14, A75.9, A79.9, A81.00-A81.9,
A83.0-A85.8, A87.2, A88.0, A88.8, A92.1-A92.2, A92.4-A92.8, A93.0,
B00.4, B00.82, B01.11-B01.12, B04, B06.01, B08.09, B08.20-B08.22,
B08.60-B08.79, B09-B10.09, B26.2, B27.00-B27.99, B33.1, B45.0,
B45.2-B45.9, B58.2, B75, G04.00-G04.01, G04.31, G04.81-G05.4,
G37.0, G37.4-G37.5, I67.3, J09.X3-J09.X9, J10.2-J10.89, J11.2-
J11.89, L44.4, M1A.10X0-M1A.19X1, P35.2-P35.9, P37.0-P37.4,
P37.8-P37.9, T56.0X1A, T56.0X2A, T56.0X3A, T56.0X4A

✓5ᵗʰ **A81.8** **Other atypical virus infections of central nervous system**

A81.81 **Kuru**   CC
CC Excl: A81.00-A81.9, I67.3

A81.82 **Gerstmann-Sträussler-Scheinker syndrome**   HIV CC
GSS syndrome
CC Excl: A81.00-A81.9, A92.30-A92.39, B97.21, I67.3

A81.83 **Fatal familial insomnia**   HIV CC
FFI
CC Excl: See code: A81.82

A81.89 **Other atypical virus infections of central nervous system**   HIV CC
CC Excl: See code: A81.82

A81.9 **Atypical virus infection of central nervous system, unspecified**   HIV CC
Prion diseases of the central nervous system NOS
CC Excl: See code: A81.81

✓4ᵗʰ **A82** **Rabies**

CC Excl: For CC codes in category A82, unless otherwise noted:
A82.0-A82.9

A82.0 **Sylvatic rabies**   CC

A82.1 **Urban rabies**   CC

A82.9 **Rabies,** unspecified   CC

✓4ᵗʰ **A83** **Mosquito-borne viral encephalitis**
INCLUDES mosquito-borne viral meningoencephalitis
EXCLUDES 2 Venezuelan equine encephalitis (A92.2)
West Nile fever (A92.3-)
West Nile virus (A92.3-)

CC Excl: For MCC codes in category A83, unless otherwise noted:
A17.82, A50.42, A52.14, A75.9, A79.9, A81.1, A81.82-A81.89, A83.0-
A85.8, A87.2, A88.0, A88.8, A92.1-A92.8, A93.0, B00.4, B00.82,
B01.11-B01.12, B04, B06.01, B08.09, B08.20-B08.22, B08.60-B08.79,
B09-B10.09, B26.2, B27.00-B27.99, B33.1, B45.0, B45.2-B45.9, B58.2,
B75, B97.10, B97.21, G04.00-G04.01, G04.31, G04.81-G05.4, G37.0,
G37.4-G37.5, J09.X3-J09.X9, J10.2-J10.89, J11.2-J11.89, L44.4,
M1A.10X0-M1A.19X1, P35.2-P35.9, P37.0-P37.4, P37.8-P37.9,
T56.0X1A, T56.0X2A, T56.0X3A, T56.0X4A

A83.0 **Japanese encephalitis**   MCC

A83.1 **Western equine encephalitis**   MCC

N Newborn: 0   P Pediatric: 0-17   M Maternity: 12-55   A Adult: 15-124   MCC Major CC Condition   PDx MCC PDx acts as own MCC   CC CC Condition   PDx CC PDx acts as own CC

A83.2 **Eastern equine encephalitis** `MCC`

A83.3 **St Louis encephalitis** `MCC`

A83.4 **Australian encephalitis** `MCC`
Kunjin virus disease

A83.5 **California encephalitis** `MCC`
California meningoencephalitis
La Crosse encephalitis

A83.6 **Rocio virus disease** `MCC`

A83.8 **Other mosquito-borne viral encephalitis** `MCC`

A83.9 **Mosquito-borne viral encephalitis, unspecified** `MCC`

✓4ᵗʰ **A84** **Tick-borne viral encephalitis**
`INCLUDES` tick-borne viral meningoencephalitis

CC Excl: For MCC codes in category A84, unless otherwise noted:
A17.82, A50.42, A52.14, A75.9, A79.9, A81.1, A81.82-A81.89, A83.0-A85.8, A87.2, A88.0, A88.8, A92.1-A92.8, A93.0, B00.4, B00.82, B01.11-B01.12, B04, B06.01, B08.09, B08.20-B08.22, B08.60-B08.79, B09-B10.09, B26.2, B27.00-B27.99, B33.1, B45.0, B45.2-B45.9, B58.2, B75, B97.10, B97.21, G04.00-G04.01, G04.31, G04.81-G05.4, G37.0, G37.4-G37.5, J09.X3-J09.X9, J10.2-J10.89, J11.2-J11.89, M1A.10X0-M1A.19X1, P35.2-P35.9, P37.0-P37.4, P37.8-P37.9, T56.0X1A, T56.0X2A, T56.0X3A, T56.0X4A

A84.0 **Far Eastern tick-borne encephalitis [Russian spring-summer encephalitis]** `MCC`

A84.1 **Central European tick-borne encephalitis** `MCC`

A84.8 **Other tick-borne viral encephalitis** `MCC`
Louping ill
Powassan virus disease

A84.9 **Tick-borne viral encephalitis, unspecified** `MCC`

✓4ᵗʰ **A85** **Other viral encephalitis, not elsewhere classified**
`INCLUDES` specified viral encephalomyelitis NEC
specified viral meningoencephalitis NEC
`EXCLUDES 1` benign myalgic encephalomyelitis (G93.3)
encephalitis due to cytomegalovirus (B25.8)
encephalitis due to herpesvirus NEC (B10.0-)
encephalitis due to herpesvirus [herpes simplex] (B00.4)
encephalitis due to measles virus (B05.0)
encephalitis due to mumps virus (B26.2)
encephalitis due to poliomyelitis virus (A80.-)
encephalitis due to zoster (B02.0)
lymphocytic choriomeningitis (A87.2)

CC Excl: For CC/MCC codes in category A85, unless otherwise noted: A17.82, A50.42, A52.14, A75.9, A79.9, A81.1, A81.82-A81.89, A83.0-A85.8, A87.2, A88.0, A88.8, A92.1-A92.8, A93.0, B00.4, B00.82, B01.11-B01.12, B04, B06.01, B08.09, B08.20-B08.22, B08.60-B08.79, B09-B10.09, B26.2, B27.00-B27.99, B33.1, B45.0, B45.2-B45.9, B58.2, B75, B97.10, B97.21, G04.00-G04.01, G04.31, G04.81-G05.4, G37.0, G37.4-G37.5, H66.40-H66.43, J09.X3-J09.X9, J10.2-J10.89, J11.2-J11.89, L44.4, M1A.10X0-M1A.19X1, M32.0-M32.9, P35.2-P35.9, P37.0-P37.4, P37.8-P37.9, T56.0X1A, T56.0X2A, T56.0X3A, T56.0X4A

A85.0 **Enteroviral encephalitis** `HIV` `CC`
Enteroviral encephalomyelitis

A85.1 **Adenoviral encephalitis** `HIV` `CC`
Adenoviral meningoencephalitis

A85.2 **Arthropod-borne viral encephalitis, unspecified** `MCC`
`EXCLUDES 1` West nile virus with encephalitis (A92.31)

A85.8 **Other specified viral encephalitis** `HIV` `CC`
Encephalitis lethargica
Von Economo-Cruchet disease

A86 **Unspecified viral encephalitis** `HIV` `CC`
Viral encephalomyelitis NOS
Viral meningoencephalitis NOS
CC Excl: A17.82, A50.42, A52.14, A75.9, A79.9, A81.1, A81.82-A81.89, A83.0-A86, A87.2, A88.0, A88.8-A89, A92.1-A92.2, A92.4-A92.8, A93.0, B00.4, B00.82, B01.11-B01.12, B04, B06.01, B08.09, B08.20-B08.22, B08.60-B08.79, B09-B10.09, B26.2, B27.00-B27.99, B33.1, B45.0, B45.2-B45.9, B58.2, B75, B97.10, G04.00-G04.01, G04.31, G04.81-G05.4, G37.0, G37.4-G37.5, H66.40-H66.43, J09.X3-J09.X9, J10.2-J10.89, J11.2-J11.89, L44.4, M1A.10X0-M1A.19X1, M32.0-M32.9, P35.2-P35.9, P37.0-P37.4, P37.8-P37.9, T56.0X1A, T56.0X2A, T56.0X3A, T56.0X4A

✓4ᵗʰ **A87** **Viral meningitis**
`EXCLUDES 1` meningitis due to herpesvirus [herpes simplex] (B00.3)
meningitis due to measles virus (B05.1)
meningitis due to mumps virus (B26.1)
meningitis due to poliomyelitis virus (A80.-)
meningitis due to zoster (B02.1)

CC Excl: For CC/MCC codes in category A87, unless otherwise noted: A02.21, A17.0-A17.1, A27.81, A39.0, A50.41, A51.41, A52.13, A54.82, A54.84, A54.89-A54.9, A74.81-A74.9, A87.0-A87.9, A96.2, A98.3-A98.4, B26.1, B33.24, B33.4-B33.8, B34.1-B34.2, B34.4-B34.8, B37.5, B38.4, B45.1, B58.2, B92, B94.2-B94.9, B97.10, B97.19, B97.29, B97.5-B97.6, B97.81-B97.89, G00.0-G03.9, G04.2, G32.89, G61.0, G96.8-G96.9, G98.0-G98.8, G99.8

A87.0 **Enteroviral meningitis** `CC`
Coxsackievirus meningitis
Echovirus meningitis

A87.1 **Adenoviral meningitis** `CC`

A87.2 **Lymphocytic choriomeningitis** `CC`
Lymphocytic meningoencephalitis
CC Excl: A02.21, A17.0-A17.1, A27.81, A39.0, A50.41, A51.41, A52.13, A54.82, A54.84, A54.89-A54.9, A74.81-A74.9, A87.0-A87.9, A92.30-A92.39, A96.2, A98.3-A98.4, B26.1, B33.24, B33.4-B33.8, B34.1-B34.2, B34.4-B34.8, B37.5, B38.4, B45.1, B58.2, B92, B94.2-B94.9, B97.10, B97.19-B97.29, B97.5-B97.6, B97.81-B97.89, G00.0-G03.9, G04.2, G32.89, G61.0, G96.8-G96.9, G98.0-G98.8, G99.8

A87.8 **Other viral meningitis** `CC`

A87.9 **Viral meningitis, unspecified** `CC`

✓4ᵗʰ **A88** **Other viral infections of central nervous system, not elsewhere classified**
`EXCLUDES 1` viral encephalitis NOS (A86)
viral meningitis NOS (A87.9)

A88.0 **Enteroviral exanthematous fever [Boston exanthem]** `CC`
CC Excl: A17.82, A50.42, A52.14, A75.9, A79.9, A81.1, A81.82-A81.89, A83.0-A85.8, A87.2, A88.0, A88.8, A92.1-A92.8, A93.0, B00.4, B00.82, B01.11-B01.12, B04, B06.01, B08.09, B08.20-B08.22, B08.60-B08.79, B09-B10.09, B26.2, B27.00-B27.99, B33.1, B45.0, B45.2-B45.9, B58.2, B75, B97.10, B97.21, G04.00-G04.01, G04.31, G04.81-G05.4, G37.0, G37.4-G37.5, J09.X3-J09.X9, J10.2-J10.89, J11.2-J11.89, L44.4, M1A.10X0-M1A.19X1, P35.2-P35.9, P37.0-P37.4, P37.8-P37.9, T56.0X1A, T56.0X2A, T56.0X3A, T56.0X4A

A88.1 **Epidemic vertigo**

A88.8 **Other specified viral infections of central nervous system** `HIV` `CC`
CC Excl: See code: A85

A89 **Unspecified viral infection of central nervous system** `HIV` `CC`
CC Excl: See code: A86

Arthropod-borne viral fevers and viral hemorrhagic fevers (A90-A99)

A90 **Dengue fever [classical dengue]** `CC`
`EXCLUDES 1` dengue hemorrhagic fever (A91)
CC Excl: A90

A91 **Dengue hemorrhagic fever** `CC`
CC Excl: A91-A94, A98.0-A98.2, A98.8-A99, B33.1

✓4ᵗʰ **A92** **Other mosquito-borne viral fevers**
`EXCLUDES 1` Ross River disease (B33.1)

A92.0 **Chikungunya virus disease** `CC`
Chikungunya (hemorrhagic) fever
CC Excl: See code: A91

A92.1 **O'nyong-nyong fever** `CC`
CC Excl: A17.82, A50.42, A52.14, A75.9, A79.9, A81.1, A81.82-A81.89, A83.0-A85.8, A87.2, A88.0, A88.8, A91-A94, A98.0-A98.2, A98.8-A99, B00.4, B00.82, B01.11-B01.12, B04, B06.01, B08.09, B08.20-B08.22, B08.60-B08.79, B09-B10.09, B26.2, B27.00-B27.99, B33.1, B45.0, B45.2-B45.9, B58.2, B75, B97.10, B97.21, G04.00-G04.01, G04.31, G04.81-G05.4, G37.0, G37.4-G37.5, J09.X3-J09.X9, J10.2-J10.89, J11.2-J11.89, L44.4, M1A.10X0-M1A.19X1, P35.2-P35.9, P37.0-P37.4, P37.8-P37.9, T56.0X1A, T56.0X2A, T56.0X3A, T56.0X4A

A92.2 **Venezuelan equine fever** `CC`
Venezuelan equine encephalitis
Venezuelan equine encephalomyelitis virus disease
CC Excl: See code: A92.1

✓ Additional Character Required ✓x7ᵗʰ Xtension Alert Unacceptable PDx Manifestation Hospital Acquired Condition `EXCLUDES 1` Not Coded Here `EXCLUDES 2` Not Included Here

✓5ᵗʰ **A92.3 West Nile virus infection**
West Nile fever

> **CC Excl:** For MCC codes in subcategory A92.3, unless otherwise noted: A17.82, A50.42, A52.14, A75.9, A79.9, A81.1, A81.82-A81.89, A83.0-A85.8, A87.2, A88.0, A88.8, A91-A92.2, A92.4-A94, A98.0-A98.2, A98.8-A99, B00.4, B00.82, B01.11-B01.12, B04, B06.01, B08.09, B08.20-B08.22, B08.60-B08.79, B09-B10.09, B26.2, B27.00-B27.99, B33.1, B45.0, B45.2-B45.9, B58.2, B75, B97.10, G04.00-G04.01, G04.31, G04.81-G05.4, G37.0, G37.4-G37.5, J09.X3-J09.X9, J10.2-J10.89, J11.2-J11.89, L44.4, P35.2-P35.9, P37.0-P37.4, P37.8-P37.9

   A92.30 West Nile virus infection, unspecified `MCC`
West Nile fever NOS
West Nile fever without complications
West Nile virus NOS

   A92.31 West Nile virus infection with encephalitis `MCC`
West Nile encephalitis
West Nile encephalomyelitis

   A92.32 West Nile virus infection with other neurologic manifestation `MCC`
Use additional code to specify the neurologic manifestation

   A92.39 West Nile virus infection with other complications `MCC`
Use additional code to specify the other conditions

A92.4 Rift Valley fever `CC`
   CC Excl: See code: A92.1

A92.8 Other specified mosquito-borne viral fevers `CC`
   CC Excl: See code: A92.1

A92.9 Mosquito-borne viral fever, unspecified `CC`
   CC Excl: See code: A91

✓4ᵗʰ **A93 Other arthropod-borne viral fevers, not elsewhere classified**

   A93.0 Oropouche virus disease `CC`
Oropouche fever
CC Excl: A17.82, A50.42, A52.14, A75.9, A79.9, A81.1, A81.82-A81.89, A83.0-A85.8, A87.2, A88.0, A88.8, A91-A94, A98.0-A98.2, A98.8-A99, B00.4, B00.82, B01.11-B01.12, B04, B06.01, B08.09, B08.20-B08.22, B08.60-B08.79, B09-B10.09, B26.2, B27.00-B27.99, B33.1, B45.0, B45.2-B45.9, B58.2, B75, B97.10, B97.21, G04.00-G04.01, G04.31, G04.81-G05.4, G37.0, G37.4-G37.5, J09.X3-J09.X9, J10.2-J10.89, J11.2-J11.89, L44.4, M1A.10-M1A.19, P35.2-P35.9, P37.0-P37.4, P37.8-P37.9, T56.0X1-T56.0X4 with 7th A

   A93.1 Sandfly fever `CC`
Pappataci fever
Phlebotomus fever
CC Excl: A91-A94, A98.0-A98.2, A98.8-A99, B33.1

   A93.2 Colorado tick fever `CC`
CC Excl: See code: A93.1

   A93.8 Other specified arthropod-borne viral fevers `CC`
Piry virus disease
Vesicular stomatitis virus disease [Indiana fever]
CC Excl: See code: A91

A94 Unspecified arthropod-borne viral fever `CC`
Arboviral fever NOS
Arbovirus infection NOS
CC Excl: A91-A94, A98.0-A98.2, A98.8-A99, B33.1

✓4ᵗʰ **A95 Yellow fever**

> **CC Excl:** For CC codes in category A95, unless otherwise noted: A95.0-A95.9

A95.0 Sylvatic yellow fever `CC`
Jungle yellow fever

A95.1 Urban yellow fever `CC`

A95.9 Yellow fever, unspecified `CC`

✓4ᵗʰ **A96 Arenaviral hemorrhagic feverr**

> **CC Excl:** For CC codes in category A96, unless otherwise noted: A74.81-A74.9, A88.1, A96.0-A96.9, A98.3-A98.5, B25.8-B25.9, B33.24-B34.2, B34.4-B34.8, B97.0-B97.89

A96.0 Junin hemorrhagic fever `CC`
Argentinian hemorrhagic fever

A96.1 Machupo hemorrhagic fever `CC`
Bolivian hemorrhagic fever

A96.2 Lassa fever

A96.8 Other arenaviral hemorrhagic fevers `CC`

A96.9 Arenaviral hemorrhagic fever, unspecified `CC`

✓4ᵗʰ **A98 Other viral hemorrhagic fevers, not elsewhere classified**
> *EXCLUDES 1* chikungunya hemorrhagic fever (A92.0)
> dengue hemorrhagic fever (A91)

> **CC Excl:** For CC codes in category A98, unless otherwise noted: A91-A94, A98.0-A98.2, A98.8-A99, B33.1

A98.0 Crimean-Congo hemorrhagic fever `CC`
Central Asian hemorrhagic fever

A98.1 Omsk hemorrhagic fever `CC`

A98.2 Kyasanur Forest disease `CC`

A98.3 Marburg virus disease

A98.4 Ebola virus disease

A98.5 Hemorrhagic fever with renal syndrome `CC`
Epidemic hemorrhagic fever
Korean hemorrhagic fever
Russian hemorrhagic fever
Hantaan virus disease
Hantavirus disease with renal manifestations
Nephropathia epidemica
Songo fever
> *EXCLUDES 1* hantavirus (cardio)-pulmonary syndrome (B33.4)

CC Excl: A17.9, A18.10-A18.11, A18.13, A18.82, A18.84, A18.89, A54.21, A54.29, A54.82, A54.84, A54.89-A54.9, A59.00, A59.8-A59.9, A98.5, B37.41-B37.49, B97.21, E08.21-E08.29, E08.618-E08.638, E08.649-E08.68, E09.21-E09.29, E09.618-E09.638, E09.649-E09.8, E10.21-E10.29, E10.618-E10.638, E10.649, E10.69-E10.8, E11.21-E11.29, E11.618-E11.638, E11.649, E11.69-E11.8, E13.21-E13.29, E13.618-E13.638, E13.649-E13.8, M10.30-M10.39, N00.0-N11.0, N11.8-N13.39, N13.6, N14.0-N17.9, N19, N25.0-N26.1, N26.9-N27.9, N28.1-N29, N36.41-N36.43, N36.8-N36.9, N39.8-N39.9, R31.0-R31.9

A98.8 Other specified viral hemorrhagic fevers `CC`

A99 Unspecified viral hemorrhagic fever `CC`
   CC Excl: See code: A98

Viral infections characterized by skin and mucous membrane lesions (B00-B09)

✓4ᵗʰ **B00 Herpesviral [herpes simplex] infections**
> *EXCLUDES 1* congenital herpesviral infections (P35.2)
> *EXCLUDES 2* anogenital herpesviral infection (A60.-)
> gammaherpesviral mononucleosis (B27.0-)
> herpangina (B08.5)

B00.0 Eczema herpeticum `HIV`
Kaposi's varicelliform eruption

B00.1 Herpesviral vesicular dermatitis `HIV`
Herpes simplex facialis   Vesicular dermatitis of ear
Herpes simplex labialis   Vesicular dermatitis of lip
Herpes simplex otitis externa

B00.2 Herpesviral gingivostomatitis and pharyngotonsillitis `HIV` `CC`
Herpesviral pharyngitis
CC Excl: B00.2

B00.3 Herpesviral meningitis `HIV` `MCC`
CC Excl: A02.21, A17.0-A17.1, A27.81, A39.0, A50.41, A51.41, A52.13, A54.82, A54.84, A54.89-A54.9, A87.0-A87.9, B00.3, B00.82-B00.9, B02.1, B10.81-B10.89, B26.1, B37.5, B38.4, B45.1, B58.2, B92, B94.2-B94.9, G00.0-G03.9, G04.2, G32.89, G61.0, G96.8-G96.9, G98.0-G98.8, G99.8

B00.4 Herpesviral encephalitis `HIV` `MCC`
Herpesviral meningoencephalitis
Simian B disease
> *EXCLUDES 1* herpesviral encephalitis due to herpesvirus 6 and 7 (B10.01, B10.09)
> non-simplex herpesviral encephalitis (B10.0-)

CC Excl: B00.4-B00.9, B10.01-B10.89, B92, B94.2-B94.9

✓5ᵗʰ **B00.5 Herpesviral ocular disease**

> **CC Excl:** For CC codes in subcategory B00.5, unless otherwise noted: B00.50-B00.59, B00.89-B00.9, B10.81-B10.89

   B00.50 Herpesviral ocular disease, unspecified `HIV` `CC`

   B00.51 Herpesviral iridocyclitis `HIV` `CC`
Herpesviral iritis
Herpesviral uveitis, anterior

   B00.52 Herpesviral keratitis `HIV` `CC`
Herpesviral keratoconjunctivitis

   B00.53 Herpesviral conjunctivitis `HIV` `CC`

   B00.59 Other herpesviral disease of eye `HIV` `CC`
Herpesviral dermatitis of eyelid

N Newborn: 0   P Pediatric: 0-17   M Maternity: 12-55   A Adult: 15-124   MCC Major CC Condition   PDx MCC PDx acts as own MCC   CC CC Condition   PDx CC PDx acts as own CC

436   ICD-10-CM Draft (2015)

B00.7 **Disseminated herpesviral disease** `HIV` `MCC`
Herpesviral sepsis
CC Excl: A02.1, A20.7, A22.7, A26.7, A32.7, A39.2-A39.4, A40.0-
A40.1, A40.8-A41.9, A42.7, A54.86, B00.7, B00.82-B00.9, B10.81-
B10.89, B37.7, B92, B94.2-B94.9, R65.10-R65.20

✓5ᵗʰ **B00.8** **Other forms of herpesviral infections**

B00.81 **Herpesviral hepatitis** `HIV` `CC`
CC Excl: B00.3, B00.81-B00.9, B10.81-B10.89, B92,
B94.2-B94.9

B00.82 **Herpes simplex myelitis** `MCC`
CC Excl: A74.81-A74.9, A96.2, A98.3-A98.4, B00.82-
B00.9, B01.12, B02.24, B10.81-B10.89, B33.24, B33.4-
B33.8, B34.1-B34.2, B34.4-B34.8, B92, B94.2-B94.9,
B97.10, B97.19, B97.29, B97.5-B97.6, B97.81-B97.89,
G04.00-G04.01, G04.31, G04.81-G04.89, G05.3-G05.4,
G37.3

B00.89 **Other herpesviral infection** `HIV` `CC`
Herpesviral whitlow
CC Excl: A74.81-A74.9, A96.2, A98.3-A98.4, B00.82-
B00.9, B10.81-B10.89, B33.24, B33.4-B33.8, B34.1-B34.2,
B34.4-B34.8, B92, B94.2-B94.9, B97.10, B97.19, B97.29,
B97.5-B97.6, B97.81-B97.89

B00.9 **Herpesviral infection, unspecified** `HIV`
Herpes simplex infection NOS

✓4ᵗʰ **B01** **Varicella [chickenpox]**

B01.0 **Varicella meningitis** `CC`
CC Excl: A74.81-A74.9, A96.2, A98.3-A98.4, B01.0, B01.12, B01.81-
B01.9, B08.04, B33.24, B33.4-B33.8, B34.1-B34.2, B34.4-B34.8, B92,
B94.2-B94.9, B97.10, B97.19, B97.29, B97.5-B97.6, B97.81-B97.89

✓5ᵗʰ **B01.1** **Varicella encephalitis, myelitis and encephalomyelitis**
Postchickenpox encephalitis, myelitis and encephalomyelitis

B01.11 **Varicella encephalitis and encephalomyelitis** `MCC`
Postchickenpox encephalitis and encephalomyelitis
CC Excl: A74.81-A74.9, A96.2, A98.3-A98.4, B01.0-
B01.12, B01.81-B01.9, B08.04, B33.24, B33.4-B33.8,
B34.1-B34.2, B34.4-B34.8, B92, B94.2-B94.9, B97.10,
B97.19, B97.29, B97.5-B97.6, B97.81-B97.89

B01.12 **Varicella myelitis** `MCC`
Postchickenpox myelitis
CC Excl: A74.81-A74.9, A96.2, A98.3-A98.4, B00.82,
B01.0, B01.12, B01.81-B01.9, B02.24, B08.04, B33.24,
B33.4-B33.8, B34.1-B34.2, B34.4-B34.8, B92, B94.2-B94.9,
B97.10, B97.19, B97.29, B97.5-B97.6, B97.81-B97.89,
G04.00-G04.01, G04.31, G04.81-G04.89, G05.3-G05.4,
G37.3

B01.2 **Varicella pneumonia** `MCC`
CC Excl: A74.81-A74.9, A96.2, A98.3-A98.4, B01.0, B01.12-B01.9,
B08.04, B33.24, B33.4-B33.8, B34.1-B34.2, B34.4-B34.8, B92, B94.2-
B94.9, B97.10, B97.19, B97.29, B97.5-B97.6, B97.81-B97.89

✓5ᵗʰ **B01.8** **Varicella with other complications**

B01.81 **Varicella keratitis** `CC`
CC Excl: See code: B01.0

B01.89 **Other varicella complications** `CC`
CC Excl: See code: B01.0

B01.9 **Varicella without complication** `CC`
Varicella NOS
CC Excl: See code: B01.0

✓4ᵗʰ **B02** **Zoster [herpes zoster]**
INCLUDES shingles
zona

B02.0 **Zoster encephalitis** `HIV` `CC`
Zoster meningoencephalitis
CC Excl: A74.81-A74.9, A96.2, A98.3-A98.4, B00.3, B00.82-B00.9,
B02.0-B02.29, B02.7-B02.9, B10.81-B10.89, B33.24, B33.4-B33.8,
B34.1-B34.2, B34.4-B34.8, B92, B94.2-B94.9, B97.10, B97.19,
B97.29, B97.5-B97.6, B97.81-B97.89

B02.1 **Zoster meningitis** `HIV` `MCC`
CC Excl: A02.21, A17.0-A17.1, A27.81, A39.0, A50.41, A51.41,
A52.13, A54.82, A54.84, A54.89-A54.9, A74.81-A74.9, A87.0-A87.9,
A96.2, A98.3-A98.4, B00.3, B00.82-B00.9, B02.0-B02.29, B02.7-
B02.9, B10.81-B10.89, B26.1, B33.24, B33.4-B33.8, B34.1-B34.2,
B34.4-B34.8, B37.5, B38.4, B45.1, B58.2, B92, B94.2-B94.9, B97.10,
B97.19, B97.29, B97.5-B97.6, B97.81-B97.89, G00.0-G03.9, G04.2,
G32.89, G61.0, G96.8-G96.9, G98.0-G98.8, G99.8

✓5ᵗʰ **B02.2** **Zoster with other nervous system involvement**

CC Excl: For CC/MCC codes in subcategory B02.2, unless
otherwise noted: A74.81-A74.9, A96.2, A98.3-A98.4, B00.3,
B00.82-B00.9, B02.0-B02.29, B02.7-B02.9, B10.81-B10.89,
B33.24, B33.4-B33.8, B34.1-B34.2, B34.4-B34.8, B92, B94.2-
B94.9, B97.10, B97.29, B97.5-B97.6, B97.81-B97.89

B02.21 **Postherpetic geniculate ganglionitis** `HIV` `CC`
B02.22 **Postherpetic trigeminal neuralgia** `HIV` `CC`

B02.23 **Postherpetic polyneuropathy** `HIV` `CC`
B02.24 **Postherpetic myelitis** `MCC`
Herpes zoster myelitis
CC Excl: A74.81-A74.9, A96.2, A98.3-A98.4, B00.3,
B00.82-B00.9, B01.12, B02.0-B02.29, B02.7-B02.9,
B10.81-B10.89, B33.24, B33.4-B33.8, B34.1-B34.2, B34.4-
B34.8, B92, B94.2-B94.9, B97.10, B97.19, B97.29, B97.5-
B97.6, B97.81-B97.89, G04.00-G04.01, G04.31, G04.81-
G04.89, G05.3-G05.4, G37.3

B02.29 **Other postherpetic nervous system** `HIV` `CC`
involvement
Postherpetic radiculopathy

✓5ᵗʰ **B02.3** **Zoster ocular disease**

CC Excl: For CC codes in subcategory B02.3, unless
otherwise noted: B02.30-B02.39

B02.30 **Zoster ocular disease, unspecified** `HIV` `CC`
B02.31 **Zoster conjunctivitis** `HIV` `CC`
B02.32 **Zoster iridocyclitis** `HIV` `CC`
B02.33 **Zoster keratitis** `HIV` `CC`
Herpes zoster keratoconjunctivitis
B02.34 **Zoster scleritis** `HIV` `CC`
B02.39 **Other herpes zoster eye disease** `HIV` `CC`
Zoster blepharitis

B02.7 **Disseminated zoster** `HIV` `CC`
CC Excl: A60.00-A60.9, A74.81-A74.9, A96.2, A98.3-A98.4, B00.0-
B00.2, B00.4-B00.9, B02.0-B02.9, B10.01-B10.89, B33.24, B33.4-
B33.8, B34.1-B34.2, B34.4-B34.8, B92, B94.2-B94.9, B97.10, B97.19,
B97.29, B97.5-B97.6, B97.81-B97.89

B02.8 **Zoster with other complications** `HIV` `CC`
Herpes zoster otitis externa
CC Excl: See code: B02.7

B02.9 **Zoster without complications** `HIV`
Zoster NOS

B03 **Smallpox** `CC`
NOTE In 1980 the 33rd World Health Assembly declared that
smallpox had been eradicated.
The classification is maintained for surveillance purposes.
CC Excl: B01.0-B01.9, B03, B08.010-B08.04

B04 **Monkeypox** `CC`
CC Excl: B04-B08.011, B08.09, B08.3, B08.60-B08.79, B09, L44.4

✓4ᵗʰ **B05** **Measles**
INCLUDES morbilli
EXCLUDES 1 subacute sclerosing panencephalitis (A81.1)

B05.0 **Measles complicated by encephalitis** `MCC`
Postmeasles encephalitis
CC Excl: A74.81-A74.9, A96.2, A98.3-A98.4, B05.0-B05.1, B05.4,
B05.89-B05.9, B33.24, B33.4-B33.8, B34.1-B34.2, B34.4-B34.8, B92,
B94.2-B94.9, B97.10, B97.19, B97.29, B97.5-B97.6, B97.81-B97.89

B05.1 **Measles complicated by meningitis** `CC`
Postmeasles meningitis
CC Excl: A74.81-A74.9, A96.2, A98.3-A98.4, B05.1, B05.4, B05.89-
B05.9, B33.24, B33.4-B33.8, B34.1-B34.2, B34.4-B34.8, B92, B94.2-
B94.9, B97.10, B97.19, B97.29, B97.5-B97.6, B97.81-B97.89

B05.2 **Measles complicated by pneumonia** `MCC`
Postmeasles pneumonia
CC Excl: A74.81-A74.9, A96.2, A98.3-A98.4, B05.1-B05.2, B05.4,
B05.89-B05.9, B33.24, B33.4-B33.8, B34.1-B34.2, B34.4-B34.8, B92,
B94.2-B94.9, B97.10, B97.19, B97.29, B97.5-B97.6, B97.81-B97.89

B05.3 **Measles complicated by otitis media**
Postmeasles otitis media

B05.4 **Measles with intestinal complications** `CC`
CC Excl: See code: B05.1

✓5ᵗʰ **B05.8** **Measles with other complications**

B05.81 **Measles keratitis and keratoconjunctivitis** `CC`
CC Excl: A74.81-A74.9, A96.2, A98.3-A98.4, B05.1, B05.4-
B05.9, B33.24, B33.4-B33.8, B34.1-B34.2, B34.4-B34.8,
B92, B94.2-B94.9, B97.10, B97.19, B97.29, B97.5-B97.6,
B97.81-B97.89

B05.89 **Other measles complications** `CC`
CC Excl: See code: B05.1

B05.9 **Measles without complication**
Measles NOS

✓ Additional Character Required   ✓x7ᵗʰ Xtension Alert   Unacceptable PDx   Manifestation   Hospital Acquired Condition   EXCLUDES 1 Not Coded Here   EXCLUDES 2 Not Included Here

Certain Infectious and Parasitic Diseases

B06–B16.2

✓4ᵗʰ **B06 Rubella [German measles]**
     EXCLUDES 1   congenital rubella (P35.0)c

✓5ᵗʰ **B06.0 Rubella with neurological complications**

> **CC Excl: For CC/MCC codes in subcategory B06.0, unless otherwise noted:** A74.81-A74.9, A96.2, A98.3-A98.4, B06.00-B06.81, B06.89-B06.9, B33.24, B33.4-B33.8, B34.1-B34.2, B34.4-B34.8, B92, B94.2-B94.9, B97.10, B97.19, B97.29, B97.5-B97.6, B97.81-B97.89

     B06.00 Rubella with neurological complication, unspecified   CC

     B06.01 Rubella encephalitis   MCC
         Rubella meningoencephalitis

     B06.02 Rubella meningitis   CC

     B06.09 Other neurological complications of rubella   CC

✓5ᵗʰ **B06.8 Rubella with other complications**

     B06.81 Rubella pneumonia   CC
         CC Excl: See code: B06.00

     B06.82 Rubella arthritis   CC
         CC Excl: A74.81-A74.9, A96.2, A98.3-A98.4, B06.81-B06.9, B33.24, B33.4-B33.8, B34.1-B34.2, B34.4-B34.8, B92, B94.2-B94.9, B97.10, B97.19, B97.29, B97.5-B97.6, B97.81-B97.89

     B06.89 Other rubella complications   CC
         CC Excl: See code: B06.0

     B06.9 Rubella without complication
         Rubella NOS

✓4ᵗʰ **B07 Viral warts**
     INCLUDES   verruca simplex
               verruca vulgaris
               viral warts due to human papillomavirus
     EXCLUDES 2   anogenital (venereal) warts (A63.0)
               papilloma of bladder (D41.4)
               papilloma of cervix (D26.0)
               papilloma larynx (D14.1)

     B07.0 Plantar wart
         Verruca plantaris

     B07.8 Other viral warts
         Common wart
         Flat wart
         Verruca plana

     B07.9 Viral wart, unspecified

✓4ᵗʰ **B08 Other viral infections characterized by skin and mucous membrane lesions, not elsewhere classified**
     EXCLUDES 1   vesicular stomatitis virus disease (A93.8)

✓5ᵗʰ **B08.0 Other orthopoxvirus infections**
     EXCLUDES 2   monkeypox (B04)

     ✓6ᵗʰ **B08.01 Cowpox and vaccinia not from vaccine**
         B08.010 Cowpox
         B08.011 Vaccinia not from vaccine
              EXCLUDES 1   vaccinia (from vaccination) (generalized) (T88.1)

     B08.02 Orf virus disease
         Contagious pustular dermatitis
         Ecthyma contagiosum

     B08.03 Pseudocowpox [milker's node]

     B08.04 Paravaccinia, unspecified

     B08.09 Other orthopoxvirus infections
         Orthopoxvirus infection NOS

     B08.1 Molluscum contagiosum

✓5ᵗʰ **B08.2 Exanthema subitum [sixth disease]**
         Roseola infantum

     B08.20 Exanthema subitum [sixth disease], unspecified   P
         Roseola infantum, unspecified

     B08.21 Exanthema subitum [sixth disease] due to human herpesvirus 6   P
         Roseola infantum due to human herpesvirus 6

     B08.22 Exanthema subitum [sixth disease] due to human herpesvirus 7   P
         Roseola infantum due to human herpesvirus 7

     B08.3 Erythema infectiosum [fifth disease]   CC
         CC Excl: B08.3-B34.3

     B08.4 Enteroviral vesicular stomatitis with exanthem
         Hand, foot and mouth disease

     B08.5 Enteroviral vesicular pharyngitis
         Herpangina

✓5ᵗʰ **B08.6 Parapoxvirus infections**

     B08.60 Parapoxvirus infection, unspecified

     B08.61 Bovine stomatitis

     B08.62 Sealpox

     B08.69 Other parapoxvirus infections

✓5ᵗʰ **B08.7 Yatapoxvirus infections**

     B08.70 Yatapoxvirus infection, unspecified

     B08.71 Tanapox virus disease   CC
         CC Excl: B04, B08.010-B08.011, B08.09, B08.3, B08.60-B08.79, B09, L44.4

     B08.72 Yaba pox virus disease
         Yaba monkey tumor disease

     B08.79 Other yatapoxvirus infections

     B08.8 Other specified viral infections characterized by skin and mucous membrane lesions
         Enteroviral lymphonodular pharyngitis
         Foot-and-mouth disease
         Poxvirus NEC

B09 Unspecified viral infection characterized by skin and mucous membrane lesions
     Viral enanthema NOS
     Viral exanthema NOS

Other human herpesviruses (B10)

✓4ᵗʰ **B10 Other human herpesviruses**
     EXCLUDES 2   cytomegalovirus (B25.9)
               Epstein-Barr virus (B27.0-)
               herpes NOS (B00.9)
               herpes simplex (B00.-)
               herpes zoster (B02.-)
               human herpesvirus NOS (B00.-)
               human herpesvirus 1 and 2 (B00.-)
               human herpesvirus 3 (B01.-, B02.-)
               human herpesvirus 4 (B27.0-)
               human herpesvirus 5 (B25.-)
               varicella (B01.-)
               zoster (B02.-)

✓5ᵗʰ **B10.0 Other human herpesvirus encephalitis**
     EXCLUDES 2   herpes encephalitis NOS (B00.4)
               herpes simplex encephalitis (B00.4)
               human herpesvirus encephalitis (B00.4)
               simian B herpes virus encephalitis (B00.4)

     B10.01 Human herpesvirus 6 encephalitis   HIV MCC
         CC Excl: B00.4, B00.82-B00.9, B10.01-B10.89, B92, B94.2-B94.9

     B10.09 Other human herpesvirus encephalitis   HIV MCC
         Human herpesvirus 7 encephalitis
         CC Excl: See code: B10.01

✓5ᵗʰ **B10.8 Other human herpesvirus infection**

     B10.81 Human herpesvirus 6 infection

     B10.82 Human herpesvirus 7 infection

     B10.89 Other human herpesvirus infection
         Human herpesvirus 8 infection
         Kaposi's sarcoma-associated herpesvirus infection

Viral hepatitis (B15-B19)

     EXCLUDES 1   sequelae of viral hepatitis (B94.2)
     EXCLUDES 2   cytomegaloviral hepatitis (B25.1)
               herpesviral [herpes simplex] hepatitis (B00.81)

✓4ᵗʰ **B15 Acute hepatitis A**

     B15.0 Hepatitis A with hepatic coma   MCC
         CC Excl: A74.81-A74.9, A96.2, A98.3-A98.4, B15.0-B19.9, B33.24, B33.4-B33.8, B34.1-B34.2, B34.4-B34.8, B92, B94.2-B94.9, B97.10, B97.19, B97.29, B97.5-B97.6, B97.81-B97.89

     B15.9 Hepatitis A without hepatic coma   CC
         Hepatitis A (acute)(viral) NOS
         CC Excl: See code: B15.0

✓4ᵗʰ **B16 Acute hepatitis B**

> **CC Excl: For CC/MCC codes in category B16, unless otherwise noted:** A74.81-A74.9, A96.2, A98.3-A98.4, B15.0-B19.9, B33.24, B33.4-B33.8, B34.1-B34.2, B34.4-B34.8, B92, B94.2-B94.9, B97.10, B97.19, B97.29, B97.5-B97.6, B97.81-B97.89

     B16.0 Acute hepatitis B with delta-agent with hepatic coma   MCC

     B16.1 Acute hepatitis B with delta-agent without hepatic coma   CC

     B16.2 Acute hepatitis B without delta-agent with hepatic coma   MCC

N Newborn: 0   P Pediatric: 0-17   M Maternity: 12-55   A Adult: 15-124   MCC Major CC Condition   PDx MCC PDx acts as own MCC   CC CC Condition   PDx CC PDx acts as own CC

438   ICD-10-CM Draft (2015)

B16.9 Acute hepatitis B without delta-agent and without hepatic coma `CC`
 Hepatitis B (acute) (viral) NOS

B17 Other acute viral hepatitis `√4th`

CC Excl: For CC/MCC codes in category B17, unless otherwise noted: A74.81-A74.9, A96.2, A98.3-A98.4, B15.0-B19.9, B33.24, B33.4-B33.8, B34.1-B34.2, B34.4-B34.8, B92, B94.2-B94.9, B97.10, B97.19, B97.29, B97.5-B97.6, B97.81-B97.89

B17.0 Acute delta-(super) infection of hepatitis B carrier `CC`

B17.1 Acute hepatitis C `√5th`
  B17.10 Acute hepatitis C without hepatic coma `CC`
   Acute hepatitis C NOS
  B17.11 Acute hepatitis C with hepatic coma `MCC`

B17.2 Acute hepatitis E `CC`

B17.8 Other specified acute viral hepatitis `CC`
  Hepatitis non-A non-B (acute) (viral) NEC

B17.9 Acute viral hepatitis, unspecified `CC`
  Acute hepatitis NOS

B18 Chronic viral hepatitis `√4th`

CC Excl: For CC codes in category B18, unless otherwise noted: A74.81-A74.9, A96.2, A98.3-A98.4, B15.0-B19.9, B33.24, B33.4-B33.8, B34.1-B34.2, B34.4-B34.8, B92, B94.2-B94.9, B97.10, B97.19, B97.29, B97.5-B97.6, B97.81-B97.89

B18.0 Chronic viral hepatitis B with delta-agent `CC`

B18.1 Chronic viral hepatitis B without delta-agent `CC`
  Chronic (viral) hepatitis B

B18.2 Chronic viral hepatitis C

B18.8 Other chronic viral hepatitis `CC`

B18.9 Chronic viral hepatitis, unspecified `CC`

B19 Unspecified viral hepatitis `√4th`

CC Excl: For CC/MCC codes in category B19, unless otherwise noted: A74.81-A74.9, A96.2, A98.3-A98.4, B15.0-B19.9, B33.24, B33.4-B33.8, B34.1-B34.2, B34.4-B34.8, B92, B94.2-B94.9, B97.10, B97.19, B97.29, B97.5-B97.6, B97.81-B97.89

B19.0 Unspecified viral hepatitis with hepatic coma `MCC`

B19.1 Unspecified viral hepatitis B `√5th`
  B19.10 Unspecified viral hepatitis B without hepatic coma `CC`
   Unspecified viral hepatitis B NOS
  B19.11 Unspecified viral hepatitis B with hepatic coma `MCC`

B19.2 Unspecified viral hepatitis C `√5th`
  B19.20 Unspecified viral hepatitis C without hepatic coma
   Viral hepatitis C NOS
  B19.21 Unspecified viral hepatitis C with hepatic coma `MCC`

B19.9 Unspecified viral hepatitis without hepatic coma `CC`
  Viral hepatitis NOS

Human immunodeficiency virus [HIV] disease (B20)

B20 Human immunodeficiency virus [HIV] disease `MCC`
  INCLUDES acquired immune deficiency syndrome [AIDS]
   AIDS-related complex [ARC]
   HIV infection, symptomatic

  Code first human immunodeficiency virus [HIV] disease complicating pregnancy, childbirth and the puerperium, if applicable (O98.7-)
  Use additional code(s) to identify all manifestations of HIV infection
  EXCLUDES1 asymptomatic human immunodeficiency virus [HIV] infection status (Z21)
   exposure to HIV virus (Z20.6)
   inconclusive serologic evidence of HIV (R75)
  CC Excl: B20, B92, B94.2-B94.9

Other viral diseases (B25-B34)

B25 Cytomegaloviral disease `√4th`
  EXCLUDES1 congenital cytomegalovirus infection (P35.1)
   cytomegaloviral mononucleosis (B27.1-)

B25.0 Cytomegaloviral pneumonitis `PDx MCC` `MCC`
  CC Excl: A15.0-A15.6, A15.8-A15.9, A17.9, A18.82, A18.84, A18.89, A21.2, A22.1, A31.0, A37.01, A37.11, A37.81, A37.91, A42.0, A43.0, A48.1, B25.0, B39.0-B39.2, B44.0, B58.3, B59, B67.1, J09.X1-J09.X2, J10.00-J10.1, J11.00-J11.1, J12.0-J12.3, J12.89-J18.1, J18.8-J18.9, J22, J44.9, J47.0-J70.4, J70.8-J70.9, J98.4, J98.8-J99, Q33.4, R91.1

B25.1 Cytomegaloviral hepatitis `PDx CC` `CC`
  CC Excl: No Excl

B25.2 Cytomegaloviral pancreatitis `PDx MCC` `MCC`
  CC Excl: B25.2, K85.0-K86.1, K86.8-K86.9

B25.8 Other cytomegaloviral diseases `HIV` `CC`
  Cytomegaloviral encephalitis
  CC Excl: A96.0-A96.9, A98.3-A98.5, B25.8-B25.9, B33.24-B34.2, B34.4-B34.8, B97.0-B97.32, B97.39, B97.5-B97.89

B25.9 Cytomegaloviral disease, unspecified `HIV` `CC`
  CC Excl: See code: B25.8

B26 Mumps `√4th`
  INCLUDES epidemic parotitis
   infectious parotitis

B26.0 Mumps orchitis `CC` ♂
  CC Excl: A74.81-A74.9, A96.2, A98.3-A98.4, B26.0, B26.82-B26.83, B26.85-B26.9, B33.24, B33.4-B33.8, B34.1-B34.2, B34.4-B34.8, B92, B94.2-B94.9, B97.10, B97.19, B97.29, B97.5-B97.6, B97.81-B97.89

B26.1 Mumps meningitis `MCC`
  CC Excl: A02.21-A17.1, A27.81, A39.0, A50.41, A51.41, A52.13, A54.82, A54.84, A54.89-A54.9, A74.81-A74.9, A87.0-A87.9, A96.2, A98.3-A98.4, B00.3, B02.1, B26.1, B26.82-B26.83, B26.85-B26.9, B33.24, B33.4-B33.8, B34.1-B34.2, B34.4-B34.8, B37.5, B38.4, B45.1, B58.2, B92, B94.2-B94.9, B97.10, B97.19, B97.29, B97.5-B97.6, B97.81-B97.89, G00.0-G03.9, G04.2, G32.89, G61.0, G96.8-G96.9, G98.0-G98.8, G99.8

B26.2 Mumps encephalitis `MCC`
  CC Excl: A74.81-A74.9, A96.2, A98.3-A98.4, B26.2, B26.82-B26.83, B26.85-B26.9, B33.24, B33.4-B33.8, B34.1-B34.2, B34.4-B34.8, B92, B94.2-B94.9, B97.10, B97.19, B97.29, B97.5-B97.6, B97.81-B97.89

B26.3 Mumps pancreatitis `CC`
  CC Excl: A74.81-A74.9, A96.2, A98.3-A98.4, B26.3, B26.82-B26.83, B26.85-B26.9, B33.24, B33.4-B33.8, B34.1-B34.2, B34.4-B34.8, B92, B94.2-B94.9, B97.10, B97.19, B97.29, B97.5-B97.6, B97.81-B97.89

B26.8 Mumps with other complications `√5th`
  B26.81 Mumps hepatitis `CC`
   CC Excl: A74.81-A74.9, A96.2, A98.3-A98.4, B26.81-B26.83, B26.85-B26.9, B33.24, B33.4-B33.8, B34.1-B34.2, B34.4-B34.8, B92, B94.2-B94.9, B97.10, B97.19, B97.29, B97.5-B97.6, B97.81-B97.89
  B26.82 Mumps myocarditis `CC`
   CC Excl: A74.81-A74.9, A96.2, A98.3-A98.4, B26.82-B26.83, B26.85-B26.9, B33.24, B33.4-B33.8, B34.1-B34.2, B34.4-B34.8, B92, B94.2-B94.9, B97.10, B97.19, B97.29, B97.5-B97.6, B97.81-B97.89
  B26.83 Mumps nephritis `CC`
   CC Excl: See code: B26.82
  B26.84 Mumps polyneuropathy `CC`
   CC Excl: A74.81-A74.9, A96.2, A98.3-A98.4, B26.82-B26.9, B33.24, B33.4-B33.8, B34.1-B34.2, B34.4-B34.8, B92, B94.2-B94.9, B97.10, B97.19, B97.29, B97.5-B97.6, B97.81-B97.89
  B26.85 Mumps arthritis `CC`
   CC Excl: See code: B26.82
  B26.89 Other mumps complications `CC`
   CC Excl: See code: B26.82

B26.9 Mumps without complication
  Mumps NOS
  Mumps parotitis NOS

B27 Infectious mononucleosis `√4th`
  INCLUDES glandular fever
   monocytic angina
   Pfeiffer's disease

B27.0 Gammaherpesviral mononucleosis `√5th`
  Mononucleosis due to Epstein-Barr virus
  B27.00 Gammaherpesviral mononucleosis without complication
  B27.01 Gammaherpesviral mononucleosis with polyneuropathy
  B27.02 Gammaherpesviral mononucleosis with meningitis
  B27.09 Gammaherpesviral mononucleosis with other complications
   Hepatomegaly in gammaherpesviral mononucleosis

B27.1 Cytomegaloviral mononucleosis `√5th`
  B27.10 Cytomegaloviral mononucleosis without complications
  B27.11 Cytomegaloviral mononucleosis with polyneuropathy
  B27.12 Cytomegaloviral mononucleosis with meningitis
  B27.19 Cytomegaloviral mononucleosis with other complication
   Hepatomegaly in cytomegaloviral mononucleosis

(Tap) – Reminder to go & see the Guidelines.

Certain Infectious and Parasitic Diseases

B27.8–B36.9

√5ᵗʰ **B27.8 Other infectious mononucleosis**

B27.80 Other infectious mononucleosis without complication

B27.81 Other infectious mononucleosis with polyneuropathy

B27.82 Other infectious mononucleosis with meningitis

B27.89 Other infectious mononucleosis with other complication
Hepatomegaly in other infectious mononucleosis

√5ᵗʰ **B27.9 Infectious mononucleosis, unspecified**

B27.90 Infectious mononucleosis, unspecified without complication

B27.91 Infectious mononucleosis, unspecified with polyneuropathy

B27.92 Infectious mononucleosis, unspecified with meningitis

B27.99 Infectious mononucleosis, unspecified with other complication
Hepatomegaly in unspecified infectious mononucleosis

√4ᵗʰ **B30 Viral conjunctivitis**
EXCLUDES 1   *herpesviral [herpes simplex] ocular disease (B00.5)*
ocular zoster (B02.3)

B30.0 Keratoconjunctivitis due to adenovirus
Epidemic keratoconjunctivitis
Shipyard eye

B30.1 Conjunctivitis due to adenovirus
Acute adenoviral follicular conjunctivitis
Swimming-pool conjunctivitis

B30.2 Viral pharyngoconjunctivitis

B30.3 Acute epidemic hemorrhagic conjunctivitis (enteroviral)
Conjunctivitis due to coxsackievirus 24
Conjunctivitis due to enterovirus 70
Hemorrhagic conjunctivitis (acute)(epidemic)

B30.8 Other viral conjunctivitis
Newcastle conjunctivitis

B30.9 Viral conjunctivitis, unspecified

√4ᵗʰ **B33 Other viral diseases, not elsewhere classified**

B33.0 Epidemic myalgia
Bornholm disease

B33.1 Ross River disease   CC
Epidemic polyarthritis and exanthema
Ross River fever
CC Excl: A17.82, A50.42, A52.14, A75.9, A79.9, A81.1, A81.82-A81.89, A83.0-A85.8, A87.2, A88.0, A88.8, A91-A94, A98.0-A98.2, A98.8-A99, B00.4, B00.82, B01.11-B01.12, B04, B06.01, B08.09, B08.20-B08.22, B08.60-B08.79, B09-B10.09, B26.2, B27.00-B27.99, B33.1, B45.0, B45.2-B45.9, B58.2, B75, B97.10, B97.21, G04.00-G04.01, G04.31, G04.81-G05.4, G37.0, G37.4-G37.5, J09.X3-J09.X9, J10.2-J10.89, J11.2-J11.89, L44.4, M1A.10X0-M1A.19X1, P35.2-P35.9, P37.0-P37.4, P37.8-P37.9, T56.0X1A, T56.0X2A, T56.0X3A, T56.0X4A

√5ᵗʰ **B33.2 Viral carditis**
Coxsackie (virus) carditis

B33.20 Viral carditis, unspecified   CC
CC Excl: A52.06, B33.20-B33.22, I00, I01.2-I01.9, I09.0, I09.9, I23.0-I23.3, I23.6-I23.8, I40.0-I41, I51.0, I51.4, I87.8, I99.8-I99.9

B33.21 Viral endocarditis   CC
CC Excl: A01.00-A01.09, A39.51, A52.03, A78, B33.21, B37.6, B40.0-B40.9, I00, I01.1, I01.8-I02.0, I05.0-I07.9, I08.1-I08.3, I08.9, I09.1, I09.89-I09.9, I33.0-I39, I42.4, I87.8, I99.8-I99.9, Q22.2, Q23.8-Q23.9, Q24.8, T82.6XXA

B33.22 Viral myocarditis   CC
CC Excl: See code: B33.20

B33.23 Viral pericarditis   CC
CC Excl: B33.23, I01.0, I09.2, I30.0-I30.9, I31.3-I32, I87.8, I99.8-I99.9

B33.24 Viral cardiomyopathy

B33.3 Retrovirus infections, not elsewhere classified
Retrovirus infection NOS

B33.4 Hantavirus (cardio)-pulmonary syndrome [HPS] [HCPS]   CC
Hantavirus disease with pulmonary manifestations
Sin nombre virus disease
Use additional code to identify any associated acute kidney failure (N17.9)
EXCLUDES 1   *hantavirus disease with renal manifestations (A98.5)*
hemorrhagic fever with renal manifestations (A98.5)
CC Excl: A74.81-A74.9, A88.1, A96.0-A96.9, A98.3-A98.5, B19.20-B19.21, B25.8-B25.9, B33.24-B34.2, B34.4-B34.8, B97.0-B97.89

B33.8 Other specified viral diseases
EXCLUDES 1   *anogenital human papillomavirus infection (A63.0)*
viral warts due to human papillomavirus infection (B07)

√4ᵗʰ **B34 Viral infection of unspecified site**
EXCLUDES 1   *anogenital human papillomavirus infection (A63.0)*
cytomegaloviral disease NOS (B25.9)
herpesvirus [herpes simplex] infection NOS (B00.9)
retrovirus infection NOS (B33.3)
viral agents as the cause of diseases classified elsewhere (B97.-)
viral warts due to human papillomavirus infection (B07)

B34.0 Adenovirus infection, unspecified

B34.1 Enterovirus infection, unspecified
Coxsackievirus infection NOS
Echovirus infection NOS

B34.2 Coronavirus infection, unspecified
EXCLUDES 1   *pneumonia due to SARS-associated coronavirus (J12.81)*

B34.3 Parvovirus infection, unspecified   CC
CC Excl: B08.3, B34.3

B34.4 Papovavirus infection, unspecified

B34.8 Other viral infections of unspecified site

B34.9 Viral infection, unspecified
Viremia NOS

Mycoses (B35-B49)

EXCLUDES 2   *hypersensitivity pneumonitis due to organic dust (J67.-)*
mycosis fungoides (C84.0-)

√4ᵗʰ **B35 Dermatophytosis**
INCLUDES   favus
infections due to species of Epidermophyton, Micro-sporum and Trichophyton
tinea, any type except those in B36-

B35.0 Tinea barbae and tinea capitis
Beard ringworm
Kerion
Scalp ringworm
Sycosis, mycotic

B35.1 Tinea unguium
Dermatophytic onychia
Dermatophytosis of nail
Onychomycosis
Ringworm of nails

B35.2 Tinea manuum
Dermatophytosis of hand
Hand ringworm

B35.3 Tinea pedis
Athlete's foot
Dermatophytosis of foot
Foot ringworm

B35.4 Tinea corporis
Ringworm of the body

B35.5 Tinea imbricata
Tokelau

B35.6 Tinea cruris
Dhobi itch
Groin ringworm
Jock itch

B35.8 Other dermatophytoses
Disseminated dermatophytosis
Granulomatous dermatophytosis

B35.9 Dermatophytosis, unspecified
Ringworm NOS

√4ᵗʰ **B36 Other superficial mycoses**

B36.0 Pityriasis versicolor
Tinea flava
Tinea versicolor

B36.1 Tinea nigra
Keratomycosis nigricans palmaris
Microsporosis nigra
Pityriasis nigra

B36.2 White piedra
Tinea blanca

B36.3 Black piedra

B36.8 Other specified superficial mycoses

B36.9 Superficial mycosis, unspecified

N Newborn: 0   P Pediatric: 0-17   M Maternity: 12-55   A Adult: 15-124   MCC Major CC Condition   PDx MCC PDx acts as own MCC   CC CC Condition   PDx CC PDx acts as own CC

440   ICD-10-CM Draft (2015)

✓4ᵗʰ B37 Candidiasis
  INCLUDES candidosis
         moniliasis
  EXCLUDES 1 neonatal candidiasis (P37.5)

B37.0 Candidal stomatitis   HIV CC
  Oral thrush
  CC Excl: B37.0-B37.9, B48.3, B49, B92, B94.2-B94.9

B37.1 Pulmonary candidiasis   HIV MCC
  Candidal bronchitis
  Candidal pneumonia
  CC Excl: See code: B37.0

B37.2 Candidiasis of skin and nail   HIV
  Candidal onychia
  Candidal paronychia
  EXCLUDES 2 diaper dermatitis (L22)

B37.3 Candidiasis of vulva and vagina   ♀
  Candidal vulvovaginitis
  Monilial vulvovaginitis
  Vaginal thrush

✓5ᵗʰ B37.4 Candidiasis of other urogenital sites
  1 B37.41 Candidal cystitis and urethritis   CC
    CC Excl: B37.1, B37.41-B37.82, B37.84-B37.9, N25.81-N25.89

  B37.42 Candidal balanitis
  1 B37.49 Other urogenital candidiasis   CC
    Candidal pyelonephritis
    CC Excl: See code: B37.41

B37.5 Candidal meningitis   HIV MCC
  CC Excl: A02.21, A17.0-A17.1, A27.81, A39.0, A50.41, A51.41, A52.13, A54.82, A54.84, A54.89-A54.9, A87.0-A87.9, B00.3, B02.1, B26.1, B37.0-B37.9, B38.4, B45.1, B48.3, B49, B58.2, B92, B94.2-B94.9, G00.0-G03.9, G04.2, G32.89, G61.0, G96.8-G96.9, G98.0-G98.8, G99.8

B37.6 Candidal endocarditis   HIV MCC
  CC Excl: B37.0-B37.9, B48.3, B49, B92, B94.2-B94.9

B37.7 Candidal sepsis   PDx MCC MCC
  Disseminated candidiasis
  Systemic candidiasis
  CC Excl: A02.1, A20.7, A22.7, A26.7, A32.7, A39.2-A39.4, A40.0-A40.1, A40.8-A41.9, A42.7, A48.2-A48.4, A48.8-A49.9, A54.86, B00.7, B37.0-B37.9, B48.3, B49, B92, B94.2-B96.89, M00.011-M00.012, M00.021-M00.022, M00.031- M00.032, M00.041-M00.042, M00.051- M00.052, M00.061-M00.062, M00.071-M00.072, R65.10-R65.20, Z16.10-Z16.39

✓5ᵗʰ B37.8 Candidiasis of other sites
  CC Excl: For CC codes in subcategory B37.8, unless otherwise noted: B37.0-B37.9, B48.3, B49, B92, B94.2-B94.9

  B37.81 Candidal esophagitis   HIV CC
  B37.82 Candidal enteritis   HIV CC
    Candidal proctitis
  B37.83 Candidal cheilitis   HIV CC
  B37.84 Candidal otitis externa   HIV CC
  B37.89 Other sites of candidiasis   HIV CC
    Candidal osteomyelitis
    CC Excl: B37.1, B37.5-B37.82, B37.84-B37.9

B37.9 Candidiasis, unspecified   HIV
  Thrush NOS

✓4ᵗʰ B38 Coccidioidomycosis

B38.0 Acute pulmonary coccidioidomycosis   HIV CC
  CC Excl: B38.0-B38.2, B38.7, B38.89-B38.9, B48.3, B49, B92, B94.2-B94.9

B38.1 Chronic pulmonary coccidioidomycosis   HIV CC
  CC Excl: B38.0-B39.9

B38.2 Pulmonary coccidioidomycosis, unspecified   HIV CC
  CC Excl: See code: B38.1

B38.3 Cutaneous coccidioidomycosis   HIV CC
  CC Excl: B38.0-B38.9

B38.4 Coccidioidomycosis meningitis   HIV MCC
  CC Excl: A02.21, A17.0-A17.1, A27.81, A39.0, A50.41, A51.41, A52.13, A54.82, A54.84, A54.89-A54.9, A87.0-A87.9, B00.3, B02.1, B26.1, B37.5, B38.4-B38.7, B38.89-B38.9, B45.1, B48.3, B49, B58.2, B92, B94.2-B94.9, G00.0-G03.9, G04.2, G32.89, G61.0, G96.8-G96.9, G98.0-G98.8, G99

B38.7 Disseminated coccidioidomycosis   HIV CC
  Generalized coccidioidomycosis
  CC Excl: B38.7, B38.89-B38.9, B48.3, B49, B92, B94.2-B94.9

✓5ᵗʰ B38.8 Other forms of coccidioidomycosis
  B38.81 Prostatic coccidioidomycosis   HIV CC ♂
    CC Excl: See code: B38.3
  B38.89 Other forms of coccidioidomycosis   HIV CC
    CC Excl: See code: B38.7

B38.9 Coccidioidomycosis, unspecified   HIV
  CC Excl: See code: B38.7

✓4ᵗʰ B39 Histoplasmosis
  Code first associated AIDS (B20)
  Use additional code for any associated manifestations, such as:
    endocarditis (I39)
    meningitis (G02)
    pericarditis (I32)
    retinitits (H32)

B39.0 Acute pulmonary histoplasmosis capsulati   HIV MCC
  CC Excl: A22.1, A37.01, A37.11, A37.81, A37.91, A48.1, B25.0, B39.0-B39.4, B39.9, B44.0, B48.3, B49, B92, B94.2-B94.9, J09.X1-J09.X2, J10.00-J10.1, J11.00-J11.1, J12.0-J12.3, J12.89-J18.1, J18.8-J18.9, J44.9, J47.0-J70.4, J70.8-J70.9, J98.4, R91.1

B39.1 Chronic pulmonary histoplasmosis capsulati   HIV MCC
  CC Excl: See code: B39.0

B39.2 Pulmonary histoplasmosis capsulati, unspecified   HIV MCC
  CC Excl: See code: B39.0

B39.3 Disseminated histoplasmosis capsulati   HIV CC
  Generalized histoplasmosis capsulati
  CC Excl: B38.0-B39.4

B39.4 Histoplasmosis capsulati, unspecified   HIV
  American histoplasmosis

B39.5 Histoplasmosis duboisii   HIV
  African histoplasmosis

B39.9 Histoplasmosis, unspecified   HIV

✓4ᵗʰ B40 Blastomycosis
  EXCLUDES 1 Brazilian blastomycosis (B41.-)
    keloidal blastomycosis (B48.0)

  CC Excl: For CC codes in category B40, unless otherwise noted: B40.0-B40.9, B48.3, B49, B92, B94.2-B94.9

B40.0 Acute pulmonary blastomycosis   CC
B40.1 Chronic pulmonary blastomycosis   CC
B40.2 Pulmonary blastomycosis, unspecified   CC
B40.3 Cutaneous blastomycosis   CC
B40.7 Disseminated blastomycosis   CC
  Generalized blastomycosis

✓5ᵗʰ B40.8 Other forms of blastomycosis
  B40.81 Blastomycotic meningoencephalitis   CC
    Meningomyelitis due to blastomycosis
  B40.89 Other forms of blastomycosis   CC

B40.9 Blastomycosis, unspecified   CC

✓4ᵗʰ B41 Paracoccidioidomycosis
  INCLUDES Brazilian blastomycosis
    Lutz' disease

  CC Excl: For CC codes in category B41, unless otherwise noted: B41.0-B41.9, B48.3, B49, B92, B94.2-B94.9

B41.0 Pulmonary paracoccidioidomycosis   CC
B41.7 Disseminated paracoccidioidomycosis   CC
  Generalized paracoccidioidomycosis
B41.8 Other forms of paracoccidioidomycosis   CC
B41.9 Paracoccidioidomycosis, unspecified   CC

✓4ᵗʰ B42 Sporotrichosis
B42.0 Pulmonary sporotrichosis
B42.1 Lymphocutaneous sporotrichosis
B42.7 Disseminated sporotrichosis
  Generalized sporotrichosis

✓5ᵗʰ B42.8 Other forms of sporotrichosis
  B42.81 Cerebral sporotrichosis
    Meningitis due to sporotrichosis
  B42.82 Sporotrichosis arthritis
  B42.89 Other forms of sporotrichosis
B42.9 Sporotrichosis, unspecified

✓4ᵗʰ B43 Chromomycosis and pheomycotic abscess
B43.0 Cutaneous chromomycosis
  Dermatitis verrucosa

---

1 HAC = as SDx not POA, in combination with SDx code T83.51XA also not POA.

Certain Infectious and Parasitic Diseases

B43.1–B52.9

B43.1 Pheomycotic brain abscess
Cerebral chromomycosis

B43.2 Subcutaneous pheomycotic abscess and cyst

B43.8 Other forms of chromomycosis

B43.9 Chromomycosis, unspecified

√4ᵗʰ **B44 Aspergillosis**
   INCLUDES   aspergilloma

> **CC Excl:** For CC/MCC codes in category B44, unless otherwise noted: B44.1-B44.7, B44.89-B44.9, B48.3-B48.4, B49, B92, B94.2-B94.9

B44.0 Invasive pulmonary aspergillosis   `PDx MCC` `MCC`
   CC Excl: A15.0-A15.6, A15.8-A15.9, A17.9, A18.82, A18.84, A18.89, A21.2, A22.1, A31.0, A37.01, A37.11, A37.81, A37.91, A42.0, A43.0, A48.1, B25.0, B39.0-B39.2, B44.0, B58.3, B59, B67.1, J09.X1-J09.X2, J10.00-J10.1, J11.00-J11.1, J12.0-J12.3, J12.89-J18.1, J18.8-J18.9, J22, J44.9, J47.0-J70.4, J70.8-J70.9, J98.4, J98.8-J99, Q33.4, R91.1

B44.1 Other pulmonary aspergillosis   `CC`

B44.2 Tonsillar aspergillosis   `CC`

B44.7 Disseminated aspergillosis   `CC`
Generalized aspergillosis

√5ᵗʰ **B44.8 Other forms of aspergillosis**

  B44.81 Allergic bronchopulmonary aspergillosis   `CC`
    CC Excl: B44.81, J22, J98.8-J98.9

  B44.89 Other forms of aspergillosis   `CC`

B44.9 Aspergillosis, unspecified   `CC`

√4ᵗʰ **B45 Cryptococcosis**

> **CC Excl:** For CC/MCC codes in category B45, unless otherwise noted: B45.0-B45.9, B48.3, B49, B92, B94.2-B94.9

B45.0 Pulmonary cryptococcosis   `HIV` `CC`
   CC Excl: B45.0, B45.2-B45.9, B48.3, B49, B92, B94.2-B94.9

B45.1 Cerebral cryptococcosis   `PDx MCC` `MCC`
Cryptococcal meningitis
Cryptococcosis meningocerebralis
   CC Excl: A02.21, A17.0-A17.1, A27.81, A39.0, A50.41, A51.41, A52.13, A54.82, A54.84, A54.89-A54.9, A87.0-A87.9, B00.3, B02.1, B26.1, B37.5, B38.4, B45.1, B58.2, E08.40-E08.49, E08.618-E08.638, E08.649-E08.8, E09.40-E09.49, E09.618-E09.638, E09.649-E09.8, E10.40-E10.49, E10.618-E10.638, E10.649, E10.69-E10.8, E11.40-E11.49, E11.618-E11.638, E11.649, E11.69-E11.8, E13.40-E13.49, E13.618-E13.638, E13.649-E13.8, G00.0-G03.9, G04.2, G32.89, G61.0, G96.8-G96.9, G98.0-G98.8, G99.8

B45.2 Cutaneous cryptococcosis   `HIV` `CC`

B45.3 Osseous cryptococcosis   `HIV` `CC`

B45.7 Disseminated cryptococcosis   `HIV` `CC`
Generalized cryptococcosis

B45.8 Other forms of cryptococcosis   `HIV` `CC`

B45.9 Cryptococcosis, unspecified   `HIV` `CC`

√4ᵗʰ **B46 Zygomycosis**

> **CC Excl:** For MCC codes in category B46, unless otherwise noted: B46.0-B46.9, B48.3, B49, B92, B94.2-B94.9

B46.0 Pulmonary mucormycosis   `MCC`

B46.1 Rhinocerebral mucormycosis   `MCC`

B46.2 Gastrointestinal mucormycosis   `MCC`

B46.3 Cutaneous mucormycosis   `MCC`
Subcutaneous mucormycosis

B46.4 Disseminated mucormycosis   `MCC`
Generalized mucormycosis

B46.5 Mucormycosis, unspecified   `MCC`

B46.8 Other zygomycoses   `MCC`
Entomophthoromycosis

B46.9 Zygomycosis, unspecified   `MCC`
Phycomycosis NOS

√4ᵗʰ **B47 Mycetoma**

B47.0 Eumycetoma   `CC`
Madura foot, mycotic
Maduromycosis
   CC Excl: B47.0, B48.3, B49, B92, B94.2-B94.9

B47.1 Actinomycetoma   `HIV` `CC`
   CC Excl: A42.0-A42.2, A42.81-A43.9, B47.1-B47.9, L08.1

B47.9 Mycetoma, unspecified   `HIV` `CC`
Madura foot NOS
   CC Excl: A42.81-A42.9, A43.8-A43.9, B47.1-B47.9

√4ᵗʰ **B48 Other mycoses, not elsewhere classified**

B48.0 Lobomycosis
Keloidal blastomycosis
Lobo's disease

B48.1 Rhinosporidiosis

B48.2 Allescheriasis   `CC`
Infection due to Pseudallescheria boydii
   EXCLUDES 1   eumycetoma (B47.0)
   CC Excl: B48.2-B48.3, B49, B92, B94.2-B94.9

B48.3 Geotrichosis   `CC`
Geotrichum stomatitis
   CC Excl: B48.3-B49

B48.4 Penicillosis   `CC`
   CC Excl: B44.1-B44.7, B44.89-B44.9, B48.3-B48.4, B49, B92, B94.2-B94.9

B48.8 Other specified mycoses   `HIV` `CC`
Adiaspiromycosis
Infection of tissue and organs by Alternaria
Infection of tissue and organs by Drechslera
Infection of tissue and organs by Fusarium
Infection of tissue and organs by saprophytic fungi NEC
   AHA: 2014, 2Q, 13
   CC Excl: B48.3, B48.8-B49, B92, B94.2-B94.9

B49 Unspecified mycosis   `CC`
Fungemia NOS
   CC Excl: See code: B48.3

Protozoal diseases (B50-B64)

   EXCLUDES 1   amebiasis (A06.-)
                  other protozoal intestinal diseases (A07.-)

√4ᵗʰ **B50 Plasmodium falciparum malaria**
   INCLUDES   mixed infections of Plasmodium falciparum with any other Plasmodium species

> **CC Excl:** For CC/MCC codes in category B50, unless otherwise noted: B50.0-B57.5

B50.0 Plasmodium falciparum malaria with cerebral complications   `CC`
Cerebral malaria NOS

B50.8 Other severe and complicated Plasmodium falciparum malaria   `CC`
Severe or complicated Plasmodium falciparum malaria NOS

B50.9 Plasmodium falciparum malaria, unspecified   `MCC`

√4ᵗʰ **B51 Plasmodium vivax malaria**
   INCLUDES   mixed infections of Plasmodium vivax with other Plasmodium species, except Plasmodium falciparum
   EXCLUDES 1   plasmodium vivax with Plasmodium falciparum (B50.-)

> **CC Excl:** For CC codes in category B51, unless otherwise noted: B50.0-B57.5

B51.0 Plasmodium vivax malaria with rupture of spleen   `CC`

B51.8 Plasmodium vivax malaria with other complications   `CC`

B51.9 Plasmodium vivax malaria without complication   `CC`
Plasmodium vivax malaria NOS
   CC Excl: A44.0-A44.9, A68.0-A68.9, A69.20-A69.29, B50.0-B57.5, B60.0

√4ᵗʰ **B52 Plasmodium malariae malaria**
   INCLUDES   mixed infections of Plasmodium malariae with other Plasmodium species, except Plasmodium falciparum and Plasmodium vivax
   EXCLUDES 1   Plasmodium falciparum (B50.-)
                   Plasmodium vivax (B51.-)

> **CC Excl:** For CC codes in category B52, unless otherwise noted: B50.0-B57.5

B52.0 Plasmodium malariae malaria with nephropathy   `PDx CC` `CC`
   CC Excl: A17.9, A18.10-A18.11, A18.13, A18.82, A18.84, A18.89, A54.21, A54.29, A54.82, A54.84, A54.89-A54.9, A59.00, A59.8-A59.9, B37.41-B37.49, B50.0-B57.5, E08.21-E08.29, E08.618-E08.638, E08.649-E08.8, E09.21-E09.29, E09.618-E09.638, E09.649-E09.8, E10.21-E10.29, E10.618-E10.638, E10.649, E10.69-E10.8, E11.21-E11.29, E11.618-E11.638, E11.649, E11.69-E11.8, E13.21-E13.29, E13.618-E13.638, E13.649-E13.8, E88.3, M10.30-M10.39, N00.0-N11.0, N11.8-N13.39, N13.6, N14.0-N19, N25.0-N26.1, N26.9-N27.9, N28.1-N29, N36.41-N36.43, N36.8-N36.9, N39.8-N39.9, R31.0-R31.9

B52.8 Plasmodium malariae malaria with other complications   `CC`

B52.9 Plasmodium malariae malaria without complication   `CC`
Plasmodium malariae malaria NOS

N Newborn: 0   P Pediatric: 0-17   M Maternity: 12-55   A Adult: 15-124   `MCC` Major CC Condition   `PDx MCC` PDx acts as own MCC   `CC` CC Condition   `PDx CC` PDx acts as own CC

442   ICD-10-CM Draft (2015)

✓4ᵗʰ B53 Other specified malaria

> **CC Excl: For CC codes in subcategory B53, unless otherwise noted:** B50.0-B57.5

B53.0 Plasmodium ovale malaria `CC`
> EXCLUDES 1   Plasmodium ovale with Plasmodium falciparum (B50.-)
> Plasmodium ovale with Plasmodium malariae (B52.-)
> Plasmodium ovale with Plasmodium vivax (B51.-)

B53.1 Malaria due to simian plasmodia `CC`
> EXCLUDES 1   Malaria due to simian plasmodia with Plasmodium falciparum (B50.-)
> Malaria due to simian plasmodia with Plasmodium malariae (B52.-)
> Malaria due to simian plasmodia with Plasmodium ovale (B53.0)
> Malaria due to simian plasmodia with Plasmodium vivax (B51.-)

B53.8 Other malaria, not elsewhere classified `CC`

B54 Unspecified malaria `CC`
> **CC Excl:** B50.0-B57.5, B97.21

✓4ᵗʰ B55 Leishmaniasis

> **CC Excl: For CC codes in category B55, unless otherwise noted:** A44.0-A44.9, A68.0-A68.9, A69.20-A69.29, A75.0-A79.9, B50.0-B57.5, B60.0

B55.0 Visceral leishmaniasis `CC`
> Kala-azar
> Post-kala-azar dermal leishmaniasis

B55.1 Cutaneous leishmaniasis `CC`

B55.2 Mucocutaneous leishmaniasis `CC`

B55.9 Leishmaniasis, unspecified `CC`

✓4ᵗʰ B56 African trypanosomiasis

> **CC Excl: For CC codes in category B56, unless otherwise noted:** A44.0-A44.9, A68.0-A68.9, A69.20-A69.29, A75.0-A79.9, B50.0-B57.5, B60.0

B56.0 Gambiense trypanosomiasis `CC`
> Infection due to Trypanosoma brucei gambiense
> West African sleeping sickness

B56.1 Rhodesiense trypanosomiasis `CC`
> East African sleeping sickness
> Infection due to Trypanosoma brucei rhodesiense

B56.9 African trypanosomiasis, unspecified `CC`
> Sleeping sickness NOS

✓4ᵗʰ B57 Chagas' disease
> INCLUDES   American trypanosomiasis
> infection due to Trypanosoma cruzi

> **CC Excl: For CC codes in category B57, unless otherwise noted:** A44.0-A44.9, A68.0-A68.9, A69.20-A69.29, A75.0-A79.9, B50.0-B57.5, B60.0

B57.0 Acute Chagas' disease with heart involvement `CC`
> Acute Chagas' disease with myocarditis
> **CC Excl:** B57.0-B57.2, B92, B94.2-B94.9

B57.1 Acute Chagas' disease without heart involvement `CC`
> Acute Chagas' disease NOS

B57.2 Chagas' disease (chronic) with heart involvement `CC`
> American trypanosomiasis NOS
> Chagas' disease (chronic) NOS
> Chagas' disease (chronic) with myocarditis
> Trypanosomiasis NOS
> **CC Excl:** See code: B57.0

✓5ᵗʰ B57.3 Chagas' disease (chronic) with digestive system involvement
> **B57.30 Chagas' disease with digestive system involvement, unspecified** `CC`
> **B57.31 Megaesophagus in Chagas' disease** `CC`
> **B57.32 Megacolon in Chagas' disease** `CC`
> **B57.39 Other digestive system involvement in Chagas' disease** `CC`

✓5ᵗʰ B57.4 Chagas' disease (chronic) with nervous system involvement
> **B57.40 Chagas' disease with nervous system involvement, unspecified** `CC`
> **B57.41 Meningitis in Chagas' disease** `CC`
> **B57.42 Meningoencephalitis in Chagas' disease** `CC`
> **B57.49 Other nervous system involvement in Chagas' disease** `CC`

B57.5 Chagas' disease (chronic) with other organ involvement `CC`

✓4ᵗʰ B58 Toxoplasmosis
> INCLUDES   infection due to Toxoplasma gondii
> EXCLUDES 1   congenital toxoplasmosis (P37.1)

✓5ᵗʰ B58.0 Toxoplasma oculopathy
> **B58.00 Toxoplasma oculopathy, unspecified** `HIV` `CC`
>   **CC Excl:** B58.00-B58.9, B92, B94.2-B94.9
> **B58.01 Toxoplasma chorioretinitis** `HIV` `CC`
>   **CC Excl:** B58.00-B58.01, B58.82-B58.9, B92, B94.2-B94.9
> **B58.09 Other toxoplasma oculopathy** `HIV` `CC`
>   Toxoplasma uveitis
>   **CC Excl:** B58.00-B58.09, B58.82-B58.9, B92, B94.2-B94.9

B58.1 Toxoplasma hepatitis `HIV` `CC`
> **CC Excl:** B58.00-B58.1, B58.82-B58.9, B92, B94.2-B94.9

B58.2 Toxoplasma meningoencephalitis `HIV` `MCC`
> **CC Excl:** B58.00-B58.2, B58.82-B58.9, B92, B94.2-B94.9

B58.3 Pulmonary toxoplasmosis `HIV` `MCC`
> **CC Excl:** A22.1, A37.01, A37.11, A37.81, A37.91, A48.1, B25.0, B44.0, B58.00, B58.3, B58.82-B58.9, B92, B94.2-B94.9, J09.X1-J09.X2, J10.00-J10.1, J11.00-J11.1, J12.0-J12.3, J12.89-J18.1, J18.8-J18.9, J44.9, J47.0-J70.4, J70.8-J70.9, J98.4, R91.1

✓5ᵗʰ B58.8 Toxoplasmosis with other organ involvement

> **CC Excl: For CC/MCC codes in subcategory B58.8, unless otherwise noted:** B58.00, B58.81-B58.9, B92, B94.2-B94.9

> **B58.81 Toxoplasma myocarditis** `HIV` `MCC`
> **B58.82 Toxoplasma myositis** `HIV` `CC`
>   **CC Excl:** B58.00, B58.82-B58.9, B92, B94.2-B94.9
> **B58.83 Toxoplasma tubulo-interstitial nephropathy** `HIV` `CC`
>   Toxoplasma pyelonephritis
> **B58.89 Toxoplasmosis with other organ involvement** `HIV` `CC`

B58.9 Toxoplasmosis, unspecified `HIV` `CC`
> **CC Excl:** B58.9

B59 Pneumocystosis `HIV` `MCC`
> Pneumonia due to Pneumocystis carinii
> Pneumonia due to Pneumocystis jiroveci
> **CC Excl:** A22.1, A37.01, A37.11, A37.81, A37.91, A48.1, B25.0, B44.0, B59, B92, B94.2-B94.9, J09.X1-J09.X2, J10.00-J10.1, J11.00-J11.1, J12.0-J12.3, J12.89-J18.1, J18.8-J18.9, J44.9, J47.0-J70.4, J70.8-J70.9, J98.4, R91.1

✓4ᵗʰ B60 Other protozoal diseases, not elsewhere classified
> EXCLUDES 1   cryptosporidiosis (A07.2)
> intestinal microsporidiosis (A07.8)
> isosporiasis (A07.3)

B60.0 Babesiosis `CC`
> Piroplasmosis
> **CC Excl:** A44.0-A44.9, A68.0-A68.9, A69.20-A69.29, A75.0-A79.9, B50.0-B57.5, B60.0

✓5ᵗʰ B60.1 Acanthamebiasis
> **B60.10 Acanthamebiasis, unspecified** `CC`
>   **CC Excl:** B59, B60.11, B60.19-B64, B89, B99.8-B99.9, L94.6, M35.2
> **B60.11 Meningoencephalitis due to Acanthamoeba (culbertsoni)**
> **B60.12 Conjunctivitis due to Acanthamoeba**
> **B60.13 Keratoconjunctivitis due to Acanthamoeba**
> **B60.19 Other acanthamebic disease** `CC`
>   **CC Excl:** See code: B60.10

B60.2 Naegleriasis `CC`
> Primary amebic meningoencephalitis
> **CC Excl:** See code: B60.10

B60.8 Other specified protozoal diseases `HIV`
> Microsporidiosis

B64 Unspecified protozoal disease

Helminthiases (B65-B83)

✓4ᵗʰ B65 Schistosomiasis [bilharziasis]
> INCLUDES   snail fever

> **CC Excl: For CC codes in category B65, unless otherwise noted:** B65.0-B65.9

B65.0 Schistosomiasis due to Schistosoma haematobium [urinary schistosomiasis] `CC`

B65.1 Schistosomiasis due to Schistosoma mansoni [intestinal schistosomiasis] `CC`

B65.2 Schistosomiasis due to Schistosoma japonicum `CC`
> Asiatic schistosomiasis

B65.3 Cercarial dermatitis `CC`
> Swimmer's itch

✔ Additional Character Required   ✔x7ᵗʰ Xtension Alert   Unacceptable PDx   Manifestation   Hospital Acquired Condition   EXCLUDES 1 Not Coded Here   EXCLUDES 2 Not Included Here

ICD-10-CM Draft (2015)   443

Certain Infectious and Parasitic Diseases

B65.8–B73.1

B65.8 **Other schistosomiasis**   CC
Infection due to Schistosoma intercalatum
Infection due to Schistosoma mattheei
Infection due to Schistosoma mekongi

B65.9 **Schistosomiasis, unspecified**   CC

✓4ᵗʰ **B66** **Other fluke infections**

CC Excl: For CC codes in category B66, unless otherwise noted:
B66.0–B66.9

B66.0 **Opisthorchiasis**   CC
Infection due to cat liver fluke
Infection due to Opisthorchis (felineus)(viverrini)

B66.1 **Clonorchiasis**   CC
Chinese liver fluke disease
Infection due to Clonorchis sinensis
Oriental liver fluke disease

B66.2 **Dicroceliasis**   CC
Infection due to Dicrocoelium dendriticum
Lancet fluke infection

B66.3 **Fascioliasis**   CC
Infection due to Fasciola gigantica
Infection due to Fasciola hepatica
Infection due to Fasciola indica
Sheep liver fluke disease

B66.4 **Paragonimiasis**   CC
Infection due to Paragonimus species
Lung fluke disease
Pulmonary distomiasis

B66.5 **Fasciolopsiasis**   CC
Infection due to Fasciolopsis buski
Intestinal distomiasis

B66.8 **Other specified fluke infections**   CC
Echinostomiasis   Nanophyetiasis
Heterophyiasis   Watsoniasis
Metagonimiasis

B66.9 **Fluke infection, unspecified**

✓4ᵗʰ **B67** **Echinococcosis**
INCLUDES hydatidosis

B67.0 **Echinococcus granulosus infection of liver**   CC
CC Excl: B67.0, B67.8-B67.99

B67.1 **Echinococcus granulosus infection of lung**   CC
CC Excl: B67.1, B67.8-B67.99, J12.81

B67.2 **Echinococcus granulosus infection of bone**   CC
CC Excl: B67.2, B67.32-B67.39, B67.8-B67.99

✓5ᵗʰ **B67.3** **Echinococcus granulosus infection, other and multiple sites**

B67.31 **Echinococcus granulosus infection, thyroid gland** CC
CC Excl: B67.31, B67.8-B67.99

B67.32 **Echinococcus granulosus infection, multiple sites** CC
CC Excl: B67.2, B67.32-B67.39, B67.8-B67.99

B67.39 **Echinococcus granulosus infection, other sites** CC
CC Excl: See code: B67.32

B67.4 **Echinococcus granulosus infection, unspecified**   CC
Dog tapeworm (infection)
CC Excl: B67.4, B67.8-B67.99

B67.5 **Echinococcus multilocularis infection of liver**   CC
CC Excl: B67.5, B67.8-B67.99

✓5ᵗʰ **B67.6** **Echinococcus multilocularis infection, other and multiple sites**

B67.61 **Echinococcus multilocularis infection, multiple sites** CC
CC Excl: B67.61-B67.69, B67.8-B67.99

B67.69 **Echinococcus multilocularis infection, other sites** CC
CC Excl: See code: B67.61

B67.7 **Echinococcus multilocularis infection, unspecified**   CC
CC Excl: B67.7-B67.99

B67.8 **Echinococcosis, unspecified, of liver**   CC
CC Excl: B67.8-B67.99

✓5ᵗʰ **B67.9** **Echinococcosis, other and unspecified**

B67.90 **Echinococcosis, unspecified**   CC
Echinococcosis NOS
CC Excl: See code: B67.8

B67.99 **Other echinococcosis**   CC
CC Excl: See code: B67.8

✓4ᵗʰ **B68** **Taeniasis**
EXCLUDES 1 cysticercosis (B69.-)

B68.0 **Taenia solium taeniasis**   CC
Pork tapeworm (infection)
CC Excl: A00.1, A01.00-A01.09, A01.4-A02.0, A03.9-A05.2, A06.0-A06.2, A06.9, A07.1-A09, A18.32-A18.39, A18.83, A48.51-A48.52, B37.82, B68.0-B71.9, B82.9, J09.X3-J09.X9, J10.2-J10.89, J11.2-J11.89, K30, K31.84, K52.1-K52.2, K52.82-K52.9, K58.0-K58.9, P76.8-P77.9, P78.1, P78.3-P78.89

B68.1 **Taenia saginata taeniasis**   CC
Beef tapeworm (infection)
Infection due to adult tapeworm Taenia saginata
CC Excl: B68.0-B71.9

B68.9 **Taeniasis, unspecified**   CC
CC Excl: See code: B68.1

✓4ᵗʰ **B69** **Cysticercosis**
INCLUDES cysticerciasis infection due to larval form of Taenia solium

CC Excl: For CC codes in category B69, unless otherwise noted:
B68.0-B71.9

B69.0 **Cysticercosis of central nervous system**   CC

B69.1 **Cysticercosis of eye**   CC

✓5ᵗʰ **B69.8** **Cysticercosis of other sites**

B69.81 **Myositis in cysticercosis**   CC

B69.89 **Cysticercosis of other sites**   CC

B69.9 **Cysticercosis, unspecified**   CC

✓4ᵗʰ **B70** **Diphyllobothriasis and sparganosis**

CC Excl: For CC codes in category B70, unless otherwise noted:
B68.0-B71.9

B70.0 **Diphyllobothriasis**   CC
Diphyllobothrium (adult) (latum) (pacificum) infection
Fish tapeworm (infection)
EXCLUDES 2 larval diphyllobothriasis (B70.1)

B70.1 **Sparganosis**   CC
Infection due to Sparganum (mansoni) (proliferum)
Infection due to Spirometra larva
Larval diphyllobothriasis
Spirometrosis

✓4ᵗʰ **B71** **Other cestode infections**

CC Excl: For CC codes in category B71, unless otherwise noted:
B68.0-B71.9

B71.0 **Hymenolepiasis**   CC
Dwarf tapeworm infection
Rat tapeworm (infection)

B71.1 **Dipylidiasis**   CC

B71.8 **Other specified cestode infections**
Coenurosis

B71.9 **Cestode infection, unspecified**
Tapeworm (infection) NOS

B72 **Dracunculiasis**   CC
INCLUDES guinea worm infection
infection due to Dracunculus medinensis
CC Excl: B72-B74.9

✓4ᵗʰ **B73** **Onchocerciasis**
INCLUDES onchocerca volvulus infection
onchocercosis
river blindness

CC Excl: For CC codes in category B73, unless otherwise noted:
B72-B74.9

✓5ᵗʰ **B73.0** **Onchocerciasis with eye disease**

B73.00 **Onchocerciasis with eye involvement, unspecified**   CC

B73.01 **Onchocerciasis with endophthalmitis**   CC

B73.02 **Onchocerciasis with glaucoma**   CC

B73.09 **Onchocerciasis with other eye involvement**   CC
Infestation of eyelid due to onchocerciasis

B73.1 **Onchocerciasis without eye disease**   CC

N Newborn: 0   P Pediatric: 0-17   M Maternity: 12-55   A Adult: 15-124   MCC Major CC Condition   PDx MCC PDx acts as own MCC   CC CC Condition   PDx CC PDx acts as own CC

444   ICD-10-CM Draft (2015)

Certain Infectious and Parasitic Diseases

B74–B87.1

✓4ᵗʰ B74 Filariasis
EXCLUDES 2 onchocerciasis (B73)
tropical (pulmonary) eosinophilia NOS (J82)

CC Excl: For CC codes in category B74, unless otherwise noted: B72-B74.9

B74.0 Filariasis due to Wuchereria bancrofti CC
Bancroftian elephantiasis
Bancroftian filariasis

B74.1 Filariasis due to Brugia malayi CC

B74.2 Filariasis due to Brugia timori CC

B74.3 Loiasis CC
Calabar swelling
Eyeworm disease of Africa
Loa loa infection

B74.4 Mansonelliasis CC
Infection due to Mansonella ozzardi
Infection due to Mansonella perstans
Infection due to Mansonella streptocerca

B74.8 Other filariases CC
Dirofilariasis

B74.9 Filariasis, unspecified CC

B75 Trichinellosis CC
INCLUDES infection due to Trichinella species
trichiniasis
CC Excl: A17.82- A50.42, A52.14, A75.9, A79.9, A81.1, A81.82-A81.89,
A83.0-A85.8, A87.2, A88.0, A88.8, A92.1-A92.8, A93.0, B00.4, B00.82,
B01.11-B01.12, B04, B06.01, B08.09, B08.20-B08.22, B08.60-B08.79, B09-
B10.09, B26.2, B33.1, B45.0, B45.2-B45.9, B58.2, B75, B97.10, B97.21,
G04.00-G04.01, G04.31, G04.81-G05.4, G37.0, G37.4-G37.5, J09.X3-J09.X9,
J10.2-J10.89, J11.2-J11.89, L44.4, M1A.10X0-M1A.19X1, P35.2-P35.9, P37.0-
P37.4, P37.8-P37.9, T56.0X1A, T56.0X2A, T56.0X3A, T56.0X4A

✓4ᵗʰ B76 Hookworm diseases
INCLUDES uncinariasis

CC Excl: For CC codes in category B76, unless otherwise noted: B76.0-B76.9

B76.0 Ancylostomiasis CC
Infection due to Ancylostoma species

B76.1 Necatoriasis CC
Infection due to Necator americanus

B76.8 Other hookworm diseases CC

B76.9 Hookworm disease, unspecified CC
Cutaneous larva migrans NOS

✓4ᵗʰ B77 Ascariasis
INCLUDES ascaridiasis
roundworm infection

B77.0 Ascariasis with intestinal complications CC
CC Excl: B77.0-B78.0, B78.7-B82.0

✓5ᵗʰ B77.8 Ascariasis with other complications

B77.81 Ascariasis pneumonia PDx MCC MCC
CC Excl: A15.0-A15.6, A15.8-A15.9, A17.9, A18.82,
A18.84, A18.89, A21.2, A22.1, A31.0, A37.01, A37.11,
A37.81, A37.91, A42.0, A43.0, A48.1, B25.0, B39.0-B39.2,
B44.0, B58.3, B59, B67.1, B77.0-B78.0, B78.7-B82.0,
J09.X1-J09.X2, J10.00-J10.1, J11.00-J11.1, J12.0-J12.3,
J12.89-J18.1, J18.8-J18.9, J22, J44.9, J47.0-J70.4, J70.8-
J70.9, J98.4, J98.8-J99, Q33.4, R91.1

B77.89 Ascariasis with other complications CC
CC Excl: B77.0-B78.0, B78.7-B82.0

B77.9 Ascariasis, unspecified CC
CC Excl: See code B77.0

✓4ᵗʰ B78 Strongyloidiasis
EXCLUDES 1 trichostrongyliasis (B81.2)

CC Excl: For CC codes in category B78, unless otherwise noted: B77.0-B78.0, B78.7-B82.0

B78.0 Intestinal strongyloidiasis HIV CC

B78.1 Cutaneous strongyloidiasis

B78.7 Disseminated strongyloidiasis HIV CC

B78.9 Strongyloidiasis, unspecified HIV CC

B79 Trichuriasis CC
INCLUDES trichocephaliasis
whipworm (disease)(infection)
CC Excl: See code: B77.89

B80 Enterobiasis CC
INCLUDES oxyuriasis
pinworm infection
threadworm infection
CC Excl: See code: B77.89

✓4ᵗʰ B81 Other intestinal helminthiases, not elsewhere classified
EXCLUDES 1 angiostrongyliasis due to Parastrongylus cantonensis (B83.2)

CC Excl: For CC codes in subcategories B81.0-B81.2, unless
otherwise noted: B77.0-B78.0, B78.7-B82.0 For CC codes in
subcategories B81.3-B81.8: B77.0-B78.0, B78.7-B83.3, B83.8-B83.9

B81.0 Anisakiasis CC
Infection due to Anisakis larva

B81.1 Intestinal capillariasis CC
Capillariasis NOS
Infection due to Capillaria philippinensis
EXCLUDES 2 hepatic capillariasis (B83.8)

B81.2 Trichostrongyliasis CC

B81.3 Intestinal angiostrongyliasis CC
Angiostrongyliasis due to Parastrongylus costaricensis

B81.4 Mixed intestinal helminthiases CC
Infection due to intestinal helminths classified to more than one
of the categories B65.0-B81.3 and B81.8
Mixed helminthiasis NOS

B81.8 Other specified intestinal helminthiases CC
Infection due to Oesophagostomum species
[esophagostomiasis]
Infection due to Ternidens diminutus [ternidensiasis]

✓4ᵗʰ B82 Unspecified intestinal parasitism

B82.0 Intestinal helminthiasis, unspecified CC
CC Excl: See code: B81.3

B82.9 Intestinal parasitism, unspecified

✓4ᵗʰ B83 Other helminthiases
EXCLUDES 1 capillariasis NOS (B81.1)
EXCLUDES 2 intestinal capillariasis (B81.1)

B83.0 Visceral larva migrans
Toxocariasis

B83.1 Gnathostomiasis
Wandering swelling

B83.2 Angiostrongyliasis due to Parastrongylus cantonensis
Eosinophilic meningoencephalitis due to Parastrongylus
cantonensis
EXCLUDES 2 intestinal angiostrongyliasis (B81.3)

B83.3 Syngamiasis
Syngamosis

B83.4 Internal hirudiniasis
EXCLUDES 2 external hirudiniasis (B88.3)

B83.8 Other specified helminthiases
Acanthocephaliasis Metastrongyliasis
Gongylonemiasis Thelaziasis
Hepatic capillariasis

B83.9 Helminthiasis, unspecified
Worms NOS
EXCLUDES 1 intestinal helminthiasis NOS (B82.0)

Pediculosis, acariasis and other infestations (B85-B89)

✓4ᵗʰ B85 Pediculosis and phthiriasis

B85.0 Pediculosis due to Pediculus humanus capitis
Head-louse infestation

B85.1 Pediculosis due to Pediculus humanus corporis
Body-louse infestation

B85.2 Pediculosis, unspecified

B85.3 Phthiriasis
Infestation by crab-louse
Infestation by Phthirus pubis

B85.4 Mixed pediculosis and phthiriasis
Infestation classifiable to more than one of the categories B85.0-
B85.3

B86 Scabies
Sarcoptic itch

✓4ᵗʰ B87 Myiasis
INCLUDES infestation by larva of flies

B87.0 Cutaneous myiasis
Creeping myiasis

B87.1 Wound myiasis
Traumatic myiasis

Certain Infectious and Parasitic Diseases

B87.2   **Ocular myiasis**

B87.3   **Nasopharyngeal myiasis**
Laryngeal myiasis

B87.4   **Aural myiasis**

√5th **B87.8**   **Myiasis of** other sites

     B87.81   **Genitourinary myiasis**

     B87.82   **Intestinal myiasis**

     B87.89   **Myiasis of** other sites

B87.9   **Myiasis, unspecified**

√4th **B88**   **Other infestations**

B88.0   **Other acariasis**
Acarine dermatitis
Dermatitis due to Demodex species
Dermatitis due to Dermanyssus gallinae
Dermatitis due to Liponyssoides sanguineus
Trombiculosis
EXCLUDES 2   scabies (B86)

B88.1   **Tungiasis [sandflea infestation]**

B88.2   **Other arthropod infestations**
Scarabiasis

B88.3   **External hirudiniasis**
Leech infestation NOS
EXCLUDES 2   internal hirudiniasis (B83.4)

B88.8   **Other specified infestations**
Ichthyoparasitism due to Vandellia cirrhosa
Linguatulosis
Porocephaliasis

B88.9   **Infestation, unspecified**
Infestation (skin) NOS   Skin parasites NOS
Infestation by mites NOS

B89   **Unspecified parasitic disease**

Sequelae of infectious and parasitic diseases (B90-B94)

NOTE   Categories B90-B94 are to be used to indicate conditions in categories A00-B89 as the cause of sequelae, which are themselves classified elsewhere. The "sequelae" include conditions specified as such; they also include residuals of diseases classifiable to the above categories if there is evidence that the disease itself is no longer present. Codes from these categories are not to be used for chronic infections. Code chronic current infections to active infectious disease as appropriate.

Code first condition resulting from (sequela) the infectious or parasitic disease

√4th **B90**   **Sequelae of** tuberculosis

B90.0   **Sequelae of** central nervous system **tuberculosis**

B90.1   **Sequelae of** genitourinary **tuberculosis**

B90.2   **Sequelae of tuberculosis of** bones and joints

B90.8   **Sequelae of tuberculosis of** other organs
EXCLUDES 2   sequelae of respiratory tuberculosis (B90.9)

B90.9   **Sequelae of** respiratory and unspecified **tuberculosis**
Sequelae of tuberculosis NOS

B91   **Sequelae of** poliomyelitis
EXCLUDES 1   postpolio syndrome (G14)

B92   **Sequelae of** leprosy

√4th **B94**   **Sequelae of** other and unspecified **infectious and parasitic diseases**

B94.0   **Sequelae of** trachoma

B94.1   **Sequelae of** viral encephalitis

B94.2   **Sequelae of** viral hepatitis

B94.8   **Sequelae of** other specified **infectious and parasitic diseases**

B94.9   **Sequelae of** unspecified **infectious and parasitic disease**

Bacterial and viral infectious agents (B95-B97)

NOTE   These categories are provided for use as supplementary or additional codes to identify the infectious agent(s) in diseases classified elsewhere.

√4th **B95**   **Streptococcus, Staphylococcus, and Enterococcus as the cause of diseases classified elsewhere**

B95.0   Streptococcus, group A, as the cause of diseases classified elsewhere

B95.1   Streptococcus, group B, as the cause of diseases classified elsewhere

B95.2   Enterococcus as the cause of diseases classified elsewhere

B95.3   Streptococcus pneumoniae as the cause of diseases classified elsewhere

B95.4   Other streptococcus as the cause of diseases classified elsewhere

B95.5   Unspecified streptococcus as the cause of diseases classified elsewhere

√5th **B95.6**   Staphylococcus aureus as the cause of diseases classified elsewhere

     B95.61   Methicillin susceptible **Staphylococcus aureus infection as the cause of diseases classified elsewhere**
Methicillin susceptible Staphylococcus aureus (MSSA) infection as the cause of diseases classified elsewhere
Staphylococcus aureus infection NOS as the cause of diseases classified elsewhere

     B95.62   Methicillin resistant **Staphylococcus aureus infection as the cause of diseases classified elsewhere**
Methicillin resistant Staphylococcus aureus (MRSA) infection as the cause of diseases classified elsewhere

B95.7   Other staphylococcus as the cause of diseases classified elsewhere

B95.8   Unspecified staphylococcus as the cause of diseases classified elsewhere

√4th **B96**   **Other bacterial agents as the cause of diseases classified elsewhere**

B96.0   Mycoplasma pneumoniae [M. pneumoniae] as the cause of diseases classified elsewhere
Pleuro-pneumonia-like-organism [PPLO]

B96.1   Klebsiella pneumoniae [K. pneumoniae] as the cause of diseases classified elsewhere

√5th **B96.2**   Escherichia coli [E. coli] as the cause of diseases classified elsewhere

     B96.20   Unspecified Escherichia coli [E. coli] as the cause of diseases classified elsewhere
Escherichia coli [E. coli] NOS

     B96.21   Shiga toxin-producing Escherichia coli [E. coli] (STEC) O157 as the cause of diseases classified elsewhere
E. coli O157:H- (nonmotile) with confirmation of Shiga toxin
E. coli O157 with confirmation of Shiga toxin when H antigen is unknown, or is not H7
O157:H7 Escherichia coli [E.coli] with or without confirmation of Shiga toxin-production
Shiga toxin-producing Escherichia coli [E.coli] O157:H7 with or without confirmation of Shiga toxin-production
STEC O157:H7 with or without confirmation of Shiga toxin-production

     B96.22   Other specified Shiga toxin-producing Escherichia coli [E. coli] (STEC) as the cause of diseases classified elsewhere
Non-O157 Shiga toxin-producing Escherichia coli [E.coli]
Non-O157 Shiga toxin-producing Escherichia coli [E.coli] with known O group

     B96.23   Unspecified Shiga toxin-producing Escherichia coli [E. coli] (STEC) as the cause of diseases classified elsewhere
Shiga toxin-producing Escherichia coli [E. coli] with unspecified O group
STEC NOS

     B96.29   Other Escherichia coli [E. coli] as the cause of diseases classified elsewhere
Non-Shiga toxin-producing E. coli

B96.3   Hemophilus influenzae [H. influenzae] as the cause of diseases classified elsewhere

B96.4   Proteus (mirabilis) (morganii) as the cause of diseases classified elsewhere

B96.5   Pseudomonas (aeruginosa) (mallei) (pseudomallei) as the cause of diseases classified elsewhere

B96.6   Bacteroides fragilis [B. fragilis] as the cause of diseases classified elsewhere

B96.7   Clostridium perfringens [C. perfringens] as the cause of diseases classified elsewhere

√5th **B96.8**   Other specified bacterial agents as the cause of diseases classified elsewhere

     B96.81   Helicobacter pylori [H. pylori] as the cause of diseases classified elsewhere

B96.82 **Vibrio vulnificus** as the cause of diseases classified elsewhere

B96.89 **Other specified bacterial agents** as the cause of diseases classified elsewhere

✓4ᵗʰ **B97 Viral agents as the cause of diseases classified elsewhere**

B97.0 Adenovirus as the cause of diseases classified elsewhere

✓5ᵗʰ B97.1 Enterovirus as the cause of diseases classified elsewhere

B97.10 **Unspecified** enterovirus as the cause of diseases classified elsewhere

B97.11 **Coxsackievirus** as the cause of diseases classified elsewhere

B97.12 **Echovirus** as the cause of diseases classified elsewhere

B97.19 **Other** enterovirus as the cause of diseases classified elsewhere

✓5ᵗʰ B97.2 Coronavirus as the cause of diseases classified elsewhere

B97.21 **SARS-associated** coronavirus as the cause of diseases classified elsewhere cc

EXCLUDES 1 pneumonia due to SARS-associated coronavirus (J12.81)

CC Excl: A15.0-A15.6, A15.8-A15.9, A17.9, A18.82, A18.84, A18.89, A21.2, A22.1, A31.0, A37.01, A37.11, A37.81, A37.91, A42.0, A43.0, A48.1, B25.0, B34.1-B34.2, B34.4-B34.8, B39.0-B39.2, B44.0, B58.3, B59, B67.1, B97.19-B97.29, B97.5-B97.6, B97.81-B97.89, J09.X1-J09.X2, J10.00-J10.1, J11.00-J11.1, J12.0-J12.3, J12.89-J18.1, J18.8-J18.9, J22, J44.9, J47.0-J70.4, J70.8-J70.9, J98.4, J98.8-J99, Q33.4, R91.1

B97.29 **Other coronavirus** as the cause of diseases classified elsewhere

✓5ᵗʰ B97.3 Retrovirus as the cause of diseases classified elsewhere

EXCLUDES 1 human immunodeficiency virus [HIV] disease (B20)

B97.30 **Unspecified** retrovirus as the cause of diseases classified elsewhere

B97.31 **Lentivirus** as the cause of diseases classified elsewhere

B97.32 **Oncovirus** as the cause of diseases classified elsewhere

B97.33 **Human T-cell lymphotrophic virus, type I [HTLV-I]** as the cause of diseases classified elsewhere cc

CC Excl: A74.81, A74.9, B33.3-B33.4, B34.1-B34.2, B34.4-B34.8, B97.10, B97.19-B97.29, B97.31-B97.39, B97.5-B97.6, B97.81-B97.89

B97.34 **Human T-cell lymphotrophic virus, type II [HTLV-II]** as the cause of diseases classified elsewhere cc

CC Excl: A74.81, A74.9, B33.3-B33.4, B34.1-B34.2, B34.4-B34.8, B97.10, B97.19-B97.39, B97.5-B97.6, B97.81-B97.89

B97.35 **Human immunodeficiency virus, type 2 [HIV 2]** as the cause of diseases classified elsewhere cc

CC Excl: A74.81, A74.9, B20, B33.3-B33.4, B34.1-B34.2, B34.4-B34.8, B97.10, B97.19-B97.39, B97.5-B97.6, B97.81-B97.89

B97.39 **Other** retrovirus as the cause of diseases classified elsewhere

B97.4 Respiratory syncytial **virus** as the cause of diseases classified elsewhere

B97.5 Reovirus as the cause of diseases classified elsewhere

B97.6 Parvovirus as the cause of diseases classified elsewhere

B97.7 Papillomavirus as the cause of diseases classified elsewhere

✓5ᵗʰ B97.8 Other **viral agents** as the cause of diseases classified elsewhere

B97.81 **Human metapneumovirus** as the cause of diseases classified elsewhere

B97.89 **Other** viral agents as the cause of diseases classified elsewhere

Other infectious diseases (B99)

✓4ᵗʰ **B99 Other and unspecified infectious diseases**

B99.8 Other infectious disease HIV

B99.9 Unspecified infectious disease

Chapter 2. Neoplasms (C00-D49)

NOTE

Functional activity

All neoplasms are classified in this chapter, whether they are functionally active or not. An additional code from Chapter 4 may be used, to identify functional activity associated with any neoplasm.

Morphology [Histology]

Chapter 2 classifies neoplasms primarily by site (topography), with broad groupings for behavior, malignant, in situ, benign, etc. The Table of Neoplasms should be used to identify the correct topography code. In a few cases, such as for malignant melanoma and certain neuroendocrine tumors, the morphology (histologic type) is included in the category and codes.

Primary malignant neoplasms overlapping site boundaries

A primary malignant neoplasm that overlaps two or more contiguous (next to each other) sites should be classified to the subcategory/code 8 ("overlapping lesion"), unless the combination is specifically indexed elsewhere. For multiple neoplasms of the same site that are not contiguous, such as tumors in different quadrants of the same breast, codes for each site should be assigned.

Malignant neoplasm of ectopic tissue

Malignant neoplasms of ectopic tissue are to be coded to the site mentioned, e.g., ectopic pancreatic malignant neoplasms are coded to pancreas, unspecified (C25.9).

This chapter contains the following blocks:

C00-C14	Malignant neoplasms of lip, oral cavity and pharynx
C15-C26	Malignant neoplasms of digestive organs
C30-C39	Malignant neoplasms of respiratory and intrathoracic organs
C40-C41	Malignant neoplasms of bone and articular cartilage
C43-C44	Melanoma and other malignant neoplasms of skin
C45-C49	Malignant neoplasms of mesothelial and soft tissue
C50	Malignant neoplasms of breast
C51-C58	Malignant neoplasms of female genital organs
C60-C63	Malignant neoplasms of male genital organs
C64-C68	Malignant neoplasms of urinary tract
C69-C72	Malignant neoplasms of eye, brain and other parts of central nervous system
C73-C75	Malignant neoplasms of thyroid and other endocrine glands
C7A	Malignant neuroendocrine tumors
C7B	Secondary neuroendocrine tumors
C76-C80	Malignant neoplasms of ill-defined, other secondary and unspecified sites
C81-C96	Malignant neoplasms of lymphoid, hematopoietic and related tissue
D00-D09	In situ neoplasms
D10-D36	Benign neoplasms, except benign neuroendocrine tumors
D3A	Benign neuroendocrine tumors
D37-D48	Neoplasms of uncertain behavior, polycythemia vera and myelodysplastic syndromes
D49	Neoplasms of unspecified behavior

MALIGNANT NEOPLASMS (C00-C96)

NOTE Malignant neoplasms, stated or presumed to be primary (of specified sites), and certain specified histologies, except neuroendocrine, and of lymphoid, hematopoietic and related tissue (C00-C75)

Malignant neoplasms of lip, oral cavity and pharynx (C00-C14)

√4ᵗʰ C00 Malignant neoplasm of lip

Use additional code to identify:
    alcohol abuse and dependence (F10.-)
    history of tobacco use (Z87.891)
    tobacco dependence (F17.-)
    tobacco use (Z72.0)
EXCLUDES 1 malignant melanoma of lip (C43.0)
    Merkel cell carcinoma of lip (C4A.0)
    other and unspecified malignant neoplasm of skin of lip (C44.0-)

C00.0 Malignant neoplasm of external upper lip
    Malignant neoplasm of lipstick area of upper lip
    Malignant neoplasm of upper lip NOS
    Malignant neoplasm of vermilion border of upper lip

C00.1 Malignant neoplasm of external lower lip
    Malignant neoplasm of lower lip NOS
    Malignant neoplasm of lipstick area of lower lip
    Malignant neoplasm of vermilion border of lower lip

C00.2 Malignant neoplasm of external lip, unspecified
    Malignant neoplasm of vermilion border of lip NOS

C00.3 Malignant neoplasm of upper lip, inner aspect
    Malignant neoplasm of buccal aspect of upper lip
    Malignant neoplasm of frenulum of upper lip
    Malignant neoplasm of mucosa of upper lip
    Malignant neoplasm of oral aspect of upper lip

C00.4 Malignant neoplasm of lower lip, inner aspect
    Malignant neoplasm of buccal aspect of lower lip
    Malignant neoplasm of frenulum of lower lip
    Malignant neoplasm of mucosa of lower lip
    Malignant neoplasm of oral aspect of lower lip

C00.5 Malignant neoplasm of lip, unspecified, inner aspect
    Malignant neoplasm of buccal aspect of lip, unspecified
    Malignant neoplasm of frenulum of lip, unspecified
    Malignant neoplasm of mucosa of lip, unspecified
    Malignant neoplasm of oral aspect of lip, unspecified

C00.6 Malignant neoplasm of commissure of lip, unspecified

C00.8 Malignant neoplasm of overlapping sites of lip

C00.9 Malignant neoplasm of lip, unspecified

C01 Malignant neoplasm of base of tongue
    Malignant neoplasm of dorsal surface of base of tongue
    Malignant neoplasm of fixed part of tongue NOS
    Malignant neoplasm of posterior third of tongue
    Use additional code to identify:
        alcohol abuse and dependence (F10.-)
        history of tobacco use (Z87.891)
        tobacco dependence (F17.-)
        tobacco use (Z72.0)

√4ᵗʰ C02 Malignant neoplasm of other and unspecified parts of tongue
    Use additional code to identify:
        alcohol abuse and dependence (F10.-)
        history of tobacco use (Z87.891)
        tobacco dependence (F17.-)
        tobacco use (Z72.0)

C02.0 Malignant neoplasm of dorsal surface of tongue
    Malignant neoplasm of anterior two-thirds of tongue, dorsal surface
    EXCLUDES 2 malignant neoplasm of dorsal surface of base of tongue (C01)

C02.1 Malignant neoplasm of border of tongue
    Malignant neoplasm of tip of tongue

C02.2 Malignant neoplasm of ventral surface of tongue
    Malignant neoplasm of anterior two-thirds of tongue, ventral surface
    Malignant neoplasm of frenulum linguae

C02.3 Malignant neoplasm of anterior two-thirds of tongue, part unspecified
    Malignant neoplasm of middle third of tongue NOS
    Malignant neoplasm of mobile part of tongue NOS

C02.4 Malignant neoplasm of lingual tonsil
    EXCLUDES 2 malignant neoplasm of tonsil NOS (C09.9)

C02.8 Malignant neoplasm of overlapping sites of tongue
    Malignant neoplasm of two or more contiguous sites of tongue

C02.9 Malignant neoplasm of tongue, unspecified

√4ᵗʰ C03 Malignant neoplasm of gum
    INCLUDES malignant neoplasm of alveolar (ridge) mucosa
        malignant neoplasm of gingiva
    Use additional code to identify:
        alcohol abuse and dependence (F10.-)
        history of tobacco use (Z87.891)
        tobacco dependence (F17.-)
        tobacco use (Z72.0)
    EXCLUDES 2 malignant odontogenic neoplasms (C41.0-C41.1)

C03.0 Malignant neoplasm of upper gum

C03.1 Malignant neoplasm of lower gum

C03.9 Malignant neoplasm of gum, unspecified

√4ᵗʰ C04 Malignant neoplasm of floor of mouth
    Use additional code to identify:
        alcohol abuse and dependence (F10.-)
        history of tobacco use (Z87.891)
        tobacco dependence (F17.-)
        tobacco use (Z72.0)

C04.0 Malignant neoplasm of anterior floor of mouth
    Malignant neoplasm of anterior to the premolar-canine junction

C04.1 Malignant neoplasm of lateral floor of mouth

C04.8 Malignant neoplasm of overlapping sites of floor of mouth

C04.9 Malignant neoplasm of floor of mouth, unspecified

N Newborn: 0   P Pediatric: 0-17   M Maternity: 12-55   A Adult: 15-124   **MCC** Major CC Condition   **PDx MCC** PDx acts as own MCC   **CC** CC Condition   **PDx CC** PDx acts as own CC

Neoplasms

✓4ᵗʰ C05 Malignant neoplasm of palate
Use additional code to identify:
alcohol abuse and dependence (F10.-)
history of tobacco use (Z87.891)
tobacco dependence (F17.-)
tobacco use (Z72.0)
EXCLUDES 1 *Kaposi's sarcoma of palate (C46.2)*

C05.0 Malignant neoplasm of hard palate

C05.1 Malignant neoplasm of soft palate
EXCLUDES 2 *malignant neoplasm of nasopharyngeal surface of soft palate (C11.3)*

C05.2 Malignant neoplasm of uvula

C05.8 Malignant neoplasm of overlapping sites of palate

C05.9 Malignant neoplasm of palate, unspecified
Malignant neoplasm of roof of mouth

✓4ᵗʰ C06 Malignant neoplasm of other and unspecified parts of mouth
Use additional code to identify:
alcohol abuse and dependence (F10.-)
history of tobacco use (Z87.891)
tobacco dependence (F17.-)
tobacco use (Z72.0)

C06.0 Malignant neoplasm of cheek mucosa
Malignant neoplasm of buccal mucosa NOS
Malignant neoplasm of internal cheek

C06.1 Malignant neoplasm of vestibule of mouth
Malignant neoplasm of buccal sulcus (upper) (lower)
Malignant neoplasm of labial sulcus (upper) (lower)

C06.2 Malignant neoplasm of retromolar area

✓5ᵗʰ C06.8 Malignant neoplasm of overlapping sites of other and unspecified parts of mouth

C06.80 Malignant neoplasm of overlapping sites of unspecified parts of mouth

C06.89 Malignant neoplasm of overlapping sites of other parts of mouth
"book leaf" neoplasm [ventral surface of tongue and floor of mouth]

C06.9 Malignant neoplasm of mouth, unspecified
Malignant neoplasm of minor salivary gland, unspecified site
Malignant neoplasm of oral cavity NOS

C07 Malignant neoplasm of parotid gland
Use additional code to identify:
alcohol abuse and dependence (F10.-)
exposure to environmental tobacco smoke (Z77.22)
exposure to tobacco smoke in the perinatal period (P96.81)
history of tobacco use (Z87.891)
occupational exposure to environmental tobacco smoke (Z57.31)
tobacco dependence (F17.-)
tobacco use (Z72.0)

✓4ᵗʰ C08 Malignant neoplasm of other and unspecified major salivary glands
INCLUDES malignant neoplasm of salivary ducts
Use additional code to identify:
alcohol abuse and dependence (F10.-)
exposure to environmental tobacco smoke (Z77.22)
exposure to tobacco smoke in the perinatal period (P96.81)
history of tobacco use (Z87.891)
occupational exposure to environmental tobacco smoke (Z57.31)
tobacco dependence (F17.-)
tobacco use (Z72.0)
EXCLUDES 1 *malignant neoplasms of specified minor salivary glands which are classified according to their anatomical location*
EXCLUDES 2 *malignant neoplasms of minor salivary glands NOS (C06.9)*
malignant neoplasm of parotid gland (C07)

C08.0 Malignant neoplasm of submandibular gland
Malignant neoplasm of submaxillary gland

C08.1 Malignant neoplasm of sublingual gland

C08.9 Malignant neoplasm of major salivary gland, unspecified
Malignant neoplasm of salivary gland (major) NOS

✓4ᵗʰ C09 Malignant neoplasm of tonsil
Use additional code to identify:
alcohol abuse and dependence (F10.-)
exposure to environmental tobacco smoke (Z77.22)
exposure to tobacco smoke in the perinatal period (P96.81)
history of tobacco use (Z87.891)
occupational exposure to environmental tobacco smoke (Z57.31)
tobacco dependence (F17.-)
tobacco use (Z72.0)
EXCLUDES 2 *malignant neoplasm of lingual tonsil (C02.4)*
malignant neoplasm of pharyngeal tonsil (C11.1)

C09.0 Malignant neoplasm of tonsillar fossa

C09.1 Malignant neoplasm of tonsillar pillar (anterior) (posterior)

C09.8 Malignant neoplasm of overlapping sites of tonsil

C09.9 Malignant neoplasm of tonsil, unspecified
Malignant neoplasm of tonsil NOS
Malignant neoplasm of faucial tonsils
Malignant neoplasm of palatine tonsils

✓4ᵗʰ C10 Malignant neoplasm of oropharynx
Use additional code to identify:
alcohol abuse and dependence (F10.-)
exposure to environmental tobacco smoke (Z77.22)
exposure to tobacco smoke in the perinatal period (P96.81)
history of tobacco use (Z87.891)
occupational exposure to environmental tobacco smoke (Z57.31)
tobacco dependence (F17.-)
tobacco use (Z72.0)
EXCLUDES 2 *malignant neoplasm of tonsil (C09.-)*

C10.0 Malignant neoplasm of vallecula

C10.1 Malignant neoplasm of anterior surface of epiglottis
Malignant neoplasm of epiglottis, free border [margin]
Malignant neoplasm of glossoepiglottic fold(s)
EXCLUDES 2 *malignant neoplasm of epiglottis (suprahyoid portion) NOS (C32.1)*

C10.2 Malignant neoplasm of lateral wall of oropharynx

C10.3 Malignant neoplasm of posterior wall of oropharynx

C10.4 Malignant neoplasm of branchial cleft
Malignant neoplasm of branchial cyst [site of neoplasm]

C10.8 Malignant neoplasm of overlapping sites of oropharynx
Malignant neoplasm of junctional region of oropharynx

C10.9 Malignant neoplasm of oropharynx, unspecified

✓4ᵗʰ C11 Malignant neoplasm of nasopharynx
Use additional code to identify:
exposure to environmental tobacco smoke (Z77.22)
exposure to tobacco smoke in the perinatal period (P96.81)
history of tobacco use (Z87.891)
occupational exposure to environmental tobacco smoke (Z57.31)
tobacco dependence (F17.-)
tobacco use (Z72.0)

C11.0 Malignant neoplasm of superior wall of nasopharynx
Malignant neoplasm of roof of nasopharynx

C11.1 Malignant neoplasm of posterior wall of nasopharynx
Malignant neoplasm of adenoid
Malignant neoplasm of pharyngeal tonsil

C11.2 Malignant neoplasm of lateral wall of nasopharynx
Malignant neoplasm of fossa of Rosenmüller
Malignant neoplasm of opening of auditory tube
Malignant neoplasm of pharyngeal recess

C11.3 Malignant neoplasm of anterior wall of nasopharynx
Malignant neoplasm of floor of nasopharynx
Malignant neoplasm of nasopharyngeal (anterior) (posterior) surface of soft palate
Malignant neoplasm of posterior margin of nasal choana
Malignant neoplasm of posterior margin of nasal septum

C11.8 Malignant neoplasm of overlapping sites of nasopharynx

C11.9 Malignant neoplasm of nasopharynx, unspecified
Malignant neoplasm of nasopharyngeal wall NOS

C12 Malignant neoplasm of pyriform sinus
Malignant neoplasm of pyriform fossa
Use additional code to identify:
exposure to environmental tobacco smoke (Z77.22)
exposure to tobacco smoke in the perinatal period (P96.81)
history of tobacco use (Z87.891)
occupational exposure to environmental tobacco smoke (Z57.31)
tobacco dependence (F17.-)
tobacco use (Z72.0)

✓ Additional Character Required   ✓x7ᵗʰ Xtension Alert   Unacceptable PDx   Manifestation   Hospital Acquired Condition   EXCLUDES1 Not Coded Here   EXCLUDES2 Not Included Here

✓4ᵗʰ C13 Malignant neoplasm of hypopharynx
Use additional code to identify:
exposure to environmental tobacco smoke (Z77.22)
exposure to tobacco smoke in the perinatal period (P96.81)
history of tobacco use (Z87.891)
occupational exposure to environmental tobacco smoke (Z57.31)
tobacco dependence (F17.-)
tobacco use (Z72.0)
EXCLUDES 2 malignant neoplasm of pyriform sinus (C12)

C13.0 Malignant neoplasm of postcricoid region

C13.1 Malignant neoplasm of aryepiglottic fold, hypopharyngeal aspect
Malignant neoplasm of aryepiglottic fold, marginal zone
Malignant neoplasm of aryepiglottic fold NOS
Malignant neoplasm of interarytenoid fold, marginal zone
Malignant neoplasm of interarytenoid fold NOS
EXCLUDES 2 malignant neoplasm of aryepiglottic fold or interarytenoid fold, laryngeal aspect (C32.1)

C13.2 Malignant neoplasm of posterior wall of hypopharynx

C13.8 Malignant neoplasm of overlapping sites of hypopharynx

C13.9 Malignant neoplasm of hypopharynx, unspecified
Malignant neoplasm of hypopharyngeal wall NOS

✓4ᵗʰ C14 Malignant neoplasm of other and ill-defined sites in the lip, oral cavity and pharynx
Use additional code to identify:
alcohol abuse and dependence (F10.-)
exposure to environmental tobacco smoke (Z77.22)
exposure to tobacco smoke in the perinatal period (P96.81)
history of tobacco use (Z87.891)
occupational exposure to environmental tobacco smoke (Z57.31)
tobacco dependence (F17.-)
tobacco use (Z72.0)
EXCLUDES 1 malignant neoplasm of oral cavity NOS (C06.9)

C14.0 Malignant neoplasm of pharynx, unspecified

C14.2 Malignant neoplasm of Waldeyer's ring

C14.8 Malignant neoplasm of overlapping sites of lip, oral cavity and pharynx
Primary malignant neoplasm of two or more contiguous sites of lip, oral cavity and pharynx
EXCLUDES 1 "book leaf" neoplasm [ventral surface of tongue and floor of mouth] (C06.89)

Malignant neoplasms of digestive organs (C15-C26)
EXCLUDES 1 Kaposi's sarcoma of gastrointestinal sites (C46.4)

✓4ᵗʰ C15 Malignant neoplasm of esophagus
Use additional code to identify:
alcohol abuse and dependence (F10.-)

CC Excl: For CC codes in category C15, unless otherwise noted:
C15.3-C15.9, C26.0, C26.9, C45.7-C45.9, C46.4, C76.8, C7A.00,
C7A.098-C7B.00, C7B.1, C80.0-C80.2, D49.0, D49.81-D49.9

C15.3 Malignant neoplasm of upper third of esophagus CC

C15.4 Malignant neoplasm of middle third of esophagus CC

C15.5 Malignant neoplasm of lower third of esophagus CC
EXCLUDES 1 malignant neoplasm of cardio-esophageal junction (C16.0)

C15.8 Malignant neoplasm of overlapping sites of esophagus CC

C15.9 Malignant neoplasm of esophagus, unspecified CC

✓4ᵗʰ C16 Malignant neoplasm of stomach
Use additional code to identify:
alcohol abuse and dependence (F10.-)
EXCLUDES 2 malignant carcinoid tumor of the stomach (C7A.092)

CC Excl: For CC codes in category C16, unless otherwise noted:
C16.0-C16.9, C26.0, C26.9, C45.7-C45.9, C46.4, C76.8, C7A.00,
C7A.092, C7A.094-C7B.00, C7B.1, C80.0-C80.2, D49.0, D49.81-D49.9

C16.0 Malignant neoplasm of cardia CC
Malignant neoplasm of cardiac orifice
Malignant neoplasm of cardio-esophageal junction
Malignant neoplasm of esophagus and stomach
Malignant neoplasm of gastro-esophageal junction

C16.1 Malignant neoplasm of fundus of stomach CC

C16.2 Malignant neoplasm of body of stomach CC

C16.3 Malignant neoplasm of pyloric antrum CC
Malignant neoplasm of gastric antrum

C16.4 Malignant neoplasm of pylorus CC
Malignant neoplasm of prepylorus
Malignant neoplasm of pyloric canal

C16.5 Malignant neoplasm of lesser curvature of stomach, unspecified CC
Malignant neoplasm of lesser curvature of stomach, not classifiable to C16.1-C16.4

C16.6 Malignant neoplasm of greater curvature of stomach, unspecified CC
Malignant neoplasm of greater curvature of stomach, not classifiable to C16.0-C16.4

C16.8 Malignant neoplasm of overlapping sites of stomach CC

C16.9 Malignant neoplasm of stomach, unspecified CC
Gastric cancer NOS

✓4ᵗʰ C17 Malignant neoplasm of small intestine
EXCLUDES 1 malignant carcinoid tumors of the small intestine (C7A.01)

C17.0 Malignant neoplasm of duodenum CC
CC Excl: C17.0, C17.8-C17.9, C26.0, C26.9, C45.7-C45.9, C46.4,
C7A.00-C7A.010, C7A.019, C7A.098-C7B.00, C7B.1, C76.8, C80.0-
C80.2, D49.0, D49.81-D49.9

C17.1 Malignant neoplasm of jejunum CC
CC Excl: C17.0, C17.8-C17.9, C26.0, C26.9, C45.7-C45.9, C46.4,
C7A.00-C7A.010, C7A.019, C7A.098-C7B.00, C7B.1, C76.8, C80.0-
C80.2, D49.0, D49.81-D49.9

C17.2 Malignant neoplasm of ileum CC
EXCLUDES 1 malignant neoplasm of ileocecal valve (C18.0)
CC Excl: C17.0, C17.8-C17.9, C26.0, C26.9, C45.7-C45.9, C46.4,
C7A.00-C7A.010, C7A.019, C7A.098-C7B.00, C7B.1, C76.8, C80.0-
C80.2, D49.0, D49.81-D49.9

C17.3 Meckel's diverticulum, malignant CC
EXCLUDES 1 Meckel's diverticulum, congenital (Q43.0)
CC Excl: C17.0, C17.8-C17.9, C26.0, C26.9, C45.7-C45.9, C46.4,
C7A.00-C7A.010, C7A.019, C7A.098-C7B.00, C7B.1, C76.8, C80.0-
C80.2, D49.0, D49.81-D49.9

C17.8 Malignant neoplasm of overlapping sites of small intestine CC
CC Excl: C17.0, C17.8-C17.9, C26.0, C26.9, C45.7-C45.9, C46.4,
C7A.00-C7A.010, C7A.019, C7A.098-C7B.00, C7B.1, C76.8, C80.0-
C80.2, D49.0, D49.81-D49.9

C17.9 Malignant neoplasm of small intestine, unspecified CC
CC Excl: See code: C17.8

✓4ᵗʰ C18 Malignant neoplasm of colon
EXCLUDES 1 malignant carcinoid tumors of the colon (C7A.02-)

C18.0 Malignant neoplasm of cecum CC
Malignant neoplasm of ileocecal valve
CC Excl: C18.0, C18.8-C18.9, C26.0, C26.9, C45.7-C45.9, C46.4,
C7A.00, C7A.021, C7A.029, C7A.098-C7B.00, C7B.1, C76.8, C80.0-
C80.2, D49.0, D49.81-D49.9

C18.1 Malignant neoplasm of appendix CC
CC Excl: C18.0, C18.8-C18.9, C26.0, C26.9, C45.7-C45.9, C46.4,
C7A.00, C7A.021, C7A.029, C7A.098-C7B.00, C7B.1, C76.8, C80.0-
C80.2, D49.0, D49.81-D49.9

C18.2 Malignant neoplasm of ascending colon CC
CC Excl: C18.0, C18.8-C18.9, C26.0, C26.9, C45.7-C45.9, C46.4,
C7A.00, C7A.021, C7A.029, C7A.098-C7B.00, C7B.1, C76.8, C80.0-
C80.2, D49.0, D49.81-D49.9

C18.3 Malignant neoplasm of hepatic flexure CC
CC Excl: C18.3, C18.8-C18.9, C26.0, C26.9, C45.7-C45.9, C46.4,
C7A.00, C7A.029, C7A.098-C7B.00, C7B.1, C76.8, C80.0-C80.2,
D49.0, D49.81-D49.9

C18.4 Malignant neoplasm of transverse colon CC
CC Excl: C18.4, C18.8-C18.9, C26.0, C26.9, C45.7-C45.9, C46.4,
C7A.00, C7A.023, C7A.029, C7A.098-C7B.00, C7B.1, C76.8, C80.0-
C80.2, D49.0, D49.81-D49.9

C18.5 Malignant neoplasm of splenic flexure CC
CC Excl: C18.5, C18.8-C18.9, C26.0, C26.9, C45.7-C45.9, C46.4,
C7A.00, C7A.029, C7A.098-C7B.00, C7B.1, C76.8, C80.0-C80.2,
D49.0, D49.81-D49.9

C18.6 Malignant neoplasm of descending colon CC
CC Excl: C18.6, C18.8-C18.9, C26.0, C26.9, C45.7-C45.9, C46.4,
C7A.00, C7A.024, C7A.029, C7A.098-C7B.00, C7B.1, C76.8, C80.0-
C80.2, D49.0, D49.81-D49.9

C18.7 Malignant neoplasm of sigmoid colon CC
Malignant neoplasm of sigmoid (flexure)
EXCLUDES 1 malignant neoplasm of rectosigmoid junction (C19)
CC Excl: C18.7-C18.9, C26.0, C26.9, C45.7-C45.9, C46.4, C7A.00,
C7A.025, C7A.029, C7A.098-C7B.00, C7B.1, C76.8, C80.0-C80.2,
D49.0, D49.81-D49.9

C18.8 Malignant neoplasm of overlapping sites of colon CC
CC Excl: C18.8-C18.9, C26.0, C26.9, C45.7-C45.9, C46.4, C7A.00,
C7A.029, C7A.098-C7B.00, C7B.1, C76.8, C80.0-C80.2, D49.0,
D49.81-D49.9

C18.9 Malignant neoplasm of colon, unspecified CC
Malignant neoplasm of large intestine NOS
CC Excl: See code: C18.8

N Newborn: 0   P Pediatric: 0-17   M Maternity: 12-55   A Adult: 15-124   MCC Major CC Condition   PDx MCC PDx acts as own MCC   CC CC Condition   PDx CC PDx acts as own CC

450   ICD-10-CM Draft (2015)

C19 Malignant neoplasm of rectosigmoid junction `CC`
Malignant neoplasm of colon with rectum
Malignant neoplasm of rectosigmoid (colon)
EXCLUDES 1   malignant carcinoid tumors of the colon (C7A.02-)
CC Excl: C19, C21.2-C21.8, C26.0, C26.9, C45.7-C45.9, C46.4, C7A.00, C7A.098-C7B.00, C7B.1, C76.8, C80.0-C80.2, D49.0, D49.81-D49.9

C20 Malignant neoplasm of rectum `CC`
Malignant neoplasm of rectal ampulla
EXCLUDES 1   malignant carcinoid tumor of the rectum (C7A.026)
CC Excl: C20, C21.2-C21.8, C26.0, C26.9, C45.7-C45.9, C46.4, C7A.00, C7A.026, C7A.098-C7B.00, C7B.1, C76.8, C80.0-C80.2, D49.0, D49.81-D49.9

☑4ᵗʰ C21 Malignant neoplasm of anus and anal canal
EXCLUDES 2   malignant carcinoid tumors of the colon (C7A.02-)
malignant melanoma of anal margin (C43.51)
malignant melanoma of anal skin (C43.51)
malignant melanoma of perianal skin (C43.51)
other and unspecified malignant neoplasm of anal margin (C44.500, C44.510, C44.520, C44.590)
other and unspecified malignant neoplasm of anal skin (C44.500, C44.510, C44.520, C44.590)
other and unspecified malignant neoplasm of perianal skin (C44.500, C44.510, C44.520, C44.590)

C21.0 Malignant neoplasm of anus, unspecified `CC`
CC Excl: C21.0-C21.8, C26.0, C26.9, C45.7-C45.9, C46.4, C76.8, C7A.00, C7A.098-C7B.00, C7B.1, C80.0-C80.2, D49.0, D49.81-D49.9

C21.1 Malignant neoplasm of anal canal `CC`
Malignant neoplasm of anal sphincter
CC Excl: See code: C21.0

C21.2 Malignant neoplasm of cloacogenic zone `CC`
CC Excl: C21.2-C21.8, C26.0, C26.9, C45.7-C45.9, C46.4, C76.8, C7A.00, C7A.098-C7B.00, C7B.1, C80.0-C80.2, D49.0, D49.81-D49.9

C21.8 Malignant neoplasm of overlapping sites of rectum, anus and anal canal `CC`
Malignant neoplasm of anorectal junction
Malignant neoplasm of anorectum
Primary malignant neoplasm of two or more contiguous sites of rectum, anus and anal canal
CC Excl: See code: C21.2

☑4ᵗʰ C22 Malignant neoplasm of liver and intrahepatic bile ducts
Use additional code to identify:
alcohol abuse and dependence (F10.-)
hepatitis B (B16.-, B18.0-B18.1)
hepatitis C (B17.1-, B18.2)
EXCLUDES 1   malignant neoplasm of biliary tract NOS (C24.9)
secondary malignant neoplasm of liver and intrahepatic bile duct (C78.7)

CC Excl: For CC codes in category C22, unless otherwise noted:
C22.0-C22.9, C26.0, C26.9, C45.7-C45.9, C46.4, C76.8, C7A.00, C7A.098-C7B.00, C7B.1, C80.0-C80.2, D49.0, D49.81-D49.9

C22.0 Liver cell carcinoma `CC`
Hepatocellular carcinoma
Hepatoma

C22.1 Intrahepatic bile duct carcinoma `CC`
Cholangiocarcinoma
EXCLUDES 1   malignant neoplasm of hepatic duct (C24.0)

C22.2 Hepatoblastoma `CC`

C22.3 Angiosarcoma of liver `CC`
Kupffer cell sarcoma

C22.4 Other sarcomas of liver `CC`

C22.7 Other specified carcinomas of liver `CC`

C22.8 Malignant neoplasm of liver, primary, unspecified as to type `CC`

C22.9 Malignant neoplasm of liver, not specified as primary or secondary `CC`

C23 Malignant neoplasm of gallbladder `CC`
CC Excl: C23, C24.8-C24.9, C26.0, C26.9, C45.7-C45.9, C46.4, C7A.00, C7A.098-C7B.00, C7B.1, C76.8, C80.0-C80.2, D49.0, D49.81-D49.9

☑4ᵗʰ C24 Malignant neoplasm of other and unspecified parts of biliary tract
EXCLUDES 1   malignant neoplasm of intrahepatic bile duct (C22.1)

C24.0 Malignant neoplasm of extrahepatic bile duct `CC`
Malignant neoplasm of biliary duct or passage NOS
Malignant neoplasm of common bile duct
Malignant neoplasm of cystic duct
Malignant neoplasm of hepatic duct
CC Excl: C24.0, C24.8-C24.9, C26.0, C26.9, C45.7-C45.9, C46.4, C7A.00, C7A.098-C7B.00, C7B.1, C76.8, C80.0-C80.2, D49.0, D49.81-D49.9

C24.1 Malignant neoplasm of ampulla of Vater `CC`
CC Excl: C24.1-C24.9, C26.0, C26.9, C45.7-C45.9, C46.4, C76.8, C7A.00, C7A.098-C7B.00, C7B.1, C80.0-C80.2, D49.0, D49.81-D49.9

C24.8 Malignant neoplasm of overlapping sites of biliary tract `CC`
Malignant neoplasm involving both intrahepatic and extrahepatic bile ducts
Primary malignant neoplasm of two or more contiguous sites of biliary tract
CC Excl: C24.8-C24.9, C26.0, C26.9, C45.7-C45.9, C46.4, C76.8, C7A.00, C7A.098-C7B.00, C7B.1, C80.0-C80.2, D49.0, D49.81-D49.9

C24.9 Malignant neoplasm of biliary tract, unspecified `CC`
CC Excl: See code: C24.8

☑4ᵗʰ C25 Malignant neoplasm of pancreas
Use additional code to identify:
alcohol abuse and dependence (F10.-)

CC Excl: For CC codes in category C25, unless otherwise noted:
C25.0-C26.0, C26.9, C45.7-C45.9, C46.4, C76.8, C7A.00, C7A.098-C7B.00, C7B.1, C80.0-C80.2, D49.0, D49.81-D49.9

C25.0 Malignant neoplasm of head of pancreas `CC`

C25.1 Malignant neoplasm of body of pancreas `CC`

C25.2 Malignant neoplasm of tail of pancreas `CC`

C25.3 Malignant neoplasm of pancreatic duct `CC`

C25.4 Malignant neoplasm of endocrine pancreas
Malignant neoplasm of islets of Langerhans
Use additional code to identify any functional activity

C25.7 Malignant neoplasm of other parts of pancreas `CC`
Malignant neoplasm of neck of pancreas

C25.8 Malignant neoplasm of overlapping sites of pancreas `CC`

C25.9 Malignant neoplasm of pancreas, unspecified `CC`

☑4ᵗʰ C26 Malignant neoplasm of other and ill-defined digestive organs
EXCLUDES 1   malignant neoplasm of peritoneum and retroperitoneum (C48.-)

C26.0 Malignant neoplasm of intestinal tract, part unspecified
Malignant neoplasm of intestine NOS

C26.1 Malignant neoplasm of spleen
EXCLUDES 1   Hodgkin lymphoma (C81.-)
non-Hodgkin lymphoma (C82-C85)

C26.9 Malignant neoplasm of ill-defined sites within the digestive system
Malignant neoplasm of alimentary canal or tract NOS
Malignant neoplasm of gastrointestinal tract NOS
EXCLUDES 1   malignant neoplasm of abdominal NOS (C76.2)
malignant neoplasm of intra-abdominal NOS (C76.2)

Malignant neoplasms of respiratory and intrathoracic organs (C30-C39)

INCLUDES   malignant neoplasm of middle ear
EXCLUDES 1   mesothelioma (C45.-)

☑4ᵗʰ C30 Malignant neoplasm of nasal cavity and middle ear

C30.0 Malignant neoplasm of nasal cavity
Malignant neoplasm of cartilage of nose
Malignant neoplasm of nasal concha
Malignant neoplasm of internal nose
Malignant neoplasm of septum of nose
Malignant neoplasm of vestibule of nose
EXCLUDES 1   malignant melanoma of skin of nose (C43.31)
malignant neoplasm of nasal bone (C41.0)
malignant neoplasm of nose NOS (C76.0)
malignant neoplasm of olfactory bulb (C72.2-)
malignant neoplasm of posterior margin of nasal septum and choana (C11.3)
malignant neoplasm of turbinates (C41.0)
other and unspecified malignant neoplasm of skin of nose (C44.301, C44.311, C44.321, C44.391)

C30.1 Malignant neoplasm of middle ear
Malignant neoplasm of antrum tympanicum
Malignant neoplasm of auditory tube
Malignant neoplasm of eustachian tube
Malignant neoplasm of inner ear
Malignant neoplasm of mastoid air cells
Malignant neoplasm of tympanic cavity
EXCLUDES 1   malignant melanoma of skin of (external) ear (C43.2-)
malignant neoplasm of auricular canal (external) (C43.2-, C44.2-)
malignant neoplasm of bone of ear (meatus) (C41.0)
malignant neoplasm of cartilage of ear (C49.0)
other and unspecified malignant neoplasm of skin of (external) ear (C44.2-)

☑ Additional Character Required   ✗7ᵗʰ Xtension Alert   Unacceptable PDx   Manifestation   Hospital Acquired Condition   *EXCLUDES 1* Not Coded Here   *EXCLUDES 2* Not Included Here

Neoplasms

C31–C38.8

✓4ᵗʰ **C31** **Malignant neoplasm of accessory sinuses**

    C31.0 **Malignant neoplasm of maxillary sinus**
        Malignant neoplasm of antrum (Highmore) (maxillary)

    C31.1 **Malignant neoplasm of ethmoidal sinus**

    C31.2 **Malignant neoplasm of frontal sinus**

    C31.3 **Malignant neoplasm of sphenoid sinus**

    C31.8 **Malignant neoplasm of overlapping sites of accessory sinuses**

    C31.9 **Malignant neoplasm of accessory sinus, unspecified**

✓4ᵗʰ **C32** **Malignant neoplasm of larynx**
    Use additional code to identify:
        alcohol abuse and dependence (F10.-)
        exposure to environmental tobacco smoke (Z77.22)
        exposure to tobacco smoke in the perinatal period (P96.81)
        history of tobacco use (Z87.891)
        occupational exposure to environmental tobacco smoke (Z57.31)
        tobacco dependence (F17.-)
        tobacco use (Z72.0)

    C32.0 **Malignant neoplasm of glottis**
        Malignant neoplasm of intrinsic larynx
        Malignant neoplasm of laryngeal commissure
          (anterior)(posterior)
        Malignant neoplasm of vocal cord (true) NOS

    C32.1 **Malignant neoplasm of supraglottis**
        Malignant neoplasm of aryepiglottic fold or interarytenoid fold,
          laryngeal aspect
        Malignant neoplasm of epiglottis (suprahyoid portion) NOS
        Malignant neoplasm of extrinsic larynx
        Malignant neoplasm of false vocal cord
        Malignant neoplasm of posterior (laryngeal) surface of epiglottis
        Malignant neoplasm of ventricular bands
        EXCLUDES 2 *malignant neoplasm of anterior surface of epiglottis*
                (C10.1)
              malignant neoplasm of aryepiglottic fold or
                interarytenoid fold, hypopharyngeal aspect
                (C13.1)
              malignant neoplasm of aryepiglottic fold or
                interarytenoid fold, marginal zone (C13.1)
              malignant neoplasm of aryepiglottic fold or
                interarytenoid fold NOS (C13.1)

    C32.2 **Malignant neoplasm of subglottis**

    C32.3 **Malignant neoplasm of laryngeal cartilage**

    C32.8 **Malignant neoplasm of overlapping sites of larynx**

    C32.9 **Malignant neoplasm of larynx, unspecified**

C33 **Malignant neoplasm of trachea**   `CC`
    Use additional code to identify:
        exposure to environmental tobacco smoke (Z77.22)
        exposure to tobacco smoke in the perinatal period (P96.81)
        history of tobacco use (Z87.891)
        occupational exposure to environmental tobacco smoke (Z57.31)
        tobacco dependence (F17.-)
        tobacco use (Z72.0)
    CC Excl: C33-C34.92, C39.9, C45.7-C45.9, C46.50-C46.52, C76.1, C76.8,
    C78.00-C78.1, C78.30-C78.39, C7A.00, C7A.090, C7A.098-C7B.00, C7B.1,
    C80.0-C80.2, D49.1, D49.81-D49.9

✓4ᵗʰ **C34** **Malignant neoplasm of bronchus and lung**
    Use additional code to identify:
        exposure to environmental tobacco smoke (Z77.22)
        exposure to tobacco smoke in the perinatal period (P96.81)
        history of tobacco use (Z87.891)
        occupational exposure to environmental tobacco smoke (Z57.31)
        tobacco dependence (F17.-)
        tobacco use (Z72.0)
        EXCLUDES 1 *Kaposi's sarcoma of lung (C46.5-)*
              malignant carcinoid tumor of the bronchus and lung (C7A.090)

    ✓5ᵗʰ **C34.0** **Malignant neoplasm of main bronchus**
        Malignant neoplasm of carina
        Malignant neoplasm of hilus (of lung)

        **CC Excl: For CC codes in subcategory C34.0, unless
        otherwise noted:** C34.00-C34.02, C34.80-C34.92, C39.9,
        C45.7-C45.9, C46.50-C46.52, C76.8, C7A.00, C7A.090,
        C7A.098-C7B.00, C7B.1, C80.0-C80.2, D49.1, D49.81-D49.9

        C34.00 **Malignant neoplasm of unspecified main** `CC`
              bronchus

        C34.01 **Malignant neoplasm of right main bronchus** `CC`

        C34.02 **Malignant neoplasm of left main bronchus** `CC`

    ✓5ᵗʰ **C34.1** **Malignant neoplasm of upper lobe, bronchus or lung**

        **CC Excl: For CC codes in subcategory C34.1, unless
        otherwise noted:** C34.10-C34.12, C34.80-C34.92, C39.9,
        C45.7-C45.9, C46.50-C46.52, C76.8, C7A.00, C7A.090,
        C7A.098-C7B.00, C7B.1, C80.0-C80.2, D49.1, D49.81-D49.9

        C34.10 **Malignant neoplasm of upper lobe, unspecified** `CC`
              bronchus or lung

        (C34.11) **Malignant neoplasm of upper lobe, right** `CC`
              bronchus or lung

        C34.12 **Malignant neoplasm of upper lobe, left** `CC`
              bronchus or lung

    C34.2 **Malignant neoplasm of middle lobe, bronchus or lung** `CC`
        CC Excl: C34.2, C34.80-C34.92, C39.9, C45.7-C45.9, C46.50-C46.52,
        C7A.00, C7A.090, C7A.098-C7B.00, C7B.1, C76.8, C80.0-C80.2,
        D49.1, D49.81-D49.9

    ✓5ᵗʰ **C34.3** **Malignant neoplasm of lower lobe, bronchus or lung**

        **CC Excl: For CC codes in subcategory C34.3, unless
        otherwise noted:** C34.30-C34.92, C39.9, C45.7-C45.9,
        C46.50-C46.52, C76.8, C7A.00, C7A.090, C7A.098-C7B.00,
        C7B.1, C80.0-C80.2, D49.1, D49.81-D49.9

        C34.30 **Malignant neoplasm of lower lobe, unspecified** `CC`
              bronchus or lung

        C34.31 **Malignant neoplasm of lower lobe, right** `CC`
              bronchus or lung

        C34.32 **Malignant neoplasm of lower lobe, left** `CC`
              bronchus or lung

    ✓5ᵗʰ **C34.8** **Malignant neoplasm of overlapping sites of bronchus and
        lung**

        **CC Excl: For CC codes in subcategory C34.8, unless
        otherwise noted:** C34.80-C34.92, C39.9, C45.7-C45.9,
        C46.50-C46.52, C76.8, C7A.00, C7A.090, C7A.098-C7B.00,
        C7B.1, C80.0-C80.2, D49.1, D49.81-D49.9

        C34.80 **Malignant neoplasm of overlapping sites of** `CC`
              unspecified bronchus and lung

        C34.81 **Malignant neoplasm of overlapping sites of** `CC`
              right bronchus and lung

        C34.82 **Malignant neoplasm of overlapping sites of** `CC`
              left bronchus and lung

    ✓5ᵗʰ **C34.9** **Malignant neoplasm of unspecified part of bronchus or lung**

        **CC Excl: For CC codes in subcategory C34.9, unless
        otherwise noted:** C34.80-C34.92, C39.9, C45.7-C45.9,
        C46.50-C46.52, C76.8, C7A.00, C7A.090, C7A.098-C7B.00,
        C7B.1, C80.0-C80.2, D49.1, D49.81-D49.9

        C34.90 **Malignant neoplasm of unspecified part of** `CC`
              unspecified bronchus or lung
              Lung cancer NOS

        C34.91 **Malignant neoplasm of unspecified part of right** `CC`
              bronchus or lung

        (C34.92) **Malignant neoplasm of unspecified part of left** `CC`
              bronchus or lung

C37 **Malignant neoplasm of thymus**   `CC`
    EXCLUDES 1 *malignant carcinoid tumor of the thymus (C7A.091)*
    CC Excl: C37, C7A.091

✓4ᵗʰ **C38** **Malignant neoplasm of heart, mediastinum and pleura**
    EXCLUDES 1 *mesothelioma (C45.-)*

    C38.0 **Malignant neoplasm of heart** `CC`
        Malignant neoplasm of pericardium
        EXCLUDES 1 *malignant neoplasm of great vessels (C49.3)*
        CC Excl: C38.0, C45.2

    C38.1 **Malignant neoplasm of anterior mediastinum** `CC`
        CC Excl: C38.1-C38.3, C38.8, C39.9, C45.7-C45.9, C76.8, C7A.00,
        C7A.098-C7B.00, C7B.1, C80.0-C80.2, D49.1, D49.81-D49.9

    C38.2 **Malignant neoplasm of posterior mediastinum** `CC`
        CC Excl: See code: C38.1

    C38.3 **Malignant neoplasm of mediastinum, part unspecified** `CC`
        CC Excl: See code: C38.1

    C38.4 **Malignant neoplasm of pleura** `CC`
        CC Excl: C38.4-C39.9, C45.0, C45.7-C45.9, C76.8, C7A.00,
        C7A.098-C7B.00, C7B.1, C80.0-C80.2, D49.1, D49.81-D49.9

    C38.8 **Malignant neoplasm of overlapping sites of heart,
        mediastinum and pleura**
        CC Excl: See code: C38.1

✅4th **C39 Malignant neoplasm of other and ill-defined sites in the respiratory system and intrathoracic organs**

Use additional code to identify:
exposure to environmental tobacco smoke (Z77.22)
exposure to tobacco smoke in the perinatal period (P96.81)
history of tobacco use (Z87.891)
occupational exposure to environmental tobacco smoke (Z57.31)
tobacco dependence (F17.-)
tobacco use (Z72.0)

EXCLUDES 1   intrathoracic malignant neoplasm NOS (C76.1)
thoracic malignant neoplasm NOS (C76.1)

C39.0 Malignant neoplasm of upper respiratory tract, part unspecified

C39.9 Malignant neoplasm of lower respiratory tract, part unspecified

Malignant neoplasm of respiratory tract NOS

Malignant neoplasms of bone and articular cartilage (C40-C41)

INCLUDES   malignant neoplasm of cartilage (articular) (joint)
malignant neoplasm of periosteum

EXCLUDES 1   malignant neoplasm of bone marrow NOS (C96.9)
malignant neoplasm of synovia (C49.-)

✅4th **C40 Malignant neoplasm of bone and articular cartilage of limbs**

Use additional code to identify major osseous defect, if applicable (M89.7-)

✅5th **C40.0 Malignant neoplasm of scapula and long bones of upper limb**

CC Excl: For CC codes in subcategory C40.0, unless otherwise noted: C40.00-C40.02, C40.80, C40.92, C41.9, Z51.0

C40.00 Malignant neoplasm of scapula and long bones of unspecified upper limb `cc`

C40.01 Malignant neoplasm of scapula and long bones of right upper limb `cc`

C40.02 Malignant neoplasm of scapula and long bones of left upper limb `cc`

✅5th **C40.1 Malignant neoplasm of short bones of upper limb**

CC Excl: For CC codes in subcategory C40.1, unless otherwise noted: C40.10-C40.12, C40.80-C40.92, C41.9, Z51.0

C40.10 Malignant neoplasm of short bones of unspecified upper limb `cc`

C40.11 Malignant neoplasm of short bones of right upper limb `cc`

C40.12 Malignant neoplasm of short bones of left upper limb `cc`

✅5th **C40.2 Malignant neoplasm of long bones of lower limb**

CC Excl: For CC codes in subcategory C40.2, unless otherwise noted: C40.20-C40.22, C40.80-C40.92, C41.9, Z51.0

C40.20 Malignant neoplasm of long bones of unspecified lower limb `cc`

C40.21 Malignant neoplasm of long bones of right lower limb `cc`

C40.22 Malignant neoplasm of long bones of left lower limb `cc`

✅5th **C40.3 Malignant neoplasm of short bones of lower limb**

CC Excl: For CC codes in subcategory C40.3, unless otherwise noted: C40.30-C40.92, C41.9, Z51.0

C40.30 Malignant neoplasm of short bones of unspecified lower limb `cc`

C40.31 Malignant neoplasm of short bones of right lower limb `cc`

C40.32 Malignant neoplasm of short bones of left lower limb `cc`

✅5th **C40.8 Malignant neoplasm of overlapping sites of bone and articular cartilage of limb**

CC Excl: For CC codes in subcategory C40.8, unless otherwise noted: C40.00-C41.9, Z51.0

C40.80 Malignant neoplasm of overlapping sites of bone and articular cartilage of unspecified limb `cc`

C40.81 Malignant neoplasm of overlapping sites of bone and articular cartilage of right limb `cc`

C40.82 Malignant neoplasm of overlapping sites of bone and articular cartilage of left limb `cc`

✅5th **C40.9 Malignant neoplasm of unspecified bones and articular cartilage of limb**

CC Excl: For CC codes in subcategory C40.9, uless otherwise noted: C40.00-C41.9, Z51.0

C40.90 Malignant neoplasm of unspecified bones and articular cartilage of unspecified limb `cc`

C40.91 Malignant neoplasm of unspecified bones and articular cartilage of right limb `cc`

C40.92 Malignant neoplasm of unspecified bones and articular cartilage of left limb `cc`

✅4th **C41 Malignant neoplasm of bone and articular cartilage of other and unspecified sites**

EXCLUDES 1   malignant neoplasm of bones of limbs (C40.-)
malignant neoplasm of cartilage of ear (C49.0)
malignant neoplasm of cartilage of eyelid (C49.0)
malignant neoplasm of cartilage of larynx (C32.3)
malignant neoplasm of cartilage of limbs (C40.-)
malignant neoplasm of cartilage of nose (C30.0)

C41.0 Malignant neoplasm of bones of skull and face `cc`

Malignant neoplasm of maxilla (superior)
Malignant neoplasm of orbital bone

EXCLUDES 2   carcinoma, any type except intraosseous or odontogenic of:
maxillary sinus (C31.0)
upper jaw (C03.0)
malignant neoplasm of jaw bone (lower) (C41.1)

CC Excl: C40.80-C41.0, C41.9, Z51.0

C41.1 Malignant neoplasm of mandible `cc`

Malignant neoplasm of inferior maxilla
Malignant neoplasm of lower jaw bone

EXCLUDES 2   carcinoma, any type except intraosseous or odontogenic of:
jaw NOS (C03.9)
lower (C03.1)
malignant neoplasm of upper jaw bone (C41.0)

CC Excl: C40.80-C40.92, C41.1, C41.9, Z51.0

C41.2 Malignant neoplasm of vertebral column `cc`

EXCLUDES 1   malignant neoplasm of sacrum and coccyx (C41.4)

CC Excl: C40.80-C40.92, C41.2, C41.9, Z51.0

C41.3 Malignant neoplasm of ribs, sternum and clavicle `cc`

CC Excl: C40.80-C40.92, C41.3, C41.9, Z51.0

C41.4 Malignant neoplasm of pelvic bones, sacrum and coccyx `cc`

CC Excl: C40.80-C40.92, C41.4-C41.9, Z51.0

C41.9 Malignant neoplasm of bone and articular cartilage, unspecified `cc`

CC Excl: C40.00-C41.9, Z51.0

Melanoma and other malignant neoplasms of skin (C43-C44)

✅4th **C43 Malignant melanoma of skin**

EXCLUDES 1   melanoma in situ (D03.-)

EXCLUDES 2   malignant melanoma of skin of genital organs (C51-C52, C60.-, C63.-)
Merkel cell carcinoma (C4A.-)
sites other than skin—code to malignant neoplasm of the site

C43.0 Malignant melanoma of lip

EXCLUDES 1   malignant neoplasm of vermilion border of lip (C00.0-C00.2)

✅5th **C43.1 Malignant melanoma of eyelid, including canthus**

C43.10 Malignant melanoma of unspecified eyelid, including canthus

C43.11 Malignant melanoma of right eyelid, including canthus

C43.12 Malignant melanoma of left eyelid, including canthus

✅5th **C43.2 Malignant melanoma of ear and external auricular canal**

C43.20 Malignant melanoma of unspecified ear and external auricular canal

C43.21 Malignant melanoma of right ear and external auricular canal

C43.22 Malignant melanoma of left ear and external auricular canal

✅5th **C43.3 Malignant melanoma of other and unspecified parts of face**

C43.30 Malignant melanoma of unspecified part of face

C43.31 Malignant melanoma of nose

C43.39 Malignant melanoma of other parts of face

C43.4 Malignant melanoma of scalp and neck

✅ Additional Character Required   ✅7th Xtension Alert   Unacceptable PDx   Manifestation   Hospital Acquired Condition   EXCLUDES 1 Not Coded Here   EXCLUDES 2 Not Included Here

Neoplasms

C43.5–C44.222

✓5ᵗʰ **C43.5 Malignant melanoma of** trunk
> EXCLUDES 2   *malignant neoplasm of anus NOS (C21.0)*
> *malignant neoplasm of scrotum (C63.2)*

     C43.51 Malignant melanoma of anal skin
> Malignant melanoma of anal margin
> Malignant melanoma of perianal skin

     C43.52 Malignant melanoma of skin of breast

     C43.59 Malignant melanoma of other part of trunk

✓5ᵗʰ **C43.6 Malignant melanoma of** upper limb, including shoulder

     C43.60 Malignant melanoma of unspecified upper limb, including shoulder

     C43.61 Malignant melanoma of right upper limb, including shoulder

     C43.62 Malignant melanoma of left upper limb, including shoulder

✓5ᵗʰ **C43.7 Malignant melanoma of** lower limb, including hip

     C43.70 Malignant melanoma of unspecified lower limb, including hip

     C43.71 Malignant melanoma of right lower limb, including hip

     C43.72 Malignant melanoma of left lower limb, including hip

     C43.8 Malignant melanoma of overlapping sites of skin

     C43.9 Malignant melanoma of skin, unspecified
> Malignant melanoma of unspecified site of skin

✓4ᵗʰ **C4A Merkel cell carcinoma**

     C4A.0 Merkel cell carcinoma of lip
> EXCLUDES 1   *malignant neoplasm of vermilion border of lip (C00.0-C00.2)*

✓5ᵗʰ **C4A.1 Merkel cell carcinoma of** eyelid, including canthus

     C4A.10 Merkel cell carcinoma of unspecified eyelid, including canthus

     C4A.11 Merkel cell carcinoma of right eyelid, including canthus

     C4A.12 Merkel cell carcinoma of left eyelid, including canthus

✓5ᵗʰ **C4A.2 Merkel cell carcinoma of** ear and external auricular canal

     C4A.20 Merkel cell carcinoma of unspecified ear and external auricular canal

     C4A.21 Merkel cell carcinoma of right ear and external auricular canal

     C4A.22 Merkel cell carcinoma of left ear and external auricular canal

✓5ᵗʰ **C4A.3 Merkel cell carcinoma of** other and unspecified parts of face

     C4A.30 Merkel cell carcinoma of unspecified part of face

     C4A.31 Merkel cell carcinoma of nose

     C4A.39 Merkel cell carcinoma of other parts of face

     C4A.4 Merkel cell carcinoma of scalp and neck

✓5ᵗʰ **C4A.5 Merkel cell carcinoma of** trunk
> EXCLUDES 2   *malignant neoplasm of anus NOS (C21.0)*
> *malignant neoplasm of scrotum (C63.2)*

     C4A.51 Merkel cell carcinoma of anal skin
> Merkel cell carcinoma of anal margin
> Merkel cell carcinoma of perianal skin

     C4A.52 Merkel cell carcinoma of skin of breast

     C4A.59 Merkel cell carcinoma of other part of trunk

✓5ᵗʰ **C4A.6 Merkel cell carcinoma of** upper limb, including shoulder

     C4A.60 Merkel cell carcinoma of unspecified upper limb, including shoulder

     C4A.61 Merkel cell carcinoma of right upper limb, including shoulder

     C4A.62 Merkel cell carcinoma of left upper limb, including shoulder

✓5ᵗʰ **C4A.7 Merkel cell carcinoma of** lower limb, including hip

     C4A.70 Merkel cell carcinoma of unspecified lower limb, including hip

     C4A.71 Merkel cell carcinoma of right lower limb, including hip

     C4A.72 Merkel cell carcinoma of left lower limb, including hip

     C4A.8 Merkel cell carcinoma of overlapping sites

     C4A.9 Merkel cell carcinoma, unspecified
> Merkel cell carcinoma of unspecified site

✓4ᵗʰ **C44 Other and unspecified malignant neoplasm of skin**
> INCLUDES   malignant neoplasm of sebaceous glands
> malignant neoplasm of sweat glands
> EXCLUDES 1   *Kaposi's sarcoma of skin (C46.0)*
> *malignant melanoma of skin (C43.-)*
> *malignant neoplasm of skin of genital organs (C51-C52, C60-, C63.2)*
> *Merkel cell carcinoma (C4A.-)*

✓5ᵗʰ **C44.0 Other and unspecified malignant neoplasm of skin of** lip
> EXCLUDES 1   *malignant neoplasm of lip (C00.-)*

     C44.00 Unspecified malignant neoplasm of skin of lip

     C44.01 Basal cell carcinoma of skin of lip

     C44.02 Squamous cell carcinoma of skin of lip

     C44.09 Other specified malignant neoplasm of skin of lip

✓5ᵗʰ **C44.1 Other and unspecified malignant neoplasm of skin of** eyelid, including canthus
> EXCLUDES 1   *connective tissue of eyelid (C49.0)*

✓6ᵗʰ **C44.10 Unspecified** malignant neoplasm of skin of eyelid, including canthus

     C44.101 Unspecified malignant neoplasm of skin of unspecified eyelid, including canthus

     C44.102 Unspecified malignant neoplasm of skin of right eyelid, including canthus

     C44.109 Unspecified malignant neoplasm of skin of left eyelid, including canthus

✓6ᵗʰ **C44.11 Basal cell carcinoma** of skin of eyelid, including canthus

     C44.111 Basal cell carcinoma of skin of unspecified eyelid, including canthus

     C44.112 Basal cell carcinoma of skin of right eyelid, including canthus

     C44.119 Basal cell carcinoma of skin of left eyelid, including canthus

✓6ᵗʰ **C44.12 Squamous cell carcinoma** of skin of eyelid, including canthus

     C44.121 Squamous cell carcinoma of skin of unspecified eyelid, including canthus

     C44.122 Squamous cell carcinoma of skin of right eyelid, including canthus

     C44.129 Squamous cell carcinoma of skin of left eyelid, including canthus

✓6ᵗʰ **C44.19 Other** specified malignant neoplasm of skin of eyelid, including canthus

     C44.191 Other specified malignant neoplasm of skin of unspecified eyelid, including canthus

     C44.192 Other specified malignant neoplasm of skin of right eyelid, including canthus

     C44.199 Other specified malignant neoplasm of skin of left eyelid, including canthus

✓5ᵗʰ **C44.2 Other and unspecified malignant neoplasm of** skin of ear and external auricular canal
> EXCLUDES 1   *connective tissue of ear (C49.0)*

✓6ᵗʰ **C44.20 Unspecified** malignant neoplasm of skin of ear and external auricular canal

     C44.201 Unspecified malignant neoplasm of skin of unspecified ear and external auricular canal

     C44.202 Unspecified malignant neoplasm of skin of right ear and external auricular canal

     C44.209 Unspecified malignant neoplasm of skin of left ear and external auricular canal

✓6ᵗʰ **C44.21 Basal cell carcinoma** of skin of ear and external auricular canal

     C44.211 Basal cell carcinoma of skin of unspecified ear and external auricular canal

     C44.212 Basal cell carcinoma of skin of right ear and external auricular canal

     C44.219 Basal cell carcinoma of skin of left ear and external auricular canal

✓6ᵗʰ **C44.22 Squamous cell carcinoma** of skin of ear and external auricular canal

     C44.221 Squamous cell carcinoma of skin of unspecified ear and external auricular canal

     C44.222 Squamous cell carcinoma of skin of right ear and external auricular canal

---

N Newborn: 0   P Pediatric: 0-17   M Maternity: 12-55   A Adult: 15-124   MCC Major CC Condition   PDx MCC PDx acts as own MCC   CC CC Condition   PDx CC PDx acts as own CC

454   ICD-10-CM Draft (2015)

C44.229 Squamous cell carcinoma of skin of left ear and external auricular canal

✓6ᵗʰ C44.29 Other specified malignant neoplasm of skin of ear and external auricular canal

C44.291 Other specified malignant neoplasm of skin of unspecified ear and external auricular canal

C44.292 Other specified malignant neoplasm of skin of right ear and external auricular canal

C44.299 Other specified malignant neoplasm of skin of left ear and external auricular canal

✓5ᵗʰ C44.3 Other and unspecified malignant neoplasm of skin of other and unspecified parts of face

✓6ᵗʰ C44.30 Unspecified malignant neoplasm of skin of other and unspecified parts of face

C44.300 Unspecified malignant neoplasm of skin of unspecified part of face

C44.301 Unspecified malignant neoplasm of skin of nose

C44.309 Unspecified malignant neoplasm of skin of other parts of face

✓6ᵗʰ C44.31 Basal cell carcinoma of skin of other and unspecified parts of face

C44.310 Basal cell carcinoma of skin of unspecified parts of face

C44.311 Basal cell carcinoma of skin of nose

C44.319 Basal cell carcinoma of skin of other parts of face

✓6ᵗʰ C44.32 Squamous cell carcinoma of skin of other and unspecified parts of face

C44.320 Squamous cell carcinoma of skin of unspecified parts of face

C44.321 Squamous cell carcinoma of skin of nose

C44.329 Squamous cell carcinoma of skin of other parts of face

✓6ᵗʰ C44.39 Other specified malignant neoplasm of skin of other and unspecified parts of face

C44.390 Other specified malignant neoplasm of skin of unspecified parts of face

C44.391 Other specified malignant neoplasm of skin of nose

C44.399 Other specified malignant neoplasm of skin of other parts of face

✓5ᵗʰ C44.4 Other and unspecified malignant neoplasm of skin of scalp and neck

C44.40 Unspecified malignant neoplasm of skin of scalp and neck

C44.41 Basal cell carcinoma of skin of scalp and neck

C44.42 Squamous cell carcinoma of skin of scalp and neck

C44.49 Other specified malignant neoplasm of skin of scalp and neck

✓5ᵗʰ C44.5 Other and unspecified malignant neoplasm of skin of trunk

EXCLUDES 1   anus NOS (C21.0)
scrotum (C63.2)

✓6ᵗʰ C44.50 Unspecified malignant neoplasm of skin of trunk

C44.500 Unspecified malignant neoplasm of anal skin
Unspecified malignant neoplasm of anal margin
Unspecified malignant neoplasm of perianal skin

C44.501 Unspecified malignant neoplasm of skin of breast

C44.509 Unspecified malignant neoplasm of skin of other part of trunk

✓6ᵗʰ C44.51 Basal cell carcinoma of skin of trunk

C44.510 Basal cell carcinoma of anal skin
Basal cell carcinoma of anal margin
Basal cell carcinoma of perianal skin

C44.511 Basal cell carcinoma of skin of breast

C44.519 Basal cell carcinoma of skin of other part of trunk

✓6ᵗʰ C44.52 Squamous cell carcinoma of skin of trunk

C44.520 Squamous cell carcinoma of anal skin
Squamous cell carcinoma of anal margin
Squamous cell carcinoma of perianal skin

C44.521 Squamous cell carcinoma of skin of breast

C44.529 Squamous cell carcinoma of skin of other part of trunk

✓6ᵗʰ C44.59 Other specified malignant neoplasm of skin of trunk

C44.590 Other specified malignant neoplasm of anal skin
Other specified malignant neoplasm of anal margin
Other specified malignant neoplasm of perianal skin

C44.591 Other specified malignant neoplasm of skin of breast

C44.599 Other specified malignant neoplasm of skin of other part of trunk

✓5ᵗʰ C44.6 Other and unspecified malignant neoplasm of skin of upper limb, including shoulder

✓6ᵗʰ C44.60 Unspecified malignant neoplasm of skin of upper limb, including shoulder

C44.601 Unspecified malignant neoplasm of skin of unspecified upper limb, including shoulder

C44.602 Unspecified malignant neoplasm of skin of right upper limb, including shoulder

C44.609 Unspecified malignant neoplasm of skin of left upper limb, including shoulder

✓6ᵗʰ C44.61 Basal cell carcinoma of skin of upper limb, including shoulder

C44.611 Basal cell carcinoma of skin of unspecified upper limb, including shoulder

C44.612 Basal cell carcinoma of skin of right upper limb, including shoulder

C44.619 Basal cell carcinoma of skin of left upper limb, including shoulder

✓6ᵗʰ C44.62 Squamous cell carcinoma of skin of upper limb, including shoulder

C44.621 Squamous cell carcinoma of skin of unspecified upper limb, including shoulder

C44.622 Squamous cell carcinoma of skin of right upper limb, including shoulder

C44.629 Squamous cell carcinoma of skin of left upper limb, including shoulder

✓6ᵗʰ C44.69 Other specified malignant neoplasm of skin of upper limb, including shoulder

C44.691 Other specified malignant neoplasm of skin of unspecified upper limb, including shoulder

C44.692 Other specified malignant neoplasm of skin of right upper limb, including shoulder

C44.699 Other specified malignant neoplasm of skin of left upper limb, including shoulder

✓5ᵗʰ C44.7 Other and unspecified malignant neoplasm of skin of lower limb, including hip

✓6ᵗʰ C44.70 Unspecified malignant neoplasm of skin of lower limb, including hip

C44.701 Unspecified malignant neoplasm of skin of unspecified lower limb, including hip

C44.702 Unspecified malignant neoplasm of skin of right lower limb, including hip

C44.709 Unspecified malignant neoplasm of skin of left lower limb, including hip

✓6ᵗʰ C44.71 Basal cell carcinoma of skin of lower limb, including hip

C44.711 Basal cell carcinoma of skin of unspecified lower limb, including hip

C44.712 Basal cell carcinoma of skin of right lower limb, including hip

C44.719 Basal cell carcinoma of skin of left lower limb, including hip

✓6ᵗʰ C44.72 Squamous cell carcinoma of skin of lower limb, including hip

C44.721 Squamous cell carcinoma of skin of unspecified lower limb, including hip

C44.722 Squamous cell carcinoma of skin of right lower limb, including hip

C44.729 Squamous cell carcinoma of skin of left lower limb, including hip

☑6ᵗʰ **C44.79** Other specified malignant neoplasm of skin of lower limb, including hip

    C44.791 Other specified malignant neoplasm of skin of unspecified lower limb, including hip

    C44.792 Other specified malignant neoplasm of skin of right lower limb, including hip

    C44.799 Other specified malignant neoplasm of skin of left lower limb, including hip

☑5ᵗʰ **C44.8** Other and unspecified malignant neoplasm of overlapping sites of skin

    C44.80 Unspecified malignant neoplasm of overlapping sites of skin

    C44.81 Basal cell carcinoma of overlapping sites of skin

    C44.82 Squamous cell carcinoma of overlapping sites of skin

    C44.89 Other specified malignant neoplasm of overlapping sites of skin

☑5ᵗʰ **C44.9** Other and unspecified malignant neoplasm of skin, unspecified

    C44.90 Unspecified malignant neoplasm of skin, unspecified

        Malignant neoplasm of unspecified site of skin

    C44.91 Basal cell carcinoma of skin, unspecified

    C44.92 Squamous cell carcinoma of skin, unspecified

    C44.99 Other specified malignant neoplasm of skin, unspecified

Malignant neoplasms of mesothelial and soft tissue (C45-C49)

☑4ᵗʰ **C45** **Mesothelioma**

    C45.0 **Mesothelioma of pleura** `CC`

        EXCLUDES 1   other malignant neoplasm of pleura (C38.4)

        CC Excl: C38.4, C39.9, C45.0, C45.7-C45.9, C76.8, C7A.0, C7A.098-C7B.00, C7B.1, C80.0-C80.2, D49.1, D49.81-D49.9

    C45.1 **Mesothelioma of peritoneum** `CC`

        Mesothelioma of cul-de-sac

        Mesothelioma of mesentery

        Mesothelioma of mesocolon

        Mesothelioma of omentum

        Mesothelioma of peritoneum (parietal) (pelvic)

        EXCLUDES 1   other malignant neoplasm of soft tissue of peritoneum (C48.-)

        CC Excl: C45.1, C48.0-C48.8, Z51.0

    C45.2 **Mesothelioma of pericardium** `CC`

        EXCLUDES 1   other malignant neoplasm of pericardium (C38.0)

        CC Excl: C38.0, C45.2

    C45.7 **Mesothelioma of other sites**

    C45.9 **Mesothelioma, unspecified**

☑4ᵗʰ **C46** **Kaposi's sarcoma**

    Code first any human immunodeficiency virus [HIV] disease (B20)

    C46.0 **Kaposi's sarcoma of skin** `HIV` `CC`

        CC Excl: C46.0, C46.7-C46.9, Z51.0

    C46.1 **Kaposi's sarcoma of soft tissue** `HIV` `CC`

        Kaposi's sarcoma of blood vessel

        Kaposi's sarcoma of connective tissue

        Kaposi's sarcoma of fascia

        Kaposi's sarcoma of ligament

        Kaposi's sarcoma of lymphatic(s) NEC

        Kaposi's sarcoma of muscle

        EXCLUDES 2   Kaposi's sarcoma of lymph glands and nodes (C46.3)

        CC Excl: C46.1, C46.7-C46.9, Z51.0

    C46.2 **Kaposi's sarcoma of palate** `HIV` `CC`

        CC Excl: C46.2, C46.7-C46.9, Z51.0

    C46.3 **Kaposi's sarcoma of lymph nodes** `HIV` `CC`

        CC Excl: C45.7-C45.9, C46.3, C76.8-C77.9, C7A.00, C7A.098-C7B.01, C7B.1, C80.0-C80.2, D49.81-D49.9

    C46.4 **Kaposi's sarcoma of gastrointestinal sites** `HIV` `CC`

        CC Excl: C46.4, C46.7-C46.9, Z51.0

☑5ᵗʰ **C46.5** **Kaposi's sarcoma of lung**

        CC Excl: For CC codes in subcategory C46.5, unless otherwise noted: C34.80-C34.92, C39.9, C45.7-C45.9, C46.50-C46.52, C76.8, C7A.00, C7A.090, C7A.098-C7B.00, C7B.1, C80.0-C80.2, D49.1, D49.81-D49.9

    C46.50 **Kaposi's sarcoma of unspecified lung** `HIV` `CC`

    C46.51 **Kaposi's sarcoma of right lung** `HIV` `CC`

    C46.52 **Kaposi's sarcoma of left lung** `HIV` `CC`

C46.7 **Kaposi's sarcoma of other sites** `HIV` `CC`

    CC Excl: See code: C46.0

C46.9 **Kaposi's sarcoma, unspecified** `HIV` `CC`

    Kaposi's sarcoma of unspecified site

    CC Excl: C45.7-C46.9, C51.0-C55, C56.1-C63.9, C64.1-C64.9, C65.1-C65.9, C66.1-C72.9, C76.0-C76.52, C76.8-C7A.00, C7A.093, C7A.098-C80.2, D00.00-D02.4, D04.0-D05.02, D05.10-D05.12, D05.80-D05.92, D06.0-D09.3, D09.8-D09.9, D37.01-D37.6, D37.8-D39.2, D39.8-D39.9, D40.0-D40.12, D40.8-D41.4, D41.8-D43.4, D43.8-D44.7, D44.9, D48.0-D48.62, D48.7-D49.9, Z51.0

☑4ᵗʰ **C47** **Malignant neoplasm of peripheral nerves and autonomic nervous system**

    INCLUDES   malignant neoplasm of sympathetic and parasympathetic nerves and ganglia

    EXCLUDES 1   Kaposi's sarcoma of soft tissue (C46.1)

    CC Excl: For CC codes in category C47, unless otherwise noted: Z51.0

    C47.0 **Malignant neoplasm of peripheral nerves of head, face and neck** `CC`

        EXCLUDES 1   malignant neoplasm of peripheral nerves of orbit (C69.6-)

☑5ᵗʰ **C47.1** **Malignant neoplasm of peripheral nerves of upper limb, including shoulder**

    C47.10 **Malignant neoplasm of peripheral nerves of unspecified upper limb, including shoulder** `CC`

    C47.11 **Malignant neoplasm of peripheral nerves of right upper limb, including shoulder** `CC`

    C47.12 **Malignant neoplasm of peripheral nerves of left upper limb, including shoulder** `CC`

☑5ᵗʰ **C47.2** **Malignant neoplasm of peripheral nerves of lower limb, including hip**

    C47.20 **Malignant neoplasm of peripheral nerves of unspecified lower limb, including hip** `CC`

    C47.21 **Malignant neoplasm of peripheral nerves of right lower limb, including hip** `CC`

    C47.22 **Malignant neoplasm of peripheral nerves of left lower limb, including hip** `CC`

    C47.3 **Malignant neoplasm of peripheral nerves of thorax** `CC`

    C47.4 **Malignant neoplasm of peripheral nerves of abdomen** `CC`

    C47.5 **Malignant neoplasm of peripheral nerves of pelvis** `CC`

    C47.6 **Malignant neoplasm of peripheral nerves of trunk, unspecified** `CC`

        Malignant neoplasm of peripheral nerves of unspecified part of trunk

    C47.8 **Malignant neoplasm of overlapping sites of peripheral nerves and autonomic nervous system** `CC`

    C47.9 **Malignant neoplasm of peripheral nerves and autonomic nervous system, unspecified** `CC`

        Malignant neoplasm of unspecified site of peripheral nerves and autonomic nervous system

☑4ᵗʰ **C48** **Malignant neoplasm of retroperitoneum and peritoneum**

    EXCLUDES 1   Kaposi's sarcoma of connective tissue (C46.1)

                 mesothelioma (C45.-)

    C48.0 **Malignant neoplasm of retroperitoneum** `CC`

        CC Excl: C48.0-Z51.0

    C48.1 **Malignant neoplasm of specified parts of peritoneum** `CC`

        Malignant neoplasm of cul-de-sac

        Malignant neoplasm of mesentery

        Malignant neoplasm of mesocolon

        Malignant neoplasm of omentum

        Malignant neoplasm of parietal peritoneum

        Malignant neoplasm of pelvic peritoneum

        CC Excl: C45.1, C48.0-C48.8, Z51.0

    C48.2 **Malignant neoplasm of peritoneum, unspecified** `CC`

        CC Excl: See code: C48.1

    C48.8 **Malignant neoplasm of overlapping sites of retroperitoneum and peritoneum** `CC`

        CC Excl: See code: C48.1

N Newborn: 0   P Pediatric: 0-17   M Maternity: 12-55   A Adult: 15-124   MCC Major CC Condition   PDx MCC PDx acts as own MCC   CC CC Condition   PDx CC PDx acts as own CC

456   ICD-10-CM Draft (2015)

✅4ᵗʰ **C49 Malignant neoplasm of other connective and soft tissue**

INCLUDES
malignant neoplasm of blood vessel
malignant neoplasm of bursa
malignant neoplasm of cartilage
malignant neoplasm of fascia
malignant neoplasm of fat
malignant neoplasm of ligament, except uterine
malignant neoplasm of lymphatic vessel
malignant neoplasm of muscle
malignant neoplasm of synovia
malignant neoplasm of tendon (sheath)

EXCLUDES 1　malignant neoplasm of cartilage (of):
　articular (C40-C41)
　larynx (C32.3)
　nose (C30.0)
malignant neoplasm of connective tissue of breast (C50.-)

EXCLUDES 2　Kaposi's sarcoma of soft tissue (C46.1)
malignant neoplasm of heart (C38.0)
malignant neoplasm of peripheral nerves and autonomic
　nervous system (C47.-)
malignant neoplasm of peritoneum (C48.2)
malignant neoplasm of retroperitoneum (C48.0)
malignant neoplasm of uterine ligament (C57.3)
mesothelioma (C45.-)

CC Excl: For CC codes in category C49, unless otherwise noted: Z51.0

C49.0 Malignant neoplasm of connective and soft tissue of head, face and neck CC
Malignant neoplasm of connective tissue of ear
Malignant neoplasm of connective tissue of eyelid
EXCLUDES 1　connective tissue of orbit (C69.6-)

✅5ᵗʰ **C49.1 Malignant neoplasm of connective and soft tissue of upper limb, including shoulder**

　C49.10 Malignant neoplasm of connective and soft tissue of unspecified upper limb, including shoulder CC

　C49.11 Malignant neoplasm of connective and soft tissue of right upper limb, including shoulder CC

　C49.12 Malignant neoplasm of connective and soft tissue of left upper limb, including shoulder CC

✅5ᵗʰ **C49.2 Malignant neoplasm of connective and soft tissue of lower limb, including hip**

　C49.20 Malignant neoplasm of connective and soft tissue of unspecified lower limb, including hip CC

　C49.21 Malignant neoplasm of connective and soft tissue of right lower limb, including hip CC

　C49.22 Malignant neoplasm of connective and soft tissue of left lower limb, including hip CC

C49.3 Malignant neoplasm of connective and soft tissue of thorax CC
Malignant neoplasm of axilla
Malignant neoplasm of diaphragm
Malignant neoplasm of great vessels
EXCLUDES 1　malignant neoplasm of breast (C50.-)
malignant neoplasm of heart (C38.0)
malignant neoplasm of mediastinum (C38.1-C38.3)
malignant neoplasm of thymus (C37)

C49.4 Malignant neoplasm of connective and soft tissue of abdomen CC
Malignant neoplasm of abdominal wall
Malignant neoplasm of hypochondrium

C49.5 Malignant neoplasm of connective and soft tissue of pelvis CC
Malignant neoplasm of buttock
Malignant neoplasm of groin
Malignant neoplasm of perineum

C49.6 Malignant neoplasm of connective and soft tissue of trunk, unspecified CC
Malignant neoplasm of back NOS

C49.8 Malignant neoplasm of overlapping sites of connective and soft tissue CC
Primary malignant neoplasm of two or more contiguous sites of connective and soft tissue

C49.9 Malignant neoplasm of connective and soft tissue, unspecified CC

Malignant neoplasms of breast (C50)

✅4ᵗʰ **C50 Malignant neoplasm of breast**
INCLUDES　connective tissue of breast
Paget's disease of breast
Paget's disease of nipple
Use additional code to identify estrogen receptor status (Z17.0, Z17.1)
EXCLUDES 1　skin of breast (C44.501, C44.511, C44.521, C44.591)

✅5ᵗʰ **C50.0 Malignant neoplasm of nipple and areola**

✅6ᵗʰ **C50.01 Malignant neoplasm of nipple and areola, female**

　C50.011 Malignant neoplasm of nipple and areola, right female breast ♀

　C50.012 Malignant neoplasm of nipple and areola, left female breast ♀

　C50.019 Malignant neoplasm of nipple and areola, unspecified female breast ♀

✅6ᵗʰ **C50.02 Malignant neoplasm of nipple and areola, male**

　C50.021 Malignant neoplasm of nipple and areola, right male breast ♂

　C50.022 Malignant neoplasm of nipple and areola, left male breast ♂

　C50.029 Malignant neoplasm of nipple and areola, unspecified male breast ♂

✅5ᵗʰ **C50.1 Malignant neoplasm of central portion of breast**

✅6ᵗʰ **C50.11 Malignant neoplasm of central portion of breast, female**

　C50.111 Malignant neoplasm of central portion of right female breast ♀

　C50.112 Malignant neoplasm of central portion of left female breast ♀

　C50.119 Malignant neoplasm of central portion of unspecified female breast ♀

✅6ᵗʰ **C50.12 Malignant neoplasm of central portion of breast, male**

　C50.121 Malignant neoplasm of central portion of right male breast ♂

　C50.122 Malignant neoplasm of central portion of left male breast ♂

　C50.129 Malignant neoplasm of central portion of unspecified male breast ♂

✅5ᵗʰ **C50.2 Malignant neoplasm of upper-inner quadrant of breast**

✅6ᵗʰ **C50.21 Malignant neoplasm of upper-inner quadrant of breast, female**

　C50.211 Malignant neoplasm of upper-inner quadrant of right female breast ♀

　C50.212 Malignant neoplasm of upper-inner quadrant of left female breast ♀

　C50.219 Malignant neoplasm of upper-inner quadrant of unspecified female breast ♀

✅6ᵗʰ **C50.22 Malignant neoplasm of upper-inner quadrant of breast, male**

　C50.221 Malignant neoplasm of upper-inner quadrant of right male breast ♂

　C50.222 Malignant neoplasm of upper-inner quadrant of left male breast ♂

　C50.229 Malignant neoplasm of upper-inner quadrant of unspecified male breast ♂

✅5ᵗʰ **C50.3 Malignant neoplasm of lower-inner quadrant of breast**

✅6ᵗʰ **C50.31 Malignant neoplasm of lower-inner quadrant of breast, female**

　C50.311 Malignant neoplasm of lower-inner quadrant of right female breast ♀

　C50.312 Malignant neoplasm of lower-inner quadrant of left female breast ♀

　C50.319 Malignant neoplasm of lower-inner quadrant of unspecified female breast ♀

✅6ᵗʰ **C50.32 Malignant neoplasm of lower-inner quadrant of breast, male**

　C50.321 Malignant neoplasm of lower-inner quadrant of right male breast ♂

　C50.322 Malignant neoplasm of lower-inner quadrant of left male breast ♂

　C50.329 Malignant neoplasm of lower-inner quadrant of unspecified male breast ♂

Neoplasms

C50.4–C57.7

√5ᵗʰ **C50.4 Malignant neoplasm of** upper-outer quadrant **of breast**

√6ᵗʰ **C50.41 Malignant neoplasm of upper-outer quadrant of breast,** female

C50.411 **Malignant neoplasm of upper-outer quadrant of** right **female breast** ♀

C50.412 **Malignant neoplasm of upper-outer quadrant of** left **female breast** ♀

C50.419 **Malignant neoplasm of upper-outer quadrant of** unspecified **female breast** ♀

√6ᵗʰ **C50.42 Malignant neoplasm of upper-outer quadrant of breast,** male

C50.421 **Malignant neoplasm of upper-outer quadrant of** right **male breast** ♂

C50.422 **Malignant neoplasm of upper-outer quadrant of** left **male breast** ♂

C50.429 **Malignant neoplasm of upper-outer quadrant of** unspecified **male breast** ♂

√5ᵗʰ **C50.5 Malignant neoplasm of** lower-outer quadrant **of breast**

√6ᵗʰ **C50.51 Malignant neoplasm of lower-outer quadrant of breast,** female

C50.511 **Malignant neoplasm of lower-outer quadrant of** right **female breast** ♀

C50.512 **Malignant neoplasm of lower-outer quadrant of** left **female breast** ♀

C50.519 **Malignant neoplasm of lower-outer quadrant of** unspecified **female breast** ♀

√6ᵗʰ **C50.52 Malignant neoplasm of lower-outer quadrant of breast,** male

C50.521 **Malignant neoplasm of lower-outer quadrant of** right **male breast** ♂

C50.522 **Malignant neoplasm of lower-outer quadrant of** left **male breast** ♂

C50.529 **Malignant neoplasm of lower-outer quadrant of** unspecified **male breast** ♂

√5ᵗʰ **C50.6 Malignant neoplasm of** axillary tail **of breast**

√6ᵗʰ **C50.61 Malignant neoplasm of axillary tail of breast,** female

C50.611 **Malignant neoplasm of axillary tail of** right **female breast** ♀

C50.612 **Malignant neoplasm of axillary tail of** left **female breast** ♀

C50.619 **Malignant neoplasm of axillary tail of** unspecified **female breast** ♀

√6ᵗʰ **C50.62 Malignant neoplasm of axillary tail of breast,** male

C50.621 **Malignant neoplasm of axillary tail of** right **male breast** ♂

C50.622 **Malignant neoplasm of axillary tail of** left **male breast** ♂

C50.629 **Malignant neoplasm of axillary tail of** unspecified **male breast** ♂

√5ᵗʰ **C50.8 Malignant neoplasm of** overlapping sites **of breast**

√6ᵗʰ **C50.81 Malignant neoplasm of overlapping sites of breast,** female

C50.811 **Malignant neoplasm of overlapping sites of** right **female breast** ♀

C50.812 **Malignant neoplasm of overlapping sites of** left **female breast** ♀

C50.819 **Malignant neoplasm of overlapping sites of** unspecified **female breast** ♀

√6ᵗʰ **C50.82 Malignant neoplasm of overlapping sites of breast,** male

C50.821 **Malignant neoplasm of overlapping sites of** right **male breast** ♂

C50.822 **Malignant neoplasm of overlapping sites of** left **male breast** ♂

C50.829 **Malignant neoplasm of overlapping sites of** unspecified **male breast** ♂

√5ᵗʰ **C50.9 Malignant neoplasm of breast of** unspecified site

√6ᵗʰ **C50.91 Malignant neoplasm of breast of unspecified site,** female

C50.911 **Malignant neoplasm of unspecified site of** right **female breast** ♀

C50.912 **Malignant neoplasm of unspecified site of** left **female breast** ♀

C50.919 **Malignant neoplasm of unspecified site of** unspecified **female breast** ♀

√6ᵗʰ **C50.92 Malignant neoplasm of breast of unspecified site,** male

C50.921 **Malignant neoplasm of unspecified site of** right **male breast** ♂

C50.922 **Malignant neoplasm of unspecified site of** left **male breast** ♂

C50.929 **Malignant neoplasm of unspecified site of** unspecified **male breast** ♂

Malignant neoplasms of female genital organs (C51-C58)

INCLUDES malignant neoplasm of skin of female genital organs

√4ᵗʰ **C51 Malignant neoplasm of** vulva

EXCLUDES 1 carcinoma in situ of vulva (D07.1)

C51.0 **Malignant neoplasm of** labium majus ♀
Malignant neoplasm of Bartholin's [greater vestibular] gland

C51.1 **Malignant neoplasm of** labium minus ♀

C51.2 **Malignant neoplasm of** clitoris ♀

C51.8 **Malignant neoplasm of** overlapping sites **of vulva** ♀

C51.9 **Malignant neoplasm of vulva,** unspecified ♀
Malignant neoplasm of external female genitalia NOS
Malignant neoplasm of pudendum

C52 Malignant neoplasm of vagina ♀
EXCLUDES 1 carcinoma in situ of vagina (D07.2)

√4ᵗʰ **C53 Malignant neoplasm of** cervix uteri
EXCLUDES 1 carcinoma in situ of cervix uteri (D06.-)

C53.0 **Malignant neoplasm of** endocervix ♀

C53.1 **Malignant neoplasm of** exocervix ♀

C53.8 **Malignant neoplasm of** overlapping sites **of cervix uteri** ♀

C53.9 **Malignant neoplasm of cervix uteri,** unspecified ♀

√4ᵗʰ **C54 Malignant neoplasm of** corpus uteri

C54.0 **Malignant neoplasm of** isthmus uteri ♀
Malignant neoplasm of lower uterine segment

C54.1 **Malignant neoplasm of** endometrium ♀

C54.2 **Malignant neoplasm of** myometrium ♀

C54.3 **Malignant neoplasm of** fundus uteri ♀

C54.8 **Malignant neoplasm of** overlapping sites **of corpus uteri** ♀

C54.9 **Malignant neoplasm of corpus uteri,** unspecified ♀

C55 Malignant neoplasm of uterus, part unspecified ♀

√4ᵗʰ **C56 Malignant neoplasm of** ovary
Use additional code to identify any functional activity

CC Excl: For CC codes in category C56, unless otherwise noted: C45.9, C56.1-C57.4, C7A.00, C7A.098-C7B.00, C7B.1, C76.3, C79.60-C79.62, C80.0-C80.2

C56.1 **Malignant neoplasm of** right **ovary** CC ♀

C56.2 **Malignant neoplasm of** left **ovary** CC ♀

C56.9 **Malignant neoplasm of** unspecified **ovary** CC ♀

√4ᵗʰ **C57 Malignant neoplasm of** other and unspecified female genital organs

√5ᵗʰ **C57.0 Malignant neoplasm of** fallopian tube
Malignant neoplasm of oviduct
Malignant neoplasm of uterine tube

C57.00 **Malignant neoplasm of** unspecified **fallopian tube** ♀

C57.01 **Malignant neoplasm of** right **fallopian tube** ♀

C57.02 **Malignant neoplasm of** left **fallopian tube** ♀

√5ᵗʰ **C57.1 Malignant neoplasm of** broad ligament

C57.10 **Malignant neoplasm of** unspecified **broad ligament** ♀

C57.11 **Malignant neoplasm of** right **broad ligament** ♀

C57.12 **Malignant neoplasm of** left **broad ligament** ♀

√5ᵗʰ **C57.2 Malignant neoplasm of** round ligament

C57.20 **Malignant neoplasm of** unspecified **round ligament** ♀

C57.21 **Malignant neoplasm of** right **round ligament** ♀

C57.22 **Malignant neoplasm of** left **round ligament** ♀

C57.3 **Malignant neoplasm of** parametrium ♀
Malignant neoplasm of uterine ligament NOS

C57.4 **Malignant neoplasm of** uterine adnexa, unspecified ♀

C57.7 **Malignant neoplasm of** other **specified female genital organs** ♀
Malignant neoplasm of wolffian body or duct

C57.8 Malignant neoplasm of overlapping sites of female genital organs ♀
Primary malignant neoplasm of two or more contiguous sites of the female genital organs whose point of origin cannot be determined
Primary tubo-ovarian malignant neoplasm whose point of origin cannot be determined
Primary utero-ovarian malignant neoplasm whose point of origin cannot be determined

C57.9 Malignant neoplasm of female genital organ, unspecified ♀
Malignant neoplasm of female genitourinary tract NOS

C58 Malignant neoplasm of placenta ♀
INCLUDES choriocarcinoma NOS
chorionepithelioma NOS
EXCLUDES 1 chorioadenoma (destruens) (D39.2)
hydatidiform mole NOS (O01.9)
invasive hydatidiform mole (D39.2)
male choriocarcinoma NOS (C62.9-)
malignant hydatidiform mole (D39.2)

Malignant neoplasms of male genital organs (C60-C63)
INCLUDES malignant neoplasm of skin of male genital organs

✓4ᵗʰ C60 Malignant neoplasm of penis

C60.0 Malignant neoplasm of prepuce ♂
Malignant neoplasm of foreskin

C60.1 Malignant neoplasm of glans penis ♂

C60.2 Malignant neoplasm of body of penis ♂
Malignant neoplasm of corpus cavernosum

C60.8 Malignant neoplasm of overlapping sites of penis ♂

C60.9 Malignant neoplasm of penis, unspecified ♂
Malignant neoplasm of skin of penis NOS

C61 Malignant neoplasm of prostate ♂
EXCLUDES 1 malignant neoplasm of seminal vesicle (C63.7)

✓4ᵗʰ C62 Malignant neoplasm of testis
Use additional code to identify any functional activity

✓5ᵗʰ C62.0 Malignant neoplasm of undescended testis
Malignant neoplasm of ectopic testis
Malignant neoplasm of retained testis

C62.00 Malignant neoplasm of unspecified undescended testis ♂

C62.01 Malignant neoplasm of undescended right testis ♂

C62.02 Malignant neoplasm of undescended left testis ♂

✓5ᵗʰ C62.1 Malignant neoplasm of descended testis
Malignant neoplasm of scrotal testis

C62.10 Malignant neoplasm of unspecified descended testis ♂

C62.11 Malignant neoplasm of descended right testis ♂

C62.12 Malignant neoplasm of descended left testis ♂

✓5ᵗʰ C62.9 Malignant neoplasm of testis, unspecified whether descended or undescended

C62.90 Malignant neoplasm of unspecified testis, unspecified whether descended or undescended ♂
Malignant neoplasm of testis NOS

C62.91 Malignant neoplasm of right testis, unspecified whether descended or undescended ♂

C62.92 Malignant neoplasm of left testis, unspecified whether descended or undescended ♂

✓4ᵗʰ C63 Malignant neoplasm of other and unspecified male genital organs

✓5ᵗʰ C63.0 Malignant neoplasm of epididymis

C63.00 Malignant neoplasm of unspecified epididymis ♂

C63.01 Malignant neoplasm of right epididymis ♂

C63.02 Malignant neoplasm of left epididymis ♂

✓5ᵗʰ C63.1 Malignant neoplasm of spermatic cord

C63.10 Malignant neoplasm of unspecified spermatic cord ♂

C63.11 Malignant neoplasm of right spermatic cord ♂

C63.12 Malignant neoplasm of left spermatic cord ♂

C63.2 Malignant neoplasm of scrotum ♂
Malignant neoplasm of skin of scrotum

C63.7 Malignant neoplasm of other specified male genital organs ♂
Malignant neoplasm of seminal vesicle
Malignant neoplasm of tunica vaginalis

C63.8 Malignant neoplasm of overlapping sites of male genital organs ♂
Primary malignant neoplasm of two or more contiguous sites of male genital organs whose point of origin cannot be determined

C63.9 Malignant neoplasm of male genital organ, unspecified ♂
Malignant neoplasm of male genitourinary tract NOS

Malignant neoplasms of urinary tract (C64-C68)

✓4ᵗʰ C64 Malignant neoplasm of kidney, except renal pelvis
EXCLUDES 1 malignant carcinoid tumor of the kidney (C7A.093)
malignant neoplasm of renal calyces (C65.-)
malignant neoplasm of renal pelvis (C65.-)

CC Excl: For CC codes in category C64, unless otherwise noted:
C45.7-C45.9, C64.1-C64.9, C65.1-C65.9, C68.8-C68.9, C76.8, C7A.00, C7A.093, C7A.098-C7B.00, C7B.1, C80.0-C80.2, D49.5, D49.81-D49.9

C64.1 Malignant neoplasm of right kidney, except renal pelvis CC

C64.2 Malignant neoplasm of left kidney, except renal pelvis CC

C64.9 Malignant neoplasm of unspecified kidney, except renal pelvis CC

✓4ᵗʰ C65 Malignant neoplasm of renal pelvis
INCLUDES malignant neoplasm of pelviureteric junction
malignant neoplasm of renal calyces

CC Excl: For CC codes in category C65, unless otherwise noted:
C45.7-C45.9, C64.1-C64.9, C65.1-C65.9, C68.8-C68.9, C76.8, C7A.00, C7A.093, C7A.098-C7B.00, C7B.1, C80.0-C80.2, D49.5, D49.81-D49.9

C65.1 Malignant neoplasm of right renal pelvis CC

C65.2 Malignant neoplasm of left renal pelvis CC

C65.9 Malignant neoplasm of unspecified renal pelvis CC

✓4ᵗʰ C66 Malignant neoplasm of ureter
EXCLUDES 1 malignant neoplasm of ureteric orifice of bladder (C67.6)

CC Excl: For CC codes in category C66, unless otherwise noted:
C45.7-C45.9, C66.1-C66.9, C68.8-C68.9, C76.8, C7A.00, C7A.098-C7B.00, C7B.1, C80.0-C80.2, D49.5, D49.81-D49.9

C66.1 Malignant neoplasm of right ureter CC

C66.2 Malignant neoplasm of left ureter CC

C66.9 Malignant neoplasm of unspecified ureter CC

✓4ᵗʰ C67 Malignant neoplasm of bladder

C67.0 Malignant neoplasm of trigone of bladder

C67.1 Malignant neoplasm of dome of bladder

C67.2 Malignant neoplasm of lateral wall of bladder

C67.3 Malignant neoplasm of anterior wall of bladder

C67.4 Malignant neoplasm of posterior wall of bladder

C67.5 Malignant neoplasm of bladder neck
Malignant neoplasm of internal urethral orifice

C67.6 Malignant neoplasm of ureteric orifice

C67.7 Malignant neoplasm of urachus

C67.8 Malignant neoplasm of overlapping sites of bladder

C67.9 Malignant neoplasm of bladder, unspecified

✓4ᵗʰ C68 Malignant neoplasm of other and unspecified urinary organs
EXCLUDES 1 malignant neoplasm of female genitourinary tract NOS (C57.9)
malignant neoplasm of male genitourinary tract NOS (C63.9)

C68.0 Malignant neoplasm of urethra CC
EXCLUDES 1 malignant neoplasm of urethral orifice of bladder (C67.5)
CC Excl: C68.0-C68.9, C79.82

C68.1 Malignant neoplasm of paraurethral glands CC
CC Excl: See code: C68.0

C68.8 Malignant neoplasm of overlapping sites of urinary organs CC
Primary malignant neoplasm of two or more contiguous sites of urinary organs whose point of origin cannot be determined
CC Excl: C64.1-C64.9, C65.1-C65.9, C66.1-C66.9, C68.0-C68.9, C76.3, C79.00-C79.19, C7A.093

C68.9 Malignant neoplasm of urinary organ, unspecified CC
Malignant neoplasm of urinary system NOS
CC Excl: See code: C68.8

✓ Additional Character Required   ✓x7ᵗʰ Xtension Alert   Unacceptable PDx   Manifestation   Hospital Acquired Condition   EXCLUDES 1 Not Coded Here   EXCLUDES 2 Not Included Here

ICD-10-CM Draft (2015)   459

C57.8-C68.9

Neoplasms

C69–C72.9

Malignant neoplasms of eye, brain and other parts of central nervous system (C69-C72)

☑4ᵗʰ **C69 Malignant neoplasm of eye and adnexa**
> EXCLUDES 1   malignant neoplasm of connective tissue of eyelid (C49.0)
> malignant neoplasm of eyelid (skin) (C43.1-, C44.1-)
> malignant neoplasm of optic nerve (C72.3-)

☑5ᵗʰ **C69.0 Malignant neoplasm of conjunctiva**
- **C69.00** Malignant neoplasm of unspecified conjunctiva
- **C69.01** Malignant neoplasm of right conjunctiva
- **C69.02** Malignant neoplasm of left conjunctiva

☑5ᵗʰ **C69.1 Malignant neoplasm of cornea**
- **C69.10** Malignant neoplasm of unspecified cornea
- **C69.11** Malignant neoplasm of right cornea
- **C69.12** Malignant neoplasm of left cornea

☑5ᵗʰ **C69.2 Malignant neoplasm of retina**
> EXCLUDES 1   dark area on retina (D49.81)
> neoplasm of unspecified behavior of retina and choroid (D49.81)
> retinal freckle (D49.81)
- **C69.20** Malignant neoplasm of unspecified retina
- **C69.21** Malignant neoplasm of right retina
- **C69.22** Malignant neoplasm of left retina

☑5ᵗʰ **C69.3 Malignant neoplasm of choroid**
- **C69.30** Malignant neoplasm of unspecified choroid
- **C69.31** Malignant neoplasm of right choroid
- **C69.32** Malignant neoplasm of left choroid

☑5ᵗʰ **C69.4 Malignant neoplasm of ciliary body**
- **C69.40** Malignant neoplasm of unspecified ciliary body
- **C69.41** Malignant neoplasm of right ciliary body
- **C69.42** Malignant neoplasm of left ciliary body

☑5ᵗʰ **C69.5 Malignant neoplasm of lacrimal gland and duct**
Malignant neoplasm of lacrimal sac
Malignant neoplasm of nasolacrimal duct
- **C69.50** Malignant neoplasm of unspecified lacrimal gland and duct
- **C69.51** Malignant neoplasm of right lacrimal gland and duct
- **C69.52** Malignant neoplasm of left lacrimal gland and duct

☑5ᵗʰ **C69.6 Malignant neoplasm of orbit**
Malignant neoplasm of connective tissue of orbit
Malignant neoplasm of extraocular muscle
Malignant neoplasm of peripheral nerves of orbit
Malignant neoplasm of retrobulbar tissue
Malignant neoplasm of retro-ocular tissue
> EXCLUDES 1   malignant neoplasm of orbital bone (C41.0)
- **C69.60** Malignant neoplasm of unspecified orbit
- **C69.61** Malignant neoplasm of right orbit
- **C69.62** Malignant neoplasm of left orbit

☑5ᵗʰ **C69.8 Malignant neoplasm of overlapping sites of eye and adnexa**
- **C69.80** Malignant neoplasm of overlapping sites of unspecified eye and adnexa
- **C69.81** Malignant neoplasm of overlapping sites of right eye and adnexa
- **C69.82** Malignant neoplasm of overlapping sites of left eye and adnexa

☑5ᵗʰ **C69.9 Malignant neoplasm of unspecified site of eye**
Malignant neoplasm of eyeball
- **C69.90** Malignant neoplasm of unspecified site of unspecified eye
- **C69.91** Malignant neoplasm of unspecified site of right eye
- **C69.92** Malignant neoplasm of unspecified site of left eye

☑4ᵗʰ **C70 Malignant neoplasm of meninges**
- **C70.0 Malignant neoplasm of cerebral meninges** CC
  CC Excl: C45.7-C45.9, C70.0, C70.9, C72.9, C76.8, C7A.00, C7A.098-C7B.00, C7B.1, C80.0-C80.2, D49.6-D49.9
- **C70.1 Malignant neoplasm of spinal meninges** CC
  CC Excl: C45.7-C45.9, C70.1, C72.9, C76.8, C7A.00, C7A.098-C7B.00, C7B.1, C80.0-C80.2, D49.6-D49.9
- **C70.9 Malignant neoplasm of meninges, unspecified** CC
  CC Excl: See code: C70.0

☑4ᵗʰ **C71 Malignant neoplasm of brain**
> EXCLUDES 1   malignant neoplasm of cranial nerves (C72.2-C72.5)
> retrobulbar malignant neoplasm (C69.6-)

CC Excl: For CC codes in category C71, unless otherwise noted:
C45.7-C45.9, C70.0, C70.9-C71.9, C72.20-C72.9, C76.8, C7A.00, C7A.098-C7B.00, C7B.1, C80.0-C80.2, D49.6-D49.9

- **C71.0 Malignant neoplasm of cerebrum, except lobes and ventricles** CC
  Malignant neoplasm of supratentorial NOS
- **C71.1 Malignant neoplasm of frontal lobe** CC
- **C71.2 Malignant neoplasm of temporal lobe** CC
- **C71.3 Malignant neoplasm of parietal lobe** CC
- **C71.4 Malignant neoplasm of occipital lobe** CC
- **C71.5 Malignant neoplasm of cerebral ventricle** CC
  > EXCLUDES 1   malignant neoplasm of fourth cerebral ventricle (C71.7)
- **C71.6 Malignant neoplasm of cerebellum** CC
- **C71.7 Malignant neoplasm of brain stem** CC
  Malignant neoplasm of fourth cerebral ventricle
  Infratentorial malignant neoplasm NOS
- **C71.8 Malignant neoplasm of overlapping sites of brain** CC
- **C71.9 Malignant neoplasm of brain, unspecified** CC

☑4ᵗʰ **C72 Malignant neoplasm of spinal cord, cranial nerves and other parts of central nervous system**
> EXCLUDES 1   malignant neoplasm of meninges (C70.-)
> malignant neoplasm of peripheral nerves and autonomic nervous system (C47.-)

- **C72.0 Malignant neoplasm of spinal cord** CC
  CC Excl: C45.7-C45.9, C72.0-C72.1, C72.9, C76.8, C7A.00, C7A.098-C7B.00, C7B.1, C80.0-C80.2, D49.6-D49.9
- **C72.1 Malignant neoplasm of cauda equina** CC
  CC Excl: See code: C72.0

☑5ᵗʰ **C72.2 Malignant neoplasm of olfactory nerve**
Malignant neoplasm of olfactory bulb

CC Excl: For CC codes in subcategory C72.2, unless otherwise noted: C45.7-C45.9, C72.20-C72.9, C76.8, C7A.00, C7A.098-C7B.00, C7B.1, C80.0-C80.2, D49.6-D49.9

- **C72.20** Malignant neoplasm of unspecified olfactory nerve CC
- **C72.21** Malignant neoplasm of right olfactory nerve CC
- **C72.22** Malignant neoplasm of left olfactory nerve CC

☑5ᵗʰ **C72.3 Malignant neoplasm of optic nerve**

CC Excl: For CC codes in subcategory C72.3, unless otherwise noted: C45.7-C45.9, C72.20-C72.9, C76.8, C7A.00, C7A.098-C7B.00, C7B.1, C80.0-C80.2, D49.6-D49.9

- **C72.30** Malignant neoplasm of unspecified optic nerve CC
- **C72.31** Malignant neoplasm of right optic nerve CC
- **C72.32** Malignant neoplasm of left optic nerve CC

☑5ᵗʰ **C72.4 Malignant neoplasm of acoustic nerve**

CC Excl: For CC codes in subcategory C72.4, unless otherwise noted: C45.7-C45.9, C72.20-C72.9, C76.8, C7A.00, C7A.098-C7B.00, C7B.1, C80.0-C80.2, D49.6-D49.9

- **C72.40** Malignant neoplasm of unspecified acoustic nerve CC
- **C72.41** Malignant neoplasm of right acoustic nerve CC
- **C72.42** Malignant neoplasm of left acoustic nerve CC

☑5ᵗʰ **C72.5 Malignant neoplasm of other and unspecified cranial nerves**

CC Excl: For CC codes in subcategory C72.5, unless otherwise noted: C45.7-C45.9, C72.20-C72.9, C76.8, C7A.00, C7A.098-C7B.00, C7B.1, C80.0-C80.2, D49.6-D49.9

- **C72.50** Malignant neoplasm of unspecified cranial nerve CC
  Malignant neoplasm of cranial nerve NOS
- **C72.59** Malignant neoplasm of other cranial nerves CC
- **C72.9 Malignant neoplasm of central nervous system, unspecified** CC
  Malignant neoplasm of unspecified site of central nervous system
  Malignant neoplasm of nervous system NOS
  CC Excl: C45.7-C45.9, C70.0-C72.9, C7A.00, C7A.098-C7B.00, C7B.1, C76.8, C79.31-C79.49, C80.0-C80.2, D49.6-D49.9

Malignant neoplasms of thyroid and other endocrine glands (C73-C75)

C73 Malignant neoplasm of thyroid gland
Use additional code to identify any functional activity

✓4th C74 Malignant neoplasm of adrenal gland

> CC Excl: For CC codes in category C74, unless otherwise noted: C45.7-C45.9, C74.00-C74.92, C75.9-C7A.00, C7A.098-C7B.00, C7B.1, C76.2, C76.8, C79.70-C79.72, C80.0-C80.2

✓5th C74.0 Malignant neoplasm of cortex of adrenal gland
- **C74.00 Malignant neoplasm of cortex of unspecified adrenal gland** CC
- **C74.01 Malignant neoplasm of cortex of right adrenal gland** CC
- **C74.02 Malignant neoplasm of cortex of left adrenal gland** CC

✓5th C74.1 Malignant neoplasm of medulla of adrenal gland
- **C74.10 Malignant neoplasm of medulla of unspecified adrenal gland** CC
- **C74.11 Malignant neoplasm of medulla of right adrenal gland** CC
- **C74.12 Malignant neoplasm of medulla of left adrenal gland** CC

✓5th C74.9 Malignant neoplasm of unspecified part of adrenal gland
- **C74.90 Malignant neoplasm of unspecified part of unspecified adrenal gland** CC
- **C74.91 Malignant neoplasm of unspecified part of right adrenal gland** CC
- **C74.92 Malignant neoplasm of unspecified part of left adrenal gland** CC

✓4th C75 Malignant neoplasm of other endocrine glands and related structures
> EXCLUDES 1 malignant carcinoid tumors (C7A.0-)
> malignant neoplasm of adrenal gland (C74.-)
> malignant neoplasm of endocrine pancreas (C25.4)
> malignant neoplasm of islets of Langerhans (C25.4)
> malignant neoplasm of ovary (C56.-)
> malignant neoplasm of testis (C62.-)
> malignant neoplasm of thymus (C37)
> malignant neoplasm of thyroid gland (C73)
> malignant neuroendocrine tumors (C7A.-)

C75.0 Malignant neoplasm of parathyroid gland CC
CC Excl: C75.0-C75.9
C75.1 Malignant neoplasm of pituitary gland CC
CC Excl: C75.1-C75.2, Z51.0
C75.2 Malignant neoplasm of craniopharyngeal duct CC
CC Excl: See code: C75.1
C75.3 Malignant neoplasm of pineal gland CC
CC Excl: C75.3-Z51.0
C75.4 Malignant neoplasm of carotid body CC
CC Excl: C75.4-C75.9
C75.5 Malignant neoplasm of aortic body and other paraganglia CC
CC Excl: See code: C75.4
C75.8 Malignant neoplasm with pluriglandular involvement, unspecified CC
CC Excl: C74.00-C75.9
C75.9 Malignant neoplasm of endocrine gland, unspecified CC
CC Excl: See code: C75.8

Malignant neuroendocrine tumors (C7A)

✓4th C7A Malignant neuroendocrine tumors
Code also any associated multiple endocrine neoplasia [MEN] syndromes (E31.2-)
Use additional code to identify any associated endocrine syndrome, such as:
carcinoid syndrome (E34.0)
> EXCLUDES 2 malignant pancreatic islet cell tumors (C25.4)
> Merkel cell carcinoma (C4A.-)

✓5th C7A.0 Malignant carcinoid tumors
- **C7A.00 Malignant carcinoid tumor of unspecified site** CC
CC Excl: C45.7-C45.9, C76.8, C79.89-C7B.00, C7B.09-C80.2, D49.81-D49.9

✓6th C7A.01 Malignant carcinoid tumors of the small intestine
- **C7A.010 Malignant carcinoid tumor of the duodenum** CC
CC Excl: C17.0-C17.9, C26.0, C26.9, C45.7-C45.9, C46.4, C76.8, C7A.00-C7B.00, C7B.1, C80.0-C80.2, D49.0, D49.81-D49.9
- **C7A.011 Malignant carcinoid tumor of the jejunum** CC
CC Excl: C17.1-C17.9, C26.0, C26.9, C45.7-C45.9, C46.4, C76.8, C7A.00-C7B.00, C7B.1, C80.0-C80.2, D49.0, D49.81-D49.9
- **C7A.012 Malignant carcinoid tumor of the ileum** CC
CC Excl: C17.2-C17.9, C26.0, C26.9, C45.7-C45.9, C46.4, C76.8, C7A.00-C7B.00, C7B.1, C80.0-C80.2, D49.0, D49.81-D49.9
- **C7A.019 Malignant carcinoid tumor of the small intestine, unspecified portion**
CC Excl: C17.8-C17.9, C26.0, C26.9, C45.7-C45.9, C46.4, C76.8, C7A.00-C7B.00, C7B.1, C80.0-C80.2, D49.0, D49.81-D49.9

✓6th C7A.02 Malignant carcinoid tumors of the appendix, large intestine, and rectum
- **C7A.020 Malignant carcinoid tumor of the appendix** CC
CC Excl: C18.1-C18.9, C26.0, C26.9, C45.7-C45.9, C46.4, C76.8, C7A.00-C7B.00, C7B.1, C80.0-C80.2, D49.0, D49.81-D49.9
- **C7A.021 Malignant carcinoid tumor of the cecum** CC
CC Excl: C18.0-C18.9, C26.0, C26.9, C45.7-C45.9, C46.4, C76.8, C7A.00-C7B.00, C7B.1, C80.0-C80.2, D49.0, D49.81-D49.9
- **C7A.022 Malignant carcinoid tumor of the ascending colon** CC
CC Excl: C18.2-C18.9, C26.0, C26.9, C45.7-C45.9, C46.4, C76.8, C7A.00-C7B.00, C7B.1, C80.0-C80.2, D49.0, D49.81-D49.9
- **C7A.023 Malignant carcinoid tumor of the transverse colon** CC
CC Excl: C18.4-C18.9, C26.0, C26.9, C45.7-C45.9, C46.4, C76.8, C7A.00-C7B.00, C7B.1, C80.0-C80.2, D49.0, D49.81-D49.9
- **C7A.024 Malignant carcinoid tumor of the descending colon** CC
CC Excl: C18.6-C18.9, C26.0, C26.9, C45.7-C45.9, C46.4, C76.8, C7A.00-C7B.00, C7B.1, C80.0-C80.2, D49.0, D49.81-D49.9
- **C7A.025 Malignant carcinoid tumor of the sigmoid colon** CC
CC Excl: C18.7-C18.9, C26.0, C26.9, C45.7-C45.9, C46.4, C76.8, C7A.00-C7B.00, C7B.1, C80.0-C80.2, D49.0, D49.81-D49.9
- **C7A.026 Malignant carcinoid tumor of the rectum** CC
CC Excl: C20-C21.8, C26.0, C26.9, C45.7-C45.9, C46.4, C76.8, C7A.00-C7B.00, C7B.1, C80.0-C80.2, D49.0, D49.81-D49.9
- **C7A.029 Malignant carcinoid tumor of the large intestine, unspecified portion** CC
Malignant carcinoid tumor of the colon NOS
CC Excl: C18.8-C18.9, C26.0, C26.9, C45.7-C45.9, C46.4, C76.8, C7A.00-C7B.00, C7B.1, C80.0-C80.2, D49.0, D49.81-D49.9

✓6th C7A.09 Malignant carcinoid tumors of other sites
- **C7A.090 Malignant carcinoid tumor of the bronchus and lung** CC
CC Excl: C34.80-C34.92, C39.9, C45.7-C45.9, C46.50-C46.52, C76.8, C7A.00-C7B.00, C7B.1, C80.0-C80.2, D49.1, D49.81-D49.9
- **C7A.091 Malignant carcinoid tumor of the thymus** CC
CC Excl: C37-C7A.8
- **C7A.092 Malignant carcinoid tumor of the stomach** CC
CC Excl: C16.0-C16.9, C26.0, C26.9, C45.7-C45.9, C46.4, C76.8, C7A.00-C7B.00, C7B.1, C80.0-C80.2, D49.0, D49.81-D49.9
- **C7A.093 Malignant carcinoid tumor of the kidney** CC
CC Excl: C45.7-C45.9, C64.1-C64.9, C65.1-C65.9, C68.8-C68.9, C76.8, C7A.00-C7B.00, C7B.1, C80.0-C80.2, D49.5, D49.81-D49.9

Neoplasms

C7A.094–C78.7

C7A.094 **Malignant carcinoid tumor of the** `CC`
foregut NOS
CC Excl: See code: C7A.092

C7A.095 **Malignant carcinoid tumor of the** `CC`
midgut NOS
CC Excl: See code: C7A.092

C7A.096 **Malignant carcinoid tumor of the** `CC`
hindgut NOS
CC Excl: See code: C7A.092

C7A.098 **Malignant carcinoid tumors of** other `CC`
sites
CC Excl: See code: C7A.00

C7A.1 **Malignant** poorly differentiated **neuroendocrine tumors** `CC`
High grade neuroendocrine carcinoma, any site
Malignant poorly differentiated neuroendocrine tumor NOS
Malignant poorly differentiated neuroendocrine carcinoma, any
site
CC Excl: See code: C7A.00

C7A.8 Other **malignant neuroendocrine tumors** `CC`
CC Excl: See code: C7A.00

Secondary neuroendocrine tumors (C7B)

√4ᵗʰ **C7B** **Secondary** neuroendocrine tumors
Use additional code to identify any functional activity

√5ᵗʰ **C7B.0** **Secondary** carcinoid tumors

C7B.00 **Secondary carcinoid tumors,** unspecified **site**

C7B.01 **Secondary carcinoid tumors of** distant lymph `CC`
nodes
CC Excl: C45.7-C45.9, C46.3, C76.8-C77.9, C7A.00,
C7A.098-C80.2, D49.81-D49.9

C7B.02 **Secondary carcinoid tumors of** liver `CC`
CC Excl: C45.7-C45.9, C76.8, C78.7-C78.89, C79.89-
C7A.00, C7A.098-C80.2, D49.81-D49.9

C7B.03 **Secondary carcinoid tumors of** bone `CC`
CC Excl: C45.7-C45.9, C76.8, C79.51-C79.52, C79.89-
C7A.00, C7A.098-C80.2, D49.81-D49.9

C7B.04 **Secondary carcinoid tumors of** peritoneum `CC`
Mesentery metastasis of carcinoid tumor
CC Excl: C45.7-C45.9, C76.8, C78.6, C78.80-C78.89,
C79.89-C7A.00, C7A.098-C80.2, D49.81-D49.9

C7B.09 **Secondary carcinoid tumors of** other **sites** `CC`
CC Excl: C45.7-C45.9, C76.8, C79.89-C7A.00, C7A.098-
C80.2, D49.81-D49.9

C7B.1 **Secondary** Merkel cell carcinoma
Merkel cell carcinoma nodal presentation
Merkel cell carcinoma visceral metastatic presentation

C7B.8 Other **secondary neuroendocrine tumors** `CC`
CC Excl: See code: C7B.09

Malignant neoplasms of ill-defined, other secondary and unspecified sites (C76-C80)

√4ᵗʰ **C76** **Malignant neoplasm of** other and ill-defined sites
EXCLUDES 1   malignant neoplasm of female genitourinary tract NOS (C57.9)
malignant neoplasm of male genitourinary tract NOS (C63.9)
malignant neoplasm of lymphoid, hematopoietic and related
tissue (C81-C96)
malignant neoplasm of skin (C44.-)
malignant neoplasm of unspecified site NOS (C80.1)

C76.0 **Malignant neoplasm of** head, face and neck
Malignant neoplasm of cheek NOS
Malignant neoplasm of nose NOS

C76.1 **Malignant neoplasm of** thorax
Intrathoracic malignant neoplasm NOS
Malignant neoplasm of axilla NOS
Thoracic malignant neoplasm NOS

C76.2 **Malignant neoplasm of** abdomen

C76.3 **Malignant neoplasm of** pelvis
Malignant neoplasm of groin NOS
Malignant neoplasm of sites overlapping systems within the
pelvis
Rectovaginal (septum) malignant neoplasm
Rectovesical (septum) malignant neoplasm

√5ᵗʰ **C76.4** **Malignant neoplasm of** upper limb

C76.40 **Malignant neoplasm of** unspecified **upper limb**

C76.41 **Malignant neoplasm of** right **upper limb**

C76.42 **Malignant neoplasm of** left **upper limb**

√5ᵗʰ **C76.5** **Malignant neoplasm of** lower limb

C76.50 **Malignant neoplasm of** unspecified **lower limb**

C76.51 **Malignant neoplasm of** right **lower limb**

C76.52 **Malignant neoplasm of** left **lower limb**

C76.8 **Malignant neoplasm of** other specified ill-defined sites
Malignant neoplasm of overlapping ill-defined sites

√4ᵗʰ **C77** **Secondary and unspecified** malignant neoplasm of lymph nodes
EXCLUDES 1   malignant neoplasm of lymph nodes, specified as primary (C81-
C86, C88, C96.-)
mesentery metastasis of carcinoid tumor (C7B.04)
secondary carcinoid tumors of distant lymph nodes (C7B.01)

CC Excl: For CC codes in category C77, unless otherwise noted:
C45.7-C45.9, C46.3, C76.8-C77.9, C7A.00, C7A.098-C7B.01, C7B.1,
C80.0-C80.2, D49.81-D49.9

C77.0 **Secondary and unspecified malignant neoplasm of** `CC`
lymph nodes of head, face and neck
Secondary and unspecified malignant neoplasm of
supraclavicular lymph nodes

C77.1 **Secondary and unspecified malignant neoplasm of** `CC`
intrathoracic **lymph nodes**

C77.2 **Secondary and unspecified malignant neoplasm of** `CC`
intra-abdominal **lymph nodes**

C77.3 **Secondary and unspecified malignant neoplasm of** axilla `CC`
and upper limb **lymph nodes**
Secondary and unspecified malignant neoplasm of pectoral
lymph nodes

C77.4 **Secondary and unspecified malignant neoplasm of** `CC`
inguinal and lower limb **lymph nodes**

C77.5 **Secondary and unspecified malignant neoplasm of** `CC`
intrapelvic **lymph nodes**

C77.8 **Secondary and unspecified malignant neoplasm of** `CC`
lymph nodes of multiple regions

C77.9 **Secondary and unspecified malignant neoplasm of** `CC`
lymph node, unspecified

√4ᵗʰ **C78** **Secondary** malignant neoplasm of respiratory and digestive
organs
EXCLUDES 1   lymph node metastases (C77.0)
secondary carcinoid tumors of liver (C7B.02)
secondary carcinoid tumors of peritoneum (C7B.04)

√5ᵗʰ **C78.0** **Secondary malignant neoplasm of** lung

C78.00 **Secondary malignant neoplasm of** unspecified `CC`
lung
CC Excl: C45.7-C45.9, C76.8, C78.00-C78.02, C78.30-
C78.39, C79.89-C7A.00, C7A.098-C7B.00, C7B.09-C80.2,
D49.81-D49.9

C78.01 **Secondary malignant neoplasm of** right **lung** `CC`
CC Excl: See code: C78.00

C78.02 **Secondary malignant neoplasm of** left lung `CC`
CC Excl: See code: C78.00

C78.1 **Secondary malignant neoplasm of** mediastinum `CC`
CC Excl: C45.7-C45.9, C76.8, C78.1, C78.30-C78.39, C79.89-C7A.00,
C7A.098-C7B.00, C7B.09-C80.2, D49.81-D49.9

C78.2 **Secondary malignant neoplasm of** pleura `CC`
CC Excl: C45.7-C45.9, C76.8, C78.2-C78.39, C79.89-C7A.00,
C7A.098-C7B.00, C7B.09-C80.2, D49.81-D49.9, J91.0

√5ᵗʰ **C78.3** **Secondary malignant neoplasm of** other and unspecified
respiratory organs

C78.30 **Secondary malignant neoplasm of** unspecified `CC`
respiratory organ
CC Excl: C45.7-C45.9, C76.8, C78.00-C78.39, C79.89-
C7A.00, C7A.098-C7B.00, C7B.09-C80.2, D49.81-D49.9

C78.39 **Secondary malignant neoplasm of** other `CC`
respiratory organs
CC Excl: See code: C78.30

C78.4 **Secondary malignant neoplasm of** small intestine `CC`
CC Excl: C45.7-C45.9, C76.8, C78.4, C78.80-C78.89, C79.89-C7A.00,
C7A.098-C7B.00, C7B.09-C80.2, D49.81-D49.9

C78.5 **Secondary malignant neoplasm of** large intestine and `CC`
rectum
CC Excl: C45.7-C45.9, C76.8, C78.5, C78.80-C78.89, C79.89-C7A.00,
C7A.098-C7B.00, C7B.09-C80.2, D49.81-D49.9

C78.6 **Secondary malignant neoplasm of** retroperitoneum and `CC`
peritoneum
CC Excl: C45.7-C45.9, C76.8, C78.6, C78.80-C78.89, C79.89-C7A.00,
C7A.098-C7B.00, C7B.04-C80.2, D49.81-D49.9

C78.7 **Secondary malignant neoplasm of** liver and intrahepatic `CC`
bile duct
CC Excl: C45.7-C45.9, C76.8, C78.7-C78.89, C79.89-C7A.00,
C7A.098-C7B.00, C7B.02, C7B.09-C80.2, D49.81-D49.9

N Newborn: 0   P Pediatric: 0-17   M Maternity: 12-55   A Adult: 15-124   MCC Major CC Condition   PDx MCC PDx acts as own MCC   CC CC Condition   PDx CC PDx acts as own CC

462   ICD-10-CM Draft (2015)

✓5ᵗʰ **C78.8** **Secondary malignant neoplasm of** other and unspecified digestive organs

     C78.80 **Secondary malignant neoplasm of** unspecified digestive organ   `cc`
         CC Excl: C45.7-C45.9, C76.8, C78.4-C78.89, C79.89-C7A.00, C7A.098-C7B.00, C7B.02, C7B.04-C80.2, D49.81-D49.9

     C78.89 **Secondary malignant neoplasm of** other digestive organs   `cc`
         CC Excl: See code: C78.80

✓4ᵗʰ **C79** **Secondary** malignant neoplasm of other and unspecified sites
     EXCLUDES 1   lymph node metastases (C77.0)
            secondary carcinoid tumors (C7B.-)
            secondary neuroendocrine tumors (C7B.-)

✓5ᵗʰ **C79.0** **Secondary malignant neoplasm of** kidney and renal pelvis

     CC Excl: For CC codes in subcategory C79.0, unless otherwise noted: C45.7-C45.9, C76.8, C79.00-C79.19, C79.89-C7A.00, C7A.098-C7B.00, C7B.09-C80.2, D49.81-D49.9

     C79.00 **Secondary malignant neoplasm of** unspecified kidney and renal pelvis   `cc`

     C79.01 **Secondary malignant neoplasm of** right kidney and renal pelvis   `cc`

     C79.02 **Secondary malignant neoplasm of** left kidney and renal pelvis   `cc`

✓5ᵗʰ **C79.1** **Secondary malignant neoplasm of** bladder and other and unspecified urinary organs

     CC Excl: For CC codes in subcategory C79.1, unless otherwise noted: C45.7-C45.9, C76.8, C79.00-C79.19, C79.89-C7A.00, C7A.098-C7B.00, C7B.09-C80.2, D49.81-D49.9

     C79.10 **Secondary malignant neoplasm of** unspecified urinary organs   `cc`

     C79.11 **Secondary malignant neoplasm of** bladder   `cc`

     C79.19 **Secondary malignant neoplasm of** other urinary organs   `cc`

✓5ᵗʰ **C79.2** **Secondary malignant neoplasm of** skin   `cc`
     EXCLUDES 1   secondary Merkel cell carcinoma (C7B.1)
     CC Excl: C45.7-C45.9, C76.8, C79.2, C79.89-C7A.00, C7A.098-C7B.00, C7B.09-C80.2, D49.81-D49.9

✓5ᵗʰ **C79.3** **Secondary malignant neoplasm of** brain and cerebral meninges

     C79.31 **Secondary malignant neoplasm of** brain   `cc`
         CC Excl: C45.7-C45.9, C76.8, C79.31, C79.89-C7A.00, C7A.098-C7B.00, C7B.09-C80.2, D49.81-D49.9

     C79.32 **Secondary malignant neoplasm of** cerebral meninges   `cc`
         CC Excl: C45.7-C45.9, C76.8, C79.32-C79.49, C79.89-C7A.00, C7A.098-C7B.00, C7B.09-C80.2, D49.81-D49.9

✓5ᵗʰ **C79.4** **Secondary malignant neoplasm of** other and unspecified parts of nervous system

     C79.40 **Secondary malignant neoplasm of** unspecified part of nervous system   `cc`
         CC Excl: See code: C79.32

     C79.49 **Secondary malignant neoplasm of** other parts of nervous system   `cc`
         CC Excl: See code: C79.32

✓5ᵗʰ **C79.5** **Secondary malignant neoplasm of** bone and bone marrow
     EXCLUDES 1   secondary carcinoid tumors of bone (C7B.03)

     C79.51 **Secondary malignant neoplasm of** bone   `cc`
         CC Excl: C45.7-C45.9, C76.8, C79.51-C79.52, C79.89-C7A.00, C7A.098-C7B.00, C7B.03, C7B.09-C80.2, D49.81-D49.9

     C79.52 **Secondary malignant neoplasm of** bone marrow   `cc`
         CC Excl: See code: C79.51

✓5ᵗʰ **C79.6** **Secondary malignant neoplasm of** ovary

     CC Excl: For CC codes in subcategory C79.6, unless otherwise noted: C45.7-C45.9, C76.8, C79.60-C79.62, C79.89-C7A.00, C7A.098-C7B.00, C7B.09-C80.2, D49.81-D49.9

     C79.60 **Secondary malignant neoplasm of** unspecified ovary   `cc` ♀

     C79.61 **Secondary malignant neoplasm of** right ovary   `cc` ♀

     C79.62 **Secondary malignant neoplasm of** left ovary   `cc` ♀

✓5ᵗʰ **C79.7** **Secondary malignant neoplasm of** adrenal gland

     CC Excl: For CC codes in subcategory C79.7, unless otherwise noted: C45.7-C45.9, C76.8, C79.70-C79.72, C79.89-C7A.00, C7A.098-C7B.00, C7B.09-C80.2, D49.81-D49.9

     C79.70 **Secondary malignant neoplasm of** unspecified adrenal gland   `cc`

     C79.71 **Secondary malignant neoplasm of** right adrenal gland   `cc`

     C79.72 **Secondary malignant neoplasm of** left adrenal gland   `cc`

✓5ᵗʰ **C79.8** **Secondary malignant neoplasm of** other specified sites

     C79.81 **Secondary malignant neoplasm of** breast   `cc`
         CC Excl: C45.7-C45.9, C76.8, C79.81, C79.89-C7A.00, C7A.098-C7B.00, C7B.09-C80.2, D49.81-D49.9

     C79.82 *(endometrium)* **Secondary malignant neoplasm of** genital organs   `cc`
         CC Excl: C45.7-C45.9, C76.8, C79.82-C7A.00, C7A.098-C7B.00, C7B.09-C80.2, D49.81-D49.9

     C79.89 **Secondary malignant neoplasm of** other specified sites   `cc`
         CC Excl: C45.7-C45.9, C76.8, C79.89-C7A.00, C7A.098-C7B.00, C7B.09-C80.2, D49.81-D49.9

C79.9 **Secondary malignant neoplasm of** unspecified site   `cc`
     Metastatic cancer NOS
     Metastatic disease NOS
     EXCLUDES 1   carcinomatosis NOS (C80.0)
            generalized cancer NOS (C80.0)
            malignant (primary) neoplasm of unspecified site (C80.1)
     CC Excl: See code: C79.89

✓4ᵗʰ **C80** **Malignant neoplasm** without specification of site
     EXCLUDES 1   malignant carcinoid tumor of unspecified site (C7A.00)
            malignant neoplasm of specified multiple sites—code to each site

C80.0 **Disseminated malignant neoplasm, unspecified**   `cc`
     Carcinomatosis NOS
     Generalized cancer, unspecified site (primary) (secondary)
     Generalized malignancy, unspecified site (primary) (secondary)
     CC Excl: See code: C79.89

C80.1 **Malignant (primary) neoplasm, unspecified**
     Cancer NOS
     Cancer unspecified site (primary)
     Carcinoma unspecified site (primary)
     Malignancy unspecified site (primary)
     EXCLUDES 1   secondary malignant neoplasm of unspecified site (C79.9)

C80.2 **Malignant neoplasm associated with** transplanted organ   `cc`
     Code first complication of transplanted organ (T86.-)
     Use additional code to identify the specific malignancy
     CC Excl: See code: C79.89

Malignant neoplasms of lymphoid, hematopoietic and related tissue (C81-C96)

     EXCLUDES 2   Kaposi's sarcoma of lymph nodes (C46.3)
            secondary and unspecified neoplasm of lymph nodes (C77.-)
            secondary neoplasm of bone marrow (C79.52)
            secondary neoplasm of spleen (C78.89)

✓4ᵗʰ **C81** **Hodgkin lymphoma**
     EXCLUDES 1   personal history of Hodgkin lymphoma (Z85.71)

✓5ᵗʰ **C81.0** **Nodular lymphocyte predominant** Hodgkin lymphoma

     C81.00 **Nodular lymphocyte predominant Hodgkin lymphoma,** unspecified site   `cc`
         CC Excl: C81.00-C81.09, C81.40-C81.49, C81.90, C81.98, D49.81-D49.9

     C81.01 **Nodular lymphocyte predominant Hodgkin lymphoma,** lymph nodes of head, face, and neck   `cc`
         CC Excl: C81.00-C81.01, C81.08-C81.09, C81.40-C81.41, C81.48-C81.49, C81.90-C81.91, C81.98, D49.81-D49.9

     C81.02 **Nodular lymphocyte predominant Hodgkin lymphoma,** intrathoracic lymph nodes   `cc`
         CC Excl: C81.00-C81.02, C81.08-C81.09, C81.40, C81.42, C81.48-C81.49, C81.90, C81.92, C81.98, D49.81-D49.9

     C81.03 **Nodular lymphocyte predominant Hodgkin lymphoma,** intra-abdominal lymph nodes   `cc`
         CC Excl: C81.00, C81.03, C81.08-C81.09, C81.40, C81.43, C81.48-C81.49, C81.90, C81.93, C81.98, D49.81-D49.9

     C81.04 **Nodular lymphocyte predominant Hodgkin lymphoma,** lymph nodes of axilla and upper limb   `cc`
         CC Excl: C81.00, C81.04, C81.08-C81.09, C81.40, C81.44, C81.48-C81.49, C81.90, C81.94, C81.98, D49.81-D49.9

✓ Additional Character Required   ✓✗7ᵗʰ Xtension Alert   Unacceptable PDx   Manifestation   Hospital Acquired Condition   *EXCLUDES 1* Not Coded Here   *EXCLUDES 2* Not Included Here

C81.05 Nodular lymphocyte predominant Hodgkin lymphoma, lymph nodes of inguinal region and lower limb CC
CC Excl: C81.00, C81.05, C81.08-C81.09, C81.40, C81.45, C81.48-C81.49, C81.90, C81.95, C81.98, D49.81-D49.9

C81.06 Nodular lymphocyte predominant Hodgkin lymphoma, intrapelvic lymph nodes CC
CC Excl: C81.00, C81.06, C81.08-C81.09, C81.40, C81.46, C81.48-C81.49, C81.90, C81.96, C81.98, D49.81-D49.9

C81.07 Nodular lymphocyte predominant Hodgkin lymphoma, spleen CC
CC Excl: C81.00, C81.07-C81.09, C81.40, C81.47-C81.49, C81.90, C81.97-C81.98, D49.81-D49.99

C81.08 Nodular lymphocyte predominant Hodgkin lymphoma, lymph nodes of multiple sites CC
CC Excl: C81.00-C81.09, C81.40-C81.49, C81.90, C81.98, D49.81-D49.9

C81.09 Nodular lymphocyte predominant Hodgkin lymphoma, extranodal and solid organ sites CC
CC Excl: See code: C81.08

✓5ᵗʰ C81.1 Nodular sclerosis classical Hodgkin lymphoma

C81.10 Nodular sclerosis classical Hodgkin lymphoma, unspecified site CC
CC Excl: C81.10-C81.19, C81.90, C81.98, D49.81-D49.9

C81.11 Nodular sclerosis classical Hodgkin lymphoma, lymph nodes of head, face, and neck CC
CC Excl: C81.10-C81.11, C81.18-C81.19, C81.90-C81.91, C81.98, D49.81-D49.9

C81.12 Nodular sclerosis classical Hodgkin lymphoma, intrathoracic lymph nodes CC
CC Excl: C81.10, C81.12, C81.18-C81.19, C81.90, C81.92, C81.98, D49.81-D49.9

C81.13 Nodular sclerosis classical Hodgkin lymphoma, intra-abdominal lymph nodes CC
CC Excl: C81.10, C81.13, C81.18-C81.19, C81.90, C81.93, C81.98, D49.81-D49.9

C81.14 Nodular sclerosis classical Hodgkin lymphoma, lymph nodes of axilla and upper limb CC
CC Excl: C81.10, C81.14, C81.18-C81.19, C81.90, C81.94, C81.98, D49.81-D49.9

C81.15 Nodular sclerosis classical Hodgkin lymphoma, lymph nodes of inguinal region and lower limb CC
CC Excl: C81.10, C81.15, C81.18-C81.19, C81.90, C81.95, C81.98, D49.81-D49.9

C81.16 Nodular sclerosis classical Hodgkin lymphoma, intrapelvic lymph nodes CC
CC Excl: C81.10, C81.16, C81.18-C81.19, C81.90, C81.96, C81.98, D49.81-D49.9

C81.17 Nodular sclerosis classical Hodgkin lymphoma, spleen CC
CC Excl: C81.10, C81.17-C81.19, C81.90, C81.97-C81.98, D49.81-D49.9

C81.18 Nodular sclerosis classical Hodgkin lymphoma, lymph nodes of multiple sites CC
CC Excl: C81.10-C81.19, C81.90, C81.98, D49.81-D49.9

C81.19 Nodular sclerosis classical Hodgkin lymphoma, extranodal and solid organ sites CC
CC Excl: See code: C81.18

✓5ᵗʰ C81.2 Mixed cellularity classical Hodgkin lymphoma

C81.20 Mixed cellularity classical Hodgkin lymphoma, unspecified site CC
CC Excl: C81.20-C81.29, C81.90, C81.98, D49.81-D49.9

C81.21 Mixed cellularity classical Hodgkin lymphoma, lymph nodes of head, face, and neck CC
CC Excl: C81.20-C81.21, C81.28-C81.29, C81.90-C81.91, C81.98, D49.81-D49.9

C81.22 Mixed cellularity classical Hodgkin lymphoma, intrathoracic lymph nodes CC
CC Excl: C81.20, C81.22, C81.28-C81.29, C81.90, C81.92, C81.98, D49.81-D49.9

C81.23 Mixed cellularity classical Hodgkin lymphoma, intra-abdominal lymph nodes CC
CC Excl: C81.20, C81.23, C81.28-C81.29, C81.90, C81.93, C81.98, D49.81-D49.9

C81.24 Mixed cellularity classical Hodgkin lymphoma, lymph nodes of axilla and upper limb CC
CC Excl: C81.20, C81.24, C81.28-C81.29, C81.90, C81.94, C81.98, D49.81-D49.9

C81.25 Mixed cellularity classical Hodgkin lymphoma, lymph nodes of inguinal region and lower limb CC
CC Excl: C81.20, C81.25, C81.28-C81.29, C81.90, C81.95, C81.98, D49.81-D49.9

C81.26 Mixed cellularity classical Hodgkin lymphoma, intrapelvic lymph nodes CC
CC Excl: C81.20, C81.26, C81.28-C81.29, C81.90, C81.96, C81.98, D49.81-D49.9

C81.27 Mixed cellularity classical Hodgkin lymphoma, spleen CC
CC Excl: C81.20, C81.27-C81.29, C81.90, C81.97-C81.98, D49.81-D49.9

C81.28 Mixed cellularity classical Hodgkin lymphoma, lymph nodes of multiple sites CC
CC Excl: See code: C81.20

C81.29 Mixed cellularity classical Hodgkin lymphoma, extranodal and solid organ sites CC
CC Excl: See code: C81.20

✓5ᵗʰ C81.3 Lymphocyte-depleted classical Hodgkin lymphoma

C81.30 Lymphocyte-depleted classical Hodgkin lymphoma, unspecified site CC
CC Excl: C81.30-C81.39, C81.90, C81.98, D49.81-D49.9

C81.31 Lymphocyte-depleted classical Hodgkin lymphoma, lymph nodes of head, face, and neck CC
CC Excl: C81.30-C81.31, C81.38-C81.39, C81.91, C81.98, D49.81-D49.9

C81.32 Lymphocyte-depleted classical Hodgkin lymphoma, intrathoracic lymph nodes CC
CC Excl: C81.30, C81.32, C81.38-C81.39, C81.92, C81.98, D49.81-D49.9

C81.33 Lymphocyte-depleted classical Hodgkin lymphoma, intra-abdominal lymph nodes CC
CC Excl: C81.30, C81.33, C81.38-C81.39, C81.93, C81.98, D49.81-D49.9

C81.34 Lymphocyte-depleted classical Hodgkin lymphoma, lymph nodes of axilla and upper limb CC
CC Excl: C81.30, C81.34, C81.38-C81.39, C81.94, C81.98, D49.81-D49.9

C81.35 Lymphocyte-depleted classical Hodgkin lymphoma, lymph nodes of inguinal region and lower limb CC
CC Excl: C81.30, C81.35, C81.38-C81.39, C81.95, C81.98, D49.81-D49.9

C81.36 Lymphocyte-depleted classical Hodgkin lymphoma, intrapelvic lymph nodes CC
CC Excl: C81.30, C81.36, C81.38-C81.39, C81.96, C81.98, D49.81-D49.9

C81.37 Lymphocyte-depleted classical Hodgkin lymphoma, spleen CC
CC Excl: C81.30, C81.37-C81.39, C81.97-C81.98, D49.81-D49.9

C81.38 Lymphocyte-depleted classical Hodgkin lymphoma, lymph nodes of multiple sites CC
CC Excl: C81.30-C81.39, C81.98, D49.81-D49.9

C81.39 Lymphocyte-depleted classical Hodgkin lymphoma, extranodal and solid organ sites CC
CC Excl: See code: C81.38

✓5ᵗʰ C81.4 Lymphocyte-rich classical Hodgkin lymphoma
EXCLUDES 1 nodular lymphocyte predominant Hodgkin lymphoma (C81.0-)

C81.40 Lymphocyte-rich classical Hodgkin lymphoma, unspecified site CC
CC Excl: C81.00-C81.09, C81.40-C81.49, C81.90, C81.98, D49.81-D49.9

C81.41 Lymphocyte-rich classical Hodgkin lymphoma, lymph nodes of head, face, and neck CC
CC Excl: C81.00-C81.01, C81.08-C81.09, C81.40-C81.41, C81.48-C81.49, C81.90-C81.91, C81.98, D49.81-D49.9

C81.42 Lymphocyte-rich classical Hodgkin lymphoma, intrathoracic lymph nodes CC
CC Excl: C81.00, C81.02, C81.08-C81.09, C81.40, C81.42, C81.48-C81.49, C81.90, C81.92, C81.98, D49.81-D49.9

C81.43 Lymphocyte-rich classical Hodgkin lymphoma, intra-abdominal lymph nodes CC
CC Excl: C81.00, C81.03, C81.08-C81.09, C81.40, C81.43, C81.48-C81.49, C81.90, C81.93, C81.98, D49.81-D49.9

C81.44 Lymphocyte-rich classical Hodgkin lymphoma, lymph nodes of axilla and upper limb CC
CC Excl: C81.00, C81.04, C81.08-C81.09, C81.40, C81.44, C81.48-C81.49, C81.90, C81.94, C81.98, D49.81-D49.9

C81.45 Lymphocyte-rich classical Hodgkin lymphoma, lymph nodes of inguinal region and lower limb CC
CC Excl: C81.00, C81.05, C81.08-C81.09, C81.40, C81.45, C81.48-C81.49, C81.90, C81.95, C81.98, D49.81-D49.9

C81.46   **Lymphocyte-rich classical Hodgkin lymphoma, intrapelvic lymph nodes** `CC`
> **CC Excl:** C81.00, C81.06, C81.08-C81.09, C81.40, C81.46, C81.48-C81.49, C81.90, C81.96, C81.98, D49.81-D49.9

C81.47   **Lymphocyte-rich classical Hodgkin lymphoma, spleen** `CC`
> **CC Excl:** C81.00, C81.07-C81.09, C81.40, C81.47-C81.49, C81.90, C81.97-C81.98, D49.81-D49.9

C81.48   **Lymphocyte-rich classical Hodgkin lymphoma, lymph nodes of multiple sites** `CC`
> **CC Excl:** See code: C81.40

C81.49   **Lymphocyte-rich classical Hodgkin lymphoma, extranodal and solid organ sites** `CC`
> **CC Excl:** See code: C81.40

√5ᵗʰ **C81.7**   **Other classical Hodgkin lymphoma**
Classical Hodgkin lymphoma NOS

C81.70   **Other classical Hodgkin lymphoma, unspecified site** `CC`
> **CC Excl:** C81.70-C81.90, C81.98, D49.81-D49.9

C81.71   **Other classical Hodgkin lymphoma, lymph nodes of head, face, and neck** `CC`
> **CC Excl:** C81.70-C81.71, C81.78-C81.91, C81.98, D49.81-D49.9

C81.72   **Other classical Hodgkin lymphoma, intrathoracic lymph nodes** `CC`
> **CC Excl:** C81.70, C81.72, C81.78-C81.90, C81.92, C81.98, D49.81-D49.9

C81.73   **Other classical Hodgkin lymphoma, intra-abdominal lymph nodes** `CC`
> **CC Excl:** C81.70, C81.73, C81.78-C81.90, C81.93, C81.98, D49.81-D49.9

C81.74   **Other classical Hodgkin lymphoma, lymph nodes of axilla and upper limb** `CC`
> **CC Excl:** C81.70, C81.74, C81.78-C81.90, C81.94, C81.98, D49.81-D49.9

C81.75   **Other classical Hodgkin lymphoma, lymph nodes of inguinal region and lower limb** `CC`
> **CC Excl:** C81.70, C81.75, C81.78-C81.90, C81.95, C81.98, D49.81-D49.9

C81.76   **Other classical Hodgkin lymphoma, intrapelvic lymph nodes** `CC`
> **CC Excl:** C81.70, C81.76, C81.78-C81.90, C81.96, C81.98, D49.81-D49.9

C81.77   **Other classical Hodgkin lymphoma, spleen** `CC`
> **CC Excl:** C81.70, C81.77-C81.90, C81.97-C81.98, D49.81-D49.

C81.78   **Other classical Hodgkin lymphoma, lymph nodes of multiple sites** `CC`
> **CC Excl:** See code: C81.70

C81.79   **Other classical Hodgkin lymphoma, extranodal and solid organ sites** `CC`
> **CC Excl:** See code: C81.70

√5ᵗʰ **C81.9**   **Hodgkin lymphoma, unspecified**

C81.90   **Hodgkin lymphoma, unspecified, unspecified site** `CC`
> **CC Excl:** C81.90-C81.98, D49.81-D49.9

C81.91   **Hodgkin lymphoma, unspecified, lymph nodes of head, face, and neck** `CC`
> **CC Excl:** C81.90-C81.91, C81.98, D49.81-D49.9

C81.92   **Hodgkin lymphoma, unspecified, intrathoracic lymph nodes** `CC`
> **CC Excl:** C81.9, C81.92, C81.98, D49.81-D49.9

C81.93   **Hodgkin lymphoma, unspecified, intra-abdominal lymph nodes** `CC`
> **CC Excl:** C81.90, C81.93, C81.98, D49.81-D49.9

C81.94   **Hodgkin lymphoma, unspecified, lymph nodes of axilla and upper limb** `CC`
> **CC Excl:** C81.90, C81.94, C81.98, D49.81-D49.9

C81.95   **Hodgkin lymphoma, unspecified, lymph nodes of inguinal region and lower limb** `CC`
> **CC Excl:** C81.90, C81.95, C81.98, D49.81-D49.9

C81.96   **Hodgkin lymphoma, unspecified, intrapelvic lymph nodes** `CC`
> **CC Excl:** C81.90, C81.96, C81.98, D49.81-D49.9

C81.97   **Hodgkin lymphoma, unspecified, spleen** `CC`
> **CC Excl:** C81.90, C81.97-C81.98, D49.81-D49.9

C81.98   **Hodgkin lymphoma, unspecified, lymph nodes of multiple sites** `CC`
> **CC Excl:** See code: C81.90

C81.99   **Hodgkin lymphoma, unspecified, extranodal and solid organ sites** `CC`
> **CC Excl:** No Excl

√4ᵗʰ **C82**   **Follicular lymphoma**
> **INCLUDES**   follicular lymphoma with or without diffuse areas
> **EXCLUDES 1**   mature T/NK-cell lymphomas (C84.-)
> personal history of non-Hodgkin lymphoma (Z85.72)

√5ᵗʰ **C82.0**   **Follicular lymphoma grade I**

C82.00   **Follicular lymphoma grade I, unspecified site** `CC`
> **CC Excl:** C82.00-C82.50, C82.59-C82.69, C82.80-C82.99, C83.10, C83.19, C84.40, C84.49, C84.60, C84.69-C84.70, C84.79-C84.90, C84.99-C84.A0, C84.A9-C84.Z0, C84.Z9, C85.10, C85.19-C85.20, C85.29, C85.80, C85.89-C85.90, C85.99, C86.4, C88.4, C96.4, C96.9, C96.Z, D49.81-D49.9

C82.01   **Follicular lymphoma grade I, lymph nodes of head, face, and neck** `CC`
> **CC Excl:** C82.00-C82.01, C82.08-C82.11, C82.18-C82.21, C82.28-C82.31, C82.38-C82.41, C82.48-C82.49, C82.51, C82.60-C82.61, C82.68-C82.69, C82.80-C82.81, C82.88-C82.91, C82.98-C82.99, C83.11, C84.41, C84.61, C84.71, C84.91, C84.A1, C84.Z1, C85.11, C85.21, C85.81, C85.91, C86.0, D49.81-D49.9

C82.02   **Follicular lymphoma grade I, intrathoracic lymph nodes** `CC`
> **CC Excl:** C82.00, C82.02, C82.08-C82.10, C82.12, C82.18-C82.20, C82.22, C82.28-C82.30, C82.32, C82.38-C82.40, C82.42 C82.48-C82.49, C82.52, C82.60, C82.62, C82.68-C82.69, C82.80, C82.82, C82.88-C82.90, C82.92, C82.98-C82.99, C83.12, C84.42, C84.62, C84.72 C84.92, C84.A2, C84.Z2, C85.12, C85.22, C85.82, C85.92, D49.81-D49.9

C82.03   **Follicular lymphoma grade I, intra-abdominal lymph nodes** `CC`
> **CC Excl:** C82.00, C82.03, C82.08-C82.10, C82.13, C82.18-C82.20, C82.23, C82.28-C82.30, C82.33, C82.38-C82.40, C82.43 C82.48-C82.49, C82.53, C82.60, C82.63, C82.68-C82.69, C82.80, C82.83, C82.88-C82.90, C82.93, C82.98-C82.99, C83.13, C84.43, C84.63, C84.73 C84.93, C84.A3, C84.Z3, C85.13, C85.23, C85.83, C85.93, C86.2-C86.3, D49.81-D49.9

C82.04   **Follicular lymphoma grade I, lymph nodes of axilla and upper limb** `CC`
> **CC Excl:** C82.00, C82.04, C82.08-C82.10, C82.14, C82.18-C82.20, C82.24, C82.28-C82.30, C82.34, C82.38-C82.40, C82.44 C82.48-C82.49, C82.54, C82.60, C82.64, C82.68-C82.69, C82.80, C82.84, C82.88-C82.90, C82.94, C82.98-C82.99, C83.14, C84.44, C84.64, C84.74 C84.94, C84.A4, C84.Z4, C85.14, C85.24, C85.84, C85.94, D49.81-D49.9

C82.05   **Follicular lymphoma grade I, lymph nodes of inguinal region and lower limb** `CC`
> **CC Excl:** C82.00, C82.05, C82.08-C82.10, C82.15, C82.18-C82.20, C82.25, C82.28-C82.30, C82.35, C82.38-C82.40, C82.45 C82.48-C82.49, C82.55, C82.60, C82.65, C82.68-C82.69, C82.80, C82.85, C82.88-C82.90, C82.95, C82.98-C82.99, C83.15, C84.45, C84.65, C84.75 C84.95, C84.A5, C84.Z5, C85.15, C85.25, C85.85, C85.95, D49.81-D49.9

C82.06   **Follicular lymphoma grade I, intrapelvic lymph nodes** `CC`
> **CC Excl:** C82.00, C82.06, C82.08-C82.10, C82.16, C82.18-C82.20, C82.26, C82.28-C82.30, C82.36, C82.38-C82.40, C82.46 C82.48-C82.49, C82.56, C82.60, C82.66, C82.68-C82.69, C82.80, C82.86, C82.88-C82.90, C82.96, C82.98-C82.99, C83.16, C84.46, C84.66, C84.76 C84.96, C84.A6, C84.Z6, C85.16, C85.26, C85.86, C85.96, D49.81-D49.9

C82.07   **Follicular lymphoma grade I, spleen** `CC`
> **CC Excl:** C82.00, C82.07-C82.10, C82.17-C82.20, C82.27-C82.30, C82.37-C82.40, C82.47-C82.49, C82.57, C82.60, C82.67-C82.80, C82.87-C82.90, C82.97-C82.99, C83.17, C84.47, C84.67, C84.77, C84.A7, C84.Z7, C84.97, C85.17, C85.27, C85.87, C85.97, C86.1, D49.81-D49.9

C82.08   **Follicular lymphoma grade I, lymph nodes of multiple sites** `CC`
> **CC Excl:** C82.00-C82.49, C82.58, C82.60-C82.69, C82.80-C82.99, C83.18, C84.48, C84.68, C84.78, C84.98, C84.A8, C84.Z8, C85.18 C85.28, C85.88, C85.98, D49.81-D49.9

C82.09   **Follicular lymphoma grade I, extranodal and solid organ sites** `CC`
> **CC Excl:** C82.00-C82.50, C82.59-C82.99, C83.10, C83.19, C84.40, C84.49-C84.60, C84.69-C84.70, C84.79-C84.A0, C84.A9-C84.Z0, C84.Z9-C84.90, C84.99-C85.10, C85.20, C85.29-C85.80, C85.89-C85.90, C85.99, C86.4, C88.4, C96.4, C96.Z-C96.9, D49.81-D49.9

√5ᵗʰ **C82.1**   **Follicular lymphoma grade II**

C82.10   **Follicular lymphoma grade II, unspecified site** `CC`
> **CC Excl:** See code: C82.00

C82.11   **Follicular lymphoma grade II, lymph nodes of head, face, and neck** `CC`
> **CC Excl:** See code: C82.01

✔ Additional Character Required   √x7ᵗʰ Xtension Alert   Unacceptable PDx   Manifestation   Hospital Acquired Condition   **EXCLUDES 1** Not Coded Here   **EXCLUDES 2** Not Included Here

C82.12 Follicular lymphoma grade II, intrathoracic lymph nodes `CC`
CC Excl: See code: C82.02

C82.13 Follicular lymphoma grade II, intra-abdominal lymph nodes `CC`
CC Excl: See code: C82.03

C82.14 Follicular lymphoma grade II, lymph nodes of axilla and upper limb `CC`
CC Excl: See code: C82.04

C82.15 Follicular lymphoma grade II, lymph nodes of inguinal region and lower limb `CC`
CC Excl: See code: C82.05

C82.16 Follicular lymphoma grade II, intrapelvic lymph nodes `CC`
CC Excl: See code: C82.06

C82.17 Follicular lymphoma grade II, spleen `CC`
CC Excl: See code: C82.07

C82.18 Follicular lymphoma grade II, lymph nodes of multiple sites `CC`
CC Excl: See code: C82.08

C82.19 Follicular lymphoma grade II, extranodal and solid organ sites `CC`
CC Excl: See code: C82.00

√5ᵗʰ **C82.2 Follicular lymphoma grade III, unspecified**

C82.20 Follicular lymphoma grade III, unspecified, unspecified site `CC`
CC Excl: See code: C82.00

C82.21 Follicular lymphoma grade III, unspecified, lymph nodes of head, face, and neck `CC`
CC Excl: See code: C82.01

C82.22 Follicular lymphoma grade III, unspecified, intrathoracic lymph nodes `CC`
CC Excl: See code: C82.02

C82.23 Follicular lymphoma grade III, unspecified, intra-abdominal lymph nodes `CC`
CC Excl: See code: C82.03

C82.24 Follicular lymphoma grade III, unspecified, lymph nodes of axilla and upper limb `CC`
CC Excl: See code: C82.04

C82.25 Follicular lymphoma grade III, unspecified, lymph nodes of inguinal region and lower limb `CC`
CC Excl: See code: C82.05

C82.26 Follicular lymphoma grade III, unspecified, intrapelvic lymph nodes `CC`
CC Excl: See code: C82.06

C82.27 Follicular lymphoma grade III, unspecified, spleen `CC`
CC Excl: See code: C82.07

C82.28 Follicular lymphoma grade III, unspecified, lymph nodes of multiple sites `CC`
CC Excl: See code: C82.08

C82.29 Follicular lymphoma grade III, unspecified, extranodal and solid organ sites `CC`
CC Excl: See code: C82.00

√5ᵗʰ **C82.3 Follicular lymphoma grade IIIa**

C82.30 Follicular lymphoma grade IIIa, unspecified sitespleen `CC`
CC Excl: See code: C82.00

C82.31 Follicular lymphoma grade IIIa, lymph nodes of head, face, and neck `CC`
CC Excl: See code: C82.01

C82.32 Follicular lymphoma grade IIIa, intrathoracic lymph nodes `CC`
CC Excl: See code: C82.02

C82.33 Follicular lymphoma grade IIIa, intra-abdominal lymph nodes `CC`
CC Excl: See code: C82.03

C82.34 Follicular lymphoma grade IIIa, lymph nodes of axilla and upper limb `CC`
CC Excl: See code: C82.04

C82.35 Follicular lymphoma grade IIIa, lymph nodes of inguinal region and lower limb `CC`
CC Excl: See code: C82.05

C82.36 Follicular lymphoma grade IIIa, intrapelvic lymph nodes `CC`
CC Excl: See code: C82.06

C82.37 Follicular lymphoma grade IIIa, spleen `CC`
CC Excl: See code: C82.07

C82.38 Follicular lymphoma grade IIIa, lymph nodes of multiple sites `CC`
CC Excl: See code: C82.08

C82.39 Follicular lymphoma grade IIIa, extranodal and solid organ sites `CC`
CC Excl: See code: C82.00

√5ᵗʰ **C82.4 Follicular lymphoma grade IIIb**

C82.40 Follicular lymphoma grade IIIb, unspecified site `CC`
CC Excl: See code: C82.00

C82.41 Follicular lymphoma grade IIIb, lymph nodes of head, face, and neck `CC`
CC Excl: See code: C82.01

C82.42 Follicular lymphoma grade IIIb, intrathoracic lymph nodes `CC`
CC Excl: See code: C82.02

C82.43 Follicular lymphoma grade IIIb, intra-abdominal lymph nodes `CC`
CC Excl: See code: C82.03

C82.44 Follicular lymphoma grade IIIb, lymph nodes of axilla and upper limb `CC`
CC Excl: See code: C82.04

C82.45 Follicular lymphoma grade IIIb, lymph nodes of inguinal region and lower limb `CC`
CC Excl: See code: C82.05

C82.46 Follicular lymphoma grade IIIb, intrapelvic lymph nodes `CC`
CC Excl: See code: C82.06

C82.47 Follicular lymphoma grade IIIb, spleen `CC`
CC Excl: See code: C82.07

C82.48 Follicular lymphoma grade IIIb, lymph nodes of multiple sites `CC`
CC Excl: See code: C82.08

C82.49 Follicular lymphoma grade IIIb, extranodal and solid organ sites `CC`
CC Excl: See code: C82.00

√5ᵗʰ **C82.5 Diffuse follicle center lymphoma**

C82.50 Diffuse follicle center lymphoma, unspecified site `HIV` `CC`
CC Excl: C82.50-C82.59, C83.10-C83.19, C84.40-C84.49, C84.60-C84.Z9, C85.10-C85.29, C85.80-C86.4, C88.4, C96.4, C96.9, C96.Z, D49.81-D49.9

C82.51 Diffuse follicle center lymphoma, lymph nodes of head, face, and neck `HIV` `CC`
CC Excl: C82.50-C82.51, C82.58-C82.59, C83.10-C83.11, C83.18-C83.19, C84.40-C84.41, C84.48-C84.49, C84.60-C84.61, C84.68-C84.71, C84.78-C84.91, C84.98-C84.A1, C84.A8-C84.Z1, C84.Z8-C84.Z9, C85.10-C85.11, C85.18-C85.21, C85.28-C85.29, C85.80-C85.81 C85.88-C85.91, C85.98-C86.0, C86.4, C88.4, D49.81-D49.9

C82.52 Diffuse follicle center lymphoma, intrathoracic lymph nodes `HIV` `CC`
CC Excl: C82.50-C82.52, C82.58-C82.59, C83.10, C83.12, C83.18-C83.19, C84.40, C84.42, C84.48-C84.49, C84.60, C84.62, C84.68-C84.70, C84.72, C84.78-C84.90, C84.92, C84.98-C84.A0, C84.A2, C84.A8-C84.Z0, C84.Z2, C84.Z8-C84.Z9, C85.10, C85.12, C85.18-C85.20, C85.22 C85.28-C85.29, C85.80, C85.82, C85.88-C85.90, C85.92, C85.98-C85.99, C86.4, C88.4, D49.81-D49.9

C82.53 Diffuse follicle center lymphoma, intra-abdominal lymph nodes `HIV` `CC`
CC Excl: C82.50-C82.53, C82.58-C82.59, C83.10, C83.13, C83.18-C83.19, C84.40, C84.43, C84.48-C84.49, C84.60, C84.63, C84.68-C84.70, C84.73, C84.78-C84.90, C84.93, C84.98-C84.A0, C84.A3, C84.A8-C84.Z0, C84.Z3, C84.Z8-C84.Z9, C85.10, C85.13, C85.18-C85.20, C85.23 C85.28-C85.29, C85.80, C85.83, C85.88-C85.90, C85.93, C85.98-C85.99, C86.2-C86.4, C88.4, D49.81-D49.9

C82.54 Diffuse follicle center lymphoma, lymph nodes of axilla and upper limb `HIV` `CC`
CC Excl: C82.50-C82.54, C82.58-C82.59, C83.10, C83.14, C83.18-C83.19, C84.40, C84.44, C84.48-C84.49, C84.60, C84.64, C84.68-C84.70, C84.74, C84.78-C84.90, C84.94, C84.98-C84.A0, C84.A4, C84.A8-C84.Z0, C84.Z4, C84.Z8-C84.Z9, C85.10, C85.14, C85.18-C85.20, C85.24 C85.28-C85.29, C85.80, C85.84, C85.88-C85.90, C85.94, C85.98-C85.99, C86.4, C88.4, D49.81-D49.9

C82.55 Diffuse follicle center lymphoma, lymph nodes of inguinal region and lower limb `HIV` `CC`
CC Excl: C82.50-C82.55, C82.58-C82.59, C83.10, C83.15, C83.18-C83.19, C84.40, C84.45, C84.48-C84.49, C84.60, C84.65, C84.68-C84.70, C84.75, C84.78-C84.90, C84.95, C84.98-C84.A0, C84.A5, C84.A8-C84.Z0, C84.Z5, C84.Z8-C84.Z9, C85.10, C85.15, C85.18-C85.20, C85.25 C85.28-C85.29, C85.80, C85.85, C85.88-C85.90, C85.95, C85.98-C85.99, C86.4, C88.4, D49.81-D49.9

C82.56 **Diffuse follicle center lymphoma, intrapelvic lymph nodes** `HIV` `CC`
  CC Excl: C82.50-C82.56, C82.58-C82.59, C83.10, C83.16, C83.18-C83.19, C84.40, C84.46, C84.48-C84.49, C84.60, C84.66, C84.68-C84.70, C84.76, C84.78-C84.90, C84.96, C84.98-C84.A0, C84.A6, C84.A8-C84.Z0, C84.Z6, C84.Z8-C84.Z9, C85.10, C85.16, C85.18-C85.20, C85.26 C85.28-C85.29, C85.80, C85.86, C85.88-C85.90, C85.96, C85.98-C85.99, C86.4, C88.4, D49.81-D49.9

C82.57 **Diffuse follicle center lymphoma, spleen** `HIV` `CC`
  CC Excl: C82.50, C82.57-C82.59, C83.10, C83.17-C83.19, C84.40, C84.47-C84.60, C84.67-C84.70, C84.77-C84.A0, C84.A7-C84.Z0, C84.Z7-C84.90, C84.97-C85.10, C85.17-C85.20, C85.27-C85.80, C85.87-C85.90, C85.97-C85.99, C86.1, C86.4, C88.4, D49.81-D49.9

C82.58 **Diffuse follicle center lymphoma, lymph nodes of multiple sites** `HIV` `CC`
  CC Excl: C82.50-C82.59, C83.10-C83.19, C84.40-C84.49, C84.60-C84.Z9, C85.10-C85.29, C85.80-C86.4, C88.4, D49.81-D49.9

C82.59 **Diffuse follicle center lymphoma, extranodal and solid organ sites** `HIV` `CC`
  CC Excl: See code: C82.50

✓5ᵗʰ C82.6 Cutaneous follicle center lymphoma

C82.60 **Cutaneous follicle center lymphoma, unspecified site** `CC`
  CC Excl: See code: C82.00

C82.61 **Cutaneous follicle center lymphoma, lymph nodes of head, face, and neck** `CC`
  CC Excl: See code: C82.01

C82.62 **Cutaneous follicle center lymphoma, intrathoracic lymph nodes** `CC`
  CC Excl: See code: C82.02

C82.63 **Cutaneous follicle center lymphoma, intra-abdominal lymph nodes** `CC`
  CC Excl: See code: C82.03

C82.64 **Cutaneous follicle center lymphoma, lymph nodes of axilla and upper limb** `CC`
  CC Excl: See code: C82.04

C82.65 **Cutaneous follicle center lymphoma, lymph nodes of inguinal region and lower limb** `CC`
  CC Excl: See code: C82.05

C82.66 **Cutaneous follicle center lymphoma, intrapelvic lymph nodes** `CC`
  CC Excl: See code: C82.06

C82.67 **Cutaneous follicle center lymphoma, spleen** `CC`
  CC Excl: See code: C82.07

C82.68 **Cutaneous follicle center lymphoma, lymph nodes of multiple sites** `CC`
  CC Excl: See code: C82.08

C82.69 **Cutaneous follicle center lymphoma, extranodal and solid organ sites** `CC`
  CC Excl: See code: C82.00

✓5ᵗʰ C82.8 Other types of follicular lymphoma

C82.80 **Other types of follicular lymphoma, unspecified site** `CC`
  CC Excl: See code: C82.00

C82.81 **Other types of follicular lymphoma, lymph nodes of head, face, and neck** `CC`
  CC Excl: See code: C82.01

C82.82 **Other types of follicular lymphoma, intrathoracic lymph nodes** `CC`
  CC Excl: See code: C82.02

C82.83 **Other types of follicular lymphoma, intra-abdominal lymph nodes** `CC`
  CC Excl: See code: C82.03

C82.84 **Other types of follicular lymphoma, lymph nodes of axilla and upper limb** `CC`
  CC Excl: See code: C82.04

C82.85 **Other types of follicular lymphoma, lymph nodes of inguinal region and lower limb** `CC`
  CC Excl: See code: C82.05

C82.86 **Other types of follicular lymphoma, intrapelvic lymph nodes** `CC`
  CC Excl: See code: C82.06

C82.87 **Other types of follicular lymphoma, spleen** `CC`
  CC Excl: See code: C82.07

C82.88 **Other types of follicular lymphoma, lymph nodes of multiple sites** `CC`
  CC Excl: See code: C82.08

C82.89 **Other types of follicular lymphoma, extranodal and solid organ sites** `CC`
  CC Excl: See code: C82.00

✓5ᵗʰ C82.9 Follicular lymphoma, unspecified

C82.90 **Follicular lymphoma, unspecified, unspecified site** `CC`
  CC Excl: See code: C82.00

C82.91 **Follicular lymphoma, unspecified, lymph nodes of head, face, and neck** `CC`
  CC Excl: See code: C82.01

C82.92 **Follicular lymphoma, unspecified, intrathoracic lymph nodes** `CC`
  CC Excl: See code: C82.02

C82.93 **Follicular lymphoma, unspecified, intra-abdominal lymph nodes** `CC`
  CC Excl: See code: C82.03

C82.94 **Follicular lymphoma, unspecified, lymph nodes of axilla and upper limb** `CC`
  CC Excl: See code: C82.04

C82.95 **Follicular lymphoma, unspecified, lymph nodes of inguinal region and lower limb** `CC`
  CC Excl: See code: C82.05

C82.96 **Follicular lymphoma, unspecified, intrapelvic lymph nodes** `CC`
  CC Excl: See code: C82.06

C82.97 **Follicular lymphoma, unspecified, spleen** `CC`
  CC Excl: See code: C82.07

C82.98 **Follicular lymphoma, unspecified, lymph nodes of multiple sites** `CC`
  CC Excl: See code: C82.08

C82.99 **Follicular lymphoma, unspecified, extranodal and solid organ sites** `CC`
  CC Excl: See code: C82.00

✓4ᵗʰ C83 Non-follicular lymphoma
  EXCLUDES 1   personal history of non-Hodgkin lymphoma (Z85.72)

✓5ᵗʰ C83.0 Small cell B-cell lymphoma
  Lymphoplasmacytic lymphoma
  Nodal marginal zone lymphoma
  Non-leukemic variant of B-CLL
  Splenic marginal zone lymphoma
  EXCLUDES 1   chronic lymphocytic leukemia (C91.1)
       mature T/NK-cell lymphomas (C84.-)
       Waldenström macroglobulinemia (C88.0)

C83.00 **Small cell B-cell lymphoma, unspecified site** `HIV` `CC`
  CC Excl: C83.00-C83.09, C83.80-C83.99, C86.5-C86.6, D49.81-D49.9

C83.01 **Small cell B-cell lymphoma, lymph nodes of head, face, and neck** `HIV` `CC`
  CC Excl: C83.00-C83.01, C83.08-C83.09, C83.80-C83.81, C83.88-C83.91, C83.98-C83.99, C86.5-C86.6, D49.81-D49.9

C83.02 **Small cell B-cell lymphoma, intrathoracic lymph nodes** `HIV` `CC`
  CC Excl: C83.00-C83.02, C83.08-C83.09, C83.80, C83.82, C83.88-C83.90, C83.92, C83.98-C83.99, C86.5-C86.6, D49.81-D49.9

C83.03 **Small cell B-cell lymphoma, intra-abdominal lymph nodes** `HIV` `CC`
  CC Excl: C83.00-C83.03, C83.08-C83.09, C83.80, C83.83, C83.88-C83.90, C83.93, C83.98-C83.99, C86.5-C86.6, D49.81-D49.9

C83.04 **Small cell B-cell lymphoma, lymph nodes of axilla and upper limb** `HIV` `CC`
  CC Excl: C83.00-C83.04, C83.08-C83.09, C83.80, C83.84, C83.88-C83.90, C83.94, C83.98-C83.99, C86.5-C86.6, D49.81-D49.9

C83.05 **Small cell B-cell lymphoma, lymph nodes of inguinal region and lower limb** `HIV` `CC`
  CC Excl: C83.00-C83.05, C83.08-C83.09, C83.80, C83.85, C83.88-C83.90, C83.95, C83.98-C83.99, C86.5-C86.6, D49.81-D49.9

C83.06 **Small cell B-cell lymphoma, intrapelvic lymph nodes** `HIV` `CC`
  CC Excl: C83.00-C83.06, C83.08-C83.09, C83.80, C83.86, C83.88-C83.90, C83.96, C83.98-C83.99, C86.5-C86.6, D49.81-D49.9

C83.07 **Small cell B-cell lymphoma, spleen** `HIV` `CC`
  CC Excl: C83.00, C83.07-C83.09, C83.80, C83.87-C83.90, C83.97-C83.99, C86.5-C86.6, D49.81-D49.9

C83.08 **Small cell B-cell lymphoma, lymph nodes of multiple sites** `HIV` `CC`
  CC Excl: C83.00-C83.09, C83.80-C83.99, C86.5-C86.6, D49.81-D49.9

C83.09 **Small cell B-cell lymphoma, extranodal and solid organ sites** `HIV` `CC`
  CC Excl: See code: C83.00

✓ Additional Character Required   ✓x7ᵗʰ Xtension Alert   Unacceptable PDx   Manifestation   Hospital Acquired Condition   *EXCLUDES 1* Not Coded Here   *EXCLUDES 2* Not Included Here

ICD-10-CM Draft (2015)   467

Neoplasms

C83.1–C83.85

√5ᵗʰ C83.1 Mantle cell lymphoma
Centrocytic lymphoma
Malignant lymphomatous polyposis

C83.10 Mantle cell lymphoma, unspecified site `HIV` `CC`
CC Excl: See code: C82.50

C83.11 Mantle cell lymphoma, lymph nodes of head, face, and neck `HIV` `CC`
CC Excl: See code: C82.51

C83.12 Mantle cell lymphoma, intrathoracic lymph nodes `HIV` `CC`
CC Excl: See code: C82.52

C83.13 Mantle cell lymphoma, intra-abdominal lymph nodes `HIV` `CC`
CC Excl: See code: C82.53

C83.14 Mantle cell lymphoma, lymph nodes of axilla and upper limb `HIV` `CC`
CC Excl: See code: C82.54

C83.15 Mantle cell lymphoma, lymph nodes of inguinal region and lower limb `HIV` `CC`
CC Excl: See code: C82.55

C83.16 Mantle cell lymphoma, intrapelvic lymph nodes `HIV` `CC`
CC Excl: See code: C82.56

C83.17 Mantle cell lymphoma, spleen `HIV` `CC`
CC Excl: See code: C82.57

C83.18 Mantle cell lymphoma, lymph nodes of multiple sites `HIV` `CC`
CC Excl: See code: C82.58

C83.19 Mantle cell lymphoma, extranodal and solid organ sites `HIV` `CC`
CC Excl: See code: C82.50

√5ᵗʰ C83.3 Diffuse large B-cell lymphoma
Anaplastic diffuse large B-cell lymphoma
CD30-positive diffuse large B-cell lymphoma
Centroblastic diffuse large B-cell lymphoma
Diffuse large B-cell lymphoma, subtype not specified
Immunoblastic diffuse large B-cell lymphoma
Plasmablastic diffuse large B-cell lymphoma
T-cell rich diffuse large B-cell lymphoma
EXCLUDES 1   mature T/NK-cell lymphomas (C84.-)
       mediastinal (thymic) large B-cell lymphoma (C85.2-)

C83.30 Diffuse large B-cell lymphoma, unspecified site `HIV` `CC`
CC Excl: C83.30-C83.39, D49.81-D49.9

C83.31 Diffuse large B-cell lymphoma, lymph nodes of head, face, and neck `HIV` `CC`
CC Excl: C83.30-C83.31, C83.38-C83.39, D49.81-D49.9

C83.32 Diffuse large B-cell lymphoma, intrathoracic lymph nodes `HIV` `CC`
CC Excl: C83.30-C83.32, C83.38-C83.39, D49.81-D49.9

C83.33 Diffuse large B-cell lymphoma, intra-abdominal lymph nodes `HIV` `CC`
CC Excl: C83.30-C83.33, C83.38-C83.39, D49.81-D49.9

C83.34 Diffuse large B-cell lymphoma, lymph nodes of axilla and upper limb `HIV` `CC`
CC Excl: C83.30-C83.34, C83.38-C83.39, D49.81-D49.9

C83.35 Diffuse large B-cell lymphoma, lymph nodes of inguinal region and lower limb `HIV` `CC`
CC Excl: C83.30-C83.35, C83.38-C83.39, D49.81-D49.9

C83.36 Diffuse large B-cell lymphoma, intrapelvic lymph nodes `HIV` `CC`
CC Excl: C83.30-C83.36, C83.38-C83.39, D49.81-D49.9

C83.37 Diffuse large B-cell lymphoma, spleen `HIV` `CC`
CC Excl: C83.30, C83.37-C83.39, D49.81-D49.9

C83.38 Diffuse large B-cell lymphoma, lymph nodes of multiple sites `HIV` `CC`
CC Excl: C83.30-C83.39, D49.81-D49.9

C83.39 Diffuse large B-cell lymphoma, extranodal and solid organ sites `HIV` `CC`
CC Excl: See code: C83.38

√5ᵗʰ C83.5 Lymphoblastic (diffuse) lymphoma
B-precursor lymphoma
Lymphoblastic B-cell lymphoma
Lymphoblastic lymphoma NOS
Lymphoblastic T-cell lymphoma
T-precursor lymphoma

C83.50 Lymphoblastic (diffuse) lymphoma, unspecified site `CC`
CC Excl: C83.50-C83.59, D49.81-D49.9

C83.51 Lymphoblastic (diffuse) lymphoma, lymph nodes of head, face, and neck `CC`
CC Excl: C83.50-C83.51, C83.58-C83.59, D49.81-D49.9

C83.52 Lymphoblastic (diffuse) lymphoma, intrathoracic lymph nodes `CC`
CC Excl: C83.50, C83.52, C83.58-C83.59, D49.81-D49.9

C83.53 Lymphoblastic (diffuse) lymphoma, intra-abdominal lymph nodes `CC`
CC Excl: C83.50, C83.53, C83.58-C83.59, D49.81-D49.9

C83.54 Lymphoblastic (diffuse) lymphoma, lymph nodes of axilla and upper limb `CC`
CC Excl: C83.50, C83.54, C83.58-C83.59, D49.81-D49.9

C83.55 Lymphoblastic (diffuse) lymphoma, lymph nodes of inguinal region and lower limb `CC`
CC Excl: C83.50, C83.55, C83.58-C83.59, D49.81-D49.9

C83.56 Lymphoblastic (diffuse) lymphoma, intrapelvic lymph nodes `CC`
CC Excl: C83.50, C83.56, C83.58-C83.59, D49.81-D49.9

C83.57 Lymphoblastic (diffuse) lymphoma, spleen `CC`
CC Excl: C83.50, C83.57-C83.59, D49.81-D49.9

C83.58 Lymphoblastic (diffuse) lymphoma, lymph nodes of multiple sites `CC`
CC Excl: See code: C83.50

C83.59 Lymphoblastic (diffuse) lymphoma, extranodal and solid organ sites `CC`
CC Excl: See code: C83.50

√5ᵗʰ C83.7 Burkitt lymphoma
Atypical Burkitt lymphoma
Burkitt-like lymphoma
EXCLUDES 1   mature B-cell leukemia Burkitt type (C91.A-)

C83.70 Burkitt lymphoma, unspecified site `HIV` `CC`
CC Excl: C83.70-C83.79, D49.81-D49.9

C83.71 Burkitt lymphoma, lymph nodes of head, face, and neck `HIV` `CC`
CC Excl: C83.70-C83.71, C83.78-C83.79, D49.81-D49.9

C83.72 Burkitt lymphoma, intrathoracic lymph nodes `HIV` `CC`
CC Excl: C83.70, C83.72, C83.78-C83.79, D49.81-D49.9

C83.73 Burkitt lymphoma, intra-abdominal lymph nodes `HIV` `CC`
CC Excl: C83.70, C83.73, C83.78-C83.79, D49.81-D49.9

C83.74 Burkitt lymphoma, lymph nodes of axilla and upper limb `HIV` `CC`
CC Excl: C83.70, C83.74, C83.78-C83.79, D49.81-D49.9

C83.75 Burkitt lymphoma, lymph nodes of inguinal region and lower limb `HIV` `CC`
CC Excl: C83.70, C83.75, C83.78-C83.79, D49.81-D49.9

C83.76 Burkitt lymphoma, intrapelvic lymph nodes `HIV` `CC`
CC Excl: C83.70, C83.76, C83.78-C83.79, D49.81-D49.9

C83.77 Burkitt lymphoma, spleen `HIV` `CC`
CC Excl: C83.70, C83.77-C83.79, D49.81-D49.9

C83.78 Burkitt lymphoma, lymph nodes of multiple sites `HIV` `CC`
CC Excl: See code: C83.70

C83.79 Burkitt lymphoma, extranodal and solid organ sites `HIV` `CC`
CC Excl: See code: C83.70

√5ᵗʰ C83.8 Other non-follicular lymphoma
Intravascular large B-cell lymphoma
Lymphoid granulomatosis
Primary effusion B-cell lymphoma
EXCLUDES 1   mediastinal (thymic) large B-cell lymphoma (C85.2-)
       T-cell rich B-cell lymphoma (C83.3-)

C83.80 Other non-follicular lymphoma, unspecified site `HIV` `CC`
CC Excl: See code: C83.00

C83.81 Other non-follicular lymphoma, lymph nodes of head, face, and neck `HIV` `CC`
CC Excl: See code: C83.01

C83.82 Other non-follicular lymphoma, intrathoracic lymph nodes `HIV` `CC`
CC Excl: See code: C83.02

C83.83 Other non-follicular lymphoma, intra-abdominal lymph nodes `HIV` `CC`
CC Excl: See code: C83.03

C83.84 Other non-follicular lymphoma, lymph nodes of axilla and upper limb `HIV` `CC`
CC Excl: See code: C83.04

C83.85 Other non-follicular lymphoma, lymph nodes of inguinal region and lower limb `HIV` `CC`
CC Excl: See code: C83.05

N Newborn: 0   P Pediatric: 0-17   M Maternity: 12-55   A Adult: 15-124   MCC Major CC Condition   PDx MCC PDx acts as own MCC   CC CC Condition   PDx CC PDx acts as own CC

468   ICD-10-CM Draft (2015)

C83.86 **Other non-follicular lymphoma, intrapelvic lymph nodes** `HIV` `CC`
CC Excl: See code: C83.06

C83.87 **Other non-follicular lymphoma, spleen** `HIV` `CC`
CC Excl: See code: C83.07

C83.88 **Other non-follicular lymphoma, lymph nodes of multiple sites** `HIV` `CC`
CC Excl: See code: C83.00

C83.89 **Other non-follicular lymphoma, extranodal and solid organ sites** `HIV` `CC`
CC Excl: See code: C83.00

✓5ᵗʰ **C83.9** **Non-follicular (diffuse) lymphoma, unspecified**

C83.90 **Non-follicular (diffuse) lymphoma, unspecified, unspecified site** `HIV` `CC`
CC Excl: See code: C83.00

C83.91 **Non-follicular (diffuse) lymphoma, unspecified, lymph nodes of head, face, and neck** `HIV` `CC`
CC Excl: See code: C83.01

C83.92 **Non-follicular (diffuse) lymphoma, unspecified, intrathoracic lymph nodes** `HIV` `CC`
CC Excl: See code: C83.02

C83.93 **Non-follicular (diffuse) lymphoma, unspecified, intra-abdominal lymph nodes** `HIV` `CC`
CC Excl: See code: C83.03

C83.94 **Non-follicular (diffuse) lymphoma, unspecified, lymph nodes of axilla and upper limb** `HIV` `CC`
CC Excl: See code: C83.04

C83.95 **Non-follicular (diffuse) lymphoma, unspecified, lymph nodes of inguinal region and lower limb** `HIV` `CC`
CC Excl: See code: C83.05

C83.96 **Non-follicular (diffuse) lymphoma, unspecified, intrapelvic lymph nodes** `HIV` `CC`
CC Excl: See code: C83.06

C83.97 **Non-follicular (diffuse) lymphoma, unspecified, spleen** `HIV` `CC`
CC Excl: See code: C83.07

C83.98 **Non-follicular (diffuse) lymphoma, unspecified, lymph nodes of multiple sites** `HIV` `CC`
CC Excl: See code: C83.00

C83.99 **Non-follicular (diffuse) lymphoma, unspecified, extranodal and solid organ sites** `HIV` `CC`
CC Excl: See code: C83.00

✓4ᵗʰ **C84** **Mature T/NK-cell lymphomas**
EXCLUDES 1 personal history of non-Hodgkin lymphoma (Z85.72)

✓5ᵗʰ **C84.0** **Mycosis fungoides**
EXCLUDES 1 peripheral T-cell lymphoma, not classified (C84.4-)

C84.00 **Mycosis fungoides, unspecified site** `CC`
CC Excl: C82.50, C82.59, C83.10, C83.19, C84.00-C84.09, C84.40, C84.49, C84.60, C84.69-C84.70, C84.79-C84.90, C84.99-C84.A0, C84.A9-C84.Z0, C84.Z9, C85.10, C85.19-C85.20, C85.29, C85.80, C85.89-C85.90, C85.99, C86.4, C88.4, C96.4, C96.9, C96.Z, D49.81-D49.9

C84.01 **Mycosis fungoides, lymph nodes of head, face, and neck** `CC`
CC Excl: C82.51, C83.11, C84.00-C84.01, C84.08-C84.09, C84.41, C84.61, C84.71, C84.91, C84.A1, C84.Z1, C85.11, C85.21, C85.81, C85.91, C86.0, D49.81-D49.9

C84.02 **Mycosis fungoides, intrathoracic lymph nodes** `CC`
CC Excl: C82.52, C83.12, C84.00, C84.02, C84.08-C84.09, C84.42, C84.62, C84.72, C84.92, C84.A2, C84.Z2, C85.12, C85.22, C85.82, C85.92, D49.81-D49.9

C84.03 **Mycosis fungoides, intra-abdominal lymph nodes** `CC`
CC Excl: C82.53, C83.13, C84.00, C84.03, C84.08-C84.09, C84.43, C84.63, C84.73, C84.93, C84.A3, C84.Z3, C85.13, C85.23, C85.83, C85.93, C86.2-C86.3, D49.81-D49.9

C84.04 **Mycosis fungoides, lymph nodes of axilla and upper limb** `CC`
CC Excl: C82.54, C83.14, C84.00, C84.04, C84.08-C84.09, C84.44, C84.64, C84.74, C84.94, C84.A4, C84.Z4, C85.14, C85.24, C85.84, C85.94, D49.81-D49.9

C84.05 **Mycosis fungoides, lymph nodes of inguinal region and lower limb** `CC`
CC Excl: C82.55, C83.15, C84.00, C84.05, C84.08-C84.09, C84.45, C84.65, C84.75, C84.95, C84.A5, C84.Z5, C85.15, C85.25, C85.85, C85.95, D49.81-D49.9

C84.06 **Mycosis fungoides, intrapelvic lymph nodes** `CC`
CC Excl: C82.56, C83.16, C84.00, C84.06, C84.08-C84.09, C84.46, C84.66, C84.76, C84.96, C84.A6, C84.Z6, C85.16, C85.26, C85.86, C85.96, D49.81-D49.9

C84.07 **Mycosis fungoides, spleen** `CC`
CC Excl: C82.57, C83.17, C84.00, C84.07-C84.09, C84.47, C84.67, C84.77, C84.97, C84.A7, C84.Z7, C85.17, C85.27, C85.87, C85.97, C86.1, D49.81-D49.9

C84.08 **Mycosis fungoides, lymph nodes of multiple sites** `CC`
CC Excl: C82.58, C83.18, C84.00-C84.09, C84.48, C84.68, C84.78, C84.98, C84.A8, C84.Z8, C85.18, C85.28, C85.88, C85.98, D49.81-D49.9

C84.09 **Mycosis fungoides, extranodal and solid organ sites** `CC`
CC Excl: See code: C84.00

✓5ᵗʰ **C84.1** **Sézary disease**

C84.10 **Sézary disease, unspecified site** `CC`
CC Excl: C82.50, C82.59, C83.10, C83.19, C84.10-C84.19, C84.40, C84.49, C84.60, C84.69-C84.70, C84.79-C84.90, C84.99-C84.A0, C84.A9-C84.Z0, C84.Z9, C85.10, C85.19-C85.20, C85.29, C85.80, C85.89-C85.90, C85.99, C86.4, C88.4, C96.4, C96.9, C96.Z, D49.81-D49.9

C84.11 **Sézary disease, lymph nodes of head, face, and neck** `CC`
CC Excl: C82.51, C83.11, C84.10-C84.11, C84.18-C84.19, C84.41, C84.61, C84.71, C84.91, C84.A1, C84.Z1, C85.11, C85.21, C85.81, C85.91, C86.0, D49.81-D49.9

C84.12 **Sézary disease, intrathoracic lymph nodes** `CC`
CC Excl: C82.52, C83.12, C84.10, C84.12, C84.18-C84.19, C84.42, C84.62, C84.72, C84.92, C84.A2, C84.Z2, C85.12, C85.22, C85.82, C85.92, D49.81-D49.9

C84.13 **Sézary disease, intra-abdominal lymph nodes** `CC`
CC Excl: C82.53, C83.13, C84.10, C84.13, C84.18-C84.19, C84.43, C84.63, C84.73, C84.93, C84.A3, C84.Z3, C85.13, C85.23, C85.83, C85.93, C86.2-C86.3, D49.81-D49.9

C84.14 **Sézary disease, lymph nodes of axilla and upper limb** `CC`
CC Excl: C82.54, C83.14, C84.10, C84.14, C84.18-C84.19, C84.44, C84.64, C84.74, C84.94, C84.A4, C84.Z4, C85.14, C85.24, C85.84, C85.94, D49.81-D49.9

C84.15 **Sézary disease, lymph nodes of inguinal region and lower limb** `CC`
CC Excl: C82.55, C83.15, C84.10, C84.15, C84.18-C84.19, C84.45, C84.65, C84.75, C84.95, C84.A5, C84.Z5, C85.15, C85.25, C85.85, C85.95, D49.81-D49.9

C84.16 **Sézary disease, intrapelvic lymph nodes** `CC`
CC Excl: C82.56, C83.16, C84.10, C84.16, C84.18-C84.19, C84.46, C84.66, C84.76, C84.96, C84.A6, C84.Z6, C85.16, C85.26, C85.86, C85.96, D49.81-D49.9

C84.17 **Sézary disease, spleen** `CC`
CC Excl: C82.57, C83.17, C84.10, C84.17-C84.19, C84.47, C84.67, C84.77, C84.97, C84.A7, C84.Z7, C85.17, C85.27, C85.87, C85.97, C86.1, D49.81-D49.9

C84.18 **Sézary disease, lymph nodes of multiple sites** `CC`
CC Excl: C82.58, C83.18, C84.10-C84.19, C84.48, C84.68, C84.78, C84.98, C84.A8, C84.Z8, C85.18, C85.28, C85.88, C85.98, D49.81-D49.9

C84.19 **Sézary disease, extranodal and solid organ sites** `CC`
CC Excl: See code: C84.10

✓5ᵗʰ **C84.4** **Peripheral T-cell lymphoma, not classified**
Lennert's lymphoma
Lymphoepithelioid lymphoma
Mature T-cell lymphoma, not elsewhere classified

C84.40 **Peripheral T-cell lymphoma, not classified, unspecified site** `HIV` `CC`
CC Excl: See code: C82.50

C84.41 **Peripheral T-cell lymphoma, not classified, lymph nodes of head, face, and neck** `HIV` `CC`
CC Excl: See code: C82.51

C84.42 **Peripheral T-cell lymphoma, not classified, intrathoracic lymph nodes** `HIV` `CC`
CC Excl: See code: C82.52

C84.43 **Peripheral T-cell lymphoma, not classified, intra-abdominal lymph nodes** `HIV` `CC`
CC Excl: See code: C82.53

C84.44 **Peripheral T-cell lymphoma, not classified, lymph nodes of axilla and upper limb** `HIV` `CC`
CC Excl: See code: C82.54

C84.45 **Peripheral T-cell lymphoma, not classified, lymph nodes of inguinal region and lower limb** `HIV` `CC`
CC Excl: See code: C82.55

C84.46 **Peripheral T-cell lymphoma, not classified, intrapelvic lymph nodes** `HIV` `CC`
CC Excl: See code: C82.56

C84.47 **Peripheral T-cell lymphoma, not classified, spleen** `HIV` `CC`
CC Excl: See code: C82.57

Neoplasms

C84.48 **Peripheral T-cell lymphoma, not classified, lymph nodes of multiple sites** HIV CC
CC Excl: See code: C82.58

C84.49 **Peripheral T-cell lymphoma, not classified, extranodal and solid organ sites** HIV CC
CC Excl: See code: C82.50

✓5th **C84.6** **Anaplastic large cell lymphoma, ALK-positive**
Anaplastic large cell lymphoma, CD30-positive

C84.60 **Anaplastic large cell lymphoma, ALK-positive,** HIV CC
unspecified site
CC Excl: See code: C82.50

C84.61 **Anaplastic large cell lymphoma, ALK-positive,** HIV CC
lymph nodes of head, face, and neck
CC Excl: See code: C82.51

C84.62 **Anaplastic large cell lymphoma, ALK-positive,** HIV CC
intrathoracic lymph nodes
CC Excl: See code: C82.52

C84.63 **Anaplastic large cell lymphoma, ALK-positive,** HIV CC
intra-abdominal lymph nodes
CC Excl: See code: C82.53

C84.64 **Anaplastic large cell lymphoma, ALK-positive,** HIV CC
lymph nodes of axilla and upper limb
CC Excl: See code: C82.54

C84.65 **Anaplastic large cell lymphoma, ALK-positive,** HIV CC
lymph nodes of inguinal region and lower limb
CC Excl: See code: C82.55

C84.66 **Anaplastic large cell lymphoma, ALK-positive,** HIV CC
intrapelvic lymph nodes
CC Excl: See code: C82.56

C84.67 **Anaplastic large cell lymphoma, ALK-positive,** HIV CC
spleen
CC Excl: See code: C82.57

C84.68 **Anaplastic large cell lymphoma, ALK-positive,** HIV CC
lymph nodes of multiple sites
CC Excl: See code: C82.58

C84.69 **Anaplastic large cell lymphoma, ALK-positive,** HIV CC
extranodal and solid organ sites
CC Excl: See code: C82.50

✓5th **C84.7** **Anaplastic large cell lymphoma, ALK-negative**
EXCLUDES 1 *primary cutaneous CD30-positive T-cell proliferations (C86.6-)*

C84.70 **Anaplastic large cell lymphoma, ALK-negative,** HIV CC
unspecified site
CC Excl: See code: C82.50

C84.71 **Anaplastic large cell lymphoma,** HIV CC
ALK-negative, lymph nodes of head, face, and neck
CC Excl: See code: C82.51

C84.72 **Anaplastic large cell lymphoma, ALK-negative,** HIV CC
intrathoracic lymph nodes
CC Excl: See code: C82.52

C84.73 **Anaplastic large cell lymphoma, ALK-negative,** HIV CC
intra-abdominal lymph nodes
CC Excl: See code: C82.53

C84.74 **Anaplastic large cell lymphoma,** HIV CC
ALK-negative, lymph nodes of axilla and upper limb
CC Excl: See code: C82.54

C84.75 **Anaplastic large cell lymphoma,** HIV CC
ALK-negative, lymph nodes of inguinal region and lower limb
CC Excl: See code: C82.55

C84.76 **Anaplastic large cell lymphoma, ALK-negative,** HIV CC
intrapelvic lymph nodes
CC Excl: See code: C82.56

C84.77 **Anaplastic large cell lymphoma,** HIV CC
ALK-negative, spleen
CC Excl: See code: C82.57

C84.78 **Anaplastic large cell lymphoma,** HIV CC
ALK-negative, lymph nodes of multiple sites
CC Excl: See code: C82.58

C84.79 **Anaplastic large cell lymphoma, ALK-negative,** HIV CC
extranodal and solid organ sites
CC Excl: See code: C82.50

✓5th **C84.A** **Cutaneous T-cell lymphoma, unspecified**

C84.A0 **Cutaneous T-cell lymphoma, unspecified,** HIV CC
unspecified site
CC Excl: See code: C82.50

C84.A1 **Cutaneous T-cell lymphoma, unspecified** HIV CC
lymph nodes of head, face, and neck
CC Excl: See code: C82.51

C84.A2 **Cutaneous T-cell lymphoma, unspecified,** HIV CC
intrathoracic lymph nodes
CC Excl: See code: C82.52

C84.A3 **Cutaneous T-cell lymphoma, unspecified,** HIV CC
intra-abdominal lymph nodes
CC Excl: See code: C82.53

C84.A4 **Cutaneous T-cell lymphoma, unspecified,** HIV CC
lymph nodes of axilla and upper limb
CC Excl: See code: C82.54

C84.A5 **Cutaneous T-cell lymphoma, unspecified,** HIV CC
lymph nodes of inguinal region and lower limb
CC Excl: See code: C82.55

C84.A6 **Cutaneous T-cell lymphoma, unspecified,** HIV CC
intrapelvic lymph nodes
CC Excl: See code: C82.56

C84.A7 **Cutaneous T-cell lymphoma, unspecified,** HIV CC
spleen
CC Excl: See code: C82.57

C84.A8 **Cutaneous T-cell lymphoma, unspecified,** HIV CC
lymph nodes of multiple sites
CC Excl: See code: C82.58

C84.A9 **Cutaneous T-cell lymphoma, unspecified,** HIV CC
extranodal and solid organ sites
CC Excl: See code: C82.50

✓5th **C84.Z** **Other mature T/NK-cell lymphomas**
NOTE   If T-cell lineage or involvement is mentioned in conjunction with a specific lymphoma, code to the more specific description.
EXCLUDES 1   *angioimmunoblastic T-cell lymphoma (C86.5)*
blastic NK-cell lymphoma (C86.4)
enteropathy-type T-cell lymphoma (C86.2)
extranodal NK-cell lymphoma, nasal type (C86.0)
hepatosplenic T-cell lymphoma (C86.1)
primary cutaneous CD30-positive T-cell proliferations (C86.6)
subcutaneous panniculitis-like T-cell lymphoma (C86.3)
T-cell leukemia (C91.1-)

C84.Z0 **Other mature T/NK-cell lymphomas,** HIV CC
unspecified site
CC Excl: See code: C82.50

C84.Z1 **Other mature T/NK-cell lymphomas, lymph** HIV CC
nodes of head, face, and neck
CC Excl: See code: C82.51

C84.Z2 **Other mature T/NK-cell lymphomas,** HIV CC
intrathoracic lymph nodes
CC Excl: See code: C82.52

C84.Z3 **Other mature T/NK-cell lymphomas, intra-** HIV CC
abdominal lymph nodes
CC Excl: See code: C82.53

C84.Z4 **Other mature T/NK-cell lymphomas, lymph** HIV CC
nodes of axilla and upper limb
CC Excl: See code: C82.54

C84.Z5 **Other mature T/NK-cell lymphomas, lymph** HIV CC
nodes of inguinal region and lower limb
CC Excl: See code: C82.55

C84.Z6 **Other mature T/NK-cell lymphomas,** HIV CC
intrapelvic lymph nodes
CC Excl: See code: C82.56

C84.Z7 **Other mature T/NK-cell lymphomas, spleen** HIV CC
CC Excl: See code: C82.57

C84.Z8 **Other mature T/NK-cell lymphomas, lymph** HIV CC
ndoes of multiple sites
CC Excl: See code: C82.58

C84.Z9 **Other mature T/NK-cell lymphomas,** HIV CC
extranodal and solid organ sites
CC Excl: See code: C82.50

✓5th **C84.9** **Mature T/NK-cell lymphomas, unspecified**
NK/T cell lymphoma NOS
EXCLUDES 1 *mature T-cell lymphoma, not elsewhere classified (C84.4-)*

C84.90 **Mature T/NK-cell lymphomas, unspecified,** HIV CC
unspecified site
CC Excl: See code: C82.50

C84.91 **Mature T/NK-cell lymphomas, unspecified,** HIV CC
lymph nodes of head, face, and neck
CC Excl: See code: C82.51

C84.92 **Mature T/NK-cell lymphomas, unspecified,** HIV CC
intrathoracic lymph nodes
CC Excl: See code: C82.52

C84.93 **Mature T/NK-cell lymphomas, unspecified,** HIV CC
intra-abdominal lymph nodes
CC Excl: See code: C82.53

C84.94 Mature T/NK-cell lymphomas, unspecified, `HIV` `CC`
lymph nodes of axilla and upper limb
CC Excl: See code: C82.54

C84.95 Mature T/NK-cell lymphomas, unspecified, `HIV` `CC`
lymph nodes of inguinal region and lower limb
CC Excl: See code: C82.55

C84.96 Mature T/NK-cell lymphomas, unspecified, `HIV` `CC`
intrapelvic lymph nodes
CC Excl: See code: C82.56

C84.97 Mature T/NK-cell lymphomas, unspecified, `HIV` `CC`
spleen
CC Excl: See code: C82.57

C84.98 Mature T/NK-cell lymphomas, unspecified, `HIV` `CC`
lymph nodes of multiple sites
CC Excl: See code: C82.58

C84.99 Mature T/NK-cell lymphomas, unspecified, `HIV` `CC`
extranodal and solid organ sites
CC Excl: See code: C82.50

`√4th` **C85** Other specified and unspecified types of non-Hodgkin
lymphoma
`EXCLUDES 1` other specified types of T/NK-cell lymphoma (C86.-)
personal history of non-Hodgkin lymphoma (Z85.72)

`√5th` **C85.1** Unspecified B-cell lymphoma
`NOTE` If B-cell lineage or involvement is mentioned in
conjunction with a specific lymphoma, code to the
more specific description.

C85.10 Unspecified B-cell lymphoma, unspecified site `HIV` `CC`
CC Excl: See code: C82.50

C85.11 Unspecified B-cell lymphoma, lymph nodes of `HIV` `CC`
head, face, and neck
CC Excl: See code: C82.51

C85.12 Unspecified B-cell lymphoma, intrathoracic `HIV` `CC`
lymph nodes
CC Excl: See code: C82.52

C85.13 Unspecified B-cell lymphoma, intra-abdominal `HIV` `CC`
lymph nodes
CC Excl: See code: C82.53

C85.14 Unspecified B-cell lymphoma, lymph nodes of `HIV` `CC`
axilla and upper limb
CC Excl: See code: C82.54

C85.15 Unspecified B-cell lymphoma, lymph nodes of `HIV` `CC`
inguinal region and lower limb
CC Excl: See code: C82.55

C85.16 Unspecified B-cell lymphoma, intrapelvic `HIV` `CC`
lymph nodes
CC Excl: See code: C82.56

C85.17 Unspecified B-cell lymphoma, spleen `HIV` `CC`
CC Excl: See code: C82.57

C85.18 Unspecified B-cell lymphoma, lymph nodes of `HIV` `CC`
multiple sites
CC Excl: See code: C82.58

C85.19 Unspecified B-cell lymphoma, extranodal and `HIV` `CC`
solid organ sites
CC Excl: See code: C82.50

`√5th` **C85.2** Mediastinal (thymic) large B-cell lymphoma

C85.20 Mediastinal (thymic) large B-cell lymphoma, `HIV` `CC`
unspecified site
CC Excl: See code: C82.50

C85.21 Mediastinal (thymic) large B-cell lymphoma, `HIV` `CC`
lymph nodes of head, face, and neck
CC Excl: See code: C82.51

C85.22 Mediastinal (thymic) large B-cell lymphoma, `HIV` `CC`
intrathoracic lymph nodes
CC Excl: See code: C82.52

C85.23 Mediastinal (thymic) large B-cell lymphoma, `HIV` `CC`
intra-abdominal lymph nodes
CC Excl: See code: C82.53

C85.24 Mediastinal (thymic) large B-cell lymphoma, `HIV` `CC`
lymph nodes of axilla and upper limb
CC Excl: See code: C82.54

C85.25 Mediastinal (thymic) large B-cell lymphoma, `HIV` `CC`
lymph nodes of inguinal region and lower limb
CC Excl: See code: C82.55

C85.26 Mediastinal (thymic) large B-cell lymphoma, `HIV` `CC`
intrapelvic lymph nodes
CC Excl: See code: C82.56

C85.27 Mediastinal (thymic) large B-cell lymphoma, `HIV` `CC`
spleen
CC Excl: See code: C82.57

C85.28 Mediastinal (thymic) large B-cell lymphoma, `HIV` `CC`
lymph nodes of multiple sites
CC Excl: See code: C82.58

C85.29 Mediastinal (thymic) large B-cell lymphoma, `HIV` `CC`
extranodal and solid organ sites
CC Excl: See code: C82.50

`√5th` **C85.8** Other specified types of non-Hodgkin lymphoma

C85.80 Other specified types of non-Hodgkin `HIV` `CC`
lymphoma, unspecified site
CC Excl: See code: C82.50

C85.81 Other specified types of non-Hodgkin `HIV` `CC`
lymphoma, lymph nodes of head, face, and neck
CC Excl: See code: C82.51

C85.82 Other specified types of non-Hodgkin `HIV` `CC`
lymphoma, intrathoracic lymph nodes
CC Excl: See code: C82.52

C85.83 Other specified types of non-Hodgkin `HIV` `CC`
lymphoma, intra-abdominal lymph nodes
CC Excl: See code: C82.53

C85.84 Other specified types of non-Hodgkin `HIV` `CC`
lymphoma, lymph nodes of axilla and upper limb
CC Excl: See code: C82.54

C85.85 Other specified types of non-Hodgkin `HIV` `CC`
lymphoma, lymph nodes of inguinal region
and lower limb
CC Excl: See code: C82.55

C85.86 Other specified types of non-Hodgkin `HIV` `CC`
lymphoma, intrapelvic lymph nodes
CC Excl: See code: C82.56

C85.87 Other specified types of non-Hodgkin `HIV` `CC`
lymphoma, spleen
CC Excl: See code: C82.57

C85.88 Other specified types of non-Hodgkin `HIV` `CC`
lymphoma, lymph nodes of multiple sites
CC Excl: See code: C82.58

C85.89 Other specified types of non-Hodgkin `HIV` `CC`
lymphoma, extranodal and solid organ sites
CC Excl: See code: C82.50

`√5th` **C85.9** Non-Hodgkin lymphoma, unspecified
Lymphoma NOS
Malignant lymphoma NOS
Non-Hodgkin lymphoma NOS

C85.90 Non-Hodgkin lymphoma, unspecified, `HIV` `CC`
unspecified site
CC Excl: See code: C82.50

C85.91 Non-Hodgkin lymphoma, unspecified, lymph `HIV` `CC`
nodes of head, face, and neck
CC Excl: See code: C82.51

C85.92 Non-Hodgkin lymphoma, unspecified, `HIV` `CC`
intrathoracic lymph nodes
CC Excl: See code: C82.52

C85.93 Non-Hodgkin lymphoma, unspecified, `HIV` `CC`
intra-abdominal lymph nodes
CC Excl: See code: C82.53

C85.94 Non-Hodgkin lymphoma, unspecified, lymph `HIV` `CC`
nodes of axilla and upper limb
CC Excl: See code: C82.54

C85.95 Non-Hodgkin lymphoma, unspecified, lymph `HIV` `CC`
nodes of inguinal region and lower limb
CC Excl: See code: C82.55

C85.96 Non-Hodgkin lymphoma, unspecified, `HIV` `CC`
intrapelvic lymph nodes
CC Excl: See code: C82.56

C85.97 Non-Hodgkin lymphoma, unspecified, spleen `HIV` `CC`
CC Excl: See code: C82.57

C85.98 Non-Hodgkin lymphoma, unspecified, lymph `HIV` `CC`
nodes of multiple sites
CC Excl: See code: C82.58

C85.99 Non-Hodgkin lymphoma, unspecified, `HIV` `CC`
extranodal and solid organ sites
CC Excl: See code: C82.50

`√4th` **C86** Other specified types of T/NK-cell lymphoma
`EXCLUDES 1` anaplastic large cell lymphoma, ALK negative (C84.7-)
anaplastic large cell lymphoma, ALK positive (C84.6-)
mature T/NK-cell lymphomas (C84.-)
other specified types of non-Hodgkin lymphoma (C85.8-)

C86.0 Extranodal NK/T-cell lymphoma, nasal type `HIV` `CC`
CC Excl: See code: C82.51

C86.1 Hepatosplenic T-cell lymphoma `HIV` `CC`
Alpha-beta and gamma delta types
CC Excl: See code: C82.57

✔ Additional Character Required   `√x7th` Xtension Alert   Unacceptable PDx   Manifestation   Hospital Acquired Condition   `EXCLUDES 1` Not Coded Here   `EXCLUDES 2` Not Included Here

Neoplasms

C86.2 Enteropathy-type (intestinal) T-cell lymphoma `HIV` `CC`
Enteropathy associated T-cell lymphoma
CC Excl: See code: C82.53

C86.3 Subcutaneous panniculitis-like T-cell lymphoma `HIV` `CC`
CC Excl: See code: C82.53

C86.4 Blastic NK-cell lymphoma `HIV` `CC`
CC Excl: See code: C82.50

C86.5 Angioimmunoblastic T-cell lymphoma `HIV` `CC`
Angioimmunoblastic lymphadenopathy with dysproteinemia [AILD]
CC Excl: See code: C83.00

C86.6 Primary cutaneous CD30-positive T-cell proliferations `HIV` `CC`
Lymphomatoid papulosis
Primary cutaneous anaplastic large cell lymphoma
Primary cutaneous CD30-positive large T-cell lymphoma
CC Excl: See code: C83.00

✓4ᵗʰ **C88 Malignant immunoproliferative diseases and certain other B-cell lymphomas**
EXCLUDES 1   *B-cell lymphoma, unspecified (C85.1-)*
personal history of other malignant neoplasms of lymphoid, hematopoietic and related tissues (Z85.79)

C88.0 Waldenström macroglobulinemia
Lymphoplasmacytic lymphoma with IgM-production
Macroglobulinemia (idiopathic) (primary)
EXCLUDES 1   *small cell B-cell lymphoma (C83.0)*

C88.2 Heavy chain disease `CC`
Franklin disease
Gamma heavy chain disease
Mu heavy chain disease
CC Excl: C88.2-C88.3, C88.8-C91.32, C91.50-C94.32, C94.80-C95.92, D49.81-D49.9

C88.3 Immunoproliferative small intestinal disease `CC`
Alpha heavy chain disease
Mediterranean lymphoma
CC Excl: See code: C88.2

C88.4 Extranodal marginal zone B-cell lymphoma of mucosa-associated lymphoid tissue [MALT-lymphoma] `HIV` `CC`
Lymphoma of skin-associated lymphoid tissue [SALT-lymphoma]
Lymphoma of bronchial-associated lymphoid tissue [BALT-lymphoma]
EXCLUDES 1   *high malignant (diffuse large B-cell) lymphoma (C83.3-)*
CC Excl: C82.50-C82.59, C83.10-C83.19, C84.40-C86.4, C88.4, C96.4, C96.Z-C96.9, D49.81-D49.9

C88.8 Other malignant immunoproliferative diseases `CC`
CC Excl: C88.2-C88.3, C88.8-C95.92, D45-D47.1, D47.3, D47.Z9-D47.9, D48.7-D48.9, D49.81-D49.9

C88.9 Malignant immunoproliferative disease, unspecified `CC`
Immunoproliferative disease NOS
CC Excl: See code: C88.2

✓4ᵗʰ **C90 Multiple myeloma and malignant plasma cell neoplasms**
EXCLUDES 1   *personal history of other malignant neoplasms of lymphoid, hematopoietic and related tissues (Z85.79)*

CC Excl: For CC codes in category C90, unless otherwise noted:
C88.2-C88.3, C88.8-C95.92, D45-D47.1, D47.3, D47.Z9-D47.9, D48.7-D48.9, D49.81-D49.9

✓5ᵗʰ **C90.0 Multiple myeloma**
Kahler's disease   Myelomatosis
Medullary plasmacytoma   Plasma cell myeloma
EXCLUDES 1   *solitary myeloma (C90.3-)*
solitary plasmactyoma (C90.3-)

C90.00 Multiple myeloma not having achieved remission `CC`
Multiple myeloma with failed remission
Multiple myeloma NOS

C90.01 Multiple myeloma in remission `CC`

C90.02 Multiple myeloma in relapse `CC`

✓5ᵗʰ **C90.1 Plasma cell leukemia**
Plasmacytic leukemia

C90.10 Plasma cell leukemia not having achieved remission `CC`
Plasma cell leukemia with failed remission
Plasma cell leukemia NOS

C90.11 Plasma cell leukemia in remission `CC`

C90.12 Plasma cell leukemia in relapse `CC`

✓5ᵗʰ **C90.2 Extramedullary plasmacytoma**

C90.20 Extramedullary plasmacytoma not having achieved remission `CC`
Extramedullary plasmacytoma with failed remission
Extramedullary plasmacytoma NOS

C90.21 Extramedullary plasmacytoma in remission `CC`

C90.22 Extramedullary plasmacytoma in relapse `CC`

✓5ᵗʰ **C90.3 Solitary plasmacytoma**
Localized malignant plasma cell tumor NOS
Plasmacytoma NOS
Solitary myeloma

C90.30 Solitary plasmacytoma not having achieved remission `CC`
Solitary plasmacytoma with failed remission
Solitary plasmacytoma NOS

C90.31 Solitary plasmacytoma in remission `CC`

C90.32 Solitary plasmacytoma in relapse `CC`

✓4ᵗʰ **C91 Lymphoid leukemia**
EXCLUDES 1   *personal history of leukemia (Z85.6)*

CC Excl: For CC codes in category C91, unless otherwise noted:
C88.2-C88.3, C88.8-C95.92, D45-D47.1, D47.3, D47.Z9-D47.9, D48.7-D48.9, D49.81-D49.9

✓5ᵗʰ **C91.0 Acute lymphoblastic leukemia [ALL]**
NOTE   Code C91.0 should only be used for T-cell and B-cell precursor leukemia

C91.00 Acute lymphoblastic leukemia not having achieved remission `CC`
Acute lymphoblastic leukemia with failed remission
Acute lymphoblastic leukemia NOS

C91.01 Acute lymphoblastic leukemia, in remission `CC`

C91.02 Acute lymphoblastic leukemia, in relapse `CC`

✓5ᵗʰ **C91.1 Chronic lymphocytic leukemia of B-cell type**
Lymphoplasmacytic leukemia
Richter syndrome
EXCLUDES 1   *lymphoplasmacytic lymphoma (C83.0-)*

C91.10 Chronic lymphocytic leukemia of B-cell type not having achieved remission `CC`
Chronic lymphocytic leukemia of B-cell type with failed remission
Chronic lymphocytic leukemia of B-cell type NOS

C91.11 Chronic lymphocytic leukemia of B-cell type in remission `CC`

C91.12 Chronic lymphocytic leukemia of B-cell type in relapse `CC`

✓5ᵗʰ **C91.3 Prolymphocytic leukemia of B-cell type**

C91.30 Prolymphocytic leukemia of B-cell type not having achieved remission `CC`
Prolymphocytic leukemia of B-cell type with failed remission
Prolymphocytic leukemia of B-cell type NOS

C91.31 Prolymphocytic leukemia of B-cell type, in remission `CC`

C91.32 Prolymphocytic leukemia of B-cell type, in relapse `CC`

✓5ᵗʰ **C91.4 Hairy cell leukemia**
Leukemic reticuloendotheliosis

C91.40 Hairy cell leukemia not having achieved remission `CC`
Hairy cell leukemia with failed remission
Hairy cell leukemia NOS
CC Excl: C82.50, C82.59, C83.10, C83.19, C84.40, C84.49, C84.60, C84.69-C84.70, C84.79-C84.90, C84.99-C84.A0, C84.A9-C84.Z0, C84.Z9, C85.10, C85.19-C85.20, C85.29, C85.80, C85.89-C85.90, C85.99, C86.4, C88.4, C91.40-C91.42, C96.4, C96.9, C96.Z, D49.81-D49.9

C91.41 Hairy cell leukemia, in remission `CC`
CC Excl: See code: C91.40

C91.42 Hairy cell leukemia, in relapse `CC`
CC Excl: See code: C91.40

Ⓝ Newborn: 0   Ⓟ Pediatric: 0-17   Ⓜ Maternity: 12-55   Ⓐ Adult: 15-124   `MCC` Major CC Condition   `PDx MCC` PDx acts as own MCC   `CC` CC Condition   `PDx CC` PDx acts as own CC

472   ICD-10-CM Draft (2015)

✓5ᵗʰ **C91.5** **Adult T-cell lymphoma/leukemia (HTLV-1-associated)**
Acute variant of adult T-cell lymphoma/leukemia (HTLV-1-associated)
Chronic variant of adult T-cell lymphoma/leukemia (HTLV-1-associated)
Lymphomatoid variant of adult T-cell lymphoma/leukemia (HTLV-1-associated)
Smouldering variant of adult T-cell lymphoma/leukemia (HTLV-1-associated)

C91.50 **Adult T-cell lymphoma/leukemia (HTLV-1-associated) not having achieved remission** cc A
Adult T-cell lymphoma/leukemia (HTLV-1-associated) with failed remission
Adult T-cell lymphoma/leukemia (HTLV-1-associated) NOS
CC Excl: C88.2-C88.3, C88.8-C91.32, C91.50-C94.32, C94.80-C95.92, D49.81-D49.9

C91.51 **Adult T-cell lymphoma/leukemia (HTLV-1-associated), in remission** cc A
CC Excl: See code: C91.50

C91.52 **Adult T-cell lymphoma/leukemia (HTLV-1-associated), in relapse** cc A
CC Excl: See code: C91.50

✓5ᵗʰ **C91.6** **Prolymphocytic leukemia of T-cell type**

C91.60 **Prolymphocytic leukemia of T-cell type not having achieved remission** cc
Prolymphocytic leukemia of T-cell type with failed remission
Prolymphocytic leukemia of T-cell type NOS
CC Excl: See code: C91.50

C91.61 **Prolymphocytic leukemia of T-cell type, in remission** cc
CC Excl: See code: C91.50

C91.62 **Prolymphocytic leukemia of T-cell type, in relapse** cc
CC Excl: See code: C91.50

✓5ᵗʰ **C91.A** **Mature B-cell leukemia Burkitt-type**
EXCLUDES1 *Burkitt lymphoma (C83.7-)*

C91.A0 **Mature B-cell leukemia Burkitt-type not having achieved remission** cc
Mature B-cell leukemia Burkitt-type with failed remission
Mature B-cell leukemia Burkitt-type NOS
CC Excl: See code: C91.50

C91.A1 **Mature B-cell leukemia Burkitt-type, in remission** cc
CC Excl: See code: C91.50

C91.A2 **Mature B-cell leukemia Burkitt-type, in relapse** cc
CC Excl: See code: C91.50

✓5ᵗʰ **C91.Z** **Other lymphoid leukemia**
T-cell large granular lymphocytic leukemia (associated with rheumatoid arthritis)

C91.Z0 **Other lymphoid leukemia not having achieved remission** cc
Other lymphoid leukemia with failed remission
Other lymphoid leukemia NOS
CC Excl: See code: C91.50

C91.Z1 **Other lymphoid leukemia, in remission** cc
CC Excl: See code: C91.50

C91.Z2 **Other lymphoid leukemia, in relapse** cc
CC Excl: See code: C91.50

✓5ᵗʰ **C91.9** **Lymphoid leukemia, unspecified**

C91.90 **Lymphoid leukemia, unspecified not having achieved remission** cc
Lymphoid leukemia with failed remission
Lymphoid leukemia NOS
CC Excl: See code: C91.50

C91.91 **Lymphoid leukemia, unspecified, in remission** cc
CC Excl: See code: C91.50

C91.92 **Lymphoid leukemia, unspecified, in relapse** cc
CC Excl: See code: C91.50

✓4ᵗʰ **C92** **Myeloid leukemia**
INCLUDES granulocytic leukemia
myelogenous leukemia
EXCLUDES1 *personal history of leukemia (Z85.6)*

CC Excl: For CC codes in category C92, unless otherwise noted: C88.2-C88.3, C88.8-C91.32, C91.50-C94.32, C94.80-C95.92, D49.81-D49.9

✓5ᵗʰ **C92.0** **Acute myeloblastic leukemia**
Acute myeloblastic leukemia, minimal differentiation
Acute myeloblastic leukemia (with maturation)
Acute myeloblastic leukemia 1/ETO
Acute myeloblastic leukemia M0
Acute myeloblastic leukemia M1
Acute myeloblastic leukemia M2
Acute myeloblastic leukemia with t(8;21)
Acute myeloblastic leukemia (without a FAB classification) NOS
Refractory anemia with excess blasts in transformation [RAEB T]
EXCLUDES1 *acute exacerbation of chronic myeloid leukemia (C92.10)*
refractory anemia with excess of blasts not in transformation (D46.2-)

C92.00 **Acute myeloblastic leukemia, not having achieved remission** cc
Acute myeloblastic leukemia with failed remission
Acute myeloblastic leukemia NOS

C92.01 **Acute myeloblastic leukemia, in remission** cc

C92.02 **Acute myeloblastic leukemia, in relapse** cc

✓5ᵗʰ **C92.1** **Chronic myeloid leukemia, BCR/ABL-positive**
Chronic myelogenous leukemia, Philadelphia chromosome (Ph1) positive
Chronic myelogenous leukemia, t(9;22) (q34;q11)
Chronic myelogenous leukemia with crisis of blast cells
EXCLUDES1 *atypical chronic myeloid leukemia BCR/ABL-negative (C92.2-)*
chronic myelomonocytic leukemia (C93.1-)
chronic myeloproliferative disease (D47.1)

C92.10 **Chronic myeloid leukemia, BCR/ABL-positive, not having achieved remission** cc
Chronic myeloid leukemia, BCR/ABL-positive with failed remission
Chronic myeloid leukemia, BCR/ABL-positive NOS

C92.11 **Chronic myeloid leukemia, BCR/ABL-positive, in remission** cc

C92.12 **Chronic myeloid leukemia, BCR/ABL-positive, in relapse** cc

✓5ᵗʰ **C92.2** **Atypical chronic myeloid leukemia, BCR/ABL-negative**

C92.20 **Atypical chronic myeloid leukemia, BCR/ABL-negative, not having achieved remission** cc
Atypical chronic myeloid leukemia, BCR/ABL-negative with failed remission
Atypical chronic myeloid leukemia, BCR/ABL-negative NOS

C92.21 **Atypical chronic myeloid leukemia, BCR/ABL-negative, in remission** cc

C92.22 **Atypical chronic myeloid leukemia, BCR/ABL-negative, in relapse** cc

✓5ᵗʰ **C92.3** **Myeloid sarcoma**
A malignant tumor of immature myeloid cells
Chloroma
Granulocytic sarcoma

C92.30 **Myeloid sarcoma, not having achieved remission** cc
Myeloid sarcoma with failed remission
Myeloid sarcoma NOS

C92.31 **Myeloid sarcoma, in remission** cc

C92.32 **Myeloid sarcoma, in relapse** cc

✓5ᵗʰ **C92.4** **Acute promyelocytic leukemia**
AML M3
AML Me with t(15;17) and variants

C92.40 **Acute promyelocytic leukemia, not having achieved remission** cc
Acute promyelocytic leukemia with failed remission
Acute promyelocytic leukemia NOS

C92.41 **Acute promyelocytic leukemia, in remission** cc

C92.42 **Acute promyelocytic leukemia, in relapse** cc

C91.5 –C92.42

✓ Additional Character Required   ✓x7ᵗʰ Xtension Alert   Unacceptable PDx   Manifestation   Hospital Acquired Condition   EXCLUDES1 Not Coded Here   EXCLUDES2 Not Included Here

Neoplasms

C92.5–C94.6

✓5th **C92.5 Acute myelomonocytic leukemia**
AML M4
AML M4 Eo with inv(16) or t(16;16)

    C92.50 Acute myelomonocytic leukemia, not having achieved remission `CC`
        Acute myelomonocytic leukemia with failed remission
        Acute myelomonocytic leukemia NOS

    C92.51 Acute myelomonocytic leukemia, in remission `CC`

    C92.52 Acute myelomonocytic leukemia, in relapse `CC`

✓5th **C92.6 Acute myeloid leukemia with 11q23-abnormality**
Acute myeloid leukemia with variation of MLL-gene

    C92.60 Acute myeloid leukemia with 11q23-abnormality not having achieved remission `CC`
        Acute myeloid leukemia with 11q23-abnormality with failed remission
        Acute myeloid leukemia with 11q23-abnormality NOS

    C92.61 Acute myeloid leukemia with 11q23-abnormality in remission `CC`

    C92.62 Acute myeloid leukemia with 11q23-abnormality in relapse `CC`

✓5th **C92.A Acute myeloid leukemia with multilineage dysplasia**
Acute myeloid leukemia with dysplasia of remaining hematopoesis and/or myelodysplastic disease in its history

    C92.A0 Acute myeloid leukemia with multilineage dysplasia, not having achieved remission `CC`
        Acute myeloid leukemia with multilineage dysplasia with failed remission
        Acute myeloid leukemia with multilineage dysplasia NOS

    C92.A1 Acute myeloid leukemia with multilineage dysplasia, in remission `CC`

    C92.A2 Acute myeloid leukemia with multilineage dysplasia, in relapse `CC`

✓5th **C92.Z Other myeloid leukemia**

    C92.Z0 Other myeloid leukemia not having achieved remission `CC`
        Myeloid leukemia NEC with failed remission
        Myeloid leukemia NEC

    C92.Z1 Other myeloid leukemia, in remission `CC`

    C92.Z2 Other myeloid leukemia, in relapse `CC`

✓5th **C92.9 Myeloid leukemia, unspecified**

    C92.90 Myeloid leukemia, unspecified, not having achieved remission `CC`
        Myeloid leukemia, unspecified with failed remission
        Myeloid leukemia, unspecified NOS

    C92.91 Myeloid leukemia, unspecified in remission `CC`

    C92.92 Myeloid leukemia, unspecified in relapse `CC`

✓4th **C93 Monocytic leukemia**
INCLUDES monocytoid leukemia
EXCLUDES 1 *personal history of leukemia (Z85.6))*

CC Excl: For CC codes in category C93, unless otherwise noted:
C88.2-C88.3, C88.8-C91.32, C91.50-C94.32, C94.80-C95.92, D49.81-D49.9

✓5th **C93.0 Acute monoblastic/monocytic leukemia**
AML M5   AML M5b
AML M5a

    C93.00 Acute monoblastic/monocytic leukemia, not having achieved remission `CC`
        Acute monoblastic/monocytic leukemia with failed remission
        Acute monoblastic/monocytic leukemia NOS

    C93.01 Acute monoblastic/monocytic leukemia, in remission `CC`

    C93.02 Acute monoblastic/monocytic leukemia, in relapse `CC`

✓5th **C93.1 Chronic myelomonocytic leukemia**
Chronic monocytic leukemia
CMML-1
CMML-2
CMML with eosinophilia

    C93.10 Chronic myelomonocytic leukemia not having achieved remission `CC`
        Chronic myelomonocytic leukemia with failed remission
        Chronic myelomonocytic leukemia NOS

    C93.11 Chronic myelomonocytic leukemia, in remission `CC`

    C93.12 Chronic myelomonocytic leukemia, in relapse `CC`

✓5th **C93.3 Juvenile myelomonocytic leukemia**

    C93.30 Juvenile myelomonocytic leukemia, not having achieved remission `CC` `P`
        Juvenile myelomonocytic leukemia with failed remission
        Juvenile myelomonocytic leukemia NOS

    C93.31 Juvenile myelomonocytic leukemia, in remission `CC` `P`

    C93.32 Juvenile myelomonocytic leukemia, in relapse `CC` `P`

✓5th **C93.Z Other monocytic leukemia**

    C93.Z0 Other monocytic leukemia, not having achieved remission `CC`
        Other monocytic leukemia NOS

    C93.Z1 Other monocytic leukemia, in remission `CC`

    C93.Z2 Other monocytic leukemia, in relapse `CC`

✓5th **C93.9 Monocytic leukemia, unspecified**

    C93.90 Monocytic leukemia, unspecified, not having achieved remission `CC`
        Monocytic leukemia, unspecified with failed remission
        Monocytic leukemia, unspecified NOS

    C93.91 Monocytic leukemia, unspecified in remission `CC`

    C93.92 Monocytic leukemia, unspecified in relapse `CC`

✓4th **C94 Other leukemias of specified cell type**
EXCLUDES 1 *leukemic reticuloendotheliosis (C91.4-)*
        myelodysplastic syndromes (D46.-)
        personal history of leukemia (Z85.6)
        plasma cell leukemia (C90.1-)

CC Excl: For CC codes in category C94, unless otherwise noted:
C88.2-C88.3, C88.8-C91.32, C91.50-C94.32, C94.80-C95.92, D49.81-D49.9

✓5th **C94.0 Acute erythroid leukemia**
Acute myeloid leukemia M6(a)(b)
Erythroleukemia

    C94.00 Acute erythroid leukemia, not having achieved remission `CC`
        Acute erythroid leukemia with failed remission
        Acute erythroid leukemia NOS

    C94.01 Acute erythroid leukemia, in remission `CC`

    C94.02 Acute erythroid leukemia, in relapse `CC`

✓5th **C94.2 Acute megakaryoblastic leukemia**
Acute myeloid leukemia M7
Acute megakaryocytic leukemia

    C94.20 Acute megakaryoblastic leukemia not having achieved remission `CC`
        Acute megakaryoblastic leukemia with failed remission
        Acute megakaryoblastic leukemia NOS

    C94.21 Acute megakaryoblastic leukemia, in remission `CC`

    C94.22 Acute megakaryoblastic leukemia, in relapse `CC`

✓5th **C94.3 Mast cell leukemia**

    C94.30 Mast cell leukemia not having achieved remission `CC`
        Mast cell leukemia with failed remission
        Mast cell leukemia NOS

    C94.31 Mast cell leukemia, in remission `CC`

    C94.32 Mast cell leukemia, in relapse `CC`

✓5th **C94.4 Acute panmyelosis with myelofibrosis**
Acute myelofibrosis
EXCLUDES 1 *myelofibrosis NOS (D75.81)*
        secondary myelofibrosis NOS (D75.81)

    C94.40 Acute panmyelosis with myelofibrosis not having achieved remission `CC`
        Acute myelofibrosis NOS
        Acute panmyelosis with myelofibrosis with failed remission
        Acute panmyelosis NOS
        CC Excl: C88.2-C88.3, C88.8-C88.9, C90.10-C90.11, C90.20-C90.21, C90.30-C90.31, C91.00-C95.92, D45-D47.1, D47.3, D47.Z9-D47.9, D48.7-D48.9

    C94.41 Acute panmyelosis with myelofibrosis, in remission `CC`
        CC Excl: See code: C94.40

    C94.42 Acute panmyelosis with myelofibrosis, in relapse `CC`
        CC Excl: See code: C94.40

C94.6 Myelodysplastic disease, not classified `CC`
Myeloproliferative disease, not classified
CC Excl: See code: C94.40

N Newborn: 0   P Pediatric: 0-17   M Maternity: 12-55   A Adult: 15-124   **MCC** Major CC Condition   **PDx MCC** PDx acts as own MCC   **CC** CC Condition   **PDx CC** PDx acts as own CC

☑5ᵗʰ **C94.8** **Other specified leukemias**
  Aggressive NK-cell leukemia
  Acute basophilic leukemia

  C94.80 **Other specified leukemias** not having achieved CC
   remission
    Other specified leukemia with failed remission
    Other specified leukemias NOS

  C94.81 **Other specified leukemias, in remission** CC

  C94.82 **Other specified leukemias, in relapse** CC

☑4ᵗʰ **C95** **Leukemia of unspecified cell type**
  EXCLUDES1 *personal history of leukemia (Z85.6)*

  CC Excl: For CC codes in category C95, unless otherwise noted:
  C88.2-C88.3, C88.8-C91.32, C91.50-C94.32, C94.80-C95.92, D49.81-
  D49.9

☑5ᵗʰ **C95.0** **Acute leukemia of unspecified cell type**
  Acute bilineal leukemia
  Acute mixed lineage leukemia
  Biphenotypic acute leukemia
  Stem cell leukemia of unclear lineage
  EXCLUDES1 *acute exacerbation of unspecified chronic leukemia*
    (C95.10)

  C95.00 **Acute leukemia of unspecified cell type** not CC
   having achieved remission
    Acute leukemia of unspecified cell type with failed
    remission
    Acute leukemia NOS

  C95.01 **Acute leukemia of unspecified cell type, in** CC
   remission

  C95.02 **Acute leukemia of unspecified cell type, in** CC
   relapse

☑5ᵗʰ **C95.1** **Chronic leukemia of unspecified cell type**

  C95.10 **Chronic leukemia of unspecified cell type** not CC
   having achieved remission
    Chronic leukemia of unspecified cell type with failed
    remission
    Chronic leukemia NOS

  C95.11 **Chronic leukemia of unspecified cell type, in** CC
   remission

  C95.12 **Chronic leukemia of unspecified cell type, in** CC
   relapse

☑5ᵗʰ **C95.9** **Leukemia, unspecified**

  C95.90 **Leukemia, unspecified** not having achieved CC
   remission
    Leukemia, unspecified with failed remission
    Leukemia NOS

  C95.91 **Leukemia, unspecified, in remission** CC

  C95.92 **Leukemia, unspecified, in relapse** CC

☑4ᵗʰ **C96** **Other and unspecified malignant neoplasms of lymphoid,**
  hematopoietic and related tissue
  EXCLUDES1 *personal history of other malignant neoplasms of lymphoid,*
    hematopoietic and related tissues (Z85.79)

  C96.0 **Multifocal and multisystemic (disseminated)** CC
   Langerhans-cell histiocytosis
   Histiocytosis X, multisystemic
   Letterer-Siwe disease
   EXCLUDES1 *adult pulmonary Langerhans cell histiocytosis (J84.82)*
    multifocal and unisystemic Langerhans-cell
     histiocytosis (C96.5)
    unifocal Langerhans-cell histiocytosis (C96.6)
   CC Excl: C82.50, C82.59, C83.10, C83.19, C84.40, C84.49, C84.60,
   C84.69-C84.70, C84.79-C84.90, C84.99-C84.A0, C84.A9-C84.Z0,
   C84.Z9, C85.10, C85.19-C85.20, C85.29, C85.80, C85.89-C85.90,
   C85.99, C86.4, C88.4, C96.0, C96.4, C96.9, C96.Z, D49.81-D49.9

  C96.2 **Malignant mast cell tumor** CC
   Aggressive systemic mastocytosis
   Mast cell sarcoma
   EXCLUDES1 *indolent mastocytosis (D47.0)*
    mast cell leukemia (C94.30)
    mastocytosis (congenital) (cutaneous) (Q82.2)
   CC Excl: C82.50, C82.59, C83.10, C83.19, C84.40, C84.49, C84.60,
   C84.69-C84.70, C84.79-C84.90, C84.99-C84.A0, C84.A9-C84.Z0,
   C84.Z9, C85.10, C85.19-C85.20, C85.29, C85.80, C85.89-C85.90,
   C85.99, C86.4, C88.4, C96.2, C96.4, C96.9, C96.Z, D49.81-D49.9

  C96.4 **Sarcoma of dendritic cells (accessory cells)** CC
   Follicular dendritic cell sarcoma
   Interdigitating dendritic cell sarcoma
   Langerhans cell sarcoma
   CC Excl: C96.4, C96.9, C96.Z, D49.81-D49.9

C96.5 **Multifocal and unisystemic Langerhans-cell histiocytosis** CC
  Hand-Schüller-Christian disease
  Histiocytosis X, multifocal
  EXCLUDES1 *multifocal and multisystemic (disseminated)*
    Langerhans-cell histiocytosis (C96.0)
   unifocal Langerhans-cell histiocytosis (C96.6)
  CC Excl: E71.310-E71.32, E71.40-E71.548, E80.4-E80.7, E88.40-
  E88.49, H49.811-H49.819

C96.6 **Unifocal Langerhans-cell histiocytosis** CC
  Eosinophilic granuloma CC
  Histiocytosis X, unifocal
  Histiocytosis X NOS
  Langerhans-cell histiocytosis NOS
  EXCLUDES1 *multifocal and multisysemic (disseminated)*
    Langerhans-cell histiocytosis (C96.0)
   multifocal and unisystemic Langerhans-cell
    histiocytosis (C96.5)
  CC Excl: See code: C96.5

C96.A **Histiocytic sarcoma** CC
  Malignant histiocytosis
  CC Excl: C82.50, C82.59, C83.10, C83.19, C84.40, C84.49, C84.60,
  C84.69-C84.70, C84.79-C84.90, C84.99-C84.A0, C84.A9-C84.Z0,
  C84.Z9, C85.10, C85.19-C85.20, C85.29, C85.80, C85.89-C85.90,
  C85.99, C86.4, C88.4, C96.4, C96.9-C96.Z, D49.81-D49.9

C96.Z **Other specified malignant neoplasms of lymphoid,** CC
 hematopoietic and related tissue
  CC Excl: See code: C96.4

C96.9 **Malignant neoplasm of lymphoid, hematopoietic and** CC
 related tissue, unspecified
  CC Excl: See code: C96.4

In situ neoplasms (D00-D09)

INCLUDES Bowen's disease
   erythroplasia
   grade III intraepithelial neoplasia
   Queyrat's erythroplasia

☑4ᵗʰ **D00** **Carcinoma in situ of oral cavity, esophagus and stomach**
  EXCLUDES1 *melanoma in situ (D03.-)*

 ☑5ᵗʰ **D00.0** **Carcinoma in situ of lip, oral cavity and pharynx**
  Use additional code to identify:
   exposure to environmental tobacco smoke (Z77.22)
   exposure to tobacco smoke in the perinatal period (P96.81)
   history of tobacco use (Z87.891)
   occupational exposure to environmental tobacco smoke
    (Z57.31)
   tobacco dependence (F17.-)
   tobacco use (Z72.0)
  EXCLUDES1 *carcinoma in situ of aryepiglottic fold or interarytenoid*
    fold, laryngeal aspect (D02.0)
   carcinoma in situ of epiglottis NOS (D02.0)
   carcinoma in situ of epiglottis suprahyoid portion
    (D02.0)
   carcinoma in situ of skin of lip (D03.0, D04.0)

  D00.00 **Carcinoma in situ of oral cavity, unspecified site**

  D00.01 **Carcinoma in situ of labial mucosa and vermilion**
   border

  D00.02 **Carcinoma in situ of buccal mucosa**

  D00.03 **Carcinoma in situ of gingiva and edentulous alveolar**
   ridge

  D00.04 **Carcinoma in situ of soft palate**

  D00.05 **Carcinoma in situ of hard palate**

  D00.06 **Carcinoma in situ of floor of mouth**

  D00.07 **Carcinoma in situ of tongue**

  D00.08 **Carcinoma in situ of pharynx**
    Carcinoma in situ of aryepiglottic fold NOS
    Carcinoma in situ of hypopharyngeal aspect of
     aryepiglottic fold
    Carcinoma in situ of marginal zone of aryepiglottic
     fold

 D00.1 **Carcinoma in situ of esophagus**

 D00.2 **Carcinoma in situ of stomach**

☑4ᵗʰ **D01** **Carcinoma in situ of other and unspecified digestive organs**
  EXCLUDES1 *melanoma in situ (D03.-)*

 D01.0 **Carcinoma in situ of colon**
  EXCLUDES1 *carcinoma in situ of rectosigmoid junction (D01.1)*

 D01.1 **Carcinoma in situ of rectosigmoid junction**

 D01.2 **Carcinoma in situ of rectum**

☑ Additional Character Required   √x7ᵗʰ *X*tension Alert   Unacceptable PDx   Manifestation   Hospital Acquired Condition   EXCLUDES1 Not Coded Here   EXCLUDES2 Not Included Here

D01.3 Carcinoma in situ of anus and anal canal
    EXCLUDES 1   carcinoma in situ of anal margin (D04.5)
        carcinoma in situ of anal skin (D04.5)
        carcinoma in situ of perianal skin (D04.5)

✓5th **D01.4 Carcinoma in situ of other and unspecified parts of** intestine
    EXCLUDES 1   carcinoma in situ of ampulla of Vater (D01.5)
    D01.40 Carcinoma in situ of unspecified **part of intestine**
    D01.49 Carcinoma in situ of other **parts of intestine**

D01.5 Carcinoma in situ of liver, gallbladder and bile ducts
    Carcinoma in situ of ampulla of Vater

D01.7 Carcinoma in situ of other **specified digestive organs**
    Carcinoma in situ of pancreas

D01.9 Carcinoma in situ of digestive organ, unspecified

✓4th **D02 Carcinoma in situ of** middle ear and respiratory system
    Use additional code to identify:
    exposure to environmental tobacco smoke (Z77.22)
    exposure to tobacco smoke in the perinatal period (P96.81)
    history of tobacco use (Z87.891)
    occupational exposure to environmental tobacco smoke (Z57.31)
    tobacco dependence (F17.-)
    tobacco use (Z72.0)
    EXCLUDES 1   melanoma in situ (D03.-)

D02.0 Carcinoma in situ of larynx
    Carcinoma in situ of aryepiglottic fold or interarytenoid fold, laryngeal aspect
    Carcinoma in situ of epiglottis (suprahyoid portion)
    EXCLUDES 1   carcinoma in situ of aryepiglottic fold or interarytenoid fold NOS (D00.08)
        carcinoma in situ of hypopharyngeal aspect (D00.08)
        carcinoma in situ of marginal zone (D00.08)

D02.1 Carcinoma in situ of trachea

✓5th **D02.2 Carcinoma in situ of** bronchus and lung
    D02.20 Carcinoma in situ of unspecified **bronchus and lung**
    D02.21 Carcinoma in situ of right **bronchus and lung**
    D02.22 Carcinoma in situ of left **bronchus and lung**

D02.3 Carcinoma in situ of other **parts of respiratory system**
    Carcinoma in situ of accessory sinuses
    Carcinoma in situ of middle ear
    Carcinoma in situ of nasal cavities
    EXCLUDES 1   carcinoma in situ of ear (external) (skin) (D04.2-)
        carcinoma in situ of nose NOS (D09.8)
        carcinoma in situ of skin of nose (D04.3)

D02.4 Carcinoma in situ of respiratory system, unspecified

✓4th **D03 Melanoma in situ**
D03.0 Melanoma in situ of lip

✓5th **D03.1 Melanoma in situ of** eyelid, including canthus
    D03.10 Melanoma in situ of unspecified **eyelid, including canthus**
    D03.11 Melanoma in situ of right **eyelid, including canthus**
    D03.12 Melanoma in situ of left **eyelid, including canthus**

✓5th **D03.2 Melanoma in situ of** ear and external auricular canal
    D03.20 Melanoma in situ of unspecified **ear and external auricular canal**
    D03.21 Melanoma in situ of right **ear and external auricular canal**
    D03.22 Melanoma in situ of left **ear and external auricular canal**

✓5th **D03.3 Melanoma in situ of** other and unspecified parts of face
    D03.30 Melanoma in situ of unspecified **part of face**
    D03.39 Melanoma in situ of other **parts of face**

D03.4 Melanoma in situ of scalp and neck

✓5th **D03.5 Melanoma in situ of** trunk
    D03.51 Melanoma in situ of anal skin
        Melanoma in situ of anal margin
        Melanoma in situ of perianal skin
    D03.52 Melanoma in situ of breast (skin) (soft tissue)
    D03.59 Melanoma in situ of other **part of trunk**

✓5th **D03.6 Melanoma in situ of** upper limb, including shoulder
    D03.60 Melanoma in situ of unspecified **upper limb, including shoulder**
    D03.61 Melanoma in situ of right **upper limb, including shoulder**
    D03.62 Melanoma in situ of left **upper limb, including shoulder**

✓5th **D03.7 Melanoma in situ of** lower limb, including hip
    D03.70 Melanoma in situ of unspecified **lower limb, including hip**
    D03.71 Melanoma in situ of right **lower limb, including hip**
    D03.72 Melanoma in situ of left **lower limb, including hip**

D03.8 Melanoma in situ of other sites
    Melanoma in situ of scrotum
    EXCLUDES 1   carcinoma in situ of scrotum (D07.61)

D03.9 Melanoma in situ, unspecified

✓4th **D04 Carcinoma in situ of** skin
    EXCLUDES 1   erythroplasia of Queyrat (penis) NOS (D07.4)
        melanoma in situ (D03.-)

D04.0 Carcinoma in situ of skin of lip
    EXCLUDES 1   carcinoma in situ of vermilion border of lip (D00.01)

✓5th **D04.1 Carcinoma in situ of skin of** eyelid, including canthus
    D04.10 Carcinoma in situ of skin of unspecified **eyelid, including canthus**
    D04.11 Carcinoma in situ of skin of right **eyelid, including canthus**
    D04.12 Carcinoma in situ of skin of left **eyelid, including canthus**

✓5th **D04.2 Carcinoma in situ of skin of** ear and external auricular canal
    D04.20 Carcinoma in situ of skin of unspecified **ear and external auricular canal**
    D04.21 Carcinoma in situ of skin of right **ear and external auricular canal**
    D04.22 Carcinoma in situ of skin of left **ear and external auricular canal**

✓5th **D04.3 Carcinoma in situ of skin of** other and unspecified parts of face
    D04.30 Carcinoma in situ of skin of unspecified **part of face**
    D04.39 Carcinoma in situ of skin of other **parts of face**

D04.4 Carcinoma in situ of skin of scalp and neck

D04.5 Carcinoma in situ of skin of trunk
    Carcinoma in situ of anal margin
    Carcinoma in situ of anal skin
    Carcinoma in situ of perianal skin
    Carcinoma in situ of skin of breast
    EXCLUDES 1   carcinoma in situ of anus NOS (D01.3)
        carcinoma in situ of scrotum (D07.61)
        carcinoma in situ of skin of genital organs (D07.-)

✓5th **D04.6 Carcinoma in situ of skin of** upper limb, including shoulder
    D04.60 Carcinoma in situ of skin of unspecified **upper limb, including shoulder**
    D04.61 Carcinoma in situ of skin of right **upper limb, including shoulder**
    D04.62 Carcinoma in situ of skin of left **upper limb, including shoulder**

✓5th **D04.7 Carcinoma in situ of skin of** lower limb, including hip
    D04.70 Carcinoma in situ of skin of unspecified **lower limb, including hip**
    D04.71 Carcinoma in situ of skin of right **lower limb, including hip**
    D04.72 Carcinoma in situ of skin of left **lower limb, including hip**

D04.8 Carcinoma in situ of skin of other sites
D04.9 Carcinoma in situ of skin, unspecified

✓4th **D05 Carcinoma in situ of** breast
    EXCLUDES 1   carcinoma in situ of skin of breast (D04.5)
        melanoma in situ of breast (skin) (D03.5)
        Paget's disease of breast or nipple (C50.-)

✓5th **D05.0 Lobular carcinoma in situ of breast**
    D05.00 Lobular carcinoma in situ of unspecified **breast**
    D05.01 Lobular carcinoma in situ of right **breast**
    D05.02 Lobular carcinoma in situ of left **breast**

✓5th **D05.1 Intraductal carcinoma in situ of breast**
    D05.10 Intraductal carcinoma in situ of unspecified **breast**
    D05.11 Intraductal carcinoma in situ of right **breast**
    D05.12 Intraductal carcinoma in situ of left **breast**

✓5th **D05.8 Other specified type of carcinoma in situ of breast**
    D05.80 Other specified type of carcinoma in situ of unspecified **breast**
    D05.81 Other specified type of carcinoma in situ of right **breast**

D05.82 Other specified type of carcinoma in situ of left breast

✓5th **D05.9 Unspecified type of carcinoma in situ of breast**

D05.90 Unspecified type of carcinoma in situ of unspecified breast

D05.91 Unspecified type of carcinoma in situ of right breast

D05.92 Unspecified type of carcinoma in situ of left breast

✓4th **D06 Carcinoma in situ of cervix uteri**
- INCLUDES cervical adenocarcinoma in situ
cervical intraepithelial glandular neoplasia
cervical intraepithelial neoplasia III [CIN III]
severe dysplasia of cervix uteri
- EXCLUDES 1 cervical intraepithelial neoplasia II [CIN II] (N87.1)
cytologic evidence of malignancy of cervix without histologic confirmation (R87.614)
high grade squamous intraepithelial lesion (HGSIL) of cervix (R87.613)
melanoma in situ of cervix (D03.5)
moderate cervical dysplasia (N87.1)

D06.0 Carcinoma in situ of endocervix ♀

D06.1 Carcinoma in situ of exocervix ♀

D06.7 Carcinoma in situ of other parts of cervix ♀

D06.9 Carcinoma in situ of cervix, unspecified ♀

✓4th **D07 Carcinoma in situ of other and unspecified genital organs**
- EXCLUDES 1 melanoma in situ of trunk (D03.5)

D07.0 Carcinoma in situ of endometrium ♀

D07.1 Carcinoma in situ of vulva ♀
Severe dysplasia of vulva
Vulvar intraepithelial neoplasia III [VIN III]
- EXCLUDES 1 moderate dysplasia of vulva (N90.1)
vulvar intraepithelial neoplasia II [VIN II] (N90.1)

D07.2 Carcinoma in situ of vagina ♀
Severe dysplasia of vagina
Vaginal intraepithelial neoplasia III [VAIN III]
- EXCLUDES 1 moderate dysplasia of vagina (N89.1)
vaginal intraepithelial neoplasia II [VIN II] (N89.1)

✓5th **D07.3 Carcinoma in situ of other and unspecified female genital organs**

D07.30 Carcinoma in situ of unspecified female genital organs ♀

D07.39 Carcinoma in situ of other female genital organs ♀

D07.4 Carcinoma in situ of penis ♂
Erythroplasia of Queyrat NOS

D07.5 Carcinoma in situ of prostate ♂
Prostatic intraepithelial neoplasia III (PIN III)
Severe dysplasia of prostate
- EXCLUDES 1 dysplasia (mild) (moderate) of prostate (N42.3)

✓5th **D07.6 Carcinoma in situ of other and unspecified male genital organs**

D07.60 Carcinoma in situ of unspecified male genital organs ♂

D07.61 Carcinoma in situ of scrotum ♂

D07.69 Carcinoma in situ of other male genital organs ♂

✓4th **D09 Carcinoma in situ of other and unspecified sites**
- EXCLUDES 1 melanoma in situ (D03.-)

D09.0 Carcinoma in situ of bladder

✓5th **D09.1 Carcinoma in situ of other and unspecified urinary organs**

D09.10 Carcinoma in situ of unspecified urinary organ

D09.19 Carcinoma in situ of other urinary organs

✓5th **D09.2 Carcinoma in situ of eye**
- EXCLUDES 1 carcinoma in situ of skin of eyelid (D04.1-)

D09.20 Carcinoma in situ of unspecified eye

D09.21 Carcinoma in situ of right eye

D09.22 Carcinoma in situ of left eye

D09.3 Carcinoma in situ of thyroid and other endocrine glands
- EXCLUDES 1 carcinoma in situ of endocrine pancreas (D01.7)
carcinoma in situ of ovary (D07.39)
carcinoma in situ of testis (D07.69)

D09.8 Carcinoma in situ of other specified sites

D09.9 Carcinoma in situ, unspecified

Benign neoplasms, except benign neuroendocrine tumors (D10-D36)

✓4th **D10 Benign neoplasm of mouth and pharynx**

D10.0 Benign neoplasm of lip
Benign neoplasm of lip (frenulum) (inner aspect) (mucosa) (vermilion border)
- EXCLUDES 1 benign neoplasm of skin of lip (D22.0, D23.0)

D10.1 Benign neoplasm of tongue
Benign neoplasm of lingual tonsil

D10.2 Benign neoplasm of floor of mouth

✓5th **D10.3 Other and unspecified parts of mouth**

D10.30 Benign neoplasm of unspecified part of mouth

D10.39 Benign neoplasm of other parts of mouth
Benign neoplasm of minor salivary gland NOS
- EXCLUDES 1 benign odontogenic neoplasms (D16.4-D16.5)
benign neoplasm of mucosa of lip (D10.0)
benign neoplasm of nasopharyngeal surface of soft palate (D10.6)

D10.4 Benign neoplasm of tonsil
Benign neoplasm of tonsil (faucial) (palatine)
- EXCLUDES 1 benign neoplasm of lingual tonsil (D10.1)
benign neoplasm of pharyngeal tonsil (D10.6)
benign neoplasm of tonsillar fossa (D10.5)
benign neoplasm of tonsillar pillars (D10.5)

D10.5 Benign neoplasm of other parts of oropharynx
Benign neoplasm of epiglottis, anterior aspect
Benign neoplasm of tonsillar fossa
Benign neoplasm of tonsillar pillars
Benign neoplasm of vallecula
- EXCLUDES 1 benign neoplasm of epiglottis NOS (D14.1)
benign neoplasm of epiglottis, suprahyoid portion (D14.1)

D10.6 Benign neoplasm of nasopharynx
Benign neoplasm of pharyngeal tonsil
Benign neoplasm of posterior margin of septum and choanae

D10.7 Benign neoplasm of hypopharynx

D10.9 Benign neoplasm of pharynx, unspecified

✓4th **D11 Benign neoplasm of major salivary glands**
- EXCLUDES 1 benign neoplasms of specified minor salivary glands which are classified according to their anatomical location
benign neoplasms of minor salivary glands NOS (D10.39)

D11.0 Benign neoplasm of parotid gland

D11.7 Benign neoplasm of other major salivary glands
Benign neoplasm of sublingual salivary gland
Benign neoplasm of submandibular salivary gland

D11.9 Benign neoplasm of major salivary gland, unspecified

✓4th **D12 Benign neoplasm of colon, rectum, anus and anal canal**
- EXCLUDES 1 benign carcinoid tumors of the large intestine, and rectum (D3A.02-)

D12.0 Benign neoplasm of cecum
Benign neoplasm of ileocecal valve

D12.1 Benign neoplasm of appendix
- EXCLUDES 1 benign carcinoid tumor of the appendix (D3A.020)

D12.2 Benign neoplasm of ascending colon

D12.3 Benign neoplasm of transverse colon
Benign neoplasm of hepatic flexure
Benign neoplasm of splenic flexure

D12.4 Benign neoplasm of descending colon

D12.5 Benign neoplasm of sigmoid colon

D12.6 Benign neoplasm of colon, unspecified
Adenomatosis of colon
Benign neoplasm of large intestine NOS
Polyposis (hereditary) of colon
- EXCLUDES 1 inflammatory polyp of colon (K51.4-)
polyp of colon NOS (K63.5)

D12.7 Benign neoplasm of rectosigmoid junction

D12.8 Benign neoplasm of rectum
- EXCLUDES 1 benign carcinoid tumor of the rectum (D3A.026)

D12.9 Benign neoplasm of anus and anal canal
Benign neoplasm of anus NOS
- EXCLUDES 1 benign neoplasm of anal margin (D22.5, D23.5)
benign neoplasm of anal skin (D22.5, D23.5)
benign neoplasm of perianal skin (D22.5, D23.5)

✓4ᵗʰ D13 Benign neoplasm of other and ill-defined parts of digestive system
> EXCLUDES 1   *benign stromal tumors of digestive system (D21.4)*

D13.0 Benign neoplasm of esophagus

D13.1 Benign neoplasm of stomach
> EXCLUDES 1   *benign carcinoid tumor of the stomach (D3A.092)*

D13.2 Benign neoplasm of duodenum
> EXCLUDES 1   *benign carcinoid tumor of the duodenum (D3A.010)*

✓5ᵗʰ D13.3 Benign neoplasm of other and unspecified parts of small intestine
> EXCLUDES 1   *benign carcinoid tumors of the small intestine (D3A.01)*
> *benign neoplasm of ileocecal valve (D12.0)*

     D13.30 Benign neoplasm of unspecified part of small intestine

     D13.39 Benign neoplasm of other parts of small intestine

D13.4 Benign neoplasm of liver
     Benign neoplasm of intrahepatic bile ducts

D13.5 Benign neoplasm of extrahepatic bile ducts

D13.6 Benign neoplasm of pancreas
> EXCLUDES 1   *benign neoplasm of endocrine pancreas (D13.7)*

D13.7 Benign neoplasm of endocrine pancreas
     Islet cell tumor
     Benign neoplasm of islets of Langerhans
     Use additional code to identify any functional activity

D13.9 Benign neoplasm of ill-defined sites within the digestive system
     Benign neoplasm of digestive system NOS
     Benign neoplasm of intestine NOS
     Benign neoplasm of spleen

✓4ᵗʰ D14 Benign neoplasm of middle ear and respiratory system

D14.0 Benign neoplasm of middle ear, nasal cavity and accessory sinuses
     Benign neoplasm of cartilage of nose
> EXCLUDES 1   *benign neoplasm of auricular canal (external) (D22.2-, D23.2-)*
> *benign neoplasm of bone of ear (D16.4)*
> *benign neoplasm of bone of nose (D16.4)*
> *benign neoplasm of cartilage of ear (D21.0)*
> *benign neoplasm of ear (external)(skin) (D22.2-, D23.2-)*
> *benign neoplasm of nose NOS (D36.7)*
> *benign neoplasm of skin of nose (D22.39, D23.39)*
> *benign neoplasm of olfactory bulb (D33.3)*
> *benign neoplasm of posterior margin of septum and choanae (D10.6)*
> *polyp of accessory sinus (J33.8)*
> *polyp of ear (middle) (H74.4)*
> *polyp of nasal (cavity) (J33.-)*

D14.1 Benign neoplasm of larynx
     Adenomatous polyp of larynx
     Benign neoplasm of epiglottis (suprahyoid portion)
> EXCLUDES 1   *benign neoplasm of epiglottis, anterior aspect (D10.5)*
> *polyp (nonadenomatous) of vocal cord or larynx (J38.1)*

D14.2 Benign neoplasm of trachea

✓5ᵗʰ D14.3 Benign neoplasm of bronchus and lung
> EXCLUDES 1   *benign carcinoid tumor of the bronchus and lung (D3A.090)*

     D14.30 Benign neoplasm of unspecified bronchus and lung
     D14.31 Benign neoplasm of right bronchus and lung
     D14.32 Benign neoplasm of left bronchus and lung

D14.4 Benign neoplasm of respiratory system, unspecified

✓4ᵗʰ D15 Benign neoplasm of other and unspecified intrathoracic organs
> EXCLUDES 1   *benign neoplasm of mesothelial tissue (D19.-)*

D15.0 Benign neoplasm of thymus
> EXCLUDES 1   *benign carcinoid tumor of the thymus (D3A.091)*

D15.1 Benign neoplasm of heart
> EXCLUDES 1   *benign neoplasm of great vessels (D21.3)*

D15.2 Benign neoplasm of mediastinum

D15.7 Benign neoplasm of other specified intrathoracic organs

D15.9 Benign neoplasm of intrathoracic organ, unspecified

✓4ᵗʰ D16 Benign neoplasm of bone and articular cartilage
> EXCLUDES 1   *benign neoplasm of connective tissue of ear (D21.0)*
> *benign neoplasm of connective tissue of eyelid (D21.0)*
> *benign neoplasm of connective tissue of larynx (D14.1)*
> *benign neoplasm of connective tissue of nose (D14.0)*
> *benign neoplasm of synovia (D21.-)*

✓5ᵗʰ D16.0 Benign neoplasm of scapula and long bones of upper limb
     D16.00 Benign neoplasm of scapula and long bones of unspecified upper limb
     D16.01 Benign neoplasm of scapula and long bones of right upper limb
     D16.02 Benign neoplasm of scapula and long bones of left upper limb

✓5ᵗʰ D16.1 Benign neoplasm of short bones of upper limb
     D16.10 Benign neoplasm of short bones of unspecified upper limb
     D16.11 Benign neoplasm of short bones of right upper limb
     D16.12 Benign neoplasm of short bones of left upper limb

✓5ᵗʰ D16.2 Benign neoplasm of long bones of lower limb
     D16.20 Benign neoplasm of long bones of unspecified lower limb
     D16.21 Benign neoplasm of long bones of right lower limb
     D16.22 Benign neoplasm of long bones of left lower limb

✓5ᵗʰ D16.3 Benign neoplasm of short bones of lower limb
     D16.30 Benign neoplasm of short bones of unspecified lower limb
     D16.31 Benign neoplasm of short bones of right lower limb
     D16.32 Benign neoplasm of short bones of left lower limb

D16.4 Benign neoplasm of bones of skull and face
     Benign neoplasm of maxilla (superior)
     Benign neoplasm of orbital bone
     Keratocyst of maxilla
     Keratocystic odontogenic tumor of maxilla
> EXCLUDES 1   *benign neoplasm of lower jaw bone (D16.5)*

D16.5 Benign neoplasm of lower jaw bone
     Keratocyst of mandible
     Keratocystic odontogenic tumor of mandible

D16.6 Benign neoplasm of vertebral column
> EXCLUDES 1   *benign neoplasm of sacrum and coccyx (D16.8)*

D16.7 Benign neoplasm of ribs, sternum and clavicle

D16.8 Benign neoplasm of pelvic bones, sacrum and coccyx

D16.9 Benign neoplasm of bone and articular cartilage, unspecified

✓4ᵗʰ D17 Benign lipomatous neoplasm

D17.0 Benign lipomatous neoplasm of skin and subcutaneous tissue of head, face and neck

D17.1 Benign lipomatous neoplasm of skin and subcutaneous tissue of trunk

✓5ᵗʰ D17.2 Benign lipomatous neoplasm of skin and subcutaneous tissue of limb
     D17.20 Benign lipomatous neoplasm of skin and subcutaneous tissue of unspecified limb
     D17.21 Benign lipomatous neoplasm of skin and subcutaneous tissue of right arm
     D17.22 Benign lipomatous neoplasm of skin and subcutaneous tissue of left arm
     D17.23 Benign lipomatous neoplasm of skin and subcutaneous tissue of right leg
     D17.24 Benign lipomatous neoplasm of skin and subcutaneous tissue of left leg

✓5ᵗʰ D17.3 Benign lipomatous neoplasm of skin and subcutaneous tissue of other and unspecified sites
     D17.30 Benign lipomatous neoplasm of skin and subcutaneous tissue of unspecified sites
     D17.39 Benign lipomatous neoplasm of skin and subcutaneous tissue of other sites

D17.4 Benign lipomatous neoplasm of intrathoracic organs

D17.5 Benign lipomatous neoplasm of intra-abdominal organs
> EXCLUDES 1   *benign lipomatous neoplasm of peritoneum and retroperitoneum (D17.79)*

D17.6 Benign lipomatous neoplasm of spermatic cord   ♂

✓5ᵗʰ D17.7 Benign lipomatous neoplasm of other sites
     D17.71 Benign lipomatous neoplasm of kidney
     D17.72 Benign lipomatous neoplasm of other genitourinary organ

---

N Newborn: 0   P Pediatric: 0-17   M Maternity: 12-55   A Adult: 15-124   MCC Major CC Condition   PDx MCC PDx acts as own MCC   CC CC Condition   PDx CC PDx acts as own CC

478   ICD-10-CM Draft (2015)

Neoplasms

D17.79   **Benign lipomatous neoplasm of** other sites
Benign lipomatous neoplasm of peritoneum
Benign lipomatous neoplasm of retroperitoneum

D17.9   **Benign lipomatous neoplasm,** unspecified
Lipoma NOS

✓4th **D18**   **Hemangioma and lymphangioma, any site**
EXCLUDES 1   *benign neoplasm of glomus jugulare (D35.6)*
blue or pigmented nevus (D22.-)
nevus NOS (D22.-)
vascular nevus (Q82.5)

✓5th **D18.0**   **Hemangioma**
Angioma NOS
Cavernous nevus

     D18.00   **Hemangioma** unspecified site

     D18.01   **Hemangioma of** skin and subcutaneous tissue

     D18.02   **Hemangioma of** intracranial structures

     D18.03   **Hemangioma of** intra-abdominal structures

     D18.09   **Hemangioma of** other sites

D18.1   **Lymphangioma, any site**

✓4th **D19**   **Benign neoplasm of** mesothelial tissue

D19.0   **Benign neoplasm of mesothelial tissue of** pleura

D19.1   **Benign neoplasm of mesothelial tissue of** peritoneum

D19.7   **Benign neoplasm of mesothelial tissue of** other sites

D19.9   **Benign neoplasm of mesothelial tissue,** unspecified
Benign mesothelioma NOS

✓4th **D20**   **Benign neoplasm of soft tissue of** retroperitoneum and peritoneum
EXCLUDES 1   *benign lipomatous neoplasm of peritoneum and retroperitoneum (D17.79)*
benign neoplasm of mesothelial tissue (D19.-)

D20.0   **Benign neoplasm of soft tissue of** retroperitoneum

D20.1   **Benign neoplasm of soft tissue of** peritoneum

✓4th **D21**   **Other benign neoplasms of** connective and other soft tissue
INCLUDES   benign neoplasm of blood vessel
benign neoplasm of bursa
benign neoplasm of cartilage
benign neoplasm of fascia
benign neoplasm of fat
benign neoplasm of ligament, except uterine
benign neoplasm of lymphatic channel
benign neoplasm of muscle
benign neoplasm of synovia
benign neoplasm of tendon (sheath)
benign stromal tumors
EXCLUDES 1   *benign neoplasm of articular cartilage (D16.-)*
benign neoplasm of cartilage of larynx (D14.1)
benign neoplasm of cartilage of nose (D14.0)
benign neoplasm of connective tissue of breast (D24.-)
benign neoplasm of peripheral nerves and autonomic nervous system (D36.1-)
benign neoplasm of peritoneum (D20.1)
benign neoplasm of retroperitoneum (D20.0)
benign neoplasm of uterine ligament, any (D28.2)
benign neoplasm of vascular tissue (D18.-)
hemangioma (D18.0-)
lipomatous neoplasm (D17.-)
lymphangioma (D18.1)
uterine leiomyoma (D25.-)

D21.0   **Benign neoplasm of connective and other soft tissue of** head, face and neck
Benign neoplasm of connective tissue of ear
Benign neoplasm of connective tissue of eyelid
EXCLUDES 1   *benign neoplasm of connective tissue of orbit (D31.6-)*

✓5th **D21.1**   **Benign neoplasm of connective and other soft tissue of** upper limb, including shoulder

     D21.10   **Benign neoplasm of connective and other soft tissue of** unspecified upper limb, including shoulder

     D21.11   **Benign neoplasm of connective and other soft tissue of** right upper limb, including shoulder

     D21.12   **Benign neoplasm of connective and other soft tissue of** left upper limb, including shoulder

✓5th **D21.2**   **Benign neoplasm of connective and other soft tissue of** lower limb, including hip

     D21.20   **Benign neoplasm of connective and other soft tissue of** unspecified lower limb, including hip

     D21.21   **Benign neoplasm of connective and other soft tissue of** right lower limb, including hip

     D21.22   **Benign neoplasm of connective and other soft tissue of** left lower limb, including hip

D21.3   **Benign neoplasm of connective and other soft tissue of** thorax
Benign neoplasm of axilla
Benign neoplasm of diaphragm
Benign neoplasm of great vessels
EXCLUDES 1   *benign neoplasm of heart (D15.1)*
benign neoplasm of mediastinum (D15.2)
benign neoplasm of thymus (D15.0)

D21.4   **Benign neoplasm of connective and other soft tissue of** abdomen
Benign stromal tumors of abdomen

D21.5   **Benign neoplasm of connective and other soft tissue of** pelvis
EXCLUDES 1   *benign neoplasm of any uterine ligament (D28.2)*
uterine leiomyoma (D25.-)

D21.6   **Benign neoplasm of connective and other soft tissue of** trunk, unspecified
Benign neoplasm of back NOS

D21.9   **Benign neoplasm of connective and other soft tissue,** unspecified

✓4th **D22**   **Melanocytic nevi**
INCLUDES   atypical nevus
blue hairy pigmented nevus
nevus NOS

D22.0   **Melanocytic nevi of** lip

✓5th **D22.1**   **Melanocytic nevi of** eyelid, including canthus

     D22.10   **Melanocytic nevi of** unspecified eyelid, including canthus

     D22.11   **Melanocytic nevi of** right eyelid, including canthus

     D22.12   **Melanocytic nevi of** left eyelid, including canthus

✓5th **D22.2**   **Melanocytic nevi of** ear and external auricular canal

     D22.20   **Melanocytic nevi of** unspecified ear and external auricular canal

     D22.21   **Melanocytic nevi of** right ear and external auricular canal

     D22.22   **Melanocytic nevi of** left ear and external auricular canal

✓5th **D22.3**   **Melanocytic nevi of** other and unspecified parts of face

     D22.30   **Melanocytic nevi of** unspecified part of face

     D22.39   **Melanocytic nevi of** other parts of face

D22.4   **Melanocytic nevi of** scalp and neck

D22.5   **Melanocytic nevi of** trunk
Melanocytic nevi of anal margin
Melanocytic nevi of anal skin
Melanocytic nevi of perianal skin
Melanocytic nevi of skin of breast

✓5th **D22.6**   **Melanocytic nevi of** upper limb, including shoulder

     D22.60   **Melanocytic nevi of** unspecified upper limb, including shoulder

     D22.61   **Melanocytic nevi of** right upper limb, including shoulder

     D22.62   **Melanocytic nevi of** left upper limb, including shoulder

✓5th **D22.7**   **Melanocytic nevi of** lower limb, including hip

     D22.70   **Melanocytic nevi of** unspecified lower limb, including hip

     D22.71   **Melanocytic nevi of** right lower limb, including hip

     D22.72   **Melanocytic nevi of** left lower limb, including hip

D22.9   **Melanocytic nevi,** unspecified

✓4th **D23**   **Other benign neoplasms of** skin
INCLUDES   benign neoplasm of hair follicles
benign neoplasm of sebaceous glands
benign neoplasm of sweat glands
EXCLUDES 1   *benign lipomatous neoplasms of skin (D17.0-D17.3)*
melanocytic nevi (D22.-)

D23.0   **Other benign neoplasm of skin of** lip
EXCLUDES 1   *benign neoplasm of vermilion border of lip (D10.0)*

✓5th **D23.1**   **Other benign neoplasm of skin of** eyelid, including canthus

     D23.10   **Other benign neoplasm of skin of** unspecified eyelid, including canthus

     D23.11   **Other benign neoplasm of skin of** right eyelid, including canthus

     D23.12   **Other benign neoplasm of skin of** left eyelid, including canthus

---

✓ Additional Character Required   ✓x7th Xtension Alert   Unacceptable PDx   Manifestation   Hospital Acquired Condition   EXCLUDES 1 Not Coded Here   EXCLUDES 2 Not Included Here

ICD-10-CM Draft (2015)   479

Neoplasms

D23.2–D31.10

√5th **D23.2** **Other benign neoplasm of skin of** ear and external auricular canal

     D23.20 Other benign neoplasm of skin of unspecified ear and external auricular canal

     D23.21 Other benign neoplasm of skin of right ear and external auricular canal

     D23.22 Other benign neoplasm of skin of left ear and external auricular canal

√5th **D23.3** **Other benign neoplasm of skin of** other and unspecified parts of face

     D23.30 Other benign neoplasm of skin of unspecified part of face

     D23.39 Other benign neoplasm of skin of other parts of face

D23.4 **Other benign neoplasm of skin of** scalp and neck

D23.5 **Other benign neoplasm of skin of** trunk

     Other benign neoplasm of anal margin
     Other benign neoplasm of anal skin
     Other benign neoplasm of perianal skin
     Other benign neoplasm of skin of breast
     EXCLUDES 1   *benign neoplasm of anus NOS (D12.9)*

√5th **D23.6** **Other benign neoplasm of skin of** upper limb, including shoulder

     D23.60 Other benign neoplasm of skin of unspecified upper limb, including shoulder

     D23.61 Other benign neoplasm of skin of right upper limb, including shoulder

     D23.62 Other benign neoplasm of skin of left upper limb, including shoulder

√5th **D23.7** **Other benign neoplasm of skin of** lower limb, including hip

     D23.70 Other benign neoplasm of skin of unspecified lower limb, including hip

     D23.71 Other benign neoplasm of skin of right lower limb, including hip

     D23.72 Other benign neoplasm of skin of left lower limb, including hip

D23.9 **Other benign neoplasm of skin,** unspecified

√4th **D24** **Benign neoplasm of** breast

     INCLUDES   benign neoplasm of connective tissue of breast
              benign neoplasm of soft parts of breast
              fibroadenoma of breast
     EXCLUDES 2   *adenofibrosis of breast (N60.2)*
              benign cyst of breast (N60.-)
              benign mammary dysplasia (N60.-)
              benign neoplasm of skin of breast (D22.5, D23.5)
              fibrocystic disease of breast (N60.-)

D24.1 **Benign neoplasm of** right breast

D24.2 **Benign neoplasm of** left breast

D24.9 **Benign neoplasm of** unspecified breast

√4th **D25** **Leiomyoma of** uterus

     INCLUDES   uterine fibroid
              uterine fibromyoma
              uterine myoma

D25.0 **Submucous leiomyoma of uterus** ♀

D25.1 **Intramural leiomyoma of uterus** ♀
     Interstitial leiomyoma of uterus

D25.2 **Subserosal leiomyoma of uterus** ♀
     Subperitoneal leiomyoma of uterus

D25.9 **Leiomyoma of uterus, unspecified** ♀

√4th **D26** **Other benign neoplasms of** uterus

D26.0 **Other benign neoplasm of** cervix uteri ♀

D26.1 **Other benign neoplasm of** corpus uteri ♀

D26.7 **Other benign neoplasm of** other parts of uterus ♀

D26.9 **Other benign neoplasm of uterus, unspecified** ♀

√4th **D27** **Benign neoplasm of** ovary

     Use additional code to identify any functional activity
     EXCLUDES 2   *corpus albicans cyst (N83.2)*
              corpus luteum cyst (N83.1)
              endometrial cyst (N80.1)
              follicular (atretic) cyst (N83.0)
              graafian follicle cyst (N83.0)
              ovarian cyst NEC (N83.2)
              ovarian retention cyst (N83.2)

D27.0 **Benign neoplasm of** right ovary ♀

D27.1 **Benign neoplasm of** left ovary ♀

D27.9 **Benign neoplasm of** unspecified ovary ♀

√4th **D28** **Benign neoplasm of** other and unspecified female genital organs

     INCLUDES   adenomatous polyp
              benign neoplasm of skin of female genital organs
              benign teratoma
     EXCLUDES 1   *epoophoron cyst (Q50.5)*
              fimbrial cyst (Q50.4)
              Gartner's duct cyst (Q52.4)
              parovarian cyst (Q50.5)

D28.0 **Benign neoplasm of** vulva ♀

D28.1 **Benign neoplasm of** vagina ♀

D28.2 **Benign neoplasm of** uterine tubes and ligaments ♀
     Benign neoplasm of fallopian tube
     Benign neoplasm of uterine ligament (broad) (round)

D28.7 **Benign neoplasm of** other specified female genital organs ♀

D28.9 **Benign neoplasm of** female genital organ, unspecified ♀

√4th **D29** **Benign neoplasm of** male genital organs

     INCLUDES   benign neoplasm of skin of male genital organs

D29.0 **Benign neoplasm of** penis ♂

D29.1 **Benign neoplasm of** prostate ♂
     EXCLUDES 1   *enlarged prostate (N40.-)*

√5th **D29.2** **Benign neoplasm of** testis
     Use additional code to identify any functional activity

     D29.20 Benign neoplasm of unspecified testis ♂

     D29.21 Benign neoplasm of right testis ♂

     D29.22 Benign neoplasm of left testis ♂

√5th **D29.3** **Benign neoplasm of** epididymis

     D29.30 Benign neoplasm of unspecified epididymis ♂

     D29.31 Benign neoplasm of right epididymis ♂

     D29.32 Benign neoplasm of left epididymis ♂

D29.4 **Benign neoplasm of** scrotum ♂
     Benign neoplasm of skin of scrotum

D29.8 **Benign neoplasm of** other specified male genital organs ♂
     Benign neoplasm of seminal vesicle
     Benign neoplasm of spermatic cord
     Benign neoplasm of tunica vaginalis

D29.9 **Benign neoplasm of** male genital organ, unspecified ♂

√4th **D30** **Benign neoplasm of** urinary organs

√5th **D30.0** **Benign neoplasm of** kidney
     EXCLUDES 1   *benign carcinoid tumor of the kidney (D3A.093)*
              benign neoplasm of renal calyces (D30.1-)
              benign neoplasm of renal pelvis (D30.1-)

     D30.00 Benign neoplasm of unspecified kidney

     D30.01 Benign neoplasm of right kidney

     D30.02 Benign neoplasm of left kidney

√5th **D30.1** **Benign neoplasm of** renal pelvis

     D30.10 Benign neoplasm of unspecified renal pelvis

     D30.11 Benign neoplasm of right renal pelvis

     D30.12 Benign neoplasm of left renal pelvis

√5th **D30.2** **Benign neoplasm of** ureter
     EXCLUDES 1   *benign neoplasm of ureteric orifice of bladder (D30.3)*

     D30.20 Benign neoplasm of unspecified ureter

     D30.21 Benign neoplasm of right ureter

     D30.22 Benign neoplasm of left ureter

D30.3 **Benign neoplasm of** bladder
     Benign neoplasm of ureteric orifice of bladder
     Benign neoplasm of urethral orifice of bladder

D30.4 **Benign neoplasm of** urethra
     EXCLUDES 1   *benign neoplasm of urethral orifice of bladder (D30.3)*

D30.8 **Benign neoplasm of** other specified urinary organs
     Benign neoplasm of paraurethral glands

D30.9 **Benign neoplasm of** urinary organ, unspecified
     Benign neoplasm of urinary system NOS

√4th **D31** **Benign neoplasm of** eye and adnexa
     EXCLUDES 1   *benign neoplasm of connective tissue of eyelid (D21.0)*
              benign neoplasm of optic nerve (D33.3)
              benign neoplasm of skin of eyelid (D22.1-, D23.1-)

√5th **D31.0** **Benign neoplasm of** conjunctiva

     D31.00 Benign neoplasm of unspecified conjunctiva

     D31.01 Benign neoplasm of right conjunctiva

     D31.02 Benign neoplasm of left conjunctiva

√5th **D31.1** **Benign neoplasm of** cornea

     D31.10 Benign neoplasm of unspecified cornea

N Newborn: 0   P Pediatric: 0-17   M Maternity: 12-55   A Adult: 15-124   MCC Major CC Condition   PDx MCC PDx acts as own MCC   CC CC Condition   PDx CC PDx acts as own CC

480   ICD-10-CM Draft (2015)

D31.11 Benign neoplasm of right cornea
D31.12 Benign neoplasm of left cornea

✓5ᵗʰ **D31.2** Benign neoplasm of retina
　EXCLUDES 1　dark area on retina (D49.81)
　　　　　　hemangioma of retina (D49.81)
　　　　　　neoplasm of unspecified behavior of retina and choroid
　　　　　　　(D49.81)
　　　　　　retinal freckle (D49.81)

D31.20 Benign neoplasm of unspecified retina
D31.21 Benign neoplasm of right retina
D31.22 Benign neoplasm of left retina

✓5ᵗʰ **D31.3** Benign neoplasm of choroid
D31.30 Benign neoplasm of unspecified choroid
D31.31 Benign neoplasm of right choroid
D31.32 Benign neoplasm of left choroid

✓5ᵗʰ **D31.4** Benign neoplasm of ciliary body
D31.40 Benign neoplasm of unspecified ciliary body
D31.41 Benign neoplasm of right ciliary body
D31.42 Benign neoplasm of left ciliary body

✓5ᵗʰ **D31.5** Benign neoplasm of lacrimal gland and duct
Benign neoplasm of lacrimal sac
Benign neoplasm of nasolacrimal duct

D31.50 Benign neoplasm of unspecified lacrimal gland and duct
D31.51 Benign neoplasm of right lacrimal gland and duct
D31.52 Benign neoplasm of left lacrimal gland and duct

✓5ᵗʰ **D31.6** Benign neoplasm of unspecified site of orbit
Benign neoplasm of connective tissue of orbit
Benign neoplasm of extraocular muscle
Benign neoplasm of peripheral nerves of orbit
Benign neoplasm of retrobulbar tissue
Benign neoplasm of retro-ocular tissue
　EXCLUDES 1　benign neoplasm of orbital bone (D16.4)

D31.60 Benign neoplasm of unspecified site of unspecified orbit
D31.61 Benign neoplasm of unspecified site of right orbit
D31.62 Benign neoplasm of unspecified site of left orbit

✓5ᵗʰ **D31.9** Benign neoplasm of unspecified part of eye
Benign neoplasm of eyeball

D31.90 Benign neoplasm of unspecified part of unspecified eye
D31.91 Benign neoplasm of unspecified part of right eye
D31.92 Benign neoplasm of unspecified part of left eye

✓4ᵗʰ **D32** Benign neoplasm of meninges
D32.0 Benign neoplasm of cerebral meninges
D32.1 Benign neoplasm of spinal meninges
D32.9 Benign neoplasm of meninges, unspecified
Meningioma NOS

✓4ᵗʰ **D33** Benign neoplasm of brain and other parts of central nervous system
　EXCLUDES 1　angioma (D18.0-)
　　　　　　benign neoplasm of meninges (D32.-)
　　　　　　benign neoplasm of peripheral nerves and autonomic nervous
　　　　　　　system (D36.1-)
　　　　　　hemangioma (D18.0-)
　　　　　　neurofibromatosis (Q85.0-)
　　　　　　retro-ocular benign neoplasm (D31.6-)

D33.0 Benign neoplasm of brain, supratentorial
Benign neoplasm of cerebral ventricle
Benign neoplasm of cerebrum
Benign neoplasm of frontal lobe
Benign neoplasm of occipital lobe
Benign neoplasm of parietal lobe
Benign neoplasm of temporal lobe
　EXCLUDES 1　benign neoplasm of fourth ventricle (D33.1)

D33.1 Benign neoplasm of brain, infratentorial
Benign neoplasm of brain stem
Benign neoplasm of cerebellum
Benign neoplasm of fourth ventricle

D33.2 Benign neoplasm of brain, unspecified
D33.3 Benign neoplasm of cranial nerves
Benign neoplasm of olfactory bulb

D33.4 Benign neoplasm of spinal cord
D33.7 Benign neoplasm of other specified parts of central nervous system

D33.9 Benign neoplasm of central nervous system, unspecified
Benign neoplasm of nervous system (central) NOS

D34 Benign neoplasm of thyroid gland
Use additional code to identify any functional activity

✓4ᵗʰ **D35** Benign neoplasm of other and unspecified endocrine glands
Use additional code to identify any functional activity
　EXCLUDES 1　benign neoplasm of endocrine pancreas (D13.7)
　　　　　　benign neoplasm of ovary (D27.-)
　　　　　　benign neoplasm of testis (D29.2-)
　　　　　　benign neoplasm of thymus (D15.0)

✓5ᵗʰ **D35.0** Benign neoplasm of adrenal gland
D35.00 Benign neoplasm of unspecified adrenal gland
D35.01 Benign neoplasm of right adrenal gland
D35.02 Benign neoplasm of left adrenal gland

D35.1 Benign neoplasm of parathyroid gland
D35.2 Benign neoplasm of pituitary gland
D35.3 Benign neoplasm of craniopharyngeal duct
D35.4 Benign neoplasm of pineal gland
D35.5 Benign neoplasm of carotid body
D35.6 Benign neoplasm of aortic body and other paraganglia
Benign tumor of glomus jugulare

D35.7 Benign neoplasm of other specified endocrine glands
D35.9 Benign neoplasm of endocrine gland, unspecified
Benign neoplasm of unspecified endocrine gland

✓4ᵗʰ **D36** Benign neoplasm of other and unspecified sites
D36.0 Benign neoplasm of lymph nodes
　EXCLUDES 1　lymphangioma (D18.1)

✓5ᵗʰ **D36.1** Benign neoplasm of peripheral nerves and autonomic nervous system
　EXCLUDES 1　benign neoplasm of peripheral nerves of orbit (D31.6-)
　　　　　　neurofibromatosis (Q85.0-)

D36.10 Benign neoplasm of peripheral nerves and autonomic nervous system, unspecified
D36.11 Benign neoplasm of peripheral nerves and autonomic nervous system of face, head, and neck
D36.12 Benign neoplasm of peripheral nerves and autonomic nervous system, upper limb, including shoulder
D36.13 Benign neoplasm of peripheral nerves and autonomic nervous system of lower limb, including hip
D36.14 Benign neoplasm of peripheral nerves and autonomic nervous system of thorax
D36.15 Benign neoplasm of peripheral nerves and autonomic nervous system of abdomen
D36.16 Benign neoplasm of peripheral nerves and autonomic nervous system of pelvis
D36.17 Benign neoplasm of peripheral nerves and autonomic nervous system of trunk, unspecified

D36.7 Benign neoplasm of other specified sites
Benign neoplasm of nose NOS
D36.9 Benign neoplasm, unspecified site

Benign neuroendocrine tumors (D3A)

✓4ᵗʰ **D3A** Benign neuroendocrine tumors
Code also any associated multiple endocrine neoplasia [MEN] syndromes (E31.2-)
Use additional code to identify any associated endocrine syndrome, such as:
carcinoid syndrome (E34.0)
　EXCLUDES 2　benign pancreatic islet cell tumors (D13.7)

✓5ᵗʰ **D3A.0** Benign carcinoid tumors
D3A.00 Benign carcinoid tumor of unspecified site
Carcinoid tumor NOS

✓6ᵗʰ **D3A.01** Benign carcinoid tumors of the small intestine
D3A.010 Benign carcinoid tumor of the duodenum
D3A.011 Benign carcinoid tumor of the jejunum
D3A.012 Benign carcinoid tumor of the ileum
D3A.019 Benign carcinoid tumor of the small intestine, unspecified portion

✓6ᵗʰ **D3A.02** Benign carcinoid tumors of the appendix, large intestine, and rectum
D3A.020 Benign carcinoid tumor of the appendix
D3A.021 Benign carcinoid tumor of the cecum

Neoplasms

D3A.Ø22–D4Ø.12

D3A.Ø22   **Benign carcinoid tumor of the** ascending colon

D3A.Ø23   **Benign carcinoid tumor of the** transverse colon

D3A.Ø24   **Benign carcinoid tumor of the** descending colon

D3A.Ø25   **Benign carcinoid tumor of the** sigmoid colon

D3A.Ø26   **Benign carcinoid tumor of the** rectum

D3A.Ø29   **Benign carcinoid tumor of the** large intestine, unspecified portion
     Benign carcinoid tumor of the colon NOS

✓6ᵗʰ   **D3A.Ø9   Benign carcinoid tumors of** other sites

D3A.Ø9Ø   **Benign carcinoid tumor of the** bronchus and lung

D3A.Ø91   **Benign carcinoid tumor of the** thymus

D3A.Ø92   **Benign carcinoid tumor of the** stomach

D3A.Ø93   **Benign carcinoid tumor of the** kidney

D3A.Ø94   **Benign carcinoid tumor of the** foregut NOS

D3A.Ø95   **Benign carcinoid tumor of the** midgut NOS

D3A.Ø96   **Benign carcinoid tumor of the** hindgut NOS

D3A.Ø98   **Benign carcinoid tumors of** other sites

D3A.8   Other benign neuroendocrine tumors
     Neuroendocrine tumor NOS

Neoplasms of uncertain behavior, polycythemia vera and myelodysplastic syndromes (D37-D48)

NOTE   Categories D37-D44, and D48 classify by site neoplasms of uncertain behavior, i.e., histologic confirmation whether the neoplasm is malignant or benign cannot be made.

EXCLUDES 1   *neoplasms of unspecified behavior (D49.-)*

✓4ᵗʰ   **D37   Neoplasm of uncertain behavior of** oral cavity and digestive organs

EXCLUDES 1   *stromal tumors of uncertain behavior of digestive system (D48.1)*

✓5ᵗʰ   **D37.Ø   Neoplasm of uncertain behavior of** lip, oral cavity and pharynx

EXCLUDES 1   *neoplasm of uncertain behavior of aryepiglottic fold or interarytenoid fold, laryngeal aspect (D38.Ø)*
neoplasm of uncertain behavior of epiglottis NOS (D38.Ø)
neoplasm of uncertain behavior of skin of lip (D48.5)
neoplasm of uncertain behavior of suprahyoid portion of epiglottis (D38.Ø)

D37.Ø1   **Neoplasm of uncertain behavior of** lip
     Neoplasm of uncertain behavior of vermilion border of lip

D37.Ø2   **Neoplasm of uncertain behavior of** tongue

✓6ᵗʰ   D37.Ø3   **Neoplasm of uncertain behavior of the** major salivary glands

D37.Ø3Ø   **Neoplasm of uncertain behavior of the** parotid salivary glands

D37.Ø31   **Neoplasm of uncertain behavior of the** sublingual salivary glands

D37.Ø32   **Neoplasm of uncertain behavior of the** submandibular salivary glands

D37.Ø39   **Neoplasm of uncertain behavior of the** major salivary glands, unspecified

D37.Ø4   **Neoplasm of uncertain behavior of the** minor salivary glands
     Neoplasm of uncertain behavior of submucosal salivary glands of lip
     Neoplasm of uncertain behavior of submucosal salivary glands of cheek
     Neoplasm of uncertain behavior of submucosal salivary glands of hard palate
     Neoplasm of uncertain behavior of submucosal salivary glands of soft palate

D37.Ø5   **Neoplasm of uncertain behavior of** pharynx
     Neoplasm of uncertain behavior of aryepiglottic fold of pharynx NOS
     Neoplasm of uncertain behavior of hypopharyngeal aspect of aryepiglottic fold of pharynx
     Neoplasm of uncertain behavior of marginal zone of aryepiglottic fold of pharynx

D37.Ø9   **Neoplasm of uncertain behavior of** other specified sites of the oral cavity

D37.1   Neoplasm of uncertain behavior of stomach

D37.2   **Neoplasm of uncertain behavior of** small intestine

D37.3   **Neoplasm of uncertain behavior of** appendix

D37.4   **Neoplasm of uncertain behavior of** colon

D37.5   **Neoplasm of uncertain behavior of** rectum
     Neoplasm of uncertain behavior of rectosigmoid junction

D37.6   **Neoplasm of uncertain behavior of** liver, gallbladder and bile ducts
     Neoplasm of uncertain behavior of ampulla of Vater

D37.8   **Neoplasm of uncertain behavior of** other specified digestive organs
     Neoplasm of uncertain behavior of anal canal
     Neoplasm of uncertain behavior of anal sphincter
     Neoplasm of uncertain behavior of anus NOS
     Neoplasm of uncertain behavior of esophagus
     Neoplasm of uncertain behavior of intestine NOS
     Neoplasm of uncertain behavior of pancreas

EXCLUDES 1   *neoplasm of uncertain behavior of anal margin (D48.5)*
neoplasm of uncertain behavior of anal skin (D48.5)
neoplasm of uncertain behavior of perianal skin (D48.5)

D37.9   **Neoplasm of uncertain behavior of** digestive organ, unspecified

✓4ᵗʰ   **D38   Neoplasm of uncertain behavior of** middle ear and respiratory and intrathoracic organs

EXCLUDES 1   *neoplasm of uncertain behavior of heart (D48.7)*

D38.Ø   **Neoplasm of uncertain behavior of** larynx
     Neoplasm of uncertain behavior of aryepiglottic fold or interarytenoid fold, laryngeal aspect
     Neoplasm of uncertain behavior of epiglottis (suprahyoid portion)

EXCLUDES 1   *neoplasm of uncertain behavior of aryepiglottic fold or interarytenoid fold NOS (D37.Ø5)*
neoplasm of uncertain behavior of hypopharyngeal aspect of aryepiglottic fold (D37.Ø5)
neoplasm of uncertain behavior of marginal zone of aryepiglottic fold (D37.Ø5)

D38.1   **Neoplasm of uncertain behavior of** trachea, bronchus and lung

D38.2   **Neoplasm of uncertain behavior of** pleura

D38.3   **Neoplasm of uncertain behavior of** mediastinum

D38.4   **Neoplasm of uncertain behavior of** thymus

D38.5   **Neoplasm of uncertain behavior of** other respiratory organs
     Neoplasm of uncertain behavior of accessory sinuses
     Neoplasm of uncertain behavior of cartilage of nose
     Neoplasm of uncertain behavior of middle ear
     Neoplasm of uncertain behavior of nasal cavities

EXCLUDES 1   *neoplasm of uncertain behavior of ear (external) (skin) (D48.5)*
neoplasm of uncertain behavior of nose NOS (D48.7)
neoplasm of uncertain behavior of skin of nose (D48.5)

D38.6   **Neoplasm of uncertain behavior of** respiratory organ, unspecified

✓4ᵗʰ   **D39   Neoplasm of uncertain behavior of** female genital organs

D39.Ø   **Neoplasm of uncertain behavior of** uterus   ♀

✓5ᵗʰ   D39.1   **Neoplasm of uncertain behavior of** ovary
     Use additional code to identify any functional activity

D39.1Ø   **Neoplasm of uncertain behavior of** unspecified ovary   ♀

D39.11   **Neoplasm of uncertain behavior of** right ovary   ♀

D39.12   **Neoplasm of uncertain behavior of** left ovary   ♀

D39.2   **Neoplasm of uncertain behavior of** placenta   ♀
     Chorioadenoma destruens
     Invasive hydatidiform mole
     Malignant hydatidiform mole

EXCLUDES 1   *hydatidiform mole NOS (OØ1.9)*

D39.8   **Neoplasm of uncertain behavior of** other specified female genital organs   ♀
     Neoplasm of uncertain behavior of skin of female genital organs

D39.9   **Neoplasm of uncertain behavior of** female genital organ, unspecified   ♀

✓4ᵗʰ   **D4Ø   Neoplasm of uncertain behavior of** male genital organs

D4Ø.Ø   **Neoplasm of uncertain behavior of** prostate   ♂

✓5ᵗʰ   D4Ø.1   **Neoplasm of uncertain behavior of** testis

D4Ø.1Ø   **Neoplasm of uncertain behavior of** unspecified testis   ♂

D4Ø.11   **Neoplasm of uncertain behavior of** right testis   ♂

D4Ø.12   **Neoplasm of uncertain behavior of** left testis   ♂

N Newborn: Ø   P Pediatric: Ø-17   M Maternity: 12-55   A Adult: 15-124   MCC Major CC Condition   PDx MCC PDx acts as own MCC   CC CC Condition   PDx CC PDx acts as own CC

482   ICD-10-CM Draft (2015)

D40.8 Neoplasm of uncertain behavior of other specified male ♂
genital organs
　　　Neoplasm of uncertain behavior of skin of male genital organs

D40.9 Neoplasm of uncertain behavior of male genital organ, ♂
unspecified

✓4th **D41** Neoplasm of uncertain behavior of urinary organs

　✓5th **D41.0** Neoplasm of uncertain behavior of kidney
　　　　EXCLUDES 1　neoplasm of uncertain behavior of renal pelvis (D41.1-)

　　　D41.00 Neoplasm of uncertain behavior of unspecified
kidney

　　　D41.01 Neoplasm of uncertain behavior of right kidney

　　　D41.02 Neoplasm of uncertain behavior of left kidney

　✓5th **D41.1** Neoplasm of uncertain behavior of renal pelvis

　　　D41.10 Neoplasm of uncertain behavior of unspecified renal
pelvis

　　　D41.11 Neoplasm of uncertain behavior of right renal pelvis

　　　D41.12 Neoplasm of uncertain behavior of left renal pelvis

　✓5th **D41.2** Neoplasm of uncertain behavior of ureter

　　　D41.20 Neoplasm of uncertain behavior of unspecified
ureter

　　　D41.21 Neoplasm of uncertain behavior of right ureter

　　　D41.22 Neoplasm of uncertain behavior of left ureter

　　D41.3 Neoplasm of uncertain behavior of urethra

　　D41.4 Neoplasm of uncertain behavior of bladder

　　D41.8 Neoplasm of uncertain behavior of other specified urinary
organs

　　D41.9 Neoplasm of uncertain behavior of unspecified urinary organ

✓4th **D42** Neoplasm of uncertain behavior of meninges

　　D42.0 Neoplasm of uncertain behavior of cerebral meninges

　　D42.1 Neoplasm of uncertain behavior of spinal meninges

　　D42.9 Neoplasm of uncertain behavior of meninges, unspecified

✓4th **D43** Neoplasm of uncertain behavior of brain and central nervous
system
　　EXCLUDES 1　neoplasm of uncertain behavior of peripheral nerves and
　　　　　　　　autonomic nervous system (D48.2)

　　D43.0 Neoplasm of uncertain behavior of brain, supratentorial
　　　Neoplasm of uncertain behavior of cerebral ventricle
　　　Neoplasm of uncertain behavior of cerebrum
　　　Neoplasm of uncertain behavior of frontal lobe
　　　Neoplasm of uncertain behavior of occipital lobe
　　　Neoplasm of uncertain behavior of parietal lobe
　　　Neoplasm of uncertain behavior of temporal lobe
　　　EXCLUDES 1　neoplasm of uncertain behavior of fourth ventricle
　　　　　　　　(D43.1)

　　D43.1 Neoplasm of uncertain behavior of brain, infratentorial
　　　Neoplasm of uncertain behavior of brain stem
　　　Neoplasm of uncertain behavior of cerebellum
　　　Neoplasm of uncertain behavior of fourth ventricle

　　D43.2 Neoplasm of uncertain behavior of brain, unspecified

　　D43.3 Neoplasm of uncertain behavior of cranial nerves

　　D43.4 Neoplasm of uncertain behavior of spinal cord

　　D43.8 Neoplasm of uncertain behavior of other specified parts of
central nervous system

　　D43.9 Neoplasm of uncertain behavior of central nervous system,
unspecified
　　　Neoplasm of uncertain behavior of nervous system (central)
　　　NOS

✓4th **D44** Neoplasm of uncertain behavior of endocrine glands
　　EXCLUDES 1　multiple endocrine adenomatosis (E31.2-)
　　　　　　　　multiple endocrine neoplasia (E31.2-)
　　　　　　　　neoplasm of uncertain behavior of endocrine pancreas (D37.8)
　　　　　　　　neoplasm of uncertain behavior of ovary (D39.1-)
　　　　　　　　neoplasm of uncertain behavior of testis (D40.1-)
　　　　　　　　neoplasm of uncertain behavior of thymus (D38.4)

　　D44.0 Neoplasm of uncertain behavior of thyroid gland

　✓5th **D44.1** Neoplasm of uncertain behavior of adrenal gland
　　　Use additional code to identify any functional activity

　　　D44.10 Neoplasm of uncertain behavior of unspecified
adrenal gland

　　　D44.11 Neoplasm of uncertain behavior of right adrenal
gland

　　　D44.12 Neoplasm of uncertain behavior of left adrenal
gland

　　D44.2 Neoplasm of uncertain behavior of parathyroid gland

　　D44.3 Neoplasm of uncertain behavior of pituitary gland
　　　Use additional code to identify any functional activity

　　D44.4 Neoplasm of uncertain behavior of craniopharyngeal duct

　　D44.5 Neoplasm of uncertain behavior of pineal gland

　　D44.6 Neoplasm of uncertain behavior of carotid body

　　D44.7 Neoplasm of uncertain behavior of aortic body and other
paraganglia

　　D44.9 Neoplasm of uncertain behavior of unspecified endocrine
gland

D45 Polycythemia vera
　　EXCLUDES 1　familial polycythemia (D75.0)
　　　　　　　　secondary polycythemia (D75.1)

✓4th **D46** Myelodysplastic syndromes
　　Use additional code for adverse effect, if applicable, to identify drug
　　(T36-T50 with fifth or sixth character 5)
　　EXCLUDES 2　drug-induced aplastic anemia (D61.1)

　　D46.0 Refractory anemia without ring sideroblasts, so stated
　　　Refractory anemia without sideroblasts, without excess of blasts

　　D46.1 Refractory anemia with ring sideroblasts
　　　RARS

　✓5th **D46.2** Refractory anemia with excess of blasts

　　　D46.20 Refractory anemia with excess of blasts, unspecified
　　　　RAEB NOS

　　　D46.21 Refractory anemia with excess of blasts 1
　　　　RAEB 1

　　　D46.22 Refractory anemia with excess of blasts 2　　CC
　　　　RAEB 2
　　　　CC Excl: C88.2-C88.3, C88.8-C88.9, C90.10-C90.11,
　　　　C90.20-C90.21, C90.30-C90.31, C91.00-C95.92, D45-
　　　　D47.1, D47.3, D47.Z9-D47.9, D48.7-D48.9

　　D46.A Refractory cytopenia with multilineage dysplasia

　　D46.B Refractory cytopenia with multilineage dysplasia and ring
sideroblasts
　　　RCMD RS

　　D46.C Myelodysplastic syndrome with isolated del(5q)　　CC
chromosomal abnormality
　　　Myelodysplastic syndrome with 5q deletion
　　　5q minus syndrome NOS
　　　CC Excl: See code: D46.22

　　D46.4 Refractory anemia, unspecified

　　D46.Z Other myelodysplastic syndromes
　　　EXCLUDES 1　chronic myelomonocytic leukemia (C93.1-)

　　D46.9 Myelodysplastic syndrome, unspecified
　　　Myelodysplasia NOS

✓4th **D47** Other neoplasms of uncertain behavior of lymphoid,
hematopoietic and related tissue

　　D47.0 Histiocytic and mast cell tumors of uncertain behavior　　CC
　　　Indolent systemic mastocytosis
　　　Mast cell tumor NOS
　　　Mastocytoma NOS
　　　EXCLUDES 1　malignant mast cell tumor (C96.2)
　　　　　　　　mastocytosis (congenital) (cutaneous) (Q82.2)
　　　CC Excl: C88.8, C94.40-C94.6, D45-D47.1, D47.3, D47.Z9-D47.9,
　　　D75.81, Z51.0

　　D47.1 Chronic myeloproliferative disease　　CC
　　　Chronic neutrophilic leukemia
　　　Myeloproliferative disease, unspecified
　　　EXCLUDES 1　atypical chronic myeloid leukemia BCR/ABL-negative
　　　　　　　　(C92.2-)
　　　　　　　　chronic myeloid leukemia BCR/ABL-positive (C92.1-)
　　　　　　　　myelofibrosis NOS (D75.81)
　　　　　　　　myelophthisic anemia (D61.82)
　　　　　　　　myelophthisis (D61.82)
　　　　　　　　secondary myelofibrosis NOS (D75.81)
　　　CC Excl: See code: D46.22

　　D47.2 Monoclonal gammopathy
　　　Monoclonal gammopathy of undetermined significance [MGUS]

　　D47.3 Essential (hemorrhagic) thrombocythemia
　　　Essential thrombocytosis
　　　Idiopathic hemorrhagic thrombocythemia

　　D47.4 Osteomyelofibrosis
　　　Chronic idiopathic myelofibrosis
　　　Myelofibrosis (idiopathic) (with myeloid metaplasia)
　　　Myelosclerosis (megakaryocytic) with myeloid metaplasia
　　　Secondary myelofibrosis in myeloproliferative disease
　　　EXCLUDES 1　acute myelofibrosis (C94.4-)

✓ Additional Character Required　✓x7th Xtension Alert　Unacceptable PDx　Manifestation　　Hospital Acquired Condition　EXCLUDES 1 Not Coded Here　EXCLUDES 2 Not Included Here

ICD-10-CM Draft (2015)　　　　　　　　　　　　　　　　　　　　　　　　　　　　483

D40.8–D47.4

Neoplasms

D47.Z–D49.9

✓5ᵗʰ **D47.Z** **Other** specified neoplasms of uncertain behavior of lymphoid, hematopoietic and related tissue

D47.Z1 **Post-transplant lymphoproliferative disorder (PTLD)**   CC
Code first complications of transplanted organs and tissue (T86.-)
CC Excl: D47.Z1, D78.81-D78.89, E89.810-E89.89, H59.011-H59.019, H59.031-H59.099, H59.811-H59.89, H95.811-H95.89, I97.3, M96.89, N98.1-N98.9, T86.850-T86.859, T86.90-T86.99

D47.Z9 **Other** specified neoplasms of uncertain behavior   CC of lymphoid, hematopoietic and related tissue
Histiocytic tumors of uncertain behavior
CC Excl: C88.2-C88.3, C88.8-C88.9, C90.10-C90.11, C90.20-C90.21, C90.30-C90.31, C91.00-C95.92, D45-D47.1, D47.3, D47.Z9-D47.9, D48.7-D48.9

D47.9 **Neoplasm** of uncertain behavior of lymphoid,   CC hematopoietic and related tissue, **unspecified**
Lymphoproliferative disease NOS
CC Excl: See code: D47.Z9

✓4ᵗʰ **D48** **Neoplasm** of uncertain behavior of other and unspecified sites
EXCLUDES 1   *neurofibromatosis (nonmalignant) (Q85.0-)*

D48.0 **Neoplasm** of uncertain behavior of **bone and articular cartilage**
EXCLUDES 1   *neoplasm of uncertain behavior of cartilage of ear (D48.1)*
neoplasm of uncertain behavior of cartilage of larynx (D38.0)
neoplasm of uncertain behavior of cartilage of nose (D38.5)
neoplasm of uncertain behavior of connective tissue of eyelid (D48.1)
neoplasm of uncertain behavior of synovia (D48.1)

D48.1 **Neoplasm** of uncertain behavior of **connective and other soft tissue**
Neoplasm of uncertain behavior of connective tissue of ear
Neoplasm of uncertain behavior of connective tissue of eyelid
Stromal tumors of uncertain behavior of digestive system
EXCLUDES 1   *neoplasm of uncertain behavior of articular cartilage (D48.0)*
neoplasm of uncertain behavior of cartilage of larynx (D38.0)
neoplasm of uncertain behavior of cartilage of nose (D38.5)
neoplasm of uncertain behavior of connective tissue of breast (D48.6-)

D48.2 **Neoplasm** of uncertain behavior of **peripheral nerves and autonomic nervous system**
EXCLUDES 1   *neoplasm of uncertain behavior of peripheral nerves of orbit (D48.7)*

D48.3 **Neoplasm** of uncertain behavior of **retroperitoneum**

D48.4 **Neoplasm** of uncertain behavior of **peritoneum**

D48.5 **Neoplasm** of uncertain behavior of **skin**
Neoplasm of uncertain behavior of anal margin
Neoplasm of uncertain behavior of anal skin
Neoplasm of uncertain behavior of perianal skin
Neoplasm of uncertain behavior of skin of breast
EXCLUDES 1   *neoplasm of uncertain behavior of anus NOS (D37.8)*
neoplasm of uncertain behavior of skin of genital organs (D39.8, D40.8)
neoplasm of uncertain behavior of vermilion border of lip (D37.0)

✓5ᵗʰ **D48.6** **Neoplasm** of uncertain behavior of **breast**
Neoplasm of uncertain behavior of connective tissue of breast
Cystosarcoma phyllodes
EXCLUDES 1   *neoplasm of uncertain behavior of skin of breast (D48.5)*

D48.60 **Neoplasm** of uncertain behavior of **unspecified breast**

D48.61 **Neoplasm** of uncertain behavior of **right breast**

D48.62 **Neoplasm** of uncertain behavior of **left breast**

D48.7 **Neoplasm** of uncertain behavior of **other** specified sites
Neoplasm of uncertain behavior of eye
Neoplasm of uncertain behavior of heart
Neoplasm of uncertain behavior of peripheral nerves of orbit
EXCLUDES 1   *neoplasm of uncertain behavior of connective tissue (D48.1)*
neoplasm of uncertain behavior of skin of eyelid (D48.5)

D48.9 **Neoplasm** of uncertain behavior, **unspecified**

Neoplasms of unspecified behavior (D49)

✓4ᵗʰ **D49** **Neoplasms** of unspecified behavior
NOTE   Category D49 classifies by site neoplasms of unspecified morphology and behavior. The term "mass", unless otherwise stated, is not to be regarded as a neoplastic growth.
INCLUDES   "growth" NOS
neoplasm NOS
new growth NOS
tumor NOS
EXCLUDES 1   *neoplasms of uncertain behavior (D37-D44, D48)*

D49.0 **Neoplasm** of unspecified behavior of **digestive system**
EXCLUDES 1   *neoplasm of unspecified behavior of margin of anus (D49.2)*
neoplasm of unspecified behavior of perianal skin (D49.2)
neoplasm of unspecified behavior of skin of anus (D49.2)

D49.1 **Neoplasm** of unspecified behavior of **respiratory system**

D49.2 **Neoplasm** of unspecified behavior of **bone, soft tissue, and skin**
EXCLUDES 1   *neoplasm of unspecified behavior of anal canal (D49.0)*
neoplasm of unspecified behavior of anus NOS (D49.0)
neoplasm of unspecified behavior of bone marrow (D49.89)
neoplasm of unspecified behavior of cartilage of larynx (D49.1)
neoplasm of unspecified behavior of cartilage of nose (D49.1)
neoplasm of unspecified behavior of connective tissue of breast (D49.3)
neoplasm of unspecified behavior of skin of genital organs (D49.5)
neoplasm of unspecified behavior of vermilion border of lip (D49.0)

D49.3 **Neoplasm** of unspecified behavior of **breast**
EXCLUDES 1   *neoplasm of unspecified behavior of skin of breast (D49.2)*

D49.4 **Neoplasm** of unspecified behavior of **bladder**

D49.5 **Neoplasm** of unspecified behavior of **other genitourinary organs**

D49.6 **Neoplasm** of unspecified behavior of **brain**
EXCLUDES 1   *neoplasm of unspecified behavior of cerebral meninges (D49.7)*
neoplasm of unspecified behavior of cranial nerves (D49.7)

D49.7 **Neoplasm** of unspecified behavior of **endocrine glands and other parts of nervous system**
EXCLUDES 1   *neoplasm of unspecified behavior of peripheral, sympathetic, and parasympathetic nerves and ganglia (D49.2)*

✓5ᵗʰ **D49.8** **Neoplasm** of unspecified behavior of **other specified sites**
EXCLUDES 1   *neoplasm of unspecified behavior of eyelid (skin) (D49.2)*
neoplasm of unspecified behavior of eyelid cartilage (D49.2)
neoplasm of unspecified behavior of great vessels (D49.2)
neoplasm of unspecified behavior of optic nerve (D49.7)

D49.81 **Neoplasm** of unspecified behavior of **retina and choroid**
Dark area on retina
Retinal freckle

D49.89 **Neoplasm** of unspecified behavior of **other specified sites**

D49.9 **Neoplasm** of unspecified behavior of **unspecified site**

N Newborn: 0   P Pediatric: 0-17   M Maternity: 12-55   A Adult: 15-124   MCC Major CC Condition   PDx MCC PDx acts as own MCC   CC CC Condition   PDx CC PDx acts as own CC

484   ICD-10-CM Draft (2015)

Chapter 3. Diseases of the Blood and Blood-forming Organs and Certain Disorders Involving the Immune Mechanism (D50-D89)

EXCLUDES 2　autoimmune disease (systemic) NOS (M35.9)
certain conditions originating in the perinatal period (P00-P96)
complications of pregnancy, childbirth and the puerperium (O00-O9A)
congenital malformations, deformations and chromosomal abnormalities (Q00-Q99)
endocrine, nutritional and metabolic diseases (E00-E88)
human immunodeficiency virus [HIV] disease (B20)
injury, poisoning and certain other consequences of external causes (S00-T88)
neoplasms (C00-D49)
symptoms, signs and abnormal clinical and laboratory findings, not elsewhere classified (R00-R94)

This chapter contains the following blocks:

D50-D53　Nutritional anemias
D55-D59　Hemolytic anemias
D60-D64　Aplastic and other anemias and other bone marrow failure syndromes
D65-D69　Coagulation defects, purpura and other hemorrhagic conditions
D70-D77　Other disorders of blood and blood-forming organs
D78　Intraoperative and postprocedural complications of the spleen
D80-D89　Certain disorders involving the immune mechanism

Nutritional anemias (D50-D53)

☑4ᵗʰ D50　Iron deficiency anemia
INCLUDES　asiderotic anemia
hypochromic anemia

D50.0　Iron deficiency anemia secondary to blood loss (chronic)
Posthemorrhagic anemia (chronic)
EXCLUDES 1　acute posthemorrhagic anemia (D62)
congenital anemia from fetal blood loss (P61.3)

D50.1　Sideropenic dysphagia
Kelly-Paterson syndrome
Plummer-Vinson syndrome

D50.8　Other iron deficiency anemias
Iron deficiency anemia due to inadequate dietary iron intake

D50.9　Iron deficiency anemia, unspecified

☑4ᵗʰ D51　Vitamin B12 deficiency anemia
EXCLUDES 1　vitamin B12 deficiency (E53.8)

D51.0　Vitamin B12 deficiency anemia due to intrinsic factor deficiency
Addison anemia
Biermer anemia
Pernicious (congenital) anemia
Congenital intrinsic factor deficiency

D51.1　Vitamin B12 deficiency anemia due to selective vitamin B12 malabsorption with proteinuria
Imerslund (Gräsbeck) syndrome
Megaloblastic hereditary anemia

D51.2　Transcobalamin II deficiency

D51.3　Other dietary vitamin B12 deficiency anemia
Vegan anemia

D51.8　Other vitamin B12 deficiency anemias

D51.9　Vitamin B12 deficiency anemia, unspecified

☑4ᵗʰ D52　Folate deficiency anemia
EXCLUDES 1　folate deficiency without anemia (E53.8)

D52.0　Dietary folate deficiency anemia
Nutritional megaloblastic anemia

D52.1　Drug-induced folate deficiency anemia
Use additional code for adverse effect, if applicable, to identify drug (T36-T50 with fifth or sixth character 5)

D52.8　Other folate deficiency anemias

D52.9　Folate deficiency anemia, unspecified
Folic acid deficiency anemia NOS

☑4ᵗʰ D53　Other nutritional anemias
INCLUDES　megaloblastic anemia unresponsive to vitamin B12 or folate therapy

D53.0　Protein deficiency anemia
Amino-acid deficiency anemia
Orotaciduric anemia
EXCLUDES 2　Lesch-Nyhan syndrome (E79.1)

D53.1　Other megaloblastic anemias, not elsewhere classified
Megaloblastic anemia NOS
EXCLUDES 1　Di Guglielmo's disease (C94.0)

D53.2　Scorbutic anemia
EXCLUDES 1　scurvy (E54)

D53.8　Other specified nutritional anemias
Anemia associated with deficiency of copper
Anemia associated with deficiency of molybdenum
Anemia associated with deficiency of zinc
EXCLUDES 1　nutritional deficiencies without anemia, such as:
copper deficiency NOS (E61.0)
molybdenum deficiency NOS (E61.5)
zinc deficiency NOS (E60)

D53.9　Nutritional anemia, unspecified
Simple chronic anemia
EXCLUDES 1　anemia NOS (D64.9)

Hemolytic anemias (D55-D59)

☑4ᵗʰ D55　Anemia due to enzyme disorders
EXCLUDES 1　drug-induced enzyme deficiency anemia (D59.2)

D55.0　Anemia due to glucose-6-phosphate dehydrogenase [G6PD] deficiency
Favism
G6PD deficiency anemia

D55.1　Anemia due to other disorders of glutathione metabolism
Anemia (due to) enzyme deficiencies, except G6PD, related to the hexose monophosphate [HMP] shunt pathway
Anemia (due to) hemolytic nonspherocytic (hereditary), type I

D55.2　Anemia due to disorders of glycolytic enzymes
Hemolytic nonspherocytic (hereditary) anemia, type II
Hexokinase deficiency anemia
Pyruvate kinase [PK] deficiency anemia
Triose-phosphate isomerase deficiency anemia
EXCLUDES 1　disorders of glycolysis not associated with anemia (E74.8)

D55.3　Anemia due to disorders of nucleotide metabolism

D55.8　Other anemias due to enzyme disorders

D55.9　Anemia due to enzyme disorder, unspecified

☑4ᵗʰ D56　Thalassemia
EXCLUDES 1　sickle-cell thalassemia (D57.4-)

D56.0　Alpha thalassemia
Alpha thalassemia major
Hemoglobin H Constant Spring
Hemoglobin H disease
Hydrops fetalis due to alpha thalassemia
Severe alpha thalassemia
Triple gene defect alpha thalassemia
Use additional code, if applicable, for hydrops fetalis due to alpha thalassemia (P56.99)
EXCLUDES 1　alpha thalassemia trait or minor (D56.3)
asymptomatic alpha thalassemia (D56.3)
hydrops fetalis due to isoimmunization (P56.0)
hydrops fetalis not due to immune hemolysis (P83.2)

D56.1　Beta thalassemia
Beta thalassemia major
Cooley's anemia
Homozygous beta thalassemia
Severe beta thalassemia
Thalassemia intermedia
Thalassemia major
EXCLUDES 1　beta thalassemia minor (D56.3)
beta thalassemia trait (D56.3)
delta-beta thalassemia (D56.2)
hemoglobin E-beta thalassemia (D56.5)
sickle-cell beta thalassemia (D57.4-)

D56.2　Delta-beta thalassemia
Homozygous delta-beta thalassemia
EXCLUDES 1　delta-beta thalassemia minor (D56.3)
delta-beta thalassemia trait (D56.3)

Diseases of the Blood and Blood-forming Organs

D56.3–D59.5

D56.3 **Thalassemia** minor
Alpha thalassemia minor
Alpha thalassemia silent carrier
Alpha thalassemia trait
Beta thalassemia minor
Beta thalassemia trait
Delta-beta thalassemia minor
Delta-beta thalassemia trait
Thalassemia trait NOS
> *EXCLUDES 1*   *alpha thalassemia (D56.0)*
> *beta thalassemia (D56.1)*
> *delta-beta thalassemia (D56.2)*
> *hemoglobin E-beta thalassemia (D56.5)*
> *sickle-cell trait (D57.3)*

D56.4 **Hereditary persistence of fetal hemoglobin [HPFH]**

D56.5 **Hemoglobin E-beta** thalassemia
> *EXCLUDES 1*   *beta thalassemia (D56.1)*
> *beta thalassemia minor (D56.3)*
> *beta thalassemia trait (D56.3)*
> *delta-beta thalassemia (D56.2)*
> *delta-beta thalassemia trait (D56.3)*
> *hemoglobin E disease (D58.2)*
> *other hemoglobinopathies (D58.2)*
> *sickle-cell beta thalassemia (D57.4-)*

D56.8 **Other** thalassemias
Dominant thalassemia
Hemoglobin C thalassemia
Mixed thalassemia
Thalassemia with other hemoglobinopathy
> *EXCLUDES 1*   *hemoglobin C disease (D58.2)*
> *hemoglobin E disease (D58.2)*
> *other hemoglobinopathies (D58.2)*
> *sickle-cell anemia (D57.-)*
> *sickle-cell thalassemia (D57.4)*

D56.9 **Thalassemia,** unspecified
Mediterranean anemia (with other hemoglobinopathy)

✓4ᵗʰ **D57** **Sickle-cell disorders**
Use additional code for any associated fever (R50.81)
> *EXCLUDES 1*   *other hemoglobinopathies (D58.-)*

> **CC Excl: For MCC codes in category D57, unless otherwise noted:**
> D47.4, D50.0-D64.9, D68.312, D68.51-D68.69, D75.81, D75.89-D75.9, D77, D89.2

✓5ᵗʰ **D57.0** **Hb-SS disease** with crisis
Sickle-cell disease NOS with crisis
Hb-SS disease with vasoocclusive pain

     D57.00 **Hb-SS disease with crisis,** unspecified   `MCC`

     D57.01 **Hb-SS disease with** acute chest syndrome   `MCC`

     D57.02 **Hb-SS disease with** splenic sequestration   `MCC`

D57.1 **Sickle-cell disease** without crisis
Hb-SS disease without crisis
Sickle-cell anemia NOS
Sickle-cell disease NOS
Sickle-cell disorder NOS

✓5ᵗʰ **D57.2** **Sickle-cell/**Hb-C **disease**
Hb-SC disease
Hb-S/Hb-C disease

     D57.20 **Sickle-cell/Hb-C disease** without crisis

✓6ᵗʰ **D57.21** **Sickle-cell/Hb-C disease** with crisis

        D57.211 **Sickle-cell/Hb-C disease with** acute chest syndrome   `PDx CC MCC`

        D57.212 **Sickle-cell/Hb-C disease with** splenic sequestration   `MCC`

        D57.219 **Sickle-cell/Hb-C disease with crisis,** unspecified   `MCC`
Sickle-cell/Hb-C disease with crisis NOS

D57.3 **Sickle-cell** trait
Hb-S trait
Heterozygous hemoglobin S

✓5ᵗʰ **D57.4** **Sickle-cell** thalassemia
Sickle-cell beta thalassemia
Thalassemia Hb-S disease

     D57.40 **Sickle-cell thalassemia** without crisis
Microdrepanocytosis
Sickle-cell thalassemia NOS

✓6ᵗʰ **D57.41** **Sickle-cell** thalassemia **with crisis**
Sickle-cell thalassemia with vasoocclusive pain

        D57.411 **Sickle-cell thalassemia with** acute chest syndrome   `PDx CC MCC`

        D57.412 **Sickle-cell thalassemia with** splenic sequestration   `MCC`

        D57.419 **Sickle-cell thalassemia with crisis,** unspecified   `MCC`
Sickle-cell thalassemia with crisis NOS

✓5ᵗʰ **D57.8** **Other** sickle-cell disorders
Hb-SD disease
Hb-SE disease

     D57.80 **Other sickle-cell disorders** without crisis

✓6ᵗʰ **D57.81** **Other sickle-cell disorders** with crisis

        D57.811 **Other sickle-cell disorders with** acute chest syndrome   `MCC`

        D57.812 **Other sickle-cell disorders with** splenic sequestration   `MCC`

        D57.819 **Other sickle-cell disorders with crisis,** unspecified   `MCC`
Other sickle-cell disorders with crisis NOS

✓4ᵗʰ **D58** **Other hereditary** hemolytic anemias
> *EXCLUDES 1*   *hemolytic anemia of the newborn (P55.-)*

D58.0 **Hereditary** spherocytosis
Acholuric (familial) jaundice
Congenital (spherocytic) hemolytic icterus
Minkowski-Chauffard syndrome

D58.1 **Hereditary** elliptocytosis
Elliptocytosis (congenital)
Ovalocytosis (congenital) (hereditary)

D58.2 **Other hemoglobinopathies**
Abnormal hemoglobin NOS
Congenital Heinz body anemia
Hb-C disease
Hb-D disease
Hb-E disease
Hemoglobinopathy NOS
Unstable hemoglobin hemolytic disease
> *EXCLUDES 1*   *familial polycythemia (D75.0)*
> *Hb-M disease (D74.0)*
> *hemoglobin E-beta thalassemia (D56.5)*
> *hereditary persistence of fetal hemoglobin [HPFH] (D56.4)*
> *high-altitude polycythemia (D75.1)*
> *methemoglobinemia (D74.-)*
> *other hemoglobinopathies with thalassemia (D56.8)*

D58.8 **Other specified hereditary hemolytic anemias**   `CC`
Stomatocytosis
CC Excl: D50.0-D64.9, D75.9, P61.2-P61.4

D58.9 **Hereditary hemolytic anemia,** unspecified   `CC`
CC Excl: See code: D58.8

✓4ᵗʰ **D59** **Acquired** hemolytic anemia

> **CC Excl: For CC/MCC codes in category D59, unless otherwise noted:** D47.4, D50.0-D64.9, D68.312, D68.51-D68.69, D75.81, D75.89-D75.9, D77, D89.2

D59.0 **Drug-induced autoimmune** hemolytic anemia   `CC`
Use additional code for adverse effect, if applicable, to identify drug (T36-T50 with fifth or sixth character 5)

D59.1 **Other autoimmune** hemolytic anemias   `CC`
Autoimmune hemolytic disease (cold type) (warm type)
Chronic cold hemagglutinin disease
Cold agglutinin disease
Cold agglutinin hemoglobinuria
Cold type (secondary) (symptomatic) hemolytic anemia
Warm type (secondary) (symptomatic) hemolytic anemia
> *EXCLUDES 1*   *Evans syndrome (D69.41)*
> *hemolytic disease of newborn (P55.-)*
> *paroxysmal cold hemoglobinuria (D59.6)*

D59.2 **Drug-induced nonautoimmune** hemolytic anemia   `CC`
Drug-induced enzyme deficiency anemia
Use additional code for adverse effect, if applicable, to identify drug (T36-T50 with fifth or sixth character 5)

D59.3 **Hemolytic-uremic syndrome**   `MCC`
Use additional code to identify associated:
   E. coli infection (B96.2-)
   Pneumococcal pneumonia (J13)
   Shigella dysenteriae (A03.9)

D59.4 **Other nonautoimmune** hemolytic anemias   `CC`
Mechanical hemolytic anemia
Microangiopathic hemolytic anemia
Toxic hemolytic anemia

D59.5 **Paroxysmal nocturnal hemoglobinuria [Marchiafava-Micheli]**
> *EXCLUDES 1*   *hemoglobinuria NOS (R82.3)*

N Newborn: 0   P Pediatric: 0-17   M Maternity: 12-55   A Adult: 15-124   MCC Major CC Condition   PDx MCC PDx acts as own MCC   CC CC Condition   PDx CC PDx acts as own CC

486   ICD-10-CM Draft (2015)

D59.6   **Hemoglobinuria** due to hemolysis from other external causes
     Hemoglobinuria from exertion
     March hemoglobinuria
     Paroxysmal cold hemoglobinuria
     Use additional code (Chapter 20) to identify external cause
     EXCLUDES 1   hemoglobinuria NOS (R82.3)

D59.8   **Other** acquired hemolytic anemias

D59.9   **Acquired hemolytic anemia, unspecified**   CC
     Idiopathic hemolytic anemia, chronic

Aplastic and other anemias and other bone marrow failure syndromes (D60-D64)

✓4ᵗʰ **D60**   **Acquired pure red cell aplasia [erythroblastopenia]**
     INCLUDES   red cell aplasia (acquired) (adult) (with thymoma)
     EXCLUDES 1   congenital red cell aplasia (D61.01)

     CC Excl: For CC/MCC codes in category D60, unless otherwise noted: D47.4, D50.0-D64.9, D68.312, D68.51-D68.69, D75.81, D75.89-D75.9, D77, D89.2

     D60.0   **Chronic** acquired pure red cell aplasia   MCC

     D60.1   **Transient** acquired pure red cell aplasia   MCC

     D60.8   **Other** acquired pure red cell aplasias   MCC

     D60.9   **Acquired pure red cell aplasia, unspecified**   MCC

✓4ᵗʰ **D61**   **Other aplastic anemias and other bone marrow failure syndromes**
     EXCLUDES 1   neutropenia (D70.-)

     ✓5ᵗʰ **D61.0**   **Constitutional** aplastic anemia

         D61.01   **Constitutional (pure)** red blood cell **aplasia**   CC
         Blackfan-Diamond syndrome
         Congenital (pure) red cell aplasia
         Familial hypoplastic anemia
         Primary (pure) red cell aplasia
         Red cell (pure) aplasia of infants
         EXCLUDES 1   acquired red cell aplasia (D60.9)
         CC Excl: D50.0-D61.3, D61.89-D64.9, D75.9, P61.2-P61.4

         D61.09   **Other constitutional aplastic anemia**   CC
         Fanconi's anemia
         Pancytopenia with malformations
         CC Excl: D50.0-D61.3, D61.89-D64.9, D69.3-D69.49, D75.9, P61.2-P61.4

     D61.1   **Drug-induced aplastic anemia**   MCC
         Use additional code for adverse effect, if applicable, to identify drug (T36-T50 with fifth or sixth character 5)
         CC Excl: D47.4, D50.0-D64.9, D68.312, D68.51-D68.69, D75.81, D75.89-D75.9, D77, D89.2

     D61.2   **Aplastic anemia** due to other external agents   MCC
         Code first, if applicable, toxic effects of substances chiefly nonmedicinal as to source (T51-T65)
         CC Excl: See code: D61.1

     D61.3   **Idiopathic aplastic anemia**   MCC
         CC Excl: See code: D61.1

     ✓5ᵗʰ **D61.8**   **Other** specified aplastic anemias and other bone marrow failure syndromes

         CC Excl: For CC/MCC codes in subcategory D61.8, unless otherwise noted: D60.0-D60.9, D61.1-D64.9, D70.0-D70.9, D72.810-D72.820, D72.823, D72.825-D72.829, D75.9, D76.1-D76.3, P61.2

         ✓6ᵗʰ **D61.81**   **Pancytopenia**
         EXCLUDES 1   pancytopenia (due to) (with) aplastic anemia (D61.9)
            pancytopenia (due to) (with) bone marrow infiltration (D61.82)
            pancytopenia (due to) (with) congenital (pure) red cell aplasia (D61.01)
            pancytopenia (due to) (with) hairy cell leukemia (C91.4-)
            pancytopenia (due to) (with) human immunodeficiency virus disease (B20)
            pancytopenia (due to) (with) leukoerythroblastic anemia (D61.82)
            pancytopenia (due to) (with) myelodysplastic syndromes (D46.-)
            pancytopenia (due to) (with) myeloproliferative disease (D47.1)

            D61.810   **Antineoplastic chemotherapy induced pancytopenia**   MCC
            EXCLUDES 2   aplastic anemia due to antineoplastic chemotherapy (D61.1)

            D61.811   **Other drug-induced pancytopenia**   MCC
            EXCLUDES 2   aplastic anemia due to drugs (D61.1)

            D61.818   **Other pancytopenia**   CC

         D61.82   **Myelophthisis**   CC
         Leukoerythroblastic anemia
         Myelophthisic anemia
         Panmyelophthisis
         Code also the underlying disorder, such as:
            malignant neoplasm of breast (C50.-)
            tuberculosis (A15.-)
         EXCLUDES 1   idiopathic myelofibrosis (D47.1)
            myelofibrosis NOS (D75.81)
            myelofibrosis with myeloid metaplasia (D47.4)
            primary myelofibrosis (D47.1)
            secondary myelofibrosis (D75.81)

         D61.89   **Other specified aplastic anemias and other bone marrow failure syndromes**   MCC
         CC Excl: See code: D61.1

     D61.9   **Aplastic anemia, unspecified**   CC
         Hypoplastic anemia NOS
         Medullary hypoplasia
         CC Excl: See code: D61.1

D62   **Acute posthemorrhagic anemia**   CC
     EXCLUDES 1   anemia due to chronic blood loss (D50.0)
         blood loss anemia NOS (D50.0)
         congenital anemia from fetal blood loss (P61.3)
     CC Excl: D47.4, D50.0-D64.9, D68.312, D68.51-D68.69, D75.81, D75.89-D75.9, D77, D89.2, T79.2XXA

✓4ᵗʰ **D63**   **Anemia in chronic diseases classified elsewhere**

     D63.0   *Anemia in neoplastic disease*
         Code first neoplasm (C00-D49)
         EXCLUDES 1   anemia due to antineoplastic chemotherapy (D64.81)
            aplastic anemia due to antineoplastic chemotherapy (D61.1)

     D63.1   *Anemia in chronic kidney disease*
         Erythropoietin resistant anemia (EPO resistant anemia)
         Code first underlying chronic kidney disease (CKD) (N18.-)

     D63.8   *Anemia in other chronic diseases classified elsewhere*
         Code first underlying disease, such as:
         diphyllobothriasis (B70.0)
         hookworm disease (B76.0-B76.9)
         hypothyroidism (E00.0-E03.9)
         malaria (B50.0-B54)
         symptomatic late syphilis (A52.79)
         tuberculosis (A18.89)

✓4ᵗʰ **D64**   **Other anemias**
     EXCLUDES 1   refractory anemia (D46.-)
         refractory anemia with excess blasts in transformation [RAEB T] (C92.0-)

     D64.0   **Hereditary sideroblastic anemia**
         Sex-linked hypochromic sideroblastic anemia

     D64.1   *Secondary sideroblastic anemia due to disease*
         Code first underlying disease

     D64.2   **Secondary sideroblastic anemia due to drugs and toxins**
         Code first poisoning due to drug or toxin, if applicable (T36-T65 with fifth or sixth character 1-4 or 6)
         Use additional code for adverse effect, if applicable, to identify drug (T36-T50 with fifth or sixth character 5)

     D64.3   **Other sideroblastic anemias**
         Sideroblastic anemia NOS
         Pyridoxine-responsive sideroblastic anemia NEC

     D64.4   **Congenital dyserythropoietic anemia**
         Dyshematopoietic anemia (congenital)
         EXCLUDES 1   Blackfan-Diamond syndrome (D61.01)
            Di Guglielmo's disease (C94.0)

     ✓5ᵗʰ **D64.8**   **Other specified anemias**

         D64.81   **Anemia due to antineoplastic chemotherapy**
         Antineoplastic chemotherapy induced anemia
         EXCLUDES 1   anemia in neoplastic disease (D63.0)
            aplastic anemia due to antineoplastic chemotherapy (D61.1)

         D64.89   **Other specified anemias**
         Infantile pseudoleukemia

     D64.9   **Anemia, unspecified**

✓ Additional Character Required   ✓x7ᵗʰ Xtension Alert   Unacceptable PDx   Manifestation   Hospital Acquired Condition   EXCLUDES 1 Not Coded Here   EXCLUDES 2 Not Included Here

Diseases of the Blood and Blood-forming Organs

D65–D68.52

Coagulation defects, purpura and other hemorrhagic conditions (D65-D69)

D65 Disseminated intravascular coagulation [defibrination syndrome] `MCC`
Afibrinogenemia, acquired
Consumption coagulopathy
Diffuse or disseminated intravascular coagulation [DIC]
Fibrinolytic hemorrhage, acquired
Fibrinolytic purpura
Purpura fulminans
EXCLUDES 1 *disseminated intravascular coagulation (complicating):*
abortion or ectopic or molar pregnancy (O00-O07, O08.1)
in newborn (P60)
pregnancy, childbirth and the puerperium (O45.0, O46.0,
O67.0, O72.3)
CC Excl: D47.4, D65-D69.9, D75.81-D75.9, D77, D89.2

D66 Hereditary factor VIII deficiency `MCC`
Classical hemophilia
Deficiency factor VIII (with functional defect)
Hemophilia A
Hemophilia NOS
EXCLUDES 1 *factor VIII deficiency with vascular defect (D68.0)*
CC Excl: See code: D65

D67 Hereditary factor IX deficiency `MCC`
Christmas disease
Factor IX deficiency (with functional defect)
Hemophilia B
Plasma thromboplastin component [PTC] deficiency
CC Excl: See code: D65

✓4ᵗʰ D68 Other coagulation defects
EXCLUDES 1 *abnormal coagulation profile (R79.1)*
coagulation defects complicating abortion or ectopic or molar
pregnancy (O00-O07, O08.1)
coagulation defects complicating pregnancy, childbirth and the
puerperium (O45.0, O46.0, O67.0, O72.3)

D68.0 Von Willebrand's disease `CC`
Angiohemophilia
Factor VIII deficiency with vascular defect
Vascular hemophilia
EXCLUDES 1 *capillary fragility (hereditary) (D69.8)*
factor VIII deficiency NOS (D66)
factor VIII deficiency with functional defect (D66)
CC Excl: See code: D65

D68.1 Hereditary factor XI deficiency `CC`
Hemophilia C
Plasma thromboplastin antecedent [PTA] deficiency
Rosenthal's disease
CC Excl: See code: D65

D68.2 Hereditary deficiency of other clotting factors `CC`
AC globulin deficiency
Congenital afibrinogenemia
Deficiency of factor I [fibrinogen]
Deficiency of factor II [prothrombin]
Deficiency of factor V [labile]
Deficiency of factor VII [stable]
Deficiency of factor X [Stuart-Prower]
Deficiency of factor XII [Hageman]
Deficiency of factor XIII [fibrin stabilizing]
Dysfibrinogenemia (congenital)
Hypoproconvertinemia
Owren's disease
Proaccelerin deficiency
CC Excl: See code: D65

✓5ᵗʰ D68.3 Hemorrhagic disorder due to circulating anticoagulants
✓6ᵗʰ D68.31 Hemorrhagic disorder due to intrinsic circulating anticoagulants, antibodies, or inhibitors
D68.311 Acquired hemophilia `CC`
Autoimmune hemophilia
Autoimmune inhibitors to clotting factors
Secondary hemophilia
CC Excl: D47.4, D65-D69.9, D75.82-D75.9, D77, D89.2

D68.312 Antiphospholipid antibody with hemorrhagic disorder `CC`
Lupus anticoagulant (LAC) with hemorrhagic disorder
Systemic lupus erythematosus [SLE] inhibitor with hemorrhagic disorder
EXCLUDES 1 *antiphospholipid antibody, finding without diagnosis (R76.0)*
antiphospholipid antibody syndrome (D68.61)
antiphospholipid antibody with hypercoagulable state (D68.61)
lupus anticoagulant (LAC) finding without diagnosis (R76.0)
lupus anticoagulant (LAC) with hypercoagulable state (D68.62)
systemic lupus erythematosus [SLE] inhibitor finding without diagnosis (R76.0)
systemic lupus erythematosus [SLE] inhibitor with hypercoagulable state (D68.62)
CC Excl: D47.4, D68.311-D68.318, D68.51-D68.69, D70.0-D72.9, D73.81, D75.81, D75.89-D77, D89.2

D68.318 Other hemorrhagic disorder due to intrinsic circulating anticoagulants, antibodies, or inhibitors `CC`
Antithromboplastinemia
Antithromboplastinogenemia
Hemorrhagic disorder due to intrinsic increase in antithrombin
Hemorrhagic disorder due to intrinsic increase in anti-VIIIa
Hemorrhagic disorder due to intrinsic increase in anti-IXa
Hemorrhagic disorder due to intrinsic increase in anti-XIa
CC Excl: See code: D68.311

D68.32 Hemorrhagic disorder due to extrinsic circulating anticoagulants `CC`
Drug-induced hemorrhagic disorder
Hemorrhagic disorder due to increase in anti-IIa
Hemorrhagic disorder due to increase in anti-Xa
Hyperheparinemia
Use additional code for adverse effect, if applicable, to identify drug (T45.515, T45.525)
CC Excl: D47.4, D65-D69.9, D75.81-D75.9, D77, D89.2

D68.4 Acquired coagulation factor deficiency `CC`
Deficiency of coagulation factor due to liver disease
Deficiency of coagulation factor due to vitamin K deficiency
EXCLUDES 1 *vitamin K deficiency of newborn (P53)*
CC Excl: See code: D68.32

✓5ᵗʰ D68.5 Primary thrombophilia
Primary hypercoagulable states
EXCLUDES 1 *antiphospholipid syndrome (D68.61)*
lupus anticoagulant (D68.62)
secondary activated protein C resistance (D68.69)
secondary antiphospholipid antibody syndrome (D68.69)
secondary lupus anticoagulant with hypercoagulable state (D68.69)
secondary systemic lupus erythematosus [SLE] inhibitor with hypercoagulable state (D68.69)
systemic lupus erythematosus [SLE] inhibitor finding without diagnosis (R76.0)
systemic lupus erythematosus [SLE] inhibitor with hemorrhagic disorder (D68.312)
thrombotic thrombocytopenic purpura (M31.1)

CC Excl: For CC codes in subcategory D68.5, unless otherwise noted: D47.4, D68.312, D68.51-D68.69, D70.0-D72.9, D73.81, D75.81, D75.89-D75.9, D76.1-D77, D89.2

D68.51 Activated protein C resistance `CC`
Factor V Leiden mutation

D68.52 Prothrombin gene mutation `CC`

D68.59　Other primary thrombophilia [CC]
Antithrombin III deficiency
Hypercoagulable state NOS
Primary hypercoagulable state NEC
Primary thrombophilia NEC
Protein C deficiency
Protein S deficiency
Thrombophilia NOS

☑5ᵗʰ **D68.6　Other thrombophilia**
Other hypercoagulable states
EXCLUDES 1　diffuse or disseminated intravascular coagulation [DIC] (D65)
heparin induced thrombocytopenia (HIT) (D75.82)
hyperhomocysteinemia (E72.11)

CC Excl: For CC codes in subcategory D68.6, unless otherwise noted: D47.4, D68.312, D68.51-D68.69, D70.0-D72.9, D73.81, D75.81, D75.89-D75.9, D76.1-D77, D89.2

D68.61　Antiphospholipid syndrome [CC]
Anticardiolipin syndrome
Antiphospholipid antibody syndrome
EXCLUDES 1　antiphospholipid antibody, finding without diagnosis (R76.0)
antiphospholipid antibody with hemorrhagic disorder (D68.312)
lupus anticoagulant syndrome (D68.62)

D68.62　Lupus anticoagulant syndrome [CC]
Lupus anticoagulant
Presence of systemic lupus erythematosus [SLE] inhibitor
EXCLUDES 1　anticardiolipin syndrome (D68.61)
antiphospholipid syndrome (D68.61)
lupus anticoagulant (LAC) finding without diagnosis (R79.0)
lupus anticoagulant (LAC) with hemorrhagic disorder (D68.312)

D68.69　Other thrombophilia [CC]
Hypercoagulable states NEC
Secondary hypercoagulable state NOS

D68.8　Other specified coagulation defects [CC]
EXCLUDES 1　hemorrhagic disease of newborn (P53)
CC Excl: See code: D68.32

D68.9　Coagulation defect, unspecified [CC]
CC Excl: See code: D68.32

☑4ᵗʰ **D69　Purpura and other hemorrhagic conditions**
EXCLUDES 1　benign hypergammaglobulinemic purpura (D89.0)
cryoglobulinemic purpura (D89.1)
essential (hemorrhagic) thrombocythemia (D47.3)
hemorrhagic thrombocythemia (D47.3)
purpura fulminans (D65)
thrombotic thrombocytopenic purpura (M31.1)
Waldenström hypergammaglobulinemic purpura (D89.0)

CC Excl: For CC codes in category D69, unless otherwise noted: D47.4, D65-D69.9, D75.81-D75.9, D77, D89.2

D69.0　Allergic purpura [CC]
Allergic vasculitis
Nonthrombocytopenic hemorrhagic purpura
Nonthrombocytopenic idiopathic purpura
Purpura anaphylactoid
Purpura Henoch(-Schönlein)
Purpura rheumatica
Vascular purpura
EXCLUDES 1　thrombocytopenic hemorrhagic purpura (D69.3)

D69.1　Qualitative platelet defects
Bernard-Soulier [giant platelet] syndrome
Glanzmann's disease
Grey platelet syndrome
Thromboasthenia (hemorrhagic) (hereditary)
Thrombocytopathy
EXCLUDES 1　von Willebrand's disease (D68.0)

D69.2　Other nonthrombocytopenic purpura
Purpura NOS
Purpura simplex
Senile purpura

D69.3　Immune thrombocytopenic purpura [CC]
Hemorrhagic (thrombocytopenic) purpura
Idiopathic thrombocytopenic purpura
Tidal platelet dysgenesis

☑5ᵗʰ **D69.4　Other primary thrombocytopenia**
EXCLUDES 1　transient neonatal thrombocytopenia (P61.0)
Wiskott-Aldrich syndrome (D82.0)

D69.41　Evans syndrome [CC]

D69.42　Congenital and hereditary thrombocytopenia purpura [CC]
Congenital thrombocytopenia
Hereditary thrombocytopenia
Code first congenital or hereditary disorder, such as: thrombocytopenia with absent radius (TAR syndrome) (Q87.2)

D69.49　Other primary thrombocytopenia
Megakaryocytic hypoplasia
Primary thrombocytopenia NOS

☑5ᵗʰ **D69.5　Secondary thrombocytopenia**
EXCLUDES 1　heparin induced thrombocytopenia (HIT) (D75.82)
transient thrombocytopenia of newborn (P61.0)

D69.51　Posttransfusion purpura
Posttransfusion purpura from whole blood (fresh) or blood products
PTP

D69.59　Other secondary thrombocytopenia

D69.6　Thrombocytopenia, unspecified

D69.8　Other specified hemorrhagic conditions
Capillary fragility (hereditary)
Vascular pseudohemophilia

D69.9　Hemorrhagic condition, unspecified

Other disorders of blood and blood-forming organs (D70-D77)

☑4ᵗʰ **D70　Neutropenia**
INCLUDES　agranulocytosis
decreased absolute neurophile count (ANC)
Use additional code for any associated:
fever (R50.81)
mucositis (J34.81, K12.3-, K92.81, N76.81)
EXCLUDES 1　neutropenic splenomegaly (D73.81)
transient neonatal neutropenia (P61.5)

always Read this

D70.0　Congenital agranulocytosis
Congenital neutropenia
Infantile genetic agranulocytosis
Kostmann's disease

D70.1　Agranulocytosis secondary to cancer chemotherapy
Code also underlying neoplasm
Use additional code for adverse effect, if applicable, to identify drug (T45.1X5)

D70.2　Other drug-induced agranulocytosis
Use additional code for adverse effect, if applicable, to identify drug (T36-T50 with fifth or sixth character 5)

D70.3　Neutropenia due to infection

D70.4　Cyclic neutropenia
Cyclic hematopoiesis
Periodic neutropenia

D70.8　Other neutropenia

D70.9　Neutropenia, unspecified　　*＊ add code R50.81*

D71　Functional disorders of polymorphonuclear neutrophils
Cell membrane receptor complex [CR3] defect
Chronic (childhood) granulomatous disease
Congenital dysphagocytosis
Progressive septic granulomatosis

☑4ᵗʰ **D72　Other disorders of white blood cells**
EXCLUDES 1　basophilia (D72.824)
immunity disorders (D80-D89)
neutropenia (D70)
preleukemia (syndrome) (D46.9)

D72.0　Genetic anomalies of leukocytes
Alder (granulation) (granulocyte) anomaly
Alder syndrome
Hereditary leukocytic hypersegmentation
Hereditary leukocytic hyposegmentation
Hereditary leukomelanopathy
May-Hegglin (granulation) (granulocyte) anomaly
May-Hegglin syndrome
Pelger-Huët (granulation) (granulocyte) anomaly
Pelger-Huët syndrome
EXCLUDES 1　Chédiak (-Steinbrinck)-Higashi syndrome (E70.330)

Diseases of the Blood and Blood-forming Organs

D72.1–D75.9

D72.1 Eosinophilia
Allergic eosinophilia
Hereditary eosinophilia
EXCLUDES 1   *Löffler's syndrome (J82)*
            pulmonary eosinophilia (J82)

√5ᵗʰ **D72.8 Other specified disorders of white blood cells**
EXCLUDES 1   *leukemia (C91-C95)*

  √6ᵗʰ **D72.81 Decreased white blood cell count**
      EXCLUDES 1   *neutropenia (D70.-)*

       D72.810 Lymphocytopenia
           Decreased lymphocytes

       D72.818 Other decreased white blood cell count
           Basophilic leukopenia
           Eosinophilic leukopenia
           Monocytopenia
           Other decreased leukocytes
           Plasmacytopenia

       D72.819 Decreased white blood cell count, unspecified
           Decreased leukocytes, unspecified
           Leukocytopenia, unspecified
           Leukopenia
           EXCLUDES 1   *malignant leukopenia (D70.9)*

  √6ᵗʰ **D72.82 Elevated white blood cell count**
      EXCLUDES 1   *eosinophilia (D72.1)*

       D72.820 Lymphocytosis (symptomatic)
           Elevated lymphocytes

       D72.821 Monocytosis (symptomatic)
           EXCLUDES 1   *infectious mononucleosis (B27.-)*

       D72.822 Plasmacytosis

       D72.823 Leukemoid reaction
           Basophilic leukemoid reaction
           Leukemoid reaction NOS
           Lymphocytic leukemoid reaction
           Monocytic leukemoid reaction
           Myelocytic leukemoid reaction
           Neutrophilic leukemoid reaction

       D72.824 Basophilia

       D72.825 Bandemia
           Bandemia without diagnosis of specific infection
           EXCLUDES 1   *confirmed infection—code to infection*
                leukemia (C91.-, C92.-, C93.-, C94.-, C95.-)

       D72.828 Other elevated white blood cell count

       D72.829 Elevated white blood cell count, unspecified
           Elevated leukocytes, unspecified
           Leukocytosis, unspecified

  D72.89 Other specified disorders of white blood cells
      Abnormality of white blood cells NEC

D72.9 Disorder of white blood cells, unspecified
      Abnormal leukocyte differential NOS

√4ᵗʰ **D73 Diseases of spleen**

D73.0 Hyposplenism
      Atrophy of spleen
      EXCLUDES 1   *asplenia (congenital) (Q89.01)*
                postsurgical absence of spleen (Z90.81)

D73.1 Hypersplenism
      EXCLUDES 1   *neutropenic splenomegaly (D73.81)*
                primary splenic neutropenia (D73.81)
                splenitis, splenomegaly in late syphilis (A52.79)
                splenitis, splenomegaly in tuberculosis (A18.85)
                splenomegaly NOS (R16.1)
                splenomegaly congenital (Q89.0)

D73.2 Chronic congestive splenomegaly

D73.3 Abscess of spleen

D73.4 Cyst of spleen

D73.5 Infarction of spleen
      Splenic rupture, nontraumatic
      Torsion of spleen
      EXCLUDES 1   *rupture of spleen due to Plasmodium vivax malaria (B51.0)*
                traumatic rupture of spleen (S36.03-)

√5ᵗʰ **D73.8 Other diseases of spleen**

D73.81 Neutropenic splenomegaly
      Werner-Schultz disease

D73.89 Other diseases of spleen
      Fibrosis of spleen NOS
      Perisplenitis
      Splenitis NOS

D73.9 Disease of spleen, unspecified

√4ᵗʰ **D74 Methemoglobinemia**

> **CC Excl: For CC codes in category D74, unless otherwise noted:**
> D56.4, D58.2-D59.2, D59.4-D59.9, D64.4-D64.9, D74.0-D74.9, D75.9

D74.0 Congenital methemoglobinemia   CC
      Congenital NADH-methemoglobin reductase deficiency
      Hemoglobin-M [Hb-M] disease
      Methemoglobinemia, hereditary

D74.8 Other methemoglobinemias   CC
      Acquired methemoglobinemia (with sulfhemoglobinemia)
      Toxic methemoglobinemia

D74.9 Methemoglobinemia, unspecified   CC

√4ᵗʰ **D75 Other and unspecified diseases of blood and blood-forming organs**
      EXCLUDES 2   *acute lymphadenitis (L04.-)*
                chronic lymphadenitis (I88.1)
                enlarged lymph nodes (R59.-)
                hypergammaglobulinemia NOS (D89.2)
                lymphadenitis NOS (I88.9)
                mesenteric lymphadenitis (acute) (chronic) (I88.0)

D75.0 Familial erythrocytosis
      Benign polycythemia
      Familial polycythemia
      EXCLUDES 1   *hereditary ovalocytosis (D58.1)*

D75.1 Secondary polycythemia
      Acquired polycythemia
      Emotional polycythemia
      Erythrocytosis NOS
      Hypoxemic polycythemia
      Nephrogenous polycythemia
      Polycythemia due to erythropoietin
      Polycythemia due to fall in plasma volume
      Polycythemia due to high altitude
      Polycythemia due to stress
      Polycythemia NOS
      Relative polycythemia
      EXCLUDES 1   *polycythemia neonatorum (P61.1)*
                polycythemia vera (D45)

√5ᵗʰ **D75.8 Other specified diseases of blood and blood-forming organs**

D75.81 Myelofibrosis   CC
      Myelofibrosis NOS
      Secondary myelofibrosis NOS
      Code first the underlying disorder, such as: malignant neoplasm of breast (C50.-)
      Use additional code, if applicable, for associated therapy-related myelodysplastic syndrome (D46.-)
      Use additional code for adverse effect, if applicable, to identify drug (T45.1X5)
      EXCLUDES 1   *acute myelofibrosis (C94.4-)*
                idiopathic myelofibrosis (D47.1)
                leukoerythroblastic anemia (D61.82)
                myelofibrosis with myeloid metaplasia (D47.4)
                myelophthisic anemia (D61.82)
                myelophthisis (D61.82)
                primary myelofibrosis (D47.1)
      CC Excl: C88.2-C88.3, C88.8-C88.9, C90.10-C90.11, C90.20-C90.21, C90.30-C90.31, C91.00-C95.92, D45-D47.1, D47.3, D47.Z9-D47.9, D48.7-D48.9

D75.82 Heparin induced thrombocytopenia (HIT)

D75.89 Other specified diseases of blood and blood-forming organs

D75.9 Disease of blood and blood-forming organs, unspecified

N Newborn: 0   P Pediatric: 0-17   M Maternity: 12-55   A Adult: 15-124   MCC Major CC Condition   PDx MCC PDx acts as own MCC   CC CC Condition   PDx CC PDx acts as own CC

490   ICD-10-CM Draft (2015)

✓4ᵗʰ **D76 Other specified diseases with participation of lymphoreticular and reticulohistiocytic tissue**

> EXCLUDES 1 (Abt-) Letterer-Siwe disease (C96.0)
> eosinophilic granuloma (C96.6)
> Hand-Schüller-Christian disease (C96.5)
> histiocytic sarcoma (C96.A)
> histiocytosis X, multifocal (C96.5)
> histiocytosis X, unifocal (C96.6)
> Langerhans-cell histiocytosis, multifocal (C96.5)
> Langerhans-cell histiocytosis NOS (C96.6)
> Langerhans-cell histiocytosis, unifocal (C96.6)
> leukemic reticuloendotheliosis or reticulosis (C91.4-)
> lipomelanotic reticuloendotheliosis or reticulosis (I89.8)
> malignant histiocytosis (C96.A)

D76.1 Hemophagocytic lymphohistiocytosis ㏄
Familial hemophagocytic reticulosis
Histiocytoses of mononuclear phagocytes
CC Excl: D60.0-D60.9, D61.1-D61.9, D65, D69.3-D70.9, D72.818-D72.819, D75.82, D75.9

D76.2 Hemophagocytic syndrome, infection-associated ㏄
Use additional code to identify infectious agent or disease
CC Excl: See code: D76.1

D76.3 Other histiocytosis syndromes ㏄
Reticulohistiocytoma (giant-cell)
Sinus histiocytosis with massive lymphadenopathy
Xanthogranuloma
CC Excl: See code: D76.1

D77 Other disorders of blood and blood-forming organs in diseases classified elsewhere

> Code first underlying disease, such as:
> amyloidosis (E85.-)
> congenital early syphilis (A50.0)
> echinococcosis (B67.0-B67.9)
> malaria (B50.0-B54)
> schistosomiasis [bilharziasis] (B65.0-B65.9)
> vitamin C deficiency (E54)

> EXCLUDES 1 rupture of spleen due to Plasmodium vivax malaria (B51.0)
> splenitis, splenomegaly in late syphilis (A52.79)
> splenitis, splenomegaly in tuberculosis (A18.85)

Intraoperative and postprocedural complications of the spleen (D78)

✓4ᵗʰ **D78 Intraoperative and postprocedural complications of the spleen**

✓5ᵗʰ **D78.0 Intraoperative hemorrhage and hematoma of the spleen complicating a procedure**
> EXCLUDES 1 intraoperative hemorrhage and hematoma of the spleen due to accidental puncture or laceration during a procedure (D78.1-)

D78.01 Intraoperative hemorrhage and hematoma of the spleen complicating a procedure on the spleen ㏄
CC Excl: D78.01-D78.02, D78.21-D78.89, H95.811-H95.89, I85.01, I85.11, I97.3, K21.9, K22.8, K23-K25.0, K25.2, K25.4, K25.6, K26.0, K26.2, K26.4, K26.6, K27.0, K27.2, K27.4, K27.6, K28.0, K28.2, K28.4, K28.6, K29.01, K29.21, K29.31, K29.41, K29.51, K29.61, K29.71, K29.81, K29.91, K31.811, K55.21, K57.01, K57.11, K57.13, K57.21, K57.31, K57.33, K57.41, K57.51, K57.53, K57.81, K57.91, K57.93, K62.5, K92.0-K92.2, M96.89, N98.1-N98.9, P54.1-P54.3, T81.10XA, T81.11XA, T81.12XA, T81.19XA, T81.82XA, T81.89XA, T81.9XXA

D78.02 Intraoperative hemorrhage and hematoma of the spleen complicating other procedure ㏄
CC Excl: See code: D78.01

✓5ᵗʰ **D78.1 Accidental puncture and laceration of the spleen during a procedure**

D78.11 Accidental puncture and laceration of the spleen during a procedure on the spleen ㏄
CC Excl: D78.11-D78.12, D78.81-D78.89, E36.11-E36.8, E89.810-E89.89, G96.11, G97.41-G97.49, H59.011-H59.019, H59.031-H59.099, H59.211-H59.229, H59.811-H59.89, H95.31-H95.32, H95.811-H95.89, I97.3, I97.51-I97.52, J95.71-J95.72, K91.71-K91.72, L76.11-L76.12, L76.81-L76.82, M96.820-M96.821, M96.89, N98.1-N98.9, N99.71-N99.72, T81.82XXA, T81.89XX1, T81.9XXA

D78.12 Accidental puncture and laceration of the spleen during other procedure ㏄
CC Excl: See code: D78.11

✓5ᵗʰ **D78.2 Postprocedural hemorrhage and hematoma of the spleen following a procedure**

D78.21 Postprocedural hemorrhage and hematoma of the spleen following a procedure on the spleen ㏄
CC Excl: See code: D78.01

D78.22 Postprocedural hemorrhage and hematoma of the spleen following other procedure ㏄
CC Excl: See code: D78.01

✓5ᵗʰ **D78.8 Other intraoperative and postprocedural complications of the spleen**
Use additional code, if applicable, to further specify disorder

D78.81 Other intraoperative complications of the spleen ㏄
CC Excl: D78.81-D78.89, H95.811-H95.89, I97.3, M96.89, N98.1-N98.9, T81.82XA, T81.89XA, T81.9XXA

D78.89 Other postprocedural complications of the spleen ㏄
CC Excl: See code: D78.81

Certain disorders involving the immune mechanism (D80-D89)

> INCLUDES defects in the complement system
> immunodeficiency disorders, except human immunodeficiency virus [HIV] disease
> sarcoidosis

> EXCLUDES 1 autoimmune disease (systemic) NOS (M35.9)
> functional disorders of polymorphonuclear neutrophils (D71)
> human immunodeficiency virus [HIV] disease (B20)

✓4ᵗʰ **D80 Immunodeficiency with predominantly antibody defects**

> CC Excl: For CC codes in category D80, unless otherwise noted:
> D80.0, D80.3-D81.2, D81.4, D81.6-D81.7, D81.89-D84.0, D84.8-D84.9, D89.3, D89.82-D89.9

D80.0 Hereditary hypogammaglobulinemia ㏄
Autosomal recessive agammaglobulinemia (Swiss type)
X-linked agammaglobulinemia [Bruton] (with growth hormone deficiency)

D80.1 Nonfamilial hypogammaglobulinemia ㏄
Agammaglobulinemia with immunoglobulin-bearing B-lymphocytes
Common variable agammaglobulinemia [CVAgamma]
Hypogammaglobulinemia NOS
CC Excl: D80.0-D81.2, D81.4, D81.6-D81.7, D81.89-D84.0, D84.8-D84.9, D89.3, D89.82-D89.9

D80.2 Selective deficiency of immunoglobulin A [IgA] ㏄

D80.3 Selective deficiency of immunoglobulin G [IgG] subclasses ㏄

D80.4 Selective deficiency of immunoglobulin M [IgM] ㏄

D80.5 Immunodeficiency with increased immunoglobulin M [IgM] ㏄

D80.6 Antibody deficiency with near-normal immunoglobulins or with hyperimmunoglobulinemia ㏄

D80.7 Transient hypogammaglobulinemia of infancy ㏄ Ⓝ

D80.8 Other immunodeficiencies with predominantly antibody defects ㏄
Kappa light chain deficiency

D80.9 Immunodeficiency with predominantly antibody defects, unspecified ㏄

✓4ᵗʰ **D81 Combined immunodeficiencies**
> EXCLUDES 1 autosomal recessive agammaglobulinemia (Swiss type) (D80.0)

> CC Excl: For CC codes in category D81, unless otherwise noted:
> D80.0, D80.3-D81.2, D81.4, D81.6-D81.7, D81.89-D84.0, D84.8-D84.9, D89.3, D89.82-D89.9

D81.0 Severe combined immunodeficiency [SCID] with reticular dysgenesis ㏄

D81.1 Severe combined immunodeficiency [SCID] with low T- and B-cell numbers ㏄

D81.2 Severe combined immunodeficiency [SCID] with low or normal B-cell numbers ㏄

D81.3 Adenosine deaminase [ADA] deficiency ㏄
CC Excl: D81.3, D81.5, D81.810, D84.1, E76.01-E76.9, E79.1-E80.29, E80.4-E80.7, E88.81

D81.4 Nezelof's syndrome ㏄

D81.5 Purine nucleoside phosphorylase [PNP] deficiency ㏄
CC Excl: See code: D81.3

D81.6 Major histocompatibility complex class I deficiency ㏄
Bare lymphocyte syndrome

D81.7 Major histocompatibility complex class II deficiency ㏄

Diseases of the Blood and Blood-forming Organs

D81.8–D89.9

✓5ᵗʰ **D81.8** Other **combined immunodeficiencies**

    ✓6ᵗʰ **D81.81** **Biotin-dependent carboxylase deficiency**
         Multiple carboxylase deficiency
         EXCLUDES 1   *biotin-dependent carboxylase deficiency due to dietary deficiency of biotin (E53.8)*

         D81.810 **Biotinidase deficiency**

         D81.818 **Other biotin-dependent carboxylase deficiency**
             Holocarboxylase synthetase deficiency
             Other multiple carboxylase deficiency

         D81.819 **Biotin-dependent carboxylase deficiency, unspecified**
             Multiple carboxylase deficiency, unspecified

     D81.89 Other **combined immunodeficiencies** `CC`

D81.9 **Combined immunodeficiency, unspecified** `CC`
     Severe combined immunodeficiency disorder [SCID] NOS

✓4ᵗʰ **D82** **Immunodeficiency associated with other major defects**
     EXCLUDES 1   *ataxia telangiectasia [Louis-Bar] (G11.3)*

D82.0 **Wiskott-Aldrich syndrome** `CC`
     Immunodeficiency with thrombocytopenia and eczema
     CC Excl: See code: D80

D82.1 **Di George's syndrome** `CC`
     Pharyngeal pouch syndrome
     Thymic alymphoplasia
     Thymic aplasia or hypoplasia with immunodeficiency
     CC Excl: See code: D80

D82.2 **Immunodeficiency with short-limbed stature**

D82.3 **Immunodeficiency following hereditary defective response to Epstein-Barr virus**
     X-linked lymphoproliferative disease

D82.4 **Hyperimmunoglobulin E [IgE] syndrome**

D82.8 **Immunodeficiency associated with other specified major defects**

D82.9 **Immunodeficiency associated with major defect, unspecified**

✓4ᵗʰ **D83** **Common variable immunodeficiency**

CC Excl: For CC codes in category D83, unless otherwise noted: D80.0, D80.3-D81.2, D81.4, D81.6-D81.7, D81.89-D84.0, D84.8-D84.9, D89.3, D89.82-D89.9

D83.0 **Common variable immunodeficiency** with predominant abnormalities of B-cell numbers and function `CC`

D83.1 **Common variable immunodeficiency** with predominant immunoregulatory T-cell disorders `CC`

D83.2 **Common variable immunodeficiency** with autoantibodies to B- or T-cells `CC`

D83.8 Other **common variable immunodeficiencies** `CC`

D83.9 **Common variable immunodeficiency, unspecified** `CC`

✓4ᵗʰ **D84** **Other immunodeficiencies**

D84.0 **Lymphocyte function antigen-1 [LFA-1] defect**

D84.1 **Defects in the complement system**
     C1 esterase inhibitor [C1-INH] deficiency

D84.8 Other **specified immunodeficiencies** `CC`
     CC Excl: See code: D83

D84.9 **Immunodeficiency, unspecified** `CC`
     CC Excl: See code: D83

✓4ᵗʰ **D86** **Sarcoidosis**

D86.0 **Sarcoidosis of lung**

D86.1 **Sarcoidosis of lymph nodes**

D86.2 **Sarcoidosis of lung with sarcoidosis of lymph nodes**

D86.3 **Sarcoidosis of skin**

✓5ᵗʰ **D86.8** **Sarcoidosis of other sites**

     D86.81 **Sarcoid meningitis**

     D86.82 **Multiple cranial nerve palsies in sarcoidosis**

     D86.83 **Sarcoid iridocyclitis**

     D86.84 **Sarcoid pyelonephritis**
         Tubulo-interstitial nephropathy in sarcoidosis

     D86.85 **Sarcoid myocarditis**

     D86.86 **Sarcoid arthropathy**
         Polyarthritis in sarcoidosis

     D86.87 **Sarcoid myositis**

     D86.89 **Sarcoidosis of other sites**
         Hepatic granuloma
         Uveoparotid fever [Heerfordt]

D86.9 **Sarcoidosis, unspecified**

✓4ᵗʰ **D89** **Other disorders involving the immune mechanism, not elsewhere classified**

     EXCLUDES 1   *hyperglobulinemia NOS (R77.1)*
                monoclonal gammopathy (of undetermined significance) (D47.2)
     EXCLUDES 2   *transplant failure and rejection (T86.-)*

D89.0 **Polyclonal hypergammaglobulinemia**
     Benign hypergammaglobulinemic purpura
     Polyclonal gammopathy NOS

D89.1 **Cryoglobulinemia**
     Cryoglobulinemic purpura
     Cryoglobulinemic vasculitis
     Essential cryoglobulinemia
     Idiopathic cryoglobulinemia
     Mixed cryoglobulinemia
     Primary cryoglobulinemia
     Secondary cryoglobulinemia

D89.2 **Hypergammaglobulinemia, unspecified**

D89.3 **Immune reconstitution syndrome**
     Immune reconstitution inflammatory syndrome [IRIS]
     Use additional code for adverse effect, if applicable, to identify drug (T36-T50 with fifth or sixth character 5)

✓5ᵗʰ **D89.8** **Other specified disorders involving the immune mechanism, not elsewhere classified**

    ✓6ᵗʰ **D89.81** **Graft-versus-host disease**
         Code first underlying cause, such as:
            complications of transplanted organs and tissue (T86.-)
            complications of blood transfusion (T80.89)
         Use additional code to identify associated manifestations, such as:
         desquamative dermatitis (L30.8)
         diarrhea (R19.7)
         elevated bilirubin (R17)
         hair loss (L65.9)

         CC Excl: For CC codes in subcategory D89.81, unless otherwise noted: D78.81-D78.89, D89.810-D89.813, E89.810-E89.89, H59.011-H59.019, H59.031-H59.099, H59.811-H59.89, H95.811-H95.89, I97.3, M96.89, N98.1-N98.9, T86.00-T86.09

         D89.810 **Acute graft-versus-host disease** `CC`

         D89.811 **Chronic graft-versus-host disease** `CC`

         D89.812 **Acute on chronic graft-versus-host disease** `CC`

         D89.813 **Graft-versus-host disease, unspecified** `CC`

     D89.82 **Autoimmune lymphoproliferative syndrome [ALPS]**

     D89.89 **Other specified disorders involving the immune mechanism, not elsewhere classified**
         EXCLUDES 1   *human immunodeficiency virus disease (B20)*

D89.9 **Disorder involving the immune mechanism, unspecified**
     Immune disease NOS

N Newborn: 0   P Pediatric: 0-17   M Maternity: 12-55   A Adult: 15-124   MCC Major CC Condition   PDx MCC PDx acts as own MCC   CC CC Condition   PDx CC PDx acts as own CC

492

ICD-10-CM Draft (2015)

Chapter 4. Endocrine, Nutritional and Metabolic Diseases (E00-E89)

NOTE   All neoplasms, whether functionally active or not, are classified in Chapter 2. Appropriate codes in this chapter (i.e. E05.8, E07.0, E16-E31, E34-) may be used as additional codes to indicate either functional activity by neoplasms and ectopic endocrine tissue or hyperfunction and hypofunction of endocrine glands associated with neoplasms and other conditions classified elsewhere.

EXCLUDES 1   *transitory endocrine and metabolic disorders specific to newborn (P70-P74)*

This chapter contains the following blocks:

E00-E07   Disorders of thyroid gland
E08-E13   Diabetes mellitus
E15-E16   Other disorders of glucose regulation and pancreatic internal secretion
E20-E35   Disorders of other endocrine glands
E36   Intraoperative complications of endocrine system
E40-E46   Malnutrition
E50-E64   Other nutritional deficiencies
E65-E68   Overweight, obesity and other hyperalimentation
E70-E88   Metabolic disorders
E89   Postprocedural endocrine and metabolic complications and disorders, not elsewhere classified

Disorders of thyroid gland (E00-E07)

✓4ᵗʰ E00   Congenital iodine-deficiency syndrome

Use additional code (F70-F79) to identify associated intellectual disabilities

EXCLUDES 1   *subclinical iodine-deficiency hypothyroidism (E02)*

E00.0   Congenital iodine-deficiency syndrome, neurological type
Endemic cretinism, neurological type

E00.1   Congenital iodine-deficiency syndrome, myxedematous type
Endemic hypothyroid cretinism
Endemic cretinism, myxedematous type

E00.2   Congenital iodine-deficiency syndrome, mixed type
Endemic cretinism, mixed type

E00.9   Congenital iodine-deficiency syndrome, unspecified
Congenital iodine-deficiency hypothyroidism NOS
Endemic cretinism NOS

✓4ᵗʰ E01   Iodine-deficiency related thyroid disorders and allied conditions

EXCLUDES 1   *congenital iodine-deficiency syndrome (E00.-)*
subclinical iodine-deficiency hypothyroidism (E02)

E01.0   Iodine-deficiency related diffuse (endemic) goiter

E01.1   Iodine-deficiency related multinodular (endemic) goiter
Iodine-deficiency related nodular goiter

E01.2   Iodine-deficiency related (endemic) goiter, unspecified
Endemic goiter NOS

E01.8   Other iodine-deficiency related thyroid disorders and allied conditions
Acquired iodine-deficiency hypothyroidism NOS

E02   Subclinical iodine-deficiency hypothyroidism

✓4ᵗʰ E03   Other hypothyroidism

EXCLUDES 1   *iodine-deficiency related hypothyroidism (E00-E02)*
postprocedural hypothyroidism (E89.0)

E03.0   Congenital hypothyroidism with diffuse goiter
Congenital parenchymatous goiter (nontoxic)
Congenital goiter (nontoxic) NOS
EXCLUDES 1   *transitory congenital goiter with normal function (P72.0)*

E03.1   Congenital hypothyroidism without goiter
Aplasia of thyroid (with myxedema)
Congenital atrophy of thyroid
Congenital hypothyroidism NOS

E03.2   Hypothyroidism due to medicaments and other exogenous substances
Code first poisoning due to drug or toxin, if applicable (T36-T65 with fifth or sixth character 1-4 or 6)
Use additional code for adverse effect, if applicable, to identify drug (T36-T50 with fifth or sixth character 5)

E03.3   Postinfectious hypothyroidism
E03.4   Atrophy of thyroid (acquired)
EXCLUDES 1   *congenital atrophy of thyroid (E03.1)*

E03.5   Myxedema coma   **MCC**
CC Excl: B15.0-B19.9, E03.5, E08.00-E08.59, E08.618-E08.638, E08.641-E09.59, E09.618-E09.638, E09.641-E10.59, E10.618-E10.638, E10.641-E10.649, E10.69-E11.59, E11.618-E11.638, E11.641-E11.649, E11.69-E13.59, E13.618-E13.638, E13.641-E16.2, E89.1, G32.89, G89.0-G89.4, G93.81-G93.9, G96.8-G96.9, G98.0-G98.8, G99.8, I60.00-I62.9, K72.91, R40.0-R40.2124, R40.2210-R40.2224, R40.2310-R40.2324, R40.2340-R40.2344, R40.3-R41.3, R41.82, R41.9-R42, R44.8-R44.9, R45.83-R45.84, R46.0-R46.89, R52, R55, R68.0-R68.19, R68.81-R68.83, R68.89-R69; S02.0XX-S06.9X9 with 7th character A

E03.8   Other specified hypothyroidism

E03.9   Hypothyroidism, unspecified
Myxedema NOS

✓4ᵗʰ E04   Other nontoxic goiter

EXCLUDES 1   *congenital goiter (NOS) (diffuse) (parenchymatous) (E03.0)*
iodine-deficiency related goiter (E00-E02)

E04.0   Nontoxic diffuse goiter
Diffuse (colloid) nontoxic goiter
Simple nontoxic goiter

E04.1   Nontoxic single thyroid nodule
Colloid nodule (cystic) (thyroid)   Thyroid (cystic) nodule NOS
Nontoxic uninodular goiter

E04.2   Non toxic multinodular goiter
Cystic goiter NOS
Multinodular (cystic) goiter NOS

E04.8   Other specified nontoxic goiter

E04.9   Nontoxic goiter, unspecified
Goiter NOS
Nodular goiter (nontoxic) NOS

✓4ᵗʰ E05   Thyrotoxicosis [hyperthyroidism]

EXCLUDES 1   *chronic thyroiditis with transient thyrotoxicosis (E06.2)*
neonatal thyrotoxicosis (P72.1)

CC Excl: For MCC codes in category E05, unless otherwise noted: A17.9-A18.82, A18.84, A18.89, E00.0-E03.4, E03.8-E07.1, E07.89-E07.9, E30.9, E34.1, E34.50-E35, E89.0

✓5ᵗʰ E05.0   Thyrotoxicosis with diffuse goiter
Exophthalmic or toxic goiter NOS
Graves' disease
Toxic diffuse goiter

     E05.00   Thyrotoxicosis with diffuse goiter without thyrotoxic crisis or storm

     E05.01   Thyrotoxicosis with diffuse goiter with thyrotoxic crisis or storm   **MCC**

✓5ᵗʰ E05.1   Thyrotoxicosis with toxic single thyroid nodule
Thyrotoxicosis with toxic uninodular goiter

     E05.10   Thyrotoxicosis with toxic single thyroid nodule without thyrotoxic crisis or storm

     E05.11   Thyrotoxicosis with toxic single thyroid nodule with thyrotoxic crisis or storm   **MCC**

✓5ᵗʰ E05.2   Thyrotoxicosis with toxic multinodular goiter
Toxic nodular goiter NOS

     E05.20   Thyrotoxicosis with toxic multinodular goiter without thyrotoxic crisis or storm

     E05.21   Thyrotoxicosis with toxic multinodular goiter with thyrotoxic crisis or storm   **MCC**

✓5ᵗʰ E05.3   Thyrotoxicosis from ectopic thyroid tissue

     E05.30   Thyrotoxicosis from ectopic thyroid tissue without thyrotoxic crisis or storm

     E05.31   Thyrotoxicosis from ectopic thyroid tissue with thyrotoxic crisis or storm   **MCC**

✓5ᵗʰ E05.4   Thyrotoxicosis factitia

     E05.40   Thyrotoxicosis factitia without thyrotoxic crisis or storm

     E05.41   Thyrotoxicosis factitia with thyrotoxic crisis or storm   **MCC**

✓5ᵗʰ E05.8   Other thyrotoxicosis
Overproduction of thyroid-stimulating hormone

     E05.80   Other thyrotoxicosis without thyrotoxic crisis or storm

     E05.81   Other thyrotoxicosis with thyrotoxic crisis or storm   **MCC**

✓5ᵗʰ E05.9   Thyrotoxicosis, unspecified
Hyperthyroidism NOS

     E05.90   Thyrotoxicosis, unspecified without thyrotoxic crisis or storm

Endocrine, Nutritional and Metabolic Diseases

E05.91–E08.36

E05.91   Thyrotoxicosis, unspecified with thyrotoxic `MCC`
crisis or storm

✓4ᵗʰ **E06   Thyroiditis**
    EXCLUDES 1 *postpartum thyroiditis (O90.5)*

  E06.0   Acute thyroiditis `CC`
    Abscess of thyroid
    Pyogenic thyroiditis
    Suppurative thyroiditis
    Use additional code (B95-B97) to identify infectious agent
    CC Excl: E06.0-E06.9

  E06.1   Subacute thyroiditis
    de Quervain thyroiditis   Nonsuppurative thyroiditis
    Giant-cell thyroiditis   Viral thyroiditis
    Granulomatous thyroiditis
      EXCLUDES 1 *autoimmune thyroiditis (E06.3)*

  E06.2   Chronic thyroiditis with transient thyrotoxicosis
      EXCLUDES 1 *autoimmune thyroiditis (E06.3)*

  E06.3   Autoimmune thyroiditis
    Hashimoto's thyroiditis
    Hashitoxicosis (transient)
    Lymphadenoid goiter
    Lymphocytic thyroiditis
    Struma lymphomatosa

  E06.4   Drug-induced thyroiditis
    Use additional code for adverse effect, if applicable, to identify
    drug (T36-T50 with fifth or sixth character 5)

  E06.5   Other chronic thyroiditis
    Chronic fibrous thyroiditis
    Chronic thyroiditis NOS
    Ligneous thyroiditis
    Riedel thyroiditis

  E06.9   Thyroiditis, unspecified

✓4ᵗʰ **E07   Other disorders of thyroid**
  E07.0   Hypersecretion of calcitonin
    C-cell hyperplasia of thyroid
    Hypersecretion of thyrocalcitonin

  E07.1   Dyshormogenetic goiter
    Familial dyshormogenetic goiter
    Pendred's syndrome
      EXCLUDES 1 *transitory congenital goiter with normal function (P72.0)*

  ✓5ᵗʰ **E07.8   Other specified disorders of thyroid**
    E07.81   Sick-euthyroid syndrome
        Euthyroid sick-syndrome
    E07.89   Other specified disorders of thyroid
        Abnormality of thyroid-binding globulin
        Hemorrhage of thyroid
        Infarction of thyroid

  E07.9   Disorder of thyroid, unspecified

Diabetes mellitus (E08-E13)

✓4ᵗʰ **E08   Diabetes mellitus due to underlying condition**
  Code first the underlying condition, such as:
    congenital rubella (P35.0)
    cushing's syndrome (E24.-)
    cystic fibrosis (E84.-)
    malignant neoplasm (C00-C96)
    malnutrition (E40-E46)
    pancreatitis and other diseases of the pancreas (K85.-, K86.-)
  Use additional code to identify any insulin use (Z79.4)
    EXCLUDES 1 *drug or chemical induced diabetes mellitus (E09.-)*
        gestational diabetes (O24.4-)
        neonatal diabetes mellitus (P70.2)
        postpancreatectomy diabetes mellitus (E13.-)
        postprocedural diabetes mellitus (E13.-)
        secondary diabetes mellitus NEC (E13.-)
        type 1 diabetes mellitus (E10.-)
        type 2 diabetes mellitus (E11.-)
  AHA: 2013, 4Q, 114; 2013, 3Q, 20

  CC Excl: For MCC codes in category E08, unless otherwise noted:
  E08.00-E08.59, E08.618-E08.638, E08.641-E09.59, E09.618-E09.638,
  E09.641-E10.59, E10.618-E10.638, E10.641-E10.649, E10.69-E11.59,
  E11.618-E11.638, E11.641-E11.649, E11.69-E13.59, E13.618-E13.638,
  E13.641-E16.2, E30.9, E34.1, E34.8-E35, E89.1

✓5ᵗʰ **E08.0   Diabetes mellitus due to underlying condition with**
hyperosmolarity
  E08.00   Diabetes mellitus due to underlying condition `MCC`
    with hyperosmolarity without nonketotic
    hyperglycemic-hyperosmolar coma (NKHHC)
  E08.01   Diabetes mellitus due to underlying condition `MCC`
    with hyperosmolarity with coma

✓5ᵗʰ **E08.1   Diabetes mellitus due to underlying condition with**
ketoacidosis
  E08.10   Diabetes mellitus due to underlying condition `MCC`
    with ketoacidosis without coma
  E08.11   Diabetes mellitus due to underlying condition `MCC`
    with ketoacidosis with coma

✓5ᵗʰ **E08.2   Diabetes mellitus due to underlying condition with kidney**
complications
  E08.21   Diabetes mellitus due to underlying condition with
    diabetic nephropathy
    Diabetes mellitus due to underlying condition with
      intercapillary glomerulosclerosis
    Diabetes mellitus due to underlying condition with
      intracapillary glomerulonephrosis
    Diabetes mellitus due to underlying condition with
      Kimmelstiel-Wilson disease
  E08.22   Diabetes mellitus due to underlying condition with
    diabetic chronic kidney disease
    Use additional code to identify stage of chronic kidney
      disease (N18.1-N18.6)
  E08.29   Diabetes mellitus due to underlying condition with
    other diabetic kidney complication
    Renal tubular degeneration in diabetes mellitus due to
      underlying condition

✓5ᵗʰ **E08.3   Diabetes mellitus due to underlying condition with**
ophthalmic complications
  ✓6ᵗʰ **E08.31   Diabetes mellitus due to underlying condition with**
    unspecified diabetic retinopathy
    E08.311   Diabetes mellitus due to underlying
        condition with unspecified diabetic
        retinopathy with macular edema
    E08.319   Diabetes mellitus due to underlying
        condition with unspecified diabetic
        retinopathy without macular edema
  ✓6ᵗʰ **E08.32   Diabetes mellitus due to underlying condition with**
    mild nonproliferative diabetic retinopathy
    Diabetes mellitus due to underlying condition with
      nonproliferative diabetic retinopathy NOS
    E08.321   Diabetes mellitus due to underlying
        condition with mild nonproliferative
        diabetic retinopathy with macular edema
    E08.329   Diabetes mellitus due to underlying
        condition with mild nonproliferative
        diabetic retinopathy without macular
        edema
  ✓6ᵗʰ **E08.33   Diabetes mellitus due to underlying condition with**
    moderate nonproliferative diabetic retinopathy
    E08.331   Diabetes mellitus due to underlying
        condition with moderate nonproliferative
        diabetic retinopathy with macular edema
    E08.339   Diabetes mellitus due to underlying
        condition with moderate nonproliferative
        diabetic retinopathy without macular
        edema
  ✓6ᵗʰ **E08.34   Diabetes mellitus due to underlying condition with**
    severe nonproliferative diabetic retinopathy
    E08.341   Diabetes mellitus due to underlying
        condition with severe nonproliferative
        diabetic retinopathy with macular edema
    E08.349   Diabetes mellitus due to underlying
        condition with severe nonproliferative
        diabetic retinopathy without macular
        edema
  ✓6ᵗʰ **E08.35   Diabetes mellitus due to underlying condition with**
    proliferative diabetic retinopathy
    E08.351   Diabetes mellitus due to underlying
        condition with proliferative diabetic
        retinopathy with macular edema
    E08.359   Diabetes mellitus due to underlying
        condition with proliferative diabetic
        retinopathy without macular edema
  E08.36   Diabetes mellitus due to underlying condition with
    diabetic cataract

E08.39 **Diabetes mellitus due to underlying condition with** other **diabetic ophthalmic complication**
> Use additional code to identify manifestation, such as: diabetic glaucoma (H40-H42)

✓5th E08.4 **Diabetes mellitus due to underlying condition with** neurological complications

E08.40 **Diabetes mellitus due to underlying condition with** diabetic neuropathy, unspecified

E08.41 **Diabetes mellitus due to underlying condition with** diabetic mononeuropathy

E08.42 **Diabetes mellitus due to underlying condition with** diabetic polyneuropathy
> Diabetes mellitus due to underlying condition with diabetic neuralgia

E08.43 **Diabetes mellitus due to underlying condition with** diabetic autonomic (poly)neuropathy
> Diabetes mellitus due to underlying condition with diabetic gastroparesis
> AHA: 2013, 4Q, 114

E08.44 **Diabetes mellitus due to underlying condition with** diabetic amyotrophy

E08.49 **Diabetes mellitus due to underlying condition with** other diabetic neurological complication

✓5th E08.5 **Diabetes mellitus due to underlying condition with** circulatory complications

E08.51 **Diabetes mellitus due to underlying condition with** diabetic peripheral angiopathy without gangrene

E08.52 **Diabetes mellitus due to underlying** `PDx CC CC` **condition with diabetic** peripheral angiopathy with gangrene
> Diabetes mellitus due to underlying condition with diabetic gangrene
> CC Excl: G89.0-G89.4, I70.261-I70.269, I96, R41.0-R41.3, R41.82, R41.9, R44.8-R44.9, R45.83-R45.84, R46.0-R46.89, R52, R68.0-R68.19, R68.81-R68.83, R68.89-R69

E08.59 **Diabetes mellitus due to underlying condition with** other circulatory complications

✓5th E08.6 **Diabetes mellitus due to underlying condition with** other specified complications

✓6th E08.61 **Diabetes mellitus due to underlying condition with** diabetic arthropathy

E08.610 **Diabetes mellitus due to underlying condition with diabetic** neuropathic arthropathy
> Diabetes mellitus due to underlying condition with Charcôt's joints

E08.618 **Diabetes mellitus due to underlying condition with** other diabetic arthropathy

✓6th E08.62 **Diabetes mellitus due to underlying condition with** skin complications

E08.620 **Diabetes mellitus due to underlying condition with** diabetic dermatitis
> Diabetes mellitus due to underlying condition with diabetic necrobiosis lipoidica

E08.621 **Diabetes mellitus due to underlying condition with** foot ulcer
> Use additional code to identify site of ulcer (L97.4-, L97.5-)

E08.622 **Diabetes mellitus due to underlying condition with** other skin ulcer
> Use additional code to identify site of ulcer (L97.1-L97.9, L98.41-L98.49)

E08.628 **Diabetes mellitus due to underlying condition with** other skin complications

✓6th E08.63 **Diabetes mellitus due to underlying condition with** oral complications

E08.630 **Diabetes mellitus due to underlying condition with** periodontal disease

E08.638 **Diabetes mellitus due to underlying condition with other** oral complications

✓6th E08.64 **Diabetes mellitus due to underlying condition with** hypoglycemia

E08.641 **Diabetes mellitus due to underlying** `MCC` **condition with hypoglycemia** with coma

E08.649 **Diabetes mellitus due to underlying condition with hypoglycemia** without coma

E08.65 **Diabetes mellitus due to underlying condition with** hyperglycemia

E08.69 **Diabetes mellitus due to underlying condition with** other specified complication
> Use additional code to identify complication

E08.8 **Diabetes mellitus due to underlying condition with** unspecified complications

E08.9 **Diabetes mellitus due to underlying condition** without complications

✓4th E09 **Drug or chemical induced diabetes mellitus**
> Code first poisoning due to drug or toxin, if applicable (T36-T65 with fifth or sixth character 1-4 or 6)
> Use additional code for adverse effect, if applicable, to identify drug (T36-T50 with fifth or sixth character 5)
> Use additional code to identify any insulin use (Z79.4)
> EXCLUDES 1 diabetes mellitus due to underlying condition (E08.-)
> gestational diabetes (O24.4-)
> neonatal diabetes mellitus (P70.2)
> postpancreatectomy diabetes mellitus (E13.-)
> postprocedural diabetes mellitus (E13.-)
> secondary diabetes mellitus NEC (E13.-)
> type 1 diabetes mellitus (E10.-)
> type 2 diabetes mellitus (E11.-)
> AHA: 2013, 4Q, 114; 2013, 3Q, 20

CC Excl: For MCC codes in category E09, unless otherwise noted: E08.00-E08.59, E08.618-E08.638, E08.641-E09.59, E09.618-E09.638, E09.641-E10.59, E10.618-E10.638, E10.641-E10.649, E10.69-E11.59, E11.618-E11.638, E11.641-E11.649, E11.69-E13.59, E13.618-E13.638, E13.641-E16.2, E30.9, E34.1, E34.8-E35, E89.1

✓5th E09.0 **Drug or chemical induced diabetes mellitus with** hyperosmolarity

E09.00 **Drug or chemical induced diabetes mellitus with hyperosmolarity** without nonketotic hyperglycemic-hyperosmolar coma (NKHHC) `MCC`

E09.01 **Drug or chemical induced diabetes mellitus with hyperosmolarity** with coma `MCC`

✓5th E09.1 **Drug or chemical induced diabetes mellitus with** ketoacidosis

E09.10 **Drug or chemical induced diabetes mellitus with ketoacidosis** without coma `MCC`

E09.11 **Drug or chemical induced diabetes mellitus with** `MCC` ketoacidosis with coma

✓5th E09.2 **Drug or chemical induced diabetes mellitus with** kidney complications

E09.21 **Drug or chemical induced diabetes mellitus with** diabetic nephropathy
> Drug or chemical induced diabetes mellitus with intercapillary glomerulosclerosis
> Drug or chemical induced diabetes mellitus with intracapillary glomerulonephrosis
> Drug or chemical induced diabetes mellitus with Kimmelstiel-Wilson disease

E09.22 **Drug or chemical induced diabetes mellitus with** diabetic chronic kidney disease
> Use additional code to identify stage of chronic kidney disease (N18.1-N18.6)

E09.29 **Drug or chemical induced diabetes mellitus with** other diabetic kidney complication
> Drug or chemical induced diabetes mellitus with renal tubular degeneration

✓5th E09.3 **Drug or chemical induced diabetes mellitus with** ophthalmic complications

✓6th E09.31 **Drug or chemical induced diabetes mellitus with** unspecified diabetic retinopathy

E09.311 **Drug or chemical induced diabetes mellitus with unspecified diabetic retinopathy** with macular edema

E09.319 **Drug or chemical induced diabetes mellitus with unspecified diabetic retinopathy** without macular edema

✓6th E09.32 **Drug or chemical induced diabetes mellitus with** mild nonproliferative diabetic retinopathy
> Drug or chemical induced diabetes mellitus with nonproliferative diabetic retinopathy NOS

E09.321 **Drug or chemical induced diabetes mellitus with mild nonproliferative diabetic retinopathy** with macular edema

E09.329 **Drug or chemical induced diabetes mellitus with mild nonproliferative diabetic retinopathy** without macular edema

✓6th E09.33 **Drug or chemical induced diabetes mellitus with** moderate nonproliferative diabetic retinopathy

E09.331 Drug or chemical induced diabetes mellitus with moderate nonproliferative diabetic retinopathy with macular edema

E09.339 Drug or chemical induced diabetes mellitus with moderate nonproliferative diabetic retinopathy without macular edema

√6th **E09.34** Drug or chemical induced diabetes mellitus with severe nonproliferative diabetic retinopathy

E09.341 Drug or chemical induced diabetes mellitus with severe nonproliferative diabetic retinopathy with macular edema

E09.349 Drug or chemical induced diabetes mellitus with severe nonproliferative diabetic retinopathy without macular edema

√6th **E09.35** Drug or chemical induced diabetes mellitus with proliferative diabetic retinopathy

E09.351 Drug or chemical induced diabetes mellitus with proliferative diabetic retinopathy with macular edema

E09.359 Drug or chemical induced diabetes mellitus with proliferative diabetic retinopathy without macular edema

E09.36 Drug or chemical induced diabetes mellitus with diabetic cataract

E09.39 Drug or chemical induced diabetes mellitus with other diabetic ophthalmic complication
Use additional code to identify manifestation, such as: diabetic glaucoma (H40-H42)

√5th **E09.4** Drug or chemical induced diabetes mellitus with neurological complications

E09.40 Drug or chemical induced diabetes mellitus with neurological complications with diabetic neuropathy, unspecified

E09.41 Drug or chemical induced diabetes mellitus with neurological complications with diabetic mononeuropathy

E09.42 Drug or chemical induced diabetes mellitus with neurological complications with diabetic polyneuropathy
Drug or chemical induced diabetes mellitus with diabetic neuralgia

E09.43 Drug or chemical induced diabetes mellitus with neurological complications with diabetic autonomic (poly)neuropathy
Drug or chemical induced diabetes mellitus with diabetic gastroparesis
AHA: 2013, 4Q, 114

E09.44 Drug or chemical induced diabetes mellitus with neurological complications with diabetic amyotrophy

E09.49 Drug or chemical induced diabetes mellitus with neurological complications with other diabetic neurological complication

√5th **E09.5** Drug or chemical induced diabetes mellitus with circulatory complications

E09.51 Drug or chemical induced diabetes mellitus with diabetic peripheral angiopathy without gangrene

E09.52 Drug or chemical induced diabetes mellitus with diabetic peripheral angiopathy with gangrene PDx CC CC
Drug or chemical induced diabetes mellitus with diabetic gangrene
CC Excl: G89.0-G89.4, I70.261-I70.269, I96, R41.0-R41.3, R41.82, R41.9, R44.8-R44.9, R45.83-R45.84, R46.0-R46.89, R52, R68.0-R68.19, R68.81-R68.83, R68.89-R69

E09.59 Drug or chemical induced diabetes mellitus with other circulatory complications

√5th **E09.6** Drug or chemical induced diabetes mellitus with other specified complications

√6th **E09.61** Drug or chemical induced diabetes mellitus with diabetic arthropathy

E09.610 Drug or chemical induced diabetes mellitus with diabetic neuropathic arthropathy
Drug or chemical induced diabetes mellitus with Charcôt's joints

E09.618 Drug or chemical induced diabetes mellitus with other diabetic arthropathy

√6th **E09.62** Drug or chemical induced diabetes mellitus with skin complications

E09.620 Drug or chemical induced diabetes mellitus with diabetic dermatitis
Drug or chemical induced diabetes mellitus with diabetic necrobiosis lipoidica

E09.621 Drug or chemical induced diabetes mellitus with foot ulcer
Use additional code to identify site of ulcer (L97.4-, L97.5-)

E09.622 Drug or chemical induced diabetes mellitus with other skin ulcer
Use additional code to identify site of ulcer (L97.1-L97.9, L98.41-L98.49)

E09.628 Drug or chemical induced diabetes mellitus with other skin complications

√6th **E09.63** Drug or chemical induced diabetes mellitus with oral complications

E09.630 Drug or chemical induced diabetes mellitus with periodontal disease

E09.638 Drug or chemical induced diabetes mellitus with other oral complications

√6th **E09.64** Drug or chemical induced diabetes mellitus with hypoglycemia

E09.641 Drug or chemical induced diabetes mellitus with hypoglycemia with coma MCC

E09.649 Drug or chemical induced diabetes mellitus with hypoglycemia without coma

E09.65 Drug or chemical induced diabetes mellitus with hyperglycemia

E09.69 Drug or chemical induced diabetes mellitus with other specified complication
Use additional code to identify complication

E09.8 Drug or chemical induced diabetes mellitus with unspecified complications

E09.9 Drug or chemical induced diabetes mellitus without complications

√4th **E10** Type 1 diabetes mellitus
INCLUDES
brittle diabetes (mellitus)
diabetes (mellitus) due to autoimmune process
diabetes (mellitus) due to immune mediated pancreatic islet beta-cell destruction
idiopathic diabetes (mellitus)
juvenile onset diabetes (mellitus)
ketosis-prone diabetes (mellitus)
EXCLUDES 1
diabetes mellitus due to underlying condition (E08.-)
drug or chemical induced diabetes mellitus (E09.-)
gestational diabetes (O24.4-)
hyperglycemia NOS (R73.9)
neonatal diabetes mellitus (P70.2)
postpancreatectomy diabetes mellitus (E13.-)
postprocedural diabetes mellitus (E13.-)
secondary diabetes mellitus NEC (E13.-)
type 2 diabetes mellitus (E11.-)
AHA: 2013, 4Q, 114; 2013, 3Q, 20

CC Excl: For MCC codes in category E10, unless otherwise noted:
E08.00-E08.59, E08.618-E08.638, E08.641-E09.59, E09.618-E09.638, E09.641-E10.59, E10.618-E10.638, E10.641-E10.649, E10.69-E11.59, E11.618-E11.638, E11.641-E11.649, E11.69-E13.59, E13.618-E13.638, E13.641-E16.2, E30.9, E34.1, E34.50-E35, E89.1

√5th **E10.1** Type 1 diabetes mellitus with ketoacidosis
AHA: 2013, 3Q, 20

E10.10 Type 1 diabetes mellitus with ketoacidosis without coma MCC

E10.11 Type 1 diabetes mellitus with ketoacidosis with coma MCC

√5th **E10.2** Type 1 diabetes mellitus with kidney complications

E10.21 Type 1 diabetes mellitus with diabetic nephropathy
Type 1 diabetes mellitus with intercapillary glomerulosclerosis
Type 1 diabetes mellitus with intracapillary glomerulonephrosis
Type 1 diabetes mellitus with Kimmelstiel-Wilson disease

E10.22 Type 1 diabetes mellitus with diabetic chronic kidney disease
Use additional code to identify stage of chronic kidney disease (N18.1-N18.6)

E10.29　Type 1 diabetes mellitus with other diabetic kidney complication
　　Type 1 diabetes mellitus with renal tubular degeneration

✓5th **E10.3　Type 1 diabetes mellitus with ophthalmic complications**

✓6th **E10.31　Type 1 diabetes mellitus with unspecified diabetic retinopathy**
　　E10.311　Type 1 diabetes mellitus with unspecified diabetic retinopathy with macular edema
　　E10.319　Type 1 diabetes mellitus with unspecified diabetic retinopathy without macular edema

✓6th **E10.32　Type 1 diabetes mellitus with mild nonproliferative diabetic retinopathy**
　　Type 1 diabetes mellitus with nonproliferative diabetic retinopathy NOS
　　E10.321　Type 1 diabetes mellitus with mild nonproliferative diabetic retinopathy with macular edema
　　E10.329　Type 1 diabetes mellitus with mild nonproliferative diabetic retinopathy without macular edema

✓6th **E10.33　Type 1 diabetes mellitus with moderate nonproliferative diabetic retinopathy**
　　E10.331　Type 1 diabetes mellitus with moderate nonproliferative diabetic retinopathy with macular edema
　　E10.339　Type 1 diabetes mellitus with moderate nonproliferative diabetic retinopathy without macular edema

✓6th **E10.34　Type 1 diabetes mellitus with severe nonproliferative diabetic retinopathy**
　　E10.341　Type 1 diabetes mellitus with severe nonproliferative diabetic retinopathy with macular edema
　　E10.349　Type 1 diabetes mellitus with severe nonproliferative diabetic retinopathy without macular edema

✓6th **E10.35　Type 1 diabetes mellitus with proliferative diabetic retinopathy**
　　E10.351　Type 1 diabetes mellitus with proliferative diabetic retinopathy with macular edema
　　E10.359　Type 1 diabetes mellitus with proliferative diabetic retinopathy without macular edema

E10.36　Type 1 diabetes mellitus with diabetic cataract

E10.39　Type 1 diabetes mellitus with other diabetic ophthalmic complication
　　Use additional code to identify manifestation, such as: diabetic glaucoma (H40-H42)

✓5th **E10.4　Type 1 diabetes mellitus with neurological complications**

E10.40　Type 1 diabetes mellitus with diabetic neuropathy, unspecified

E10.41　Type 1 diabetes mellitus with diabetic mononeuropathy

E10.42　Type 1 diabetes mellitus with diabetic polyneuropathy
　　Type 1 diabetes mellitus with diabetic neuralgia

E10.43　Type 1 diabetes mellitus with diabetic autonomic (poly)neuropathy
　　Type 1 diabetes mellitus with diabetic gastroparesis
　　AHA: 2013, 4Q, 114

E10.44　Type 1 diabetes mellitus with diabetic amyotrophy

E10.49　Type 1 diabetes mellitus with other diabetic neurological complication

✓5th **E10.5　Type 1 diabetes mellitus with circulatory complications**

E10.51　Type 1 diabetes mellitus with diabetic peripheral angiopathy without gangrene

E10.52　Type 1 diabetes mellitus with diabetic peripheral angiopathy with gangrene `PDx` `CC` `CC`
　　Type 1 diabetes mellitus with diabetic gangrene
　　CC Excl: G89.0-G89.4, I70.261-I70.269, I96, R41.0-R41.3, R41.82, R41.9, R44.8-R44.9, R45.83-R45.84, R46.0-R46.89, R52, R68.0-R68.19, R68.81-R68.83, R68.89-R69

E10.59　Type 1 diabetes mellitus with other circulatory complications

---

✓5th **E10.6　Type 1 diabetes mellitus with other specified complications**

✓6th **E10.61　Type 1 diabetes mellitus with diabetic arthropathy**
　　E10.610　Type 1 diabetes mellitus with diabetic neuropathic arthropathy
　　　Type 1 diabetes mellitus with Charcôt's joints
　　E10.618　Type 1 diabetes mellitus with other diabetic arthropathy

✓6th **E10.62　Type 1 diabetes mellitus with skin complications**
　　E10.620　Type 1 diabetes mellitus with diabetic dermatitis
　　　Type 1 diabetes mellitus with diabetic necrobiosis lipoidica
　　E10.621　Type 1 diabetes mellitus with foot ulcer
　　　Use additional code to identify site of ulcer (L97.4-, L97.5-)
　　E10.622　Type 1 diabetes mellitus with other skin ulcer
　　　Use additional code to identify site of ulcer (L97.1-L97.9, L98.41-L98.49)
　　E10.628　Type 1 diabetes mellitus with other skin complications

✓6th **E10.63　Type 1 diabetes mellitus with oral complications**
　　E10.630　Type 1 diabetes mellitus with periodontal disease
　　E10.638　Type 1 diabetes mellitus with other oral complications

✓6th **E10.64　Type 1 diabetes mellitus with hypoglycemia**
　　E10.641　Type 1 diabetes mellitus with hypoglycemia with coma `MCC`
　　E10.649　Type 1 diabetes mellitus with hypoglycemia without coma

E10.65　Type 1 diabetes mellitus with hyperglycemia
　　AHA: 2013, 3Q, 20

E10.69　Type 1 diabetes mellitus with other specified complication
　　Use additional code to identify complication

E10.8　Type 1 diabetes mellitus with unspecified complications

E10.9　Type 1 diabetes mellitus without complications

✓4th **E11　Type 2 diabetes mellitus**
　　`INCLUDES` diabetes (mellitus) due to insulin secretory defect
　　　diabetes NOS
　　　insulin resistant diabetes (mellitus)
　　Use additional code to identify any insulin use (Z79.4)
　　`EXCLUDES 1` diabetes mellitus due to underlying condition (E08.-)
　　　drug or chemical induced diabetes mellitus (E09.-)
　　　gestational diabetes (O24.4-)
　　　neonatal diabetes mellitus (P70.2)
　　　postpancreatectomy diabetes mellitus (E13.-)
　　　postprocedural diabetes mellitus (E13.-)
　　　secondary diabetes mellitus NEC (E13.-)
　　　type 1 diabetes mellitus (E10.-)
　　AHA: 2013, 4Q, 114; 2013, 3Q, 20; 2013, 1Q, 26

　　CC Excl: For MCC codes in category E11, unless otherwise noted:
　　E08.00-E08.59, E08.618-E08.638, E08.641-E09.59, E09.618-E09.638, E09.641-E10.59, E10.618-E10.638, E10.641-E10.649, E10.69-E11.59, E11.618-E11.638, E11.641-E11.649, E11.69-E13.59, E13.618-E13.638, E13.641-E16.2, E30.9, E34.1, E34.8-E35, E89.1

✓5th **E11.0　Type 2 diabetes mellitus with hyperosmolarity**
　　E11.00　Type 2 diabetes mellitus with hyperosmolarity without nonketotic hyperglycemic-hyperosmolar coma (NKHHC) `MCC`
　　E11.01　Type 2 diabetes mellitus with hyperosmolarity with coma `MCC`

✓5th **E11.2　Type 2 diabetes mellitus with kidney complications**
　　E11.21　Type 2 diabetes mellitus with diabetic nephropathy
　　　Type 2 diabetes mellitus with intercapillary glomerulosclerosis
　　　Type 2 diabetes mellitus with intracapillary glomerulonephrosis
　　　Type 2 diabetes mellitus with Kimmelstiel-Wilson disease
　　E11.22　Type 2 diabetes mellitus with diabetic chronic kidney disease
　　　Use additional code to identify stage of chronic kidney disease (N18.1-N18.6)

N18.2 for stage II
Z79.4 (insuline)
deg

✔ Additional Character Required　`x7th` Xtension Alert　Unacceptable PDx　Manifestation　Hospital Acquired Condition　`EXCLUDES 1` Not Coded Here　`EXCLUDES 2` Not Included Here

E11.29 Type 2 diabetes mellitus with other diabetic kidney complication
Type 2 diabetes mellitus with renal tubular degeneration

✓5ᵗʰ **E11.3 Type 2 diabetes mellitus with ophthalmic complications**

✓6ᵗʰ **E11.31 Type 2 diabetes mellitus with unspecified diabetic retinopathy**
E11.311 Type 2 diabetes mellitus with unspecified diabetic retinopathy with macular edema
E11.319 Type 2 diabetes mellitus with unspecified diabetic retinopathy without macular edema

✓6ᵗʰ **E11.32 Type 2 diabetes mellitus with mild nonproliferative diabetic retinopathy**
Type 2 diabetes mellitus with nonproliferative diabetic retinopathy NOS
E11.321 Type 2 diabetes mellitus with mild nonproliferative diabetic retinopathy with macular edema
E11.329 Type 2 diabetes mellitus with mild nonproliferative diabetic retinopathy without macular edema

✓6ᵗʰ **E11.33 Type 2 diabetes mellitus with moderate nonproliferative diabetic retinopathy**
E11.331 Type 2 diabetes mellitus with moderate nonproliferative diabetic retinopathy with macular edema
E11.339 Type 2 diabetes mellitus with moderate nonproliferative diabetic retinopathy without macular edema

✓6ᵗʰ **E11.34 Type 2 diabetes mellitus with severe nonproliferative diabetic retinopathy**
E11.341 Type 2 diabetes mellitus with severe nonproliferative diabetic retinopathy with macular edema
E11.349 Type 2 diabetes mellitus with severe nonproliferative diabetic retinopathy without macular edema

✓6ᵗʰ **E11.35 Type 2 diabetes mellitus with proliferative diabetic retinopathy**
E11.351 Type 2 diabetes mellitus with proliferative diabetic retinopathy with macular edema
E11.359 Type 2 diabetes mellitus with proliferative diabetic retinopathy without macular edema

E11.36 Type 2 diabetes mellitus with diabetic cataract
E11.39 Type 2 diabetes mellitus with other diabetic ophthalmic complication
Use additional code to identify manifestation, such as: diabetic glaucoma (H40-H42)

✓5ᵗʰ **E11.4 Type 2 diabetes mellitus with neurological complications**
E11.40 Type 2 diabetes mellitus with diabetic neuropathy, unspecified
AHA: 2013, 4Q, 129
E11.41 Type 2 diabetes mellitus with diabetic mononeuropathy
E11.42 Type 2 diabetes mellitus with diabetic polyneuropathy
Type 2 diabetes mellitus with diabetic neuralgia
E11.43 Type 2 diabetes mellitus with diabetic autonomic (poly)neuropathy
Type 2 diabetes mellitus with diabetic gastroparesis
AHA: 2013, 4Q, 114
E11.44 Type 2 diabetes mellitus with diabetic amyotrophy
E11.49 Type 2 diabetes mellitus with other diabetic neurological complication

✓5ᵗʰ **E11.5 Type 2 diabetes mellitus with circulatory complications**
E11.51 Type 2 diabetes mellitus with diabetic peripheral angiopathy without gangrene
E11.52 Type 2 diabetes mellitus with diabetic peripheral angiopathy with gangrene PDx CC CC
Type 2 diabetes mellitus with diabetic gangrene
CC Excl: G89.0-G89.4, I70.261-I70.269, I96, R41.0-R41.3, R41.82, R41.9, R44.8-R44.9, R45.83-R45.84, R46.0-R46.89, R52, R68.0-R68.19, R68.81-R68.83, R68.89-R69
E11.59 Type 2 diabetes mellitus with other circulatory complications

✓5ᵗʰ **E11.6 Type 2 diabetes mellitus with other specified complications**
✓6ᵗʰ **E11.61 Type 2 diabetes mellitus with diabetic arthropathy**
E11.610 Type 2 diabetes mellitus with diabetic neuropathic arthropathy
Type 2 diabetes mellitus with Charcôt's joints
E11.618 Type 2 diabetes mellitus with other diabetic arthropathy

✓6ᵗʰ **E11.62 Type 2 diabetes mellitus with skin complications**
E11.620 Type 2 diabetes mellitus with diabetic dermatitis
Type 2 diabetes mellitus with diabetic necrobiosis lipoidica
E11.621 Type 2 diabetes mellitus with foot ulcer
Use additional code to identify site of ulcer (L97.4-, L97.5-)
E11.622 Type 2 diabetes mellitus with other skin ulcer
Use additional code to identify site of ulcer (L97.1-L97.9, L98.41-L98.49)
E11.628 Type 2 diabetes mellitus with other skin complications

✓6ᵗʰ **E11.63 Type 2 diabetes mellitus with oral complications**
E11.630 Type 2 diabetes mellitus with periodontal disease
E11.638 Type 2 diabetes mellitus with other oral complications

✓6ᵗʰ **E11.64 Type 2 diabetes mellitus with hypoglycemia**
E11.641 Type 2 diabetes mellitus with hypoglycemia with coma MCC
E11.649 Type 2 diabetes mellitus with hypoglycemia without coma

E11.65 Type 2 diabetes mellitus with hyperglycemia
AHA: 2013, 3Q, 20
E11.69 Type 2 diabetes mellitus with other specified complication
Use additional code to identify complication

E11.8 Type 2 diabetes mellitus with unspecified complications
13 **E11.9 Type 2 diabetes mellitus without complications**

✓4ᵗʰ **E13 Other specified diabetes mellitus**
Diabetes mellitus due to genetic defects of beta-cell function
Diabetes mellitus due to genetic defects in insulin action
Postpancreatectomy diabetes mellitus
Postprocedural diabetes mellitus
Secondary diabetes mellitus NEC
Use additional code to identify any insulin use (Z79.4)
EXCLUDES 1 diabetes (mellitus) due to autoimmune process (E10.-)
diabetes (mellitus) due to immune mediated pancreatic islet beta-cell destruction (E10.-)
diabetes mellitus due to underlying condition (E08.-)
drug or chemical induced diabetes mellitus (E09.-)
gestational diabetes (O24.4-)
neonatal diabetes mellitus (P70.2)
type 2 diabetes mellitus (E11.-)
AHA: 2013, 4Q, 114; 2013, 3Q, 20

CC Excl: For MCC codes in category E13, unless otherwise noted: E08.00-E08.59, E08.618-E08.638, E08.641-E09.59, E09.618-E09.638, E09.641-E10.59, E10.618-E10.638, E10.641-E10.649, E10.69-E11.59, E11.618-E11.638, E11.641-E11.649, E11.69-E13.59, E13.618-E13.638, E13.641-E16.2, E30.9, E34.1, E34.8-E35, E89.1

✓5ᵗʰ **E13.0 Other specified diabetes mellitus with hyperosmolarity**
E13.00 Other specified diabetes mellitus with hyperosmolarity without nonketotic hyperglycemic-hyperosmolar coma (NKHHC) MCC
E13.01 Other specified diabetes mellitus with hyperosmolarity with coma MCC

✓5ᵗʰ **E13.1 Other specified diabetes mellitus with ketoacidosis**
AHA: 2013, 1Q, 26
E13.10 Other specified diabetes mellitus with ketoacidosis without coma MCC
E13.11 Other specified diabetes mellitus with ketoacidosis with coma MCC

13 Questionable admission when used as PDx.

N Newborn: 0   P Pediatric: 0-17   M Maternity: 12-55   A Adult: 15-124   MCC Major CC Condition   PDx MCC PDx acts as own MCC   CC CC Condition   PDx CC PDx acts as own CC
498   ICD-10-CM Draft (2015)

√5ᵗʰ E13.2 Other specified diabetes mellitus with kidney complications

E13.21 Other specified diabetes mellitus with diabetic nephropathy
Other specified diabetes mellitus with intercapillary glomerulosclerosis
Other specified diabetes mellitus with intracapillary glomerulonephrosis
Other specified diabetes mellitus with Kimmelstiel-Wilson disease

E13.22 Other specified diabetes mellitus with diabetic chronic kidney disease
Use additional code to identify stage of chronic kidney disease (N18.1-N18.6)

E13.29 Other specified diabetes mellitus with other diabetic kidney complication
Other specified diabetes mellitus with renal tubular degeneration

√5ᵗʰ E13.3 Other specified diabetes mellitus with ophthalmic complications

√6ᵗʰ E13.31 Other specified diabetes mellitus with unspecified diabetic retinopathy

E13.311 Other specified diabetes mellitus with unspecified diabetic retinopathy with macular edema

E13.319 Other specified diabetes mellitus with unspecified diabetic retinopathy without macular edema

√6ᵗʰ E13.32 Other specified diabetes mellitus with mild nonproliferative diabetic retinopathy
Other specified diabetes mellitus with nonproliferative diabetic retinopathy NOS

E13.321 Other specified diabetes mellitus with mild nonproliferative diabetic retinopathy with macular edema

E13.329 Other specified diabetes mellitus with mild nonproliferative diabetic retinopathy without macular edema

√6ᵗʰ E13.33 Other specified diabetes mellitus with moderate nonproliferative diabetic retinopathy

E13.331 Other specified diabetes mellitus with moderate nonproliferative diabetic retinopathy with macular edema

E13.339 Other specified diabetes mellitus with moderate nonproliferative diabetic retinopathy without macular edema

√6ᵗʰ E13.34 Other specified diabetes mellitus with severe nonproliferative diabetic retinopathy

E13.341 Other specified diabetes mellitus with severe nonproliferative diabetic retinopathy with macular edema

E13.349 Other specified diabetes mellitus with severe nonproliferative diabetic retinopathy without macular edema

√6ᵗʰ E13.35 Other specified diabetes mellitus with proliferative diabetic retinopathy

E13.351 Other specified diabetes mellitus with proliferative diabetic retinopathy with macular edema

E13.359 Other specified diabetes mellitus with proliferative diabetic retinopathy without macular edema

E13.36 Other specified diabetes mellitus with diabetic cataract

E13.39 Other specified diabetes mellitus with other diabetic ophthalmic complication
Use additional code to identify manifestation, such as: diabetic glaucoma (H40-H42)

√5ᵗʰ E13.4 Other specified diabetes mellitus with neurological complications

E13.40 Other specified diabetes mellitus with diabetic neuropathy, unspecified

E13.41 Other specified diabetes mellitus with diabetic mononeuropathy

E13.42 Other specified diabetes mellitus with diabetic polyneuropathy
Other specified diabetes mellitus with diabetic neuralgia

E13.43 Other specified diabetes mellitus with diabetic autonomic (poly)neuropathy
Other specified diabetes mellitus with diabetic gastroparesis
AHA: 2013, 4Q, 114

E13.44 Other specified diabetes mellitus with diabetic amyotrophy

E13.49 Other specified diabetes mellitus with other diabetic neurological complication

√5ᵗʰ E13.5 Other specified diabetes mellitus with circulatory complications

E13.51 Other specified diabetes mellitus with diabetic peripheral angiopathy without gangrene

E13.52 Other specified diabetes mellitus with diabetic peripheral angiopathy with gangrene   `PDx CC` `CC`
Other specified diabetes mellitus with diabetic gangrene
CC Excl: G89.0-G89.4, I70.261-I70.269, I96, R41.0-R41.3, R41.82, R41.9, R44.8-R44.9, R45.83-R45.84, R46.0-R46.89, R52, R68.0-R68.19, R68.81-R68.83, R68.89-R69

E13.59 Other specified diabetes mellitus with other circulatory complications

√5ᵗʰ E13.6 Other specified diabetes mellitus with other specified complications

√6ᵗʰ E13.61 Other specified diabetes mellitus with diabetic arthropathy

E13.610 Other specified diabetes mellitus with diabetic neuropathic arthropathy
Other specified diabetes mellitus with Charcôt's joints

E13.618 Other specified diabetes mellitus with other diabetic arthropathy

√6ᵗʰ E13.62 Other specified diabetes mellitus with skin complications

E13.620 Other specified diabetes mellitus with diabetic dermatitis
Other specified diabetes mellitus with diabetic necrobiosis lipoidica

E13.621 Other specified diabetes mellitus with foot ulcer
Use additional code to identify site of ulcer (L97.4-, L97.5-)

E13.622 Other specified diabetes mellitus with other skin ulcer
Use additional code to identify site of ulcer (L97.1-L97.9, L98.41-L98.49)

E13.628 Other specified diabetes mellitus with other skin complications

√6ᵗʰ E13.63 Other specified diabetes mellitus with oral complications

E13.630 Other specified diabetes mellitus with periodontal disease

E13.638 Other specified diabetes mellitus with other oral complications

√6ᵗʰ E13.64 Other specified diabetes mellitus with hypoglycemia

E13.641 Other specified diabetes mellitus with hypoglycemia with coma   `MCC`

E13.649 Other specified diabetes mellitus with hypoglycemia without coma

E13.65 Other specified diabetes mellitus with hyperglycemia

E13.69 Other specified diabetes mellitus with other specified complication
Use additional code to identify complication

E13.8 Other specified diabetes mellitus with unspecified complications

¹³ **E13.9 Other specified diabetes mellitus without complications**

---

¹³ Questionable admission when used as PDx.

✔ Additional Character Required   ✔x7ᵗʰ Xtension Alert   Unacceptable PDx   Manifestation   Hospital Acquired Condition   EXCLUDES1 Not Coded Here   EXCLUDES2 Not Included Here

ICD-10-CM Draft (2015)   499

Endocrine, Nutritional and Metabolic Diseases

E15–E24.9

Other disorders of glucose regulation and pancreatic internal secretion (E15-E16)

E15   Nondiabetic hypoglycemic coma   CC
  INCLUDES drug-induced insulin coma in nondiabetic
          hyperinsulinism with hypoglycemic coma
          hypoglycemic coma NOS
  CC Excl: E08.00-E08.59, E08.618-E08.638, E08.641-E09.59, E09.618-
          E09.638, E09.641-E10.59, E10.618-E10.638, E10.641-E10.649, E10.69-
          E11.59, E11.618-E11.638, E11.641-E11.649, E11.69-E13.59, E13.618-
          E13.638, E13.641-E16.2, E30.9, E34.1, E34.50-E35, E89.1

✓4ᵗʰ **E16   Other disorders of pancreatic internal secretion**
  E16.0   Drug-induced hypoglycemia without coma
          Use additional code for adverse effect, if applicable, to identify
              drug (T36-T50 with fifth or sixth character 5)

  E16.1   Other hypoglycemia
          Functional hyperinsulinism
          Functional nonhyperinsulinemic hypoglycemia
          Hyperinsulinism NOS
          Hyperplasia of pancreatic islet beta cells NOS
          EXCLUDES 1 hypoglycemia in infant of diabetic mother (P70.1)
                    neonatal hypoglycemia (P70.4)

  E16.2   Hypoglycemia, unspecified

  E16.3   Increased secretion of glucagon
          Hyperplasia of pancreatic endocrine cells with glucagon excess

  E16.4   Increased secretion of gastrin
          Hypergastrinemia
          Hyperplasia of pancreatic endocrine cells with gastrin excess
          Zollinger-Ellison syndrome

  E16.8   Other specified disorders of pancreatic internal secretion
          Increased secretion from endocrine pancreas of growth
              hormone-releasing hormone
          Increased secretion from endocrine pancreas of pancreatic
              polypeptide
          Increased secretion from endocrine pancreas of somatostatin
          Increased secretion from endocrine pancreas of vasoactive-
              intestinal polypeptide

  E16.9   Disorder of pancreatic internal secretion, unspecified
          Islet-cell hyperplasia NOS
          Pancreatic endocrine cell hyperplasia NOS

Disorders of other endocrine glands (E20-E35)

  EXCLUDES 1 galactorrhea (N64.3)
            gynecomastia (N62)

✓4ᵗʰ **E20   Hypoparathyroidism**
  EXCLUDES 1 Di George's syndrome (D82.1)
            postprocedural hypoparathyroidism (E89.2)
            tetany NOS (R29.0)
            transitory neonatal hypoparathyroidism (P71.4)

  E20.0   Idiopathic hypoparathyroidism
  E20.1   Pseudohypoparathyroidism
  E20.8   Other hypoparathyroidism
  E20.9   Hypoparathyroidism, unspecified
          Parathyroid tetany

✓4ᵗʰ **E21   Hyperparathyroidism and other disorders of parathyroid gland**
  EXCLUDES 1 adult osteomalacia (M83.-)
            ectopic hyperparathyroidism (E34.2)
            familial hypocalciuric hypercalcemia (E83.52)
            hungry bone syndrome (E83.81)
            infantile and juvenile osteomalacia (E55.0)

  E21.0   Primary hyperparathyroidism
          Hyperplasia of parathyroid
          Osteitis fibrosa cystica generalisata [von Recklinghausen's
              disease of bone]

  E21.1   Secondary hyperparathyroidism, not elsewhere classified
          EXCLUDES 1 secondary hyperparathyroidism of renal origin (N25.81)

  E21.2   Other hyperparathyroidism
          Tertiary hyperparathyroidism
          EXCLUDES 1 familial hypocalciuric hypercalcemia (E83.52)

  E21.3   Hyperparathyroidism, unspecified
  E21.4   Other specified disorders of parathyroid gland
  E21.5   Disorder of parathyroid gland, unspecified

✓4ᵗʰ **E22   Hyperfunction of pituitary gland**
  EXCLUDES 1 Cushing's syndrome (E24.-)
            Nelson's syndrome (E24.1)
            overproduction of ACTH not associated with Cushing's disease
                (E27.0)
            overproduction of pituitary ACTH (E24.0)
            overproduction of thyroid-stimulating hormone (E05.8-)

  E22.0   Acromegaly and pituitary gigantism
          Overproduction of growth hormone
          EXCLUDES 1 constitutional gigantism (E34.4)
                    constitutional tall stature (E34.4)
                    increased secretion from endocrine pancreas of growth
                        hormone-releasing hormone (E16.8)

  E22.1   Hyperprolactinemia   CC
          Use additional code for adverse effect, if applicable, to identify
              drug (T36-T50 with fifth or sixth character 5)
          CC Excl: E22.1-E22.9

  E22.2   Syndrome of inappropriate secretion of antidiuretic   CC
          hormone
          CC Excl: E22.0-E23.7, E24.1, E30.9, E34.1, E34.4, E34.8-E35, E89.3

  E22.8   Other hyperfunction of pituitary gland   CC
          Central precocious puberty
          CC Excl: See code: E22.1

  E22.9   Hyperfunction of pituitary gland, unspecified   CC
          CC Excl: See code: E22.1

✓4ᵗʰ **E23   Hypofunction and other disorders of the pituitary gland**
  INCLUDES the listed conditions whether the disorder is in the pituitary
          or the hypothalamus
  EXCLUDES 1 postprocedural hypopituitarism (E89.3)

  E23.0   Hypopituitarism   CC
          Fertile eunuch syndrome
          Hypogonadotropic hypogonadism
          Idiopathic growth hormone deficiency
          Isolated deficiency of gonadotropin
          Isolated deficiency of growth hormone
          Isolated deficiency of pituitary hormone
          Kallmann's syndrome
          Lorain-Levi short stature
          Necrosis of pituitary gland (postpartum)
          Panhypopituitarism
          Pituitary cachexia
          Pituitary insufficiency NOS
          Pituitary short stature
          Sheehan's syndrome
          Simmonds' disease
          CC Excl: E22.0-E23.7, E24.1, E30.9, E34.1, E34.4-E35, E89.3

  E23.1   Drug-induced hypopituitarism
          Use additional code for adverse effect, if applicable, to identify
              drug (T36-T50 with fifth or sixth character 5)

  E23.2   Diabetes insipidus   CC
          EXCLUDES 1 nephrogenic diabetes insipidus (N25.1)
          CC Excl: E22.1-E23.7, E24.1, E30.9, E34.1, E34.50-E35, E89.3

  E23.3   Hypothalamic dysfunction, not elsewhere classified
          EXCLUDES 1 Prader-Willi syndrome (Q87.1)
                    Russell-Silver syndrome (Q87.1)

  E23.6   Other disorders of pituitary gland
          Abscess of pituitary
          Adiposogenital dystrophy

  E23.7   Disorder of pituitary gland, unspecified

✓4ᵗʰ **E24   Cushing's syndrome**
  EXCLUDES 1 congenital adrenal hyperplasia (E25.0)

  CC Excl: For CC codes in category E24, unless otherwise noted:
  E24.0, E24.2-E26.9, E30.9, E34.1, E34.50-E35

  E24.0   Pituitary-dependent Cushing's disease   CC
          Overproduction of pituitary ACTH
          Pituitary-dependent hypercorticalism

  E24.1   Nelson's syndrome

  E24.2   Drug-induced Cushing's syndrome   CC
          Use additional code for adverse effect, if applicable, to identify
              drug (T36-T50 with fifth or sixth character 5)

  E24.3   Ectopic ACTH syndrome   CC
  E24.4   Alcohol-induced pseudo-Cushing's syndrome   CC
  E24.8   Other Cushing's syndrome   CC
  E24.9   Cushing's syndrome, unspecified   CC

N Newborn: 0   P Pediatric: 0-17   M Maternity: 12-55   A Adult: 15-124   MCC Major CC Condition   PDx MCC PDx acts as own MCC   CC CC Condition   PDx CC PDx acts as own CC

500   ICD-10-CM Draft (2015)

√4ᵗʰ **E25　Adrenogenital disorders**

INCLUDES　adrenogenital syndromes, virilizing or feminizing, whether acquired or due to adrenal hyperplasia consequent on inborn enzyme defects in hormone synthesis
female adrenal pseudohermaphroditism
female heterosexual precocious pseudopuberty
male isosexual precocious pseudopuberty
male macrogenitosomia praecox
male sexual precocity with adrenal hyperplasia
male virilization (female)

EXCLUDES 1　*indeterminate sex and pseudohermaphroditism (Q56)*
chromosomal abnormalities (Q90-Q99)

E25.0　Congenital adrenogenital disorders associated with enzyme deficiency
Congenital adrenal hyperplasia
21-Hydroxylase deficiency
Salt-losing congenital adrenal hyperplasia

E25.8　Other adrenogenital disorders
Idiopathic adrenogenital disorder
Use additional code for adverse effect, if applicable, to identify drug (T36-T50 with fifth or sixth character 5)

E25.9　Adrenogenital disorder, unspecified
Adrenogenital syndrome NOS

√4ᵗʰ **E26　Hyperaldosteronism**

√5ᵗʰ **E26.0　Primary hyperaldosteronism**

　　E26.01　Conn's syndrome ✓
Code also adrenal adenoma (D35.0-)

　　E26.02　Glucocorticoid-remediable aldosteronism
Familial aldosteronism type I

　　E26.09　Other primary hyperaldosteronism
Primary aldosteronism due to adrenal hyperplasia (bilateral)

E26.1　Secondary hyperaldosteronism

√5ᵗʰ **E26.8　Other hyperaldosteronism**

　　E26.81　Bartter's syndrome

　　E26.89　Other hyperaldosteronism

E26.9　Hyperaldosteronism, unspecified
Aldosteronism NOS
Hyperaldosteronism NOS

√4ᵗʰ **E27　Other disorders of adrenal gland**

CC Excl: For CC codes in category E27, unless otherwise noted:
A17.9, A18.7, A18.82, A18.84, A18.89, E27.0-E27.9, E30.9, E34.1, E34.50-E35, E89.6

E27.0　Other adrenocortical overactivity　CC
Overproduction of ACTH, not associated with Cushing's disease
Premature adrenarche
EXCLUDES 1　*Cushing's syndrome (E24.-)*

E27.1　Primary adrenocortical insufficiency　CC
Addison's disease
Autoimmune adrenalitis
EXCLUDES 1　*Addison only phenotype adrenoleukodystrophy (E71.528)*
amyloidosis (E85.-)
tuberculous Addison's disease (A18.7)
Waterhouse-Friderichsen syndrome (A39.1)

E27.2　Addisonian crisis　CC
Adrenal crisis
Adrenocortical crisis

E27.3　Drug-induced adrenocortical insufficiency　CC
Use additional code for adverse effect, if applicable, to identify drug (T36-T50 with fifth or sixth character 5)

√5ᵗʰ **E27.4　Other and unspecified adrenocortical insufficiency**
EXCLUDES 1　*adrenoleukodystrophy [Addison-Schilder] (E71.528)*
Waterhouse-Friderichsen syndrome (A39.1)

　　E27.40　Unspecified adrenocortical insufficiency　CC
Adrenocortical insufficiency NOS
Hypoaldosteronism

　　E27.49　Other adrenocortical insufficiency　CC
Adrenal hemorrhage
Adrenal infarction

E27.5　Adrenomedullary hyperfunction　CC
Adrenomedullary hyperplasia
Catecholamine hypersecretion

E27.8　Other specified disorders of adrenal gland
Abnormality of cortisol-binding globulin

E27.9　Disorder of adrenal gland, unspecified

√4ᵗʰ **E28　Ovarian dysfunction**
EXCLUDES 1　*isolated gonadotropin deficiency (E23.0)*
postprocedural ovarian failure (E89.4-)

E28.0　Estrogen excess　♀
Use additional code for adverse effect, if applicable, to identify drug (T36-T50 with fifth or sixth character 5)

E28.1　Androgen excess　♀
Hypersecretion of ovarian androgens
Use additional code for adverse effect, if applicable, to identify drug (T36-T50 with fifth or sixth character 5)

E28.2　Polycystic ovarian syndrome　♀
Sclerocystic ovary syndrome
Stein-Leventhal syndrome

√5ᵗʰ **E28.3　Primary ovarian failure**
EXCLUDES 1　*pure gonadal dysgenesis (Q99.1)*
Turner's syndrome (Q96.-)

　√6ᵗʰ **E28.31　Premature menopause**

　　　E28.310　Symptomatic premature menopause　A ♀
Symptoms such as flushing, sleeplessness, headache, lack of concentration, associated with premature menopause

　　　E28.319　Asymptomatic premature menopause　A ♀
Premature menopause NOS

　　E28.39　Other primary ovarian failure　♀
Decreased estrogen
Resistant ovary syndrome

E28.8　Other ovarian dysfunction　♀
Ovarian hyperfunction NOS
EXCLUDES 1　*postprocedural ovarian failure (E89.4-)*

E28.9　Ovarian dysfunction, unspecified　♀

√4ᵗʰ **E29　Testicular dysfunction**
EXCLUDES 1　*androgen insensitivity syndrome (E34.5-)*
azoospermia or oligospermia NOS (N46.0-N46.1)
isolated gonadotropin deficiency (E23.0)
Klinefelter's syndrome (Q98.0-Q98.2, Q98.4)

E29.0　Testicular hyperfunction　♂
Hypersecretion of testicular hormones

E29.1　Testicular hypofunction　♂
Defective biosynthesis of testicular androgen NOS
5-delta-Reductase deficiency (with male pseudohermaphroditism)
Testicular hypogonadism NOS
Use additional code for adverse effect, if applicable, to identify drug (T36-T50 with fifth or sixth character 5)
EXCLUDES 1　*postprocedural testicular hypofunction (E89.5)*

E29.8　Other testicular dysfunction　♂

E29.9　Testicular dysfunction, unspecified　♂

√4ᵗʰ **E30　Disorders of puberty, not elsewhere classified**

E30.0　Delayed puberty
Constitutional delay of puberty
Delayed sexual development

E30.1　Precocious puberty　P
Precocious menstruation
EXCLUDES 1　*Albright (-McCune) (-Sternberg) syndrome (Q78.1)*
central precocious puberty (E22.8)
congenital adrenal hyperplasia (E25.0)
female heterosexual precocious pseudopuberty (E25.-)
male isosexual precocious pseudopuberty (E25.-)

E30.8　Other disorders of puberty　P
Premature thelarche

E30.9　Disorder of puberty, unspecified

√4ᵗʰ **E31　Polyglandular dysfunction**
EXCLUDES 1　*ataxia telangiectasia [Louis-Bar] (G11.3)*
dystrophia myotonica [Steinert] (G71.11)
pseudohypoparathyroidism (E20.1)

E31.0　Autoimmune polyglandular failure
Schmidt's syndrome

E31.1　Polyglandular hyperfunction
EXCLUDES 1　*multiple endocrine adenomatosis (E31.2-)*
multiple endocrine neoplasia (E31.2-)

✓ Additional Character Required　　√x7ᵗʰ Xtension Alert　　Unacceptable PDx　　Manifestation　　Hospital Acquired Condition　　EXCLUDES 1 Not Coded Here　　EXCLUDES 2 Not Included Here

ICD-10-CM Draft (2015)

501

Endocrine, Nutritional and Metabolic Diseases

E31.2–E43

✓5th **E31.2 Multiple endocrine neoplasia [MEN] syndromes**
Multiple endocrine adenomatosis
Code also any associated malignancies and other conditions associated with the syndromes

    E31.20 Multiple endocrine neoplasia [MEN] syndrome, unspecified
Multiple endocrine adenomatosis NOS
Multiple endocrine neoplasia [MEN] syndrome NOS

    E31.21 Multiple endocrine neoplasia [MEN] type I
Wermer's syndrome

    E31.22 Multiple endocrine neoplasia [MEN] type IIA
Sipple's syndrome

    E31.23 Multiple endocrine neoplasia [MEN] type IIB

E31.8 Other polyglandular dysfunction

E31.9 Polyglandular dysfunction, unspecified

✓4th **E32 Diseases of thymus**
   EXCLUDES 1   aplasia or hypoplasia of thymus with immunodeficiency (D82.1)
           myasthenia gravis (G70.0)

E32.0 Persistent hyperplasia of thymus
Hypertrophy of thymus

E32.1 Abscess of thymus   CC
CC Excl: E30.9, E32.0-E32.9, E34.1, E34.50-E35

E32.8 Other diseases of thymus
   EXCLUDES 1   aplasia or hypoplasia with immunodeficiency (D82.1)
           thymoma (D15.0)

E32.9 Disease of thymus, unspecified

✓4th **E34 Other endocrine disorders**
   EXCLUDES 1   pseudohypoparathyroidism (E20.1)

E34.0 Carcinoid syndrome   CC
   NOTE   May be used as an additional code to identify functional activity associated with a carcinoid tumor.
CC Excl: E30.9, E34.0-E34.2, E34.50-E35

E34.1 Other hypersecretion of intestinal hormones

E34.2 Ectopic hormone secretion, not elsewhere classified
   EXCLUDES 1   ectopic ACTH syndrome (E24.3)

E34.3 Short stature due to endocrine disorder
Constitutional short stature
Laron-type short stature
   EXCLUDES 1   achondroplastic short stature (Q77.4)
           hypochondroplastic short stature (Q77.4)
           nutritional short stature (E45)
           pituitary short stature (E23.0)
           progeria (E34.8)
           renal short stature (N25.0)
           Russell-Silver syndrome (Q87.1)
           short-limbed stature with immunodeficiency (D82.2)
           short stature in specific dysmorphic syndromes— code to syndrome—see Alphabetical Index
           short stature NOS (R62.52)

E34.4 Constitutional tall stature
Constitutional gigantism

✓5th **E34.5 Androgen insensitivity syndrome**

    E34.50 Androgen insensitivity syndrome, unspecified
Androgen insensitivity NOS

    E34.51 Complete androgen insensitivity syndrome
Complete androgen insensitivity
de Quervain syndrome
Goldberg-Maxwell syndrome

    E34.52 Partial androgen insensitivity syndrome
Partial androgen insensitivity
Reifenstein syndrome

E34.8 Other specified endocrine disorders
Pineal gland dysfunction   Progeria
   EXCLUDES 2   pseudohypoparathyroidism (E20.1)

E34.9 Endocrine disorder, unspecified
Endocrine disturbance NOS
Hormone disturbance NOS

E35 Disorders of endocrine glands in diseases classified elsewhere
Code first underlying disease, such as:
   late congenital syphilis of thymus gland [Dubois disease] (A50.5)
Use additional code, if applicable, to identify:
   sequelae of tuberculosis of other organs (B90.8)
   EXCLUDES 1   Echinococcus granulosus infection of thyroid gland (B67.3)
           meningococcal hemorrhagic adrenalitis (A39.1)
           syphilis of endocrine gland (A52.79)
           tuberculosis of adrenal gland, except calcification (A18.7)
           tuberculosis of endocrine gland NEC (A18.82)
           tuberculosis of thyroid gland (A18.81)
           Waterhouse-Friderichsen syndrome (A39.1)

✓4th **E36 Intraoperative complications of endocrine system**
   EXCLUDES 2   postprocedural endocrine and metabolic complications and disorders, not elsewhere classified (E89.-)

✓5th **E36.0 Intraoperative hemorrhage and hematoma of an endocrine system organ or structure complicating a procedure**
   EXCLUDES 1   intraoperative hemorrhage and hematoma of an endocrine system organ or structure due to accidental puncture or laceration during a procedure (E36.1-)

    E36.01 Intraoperative hemorrhage and hematoma of an endocrine system organ or structure complicating an endocrine system procedure   CC
CC Excl: E36.01-E36.02, E36.8, E89.810-E89.89, H95.811-H95.89, I85.01, I85.11, I97.3, K21.9, K22.8, K23-K25.0, K25.2, K25.4, K25.6, K26.0, K26.2, K26.4, K26.6, K27.0, K27.2, K27.4, K27.6, K28.0, K28.2, K28.4, K28.6, K29.01, K29.21, K29.31, K29.41, K29.51, K29.61, K29.71, K29.81, K29.91, K31.811, K55.21, K57.01, K57.11, K57.13, K57.21, K57.31, K57.33, K57.41, K57.51, K57.53, K57.81, K57.91, K57.93, K62.5, K92.0-K92.2, M96.89, N98.1-N98.9, P54.1-P54.3, T81.10XA, T81.11XA, T81.12XA, T81.19XA, T81.82XA, T81.89XA, T81.9XXA

    E36.02 Intraoperative hemorrhage and hematoma of an endocrine system organ or structure complicating other procedure   CC
CC Excl: See code: E36.01

✓5th **E36.1 Accidental puncture and laceration of an endocrine system organ or structure during a procedure**

    E36.11 Accidental puncture and laceration of an endocrine system organ or structure during an endocrine system procedure   CC
CC Excl: D78.11-D78.12, D78.81-D78.89, E36.11-E36.8, E89.810-E89.89, G96.11, G97.41, G97.48-G97.49, H59.011-H59.019, H59.031-H59.099, H59.211-H59.229, H59.811-H59.89, H95.31-H95.32, H95.811-H95.89, I97.3, I97.51-I97.52, J95.71-J95.72, K91.71-K91.72, L76.11-L76.12, L76.81-L76.82, M96.820-M96.821, M96.89, N98.1-N98.9, N99.71-N99.72, T81.82XA, T81.89XA, T81.9XXA

    E36.12 Accidental puncture and laceration of an endocrine system organ or structure during other procedure   CC
CC Excl: See code: E36.11

E36.8 Other intraoperative complications of endocrine system
Use additional code, if applicable, to further specify disorder

Malnutrition (E40-E46)

   EXCLUDES 1   intestinal malabsorption (K90.-)
           sequelae of protein-calorie malnutrition (E64.0)
   EXCLUDES 2   nutritional anemias (D50-D53)
           starvation (T73.0)

E40 Kwashiorkor   MCC
Severe malnutrition with nutritional edema with dyspigmentation of skin and hair
   EXCLUDES 1   marasmic kwashiorkor (E42)
CC Excl: E40-E46, E64.0

E41 Nutritional marasmus   MCC
Severe malnutrition with marasmus
   EXCLUDES 1   marasmic kwashiorkor (E42)
CC Excl: See code: E40

E42 Marasmic kwashiorkor   MCC
Intermediate form severe protein-calorie malnutrition
Severe protein-calorie malnutrition with signs of both kwashiorkor and marasmus
CC Excl: See code: E40

E43 Unspecified severe protein-calorie malnutrition   MCC
Starvation edema
CC Excl: See code: E40

N Newborn: 0   P Pediatric: 0-17   M Maternity: 12-55   A Adult: 15-124   MCC Major CC Condition   PDx MCC PDx acts as own MCC   CC CC Condition   PDx CC PDx acts as own CC

502   ICD-10-CM Draft (2015)

✓4th **E44** **Protein-calorie malnutrition of moderate and mild degree**
     E44.0 **Moderate** protein-calorie malnutrition `cc`
     E44.1 **Mild** protein-calorie malnutrition `cc`

E45 **Retarded development following protein-calorie** `cc`
malnutrition
     Nutritional short stature
     Nutritional stunting
     Physical retardation due to malnutrition
     CC Excl: See code: E40

E46 **Unspecified protein-calorie malnutrition** `cc`
     Malnutrition NOS
     Protein-calorie imbalance NOS
     EXCLUDES 1   *nutritional deficiency NOS (E63.9)*
     CC Excl: See code: E40

Other nutritional deficiencies (E50-E64)

EXCLUDES 2   *nutritional anemias (D50-D53)*

✓4th **E50** **Vitamin A deficiency**
     EXCLUDES 1   *sequelae of vitamin A deficiency (E64.1)*

     E50.0 **Vitamin A deficiency with** conjunctival xerosis
     E50.1 **Vitamin A deficiency with** Bitot's spot and conjunctival
          xerosis
           Bitot's spot in the young child
     E50.2 **Vitamin A deficiency with** corneal xerosis
     E50.3 **Vitamin A deficiency with** corneal ulceration and xerosis
     E50.4 **Vitamin A deficiency with** keratomalacia
     E50.5 **Vitamin A deficiency with** night blindness
     E50.6 **Vitamin A deficiency with** xerophthalmic scars of cornea
     E50.7 **Other ocular manifestations** of vitamin A deficiency
          Xerophthalmia NOS
     E50.8 **Other manifestations of vitamin A deficiency**
          Follicular keratosis
          Xeroderma
     E50.9 **Vitamin A deficiency,** unspecified
          Hypovitaminosis A NOS

✓4th **E51** **Thiamine deficiency**
     EXCLUDES 1   *sequelae of thiamine deficiency (E64.8)*

     CC Excl: For CC codes in category E51, unless otherwise noted:
     D81.818-D81.819, E51.11-E53.9, E56.0, E56.8-E63.9, E64.8-E64.9

     ✓5th **E51.1** **Beriberi**
          E51.11 **Dry beriberi** `cc`
              Beriberi NOS
              Beriberi with polyneuropathy
          E51.12 **Wet beriberi** `cc`
              Beriberi with cardiovascular manifestations
              Cardiovascular beriberi
              Shoshin disease
     E51.2 **Wernicke's encephalopathy** `cc`
     E51.8 **Other manifestations** of thiamine deficiency `cc`
     E51.9 **Thiamine deficiency,** unspecified `cc`

E52 **Niacin deficiency [pellagra]**
     Niacin (-tryptophan) deficiency
     Nicotinamide deficiency
     Pellagra (alcoholic)
     EXCLUDES 1   *sequelae of niacin deficiency (E64.8)*

✓4th **E53** **Deficiency of other B group vitamins**
     EXCLUDES 1   *sequelae of vitamin B deficiency (E64.8)*

     E53.0 **Riboflavin deficiency** `cc`
          Ariboflavinosis
          Vitamin B2 deficiency
          CC Excl: See code: E51
     E53.1 **Pyridoxine deficiency**
          Vitamin B6 deficiency
          EXCLUDES 1   *pyridoxine-responsive sideroblastic anemia (D64.3)*
     E53.8 **Deficiency of** other specified B group vitamins
          Biotin deficiency
          Cyanocobalamin deficiency
          Folate deficiency
          Folic acid deficiency
          Pantothenic acid deficiency
          Vitamin B12 deficiency
          EXCLUDES 1   *folate deficiency anemia (D52.-)*
                        vitamin B12 deficiency anemia (D51.-)
     E53.9 **Vitamin B deficiency,** unspecified

E54 **Ascorbic acid deficiency**
     Deficiency of vitamin C
     Scurvy
     EXCLUDES 1   *scorbutic anemia (D53.2)*
                  sequelae of vitamin C deficiency (E64.2)

✓4th **E55** **Vitamin D deficiency**
     EXCLUDES 1   *adult osteomalacia (M83.-)*
                  osteoporosis (M80.-)
                  sequelae of rickets (E64.3)

     E55.0 **Rickets, active** `cc`
          Infantile osteomalacia
          Juvenile osteomalacia
          EXCLUDES 1   *celiac rickets (K90.0)*
                  Crohn's rickets (K50.-)
                  hereditary vitamin D-dependent rickets (E83.32)
                  inactive rickets (E64.3)
                  renal rickets (N25.0)
                  sequelae of rickets (E64.3)
                  vitamin D-resistant rickets (E83.31)
          CC Excl: E55.0-E63.9, E64.3-E64.9, M83.0-M83.9
     E55.9 **Vitamin D deficiency, unspecified**
          Avitaminosis D

✓4th **E56** **Other vitamin deficiencies**
     EXCLUDES 1   *sequelae of other vitamin deficiencies (E64.8)*

     E56.0 **Deficiency of** vitamin E
     E56.1 **Deficiency of** vitamin K
          EXCLUDES 1   *deficiency of coagulation factor due to vitamin K*
                      deficiency (D68.4)
                  vitamin K deficiency of newborn (P53)
     E56.8 **Deficiency of** other vitamins
     E56.9 **Vitamin deficiency,** unspecified

E58 **Dietary calcium deficiency**
     EXCLUDES 1   *disorders of calcium metabolism (E83.5-)*
                  sequelae of calcium deficiency (E64.8)

E59 **Dietary selenium deficiency**
     Keshan disease
     EXCLUDES 1   *sequelae of selenium deficiency (E64.8)*

E60 **Dietary zinc deficiency**

✓4th **E61** **Deficiency of other nutrient elements**
     Use additional code for adverse effect, if applicable, to identify drug
     (T36-T50 with fifth or sixth character 5)
     EXCLUDES 1   *disorders of mineral metabolism (E83.-)*
                  iodine deficiency related thyroid disorders (E00-E02)
                  sequelae of malnutrition and other nutritional deficiencies
                      (E64.-)
     E61.0 **Copper deficiency**
     E61.1 **Iron deficiency**
          EXCLUDES 1   *iron deficiency anemia (D50.-)*
     E61.2 **Magnesium deficiency**
     E61.3 **Manganese deficiency**
     E61.4 **Chromium deficiency**
     E61.5 **Molybdenum deficiency**
     E61.6 **Vanadium deficiency**
     E61.7 **Deficiency of** multiple nutrient elements
     E61.8 **Deficiency of** other specified nutrient elements
     E61.9 **Deficiency of nutrient element,** unspecified

✓4th **E63** **Other nutritional deficiencies**
     EXCLUDES 1   *dehydration (E86.0)*
                  failure to thrive, adult (R62.7)
                  failure to thrive, child (R62.51)
                  feeding problems in newborn (P92.-)
                  sequelae of malnutrition and other nutritional deficiencies
                      (E64.-)
     E63.0 **Essential fatty acid [EFA] deficiency**
     E63.1 **Imbalance of constituents of food intake**
     E63.8 **Other specified nutritional deficiencies**
     E63.9 **Nutritional deficiency,** unspecified

✓ Additional Character Required   ✓x7th Xtension Alert   Unacceptable PDx   Manifestation   Hospital Acquired Condition   *EXCLUDES 1* Not Coded Here   *EXCLUDES 2* Not Included Here

Endocrine, Nutritional and Metabolic Diseases

E64–E71.2

✓4ᵗʰ E64 Sequelae of malnutrition and other nutritional deficiencies

NOTE This category is to be used to indicate conditions in categories E43, E44, E46, E50-E63 as the cause of sequelae, which are themselves classified elsewhere. The 'sequelae' include conditions specified as such; they also include the late effects of diseases classifiable to the above categories if the disease itself is no longer present

Code first condition resulting from (sequela) of malnutrition and other nutritional deficiencies

E64.0 Sequelae of protein-calorie malnutrition `CC`
> **EXCLUDES 2** retarded development following protein-calorie malnutrition (E45)
> **CC Excl:** E40-E46, E64.0

E64.1 Sequelae of vitamin A deficiency

E64.2 Sequelae of vitamin C deficiency

E64.3 Sequelae of rickets

E64.8 Sequelae of other nutritional deficiencies

E64.9 Sequelae of unspecified nutritional deficiency

Overweight, obesity and other hyperalimentation (E65-E68)

E65 Localized adiposity
Fat pad

✓4ᵗʰ E66 Overweight and obesity
Code first obesity complicating pregnancy, childbirth and the puerperium, if applicable (O99.21-)
Use additional code to identify body mass index (BMI), if known (Z68.-)
> **EXCLUDES 1** adiposogenital dystrophy (E23.6)
> lipomatosis NOS (E88.2)
> lipomatosis dolorosa [Dercum] (E88.2)
> Prader-Willi syndrome (Q87.1)

✓5ᵗʰ E66.0 Obesity due to excess calories
   2 **E66.01 Morbid (severe) obesity due to excess calories**
> **EXCLUDES 1** morbid (severe) obesity with alveolar hypoventilation (E66.2)

   13 **E66.09 Other obesity due to excess calories**

13 **E66.1 Drug-induced obesity**
Use additional code for adverse effect, if applicable, to identify drug (T36-T50 with fifth or sixth character 5)

E66.2 Morbid (severe) obesity with alveolar hypoventilation `CC`
Pickwickian syndrome
CC Excl: E66.2-I27.81, I27.89-I27.9

E66.3 Overweight

13 **E66.8 Other obesity**

13 **E66.9 Obesity, unspecified**
Obesity NOS

✓4ᵗʰ E67 Other hyperalimentation
> **EXCLUDES 1** hyperalimentation NOS (R63.2)
> sequelae of hyperalimentation (E68)

E67.0 Hypervitaminosis A

E67.1 Hypercarotinemia

E67.2 Megavitamin-B6 syndrome

E67.3 Hypervitaminosis D

E67.8 Other specified hyperalimentation

E68 Sequelae of hyperalimentation
Code first condition resulting from (sequela) of hyperalimentation

Metabolic disorders (E70-E88)

> **EXCLUDES 1** androgen insensitivity syndrome (E34.5-)
> congenital adrenal hyperplasia (E25.0)
> Ehlers-Danlos syndrome (Q79.6)
> hemolytic anemias attributable to enzyme disorders (D55.-)
> Marfan's syndrome (Q87.4)
> 5-alpha-reductase deficiency (E29.1)

✓4ᵗʰ E70 Disorders of aromatic amino-acid metabolism

CC Excl: For CC codes in category E70, unless otherwise noted: C88.0, D47.2, D89.0-D89.1, E70.0-E71.30, E72.00-E72.02, E72.04-E74.9, E75.21-E75.22, E75.240-E75.249, E75.3, E75.5-E75.6, E77.0-E78.70, E78.79-E78.9, E88.09-E88.2, E88.89

E70.0 Classical phenylketonuria `CC`

E70.1 Other hyperphenylalaninemias `CC`

✓5ᵗʰ E70.2 Disorders of tyrosine metabolism
> **EXCLUDES 1** transitory tyrosinemia of newborn (P74.5)

E70.20 Disorder of tyrosine metabolism, unspecified `CC`

E70.21 Tyrosinemia `CC`
Hypertyrosinemia

E70.29 Other disorders of tyrosine metabolism
Alkaptonuria
Ochronosis

✓5ᵗʰ E70.3 Albinism

E70.30 Albinism, unspecified `CC`

✓6ᵗʰ E70.31 Ocular albinism
E70.310 X-linked ocular albinism `CC`
E70.311 Autosomal recessive ocular albinism `CC`
E70.318 Other ocular albinism `CC`
E70.319 Ocular albinism, unspecified `CC`

✓6ᵗʰ E70.32 Oculocutaneous albinism
> **EXCLUDES 1** Chediak-Higashi syndrome (E70.330)
> Hermansky-Pudlak syndrome (E70.331)

E70.320 Tyrosinase negative oculocutaneous albinism `CC`
Albinism I
Oculocutaneous albinism ty-neg

E70.321 Tyrosinase positive oculocutaneous albinism `CC`
Albinism II
Oculocutaneous albinism ty-pos

E70.328 Other oculocutaneous albinism `CC`
Cross syndrome

E70.329 Oculocutaneous albinism, unspecified `CC`

✓6ᵗʰ E70.33 Albinism with hematologic abnormality
E70.330 Chediak-Higashi syndrome `CC`
E70.331 Hermansky-Pudlak syndrome `CC`
E70.338 Other albinism with hematologic abnormality `CC`
E70.339 Albinism with hematologic abnormality, unspecified `CC`

E70.39 Other specified albinism `CC`
Piebaldism

✓5ᵗʰ E70.4 Disorders of histidine metabolism
E70.40 Disorders of histidine metabolism, unspecified `CC`
E70.41 Histidinemia `CC`
E70.49 Other disorders of histidine metabolism `CC`

E70.5 Disorders of tryptophan metabolism `CC`

E70.8 Other disorders of aromatic amino-acid metabolism `CC`

E70.9 Disorder of aromatic amino-acid metabolism, unspecified `CC`

✓4ᵗʰ E71 Disorders of branched-chain amino-acid metabolism and fatty-acid metabolism

E71.0 Maple-syrup-urine disease `CC`
CC Excl: See code: E70

✓5ᵗʰ E71.1 Other disorders of branched-chain amino-acid metabolism

CC Excl: For CC codes in subcategory E71.1, unless otherwise noted: C88.0, D47.2, D89.0-D89.1, E70.0-E71.30, E72.00-E72.02, E72.04-E74.9, E75.21-E75.22, E75.240-E75.249, E75.3, E75.5-E75.6, E77.0-E78.70, E78.79-E78.9, E88.09-E88.2, E88.89

✓6ᵗʰ E71.11 Branched-chain organic acidurias
E71.110 Isovaleric acidemia `CC`
E71.111 3-methylglutaconic aciduria `CC`
E71.118 Other branched-chain organic acidurias

✓6ᵗʰ E71.12 Disorders of propionate metabolism
E71.120 Methylmalonic acidemia `CC`
E71.121 Propionic acidemia `CC`
E71.128 Other disorders of propionate metabolism `CC`

E71.19 Other disorders of branched-chain amino-acid metabolism `CC`
Hyperleucine-isoleucinemia
Hypervalinemia

E71.2 Disorder of branched-chain amino-acid metabolism, unspecified `CC`
CC Excl: See code: E70

---

2 HAC = as PDx in combination with one of the following procedure codes: 0D16[0,4,8][7,J,K,Z][9,A,B,L] or 0DV64CZ **AND** in combination with SDx, not POA, of K68.11, K95.01, K95.81 or T81.4XXA.

13 Questionable admission when used as PDx.

N Newborn: 0   P Pediatric: 0-17   M Maternity: 12-55   A Adult: 15-124   **MCC** Major CC Condition   **PDx MCC** PDx acts as own MCC   **CC** CC Condition   **PDx CC** PDx acts as own CC

504   ICD-10-CM Draft (2015)

√5th **E71.3 Disorders of fatty-acid metabolism**

EXCLUDES 1 *peroxisomal disorders (E71.5)*
Refsum's disease (G60.1)
Schilder's disease (G37.0)

EXCLUDES 2 *carnitine deficiency due to inborn error of metabolism (E71.42)*

CC Excl: For CC codes in subcategory E71.3, unless otherwise noted: C96.5-C96.6, E71.39-E71.548, E80.3, E88.40-E88.49, E88.89, H49.811-H49.819

E71.30 Disorder of fatty-acid metabolism, unspecified

√6th **E71.31 Disorders of fatty-acid oxidation**

     E71.310 Long chain/very long chain acyl CoA dehydrogenase deficiency CC
         LCAD
         VLCAD

     E71.311 Medium chain acyl CoA dehydrogenase deficiency CC
         MCAD

     E71.312 Short chain acyl CoA dehydrogenase deficiency CC
         SCAD

     E71.313 Glutaric aciduria type II CC
         Glutaric aciduria type II A
         Glutaric aciduria type II B
         Glutaric aciduria type II C
         EXCLUDES 1 *glutaric aciduria (type 1) NOS (E72.3)*

     E71.314 Muscle carnitine palmitoyltransferase deficiency CC

     E71.318 Other disorders of fatty-acid oxidation CC

E71.32 Disorders of ketone metabolism CC

E71.39 Other disorders of fatty-acid metabolism CC
     CC Excl: E71.310-E71.32, E71.40-E71.548, E80.4-E80.7, E88.40-E88.49, H49.811-H49.819

√5th **E71.4 Disorders of carnitine metabolism**

EXCLUDES 1 *muscle carnitine palmitoyltransferase deficiency (E71.314)*

E71.40 Disorder of carnitine metabolism, unspecified

E71.41 Primary carnitine deficiency

E71.42 Carnitine deficiency due to inborn errors of metabolism
     Code also associated inborn error or metabolism

E71.43 Iatrogenic carnitine deficiency
     Carnitine deficiency due to hemodialysis
     Carnitine deficiency due to Valproic acid therapy

√6th **E71.44 Other secondary carnitine deficiency**

     E71.440 Ruvalcaba-Myhre-Smith syndrome

     E71.448 Other secondary carnitine deficiency

√5th **E71.5 Peroxisomal disorders**

EXCLUDES 1 *Schilder's disease (G37.0)*

CC Excl: For CC codes in subcategory E71.5, unless otherwise noted: C96.5-C96.6, E71.310-E71.448, E80.3-E80.7, E88.40-E88.49, E88.89, H49.811-H49.819

E71.50 Peroxisomal disorder, unspecified CC

√6th **E71.51 Disorders of peroxisome biogenesis**
     Group 1 peroxisomal disorders
     EXCLUDES 1 *Refsum's disease (G60.1)*

     E71.510 Zellweger syndrome CC

     E71.511 Neonatal adrenoleukodystrophy CC N
         EXCLUDES 1 *X-linked adrenoleukodystrophy (E71.52-)*

     E71.518 Other disorders of peroxisome biogenesis CC

√6th **E71.52 X-linked adrenoleukodystrophy**

     E71.520 Childhood cerebral X-linked adrenoleukodystrophy CC

     E71.521 Adolescent X-linked adrenoleukodystrophy CC

     E71.522 Adrenomyeloneuropathy CC

     E71.528 Other X-linked adrenoleukodystrophy CC
         Addison only phenotype adrenoleukodystrophy
         Addison-Schilder adrenoleukodystrophy

     E71.529 X-linked adrenoleukodystrophy, unspecified type CC

E71.53 Other group 2 peroxisomal disorders CC

√6th **E71.54 Other peroxisomal disorders**

     E71.540 Rhizomelic chondrodysplasia punctata CC
         EXCLUDES 1 *chondrodysplasia punctata NOS (Q77.3)*

     E71.541 Zellweger-like syndrome CC

     E71.542 Other group 3 peroxisomal disorders CC

     E71.548 Other peroxisomal disorders CC

√4th **E72 Other disorders of amino-acid metabolism**

EXCLUDES 1 *disorders of:*
     aromatic amino-acid metabolism (E70.-)
     branched-chain amino-acid metabolism (E71.0-E71.2)
     fatty-acid metabolism (E71.3)
     purine and pyrimidine metabolism (E79.-)
     gout (M1A.-, M10.-)

CC Excl: For CC codes in category E72, unless otherwise noted: C88.0, D47.2, D89.0-D89.1, E70.0-E71.30, E72.00-E72.02, E72.04-E74.9, E75.21-E75.22, E75.240-E75.249, E75.3, E75.5-E75.6, E77.0-E78.70, E78.79-E78.9, E88.09-E88.2, E88.89

√5th **E72.0 Disorders of amino-acid transport**

EXCLUDES 1 *disorders of tryptophan metabolism (E70.5)*

E72.00 Disorders of amino-acid transport, unspecified CC

E72.01 Cystinuria CC

E72.02 Hartnup's disease CC

E72.03 Lowe's syndrome CC
     Use additional code for associated glaucoma (H42)
     CC Excl: No Excl

E72.04 Cystinosis CC
     Fanconi (-de Toni) (-Debré) syndrome with cystinosis
     EXCLUDES 1 *Fanconi (-de Toni) (-Debré) syndrome without cystinosis (E72.09)*

E72.09 Other disorders of amino-acid transport CC
     Fanconi (-de Toni) (-Debré) syndrome, unspecified

√5th **E72.1 Disorders of sulfur-bearing amino-acid metabolism**

EXCLUDES 1 *cystinosis (E72.04)*
cystinuria (E72.01)
transcobalamin II deficiency (D51.2)

E72.10 Disorders of sulfur-bearing amino-acid metabolism, unspecified CC

E72.11 Homocystinuria CC
     Cystathionine synthase deficiency

E72.12 Methylenetetrahydrofolate reductase deficiency CC

E72.19 Other disorders of sulfur-bearing amino-acid metabolism CC
     Cystathioninuria
     Methioninemia
     Sulfite oxidase deficiency

√5th **E72.2 Disorders of urea cycle metabolism**

EXCLUDES 1 *disorders of ornithine metabolism (E72.4)*

E72.20 Disorder of urea cycle metabolism, unspecified CC
     Hyperammonemia
     EXCLUDES 1 *hyperammonemia- hyperornithinemia- homocitrullinemia syndrome (E72.4)*
         transient hyperammonemia of newborn (P74.6)

E72.21 Argininemia CC

E72.22 Arginosuccinic aciduria CC

E72.23 Citrullinemia CC

E72.29 Other disorders of urea cycle metabolism CC

E72.3 Disorders of lysine and hydroxylysine metabolism CC
     Glutaric aciduria NOS
     Glutaric aciduria (type I)
     Hydroxylysinemia
     Hyperlysinemia
     EXCLUDES 1 *glutaric aciduria type II (E71.313)*
         Refsum's disease (G60.1)
         Zellweger syndrome (E71.510)

E72.4 Disorders of ornithine metabolism CC
     Hyperammonemia-hyperornithinemia-homocitrullinemia syndrome
     Ornithinemia (types I, II)
     Ornithine transcarbamylase deficiency
     EXCLUDES 1 *hereditary choroidal dystrophy (H31.2-)*

√5th **E72.5 Disorders of glycine metabolism**

E72.50 Disorder of glycine metabolism, unspecified CC

E72.51 Non-ketotic hyperglycinemia CC

E72.52 Trimethylaminuria CC

√ Additional Character Required   √x7th Xtension Alert   <u>Unacceptable PDx</u>   Manifestation   Hospital Acquired Condition   **EXCLUDES 1** Not Coded Here   **EXCLUDES 2** Not Included Here

ICD-10-CM Draft (2015)   505

E72.53 Hyperoxaluria CC
Oxalosis
Oxaluria

E72.59 Other disorders of glycine metabolism CC
D-glycericacidemia
Hyperhydroxyprolinemia
Hyperprolinemia (types I, II)
Sarcosinemia

E72.8 Other specified disorders of amino-acid metabolism CC
Disorders of beta-amino-acid metabolism
Disorders of gamma-glutamyl cycle

E72.9 Disorder of amino-acid metabolism, unspecified CC

√4th **E73 Lactose intolerance**

E73.0 Congenital lactase deficiency

E73.1 Secondary lactase deficiency

E73.8 Other lactose intolerance

E73.9 Lactose intolerance, unspecified

√4th **E74 Other disorders of carbohydrate metabolism**
EXCLUDES 1 diabetes mellitus (E08-E13)
hypoglycemia NOS (E16.2)
increased secretion of glucagon (E16.3)
mucopolysaccharidosis (E76.0-E76.3)

CC Excl: For CC codes in category E74, unless otherwise noted:
C88.0, D47.2, D89.0-D89.1, E70.0-E71.30, E72.00-E72.02, E72.04-E74.9, E75.21-E75.22, E75.240-E75.249, E75.3, E75.5-E75.6, E77.0-E78.70, E78.79-E78.9, E88.09-E88.2, E88.89

√5th **E74.0 Glycogen storage disease**

E74.00 Glycogen storage disease, unspecified CC
E74.01 von Gierke disease CC
Type I glycogen storage disease
E74.02 Pompe disease CC
Cardiac glycogenosis
Type II glycogen storage disease
E74.03 Cori disease CC
Forbes disease
Type III glycogen storage disease
E74.04 McArdle disease CC
Type V glycogen storage disease
E74.09 Other glycogen storage disease CC
Andersen disease
Hers disease
Tauri disease
Glycogen storage disease, types 0, IV, VI-XI
Liver phosphorylase deficiency
Muscle phosphofructokinase deficiency

√5th **E74.1 Disorders of fructose metabolism**
EXCLUDES 1 muscle phosphofructokinase deficiency (E74.09)
E74.10 Disorder of fructose metabolism, unspecified
E74.11 Essential fructosuria
Fructokinase deficiency
E74.12 Hereditary fructose intolerance
Fructosemia
E74.19 Other disorders of fructose metabolism
Fructose-1, 6-diphosphatase deficiency

√5th **E74.2 Disorders of galactose metabolism**
E74.20 Disorders of galactose metabolism, unspecified CC
E74.21 Galactosemia CC
E74.29 Other disorders of galactose metabolism CC
Galactokinase deficiency

√5th **E74.3 Other disorders of intestinal carbohydrate absorption**
EXCLUDES 2 lactose intolerance (E73.-)
E74.31 Sucrase-isomaltase deficiency
E74.39 Other disorders of intestinal carbohydrate absorption
Disorder of intestinal carbohydrate absorption NOS
Glucose-galactose malabsorption
Sucrase deficiency

E74.4 Disorders of pyruvate metabolism and gluconeogenesis CC
Deficiency of phosphoenolpyruvate carboxykinase
Deficiency of pyruvate carboxylase
Deficiency of pyruvate dehydrogenase
EXCLUDES 1 disorders of pyruvate metabolism and gluconeogenesis with anemia (D55.-)
Leigh's syndrome (G31.82)

E74.8 Other specified disorders of carbohydrate metabolism CC
Essential pentosuria
Renal glycosuria

E74.9 Disorder of carbohydrate metabolism, unspecified

√4th **E75 Disorders of sphingolipid metabolism and other lipid storage disorders**
EXCLUDES 1 mucolipidosis, types I-III (E77.0-E77.1)
Refsum's disease (G60.1)

√5th **E75.0 GM2 gangliosidosis**

CC Excl: For CC codes in subcategory E75.0, unless otherwise noted: E75.00-E75.19, E75.4, F84.2, G13.2-G13.8, G30.0-G31.82, G31.84-G31.9, G91.4, G94

E75.00 GM2 gangliosidosis, unspecified CC
E75.01 Sandhoff disease CC
E75.02 Tay-Sachs disease CC
E75.09 Other GM2 gangliosidosis CC
Adult GM2 gangliosidosis
Juvenile GM2 gangliosidosis

√5th **E75.1 Other and unspecified gangliosidosis**

CC Excl: For CC codes in subcategory E75.1, unless otherwise noted: E75.00-E75.19, E75.4, F84.2, G13.2-G13.8, G30.0-G31.82, G31.84-G31.9, G91.4, G94

E75.10 Unspecified gangliosidosis CC
Gangliosidosis NOS
E75.11 Mucolipidosis IV CC
E75.19 Other gangliosidosis
GM1 gangliosidosis
GM3 gangliosidosis

√5th **E75.2 Other sphingolipidosis**
EXCLUDES 1 adrenoleukodystrophy [Addison-Schilder] (E71.528)

CC Excl: For CC codes in subcategory E75.2, unless otherwise noted: E75.00-E75.19, E75.23, E75.25-E75.29, E75.4, F84.2, G13.2-G13.8, G31.2-G31.82, G32.89, G91.4, G93.81, G93.89-G94, G96.8-G96.9, G98.0-G98.8, G99.8

E75.21 Fabry (-Anderson) disease
E75.22 Gaucher disease
E75.23 Krabbe disease CC
√6th **E75.24 Niemann-Pick disease**
E75.240 Niemann-Pick disease type A
E75.241 Niemann-Pick disease type B
E75.242 Niemann-Pick disease type C
E75.243 Niemann-Pick disease type D
E75.248 Other Niemann-Pick disease
E75.249 Niemann-Pick disease, unspecified
E75.25 Metachromatic leukodystrophy CC
E75.29 Other sphingolipidosis CC
Farber's syndrome
Sulfatase deficiency
Sulfatide lipidosis

E75.3 Sphingolipidosis, unspecified
E75.4 Neuronal ceroid lipofuscinosis CC
Batten disease
Bielschowsky-Jansky disease
Kufs disease
Spielmeyer-Vogt disease
CC Excl: See code: E75.0
E75.5 Other lipid storage disorders
Cerebrotendinous cholesterosis [van Bogaert-Scherer-Epstein]
Wolman's disease
E75.6 Lipid storage disorder, unspecified

√4th **E76 Disorders of glycosaminoglycan metabolism**

CC Excl: For CC codes in category E76, unless otherwise noted: D81.3, D81.5, D81.810, D84.1, E76.01-E76.9, E79.1-E80.29, E80.4-E80.7, E85.0, E85.9, E88.81

√5th **E76.0 Mucopolysaccharidosis, type I**
E76.01 Hurler's syndrome CC
E76.02 Hurler-Scheie syndrome CC
E76.03 Scheie's syndrome CC
E76.1 Mucopolysaccharidosis, type II CC
Hunter's syndrome
√5th **E76.2 Other mucopolysaccharidoses**
√6th **E76.21 Morquio mucopolysaccharidoses**
E76.210 Morquio A mucopolysaccharidoses CC
Classic Morquio syndrome
Morquio syndrome A
Mucopolysaccharidosis, type IVA

E76.211   **Morquio B mucopolysaccharidoses**   `cc`
Morquio-like mucopolysaccharidoses
Morquio-like syndrome
Morquio syndrome B
Mucopolysaccharidosis, type IVB

E76.219   **Morquio mucopolysaccharidoses, unspecified**   `cc`
Morquio syndrome
Mucopolysaccharidosis, type IV

E76.22   Sanfilippo **mucopolysaccharidoses**   `cc`
Mucopolysaccharidosis, type III (A) (B) (C) (D)
Sanfilippo A syndrome
Sanfilippo B syndrome
Sanfilippo C syndrome
Sanfilippo D syndrome

E76.29   Other **mucopolysaccharidoses**   `cc`
beta-Glucuronidase deficiency
Maroteaux-Lamy (mild) (severe) syndrome
Mucopolysaccharidosis, types VI, VII

E76.3   Mucopolysaccharidosis, unspecified   `cc`

E76.8   Other **disorders of glucosaminoglycan metabolism**   `cc`

E76.9   Glucosaminoglycan metabolism disorder, unspecified   `cc`

☑4ᵗʰ **E77**   **Disorders of glycoprotein metabolism**

E77.0   **Defects in post-translational modification of lysosomal enzymes**
Mucolipidosis II [I-cell disease]
Mucolipidosis III [pseudo-Hurler polydystrophy]

E77.1   **Defects in glycoprotein degradation**
Aspartylglucosaminuria
Fucosidosis
Mannosidosis
Sialidosis [mucolipidosis I]
CC Excl: See code: E76

E77.8   Other **disorders of glycoprotein metabolism**

E77.9   Disorder of glycoprotein metabolism, unspecified

☑4ᵗʰ **E78**   **Disorders of lipoprotein metabolism and other lipidemias**
EXCLUDES 1   *sphingolipidosis (E75.0-E75.3)*

E78.0   **Pure hypercholesterolemia**
Familial hypercholesterolemia
Fredrickson's hyperlipoproteinemia, type IIa
Hyperbetalipoproteinemia
Hyperlipidemia, Group A
Low-density-lipoprotein-type [LDL] hyperlipoproteinemia

E78.1   **Pure hyperglyceridemia**
Elevated fasting triglycerides
Endogenous hyperglyceridemia
Fredrickson's hyperlipoproteinemia, type IV
Hyperlipidemia, group B
Hyperprebetalipoproteinemia
Very-low-density-lipoprotein-type [VLDL] hyperlipoproteinemia

E78.2   **Mixed hyperlipidemia**
Broad- or floating-betalipoproteinemia
Combined hyperlipidemia NOS
Elevated cholesterol with elevated triglycerides NEC
Fredrickson's hyperlipoproteinemia, type IIb or III
Hyperbetalipoproteinemia with prebetalipoproteinemia
Hypercholesteremia with endogenous hyperglyceridemia
Hyperlipidemia, group C
Tubo-eruptive xanthoma
Xanthoma tuberosum
EXCLUDES 1   *cerebrotendinous cholesterosis [van Bogaert-Scherer-Epstein] (E75.5)*
familial combined hyperlipidemia (E78.4)

E78.3   **Hyperchylomicronemia**
Chylomicron retention disease
Fredrickson's hyperlipoproteinemia, type I or V
Hyperlipidemia, group D
Mixed hyperglyceridemia

E78.4   **Other hyperlipidemia**
Familial combined hyperlipidemia

E78.5   **Hyperlipidemia, unspecified**

E78.6   **Lipoprotein deficiency**
Abetalipoproteinemia
Depressed HDL cholesterol
High-density lipoprotein deficiency
Hypoalphalipoproteinemia
Hypobetalipoproteinemia (familial)
Lecithin cholesterol acyltransferase deficiency
Tangier disease

☑5ᵗʰ E78.7   **Disorders of bile acid and cholesterol metabolism**
EXCLUDES 1   *Niemann-Pick disease type C (E75.242)*

E78.70   **Disorder of bile acid and cholesterol metabolism, unspecified**

E78.71   **Barth syndrome**   `cc`
CC Excl: E78.71-E78.72, Q87.1-Q87.89, Q89.8, Q99.2

E78.72   **Smith-Lemli-Opitz syndrome**   `cc`
CC Excl: See code: E78.71

E78.79   **Other disorders of bile acid and cholesterol metabolism**

☑5ᵗʰ E78.8   **Other disorders of lipoprotein metabolism**

E78.81   **Lipoid dermatoarthritis**

E78.89   **Other lipoprotein metabolism disorders**

E78.9   **Disorder of lipoprotein metabolism, unspecified**

☑4ᵗʰ **E79**   **Disorders of purine and pyrimidine metabolism**
EXCLUDES 1   *Ataxia-telangiectasia (Q87.1)*
Bloom's syndrome (Q82.8)
Cockayne's syndrome (Q87.1)
calculus of kidney (N20.0)
combined immunodeficiency disorders (D81.-)
Fanconi's anemia (D61.09)
gout (M1A.-, M10.-)
orotaciduric anemia (D53.0)
progeria (E34.8)
Werner's syndrome (E34.8)
xeroderma pigmentosum (Q82.1)

CC Excl: For CC codes in category E79, unless otherwise noted:
D81.3, D81.5, D81.810, D84.1, E76.01-E76.9, E79.1-E80.29, E80.4-E80.7, E88.81

E79.0   **Hyperuricemia without signs of inflammatory arthritis and tophaceous disease**
Asymptomatic hyperuricemia

E79.1   **Lesch-Nyhan syndrome**   `cc`
HGPRT deficiency

E79.2   **Myoadenylate deaminase deficiency**   `cc`

E79.8   **Other disorders of purine and pyrimidine metabolism**   `cc`
Hereditary xanthinuria

E79.9   **Disorder of purine and pyrimidine metabolism, unspecified**   `cc`

☑4ᵗʰ **E80**   **Disorders of porphyrin and bilirubin metabolism**
INCLUDES   defects of catalase and peroxidase

CC Excl: For CC codes in category E80, unless otherwise noted:
D81.3, D81.5, D81.810, D84.1, E76.01-E76.9, E79.1-E80.29, E80.4-E80.7, E88.81

E80.0   **Hereditary erythropoietic porphyria**   `cc`
Congenital erythropoietic porphyria
Erythropoietic protoporphyria

E80.1   **Porphyria cutanea tarda**   `cc`

☑5ᵗʰ E80.2   **Other and unspecified porphyria**

E80.20   **Unspecified porphyria**   `cc`
Porphyria NOS

E80.21   **Acute intermittent (hepatic) porphyria**   `cc`

E80.29   **Other porphyria**   `cc`
Hereditary coproporphyria

E80.3   **Defects of catalase and peroxidase**   `cc`
Acatalasia [Takahara]
CC Excl: E71.310-E71.32, E71.40-E71.548, E80.4-E80.7, E88.40-E88.49, H49.811-H49.819

E80.4   **Gilbert syndrome**

E80.5   **Crigler-Najjar syndrome**

E80.6   **Other disorders of bilirubin metabolism**
Dubin-Johnson syndrome
Rotor's syndrome

E80.7   **Disorder of bilirubin metabolism, unspecified**

☑4ᵗʰ **E83**   **Disorders of mineral metabolism**
EXCLUDES 1   *dietary mineral deficiency (E58-E61)*
parathyroid disorders (E20-E21)
vitamin D deficiency (E55.-)

☑5ᵗʰ E83.0   **Disorders of copper metabolism**

E83.00   **Disorder of copper metabolism, unspecified**

E83.01   **Wilson's disease**
Code also associated Kayser Fleischer ring (H18.04-)

E83.09   **Other disorders of copper metabolism**
Menkes' (kinky hair) (steely hair) disease

☑ Additional Character Required   ☑x7ᵗʰ *X*tension Alert   **Unacceptable PDx**   **Manifestation**   **Hospital Acquired Condition**   *EXCLUDES 1* Not Coded Here   *EXCLUDES 2* Not Included Here

Endocrine, Nutritional and Metabolic Diseases

E83.1–E87.8

✓5th **E83.1** **Disorders of iron metabolism**
     EXCLUDES 1   *iron deficiency anemia (D50.-)*
                sideroblastic anemia (D64.0-D64.3)

     E83.10 **Disorder of iron metabolism, unspecified**

     ✓6th **E83.11** **Hemochromatosis**

         E83.110 **Hereditary hemochromatosis**
             Bronzed diabetes
             Pigmentary cirrhosis (of liver)
             Primary (hereditary) hemochromatosis

         E83.111 **Hemochromatosis due to repeated red blood cell transfusions**
             Iron overload due to repeated red blood cell transfusions
             Transfusion (red blood cell) associated hemochromatosis

         E83.118 **Other hemochromatosis**

         E83.119 **Hemochromatosis, unspecified**

     E83.19 **Other disorders of iron metabolism**
         Use additional code, if applicable, for idiopathic pulmonary hemosiderosis (J84.03)

E83.2 **Disorders of zinc metabolism**
     Acrodermatitis enteropathica

✓5th **E83.3** **Disorders of phosphorus metabolism and phosphatases**
     EXCLUDES 1   *adult osteomalacia (M83.-)*
                osteoporosis (M80.-)

     E83.30 **Disorder of phosphorus metabolism, unspecified**

     E83.31 **Familial hypophosphatemia**
         Vitamin D-resistant osteomalacia
         Vitamin D-resistant rickets
         EXCLUDES 1   *vitamin D-deficiency rickets (E55.0)*

     E83.32 **Hereditary vitamin D-dependent rickets (type 1) (type 2)**
         25-hydroxyvitamin D 1-alpha-hydroxylase deficiency
         Pseudovitamin D deficiency
         Vitamin D receptor defect

     E83.39 **Other disorders of phosphorus metabolism**
         Acid phosphatase deficiency
         Hypophosphatasia

✓5th **E83.4** **Disorders of magnesium metabolism**

     E83.40 **Disorders of magnesium metabolism, unspecified**

     E83.41 **Hypermagnesemia**

     E83.42 **Hypomagnesemia**

     E83.49 **Other disorders of magnesium metabolism**

✓5th **E83.5** **Disorders of calcium metabolism**
     EXCLUDES 1   *chondrocalcinosis (M11.1-M11.2)*
                hungry bone syndrome (E83.81)
                hyperparathyroidism (E21.0-E21.3)

     E83.50 **Unspecified disorder of calcium metabolism**

     E83.51 **Hypocalcemia**

     E83.52 **Hypercalcemia**
         Familial hypocalciuric hypercalcemia

     E83.59 **Other disorders of calcium metabolism**
         Idiopathic hypercalciuria

✓5th **E83.8** **Other disorders of mineral metabolism**

     E83.81 **Hungry bone syndrome**

     E83.89 **Other disorders of mineral metabolism**

E83.9 **Disorder of mineral metabolism, unspecified**

✓4th **E84** **Cystic fibrosis**
     INCLUDES   mucoviscidosis

     CC Excl: For CC/MCC codes in category E84, unless otherwise noted: E84.0-E84.9

     E84.0 **Cystic fibrosis with pulmonary manifestations**   MCC
         Use additional code to identify any infectious organism present, such as:
         Pseudomonas (B96.5)

     ✓5th **E84.1** **Cystic fibrosis with intestinal manifestations**

         E84.11 **Meconium ileus in cystic fibrosis**   MCC N
             EXCLUDES 1   *meconium ileus not due to cystic fibrosis (P76.0)*

         E84.19 **Cystic fibrosis with other intestinal manifestations**   CC
             Distal intestinal obstruction syndrome

     E84.8 **Cystic fibrosis with other manifestations**   CC

     E84.9 **Cystic fibrosis, unspecified**   CC

✓4th **E85** **Amyloidosis**
     EXCLUDES 1   *Alzheimer's disease (G30.0-)*

     CC Excl: For CC codes in category E85, unless otherwise noted: E85.0-E85.9, E88.81

     E85.0 **Non-neuropathic heredofamilial amyloidosis**   CC
         Familial Mediterranean fever
         Hereditary amyloid nephropathy
         AHA: 2012, 4Q, 99

     E85.1 **Neuropathic heredofamilial amyloidosis**   CC
         Amyloid polyneuropathy (Portuguese)

     E85.2 **Heredofamilial amyloidosis, unspecified**   CC

     E85.3 **Secondary systemic amyloidosis**   CC
         Hemodialysis-associated amyloidosis

     E85.4 **Organ-limited amyloidosis**   CC
         Localized amyloidosis

     E85.8 **Other amyloidosis**   CC

     E85.9 **Amyloidosis, unspecified**   CC

✓4th **E86** **Volume depletion**
     EXCLUDES 1   *dehydration of newborn (P74.1)*
                hypovolemic shock NOS (R57.1)
                postprocedural hypovolemic shock (T81.19)
                traumatic hypovolemic shock (T79.4)

     E86.0 **Dehydration**
         AHA: 2014, 1Q, 7

     E86.1 **Hypovolemia**
         Depletion of volume of plasma

     E86.9 **Volume depletion, unspecified**

✓4th **E87** **Other disorders of fluid, electrolyte and acid-base balance**
     EXCLUDES 1   *diabetes insipidus (E23.2)*
                electrolyte imbalance associated with hyperemesis gravidarum (O21.1)
                electrolyte imbalance following ectopic or molar pregnancy (O08.5)
                familial periodic paralysis (G72.3)

     CC Excl: For CC codes in category E87, unless otherwise noted: E86.0-E87.8

     E87.0 **Hyperosmolality and hypernatremia**   CC
         Sodium [Na] excess
         Sodium [Na] overload
         AHA: 2014, 1Q, 7

     E87.1 **Hypo-osmolality and hyponatremia**   CC
         Sodium [Na] deficiency
         EXCLUDES 1   *syndrome of inappropriate secretion of antidiuretic hormone (E22.2)*
         AHA: 2014, 1Q, 7

     E87.2 **Acidosis**   CC
         Acidosis NOS
         Lactic acidosis
         Metabolic acidosis
         Respiratory acidosis
         EXCLUDES 1   *diabetic acidosis—see categories E08-E10, E13 with ketoacidosis*

     E87.3 **Alkalosis**   CC
         Alkalosis NOS
         Metabolic alkalosis
         Respiratory alkalosis

     E87.4 **Mixed disorder of acid-base balance**   CC

     E87.5 **Hyperkalemia**
         Potassium [K] excess
         Potassium [K] overload

     E87.6 **Hypokalemia**
         Potassium [K] deficiency

     ✓5th **E87.7** **Fluid overload**
         EXCLUDES 1   *edema NOS (R60.9)*
                 fluid retention (R60.9)

         E87.70 **Fluid overload, unspecified**

         E87.71 **Transfusion associated circulatory overload**
             Fluid overload due to transfusion (blood) (blood components)
             TACO

         E87.79 **Other fluid overload**

     E87.8 **Other disorders of electrolyte and fluid balance, not elsewhere classified**
         Electrolyte imbalance NOS
         Hyperchloremia
         Hypochloremia

N Newborn: 0   P Pediatric: 0-17   M Maternity: 12-55   A Adult: 15-124   MCC Major CC Condition   PDx MCC PDx acts as own MCC   CC CC Condition   PDx CC PDx acts as own CC

508   ICD-10-CM Draft (2015)

✓4th **E88 Other and unspecified metabolic disorders**
Use additional codes for associated conditions
EXCLUDES 1 *histiocytosis X (chronic) (C96.6)*

✓5th **E88.0 Disorders of plasma-protein metabolism, not elsewhere classified**
EXCLUDES 1 *disorder of lipoprotein metabolism (E78.-)*
monoclonal gammopathy (of undetermined significance) (D47.2)
polyclonal hypergammaglobulinemia (D89.0)
Waldenström's macroglobulinemia (C88.0)

E88.01 Alpha-1-antitrypsin deficiency
AAT deficiency

E88.09 Other disorders of plasma-protein metabolism, not elsewhere classified
Bisalbuminemia

E88.1 Lipodystrophy, not elsewhere classified
Lipodystrophy NOS
EXCLUDES 1 *Whipple's disease (K90.81)*

E88.2 Lipomatosis, not elsewhere classified
Lipomatosis NOS
Lipomatosis (Check) dolorosa [Dercum]

E88.3 Tumor lysis syndrome MCC
Tumor lysis syndrome (spontaneous)
Tumor lysis syndrome following antineoplastic drug chemotherapy
Use additional code for adverse effect, if applicable, to identify drug (T45.1X5)
CC Excl: E08.21-E08.29, E09.21-E09.29, E88.3, N00.0-N01.9, N02.8-N02.9, N04.7-N05.1, N05.6-N06.1, N06.6-N07.1, N07.6-N08, N14.0-N15.0, N15.8-N17.9

✓5th **E88.4 Mitochondrial metabolism disorders**
EXCLUDES 1 *disorders of pyruvate metabolism (E74.4)*
Kearns-Sayre syndrome (H49.81)
Leber's disease (H47.22)
Leigh's encephalopathy (G31.82)
Mitochondrial myopathy, NEC (G71.3)
Reye's syndrome (G93.7)

CC Excl: For CC codes in subcategory E88.4, unless otherwise noted: C96.5-C96.6, E71.310-E71.548, E80.3-E80.7, E88.89

E88.40 Mitochondrial metabolism disorder, unspecified CC

E88.41 MELAS syndrome CC
Mitochondrial myopathy, encephalopathy, lactic acidosis and stroke-like episodes

E88.42 MERRF syndrome CC
Myoclonic epilepsy associated with ragged-red fibers
Code also myoclonic epilepsy (G40.3-)

E88.49 Other mitochondrial metabolism disorders CC

✓5th **E88.8 Other specified metabolic disorders**

E88.81 Metabolic syndrome
Dysmetabolic syndrome X
Use additional codes for associated manifestations, such as:
obesity (E66.-)

E88.89 Other specified metabolic disorders CC
Launois-Bensaude adenolipomatosis
EXCLUDES 1 *adult pulmonary Langerhans cell histiocytosis (J84.82)*
CC Excl: E71.310-E71.32, E71.40-E71.548, E80.4-E80.7, E88.40-E88.49, H49.811-H49.819

E88.9 Metabolic disorder, unspecified

✓4th **E89 Postprocedural endocrine and metabolic complications and disorders, not elsewhere classified**
EXCLUDES 2 *intraoperative complications of endocrine system organ or structure (E36.0-, E36.1-, E36.8)*

E89.0 Postprocedural hypothyroidism
Postirradiation hypothyroidism
Postsurgical hypothyroidism

E89.1 Postprocedural hypoinsulinemia CC
Postpancreatectomy hyperglycemia
Postsurgical hypoinsulinemia
Use additional code, if applicable, to identify:
acquired absence of pancreas (Z90.41-)
diabetes mellitus (postpancreatectomy) (postprocedural) (E13.-)
insulin use (Z79.4)
EXCLUDES 1 *transient postprocedural hyperglycemia (R73.9)*
transient postprocedural hypoglycemia (E16.2)
CC Excl: E08.00-E08.59, E08.618-E08.638, E08.641-E09.59, E09.618-E09.638, E09.641-E10.59, E10.618-E10.638, E10.641-E10.649, E10.69-E11.59, E11.618-E11.638, E11.641-E11.649, E11.69-E13.59, E13.618-E13.638, E13.641-E16.2, E30.9, E34.1, E34.50-E35, E89.1

E89.2 Postprocedural hypoparathyroidism
Parathyroprival tetany

E89.3 Postprocedural hypopituitarism
Postirradiation hypopituitarism

✓5th **E89.4 Postprocedural ovarian failure**

E89.40 Asymptomatic postprocedural ovarian failure ♀
Postprocedural ovarian failure NOS

E89.41 Symptomatic postprocedural ovarian failure ♀
Symptoms such as flushing, sleeplessness, headache, lack of concentration, associated with postprocedural menopause

E89.5 Postprocedural testicular hypofunction ♂

E89.6 Postprocedural adrenocortical (-medullary) hypofunction CC
CC Excl: A17.9, A18.7, A18.82, A18.84, A18.89, E27.0-E27.9, E30.9, E34.1, E34.50-E35, E89.6

✓5th **E89.8 Other postprocedural endocrine and metabolic complications and disordersd**

✓6th **E89.81 Postprocedural hemorrhage and hematoma of an endocrine system organ or structure following a procedure**

E89.810 Postprocedural hemorrhage and hematoma of an endocrine system organ or structure following an endocrine system procedure CC
CC Excl: E36.8, E89.810-E89.89, H95.811-H95.89, I97.3, M96.89, N98.1-N98.9, T81.82 with 7th character A, T81.89X-T81.9XX with 7th A

E89.811 Postprocedural hemorrhage and hematoma of an endocrine system organ or structure following other procedure CC
CC Excl: See code E89.810

E89.89 Other postprocedural endocrine and metabolic complications and disorders CC
Use additional code, if applicable, to further specify disorder
CC Excl: See code E89.810

Mental, Behavioral, and Neurodevelopmental Disorders

F01–F06.0

Chapter 5. Mental, Behavioral, and Neurodevelopmental Disorders (F01-F99)

INCLUDES disorders of psychological development

EXCLUDES 2 symptoms, signs and abnormal clinical laboratory findings, not elsewhere classified (R00-R99)

This chapter contains the following blocks:

F01-F09	Mental disorders due to known physiological conditions
F10-F19	Mental and behavioral disorders due to psychoactive substance use
F20-F29	Schizophrenia, schizotypal, delusional, and other non-mood psychotic disorders
F30-F39	Mood [affective] disorders
F40-F48	Anxiety, dissociative, stress-related, somatoform and other nonpsychotic mental disorders
F50-F59	Behavioral syndromes associated with physiological disturbances and physical factors
F60-F69	Disorders of adult personality and behavior
F70-F79	Intellectual disabilities
F80-F89	Pervasive and specific developmental disorders
F90-F98	Behavioral and emotional disorders with onset usually occurring in childhood and adolescence
F99	Unspecified mental disorder

Mental disorders due to known physiological conditions (F01-F09)

NOTE This block comprises a range of mental disorders grouped together on the basis of their having in common a demonstrable etiology in cerebral disease, brain injury, or other insult leading to cerebral dysfunction. The dysfunction may be primary, as in diseases, injuries, and insults that affect the brain directly and selectively; or secondary, as in systemic diseases and disorders that attack the brain only as one of the multiple organs or systems of the body that are involved.

✓4th F01   Vascular dementia

Vascular demdentia as a result of infarction of the brain due to vascular disease, including hypertensive cerebrovascular disease.

INCLUDES arteriosclerotic dementia

Code first the underlying physiological condition or sequelae of cerebrovascular disease.

✓5th F01.5   Vascular dementia

F01.50   Vascular dementia without behavioral **A**
disturbance

F01.51   Vascular dementia with behavioral **CC A**
disturbance

Vascular dementia with aggressive behavior
Vascular dementia with combative behavior
Vascular dementia with violent behavior
Use additional code, if applicable, to identify
wandering in vascular dementia (Z91.83)
CC Excl: F01.51

✓4th F02   Dementia in other diseases classified elsewhere

Code first the underlying physiological condition, such as:
Alzheimer's (G30.-)
cerebral lipidosis (E75.4)
Creutzfeldt-Jakob disease (A81.0-)
dementia with Lewy bodies (G31.83)
epilepsy and recurrent seizures (G40.-)
frontotemporal dementia (G31.09)
hepatolenticular degeneration (E83.0)
human immunodeficiency virus [HIV] disease (B20)
hypercalcemia (E83.52)
hypothyroidism, acquired (E00-E03.-)
intoxications (T36-T65)
Jakob-Creutzfeldt disease (A81.0-)
multiple sclerosis (G35)
neurosyphilis (A52.17)
niacin deficiency [pellagra] (E52)
Parkinson's disease (G20)
Pick's disease (G31.01)
polyarteritis nodosa (M30.0)
systemic lupus erythematosus (M32.-)
trypanosomiasis (B56.-, B57.-)
vitamin B deficiency (E53.8)

EXCLUDES 1 dementia with Parkinsonism (G31.83)

EXCLUDES 2 dementia in alcohol and psychoactive substance disorders (F10-F19, with .17, .27, .97)
vascular dementia (F01.5-)

✓5th F02.8   Dementia in other diseases classified elsewhere

F02.80   Dementia in other diseases classified elsewhere without behavioral disturbance
Dementia in other diseases classified elsewhere NOS

F02.81   Dementia in other diseases classified elsewhere with behavioral disturbance   **CC**

Dementia in other diseases classified elsewhere with aggressive behavior
Dementia in other diseases classified elsewhere with combative behavior
Dementia in other diseases classified elsewhere with violent behavior
Use additional code, if applicable, to identify wandering in dementia in conditions classified elsewhere (Z91.83)
CC Excl: F02.81, F03.91

✓4th F03   Unspecified dementia

Presenile dementia NOS	Senile dementia NOS
Presenile psychosis NOS	Senile dementia depressed
Primary degenerative dementia NOS	or paranoid type
Senile dementia NOS	Senile psychosis NOS

EXCLUDES 1 senility NOS (R41.81)

EXCLUDES 2 mild memory disturbance due to known physiological condition (F06.8)
senile dementia with delirium or acute confusional state (F05)

✓5th F03.9   Unspecified dementia

F03.90   Unspecified dementia without behavioral **HIV A**
disturbance
Dementia NOS
AHA: 2012, 4Q, 92

F03.91   Unspecified dementia with behavioral **CC A**
disturbance
Unspecified dementia with aggressive behavior
Unspecified dementia with combative behavior
Unspecified dementia with violent behavior
Use additional code, if applicable, to identify wandering in unspecified dementia (Z91.83)
CC Excl: See code: F02.81

F04   Amnestic disorder due to known physiological condition

Korsakov's psychosis or syndrome, nonalcoholic
Code first the underlying physiological condition

EXCLUDES 1 amnesia NOS (R41.3)
anterograde amnesia (R41.1)
dissociative amnesia (F44.0)
retrograde amnesia (R41.2)

EXCLUDES 2 alcohol-induced or unspecified Korsakov's syndrome (F10.26, F10.96)
Korsakov's syndrome induced by other psychoactive substances (F13.26, F13.96, F19.16, F19.26, F19.96)

F05   Delirium due to known physiological condition   **CC**

Acute or subacute brain syndrome
Acute or subacute confusional state (nonalcoholic)
Acute or subacute infective psychosis
Acute or subacute organic reaction
Acute or subacute psycho-organic syndrome
Delirium of mixed etiology
Delirium superimposed on dementia
Sundowning
Code first the underlying physiological condition

EXCLUDES 1 delirium NOS (R41.0)

EXCLUDES 2 delirium tremens alcohol-induced or unspecified (F10.231, F10.921)
CC Excl: F05, R45.851

✓4th F06   Other mental disorders due to known physiological condition

INCLUDES mental disorders due to endocrine disorder
mental disorders due to exogenous hormone
mental disorders due to exogenous toxic substance
mental disorders due to primary cerebral disease
mental disorders due to somatic illness
mental disorders due to systemic disease affecting the brain

Code first the underlying physiological condition

EXCLUDES 1 unspecified dementia (F03)

EXCLUDES 2 delirium due to known physiological condition (F05)
dementia as classified in F01-F02
other mental disorders associated with alcohol and other psychoactive substances (F10-F19)

F06.0   Psychotic disorder with hallucinations **due to known**   **CC**
physiological condition
Organic hallucinatory state (nonalcoholic)

EXCLUDES 2 hallucinations and perceptual disturbance induced by alcohol and other psychoactive substances (F10-F19 with .151, .251, .951)
schizophrenia (F20.-)

CC Excl: F02.80-F02.81, F04-F06.8, F10.10-F11.19, F11.21-F13.19, F13.21-F14.19, F14.21-F15.19, F15.21-F16.19, F16.21-F16.99, F17.203-F17.209, F17.213-F17.219, F17.223-F17.229, F17.293-F18.19, F18.21-F19.19, F19.21-F19.99, F53, F55.0-F55.8, R78.0

N Newborn: 0   **P** Pediatric: 0-17   **M** Maternity: 12-55   **A** Adult: 15-124   **MCC** Major CC Condition   **PDx MCC** PDx acts as own MCC   **CC** CC Condition   **PDx CC** PDx acts as own CC

F06.1 Catatonic disorder due to known physiological condition
> EXCLUDES 1 catatonic stupor (R40.1)
> stupor NOS (R40.1)
> EXCLUDES 2 catatonic schizophrenia (F20.2)
> dissociative stupor (F44.2)

F06.2 Psychotic disorder with delusions due to known physiological condition CC
> Paranoid and paranoid-hallucinatory organic states
> Schizophrenia-like psychosis in epilepsy
> EXCLUDES 2 alcohol and drug-induced psychotic disorder (F10-F19 with .150, .250, .950)
> brief psychotic disorder (F23)
> delusional disorder (F22)
> schizophrenia (F20.-)
> CC Excl: See code: F06.0

✓5ᵗʰ **F06.3 Mood disorder due to known physiological condition**
> EXCLUDES 2 mood disorders due to alcohol and other psychoactive substances (F10-F19 with .14, .24, .94)
> mood disorders, not due to known physiological condition or unspecified (F30-F39)

F06.30 Mood disorder due to known physiological condition, unspecified

F06.31 Mood disorder due to known physiological condition with depressive features

F06.32 Mood disorder due to known physiological condition with major depressive-like episode

F06.33 Mood disorder due to known physiological condition with manic features

F06.34 Mood disorder due to known physiological condition with mixed features

F06.4 Anxiety disorder due to known physiological condition
> EXCLUDES 2 anxiety disorders due to alcohol and other psychoactive substances (F10-F19 with .180, .280, .980)
> anxiety disorders, not due to known physiological condition or unspecified (F40.-, F41.-)

F06.8 Other specified mental disorders due to known physiological condition HIV
> Epileptic psychosis NOS
> Organic dissociative disorder
> Organic emotionally labile [asthenic] disorder

✓4ᵗʰ **F07 Personality and behavioral disorders due to known physiological condition**
> Code first the underlying physiological condition

F07.0 Personality change due to known physiological condition
> Frontal lobe syndrome
> Limbic epilepsy personality syndrome
> Lobotomy syndrome
> Organic personality disorder
> Organic pseudopsychopathic personality
> Organic pseudoretarded personality
> Postleucotomy syndrome
> Code first underlying physiological condition
> EXCLUDES 1 mild cognitive impairment (G31.84)
> postconcussional syndrome (F07.81)
> postencephalitic syndrome (F07.89)
> signs and symptoms involving emotional state (R45.-)
> EXCLUDES 2 specific personality disorder (F60.-)

✓5ᵗʰ **F07.8 Other personality and behavioral disorders due to known physiological condition**

F07.81 Postconcussional syndrome
> Postcontusional syndrome (encephalopathy)
> Post-traumatic brain syndrome, nonpsychotic
> Use additional code to identify associated post-traumatic headache, if applicable (G44.3-)
> EXCLUDES 1 current concussion (brain) (S06.0-)
> postencephalitic syndrome (F07.89)

F07.89 Other personality and behavioral disorders due to known physiological condition
> Postencephalitic syndrome
> Right hemispheric organic affective disorder

F07.9 Unspecified personality and behavioral disorder due to known physiological condition HIV
> Organic psychosyndrome

F09 Unspecified mental disorder due to known physiological condition HIV
> Mental disorder NOS due to known physiological condition
> Organic brain syndrome NOS
> Organic mental disorder NOS
> Organic psychosis NOS
> Symptomatic psychosis NOS
> Code first the underlying physiological condition
> EXCLUDES 1 psychosis NOS (F29)

Mental and behavioral disorders due to psychoactive substance use (F10-F19)

✓4ᵗʰ **F10 Alcohol related disorders**
> Use additional code for blood alcohol level, if applicable (Y90.-)

> CC Excl: For CC codes in category F10, unless otherwise noted: F02.80-F02.81, F04-F06.8, F10.10-F11.19, F11.21-F13.19, F13.21-F14.19, F14.21-F15.19, F15.21-F16.19, F16.21-F16.99, F17.203-F17.209, F17.213-F17.219, F17.223-F17.229, F17.293-F18.19, F18.21-F19.19, F19.21-F19.99, F53, F55.0-F55.8, R78.0

✓5ᵗʰ **F10.1 Alcohol abuse**
> EXCLUDES 1 alcohol dependence (F10.2-)
> alcohol use, unspecified (F10.9-)

F10.10 Alcohol abuse, uncomplicated

✓6ᵗʰ **F10.12 Alcohol abuse with intoxication**

F10.120 Alcohol abuse with intoxication, uncomplicated

F10.121 Alcohol abuse with intoxication delirium CC

F10.129 Alcohol abuse with intoxication, unspecified

F10.14 Alcohol abuse with alcohol-induced mood disorder CC

✓6ᵗʰ **F10.15 Alcohol abuse with alcohol-induced psychotic disorder**

F10.150 Alcohol abuse with alcohol-induced psychotic disorder with delusions

F10.151 Alcohol abuse with alcohol-induced psychotic disorder with hallucinations CC

F10.159 Alcohol abuse with alcohol-induced psychotic disorder, unspecified CC

✓6ᵗʰ **F10.18 Alcohol abuse with other alcohol-induced disorders**

F10.180 Alcohol abuse with alcohol-induced anxiety disorder CC

F10.181 Alcohol abuse with alcohol-induced sexual dysfunction CC

F10.182 Alcohol abuse with alcohol-induced sleep disorder

F10.188 Alcohol abuse with other alcohol-induced disorder CC

F10.19 Alcohol abuse with unspecified alcohol-induced disorder CC

✓5ᵗʰ **F10.2 Alcohol dependence**
> EXCLUDES 1 alcohol abuse (F10.1-)
> alcohol use, unspecified (F10.9-)
> EXCLUDES 2 toxic effect of alcohol (T51.0-)

F10.20 Alcohol dependence, uncomplicated

F10.21 Alcohol dependence, in remission

✓6ᵗʰ **F10.22 Alcohol dependence with intoxication**
> Acute drunkenness (in alcoholism)
> EXCLUDES 1 alcohol dependence with withdrawal (F10.23-)

F10.220 Alcohol dependence with intoxication, uncomplicated

F10.221 Alcohol dependence with intoxication delirium CC

F10.229 Alcohol dependence with intoxication, unspecified

✓6ᵗʰ **F10.23 Alcohol dependence with withdrawal**
> EXCLUDES 1 Alcohol dependence with intoxication (F10.22-)

F10.230 Alcohol dependence with withdrawal, uncomplicated CC

F10.231 Alcohol dependence with withdrawal delirium CC

F10.232 Alcohol dependence with withdrawal with perceptual disturbance CC

✓ Additional Character Required   ✓x7ᵗʰ Xtension Alert   Unacceptable PDx   Manifestation   Hospital Acquired Condition   EXCLUDES 1 Not Coded Here   EXCLUDES 2 Not Included Here

ICD-10-CM Draft (2015) 511

Mental, Behavioral, and Neurodevelopmental Disorders

F10.239–F11.250

F10.239 Alcohol dependence with withdrawal, unspecified   `CC`

F10.24 Alcohol dependence with alcohol-induced mood disorder   `CC`

✓6th **F10.25** Alcohol dependence with alcohol-induced psychotic disorder

     F10.250 Alcohol dependence with alcohol-induced psychotic disorder with delusions

     F10.251 Alcohol dependence with alcohol-induced psychotic disorder with hallucinations   `CC`

     F10.259 Alcohol dependence with alcohol-induced psychotic disorder, unspecified   `CC`

F10.26 Alcohol dependence with alcohol-induced persisting amnestic disorder

F10.27 Alcohol dependence with alcohol-induced persisting dementia   `CC`

✓6th **F10.28** Alcohol dependence with other alcohol-induced disorders

     F10.280 Alcohol dependence with alcohol-induced anxiety disorder   `CC`

     F10.281 Alcohol dependence with alcohol-induced sexual dysfunction   `CC`

     F10.282 Alcohol dependence with alcohol-induced sleep disorder

     F10.288 Alcohol dependence with other alcohol-induced disorder   `CC`

F10.29 Alcohol dependence with unspecified alcohol-induced disorder   `CC`

✓5th **F10.9** Alcohol use, unspecified

     EXCLUDES 1   alcohol abuse (F10.1-)
                  alcohol dependence (F10.2-)

✓6th **F10.92** Alcohol use, unspecified with intoxication

     F10.920 Alcohol use, unspecified with intoxication, uncomplicated

     F10.921 Alcohol use, unspecified with intoxication delirium   `CC`

     F10.929 Alcohol use, unspecified with intoxication, unspecified

F10.94 Alcohol use, unspecified with alcohol-induced mood disorder   `CC`

✓6th **F10.95** Alcohol use, unspecified with alcohol-induced psychotic disorder

     F10.950 Alcohol use, unspecified with alcohol-induced psychotic disorder with delusions

     F10.951 Alcohol use, unspecified with alcohol-induced psychotic disorder with hallucinations   `CC`

     F10.959 Alcohol use, unspecified with alcohol-induced psychotic disorder, unspecified   `CC`

F10.96 Alcohol use, unspecified with alcohol-induced persisting amnestic disorder

F10.97 Alcohol use, unspecified with alcohol-induced persisting dementia

✓6th **F10.98** Alcohol use, unspecified with other alcohol-induced disorders

     F10.980 Alcohol use, unspecified with alcohol-induced anxiety disorder   `CC`

     F10.981 Alcohol use, unspecified with alcohol-induced sexual dysfunction   `CC`

     F10.982 Alcohol use, unspecified with alcohol-induced sleep disorder

     F10.988 Alcohol use, unspecified with other alcohol-induced disorder   `CC`

F10.99 Alcohol use, unspecified with unspecified alcohol-induced disorder   `CC`

✓4th **F11** Opioid related disorders

     CC Excl: For CC codes in category F11, unless otherwise noted:
     F02.80-F02.81, F04-F06.8, F10.10-F11.19, F11.21-F13.19, F13.21-
     F14.19, F14.21-F15.19, F15.21-F16.19, F16.21-F16.99, F17.203-
     F17.209, F17.213-F17.219, F17.223-F17.229, F17.293-F18.19, F18.21-
     F19.19, F19.21-F19.99, F53, F55.0-F55.8, R78.0

✓5th **F11.1** Opioid abuse

     EXCLUDES 1   opioid dependence (F11.2-)
                  opioid use, unspecified (F11.9-)

     F11.10 Opioid abuse, uncomplicated

✓6th **F11.12** Opioid abuse with intoxication

     F11.120 Opioid abuse with intoxication, uncomplicated

     F11.121 Opioid abuse with intoxication delirium   `CC`

     F11.122 Opioid abuse with intoxication with perceptual disturbance

     F11.129 Opioid abuse with intoxication, unspecified

F11.14 Opioid abuse with opioid-induced mood disorder

✓6th **F11.15** Opioid abuse with opioid-induced psychotic disorder

     F11.150 Opioid abuse with opioid-induced psychotic disorder with delusions   `CC`

     F11.151 Opioid abuse with opioid-induced psychotic disorder with hallucinations   `CC`

     F11.159 Opioid abuse with opioid-induced psychotic disorder, unspecified

✓6th **F11.18** Opioid abuse with other opioid-induced disorder

     F11.181 Opioid abuse with opioid-induced sexual dysfunction

     F11.182 Opioid abuse with opioid-induced sleep disorder

     F11.188 Opioid abuse with other opioid-induced disorder

F11.19 Opioid abuse with unspecified opioid-induced disorder

✓5th **F11.2** Opioid dependence

     EXCLUDES 1   opioid abuse (F11.1-)
                  opioid use, unspecified (F11.9-)
     EXCLUDES 2   opioid poisoning (T40.0-T40.2-)

     F11.20 Opioid dependence, uncomplicated   `CC`
         CC Excl: No excl

     F11.21 Opioid dependence, in remission

✓6th **F11.22** Opioid dependence with intoxication
     EXCLUDES 1   opioid dependence with withdrawal (F11.23)

     F11.220 Opioid dependence with intoxication, uncomplicated
         CC Excl: No excl

     F11.221 Opioid dependence with intoxication delirium   `CC`
         CC Excl: F02.80-F02.81, F04- F06.8, F10.10-
         F11.19, F11.21-F13.19, F13.21- F14.19,
         F14.21-F15.19, F15.21-F16.19, F16.21-
         F16.99, F17.203-F17.209, F17.213- F17.219,
         F17.223-F17.229, F17.293-F18.19, F18.21-
         F19.19, F19.21-F19.99, F53, F55.0-F55.8,
         R78.0

     F11.222 Opioid dependence with intoxication with perceptual disturbance   `CC`
         CC Excl: No excl

     F11.229 Opioid dependence with intoxication, unspecified
         CC Excl: No excl

     F11.23 Opioid dependence with withdrawal   `CC`
     EXCLUDES 1   opioid dependence with intoxication (F11.22-)
         CC Excl: See code: F11.221

     F11.24 Opioid dependence with opioid-induced mood disorder

✓6th **F11.25** Opioid dependence with opioid-induced psychotic disorder

     F11.250 Opioid dependence with opioid-induced psychotic disorder with delusions   `CC`
         CC Excl: See code: F11.221

N Newborn: 0   P Pediatric: 0-17   M Maternity: 12-55   A Adult: 15-124   MCC Major CC Condition   PDx MCC PDx acts as own MCC   CC CC Condition   PDx CC PDx acts as own CC

512   ICD-10-CM Draft (2015)

F11.251   Opioid dependence with opioid-induced psychotic disorder with hallucinations   CC
        CC Excl: See code: F11.221

F11.259   Opioid dependence with opioid-induced psychotic disorder, unspecified   CC
        CC Excl: No excl

√6ᵗʰ   F11.28   Opioid dependence with other opioid-induced disorder

F11.281   Opioid dependence with opioid-induced sexual dysfunction   CC
        CC Excl: No excl

F11.282   Opioid dependence with opioid-induced sleep disorder   CC
        CC Excl: No excl

F11.288   Opioid dependence with other opioid-induced disorder   CC
        CC Excl: No excl

F11.29   Opioid dependence with unspecified opioid-induced disorder
        CC Excl: No excl

√5ᵗʰ   F11.9   Opioid use, unspecified
        EXCLUDES 1   opioid abuse (F11.1-)
                    opioid dependence (F11.2-)

F11.90   Opioid use, unspecified, uncomplicated

√6ᵗʰ   F11.92   Opioid use, unspecified with intoxication
        EXCLUDES 1   opioid use, unspecified with withdrawal (F11.93)

F11.920   Opioid use, unspecified with intoxication, uncomplicated

F11.921   Opioid use, unspecified with intoxication delirium   CC
        CC Excl: See code: F11.221

F11.922   Opioid use, unspecified with intoxication with perceptual disturbance

F11.929   Opioid use, unspecified with intoxication, unspecified

F11.93   Opioid use, unspecified with withdrawal   CC
        EXCLUDES 1   opioid use, unspecified with intoxication (F11.92-)
        CC Excl: See code: F11.221

F11.94   Opioid use, unspecified with opioid-induced mood disorder

√6ᵗʰ   F11.95   Opioid use, unspecified with opioid-induced psychotic disorder

F11.950   Opioid use, unspecified with opioid-induced psychotic disorder with delusions   CC
        CC Excl: See code: F11.221

F11.951   Opioid use, unspecified with opioid-induced psychotic disorder with hallucinations   CC
        CC Excl: See code: F11.221

F11.959   Opioid use, unspecified with opioid-induced psychotic disorder, unspecified

√6ᵗʰ   F11.98   Opioid use, unspecified with other specified opioid-induced disorder

F11.981   Opioid use, unspecified with opioid-induced sexual dysfunction

F11.982   Opioid use, unspecified with opioid-induced sleep disorder

F11.988   Opioid use, unspecified with other opioid-induced disorder

F11.99   Opioid use, unspecified with unspecified opioid-induced disorder

√4ᵗʰ   F12   Cannabis related disorders
        INCLUDES   marijuana

        CC Excl: For CC codes in category F12, unless otherwise noted:
        F02.80-F02.81, F04-F06.8, F10.10-F11.19, F11.21-F13.19, F13.21-
        F14.19, F14.21-F15.19, F15.21-F16.19, F16.21-F16.99, F17.203-
        F17.209, F17.213-F17.219, F17.223-F17.229, F17.293-F18.19, F18.21-
        F19.19, F19.21-F19.99, F53, F55.0-F55.8, R78.0

√5ᵗʰ   F12.1   Cannabis abuse
        EXCLUDES 1   cannabis dependence (F12.2-)
                    cannabis use, unspecified (F12.9-)

F12.10   Cannabis abuse, uncomplicated

√6ᵗʰ   F12.12   Cannabis abuse with intoxication

F12.120   Cannabis abuse with intoxication, uncomplicated

F12.121   Cannabis abuse with intoxication delirium   CC

F12.122   Cannabis abuse with intoxication with perceptual disturbance

F12.129   Cannabis abuse with intoxication, unspecified

√6ᵗʰ   F12.15   Cannabis abuse with psychotic disorder

F12.150   Cannabis abuse with psychotic disorder with delusions   CC

F12.151   Cannabis abuse with psychotic disorder with hallucinations   CC

F12.159   Cannabis abuse with psychotic disorder, unspecified

√6ᵗʰ   F12.18   Cannabis abuse with other cannabis-induced disorder

F12.180   Cannabis abuse with cannabis-induced anxiety disorder

F12.188   Cannabis abuse with other cannabis-induced disorder

F12.19   Cannabis abuse with unspecified cannabis-induced disorder

√5ᵗʰ   F12.2   Cannabis dependence
        EXCLUDES 1   cannabis abuse (F12.1-)
                    cannabis use, unspecified (F12.9-)
        EXCLUDES 2   cannabis poisoning (T40.7-)

F12.20   Cannabis dependence, uncomplicated

F12.21   Cannabis dependence, in remission

√6ᵗʰ   F12.22   Cannabis dependence with intoxication

F12.220   Cannabis dependence with intoxication, uncomplicated

F12.221   Cannabis dependence with intoxication delirium   CC

F12.222   Cannabis dependence with intoxication with perceptual disturbance

F12.229   Cannabis dependence with intoxication, unspecified

√6ᵗʰ   F12.25   Cannabis dependence with psychotic disorder

F12.250   Cannabis dependence with psychotic disorder with delusions   CC

F12.251   Cannabis dependence with psychotic disorder with hallucinations   CC

F12.259   Cannabis dependence with psychotic disorder, unspecified

√6ᵗʰ   F12.28   Cannabis dependence with other cannabis-induced disorder

F12.280   Cannabis dependence with cannabis-induced anxiety disorder

F12.288   Cannabis dependence with other cannabis-induced disorder

F12.29   Cannabis dependence with unspecified cannabis-induced disorder

√5ᵗʰ   F12.9   Cannabis use, unspecified
        EXCLUDES 1   cannabis abuse (F12.1-)
                    cannabis dependence (F12.2-)

F12.90   Cannabis use, unspecified, uncomplicated

√6ᵗʰ   F12.92   Cannabis use, unspecified with intoxication

F12.920   Cannabis use, unspecified with intoxication, uncomplicated

F12.921   Cannabis use, unspecified with intoxication delirium   CC

F12.922   Cannabis use, unspecified with intoxication with perceptual disturbance

F12.929   Cannabis use, unspecified with intoxication, unspecified

√6ᵗʰ   F12.95   Cannabis use, unspecified with psychotic disorder

F12.950   Cannabis use, unspecified with psychotic disorder with delusions   CC

F12.951   Cannabis use, unspecified with psychotic disorder with hallucinations   CC

F12.959   Cannabis use, unspecified with psychotic disorder, unspecified

√6ᵗʰ   F12.98   Cannabis use, unspecified with other cannabis-induced disorder

F12.980   Cannabis use, unspecified with anxiety disorder

F12.988   Cannabis use, unspecified with other cannabis-induced disorder

Mental, Behavioral, and Neurodevelopmental Disorders

F12.99–F13.90

F12.99   **Cannabis use, unspecified with unspecified cannabis-induced disorder**

✓4th **F13**   **Sedative, hypnotic, or anxiolytic related disorders**

CC Excl: For CC codes in category F13, unless otherwise noted: F02.80-F02.81, F04-F06.8, F10.10-F11.19, F11.21-F13.19, F13.21-F14.19, F14.21-F15.19, F15.21-F16.19, F16.21-F16.99, F17.203-F17.209, F17.213-F17.219, F17.223-F17.229, F17.293- F18.19, F18.21-F19.19, F19.21-F19.99, F53, F55.0-F55.8, R78.0

✓5th **F13.1**   **Sedative, hypnotic or anxiolytic-related abuse**
> EXCLUDES 1   sedative, hypnotic or anxiolytic-related dependence (F13.2-)
> sedative, hypnotic, or anxiolytic use, unspecified (F13.9-)

F13.10   **Sedative, hypnotic or anxiolytic abuse, uncomplicated**

✓6th **F13.12**   **Sedative, hypnotic or anxiolytic abuse with intoxication**

F13.120   **Sedative, hypnotic or anxiolytic abuse with intoxication, uncomplicated**

F13.121   **Sedative, hypnotic or anxiolytic abuse** CC **with intoxication delirium**

F13.129   **Sedative, hypnotic or anxiolytic abuse with intoxication, unspecified**

F13.14   **Sedative, hypnotic or anxiolytic abuse with sedative, hypnotic or anxiolytic-induced mood disorder**

✓6th **F13.15**   **Sedative, hypnotic or anxiolytic abuse with sedative, hypnotic or anxiolytic-induced psychotic disorder**

F13.150   **Sedative, hypnotic or anxiolytic** CC **abuse with sedative, hypnotic or anxiolytic-induced psychotic disorder with delusions**

F13.151   **Sedative, hypnotic or anxiolytic** CC **abuse with sedative, hypnotic or anxiolytic-induced psychotic disorder with hallucinations**

F13.159   **Sedative, hypnotic or anxiolytic abuse with sedative, hypnotic or anxiolytic-induced psychotic disorder, unspecified**

✓6th **F13.18**   **Sedative, hypnotic or anxiolytic abuse with other sedative, hypnotic or anxiolytic-induced disorders**

F13.180   **Sedative, hypnotic or anxiolytic abuse with sedative, hypnotic or anxiolytic-induced anxiety disorder**

F13.181   **Sedative, hypnotic or anxiolytic abuse with sedative, hypnotic or anxiolytic-induced sexual dysfunction**

F13.182   **Sedative, hypnotic or anxiolytic abuse with sedative, hypnotic or anxiolytic-induced sleep disorder**

F13.188   **Sedative, hypnotic or anxiolytic abuse with other sedative, hypnotic or anxiolytic-induced disorder**

F13.19   **Sedative, hypnotic or anxiolytic abuse with unspecified sedative, hypnotic or anxiolytic-induced disorder**

✓5th **F13.2**   **Sedative, hypnotic or anxiolytic-related dependence**
> EXCLUDES 1   sedative, hypnotic or anxiolytic-related abuse (F13.1-)
> sedative, hypnotic, or anxiolytic use, unspecified (F13.9-)
> EXCLUDES 2   sedative, hypnotic, or anxiolytic poisoning (T42.-)

F13.20   **Sedative, hypnotic or anxiolytic dependence,** CC **uncomplicated**
> CC Excl: No excl

F13.21   **Sedative, hypnotic or anxiolytic dependence, in remission**

✓6th **F13.22**   **Sedative, hypnotic or anxiolytic dependence with intoxication**
> EXCLUDES 1   sedative, hypnotic or anxiolytic dependence with withdrawal (F13.23-)

F13.220   **Sedative, hypnotic or anxiolytic dependence with intoxication, uncomplicated**

F13.221   **Sedative, hypnotic or anxiolytic** CC **dependence with intoxication delirium**
> CC Excl: See code: F13

F13.229   **Sedative, hypnotic or anxiolytic dependence with intoxication, unspecified**
> CC Excl: No Excl

✓6th **F13.23**   **Sedative, hypnotic or anxiolytic dependence with withdrawal**
> EXCLUDES 1   sedative, hypnotic or anxiolytic dependence with intoxication (F13.22-)

F13.230   **Sedative, hypnotic or anxiolytic** CC **dependence with withdrawal, uncomplicated**
> CC Excl: See code: F13

F13.231   **Sedative, hypnotic or anxiolytic** CC **dependence with withdrawal delirium**
> CC Excl: See code: F13

F13.232   **Sedative, hypnotic or anxiolytic** CC **dependence with withdrawal with perceptual disturbance**
> CC Excl: See code: F13

F13.239   **Sedative, hypnotic or anxiolytic** CC **dependence with withdrawal, unspecified**
> CC Excl: See code: F13

F13.24   **Sedative, hypnotic or anxiolytic dependence with sedative, hypnotic or anxiolytic-induced mood disorder**

✓6th **F13.25**   **Sedative, hypnotic or anxiolytic dependence with sedative, hypnotic or anxiolytic-induced psychotic disorder**

F13.250   **Sedative, hypnotic or anxiolytic** CC **dependence with sedative, hypnotic or anxiolytic-induced psychotic disorder with delusions**
> CC Excl: See code: F13

F13.251   **Sedative, hypnotic or anxiolytic** CC **dependence with sedative, hypnotic or anxiolytic-induced psychotic disorder with hallucinations**
> CC Excl: See code: F13

F13.259   **Sedative, hypnotic or anxiolytic** CC **dependence with sedative, hypnotic or anxiolytic-induced psychotic disorder, unspecified**
> CC Excl: No Excl

F13.26   **Sedative, hypnotic or anxiolytic dependence** CC **with sedative, hypnotic or anxiolytic-induced persisting amnestic disorder**
> CC Excl: No Excl

F13.27   **Sedative, hypnotic or anxiolytic dependence** CC **with sedative, hypnotic or anxiolytic-induced persisting dementia**
> CC Excl: See code: F13

✓6th **F13.28**   **Sedative, hypnotic or anxiolytic dependence with other sedative, hypnotic or anxiolytic-induced disorders**

F13.280   **Sedative, hypnotic or anxiolytic** CC **dependence with sedative, hypnotic or anxiolytic-induced anxiety disorder**
> CC Excl: No Excl

F13.281   **Sedative, hypnotic or anxiolytic** CC **dependence with sedative, hypnotic or anxiolytic-induced sexual dysfunction**
> CC Excl: No Excl

F13.282   **Sedative, hypnotic or anxiolytic** CC **dependence with sedative, hypnotic or anxiolytic-induced sleep disorder**
> CC Excl: No Excl

F13.288   **Sedative, hypnotic or anxiolytic** CC **dependence with other sedative, hypnotic or anxiolytic-induced disorder**
> CC Excl: No Excl

F13.29   **Sedative, hypnotic or anxiolytic dependence with unspecified sedative, hypnotic or anxiolytic-induced disorder**
> CC Excl: No Excl

✓5th **F13.9**   **Sedative, hypnotic or anxiolytic-related use, unspecified**
> EXCLUDES 1   sedative, hypnotic or anxiolytic-related abuse (F13.1-)
> sedative, hypnotic or anxiolytic-related dependence (F13.2-)

F13.90   **Sedative, hypnotic, or anxiolytic use, unspecified, uncomplicated**

N Newborn: 0   P Pediatric: 0-17   M Maternity: 12-55   A Adult: 15-124   MCC Major CC Condition   PDx MCC PDx acts as own MCC   CC CC Condition   PDx CC PDx acts as own CC

514   ICD-10-CM Draft (2015)

✓6th **F13.92 Sedative, hypnotic or anxiolytic use, unspecified with intoxication**
    EXCLUDES 1 *sedative, hypnotic or anxiolytic use, unspecified with withdrawal (F13.93-)*

F13.920 Sedative, hypnotic or anxiolytic use, unspecified with intoxication, uncomplicated

F13.921 Sedative, hypnotic or anxiolytic use, unspecified with intoxication delirium CC

F13.929 Sedative, hypnotic or anxiolytic use, unspecified with intoxication, unspecified

✓6th **F13.93 Sedative, hypnotic or anxiolytic use, unspecified with withdrawal**
    EXCLUDES 1 *sedative, hypnotic or anxiolytic use, unspecified with intoxication (F13.92-)*

F13.930 Sedative, hypnotic or anxiolytic use, unspecified with withdrawal, uncomplicated CC

F13.931 Sedative, hypnotic or anxiolytic use, unspecified with withdrawal delirium CC

F13.932 Sedative, hypnotic or anxiolytic use, unspecified with withdrawal with perceptual disturbances CC

F13.939 Sedative, hypnotic or anxiolytic use, unspecified with withdrawal, unspecified CC

F13.94 Sedative, hypnotic or anxiolytic use, unspecified with sedative, hypnotic or anxiolytic-induced mood disorder

✓6th **F13.95 Sedative, hypnotic or anxiolytic use, unspecified with sedative, hypnotic or anxiolytic-induced psychotic disorder**

F13.950 Sedative, hypnotic or anxiolytic use, unspecified with sedative, hypnotic or anxiolytic-induced psychotic disorder with delusions CC

F13.951 Sedative, hypnotic or anxiolytic use, unspecified with sedative, hypnotic or anxiolytic-induced psychotic disorder with hallucinations CC

F13.959 Sedative, hypnotic or anxiolytic use, unspecified with sedative, hypnotic or anxiolytic-induced psychotic disorder, unspecified

F13.96 Sedative, hypnotic or anxiolytic use, unspecified with sedative, hypnotic or anxiolytic-induced persisting amnestic disorder

F13.97 Sedative, hypnotic or anxiolytic use, unspecified with sedative, hypnotic or anxiolytic-induced persisting dementia CC

✓6th **F13.98 Sedative, hypnotic or anxiolytic use, unspecified with other sedative, hypnotic or anxiolytic-induced disorders**

F13.980 Sedative, hypnotic or anxiolytic use, unspecified with sedative, hypnotic or anxiolytic-induced anxiety disorder

F13.981 Sedative, hypnotic or anxiolytic use, unspecified with sedative, hypnotic or anxiolytic-induced sexual dysfunction

F13.982 Sedative, hypnotic or anxiolytic use, unspecified with sedative, hypnotic or anxiolytic-induced sleep disorder

F13.988 Sedative, hypnotic or anxiolytic use, unspecified with other sedative, hypnotic or anxiolytic-induced disorder

F13.99 Sedative, hypnotic or anxiolytic use, unspecified with unspecified sedative, hypnotic or anxiolytic-induced disorder

✓4th **F14 Cocaine related disorders**
    EXCLUDES 2 *other stimulant-related disorders (F15.-)*

CC Excl: For CC codes in category F14, unless otherwise noted: F02.80-F02.81, F04-F06.8, F10.10-F11.19, F11.21-F13.19, F13.21-F14.19, F14.21-F15.19, F15.21-F16.19, F16.21-F16.99, F17.203-F17.209, F17.213-F17.219, F17.223-F17.229, F17.293-F18.19, F18.21-F19.19, F19.21-F19.99, F53, F55.0-F55.8, R78.0

✓5th **F14.1 Cocaine abuse**
    EXCLUDES 1 *cocaine dependence (F14.2-)*
            cocaine use, unspecified (F14.9-)

F14.10 Cocaine abuse, uncomplicated

✓6th **F14.12 Cocaine abuse with intoxication**

F14.120 Cocaine abuse with intoxication, uncomplicated

F14.121 Cocaine abuse with intoxication with delirium CC

F14.122 Cocaine abuse with intoxication with perceptual disturbance

F14.129 Cocaine abuse with intoxication, unspecified

F14.14 Cocaine abuse with cocaine-induced mood disorder

✓6th **F14.15 Cocaine abuse with cocaine-induced psychotic disorder**

F14.150 Cocaine abuse with cocaine-induced psychotic disorder with delusions CC

F14.151 Cocaine abuse with cocaine-induced psychotic disorder with hallucinations CC

F14.159 Cocaine abuse with cocaine-induced psychotic disorder, unspecified

✓6th **F14.18 Cocaine abuse with other cocaine-induced disorder**

F14.180 Cocaine abuse with cocaine-induced anxiety disorder

F14.181 Cocaine abuse with cocaine-induced sexual dysfunction

F14.182 Cocaine abuse with cocaine-induced sleep disorder

F14.188 Cocaine abuse with other cocaine-induced disorder

F14.19 Cocaine abuse with unspecified cocaine-induced disorder

✓5th **F14.2 Cocaine dependence**
    EXCLUDES 1 *cocaine abuse (F14.1-)*
            cocaine use, unspecified (F14.9-)
    EXCLUDES 2 *cocaine poisoning (T40.5-)*

F14.20 Cocaine dependence, uncomplicated CC
    CC Excl: No Excl

F14.21 Cocaine dependence, in remission

✓6th **F14.22 Cocaine dependence with intoxication**
    EXCLUDES 1 *cocaine dependence with withdrawal (F14.23)*

F14.220 Cocaine dependence with intoxication, uncomplicated

F14.221 Cocaine dependence with intoxication delirium CC

F14.222 Cocaine dependence with intoxication with perceptual disturbance CC
    CC Excl: No Excl

F14.229 Cocaine dependence with intoxication, unspecified CC
    CC Excl: No Excl

F14.23 Cocaine dependence with withdrawal CC
    EXCLUDES 1 *cocaine dependence with intoxication (F14.22-)*

F14.24 Cocaine dependence with cocaine-induced mood disorder

✓6th **F14.25 Cocaine dependence with cocaine-induced psychotic disorder**

F14.250 Cocaine dependence with cocaine-induced psychotic disorder with delusions CC

F14.251 Cocaine dependence with cocaine-induced psychotic disorder with hallucinations CC

F14.259 Cocaine dependence with cocaine-induced psychotic disorder, unspecified CC
    CC Excl: No Excl

✓6th **F14.28 Cocaine dependence with other cocaine-induced disorder**

F14.280 Cocaine dependence with cocaine-induced anxiety disorder CC
    CC Excl: No Excl

F14.281 Cocaine dependence with cocaine-induced sexual dysfunction CC
    CC Excl: No Excl

F14.282 Cocaine dependence with cocaine-induced sleep disorder CC
    CC Excl: No Excl

✓ Additional Character Required   ✓x7th Xtension Alert   Unacceptable PDx   Manifestation   Hospital Acquired Condition   EXCLUDES 1 Not Coded Here   EXCLUDES 2 Not Included Here

Mental, Behavioral, and Neurodevelopmental Disorders

F14.288–F15.929

F14.288 **Cocaine dependence with** other **cocaine-induced disorder**   **CC**
     CC Excl: No Excl

F14.29 **Cocaine dependence with** unspecified **cocaine-induced disorder**

✓5ᵗʰ **F14.9** **Cocaine use,** unspecified
     EXCLUDES 1   cocaine abuse (F14.1-)
                cocaine dependence (F14.2-)

F14.90 **Cocaine use, unspecified,** uncomplicated

✓6ᵗʰ **F14.92** **Cocaine use, unspecified with** intoxication

     F14.920 **Cocaine use, unspecified with intoxication,** uncomplicated

     F14.921 **Cocaine use, unspecified with intoxication** delirium   **CC**

     F14.922 **Cocaine use, unspecified with intoxication with** perceptual disturbance

     F14.929 **Cocaine use, unspecified with intoxication,** unspecified

F14.94 **Cocaine use, unspecified with cocaine-induced** mood disorder

✓6ᵗʰ **F14.95** **Cocaine use, unspecified with cocaine-induced** psychotic disorder

     F14.950 **Cocaine use, unspecified with cocaine-induced psychotic disorder with** delusions   **CC**

     F14.951 **Cocaine use, unspecified with cocaine-induced psychotic disorder with** hallucinations   **CC**

     F14.959 **Cocaine use, unspecified with cocaine-induced psychotic disorder,** unspecified

✓6ᵗʰ **F14.98** **Cocaine use, unspecified with** other specified **cocaine-induced disorder**

     F14.980 **Cocaine use, unspecified with cocaine-induced** anxiety disorder

     F14.981 **Cocaine use, unspecified with cocaine-induced** sexual dysfunction

     F14.982 **Cocaine use, unspecified with cocaine-induced** sleep disorder

     F14.988 **Cocaine use, unspecified with** other **cocaine-induced disorder**

F14.99 **Cocaine use, unspecified with** unspecified **cocaine-induced disorder**

✓4ᵗʰ **F15** **Other stimulant** related disorders
     INCLUDES   amphetamine-related disorders
                 caffeine
     EXCLUDES 2   cocaine-related disorders (F14.-)

     CC Excl: For CC codes in category F15, unless otherwise noted:
     F02.80-F02.81, F04-F06.8, F10.10-F11.19, F11.21-F13.19, F13.21-
     F14.19, F14.21-F15.19, F15.21-F16.19, F16.21-F16.99, F17.203-
     F17.209, F17.213-F17.219, F17.223-F17.229, F17.293-F18.19, F18.21-
     F19.19, F19.21-F19.99, F53, F55.0-F55.8, R78.0

✓5ᵗʰ **F15.1** **Other stimulant** abuse
     EXCLUDES 1   other stimulant dependence (F15.2-)
                other stimulant use, unspecified (F15.9-)

F15.10 **Other stimulant abuse,** uncomplicated

✓6ᵗʰ **F15.12** **Other stimulant abuse with** intoxication

     F15.120 **Other stimulant abuse with intoxication,** uncomplicated

     F15.121 **Other stimulant abuse with intoxication** delirium   **CC**

     F15.122 **Other stimulant abuse with intoxication with** perceptual disturbance

     F15.129 **Other stimulant abuse with intoxication,** unspecified

F15.14 **Other stimulant abuse with stimulant-induced** mood disorder

✓6ᵗʰ **F15.15** **Other stimulant abuse with stimulant-induced** psychotic disorder

     F15.150 **Other stimulant abuse with stimulant-induced psychotic disorder with** delusions   **CC**

     F15.151 **Other stimulant abuse with stimulant-induced psychotic disorder with** hallucinations   **CC**

     F15.159 **Other stimulant abuse with stimulant-induced psychotic disorder,** unspecified

F15.18 **Other stimulant abuse with** other **stimulant-induced disorder**

     F15.180 **Other stimulant abuse with stimulant-induced** anxiety disorder

     F15.181 **Other stimulant abuse with stimulant-induced** sexual dysfunction

     F15.182 **Other stimulant abuse with stimulant-induced** sleep disorder

     F15.188 **Other stimulant abuse with** other **stimulant-induced disorder**

F15.19 **Other stimulant abuse with** unspecified **stimulant-induced disorder**

✓5ᵗʰ **F15.2** **Other stimulant** dependence
     EXCLUDES 1   other stimulant abuse (F15.1-)
                other stimulant use, unspecified (F15.9-)

F15.20 **Other stimulant dependence,** uncomplicated   **CC**
     CC Excl: No Excl

F15.21 **Other stimulant dependence, in remission**

✓6ᵗʰ **F15.22** **Other stimulant dependence with** intoxication
     EXCLUDES 1   other stimulant dependence with withdrawal
                (F15.23)

     F15.220 **Other stimulant dependence with intoxication,** uncomplicated

     F15.221 **Other stimulant dependence with intoxication** delirium   **CC**

     F15.222 **Other stimulant dependence with intoxication with** perceptual disturbance   **CC**
         CC Excl: No Excl

     F15.229 **Other stimulant dependence with intoxication,** unspecified

F15.23 **Other stimulant dependence with** withdrawal   **CC**
     EXCLUDES 1   other stimulant dependence with
                intoxication (F15.22-)

F15.24 **Other stimulant dependence with stimulant-induced** mood disorder

✓6ᵗʰ **F15.25** **Other stimulant dependence with stimulant-induced** psychotic disorder

     F15.250 **Other stimulant dependence with stimulant-induced psychotic disorder with** delusions   **CC**

     F15.251 **Other stimulant dependence with stimulant-induced psychotic disorder with** hallucinations   **CC**

     F15.259 **Other stimulant dependence with stimulant-induced psychotic disorder,** unspecified   **CC**
         CC Excl: No Excl

✓6ᵗʰ **F15.28** **Other stimulant dependence with** other **stimulant-induced disorder**

     F15.280 **Other stimulant dependence with stimulant-induced** anxiety disorder   **CC**
         CC Excl: No Excl

     F15.281 **Other stimulant dependence with stimulant-induced** sexual dysfunction   **CC**
         CC Excl: No Excl

     F15.282 **Other stimulant dependence with stimulant-induced** sleep disorder   **CC**
         CC Excl: No Excl

     F15.288 **Other stimulant dependence with** other **stimulant-induced disorder**   **CC**
         CC Excl: No Excl

F15.29 **Other stimulant dependence with** unspecified **stimulant-induced disorder**

✓5ᵗʰ **F15.9** **Other stimulant use,** unspecified
     EXCLUDES 1   other stimulant abuse (F15.1-)
                other stimulant dependence (F15.2-)

F15.90 **Other stimulant use, unspecified,** uncomplicated

✓6ᵗʰ **F15.92** **Other stimulant use, unspecified** with intoxication
     EXCLUDES 1   other stimulant use, unspecified with
                withdrawal (F15.93)

     F15.920 **Other stimulant use, unspecified with intoxication,** uncomplicated

     F15.921 **Other stimulant use, unspecified with intoxication** delirium   **CC**

     F15.922 **Other stimulant use, unspecified with intoxication with** perceptual disturbance

     F15.929 **Other stimulant use, unspecified with intoxication,** unspecified

---

N Newborn: 0   **P** Pediatric: 0-17   **M** Maternity: 12-55   **A** Adult: 15-124   **MCC** Major CC Condition   **PDx MCC** PDx acts as own MCC   **CC** CC Condition   **PDx CC** PDx acts as own CC

516   ICD-10-CM Draft (2015)

F15.93 Other stimulant use, unspecified with withdrawal `cc`
EXCLUDES 1 *other stimulant use, unspecified with intoxication (F15.92-)*

F15.94 Other stimulant use, unspecified with stimulant-induced mood disorder

✓6th **F15.95 Other stimulant use, unspecified with stimulant-induced psychotic disorder**
- **F15.950 Other stimulant use, unspecified with stimulant-induced psychotic disorder with delusions** `cc`
- **F15.951 Other stimulant use, unspecified with stimulant-induced psychotic disorder with hallucinations** `cc`
- **F15.959 Other stimulant use, unspecified with stimulant-induced psychotic disorder, unspecified**

✓6th **F15.98 Other stimulant use, unspecified with other stimulant-induced disorder**
- **F15.980 Other stimulant use, unspecified with stimulant-induced anxiety disorder**
- **F15.981 Other stimulant use, unspecified with stimulant-induced sexual dysfunction**
- **F15.982 Other stimulant use, unspecified with stimulant-induced sleep disorder**
- **F15.988 Other stimulant use, unspecified with other stimulant-induced disorder**

F15.99 Other stimulant use, unspecified with unspecified stimulant-induced disorder

✓4th **F16 Hallucinogen related disorders**
INCLUDES ecstasy
PCP
phencyclidine

CC Excl: For CC codes in category F16, unless otherwise noted: F02.80-F02.81, F04-F06.8, F10.10-F11.19, F11.21-F13.19, F13.21-F14.19, F14.21-F15.19, F15.21-F16.19, F16.21-F16.99, F17.203-F17.209, F17.213-F17.219, F17.223-F17.229, F17.293-F18.19, F18.21-F19.19, F19.21-F19.99, F53, F55.0-F55.8, R78.0

✓5th **F16.1 Hallucinogen abuse**
EXCLUDES 1 *hallucinogen dependence (F16.2-)*
hallucinogen use, unspecified (F16.9-)
- **F16.10 Hallucinogen abuse, uncomplicated**
- ✓6th **F16.12 Hallucinogen abuse with intoxication**
  - **F16.120 Hallucinogen abuse with intoxication, uncomplicated**
  - **F16.121 Hallucinogen abuse with intoxication with delirium** `cc`
  - **F16.122 Hallucinogen abuse with intoxication with perceptual disturbance**
  - **F16.129 Hallucinogen abuse with intoxication, unspecified**
- **F16.14 Hallucinogen abuse with hallucinogen-induced mood disorder**
- ✓6th **F16.15 Hallucinogen abuse with hallucinogen-induced psychotic disorder**
  - **F16.150 Hallucinogen abuse with hallucinogen-induced psychotic disorder with delusions** `cc`
  - **F16.151 Hallucinogen abuse with hallucinogen-induced psychotic disorder with hallucinations** `cc`
  - **F16.159 Hallucinogen abuse with hallucinogen-induced psychotic disorder, unspecified**
- ✓6th **F16.18 Hallucinogen abuse with other hallucinogen-induced disorder**
  - **F16.180 Hallucinogen abuse with hallucinogen-induced anxiety disorder**
  - **F16.183 Hallucinogen abuse with hallucinogen-induced persisting perception disorder (flashbacks)**
  - **F16.188 Hallucinogen abuse with other hallucinogen-induced disorder**
- **F16.19 Hallucinogen abuse with unspecified hallucinogen-induced disorder**

✓5th **F16.2 Hallucinogen dependence**
EXCLUDES 1 *hallucinogen abuse (F16.1-)*
hallucinogen use, unspecified (F16.9-)
- **F16.20 Hallucinogen dependence, uncomplicated** `cc`
  CC Excl: No Excl
- **F16.21 Hallucinogen dependence, in remission**
- ✓6th **F16.22 Hallucinogen dependence with intoxication**
  - **F16.220 Hallucinogen dependence with intoxication, uncomplicated**
  - **F16.221 Hallucinogen dependence with intoxication with delirium** `cc`
  - **F16.229 Hallucinogen dependence with intoxication, unspecified**
- **F16.24 Hallucinogen dependence with hallucinogen-induced mood disorder**
- ✓6th **F16.25 Hallucinogen dependence with hallucinogen-induced psychotic disorder**
  - **F16.250 Hallucinogen dependence with hallucinogen-induced psychotic disorder with delusions** `cc`
  - **F16.251 Hallucinogen dependence with hallucinogen-induced psychotic disorder with hallucinations** `cc`
  - **F16.259 Hallucinogen dependence with hallucinogen-induced psychotic disorder, unspecified** `cc`
    CC Excl: No Excl
- ✓6th **F16.28 Hallucinogen dependence with other hallucinogen-induced disorder**
  - **F16.280 Hallucinogen dependence with hallucinogen-induced anxiety disorder** `cc`
    CC Excl: No Excl
  - **F16.283 Hallucinogen dependence with hallucinogen persisting perception disorder (flashbacks)** `cc`
    CC Excl: No Excl
  - **F16.288 Hallucinogen dependence with other hallucinogen-induced disorder** `cc`
    CC Excl: No Excl
- **F16.29 Hallucinogen dependence with unspecified hallucinogen-induced disorder**

✓5th **F16.9 Hallucinogen use, unspecified**
EXCLUDES 1 *hallucinogen abuse (F16.1-)*
hallucinogen dependence (F16.2-)
- **F16.90 Hallucinogen use, unspecified, uncomplicated**
- ✓6th **F16.92 Hallucinogen use, unspecified with intoxication**
  - **F16.920 Hallucinogen use, unspecified with intoxication, uncomplicated**
  - **F16.921 Hallucinogen use, unspecified with intoxication with delirium** `cc`
  - **F16.929 Hallucinogen use, unspecified with intoxication, unspecified**
- **F16.94 Hallucinogen use, unspecified with hallucinogen-induced mood disorder**
- ✓6th **F16.95 Hallucinogen use, unspecified with hallucinogen-induced psychotic disorder**
  - **F16.950 Hallucinogen use, unspecified with hallucinogen-induced psychotic disorder with delusions** `cc`
  - **F16.951 Hallucinogen use, unspecified with hallucinogen-induced psychotic disorder with hallucinations** `cc`
  - **F16.959 Hallucinogen use, unspecified with hallucinogen-induced psychotic disorder, unspecified**
- ✓6th **F16.98 Hallucinogen use, unspecified with other specified hallucinogen-induced disorder**
  - **F16.980 Hallucinogen use, unspecified with hallucinogen-induced anxiety disorder**
  - **F16.983 Hallucinogen use, unspecified with hallucinogen persisting perception disorder (flashbacks)**
  - **F16.988 Hallucinogen use, unspecified with other hallucinogen-induced disorder**
- **F16.99 Hallucinogen use, unspecified with unspecified hallucinogen-induced disorder**

✓4ᵗʰ **F17 Nicotine dependence**

   EXCLUDES 1   history of tobacco dependence (Z87.891)
             tobacco use NOS (Z72.0)
   EXCLUDES 2   tobacco use (smoking) during pregnancy, childbirth and the
             puerperium (O99.33-)
             toxic effect of nicotine (T65.2-)
   AHA: 2013, 4Q, 108-109

CC Excl: For CC codes in category F17, unless otherwise noted:
F02.80-F02.81, F04-F06.8, F10.10-F11.19, F11.21-F13.19, F13.21-
F14.19, F14.21-F15.19, F15.21-F16.19, F16.21-F16.99, F17.203-
F17.209, F17.213-F17.219, F17.223-F17.229, F17.293-F18.19, F18.21-
F19.19, F19.21-F19.99, F53, F55.0-F55.8, R78.0

   ✓5ᵗʰ **F17.2 Nicotine dependence**

     ✓6ᵗʰ **F17.20 Nicotine dependence, unspecified**
         F17.200 Nicotine dependence, unspecified, uncomplicated
         F17.201 Nicotine dependence, unspecified, in remission
         F17.203 Nicotine dependence unspecified, withdrawal CC
         F17.208 Nicotine dependence, unspecified, with other nicotine-induced disorders
         F17.209 Nicotine dependence, unspecified, with unspecified nicotine-induced disorders

     ✓6ᵗʰ **F17.21 Nicotine dependence, cigarettes**
         F17.210 Nicotine dependence, cigarettes, uncomplicated
         F17.211 Nicotine dependence, cigarettes, in remission
         F17.213 Nicotine dependence, cigarettes, with withdrawal CC
         F17.218 Nicotine dependence, cigarettes, with other nicotine-induced disorders
         F17.219 Nicotine dependence, cigarettes, with unspecified nicotine-induced disorders

     ✓6ᵗʰ **F17.22 Nicotine dependence, chewing tobacco**
         F17.220 Nicotine dependence, chewing tobacco, uncomplicated
         F17.221 Nicotine dependence, chewing tobacco, in remission
         F17.223 Nicotine dependence, chewing tobacco, with withdrawal CC
         F17.228 Nicotine dependence, chewing tobacco, with other nicotine-induced disorders
         F17.229 Nicotine dependence, chewing tobacco, with unspecified nicotine-induced disorders

     ✓6ᵗʰ **F17.29 Nicotine dependence, other tobacco product**
         F17.290 Nicotine dependence, other tobacco product, uncomplicated
         F17.291 Nicotine dependence, other tobacco product, in remission
         F17.293 Nicotine dependence, other tobacco product, with withdrawal CC
         F17.298 Nicotine dependence, other tobacco product, with other nicotine-induced disorders
         F17.299 Nicotine dependence, other tobacco product, with unspecified nicotine-induced disorders

✓4ᵗʰ **F18 Inhalant related disorders**

   INCLUDES   volatile solvents

CC Excl: For CC codes in category F18, unless otherwise noted:
F02.80-F02.81, F04-F06.8, F10.10-F11.19, F11.21-F13.19, F13.21-
F14.19, F14.21-F15.19, F15.21-F16.19, F16.21-F16.99, F17.203-
F17.209, F17.213-F17.219, F17.223-F17.229, F17.293-F18.19, F18.21-
F19.19, F19.21-F19.99, F53, F55.0-F55.8, R78.0

   ✓5ᵗʰ **F18.1 Inhalant abuse**
    EXCLUDES 1   inhalant dependence (F18.2-)
             inhalant use, unspecified (F18.9-)
     F18.10 Inhalant abuse, uncomplicated
     ✓6ᵗʰ **F18.12 Inhalant abuse with intoxication**
         F18.120 Inhalant abuse with intoxication, uncomplicated
         F18.121 Inhalant abuse with intoxication delirium CC

         F18.129 Inhalant abuse with intoxication, unspecified
     F18.14 Inhalant abuse with inhalant-induced mood disorder
     ✓6ᵗʰ **F18.15 Inhalant abuse with inhalant-induced psychotic disorder**
         F18.150 Inhalant abuse with inhalant-induced psychotic disorder with delusions CC
         F18.151 Inhalant abuse with inhalant-induced psychotic disorder with hallucinations CC
         F18.159 Inhalant abuse with inhalant-induced psychotic disorder, unspecified
     F18.17 Inhalant abuse with inhalant-induced dementia CC
     ✓6ᵗʰ **F18.18 Inhalant abuse with other inhalant-induced disorders**
         F18.180 Inhalant abuse with inhalant-induced anxiety disorder
         F18.188 Inhalant abuse with other inhalant-induced disorder
     F18.19 Inhalant abuse with unspecified inhalant-induced disorder

   ✓5ᵗʰ **F18.2 Inhalant dependence**
    EXCLUDES 1   inhalant abuse (F18.1-)
             inhalant use, unspecified (F18.9-)
     F18.20 Inhalant dependence, uncomplicated CC
       CC Excl: No Excl
     F18.21 Inhalant dependence, in remission
     ✓6ᵗʰ **F18.22 Inhalant dependence with intoxication**
         F18.220 Inhalant dependence with intoxication, uncomplicated
         F18.221 Inhalant dependence with intoxication delirium CC
         F18.229 Inhalant dependence with intoxication, unspecified
     F18.24 Inhalant dependence with inhalant-induced mood disorder
     ✓6ᵗʰ **F18.25 Inhalant dependence with inhalant-induced psychotic disorder**
         F18.250 Inhalant dependence with inhalant-induced psychotic disorder with delusions CC
         F18.251 Inhalant dependence with inhalant-induced psychotic disorder with hallucinations CC
         F18.259 Inhalant dependence with inhalant-induced psychotic disorder, unspecified CC
           CC Excl: No Excl
     F18.27 Inhalant dependence with inhalant-induced dementia CC
     ✓6ᵗʰ **F18.28 Inhalant dependence with other inhalant-induced disorders**
         F18.280 Inhalant dependence with inhalant-induced anxiety disorder CC
           CC Excl: No Excl
         F18.288 Inhalant dependence with other inhalant-induced disorder CC
           CC Excl: No Excl
     F18.29 Inhalant dependence with unspecified inhalant-induced disorder
       CC Excl: No Excl

   ✓5ᵗʰ **F18.9 Inhalant use, unspecified**
    EXCLUDES 1   inhalant abuse (F18.1-)
             inhalant dependence (F18.2-)
     F18.90 Inhalant use, unspecified, uncomplicated
     ✓6ᵗʰ **F18.92 Inhalant use, unspecified with intoxication**
         F18.920 Inhalant use, unspecified with intoxication, uncomplicated
         F18.921 Inhalant use, unspecified with intoxication with delirium CC
         F18.929 Inhalant use, unspecified with intoxication, unspecified
     F18.94 Inhalant use, unspecified with inhalant-induced mood disorder
     ✓6ᵗʰ **F18.95 Inhalant use, unspecified with inhalant-induced psychotic disorder**
         F18.950 Inhalant use, unspecified with inhalant-induced psychotic disorder with delusions CC

N Newborn: 0   P Pediatric: 0-17   M Maternity: 12-55   A Adult: 15-124   MCC Major CC Condition   PDx MCC PDx acts as own MCC   CC CC Condition   PDx CC PDx acts as own CC

F18.951 **Inhalant use, unspecified with inhalant-induced psychotic disorder with hallucinations** `CC`

F18.959 **Inhalant use, unspecified with inhalant-induced psychotic disorder, unspecified**

F18.97 **Inhalant use, unspecified with inhalant-induced persisting dementia** `CC`

√6ᵗʰ F18.98 **Inhalant use, unspecified with other inhalant-induced disorders**

F18.980 **Inhalant use, unspecified with inhalant-induced anxiety disorder**

F18.988 **Inhalant use, unspecified with other inhalant-induced disorder**

F18.99 **Inhalant use, unspecified with unspecified inhalant-induced disorder**

√4ᵗʰ **F19 Other psychoactive substance related disorders**

INCLUDES polysubstance drug use (indiscriminate drug use)

CC Excl: For CC codes in category F19, unless otherwise noted: F02.80-F02.81, F04-F06.8, F10.10-F11.19, F11.21-F13.19, F13.21-F14.19, F14.21-F15.19, F15.21-F16.19, F16.21-F16.99, F17.203-F17.209, F17.213-F17.219, F17.223-F17.229, F17.293-F18.19, F18.21-F19.19, F19.21-F19.99, F53, F55.0-F55.8, R78.0

√5ᵗʰ F19.1 **Other psychoactive substance abuse**

EXCLUDES1 other psychoactive substance dependence (F19.2-)
other psychoactive substance use, unspecified (F19.9-)

F19.10 **Other psychoactive substance abuse, uncomplicated**

√6ᵗʰ F19.12 **Other psychoactive substance abuse with intoxication**

F19.120 **Other psychoactive substance abuse with intoxication, uncomplicated**

F19.121 **Other psychoactive substance abuse with intoxication delirium** `CC`

F19.122 **Other psychoactive substance abuse with intoxication with perceptual disturbances**

F19.129 **Other psychoactive substance abuse with intoxication, unspecified**

F19.14 **Other psychoactive substance abuse with psychoactive substance-induced mood disorder**

√6ᵗʰ F19.15 **Other psychoactive substance abuse with psychoactive substance-induced psychotic disorder**

F19.150 **Other psychoactive substance abuse with psychoactive substance-induced psychotic disorder with delusions** `CC`

F19.151 **Other psychoactive substance abuse with psychoactive substance-induced psychotic disorder with hallucinations** `CC`

F19.159 **Other psychoactive substance abuse with psychoactive substance-induced psychotic disorder, unspecified**

F19.16 **Other psychoactive substance abuse with psychoactive substance-induced persisting amnestic disorder**

F19.17 **Other psychoactive substance abuse with psychoactive substance-induced persisting dementia** `CC`

√6ᵗʰ F19.18 **Other psychoactive substance abuse with other psychoactive substance-induced disorders**

F19.180 **Other psychoactive substance abuse with psychoactive substance-induced anxiety disorder**

F19.181 **Other psychoactive substance abuse with psychoactive substance-induced sexual dysfunction**

F19.182 **Other psychoactive substance abuse with psychoactive substance-induced sleep disorder**

F19.188 **Other psychoactive substance abuse with other psychoactive substance-induced disorder**

F19.19 **Other psychoactive substance abuse with unspecified psychoactive substance-induced disorder**

√5ᵗʰ F19.2 **Other psychoactive substance dependence**

EXCLUDES1 other psychoactive substance abuse (F19.1-)
other psychoactive substance use, unspecified (F19.9-)

F19.20 **Other psychoactive substance dependence, uncomplicated** `CC`
CC Excl: No Excl

F19.21 **Other psychoactive substance dependence, in remission**

√6ᵗʰ F19.22 **Other psychoactive substance dependence with intoxication**

EXCLUDES1 other psychoactive substance dependence with withdrawal (F19.23-)

F19.220 **Other psychoactive substance dependence with intoxication, uncomplicated**

F19.221 **Other psychoactive substance dependence with intoxication delirium** `CC`

F19.222 **Other psychoactive substance dependence with intoxication with perceptual disturbance** `CC`
CC Excl: No Excl

F19.229 **Other psychoactive substance dependence with intoxication, unspecified**

√6ᵗʰ F19.23 **Other psychoactive substance dependence with withdrawal**

EXCLUDES1 other psychoactive substance dependence with intoxication (F19.22-)

F19.230 **Other psychoactive substance dependence with withdrawal, uncomplicated** `CC`

F19.231 **Other psychoactive substance dependence with withdrawal delirium** `CC`

F19.232 **Other psychoactive substance dependence with withdrawal with perceptual disturbance** `CC`

F19.239 **Other psychoactive substance dependence with withdrawal, unspecified** `CC`

F19.24 **Other psychoactive substance dependence with psychoactive substance-induced mood disorder**

√6ᵗʰ F19.25 **Other psychoactive substance dependence with psychoactive substance-induced psychotic disorder**

F19.250 **Other psychoactive substance dependence with psychoactive substance-induced psychotic disorder with delusions** `CC`

F19.251 **Other psychoactive substance dependence with psychoactive substance-induced psychotic disorder with hallucinations** `CC`

F19.259 **Other psychoactive substance dependence with psychoactive substance-induced psychotic disorder, unspecified** `CC`
CC Excl: No Excl

F19.26 **Other psychoactive substance dependence with psychoactive substance-induced persisting amnestic disorder** `CC`
CC Excl: No Excl

F19.27 **Other psychoactive substance dependence with psychoactive substance-induced persisting dementia** `CC`

√6ᵗʰ F19.28 **Other psychoactive substance dependence with other psychoactive substance-induced disorders**

F19.280 **Other psychoactive substance dependence with psychoactive substance-induced anxiety disorder** `CC`
CC Excl: No Excl

F19.281 **Other psychoactive substance dependence with psychoactive substance-induced sexual dysfunction** `CC`
CC Excl: No Excl

F19.282 **Other psychoactive substance dependence with psychoactive substance-induced sleep disorder** `CC`
CC Excl: No Excl

F19.288 **Other psychoactive substance dependence with other psychoactive substance-induced disorder** `CC`
CC Excl: No Excl

F19.29 **Other psychoactive substance dependence with unspecified psychoactive substance-induced disorder**

√5th **F19.9 Other psychoactive substance use, unspecified**
- EXCLUDES 1 *other psychoactive substance abuse (F19.1-)*
  other psychoactive substance dependence (F19.2-)

F19.90 Other psychoactive substance use, unspecified, uncomplicated

√6th **F19.92 Other psychoactive substance use, unspecified with intoxication**
- EXCLUDES 1 *other psychoactive substance use, unspecified with withdrawal (F19.93)*

  F19.920 Other psychoactive substance use, unspecified with intoxication, uncomplicated

  F19.921 Other psychoactive substance use, unspecified with intoxication with delirium CC

  F19.922 Other psychoactive substance use, unspecified with intoxication with perceptual disturbance

  F19.929 Other psychoactive substance use, unspecified with intoxication, unspecified

√6th **F19.93 Other psychoactive substance use, unspecified with withdrawal**
- EXCLUDES 1 *other psychoactive substance use, unspecified with intoxication (F19.92-)*

  F19.930 Other psychoactive substance use, unspecified with withdrawal, uncomplicated CC

  F19.931 Other psychoactive substance use, unspecified with withdrawal delirium CC

  F19.932 Other psychoactive substance use, unspecified with withdrawal with perceptual disturbance CC

  F19.939 Other psychoactive substance use, unspecified with withdrawal, unspecified CC

F19.94 Other psychoactive substance use, unspecified with psychoactive substance-induced mood disorder

√6th **F19.95 Other psychoactive substance use, unspecified with psychoactive substance-induced psychotic disorder**

  F19.950 Other psychoactive substance use, unspecified with psychoactive substance-induced psychotic disorder with delusions CC

  F19.951 Other psychoactive substance use, unspecified with psychoactive substance-induced psychotic disorder with hallucinations CC

  F19.959 Other psychoactive substance use, unspecified with psychoactive substance-induced psychotic disorder, unspecified

F19.96 Other psychoactive substance use, unspecified with psychoactive substance-induced persisting amnestic disorder

F19.97 Other psychoactive substance use, unspecified with psychoactive substance-induced persisting dementia CC

√6th **F19.98 Other psychoactive substance use, unspecified with other psychoactive substance-induced disorders**

  F19.980 Other psychoactive substance use, unspecified with psychoactive substance-induced anxiety disorder

  F19.981 Other psychoactive substance use, unspecified with psychoactive substance-induced sexual dysfunction

  F19.982 Other psychoactive substance use, unspecified with psychoactive substance-induced sleep disorder

  F19.988 Other psychoactive substance use, unspecified with other psychoactive substance-induced disorder

F19.99 Other psychoactive substance use, unspecified with unspecified psychoactive substance-induced disorder

Schizophrenia, schizotypal, delusional, and other non-mood psychotic disorders (F20-F29)

√4th **F20 Schizophrenia**
- EXCLUDES 1 *brief psychotic disorder (F23)*
  cyclic schizophrenia (F25.0)
  mood [affective] disorders with psychotic symptoms (F30.2, F31.2, F31.5, F31.64, F32.3, F33.3)
  schizoaffective disorder (F25.-)
  schizophrenic reaction NOS (F23)
- EXCLUDES 2 *schizophrenic reaction in:*
  alcoholism (F10.15-, F10.25-, F10.95-)
  brain disease (F06.2)
  epilepsy (F06.2)
  psychoactive drug use (F11-F19 with .15. .25, .95)
  schizotypal disorder (F21)

> **CC Excl: For CC codes in category F20, unless otherwise noted:** F07.0-F07.81, F07.9-F09, F20.0-F48.1, F48.8-F51.03, F51.12, F51.19, F51.3-F51.9, F52.5, F54, F59-F63.2, F63.81-F63.9, F68.10-F80.2, F80.4, F80.89-F84.0, F84.3-F99, G44.201-G44.229, H93.25, R45.1-R45.2, R45.5-R45.82, R45.86-R45.87

F20.0 Paranoid schizophrenia CC
Paraphrenic schizophrenia
- EXCLUDES 1 *involutional paranoid state (F22)*
  paranoia (F22)

F20.1 Disorganized schizophrenia CC
Hebephrenic schizophrenia
Hebephrenia

F20.2 Catatonic schizophrenia CC
Schizophrenic catalepsy
Schizophrenic catatonia
Schizophrenic flexibilitas cerea
- EXCLUDES 1 *catatonic stupor (R40.1)*

F20.3 Undifferentiated schizophrenia
Atypical schizophrenia
- EXCLUDES 1 *acute schizophrenia-like psychotic disorder (F23)*
- EXCLUDES 2 *post-schizophrenic depression (F32.8)*

F20.5 Residual schizophrenia CC
Restzustand (schizophrenic)
Schizophrenic residual state

√5th **F20.8 Other schizophrenia**

  F20.81 Schizophreniform disorder CC
  Schizophreniform psychosis NOS

  F20.89 Other schizophrenia CC
  Cenesthopathic schizophrenia
  Simple schizophrenia

F20.9 Schizophrenia, unspecified

F21 Schizotypal disorder
Borderline schizophrenia
Latent schizophrenia
Latent schizophrenic reaction
Prepsychotic schizophrenia
Prodromal schizophrenia
Pseudoneurotic schizophrenia
Pseudopsychopathic schizophrenia
Schizotypal personality disorder
- EXCLUDES 2 *Asperger's syndrome (F84.5)*
  schizoid personality disorder (F60.1)

F22 Delusional disorders
Delusional dysmorphophobia
Involutional paranoid state
Paranoia
Paranoia querulans
Paranoid psychosis
Paranoid state
Paraphrenia (late)
Sensitiver Beziehungswahn
- EXCLUDES 1 *mood [affective] disorders with psychotic symptoms (F30.2, F31.2, F31.5, F31.64, F32.3, F33.3)*
  paranoid schizophrenia (F20.0)
- EXCLUDES 2 *paranoid personality disorder (F60.0)*
  paranoid psychosis, psychogenic (F23)
  paranoid reaction (F23)

F23 Brief psychotic disorder CC
Paranoid reaction
Psychogenic paranoid psychosis
- EXCLUDES 2 *mood [affective] disorders with psychotic symptoms (F30.2, F31.2, F31.5, F31.64, F32.3, F33.3)*

CC Excl: No Excl

N Newborn: 0   P Pediatric: 0-17   M Maternity: 12-55   A Adult: 15-124   MCC Major CC Condition   PDx MCC PDx acts as own MCC   CC CC Condition   PDx CC PDx acts as own CC

520   ICD-10-CM Draft (2015)

F24 Shared psychotic disorder
Folie à deux
Induced paranoid disorder
Induced psychotic disorder

✓4ᵗʰ F25 Schizoaffective disorders
EXCLUDES 1 mood [affective] disorders with psychotic symptoms (F30.2, F31.2, F31.5, F31.64, F32.3, F33.3)
schizophrenia (F20.-)

F25.0 Schizoaffective disorder, bipolar type
Cyclic schizophrenia
Schizoaffective disorder, manic type
Schizoaffective disorder, mixed type
Schizoaffective psychosis, bipolar type
Schizophreniform psychosis, manic type

F25.1 Schizoaffective disorder, depressive type
Schizoaffective psychosis, depressive type
Schizophreniform psychosis, depressive type

F25.8 Other schizoaffective disorders

F25.9 Schizoaffective disorder, unspecified
Schizoaffective psychosis NOS

F28 Other psychotic disorder not due to a substance or known physiological condition [HIV]
Chronic hallucinatory psychosis

F29 Unspecified psychosis not due to a substance or known physiological condition [HIV]
Psychosis NOS
EXCLUDES 1 mental disorder NOS (F99)
unspecified mental disorder due to known physiological condition (F09)

Mood [affective] disorders (F30-F39)

✓4ᵗʰ F30 Manic episode
INCLUDES bipolar disorder, single manic episode
mixed affective episode
EXCLUDES 1 bipolar disorder (F31.-)
major depressive disorder, recurrent (F33.-)
major depressive disorder, single episode (F32.-)

CC Excl: For CC codes in category F30, unless otherwise noted:
F07.0-F07.81, F07.9-F09, F20.0-F48.1, F48.8-F51.03, F51.12, F51.19, F51.3-F51.9, F52.5, F54, F59-F63.2, F63.81-F63.9, F68.10-F80.2, F80.4, F80.89-F84.0, F84.3-F99, G44.201-G44.229, H93.25, R45.1-R45.2, R45.5-R45.82, R45.86-R45.87

✓5ᵗʰ F30.1 Manic episode without psychotic symptoms
F30.10 Manic episode without psychotic symptoms, unspecified [CC]
F30.11 Manic episode without psychotic symptoms, mild [CC]
F30.12 Manic episode without psychotic symptoms, moderate [CC]
F30.13 Manic episode, severe, without psychotic symptoms [CC]
CC Excl: F30.13-F30.2, F31.13-F31.2, F31.4-F31.5, F31.63-F31.64

F30.2 Manic episode, severe with psychotic symptoms [CC]
Manic stupor
Mania with mood-congruent psychotic symptoms
Mania with mood-incongruent psychotic symptoms

F30.3 Manic episode in partial remission

F30.4 Manic episode in full remission

F30.8 Other manic episodes
Hypomania

F30.9 Manic episode, unspecified [CC]
Mania NOS

✓4ᵗʰ F31 Bipolar disorder
INCLUDES manic-depressive illness
manic-depressive psychosis
manic-depressive reaction
EXCLUDES 1 bipolar disorder, single manic episode (F30.-)
major depressive disorder, single episode (F32.-)
major depressive disorder, recurrent (F33.-)
EXCLUDES 2 cyclothymia (F34.0)

CC Excl: For CC codes in category F31, unless otherwise noted:
F07.0-F07.81, F07.9-F09, F20.0-F48.1, F48.8-F51.03, F51.12, F51.19, F51.3-F51.9, F52.5, F54, F59-F63.2, F63.81-F63.9, F68.10-F80.2, F80.4, F80.89-F84.0, F84.3-F99, G44.201-G44.229, H93.25, R45.1-R45.2, R45.5-R45.82, R45.86-R45.87

F31.0 Bipolar disorder, current episode hypomanic [CC]

✓5ᵗʰ F31.1 Bipolar disorder, current episode manic without psychotic features
F31.10 Bipolar disorder, current episode manic without psychotic features, unspecified [CC]
F31.11 Bipolar disorder, current episode manic without psychotic features, mild [CC]
F31.12 Bipolar disorder, current episode manic without psychotic features, moderate [CC]
F31.13 Bipolar disorder, current episode manic without psychotic features, severe [CC]
CC Excl: F31.13-F31.2, F31.63-F31.64

F31.2 Bipolar disorder, current episode manic severe with psychotic features [CC]
Bipolar disorder, current episode manic with mood-congruent psychotic symptoms
Bipolar disorder, current episode manic with mood-incongruent psychotic symptoms

✓5ᵗʰ F31.3 Bipolar disorder, current episode depressed, mild or moderate severity
F31.30 Bipolar disorder, current episode depressed, mild or moderate severity, unspecified [CC]
F31.31 Bipolar disorder, current episode depressed, mild [CC]
F31.32 Bipolar disorder, current episode depressed, moderate [CC]

F31.4 Bipolar disorder, current episode depressed, severe, without psychotic features [CC]
CC Excl: F31.13-F31.2, F31.4-F31.5, F31.63-F31.64

F31.5 Bipolar disorder, current episode depressed, severe, with psychotic features [CC]
Bipolar disorder, current episode depressed with mood-incongruent psychotic symptoms
Bipolar disorder, current episode depressed with mood-congruent psychotic symptoms

✓5ᵗʰ F31.6 Bipolar disorder, current episode mixed
F31.60 Bipolar disorder, current episode mixed, unspecified [CC]
F31.61 Bipolar disorder, current episode mixed, mild [CC]
F31.62 Bipolar disorder, current episode mixed, moderate [CC]
F31.63 Bipolar disorder, current episode mixed, severe, without psychotic features [CC]
CC Excl: See code: F31.4
F31.64 Bipolar disorder, current episode mixed, severe, with psychotic features [CC]
Bipolar disorder, current episode mixed with mood-congruent psychotic symptoms
Bipolar disorder, current episode mixed with mood-incongruent psychotic symptoms

✓5ᵗʰ F31.7 Bipolar disorder, currently in remission
F31.70 Bipolar disorder, currently in remission, most recent episode unspecified
F31.71 Bipolar disorder, in partial remission, most recent episode hypomanic
F31.72 Bipolar disorder, in full remission, most recent episode hypomanic
F31.73 Bipolar disorder, in partial remission, most recent episode manic
F31.74 Bipolar disorder, in full remission, most recent episode manic
F31.75 Bipolar disorder, in partial remission, most recent episode depressed
F31.76 Bipolar disorder, in full remission, most recent episode depressed
F31.77 Bipolar disorder, in partial remission, most recent episode mixed
F31.78 Bipolar disorder, in full remission, most recent episode mixed

✓5ᵗʰ F31.8 Other bipolar disorders
F31.81 Bipolar II disorder [CC]
F31.89 Other bipolar disorder [CC]
Recurrent manic episodes NOS

F31.9 Bipolar disorder, unspecified

✓4th **F32	Major depressive disorder, single episode**
INCLUDES	single episode of agitated depression
single episode of depressive reaction
single episode of major depression
single episode of psychogenic depression
single episode of reactive depression
single episode of vital depression
EXCLUDES 1	*bipolar disorder (F31.-)*
manic episode (F30.-)
recurrent depressive disorder (F33.-)
EXCLUDES 2	*adjustment disorder (F43.2)*

CC Excl: For CC codes in category F32, unless otherwise noted:
F32.0-F32.3, F33.0-F33.40, F33.9

**F32.0	Major depressive disorder, single episode, mild**	CC
**F32.1	Major depressive disorder, single episode, moderate**	CC
**F32.2	Major depressive disorder, single episode, severe without psychotic features**	CC
**F32.3	Major depressive disorder, single episode, severe with psychotic features**	CC
Single episode of major depression with mood-congruent psychotic symptoms
Single episode of major depression with mood-incongruent psychotic symptoms
Single episode of major depression with psychotic symptoms
Single episode of psychogenic depressive psychosis
Single episode of psychotic depression
Single episode of reactive depressive psychosis
**F32.4	Major depressive disorder, single episode, in partial remission**
**F32.5	Major depressive disorder, single episode, in full remission**
**F32.8	Other depressive episodes**
Atypical depression
Post-schizophrenic depression
Single episode of 'masked' depression NOS
**F32.9	Major depressive disorder, single episode, unspecified**
Depression NOS
Depressive disorder NOS
Major depression NOS
AHA: 2013, 4Q, 107

✓4th **F33	Major depressive disorder, recurrent**
Recurrent episodes of depressive reaction
Recurrent episodes of endogenous depression
Recurrent episodes of major depression
Recurrent episodes of psychogenic depression
Recurrent episodes of reactive depression
Recurrent episodes of seasonal depressive disorder
Recurrent episodes of vital depression
EXCLUDES 1	*bipolar disorder (F31.-)*
manic episode (F30.-)

**F33.0	Major depressive disorder, recurrent, mild**	CC
CC Excl: See code: F32
**F33.1	Major depressive disorder, recurrent, moderate**	CC
CC Excl: See code: F32
**F33.2	Major depressive disorder, recurrent, severe without psychotic features**	CC
CC Excl: See code: F32
**F33.3	Major depressive disorder, recurrent, severe with psychotic symptoms**	CC
Endogenous depression with psychotic symptoms
Recurrent severe episodes of major depression with mood-congruent psychotic symptoms
Recurrent severe episodes of major depression with mood-incongruent psychotic symptoms
Recurrent severe episodes of major depression with psychotic symptoms
Recurrent severe episodes of psychogenic depressive psychosis
Recurrent severe episodes of psychotic depression
Recurrent severe episodes of reactive depressive psychosis
CC Excl: F07.0-F07.81, F07.9-F09, F20.0-F48.1, F48.8-F51.03,
F51.12, F51.19, F51.3-F51.9, F52.5, F54, F59-F63.2, F63.81-F63.9,
F68.10-F80.4, F80.89-F84.0, F84.3-F99, G44.201-G44.229, H93.25,
R45.1-R45.2, R45.5-R45.82, R45.86-R45.87

✓5th **F33.4	Major depressive disorder, recurrent, in remission**
**F33.40	Major depressive disorder, recurrent, in remission, unspecified**	CC
CC Excl: See code: F32
**F33.41	Major depressive disorder, recurrent, in partial remission**
**F33.42	Major depressive disorder, recurrent, in full remission**

**F33.8	Other recurrent depressive disorders**	CC
Recurrent brief depressive episodes
CC Excl: See code: F33.3
**F33.9	Major depressive disorder, recurrent, unspecified**	CC
Monopolar depression NOS
CC Excl: See code: F32

✓4th **F34	Persistent mood [affective] disorders**
**F34.0	Cyclothymic disorder**
Affective personality disorder
Cycloid personality
Cyclothymia
Cyclothymic personality
**F34.1	Dysthymic disorder**
Depressive neurosis
Depressive personality disorder
Dysthymia
Neurotic depression
Persistent anxiety depression
EXCLUDES 2	*anxiety depression (mild or not persistent) (F41.8)*
**F34.8	Other persistent mood [affective] disorders**	CC
CC Excl: See code: F33.3
**F34.9	Persistent mood [affective] disorder, unspecified**	CC
CC Excl: See code: F33.3

**F39	Unspecified mood [affective] disorder**
Affective psychosis NOS

Anxiety, dissociative, stress-related, somatoform and other nonpsychotic mental disorders (F40-F48)

✓4th **F40	Phobic anxiety disorders**
✓5th **F40.0	Agoraphobia**
**F40.00	Agoraphobia, unspecified**
**F40.01	Agoraphobia with panic disorder**
Panic disorder with agoraphobia
EXCLUDES 1	*panic disorder without agoraphobia (F41.0)*
**F40.02	Agoraphobia without panic disorder**
✓5th **F40.1	Social phobias**
Anthropophobia
Social anxiety disorder of childhood
Social neurosis
**F40.10	Social phobia, unspecified**
**F40.11	Social phobia, generalized**
✓5th **F40.2	Specific (isolated) phobias**
EXCLUDES 2	*dysmorphophobia (nondelusional) (F45.22)*
nosophobia (F45.22)
✓6th **F40.21	Animal type phobia**
**F40.210	Arachnophobia**
Fear of spiders
**F40.218	Other animal type phobia**
✓6th **F40.22	Natural environment type phobia**
**F40.220	Fear of thunderstorms**
**F40.228	Other natural environment type phobia**
✓6th **F40.23	Blood, injection, injury type phobia**
**F40.230	Fear of blood**
**F40.231	Fear of injections and transfusions**
**F40.232	Fear of other medical care**
**F40.233	Fear of injury**
✓6th **F40.24	Situational type phobia**
**F40.240	Claustrophobia**
**F40.241	Acrophobia**
**F40.242	Fear of bridges**
**F40.243	Fear of flying**
**F40.248	Other situational type phobia**
✓6th **F40.29	Other specified phobia**
**F40.290	Androphobia**
Fear of men
**F40.291	Gynephobia**
Fear of women
**F40.298	Other specified phobia**
**F40.8	Other phobic anxiety disorders**
Phobic anxiety disorder of childhood
**F40.9	Phobic anxiety disorder, unspecified**
Phobia NOS
Phobic state NOS

N Newborn: 0	P Pediatric: 0-17	M Maternity: 12-55	A Adult: 15-124	MCC Major CC Condition	PDx MCC PDx acts as own MCC	CC CC Condition	PDx CC PDx acts as own CC

522	ICD-10-CM Draft (2015)

✓4th **F41　Other anxiety disorders**

　　EXCLUDES 2　*anxiety in:*
　　　　acute stress reaction (F43.0)
　　　　transient adjustment reaction (F43.2)
　　　　neurasthenia (F48.8)
　　　　psychophysiologic disorders (F45.-)
　　　　separation anxiety (F93.0)

F41.0　Panic disorder [episodic paroxysmal anxiety] without agoraphobia
　　Panic attack
　　Panic state
　　EXCLUDES 1　*panic disorder with agoraphobia (F40.01)*

F41.1　Generalized anxiety disorder
　　Anxiety neurosis
　　Anxiety reaction
　　Anxiety state
　　Overanxious disorder
　　EXCLUDES 2　*neurasthenia (F48.8)*

F41.3　Other mixed anxiety disorders

F41.8　Other specified anxiety disorders
　　Anxiety depression (mild or not persistent)
　　Anxiety hysteria
　　Mixed anxiety and depressive disorder

F41.9　Anxiety disorder, unspecified
　　Anxiety NOS

F42　Obsessive-compulsive disorder
　　Anancastic neurosis
　　Obsessive-compulsive neurosis
　　EXCLUDES 2　*obsessive-compulsive personality (disorder) (F60.5)*
　　　　obsessive-compulsive symptoms occurring in depression (F32-F33)
　　　　obsessive-compulsive symptoms occurring in schizophrenia (F20.-)

✓4th **F43　Reaction to severe stress, and adjustment disorders**

F43.0　Acute stress reaction
　　Acute crisis reaction
　　Acute reaction to stress
　　Combat and operational stress reaction
　　Combat fatigue
　　Crisis state
　　Psychic shock

✓5th **F43.1　Post-traumatic stress disorder (PTSD)**
　　Traumatic neurosis

　　F43.10　Post-traumatic stress disorder, unspecified

　　F43.11　Post-traumatic stress disorder, acute

　　F43.12　Post-traumatic stress disorder, chronic

✓5th **F43.2　Adjustment disorders**
　　Culture shock
　　Grief reaction
　　Hospitalism in children
　　EXCLUDES 2　*separation anxiety disorder of childhood (F93.0)*

　　F43.20　Adjustment disorder, unspecified

　　F43.21　Adjustment disorder with depressed mood
　　　　AHA: 2014, 1Q, 25

　　F43.22　Adjustment disorder with anxiety

　　F43.23　Adjustment disorder with mixed anxiety and depressed mood

　　F43.24　Adjustment disorder with disturbance of conduct

　　F43.25　Adjustment disorder with mixed disturbance of emotions and conduct

　　F43.29　Adjustment disorder with other symptoms

F43.8　Other reactions to severe stress

F43.9　Reaction to severe stress, unspecified

✓4th **F44　Dissociative and conversion disorders**
　　INCLUDES　conversion hysteria
　　　　conversion reaction
　　　　hysteria
　　　　hysterical psychosis
　　EXCLUDES 2　*malingering [conscious simulation] (Z76.5)*

F44.0　Dissociative amnesia
　　EXCLUDES 1　*amnesia NOS (R41.3)*
　　　　anterograde amnesia (R41.1)
　　　　retrograde amnesia (R41.2)
　　EXCLUDES 2　*alcohol-or other psychoactive substance-induced amnestic disorder (F10, F13, F19 with .26, .96)*
　　　　amnestic disorder due to known physiological condition (F04)
　　　　postictal amnesia in epilepsy (G40.-)

F44.1　Dissociative fugue
　　EXCLUDES 2　*postictal fugue in epilepsy (G40.-)*

F44.2　Dissociative stupor
　　EXCLUDES 1　*catatonic stupor (R40.1)*
　　　　stupor NOS (R40.1)
　　EXCLUDES 2　*catatonic disorder due to known physiological condition (F06.1)*
　　　　depressive stupor (F32, F33)
　　　　manic stupor (F30, F31)

F44.4　Conversion disorder with motor symptom or deficit
　　Dissociative motor disorders
　　Psychogenic aphonia
　　Psychogenic dysphonia

F44.5　Conversion disorder with seizures or convulsions
　　Dissociative convulsions

F44.6　Conversion disorder with sensory symptom or deficit
　　Dissociative anesthesia and sensory loss
　　Psychogenic deafness

F44.7　Conversion disorder with mixed symptom presentation

✓5th **F44.8　Other dissociative and conversion disorders**

　　F44.81　Dissociative identity disorder
　　　　Multiple personality disorder

　　F44.89　Other dissociative and conversion disorders
　　　　Ganser's syndrome
　　　　Psychogenic confusion
　　　　Psychogenic twilight state
　　　　Trance and possession disorders

F44.9　Dissociative and conversion disorder, unspecified
　　Dissociative disorder NOS

✓4th **F45　Somatoform disorders**
　　EXCLUDES 2　*dissociative and conversion disorders (F44.-)*
　　　　factitious disorders (F68.1-)
　　　　hair-plucking (F63.3)
　　　　lalling (F80.0)
　　　　lisping (F80.0)
　　　　malingering [conscious simulation] (Z76.5)
　　　　nail-biting (F98.8)
　　　　psychological or behavioral factors associated with disorders or diseases classified elsewhere (F54)
　　　　sexual dysfunction, not due to a substance or known physiological condition (F52.-)
　　　　thumb-sucking (F98.8)
　　　　tic disorders (in childhood and adolescence) (F95.-)
　　　　Tourette's syndrome (F95.2)
　　　　trichotillomania (F63.3)

F45.0　Somatization disorder
　　Briquet's disorder
　　Multiple psychosomatic disorder

F45.1　Undifferentiated somatoform disorder
　　Undifferentiated psychosomatic disorder

✓5th **F45.2　Hypochondriacal disorders**
　　EXCLUDES 2　*delusional dysmorphophobia (F22)*
　　　　fixed delusions about bodily functions or shape (F22)

　　F45.20　Hypochondriacal disorder, unspecified

　　F45.21　Hypochondriasis
　　　　Hypochondriacal neurosis

　　F45.22　Body dysmorphic disorder
　　　　Dysmorphophobia (nondelusional)
　　　　Nosophobia

　　F45.29　Other hypochondriacal disorders

✓5th **F45.4　Pain disorders related to psychological factors**
　　EXCLUDES 1　*pain NOS (R52)*

　　F45.41　Pain disorder exclusively related to psychological factors
　　　　Somatoform pain disorder (persistent)

　　F45.42　Pain disorder with related psychological factors
　　　　Code also associated acute or chronic pain (G89.-)

F45.8　Other somatoform disorders
　　Psychogenic dysmenorrhea
　　Psychogenic dysphagia, including "globus hystericus"
　　Psychogenic pruritus
　　Psychogenic torticollis
　　Somatoform autonomic dysfunction
　　Teeth grinding
　　EXCLUDES 1　*sleep related teeth grinding (G47.63)*

F45.9　Somatoform disorder, unspecified
　　Psychosomatic disorder NOS

✓ Additional Character Required　　✓x7th Xtension Alert　　Unacceptable PDx　　Manifestation　　Hospital Acquired Condition　　EXCLUDES 1 Not Coded Here　　EXCLUDES 2 Not Included Here

ICD-10-CM Draft (2015)

523

Mental, Behavioral, and Neurodevelopmental Disorders

F41–F45.9

Mental, Behavioral, and Neurodevelopmental Disorders

F48–F53

✓4th **F48   Other nonpsychotic mental disorders**

    F48.1   Depersonalization-derealization syndrome

    F48.2   Pseudobulbar affect
        Involuntary emotional expression disorder
        Code first underlying cause, if known, such as:
          amyotrophic lateral sclerosis (G12.21)
          multiple sclerosis (G35)
          sequelae of cerebrovascular disease (I69.-)
          sequelae of traumatic intracranial injury (S06.-)

    F48.8   Other specified nonpsychotic mental disorders
        Dhat syndrome
        Neurasthenia
        Occupational neurosis, including writer's cramp
        Psychasthenia
        Psychasthenic neurosis
        Psychogenic syncope

    F48.9   Nonpsychotic mental disorder, unspecified
        Neurosis NOS

Behavioral syndromes associated with physiological disturbances and physical factors (F50-F59)

✓4th **F50   Eating disorders**
    EXCLUDES 1   anorexia NOS (R63.0)
          feeding difficulties (R63.3)
          polyphagia (R63.2)
    EXCLUDES 2   feeding disorder in infancy or childhood (F98.2-)

    CC Excl: For CC codes in category F50, unless otherwise noted:
    F45.9, F50.00-F50.9, F59, F98.21-F98.3

  ✓5th **F50.0   Anorexia nervosa**
      EXCLUDES 1   loss of appetite (R63.0)
            psychogenic loss of appetite (F50.8)

      F50.00   Anorexia nervosa, unspecified   CC

      F50.01   Anorexia nervosa, restricting type   CC

      F50.02   Anorexia nervosa, binge eating/purging type   CC
        EXCLUDES 1   bulimia nervosa (F50.2)

    F50.2   Bulimia nervosa   CC
        Bulimia NOS
        Hyperorexia nervosa
      EXCLUDES 1   anorexia nervosa, binge eating/purging type (F50.02)
      CC Excl: F50.00-F50.9, F98.21-F98.29

    F50.8   Other eating disorders
        Pica in adults
        Psychogenic loss of appetite
      EXCLUDES 2   pica of infancy and childhood (F98.3)

    F50.9   Eating disorder, unspecified
        Atypical anorexia nervosa
        Atypical bulimia nervosa

✓4th **F51   Sleep disorders not due to a substance or known physiological condition**
    EXCLUDES 2   organic sleep disorders (G47.-)

  ✓5th **F51.0   Insomnia not due to a substance or known physiological condition**
      EXCLUDES 2   alcohol related insomnia (F10.182, F10.282, F10.982)
            drug-related insomnia (F11.182, F11.282, F11.982, F13.182, F13.282, F13.982, F14.182, F14.282, F14.982, F15.182, F15.282, F15.982, F19.182, F19.282, F19.982)
            insomnia NOS (G47.0-)
            insomnia due to known physiological condition (G47.0-)
            organic insomnia (G47.0-)
            sleep deprivation (Z72.820)

      F51.01   Primary insomnia
        Idiopathic insomnia

      F51.02   Adjustment insomnia

      F51.03   Paradoxical insomnia

      F51.04   Psychophysiologic insomnia

      F51.05   Insomnia due to other mental disorder
        Code also associated mental disorder

      F51.09   Other insomnia not due to a substance or known physiological condition

  ✓5th **F51.1   Hypersomnia not due to a substance or known physiological condition**
      EXCLUDES 2   alcohol related hypersomnia (F10.182, F10.282, F10.982)
            drug-related hypersomnia (F11.182, F11.282, F11.982, F13.182, F13.282, F13.982, F14.182, F14.282, F14.982, F15.182, F15.282, F15.982, F19.182, F19.282, F19.982)
            hypersomnia NOS (G47.10)
            hypersomnia due to known physiological condition (G47.10)
            idiopathic hypersomnia (G47.11, G47.12)
            narcolepsy (G47.4-)

      F51.11   Primary hypersomnia

      F51.12   Insufficient sleep syndrome
        EXCLUDES 1   sleep deprivation (Z72.820)

      F51.13   Hypersomnia due to other mental disorder
        Code also associated mental disorder

      F51.19   Other hypersomnia not due to a substance or known physiological condition

    F51.3   Sleepwalking [somnambulism]

    F51.4   Sleep terrors [night terrors]

    F51.5   Nightmare disorder
        Dream anxiety disorder

    F51.8   Other sleep disorders not due to a substance or known physiological condition

    F51.9   Sleep disorder not due to a substance or known physiological condition, unspecified
        Emotional sleep disorder NOS

✓4th **F52   Sexual dysfunction not due to a substance or known physiological condition**
    EXCLUDES 2   Dhat syndrome (F48.8)

    F52.0   Hypoactive sexual desire disorder
        Anhedonia (sexual)
        Lack or loss of sexual desire
      EXCLUDES 1   decreased libido (R68.82)

    F52.1   Sexual aversion disorder
        Sexual aversion and lack of sexual enjoyment

  ✓5th **F52.2   Sexual arousal disorders**
        Failure of genital response

      F52.21   Male erectile disorder   ♂
        Psychogenic impotence
        EXCLUDES 1   impotence of organic origin (N52.-)
            impotence NOS (N52.-)

      F52.22   Female sexual arousal disorder   ♀
        Frigidity

  ✓5th **F52.3   Orgasmic disorder**
        Inhibited orgasm
        Psychogenic anorgasmy

      F52.31   Female orgasmic disorder   ♀

      F52.32   Male orgasmic disorder   ♂

    F52.4   Premature ejaculation   ♂

    F52.5   Vaginismus not due to a substance or known physiological condition   ♀
        Psychogenic vaginismus
      EXCLUDES 2   vaginismus (due to a known physiological condition) (N94.2)

    F52.6   Dyspareunia not due to a substance or known physiological condition   ♀
        Psychogenic dyspareunia
      EXCLUDES 2   dyspareunia (due to a known physiological condition) (N94.1)

    F52.8   Other sexual dysfunction not due to a substance or known physiological condition
        Excessive sexual drive
        Nymphomania
        Satyriasis

    F52.9   Unspecified sexual dysfunction not due to a substance or known physiological condition
        Sexual dysfunction NOS

F53   Puerperal psychosis   ♀
    Postpartum depression
    EXCLUDES 1   mood disorders with psychotic features (F30.2, F31.2, F31.5, F31.64, F32.3, F33.3)
          postpartum dysphoria (O90.6)
          psychosis in schizophrenia, schizotypal, delusional, and other psychotic disorders (F20-F29)

N Newborn: 0   P Pediatric: 0-17   M Maternity: 12-55   A Adult: 15-124   MCC Major CC Condition   PDx MCC PDx acts as own MCC   CC CC Condition   PDx CC PDx acts as own CC

524   ICD-10-CM Draft (2015)

F54   ***Psychological and behavioral factors associated with disorders or diseases classified elsewhere***

Psychological factors affecting physical conditions

Code first the associated physical disorder, such as:
asthma (J45.-)
dermatitis (L23-L25)
gastric ulcer (K25.-)
mucous colitis (K58.-)
ulcerative colitis (K51.-)
urticaria (L50.-)
    EXCLUDES 2   *tension-type headache (G44.2)*

✓4ᵗʰ **F55**   **Abuse of non-psychoactive substances**
    EXCLUDES 2   *abuse of psychoactive substances (F10-F19)*

   F55.0   **Abuse of** antacids

   F55.1   **Abuse of** herbal or folk remedies

   F55.2   **Abuse of** laxatives

   F55.3   **Abuse of** steroids or hormones

   F55.4   **Abuse of** vitamins

   F55.8   **Abuse of** other non-psychoactive substances

F59   **Unspecified behavioral syndromes associated with physiological disturbances and physical factors**

Psychogenic physiological dysfunction NOS

Disorders of adult personality and behavior (F60-F69)

✓4ᵗʰ **F60**   **Specific personality disorders**

   F60.0   **Paranoid** personality disorder
     Expansive paranoid personality (disorder)
     Fanatic personality (disorder)
     Paranoid personality (disorder)
     Querulant personality (disorder)
     Sensitive paranoid personality (disorder)
      EXCLUDES 2   *paranoia (F22)*
         paranoia querulans (F22)
         paranoid psychosis (F22)
         paranoid schizophrenia (F20.0)
         paranoid state (F22)

   F60.1   **Schizoid** personality disorder
      EXCLUDES 2   *Asperger's syndrome (F84.5)*
         delusional disorder (F22)
         schizoid disorder of childhood (F84.5)
         schizophrenia (F20.-)
         schizotypal disorder (F21)

   F60.2   **Antisocial** personality disorder
     Amoral personality (disorder)
     Asocial personality (disorder)
     Dissocial personality disorder
     Psychopathic personality (disorder)
     Sociopathic personality (disorder)
      EXCLUDES 1   *conduct disorders (F91.-)*
      EXCLUDES 2   *borderline personality disorder (F60.3)*

   F60.3   **Borderline** personality disorder
     Aggressive personality (disorder)
     Emotionally unstable personality (disorder)
     Explosive personality (disorder)
      EXCLUDES 2   *antisocial personality disorder (F60.2)*

   F60.4   **Histrionic** personality disorder
     Hysterical personality (disorder)
     Psychoinfantile personality (disorder)

   F60.5   **Obsessive-compulsive** personality disorder
     Anankastic personality (disorder)
     Compulsive personality (disorder)
     Obsessional personality (disorder)
      EXCLUDES 2   *obsessive-compulsive disorder (F42)*

   F60.6   **Avoidant** personality disorder
     Anxious personality disorder

   F60.7   **Dependent** personality disorder
     Asthenic personality (disorder)
     Inadequate personality (disorder)
     Passive personality (disorder)

✓5ᵗʰ   **F60.8**   **Other specific personality disorders**

     F60.81   **Narcissistic personality disorder**

     F60.89   **Other specific personality disorders**
       Eccentric personality disorder
       "Haltlose" type personality disorder
       Immature personality disorder
       Passive-aggressive personality disorder
       Psychoneurotic personality disorder
       Self-defeating personality disorder

   F60.9   **Personality disorder, unspecified**
     Character disorder NOS
     Character neurosis NOS
     Pathological personality NOS

✓4ᵗʰ **F63**   **Impulse disorders**
    EXCLUDES 2   *habitual excessive use of alcohol or psychoactive substances (F10-F19)*
          impulse disorders involving sexual behavior (F65.-)

   F63.0   **Pathological gambling**
     Compulsive gambling
      EXCLUDES 1   *gambling and betting NOS (Z72.6)*
      EXCLUDES 2   *excessive gambling by manic patients (F30, F31)*
         gambling in antisocial personality disorder (F60.2)

   F63.1   **Pyromania**
     Pathological fire-setting
      EXCLUDES 2   *fire-setting (by) (in):*
        adult with antisocial personality disorder (F60.2)
        alcohol or psychoactive substance intoxication (F10-F19)
        conduct disorders (F91.-)
        mental disorders due to known physiological condition (F01-F09)
        schizophrenia (F20.-)

   F63.2   **Kleptomania**
     Pathological stealing
      EXCLUDES 1   *shoplifting as the reason for observation for suspected mental disorder (Z03.8)*
      EXCLUDES 2   *depressive disorder with stealing (F31-F33)*
        stealing due to underlying mental condition—code to mental condition
        stealing in mental disorders due to known physiological condition (F01-F09)

   F63.3   **Trichotillomania**
     Hair plucking
      EXCLUDES 2   *other stereotyped movement disorder (F98.4)*

✓5ᵗʰ   **F63.8**   **Other impulse disorders**

     F63.81   **Intermittent explosive disorder**

     F63.89   **Other impulse disorders**

   F63.9   **Impulse disorder, unspecified**
     Impulse control disorder NOS

✓4ᵗʰ **F64**   **Gender identity disorders**

   F64.1   **Gender identity disorder in** adolescence and adulthood
     Dual role transvestism
     Transsexualism
     Use additional code to identify sex reassignment status (Z87.890)
      EXCLUDES 1   *gender identity disorder in childhood (F64.2)*
      EXCLUDES 2   *fetishistic transvestism (F65.1)*

   F64.2   **Gender identity disorder of** childhood   P
      EXCLUDES 1   *gender identity disorder in adolescence and adulthood (F64.1)*
      EXCLUDES 2   *sexual maturation disorder (F66)*

   F64.8   **Other gender identity disorders**

   F64.9   **Gender identity disorder,** unspecified
     Gender-role disorder NOS

✓4ᵗʰ **F65**   **Paraphilias**

   F65.0   **Fetishism**

   F65.1   **Transvestic fetishism**
     Fetishistic transvestism

   F65.2   **Exhibitionism**

   F65.3   **Voyeurism**

   F65.4   **Pedophilia**

✓5ᵗʰ   **F65.5**   **Sadomasochism**

     F65.50   **Sadomasochism, unspecified**

     F65.51   **Sexual masochism**

     F65.52   **Sexual sadism**

✓5ᵗʰ   **F65.8**   **Other paraphilias**

     F65.81   **Frotteurism**

     F65.89   **Other paraphilias**
       Necrophilia

   F65.9   **Paraphilia, unspecified**
     Sexual deviation NOS

F66   **Other sexual disorders**
    Sexual maturation disorder
    Sexual relationship disorder

☑ Additional Character Required   ✓x7ᵗʰ *X*tension Alert   Unacceptable PDx   Manifestation   Hospital Acquired Condition   EXCLUDES 1 Not Coded Here   EXCLUDES 2 Not Included Here

Mental, Behavioral, and Neurodevelopmental Disorders

F68–F84.0

√4ᵗʰ **F68 Other disorders of adult personality and behavior**

√5ᵗʰ **F68.1 Factitious disorder**
Compensation neurosis
Elaboration of physical symptoms for psychological reasons
Hospital hopper syndrome
Münchhausen's syndrome
Peregrinating patient
EXCLUDES 2   *factitial dermatitis (L98.1)*
      person feigning illness (with obvious motivation) (Z76.5)

     F68.10 Factitious disorder, unspecified   CC
         CC Excl: F07.0-F07.81, F07.9-F09, F20.0-F48.1, F48.8-F51.03, F51.12, F51.19, F51.3-F51.9, F52.5, F54, F59-F63.2, F63.81-F63.9, F68.10-F80.2, F80.4, F80.89-F84.0, F84.3-F99, G44.201-G44.229, H93.25, R45.1-R45.2, R45.5-R45.82, R45.86-R45.87

     F68.11 Factitious disorder with predominantly psychological signs and symptoms

     F68.12 Factitious disorder with predominantly physical signs and symptoms   CC
         CC Excl: See code: F68.10

     F68.13 Factitious disorder with combined psychological and physical signs and symptoms

   F68.8 Other specified disorders of adult personality and behavior

F69 Unspecified disorder of adult personality and behavior   A

Intellectual Disabilities (F70-F79)

Code first any associated physical or developmental disorders
EXCLUDES 1   *borderline intellectual functioning, IQ above 70 to 84 (R41.83)*

F70 Mild intellectual disabilities
IQ level 50-55 to approximately 70
Mild mental subnormality

F71 Moderate intellectual disabilities
IQ level 35-40 to 50-55
Moderate mental subnormality

F72 Severe intellectual disabilities   CC
IQ 20-25 to 35-40
Severe mental subnormality
CC Excl: F72-F73

F73 Profound intellectual disabilities   CC
IQ level below 20-25
Profound mental subnormality
CC Excl: See code: F72

F78 Other intellectual disabilities

F79 Unspecified intellectual disabilities
Mental deficiency NOS
Mental subnormality NOS

Pervasive and specific developmental disorders (F80-F89)

√4ᵗʰ **F80 Specific developmental disorders of speech and language**

   F80.0 Phonological disorder
Dyslalia
Functional speech articulation disorder
Lalling
Lisping
Phonological developmental disorder
Speech articulation developmental disorder
EXCLUDES 1   *speech articulation impairment due to aphasia NOS (R47.01)*
      speech articulation impairment due to apraxia (R48.2)
EXCLUDES 2   *speech articulation impairment due to hearing loss (F80.4)*
      speech articulation impairment due to intellectual disabilities (F70-F79)
      speech articulation impairment with expressive language developmental disorder (F80.1)
      speech articulation impairment with mixed receptive expressive language developmental disorder (F80.2)

   F80.1 Expressive language disorder
Developmental dysphasia or aphasia, expressive type
EXCLUDES 1   *dysphasia and aphasia NOS (R47.-)*
      mixed receptive-expressive language disorder (F80.2)
EXCLUDES 2   *acquired aphasia with epilepsy [Landau-Kleffner] (G40.80-)*
      intellectual disabilities (F70-F79)
      pervasive developmental disorders (F84.-)
      selective mutism (F94.0)

   F80.2 Mixed receptive-expressive language disorder
Developmental dysphasia or aphasia, receptive type
Developmental Wernicke's aphasia
EXCLUDES 1   *central auditory processing disorder (H93.25)*
      dysphasia or aphasia NOS (R47.-)
      expressive language disorder (F80.1)
      expressive type dysphasia or aphasia (F80.1)
      word deafness (H93.25)
EXCLUDES 2   *acquired aphasia with epilepsy [Landau-Kleffner] (G40.80-)*
      intellectual disabilities (F70-F79)
      pervasive developmental disorders (F84.-)
      selective mutism (F94.0)

   F80.4 Speech and language development delay due to hearing loss
Code also type of hearing loss (H90.-, H91.-)

√5ᵗʰ **F80.8 Other developmental disorders of speech and language**

     F80.81 Childhood onset fluency disorder
Cluttering NOS
Stuttering NOS
EXCLUDES 1   *adult onset fluency disorder (F98.5)*
      fluency disorder in conditions classified elsewhere (R47.82)
      fluency disorder (stuttering) following cerebrovascular disease (I69. with final characters-23)

     F80.89 Other developmental disorders of speech and language

   F80.9 Developmental disorder of speech and language, unspecified
Communication disorder NOS
Language disorder NOS

√4ᵗʰ **F81 Specific developmental disorders of scholastic skills**

   F81.0 Specific reading disorder
"Backward reading"
Developmental dyslexia
Specific reading retardation
EXCLUDES 1   *alexia NOS (R48.0)*
      dyslexia NOS (R48.0)

   F81.2 Mathematics disorder
Developmental acalculia
Developmental arithmetical disorder
Developmental Gerstmann's syndrome
EXCLUDES 1   *acalculia NOS (R48.8)*
EXCLUDES 2   *arithmetical difficulties associated with a reading disorder (F81.0)*
      arithmetical difficulties associated with a spelling disorder (F81.81)
      arithmetical difficulties due to inadequate teaching (Z55.8)

√5ᵗʰ **F81.8 Other developmental disorders of scholastic skills**

     F81.81 Disorder of written expression
Specific spelling disorder

     F81.89 Other developmental disorders of scholastic skills

   F81.9 Developmental disorder of scholastic skills, unspecified
Knowledge acquisition disability NOS
Learning disability NOS
Learning disorder NOS

F82 Specific developmental disorder of motor function
Clumsy child syndrome
Developmental coordination disorder
Developmental dyspraxia
EXCLUDES 1   *abnormalities of gait and mobility (R26.-)*
      lack of coordination (R27.-)
EXCLUDES 2   *lack of coordination secondary to intellectual disabilities (F70-F79)*

√4ᵗʰ **F84 Pervasive developmental disorders**
Use additional code to identify any associated medical condition and intellectual disabilities

CC Excl: For CC codes in category F84, unless otherwise noted:
F07.0-F07.81, F07.9-F09, F20.0-F48.1, F48.8-F51.03, F51.12, F51.19, F51.3-F51.9, F52.5, F54, F59-F63.2, F63.81-F63.9, F68.10-F80.2, F80.4, F80.89-F84.0, F84.3-F99, G44.201-G44.229, H93.25, R45.1-R45.2, R45.5-R45.82, R45.86-R45.87

   F84.0 Autistic disorder   CC
Infantile autism
Infantile psychosis
Kanner's syndrome
EXCLUDES 1   *Asperger's syndrome (F84.5)*

N Newborn: 0   P Pediatric: 0-17   M Maternity: 12-55   A Adult: 15-124   MCC Major CC Condition   PDx MCC PDx acts as own MCC   CC CC Condition   PDx CC PDx acts as own CC

526   ICD-10-CM Draft (2015)

F84.2 Rett's syndrome `CC`
> **EXCLUDES 1** Asperger's syndrome (F84.5)
> Autistic disorder (F84.0)
> Other childhood disintegrative disorder (F84.3)
> **CC Excl:** E75.00-E75.19, E75.4, F84.2, G13.2-G13.8, G30.0-G31.82, G31.84-G31.9, G91.4, G94

F84.3 Other childhood disintegrative disorder `CC` `P`
> Dementia infantilis
> Disintegrative psychosis
> Heller's syndrome
> Symbiotic psychosis
> Use additional code to identify any associated neurological condition
> **EXCLUDES 1** Asperger's syndrome (F84.5)
> Autistic disorder (F84.0)
> Rett's syndrome (F84.2)

F84.5 Asperger's syndrome `CC`
> Asperger's disorder
> Autistic psychopathy
> Schizoid disorder of childhood

F84.8 Other pervasive developmental disorders `CC`
> Overactive disorder associated with intellectual disabilities and stereotyped movements

F84.9 Pervasive developmental disorder, unspecified `CC`
> Atypical autism

F88 Other disorders of psychological development
> Developmental agnosia

F89 Unspecified disorder of psychological development
> Developmental disorder NOS

Behavioral and emotional disorders with onset usually occurring in childhood and adolescence (F90-F98)

> **NOTE** Codes within categories F90-F98 may be used regardless of the age of a patient. These disorders generally have onset within the childhood or adolescent years, but may continue throughout life or not be diagnosed until adulthood

✓4th F90 Attention-deficit hyperactivity disorders
> **INCLUDES** attention deficit disorder with hyperactivity
> attention deficit syndrome with hyperactivity
> **EXCLUDES 2** anxiety disorders (F40.-, F41.-)
> mood [affective] disorders (F30-F39)
> pervasive developmental disorders (F84.-)
> schizophrenia (F20.-)

F90.0 Attention-deficit hyperactivity disorder, predominantly inattentive type

F90.1 Attention-deficit hyperactivity disorder, predominantly hyperactive type

F90.2 Attention-deficit hyperactivity disorder, combined type

F90.8 Attention-deficit hyperactivity disorder, other type

F90.9 Attention-deficit hyperactivity disorder, unspecified type
> Attention-deficit hyperactivity disorder of childhood or adolescence NOS
> Attention-deficit hyperactivity disorder NOS

✓4th F91 Conduct disorders
> **EXCLUDES 1** antisocial behavior (Z72.81-)
> antisocial personality disorder (F60.2)
> **EXCLUDES 2** conduct problems associated with attention-deficit hyperactivity disorder (F90.-)
> mood [affective] disorders (F30-F39)
> pervasive developmental disorders (F84.-)
> schizophrenia (F20.-)

F91.0 Conduct disorder confined to family context

F91.1 Conduct disorder, childhood-onset type
> Unsocialized conduct disorder
> Conduct disorder, solitary aggressive type
> Unsocialized aggressive disorder

F91.2 Conduct disorder, adolescent-onset type
> Socialized conduct disorder
> Conduct disorder, group type

F91.3 Oppositional defiant disorder

F91.8 Other conduct disorders

F91.9 Conduct disorder, unspecified
> Behavioral disorder NOS
> Conduct disorder NOS
> Disruptive behavior disorder NOS

✓4th F93 Emotional disorders with onset specific to childhood

F93.0 Separation anxiety disorder of childhood `P`
> **EXCLUDES 2** mood [affective] disorders (F30-F39)
> nonpsychotic mental disorders (F40-F48)
> phobic anxiety disorder of childhood (F40.8)
> social phobia (F40.1)

F93.8 Other childhood emotional disorders `P`
> Identity disorder
> **EXCLUDES 2** gender identity disorder of childhood (F64.2)

F93.9 Childhood emotional disorder, unspecified `P`

✓4th F94 Disorders of social functioning with onset specific to childhood and adolescence

F94.0 Selective mutism
> Elective mutism
> **EXCLUDES 2** pervasive developmental disorders (F84.-)
> schizophrenia (F20.-)
> specific developmental disorders of speech and language (F80.-)
> transient mutism as part of separation anxiety in young children (F93.0)

F94.1 Reactive attachment disorder of childhood `P`
> Use additional code to identify any associated failure to thrive or growth retardation
> **EXCLUDES 1** disinhibited attachment disorder of childhood (F94.1)
> normal variation in pattern of selective attachment
> **EXCLUDES 2** Asperger's syndrome (F84.5)
> maltreatment syndromes (T74.-)
> sexual or physical abuse in childhood, resulting in psychosocial problems (Z62.81-)

F94.2 Disinhibited attachment disorder of childhood `P`
> Affectionless psychopathy
> Institutional syndrome
> **EXCLUDES 1** reactive attachment disorder of childhood (F94.1)
> **EXCLUDES 2** Asperger's syndrome (F84.5)
> attention-deficit hyperactivity disorders (F90.-)
> hospitalism in children (F43.2-)

F94.8 Other childhood disorders of social functioning `P`

F94.9 Childhood disorder of social functioning, unspecified `P`

✓4th F95 Tic disorder

F95.0 Transient tic disorder

F95.1 Chronic motor or vocal tic disorder

F95.2 Tourette's disorder
> Combined vocal and multiple motor tic disorder [de la Tourette]
> Tourette's syndrome

F95.8 Other tic disorders

F95.9 Tic disorder, unspecified
> Tic NOS

✓4th F98 Other behavioral and emotional disorders with onset usually occurring in childhood and adolescence
> **EXCLUDES 2** breath-holding spells (R06.89)
> gender identity disorder of childhood (F64.2)
> Kleine-Levin syndrome (G47.13)
> obsessive-compulsive disorder (F42)
> sleep disorders not due to a substance or known physiological condition (F51.-)

F98.0 Enuresis not due to a substance or known physiological condition
> Enuresis (primary) (secondary) of nonorganic origin
> Functional enuresis
> Psychogenic enuresis
> Urinary incontinence of nonorganic origin
> **EXCLUDES 1** enuresis NOS (R32)

F98.1 Encopresis not due to a substance or known physiological condition
> Functional encopresis
> Incontinence of feces of nonorganic origin
> Psychogenic encopresis
> Use additional code to identify the cause of any coexisting constipation
> **EXCLUDES 1** encopresis NOS (R15.-)

✓5th F98.2 Other feeding disorders of infancy and childhood
> **EXCLUDES 1** feeding difficulties (R63.3)
> **EXCLUDES 2** anorexia nervosa and other eating disorders (F50.-)
> feeding problems of newborn (P92.-)
> pica of infancy or childhood (F98.3)

F98.21 Rumination disorder of infancy `P`

F98.29 Other feeding disorders of infancy and early childhood `P`

✓ Additional Character Required ✓x7th Xtension Alert Unacceptable PDx Manifestation Hospital Acquired Condition **EXCLUDES 1** Not Coded Here **EXCLUDES 2** Not Included Here

Mental, Behavioral, and Neurodevelopmental Disorders

F98.3–F99

F98.3 Pica of infancy and childhood   **P**

F98.4 Stereotyped movement disorders
Stereotype/habit disorder
EXCLUDES 1   *abnormal involuntary movements (R25.-)*
EXCLUDES 2   *compulsions in obsessive-compulsive disorder (F42)*
    hair plucking (F63.3)
    movement disorders of organic origin (G20-G25)
    nail-biting (F98.8)
    nose-picking (F98.8)
    stereotypies that are part of a broader psychiatric
       condition (F01-F95)
    thumb-sucking (F98.8)
    tic disorders (F95.-)
    trichotillomania (F63.3)

F98.5 Adult onset fluency disorder
EXCLUDES 1   *childhood onset fluency disorder (F80.81)*
    dysphasia (R47.02)
    fluency disorder in conditions classified elsewhere
       (R47.82)
    fluency disorder (stuttering) following cerebrovascular
       disease (I69. with final characters -23)
    tic disorders (F95.-)

F98.8 Other specified behavioral and emotional disorders with onset usually occurring in childhood and adolescence   **P**
Excessive masturbation
Nail-biting
Nose-picking
Thumb-sucking

F98.9 Unspecified behavioral and emotional disorders with onset usually occurring in childhood and adolescence   **P**

Unspecified mental disorder (F99)

F99 Mental disorder, not otherwise specified
Mental illness NOS
EXCLUDES 1   *unspecified mental disorder due to known physiological condition (F09)*

N Newborn: 0   P Pediatric: 0-17   M Maternity: 12-55   A Adult: 15-124   MCC Major CC Condition   PDx MCC PDx acts as own MCC   CC CC Condition   PDx CC PDx acts as own CC

528   ICD-10-CM Draft (2015)

Chapter 6. Diseases of the Nervous System (G00-G99)

EXCLUDES 2 certain conditions originating in the perinatal period (P04-P96)
certain infectious and parasitic diseases (A00-B99)
complications of pregnancy, childbirth and the puerperium (O00-O9A)
congenital malformations, deformations, and chromosomal abnormalities (Q00-Q99)
endocrine, nutritional and metabolic diseases (E00-E88)
injury, poisoning and certain other consequences of external causes (S00-T88)
neoplasms (C00-D49)
symptoms, signs and abnormal clinical and laboratory findings, not elsewhere classified (R00-R94)

This chapter contains the following blocks:

G00-G09 Inflammatory diseases of the central nervous system
G10-G14 Systemic atrophies primarily affecting the central nervous system
G20-G26 Extrapyramidal and movement disorders
G30-G32 Other degenerative diseases of the nervous system
G35-G37 Demyelinating diseases of the central nervous system
G40-G47 Episodic and paroxysmal disorders
G50-G59 Nerve, nerve root and plexus disorders
G60-G65 Polyneuropathies and other disorders of the peripheral nervous system
G70-G73 Diseases of myoneural junction and muscle
G80-G83 Cerebral palsy and other paralytic syndromes
G89-G99 Other disorders of the nervous system

Inflammatory diseases of the central nervous system (G00-G09)

✓4ᵗʰ G00 Bacterial meningitis, not elsewhere classified

INCLUDES bacterial arachnoiditis
bacterial leptomeningitis
bacterial meningitis
bacterial pachymeningitis

EXCLUDES 1 bacterial:
meningoencephalitis (G04.2)
meningomyelitis (G04.2)

CC Excl: For MCC codes in category G00, unless otherwise noted:
A02.21, A17.0-A17.1, A27.81, A39.0, A50.41, A51.41, A52.13, A54.82, A54.84, A54.89-A54.9, A87.0-A87.9, B00.3, B02.1, B26.1, B37.5, B38.4, B45.1, B58.2, E08.40-E08.49, E08.618-E08.638, E08.649-E08.8, E09.40-E09.49, E09.618-E09.638, E09.649-E09.8, E10.40-E10.49, E10.618-E10.638, E10.649, E10.69-E10.8, E11.40-E11.49, E11.618-E11.638, E11.649, E11.69-E11.8, E13.40-E13.49, E13.618-E13.638, E13.649-E13.8, G00.0-G03.9, G04.2, G32.89, G61.0, G96.8-G96.9, G98.0-G98.8, G99.8

G00.0 Hemophilus meningitis MCC
Meningitis due to Hemophilus influenzae

G00.1 Pneumococcal meningitis MCC

G00.2 Streptococcal meningitis MCC
Use additional code to further identify organism (B95.0-B95.5)

G00.3 Staphylococcal meningitis MCC
Use additional code to further identify organism (B95.61-B95.8)

G00.8 Other bacterial meningitis MCC
Meningitis due to Escherichia coli
Meningitis due to Friedländer's bacillus
Meningitis due to Klebsiella
Use additional code to further identify organism (B96.-)

G00.9 Bacterial meningitis, unspecified MCC
Meningitis due to gram-negative bacteria, unspecified
Purulent meningitis NOS
Pyogenic meningitis NOS
Suppurative meningitis NOS

G01 Meningitis in bacterial diseases classified elsewhere MCC
Code first underlying disease
EXCLUDES 1 meningitis (in):
gonococcal (A54.81)
leptospirosis (A27.81)
listeriosis (A32.11)
Lyme disease (A69.21)
meningococcal (A39.0)
neurosyphilis (A52.13)
tuberculosis (A17.0)
meningoencephalitis and meningomyelitis in bacterial diseases classified elsewhere (G05)
CC Excl: See code: G00

G02 Meningitis in other infectious and parasitic diseases classified elsewhere MCC
Code first underlying disease, such as:
African trypanosomiasis (B56.-)
poliovirus infection (A80.-)
EXCLUDES 1 candidal meningitis (B37.5)
coccidioidomycosis meningitis (B38.4)
cryptococcal meningitis (B45.1)
herpesviral [herpes simplex] meningitis (B00.3)
infectious mononucleosis complicated by meningitis (B27.- with fourth character 2)
measles complicated by meningitis (B05.1)
meningoencephalitis and meningomyelitis in other infectious and parasitic diseases classified elsewhere (G05)
mumps meningitis (B26.1)
rubella meningitis (B06.02)
varicella [chickenpox] meningitis (B01.0)
zoster meningitis (B02.1)
CC Excl: A02.21, A17.0-A17.1, A27.81, A39.0, A50.41, A51.41, A52.13, A54.82, A54.84, A54.89-A54.9, A87.0-A87.9, B00.3, B02.1, B26.1, B37.5, B38.4, B45.1, B58.2, G00.0-G03.9, G04.2, G32.89, G61.0, G96.8-G96.9, G98.0-G98.8, G99.8

✓4ᵗʰ G03 Meningitis due to other and unspecified causes
INCLUDES arachnoiditis NOS
leptomeningitis NOS
meningitis NOS
pachymeningitis NOS
EXCLUDES 1 meningoencephalitis (G04.-)
meningomyelitis (G04.-)

G03.0 Nonpyogenic meningitis MCC
Aseptic meningitis
Nonbacterial meningitis
CC Excl: See code: G00

G03.1 Chronic meningitis CC
CC Excl: See code: G00

G03.2 Benign recurrent meningitis [Mollaret] CC
CC Excl: A02.21, A17.0-A17.1, A27.81, A39.0, A50.41, A51.41, A52.13, A54.82, A54.84, A54.89-A54.9, A74.81-A74.9, A87.0-A87.9, A96.2, A98.3-A98.4, B26.1, B33.24, B33.4-B33.8, B34.1-B34.2, B34.4-B34.8, B37.5, B38.4, B45.1, B58.2, B92, B94.2-B94.9, B97.10, B97.19, B97.29, B97.5-B97.6, B97.81-B97.89, G00.0-G03.9, G04.2, G32.89, G61.0, G96.8-G96.9, G98.0-G98.8, G99.8

G03.8 Meningitis due to other specified causes MCC
CC Excl: See code: G00

G03.9 Meningitis, unspecified MCC
Arachnoiditis (spinal) NOS
CC Excl: See code: G00

✓4ᵗʰ G04 Encephalitis, myelitis and encephalomyelitis
INCLUDES acute ascending myelitis
meningoencephalitis
meningomyelitis
EXCLUDES 1 encephalopathy NOS (G93.40)
EXCLUDES 2 acute transverse myelitis (G37.3-)
alcoholic encephalopathy (G31.2)
benign myalgic encephalomyelitis (G93.3)
multiple sclerosis (G35)
subacute necrotizing myelitis (G37.4)
toxic encephalitis (G92)
toxic encephalopathy (G92)

✓5ᵗʰ G04.0 Acute disseminated encephalitis and encephalomyelitis (ADEM)
EXCLUDES 1 acute necrotizing hemorrhagic encephalopathy (G04.3-)
other noninfectious acute disseminated encephalomyelitis (noninfectious ADEM) (G04.81)

G04.00 Acute disseminated encephalitis and encephalomyelitis, unspecified MCC
CC Excl: A02.21, A17.0-A17.1, A17.82, A27.81, A39.0, A50.41-A50.42, A51.41, A52.13-A52.14, A54.82, A54.84, A54.89-A54.9, A81.1, A81.82-A81.89, A83.0-A85.8, A87.0-A88.0, A88.8, A92.1-A92.8, A93.0, A96.2, A98.3-A98.4, B00.3-B00.4, B00.89-B01.11, B01.81-B02.23, B02.29, B02.7-B02.9, B04, B06.01, B08.04-B08.09, B08.20-B08.22, B08.60-B08.79, B09-B10.89, B26.1-B26.2, B27.00-B27.99, B33.1, B33.24, B33.4-B33.8, B34.1-B34.2, B34.4-B34.8, B37.5, B38.4, B45.1, B58.2, B92, B94.2-B94.9, B97.10, B97.19-B97.29, B97.5-B97.6, B97.81-B97.89, G00.0-G04.01, G04.2, G04.31, G04.81-G05.4, G32.89, G37.0, G37.4-G37.5, G61.0, G96.8-G96.9, G98.0-G98.8, G99.8, J09.X3-J09.X9, J10.2-J10.89, J11.2-J11.89, L44.4, P35.2-P35.9, P37.0-P37.4, P37.8-P37.9

Diseases of the Nervous System

G04.01–G07

G04.01 Postinfectious acute disseminated encephalitis and encephalomyelitis (postinfectious ADEM) `MCC`
> EXCLUDES 1   post chickenpox encephalitis (B01.1)
> post measles encephalitis (B05.0)
> post measles myelitis (B05.1)
> **CC Excl:** See code: G04.00

G04.02 Postimmunization acute disseminated encephalitis, myelitis and encephalomyelitis `MCC`
Encephalitis, postimmunization
Encephalomyelitis, postimmunization
Use additional code to identify the vaccine (T50.A-, T50.B-, T50Z-)
CC Excl: No Excl

G04.1 Tropical spastic paraplegia `CC`
CC Excl: G04.1, G11.0-G12.9, G32.0-G37.3, G37.5-G37.9, G80.0-G80.2, G80.4-G83.9, G90.01-G90.09, G90.2, G90.4-G90.9, G92, G93.40-G93.49, G93.81, G93.89-G93.9, G95.0-G95.9, G96.8-G96.9, G98.0-G99.8, I67.83, R53.2

G04.2 Bacterial meningoencephalitis and meningomyelitis, not elsewhere classified `MCC`
CC Excl: See code: G00

G04.3 Acute necrotizing hemorrhagic encephalopathy ✓5th
> EXCLUDES 1   acute disseminated encephalitis and encephalomyelitis (G04.0-)

G04.30 Acute necrotizing hemorrhagic encephalopathy, unspecified `MCC`
CC Excl: No Excl

G04.31 Postinfectious acute necrotizing hemorrhagic encephalopathy `MCC`
CC Excl: See code: G04.00

G04.32 Postimmunization acute necrotizing hemorrhagic encephalopathy `MCC`
Use additional code to identify the vaccine (T50.A-, T50.B-, T50Z-)
CC Excl: No Excl

G04.39 Other acute necrotizing hemorrhagic encephalopathy `MCC`
Code also underlying etiology, if applicable
CC Excl: No Excl

G04.8 Other encephalitis, myelitis and encephalomyelitis ✓5th
Code also any associated seizure (G40.-, R56.9)

G04.81 Other encephalitis, myelitis and encephalomyelitis `HIV` `MCC`
Noninfectious acute disseminated encephalomyelitis (noninfectious ADEM)
CC Excl: See code: G04.00

G04.89 Other myelitis `HIV` `MCC`
CC Excl: See code: G04.00

G04.9 Encephalitis, myelitis and encephalomyelitis, unspecified ✓5th

G04.90 Encephalitis and encephalomyelitis, unspecified `HIV` `MCC`
Ventriculitis (cerebral) NOS
CC Excl: A17.82, A28.1, A50.42, A52.14, A75.9, A79.9, A81.1, A81.82-A81.89, A83.0-A85.8, A87.2, A88.0, A88.8, A92.1-A92.8, A93.0, B00.4, B00.82, B01.11-B01.12, B04, B06.01, B08.09, B08.20-B08.22, B08.60-B08.79, B09-B10.09, B26.2, B27.00-B27.99, B33.1, B45.0, B45.2-B45.9, B54, B58.2, B75, B97.10, B97.21, G04.00-G04.01, G04.31, G04.81-G05.4, G37.0, G37.4-G37.5, H66.40-H66.43, J09.X3-J09.X9, J10.2-J10.89, J11.2-J11.89, L44.4, M1A.10X0-M1A.19X1, M32.0-M32.9, P35.2-P35.9, P37.0-P37.4, P37.8-P37.9, T56.0X1A, T56.0X2A, T56.0X3A, T56.0X4A

G04.91 Myelitis, unspecified `HIV` `MCC`
CC Excl: See code: G04.90

G05 Encephalitis, myelitis and encephalomyelitis in diseases classified elsewhere ✓4th
Code first underlying disease, such as:
human immunodeficiency virus [HIV] disease (B20)
poliovirus (A80.-)
suppurative otitis media (H66.01-H66.4)
trichinellosis (B75)
> EXCLUDES 1   adenoviral encephalitis, myelitis and encephalomyelitis (A85.1)
> congenital toxoplasmosis encephalitis, myelitis and encephalomyelitis (P37.1)
> cytomegaloviral encephalitis, myelitis and encephalomyelitis (B25.8)
> encephalitis, myelitis and encephalomyelitis (in) measles (B05.0)
> encephalitis, myelitis and encephalomyelitis (in) systemic lupus erythematosus (M32.19)
> enteroviral encephalitis, myelitis and encephalomyelitis (A85.0)
> eosinophilic meningoencephalitis (B83.2)
> herpesviral [herpes simplex] encephalitis, myelitis and encephalomyelitis (B00.4)
> listerial encephalitis, myelitis and encephalomyelitis (A32.12)
> meningococcal encephalitis, myelitis and encephalomyelitis (A39.81)
> mumps encephalitis, myelitis and encephalomyelitis (B26.2)
> postchickenpox encephalitis, myelitis and encephalomyelitis (B01.1-)
> rubella encephalitis, myelitis and encephalomyelitis (B06.01)
> toxoplasmosis encephalitis, myelitis and encephalomyelitis (B58.2)
> zoster encephalitis, myelitis and encephalomyelitis (B02.0)

G05.3 Encephalitis and encephalomyelitis in diseases classified elsewhere `MCC`
Meningoencephalitis in diseases classified elsewhere
CC Excl: See code: G04.00

G05.4 Myelitis in diseases classified elsewhere `MCC`
Meningomyelitis in diseases classified elsewhere
CC Excl: See code: G04.00

G06 Intracranial and intraspinal abscess and granuloma ✓4th
Use additional code (B95-B97) to identify infectious agent

G06.0 Intracranial abscess and granuloma `MCC`
Brain [any part] abscess (embolic)
Cerebellar abscess (embolic)
Cerebral abscess (embolic)
Intracranial epidural abscess or granuloma
Intracranial extradural abscess or granuloma
Intracranial subdural abscess or granuloma
Otogenic abscess (embolic)
> EXCLUDES 1   tuberculous intracranial abscess and granuloma (A17.81)
CC Excl: A06.6, A17.81, E08.40-E08.49, E08.618-E08.638, E08.649-E08.8, E09.40-E09.49, E09.618-E09.638, E09.649-E09.8, E10.40-E10.49, E10.618-E10.638, E10.649, E10.69-E10.8, E11.40-E11.49, E11.618-E11.638, E11.649, E11.69-E11.8, E13.40-E13.49, E13.618-E13.638, E13.649-E13.8, G06.0-G08, G93.81, G93.89-G93.9

G06.1 Intraspinal abscess and granulom `MCC`
Abscess (embolic) of spinal cord [any part]
Intraspinal epidural abscess or granuloma
Intraspinal extradural abscess or granuloma
Intraspinal subdural abscess or granuloma
> EXCLUDES 1   tuberculous intraspinal abscess and granuloma (A17.81)
CC Excl: A06.6, A17.81, E08.40-E08.49, E08.618-E08.638, E08.649-E08.8, E09.40-E09.49, E09.618-E09.638, E09.649-E09.8, E10.40-E10.49, E10.618-E10.638, E10.649, E10.69-E10.8, E11.40-E11.49, E11.618-E11.638, E11.649, E11.69-E11.8, E13.40-E13.49, E13.618-E13.638, E13.649-E13.8, G06.1

G06.2 Extradural and subdural abscess, unspecified `MCC`
CC Excl: A06.6, A17.81, E08.40-E08.49, E08.618-E08.638, E08.649-E08.8, E09.40-E09.49, E09.618-E09.638, E09.649-E09.8, E10.40-E10.49, E10.618-E10.638, E10.649, E10.69-E10.8, E11.40-E11.49, E11.618-E11.638, E11.649, E11.69-E11.8, E13.40-E13.49, E13.618-E13.638, E13.649-E13.8, G06.0-G08

G07 Intracranial and intraspinal abscess and granuloma in diseases classified elsewhere `MCC`
Code first underlying disease, such as:
schistosomiasis granuloma of brain (B65.-)
> EXCLUDES 1   abscess of brain:
> amebic (A06.6)
> chromomycotic (B43.1)
> gonococcal (A54.82)
> tuberculous (A17.81)
> tuberculoma of meninges (A17.1)
CC Excl: See code: G06.2

G08   Intracranial and intraspinal phlebitis and thrombophlebitis `MCC`
Septic embolism of intracranial or intraspinal venous sinuses and veins
Septic endophlebitis of intracranial or intraspinal venous sinuses and veins
Septic phlebitis of intracranial or intraspinal venous sinuses and veins
Septic thrombophlebitis of intracranial or intraspinal venous sinuses and veins
Septic thrombosis of intracranial or intraspinal venous sinuses and veins
EXCLUDES 1   intracranial phlebitis and thrombophlebitis complicating: abortion, ectopic or molar pregnancy (O00-O07, O08.7) pregnancy, childbirth and the puerperium (O22.5, O87.3) nonpyogenic intracranial phlebitis and thrombophlebitis (I67.6)
EXCLUDES 2   intracranial phlebitis and thrombophlebitis complicating nonpyogenic intraspinal phlebitis and thrombophlebitis (G95.1)
CC Excl: See code: G06.2

G09   Sequelae of inflammatory diseases of central nervous system
`NOTE`   Category G09 is to be used to indicate conditions whose primary classification is to G00-G08 as the cause of sequelae, themselves classifiable elsewhere. The "sequelae" include conditions specified as residuals.
Code first condition resulting from (sequela) of inflammatory diseases of central nervous system

Systemic atrophies primarily affecting the central nervous system (G10-G14)

G10   Huntington's disease `CC`
Huntington's chorea
Huntington's dementia
CC Excl: G04.1, G20, G21.11-G21.9, G32.89-G37.2, G37.5-G37.9, G80.0-G80.2, G80.4-G80.9, G82.20-G83.0, G92, G93.1, G93.40-G93.6, G93.81, G93.89-G93.9, G96.8-G96.9, G98.0-G98.8, G99.8, I67.83, R53.2

`✓4ᵗʰ` **G11   Hereditary ataxia**
EXCLUDES 2   cerebral palsy (G80.-) hereditary and idiopathic neuropathy (G60.-) metabolic disorders (E70-E88)

CC Excl: For CC codes in category G11, unless otherwise noted:
G04.1, G10-G12.9, G21.0, G23.0-G25.79, G25.82-G26, G32.0-G37.3, G37.5-G37.9, G80.0-G83.9, G90.01-G90.09, G90.2-G90.9, G92-G93.1, G93.40-G93.49, G93.81, G93.89-G93.9, G95.0-G95.9, G96.8-G96.9, G98.0-G99.8, I67.83, R53.2

G11.0   Congenital nonprogressive ataxia `CC`
G11.1   Early-onset cerebellar ataxia `CC`
Early-onset cerebellar ataxia with essential tremor
Early-onset cerebellar ataxia with myoclonus [Hunt's ataxia]
Early-onset cerebellar ataxia with retained tendon reflexes
Friedreich's ataxia (autosomal recessive)
X-linked recessive spinocerebellar ataxia
G11.2   Late-onset cerebellar ataxia `CC` `A`
G11.3   Cerebellar ataxia with defective DNA repair `CC`
Ataxia telangiectasia [Louis-Bar]
EXCLUDES 2   Cockayne's syndrome (Q87.1) other disorders of purine and pyrimidine metabolism (E79.-) xeroderma pigmentosum (Q82.1)
G11.4   Hereditary spastic paraplegia `CC`
CC Excl: G04.1, G10-G12.9, G21.0, G23.0-G25.79, G25.82-G26, G32.0-G37.3, G37.5-G37.9, G80.0-G83.9, G90.01-G90.09, G90.2-G90.9, G92, G93.1, G93.40-G93.49, G93.81, G93.89-G93.9, G95.0-G95.9, G96.12-G96.9, G97.1, G98.0-G99.8, I67.83, R53.2
G11.8   Other hereditary ataxias `CC`
G11.9   Hereditary ataxia, unspecified `CC`
Hereditary cerebellar ataxia NOS
Hereditary cerebellar degeneration
Hereditary cerebellar disease
Hereditary cerebellar syndrome
CC Excl: G11.0-G11.9, G32.81

`✓4ᵗʰ` **G12   Spinal muscular atrophy and related syndromes**
CC Excl: For CC codes in category G12, unless otherwise noted:
E08.40-E08.49, E08.618-E08.638, E08.649-E08.8, E09.40-E09.49, E09.618-E09.638, E09.649-E09.8, E10.40-E10.49, E10.618-E10.638, E10.649, E10.69-E10.8, E11.40-E11.49, E11.618-E11.638, E11.649, E11.69-E11.8, E13.40-E13.49, E13.618-E13.638, E13.649-E13.8, G11.3, G11.8-G12.9, G32.0, G32.89, G90.01-G90.09, G90.2, G90.4-G90.9, G95.0-G95.9, G96.8-G96.9, G98.0-G99.8

G12.0   Infantile spinal muscular atrophy, type I [Werdnig-Hoffman] `CC`

G12.1   Other inherited spinal muscular atrophy `CC`
Adult form spinal muscular atrophy
Childhood form, type II spinal muscular atrophy
Distal spinal muscular atrophy
Juvenile form, type III spinal muscular atrophy [Kugelberg-Welander]
Progressive bulbar palsy of childhood [Fazio-Londe]
Scapuloperoneal form spinal muscular atrophy
`✓5ᵗʰ` **G12.2   Motor neuron disease**
G12.20   Motor neuron disease, unspecified `CC`
G12.21   Amyotrophic lateral sclerosis `CC` `A`
Progressive spinal muscle atrophy
G12.22   Progressive bulbar palsy `CC`
G12.29   Other motor neuron disease `CC`
Familial motor neuron disease
Primary lateral sclerosis
G12.8   Other spinal muscular atrophies and related syndromes `CC`
G12.9   Spinal muscular atrophy, unspecified `CC`

`✓4ᵗʰ` **G13   Systemic atrophies primarily affecting central nervous system in diseases classified elsewhere**
G13.0   Paraneoplastic neuromyopathy and neuropathy
Carcinomatous neuromyopathy
Sensorial paraneoplastic neuropathy [Denny Brown]
Code first underlying neoplasm (C00-D49)
G13.1   Other systemic atrophy primarily affecting central nervous system in neoplastic disease
Paraneoplastic limbic encephalopathy
Code first underlying neoplasm (C00-D49)
G13.2   Systemic atrophy primarily affecting the central nervous system in myxedema
Code first underlying disease, such as:
hypothyroidism (E03.-)
myxedematous congenital iodine deficiency (E00.1)
G13.8   Systemic atrophy primarily affecting central nervous system in other diseases classified elsewhere
Code first underlying disease

G14   Postpolio syndrome
Postpolio myelitic syndrome
EXCLUDES 1   sequelae of poliomyelitis (B91)

Extrapyramidal and movement disorders (G20-G26)

G20   Parkinson's disease
Hemiparkinsonism
Idiopathic Parkinsonism or Parkinson's disease
Paralysis agitans
Parkinsonism or Parkinson's disease NOS
Primary Parkinsonism or Parkinson's disease
EXCLUDES 1   dementia with Parkinsonism (G31.83)

`✓4ᵗʰ` **G21   Secondary parkinsonism**
EXCLUDES 1   dementia with Parkinsonism (G31.83) Huntington's disease (G10) Shy-Drager syndrome (G90.3) syphilitic Parkinsonism (A52.19)
G21.0   Malignant neuroleptic syndrome `MCC`
Use additional code for adverse effect, if applicable, to identify drug (T43.3X5, T43.4X5, T43.5Ø5, T43.595)
EXCLUDES 1   neuroleptic induced parkinsonism (G21.11)
CC Excl: G10, G21.0, G23.0-G25.79, G25.82-G26, G80.3, G81.00-G81.94, G90.3, G93.2, G93.40-G93.49, I67.83
`✓5ᵗʰ` **G21.1   Other drug-induced secondary parkinsonism***
G21.11   Neuroleptic induced parkinsonism `CC`
Use additional code for adverse effect, if applicable, to identify drug (T43.3X5, T43.4X5, T43.5Ø5, T43.595)
EXCLUDES 1   malignant neuroleptic syndrome (G21.0)
CC Excl: G20-G21.9
G21.19   Other drug induced secondary parkinsonism `CC`
Use additional code for adverse effect, if applicable, to identify drug (T36-T50 with fifth or sixth character 5)
CC Excl: See code: G21.11
G21.2   Secondary parkinsonism due to other external agents `CC`
Code first (T51-T65) to identify external agent
CC Excl: See code: G21.11
G21.3   Postencephalitic parkinsonism `CC`
CC Excl: See code: G21.11
G21.4   Vascular parkinsonism

Diseases of the Nervous System

G21.8–G31.1

G21.8 **Other secondary parkinsonism** `CC`
CC Excl: See code: G21.11

G21.9 **Secondary parkinsonism,** unspecified `CC`
CC Excl: See code: G21.11

✓4ᵗʰ **G23** **Other degenerative diseases of basal ganglia**
EXCLUDES 2 *multi-system degeneration of the autonomic nervous system (G90.3)*

CC Excl: For CC codes in category G23, unless otherwise noted:
G20, G21.11-G21.9, G90.01-G90.09, G93.40-G93.49, I67.83

G23.0 **Hallervorden-Spatz disease** `CC`
Pigmentary pallidal degeneration

G23.1 **Progressive supranuclear ophthalmoplegia [Steele-Richardson-Olszewski]** `CC`
Progressive supranuclear palsy

G23.2 **Striatonigral degeneration** `CC`

G23.8 **Other specified degenerative diseases of basal ganglia** `CC`
Calcification of basal ganglia

G23.9 **Degenerative disease of basal ganglia, unspecified** `CC`

✓4ᵗʰ **G24** **Dystonia**
INCLUDES dyskinesia
EXCLUDES 2 *athetoid cerebral palsy (G80.3)*

CC Excl: For CC codes in category G24, unless otherwise noted:
G20, G21.11-G21.9, G25.70-G25.79, G25.89-G26, G80.3, G93.40-G93.49, I67.8

✓5ᵗʰ **G24.0** **Drug induced dystonia**
Use additional code code for adverse effect, if applicable, to identify drug (T36-T50 with fifth or sixth character5)

G24.01 **Drug induced subacute dyskinesia**
Drug induced blepharospasm
Drug induced orofacial dyskinesia
Neuroleptic induced tardive dyskinesia
Tardive dyskinesia

G24.02 **Drug induced acute dystonia** `CC`
Acute dystonic reaction to drugs
Neuroleptic induced acute dystonia

G24.09 **Other drug induced dystonia** `CC`

G24.1 **Genetic torsion dystonia**
Dystonia deformans progressiva
Dystonia musculorum deformans
Familial torsion dystonia
Idiopathic familial dystonia
Idiopathic (torsion) dystonia NOS
(Schwalbe-) Ziehen-Oppenheim disease

G24.2 **Idiopathic nonfamilial dystonia** `CC`

G24.3 **Spasmodic torticollis**
EXCLUDES 1 *congenital torticollis (Q68.0)*
hysterical torticollis (F44.4)
ocular torticollis (R29.891)
psychogenic torticollis (F45.8)
torticollis NOS (M43.6)
traumatic recurrent torticollis (S13.4)

G24.4 **Idiopathic orofacial dystonia**
Orofacial dyskinesia
EXCLUDES 1 *drug induced orofacial dyskinesia (G24.01)*

G24.5 **Blepharospasm**
EXCLUDES 1 *drug induced blepharospasm (G24.01)*

G24.8 **Other dystonia** `CC`
Acquired torsion dystonia NOS

G24.9 **Dystonia, unspecified**
Dyskinesia NOS

✓4ᵗʰ **G25** **Other extrapyramidal and movement disorders**
EXCLUDES 2 *sleep related movement disorders (G47.6-)*

G25.0 **Essential tremor**
Familial tremor
EXCLUDES 1 *tremor NOS (R25.1)*

G25.1 **Drug-induced tremor**
Use additional code for adverse effect, if applicable, to identify drug (T36-T50 with fifth or sixth character 5)

G25.2 **Other specified forms of tremor**
Intention tremor

G25.3 **Myoclonus**
Drug-induced myoclonus
Palatal myoclonus
Use additional code for adverse effect, if applicable, to identify drug (T36-T50 with fifth or sixth character 5)
EXCLUDES 1 *facial myokymia (G51.4)*
myoclonic epilepsy (G40.-)

G25.4 **Drug-induced chorea**
Use additional code for adverse effect, if applicable, to identify drug (T36-T50 with fifth or sixth character 5)

G25.5 **Other chorea**
Chorea NOS
EXCLUDES 1 *chorea NOS with heart involvement (I02.0)*
Huntington's chorea (G10)
rheumatic chorea (I02.-)
Sydenham's chorea (I02.-)

✓5ᵗʰ **G25.6** **Drug induced tics and other tics of organic origin**

G25.61 **Drug induced tics**
Use additional code for adverse effect, if applicable, to identify drug (T36-T50 with fifth or sixth character 5)

G25.69 **Other tics of organic origin**
EXCLUDES 1 *habit spasm (F95.9)*
tic NOS (F95.9)
Tourette's syndrome (F95.2)

✓5ᵗʰ **G25.7** **Other and unspecified drug induced movement disorders**
Use additional code for adverse effect, if applicable, to identify drug (T36-T50 with fifth or sixth character 5)

G25.70 **Drug induced movement disorder, unspecified**

G25.71 **Drug induced akathisia**
Drug induced acathisia
Neuroleptic induced acute akathisia

G25.79 **Other drug induced movement disorders**

✓5ᵗʰ **G25.8** **Other specified extrapyramidal and movement disorders**

G25.81 **Restless legs syndrome**

G25.82 **Stiff-man syndrome** `CC`
CC Excl: G04.1, G10, G12.22, G20-G21.9, G24.01-G25.79, G25.82-G26, G32.89-G37.2, G37.5-G37.9, G80.0-G80.9, G82.20-G83.0, G92, G93.1, G93.40-G93.6, G93.81, G93.89-G93.9, G96.8-G96.9

G25.83 **Benign shuddering attacks**

G25.89 **Other specified extrapyramidal and movement disorders**

G25.9 **Extrapyramidal and movement disorder, unspecified** `CC`
CC Excl: See code: G25.82

G26 *Extrapyramidal and movement disorders in diseases classified elsewhere*
Code first underlying disease

Other degenerative diseases of the nervous system (G30-G32)

✓4ᵗʰ **G30** **Alzheimer's disease**
INCLUDES Alzheimer's dementia senile and presenile forms
Use additional code to identify:
delirium, if applicable (F05)
dementia with behavioral disturbance (F02.81)
dementia without behavioral disturbance (F02.80)
EXCLUDES 1 *senile degeneration of brain NEC (G31.1)*
senile dementia NOS (F03)
senility NOS (R41.81)

G30.0 **Alzheimer's disease with early onset**

G30.1 **Alzheimer's disease with late onset** `A`

G30.8 **Other Alzheimer's disease**

G30.9 **Alzheimer's disease, unspecified**
AHA: 2012, 4Q, 95

✓4ᵗʰ **G31** **Other degenerative diseases of nervous system, not elsewhere classified**
Use additional code to identify:
dementia with behavioral disturbance (F02.81)
dementia without behavioral disturbance (F02.80)
EXCLUDES 2 *Reye's syndrome (G93.7)*

✓5ᵗʰ **G31.0** **Frontotemporal dementia**

G31.01 **Pick's disease**
Primary progressive aphasia
Progressive isolated aphasia

G31.09 **Other frontotemporal dementia**
Frontal dementia

G31.1 **Senile degeneration of brain, not elsewhere classified**
EXCLUDES 1 *Alzheimer's disease (G30.-)*
senility NOS (R41.81)

Ⓝ Newborn: 0   Ⓟ Pediatric: 0-17   Ⓜ Maternity: 12-55   Ⓐ Adult: 15-124   MCC Major CC Condition   PDx MCC PDx acts as own MCC   CC CC Condition   PDx CC PDx acts as own CC

532   ICD-10-CM Draft (2015)

G31.2 Degeneration of nervous system due to alcohol
Alcoholic cerebellar ataxia
Alcoholic cerebellar degeneration
Alcoholic cerebral degeneration
Alcoholic encephalopathy
Dysfunction of the autonomic nervous system due to alcohol
Code also associated alcoholism (F10.-)

✓5th **G31.8 Other specified degenerative diseases of nervous system**

> **CC Excl:** For CC codes in subcategory G31.8, unless otherwise noted: E75.00-E75.19, E75.4, F84.2, G13.2-G13.8, G30.0-G31.82, G31.84-G31.9, G91.4, G94

G31.81 Alpers disease `CC`
Grey-matter degeneration

G31.82 Leigh's disease `CC`
Subacute necrotizing encephalopathy

G31.83 Dementia with Lewy bodies
Dementia with Parkinsonism   Lewy body disease
Lewy body dementia

G31.84 Mild cognitive impairment, so stated
> **EXCLUDES 1** age related cognitive decline (R41.81)
> altered mental status (R41.82)
> cerebral degeneration (G31.9)
> change in mental status (R41.82)
> cognitive deficits following (sequelae of) cerebral hemorrhage or infarction (I69.01, I69.11, I69.21, I69.31, I69.81, I69.91)
> cognitive impairment due to intracranial or head injury (S06.-)
> dementia (F01.-, F02.-, F03)
> mild memory disturbance (F06.8)
> neurologic neglect syndrome (R41.4)
> personality change, nonpsychotic (F68.8)

G31.85 Corticobasal degeneration

G31.89 Other specified degenerative diseases of nervous system

G31.9 Degenerative disease of nervous system, unspecified

✓4th **G32 Other degenerative disorders of nervous system in diseases classified elsewhere**

G32.0 Subacute combined degeneration of spinal cord in diseases elsewhere `CC`
Dana-Putnam syndrome
Sclerosis of spinal cord (combined) (dorsolateral) (posterolateral)
Code first underlying disease, such as:
vitamin B12 deficiency (E53.8)
vitamin B12 deficiency:
anemia (D51.9)
dietary (D51.3)
pernicious (D51.0)
> **EXCLUDES 1** syphilitic combined degeneration of spinal cord (A52.11)
CC Excl: G04.1, G11.3, G11.8-G12.9, G32.0, G32.89-G37.3, G37.5-G37.9, G80.0-G80.2, G80.4-G83.9, G90.01-G90.09, G90.2, G90.4-G90.9, G93.1, G93.40-G93.49, G95.0-G95.9, G96.12-G96.9, G97.1, G98.0-G99.8, I67.83, R53.2

✓5th **G32.8 Other specified degenerative disorders of nervous system in diseases classified elsewhere**
Code first underlying disease, such as:
amyloidosis cerebral degeneration (E85.-)
cerebral degeneration (due to) hypothyroidism (E00.0-E03.9)
cerebral degeneration (due to) neoplasm (C00-D49)
cerebral degeneration (due to) vitamin B deficiency, except thiamine (E52-E53.-)
> **EXCLUDES 1** superior hemorrhagic polioencephalitis [Wernicke's encephalopathy] (E51.2)

G32.81 Cerebellar ataxia in diseases classified elsewhere `CC`
Code first underlying disease, such as:
celiac disease (with gluten ataxia) (K90.0)
cerebellar ataxia (in) neoplastic disease (paraneoplastic cerebellar degeneration) (C00-D49)
non-celiac gluten ataxia (M35.9)
> **EXCLUDES 1** systemic atrophy primarily affecting the central nervous system in alcoholic cerebellar ataxia (G31.2)
> systemic atrophy primarily affecting the central nervous system in myxedema (G13.2)
CC Excl: G04.1, G10-G12.9, G21.0, G23.0-G25.79, G25.82-G26, G32.0-G37.3, G37.5-G37.9, G80.0-G83.9, G90.01-G90.09, G90.2-G90.9, G92-G93.1, G93.40-G93.49, G93.81, G93.89-G93.9, G95.0-G95.9, G96.8-G96.9, G98.0-G99.8, I67.83, R53.2

G32.89 Other specified degenerative disorders of nervous system in diseases classified elsewhere
Degenerative encephalopathy in diseases classified elsewhere

Demyelinating diseases of the central nervous system (G35-G37)

G35 Multiple sclerosis
Disseminated multiple sclerosis
Generalized multiple sclerosis
Multiple sclerosis NOS
Multiple sclerosis of brain stem
Multiple sclerosis of cord

✓4th **G36 Other acute disseminated demyelination**
> **EXCLUDES 1** postinfectious encephalitis and encephalomyelitis NOS (G04.01)

G36.0 Neuromyelitis optica [Devic] `CC`
Demyelination in optic neuritis
> **EXCLUDES 1** optic neuritis NOS (H46)
CC Excl: G36.0, G93.40-G93.49, I67.83

G36.1 Acute and subacute hemorrhagic leuko encephalitis [Hurst] `CC`
CC Excl: G04.1, G10-G12.9, G21.0, G24.01-G25.79, G25.82-G26, G32.0-G37.3, G37.5-G37.9, G80.0-G83.9, G90.01-G90.09, G90.2, G90.4-G90.9, G92, G93.40-G93.49, G93.81, G93.89-G93.9, G95.0-G95.9, G96.8-G96.9, G98.0-G99.8, I67.83, R53.2

G36.8 Other specified acute disseminated demyelination `CC`
CC Excl: See code: G36.1

G36.9 Acute disseminated demyelination, unspecified `HIV` `CC`
CC Excl: See code: G36.1

✓4th **G37 Other demyelinating diseases of central nervous system**

G37.0 Diffuse sclerosis of central nervous system `CC`
Periaxial encephalitis
Schilder's disease
> **EXCLUDES 1** X linked adrenoleukodystrophy (E71.52-)
CC Excl: A92.30-A92.39, B97.21, G93.40-G93.49, I67.83

G37.1 Central demyelination of corpus callosum `CC`
CC Excl: See code: G36.1

G37.2 Central pontine myelinolysis `CC`
CC Excl: See code: G36.1

G37.3 Acute transverse myelitis in demyelinating disease of central nervous system `CC`
Acute transverse myelitis NOS
Acute transverse myelopathy
> **EXCLUDES 1** multiple sclerosis (G35)
> neuromyelitis optica [Devic] (G36.0)
CC Excl: A02.21, A17.0-A17.1, A27.81, A39.0, A50.41, A51.41, A52.13, A54.82, A54.84, A54.89-A54.9, A87.0-A87.9, A96.2, A98.3-A98.4, B00.3, B00.89-B00.9, B02.0-B02.23, B02.29, B02.7-B02.9, B10.81-B10.89, B26.1, B33.24, B33.4-B33.8, B34.1-B34.2, B34.4-B34.8, B37.5, B38.4, B45.1, B58.2, B92, B94.2-B94.9, B97.10, B97.19, B97.29, B97.5-B97.6, B97.81-B97.89, E08.40-E08.49, E09.40-E09.49, E10.40-E10.49, E11.40-E11.49, E13.40-E13.49, G00.0-G03.9, G04.1-G04.2, G11.3, G11.8-G12.9, G32.0, G32.89-G37.2, G37.5-G37.9, G61.0, G80.0-G80.2, G80.4-G83.9, G90.01-G90.09, G90.2, G90.4-G90.9, G93.1, G93.40-G93.49, G95.0-G95.9, G96.12-G96.9, G97.1, G98.0-G99.8, I67.83, R53.2

G37.4 Subacute necrotizing myelitis of central nervous system `HIV` `MCC`
CC Excl: A17.82, A28.1, A50.42, A52.14, A75.9, A79.9, A81.1, A81.82-A81.89, A83.0-A85.8, A87.2, A88.0, A88.8, A92.1-A92.8, A93.0, B00.4, B00.82, B01.11-B01.12, B04, B06.01, B08.09, B08.20-B08.22, B08.60-B08.79, B09-B10.09, B26.2, B27.00-B27.99, B33.1, B45.0, B45.2-B45.9, B54, B58.2, B75, B97.10, B97.21, G04.00-G04.01, G04.31, G04.81-G05.4, G37.0, G37.4-G37.5, H66.40-H66.43, J09.X3-J09.X9, J10.2-J10.89, J11.2-J11.89, L44.4, M1A.10X0-M1A.19X1, M32.0-M32.9, P35.2-P35.9, P37.0-P37.4, P37.8-P37.9, T56.0X1A, T56.0X2A, T56.0X3A, T56.0X4A

Diseases of the Nervous System

G37.5–G40.211

G37.5 Concentric sclerosis [Balo] of central nervous system `CC`
    CC Excl: See code: G37.0

G37.8 Other specified demyelinating diseases of central nervous system `CC`
    CC Excl: See code: G36.1

G37.9 Demyelinating disease of central nervous system, unspecified `HIV` `CC`
    CC Excl: See code: G36.1

Episodic and paroxysmal disorders (G40-G47)

√4ᵗʰ G40 Epilepsy and recurrent seizures
> **NOTE** The following terms are to be considered equivalent to intractable: pharmacoresistant (pharmacologically resistant), treatment resistant, refractory (medically) and poorly controlled
>
> **EXCLUDES 1** conversion disorder with seizures (F44.5)
> convulsions NOS (R56.9)
> hippocampal sclerosis (G93.81)
> mesial temporal sclerosis (G93.81)
> post traumatic seizures (R56.1)
> seizure (convulsive) NOS (R56.9)
> seizure of newborn (P90)
> temporal sclerosis (G93.81)
> Todd's paralysis (G83.8)

√5ᵗʰ G40.0 Localization-related (focal) (partial) idiopathic epilepsy and epileptic syndromes with seizures of localized onset
> Benign childhood epilepsy with centrotemporal EEG spikes
> Childhood epilepsy with occipital EEG paroxysms
> **EXCLUDES 1** adult onset localization-related epilepsy (G40.1-, G40.2-)

√6ᵗʰ G40.00 Localization-related (focal) (partial) idiopathic epilepsy and epileptic syndromes with seizures of localized onset, not intractable
> Localization-related (focal) (partial) idiopathic epilepsy and epileptic syndromes with seizures of localized onset without intractability

    G40.001 Localization-related (focal) (partial) idiopathic epilepsy and epileptic syndromes with seizures of localized onset, not intractable, with status epilepticus `CC`
> CC Excl: G32.89, G40.001-G40.919, G93.40-G93.49, G93.9, G96.8-G96.9, G98.0-G98.8, G99.8, I67.83, R56.1

    G40.009 Localization-related (focal) (partial) idiopathic epilepsy and epileptic syndromes with seizures of localized onset, not intractable, without status epilepticus `CC`
> Localization-related (focal) (partial) idiopathic epilepsy and epileptic syndromes with seizures of localized onset NOS
> CC Excl: See code: G40.001

√6ᵗʰ G40.01 Localization-related (focal) (partial) idiopathic epilepsy and epileptic syndromes with seizures of localized onset, intractable
> CC Excl: For CC codes in subcategory G40.01, unless otherwise noted: E08.40-E08.49, E09.40-E09.49, E10.40-E10.49, E11.40-E11.49, E13.40-E13.49, G32.89, G40.001-G40.919, G93.81, G93.89-G93.9, G96.8-G96.9, G98.0-G98.8, G99.8, R56.1

    G40.011 Localization-related (focal) (partial) idiopathic epilepsy and epileptic syndromes with seizures of localized onset, intractable, with status epilepticus `CC`

    G40.019 Localization-related (focal) (partial) idiopathic epilepsy and epileptic syndromes with seizures of localized onset, intractable, without status epilepticus `CC`

√5ᵗʰ G40.1 Localization-related (focal) (partial) symptomatic epilepsy and epileptic syndromes with simple partial seizures
> Attacks without alteration of consciousness
> Epilepsia partialis continua [Kozhevnikof]
> Simple partial seizures developing into secondarily generalized seizures

√6ᵗʰ G40.10 Localization-related (focal) (partial) symptomatic epilepsy and epileptic syndromes with simple partial seizures, not intractable
> Localization-related (focal) (partial) symptomatic epilepsy and epileptic syndromes with simple partial seizures without intractability
>
> CC Excl: For CC codes in subcategory G40.10, unless otherwise noted: G32.89, G40.001-G40.919, G93.40-G93.49, G93.9, G96.8-G96.9, G98.0-G98.8, G99.8, I67.83, R56.1

    G40.101 Localization-related (focal) (partial) symptomatic epilepsy and epileptic syndromes with simple partial seizures, not intractable, with status epilepticus `CC`

    G40.109 Localization-related (focal) (partial) symptomatic epilepsy and epileptic syndromes with simple partial seizures, not intractable, without status epilepticus `CC`
> Localization-related (focal) (partial) symptomatic epilepsy and epileptic syndromes with simple partial seizures NOS

√6ᵗʰ G40.11 Localization-related (focal) (partial) symptomatic epilepsy and epileptic syndromes with simple partial seizures, intractable
> CC Excl: For CC codes in subcategory G40.11, unless otherwise noted: E08.40-E08.49, E09.40-E09.49, E10.40-E10.49, E11.40-E11.49, E13.40-E13.49, G32.89, G40.001-G40.919, G93.81, G93.89-G93.9, G96.8-G96.9, G98.0-G98.8, G99.8, R56.1

    G40.111 Localization-related (focal) (partial) symptomatic epilepsy and epileptic syndromes with simple partial seizures, intractable, with status epilepticus `CC`

    G40.119 Localization-related (focal) (partial) symptomatic epilepsy and epileptic syndromes with simple partial seizures, intractable, without status epilepticus `CC`

√5ᵗʰ G40.2 Localization-related (focal) (partial) symptomatic epilepsy and epileptic syndromes with complex partial seizures
> Attacks with alteration of consciousness, often with automatisms
> Complex partial seizures developing into secondarily generalized seizures

√6ᵗʰ G40.20 Localization-related (focal) (partial) symptomatic epilepsy and epileptic syndromes with complex partial seizures, not intractable
> Localization-related (focal) (partial) symptomatic epilepsy and epileptic syndromes with complex partial seizures without intractability
>
> CC Excl: For CC codes in subcategory G40.20, unless otherwise noted: G32.89, G40.001-G40.919, G93.40-G93.49, G93.9, G96.8-G96.9, G98.0-G98.8, G99.8, I67.83, R56.1

    G40.201 Localization-related (focal) (partial) symptomatic epilepsy and epileptic syndromes with complex partial seizures, not intractable, with status epilepticus `CC`

    G40.209 Localization-related (focal) (partial) symptomatic epilepsy and epileptic syndromes with complex partial seizures, not intractable, without status epilepticus `CC`
> Localization-related (focal) (partial) symptomatic epilepsy and epileptic syndromes with complex partial seizures NOS

√6ᵗʰ G40.21 Localization-related (focal) (partial) symptomatic epilepsy and epileptic syndromes with complex partial seizures, intractable
> CC Excl: For CC codes in subcategory G40.21, unless otherwise noted: E08.40-E08.49, E09.40-E09.49, E10.40-E10.49, E11.40-E11.49, E13.40-E13.49, G32.89, G40.001-G40.919, G93.81, G93.89-G93.9, G96.8-G96.9, G98.0-G98.8, G99.8, R56.1

    G40.211 Localization-related (focal) (partial) symptomatic epilepsy and epileptic syndromes with complex partial seizures, intractable, with status epilepticus `CC`

N Newborn: 0   P Pediatric: 0-17   M Maternity: 12-55   A Adult: 15-124   MCC Major CC Condition   PDx MCC PDx acts as own MCC   CC CC Condition   PDx CC PDx acts as own CC

534   ICD-10-CM Draft (2015)

G40.219 Localization-related (focal) (partial) symptomatic epilepsy and epileptic syndromes with complex partial seizures, intractable, without status epilepticus `CC`

✓5th **G40.3** Generalized **idiopathic epilepsy and epileptic syndromes**
Code also MERRF syndrome, if applicable (E88.42)

> **CC Excl:** For MCC codes in subcategory G40.3, unless otherwise noted: E08.40-E08.49, E08.618-E08.638, E08.649-E08.8, E09.40-E09.49, E09.618-E09.638, E09.649-E09.8, E10.40-E10.49, E10.618-E10.638, E10.649, E10.69-E10.8, E11.40-E11.49, E11.618-E11.638, E11.649, E11.69-E11.8, E13.40-E13.49, E13.618-E13.638, E13.649-E13.8, G32.89, G40.001-G40.919, G93.81, G93.89-G93.9, G96.8-G96.9, G98.0-G98.8, G99.8, R56.1

✓6th **G40.30** Generalized idiopathic epilepsy and epileptic syndromes, **not intractable**
Generalized idiopathic epilepsy and epileptic syndromes without intractability

G40.301 Generalized idiopathic epilepsy and epileptic syndromes, not intractable, with status epilepticus `MCC`

G40.309 Generalized idiopathic epilepsy and epileptic syndromes, not intractable, without status epilepticus
Generalized idiopathic epilepsy and epileptic syndromes NOS

✓6th **G40.31** Generalized idiopathic epilepsy and epileptic syndromes, **intractable**

G40.311 Generalized idiopathic epilepsy and epileptic syndromes, intractable, with status epilepticus `MCC`

G40.319 Generalized idiopathic epilepsy and epileptic syndromes, intractable, without status epilepticus `MCC`

✓5th **G40.A** Absence **epileptic syndrome**
Childhood absence epilepsy [pyknolepsy]
Juvenile absence epilepsy
Absence epileptic syndrome, NOS

> **CC Excl:** For CC codes in subcategory G40.A, unless otherwise noted: E08.40-E08.49, E09.40-E09.49, E10.40-E10.49, E11.40-E11.49, E13.40-E13.49, G32.89, G40.001-G40.919, G93.81, G93.89-G93.9, G96.8-G96.9, G98.0-G98.8, G99.8, R56.1

✓6th **G40.A0** Absence epileptic syndrome, **not intractable**
G40.A01 Absence epileptic syndrome, not intractable, with status epilepticus
G40.A09 Absence epileptic syndrome, not intractable, without status epilepticus

✓6th **G40.A1** Absence epileptic syndrome, **intractable**
G40.A11 Absence epileptic syndrome, intractable, with status epilepticus `CC`
G40.A19 Absence epileptic syndrome, intractable, without status epilepticus `CC`

✓5th **G40.B** Juvenile myoclonic epilepsy [impulsive petit mal]

> **CC Excl:** For CC codes in subcategory G40.B, unless otherwise noted: E08.40-E08.49, E09.40-E09.49, E10.40-E10.49, E11.40-E11.49, E13.40-E13.49, G32.89, G40.001-G40.919, G93.81, G93.89-G93.9, G96.8-G96.9, G98.0-G98.8, G99.8, R56.1

✓6th **G40.B0** Juvenile myoclonic epilepsy, **not intractable**
G40.B01 Juvenile myoclonic epilepsy, not intractable, with status epilepticus `CC`
G40.B09 Juvenile myoclonic epilepsy, not intractable, without status epilepticus `CC`

✓6th **G40.B1** Juvenile myoclonic epilepsy, **intractable**
G40.B11 Juvenile myoclonic epilepsy, intractable, with status epilepticus `CC`
G40.B19 Juvenile myoclonic epilepsy, intractable, without status epilepticus `CC`

✓5th **G40.4** Other generalized **epilepsy and epileptic syndromes**
Epilepsy with grand mal seizures on awakening
Epilepsy with myoclonic absences
Epilepsy with myoclonic-astatic seizures
Grand mal seizure NOS
Nonspecific atonic epileptic seizures
Nonspecific clonic epileptic seizures
Nonspecific myoclonic epileptic seizures
Nonspecific tonic epileptic seizures
Nonspecific tonic-clonic epileptic seizures
Symptomatic early myoclonic encephalopathy

✓6th **G40.40** Other generalized epilepsy and epileptic syndromes, **not intractable**
Other generalized epilepsy and epileptic syndromes without intractability
Other generalized epilepsy and epileptic syndromes NOS

G40.401 Other generalized epilepsy and epileptic syndromes, not intractable, with status epilepticus
CC Excl: See code: G40.001

G40.409 Other generalized epilepsy and epileptic syndromes, not intractable, without status epilepticus
CC Excl: See code: G40.001

✓6th **G40.41** Other generalized epilepsy and epileptic syndromes, **intractable**

> **CC Excl:** For CC codes in subcategory G40.41, unless otherwise noted: E08.40-E08.49, E09.40-E09.49, E10.40-E10.49, E11.40-E11.49, E13.40-E13.49, G32.89, G40.001-G40.919, G93.81, G93.89-G93.9, G96.8-G96.9, G98.0-G98.8, G99.8, R56.1

G40.411 Other generalized epilepsy and epileptic syndromes, intractable, with status epilepticus `CC`

G40.419 Other generalized epilepsy and epileptic syndromes, intractable, without status epilepticus `CC`

✓5th **G40.5** Epileptic **seizures related to external causes**
Epileptic seizures related to alcohol
Epileptic seizures related to drugs
Epileptic seizures related to hormonal changes
Epileptic seizures related to sleep deprivation
Epileptic seizures related to stress
Use additional code for adverse effect, if applicable, to identify drug (T36-T50 with fifth or sixth character 5)
Code also, if applicable, associated epilepsy and recurrent seizures (G40.-)

> **CC Excl:** For CC codes in subcategory G40.5, unless otherwise noted: E08.40-E08.49, E09.40-E09.49, E10.40-E10.49, E11.40-E11.49, E13.40-E13.49, G32.89, G40.001-G40.919, G93.81, G93.89-G93.9, G96.8-G96.9, G98.0-G98.8, G99.8, R56.1

✓6th **G40.50** Epileptic seizures related to external causes, **not intractable**
G40.501 Epileptic seizures related to external causes, not intractable, with status epilepticus `CC`
G40.509 Epileptic seizures related to external causes, not intractable, without status epilepticus `CC`
Epileptic seizures related to external causes, NOS

✓5th **G40.8** Other **epilepsy and recurrent seizures**
Epilepsies and epileptic syndromes undetermined as to whether they are focal or generalized
Landau-Kleffner syndrome

> **CC Excl:** For CC codes in subcategory G40.8, unless otherwise noted: E08.40-E08.49, E09.40-E09.49, E10.40-E10.49, E11.40-E11.49, E13.40-E13.49, G32.89, G40.001-G40.919, G93.81, G93.89-G93.9, G96.8-G96.9, G98.0-G98.8, G99.8, R56.1

✓6th **G40.80** Other **epilepsy**
G40.801 Other epilepsy, not intractable, with status epilepticus `CC`
Other epilepsy without intractability with status epilepticus

---

✓ Additional Character Required   ✓x7th Xtension Alert   <u>Unacceptable PDx</u>   Manifestation   Hospital Acquired Condition   **EXCLUDES 1** Not Coded Here   **EXCLUDES 2** Not Included Here

Diseases of the Nervous System

G40.802–G43.519

G40.802 **Other epilepsy, not intractable, without status epilepticus** `CC`
Other epilepsy without intractability without status epilepticus

G40.803 **Other epilepsy, intractable, with status epilepticus** `CC`

G40.804 **Other epilepsy, intractable, without status epilepticus** `CC`

√6ᵗʰ **G40.81** **Lennox-Gastaut syndrome**

G40.811 **Lennox-Gastaut syndrome, not intractable, with status epilepticus** `CC`

G40.812 **Lennox-Gastaut syndrome, not intractable, without status epilepticus** `CC`

G40.813 **Lennox-Gastaut syndrome, intractable, with status epilepticus** `CC`

G40.814 **Lennox-Gastaut syndrome, intractable, without status epilepticus** `CC`

√6ᵗʰ **G40.82** **Epileptic spasms**
Infantile spasms
Salaam attacks
West's syndrome

G40.821 **Epileptic spasms, not intractable, with status epilepticus** `CC`

G40.822 **Epileptic spasms, not intractable, without status epilepticus** `CC`

G40.823 **Epileptic spasms, intractable, with status epilepticus** `CC`

G40.824 **Epileptic spasms, intractable, without status epilepticus** `CC`

G40.89 **Other seizures** `CC`
EXCLUDES 1   *post traumatic seizures (R56.1)*
recurrent seizures NOS (G40.909)
seizure NOS (R56.9)

√5ᵗʰ **G40.9** **Epilepsy, unspecified**

> **CC Excl: For CC codes in subcategory G40.9, unless otherwise noted:** E08.40-E08.49, E09.40-E09.49, E10.40-E10.49, E11.40-E11.49, E13.40-E13.49, G32.89, G40.001-G40.919, G93.81, G93.89-G93.9, G96.8-G96.9, G98.0-G98.8, G99.8, R56.1

√6ᵗʰ **G40.90** **Epilepsy, unspecified, not intractable**
Epilepsy, unspecified, without intractability

G40.901 **Epilepsy, unspecified, not intractable, with status epilepticus**

G40.909 **Epilepsy, unspecified, not intractable, without status epilepticus**
Epilepsy NOS
Epileptic convulsions NOS
Epileptic fits NOS
Epileptic seizures NOS
Recurrent seizures NOS
Seizure disorder NOS

√6ᵗʰ **G40.91** **Epilepsy, unspecified, intractable**
Intractable seizure disorder NOS

G40.911 **Epilepsy, unspecified, intractable, with status epilepticus** `CC`

G40.919 **Epilepsy, unspecified, intractable, without status epilepticus** `CC`

√4ᵗʰ **G43** **Migraine**
NOTE   The following terms are to be considered equivalent to intractable: pharmacoresistant (pharmacologically resistant), treatment resistant, refractory (medically) and poorly controlled
Use additional code for adverse effect, if applicable, to identify drug (T36-T50 with fifth or sixth character 5)
EXCLUDES 1   *headache NOS (R51)*
lower half migraine (G44.00)
EXCLUDES 2   *headache syndromes (G44.-)*

√5ᵗʰ **G43.0** **Migraine without aura**
Common migraine
EXCLUDES 1   *chronic migraine without aura (G43.7-)*

√6ᵗʰ **G43.00** **Migraine without aura, not intractable**
Migraine without aura without mention of refractory migraine

G43.001 **Migraine without aura, not intractable, with status migrainosus**

G43.009 **Migraine without aura, not intractable, without status migrainosus**
Migraine without aura NOS

√6ᵗʰ **G43.01** **Migraine without aura, intractable**
Migraine without aura with refractory migraine

G43.011 **Migraine without aura, intractable, with status migrainosus**

G43.019 **Migraine without aura, intractable, without status migrainosus**

√5ᵗʰ **G43.1** **Migraine with aura**
Basilar migraine
Classical migraine
Migraine equivalents
Migraine preceded or accompanied by transient focal neurological phenomena
Migraine triggered seizures
Migraine with acute-onset aura
Migraine with aura without headache (migraine equivalents)
Migraine with prolonged aura
Migraine with typical aura
Retinal migraine
Code also any associated seizure (G40.-, R56.9)
EXCLUDES 1   *persistent migraine aura (G43.5-, G43.6-)*

√6ᵗʰ **G43.10** **Migraine with aura, not intractable**
Migraine with aura without mention of refractory migraine

G43.101 **Migraine with aura, not intractable, with status migrainosus**

G43.109 **Migraine with aura, not intractable, without status migrainosus**
Migraine with aura NOS

√6ᵗʰ **G43.11** **Migraine with aura, intractable**
Migraine with aura with refractory migraine

G43.111 **Migraine with aura, intractable, with status migrainosus**

G43.119 **Migraine with aura, intractable, without status migrainosus**

√5ᵗʰ **G43.4** **Hemiplegic migraine**
Familial migraine
Sporadic migraine

√6ᵗʰ **G43.40** **Hemiplegic migraine, not intractable**
Hemiplegic migraine without refractory migraine

G43.401 **Hemiplegic migraine, not intractable, with status migrainosus**

G43.409 **Hemiplegic migraine, not intractable, without status migrainosus**
Hemiplegic migraine NOS

√6ᵗʰ **G43.41** **Hemiplegic migraine, intractable**
Hemiplegic migraine with refractory migraine

G43.411 **Hemiplegic migraine, intractable, with status migrainosus**

G43.419 **Hemiplegic migraine, intractable, without status migrainosus**

√5ᵗʰ **G43.5** **Persistent migraine aura without cerebral infarction**

√6ᵗʰ **G43.50** **Persistent migraine aura without cerebral infarction, not intractable**
Persistent migraine aura without cerebral infarction, without refractory migraine

G43.501 **Persistent migraine aura without cerebral infarction, not intractable, with status migrainosus**

G43.509 **Persistent migraine aura without cerebral infarction, not intractable, without status migrainosus**
Persistent migraine aura NOS

√6ᵗʰ **G43.51** **Persistent migraine aura without cerebral infarction, intractable**
Persistent migraine aura without cerebral infarction, with refractory migraine

G43.511 **Persistent migraine aura without cerebral infarction, intractable, with status migrainosus**

G43.519 **Persistent migraine aura without cerebral infarction, intractable, without status migrainosus**

N Newborn: 0   P Pediatric: 0-17   M Maternity: 12-55   A Adult: 15-124   MCC Major CC Condition   PDx MCC PDx acts as own MCC   CC CC Condition   PDx CC PDx acts as own CC

536   ICD-10-CM Draft (2015)

Diseases of the Nervous System

G43.6–G44.031

√5th **G43.6 Persistent migraine aura with cerebral infarction**
Code also the type of cerebral infarction (I63.-)

CC Excl: For CC codes in subcategory G43.6, unless otherwise noted: G43.601-G43.619, I63.00-I66.9

√6th **G43.60 Persistent migraine aura with cerebral infarction, not intractable**
Persistent migraine aura with cerebral infarction, without refractory migraine

G43.601 Persistent migraine aura with cerebral CC
infarction, not intractable, with status migrainosus

G43.609 Persistent migraine aura with cerebral CC
infarction, not intractable, without status migrainosus

√6th **G43.61 Persistent migraine aura with cerebral infarction, intractable**
Persistent migraine aura with cerebral infarction, with refractory migraine

G43.611 Persistent migraine aura with cerebral CC
infarction, intractable, with status migrainosus

G43.619 Persistent migraine aura with cerebral CC
infarction, intractable, without status migrainosus

√5th **G43.7 Chronic migraine without aura**
Transformed migraine
EXCLUDES 1 *migraine without aura (G43.0-)*

√6th **G43.70 Chronic migraine without aura, not intractable**
Chronic migraine without aura, without refractory migraine

G43.701 Chronic migraine without aura, not intractable, with status migrainosus

G43.709 Chronic migraine without aura, not intractable, without status migrainosus
Chronic migraine without aura NOS

√6th **G43.71 Chronic migraine without aura, intractable**
Chronic migraine without aura, with refractory migraine

G43.711 Chronic migraine without aura, intractable, with status migrainosus

G43.719 Chronic migraine without aura, intractable, without status migrainosus

√5th **G43.A Cyclical vomiting**

G43.A0 Cyclical vomiting, not intractable
Cyclical vomiting, without refractory migraine

G43.A1 Cyclical vomiting, intractable
Cyclical vomiting, with refractory migraine

√5th **G43.B Ophthalmoplegic migraine**

G43.B0 Ophthalmoplegic migraine, not intractable
Ophthalmoplegic migraine, without refractory migraine

G43.B1 Ophthalmoplegic migraine, intractable
Ophthalmoplegic migraine, with refractory migraine

√5th **G43.C Periodic headache syndromes in child or adult**

G43.C0 Periodic headache syndromes in child or adult, not intractable
Periodic headache syndromes in child or adult, without refractory migraine

G43.C1 Periodic headache syndromes in child or adult, intractable
Periodic headache syndromes in child or adult, with refractory migraine

√5th **G43.D Abdominal migraine**

G43.D0 Abdominal migraine, not intractable
Abdominal migraine, without refractory migraine

G43.D1 Abdominal migraine, intractable
Abdominal migraine, with refractory migraine

√5th **G43.8 Other migraine**

√6th **G43.80 Other migraine, not intractable**
Other migraine, without refractory migraine

G43.801 Other migraine, not intractable, with status migrainosus

G43.809 Other migraine, not intractable, without status migrainosus

√6th **G43.81 Other migraine, intractable**
Other migraine, with refractory migraine

G43.811 Other migraine, intractable, with status migrainosus

G43.819 Other migraine, intractable, without status migrainosus

√6th **G43.82 Menstrual migraine, not intractable**
Menstrual headache, not intractable
Menstrual migraine, without refractory migraine
Menstrually related migraine, not intractable
Pre-menstrual headache, not intractable
Pre-menstrual migraine, not intractable
Pure menstrual migraine, not intractable
Code also associated premenstrual tension syndrome (N94.3)

G43.821 Menstrual migraine, not intractable, ♀
with status migrainosus

G43.829 Menstrual migraine, not intractable, ♀
without status migrainosus
Menstrual migraine NOS

√6th **G43.83 Menstrual migraine, intractable**
Menstrual headache, intractable
Menstrual migraine, with refractory migraine
Menstrually related migraine, intractable
Pre-menstrual headache, intractable
Pre-menstrual migraine, intractable
Pure menstrual migraine, intractable
Code also associated premenstrual tension syndrome (N94.3)

G43.831 Menstrual migraine, intractable, with ♀
status migrainosus

G43.839 Menstrual migraine, intractable, ♀
without status migrainosus

√5th **G43.9 Migraine, unspecified**

√6th **G43.90 Migraine, unspecified, not intractable**
Migraine, unspecified, without refractory migraine

G43.901 Migraine, unspecified, not intractable, with status migrainosus
Status migrainosus NOS

G43.909 Migraine, unspecified, not intractable, without status migrainosus
Migraine NOS

√6th **G43.91 Migraine, unspecified, intractable**
Migraine, unspecified, with refractory migraine

G43.911 Migraine, unspecified, intractable, with status migrainosus

G43.919 Migraine, unspecified, intractable, without status migrainosus

√4th **G44 Other headache syndromes**
EXCLUDES 1 *headache NOS (R51)*
EXCLUDES 2 *atypical facial pain (G50.1)*
headache due to lumbar puncture (G97.1)
migraines (G43.-)
trigeminal neuralgia (G50.0)

√5th **G44.0 Cluster headaches and other trigeminal autonomic cephalgias (TAC)**

√6th **G44.00 Cluster headache syndrome, unspecified**
Ciliary neuralgia   Lower half migraine
Cluster headache NOS   Migrainous neuralgia
Histamine cephalgia

G44.001 Cluster headache syndrome, unspecified, intractable

G44.009 Cluster headache syndrome, unspecified, not intractable
Cluster headache syndrome NOS

√6th **G44.01 Episodic cluster headache**

G44.011 Episodic cluster headache, intractable

G44.019 Episodic cluster headache, not intractable
Episodic cluster headache NOS

√6th **G44.02 Chronic cluster headache**

G44.021 Chronic cluster headache, intractable

G44.029 Chronic cluster headache, not intractable
Chronic cluster headache NOS

√6th **G44.03 Episodic paroxysmal hemicrania**
Paroxysmal hemicrania NOS

G44.031 Episodic paroxysmal hemicrania, intractable

✓ Additional Character Required   ✓x7th Xtension Alert   Unacceptable PDx   Manifestation   Hospital Acquired Condition   EXCLUDES 1 Not Coded Here   EXCLUDES 2 Not Included Here

ICD-10-CM Draft (2015)   537

G44.039 Episodic paroxysmal hemicrania, not intractable
Episodic paroxysmal hemicrania NOS

√6ᵗʰ **G44.04 Chronic paroxysmal hemicrania**
G44.041 Chronic paroxysmal hemicrania, intractable
G44.049 Chronic paroxysmal hemicrania, not intractable
Chronic paroxysmal hemicrania NOS

√6ᵗʰ **G44.05 Short lasting unilateral neuralgiform headache with conjunctival injection and tearing (SUNCT)**
G44.051 Short lasting unilateral neuralgiform headache with conjunctival injection and tearing (SUNCT), intractable
G44.059 Short lasting unilateral neuralgiform headache with conjunctival injection and tearing (SUNCT), not intractable
Short lasting unilateral neuralgiform headache with conjunctival injection and tearing (SUNCT) NOS

√6ᵗʰ **G44.09 Other trigeminal autonomic cephalgias (TAC)**
G44.091 Other trigeminal autonomic cephalgias (TAC), intractable
G44.099 Other trigeminal autonomic cephalgias syndrome (TAC), not intractable

G44.1 Vascular headache, not elsewhere classified
EXCLUDES 2 cluster headache (G44.0)
complicated headache syndromes (G44.5-)
drug-induced headache (G44.4-)
migraine (G43.-)
other specified headache syndromes (G44.8-)
post-traumatic headache (G44.3-)
tension-type headache (G44.2-)

√5ᵗʰ **G44.2 Tension-type headache**
√6ᵗʰ **G44.20 Tension-type headache, unspecified**
G44.201 Tension-type headache, unspecified, intractable
G44.209 Tension-type headache, unspecified, not intractable
Tension headache NOS

√6ᵗʰ **G44.21 Episodic tension-type headache**
G44.211 Episodic tension-type headache, intractable
G44.219 Episodic tension-type headache, not intractable
Episodic tension-type headache NOS

√6ᵗʰ **G44.22 Chronic tension-type headache**
G44.221 Chronic tension-type headache, intractable
G44.229 Chronic tension-type headache, not intractable
Chronic tension-type headache NOS

√5ᵗʰ **G44.3 Post-traumatic headache**
√6ᵗʰ **G44.30 Post-traumatic headache, unspecified**
G44.301 Post-traumatic headache, unspecified, intractable
G44.309 Post-traumatic headache, unspecified, not intractable
Post-traumatic headache NOS

√6ᵗʰ **G44.31 Acute post-traumatic headache**
G44.311 Acute post-traumatic headache, intractable
G44.319 Acute post-traumatic headache, not intractable
Acute post-traumatic headache NOS

√6ᵗʰ **G44.32 Chronic post-traumatic headache**
G44.321 Chronic post-traumatic headache, intractable
G44.329 Chronic post-traumatic headache, not intractable
Chronic post-traumatic headache NOS

√5ᵗʰ **G44.4 Drug-induced headache, not elsewhere classified**
Medication overuse headache
Use additional code for adverse effect, if applicable, to identify drug (T36-T50 with fifth or sixth character 5)
G44.40 Drug-induced headache, not elsewhere classified, not intractable

G44.41 Drug-induced headache, not elsewhere classified, intractable

√5ᵗʰ **G44.5 Complicated headache syndromes**
G44.51 Hemicrania continua
G44.52 New daily persistent headache (NDPH)
G44.53 Primary thunderclap headache
G44.59 Other complicated headache syndrome

√5ᵗʰ **G44.8 Other specified headache syndromes**
G44.81 Hypnic headache
G44.82 Headache associated with sexual activity
Orgasmic headache
Preorgasmic headache
G44.83 Primary cough headache
G44.84 Primary exertional headache
G44.85 Primary stabbing headache
G44.89 Other headache syndrome

√4ᵗʰ **G45 Transient cerebral ischemic attacks and related syndromes**
EXCLUDES 1 neonatal cerebral ischemia (P91.0)
transient retinal artery occlusion (H34.0-)

CC Excl: For CC codes in category G45, unless otherwise noted:
E08.51-E08.59, E08.618-E08.638, E08.649-E08.8, E09.51-E09.59, E09.618-E09.638, E09.649-E09.8, E10.51-E10.59, E10.618-E10.638, E10.649, E10.69-E10.8, E11.51-E11.59, E11.618-E11.638, E11.649, E11.69-E11.8, E13.51-E13.59, E13.618-E13.638, E13.649-E13.8, G45.0-G45.2, G45.8-G46.2, I63.00-I63.29, I65.01-I65.9, I67.841-I67.848, I87.8, I99.8-I99.9

G45.0 Vertebro-basilar artery syndrome CC
G45.1 Carotid artery syndrome (hemispheric) CC
G45.2 Multiple and bilateral precerebral artery syndromes CC
G45.3 Amaurosis fugax CC
CC Excl: G45.3-H34.9
G45.4 Transient global amnesia
EXCLUDES 1 amnesia NOS (R41.3)
G45.8 Other transient cerebral ischemic attacks and related syndromes CC
G45.9 Transient cerebral ischemic attack, unspecified CC
Spasm of cerebral artery
TIA
Transient cerebral ischemia NOS

√4ᵗʰ **G46 Vascular syndromes of brain in cerebrovascular diseases**
Code first underlying cerebrovascular disease (I60-I69)

CC Excl: For CC codes in category G46, unless otherwise noted:
E08.51-E08.59, E08.618-E08.638, E08.649-E08.8, E09.51-E09.59, E09.618-E09.638, E09.649-E09.8, E10.51-E10.59, E10.618-E10.638, E10.649, E10.69-E10.8, E11.51-E11.59, E11.618-E11.638, E11.649, E11.69-E11.8, E13.51-E13.59, E13.618-E13.638, E13.649-E13.8, G45.0-G45.2, G45.8-G46.2, I63.00-I63.29, I65.01-I65.9, I67.841-I67.848, I87.8, I99.8-I99.9

G46.0 Middle cerebral artery syndrome CC
G46.1 Anterior cerebral artery syndrome CC
G46.2 Posterior cerebral artery syndrome CC
G46.3 Brain stem stroke syndrome
Benedikt syndrome   Millard-Gubler syndrome
Claude syndrome   Wallenberg syndrome
Foville syndrome   Weber syndrome
G46.4 Cerebellar stroke syndrome
G46.5 Pure motor lacunar syndrome
G46.6 Pure sensory lacunar syndrome
G46.7 Other lacunar syndromes
G46.8 Other vascular syndromes of brain in cerebrovascular diseases

√4ᵗʰ **G47 Sleep disorders**
EXCLUDES 2 nightmares (F51.5)
nonorganic sleep disorders (F51.-)
sleep terrors (F51.4)
sleepwalking (F51.3)

✓5ᵗʰ **G47.0 Insomnia**
    EXCLUDES 2   *alcohol related insomnia (F10.182, F10.282, F10.982)*
            drug-related insomnia (F11.182, F11.282, F11.982,
                F13.182, F13.282, F13.982, F14.182,
                F14.282, F14.982, F15.182, F15.282, F15.982,
                F19.182, F19.282, F19.982)
            idiopathic insomnia (F51.01)
            insomnia due to a mental disorder (F51.05)
            insomnia not due to a substance or known
                physiological condition (F51.0-)
            nonorganic insomnia (F51.0-)
            primary insomnia (F51.01)
            sleep apnea (G47.3-)

     G47.00 Insomnia, unspecified
            Insomnia NOS

     G47.01 Insomnia due to medical condition
            Code also associated medical condition

     G47.09 Other insomnia

✓5ᵗʰ **G47.1 Hypersomnia**
    EXCLUDES 2   *alcohol-related hypersomnia (F10.182, F10.282,*
                F10.982)
            drug-related hypersomnia (F11.182, F11.282, F11.982,
                F13.182, F13.282, F13.982, F14.182, F14.282,
                F14.982, F15.182, F15.282, F15.982, F19.182,
                F19.282, F19.982)
            hypersomnia due to a mental disorder (F51.13)
            hypersomnia not due to a substance or known
                physiological condition (F51.1-)
            primary hypersomnia (F51.11)
            sleep apnea (G47.3-)

     G47.10 Hypersomnia, unspecified
            Hypersomnia NOS

     G47.11 Idiopathic hypersomnia with long sleep time
            Idiopathic hypersomnia NOS

     G47.12 Idiopathic hypersomnia without long sleep time

     G47.13 Recurrent hypersomnia
            Kleine-Levin syndrome
            Menstrual related hypersomnia

     G47.14 Hypersomnia due to medical condition
            Code also associated medical condition

     G47.19 Other hypersomnia

✓5ᵗʰ **G47.2 Circadian rhythm sleep disorders**
            Disorders of the sleep wake schedule
            Inversion of nyctohemeral rhythm
            Inversion of sleep rhythm

     G47.20 Circadian rhythm sleep disorder, unspecified type
            Sleep wake schedule disorder NOS

     G47.21 Circadian rhythm sleep disorder, delayed sleep phase type
            Delayed sleep phase syndrome

     G47.22 Circadian rhythm sleep disorder, advanced sleep phase type

     G47.23 Circadian rhythm sleep disorder, irregular sleep wake type
            Irregular sleep-wake pattern

     G47.24 Circadian rhythm sleep disorder, free running type

     G47.25 Circadian rhythm sleep disorder, jet lag type

     G47.26 Circadian rhythm sleep disorder, shift work type

     G47.27 Circadian rhythm sleep disorder in conditions classified elsewhere
            Code first underlying condition

     G47.29 Other circadian rhythm sleep disorder

✓5ᵗʰ **G47.3 Sleep apnea**
            Code also any associated underlying condition
    EXCLUDES 1   *apnea NOS (R06.81)*
            Cheyne-Stokes breathing (R06.3)
            pickwickian syndrome (E66.2)
            sleep apnea of newborn (P28.3)

     G47.30 Sleep apnea, unspecified
            Sleep apnea NOS

     G47.31 Primary central sleep apnea

     G47.32 High altitude periodic breathing

     G47.33 Obstructive sleep apnea (adult) (pediatric)
        EXCLUDES 1   *obstructive sleep apnea of newborn (P28.3)*

     G47.34 Idiopathic sleep related nonobstructive alveolar hypoventilation
            Sleep related hypoxia

     G47.35 Congenital central alveolar hypoventilation syndrome

     G47.36 Sleep related hypoventilation in conditions classified elsewhere
            Sleep related hypoxemia in conditions classified elsewhere
            Code first underlying condition

     G47.37 Central sleep apnea in conditions classified elsewhere
            Code first underlying condition

     G47.39 Other sleep apnea

✓5ᵗʰ **G47.4 Narcolepsy and cataplexy**

     ✓6ᵗʰ **G47.41 Narcolepsy**

         G47.411 Narcolepsy with cataplexy

         G47.419 Narcolepsy without cataplexy
            Narcolepsy NOS

     ✓6ᵗʰ **G47.42 Narcolepsy in conditions classified elsewhere**
            Code first underlying condition

         G47.421 Narcolepsy in conditions classified elsewhere with cataplexy

         G47.429 Narcolepsy in conditions classified elsewhere without cataplexy

✓5ᵗʰ **G47.5 Parasomnia**
    EXCLUDES 1   *alcohol induced parasomnia (F10.182, F10.282,*
                F10.982)
            drug induced parasomnia (F11.182, F11.282, F11.982,
                F13.182, F13.282, F13.982, F14.182, F14.282,
                F14.982, F15.182, F15.282, F15.982, F19.182,
                F19.282, F19.982)
            parasomnia not due to a substance or known
                physiological condition (F51.8)

     G47.50 Parasomnia, unspecified
            Parasomnia NOS

     G47.51 Confusional arousals

     G47.52 REM sleep behavior disorder

     G47.53 Recurrent isolated sleep paralysis

     G47.54 Parasomnia in conditions classified elsewhere
            Code first underlying condition

     G47.59 Other parasomnia

✓5ᵗʰ **G47.6 Sleep related movement disorders**
    EXCLUDES 2   *restless legs syndrome (G25.81)*

     G47.61 Periodic limb movement disorder

     G47.62 Sleep related leg cramps

     G47.63 Sleep related bruxism
        EXCLUDES 1   *psychogenic bruxism (F45.8)*

     G47.69 Other sleep related movement disorders

     G47.8 Other sleep disorders

     G47.9 Sleep disorder, unspecified
            Sleep disorder NOS

Nerve, nerve root and plexus disorders (G50-G59)

EXCLUDES 1   *current traumatic nerve, nerve root and plexus disorders—see Injury,*
            nerve by body region
         neuralgia NOS (M79.2)
         neuritis NOS (M79.2)
         peripheral neuritis in pregnancy (O26.82-)
         radiculitis NOS (M54.1-)

✓4ᵗʰ **G50 Disorders of trigeminal nerve**
    INCLUDES   disorders of 5th cranial nerve

     G50.0 Trigeminal neuralgia
            Syndrome of paroxysmal facial pain
            Tic douloureux

     G50.1 Atypical facial pain

     G50.8 Other disorders of trigeminal nerve

     G50.9 Disorder of trigeminal nerve, unspecified

✓4ᵗʰ **G51 Facial nerve disorders**
    INCLUDES   disorders of 7th cranial nerve

     G51.0 Bell's palsy
            Facial palsy

     G51.1 Geniculate ganglionitis
        EXCLUDES 1   *postherpetic geniculate ganglionitis (B02.21)*

     G51.2 Melkersson's syndrome
            Melkersson-Rosenthal syndrome

     G51.3 Clonic hemifacial spasm

     G51.4 Facial myokymia

     G51.8 Other disorders of facial nerve

     G51.9 Disorder of facial nerve, unspecified

✓ Additional Character Required   ✓x7ᵗʰ Xtension Alert   Unacceptable PDx   Manifestation   Hospital Acquired Condition   EXCLUDES 1 Not Coded Here   EXCLUDES 2 Not Included Here

Diseases of the Nervous System

G52–G57.61

✓4ᵗʰ **G52   Disorders of other cranial nerves**

> EXCLUDES 2   *disorders of acoustic [8th] nerve (H93.3)*
> *disorders of optic [2nd] nerve (H46, H47.0)*
> *paralytic strabismus due to nerve palsy (H49.0–H49.2)*

G52.0   Disorders of olfactory nerve
Disorders of 1st cranial nerve

G52.1   Disorders of glossopharyngeal nerve
Disorder of 9th cranial nerve
Glossopharyngeal neuralgia

G52.2   Disorders of vagus nerve
Disorders of pneumogastric [10th] nerve

G52.3   Disorders of hypoglossal nerve
Disorders of 12th cranial nerve

G52.7   Disorders of multiple cranial nerves
Polyneuritis cranialis

G52.8   Disorders of other specified cranial nerves

G52.9   Cranial nerve disorder, unspecified

G53   *Cranial nerve disorders in diseases classified elsewhere*

> *Code first underlying disease, such as:*
> *neoplasm (C00-D49)*
>
> EXCLUDES 1   *multiple cranial nerve palsy in sarcoidosis (D86.82)*
> *multiple cranial nerve palsy in syphilis (A52.15)*
> *postherpetic geniculate ganglionitis (B02.21)*
> *postherpetic trigeminal neuralgia (B02.22)*

✓4ᵗʰ **G54   Nerve root and plexus disorders**

> EXCLUDES 1   *current traumatic nerve root and plexus disorders—see nerve*
> *injury by body region*
> *intervertebral disc disorders (M50-M51)*
> *neuritis or radiculitis brachial NOS (M54.13)*
> *neuritis or radiculitis lumbar NOS (M54.16)*
> *neuritis or radiculitis lumbosacral NOS (M54.17)*
> *neuritis or radiculitis thoracic NOS (M54.14)*
> *radiculitis NOS (M54.10)*
> *radiculopathy NOS (M54.10)*
> *spondylosis (M47.-)*

G54.0   Brachial plexus disorders
Thoracic outlet syndrome

G54.1   Lumbosacral plexus disorders

G54.2   Cervical root disorders, not elsewhere classified

G54.3   Thoracic root disorders, not elsewhere classified

G54.4   Lumbosacral root disorders, not elsewhere classified

G54.5   Neuralgic amyotrophy
Parsonage-Aldren-Turner syndrome
Shoulder-girdle neuritis

> EXCLUDES 1   *neuralgic amyotrophy in diabetes mellitus (E08-E13*
> *with .44)*

G54.6   Phantom limb syndrome with pain

G54.7   Phantom limb syndrome without pain
Phantom limb syndrome NOS

G54.8   Other nerve root and plexus disorders

G54.9   Nerve root and plexus disorder, unspecified

G55   *Nerve root and plexus compressions in diseases classified elsewhere*

> *Code first underlying disease, such as:*
> *neoplasm (C00-D49)*
>
> EXCLUDES 1   *nerve root compression (due to) (in) ankylosing spondylitis*
> *(M45.-)*
> *nerve root compression (due to) (in) dorsopathies (M53.-, M54.-)*
> *nerve root compression (due to) (in) intervertebral disc disorders*
> *(M50.1-, M51.1-)*
> *nerve root compression (due to) (in) spondylopathies (M46.-,*
> *M48.-)*

✓4ᵗʰ **G56   Mononeuropathies of upper limb**

> EXCLUDES 1   *current traumatic nerve disorder—see nerve injury by body*
> *region*

✓5ᵗʰ **G56.0   Carpal tunnel syndrome**

G56.00   Carpal tunnel syndrome, unspecified upper limb

G56.01   Carpal tunnel syndrome, right upper limb

G56.02   Carpal tunnel syndrome, left upper limb

✓5ᵗʰ **G56.1   Other lesions of median nerve**

G56.10   Other lesions of median nerve, unspecified upper limb

G56.11   Other lesions of median nerve, right upper limb

G56.12   Other lesions of median nerve, left upper limb

✓5ᵗʰ **G56.2   Lesion of ulnar nerve**
Tardy ulnar nerve palsy

G56.20   Lesion of ulnar nerve, unspecified upper limb

G56.21   Lesion of ulnar nerve, right upper limb

G56.22   Lesion of ulnar nerve, left upper limb

✓5ᵗʰ **G56.3   Lesion of radial nerve**

G56.30   Lesion of radial nerve, unspecified upper limb

G56.31   Lesion of radial nerve, right upper limb

G56.32   Lesion of radial nerve, left upper limb

✓5ᵗʰ **G56.4   Causalgia of upper limb**
Complex regional pain syndrome II of upper limb

> EXCLUDES 1   *complex regional pain syndrome I of lower limb*
> *(G90.52-)*
> *complex regional pain syndrome I of upper limb*
> *(G90.51-)*
> *complex regional pain syndrome II of lower limb*
> *(G57.7-)*
> *reflex sympathetic dystrophy of lower limb (G90.52-)*
> *reflex sympathetic dystrophy of upper limb (G90.51-)*

G56.40   Causalgia of unspecified upper limb

G56.41   Causalgia of right upper limb

G56.42   Causalgia of left upper limb

✓5ᵗʰ **G56.8   Other specified mononeuropathies of upper limb**
Interdigital neuroma of upper limb

G56.80   Other specified mononeuropathies of unspecified upper limb

G56.81   Other specified mononeuropathies of right upper limb

G56.82   Other specified mononeuropathies of left upper limb

✓5ᵗʰ **G56.9   Unspecified mononeuropathy of upper limb**

G56.90   Unspecified mononeuropathy of unspecified upper limb

G56.91   Unspecified mononeuropathy of right upper limb

G56.92   Unspecified mononeuropathy of left upper limb

✓4ᵗʰ **G57   Mononeuropathies of lower limb**

> EXCLUDES 1   *current traumatic nerve disorder—see nerve injury by body*
> *region*

✓5ᵗʰ **G57.0   Lesion of sciatic nerve**

> EXCLUDES 1   *sciatica NOS (M54.3-)*
> EXCLUDES 2   *sciatica attributed to intervertebral disc disorder*
> *(M51.1-)*

G57.00   Lesion of sciatic nerve, unspecified lower limb

G57.01   Lesion of sciatic nerve, right lower limb

G57.02   Lesion of sciatic nerve, left lower limb

✓5ᵗʰ **G57.1   Meralgia paresthetica**
Lateral cutaneous nerve of thigh syndrome

G57.10   Meralgia paresthetica, unspecified lower limb

G57.11   Meralgia paresthetica, right lower limb

G57.12   Meralgia paresthetica, left lower limb

✓5ᵗʰ **G57.2   Lesion of femoral nerve**

G57.20   Lesion of femoral nerve, unspecified lower limb

G57.21   Lesion of femoral nerve, right lower limb

G57.22   Lesion of femoral nerve, left lower limb

✓5ᵗʰ **G57.3   Lesion of lateral popliteal nerve**
Peroneal nerve palsy

G57.30   Lesion of lateral popliteal nerve, unspecified lower limb

G57.31   Lesion of lateral popliteal nerve, right lower limb

G57.32   Lesion of lateral popliteal nerve, left lower limb

✓5ᵗʰ **G57.4   Lesion of medial popliteal nerve**

G57.40   Lesion of medial popliteal nerve, unspecified lower limb

G57.41   Lesion of medial popliteal nerve, right lower limb

G57.42   Lesion of medial popliteal nerve, left lower limb

✓5ᵗʰ **G57.5   Tarsal tunnel syndrome**

G57.50   Tarsal tunnel syndrome, unspecified lower limb

G57.51   Tarsal tunnel syndrome, right lower limb

G57.52   Tarsal tunnel syndrome, left lower limb

✓5ᵗʰ **G57.6   Lesion of plantar nerve**
Morton's metatarsalgia

G57.60   Lesion of plantar nerve, unspecified lower limb

G57.61   Lesion of plantar nerve, right lower limb

N Newborn: 0   P Pediatric: 0-17   M Maternity: 12-55   A Adult: 15-124   MCC Major CC Condition   PDx MCC PDx acts as own MCC   CC CC Condition   PDx CC PDx acts as own CC

540   ICD-10-CM Draft (2015)

Diseases of the Nervous System

G57.62–G70.80

    G57.62   **Lesion of plantar nerve, left lower limb**

✓5ᵗʰ **G57.7** **Causalgia of lower limb**
        Complex regional pain syndrome II of lower limb
        EXCLUDES 1   *complex regional pain syndrome I of lower limb (G90.52-)*
                  complex regional pain syndrome I of upper limb (G90.51-)
                  complex regional pain syndrome II of upper limb (G56.4-)
                  reflex sympathetic dystrophy of lower limb (G90.52-)
                  reflex sympathetic dystrophy of upper limb (G90.51-)

        G57.70   **Causalgia of unspecified lower limb**
        G57.71   **Causalgia of right lower limb**
        G57.72   **Causalgia of left lower limb**

✓5ᵗʰ **G57.8** **Other specified mononeuropathies of lower limb**
        Interdigital neuroma of lower limb

        G57.80   **Other specified mononeuropathies of unspecified lower limb**
        G57.81   **Other specified mononeuropathies of right lower limb**
        G57.82   **Other specified mononeuropathies of left lower limb**

✓5ᵗʰ **G57.9** **Unspecified mononeuropathy of lower limb**

        G57.90   **Unspecified mononeuropathy of unspecified lower limb**
        G57.91   **Unspecified mononeuropathy of right lower limb**
        G57.92   **Unspecified mononeuropathy of left lower limb**

✓4ᵗʰ **G58** **Other mononeuropathies**
    G58.0 **Intercostal neuropathy**
    G58.7 **Mononeuritis multiplex**
    G58.8 **Other specified mononeuropathies**
    G58.9 **Mononeuropathy, unspecified**

G59 *Mononeuropathy in diseases classified elsewhere*
    Code first underlying disease
    EXCLUDES 1 *diabetic mononeuropathy (E08-E13 with .41)*
             syphilitic nerve paralysis (A52.19)
             syphilitic neuritis (A52.15)
             tuberculous mononeuropathy (A17.83)

Polyneuropathies and other disorders of the peripheral nervous system (G60-G65)

    EXCLUDES 1 *neuralgia NOS (M79.2)*
             neuritis NOS (M79.2)
             peripheral neuritis in pregnancy (O26.82-)
             radiculitis NOS (M54.10)

✓4ᵗʰ **G60** **Hereditary and idiopathic neuropathy**
    G60.0 **Hereditary motor and sensory neuropathy**
        Charcôt-Marie-Tooth disease
        Déjérine-Sottas disease
        Hereditary motor and sensory neuropathy, types I-IV
        Hypertrophic neuropathy of infancy
        Peroneal muscular atrophy (axonal type) (hypertrophic type)
        Roussy-Levy syndrome

    G60.1 **Refsum's disease**   CC
        Infantile Refsum disease
        AHA: 2014, 2Q, 4
        CC Excl: E11.42, G13.0-G13.1, G50.0-G65.2, M34.83

    G60.2 **Neuropathy in association with hereditary ataxia**
    G60.3 **Idiopathic progressive neuropathy**
    G60.8 **Other hereditary and idiopathic neuropathies**
        Dominantly inherited sensory neuropathy
        Morvan's disease
        Nelaton's syndrome
        Recessively inherited sensory neuropathy

    G60.9 **Hereditary and idiopathic neuropathy, unspecified**

✓4ᵗʰ **G61** **Inflammatory polyneuropathy**
    G61.0 **Guillain-Barre syndrome**   CC
        Acute (post-)infective polyneuritis
        Miller Fisher syndrome
        AHA: 2014, 2Q, 4
        CC Excl: A02.21, A17.0-A17.1, A27.81, A39.0, A39.89-A39.9, A49.3-A49.9, A50.41, A51.41, A52.13, A54.82, A54.84, A54.89-A54.9, A87.0-A87.9, B00.3, B02.1, B26.1, B37.5, B38.4, B45.1, B58.2, B92, B94.2-B94.9, B96.0, B96.6-B96.89, G00.0-G03.9, G04.2, G32.89, G61.0, G96.8-G96.9, G98.0-G98.8, G99.8

    G61.1 **Serum neuropathy**
        Use additional code for adverse effect, if applicable, to identify serum (T50.-)

✓5ᵗʰ **G61.8** **Other inflammatory polyneuropathies**
        G61.81   **Chronic inflammatory demyelinating polyneuritis**   CC
               CC Excl: G51.0-G54.5, G54.8-G60.9, G61.81-G61.89, G62.81, G62.89, G64
        G61.89   **Other inflammatory polyneuropathies**
    G61.9 **Inflammatory polyneuropathy, unspecified**

✓4ᵗʰ **G62** **Other and unspecified polyneuropathies**
    G62.0 **Drug-induced polyneuropathy**
        Use additional code for adverse effect, if applicable, to identify drug (T36-T50 with fifth or sixth character 5)

    G62.1 **Alcoholic polyneuropathy**
    G62.2 **Polyneuropathy due to other toxic agents**
        Code first (T51-T65) to identify toxic agent

✓5ᵗʰ **G62.8** **Other specified polyneuropathies**
        G62.81   **Critical illness polyneuropathy**   CC
               Acute motor neuropathy
               CC Excl: G51.0-G54.5, G54.8-G60.9, G61.81-G61.9, G62.81, G62.89-G62.9, G64
        G62.82   **Radiation-induced polyneuropathy**
               Use additional external cause code (W88-W90, X39.0-) to identify cause
        G62.89   **Other specified polyneuropathies**
    G62.9 **Polyneuropathy, unspecified**
        Neuropathy NOS

G63 *Polyneuropathy in diseases classified elsewhere*
    Code first underlying disease, such as:
      amyloidosis (E85.-)
      endocrine disease, except diabetes (E00-E07, E15-E16, E20-E34)
      metabolic diseases (E70-E88)
      neoplasm (C00-D49)
      nutritional deficiency (E40-E64)
    EXCLUDES 1 *polyneuropathy (in):*
      diabetes mellitus (E08-E13 with .42)
      diphtheria (A36.83)
      infectious mononucleosis (B27.0-B27.9 with 1)
      Lyme disease (A69.22)
      mumps (B26.84)
      postherpetic (B02.23)
      rheumatoid arthritis (M05.33)
      scleroderma (M34.83)
      systemic lupus erythematosus (M32.19)
    AHA: 2012, 4Q, 99

G64 **Other disorders of peripheral nervous system**
    Disorder of peripheral nervous system NOS

✓4ᵗʰ **G65** **Sequelae of inflammatory and toxic polyneuropathies**
    Code first condition resulting from (sequela) of inflammatory and toxic polyneuropathies
    G65.0 **Sequelae of Guillain-Barré syndrome**
    G65.1 **Sequelae of other inflammatory polyneuropathy**
    G65.2 **Sequelae of toxic polyneuropathy**

Diseases of myoneural junction and muscle (G70-G73)

✓4ᵗʰ **G70** **Myasthenia gravis and other myoneural disorders**
    EXCLUDES 1 *botulism (A05.1, A48.51-A48.52)*
             transient neonatal myasthenia gravis (P94.0)

    CC Excl: For CC/MCC codes in category G70, unless otherwise noted: E08.40-E08.49, E08.618-E08.638, E08.649-E08.8, E09.40-E09.49, E09.618-E09.638, E09.649-E09.8, E10.40-E10.49, E10.618-E10.638, E10.649, E10.69-E10.8, E11.40-E11.49, E11.618-E11.638, E11.649, E11.69-E11.8, E13.40-E13.49, E13.618-E13.638, E13.649-E13.8, G32.89, G70.00-G70.01, G70.80-G70.81, G73.1-G73.3, G96.8-G96.9, G98.0-G98.8, G99.8

✓5ᵗʰ **G70.0** **Myasthenia gravis**
        G70.00   **Myasthenia gravis without (acute) exacerbation**
               Myasthenia gravis NOS
        G70.01   **Myasthenia gravis with (acute) exacerbation**   MCC
               Myasthenia gravis in crisis

    G70.1 **Toxic myoneural disorders**
        Code first (T51-T65) to identify toxic agent

    G70.2 **Congenital and developmental myasthenia**

✓5ᵗʰ **G70.8** **Other specified myoneural disorders**
        G70.80   **Lambert-Eaton syndrome, unspecified**   CC
               Lambert-Eaton syndrome NOS

G70.81 Lambert-Eaton syndrome in disease classified elsewhere [CC]
  Code first underlying disease
  EXCLUDES 1 Lambert-Eaton syndrome in neoplastic disease (G73.1)

G70.89 Other specified myoneural disorders

G70.9 Myoneural disorder, unspecified

✓4th **G71 Primary disorders of muscles**
  EXCLUDES 2 arthrogryposis multiplex congenita (Q74.3)
    metabolic disorders (E70-E88)
    myositis (M60.-)

G71.0 Muscular dystrophy [CC]
  Autosomal recessive, childhood type, muscular dystrophy resembling Duchenne or Becker muscular dystrophy
  Benign [Becker] muscular dystrophy
  Benign scapuloperoneal muscular dystrophy with early contractures [Emery-Dreifuss]
  Congenital muscular dystrophy NOS
  Congenital muscular dystrophy with specific morphological abnormalities of the muscle fiber
  Distal muscular dystrophy
  Facioscapulohumeral muscular dystrophy
  Limb-girdle muscular dystrophy
  Ocular muscular dystrophy
  Oculopharyngeal muscular dystrophy
  Scapuloperoneal muscular dystrophy
  Severe [Duchenne] muscular dystrophy
  CC Excl: E08.40-E08.49, E08.618-E08.638, E08.649-E08.8, E09.40-E09.49, E09.618-E09.638, E09.649-E09.8, E10.40-E10.49, E10.618-E10.638, E10.649, E10.69-E10.8, E11.40-E11.49, E11.618-E11.638, E11.649, E11.69-E11.8, E13.40-E13.49, E13.618-E13.638, E13.649-E13.8, G32.89, G71.0, G71.2, G96.8-G96.9, G98.0-G98.8, G99.8

✓5th **G71.1 Myotonic disorders**

  G71.11 Myotonic muscular dystrophy
    Dystrophia myotonica [Steinert]
    Myotonia atrophica
    Myotonic dystrophy
    Proximal myotonic myopathy (PROMM)
    Steinert disease

  G71.12 Myotonia congenita
    Acetazolamide responsive myotonia congenita
    Dominant myotonia congenita [Thomsen disease]
    Myotonia levior
    Recessive myotonia congenita [Becker disease]

  G71.13 Myotonic chondrodystrophy
    Chondrodystrophic myotonia
    Congenital myotonic chondrodystrophy
    Schwartz-Jampel disease

  G71.14 Drug induced myotonia
    Use additional code for adverse effect, if applicable, to identify drug (T36-T50 with fifth or sixth character 5)

  G71.19 Other specified myotonic disorders
    Myotonia fluctuans
    Myotonia permanens
    Neuromyotonia [Isaacs]
    Paramyotonia congenita (of von Eulenburg)
    Pseudomyotonia
    Symptomatic myotonia

G71.2 Congenital myopathies [CC]
  Central core disease   Myotubular (centronuclear)
  Fiber-type disproportion   myopathy
  Minicore disease   Nemaline myopathy
  Multicore disease
  EXCLUDES 1 arthrogryposis multiplex congenita (Q74.3)
  CC Excl: See code: G71.0

G71.3 Mitochondrial myopathy, not elsewhere classified
  EXCLUDES 1 Kearns-Sayre syndrome (H49.81)
    Leber's disease (H47.21)
    Leigh's encephalopathy (G31.82)
    mitochondrial metabolism disorders (E88.4-)
    Reye's syndrome (G93.7)

G71.8 Other primary disorders of muscles

G71.9 Primary disorder of muscle, unspecified
  Hereditary myopathy NOS

✓4th **G72 Other and unspecified myopathies**
  EXCLUDES 1 arthrogryposis multiplex congenita (Q74.3)
    dermatopolymyositis (M33.-)
    ischemic infarction of muscle (M62.2-)
    myositis (M60.-)
    polymyositis (M33.2-)

G72.0 Drug-induced myopathy [CC]
  Use additional code for adverse effect, if applicable, to identify drug (T36-T50 with fifth or sixth character 5)
  CC Excl: G32.89, G70.00-G72.3, G72.81-G73.7, G96.8-G96.9, G98.0-G98.8, G99.8

G72.1 Alcoholic myopathy [CC]
  Use additional code to identify alcoholism (F10.-)
  CC Excl: See code: G72.0

G72.2 Myopathy due to other toxic agents [CC]
  Code first (T51-T65) to identify toxic agent
  CC Excl: See code: G72.0

G72.3 Periodic paralysis
  Familial periodic paralysis
  Hyperkalemic periodic paralysis (familial)
  Hypokalemic periodic paralysis (familial)
  Myotonic periodic paralysis (familial)
  Normokalemic paralysis (familial)
  Potassium sensitive periodic paralysis
  EXCLUDES 1 paramyotonia congenita (of von Eulenburg) (G71.19)

✓5th **G72.4 Inflammatory and immune myopathies, not elsewhere classified**

  G72.41 Inclusion body myositis [IBM]

  G72.49 Other inflammatory and immune myopathies, not elsewhere classified
    Inflammatory myopathy NOS

✓5th **G72.8 Other specified myopathies**

  G72.81 Critical illness myopathy [CC]
    Acute necrotizing myopathy
    Acute quadriplegic myopathy
    Intensive care (ICU) myopathy
    Myopathy of critical illness
    CC Excl: G70.1-G72.3, G72.81-G73.7

  G72.89 Other specified myopathies

G72.9 Myopathy, unspecified

✓4th **G73 Disorders of myoneural junction and muscle in diseases classified elsewhere**

G73.1 Lambert-Eaton syndrome in neoplastic disease [CC]
  Code first underlying neoplasm (C00-D49)
  EXCLUDES 1 Lambert-Eaton syndrome not associated with neoplasm (G70.80-G70.81)
  CC Excl: E08.40-E08.49, E08.618-E08.638, E08.649-E08.8, E09.40-E09.49, E09.618-E09.638, E09.649-E09.8, E10.40-E10.49, E10.618-E10.638, E10.649, E10.69-E10.8, E11.40-E11.49, E11.618-E11.638, E11.649, E11.69-E11.8, E13.40-E13.49, E13.618-E13.638, E13.649-E13.8, G32.89, G70.00-G70.01, G70.80-G70.81, G73.1-G73.3, G96.8-G96.9, G98.0-G98.8, G99.8

G73.3 Myasthenic syndromes in other diseases classified elsewhere [CC]
  Code first underlying disease, such as:
    neoplasm (C00-D49)
    thyrotoxicosis (E05.-)
  CC Excl: See code: G73.1

G73.7 Myopathy in diseases classified elsewhere
  Code first underlying disease, such as:
    hyperparathyroidism (E21.0, E21.3)
    hypoparathyroidism (E20.-)
    glycogen storage disease (E74.0)
    lipid storage disorders (E75.-)
  EXCLUDES 1 myopathy in:
    rheumatoid arthritis (M05.4-)
    sarcoidosis (D86.87)
    scleroderma (M34.82)
    sicca syndrome [Sjögren] (M35.03)
    systemic lupus erythematosus (M32.19)

Cerebral palsy and other paralytic syndromes (G80-G83)

✓4th **G80 Cerebral palsy**
  EXCLUDES 1 hereditary spastic paraplegia (G11.4)

G80.0 Spastic quadriplegic cerebral palsy [MCC]
  Congenital spastic paralysis (cerebral)
  CC Excl: E08.40-E08.49, E08.618-E08.638, E08.649-E08.8, E09.40-E09.49, E09.618-E09.638, E09.649-E09.8, E10.40-E10.49, E10.618-E10.638, E10.649, E10.69-E10.8, E11.40-E11.49, E11.618-E11.638, E11.649, E11.69-E11.8, E13.40-E13.49, E13.618-E13.638, E13.649-E13.8, G04.1, G32.89, G80.0-G80.2, G80.4-G83.9, G90.1, G93.81, G93.89-G93.9, G96.8-G96.9, G98.0-G98.8, G99.8, Q06.0-Q06.1, Q06.3, Q06.8-Q06.9, Q07.8-Q07.9, R53.2

G80.1 Spastic diplegic cerebral palsy [CC]
  Spastic cerebral palsy NOS
  CC Excl: G80.1, G93.40-G93.49, I67.83

G80.2 Spastic hemiplegic **cerebral palsy** `CC`
CC Excl: G80.2, G93.40-G93.49, I67.83

G80.3 Athetoid **cerebral palsy** `CC`
Double athetosis (syndrome)
Dyskinetic cerebral palsy
Dystonic cerebral palsy
Vogt disease
CC Excl: G20, G21.11-G21.9, G25.70-G25.79, G25.89-G26, G80.0-G80.9, G93.40-G93.49, I67.83

G80.4 Ataxic **cerebral palsy**

G80.8 Other **cerebral palsy**
Mixed cerebral palsy syndromes

G80.9 **Cerebral palsy,** unspecified
Cerebral palsy NOS

✓4ᵗʰ **G81** **Hemiplegia and hemiparesis**
NOTE This category is to be used only when hemiplegia (complete)(incomplete) is reported without further specification, or is stated to be old or longstanding but of unspecified cause. The category is also for use in multiple coding to identify these types of hemiplegia resulting from any cause.
EXCLUDES 1 congenital cerebral palsy (G80.-)
hemiplegia and hemiparesis due to sequela of cerebrovascular disease (I69.05-, I69.15-, I69.25-, I69.35-, I69.85-, I69.95-)

CC Excl: For CC codes in category G81, unless otherwise noted:
G04.1, G11.0-G12.9, G32.0-G37.3, G37.5-G37.9, G80.0-G80.2, G80.4-G83.9, G90.01-G90.09, G90.2, G90.4-G90.9, G92, G93.40-G93.49, G93.81, G93.89-G93.9, G95.0-G95.9, G96.8-G96.9, G98.0-G99.8, I67.83, R53.2

✓5ᵗʰ **G81.0** **Flaccid hemiplegia**
G81.00 **Flaccid hemiplegia affecting** unspecified **side** `CC`
G81.01 **Flaccid hemiplegia affecting** right dominant **side** `CC`
G81.02 **Flaccid hemiplegia affecting** left dominant **side** `CC`
G81.03 **Flaccid hemiplegia affecting** right nondominant **side** `CC`
G81.04 **Flaccid hemiplegia affecting** left nondominant **side** `CC`

✓5ᵗʰ **G81.1** **Spastic hemiplegia**
G81.10 **Spastic hemiplegia affecting** unspecified **side** `CC`
G81.11 **Spastic hemiplegia affecting** right dominant **side** `CC`
G81.12 **Spastic hemiplegia affecting** left dominant **side** `CC`
G81.13 **Spastic hemiplegia affecting** right nondominant **side** `CC`
G81.14 **Spastic hemiplegia affecting** left nondominant **side** `CC`

✓5ᵗʰ **G81.9** **Hemiplegia,** unspecified
AHA: 2014, 1Q, 23
G81.90 **Hemiplegia, unspecified affecting** unspecified **side** `CC`
G81.91 **Hemiplegia, unspecified affecting** right dominant **side** `CC`
G81.92 **Hemiplegia, unspecified affecting** left dominant **side** `CC`
G81.93 **Hemiplegia, unspecified affecting** right nondominant **side** `CC`
G81.94 **Hemiplegia, unspecified affecting** left nondominant **side** `CC`

✓4ᵗʰ **G82** **Paraplegia (paraparesis) and quadriplegia (quadriparesis)**
NOTE This category is to be used only when the listed conditions are reported without further specification, or are stated to be old or longstanding but of unspecified cause. The category is also for use in multiple coding to identify these conditions resulting from any cause
EXCLUDES 1 congenital cerebral palsy (G80.-)
functional quadriplegia (R53.2)
hysterical paralysis (F44.4)

✓5ᵗʰ **G82.2** **Paraplegia**
Paralysis of both lower limbs NOS
Paraparesis (lower) NOS
Paraplegia (lower) NOS

CC Excl: For CC codes in subcategory G82.2, unless otherwise noted: See code: G81

G82.20 **Paraplegia,** unspecified `CC`
G82.21 **Paraplegia,** complete `CC`
G82.22 **Paraplegia,** incomplete `CC`

✓5ᵗʰ **G82.5** **Quadriplegia**

CC Excl: For MCC codes in subcategory G82.5, unless otherwise noted: See code: G80.0

G82.50 **Quadriplegia,** unspecified `MCC`
G82.51 **Quadriplegia,** C1-C4 complete `MCC`
G82.52 **Quadriplegia,** C1-C4 incomplete `MCC`
G82.53 **Quadriplegia,** C5-C7 complete `MCC`
G82.54 **Quadriplegia,** C5-C7 incomplete `MCC`

✓4ᵗʰ **G83** **Other paralytic syndromes**
NOTE This category is to be used only when the listed conditions are reported without further specification, or are stated to be old or longstanding but of unspecified cause. The category is also for use in multiple coding to identify these conditions resulting from any cause.
INCLUDES paralysis (complete) (incomplete), except as in G80-G82

G83.0 **Diplegia** of upper limbs `CC`
Diplegia (upper)   Paralysis of both upper limbs
CC Excl: G32.89, G82.50-G83.0, G83.5-G83.9, G96.8-G96.9, G98.0-G98.8, G99.8, R53.2

✓5ᵗʰ **G83.1** **Monoplegia of lower limb**
Paralysis of lower limb
EXCLUDES 1 monoplegia of lower limbs due to sequela of cerebrovascular disease (I69.04-, I69.14-, I69.24-, I69.34-, I69.84-, I69.94-)
G83.10 **Monoplegia of lower limb affecting** unspecified **side**
G83.11 **Monoplegia of lower limb affecting** right dominant **side**
G83.12 **Monoplegia of lower limb affecting** left dominant **side**
G83.13 **Monoplegia of lower limb affecting** right nondominant **side**
G83.14 **Monoplegia of lower limb affecting** left nondominant **side**

✓5ᵗʰ **G83.2** **Monoplegia** of upper limb
Paralysis of upper limb
EXCLUDES 1 monoplegia of upper limbs due to sequela of cerebrovascular disease (I69.03-, I69.13-, I69.23-, I69.33-, I69.83-, I69.93-)
G83.20 **Monoplegia of upper limb affecting** unspecified **side**
G83.21 **Monoplegia of upper limb affecting** right dominant **side**
G83.22 **Monoplegia of upper limb affecting** left dominant **side**
G83.23 **Monoplegia of upper limb affecting** right nondominant **side**
G83.24 **Monoplegia of upper limb affecting** left nondominant **side**

✓5ᵗʰ **G83.3** **Monoplegia,** unspecified
G83.30 **Monoplegia, unspecified affecting** unspecified **side**
G83.31 **Monoplegia, unspecified affecting** right dominant **side**
G83.32 **Monoplegia, unspecified affecting** left dominant **side**
G83.33 **Monoplegia, unspecified affecting** right nondominant **side**
G83.34 **Monoplegia, unspecified affecting** left nondominant **side**

G83.4 **Cauda equina syndrome** `CC`
Neurogenic bladder due to cauda equina syndrome
EXCLUDES 1 cord bladder NOS (G95.89)
neurogenic bladder NOS (N31.9)
CC Excl: G04.1, G32.89, G82.20-G82.54, G83.10-G83.14, G83.4-G83.9, G96.8-G96.9, G98.0-G98.8, G99.8, R53.2

G83.5 **Locked-in state** `MCC`
CC Excl: G04.1, G32.89, G80.0-G80.2, G80.4-G83.9, G92, G93.40-G93.49, G93.81, G93.89-G93.9, G96.8-G96.9, G98.0-G98.8, G99.8, I67.83, R53.2

✓5ᵗʰ **G83.8** **Other specified paralytic syndromes**
EXCLUDES 1 paralytic syndromes due to current spinal cord injury—code to spinal cord injury (S14, S24, S34)
G83.81 **Brown-Séquard syndrome**
G83.82 **Anterior cord syndrome**
G83.83 **Posterior cord syndrome**
G83.84 **Todd's paralysis (postepileptic)**
G83.89 **Other specified paralytic syndromes**

G83.9 **Paralytic syndrome, unspecified**

✓ Additional Character Required   ✓x7ᵗʰ Xtension Alert   Unacceptable PDx   Manifestation   Hospital Acquired Condition   **EXCLUDES 1** Not Coded Here   **EXCLUDES 2** Not Included Here

Diseases of the Nervous System

G89–G91.2

Other disorders of the nervous system (G89-G99)

☑4ᵗʰ **G89 Pain, not elsewhere classified**
Code also related psychological factors associated with pain (F45.42)
EXCLUDES 1 *generalized pain NOS (R52)*
pain disorders exclusively related to psychological factors (F45.41)
pain NOS (R52)
EXCLUDES 2 *atypical face pain (G50.1)*
headache syndromes (G44.-)
localized pain, unspecified type—code to pain by site, such as:
  abdomen pain (R10.-)
  back pain (M54.9)
  breast pain (N64.4)
  chest pain (R07.1-R07.9)
  ear pain (H92.0-)
  eye pain (H57.1)
  headache (R51)
  joint pain (M25.5-)
  limb pain (M79.6-)
  lumbar region pain (M54.5)
  painful urination (R30.9)
  pelvic and perineal pain (R10.2)
  renal colic (N23)
  shoulder pain (M25.51-)
  spine pain (M54.-)
  throat pain (R07.0)
  tongue pain (K14.6)
  tooth pain (K08.8)
migraines (G43.-)
myalgia (M79.1)
pain from prosthetic devices, implants, and grafts (T82.84, T83.84, T84.84, T85.84)
phantom limb syndrome with pain (G54.6)
vulvar vestibulitis (N94.810)
vulvodynia (N94.81-)

G89.0 Central pain syndrome
Déjérine-Roussy syndrome
Myelopathic pain syndrome
Thalamic pain syndrome (hyperesthetic)

☑5ᵗʰ **G89.1 Acute pain, not elsewhere classified**
  G89.11 Acute pain due to trauma
  G89.12 Acute post-thoracotomy pain
    Post-thoracotomy pain NOS
  G89.18 Other acute postprocedural pain
    Postoperative pain NOS
    Postprocedural pain NOS

☑5ᵗʰ **G89.2 Chronic pain, not elsewhere classified**
EXCLUDES 1 *causalgia, lower limb (G57.7-)*
causalgia, upper limb (G56.4-)
central pain syndrome (G89.0)
chronic pain syndrome (G89.4)
complex regional pain syndrome II, lower limb (G57.7-)
complex regional pain syndrome II, upper limb (G56.4-)
neoplasm related chronic pain (G89.3)
reflex sympathetic dystrophy (G90.5-)
  G89.21 Chronic pain due to trauma
  G89.22 Chronic post-thoracotomy pain
  G89.28 Other chronic postprocedural pain
    Other chronic postoperative pain
  G89.29 Other chronic pain

G89.3 Neoplasm related pain (acute) (chronic)
Cancer associated pain
Pain due to malignancy (primary) (secondary)
Tumor associated pain

G89.4 Chronic pain syndrome
Chronic pain associated with significant psychosocial dysfunction

☑4ᵗʰ **G90 Disorders of autonomic nervous system**
EXCLUDES 1 *dysfunction of the autonomic nervous system due to alcohol (G31.2)*

☑5ᵗʰ **G90.0 Idiopathic peripheral autonomic neuropathy**
  G90.01 Carotid sinus syncope
    Carotid sinus syndrome
  G90.09 Other idiopathic peripheral autonomic neuropathy
    Idiopathic peripheral autonomic neuropathy NOS

G90.1 Familial dysautonomia [Riley-Day]

G90.2 Horner's syndrome
Bernard(-Horner) syndrome
Cervical sympathetic dystrophy or paralysis

G90.3 Multi-system degeneration of the autonomic nervous system CC
Neurogenic orthostatic hypotension [Shy-Drager]
EXCLUDES 1 *orthostatic hypotension NOS (I95.1)*
CC Excl: G20-G21.9, G90.01-G90.09, G93.40-G93.49, I67.83

G90.4 Autonomic dysreflexia
Use additional code to identify the cause, such as:
fecal impaction (K56.41)
pressure ulcer (pressure area) (L89.-)
urinary tract infection (N39.0)

☑5ᵗʰ **G90.5 Complex regional pain syndrome I (CRPS I)**
Reflex sympathetic dystrophy
EXCLUDES 1 *causalgia of lower limb (G57.7-)*
causalgia of upper limb (G56.4-)
complex regional pain syndrome II of lower limb (G57.7-)
complex regional pain syndrome II of upper limb (G56.4-)

  G90.50 Complex regional pain syndrome I, unspecified CC
    CC Excl: G90.50-G90.59

☑6ᵗʰ   **G90.51 Complex regional pain syndrome I of upper limb**

CC Excl: For CC codes in subcategory G90.51, unless otherwise noted: E08.40-E08.49, E09.40-E09.49, E10.40-E10.49, E11.40-E11.49, E13.40-E13.49, G04.1, G11.3, G11.8-G12.9, G32.0, G32.89-G37.3, G37.5-G37.9, G80.0-G80.2, G80.4-G83.9, G90.01-G90.09, G90.2, G90.4-G90.9, G93.1, G93.40-G93.49, G95.0-G95.9, G96.12-G96.9, G97.1, G98.0-G99.8, I67.83, R53.2

    G90.511 Complex regional pain syndrome I of right upper limb CC
    G90.512 Complex regional pain syndrome I of left upper limb CC
    G90.513 Complex regional pain syndrome I of upper limb, bilateral CC
    G90.519 Complex regional pain syndrome I of unspecified upper limb CC

☑6ᵗʰ   **G90.52 Complex regional pain syndrome I of lower limb**

CC Excl: For CC codes in subcategory G90.52, unless otherwise noted: E08.40-E08.49, E09.40-E09.49, E10.40-E10.49, E11.40-E11.49, E13.40-E13.49, G04.1, G11.3, G11.8-G12.9, G32.0, G32.89-G37.3, G37.5-G37.9, G80.0-G80.2, G80.4-G83.9, G90.01-G90.09, G90.2, G90.4-G90.9, G93.1, G93.40-G93.49, G95.0-G95.9, G96.12-G96.9, G97.1, G98.0-G99.8, I67.83, R53.2

    G90.521 Complex regional pain syndrome I of right lower limb CC
    G90.522 Complex regional pain syndrome I of left lower limb CC
    G90.523 Complex regional pain syndrome I of lower limb, bilateral CC
    G90.529 Complex regional pain syndrome I of unspecified lower limb CC

  G90.59 Complex regional pain syndrome I of other specified site CC
    CC Excl: See code: G90.52

G90.8 Other disorders of autonomic nervous system

G90.9 Disorder of the autonomic nervous system, unspecified

☑4ᵗʰ **G91 Hydrocephalus**
INCLUDES acquired hydrocephalus
EXCLUDES 1 *Arnold-Chiari syndrome with hydrocephalus (Q07.-)*
congenital hydrocephalus (Q03.-)
spina bifida with hydrocephalus (Q05.-)

CC Excl: For CC codes in subcategories G91.0 & G91.2, unless otherwise noted: G91.0-G91.3, G91.8-G91.9
For CC codes in subcategories G91.1, G91.3-G91.9, unless otherwise noted: E08.40-E08.49, E08.618-E08.638, E08.649-E08.8, E09.40-E09.49, E09.618-E09.638, E09.649-E09.8, E10.40-E10.49, E10.618-E10.638, E10.649, E10.69-E10.8, E11.40-E11.49, E11.618-E11.638, E11.649, E11.69-E11.8, E13.40-E13.49, E13.618-E13.638, E13.649-E13.8, G13.2-G13.8, G31.2, G31.83-G31.9, G90.1, G90.1-G91.9, G93.81, G93.89-G94, Q03.0-Q03.9, Q04.4-Q04.8, Q05.0-Q05.4, Q05.9-Q06.1, Q06.3, Q06.8-Q06.9, Q07.02-Q07.9

G91.0 Communicating hydrocephalus CC
Secondary normal pressure hydrocephalus

G91.1 Obstructive hydrocephalus CC

G91.2 (Idiopathic) normal pressure hydrocephalus CC
Normal pressure hydrocephalus NOS

G91.3 Post-traumatic **hydrocephalus, unspecified** `CC`

G91.4 *Hydrocephalus in diseases classified elsewhere*
    Code first underlying condition, such as:
      congenital syphilis (A50.4-)
      neoplasm (C00-D49)
    `EXCLUDES 1` *hydrocephalus due to congenital toxoplasmosis (P37.1)*

G91.8 Other **hydrocephalus** `CC`

G91.9 **Hydrocephalus,** unspecified `CC`

G92 **Toxic encephalopathy** `MCC`
    Toxic encephalitis
    Toxic metabolic encephalopathy
    Code first (T51-T65) to identify toxic agent
    CC Excl: A17.82, A17.9, A18.82, A18.84, A18.89, A39.81, A50.42, A52.14,
    A83.0-A85.1, A85.8-A86, A88.8-A89, B00.4, B01.11, B10.01-B10.09, B26.2,
    B58.2, E08.40-E08.49, E08.618-E08.638, E08.649-E08.8, E09.40-E09.49,
    E09.618-E09.638, E09.649-E09.8, E10.40-E10.49, E10.618-E10.638, E10.649,
    E10.69-E10.8, E11.40-E11.49, E11.618-E11.638, E11.649, E11.69- E11.8,
    E13.40-E13.49, E13.618-E13.638, E13.649-E13.8, G04.00-G04.01, G04.31,
    G04.81-G05.4, G32.89, G37.3-G37.4, G92, G93.40-G93.49, G93.81, G93.89-
    G93.9, G96.8-G96.9, G98.0-G98.8, G99.8, I67.83

`✓4th` **G93** **Other disorders of brain**

    G93.0 **Cerebral cysts**
        Arachnoid cyst
        Porencephalic cyst, acquired
        `EXCLUDES 1` *acquired periventricular cysts of newborn (P91.1)*
                   congenital cerebral cysts (Q04.6)

    G93.1 **Anoxic brain damage, not elsewhere classified** `CC`
        `EXCLUDES 1` *cerebral anoxia due to anesthesia during labor and*
                   delivery (O74.3)
                  cerebral anoxia due to anesthesia during the
                   puerperium (O89.2)
                  neonatal anoxia (P84)
        CC Excl: E08.40-E08.49, E08.618-E08.638, E08.649-E08.8, E09.40-
        E09.49, E09.618-E09.638, E09.649-E09.8, E10.40-E10.49, E10.618-
        E10.638, E10.649, E10.69-E10.8, E11.40-E11.49, E11.618-E11.638,
        E11.649, E11.69-E11.8, E13.40-E13.49, E13.618-E13.638, E13.649-
        E13.8, G32.89, G93.1-G93.2, G96.8-G96.9, G98.0-G98.8, G99.8

    G93.2 **Benign intracranial hypertension**
        `EXCLUDES 1` *hypertensive encephalopathy (I67.4)*

    G93.3 **Postviral fatigue syndrome**
        Benign myalgic encephalomyelitis
        `EXCLUDES 1` *chronic fatigue syndrome NOS (R53.82)*

  `✓5th` **G93.4** **Other and unspecified encephalopathy**
        `EXCLUDES 1` *alcoholic encephalopathy (G31.2)*
                 encephalopathy in diseases classified elsewhere (G94)
                 hypertensive encephalopathy (I67.4)
                 toxic (metabolic) encephalopathy (G92)

        G93.40 **Encephalopathy,** unspecified `HIV` `MCC`
            CC Excl: G21.0, G83.5, G93.41-G93.49, I67.83

        G93.41 **Metabolic encephalopathy** `HIV` `MCC`
            Septic encephalopathy
            CC Excl: G21.0, G83.5, G93.40, G93.49, I67.83

        G93.49 **Other encephalopathy** `HIV` `MCC`
            Encephalopathy NEC
            CC Excl: G21.0, G83.5, G93.40-G93.41

    G93.5 **Compression of brain** `MCC`
        Arnold-Chiari type 1 compression of brain
        Compression of brain (stem)
        Herniation of brain (stem)
        `EXCLUDES 1` *diffuse traumatic compression of brain (S06.2-)*
                 focal traumatic compression of brain (S06.3-)
        CC Excl: G81.90, G93.82

    G93.6 **Cerebral edema** `MCC`
        `EXCLUDES 1` *cerebral edema due to birth injury (P11.0)*
                 traumatic cerebral edema (S06.1-)
        CC Excl: G93.6, G93.82

    G93.7 **Reye's syndrome** `MCC` `P`
        Code first (T39.0-), if salicylates-induced
        CC Excl: G93.7

  `✓5th` **G93.8** **Other specified disorders of brain**
        G93.81 **Temporal sclerosis**
            Hippocampal sclerosis
            Mesial temporal sclerosis

        G93.82 **Brain death** `MCC`
            CC Excl: B15.0-B19.9, E03.5, E08.00-E08.59, E08.618-
            E09.59, E09.618-E10.59, E10.618-E10.649, E10.69-
            E11.59, E11.618-E11.649, E11.69-E13.59, E13.618-E16.2,
            E89.1, G32.89, G89.0-G89.4, G93.81-G93.9, G96.8-G96.9,
            G98.0-G98.8, G99.8, I60.00-I62.9, K72.91, R40.0-
            R40.2124, R40.2210-R40.2224, R40.2310-R40.2324,
            R40.2340-R40.2344, R40.3-R41.3, R41.82, R41.9-R42,
            R44.8-R44.9, R45.83-R45.84, R46.0-R46.89, R52, R55,
            R68.0-R68.19, R68.81-R68.83, R68.89-R69, S02.0XX-
            S02.19X with 7th [A, B], S02.91X with 7th [A, B], S06.0X0-
            S06.9X9 with 7th A

        G93.89 **Other specified disorders of brain**
            Postradiation encephalopathy

    G93.9 **Disorder of brain, unspecified** `HIV`

`G94` *Other disorders of brain in diseases classified elsewhere*
    Code first underlying disease
    `EXCLUDES 1` *encephalopathy in congenital syphilis (A50.49)*
            encephalopathy in influenza (J09.X9, J10.81, J11.81)
            encephalopathy in syphilis (A52.19)
            hydrocephalus in diseases classified elsewhere (G91.4)

`✓4th` **G95** **Other and unspecified diseases of spinal cord**
    `EXCLUDES 2` *myelitis (G04.-)*

    G95.0 **Syringomyelia and syringobulbia** `CC`
        CC Excl: G04.1, G11.3, G11.8-G12.9, G32.0, G32.89-G37.3, G37.5-
        G37.9, G80.0-G80.2, G80.4-G83.9, G90.01-G90.09, G90.2, G90.4-
        G90.9, G93.40-G93.49, G93.81, G93.89-G93.9, G95.0-G95.9,
        G96.12-G96.9, G97.1, G98.0-G99.8, I67.83, R53.2

  `✓5th` **G95.1** **Vascular myelopathies**
        `EXCLUDES 2` *intraspinal phlebitis and thrombophlebitis, except non-*
                 pyogenic (G08)

        G95.11 **Acute infarction of spinal cord (embolic)** `MCC`
            (nonembolic)
            Anoxia of spinal cord
            Arterial thrombosis of spinal cord
            CC Excl: E08.40-E08.49, E09.40-E09.49, E10.40-E10.49,
            E11.40-E11.49, E13.40-E13.49, G04.1, G11.3, G11.8-
            G12.9, G32.0, G32.89-G37.3, G37.5-G37.9, G80.0-G80.2,
            G80.4-G83.9, G90.01-G90.09, G90.2, G90.4-G90.9, G93.1,
            G93.40-G93.49, G95.0-G95.9, G96.12-G96.9, G97.1,
            G98.0-G99.8, I67.83, R53.2

        G95.19 **Other vascular myelopathies** `MCC`
            Edema of spinal cord
            Hematomyelia
            Nonpyogenic intraspinal phlebitis and
              thrombophlebitis
            Subacute necrotic myelopathy
            CC Excl: See code: G95.11

  `✓5th` **G95.2** **Other and unspecified cord compression**
        G95.20 **Unspecified cord compression** `HIV` `CC`
            CC Excl: E08.40-E08.49, E09.40-E09.49, E10.40-E10.49,
            E11.40-E11.49, E13.40-E13.49, G04.1, G11.3-G12.9,
            G32.0, G32.89-G37.3, G37.5-G37.9, G80.0-G80.2, G80.4-
            G83.9, G90.01-G90.09, G90.2, G90.4-G90.9, G93.1,
            G93.40-G93.49, G95.0-G95.9, G96.12-G96.9, G97.1,
            G98.0-G99.8, I67.83, R53.2

        G95.29 **Other cord compression** `HIV` `CC`
            CC Excl: See code: G95.20

  `✓5th` **G95.8** **Other specified diseases of spinal cord**
        `EXCLUDES 1` *neurogenic bladder NOS (N31.9)*
                 neurogenic bladder due to cauda equina syndrome
                   (G83.4)
                 neuromuscular dysfunction of bladder without spinal
                   cord lesion (N31.-)

        G95.81 **Conus medullaris syndrome** `CC`
            CC Excl: See code: G90.51

        G95.89 **Other specified diseases of spinal cord** `CC`
            Cord bladder NOS
            Drug-induced myelopathy
            Radiation-induced myelopathy
            `EXCLUDES 1` *myelopathy NOS (G95.9)*
            CC Excl: See code: G90.51

    G95.9 **Disease of spinal cord, unspecified** `HIV` `CC`
        Myelopathy NOS
        CC Excl: See code: G95.20

`✓` Additional Character Required   `✓x7th` Xtension Alert   Unacceptable PDx   Manifestation   Hospital Acquired Condition   `EXCLUDES 1` Not Coded Here   `EXCLUDES 2` Not Included Here

Diseases of the Nervous System

G96–G99.8

√4th **G96 Other disorders of central nervous system**

G96.0 Cerebrospinal fluid leak cc
EXCLUDES 1 *cerebrospinal fluid leak from spinal puncture (G97.0)*
CC Excl: E08.40-E08.49, E08.618-E08.638, E08.649-E08.8, E09.40-
E09.49, E09.618-E09.638, E09.649-E09.8, E10.40-E10.49, E10.618-
E10.638, E10.649, E10.69-E10.8, E11.40-E11.49, E11.618-E11.638,
E11.649, E11.69-E11.8, E13.40-E13.49, E13.618-E13.638, E13.649-
E13.8, G32.89, G96.0, G96.8-G96.9, G98.0-G98.8, G99.8

√5th **G96.1 Disorders of meninges, not elsewhere classified**

G96.11 Dural tear cc
EXCLUDES 1 *accidental puncture or laceration of dura
during a procedure (G97.41)*
CC Excl: D78.11-D78.12, D78.81-D78.89, E36.11-E36.8,
E89.810-E89.89, G96.11, G97.41, G97.48-G97.49,
H59.011-H59.019, H59.031-H59.099, H59.211-H59.229,
H59.811-H59.89, H95.31-H95.32, H95.811-H95.89, I97.3,
I97.51-I97.52, J95.71-J95.72, K91.71-K91.72, L76.11-
L76.12, L76.81-L76.82, M96.820-M96.821, M96.89,
N98.1-N98.9, N99.71-N99.72, T81.82XA, T81.89XA,
T81.9XXA

G96.12 Meningeal adhesions (cerebral) (spinal)

**G96.19 Other disorders of meninges, not elsewhere
classified**

G96.8 Other specified disorders of central nervous system

G96.9 Disorder of central nervous system, unspecified HIV

√4th **G97 Intraoperative and postprocedural complications and disorders
of nervous system, not elsewhere classified**
EXCLUDES 2 *intraoperative and postprocedural cerebrovascular infarction
(I97.81-, I97.82-)*

G97.0 Cerebrospinal fluid leak from spinal puncture cc
CC Excl: D78.81-D78.89, E36.8, E89.810-E89.89, G97.0, G97.2-
G97.32, G97.81-G97.82, H59.011-H59.019, H59.031-H59.099,
H59.811-H59.89, H95.811-H95.89, I97.3, I97.810-I97.821, L76.81-
L76.82, M96.89, N98.1-N98.9, T81.82XA, T81.89XA, T81.9XXA

G97.1 Other reaction to spinal and lumbar puncture
Headache due to lumbar puncture

G97.2 Intracranial hypotension following ventricular shunting cc
CC Excl: See code: G97.0

√5th **G97.3 Intraoperative hemorrhage and hematoma of a nervous
system organ or structure complicating a procedure**
EXCLUDES 1 *intraoperative hemorrhage and hematoma of a
nervous system organ or structure due to
accidental puncture and laceration during a
procedure (G97.4-)*

**G97.31 Intraoperative hemorrhage and hematoma of a
nervous system organ or structure complicating a
nervous system procedure** cc
CC Excl: G97.4, G97.2-G97.32, G97.81-G97.82, H95.811-
H95.89, I97.3, I97.810-I97.821, M96.89, N98.1-N98.9,
T81.82XA, T81.89XA, T81.9XXA

**G97.32 Intraoperative hemorrhage and hematoma of a
nervous system organ or structure complicating
other procedure** cc
CC Excl: See code: G97.31

√5th **G97.4 Accidental puncture and laceration of a nervous system organ
or structure during a procedure**

**CC Excl: For CC codes in subcategory G97.4, unless
otherwise noted:** D78.11-D78.12, D78.81-D78.89, E36.11-
E36.8, E89.810-E89.89, G96.11, G97.41, G97.48-G97.49,
H59.011-H59.019, H59.031-H59.099, H59.211-H59.229,
H59.811-H59.89, H95.31-H95.32, H95.811-H95.89, I97.3,
I97.51-I97.52, J95.71-J95.72, K91.71-K91.72, L76.11-L76.12,
L76.81-L76.82, M96.820-M96.821, M96.89, N98.1-N98.9,
N99.71-N99.72, T81.82XA, T81.89XA, T81.9XXA

**G97.41 Accidental puncture or laceration of dura
during a procedure** cc
Incidental (inadvertent) durotomy

**G97.48 Accidental puncture and laceration of other
nervous system organ or structure during a
nervous system procedure** cc

**G97.49 Accidental puncture and laceration of other
nervous system organ or structure during
other procedure** cc

√5th **G97.5 Postprocedural hemorrhage and hematoma of a nervous
system organ or structure following a procedure**

**G97.51 Postprocedural hemorrhage and hematoma
of a nervous system organ or structure following
a nervous system procedure** cc
CC Excl: G97.51-G97.52, H95.811-H95.89, I85.01, I85.11,
I97.3, K21.9, K22.8, K23-K25.0, K25.2, K25.4, K25.6, K26.0,
K26.2, K26.4, K26.6, K27.0, K27.2, K27.4, K27.6, K28.0,
K28.2, K28.4, K28.6, K29.01, K29.21, K29.31, K29.41,
K29.51, K29.61, K29.71, K29.81, K29.91, K31.811, K55.21,
K57.01, K57.11, K57.13, K57.21, K57.31, K57.33, K57.41,
K57.51, K57.53, K57.81, K57.91, K57.93, K62.5, K92.0-
K92.2, M96.89, N98.1-N98.9, P54.1-P54.3, T81.10XA,
T81.11XA, T81.12XA, T81.19XA, T81.82XA, T81.89XA,
T81.9XXA

**G97.52 Postprocedural hemorrhage and hematoma
of a nervous system organ or structure following
other procedure** cc
CC Excl: See code: G97.51

√5th **G97.8 Other intraoperative and postprocedural complications and
disorders of nervous system**
Use additional code to further specify disorder

**G97.81 Other intraoperative complications of nervous
system** cc
CC Excl: See code: G97.0

**G97.82 Other postprocedural complications and
disorders of nervous system** cc
CC Excl: See code: G97.0

√4th **G98 Other disorders of nervous system not elsewhere classified**
INCLUDES nervous system disorder NOS

G98.0 Neurogenic arthritis, not elsewhere classified
Nonsyphilitic neurogenic arthropathy NEC
Nonsyphilitic neurogenic spondylopathy NEC
EXCLUDES 1 *spondylopathy (in):*
syringomyelia and syringobulbia (G95.0)
tabes dorsalis (A52.11)

G98.8 Other disorders of nervous system HIV
Nervous system disorder NOS

√4th **G99 Other disorders of nervous system in diseases classified
elsewhere**

G99.0 Autonomic neuropathy in diseases classified elsewhere cc
Code first underlying disease, such as:
amyloidosis (E85.-)
gout (M1A.-, M10.-)
hyperthyroidism (E05.-)
EXCLUDES 1 *diabetic autonomic neuropathy (E08-E13 with .43)*
CC Excl: G90.01-G90.09, G90.2, G90.50-G90.9, G93.40-G93.49,
G99.0, I67.83

G99.2 Myelopathy in diseases classified elsewhere cc
Code first underlying disease, such as:
neoplasm (C00-D49)
EXCLUDES 1 *myelopathy in:*
intervertebral disease (M50.0-, M51.0-)
spondylosis (M47.0-, M47.1-)
CC Excl: E08.40-E08.49, E09.40-E09.49, E10.40-E10.49, E11.40-
E11.49, E13.40-E13.49, G04.1, G11.3, G11.8-G12.9, G32.0, G32.89-
G37.3, G37.5-G37.9, G80.0-G80.2, G80.4-G83.9, G90.01-G90.09,
G90.2, G90.4-G90.9, G93.1, G93.40-G93.49, G95.0-G95.9, G96.12-
G96.9, G97.1, G98.0-G98.8, I67.83, R53.2

**G99.8 Other specified disorders of nervous system in diseases
classified elsewhere**
Code first underlying disorder, such as:
amyloidosis (E85.-)
avitaminosis (E56.9)
EXCLUDES 1 *nervous system involvement in:*
cysticercosis (B69.0)
rubella (B06.0-)
syphilis (A52.1-)

N Newborn: 0   P Pediatric: 0-17   M Maternity: 12-55   A Adult: 15-124   MCC Major CC Condition   PDx MCC PDx acts as own MCC   CC CC Condition   PDx CC PDx acts as own CC

546   ICD-10-CM Draft (2015)

Chapter 7. Diseases of the Eye and Adnexa (H00-H59)

NOTE   Use an external cause code following the code for the eye condition, if applicable, to identify the cause of the eye condition.

EXCLUDES 2   certain conditions originating in the perinatal period (P04-P96)
certain infectious and parasitic diseases (A00-B99)
complications of pregnancy, childbirth and the puerperium (O00-O9A)
congenital malformations, deformations, and chromosomal abnormalities (Q00-Q99)
diabetes mellitus related eye conditions (E09.3-, E10.3-, E11.3-, E13.3-)
endocrine, nutritional and metabolic diseases (E00-E88)
injury (trauma) of eye and orbit (S05.-)
injury, poisoning and certain other consequences of external causes (S00-T88)
neoplasms (C00-D49)
symptoms, signs and abnormal clinical and laboratory findings, not elsewhere classified (R00-R94)
syphilis related eye disorders (A50.01, A50.3-, A51.43, A52.71)

This chapter contains the following blocks:

H00-H05   Disorders of eyelid, lacrimal system and orbit
H10-H11   Disorders of conjunctiva
H15-H22   Disorders of sclera, cornea, iris and ciliary body
H25-H28   Disorders of lens
H30-H36   Disorders of choroid and retina
H40-H42   Glaucoma
H43-H44   Disorders of vitreous body and globe
H46-H47   Disorders of optic nerve and visual pathways
H49-H52   Disorders of ocular muscles, binocular movement, accommodation and refraction
H53-H54   Visual disturbances and blindness
H55-H57   Other disorders of eye and adnexa
H59   Intraoperative and postprocedural complications and disorders of eye and adnexa, not elsewhere classified

Disorders of eyelid, lacrimal system and orbit (H00-H05)

EXCLUDES 2   open wound of eyelid (S01.1-)
superficial injury of eyelid (S00.1-, S00.2-)

✓4th H00   Hordeolum and chalazion

✓5th   H00.0   Hordeolum (externum) (internum) of eyelid

✓6th   H00.01   Hordeolum externum
Hordeolum NOS
Stye

H00.011   Hordeolum externum right upper eyelid
H00.012   Hordeolum externum right lower eyelid
H00.013   Hordeolum externum right eye, unspecified eyelid
H00.014   Hordeolum externum left upper eyelid
H00.015   Hordeolum externum left lower eyelid
H00.016   Hordeolum externum left eye, unspecified eyelid
H00.019   Hordeolum externum unspecified eye, unspecified eyelid

✓6th   H00.02   Hordeolum internum
Infection of meibomian gland

H00.021   Hordeolum internum right upper eyelid
H00.022   Hordeolum internum right lower eyelid
H00.023   Hordeolum internum right eye, unspecified eyelid
H00.024   Hordeolum internum left upper eyelid
H00.025   Hordeolum internum left lower eyelid
H00.026   Hordeolum internum left eye, unspecified eyelid
H00.029   Hordeolum internum unspecified eye, unspecified eyelid

✓6th   H00.03   Abscess of eyelid
Furuncle of eyelid

H00.031   Abscess of right upper eyelid
H00.032   Abscess of right lower eyelid
H00.033   Abscess of eyelid right eye, unspecified eyelid
H00.034   Abscess of left upper eyelid
H00.035   Abscess of left lower eyelid
H00.036   Abscess of eyelid left eye, unspecified eyelid
H00.039   Abscess of eyelid unspecified eye, unspecified eyelid

✓5th   H00.1   Chalazion
Meibomian (gland) cyst
EXCLUDES 2   infected meibomian gland (H00.02-)

H00.11   Chalazion right upper eyelid
H00.12   Chalazion right lower eyelid
H00.13   Chalazion right eye, unspecified eyelid
H00.14   Chalazion left upper eyelid
H00.15   Chalazion left lower eyelid
H00.16   Chalazion left eye, unspecified eyelid
H00.19   Chalazion unspecified eye, unspecified eyelid

✓4th H01   Other inflammation of eyelid

✓5th   H01.0   Blepharitis
EXCLUDES 1   blepharoconjunctivitis (H10.5-)

✓6th   H01.00   Unspecified blepharitis
H01.001   Unspecified blepharitis right upper eyelid
H01.002   Unspecified blepharitis right lower eyelid
H01.003   Unspecified blepharitis right eye, unspecified eyelid
H01.004   Unspecified blepharitis left upper eyelid
H01.005   Unspecified blepharitis left lower eyelid
H01.006   Unspecified blepharitis left eye, unspecified eyelid
H01.009   Unspecified blepharitis unspecified eye, unspecified eyelid

✓6th   H01.01   Ulcerative blepharitis
H01.011   Ulcerative blepharitis right upper eyelid
H01.012   Ulcerative blepharitis right lower eyelid
H01.013   Ulcerative blepharitis right eye, unspecified eyelid
H01.014   Ulcerative blepharitis left upper eyelid
H01.015   Ulcerative blepharitis left lower eyelid
H01.016   Ulcerative blepharitis left eye, unspecified eyelid
H01.019   Ulcerative blepharitis unspecified eye, unspecified eyelid

✓6th   H01.02   Squamous blepharitis
H01.021   Squamous blepharitis right upper eyelid
H01.022   Squamous blepharitis right lower eyelid
H01.023   Squamous blepharitis right eye, unspecified eyelid
H01.024   Squamous blepharitis left upper eyelid
H01.025   Squamous blepharitis left lower eyelid
H01.026   Squamous blepharitis left eye, unspecified eyelid
H01.029   Squamous blepharitis unspecified eye, unspecified eyelid

✓5th   H01.1   Noninfectious dermatoses of eyelid

✓6th   H01.11   Allergic dermatitis of eyelid
Contact dermatitis of eyelid

H01.111   Allergic dermatitis of right upper eyelid
H01.112   Allergic dermatitis of right lower eyelid
H01.113   Allergic dermatitis of right eye, unspecified eyelid
H01.114   Allergic dermatitis of left upper eyelid
H01.115   Allergic dermatitis of left lower eyelid
H01.116   Allergic dermatitis of left eye, unspecified eyelid
H01.119   Allergic dermatitis of unspecified eye, unspecified eyelid

✓6th   H01.12   Discoid lupus erythematosus of eyelid
H01.121   Discoid lupus erythematosus of right upper eyelid
H01.122   Discoid lupus erythematosus of right lower eyelid
H01.123   Discoid lupus erythematosus of right eye, unspecified eyelid
H01.124   Discoid lupus erythematosus of left upper eyelid
H01.125   Discoid lupus erythematosus of left lower eyelid
H01.126   Discoid lupus erythematosus of left eye, unspecified eyelid
H01.129   Discoid lupus erythematosus of unspecified eye, unspecified eyelid

√6th **H01.13** **Eczematous dermatitis of eyelid**

 H01.131 Eczematous dermatitis of right upper eyelid

 H01.132 Eczematous dermatitis of right lower eyelid

 H01.133 Eczematous dermatitis of right eye, unspecified eyelid

 H01.134 Eczematous dermatitis of left upper eyelid

 H01.135 Eczematous dermatitis of left lower eyelid

 H01.136 Eczematous dermatitis of left eye, unspecified eyelid

 H01.139 Eczematous dermatitis of unspecified eye, unspecified eyelid

√6th **H01.14** **Xeroderma of eyelid**

 H01.141 Xeroderma of right upper eyelid

 H01.142 Xeroderma of right lower eyelid

 H01.143 Xeroderma of right eye, unspecified eyelid

 H01.144 Xeroderma of left upper eyelid

 H01.145 Xeroderma of left lower eyelid

 H01.146 Xeroderma of left eye, unspecified eyelid

 H01.149 Xeroderma of unspecified eye, unspecified eyelid

H01.8 Other specified inflammations of eyelid

H01.9 Unspecified inflammation of eyelid

 Inflammation of eyelid NOS

√4th **H02** **Other disorders of eyelid**

 EXCLUDES 1 *congenital malformations of eyelid (Q10.0-Q10.3)*

√5th **H02.0** **Entropion and trichiasis of eyelid**

√6th **H02.00** **Unspecified entropion of eyelid**

 H02.001 Unspecified entropion of right upper eyelid

 H02.002 Unspecified entropion of right lower eyelid

 H02.003 Unspecified entropion of right eye, unspecified eyelid

 H02.004 Unspecified entropion of left upper eyelid

 H02.005 Unspecified entropion of left lower eyelid

 H02.006 Unspecified entropion of left eye, unspecified eyelid

 H02.009 Unspecified entropion of unspecified eye, unspecified eyelid

√6th **H02.01** **Cicatricial entropion of eyelid**

 H02.011 Cicatricial entropion of right upper eyelid

 H02.012 Cicatricial entropion of right lower eyelid

 H02.013 Cicatricial entropion of right eye, unspecified eyelid

 H02.014 Cicatricial entropion of left upper eyelid

 H02.015 Cicatricial entropion of left lower eyelid

 H02.016 Cicatricial entropion of left eye, unspecified eyelid

 H02.019 Cicatricial entropion of unspecified eye, unspecified eyelid

√6th **H02.02** **Mechanical entropion of eyelid**

 H02.021 Mechanical entropion of right upper eyelid

 H02.022 Mechanical entropion of right lower eyelid

 H02.023 Mechanical entropion of right eye, unspecified eyelid

 H02.024 Mechanical entropion of left upper eyelid

 H02.025 Mechanical entropion of left lower eyelid

 H02.026 Mechanical entropion of left eye, unspecified eyelid

 H02.029 Mechanical entropion of unspecified eye, unspecified eyelid

√6th **H02.03** **Senile entropion of eyelid**

 H02.031 Senile entropion of right upper eyelid Ⓐ

 H02.032 Senile entropion of right lower eyelid Ⓐ

 H02.033 Senile entropion of right eye, unspecified eyelid Ⓐ

 H02.034 Senile entropion of left upper eyelid Ⓐ

 H02.035 Senile entropion of left lower eyelid Ⓐ

 H02.036 Senile entropion of left eye, unspecified eyelid Ⓐ

 H02.039 Senile entropion of unspecified eye, unspecified eyelid Ⓐ

√6th **H02.04** **Spastic entropion of eyelid**

 H02.041 Spastic entropion of right upper eyelid

 H02.042 Spastic entropion of right lower eyelid

 H02.043 Spastic entropion of right eye, unspecified eyelid

 H02.044 Spastic entropion of left upper eyelid

 H02.045 Spastic entropion of left lower eyelid

 H02.046 Spastic entropion of left eye, unspecified eyelid

 H02.049 Spastic entropion of unspecified eye, unspecified eyelid

√6th **H02.05** **Trichiasis without entropian**

 H02.051 Trichiasis without entropian right upper eyelid

 H02.052 Trichiasis without entropian right lower eyelid

 H02.053 Trichiasis without entropian right eye, unspecified eyelid

 H02.054 Trichiasis without entropian left upper eyelid

 H02.055 Trichiasis without entropian left lower eyelid

 H02.056 Trichiasis without entropian left eye, unspecified eyelid

 H02.059 Trichiasis without entropian unspecified eye, unspecified eyelid

√5th **H02.1** **Ectropion of eyelid**

√6th **H02.10** **Unspecified ectropion of eyelid**

 H02.101 Unspecified ectropion of right upper eyelid

 H02.102 Unspecified ectropion of right lower eyelid

 H02.103 Unspecified ectropion of right eye, unspecified eyelid

 H02.104 Unspecified ectropion of left upper eyelid

 H02.105 Unspecified ectropion of left lower eyelid

 H02.106 Unspecified ectropion of left eye, unspecified eyelid

 H02.109 Unspecified ectropion of unspecified eye, unspecified eyelid

√6th **H02.11** **Cicatricial ectropion of eyelid**

 H02.111 Cicatricial ectropion of right upper eyelid

 H02.112 Cicatricial ectropion of right lower eyelid

 H02.113 Cicatricial ectropion of right eye, unspecified eyelid

 H02.114 Cicatricial ectropion of left upper eyelid

 H02.115 Cicatricial ectropion of left lower eyelid

 H02.116 Cicatricial ectropion of left eye, unspecified eyelid

 H02.119 Cicatricial ectropion of unspecified eye, unspecified eyelid

√6th **H02.12** **Mechanical ectropion of eyelid**

 H02.121 Mechanical ectropion of right upper eyelid

 H02.122 Mechanical ectropion of right lower eyelid

 H02.123 Mechanical ectropion of right eye, unspecified eyelid

 H02.124 Mechanical ectropion of left upper eyelid

 H02.125 Mechanical ectropion of left lower eyelid

 H02.126 Mechanical ectropion of left eye, unspecified eyelid

 H02.129 Mechanical ectropion of unspecified eye, unspecified eyelid

√6th **H02.13** **Senile ectropion of eyelid**

 H02.131 Senile ectropion of right upper eyelid Ⓐ

 H02.132 Senile ectropion of right lower eyelid Ⓐ

 H02.133 Senile ectropion of right eye, unspecified eyelid Ⓐ

 H02.134 Senile ectropion of left upper eyelid Ⓐ

 H02.135 Senile ectropion of left lower eyelid Ⓐ

 H02.136 Senile ectropion of left eye, unspecified eyelid Ⓐ

 H02.139 Senile ectropion of unspecified eye, unspecified eyelid Ⓐ

√6th **H02.14** **Spastic ectropion of eyelid**

 H02.141 Spastic ectropion of right upper eyelid

 H02.142 Spastic ectropion of right lower eyelid

Ⓝ Newborn: 0   Ⓟ Pediatric: 0-17   Ⓜ Maternity: 12-55   Ⓐ Adult: 15-124   **MCC** Major CC Condition   **PDx MCC** PDx acts as own MCC   **CC** CC Condition   **PDx CC** PDx acts as own CC

548   ICD-10-CM Draft (2015)

H02.143 Spastic ectropion of right eye, unspecified eyelid
H02.144 Spastic ectropion of left upper eyelid
H02.145 Spastic ectropion of left lower eyelid
H02.146 Spastic ectropion of left eye, unspecified eyelid
H02.149 Spastic ectropion of unspecified eye, unspecified eyelid

✓5th **H02.2 Lagophthalmos**

✓6th **H02.20 Unspecified lagophthalmos**
H02.201 Unspecified lagophthalmos right upper eyelid
H02.202 Unspecified lagophthalmos right lower eyelid
H02.203 Unspecified lagophthalmos right eye, unspecified eyelid
H02.204 Unspecified lagophthalmos left upper eyelid
H02.205 Unspecified lagophthalmos left lower eyelid
H02.206 Unspecified lagophthalmos left eye, unspecified eyelid
H02.209 Unspecified lagophthalmos unspecified eye, unspecified eyelid

✓6th **H02.21 Cicatricial lagophthalmos**
H02.211 Cicatricial lagophthalmos right upper eyelid
H02.212 Cicatricial lagophthalmos right lower eyelid
H02.213 Cicatricial lagophthalmos right eye, unspecified eyelid
H02.214 Cicatricial lagophthalmos left upper eyelid
H02.215 Cicatricial lagophthalmos left lower eyelid
H02.216 Cicatricial lagophthalmos left eye, unspecified eyelid
H02.219 Cicatricial lagophthalmos unspecified eye, unspecified eyelid

✓6th **H02.22 Mechanical lagophthalmos**
H02.221 Mechanical lagophthalmos right upper eyelid
H02.222 Mechanical lagophthalmos right lower eyelid
H02.223 Mechanical lagophthalmos right eye, unspecified eyelid
H02.224 Mechanical lagophthalmos left upper eyelid
H02.225 Mechanical lagophthalmos left lower eyelid
H02.226 Mechanical lagophthalmos left eye, unspecified eyelid
H02.229 Mechanical lagophthalmos unspecified eye, unspecified eyelid

✓6th **H02.23 Paralytic lagophthalmos**
H02.231 Paralytic lagophthalmos right upper eyelid
H02.232 Paralytic lagophthalmos right lower eyelid
H02.233 Paralytic lagophthalmos right eye, unspecified eyelid
H02.234 Paralytic lagophthalmos left upper eyelid
H02.235 Paralytic lagophthalmos left lower eyelid
H02.236 Paralytic lagophthalmos left eye, unspecified eyelid
H02.239 Paralytic lagophthalmos unspecified eye, unspecified eyelid

✓5th **H02.3 Blepharochalasis**
Pseudoptosis
H02.30 Blepharochalasis unspecified eye, unspecified eyelid
H02.31 Blepharochalasis right upper eyelid
H02.32 Blepharochalasis right lower eyelid
H02.33 Blepharochalasis right eye, unspecified eyelid
H02.34 Blepharochalasis left upper eyelid
H02.35 Blepharochalasis left lower eyelid
H02.36 Blepharochalasis left eye, unspecified eyelid

✓5th **H02.4 Ptosis of eyelid**

✓6th **H02.40 Unspecified ptosis of eyelid**
H02.401 Unspecified ptosis of right eyelid
H02.402 Unspecified ptosis of left eyelid
H02.403 Unspecified ptosis of bilateral eyelids
H02.409 Unspecified ptosis of unspecified eyelid

✓6th **H02.41 Mechanical ptosis of eyelid**
H02.411 Mechanical ptosis of right eyelid
H02.412 Mechanical ptosis of left eyelid
H02.413 Mechanical ptosis of bilateral eyelids
H02.419 Mechanical ptosis of unspecified eyelid

✓6th **H02.42 Myogenic ptosis of eyelid**
H02.421 Myogenic ptosis of right eyelid
H02.422 Myogenic ptosis of left eyelid
H02.423 Myogenic ptosis of bilateral eyelids
H02.429 Myogenic ptosis of unspecified eyelid

✓6th **H02.43 Paralytic ptosis of eyelid**
Neurogenic ptosis of eyelid
H02.431 Paralytic ptosis of right eyelid
H02.432 Paralytic ptosis of left eyelid
H02.433 Paralytic ptosis of bilateral eyelids
H02.439 Paralytic ptosis unspecified eyelid

✓5th **H02.5 Other disorders affecting eyelid function**
EXCLUDES 2 blepharospasm (G24.5)
organic tic (G25.69)
psychogenic tic (F95.-)

✓6th **H02.51 Abnormal innervation syndrome**
H02.511 Abnormal innervation syndrome right upper eyelid
H02.512 Abnormal innervation syndrome right lower eyelid
H02.513 Abnormal innervation syndrome right eye, unspecified eyelid
H02.514 Abnormal innervation syndrome left upper eyelid
H02.515 Abnormal innervation syndrome left lower eyelid
H02.516 Abnormal innervation syndrome left eye, unspecified eyelid
H02.519 Abnormal innervation syndrome unspecified eye, unspecified eyelid

✓6th **H02.52 Blepharophimosis**
Ankyloblepharon
H02.521 Blepharophimosis right upper eyelid
H02.522 Blepharophimosis right lower eyelid
H02.523 Blepharophimosis right eye, unspecified eyelid
H02.524 Blepharophimosis left upper eyelid
H02.525 Blepharophimosis left lower eyelid
H02.526 Blepharophimosis left eye, unspecified eyelid
H02.529 Blepharophimosis unspecified eye, unspecified lid

✓6th **H02.53 Eyelid retraction**
Eyelid lag
H02.531 Eyelid retraction right upper eyelid
H02.532 Eyelid retraction right lower eyelid
H02.533 Eyelid retraction right eye, unspecified eyelid
H02.534 Eyelid retraction left upper eyelid
H02.535 Eyelid retraction left lower eyelid
H02.536 Eyelid retraction left eye, unspecified eyelid
H02.539 Eyelid retraction unspecified eye, unspecified lid

H02.59 Other disorders affecting eyelid function
Deficient blink reflex
Sensory disorders

✓5th **H02.6 Xanthelasma of eyelid**
H02.60 Xanthelasma of unspecified eye, unspecified eyelid
H02.61 Xanthelasma of right upper eyelid
H02.62 Xanthelasma of right lower eyelid
H02.63 Xanthelasma of right eye, unspecified eyelid
H02.64 Xanthelasma of left upper eyelid

Diseases of the Eye and Adnexa

H02.65–H04.001

H02.65   Xanthelasma of left lower eyelid

H02.66   Xanthelasma of left eye, unspecified eyelid

√5th   **H02.7**   **Other and unspecified degenerative disorders of eyelid and periocular area**

H02.70   Unspecified degenerative disorders of eyelid and periocular area

√6th   H02.71   **Chloasma of eyelid and periocular area**
Dyspigmentation of eyelid
Hyperpigmentation of eyelid

    H02.711   Chloasma of right upper eyelid and periocular area

    H02.712   Chloasma of right lower eyelid and periocular area

    H02.713   Chloasma of right eye, unspecified eyelid and periocular area

    H02.714   Chloasma of left upper eyelid and periocular area

    H02.715   Chloasma of left lower eyelid and periocular area

    H02.716   Chloasma of left eye, unspecified eyelid and periocular area

    H02.719   Chloasma of unspecified eye, unspecified eyelid and periocular area

√6th   H02.72   **Madarosis of eyelid and periocular area**
Hypotrichosis of eyelid

    H02.721   Madarosis of right upper eyelid and periocular area

    H02.722   Madarosis of right lower eyelid and periocular area

    H02.723   Madarosis of right eye, unspecified eyelid and periocular area

    H02.724   Madarosis of left upper eyelid and periocular area

    H02.725   Madarosis of left lower eyelid and periocular area

    H02.726   Madarosis of left eye, unspecified eyelid and periocular area

    H02.729   Madarosis of unspecified eye, unspecified eyelid and periocular area

√6th   H02.73   **Vitiligo of eyelid and periocular area**
Hypopigmentation of eyelid

    H02.731   Vitiligo of right upper eyelid and periocular area

    H02.732   Vitiligo of right lower eyelid and periocular area

    H02.733   Vitiligo of right eye, unspecified eyelid and periocular area

    H02.734   Vitiligo of left upper eyelid and periocular area

    H02.735   Vitiligo of left lower eyelid and periocular area

    H02.736   Vitiligo of left eye, unspecified eyelid and periocular area

    H02.739   Vitiligo of unspecified eye, unspecified eyelid and periocular area

H02.79   Other degenerative disorders of eyelid and periocular area

√5th   **H02.8**   **Other specified disorders of eyelid**

√6th   H02.81   **Retained foreign body in eyelid**
Use additional code to identify the type of retained foreign body (Z18.-)

    EXCLUDES 1   laceration of eyelid with foreign body (S01.12-)
retained intraocular foreign body (H44.6-, H44.7-)
superficial foreign body of eyelid and periocular area (S00.25-)

    H02.811   Retained foreign body in right upper eyelid

    H02.812   Retained foreign body in right lower eyelid

    H02.813   Retained foreign body in right eye, unspecified eyelid

    H02.814   Retained foreign body in left upper eyelid

    H02.815   Retained foreign body in left lower eyelid

    H02.816   Retained foreign body in left eye, unspecified eyelid

    H02.819   Retained foreign body in unspecified eye, unspecified eyelid

√6th   H02.82   **Cysts of eyelid**
Sebaceous cyst of eyelid

    H02.821   Cysts of right upper eyelid

    H02.822   Cysts of right lower eyelid

    H02.823   Cysts of right eye, unspecified eyelid

    H02.824   Cysts of left upper eyelid

    H02.825   Cysts of left lower eyelid

    H02.826   Cysts of left eye, unspecified eyelid

    H02.829   Cysts of unspecified eye, unspecified eyelid

√6th   H02.83   **Dermatochalasis of eyelid**

    H02.831   Dermatochalasis of right upper eyelid

    H02.832   Dermatochalasis of right lower eyelid

    H02.833   Dermatochalasis of right eye, unspecified eyelid

    H02.834   Dermatochalasis of left upper eyelid

    H02.835   Dermatochalasis of left lower eyelid

    H02.836   Dermatochalasis of left eye, unspecified eyelid

    H02.839   Dermatochalasis of unspecified eye, unspecified eyelid

√6th   H02.84   **Edema of eyelid**
Hyperemia of eyelid

    H02.841   Edema of right upper eyelid

    H02.842   Edema of right lower eyelid

    H02.843   Edema of right eye, unspecified eyelid

    H02.844   Edema of left upper eyelid

    H02.845   Edema of left lower eyelid

    H02.846   Edema of left eye, unspecified eyelid

    H02.849   Edema of unspecified eye, unspecified eyelid

√6th   H02.85   **Elephantiasis of eyelid**

    H02.851   Elephantiasis of right upper eyelid

    H02.852   Elephantiasis of right lower eyelid

    H02.853   Elephantiasis of right eye, unspecified eyelid

    H02.854   Elephantiasis of left upper eyelid

    H02.855   Elephantiasis of left lower eyelid

    H02.856   Elephantiasis of left eye, unspecified eyelid

    H02.859   Elephantiasis of unspecified eye, unspecified eyelid

√6th   H02.86   **Hypertrichosis of eyelid**

    H02.861   Hypertrichosis of right upper eyelid

    H02.862   Hypertrichosis of right lower eyelid

    H02.863   Hypertrichosis of right eye, unspecified eyelid

    H02.864   Hypertrichosis of left upper eyelid

    H02.865   Hypertrichosis of left lower eyelid

    H02.866   Hypertrichosis of left eye, unspecified eyelid

    H02.869   Hypertrichosis of unspecified eye, unspecified eyelid

√6th   H02.87   **Vascular anomalies of eyelid**

    H02.871   Vascular anomalies of right upper eyelid

    H02.872   Vascular anomalies of right lower eyelid

    H02.873   Vascular anomalies of right eye, unspecified eyelid

    H02.874   Vascular anomalies of left upper eyelid

    H02.875   Vascular anomalies of left lower eyelid

    H02.876   Vascular anomalies of left eye, unspecified eyelid

    H02.879   Vascular anomalies of unspecified eye, unspecified eyelid

H02.89   Other specified disorders of eyelid
Hemorrhage of eyelid

H02.9   **Unspecified disorder of eyelid**
Disorder of eyelid NOS

√4th   **H04**   **Disorders of lacrimal system**

    EXCLUDES 1   congenital malformations of lacrimal system (Q10.4-Q10.6)

√5th   **H04.0**   **Dacryoadenitis**

√6th   H04.00   Unspecified dacryoadenitis

    H04.001   Unspecified dacryoadenitis, right lacrimal gland

N Newborn: 0   P Pediatric: 0-17   M Maternity: 12-55   A Adult: 15-124   MCC Major CC Condition   PDx MCC PDx acts as own MCC   CC CC Condition   PDx CC PDx acts as own CC

550   ICD-10-CM Draft (2015)

Diseases of the Eye and Adnexa

H04.002   Unspecified dacryoadenitis, left lacrimal gland
H04.003   Unspecified dacryoadenitis, bilateral lacrimal glands
H04.009   Unspecified dacryoadenitis, unspecified lacrimal gland

✓6ᵗʰ H04.01   Acute dacryoadenitis
H04.011   Acute dacryoadenitis, right lacrimal gland
H04.012   Acute dacryoadenitis, left lacrimal gland
H04.013   Acute dacryoadenitis, bilateral lacrimal glands
H04.019   Acute dacryoadenitis, unspecified lacrimal gland

✓6ᵗʰ H04.02   Chronic dacryoadenitis
H04.021   Chronic dacryoadenitis, right lacrimal gland
H04.022   Chronic dacryoadenitis, left lacrimal gland
H04.023   Chronic dacryoadenitis, bilateral lacrimal glands
H04.029   Chronic dacryoadenitis, unspecified lacrimal gland

✓6ᵗʰ H04.03   Chronic enlargement of lacrimal gland
H04.031   Chronic enlargement of right lacrimal gland
H04.032   Chronic enlargement of left lacrimal gland
H04.033   Chronic enlargement of bilateral lacrimal glands
H04.039   Chronic enlargement of unspecified lacrimal gland

✓5ᵗʰ H04.1   Other disorders of lacrimal gland
✓6ᵗʰ H04.11   Dacryops
H04.111   Dacryops of right lacrimal gland
H04.112   Dacryops of left lacrimal gland
H04.113   Dacryops of bilateral lacrimal glands
H04.119   Dacryops of unspecified lacrimal gland

✓6ᵗʰ H04.12   Dry eye syndrome
Tear film insufficiency, NOS
H04.121   Dry eye syndrome of right lacrimal gland
H04.122   Dry eye syndrome of left lacrimal gland
H04.123   Dry eye syndrome of bilateral lacrimal glands
H04.129   Dry eye syndrome of unspecified lacrimal gland

✓6ᵗʰ H04.13   Lacrimal cyst
Lacrimal cystic degeneration
H04.131   Lacrimal cyst, right lacrimal gland
H04.132   Lacrimal cyst, left lacrimal gland
H04.133   Lacrimal cyst, bilateral lacrimal glands
H04.139   Lacrimal cyst, unspecified lacrimal gland

✓6ᵗʰ H04.14   Primary lacrimal gland atrophy
H04.141   Primary lacrimal gland atrophy, right lacrimal gland
H04.142   Primary lacrimal gland atrophy, left lacrimal gland
H04.143   Primary lacrimal gland atrophy, bilateral lacrimal glands
H04.149   Primary lacrimal gland atrophy, unspecified lacrimal gland

✓6ᵗʰ H04.15   Secondary lacrimal gland atrophy
H04.151   Secondary lacrimal gland atrophy, right lacrimal gland
H04.152   Secondary lacrimal gland atrophy, left lacrimal gland
H04.153   Secondary lacrimal gland atrophy, bilateral lacrimal glands
H04.159   Secondary lacrimal gland atrophy, unspecified lacrimal gland

✓6ᵗʰ H04.16   Lacrimal gland dislocation
H04.161   Lacrimal gland dislocation, right lacrimal gland
H04.162   Lacrimal gland dislocation, left lacrimal gland
H04.163   Lacrimal gland dislocation, bilateral lacrimal glands

H04.169   Lacrimal gland dislocation, unspecified lacrimal gland
H04.19   Other specified disorders of lacrimal gland

✓5ᵗʰ H04.2   Epiphora
✓6ᵗʰ H04.20   Unspecified epiphora
H04.201   Unspecified epiphora, right lacrimal gland
H04.202   Unspecified epiphora, left lacrimal gland
H04.203   Unspecified epiphora, bilateral lacrimal glands
H04.209   Unspecified epiphora, unspecified lacrimal gland

✓6ᵗʰ H04.21   Epiphora due to excess lacrimation
H04.211   Epiphora due to excess lacrimation, right lacrimal gland
H04.212   Epiphora due to excess lacrimation, left lacrimal gland
H04.213   Epiphora due to excess lacrimation, bilateral lacrimal glands
H04.219   Epiphora due to excess lacrimation, unspecified lacrimal gland

✓6ᵗʰ H04.22   Epiphora due to insufficient drainage
H04.221   Epiphora due to insufficient drainage, right lacrimal gland
H04.222   Epiphora due to insufficient drainage, left lacrimal gland
H04.223   Epiphora due to insufficient drainage, bilateral lacrimal glands
H04.229   Epiphora due to insufficient drainage, unspecified lacrimal gland

✓5ᵗʰ H04.3   Acute and unspecified inflammation of lacrimal passages
EXCLUDES 1   neonatal dacryocystitis (P39.1)
✓6ᵗʰ H04.30   Unspecified dacryocystitis
H04.301   Unspecified dacryocystitis of right lacrimal passage
H04.302   Unspecified dacryocystitis of left lacrimal passage
H04.303   Unspecified dacryocystitis of bilateral lacrimal passages
H04.309   Unspecified dacryocystitis of unspecified lacrimal passage

✓6ᵗʰ H04.31   Phlegmonous dacryocystitis
H04.311   Phlegmonous dacryocystitis of right lacrimal passage
H04.312   Phlegmonous dacryocystitis of left lacrimal passage
H04.313   Phlegmonous dacryocystitis of bilateral lacrimal passages
H04.319   Phlegmonous dacryocystitis of unspecified lacrimal passage

✓6ᵗʰ H04.32   Acute dacryocystitis
Acute dacryopericystitis
H04.321   Acute dacryocystitis of right lacrimal passage
H04.322   Acute dacryocystitis of left lacrimal passage
H04.323   Acute dacryocystitis of bilateral lacrimal passages
H04.329   Acute dacryocystitis of unspecified lacrimal passage

✓6ᵗʰ H04.33   Acute lacrimal canaliculitis
H04.331   Acute lacrimal canaliculitis of right lacrimal passage
H04.332   Acute lacrimal canaliculitis of left lacrimal passage
H04.333   Acute lacrimal canaliculitis of bilateral lacrimal passages
H04.339   Acute lacrimal canaliculitis of unspecified lacrimal passage

✓5ᵗʰ H04.4   Chronic inflammation of lacrimal passages
✓6ᵗʰ H04.41   Chronic dacryocystitis
H04.411   Chronic dacryocystitis of right lacrimal passage
H04.412   Chronic dacryocystitis of left lacrimal passage

H04.002–H04.412

Diseases of the Eye and Adnexa

H04.413–H05.229

H04.413   **Chronic dacryocystitis of bilateral lacrimal passages**

H04.419   **Chronic dacryocystitis of unspecified lacrimal passage**

✓6th **H04.42**   **Chronic lacrimal canaliculitis**

H04.421   **Chronic lacrimal canaliculitis of right lacrimal passage**

H04.422   **Chronic lacrimal canaliculitis of left lacrimal passage**

H04.423   **Chronic lacrimal canaliculitis of bilateral lacrimal passages**

H04.429   **Chronic lacrimal canaliculitis of unspecified lacrimal passage**

✓6th **H04.43**   **Chronic lacrimal mucocele**

H04.431   **Chronic lacrimal mucocele of right lacrimal passage**

H04.432   **Chronic lacrimal mucocele of left lacrimal passage**

H04.433   **Chronic lacrimal mucocele of bilateral lacrimal passages**

H04.439   **Chronic lacrimal mucocele of unspecified lacrimal passage**

✓5th **H04.5**   **Stenosis and insufficiency of lacrimal passages**

✓6th **H04.51**   **Dacryolith**

H04.511   **Dacryolith of right lacrimal passage**

H04.512   **Dacryolith of left lacrimal passage**

H04.513   **Dacryolith of bilateral lacrimal passages**

H04.519   **Dacryolith of unspecified lacrimal passage**

✓6th **H04.52**   **Eversion of lacrimal punctum**

H04.521   **Eversion of right lacrimal punctum**

H04.522   **Eversion of left lacrimal punctum**

H04.523   **Eversion of bilateral lacrimal punctum**

H04.529   **Eversion of unspecified lacrimal punctum**

✓6th **H04.53**   **Neonatal obstruction of nasolacrimal duct**

EXCLUDES 1   *congenital stenosis and stricture of lacrimal duct (Q10.5)*

H04.531   **Neonatal obstruction of right nasolacrimal duct**   N

H04.532   **Neonatal obstruction of left nasolacrimal duct**   N

H04.533   **Neonatal obstruction of bilateral nasolacrimal duct**   N

H04.539   **Neonatal obstruction of unspecified nasolacrimal duct**   N

✓6th **H04.54**   **Stenosis of lacrimal canaliculi**

H04.541   **Stenosis of right lacrimal canaliculi**

H04.542   **Stenosis of left lacrimal canaliculi**

H04.543   **Stenosis of bilateral lacrimal canaliculi**

H04.549   **Stenosis of unspecified lacrimal canaliculi**

✓6th **H04.55**   **Acquired stenosis of nasolacrimal duct**

H04.551   **Acquired stenosis of right nasolacrimal duct**

H04.552   **Acquired stenosis of left nasolacrimal duct**

H04.553   **Acquired stenosis of bilateral nasolacrimal duct**

H04.559   **Acquired stenosis of unspecified nasolacrimal duct**

✓6th **H04.56**   **Stenosis of lacrimal punctum**

H04.561   **Stenosis of right lacrimal punctum**

H04.562   **Stenosis of left lacrimal punctum**

H04.563   **Stenosis of bilateral lacrimal punctum**

H04.569   **Stenosis of unspecified lacrimal punctum**

✓6th **H04.57**   **Stenosis of lacrimal sac**

H04.571   **Stenosis of right lacrimal sac**

H04.572   **Stenosis of left lacrimal sac**

H04.573   **Stenosis of bilateral lacrimal sac**

H04.579   **Stenosis of unspecified lacrimal sac**

✓5th **H04.6**   **Other changes of lacrimal passages**

✓6th **H04.61**   **Lacrimal fistula**

H04.611   **Lacrimal fistula right lacrimal passage**

H04.612   **Lacrimal fistula left lacrimal passage**

H04.613   **Lacrimal fistula bilateral lacrimal passages**

H04.619   **Lacrimal fistula unspecified lacrimal passage**

H04.69   **Other changes of lacrimal passages**

✓5th **H04.8**   **Other disorders of lacrimal system**

✓6th **H04.81**   **Granuloma of lacrimal passages**

H04.811   **Granuloma of right lacrimal passage**

H04.812   **Granuloma of left lacrimal passage**

H04.813   **Granuloma of bilateral lacrimal passages**

H04.819   **Granuloma of unspecified lacrimal passage**

H04.89   **Other disorders of lacrimal system**

H04.9   **Disorder of lacrimal system, unspecified**

✓4th **H05**   **Disorders of orbit**

EXCLUDES 1   *congenital malformation of orbit (Q10.7)*

✓5th **H05.0**   **Acute inflammation of orbit**

H05.00   **Unspecified acute inflammation of orbit**

✓6th **H05.01**   **Cellulitis of orbit**

Abscess of orbit

> **CC Excl: For CC codes in subcategory H05.01, unless otherwise noted: H05.00–H05.049**

H05.011   **Cellulitis of right orbit**   CC

H05.012   **Cellulitis of left orbit**   CC

H05.013   **Cellulitis of bilateral orbits**   CC

H05.019   **Cellulitis of unspecified orbit**   CC

✓6th **H05.02**   **Osteomyelitis of orbit**

> **CC Excl: For CC codes in subcategory H05.02, unless otherwise noted: A02.24, A17.9, A18.03-A18.09, A18.82, A18.84, A18.89, H05.021-H05.029, M46.20-M46.39, M86.00-M86.9**

H05.021   **Osteomyelitis of right orbit**   CC

H05.022   **Osteomyelitis of left orbit**   CC

H05.023   **Osteomyelitis of bilateral orbits**   CC

H05.029   **Osteomyelitis of unspecified orbit**   CC

✓6th **H05.03**   **Periostitis of orbit**

> **CC Excl: For CC codes in subcategory H05.03, unless otherwise noted: A02.24, A17.9, A18.03-A18.09, A18.82, A18.84, A18.89, H05.031-H05.039, M46.20-M46.39, M86.00-M86.9**

H05.031   **Periostitis of right orbit**   CC

H05.032   **Periostitis of left orbit**   CC

H05.033   **Periostitis of bilateral orbits**   CC

H05.039   **Periostitis of unspecified orbit**   CC

✓6th **H05.04**   **Tenonitis of orbit**

H05.041   **Tenonitis of right orbit**

H05.042   **Tenonitis of left orbit**

H05.043   **Tenonitis of bilateral orbits**

H05.049   **Tenonitis of unspecified orbit**

✓5th **H05.1**   **Chronic inflammatory disorders of orbit**

H05.10   **Unspecified chronic inflammatory disorders of orbit**

✓6th **H05.11**   **Granuloma of orbit**

Pseudotumor (inflammatory) of orbit

H05.111   **Granuloma of right orbit**

H05.112   **Granuloma of left orbit**

H05.113   **Granuloma of bilateral orbits**

H05.119   **Granuloma of unspecified orbit**

✓6th **H05.12**   **Orbital myositis**

H05.121   **Orbital myositis, right orbit**

H05.122   **Orbital myositis, left orbit**

H05.123   **Orbital myositis, bilateral**

H05.129   **Orbital myositis, unspecified orbit**

✓5th **H05.2**   **Exophthalmic conditions**

H05.20   **Unspecified exophthalmos**

✓6th **H05.21**   **Displacement (lateral) of globe**

H05.211   **Displacement (lateral) of globe, right eye**

H05.212   **Displacement (lateral) of globe, left eye**

H05.213   **Displacement (lateral) of globe, bilateral**

H05.219   **Displacement (lateral) of globe, unspecified eye**

✓6th **H05.22**   **Edema of orbit**

Orbital congestion

H05.221   **Edema of right orbit**

H05.222   **Edema of left orbit**

H05.223   **Edema of bilateral orbit**

H05.229   **Edema of unspecified orbit**

N Newborn: 0   P Pediatric: 0-17   M Maternity: 12-55   A Adult: 15-124   MCC Major CC Condition   PDx MCC PDx acts as own MCC   CC CC Condition   PDx CC PDx acts as own CC

552   ICD-10-CM Draft (2015)

✓6th **H05.23 Hemorrhage of orbit**
- H05.231 Hemorrhage of right orbit
- H05.232 Hemorrhage of left orbit
- H05.233 Hemorrhage of bilateral orbit
- H05.239 Hemorrhage of unspecified orbit

✓6th **H05.24 Constant exophthalmos**
- H05.241 Constant exophthalmos, right eye
- H05.242 Constant exophthalmos, left eye
- H05.243 Constant exophthalmos, bilateral
- H05.249 Constant exophthalmos, unspecified eye

✓6th **H05.25 Intermittent exophthalmos**
- H05.251 Intermittent exophthalmos, right eye
- H05.252 Intermittent exophthalmos, left eye
- H05.253 Intermittent exophthalmos, bilateral
- H05.259 Intermittent exophthalmos, unspecified eye

✓6th **H05.26 Pulsating exophthalmos**
- H05.261 Pulsating exophthalmos, right eye
- H05.262 Pulsating exophthalmos, left eye
- H05.263 Pulsating exophthalmos, bilateral
- H05.269 Pulsating exophthalmos, unspecified eye

✓5th **H05.3 Deformity of orbit**

    EXCLUDES 1   congenital deformity of orbit (Q10.7)
                hypertelorism (Q75.2)

- H05.30 Unspecified deformity of orbit

✓6th **H05.31 Atrophy of orbit**
- H05.311 Atrophy of right orbit
- H05.312 Atrophy of left orbit
- H05.313 Atrophy of bilateral orbit
- H05.319 Atrophy of unspecified orbit

✓6th **H05.32 Deformity of orbit due to bone disease**

    Code also associated bone disease
- H05.321 Deformity of right orbit due to bone disease
- H05.322 Deformity of left orbit due to bone disease
- H05.323 Deformity of bilateral orbits due to bone disease
- H05.329 Deformity of unspecified orbit due to bone disease

✓6th **H05.33 Deformity of orbit due to trauma or surgery**
- H05.331 Deformity of right orbit due to trauma or surgery
- H05.332 Deformity of left orbit due to trauma or surgery
- H05.333 Deformity of bilateral orbits due to trauma or surgery
- H05.339 Deformity of unspecified orbit due to trauma or surgery

✓6th **H05.34 Enlargement of orbit**
- H05.341 Enlargement of right orbit
- H05.342 Enlargement of left orbit
- H05.343 Enlargement of bilateral orbits
- H05.349 Enlargement of unspecified orbit

✓6th **H05.35 Exostosis of orbit**
- H05.351 Exostosis of right orbit
- H05.352 Exostosis of left orbit
- H05.353 Exostosis of bilateral orbits
- H05.359 Exostosis of unspecified orbit

✓5th **H05.4 Enophthalmos**

✓6th **H05.40 Unspecified enophthalmos**
- H05.401 Unspecified enophthalmos, right eye
- H05.402 Unspecified enophthalmos, left eye
- H05.403 Unspecified enophthalmos, bilateral
- H05.409 Unspecified enophthalmos, unspecified eye

✓6th **H05.41 Enophthalmos due to atrophy of orbital tissue**
- H05.411 Enophthalmos due to atrophy of orbital tissue, right eye
- H05.412 Enophthalmos due to atrophy of orbital tissue, left eye
- H05.413 Enophthalmos due to atrophy of orbital tissue, bilateral
- H05.419 Enophthalmos due to atrophy of orbital tissue, unspecified eye

✓6th **H05.42 Enophthalmos due to trauma or surgery**
- H05.421 Enophthalmos due to trauma or surgery, right eye
- H05.422 Enophthalmos due to trauma or surgery, left eye
- H05.423 Enophthalmos due to trauma or surgery, bilateral
- H05.429 Enophthalmos due to trauma or surgery, unspecified eye

✓5th **H05.5 Retained (old) foreign body following penetrating wound of orbit**

    Retrobulbar foreign body
    Use additional code to identify the type of retained foreign body (Z18.-)

    EXCLUDES 1   current penetrating wound of orbit (S05.4-)
    EXCLUDES 2   retained foreign body of eyelid (H02.81-)
                retained intraocular foreign body (H44.6-, H44.7-)

- H05.50 Retained (old) foreign body following penetrating wound of unspecified orbit
- H05.51 Retained (old) foreign body following penetrating wound of right orbit
- H05.52 Retained (old) foreign body following penetrating wound of left orbit
- H05.53 Retained (old) foreign body following penetrating wound of bilateral orbits

✓5th **H05.8 Other disorders of orbit**

✓6th **H05.81 Cyst of orbit**

    Encephalocele of orbit
- H05.811 Cyst of right orbit
- H05.812 Cyst of left orbit
- H05.813 Cyst of bilateral orbits
- H05.819 Cyst of unspecified orbit

✓6th **H05.82 Myopathy of extraocular muscles**
- H05.821 Myopathy of extraocular muscles, right orbit
- H05.822 Myopathy of extraocular muscles, left orbit
- H05.823 Myopathy of extraocular muscles, bilateral
- H05.829 Myopathy of extraocular muscles, unspecified orbit

- H05.89 Other disorders of orbit

H05.9 Unspecified disorder of orbit

Disorders of conjunctiva (H10-H11)

✓4th **H10 Conjunctivitis**

    EXCLUDES 1   keratoconjunctivitis (H16.2-)

✓5th **H10.0 Mucopurulent conjunctivitis**

✓6th **H10.01 Acute follicular conjunctivitis**
- H10.011 Acute follicular conjunctivitis, right eye
- H10.012 Acute follicular conjunctivitis, left eye
- H10.013 Acute follicular conjunctivitis, bilateral
- H10.019 Acute follicular conjunctivitis, unspecified eye

✓6th **H10.02 Other mucopurulent conjunctivitis**
- H10.021 Other mucopurulent conjunctivitis, right eye
- H10.022 Other mucopurulent conjunctivitis, left eye
- H10.023 Other mucopurulent conjunctivitis, bilateral
- H10.029 Other mucopurulent conjunctivitis, unspecified eye

✓5th **H10.1 Acute atopic conjunctivitis**

    Acute papillary conjunctivitis
- H10.10 Acute atopic conjunctivitis, unspecified eye
- H10.11 Acute atopic conjunctivitis, right eye
- H10.12 Acute atopic conjunctivitis, left eye
- H10.13 Acute atopic conjunctivitis, bilateral

✓ Additional Character Required   ✓x7th Xtension Alert   Unacceptable PDx   Manifestation   Hospital Acquired Condition   EXCLUDES 1 Not Coded Here   EXCLUDES 2 Not Included Here

Diseases of the Eye and Adnexa

H10.2–H11.059

✓5th **H10.2 Other acute conjunctivitis**
  ✓6th **H10.21 Acute toxic conjunctivitis**
        Acute chemical conjunctivitis
        Code first (T51-T65) to identify chemical and intent
        EXCLUDES 1 *burn and corrosion of eye and adnexa (T26.-)*
        H10.211 Acute toxic conjunctivitis, right eye
        H10.212 Acute toxic conjunctivitis, left eye
        H10.213 Acute toxic conjunctivitis, bilateral
        H10.219 Acute toxic conjunctivitis, unspecified eye
  ✓6th **H10.22 Pseudomembranous conjunctivitis**
        H10.221 Pseudomembranous conjunctivitis, right eye
        H10.222 Pseudomembranous conjunctivitis, left eye
        H10.223 Pseudomembranous conjunctivitis, bilateral
        H10.229 Pseudomembranous conjunctivitis, unspecified eye
  ✓6th **H10.23 Serous conjunctivitis, except viral**
        EXCLUDES 1 *viral conjunctivitis (B30.-)*
        H10.231 Serous conjunctivitis, except viral, right eye
        H10.232 Serous conjunctivitis, except viral, left eye
        H10.233 Serous conjunctivitis, except viral, bilateral
        H10.239 Serous conjunctivitis, except viral, unspecified eye
✓5th **H10.3 Unspecified acute conjunctivitis**
      EXCLUDES 1 *ophthalmia neonatorum NOS (P39.1)*
      H10.30 Unspecified acute conjunctivitis, unspecified eye
      H10.31 Unspecified acute conjunctivitis, right eye
      H10.32 Unspecified acute conjunctivitis, left eye
      H10.33 Unspecified acute conjunctivitis, bilateral
✓5th **H10.4 Chronic conjunctivitis**
  ✓6th **H10.40 Unspecified chronic conjunctivitis**
        H10.401 Unspecified chronic conjunctivitis, right eye
        H10.402 Unspecified chronic conjunctivitis, left eye
        H10.403 Unspecified chronic conjunctivitis, bilateral
        H10.409 Unspecified chronic conjunctivitis, unspecified eye
  ✓6th **H10.41 Chronic giant papillary conjunctivitis**
        H10.411 Chronic giant papillary conjunctivitis, right eye
        H10.412 Chronic giant papillary conjunctivitis, left eye
        H10.413 Chronic giant papillary conjunctivitis, bilateral
        H10.419 Chronic giant papillary conjunctivitis, unspecified eye
  ✓6th **H10.42 Simple chronic conjunctivitis**
        H10.421 Simple chronic conjunctivitis, right eye
        H10.422 Simple chronic conjunctivitis, left eye
        H10.423 Simple chronic conjunctivitis, bilateral
        H10.429 Simple chronic conjunctivitis, unspecified eye
  ✓6th **H10.43 Chronic follicular conjunctivitis**
        H10.431 Chronic follicular conjunctivitis, right eye
        H10.432 Chronic follicular conjunctivitis, left eye
        H10.433 Chronic follicular conjunctivitis, bilateral
        H10.439 Chronic follicular conjunctivitis, unspecified eye
      H10.44 Vernal conjunctivitis
            EXCLUDES 1 *vernal keratoconjunctivitis with limbar and corneal involvement (H16.26-)*
      H10.45 Other chronic allergic conjunctivitis
✓5th **H10.5 Blepharoconjunctivitis**
  ✓6th **H10.50 Unspecified blepharoconjunctivitis**
        H10.501 Unspecified blepharoconjunctivitis, right eye
        H10.502 Unspecified blepharoconjunctivitis, left eye

        H10.503 Unspecified blepharoconjunctivitis, bilateral
        H10.509 Unspecified blepharoconjunctivitis, unspecified eye
  ✓6th **H10.51 Ligneous conjunctivitis**
        H10.511 Ligneous conjunctivitis, right eye
        H10.512 Ligneous conjunctivitis, left eye
        H10.513 Ligneous conjunctivitis, bilateral
        H10.519 Ligneous conjunctivitis, unspecified eye
  ✓6th **H10.52 Angular blepharoconjunctivitis**
        H10.521 Angular blepharoconjunctivitis, right eye
        H10.522 Angular blepharoconjunctivitis, left eye
        H10.523 Angular blepharoconjunctivitis, bilateral
        H10.529 Angular blepharoconjunctivitis, unspecified eye
  ✓6th **H10.53 Contact blepharoconjunctivitis**
        H10.531 Contact blepharoconjunctivitis, right eye
        H10.532 Contact blepharoconjunctivitis, left eye
        H10.533 Contact blepharoconjunctivitis, bilateral
        H10.539 Contact blepharoconjunctivitis, unspecified eye
✓5th **H10.8 Other conjunctivitis**
  ✓6th **H10.81 Pingueculitis**
        EXCLUDES 1 *pinguecula (H11.15-)*
        H10.811 Pingueculitis, right eye
        H10.812 Pingueculitis, left eye
        H10.813 Pingueculitis, bilateral
        H10.819 Pingueculitis, unspecified eye
      H10.89 Other conjunctivitis
  H10.9 Unspecified conjunctivitis
✓4th **H11 Other disorders of conjunctiva**
      EXCLUDES 1 *keratoconjunctivitis (H16.2-)*
  ✓5th **H11.0 Pterygium of eye**
        EXCLUDES 1 *pseudopterygium (H11.81-)*
    ✓6th **H11.00 Unspecified pterygium of eye**
          H11.001 Unspecified pterygium of right eye
          H11.002 Unspecified pterygium of left eye
          H11.003 Unspecified pterygium of eye, bilateral
          H11.009 Unspecified pterygium of unspecified eye
    ✓6th **H11.01 Amyloid pterygium**
          H11.011 Amyloid pterygium of right eye
          H11.012 Amyloid pterygium of left eye
          H11.013 Amyloid pterygium of eye, bilateral
          H11.019 Amyloid pterygium of unspecified eye
    ✓6th **H11.02 Central pterygium of eye**
          H11.021 Central pterygium of right eye
          H11.022 Central pterygium of left eye
          H11.023 Central pterygium of eye, bilateral
          H11.029 Central pterygium of unspecified eye
    ✓6th **H11.03 Double pterygium of eye**
          H11.031 Double pterygium of right eye
          H11.032 Double pterygium of left eye
          H11.033 Double pterygium of eye, bilateral
          H11.039 Double pterygium of unspecified eye
    ✓6th **H11.04 Peripheral pterygium of eye, stationary**
          H11.041 Peripheral pterygium, stationary, right eye
          H11.042 Peripheral pterygium, stationary, left eye
          H11.043 Peripheral pterygium, stationary, bilateral
          H11.049 Peripheral pterygium, stationary, unspecified eye
    ✓6th **H11.05 Peripheral pterygium of eye, progressive**
          H11.051 Peripheral pterygium, progressive, right eye
          H11.052 Peripheral pterygium, progressive, left eye
          H11.053 Peripheral pterygium, progressive, bilateral
          H11.059 Peripheral pterygium, progressive, unspecified eye

√6ᵗʰ **H11.06 Recurrent pterygium of eye**
    H11.061 Recurrent pterygium of right eye
    H11.062 Recurrent pterygium of left eye
    H11.063 Recurrent pterygium of eye, bilateral
    H11.069 Recurrent pterygium of unspecified eye

√5ᵗʰ **H11.1 Conjunctival degenerations and deposits**
    EXCLUDES 2   pseudopterygium (H11.81)
    H11.10 Unspecified conjunctival degenerations

√6ᵗʰ **H11.11 Conjunctival deposits**
    H11.111 Conjunctival deposits, right eye
    H11.112 Conjunctival deposits, left eye
    H11.113 Conjunctival deposits, bilateral
    H11.119 Conjunctival deposits, unspecified eye

√6ᵗʰ **H11.12 Conjunctival concretions**
    H11.121 Conjunctival concretions, right eye
    H11.122 Conjunctival concretions, left eye
    H11.123 Conjunctival concretions, bilateral
    H11.129 Conjunctival concretions, unspecified eye

√6ᵗʰ **H11.13 Conjunctival pigmentations**
    Conjunctival argyrosis [argyria]
    H11.131 Conjunctival pigmentations, right eye
    H11.132 Conjunctival pigmentations, left eye
    H11.133 Conjunctival pigmentations, bilateral
    H11.139 Conjunctival pigmentations, unspecified eye

√6ᵗʰ **H11.14 Conjunctival xerosis, unspecified**
    EXCLUDES 1   xerosis of conjunctiva due to vitamin A deficiency (E50.0, E50.1)
    H11.141 Conjunctival xerosis, unspecified, right eye
    H11.142 Conjunctival xerosis , unspecified, left eye
    H11.143 Conjunctival xerosis, unspecified, bilateral
    H11.149 Conjunctival xerosis, unspecified, unspecified eye

√6ᵗʰ **H11.15 Pinguecula**
    EXCLUDES 1   pingueculitis (H10.81-)
    H11.151 Pinguecula, right eye
    H11.152 Pinguecula, left eye
    H11.153 Pinguecula, bilateral
    H11.159 Pinguecula, unspecified eye

√5ᵗʰ **H11.2 Conjunctival scars**

√6ᵗʰ **H11.21 Conjunctival adhesions and strands (localized)**
    H11.211 Conjunctival adhesions and strands (localized), right eye
    H11.212 Conjunctival adhesions and strands (localized), left eye
    H11.213 Conjunctival adhesions and strands (localized), bilateral
    H11.219 Conjunctival adhesions and strands (localized), unspecified eye

√6ᵗʰ **H11.22 Conjunctival granuloma**
    H11.221 Conjunctival granuloma, right eye
    H11.222 Conjunctival granuloma, left eye
    H11.223 Conjunctival granuloma, bilateral
    H11.229 Conjunctival granuloma, unspecified

√6ᵗʰ **H11.23 Symblepharon**
    H11.231 Symblepharon, right eye
    H11.232 Symblepharon, left eye
    H11.233 Symblepharon, bilateral
    H11.239 Symblepharon, unspecified eye

√6ᵗʰ **H11.24 Scarring of conjunctiva**
    H11.241 Scarring of conjunctiva, right eye
    H11.242 Scarring of conjunctiva, left eye
    H11.243 Scarring of conjunctiva, bilateral
    H11.249 Scarring of conjunctiva, unspecified eye

√5ᵗʰ **H11.3 Conjunctival hemorrhage**
    Subconjunctival hemorrhage
    H11.30 Conjunctival hemorrhage, unspecified eye
    H11.31 Conjunctival hemorrhage, right eye
    H11.32 Conjunctival hemorrhage, left eye
    H11.33 Conjunctival hemorrhage, bilateral

√5ᵗʰ **H11.4 Other conjunctival vascular disorders and cysts**

√6ᵗʰ **H11.41 Vascular abnormalities of conjunctiva**
    Conjunctival aneurysm
    H11.411 Vascular abnormalities of conjunctiva, right eye
    H11.412 Vascular abnormalities of conjunctiva, left eye
    H11.413 Vascular abnormalities of conjunctiva, bilateral
    H11.419 Vascular abnormalities of conjunctiva, unspecified eye

√6ᵗʰ **H11.42 Conjunctival edema**
    H11.421 Conjunctival edema, right eye
    H11.422 Conjunctival edema, left eye
    H11.423 Conjunctival edema, bilateral
    H11.429 Conjunctival edema, unspecified eye

√6ᵗʰ **H11.43 Conjunctival hyperemia**
    H11.431 Conjunctival hyperemia, right eye
    H11.432 Conjunctival hyperemia, left eye
    H11.433 Conjunctival hyperemia, bilateral
    H11.439 Conjunctival hyperemia, unspecified eye

√6ᵗʰ **H11.44 Conjunctival cysts**
    H11.441 Conjunctival cysts, right eye
    H11.442 Conjunctival cysts, left eye
    H11.443 Conjunctival cysts, bilateral
    H11.449 Conjunctival cysts, unspecified eye

√5ᵗʰ **H11.8 Other specified disorders of conjunctiva**

√6ᵗʰ **H11.81 Pseudopterygium of conjunctiva**
    H11.811 Pseudopterygium of conjunctiva, right eye
    H11.812 Pseudopterygium of conjunctiva, left eye
    H11.813 Pseudopterygium of conjunctiva, bilateral
    H11.819 Pseudopterygium of conjunctiva, unspecified eye

√6ᵗʰ **H11.82 Conjunctivochalasis**
    H11.821 Conjunctivochalasis, right eye
    H11.822 Conjunctivochalasis, left eye
    H11.823 Conjunctivochalasis, bilateral
    H11.829 Conjunctivochalasis, unspecified eye
    H11.89 Other specified disorders of conjunctiva
    H11.9 Unspecified disorder of conjunctiva

Disorders of sclera, cornea, iris and ciliary body (H15-H22)

√4ᵗʰ **H15 Disorders of sclera**

√5ᵗʰ **H15.0 Scleritis**

√6ᵗʰ **H15.00 Unspecified scleritis**
    H15.001 Unspecified scleritis, right eye
    H15.002 Unspecified scleritis, left eye
    H15.003 Unspecified scleritis, bilateral
    H15.009 Unspecified scleritis, unspecified eye

√6ᵗʰ **H15.01 Anterior scleritis**
    H15.011 Anterior scleritis, right eye
    H15.012 Anterior scleritis, left eye
    H15.013 Anterior scleritis, bilateral
    H15.019 Anterior scleritis, unspecified eye

√6ᵗʰ **H15.02 Brawny scleritis**
    H15.021 Brawny scleritis, right eye
    H15.022 Brawny scleritis, left eye
    H15.023 Brawny scleritis, bilateral
    H15.029 Brawny scleritis, unspecified eye

√6ᵗʰ **H15.03 Posterior scleritis**
    Sclerotenonitis
    H15.031 Posterior scleritis, right eye
    H15.032 Posterior scleritis, left eye
    H15.033 Posterior scleritis, bilateral
    H15.039 Posterior scleritis, unspecified eye

√6ᵗʰ **H15.04 Scleritis with corneal involvement**
    H15.041 Scleritis with corneal involvement, right eye
    H15.042 Scleritis with corneal involvement, left eye
    H15.043 Scleritis with corneal involvement, bilateral

☑ Additional Character Required   √x7ᵗʰ Xtension Alert   Unacceptable PDx   Manifestation   Hospital Acquired Condition   *EXCLUDES 1* Not Coded Here   *EXCLUDES 2* Not Included Here

Diseases of the Eye and Adnexa

H15.049–H16.202

H15.049   Scleritis with corneal involvement, unspecified eye

✓6th **H15.05**   Scleromalacia perforans
- **H15.051**   Scleromalacia perforans, right eye
- **H15.052**   Scleromalacia perforans, left eye
- **H15.053**   Scleromalacia perforans, bilateral
- **H15.059**   Scleromalacia perforans, unspecified eye

✓6th **H15.09**   Other scleritis
     Scleral abscess
- **H15.091**   Other scleritis, right eye
- **H15.092**   Other scleritis, left eye
- **H15.093**   Other scleritis, bilateral
- **H15.099**   Other scleritis, unspecified eye

✓5th **H15.1**   Episcleritis

✓6th **H15.10**   Unspecified episcleritis
- **H15.101**   Unspecified episcleritis, right eye
- **H15.102**   Unspecified episcleritis, left eye
- **H15.103**   Unspecified episcleritis, bilateral
- **H15.109**   Unspecified episcleritis, unspecified eye

✓6th **H15.11**   Episcleritis periodica fugax
- **H15.111**   Episcleritis periodica fugax, right eye
- **H15.112**   Episcleritis periodica fugax, left eye
- **H15.113**   Episcleritis periodica fugax, bilateral
- **H15.119**   Episcleritis periodica fugax, unspecified eye

✓6th **H15.12**   Nodular episcleritis
- **H15.121**   Nodular episcleritis, right eye
- **H15.122**   Nodular episcleritis, left eye
- **H15.123**   Nodular episcleritis, bilateral
- **H15.129**   Nodular episcleritis, unspecified eye

✓5th **H15.8**   Other disorders of sclera
     EXCLUDES 2   blue sclera (Q13.5)
                 degenerative myopia (H44.2-)

✓6th **H15.81**   Equatorial staphyloma
- **H15.811**   Equatorial staphyloma, right eye
- **H15.812**   Equatorial staphyloma, left eye
- **H15.813**   Equatorial staphyloma, bilateral
- **H15.819**   Equatorial staphyloma, unspecified eye

✓6th **H15.82**   Localized anterior staphyloma
- **H15.821**   Localized anterior staphyloma, right eye
- **H15.822**   Localized anterior staphyloma, left eye
- **H15.823**   Localized anterior staphyloma, bilateral
- **H15.829**   Localized anterior staphyloma, unspecified eye

✓6th **H15.83**   Staphyloma posticum
- **H15.831**   Staphyloma posticum, right eye
- **H15.832**   Staphyloma posticum, left eye
- **H15.833**   Staphyloma posticum, bilateral
- **H15.839**   Staphyloma posticum, unspecified eye

✓6th **H15.84**   Scleral ectasia
- **H15.841**   Scleral ectasia, right eye
- **H15.842**   Scleral ectasia, left eye
- **H15.843**   Scleral ectasia, bilateral
- **H15.849**   Scleral ectasia, unspecified eye

✓6th **H15.85**   Ring staphyloma
- **H15.851**   Ring staphyloma, right eye
- **H15.852**   Ring staphyloma, left eye
- **H15.853**   Ring staphyloma, bilateral
- **H15.859**   Ring staphyloma, unspecified eye

H15.89   Other disorders of sclera

H15.9   Unspecified disorder of sclera

✓4th **H16**   Keratitis

✓5th **H16.0**   Corneal ulcer

✓6th **H16.00**   Unspecified corneal ulcer
- **H16.001**   Unspecified corneal ulcer, right eye
- **H16.002**   Unspecified corneal ulcer, left eye
- **H16.003**   Unspecified corneal ulcer, bilateral
- **H16.009**   Unspecified corneal ulcer, unspecified eye

✓6th **H16.01**   Central corneal ulcer
- **H16.011**   Central corneal ulcer, right eye
- **H16.012**   Central corneal ulcer, left eye
- **H16.013**   Central corneal ulcer, bilateral
- **H16.019**   Central corneal ulcer, unspecified eye

✓6th **H16.02**   Ring corneal ulcer
- **H16.021**   Ring corneal ulcer, right eye
- **H16.022**   Ring corneal ulcer, left eye
- **H16.023**   Ring corneal ulcer, bilateral
- **H16.029**   Ring corneal ulcer, unspecified eye

✓6th **H16.03**   Corneal ulcer with hypopyon
- **H16.031**   Corneal ulcer with hypopyon, right eye
- **H16.032**   Corneal ulcer with hypopyon, left eye
- **H16.033**   Corneal ulcer with hypopyon, bilateral
- **H16.039**   Corneal ulcer with hypopyon, unspecified eye

✓6th **H16.04**   Marginal corneal ulcer
- **H16.041**   Marginal corneal ulcer, right eye
- **H16.042**   Marginal corneal ulcer, left eye
- **H16.043**   Marginal corneal ulcer, bilateral
- **H16.049**   Marginal corneal ulcer, unspecified eye

✓6th **H16.05**   Mooren's corneal ulcer
- **H16.051**   Mooren's corneal ulcer, right eye
- **H16.052**   Mooren's corneal ulcer, left eye
- **H16.053**   Mooren's corneal ulcer, bilateral
- **H16.059**   Mooren's corneal ulcer, unspecified eye

✓6th **H16.06**   Mycotic corneal ulcer
- **H16.061**   Mycotic corneal ulcer, right eye
- **H16.062**   Mycotic corneal ulcer, left eye
- **H16.063**   Mycotic corneal ulcer, bilateral
- **H16.069**   Mycotic corneal ulcer, unspecified eye

✓6th **H16.07**   Perforated corneal ulcer
- **H16.071**   Perforated corneal ulcer, right eye
- **H16.072**   Perforated corneal ulcer, left eye
- **H16.073**   Perforated corneal ulcer, bilateral
- **H16.079**   Perforated corneal ulcer, unspecified eye

✓5th **H16.1**   Other and unspecified superficial keratitis without conjunctivitis

✓6th **H16.10**   Unspecified superficial keratitis
- **H16.101**   Unspecified superficial keratitis, right eye
- **H16.102**   Unspecified superficial keratitis, left eye
- **H16.103**   Unspecified superficial keratitis, bilateral
- **H16.109**   Unspecified superficial keratitis, unspecified eye

✓6th **H16.11**   Macular keratitis
     Areolar keratitis
     Nummular keratitis
     Stellate keratitis
     Striate keratitis
- **H16.111**   Macular keratitis, right eye
- **H16.112**   Macular keratitis, left eye
- **H16.113**   Macular keratitis, bilateral
- **H16.119**   Macular keratitis, unspecified eye

✓6th **H16.12**   Filamentary keratitis
- **H16.121**   Filamentary keratitis, right eye
- **H16.122**   Filamentary keratitis, left eye
- **H16.123**   Filamentary keratitis, bilateral
- **H16.129**   Filamentary keratitis, unspecified eye

✓6th **H16.13**   Photokeratitis
     Snow blindness
     Welders keratitis
- **H16.131**   Photokeratitis, right eye
- **H16.132**   Photokeratitis, left eye
- **H16.133**   Photokeratitis, bilateral
- **H16.139**   Photokeratitis, unspecified eye

✓6th **H16.14**   Punctate keratitis
- **H16.141**   Punctate keratitis, right eye
- **H16.142**   Punctate keratitis, left eye
- **H16.143**   Punctate keratitis, bilateral
- **H16.149**   Punctate keratitis, unspecified eye

✓5th **H16.2**   Keratoconjunctivitis

✓6th **H16.20**   Unspecified keratoconjunctivitis
     Superficial keratitis with conjunctivitis NOS
- **H16.201**   Unspecified keratoconjunctivitis, right eye
- **H16.202**   Unspecified keratoconjunctivitis, left eye

N Newborn: 0   P Pediatric: 0-17   M Maternity: 12-55   A Adult: 15-124   MCC Major CC Condition   PDx MCC PDx acts as own MCC   CC CC Condition   PDx CC PDx acts as own CC

556   ICD-10-CM Draft (2015)

H16.203 Unspecified keratoconjunctivitis, bilateral
H16.209 Unspecified keratoconjunctivitis, unspecified eye

√6ᵗʰ H16.21 Exposure keratoconjunctivitis
H16.211 Exposure keratoconjunctivitis, right eye
H16.212 Exposure keratoconjunctivitis, left eye
H16.213 Exposure keratoconjunctivitis, bilateral
H16.219 Exposure keratoconjunctivitis, unspecified eye

√6ᵗʰ H16.22 Keratoconjunctivitis sicca, not specified as Sjögren's
EXCLUDES 1 Sjögren's syndrome (M35.01)
H16.221 Keratoconjunctivitis sicca, not specified as Sjögren's, right eye
H16.222 Keratoconjunctivitis sicca, not specified as Sjögren's, left eye
H16.223 Keratoconjunctivitis sicca, not specified as Sjögren's, bilateral
H16.229 Keratoconjunctivitis sicca, not specified as Sjögren's, unspecified eye

√6ᵗʰ H16.23 Neurotrophic keratoconjunctivitis
H16.231 Neurotrophic keratoconjunctivitis, right eye
H16.232 Neurotrophic keratoconjunctivitis, left eye
H16.233 Neurotrophic keratoconjunctivitis, bilateral
H16.239 Neurotrophic keratoconjunctivitis, unspecified eye

√6ᵗʰ H16.24 Ophthalmia nodosa
H16.241 Ophthalmia nodosa, right eye
H16.242 Ophthalmia nodosa, left eye
H16.243 Ophthalmia nodosa, bilateral
H16.249 Ophthalmia nodosa, unspecified eye

√6ᵗʰ H16.25 Phlyctenular keratoconjunctivitis
H16.251 Phlyctenular keratoconjunctivitis, right eye
H16.252 Phlyctenular keratoconjunctivitis, left eye
H16.253 Phlyctenular keratoconjunctivitis, bilateral
H16.259 Phlyctenular keratoconjunctivitis, unspecified eye

√6ᵗʰ H16.26 Vernal keratoconjunctivitis, with limbar and corneal involvement
EXCLUDES 1 vernal conjunctivitis without limbar and corneal involvement (H10.44)
H16.261 Vernal keratoconjunctivitis, with limbar and corneal involvement, right eye
H16.262 Vernal keratoconjunctivitis, with limbar and corneal involvement, left eye
H16.263 Vernal keratoconjunctivitis, with limbar and corneal involvement, bilateral
H16.269 Vernal keratoconjunctivitis, with limbar and corneal involvement, unspecified eye

√6ᵗʰ H16.29 Other keratoconjunctivitis
H16.291 Other keratoconjunctivitis, right eye
H16.292 Other keratoconjunctivitis, left eye
H16.293 Other keratoconjunctivitis, bilateral
H16.299 Other keratoconjunctivitis, unspecified eye

√5ᵗʰ H16.3 Interstitial and deep keratitis
√6ᵗʰ H16.30 Unspecified interstitial keratitis
H16.301 Unspecified interstitial keratitis, right eye
H16.302 Unspecified interstitial keratitis, left eye
H16.303 Unspecified interstitial keratitis, bilateral
H16.309 Unspecified interstitial keratitis, unspecified eye

√6ᵗʰ H16.31 Corneal abscess
H16.311 Corneal abscess, right eye
H16.312 Corneal abscess, left eye
H16.313 Corneal abscess, bilateral
H16.319 Corneal abscess, unspecified eye

√6ᵗʰ H16.32 Diffuse interstitial keratitis
Cogan's syndrome
H16.321 Diffuse interstitial keratitis, right eye
H16.322 Diffuse interstitial keratitis, left eye

H16.323 Diffuse interstitial keratitis, bilateral
H16.329 Diffuse interstitial keratitis, unspecified eye

√6ᵗʰ H16.33 Sclerosing keratitis
H16.331 Sclerosing keratitis, right eye
H16.332 Sclerosing keratitis, left eye
H16.333 Sclerosing keratitis, bilateral
H16.339 Sclerosing keratitis, unspecified eye

√6ᵗʰ H16.39 Other interstitial and deep keratitis
H16.391 Other interstitial and deep keratitis, right eye
H16.392 Other interstitial and deep keratitis, left eye
H16.393 Other interstitial and deep keratitis, bilateral
H16.399 Other interstitial and deep keratitis, unspecified eye

√5ᵗʰ H16.4 Corneal neovascularization
√6ᵗʰ H16.40 Unspecified corneal neovascularization
H16.401 Unspecified corneal neovascularization, right eye
H16.402 Unspecified corneal neovascularization, left eye
H16.403 Unspecified corneal neovascularization, bilateral
H16.409 Unspecified corneal neovascularization, unspecified eye

√6ᵗʰ H16.41 Ghost vessels (corneal)
H16.411 Ghost vessels (corneal), right eye
H16.412 Ghost vessels (corneal), left eye
H16.413 Ghost vessels (corneal), bilateral
H16.419 Ghost vessels (corneal), unspecified eye

√6ᵗʰ H16.42 Pannus (corneal)
H16.421 Pannus (corneal), right eye
H16.422 Pannus (corneal), left eye
H16.423 Pannus (corneal), bilateral
H16.429 Pannus (corneal), unspecified eye

√6ᵗʰ H16.43 Localized vascularization of cornea
H16.431 Localized vascularization of cornea, right eye
H16.432 Localized vascularization of cornea, left eye
H16.433 Localized vascularization of cornea, bilateral
H16.439 Localized vascularization of cornea, unspecified eye

√6ᵗʰ H16.44 Deep vascularization of cornea
H16.441 Deep vascularization of cornea, right eye
H16.442 Deep vascularization of cornea, left eye
H16.443 Deep vascularization of cornea, bilateral
H16.449 Deep vascularization of cornea, unspecified eye

H16.8 Other keratitis
H16.9 Unspecified keratitis

√4ᵗʰ H17 Corneal scars and opacities
√5ᵗʰ H17.0 Adherent leukoma
H17.00 Adherent leukoma, unspecified eye
H17.01 Adherent leukoma, right eye
H17.02 Adherent leukoma, left eye
H17.03 Adherent leukoma, bilateral

√5ᵗʰ H17.1 Central corneal opacity
H17.10 Central corneal opacity, unspecified eye
H17.11 Central corneal opacity, right eye
H17.12 Central corneal opacity, left eye
H17.13 Central corneal opacity, bilateral

√5ᵗʰ H17.8 Other corneal scars and opacities
√6ᵗʰ H17.81 Minor opacity of cornea
Corneal nebula
H17.811 Minor opacity of cornea, right eye
H17.812 Minor opacity of cornea, left eye
H17.813 Minor opacity of cornea, bilateral
H17.819 Minor opacity of cornea, unspecified eye

✔ Additional Character Required   √x7ᵗʰ Xtension Alert   Unacceptable PDx   Manifestation   Hospital Acquired Condition   EXCLUDES 1 Not Coded Here   EXCLUDES 2 Not Included Here

Diseases of the Eye and Adnexa

H17.82–H18.463

√6ᵗʰ **H17.82** Peripheral opacity of cornea
    H17.821 Peripheral opacity of cornea, right eye
    H17.822 Peripheral opacity of cornea, left eye
    H17.823 Peripheral opacity of cornea, bilateral
    H17.829 Peripheral opacity of cornea, unspecified eye
  H17.89 Other corneal scars and opacities
 H17.9 Unspecified corneal scar and opacity

√4ᵗʰ **H18** Other disorders of cornea
 √5ᵗʰ **H18.0** Corneal pigmentations and deposits
  √6ᵗʰ **H18.00** Unspecified corneal deposit
   H18.001 Unspecified corneal deposit, right eye
   H18.002 Unspecified corneal deposit, left eye
   H18.003 Unspecified corneal deposit, bilateral
   H18.009 Unspecified corneal deposit, unspecified eye
  √6ᵗʰ **H18.01** Anterior corneal pigmentations
   Staehli's line
   H18.011 Anterior corneal pigmentations, right eye
   H18.012 Anterior corneal pigmentations, left eye
   H18.013 Anterior corneal pigmentations, bilateral
   H18.019 Anterior corneal pigmentations, unspecified eye
  √6ᵗʰ **H18.02** Argentous corneal deposits
   H18.021 Argentous corneal deposits, right eye
   H18.022 Argentous corneal deposits, left eye
   H18.023 Argentous corneal deposits, bilateral
   H18.029 Argentous corneal deposits, unspecified eye
  √6ᵗʰ **H18.03** Corneal deposits in metabolic disorders
   Code also associated metabolic disorder
   H18.031 Corneal deposits in metabolic disorders, right eye
   H18.032 Corneal deposits in metabolic disorders, left eye
   H18.033 Corneal deposits in metabolic disorders, bilateral
   H18.039 Corneal deposits in metabolic disorders, unspecified eye
  √6ᵗʰ **H18.04** Kayser-Fleischer ring
   Code also associated Wilson's disease (E83.01)
   H18.041 Kayser-Fleischer ring, right eye
   H18.042 Kayser-Fleischer ring, left eye
   H18.043 Kayser-Fleischer ring, bilateral
   H18.049 Kayser-Fleischer ring, unspecified eye
  √6ᵗʰ **H18.05** Posterior corneal pigmentations
   Krukenberg's spindle
   H18.051 Posterior corneal pigmentations, right eye
   H18.052 Posterior corneal pigmentations, left eye
   H18.053 Posterior corneal pigmentations, bilateral
   H18.059 Posterior corneal pigmentations, unspecified eye
  √6ᵗʰ **H18.06** Stromal corneal pigmentations
   Hematocornea
   H18.061 Stromal corneal pigmentations, right eye
   H18.062 Stromal corneal pigmentations, left eye
   H18.063 Stromal corneal pigmentations, bilateral
   H18.069 Stromal corneal pigmentations, unspecified eye
 √5ᵗʰ **H18.1** Bullous keratopathy
  H18.10 Bullous keratopathy, unspecified eye
  H18.11 Bullous keratopathy, right eye
  H18.12 Bullous keratopathy, left eye
  H18.13 Bullous keratopathy, bilateral
 √5ᵗʰ **H18.2** Other and unspecified corneal edema
  H18.20 Unspecified corneal edema
  √6ᵗʰ **H18.21** Corneal edema secondary to contact lens
   EXCLUDES 2 other corneal disorders due to contact lens (H18.82-)
   H18.211 Corneal edema secondary to contact lens, right eye
   H18.212 Corneal edema secondary to contact lens, left eye

   H18.213 Corneal edema secondary to contact lens, bilateral
   H18.219 Corneal edema secondary to contact lens, unspecified eye
  √6ᵗʰ **H18.22** Idiopathic corneal edema
   H18.221 Idiopathic corneal edema, right eye
   H18.222 Idiopathic corneal edema, left eye
   H18.223 Idiopathic corneal edema, bilateral
   H18.229 Idiopathic corneal edema, unspecified eye
  √6ᵗʰ **H18.23** Secondary corneal edema
   H18.231 Secondary corneal edema, right eye
   H18.232 Secondary corneal edema, left eye
   H18.233 Secondary corneal edema, bilateral
   H18.239 Secondary corneal edema, unspecified eye
 √5ᵗʰ **H18.3** Changes of corneal membranes
  H18.30 Unspecified corneal membrane change
  √6ᵗʰ **H18.31** Folds and rupture in Bowman's membrane
   H18.311 Folds and rupture in Bowman's membrane, right eye
   H18.312 Folds and rupture in Bowman's membrane, left eye
   H18.313 Folds and rupture in Bowman's membrane, bilateral
   H18.319 Folds and rupture in Bowman's membrane, unspecified eye
  √6ᵗʰ **H18.32** Folds in Descemet's membrane
   H18.321 Folds in Descemet's membrane, right eye
   H18.322 Folds in Descemet's membrane, left eye
   H18.323 Folds in Descemet's membrane, bilateral
   H18.329 Folds in Descemet's membrane, unspecified eye
  √6ᵗʰ **H18.33** Rupture in Descemet's membrane
   H18.331 Rupture in Descemet's membrane, right eye
   H18.332 Rupture in Descemet's membrane, left eye
   H18.333 Rupture in Descemet's membrane, bilateral
   H18.339 Rupture in Descemet's membrane, unspecified eye
 √5ᵗʰ **H18.4** Corneal degeneration
  EXCLUDES 1 Mooren's ulcer (H16.0-)
   recurrent erosion of cornea (H18.83-)
  H18.40 Unspecified corneal degeneration
  √6ᵗʰ **H18.41** Arcus senilis
   Senile corneal changes
   H18.411 Arcus senilis, right eye
   H18.412 Arcus senilis, left eye
   H18.413 Arcus senilis, bilateral
   H18.419 Arcus senilis, unspecified eye
  √6ᵗʰ **H18.42** Band keratopathy
   H18.421 Band keratopathy, right eye
   H18.422 Band keratopathy, left eye
   H18.423 Band keratopathy, bilateral
   H18.429 Band keratopathy, unspecified eye
  H18.43 Other calcerous corneal degeneration
  √6ᵗʰ **H18.44** Keratomalacia
   EXCLUDES 1 keratomalacia due to vitamin A deficiency (E50.4)
   H18.441 Keratomalacia, right eye
   H18.442 Keratomalacia, left eye
   H18.443 Keratomalacia, bilateral
   H18.449 Keratomalacia, unspecified eye
  √6ᵗʰ **H18.45** Nodular corneal degeneration
   H18.451 Nodular corneal degeneration, right eye
   H18.452 Nodular corneal degeneration, left eye
   H18.453 Nodular corneal degeneration, bilateral
   H18.459 Nodular corneal degeneration, unspecified eye
  √6ᵗʰ **H18.46** Peripheral corneal degeneration
   H18.461 Peripheral corneal degeneration, right eye
   H18.462 Peripheral corneal degeneration, left eye
   H18.463 Peripheral corneal degeneration, bilateral

N Newborn: 0 P Pediatric: 0-17 M Maternity: 12-55 A Adult: 15-124 MCC Major CC Condition PDx MCC PDx acts as own MCC CC CC Condition PDx CC PDx acts as own CC

558   ICD-10-CM Draft (2015)

H18.469   Peripheral corneal degeneration, unspecified eye

H18.49   Other corneal degeneration

✓5th H18.5   Hereditary corneal dystrophies

H18.50   Unspecified hereditary corneal dystrophies

H18.51   Endothelial corneal dystrophy
Fuchs' dystrophy

H18.52   Epithelial (juvenile) corneal dystrophy

H18.53   Granular corneal dystrophy

H18.54   Lattice corneal dystrophy

H18.55   Macular corneal dystrophy

H18.59   Other hereditary corneal dystrophies

✓5th H18.6   Keratoconus

✓6th H18.60   Keratoconus, unspecified
H18.601   Keratoconus, unspecified, right eye
H18.602   Keratoconus, unspecified, left eye
H18.603   Keratoconus, unspecified, bilateral
H18.609   Keratoconus, unspecified, unspecified eye

✓6th H18.61   Keratoconus, stable
H18.611   Keratoconus, stable, right eye
H18.612   Keratoconus, stable, left eye
H18.613   Keratoconus, stable, bilateral
H18.619   Keratoconus, stable, unspecified eye

✓6th H18.62   Keratoconus, unstable
Acute hydrops
H18.621   Keratoconus, unstable, right eye
H18.622   Keratoconus, unstable, left eye
H18.623   Keratoconus, unstable, bilateral
H18.629   Keratoconus, unstable, unspecified eye

✓5th H18.7   Other and unspecified corneal deformities
EXCLUDES 1   congenital malformations of cornea (Q13.3-Q13.4)

H18.70   Unspecified corneal deformity

✓6th H18.71   Corneal ectasia
H18.711   Corneal ectasia, right eye
H18.712   Corneal ectasia, left eye
H18.713   Corneal ectasia, bilateral
H18.719   Corneal ectasia, unspecified eye

✓6th H18.72   Corneal staphyloma
H18.721   Corneal staphyloma, right eye
H18.722   Corneal staphyloma, left eye
H18.723   Corneal staphyloma, bilateral
H18.729   Corneal staphyloma, unspecified eye

✓6th H18.73   Descemetocele
H18.731   Descemetocele, right eye
H18.732   Descemetocele, left eye
H18.733   Descemetocele, bilateral
H18.739   Descemetocele, unspecified eye

✓6th H18.79   Other corneal deformities
H18.791   Other corneal deformities, right eye
H18.792   Other corneal deformities, left eye
H18.793   Other corneal deformities, bilateral
H18.799   Other corneal deformities, unspecified eye

✓5th H18.8   Other specified disorders of cornea

✓6th H18.81   Anesthesia and hypoesthesia of cornea
H18.811   Anesthesia and hypoesthesia of cornea, right eye
H18.812   Anesthesia and hypoesthesia of cornea, left eye
H18.813   Anesthesia and hypoesthesia of cornea, bilateral
H18.819   Anesthesia and hypoesthesia of cornea, unspecified eye

✓6th H18.82   Corneal disorder due to contact lens
EXCLUDES 2   corneal edema due to contact lens (H18.21-)
H18.821   Corneal disorder due to contact lens, right eye
H18.822   Corneal disorder due to contact lens, left eye
H18.823   Corneal disorder due to contact lens, bilateral
H18.829   Corneal disorder due to contact lens, unspecified eye

✓6th H18.83   Recurrent erosion of cornea
H18.831   Recurrent erosion of cornea, right eye
H18.832   Recurrent erosion of cornea, left eye
H18.833   Recurrent erosion of cornea, bilateral
H18.839   Recurrent erosion of cornea, unspecified eye

✓6th H18.89   Other specified disorders of cornea
H18.891   Other specified disorders of cornea, right eye
H18.892   Other specified disorders of cornea, left eye
H18.893   Other specified disorders of cornea, bilateral
H18.899   Other specified disorders of cornea, unspecified eye

H18.9   Unspecified disorder of cornea

✓4th H20   Iridocyclitis

CC Excl: For CC codes in category H20, unless otherwise noted: A18.54, H20.00-H20.9

✓5th H20.0   Acute and subacute iridocyclitis
Acute anterior uveitis
Acute cyclitis
Acute iritis
Subacute anterior uveitis
Subacute cyclitis
Subacute iritis
EXCLUDES 1   iridocyclitis, iritis, uveitis (due to) (in) diabetes mellitus (E08-E13 with .39)
iridocyclitis, iritis, uveitis (due to) (in) diphtheria (A36.89)
iridocyclitis, iritis, uveitis (due to) (in) gonococcal (A54.32)
iridocyclitis, iritis, uveitis (due to) (in) herpes (simplex) (B00.51)
iridocyclitis, iritis, uveitis (due to) (in) herpes zoster (B02.32)
iridocyclitis, iritis, uveitis (due to) (in) late congenital syphilis (A50.39)
iridocyclitis, iritis, uveitis (due to) (in) late syphilis (A52.71)
iridocyclitis, iritis, uveitis (due to) (in) sarcoidosis (D86.83)
iridocyclitis, iritis, uveitis (due to) (in) syphilis (A51.43)
iridocyclitis, iritis, uveitis (due to) (in) toxoplasmosis (B58.09)
iridocyclitis, iritis, uveitis (due to) (in) tuberculosis (A18.54)

H20.00   Unspecified acute and subacute iridocyclitis   CC

✓6th H20.01   Primary iridocyclitis
H20.011   Primary iridocyclitis, right eye   CC
H20.012   Primary iridocyclitis, left eye   CC
H20.013   Primary iridocyclitis, bilateral   CC
H20.019   Primary iridocyclitis, unspecified eye   CC

✓6th H20.02   Recurrent acute iridocyclitis
H20.021   Recurrent acute iridocyclitis, right eye   CC
H20.022   Recurrent acute iridocyclitis, left eye   CC
H20.023   Recurrent acute iridocyclitis, bilateral   CC
H20.029   Recurrent acute iridocyclitis, unspecified eye   CC

✓6th H20.03   Secondary infectious iridocyclitis
H20.031   Secondary infectious iridocyclitis, right eye   CC
H20.032   Secondary infectious iridocyclitis, left eye   CC
H20.033   Secondary infectious iridocyclitis, bilateral   CC
H20.039   Secondary infectious iridocyclitis, unspecified eye   CC

✓6th H20.04   Secondary noninfectious iridocyclitis
H20.041   Secondary noninfectious iridocyclitis, right eye
H20.042   Secondary noninfectious iridocyclitis, left eye
H20.043   Secondary noninfectious iridocyclitis, bilateral
H20.049   Secondary noninfectious iridocyclitis, unspecified eye

✓ Additional Character Required   ✓x7th Xtension Alert   Unacceptable PDx   Manifestation   Hospital Acquired Condition   EXCLUDES 1 Not Coded Here   EXCLUDES 2 Not Included Here

ICD-10-CM Draft (2015)   559

✓6ᵗʰ **H20.05** **Hypopyon**
- **H20.051** Hypopyon, right eye
- **H20.052** Hypopyon, left eye
- **H20.053** Hypopyon, bilateral
- **H20.059** Hypopyon, unspecified eye

✓5ᵗʰ **H20.1** **Chronic iridocyclitis**
Use additional code for any associated cataract (H26.21-)
EXCLUDES 2   posterior cyclitis (H30.2-)
- **H20.10** Chronic iridocyclitis, unspecified eye
- **H20.11** Chronic iridocyclitis, right eye
- **H20.12** Chronic iridocyclitis, left eye
- **H20.13** Chronic iridocyclitis, bilateral

✓5ᵗʰ **H20.2** **Lens-induced iridocyclitis**
- **H20.20** Lens-induced iridocyclitis, unspecified eye
- **H20.21** Lens-induced iridocyclitis, right eye
- **H20.22** Lens-induced iridocyclitis, left eye
- **H20.23** Lens-induced iridocyclitis, bilateral

✓5ᵗʰ **H20.8** **Other iridocyclitis**
EXCLUDES 2   glaucomatocyclitis crises (H40.4-)
     posterior cyclitis (H30.2-)
     sympathetic uveitis (H44.13-)

     ✓6ᵗʰ **H20.81** **Fuchs' heterochromic cyclitis**
- **H20.811** Fuchs' heterochromic cyclitis, right eye
- **H20.812** Fuchs' heterochromic cyclitis, left eye
- **H20.813** Fuchs' heterochromic cyclitis, bilateral
- **H20.819** Fuchs' heterochromic cyclitis, unspecified eye

     ✓6ᵗʰ **H20.82** **Vogt-Koyanagi syndrome**
- **H20.821** Vogt-Koyanagi syndrome, right eye
- **H20.822** Vogt-Koyanagi syndrome, left eye
- **H20.823** Vogt-Koyanagi syndrome, bilateral
- **H20.829** Vogt-Koyanagi syndrome, unspecified eye

H20.9 **Unspecified iridocyclitis**   CC
Uveitis NOS

✓4ᵗʰ **H21** **Other disorders of iris and ciliary body**
EXCLUDES 2   sympathetic uveitis (H44.1-)

✓5ᵗʰ **H21.0** **Hyphema**
EXCLUDES 1   traumatic hyphema (S05.1-)
- **H21.00** Hyphema, unspecified eye
- **H21.01** Hyphema, right eye
- **H21.02** Hyphema, left eye
- **H21.03** Hyphema, bilateral

✓5ᵗʰ **H21.1** **Other vascular disorders of iris and ciliary body**
Neovascularization of iris or ciliary body
Rubeosis iridis
Rubeosis of iris

     ✓6ᵗʰ **H21.1X** **Other vascular disorders of iris and ciliary body**
- **H21.1X1** Other vascular disorders of iris and ciliary body, right eye
- **H21.1X2** Other vascular disorders of iris and ciliary body, left eye
- **H21.1X3** Other vascular disorders of iris and ciliary body, bilateral
- **H21.1X9** Other vascular disorders of iris and ciliary body, unspecified eye

✓5ᵗʰ **H21.2** **Degeneration of iris and ciliary body**

     ✓6ᵗʰ **H21.21** **Degeneration of chamber angle**
- **H21.211** Degeneration of chamber angle, right eye
- **H21.212** Degeneration of chamber angle, left eye
- **H21.213** Degeneration of chamber angle, bilateral
- **H21.219** Degeneration of chamber angle, unspecified eye

     ✓6ᵗʰ **H21.22** **Degeneration of ciliary body**
- **H21.221** Degeneration of ciliary body, right eye
- **H21.222** Degeneration of ciliary body, left eye
- **H21.223** Degeneration of ciliary body, bilateral
- **H21.229** Degeneration of ciliary body, unspecified eye

     ✓6ᵗʰ **H21.23** **Degeneration of iris (pigmentary)**
Translucency of iris
- **H21.231** Degeneration of iris (pigmentary), right eye

- **H21.232** Degeneration of iris (pigmentary), left eye
- **H21.233** Degeneration of iris (pigmentary), bilateral
- **H21.239** Degeneration of iris (pigmentary), unspecified eye

✓6ᵗʰ **H21.24** **Degeneration of pupillary margin**
- **H21.241** Degeneration of pupillary margin, right eye
- **H21.242** Degeneration of pupillary margin, left eye
- **H21.243** Degeneration of pupillary margin, bilateral
- **H21.249** Degeneration of pupillary margin, unspecified eye

✓6ᵗʰ **H21.25** **Iridoschisis**
- **H21.251** Iridoschisis, right eye
- **H21.252** Iridoschisis, left eye
- **H21.253** Iridoschisis, bilateral
- **H21.259** Iridoschisis, unspecified eye

✓6ᵗʰ **H21.26** **Iris atrophy (essential) (progressive)**
- **H21.261** Iris atrophy (essential) (progressive), right eye
- **H21.262** Iris atrophy (essential) (progressive), left eye
- **H21.263** Iris atrophy (essential) (progressive), bilateral
- **H21.269** Iris atrophy (essential) (progressive), unspecified eye

✓6ᵗʰ **H21.27** **Miotic pupillary cyst**
- **H21.271** Miotic pupillary cyst, right eye
- **H21.272** Miotic pupillary cyst, left eye
- **H21.273** Miotic pupillary cyst, bilateral
- **H21.279** Miotic pupillary cyst, unspecified eye

H21.29 **Other iris atrophy**

✓5ᵗʰ **H21.3** **Cyst of iris, ciliary body and anterior chamber**
EXCLUDES 2   miotic pupillary cyst (H21.27-)

     ✓6ᵗʰ **H21.30** **Idiopathic cysts of iris, ciliary body or anterior chamber**
Cyst of iris, ciliary body or anterior chamber NOS
- **H21.301** Idiopathic cysts of iris, ciliary body or anterior chamber, right eye
- **H21.302** Idiopathic cysts of iris, ciliary body or anterior chamber, left eye
- **H21.303** Idiopathic cysts of iris, ciliary body or anterior chamber, bilateral
- **H21.309** Idiopathic cysts of iris, ciliary body or anterior chamber, unspecified eye

     ✓6ᵗʰ **H21.31** **Exudative cysts of iris or anterior chamber**
- **H21.311** Exudative cysts of iris or anterior chamber, right eye
- **H21.312** Exudative cysts of iris or anterior chamber, left eye
- **H21.313** Exudative cysts of iris or anterior chamber, bilateral
- **H21.319** Exudative cysts of iris or anterior chamber, unspecified eye

     ✓6ᵗʰ **H21.32** **Implantation cysts of iris, ciliary body or anterior chamber**
- **H21.321** Implantation cysts of iris, ciliary body or anterior chamber, right eye
- **H21.322** Implantation cysts of iris, ciliary body or anterior chamber, left eye
- **H21.323** Implantation cysts of iris, ciliary body or anterior chamber, bilateral
- **H21.329** Implantation cysts of iris, ciliary body or anterior chamber, unspecified eye

     ✓6ᵗʰ **H21.33** **Parasitic cyst of iris, ciliary body or anterior chamber**

> **CC Excl:** For CC codes in subcategory H21.33, unless otherwise noted: H20.051-H20.059, H21.331-H21.339, H33.121-H33.129, H44.001-H44.029, H44.121-H44.129, H44.19

- **H21.331** Parasitic cyst of iris, ciliary body or anterior chamber, right eye   CC
- **H21.332** Parasitic cyst of iris, ciliary body or anterior chamber, left eye   CC

N Newborn: 0   P Pediatric: 0-17   M Maternity: 12-55   A Adult: 15-124   MCC Major CC Condition   PDx MCC PDx acts as own MCC   CC CC Condition   PDx CC PDx acts as own CC

560   ICD-10-CM Draft (2015)

H21.333   **Parasitic cyst of iris, ciliary body or anterior chamber,** bilateral   `CC`

H21.339   **Parasitic cyst of iris, ciliary body or anterior chamber,** unspecified eye   `CC`

✓⁶ᵗʰ **H21.34 Primary** cyst of **pars plana**

H21.341   **Primary cyst of pars plana,** right eye

H21.342   **Primary cyst of pars plana,** left eye

H21.343   **Primary cyst of pars plana,** bilateral

H21.349   **Primary cyst of pars plana,** unspecified eye

✓⁶ᵗʰ **H21.35 Exudative** cyst of **pars plana**

H21.351   **Exudative cyst of pars plana,** right eye

H21.352   **Exudative cyst of pars plana,** left eye

H21.353   **Exudative cyst of pars plana,** bilateral

H21.359   **Exudative cyst of pars plana,** unspecified eye

✓⁵ᵗʰ **H21.4 Pupillary membranes**
Iris bombé
Pupillary occlusion
Pupillary seclusion
> **EXCLUDES 1**   *congenital pupillary membranes (Q13.8)*

H21.40   **Pupillary membranes,** unspecified eye

H21.41   **Pupillary membranes,** right eye

H21.42   **Pupillary membranes,** left eye

H21.43   **Pupillary membranes,** bilateral

✓⁵ᵗʰ **H21.5 Other and unspecified adhesions and disruptions of iris and ciliary body**
> **EXCLUDES 1**   *corectopia (Q13.2)*

✓⁶ᵗʰ **H21.50 Unspecified adhesions of iris**
Synechia (iris) NOS

H21.501   **Unspecified adhesions of iris,** right eye

H21.502   **Unspecified adhesions of iris,** left eye

H21.503   **Unspecified adhesions of iris,** bilateral

H21.509   **Unspecified adhesions of iris and ciliary body,** unspecified eye

✓⁶ᵗʰ **H21.51 Anterior synechiae (iris)**

H21.511   **Anterior synechiae (iris),** right eye

H21.512   **Anterior synechiae (iris),** left eye

H21.513   **Anterior synechiae (iris),** bilateral

H21.519   **Anterior synechiae (iris),** unspecified eye

✓⁶ᵗʰ **H21.52 Goniosynechiae**

H21.521   **Goniosynechiae,** right eye

H21.522   **Goniosynechiae,** left eye

H21.523   **Goniosynechiae,** bilateral

H21.529   **Goniosynechiae,** unspecified eye

✓⁶ᵗʰ **H21.53 Iridodialysis**

H21.531   **Iridodialysis,** right eye

H21.532   **Iridodialysis,** left eye

H21.533   **Iridodialysis,** bilateral

H21.539   **Iridodialysis,** unspecified eye

✓⁶ᵗʰ **H21.54 Posterior synechiae (iris)**

H21.541   **Posterior synechiae (iris),** right eye

H21.542   **Posterior synechiae (iris),** left eye

H21.543   **Posterior synechiae (iris),** bilateral

H21.549   **Posterior synechiae (iris),** unspecified eye

✓⁶ᵗʰ **H21.55 Recession of chamber angle**

H21.551   **Recession of chamber angle,** right eye

H21.552   **Recession of chamber angle,** left eye

H21.553   **Recession of chamber angle,** bilateral

H21.559   **Recession of chamber angle,** unspecified eye

✓⁶ᵗʰ **H21.56 Pupillary abnormalities**
Deformed pupil
Ectopic pupil
Rupture of sphincter, pupil
> **EXCLUDES 1**   *congenital deformity of pupil (Q13.2-)*

H21.561   **Pupillary abnormality,** right eye

H21.562   **Pupillary abnormality,** left eye

H21.563   **Pupillary abnormality,** bilateral

H21.569   **Pupillary abnormality,** unspecified eye

✓⁵ᵗʰ **H21.8 Other specified disorders of iris and ciliary body**

H21.81   **Floppy iris syndrome**
Intraoperative floppy iris syndrome (IFIS)
Use additional code for adverse effect, if applicable, to identify drug (T36-T50 with fifth or sixth character 5)

H21.82   **Plateau iris syndrome (post-iridectomy) (postprocedural)**

H21.89   **Other specified disorders of iris and ciliary body**

H21.9   **Unspecified disorder of iris and ciliary body**

H22   *Disorders of iris and ciliary body in diseases classified elsewhere*
Code first underlying disease, such as:
   gout (M1A.-, M10.-)
   leprosy (A30.-)
   parasitic disease (B89)

Disorders of lens (H25-H28)

✓⁴ᵗʰ **H25 Age-related cataract**
Senile cataract
> **EXCLUDES 2**   *capsular glaucoma with pseudoexfoliation of lens (H40.1-)*

✓⁵ᵗʰ **H25.0 Age-related incipient cataract**

✓⁶ᵗʰ **H25.01 Cortical age-related cataract**

H25.011   **Cortical age-related cataract,** right eye   `A`

H25.012   **Cortical age-related cataract,** left eye   `A`

H25.013   **Cortical age-related cataract,** bilateral   `A`

H25.019   **Cortical age-related cataract,** unspecified eye   `A`

✓⁶ᵗʰ **H25.03 Anterior subcapsular polar age-related cataract**

H25.031   **Anterior subcapsular polar age-related cataract,** right eye   `A`

H25.032   **Anterior subcapsular polar age-related cataract,** left eye   `A`

H25.033   **Anterior subcapsular polar age-related cataract,** bilateral   `A`

H25.039   **Anterior subcapsular polar age-related cataract,** unspecified eye   `A`

✓⁶ᵗʰ **H25.04 Posterior subcapsular polar age-related cataract**

H25.041   **Posterior subcapsular polar age-related cataract,** right eye   `A`

H25.042   **Posterior subcapsular polar age-related cataract,** left eye   `A`

H25.043   **Posterior subcapsular polar age-related cataract,** bilateral   `A`

H25.049   **Posterior subcapsular polar age-related cataract,** unspecified eye   `A`

✓⁶ᵗʰ **H25.09 Other age-related incipient cataract**
Coronary age-related cataract
Punctate age-related cataract
Water clefts

H25.091   **Other age-related incipient cataract,** right eye   `A`

H25.092   **Other age-related incipient cataract,** left eye   `A`

H25.093   **Other age-related incipient cataract,** bilateral   `A`

H25.099   **Other age-related incipient cataract,** unspecified eye   `A`

✓⁵ᵗʰ **H25.1 Age-related nuclear cataract**
Cataracta brunescens
Nuclear sclerosis cataract

H25.10   **Age-related nuclear cataract,** unspecified eye   `A`

H25.11   **Age-related nuclear cataract,** right eye   `A`

H25.12   **Age-related nuclear cataract,** left eye   `A`

H25.13   **Age-related nuclear cataract,** bilateral   `A`

✓⁵ᵗʰ **H25.2 Age-related cataract, morgagnian type**
Age-related hypermature cataract

H25.20   **Age-related cataract, morgagnian type,** unspecified eye   `A`

H25.21   **Age-related cataract, morgagnian type,** right eye   `A`

H25.22   **Age-related cataract, morgagnian type,** left eye   `A`

H25.23   **Age-related cataract, morgagnian type,** bilateral   `A`

✓ Additional Character Required   ✓x7ᵗʰ Xtension Alert   Unacceptable PDx   Manifestation   Hospital Acquired Condition   **EXCLUDES 1** Not Coded Here   **EXCLUDES 2** Not Included Here

ICD-10-CM Draft (2015)   561

✓5ᵗʰ **H25.8** Other age-related cataract

    ✓6ᵗʰ **H25.81** Combined forms of age-related cataract

        H25.811 Combined forms of age-related cataract, right eye Ⓐ

        H25.812 Combined forms of age-related cataract, left eye Ⓐ

        H25.813 Combined forms of age-related cataract, bilateral Ⓐ

        H25.819 Combined forms of age-related cataract, unspecified eye Ⓐ

    H25.89 Other age-related cataract Ⓐ

  H25.9 Unspecified age-related cataract Ⓐ

✓4ᵗʰ **H26** Other cataract

    EXCLUDES 1 congenital cataract (Q12.0)

  ✓5ᵗʰ **H26.0** Infantile and juvenile cataract

    ✓6ᵗʰ **H26.00** Unspecified infantile and juvenile cataract

        H26.001 Unspecified infantile and juvenile cataract, right eye Ⓟ

        H26.002 Unspecified infantile and juvenile cataract, left eye Ⓟ

        H26.003 Unspecified infantile and juvenile cataract, bilateral Ⓟ

        H26.009 Unspecified infantile and juvenile cataract, unspecified eye Ⓟ

    ✓6ᵗʰ **H26.01** Infantile and juvenile cortical, lamellar, or zonular cataract

        H26.011 Infantile and juvenile cortical, lamellar, or zonular cataract, right eye Ⓟ

        H26.012 Infantile and juvenile cortical, lamellar, or zonular cataract, left eye Ⓟ

        H26.013 Infantile and juvenile cortical, lamellar, or zonular cataract, bilateral Ⓟ

        H26.019 Infantile and juvenile cortical, lamellar, or zonular cataract, unspecified eye Ⓟ

    ✓6ᵗʰ **H26.03** Infantile and juvenile nuclear cataract

        H26.031 Infantile and juvenile nuclear cataract, right eye Ⓟ

        H26.032 Infantile and juvenile nuclear cataract, left eye Ⓟ

        H26.033 Infantile and juvenile nuclear cataract, bilateral Ⓟ

        H26.039 Infantile and juvenile nuclear cataract, unspecified eye Ⓟ

    ✓6ᵗʰ **H26.04** Anterior subcapsular polar infantile and juvenile cataract

        H26.041 Anterior subcapsular polar infantile and juvenile cataract, right eye Ⓟ

        H26.042 Anterior subcapsular polar infantile and juvenile cataract, left eye Ⓟ

        H26.043 Anterior subcapsular polar infantile and juvenile cataract, bilateral Ⓟ

        H26.049 Anterior subcapsular polar infantile and juvenile cataract, unspecified eye Ⓟ

    ✓6ᵗʰ **H26.05** Posterior subcapsular polar infantile and juvenile cataract

        H26.051 Posterior subcapsular polar infantile and juvenile cataract, right eye Ⓟ

        H26.052 Posterior subcapsular polar infantile and juvenile cataract, left eye Ⓟ

        H26.053 Posterior subcapsular polar infantile and juvenile cataract, bilateral Ⓟ

        H26.059 Posterior subcapsular polar infantile and juvenile cataract, unspecified eye Ⓟ

    ✓6ᵗʰ **H26.06** Combined forms of infantile and juvenile cataract

        H26.061 Combined forms of infantile and juvenile cataract, right eye Ⓟ

        H26.062 Combined forms of infantile and juvenile cataract, left eye Ⓟ

        H26.063 Combined forms of infantile and juvenile cataract, bilateral Ⓟ

        H26.069 Combined forms of infantile and juvenile cataract, unspecified eye Ⓟ

    H26.09 Other infantile and juvenile cataract Ⓟ

✓5ᵗʰ **H26.1** Traumatic cataract

    Use additional code (Chapter 20) to identify external cause

  ✓6ᵗʰ **H26.10** Unspecified traumatic cataract

    H26.101 Unspecified traumatic cataract, right eye

    H26.102 Unspecified traumatic cataract, left eye

    H26.103 Unspecified traumatic cataract, bilateral

    H26.109 Unspecified traumatic cataract, unspecified eye

  ✓6ᵗʰ **H26.11** Localized traumatic opacities

    H26.111 Localized traumatic opacities, right eye

    H26.112 Localized traumatic opacities, left eye

    H26.113 Localized traumatic opacities, bilateral

    H26.119 Localized traumatic opacities, unspecified eye

  ✓6ᵗʰ **H26.12** Partially resolved traumatic cataract

    H26.121 Partially resolved traumatic cataract, right eye

    H26.122 Partially resolved traumatic cataract, left eye

    H26.123 Partially resolved traumatic cataract, bilateral

    H26.129 Partially resolved traumatic cataract, unspecified eye

  ✓6ᵗʰ **H26.13** Total traumatic cataract

    H26.131 Total traumatic cataract, right eye

    H26.132 Total traumatic cataract, left eye

    H26.133 Total traumatic cataract, bilateral

    H26.139 Total traumatic cataract, unspecified eye

✓5ᵗʰ **H26.2** Complicated cataract

  H26.20 Unspecified complicated cataract

    Cataracta complicata NOS

  ✓6ᵗʰ **H26.21** Cataract with neovascularization

    Code also associated condition, such as: chronic iridocyclitis (H20.1-)

    H26.211 Cataract with neovascularization, right eye

    H26.212 Cataract with neovascularization, left eye

    H26.213 Cataract with neovascularization, bilateral

    H26.219 Cataract with neovascularization, unspecified eye

  ✓6ᵗʰ **H26.22** Cataract secondary to ocular disorders (degenerative) (inflammatory)

    Code also associated ocular disorder

    H26.221 Cataract secondary to ocular disorders (degenerative) (inflammatory), right eye

    H26.222 Cataract secondary to ocular disorders (degenerative) (inflammatory), left eye

    H26.223 Cataract secondary to ocular disorders (degenerative) (inflammatory), bilateral

    H26.229 Cataract secondary to ocular disorders (degenerative) (inflammatory), unspecified eye

  ✓6ᵗʰ **H26.23** Glaucomatous flecks (subcapsular)

    Code first underlying glaucoma (H40-H42)

    H26.231 Glaucomatous flecks (subcapsular), right eye

    H26.232 Glaucomatous flecks (subcapsular), left eye

    H26.233 Glaucomatous flecks (subcapsular), bilateral

    H26.239 Glaucomatous flecks (subcapsular), unspecified eye

✓5ᵗʰ **H26.3** Drug-induced cataract

    Toxic cataract

    Use additional code for adverse effect, if applicable, to identify drug (T36-T50 with fifth or sixth character 5)

    H26.30 Drug-induced cataract, unspecified eye

    H26.31 Drug-induced cataract, right eye

    H26.32 Drug-induced cataract, left eye

    H26.33 Drug-induced cataract, bilateral

✓5ᵗʰ **H26.4** Secondary cataract

    H26.40 Unspecified secondary cataract

  ✓6ᵗʰ **H26.41** Soemmering's ring

    H26.411 Soemmering's ring, right eye

    H26.412 Soemmering's ring, left eye

Ⓝ Newborn: 0   Ⓟ Pediatric: 0-17   Ⓜ Maternity: 12-55   Ⓐ Adult: 15-124   MCC Major CC Condition   PDx MCC PDx acts as own MCC   CC CC Condition   PDx CC PDx acts as own CC

562   ICD-10-CM Draft (2015)

	H26.413	Soemmering's ring, bilateral
	H26.419	Soemmering's ring, unspecified eye
√6th H26.49	Other secondary cataract	
	H26.491	Other secondary cataract, right eye
	H26.492	Other secondary cataract, left eye
	H26.493	Other secondary cataract, bilateral
	H26.499	Other secondary cataract, unspecified eye

H26.8 Other specified cataract

H26.9 Unspecified cataract

√4th H27 Other disorders of lens

EXCLUDES 1   congenital lens malformations (Q12.-)
mechanical complications of intraocular lens implant (T85.2)
pseudophakia (Z96.1)

√5th **H27.0 Aphakia**
Acquired absence of lens
Acquired aphakia
Aphakia due to trauma
EXCLUDES 1   cataract extraction status (Z98.4-)
congenital absence of lens (Q12.3)
congenital aphakia (Q12.3)

	H27.00	Aphakia, unspecified eye
	H27.01	Aphakia, right eye
	H27.02	Aphakia, left eye
	H27.03	Aphakia, bilateral

√5th **H27.1 Dislocation of lens**

	H27.10	Unspecified dislocation of lens
√6th H27.11	Subluxation of lens	
	H27.111	Subluxation of lens, right eye
	H27.112	Subluxation of lens, left eye
	H27.113	Subluxation of lens, bilateral
	H27.119	Subluxation of lens, unspecified eye
√6th H27.12	Anterior dislocation of lens	
	H27.121	Anterior dislocation of lens, right eye
	H27.122	Anterior dislocation of lens, left eye
	H27.123	Anterior dislocation of lens, bilateral
	H27.129	Anterior dislocation of lens, unspecified eye
√6th H27.13	Posterior dislocation of lens	
	H27.131	Posterior dislocation of lens, right eye
	H27.132	Posterior dislocation of lens, left eye
	H27.133	Posterior dislocation of lens, bilateral
	H27.139	Posterior dislocation of lens, unspecified eye

H27.8 Other specified disorders of lens

H27.9 Unspecified disorder of lens

H28 *Cataract in diseases classified elsewhere*

Code first underlying disease, such as:
hypoparathyroidism (E20.-)
myotonia (G71.1-)
myxedema (E03.-)
protein-calorie malnutrition (E40-E46)
EXCLUDES 1   *cataract in diabetes mellitus (E08.36, E09.36, E10.36, E11.36, E13.36)*

Disorders of choroid and retina (H30-H36)

√4th H30 Chorioretinal inflammation

CC Excl: For CC codes in category H30, unless otherwise noted: H30.001–H30.93

√5th **H30.0 Focal chorioretinal inflammation**
Focal chorioretinitis
Focal choroiditis
Focal retinitis
Focal retinochoroiditis

√6th H30.00	Unspecified focal chorioretinal inflammation	
	Focal chorioretinitis NOS	
	Focal choroiditis NOS	
	Focal retinitis NOS	
	Focal retinochoroiditis NOS	
	H30.001	Unspecified focal chorioretinal inflammation, right eye
	H30.002	Unspecified focal chorioretinal inflammation, left eye
	H30.003	Unspecified focal chorioretinal inflammation, bilateral

	H30.009	Unspecified focal chorioretinal inflammation, unspecified eye
√6th H30.01	Focal chorioretinal inflammation, juxtapapillary	
	H30.011	Focal chorioretinal inflammation, juxtapapillary, right eye
	H30.012	Focal chorioretinal inflammation, juxtapapillary, left eye
	H30.013	Focal chorioretinal inflammation, juxtapapillary, bilateral
	H30.019	Focal chorioretinal inflammation, juxtapapillary, unspecified eye
√6th H30.02	Focal chorioretinal inflammation of posterior pole	
	H30.021	Focal chorioretinal inflammation of posterior pole, right eye
	H30.022	Focal chorioretinal inflammation of posterior pole, left eye
	H30.023	Focal chorioretinal inflammation of posterior pole, bilateral
	H30.029	Focal chorioretinal inflammation of posterior pole, unspecified eye
√6th H30.03	Focal chorioretinal inflammation, peripheral	
	H30.031	Focal chorioretinal inflammation, peripheral, right eye
	H30.032	Focal chorioretinal inflammation, peripheral, left eye
	H30.033	Focal chorioretinal inflammation, peripheral, bilateral
	H30.039	Focal chorioretinal inflammation, peripheral, unspecified eye
√6th H30.04	Focal chorioretinal inflammation, macular or paramacular	
	H30.041	Focal chorioretinal inflammation, macular or paramacular, right eye
	H30.042	Focal chorioretinal inflammation, macular or paramacular, left eye
	H30.043	Focal chorioretinal inflammation, macular or paramacular, bilateral
	H30.049	Focal chorioretinal inflammation, macular or paramacular, unspecified eye

√5th **H30.1 Disseminated chorioretinal inflammation**
Disseminated chorioretinitis
Disseminated choroiditis
Disseminated retinitis
Disseminated retinochoroiditis
EXCLUDES 2   *exudative retinopathy (H35.02-)*

√6th H30.10	Unspecified disseminated chorioretinal inflammation		
	Disseminated chorioretinitis NOS		
	Disseminated choroiditis NOS		
	Disseminated retinitis NOS		
	Disseminated retinochoroiditis NOS		
	H30.101	Unspecified disseminated chorioretinal inflammation, right eye	CC
	H30.102	Unspecified disseminated chorioretinal inflammation, left eye	CC
	H30.103	Unspecified disseminated chorioretinal inflammation, bilateral	CC
	H30.109	Unspecified disseminated chorioretinal inflammation, unspecified eye	CC
√6th H30.11	Disseminated chorioretinal inflammation of posterior pole		
	H30.111	Disseminated chorioretinal inflammation of posterior pole, right eye	CC
	H30.112	Disseminated chorioretinal inflammation of posterior pole, left eye	CC
	H30.113	Disseminated chorioretinal inflammation of posterior pole, bilateral	CC
	H30.119	Disseminated chorioretinal inflammation of posterior pole, unspecified eye	CC
√6th H30.12	Disseminated chorioretinal inflammation, peripheral		
	H30.121	Disseminated chorioretinal inflammation, peripheral right eye	CC

Diseases of the Eye and Adnexa

H30.122–H31.312

H30.122   **Disseminated chorioretinal inflammation, peripheral, left eye**   CC

H30.123   **Disseminated chorioretinal inflammation, peripheral, bilateral**   CC

H30.129   **Disseminated chorioretinal inflammation, peripheral, unspecified eye**   CC

✓6th **H30.13**   **Disseminated chorioretinal inflammation, generalized**

H30.131   **Disseminated chorioretinal inflammation, generalized, right eye**   CC

H30.132   **Disseminated chorioretinal inflammation, generalized, left eye**   CC

H30.133   **Disseminated chorioretinal inflammation, generalized, bilateral**   CC

H30.139   **Disseminated chorioretinal inflammation, generalized, unspecified eye**   CC

✓6th **H30.14**   **Acute posterior multifocal placoid pigment epitheliopathy**

H30.141   **Acute posterior multifocal placoid pigment epitheliopathy, right eye**   CC

H30.142   **Acute posterior multifocal placoid pigment epitheliopathy, left eye**   CC

H30.143   **Acute posterior multifocal placoid pigment epitheliopathy, bilateral**   CC

H30.149   **Acute posterior multifocal placoid pigment epitheliopathy, unspecified eye**   CC

✓5th **H30.2**   **Posterior cyclitis**
Pars planitis

H30.20   **Posterior cyclitis, unspecified eye**

H30.21   **Posterior cyclitis, right eye**

H30.22   **Posterior cyclitis, left eye**

H30.23   **Posterior cyclitis, bilateral**

✓5th **H30.8**   **Other chorioretinal inflammations**

✓6th **H30.81**   **Harada's disease**

H30.811   **Harada's disease, right eye**

H30.812   **Harada's disease, left eye**

H30.813   **Harada's disease, bilateral**

H30.819   **Harada's disease, unspecified eye**

✓6th **H30.89**   **Other chorioretinal inflammations**

H30.891   **Other chorioretinal inflammations, right eye**   CC

H30.892   **Other chorioretinal inflammations, left eye**   CC

H30.893   **Other chorioretinal inflammations, bilateral**   CC

H30.899   **Other chorioretinal inflammations, unspecified eye**   CC

✓5th **H30.9**   **Unspecified chorioretinal inflammation**
Chorioretinitis NOS
Choroiditis NOS
Neuroretinitis NOS
Retinitis NOS
Retinochoroiditis NOS

H30.90   **Unspecified chorioretinal inflammation, unspecified eye**   CC

H30.91   **Unspecified chorioretinal inflammation, right eye**   CC

H30.92   **Unspecified chorioretinal inflammation, left eye**   CC

H30.93   **Unspecified chorioretinal inflammation, bilateral**   CC

✓4th **H31**   **Other disorders of choroid**

> **CC Excl: For CC codes in category H31, unless otherwise noted:** H31.301-H32

✓5th **H31.0**   **Chorioretinal scars**
EXCLUDES 2   *postsurgical chorioretinal scars (H59.81-)*

✓6th **H31.00**   **Unspecified chorioretinal scars**

H31.001   **Unspecified chorioretinal scars, right eye**

H31.002   **Unspecified chorioretinal scars, left eye**

H31.003   **Unspecified chorioretinal scars, bilateral**

H31.009   **Unspecified chorioretinal scars, unspecified eye**

✓6th **H31.01**   **Macula scars of posterior pole (postinflammatory) (post-traumatic)**
EXCLUDES 1   *postprocedural chorioretinal scar (H59.81-)*

H31.011   **Macula scars of posterior pole (postinflammatory) (post-traumatic), right eye**

H31.012   **Macula scars of posterior pole (postinflammatory) (post-traumatic), left eye**

H31.013   **Macula scars of posterior pole (postinflammatory) (post-traumatic), bilateral**

H31.019   **Macula scars of posterior pole (postinflammatory) (post-traumatic), unspecified eye**

✓6th **H31.02**   **Solar retinopathy**

H31.021   **Solar retinopathy, right eye**

H31.022   **Solar retinopathy, left eye**

H31.023   **Solar retinopathy, bilateral**

H31.029   **Solar retinopathy, unspecified eye**

✓6th **H31.09**   **Other chorioretinal scars**

H31.091   **Other chorioretinal scars, right eye**

H31.092   **Other chorioretinal scars, left eye**

H31.093   **Other chorioretinal scars, bilateral**

H31.099   **Other chorioretinal scars, unspecified eye**

✓5th **H31.1**   **Choroidal degeneration**
EXCLUDES 2   *angioid streaks of macula (H35.33)*

✓6th **H31.10**   **Unspecified choroidal degeneration**
Choroidal sclerosis NOS

H31.101   **Choroidal degeneration, unspecified, right eye**

H31.102   **Choroidal degeneration, unspecified, left eye**

H31.103   **Choroidal degeneration, unspecified, bilateral**

H31.109   **Choroidal degeneration, unspecified, unspecified eye**

✓6th **H31.11**   **Age-related choroidal atrophy**

H31.111   **Age-related choroidal atrophy, right eye**   A

H31.112   **Age-related choroidal atrophy, left eye**   A

H31.113   **Age-related choroidal atrophy, bilateral**   A

H31.119   **Age-related choroidal atrophy, unspecified eye**   A

✓6th **H31.12**   **Diffuse secondary atrophy of choroid**

H31.121   **Diffuse secondary atrophy of choroid, right eye**

H31.122   **Diffuse secondary atrophy of choroid, left eye**

H31.123   **Diffuse secondary atrophy of choroid, bilateral**

H31.129   **Diffuse secondary atrophy of choroid, unspecified eye**

✓5th **H31.2**   **Hereditary choroidal dystrophy**
EXCLUDES 2   *hyperornithinemia (E72.4)*
          ornithinemia (E72.4)

H31.20   **Hereditary choroidal dystrophy, unspecified**

H31.21   **Choroideremia**

H31.22   **Choroidal dystrophy (central areolar) (generalized) (peripapillary)**

H31.23   **Gyrate atrophy, choroid**

H31.29   **Other hereditary choroidal dystrophy**

✓5th **H31.3**   **Choroidal hemorrhage and rupture**

✓6th **H31.30**   **Unspecified choroidal hemorrhage**

H31.301   **Unspecified choroidal hemorrhage, right eye**

H31.302   **Unspecified choroidal hemorrhage, left eye**

H31.303   **Unspecified choroidal hemorrhage, bilateral**

H31.309   **Unspecified choroidal hemorrhage, unspecified eye**

✓6th **H31.31**   **Expulsive choroidal hemorrhage**

H31.311   **Expulsive choroidal hemorrhage, right eye**

H31.312   **Expulsive choroidal hemorrhage, left eye**

N Newborn: 0   P Pediatric: 0-17   M Maternity: 12-55   A Adult: 15-124   MCC Major CC Condition   PDx MCC PDx acts as own MCC   CC CC Condition   PDx CC PDx acts as own CC

564   ICD-10-CM Draft (2015)

Diseases of the Eye and Adnexa

H31.313　Expulsive choroidal hemorrhage, bilateral

H31.319　Expulsive choroidal hemorrhage, unspecified eye

√6th H31.32　Choroidal rupture

H31.321　Choroidal rupture, right eye　CC

H31.322　Choroidal rupture, left eye　CC

H31.323　Choroidal rupture, bilateral　CC

H31.329　Choroidal rupture, unspecified eye　CC

√5th H31.4　Choroidal detachment

√6th H31.40　Unspecified choroidal detachment

H31.401　Unspecified choroidal detachment, right eye

H31.402　Unspecified choroidal detachment, left eye　CC

H31.403　Unspecified choroidal detachment, bilateral　CC

H31.409　Unspecified choroidal detachment, unspecified eye

√6th H31.41　Hemorrhagic choroidal detachment

H31.411　Hemorrhagic choroidal detachment, right eye　CC

H31.412　Hemorrhagic choroidal detachment, left eye　CC

H31.413　Hemorrhagic choroidal detachment, bilateral　CC

H31.419　Hemorrhagic choroidal detachment, unspecified eye　CC

√6th H31.42　Serous choroidal detachment

H31.421　Serous choroidal detachment, right eye　CC

H31.422　Serous choroidal detachment, left eye　CC

H31.423　Serous choroidal detachment, bilateral　CC

H31.429　Serous choroidal detachment, unspecified eye　CC

H31.8　Other specified disorders of choroid

H31.9　Unspecified disorder of choroid

H32　Chorioretinal disorders in diseases classified elsewhere

Code first underlying disease, such as:
congenital toxoplasmosis (P37.1)
histoplasmosis (B39.-)
leprosy (A30.-)

EXCLUDES 1　chorioretinitis (in):
toxoplasmosis (acquired) (B58.01)
tuberculosis (A18.53)

√4th H33　Retinal detachments and breaks

CC Excl: For CC codes in category H33, unless otherwise noted: H33.001-H33.119, H33.191-H33.8, H35.70-H35.739

EXCLUDES 1　detachment of retinal pigment epithelium (H35.72-, H35.73-)

√5th H33.0　Retinal detachment with retinal break
Rhegmatogenous retinal detachment

EXCLUDES 1　serous retinal detachment (without retinal break) (H33.2-)

√6th H33.00　Unspecified retinal detachment with retinal break

H33.001　Unspecified retinal detachment with retinal break, right eye

H33.002　Unspecified retinal detachment with retinal break, left eye

H33.003　Unspecified retinal detachment with retinal break, bilateral

H33.009　Unspecified retinal detachment with retinal break, unspecified eye

√6th H33.01　Retinal detachment with single break

H33.011　Retinal detachment with single break, right eye

H33.012　Retinal detachment with single break, left eye

H33.013　Retinal detachment with single break, bilateral

H33.019　Retinal detachment with single break, unspecified eye

√6th H33.02　Retinal detachment with multiple breaks

H33.021　Retinal detachment with multiple breaks, right eye

H33.022　Retinal detachment with multiple breaks, left eye

H33.023　Retinal detachment with multiple breaks, bilateral

H33.029　Retinal detachment with multiple breaks, unspecified eye

√6th H33.03　Retinal detachment with giant retinal tear

H33.031　Retinal detachment with giant retinal tear, right eye

H33.032　Retinal detachment with giant retinal tear, left eye

H33.033　Retinal detachment with giant retinal tear, bilateral

H33.039　Retinal detachment with giant retinal tear, unspecified eye

√6th H33.04　Retinal detachment with retinal dialysis

H33.041　Retinal detachment with retinal dialysis, right eye

H33.042　Retinal detachment with retinal dialysis, left eye

H33.043　Retinal detachment with retinal dialysis, bilateral

H33.049　Retinal detachment with retinal dialysis, unspecified eye

√6th H33.05　Total retinal detachment

H33.051　Total retinal detachment, right eye

H33.052　Total retinal detachment, left eye

H33.053　Total retinal detachment, bilateral

H33.059　Total retinal detachment, unspecified eye

√5th H33.1　Retinoschisis and retinal cysts

EXCLUDES 1　congenital retinoschisis (Q14.1)
microcystoid degeneration of retina (H35.42-)

√6th H33.10　Unspecified retinoschisis

H33.101　Unspecified retinoschisis, right eye

H33.102　Unspecified retinoschisis, left eye

H33.103　Unspecified retinoschisis, bilateral

H33.109　Unspecified retinoschisis, unspecified eye

√6th H33.11　Cyst of ora serrata

H33.111　Cyst of ora serrata, right eye

H33.112　Cyst of ora serrata, left eye

H33.113　Cyst of ora serrata, bilateral

H33.119　Cyst of ora serrata, unspecified eye

√6th H33.12　Parasitic cyst of retina

CC Excl: For CC codes in subcategory H33.12, unless otherwise noted: H20.051-H20.059, H21.331-H21.339, H33.121-H33.129, H44.001-H44.029, H44.121-H44.129, H44.19

H33.121　Parasitic cyst of retina, right eye　CC

H33.122　Parasitic cyst of retina, left eye　CC

H33.123　Parasitic cyst of retina, bilateral　CC

H33.129　Parasitic cyst of retina, unspecified eye　CC

√6th H33.19　Other retinoschisis and retinal cysts
Pseudocyst of retina

H33.191　Other retinoschisis and retinal cysts, right eye

H33.192　Other retinoschisis and retinal cysts, left eye

H33.193　Other retinoschisis and retinal cysts, bilateral

H33.199　Other retinoschisis and retinal cysts, unspecified eye

√5th H33.2　Serous retinal detachment
Retinal detachment NOS
Retinal detachment without retinal break

EXCLUDES 1　central serous chorioretinopathy (H35.71-)

H33.20　Serous retinal detachment, unspecified eye　CC

H33.21　Serous retinal detachment, right eye　CC

H33.22　Serous retinal detachment, left eye　CC

H33.23　Serous retinal detachment, bilateral　CC

☑ Additional Character Required　√x7th Xtension Alert　Unacceptable PDx　Manifestation　Hospital Acquired Condition　EXCLUDES 1 Not Coded Here　EXCLUDES 2 Not Included Here

ICD-10-CM Draft (2015)　　　　　565

Diseases of the Eye and Adnexa

H33.3–H35.059

✓5th **H33.3 Retinal breaks** without detachment

    EXCLUDES 1 *chorioretinal scars after surgery for detachment (H59.81-)*
    peripheral retinal degeneration without break (H35.4-)

  ✓6th **H33.30 Unspecified** retinal break

    H33.301 Unspecified retinal break, right eye
    H33.302 Unspecified retinal break, left eye
    H33.303 Unspecified retinal break, bilateral
    H33.309 Unspecified retinal break, unspecified eye

  ✓6th **H33.31 Horseshoe tear of retina without detachment**
    Operculum of retina without detachment

    H33.311 Horseshoe tear of retina without detachment, right eye
    H33.312 Horseshoe tear of retina without detachment, left eye
    H33.313 Horseshoe tear of retina without detachment, bilateral
    H33.319 Horseshoe tear of retina without detachment, unspecified eye

  ✓6th **H33.32 Round hole of retina without detachment**
    H33.321 Round hole, right eye
    H33.322 Round hole, left eye
    H33.323 Round hole, bilateral
    H33.329 Round hole, unspecified eye

  ✓6th **H33.33 Multiple defects of retina without detachment**
    H33.331 Multiple defects of retina without detachment, right eye
    H33.332 Multiple defects of retina without detachment, left eye
    H33.333 Multiple defects of retina without detachment, bilateral
    H33.339 Multiple defects of retina without detachment, unspecified eye

✓5th **H33.4 Traction detachment of retina**
    Proliferative vitreo-retinopathy with retinal detachment

    H33.40 Traction detachment of retina, unspecified eye CC
    H33.41 Traction detachment of retina, right eye CC
    H33.42 Traction detachment of retina, left eye CC
    H33.43 Traction detachment of retina, bilateral CC

  H33.8 Other retinal detachments CC

✓4th **H34 Retinal vascular occlusions**

    CC Excl: For CC codes in category H34, unless otherwise noted: G45.3, H34.00-H34.9

    EXCLUDES 1 *amaurosis fugax (G45.3)*

✓5th **H34.0 Transient retinal artery occlusion**
    H34.00 Transient retinal artery occlusion, unspecified eye CC
    H34.01 Transient retinal artery occlusion, right eye CC
    H34.02 Transient retinal artery occlusion, left eye CC
    H34.03 Transient retinal artery occlusion, bilateral CC

✓5th **H34.1 Central retinal artery occlusion**
    H34.10 Central retinal artery occlusion, unspecified eye CC
    H34.11 Central retinal artery occlusion, right eye CC
    H34.12 Central retinal artery occlusion, left eye CC
    H34.13 Central retinal artery occlusion, bilateral CC

✓5th **H34.2 Other retinal artery occlusions**

  ✓6th **H34.21 Partial retinal artery occlusion**
    Hollenhorst's plaque
    Retinal microembolism

    H34.211 Partial retinal artery occlusion, right eye CC
    H34.212 Partial retinal artery occlusion, left eye CC
    H34.213 Partial retinal artery occlusion, bilateral CC
    H34.219 Partial retinal artery occlusion, unspecified eye CC

  ✓6th **H34.23 Retinal artery branch occlusion**
    H34.231 Retinal artery branch occlusion, right eye CC
    H34.232 Retinal artery branch occlusion, left eye CC
    H34.233 Retinal artery branch occlusion, bilateral CC

    H34.239 Retinal artery branch occlusion, unspecified eye CC

✓5th **H34.8 Other retinal vascular occlusions**

  ✓6th **H34.81 Central retinal vein occlusion**
    H34.811 Central retinal vein occlusion, right eye CC
    H34.812 Central retinal vein occlusion, left eye CC
    H34.813 Central retinal vein occlusion, bilateral CC
    H34.819 Central retinal vein occlusion, unspecified eye CC

  ✓6th **H34.82 Venous engorgement**
    Incipient retinal vein occlusion
    Partial retinal vein occlusion

    H34.821 Venous engorgement, right eye
    H34.822 Venous engorgement, left eye
    H34.823 Venous engorgement, bilateral
    H34.829 Venous engorgement, unspecified eye

  ✓6th **H34.83 Tributary (branch) retinal vein occlusion**
    H34.831 Tributary (branch) retinal vein occlusion, right eye
    H34.832 Tributary (branch) retinal vein occlusion, left eye
    H34.833 Tributary (branch) retinal vein occlusion, bilateral
    H34.839 Tributary (branch) retinal vein occlusion, unspecified eye

  H34.9 Unspecified retinal vascular occlusion CC

✓4th **H35 Other retinal disorders**

    EXCLUDES 2 *diabetic retinal disorders (E08.311- E08.359, E09.311- E09.359, E10.311- E10.359, E11.311- E11.359, E13.311- E13.359)*

✓5th **H35.0 Background retinopathy and retinal vascular changes**
    Code also any associated hypertension (I10.-)

  H35.00 Unspecified background retinopathy

  ✓6th **H35.01 Changes in retinal vascular appearance**
    Retinal vascular sheathing

    H35.011 Changes in retinal vascular appearance, right eye
    H35.012 Changes in retinal vascular appearance, left eye
    H35.013 Changes in retinal vascular appearance, bilateral
    H35.019 Changes in retinal vascular appearance, unspecified eye

  ✓6th **H35.02 Exudative retinopathy**
    Coats retinopathy

    H35.021 Exudative retinopathy, right eye
    H35.022 Exudative retinopathy, left eye
    H35.023 Exudative retinopathy, bilateral
    H35.029 Exudative retinopathy, unspecified eye

  ✓6th **H35.03 Hypertensive retinopathy**
    H35.031 Hypertensive retinopathy, right eye
    H35.032 Hypertensive retinopathy, left eye
    H35.033 Hypertensive retinopathy, bilateral
    H35.039 Hypertensive retinopathy, unspecified eye

  ✓6th **H35.04 Retinal micro-aneurysms, unspecified**
    H35.041 Retinal micro-aneurysms, unspecified, right eye
    H35.042 Retinal micro-aneurysms, unspecified, left eye
    H35.043 Retinal micro-aneurysms, unspecified, bilateral
    H35.049 Retinal micro-aneurysms, unspecified, unspecified eye

  ✓6th **H35.05 Retinal neovascularization, unspecified**
    H35.051 Retinal neovascularization, unspecified, right eye
    H35.052 Retinal neovascularization, unspecified, left eye
    H35.053 Retinal neovascularization, unspecified, bilateral
    H35.059 Retinal neovascularization, unspecified, unspecified eye

N Newborn: 0   **P** Pediatric: 0-17   **M** Maternity: 12-55   **A** Adult: 15-124   **MCC** Major CC Condition   **PDx MCC** PDx acts as own MCC   **CC** CC Condition   **PDx CC** PDx acts as own CC

566   ICD-10-CM Draft (2015)

✓6th **H35.06** **Retinal** vasculitis
Eales disease
Retinal perivasculitis
　　H35.061 **Retinal vasculitis,** right **eye**
　　H35.062 **Retinal vasculitis,** left **eye**
　　H35.063 **Retinal vasculitis,** bilateral
　　H35.069 **Retinal vasculitis,** unspecified **eye**

✓6th **H35.07** **Retinal** telangiectasis
　　H35.071 **Retinal telangiectasis,** right **eye**
　　H35.072 **Retinal telangiectasis,** left **eye**
　　H35.073 **Retinal telangiectasis,** bilateral
　　H35.079 **Retinal telangiectasis,** unspecified **eye**

　　H35.09 **Other intraretinal microvascular abnormalities**
Retinal varices

✓5th **H35.1** **Retinopathy of prematurity**

✓6th **H35.10** **Retinopathy of prematurity,** unspecified
Retinopathy of prematurity NOS
　　H35.101 **Retinopathy of prematurity, unspecified,** right **eye**
　　H35.102 **Retinopathy of prematurity, unspecified,** left **eye**
　　H35.103 **Retinopathy of prematurity, unspecified,** bilateral
　　H35.109 **Retinopathy of prematurity, unspecified,** unspecified **eye**

✓6th **H35.11** **Retinopathy of prematurity,** stage 0
　　H35.111 **Retinopathy of prematurity, stage 0,** right **eye**
　　H35.112 **Retinopathy of prematurity, stage 0,** left **eye**
　　H35.113 **Retinopathy of prematurity, stage 0,** bilateral
　　H35.119 **Retinopathy of prematurity, stage 0,** unspecified **eye**

✓6th **H35.12** **Retinopathy of prematurity,** stage 1
　　H35.121 **Retinopathy of prematurity, stage 1,** right **eye**
　　H35.122 **Retinopathy of prematurity, stage 1,** left **eye**
　　H35.123 **Retinopathy of prematurity, stage 1,** bilateral
　　H35.129 **Retinopathy of prematurity, stage 1,** unspecified **eye**

✓6th **H35.13** **Retinopathy of prematurity,** stage 2
　　H35.131 **Retinopathy of prematurity, stage 2,** right **eye**
　　H35.132 **Retinopathy of prematurity, stage 2,** left **eye**
　　H35.133 **Retinopathy of prematurity, stage 2,** bilateral
　　H35.139 **Retinopathy of prematurity, stage 2,** unspecified **eye**

✓6th **H35.14** **Retinopathy of prematurity,** stage 3
　　H35.141 **Retinopathy of prematurity, stage 3,** right **eye**
　　H35.142 **Retinopathy of prematurity, stage 3,** left **eye**
　　H35.143 **Retinopathy of prematurity, stage 3,** bilateral
　　H35.149 **Retinopathy of prematurity, stage 3,** unspecified **eye**

✓6th **H35.15** **Retinopathy of prematurity,** stage 4
　　H35.151 **Retinopathy of prematurity, stage 4,** right **eye**
　　H35.152 **Retinopathy of prematurity, stage 4,** left **eye**
　　H35.153 **Retinopathy of prematurity, stage 4,** bilateral
　　H35.159 **Retinopathy of prematurity, stage 4,** unspecified **eye**

✓6th **H35.16** **Retinopathy of prematurity,** stage 5
　　H35.161 **Retinopathy of prematurity, stage 5,** right **eye**
　　H35.162 **Retinopathy of prematurity, stage 5,** left **eye**
　　H35.163 **Retinopathy of prematurity, stage 5,** bilateral

　　H35.169 **Retinopathy of prematurity, stage 5,** unspecified **eye**

✓6th **H35.17** **Retrolental fibroplasia**
　　H35.171 **Retrolental fibroplasia,** right **eye**
　　H35.172 **Retrolental fibroplasia,** left **eye**
　　H35.173 **Retrolental fibroplasia,** bilateral
　　H35.179 **Retrolental fibroplasia,** unspecified **eye**

✓5th **H35.2** **Other non-diabetic proliferative retinopathy**
Proliferative vitreo-retinopathy
EXCLUDES 1 *proliferative vitreo-retinopathy with retinal detachment (H33.4-)*
　　H35.20 **Other non-diabetic proliferative retinopathy,** unspecified **eye**
　　H35.21 **Other non-diabetic proliferative retinopathy,** right **eye**
　　H35.22 **Other non-diabetic proliferative retinopathy,** left **eye**
　　H35.23 **Other non-diabetic proliferative retinopathy,** bilateral

✓5th **H35.3** **Degeneration of macula and posterior pole**
　　H35.30 **Unspecified macular degeneration** Ⓐ
Age-related macular degeneration
　　H35.31 **Nonexudative age-related macular degeneration** Ⓐ
Atrophic age-related macular degeneration
　　H35.32 **Exudative age-related macular degeneration** Ⓐ
　　H35.33 **Angioid streaks of macula**

✓6th **H35.34** **Macular cyst, hole, or pseudohole**
　　H35.341 **Macular cyst, hole, or pseudohole,** right **eye**
　　H35.342 **Macular cyst, hole, or pseudohole,** left **eye**
　　H35.343 **Macular cyst, hole, or pseudohole,** bilateral
　　H35.349 **Macular cyst, hole, or pseudohole,** unspecified **eye**

✓6th **H35.35** **Cystoid macular degeneration**
EXCLUDES 1 *cystoid macular edema following cataract surgery (H59.03-)*
　　H35.351 **Cystoid macular degeneration,** right **eye**
　　H35.352 **Cystoid macular degeneration,** left **eye**
　　H35.353 **Cystoid macular degeneration,** bilateral
　　H35.359 **Cystoid macular degeneration,** unspecified **eye**

✓6th **H35.36** **Drusen (degenerative) of macula**
　　H35.361 **Drusen (degenerative) of macula,** right **eye**
　　H35.362 **Drusen (degenerative) of macula,** left **eye**
　　H35.363 **Drusen (degenerative) of macula,** bilateral
　　H35.369 **Drusen (degenerative) of macula,** unspecified **eye**

✓6th **H35.37** **Puckering of macula**
　　H35.371 **Puckering of macula,** right **eye**
　　H35.372 **Puckering of macula,** left **eye**
　　H35.373 **Puckering of macula,** bilateral
　　H35.379 **Puckering of macula,** unspecified **eye**

✓6th **H35.38** **Toxic maculopathy**
Code first poisoning due to drug or toxin, if applicable (T36-T65 with fifth or sixth character 1-4 or 6)
Use additional code for adverse effect, if applicable, to identify drug (T36-T50 with fifth or sixth character 5)
　　H35.381 **Toxic maculopathy,** right **eye**
　　H35.382 **Toxic maculopathy,** left **eye**
　　H35.383 **Toxic maculopathy,** bilateral
　　H35.389 **Toxic maculopathy,** unspecified **eye**

✓5th **H35.4** **Peripheral retinal degeneration**
EXCLUDES 1 *hereditary retinal degeneration (dystrophy) (H35.5-)*
peripheral retinal degeneration with retinal break (H33.3-)
　　H35.40 **Unspecified peripheral retinal degeneration**

✓6th **H35.41** **Lattice degeneration of retina**
Palisade degeneration of retina
　　H35.411 **Lattice degeneration of retina,** right **eye**
　　H35.412 **Lattice degeneration of retina,** left **eye**
　　H35.413 **Lattice degeneration of retina,** bilateral

H35.419   **Lattice** degeneration of retina, **unspecified eye**

✓6ᵗʰ **H35.42**   **Microcystoid** degeneration of retina

H35.421   **Microcystoid** degeneration of retina, **right eye**

H35.422   **Microcystoid** degeneration of retina, **left eye**

H35.423   **Microcystoid** degeneration of retina, **bilateral**

H35.429   **Microcystoid** degeneration of retina, **unspecified eye**

✓6ᵗʰ **H35.43**   **Paving stone** degeneration of retina

H35.431   **Paving stone** degeneration of retina, **right eye**

H35.432   **Paving stone** degeneration of retina, **left eye**

H35.433   **Paving stone** degeneration of retina, **bilateral**

H35.439   **Paving stone** degeneration of retina, **unspecified eye**

✓6ᵗʰ **H35.44**   **Age-related reticular** degeneration of retina

H35.441   **Age-related reticular** degeneration of retina, **right eye**   Ⓐ

H35.442   **Age-related reticular** degeneration of retina, **left eye**   Ⓐ

H35.443   **Age-related reticular** degeneration of retina, **bilateral**   Ⓐ

H35.449   **Age-related reticular** degeneration of retina, **unspecified eye**   Ⓐ

✓6ᵗʰ **H35.45**   **Secondary pigmentary** degeneration

H35.451   **Secondary pigmentary** degeneration, **right eye**

H35.452   **Secondary pigmentary** degeneration, **left eye**

H35.453   **Secondary pigmentary** degeneration, **bilateral**

H35.459   **Secondary pigmentary** degeneration, **unspecified eye**

✓6ᵗʰ **H35.46**   **Secondary vitreoretinal** degeneration

H35.461   **Secondary vitreoretinal** degeneration, **right eye**

H35.462   **Secondary vitreoretinal** degeneration, **left eye**

H35.463   **Secondary vitreoretinal** degeneration, **bilateral**

H35.469   **Secondary vitreoretinal** degeneration, **unspecified eye**

✓5ᵗʰ **H35.5**   **Hereditary retinal dystrophy**

EXCLUDES 1   *dystrophies primarily involving Bruch's membrane (H31.1-)*

H35.50   **Unspecified hereditary retinal dystrophy**

H35.51   **Vitreoretinal dystrophy**

H35.52   **Pigmentary retinal dystrophy**
Albipunctate retinal dystrophy
Retinitis pigmentosa
Tapetoretinal dystrophy

H35.53   **Other dystrophies primarily involving the sensory retina**
Stargardt's disease

H35.54   **Dystrophies primarily involving the retinal pigment epithelium**
Vitelliform retinal dystrophy

✓5ᵗʰ **H35.6**   **Retinal hemorrhage**

H35.60   **Retinal hemorrhage, unspecified eye**

H35.61   **Retinal hemorrhage, right eye**

H35.62   **Retinal hemorrhage, left eye**

H35.63   **Retinal hemorrhage, bilateral**

✓5ᵗʰ **H35.7**   **Separation of retinal layers**

EXCLUDES 1   *retinal detachment (serous) (H33.2-)*
rhegmatogenous retinal detachment (H33.0-)

CC Excl: For CC codes in subcategory H35.7, unless otherwise noted: H33.001-H33.119, H33.191-H33.8, H35.70-H35.739

H35.70   **Unspecified separation of retinal layers**   cc

✓6ᵗʰ **H35.71**   **Central serous chorioretinopathy**

H35.711   **Central serous chorioretinopathy, right eye**

H35.712   **Central serous chorioretinopathy, left eye**

H35.713   **Central serous chorioretinopathy, bilateral**

H35.719   **Central serous chorioretinopathy, unspecified eye**

✓6ᵗʰ **H35.72**   **Serous detachment of retinal pigment epithelium**

H35.721   **Serous detachment of retinal pigment epithelium, right eye**   cc

H35.722   **Serous detachment of retinal pigment epithelium, left eye**   cc

H35.723   **Serous detachment of retinal pigment epithelium, bilateral**   cc

H35.729   **Serous detachment of retinal pigment epithelium, unspecified eye**   cc

✓6ᵗʰ **H35.73**   **Hemorrhagic detachment of retinal pigment epithelium**

H35.731   **Hemorrhagic detachment of retinal pigment epithelium, right eye**   cc

H35.732   **Hemorrhagic detachment of retinal pigment epithelium, left eye**   cc

H35.733   **Hemorrhagic detachment of retinal pigment epithelium, bilateral**   cc

H35.739   **Hemorrhagic detachment of retinal pigment epithelium, unspecified eye**   cc

✓5ᵗʰ **H35.8**   **Other specified retinal disorders**

EXCLUDES 2   *retinal hemorrhage (H35.6-)*

H35.81   **Retinal edema**
Retinal cotton wool spots

H35.82   **Retinal ischemia**   cc
CC Excl: H35.60-H35.63, H35.81-H35.89

H35.89   **Other specified retinal disorders**

H35.9   **Unspecified retinal disorder**

H36   **Retinal disorders in diseases classified elsewhere**
Code first underlying disease, such as:
  lipid storage disorders (E75.-)
  sickle-cell disorders (D57.-)

EXCLUDES 1   *arteriosclerotic retinopathy (H35.0-)*
diabetic retinopathy (E08.3-, E09.3-, E10.3-, E11.3-, E13.3-)

Glaucoma (H40-H42)

✓4ᵗʰ **H40**   **Glaucoma**

EXCLUDES 1   *absolute glaucoma (H44.51-)*
congenital glaucoma (Q15.0)
traumatic glaucoma due to birth injury (P15.3)

✓5ᵗʰ **H40.0**   **Glaucoma suspect**

✓6ᵗʰ **H40.00**   **Preglaucoma, unspecified**

H40.001   **Preglaucoma, unspecified, right eye**

H40.002   **Preglaucoma, unspecified, left eye**

H40.003   **Preglaucoma, unspecified, bilateral**

H40.009   **Preglaucoma, unspecified, unspecified eye**

✓6ᵗʰ **H40.01**   **Open angle with borderline findings, low risk**
Open angle, low risk

H40.011   **Open angle with borderline findings, low risk, right eye**

H40.012   **Open angle with borderline findings, low risk, left eye**

H40.013   **Open angle with borderline findings, low risk, bilateral**

H40.019   **Open angle with borderline findings, low risk, unspecified eye**

✓6ᵗʰ **H40.02**   **Open angle with borderline findings, high risk**
Open angle, high risk

H40.021   **Open angle with borderline findings, high risk, right eye**

H40.022   **Open angle with borderline findings, high risk, left eye**

H40.023   **Open angle with borderline findings, high risk, bilateral**

H40.029   **Open angle with borderline findings, high risk, unspecified eye**

Ⓝ Newborn: 0   Ⓟ Pediatric: 0-17   Ⓜ Maternity: 12-55   Ⓐ Adult: 15-124   **MCC** Major CC Condition   **PDx MCC** PDx acts as own MCC   **CC** CC Condition   **PDx CC** PDx acts as own CC

568   ICD-10-CM Draft (2015)

✓6ᵗʰ **H40.03** Anatomical narrow angle
　　　Primary angle closure suspect
　　　H40.031 Anatomical narrow angle, right eye
　　　H40.032 Anatomical narrow angle, left eye
　　　H40.033 Anatomical narrow angle, bilateral
　　　H40.039 Anatomical narrow angle, unspecified eye

✓6ᵗʰ **H40.04** Steroid responder
　　　H40.041 Steroid responder, right eye
　　　H40.042 Steroid responder, left eye
　　　H40.043 Steroid responder, bilateral
　　　H40.049 Steroid responder, unspecified eye

✓6ᵗʰ **H40.05** Ocular hypertension
　　　H40.051 Ocular hypertension, right eye
　　　H40.052 Ocular hypertension, left eye
　　　H40.053 Ocular hypertension, bilateral
　　　H40.059 Ocular hypertension, unspecified eye

✓6ᵗʰ **H40.06** Primary angle closure without glaucoma damage
　　　H40.061 Primary angle closure without glaucoma damage, right eye
　　　H40.062 Primary angle closure without glaucoma damage, left eye
　　　H40.063 Primary angle closure without glaucoma damage, bilateral
　　　H40.069 Primary angle closure without glaucoma damage, unspecified eye

✓5ᵗʰ **H40.1** Open-angle glaucoma

> One of the following 7th characters is to be assigned to each code in subcategories H40.10, H40.11, H40.12-, H40.13-, and H40.14- to designate the stage of glaucoma.
> Ø　stage unspecified
> 1　mild stage
> 2　moderate stage
> 3　severe stage
> 4　indeterminate stage

✓x7ᵗʰ **H40.10** Unspecified open-angle glaucoma

✓x7ᵗʰ **H40.11** Primary open-angle glaucoma
　　　Chronic simple glaucoma

✓6ᵗʰ **H40.12** Low-tension glaucoma
　✓7ᵗʰ **H40.121** Low-tension glaucoma, right eye
　✓7ᵗʰ **H40.122** Low-tension glaucoma, left eye
　✓7ᵗʰ **H40.123** Low-tension glaucoma, bilateral
　✓7ᵗʰ **H40.129** Low-tension glaucoma, unspecified eye

✓6ᵗʰ **H40.13** Pigmentary glaucoma
　✓7ᵗʰ **H40.131** Pigmentary glaucoma, right eye
　✓7ᵗʰ **H40.132** Pigmentary glaucoma, left eye
　✓7ᵗʰ **H40.133** Pigmentary glaucoma, bilateral
　✓7ᵗʰ **H40.139** Pigmentary glaucoma, unspecified eye

✓6ᵗʰ **H40.14** Capsular glaucoma with pseudoexfoliation of lens
　✓7ᵗʰ **H40.141** Capsular glaucoma with pseudoexfoliation of lens, right eye
　✓7ᵗʰ **H40.142** Capsular glaucoma with pseudoexfoliation of lens, left eye
　✓7ᵗʰ **H40.143** Capsular glaucoma with pseudoexfoliation of lens, bilateral
　✓7ᵗʰ **H40.149** Capsular glaucoma with pseudoexfoliation of lens, unspecified eye

✓6ᵗʰ **H40.15** Residual stage of open-angle glaucoma
　　　H40.151 Residual stage of open-angle glaucoma, right eye
　　　H40.152 Residual stage of open-angle glaucoma, left eye
　　　H40.153 Residual stage of open-angle glaucoma, bilateral
　　　H40.159 Residual stage of open-angle glaucoma, unspecified eye

✓5ᵗʰ **H40.2** Primary angle-closure glaucoma

> **EXCLUDES 1**　aqueous misdirection (H40.83-)
> 　　　　　　malignant glaucoma (H40.83-)

> One of the following 7th characters is to be assigned to each code in subcategories H40.20 and H40.22- to designate the stage of glaucoma.
> Ø　stage unspecified
> 1　mild stage
> 2　moderate stage
> 3　severe stage
> 4　indeterminate stage

> **CC Excl:** For CC codes in subcategory H40.2, unless otherwise noted: H40.211-H40.219

✓x7ᵗʰ **H40.20** Unspecified primary angle-closure glaucoma

✓6ᵗʰ **H40.21** Acute angle-closure glaucoma
　　　Acute angle-closure glaucoma attack
　　　Acute angle-closure glaucoma crisis
　　　H40.211 Acute angle-closure glaucoma, right eye　**CC**
　　　H40.212 Acute angle-closure glaucoma, left eye　**CC**
　　　H40.213 Acute angle-closure glaucoma, bilateral　**CC**
　　　H40.219 Acute angle-closure glaucoma, unspecified eye　**CC**

✓6ᵗʰ **H40.22** Chronic angle-closure glaucoma
　　　Chronic primary angle-closure glaucoma
　✓7ᵗʰ **H40.221** Chronic angle-closure glaucoma, right eye
　✓7ᵗʰ **H40.222** Chronic angle-closure glaucoma, left eye
　✓7ᵗʰ **H40.223** Chronic angle-closure glaucoma, bilateral
　✓7ᵗʰ **H40.229** Chronic angle-closure glaucoma, unspecified eye

✓6ᵗʰ **H40.23** Intermittent angle-closure glaucoma
　　　H40.231 Intermittent angle-closure glaucoma, right eye
　　　H40.232 Intermittent angle-closure glaucoma, left eye
　　　H40.233 Intermittent angle-closure glaucoma, bilateral
　　　H40.239 Intermittent angle-closure glaucoma, unspecified eye

✓6ᵗʰ **H40.24** Residual stage of angle-closure glaucoma
　　　H40.241 Residual stage of angle-closure glaucoma, right eye
　　　H40.242 Residual stage of angle-closure glaucoma, left eye
　　　H40.243 Residual stage of angle-closure glaucoma, bilateral
　　　H40.249 Residual stage of angle-closure glaucoma, unspecified eye

✓5ᵗʰ **H40.3** Glaucoma secondary to eye trauma
　　　Code also underlying condition

> One of the following 7th characters is to be assigned to each code in subcategory H40.3- to designate the stage of glaucoma.
> Ø　stage unspecified
> 1　mild stage
> 2　moderate stage
> 3　severe stage
> 4　indeterminate stage

✓x7ᵗʰ **H40.30** Glaucoma secondary to eye trauma, unspecified eye
✓x7ᵗʰ **H40.31** Glaucoma secondary to eye trauma, right eye
✓x7ᵗʰ **H40.32** Glaucoma secondary to eye trauma, left eye
✓x7ᵗʰ **H40.33** Glaucoma secondary to eye trauma, bilateral

✓5ᵗʰ **H40.4** Glaucoma secondary to eye inflammation
　　　Code also underlying condition

> One of the following 7th characters is to be assigned to each code in subcategory H40.4- to designate the stage of glaucoma.
> Ø　stage unspecified
> 1　mild stage
> 2　moderate stage
> 3　severe stage
> 4　indeterminate stage

☑ Additional Character Required　✓x7ᵗʰ Xtension Alert　Unacceptable PDx　Manifestation　Hospital Acquired Condition　**EXCLUDES 1** Not Coded Here　**EXCLUDES 2** Not Included Here

√x7ᵗʰ **H40.40 Glaucoma secondary to eye inflammation, unspecified eye**

√x7ᵗʰ **H40.41 Glaucoma secondary to eye inflammation, right eye**

√x7ᵗʰ **H40.42 Glaucoma secondary to eye inflammation, left eye**

√x7ᵗʰ **H40.43 Glaucoma secondary to eye inflammation, bilateral**

√5ᵗʰ **H40.5 Glaucoma secondary to other eye disorders**
Code also underlying eye disorder

One of the following 7th characters is to be assigned to each code in subcategory H40.5- to designate the stage of glaucoma.
Ø stage unspecified
1 mild stage
2 moderate stage
3 severe stage
4 indeterminate stage

√x7ᵗʰ **H40.50 Glaucoma secondary to other eye disorders, unspecified eye**

√x7ᵗʰ **H40.51 Glaucoma secondary to other eye disorders, right eye**

√x7ᵗʰ **H40.52 Glaucoma secondary to other eye disorders, left eye**

√x7ᵗʰ **H40.53 Glaucoma secondary to other eye disorders, bilateral**

√5ᵗʰ **H40.6 Glaucoma secondary to drugs**
Use additional code for adverse effect, if applicable, to identify drug (T36-T50 with fifth or sixth character 5)

One of the following 7th characters is to be assigned to each code in subcategory H40.6- to designate the stage of glaucoma.
Ø stage unspecified
1 mild stage
2 moderate stage
3 severe stage
4 indeterminate stage

√x7ᵗʰ **H40.60 Glaucoma secondary to drugs, unspecified eye**

√x7ᵗʰ **H40.61 Glaucoma secondary to drugs, right eye**

√x7ᵗʰ **H40.62 Glaucoma secondary to drugs, left eye**

√x7ᵗʰ **H40.63 Glaucoma secondary to drugs, bilateral**

√5ᵗʰ **H40.8 Other glaucoma**

√6ᵗʰ **H40.81 Glaucoma with increased episcleral venous pressure**

H40.811 Glaucoma with increased episcleral venous pressure, right eye

H40.812 Glaucoma with increased episcleral venous pressure, left eye

H40.813 Glaucoma with increased episcleral venous pressure, bilateral

H40.819 Glaucoma with increased episcleral venous pressure, unspecified eye

√6ᵗʰ **H40.82 Hypersecretion glaucoma**

H40.821 Hypersecretion glaucoma, right eye

H40.822 Hypersecretion glaucoma, left eye

H40.823 Hypersecretion glaucoma, bilateral

H40.829 Hypersecretion glaucoma, unspecified eye

√6ᵗʰ **H40.83 Aqueous misdirection**
Malignant glaucoma

H40.831 Aqueous misdirection, right eye

H40.832 Aqueous misdirection, left eye

H40.833 Aqueous misdirection, bilateral

H40.839 Aqueous misdirection, unspecified eye

H40.89 Other specified glaucoma

H40.9 Unspecified glaucoma

H42 *Glaucoma in diseases classified elsewhere*
Code first underlying condition, such as:
amyloidosis (E85.-)
aniridia (Q13.1)
Lowe's syndrome (E72.03)
Reiger's anomaly (Q13.81)
specified metabolic disorder (E70-E88)
EXCLUDES 1 *glaucoma (in):*
diabetes mellitus (E08.39, E09.39, E10.39, E11.39, E13.39)
onchocerciasis (B73.02)
syphilis (A52.71)
tuberculous (A18.59)

Disorders of vitreous body and globe (H43-H44)

√4ᵗʰ **H43 Disorders of vitreous body**

√5ᵗʰ **H43.0 Vitreous prolapse**
EXCLUDES 1 *traumatic vitreous prolapse (S05.2-)*
vitreous syndrome following cataract surgery (H59.0-)

H43.00 Vitreous prolapse, unspecified eye

H43.01 Vitreous prolapse, right eye

H43.02 Vitreous prolapse, left eye

H43.03 Vitreous prolapse, bilateral

√5ᵗʰ **H43.1 Vitreous hemorrhage**

H43.10 Vitreous hemorrhage, unspecified eye

H43.11 Vitreous hemorrhage, right eye

H43.12 Vitreous hemorrhage, left eye

H43.13 Vitreous hemorrhage, bilateral

√5ᵗʰ **H43.2 Crystalline deposits in vitreous body**

H43.20 Crystalline deposits in vitreous body, unspecified eye

H43.21 Crystalline deposits in vitreous body, right eye

H43.22 Crystalline deposits in vitreous body, left eye

H43.23 Crystalline deposits in vitreous body, bilateral

√5ᵗʰ **H43.3 Other vitreous opacities**

√6ᵗʰ **H43.31 Vitreous membranes and strands**

H43.311 Vitreous membranes and strands, right eye

H43.312 Vitreous membranes and strands, left eye

H43.313 Vitreous membranes and strands, bilateral

H43.319 Vitreous membranes and strands, unspecified eye

√6ᵗʰ **H43.39 Other vitreous opacities**
Vitreous floaters

H43.391 Other vitreous opacities, right eye

H43.392 Other vitreous opacities, left eye

H43.393 Other vitreous opacities, bilateral

H43.399 Other vitreous opacities, unspecified eye

√5ᵗʰ **H43.8 Other disorders of vitreous body**
EXCLUDES 1 *proliferative vitreo-retinopathy with retinal detachment (H33.4-)*
EXCLUDES 2 *vitreous abscess (H44.02-)*

√6ᵗʰ **H43.81 Vitreous degeneration**
Vitreous detachment

H43.811 Vitreous degeneration, right eye

H43.812 Vitreous degeneration, left eye

H43.813 Vitreous degeneration, bilateral

H43.819 Vitreous degeneration, unspecified eye

√6ᵗʰ **H43.82 Vitreomacular adhesion**
Vitreomacular traction

H43.821 Vitreomacular adhesion, right eye A

H43.822 Vitreomacular adhesion, left eye A

H43.823 Vitreomacular adhesion, bilateral A

H43.829 Vitreomacular adhesion, unspecified eye A

H43.89 Other disorders of vitreous body

H43.9 Unspecified disorder of vitreous body

√4ᵗʰ **H44 Disorders of globe**
INCLUDES disorders affecting multiple structures of eye

√5ᵗʰ **H44.0 Purulent endophthalmitis**
Use additional code to identify organism
EXCLUDES 1 *bleb associated endophthalmitis (H59.4-)*

√6ᵗʰ **H44.00 Unspecified purulent endophthalmitis**

CC Excl: For CC codes in subcategory H44.00, unless otherwise noted: H20.051-H20.059, H21.331-H21.339, H33.121-H33.129, H44.001-H44.029, H44.121-H44.129, H44.19

H44.001 Unspecified purulent endophthalmitis, right eye CC

H44.002 Unspecified purulent endophthalmitis, left eye CC

H44.003 Unspecified purulent endophthalmitis, bilateral CC

H44.009 Unspecified purulent endophthalmitis, unspecified eye CC

N Newborn: Ø   P Pediatric: Ø-17   M Maternity: 12-55   A Adult: 15-124   MCC Major CC Condition   PDx MCC PDx acts as own MCC   CC CC Condition   PDx CC PDx acts as own CC

570   ICD-10-CM Draft (2015)

√6ᵗʰ **H44.01 Panophthalmitis (acute)**

> **CC Excl:** For CC codes in subcategory H44.01, unless otherwise noted: H20.051-H20.059, H21.331-H21.339, H33.121-H33.129, H44.001-H44.029, H44.121-H44.129, H44.19

  H44.011 Panophthalmitis (acute), right eye `CC`
  H44.012 Panophthalmitis (acute), left eye `CC`
  H44.013 Panophthalmitis (acute), bilateral `CC`
  H44.019 Panophthalmitis (acute), unspecified eye `CC`

√6ᵗʰ **H44.02 Vitreous abscess (chronic)**

> **CC Excl:** For CC codes in subcategory H44.02, unless otherwise noted: H16.241-H16.249, H21.331-H21.339, H33.121-H33.129, H44.001-H44.19

  H44.021 Vitreous abscess (chronic), right eye `CC`
  H44.022 Vitreous abscess (chronic), left eye `CC`
  H44.023 Vitreous abscess (chronic), bilateral `CC`
  H44.029 Vitreous abscess (chronic), unspecified eye `CC`

√5ᵗʰ **H44.1 Other endophthalmitis**
  EXCLUDES 1 bleb associated endophthalmitis (H59.4-)
  EXCLUDES 2 ophthalmia nodosa (H16.2-)

√6ᵗʰ **H44.11 Panuveitis**

> **CC Excl:** For CC codes in subcategory H44.11, unless otherwise noted: H44.111-H44.119, H44.131-H44.139

  H44.111 Panuveitis, right eye `CC`
  H44.112 Panuveitis, left eye `CC`
  H44.113 Panuveitis, bilateral `CC`
  H44.119 Panuveitis, unspecified eye `CC`

√6ᵗʰ **H44.12 Parasitic endophthalmitis, unspecified**

> **CC Excl:** For CC codes in subcategory H44.12, unless otherwise noted: H20.051-H20.059, H21.331-H21.339, H33.121-H33.129, H44.001-H44.029, H44.121-H44.129, H44.19

  H44.121 Parasitic endophthalmitis, unspecified, right eye `CC`
  H44.122 Parasitic endophthalmitis, unspecified, left eye `CC`
  H44.123 Parasitic endophthalmitis, unspecified, bilateral `CC`
  H44.129 Parasitic endophthalmitis, unspecified, unspecified eye `CC`

√6ᵗʰ **H44.13 Sympathetic uveitis**

> **CC Excl:** For CC codes in subcategory H44.13 unless otherwise noted: H44.111-H44.119, H44.131-H44.139

  H44.131 Sympathetic uveitis, right eye `CC`
  H44.132 Sympathetic uveitis, left eye `CC`
  H44.133 Sympathetic uveitis, bilateral `CC`
  H44.139 Sympathetic uveitis, unspecified eye `CC`

  H44.19 Other endophthalmitis `CC`
  CC Excl: H20.051-H20.059, H21.331-H21.339, H33.121-H33.129, H44.001-H44.029, H44.121-H44.129, H44.19

√5ᵗʰ **H44.2 Degenerative myopia**
  Malignant myopia
  H44.20 Degenerative myopia, unspecified eye
  H44.21 Degenerative myopia, right eye
  H44.22 Degenerative myopia, left eye
  H44.23 Degenerative myopia, bilateral

√5ᵗʰ **H44.3 Other and unspecified degenerative disorders of globe**
  H44.30 Unspecified degenerative disorder of globe
√6ᵗʰ **H44.31 Chalcosis**
  H44.311 Chalcosis, right eye
  H44.312 Chalcosis, left eye
  H44.313 Chalcosis, bilateral
  H44.319 Chalcosis, unspecified eye

√6ᵗʰ **H44.32 Siderosis of eye**
  H44.321 Siderosis of eye, right eye
  H44.322 Siderosis of eye, left eye
  H44.323 Siderosis of eye, bilateral
  H44.329 Siderosis of eye, unspecified eye
√6ᵗʰ **H44.39 Other degenerative disorders of globe**
  H44.391 Other degenerative disorders of globe, right eye
  H44.392 Other degenerative disorders of globe, left eye
  H44.393 Other degenerative disorders of globe, bilateral
  H44.399 Other degenerative disorders of globe, unspecified eye

√5ᵗʰ **H44.4 Hypotony of eye**
  H44.40 Unspecified hypotony of eye
√6ᵗʰ **H44.41 Flat anterior chamber hypotony of eye**
  H44.411 Flat anterior chamber hypotony of right eye
  H44.412 Flat anterior chamber hypotony of left eye
  H44.413 Flat anterior chamber hypotony of eye, bilateral
  H44.419 Flat anterior chamber hypotony of unspecified eye
√6ᵗʰ **H44.42 Hypotony of eye due to ocular fistula**
  H44.421 Hypotony of right eye due to ocular fistula
  H44.422 Hypotony of left eye due to ocular fistula
  H44.423 Hypotony of eye due to ocular fistula, bilateral
  H44.429 Hypotony of unspecified eye due to ocular fistula
√6ᵗʰ **H44.43 Hypotony of eye due to other ocular disorders**
  H44.431 Hypotony of eye due to other ocular disorders, right eye
  H44.432 Hypotony of eye due to other ocular disorders, left eye
  H44.433 Hypotony of eye due to other ocular disorders, bilateral
  H44.439 Hypotony of eye due to other ocular disorders, unspecified eye
√6ᵗʰ **H44.44 Primary hypotony of eye**
  H44.441 Primary hypotony of right eye
  H44.442 Primary hypotony of left eye
  H44.443 Primary hypotony of eye, bilateral
  H44.449 Primary hypotony of unspecified eye

√5ᵗʰ **H44.5 Degenerated conditions of globe**
  H44.50 Unspecified degenerated conditions of globe
√6ᵗʰ **H44.51 Absolute glaucoma**
  H44.511 Absolute glaucoma, right eye
  H44.512 Absolute glaucoma, left eye
  H44.513 Absolute glaucoma, bilateral
  H44.519 Absolute glaucoma, unspecified eye
√6ᵗʰ **H44.52 Atrophy of globe**
  Phthisis bulbi
  H44.521 Atrophy of globe, right eye
  H44.522 Atrophy of globe, left eye
  H44.523 Atrophy of globe, bilateral
  H44.529 Atrophy of globe, unspecified eye
√6ᵗʰ **H44.53 Leucocoria**
  H44.531 Leucocoria, right eye
  H44.532 Leucocoria, left eye
  H44.533 Leucocoria, bilateral
  H44.539 Leucocoria, unspecified eye

√5ᵗʰ **H44.6 Retained (old) intraocular foreign body, magnetic**
  Use additional code to identify magnetic foreign body (Z18.11)
  EXCLUDES 1 current intraocular foreign body (S05.-)
  EXCLUDES 2 retained foreign body in eyelid (H02.81-)
        retained (old) foreign body following penetrating wound of orbit (H05.5-)
        retained (old) intraocular foreign body, nonmagnetic (H44.7-)

√6ᵗʰ **H44.60 Unspecified retained (old) intraocular foreign body, magnetic**
  H44.601 Unspecified retained (old) intraocular foreign body, magnetic, right eye

H44.602   Unspecified retained (old) intraocular foreign body, magnetic, left eye

H44.603   Unspecified retained (old) intraocular foreign body, magnetic, bilateral

H44.609   Unspecified retained (old) intraocular foreign body, magnetic, unspecified eye

✓6th H44.61   Retained (old) magnetic foreign body in anterior chamber

    H44.611   Retained (old) magnetic foreign body in anterior chamber, right eye

    H44.612   Retained (old) magnetic foreign body in anterior chamber, left eye

    H44.613   Retained (old) magnetic foreign body in anterior chamber, bilateral

    H44.619   Retained (old) magnetic foreign body in anterior chamber, unspecified eye

✓6th H44.62   Retained (old) magnetic foreign body in iris or ciliary body

    H44.621   Retained (old) magnetic foreign body in iris or ciliary body, right eye

    H44.622   Retained (old) magnetic foreign body in iris or ciliary body, left eye

    H44.623   Retained (old) magnetic foreign body in iris or ciliary body, bilateral

    H44.629   Retained (old) magnetic foreign body in iris or ciliary body, unspecified eye

✓6th H44.63   Retained (old) magnetic foreign body in lens

    H44.631   Retained (old) magnetic foreign body in lens, right eye

    H44.632   Retained (old) magnetic foreign body in lens, left eye

    H44.633   Retained (old) magnetic foreign body in lens, bilateral

    H44.639   Retained (old) magnetic foreign body in lens, unspecified eye

✓6th H44.64   Retained (old) magnetic foreign body in posterior wall of globe

    H44.641   Retained (old) magnetic foreign body in posterior wall of globe, right eye

    H44.642   Retained (old) magnetic foreign body in posterior wall of globe, left eye

    H44.643   Retained (old) magnetic foreign body in posterior wall of globe, bilateral

    H44.649   Retained (old) magnetic foreign body in posterior wall of globe, unspecified eye

✓6th H44.65   Retained (old) magnetic foreign body in vitreous body

    H44.651   Retained (old) magnetic foreign body in vitreous body, right eye

    H44.652   Retained (old) magnetic foreign body in vitreous body, left eye

    H44.653   Retained (old) magnetic foreign body in vitreous body, bilateral

    H44.659   Retained (old) magnetic foreign body in vitreous body, unspecified eye

✓6th H44.69   Retained (old) intraocular foreign body, magnetic, in other or multiple sites

    H44.691   Retained (old) intraocular foreign body, magnetic, in other or multiple sites, right eye

    H44.692   Retained (old) intraocular foreign body, magnetic, in other or multiple sites, left eye

    H44.693   Retained (old) intraocular foreign body, magnetic, in other or multiple sites, bilateral

    H44.699   Retained (old) intraocular foreign body, magnetic, in other or multiple sites, unspecified eye

✓5th H44.7   Retained (old) intraocular foreign body, nonmagnetic

Use additional code to identify nonmagnetic foreign body (Z18.01-Z18.10, Z18.12, Z18.2-Z18.9)

EXCLUDES 1   current intraocular foreign body (S05.-)

EXCLUDES 2   retained foreign body in eyelid (H02.81-)
           retained (old) foreign body following penetrating wound of orbit (H05.5-)
           retained (old) intraocular foreign body, magnetic (H44.6-)

✓6th H44.70   Unspecified retained (old) intraocular foreign body, nonmagnetic

    H44.701   Unspecified retained (old) intraocular foreign body, nonmagnetic, right eye

    H44.702   Unspecified retained (old) intraocular foreign body, nonmagnetic, left eye

    H44.703   Unspecified retained (old) intraocular foreign body, nonmagnetic, bilateral

    H44.709   Unspecified retained (old) intraocular foreign body, nonmagnetic, unspecified eye

          Retained (old) intraocular foreign body NOS

✓6th H44.71   Retained (nonmagnetic) (old) foreign body in anterior chamber

    H44.711   Retained (nonmagnetic) (old) foreign body in anterior chamber, right eye

    H44.712   Retained (nonmagnetic) (old) foreign body in anterior chamber, left eye

    H44.713   Retained (nonmagnetic) (old) foreign body in anterior chamber, bilateral

    H44.719   Retained (nonmagnetic) (old) foreign body in anterior chamber, unspecified eye

✓6th H44.72   Retained (nonmagnetic) (old) foreign body in iris or ciliary body

    H44.721   Retained (nonmagnetic) (old) foreign body in iris or ciliary body, right eye

    H44.722   Retained (nonmagnetic) (old) foreign body in iris or ciliary body, left eye

    H44.723   Retained (nonmagnetic) (old) foreign body in iris or ciliary body, bilateral

    H44.729   Retained (nonmagnetic) (old) foreign body in iris or ciliary body, unspecified eye

✓6th H44.73   Retained (nonmagnetic) (old) foreign body in lens

    H44.731   Retained (nonmagnetic) (old) foreign body in lens, right eye

    H44.732   Retained (nonmagnetic) (old) foreign body in lens, left eye

    H44.733   Retained (nonmagnetic) (old) foreign body in lens, bilateral

    H44.739   Retained (nonmagnetic) (old) foreign body in lens, unspecified eye

✓6th H44.74   Retained (nonmagnetic) (old) foreign body in posterior wall of globe

    H44.741   Retained (nonmagnetic) (old) foreign body in posterior wall of globe, right eye

    H44.742   Retained (nonmagnetic) (old) foreign body in posterior wall of globe, left eye

    H44.743   Retained (nonmagnetic) (old) foreign body in posterior wall of globe, bilateral

    H44.749   Retained (nonmagnetic) (old) foreign body in posterior wall of globe, unspecified eye

✓6th H44.75   Retained (nonmagnetic) (old) foreign body in vitreous body

    H44.751   Retained (nonmagnetic) (old) foreign body in vitreous body, right eye

    H44.752   Retained (nonmagnetic) (old) foreign body in vitreous body, left eye

    H44.753   Retained (nonmagnetic) (old) foreign body in vitreous body, bilateral

    H44.759   Retained (nonmagnetic) (old) foreign body in vitreous body, unspecified eye

✓6th H44.79   Retained (old) intraocular foreign body, nonmagnetic, in other or multiple sites

    H44.791   Retained (old) intraocular foreign body, nonmagnetic, in other or multiple sites, right eye

N Newborn: 0   P Pediatric: 0-17   M Maternity: 12-55   A Adult: 15-124   MCC Major CC Condition   PDx MCC PDx acts as own MCC   CC CC Condition   PDx CC PDx acts as own CC

572   ICD-10-CM Draft (2015)

H44.792 Retained (old) intraocular foreign body, nonmagnetic, in other or multiple sites, left eye

H44.793 Retained (old) intraocular foreign body, nonmagnetic, in other or multiple sites, bilateral

H44.799 Retained (old) intraocular foreign body, nonmagnetic, in other or multiple sites, unspecified eye

√5th **H44.8 Other disorders of globe**

√6th **H44.81 Hemophthalmos**

H44.811 Hemophthalmos, right eye

H44.812 Hemophthalmos, left eye

H44.813 Hemophthalmos, bilateral

H44.819 Hemophthalmos, unspecified eye

√6th **H44.82 Luxation of globe**

H44.821 Luxation of globe, right eye

H44.822 Luxation of globe, left eye

H44.823 Luxation of globe, bilateral

H44.829 Luxation of globe, unspecified eye

H44.89 Other disorders of globe

H44.9 Unspecified disorder of globe

Disorders of optic nerve and visual pathways (H46-H47)

√4th **H46 Optic neuritis**

EXCLUDES 2 ischemic optic neuropathy (H47.01-)
neuromyelitis optica [Devic] (G36.0)

CC Excl: For CC codes in category H46, unless otherwise noted: H46.00-H46.9

√5th **H46.0 Optic papillitis**

H46.00 Optic papillitis, unspecified eye CC

H46.01 Optic papillitis, right eye CC

H46.02 Optic papillitis, left eye CC

H46.03 Optic papillitis, bilateral CC

√5th **H46.1 Retrobulbar neuritis**

Retrobulbar neuritis NOS

EXCLUDES 1 syphilitic retrobulbar neuritis (A52.15)

H46.10 Retrobulbar neuritis, unspecified eye CC

H46.11 Retrobulbar neuritis, right eye CC

H46.12 Retrobulbar neuritis, left eye CC

H46.13 Retrobulbar neuritis, bilateral CC

H46.2 Nutritional optic neuropathy

H46.3 Toxic optic neuropathy

Code first (T51-T65) to identify cause

H46.8 Other optic neuritis CC

H46.9 Unspecified optic neuritis CC

√4th **H47 Other disorders of optic [2nd] nerve and visual pathways**

√5th **H47.0 Disorders of optic nerve, not elsewhere classified**

√6th **H47.01 Ischemic optic neuropathy**

H47.011 Ischemic optic neuropathy, right eye

H47.012 Ischemic optic neuropathy, left eye

H47.013 Ischemic optic neuropathy, bilateral

H47.019 Ischemic optic neuropathy, unspecified eye

√6th **H47.02 Hemorrhage in optic nerve sheath**

H47.021 Hemorrhage in optic nerve sheath, right eye

H47.022 Hemorrhage in optic nerve sheath, left eye

H47.023 Hemorrhage in optic nerve sheath, bilateral

H47.029 Hemorrhage in optic nerve sheath, unspecified eye

√6th **H47.03 Optic nerve hypoplasia**

H47.031 Optic nerve hypoplasia, right eye

H47.032 Optic nerve hypoplasia, left eye

H47.033 Optic nerve hypoplasia, bilateral

H47.039 Optic nerve hypoplasia, unspecified eye

√6th **H47.09 Other disorders of optic nerve, not elsewhere classified**

Compression of optic nerve

H47.091 Other disorders of optic nerve, not elsewhere classified, right eye

H47.092 Other disorders of optic nerve, not elsewhere classified, left eye

H47.093 Other disorders of optic nerve, not elsewhere classified, bilateral

H47.099 Other disorders of optic nerve, not elsewhere classified, unspecified eye

√5th **H47.1 Papilledema**

H47.10 Unspecified papilledema CC
CC Excl: A17.9, A18.50-A18.59, A18.82, A18.84, A18.89, A39.82, E08.311-E08.39, E08.618-E08.638, E08.649-E08.8, E09.311-E09.39, E09.618-E09.638, E09.649-E09.8, E10.311-E10.39, E10.618-E10.638, E10.649, E10.69-E10.8, E11.311-E11.39, E11.618-E11.638, E11.649, E11.69-E11.8, E13.311-E13.39, E13.618-E13.638, E13.649-E13.8, H47.10-H47.13, H47.231-H47.239, H47.331-H47.339, H57.8-H57.9, H59.40-H59.43, Q11.3, Q15.8-Q15.9

H47.11 Papilledema associated with increased intracranial pressure CC
CC Excl: See code: H47.10

H47.12 Papilledema associated with decreased ocular pressure

H47.13 Papilledema associated with retinal disorder

√6th **H47.14 Foster-Kennedy syndrome**

H47.141 Foster-Kennedy syndrome, right eye

H47.142 Foster-Kennedy syndrome, left eye

H47.143 Foster-Kennedy syndrome, bilateral

H47.149 Foster-Kennedy syndrome, unspecified eye

√5th **H47.2 Optic atrophy**

H47.20 Unspecified optic atrophy

√6th **H47.21 Primary optic atrophy**

H47.211 Primary optic atrophy, right eye

H47.212 Primary optic atrophy, left eye

H47.213 Primary optic atrophy, bilateral

H47.219 Primary optic atrophy, unspecified eye

H47.22 Hereditary optic atrophy

Leber's optic atrophy

√6th **H47.23 Glaucomatous optic atrophy**

H47.231 Glaucomatous optic atrophy, right eye

H47.232 Glaucomatous optic atrophy, left eye

H47.233 Glaucomatous optic atrophy, bilateral

H47.239 Glaucomatous optic atrophy, unspecified eye

√6th **H47.29 Other optic atrophy**

Temporal pallor of optic disc

H47.291 Other optic atrophy, right eye

H47.292 Other optic atrophy, left eye

H47.293 Other optic atrophy, bilateral

H47.299 Other optic atrophy, unspecified eye

√5th **H47.3 Other disorders of optic disc**

√6th **H47.31 Coloboma of optic disc**

H47.311 Coloboma of optic disc, right eye

H47.312 Coloboma of optic disc, left eye

H47.313 Coloboma of optic disc, bilateral

H47.319 Coloboma of optic disc, unspecified eye

√6th **H47.32 Drusen of optic disc**

H47.321 Drusen of optic disc, right eye

H47.322 Drusen of optic disc, left eye

H47.323 Drusen of optic disc, bilateral

H47.329 Drusen of optic disc, unspecified eye

√6th **H47.33 Pseudopapilledema of optic disc**

H47.331 Pseudopapilledema of optic disc, right eye

H47.332 Pseudopapilledema of optic disc, left eye

H47.333 Pseudopapilledema of optic disc, bilateral

H47.339 Pseudopapilledema of optic disc, unspecified eye

√6th **H47.39 Other disorders of optic disc**

H47.391 Other disorders of optic disc, right eye

H47.392 Other disorders of optic disc, left eye

H47.393 Other disorders of optic disc, bilateral

H47.399 Other disorders of optic disc, unspecified eye

☑ Additional Character Required   √x7th Xtension Alert   Unacceptable PDx   Manifestation   Hospital Acquired Condition   EXCLUDES1 Not Coded Here   EXCLUDES2 Not Included Here

ICD-10-CM Draft (2015)   573

√5th **H47.4 Disorders of optic chiasm**
Code also underlying condition

CC Excl: For CC codes in subcategory H47.4, unless otherwise noted: H47.41-H47.539

H47.41 Disorders of optic chiasm in (due to) inflammatory disorders CC

H47.42 Disorders of optic chiasm in (due to) neoplasm CC

H47.43 Disorders of optic chiasm in (due to) vascular disorders CC

H47.49 Disorders of optic chiasm in (due to) other disorders CC

√5th **H47.5 Disorders of other visual pathways**
Disorders of optic tracts, geniculate nuclei and optic radiations
Code also underlying condition

CC Excl: For CC codes in subcategory H47.5, unless otherwise noted: H47.41-H47.539

√6th **H47.51 Disorders of visual pathways in (due to) inflammatory disorders**

H47.511 Disorders of visual pathways in (due to) inflammatory disorders, right side CC

H47.512 Disorders of visual pathways in (due to) inflammatory disorders, left side CC

H47.519 Disorders of visual pathways in (due to) inflammatory disorders, unspecified side CC

√6th **H47.52 Disorders of visual pathways in (due to)** neoplasm

H47.521 Disorders of visual pathways in (due to) neoplasm, right side CC

H47.522 Disorders of visual pathways in (due to) neoplasm, left side CC

H47.529 Disorders of visual pathways in (due to) neoplasm, unspecified side CC

√6th **H47.53 Disorders of visual pathways in (due to)** vascular disorders

H47.531 Disorders of visual pathways in (due to) vascular disorders, right side CC

H47.532 Disorders of visual pathways in (due to) vascular disorders, left side CC

H47.539 Disorders of visual pathways in (due to) vascular disorders, unspecified side CC

√5th **H47.6 Disorders of visual cortex**
Code also underlying condition
EXCLUDES 1 injury to visual cortex S04.04

CC Excl: For CC codes in subcategory H47.6, unless otherwise noted: H47.611-H47.9

√6th **H47.61 Cortical blindness**

H47.611 Cortical blindness, right side of brain

H47.612 Cortical blindness, left side of brain

H47.619 Cortical blindness, unspecified side of brain

√6th **H47.62 Disorders of visual cortex in (due to)** inflammatory disorders

H47.621 Disorders of visual cortex in (due to) inflammatory disorders, right side of brain CC

H47.622 Disorders of visual cortex in (due to) inflammatory disorders, left side of brain CC

H47.629 Disorders of visual cortex in (due to) inflammatory disorders, unspecified side of brain CC

√6th **H47.63 Disorders of visual cortex in (due to)** neoplasm

H47.631 Disorders of visual cortex in (due to) neoplasm, right side of brain CC

H47.632 Disorders of visual cortex in (due to) neoplasm, left side of brain CC

H47.639 Disorders of visual cortex in (due to) neoplasm, unspecified side of brain CC

√6th **H47.64 Disorders of visual cortex in (due to)** vascular disorders

H47.641 Disorders of visual cortex in (due to) vascular disorders, right side of brain CC

H47.642 Disorders of visual cortex in (due to) vascular disorders, left side of brain CC

H47.649 Disorders of visual cortex in (due to) vascular disorders, unspecified side of brain CC

H47.9 Unspecified disorder of visual pathways

Disorders of ocular muscles, binocular movement, accommodation and refraction (H49-H52)
EXCLUDES 2 nystagmus and other irregular eye movements (H55)

√4th **H49 Paralytic strabismus**
EXCLUDES 2 internal ophthalmoplegia (H52.51-)
internuclear ophthalmoplegia (H51.2-)
progressive supranuclear ophthalmoplegia (G23.1)

√5th **H49.0 Third [oculomotor] nerve palsy**

H49.00 Third [oculomotor] nerve palsy, unspecified eye

H49.01 Third [oculomotor] nerve palsy, right eye

H49.02 Third [oculomotor] nerve palsy, left eye

H49.03 Third [oculomotor] nerve palsy, bilateral

√5th **H49.1 Fourth [trochlear] nerve palsy**

H49.10 Fourth [trochlear] nerve palsy, unspecified eye

H49.11 Fourth [trochlear] nerve palsy, right eye

H49.12 Fourth [trochlear] nerve palsy, left eye

H49.13 Fourth [trochlear] nerve palsy, bilateral

√5th **H49.2 Sixth [abducent] nerve palsy**

H49.20 Sixth [abducent] nerve palsy, unspecified eye

H49.21 Sixth [abducent] nerve palsy, right eye

H49.22 Sixth [abducent] nerve palsy, left eye

H49.23 Sixth [abducent] nerve palsy, bilateral

√5th **H49.3 Total (external) ophthalmoplegia**

H49.30 Total (external) ophthalmoplegia, unspecified eye

H49.31 Total (external) ophthalmoplegia, right eye

H49.32 Total (external) ophthalmoplegia, left eye

H49.33 Total (external) ophthalmoplegia, bilateral

√5th **H49.4 Progressive external ophthalmoplegia**
EXCLUDES 1 Kearns-Sayre syndrome (H49.81-)

H49.40 Progressive external ophthalmoplegia, unspecified eye

H49.41 Progressive external ophthalmoplegia, right eye

H49.42 Progressive external ophthalmoplegia, left eye

H49.43 Progressive external ophthalmoplegia, bilateral

√5th **H49.8 Other paralytic strabismus**

CC Excl: For CC codes in subcategory H49.8, unless otherwise noted: C96.5-C96.6, E71.310-E71.548, E80.3-E80.7, E88.89

√6th **H49.81 Kearns-Sayre syndrome**
Progressive external ophthalmoplegia with pigmentary retinopathy
Use additional code for other manifestation, such as: heart block (I45.9)

H49.811 Kearns-Sayre syndrome, right eye CC

H49.812 Kearns-Sayre syndrome, left eye CC

H49.813 Kearns-Sayre syndrome, bilateral CC

H49.819 Kearns-Sayre syndrome, unspecified eye CC

√6th **H49.88 Other paralytic strabismus**
External ophthalmoplegia NOS

H49.881 Other paralytic strabismus, right eye

H49.882 Other paralytic strabismus, left eye

H49.883 Other paralytic strabismus, bilateral

H49.889 Other paralytic strabismus, unspecified eye

H49.9 Unspecified paralytic strabismus

√4th **H50 Other strabismus**

√5th **H50.0 Esotropia**
Convergent concomitant strabismus
EXCLUDES 1 intermittent esotropia (H50.31-, H50.32)

H50.00 Unspecified esotropia

√6th **H50.01 Monocular esotropia**

H50.011 Monocular esotropia, right eye

H50.012 Monocular esotropia, left eye

✓6ᵗʰ **H50.02 Monocular esotropia with** A **pattern**
　　　H50.021 **Monocular esotropia with A pattern, right eye**
　　　H50.022 **Monocular esotropia with A pattern, left eye**

✓6ᵗʰ **H50.03 Monocular esotropia with** V **pattern**
　　　H50.031 **Monocular esotropia with V pattern, right eye**
　　　H50.032 **Monocular esotropia with V pattern, left eye**

✓6ᵗʰ **H50.04 Monocular esotropia with** other noncomitancies
　　　H50.041 **Monocular esotropia with other noncomitancies, right eye**
　　　H50.042 **Monocular esotropia with other noncomitancies, left eye**

H50.05 Alternating **esotropia**
H50.06 Alternating **esotropia with** A **pattern**
H50.07 Alternating **esotropia with** V **pattern**
H50.08 Alternating **esotropia with** other noncomitancies

✓5ᵗʰ **H50.1 Exotropia**
　　Divergent concomitant strabismus
　　EXCLUDES 1　intermittent exotropia (H50.33-, H50.34)
H50.10 Unspecified **exotropia**

✓6ᵗʰ **H50.11** Monocular **exotropia**
　　　H50.111 **Monocular exotropia, right eye**
　　　H50.112 **Monocular exotropia, left eye**

✓6ᵗʰ **H50.12 Monocular exotropia with** A **pattern**
　　　H50.121 **Monocular exotropia with A pattern, right eye**
　　　H50.122 **Monocular exotropia with A pattern, left eye**

✓6ᵗʰ **H50.13 Monocular exotropia with** V pattern
　　　H50.131 **Monocular exotropia with V pattern, right eye**
　　　H50.132 **Monocular exotropia with V pattern, left eye**

✓6ᵗʰ **H50.14 Monocular exotropia with** other noncomitancies
　　　H50.141 **Monocular exotropia with other noncomitancies, right eye**
　　　H50.142 **Monocular exotropia with other noncomitancies, left eye**

H50.15 Alternating **exotropia**
H50.16 Alternating **exotropia with** A **pattern**
H50.17 Alternating **exotropia with** V **pattern**
H50.18 Alternating **exotropia with** other noncomitancies

✓5ᵗʰ **H50.2 Vertical strabismus**
　　Hypertropia
H50.21 Vertical strabismus, right eye
H50.22 Vertical strabismus, left eye

✓5ᵗʰ **H50.3 Intermittent heterotropia**
H50.30 Unspecified **intermittent heterotropia**

✓6ᵗʰ **H50.31 Intermittent** monocular esotropia
　　　H50.311 **Intermittent monocular esotropia, right eye**
　　　H50.312 **Intermittent monocular esotropia, left eye**

H50.32 Intermittent alternating **esotropia**

✓6ᵗʰ **H50.33 Intermittent** monocular exotropia
　　　H50.331 **Intermittent monocular exotropia, right eye**
　　　H50.332 **Intermittent monocular exotropia, left eye**

H50.34 Intermittent alternating **exotropia**

✓5ᵗʰ **H50.4 Other and unspecified heterotropia**
H50.40 Unspecified **heterotropia**

✓6ᵗʰ **H50.41** Cyclotropia
　　　H50.411 **Cyclotropia, right eye**
　　　H50.412 **Cyclotropia, left eye**

H50.42 Monofixation **syndrome**
H50.43 Accommodative component in esotropia

✓5ᵗʰ **H50.5 Heterophoria**
H50.50 Unspecified **heterophoria**
H50.51 Esophoria
H50.52 Exophoria
H50.53 Vertical **heterophoria**

H50.54 Cyclophoria
H50.55 Alternating **heterophoria**

✓5ᵗʰ **H50.6 Mechanical strabismus**
H50.60 Mechanical strabismus, unspecified

✓6ᵗʰ **H50.61** Brown's sheath **syndrome**
　　　H50.611 **Brown's sheath syndrome, right eye**
　　　H50.612 **Brown's sheath syndrome, left eye**

H50.69 Other **mechanical strabismus**
　　Strabismus due to adhesions
　　Traumatic limitation of duction of eye muscle

✓5ᵗʰ **H50.8 Other specified strabismus**

✓6ᵗʰ **H50.81** Duane's **syndrome**
　　　H50.811 **Duane's syndrome, right eye**
　　　H50.812 **Duane's syndrome, left eye**

H50.89 Other specified strabismus
H50.9 Unspecified strabismus

✓4ᵗʰ **H51 Other disorders of binocular movement**
H51.0 Palsy (spasm) of conjugate gaze

✓5ᵗʰ **H51.1 Convergence insufficiency and excess**
H51.11 Convergence insufficiency
H51.12 Convergence excess

✓5ᵗʰ **H51.2 Internuclear ophthalmoplegia**
H51.20 Internuclear ophthalmoplegia, unspecified eye
H51.21 Internuclear ophthalmoplegia, right eye
H51.22 Internuclear ophthalmoplegia, left eye
H51.23 Internuclear ophthalmoplegia, bilateral

H51.8 Other specified **disorders of binocular movement**
H51.9 Unspecified **disorder of binocular movement**

✓4ᵗʰ **H52 Disorders of refraction and accommodation**

✓5ᵗʰ **H52.0 Hypermetropia**
H52.00 Hypermetropia, unspecified eye
H52.01 Hypermetropia, right eye
H52.02 Hypermetropia, left eye
H52.03 Hypermetropia, bilateral

✓5ᵗʰ **H52.1 Myopia**
　　EXCLUDES 1　degenerative myopia (H44.2-)
H52.10 Myopia, unspecified eye
H52.11 Myopia, right eye
H52.12 Myopia, left eye
H52.13 Myopia, bilateral

✓5ᵗʰ **H52.2 Astigmatism**

✓6ᵗʰ **H52.20** Unspecified astigmatism
　　　H52.201 **Unspecified astigmatism, right eye**
　　　H52.202 **Unspecified astigmatism, left eye**
　　　H52.203 **Unspecified astigmatism, bilateral**
　　　H52.209 **Unspecified astigmatism, unspecified eye**

✓6ᵗʰ **H52.21** Irregular astigmatism
　　　H52.211 **Irregular astigmatism, right eye**
　　　H52.212 **Irregular astigmatism, left eye**
　　　H52.213 **Irregular astigmatism, bilateral**
　　　H52.219 **Irregular astigmatism, unspecified eye**

✓6ᵗʰ **H52.22** Regular astigmatism
　　　H52.221 **Regular astigmatism, right eye**
　　　H52.222 **Regular astigmatism, left eye**
　　　H52.223 **Regular astigmatism, bilateral**
　　　H52.229 **Regular astigmatism, unspecified eye**

✓5ᵗʰ **H52.3 Anisometropia and aniseikonia**
H52.31 Anisometropia
H52.32 Aniseikonia

H52.4 Presbyopia

✓5ᵗʰ **H52.5 Disorders of accommodation**

✓6ᵗʰ **H52.51** Internal ophthalmoplegia (complete) (total)
　　　H52.511 **Internal ophthalmoplegia (complete) (total), right eye**
　　　H52.512 **Internal ophthalmoplegia (complete) (total), left eye**
　　　H52.513 **Internal ophthalmoplegia (complete) (total), bilateral**
　　　H52.519 **Internal ophthalmoplegia (complete) (total), unspecified eye**

Diseases of the Eye and Adnexa

H52.52–H53.53

✓6th **H52.52 Paresis of accommodation**
    H52.521 Paresis of accommodation, right eye
    H52.522 Paresis of accommodation, left eye
    H52.523 Paresis of accommodation, bilateral
    H52.529 Paresis of accommodation, unspecified eye

✓6th **H52.53 Spasm of accommodation**
    H52.531 Spasm of accommodation, right eye
    H52.532 Spasm of accommodation, left eye
    H52.533 Spasm of accommodation, bilateral
    H52.539 Spasm of accommodation, unspecified eye

H52.6 Other disorders of refraction

H52.7 Unspecified disorder of refraction

Visual disturbances and blindness (H53-H54)

✓4th **H53 Visual disturbances**

✓5th **H53.0 Amblyopia ex anopsia**
    EXCLUDES 1 *amblyopia due to vitamin A deficiency (E50.5)*

✓6th **H53.00 Unspecified amblyopia**
    H53.001 Unspecified amblyopia, right eye
    H53.002 Unspecified amblyopia, left eye
    H53.003 Unspecified amblyopia, bilateral
    H53.009 Unspecified amblyopia, unspecified eye

✓6th **H53.01 Deprivation amblyopia**
    H53.011 Deprivation amblyopia, right eye
    H53.012 Deprivation amblyopia, left eye
    H53.013 Deprivation amblyopia, bilateral
    H53.019 Deprivation amblyopia, unspecified eye

✓6th **H53.02 Refractive amblyopia**
    H53.021 Refractive amblyopia, right eye
    H53.022 Refractive amblyopia, left eye
    H53.023 Refractive amblyopia, bilateral
    H53.029 Refractive amblyopia, unspecified eye

✓6th **H53.03 Strabismic amblyopia**
    EXCLUDES 1 *strabismus (H50.-)*
    H53.031 Strabismic amblyopia, right eye
    H53.032 Strabismic amblyopia, left eye
    H53.033 Strabismic amblyopia, bilateral
    H53.039 Strabismic amblyopia, unspecified eye

✓5th **H53.1 Subjective visual disturbances**

    CC Excl: For CC codes in subcategory H53.1, unless otherwise noted: H53.10-H53.139, H53.16, R44.1, R48.3

    EXCLUDES 1 *subjective visual disturbances due to vitamin A deficiency (E50.5)*
    visual hallucinations (R44.1)

    H53.10 Unspecified subjective visual disturbances

    H53.11 Day blindness
        Hemeralopia

✓6th **H53.12 Transient visual loss**
    Scintillating scotoma
    EXCLUDES 1 *amaurosis fugax (G45.3-)*
    transient retinal artery occlusion (H34.0-)
    H53.121 Transient visual loss, right eye — CC
    H53.122 Transient visual loss, left eye — CC
    H53.123 Transient visual loss, bilateral — CC
    H53.129 Transient visual loss, unspecified eye — CC

✓6th **H53.13 Sudden visual loss**
    H53.131 Sudden visual loss, right eye — CC
    H53.132 Sudden visual loss, left eye — CC
    H53.133 Sudden visual loss, bilateral — CC
    H53.139 Sudden visual loss, unspecified eye — CC

✓6th **H53.14 Visual discomfort**
    Asthenopia
    Photophobia
    H53.141 Visual discomfort, right eye
    H53.142 Visual discomfort, left eye
    H53.143 Visual discomfort, bilateral
    H53.149 Visual discomfort, unspecified

    H53.15 Visual distortions of shape and size
        Metamorphopsia

    H53.16 Psychophysical visual disturbances

    H53.19 Other subjective visual disturbances
        Visual halos

H53.2 Diplopia
    Double vision

✓5th **H53.3 Other and unspecified disorders of binocular vision**
    H53.30 Unspecified disorder of binocular vision
    H53.31 Abnormal retinal correspondence
    H53.32 Fusion with defective stereopsis
    H53.33 Simultaneous visual perception without fusion
    H53.34 Suppression of binocular vision

✓5th **H53.4 Visual field defects**
    H53.40 Unspecified visual field defects

✓6th **H53.41 Scotoma involving central area**
    Central scotoma
    H53.411 Scotoma involving central area, right eye
    H53.412 Scotoma involving central area, left eye
    H53.413 Scotoma involving central area, bilateral
    H53.419 Scotoma involving central area, unspecified eye

✓6th **H53.42 Scotoma of blind spot area**
    Enlarged blind spot
    H53.421 Scotoma of blind spot area, right eye
    H53.422 Scotoma of blind spot area, left eye
    H53.423 Scotoma of blind spot area, bilateral
    H53.429 Scotoma of blind spot area, unspecified eye

✓6th **H53.43 Sector or arcuate defects**
    Arcuate scotoma
    Bjerrum scotoma
    H53.431 Sector or arcuate defects, right eye
    H53.432 Sector or arcuate defects, left eye
    H53.433 Sector or arcuate defects, bilateral
    H53.439 Sector or arcuate defects, unspecified eye

✓6th **H53.45 Other localized visual field defect**
    Peripheral visual field defect
    Ring scotoma NOS
    Scotoma NOS
    H53.451 Other localized visual field defect, right eye
    H53.452 Other localized visual field defect, left eye
    H53.453 Other localized visual field defect, bilateral
    H53.459 Other localized visual field defect, unspecified eye

✓6th **H53.46 Homonymous bilateral field defects**
    Homonymous hemianopia
    Homonymous hemianopsia
    Quadrant anopia
    Quadrant anopsia
    H53.461 Homonymous bilateral field defects, right side
    H53.462 Homonymous bilateral field defects, left side
    H53.469 Homonymous bilateral field defects, unspecified side
        Homonymous bilateral field defects NOS

    H53.47 Heteronymous bilateral field defects
        Heteronymous hemianop(s)ia

✓6th **H53.48 Generalized contraction of visual field**
    H53.481 Generalized contraction of visual field, right eye
    H53.482 Generalized contraction of visual field, left eye
    H53.483 Generalized contraction of visual field, bilateral
    H53.489 Generalized contraction of visual field, unspecified eye

✓5th **H53.5 Color vision deficiencies**
    Color blindness
    EXCLUDES 2 *day blindness (H53.11)*
    H53.50 Unspecified color vision deficiencies
        Color blindness NOS
    H53.51 Achromatopsia
    H53.52 Acquired color vision deficiency
    H53.53 Deuteranomaly
        Deuteranopia

N Newborn: 0   P Pediatric: 0-17   M Maternity: 12-55   A Adult: 15-124   MCC Major CC Condition   PDx MCC PDx acts as own MCC   CC CC Condition   PDx CC PDx acts as own CC

576   ICD-10-CM Draft (2015)

H53.54　**Protanomaly**
　　　　　Protanopia

H53.55　**Tritanomaly**
　　　　　Tritanopia

H53.59　**Other color vision deficiencies**

✓5ᵗʰ　**H53.6**　**Night blindness**
　　EXCLUDES 1　*night blindness due to vitamin A deficiency (E50.5)*

H53.60　**Unspecified** night blindness

H53.61　**Abnormal dark adaptation curve**

H53.62　**Acquired** night blindness

H53.63　**Congenital** night blindness

H53.69　**Other** night blindness

✓5ᵗʰ　**H53.7**　**Vision** sensitivity **deficiencies**

H53.71　**Glare** sensitivity

H53.72　**Impaired contrast** sensitivity

H53.8　Other visual disturbances

H53.9　Unspecified visual disturbance

✓4ᵗʰ　**H54**　**Blindness and low vision**
　　NOTE　For definition of visual impairment categories see table below
　　Code first any associated underlying cause of the blindness
　　EXCLUDES 1　*amaurosis fugax (G45.3)*

H54.0　**Blindness, both eyes**
　　　Visual impairment categories 3, 4, 5 in both eyes.

✓5ᵗʰ　**H54.1**　**Blindness, one eye, low vision other eye**
　　　Visual impairment categories 3, 4, 5 in one eye, with categories 1 or 2 in the other eye.

H54.10　**Blindness, one eye, low vision other eye, unspecified eyes**

H54.11　**Blindness, right eye, low vision left eye**

H54.12　**Blindness, left eye, low vision right eye**

H54.2　**Low vision, both eyes**
　　　Visual impairment categories 1 or 2 in both eyes.

H54.3　Unqualified **visual loss, both eyes**
　　　Visual impairment category 9 in both eyes.

✓5ᵗʰ　**H54.4**　Blindness, **one eye**
　　　Visual impairment categories 3, 4, 5 in one eye [normal vision in other eye]

H54.40　**Blindness, one eye, unspecified eye**

H54.41　**Blindness, right eye, normal vision left eye**

H54.42　**Blindness, left eye, normal vision right eye**

✓5ᵗʰ　**H54.5**　Low vision, **one eye**
　　　Visual impairment categories 1 or 2 in one eye [normal vision in other eye].

H54.50　**Low vision, one eye, unspecified eye**

H54.51　**Low vision, right eye, normal vision left eye**

H54.52　**Low vision, left eye, normal vision right eye**

✓5ᵗʰ　**H54.6**　Unqualified **visual loss, one eye**
　　　Visual impairment category 9 in one eye [normal vision in other eye].

H54.60　**Unqualified visual loss, one eye, unspecified**

H54.61　**Unqualified visual loss, right eye, normal vision left eye**

H54.62　**Unqualified visual loss, left eye, normal vision right eye**

H54.7　Unspecified **visual loss**
　　　Visual impairment category 9 NOS

H54.8　**Legal blindness, as defined in USA**
　　　Blindness NOS according to USA definition
　　　EXCLUDES 1　*legal blindness with specification of impairment level (H54.0-H54.7)*

NOTE　The following table gives a classification of severity of visual impairment recommended by a WHO Study Group on the Prevention of Blindness, Geneva, 6-10 November l972.

The term "low vision" in category H54 comprises categories 1 and 2 of the table, the term "blindness" categories 3, 4 and 5, and the term "unqualified visual loss" category 9.

If the extent of the visual field is taken into account, patients with a field no greater than 10 but greater than 5 around central fixation should be placed in category 3 and patients with a field nocategory greater than 5 around central fixation should be placed in 4, even if the central acuity is not impaired.

Category of visual impairment	Visual acuity with best possible correction	
	Maximum less than:	Minimum equal to or better than:
1	6/18 3/10 (0.3) 20/70	6/60 1/10 (0.1) 20/200
2	6/60 1/10 (0.1) 20/200	3/60 1/20 (0.5) 20/400
3	3/60 1/20 (0.05) 20/400	1/60 (finger counting at one meter) 1/50 (0.02) 5/300 (20/1200)
4	1/60 (finger counting at one meter) 1/50 (0.02) 5/300	Light perception
5	No light perception	
9	Undetermined or unspecified	

Other disorders of eye and adnexa (H55-H59)

✓4ᵗʰ　**H55**　**Nystagmus and other** irregular eye movements

✓5ᵗʰ　**H55.0**　**Nystagmus**

H55.00　**Unspecified** nystagmus

H55.01　**Congenital** nystagmus

H55.02　**Latent** nystagmus

H55.03　**Visual deprivation** nystagmus

H55.04　**Dissociated** nystagmus

H55.09　**Other** forms of nystagmus

✓5ᵗʰ　**H55.8**　**Other irregular eye movements**

H55.81　**Saccadic** eye movements

H55.89　**Other** irregular eye movements

✓4ᵗʰ　**H57**　**Other disorders of eye and adnexa**

✓5ᵗʰ　**H57.0**　**Anomalies of pupillary function**

H57.00　**Unspecified anomaly of pupillary function**

H57.01　**Argyll Robertson pupil, atypical**
　　　EXCLUDES 1　*syphilitic Argyll Robertson pupil (A52.19)*

H57.02　**Anisocoria**

H57.03　**Miosis**

H57.04　**Mydriasis**

✓6ᵗʰ　H57.05　**Tonic pupil**

H57.051　**Tonic pupil, right eye**

H57.052　**Tonic pupil, left eye**

H57.053　**Tonic pupil, bilateral**

H57.059　**Tonic pupil, unspecified eye**

H57.09　**Other anomalies of pupillary function**

✓5ᵗʰ　**H57.1**　**Ocular pain**

H57.10　**Ocular pain, unspecified eye**

H57.11　**Ocular pain, right eye**

H57.12　**Ocular pain, left eye**

H57.13　**Ocular pain, bilateral**

H57.8　Other specified disorders of eye and adnexa

H57.9　Unspecified disorder of eye and adnexa

✓ Additional Character Required　✓x7ᵗʰ Xtension Alert　Unacceptable PDx　Manifestation　　Hospital Acquired Condition　　EXCLUDES 1 Not Coded Here　EXCLUDES 2 Not Included Here

✓4ᵗʰ **H59 Intraoperative and postprocedural complications and disorders of eye and adnexa, not elsewhere classified**

EXCLUDES 1 *mechanical complication of intraocular lens (T85.2)*
mechanical complication of other ocular prosthetic devices, implants and grafts (T85.3)
pseudophakia (Z96.1)
secondary cataracts (H26.4-)

✓5ᵗʰ **H59.0 Disorders of the eye** following cataract surgery

> **CC Excl: For CC codes in subcategory H59.0, unless otherwise noted:** H59.011-H59.019, H59.031-H59.099, H59.811-H59.89, H95.811-H95.89, I97.3, M96.89, N98.1-N98.9, T81.82XA, T81.89XA, T81.9XXA

✓6ᵗʰ **H59.01 Keratopathy (bullous aphakic) following cataract surgery**
Vitreal corneal syndrome
Vitreous (touch) syndrome

H59.011 **Keratopathy (bullous aphakic) following cataract surgery, right eye** CC

H59.012 **Keratopathy (bullous aphakic) following cataract surgery, left eye** CC

H59.013 **Keratopathy (bullous aphakic) following cataract surgery, bilateral** CC

H59.019 **Keratopathy (bullous aphakic) following cataract surgery, unspecified eye** CC

✓6ᵗʰ **H59.02 Cataract (lens) fragments in eye following cataract surgery**

H59.021 **Cataract (lens) fragments in eye following cataract surgery, right eye**

H59.022 **Cataract (lens) fragments in eye following cataract surgery, left eye**

H59.023 **Cataract (lens) fragments in eye following cataract surgery, bilateral**

H59.029 **Cataract (lens) fragments in eye following cataract surgery, unspecified eye**

✓6ᵗʰ **H59.03 Cystoid macular edema following cataract surgery**

H59.031 **Cystoid macular edema following cataract surgery, right eye** CC

H59.032 **Cystoid macular edema following cataract surgery, left eye** CC

H59.033 **Cystoid macular edema following cataract surgery, bilateral** CC

H59.039 **Cystoid macular edema following cataract surgery, unspecified eye** CC

✓6ᵗʰ **H59.09 Other disorders of the eye following cataract surgery**

H59.091 **Other disorders of the right eye following cataract surgery** CC

H59.092 **Other disorders of the left eye following cataract surgery** CC

H59.093 **Other disorders of the eye following cataract surgery, bilateral** CC

H59.099 **Other disorders of unspecified eye following cataract surgery** CC

✓5ᵗʰ **H59.1 Intraoperative hemorrhage and hematoma** of eye and adnexa complicating a procedure

EXCLUDES 1 *intraoperative hemorrhage and hematoma of eye and adnexa due to accidental puncture or laceration during a procedure (H59.2-)*

> **CC Excl: For CC codes in subcategory H59.1, unless otherwise noted:** H59.011-H59.019, H59.031-H59.129, H59.311-H59.329, H59.811-H59.89, H95.811-H95.89, I85.01, I85.11, I97.3, K21.9, K22.8, K23-K25.0, K25.2, K25.4, K25.6, K26.0, K26.2, K26.4, K26.6, K27.0, K27.2, K27.4, K27.6, K28.0, K28.2, K28.4, K28.6, K29.01, K29.21, K29.31, K29.41, K29.51, K29.61, K29.71, K29.81, K29.91, K31.811, K55.21, K57.01, K57.11, K57.13, K57.21, K57.31, K57.33, K57.41, K57.51, K57.53, K57.81, K57.91, K57.93, K62.5, K92.0-K92.2, M96.89, N98.1-N98.9, P54.1-P54.3, T81.10XA, T81.11XA, T81.12XA, T81.19XA, T81.82XA, T81.89XA, T81.9XXA

✓6ᵗʰ **H59.11 Intraoperative hemorrhage and hematoma of eye and adnexa complicating an ophthalmic procedure**

H59.111 **Intraoperative hemorrhage and hematoma of right eye and adnexa complicating an ophthalmic procedure** CC

H59.112 **Intraoperative hemorrhage and hematoma of left eye and adnexa complicating an ophthalmic procedure** CC

H59.113 **Intraoperative hemorrhage and hematoma of eye and adnexa complicating an ophthalmic procedure, bilateral** CC

H59.119 **Intraoperative hemorrhage and hematoma of unspecified eye and adnexa complicating an ophthalmic procedure** CC

✓6ᵗʰ **H59.12 Intraoperative hemorrhage and hematoma of eye and adnexa complicating other procedure**

H59.121 **Intraoperative hemorrhage and hematoma of right eye and adnexa complicating other procedure** CC

H59.122 **Intraoperative hemorrhage and hematoma of left eye and adnexa complicating other procedure** CC

H59.123 **Intraoperative hemorrhage and hematoma of eye and adnexa complicating other procedure, bilateral** CC

H59.129 **Intraoperative hemorrhage and hematoma of unspecified eye and adnexa complicating other procedure** CC

✓5ᵗʰ **H59.2 Accidental puncture and laceration** of eye and adnexa during a procedure

> **CC Excl: For CC codes in subcategory H59.2, unless otherwise noted:** D78.11-D78.12, D78.81-D78.89, E36.11-E36.8, E89.810-E89.89, G96.11, G97.41, G97.48-G97.49, H59.011-H59.019, H59.031-H59.099, H59.211-H59.229, H59.811-H59.89, H95.31-H95.32, H95.811-H95.89, I97.3, I97.51-I97.52, J95.71-J95.72, K91.71-K91.72, L76.11-L76.12, L76.81-L76.82, M96.820-M96.821, M96.89, N98.1-N98.9, N99.71-N99.72, T81.82XA, T81.89XA, T81.9XXA

✓6ᵗʰ **H59.21 Accidental puncture and laceration of eye and adnexa during an ophthalmic procedure**

H59.211 **Accidental puncture and laceration of right eye and adnexa during an ophthalmic procedure** CC

H59.212 **Accidental puncture and laceration of left eye and adnexa during an ophthalmic procedure** CC

H59.213 **Accidental puncture and laceration of eye and adnexa during an ophthalmic procedure, bilateral** CC

H59.219 **Accidental puncture and laceration of unspecified eye and adnexa during an ophthalmic procedure** CC

✓6ᵗʰ **H59.22 Accidental puncture and laceration of eye and adnexa during other procedure**

H59.221 **Accidental puncture and laceration of right eye and adnexa during other procedure** CC

H59.222 **Accidental puncture and laceration of left eye and adnexa during other procedure** CC

H59.223 **Accidental puncture and laceration of eye and adnexa during other procedure, bilateral** CC

H59.229 **Accidental puncture and laceration of unspecified eye and adnexa during other procedure** CC

✓5ᵗʰ **H59.3 Postprocedural hemorrhage and hematoma** of eye and adnexa following a procedure

> **CC Excl: For CC codes in subcategory H59.3, unless otherwise noted:** See code: H59.1

✓6ᵗʰ **H59.31 Postprocedural hemorrhage and hematoma of eye and adnexa following an ophthalmic procedure**

H59.311 **Postprocedural hemorrhage and hematoma of right eye and adnexa following an ophthalmic procedure** CC

H59.312 **Postprocedural hemorrhage and hematoma of left eye and adnexa following an ophthalmic procedure** CC

H59.313 **Postprocedural hemorrhage and hematoma of eye and adnexa following an ophthalmic procedure, bilateral** CC

H59.319 **Postprocedural hemorrhage and hematoma of unspecified eye and adnexa following an ophthalmic procedure** CC

N Newborn: 0 P Pediatric: 0-17 M Maternity: 12-55 A Adult: 15-124 MCC Major CC Condition PDx MCC PDx acts as own MCC CC CC Condition PDx CC PDx acts as own CC

578   ICD-10-CM Draft (2015)

✓6ᵗʰ **H59.32**　**Postprocedural hemorrhage and hematoma of eye and adnexa following** other procedure

　　　　H59.321　Postprocedural hemorrhage and　　　CC
　　　　　　hematoma of right eye and adnexa
　　　　　　following other procedure

　　　　H59.322　Postprocedural hemorrhage and　　　CC
　　　　　　hematoma of left eye and adnexa
　　　　　　following other procedure

　　　　H59.323　Postprocedural hemorrhage and　　　CC
　　　　　　hematoma of eye and adnexa following
　　　　　　other procedure, bilateral

　　　　H59.329　Postprocedural hemorrhage and　　　CC
　　　　　　hematoma of unspecified eye and
　　　　　　adnexa following other procedure

✓5ᵗʰ **H59.4**　**Inflammation (infection) of** postprocedural bleb
　　　Postprocedural blebitis
　　　EXCLUDES 1　*filtering (vitreous) bleb after glaucoma surgery status*
　　　　　　(Z98.83)

　　　H59.40　**Inflammation (infection) of postprocedural bleb,
　　　　unspecified**

　　　H59.41　**Inflammation (infection) of postprocedural bleb,
　　　　stage 1**

　　　H59.42　**Inflammation (infection) of postprocedural bleb,
　　　　stage 2**

　　　H59.43　**Inflammation (infection) of postprocedural bleb,
　　　　stage 3**
　　　　　Bleb endophthalmitis

✓5ᵗʰ **H59.8**　**Other intraoperative and postprocedural complications and
　　　disorders of eye and adnexa, not elsewhere classified**

CC Excl: For CC codes in subcategory H59.8, unless
otherwise noted: H59.011-H59.019, H59.031-H59.099,
H59.811-H59.89, H95.811-H95.89, I97.3, M96.89, N98.1-
N98.9, T81.82XA, T81.89XA, T81.9XXA

✓6ᵗʰ **H59.81**　**Chorioretinal scars after surgery for detachment**

　　　　H59.811　Chorioretinal scars after surgery for　　CC
　　　　　　detachment, right eye

　　　　H59.812　Chorioretinal scars after surgery for　　CC
　　　　　　detachment, left eye

　　　　H59.813　Chorioretinal scars after surgery for　　CC
　　　　　　detachment, bilateral

　　　　H59.819　Chorioretinal scars after surgery for　　CC
　　　　　　detachment, unspecified eye

　　　H59.88　**Other intraoperative complications of eye and**　　CC
　　　　adnexa, not elsewhere classified

　　　H59.89　**Other postprocedural complications and**　　　CC
　　　　disorders of eye and adnexa, not elsewhere
　　　　classified

Chapter 8. Diseases of the Ear and Mastoid Process (H60-H95)

NOTE Use an external cause code following the code for the ear condition, if applicable, to identify the cause of the ear condition.

EXCLUDES 2 certain conditions originating in the perinatal period (P04-P96)
certain infectious and parasitic diseases (A00-B99)
complications of pregnancy, childbirth and the puerperium (O00-O9A)
congenital malformations, deformations and chromosomal abnormalities (Q00-Q99)
endocrine, nutritional and metabolic diseases (E00-E88)
injury, poisoning and certain other consequences of external causes (S00-T88)
neoplasms (C00-D49)
symptoms, signs and abnormal clinical and laboratory findings, not elsewhere classified (R00-R94)

This chapter contains the following blocks:

H60-H62 Diseases of external ear
H65-H75 Diseases of middle ear and mastoid
H80-H83 Diseases of inner ear
H90-H94 Other disorders of ear
H95 Intraoperative and postprocedural complications and disorders of ear and mastoid process, not elsewhere classified

Diseases of external ear (H60-H62)

H60 Otitis externa

H60.0 Abscess of external ear
Boil of external ear
Carbuncle of auricle or external auditory canal
Furuncle of external ear

H60.00 Abscess of external ear, unspecified ear
H60.01 Abscess of right external ear
H60.02 Abscess of left external ear
H60.03 Abscess of external ear, bilateral

H60.1 Cellulitis of external ear
Cellulitis of auricle
Cellulitis of external auditory canal

H60.10 Cellulitis of external ear, unspecified ear
H60.11 Cellulitis of right external ear
H60.12 Cellulitis of left external ear
H60.13 Cellulitis of external ear, bilateral

H60.2 Malignant otitis externa

CC Excl: For CC codes in subcategory H60.2, unless otherwise noted: H60.20-H60.23, H70.001-H70.13

H60.20 Malignant otitis externa, unspecified ear **CC**
H60.21 Malignant otitis externa, right ear **CC**
H60.22 Malignant otitis externa, left ear **CC**
H60.23 Malignant otitis externa, bilateral **CC**

H60.3 Other infective otitis externa
H60.31 Diffuse otitis externa
H60.311 Diffuse otitis externa, right ear
H60.312 Diffuse otitis externa, left ear
H60.313 Diffuse otitis externa, bilateral
H60.319 Diffuse otitis externa, unspecified ear
H60.32 Hemorrhagic otitis externa
H60.321 Hemorrhagic otitis externa, right ear
H60.322 Hemorrhagic otitis externa, left ear
H60.323 Hemorrhagic otitis externa, bilateral
H60.329 Hemorrhagic otitis externa, unspecified ear
H60.33 Swimmer's ear
H60.331 Swimmer's ear, right ear
H60.332 Swimmer's ear, left ear
H60.333 Swimmer's ear, bilateral
H60.339 Swimmer's ear, unspecified ear
H60.39 Other infective otitis externa
H60.391 Other infective otitis externa, right ear
H60.392 Other infective otitis externa, left ear
H60.393 Other infective otitis externa, bilateral
H60.399 Other infective otitis externa, unspecified ear

H60.4 Cholesteatoma of external ear
Keratosis obturans of external ear (canal)
EXCLUDES 2 cholesteatoma of middle ear (H71.-)
recurrent cholesteatoma of postmastoidectomy cavity (H95.0-)
H60.40 Cholesteatoma of external ear, unspecified ear
H60.41 Cholesteatoma of right external ear
H60.42 Cholesteatoma of left external ear
H60.43 Cholesteatoma of external ear, bilateral

H60.5 Acute noninfective otitis externa
H60.50 Unspecified acute noninfective otitis externa
Acute otitis externa NOS
H60.501 Unspecified acute noninfective otitis externa, right ear
H60.502 Unspecified acute noninfective otitis externa, left ear
H60.503 Unspecified acute noninfective otitis externa, bilateral
H60.509 Unspecified acute noninfective otitis externa, unspecified ear
H60.51 Acute actinic otitis externa
H60.511 Acute actinic otitis externa, right ear
H60.512 Acute actinic otitis externa, left ear
H60.513 Acute actinic otitis externa, bilateral
H60.519 Acute actinic otitis externa, unspecified ear
H60.52 Acute chemical otitis externa
H60.521 Acute chemical otitis externa, right ear
H60.522 Acute chemical otitis externa, left ear
H60.523 Acute chemical otitis externa, bilateral
H60.529 Acute chemical otitis externa, unspecified ear
H60.53 Acute contact otitis externa
H60.531 Acute contact otitis externa, right ear
H60.532 Acute contact otitis externa, left ear
H60.533 Acute contact otitis externa, bilateral
H60.539 Acute contact otitis externa, unspecified ear
H60.54 Acute eczematoid otitis externa
H60.541 Acute eczematoid otitis externa, right ear
H60.542 Acute eczematoid otitis externa, left ear
H60.543 Acute eczematoid otitis externa, bilateral
H60.549 Acute eczematoid otitis externa, unspecified ear
H60.55 Acute reactive otitis externa
H60.551 Acute reactive otitis externa, right ear
H60.552 Acute reactive otitis externa, left ear
H60.553 Acute reactive otitis externa, bilateral
H60.559 Acute reactive otitis externa, unspecified ear
H60.59 Other noninfective acute otitis externa
H60.591 Other noninfective acute otitis externa, right ear
H60.592 Other noninfective acute otitis externa, left ear
H60.593 Other noninfective acute otitis externa, bilateral
H60.599 Other noninfective acute otitis externa, unspecified ear

H60.6 Unspecified chronic otitis externa
H60.60 Unspecified chronic otitis externa, unspecified ear
H60.61 Unspecified chronic otitis externa, right ear
H60.62 Unspecified chronic otitis externa, left ear
H60.63 Unspecified chronic otitis externa, bilateral

H60.8 Other otitis externa
H60.8X Other otitis externa
H60.8X1 Other otitis externa, right ear
H60.8X2 Other otitis externa, left ear
H60.8X3 Other otitis externa, bilateral
H60.8X9 Other otitis externa, unspecified ear

H60.9 Unspecified otitis externa
H60.90 Unspecified otitis externa, unspecified ear
H60.91 Unspecified otitis externa, right ear

H60.92   Unspecified otitis externa, left ear
H60.93   Unspecified otitis externa, bilateral

✓4ᵗʰ **H61   Other disorders of external ear**

✓5ᵗʰ **H61.0   Chondritis and perichondritis of external ear**
Chondrodermatitis nodularis chronica helicis
Perichondritis of auricle
Perichondritis of pinna

✓6ᵗʰ **H61.00   Unspecified perichondritis of external ear**
H61.001   Unspecified perichondritis of right external ear
H61.002   Unspecified perichondritis of left external ear
H61.003   Unspecified perichondritis of external ear, bilateral
H61.009   Unspecified perichondritis of external ear, unspecified ear

✓6ᵗʰ **H61.01   Acute perichondritis of external ear**
H61.011   Acute perichondritis of right external ear
H61.012   Acute perichondritis of left external ear
H61.013   Acute perichondritis of external ear, bilateral
H61.019   Acute perichondritis of external ear, unspecified ear

✓6ᵗʰ **H61.02   Chronic perichondritis of external ear**
H61.021   Chronic perichondritis of right external ear
H61.022   Chronic perichondritis of left external ear
H61.023   Chronic perichondritis of external ear, bilateral
H61.029   Chronic perichondritis of external ear, unspecified ear

✓6ᵗʰ **H61.03   Chondritis of external ear**
Chondritis of auricle   Chondritis of pinna
H61.031   Chondritis of right external ear
H61.032   Chondritis of left external ear
H61.033   Chondritis of external ear, bilateral
H61.039   Chondritis of external ear, unspecified ear

✓5ᵗʰ **H61.1   Noninfective disorders of pinna**
EXCLUDES 2   cauliflower ear (M95.1-)
gouty tophi of ear (M1A.-)

✓6ᵗʰ **H61.10   Unspecified noninfective disorders of pinna**
Disorder of pinna NOS
H61.101   Unspecified noninfective disorders of pinna, right ear
H61.102   Unspecified noninfective disorders of pinna, left ear
H61.103   Unspecified noninfective disorders of pinna, bilateral
H61.109   Unspecified noninfective disorders of pinna, unspecified ear

✓6ᵗʰ **H61.11   Acquired deformity of pinna**
Acquired deformity of auricle
EXCLUDES 2   cauliflower ear (M95.1-)
H61.111   Acquired deformity of pinna, right ear
H61.112   Acquired deformity of pinna, left ear
H61.113   Acquired deformity of pinna, bilateral
H61.119   Acquired deformity of pinna, unspecified ear

✓6ᵗʰ **H61.12   Hematoma of pinna**
Hematoma of auricle
H61.121   Hematoma of pinna, right ear
H61.122   Hematoma of pinna, left ear
H61.123   Hematoma of pinna, bilateral
H61.129   Hematoma of pinna, unspecified ear

✓6ᵗʰ **H61.19   Other noninfective disorders of pinna**
H61.191   Noninfective disorders of pinna, right ear
H61.192   Noninfective disorders of pinna, left ear
H61.193   Noninfective disorders of pinna, bilateral
H61.199   Noninfective disorders of pinna, unspecified ear

✓5ᵗʰ **H61.2   Impacted cerumen**
Wax in ear
13 **H61.20   Impacted cerumen, unspecified ear**
13 **H61.21   Impacted cerumen, right ear**
13 **H61.22   Impacted cerumen, left ear**
13 **H61.23   Impacted cerumen, bilateral**

✓5ᵗʰ **H61.3   Acquired stenosis of external ear canal**
Collapse of external ear canal
EXCLUDES 1   postprocedural stenosis of external ear canal (H95.81-)

✓6ᵗʰ **H61.30   Acquired stenosis of external ear canal, unspecified**
H61.301   Acquired stenosis of right external ear canal, unspecified
H61.302   Acquired stenosis of left external ear canal, unspecified
H61.303   Acquired stenosis of external ear canal, unspecified, bilateral
H61.309   Acquired stenosis of external ear canal, unspecified, unspecified ear

✓6ᵗʰ **H61.31   Acquired stenosis of external ear canal secondary to trauma**
H61.311   Acquired stenosis of right external ear canal secondary to trauma
H61.312   Acquired stenosis of left external ear canal secondary to trauma
H61.313   Acquired stenosis of external ear canal secondary to trauma, bilateral
H61.319   Acquired stenosis of external ear canal secondary to trauma, unspecified ear

✓6ᵗʰ **H61.32   Acquired stenosis of external ear canal secondary to inflammation and infection**
H61.321   Acquired stenosis of right external ear canal secondary to inflammation and infection
H61.322   Acquired stenosis of left external ear canal secondary to inflammation and infection
H61.323   Acquired stenosis of external ear canal secondary to inflammation and infection, bilateral
H61.329   Acquired stenosis of external ear canal secondary to inflammation and infection, unspecified ear

✓6ᵗʰ **H61.39   Other acquired stenosis of external ear canal**
H61.391   Other acquired stenosis of right external ear canal
H61.392   Other acquired stenosis of left external ear canal
H61.393   Other acquired stenosis of external ear canal, bilateral
H61.399   Other acquired stenosis of external ear canal, unspecified ear

✓5ᵗʰ **H61.8   Other specified disorders of external ear**

✓6ᵗʰ **H61.81   Exostosis of external canal**
H61.811   Exostosis of right external canal
H61.812   Exostosis of left external canal
H61.813   Exostosis of external canal, bilateral
H61.819   Exostosis of external canal, unspecified ear

✓6ᵗʰ **H61.89   Other specified disorders of external ear**
H61.891   Other specified disorders of right external ear
H61.892   Other specified disorders of left external ear
H61.893   Other specified disorders of external ear, bilateral
H61.899   Other specified disorders of external ear, unspecified ear

✓5ᵗʰ **H61.9   Disorder of external ear, unspecified**
H61.90   Disorder of external ear, unspecified, unspecified ear
H61.91   Disorder of right external ear, unspecified
H61.92   Disorder of left external ear, unspecified
H61.93   Disorder of external ear, unspecified, bilateral

---

13 Questionable admission when used as PDx.

✓ Additional Character Required   √x7ᵗʰ Xtension Alert   Unacceptable PDx   Manifestation   Hospital Acquired Condition   EXCLUDES 1 Not Coded Here   EXCLUDES 2 Not Included Here

Diseases of the Ear and Mastoid Process

H62–H65.93

☑4ᵗʰ H62 Disorders of external ear in diseases classified elsewhere

  ☑5ᵗʰ H62.4 Otitis externa in other diseases classified elsewhere

    Code first underlying disease, such as:
      erysipelas (A46)
      impetigo (L01.0)

    EXCLUDES 1   *otitis externa (in):*
        candidiasis (B37.84)
        herpes viral [herpes simplex] (B00.1)
        herpes zoster (B02.8)

    H62.40 Otitis externa in other diseases classified elsewhere, unspecified ear

    H62.41 Otitis externa in other diseases classified elsewhere, right ear

    H62.42 Otitis externa in other diseases classified elsewhere, left ear

    H62.43 Otitis externa in other diseases classified elsewhere, bilateral

  ☑5ᵗʰ H62.8 Other disorders of external ear in diseases classified elsewhere

    Code first underlying disease, such as:
      gout (M1A.-, M10.-)

    ☑6ᵗʰ H62.8X Other disorders of external ear in diseases classified elsewhere

      H62.8X1 Other disorders of right external ear in diseases classified elsewhere

      H62.8X2 Other disorders of left external ear in diseases classified elsewhere

      H62.8X3 Other disorders of external ear in diseases classified elsewhere, bilateral

      H62.8X9 Other disorders of external ear in diseases classified elsewhere, unspecified ear

Diseases of middle ear and mastoid (H65-H75)

☑4ᵗʰ H65 Nonsuppurative otitis media

  INCLUDES   nonsuppurative otitis media with myringitis

  Use additional code for any associated perforated tympanic membrane (H72.-)

  Use additional code to identify:
    exposure to environmental tobacco smoke (Z77.22)
    exposure to tobacco smoke in the perinatal period (P96.81)
    history of tobacco use (Z87.891)
    occupational exposure to environmental tobacco smoke (Z57.31)
    tobacco dependence (F17.-)
    tobacco use (Z72.0)

  ☑5ᵗʰ H65.0 Acute serous otitis media

    Acute and subacute secretory otitis

    H65.00 Acute serous otitis media, unspecified ear

    H65.01 Acute serous otitis media, right ear

    H65.02 Acute serous otitis media, left ear

    H65.03 Acute serous otitis media, bilateral

    H65.04 Acute serous otitis media, recurrent, right ear

    H65.05 Acute serous otitis media, recurrent, left ear

    H65.06 Acute serous otitis media, recurrent, bilateral

    H65.07 Acute serous otitis media, recurrent, unspecified ear

  ☑5ᵗʰ H65.1 Other acute nonsuppurative otitis media

    EXCLUDES 1   *otitic barotrauma (T70.0)*
           otitis media (acute) NOS (H66.9)

    ☑6ᵗʰ H65.11 Acute and subacute allergic otitis media (mucoid) (sanguinous) (serous)

      H65.111 Acute and subacute allergic otitis media (mucoid) (sanguinous) (serous), right ear

      H65.112 Acute and subacute allergic otitis media (mucoid) (sanguinous) (serous), left ear

      H65.113 Acute and subacute allergic otitis media (mucoid) (sanguinous) (serous), bilateral

      H65.114 Acute and subacute allergic otitis media (mucoid) (sanguinous) (serous), recurrent, right ear

      H65.115 Acute and subacute allergic otitis media (mucoid) (sanguinous) (serous), recurrent, left ear

      H65.116 Acute and subacute allergic otitis media (mucoid) (sanguinous) (serous), recurrent, bilateral

      H65.117 Acute and subacute allergic otitis media (mucoid) (sanguinous) (serous), recurrent, unspecified ear

      H65.119 Acute and subacute allergic otitis media (mucoid) (sanguinous) (serous), unspecified ear

    ☑6ᵗʰ H65.19 Other acute nonsuppurative otitis media

      Acute and subacute mucoid otitis media
      Acute and subacute nonsuppurative otitis media NOS
      Acute and subacute sanguinous otitis media
      Acute and subacute seromucinous otitis media

      H65.191 Other acute nonsuppurative otitis media, right ear

      H65.192 Other acute nonsuppurative otitis media, left ear

      H65.193 Other acute nonsuppurative otitis media, bilateral

      H65.194 Other acute nonsuppurative otitis media, recurrent, right ear

      H65.195 Other acute nonsuppurative otitis media, recurrent, left ear

      H65.196 Other acute nonsuppurative otitis media, recurrent, bilateral

      H65.197 Other acute nonsuppurative otitis media, recurrent, unspecified ear

      H65.199 Other acute nonsuppurative otitis media, unspecified ear

  ☑5ᵗʰ H65.2 Chronic serous otitis media

    Chronic tubotympanal catarrh

    H65.20 Chronic serous otitis media, unspecified ear

    H65.21 Chronic serous otitis media, right ear

    H65.22 Chronic serous otitis media, left ear

    H65.23 Chronic serous otitis media, bilateral

  ☑5ᵗʰ H65.3 Chronic mucoid otitis media

    Chronic mucinous otitis media
    Chronic secretory otitis media
    Chronic transudative otitis media
    Glue ear

    EXCLUDES 1   *adhesive middle ear disease (H74.1)*

    H65.30 Chronic mucoid otitis media, unspecified ear

    H65.31 Chronic mucoid otitis media, right ear

    H65.32 Chronic mucoid otitis media, left ear

    H65.33 Chronic mucoid otitis media, bilateral

  ☑5ᵗʰ H65.4 Other chronic nonsuppurative otitis media

    ☑6ᵗʰ H65.41 Chronic allergic otitis media

      H65.411 Chronic allergic otitis media, right ear

      H65.412 Chronic allergic otitis media, left ear

      H65.413 Chronic allergic otitis media, bilateral

      H65.419 Chronic allergic otitis media, unspecified ear

    ☑6ᵗʰ H65.49 Other chronic nonsuppurative otitis media

      Chronic exudative otitis media
      Chronic nonsuppurative otitis media NOS
      Chronic otitis media with effusion (nonpurulent)
      Chronic seromucinous otitis media

      H65.491 Other chronic nonsuppurative otitis media, right ear

      H65.492 Other chronic nonsuppurative otitis media, left ear

      H65.493 Other chronic nonsuppurative otitis media, bilateral

      H65.499 Other chronic nonsuppurative otitis media, unspecified ear

  ☑5ᵗʰ H65.9 Unspecified nonsuppurative otitis media

    Allergic otitis media NOS
    Catarrhal otitis media NOS
    Exudative otitis media NOS
    Mucoid otitis media NOS
    Otitis media with effusion (nonpurulent) NOS
    Secretory otitis media NOS
    Seromucinous otitis media NOS
    Serous otitis media NOS
    Transudative otitis media NOS

    H65.90 Unspecified nonsuppurative otitis media, unspecified ear

    H65.91 Unspecified nonsuppurative otitis media, right ear

    H65.92 Unspecified nonsuppurative otitis media, left ear

    H65.93 Unspecified nonsuppurative otitis media, bilateral

N Newborn: 0   **P** Pediatric: 0-17   **M** Maternity: 12-55   **A** Adult: 15-124   **MCC** Major CC Condition   **PDx MCC** PDx acts as own MCC   **CC** CC Condition   **PDx CC** PDx acts as own CC

582   ICD-10-CM Draft (2015)

√4th **H66 Suppurative and unspecified otitis media**
INCLUDES suppurative and unspecified otitis media with myringitis
Use additional code to identify:
exposure to environmental tobacco smoke (Z77.22)
exposure to tobacco smoke in the perinatal period (P96.81)
history of tobacco use (Z87.891)
occupational exposure to environmental tobacco smoke (Z57.31)
tobacco dependence (F17.-)
tobacco use (Z72.0)

√5th **H66.0 Acute suppurative otitis media**

√6th **H66.00 Acute suppurative otitis media without spontaneous rupture of ear drum**

H66.001 Acute suppurative otitis media without spontaneous rupture of ear drum, right ear

H66.002 Acute suppurative otitis media without spontaneous rupture of ear drum, left ear

H66.003 Acute suppurative otitis media without spontaneous rupture of ear drum, bilateral

H66.004 Acute suppurative otitis media without spontaneous rupture of ear drum, recurrent, right ear

H66.005 Acute suppurative otitis media without spontaneous rupture of ear drum, recurrent, left ear

H66.006 Acute suppurative otitis media without spontaneous rupture of ear drum, recurrent, bilateral

H66.007 Acute suppurative otitis media without spontaneous rupture of ear drum, recurrent, unspecified ear

H66.009 Acute suppurative otitis media without spontaneous rupture of ear drum, unspecified ear

√6th **H66.01 Acute suppurative otitis media with spontaneous rupture of ear drum**

H66.011 Acute suppurative otitis media with spontaneous rupture of ear drum, right ear

H66.012 Acute suppurative otitis media with spontaneous rupture of ear drum, left ear

H66.013 Acute suppurative otitis media with spontaneous rupture of ear drum, bilateral

H66.014 Acute suppurative otitis media with spontaneous rupture of ear drum, recurrent, right ear

H66.015 Acute suppurative otitis media with spontaneous rupture of ear drum, recurrent, left ear

H66.016 Acute suppurative otitis media with spontaneous rupture of ear drum, recurrent, bilateral

H66.017 Acute suppurative otitis media with spontaneous rupture of ear drum, recurrent, unspecified ear

H66.019 Acute suppurative otitis media with spontaneous rupture of ear drum, unspecified ear

√5th **H66.1 Chronic tubotympanic suppurative otitis media**
Benign chronic suppurative otitis media
Chronic tubotympanic disease
Use additional code for any associated perforated tympanic membrane (H72.-)

H66.10 Chronic tubotympanic suppurative otitis media, unspecified

H66.11 Chronic tubotympanic suppurative otitis media, right ear

H66.12 Chronic tubotympanic suppurative otitis media, left ear

H66.13 Chronic tubotympanic suppurative otitis media, bilateral

√5th **H66.2 Chronic atticoantral suppurative otitis media**
Chronic atticoantral disease
Use additional code for any associated perforated tympanic membrane (H72.-)

H66.20 Chronic atticoantral suppurative otitis media, unspecified ear

H66.21 Chronic atticoantral suppurative otitis media, right ear

H66.22 Chronic atticoantral suppurative otitis media, left ear

H66.23 Chronic atticoantral suppurative otitis media, bilateral

√5th **H66.3 Other chronic suppurative otitis media**
Chronic suppurative otitis media NOS
Use additional code for any associated perforated tympanic membrane (H72.-)
EXCLUDES 1 tuberculous otitis media (A18.6)

√6th **H66.3X Other chronic suppurative otitis media**

H66.3X1 Other chronic suppurative otitis media, right ear

H66.3X2 Other chronic suppurative otitis media, left ear

H66.3X3 Other chronic suppurative otitis media, bilateral

H66.3X9 Other chronic suppurative otitis media, unspecified ear

√5th **H66.4 Suppurative otitis media, unspecified**
Purulent otitis media NOS
Use additional code for any associated perforated tympanic membrane (H72.-)

H66.40 Suppurative otitis media, unspecified, unspecified ear

H66.41 Suppurative otitis media, unspecified, right ear

H66.42 Suppurative otitis media, unspecified, left ear

H66.43 Suppurative otitis media, unspecified, bilateral

√5th **H66.9 Otitis media, unspecified**
Otitis media NOS
Acute otitis media NOS
Chronic otitis media NOS
Use additional code for any associated perforated tympanic membrane (H72.-)

H66.90 Otitis media, unspecified, unspecified ear

H66.91 Otitis media, unspecified, right ear

H66.92 Otitis media, unspecified, left ear

H66.93 Otitis media, unspecified, bilateral

√4th **H67 Otitis media in diseases classified elsewhere**
Code first underlying disease, such as:
viral disease NEC (B00-B34)
Use additional code for any associated perforated tympanic membrane (H72.-)
EXCLUDES 1 otitis media in:
influenza (J09.X9, J10.83, J11.83)
measles (B05.3)
scarlet fever (A38.0)
tuberculosis (A18.6)

H67.1 *Otitis media in diseases classified elsewhere, right ear*

H67.2 *Otitis media in diseases classified elsewhere, left ear*

H67.3 *Otitis media in diseases classified elsewhere, bilateral*

H67.9 *Otitis media in diseases classified elsewhere, unspecified ear*

√4th **H68 Eustachian salpingitis and obstruction**

√5th **H68.0 Eustachian salpingitis**

√6th **H68.00 Unspecified Eustachian salpingitis**

H68.001 Unspecified Eustachian salpingitis, right ear

H68.002 Unspecified Eustachian salpingitis, left ear

H68.003 Unspecified Eustachian salpingitis, bilateral

H68.009 Unspecified Eustachian salpingitis, unspecified ear

√6th **H68.01 Acute Eustachian salpingitis**

H68.011 Acute Eustachian salpingitis, right ear

H68.012 Acute Eustachian salpingitis, left ear

H68.013 Acute Eustachian salpingitis, bilateral

H68.019 Acute Eustachian salpingitis, unspecified ear

√6th **H68.02 Chronic Eustachian salpingitis**

H68.021 Chronic Eustachian salpingitis, right ear

H68.022 Chronic Eustachian salpingitis, left ear

H68.023 Chronic Eustachian salpingitis, bilateral

H68.029 Chronic Eustachian salpingitis, unspecified ear

✓ Additional Character Required √x7th Xtension Alert Unacceptable PDx Manifestation Hospital Acquired Condition EXCLUDES 1 Not Coded Here EXCLUDES 2 Not Included Here

Diseases of the Ear and Mastoid Process

H68.1–H70.93

✓5ᵗʰ **H68.1** **Obstruction** of Eustachian tube
Stenosis of Eustachian tube
Stricture of Eustachian tube

    ✓6ᵗʰ **H68.10** **Unspecified** obstruction of Eustachian tube
        H68.101 Unspecified obstruction of Eustachian tube, **right** ear
        H68.102 Unspecified obstruction of Eustachian tube, **left** ear
        H68.103 Unspecified obstruction of Eustachian tube, **bilateral**
        H68.109 Unspecified obstruction of Eustachian tube, **unspecified** ear

    ✓6ᵗʰ **H68.11** **Osseous** obstruction of Eustachian tube
        H68.111 Osseous obstruction of Eustachian tube, **right** ear
        H68.112 Osseous obstruction of Eustachian tube, **left** ear
        H68.113 Osseous obstruction of Eustachian tube, **bilateral**
        H68.119 Osseous obstruction of Eustachian tube, **unspecified** ear

    ✓6ᵗʰ **H68.12** **Intrinsic cartilagenous** obstruction of Eustachian tube
        H68.121 Intrinsic cartilagenous obstruction of Eustachian tube, **right** ear
        H68.122 Intrinsic cartilagenous obstruction of Eustachian tube, **left** ear
        H68.123 Intrinsic cartilagenous obstruction of Eustachian tube, **bilateral**
        H68.129 Intrinsic cartilagenous obstruction of Eustachian tube, **unspecified** ear

    ✓6ᵗʰ **H68.13** **Extrinsic cartilagenous** obstruction of Eustachian tube
        Compression of Eustachian tube
        H68.131 Extrinsic cartilagenous obstruction of Eustachian tube, **right** ear
        H68.132 Extrinsic cartilagenous obstruction of Eustachian tube, **left** ear
        H68.133 Extrinsic cartilagenous obstruction of Eustachian tube, **bilateral**
        H68.139 Extrinsic cartilagenous obstruction of Eustachian tube, **unspecified** ear

✓4ᵗʰ **H69** **Other and unspecified disorders of Eustachian tube**

    ✓5ᵗʰ **H69.0** **Patulous** Eustachian tube
        H69.00 Patulous Eustachian tube, **unspecified** ear
        H69.01 Patulous Eustachian tube, **right** ear
        H69.02 Patulous Eustachian tube, **left** ear
        H69.03 Patulous Eustachian tube, **bilateral**

    ✓5ᵗʰ **H69.8** **Other specified** disorders of Eustachian tube
        H69.80 Other specified disorders of Eustachian tube, **unspecified** ear
        H69.81 Other specified disorders of Eustachian tube, **right** ear
        H69.82 Other specified disorders of Eustachian tube, **left** ear
        H69.83 Other specified disorders of Eustachian tube, **bilateral**

    ✓5ᵗʰ **H69.9** **Unspecified** Eustachian tube disorder
        H69.90 Unspecified Eustachian tube disorder, **unspecified** ear
        H69.91 Unspecified Eustachian tube disorder, **right** ear
        H69.92 Unspecified Eustachian tube disorder, **left** ear
        H69.93 Unspecified Eustachian tube disorder, **bilateral**

✓4ᵗʰ **H70** **Mastoiditis and related conditions**

    ✓5ᵗʰ **H70.0** **Acute mastoiditis**
        Abscess of mastoid
        Empyema of mastoid

        CC Excl: For CC codes in subcategory H70.0, unless otherwise noted: A17.9, A18.6, A18.82, A18.84, A18.89, H70.001-H70.93, H75.00-H75.83, H93.8X1-H93.93, H94.80-H95.199, Q16.1, Q16.9, Q17.3-Q17.9

    ✓6ᵗʰ **H70.00** **Acute mastoiditis** without complications
        H70.001 Acute mastoiditis without complications, **right** ear   CC
        H70.002 Acute mastoiditis without complications, **left** ear   CC

        H70.003 Acute mastoiditis without complications, **bilateral**   CC
        H70.009 Acute mastoiditis without complications, **unspecified** eard   CC

    ✓6ᵗʰ **H70.01** **Subperiosteal abscess** of mastoid
        H70.011 Subperiosteal abscess of mastoid, **right** ear   CC
        H70.012 Subperiosteal abscess of mastoid, **left** ear   CC
        H70.013 Subperiosteal abscess of mastoid, **bilateral**   CC
        H70.019 Subperiosteal abscess of mastoid, **unspecified** ear   CC

    ✓6ᵗʰ **H70.09** **Acute mastoiditis** with other complications
        H70.091 Acute mastoiditis with other complications, **right** ear   CC
        H70.092 Acute mastoiditis with other complications, **left** ear   CC
        H70.093 Acute mastoiditis with other complications, **bilateral**   CC
        H70.099 Acute mastoiditis with other complications, **unspecified** ear   CC

    ✓5ᵗʰ **H70.1** **Chronic mastoiditis**
        Caries of mastoid
        Fistula of mastoid
        EXCLUDES 1   *tuberculous mastoiditis (A18.03)*
        H70.10 Chronic mastoiditis, **unspecified** ear
        H70.11 Chronic mastoiditis, **right** ear
        H70.12 Chronic mastoiditis, **left** ear
        H70.13 Chronic mastoiditis, **bilateral**

    ✓5ᵗʰ **H70.2** **Petrositis**
        Inflammation of petrous bone
    ✓6ᵗʰ **H70.20** **Unspecified** petrositis
        H70.201 Unspecified petrositis, **right** ear
        H70.202 Unspecified petrositis, **left** ear
        H70.203 Unspecified petrositis, **bilateral**
        H70.209 Unspecified petrositis, **unspecified** ear

    ✓6ᵗʰ **H70.21** **Acute** petrositis
        H70.211 Acute petrositis, **right** ear
        H70.212 Acute petrositis, **left** ear
        H70.213 Acute petrositis, **bilateral**
        H70.219 Acute petrositis, **unspecified** ear

    ✓6ᵗʰ **H70.22** **Chronic** petrositis
        H70.221 Chronic petrositis, **right** ear
        H70.222 Chronic petrositis, **left** ear
        H70.223 Chronic petrositis, **bilateral**
        H70.229 Chronic petrositis, **unspecified** ear

    ✓5ᵗʰ **H70.8** **Other mastoiditis and related conditions**
        EXCLUDES 1   *preauricular sinus and cyst (Q18.1)*
                sinus, fistula, and cyst of branchial cleft (Q18.0)

    ✓6ᵗʰ **H70.81** **Postauricular fistula**
        H70.811 Postauricular fistula, **right** ear
        H70.812 Postauricular fistula, **left** ear
        H70.813 Postauricular fistula, **bilateral**
        H70.819 Postauricular fistula, **unspecified** ear

    ✓6ᵗʰ **H70.89** **Other mastoiditis and related conditions**
        H70.891 Other mastoiditis and related conditions, **right** ear
        H70.892 Other mastoiditis and related conditions, **left** ear
        H70.893 Other mastoiditis and related conditions, **bilateral**
        H70.899 Other mastoiditis and related conditions, **unspecified** ear

    ✓5ᵗʰ **H70.9** **Unspecified mastoiditis**
        H70.90 Unspecified mastoiditis, **unspecified** ear
        H70.91 Unspecified mastoiditis, **right** ear
        H70.92 Unspecified mastoiditis, **left** ear
        H70.93 Unspecified mastoiditis, **bilateral**

N Newborn: 0   **P** Pediatric: 0-17   **M** Maternity: 12-55   **A** Adult: 15-124   **MCC** Major CC Condition   **PDx MCC** PDx acts as own MCC   **CC** CC Condition   **PDx CC** PDx acts as own CC

584   ICD-10-CM Draft (2015)

☑4ᵗʰ **H71 Cholesteatoma of middle ear**

EXCLUDES 2   *cholesteatoma of external ear (H60.4-)*
         recurrent cholesteatoma of postmastoidectomy cavity (H95.0-)

☑5ᵗʰ **H71.0 Cholesteatoma of attic**

    H71.00 Cholesteatoma of attic, unspecified ear
    H71.01 Cholesteatoma of attic, right ear
    H71.02 Cholesteatoma of attic, left ear
    H71.03 Cholesteatoma of attic, bilateral

☑5ᵗʰ **H71.1 Cholesteatoma of tympanum**

    H71.10 Cholesteatoma of tympanum, unspecified ear
    H71.11 Cholesteatoma of tympanum, right ear
    H71.12 Cholesteatoma of tympanum, left ear
    H71.13 Cholesteatoma of tympanum, bilateral

☑5ᵗʰ **H71.2 Cholesteatoma of mastoid**

    H71.20 Cholesteatoma of mastoid, unspecified ear
    H71.21 Cholesteatoma of mastoid, right ear
    H71.22 Cholesteatoma of mastoid, left ear
    H71.23 Cholesteatoma of mastoid, bilateral

☑5ᵗʰ **H71.3 Diffuse cholesteatosis**

    H71.30 Diffuse cholesteatosis, unspecified ear
    H71.31 Diffuse cholesteatosis, right ear
    H71.32 Diffuse cholesteatosis, left ear
    H71.33 Diffuse cholesteatosis, bilateral

☑5ᵗʰ **H71.9 Unspecified cholesteatoma**

    H71.90 Unspecified cholesteatoma, unspecified ear
    H71.91 Unspecified cholesteatoma, right ear
    H71.92 Unspecified cholesteatoma, left ear
    H71.93 Unspecified cholesteatoma, bilateral

☑4ᵗʰ **H72 Perforation of tympanic membrane**

INCLUDES   persistent post-traumatic perforation of ear drum
         postinflammatory perforation of ear drum

Code first any associated otitis media (H65.-, H66.1-, H66.2-, H66.3-, H66.4-, H66.9-, H67.-)

EXCLUDES 1   *acute suppurative otitis media with rupture of the tympanic membrane (H66.01-)*
         traumatic rupture of ear drum (S09.2-)

☑5ᵗʰ **H72.0 Central perforation of tympanic membrane**

    H72.00 Central perforation of tympanic membrane, unspecified ear
    H72.01 Central perforation of tympanic membrane, right ear
    H72.02 Central perforation of tympanic membrane, left ear
    H72.03 Central perforation of tympanic membrane, bilateral

☑5ᵗʰ **H72.1 Attic perforation of tympanic membrane**

    Perforation of pars flaccida

    H72.10 Attic perforation of tympanic membrane, unspecified ear
    H72.11 Attic perforation of tympanic membrane, right ear
    H72.12 Attic perforation of tympanic membrane, left ear
    H72.13 Attic perforation of tympanic membrane, bilateral

☑5ᵗʰ **H72.2 Other marginal perforations of tympanic membrane**

  ☑6ᵗʰ **H72.2X Other marginal perforations of tympanic membrane**

    H72.2X1 Other marginal perforations of tympanic membrane, right ear
    H72.2X2 Other marginal perforations of tympanic membrane, left ear
    H72.2X3 Other marginal perforations of tympanic membrane, bilateral
    H72.2X9 Other marginal perforations of tympanic membrane, unspecified ear

☑5ᵗʰ **H72.8 Other perforations of tympanic membrane**

  ☑6ᵗʰ **H72.81 Multiple perforations of tympanic membrane**

    H72.811 Multiple perforations of tympanic membrane, right ear
    H72.812 Multiple perforations of tympanic membrane, left ear
    H72.813 Multiple perforations of tympanic membrane, bilateral
    H72.819 Multiple perforations of tympanic membrane, unspecified ear

☑6ᵗʰ **H72.82 Total perforations of tympanic membrane**

    H72.821 Total perforations of tympanic membrane, right ear
    H72.822 Total perforations of tympanic membrane, left ear
    H72.823 Total perforations of tympanic membrane, bilateral
    H72.829 Total perforations of tympanic membrane, unspecified ear

☑5ᵗʰ **H72.9 Unspecified perforation of tympanic membrane**

    H72.90 Unspecified perforation of tympanic membrane, unspecified ear
    H72.91 Unspecified perforation of tympanic membrane, right ear
    H72.92 Unspecified perforation of tympanic membrane, left ear
    H72.93 Unspecified perforation of tympanic membrane, bilateral

☑4ᵗʰ **H73 Other disorders of tympanic membrane**

☑5ᵗʰ **H73.0 Acute myringitis**

EXCLUDES 1   *acute myringitis with otitis media (H65, H66)*

  ☑6ᵗʰ **H73.00 Unspecified acute myringitis**
    Acute tympanitis NOS
    H73.001 Acute myringitis, right ear
    H73.002 Acute myringitis, left ear
    H73.003 Acute myringitis, bilateral
    H73.009 Acute myringitis, unspecified ear

  ☑6ᵗʰ **H73.01 Bullous myringitis**
    H73.011 Bullous myringitis, right ear
    H73.012 Bullous myringitis, left ear
    H73.013 Bullous myringitis, bilateral
    H73.019 Bullous myringitis, unspecified ear

  ☑6ᵗʰ **H73.09 Other acute myringitis**
    H73.091 Other acute myringitis, right ear
    H73.092 Other acute myringitis, left ear
    H73.093 Other acute myringitis, bilateral
    H73.099 Other acute myringitis, unspecified ear

☑5ᵗʰ **H73.1 Chronic myringitis**

    Chronic tympanitis

EXCLUDES 1   *chronic myringitis with otitis media (H65, H66)*

    H73.10 Chronic myringitis, unspecified ear
    H73.11 Chronic myringitis, right ear
    H73.12 Chronic myringitis, left ear
    H73.13 Chronic myringitis, bilateral

☑5ᵗʰ **H73.2 Unspecified myringitis**

    H73.20 Unspecified myringitis, unspecified ear
    H73.21 Unspecified myringitis, right ear
    H73.22 Unspecified myringitis, left ear
    H73.23 Unspecified myringitis, bilateral

☑5ᵗʰ **H73.8 Other specified disorders of tympanic membrane**

  ☑6ᵗʰ **H73.81 Atrophic flaccid tympanic membrane**
    H73.811 Atrophic flaccid tympanic membrane, right ear
    H73.812 Atrophic flaccid tympanic membrane, left ear
    H73.813 Atrophic flaccid tympanic membrane, bilateral
    H73.819 Atrophic flaccid tympanic membrane, unspecified ear

  ☑6ᵗʰ **H73.82 Atrophic nonflaccid tympanic membrane**
    H73.821 Atrophic nonflaccid tympanic membrane, right ear
    H73.822 Atrophic nonflaccid tympanic membrane, left ear
    H73.823 Atrophic nonflaccid tympanic membrane, bilateral
    H73.829 Atrophic nonflaccid tympanic membrane, unspecified ear

  ☑6ᵗʰ **H73.89 Other specified disorders of tympanic membrane**
    H73.891 Other specified disorders of tympanic membrane, right ear
    H73.892 Other specified disorders of tympanic membrane, left ear

---

☑ Additional Character Required ☑x7ᵗʰ Xtension Alert Unacceptable PDx Manifestation   Hospital Acquired Condition EXCLUDES 1 Not Coded Here EXCLUDES 2 Not Included Here

H73.893 **Other specified disorders of tympanic membrane, bilateral**

H73.899 **Other specified disorders of tympanic membrane, unspecified ear**

√5th **H73.9 Unspecified disorder of tympanic membrane**

H73.90 **Unspecified disorder of tympanic membrane, unspecified ear**

H73.91 **Unspecified disorder of tympanic membrane, right ear**

H73.92 **Unspecified disorder of tympanic membrane, left ear**

H73.93 **Unspecified disorder of tympanic membrane, bilateral**

√4th **H74 Other disorders of middle ear mastoid**

EXCLUDES 2   *mastoiditis (H70.-)*

√5th **H74.0 Tympanosclerosis**

H74.01 **Tympanosclerosis, right ear**

H74.02 **Tympanosclerosis, left ear**

H74.03 **Tympanosclerosis, bilateral**

H74.09 **Tympanosclerosis, unspecified ear**

√5th **H74.1 Adhesive middle ear disease**

Adhesive otitis

EXCLUDES 1   *glue ear (H65.3-)*

H74.11 **Adhesive right middle ear disease**

H74.12 **Adhesive left middle ear disease**

H74.13 **Adhesive middle ear disease, bilateral**

H74.19 **Adhesive middle ear disease, unspecified ear**

√5th **H74.2 Discontinuity and dislocation of ear ossicles**

H74.20 **Discontinuity and dislocation of ear ossicles, unspecified ear**

H74.21 **Discontinuity and dislocation of right ear ossicles**

H74.22 **Discontinuity and dislocation of left ear ossicles**

H74.23 **Discontinuity and dislocation of ear ossicles, bilateral**

√5th **H74.3 Other acquired abnormalities of ear ossicles**

√6th **H74.31 Ankylosis of ear ossicles**

H74.311 **Ankylosis of ear ossicles, right ear**

H74.312 **Ankylosis of ear ossicles, left ear**

H74.313 **Ankylosis of ear ossicles, bilateral**

H74.319 **Ankylosis of ear ossicles, unspecified ear**

√6th **H74.32 Partial loss of ear ossicles**

H74.321 **Partial loss of ear ossicles, right ear**

H74.322 **Partial loss of ear ossicles, left ear**

H74.323 **Partial loss of ear ossicles, bilateral**

H74.329 **Partial loss of ear ossicles, unspecified ear**

√6th **H74.39 Other acquired abnormalities of ear ossicles**

H74.391 **Other acquired abnormalities of right ear ossicles**

H74.392 **Other acquired abnormalities of left ear ossicles**

H74.393 **Other acquired abnormalities of ear ossicles, bilateral**

H74.399 **Other acquired abnormalities of ear ossicles, unspecified ear**

√5th **H74.4 Polyp of middle ear**

H74.40 **Polyp of middle ear, unspecified ear**

H74.41 **Polyp of right middle ear**

H74.42 **Polyp of left middle ear**

H74.43 **Polyp of middle ear, bilateral**

√5th **H74.8 Other specified disorders of middle ear and mastoid**

√6th **H74.8X Other specified disorders of middle ear and mastoid**

H74.8X1 **Other specified disorders of right middle ear and mastoid**

H74.8X2 **Other specified disorders of left middle ear and mastoid**

H74.8X3 **Other specified disorders of middle ear and mastoid, bilateral**

H74.8X9 **Other specified disorders of middle ear and mastoid, unspecified ear**

√5th **H74.9 Unspecified disorder of middle ear and mastoid**

H74.90 **Unspecified disorder of middle ear and mastoid, unspecified ear**

H74.91 **Unspecified disorder of right middle ear and mastoid**

H74.92 **Unspecified disorder of left middle ear and mastoid**

H74.93 **Unspecified disorder of middle ear and mastoid, bilateral**

√4th **H75 Other disorders of middle ear and mastoid in diseases classified elsewhere**

Code first underlying disease

√5th **H75.0 Mastoiditis in infectious and parasitic diseases classified elsewhere**

EXCLUDES 1   *mastoiditis (in):*
syphilis (A52.77)
tuberculosis (A18.03)

H75.00 *Mastoiditis in infectious and parasitic diseases classified elsewhere, unspecified ear*

H75.01 *Mastoiditis in infectious and parasitic diseases classified elsewhere, right ear*

H75.02 *Mastoiditis in infectious and parasitic diseases classified elsewhere, left ear*

H75.03 *Mastoiditis in infectious and parasitic diseases classified elsewhere, bilateral*

√5th **H75.8 Other specified disorders of middle ear and mastoid in diseases classified elsewhere**

H75.80 *Other specified disorders of middle ear and mastoid in diseases classified elsewhere, unspecified ear*

H75.81 *Other specified disorders of right middle ear and mastoid in diseases classified elsewhere*

H75.82 *Other specified disorders of left middle ear and mastoid in diseases classified elsewhere*

H75.83 *Other specified disorders of middle ear and mastoid in diseases classified elsewhere, bilateral*

Diseases of inner ear (H80-H83)

√4th **H80 Otosclerosis**

INCLUDES   Otospongiosis

√5th **H80.0 Otosclerosis involving oval window, nonobliterative**

H80.00 **Otosclerosis involving oval window, nonobliterative, unspecified ear**

H80.01 **Otosclerosis involving oval window, nonobliterative, right ear**

H80.02 **Otosclerosis involving oval window, nonobliterative, left ear**

H80.03 **Otosclerosis involving oval window, nonobliterative, bilateral**

√5th **H80.1 Otosclerosis involving oval window, obliterative**

H80.10 **Otosclerosis involving oval window, obliterative, unspecified ear**

H80.11 **Otosclerosis involving oval window, obliterative, right ear**

H80.12 **Otosclerosis involving oval window, obliterative, left ear**

H80.13 **Otosclerosis involving oval window, obliterative, bilateral**

√5th **H80.2 Cochlear otosclerosis**

Otosclerosis involving otic capsule
Otosclerosis involving round window

H80.20 **Cochlear otosclerosis, unspecified ear**

H80.21 **Cochlear otosclerosis, right ear**

H80.22 **Cochlear otosclerosis, left ear**

H80.23 **Cochlear otosclerosis, bilateral**

√5th **H80.8 Other otosclerosis**

H80.80 **Other otosclerosis, unspecified ear**

H80.81 **Other otosclerosis, right ear**

H80.82 **Other otosclerosis, left ear**

H80.83 **Other otosclerosis, bilateral**

√5th **H80.9 Unspecified otosclerosis**

H80.90 **Unspecified otosclerosis, unspecified ear**

H80.91 **Unspecified otosclerosis, right ear**

H80.92 **Unspecified otosclerosis, left ear**

H80.93 **Unspecified otosclerosis, bilateral**

N Newborn: 0   P Pediatric: 0-17   M Maternity: 12-55   A Adult: 15-124   MCC Major CC Condition   PDx MCC PDx acts as own MCC   CC CC Condition   PDx CC PDx acts as own CC

586   ICD-10-CM Draft (2015)

☑4ᵗʰ H81 Disorders of vestibular function
> *EXCLUDES 1* epidemic vertigo (A88.1)
> vertigo NOS (R42)

☑5ᵗʰ H81.0 Ménière's disease
> Labyrinthine hydrops
> Ménière's syndrome or vertigo

    H81.01 Ménière's disease, right ear
    H81.02 Ménière's disease, left ear
    H81.03 Ménière's disease, bilateral
    H81.09 Ménière's disease, unspecified ear

☑5ᵗʰ H81.1 Benign paroxysmal vertigo
    H81.10 Benign paroxysmal vertigo, unspecified ear
    H81.11 Benign paroxysmal vertigo, right ear
    H81.12 Benign paroxysmal vertigo, left ear
    H81.13 Benign paroxysmal vertigo, bilateral

☑5ᵗʰ H81.2 Vestibular neuronitis
    H81.20 Vestibular neuronitis, unspecified ear
    H81.21 Vestibular neuronitis, right ear
    H81.22 Vestibular neuronitis, left ear
    H81.23 Vestibular neuronitis, bilateral

☑5ᵗʰ H81.3 Other peripheral vertigo
  ☑6ᵗʰ H81.31 Aural vertigo
    H81.311 Aural vertigo, right ear
    H81.312 Aural vertigo, left ear
    H81.313 Aural vertigo, bilateral
    H81.319 Aural vertigo, unspecified ear

  ☑6ᵗʰ H81.39 Other peripheral vertigo
> Lermoyez' syndrome
> Otogenic vertigo
> Peripheral vertigo NOS

    H81.391 Other peripheral vertigo, right ear
    H81.392 Other peripheral vertigo, left ear
    H81.393 Other peripheral vertigo, bilateral
    H81.399 Other peripheral vertigo, unspecified ear

☑5ᵗʰ H81.4 Vertigo of central origin
> Central positional nystagmus

    H81.41 Vertigo of central origin, right ear
    H81.42 Vertigo of central origin, left ear
    H81.43 Vertigo of central origin, bilateral
    H81.49 Vertigo of central origin, unspecified ear

☑5ᵗʰ H81.8 Other disorders of vestibular function
  ☑6ᵗʰ H81.8X Other disorders of vestibular function
    H81.8X1 Other disorders of vestibular function, right ear
    H81.8X2 Other disorders of vestibular function, left ear
    H81.8X3 Other disorders of vestibular function, bilateral
    H81.8X9 Other disorders of vestibular function, unspecified ear

☑5ᵗʰ H81.9 Unspecified disorder of vestibular function
> Vertiginous syndrome NOS

    H81.90 Unspecified disorder of vestibular function, unspecified ear
    H81.91 Unspecified disorder of vestibular function, right ear
    H81.92 Unspecified disorder of vestibular function, left ear
    H81.93 Unspecified disorder of vestibular function, bilateral

☑4ᵗʰ H82 Vertiginous syndromes in diseases classified elsewhere
> *Code first underlying disease*
> *EXCLUDES 1* epidemic vertigo (A88.1)

    H82.1 *Vertiginous syndromes in diseases classified elsewhere, right ear*
    H82.2 *Vertiginous syndromes in diseases classified elsewhere, left ear*
    H82.3 *Vertiginous syndromes in diseases classified elsewhere, bilateral*
    H82.9 *Vertiginous syndromes in diseases classified elsewhere, unspecified ear*

☑4ᵗʰ H83 Other diseases of inner ear
☑5ᵗʰ H83.0 Labyrinthitis
    H83.01 Labyrinthitis, right ear
    H83.02 Labyrinthitis, left ear

    H83.03 Labyrinthitis, bilateral
    H83.09 Labyrinthitis, unspecified ear

☑5ᵗʰ H83.1 Labyrinthine fistula
    H83.11 Labyrinthine fistula, right ear
    H83.12 Labyrinthine fistula, left ear
    H83.13 Labyrinthine fistula, bilateral
    H83.19 Labyrinthine fistula, unspecified ear

☑5ᵗʰ H83.2 Labyrinthine dysfunction
> Labyrinthine hypersensitivity
> Labyrinthine hypofunction
> Labyrinthine loss of function

  ☑6ᵗʰ H83.2X Labyrinthine dysfunction
    H83.2X1 Labyrinthine dysfunction, right ear
    H83.2X2 Labyrinthine dysfunction, left ear
    H83.2X3 Labyrinthine dysfunction, bilateral
    H83.2X9 Labyrinthine dysfunction, unspecified ear

☑5ᵗʰ H83.3 Noise effects on inner ear
> Acoustic trauma of inner ear
> Noise-induced hearing loss of inner ear

  ☑6ᵗʰ H83.3X Noise effects on inner ear
    H83.3X1 Noise effects on right inner ear
    H83.3X2 Noise effects on left inner ear
    H83.3X3 Noise effects on inner ear, bilateral
    H83.3X9 Noise effects on inner ear, unspecified ear

☑5ᵗʰ H83.8 Other specified diseases of inner ear
  ☑6ᵗʰ H83.8X Other specified diseases of inner ear
    H83.8X1 Other specified diseases of right inner ear
    H83.8X2 Other specified diseases of left inner ear
    H83.8X3 Other specified diseases of inner ear, bilateral
    H83.8X9 Other specified diseases of inner ear, unspecified ear

☑5ᵗʰ H83.9 Unspecified disease of inner ear
    H83.90 Unspecified disease of inner ear, unspecified ear
    H83.91 Unspecified disease of right inner ear
    H83.92 Unspecified disease of left inner ear
    H83.93 Unspecified disease of inner ear, bilateral

Other disorders of ear (H90-H94)

☑4ᵗʰ H90 Conductive and sensorineural hearing loss
> *EXCLUDES 1* deaf nonspeaking NEC (H91.3)
> deafness NOS (H91.9-)
> hearing loss NOS (H91.9-)
> noise-induced hearing loss (H83.3-)
> ototoxic hearing loss (H91.0-)
> sudden (idiopathic) hearing loss (H91.2-)

H90.0 Conductive hearing loss, bilateral

☑5ᵗʰ H90.1 Conductive hearing loss, unilateral with unrestricted hearing on the contralateral side
    H90.11 Conductive hearing loss, unilateral, right ear, with unrestricted hearing on the contralateral side
    H90.12 Conductive hearing loss, unilateral, left ear, with unrestricted hearing on the contralateral side

H90.2 Conductive hearing loss, unspecified
> Conductive deafness NOS

H90.3 Sensorineural hearing loss, bilateral

☑5ᵗʰ H90.4 Sensorineural hearing loss, unilateral with unrestricted hearing on the contralateral side
    H90.41 Sensorineural hearing loss, unilateral, right ear, with unrestricted hearing on the contralateral side
    H90.42 Sensorineural hearing loss, unilateral, left ear, with unrestricted hearing on the contralateral side

H90.5 Unspecified sensorineural hearing loss
> Central hearing loss NOS   Perceptive hearing loss NOS
> Congenital deafness NOS   Sensorineural deafness NOS
> Neural hearing loss NOS   Sensory hearing loss NOS
> *EXCLUDES 1* abnormal auditory perception (H93.2-)
> psychogenic deafness (F44.6)

H90.6 Mixed conductive and sensorineural hearing loss, bilateral

☑5ᵗʰ H90.7 Mixed conductive and sensorineural hearing loss, unilateral with unrestricted hearing on the contralateral side
    H90.71 Mixed conductive and sensorineural hearing loss, unilateral, right ear, with unrestricted hearing on the contralateral side

---

☑ Additional Character Required   ☑x7ᵗʰ Xtension Alert   Unacceptable PDx   Manifestation   Hospital Acquired Condition   *EXCLUDES 1* Not Coded Here   *EXCLUDES 2* Not Included Here

Diseases of the Ear and Mastoid Process

H90.72–H93.8X9

H90.72   **Mixed conductive and sensorineural hearing loss, unilateral, left ear, with unrestricted hearing on the contralateral side**

H90.8   Mixed conductive and sensorineural hearing loss, unspecified

✓4ᵗʰ **H91**   **Other and unspecified hearing loss**
> EXCLUDES 1   abnormal auditory perception (H93.2-)
> hearing loss as classified in H90-
> impacted cerumen (H61.2-)
> noise-induced hearing loss (H83.3-)
> psychogenic deafness (F44.6)
> transient ischemic deafness (H93.01-)

✓5ᵗʰ **H91.0**   **Ototoxic hearing loss**
> Code first poisoning due to drug or toxin, if applicable (T36-T65 with fifth or sixth character 1-4 or 6)
> Use additional code for adverse effect, if applicable, to identify drug (T36-T50 with fifth or sixth character 5)

     H91.01   Ototoxic hearing loss, right ear
     H91.02   Ototoxic hearing loss, left ear
     H91.03   Ototoxic hearing loss, bilateral
     H91.09   Ototoxic hearing loss, unspecified ear

✓5ᵗʰ **H91.1**   **Presbycusis**
> Presbyacusis

     H91.10   Presbycusis, unspecified ear
     H91.11   Presbycusis, right ear
     H91.12   Presbycusis, left ear
     H91.13   Presbycusis, bilateral

✓5ᵗʰ **H91.2**   **Sudden idiopathic hearing loss**
> Sudden hearing loss NOS

     H91.20   Sudden idiopathic hearing loss, unspecified ear
     H91.21   Sudden idiopathic hearing loss, right ear
     H91.22   Sudden idiopathic hearing loss, left ear
     H91.23   Sudden idiopathic hearing loss, bilateral

     H91.3   Deaf nonspeaking, not elsewhere classified

✓5ᵗʰ **H91.8**   **Other specified hearing loss**
    ✓6ᵗʰ **H91.8X**   **Other specified hearing loss**
       H91.8X1   Other specified hearing loss, right ear
       H91.8X2   Other specified hearing loss, left ear
       H91.8X3   Other specified hearing loss, bilateral
       H91.8X9   Other specified hearing loss, unspecified ear

✓5ᵗʰ **H91.9**   **Unspecified hearing loss**
> Deafness NOS
> High frequency deafness
> Low frequency deafness

     H91.90   Unspecified hearing loss, unspecified ear
     H91.91   Unspecified hearing loss, right ear
     H91.92   Unspecified hearing loss, left ear
     H91.93   Unspecified hearing loss, bilateral

✓4ᵗʰ **H92**   **Otalgia and effusion of ear**

✓5ᵗʰ **H92.0**   **Otalgia**
     H92.01   Otalgia, right ear
     H92.02   Otalgia, left ear
     H92.03   Otalgia, bilateral
     H92.09   Otalgia, unspecified ear

✓5ᵗʰ **H92.1**   **Otorrhea**
> EXCLUDES 1   leakage of cerebrospinal fluid through ear (G96.0)

     H92.10   Otorrhea, unspecified ear
     H92.11   Otorrhea, right ear
     H92.12   Otorrhea, left ear
     H92.13   Otorrhea, bilateral

✓5ᵗʰ **H92.2**   **Otorrhagia**
> EXCLUDES 1   traumatic otorrhagia—code to injury

     H92.20   Otorrhagia, unspecified ear
     H92.21   Otorrhagia, right ear
     H92.22   Otorrhagia, left ear
     H92.23   Otorrhagia, bilateral

✓4ᵗʰ **H93**   **Other disorders of ear, not elsewhere classified**

✓5ᵗʰ **H93.0**   **Degenerative and vascular disorders of ear**
> EXCLUDES 1   presbycusis (H91.1)

    ✓6ᵗʰ **H93.01**   **Transient ischemic deafness**
       H93.011   Transient ischemic deafness, right ear
       H93.012   Transient ischemic deafness, left ear

       H93.013   Transient ischemic deafness, bilateral
       H93.019   Transient ischemic deafness, unspecified ear

    ✓6ᵗʰ **H93.09**   **Unspecified degenerative and vascular disorders of ear**
       H93.091   Unspecified degenerative and vascular disorders of right ear
       H93.092   Unspecified degenerative and vascular disorders of left ear
       H93.093   Unspecified degenerative and vascular disorders of ear, bilateral
       H93.099   Unspecified degenerative and vascular disorders of unspecified ear

✓5ᵗʰ **H93.1**   **Tinnitus**
     H93.11   Tinnitus, right ear
     H93.12   Tinnitus, left ear
     H93.13   Tinnitus, bilateral
     H93.19   Tinnitus, unspecified ear

✓5ᵗʰ **H93.2**   **Other abnormal auditory perceptions**
> EXCLUDES 2   auditory hallucinations (R44.0)

    ✓6ᵗʰ **H93.21**   **Auditory recruitment**
       H93.211   Auditory recruitment, right ear
       H93.212   Auditory recruitment, left ear
       H93.213   Auditory recruitment, bilateral
       H93.219   Auditory recruitment, unspecified ear

    ✓6ᵗʰ **H93.22**   **Diplacusis**
       H93.221   Diplacusis, right ear
       H93.222   Diplacusis, left ear
       H93.223   Diplacusis, bilateral
       H93.229   Diplacusis, unspecified ear

    ✓6ᵗʰ **H93.23**   **Hyperacusis**
       H93.231   Hyperacusis, right ear
       H93.232   Hyperacusis, left ear
       H93.233   Hyperacusis, bilateral
       H93.239   Hyperacusis, unspecified ear

    ✓6ᵗʰ **H93.24**   **Temporary auditory threshold shift**
       H93.241   Temporary auditory threshold shift, right ear
       H93.242   Temporary auditory threshold shift, left ear
       H93.243   Temporary auditory threshold shift, bilateral
       H93.249   Temporary auditory threshold shift, unspecified ear

     H93.25   Central auditory processing disorder
> Congenital auditory imperception
> Word deafness
> EXCLUDES 1   mixed receptive-expressive language disorder (F80.2)

    ✓6ᵗʰ **H93.29**   **Other abnormal auditory perceptions**
       H93.291   Other abnormal auditory perceptions, right ear
       H93.292   Other abnormal auditory perceptions, left ear
       H93.293   Other abnormal auditory perceptions, bilateral
       H93.299   Other abnormal auditory perceptions, unspecified ear

✓5ᵗʰ **H93.3**   **Disorders of acoustic nerve**
> Disorder of 8th cranial nerve
> EXCLUDES 1   acoustic neuroma (D33.3)
> syphilitic acoustic neuritis (A52.15)

    ✓6ᵗʰ **H93.3X**   **Disorders of acoustic nerve**
       H93.3X1   Disorders of right acoustic nerve
       H93.3X2   Disorders of left acoustic nerve
       H93.3X3   Disorders of bilateral acoustic nerves
       H93.3X9   Disorders of unspecified acoustic nerve

✓5ᵗʰ **H93.8**   **Other specified disorders of ear**
    ✓6ᵗʰ **H93.8X**   **Other specified disorders of ear**
       H93.8X1   Other specified disorders of right ear
       H93.8X2   Other specified disorders of left ear
       H93.8X3   Other specified disorders of ear, bilateral
       H93.8X9   Other specified disorders of ear, unspecified ear

---

Ⓝ Newborn: 0   Ⓟ Pediatric: 0-17   Ⓜ Maternity: 12-55   Ⓐ Adult: 15-124   MCC Major CC Condition   PDx MCC PDx acts as own MCC   CC CC Condition   PDx CC PDx acts as own CC

588   ICD-10-CM Draft (2015)

✓5ᵗʰ **H93.9** **Unspecified disorder of ear**
    H93.90 **Unspecified disorder of ear, unspecified ear**
    H93.91 **Unspecified disorder of right ear**
    H93.92 **Unspecified disorder of left ear**
    H93.93 **Unspecified disorder of ear, bilateral**

✓4ᵗʰ **H94** **Other disorders of ear in diseases classified elsewhere**
   ✓5ᵗʰ **H94.0** **Acoustic neuritis in infectious and parasitic diseases classified elsewhere**
      Code first underlying disease, such as:
       parasitic disease (B65-B89)
      EXCLUDES 1   *acoustic neuritis (in):*
         herpes zoster (B02.29)
         syphilis (A52.15)
      H94.00 **Acoustic neuritis in infectious and parasitic diseases classified elsewhere, unspecified ear**
      H94.01 **Acoustic neuritis in infectious and parasitic diseases classified elsewhere, right ear**
      H94.02 **Acoustic neuritis in infectious and parasitic diseases classified elsewhere, left ear**
      H94.03 **Acoustic neuritis in infectious and parasitic diseases classified elsewhere, bilateral**
   ✓5ᵗʰ **H94.8** **Other specified disorders of ear in diseases classified elsewhere**
      Code first underlying disease, such as:
       congenital syphilis (A50.0)
      EXCLUDES 1   *aural myiasis (B87.4)*
         syphilitic labyrinthitis (A52.79)
      H94.80 **Other specified disorders of ear in diseases classified elsewhere, unspecified ear**
      H94.81 **Other specified disorders of right ear in diseases classified elsewhere**
      H94.82 **Other specified disorders of left ear in diseases classified elsewhere**
      H94.83 **Other specified disorders of ear in diseases classified elsewhere, bilateral**

Intraoperative and postprocedural complications and disorders of ear and mastoid process, not elsewhere classified (H95)

✓4ᵗʰ **H95** **Intraoperative and postprocedural complications and disorders of ear and mastoid process, not elsewhere classified**
   ✓5ᵗʰ **H95.0** **Recurrent cholesteatoma of postmastoidectomy cavity**
      H95.00 **Recurrent cholesteatoma of postmastoidectomy cavity, unspecified ear**
      H95.01 **Recurrent cholesteatoma of postmastoidectomy cavity, right ear**
      H95.02 **Recurrent cholesteatoma of postmastoidectomy cavity, left ear**
      H95.03 **Recurrent cholesteatoma of postmastoidectomy cavity, bilateral ears**
   ✓5ᵗʰ **H95.1** **Other disorders of ear and mastoid process following mastoidectomy**
    ✓6ᵗʰ **H95.11** **Chronic inflammation of postmastoidectomy cavity**
      H95.111 **Chronic inflammation of postmastoidectomy cavity, right ear**
      H95.112 **Chronic inflammation of postmastoidectomy cavity, left ear**
      H95.113 **Chronic inflammation of postmastoidectomy cavity, bilateral ears**
      H95.119 **Chronic inflammation of postmastoidectomy cavity, unspecified ear**
    ✓6ᵗʰ **H95.12** **Granulation of postmastoidectomy cavity**
      H95.121 **Granulation of postmastoidectomy cavity, right ear**
      H95.122 **Granulation of postmastoidectomy cavity, left ear**
      H95.123 **Granulation of postmastoidectomy cavity, bilateral ears**
      H95.129 **Granulation of postmastoidectomy cavity, unspecified ear**
    ✓6ᵗʰ **H95.13** **Mucosal cyst of postmastoidectomy cavity**
      H95.131 **Mucosal cyst of postmastoidectomy cavity, right ear**
      H95.132 **Mucosal cyst of postmastoidectomy cavity, left ear**

      H95.133 **Mucosal cyst of postmastoidectomy cavity, bilateral ears**
      H95.139 **Mucosal cyst of postmastoidectomy cavity, unspecified ear**
    ✓6ᵗʰ **H95.19** **Other disorders following mastoidectomy**
      H95.191 **Other disorders following mastoidectomy, right ear**
      H95.192 **Other disorders following mastoidectomy, left ear**
      H95.193 **Other disorders following mastoidectomy, bilateral ears**
      H95.199 **Other disorders following mastoidectomy, unspecified ear**
   ✓5ᵗʰ **H95.2** **Intraoperative hemorrhage and hematoma of ear and mastoid process complicating a procedure**
      EXCLUDES 1   *intraoperative hemorrhage and hematoma of ear and mastoid process due to accidental puncture or laceration during a procedure (H95.3-)*
      H95.21 **Intraoperative hemorrhage and hematoma of** CC **ear and mastoid process complicating a procedure on the ear and mastoid process**
        CC Excl: H95.21-H95.22, H95.41-H95.89, I85.01, I85.11, I97.3, K21.9, K22.8, K23-K25.0, K25.2, K25.4, K25.6, K26.0, K26.2, K26.4, K26.6, K27.0, K27.2, K27.4, K27.6, K28.0, K28.2, K28.4, K28.6, K29.01, K29.21, K29.31, K29.41, K29.51, K29.61, K29.71, K29.81, K29.91, K31.811, K55.21, K57.01, K57.11, K57.13, K57.21, K57.31, K57.33, K57.41, K57.51, K57.53, K57.81, K57.91, K57.93, K62.5, K92.0-K92.2, M96.89, N98.1-N98.9, P54.1-P54.3, T81.10XA, T81.11XA, T81.12XA, T81.19XA, T81.82XA, T81.89XA, T81.9XXA
      H95.22 **Intraoperative hemorrhage and hematoma of** CC **of ear and mastoid process complicating other procedure**
        CC Excl: See code: H95.21
   ✓5ᵗʰ **H95.3** **Accidental puncture and laceration of ear and mastoid process during a procedure**
      CC Excl: For CC codes in subcategory H95.3, unless otherwise noted: D78.11-D78.12, D78.81-D78.89, E36.11-E36.8, E89.810-E89.89, G96.11, G97.41, G97.48-G97.49, H59.011-H59.019, H59.031-H59.099, H59.211-H59.229, H59.811-H59.89, H95.31-H95.32, H95.811-H95.89, I97.3, I97.51-I97.52, J95.71-J95.72, K91.71-K91.72, L76.11-L76.12, L76.81-L76.82, M96.820-M96.821, M96.89, N98.1-N98.9, N99.71-N99.72, T81.82XA, T81.89XA, T81.9XXA
      H95.31 **Accidental puncture and laceration of the ear** CC **and mastoid process during a procedure on the ear and mastoid process**
      H95.32 **Accidental puncture and laceration of the ear** CC **and mastoid process during other procedure**
   ✓5ᵗʰ **H95.4** **Postprocedural hemorrhage and hematoma of ear and mastoid process following a procedure**
      H95.41 **Postprocedural hemorrhage and hematoma of** CC **ear and mastoid process following a procedure on the ear and mastoid process**
        CC Excl: See code: H95.21
      H95.42 **Postprocedural hemorrhage and hematoma of** CC **ear and mastoid process following other procedure**
        CC Excl: See code: H95.21
   ✓5ᵗʰ **H95.8** **Other intraoperative and postprocedural complications and disorders of the ear and mastoid process, not elsewhere classified**
      EXCLUDES 2   *postprocedural complications and disorders following mastoidectomy (H95.0-, H95.1-)*
      CC Excl: For CC codes in subcategory H95.8, unless otherwise noted: D78.81-D78.89, E36.8, E89.810-E89.89, H59.011-H59.019, H59.031-H59.099, H59.811-H59.89, H95.811-H95.89, I97.3, L76.81-L76.82, M96.89, N98.1-N98.9, T81.82XA, T81.89XA, T81.9XXA
    ✓6ᵗʰ **H95.81** **Postprocedural stenosis of external ear canal**
      H95.811 **Postprocedural stenosis of right** CC **external ear canal**
      H95.812 **Postprocedural stenosis of left** CC **external ear canal**
      H95.813 **Postprocedural stenosis of external** CC **ear canal, bilateral**
      H95.819 **Postprocedural stenosis of** CC **unspecified external ear canal**

✓ Additional Character Required   ✓x7ᵗʰ Xtension Alert   Unacceptable PDx   Manifestation   Hospital Acquired Condition   EXCLUDES 1 Not Coded Here   EXCLUDES 2 Not Included Here

H95.88   **Other intraoperative complications and disorders of the ear and mastoid process, not elsewhere classified**   `CC`
Use additional code, if applicable, to further specify disorder

H95.89   **Other postprocedural complications and disorders of the ear and mastoid process, not elsewhere classified**   `CC`
Use additional code, if applicable, to further specify disorder

H95.88–H95.89

N Newborn: 0   **P** Pediatric: 0-17   **M** Maternity: 12-55   **A** Adult: 15-124   **MCC** Major CC Condition   **PDx MCC** PDx acts as own MCC   **CC** CC Condition   **PDx CC** PDx acts as own CC

590   ICD-10-CM Draft (2015)

Chapter 9. Diseases of the Circulatory System (I00-I99)

EXCLUDES 2 *certain conditions originating in the perinatal period (P04-P96)*
certain infectious and parasitic diseases (A00-B99)
complications of pregnancy, childbirth and the puerperium (O00-O9A)
congenital malformations, deformations, and chromosomal abnormalities (Q00-Q99)
endocrine, nutritional and metabolic diseases (E00-E88)
injury, poisoning and certain other consequences of external causes (S00-T88)
neoplasms (C00-D49)
symptoms, signs and abnormal clinical and laboratory findings, not elsewhere classified (R00-R94)
systemic connective tissue disorders (M30-M36)
transient cerebral ischemic attacks and related syndromes (G45.-)

This chapter contains the following blocks:

I00-I02   Acute rheumatic fever
I05-I09   Chronic rheumatic heart diseases
I10-I15   Hypertensive diseases
I20-I25   Ischemic heart diseases
I26-I28   Pulmonary heart disease and diseases of pulmonary circulation
I30-I52   Other forms of heart disease
I60-I69   Cerebrovascular diseases
I70-I79   Diseases of arteries, arterioles and capillaries
I80-I89   Diseases of veins, lymphatic vessels and lymph nodes, not elsewhere classified
I95-I99   Other and unspecified disorders of the circulatory system

Acute rheumatic fever (I00-I02)

I00   Rheumatic fever without heart involvement
  INCLUDES arthritis, rheumatic, acute or subacute
  EXCLUDES 1 *rheumatic fever with heart involvement (I01.0-I01.9)*

✓4th I01   Rheumatic fever with heart involvement
  EXCLUDES 1 *chronic diseases of rheumatic origin (I05-I09) unless rheumatic fever is also present or there is evidence of reactivation or activity of the rheumatic process.*

  I01.0   Acute rheumatic pericarditis `cc`
    Any condition in I00 with pericarditis
    Rheumatic pericarditis (acute)
    EXCLUDES 1 *acute pericarditis not specified as rheumatic (I30.-)*
    CC Excl: B33.23, I01.0, I09.2, I30.0-I30.9, I31.3-I32, I87.8, I99.8-I99.9

  I01.1   Acute rheumatic endocarditis `cc`
    Any condition in I00 with endocarditis or valvulitis
    Acute rheumatic valvulitis
    CC Excl: A01.00-A01.09, A39.51, A52.03, A78, B33.21, B37.6, I00, I01.1, I01.8-I02.0, I05.0-I07.9, I08.1-I08.3, I08.9, I09.1, I09.89-I09.9, I33.0-I39, I42.4, I87.8, I99.8-I99.9, Q22.2, Q23.8-Q23.9, Q24.8, T82.6XXA

  I01.2   Acute rheumatic myocarditis `cc`
    Any condition in I00 with myocarditis
    CC Excl: A52.06, B33.22, I00, I01.2-I01.9, I09.0, I09.9, I23.0-I23.3, I23.6-I23.8, I40.0-I41, I51.0, I51.4, I87.8, I99.8-I99.9

  I01.8   Other acute rheumatic heart disease `cc`
    Any condition in I00 with other or multiple types of heart involvement
    Acute rheumatic pancarditis
    CC Excl: I01.0-I09.9, I50.20-I50.43

  I01.9   Acute rheumatic heart disease, unspecified `cc`
    Any condition in I00 with unspecified type of heart involvement
    Rheumatic carditis, acute
    Rheumatic heart disease, active or acute
    CC Excl: I01.0-I09.9

✓4th I02   Rheumatic chorea
  INCLUDES Sydenham's chorea
  EXCLUDES 1 *chorea NOS (G25.5)*
    Huntington's chorea (G10)

  I02.0   Rheumatic chorea with heart involvement `cc`
    Chorea NOS with heart involvement
    Rheumatic chorea with heart involvement of any type classifiable under I01-
    CC Excl: See code: I01.8

  I02.9   Rheumatic chorea without heart involvement `cc`
    Rheumatic chorea NOS
    CC Excl: See code: I01.9

Chronic rheumatic heart diseases (I05-I09)

✓4th I05   Rheumatic mitral valve diseases
  INCLUDES conditions classifiable to both I05.0 and I05.2-I05.9, whether specified as rheumatic or not
  EXCLUDES 1 *mitral valve disease specified as nonrheumatic (I34.-)*
    mitral valve disease with aortic and/or tricuspid valve involvement (I08.-)

  I05.0   Rheumatic mitral stenosis
    Mitral (valve) obstruction (rheumatic)

  I05.1   Rheumatic mitral insufficiency
    Rheumatic mitral incompetence
    Rheumatic mitral regurgitation
    EXCLUDES 1 *mitral insufficiency not specified as rheumatic (I34.0)*

  I05.2   Rheumatic mitral stenosis with insufficiency
    Rheumatic mitral stenosis with incompetence or regurgitation

  I05.8   Other rheumatic mitral valve diseases
    Rheumatic mitral (valve) failure

  I05.9   Rheumatic mitral valve disease, unspecified
    Rheumatic mitral (valve) disorder (chronic) NOS

✓4th I06   Rheumatic aortic valve diseases
  EXCLUDES 1 *aortic valve disease not specified as rheumatic (I35.-)*
    aortic valve disease with mitral and/or tricuspid valve involvement (I08.-)

  I06.0   Rheumatic aortic stenosis
    Rheumatic aortic (valve) obstruction

  I06.1   Rheumatic aortic insufficiency
    Rheumatic aortic incompetence
    Rheumatic aortic regurgitation

  I06.2   Rheumatic aortic stenosis with insufficiency
    Rheumatic aortic stenosis with incompetence or regurgitation

  I06.8   Other rheumatic aortic valve diseases

  I06.9   Rheumatic aortic valve disease, unspecified
    Rheumatic aortic (valve) disease NOS

✓4th I07   Rheumatic tricuspid valve diseases
  INCLUDES rheumatic tricuspid valve diseases specified as rheumatic or unspecified
  EXCLUDES 1 *tricuspid valve disease specified as nonrheumatic (I36.-)*
    tricuspid valve disease with aortic and/or mitral valve involvement (I08.-)

  I07.0   Rheumatic tricuspid stenosis
    Tricuspid (valve) stenosis (rheumatic)

  I07.1   Rheumatic tricuspid insufficiency
    Tricuspid (valve) insufficiency (rheumatic)

  I07.2   Rheumatic tricuspid stenosis and insufficiency

  I07.8   Other rheumatic tricuspid valve diseases

  I07.9   Rheumatic tricuspid valve disease, unspecified
    Rheumatic tricuspid valve disorder NOS

✓4th I08   Multiple valve diseases
  INCLUDES multiple valve diseases specified as rheumatic or unspecified
  EXCLUDES 1 *endocarditis, valve unspecified (I38)*
    multiple valve disease specified a nonrheumatic (I34.-, I35.-, I36.-, I37.-, I38.-, Q22.-, Q23.-, Q24.8-)
    rheumatic valve disease NOS (I09.1)

  I08.0   Rheumatic disorders of both mitral and aortic valves
    Involvement of both mitral and aortic valves specified as rheumatic or unspecified

  I08.1   Rheumatic disorders of both mitral and tricuspid valves

  I08.2   Rheumatic disorders of both aortic and tricuspid valves

  I08.3   Combined rheumatic disorders of mitral, aortic and tricuspid valves

  I08.8   Other rheumatic multiple valve diseases

  I08.9   Rheumatic multiple valve disease, unspecified

✓4th I09   Other rheumatic heart diseases

  I09.0   Rheumatic myocarditis `cc`
    EXCLUDES 1 *myocarditis not specified as rheumatic (I51.4)*
    CC Excl: I00, I01.2-I01.9, I09.0, I09.9, I23.0-I23.3, I23.6-I23.8, I40.0-I41, I51.0, I51.4, I87.8, I99.8-I99.9

  I09.1   Rheumatic diseases of endocardium, valve unspecified
    Rheumatic endocarditis (chronic)
    Rheumatic valvulitis (chronic)
    EXCLUDES 1 *endocarditis, valve unspecified (I38)*

  I09.2   Chronic rheumatic pericarditis `cc`
    Adherent pericardium, rheumatic
    Chronic rheumatic mediastinopericarditis
    Chronic rheumatic myopericarditis
    EXCLUDES 1 *chronic pericarditis not specified as rheumatic (I31.-)*
    CC Excl: B33.23, I01.0, I09.2, I30.0-I30.9, I31.3-I32, I87.8, I99.8-I99.9

Diseases of the Circulatory System

I09.8–I20.9

√5ᵗʰ **I09.8 Other specified rheumatic heart diseases**

  I09.81 Rheumatic heart failure `CC`
    Use additional code to identify type of heart failure (I50.-)
    CC Excl: I09.81, I09.9, I11.0, I50.1-I50.9, I87.8, I99.8-I99.9

  I09.89 Other specified rheumatic heart diseases
    Rheumatic disease of pulmonary valve

I09.9 Rheumatic heart disease, unspecified
  Rheumatic carditis
  EXCLUDES 1 rheumatoid carditis (M05.31)

Hypertensive diseases (I10-I15)

Use additional code to identify:
  exposure to environmental tobacco smoke (Z77.22)
  history of tobacco use (Z87.891)
  occupational exposure to environmental tobacco smoke (Z57.31)
  tobacco dependence (F17.-)
  tobacco use (Z72.0)
EXCLUDES 1 hypertensive disease complicating pregnancy, childbirth and the puerperium (O10-O11, O13-O16)
  neonatal hypertension (P29.2)
  primary pulmonary hypertension (I27.0)

13 **I10 Essential (primary) hypertension**
  INCLUDES high blood pressure
    hypertension (arterial) (benign) (essential) (malignant) (primary) (systemic)
  EXCLUDES 1 hypertensive disease complicating pregnancy, childbirth and the puerperium (O10-O11, O13-O16)
  EXCLUDES 2 essential (primary) hypertension involving vessels of brain (I60-I69)
    essential (primary) hypertension involving vessels of eye (H35.0-)

√4ᵗʰ **I11 Hypertensive heart disease**
  INCLUDES any condition in I51.4-I51.9 due to hypertension

  I11.0 Hypertensive heart disease with heart failure
    Hypertensive heart failure
    Use additional code to identify type of heart failure (I50.-)

  I11.9 Hypertensive heart disease without heart failure
    Hypertensive heart disease NOS

√4ᵗʰ **I12 Hypertensive chronic kidney disease**
  INCLUDES any condition in N18- and N26- due to hypertension
    arteriosclerosis of kidney
    arteriosclerotic nephritis (chronic) (interstitial)
    hypertensive nephropathy
    nephrosclerosis
  EXCLUDES 1 hypertension due to kidney disease (I15.0, I15.1)
    renovascular hypertension (I15.0)
    secondary hypertension (I15.-)
  EXCLUDES 2 acute kidney failure (N17.-)

  I12.0 Hypertensive chronic kidney disease with stage 5 chronic kidney disease or end stage renal disease `CC`
    Use additional code to identify the stage of chronic kidney disease (N18.5, N18.6)
    CC Excl: I10-I15.9, I87.8, I99.8-I99.9, N18.6, N26.2

  I12.9 Hypertensive chronic kidney disease with stage 1 through stage 4 chronic kidney disease, or unspecified chronic kidney disease
    Hypertensive chronic kidney disease NOS
    Hypertensive renal disease NOS
    Use additional code to identify the stage of chronic kidney disease (N18.1-N18.4, N18.9)

√4ᵗʰ **I13 Hypertensive heart and chronic kidney disease**
  INCLUDES any condition in I11- with any condition in I12-
    cardiorenal disease
    cardiovascular renal disease

  CC Excl: For CC codes in category I13, unless otherwise noted: I10-I15.9, I87.8, I99.8-I99.9, N26.2

  I13.0 Hypertensive heart and chronic kidney disease with heart failure and stage 1 through stage 4 chronic kidney disease, or unspecified chronic kidney disease `CC`
    Use additional code to identify type of heart failure (I50.-)
    Use additional code to identify stage of chronic kidney disease (N18.1-N18.4, N18.9)

√5ᵗʰ **I13.1 Hypertensive heart and chronic kidney disease without heart failure**

  I13.10 Hypertensive heart and chronic kidney disease without heart failure, with stage 1 through stage 4 chronic kidney disease, or unspecified chronic kidney disease
    Hypertensive heart disease and hypertensive chronic kidney disease NOS
    Use additional code to identify the stage of chronic kidney disease (N18.1-N18.4, N18.9)

  I13.11 Hypertensive heart and chronic kidney disease without heart failure, with stage 5 chronic kidney disease, or end stage renal disease `CC`
    Use additional code to identify the stage of chronic kidney disease (N18.5, N18.6)

  I13.2 Hypertensive heart and chronic kidney disease with heart failure and with stage 5 chronic kidney disease, or end stage renal disease `CC`
    Use additional code to identify type of heart failure (I50.-)
    Use additional code to identify the stage of chronic kidney disease (N18.5, N18.6)

√4ᵗʰ **I15 Secondary hypertension**
  Code also underlying condition
  EXCLUDES 1 postprocedural hypertension (I97.3)
  EXCLUDES 2 secondary hypertension involving vessels of brain (I60-I69)
    secondary hypertension involving vessels of eye (H35.0-)

  I15.0 Renovascular hypertension
  I15.1 Hypertension secondary to other renal disorders
  I15.2 Hypertension secondary to endocrine disorders
  I15.8 Other secondary hypertension
  I15.9 Secondary hypertension, unspecified

Ischemic heart diseases (I20-I25)

Use additional code to identify presence of hypertension (I10-I15)

√4ᵗʰ **I20 Angina pectoris**
  Use additional code to identify:
    exposure to environmental tobacco smoke (Z77.22)
    history of tobacco use (Z87.891)
    occupational exposure to environmental tobacco smoke (Z57.31)
    tobacco dependence (F17.-)
    tobacco use (Z72.0)
  EXCLUDES 1 angina pectoris with atherosclerotic heart disease of native coronary arteries (I25.1-)
    atherosclerosis of coronary artery bypass graft(s) and coronary artery of transplanted heart with angina pectoris (I25.7-)
    postinfarction angina (I23.7)

  I20.0 Unstable angina `CC`
    Accelerated angina
    Crescendo angina
    De novo effort angina
    Intermediate coronary syndrome
    Preinfarction syndrome
    Worsening effort angina
    CC Excl: I09.81, I11.0, I13.0, I13.2, I20.0-I22.9, I24.0, I24.8-I24.9, I25.5-I25.6, I25.82-I25.83, I25.89-I25.9, I50.1, I50.9, I87.8, I99.8-I99.9, R57.0, R57.9

  I20.1 Angina pectoris with documented spasm `CC`
    Angiospastic angina
    Prinzmetal angina
    Spasm-induced angina
    Variant angina
    CC Excl: I20.0-I22.9, I24.0, I24.8-I24.9, I25.5-I25.6, I25.89-I25.9, I87.8, I99.8-I99.9

  I20.8 Other forms of angina pectoris
    Angina equivalent
    Angina of effort
    Coronary slow flow syndrome
    Stenocardia
    Use additional code(s) for symptoms associated with angina equivalent

  I20.9 Angina pectoris, unspecified
    Angina NOS
    Anginal syndrome
    Cardiac angina
    Ischemic chest pain

---

13 Questionable admission when used as PDx.

N Newborn: 0   P Pediatric: 0-17   M Maternity: 12-55   A Adult: 15-124   MCC Major CC Condition   PDx MCC PDx acts as own MCC   CC CC Condition   PDx CC PDx acts as own CC

592   ICD-10-CM Draft (2015)

✓4th **I21** **ST elevation (STEMI) and non-ST elevation (NSTEMI) myocardial infarction**

INCLUDES   cardiac infarction
coronary (artery) embolism
coronary (artery) occlusion
coronary (artery) rupture
coronary (artery) thrombosis
infarction of heart, myocardium, or ventricle
myocardial infarction specified as acute or with a stated duration of 4 weeks (28 days) or less from onset

Use additional code, if applicable, to identify:
exposure to environmental tobacco smoke (Z77.22)
history of tobacco use (Z87.891)
occupational exposure to environmental tobacco smoke (Z57.31)
status post administration of tPA (rtPA) in a different facility within the last 24 hours prior to admission to current facility (Z92.82)
tobacco dependence (F17.-)
tobacco use (Z72.0)

EXCLUDES 2 *old myocardial infarction (I25.2)*
postmyocardial infarction syndrome (I24.1)
subsequent myocardial infarction (I22.-)

AHA: 2013, 1Q, 25; 2012, 4Q, 96, 102-103

CC Excl: For MCC codes in category I21, unless otherwise noted:
I21.01-I22.9, I87.8, I99.8-I99.9

✓5th **I21.0** **ST elevation (STEMI) myocardial infarction of anterior wall**

I21.01 **ST elevation (STEMI) myocardial infarction involving left main coronary artery** MCC

I21.02 **ST elevation (STEMI) myocardial infarction involving left anterior descending coronary artery** MCC
ST elevation (STEMI) myocardial infarction involving diagonal coronary artery
AHA: 2013, 1Q, 25

I21.09 **ST elevation (STEMI) myocardial infarction involving other coronary artery of anterior wall** MCC
Acute transmural myocardial infarction of anterior wall
Anteroapical transmural (Q wave) infarction (acute)
Anterolateral transmural (Q wave) infarction (acute)
Anteroseptal transmural (Q wave) infarction (acute)
Transmural (Q wave) infarction (acute) (of) anterior (wall) NOS
AHA: 2012, 4Q, 102-103

✓5th **I21.1** **ST elevation (STEMI) myocardial infarction of inferior wall**

I21.11 **ST elevation (STEMI) myocardial infarction involving right coronary artery** MCC
Inferoposterior transmural (Q wave) infarction (acute)

I21.19 **ST elevation (STEMI) myocardial infarction involving other coronary artery of inferior wall** MCC
Acute transmural myocardial infarction of inferior wall
Inferolateral transmural (Q wave) infarction (acute)
Transmural (Q wave) infarction (acute) (of) diaphragmatic wall
Transmural (Q wave) infarction (acute) (of) inferior (wall) NOS
EXCLUDES 2 *ST elevation (STEMI) myocardial infarction involving left circumflex coronary artery (I21.21)*
AHA: 2012, 4Q, 96

✓5th **I21.2** **ST elevation (STEMI) myocardial infarction of other sites**

I21.21 **ST elevation (STEMI) myocardial infarction involving left circumflex coronary artery** MCC
ST elevation (STEMI) myocardial infarction involving oblique marginal coronary artery

I21.29 **ST elevation (STEMI) myocardial infarction involving other sites** MCC
Acute transmural myocardial infarction of other sites
Apical-lateral transmural (Q wave) infarction (acute)
Basal-lateral transmural (Q wave) infarction (acute)
High lateral transmural (Q wave) infarction (acute)
Lateral (wall) NOS transmural (Q wave) infarction (acute)
Posterior (true) transmural (Q wave) infarction (acute)
Posterobasal transmural (Q wave) infarction (acute)
Posterolateral transmural (Q wave) infarction (acute)
Posteroseptal transmural (Q wave) infarction (acute)
Septal transmural (Q wave) infarction (acute) NOS

I21.3 **ST elevation (STEMI) myocardial infarction of unspecified site** MCC
Acute transmural myocardial infarction of unspecified site
Myocardial infarction (acute) NOS
Transmural (Q wave) myocardial infarction NOS

I21.4 **Non-ST elevation (NSTEMI) myocardial infarction** MCC
Acute subendocardial myocardial infarction
Non-Q wave myocardial infarction NOS
Nontransmural myocardial infarction NOS

✓4th **I22** **Subsequent ST elevation (STEMI) and non-ST elevation (NSTEMI) myocardial infarction**

INCLUDES   acute myocardial infarction occurring within four weeks (28 days) of a previous acute myocardial infarction, regardless of site
cardiac infarction
coronary (artery) embolism
coronary (artery) occlusion
coronary (artery) rupture
coronary (artery) thrombosis
infarction of heart, myocardium, or ventricle
recurrent myocardial infarction
reinfarction of myocardium
rupture of heart, myocardium, or ventricle

Use additional code, if applicable, to identify:
exposure to environmental tobacco smoke (Z77.22)
history of tobacco use (Z87.891)
occupational exposure to environmental tobacco smoke (Z57.31)
status post administration of tPA (rtPA) in a different facility within the last 24 hours prior to admission to current facility (Z92.82)
tobacco dependence (F17.-)
tobacco use (Z72.0))
AHA: 2013, 1Q, 25; 2012, 4Q, 97, 102-103

CC Excl: For MCC codes in category I22, unless otherwise noted:
See code: I21

I22.0 **Subsequent ST elevation (STEMI) myocardial infarction of anterior wall** MCC
Subsequent acute transmural myocardial infarction of anterior wall
Subsequent transmural (Q wave) infarction (acute)(of) anterior (wall) NOS
Subsequent anteroapical transmural (Q wave) infarction (acute)
Subsequent anterolateral transmural (Q wave) infarction (acute)
Subsequent anteroseptal transmural (Q wave) infarction (acute)

I22.1 **Subsequent ST elevation (STEMI) myocardial infarction of inferior wall** MCC
Subsequent acute transmural myocardial infarction of inferior wall
Subsequent transmural (Q wave) infarction (acute)(of) diaphragmatic wall
Subsequent transmural (Q wave) infarction (acute)(of) inferior (wall) NOS
Subsequent inferolateral transmural (Q wave) infarction (acute)
Subsequent inferoposterior transmural (Q wave) infarction (acute)
AHA: 2012, 4Q, 102

I22.2 **Subsequent non-ST elevation (NSTEMI) myocardial infarction** MCC
Subsequent acute subendocardial myocardial infarction
Subsequent non-Q wave myocardial infarction NOS
Subsequent nontransmural myocardial infarction NOS

I22.8 **Subsequent ST elevation (STEMI) myocardial infarction of other sites** MCC
Subsequent acute transmural myocardial infarction of other sites
Subsequent apical-lateral transmural (Q wave) myocardial infarction (acute)
Subsequent basal-lateral transmural (Q wave) myocardial infarction (acute)
Subsequent high lateral transmural (Q wave) myocardial infarction (acute)
Subsequent transmural (Q wave) myocardial infarction (acute)(of) lateral (wall) NOS
Subsequent posterior (true)transmural (Q wave) myocardial infarction (acute)
Subsequent posterobasal transmural (Q wave) myocardial infarction (acute)
Subsequent posterolateral transmural (Q wave) myocardial infarction (acute)
Subsequent posteroseptal transmural (Q wave) myocardial infarction (acute)
Subsequent septal NOS transmural (Q wave) myocardial infarction (acute)

I22.9 **Subsequent ST elevation (STEMI) myocardial infarction of unspecified site** MCC
Subsequent acute myocardial infarction of unspecified site
Subsequent myocardial infarction (acute) NOS

Diseases of the Circulatory System

I23–I25.6

✓4ᵗʰ **I23**   **Certain current complications following ST elevation (STEMI) and non-ST elevation (NSTEMI) myocardial infarction (within the 28 day period)**

> **CC Excl:** For CC/MCC codes in category I23, unless otherwise noted: E78.71-E78.72, I23.0-I23.8, I40.0-I41, I51.0-I51.2, I51.4, I87.8, I97.0-I97.191, I99.8-I99.9, P29.3, Q20.0-Q21.9, Q23.8-Q23.9, Q24.8-Q24.9, Q27.30, Q27.4, Q28.0-Q28.1, Q28.8-Q28.9, Q87.1-Q87.89, Q89.7-Q89.8, Q99.2

I23.0   **Hemopericardium as current complication following acute myocardial infarction**   [CC][A]
> *EXCLUDES 1*   hemopericardium not specified as current complication following acute myocardial infarction (I31.2)

I23.1   **Atrial septal defect as current complication following acute myocardial infarction**   [CC][A]
> *EXCLUDES 1*   acquired atrial septal defect not specified as current complication following acute myocardial infarction (I51.0)

I23.2   **Ventricular septal defect as current complication following acute myocardial infarction**   [CC][A]
> *EXCLUDES 1*   acquired ventricular septal defect not specified as current complication following acute myocardial infarction (I51.0)

I23.3   **Rupture of cardiac wall without hemopericardium as current complication following acute myocardial infarction**   [CC][A]

I23.4   **Rupture of chordae tendineae as current complication following acute myocardial infarction**   [MCC]
> *EXCLUDES 1*   rupture of chordae tendineae not specified as current complication following acute myocardial infarction (I51.1)
>
> **CC Excl:** I23.0-I23.4, I23.6-I23.8, I51.0-I51.1, I87.8, I99.8-I99.9

I23.5   **Rupture of papillary muscle as current complication following acute myocardial infarction**   [MCC]
> *EXCLUDES 1*   rupture of papillary muscle not specified as current complication following acute myocardial infarction (I51.2)
>
> **CC Excl:** I23.0-I23.3, I23.5-I23.8, I51.0, I51.2, I87.8, I99.8-I99.9

I23.6   **Thrombosis of atrium, auricular appendage, and ventricle as current complications following acute myocardial infarction**   [CC][A]
> *EXCLUDES 1*   thrombosis of atrium, auricular appendage, and ventricle not specified as current complication following acute myocardial infarction (I51.3)

I23.7   **Postinfarction angina**   [CC][A]

I23.8   **Other current complications following acute myocardial infarction**   [CC][A]

✓4ᵗʰ **I24**   **Other acute ischemic heart diseases**
> *EXCLUDES 1*   angina pectoris (I20.-)
>   transient myocardial ischemia in newborn (P29.4)

> **CC Excl:** For CC codes in category I24, unless otherwise noted: I20.0-I22.9, I24.0-I24.9, I25.5-I25.6, I25.89-I25.9, I87.8, I99.8-I99.9

I24.0   **Acute coronary thrombosis not resulting in myocardial infarction**   [CC]
> Acute coronary (artery) (vein) embolism not resulting in myocardial infarction
> Acute coronary (artery) (vein) occlusion not resulting in myocardial infarction
> Acute coronary (artery) (vein) thromboembolism not resulting in myocardial infarction
> *EXCLUDES 1*   atherosclerotic heart disease (I25.1-)
> **AHA:** 2013, 1Q, 24

I24.1   **Dressler's syndrome**   [CC]
> Postmyocardial infarction syndrome
> *EXCLUDES 1*   postinfarction angina (I23.7)
> **CC Excl:** I24.0-I24.9, I87.8, I99.8-I99.9

I24.8   **Other forms of acute ischemic heart disease**   [CC]

I24.9   **Acute ischemic heart disease, unspecified**   [CC]
> *EXCLUDES 1*   ischemic heart disease (chronic) NOS (I25.9)

✓4ᵗʰ **I25**   **Chronic ischemic heart disease**
> Use additional code to identify:
> chronic total occlusion of coronary artery (I25.82)
> exposure to environmental tobacco smoke (Z77.22)
> history of tobacco use (Z87.891)
> occupational exposure to environmental tobacco smoke (Z57.31)
> tobacco dependence (F17.-)
> tobacco use (Z72.0)

I25.1   **Atherosclerotic heart disease of native coronary artery**
> Atherosclerotic cardiovascular disease
> Coronary (artery) atheroma
> Coronary (artery) atherosclerosis
> Coronary (artery) disease
> Coronary (artery) sclerosis
> Use additional code, if applicable, to identify:
> coronary atherosclerosis due to calcified coronary lesion (I25.84)
> coronary atherosclerosis due to lipid rich plaque (I25.83)
> *EXCLUDES 2*   atheroembolism (I75.-)
>   atherosclerosis of coronary artery bypass graft(s) and transplanted heart (I25.7-)

I25.10   **Atherosclerotic heart disease of native coronary artery without angina pectoris**   [A]
> Atherosclerotic heart disease NOS
> **AHA:** 2012, 4Q, 92

✓6ᵗʰ **I25.11**   **Atherosclerotic heart disease of native coronary artery with angina pectoris**

     I25.110   **Atherosclerotic heart disease of native coronary artery with unstable angina pectoris**   [PDx CC][CC][A]
> *EXCLUDES 1*   unstable angina without atherosclerotic heart disease (I20.0)
> **CC Excl:** I09.81, I11.0, I13.0, I13.2, I20.0-I22.9, I24.0, I24.8-I24.9, I25.5-I25.6, I25.82-I25.83, I25.89-I25.9, I50.1, I50.9, I87.8, I99.8-I99.9, R57.0, R57.9

     I25.111   **Atherosclerotic heart disease of native coronary artery with angina pectoris with documented spasm**   [A]
> *EXCLUDES 1*   angina pectoris with documented spasm without atherosclerotic heart disease (I20.1)

     I25.118   **Atherosclerotic heart disease of native coronary artery with other forms of angina pectoris**   [A]
> *EXCLUDES 1*   other forms of angina pectoris without atherosclerotic heart disease (I20.8)

     I25.119   **Atherosclerotic heart disease of native coronary artery with unspecified angina pectoris**   [A]
> Atherosclerotic heart disease with angina NOS
> Atherosclerotic heart disease with ischemic chest pain
> *EXCLUDES 1*   unspecified angina pectoris without atherosclerotic heart disease (I20.9)

I25.2   **Old myocardial infarction**
> Healed myocardial infarction
> Past myocardial infarction diagnosed by ECG or other investigation, but currently presenting no symptoms

I25.3   **Aneurysm of heart**   [CC]
> Mural aneurysm
> Ventricular aneurysm
> **CC Excl:** I25.3-I25.41

✓5ᵗʰ **I25.4**   **Coronary artery aneurysm and dissection**

     I25.41   **Coronary artery aneurysm**
> Coronary arteriovenous fistula, acquired
> *EXCLUDES 1*   congenital coronary (artery) aneurysm (Q24.5)

     I25.42   **Coronary artery dissection**   [MCC]
> **CC Excl:** I25.42, I67.0, I77.2-I77.3, I77.5-I77.6, I77.79, I77.89-I77.9, M31.8-M31.9

I25.5   **Ischemic cardiomyopathy**
> *EXCLUDES 2*   coronary atherosclerosis (I25.1-, I25.7-)

I25.6   **Silent myocardial ischemia**

[N] Newborn: 0   [P] Pediatric: 0-17   [M] Maternity: 12-55   [A] Adult: 15-124   [MCC] Major CC Condition   [PDx MCC] PDx acts as own MCC   [CC] CC Condition   [PDx CC] PDx acts as own CC

594   ICD-10-CM Draft (2015)

PDx unacceptable (handwritten margin note)

√5ᵗʰ I25.7　Atherosclerosis of coronary artery bypass graft(s) and coronary artery of transplanted heart with angina pectoris
Use additional code, if applicable, to identify:
coronary atherosclerosis due to calcified coronary lesion (I25.84)
coronary atherosclerosis due to lipid rich plaque (I25.83)
EXCLUDES 1　atherosclerosis of bypass graft(s) of transplanted heart without angina pectoris (I25.812)
atherosclerosis of coronary artery bypass graft(s) without angina pectoris (I25.810)
atherosclerosis of native coronary artery of transplanted heart without angina pectoris (I25.811)
embolism or thrombus of coronary artery bypass graft(s) (T82.8-)

√6ᵗʰ I25.70　Atherosclerosis of coronary artery bypass graft(s), unspecified, with angina pectoris

I25.700　Atherosclerosis of coronary artery bypass graft(s), unspecified, with unstable angina pectoris PDx CC　CC　A
EXCLUDES 1　unstable angina pectoris without atherosclerosis of coronary artery bypass graft (I20.0)
CC Excl: I09.81, I11.0, I13.0, I13.2, I20.0-I22.9, I24.0, I24.8-I24.9, I25.5-I25.6, I25.82-I25.83, I25.89-I25.9, I50.1, I50.9, I87.8, I99.8-I99.9, R57.0, R57.9

I25.701　Atherosclerosis of coronary artery bypass graft(s), unspecified, with angina pectoris with documented spasm A
EXCLUDES 1　angina pectoris with documented spasm without atherosclerosis of coronary artery bypass graft (I20.1)

I25.708　Atherosclerosis of coronary artery bypass graft(s), unspecified, with other forms of angina pectoris A
EXCLUDES 1　other forms of angina pectoris without atherosclerosis of coronary artery bypass graft (I20.8)

I25.709　Atherosclerosis of coronary artery bypass graft(s), unspecified, with unspecified angina pectoris A
EXCLUDES 1　unspecified angina pectoris without atherosclerosis of coronary artery bypass graft (I20.9)

√6ᵗʰ I25.71　Atherosclerosis of autologous vein coronary artery bypass graft(s) with angina pectoris

CC Excl: For CC codes in subcategory I25.71, unless otherwise noted: I25.10-I25.119, I25.700-I25.799, I25.811-I25.84

I25.710　Atherosclerosis of autologous vein coronary artery bypass graft(s) with unstable angina pectoris PDx CC　CC　A
EXCLUDES 1　unstable angina without atherosclerosis of autologous vein coronary artery bypass graft(s) (I20.0)
CC Excl: I09.81-I11.0, I13.0, I13.2, I20.0-I22.9, I24.0, I24.8-I25.119, I25.5-I25.739, I25.760-I25.799, I25.812-I25.9, I50.1, I50.9, I87.8, I99.8-I99.9, R57.0, R57.9

I25.711　Atherosclerosis of autologous vein coronary artery bypass graft(s) with angina pectoris with documented spasm CC　A
EXCLUDES 1　angina pectoris with documented spasm without atherosclerosis of autologous vein coronary artery bypass graft(s) (I20.1)

I25.718　Atherosclerosis of autologous vein coronary artery bypass graft(s) with other forms of angina pectoris CC　A
EXCLUDES 1　other forms of angina pectoris without atherosclerosis of autologous vein coronary artery bypass graft(s) (I20.8)

I25.719　Atherosclerosis of autologous vein coronary artery bypass graft(s) with unspecified angina pectoris CC　A
EXCLUDES 1　unspecified angina pectoris without atherosclerosis of autologous vein coronary artery bypass graft(s) (I20.9)

√6ᵗʰ I25.72　Atherosclerosis of autologous artery coronary artery bypass graft(s) with angina pectoris
Atherosclerosis of internal mammary artery graft with angina pectoris

CC Excl: For CC codes in subcategories I25.72, unless otherwise noted: I25.10-I25.119, I25.700-I25.738

I25.720　Atherosclerosis of autologous artery coronary artery bypass graft(s) with unstable angina pectoris PDx CC　CC　A
EXCLUDES 1　unstable angina without atherosclerosis of autologous artery coronary artery bypass graft(s) (I20.0)
CC Excl: See code: I25.710

I25.721　Atherosclerosis of autologous artery coronary artery bypass graft(s) with angina pectoris with documented spasm CC　A
EXCLUDES 1　angina pectoris with documented spasm without atherosclerosis of autologous artery coronary artery bypass graft(s) (I20.1)

I25.728　Atherosclerosis of autologous artery coronary artery bypass graft(s) with other forms of angina pectoris CC　A
EXCLUDES 1　other forms of angina pectoris without atherosclerosis of autologous artery coronary artery bypass graft(s) (I20.8)

I25.729　Atherosclerosis of autologous artery coronary artery bypass graft(s) with unspecified angina pectoris CC　A
EXCLUDES 1　unspecified angina pectoris without atherosclerosis of autologous artery coronary artery bypass graft(s) (I20.9)

√6ᵗʰ I25.73　Atherosclerosis of nonautologous biological coronary artery bypass graft(s) with angina pectoris

CC Excl: For CC codes in subcategories I25.73, unless otherwise noted: I25.10-I25.119, I25.700-I25.738

I25.730　Atherosclerosis of nonautologous biological coronary artery bypass graft(s) with unstable angina pectoris PDx CC　CC　A
EXCLUDES 1　unstable angina without atherosclerosis of nonautologous biological coronary artery bypass graft(s) (I20.0)
CC Excl: See code: I25.710

I25.731　Atherosclerosis of nonautologous biological coronary artery bypass graft(s) with angina pectoris with documented spasm CC　A
EXCLUDES 1　angina pectoris with documented spasm without atherosclerosis of nonautologous biological coronary artery bypass graft(s) (I20.1)

I25.738　Atherosclerosis of nonautologous biological coronary artery bypass graft(s) with other forms of angina pectoris CC　A
EXCLUDES 1　other forms of angina pectoris without atherosclerosis of nonautologous biological coronary artery bypass graft(s) (I20.8)

✔ Additional Character Required　　√x7ᵗʰ Xtension Alert　　Unacceptable PDx　　Manifestation　　Hospital Acquired Condition　　EXCLUDES 1 Not Coded Here　　EXCLUDES 2 Not Included Here

Diseases of the Circulatory System

I25.739–I25.9

I25.739 Atherosclerosis of nonautologous biological coronary artery bypass graft(s) with **unspecified** angina pectoris `CC` `A`
> **EXCLUDES 1**   unspecified angina pectoris without atherosclerosis of nonautologous biological coronary artery bypass graft(s) (I20.9)

✓6ᵗʰ **I25.75** Atherosclerosis of **native** coronary artery of **transplanted heart** with angina pectoris
> **EXCLUDES 1**   atherosclerosis of native coronary artery of transplanted heart without angina pectoris (I25.811)

> **CC Excl:** For CC codes in subcategory I25.75, unless otherwise noted: I25.10-I25.119, I25.700-I25.799, I25.811-I25.84

I25.750 Atherosclerosis of native coronary artery of transplanted heart with **unstable** angina `PDx CC` `CC`
> **CC Excl:** I09.81, I11.0, I13.0, I13.2, I20.0-I22.9, I24.0, I24.8-I25.119, I25.5-I25.799, I25.811-I25.9, I50.1, I50.9, I87.8, I99.8-I99.9, R57.0, R57.9

I25.751 Atherosclerosis of native coronary artery of transplanted heart with angina pectoris with **documented spasm** `CC`

I25.758 Atherosclerosis of native coronary artery of transplanted heart with **other forms** of angina pectoris `CC`

I25.759 Atherosclerosis of native coronary artery of transplanted heart with **unspecified** angina pectoris `CC`

✓6ᵗʰ **I25.76** Atherosclerosis of **bypass graft** of coronary artery of **transplanted heart** with angina pectoris
> **EXCLUDES 1**   atherosclerosis of bypass graft of coronary artery of transplanted heart without angina pectoris (I25.812)

> **CC Excl:** For CC codes in subcategory I25.76, unless otherwise noted: I25.10-I25.119, I25.700-I25.759, I25.790-I25.799, I25.811, I25.82-I25.84

I25.760 Atherosclerosis of bypass graft of coronary artery of transplanted heart with **unstable** angina `PDx CC` `CC` `A`
> **CC Excl:** I09.81-I11.0, I13.0, I13.2, I20.0-I22.9, I24.0, I24.8-I25.119, I25.5-I25.759, I25.790-I25.799, I25.811, I25.82-I25.9, I50.1, I50.9, I87.8, I99.8-I99.9, R57.0, R57.9

I25.761 Atherosclerosis of bypass graft of coronary artery of transplanted heart with angina pectoris with **documented spasm** `CC` `A`

I25.768 Atherosclerosis of bypass graft of coronary artery of transplanted heart with **other forms** of angina pectoris `CC` `A`

I25.769 Atherosclerosis of bypass graft of coronary artery of transplanted heart with **unspecified** angina pectoris `CC` `A`

✓6ᵗʰ **I25.79** Atherosclerosis of **other** coronary artery bypass graft(s) with angina pectoris

> **CC Excl:** For CC codes in subcategory I25.79, unless otherwise noted: No exclusion

I25.790 Atherosclerosis of other coronary artery bypass graft(s) with **unstable** angina pectoris `PDx CC` `CC` `A`
> **EXCLUDES 1**   unstable angina without atherosclerosis of other coronary artery bypass graft(s) (I20.0)
>
> **CC Excl:** I09.81, I11.0, I13.0, I13.2, I20.0-I22.9, I24.0, I24.8-I24.9, I25.5-I25.6, I25.82-I25.83, I25.89-I25.9, I50.1, I50.9, I87.8, I99.8-I99.9, R57.0, R57.9

I25.791 Atherosclerosis of other coronary artery bypass graft(s) with angina pectoris with **documented spasm** `CC` `A`
> **EXCLUDES 1**   angina pectoris with documented spasm without atherosclerosis of other coronary artery bypass graft(s) (I20.1)

I25.798 Atherosclerosis of other coronary artery bypass graft(s) with **other forms** of angina pectoris `CC` `A`
> **EXCLUDES 1**   other forms of angina pectoris without atherosclerosis of other coronary artery bypass graft(s) (I20.8)

I25.799 Atherosclerosis of other coronary artery bypass graft(s) with **unspecified** angina pectoris `CC` `A`
> **EXCLUDES 1**   unspecified angina pectoris without atherosclerosis of other coronary artery bypass graft(s) (I20.9)

✓5ᵗʰ **I25.8** Other forms of chronic ischemic heart disease

✓6ᵗʰ **I25.81** Atherosclerosis of **other coronary vessels** without angina pectoris
> Use additional code, if applicable, to identify:
> coronary atherosclerosis due to calcified coronary lesion (I25.84)
> coronary atherosclerosis due to lipid rich plaque (I25.83)
>
> **EXCLUDES 1**   atherosclerotic heart disease of native coronary artery without angina pectoris (I25.10)

I25.810 Atherosclerosis of coronary artery bypass graft(s) without angina pectoris `CC` `A`
> Atherosclerosis of coronary artery bypass graft NOS
> **EXCLUDES 1**   atherosclerosis of coronary bypass graft(s) with angina pectoris (I25.70--I25.73-, I25.79-)
>
> **CC Excl:** No excl

I25.811 Atherosclerosis of **native coronary** artery of **transplanted heart** without angina pectoris `CC`
> Atherosclerosis of native coronary artery of transplanted heart NOS
> **EXCLUDES 1**   atherosclerosis of native coronary artery of transplanted heart with angina pectoris (I25.75-)
>
> **CC Excl:** See code: I25.75

I25.812 Atherosclerosis of **bypass graft** of coronary artery of **transplanted heart** without angina pectoris `CC` `A`
> Atherosclerosis of bypass graft of transplanted heart NOS
> **EXCLUDES 1**   atherosclerosis of bypass graft of transplanted heart with angina pectoris (I25.76)
>
> **CC Excl:** See code: I25.76

I25.82 Chronic total occlusion of coronary artery
> Complete occlusion of coronary artery
> Total occlusion of coronary artery
> Code first coronary atherosclerosis (I25.1-, I25.7-, I25.81-)
> **EXCLUDES 1**   acute coronary occlusion with myocardial infarction (I21.-, I22.-)
> acute coronary occlusion without myocardial infarction (I24.0)

I25.83 Coronary atherosclerosis due to lipid rich plaque `A`
> Code first coronary atherosclerosis (I25.1-, I25.7-, I25.81-)

I25.84 Coronary atherosclerosis due to calcified coronary lesion
> Coronary atherosclerosis due to severely calcified coronary lesion
> Code first coronary atherosclerosis (I25.1-, I25.7-, I25.81-)

I25.89 Other forms of chronic ischemic heart disease

I25.9 Chronic ischemic heart disease, **unspecified**
> Ischemic heart disease (chronic) NOS

`N` Newborn: 0   `P` Pediatric: 0-17   `M` Maternity: 12-55   `A` Adult: 15-124   `MCC` Major CC Condition   `PDx MCC` PDx acts as own MCC   `CC` CC Condition   `PDx CC` PDx acts as own CC

596   ICD-10-CM Draft (2015)

Pulmonary heart disease and diseases of pulmonary circulation (I26-I28)

✓4th **I26 Pulmonary embolism**
Pulmonary (acute) (artery)(vein) infarction
Pulmonary (acute) (artery)(vein) thromboembolism
Pulmonary (acute) (artery)(vein) thrombosis
EXCLUDES 2   *chronic pulmonary embolism (I27.82)*
personal history of pulmonary embolism (Z86.711)
pulmonary embolism due to trauma (T79.0, T79.1)
pulmonary embolism due to complications of surgical and medical care (T80.0, T81.7-, T82.8-)
pulmonary embolism complicating abortion, ectopic or molar pregnancy (O00-O07, O08.2)
pulmonary embolism complicating pregnancy, childbirth and the puerperium (O88.-)
septic (non-pulmonary) arterial embolism (I76)

✓5th **I26.0 Pulmonary embolism with acute cor pulmonale**

    I26.01 Septic pulmonary embolism with acute cor pulmonale   PDx MCC MCC
Code first underlying infection
CC Excl: I26.01-I26.99, I27.2-I27.9, I74.01-I74.10, I74.19, I87.8, I99.8-I99.9

    3 **I26.02 Saddle embolus of pulmonary artery with acute cor pulmonale**   PDx MCC MCC
CC Excl: See code: I26.01

    3 **I26.09 Other pulmonary embolism with acute cor pulmonale**   PDx MCC MCC
Acute cor pulmonale NOS
CC Excl: See code: I26.01

✓5th **I26.9 Pulmonary embolism without acute cor pulmonale**

    I26.90 Septic pulmonary embolism without acute cor pulmonale   MCC
Code first underlying infection
CC Excl: I26.01-I26.99, I27.82, I74.01-I74.10, I74.19, I87.8, I99.8-I99.9, T80.0XXA, T81.718A, T81.72XA, T82.817A, T82.818A

    3 **I26.92 Saddle embolus of pulmonary artery without acute cor pulmonale**   MCC
CC Excl: I26.01-I26.99, I27.82, I74.01-I74.10, I74.19, I87.8, I99.8-I99.9

    3 **I26.99 Other pulmonary embolism without acute cor pulmonale**   MCC
Acute pulmonary embolism NOS
Pulmonary embolism NOS
CC Excl: See code: I26.90

✓4th **I27 Other pulmonary heart diseases**

I27.0 Primary pulmonary hypertension   CC
EXCLUDES 1   *pulmonary hypertension NOS (I27.2)*
secondary pulmonary hypertension (I27.2)
CC Excl: E66.2, I27.0, I27.2-I27.81, I27.89-I27.9, I28.8-I28.9, I87.8, I99.8-I99.9

I27.1 Kyphoscoliotic heart disease   CC
CC Excl: E66.2, I27.0-I27.81, I27.89-I27.9

I27.2 Other secondary pulmonary hypertension
Pulmonary hypertension NOS
Code also associated underlying condition

✓5th **I27.8 Other specified pulmonary heart diseases**

    I27.81 Cor pulmonale (chronic)
Cor pulmonale NOS
EXCLUDES 1   *acute cor pulmonale (I26.0-)*

    I27.82 Chronic pulmonary embolism   CC
Use additional code, if applicable, for associated long-term (current) use of anticoagulants (Z79.01)
EXCLUDES 1   *personal history of pulmonary embolism (Z86.711)*
CC Excl: I26.01-I26.99, I27.82, I74.01-I74.10, I74.19, I87.8, I99.8-I99.9

    I27.89 Other specified pulmonary heart diseases
Eisenmenger's complex
Eisenmenger's syndrome
EXCLUDES 1   *Eisenmenger's defect (Q21.8)*

I27.9 Pulmonary heart disease, unspecified
Chronic cardiopulmonary disease

✓4th **I28 Other diseases of pulmonary vessels**

I28.0 Arteriovenous fistula of pulmonary vessels   CC
EXCLUDES 1   *congenital arteriovenous fistula (Q25.72)*
CC Excl: I28.0-I28.9

I28.1 Aneurysm of pulmonary artery   CC
EXCLUDES 1   *congenital aneurysm (Q25.79)*
congenital arteriovenous aneurysm (Q25.72)
CC Excl: See code: I28.0

I28.8 Other diseases of pulmonary vessels
Pulmonary arteritis
Pulmonary endarteritis
Rupture of pulmonary vessels
Stenosis of pulmonary vessels
Stricture of pulmonary vessels

I28.9 Disease of pulmonary vessels, unspecified

Other forms of heart disease (I30-I52)

✓4th **I30 Acute pericarditis**
INCLUDES   acute mediastinopericarditis
acute myopericarditis
acute pericardial effusion
acute pleuropericarditis
acute pneumopericarditis
EXCLUDES 1   *Dressler's syndrome (I24.1)*
rheumatic pericarditis (acute) (I01.0)

CC Excl: For CC codes in category I30, unless otherwise noted: I01.0, I09.2, I30.0-I30.9, I31.1-I32, I87.8, I99.8-I99.9

I30.0 Acute nonspecific idiopathic pericarditis   CC

I30.1 Infective pericarditis   CC
Pneumococcal pericarditis
Pneumopyopericardium
Purulent pericarditis
Pyopericarditis
Pyopericardium
Pyopneumopericardium
Staphylococcal pericarditis
Streptococcal pericarditis
Suppurative pericarditis
Viral pericarditis
Use additional code (B95-B97) to identify infectious agent

I30.8 Other forms of acute pericarditis   CC

I30.9 Acute pericarditis, unspecified   CC

✓4th **I31 Other diseases of pericardium**
EXCLUDES 1   *diseases of pericardium specified as rheumatic (I09.2)*
postcardiotomy syndrome (I97.0)
traumatic injury to pericardium (S26.-)

I31.0 Chronic adhesive pericarditis   CC
Accretio cordis   Adhesive mediastinopericarditis
Adherent pericardium
CC Excl: I31.0-I31.9, I87.8, I99.8-I99.9

I31.1 Chronic constrictive pericarditis   CC
Concretio cordis   Pericardial calcification
CC Excl: See code: I31.0

I31.2 Hemopericardium, not elsewhere classified   CC
EXCLUDES 1   *hemopericardium as current complication following acute myocardial infarction (I23.0)*
CC Excl: See code: I31.0

I31.3 Pericardial effusion (noninflammatory)   CC
Chylopericardium
EXCLUDES 1   *acute pericardial effusion (I30.9)*
CC Excl: B33.23, I01.0, I09.2, I30.0-I30.9, I31.3-I32, I87.8, I99.8-I99.9

I31.4 Cardiac tamponade   CC
Code first underlying cause
CC Excl: See code: I31.3

I31.8 Other specified diseases of pericardium   CC
Epicardial plaques   Focal pericardial adhesions
CC Excl: See code: I31.3

I31.9 Disease of pericardium, unspecified   CC
Pericarditis (chronic) NOS
CC Excl: See code: I31.3

I32 Pericarditis in diseases classified elsewhere   CC
Code first underlying disease
EXCLUDES 1   *pericarditis (in):*
coxsackie (virus) (B33.23)
gonococcal (A54.83)
meningococcal (A39.53)
rheumatoid (arthritis) (M05.31)
syphilitic (A52.06)
systemic lupus erythematosus (M32.12)
tuberculosis (A18.84)
CC Excl: I01.0, I09.2, I30.0-I30.9, I31.3-I32, I87.8, I99.8-I99.9

---

3 These codes, although not unacceptable as PDx, would be considered questionable as a PDx for acute care hospital admissions.

✓ Additional Character Required   ✓x7th *Xtension* Alert   Unacceptable PDx   Manifestation   Hospital Acquired Condition   *EXCLUDES 1* Not Coded Here   *EXCLUDES 2* Not Included Here

Diseases of the Circulatory System

I33–I42.2

✓4ᵗʰ I33 Acute and subacute endocarditis

> EXCLUDES 1   acute rheumatic endocarditis (I01.1)
> endocarditis NOS (I38)

I33.0 Acute and subacute infective endocarditis   HIV MCC
Bacterial endocarditis (acute) (subacute)
Infective endocarditis (acute) (subacute) NOS
Endocarditis lenta (acute) (subacute)
Malignant endocarditis (acute) (subacute)
Purulent endocarditis (acute) (subacute)
Septic endocarditis (acute) (subacute)
Ulcerative endocarditis (acute) (subacute)
Vegetative endocarditis (acute) (subacute)
Use additional code (B95-B97) to identify infectious agent
CC Excl: I01.1-I08.3, I09.1, I33.0-I33.9, I38-I39, I87.8, I99.8-I99.9

I33.9 Acute and subacute endocarditis, unspecified   HIV MCC
Acute endocarditis NOS
Acute myoendocarditis NOS
Acute periendocarditis NOS
Subacute endocarditis NOS
Subacute myoendocarditis NOS
Subacute periendocarditis NOS
CC Excl: See code: I33.0

✓4ᵗʰ I34 Nonrheumatic mitral valve disorders

> EXCLUDES 1   mitral valve disease (I05.9)
> mitral valve failure (I05.8)
> mitral valve stenosis (I05.0)
> mitral valve disorder of unspecified cause with diseases of aortic and/or tricuspid valve(s) (I08.-)
> mitral valve disorder of unspecified cause with mitral stenosis or obstruction (I05.0)
> mitral valve disorder specified as congenital (Q23.2, Q23.3)
> mitral valve disorder specified as rheumatic (I05.-)

I34.0 Nonrheumatic mitral (valve) insufficiency
Nonrheumatic mitral (valve) incompetence NOS
Nonrheumatic mitral (valve) regurgitation NOS

I34.1 Nonrheumatic mitral (valve) prolapse
Floppy nonrheumatic mitral valve syndrome

> EXCLUDES 1   Marfan's syndrome (Q87.4-)

I34.2 Nonrheumatic mitral (valve) stenosis

I34.8 Other nonrheumatic mitral valve disorders

I34.9 Nonrheumatic mitral valve disorder, unspecified

✓4ᵗʰ I35 Nonrheumatic aortic valve disorders

> EXCLUDES 1   aortic valve disorder of unspecified cause but with diseases of mitral and/or tricuspid valve(s) (I08.-)
> aortic valve disorder specified as congenital (Q23.0, Q23.1)
> aortic valve disorder specified as rheumatic (I06.-)
> hypertrophic subaortic stenosis (I42.1)

I35.0 Nonrheumatic aortic (valve) stenosis

I35.1 Nonrheumatic aortic (valve) insufficiency
Nonrheumatic aortic (valve) incompetence NOS
Nonrheumatic aortic (valve) regurgitation NOS

I35.2 Nonrheumatic aortic (valve) stenosis with insufficiency

I35.8 Other nonrheumatic aortic valve disorders

I35.9 Nonrheumatic aortic valve disorder, unspecified

✓4ᵗʰ I36 Nonrheumatic tricuspid valve disorders

> EXCLUDES 1   tricuspid valve disorders of unspecified cause (I07.-)
> tricuspid valve disorders specified as congenital (Q22.4, Q22.8, Q22.9)
> tricuspid valve disorders specified as rheumatic (I07.-)
> tricuspid valve disorders with aortic and/or mitral valve involvement (I08.-)

I36.0 Nonrheumatic tricuspid (valve) stenosis

I36.1 Nonrheumatic tricuspid (valve) insufficiency
Nonrheumatic tricuspid (valve) incompetence
Nonrheumatic tricuspid (valve) regurgitation

I36.2 Nonrheumatic tricuspid (valve) stenosis with insufficiency

I36.8 Other nonrheumatic tricuspid valve disorders

I36.9 Nonrheumatic tricuspid valve disorder, unspecified

✓4ᵗʰ I37 Nonrheumatic pulmonary valve disorders

> EXCLUDES 1   pulmonary valve disorder specified as congenital (Q22.1, Q22.2, Q22.3)
> pulmonary valve disorder specified as rheumatic (I09.89)

I37.0 Nonrheumatic pulmonary valve stenosis

I37.1 Nonrheumatic pulmonary valve insufficiency
Nonrheumatic pulmonary valve incompetence
Nonrheumatic pulmonary valve regurgitation

I37.2 Nonrheumatic pulmonary valve stenosis with insufficiency

I37.8 Other nonrheumatic pulmonary valve disorders

I37.9 Nonrheumatic pulmonary valve disorder, unspecified

I38 Endocarditis, valve unspecified   CC

> INCLUDES   endocarditis (chronic) NOS
> valvular incompetence NOS
> valvular insufficiency NOS
> valvular regurgitation NOS
> valvular stenosis NOS
> valvulitis (chronic) NOS

> EXCLUDES 1   congenital insufficiency of cardiac valve NOS (Q24.8)
> congenital stenosis of cardiac valve NOS (Q24.8)
> endocardial fibroelastosis (I42.4)
> endocarditis specified as rheumatic (I09.1)

CC Excl: I38-I39, I87.8, I99.8-I99.9

I39 Endocarditis and heart valve disorders in diseases classified elsewhere   CC

> Code first underlying disease, such as:
> Q fever (A78)

> EXCLUDES 1   endocardial involvement in:
> candidiasis (B37.6)
> gonococcal infection (A54.83)
> Libman-Sacks disease (M32.11)
> listerosis (A32.82)
> meningococcal infection (A39.51)
> rheumatoid arthritis (M05.31)
> syphilis (A52.03)
> tuberculosis (A18.84)
> typhoid fever (A01.02)

CC Excl: See code: I38

✓4ᵗʰ I40 Acute myocarditis

> INCLUDES   subacute myocarditis

> EXCLUDES 1   acute rheumatic myocarditis (I01.2)

CC Excl: For MCC codes in category I40, unless otherwise noted: I01.2, I09.0, I23.0-I23.3, I23.6-I23.8, I40.0-I41, I51.0, I51.4, I87.8, I99.8-I99.9

I40.0 Infective myocarditis   HIV MCC
Septic myocarditis
Use additional code (B95-B97) to identify infectious agent

I40.1 Isolated myocarditis   HIV MCC
Fiedler's myocarditis
Giant cell myocarditis
Idiopathic myocarditis

I40.8 Other acute myocarditis   HIV MCC

I40.9 Acute myocarditis, unspecified   HIV MCC

I41 Myocarditis in diseases classified elsewhere   MCC

> Code first underlying disease, such as:
> typhus (A75.0-A75.9):

> EXCLUDES 1   myocarditis (in):
> Chagas' disease (chronic) (B57.2)
>   acute (B57.0)
> coxsackie (virus) infection (B33.22)
> diphtheritic (A36.81)
> gonococcal (A54.83)
> influenzal (J09.X9, J10.82, J11.82)
> meningococcal (A39.52)
> mumps (B26.82)
> rheumatoid arthritis (M05.31)
> sarcoid (D86.85)
> syphilis (A52.06)
> toxoplasmosis (B58.81)
> tuberculous (A18.84)

CC Excl: See code: I40

✓4ᵗʰ I42 Cardiomyopathy

> INCLUDES   myocardiopathy

> Code first pre-existing cardiomyopathy complicating pregnancy and puerperium (O99.4)

> EXCLUDES 1   ischemic cardiomyopathy (I25.5)
> peripartum cardiomyopathy (O90.3)

> EXCLUDES 2   ventricular hypertrophy (I51.7)

CC Excl: For CC codes in category I42, unless otherwise noted: I09.81, I11.0, I13.0, I13.2, I25.10-I25.119, I25.5-I25.799, I25.811-I25.9, I42.0-I44.1, I44.30-I44.39, I45.2-I45.4, I45.81-I45.89, I48.0-I49.1, I49.3-I49.8, I50.1, I50.9, I87.8, I99.8-I99.9, Q24.6, R00.0-R00.2, R57.0, R57.9

I42.0 Dilated cardiomyopathy   CC
Congestive cardiomyopathy

I42.1 Obstructive hypertrophic cardiomyopathy   CC
Hypertrophic subaortic stenosis (idiopathic)

I42.2 Other hypertrophic cardiomyopathy   CC
Nonobstructive hypertrophic cardiomyopathy

N Newborn: 0   P Pediatric: 0-17   M Maternity: 12-55   A Adult: 15-124   MCC Major CC Condition   PDx MCC PDx acts as own MCC   CC CC Condition   PDx CC PDx acts as own CC

598   ICD-10-CM Draft (2015)

I42.3   **Endomyocardial (eosinophilic) disease**   `CC`
Endomyocardial (tropical) fibrosis
Löffler's endocarditis

I42.4   **Endocardial fibroelastosis**   `CC`
Congenital cardiomyopathy
Elastomyofibrosis

I42.5   **Other restrictive cardiomyopathy**   `CC`
Constrictive cardiomyopathy NOS

I42.6   **Alcoholic cardiomyopathy**   `CC`
Code also presence of alcoholism (F10.-)

I42.7   **Cardiomyopathy due to drug and external agent**   `CC`
Code first poisoning due to drug or toxin, if applicable (T36-T65 with fifth or sixth character 1-4 or 6)
Use additional code for adverse effect, if applicable, to identify drug (T36-T50 with fifth or sixth character 5)

I42.8   **Other cardiomyopathies**   `CC`

I42.9   **Cardiomyopathy, unspecified**   `CC`
Cardiomyopathy (primary) (secondary) NOS

I43   *Cardiomyopathy in diseases classified elsewhere*   `CC`
Code first underlying disease, such as:
amyloidosis (E85.-)
glycogen storage disease (E74.0)
gout (M10.0-)
thyrotoxicosis (E05.0-E05.9-)
EXCLUDES 1   *cardiomyopathy (in):*
coxsackie (virus) (B33.24)
diphtheria (A36.81)
sarcoidosis (D86.85)
tuberculosis (A18.84)
CC Excl: See code: I42

✓4ᵗʰ **I44**   **Atrioventricular and left bundle-branch block**

I44.0   **Atrioventricular block, first degree**

I44.1   **Atrioventricular block, second degree**
Atrioventricular block, type I and II
Möbitz block, type I and II ✓
Second degree block, type I and II
Wenckebach's block

I44.2   **Atrioventricular block, complete**   `CC`
Complete heart block NOS
Third degree block
CC Excl: I44.0-I49.02, I49.2, I49.8, I87.8, I99.8-I99.9, R00.1

✓5ᵗʰ **I44.3**   **Other and unspecified atrioventricular block**
Atrioventricular block NOS

I44.30   **Unspecified atrioventricular block**

I44.39   **Other atrioventricular block**

¹³ **I44.4**   **Left anterior fascicular block**

¹³ **I44.5**   **Left posterior fascicular block**

✓5ᵗʰ **I44.6**   **Other and unspecified fascicular block**

¹³ **I44.60**   **Unspecified fascicular block**
Left bundle-branch hemiblock NOS

¹³ **I44.69**   **Other fascicular block**

✗ ¹³ **I44.7**   **Left bundle-branch block, unspecified**

✓4ᵗʰ **I45**   **Other conduction disorders**

CC Excl: For CC codes in category I45, unless otherwise noted: I44.0-I49.02, I49.2, I49.8, I87.8, I99.8-I99.9, R00.1

¹³ **I45.0**   **Right fascicular block**

✓5ᵗʰ **I45.1**   **Other and unspecified right bundle-branch block**

✗ ¹³ **I45.10**   **Unspecified right bundle-branch block**
Right bundle-branch block NOS

¹³ **I45.19**   **Other right bundle-branch block**

I45.2   **Bifascicular block**   `CC`

I45.3   **Trifascicular block**   `CC`

I45.4   **Nonspecific intraventricular block**
Bundle-branch block NOS

I45.5   **Other specified heart block**
Sinoatrial block   Sinoauricular block
EXCLUDES 1   *heart block NOS (I45.9)*

I45.6   **Pre-excitation syndrome**
Accelerated atrioventricular conduction
Accessory atrioventricular conduction
Anomalous atrioventricular excitation
Lown-Ganong-Levine syndrome
Pre-excitation atrioventricular conduction
Wolff-Parkinson-White syndrome

✓5ᵗʰ **I45.8**   **Other specified conduction disorders**

I45.81   **Long QT syndrome**

I45.89   **Other specified conduction disorders**   `CC`
Atrioventricular [AV] dissociation
Interference dissociation
Isorhythmic dissociation
Nonparoxysmal AV nodal tachycardia
AHA: 2013, 2Q, 31

I45.9   **Conduction disorder, unspecified**
Heart block NOS
Stokes-Adams syndrome

✓4ᵗʰ **I46**   **Cardiac arrest**
EXCLUDES 1   *cardiogenic shock (R57.0)*

CC Excl: For MCC codes in category I46, unless otherwise noted: I46.2-I49.02, I49.2, I87.8, I99.8-I99.9

¹⁰ **I46.2**   **Cardiac arrest due to underlying cardiac condition**   `MCC`
Code first underlying cardiac condition

¹⁰ **I46.8**   **Cardiac arrest due to other underlying condition**   `MCC`
Code first underlying condition

¹⁰ **I46.9**   **Cardiac arrest, cause unspecified**   `MCC`

✓4ᵗʰ **I47**   **Paroxysmal tachycardia**
Code first tachycardia complicating:
abortion or ectopic or molar pregnancy (O00-O07, O08.8)
obstetric surgery and procedures (O75.4)
EXCLUDES 1   *tachycardia NOS (R00.0)*
sinoauricular tachycardia NOS (R00.0)
sinus [sinusal] tachycardia NOS (R00.0)

CC Excl: For CC codes in category I47, unless otherwise noted: See code: I45

I47.0   **Re-entry ventricular arrhythmia**   `CC`

I47.1   **Supraventricular tachycardia**   `CC`
Atrial (paroxysmal) tachycardia
Atrioventricular [AV] (paroxysmal) tachycardia
Atrioventricular re-entrant (nodal) tachycardia [AVNRT] [AVRT]
Junctional (paroxysmal) tachycardia
Nodal (paroxysmal) tachycardia

I47.2   **Ventricular tachycardia**   `CC`
AHA: 2013, 3Q, 23

I47.9   **Paroxysmal tachycardia, unspecified**
Bouveret (-Hoffman) syndrome

✓4ᵗʰ **I48**   **Atrial fibrillation and flutter**

CC Excl: For CC codes in category I48, unless otherwise noted: See code: I45

I48.0   **Paroxysmal atrial fibrillation**

I48.1   **Persistent atrial fibrillation**   `CC`

I48.2   **Chronic atrial fibrillation**
Permanent atrial fibrillation

I48.3   **Typical atrial flutter**   `CC`
Type I atrial flutter

I48.4   **Atypical atrial flutter**   `CC`
Type II atrial flutter

✓5ᵗʰ **I48.9**   **Unspecified atrial fibrillation and atrial flutter**

I48.91   **Unspecified atrial fibrillation**

I48.92   **Unspecified atrial flutter**   `CC`

✓4ᵗʰ **I49**   **Other cardiac arrhythmias**

CC Excl: For MCC codes in category I49, unless otherwise noted: See code: I45

Code first cardiac arrhythmia complicating:
abortion or ectopic or molar pregnancy (O00-O07, O08.8)
obstetric surgery and procedures (O75.4)
EXCLUDES 1   *bradycardia NOS (R00.1)*
neonatal dysrhythmia (P29.1-)
sinoatrial bradycardia (R00.1)
sinus bradycardia (R00.1)
vagal bradycardia (R00.1)

✓5ᵗʰ **I49.0**   **Ventricular fibrillation and flutter**

¹⁰ **I49.01**   **Ventricular fibrillation**   `MCC`

I49.02   **Ventricular flutter**   `MCC`

I49.1   **Atrial premature depolarization**
Atrial premature beats

I49.2   **Junctional premature depolarization**   `CC`

---

¹⁰ MCC only if patient is discharged alive.
¹³ Questionable admission when used as PDx.

☑ Additional Character Required   **✗⁷ᵗʰ** Xtension Alert   Unacceptable PDx   Manifestation   Hospital Acquired Condition   **EXCLUDES 1** Not Coded Here   **EXCLUDES 2** Not Included Here

Diseases of the Circulatory System

I49.3 — Ventricular premature depolarization

✓5ᵗʰ **I49.4 Other and unspecified premature depolarization**

I49.40 Unspecified premature depolarization
Premature beats NOS

I49.49 Other premature depolarization
Ectopic beats   Extrasystolic arrhythmias
Extrasystoles   Premature contractions

I49.5 Sick sinus syndrome
Tachycardia-bradycardia syndrome

I49.8 Other specified cardiac arrhythmias
Coronary sinus rhythm disorder
Ectopic rhythm disorder
Nodal rhythm disorder

I49.9 Cardiac arrhythmia, unspecified
Arrhythmia (cardiac) NOS

✓4ᵗʰ **I50 Heart failure**
Code first:
heart failure complicating abortion or ectopic or molar pregnancy
(O00-O07, O08.8)
heart failure following surgery (I97.13-)
heart failure due to hypertension (I11.0)
heart failure due to hypertension with chronic kidney disease (I13.-)
obstetric surgery and procedures (O75.4)
rheumatic heart failure (I09.81)
EXCLUDES 1 *cardiac arrest (I46.-)*
neonatal cardiac failure (P29.0)
AHA: 2014, 1Q, 25; 2013, 2Q, 33

CC Excl: For CC/MCC codes in category I50, unless
otherwise noted: I09.81, I11.0, I50.1-I50.9, I87.8, I99.8-I99.9,
J81.0

I50.1 Left ventricular failure CC
Cardiac asthma
Edema of lung with heart disease NOS
Edema of lung with heart failure
Left heart failure
Pulmonary edema with heart disease NOS
Pulmonary edema with heart failure
EXCLUDES 1 *edema of lung without heart disease or heart failure*
(J81.-)
pulmonary edema without heart disease or failure
(J81.-)
CC Excl: I09.81, I11.0, I50.1-I50.9, I87.8, I99.8-I99.9

✓5ᵗʰ **I50.2 Systolic (congestive) heart failure**
EXCLUDES 1 *combined systolic (congestive) and diastolic*
(congestive) heart failure (I50.4-)

I50.20 Unspecified systolic (congestive) heart failure CC
I50.21 Acute systolic (congestive) heart failure MCC
I50.22 Chronic systolic (congestive) heart failure CC
I50.23 Acute on chronic systolic (congestive) heart failure MCC

✓5ᵗʰ **I50.3 Diastolic (congestive) heart failure**
EXCLUDES 1 *combined systolic (congestive) and diastolic*
(congestive) heart failure (I50.4-)

I50.30 Unspecified diastolic (congestive) heart failure CC
I50.31 Acute diastolic (congestive) heart failure MCC
I50.32 Chronic diastolic (congestive) heart failure CC
I50.33 Acute on chronic diastolic (congestive) heart failure MCC

✓5ᵗʰ **I50.4 Combined systolic (congestive) and diastolic (congestive) heart failure**

I50.40 Unspecified combined systolic (congestive) and diastolic (congestive) heart failure CC
I50.41 Acute combined systolic (congestive) and diastolic (congestive) heart failure MCC
I50.42 Chronic combined systolic (congestive) and diastolic (congestive) heart failure CC
I50.43 Acute on chronic combined systolic (congestive) and diastolic (congestive) heart failure MCC

I50.9 Heart failure, unspecified
Biventricular (heart) failure NOS
Cardiac, heart or myocardial failure NOS
Congestive heart disease
Congestive heart failure NOS
Right ventricular failure (secondary to left heart failure)
EXCLUDES 1 *fluid overload (E87.70)*
AHA: 2012, 4Q, 92

✓4ᵗʰ **I51 Complications and ill-defined descriptions of heart disease**
EXCLUDES 1 *any condition in I51.4-I51.9 due to hypertension (I11.-)*
any condition in I51.4-I51.9 due to hypertension and chronic
kidney disease (I13.-)
heart disease specified as rheumatic (I00-I09)

I51.0 Cardiac septal defect, acquired CC A
Acquired septal atrial defect (old)
Acquired septal auricular defect (old)
Acquired septal ventricular defect (old)
EXCLUDES 1 *cardiac septal defect as current complication following*
acute myocardial infarction (I23.1, I23.2)
CC Excl: E78.71-E78.72, I23.0-I23.8, I40.0-I41, I51.0-I51.2, I51.4,
I87.8, I97.0-I97.191, I99.8-I99.9, P29.3, Q20.0-Q21.9, Q23.8-Q23.9,
Q24.8-Q24.9, Q27.30, Q27.4, Q28.0-Q28.1, Q28.8-Q28.9, Q87.1-
Q87.89, Q89.7-Q89.8, Q99.2

I51.1 Rupture of chordae tendineae, not elsewhere classified MCC
EXCLUDES 1 *rupture of chordae tendineae as current complication*
following acute myocardial infarction (I23.4)
CC Excl: I23.0-I23.4, I23.6-I23.8, I51.0-I51.1, I87.8, I99.8-I99.9

I51.2 Rupture of papillary muscle, not elsewhere classified MCC
EXCLUDES 1 *rupture of papillary muscle as current complication*
following acute myocardial infarction (I23.5)
CC Excl: I23.0-I23.3, I23.5-I23.8, I51.0, I51.2, I87.8, I99.8-I99.9

I51.3 Intracardiac thrombosis, not elsewhere classified A
Apical thrombosis (old)   Mural thrombosis (old)
Atrial thrombosis (old)   Ventricular thrombosis (old)
Auricular thrombosis (old)
EXCLUDES 1 *intracardiac thrombosis as current complication*
following acute myocardial infarction (I23.6)
AHA: 2013, 1Q, 24

I51.4 Myocarditis, unspecified
Chronic (interstitial) myocarditis   Myocarditis NOS
Myocardial fibrosis
EXCLUDES 1 *acute or subacute myocarditis (I40.-)*

I51.5 Myocardial degeneration
Fatty degeneration of heart or myocardium
Myocardial disease
Senile degeneration of heart or myocardium

I51.7 Cardiomegaly
Cardiac dilatation   Ventricular dilatation
Cardiac hypertrophy

✓5ᵗʰ **I51.8 Other ill-defined heart diseases**

I51.81 Takotsubo syndrome CC
Reversible left ventricular dysfunction following
sudden emotional stress
Stress induced cardiomyopathy
Takotsubo cardiomyopathy
Transient left ventricular apical ballooning syndrome
CC Excl: I09.81, I11.0, I50.1-I50.9, I51.81, I51.9-I52, I87.8,
I99.8-I99.9

I51.89 Other ill-defined heart diseases
Carditis (acute)(chronic)
Pancarditis (acute)(chronic)

I51.9 Heart disease, unspecified

I52 Other heart disorders in diseases classified elsewhere
Code first underlying disease, such as:
congenital syphilis (A50.5)
mucopolysaccharidosis (E76.3)
schistosomiasis (B65.0-B65.9)
EXCLUDES 1 *heart disease (in):*
gonococcal infection (A54.83)
meningococcal infection (A39.50)
rheumatoid arthritis (M05.31)
syphilis (A52.06)

Cerebrovascular diseases (I60-I69)

Use additional code to identify presence of:
alcohol abuse and dependence (F10.-)
exposure to environmental tobacco smoke (Z77.22)
history of tobacco use (Z87.891)
hypertension (I10-I15)
occupational exposure to environmental tobacco smoke (Z57.31)
tobacco dependence (F17.-)
tobacco use (Z72.0)
EXCLUDES 1 *transient cerebral ischemic attacks and related syndromes (G45.-)*
traumatic intracranial hemorrhage (S06.-)
AHA: 2012, 4Q, 91-92

N Newborn: 0   P Pediatric: 0-17   M Maternity: 12-55   A Adult: 15-124   MCC Major CC Condition   PDx MCC PDx acts as own MCC   CC CC Condition   PDx CC PDx acts as own CC

600   ICD-10-CM Draft (2015)

✓4th **I60** **Nontraumatic subarachnoid hemorrhage**

INCLUDES ruptured cerebral aneurysm

EXCLUDES 1 sequelae of subarachnoid hemorrhage (I69.0-)
syphilitic ruptured cerebral aneurysm (A52.05)

CC Excl: For MCC codes in category I60, unless otherwise noted:
E03.5, G93.82, I60.00-I62.9, I87.8, I99.8-I99.9, R40.0-R40.2124,
R40.2210-R40.2224, R40.2310-R40.2324, R40.2340-R40.2344, R40.3-
R40.4, S02.0XX-S02.19X with 7th [A, B], S02.91X with 7th [A, B],
S06.0X0-S06.9X9 with 7th A

✓5th **I60.0** **Nontraumatic subarachnoid hemorrhage from** carotid siphon and bifurcation

   I60.00 **Nontraumatic subarachnoid hemorrhage from** MCC unspecified **carotid siphon and bifurcation**

   I60.01 **Nontraumatic subarachnoid hemorrhage from** MCC right **carotid siphon and bifurcation**

   I60.02 **Nontraumatic subarachnoid hemorrhage from** MCC left **carotid siphon and bifurcation**

✓5th **I60.1** **Nontraumatic subarachnoid hemorrhage from** middle cerebral artery

   I60.10 **Nontraumatic subarachnoid hemorrhage from** MCC unspecified **middle cerebral artery**

   I60.11 **Nontraumatic subarachnoid hemorrhage from** MCC right **middle cerebral artery**

   I60.12 **Nontraumatic subarachnoid hemorrhage from** MCC left **middle cerebral artery**

✓5th **I60.2** **Nontraumatic subarachnoid hemorrhage from** anterior communicating artery

   I60.20 **Nontraumatic subarachnoid hemorrhage from** MCC unspecified **anterior communicating artery**

   I60.21 **Nontraumatic subarachnoid hemorrhage from** MCC right **anterior communicating artery**

   I60.22 **Nontraumatic subarachnoid hemorrhage from** MCC left **anterior communicating artery**

✓5th **I60.3** **Nontraumatic subarachnoid hemorrhage from** posterior communicating artery

   I60.30 **Nontraumatic subarachnoid hemorrhage from** MCC unspecified **posterior communicating artery**

   I60.31 **Nontraumatic subarachnoid hemorrhage from** MCC right **posterior communicating artery**

   I60.32 **Nontraumatic subarachnoid hemorrhage from** MCC left **posterior communicating artery**

  I60.4 **Nontraumatic subarachnoid hemorrhage from** basilar MCC artery

✓5th **I60.5** **Nontraumatic subarachnoid hemorrhage from** vertebral artery

   I60.50 **Nontraumatic subarachnoid hemorrhage from** MCC unspecified **vertebral artery**

   I60.51 **Nontraumatic subarachnoid hemorrhage from** MCC right **vertebral artery**

   I60.52 **Nontraumatic subarachnoid hemorrhage from** MCC left **vertebral artery**

  I60.6 **Nontraumatic subarachnoid hemorrhage from** other MCC intracranial arteries

  I60.7 **Nontraumatic subarachnoid hemorrhage from** MCC unspecified intracranial artery

   Ruptured (congenital) berry aneurysm
   Ruptured (congenital) cerebral aneurysm
   Subarachnoid hemorrhage (nontraumatic) from cerebral artery NOS
   Subarachnoid hemorrhage (nontraumatic) from communicating artery NOS

   EXCLUDES 1 berry aneurysm, nonruptured (I67.1)

  I60.8 **Other nontraumatic subarachnoid hemorrhage** MCC
   Meningeal hemorrhage
   Rupture of cerebral arteriovenous malformation

  I60.9 **Nontraumatic subarachnoid hemorrhage,** unspecified MCC

✓4th **I61** **Nontraumatic intracerebral hemorrhage**

EXCLUDES 1 sequelae of intracerebral hemorrhage (I69.1-)

CC Excl: For MCC codes in category I61, unless otherwise noted:
See code: I60

  I61.0 **Nontraumatic intracerebral hemorrhage in** hemisphere, MCC subcortical
   Deep intracerebral hemorrhage (nontraumatic)

  I61.1 **Nontraumatic intracerebral hemorrhage in** hemisphere, MCC cortical
   Cerebral lobe hemorrhage (nontraumatic)
   Superficial intracerebral hemorrhage (nontraumatic)

  I61.2 **Nontraumatic intracerebral hemorrhage in** hemisphere, MCC unspecified

  I61.3 **Nontraumatic intracerebral hemorrhage in** brain stem MCC

  I61.4 **Nontraumatic intracerebral hemorrhage in** cerebellum MCC

  I61.5 **Nontraumatic intracerebral hemorrhage,** intraventricular MCC

  I61.6 **Nontraumatic intracerebral hemorrhage,** multiple MCC localized

  I61.8 **Other** nontraumatic intracerebral hemorrhage MCC

  I61.9 **Nontraumatic intracerebral hemorrhage,** unspecified MCC

✓4th **I62** **Other and unspecified nontraumatic intracranial hemorrhage**

EXCLUDES 1 sequelae of intracranial hemorrhage (I69.2)

CC Excl: For CC/MCC codes in category I62, unless otherwise noted: See code: I60

✓5th **I62.0** **Nontraumatic** subdural **hemorrhage**

   I62.00 **Nontraumatic subdural hemorrhage,** MCC unspecified

   I62.01 **Nontraumatic** acute **subdural hemorrhage** MCC

   I62.02 **Nontraumatic** subacute **subdural hemorrhage** MCC

   I62.03 **Nontraumatic** chronic **subdural hemorrhage** MCC

  I62.1 **Nontraumatic** extradural **hemorrhage** MCC
   Nontraumatic epidural hemorrhage

  I62.9 **Nontraumatic intracranial hemorrhage,** unspecified CC

✓4th **I63** **Cerebral infarction**

INCLUDES occlusion and stenosis of cerebral and precerebral arteries, resulting in cerebral infarction

Use additional code, if applicable, to identify status post administration of tPA (rtPA) in a different facility within the last 24 hours prior to admission to current facility (Z92.82)

EXCLUDES 1 sequelae of cerebral infarction (I69.3-)

AHA: 2014, 1Q, 23

✓5th **I63.0** **Cerebral infarction due to** thrombosis **of precerebral arteries**

CC Excl: For MCC codes in subcategory I63.0, unless otherwise noted: E08.51-E08.59, E08.618-E08.638,
E08.649-E08.8, E09.51-E09.59, E09.618-E09.638, E09.649-
E09.8, E10.51-E10.59, E10.618-E10.638, E10.649, E10.69-
E10.8, E11.51-E11.59, E11.618-E11.638, E11.649, E11.69-
E11.8, E13.51-E13.59, E13.618-E13.638, E13.649-E13.8,
G43.601-G43.619, I63.00-I63.29, I65.01-I65.9, I87.8, I99.8-
I99.9

   I63.00 **Cerebral infarction due to thrombosis of** MCC unspecified **precerebral artery**

✓6th   **I63.01** **Cerebral infarction due to thrombosis of** vertebral artery

     I63.011 **Cerebral infarction due to thrombosis** MCC **of** right **vertebral artery**

     I63.012 **Cerebral infarction due to thrombosis** MCC **of** left **vertebral artery**

     I63.019 **Cerebral infarction due to thrombosis** MCC **of** unspecified **vertebral artery**

   I63.02 **Cerebral infarction due to thrombosis of** basilar MCC artery

✓6th   **I63.03** **Cerebral infarction due to thrombosis of** carotid artery

     I63.031 **Cerebral infarction due to thrombosis** MCC **of** right **carotid artery**

     I63.032 **Cerebral infarction due to thrombosis** MCC **of** left **carotid artery**

     I63.039 **Cerebral infarction due to thrombosis** MCC **of** unspecified **carotid artery**

   I63.09 **Cerebral infarction due to thrombosis of** other MCC precerebral **artery**

✓5th **I63.1** **Cerebral infarction due to** embolism **of** precerebral **arteries**

CC Excl: For MCC codes in subcategory I63.1, unless otherwise noted: E08.51-E08.59, E08.618-E08.638,
E08.649-E08.8, E09.51-E09.59, E09.618-E09.638, E09.649-
E09.8, E10.51-E10.59, E10.618-E10.638, E10.649, E10.69-
E10.8, E11.51-E11.59, E11.618-E11.638, E11.649, E11.69-
E11.8, E13.51-E13.59, E13.618-E13.638, E13.649-E13.8,
G43.601-G43.619, I63.00-I63.29, I65.01-I65.9, I87.8, I99.8-
I99.9

   I63.10 **Cerebral infarction due to embolism of** MCC unspecified **precerebral artery**

✓6th   **I63.11** **Cerebral infarction due to embolism of** vertebral artery

     I63.111 **Cerebral infarction due to embolism** MCC **of** right **vertebral artery**

✓ Additional Character Required   ✓x7th Xtension Alert   Unacceptable PDx   Manifestation   Hospital Acquired Condition   EXCLUDES 1 Not Coded Here   EXCLUDES 2 Not Included Here

ICD-10-CM Draft (2015)   601

Diseases of the Circulatory System

I63.112–I63.50

I63.112   Cerebral infarction due to embolism of left vertebral artery `MCC`

I63.119   Cerebral infarction due to embolism of unspecified vertebral artery `MCC`

I63.12   Cerebral infarction due to embolism of basilar artery `MCC`

✓6th   I63.13   Cerebral infarction due to embolism of carotid artery

I63.131   Cerebral infarction due to embolism of right carotid artery `MCC`

I63.132   Cerebral infarction due to embolism of left carotid artery `MCC`

I63.139   Cerebral infarction due to embolism of unspecified carotid artery `MCC`

I63.19   Cerebral infarction due to embolism of other precerebral artery `MCC`

✓5th   I63.2   Cerebral infarction due to unspecified occlusion or stenosis of precerebral arteries

> CC Excl: For MCC codes in subcategory I63.2, unless otherwise noted: E08.51-E08.59, E08.618-E08.638, E08.649-E08.8, E09.51-E09.59, E09.618-E09.638, E09.649-E09.8, E10.51-E10.59, E10.618-E10.638, E10.649, E10.69-E10.8, E11.51-E11.59, E11.618-E11.638, E11.649, E11.69-E11.8, E13.51-E13.59, E13.618-E13.638, E13.649-E13.8, G43.601-G43.619, I63.00-I63.29, I65.01-I65.9, I87.8, I99.8-I99.9

I63.20   Cerebral infarction due to unspecified occlusion or stenosis of unspecified precerebral arteries `MCC`

✓6th   I63.21   Cerebral infarction due to unspecified occlusion or stenosis of vertebral arteries

I63.211   Cerebral infarction due to unspecified occlusion or stenosis of right vertebral arteries `MCC`

I63.212   Cerebral infarction due to unspecified occlusion or stenosis of left vertebral arteries `MCC`

I63.219   Cerebral infarction due to unspecified occlusion or stenosis of unspecified vertebral arteries `MCC`

I63.22   Cerebral infarction due to unspecified occlusion or stenosis of basilar arteries `MCC`

✓6th   I63.23   Cerebral infarction due to unspecified occlusion or stenosis of carotid arteries

I63.231   Cerebral infarction due to unspecified occlusion or stenosis of right carotid arteries `MCC`

I63.232   Cerebral infarction due to unspecified occlusion or stenosis of left carotid arteries `MCC`

I63.239   Cerebral infarction due to unspecified occlusion or stenosis of unspecified carotid arteries `MCC`

I63.29   Cerebral infarction due to unspecified occlusion or stenosis of other precerebral arteries `MCC`

✓5th   I63.3   Cerebral infarction due to thrombosis of cerebral arteries

> CC Excl: For MCC codes in subcategory I63.3, unless otherwise noted: E08.51-E08.59, E08.618-E08.638, E08.649-E08.8, E09.51-E09.59, E09.618-E09.638, E09.649-E09.8, E10.51-E10.59, E10.618-E10.638, E10.649, E10.69-E10.8, E11.51-E11.59, E11.618-E11.638, E11.649, E11.69-E11.8, E13.51-E13.59, E13.618-E13.638, E13.649-E13.8, G43.601-G43.619, I63.30-I63.9, I66.01-I66.9, I87.8, I99.8-I99.9

I63.30   Cerebral infarction due to thrombosis of unspecified cerebral artery `MCC`

✓6th   I63.31   Cerebral infarction due to thrombosis of middle cerebral artery

I63.311   Cerebral infarction due to thrombosis of right middle cerebral artery `MCC`

I63.312   Cerebral infarction due to thrombosis of left middle cerebral artery `MCC`

I63.319   Cerebral infarction due to thrombosis of unspecified middle cerebral artery `MCC`

✓6th   I63.32   Cerebral infarction due to thrombosis of anterior cerebral artery

I63.321   Cerebral infarction due to thrombosis of right anterior cerebral artery `MCC`

I63.322   Cerebral infarction due to thrombosis of left anterior cerebral artery `MCC`

I63.329   Cerebral infarction due to thrombosis of unspecified anterior cerebral artery `MCC`

✓6th   I63.33   Cerebral infarction due to thrombosis of posterior cerebral artery

I63.331   Cerebral infarction due to thrombosis of right posterior cerebral artery `MCC`

I63.332   Cerebral infarction due to thrombosis of left posterior cerebral artery `MCC`

I63.339   Cerebral infarction due to thrombosis of unspecified posterior cerebral artery `MCC`

✓6th   I63.34   Cerebral infarction due to thrombosis of cerebellar artery

I63.341   Cerebral infarction due to thrombosis of right cerebellar artery `MCC`

I63.342   Cerebral infarction due to thrombosis of left cerebellar artery `MCC`

I63.349   Cerebral infarction due to thrombosis of unspecified cerebellar artery `MCC`

I63.39   Cerebral infarction due to thrombosis of other cerebral artery `MCC`

✓5th   I63.4   Cerebral infarction due to embolism of cerebral arteries

> CC Excl: For MCC codes in subcategory I63.4, unless otherwise noted: E08.51-E08.59, E08.618-E08.638, E08.649-E08.8, E09.51-E09.59, E09.618-E09.638, E09.649-E09.8, E10.51-E10.59, E10.618-E10.638, E10.649, E10.69-E10.8, E11.51-E11.59, E11.618-E11.638, E11.649, E11.69-E11.8, E13.51-E13.59, E13.618-E13.638, E13.649-E13.8, G43.601-G43.619, I63.30-I63.9, I66.01-I66.9, I87.8, I99.8-I99.9

I63.40   Cerebral infarction due to embolism of unspecified cerebral artery `MCC`

✓6th   I63.41   Cerebral infarction due to embolism of middle cerebral artery

I63.411   Cerebral infarction due to embolism of right middle cerebral artery `MCC`

I63.412   Cerebral infarction due to embolism of left middle cerebral artery `MCC`

I63.419   Cerebral infarction due to embolism of unspecified middle cerebral artery `MCC`

✓6th   I63.42   Cerebral infarction due to embolism of anterior cerebral artery

I63.421   Cerebral infarction due to embolism of right anterior cerebral artery `MCC`

I63.422   Cerebral infarction due to embolism of left anterior cerebral artery `MCC`

I63.429   Cerebral infarction due to embolism of unspecified anterior cerebral artery `MCC`

✓6th   I63.43   Cerebral infarction due to embolism of posterior cerebral artery

I63.431   Cerebral infarction due to embolism of right posterior cerebral artery `MCC`

I63.432   Cerebral infarction due to embolism of left posterior cerebral artery `MCC`

I63.439   Cerebral infarction due to embolism of unspecified posterior cerebral artery `MCC`

✓6th   I63.44   Cerebral infarction due to embolism of cerebellar artery

I63.441   Cerebral infarction due to embolism of right cerebellar artery `MCC`

I63.442   Cerebral infarction due to embolism of left cerebellar artery `MCC`

I63.449   Cerebral infarction due to embolism of unspecified cerebellar artery `MCC`

I63.49   Cerebral infarction due to embolism of other cerebral artery `MCC`

✓5th   I63.5   Cerebral infarction due to unspecified occlusion or stenosis of cerebral arteries

> CC Excl: For MCC codes in subcategory I63.5, unless otherwise noted: E08.51-E08.59, E08.618-E08.638, E08.649-E08.8, E09.51-E09.59, E09.618-E09.638, E09.649-E09.8, E10.51-E10.59, E10.618-E10.638, E10.649, E10.69-E10.8, E11.51-E11.59, E11.618-E11.638, E11.649, E11.69-E11.8, E13.51-E13.59, E13.618-E13.638, E13.649-E13.8, G43.601-G43.619, I63.30-I63.9, I66.01-I66.9, I87.8, I99.8-I99.9

I63.50   Cerebral infarction due to unspecified occlusion or stenosis of unspecified cerebral artery `MCC`

N Newborn: 0   P Pediatric: 0-17   M Maternity: 12-55   A Adult: 15-124   MCC Major CC Condition   PDx MCC PDx acts as own MCC   CC CC Condition   PDx CC PDx acts as own CC

602   ICD-10-CM Draft (2015)

√6th **I63.51**   **Cerebral infarction due to unspecified occlusion or stenosis of middle cerebral artery**

   I63.511   Cerebral infarction due to unspecified MCC occlusion or stenosis of right middle cerebral artery

   I63.512   Cerebral infarction due to unspecified MCC occlusion or stenosis of left middle cerebral artery

   I63.519   Cerebral infarction due to unspecified MCC occlusion or stenosis of unspecified middle cerebral artery

√6th **I63.52**   **Cerebral infarction due to unspecified occlusion or stenosis of anterior cerebral artery**

   I63.521   Cerebral infarction due to unspecified MCC occlusion or stenosis of right anterior cerebral artery

   I63.522   Cerebral infarction due to unspecified MCC occlusion or stenosis of left anterior cerebral artery

   I63.529   Cerebral infarction due to unspecified MCC occlusion or stenosis of unspecified anterior cerebral artery

√6th **I63.53**   **Cerebral infarction due to unspecified occlusion or stenosis of posterior cerebral artery**

   I63.531   Cerebral infarction due to unspecified MCC occlusion or stenosis of right posterior cerebral artery

   I63.532   Cerebral infarction due to unspecified MCC occlusion or stenosis of left posterior cerebral artery

   I63.539   Cerebral infarction due to unspecified MCC occlusion or stenosis of unspecified posterior cerebral artery

√6th **I63.54**   **Cerebral infarction due to unspecified occlusion or stenosis of cerebellar artery**

   I63.541   Cerebral infarction due to unspecified MCC occlusion or stenosis of right cerebellar artery

   I63.542   Cerebral infarction due to unspecified MCC occlusion or stenosis of left cerebellar artery

   I63.549   Cerebral infarction due to unspecified MCC occlusion or stenosis of unspecified cerebellar artery

   I63.59   Cerebral infarction due to unspecified occlusion MCC or stenosis of other cerebral artery

I63.6   **Cerebral infarction due to cerebral venous thrombosis,** MCC **nonpyogenic**
   CC Excl: See code: I63.5

I63.8   **Other cerebral infarction** MCC
   CC Excl: See code: I63.5

I63.9   **Cerebral infarction, unspecified** MCC
   Stroke NOS
   CC Excl: See code: I63.5

√4th **I65**   **Occlusion and stenosis of precerebral arteries, not resulting in cerebral infarction**
   INCLUDES embolism of precerebral artery
            narrowing of precerebral artery
            obstruction (complete) (partial) of precerebral artery
            thrombosis of precerebral artery
   EXCLUDES 1 insufficiency, NOS, of precerebral artery (G45.-)
            insufficiency of precerebral arteries causing cerebral infarction (I63.0-I63.2)

√5th **I65.0**   **Occlusion and stenosis of vertebral artery**

   I65.01   Occlusion and stenosis of right vertebral artery

   I65.02   Occlusion and stenosis of left vertebral artery

   I65.03   Occlusion and stenosis of bilateral vertebral arteries

   I65.09   Occlusion and stenosis of unspecified vertebral artery

I65.1   **Occlusion and stenosis of basilar artery**

√5th **I65.2**   **Occlusion and stenosis of carotid artery**

   I65.21   Occlusion and stenosis of right carotid artery

   I65.22   Occlusion and stenosis of left carotid artery

   I65.23   Occlusion and stenosis of bilateral carotid arteries

   I65.29   Occlusion and stenosis of unspecified carotid artery

I65.8   **Occlusion and stenosis of other precerebral arteries**

I65.9   **Occlusion and stenosis of unspecified precerebral artery**
   Occlusion and stenosis of precerebral artery NOS

√4th **I66**   **Occlusion and stenosis of cerebral arteries, not resulting in cerebral infarction**
   INCLUDES embolism of cerebral artery
            narrowing of cerebral artery
            obstruction (complete) (partial) of cerebral artery
            thrombosis of cerebral artery
   EXCLUDES 1 occlusion and stenosis of cerebral artery causing cerebral infarction (I63.3-I63.5)

√5th **I66.0**   **Occlusion and stenosis of middle cerebral artery**

   I66.01   Occlusion and stenosis of right middle cerebral artery

   I66.02   Occlusion and stenosis of left middle cerebral artery

   I66.03   Occlusion and stenosis of bilateral middle cerebral arteries

   I66.09   Occlusion and stenosis of unspecified middle cerebral artery

√5th **I66.1**   **Occlusion and stenosis of anterior cerebral artery**

   I66.11   Occlusion and stenosis of right anterior cerebral artery

   I66.12   Occlusion and stenosis of left anterior cerebral artery

   I66.13   Occlusion and stenosis of bilateral anterior cerebral arteries

   I66.19   Occlusion and stenosis of unspecified anterior cerebral artery

√5th **I66.2**   **Occlusion and stenosis of posterior cerebral artery**

   I66.21   Occlusion and stenosis of right posterior cerebral artery

   I66.22   Occlusion and stenosis of left posterior cerebral artery

   I66.23   Occlusion and stenosis of bilateral posterior cerebral arteries

   I66.29   Occlusion and stenosis of unspecified posterior cerebral artery

I66.3   **Occlusion and stenosis of cerebellar arteries**

I66.8   **Occlusion and stenosis of other cerebral arteries**
   Occlusion and stenosis of perforating arteries

I66.9   **Occlusion and stenosis of unspecified cerebral artery**

√4th **I67**   **Other cerebrovascular diseases**
   EXCLUDES 1 sequelae of the listed conditions (I69.8)

I67.0   **Dissection of cerebral arteries, nonruptured** MCC
   EXCLUDES 1 ruptured cerebral arteries (I60.7)
   CC Excl: I77.2-I77.3, I77.5-I77.6, I77.89-I77.9, M31.8-M31.9

I67.1   **Cerebral aneurysm, nonruptured**
   Cerebral aneurysm NOS
   Cerebral arteriovenous fistula, acquired
   Internal carotid artery aneurysm, intracranial portion
   Internal carotid artery aneurysm, NOS
   EXCLUDES 1 congenital cerebral aneurysm, nonruptured (Q28.-)
            ruptured cerebral aneurysm (I60.7)

I67.2   **Cerebral atherosclerosis** A
   Atheroma of cerebral and precerebral arteries

I67.3   **Progressive vascular leukoencephalopathy** HIV CC
   Binswanger's disease
   CC Excl: A17.82, A50.42, A52.14, A75.9, A79.9, A81.00-A81.9, A83.0-A85.8, A87.2, A88.0, A88.8, A92.1-A92.2, A92.4-A92.8, A93.0, B00.4, B00.82, B01.11-B01.12, B04, B06.01, B08.09, B08.20-B08.22, B08.60-B08.79, B09-B10.09, B26.2, B27.00-B27.99, B33.1, B45.0, B45.2-B45.9, B58.2, B75, G04.00-G04.01, G04.31, G04.81-G05.4, G37.0, G37.4-G37.5, I67.3, J09.X3-J09.X9, J10.2-J10.89, J11.2-J11.89, L44.4, M1A.10X0-M1A.19X1, P35.2-P35.9, P37.0-P37.4, P37.8-P37.9, T56.0X1A, T56.0X2A, T56.0X3A, T56.0X4A

I67.4   **Hypertensive encephalopathy** CC
   CC Excl: E08.51-E08.59, E08.618-E08.638, E08.649-E08.8, E09.51-E09.59, E09.618-E09.638, E09.649-E09.8, E10.51-E10.59, E10.618-E10.638, E10.649, E10.69-E10.8, E11.51-E11.59, E11.618-E11.638, E11.649, E11.69-E11.8, E13.51-E13.59, E13.618-E13.638, E13.649-E13.8, I67.4, I87.8, I99.8-I99.9

I67.5   **Moyamoya disease** CC
   CC Excl: E08.51-E08.59, E08.618-E08.638, E08.649-E08.8, E09.51-E09.59, E09.618-E09.638, E09.649-E09.8, E10.51-E10.59, E10.618-E10.638, E10.649, E10.69-E10.8, E11.51-E11.59, E11.618-E11.638, E11.649, E11.69-E11.8, E13.51-E13.59, E13.618-E13.638, E13.649-E13.8, I67.5, I87.8, I99.8-I99.9

√ Additional Character Required   √x7th Xtension Alert   Unacceptable PDx   Manifestation   Hospital Acquired Condition   EXCLUDES 1 Not Coded Here   EXCLUDES 2 Not Included Here

I67.6 **Nonpyogenic thrombosis of intracranial venous system** `CC`
Nonpyogenic thrombosis of cerebral vein
Nonpyogenic thrombosis of intracranial venous sinus
EXCLUDES 1   *nonpyogenic thrombosis of intracranial venous system causing infarction (I63.6)*
CC Excl: E08.51-E08.59, E08.618-E08.638, E08.649-E08.8, E09.51-E09.59, E09.618-E09.638, E09.649-E09.8, E10.51-E10.59, E10.618-E10.638, E10.649, E10.69-E10.8, E11.51-E11.59, E11.618-E11.638, E11.649, E11.69-E11.8, E13.51-E13.59, E13.618-E13.638, E13.649-E13.8, I67.6, I87.8, I99.8-I99.9

I67.7 **Cerebral arteritis, not elsewhere classified** `CC`
Granulomatous angiitis of the nervous system
EXCLUDES 1   *allergic granulomatous angiitis (M30.1)*
CC Excl: E08.51-E08.59, E08.618-E08.638, E08.649-E08.8, E09.51-E09.59, E09.618-E09.638, E09.649-E09.8, E10.51-E10.59, E10.618-E10.638, E10.649, E10.69-E10.8, E11.51-E11.59, E11.618-E11.638, E11.649, E11.69-E11.8, E13.51-E13.59, E13.618-E13.638, E13.649-E13.8, I67.7, I68.2, I87.8, I99.8-I99.9

√5th **I67.8** **Other specified cerebrovascular diseases**

I67.81 **Acute cerebrovascular insufficiency** `CC`
Acute cerebrovascular insufficiency unspecified as to location or reversibility
CC Excl: E08.51-E08.59, E08.618-E08.638, E08.649-E08.8, E09.51-E09.59, E09.618-E09.638, E09.649-E09.8, E10.51-E10.59, E10.618-E10.638, E10.649, E10.69-E10.8, E11.51-E11.59, E11.618-E11.638, E11.649, E11.69-E11.8, E13.51-E13.59, E13.618-E13.638, E13.649-E13.8, G45.0-G45.2, G45.8-G46.2, I60.00-I62.9, I63.30-I63.9, I66.01-I66.9, I67.81-I67.82, I67.841-I67.89, I87.8, I99.8-I99.9

I67.82 **Cerebral ischemia** `CC`
Chronic cerebral ischemia
CC Excl: See code: I67.81

I67.83 **Posterior reversible encephalopathy syndrome** `HIV` `MCC`
PRES
CC Excl: G21.0, G83.5, G93.40-G93.41

√6th **I67.84** **Cerebral vasospasm and vasoconstriction**

I67.841 **Reversible cerebrovascular vasoconstriction syndrome** `CC`
Call-Fleming syndrome
Code first underlying condition, if applicable, such as eclampsia (O15.00-O15.9)
CC Excl: E08.51-E08.59, E08.618-E08.638, E08.649-E08.8, E09.51-E09.59, E09.618-E09.638, E09.649-E09.8, E10.51-E10.59, E10.618-E10.638, E10.649, E10.69-E10.8, E11.51-E11.59, E11.618-E11.638, E11.649, E11.69-E11.8, E13.51-E13.59, E13.618-E13.638, E13.649-E13.8, G45.0-G45.2, G45.8-G46.2, I63.00-I63.29, I65.01-I65.9, I67.841-I67.848, I87.8, I99.8-I99.9

I67.848 **Other cerebrovascular vasospasm and vasoconstriction** `CC`
CC Excl: See code: I67.841

I67.89 **Other cerebrovascular disease** `CC`
CC Excl: See code: I67.81

I67.9 **Cerebrovascular disease, unspecified**

√4th **I68** **Cerebrovascular disorders in diseases classified elsewhere**

I68.0 *Cerebral amyloid angiopathy*
Code first underlying amyloidosis (E85.-)

I68.2 *Cerebral arteritis in other diseases classified elsewhere* `CC`
Code first underlying disease
EXCLUDES 1   *cerebral arteritis (in):*
listerosis (A32.89)
systemic lupus erythematosus (M32.19)
syphilis (A52.04)
tuberculosis (A18.89)
CC Excl: See code: I67.7

I68.8 *Other cerebrovascular disorders in diseases classified elsewhere*
Code first underlying disease
EXCLUDES 1   *syphilitic cerebral aneurysm (A52.05)*

√4th **I69** **Sequelae of cerebrovascular disease**
`NOTE`   Category I69 is to be used to indicate conditions in I60-I67 as the cause of sequelae. The "sequelae" include conditions specified as such or as residuals which may occur at any time after the onset of the causal condition
EXCLUDES 1   *personal history of cerebral infarction without residual deficit (Z86.73)*
personal history of prolonged reversible ischemic neurologic deficit (PRIND) (Z86.73)
personal history of reversible ischemic neurologcial deficit (RIND) (Z86.73)
sequelae of traumatic intracranial injury (S06.-)
transient ischemic attack (TIA) (G45.9)
AHA: 2012, 4Q, 106

√5th **I69.0** **Sequelae of nontraumatic subarachnoid hemorrhage**

I69.00 **Unspecified sequelae of nontraumatic subarachnoid hemorrhage**

I69.01 **Cognitive deficits following nontraumatic subarachnoid hemorrhage**

√6th **I69.02** **Speech and language deficits following nontraumatic subarachnoid hemorrhage**

I69.020 **Aphasia following nontraumatic subarachnoid hemorrhage**

I69.021 **Dysphasia following nontraumatic subarachnoid hemorrhage**

I69.022 **Dysarthria following nontraumatic subarachnoid hemorrhage**

I69.023 **Fluency disorder following nontraumatic subarachnoid hemorrhage**
Stuttering following nontraumatic subarachnoid hemorrhage

I69.028 **Other speech and language deficits following nontraumatic subarachnoid hemorrhage**

√6th **I69.03** **Monoplegia of upper limb following nontraumatic subarachnoid hemorrhage**

I69.031 **Monoplegia of upper limb following nontraumatic subarachnoid hemorrhage affecting right dominant side**

I69.032 **Monoplegia of upper limb following nontraumatic subarachnoid hemorrhage affecting left dominant side**

I69.033 **Monoplegia of upper limb following nontraumatic subarachnoid hemorrhage affecting right non-dominant side**

I69.034 **Monoplegia of upper limb following nontraumatic subarachnoid hemorrhage affecting left non-dominant side**

I69.039 **Monoplegia of upper limb following nontraumatic subarachnoid hemorrhage affecting unspecified side**

√6th **I69.04** **Monoplegia of lower limb following nontraumatic subarachnoid hemorrhage**

I69.041 **Monoplegia of lower limb following nontraumatic subarachnoid hemorrhage affecting right dominant side**

I69.042 **Monoplegia of lower limb following nontraumatic subarachnoid hemorrhage affecting left dominant side**

I69.043 **Monoplegia of lower limb following nontraumatic subarachnoid hemorrhage affecting right non-dominant side**

I69.044 **Monoplegia of lower limb following nontraumatic subarachnoid hemorrhage affecting left non-dominant side**

I69.049 **Monoplegia of lower limb following nontraumatic subarachnoid hemorrhage affecting unspecified side**

√6th **I69.05** **Hemiplegia and hemiparesis following nontraumatic subarachnoid hemorrhage**

I69.051 **Hemiplegia and hemiparesis following nontraumatic subarachnoid hemorrhage affecting right dominant side** `CC`
CC Excl: I69.051-I69.052, I69.151-I69.152, I69.251-I69.252, I69.351-I69.352, I69.851-I69.852, I69.951-I69.952

I69.052 **Hemiplegia and hemiparesis following nontraumatic subarachnoid hemorrhage affecting left dominant side** `CC`
CC Excl: See code: I69.051

`N` Newborn: 0   `P` Pediatric: 0-17   `M` Maternity: 12-55   `A` Adult: 15-124   `MCC` Major CC Condition   `PDx MCC` PDx acts as own MCC   `CC` CC Condition   `PDx CC` PDx acts as own CC

604   ICD-10-CM Draft (2015)

I69.053 **Hemiplegia and hemiparesis following** cc **nontraumatic subarachnoid hemorrhage affecting right non-dominant side**
  CC Excl: I69.053-I69.054, I69.153-I69.154, I69.253-I69.254, I69.353-I69.354, I69.853-I69.854, I69.953-I69.954

I69.054 **Hemiplegia and hemiparesis following** cc **nontraumatic subarachnoid hemorrhage affecting left non-dominant side**
  CC Excl: See code: I69.053

I69.059 **Hemiplegia and hemiparesis following** cc **nontraumatic subarachnoid hemorrhage affecting unspecified side**
  CC Excl: I69.059-I69.159, I69.259, I69.359, I69.859, I69.959

☑6th **I69.06** **Other paralytic syndrome following nontraumatic subarachnoid hemorrhage**
  Use additional code to identify type of paralytic syndrome, such as:
  locked-in state (G83.5)
  quadriplegia (G82.5-)
  EXCLUDES 1 *hemiplegia/hemiparesis following nontraumatic subarachnoid hemorrhage (I69.05-)*
  monoplegia of lower limb following nontraumatic subarachnoid hemorrhage (I69.04-)
  monoplegia of upper limb following nontraumatic subarachnoid hemorrhage (I69.03-)

I69.061 **Other paralytic syndrome following nontraumatic subarachnoid hemorrhage affecting right dominant side**

I69.062 **Other paralytic syndrome following nontraumatic subarachnoid hemorrhage affecting left dominant side**

I69.063 **Other paralytic syndrome following nontraumatic subarachnoid hemorrhage affecting right non-dominant side**

I69.064 **Other paralytic syndrome following nontraumatic subarachnoid hemorrhage affecting left non-dominant side**

I69.065 **Other paralytic syndrome following nontraumatic subarachnoid hemorrhage, bilateral**

I69.069 **Other paralytic syndrome following nontraumatic subarachnoid hemorrhage affecting unspecified side**

☑6th **I69.09** **Other sequelae of nontraumatic subarachnoid hemorrhage**

I69.090 **Apraxia following nontraumatic subarachnoid hemorrhage**

I69.091 **Dysphagia following nontraumatic subarachnoid hemorrhage**
  Use additional code to identify the type of dysphagia, if known (R13.1-)

I69.092 **Facial weakness following nontraumatic subarachnoid hemorrhage**
  Facial droop following nontraumatic subarachnoid hemorrhage

I69.093 **Ataxia following nontraumatic subarachnoid hemorrhage**

I69.098 **Other sequelae following nontraumatic subarachnoid hemorrhage**
  Alterations of sensation following nontraumatic subarachnoid hemorrhage
  Disturbance of vision following nontraumatic subarachnoid hemorrhage
  Use additional code to identify the sequelae

☑5th **I69.1** **Sequelae of nontraumatic intracerebral hemorrhage**

I69.10 **Unspecified sequelae of nontraumatic intracerebral hemorrhage**

I69.11 **Cognitive deficits following nontraumatic intracerebral hemorrhage**

☑6th **I69.12** **Speech and language deficits following nontraumatic intracerebral hemorrhage**

I69.120 **Aphasia following nontraumatic intracerebral hemorrhage**

I69.121 **Dysphasia following nontraumatic intracerebral hemorrhage**

I69.122 **Dysarthria following nontraumatic intracerebral hemorrhage**

I69.123 **Fluency disorder following nontraumatic intracerebral hemorrhage**
  Stuttering following nontraumatic subarachnoid hemorrhage

I69.128 **Other speech and language deficits following nontraumatic intracerebral hemorrhage**

☑6th **I69.13** **Monoplegia of upper limb following nontraumatic intracerebral hemorrhage**

I69.131 **Monoplegia of upper limb following nontraumatic intracerebral hemorrhage affecting right dominant side**

I69.132 **Monoplegia of upper limb following nontraumatic intracerebral hemorrhage affecting left dominant side**

I69.133 **Monoplegia of upper limb following nontraumatic intracerebral hemorrhage affecting right non-dominant side**

I69.134 **Monoplegia of upper limb following nontraumatic intracerebral hemorrhage affecting left non-dominant side**

I69.139 **Monoplegia of upper limb following nontraumatic intracerebral hemorrhage affecting unspecified side**

☑6th **I69.14** **Monoplegia of lower limb following nontraumatic intracerebral hemorrhage**

I69.141 **Monoplegia of lower limb following nontraumatic intracerebral hemorrhage affecting right dominant side**

I69.142 **Monoplegia of lower limb following nontraumatic intracerebral hemorrhage affecting left dominant side**

I69.143 **Monoplegia of lower limb following nontraumatic intracerebral hemorrhage affecting right non-dominant side**

I69.144 **Monoplegia of lower limb following nontraumatic intracerebral hemorrhage affecting left non-dominant side**

I69.149 **Monoplegia of lower limb following nontraumatic intracerebral hemorrhage affecting unspecified side**

☑6th **I69.15** **Hemiplegia and hemiparesis following nontraumatic intracerebral hemorrhage**

I69.151 **Hemiplegia and hemiparesis following** cc **nontraumatic intracerebral hemorrhage affecting right dominant side**
  CC Excl: I69.051-I69.052, I69.151-I69.152, I69.251-I69.252, I69.351-I69.352, I69.851-I69.852, I69.951-I69.952

I69.152 **Hemiplegia and hemiparesis following** cc **nontraumatic intracerebral hemorrhage affecting left dominant side**
  CC Excl: See code: I69.151

I69.153 **Hemiplegia and hemiparesis following** cc **nontraumatic intracerebral hemorrhage affecting right non-dominant side**
  CC Excl: I69.053-I69.054, I69.153-I69.154, I69.253-I69.254, I69.353-I69.354, I69.853-I69.854, I69.953-I69.954

I69.154 **Hemiplegia and hemiparesis following** cc **nontraumatic intracerebral hemorrhage affecting left non-dominant side**
  CC Excl: See code: I69.153

I69.159 **Hemiplegia and hemiparesis following** cc **nontraumatic intracerebral hemorrhage affecting unspecified side**
  CC Excl: I69.059, I69.159, I69.259, I69.359, I69.859, I69.959

━━
☑ Additional Character Required   ☑x7th Xtension Alert   Unacceptable PDx   Manifestation   Hospital Acquired Condition   EXCLUDES 1 Not Coded Here   EXCLUDES 2 Not Included Here
ICD-10-CM Draft (2015)   605

✓6ᵗʰ **I69.16** **Other paralytic syndrome following nontraumatic intracerebral hemorrhage**
Use additional code to identify type of paralytic syndrome, such as:
locked-in state (G83.5)
quadriplegia (G82.5-)

EXCLUDES 1 *hemiplegia/hemiparesis following nontraumatic intracerebral hemorrhage (I69.15-)*
monoplegia of lower limb following nontraumatic intracerebral hemorrhage (I69.14-)
monoplegia of upper limb following nontraumatic intracerebral hemorrhage (I69.13-)

I69.161 **Other paralytic syndrome following nontraumatic intracerebral hemorrhage affecting right dominant side**

I69.162 **Other paralytic syndrome following nontraumatic intracerebral hemorrhage affecting left dominant side**

I69.163 **Other paralytic syndrome following nontraumatic intracerebral hemorrhage affecting right non-dominant side**

I69.164 **Other paralytic syndrome following nontraumatic intracerebral hemorrhage affecting left non-dominant side**

I69.165 **Other paralytic syndrome following nontraumatic intracerebral hemorrhage, bilateral**

I69.169 **Other paralytic syndrome following nontraumatic intracerebral hemorrhage affecting unspecified side**

✓6ᵗʰ **I69.19** **Other sequelae of nontraumatic intracerebral hemorrhage**

I69.190 **Apraxia following nontraumatic intracerebral hemorrhage**

I69.191 **Dysphagia following nontraumatic intracerebral hemorrhage**
Use additional code to identify the type of dysphagia, if known (R13.1-)

I69.192 **Facial weakness following nontraumatic intracerebral hemorrhage**
Facial droop following nontraumatic intracerebral hemorrhage

I69.193 **Ataxia following nontraumatic intracerebral hemorrhage**

I69.198 **Other sequelae of nontraumatic intracerebral hemorrhage**
Alteration of sensations following nontraumatic intracerebral hemorrhage
Disturbance of vision following nontraumatic intracerebral hemorrhage
Use additional code to identify the sequelae

✓5ᵗʰ **I69.2** **Sequelae of other nontraumatic intracranial hemorrhage**

I69.20 **Unspecified sequelae of other nontraumatic intracranial hemorrhage**

I69.21 **Cognitive deficits following other nontraumatic intracranial hemorrhage**

✓6ᵗʰ **I69.22** **Speech and language deficits following other nontraumatic intracranial hemorrhage**

I69.220 **Aphasia following other nontraumatic intracranial hemorrhage**

I69.221 **Dysphasia following other nontraumatic intracranial hemorrhage**

I69.222 **Dysarthria following other nontraumatic intracranial hemorrhage**

I69.223 **Fluency disorder following other nontraumatic intracranial hemorrhage**
Stuttering following nontraumatic subarachnoid hemorrhage

I69.228 **Other speech and language deficits following other nontraumatic intracranial hemorrhage**

✓6ᵗʰ **I69.23** **Monoplegia of upper limb following other nontraumatic intracranial hemorrhage**

I69.231 **Monoplegia of upper limb following other nontraumatic intracranial hemorrhage affecting right dominant side**

I69.232 **Monoplegia of upper limb following other nontraumatic intracranial hemorrhage affecting left dominant side**

I69.233 **Monoplegia of upper limb following other nontraumatic intracranial hemorrhage affecting right non-dominant side**

I69.234 **Monoplegia of upper limb following other nontraumatic intracranial hemorrhage affecting left non-dominant side**

I69.239 **Monoplegia of upper limb following other nontraumatic intracranial hemorrhage affecting unspecified side**

✓6ᵗʰ **I69.24** **Monoplegia of lower limb following other nontraumatic intracranial hemorrhage**

I69.241 **Monoplegia of lower limb following other nontraumatic intracranial hemorrhage affecting right dominant side**

I69.242 **Monoplegia of lower limb following other nontraumatic intracranial hemorrhage affecting left dominant side**

I69.243 **Monoplegia of lower limb following other nontraumatic intracranial hemorrhage affecting right non-dominant side**

I69.244 **Monoplegia of lower limb following other nontraumatic intracranial hemorrhage affecting left non-dominant side**

I69.249 **Monoplegia of lower limb following other nontraumatic intracranial hemorrhage affecting unspecified side**

✓6ᵗʰ **I69.25** **Hemiplegia and hemiparesis following other nontraumatic intracranial hemorrhage**

I69.251 **Hemiplegia and hemiparesis following other nontraumatic intracranial hemorrhage affecting right dominant side** CC
CC Excl: See code: I69.151

I69.252 **Hemiplegia and hemiparesis following other nontraumatic intracranial hemorrhage affecting left dominant side** CC
CC Excl: See code: I69.151

I69.253 **Hemiplegia and hemiparesis following other nontraumatic intracranial hemorrhage affecting right non-dominant side** CC
CC Excl: See code: I69.153

I69.254 **Hemiplegia and hemiparesis following other nontraumatic intracranial hemorrhage affecting left non-dominant side** CC
CC Excl: See code: I69.153

I69.259 **Hemiplegia and hemiparesis following other nontraumatic intracranial hemorrhage affecting unspecified side** CC
CC Excl: See code: I69.159

✓6ᵗʰ **I69.26** **Other paralytic syndrome following other nontraumatic intracranial hemorrhage**
Use additional code to identify type of paralytic syndrome, such as:
locked-in state (G83.5)
quadriplegia (G82.5-)

EXCLUDES 1 *hemiplegia/hemiparesis following other nontraumatic intracranial hemorrhage (I69.25-)*
monoplegia of lower limb following other nontraumatic intracranial hemorrhage (I69.24-)
monoplegia of upper limb following other nontraumatic intracranial hemorrhage (I69.23-)

I69.261 **Other paralytic syndrome following other nontraumatic intracranial hemorrhage affecting right dominant side**

I69.262 **Other paralytic syndrome following other nontraumatic intracranial hemorrhage affecting left dominant side**

N Newborn: 0   P Pediatric: 0-17   M Maternity: 12-55   A Adult: 15-124   MCC Major CC Condition   PDx MCC PDx acts as own MCC   CC CC Condition   PDx CC PDx acts as own CC

606   ICD-10-CM Draft (2015)

I69.263 Other paralytic syndrome following other nontraumatic intracranial hemorrhage affecting right non-dominant side

I69.264 Other paralytic syndrome following other nontraumatic intracranial hemorrhage affecting left non-dominant side

I69.265 Other paralytic syndrome following other nontraumatic intracranial hemorrhage, bilateral

I69.269 Other paralytic syndrome following other nontraumatic intracranial hemorrhage affecting unspecified side

✓6ᵗʰ **I69.29** Other sequelae of other nontraumatic intracranial hemorrhage

I69.290 Apraxia following other nontraumatic intracranial hemorrhage

I69.291 Dysphagia following other nontraumatic intracranial hemorrhage
Use additional code to identify the type of dysphagia, if known (R13.1-)

I69.292 Facial weakness following other nontraumatic intracranial hemorrhage
Facial droop following other nontraumatic intracranial hemorrhage

I69.293 Ataxia following other nontraumatic intracranial hemorrhage

I69.298 Other sequelae of other nontraumatic intracranial hemorrhage
Alteration of sensation following other nontraumatic intracranial hemorrhage
Disturbance of vision following other nontraumatic intracranial hemorrhage
Use additional code to identify the sequelae

✓5ᵗʰ **I69.3** Sequelae of cerebral infarction
Sequelae of stroke NOS
AHA: 2013, 4Q, 127-128; 2012, 4Q, 92, 94

I69.30 Unspecified sequelae of cerebral infarction

I69.31 Cognitive deficits following cerebral infarction

✓6ᵗʰ **I69.32** Speech and language deficits following cerebral infarction

I69.320 Aphasia following cerebral infarction

I69.321 Dysphasia following cerebral infarction
AHA: 2012, 4Q, 91

I69.322 Dysarthria following cerebral infarction

I69.323 Fluency disorder following cerebral infarction
Stuttering following nontraumatic subarachnoid hemorrhage

I69.328 Other speech and language deficits following cerebral infarction

✓6ᵗʰ **I69.33** Monoplegia of upper limb following cerebral infarction

I69.331 Monoplegia of upper limb following cerebral infarction affecting right dominant side

I69.332 Monoplegia of upper limb following cerebral infarction affecting left dominant side

I69.333 Monoplegia of upper limb following cerebral infarction affecting right non-dominant side

I69.334 Monoplegia of upper limb following cerebral infarction affecting left non-dominant side

I69.339 Monoplegia of upper limb following cerebral infarction affecting unspecified side

✓6ᵗʰ **I69.34** Monoplegia of lower limb following cerebral infarction

I69.341 Monoplegia of lower limb following cerebral infarction affecting right dominant side

I69.342 Monoplegia of lower limb following cerebral infarction affecting left dominant side

I69.343 Monoplegia of lower limb following cerebral infarction affecting right non-dominant side

I69.344 Monoplegia of lower limb following cerebral infarction affecting left non-dominant side

I69.349 Monoplegia of lower limb following cerebral infarction affecting unspecified side

✓6ᵗʰ **I69.35** Hemiplegia and hemiparesis following cerebral infarction

I69.351 Hemiplegia and hemiparesis following cerebral infarction affecting right dominant side ㏄
CC Excl: I69.051-I69.052, I69.151-I69.152, I69.251-I69.252, I69.351-I69.352, I69.851-I69.852, I69.951-I69.952

I69.352 Hemiplegia and hemiparesis following cerebral infarction affecting left dominant side ㏄
CC Excl: See code: I69.351

I69.353 Hemiplegia and hemiparesis following cerebral infarction affecting right non-dominant side ㏄
CC Excl: I69.053-I69.054, I69.153-I69.154, I69.253-I69.254, I69.353-I69.354, I69.853-I69.854, I69.953-I69.954

I69.354 Hemiplegia and hemiparesis following cerebral infarction affecting left non-dominant side ㏄
CC Excl: See code: I69.353
AHA: 2012, 4Q, 91

I69.359 Hemiplegia and hemiparesis following cerebral infarction affecting unspecified side ㏄
CC Excl: I69.059, I69.159, I69.259, I69.359, I69.859, I69.959

✓6ᵗʰ **I69.36** Other paralytic syndrome following cerebral infarction
Use additional code to identify type of paralytic syndrome, such as:
locked-in state (G83.5)
quadriplegia (G82.5-)
EXCLUDES 1 hemiplegia/hemiparesis following cerebral infarction (I69.35-)
monoplegia of lower limb following cerebral infarction (I69.34-)
monoplegia of upper limb following cerebral infarction (I69.33-)

I69.361 Other paralytic syndrome following cerebral infarction affecting right dominant side

I69.362 Other paralytic syndrome following cerebral infarction affecting left dominant side

I69.363 Other paralytic syndrome following cerebral infarction affecting right non-dominant side

I69.364 Other paralytic syndrome following cerebral infarction affecting left non-dominant side

I69.365 Other paralytic syndrome following cerebral infarction, bilateral

I69.369 Other paralytic syndrome following cerebral infarction affecting unspecified side

✓6ᵗʰ **I69.39** Other sequelae of cerebral infarction

I69.390 Apraxia following cerebral infarction

I69.391 Dysphagia following cerebral infarction
Use additional code to identify the type of dysphagia, if known (R13.1-)

I69.392 Facial weakness following cerebral infarction
Facial droop following cerebral infarction

I69.393 Ataxia following cerebral infarction

I69.398 Other sequelae of cerebral infarction
Alteration of sensation following cerebral infarction
Disturbance of vision following cerebral infarction
Use additional code to identify the sequelae

✓ Additional Character Required   ✓x7ᵗʰ Xtension Alert   Unacceptable PDx   Manifestation   Hospital Acquired Condition   EXCLUDES 1 Not Coded Here   EXCLUDES 2 Not Included Here

Diseases of the Circulatory System

I69.8–I69.932

☑5th **I69.8** **Sequelae of** other cerebrovascular diseases

> EXCLUDES 1   *sequelae of traumatic intracranial injury (S06.-)*

I69.80 **Unspecified sequelae of other cerebrovascular** disease

I69.81 **Cognitive deficits following other cerebrovascular** disease

☑6th **I69.82** **Speech** and language deficits following other cerebrovascular disease

I69.820 **Aphasia following other cerebrovascular** disease

I69.821 **Dysphasia following other** cerebrovascular disease

I69.822 **Dysarthria following other** cerebrovascular disease

I69.823 **Fluency disorder following other** cerebrovascular disease
> Stuttering following nontraumatic subarachnoid hemorrhage

I69.828 **Other speech and language deficits following other cerebrovascular disease**

☑6th **I69.83** **Monoplegia of** upper limb following other cerebrovascular disease

I69.831 **Monoplegia of upper limb following other cerebrovascular disease affecting** right **dominant** side

I69.832 **Monoplegia of upper limb following other cerebrovascular disease affecting** left **dominant** side

I69.833 **Monoplegia of upper limb following other cerebrovascular disease affecting** right **non-dominant** side

I69.834 **Monoplegia of upper limb following other cerebrovascular disease affecting** left **non-dominant** side

I69.839 **Monoplegia of upper limb following other cerebrovascular disease affecting** unspecified side

☑6th **I69.84** **Monoplegia of** lower limb following other cerebrovascular disease

I69.841 **Monoplegia of lower limb following other cerebrovascular disease affecting** right **dominant** side

I69.842 **Monoplegia of lower limb following other cerebrovascular disease affecting** left **dominant** side

I69.843 **Monoplegia of lower limb following other cerebrovascular disease affecting** right **non-dominant** side

I69.844 **Monoplegia of lower limb following other cerebrovascular disease affecting** left **non-dominant** side

I69.849 **Monoplegia of lower limb following other cerebrovascular disease affecting** unspecified side

☑6th **I69.85** **Hemiplegia** and hemiparesis following other cerebrovascular disease

I69.851 **Hemiplegia and hemiparesis following** ᴄᴄ **other cerebrovascular disease affecting** right dominant side
> CC Excl: See code: I69.051

I69.852 **Hemiplegia and hemiparesis following** ᴄᴄ **other cerebrovascular disease affecting** left dominant side
> CC Excl: See code: I69.051

I69.853 **Hemiplegia and hemiparesis following** ᴄᴄ **other cerebrovascular disease affecting** right non-dominant side
> CC Excl: See code: I69.053

I69.854 **Hemiplegia and hemiparesis following** ᴄᴄ **other cerebrovascular disease affecting** left non-dominant side
> CC Excl: See code: I69.053

I69.859 **Hemiplegia and hemiparesis following** ᴄᴄ **other cerebrovascular disease affecting** unspecified side
> CC Excl: See code: I69.059

☑6th **I69.86** **Other paralytic syndrome following other** cerebrovascular disease
> Use additional code to identify type of paralytic syndrome, such as:
> locked-in state (G83.5)
> quadriplegia (G82.5-)
>
> EXCLUDES 1   *hemiplegia/hemiparesis following other cerebrovascular disease (I69.85-)*
> *monoplegia of lower limb following other cerebrovascular disease (I69.84-)*
> *monoplegia of upper limb following other cerebrovascular disease (I69.83-)*

I69.861 **Other paralytic syndrome following other cerebrovascular disease affecting** right dominant **side**

I69.862 **Other paralytic syndrome following other cerebrovascular disease affecting** left dominant **side**

I69.863 **Other paralytic syndrome following other cerebrovascular disease affecting** right non-dominant **side**

I69.864 **Other paralytic syndrome following other cerebrovascular disease affecting** left non-dominant **side**

I69.865 **Other paralytic syndrome following other cerebrovascular disease, bilateral**

I69.869 **Other paralytic syndrome following other cerebrovascular disease affecting** unspecified **side**

☑6th **I69.89** **Other sequelae of other cerebrovascular disease**

I69.890 **Apraxia following other cerebrovascular** disease

I69.891 **Dysphagia following other** cerebrovascular disease
> Use additional code to identify the type of dysphagia, if known (R13.1-)

I69.892 **Facial weakness following other** cerebrovascular disease
> Facial droop following other cerebrovascular disease

I69.893 **Ataxia following other cerebrovascular** disease

I69.898 **Other sequelae of other cerebrovascular** disease
> Alteration of sensation following other cerebrovascular disease
> Disturbance of vision following other cerebrovascular disease
> Use additional code to identify the sequelae

☑5th **I69.9** **Sequelae of** unspecified cerebrovascular diseases
> EXCLUDES 1   *sequelae of stroke (I69.3)*
> *sequelae of traumatic intracranial injury (S06.-)*

I69.90 **Unspecified sequelae of unspecified cerebrovascular** disease

I69.91 **Cognitive deficits following unspecified** cerebrovascular disease

☑6th **I69.92** **Speech and language deficits following unspecified** cerebrovascular disease

I69.920 **Aphasia following unspecified** cerebrovascular disease

I69.921 **Dysphasia following unspecified** cerebrovascular disease

I69.922 **Dysarthria following unspecified** cerebrovascular disease

I69.923 **Fluency disorder following unspecified** cerebrovascular disease
> Stuttering following nontraumatic subarachnoid hemorrhage

I69.928 **Other speech and language deficits following unspecified cerebrovascular** disease

☑6th **I69.93** **Monoplegia of** upper limb following unspecified cerebrovascular disease

I69.931 **Monoplegia of upper limb following unspecified cerebrovascular disease affecting** right dominant side

I69.932 **Monoplegia of upper limb following unspecified cerebrovascular disease affecting** left dominant side

---

Ⓝ Newborn: 0   Ⓟ Pediatric: 0-17   Ⓜ Maternity: 12-55   Ⓐ Adult: 15-124   ᴹᶜᶜ Major CC Condition   ᴾᴰˣ ᴹᶜᶜ PDx acts as own MCC   ᴄᴄ CC Condition   ᴾᴰˣ ᴄᴄ PDx acts as own CC

I69.933 Monoplegia of upper limb following unspecified cerebrovascular disease affecting right non-dominant side

I69.934 Monoplegia of upper limb following unspecified cerebrovascular disease affecting left non-dominant side

I69.939 Monoplegia of upper limb following unspecified cerebrovascular disease affecting unspecified side

✓6ᵗʰ **I69.94** Monoplegia of lower limb following unspecified cerebrovascular disease

I69.941 Monoplegia of lower limb following unspecified cerebrovascular disease affecting right dominant side

I69.942 Monoplegia of lower limb following unspecified cerebrovascular disease affecting left dominant side

I69.943 Monoplegia of lower limb following unspecified cerebrovascular disease affecting right non-dominant side

I69.944 Monoplegia of lower limb following unspecified cerebrovascular disease affecting left non-dominant side

I69.949 Monoplegia of lower limb following unspecified cerebrovascular disease affecting unspecified side

✓6ᵗʰ **I69.95** Hemiplegia and hemiparesis following unspecified cerebrovascular disease

I69.951 Hemiplegia and hemiparesis following unspecified cerebrovascular disease affecting right dominant side `CC`
CC Excl: I69.051-I69.052, I69.151-I69.152, I69.251-I69.252, I69.351-I69.352, I69.851-I69.852, I69.951-I69.952

I69.952 Hemiplegia and hemiparesis following unspecified cerebrovascular disease affecting left dominant side `CC`
CC Excl: See code: I69.951

I69.953 Hemiplegia and hemiparesis following unspecified cerebrovascular disease affecting right non-dominant side `CC`
CC Excl: I69.053-I69.054, I69.153-I69.154, I69.253-I69.254, I69.353-I69.354, I69.853-I69.854, I69.953-I69.954

I69.954 Hemiplegia and hemiparesis following unspecified cerebrovascular disease affecting left non-dominant side `CC`
CC Excl: See code: I69.953

I69.959 Hemiplegia and hemiparesis following unspecified cerebrovascular disease affecting unspecified side `CC`
CC Excl: I69.059, I69.159, I69.259, I69.359, I69.859, I69.959

✓6ᵗʰ **I69.96** Other paralytic syndrome following unspecified cerebrovascular disease
Use additional code to identify type of paralytic syndrome, such as:
locked-in state (G83.5)
quadriplegia (G82.5-)
EXCLUDES 1 hemiplegia/hemiparesis following unspecified cerebrovascular disease (I69.95-)
monoplegia of lower limb following unspecified cerebrovascular disease (I69.94-)
monoplegia of upper limb following unspecified cerebrovascular disease (I69.93-)

I69.961 Other paralytic syndrome following unspecified cerebrovascular disease affecting right dominant side

I69.962 Other paralytic syndrome following unspecified cerebrovascular disease affecting left dominant side

I69.963 Other paralytic syndrome following unspecified cerebrovascular disease affecting right non-dominant side

I69.964 Other paralytic syndrome following unspecified cerebrovascular disease affecting left non-dominant side

I69.965 Other paralytic syndrome following unspecified cerebrovascular disease, bilateral

I69.969 Other paralytic syndrome following unspecified cerebrovascular disease affecting unspecified side

✓6ᵗʰ **I69.99** Other sequelae of unspecified cerebrovascular disease

I69.990 Apraxia following unspecified cerebrovascular disease

I69.991 Dysphagia following unspecified cerebrovascular disease
Use additional code to identify the type of dysphagia, if known (R13.1-)

I69.992 Facial weakness following unspecified cerebrovascular disease
Facial droop following unspecified cerebrovascular disease

I69.993 Ataxia following unspecified cerebrovascular disease

I69.998 Other sequelae following unspecified cerebrovascular disease
Alteration in sensation following unspecified cerebrovascular disease
Disturbance of vision following unspecified cerebrovascular disease
Use additional code to identify the sequelae

Diseases of arteries, arterioles and capillaries (I70-I79)

✓4ᵗʰ **I70** **Atherosclerosis**
INCLUDES arteriolosclerosis
arterial degeneration
arteriosclerosis
arteriosclerotic vascular disease
arteriovascular degeneration
atheroma
endarteritis deformans or obliterans
senile arteritis
senile endarteritis
vascular degeneration
Use additional code to identify:
exposure to environmental tobacco smoke (Z77.22)
history of tobacco use (Z87.891)
occupational exposure to environmental tobacco smoke (Z57.31)
tobacco dependence (F17.-)
tobacco use (Z72.0)
EXCLUDES 2 arteriosclerotic cardiovascular disease (I25.1-)
arteriosclerotic heart disease (I25.1-)
atheroembolism (I75.-)
cerebral atherosclerosis (I67.2)
coronary atherosclerosis (I25.1-)
mesenteric atherosclerosis (K55.1)
precerebral atherosclerosis (I67.2)
primary pulmonary atherosclerosis (I27.0)

I70.0 Atherosclerosis of aorta `A`

I70.1 Atherosclerosis of renal artery `A`
Goldblatt's kidney
EXCLUDES 2 atherosclerosis of renal arterioles (I12.-)

✓5ᵗʰ **I70.2** Atherosclerosis of native arteries of the extremities
Mönckeberg's (medial) sclerosis
Use additional code, if applicable, to identify chronic total occlusion of artery of extremity (I70.92)
EXCLUDES 2 atherosclerosis of bypass graft of extremities (I70.30-I70.79)

✓6ᵗʰ **I70.20** Unspecified atherosclerosis of native arteries of extremities

I70.201 Unspecified atherosclerosis of native arteries of extremities, right leg `A`

I70.202 Unspecified atherosclerosis of native arteries of extremities, left leg `A`

I70.203 Unspecified atherosclerosis of native arteries of extremities, bilateral legs `A`

I70.208 Unspecified atherosclerosis of native arteries of extremities, other extremity `A`

I70.209 Unspecified atherosclerosis of native arteries of extremities, unspecified extremity `A`

✓6ᵗʰ **I70.21** Atherosclerosis of native arteries of extremities with intermittent claudication

I70.211 Atherosclerosis of native arteries of extremities with intermittent claudication, right leg `A`

✓ Additional Character Required   ✓x7ᵗʰ Xtension Alert   Unacceptable PDx   Manifestation   Hospital Acquired Condition   EXCLUDES 1 Not Coded Here   EXCLUDES 2 Not Included Here

I70.212 Atherosclerosis of native arteries of extremities with intermittent claudication, **left leg** ▢A

I70.213 Atherosclerosis of native arteries of extremities with intermittent claudication, **bilateral legs** ▢A

I70.218 Atherosclerosis of native arteries of extremities with intermittent claudication, **other extremity** ▢A

I70.219 Atherosclerosis of native arteries of extremities with intermittent claudication, **unspecified extremity** ▢A

✓6ᵗʰ **I70.22** Atherosclerosis of native arteries of extremities with **rest pain**

INCLUDES   any condition classifiable to I70.21-

I70.221 Atherosclerosis of native arteries of extremities with rest pain, **right leg** ▢A

I70.222 Atherosclerosis of native arteries of extremities with rest pain, **left leg** ▢A

I70.223 Atherosclerosis of native arteries of extremities with rest pain, **bilateral legs** ▢A

I70.228 Atherosclerosis of native arteries of extremities with rest pain, **other extremity** ▢A

I70.229 Atherosclerosis of native arteries of extremities with rest pain, **unspecified extremity** ▢A

✓6ᵗʰ **I70.23** Atherosclerosis of native arteries of **right leg with ulceration**

INCLUDES   any condition classifiable to I70.211 and I70.221

Use additional code to identify severity of ulcer (L97.-)

I70.231 Atherosclerosis of native arteries of right leg with ulceration of **thigh** ▢A

I70.232 Atherosclerosis of native arteries of right leg with ulceration of **calf** ▢A

I70.233 Atherosclerosis of native arteries of right leg with ulceration of **ankle** ▢A

I70.234 Atherosclerosis of native arteries of right leg with ulceration of **heel and midfoot** ▢A

Atherosclerosis of native arteries of right leg with ulceration of plantar surface of midfoot

I70.235 Atherosclerosis of native arteries of right leg with ulceration of **other part of foot** ▢A

Atherosclerosis of native arteries of right leg extremities with ulceration of toe

I70.238 Atherosclerosis of native arteries of right leg with ulceration of **other part of lower right leg** ▢A

I70.239 Atherosclerosis of native arteries of right leg with ulceration of **unspecified site** ▢A

✓6ᵗʰ **I70.24** Atherosclerosis of native arteries of **left leg with ulceration**

INCLUDES   any condition classifiable to I70.212 and I70.222

Use additional code to identify severity of ulcer (L97.-)

I70.241 Atherosclerosis of native arteries of left leg with ulceration of **thigh** ▢A

I70.242 Atherosclerosis of native arteries of left leg with ulceration of **calf** ▢A

I70.243 Atherosclerosis of native arteries of left leg with ulceration of **ankle** ▢A

I70.244 Atherosclerosis of native arteries of left leg with ulceration of **heel and midfoot** ▢A

Atherosclerosis of native arteries of left leg with ulceration of plantar surface of midfoot

I70.245 Atherosclerosis of native arteries of left leg with ulceration of **other part of foot** ▢A

Atherosclerosis of native arteries of left leg extremities with ulceration of toe

I70.248 Atherosclerosis of native arteries of left leg with ulceration of **other part of lower left leg** ▢A

I70.249 Atherosclerosis of native arteries of left leg with ulceration of **unspecified site** ▢A

I70.25 Atherosclerosis of native arteries of **other extremities** with **ulceration** ▢A

INCLUDES   any condition classifiable to I70.218 and I70.228

Use additional code to identify the severity of the ulcer (L98.49-)

✓6ᵗʰ **I70.26** Atherosclerosis of native arteries of extremities with **gangrene**

INCLUDES   any condition classifiable to I70.21-, I70.22-, I70.23-, I70.24-, and I70.25-

Use additional code to identify the severity of any ulcer (L97.-, L98.49-), if applicable

CC Excl: For CC codes in subcategory I70.26, unless otherwise noted: G89.0-G89.4, I70.261-I70.269, I96, R41.0-R41.3, R41.82, R41.9, R44.8-R44.9, R45.83-R45.84, R46.0-R46.89, R52, R68.0-R68.19, R68.81-R68.83, R68.89-R69

I70.261 Atherosclerosis of native arteries of extremities with gangrene, **right leg** CC ▢A

I70.262 Atherosclerosis of native arteries of extremities with gangrene, **left leg** CC ▢A

I70.263 Atherosclerosis of native arteries of extremities with gangrene, **bilateral legs** CC ▢A

I70.268 Atherosclerosis of native arteries of extremities with gangrene, **other extremity** CC ▢A

I70.269 Atherosclerosis of native arteries of extremities with gangrene, **unspecified extremity** CC ▢A

✓6ᵗʰ **I70.29** **Other** atherosclerosis of native arteries of extremities

I70.291 Other atherosclerosis of native arteries of extremities, **right leg** ▢A

I70.292 Other atherosclerosis of native arteries of extremities, **left leg** ▢A

I70.293 Other atherosclerosis of native arteries of extremities, **bilateral legs** ▢A

I70.298 Other atherosclerosis of native arteries of extremities, **other extremity** ▢A

I70.299 Other atherosclerosis of native arteries of extremities, **unspecified extremity** ▢A

✓5ᵗʰ **I70.3** Atherosclerosis of **unspecified type of bypass graft(s) of the extremities**

Use additional code, if applicable, to identify chronic total occlusion of artery of extremity (I70.92)

EXCLUDES 1   embolism or thrombus of bypass graft(s) of extremities (T82.8-)

✓6ᵗʰ **I70.30** **Unspecified** atherosclerosis of unspecified type of bypass graft(s) of the extremities

I70.301 Unspecified atherosclerosis of unspecified type of bypass graft(s) of the extremities, **right leg** ▢A

I70.302 Unspecified atherosclerosis of unspecified type of bypass graft(s) of the extremities, **left leg** ▢A

I70.303 Unspecified atherosclerosis of unspecified type of bypass graft(s) of the extremities, **bilateral legs** ▢A

I70.308 Unspecified atherosclerosis of unspecified type of bypass graft(s) of the extremities, **other extremity** ▢A

I70.309 Unspecified atherosclerosis of unspecified type of bypass graft(s) of the extremities, **unspecified extremity** ▢A

✓6ᵗʰ **I70.31** Atherosclerosis of unspecified type of bypass graft(s) of the extremities with **intermittent claudication**

I70.311 Atherosclerosis of unspecified type of bypass graft(s) of the extremities with intermittent claudication, **right leg** ▢A

I70.312 Atherosclerosis of unspecified type of bypass graft(s) of the extremities with intermittent claudication, **left leg** ▢A

N Newborn: 0   P Pediatric: 0-17   M Maternity: 12-55   A Adult: 15-124   MCC Major CC Condition   PDx MCC PDx acts as own MCC   CC CC Condition   PDx CC PDx acts as own CC

610   ICD-10-CM Draft (2015)

I70.313	Atherosclerosis of unspecified type of bypass graft(s) of the extremities with intermittent claudication, bilateral legs Ⓐ
I70.318	Atherosclerosis of unspecified type of bypass graft(s) of the extremities with intermittent claudication, other extremity Ⓐ
I70.319	Atherosclerosis of unspecified type of bypass graft(s) of the extremities with intermittent claudication, unspecified extremity Ⓐ

✓6ᵗʰ **I70.32**   Atherosclerosis of unspecified type of bypass graft(s) of the extremities with rest pain
     INCLUDES   any condition classifiable to I70.31-

I70.321	Atherosclerosis of unspecified type of bypass graft(s) of the extremities with rest pain, right leg Ⓐ
I70.322	Atherosclerosis of unspecified type of bypass graft(s) of the extremities with rest pain, left leg Ⓐ
I70.323	Atherosclerosis of unspecified type of bypass graft(s) of the extremities with rest pain, bilateral legs Ⓐ
I70.328	Atherosclerosis of unspecified type of bypass graft(s) of the extremities with rest pain, other extremity Ⓐ
I70.329	Atherosclerosis of unspecified type of bypass graft(s) of the extremities with rest pain, unspecified extremity Ⓐ

✓6ᵗʰ **I70.33**   Atherosclerosis of unspecified type of bypass graft(s) of the right leg with ulceration
     INCLUDES   any condition classifiable to I70.311 and I70.321
     Use additional code to identify severity of ulcer (L97.-)

> **CC Excl:** For CC codes in subcategory I70.33, unless otherwise noted: I70.231-I70.25, L44.8-L45, L94.2, L94.4, L97.101-L97.929, L98.411-L98.499, L98.8, L99

I70.331	Atherosclerosis of unspecified type of bypass graft(s) of the right leg with ulceration of thigh PDx CC CC Ⓐ
I70.332	Atherosclerosis of unspecified type of bypass graft(s) of the right leg with ulceration of calf PDx CC CC Ⓐ
I70.333	Atherosclerosis of unspecified type of bypass graft(s) of the right leg with ulceration of ankle PDx CC CC Ⓐ
I70.334	Atherosclerosis of unspecified type of bypass graft(s) of the right leg with ulceration of heel and midfoot PDx CC CC Ⓐ Atherosclerosis of unspecified type of bypass graft(s) of right leg with ulceration of plantar surface of midfoot
I70.335	Atherosclerosis of unspecified type of bypass graft(s) of the right leg with ulceration of other part of foot Ⓐ Atherosclerosis of unspecified type of bypass graft(s) of the right leg with ulceration of toe
I70.338	Atherosclerosis of unspecified type of bypass graft(s) of the right leg with ulceration of other part of lower leg PDx CC CC Ⓐ
I70.339	Atherosclerosis of unspecified type of bypass graft(s) of the right leg with ulceration of unspecified site PDx CC CC Ⓐ

✓6ᵗʰ **I70.34**   Atherosclerosis of unspecified type of bypass graft(s) of the left leg with ulceration
     INCLUDES   any condition classifiable to I70.312 and I70.322
     Use additional code to identify severity of ulcer (L97.-)

I70.341	Atherosclerosis of unspecified type of bypass graft(s) of the left leg with ulceration of thigh PDx CC CC Ⓐ
I70.342	Atherosclerosis of unspecified type of bypass graft(s) of the left leg with ulceration of calf PDx CC CC Ⓐ
I70.343	Atherosclerosis of unspecified type of bypass graft(s) of the left leg with ulceration of ankle PDx CC CC Ⓐ
I70.344	Atherosclerosis of unspecified type of bypass graft(s) of the left leg with ulceration of heel and midfoot PDx CC CC Ⓐ Atherosclerosis of unspecified type of bypass graft(s) of left leg with ulceration of plantar surface of midfoot
I70.345	Atherosclerosis of unspecified type of bypass graft(s) of the left leg with ulceration of other part of foot Ⓐ Atherosclerosis of unspecified type of bypass graft(s) of the left leg with ulceration of toe
I70.348	Atherosclerosis of unspecified type of bypass graft(s) of the left leg with ulceration of other part of lower leg PDx CC CC Ⓐ
I70.349	Atherosclerosis of unspecified type of bypass graft(s) of the left leg with ulceration of unspecified site PDx CC CC Ⓐ

I70.35   Atherosclerosis of unspecified type of bypass graft(s) of other extremity with ulceration   Ⓐ
     INCLUDES   any condition classifiable to I70.318 and I70.328
     Use additional code to identify severity of ulcer (L98.49-)

✓6ᵗʰ **I70.36**   Atherosclerosis of unspecified type of bypass graft(s) of the extremities with gangrene
     INCLUDES   any condition classifiable to I70.31-, I70.32-, I70.33-, I70.34-, I70.35
     Use additional code to identify the severity of any ulcer (L97.-, L98.49-), if applicable

I70.361	Atherosclerosis of unspecified type of bypass graft(s) of the extremities with gangrene, right leg PDx CC CC Ⓐ CC Excl: G89.0-G89.4, I70.261-I70.269, I96, R41.0-R41.3, R41.82, R41.9, R44.8-R44.9, R45.83-R45.84, R46.0-R46.89, R52, R68.0-R68.19, R68.81-R68.83, R68.89-R69
I70.362	Atherosclerosis of unspecified type of bypass graft(s) of the extremities with gangrene, left leg PDx CC CC Ⓐ CC Excl: See code: I70.361
I70.363	Atherosclerosis of unspecified type of bypass graft(s) of the extremities with gangrene, bilateral legs PDx CC CC Ⓐ CC Excl: See code: I70.361
I70.368	Atherosclerosis of unspecified type of bypass graft(s) of the extremities with gangrene, other extremity PDx CC CC Ⓐ CC Excl: See code: I70.361
I70.369	Atherosclerosis of unspecified type of bypass graft(s) of the extremities with gangrene, unspecified extremity PDx CC CC Ⓐ CC Excl: See code: I70.361

✓6ᵗʰ **I70.39**   Other atherosclerosis of unspecified type of bypass graft(s) of the extremities

I70.391	Other atherosclerosis of unspecified type of bypass graft(s) of the extremities, right leg Ⓐ
I70.392	Other atherosclerosis of unspecified type of bypass graft(s) of the extremities, left leg Ⓐ
I70.393	Other atherosclerosis of unspecified type of bypass graft(s) of the extremities, bilateral legs Ⓐ
I70.398	Other atherosclerosis of unspecified type of bypass graft(s) of the extremities, other extremity Ⓐ
I70.399	Other atherosclerosis of unspecified type of bypass graft(s) of the extremities, unspecified extremity Ⓐ

☑ Additional Character Required   ✓x7ᵗʰ Xtension Alert   Unacceptable PDx   Manifestation   Hospital Acquired Condition   EXCLUDES 1 Not Coded Here   EXCLUDES 2 Not Included Here

Diseases of the Circulatory System

I70.4–I70.468

√5ᵗʰ **I70.4 Atherosclerosis of autologous vein bypass graft(s) of the extremities**
  Use additional code, if applicable, to identify chronic total occlusion of artery of extremity (I70.92)

√6ᵗʰ **I70.40 Unspecified atherosclerosis of autologous vein bypass graft(s) of the extremities**

I70.401 Unspecified atherosclerosis of autologous vein bypass graft(s) of the extremities, right leg Ⓐ

I70.402 Unspecified atherosclerosis of autologous vein bypass graft(s) of the extremities, left leg Ⓐ

I70.403 Unspecified atherosclerosis of autologous vein bypass graft(s) of the extremities, bilateral legs Ⓐ

I70.408 Unspecified atherosclerosis of autologous vein bypass graft(s) of the extremities, other extremity Ⓐ

I70.409 Unspecified atherosclerosis of autologous vein bypass graft(s) of the extremities, unspecified extremity Ⓐ

√6ᵗʰ **I70.41 Atherosclerosis of autologous vein bypass graft(s) of the extremities with intermittent claudication**

I70.411 Atherosclerosis of autologous vein bypass graft(s) of the extremities with intermittent claudication, right leg Ⓐ

I70.412 Atherosclerosis of autologous vein bypass graft(s) of the extremities with intermittent claudication, left leg Ⓐ

I70.413 Atherosclerosis of autologous vein bypass graft(s) of the extremities with intermittent claudication, bilateral legs Ⓐ

I70.418 Atherosclerosis of autologous vein bypass graft(s) of the extremities with intermittent claudication, other extremity Ⓐ

I70.419 Atherosclerosis of autologous vein bypass graft(s) of the extremities with intermittent claudication, unspecified extremity Ⓐ

√6ᵗʰ **I70.42 Atherosclerosis of autologous vein bypass graft(s) of the extremities with rest pain**
  INCLUDES any condition classifiable to I70.41-

I70.421 Atherosclerosis of autologous vein bypass graft(s) of the extremities with rest pain, right leg Ⓐ

I70.422 Atherosclerosis of autologous vein bypass graft(s) of the extremities with rest pain, left leg Ⓐ

I70.423 Atherosclerosis of autologous vein bypass graft(s) of the extremities with rest pain, bilateral legs Ⓐ

I70.428 Atherosclerosis of autologous vein bypass graft(s) of the extremities with rest pain, other extremity Ⓐ

I70.429 Atherosclerosis of autologous vein bypass graft(s) of the extremities with rest pain, unspecified extremity Ⓐ

√6ᵗʰ **I70.43 Atherosclerosis of autologous vein bypass graft(s) of the right leg with ulceration**
  INCLUDES any condition classifiable to I70.411 and I70.421
  Use additional code to identify severity of ulcer (L97.-)

  CC Excl: For CC codes in subcategory I70.43, unless otherwise noted: I70.231-I70.25, L44.8-L45, L94.2, L94.4, L97.101-L97.929, L98.411-L98.499, L98.8, L99

I70.431 Atherosclerosis of autologous vein bypass graft(s) of the right leg with ulceration of thigh PDx CC CC Ⓐ

I70.432 Atherosclerosis of autologous vein bypass graft(s) of the right leg with ulceration of calf PDx CC CC Ⓐ

I70.433 Atherosclerosis of autologous vein bypass graft(s) of the right leg with ulceration of ankle PDx CC CC Ⓐ

I70.434 Atherosclerosis of autologous vein bypass graft(s) of the right leg with ulceration of heel and midfoot PDx CC CC Ⓐ
  Atherosclerosis of autologous vein bypass graft(s) of right leg with ulceration of plantar surface of midfoot

I70.435 Atherosclerosis of autologous vein bypass graft(s) of the right leg with ulceration of other part of foot Ⓐ
  Atherosclerosis of autologous vein bypass graft(s) of right leg with ulceration of toe

I70.438 Atherosclerosis of autologous vein bypass graft(s) of the right leg with ulceration of other part of lower leg PDx CC CC Ⓐ

I70.439 Atherosclerosis of autologous vein bypass graft(s) of the right leg with ulceration of unspecified site PDx CC Ⓐ

√6ᵗʰ **I70.44 Atherosclerosis of autologous vein bypass graft(s) of the left leg with ulceration**
  INCLUDES any condition classifiable to I70.412 and I70.422
  Use additional code to identify severity of ulcer (L97.-)

I70.441 Atherosclerosis of autologous vein bypass graft(s) of the left leg with ulceration of thigh PDx CC CC Ⓐ

I70.442 Atherosclerosis of autologous vein bypass graft(s) of the left leg with ulceration of calf PDx CC CC Ⓐ

I70.443 Atherosclerosis of autologous vein bypass graft(s) of the left leg with ulceration of ankle PDx CC CC Ⓐ

I70.444 Atherosclerosis of autologous vein bypass graft(s) of the left leg with ulceration of heel and midfoot PDx CC CC Ⓐ
  Atherosclerosis of autologous vein bypass graft(s) of left leg with ulceration of plantar surface of midfoot

I70.445 Atherosclerosis of autologous vein bypass graft(s) of the left leg with ulceration of other part of foot Ⓐ
  Atherosclerosis of autologous vein bypass graft(s) of left leg with ulceration of toe

I70.448 Atherosclerosis of autologous vein bypass graft(s) of the left leg with ulceration of other part of lower leg PDx CC CC Ⓐ

I70.449 Atherosclerosis of autologous vein bypass graft(s) of the left leg with ulceration of unspecified site PDx CC CC Ⓐ

I70.45 Atherosclerosis of autologous vein bypass graft(s) of other extremity with ulceration Ⓐ
  INCLUDES any condition classifiable to I70.418, I70.428, and I70.438
  Use additional code to identify severity of ulcer (L98.49)

√6ᵗʰ **I70.46 Atherosclerosis of autologous vein bypass graft(s) of the extremities with gangrene**
  INCLUDES any condition classifiable to I70.41-, I70.42-, and I70.43-, I70.44-, I70.45
  Use additional code to identify the severity of any ulcer (L97.-, L98.49-), if applicable

I70.461 Atherosclerosis of autologous vein bypass graft(s) of the extremities with gangrene, right leg PDx CC CC Ⓐ
  CC Excl: G89.0-G89.4, I70.261-I70.269, I96, R41.0-R41.3, R41.82, R41.9, R44.8-R44.9, R45.83-R45.84, R46.0-R46.89, R52, R68.0-R68.19, R68.81-R68.83, R68.89-R69

I70.462 Atherosclerosis of autologous vein bypass graft(s) of the extremities with gangrene, left leg PDx CC CC Ⓐ
  CC Excl: See code: I70.461

I70.463 Atherosclerosis of autologous vein bypass graft(s) of the extremities with gangrene, bilateral legs PDx CC CC Ⓐ
  CC Excl: See code: I70.461

I70.468 Atherosclerosis of autologous vein bypass graft(s) of the extremities with gangrene, other extremity PDx CC CC Ⓐ
  CC Excl: See code: I70.461

I70.469   **Atherosclerosis of autologous** `PDx` `CC` `CC` `A`
          vein bypass graft(s) of the extremities
          with gangrene, unspecified extremity
          CC Excl: See code: I70.461

✓6ᵗʰ I70.49   Other **atherosclerosis of autologous vein bypass**
          graft(s) of the extremities

I70.491   **Other atherosclerosis of autologous** `A`
          vein bypass graft(s) of the extremities,
          right leg

I70.492   **Other atherosclerosis of autologous** `A`
          vein bypass graft(s) of the extremities,
          left leg

I70.493   **Other atherosclerosis of autologous** `A`
          vein bypass graft(s) of the extremities,
          bilateral legs

I70.498   **Other atherosclerosis of autologous** `A`
          vein bypass graft(s) of the extremities,
          other extremity

I70.499   **Other atherosclerosis of autologous** `A`
          vein bypass graft(s) of the extremities,
          unspecified extremity

✓5ᵗʰ I70.5   **Atherosclerosis of** nonautologous biological bypass graft(s)
          of the extremities
          Use additional code, if applicable, to identify chronic total
          occlusion of artery of extremity (I70.92)

✓6ᵗʰ I70.50   Unspecified **atherosclerosis of nonautologous**
          biological bypass graft(s) of the extremities

I70.501   **Unspecified atherosclerosis of** `A`
          nonautologous biological bypass graft(s)
          of the extremities, right leg

I70.502   **Unspecified atherosclerosis of** `A`
          nonautologous biological bypass graft(s)
          of the extremities, left leg

I70.503   **Unspecified atherosclerosis of** `A`
          nonautologous biological bypass graft(s)
          of the extremities, bilateral legs

I70.508   **Unspecified atherosclerosis of** `A`
          nonautologous biological bypass graft(s)
          of the extremities, other extremity

I70.509   **Unspecified atherosclerosis of** `A`
          nonautologous biological bypass graft(s)
          of the extremities, unspecified extremity

✓6ᵗʰ I70.51   **Atherosclerosis of nonautologous biological bypass**
          graft(s) of the extremities with intermittent
          claudication

I70.511   **Atherosclerosis of nonautologous** `A`
          biological bypass graft(s) of the
          extremities with intermittent
          claudication, right leg

I70.512   **Atherosclerosis of nonautologous** `A`
          biological bypass graft(s) of the
          extremities with intermittent
          claudication, left leg

I70.513   **Atherosclerosis of nonautologous** `A`
          biological bypass graft(s) of the
          extremities with intermittent
          claudication, bilateral legs

I70.518   **Atherosclerosis of nonautologous** `A`
          biological bypass graft(s) of the
          extremities with intermittent
          claudication, other extremity

I70.519   **Atherosclerosis of nonautologous** `A`
          biological bypass graft(s) of the
          extremities with intermittent
          claudication, unspecified extremity

✓6ᵗʰ I70.52   **Atherosclerosis of nonautologous biological bypass**
          graft(s) of the extremities with rest pain
          INCLUDES   any condition classifiable to I70.51-

I70.521   **Atherosclerosis of nonautologous** `A`
          biological bypass graft(s) of the
          extremities with rest pain, right leg

I70.522   **Atherosclerosis of nonautologous** `A`
          biological bypass graft(s) of the
          extremities with rest pain, left leg

I70.523   **Atherosclerosis of nonautologous** `A`
          biological bypass graft(s) of the
          extremities with rest pain, bilateral legs

I70.528   **Atherosclerosis of nonautologous**
          biological bypass graft(s) of the
          extremities with rest pain, other extremity

I70.529   **Atherosclerosis of nonautologous** `A`
          biological bypass graft(s) of the
          extremities with rest pain, unspecified
          extremity

✓6ᵗʰ I70.53   **Atherosclerosis of nonautologous biological bypass**
          graft(s) of the right leg **with** ulceration
          INCLUDES   any condition classifiable to I70.511 and
          I70.521
          Use additional code to identify severity of ulcer (L97.-)

          CC Excl: For CC codes in subcategory I70.53,
          unless otherwise noted: I70.231-I70.25, L44.8-
          L45, L94.2, L94.4, L97.101-L97.929, L98.411-
          L98.499, L98.8, L99

I70.531   **Atherosclerosis of** `PDx` `CC` `CC` `A`
          biological nonautologous bypass graft(s)
          of the right leg with ulceration of thigh

I70.532   **Atherosclerosis of** `PDx` `CC` `CC` `A`
          biological nonautologous bypass graft(s)
          of the right leg with ulceration of calf

I70.533   **Atherosclerosis of** `PDx` `CC` `CC` `A`
          nonautologous biological bypass graft(s)
          of the right leg with ulceration of ankle

I70.534   **Atherosclerosis of** `PDx` `CC` `CC` `A`
          nonautologous biological bypass graft(s)
          of the right leg with ulceration of heel and
          midfoot
          Atherosclerosis of nonautologous
              biological bypass graft(s) of right leg
              with ulceration of plantar surface of
              midfoot

I70.535   **Atherosclerosis of nonautologous** `A`
          biological bypass graft(s) of the right leg
          with ulceration of other part of foot
          Atherosclerosis of nonautologous
              biological bypass graft(s) of the right
              leg with ulceration of toe

I70.538   **Atherosclerosis of** `PDx` `CC` `CC` `A`
          nonautologous biological bypass graft(s)
          of the right leg with ulceration of other
          part of lower leg

I70.539   **Atherosclerosis of** `PDx` `CC` `CC` `A`
          nonautologous biological bypass graft(s)
          of the right leg with ulceration of
          unspecified site

✓6ᵗʰ I70.54   **Atherosclerosis of nonautologous biological bypass**
          graft(s) of the left leg **with** ulceration
          INCLUDES   any condition classifiable to I70.512 and
          I70.522
          Use additional code to identify severity of ulcer (L97.-)

I70.541   **Atherosclerosis of** `PDx` `CC` `CC` `A`
          nonautologous biological bypass graft(s)
          of the left leg with ulceration of thigh

I70.542   **Atherosclerosis of** `PDx` `CC` `CC` `A`
          nonautologous biological bypass graft(s)
          of the left leg with ulceration of calf

I70.543   **Atherosclerosis of** `PDx` `CC` `CC` `A`
          nonautologous biological bypass graft(s)
          of the left leg with ulceration of ankle

I70.544   **Atherosclerosis of** `PDx` `CC` `CC` `A`
          nonautologous biological bypass graft(s)
          of the left leg with ulceration of heel and
          midfoot
          Atherosclerosis of nonautologous
              biological bypass graft(s) of left leg
              with ulceration of plantar surface of
              midfoot

I70.545   **Atherosclerosis of nonautologous** `A`
          biological bypass graft(s) of the left leg
          with ulceration of other part of foot
          Atherosclerosis of nonautologous
              biological bypass graft(s) of the left leg
              with ulceration of toe

I70.548   **Atherosclerosis of** `PDx` `CC` `CC` `A`
          nonautologous biological bypass graft(s)
          of the left leg with ulceration of other part
          of lower leg

I70.549   **Atherosclerosis of** `PDx` `CC` `CC` `A`
          nonautologous biological bypass graft(s)
          of the left leg with ulceration of
          unspecified site

✓ Additional Character Required   ✓x7ᵗʰ Xtension Alert   Unacceptable PDx   Manifestation   Hospital Acquired Condition   **EXCLUDES 1** Not Coded Here   **EXCLUDES 2** Not Included Here

I70.55 Atherosclerosis of nonautologous biological bypass graft(s) of other extremity with ulceration A
INCLUDES any condition classifiable to I70.518, I70.528, and I70.538
Use additional code to identify severity of ulcer (L98.49)

✓6ᵗʰ **I70.56 Atherosclerosis of nonautologous biological bypass graft(s) of the extremities with gangrene**
INCLUDES any condition classifiable to I70.51-, I70.52-, and I70.53-, I70.54-, I70.55
Use additional code to identify the severity of any ulcer (L97.-, L98.49-), if applicable

I70.561 Atherosclerosis of nonautologous biological bypass graft(s) of the extremities with gangrene, right leg [PDx CC CC A]
CC Excl: G89.0-G89.4, I70.261-I70.269, I96, R41.0-R41.3, R41.82, R41.9, R44.8-R44.9, R45.83-R45.84, R46.0-R46.89, R52, R68.0-R68.19, R68.81-R68.83, R68.89-R69

I70.562 Atherosclerosis of nonautologous biological bypass graft(s) of the extremities with gangrene, left leg [PDx CC CC A]
CC Excl: See code: I70.561

I70.563 Atherosclerosis of nonautologous biological bypass graft(s) of the extremities with gangrene, bilateral legs [PDx CC CC A]
CC Excl: See code: I70.561

I70.568 Atherosclerosis of nonautologous biological bypass graft(s) of the extremities with gangrene, other extremity [PDx CC CC A]
CC Excl: See code: I70.561

I70.569 Atherosclerosis of nonautologous biological bypass graft(s) of the extremities with gangrene, unspecified extremity [PDx CC CC A]
CC Excl: See code: I70.561

✓6ᵗʰ **I70.59 Other atherosclerosis of nonautologous biological bypass graft(s) of the extremities**

I70.591 Other atherosclerosis of biological nonautologous bypass graft(s) of the extremities, right leg A

I70.592 Other atherosclerosis of nonautologous biological bypass graft(s) of the extremities, left leg A

I70.593 Other atherosclerosis of nonautologous biological bypass graft(s) of the extremities, bilateral legs A

I70.598 Other atherosclerosis of nonautologous biological bypass graft(s) of the extremities, other extremity A

I70.599 Other atherosclerosis of nonautologous biological bypass graft(s) of the extremities, unspecified extremity A

✓5ᵗʰ **I70.6 Atherosclerosis of nonbiological bypass graft(s) of the extremities**
Use additional code, if applicable, to identify chronic total occlusion of artery of extremity (I70.92)

✓6ᵗʰ **I70.60 Unspecified atherosclerosis of nonbiological bypass graft(s) of the extremities**

I70.601 Unspecified atherosclerosis of nonbiological bypass graft(s) of the extremities, right leg A

I70.602 Unspecified atherosclerosis of nonbiological bypass graft(s) of the extremities, left leg A

I70.603 Unspecified atherosclerosis of nonbiological bypass graft(s) of the extremities, bilateral legs A

I70.608 Unspecified atherosclerosis of nonbiological bypass graft(s) of the extremities, other extremity A

I70.609 Unspecified atherosclerosis of nonbiological bypass graft(s) of the extremities, unspecified extremity A

✓6ᵗʰ **I70.61 Atherosclerosis of nonbiological bypass graft(s) of the extremities with intermittent claudication**

I70.611 Atherosclerosis of nonbiological bypass graft(s) of the extremities with intermittent claudication, right leg A

I70.612 Atherosclerosis of nonbiological bypass graft(s) of the extremities with intermittent claudication, left leg A

I70.613 Atherosclerosis of nonbiological bypass graft(s) of the extremities with intermittent claudication, bilateral legs A

I70.618 Atherosclerosis of nonbiological bypass graft(s) of the extremities with intermittent claudication, other extremity A

I70.619 Atherosclerosis of nonbiological bypass graft(s) of the extremities with intermittent claudication, unspecified extremity A

✓6ᵗʰ **I70.62 Atherosclerosis of nonbiological bypass graft(s) of the extremities with rest pain**
INCLUDES any condition classifiable to I70.61-

I70.621 Atherosclerosis of nonbiological bypass graft(s) of the extremities with rest pain, right leg A

I70.622 Atherosclerosis of nonbiological bypass graft(s) of the extremities with rest pain, left leg A

I70.623 Atherosclerosis of nonbiological bypass graft(s) of the extremities with rest pain, bilateral legs A

I70.628 Atherosclerosis of nonbiological bypass graft(s) of the extremities with rest pain, other extremity A

I70.629 Atherosclerosis of nonbiological bypass graft(s) of the extremities with rest pain, unspecified extremity A

✓6ᵗʰ **I70.63 Atherosclerosis of nonbiological bypass graft(s) of the right leg with ulceration**
INCLUDES any condition classifiable to I70.611 and I70.621
Use additional code to identify severity of ulcer (L97.-)

CC Excl: For CC codes in subcategory I70.63, unless otherwise noted: I70.231-I70.25, L44.8-L45, L94.2, L94.4, L97.101-L97.929, L98.411-L98.499, L98.8, L99

I70.631 Atherosclerosis of nonbiological bypass graft(s) of the right leg with ulceration of thigh [PDx CC CC A]

I70.632 Atherosclerosis of nonbiological bypass graft(s) of the right leg with ulceration of calf [PDx CC CC A]

I70.633 Atherosclerosis of nonbiological bypass graft(s) of the right leg with ulceration of ankle [PDx CC CC A]

I70.634 Atherosclerosis of nonbiological bypass graft(s) of the right leg with ulceration of heel and midfoot [PDx CC CC A]
Atherosclerosis of nonbiological bypass graft(s) of right leg with ulceration of plantar surface of midfoot

I70.635 Atherosclerosis of nonbiological bypass graft(s) of the right leg with ulceration of other part of foot A
Atherosclerosis of nonbiological bypass graft(s) of the right leg with ulceration of toe

I70.638 Atherosclerosis of nonbiological bypass graft(s) of the right leg with ulceration of other part of lower leg [PDx CC CC A]

I70.639 Atherosclerosis of nonbiological bypass graft(s) of the right leg with ulceration of unspecified site [PDx CC CC A]

√6ᵗʰ **I70.64　Atherosclerosis of nonbiological bypass graft(s) of the left leg with ulceration**
　　INCLUDES　any condition classifiable to I70.612 and I70.622
　　Use additional code to identify severity of ulcer (L97.-)

　　I70.641　Atherosclerosis of nonbiological bypass graft(s) of the left leg with ulceration of thigh PDx CC CC A

　　I70.642　Atherosclerosis of nonbiological bypass graft(s) of the left leg with ulceration of calf PDx CC CC A

　　I70.643　Atherosclerosis of nonbiological bypass graft(s) of the left leg with ulceration of ankle PDx CC CC A

　　I70.644　Atherosclerosis of nonbiological bypass graft(s) of the left leg with ulceration of heel and midfoot PDx CC CC A
　　　　Atherosclerosis of nonbiological bypass graft(s) of left leg with ulceration of plantar surface of midfoot

　　I70.645　Atherosclerosis of nonbiological bypass graft(s) of the left leg with ulceration of other part of foot A
　　　　Atherosclerosis of nonbiological bypass graft(s) of the left leg with ulceration of toe

　　I70.648　Atherosclerosis of nonbiological bypass graft(s) of the left leg with ulceration of other part of lower leg PDx CC CC A

　　I70.649　Atherosclerosis of nonbiological bypass graft(s) of the left leg with ulceration of unspecified site PDx CC CC A

I70.65　Atherosclerosis of nonbiological bypass graft(s) of other extremity with ulceration A
　　INCLUDES　any condition classifiable to I70.618 and I70.628
　　Use additional code to identify severity of ulcer (L98.49)

√6ᵗʰ **I70.66　Atherosclerosis of nonbiological bypass graft(s) of the extremities with gangrene**
　　INCLUDES　any condition classifiable to I70.61-, I70.62-, I70.63-, I70.64-, I70.65
　　Use additional code to identify the severity of any ulcer (L97.-, L98.49-), if applicable

　　I70.661　Atherosclerosis of nonbiological bypass graft(s) of the extremities with gangrene, right leg PDx CC CC A
　　　　CC Excl: G89.0-G89.4, I70.261-I70.269, I96, R41.0-R41.3, R41.82, R41.9, R44.8-R44.9, R45.83-R45.84, R46.0-R46.89, R52, R68.0-R68.19, R68.81-R68.83, R68.89-R69

　　I70.662　Atherosclerosis of nonbiological bypass graft(s) of the extremities with gangrene, left leg PDx CC CC A
　　　　CC Excl: See code: I70.661

　　I70.663　Atherosclerosis of nonbiological bypass graft(s) of the extremities with gangrene, bilateral legs PDx CC CC A
　　　　CC Excl: See code: I70.661

　　I70.668　Atherosclerosis of nonbiological bypass graft(s) of the extremities with gangrene, other extremity PDx CC CC A
　　　　CC Excl: See code: I70.661

　　I70.669　Atherosclerosis of nonbiological bypass graft(s) of the extremities with gangrene, unspecified extremity PDx CC CC A
　　　　CC Excl: See code: I70.661

√6ᵗʰ **I70.69　Other atherosclerosis of nonbiological bypass graft(s) of the extremities**

　　I70.691　Other atherosclerosis of nonbiological bypass graft(s) of the extremities, right leg A

　　I70.692　Other atherosclerosis of nonbiological bypass graft(s) of the extremities, left leg A

　　I70.693　Other atherosclerosis of nonbiological bypass graft(s) of the extremities, bilateral legs A

　　I70.698　Other atherosclerosis of nonbiological bypass graft(s) of the extremities, other extremity A

　　I70.699　Other atherosclerosis of nonbiological bypass graft(s) of the extremities, unspecified extremity A

√5ᵗʰ **I70.7　Atherosclerosis of other type of bypass graft(s) of the extremities**
　　Use additional code, if applicable, to identify chronic total occlusion of artery of extremity (I70.92)

√6ᵗʰ **I70.70　Unspecified atherosclerosis of other type of bypass graft(s) of the extremities**

　　I70.701　Unspecified atherosclerosis of other type of bypass graft(s) of the extremities, right leg A

　　I70.702　Unspecified atherosclerosis of other type of bypass graft(s) of the extremities, left leg A

　　I70.703　Unspecified atherosclerosis of other type of bypass graft(s) of the extremities, bilateral legs A

　　I70.708　Unspecified atherosclerosis of other type of bypass graft(s) of the extremities, other extremity A

　　I70.709　Unspecified atherosclerosis of other type of bypass graft(s) of the extremities, unspecified extremity A

√6ᵗʰ **I70.71　Atherosclerosis of other type of bypass graft(s) of the extremities with intermittent claudication**

　　I70.711　Atherosclerosis of other type of bypass graft(s) of the extremities with intermittent claudication, right leg A

　　I70.712　Atherosclerosis of other type of bypass graft(s) of the extremities with intermittent claudication, left leg A

　　I70.713　Atherosclerosis of other type of bypass graft(s) of the extremities with intermittent claudication, bilateral legs A

　　I70.718　Atherosclerosis of other type of bypass graft(s) of the extremities with intermittent claudication, other extremity A

　　I70.719　Atherosclerosis of other type of bypass graft(s) of the extremities with intermittent claudication, unspecified extremity A

√6ᵗʰ **I70.72　Atherosclerosis of other type of bypass graft(s) of the extremities with rest pain**
　　INCLUDES　any condition classifiable to I70.71-

　　I70.721　Atherosclerosis of other type of bypass graft(s) of the extremities with rest pain, right leg A

　　I70.722　Atherosclerosis of other type of bypass graft(s) of the extremities with rest pain, left leg A

　　I70.723　Atherosclerosis of other type of bypass graft(s) of the extremities with rest pain, bilateral legs A

　　I70.728　Atherosclerosis of other type of bypass graft(s) of the extremities with rest pain, other extremity A

　　I70.729　Atherosclerosis of other type of bypass graft(s) of the extremities with rest pain, unspecified extremity A

√6ᵗʰ **I70.73　Atherosclerosis of other type of bypass graft(s) of the right leg with ulceration**
　　INCLUDES　any condition classifiable to I70.711 and I70.721
　　Use additional code to identify severity of ulcer (L97.-)

　　CC Excl: For CC codes in subcategory I70.73, unless otherwise noted:I70.231-I70.25, L44.8-L45, L94.2, L94.4, L97.101-L97.929, L98.411-L98.499, L98.8, L99

　　I70.731　Atherosclerosis of other type of bypass graft(s) of the right leg with ulceration of thigh PDx CC CC A

　　I70.732　Atherosclerosis of other type of bypass graft(s) of the right leg with ulceration of calf PDx CC CC A

　　I70.733　Atherosclerosis of other type of bypass graft(s) of the right leg with ulceration of ankle PDx CC CC A

I70.734 Atherosclerosis of other type `PDx CC` `CC` `A`
of bypass graft(s) of the right leg with
ulceration of heel and midfoot
　　Atherosclerosis of other type of bypass
　　graft(s) of right leg with ulceration of
　　plantar surface of midfoot

I70.735 Atherosclerosis of other type of bypass `A`
graft(s) of the right leg with ulceration of
other part of foot
　　Atherosclerosis of other type of bypass
　　graft(s) of right leg with ulceration of
　　toe

I70.738 Atherosclerosis of other type `PDx CC` `CC` `A`
of bypass graft(s) of the right leg with
ulceration of other part of lower leg

I70.739 Atherosclerosis of other type `PDx CC` `CC` `A`
of bypass graft(s) of the right leg with
ulceration of unspecified site

√6ᵗʰ **I70.74** Atherosclerosis of other type of bypass graft(s) of
the left leg with ulceration
　　INCLUDES　any condition classifiable to I70.712 and
　　　　　　　I70.722
　　Use additional code to identify severity of ulcer (L97.-)

I70.741 Atherosclerosis of other type `PDx CC` `CC` `A`
of bypass graft(s) of the left leg with
ulceration of thigh

I70.742 Atherosclerosis of other type `PDx CC` `CC` `A`
of bypass graft(s) of the left leg with
ulceration of calf

I70.743 Atherosclerosis of other type `PDx CC` `CC` `A`
of bypass graft(s) of the left leg with
ulceration of ankle

I70.744 Atherosclerosis of other type `PDx CC` `CC` `A`
of bypass raft(s) of the left leg with
ulceration of heel and midfoot
　　Atherosclerosis of other type of bypass
　　graft(s) of left leg with ulceration of
　　plantar surface of midfoot

I70.745 Atherosclerosis of other type of bypass `A`
graft(s) of the left leg with ulceration of
other part of foot
　　Atherosclerosis of other type of bypass
　　graft(s) of left leg with ulceration of
　　toe

I70.748 Atherosclerosis of other type `PDx CC` `CC` `A`
of bypass graft(s) of the left leg with
ulceration of other part of lower leg

I70.749 Atherosclerosis of other type `PDx CC` `CC` `A`
of bypass graft(s) of the left leg with
ulceration of unspecified site

I70.75 Atherosclerosis of other type of bypass graft(s) `A`
of other extremity with ulceration
　　INCLUDES　any condition classifiable to I70.718 and
　　　　　　　I70.728
　　Use additional code to identify severity of ulcer
　　　　(L98.49)

√6ᵗʰ **I70.76** Atherosclerosis of other type of bypass graft(s) of
the extremities with gangrene
　　INCLUDES　any condition classifiable to I70.71-, I70.72-,
　　　　　　　I70.73-, I70.74-, I70.75
　　Use additional code to identify the severity of any
　　　　ulcer (L97.-, L98.49-), if applicable

I70.761 Atherosclerosis of other type `PDx CC` `CC` `A`
of bypass graft(s) of the extremities with
gangrene, right leg
　　CC Excl: G89.0-G89.4, I70.261-I70.269, I96,
　　R41.0-R41.3, R41.82, R41.9, R44.8-R44.9,
　　R45.83-R45.84, R46.0-R46.89, R52, R68.0-
　　R68.19, R68.81-R68.83, R68.89-R69

I70.762 Atherosclerosis of other type `PDx CC` `CC` `A`
of bypass graft(s) of the extremities with
gangrene, left leg
　　CC Excl: See code: I70.761

I70.763 Atherosclerosis of other type `PDx CC` `CC` `A`
of bypass graft(s) of the extremities with
gangrene, bilateral legs
　　CC Excl: See code: I70.761

I70.768 Atherosclerosis of other type `PDx CC` `CC` `A`
of bypass graft(s) of the extremities with
gangrene, other extremity
　　CC Excl: See code: I70.761

I70.769 Atherosclerosis of other type `PDx CC` `CC` `A`
of bypass graft(s) of the extremities with
gangrene, unspecified extremity
　　CC Excl: See code: I70.761

√6ᵗʰ **I70.79** Other atherosclerosis of other type of bypass graft(s)
of the extremities

I70.791 Other atherosclerosis of other type of `A`
bypass graft(s) of the extremities, right
leg

I70.792 Other atherosclerosis of other type of `A`
bypass graft(s) of the extremities, left leg

I70.793 Other atherosclerosis of other type of `A`
bypass graft(s) of the extremities,
bilateral legs

I70.798 Other atherosclerosis of other type of `A`
bypass graft(s) of the extremities, other
extremity

I70.799 Other atherosclerosis of other type of `A`
bypass graft(s) of the extremities,
unspecified extremity

I70.8 Atherosclerosis of other arteries `A`

√5ᵗʰ **I70.9** Other and unspecified atherosclerosis

I70.90 Unspecified atherosclerosis `A`

I70.91 Generalized atherosclerosis `A`

I70.92 Chronic total occlusion of artery of the `CC` `A`
extremities
　　Complete occlusion of artery of the extremities
　　Total occlusion of artery of the extremities
　　Code first atherosclerosis of arteries of the extremities
　　　　(I70.2-, I70.3-, I70.4-, I70.5-, I70.6-, I70.7-)
　　CC Excl: I67.0, I70.201-I70.799, I70.92-I71.9, I72.1,
　　I72.3-I72.4, I72.9, I73.81-I77.2, I77.5-I77.6, I77.72,
　　I77.79-I77.819, I79.0-I79.8, M31.8-M31.9

√4ᵗʰ **I71** Aortic aneurysm and dissection
　　EXCLUDES 1　aortic ectasia (I77.81-)
　　　　　　　syphilitic aortic aneurysm (A52.01)
　　　　　　　traumatic aortic aneurysm (S25.09, S35.09)

　　CC Excl: For MCC codes in category I71, unless otherwise noted:
　　E08.51-E08.59, E08.618-E08.638, E08.649-E08.8, E09.51-E09.59,
　　E09.618-E09.638, E09.649-E09.8, E10.51-E10.59, E10.618-E10.638,
　　E10.649, E10.69-E10.8, E11.51-E11.59, E11.618-E11.638, E11.649,
　　E11.69-E11.8, E13.51-E13.59, E13.618-E13.638, E13.649-E13.8, I71.00-
　　I71.9, I77.810-I77.819, I79.0, I87.8, I99.8-I99.9

√5ᵗʰ **I71.0** Dissection of aorta

I71.00 Dissection of unspecified site of aorta `MCC`

I71.01 Dissection of thoracic aorta `MCC`

I71.02 Dissection of abdominal aorta `MCC`

I71.03 Dissection of thoracoabdominal aorta `MCC`

I71.1 Thoracic aortic aneurysm, ruptured `MCC`

I71.2 Thoracic aortic aneurysm, without rupture

I71.3 Abdominal aortic aneurysm, ruptured `MCC`

I71.4 Abdominal aortic aneurysm, without rupture

I71.5 Thoracoabdominal aortic aneurysm, ruptured `MCC`

I71.6 Thoracoabdominal aortic aneurysm, without rupture

I71.8 Aortic aneurysm of unspecified site, ruptured `MCC`
　　Rupture of aorta NOS

I71.9 Aortic aneurysm of unspecified site, without rupture
　　Aneurysm of aorta
　　Dilatation of aorta
　　Hyaline necrosis of aorta

`N` Newborn: 0　`P` Pediatric: 0-17　`M` Maternity: 12-55　`A` Adult: 15-124　`MCC` Major CC Condition　`PDx MCC` PDx acts as own MCC　`CC` CC Condition　`PDx CC` PDx acts as own CC

616　　　　　　　　　　　　　　　　　　　　　　　　　　　　　　　　　　　　　　　ICD-10-CM Draft (2015)

✓4ᵗʰ I72 Other aneurysm

INCLUDES aneurysm (cirsoid) (false) (ruptured)
EXCLUDES 2 acquired aneurysm (I77.0)
aneurysm (of) aorta (I71.-)
aneurysm (of) arteriovenous NOS (Q27.3-)
carotid artery dissection (I77.71)
cerebral (nonruptured) aneurysm (I67.1)
coronary aneurysm (I25.4)
coronary artery dissection (I25.42)
dissection of artery NEC (I77.79)
heart aneurysm (I25.3)
iliac artery dissection (I77.72)
pulmonary artery aneurysm (I28.1)
renal artery dissection (I77.73)
retinal aneurysm (H35.0)
ruptured cerebral aneurysm (I60.7)
varicose aneurysm (I77.0)
vertebral artery dissection (I77.74)

I72.0 Aneurysm of carotid artery
Aneurysm of common carotid artery
Aneurysm of external carotid artery
Aneurysm of internal carotid artery, extracranial portion
EXCLUDES 1 aneurysm of internal carotid artery, intracranial portion (I67.1)
aneurysm of internal carotid artery NOS (I67.1)

I72.1 Aneurysm of artery of upper extremity
I72.2 Aneurysm of renal artery
I72.3 Aneurysm of iliac artery
I72.4 Aneurysm of artery of lower extremity
I72.8 Aneurysm of other specified arteries
I72.9 Aneurysm of unspecified site

✓4ᵗʰ I73 Other peripheral vascular diseases
EXCLUDES 2 chilblains (T69.1)
frostbite (T33- T34)
immersion hand or foot (T69.0-)
spasm of cerebral artery (G45.9)

✓5ᵗʰ I73.0 Raynaud's syndrome
Raynaud's disease
Raynaud's phenomenon (secondary)
I73.00 Raynaud's syndrome without gangrene
I73.01 Raynaud's syndrome with gangrene   PDx CC CC
CC Excl: G89.0-G89.4, I70.261-I70.269, I96, R41.0-R41.3, R41.82, R41.9, R44.8-R44.9, R45.83-R45.84, R46.0-R46.89, R52, R68.0-R68.19, R68.81-R68.83, R68.89-R69

I73.1 Thromboangiitis obliterans [Buerger's disease]
✓5ᵗʰ I73.8 Other specified peripheral vascular diseases
EXCLUDES 1 diabetic (peripheral) angiopathy (E08-E13 with .51-.52)
I73.81 Erythromelalgia
I73.89 Other specified peripheral vascular diseases
Acrocyanosis
Erythrocyanosis
Simple acroparesthesia [Schultze's type]
Vasomotor acroparesthesia [Nothnagel's type]

I73.9 Peripheral vascular disease, unspecified
Intermittent claudication
Peripheral angiopathy NOS
Spasm of artery
EXCLUDES 1 atherosclerosis of the extremities (I70.2--I70.7-)

✓4ᵗʰ I74 Arterial embolism and thrombosis
Embolic infarction
Embolic occlusion
Thrombotic infarction
Thrombotic occlusion
Code first:
embolism and thrombosis complicating abortion or ectopic or molar pregnancy (O00-O07, O08.2)
embolism and thrombosis complicating pregnancy, childbirth and the puerperium (O88.-)
EXCLUDES 2 atheroembolism (I75.-)
basilar embolism and thrombosis (I63.0-I63.2, I65.1)
carotid embolism and thrombosis (I63.0-I63.2, I65.2)
cerebral embolism and thrombosis (I63.3-I63.5, I66-)
coronary embolism and thrombosis (I21-I25)
mesenteric embolism and thrombosis (K55.0)
ophthalmic embolism and thrombosis (H34.-)
precerebral embolism and thrombosis NOS (I63.0-I63.2, I65.9)
pulmonary embolism and thrombosis (I26.-)
renal embolism and thrombosis (N28.0)
retinal embolism and thrombosis (H34.-)
septic embolism and thrombosis (I76)
vertebral embolism and thrombosis (I63.0-I63.2, I65.0)

✓5ᵗʰ I74.0 Embolism and thrombosis of abdominal aorta
I74.01 Saddle embolus of abdominal aorta   MCC
CC Excl: I26.01-I26.99, I27.82, I74.01-I74.10, I74.19, I87.8, I99.8-I99.9
I74.09 Other arterial embolism and thrombosis of abdominal aorta   CC
Aortic bifurcation syndrome   Leriche's syndrome
Aortoiliac obstruction
CC Excl: See code: I74.01

✓5ᵗʰ I74.1 Embolism and thrombosis of other and unspecified parts of aorta
I74.10 Embolism and thrombosis of unspecified parts of aorta   CC
CC Excl: See code: I74.01
I74.11 Embolism and thrombosis of thoracic aorta   CC
CC Excl: E08.51-E08.59, E08.618-E08.638, E08.649-E08.8, E09.51-E09.59, E09.618-E09.638, E09.649-E09.8, E10.51-E10.59, E10.618-E10.638, E10.649, E10.69-E10.8, E11.51-E11.59, E11.618-E11.638, E11.649, E11.69-E11.8, E13.51-E13.59, E13.618-E13.638, E13.649-E13.8, I74.11, I74.8-I74.9, I76, I87.8, I99.8-I99.9
I74.19 Embolism and thrombosis of other parts of aorta   CC
CC Excl: I26.01-I26.99, I27.82, I74.01-I74.10, I74.19, I87.8, I99.8-I99.9

I74.2 Embolism and thrombosis of arteries of the upper extremities   CC
CC Excl: E08.51-E08.59, E08.618-E08.638, E08.649-E08.8, E09.51-E09.59, E09.618-E09.638, E09.649-E09.8, E10.51-E10.59, E10.618-E10.638, E10.649, E10.69-E10.8, E11.51-E11.59, E11.618-E11.638, E11.649, E11.69-E11.8, E13.51-E13.59, E13.618-E13.638, E13.649-E13.8, I74.2, I74.8-I74.9, I76, I87.8, I99.8-I99.9

I74.3 Embolism and thrombosis of arteries of the lower extremities   CC
CC Excl: E08.51-E08.59, E08.618-E08.638, E08.649-E08.8, E09.51-E09.59, E09.618-E09.638, E09.649-E09.8, E10.51-E10.59, E10.618-E10.638, E10.649, E10.69-E10.8, E11.51-E11.59, E11.618-E11.638, E11.649, E11.69-E11.8, E13.51-E13.59, E13.618-E13.638, E13.649-E13.8, I74.3-I74.4, I74.8-I74.9, I76, I87.8, I99.8-I99.9

I74.4 Embolism and thrombosis of arteries of extremities, unspecified   CC
Peripheral arterial embolism NOS
CC Excl: See code: I74.3

I74.5 Embolism and thrombosis of iliac artery   CC
CC Excl: E08.51-E08.59, E08.618-E08.638, E08.649-E08.8, E09.51-E09.59, E09.618-E09.638, E09.649-E09.8, E10.51-E10.59, E10.618-E10.638, E10.649, E10.69-E10.8, E11.51-E11.59, E11.618-E11.638, E11.649, E11.69-E11.8, E13.51-E13.59, E13.618-E13.638, E13.649-E13.8, I74.5-I74.9, I76, I87.8, I99.8-I99.9

I74.8 Embolism and thrombosis of other arteries   CC
CC Excl: E08.51-E08.59, E08.618-E08.638, E08.649-E08.8, E09.51-E09.59, E09.618-E09.638, E09.649-E09.8, E10.51-E10.59, E10.618-E10.638, E10.649, E10.69-E10.8, E11.51-E11.59, E11.618-E11.638, E11.649, E11.69-E11.8, E13.51-E13.59, E13.618-E13.638, E13.649-E13.8, I74.8, I74.8-I74.9, I76, I87.8, I99.8-I99.9

I74.9 Embolism and thrombosis of unspecified artery   CC
CC Excl: See code: I74.8

✓4ᵗʰ I75 Atheroembolism
Atherothrombotic microembolism
Cholesterol embolism

✓5ᵗʰ I75.0 Atheroembolism of extremities
✓6ᵗʰ I75.01 Atheroembolism of upper extremity
CC Excl: For CC codes in subcategory I75.01, unless otherwise noted: E08.51-E08.59, E08.618-E08.638, E08.649-E08.8, E09.51-E09.59, E09.618-E09.638, E09.649-E09.8, E10.51-E10.59, E10.618-E10.638, E10.649, E10.69-E10.8, E11.51-E11.59, E11.618-E11.638, E11.649, E11.69-E11.8, E13.51-E13.59, E13.618-E13.638, E13.649-E13.8, I74.8-I75.019, I76, I87.8, I99.8-I99.9
I75.011 Atheroembolism of right upper extremity   CC
I75.012 Atheroembolism of left upper extremity   CC
I75.013 Atheroembolism of bilateral upper extremities   CC
I75.019 Atheroembolism of unspecified upper extremity   CC

Diseases of the Circulatory System

I75.02–I79.8

✓6th **I75.02 Atheroembolism of lower extremity**

CC Excl: For CC codes in subcategory I75.02, unless otherwise noted: E08.51-E08.59, E08.618-E08.638, E08.649-E08.8, E09.51-E09.59, E09.618-E09.638, E09.649-E09.8, E10.51-E10.59, E10.618-E10.638, E10.649, E10.69-E10.8, E11.51-E11.59, E11.618-E11.638, E11.649, E11.69-E11.8, E13.51-E13.59, E13.618-E13.638, E13.649-E13.8, I74.8-I74.9, I75.021-I75.029, I76, I87.8, I99.8-I99.9

I75.021 Atheroembolism of right lower extremity CC

I75.022 Atheroembolism of left lower extremity CC

I75.023 Atheroembolism of bilateral lower extremities CC

I75.029 Atheroembolism of unspecified lower extremity CC

✓5th **I75.8 Atheroembolism of other sites**

I75.81 Atheroembolism of kidney CC
Use additional code for any associated acute kidney failure and chronic kidney disease (N17.-, N18.-)
CC Excl: E08.51-E08.59, E08.618-E08.638, E08.649-E08.8, E09.51-E09.59, E09.618-E09.638, E09.649-E09.8, E10.51-E10.59, E10.618-E10.638, E10.649, E10.69-E10.8, E11.51-E11.59, E11.618-E11.638, E11.649, E11.69-E11.8, E13.51-E13.59, E13.618-E13.638, E13.649-E13.8, I74.8-I74.9, I75.81, I76, I87.8, I99.8-I99.9

I75.89 Atheroembolism of other site CC
CC Excl: E08.51-E08.59, E08.618-E08.638, E08.649-E08.8, E09.51-E09.59, E09.618-E09.638, E09.649-E09.8, E10.51-E10.59, E10.618-E10.638, E10.649, E10.69-E10.8, E11.51-E11.59, E11.618-E11.638, E11.649, E11.69-E11.8, E13.51-E13.59, E13.618-E13.638, E13.649-E13.8, I74.8-I74.9, I75.89-I76, I87.8, I99.8-I99.9

I76 Septic arterial embolism CC
Code first underlying infection, such as:
infective endocarditis (I33.0)
lung abscess (J85.-)
Use additional code to identify the site of the embolism (I74.-)
EXCLUDES 2 septic pulmonary embolism (I26.01, I26.90)
CC Excl: See code: I74.8

✓4th **I77 Other disorders of arteries and arterioles**
EXCLUDES 2 collagen (vascular) diseases (M30-M36)
hypersensitivity angiitis (M31.0)
pulmonary artery (I28.-)

I77.0 Arteriovenous fistula, acquired
Aneurysmal varix
Arteriovenous aneurysm, acquired
EXCLUDES 1 arteriovenous aneurysm NOS (Q27.3-)
presence of arteriovenous shunt (fistula) for dialysis (Z99.2)
traumatic—see injury of blood vessel by body region
EXCLUDES 2 cerebral (I67.1)
coronary (I25.4)

I77.1 Stricture of artery
Narrowing of artery

I77.2 Rupture of artery CC
Erosion of artery
Fistula of artery
Ulcer of artery
EXCLUDES 1 traumatic rupture of artery—see injury of blood vessel by body region
CC Excl: I25.42, I67.0, I77.2, I77.72-I77.79

I77.3 Arterial fibromuscular dysplasia
Fibromuscular hyperplasia (of) carotid artery
Fibromuscular hyperplasia (of) renal artery

I77.4 Celiac artery compression syndrome CC
CC Excl: I77.4

I77.5 Necrosis of artery CC
CC Excl: I77.5, M31.8-M31.9

I77.6 Arteritis, unspecified
Aortitis NOS
Endarteritis NOS
EXCLUDES 1 arteritis or endarteritis:
aortic arch (M31.4)
cerebral NEC (I67.7)
coronary (I25.89)
deformans (I70.-)
giant cell (M31.5., M31.6)
obliterans (I70.-)
senile (I70.-)

✓5th **I77.7 Other arterial dissection**
EXCLUDES 2 dissection of aorta (I71.0-)
dissection of coronary artery (I25.42)

CC Excl: For MCC codes in subcategory I77.7, unless otherwise noted: I77.2-I77.3, I77.5-I77.6, I77.89-I77.9, M31.8-M31.9

I77.71 Dissection of carotid artery MCC
I77.72 Dissection of iliac artery MCC
I77.73 Dissection of renal artery MCC
I77.74 Dissection of vertebral artery MCC
I77.79 Dissection of other artery MCC

✓5th **I77.8 Other specified disorders of arteries and arterioles**

✓6th **I77.81 Aortic ectasia**
Ectasis aorta
EXCLUDES 1 aortic aneurysm and dissection (I71.0-)
I77.810 Thoracic aortic ectasia
I77.811 Abdominal aortic ectasia
I77.812 Thoracoabdominal aortic ectasia
I77.819 Aortic ectasia, unspecified site

I77.89 Other specified disorders of arteries and arterioles

I77.9 Disorder of arteries and arterioles, unspecified

✓4th **I78 Diseases of capillaries**

I78.0 Hereditary hemorrhagic telangiectasia
Rendu-Osler-Weber disease

I78.1 Nevus, non-neoplastic
Araneus nevus
Senile nevus
Spider nevus
Stellar nevus
EXCLUDES 1 nevus NOS (D22.-)
vascular NOS (Q82.5)
EXCLUDES 2 blue nevus (D22.-)
flammeus nevus (Q82.5)
hairy nevus (D22.-)
melanocytic nevus (D22.-)
pigmented nevus (D22.-)
portwine nevus (Q82.5)
sanguineous nevus (Q82.5)
strawberry nevus (Q82.5)
verrucous nevus (Q82.5)

I78.8 Other diseases of capillaries
I78.9 Disease of capillaries, unspecified

✓4th **I79 Disorders of arteries, arterioles and capillaries in diseases classified elsewhere**

I79.0 Aneurysm of aorta in diseases classified elsewhere
Code first underlying disease
EXCLUDES 1 syphilitic aneurysm (A52.01)

I79.1 Aortitis in diseases classified elsewhere
Code first underlying disease
EXCLUDES 1 syphilitic aortitis (A52.02)

I79.8 Other disorders of arteries, arterioles and capillaries in diseases classified elsewhere
Code first underlying disease, such as:
amyloidosis (E85.-)
EXCLUDES 1 diabetic (peripheral) angiopathy (E08-E13 with .51-.52)
syphilitic endarteritis (A52.09)
tuberculous endarteritis (A18.89)

Diseases of veins, lymphatic vessels and lymph nodes, not elsewhere classified. (I80-I89)

✓4th I80   Phlebitis and thrombophlebitis

INCLUDES   endophlebitis
inflammation, vein
periphlebitis
suppurative phlebitis

Code first:
phlebitis and thrombophlebitis complicating abortion, ectopic or molar pregnancy (O00-O07, O08.7)
phlebitis and thrombophlebitis complicating pregnancy, childbirth and the puerperium (O22.-, O87.-)

EXCLUDES 1 *venous embolism and thrombosis of lower extremities ((I82.4-, I82.5-, I82.81-)*

CC Excl: For CC codes in category I80, unless otherwise noted:
E08.51-E08.59, E08.618-E08.638, E08.649-E08.8, E09.51-E09.59, E09.618-E09.638, E09.649-E09.8, E10.51-E10.59, E10.618-E10.638, E10.649, E10.69-E10.8, E11.51-E11.59, E11.618-E11.638, E11.649, E11.69-E11.8, E13.51-E13.59, E13.618-E13.638, E13.649-E13.8, I80.00-I80.9, I87.8, I99.8-I99.9

✓5th I80.0   Phlebitis and thrombophlebitis of superficial vessels of lower extremities
Phlebitis and thrombophlebitis of femoropopliteal vein

- **I80.00**   Phlebitis and thrombophlebitis of superficial vessels of unspecified lower extremity
- **I80.01**   Phlebitis and thrombophlebitis of superficial vessels of right lower extremity
- **I80.02**   Phlebitis and thrombophlebitis of superficial vessels of left lower extremity
- **I80.03**   Phlebitis and thrombophlebitis of superficial vessels of lower extremities, bilateral

✓5th I80.1   Phlebitis and thrombophlebitis of femoral vein

- **I80.10**   Phlebitis and thrombophlebitis of unspecified femoral vein   CC
- **I80.11**   Phlebitis and thrombophlebitis of right femoral vein   CC
- **I80.12**   Phlebitis and thrombophlebitis of left femoral vein   CC
- **I80.13**   Phlebitis and thrombophlebitis of femoral vein, bilateral   CC

✓5th I80.2   Phlebitis and thrombophlebitis of other and unspecified deep vessels of lower extremities

- **✓6th I80.20**   Phlebitis and thrombophlebitis of unspecified deep vessels of lower extremities
  - **I80.201**   Phlebitis and thrombophlebitis of unspecified deep vessels of right lower extremity   CC
  - **I80.202**   Phlebitis and thrombophlebitis of unspecified deep vessels of left lower extremity   CC
  - **I80.203**   Phlebitis and thrombophlebitis of unspecified deep vessels of lower extremities, bilateral   CC
  - **I80.209**   Phlebitis and thrombophlebitis of unspecified deep vessels of unspecified lower extremity   CC
- **✓6th I80.21**   Phlebitis and thrombophlebitis of iliac vein
  - **I80.211**   Phlebitis and thrombophlebitis of right iliac vein   CC
  - **I80.212**   Phlebitis and thrombophlebitis of left iliac vein   CC
  - **I80.213**   Phlebitis and thrombophlebitis of iliac vein, bilateral   CC
  - **I80.219**   Phlebitis and thrombophlebitis of unspecified iliac vein   CC
- **✓6th I80.22**   Phlebitis and thrombophlebitis of popliteal vein
  - **I80.221**   Phlebitis and thrombophlebitis of right popliteal vein   CC
  - **I80.222**   Phlebitis and thrombophlebitis of left popliteal vein   CC
  - **I80.223**   Phlebitis and thrombophlebitis of popliteal vein, bilateral   CC
  - **I80.229**   Phlebitis and thrombophlebitis of unspecified popliteal vein   CC
- **✓6th I80.23**   Phlebitis and thrombophlebitis of tibial vein
  - **I80.231**   Phlebitis and thrombophlebitis of right tibial vein   CC
  - **I80.232**   Phlebitis and thrombophlebitis of left tibial vein   CC
  - **I80.233**   Phlebitis and thrombophlebitis of tibial vein, bilateral   CC
  - **I80.239**   Phlebitis and thrombophlebitis of unspecified tibial vein   CC
- **✓6th I80.29**   Phlebitis and thrombophlebitis of other deep vessels of lower extremities
  - **I80.291**   Phlebitis and thrombophlebitis of other deep vessels of right lower extremity   CC
  - **I80.292**   Phlebitis and thrombophlebitis of other deep vessels of left lower extremity   CC
  - **I80.293**   Phlebitis and thrombophlebitis of other deep vessels of lower extremity, bilateral   CC
  - **I80.299**   Phlebitis and thrombophlebitis of other deep vessels of unspecified lower extremity   CC

I80.3   Phlebitis and thrombophlebitis of lower extremities, unspecified
I80.8   Phlebitis and thrombophlebitis of other sites
I80.9   Phlebitis and thrombophlebitis of unspecified site

I81   Portal vein thrombosis   MCC
Portal (vein) obstruction

EXCLUDES 2 *hepatic vein thrombosis (I82.0)*
phlebitis of portal vein (K75.1)

CC Excl: E08.51-E08.59, E08.618-E08.638, E08.649-E08.8, E09.51-E09.59, E09.618-E09.638, E09.649-E09.8, E10.51-E10.59, E10.618-E10.638, E10.649, E10.69-E10.8, E11.51-E11.59, E11.618-E11.638, E11.649, E11.69-E11.8, E13.51-E13.59, E13.618-E13.638, E13.649-E13.8, I81, I82.210-I82.211, I82.290-I82.291, I82.401-I82.91, I87.8, I99.8-I99.9

✓4th I82   Other venous embolism and thrombosis
Code first venous embolism and thrombosis complicating:
abortion, ectopic or molar pregnancy (O00-O07, O08.7)
pregnancy, childbirth and the puerperium (O22.-, O87.-)

EXCLUDES 2 *venous embolism and thrombosis (of):*
cerebral (I63.6, I67.6)
coronary (I21-I25)
intracranial and intraspinal, septic or NOS (G08)
intracranial, nonpyogenic (I67.6)
intraspinal, nonpyogenic (G95.1)
mesenteric (K55.0)
portal (I81)
pulmonary (I26.-)

I82.0   Budd-Chiari syndrome   MCC
Hepatic vein thrombosis
CC Excl: E08.51-E08.59, E08.618-E08.638, E08.649-E08.8, E09.51-E09.59, E09.618-E09.638, E09.649-E09.8, E10.51-E10.59, E10.618-E10.638, E10.649, E10.69-E10.8, E11.51-E11.59, E11.618-E11.638, E11.649, E11.69-E11.8, E13.51-E13.59, E13.618-E13.638, E13.649-E13.8, I82.0, I82.210-I82.211, I82.290-I82.291, I82.401-I82.91, I87.8, I99.8-I99.9

I82.1   Thrombophlebitis migrans   CC
CC Excl: E08.51-E08.59, E08.618-E08.638, E08.649-E08.8, E09.51-E09.59, E09.618-E09.638, E09.649-E09.8, E10.51-E10.59, E10.618-E10.638, E10.649, E10.69-E10.8, E11.51-E11.59, E11.618-E11.638, E11.649, E11.69-E11.8, E13.51-E13.59, E13.618-E13.638, E13.649-E13.8, I82.1-I82.211, I82.290-I82.291, I82.401-I82.91, I87.8, I99.8-I99.9

✓5th I82.2   Embolism and thrombosis of vena cava and other thoracic veins

- **✓6th I82.21**   Embolism and thrombosis of superior vena cava
  - **I82.210**   Acute embolism and thrombosis of superior vena cava   CC
    Embolism and thrombosis of superior vena cava NOS
    CC Excl: E08.51-E08.59, E08.618-E08.638, E08.649-E08.8, E09.51-E09.59, E09.618-E09.638, E09.649-E09.8, E10.51-E10.59, E10.618-E10.638, E10.649, E10.69-E10.8, E11.51-E11.59, E11.618-E11.638, E11.649, E11.69-E11.8, E13.51-E13.59, E13.618-E13.638, E13.649-E13.8, I82.210-I82.211, I82.290-I82.291, I82.401-I82.91, I87.8, I99.8-I99.9
  - **I82.211**   Chronic embolism and thrombosis of superior vena cava   CC
    CC Excl: See code: I82.210

✓ Additional Character Required   ✓x7th Xtension Alert   Unacceptable PDx   Manifestation   Hospital Acquired Condition   EXCLUDES1 Not Coded Here   EXCLUDES2 Not Included Here

ICD-10-CM Draft (2015)   619

√6ᵗʰ **I82.22** **Embolism and thrombosis of** inferior vena cava

I82.220 **Acute embolism and thrombosis of** MCC
inferior vena cava
Embolism and thrombosis of inferior vena
cava NOS
CC Excl: E08.51-E08.59, E08.618-E08.638,
E08.649-E08.8, E09.51-E09.59, E09.618-
E09.638, E09.649-E09.8, E10.51-E10.59,
E10.618-E10.638, E10.649, E10.69-E10.8,
E11.51-E11.59, E11.618-E11.638, E11.649,
E11.69-E11.8, E13.51-E13.59, E13.618-
E13.638, E13.649-E13.8, I82.210-I82.291,
I82.401-I82.91, I87.8, I99.8-I99.9

I82.221 **Chronic embolism and thrombosis of** MCC
inferior vena cava
CC Excl: See code: I82.220

√6ᵗʰ **I82.29** **Embolism and thrombosis of** other thoracic veins
Embolism and thrombosis of brachiocephalic
(innominate) vein

I82.290 **Acute embolism and thrombosis of** CC
other thoracic veins
CC Excl: See code: I82.210

I82.291 **Chronic embolism and thrombosis of** CC
other thoracic veins
CC Excl: See code: I82.210

I82.3 **Embolism and thrombosis of** renal vein   CC
CC Excl: E08.51-E08.59, E08.618-E08.638, E08.649-E08.8, E09.51-
E09.59, E09.618-E09.638, E09.649-E09.8, E10.51-E10.59, E10.618-
E10.638, E10.649, E10.69-E10.8, E11.51-E11.59, E11.618-E11.638,
E11.649, E11.69-E11.8, E13.51-E13.59, E13.618-E13.638, E13.649-
E13.8, I82.210-I82.211, I82.290-I82.91, I87.8, I99.8-I99.9

√5ᵗʰ **I82.4** **Acute embolism and thrombosis of** deep veins of lower
extremity

CC Excl: For CC codes in subcategory I82.4, unless
otherwise noted: E08.51-E08.59, E08.618-E08.638,
E08.649-E08.8, E09.51-E09.59, E09.618-E09.638, E09.649-
E09.8, E10.51-E10.59, E10.618-E10.638, E10.649, E10.69-
E10.8, E11.51-E11.59, E11.618-E11.638, E11.649, E11.69-
E11.8, E13.51-E13.59, E13.618-E13.638, E13.649-E13.8,
I82.210-I82.211, I82.290-I82.291, I82.401-I82.91, I87.8,
I99.8-I99.9

√6ᵗʰ **I82.40** **Acute embolism and thrombosis of** unspecified deep
veins of lower extremity
Deep vein thrombosis NOS
DVT NOS
EXCLUDES 1 *acute embolism and thrombosis of
unspecified deep veins of distal lower
extremity (I82.4Z-)*
*acute embolism and thrombosis of
unspecified deep veins of proximal lower
extremity (I82.4Y-)*

3 **I82.401** **Acute embolism and thrombosis of** CC
unspecified deep veins of right **lower**
extremity

3 **I82.402** **Acute embolism and thrombosis of** CC
unspecified deep veins of left **lower**
extremity

3 **I82.403** **Acute embolism and thrombosis of** CC
unspecified deep veins of lower
extremity, bilateral

3 **I82.409** **Acute embolism and thrombosis of** CC
unspecified deep veins of unspecified
lower extremity

√6ᵗʰ **I82.41** **Acute embolism and thrombosis of** femoral vein

3 **I82.411** **Acute embolism and thrombosis of** CC
right **femoral vein**

3 **I82.412** **Acute embolism and thrombosis of** left CC
femoral vein

3 **I82.413** **Acute embolism and thrombosis of** CC
femoral vein, bilateral

3 **I82.419** **Acute embolism and thrombosis of** CC
unspecified **femoral vein**

√6ᵗʰ **I82.42** **Acute embolism and thrombosis of** iliac vein

3 **I82.421** **Acute embolism and thrombosis of** CC
right **iliac vein**

3 **I82.422** **Acute embolism and thrombosis of** CC
left **iliac vein**

3 **I82.423** **Acute embolism and thrombosis of** CC
iliac vein, bilateral

3 **I82.429** **Acute embolism and thrombosis of** CC
unspecified **iliac vein**

√6ᵗʰ **I82.43** **Acute embolism and thrombosis of** popliteal vein

3 **I82.431** **Acute embolism and thrombosis of** CC
right **popliteal vein**

3 **I82.432** **Acute embolism and thrombosis of** left CC
popliteal vein

3 **I82.433** **Acute embolism and thrombosis of** CC
popliteal vein, bilateral

3 **I82.439** **Acute embolism and thrombosis of** CC
unspecified **popliteal vein**

√6ᵗʰ **I82.44** **Acute embolism and thrombosis of** tibial vein

3 **I82.441** **Acute embolism and thrombosis of** CC
right **tibial vein**

3 **I82.442** **Acute embolism and thrombosis of** CC
left **tibial vein**

3 **I82.443** **Acute embolism and thrombosis of** CC
tibial vein, bilateral

3 **I82.449** **Acute embolism and thrombosis of** CC
unspecified **tibial vein**

√6ᵗʰ **I82.49** **Acute embolism and thrombosis of** other specified
deep vein of lower extremity

3 **I82.491** **Acute embolism and thrombosis of** CC
other specified deep vein of right
lower extremity

3 **I82.492** **Acute embolism and thrombosis of** CC
other specified deep vein of left
lower extremity

3 **I82.493** **Acute embolism and thrombosis of** CC
other specified deep vein of lower
extremity, bilateral

3 **I82.499** **Acute embolism and thrombosis of** CC
other specified deep vein of unspecified
lower extremity

√6ᵗʰ **I82.4Y** **Acute embolism and thrombosis of** unspecified deep
veins of proximal lower extremity
Acute embolism and thrombosis of deep vein of thigh
NOS
Acute embolism and thrombosis of deep vein of upper
leg NOS

3 **I82.4Y1** **Acute embolism and thrombosis of** CC
unspecified deep veins of right **proximal**
lower extremity

3 **I82.4Y2** **Acute embolism and thrombosis of** CC
unspecified deep veins of left **proximal**
lower extremity

3 **I82.4Y3** **Acute embolism and thrombosis of** CC
unspecified deep veins of proximal lower
extremity, bilateral

3 **I82.4Y9** **Acute embolism and thrombosis of** CC
unspecified deep veins of unspecified
proximal lower extremity

√6ᵗʰ **I82.4Z** **Acute embolism and thrombosis of** unspecified deep
veins of distal lower extremity
Acute embolism and thrombosis of deep vein of calf
NOS
Acute embolism and thrombosis of deep vein of lower
leg NOS

3 **I82.4Z1** **Acute embolism and thrombosis of** CC
unspecified deep veins of right **distal**
lower extremity

3 **I82.4Z2** **Acute embolism and thrombosis of** CC
unspecified deep veins of left **distal**
lower extremity

3 **I82.4Z3** **Acute embolism and thrombosis of** CC
unspecified deep veins of distal lower
extremity, bilateral

3 **I82.4Z9** **Acute embolism and thrombosis of** CC
unspecified deep veins of unspecified
distal lower extremity

---

3 HAC = as SDx not POA, in combination with one of the following procedure codes: ØSR[9,B]Ø[1,2,3,4,J][9,A,Z]; ØSR[9,B]Ø[7,K]Z; ØSR[A,E]Ø[Ø,1,3,J][9,A,Z]; ØSR[A,E]Ø[7,K]Z;
ØSR[C,D,T,U,V,W]Ø[7,K]Z; ØSR[C,D,T,U,V,W]ØJ[9,A,Z]; ØSR[R,S]Ø[1,3,J][9,A,Z]; ØSR[R,S]Ø[7,K]Z; ØSU[9,B]ØBZ; ØSU[A,E,R,S]ØBZ.

✓5ᵗʰ I82.5 Chronic embolism and thrombosis of deep veins of lower extremity

Use additional code, if applicable, for associated long-term (current) use of anticoagulants (Z79.01)

EXCLUDES 1 personal history of venous embolism and thrombosis (Z86.718)

CC Excl: For CC codes in subcategory I82.5, unless otherwise noted: See code: I82.4

✓6ᵗʰ I82.50 Chronic embolism and thrombosis of unspecified deep veins of lower extremity

EXCLUDES 1 chronic embolism and thrombosis of unspecified deep veins of distal lower extremity (I82.5Z-)
chronic embolism and thrombosis of unspecified deep veins of proximal lower extremity (I82.5Y-)

I82.501 Chronic embolism and thrombosis of unspecified deep veins of right lower extremity CC

I82.502 Chronic embolism and thrombosis of unspecified deep veins of left lower extremity CC

I82.503 Chronic embolism and thrombosis of unspecified deep veins of lower extremity, bilateral CC

I82.509 Chronic embolism and thrombosis of unspecified deep veins of unspecified lower extremity CC

✓6ᵗʰ I82.51 Chronic embolism and thrombosis of femoral vein

I82.511 Chronic embolism and thrombosis of right femoral vein CC

I82.512 Chronic embolism and thrombosis of left femoral vein CC

I82.513 Chronic embolism and thrombosis of femoral vein, bilateral CC

I82.519 Chronic embolism and thrombosis of unspecified femoral vein CC

✓6ᵗʰ I82.52 Chronic embolism and thrombosis of iliac vein

I82.521 Chronic embolism and thrombosis of right iliac vein CC

I82.522 Chronic embolism and thrombosis of left iliac vein CC

I82.523 Chronic embolism and thrombosis of iliac vein, bilateral CC

I82.529 Chronic embolism and thrombosis of unspecified iliac vein CC

✓6ᵗʰ I82.53 Chronic embolism and thrombosis of popliteal vein

I82.531 Chronic embolism and thrombosis of right popliteal vein CC

I82.532 Chronic embolism and thrombosis of left popliteal vein CC

I82.533 Chronic embolism and thrombosis of popliteal vein, bilateral CC

I82.539 Chronic embolism and thrombosis of unspecified popliteal vein CC

✓6ᵗʰ I82.54 Chronic embolism and thrombosis of tibial vein

I82.541 Chronic embolism and thrombosis of right tibial vein CC

I82.542 Chronic embolism and thrombosis of left tibial vein CC

I82.543 Chronic embolism and thrombosis of tibial vein, bilateral CC

I82.549 Chronic embolism and thrombosis of unspecified tibial vein CC

✓6ᵗʰ I82.59 Chronic embolism and thrombosis of other specified deep vein of lower extremity

I82.591 Chronic embolism and thrombosis of other specified deep vein of right lower extremity CC

I82.592 Chronic embolism and thrombosis of other specified deep vein of left lower extremity CC

I82.593 Chronic embolism and thrombosis of other specified deep vein of lower extremity, bilateral CC

I82.599 Chronic embolism and thrombosis of other specified deep vein of unspecified lower extremity CC

✓6ᵗʰ I82.5Y Chronic embolism and thrombosis of unspecified deep veins of proximal lower extremity

Chronic embolism and thrombosis of deep veins of thigh NOS
Chronic embolism and thrombosis of deep veins of upper leg NOS

I82.5Y1 Chronic embolism and thrombosis of unspecified deep veins of right proximal lower extremity CC

I82.5Y2 Chronic embolism and thrombosis of unspecified deep veins of left proximal lower extremity CC

I82.5Y3 Chronic embolism and thrombosis of unspecified deep veins of proximal lower extremity, bilateral CC

I82.5Y9 Chronic embolism and thrombosis of unspecified deep veins of unspecified proximal lower extremity CC

✓6ᵗʰ I82.5Z Chronic embolism and thrombosis of unspecified deep veins of distal lower extremity

Chronic embolism and thrombosis of deep veins of calf NOS
Chronic embolism and thrombosis of deep veins of lower leg NOS

I82.5Z1 Chronic embolism and thrombosis of unspecified deep veins of right distal lower extremity CC

I82.5Z2 Chronic embolism and thrombosis of unspecified deep veins of left distal lower extremity CC

I82.5Z3 Chronic embolism and thrombosis of unspecified deep veins of distal lower extremity, bilateral CC

I82.5Z9 Chronic embolism and thrombosis of unspecified deep veins of unspecified distal lower extremity CC

✓5ᵗʰ I82.6 Acute embolism and thrombosis of veins of upper extremity

CC Excl: For CC codes in subcategory I82.6, unless otherwise noted: See code: I82.4

✓6ᵗʰ I82.60 Acute embolism and thrombosis of unspecified veins of upper extremity

I82.601 Acute embolism and thrombosis of unspecified veins of right upper extremity CC

I82.602 Acute embolism and thrombosis of unspecified veins of left upper extremity CC

I82.603 Acute embolism and thrombosis of unspecified veins of upper extremity, bilateral CC

I82.609 Acute embolism and thrombosis of unspecified veins of unspecified upper extremity CC

✓6ᵗʰ I82.61 Acute embolism and thrombosis of superficial veins of upper extremity

Acute embolism and thrombosis of antecubital vein
Acute embolism and thrombosis of basilic vein
Acute embolism and thrombosis of cephalic vein

I82.611 Acute embolism and thrombosis of superficial veins of right upper extremity CC

I82.612 Acute embolism and thrombosis of superficial veins of left upper extremity CC

I82.613 Acute embolism and thrombosis of superficial veins of upper extremity, bilateral CC

I82.619 Acute embolism and thrombosis of superficial veins of unspecified upper extremity CC

✓6ᵗʰ I82.62 Acute embolism and thrombosis of deep veins of upper extremity

Acute embolism and thrombosis of brachial vein
Acute embolism and thrombosis of radial vein
Acute embolism and thrombosis of ulnar vein

I82.621 Acute embolism and thrombosis of deep veins of right upper extremity CC

I82.622 Acute embolism and thrombosis of deep veins of left upper extremity CC

I82.623 **Acute embolism and thrombosis of deep veins of upper extremity, bilateral** `CC`

I82.629 **Acute embolism and thrombosis of deep veins of unspecified upper extremity** `CC`

✓5th **I82.7** **Chronic embolism and thrombosis of veins of upper extremity**
Use additional code, if applicable, for associated long-term (current) use of anticoagulants (Z79.01)
EXCLUDES 1 personal history of venous embolism and thrombosis (Z86.718)

CC Excl: For CC codes in subcategory I82.7, unless otherwise noted: See code: I82.4

✓6th **I82.70** **Chronic embolism and thrombosis of unspecified veins of upper extremity**

I82.701 **Chronic embolism and thrombosis of unspecified veins of right upper extremity** `CC`

I82.702 **Chronic embolism and thrombosis of unspecified veins of left upper extremity** `CC`

I82.703 **Chronic embolism and thrombosis of unspecified veins of upper extremity, bilateral** `CC`

I82.709 **Chronic embolism and thrombosis of unspecified veins of unspecified upper extremity** `CC`

✓6th **I82.71** **Chronic embolism and thrombosis of superficial veins of upper extremity**
Chronic embolism and thrombosis of antecubital vein
Chronic embolism and thrombosis of basilic vein
Chronic embolism and thrombosis of cephalic vein

I82.711 **Chronic embolism and thrombosis of superficial veins of right upper extremity** `CC`

I82.712 **Chronic embolism and thrombosis of superficial veins of left upper extremity** `CC`

I82.713 **Chronic embolism and thrombosis of superficial veins of upper extremity, bilateral** `CC`

I82.719 **Chronic embolism and thrombosis of superficial veins of unspecified upper extremity** `CC`

✓6th **I82.72** **Chronic embolism and thrombosis of deep veins of upper extremity**
Chronic embolism and thrombosis of brachial vein
Chronic embolism and thrombosis of radial vein
Chronic embolism and thrombosis of ulnar vein

I82.721 **Chronic embolism and thrombosis of deep veins of right upper extremity** `CC`

I82.722 **Chronic embolism and thrombosis of deep veins of left upper extremity** `CC`

I82.723 **Chronic embolism and thrombosis of deep veins of upper extremity, bilateral** `CC`

I82.729 **Chronic embolism and thrombosis of deep veins of unspecified upper extremity** `CC`

✓5th **I82.A** **Embolism and thrombosis of axillary vein**

CC Excl: For CC codes in subcategory I82.A, unless otherwise noted: See code: I82.4

✓6th **I82.A1** **Acute embolism and thrombosis of axillary vein**

I82.A11 **Acute embolism and thrombosis of right axillary vein** `CC`

I82.A12 **Acute embolism and thrombosis of left axillary vein** `CC`

I82.A13 **Acute embolism and thrombosis of axillary vein, bilateral** `CC`

I82.A19 **Acute embolism and thrombosis of unspecified axillary vein** `CC`

✓6th **I82.A2** **Chronic embolism and thrombosis of axillary vein**

I82.A21 **Chronic embolism and thrombosis of right axillary vein** `CC`

I82.A22 **Chronic embolism and thrombosis of left axillary vein** `CC`

I82.A23 **Chronic embolism and thrombosis of axillary vein, bilateral** `CC`

I82.A29 **Chronic embolism and thrombosis of unspecified axillary vein** `CC`

✓5th **I82.B** **Embolism and thrombosis of subclavian vein**

CC Excl: For CC codes in subcategory I82.B, unless otherwise noted: E08.51-E08.59, E08.618-E08.638, E08.649-E08.8, E09.51-E09.59, E09.618-E09.638, E09.649-E09.8, E10.51-E10.59, E10.618-E10.638, E10.649, E10.69-E10.8, E11.51-E11.59, E11.618-E11.638, E11.649, E11.69-E11.8, E13.51-E13.59, E13.618-E13.638, E13.649-E13.8, I82.210-I82.211, I82.290-I82.291, I82.401-I82.91, I87.8, I99.8-I99.9

✓6th **I82.B1** **Acute embolism and thrombosis of subclavian vein**

I82.B11 **Acute embolism and thrombosis of right subclavian vein** `CC`

I82.B12 **Acute embolism and thrombosis of left subclavian vein** `CC`

I82.B13 **Acute embolism and thrombosis of subclavian vein, bilateral** `CC`

I82.B19 **Acute embolism and thrombosis of unspecified subclavian vein** `CC`

✓6th **I82.B2** **Chronic embolism and thrombosis of subclavian vein**

I82.B21 **Chronic embolism and thrombosis of right subclavian vein** `CC`

I82.B22 **Chronic embolism and thrombosis of left subclavian vein** `CC`

I82.B23 **Chronic embolism and thrombosis of subclavian vein, bilateral** `CC`

I82.B29 **Chronic embolism and thrombosis of unspecified subclavian vein** `CC`

✓5th **I82.C** **Embolism and thrombosis of internal jugular vein**

CC Excl: For CC codes in subcategory I82.C, unless otherwise noted: See code: I82.B

✓6th **I82.C1** **Acute embolism and thrombosis of internal jugular vein**

I82.C11 **Acute embolism and thrombosis of right internal jugular vein** `CC`

I82.C12 **Acute embolism and thrombosis of left internal jugular vein** `CC`

I82.C13 **Acute embolism and thrombosis of internal jugular vein, bilateral** `CC`

I82.C19 **Acute embolism and thrombosis of unspecified internal jugular vein** `CC`

✓6th **I82.C2** **Chronic embolism and thrombosis of internal jugular vein**

I82.C21 **Chronic embolism and thrombosis of right internal jugular vein** `CC`

I82.C22 **Chronic embolism and thrombosis of left internal jugular vein** `CC`

I82.C23 **Chronic embolism and thrombosis of internal jugular vein, bilateral** `CC`

I82.C29 **Chronic embolism and thrombosis of unspecified internal jugular vein** `CC`

✓5th **I82.8** **Embolism and thrombosis of other specified veins**
Use additional code, if applicable, for associated long-term (current) use of anticoagulants (Z79.01)

CC Excl: For CC codes in subcategory I82.8, unless otherwise noted: See code: I82.B

✓6th **I82.81** **Embolism and thrombosis of superficial veins of lower extremities**
Embolism and thrombosis of saphenous vein (greater) (lesser)

I82.811 **Embolism and thrombosis of superficial veins of right lower extremities** `CC`

I82.812 **Embolism and thrombosis of superficial veins of left lower extremities** `CC`

I82.813 **Embolism and thrombosis of superficial veins of lower extremities, bilateral** `CC`

I82.819 **Embolism and thrombosis of superficial veins of unspecified lower extremities** `CC`

✓6th **I82.89** **Embolism and thrombosis of other specified veins**

I82.890 **Acute embolism and thrombosis of other specified veins** `CC`

N Newborn: 0   P Pediatric: 0-17   M Maternity: 12-55   A Adult: 15-124   MCC Major CC Condition   PDx MCC PDx acts as own MCC   CC CC Condition   PDx CC PDx acts as own CC

622   ICD-10-CM Draft (2015)

I82.891   Chronic embolism and thrombosis of other specified veins   `CC`

√5ᵗʰ **I82.9**   Embolism and thrombosis of unspecified vein

> **CC Excl: For CC codes in subcategory I82.9, unless otherwise noted:** See code: I82B

I82.90   Acute embolism and thrombosis of unspecified vein   `CC`
Embolism of vein NOS
Thrombosis (vein) NOS

I82.91   Chronic embolism and thrombosis of unspecified vein   `CC`

√4ᵗʰ **I83**   **Varicose veins of lower extremities**

> EXCLUDES 1   varicose veins complicating pregnancy (O22.0-)
> varicose veins complicating the puerperium (O87.4)

√5ᵗʰ **I83.0**   Varicose veins of lower extremities with ulcer
Use additional code to identify severity of ulcer (L97.-)

√6ᵗʰ **I83.00**   Varicose veins of unspecified lower extremity with ulcer

I83.001   Varicose veins of unspecified lower extremity with ulcer of thigh   `A`

I83.002   Varicose veins of unspecified lower extremity with ulcer of calf   `A`

I83.003   Varicose veins of unspecified lower extremity with ulcer of ankle   `A`

I83.004   Varicose veins of unspecified lower extremity with ulcer of heel and midfoot   `A`
Varicose veins of unspecified lower extremity with ulcer of plantar surface of midfoot

I83.005   Varicose veins of unspecified lower extremity with ulcer other part of foot   `A`
Varicose veins of unspecified lower extremity with ulcer of toe

I83.008   Varicose veins of unspecified lower extremity with ulcer other part of lower leg   `A`

I83.009   Varicose veins of unspecified lower extremity with ulcer of unspecified site   `A`

√6ᵗʰ **I83.01**   Varicose veins of right lower extremity with ulcer

I83.011   Varicose veins of right lower extremity with ulcer of thigh   `A`

I83.012   Varicose veins of right lower extremity with ulcer of calf   `A`

I83.013   Varicose veins of right lower extremity with ulcer of ankle   `A`

I83.014   Varicose veins of right lower extremity with ulcer of heel and midfoot   `A`
Varicose veins of right lower extremity with ulcer of plantar surface of midfoot

I83.015   Varicose veins of right lower extremity with ulcer other part of foot   `A`
Varicose veins of right lower extremity with ulcer of toe

I83.018   Varicose veins of right lower extremity with ulcer other part of lower leg   `A`

I83.019   Varicose veins of right lower extremity with ulcer of unspecified site   `A`

√6ᵗʰ **I83.02**   Varicose veins of left lower extremity with ulcer

I83.021   Varicose veins of left lower extremity with ulcer of thigh   `A`

I83.022   Varicose veins of left lower extremity with ulcer of calf   `A`

I83.023   Varicose veins of left lower extremity with ulcer of ankle   `A`

I83.024   Varicose veins of left lower extremity with ulcer of heel and midfoot   `A`
Varicose veins of left lower extremity with ulcer of plantar surface of midfoot

I83.025   Varicose veins of left lower extremity with ulcer other part of foot   `A`
Varicose veins of left lower extremity with ulcer of toe

I83.028   Varicose veins of left lower extremity with ulcer other part of lower leg   `A`

I83.029   Varicose veins of left lower extremity with ulcer of unspecified site   `A`

√5ᵗʰ **I83.1**   Varicose veins of lower extremities with inflammation
Stasis dermatitis

I83.10   Varicose veins of unspecified lower extremity with inflammation   `A`

I83.11   Varicose veins of right lower extremity with inflammation   `A`

I83.12   Varicose veins of left lower extremity with inflammation   `A`

√5ᵗʰ **I83.2**   Varicose veins of lower extremities with both ulcer and inflammation

> **CC Excl: For CC codes in subcategory I83.2, unless otherwise noted:** I83.001-I83.229, I83.90-I83.93

Use additional code to identify severity of ulcer (L97.-)

√6ᵗʰ **I83.20**   Varicose veins of unspecified lower extremity with both ulcer and inflammation

I83.201   Varicose veins of unspecified lower extremity with both ulcer of thigh and inflammation   `CC` `A`

I83.202   Varicose veins of unspecified lower extremity with both ulcer of calf and inflammation   `CC` `A`

I83.203   Varicose veins of unspecified lower extremity with both ulcer of ankle and inflammation   `CC` `A`

I83.204   Varicose veins of unspecified lower extremity with both ulcer of heel and midfoot and inflammation   `CC` `A`
Varicose veins of unspecified lower extremity with both ulcer of plantar surface of midfoot and inflammation

I83.205   Varicose veins of unspecified lower extremity with both ulcer of other part of foot and inflammation   `CC` `A`
Varicose veins of unspecified lower extremity with both ulcer of toe and inflammation

I83.208   Varicose veins of unspecified lower extremity with both ulcer of other part of lower extremity and inflammation   `CC` `A`

I83.209   Varicose veins of unspecified lower extremity with both ulcer of unspecified site and inflammation   `CC` `A`

√6ᵗʰ **I83.21**   Varicose veins of right lower extremity with both ulcer and inflammation

I83.211   Varicose veins of right lower extremity with both ulcer of thigh and inflammation   `CC` `A`

I83.212   Varicose veins of right lower extremity with both ulcer of calf and inflammation   `CC` `A`

I83.213   Varicose veins of right lower extremity with both ulcer of ankle and inflammation   `CC` `A`

I83.214   Varicose veins of right lower extremity with both ulcer of heel and midfoot and inflammation   `CC` `A`
Varicose veins of right lower extremity with both ulcer of plantar surface of midfoot and inflammation

I83.215   Varicose veins of right lower extremity with both ulcer other part of foot and inflammation   `CC` `A`
Varicose veins of right lower extremity with both ulcer of toe and inflammation

I83.218   Varicose veins of right lower extremity with both ulcer of other part of lower extremity and inflammation   `CC` `A`

I83.219   Varicose veins of right lower extremity with both ulcer of unspecified site and inflammation   `CC` `A`

√6ᵗʰ **I83.22**   Varicose veins of left lower extremity with both ulcer and inflammation

I83.221   Varicose veins of left lower extremity with both ulcer of thigh and inflammation   `CC` `A`

I83.222   Varicose veins of left lower extremity with both ulcer of calf and inflammation   `CC` `A`

✅ Additional Character Required   √xⁿ Xtension Alert   Unacceptable PDx   Manifestation   Hospital Acquired Condition   EXCLUDES 1 Not Coded Here   EXCLUDES 2 Not Included Here

Diseases of the Circulatory System

I83.223–I87.091

I83.223 Varicose veins of left lower extremity with both ulcer of ankle and inflammation `CC` `A`

I83.224 Varicose veins of left lower extremity with both ulcer of heel and midfoot and inflammation `CC` `A`
Varicose veins of left lower extremity with both ulcer of plantar surface of midfoot and inflammation

I83.225 Varicose veins of left lower extremity with both ulcer other part of foot and inflammation `CC` `A`
Varicose veins of left lower extremity with both ulcer of toe and inflammation

I83.228 Varicose veins of left lower extremity with both ulcer of other part of lower extremity and inflammation `CC` `A`

I83.229 Varicose veins of left lower extremity with both ulcer of unspecified site and inflammation `CC` `A`

I83.8 Varicose veins of lower extremities with other complications

I83.81 Varicose veins of lower extremities with pain

I83.811 Varicose veins of right lower extremities with pain `A`

I83.812 Varicose veins of left lower extremities with pain `A`

I83.813 Varicose veins of bilateral lower extremities with pain `A`

I83.819 Varicose veins of unspecified lower extremities with pain `A`

I83.89 Varicose veins of lower extremities with other complications
Varicose veins of lower extremities with edema
Varicose veins of lower extremities with swelling

I83.891 Varicose veins of right lower extremities with other complications `A`

I83.892 Varicose veins of left lower extremities with other complications `A`

I83.893 Varicose veins of bilateral lower extremities with other complications `A`

I83.899 Varicose veins of unspecified lower extremities with other complications `A`

I83.9 Asymptomatic varicose veins of lower extremities
Phlebectasia of lower extremities
Varicose veins of lower extremities
Varix of lower extremities

I83.90 Asymptomatic varicose veins of unspecified lower extremity `A`
Varicose veins NOS

I83.91 Asymptomatic varicose veins of right lower extremity `A`

I83.92 Asymptomatic varicose veins of left lower extremity `A`

I83.93 Asymptomatic varicose veins of bilateral lower extremities `A`

I85 Esophageal varices
Use additional code to identify:
alcohol abuse and dependence (F10.-)

I85.0 Esophageal varices
Idiopathic esophageal varices
Primary esophageal varices

I85.00 Esophageal varices without bleeding `CC`
Esophageal varices NOS
CC Excl: E16.4, I85.00-I85.01, I85.11, I87.8, I99.8-I99.9, K22.6, K25.0-K28.9, K29.01, K29.21, K29.31, K29.41, K29.51, K29.61, K29.71, K29.81, K29.91, K31.811, K92.0-K92.2

I85.01 Esophageal varices with bleeding `MCC`
CC Excl: E16.4, I85.01, I85.11, I87.8, I99.8-I99.9, K22.10-K22.11, K22.6-K22.719, K25.0-K28.9, K29.01, K29.21, K29.31, K29.41, K29.51, K29.61, K29.71, K29.81, K29.91, K31.811, K55.21, K57.01, K57.11, K57.13, K57.21, K57.31, K57.33, K57.41, K57.51, K57.53, K57.81, K57.91, K57.93, K62.5, K92.0-K92.2

I85.1 Secondary esophageal varices
Esophageal varices secondary to alcoholic liver disease
Esophageal varices secondary to cirrhosis of liver
Esophageal varices secondary to schistosomiasis
Esophageal varices secondary to toxic liver disease
Code first underlying disease

I85.10 Secondary esophageal varices without bleeding `CC`
CC Excl: E16.4, I85.01-I85.11, I87.8, I99.8-I99.9, K22.6, K25.0-K28.9, K29.01, K29.21, K29.31, K29.41, K29.51, K29.61, K29.71, K29.81, K29.91, K31.811, K92.0-K92.2

I85.11 Secondary esophageal varices with bleeding `MCC`
CC Excl: I85.01, I85.11, I87.8, I99.8-I99.9

I86 Varicose veins of other sites
EXCLUDES 1 varicose veins of unspecified site (I83.9-)
EXCLUDES 2 retinal varices (H35.0-)

I86.0 Sublingual varices

I86.1 Scrotal varices ♂
Varicocele

I86.2 Pelvic varices

I86.3 Vulval varices ♀
EXCLUDES 1 vulval varices complicating childbirth and the puerperium (O87.8)
vulval varices complicating pregnancy (O22.1-)

I86.4 Gastric varices

I86.8 Varicose veins of other specified sites `A`
Varicose ulcer of nasal septum

I87 Other disorders of veins

I87.0 Postthrombotic syndrome
Chronic venous hypertension due to deep vein thrombosis
Postphlebitic syndrome
EXCLUDES 1 chronic venous hypertension without deep vein thrombosis (I87.3-)

CC Excl: For CC codes in subcategory I87.0, unless otherwise noted: I80.00-I80.9

I87.00 Postthrombotic syndrome without complications
Asymptomatic postthrombotic syndrome

I87.001 Postthrombotic syndrome without complications of right lower extremity

I87.002 Postthrombotic syndrome without complications of left lower extremity

I87.003 Postthrombotic syndrome without complications of bilateral lower extremity

I87.009 Postthrombotic syndrome without complications of unspecified extremity
Postthrombotic syndrome NOS

I87.01 Postthrombotic syndrome with ulcer
Use additional code to specify site and severity of ulcer (L97.-)

I87.011 Postthrombotic syndrome with ulcer of right lower extremity `CC`

I87.012 Postthrombotic syndrome with ulcer of left lower extremity `CC`

I87.013 Postthrombotic syndrome with ulcer of bilateral lower extremity `CC`

I87.019 Postthrombotic syndrome with ulcer of unspecified lower extremity `CC`

I87.02 Postthrombotic syndrome with inflammation

I87.021 Postthrombotic syndrome with inflammation of right lower extremity

I87.022 Postthrombotic syndrome with inflammation of left lower extremity

I87.023 Postthrombotic syndrome with inflammation of bilateral lower extremity

I87.029 Postthrombotic syndrome with inflammation of unspecified lower extremity

I87.03 Postthrombotic syndrome with ulcer and inflammation
Use additional code to specify site and severity of ulcer (L97.-)

I87.031 Postthrombotic syndrome with ulcer and inflammation of right lower extremity `CC`

I87.032 Postthrombotic syndrome with ulcer and inflammation of left lower extremity `CC`

I87.033 Postthrombotic syndrome with ulcer and inflammation of bilateral lower extremity `CC`

I87.039 Postthrombotic syndrome with ulcer and inflammation of unspecified lower extremity `CC`

I87.09 Postthrombotic syndrome with other complications

I87.091 Postthrombotic syndrome with other complications of right lower extremity

I87.Ø92   **Postthrombotic syndrome with other complications of** left lower **extremity**

I87.Ø93   **Postthrombotic syndrome with other complications of** bilateral lower **extremity**

I87.Ø99   **Postthrombotic syndrome with other complications of** unspecified lower **extremity**

I87.1   **Compression of vein**   `CC`
Stricture of vein
Vena cava syndrome (inferior) (superior)
EXCLUDES 2   compression of pulmonary vein (I28.8)
CC Excl: I87.1

I87.2   **Venous insufficiency (chronic) (peripheral)**

✓5ᵗʰ I87.3   **Chronic venous hypertension (idiopathic)**
Stasis edema
EXCLUDES 1   chronic venous hypertension due to deep vein thrombosis (I87.Ø-)
varicose veins of lower extremities (I83.-)

CC Excl: For CC codes in subcategory I87.3, unless otherwise noted: I83.ØØ1-I83.229, I83.9Ø-I83.93, I87.2, I87.8-I87.9, I99.8-I99.9

✓6ᵗʰ I87.3Ø   **Chronic venous hypertension (idiopathic)** without complications
Asymptomatic chronic venous hypertension (idiopathic)

I87.3Ø1   **Chronic venous hypertension (idiopathic) without complications of** right lower **extremity**

I87.3Ø2   **Chronic venous hypertension (idiopathic) without complications of** left lower **extremity**

I87.3Ø3   **Chronic venous hypertension (idiopathic) without complications of** bilateral lower **extremity**

I87.3Ø9   **Chronic venous hypertension (idiopathic) without complications of** unspecified lower **extremity**
Chronic venous hypertension NOS

✓6ᵗʰ I87.31   **Chronic venous hypertension (idiopathic)** with ulcer
Use additional code to specify site and severity of ulcer (L97.-)

I87.311   **Chronic venous hypertension (idiopathic) with ulcer of** right lower **extremity**   `CC`

I87.312   **Chronic venous hypertension (idiopathic) with ulcer of** left lower **extremity**   `CC`

I87.313   **Chronic venous hypertension (idiopathic) with ulcer of** bilateral lower **extremity**   `CC`

I87.319   **Chronic venous hypertension (idiopathic) with ulcer of** unspecified lower **extremity**   `CC`

✓6ᵗʰ I87.32   **Chronic venous hypertension (idiopathic) with** inflammation

I87.321   **Chronic venous hypertension (idiopathic) with inflammation of** right lower **extremity**

I87.322   **Chronic venous hypertension (idiopathic) with inflammation of** left lower **extremity**

I87.323   **Chronic venous hypertension (idiopathic) with inflammation of** bilateral lower **extremity**

I87.329   **Chronic venous hypertension (idiopathic) with inflammation of** unspecified lower **extremity**

✓6ᵗʰ I87.33   **Chronic venous hypertension (idiopathic) with** ulcer and inflammation
Use additional code to specify site and severity of ulcer (L97.-)

I87.331   **Chronic venous hypertension (idiopathic) with ulcer and inflammation of** right lower **extremity**   `CC`

I87.332   **Chronic venous hypertension (idiopathic) with ulcer and inflammation of** left lower **extremity**   `CC`

I87.333   **Chronic venous hypertension (idiopathic) with ulcer and inflammation of** bilateral lower **extremity**   `CC`

I87.339   **Chronic venous hypertension (idiopathic) with ulcer and inflammation of** unspecified lower **extremity**   `CC`

✓6ᵗʰ I87.39   **Chronic venous hypertension (idiopathic) with** other complications

I87.391   **Chronic venous hypertension (idiopathic) with other complications of** right lower **extremity**

I87.392   **Chronic venous hypertension (idiopathic) with other complications of** left lower **extremity**

I87.393   **Chronic venous hypertension (idiopathic) with other complications of** bilateral lower **extremity**

I87.399   **Chronic venous hypertension (idiopathic) with other complications of** unspecified lower **extremity**

I87.8   **Other specified disorders of veins**
Phlebosclerosis
Venofibrosis

I87.9   **Disorder of vein, unspecified**

✓4ᵗʰ I88   **Nonspecific lymphadenitis**
EXCLUDES 1   acute lymphadenitis, except mesenteric (LØ4.-)
enlarged lymph nodes NOS (R59.-)
human immunodeficiency virus [HIV] disease resulting in generalized lymphadenopathy (B2Ø)

I88.Ø   **Nonspecific mesenteric lymphadenitis**
Mesenteric lymphadenitis (acute)(chronic)

I88.1   **Chronic lymphadenitis, except mesenteric**
Adenitis
Lymphadenitis

I88.8   **Other nonspecific lymphadenitis**

I88.9   **Nonspecific lymphadenitis, unspecified**
Lymphadenitis NOS

✓4ᵗʰ I89   **Other noninfective disorders of lymphatic vessels and lymph nodes**
EXCLUDES 1   chylocele, tunica vaginalis (nonfilarial) NOS (N5Ø.8)
enlarged lymph nodes NOS (R59.-)
filarial chylocele (B74.-)
hereditary lymphedema (Q82.Ø)

I89.Ø   **Lymphedema, not elsewhere classified**
Elephantiasis (nonfilarial) NOS
Lymphangiectasis
Obliteration, lymphatic vessel
Praecox lymphedema
Secondary lymphedema
EXCLUDES 1   postmastectomy lymphedema (I97.2)

I89.1   **Lymphangitis**
Chronic lymphangitis
Lymphangitis NOS
Subacute lymphangitis
EXCLUDES 1   acute lymphangitis (LØ3.-)

I89.8   **Other specified noninfective disorders of lymphatic vessels and lymph nodes**
Chylocele (nonfilarial)
Chylous ascites
Chylous cyst
Lipomelanotic reticulosis
Lymph node or vessel fistula
Lymph node or vessel infarction
Lymph node or vessel rupture

I89.9   **Noninfective disorder of lymphatic vessels and lymph nodes, unspecified**
Disease of lymphatic vessels NOS

Other and unspecified disorders of the circulatory system (I95-I99)

✓4ᵗʰ I95   **Hypotension**
EXCLUDES 1   cardiovascular collapse (R57.9)
maternal hypotension syndrome (O26.5-)
nonspecific low blood pressure reading NOS (RØ3.1)

I95.Ø   **Idiopathic hypotension**

I95.1   **Orthostatic hypotension**
Hypotension, postural
EXCLUDES 1   neurogenic orthostatic hypotension [Shy-Drager] (G9Ø.3)
orthostatic hypotension due to drugs (I95.2)

Diseases of the Circulatory System

I95.2   **Hypotension** due to drugs
Orthostatic hypotension due to drugs
Use additional code for adverse effect, if applicable, to identify drug (T36-T50 with fifth or sixth character 5)

I95.3   **Hypotension of** hemodialysis
Intra-dialytic hypotension

✓5th **I95.8**   **Other hypotension**

    I95.81   **Postprocedural** hypotension

    I95.89   **Other** hypotension
       Chronic hypotension

I95.9   **Hypotension,** unspecified

I96   **Gangrene, not elsewhere classified**   `CC`
Gangrenous cellulitis
EXCLUDES 1   *gangrene in atherosclerosis of native arteries of the extremities (I70.26)*
gangrene in diabetes mellitus (E08-E13)
gangrene in hernia (K40.1, K40.4, K41.1, K41.4, K42.1, K43.1-, K44.1, K45.1, K46.1)
gangrene in other peripheral vascular diseases (I73.-)
gangrene of certain specified sites—see Alphabetical Index
gas gangrene (A48.0)
pyoderma gangrenosum (L88)
AHA: 2013, 2Q, 34
CC Excl: G89.0-G89.4, I70.261-I70.269, I96, R41.0-R41.3, R41.82, R41.9, R44.8-R44.9, R45.83-R45.84, R46.0-R46.89, R52, R68.0-R68.19, R68.81-R68.83, R68.89-R69

✓4th **I97**   **Intraoperative and postprocedural complications and disorders of circulatory system, not elsewhere classified**
EXCLUDES 2   *postprocedural shock (T81.1-)*

I97.0   **Postcardiotomy syndrome**

✓5th **I97.1**   **Other** postprocedural cardiac **functional disturbances**
EXCLUDES 2   *acute pulmonary insufficiency following thoracic surgery (J95.1)*
intraoperative cardiac functional disturbances (I97.7-)

> **CC Excl: For CC codes in subcategory I97.1, unless otherwise noted:** D78.81-D78.89, E36.8, E89.810-E89.89, H59.011-H59.019, H59.031-H59.099, H59.811-H59.89, H95.811-H95.89, I97.110-I97.191, I97.3, I97.710-I97.791, I97.88-I97.89, L76.81-L76.82, M96.89, N98.1-N98.9, T81.82XA, T81.89XA, T81.9XXA

   ✓6th **I97.11**   **Postprocedural** cardiac insufficiency

     I97.110   **Postprocedural cardiac insufficiency following** cardiac surgery   `CC`

     I97.111   **Postprocedural cardiac insufficiency following** other surgery   `CC`

   ✓6th **I97.12**   **Postprocedural** cardiac arrest

     I97.120   **Postprocedural cardiac arrest following** cardiac surgery   `CC`

     I97.121   **Postprocedural cardiac arrest following** other surgery   `CC`

   ✓6th **I97.13**   **Postprocedural** heart failure
      Use additional code to identify the heart failure (I50.-)

     I97.130   **Postprocedural heart failure following** cardiac surgery   `CC`

     I97.131   **Postprocedural heart failure following** other surgery   `CC`

   ✓6th **I97.19**   **Other** postprocedural cardiac **functional disturbances**
      Use additional code, if applicable, to further specify disorder

     I97.190   **Other postprocedural cardiac functional disturbances following** cardiac surgery   `CC`

     I97.191   **Other postprocedural cardiac functional disturbances following** other surgery   `CC`

I97.2   **Postmastectomy lymphedema syndrome**   `A`
Elephantiasis due to mastectomy
Obliteration of lymphatic vessels

I97.3   **Postprocedural hypertension**

✓5th **I97.4**   **Intraoperative hemorrhage and hematoma** of a circulatory system organ or structure complicating a procedure
EXCLUDES 1   *intraoperative hemorrhage and hematoma of a circulatory system organ or structure due to accidental puncture and laceration during a procedure (I97.5-)*
EXCLUDES 2   *intraoperative cerebrovascular hemorrhage complicating a procedure (G97.3-)*

> **CC Excl: For CC codes in subcategory I97.4, unless otherwise noted:** H95.811-H95.89, I85.01, I85.11, I97.3-I97.42, I97.610-I97.62, K21.9, K22.8, K23-K25.0, K25.2, K25.4, K25.6, K26.0, K26.2, K26.4, K26.6, K27.0, K27.2, K27.4, K27.6, K28.0, K28.2, K28.4, K28.6, K29.01, K29.21, K29.31, K29.41, K29.51, K29.61, K29.71, K29.81, K29.91, K31.811, K55.21, K57.01, K57.11, K57.13, K57.21, K57.31, K57.41, K57.51, K57.53, K57.81, K57.91, K57.93, K62.5, K92.0-K92.2, M96.89, N98.1-N98.9, P54.1-P54.3, T81.10XA, T81.11XA, T81.12XA, T81.19XA, T81.82XA, T81.89XA, T81.9XXA

   ✓6th **I97.41**   **Intraoperative hemorrhage and hematoma of a circulatory system organ or structure complicating a circulatory system procedure**

     I97.410   **Intraoperative hemorrhage and hematoma of a circulatory system organ or structure complicating a cardiac catheterization**   `CC`

     I97.411   **Intraoperative hemorrhage and hematoma of a circulatory system organ or structure complicating a cardiac bypass**   `CC`

     I97.418   **Intraoperative hemorrhage and hematoma of a circulatory system organ or structure complicating** other circulatory system procedure   `CC`

   I97.42   **Intraoperative hemorrhage and hematoma of a circulatory system organ or structure complicating** other procedure   `CC`

✓5th **I97.5**   **Accidental puncture and laceration** of a circulatory system organ or structure during a procedure
EXCLUDES 2   *accidental puncture and laceration of brain during a procedure (G97.4-)*

   I97.51   **Accidental puncture and laceration of a circulatory system organ or structure during a** circulatory system procedure   `CC`
CC Excl: D78.11-D78.12, D78.81-D78.89, E36.11-E36.8, E89.810-E89.89, G96.11, G97.41-G97.49, H59.011-H59.019, H59.031-H59.099, H59.211-H59.229, H59.811-H59.89, H95.31-H95.32, H95.811-H95.89, I97.3, I97.51-I97.52, J95.71-J95.72, K91.71-K91.72, L76.11-L76.12, L76.81-L76.82, M96.820-M96.821, M96.89, N98.1-N98.9, N99.71-N99.72, T81.10XA, T81.11XA, T81.12XA, T81.19XA, T81.82XA, T81.89XA, T81.9XXA

   I97.52   **Accidental puncture and laceration of a circulatory system organ or structure during** other procedure   `CC`
CC Excl: See code: I97.51

✓5th **I97.6**   **Postprocedural hemorrhage and hematoma** of a circulatory system organ or structure following a procedure
EXCLUDES 2   *postprocedural cerebrovascular hemorrhage complicating a procedure (G97.5-)*

> **CC Excl: For CC codes in subcategory I97.6, unless otherwise noted:** See code: I97.4

   ✓6th **I97.61**   **Postprocedural hemorrhage and hematoma of a circulatory system organ or structure following a circulatory system procedure**

     I97.610   **Postprocedural hemorrhage and hematoma of a circulatory system organ or structure following a** cardiac catheterization   `CC`

     I97.611   **Postprocedural hemorrhage and hematoma of a circulatory system organ or structure following** cardiac bypass   `CC`

     I97.618   **Postprocedural hemorrhage and hematoma of a circulatory system organ or structure following** other circulatory system procedure   `CC`

   I97.62   **Postprocedural hemorrhage and hematoma of a circulatory system organ or structure following** other procedure   `CC`

☑️5ᵗʰ **I97.7   Intraoperative cardiac functional disturbances**

EXCLUDES 2 *acute pulmonary insufficiency following thoracic surgery (J95.1)*
postprocedural cardiac functional disturbances (I97.1-)

CC Excl: For CC codes in subcategory I97.7, unless otherwise noted: D78.81-D78.89, E36.8, E89.810-E89.89, H59.011-H59.019, H59.031-H59.099, H59.811-H59.89, H95.811-H95.89, I97.110-I97.191, I97.3, I97.710-I97.791, I97.88-I97.89, L76.81-L76.82, M96.89, N98.1-N98.9, T81.82XA,T81.89XA,T81.9XXA

☑️6ᵗʰ **I97.71   Intraoperative cardiac arrest**

    I97.710   Intraoperative cardiac arrest during cardiac surgery   `CC`

    I97.711   Intraoperative cardiac arrest during other surgery   `CC`

☑️6ᵗʰ **I97.79   Other intraoperative cardiac functional disturbances**
    Use additional code, if applicable, to further specify disorder

    I97.790   Other intraoperative cardiac functional disturbances during cardiac surgery   `CC`

    I97.791   Other intraoperative cardiac functional disturbances during other surgery   `CC`

☑️5ᵗʰ **I97.8   Other intraoperative and postprocedural complications and disorders of the circulatory system, not elsewhere classified**
    Use additional code, if applicable, to further specify disorder

☑️6ᵗʰ **I97.81   Intraoperative cerebrovascular infarction**

    I97.810   Intraoperative cerebrovascular infarction during cardiac surgery   `CC`
        CC Excl: D78.81-D78.89, E36.8, E89.810-E89.89, G97.0, G97.2-G97.32, G97.81-G97.82, H59.011-H59.019, H59.031-H59.099, H59.811-H59.89, H95.811-H95.89, I97.3, I97.810-I97.821, L76.81-L76.82, M96.89, N98.1-N98.9, T81.10XA, T81.11XA,T81.12XA, T81.19XA,T81.82XA, T81.89XA, T81.9XXA

    I97.811   Intraoperative cerebrovascular infarction during other surgery   `CC`
        CC Excl: See code: I97.810

☑️6ᵗʰ **I97.82   Postprocedural cerebrovascular infarction**

    I97.820   Postprocedural cerebrovascular infarction during cardiac surgery   `CC`
        CC Excl: See code: I97.810

    I97.821   Postprocedural cerebrovascular infarction during other surgery   `CC`
        CC Excl: See code: I97.810

    I97.88   Other intraoperative complications of the circulatory system, not elsewhere classified   `CC`
        CC Excl: See code: I97.1

    I97.89   Other postprocedural complications and disorders of the circulatory system, not elsewhere classified   `CC`
        CC Excl: See code: I97.1

☑️4ᵗʰ **I99   Other and unspecified disorders of circulatory system**

    I99.8   Other disorder of circulatory system

    I99.9   Unspecified disorder of circulatory system

Chapter 10. Diseases of the Respiratory System (J00-J99)

NOTE   When a respiratory condition is described as occurring in more than one site and is not specifically indexed, it should be classified to the lower anatomic site (e.g. tracheobronchitis to bronchitis in J40).

Use additional code, where applicable, to identify:
exposure to environmental tobacco smoke (Z77.22)
exposure to tobacco smoke in the perinatal period (P96.81)
history of tobacco use (Z87.891)
occupational exposure to environmental tobacco smoke (Z57.31)
tobacco dependence (F17.-)
tobacco use (Z72.0)

EXCLUDES 2   *certain conditions originating in the perinatal period (P04-P96)*
certain infectious and parasitic diseases (A00-B99)
complications of pregnancy, childbirth and the puerperium (O00-O9A)
congenital malformations, deformations and chromosomal abnormalities (Q00-Q99)
endocrine, nutritional and metabolic diseases (E00-E88)
injury, poisoning and certain other consequences of external causes (S00-T88)
neoplasms (C00-D49)
smoke inhalation (T59.81-)
symptoms, signs and abnormal clinical and laboratory findings, not elsewhere classified (R00-R94)

This chapter contains the following blocks:

J00-J06	Acute upper respiratory infections
J09-J18	Influenza and pneumonia
J20-J22	Other acute lower respiratory infections
J30-J39	Other diseases of upper respiratory tract
J40-J47	Chronic lower respiratory diseases
J60-J70	Lung diseases due to external agents
J80-J84	Other respiratory diseases principally affecting the interstitium
J85-J86	Suppurative and necrotic conditions of the lower respiratory tract
J90-J94	Other diseases of the pleura
J95	Intraoperative and postprocedural complications and disorders of respiratory system, not elsewhere classified
J96-J99	Other diseases of the respiratory system

Acute upper respiratory infections (J00-J06)

EXCLUDES 1   *chronic obstructive pulmonary disease with acute lower respiratory infection (J44.0)*
influenza virus with other respiratory manifestations (J09.X2, J10.1, J11.1)

J00   **Acute nasopharyngitis (common cold)**
Acute rhinitis   Infective rhinitis
Coryza (acute)   Nasal catarrh, acute
Infective nasopharyngitis NOS   Nasopharyngitis NOS
   EXCLUDES 1   *acute pharyngitis (J02.-)*
acute sore throat NOS (J02.9)
pharyngitis NOS (J02.9)
rhinitis NOS (J31.0)
sore throat NOS (J02.9)
   EXCLUDES 2   *allergic rhinitis (J30.1-J30.9)*
chronic pharyngitis (J31.2)
chronic rhinitis (J31.0)
chronic sore throat (J31.2)
nasopharyngitis, chronic (J31.1)
vasomotor rhinitis (J30.0)

√4ᵗʰ J01   **Acute sinusitis**
   INCLUDES   acute abscess of sinus
acute empyema of sinus
acute infection of sinus
acute inflammation of sinus
acute suppuration of sinus
Use additional code (B95-B97) to identify infectious agent
   EXCLUDES 1   *sinusitis NOS (J32.9)*
   EXCLUDES 2   *chronic sinusitis (J32.0-J32.8)*

   √5ᵗʰ J01.0   **Acute maxillary sinusitis**
     Acute antritis
     J01.00   **Acute maxillary sinusitis, unspecified**
     J01.01   **Acute recurrent maxillary sinusitis**

   √5ᵗʰ J01.1   **Acute frontal sinusitis**
     J01.10   **Acute frontal sinusitis, unspecified**
     J01.11   **Acute recurrent frontal sinusitis**

   √5ᵗʰ J01.2   **Acute ethmoidal sinusitis**
     J01.20   **Acute ethmoidal sinusitis, unspecified**
     J01.21   **Acute recurrent ethmoidal sinusitis**

   √5ᵗʰ J01.3   **Acute sphenoidal sinusitis**
     J01.30   **Acute sphenoidal sinusitis, unspecified**
     J01.31   **Acute recurrent sphenoidal sinusitis**

   √5ᵗʰ J01.4   **Acute pansinusitis**
     J01.40   **Acute pansinusitis, unspecified**
     J01.41   **Acute recurrent pansinusitis**

   √5ᵗʰ J01.8   **Other acute sinusitis**
     J01.80   **Other acute sinusitis**
       Acute sinusitis involving more than one sinus but not pansinusitis
     J01.81   **Other acute recurrent sinusitis**
       Acute recurrent sinusitis involving more than one sinus but not pansinusitis

   √5ᵗʰ J01.9   **Acute sinusitis, unspecified**
     J01.90   **Acute sinusitis, unspecified**
     J01.91   **Acute recurrent sinusitis, unspecified**

√4ᵗʰ J02   **Acute pharyngitis**
   INCLUDES   acute sore throat
   EXCLUDES 1   *acute laryngopharyngitis (J06.0)*
peritonsillar abscess (J36)
pharyngeal abscess (J39.1)
retropharyngeal abscess (J39.0)
   EXCLUDES 2   *chronic pharyngitis (J31.2)*

   J02.0   **Streptococcal pharyngitis**
     Septic pharyngitis
     Streptococcal sore throat
     EXCLUDES 2   *scarlet fever (A38.-)*

   J02.8   **Acute pharyngitis due to other specified organisms**
     Use additional code (B95-B97) to identify infectious agent
     EXCLUDES 1   *acute pharyngitis due to coxsackie virus (B08.5)*
acute pharyngitis due to gonococcus (A54.5)
acute pharyngitis due to herpes [simplex] virus (B00.2)
acute pharyngitis due to infectious mononucleosis (B27.-)
enteroviral vesicular pharyngitis (B08.5)

   J02.9   **Acute pharyngitis, unspecified**
     Gangrenous pharyngitis (acute)
     Infective pharyngitis (acute) NOS
     Pharyngitis (acute) NOS
     Sore throat (acute) NOS
     Suppurative pharyngitis (acute)
     Ulcerative pharyngitis (acute)

√4ᵗʰ J03   **Acute tonsillitis**
   EXCLUDES 1   *acute sore throat (J02.-)*
hypertrophy of tonsils (J35.1)
peritonsillar abscess (J36)
sore throat NOS (J02.9)
streptococcal sore throat (J02.0)
   EXCLUDES 2   *chronic tonsillitis (J35.0)*

   √5ᵗʰ J03.0   **Streptococcal tonsillitis**
     J03.00   **Acute streptococcal tonsillitis, unspecified**
     J03.01   **Acute recurrent streptococcal tonsillitis**

   √5ᵗʰ J03.8   **Acute tonsillitis due to other specified organisms**
     Use additional code (B95-B97) to identify infectious agent
     EXCLUDES 1   *diphtheritic tonsillitis (A36.0)*
herpesviral pharyngotonsillitis (B00.2)
streptococcal tonsillitis (J03.0)
tuberculous tonsillitis (A15.8)
Vincent's tonsillitis (A69.1)
     J03.80   **Acute tonsillitis due to other specified organisms**
     J03.81   **Acute recurrent tonsillitis due to other specified organisms**

   √5ᵗʰ J03.9   **Acute tonsillitis, unspecified**
     Follicular tonsillitis (acute)   Tonsillitis (acute) NOS
     Gangrenous tonsillitis (acute)   Ulcerative tonsillitis (acute)
     Infective tonsillitis (acute)
     J03.90   **Acute tonsillitis, unspecified**
     J03.91   **Acute recurrent tonsillitis, unspecified**

√4ᵗʰ J04   **Acute laryngitis and tracheitis**
   Use additional code (B95-B97) to identify infectious agent
   EXCLUDES 1   *acute obstructive laryngitis [croup] and epiglottitis (J05.-)*
   EXCLUDES 2   *laryngismus (stridulus) (J38.5)*

N Newborn: 0   **P** Pediatric: 0-17   **M** Maternity: 12-55   **A** Adult: 15-124   **MCC** Major CC Condition   **PDx MCC** PDx acts as own MCC   **CC** CC Condition   **PDx CC** PDx acts as own CC

628   ICD-10-CM Draft (2015)

J04.0 Acute laryngitis
Edematous laryngitis (acute)   Suppurative laryngitis (acute)
Laryngitis (acute) NOS   Ulcerative laryngitis (acute)
Subglottic laryngitis (acute)
EXCLUDES 1   acute obstructive laryngitis (J05.0)
EXCLUDES 2   chronic laryngitis (J37.0)

✓5ᵗʰ **J04.1 Acute tracheitis**
Acute viral tracheitis   Tracheitis (acute) NOS
Catarrhal tracheitis (acute)
EXCLUDES 2   chronic tracheitis (J42)

   J04.10 Acute tracheitis without obstruction

   J04.11 Acute tracheitis with obstruction   MCC
     CC Excl: A15.8-A15.9, A17.9, A18.82, A18.84, A18.89,
     J04.10-J04.2, J05.10-J05.11, J22, J98.8-J98.9

J04.2 Acute laryngotracheitis
Laryngotracheitis NOS
Tracheitis (acute) with laryngitis (acute)
EXCLUDES 1   acute obstructive laryngotracheitis (J05.0)
EXCLUDES 2   chronic laryngotracheitis (J37.1)

✓5ᵗʰ **J04.3 Supraglottitis, unspecified**

   J04.30 Supraglottitis, unspecified, without obstruction

   J04.31 Supraglottitis, unspecified, with obstruction   MCC
     CC Excl: A15.8-A15.9, A17.9, A18.82, A18.84, A18.89,
     J04.0-J04.2, J05.10-J05.11, J22, J98.8-J98.9

✓4ᵗʰ **J05 Acute obstructive laryngitis [croup] and epiglottitis**
Use additional code (B95-B97) to identify infectious agent

J05.0 Acute obstructive laryngitis [croup]
Obstructive laryngitis (acute) NOS
Obstructive laryngotracheitis NOS

✓5ᵗʰ **J05.1 Acute epiglottitis**
EXCLUDES 2   epiglottitis, chronic (J37.0)

   J05.10 Acute epiglottitis without obstruction   CC
     Epiglottitis NOS
     CC Excl: J04.31, J05.10-J05.11

   J05.11 Acute epiglottitis with obstruction   MCC
     CC Excl: See code: J04.31

✓4ᵗʰ **J06 Acute upper respiratory infections of multiple and unspecified sites**
EXCLUDES 1   acute respiratory infection NOS (J22)
         streptococcal pharyngitis (J02.0)3

J06.0 Acute laryngopharyngitis

J06.9 Acute upper respiratory infection, unspecified
Upper respiratory disease, acute
Upper respiratory infection NOS

Influenza and pneumonia (J09-J18)
EXCLUDES 2   allergic or eosinophilic pneumonia (J82)
         aspiration pneumonia NOS (J69.0)
         congenital pneumonia (P23.9)
         lipid pneumonia (J69.1)
         meconium pneumonia (P24.01)
         neonatal aspiration pneumonia (P24.-)
         pneumonia due to solids and liquids (J69.-)
         rheumatic pneumonia (I00)
         ventilator associated pneumonia (J95.851)

✓4ᵗʰ **J09 Influenza due to certain identified influenza viruses**
EXCLUDES 1   seasonal influenza due to other identified influenza virus (J10.-)
         seasonal influenza due to unidentified influenza virus (J11.-)

✓5ᵗʰ **J09.X Influenza due to identified novel influenza A virus**
Avian influenza
Bird influenza
Influenza A/H5N1
Influenza of other animal origin, not bird or swine
Swine influenza virus (viruses that normally cause infections in pigs)

   J09.X1 Influenza due to identified novel influenza A   HIV MCC
     virus with pneumonia
     Code also, if applicable, associated:
       lung abscess (J85.1)
       other specified type of pneumonia
     CC Excl: A15.0-A15.6, A15.8-A15.9, A17.9, A18.82,
     A18.84, A18.89, A21.2, A22.1, A31.0, A37.01, A37.11,
     A37.81, A37.91, A42.0, A43.0, A48.1, B25.0, B39.0-B39.2,
     B44.0, B58.3, B59, B67.1, J09.X1-J09.X2, J10.00-J10.1,
     J11.00-J11.1, J12.0-J12.3, J12.89-J18.1, J18.8-J18.9, J22,
     J44.9, J47.0-J70.4, J70.8-J70.9, J98.4, J98.8-J99, Q33.4,
     R91.1

   J09.X2 Influenza due to identified novel influenza A virus with other respiratory manifestations
     Influenza due to identified novel influenza A virus NOS
     Influenza due to identified novel influenza A virus with laryngitis
     Influenza due to identified novel influenza A virus with pharyngitis
     Influenza due to identified novel influenza A virus with upper respiratory symptoms
     Use additional code, if applicable, for associated:
       pleural effusion (J91.8)
       sinusitis (J01.-)

   J09.X3 Influenza due to identified novel influenza A virus with gastrointestinal manifestations
     Influenza due to identified novel influenza A virus gastroenteritis
     EXCLUDES 1   'intestinal flu' [viral gastroenteritis] (A08.-)

   J09.X9 Influenza due to identified novel influenza A virus with other manifestations
     Influenza due to identified novel influenza A virus with encephalopathy
     Influenza due to identified novel influenza A virus with myocarditis
     Influenza due to identified novel influenza A virus with otitis media
     Use additional code to identify manifestation

✓4ᵗʰ **J10 Influenza due to other identified influenza virus**
EXCLUDES 1   influenza due to avian influenza virus (J09.X-)
         influenza due to swine flu (J09.X-)
         influenza due to unidentifed influenza virus (J11.-)

✓5ᵗʰ **J10.0 Influenza due to other identified influenza virus with pneumonia**
Code also associated lung abscess, if applicable (J85.1)

   J10.00 Influenza due to other identified influenza virus with unspecified type of pneumonia   MCC
     CC Excl: See code: J09.X1

   J10.01 Influenza due to other identified influenza virus with the same other identified influenza virus pneumonia   MCC
     CC Excl: See code: J09.X1

   J10.08 Influenza due to other identified influenza virus with other specified pneumonia   HIV MCC
     Code also other specified type of pneumonia
     CC Excl: See code: J09.X1

J10.1 Influenza due to other identified influenza virus with other respiratory manifestations
Influenza due to other identified influenza virus NOS
Influenza due to other identified influenza virus with laryngitis
Influenza due to other identified influenza virus with pharyngitis
Influenza due to other identified influenza virus with upper respiratory symptoms
Use additional code for associated pleural effusion, if applicable (J91.8)
Use additional code for associated sinusitis, if applicable (J01.-)

J10.2 Influenza due to other identified influenza virus with gastrointestinal manifestations
Influenza due to other identified influenza virus gastroenteritis
EXCLUDES 1   'intestinal flu' [viral gastroenteritis] (A08.-)

✓5ᵗʰ **J10.8 Influenza due to other identified influenza virus with other manifestations**

   J10.81 Influenza due to other identified influenza virus with encephalopathy

   J10.82 Influenza due to other identified influenza virus with myocarditis

   J10.83 Influenza due to other identified influenza virus with otitis media
     Use additional code for any associated perforated tympanic membrane (H72.-)

   J10.89 Influenza due to other identified influenza virus with other manifestations
     Use additional codes to identify the manifestations

✓4ᵗʰ **J11 Influenza due to unidentified influenza virus**

✓5ᵗʰ **J11.0 Influenza due to unidentified influenza virus with pneumonia**
Code also associated lung abscess, if applicable (J85.1)

   J11.00 Influenza due to unidentified influenza virus with unspecified type of pneumonia   MCC
     Influenza with pneumonia NOS
     CC Excl: See code: J09.X1

✓ Additional Character Required   ✓x7ᵗʰ Xtension Alert   Unacceptable PDx   Manifestation   Hospital Acquired Condition   *EXCLUDES 1* Not Coded Here   *EXCLUDES 2* Not Included Here

ICD-10-CM Draft (2015)   629

Diseases of the Respiratory System

J11.Ø8–J16.8

J11.Ø8   **Influenza due to unidentified influenza virus with specified pneumonia**   `MCC`
Code also other specified type of pneumonia
CC Excl: See code: JØ9.X1

J11.1   **Influenza due to unidentified influenza virus with other respiratory manifestations**
Influenza NOS
Influenzal laryngitis NOS
Influenzal pharyngitis NOS
Influenza with upper respiratory symptoms NOS
Use additional code for associated pleural effusion, if applicable (J91.8)
Use additional code for associated sinusitis, if applicable (JØ1.-)

J11.2   **Influenza due to unidentified influenza virus with gastrointestinal manifestations**
Influenza gastroenteritis NOS
EXCLUDES 1   'intestinal flu' [viral gastroenteritis] (AØ8.-)

√5ᵗʰ **J11.8**   **Influenza due to unidentified influenza virus with other manifestations**

J11.81   **Influenza due to unidentified influenza virus with encephalopathy**
Influenzal encephalopathy NOS

J11.82   **Influenza due to unidentified influenza virus with myocarditis**
Influenzal myocarditis NOS

J11.83   **Influenza due to unidentified influenza virus with otitis media**
Influenzal otitis media NOS
Use additional code for any associated perforated tympanic membrane (H72.-)

J11.89   **Influenza due to unidentified influenza virus with other manifestations**
Use additional codes to identify the manifestations

√4ᵗʰ **J12**   **Viral pneumonia, not elsewhere classified**
INCLUDES   bronchopneumonia due to viruses other than influenza viruses
Code first associated influenza, if applicable (JØ9.X1, J1Ø.Ø-, J11.Ø-)
Code also associated abscess, if applicable (J85.1)
EXCLUDES 1   aspiration pneumonia due to anesthesia during labor and delivery (O74.Ø)
aspiration pneumonia due to anesthesia during pregnancy (O29)
aspiration pneumonia due to anesthesia during puerperium (O89.Ø)
aspiration pneumonia due to solids and liquids (J69.-)
aspiration pneumonia NOS (J69.Ø)
congenital pneumonia (P23.Ø)
congenital rubella pneumonitis (P35.Ø)
interstitial pneumonia NOS (J84.9)
lipid pneumonia (J69.1)
neonatal aspiration pneumonia (P24.-)
AHA: 2Ø13, 4Q, 118

CC Excl: For MCC codes in category J12, unless otherwise noted: A15.Ø-A15.6, A15.8-A15.9, A17.9, A18.82, A18.84, A18.89, A2Ø.2, A21.1, A22.1, A31.Ø, A37.Ø1, A37.11, A37.81, A37.91, A42.Ø, A43.Ø, A48.1, B25.Ø, B39.Ø-B39.2, B44.Ø, B58.3, B59, B67.1, JØ9.X1-JØ9.X2, J1Ø.ØØ-J1Ø.1, J11.ØØ-J11.1, J12.Ø-J18.1, J18.8-J18.9, J22, J6Ø-J7Ø.4, J7Ø.8-J7Ø.9, J98.4, J98.8-J99, R91.1

J12.Ø   **Adenoviral pneumonia**   `MCC`

J12.1   **Respiratory syncytial virus pneumonia**   `MCC`

J12.2   **Parainfluenza virus pneumonia**   `MCC`

J12.3   **Human metapneumovirus pneumonia**   `HIV` `MCC`

√5ᵗʰ **J12.8**   **Other viral pneumonia**

J12.81   **Pneumonia due to SARS-associated coronavirus**   `HIV` `MCC`
Severe acute respiratory syndrome NOS
CC Excl: A15.Ø-A15.6, A15.8-A15.9, A17.9, A18.82, A18.84, A18.89, A21.2, A22.1, A31.Ø, A37.Ø1, A37.11, A37.81, A37.91, A42.Ø, A43.Ø, A48.1, B25.Ø, B39.Ø-B39.2, B44.Ø, B58.3, B59, B67.1, JØ9.X1-JØ9.X2, J1Ø.ØØ-J1Ø.1, J11.ØØ-J11.1, J12.Ø-J18.1, J18.8-J18.9, J22, J44.9, J47.Ø-J7Ø.4, J7Ø.8-J7Ø.9, J98.4, J98.8-J99, Q33.4, R91.1

J12.89   **Other viral pneumonia**   `HIV` `MCC`

J12.9   **Viral pneumonia, unspecified**   `HIV` `MCC`

J13   **Pneumonia due to Streptococcus pneumoniae**   `HIV` `MCC`
Bronchopneumonia due to S. pneumoniae
Code first associated influenza, if applicable (JØ9.X1, J1Ø.Ø-, J11.Ø-)
Code also associated lung abscess, if applicable (J85.1)
EXCLUDES 1   congenital pneumonia due to S. pneumoniae (P23.6)
lobar pneumonia, unspecified organism (J18.1)
pneumonia due to other streptococci (J15.3-J15.4)
AHA: 2Ø13, 4Q, 118
CC Excl: See code: JØ9.X1

J14   **Pneumonia due to Hemophilus influenzae**   `HIV` `MCC`
Bronchopneumonia due to H. influenzae
Code first associated influenza, if applicable (JØ9.X1, J1Ø.Ø-, J11.Ø-)
Code also associated lung abscess, if applicable (J85.1)
EXCLUDES 1   congenital pneumonia due to H. influenzae (P23.6)
AHA: 2Ø13, 4Q, 118
CC Excl: See code: JØ9.X1

√4ᵗʰ **J15**   **Bacterial pneumonia, not elsewhere classified**
Bronchopneumonia due to bacteria other than S. pneumoniae and H. influenzae
Code first associated influenza, if applicable (JØ9.X1, J1Ø.Ø-, J11.Ø-)
Code also associated lung abscess, if applicable (J85.1)
EXCLUDES 1   chlamydial pneumonia (J16.Ø)
congenital pneumonia (P23.-)
Legionnaires' disease (A48.1)
spirochetal pneumonia (A69.8)
AHA: 2Ø13, 4Q, 118

CC Excl: For MCC codes in category J15, unless otherwise noted: See code: JØ9.X1

J15.Ø   **Pneumonia due to Klebsiella pneumoniae**   `HIV` `MCC`

J15.1   **Pneumonia due to Pseudomonas**   `HIV` `MCC`

√5ᵗʰ **J15.2**   **Pneumonia due to staphylococcus**

J15.2Ø   **Pneumonia due to staphylococcus, unspecified**   `HIV` `MCC`

√6ᵗʰ **J15.21**   **Pneumonia due to Staphylococcus aureus**

J15.211   **Pneumonia due to methicillin susceptible Staphylococcus aureus**   `HIV` `MCC`
MSSA pneumonia
Pneumonia due to Staphylococcus aureus NOS

J15.212   **Pneumonia due to methicillin resistant Staphylococcus aureus**   `HIV` `MCC`

J15.29   **Pneumonia due to other staphylococcus**   `HIV` `MCC`

J15.3   **Pneumonia due to streptococcus, group**   `HIV` `MCC`

J15.4   **Pneumonia due to other streptococci**   `HIV` `MCC`
EXCLUDES 1   pneumonia due to streptococcus, group B (J15.3)
pneumonia due to Streptococcus pneumoniae (J13)

J15.5   **Pneumonia due to Escherichia coli**   `HIV` `MCC`

J15.6   **Pneumonia due to other aerobic Gram-negative bacteria**   `HIV` `MCC`
Pneumonia due to Serratia marcescens

J15.7   **Pneumonia due to Mycoplasma pneumoniae**   `MCC`

J15.8   **Pneumonia due to other specified bacteria**   `HIV` `MCC`

J15.9   **Unspecified bacterial pneumonia**   `HIV` `MCC`
Pneumonia due to gram-positive bacteria

√4ᵗʰ **J16**   **Pneumonia due to other infectious organisms, not elsewhere classified**
Code first associated influenza, if applicable (JØ9.X1, J1Ø.Ø-, J11.Ø-)
Code also associated lung abscess, if applicable (J85.1)
EXCLUDES 1   congenital pneumonia (P23.-)
ornithosis (A7Ø)
pneumocystosis (B59)
pneumonia NOS (J18.9)
AHA: 2Ø13, 4Q, 118

J16.Ø   **Chlamydial pneumonia**   `MCC`
CC Excl: See code: JØ9.X1

J16.8   **Pneumonia due to other specified infectious organisms**   `MCC`
CC Excl: See code: JØ9.X1

J17   *Pneumonia in diseases classified elsewhere*   `MCC`

    Code first underlying disease, such as:
      Q fever (A78)
      rheumatic fever (I00)
      schistosomiasis (B65.0-B65.9)

    `EXCLUDES 1` *candidial pneumonia (B37.1)*
      chlamydial pneumonia (J16.0)
      gonorrheal pneumonia (A54.84)
      histoplasmosis pneumonia (B39.0-B39.2)
      measles pneumonia (B05.2)
      nocardiosis pneumonia (A43.0)
      pneumocystosis (B59)
      pneumonia due to Pneumocystis carinii (B59)
      pneumonia due to Pneumocystis jiroveci (B59)
      pneumonia in actinomycosis (A42.0)
      pneumonia in anthrax (A22.1)
      pneumonia in ascariasis (B77.81)
      pneumonia in aspergillosis (B44.0-B44.1)
      pneumonia in coccidioidomycosis (B38.0-B38.2)
      pneumonia in cytomegalovirus disease (B25.0)
      pneumonia in toxoplasmosis (B58.3)
      rubella pneumonia (B06.81)
      salmonella pneumonia (A02.22)
      spirochetal infection NEC with pneumonia (A69.8)
      tularemia pneumonia (A21.2)
      typhoid fever with pneumonia (A01.03)
      varicella pneumonia (B01.2)
      whooping cough with pneumonia (A37 with fifth-character 1)

    AHA: 2013, 4Q, 118
    CC Excl: A15.0-A15.6, A15.8-A15.9, A17.9, A18.82, A18.84, A18.89, A21.2, A22.1, A31.0, A37.01, A37.11, A37.81, A37.91, A42.0, A43.0, A48.1, B25.0, B39.0-B39.2, B44.0, B58.3, B59, B67.1, J09.X1-J09.X2, J10.00-J10.1, J11.00-J11.1, J12.0-J12.3, J12.89-J18.1, J18.8-J18.9, J22, J44.9, J47.0-J70.4, J70.8-J70.9, J98.4, J98.8-J99, Q33.4, R91.1

`✓4ᵗʰ` **J18**   **Pneumonia, unspecified organism**

    Code first associated influenza, if applicable (J09.X1, J10.0-, J11.0-)

    `EXCLUDES 1` *abscess of lung with pneumonia (J85.1)*
      aspiration pneumonia due to anesthesia during labor and
        delivery (O74.0)
      aspiration pneumonia due to anesthesia during pregnancy
        (O29)
      aspiration pneumonia due to anesthesia during puerperium
        (O89.0)
      aspiration pneumonia due to solids and liquids (J69.-)
      aspiration pneumonia NOS (J69.0)
      congenital pneumonia (P23.0)
      drug-induced interstitial lung disorder (J70.2-J70.4)
      interstitial pneumonia NOS (J84.9)
      lipid pneumonia (J69.1)
      neonatal aspiration pneumonia (P24.-)
      pneumonitis due to external agents (J67-J70)
      pneumonitis due to fumes and vapors (J68.0)
      usual interstitial pneumonia (J84.17)

    AHA: 2013, 4Q, 118

    CC Excl: For CC/MCC codes in category J18, unless otherwise noted: See code: J17

    J18.0   **Bronchopneumonia, unspecified organism**   `MCC`
        `EXCLUDES 1` *hypostatic bronchopneumonia (J18.2)*
          lipid pneumonia (J69.1)
        `EXCLUDES 2` *acute bronchiolitis (J21.-)*
          chronic bronchiolitis (J44.9)

    J18.1   **Lobar pneumonia, unspecified organism**   `HIV` `MCC`

    J18.2   **Hypostatic pneumonia, unspecified organism**   `CC`
        Hypostatic bronchopneumonia
        Passive pneumonia
        CC Excl: J18.2, J22, J81.1, J98.4, J98.8-J99, R91.1

    J18.8   **Other pneumonia, unspecified organism**   `HIV` `MCC`

    (**J18.9**   **Pneumonia, unspecified organism**)   `HIV` `MCC`
        AHA: 2013, 4Q, 119; 2012, 4Q, 94

Other acute lower respiratory infections (J20-J22)

`EXCLUDES 2` *chronic obstructive pulmonary disease with acute lower respiratory infection (J44.0)*

`✓4ᵗʰ` **J20**   **Acute bronchitis**

    `INCLUDES` acute and subacute bronchitis (with) bronchospasm
      acute and subacute bronchitis (with) tracheitis
      acute and subacute bronchitis (with) tracheobronchitis, acute
      acute and subacute fibrinous bronchitis
      acute and subacute membranous bronchitis
      acute and subacute purulent bronchitis
      acute and subacute septic bronchitis

    `EXCLUDES 1` *bronchitis NOS (J40)*
      tracheobronchitis NOS (J40)

    `EXCLUDES 2` *acute bronchitis with bronchiectasis (J47.0)*
      acute bronchitis with chronic obstructive asthma (J44.0)
      acute bronchitis with chronic obstructive pulmonary disease (J44.0)
      allergic bronchitis NOS (J45.909)
      bronchitis due to chemicals, fumes and vapors (J68.0)
      chronic bronchitis NOS (J42)
      chronic mucopurulent bronchitis (J41.1)
      chronic obstructive bronchitis (J44.-)
      chronic obstructive tracheobronchitis (J44.-)
      chronic simple bronchitis (J41.0)
      chronic tracheobronchitis (J42)

    J20.0   **Acute bronchitis due to Mycoplasma pneumoniae**
    J20.1   **Acute bronchitis due to Hemophilus influenzae**
    J20.2   **Acute bronchitis due to streptococcus**
    J20.3   **Acute bronchitis due to coxsackievirus**
    J20.4   **Acute bronchitis due to parainfluenza virus**
    J20.5   **Acute bronchitis due to respiratory syncytial virus**
    J20.6   **Acute bronchitis due to rhinovirus**
    J20.7   **Acute bronchitis due to echovirus**
    J20.8   **Acute bronchitis due to other specified organisms**
    J20.9   **Acute bronchitis, unspecified**

`✓4ᵗʰ` **J21**   **Acute bronchiolitis**
    Acute bronchiolitis with bronchospasm
    `EXCLUDES 2` *respiratory bronchiolitis interstitial lung disease (J84.115)*

    CC Excl: For CC codes in category J21, unless otherwise noted: J20.0-J21.9

    J21.0   **Acute bronchiolitis due to respiratory syncytial virus**   `CC`
        CC Excl: J21.0
    J21.1   **Acute bronchiolitis due to human metapneumovirus**   `CC`
    J21.8   **Acute bronchiolitis due to other specified organisms**   `CC`
    J21.9   **Acute bronchiolitis, unspecified**   `CC`
        Bronchiolitis (acute)
        `EXCLUDES 1` *chronic bronchiolitis (J44.-)*

    J22   **Unspecified acute lower respiratory infection**
        Acute (lower) respiratory (tract) infection NOS
        `EXCLUDES 1` *upper respiratory infection (acute) (J06.9)*

Other diseases of upper respiratory tract (J30-J39)

`✓4ᵗʰ` **J30**   **Vasomotor and allergic rhinitis**
    `INCLUDES` spasmodic rhinorrhea
    `EXCLUDES 1` *allergic rhinitis with asthma (bronchial) (J45.909)*
      rhinitis NOS (J31.0)

    J30.0   **Vasomotor rhinitis**
    J30.1   **Allergic rhinitis due to pollen**
        Allergy NOS due to pollen
        Hay fever
        Pollinosis
    J30.2   **Other seasonal allergic rhinitis**
    J30.5   **Allergic rhinitis due to food**
    `✓5ᵗʰ` **J30.8**   **Other allergic rhinitis**
        J30.81   **Allergic rhinitis due to animal (cat) (dog) hair and dander**
        J30.89   **Other allergic rhinitis**
          Perennial allergic rhinitis
    J30.9   **Allergic rhinitis, unspecified**

Diseases of the Respiratory System

J31–J37.0

✓4ᵗʰ **J31 Chronic rhinitis, nasopharyngitis and pharyngitis**

Use additional code to identify:
exposure to environmental tobacco smoke (Z77.22)
exposure to tobacco smoke in the perinatal period (P96.81)
history of tobacco use (Z87.891)
occupational exposure to environmental tobacco smoke (Z57.31)
tobacco dependence (F17.-)
tobacco use (Z72.0)

J31.0 Chronic rhinitis
Atrophic rhinitis (chronic)
Granulomatous rhinitis (chronic)
Hypertrophic rhinitis (chronic)
Obstructive rhinitis (chronic)
Ozena
Purulent rhinitis (chronic)
Rhinitis (chronic) NOS
Ulcerative rhinitis (chronic)
EXCLUDES 1   *allergic rhinitis (J30.1-J30.9)*
                vasomotor rhinitis (J30.0)

J31.1 Chronic nasopharyngitis
EXCLUDES 2   *acute nasopharyngitis (J00)*

J31.2 Chronic pharyngitis
Atrophic pharyngitis (chronic)
Chronic sore throat
Granular pharyngitis (chronic)
Hypertrophic pharyngitis (chronic)
EXCLUDES 2   *acute pharyngitis (J02.9)*

✓4ᵗʰ **J32 Chronic sinusitis**

INCLUDES   sinus abscess
           sinus empyema
           sinus infection
           sinus suppuration
Use additional code to identify:
exposure to environmental tobacco smoke (Z77.22)
exposure to tobacco smoke in the perinatal period (P96.81)
history of tobacco use (Z87.891)
infectious agent (B95-B97)
occupational exposure to environmental tobacco smoke (Z57.31)
tobacco dependence (F17.-)
tobacco use (Z72.0)
EXCLUDES 2   *acute sinusitis (J01.-)*

J32.0 Chronic maxillary sinusitis
Antritis (chronic)
Maxillary sinusitis NOS

J32.1 Chronic frontal sinusitis
Frontal sinusitis NOS

J32.2 Chronic ethmoidal sinusitis
Ethmoidal sinusitis NOS
EXCLUDES 1   *Woakes' ethmoiditis (J33.1)*

J32.3 Chronic sphenoidal sinusitis
Sphenoidal sinusitis NOS

J32.4 Chronic pansinusitis
Pansinusitis NOS

J32.8 Other chronic sinusitis
Sinusitis (chronic) involving more than one sinus but not pansinusitis

J32.9 Chronic sinusitis, unspecified
Sinusitis (chronic) NOS

✓4ᵗʰ **J33 Nasal polyp**

Use additional code to identify:
exposure to environmental tobacco smoke (Z77.22)
exposure to tobacco smoke in the perinatal period (P96.81)
history of tobacco use (Z87.891)
occupational exposure to environmental tobacco smoke (Z57.31)
tobacco dependence (F17.-)
tobacco use (Z72.0)
EXCLUDES 1   *adenomatous polyps (D14.0)*

J33.0 Polyp of nasal cavity
Choanal polyp
Nasopharyngeal polyp

J33.1 Polypoid sinus degeneration
Woakes' syndrome or ethmoiditis

J33.8 Other polyp of sinus
Accessory polyp of sinus
Ethmoidal polyp of sinus
Maxillary polyp of sinus
Sphenoidal polyp of sinus

J33.9 Nasal polyp, unspecified

✓4ᵗʰ **J34 Other and unspecified disorders of nose and nasal sinuses**

EXCLUDES 2   *varicose ulcer of nasal septum (I86.8)*

J34.0 Abscess, furuncle and carbuncle of nose
Cellulitis of nose   Ulceration of nose
Necrosis of nose

J34.1 Cyst and mucocele of nose and nasal sinus

J34.2 Deviated nasal septum
Deflection or deviation of septum (nasal) (acquired)
EXCLUDES 1   *congenital deviated nasal septum (Q67.4)*

J34.3 Hypertrophy of nasal turbinates

✓5ᵗʰ **J34.8 Other specified disorders of nose and nasal sinuses**

J34.81 Nasal mucositis (ulcerative)
Code also type of associated therapy, such as:
antineoplastic and immunosuppressive drugs (T45.1X-)
radiological procedure and radiotherapy (Y84.2)
EXCLUDES 2   *gastrointestinal mucositis (ulcerative) (K92.81)*
               mucositis (ulcerative) of vagina and vulva (N76.81)
               oral mucositis (ulcerative) (K12.3-)

J34.89 Other specified disorders of nose and nasal sinuses
Perforation of nasal septum NOS
Rhinolith

J34.9 Unspecified disorder of nose and nasal sinuses

✓4ᵗʰ **J35 Chronic diseases of tonsils and adenoids**

Use additional code to identify:
exposure to environmental tobacco smoke (Z77.22)
exposure to tobacco smoke in the perinatal period (P96.81)
history of tobacco use (Z87.891)
occupational exposure to environmental tobacco smoke (Z57.31)
tobacco dependence (F17.-)
tobacco use (Z72.0)

✓5ᵗʰ **J35.0 Chronic tonsillitis and adenoiditis**
EXCLUDES 2   *acute tonsillitis (J03.-)*

J35.01 Chronic tonsillitis

J35.02 Chronic adenoiditis

J35.03 Chronic tonsillitis and adenoiditis

J35.1 Hypertrophy of tonsils
Enlargement of tonsils
EXCLUDES 1   *hypertrophy of tonsils with tonsillitis (J35.0-)*

J35.2 Hypertrophy of adenoids
Enlargement of adenoids
EXCLUDES 1   *hypertrophy of adenoids with adenoiditis (J35.0-)*

J35.3 Hypertrophy of tonsils with hypertrophy of adenoids
EXCLUDES 1   *hypertrophy of tonsils and adenoids with tonsillitis and adenoiditis (J35.03)*

J35.8 Other chronic diseases of tonsils and adenoids
Adenoid vegetations   Tonsillar tag
Amygdalolith   Ulcer of tonsil
Calculus, tonsil
Cicatrix of tonsil (and adenoid)

J35.9 Chronic disease of tonsils and adenoids, unspecified
Disease (chronic) of tonsils and adenoids NOS

J36 Peritonsillar abscess   CC
INCLUDES   abscess of tonsil
           peritonsillar cellulitis
           quinsy
Use additional code (B95-B97) to identify infectious agent
EXCLUDES 1   *acute tonsillitis (J03.-)*
               chronic tonsillitis (J35.0)
               retropharyngeal abscess (J39.0)
               tonsillitis NOS (J03.9-)
CC Excl: J22, J36, J98.8-J98.9

✓4ᵗʰ **J37 Chronic laryngitis and laryngotracheitis**

Use additional code to identify:
exposure to environmental tobacco smoke (Z77.22)
exposure to tobacco smoke in the perinatal period (P96.81)
history of tobacco use (Z87.891)
infectious agent (B95-B97)
occupational exposure to environmental tobacco smoke (Z57.31)
tobacco dependence (F17.-)
tobacco use (Z72.0)

J37.0 Chronic laryngitis
Catarrhal laryngitis
Hypertrophic laryngitis
Sicca laryngitis
EXCLUDES 2   *acute laryngitis (J04.0)*
               obstructive (acute) laryngitis (J05.0)

N Newborn: 0   P Pediatric: 0-17   M Maternity: 12-55   A Adult: 15-124   MCC Major CC Condition   PDx MCC PDx acts as own MCC   CC CC Condition   PDx CC PDx acts as own CC

632   ICD-10-CM Draft (2015)

J37.1　**Chronic laryngotracheitis**
Laryngitis, chronic, with tracheitis (chronic)
Tracheitis, chronic, with laryngitis
EXCLUDES 1　*chronic tracheitis (J42)*
EXCLUDES 2　*acute laryngotracheitis (J04.2)*
acute tracheitis (J04.1)

✓4ᵗʰ **J38**　**Diseases of vocal cords and larynx, not elsewhere classified**
Use additional code to identify:
exposure to environmental tobacco smoke (Z77.22)
exposure to tobacco smoke in the perinatal period (P96.81)
history of tobacco use (Z87.891)
occupational exposure to environmental tobacco smoke (Z57.31)
tobacco dependence (F17.-)
tobacco use (Z72.0)
EXCLUDES 1　*congenital laryngeal stridor (P28.89)*
obstructive laryngitis (acute) (J05.0)
postprocedural subglottic stenosis (J95.5)
stridor (R06.1)
ulcerative laryngitis (J04.0)

✓5ᵗʰ **J38.0**　**Paralysis of vocal cords and larynx**
Laryngoplegia
Paralysis of glottis

　　J38.00　**Paralysis of vocal cords and larynx, unspecified**
　　J38.01　**Paralysis of vocal cords and larynx, unilateral**
　　J38.02　**Paralysis of vocal cords and larynx, bilateral**

J38.1　**Polyp of vocal cord and larynx**
EXCLUDES 1　*adenomatous polyps (D14.1)*

J38.2　**Nodules of vocal cords**
Chorditis (fibrinous)(nodosa)(tuberosa)
Singer's nodes
Teacher's nodes

J38.3　**Other diseases of vocal cords**
Abscess of vocal cords
Cellulitis of vocal cords
Granuloma of vocal cords
Leukokeratosis of vocal cords
Leukoplakia of vocal cords

J38.4　**Edema of larynx**
Edema (of) glottis
Subglottic edema
Supraglottic edema
EXCLUDES 1　*acute obstructive laryngitis [croup] (J05.0)*
edematous laryngitis (J04.0)

J38.5　**Laryngeal spasm**
Laryngismus (stridulus)

J38.6　**Stenosis of larynx**

J38.7　**Other diseases of larynx**
Abscess of larynx　　　　Pachyderma of larynx
Cellulitis of larynx　　　　Perichondritis of larynx
Disease of larynx NOS　　Ulcer of larynx
Necrosis of larynx

✓4ᵗʰ **J39**　**Other diseases of upper respiratory tract**
EXCLUDES 1　*acute respiratory infection NOS (J22)*
acute upper respiratory infection (J06.9)
upper respiratory inflammation due to chemicals, gases, fumes or vapors (J68.2)

J39.0　**Retropharyngeal and parapharyngeal abscess**　CC
Peripharyngeal abscess
EXCLUDES 1　*peritonsillar abscess (J36)*
CC Excl: J22, J39.0-J39.1, J98.8-J98.9

J39.1　**Other abscess of pharynx**　CC
Cellulitis of pharynx
Nasopharyngeal abscess
CC Excl: See code: J39.0

J39.2　**Other diseases of pharynx**
Cyst of pharynx
Edema of pharynx
EXCLUDES 2　*chronic pharyngitis (J31.2)*
ulcerative pharyngitis (J02.9)

J39.3　**Upper respiratory tract hypersensitivity reaction, site unspecified**
EXCLUDES 1　*hypersensitivity reaction of upper respiratory tract, such as:*
extrinsic allergic alveolitis (J67.9)
pneumoconiosis (J60-J67.9)

J39.8　**Other specified diseases of upper respiratory tract**

J39.9　**Disease of upper respiratory tract, unspecified**

Chronic lower respiratory diseases (J40-J47)

EXCLUDES 1　*bronchitis due to chemicals, gases, fumes and vapors (J68.0)*
EXCLUDES 2　*cystic fibrosis (E84.-)*

J40　**Bronchitis, not specified as acute or chronic**
Bronchitis NOS
Bronchitis with tracheitis NOS
Catarrhal bronchitis
Tracheobronchitis NOS
Use additional code to identify:
exposure to environmental tobacco smoke (Z77.22)
exposure to tobacco smoke in the perinatal period (P96.81)
history of tobacco use (Z87.891)
occupational exposure to environmental tobacco smoke (Z57.31)
tobacco dependence (F17.-)
tobacco use (Z72.0)
EXCLUDES 1　*acute bronchitis (J20.-)*
allergic bronchitis NOS (J45.909)
asthmatic bronchitis NOS (J45.9-)
bronchitis due to chemicals, gases, fumes and vapors (J68.0)

✓4ᵗʰ **J41**　**Simple and mucopurulent chronic bronchitis**
Use additional code to identify:
exposure to environmental tobacco smoke (Z77.22)
exposure to tobacco smoke in the perinatal period (P96.81)
history of tobacco use (Z87.891)
occupational exposure to environmental tobacco smoke (Z57.31)
tobacco dependence (F17.-)
tobacco use (Z72.0)
EXCLUDES 1　*chronic bronchitis NOS (J42)*
chronic obstructive bronchitis (J44.-)

J41.0　**Simple chronic bronchitis**
J41.1　**Mucopurulent chronic bronchitis**
J41.8　**Mixed simple and mucopurulent chronic bronchitis**

J42　**Unspecified chronic bronchitis**
Chronic bronchitis NOS
Chronic tracheitis
Chronic tracheobronchitis
Use additional code to identify:
exposure to environmental tobacco smoke (Z77.22)
exposure to tobacco smoke in the perinatal period (P96.81)
history of tobacco use (Z87.891)
occupational exposure to environmental tobacco smoke (Z57.31)
tobacco dependence (F17.-)
tobacco use (Z72.0)
EXCLUDES 1　*chronic asthmatic bronchitis (J44.-)*
chronic bronchitis with airways obstruction (J44.-)
chronic emphysematous bronchitis (J44.-)
chronic obstructive pulmonary disease NOS (J44.9)
simple and mucopurulent chronic bronchitis (J41.-)

✓4ᵗʰ **J43**　**Emphysema**
Use additional code to identify:
exposure to environmental tobacco smoke (Z77.22)
history of tobacco use (Z87.891)
occupational exposure to environmental tobacco smoke (Z57.31)
tobacco dependence (F17.-)
tobacco use (Z72.0)
EXCLUDES 1　*compensatory emphysema (J98.3)*
emphysema due to inhalation of chemicals, gases, fumes or vapors (J68.4)
emphysema with chronic (obstructive) bronchitis (J44.-)
emphysematous (obstructive) bronchitis (J44.-)
interstitial emphysema (J98.2)
mediastinal emphysema (J98.2)
neonatal interstitial emphysema (P25.0)
surgical (subcutaneous) emphysema (T81.82)
traumatic subcutaneous emphysema (T79.7)

J43.0　**Unilateral pulmonary emphysema [MacLeod's syndrome]**
Swyer-James syndrome
Unilateral emphysema
Unilateral hyperlucent lung
Unilateral pulmonary artery functional hypoplasia
Unilateral transparency of lung

J43.1　**Panlobular emphysema**
Panacinar emphysema

J43.2　**Centrilobular emphysema**

J43.8　**Other emphysema**

J43.9　**Emphysema, unspecified**
Bullous emphysema (lung)(pulmonary)
Emphysema (lung)(pulmonary) NOS
Emphysematous bleb
Vesicular emphysema (lung)(pulmonary)

☑ Additional Character Required　✓x7ᵗʰ Xtension Alert　Unacceptable PDx　Manifestation　Hospital Acquired Condition　EXCLUDES 1 Not Coded Here　EXCLUDES 2 Not Included Here

Diseases of the Respiratory System

J44–J63.4

✓4th **J44 Other chronic obstructive pulmonary disease**
INCLUDES asthma with chronic obstructive pulmonary disease
chronic asthmatic (obstructive) bronchitis
chronic bronchitis with airways obstruction
chronic bronchitis with emphysema
chronic emphysematous bronchitis
chronic obstructive asthma
chronic obstructive bronchitis
chronic obstructive tracheobronchitis
Code also type of asthma, if applicable (J45.-)
Use additional code to identify:
exposure to environmental tobacco smoke (Z77.22)
history of tobacco use (Z87.891)
occupational exposure to environmental tobacco smoke (Z57.31)
tobacco dependence (F17.-)
tobacco use (Z72.0)
EXCLUDES 1 bronchiectasis (J47.-)
chronic bronchitis NOS (J42)
chronic simple and mucopurulent bronchitis (J41.-)
chronic tracheitis (J42)
chronic tracheobronchitis (J42)
emphysema without chronic bronchitis (J43.-)
lung diseases due to external agents (J60-J70)
AHA: 2013, 4Q, 109

J44.0 Chronic obstructive pulmonary disease with acute lower CC
respiratory infection
Use additional code to identify the infection
CC Excl: J10.08, J41.1-J42, J44.0-J44.1

J44.1 Chronic obstructive pulmonary disease with (acute) CC
exacerbation
Decompensated COPD
Decompensated COPD with (acute) exacerbation
EXCLUDES 2 chronic obstructive pulmonary disease [COPD] with
acute bronchitis (J44.0)
CC Excl: See code: J44.0

J44.9 Chronic obstructive pulmonary disease, unspecified
Chronic obstructive airway disease NOS
Chronic obstructive lung disease NOS
AHA: 2013, 4Q, 129

✓4th **J45 Asthma**
INCLUDES allergic (predominantly) asthma
allergic bronchitis NOS
allergic rhinitis with asthma
atopic asthma
extrinsic allergic asthma
hay fever with asthma
idiosyncratic asthma
intrinsic nonallergic asthma
nonallergic asthma
Use additional code to identify:
exposure to environmental tobacco smoke (Z77.22)
exposure to tobacco smoke in the perinatal period (P96.81)
history of tobacco use (Z87.891)
occupational exposure to environmental tobacco smoke (Z57.31)
tobacco dependence (F17.-)
tobacco use (Z72.0)
EXCLUDES 1 detergent asthma (J69.8)
eosinophilic asthma (J82)
lung diseases due to external agents (J60-J70)
miner's asthma (J60)
wheezing NOS (R06.2)
wood asthma (J67.8)
EXCLUDES 2 asthma with chronic obstructive pulmonary disease (J44.9)
chronic asthmatic (obstructive) bronchitis (J44.9)
chronic obstructive asthma (J44.9)

CC Excl: For CC codes in category J45, unless otherwise noted:
J10.08, J22, J45.998, J98.4, J98.8-J99, R91.1

✓5th **J45.2 Mild intermittent asthma**
J45.20 Mild intermittent asthma, uncomplicated
Mild intermittent asthma NOS
J45.21 Mild intermittent asthma with (acute) CC
exacerbation
J45.22 Mild intermittent asthma with status CC
asthmaticus

✓5th **J45.3 Mild persistent asthma**
J45.30 Mild persistent asthma, uncomplicated
Mild persistent asthma NOS
J45.31 Mild persistent asthma with (acute) exacerbation CC
J45.32 Mild persistent asthma with status asthmaticus CC

✓5th **J45.4 Moderate persistent asthma**
J45.40 Moderate persistent asthma, uncomplicated
Moderate persistent asthma NOS
J45.41 Moderate persistent asthma with (acute) CC
exacerbation
J45.42 Moderate persistent asthma with status CC
asthmaticus

✓5th **J45.5 Severe persistent asthma**
J45.50 Severe persistent asthma, uncomplicated
Severe persistent asthma NOS
J45.51 Severe persistent asthma with (acute) CC
exacerbation
J45.52 Severe persistent asthma with status CC
asthmaticus

✓5th **J45.9 Other and unspecified asthma**
✓6th **J45.90 Unspecified asthma**
Asthmatic bronchitis NOS
Childhood asthma NOS
Late onset asthma
J45.901 Unspecified asthma with (acute) CC
exacerbation
J45.902 Unspecified asthma with status CC
asthmaticus
J45.909 Unspecified asthma, uncomplicated
Asthma NOS
✓6th **J45.99 Other asthma**
J45.990 Exercise induced bronchospasm
J45.991 Cough variant asthma
J45.998 Other asthma

✓4th **J47 Bronchiectasis**
INCLUDES bronchiolectasis
Use additional code to identify:
exposure to environmental tobacco smoke (Z77.22)
exposure to tobacco smoke in the perinatal period (P96.81)
history of tobacco use (Z87.891)
occupational exposure to environmental tobacco smoke (Z57.31)
tobacco dependence (F17.-)
tobacco use (Z72.0)
EXCLUDES 1 congenital bronchiectasis (Q33.4)
tuberculous bronchiectasis (current disease) (A15.0)

J47.0 Bronchiectasis with acute lower respiratory infection CC
Bronchiectasis with acute bronchitis
CC Excl: A17.9, A18.82, A18.84, A18.89, J09.X2, J10.1, J11.1, J44.9,
J47.0-J47.1, J68.1, J68.4-J68.9, Q33.4

J47.1 Bronchiectasis with (acute) exacerbation CC
CC Excl: See code: J47.0

J47.9 Bronchiectasis, uncomplicated
Bronchiectasis NOS

Lung diseases due to external agents (J60-J70)
EXCLUDES 2 asthma (J45.-)
malignant neoplasm of bronchus and lung (C34.-)

J60 Coalworker's pneumoconiosis A
Anthracosilicosis
Anthracosis
Black lung disease
Coalworker's lung
EXCLUDES 1 coalworker pneumoconiosis with tuberculosis, any type in A15
(J65)

J61 Pneumoconiosis due to asbestos and other mineral fibers A
Asbestosis
EXCLUDES 1 pleural plaque with asbestosis (J92.0)
pneumoconiosis with tuberculosis, any type in A15 (J65)

✓4th **J62 Pneumoconiosis due to dust containing silica**
INCLUDES silicotic fibrosis (massive) of lung
EXCLUDES 1 pneumoconiosis with tuberculosis, any type in A15 (J65)
J62.0 Pneumoconiosis due to talc dust
J62.8 Pneumoconiosis due to other dust containing silica
Silicosis NOS

✓4th **J63 Pneumoconiosis due to other inorganic dusts**
EXCLUDES 1 pneumoconiosis with tuberculosis, any type in A15 (J65)
J63.0 Aluminosis (of lung)
J63.1 Bauxite fibrosis (of lung)
J63.2 Berylliosis
J63.3 Graphite fibrosis (of lung)
J63.4 Siderosis

N Newborn: 0   P Pediatric: 0-17   M Maternity: 12-55   A Adult: 15-124   MCC Major CC Condition   PDx MCC PDx acts as own MCC   CC CC Condition   PDx CC PDx acts as own CC

634   ICD-10-CM Draft (2015)

J63.5 **Stannosis**

J63.6 **Pneumoconiosis due to other specified inorganic dusts**

J64 **Unspecified pneumoconiosis**
  EXCLUDES 1 *pneumoconiosis with tuberculosis, any type in A15 (J65)*

J65 **Pneumoconiosis associated with tuberculosis**
  Any condition in J60-J64 with tuberculosis, any type in A15
  Silicotuberculosis

✓4th **J66 Airway disease due to specific organic dust**
  EXCLUDES 2 *allergic alveolitis (J67.-)*
         asbestosis (J61)
         bagassosis (J67.1)
         farmer's lung (J67.0)
         hypersensitivity pneumonitis due to organic dust (J67.-)
         reactive airways dysfunction syndrome (J68.3)

  J66.0 **Byssinosis**
       Airway disease due to cotton dust

  J66.1 **Flax-dressers' disease**

  J66.2 **Cannabinosis**

  J66.8 **Airway disease due to other specific organic dusts**

✓4th **J67 Hypersensitivity pneumonitis due to organic dust**
  INCLUDES allergic alveolitis and pneumonitis due to inhaled organic
         dust and particles of fungal, actinomycetic or other
         origin
  EXCLUDES 1 *pneumonitis due to inhalation of chemicals, gases, fumes or*
         vapors (J68.0)

  CC Excl: For CC codes in category J67, unless otherwise noted:
  A15.0-A15.6, A15.8-A15.9, A17.9, A18.82, A18.84, A18.89, A21.2,
  A22.1, A31.0, A37.01, A37.11, A37.81, A37.91, A42.0, A43.0, A48.1,
  B25.0, B39.0-B39.2, B44.0, B58.3, B59, B67.1, J09.X1-J09.X2, J10.00-
  J10.1, J11.00-J11.1, J12.0-J12.3, J12.89-J18.1, J18.8-J18.9, J22, J44.9,
  J47.0-J70.4, J70.8-J70.9, J98.4, J98.8-J99, Q33.4, R91.1

  J67.0 **Farmer's lung**
       Harvester's lung
       Haymaker's lung
       Moldy hay disease

  J67.1 **Bagassosis**
       Bagasse disease
       Bagasse pneumonitis

  J67.2 **Bird fancier's lung**
       Budgerigar fancier's disease or lung
       Pigeon fancier's disease or lung

  J67.3 **Suberosis**
       Corkhandler's disease or lung
       Corkworker's disease or lung

  J67.4 **Maltworker's lung**
       Alveolitis due to Aspergillus clavatus

  J67.5 **Mushroom-worker's lung**

  J67.6 **Maple-bark-stripper's lung**
       Alveolitis due to Cryptostroma corticale
       Cryptostromosis

  J67.7 **Air conditioner and humidifier lung** `CC`
       Allergic alveolitis due to fungal, thermophilic actinomycetes and
           other organisms growing in ventilation [air conditioning]
           systems

  J67.8 **Hypersensitivity pneumonitis due to other organic dusts** `CC`
       Cheese-washer's lung
       Coffee-worker's lung
       Fish-meal worker's lung
       Furrier's lung
       Sequoiosis

  J67.9 **Hypersensitivity pneumonitis due to unspecified organic dust** `CC`
       Allergic alveolitis (extrinsic) NOS
       Hypersensitivity pneumonitis NOS

✓4th **J68 Respiratory conditions due to inhalation of chemicals, gases, fumes and vapors**
  Code first (T51-T65) to identify cause
  Use additional code to identify associated respiratory conditions, such
     as:
     acute respiratory failure (J96.0-)

  CC Excl: For CC/MCC codes in category J68, unless otherwise noted: See code: J67

  J68.0 **Bronchitis and pneumonitis due to chemicals, gases, fumes and vapors** `CC`
       Chemical bronchitis (acute)

  J68.1 **Pulmonary edema due to chemicals, gases, fumes and vapors** `MCC`
       Chemical pulmonary edema (acute) (chronic)
       EXCLUDES 1 *pulmonary edema (acute) (chronic) NOS (J81.-)*

  J68.2 **Upper respiratory inflammation due to chemicals, gases, fumes and vapors, not elsewhere classified**

  J68.3 **Other acute and subacute respiratory conditions due to chemicals, gases, fumes and vapors**
       Reactive airways dysfunction syndrome

  J68.4 **Chronic respiratory conditions due to chemicals, gases, fumes and vapors**
       Emphysema (diffuse) (chronic) due to inhalation of chemicals,
           gases, fumes and vapors
       Obliterative bronchiolitis (chronic) (subacute) due to inhalation
           of chemicals, gases, fumes and vapors
       Pulmonary fibrosis (chronic) due to inhalation of chemicals,
           gases, fumes and vapors
       EXCLUDES 1 *chronic pulmonary edema due to chemicals, gases,*
              fumes and vapors (J68.1)

  J68.8 **Other respiratory conditions due to chemicals, gases, fumes and vapors**

  J68.9 **Unspecified respiratory condition due to chemicals, gases, fumes and vapors**

✓4th **J69 Pneumonitis due to solids and liquids**
  EXCLUDES 1 *neonatal aspiration syndromes (P24.-)*
         postprocedural pneumonitis (J95.4)

  CC Excl: For MCC codes in category J69, unless otherwise noted: See code: J67

  J69.0 **Pneumonitis due to inhalation of food and vomit** `MCC`
       Aspiration pneumonia NOS
       Aspiration pneumonia (due to) food (regurgitated)
       Aspiration pneumonia (due to) gastric secretions
       Aspiration pneumonia (due to) milk
       Aspiration pneumonia (due to) vomit
       Code also any associated foreign body in respiratory tract (T17.-)
       EXCLUDES 1 *chemical pneumonitis due to anesthesia (J95.4)*
              obstetric aspiration pneumonia (O74.0)

  J69.1 **Pneumonitis due to inhalation of oils and essences** `MCC`
       Exogenous lipoid pneumonia
       Lipid pneumonia NOS
       Code first (T51-T65) to identify substance
       EXCLUDES 1 *endogenous lipoid pneumonia (J84.89)*

  J69.8 **Pneumonitis due to inhalation of other solids and liquids** `MCC`
       Pneumonitis due to aspiration of blood
       Pneumonitis due to aspiration of detergent
       Code first (T51-T65) to identify substance

✓4th **J70 Respiratory conditions due to other external agents**

  CC Excl: For CC codes in category J70, unless otherwise noted: See code: J67

  J70.0 **Acute pulmonary manifestations due to radiation** `CC`
       Radiation pneumonitis
       Use additional code (W88-W90, X39.0-) to identify the external
           cause

  J70.1 **Chronic and other pulmonary manifestations due to radiation** `CC`
       Fibrosis of lung following radiation
       Use additional code (W88-W90, X39.0-) to identify the external
           cause

  J70.2 **Acute drug-induced interstitial lung disorders**
       Use additional code for adverse effect, if applicable, to identify
           drug (T36-T50 with fifth or sixth character 5)
       EXCLUDES 1 *interstitial pneumonia NOS (J84.9)*
              lymphoid interstitial pneumonia (J84.2)

  J70.3 **Chronic drug-induced interstitial lung disorders**
       Use additional code for adverse effect, if applicable, to identify
           drug (T36-T50 with fifth or sixth character 5)
       EXCLUDES 1 *interstitial pneumonia NOS (J84.9)*
              lymphoid interstitial pneumonia (J84.2)

  J70.4 **Drug-induced interstitial lung disorders, unspecified**
       Use additional code for adverse effect, if applicable, to identify
           drug (T36-T50 with fifth or sixth character 5)
       EXCLUDES 1 *interstitial pneumonia NOS (J84.9)*
              lymphoid interstitial pneumonia (J84.2)

  J70.5 **Respiratory conditions due to smoke inhalation**
       Smoke inhalation NOS
       EXCLUDES 1 *smoke inhalation due to chemicals, gases, fumes and*
              vapors (J68.9)
       AHA: 2013, 4Q, 121

Diseases of the Respiratory System

J70.8–J84.848

J70.8   **Respiratory conditions due to other specified external agents**
Code first (T51-T65) to identify the external agent

J70.9   **Respiratory conditions due to unspecified external agent**
Code first (T51-T65) to identify the external agent

Other respiratory diseases principally affecting the interstitium (J80-J84)

J80   **Acute respiratory distress syndrome**   `cc`
Acute respiratory distress syndrome in adult or child
Adult hyaline membrane disease
EXCLUDES1   *respiratory distress syndrome in newborn (perinatal) (P22.0)*
CC Excl: J22, J80, J96.00-J96.92, J98.8-J98.9, R09.2

√4th J81   **Pulmonary edema**
Use additional code to identify:
exposure to environmental tobacco smoke (Z77.22)
history of tobacco use (Z87.891)
occupational exposure to environmental tobacco smoke (Z57.31)
tobacco dependence (F17.-)
tobacco use (Z72.0)
EXCLUDES1   *chemical (acute) pulmonary edema (J68.1)*
hypostatic pneumonia (J18.2)
passive pneumonia (J18.2)
pulmonary edema due to external agents (J60-J70)
pulmonary edema with heart disease NOS (I50.1)
pulmonary edema with heart failure (I50.1)

   J81.0   **Acute pulmonary edema**   `MCC`
Acute edema of lung
CC Excl: I09.81, I50.9, J22, J81.0, J98.8-J98.9

   J81.1   **Chronic pulmonary edema**   `cc`
Pulmonary congestion (chronic) (passive)
Pulmonary edema NOS
CC Excl: J18.2, J22, J81.1, J98.4, J98.8-J99, R91.1

J82   **Pulmonary eosinophilia, not elsewhere classified**   `cc`
Allergic pneumonia
Eosinophilic asthma
Eosinophilic pneumonia
Löffler's pneumonia
Tropical (pulmonary) eosinophilia NOS
EXCLUDES1   *pulmonary eosinophilia due to aspergillosis (B44.-)*
pulmonary eosinophilia due to drugs (J70.2-J70.4)
pulmonary eosinophilia due to specified parasitic infection (B50-B83)
pulmonary eosinophilia due to systemic connective tissue disorders (M30-M36)
pulmonary infiltrate NOS (R91.8)
CC Excl: A15.0-A15.6, A15.8-A15.9, A17.9, A18.82, A18.84, A18.89, A20.2, A21.1, A22.1, A31.0, A37.01, A37.11, A37.81, A37.91, A42.0, A43.0, A48.1, B25.0, B39.0-B39.2, B44.0, B58.3, B59, B67.1, J09.X1-J09.X2, J10.00-J10.1, J11.00-J11.1, J12.0-J12.3, J12.89-J18.1, J18.8-J18.9, J22, J47.0-J70.4, J70.8-J70.9, J82, J98.4, J98.8-J99, Q33.4, R91.1

√4th J84   **Other interstitial pulmonary diseases**
EXCLUDES1   *drug-induced interstitial lung disorders (J70.2-J70.4)*
interstitial emphysema (J98.2)
lung diseases due to external agents (J60-J70)

   √5th J84.0   **Alveolar and parieto-alveolar conditions**

     CC Excl: For CC codes in subcategory J84.0, unless otherwise noted: A15.0-A15.6, A15.8-A15.9, A17.9, A18.82, A18.84, A18.89, J22, J44.9, J47.0-J70.4, J70.8-J70.9, J84.01-J84.82, J84.89-J84.9, J98.4, J98.8-J99, Q33.4, R91.1

     J84.01   **Alveolar proteinosis**   `cc`
     J84.02   **Pulmonary alveolar microlithiasis**   `cc`
     J84.03   *Idiopathic pulmonary hemosiderosis*   `cc`
Essential brown induration of lung
Code first underlying disease, such as:
disorders of iron metabolism (E83.1-)
EXCLUDES1   *acute idiopathic pulmonary hemorrhage in infants [AIPHI] (R04.81)*
     J84.09   **Other alveolar and parieto-alveolar conditions**   `cc`

   √5th J84.1   **Other interstitial pulmonary diseases with fibrosis**
EXCLUDES1   *pulmonary fibrosis (chronic) due to inhalation of chemicals, gases, fumes or vapors (J68.4)*
pulmonary fibrosis (chronic) following radiation (J70.1)

     CC Excl: For CC codes in subcategory J84.1, unless otherwise noted: See code: J84.0

     J84.10   **Pulmonary fibrosis, unspecified**
Capillary fibrosis of lung
Cirrhosis of lung (chronic) NOS
Fibrosis of lung (atrophic) (chronic) (confluent) (massive) (perialveolar) (peribronchial) NOS
Induration of lung (chronic) NOS
Postinflammatory pulmonary fibrosis

     √6th J84.11   **Idiopathic interstitial pneumonia**
EXCLUDES1   *lymphoid interstitial pneumonia (J84.2)*
pneumocystis pneumonia (B59)

       J84.111   **Idiopathic interstitial pneumonia, not otherwise specified**
       J84.112   **Idiopathic pulmonary fibrosis**
Cryptogenic fibrosing alveolitis
Idiopathic fibrosing alveolitis
       J84.113   **Idiopathic non-specific interstitial pneumonitis**
EXCLUDES1   *non-specific interstitial pneumonia NOS, or due to known underlying cause (J84.89)*
       J84.114   **Acute interstitial pneumonitis**   `cc`
Hamman-Rich syndrome
EXCLUDES1   *pneumocystis pneumonia (B59)*
       J84.115   **Respiratory bronchiolitis interstitial lung disease**
       J84.116   **Cryptogenic organizing pneumonia**   `cc`
EXCLUDES1   *organizing pneumonia NOS, or due to known underlying cause (J84.89)*
       J84.117   **Desquamative interstitial pneumonia**   `cc`

     J84.17   *Other interstitial pulmonary diseases with fibrosis in diseases classified elsewhere*
Interstitial pneumonia (nonspecific) (usual) due to collagen vascular disease
Interstitial pneumonia (nonspecific) (usual) in diseases classified elsewhere
Organizing pneumonia due to collagen vascular disease
Organizing pneumonia in diseases classified elsewhere
Code first underlying disease, such as:
progressive systemic sclerosis (M34.0)
rheumatoid arthritis (M05.00-M06.9)
systemic lupus erythematosis (M32.0-M32.9)

   J84.2   **Lymphoid interstitial pneumonia**   `cc`
Lymphoid interstitial pneumonitis
CC Excl: See code: J84.0

   √5th J84.8   **Other specified interstitial pulmonary diseases**
EXCLUDES1   *exogenous lipoid pneumonia (J69.1)*
unspecified lipoid pneumonia (J69.1)

     J84.81   **Lymphangioleiomyomatosis**   `MCC` ♀
Lymphangiomyomatosis
CC Excl: See code: J84.0
     J84.82   **Adult pulmonary Langerhans cell histiocytosis**   `cc` `A`
Adult PLCH
CC Excl: See code: J84.0
     J84.83   **Surfactant mutations of the lung**   `MCC`
CC Excl: J84.83-J84.848, P22.0-P28.5, P28.89-P29.2, P29.4, P29.89-P29.9, P84, P94.1-P94.9, P96.0, P96.3-P96.5, P96.82-P96.89

   √6th J84.84   **Other interstitial lung diseases of childhood**

     CC Excl: For MCC codes in subcategory J84.84, unless otherwise noted: See code: J84.83

     J84.841   **Neuroendocrine cell hyperplasia of infancy**   `MCC`
     J84.842   **Pulmonary interstitial glycogenosis**   `MCC`
     J84.843   **Alveolar capillary dysplasia with vein misalignment**   `MCC`
     J84.848   **Other interstitial lung diseases of childhood**   `MCC`

N Newborn: 0   P Pediatric: 0-17   M Maternity: 12-55   A Adult: 15-124   `MCC` Major CC Condition   `PDx MCC` PDx acts as own MCC   `cc` CC Condition   `PDx CC` PDx acts as own CC

636   ICD-10-CM Draft (2015)

J84.89   **Other specified interstitial pulmonary diseases**
   Endogenous lipoid pneumonia
   Interstitial pneumonitis
   Non-specific interstitial pneumonitis NOS
   Organizing pneumonia due to known underlying cause
   Organizing pneumonia NOS
   Code first, if applicable:
    poisoning due to drug or toxin (T51-T65 with fifth or sixth character to indicate intent), for toxic pneumonopathy
    underlying cause of pneumonopathy, if known
   Use additional code, for adverse effect, to identify drug (T36-T50 with fifth or sixth character 5), if drug-induced
   EXCLUDES 1   *cryptogenic organizing pneumonia (J84.116)*
      idiopathic non-specific interstitial pneumonitis (J84.113)
      lipoid pneumonia, exogenous or unspecified (J69.1)
      lymphoid interstitial pneumonia (J84.2)

J84.9   **Interstitial pulmonary disease, unspecified**   `CC`
   Interstitial pneumonia NOS
   CC Excl: See code: J84.0

Suppurative and necrotic conditions of the lower respiratory tract (J85-J86)

✓4ᵗʰ **J85**   **Abscess of lung and mediastinum**
   Use additional code (B95-B97) to identify infectious agent.

   J85.0   **Gangrene and necrosis of lung**   `MCC`
    CC Excl: A06.5, A15.6, A15.8-A15.9, A17.9, A18.82, A18.84, A18.89, J22, J85.0-J85.2, J98.8-J98.9

   J85.1   **Abscess of lung with pneumonia**   `MCC`
    Code also the type of pneumonia
    CC Excl: See code: J85.0

   J85.2   **Abscess of lung without pneumonia**   `MCC`
    Abscess of lung NOS
    CC Excl: See code: J85.0

   J85.3   **Abscess of mediastinum**   `MCC`
    CC Excl: J22, J85.3, J98.8-J98.9

✓4ᵗʰ **J86**   **Pyothorax**
   Use additional code (B95-B97) to identify infectious agent
   EXCLUDES 1   *abscess of lung (J85.-)*
      pyothorax due to tuberculosis (A15.6)

   J86.0   **Pyothorax with fistula**   `MCC`
    Bronchocutaneous fistula
    Bronchopleural fistula
    Hepatopleural fistula
    Mediastinal fistula
    Pleural fistula
    Thoracic fistula
    Any condition classifiable to J86.9 with fistula
    CC Excl: J22-J86.9, J98.4, J98.8-J99, R91.1

   J86.9   **Pyothorax without fistula**   `MCC`
    Abscess of pleura
    Abscess of thorax
    Empyema (chest) (lung) (pleura)
    Fibrinopurulent pleurisy
    Purulent pleurisy
    Pyopneumothorax
    Septic pleurisy
    Seropurulent pleurisy
    Suppurative pleurisy
    CC Excl: See code: J86.0

Other diseases of the pleura (J90-J94)

J90   **Pleural effusion, not elsewhere classified**   `CC`
   Encysted pleurisy
   Pleural effusion NOS
   Pleurisy with effusion (exudative) (serous)
   EXCLUDES 1   *chylous (pleural) effusion (J94.0)*
      malignant pleural effusion (J91.0))
      pleurisy NOS (R09.1)
      tuberculous pleural effusion (A15.6)
   CC Excl: A15.0-A15.6, A15.8-A15.9, A17.9, A18.82, A18.84, A18.89, J22, J90-J92.9, J94.0-J94.9, J98.4, J98.8-J99, R09.1, R91.1

✓4ᵗʰ **J91**   **Pleural effusion in conditions classified elsewhere**
   EXCLUDES 2   *pleural effusion in heart failure (I50.-)*
      pleural effusion in systemic lupus erythematosus (M32.13)

   J91.0   ***Malignant pleural effusion***   `CC`
    Code first underlying neoplasm
    CC Excl: C45.7-C45.9, C76.8, C78.2-C78.39, C79.89-C7A.00, C7A.098-C7B.00, C7B.09-C80.2, D49.81-D49.9, J90-J91.0, J94.0, J94.2

   J91.8   ***Pleural effusion in other conditions classified elsewhere***   `CC`
    Code first underlying disease, such as:
     filariasis (B74.0-B74.9)
     influenza (J09.X2, J10.1, J11.1)
    CC Excl: See code: J90

✓4ᵗʰ **J92**   **Pleural plaque**
   `INCLUDES`   pleural thickening

   J92.0   **Pleural plaque with presence of asbestos**

   J92.9   **Pleural plaque without asbestos**
    Pleural plaque NOS

✓4ᵗʰ **J93**   **Pneumothorax and air leak**
   EXCLUDES 1   *congenital or perinatal pneumothorax (P25.1)*
      postprocedural air leak (J95.812)
      postprocedural pneumothorax (J95.811)
      traumatic pneumothorax (S27.0)
      tuberculous (current disease) pneumothorax (A15.-)
      pyopneumothorax (J86.-)

   CC Excl: For CC/MCC codes in category J93, unless otherwise noted: J22, J93.9, J95.811-J95.812, J98.4, J98.8-J99, R91.1

   J93.0   **Spontaneous tension pneumothorax**   `MCC`

   ✓5ᵗʰ **J93.1**   **Other spontaneous pneumothorax**

    J93.11   **Primary spontaneous pneumothorax**   `CC`

    J93.12   **Secondary spontaneous pneumothorax**   `CC`
     Code first underlying condition, such as:
      catamenial pneumothorax due to endometriosis (N80.8)
      cystic fibrosis (E84.-)
      eosinophilic pneumonia (J82)
      lymphangioleiomyomatosis (J84.81)
      malignant neoplasm of bronchus and lung (C34.-)
      Marfan's syndrome (Q87.4)
      pneumonia due to Pneumocystis carinii (B59)
      secondary malignant neoplasm of lung (C78.0-)
      spontaneous rupture of the esophagus (K22.3)

   ✓5ᵗʰ **J93.8**   **Other pneumothorax and air leak**

    J93.81   **Chronic pneumothorax**   `CC`

    J93.82   **Other air leak**   `CC`
     Persistent air leak

    J93.83   **Other pneumothorax**   `CC`
     Acute pneumothorax
     Spontaneous pneumothorax NOS

   J93.9   **Pneumothorax, unspecified**   `CC`
    Pneumothorax NOS

✓4ᵗʰ **J94**   **Other pleural conditions**
   EXCLUDES 1   *pleurisy NOS (R09.1)*
      traumatic hemopneumothorax (S27.2)
      traumatic hemothorax (S27.1)
      tuberculous pleural conditions (current disease) (A15.-)

   J94.0   **Chylous effusion**   `CC`
    Chyliform effusion
    CC Excl: See code: J90

   J94.1   **Fibrothorax**

   J94.2   **Hemothorax**   `CC`
    Hemopneumothorax
    CC Excl: See code: J90

   J94.8   **Other specified pleural conditions**   `CC`
    Hydropneumothorax
    Hydrothorax
    CC Excl: No excl

   J94.9   **Pleural condition, unspecified**

✓ Additional Character Required   √x7ᵗʰ Xtension Alert   Unacceptable PDx   Manifestation   Hospital Acquired Condition   *EXCLUDES 1* Not Coded Here   *EXCLUDES 2* Not Included Here

Intraoperative and postprocedural complications and disorders of respiratory system, not elsewhere classified (J95)

✓4ᵗʰ J95 Intraoperative and postprocedural complications and disorders of respiratory system, not elsewhere classified
EXCLUDES 2 aspiration pneumonia (J69.-)
emphysema (subcutaneous) resulting from a procedure (T81.82)
hypostatic pneumonia (J18.2)
pulmonary manifestations due to radiation (J70.0- J70.1)

✓5ᵗʰ J95.0 Tracheostomy complications
CC Excl: For CC codes in subcategory J95.0, unless otherwise noted: J22, J39.8, J95.00-J95.09, J98.01-J98.09, J98.8-J98.9

J95.00 Unspecified tracheostomy complication   CC
J95.01 Hemorrhage from tracheostomy stoma   CC
J95.02 Infection of tracheostomy stoma   CC
Use additional code to identify type of infection, such as:
cellulitis of neck (L03.8)
sepsis (A40, A41-)
J95.03 Malfunction of tracheostomy stoma   CC
Mechanical complication of tracheostomy stoma
Obstruction of tracheostomy airway
Tracheal stenosis due to tracheostomy
J95.04 Tracheo-esophageal fistula following tracheostomy   CC
J95.09 Other tracheostomy complication   CC

J95.1 Acute pulmonary insufficiency following thoracic surgery   MCC
EXCLUDES 2 functional disturbances following cardiac surgery (I97.0, I97.1-)
CC Excl: J22, J95.3, J95.821-J95.822, J98.8-J98.9

J95.2 Acute pulmonary insufficiency following nonthoracic surgery   MCC
EXCLUDES 2 functional disturbances following cardiac surgery (I97.0, I97.1-)
CC Excl: See code: J95.1

J95.3 Chronic pulmonary insufficiency following surgery   MCC
EXCLUDES 2 functional disturbances following cardiac surgery (I97.0, I97.1-)
CC Excl: See code: J95.1

J95.4 Chemical pneumonitis due to anesthesia   CC
Mendelson's syndrome
Postprocedural aspiration pneumonia
Use additional code for adverse effect, if applicable, to identify drug (T41.- with fifth or sixth character 5)
EXCLUDES 1 aspiration pneumonitis due to anesthesia complicating labor and delivery (O74.0)
aspiration pneumonitis due to anesthesia complicating pregnancy (O29)
aspiration pneumonitis due to anesthesia complicating the puerperium (O89.01)
CC Excl: D78.81-D78.89, E36.8, E89.810-E89.89, H59.011-H59.019, H59.031-H59.099, H59.811-H59.89, H95.811-H95.89, I97.3, J95.4-J95.5, J95.84, J95.851-J95.89, L76.81-L76.82, M96.89, N98.1-N98.9, T81.82XA, T81.89XA, T81.9XXA

J95.5 Postprocedural subglottic stenosis   CC
CC Excl: See code: J95.4

✓5ᵗʰ J95.6 Intraoperative hemorrhage and hematoma of a respiratory system organ or structure complicating a procedure
EXCLUDES 1 intraoperative hemorrhage and hematoma of a respiratory system organ or structure due to accidental puncture and laceration during procedure (J95.7-)
J95.61 Intraoperative hemorrhage and hematoma of a respiratory system organ or structure complicating a respiratory system procedure   CC
CC Excl: H95.811-H95.89, I85.01, I85.11, I97.3, J95.61-J95.62, J95.830-J95.831, K21.9, K22.8, K23-K25.0, K25.2, K25.4, K25.6, K26.0, K26.2, K26.4, K26.6, K27.0, K27.2, K27.4, K27.6, K28.0, K28.2, K28.4, K28.6, K29.01, K29.21, K29.31, K29.41, K29.51, K29.61, K29.71, K29.81, K29.91, K31.811, K55.21, K57.01, K57.11, K57.13, K57.21, K57.31, K57.33, K57.41, K57.51, K57.53, K57.81, K57.91, K57.93, K62.5, K92.0-K92.2, M96.89, N98.1-N98.9, P54.1-P54.3, T81.10XA, T81.11XA, T81.12XA, T81.19XA, T81.82XA, T81.89XA, T81.9XXA

J95.62 Intraoperative hemorrhage and hematoma of a respiratory system organ or structure complicating other procedure   CC
CC Excl: See code: J95.61

✓5ᵗʰ J95.7 Accidental puncture and laceration of a respiratory system organ or structure during a procedure
EXCLUDES 2 postprocedural pneumothorax (J95.811)
J95.71 Accidental puncture and laceration of a respiratory system organ or structure during a respiratory system procedure   CC
CC Excl: D78.11-D78.12, D78.81-D78.89, E36.11-E36.8, E89.810-E89.89, G96.11, G97.41-G97.49, H59.011-H59.019, H59.031-H59.099, H59.211-H59.229, H59.811-H59.89, H95.31-H95.32, H95.811-H95.89, I97.3, I97.51-I97.52, J95.71-J95.72, K91.71-K91.72, L76.11-L76.12, L76.81-L76.82, M96.820-M96.821, M96.89, N98.1-N98.9, N99.71-N99.72, T81.10XA, T81.11XA, T81.12XA, T81.19XA, T81.82XA, T81.89XA, T81.9XXA
J95.72 Accidental puncture and laceration of a respiratory system organ or structure during other procedure   CC
CC Excl: See code: J95.71

✓5ᵗʰ J95.8 Other intraoperative and postprocedural complications and disorders of respiratory system, not elsewhere classified
✓6ᵗʰ J95.81 Postprocedural pneumothorax and air leak
[9] J95.811 Postprocedural pneumothorax   CC
CC Excl: J22, J93.9, J95.811-J95.812, J98.4, J98.8-J99, R91.1
J95.812 Postprocedural air leak   CC
CC Excl: See code: J95.811
✓6ᵗʰ J95.82 Postprocedural respiratory failure
EXCLUDES 1 respiratory failure in other conditions (J96.-)
J95.821 Acute postprocedural respiratory failure   MCC
Postprocedural respiratory failure NOS
CC Excl: See code: J95.1
J95.822 Acute and chronic postprocedural respiratory failure   MCC
CC Excl: See code: J95.1
✓6ᵗʰ J95.83 Postprocedural hemorrhage and hematoma of a respiratory system organ or structure following a procedure
J95.830 Postprocedural hemorrhage and hematoma of a respiratory system organ or structure following a respiratory system procedure   CC
CC Excl: See code: J95.61
J95.831 Postprocedural hemorrhage and hematoma of a respiratory system organ or structure following other procedure   CC
CC Excl: See code: J95.61
J95.84 Transfusion-related acute lung injury (TRALI)   CC
CC Excl: See code: J95.4
✓6ᵗʰ J95.85 Complication of respirator [ventilator]
CC Excl: For CC codes in subcategory J95.0, unless otherwise noted: See code: J95.4
J95.850 Mechanical complication of respirator   CC
EXCLUDES 1 encounter for respirator [ventilator] dependence during power failure (Z99.12)
CC Excl: J95.850, Z99.12, Z99.81-Z99.89
J95.851 Ventilator associated pneumonia   CC
Ventilator associated pneumonitis
Use additional code to identify the organism, if known (B95.-, B96.-, B97.-)
EXCLUDES 1 ventilator lung in newborn (P27.8)
J95.859 Other complication of respirator [ventilator]   CC
J95.88 Other intraoperative complications of respiratory system, not elsewhere classified   CC
CC Excl: See code: J95.4

[9] HAC = as SDx not POA, in combination with one of the following procedure codes: 05H[M,N,P,Q]33Z or 0JH63XZ.

N Newborn: 0   P Pediatric: 0-17   M Maternity: 12-55   A Adult: 15-124   MCC Major CC Condition   PDx MCC PDx acts as own MCC   CC CC Condition   PDx CC PDx acts as own CC

638   ICD-10-CM Draft (2015)

J95.89   Other postprocedural complications and disorders of respiratory system, not elsewhere classified   CC

Use additional code to identify disorder, such as:
aspiration pneumonia (J69.-)
bacterial or viral pneumonia (J12-J18)
EXCLUDES 2   *acute pulmonary insufficiency following thoracic surgery (J95.1)*
postprocedural subglottic stenosis (J95.5)
CC Excl: See code: J95.4

Other diseases of the respiratory system (J96-J99)

J96   Respiratory failure, not elsewhere classified
EXCLUDES 1   *acute respiratory distress syndrome (J80)*
cardiorespiratory failure (R09.2)
newborn respiratory distress syndrome (P22.0)
postprocedural respiratory failure (J95.82-)
respiratory arrest (R09.2)
respiratory arrest of newborn (P28.81)
respiratory failure of newborn (P28.5)

CC Excl: For CC/MCC codes in category J96, unless otherwise noted: J22, J80, J96.00-J96.92, J98.8-J98.9, R09.2

J96.0   Acute respiratory failure
J96.00   Acute respiratory failure, unspecified whether with hypoxia or hypercapnia   MCC
AHA: 2013, 4Q, 121
J96.01   Acute respiratory failure with hypoxia   MCC
J96.02   Acute respiratory failure with hypercapnia   MCC

J96.1   Chronic respiratory failure
J96.10   Chronic respiratory failure, unspecified whether with hypoxia or hypercapnia   CC
J96.11   Chronic respiratory failure with hypoxia   CC
AHA: 2013, 4Q, 129
J96.12   Chronic respiratory failure with hypercapnia   CC

J96.2   Acute and chronic respiratory failure
Acute on chronic respiratory failure
J96.20   Acute and chronic respiratory failure, unspecified whether with hypoxia or hypercapnia   MCC
J96.21   Acute and chronic respiratory failure with hypoxia   MCC
J96.22   Acute and chronic respiratory failure with hypercapnia   MCC

J96.9   Respiratory failure, unspecified
J96.90   Respiratory failure, unspecified, unspecified whether with hypoxia or hypercapnia   MCC
J96.91   Respiratory failure, unspecified with hypoxia   MCC
J96.92   Respiratory failure, unspecified with hypercapnia   MCC

J98   Other respiratory disorders
Use additional code to identify:
exposure to environmental tobacco smoke (Z77.22)
exposure to tobacco smoke in the perinatal period (P96.81)
history of tobacco use (Z87.891)
occupational exposure to environmental tobacco smoke (Z57.31)
tobacco dependence (F17.-)
tobacco use (Z72.0)
EXCLUDES 1   *newborn apnea (P28.4)*
newborn sleep apnea (P28.3)
EXCLUDES 2   *apnea NOS (R06.81)*
sleep apnea (G47.3-)

J98.0   Diseases of bronchus, not elsewhere classified
J98.01   Acute bronchospasm
EXCLUDES 1   *acute bronchiolitis with bronchospasm (J21.-)*
acute bronchitis with bronchospasm (J20.-)
asthma (J45.-)
exercise induced bronchospasm (J45.990)
J98.09   Other diseases of bronchus, not elsewhere classified
Broncholithiasis
Calcification of bronchus
Stenosis of bronchus
Tracheobronchial collapse
Tracheobronchial dyskinesia
Ulcer of bronchus

J98.1   Pulmonary collapse
EXCLUDES 1   *therapeutic collapse of lung status (Z98.3)*
J98.11   Atelectasis   CC
EXCLUDES 1   *newborn atelectasis*
tuberculous atelectasis (current disease) (A15)
CC Excl: J22, J98.19, J98.8-J98.9
J98.19   Other pulmonary collapse   CC
CC Excl: See code: J98.11

J98.2   Interstitial emphysema
Mediastinal emphysema
EXCLUDES 1   *emphysema NOS (J43.9)*
emphysema in newborn (P25.0)
surgical emphysema (subcutaneous) (T81.82)
traumatic subcutaneous emphysema (T79.7)

J98.3   Compensatory emphysema

J98.4   Other disorders of lung
Calcification of lung
Cystic lung disease (acquired)
Lung disease NOS
Pulmolithiasis
EXCLUDES 1   *acute interstitial pneumonitis (J84.114)*
pulmonary insufficiency following surgery (J95.1-J95.2)

J98.5   Diseases of mediastinum, not elsewhere classified   MCC
Fibrosis of mediastinum
Hernia of mediastinum
Retraction of mediastinum
Mediastinitis
EXCLUDES 2   *abscess of mediastinum (J85.3)*
CC Excl: No excl

J98.6   Disorders of diaphragm
Diaphragmatitis
Paralysis of diaphragm
Relaxation of diaphragm
EXCLUDES 1   *congenital malformation of diaphragm NEC (Q79.1)*
congenital diaphragmatic hernia (Q79.0)
EXCLUDES 2   *diaphragmatic hernia (K44.-)*

J98.8   Other specified respiratory disorders
J98.9   Respiratory disorder, unspecified
Respiratory disease (chronic) NOS

J99   *Respiratory disorders in diseases classified elsewhere*
Code first underlying disease, such as:
amyloidosis (E85.-)
ankylosing spondylitis (M45)
congenital syphilis (A50.5)
cryoglobulinemia (D89.1)
early congenital syphilis (A50.0)
schistosomiasis (B65.0-B65.9)
EXCLUDES 1   *respiratory disorders in:*
amebiasis (A06.5)
blastomycosis (B40.0-B40.2)
candidiasis (B37.1)
coccidioidomycosis (B38.0-B38.2)
cystic fibrosis with pulmonary manifestations (E84.0)
dermatomyositis (M33.01, M33.11)
histoplasmosis (B39.0-B39.2)
late syphilis (A52.72, A52.73)
polymyositis (M33.21)
sicca syndrome (M35.02)
systemic lupus erythematosus (M32.13)
systemic sclerosis (M34.81)
Wegener's granulomatosis (M31.30-M31.31)

---

5 HAC = as SDx not POA, in combination with one of the following procedure codes: 021[0,1,2,3][0,4][9,A,J,K][3,8,9,C,F,W]; 021[0,1,2,3][0,4]Z[3,8,9,C,F].

✓ Additional Character Required   ✓x7th Xtension Alert   Unacceptable PDx   Manifestation   Hospital Acquired Condition   EXCLUDES 1 Not Coded Here   EXCLUDES 2 Not Included Here

Chapter 11. Diseases of the Digestive System (K00-K95)

EXCLUDES 2 certain conditions originating in the perinatal period (P04-P96)
certain infectious and parasitic diseases (A00-B99)
complications of pregnancy, childbirth and the puerperium (O00-O9A)
congenital malformations, deformations and chromosomal abnormalities (Q00-Q99)
endocrine, nutritional and metabolic diseases (E00-E88)
injury, poisoning and certain other consequences of external causes (S00-T88)
neoplasms (C00-D49)
symptoms, signs and abnormal clinical and laboratory findings, not elsewhere classified (R00-R94)

This chapter contains the following blocks:

K00-K14 Diseases of oral cavity and salivary glands
K20-K31 Diseases of esophagus, stomach and duodenum
K35-K38 Diseases of appendix
K40-K46 Hernia
K50-K52 Noninfective enteritis and colitis
K55-K64 Other diseases of intestines
K65-K68 Diseases of peritoneum and retroperitoneum
K70-K77 Diseases of liver
K80-K87 Disorders of gallbladder, biliary tract and pancreas
K90-K95 Other diseases of the digestive system

Diseases of oral cavity and salivary glands (K00-K14)

✓4th K00 Disorders of tooth development and eruption
EXCLUDES 2 embedded and impacted teeth (K01.-)

K00.0 Anodontia
Hypodontia
Oligodontia
EXCLUDES 1 acquired absence of teeth (K08.1-)

K00.1 Supernumerary teeth
Distomolar
Fourth molar
Mesiodens
Paramolar
Supplementary teeth
EXCLUDES 2 supernumerary roots (K00.2)

K00.2 Abnormalities of size and form of teeth
Concrescence of teeth
Dens evaginatus
Dens in dente
Dens invaginatus
Enamel pearls
Fusion of teeth
Gemination of teeth
Macrodontia
Microdontia
Peg-shaped [conical] teeth
Supernumerary roots
Taurodontism
Tuberculum paramolare
EXCLUDES 1 abnormalities of teeth due to congenital syphilis (A50.5)
tuberculum Carabelli, which is regarded as a normal variation and should not be coded

K00.3 Mottled teeth
Dental fluorosis
Mottling of enamel
Nonfluoride enamel opacities
EXCLUDES 2 deposits [accretions] on teeth (K03.6)

K00.4 Disturbances in tooth formation
Aplasia and hypoplasia of cementum
Dilaceration of tooth
Enamel hypoplasia (neonatal) (postnatal) (prenatal)
Regional odontodysplasia
Turner's tooth
EXCLUDES 1 Hutchinson's teeth and mulberry molars in congenital syphilis (A50.5)
EXCLUDES 2 mottled teeth (K00.3)

K00.5 Hereditary disturbances in tooth structure, not elsewhere classified
Amelogenesis imperfecta
Dentinogenesis imperfecta
Odontogenesis imperfecta
Dentinal dysplasia
Shell teeth

K00.6 Disturbances in tooth eruption
Dentia praecox
Natal tooth
Neonatal tooth
Premature eruption of tooth
Premature shedding of primary [deciduous] tooth
Prenatal teeth
Retained [persistent] primary tooth
EXCLUDES 2 embedded and impacted teeth (K01.-)

K00.7 Teething syndrome

K00.8 Other disorders of tooth development
Color changes during tooth formation
Intrinsic staining of teeth NOS
EXCLUDES 2 posteruptive color changes (K03.7)

K00.9 Disorder of tooth development, unspecified
Disorder of odontogenesis NOS

✓4th K01 Embedded and impacted teeth
EXCLUDES 1 abnormal position of fully erupted teeth (M26.3-)

K01.0 Embedded teeth

K01.1 Impacted teeth

✓4th K02 Dental caries
Dental cavities
Tooth decay

K02.3 Arrested dental caries
Arrested coronal and root caries

✓5th K02.5 Dental caries on pit and fissure surface
Dental caries on chewing surface of tooth

K02.51 Dental caries on pit and fissure surface limited to enamel
White spot lesions [initial caries] on pit and fissure surface of tooth

K02.52 Dental caries on pit and fissure surface penetrating into dentin

K02.53 Dental caries on pit and fissure surface penetrating into pulp

✓5th K02.6 Dental caries on smooth surface

K02.61 Dental caries on smooth surface limited to enamel
White spot lesions [initial caries] on smooth surface of tooth

K02.62 Dental caries on smooth surface penetrating into dentin

K02.63 Dental caries on smooth surface penetrating into pulp

K02.7 Dental root caries

K02.9 Dental caries, unspecified

✓4th K03 Other diseases of hard tissues of teeth
EXCLUDES 2 bruxism (F45.8)
dental caries (K02.-)
teeth-grinding NOS (F45.8)

K03.0 Excessive attrition of teeth
Approximal wear of teeth
Occlusal wear of teeth

K03.1 Abrasion of teeth
Dentifrice abrasion of teeth
Habitual abrasion of teeth
Occupational abrasion of teeth
Ritual abrasion of teeth
Traditional abrasion of teeth
Wedge defect NOS

K03.2 Erosion of teeth
Erosion of teeth due to diet
Erosion of teeth due to drugs and medicaments
Erosion of teeth due to persistent vomiting
Erosion of teeth NOS
Idiopathic erosion of teeth
Occupational erosion of teeth

K03.3 Pathological resorption of teeth
Internal granuloma of pulp
Resorption of teeth (external)

K03.4 Hypercementosis
Cementation hyperplasia

K03.5 Ankylosis of teeth

K03.6 Deposits [accretions] on teeth
Betel deposits [accretions] on teeth
Black deposits [accretions] on teeth
Extrinsic staining of teeth NOS
Green deposits [accretions] on teeth
Materia alba deposits [accretions] on teeth
Orange deposits [accretions] on teeth
Staining of teeth NOS
Subgingival dental calculus
Supragingival dental calculus
Tobacco deposits [accretions] on teeth

K03.7 Posteruptive color changes of dental hard tissues
EXCLUDES 2 deposits [accretions] on teeth (K03.6)

√5ᵗʰ **K03.8 Other specified diseases of hard tissues of teeth**
K03.81 Cracked tooth
EXCLUDES 1 asymptomatic craze lines in enamel—omit code
broken or fractured tooth due to trauma (S02.5)
K03.89 Other specified diseases of hard tissues of teeth
K03.9 Disease of hard tissues of teeth, unspecified

√4ᵗʰ **K04 Diseases of pulp and periapical tissues**
K04.0 Pulpitis   CC
Acute pulpitis
Chronic (hyperplastic) (ulcerative) pulpitis
Irreversible pulpitis
Reversible pulpitis
CC Excl: K00.0-K08.9, M26.00-M26.9, M27.61-M27.69

K04.1 Necrosis of pulp
Pulpal gangrene

K04.2 Pulp degeneration
Denticles
Pulpal calcifications
Pulpal stones

K04.3 Abnormal hard tissue formation in pulp
Secondary or irregular dentine

K04.4 Acute apical periodontitis of pulpal origin   CC
Acute apical periodontitis NOS
EXCLUDES 1 acute periodontitis (K05.2-)
CC Excl: See code: K04.0

K04.5 Chronic apical periodontitis
Apical or periapical granuloma
Apical periodontitis NOS
EXCLUDES 1 chronic periodontitis (K05.3-)

K04.6 Periapical abscess with sinus
Dental abscess with sinus
Dentoalveolar abscess with sinus

K04.7 Periapical abscess without sinus
Dental abscess without sinus
Dentoalveolar abscess without sinus
Periapical abscess without sinus

K04.8 Radicular cyst
Apical (periodontal) cyst
Periapical cyst
Residual radicular cyst
EXCLUDES 2 lateral periodontal cyst (K09.0)

√5ᵗʰ **K04.9 Other and unspecified diseases of pulp and periapical tissues**
K04.90 Unspecified diseases of pulp and periapical tissues
K04.99 Other diseases of pulp and periapical tissues

√4ᵗʰ **K05 Gingivitis and periodontal diseases**
Use additional code to identify:
alcohol abuse and dependence (F10.-)
exposure to environmental tobacco smoke (Z77.22)
exposure to tobacco smoke in the perinatal period (P96.81)
history of tobacco use (Z87.891)
occupational exposure to environmental tobacco smoke (Z57.31)
tobacco dependence (F17.-)
tobacco use (Z72.0)

√5ᵗʰ **K05.0 Acute gingivitis**
EXCLUDES 1 acute necrotizing ulcerative gingivitis (A69.1)
herpesviral [herpes simplex] gingivostomatitis (B00.2)
K05.00 Acute gingivitis, plaque induced
Acute gingivitis NOS
K05.01 Acute gingivitis, non-plaque induced

√5ᵗʰ **K05.1 Chronic gingivitis**
Desquamative gingivitis (chronic)
Gingivitis (chronic) NOS
Hyperplastic gingivitis (chronic)
Simple marginal gingivitis (chronic)
Ulcerative gingivitis (chronic)
K05.10 Chronic gingivitis, plaque induced
Chronic gingivitis NOS
Gingivitis NOS
K05.11 Chronic gingivitis, non-plaque induced

√5ᵗʰ **K05.2 Aggressive periodontitis**
Acute pericoronitis
EXCLUDES 1 acute apical periodontitis (K04.4)
periapical abscess (K04.7)
periapical abscess with sinus (K04.6)
K05.20 Aggressive periodontitis, unspecified
K05.21 Aggressive periodontitis, localized
Periodontal abscess
K05.22 Aggressive periodontitis, generalized

√5ᵗʰ **K05.3 Chronic periodontitis**
Chronic pericoronitis
Complex periodontitis
Periodontitis NOS
Simplex periodontitis
EXCLUDES 1 chronic apical periodontitis (K04.5)
K05.30 Chronic periodontitis, unspecified
K05.31 Chronic periodontitis, localized
K05.32 Chronic periodontitis, generalized

K05.4 Periodontosis
Juvenile periodontosis

K05.5 Other periodontal diseases
EXCLUDES 2 leukoplakia of gingiva (K13.21)

K05.6 Periodontal disease, unspecified

√4ᵗʰ **K06 Other disorders of gingiva and edentulous alveolar ridge**
EXCLUDES 2 acute gingivitis (K05.0)
atrophy of edentulous alveolar ridge (K08.2)
chronic gingivitis (K05.1)
gingivitis NOS (K05.1)

K06.0 Gingival recession
Gingival recession (generalized) (localized) (postinfective) (postprocedural)

K06.1 Gingival enlargement
Gingival fibromatosis

K06.2 Gingival and edentulous alveolar ridge lesions associated with trauma
Irritative hyperplasia of edentulous ridge [denture hyperplasia]
Use additional code (Chapter 20) to identify external cause or denture status (Z97.2)

K06.8 Other specified disorders of gingiva and edentulous alveolar ridge
Fibrous epulis
Flabby alveolar ridge
Giant cell epulis
Peripheral giant cell granuloma of gingiva
Pyogenic granuloma of gingiva
EXCLUDES 2 gingival cyst (K09.0)

K06.9 Disorder of gingiva and edentulous alveolar ridge, unspecified

√4ᵗʰ **K08 Other disorders of teeth and supporting structures**
EXCLUDES 2 dentofacial anomalies [including malocclusion] (M26.-)
disorders of jaw (M27.-)

K08.0 Exfoliation of teeth due to systemic causes
Code also underlying systemic condition

√5ᵗʰ **K08.1 Complete loss of teeth**
Acquired loss of teeth, complete
EXCLUDES 1 congenital absence of teeth (K00.0)
exfoliation of teeth due to systemic causes (K08.0)
partial loss of teeth (K08.4-)
√6ᵗʰ **K08.10 Complete loss of teeth, unspecified cause**
K08.101 Complete loss of teeth, unspecified cause, class I
K08.102 Complete loss of teeth, unspecified cause, class II
K08.103 Complete loss of teeth, unspecified cause, class III
K08.104 Complete loss of teeth, unspecified cause, class IV

K08.109　Complete loss of teeth, unspecified cause, unspecified class
Edentulism NOS

✓6th　K08.11　Complete loss of teeth due to trauma
K08.111　Complete loss of teeth due to trauma, class I
K08.112　Complete loss of teeth due to trauma, class II
K08.113　Complete loss of teeth due to trauma, class III
K08.114　Complete loss of teeth due to trauma, class IV
K08.119　Complete loss of teeth due to trauma, unspecified class

✓6th　K08.12　Complete loss of teeth due to periodontal diseases
K08.121　Complete loss of teeth due to periodontal diseases, class I
K08.122　Complete loss of teeth due to periodontal diseases, class II
K08.123　Complete loss of teeth due to periodontal diseases, class III
K08.124　Complete loss of teeth due to periodontal diseases, class IV
K08.129　Complete loss of teeth due to periodontal diseases, unspecified class

✓6th　K08.13　Complete loss of teeth due to caries
K08.131　Complete loss of teeth due to caries, class I
K08.132　Complete loss of teeth due to caries, class II
K08.133　Complete loss of teeth due to caries, class III
K08.134　Complete loss of teeth due to caries, class IV
K08.139　Complete loss of teeth due to caries, unspecified class

✓6th　K08.19　Complete loss of teeth due to other specified cause
K08.191　Complete loss of teeth due to other specified cause, class I
K08.192　Complete loss of teeth due to other specified cause, class II
K08.193　Complete loss of teeth due to other specified cause, class III
K08.194　Complete loss of teeth due to other specified cause, class IV
K08.199　Complete loss of teeth due to other specified cause, unspecified class

✓5th　K08.2　Atrophy of edentulous alveolar ridge
K08.20　Unspecified atrophy of edentulous alveolar ridge
Atrophy of the mandible NOS
Atrophy of the maxilla NOS
K08.21　Minimal atrophy of the mandible
Minimal atrophy of the edentulous mandible
K08.22　Moderate atrophy of the mandible
Moderate atrophy of the edentulous mandible
K08.23　Severe atrophy of the mandible
Severe atrophy of the edentulous mandible
K08.24　Minimal atrophy of maxilla
Minimal atrophy of the edentulous maxilla
K08.25　Moderate atrophy of maxilla
Moderate atrophy of the edentulous maxilla
K08.26　Severe atrophy of maxilla
Severe atrophy of the edentulous maxilla

K08.3　Retained dental root

✓5th　K08.4　Partial loss of teeth
Acquired loss of teeth, partial
EXCLUDES 1　complete loss of teeth (K08.1-)
congenital absence of teeth (K00.0)
EXCLUDES 2　exfoliation of teeth due to systemic causes (K08.0)

✓6th　K08.40　Partial loss of teeth, unspecified cause
K08.401　Partial loss of teeth, unspecified cause, class I
K08.402　Partial loss of teeth, unspecified cause, class II
K08.403　Partial loss of teeth, unspecified cause, class III
K08.404　Partial loss of teeth, unspecified cause, class IV

K08.409　Partial loss of teeth, unspecified cause, unspecified class
Tooth extraction status NOS

✓6th　K08.41　Partial loss of teeth due to trauma
K08.411　Partial loss of teeth due to trauma, class I
K08.412　Partial loss of teeth due to trauma, class II
K08.413　Partial loss of teeth due to trauma, class III
K08.414　Partial loss of teeth due to trauma, class IV
K08.419　Partial loss of teeth due to trauma, unspecified class

✓6th　K08.42　Partial loss of teeth due to periodontal diseases
K08.421　Partial loss of teeth due to periodontal diseases, class I
K08.422　Partial loss of teeth due to periodontal diseases, class II
K08.423　Partial loss of teeth due to periodontal diseases, class III
K08.424　Partial loss of teeth due to periodontal diseases, class IV
K08.429　Partial loss of teeth due to periodontal diseases, unspecified class

✓6th　K08.43　Partial loss of teeth due to caries
K08.431　Partial loss of teeth due to caries, class I
K08.432　Partial loss of teeth due to caries, class II
K08.433　Partial loss of teeth due to caries, class III
K08.434　Partial loss of teeth due to caries, class IV
K08.439　Partial loss of teeth due to caries, unspecified class

✓6th　K08.49　Partial loss of teeth due to other specified cause
K08.491　Partial loss of teeth due to other specified cause, class I
K08.492　Partial loss of teeth due to other specified cause, class II
K08.493　Partial loss of teeth due to other specified cause, class III
K08.494　Partial loss of teeth due to other specified cause, class IV
K08.499　Partial loss of teeth due to other specified cause, unspecified class

✓5th　K08.5　Unsatisfactory restoration of tooth
Defective bridge, crown, filling
Defective dental restoration
EXCLUDES 1　dental restoration status (Z98.811)
EXCLUDES 2　endosseous dental implant failure (M27.6-)
unsatisfactory endodontic treatment (M27.5-)

K08.50　Unsatisfactory restoration of tooth, unspecified
Defective dental restoration NOS

K08.51　Open restoration margins of tooth
Dental restoration failure of marginal integrity
Open margin on tooth restoration
Poor gingival margin to tooth restoration

K08.52　Unrepairable overhanging of dental restorative materials
Overhanging of tooth restoration

✓6th　K08.53　Fractured dental restorative material
EXCLUDES 1　cracked tooth (K03.81)
traumatic fracture of tooth (S02.5)
K08.530　Fractured dental restorative material without loss of material
K08.531　Fractured dental restorative material with loss of material
K08.539　Fractured dental restorative material, unspecified

K08.54　Contour of existing restoration of tooth biologically incompatible with oral health
Dental restoration failure of periodontal anatomical integrity
Unacceptable contours of existing restoration of tooth
Unacceptable morphology of existing restoration of tooth

K08.55　Allergy to existing dental restorative material
Use additional code to identify the specific type of allergy

N Newborn: 0　P Pediatric: 0-17　M Maternity: 12-55　A Adult: 15-124　MCC Major CC Condition　PDx MCC PDx acts as own MCC　CC CC Condition　PDx CC PDx acts as own CC

642

ICD-10-CM Draft (2015)

K08.56 Poor aesthetic of existing restoration of tooth
Dental restoration aesthetically inadequate or displeasing

K08.59 Other unsatisfactory restoration of tooth
Other defective dental restoration

K08.8 Other specified disorders of teeth and supporting structures
Enlargement of alveolar ridge NOS
Irregular alveolar process
Toothache NOS

K08.9 Disorder of teeth and supporting structures, unspecified

✓4ᵗʰ **K09 Cysts of oral region, not elsewhere classified**
INCLUDES lesions showing histological features both of aneurysmal cyst and of another fibro-osseous lesion
EXCLUDES 2 cysts of jaw (M27.0-, M27.4-)
radicular cyst (K04.8)

K09.0 Developmental odontogenic cysts
Dentigerous cyst
Eruption cyst
Follicular cyst
Gingival cyst
Lateral periodontal cyst
Primordial cyst
EXCLUDES 2 keratocysts (D16.4, D16.5)
odontogenic keratocystic tumors (D16.4, D16.5)

K09.1 Developmental (nonodontogenic) cysts of oral region
Cyst (of) incisive canal
Cyst (of) palatine of papilla
Globulomaxillary cyst
Median palatal cyst
Nasoalveolar cyst
Nasolabial cyst
Nasopalatine duct cyst

K09.8 Other cysts of oral region, not elsewhere classified
Dermoid cyst
Epidermoid cyst
Lymphoepithelial cyst
Epstein's pearl

K09.9 Cyst of oral region, unspecified

✓4ᵗʰ **K11 Diseases of salivary glands**
Use additional code to identify:
alcohol abuse and dependence (F10.-)
exposure to environmental tobacco smoke (Z77.22)
exposure to tobacco smoke in the perinatal period (P96.81)
history of tobacco use (Z87.891)
occupational exposure to environmental tobacco smoke (Z57.31)
tobacco dependence (F17.-)
tobacco use (Z72.0)

K11.0 Atrophy of salivary gland

K11.1 Hypertrophy of salivary gland

✓5ᵗʰ **K11.2 Sialoadenitis**
Parotitis
EXCLUDES 1 epidemic parotitis (B26.-)
mumps (B26.-)
uveoparotid fever [Heerfordt] (D86.89)

K11.20 Sialoadenitis, unspecified

K11.21 Acute sialoadenitis
EXCLUDES 1 acute recurrent sialoadenitis (K11.22)

K11.22 Acute recurrent sialoadenitis

K11.23 Chronic sialoadenitis

K11.3 Abscess of salivary gland   cc
CC Excl: K11.0-K11.9, K31.89-K31.9, K92.81, R68.2

K11.4 Fistula of salivary gland   cc
EXCLUDES 1 congenital fistula of salivary gland (Q38.4)
CC Excl: See code: K11.3

K11.5 Sialolithiasis
Calculus of salivary gland or duct
Stone of salivary gland or duct

K11.6 Mucocele of salivary gland
Mucous extravasation cyst of salivary gland
Mucous retention cyst of salivary gland
Ranula

K11.7 Disturbances of salivary secretion
Hypoptyalism
Ptyalism
Xerostomia
EXCLUDES 2 dry mouth NOS (R68.2)

K11.8 Other diseases of salivary glands
Benign lymphoepithelial lesion of salivary gland
Mikulicz' disease
Necrotizing sialometaplasia
Sialectasia
Stenosis of salivary duct
Stricture of salivary duct
EXCLUDES 1 sicca syndrome [Sjögren] (M35.0-)

K11.9 Disease of salivary gland, unspecified
Sialoadenopathy NOS

✓4ᵗʰ **K12 Stomatitis and related lesions**
Use additional code to identify:
alcohol abuse and dependence (F10.-)
exposure to environmental tobacco smoke (Z77.22)
exposure to tobacco smoke in the perinatal period (P96.81)
history of tobacco use (Z87.891)
occupational exposure to environmental tobacco smoke (Z57.31)
tobacco dependence (F17.-)
tobacco use (Z72.0)
EXCLUDES 1 cancrum oris (A69.0)
cheilitis (K13.0)
gangrenous stomatitis (A69.0)
herpesviral [herpes simplex] gingivostomatitis (B00.2)
noma (A69.0)

K12.0 Recurrent oral aphthae
Aphthous stomatitis (major) (minor)
Bednar's aphthae
Periadenitis mucosa necrotica recurrens
Recurrent aphthous ulcer
Stomatitis herpetiformis

K12.1 Other forms of stomatitis
Stomatitis NOS
Denture stomatitis
Ulcerative stomatitis
Vesicular stomatitis
EXCLUDES 1 acute necrotizing ulcerative stomatitis (A69.1)
Vincent's stomatitis (A69.1)

K12.2 Cellulitis and abscess of mouth   cc
Cellulitis of mouth (floor)
Submandibular abscess
EXCLUDES 2 abscess of salivary gland (K11.3)
abscess of tongue (K14.0)
periapical abscess (K04.6-K04.7)
periodontal abscess (K05.21)
peritonsillar abscess (J36)
CC Excl: K12.1-K12.39, K14.0, K14.2

✓5ᵗʰ **K12.3 Oral mucositis (ulcerative)**
Mucositis (oral) (oropharyneal)
EXCLUDES 2 gastrointestinal mucositis (ulcerative) (K92.81)
mucositis (ulcerative) of vagina and vulva (N76.81)
nasal mucositis (ulcerative) (J34.81)

K12.30 Oral mucositis (ulcerative), unspecified

K12.31 Oral mucositis (ulcerative) due to antineoplastic therapy
Use additional code for adverse effect, if applicable, to identify antineoplastic and immunosuppressive drugs (T45.1X5)
Use additional code for other antineoplastic therapy, such as:
radiological procedure and radiotherapy (Y84.2)

K12.32 Oral mucositis (ulcerative) due to other drugs
Use additional code for adverse effect, if applicable, to identify drug (T36-T50 with fifth or sixth character 5)

K12.33 Oral mucositis (ulcerative) due to radiation
Use additional external cause code (W88-W90, X39.0-) to identify cause

K12.39 Other oral mucositis (ulcerative)
Viral oral mucositis (ulcerative)

✓ Additional Character Required   ✓×7ᵗʰ Xtension Alert   Unacceptable PDx   Manifestation   Hospital Acquired Condition   EXCLUDES 1 Not Coded Here   EXCLUDES 2 Not Included Here

Diseases of the Digestive System

K13–K22.0

✓4th K13 Other diseases of lip and oral mucosa
INCLUDES epithelial disturbances of tongue
Use additional code to identify:
alcohol abuse and dependence (F10.-)
exposure to environmental tobacco smoke (Z77.22)
exposure to tobacco smoke in the perinatal period (P96.81)
history of tobacco use (Z87.891)
occupational exposure to environmental tobacco smoke (Z57.31)
tobacco dependence (F17.-)
tobacco use (Z72.0)
EXCLUDES2 certain disorders of gingiva and edentulous alveolar ridge (K05-K06)
cysts of oral region (K09.-)
diseases of tongue (K14.-)
stomatitis and related lesions (K12.-)

K13.0 Diseases of lips
Abscess of lips
Angular cheilitis
Cellulitis of lips
Cheilitis NOS
Cheilodynia
Cheilosis
Exfoliative cheilitis
Fistula of lips
Glandular cheilitis
Hypertrophy of lips
Perlèche NEC
EXCLUDES1 ariboflavinosis (E53.0)
cheilitis due to radiation-related disorders (L55-L59)
congenital fistula of lips (Q38.0)
congenital hypertrophy of lips (Q18.6)
Perlèche due to candidiasis (B37.83)
Perlèche due to riboflavin deficiency (E53.0)

K13.1 Cheek and lip biting

✓5th K13.2 Leukoplakia and other disturbances of oral epithelium, including tongue
EXCLUDES1 carcinoma in situ of oral epithelium (D00.0-)
hairy leukoplakia (K13.3)

K13.21 Leukoplakia of oral mucosa, including tongue
Leukokeratosis of oral mucosa
Leukoplakia of gingiva, lips, tongue
EXCLUDES1 hairy leukoplakia (K13.3)
leukokeratosis nicotina palati (K13.24)

K13.22 Minimal keratinized residual ridge mucosa
Minimal keratinization of alveolar ridge mucosa

K13.23 Excessive keratinized residual ridge mucosa
Excessive keratinization of alveolar ridge mucosa

K13.24 Leukokeratosis nicotina palati
Smoker's palate

K13.29 Other disturbances of oral epithelium, including tongue
Erythroplakia of mouth or tongue
Focal epithelial hyperplasia of mouth or tongue
Leukoedema of mouth or tongue
Other oral epithelium disturbances

K13.3 Hairy leukoplakia

K13.4 Granuloma and granuloma-like lesions of oral mucosa
Eosinophilic granuloma
Granuloma pyogenicum
Verrucous xanthoma

K13.5 Oral submucous fibrosis
Submucous fibrosis of tongue

K13.6 Irritative hyperplasia of oral mucosa
EXCLUDES2 irritative hyperplasia of edentulous ridge [denture hyperplasia] (K06.2)

✓5th K13.7 Other and unspecified lesions of oral mucosa
K13.70 Unspecified lesions of oral mucosa
K13.79 Other lesions of oral mucosa
Focal oral mucinosis

✓4th K14 Diseases of tongue
Use additional code to identify:
alcohol abuse and dependence (F10.-)
exposure to environmental tobacco smoke (Z77.22)
history of tobacco use (Z87.891)
occupational exposure to environmental tobacco smoke (Z57.31)
tobacco dependence (F17.-)
tobacco use (Z72.0)
EXCLUDES2 erythroplakia (K13.29)
focal epithelial hyperplasia (K13.29)
leukedema of tongue (K13.29)
leukoplakia of tongue (K13.21)
hairy leukoplakia (K13.3)
macroglossia (congenital) (Q38.2)
submucous fibrosis of tongue (K13.5)

K14.0 Glossitis
Abscess of tongue
Ulceration (traumatic) of tongue
EXCLUDES1 atrophic glossitis (K14.4)

K14.1 Geographic tongue
Benign migratory glossitis
Glossitis areata exfoliativa

K14.2 Median rhomboid glossitis

K14.3 Hypertrophy of tongue papillae
Black hairy tongue
Coated tongue
Hypertrophy of foliate papillae
Lingua villosa nigra

K14.4 Atrophy of tongue papillae
Atrophic glossitis

K14.5 Plicated tongue
Fissured tongue
Furrowed tongue
Scrotal tongue
EXCLUDES1 fissured tongue, congenital (Q38.3)

K14.6 Glossodynia
Glossopyrosis
Painful tongue

K14.8 Other diseases of tongue
Atrophy of tongue
Crenated tongue
Enlargement of tongue
Glossocele
Glossoptosis
Hypertrophy of tongue

K14.9 Disease of tongue, unspecified
Glossopathy NOS

Diseases of esophagus, stomach and duodenum (K20-K31)
EXCLUDES2 hiatus hernia (K44.-)

✓4th K20 Esophagitis
Use additional code to identify:
alcohol abuse and dependence (F10.-)
EXCLUDES1 erosion of esophagus (K22.1-)
esophagitis with gastro-esophageal reflux disease (K21.0)
reflux esophagitis (K21.0)
ulcerative esophagitis (K22.1-)
EXCLUDES2 eosinophilic gastritis or gastroenteritis (K52.81)

K20.0 Eosinophilic esophagitis
K20.8 Other esophagitis
Abscess of esophagus
K20.9 Esophagitis, unspecified
Esophagitis NOS

✓4th K21 Gastro-esophageal reflux disease
EXCLUDES1 newborn esophageal reflux (P78.83)

K21.0 Gastro-esophageal reflux disease with esophagitis
Reflux esophagitis

K21.9 Gastro-esophageal reflux disease without esophagitis
Esophageal reflux NOS

✓4th K22 Other diseases of esophagus
EXCLUDES2 esophageal varices (I85.-)

K22.0 Achalasia of cardia
Achalasia NOS
Cardiospasm
EXCLUDES1 congenital cardiospasm (Q39.5)

K22.1 ✓5th **Ulcer of esophagus**
Barrett's ulcer
Erosion of esophagus
Fungal ulcer of esophagus
Peptic ulcer of esophagus
Ulcer of esophagus due to ingestion of chemicals
Ulcer of esophagus due to ingestion of drugs and medicaments
Ulcerative esophagitis
Code first poisoning due to drug or toxin, if applicable (T36-T65 with fifth or sixth character 1-4 or 6)
Use additional code for adverse effect, if applicable, to identify drug (T36-T50 with fifth or sixth character 5)
EXCLUDES 1   *Barrett's esophagus (K22.7-)*

K22.10   **Ulcer of esophagus without bleeding**   CC
Ulcer of esophagus NOS
CC Excl: K22.11, K22.8-K23, K31.82

K22.11   **Ulcer of esophagus with bleeding**   MCC
EXCLUDES 2   *bleeding esophageal varices (I85.01, I85.11)*
CC Excl: E16.4, I85.01, K22.10-K22.11, K22.6-K22.719, K25.0-K28.9, K29.01, K29.21, K29.31, K29.41, K29.51, K29.61, K29.71, K29.81, K29.91, K31.811, K31.89-K31.9, K55.21, K57.01, K57.11, K57.13, K57.21, K57.31, K57.33, K57.41, K57.51, K57.53, K57.81, K57.91, K57.93, K62.5, K92.0-K92.81

K22.2   **Esophageal obstruction**
Compression of esophagus
Constriction of esophagus
Stenosis of esophagus
Stricture of esophagus
EXCLUDES 1   *congenital stenosis or stricture of esophagus (Q39.3)*

K22.3   **Perforation of esophagus**   MCC
Rupture of esophagus
EXCLUDES 1   *traumatic perforation of (thoracic) esophagus (S27.8-)*
CC Excl: K21.9, K22.3, K22.6, K22.8-K23

K22.4   **Dyskinesia of esophagus**
Corkscrew esophagus
Diffuse esophageal spasm
Spasm of esophagus
EXCLUDES 1   *cardiospasm (K22.0)*

K22.5   **Diverticulum of esophagus, acquired**
Esophageal pouch, acquired
EXCLUDES 1   *diverticulum of esophagus (congenital) (Q39.6)*

K22.6   **Gastro-esophageal laceration-hemorrhage syndrome**   MCC
Mallory-Weiss syndrome
CC Excl: E16.4, I85.01, K21.9, K22.10-K22.11, K22.3, K22.6-K28.9, K29.01, K29.21, K29.31, K29.41, K29.51, K29.61, K29.71, K29.81, K29.91, K31.811, K55.21, K57.01, K57.11, K57.13, K57.21, K57.31, K57.33, K57.41, K57.51, K57.53, K57.81, K57.91, K57.93, K62.5, K92.0-K92.2

K22.7 ✓5th **Barrett's esophagus**
Barrett's disease
Barrett's syndrome
EXCLUDES 1   *Barrett's ulcer (K22.1)*
malignant neoplasm of esophagus (C15.-)

K22.70   **Barrett's esophagus without dysplasia**
Barrett's esophagus NOS

K22.71 ✓6th **Barrett's esophagus with dysplasia**

K22.710   **Barrett's esophagus with low grade dysplasia**

K22.711   **Barrett's esophagus with high grade dysplasia**

K22.719   **Barrett's esophagus with dysplasia, unspecified**

K22.8   **Other specified diseases of esophagus**
Hemorrhage of esophagus NOS
EXCLUDES 2   *esophageal varices (I85.-)*
Paterson-Kelly syndrome (D50.1)

K22.9   **Disease of esophagus, unspecified**

K23   *Disorders of esophagus in diseases classified elsewhere*
Code first underlying disease, such as:
congenital syphilis (A50.5)
EXCLUDES 1   *late syphilis (A52.79)*
megaesophagus due to Chagas' disease (B57.31)
tuberculosis (A18.83)

K25 ✓4th **Gastric ulcer**
INCLUDES   erosion (acute) of stomach
pylorus ulcer (peptic)
stomach ulcer (peptic)
Use additional code to identify:
alcohol abuse and dependence (F10.-)
EXCLUDES 1   *acute gastritis (K29.0-)*
peptic ulcer NOS (K27.-)

CC Excl: For CC/MCC codes in category K25, unless otherwise noted: See code: K22.11

K25.0   **Acute gastric ulcer with hemorrhage**   MCC
K25.1   **Acute gastric ulcer with perforation**   MCC
K25.2   **Acute gastric ulcer with both hemorrhage and perforation**   MCC
K25.3   **Acute gastric ulcer without hemorrhage or perforation**   CC
K25.4   **Chronic or unspecified gastric ulcer with hemorrhage**   MCC
K25.5   **Chronic or unspecified gastric ulcer with perforation**   MCC
K25.6   **Chronic or unspecified gastric ulcer with both hemorrhage and perforation**   MCC
K25.7   **Chronic gastric ulcer without hemorrhage or perforation**
K25.9   **Gastric ulcer, unspecified as acute or chronic, without hemorrhage or perforation**

K26 ✓4th **Duodenal ulcer**
INCLUDES   erosion (acute) of duodenum
duodenum ulcer (peptic)
postpyloric ulcer (peptic)
Use additional code to identify:
alcohol abuse and dependence (F10.-)
EXCLUDES 1   *peptic ulcer NOS (K27.-)*

CC Excl: For CC/MCC codes in category K26, unless otherwise noted: E16.4, I85.01, K22.10-K22.11, K22.6-K22.719, K25.0-K28.9, K29.01, K29.21, K29.31, K29.41, K29.51, K29.61, K29.71, K29.81, K29.91, K31.5, K31.811, K31.89-K31.9, K55.21, K57.01, K57.11, K57.13, K57.21, K57.31, K57.33, K57.41, K57.51, K57.53, K57.81, K57.91, K57.93, K62.5, K92.0-K92.81

K26.0   **Acute duodenal ulcer with hemorrhage**   MCC
K26.1   **Acute duodenal ulcer with perforation**   MCC
K26.2   **Acute duodenal ulcer with both hemorrhage and perforation**   MCC
K26.3   **Acute duodenal ulcer without hemorrhage or perforation**   CC
CC Excl: E16.4, I85.01, K22.6, K25.0-K28.9, K29.01, K29.21, K29.31, K29.41, K29.51, K29.61, K29.71, K29.81, K29.91, K31.5, K31.811, K31.82, K31.89-K31.9, K55.21, K57.01, K57.11, K57.13, K57.21, K57.31, K57.33, K57.41, K57.51, K57.53, K57.81, K57.91, K57.93, K62.5, K92.0-K92.81
K26.4   **Chronic or unspecified duodenal ulcer with hemorrhage**   MCC
K26.5   **Chronic or unspecified duodenal ulcer with perforation**   MCC
K26.6   **Chronic or unspecified duodenal ulcer with both hemorrhage and perforation**   MCC
K26.7   **Chronic duodenal ulcer without hemorrhage or perforation**
K26.9   **Duodenal ulcer, unspecified as acute or chronic, without hemorrhage or perforation**

K27 ✓4th **Peptic ulcer, site unspecified**
INCLUDES   gastroduodenal ulcer NOS
peptic ulcer NOS
Use additional code to identify:
alcohol abuse and dependence (F10.-)
EXCLUDES 1   *peptic ulcer of newborn (P78.82)*

CC Excl: For CC/MCC codes in category K27, unless otherwise noted: See code: K26

K27.0   **Acute peptic ulcer, site unspecified, with hemorrhage**   MCC
K27.1   **Acute peptic ulcer, site unspecified, with perforation**   MCC
K27.2   **Acute peptic ulcer, site unspecified, with both hemorrhage and perforation**   MCC
K27.3   **Acute peptic ulcer, site unspecified, without hemorrhage or perforation**   CC
K27.4   **Chronic or unspecified peptic ulcer, site unspecified, with hemorrhage**   MCC
K27.5   **Chronic or unspecified peptic ulcer, site unspecified, with perforation**   MCC
K27.6   **Chronic or unspecified peptic ulcer, site unspecified, with both hemorrhage and perforation**   MCC
K27.7   **Chronic peptic ulcer, site unspecified, without hemorrhage or perforation**
K27.9   **Peptic ulcer, site unspecified, unspecified as acute or chronic, without hemorrhage or perforation**

☑ Additional Character Required   ✓x7th Xtension Alert   Unacceptable PDx   Manifestation   Hospital Acquired Condition   *EXCLUDES 1* Not Coded Here   *EXCLUDES 2* Not Included Here

Diseases of the Digestive System

K28–K31.9

✓4ᵗʰ **K28** **Gastrojejunal ulcer**

> **INCLUDES**   anastomotic ulcer (peptic) or erosion
> gastrocolic ulcer (peptic) or erosion
> gastrointestinal ulcer (peptic) or erosion
> gastrojejunal ulcer (peptic) or erosion
> jejunal ulcer (peptic) or erosion
> marginal ulcer (peptic) or erosion
> stomal ulcer (peptic) or erosion
>
> Use additional code to identify:
>   alcohol abuse and dependence (F10.-)
> **EXCLUDES 1**   primary ulcer of small intestine (K63.3)

> **CC Excl: For CC/MCC codes in category K28, unless otherwise noted:** See code: K22.11

K28.0   Acute **gastrojejunal ulcer** with hemorrhage   MCC

K28.1   Acute **gastrojejunal ulcer** with perforation   MCC

K28.2   Acute **gastrojejunal ulcer** with both hemorrhage and perforation   MCC

K28.3   Acute **gastrojejunal ulcer** without hemorrhage or perforation   CC

K28.4   Chronic or unspecified **gastrojejunal ulcer** with hemorrhage   MCC

K28.5   Chronic or unspecified **gastrojejunal ulcer** with perforation   MCC

K28.6   Chronic or unspecified **gastrojejunal ulcer** with both hemorrhage and perforation   MCC

K28.7   Chronic **gastrojejunal ulcer** without hemorrhage or perforation

K28.9   Gastrojejunal ulcer, unspecified as acute or chronic, without hemorrhage or perforation

✓4ᵗʰ **K29** **Gastritis and duodenitis**

> **EXCLUDES 1**   eosinophilic gastritis or gastroenteritis (K52.81)
> Zollinger-Ellison syndrome (E16.4)

> **CC Excl: For MCC codes in category K29, unless otherwise noted:** E16.4, I85.01, K22.10-K22.11, K22.6-K22.719, K25.0-K28.9, K29.01, K29.21, K29.31, K29.41, K29.51, K29.61, K29.71, K29.81, K29.91, K31.811, K55.21, K57.01, K57.11, K57.13, K57.21, K57.31, K57.33, K57.41, K57.51, K57.53, K57.81, K57.91, K57.93, K62.5, K92.0-K92.2

✓5ᵗʰ **K29.0**   Acute **gastritis**

> Use additional code to identify:
>   alcohol abuse and dependence (F10.-)
> **EXCLUDES 1**   erosion (acute) of stomach (K25.-)

K29.00   Acute gastritis without bleeding

K29.01   Acute gastritis with bleeding   MCC

✓5ᵗʰ **K29.2**   Alcoholic **gastritis**

> Use additional code to identify:
>   alcohol abuse and dependence (F10.-)

K29.20   Alcoholic gastritis without bleeding

K29.21   Alcoholic gastritis with bleeding   MCC

✓5ᵗʰ **K29.3**   Chronic superficial **gastritis**

K29.30   Chronic superficial gastritis without bleeding

K29.31   Chronic superficial gastritis with bleeding   MCC

✓5ᵗʰ **K29.4**   Chronic atrophic **gastritis**

> Gastric atrophy

K29.40   Chronic atrophic gastritis without bleeding

K29.41   Chronic atrophic gastritis with bleeding   MCC

✓5ᵗʰ **K29.5**   Unspecified chronic **gastritis**

> Chronic antral gastritis
> Chronic fundal gastritis

K29.50   Unspecified chronic gastritis without bleeding

K29.51   Unspecified chronic gastritis with bleeding   MCC

✓5ᵗʰ **K29.6**   Other **gastritis**

> Giant hypertrophic gastritis
> Granulomatous gastritis
> Ménétrier's disease

K29.60   Other gastritis without bleeding

K29.61   Other gastritis with bleeding   MCC

✓5ᵗʰ **K29.7**   Gastritis, unspecified

K29.70   Gastritis, unspecified, without bleeding

K29.71   Gastritis, unspecified, with bleeding   MCC

✓5ᵗʰ **K29.8**   Duodenitis

K29.80   Duodenitis without bleeding

K29.81   Duodenitis with bleeding   MCC

✓5ᵗʰ **K29.9**   Gastroduodenitis, unspecified

K29.90   Gastroduodenitis, unspecified, without bleeding

K29.91   Gastroduodenitis, unspecified, with bleeding   MCC

K30 **Functional dyspepsia**

> Indigestion
> **EXCLUDES 1**   dyspepsia NOS (R10.13)
> heartburn (R12)
> nervous dyspepsia (F45.8)
> neurotic dyspepsia (F45.8)
> psychogenic dyspepsia (F45.8)

✓4ᵗʰ **K31** **Other diseases of stomach and duodenum**

> **INCLUDES**   functional disorders of stomach
> **EXCLUDES 2**   diabetic gastroparesis (E08.43, E09.43, E10.43, E11.43, E13.43)
> diverticulum of duodenum (K57.00-K57.13)

K31.0   Acute dilatation of stomach   CC

> Acute distention of stomach
> **CC Excl:** K31.0

K31.1   Adult hypertrophic pyloric stenosis   CC A

> Pyloric stenosis NOS
> **EXCLUDES 1**   congenital or infantile pyloric stenosis (Q40.0)
> **CC Excl:** K30, K31.1, K31.5, K31.84, Q38.5, Q40.0, Q40.8-Q41.9, Q43.4-Q43.9

K31.2   Hourglass stricture and stenosis of stomach

> **EXCLUDES 1**   congenital hourglass stomach (Q40.2)
> hourglass contraction of stomach (K31.89)

K31.3   Pylorospasm, not elsewhere classified

> **EXCLUDES 1**   congenital or infantile pylorospasm (Q40.0)
> neurotic pylorospasm (F45.8)
> psychogenic pylorospasm (F45.8)

K31.4   Gastric diverticulum

> **EXCLUDES 1**   congenital diverticulum of stomach (Q40.2)

K31.5   Obstruction of duodenum   CC

> Constriction of duodenum
> Duodenal ileus (chronic)
> Stenosis of duodenum
> Stricture of duodenum
> Volvulus of duodenum
> **EXCLUDES 1**   congenital stenosis of duodenum (Q41.0)
> **CC Excl:** K31.5, Q38.5, Q40.8-Q41.9, Q43.4-Q43.9

K31.6   Fistula of stomach and duodenum   CC

> Gastrocolic fistula
> Gastrojejunocolic fistula
> **CC Excl:** K31.6, Q38.5, Q40.8-Q40.9, Q43.4-Q43.9

K31.7   Polyp of stomach and duodenum

> **EXCLUDES 1**   adenomatous polyp of stomach (D13.1)

✓5ᵗʰ **K31.8**   Other specified diseases of stomach and duodenum

✓6ᵗʰ **K31.81**   Angiodysplasia of stomach and duodenum

K31.811   Angiodysplasia of stomach and duodenum with bleeding   MCC

> **CC Excl:** See code: K29

K31.819   Angiodysplasia of stomach and duodenum without bleeding

> Angiodysplasia of stomach and duodenum NOS

K31.82   Dieulafoy lesion (hemorrhagic) of stomach and duodenum   MCC

> **EXCLUDES 2**   Dieulafoy lesion of intestine (K63.81)
> **CC Excl:** E16.4, I85.01, K22.10-K22.11, K22.6-K22.719, K25.0-K28.9, K29.01, K29.21, K29.31, K29.41, K29.51, K29.61, K29.71, K29.81, K29.91, K31.811, K31.82, K55.21, K57.01, K57.11, K57.13, K57.21, K57.31, K57.33, K57.41, K57.51, K57.53, K57.81, K57.91, K57.93, K62.5, K92.0-K92.2

K31.83   Achlorhydria

K31.84   Gastroparesis

> Gastroparalysis
> Code first underlying disease, if known, such as:
>   anorexia nervosa (F50.0-)
>   diabetes mellitus (E08.43, E09.43, E10.43, E11.43, E13.43)
>   scleroderma (M34.-)
> **AHA:** 2013, 4Q, 114

K31.89   Other diseases of stomach and duodenum

K31.9   Disease of stomach and duodenum, unspecified

N Newborn: 0   P Pediatric: 0-17   M Maternity: 12-55   A Adult: 15-124   MCC Major CC Condition   PDx MCC PDx acts as own MCC   CC CC Condition   PDx CC PDx acts as own CC

646   ICD-10-CM Draft (2015)

Diseases of appendix (K35-K38)

✓4ᵗʰ K35 Acute **appendicitis**

CC Excl: For CC/MCC codes in category K35, unless otherwise noted: K31.89-K38.9, K92.81

K35.2 Acute appendicitis with generalized peritonitis MCC
Appendicitis (acute) with generalized (diffuse) peritonitis following rupture or perforation of appendix
Perforated appendix NOS
Ruptured appendix NOS

K35.3 Acute appendicitis with localized peritonitis MCC
Acute appendicitis with or without perforation or rupture NOS
Acute appendicitis with or without perforation or rupture with localized peritonitis
Acute appendicitis with peritoneal abscess

✓5ᵗʰ **K35.8 Other and unspecified acute appendicitis**
K35.80 Unspecified acute appendicitis CC
Acute appendicitis NOS
Acute appendicitis without (localized) (generalized) peritonitis
K35.89 Other acute appendicitis CC

K36 Other **appendicitis**
Chronic appendicitis
Recurrent appendicitis

K37 Unspecified **appendicitis**
EXCLUDES 1 unspecified appendicitis with peritonitis (K35.2-K35.3)

✓4ᵗʰ K38 Other diseases of appendix
K38.0 Hyperplasia of appendix
K38.1 Appendicular concretions
Fecalith of appendix
Stercolith of appendix
K38.2 Diverticulum of appendix
K38.3 Fistula of appendix
K38.8 Other specified diseases of appendix
Intussusception of appendix
K38.9 Disease of appendix, unspecified

Hernia (K40-K46)

NOTE   Hernia with both gangrene and obstruction is classified to hernia with gangrene.
INCLUDES   acquired hernia
congenital [except diaphragmatic or hiatus] hernia
recurrent hernia

✓4ᵗʰ K40 Inguinal **hernia**
INCLUDES bubonocele
direct inguinal hernia
double inguinal hernia
indirect inguinal hernia
inguinal hernia NOS
oblique inguinal hernia
scrotal hernia

CC Excl: For CC/MCC codes in category K40, unless otherwise noted: K31.89-K31.9, K40.00-K40.91, K45.0, K45.8-K46.0, K92.81

✓5ᵗʰ **K40.0 Bilateral inguinal hernia, with obstruction, without gangrene**
Inguinal hernia (bilateral) causing obstruction without gangrene
Incarcerated inguinal hernia (bilateral) without gangrene
Irreducible inguinal hernia (bilateral) without gangrene
Strangulated inguinal hernia (bilateral) without gangrene
K40.00 Bilateral inguinal hernia, with obstruction, without gangrene, not specified as recurrent CC
Bilateral inguinal hernia, with obstruction, without gangrene NOS
K40.01 Bilateral inguinal hernia, with obstruction, without gangrene, recurrent CC

✓5ᵗʰ **K40.1 Bilateral inguinal hernia, with gangrene**
K40.10 Bilateral inguinal hernia, with gangrene, not specified as recurrent MCC
Bilateral inguinal hernia, with gangrene NOS
K40.11 Bilateral inguinal hernia, with gangrene, recurrent MCC

✓5ᵗʰ **K40.2 Bilateral inguinal hernia, without obstruction or gangrene**
K40.20 Bilateral inguinal hernia, without obstruction or gangrene, not specified as recurrent
Bilateral inguinal hernia NOS
K40.21 Bilateral inguinal hernia, without obstruction or gangrene, recurrent

✓5ᵗʰ **K40.3 Unilateral inguinal hernia, with obstruction, without gangrene**
Inguinal hernia (unilateral) causing obstruction without gangrene
Incarcerated inguinal hernia (unilateral) without gangrene
Irreducible inguinal hernia (unilateral) without gangrene
Strangulated inguinal hernia (unilateral) without gangrene
K40.30 Unilateral inguinal hernia, with obstruction, without gangrene, not specified as recurrent CC
Inguinal hernia, with obstruction NOS
Unilateral inguinal hernia, with obstruction, without gangrene NOS
K40.31 Unilateral inguinal hernia, with obstruction, without gangrene, recurrent CC

✓5ᵗʰ **K40.4 Unilateral inguinal hernia, with gangrene**
K40.40 Unilateral inguinal hernia, with gangrene, not specified as recurrent MCC
Inguinal hernia with gangrene NOS
Unilateral inguinal hernia with gangrene NOS
K40.41 Unilateral inguinal hernia, with gangrene, recurrent MCC

✓5ᵗʰ **K40.9 Unilateral inguinal hernia, without obstruction or gangrene**
K40.90 Unilateral inguinal hernia, without obstruction or gangrene, not specified as recurrent
Inguinal hernia NOS
Unilateral inguinal hernia NOS
K40.91 Unilateral inguinal hernia, without obstruction or gangrene, recurrent

✓4ᵗʰ K41 Femoral **hernia**
CC Excl: For CC/MCC codes in category K41, unless otherwise noted: K31.89-K31.9, K41.00-K41.91, K45.0, K45.8-K46.0, K92.81

✓5ᵗʰ **K41.0 Bilateral femoral hernia, with obstruction, without gangrene**
Femoral hernia (bilateral) causing obstruction, without gangrene
Incarcerated femoral hernia (bilateral), without gangrene
Irreducible femoral hernia (bilateral), without gangrene
Strangulated femoral hernia (bilateral), without gangrene
K41.00 Bilateral femoral hernia, with obstruction, without gangrene, not specified as recurrent CC
Bilateral femoral hernia, with obstruction, without gangrene NOS
K41.01 Bilateral femoral hernia, with obstruction, without gangrene, recurrent CC

✓5ᵗʰ **K41.1 Bilateral femoral hernia, with gangrene**
K41.10 Bilateral femoral hernia, with gangrene, not specified as recurrent MCC
Bilateral femoral hernia, with gangrene NOS
CC Excl: K31.89-K31.9, K41.10-K41.21, K41.40-K41.91, K45.0, K45.8-K46.0, K92.81
K41.11 Bilateral femoral hernia, with gangrene, recurrent MCC
CC Excl: See code: K41.10

✓5ᵗʰ **K41.2 Bilateral femoral hernia, without obstruction or gangrene**
K41.20 Bilateral femoral hernia, without obstruction or gangrene, not specified as recurrent
Bilateral femoral hernia NOS
K41.21 Bilateral femoral hernia, without obstruction or gangrene, recurrent

✓5ᵗʰ **K41.3 Unilateral femoral hernia, with obstruction, without gangrene**
Femoral hernia (unilateral) causing obstruction, without gangrene
Incarcerated femoral hernia (unilateral), without gangrene
Irreducible femoral hernia (unilateral), without gangrene
Strangulated femoral hernia (unilateral), without gangrene
K41.30 Unilateral femoral hernia, with obstruction, without gangrene, not specified as recurrent CC
Femoral hernia, with obstruction NOS
Unilateral femoral hernia, with obstruction NOS
K41.31 Unilateral femoral hernia, with obstruction, without gangrene, recurrent CC

✓5ᵗʰ **K41.4 Unilateral femoral hernia, with gangrene**
K41.40 Unilateral femoral hernia, with gangrene, not specified as recurrent MCC
Femoral hernia, with gangrene NOS
Unilateral femoral hernia, with gangrene NOS
CC Excl: See code: K41.10

Diseases of the Digestive System

K41.41–K50.0

K41.41 Unilateral femoral hernia, with gangrene, recurrent   `MCC`
CC Excl: See code: K41.10

✓5ᵗʰ K41.9 Unilateral femoral hernia, without obstruction or gangrene

K41.90 Unilateral femoral hernia, without obstruction or gangrene, not specified as recurrent
Femoral hernia NOS
Unilateral femoral hernia NOS

K41.91 Unilateral femoral hernia, without obstruction or gangrene, recurrent

✓4ᵗʰ K42 Umbilical hernia
INCLUDES paraumbilical hernia
EXCLUDES 1 omphalocele (Q79.2)

K42.0 Umbilical hernia with obstruction, without gangrene   `CC`
Umbilical hernia causing obstruction, without gangrene
Incarcerated umbilical hernia, without gangrene
Irreducible umbilical hernia, without gangrene
Strangulated umbilical hernia, without gangrene
CC Excl: K42.0-K42.1, K43.0, K43.1, K43.3-K43.4, K43.6-K43.7, K45.0, K45.8-K46.0

K42.1 Umbilical hernia with gangrene   `MCC`
Gangrenous umbilical hernia
CC Excl: K31.89-K31.9, K42.0-K43.0, K43.1, K43.2-K43.9, K45.0, K45.8-K46.0, K46.9, K92.81

K42.9 Umbilical hernia without obstruction or gangrene
Umbilical hernia NOS

✓4ᵗʰ K43 Ventral hernia

K43.0 Incisional hernia with obstruction, without gangrene   `CC`
Incisional hernia causing obstruction, without gangrene
Incarcerated incisional hernia, without gangrene
Irreducible incisional hernia, without gangrene
Strangulated incisional hernia, without gangrene
CC Excl: See code: K42.0

K43.1 Incisional hernia with gangrene   `MCC`
Gangrenous incisional hernia
CC Excl: See code: K42.1

K43.2 Incisional hernia without obstruction or gangrene
Incisional hernia NOS

K43.3 Parastomal hernia with obstruction, without gangrene   `CC`
Incarcerated parastomal hernia, without gangrene
Irreducible parastomal hernia, without gangrene
Parastomal hernia causing obstruction, without gangrene
Strangulated parastomal hernia, without gangrene
CC Excl: See code: K42.0

K43.4 Parastomal hernia with gangrene   `MCC`
Gangrenous parastomal hernia
CC Excl: See code: K42.1

K43.5 Parastomal hernia without obstruction or gangrene
Parastomal hernia NOS

K43.6 Other and unspecified ventral hernia with obstruction, without gangrene   `CC`
Epigastric hernia causing obstruction, without gangrene
Hypogastric hernia causing obstruction, without gangrene
Incarcerated epigastric hernia without gangrene
Incarcerated hypogastric hernia without gangrene
Incarcerated midline hernia without gangrene
Incarcerated spigelian hernia without gangrene
Incarcerated subxiphoid hernia without gangrene
Irreducible epigastric hernia without gangrene
Irreducible hypogastric hernia without gangrene
Irreducible midline hernia without gangrene
Irreducible spigelian hernia without gangrene
Irreducible subxiphoid hernia without gangrene
Midline hernia causing obstruction, without gangrene
Spigelian hernia causing obstruction, without gangrene
Strangulated epigastric hernia without gangrene
Strangulated hypogastric hernia without gangrene
Strangulated midline hernia without gangrene
Strangulated spigelian hernia without gangrene
Strangulated subxiphoid hernia without gangrene
Subxiphoid hernia causing obstruction, without gangrene
CC Excl: See code: K42.0

K43.7 Other and unspecified ventral hernia with gangrene   `MCC`
Any condition listed under K43.6 specified as gangrenous
CC Excl: See code: K42.1

K43.9 Ventral hernia without obstruction or gangrene
Epigastric hernia
Ventral hernia NOS

✓4ᵗʰ K44 Diaphragmatic hernia
INCLUDES hiatus hernia (esophageal) (sliding)
paraesophageal hernia
EXCLUDES 1 congenital diaphragmatic hernia (Q79.0)
congenital hiatus hernia (Q40.1)

K44.0 Diaphragmatic hernia with obstruction, without gangrene   `CC`
Diaphragmatic hernia causing obstruction
Incarcerated diaphragmatic hernia
Irreducible diaphragmatic hernia
Strangulated diaphragmatic hernia
CC Excl: K44.0-K45.0, K45.8-K46.0

K44.1 Diaphragmatic hernia with gangrene   `MCC`
Gangrenous diaphragmatic hernia
CC Excl: See code: K44.0

K44.9 Diaphragmatic hernia without obstruction or gangrene
Diaphragmatic hernia NOS

✓4ᵗʰ K45 Other abdominal hernia
INCLUDES abdominal hernia, specified site NEC
lumbar hernia
obturator hernia
pudendal hernia
retroperitoneal hernia
sciatic hernia

K45.0 Other specified abdominal hernia with obstruction, without gangrene   `CC`
Other specified abdominal hernia causing obstruction
Other specified incarcerated abdominal hernia
Other specified irreducible abdominal hernia
Other specified strangulated abdominal hernia
CC Excl: K40.00-K43.0, K43.1, K43.2-K43.9, K44.0-K46.9

K45.1 Other specified abdominal hernia with gangrene   `MCC`
Any condition listed under K45 specified as gangrenous
CC Excl: K31.89-K31.9, K40.00-K43.0, K43.1, K43.2-K43.9, K44.0-K46.9, K92.81

K45.8 Other specified abdominal hernia without obstruction or gangrene

✓4ᵗʰ K46 Unspecified abdominal hernia
INCLUDES enterocele
epiplocele
hernia NOS
interstitial hernia
intestinal hernia
intra-abdominal hernia
EXCLUDES 1 vaginal enterocele (N81.5)

K46.0 Unspecified abdominal hernia with obstruction, without gangrene   `CC`
Unspecified abdominal hernia causing obstruction
Unspecified incarcerated abdominal hernia
Unspecified irreducible abdominal hernia
Unspecified strangulated abdominal hernia
CC Excl: See code: K45.0

K46.1 Unspecified abdominal hernia with gangrene   `MCC`
Any condition listed under K46 specified as gangrenous
CC Excl: See code: K45.1

K46.9 Unspecified abdominal hernia without obstruction or gangrene
Abdominal hernia NOS

Noninfective enteritis and colitis (K50-K52)

INCLUDES noninfective inflammatory bowel disease
EXCLUDES 1 irritable bowel syndrome (K58.-)
megacolon (K59.3)

✓4ᵗʰ K50 Crohn's disease [regional enteritis]
INCLUDES granulomatous enteritis
Use additional code to identify manifestations, such as:
pyoderma gangrenosum (L88)
EXCLUDES 1 ulcerative colitis (K51.-)
AHA: 2012, 4Q, 104

CC Excl: For CC codes in category K50, unless otherwise noted:
K50.00-K51.919

✓5ᵗʰ K50.0 Crohn's disease of small intestine
Crohn's disease [regional enteritis] of duodenum
Crohn's disease [regional enteritis] of ileum
Crohn's disease [regional enteritis] of jejunum
Regional ileitis
Terminal ileitis
EXCLUDES 1 Crohn's disease of both small and large intestine (K50.8-)

N Newborn: 0   P Pediatric: 0-17   M Maternity: 12-55   A Adult: 15-124   MCC Major CC Condition   PDx MCC PDx acts as own MCC   CC CC Condition   PDx CC PDx acts as own CC

K50.00   Crohn's disease of small intestine *without complications*   `CC`

✓6th **K50.01**   Crohn's disease of small intestine *with complications*

     K50.011   Crohn's disease of small intestine with *rectal bleeding*   `CC`

     K50.012   Crohn's disease of small intestine with *intestinal obstruction*   `PDx CC` `CC`

     K50.013   Crohn's disease of small intestine with *fistula*   `PDx CC` `CC`

     K50.014   Crohn's disease of small intestine with *abscess*   `PDx CC` `CC`
          AHA: 2012, 4Q, 104

     K50.018   Crohn's disease of small intestine with *other complication*   `CC`

     K50.019   Crohn's disease of small intestine with *unspecified complications*   `CC`

✓5th **K50.1**   Crohn's disease of *large intestine*
     Crohn's disease [regional enteritis] of colon
     Crohn's disease [regional enteritis] of large bowel
     Crohn's disease [regional enteritis] of rectum
     Granulomatous colitis
     Regional colitis
     EXCLUDES 1   Crohn's disease of both small and large intestine (K50.8)

     K50.10   Crohn's disease of large intestine *without complications*   `CC`

✓6th   **K50.11**   Crohn's disease of large intestine *with complications*

     K50.111   Crohn's disease of large intestine with *rectal bleeding*   `CC`

     K50.112   Crohn's disease of large intestine with *intestinal obstruction*   `PDx CC` `CC`

     K50.113   Crohn's disease of large intestine with *fistula*   `PDx CC` `CC`

     K50.114   Crohn's disease of large intestine with *abscess*   `PDx CC` `CC`

     K50.118   Crohn's disease of large intestine with *other complication*   `CC`

     K50.119   Crohn's disease of large intestine with *unspecified complications*   `CC`

✓5th **K50.8**   Crohn's disease of *both small and large intestine*

     K50.80   Crohn's disease of both small and large intestine *without complications*   `CC`

✓6th   **K50.81**   Crohn's disease of both small and large intestine *with complications*

     K50.811   Crohn's disease of both small and large intestine with *rectal bleeding*   `CC`

     K50.812   Crohn's disease of both small and large intestine with *intestinal obstruction*   `PDx CC` `CC`

     K50.813   Crohn's disease of both small and large intestine with *fistula*   `PDx CC` `CC`

     K50.814   Crohn's disease of both small and large intestine with *abscess*   `PDx CC` `CC`

     K50.818   Crohn's disease of both small and large intestine with *other complication*   `CC`

     K50.819   Crohn's disease of both small and large intestine with *unspecified complications*   `CC`

✓5th **K50.9**   Crohn's disease, *unspecified*

> **CC Excl: For CC codes in subcategory K50.9, unless otherwise noted:** K50.00-K50.919

     K50.90   Crohn's disease, unspecified, *without complications*   `CC`
          Crohn's disease NOS
          Regional enteritis NOS

✓6th   **K50.91**   Crohn's disease, unspecified, *with complications*

     K50.911   Crohn's disease, unspecified, with *rectal bleeding*   `CC`

     K50.912   Crohn's disease, unspecified, with *intestinal obstruction*   `PDx CC` `CC`

     K50.913   Crohn's disease, unspecified, with *fistula*   `PDx CC` `CC`

     K50.914   Crohn's disease, unspecified, with *abscess*   `PDx CC` `CC`

     K50.918   Crohn's disease, unspecified, with *other complication*   `CC`

     K50.919   Crohn's disease, unspecified, with *unspecified complications*   `CC`

✓4th **K51**   **Ulcerative colitis**
     Use additional code to identify manifestations, such as:
     pyoderma gangrenosum (L88)
     EXCLUDES 1   Crohn's disease [regional enteritis] (K50.-)

> **CC Excl: For CC codes in category K51, unless otherwise noted:** See code: K50.9

✓5th **K51.0**   Ulcerative (chronic) *pancolitis*
     Backwash ileitis

     K51.00   Ulcerative (chronic) pancolitis *without complications*   `CC`
          Ulcerative (chronic) pancolitis NOS

✓6th   **K51.01**   Ulcerative (chronic) pancolitis *with complications*

     K51.011   Ulcerative (chronic) pancolitis with *rectal bleeding*   `CC`

     K51.012   Ulcerative (chronic) pancolitis with *intestinal obstruction*   `PDx CC` `CC`

     K51.013   Ulcerative (chronic) pancolitis with *fistula*   `PDx CC` `CC`

     K51.014   Ulcerative (chronic) pancolitis with *abscess*   `PDx CC` `CC`

     K51.018   Ulcerative (chronic) pancolitis with *other complication*   `CC`

     K51.019   Ulcerative (chronic) pancolitis with *unspecified complications*   `CC`

✓5th **K51.2**   Ulcerative (chronic) *proctitis*

     K51.20   Ulcerative (chronic) proctitis *without complications*   `CC`
          Ulcerative (chronic) proctitis NOS

✓6th   **K51.21**   Ulcerative (chronic) proctitis *with complications*

     K51.211   Ulcerative (chronic) proctitis with *rectal bleeding*   `CC`

     K51.212   Ulcerative (chronic) proctitis with *intestinal obstruction*   `PDx CC` `CC`

     K51.213   Ulcerative (chronic) proctitis with *fistula*   `PDx CC` `CC`

     K51.214   Ulcerative (chronic) proctitis with *abscess*   `PDx CC` `CC`

     K51.218   Ulcerative (chronic) proctitis with *other complication*   `CC`

     K51.219   Ulcerative (chronic) proctitis with *unspecified complications*   `CC`

✓5th **K51.3**   Ulcerative (chronic) *rectosigmoiditis*

     K51.30   Ulcerative (chronic) rectosigmoiditis *without complications*   `CC`
          Ulcerative (chronic) rectosigmoiditis NOS

✓6th   **K51.31**   Ulcerative (chronic) rectosigmoiditis *with complications*

     K51.311   Ulcerative (chronic) rectosigmoiditis with *rectal bleeding*   `CC`

     K51.312   Ulcerative (chronic) rectosigmoiditis with *intestinal obstruction*   `PDx CC` `CC`

     K51.313   Ulcerative (chronic) rectosigmoiditis with *fistula*   `PDx CC` `CC`

     K51.314   Ulcerative (chronic) rectosigmoiditis with *abscess*   `PDx CC` `CC`

     K51.318   Ulcerative (chronic) rectosigmoiditis with *other complication*   `CC`

     K51.319   Ulcerative (chronic) rectosigmoiditis with *unspecified complications*   `CC`

✓5th **K51.4**   Inflammatory polyps of colon
     EXCLUDES 1   adenomatous polyp of colon (D12.6)
          polyposis of colon (D12.6)
          polyps of colon NOS (K63.5)

     K51.40   Inflammatory polyps of colon *without complications*   `CC`
          Inflammatory polyps of colon NOS

✓6th   **K51.41**   Inflammatory polyps of colon *with complications*

     K51.411   Inflammatory polyps of colon with *rectal bleeding*   `CC`

     K51.412   Inflammatory polyps of colon with *intestinal obstruction*   `PDx CC` `CC`

     K51.413   Inflammatory polyps of colon with *fistula*   `PDx CC` `CC`

     K51.414   Inflammatory polyps of colon with *abscess*   `PDx CC` `CC`

✓ Additional Character Required   ✓x7th *Xtension Alert*   Unacceptable PDx   Manifestation   Hospital Acquired Condition   *EXCLUDES 1* Not Coded Here   *EXCLUDES 2* Not Included Here

K51.418 Inflammatory polyps of colon with other complication `CC`

K51.419 Inflammatory polyps of colon with unspecified complications `CC`

✓5th **K51.5 Left sided colitis**
Left hemicolitis

K51.50 Left sided colitis without complications `CC`
Left sided colitis NOS

✓6th **K51.51 Left sided colitis** with complications

K51.511 Left sided colitis with rectal bleeding `CC`

K51.512 Left sided colitis with intestinal obstruction `PDx CC` `CC`

K51.513 Left sided colitis with fistula `PDx CC` `CC`

K51.514 Left sided colitis with abscess `PDx CC` `CC`

K51.518 Left sided colitis with other complication `CC`

K51.519 Left sided colitis with unspecified complications `CC`

✓5th **K51.8 Other ulcerative colitis**

K51.80 Other ulcerative colitis without complications `CC`

✓6th **K51.81 Other ulcerative colitis** with complications

K51.811 Other ulcerative colitis with rectal bleeding `CC`

K51.812 Other ulcerative colitis with intestinal obstruction `PDx CC` `CC`

K51.813 Other ulcerative colitis with fistula `PDx CC` `CC`

K51.814 Other ulcerative colitis with abscess `PDx CC` `CC`

K51.818 Other ulcerative colitis with other complication `CC`

K51.819 Other ulcerative colitis with unspecified complications `CC`

✓5th **K51.9 Ulcerative colitis, unspecified**

CC Excl: For CC codes in subcategory K51.9, unless otherwise noted: K51.00-K51.919

K51.90 Ulcerative colitis, unspecified, without complications `CC`

✓6th **K51.91 Ulcerative colitis, unspecified,** with complications

K51.911 Ulcerative colitis, unspecified with rectal bleeding `CC`

K51.912 Ulcerative colitis, unspecified with intestinal obstruction `PDx CC` `CC`

K51.913 Ulcerative colitis, unspecified with fistula `PDx CC` `CC`

K51.914 Ulcerative colitis, unspecified with abscess `PDx CC` `CC`

K51.918 Ulcerative colitis, unspecified with other complication `CC`

K51.919 Ulcerative colitis, unspecified with unspecified complications `CC`

✓4th **K52 Other and unspecified noninfective gastroenteritis and colitis**

K52.0 Gastroenteritis and colitis due to radiation `CC`
CC Excl: K52.0

K52.1 Toxic gastroenteritis and colitis `CC`
Drug-induced gastroenteritis and colitis
Code first (T51-T65) to identify toxic agent
Use additional code for adverse effect, if applicable, to identify drug (T36-T50 with fifth or sixth character 5)
CC Excl: K52.1

K52.2 Allergic and dietetic gastroenteritis and colitis
Food hypersensitivity gastroenteritis or colitis
Use additional code to identify type of food allergy (Z91.01-, Z91.02-)

✓5th **K52.8 Other specified noninfective gastroenteritis and colitis**

K52.81 Eosinophilic gastritis or gastroenteritis
Eosinophilic enteritis
EXCLUDES 1 eosinophilic esophagitis (K20.0)

K52.82 Eosinophilic colitis

K52.89 Other specified noninfective gastroenteritis and colitis
Collagenous colitis
Lymphocytic colitis
Microscopic colitis (collagenous or lymphocytic)

K52.9 Noninfective gastroenteritis and colitis, unspecified
Colitis NOS   Ileitis NOS
Enteritis NOS   Jejunitis NOS
Gastroenteritis NOS   Sigmoiditis NOS
EXCLUDES 1 diarrhea NOS (R19.7)
functional diarrhea (K59.1)
infectious gastroenteritis and colitis NOS (A09)
neonatal diarrhea (noninfective) (P78.3)
psychogenic diarrhea (F45.8)

Other diseases of intestines (K55-K64)

✓4th **K55 Vascular disorders of intestine**
EXCLUDES 1 necrotizing enterocolitis of newborn (P77.-)

K55.0 Acute vascular disorders of intestine `MCC`
Acute fulminant ischemic colitis
Acute intestinal infarction
Acute small intestine ischemia
Infarction of appendices epiploicae
Mesenteric (artery) (vein) embolism
Mesenteric (artery) (vein) infarction
Mesenteric (artery) (vein) thrombosis
Necrosis of intestine
Subacute ischemic colitis
CC Excl: K55.0-K55.1

K55.1 Chronic vascular disorders of intestine `CC`
Chronic ischemic colitis
Chronic ischemic enteritis
Chronic ischemic enterocolitis
Ischemic stricture of intestine
Mesenteric atherosclerosis
Mesenteric vascular insufficiency
CC Excl: K55.0-K55.1, K55.8-K55.9

✓5th **K55.2 Angiodysplasia of colon**

K55.20 Angiodysplasia of colon without hemorrhage

K55.21 Angiodysplasia of colon with hemorrhage `MCC`
CC Excl: E16.4, I85.01, K22.10-K22.11, K22.6-K22.719, K25.0-K28.9, K29.01, K29.21, K29.31, K29.41, K29.51, K29.61, K29.71, K29.81, K29.91, K31.811, K55.21, K57.01, K57.11, K57.13, K57.21, K57.31, K57.33, K57.41, K57.51, K57.53, K57.81, K57.91, K57.93, K62.5, K92.0-K92.2

K55.8 Other vascular disorders of intestine `CC`
CC Excl: See code: K55.1

K55.9 Vascular disorder of intestine, unspecified `CC`
Ischemic colitis
Ischemic enteritis
Ischemic enterocolitis
CC Excl: See code: K55.1

✓4th **K56 Paralytic ileus and intestinal obstruction without hernia**
EXCLUDES 1 congenital stricture or stenosis of intestine (Q41-Q42)
cystic fibrosis with meconium ileus (E84.11)
intestinal obstruction with hernia (K40-K46)
ischemic stricture of intestine (K55.1)
meconium ileus NOS (P76.0)
neonatal intestinal obstructions classifiable to P76-
obstruction of duodenum (K31.5)
postprocedural intestinal obstruction (K91.3)
stenosis of anus or rectum (K62.4)

CC Excl: For CC/MCC codes in category K56, unless otherwise noted: K56.0-K56.3, K56.49-K56.7, K63.4, K63.89-K63.9, K92.89-K92.9, R11.13

K56.0 Paralytic ileus `CC`
Paralysis of bowel   Paralysis of intestine
Paralysis of colon
EXCLUDES 1 gallstone ileus (K56.3)
ileus NOS (K56.7)
obstructive ileus NOS (K56.69)

K56.1 Intussusception `CC`
Intussusception or invagination of bowel
Intussusception or invagination of colon
Intussusception or invagination of intestine
Intussusception or invagination of rectum
EXCLUDES 2 intussusception of appendix (K38.8)

K56.2 Volvulus `MCC`
Strangulation of colon or intestine
Torsion of colon or intestine
Twist of colon or intestine
EXCLUDES 2 volvulus of duodenum (K31.5)

K56.3 Gallstone ileus `CC`
Obstruction of intestine by gallstone

Diseases of the Digestive System

✓5ᵗʰ **K56.4 Other impaction of intestine**

  K56.41 Fecal impaction
    EXCLUDES 1   constipation (K59.0-)
             incomplete defecation (R15.0)

  K56.49 Other impaction of intestine `CC`

K56.5 Intestinal adhesions [bands] with obstruction (postprocedural) (postinfection) `CC`
  Abdominal hernia due to adhesions with obstruction
  Peritoneal adhesions [bands] with intestinal obstruction (postprocedural) (postinfection)

✓5ᵗʰ **K56.6 Other and unspecified intestinal obstruction**

  K56.60 Unspecified intestinal obstruction `CC`
    Intestinal obstruction NOS
    EXCLUDES 1 intestinal obstruction due to specified condition—code to condition

  K56.69 Other intestinal obstruction `CC`
    Enterostenosis NOS
    Obstructive ileus NOS
    Occlusion of colon or intestine NOS
    Stenosis of colon or intestine NOS
    Stricture of colon or intestine NOS
    EXCLUDES 1 intestinal obstruction due to specified condition—code to condition

K56.7 Ileus, unspecified `CC`
  EXCLUDES 1 obstructive ileus (K56.69)

✓4ᵗʰ **K57 Diverticular disease of intestine**
  EXCLUDES 1 congenital diverticulum of intestine (Q43.8)
          Meckel's diverticulum (Q43.0)
  EXCLUDES 2 diverticulum of appendix (K38.2)

> CC Excl: For CC/MCC codes in category K57, unless otherwise noted: E16.4, I85.01, K22.10-K22.11, K22.6-K22.719, K25.0-K28.9, K29.01, K29.21, K29.31, K29.41, K29.51, K29.61, K29.71, K29.81, K29.91, K31.811, K55.21, K57.01, K57.11, K57.13, K57.21, K57.31, K57.33, K57.41, K57.51, K57.53, K57.81, K57.91, K57.93, K62.5, K92.0-K92.2

✓5ᵗʰ **K57.0 Diverticulitis of small intestine with perforation and abscess**
  Diverticulitis of small intestine with peritonitis
  EXCLUDES 1 diverticulitis of both small and large intestine with perforation and abscess (K57.4-)

  K57.00 Diverticulitis of small intestine with perforation and abscess without bleeding `PDx CC` `CC`
    CC Excl: K57.00-K57.13

  K57.01 Diverticulitis of small intestine with perforation and abscess with bleeding `PDx CC` `MCC`

✓5ᵗʰ **K57.1 Diverticular disease of small intestine without perforation or abscess**
  EXCLUDES 1 diverticular disease of both small and large intestine without perforation or abscess (K57.5-)

  K57.10 Diverticulosis of small intestine without perforation or abscess without bleeding
    Diverticular disease of small intestine NOS

  K57.11 Diverticulosis of small intestine without perforation or abscess with bleeding `MCC`

  K57.12 Diverticulitis of small intestine without perforation or abscess without bleeding `CC`
    CC Excl: See code: K57.00

  K57.13 Diverticulitis of small intestine without perforation or abscess with bleeding `MCC`

✓5ᵗʰ **K57.2 Diverticulitis of large intestine with perforation and abscess**
  Diverticulitis of colon with peritonitis
  EXCLUDES 1 diverticulitis of both small and large intestine with perforation and abscess (K57.4-)

  K57.20 Diverticulitis of large intestine with perforation and abscess without bleeding `PDx CC` `CC`
    CC Excl: K57.20-K57.93

  K57.21 Diverticulitis of large intestine with perforation and abscess with bleeding `PDx CC` `MCC`

✓5ᵗʰ **K57.3 Diverticular disease of large intestine without perforation or abscess**
  EXCLUDES 1 diverticular disease of both small and large intestine without perforation or abscess (K57.5-)

  K57.30 Diverticulosis of large intestine without perforation or abscess without bleeding
    Diverticular disease of colon NOS

  K57.31 Diverticulosis of large intestine without perforation or abscess with bleeding `MCC`

  K57.32 Diverticulitis of large intestine without perforation or abscess without bleeding `CC`
    CC Excl: See code: K57.20

  K57.33 Diverticulitis of large intestine without perforation or abscess with bleeding `MCC`

✓5ᵗʰ **K57.4 Diverticulitis of both small and large intestine with perforation and abscess**
  Diverticulitis of both small and large intestine with peritonitis

  K57.40 Diverticulitis of both small and large intestine with perforation and abscess without bleeding `PDx CC` `CC`
    CC Excl: See code: K57.20

  K57.41 Diverticulitis of both small and large intestine with perforation and abscess with bleeding `PDx CC` `MCC`

✓5ᵗʰ **K57.5 Diverticular disease of both small and large intestine without perforation or abscess**

  K57.50 Diverticulosis of both small and large intestine without perforation or abscess without bleeding
    Diverticular disease of both small and large intestine NOS

  K57.51 Diverticulitis of both small and large intestine without perforation or abscess with bleeding `MCC`

  K57.52 Diverticulitis of both small and large intestine without perforation or abscess without bleeding `PDx CC` `CC`
    CC Excl: See code: K57.20

  K57.53 Diverticulitis of both small and large intestine without perforation or abscess with bleeding `MCC`

✓5ᵗʰ **K57.8 Diverticulitis of intestine, part unspecified, with perforation and abscess**
  Diverticulitis of intestine NOS with peritonitis

  K57.80 Diverticulitis of intestine, part unspecified, with perforation and abscess without bleeding `PDx CC` `CC`
    CC Excl: See code: K57.20

  K57.81 Diverticulitis of intestine, part unspecified, with perforation and abscess with bleeding `PDx CC` `MCC`

✓5ᵗʰ **K57.9 Diverticular disease of intestine, part unspecified, without perforation or abscess**

  K57.90 Diverticulosis of intestine, part unspecified, without perforation or abscess without bleeding
    Diverticular disease of intestine NOS

  K57.91 Diverticulosis of intestine, part unspecified, without perforation or abscess with bleeding `MCC`

  (**K57.92**) **Diverticulitis of intestine, part unspecified, without perforation or abscess without bleeding** `CC`
    CC Excl: See code: K57.20

  K57.93 Diverticulitis of intestine, part unspecified, without perforation or abscess with bleeding `MCC`

✓4ᵗʰ **K58 Irritable bowel syndrome**
  INCLUDES irritable colon
         spastic colon

  K58.0 Irritable bowel syndrome with diarrhea

  K58.9 Irritable bowel syndrome without diarrhea
    Irritable bowel syndrome NOS

✓4ᵗʰ **K59 Other functional intestinal disorders**
  EXCLUDES 1 change in bowel habit NOS (R19.4)
          intestinal malabsorption (K90.-)
          psychogenic intestinal disorders (F45.8)
  EXCLUDES 2 functional disorders of stomach (K31.-)

✓5ᵗʰ **K59.0 Constipation**
  EXCLUDES 1 fecal impaction (K56.41)
          incomplete defecation (R15.0)

  K59.00 Constipation, unspecified

  K59.01 Slow transit constipation

  K59.02 Outlet dysfunction constipation

  K59.09 Other constipation

  K59.1 Functional diarrhea
    EXCLUDES 1 diarrhea NOS (R19.7)
           irritable bowel syndrome with diarrhea (K58.0)

  K59.2 Neurogenic bowel, not elsewhere classified `CC`
    CC Excl: K58.0-K58.9, K59.1-K59.9, K91.0-K91.1

✓ Additional Character Required   ✓x7ᵗʰ Xtension Alert   Unacceptable PDx   Manifestation   Hospital Acquired Condition   *EXCLUDES 1* Not Coded Here   *EXCLUDES 2* Not Included Here

ICD-10-CM Draft (2015)   651

Diseases of the Digestive System

K59.3–K63.5

K59.3 Megacolon, not elsewhere classified `CC`
Dilatation of colon
Toxic megacolon
Code first (T51-T65) to identify toxic agent
EXCLUDES 1   congenital megacolon (aganglionic) (Q43.1)
megacolon (due to) (in) Chagas' disease (B57.32)
megacolon (due to) (in) Clostridium difficile (A04.7)
megacolon (due to) (in) Hirschsprung's disease (Q43.1)
CC Excl: See code: K59.2

K59.4 Anal spasm
Proctalgia fugax

K59.8 Other specified functional intestinal disorders
Atony of colon
Pseudo-obstruction (acute) (chronic) of intestine

K59.9 Functional intestinal disorder, unspecified

✓4ᵗʰ K60 Fissure and fistula of anal and rectal regions
EXCLUDES 1   fissure and fistula of anal and rectal regions with abscess or
cellulitis (K61.-)
EXCLUDES 2   anal sphincter tear (healed) (nontraumatic) (old) (K62.81)

K60.0 Acute anal fissure

K60.1 Chronic anal fissure

K60.2 Anal fissure, unspecified

K60.3 Anal fistula

K60.4 Rectal fistula
Fistula of rectum to skin
EXCLUDES 1   rectovaginal fistula (N82.3)
vesicorectal fistual (N32.1)

K60.5 Anorectal fistula

✓4ᵗʰ K61 Abscess of anal and rectal regions
INCLUDES   abscess of anal and rectal regions
cellulitis of anal and rectal regions

**CC Excl: For CC codes in category K61, unless otherwise
noted:** K61.0-K61.4

K61.0 Anal abscess `CC`
Perianal abscess
EXCLUDES 1   intrasphincteric abscess (K61.4)

K61.1 Rectal abscess `CC`
Perirectal abscess
EXCLUDES 1   ischiorectal abscess (K61.3)
AHA: 2012, 4Q, 104

K61.2 Anorectal abscess `CC`

K61.3 Ischiorectal abscess `CC`
Abscess of ischiorectal fossa

K61.4 Intrasphincteric abscess `CC`

✓4ᵗʰ K62 Other diseases of anus and rectum
INCLUDES   anal canal
EXCLUDES 2   colostomy and enterostomy malfunction (K94.0-, K94.1-)
fecal incontinence (R15.-)
hemorrhoids (K64.-)

K62.0 Anal polyp

K62.1 Rectal polyp
EXCLUDES 1   adenomatous polyp (D12.8)

K62.2 Anal prolapse
Prolapse of anal canal

K62.3 Rectal prolapse
Prolapse of rectal mucosa

K62.4 Stenosis of anus and rectum
Stricture of anus (sphincter)

K62.5 Hemorrhage of anus and rectum `CC`
EXCLUDES 1   gastrointestinal bleeding NOS (K92.2)
melena (K92.1)
neonatal rectal hemorrhage (P54.2)
CC Excl: E16.4, I85.01, K22.10-K22.11, K22.6-K22.719, K25.0-K28.9,
K29.01, K29.21, K29.31, K29.41, K29.51, K29.61, K29.71, K29.81,
K29.91, K31.811, K55.21, K57.01, K57.11, K57.13, K57.21, K57.31,
K57.33, K57.41, K57.51, K57.53, K57.81, K57.91, K57.93, K62.5,
K92.0-K92.2

K62.6 Ulcer of anus and rectum `CC`
Solitary ulcer of anus and rectum
Stercoral ulcer of anus and rectum
EXCLUDES 1   fissure and fistula of anus and rectum (K60.-)
ulcerative colitis (K51.-)
CC Excl: K62.6

K62.7 Radiation proctitis
Use additional code to identify the type of radiation (W90.-)

✓5ᵗʰ K62.8 Other specified diseases of anus and rectum
EXCLUDES 2   ulcerative proctitis (K51.2)

K62.81 Anal sphincter tear (healed) (nontraumatic) (old)
Tear of anus, nontraumatic
Use additional code for any associated fecal
incontinence (R15.-)
EXCLUDES 2   anal fissure (K60.-)
anal sphincter tear (healed) (old)
complicating delivery (O34.7-)
traumatic tear of anal sphincter (S31.831)

K62.82 Dysplasia of anus
Anal intraepithelial neoplasia I and II (AIN I and II)
(histologically confirmed)
Dysplasia of anus NOS
Mild and moderate dysplasia of anus (histologically
confirmed)
EXCLUDES 1   abnormal results from anal cytologic
examination without histologic
confirmation (R85.61-)
anal intraepithelial neoplasia III (D01.3)
carcinoma in situ of anus (D01.3)
HGSIL of anus (R85.613)
severe dysplasia of anus (D01.3)

K62.89 Other specified diseases of anus and rectum
Proctitis NOS
Use additional code for any associated fecal
incontinence (R15.-)

K62.9 Disease of anus and rectum, unspecified

✓4ᵗʰ K63 Other diseases of intestine

K63.0 Abscess of intestine `CC`
EXCLUDES 1   abscess of intestine with Crohn's disease (K50.014,
K50.114, K50.814, K50.914)
abscess of intestine with diverticular disease (K57.0,
K57.2, K57.4, K57.8)
abscess of intestine with ulcerative colitis (K51.014,
K51.214, K51.314, K51.414, K51.514, K51.814,
K51.914)
EXCLUDES 2   abscess of anal and rectal regions (K61.-)
abscess of appendix (K35.3)
CC Excl: K63.0

K63.1 Perforation of intestine (nontraumatic) `MCC`
Perforation (nontraumatic) of rectum
EXCLUDES 1   perforation (nontraumatic) of duodenum (K26.-)
perforation (nontraumatic) of intestine with
diverticular disease (K57.0, K57.2, K57.4, K57.8)
EXCLUDES 2   perforation (nontraumatic) of appendix (K35.2, K35.3)
CC Excl: K63.1

K63.2 Fistula of intestine `CC`
EXCLUDES 1   fistula of duodenum (K31.6)
fistula of intestine with Crohn's disease (K50.013,
K50.113, K50.813, K50.913)
fistula of intestine with ulcerative colitis (K51.013,
K51.213, K51.313, K51.413, K51.513, K51.813,
K51.913)
EXCLUDES 2   fistula of anal and rectal regions (K60.-)
fistula of appendix (K38.3)
intestinal-genital fistula, female (N82.2-N82.4)
vesicointestinal fistula (N32.1)
CC Excl: K63.2

K63.3 Ulcer of intestine `CC`
Primary ulcer of small intestine
EXCLUDES 1   duodenal ulcer (K26.-)
gastrointestinal ulcer (K28.-)
gastrojejunal ulcer (K28.-)
jejunal ulcer (K28.-)
peptic ulcer, site unspecified (K27.-)
ulcer of intestine with perforation (K63.1)
ulcer of anus or rectum (K62.6)
ulcerative colitis (K51.-)
CC Excl: K63.3

K63.4 Enteroptosis

K63.5 Polyp of colon
EXCLUDES 1   adenomatous polyp of colon (D12.6)
inflammatory polyp of colon (K51.4-)
polyposis of colon (D12.6)

N Newborn: 0   **P** Pediatric: 0-17   **M** Maternity: 12-55   **A** Adult: 15-124   **MCC** Major CC Condition   **PDx MCC** PDx acts as own MCC   **CC** CC Condition   **PDx CC** PDx acts as own CC

652   ICD-10-CM Draft (2015)

✓5ᵗʰ K63.8 Other specified diseases of intestine

K63.81 Dieulafoy lesion of intestine `MCC`
    `EXCLUDES 2` *Dieulafoy lesion of stomach and duodenum (K31.82)*
    CC Excl: E16.4, I85.01, K22.10-K22.11, K22.6-K22.719, K25.0-K28.9, K29.01, K29.21, K29.31, K29.41, K29.51, K29.61, K29.71, K29.81, K29.91, K31.811, K55.21, K57.01, K57.11, K57.13, K57.21, K57.31, K57.33, K57.41, K57.51, K57.53, K57.81, K57.91, K57.93, K62.5, K63.81, K92.0-K92.2

K63.89 Other specified diseases of intestine
    AHA: 2013, 2Q, 31

K63.9 Disease of intestine, unspecified

✓4ᵗʰ K64 Hemorrhoids and perianal venous thrombosis
    `INCLUDES` piles
    `EXCLUDES 1` *hemorrhoids complicating childbirth and the puerperium (O87.2)*
                hemorrhoids complicating pregnancy (O22.4)

K64.0 First degree hemorrhoids
    Grade/stage I hemorrhoids
    Hemorrhoids (bleeding) without prolapse outside of anal canal

K64.1 Second degree hemorrhoids
    Grade/stage II hemorrhoids
    Hemorrhoids (bleeding) that prolapse with straining, but retract spontaneously

K64.2 Third degree hemorrhoids
    Grade/stage III hemorrhoids
    Hemorrhoids (bleeding) that prolapse with straining and require manual replacement back inside anal canal

K64.3 Fourth degree hemorrhoids
    Grade/stage IV hemorrhoids
    Hemorrhoids (bleeding) with prolapsed tissue that cannot be manually replaced

K64.4 Residual hemorrhoidal skin tags
    External hemorrhoids, NOS   Skin tags of anus

K64.5 Perianal venous thrombosis
    External hemorrhoids with thrombosis
    Perianal hematoma
    Thrombosed hemorrhoids NOS

K64.8 Other hemorrhoids
    Internal hemorrhoids, without mention of degree
    Prolapsed hemorrhoids, degree not specified

K64.9 Unspecified hemorrhoids
    Hemorrhoids (bleeding) NOS
    Hemorrhoids (bleeding) without mention of degree

Diseases of peritoneum and retroperitoneum (K65-K68)

✓4ᵗʰ K65 Peritonitis
    Use additional code (B95-B97), to identify infectious agent
    `EXCLUDES 1` *acute appendicitis with generalized peritonitis (K35.2)*
                aseptic peritonitis (T81.6)
                benign paroxysmal peritonitis (E85.0)
                chemical peritonitis (T81.6)
                diverticulitis of both small and large intestine with peritonitis (K57.4-)
                diverticulitis of colon with peritonitis (K57.2-)
                diverticulitis of intestine, NOS, with peritonitis (K57.8-)
                diverticulitis of small intestine with peritonitis (K57.0-)
                gonococcal peritonitis (A54.85)
                neonatal peritonitis (P78.0-P78.1)
                pelvic peritonitis, female (N73.3-N73.5)
                periodic familial peritonitis (E85.0)
                peritonitis due to talc or other foreign substance (T81.6)
                peritonitis in chlamydia (A74.81)
                peritonitis in diphtheria (A36.89)
                peritonitis in syphilis (late) (A52.74)
                peritonitis in tuberculosis (A18.31)
                peritonitis with or following abortion or ectopic or molar pregnancy (O00-O07, O08.0)
                peritonitis with or following appendicitis (K35.-)
                peritonitis with or following diverticular disease of intestine (K57.-)
                puerperal peritonitis (O85)
                retroperitoneal infections (K68.-)

> **CC Excl: For MCC codes in category K65, unless otherwise noted:**
> K63.4, K63.89-K63.9, K65.0-K65.9, K67, K68.19-K68.9, K92.89-K92.9, R11.13

K65.0 Generalized (acute) peritonitis `MCC`
    Pelvic peritonitis (acute), male
    Subphrenic peritonitis (acute)
    Suppurative peritonitis (acute)

K65.1 Peritoneal abscess `MCC`
    Abdominopelvic abscess   Subdiaphragmatic abscess
    Abscess (of) omentum   Subhepatic abscess
    Abscess (of) peritoneum   Subphrenic abscess
    Mesenteric abscess
    Retrocecal abscess

K65.2 Spontaneous bacterial peritonitis `MCC`
    `EXCLUDES 1` *bacterial peritonitis NOS (K65.9)*

K65.3 Choleperitonitis `MCC`
    Peritonitis due to bile

K65.4 Sclerosing mesenteritis `CC`
    Fat necrosis of peritoneum
    (Idiopathic) sclerosing mesenteric fibrosis
    Mesenteric lipodystrophy
    Mesenteric panniculitis
    Retractile mesenteritis

K65.8 Other peritonitis `MCC`
    Chronic proliferative peritonitis   Peritonitis due to urine

K65.9 Peritonitis, unspecified `MCC`
    Bacterial peritonitis NOS
    AHA: 2013, 2Q, 31

✓4ᵗʰ K66 Other disorders of peritoneum
    `EXCLUDES 2` *ascites (R18.-)*
                peritoneal effusion (chronic) (R18.8)

K66.0 Peritoneal adhesions (postprocedural) (postinfection)
    Adhesions (of) abdominal (wall)   Adhesions (of) omentum
    Adhesions (of) diaphragm   Adhesions (of) stomach
    Adhesions (of) intestine   Adhesive bands
    Adhesions (of) male pelvis   Mesenteric adhesions
    `EXCLUDES 1` *female pelvic adhesions [bands] (N73.6)*
                peritoneal adhesions with intestinal obstruction (K56.5)

K66.1 Hemoperitoneum `MCC`
    `EXCLUDES 1` *traumatic hemoperitoneum (S36.8-)*
    CC Excl: K66.1

K66.8 Other specified disorders of peritoneum

K66.9 Disorder of peritoneum, unspecified

K67 Disorders of peritoneum in infectious diseases classified elsewhere `MCC`
    Code first underlying disease, such as:
      congenital syphilis (A50.0)
      helminthiasis (B65.0-B83.9)
    `EXCLUDES 1` *peritonitis in chlamydia (A74.81)*
                peritonitis in diphtheria (A36.89)
                peritonitis in gonococcal (A54.85)
                peritonitis in syphilis (late) (A52.74)
                peritonitis in tuberculosis (A18.31)
    CC Excl: See code: K65

✓4ᵗʰ K68 Disorders of retroperitoneum

✓5ᵗʰ K68.1 Retroperitoneal abscess

4, 6, 8 K68.11 Postprocedural retroperitoneal abscess `CC`
    CC Excl: D78.81-D78.89, E36.8, E89.810-E89.89, H59.011-H59.019, H59.031-H59.099, H59.811-H59.89, H95.811-H95.89, I97.3, K68.11, L76.81-L76.82, M96.89, N98.1-N98.9, T81.4XXA, T81.82XA, T81.89XA, T81.9XXA

K68.12 Psoas muscle abscess `MCC`
    CC Excl: K68.12, M60.000-M60.19, M61.00-M61.19, M61.30-M61.59, M62.3, M62.50-M62.59, M62.89, M72.6

K68.19 Other retroperitoneal abscess `MCC`
    CC Excl: See code: K65

K68.9 Other disorders of retroperitoneum `MCC`
    CC Excl: See code: K65

---

4 HAC = as SDx not POA, in combination with PDx E66.01 **AND** one of the following procedure codes: 0D16[0,4,8][7,J,K,Z][9,A,B,L] or 0DV64CZ.

6 HAC = as SDx not POA, in combination with one of the following procedure codes: 0RG[0,1,2,4,6,7,8,A][0,3,4][7,A,J,K,Z][0,1,J]; 0RG[E,F,G,H,J,K][0,3,4][4,7,J,K,Z]; 0RG[L,M][0,3,4][4,5,7,J,K,Z]; 0RQ[E,F,G,H,J,K,L,M][0,3,4,X]ZZ; 0RU[E,F,G,H,J,K,L,M][0,3,4][7,J,K]Z; 0SG[0,1,3][0,3,4][7,A,J,K,Z][0,1,J]; 0SG[7,8][0,3,4[4,7,J,K,Z]Z.

8 HAC = as SDx not POA, in combination with one of the following procedure codes: 02H43[J,K,M]Z; 02H[6,7]3[J,M]Z; 02H[K,L]3JZ; 02HN[0,3,4][J,M]Z; 02PA[0,3,4]MZ; 02PAXMZ; 02WA[0,3,4]MZ; 0JH[6,8][0,3][4,5,6,7,8,9,P]Z; 0J[P,W]T[0,3]PZ.

✓ Additional Character Required   ✓x7ᵗʰ Xtension Alert   Unacceptable PDx   Manifestation   Hospital Acquired Condition   `EXCLUDES 1` Not Coded Here   `EXCLUDES 2` Not Included Here

Diseases of the Digestive System

K70–K74.69

Diseases of liver (K70-K77)

EXCLUDES 1   *jaundice NOS (R17)*
EXCLUDES 2   *hemochromatosis (E83.11-)*
          Reye's syndrome (G93.7)
          viral hepatitis (B15-B19)
          Wilson's disease (E83.0)

✓4th **K70   Alcoholic liver disease**
     Use additional code to identify:
         alcohol abuse and dependence (F10.-)

     K70.0   Alcoholic fatty liver   A

  ✓5th **K70.1   Alcoholic hepatitis**
        K70.10   Alcoholic hepatitis without ascites   A
        K70.11   Alcoholic hepatitis with ascites   A

     K70.2   Alcoholic fibrosis and sclerosis of liver   A

  ✓5th **K70.3   Alcoholic cirrhosis of liver**
        Alcoholic cirrhosis NOS
        K70.30   Alcoholic cirrhosis of liver without ascites   A
        K70.31   Alcoholic cirrhosis of liver with ascites   A

  ✓5th **K70.4   Alcoholic hepatic failure**
        Acute alcoholic hepatic failure
        Alcoholic hepatic failure NOS
        Chronic alcoholic hepatic failure
        Subacute alcoholic hepatic failure
        K70.40   Alcoholic hepatic failure without coma   A
        K70.41   Alcoholic hepatic failure with coma   PDx MCC   MCC   A
            CC Excl: K72.91, K76.5, K76.89-K76.9

     K70.9   Alcoholic liver disease, unspecified   A

✓4th **K71   Toxic liver disease**
     INCLUDES   drug-induced idiosyncratic (unpredictable) liver disease
               drug-induced toxic (predictable) liver disease
     Code first poisoning due to drug or toxin, if applicable (T36-T65 with fifth or sixth character 1-4 or 6)
     Use additional code for adverse effect, if applicable, to identify drug (T36-T50 with fifth or sixth character 5)
     EXCLUDES 2   *alcoholic liver disease (K70.-)*
              Budd-Chiari syndrome (I82.0)

     K71.0   Toxic liver disease with cholestasis
        Cholestasis with hepatocyte injury
        "Pure" cholestasis

  ✓5th **K71.1   Toxic liver disease with hepatic necrosis**
        Hepatic failure (acute) (chronic) due to drugs
        K71.10   Toxic liver disease with hepatic necrosis, without coma
        K71.11   Toxic liver disease with hepatic necrosis, with coma   PDx MCC   MCC
            CC Excl: See code: K70.41

     K71.2   Toxic liver disease with acute hepatitis

     K71.3   Toxic liver disease with chronic persistent hepatitis

     K71.4   Toxic liver disease with chronic lobular hepatitis

  ✓5th **K71.5   Toxic liver disease with chronic active hepatitis**
        Toxic liver disease with lupoid hepatitis
        K71.50   Toxic liver disease with chronic active hepatitis without ascites
        K71.51   Toxic liver disease with chronic active hepatitis with ascites

     K71.6   Toxic liver disease with hepatitis, not elsewhere classified

     K71.7   Toxic liver disease with fibrosis and cirrhosis of liver

     K71.8   Toxic liver disease with other disorders of liver
        Toxic liver disease with focal nodular hyperplasia
        Toxic liver disease with hepatic granulomas
        Toxic liver disease with peliosis hepatis
        Toxic liver disease with veno-occlusive disease of liver

     K71.9   Toxic liver disease, unspecified

✓4th **K72   Hepatic failure, not elsewhere classified**
     INCLUDES   acute hepatitis NEC, with hepatic failure
               fulminant hepatitis NEC, with hepatic failure
               hepatic encephalopathy NOS
               liver (cell) necrosis with hepatic failure
               malignant hepatitis NEC, with hepatic failure
               yellow liver atrophy or dystrophy
     EXCLUDES 1   *alcoholic hepatic failure (K70.4)*
              hepatic failure with toxic liver disease (K71.1-)
              icterus of newborn (P55-P59)
              postprocedural hepatic failure (K91.82)
              viral hepatitis with hepatic coma (B15-B19)
     EXCLUDES 2   *hepatic failure complicating abortion or ectopic or molar pregnancy (O00-O07, O08.8)*
              hepatic failure complicating pregnancy, childbirth and the puerperium (O26.6-)

  ✓5th **K72.0   Acute and subacute hepatic failure**
        AHA: 2014, 2Q, 13
        K72.00   Acute and subacute hepatic failure without coma   MCC
            CC Excl: K72.00-K72.01, K76.2-K76.3, K76.5, K76.89-K76.9
        K72.01   Acute and subacute hepatic failure with coma   PDx MCC   MCC
            CC Excl: See code: K72.00

  ✓5th **K72.1   Chronic hepatic failure**
        K72.10   Chronic hepatic failure without coma
        K72.11   Chronic hepatic failure with coma   PDx MCC   MCC
            CC Excl: K72.91, K76.5, K76.89-K76.9

  ✓5th **K72.9   Hepatic failure, unspecified**
        K72.90   Hepatic failure, unspecified without coma
            CC Excl: No Excl
        K72.91   Hepatic failure, unspecified with coma   MCC
            Hepatic coma NOS
            CC Excl: K72.91-K76.5, K76.89-K76.9

✓4th **K73   Chronic hepatitis, not elsewhere classified**
     EXCLUDES 1   *alcoholic hepatitis (chronic) (K70.1-)*
              drug-induced hepatitis (chronic) (K71.-)
              granulomatous hepatitis (chronic) NEC (K75.3)
              reactive, nonspecific hepatitis (chronic) (K75.2)
              viral hepatitis (chronic) (B15-B19)

     K73.0   Chronic persistent hepatitis, not elsewhere classified

     K73.1   Chronic lobular hepatitis, not elsewhere classified

     K73.2   Chronic active hepatitis, not elsewhere classified

     K73.8   Other chronic hepatitis, not elsewhere classified

     K73.9   Chronic hepatitis, unspecified

✓4th **K74   Fibrosis and cirrhosis of liver**
     Code also, if applicable, viral hepatitis (acute) (chronic) (B15-B19)
     EXCLUDES 1   *alcoholic cirrhosis (of liver) (K70.3)*
              alcoholic fibrosis of liver (K70.2)
              cardiac sclerosis of liver (K76.1)
              cirrhosis (of liver) with toxic liver disease (K71.7)
              congenital cirrhosis (of liver) (P78.81)
              pigmentary cirrhosis (of liver) (E83.110)

     K74.0   Hepatic fibrosis

     K74.1   Hepatic sclerosis

     K74.2   Hepatic fibrosis with hepatic sclerosis

     K74.3   Primary biliary cirrhosis
        Chronic nonsuppurative destructive cholangitis

     K74.4   Secondary biliary cirrhosis

     K74.5   Biliary cirrhosis, unspecified

  ✓5th **K74.6   Other and unspecified cirrhosis of liver**
        K74.60   Unspecified cirrhosis of liver
            Cirrhosis (of liver) NOS
        K74.69   Other cirrhosis of liver
            Cryptogenic cirrhosis (of liver)
            Macronodular cirrhosis (of liver)
            Micronodular cirrhosis (of liver)
            Mixed type cirrhosis (of liver)
            Portal cirrhosis (of liver)
            Postnecrotic cirrhosis (of liver)

N Newborn: 0   P Pediatric: 0-17   M Maternity: 12-55   A Adult: 15-124   MCC Major CC Condition   PDx MCC PDx acts as own MCC   CC CC Condition   PDx CC PDx acts as own CC

654   ICD-10-CM Draft (2015)

K75 Other inflammatory liver diseases
EXCLUDES 2 *toxic liver disease (K71.-)*

K75.0 Abscess of liver   MCC
Cholangitic hepatic abscess
Hematogenic hepatic abscess
Hepatic abscess NOS
Lymphogenic hepatic abscess
Pylephlebitic hepatic abscess
EXCLUDES 1 *amebic liver abscess (A06.4)*
cholangitis without liver abscess (K83.0)
pylephlebitis without liver abscess (K75.1)
CC Excl: A06.4, K75.1, K76.5, K76.89-K76.9

K75.1 Phlebitis of portal vein   MCC
Pylephlebitis
EXCLUDES 1 *pylephlebitic liver abscess (K75.0)*
CC Excl: See code: K75.0

K75.2 Nonspecific reactive hepatitis
EXCLUDES 1 *acute or subacute hepatitis (K72.0-)*
chronic hepatitis NEC (K73.-)
viral hepatitis (B15-B19)

K75.3 Granulomatous hepatitis, not elsewhere classified
EXCLUDES 1 *acute or subacute hepatitis (K72.0-)*
chronic hepatitis NEC (K73.-)
viral hepatitis (B15-B19)

K75.4 Autoimmune hepatitis
Lupoid hepatitis NEC

K75.8 Other specified inflammatory liver diseases
K75.81 Nonalcoholic steatohepatitis (NASH)
K75.89 Other specified inflammatory liver diseases

K75.9 Inflammatory liver disease, unspecified
Hepatitis NOS
EXCLUDES 1 *acute or subacute hepatitis (K72.0-)*
chronic hepatitis NEC (K73.-)
viral hepatitis (B15-B19)

K76 Other diseases of liver
EXCLUDES 2 *alcoholic liver disease (K70.-)*
amyloid degeneration of liver (E85.-)
cystic disease of liver (congenital) (Q44.6)
hepatic vein thrombosis (I82.0)
hepatomegaly NOS (R16.0)
pigmentary cirrhosis (of liver) (E83.110)
portal vein thrombosis (I81)
toxic liver disease (K71.-)

K76.0 Fatty (change of) liver, not elsewhere classified
Nonalcoholic fatty liver disease (NAFLD)
EXCLUDES 1 *nonalcoholic steatohepatitis (NASH) (K75.81)*

K76.1 Chronic passive congestion of liver
Cardiac cirrhosis
Cardiac sclerosis

K76.2 Central hemorrhagic necrosis of liver   MCC
EXCLUDES 1 *liver necrosis with hepatic failure (K72.-)*
CC Excl: K72.00-K72.01, K76.2-K76.3, K76.5, K76.89-K76.9

K76.3 Infarction of liver   MCC
CC Excl: See code: K76.2

K76.4 Peliosis hepatis
Hepatic angiomatosis

K76.5 Hepatic veno-occlusive disease
EXCLUDES 1 *Budd-Chiari syndrome (I82.0)*

K76.6 Portal hypertension   CC
Use additional code for any associated complications, such as:
portal hypertensive gastropathy (K31.89)
CC Excl: K72.91-K76.6, K76.89-K76.9

K76.7 Hepatorenal syndrome   MCC
EXCLUDES 1 *hepatorenal syndrome following labor and delivery (O90.4)*
postprocedural hepatorenal syndrome (K91.82)
CC Excl: K76.5-K76.7, K76.89-K76.9

K76.8 Other specified diseases of liver
K76.81 Hepatopulmonary syndrome
Code first underlying liver disease, such as:
alcoholic cirrhosis of liver (K70.3-)
cirrhosis of liver without mention of alcohol (K74.6-)
K76.89 Other specified diseases of liver
Cyst (simple) of liver
Focal nodular hyperplasia of liver
Hepatoptosis

K76.9 Liver disease, unspecified

K77 Liver disorders in diseases classified elsewhere   CC
Code first underlying disease, such as:
amyloidosis (E85.-)
congenital syphilis (A50.0, A50.5)
congenital toxoplasmosis (P37.1)
schistosomiasis (B65.0-B65.9)
EXCLUDES 1 *alcoholic hepatitis (K70.1-)*
alcoholic liver disease (K70-.)
cytomegaloviral hepatitis (B25.1)
herpesviral [herpes simplex] hepatitis (B00.81)
infectious mononucleosis with liver disease (B27.0-B27.9 with .9)
mumps hepatitis (B26.81)
sarcoidosis with liver disease (D86.89)
secondary syphilis with liver disease (A51.45)
syphilis (late) with liver disease (A52.74)
toxoplasmosis (acquired) hepatitis (B58.1)
tuberculosis with liver disease (A18.83)
CC Excl: No Excl

Disorders of gallbladder, biliary tract and pancreas (K80-K87)

K80 Cholelithiasis
EXCLUDES 1 *retained cholelithiasis following cholecystectomy (K91.86)*

K80.0 Calculus of gallbladder with acute cholecystitis
Any condition listed in K80.2 with acute cholecystitis

K80.00 Calculus of gallbladder with acute cholecystitis without obstruction   CC
CC Excl: K80.00-K80.21, K80.40, K80.44, K80.62-K80.63, K80.66-K80.67, K80.80, K81.0-K81.9, K82.9, K83.5-K83.9, K87

K80.01 Calculus of gallbladder with acute cholecystitis with obstruction   CC
CC Excl: K80.00-K80.21, K80.62-K80.63, K80.66-K80.67, K80.80, K81.0-K81.9, K82.9, K83.5-K83.9, K87

K80.1 Calculus of gallbladder with other cholecystitis
CC Excl: For CC codes in subcategory K80.1, unless otherwise noted: See code: K80.01

K80.10 Calculus of gallbladder with chronic cholecystitis without obstruction   CC
Cholelithiasis with cholecystitis NOS

K80.11 Calculus of gallbladder with chronic cholecystitis with obstruction   CC

K80.12 Calculus of gallbladder with acute and chronic cholecystitis without obstruction   CC
CC Excl: See code: K80.00

K80.13 Calculus of gallbladder with acute and chronic cholecystitis with obstruction   CC

K80.18 Calculus of gallbladder with other cholecystitis without obstruction   CC

K80.19 Calculus of gallbladder with other cholecystitis with obstruction   CC

K80.2 Calculus of gallbladder without cholecystitis
Cholecystolithiasis without cholecystitis
Cholelithiasis (without cholecystitis)
Colic (recurrent) of gallbladder (without cholecystitis)
Gallstone (impacted) of cystic duct (without cholecystitis)
Gallstone (impacted) of gallbladder (without cholecystitis)

K80.20 Calculus of gallbladder without cholecystitis without obstruction

K80.21 Calculus of gallbladder without cholecystitis with obstruction   CC
CC Excl: See code: K80.01

K80.3 Calculus of bile duct with cholangitis
Any condition listed in K80.5 with cholangitis
CC Excl: For CC codes in subcategory K80.3, unless otherwise noted: K83.0, K83.5-K83.9, K87

K80.30 Calculus of bile duct with cholangitis, unspecified, without obstruction   PDx CC

K80.31 Calculus of bile duct with cholangitis, unspecified, with obstruction   PDx CC CC
CC Excl: K80.30-K80.71, K80.81-K81.9, K83.5-K83.9, K87

K80.32 Calculus of bile duct with acute cholangitis without obstruction   PDx CC

K80.33 Calculus of bile duct with acute cholangitis with obstruction   PDx CC CC
CC Excl: See code: K80.31

K80.34 Calculus of bile duct with chronic cholangitis without obstruction   PDx CC

K80.35 Calculus of bile duct with chronic cholangitis with obstruction `PDx CC` `CC`
CC Excl: See code: K80.31

K80.36 Calculus of bile duct with acute and chronic cholangitis without obstruction `PDx CC`

K80.37 Calculus of bile duct with acute and chronic cholangitis with obstruction `PDx CC` `CC`
CC Excl: See code: K80.31

K80.4 Calculus of bile duct with cholecystitis
Any condition listed in K80.5 with cholecystitis (with cholangitis)

CC Excl: For CC codes in subcategory K80.4, unless otherwise noted: K80.30-K80.71, K80.81-K81.9, K83.5-K83.9, K87

K80.40 Calculus of bile duct with cholecystitis, unspecified, without obstruction `CC`

K80.41 Calculus of bile duct with cholecystitis, unspecified, with obstruction `CC`

K80.42 Calculus of bile duct with acute cholecystitis without obstruction `CC`

K80.43 Calculus of bile duct with acute cholecystitis with obstruction `CC`

K80.44 Calculus of bile duct with chronic cholecystitis without obstruction `CC`

K80.45 Calculus of bile duct with chronic cholecystitis with obstruction `CC`

K80.46 Calculus of bile duct with acute and chronic cholecystitis without obstruction `CC`

K80.47 Calculus of bile duct with acute and chronic cholecystitis with obstruction `CC`

K80.5 Calculus of bile duct without cholangitis or cholecystitis
Choledocholithiasis (without cholangitis or cholecystitis)
Gallstone (impacted) of bile duct NOS (without cholangitis or cholecystitis)
Gallstone (impacted) of common duct (without cholangitis or cholecystitis)
Gallstone (impacted) of hepatic duct (without cholangitis or cholecystitis)
Hepatic cholelithiasis (without cholangitis or cholecystitis)
Hepatic colic (recurrent) (without cholangitis or cholecystitis)

K80.50 Calculus of bile duct without cholangitis or cholecystitis without obstruction

K80.51 Calculus of bile duct without cholangitis or cholecystitis with obstruction `CC`
CC Excl: K80.30-K80.71, K80.81-K81.9, K83.5-K83.9, K87

K80.6 Calculus of gallbladder and bile duct with cholecystitis

CC Excl: For CC codes in subcategory K80.6, unless otherwise noted: See code: K80.51

K80.60 Calculus of gallbladder and bile duct with cholecystitis, unspecified, without obstruction `CC`

K80.61 Calculus of gallbladder and bile duct with cholecystitis, unspecified, with obstruction `CC`

K80.62 Calculus of gallbladder and bile duct with acute cholecystitis without obstruction `CC`
CC Excl: K80.62-K80.63, K81.0-K81.9, K82.9, K83.5-K83.9, K87

K80.63 Calculus of gallbladder and bile duct with acute cholecystitis with obstruction `CC`
CC Excl: See code: K80.62

K80.64 Calculus of gallbladder and bile duct with chronic cholecystitis without obstruction `CC`

K80.65 Calculus of gallbladder and bile duct with chronic cholecystitis with obstruction `CC`

K80.66 Calculus of gallbladder and bile duct with acute and chronic cholecystitis without obstruction `CC`
CC Excl: K80.66-K80.67, K81.0-K81.9, K82.9, K83.5-K83.9, K87

K80.67 Calculus of gallbladder and bile duct with acute and chronic cholecystitis with obstruction `MCC`
CC Excl: See code: K80.66

K80.7 Calculus of gallbladder and bile duct without cholecystitis

K80.70 Calculus of gallbladder and bile duct without cholecystitis without obstruction

K80.71 Calculus of gallbladder and bile duct without cholecystitis with obstruction `CC`
CC Excl: See code: K80.51

K80.8 Other cholelithiasis

K80.80 Other cholelithiasis without obstruction

K80.81 Other cholelithiasis with obstruction `CC`
CC Excl: See code: K80.51

K81 Cholecystitis
EXCLUDES 1 cholecystitis with cholelithiasis (K80.-)

K81.0 Acute cholecystitis `CC`
Abscess of gallbladder
Angiocholecystitis
Emphysematous (acute) cholecystitis
Empyema of gallbladder
Gangrene of gallbladder
Gangrenous cholecystitis
Suppurative cholecystitis
CC Excl: K80.62-K80.63, K80.66-K80.67, K81.0-K81.9, K82.9, K83.5-K83.9, K87

K81.1 Chronic cholecystitis

K81.2 Acute cholecystitis with chronic cholecystitis `CC`
CC Excl: K81.0-K81.9, K82.9, K83.5-K83.9, K87

K81.9 Cholecystitis, unspecified

K82 Other diseases of gallbladder
EXCLUDES 1 nonvisualization of gallbladder (R93.2)
postcholecystectomy syndrome (K91.5)

CC Excl: For CC/MCC codes in category K82, unless otherwise noted: K82.0-K82.9, K83.5-K83.9, K87

K82.0 Obstruction of gallbladder `CC`
Occlusion of cystic duct or gallbladder without cholelithiasis
Stenosis of cystic duct or gallbladder without cholelithiasis
Stricture of cystic duct or gallbladder without cholelithiasis
EXCLUDES 1 obstruction of gallbladder with cholelithiasis (K80.-)

K82.1 Hydrops of gallbladder `CC`
Mucocele of gallbladder

K82.2 Perforation of gallbladder `MCC`
Rupture of cystic duct or gallbladder

K82.3 Fistula of gallbladder `CC`
Cholecystocolic fistula
Cholecystoduodenal fistula

K82.4 Cholesterolosis of gallbladder
Strawberry gallbladder
EXCLUDES 1 cholesterolosis of gallbladder with cholecystitis (K81.-)
cholesterolosis of gallbladder with cholelithiasis (K80.-)

K82.8 Other specified diseases of gallbladder
Adhesions of cystic duct or gallbladder
Atrophy of cystic duct or gallbladder
Cyst of cystic duct or gallbladder
Dyskinesia of cystic duct or gallbladder
Hypertrophy of cystic duct or gallbladder
Nonfunctioning of cystic duct or gallbladder
Ulcer of cystic duct or gallbladder

K82.9 Disease of gallbladder, unspecified

K83 Other diseases of biliary tract
EXCLUDES 1 postcholecystectomy syndrome (K91.5)
EXCLUDES 2 conditions involving the gallbladder (K81-K82)
conditions involving the cystic duct (K81-K82)

K83.0 Cholangitis `CC`
Ascending cholangitis
Cholangitis NOS
Primary cholangitis
Recurrent cholangitis
Sclerosing cholangitis
Secondary cholangitis
Stenosing cholangitis
Suppurative cholangitis
EXCLUDES 1 cholangitic liver abscess (K75.0)
cholangitis with choledocholithiasis (K80.3-, K80.4-)
chronic nonsuppurative destructive cholangitis (K74.3)
CC Excl: K83.0, K83.5-K83.9, K87

main term

K83.1 Obstruction of bile duct `MCC`
Occlusion of bile duct without cholelithiasis
Stenosis of bile duct without cholelithiasis
Stricture of bile duct without cholelithiasis
EXCLUDES 1 congenital obstruction of bile duct (Q44.3)
obstruction of bile duct with cholelithiasis (K80.-)
CC Excl: K80.31, K80.33, K80.35, K80.37, K80.41, K80.43, K80.45, K80.47, K80.51, K80.81, K83.1, K83.5-K83.9, K87, Q44.2-Q44.3

K83.2 Perforation of bile duct `MCC`
Rupture of bile duct
CC Excl: K83.2-K83.3, K83.5-K83.9, K87

K83.3 Fistula of bile duct `CC`
Choledochoduodenal fistula
CC Excl: See code: K83.2

K83.4 Spasm of sphincter of Oddi

K83.5 **Biliary cyst**

K83.8 **Other specified diseases of biliary tract**
Adhesions of biliary tract
Atrophy of biliary tract
Hypertrophy of biliary tract
Ulcer of biliary tract

K83.9 **Disease of biliary tract, unspecified**

✓4ᵗʰ **K85 Acute pancreatitis**
Abscess of pancreas
Acute necrosis of pancreas
Acute (recurrent) pancreatitis
Gangrene of (gangrenous) pancreas
Hemorrhagic pancreatitis
Infective necrosis of pancreas
Subacute pancreatitis
Suppurative pancreatitis

CC Excl: For MCC codes in category K85, unless otherwise noted:
B25.2, K86.1, K86.8-K86.9

K85.0 **Idiopathic acute pancreatitis** `MCC`

K85.1 **Biliary acute pancreatitis** `MCC`
Gallstone pancreatitis

K85.2 **Alcohol induced acute pancreatitis** `MCC`
EXCLUDES 2 *alcohol induced chronic pancreatitis (K86.0)*

K85.3 **Drug induced acute pancreatitis** `MCC`
Use additional code for adverse effect, if applicable, to identify drug (T36-T50 with fifth or sixth character 5)
Use additional code to identify drug abuse and dependence (F11. – F17.-)

K85.8 **Other acute pancreatitis** `MCC`

K85.9 **Acute pancreatitis, unspecified** `MCC`
Pancreatitis NOS

✓4ᵗʰ **K86 Other diseases of pancreas**
EXCLUDES 2 *fibrocystic disease of pancreas (E84.-)*
islet cell tumor (of pancreas) (D13.7)
pancreatic steatorrhea (K90.3)

K86.0 **Alcohol-induced chronic pancreatitis** `CC`
Use additional code to identify:
alcohol abuse and dependence (F10.-)
EXCLUDES 2 *alcohol induced acute pancreatitis (K85.2)*
CC Excl: B25.2, E16.8, K85.0-K86.9

K86.1 **Other chronic pancreatitis** `CC`
Chronic pancreatitis NOS
Infectious chronic pancreatitis
Recurrent chronic pancreatitis
Relapsing chronic pancreatitis
CC Excl: See code: K86.0

K86.2 **Cyst of pancreas** `CC`
CC Excl: K86.2-K86.9

K86.3 **Pseudocyst of pancreas** `CC`
CC Excl: See code: K86.2

K86.8 **Other specified diseases of pancreas**
Aseptic pancreatic necrosis
Atrophy of pancreas
Calculus of pancreas
Cirrhosis of pancreas
Fibrosis of pancreas
Pancreatic fat necrosis
Pancreatic infantilism
Pancreatic necrosis NOS

K86.9 **Disease of pancreas, unspecified**

K87 *Disorders of gallbladder, biliary tract and pancreas in diseases classified elsewhere*
Code first underlying disease
EXCLUDES 1 *cytomegaloviral pancreatitis (B25.2)*
mumps pancreatitis (B26.3)
syphilitic gallbladder (A52.74)
syphilitic pancreas (A52.74)
tuberculosis of gallbladder (A18.83)
tuberculosis of pancreas (A18.83)

Other diseases of the digestive system (K90-K95)

✓4ᵗʰ **K90 Intestinal malabsorption**
EXCLUDES 1 *intestinal malabsorption following gastrointestinal surgery (K91.2)*

CC Excl: For CC codes in category K90, unless otherwise noted:
E84.19, K90.0-K90.4, K90.89-K90.9, K91.2

K90.0 **Celiac disease**
Gluten-sensitive enteropathy
Idiopathic steatorrhea
Nontropical sprue
Use additional code for associated disorders including:
dermatitis herpetiformis (L13.0)
gluten ataxia (G32.81)

K90.1 **Tropical sprue** `CC`
Sprue NOS
Tropical steatorrhea

K90.2 **Blind loop syndrome, not elsewhere classified** `CC`
Blind loop syndrome NOS
EXCLUDES 1 *congenital blind loop syndrome (Q43.8)*
postsurgical blind loop syndrome (K91.2)

K90.3 **Pancreatic steatorrhea** `CC`

K90.4 **Malabsorption due to intolerance, not elsewhere classified** `CC`
Malabsorption due to intolerance to carbohydrate
Malabsorption due to intolerance to fat
Malabsorption due to intolerance to protein
Malabsorption due to intolerance to starch
EXCLUDES 2 *gluten-sensitive enteropathy (K90.0)*
lactose intolerance (E73.-)

✓5ᵗʰ K90.8 **Other intestinal malabsorption**

K90.81 **Whipple's disease** `CC`
CC Excl: K90.81

K90.89 **Other intestinal malabsorption** `CC`

K90.9 **Intestinal malabsorption, unspecified** `CC`

✓4ᵗʰ **K91 Intraoperative and postprocedural complications and disorders of digestive system, not elsewhere classified**
EXCLUDES 2 *complications of artificial opening of digestive system (K94.-)*
complications of bariatric procedures (K95.-)
gastrojejunal ulcer (K28.-)
postprocedural (radiation) retroperitoneal abscess (K68.11)
radiation colitis (K52.0)
radiation gastroenteritis (K52.0)
radiation proctitis (K62.7)

K91.0 **Vomiting following gastrointestinal surgery**

K91.1 **Postgastric surgery syndromes**
Dumping syndrome
Postgastrectomy syndrome
Postvagotomy syndrome

K91.2 **Postsurgical malabsorption, not elsewhere classified** `CC`
Postsurgical blind loop syndrome
EXCLUDES 1 *malabsorption osteomalacia in adults (M83.2)*
malabsorption osteoporosis, postsurgical (M80.8-, M81.8)
CC Excl: K90.3-K90.4, K90.89-K90.9, K91.2

K91.3 **Postprocedural intestinal obstruction** `CC`
CC Excl: D78.81-D78.89, E36.8, E89.810-E89.89, H59.011-H59.019, H59.031-H59.099, H59.811-H59.89, H95.811-H95.89, I97.3, K91.3, K91.81-K91.83, K91.850-K91.89, K94.20-K95.89, L76.81-L76.82, M96.89, N98.1-N98.9, T81.710A, T81.82XA, T81.89XA, T81.9XXA

K91.5 **Postcholecystectomy syndrome**

✓5ᵗʰ K91.6 **Intraoperative hemorrhage and hematoma of a digestive system organ or structure complicating a procedure**
EXCLUDES 1 *intraoperative hemorrhage and hematoma of a digestive system organ or structure due to accidental puncture and laceration during a procedure (K91.7-)*

K91.61 **Intraoperative hemorrhage and hematoma of a digestive system organ or structure complicating a digestive sytem procedure** `CC`
CC Excl: H95.811-H95.89, I85.01, I85.11, I97.3, K21.9, K22.8, K23-K25.0, K25.2, K25.4, K25.6, K26.0, K26.2, K26.4, K26.6, K27.0, K27.2, K27.4, K27.6, K28.0, K28.2, K28.4, K28.6, K29.01, K29.21, K29.31, K29.41, K29.51, K29.61, K29.71, K29.81, K29.91, K31.811, K55.21, K57.01, K57.11, K57.13, K57.21, K57.31, K57.33, K57.41, K57.51, K57.53, K57.81, K57.91, K57.93, K62.5, K91.61-K91.62, K91.840-K91.841, K92.0-K92.2, M96.89, N98.1-N98.9, P54.1-P54.3, T81.10XA, T81.11XA, T81.12XA, T81.19XA, T81.82XA, T81.89XA, T81.9XXA

✅ Additional Character Required   ✓x7ᵗʰ Xtension Alert   Unacceptable PDx   Manifestation   Hospital Acquired Condition   _EXCLUDES 1_ Not Coded Here   _EXCLUDES 2_ Not Included Here

Diseases of the Digestive System

K91.62–K94.39

K91.62   **Intraoperative hemorrhage and hematoma of a** `CC`
digestive system organ or structure complicating other procedure
    CC Excl: See code: K91.61

✓5ᵗʰ **K91.7**   **Accidental puncture and laceration of a digestive system organ or structure during a procedure**

K91.71   **Accidental puncture and laceration of a digestive** `CC`
system organ or structure during a digestive system procedure
    CC Excl: D78.11-D78.12, D78.81-D78.89, E36.11-E36.8,
E89.810-E89.89, G96.11, G97.41-G97.49, H59.011-
H59.019, H59.031-H59.099, H59.211-H59.229, H59.811-
H59.89, H95.31-H95.32, H95.811-H95.89, I97.3, I97.51-
I97.52, J95.71-J95.72, K91.71-K91.72, L76.11-L76.12,
L76.81-L76.82, M96.820-M96.821, M96.89, N98.1-N98.9,
N99.71-N99.72, T81.82XA, T81.89XA, T81.9XXA

K91.72   **Accidental puncture and laceration of a digestive** `CC`
system organ or structure during other procedure
    CC Excl: See code: K91.71

✓5ᵗʰ **K91.8**   **Other intraoperative and postprocedural complications and disorders of digestive system**

> **CC Excl: For CC codes in subcategory K91.8, unless otherwise noted:** See code: K91.3

K91.81   **Other intraoperative complications of digestive** `CC`
system

K91.82   **Postprocedural hepatic failure** `CC`

K91.83   **Postprocedural hepatorenal syndrome** `CC`

✓6ᵗʰ **K91.84**   **Postprocedural hemorrhage and hematoma of a digestive system organ or structure following a procedure**

K91.840   **Postprocedural hemorrhage and** `CC`
hematoma of a digestive system organ or structure following a digestive system procedure
    CC Excl: See code: K91.61

K91.841   **Postprocedural hemorrhage and** `CC`
hematoma of a digestive system organ or structure following other procedure
    CC Excl: See code: K91.61

✓6ᵗʰ **K91.85**   **Complications of intestinal pouch**

K91.850   **Pouchitis** `CC`
    Inflammation of internal ileoanal pouch

K91.858   **Other complications of intestinal** `CC`
pouch

K91.86   **Retained cholelithiasis following** `CC`
cholecystectomy

K91.89   **Other postprocedural complications and** `CC`
disorders of digestive system
    Use additional code, if applicable, to further specify disorder
    EXCLUDES 2   *postprocedural retroperitoneal abscess (K68.11)*

✓4ᵗʰ **K92**   **Other diseases of digestive system**
    EXCLUDES 1   *neonatal gastrointestinal hemorrhage (P54.0-P54.3)*

K92.0   **Hematemesis** `CC`
    CC Excl: E16.4, I85.01, K22.10-K22.11, K22.6-K22.719, K25.0-K28.9,
K29.01, K29.21, K29.31, K29.41, K29.51, K29.61, K29.71, K29.81,
K29.91, K31.811, K55.21, K57.01, K57.11, K57.13, K57.21, K57.31,
K57.33, K57.41, K57.51, K57.53, K57.81, K57.91, K57.93, K62.5,
K92.0-K92.2

K92.1   **Melena** `CC`
    EXCLUDES 1   *occult blood in feces (R19.5)*
    CC Excl: See code: K92.0

K92.2   **Gastrointestinal hemorrhage, unspecified** `CC`
    Gastric hemorrhage NOS
    Intestinal hemorrhage NOS
    EXCLUDES 1   *acute hemorrhagic gastritis (K29.01)*
              hemorrhage of anus and rectum (K62.5)
              angiodysplasia of stomach with hemorrhage (K31.811)
              diverticular disease with hemorrhage (K57.-)
              gastritis and duodenitis with hemorrhage (K29.-)
              peptic ulcer with hemorrhage (K25-K28)
    CC Excl: See code: K92.0

✓5ᵗʰ **K92.8**   **Other specified diseases of the digestive system**

K92.81   **Gastrointestinal mucositis (ulcerative)** `CC`
    Code also type of associated therapy, such as:
    antineoplastic and immunosuppressive drugs (T45.1X-)
    radiological procedure and radiotherapy (Y84.2)
    EXCLUDES 2   *mucositis (ulcerative) of vagina and vulva (N76.81)*
              nasal mucositis (ulcerative) (J34.81)
              oral mucositis (ulcerative) (K12.3-)
    CC Excl: E16.4, I85.01, K22.10-K22.11, K22.6-K22.719,
K25.0-K28.9, K29.01, K29.21, K29.31, K29.41, K29.51,
K29.61, K29.71, K29.81, K29.91, K31.811, K31.89-K31.9,
K55.21, K57.01, K57.11, K57.13, K57.21, K57.31, K57.33,
K57.41, K57.51, K57.53, K57.81, K57.91, K57.93, K62.5,
K92.0-K92.81

K92.89   **Other specified diseases of the digestive system**

K92.9   **Disease of digestive system, unspecified**

✓4ᵗʰ **K94**   **Complications of artificial openings of the digestive system**

✓5ᵗʰ **K94.0**   **Colostomy complications**

K94.00   **Colostomy complication, unspecified**

K94.01   **Colostomy hemorrhage** `CC`
    CC Excl: K94.00-K94.19

K94.02   **Colostomy infection** `CC`
    Use additional code to specify type of infection, such as:
    cellulitis of abdominal wall (L03.311)
    sepsis (A40-, A41-)
    CC Excl: See code: K94.01

K94.03   **Colostomy malfunction** `CC`
    Mechanical complication of colostomy
    CC Excl: D78.81-D78.89, E36.8, E89.810-E89.89,
H59.011-H59.019, H59.031-H59.099, H59.811-H59.89,
H95.811-H95.89, I97.3, K91.3, K91.81-K91.83, K91.850-
K91.89, K94.00-K95.89, L76.81-L76.82, M96.89, N98.1-
N98.9, T81.710A, T81.82XA, T81.89XA, T81.9XXA

K94.09   **Other complications of colostomy** `CC`
    CC Excl: See code: K94.01

✓5ᵗʰ **K94.1**   **Enterostomy complications**

K94.10   **Enterostomy complication, unspecified**

K94.11   **Enterostomy hemorrhage** `CC`
    CC Excl: See code: K94.01

K94.12   **Enterostomy infection** `CC`
    Use additional code to specify type of infection, such as:
    cellulitis of abdominal wall (L03.311)
    sepsis (A40-, A41-)
    CC Excl: See code: K94.01

K94.13   **Enterostomy malfunction** `CC`
    Mechanical complication of enterostomy
    CC Excl: See code: K94.03

K94.19   **Other complications of enterostomy** `CC`
    CC Excl: See code: K94.01

✓5ᵗʰ **K94.2**   **Gastrostomy complications**

K94.20   **Gastrostomy complication, unspecified**

K94.21   **Gastrostomy hemorrhage**

K94.22   **Gastrostomy infection** `CC`
    Use additional code to specify type of infection, such as:
    cellulitis of abdominal wall (L03.311)
    sepsis (A40-, A41-)
    CC Excl: See code: K91.3

K94.23   **Gastrostomy malfunction** `CC`
    Mechanical complication of gastrostomy
    CC Excl: See code: K91.3

K94.29   **Other complications of gastrostomy**

✓5ᵗʰ **K94.3**   **Esophagostomy complications**

> **CC Excl: For CC codes in subcategory K94.3, unless otherwise noted:** D78.81-D78.89, E36.8, E89.810-E89.89,
> H59.011-H59.019, H59.031-H59.099, H59.811-H59.89,
> H95.811-H95.89, I97.3, K91.3, K91.81-K91.83, K91.850-K91.89,
> K94.20-K95.89, L76.81-L76.82, M96.89, N98.1-N98.9, T81.710A,
> T81.82XA, T81.89XA, T81.9XXA

K94.30   **Esophagostomy complications, unspecified** `CC`

K94.31   **Esophagostomy hemorrhage** `CC`

K94.32   **Esophagostomy infection** `CC`
    Use additional code to identify the infection

K94.33   **Esophagostomy malfunction** `CC`
    Mechanical complication of esophagostomy

K94.39   **Other complications of esophagostom** `CC`

Ⓝ Newborn: 0   Ⓟ Pediatric: 0-17   Ⓜ Maternity: 12-55   Ⓐ Adult: 15-124   `MCC` Major CC Condition   `PDx MCC` PDx acts as own MCC   `CC` CC Condition   `PDx CC` PDx acts as own CC

658   ICD-10-CM Draft (2015)

K95 ☑4th **Complications of bariatric procedures**

> **CC Excl: For CC codes in category K95, unless otherwise noted:**
> See code: K94.3

☑5th **K95.0 Complications of gastric band procedure**

4 **K95.01 Infection due to gastric band procedure** `CC`
> Use additional code to specify type of infection or
> organism, such as:
> bacterial and viral infectious agents (B95.-, B96.-)
> cellulitis of abdominal wall (L03.311)
> sepsis (A40.-, A41.-)

K95.09 Other complications of gastric band procedure `CC`
> Use additional code, if applicable, to further specify
> complication

☑5th **K95.8 Complications of other bariatric procedure**
> *EXCLUDES 1* complications of gastric band surgery (K95.0-)

4 **K95.81 Infection due to other bariatric procedure** `CC`
> Use additional code to specify type of infection or
> organism, such as:
> bacterial and viral infectious agents (B95.-, B96.-)
> cellulitis of abdominal wall (L03.311)
> sepsis (A40.-, A41.-)

K95.89 Other complications of other bariatric procedure `CC`
> Use additional code, if applicable, to further specify
> complication

(?) Branchio with (Tor current)
is
explanation

4 HAC = as SDx not POA, in combination with PDx E66.01 **AND** one of the following procedure codes: 0D16[0,4,8][7,J,K,Z][9,A,B,L] or 0DV64CZ.

☑ Additional Character Required   ☑x7th *Xtension* Alert   Unacceptable PDx   Manifestation   Hospital Acquired Condition   *EXCLUDES 1* Not Coded Here   *EXCLUDES 2* Not Included Here

Diseases of the Skin and Subcutaneous Tissue

L00–L02.31

Chapter 12. Diseases of the Skin and Subcutaneous Tissue (L00-L99)

> EXCLUDES 2   certain conditions originating in the perinatal period (P04-P96)
> certain infectious and parasitic diseases (A00-B99)
> complications of pregnancy, childbirth and the puerperium (O00-O9A)
> congenital malformations, deformations, and chromosomal
>   abnormalities (Q00-Q99)
> endocrine, nutritional and metabolic diseases (E00-E88)
> lipomelanotic reticulosis (I89.8)
> neoplasms (C00-D49)
> symptoms, signs and abnormal clinical and laboratory findings, not
>   elsewhere classified (R00-R94)
> systemic connective tissue disorders (M30-M36)
> viral warts (B07.-)

This chapter contains the following blocks:

L00-L08   Infections of the skin and subcutaneous tissue
L10-L14   Bullous disorders
L20-L30   Dermatitis and eczema
L40-L45   Papulosquamous disorders
L49-L54   Urticaria and erythema
L55-L59   Radiation-related disorders of the skin and subcutaneous tissue
L60-L75   Disorders of skin appendages
L76   Intraoperative and postprocedural complications of skin and
            subcutaneous tissue
L80-L99   Other disorders of the skin and subcutaneous tissue

Infections of the skin and subcutaneous tissue (L00-L08)

Use additional code (B95-B97) to identify infectious agent

> EXCLUDES 2   hordeolum (H00.0)
> infective dermatitis (L30.3)
> local infections of skin classified in Chapter 1
> lupus panniculitis (L93.2)
> panniculitis NOS (M79.3)
> panniculitis of neck and back (M54.0-)
> Perlèche NOS (K13.0)
> Perlèche due to candidiasis (B37.0)
> Perlèche due to riboflavin deficiency (E53.0)
> pyogenic granuloma (L98.0)
> relapsing panniculitis [Weber-Christian] (M35.6)
> viral warts (B07.-)
> zoster (B02.-)

L00   Staphylococcal scalded skin syndrome
     Ritter's disease
     Use additional code to identify percentage of skin exfoliation (L49.-)

> EXCLUDES 1   bullous impetigo (L01.03)
> pemphigus neonatorum (L01.03)
> toxic epidermal necrolysis [Lyell] (L51.2)

✓4th **L01   Impetigo**

> EXCLUDES 1   impetigo herpetiformis (L40.1)

   ✓5th **L01.0   Impetigo**
         Impetigo contagiosa   Impetigo vulgaris

       L01.00   Impetigo, unspecified
              Impetigo NOS

       L01.01   Non-bullous impetigo

       L01.02   Bockhart's impetigo
              Impetigo follicularis
              Perifolliculitis NOS
              Superficial pustular perifolliculitis

       L01.03   Bullous impetigo
              Impetigo neonatorum   Pemphigus neonatorum

       L01.09   Other impetigo
              Ulcerative impetigo

   L01.1   Impetiginization of other dermatoses

✓4th **L02   Cutaneous abscess, furuncle and carbuncle**
     Use additional code to identify organism (B95-B96)

> EXCLUDES 2   abscess of anus and rectal regions (K61.-)
> abscess of female genital organs (external) (N76.4)
> abscess of male genital organs (external) (N48.2, N49-)

   ✓5th **L02.0   Cutaneous abscess, furuncle and carbuncle of face**

> EXCLUDES 2   abscess of ear, external (H60.0)
> abscess of eyelid (H00.0)
> abscess of head [any part, except face] (L02.8)
> abscess of lacrimal gland (H04.0)
> abscess of lacrimal passages (H04.3)
> abscess of mouth (K12.2)
> abscess of nose (J34.0)
> abscess of orbit (H05.0)
> submandibular abscess (K12.2)

       L02.01   Cutaneous abscess of face   CC

       L02.02   Furuncle of face
              Boil of face Folliculitis of face

       L02.03   Carbuncle of face

   ✓5th **L02.1   Cutaneous abscess, furuncle and carbuncle of neck**
       CC Excl: No Excl

       L02.11   Cutaneous abscess of neck   CC
              CC Excl: A17.9, A18.4, A18.82, A18.84, A18.89, A48.2-
              A48.4, A48.8-A49.9, B78.1, B95.0-B96.89, E83.2, L02.11,
              L02.811-L02.818, L02.91, L03.221-L03.222, L03.811-
              L03.91, L08.0, L08.81-L08.9, L44.8-L45, L73.2, L88, L92.8,
              L94.2, L94.4, L98.0, L98.3, L98.8, L99, M00.011-M00.012,
              M00.021-M00.022, M00.031-M00.032, M00.041-
              M00.042, M00.051-M00.052, M00.061-M00.062,
              M00.071-M00.072, Z16.10-Z16.39

       L02.12   Furuncle of neck
              Boil of neck
              Folliculitis of neck

       L02.13   Carbuncle of neck

   ✓5th **L02.2   Cutaneous abscess, furuncle and carbuncle of trunk**

> EXCLUDES 1   non-newborn omphalitis (L08.82)
> omphalitis of newborn (P38.-)

> EXCLUDES 2   abscess of breast (N61)
> abscess of buttocks (L02.3)
> abscess of female external genital organs (N76.4)
> abscess of hip (L02.4)
> abscess of male external genital organs (N48.2, N49-)

> **CC Excl:** For CC codes in subcategory L02.2, unless
> otherwise noted: A17.9, A18.4, A18.82, A18.84, A18.89,
> A48.2-A48.4, A48.8-A49.9, B78.1, B95.0-B96.89, E83.2, L02.211-
> L02.219, L02.811-L02.818, L02.91, L03.311-L03.316, L03.319-
> L03.326, L03.329-L03.91, L08.0, L08.81-L08.9, L44.8-L45, L73.2,
> L88, L92.8, L94.2, L94.4, L98.0, L98.3, L98.8, L99, M00.011-
> M00.012, M00.021-M00.022, M00.031-M00.032, M00.041-
> M00.042, M00.051-M00.052, M00.061-M00.062, M00.071-
> M00.072, Z16.10-Z16.39

    ✓6th **L02.21   Cutaneous abscess of trunk**

          L02.211   Cutaneous abscess of abdominal wall   CC
          L02.212   Cutaneous abscess of back [any part, except buttock]   CC
          L02.213   Cutaneous abscess of chest wall   CC
          L02.214   Cutaneous abscess of groin   CC
          L02.215   Cutaneous abscess of perineum   CC
          L02.216   Cutaneous abscess of umbilicus   CC
          L02.219   Cutaneous abscess of trunk, unspecified   CC

    ✓6th **L02.22   Furuncle of trunk**
          Boil of trunk Folliculitis of trunk

          L02.221   Furuncle of abdominal wall
          L02.222   Furuncle of back [any part, except buttock]
          L02.223   Furuncle of chest wall
          L02.224   Furuncle of groin
          L02.225   Furuncle of perineum
          L02.226   Furuncle of umbilicus
          L02.229   Furuncle of trunk, unspecified

    ✓6th **L02.23   Carbuncle of trunk**

          L02.231   Carbuncle of abdominal wall
          L02.232   Carbuncle of back [any part, except buttock]
          L02.233   Carbuncle of chest wall
          L02.234   Carbuncle of groin
          L02.235   Carbuncle of perineum
          L02.236   Carbuncle of umbilicus
          L02.239   Carbuncle of trunk, unspecified

   ✓5th **L02.3   Cutaneous abscess, furuncle and carbuncle of buttock**

> EXCLUDES 1   pilonidal cyst with abscess (L05.01)

       L02.31   Cutaneous abscess of buttock   CC
              Cutaneous abscess of gluteal region
              CC Excl: A17.9, A18.4, A18.82, A18.84, A18.89, A48.2-
              A48.4, A48.8-A49.9, B78.1, B95.0-B96.89, E83.2, L02.31,
              L02.811-L02.818, L02.91, L03.317, L03.327, L03.811-
              L03.91, L08.0, L08.81-L08.9, L44.8-L45, L73.2, L88, L92.8,
              L94.2, L94.4, L98.0, L98.3, L98.8, L99, M00.011-M00.012,
              M00.021-M00.022, M00.031-M00.032, M00.041-
              M00.042, M00.051-M00.052, M00.061-M00.062,
              M00.071-M00.072, Z16.10-Z16.39

N Newborn: 0   P Pediatric: 0-17   M Maternity: 12-55   A Adult: 15-124   MCC Major CC Condition   PDx MCC PDx acts as own MCC   CC CC Condition   PDx CC PDx acts as own CC

660   ICD-10-CM Draft (2015)

L02.32 **Furuncle of buttock**
Boil of buttock   Furuncle of gluteal region
Folliculitis of buttock

L02.33 **Carbuncle of buttock**
Carbuncle of gluteal region

✓5th **L02.4** **Cutaneous abscess, furuncle and carbuncle of limb**
EXCLUDES 2 cutaneous abscess, furuncle and carbuncle of groin
(L02.214, L02.224, L02.234)
cutaneous abscess, furuncle and carbuncle of hand
(L02.5-)
cutaneous abscess, furuncle and carbuncle of foot
(L02.6-)

CC Excl: For CC codes in subcategory L02.4, unless
otherwise noted: A17.9, A18.4, A18.82, A18.84, A18.89,
A48.2-A48.4, A48.8-A49.9, B78.1, B95.0-B96.89, E83.2, L02.411-
L02.414, L02.811-L02.818, L02.91, L03.111-L03.114, L03.121-
L03.124, L03.811-L03.91, L08.0, L08.81-L08.9, L44.8-L45, L73.2,
L88, L92.8, L94.2, L94.4, L98.0, L98.3, L98.8, L99, M00.011-
M00.012, M00.021-M00.022, M00.031-M00.032, M00.041-
M00.042, M00.051-M00.052, M00.061-M00.062, M00.071-
M00.072, Z16.10-Z16.39

✓6th **L02.41** **Cutaneous abscess of limb**
L02.411 **Cutaneous abscess of right axilla** CC
L02.412 **Cutaneous abscess of left axilla** CC
L02.413 **Cutaneous abscess of right upper limb** CC
L02.414 **Cutaneous abscess of left upper limb** CC
L02.415 **Cutaneous abscess of right lower limb** CC
CC Excl: A17.9-A18.4, A18.82, A18.84,
A18.89, A48.2-A48.4, A48.8-A49.9, B78.1,
B95.0-B96.89, E83.2, L02.415-L02.419,
L02.811-L02.818, L02.91, L03.115-L03.119,
L03.125-L03.129, L03.811-L03.91, L08.0,
L08.81-L08.9, L44.8-L45, L73.2, L88, L92.8,
L94.2, L94.4, L98.0, L98.3, L98.8, L99,
M00.011-M00.012, M00.021-M00.022,
M00.031-M00.032, M00.041-M00.042,
M00.051-M00.052, M00.061-M00.062,
M00.071-M00.072, Z16.10-Z16.39
L02.416 **Cutaneous abscess of left lower limb** CC
CC Excl: See code: L02.415
L02.419 **Cutaneous abscess of limb,** CC
unspecified
CC Excl: See code: L02.415

✓6th **L02.42** **Furuncle of limb**
Boil of limb Folliculitis of limb
L02.421 **Furuncle of right axilla**
L02.422 **Furuncle of left axilla**
L02.423 **Furuncle of right upper limb**
L02.424 **Furuncle of left upper limb**
L02.425 **Furuncle of right lower limb**
L02.426 **Furuncle of left lower limb**
L02.429 **Furuncle of limb, unspecified**

✓6th **L02.43** **Carbuncle of limb**
L02.431 **Carbuncle of right axilla**
L02.432 **Carbuncle of left axilla**
L02.433 **Carbuncle of right upper limb**
L02.434 **Carbuncle of left upper limb**
L02.435 **Carbuncle of right lower limb**
L02.436 **Carbuncle of left lower limb**
L02.439 **Carbuncle of limb, unspecified**

✓5th **L02.5** **Cutaneous abscess, furuncle and carbuncle of hand**

CC Excl: For CC codes in subcategory L02.5, unless
otherwise noted: A17.9, A18.4, A18.82, A18.84, A18.89,
A48.2-A48.4, A48.8-A49.9, B78.1, B95.0-B96.89, E83.2, L02.511-
L02.519, L02.811-L02.818, L02.91, L03.811-L03.91, L08.0,
L08.81-L08.9, L44.8-L45, L73.2, L88, L92.8, L94.2, L94.4, L98.0,
L98.3, L98.8, L99, M00.011-M00.012, M00.021-M00.022,
M00.031-M00.032, M00.041-M00.042, M00.051-M00.052,
M00.061-M00.062, M00.071-M00.072, Z16.10-Z16.39

✓6th **L02.51** **Cutaneous abscess of hand**
L02.511 **Cutaneous abscess of right hand** CC
L02.512 **Cutaneous abscess of left hand** CC
L02.519 **Cutaneous abscess of unspecified** CC
hand

✓6th **L02.52** **Furuncle hand**
Boil of hand Folliculitis of hand
L02.521 **Furuncle right hand**
L02.522 **Furuncle left hand**
L02.529 **Furuncle unspecified hand**

✓6th **L02.53** **Carbuncle of hand**
L02.531 **Carbuncle of right hand**
L02.532 **Carbuncle of left hand**
L02.539 **Carbuncle of unspecified hand**

✓5th **L02.6** **Cutaneous abscess, furuncle and carbuncle of foot**

CC Excl: For CC codes in subcategory L02.6, unless
otherwise noted: A17.9, A18.4, A18.82, A18.84, A18.89,
A48.2-A48.4, A48.8-A49.9, B78.1, B95.0-B96.89, E83.2, L02.611-
L02.619, L02.811-L02.818, L02.91, L03.811-L03.91, L08.0,
L08.81-L08.9, L44.8-L45, L73.2, L88, L92.8, L94.2, L94.4, L98.0,
L98.3, L98.8, L99, M00.011-M00.012, M00.021-M00.022,
M00.031-M00.032, M00.041-M00.042, M00.051-M00.052,
M00.061-M00.062, M00.071-M00.072, Z16.10-Z16.39

✓6th **L02.61** **Cutaneous abscess of foot**
L02.611 **Cutaneous abscess of right foot** CC
L02.612 **Cutaneous abscess of left foot** CC
L02.619 **Cutaneous abscess of unspecified** CC
foot

✓6th **L02.62** **Furuncle of foot**
Boil of foot Folliculitis of foot
L02.621 **Furuncle of right foot**
L02.622 **Furuncle of left foot**
L02.629 **Furuncle of unspecified foot**

✓6th **L02.63** **Carbuncle of foot**
L02.631 **Carbuncle of right foot**
L02.632 **Carbuncle of left foot**
L02.639 **Carbuncle of unspecified foot**

✓5th **L02.8** **Cutaneous abscess, furuncle and carbuncle of other sites**
✓6th **L02.81** **Cutaneous abscess of other sites**
L02.811 **Cutaneous abscess of head [any part,** CC
except face]
CC Excl: A17.9, A18.4, A18.82, A18.84,
A18.89, A48.2-A48.4, A48.8-A49.9, B78.1,
B95.0-B96.89, E83.2, L02.811-L02.818,
L02.91, L03.811-L03.91, L08.0, L08.81-L08.9,
L44.8-L45, L73.2, L88, L92.8, L94.2, L94.4,
L98.0, L98.3, L98.8, L99, M00.011-M00.012,
M00.021-M00.022, M00.031-M00.032,
M00.041-M00.042, M00.051-M00.052,
M00.061-M00.062, M00.071-M00.07,
Z16.10-Z16.39
L02.818 **Cutaneous abscess of other sites** CC
CC Excl: See code: L02.811

✓6th **L02.82** **Furuncle of other sites**
Boil of other sites Folliculitis of other sites
L02.821 **Furuncle of head [any part, except face]**
L02.828 **Furuncle of other sites**

✓6th **L02.83** **Carbuncle of other sites**
L02.831 **Carbuncle of head [any part, except face]**
L02.838 **Carbuncle of other sites**

✓5th **L02.9** **Cutaneous abscess, furuncle and carbuncle, unspecified**
L02.91 **Cutaneous abscess, unspecified** CC
CC Excl: See code: L02.811
L02.92 **Furuncle, unspecified**
Boil NOS   Furunculosis NOS
L02.93 **Carbuncle, unspecified**

✓4th **L03** **Cellulitis and acute lymphangitis**
EXCLUDES 2 cellulitis of anal and rectal region (K61.-)
cellulitis of external auditory canal (H60.1)
cellulitis of eyelid (H00.03-)
cellulitis of female external genital organs (N76.4)
cellulitis of lacrimal apparatus (H04.3)
cellulitis of male external genital organs (N48.2, N49-)
cellulitis of mouth (K12.2)
cellulitis of nose (J34.0)
eosinophilic cellulitis [Wells] (L98.3)
febrile neutrophilic dermatosis [Sweet] (L98.2)
lymphangitis (chronic) (subacute) (I89.1)

✓5th **L03.0** **Cellulitis and acute lymphangitis of finger and toe**
Infection of nail   Paronychia
Onychia   Perionychia

✓6th **L03.01** **Cellulitis of finger**
Felon
Whitlow
EXCLUDES 1 herpetic whitlow (B00.89)
L03.011 **Cellulitis of right finger**
L03.012 **Cellulitis of left finger**
L03.019 **Cellulitis of unspecified finger**

Diseases of the Skin and Subcutaneous Tissue

L03.02–L03.818

✓6ᵗʰ **L03.02** **Acute lymphangitis of finger**
Hangnail with lymphangitis of finger

    L03.021 Acute lymphangitis of right finger
    L03.022 Acute lymphangitis of left finger
    L03.029 Acute lymphangitis of unspecified finger

✓6ᵗʰ **L03.03** **Cellulitis of toe**
    L03.031 Cellulitis of right toe
    L03.032 Cellulitis of left toe
    L03.039 Cellulitis of unspecified toe

✓6ᵗʰ **L03.04** **Acute lymphangitis of toe**
Hangnail with lymphangitis of toe

    L03.041 Acute lymphangitis of right toe
    L03.042 Acute lymphangitis of left toe
    L03.049 Acute lymphangitis of unspecified toe

✓5ᵗʰ **L03.1** **Cellulitis and acute lymphangitis of other parts of limb**

> **CC Excl:** For CC codes in subcategory L03.1, unless otherwise noted: A17.9, A18.4, A18.82, A18.84, A18.89, A48.2-A48.4, A48.8-A49.9, B78.1, B95.0-B96.89, E83.2, L02.411-L02.414, L02.811-L02.818, L02.91, L03.111-L03.114, L03.121-L03.124, L03.811-L03.91, L08.0, L08.81-L08.9, L44.8-L45, L73.2, L88, L92.8, L94.2, L94.4, L98.0, L98.3, L98.8, L99, M00.011-M00.012, M00.021-M00.022, M00.031-M00.032, M00.041-M00.042, M00.051-M00.052, M00.061-M00.062, M00.071-M00.072, Z16.10-Z16.39

✓6ᵗʰ **L03.11** **Cellulitis of other parts of limb**
> EXCLUDES 2   cellulitis of fingers (L03.01-)
>   cellulitis of toes (L03.03-)
>   groin (L03.314)

    L03.111 Cellulitis of right axilla   CC
    L03.112 Cellulitis of left axilla   CC
    L03.113 Cellulitis of right upper limb   CC
    L03.114 Cellulitis of left upper limb   CC
    L03.115 Cellulitis of right lower limb   CC
        CC Excl: See code: L02.415
    L03.116 Cellulitis of left lower limb   CC
        CC Excl: See code: L02.415
    L03.119 Cellulitis of unspecified part of limb   CC
        CC Excl: See code: L02.415

✓6ᵗʰ **L03.12** **Acute lymphangitis of other parts of limb**
> EXCLUDES 2   acute lymphangitis of fingers (L03.02-)
>   acute lymphangitis of groin (L03.324)
>   acute lymphangitis of toes (L03.04-)

    L03.121 Acute lymphangitis of right axilla   CC
    L03.122 Acute lymphangitis of left axilla   CC
    L03.123 Acute lymphangitis of right upper limb   CC
    L03.124 Acute lymphangitis of left upper limb   CC
    L03.125 Acute lymphangitis of right lower limb   CC
        CC Excl: See code: L02.415
    L03.126 Acute lymphangitis of left lower limb   CC
        CC Excl: See code: L02.415
    L03.129 Acute lymphangitis of unspecified part of limb   CC
        CC Excl: See code: L02.415

✓5ᵗʰ **L03.2** **Cellulitis and acute lymphangitis of face and neck**

✓6ᵗʰ **L03.21** **Cellulitis and acute lymphangitis of face**
    L03.211 **Cellulitis of face**   CC
> EXCLUDES 2   cellulitis of ear (H60.1-)
>   cellulitis of eyelid (H00.03-)
>   cellulitis of head (L03.811)
>   cellulitis of lacrimal apparatus
>   (H04.3)
>   cellulitis of lip (K13.0)
>   cellulitis of mouth (K12.2)
>   cellulitis of nose (internal) (J34.0)
>   cellulitis of orbit (H05.0)
>   cellulitis of scalp (L03.811)

        AHA: 2013, 4Q, 123
        CC Excl: A17.9, A18.4, A18.82, A18.84, A18.89, A48.2-A48.4, A48.8-A49.9, B78.1, B95.0-B96.89, E83.2, L02.811-L02.818, L02.91, L03.211, L03.811-L03.91, L08.0, L08.81-L08.9, L44.8-L45, L73.2, L88, L92.8, L94.2, L94.4, L98.0, L98.3, L98.8, L99, M00.011-M00.012, M00.021-M00.022, M00.031-M00.032, M00.041-M00.042, M00.051-M00.052, M00.061-M00.062, M00.071-M00.072, Z16.10-Z16.39

    L03.212 **Acute lymphangitis of face**   CC
        CC Excl: No Excl

✓6ᵗʰ **L03.22** **Cellulitis and acute lymphangitis of neck**
    L03.221 **Cellulitis of neck**   CC
        CC Excl: A17.9, A18.4, A18.82, A18.84, A18.89, A48.2-A48.4, A48.8-A49.9, B78.1, B95.0-B96.89, E83.2, L02.11, L02.811-L02.818, L02.91, L03.221-L03.222, L03.811-L03.91, L08.0, L08.81-L08.9, L44.8-L45, L73.2, L88, L92.8, L94.2, L94.4, L98.0, L98.3, L98.8, L99, M00.011-M00.012, M00.021-M00.022, M00.031-M00.032, M00.041-M00.042, M00.051-M00.052, M00.061-M00.062, M00.071-M00.072, Z16.10-Z16.39
    L03.222 **Acute lymphangitis of neck**   CC
        CC Excl: See code: L03.221

✓5ᵗʰ **L03.3** **Cellulitis and acute lymphangitis of trunk**

> **CC Excl:** For CC codes in subcategory L03.3, unless otherwise noted: A17.9, A18.4, A18.82, A18.84, A18.89, A48.2-A48.4, A48.8-A49.9, B78.1, B95.0-B96.89, E83.2, L02.211-L02.219, L02.811-L02.818, L02.91, L03.311-L03.316, L03.319-L03.326, L03.329-L03.91, L08.0, L08.81-L08.9, L44.8-L45, L73.2, L88, L92.8, L94.2, L94.4, L98.0, L98.3, L98.8, L99, M00.011-M00.012, M00.021-M00.022, M00.031-M00.032, M00.041-M00.042, M00.051-M00.052, M00.061-M00.062, M00.071-M00.072, Z16.10-Z16.39

✓6ᵗʰ **L03.31** **Cellulitis of trunk**
> EXCLUDES 2   cellulitis of anal and rectal regions (K61.-)
>   cellulitis of breast NOS (N61)
>   cellulitis of female external genital organs
>   (N76.4)
>   cellulitis of male external genital organs
>   (N48.2, N49-)
>   omphalitis of newborn (P38.-)
>   puerperal cellulitis of breast (O91.2)

    L03.311 **Cellulitis of abdominal wall**   CC
> EXCLUDES 2   cellulitis of umbilicus (L03.316)
>   cellulitis of groin (L03.314)

    L03.312 **Cellulitis of back [any part except buttock]**   CC
    L03.313 **Cellulitis of chest wall**   CC
    L03.314 **Cellulitis of groin**   CC
    L03.315 **Cellulitis of perineum**   CC
    L03.316 **Cellulitis of umbilicus**   CC
    L03.317 **Cellulitis of buttock**   CC
        CC Excl: A17.9, A18.4, A18.82, A18.84, A18.89, A48.2-A48.4, A48.8-A49.9, B78.1, B95.0-B96.89, E83.2, L02.31, L02.811-L02.818, L02.91, L03.317, L03.327, L03.811-L03.91, L08.0, L08.81-L08.9, L44.8-L45, L73.2, L88, L92.8, L94.2, L94.4, L98.0, L98.3, L98.8, L99, M00.011-M00.012, M00.021-M00.022, M00.031-M00.032, M00.041-M00.042, M00.051-M00.052, M00.061-M00.062, M00.071-M00.072, Z16.10-Z16.39
    L03.319 **Cellulitis of trunk, unspecified**   CC

✓6ᵗʰ **L03.32** **Acute lymphangitis of trunk**
    L03.321 Acute lymphangitis of abdominal wall   CC
    L03.322 Acute lymphangitis of back [any part except buttock]   CC
    L03.323 Acute lymphangitis of chest wall   CC
    L03.324 Acute lymphangitis of groin   CC
    L03.325 Acute lymphangitis of perineum   CC
    L03.326 Acute lymphangitis of umbilicus   CC
    L03.327 Acute lymphangitis of buttock   CC
        CC Excl: See code: L03.317
    L03.329 Acute lymphangitis of trunk, unspecified

✓5ᵗʰ **L03.8** **Cellulitis and acute lymphangitis of other sites**

> **CC Excl:** For CC codes in subcategory L03.8, unless otherwise noted: A17.9, A18.4, A18.82, A18.84, A18.89, A48.2-A48.4, A48.8-A49.9, B78.1, B95.0-B96.89, E83.2, L02.811-L02.818, L02.91, L03.811-L03.91, L08.0, L08.81-L08.9, L44.8-L45, L73.2, L88, L92.8, L94.2, L94.4, L98.0, L98.3, L98.8, L99, M00.011-M00.012, M00.021-M00.022, M00.031-M00.032, M00.041-M00.042, M00.051-M00.052, M00.061-M00.062, M00.071-M00.072, Z16.10-Z16.39

✓6ᵗʰ **L03.81** **Cellulitis of other sites**
    L03.811 **Cellulitis of head [any part, except face]**   CC
        Cellulitis of scalp
>   EXCLUDES 2   cellulitis of face (L03.211)

    L03.818 **Cellulitis of other sites**   CC

N Newborn: 0   P Pediatric: 0-17   M Maternity: 12-55   A Adult: 15-124   MCC Major CC Condition   PDx MCC PDx acts as own MCC   CC CC Condition   PDx CC PDx acts as own CC

662   ICD-10-CM Draft (2015)

✓6ᵗʰ **L03.89** Acute lymphangitis of other sites

　　L03.891 Acute lymphangitis of head [any part, except face] `CC`

　　L03.898 Acute lymphangitis of other sites `CC`

✓5ᵗʰ **L03.9** Cellulitis and acute lymphangitis, unspecified

> **CC Excl: For CC codes in subcategory L03.9, unless otherwise noted:** See code: L03.8

　　L03.90 Cellulitis, unspecified `CC`

　　L03.91 Acute lymphangitis, unspecified `CC`
　　　EXCLUDES 1 lymphangitis NOS (I89.1)

✓4ᵗʰ **L04 Acute lymphadenitis**

INCLUDES abscess (acute) of lymph nodes, except mesenteric
acute lymphadenitis, except mesenteric

EXCLUDES 1 chronic or subacute lymphadenitis, except mesenteric (I88.1)
enlarged lymph nodes (R59.-)
human immunodeficiency virus [HIV] disease resulting in
　generalized lymphadenopathy (B20)
lymphadenitis NOS (I88.9)
nonspecific mesenteric lymphadenitis (I88.0)

L04.0 Acute lymphadenitis of face, head and neck

L04.1 Acute lymphadenitis of trunk

L04.2 Acute lymphadenitis of upper limb
Acute lymphadenitis of axilla　　Acute lymphadenitis of shoulder

L04.3 Acute lymphadenitis of lower limb
Acute lymphadenitis of hip
EXCLUDES 2 acute lymphadenitis of groin (L04.1)

L04.8 Acute lymphadenitis of other sites

L04.9 Acute lymphadenitis, unspecified

✓4ᵗʰ **L05 Pilonidal cyst and sinus**

✓5ᵗʰ **L05.0** Pilonidal cyst and sinus with abscess

　　L05.01 Pilonidal cyst with abscess `CC`
　　　Parasacral dimple with abscess
　　　Pilonidal abscess
　　　Pilonidal dimple with abscess
　　　Postanal dimple with abscess
　　　CC Excl: L05.01-L05.92, L44.8-L45, L94.2, L94.4, L98.8, L99

　　L05.02 Pilonidal sinus with abscess `CC`
　　　Coccygeal fistula with abscess
　　　Coccygeal sinus with abscess
　　　Pilonidal fistula with abscess
　　　CC Excl: See code: L05.01

✓5ᵗʰ **L05.9** Pilonidal cyst and sinus without abscess

　　L05.91 Pilonidal cyst without abscess
　　　Parasacral dimple　　Postanal dimple
　　　Pilonidal dimple　Pilonidal cyst NOS

　　L05.92 Pilonidal sinus without abscess
　　　Coccygeal fistula
　　　Coccygeal sinus without abscess
　　　Pilonidal fistula

✓4ᵗʰ **L08 Other local infections of skin and subcutaneous tissue**

L08.0 Pyoderma
Dermatitis gangrenosa　　　Septic dermatitis
Purulent dermatitis　　　　Suppurative dermatitis
EXCLUDES 1 pyoderma gangrenosum (L88)
　　pyoderma vegetans (L08.81)

L08.1 Erythrasma `HIV` `CC`
CC Excl: A42.81-A42.9, A43.1-A43.9, B47.1, L08.1

✓5ᵗʰ **L08.8** Other specified local infections of the skin and subcutaneous tissue

　　L08.81 Pyoderma vegetans
　　　EXCLUDES 1 pyoderma gangrenosum (L88)
　　　　pyoderma NOS (L08.0)

　　L08.82 Omphalitis not of newborn
　　　EXCLUDES 1 omphalitis of newborn (P38.-)

　　L08.89 Other specified local infections of the skin and subcutaneous tissue

L08.9 Local infection of the skin and subcutaneous tissue, unspecified

Bullous disorders (L10-L14)

EXCLUDES 1 benign familial pemphigus [Hailey-Hailey] (Q82.8)
staphylococcal scalded skin syndrome (L00)
toxic epidermal necrolysis [Lyell] (L51.2)

✓4ᵗʰ **L10 Pemphigus**
EXCLUDES 1 pemphigus neonatorum (L01.03)

> **CC Excl: For CC codes in category L10, unless otherwise noted:**
> L10.0-L10.9, L12.0-L12.1, L12.8-L12.9, L13.8-L14, L44.8-L45, L94.2, L94.4, L98.8, L99

L10.0 Pemphigus vulgaris `CC`

L10.1 Pemphigus vegetans `CC`

L10.2 Pemphigus foliaceous `CC`

L10.3 Brazilian pemphigus [fogo selvagem] `CC`

L10.4 Pemphigus erythematosus `CC`
Senear-Usher syndrome

L10.5 Drug-induced pemphigus
Use additional code for adverse effect, if applicable, to identify
　drug (T36-T50 with fifth or sixth character 5)

✓5ᵗʰ **L10.8** Other pemphigus

　　L10.81 Paraneoplastic pemphigus `CC`

　　L10.89 Other pemphigus `CC`

L10.9 Pemphigus, unspecified `CC`

✓4ᵗʰ **L11 Other acantholytic disorders**

L11.0 Acquired keratosis follicularis
EXCLUDES 1 keratosis follicularis (congenital) [Darier-White] (Q82.8)

L11.1 Transient acantholytic dermatosis [Grover]

L11.8 Other specified acantholytic disorders

L11.9 Acantholytic disorder, unspecified

✓4ᵗʰ **L12 Pemphigoid**
EXCLUDES 1 herpes gestationis (O26.4-)
impetigo herpetiformis (L40.1)

> **CC Excl: For CC codes in category L12, unless otherwise noted:**
> See code: L10

L12.0 Bullous pemphigoid `CC`

L12.1 Cicatricial pemphigoid
Benign mucous membrane pemphigoid

L12.2 Chronic bullous disease of childhood `P`
Juvenile dermatitis herpetiformis

✓5ᵗʰ **L12.3** Acquired epidermolysis bullosa
EXCLUDES 1 epidermolysis bullosa (congenital) (Q81.-)

　　L12.30 Acquired epidermolysis bullosa, unspecified `CC`
　　　CC Excl: L00, L12.30-L12.35, L26, L30.4, L44.8-L45,
　　　L51.0-L54, L71.0-L71.9, L92.0, L93.0-L93.2, L94.2, L94.4,
　　　L95.1, L98.2, L98.8, L99

　　L12.31 Epidermolysis bullosa due to drug `CC`
　　　Use additional code for adverse effect, if applicable, to
　　　identify drug (T36-T50 with fifth or sixth
　　　character 5)
　　　CC Excl: See code: L12.30

　　L12.35 Other acquired epidermolysis bullosa `CC`
　　　CC Excl: See code: L12.30

L12.8 Other pemphigoid `CC`

L12.9 Pemphigoid, unspecified `CC`

✓4ᵗʰ **L13 Other bullous disorders**

L13.0 Dermatitis herpetiformis
Duhring's disease
Hydroa herpetiformis
EXCLUDES 1 juvenile dermatitis herpetiformis (L12.2)
　　senile dermatitis herpetiformis (L13.0)

L13.1 Subcorneal pustular dermatitis
Sneddon-Wilkinson disease

L13.8 Other specified bullous disorders

L13.9 Bullous disorder, unspecified

✓ **L14 Bullous disorders in diseases classified elsewhere**
Code first underlying disease

✓ Additional Character Required　✓7ᵗʰ Xtension Alert　Unacceptable PDx　Manifestation　　Hospital Acquired Condition　*EXCLUDES 1* Not Coded Here　*EXCLUDES 2* Not Included Here

Diseases of the Skin and Subcutaneous Tissue

L20–L26

Dermatitis and eczema (L20-L30)

NOTE   In this block the terms dermatitis and eczema are used synonymously and interchangeably.

EXCLUDES 2   chronic (childhood) granulomatous disease (D71)
dermatitis gangrenosa (L08.0)
dermatitis herpetiformis (L13.0)
dry skin dermatitis (L85.3)
factitial dermatitis (L98.1)
perioral dermatitis (L71.0)
radiation-related disorders of the skin and subcutaneous tissue (L55-L59)
stasis dermatitis (I83.1-I83.2)

✓4ᵗʰ **L20   Atopic dermatitis**

L20.0   Besnier's prurigo

✓5ᵗʰ **L20.8   Other atopic dermatitis**
EXCLUDES 2   circumscribed neurodermatitis (L28.0)

L20.81   Atopic neurodermatitis
Diffuse neurodermatitis

L20.82   Flexural eczema

L20.83   Infantile (acute) (chronic) eczema   **P**

L20.84   Intrinsic (allergic) eczema

L20.89   Other atopic dermatitis

L20.9   Atopic dermatitis, unspecified

✓4ᵗʰ **L21   Seborrheic dermatitis**
EXCLUDES 2   infective dermatitis (L30.3)
seborrheic keratosis (L82.-)

L21.0   Seborrhea capitis   **P**
Cradle cap

L21.1   Seborrheic infantile dermatitis   **P**

L21.8   Other seborrheic dermatitis

L21.9   Seborrheic dermatitis, unspecified
Seborrhea NOS

L22   Diaper dermatitis
Diaper erythema   Psoriasiform diaper rash
Diaper rash

✓4ᵗʰ **L23   Allergic contact dermatitis**
EXCLUDES 1   allergy NOS (T78.40)
contact dermatitis NOS (L25.9)
dermatitis NOS (L30.9)
EXCLUDES 2   dermatitis due to substances taken internally (L27.-)
dermatitis of eyelid (H01.1-)
diaper dermatitis (L22)
eczema of external ear (H60.5-)
irritant contact dermatitis (L24.-)
perioral dermatitis (L71.0)
radiation-related disorders of the skin and subcutaneous tissue (L55-L59)

L23.0   Allergic contact dermatitis due to metals
Allergic contact dermatitis due to chromium
Allergic contact dermatitis due to nickel

L23.1   Allergic contact dermatitis due to adhesives

L23.2   Allergic contact dermatitis due to cosmetics

L23.3   Allergic contact dermatitis due to drugs in contact with skin
Use additional code for adverse effect, if applicable, to identify drug (T36-T50 with fifth or sixth character 5)
EXCLUDES 2   dermatitis due to ingested drugs and medicaments (L27.0-L27.1)

L23.4   Allergic contact dermatitis due to dyes

L23.5   Allergic contact dermatitis due to other chemical products
Allergic contact dermatitis due to cement
Allergic contact dermatitis due to insecticide
Allergic contact dermatitis due to plastic
Allergic contact dermatitis due to rubber

L23.6   Allergic contact dermatitis due to food in contact with the skin
EXCLUDES 2   dermatitis due to ingested food (L27.2)

L23.7   Allergic contact dermatitis due to plants, except food
EXCLUDES 2   allergy NOS due to pollen (J30.1)

✓5ᵗʰ **L23.8   Allergic contact dermatitis due to other agents**

L23.81   Allergic contact dermatitis due to animal (cat) (dog) dander
Allergic contact dermatitis due to animal (cat) (dog) hair

L23.89   Allergic contact dermatitis due to other agents

L23.9   Allergic contact dermatitis, unspecified cause
Allergic contact eczema NOS

✓4ᵗʰ **L24   Irritant contact dermatitis**
EXCLUDES 1   allergy NOS (T78.40)
contact dermatitis NOS (L25.9)
dermatitis NOS (L30.9)
EXCLUDES 2   allergic contact dermatitis (L23.-)
dermatitis due to substances taken internally (L27.-)
dermatitis of eyelid (H01.1-)
diaper dermatitis (L22)
eczema of external ear (H60.5-)
perioral dermatitis (L71.0)
radiation-related disorders of the skin and subcutaneous tissue (L55-L59)

L24.0   Irritant contact dermatitis due to detergents

L24.1   Irritant contact dermatitis due to oils and greases

L24.2   Irritant contact dermatitis due to solvents
Irritant contact dermatitis due to chlorocompound
Irritant contact dermatitis due to cyclohexane
Irritant contact dermatitis due to ester
Irritant contact dermatitis due to glycol
Irritant contact dermatitis due to hydrocarbon
Irritant contact dermatitis due to ketone

L24.3   Irritant contact dermatitis due to cosmetics

L24.4   Irritant contact dermatitis due to drugs in contact with skin
Use additional code for adverse effect, if applicable, to identify drug (T36-T50 with fifth or sixth character 5)

L24.5   Irritant contact dermatitis due to other chemical products
Irritant contact dermatitis due to cement
Irritant contact dermatitis due to insecticide
Irritant contact dermatitis due to plastic
Irritant contact dermatitis due to rubber

L24.6   Irritant contact dermatitis due to food in contact with skin
EXCLUDES 2   dermatitis due to ingested food (L27.2)

L24.7   Irritant contact dermatitis due to plants, except food
EXCLUDES 2   allergy NOS to pollen (J30.1)

✓5ᵗʰ **L24.8   Irritant contact dermatitis due to other agents**

L24.81   Irritant contact dermatitis due to metals
Irritant contact dermatitis due to chromium
Irritant contact dermatitis due to nickel

L24.89   Irritant contact dermatitis due to other agents
Irritant contact dermatitis due to dyes

L24.9   Irritant contact dermatitis, unspecified cause
Irritant contact eczema NOS

✓4ᵗʰ **L25   Unspecified contact dermatitis**
EXCLUDES 1   allergic contact dermatitis (L23.-)
allergy NOS (T78.40)
dermatitis NOS (L30.9)
irritant contact dermatitis (L24.-)
EXCLUDES 2   dermatitis due to ingested substances (L27.-)
dermatitis of eyelid (H01.1-)
eczema of external ear (H60.5-)
perioral dermatitis (L71.0)
radiation-related disorders of the skin and subcutaneous tissue (L55-L59)

L25.0   Unspecified contact dermatitis due to cosmetics

L25.1   Unspecified contact dermatitis due to drugs in contact with skin
Use additional code for adverse effect, if applicable, to identify drug (T36-T50 with fifth or sixth character 5)
EXCLUDES 2   dermatitis due to ingested drugs and medicaments (L27.0-L27.1)

L25.2   Unspecified contact dermatitis due to dyes

L25.3   Unspecified contact dermatitis due to other chemical products
Unspecified contact dermatitis due to cement
Unspecified contact dermatitis due to insecticide

L25.4   Unspecified contact dermatitis due to food in contact with skin
EXCLUDES 2   dermatitis due to ingested food (L27.2)

L25.5   Unspecified contact dermatitis due to plants, except food
EXCLUDES 1   nettle rash (L50.9)
EXCLUDES 2   allergy NOS due to pollen (J30.1)

L25.8   Unspecified contact dermatitis due to other agents

L25.9   Unspecified contact dermatitis, unspecified cause
Contact dermatitis (occupational) NOS
Contact eczema (occupational) NOS

L26   Exfoliative dermatitis
Hebra's pityriasis
EXCLUDES 1   Ritter's disease (L00)

☑4th **L27**   **Dermatitis** due to substances taken internally
- EXCLUDES 1   *allergy NOS (T78.40)*
- EXCLUDES 2   *adverse food reaction, except dermatitis (T78.0-T78.1)*
  - *contact dermatitis (L23-L25)*
  - *drug photoallergic response (L56.1)*
  - *drug phototoxic response (L56.0)*
  - *urticaria (L50.-)*

L27.0   Generalized **skin eruption due to** drugs and medicaments **taken internally**
> Use additional code for adverse effect, if applicable, to identify drug (T36-T50 with fifth or sixth character 5)

L27.1   Localized **skin eruption due to** drugs and medicaments **taken internally**
> Use additional code for adverse effect, if applicable, to identify drug (T36-T50 with fifth or sixth character 5)

L27.2   **Dermatitis** due to ingested food
- EXCLUDES 2   *dermatitis due to food in contact with skin (L23.6, L24.6, L25.4)*

L27.8   **Dermatitis** due to other substances taken internally

L27.9   **Dermatitis** due to unspecified substance taken internally

☑4th **L28**   **Lichen simplex chronicus and prurigo**

L28.0   **Lichen simplex chronicus**
> Circumscribed neurodermatitis   Lichen NOS

L28.1   **Prurigo nodularis**

L28.2   **Other prurigo**
> Prurigo NOS   Prurigo mitis
> Prurigo Hebra   Urticaria papulosa

☑4th **L29**   **Pruritus**
- EXCLUDES 1   *neurotic excoriation (L98.1)*
  - *psychogenic pruritus (F45.8)*

L29.0   **Pruritus** ani

L29.1   **Pruritus** scroti   ♂

L29.2   **Pruritus** vulvae   ♀

L29.3   **Anogenital** pruritus, unspecified

L29.8   **Other** pruritus

L29.9   **Pruritus,** unspecified
> Itch NOS

☑4th **L30**   **Other and unspecified dermatitis**
- EXCLUDES 2   *contact dermatitis (L23-L25)*
  - *dry skin dermatitis (L85.3)*
  - *small plaque parapsoriasis (L41.3)*
  - *stasis dermatitis (I83.1-.2)*

L30.0   **Nummular dermatitis**

L30.1   **Dyshidrosis [pompholyx]**

L30.2   **Cutaneous autosensitization**
> Candidid [levurid]   Eczematid
> Dermatophytid

L30.3   **Infective dermatitis**
> Infectious eczematoid dermatitis

L30.4   **Erythema intertrigo**

L30.5   **Pityriasis alba**

L30.8   **Other specified dermatitis**

L30.9   **Dermatitis, unspecified**
> Eczema NOS

Papulosquamous disorders (L40-L45)

☑4th **L40**   **Psoriasis**

L40.0   **Psoriasis** vulgaris
> Nummular psoriasis   Plaque psoriasis

L40.1   **Generalized pustular** psoriasis
> Impetigo herpetiformis   Von Zumbusch's disease

L40.2   **Acrodermatitis continua**

L40.3   **Pustulosis palmaris et plantaris**

L40.4   **Guttate** psoriasis

☑5th **L40.5**   **Arthropathic** psoriasis

     L40.50   **Arthropathic psoriasis,** unspecified

     L40.51   **Distal interphalangeal** psoriatic arthropathy

     L40.52   **Psoriatic arthritis** mutilans

     L40.53   **Psoriatic** spondylitis

     L40.54   **Psoriatic** juvenile **arthropathy**

     L40.59   **Other** psoriatic arthropathy

L40.8   **Other** psoriasis
> Flexural psoriasis

L40.9   **Psoriasis,** unspecified

☑4th **L41**   **Parapsoriasis**
- EXCLUDES 1   *poikiloderma vasculare atrophicans (L94.5)*

L41.0   **Pityriasis lichenoides et varioliformis acuta**
> Mucha-Habermann disease

L41.1   **Pityriasis lichenoides chronica**

L41.3   **Small plaque** parapsoriasis

L41.4   **Large plaque** parapsoriasis

L41.5   **Retiform** parapsoriasis

L41.8   **Other** parapsoriasis

L41.9   **Parapsoriasis,** unspecified

L42   **Pityriasis rosea**

☑4th **L43**   **Lichen planus**
- EXCLUDES 1   *lichen planopilaris (L66.1)*

L43.0   **Hypertrophic** lichen planus

L43.1   **Bullous** lichen planus

L43.2   **Lichenoid** drug reaction
> Use additional code for adverse effect, if applicable, to identify drug (T36-T50 with fifth or sixth character 5)

L43.3   **Subacute (active) lichen planus**
> Lichen planus tropicus

L43.8   **Other** lichen planus

L43.9   **Lichen planus,** unspecified

☑4th **L44**   **Other papulosquamous disorders**

L44.0   **Pityriasis rubra pilaris**

L44.1   **Lichen nitidus**

L44.3   **Lichen ruber moniliformis**

L44.4   **Infantile papular acrodermatitis [Gianotti-Crosti]**   P

L44.8   **Other specified papulosquamous disorders**

L44.9   **Papulosquamous disorder,** unspecified

L45   *Papulosquamous disorders in diseases classified elsewhere*
> *Code first underlying disease*

Urticaria and erythema (L49-L54)

- EXCLUDES 1   *Lyme disease (A69.2-)*
  - *rosacea (L71.-)*

☑4th **L49**   **Exfoliation due to erythematous conditions according to extent of body surface involved**
> Code first erythematous condition causing exfoliation, such as:
> Ritter's disease (L00)
> (Staphylococcal) scalded skin syndrom (L00)
> Stevens-Johnson syndrome (L51.1)
> Stevens-Johnson syndrome-toxic epidermal necrolysis overlap syndrome (L51.3)
> toxic epidermal necrolysis (L51.2)

L49.0   **Exfoliation due to erythematous condition involving less than 10 percent of body surface**
> Exfoliation due to erythematous condition NOS

L49.1   **Exfoliation due to erythematous condition involving 10-19 percent of body surface**

L49.2   **Exfoliation due to erythematous condition involving 20-29 percent of body surface**

L49.3   **Exfoliation due to erythematous condition involving 30-39 percent of body surface**   CC
> CC Excl: L49.3

L49.4   **Exfoliation due to erythematous condition involving 40-49 percent of body surface**   CC
> CC Excl: L49.4

L49.5   **Exfoliation due to erythematous condition involving 50-59 percent of body surface**   CC
> CC Excl: L49.5

L49.6   **Exfoliation due to erythematous condition involving 60-69 percent of body surface**   CC
> CC Excl: L49.6

L49.7   **Exfoliation due to erythematous condition involving 70-79 percent of body surface**   CC
> CC Excl: L49.7

L49.8   **Exfoliation due to erythematous condition involving 80-89 percent of body surface**   CC
> CC Excl: L49.8

L49.9   **Exfoliation due to erythematous condition involving 90 or more percent of body surface**   CC
> CC Excl: L49.9

☑ Additional Character Required   ☑7th Xtension Alert   Unacceptable PDx   Manifestation   Hospital Acquired Condition   EXCLUDES 1 Not Coded Here   EXCLUDES 2 Not Included Here

Diseases of the Skin and Subcutaneous Tissue

L50–L60.9

✓4ᵗʰ **L50 Urticaria**
> **EXCLUDES 1**   *allergic contact dermatitis (L23.-)*
> *angioneurotic edema (T78.3)*
> *giant urticaria (T78.3)*
> *hereditary angio-edema (D84.1)*
> *Quincke's edema (T78.3)*
> *serum urticaria (T80.6-)*
> *solar urticaria (L56.3)*
> *urticaria neonatorum (P83.8)*
> *urticaria papulosa (L28.2)*
> *urticaria pigmentosa (Q82.2)*

  L50.0 Allergic urticaria

  L50.1 Idiopathic urticaria

  L50.2 Urticaria due to cold and heat

  L50.3 Dermatographic urticaria

  L50.4 Vibratory urticaria

  L50.5 Cholinergic urticaria

  L50.6 Contact urticaria

  L50.8 Other urticaria
> Chronic urticaria   Recurrent periodic urticaria

  L50.9 Urticaria, unspecified

✓4ᵗʰ **L51 Erythema multiforme**
> Use additional code for adverse effect, if applicable, to identify drug (T36-T50 with fifth or sixth character 5)
> Use additional code to identify associated manifestations, such as:
> arthropathy associated with dermatological disorders (M14.8-)
> conjunctival edema (H11.42)
> conjunctivitis (H10.22-)
> corneal scars and opacities (H17.-)
> corneal ulcer (H16.0-)
> edema of eyelid (H02.84)
> inflammation of eyelid (H01.8)
> keratoconjunctivitis sicca (H16.22-)
> mechanical lagophthalmos (H02.22-)
> stomatitis (K12.-)
> symblepharon (H11.23-)
> Use additional code to identify percentage of skin exfoliation (L49.-)

> **EXCLUDES 1**   *staphylococcal scalded skin syndrome (L00)*
> *Ritter's disease (L00)*

  L51.0 Nonbullous erythema multiforme

  L51.1 Stevens-Johnson syndrome   CC
> **CC Excl:** L00, L12.30-L12.35, L26, L30.4, L44.8-L45, L51.0-L54, L71.0-L71.9, L92.0, L93.0-L93.2, L94.2, L94.4, L95.1, L98.2, L98.8, L99

  L51.2 Toxic epidermal necrolysis [Lyell]   CC
> **CC Excl:** See code: L51.1

  L51.3 Stevens-Johnson syndrome-toxic epidermal necrolysis overlap syndrome   CC
> SJS-TEN overlap syndrome
> **CC Excl:** See code: L51.1

  L51.8 Other erythema multiforme

  L51.9 Erythema multiforme, unspecified
> Erythema iris   Herpes iris
> Erythema multiforme major NOS
> Erythema multiforme minor NOS

  L52 Erythema nodosum
> **EXCLUDES 1**   *tuberculous erythema nodosum (A18.4)*

✓4ᵗʰ **L53 Other erythematous conditions**
> **EXCLUDES 1**   *erythema ab igne (L59.0)*
> *erythema due to external agents in contact with skin (L23-L25)*
> *erythema intertrigo (L30.4)*

> **CC Excl: For CC codes in category L53, unless otherwise noted:**
> L12.30-L12.35, L44.8-L45, L51.0-L53.3, L71.0-L71.9, L93.0-L93.2, L94.2, L94.4, L98.8, L99

  L53.0 Toxic erythema   CC
> Code first poisoning due to drug or toxin, if applicable (T36-T65 with fifth or sixth character 1-4 or 6)
> Use additional code for adverse effect, if applicable, to identify drug (T36-T50 with fifth or sixth character 5)
> **EXCLUDES 1**   *neonatal erythema toxicum (P83.1)*

  L53.1 Erythema annulare centrifugum   CC

  L53.2 Erythema marginatum   CC

  L53.3 Other chronic figurate erythema   CC

  L53.8 Other specified erythematous conditions

  L53.9 Erythematous condition, unspecified
> Erythema NOS   Erythroderma NOS

L54 ***Erythema in diseases classified elsewhere***
> *Code first underlying disease*

Radiation-related disorders of the skin and subcutaneous tissue (L55-L59)

✓4ᵗʰ **L55 Sunburn**

  L55.0 Sunburn of first degree

  L55.1 Sunburn of second degree

  L55.2 Sunburn of third degree

  L55.9 Sunburn, unspecified

✓4ᵗʰ **L56 Other acute skin changes due to ultraviolet radiation**
> Use additional code to identify the source of the ultraviolet radiation (W89, X32)

  L56.0 Drug phototoxic response
> Use additional code for adverse effect, if applicable, to identify drug (T36-T50 with fifth or sixth character 5)

  L56.1 Drug photoallergic response
> Use additional code for adverse effect, if applicable, to identify drug (T36-T50 with fifth or sixth character 5)

  L56.2 Photocontact dermatitis [berloque dermatitis]

  L56.3 Solar urticaria

  L56.4 Polymorphous light eruption

  L56.5 Disseminated superficial actinic porokeratosis (DSAP)

  L56.8 Other specified acute skin changes due to ultraviolet radiation

  L56.9 Acute skin change due to ultraviolet radiation, unspecified

✓4ᵗʰ **L57 Skin changes due to chronic exposure to nonionizing radiation**
> Use additional code to identify the source of the ultraviolet radiation (W89, X32)

  L57.0 Actinic keratosis
> Keratosis NOS   Solar keratosis
> Senile keratosis

  L57.1 Actinic reticuloid

  L57.2 Cutis rhomboidalis nuchae

  L57.3 Poikiloderma of Civatte

  L57.4 Cutis laxa senilis
> Elastosis senilis

  L57.5 Actinic granuloma

  L57.8 Other skin changes due to chronic exposure to nonionizing radiation
> Farmer's skin   Solar dermatitis
> Sailor's skin

  L57.9 Skin changes due to chronic exposure to nonionizing radiation, unspecified

✓4ᵗʰ **L58 Radiodermatitis**
> Use additional code to identify the source of the radiation (W88, W90)

  L58.0 Acute radiodermatitis

  L58.1 Chronic radiodermatitis

  L58.9 Radiodermatitis, unspecified

✓4ᵗʰ **L59 Other disorders of skin and subcutaneous tissue related to radiation**

  L59.0 Erythema ab igne [dermatitis ab igne]

  L59.8 Other specified disorders of the skin and subcutaneous tissue related to radiation

  L59.9 Disorder of the skin and subcutaneous tissue related to radiation, unspecified

Disorders of skin appendages (L60-L75)
> **EXCLUDES 1**   *congenital malformations of integument (Q84.-)*

✓4ᵗʰ **L60 Nail disorders**
> **EXCLUDES 2**   *clubbing of nails (R68.3)*
> *onychia and paronychia (L03.0-)*

  L60.0 Ingrowing nail

  L60.1 Onycholysis

  L60.2 Onychogryphosis

  L60.3 Nail dystrophy

  L60.4 Beau's lines

  L60.5 Yellow nail syndrome

  L60.8 Other nail disorders

  L60.9 Nail disorder, unspecified

N Newborn: 0   P Pediatric: 0-17   M Maternity: 12-55   A Adult: 15-124   MCC Major CC Condition   PDx MCC PDx acts as own MCC   CC CC Condition   PDx CC PDx acts as own CC

666   ICD-10-CM Draft (2015)

L62   *Nail disorders in diseases classified elsewhere*
  Code first underlying disease, such as:
  pachydermoperiostosis (M89.4-)

✓4ᵗʰ **L63**   **Alopecia areata**
  L63.0   **Alopecia (capitis) totalis**
  L63.1   **Alopecia universalis**
  L63.2   **Ophiasis**
  L63.8   **Other alopecia areata**
  L63.9   **Alopecia areata, unspecified**

✓4ᵗʰ **L64**   **Androgenic alopecia**
  INCLUDES   male-pattern baldness
  L64.0   **Drug-induced androgenic alopecia**
      Use additional code for adverse effect, if applicable, to identify drug (T36-T50 with fifth or sixth character 5)
  L64.8   **Other androgenic alopecia**
  L64.9   **Androgenic alopecia, unspecified**

✓4ᵗʰ **L65**   **Other nonscarring hair loss**
      Use additional code for adverse effect, if applicable, to identify drug (T36-T50 with fifth or sixth character 5)
  EXCLUDES 1   trichotillomania (F63.3)
  L65.0   **Telogen effluvium**
  L65.1   **Anagen effluvium**
  L65.2   **Alopecia mucinosa**
  L65.8   **Other specified nonscarring hair loss**
  L65.9   **Nonscarring hair loss, unspecified**
      Alopecia NOS

✓4ᵗʰ **L66**   **Cicatricial alopecia [scarring hair loss]**
  L66.0   **Pseudopelade**
  L66.1   **Lichen planopilaris**
      Follicular lichen planus
  L66.2   **Folliculitis decalvans**
  L66.3   **Perifolliculitis capitis abscedens**
  L66.4   **Folliculitis ulerythematosa reticulata**
  L66.8   **Other cicatricial alopecia**
  L66.9   **Cicatricial alopecia, unspecified**

✓4ᵗʰ **L67**   **Hair color and hair shaft abnormalities**
  EXCLUDES 1   monilethrix (Q84.1)
      pili annulati (Q84.1)
      telogen effluvium (L65.0)
  L67.0   **Trichorrhexis nodosa**
  L67.1   **Variations in hair color**
      Canities
      Greyness, hair (premature)
      Heterochromia of hair
      Poliosis circumscripta, acquired
      Poliosis NOS
  L67.8   **Other hair color and hair shaft abnormalities**
      Fragilitas crinium
  L67.9   **Hair color and hair shaft abnormality, unspecified**

✓4ᵗʰ **L68**   **Hypertrichosis**
  INCLUDES   excess hair
  EXCLUDES 1   congenital hypertrichosis (Q84.2)
      persistent lanugo (Q84.2)
  L68.0   **Hirsutism**
  L68.1   **Acquired hypertrichosis lanuginosa**
  L68.2   **Localized hypertrichosis**
  L68.3   **Polytrichia**
  L68.8   **Other hypertrichosis**
  L68.9   **Hypertrichosis, unspecified**

✓4ᵗʰ **L70**   **Acne**
  EXCLUDES 2   acne keloid (L73.0)
  L70.0   **Acne vulgaris**
  L70.1   **Acne conglobata**
  L70.2   **Acne varioliformis**
      Acne necrotica miliaris
  L70.3   **Acne tropica**
  L70.4   **Infantile acne**   Ⓟ
  L70.5   **Acné excoriée des jeunes filles**
      Picker's acne
  L70.8   **Other acne**
  L70.9   **Acne, unspecified**

✓4ᵗʰ **L71**   **Rosacea**
      Use additional code for adverse effect, if applicable, to identify drug (T36-T50 with fifth or sixth character 5)
  L71.0   **Perioral dermatitis**
  L71.1   **Rhinophyma**
  L71.8   **Other rosacea**
  L71.9   **Rosacea, unspecified**

✓4ᵗʰ **L72**   **Follicular cysts of skin and subcutaneous tissue**
  L72.0   **Epidermal cyst**
  ✓5ᵗʰ **L72.1**   **Pilar and trichodermal cyst**
      L72.11   **Pilar cyst**
      L72.12   **Trichodermal cyst**
          Trichilemmal (proliferating) cyst
  L72.2   **Steatocystoma multiplex**
  L72.3   **Sebaceous cyst**
      EXCLUDES 2   pilar cyst (L72.11)
          trichilemmal (proliferating) cyst (L72.12)
  L72.8   **Other follicular cysts of the skin and subcutaneous tissue**
  L72.9   **Follicular cyst of the skin and subcutaneous tissue, unspecified**

✓4ᵗʰ **L73**   **Other follicular disorders**
  L73.0   **Acne keloid**
  L73.1   **Pseudofolliculitis barbae**
  L73.2   **Hidradenitis suppurativa**
  L73.8   **Other specified follicular disorders**
      Sycosis barbae
  L73.9   **Follicular disorder, unspecified**

✓4ᵗʰ **L74**   **Eccrine sweat disorders**
  EXCLUDES 2   generalized hyperhidrosis (R61)
  L74.0   **Miliaria rubra**
  L74.1   **Miliaria crystallina**
  L74.2   **Miliaria profunda**
      Miliaria tropicalis
  L74.3   **Miliaria, unspecified**
  L74.4   **Anhidrosis**
      Hypohidrosis
  ✓5ᵗʰ **L74.5**   **Focal hyperhidrosis**
      ✓6ᵗʰ **L74.51**   **Primary focal hyperhidrosis**
          L74.510   **Primary focal hyperhidrosis, axilla**
          L74.511   **Primary focal hyperhidrosis, face**
          L74.512   **Primary focal hyperhidrosis, palms**
          L74.513   **Primary focal hyperhidrosis, soles**
          L74.519   **Primary focal hyperhidrosis, unspecified**
      L74.52   **Secondary focal hyperhidrosis**
          Frey's syndrome
  L74.8   **Other eccrine sweat disorders**
  L74.9   **Eccrine sweat disorder, unspecified**
      Sweat gland disorder NOS

✓4ᵗʰ **L75**   **Apocrine sweat disorders**
  EXCLUDES 1   dyshidrosis (L30.1)
      hidradenitis suppurativa (L73.2)
  L75.0   **Bromhidrosis**
  L75.1   **Chromhidrosis**
  L75.2   **Apocrine miliaria**
      Fox-Fordyce disease
  L75.8   **Other apocrine sweat disorders**
  L75.9   **Apocrine sweat disorder, unspecified**

Intraoperative and postprocedural complications of skin and subcutaneous tissue (L76)

✓4ᵗʰ **L76**   **Intraoperative and postprocedural complications of skin and subcutaneous tissue**

> **CC Excl: For CC codes in category L76, unless otherwise noted:**
> H95.811-H95.89, I85.01, I85.11, I97.3, K21.9, K22.8, K23-K25.0, K25.2, K25.4, K25.6, K26.0, K26.2, K26.4, K26.6, K27.0, K27.2, K27.4, K27.6, K28.0, K28.2, K28.4, K28.6, K29.01, K29.21, K29.31, K29.41, K29.51, K29.61, K29.71, K29.81, K29.91, K31.811, K55.21, K57.01, K57.11, K57.13, K57.21, K57.31, K57.33, K57.41, K57.51, K57.53, K57.81, K57.91, K57.93, K62.5, K92.0-K92.2, L76.01-L76.02, L76.21-L76.82, M96.89, N98.1-N98.9, P54.1-P54.3, T81.10XA, T81.11XA, T81.12XA, T81.19XA, T81.82XA, T81.89XA, T81.9XXA

✓ Additional Character Required   ✓x7ᵗʰ Xtension Alert   Unacceptable PDx   Manifestation   Hospital Acquired Condition   EXCLUDES 1 Not Coded Here   EXCLUDES 2 Not Included Here

ICD-10-CM Draft (2015)   667

Diseases of the Skin and Subcutaneous Tissue

L76.0–L89.003

√5ᵗʰ **L76.0** **Intraoperative hemorrhage and hematoma** of skin and subcutaneous tissue complicating a procedure

     EXCLUDES 1 *intraoperative hemorrhage and hematoma of skin and subcutaneous tissue due to accidental puncture and laceration during a procedure (L76.1-)*

     L76.01 **Intraoperative hemorrhage and hematoma of**   CC **skin and subcutaneous tissue complicating a dermatologic procedure**

     L76.02 **Intraoperative hemorrhage and hematoma of**   CC **skin and subcutaneous tissue complicating** other **procedure**

√5ᵗʰ **L76.1** **Accidental puncture and laceration** of skin and subcutaneous tissue during a procedure

     L76.11 **Accidental puncture and laceration of skin and**   CC **subcutaneous tissue during a** dermatologic **procedure**

        CC Excl: D78.11-D78.12, D78.81-D78.89, E36.11-E36.8, E89.810-E89.89, G96.11, G97.41, G97.48-G97.49, H59.011-H59.019, H59.031-H59.099, H59.211-H59.229, H59.811-H59.89, H95.31-H95.32, H95.811-H95.89, I97.3, I97.51-I97.52, J95.71-J95.72, K91.71-K91.72, L76.11-L76.12, L76.81-L76.82, M96.820-M96.821, M96.89, N98.1-N98.9, N99.71-N99.72, T81.82XA, T81.89XA, T81.9XXA

     L76.12 **Accidental puncture and laceration of skin and**   CC **subcutaneous tissue during** other procedure

        CC Excl: See code: D76.11

√5ᵗʰ **L76.2** **Postprocedural hemorrhage and hematoma** of skin and subcutaneous tissue following a procedure

     L76.21 **Postprocedural hemorrhage and hematoma of**   CC **skin and subcutaneous tissue following a dermatologic procedure**

     L76.22 **Postprocedural hemorrhage and hematoma of**   CC **skin and subcutaneous tissue following** other **procedure**

√5ᵗʰ **L76.8** **Other** intraoperative and postprocedural complications of skin and subcutaneous tissue

     Use additional code, if applicable, to further specify disorder

     L76.81 **Other** intraoperative **complications of skin and subcutaneous tissue**

     L76.82 **Other** postprocedural **complications of skin and subcutaneous tissue**

Other disorders of the skin and subcutaneous tissue (L80-L99)

L80 **Vitiligo**

     EXCLUDES 2 *vitiligo of eyelids (H02.73-)*
                   vitiligo of vulva (N90.89)

√4ᵗʰ **L81** **Other disorders of pigmentation**

     EXCLUDES 1 *birthmark NOS (Q82.5)*
                   Peutz-Jeghers syndrome (Q85.8)

     EXCLUDES 2 *nevus—see Alphabetical Index*

     L81.0 **Postinflammatory hyperpigmentation**

     L81.1 **Chloasma**

     L81.2 **Freckles**

     L81.3 **Café au lait spots**

     L81.4 **Other melanin hyperpigmentation**
           Lentigo

     L81.5 **Leukoderma, not elsewhere classified**

     L81.6 **Other disorders of diminished melanin formation**

     L81.7 **Pigmented purpuric dermatosis**
           Angioma serpiginosum

     L81.8 **Other specified disorders of pigmentation**
           Iron pigmentation   Tattoo pigmentation

     L81.9 **Disorder of pigmentation, unspecified**

√4ᵗʰ **L82** **Seborrheic keratosis**

     INCLUDES dermatosis papulosa nigra
                 Leser-Trélat disease

     EXCLUDES 2 *seborrheic dermatitis (L21.-)*

     L82.0 Inflamed **seborrheic keratosis**

     L82.1 Other **seborrheic keratosis**
           Seborrheic keratosis NOS

L83 **Acanthosis nigricans**
     Confluent and reticulated papillomatosis

L84 **Corns and callosities**
     Callus   Clavus

√4ᵗʰ **L85** **Other epidermal thickening**

     EXCLUDES 2 *hypertrophic disorders of the skin (L91.-)*

     L85.0 **Acquired ichthyosis**
        EXCLUDES 1 *congenital ichthyosis (Q80.-)*

     L85.1 **Acquired keratosis [keratoderma] palmaris et plantaris**
        EXCLUDES 1 *inherited keratosis palmaris et plantaris (Q82.8)*

     L85.2 **Keratosis punctata (palmaris et plantaris)**

     L85.3 **Xerosis cutis**
        Dry skin dermatitis

     L85.8 **Other specified epidermal thickening**
        Cutaneous horn

     L85.9 **Epidermal thickening, unspecified**

L86 ***Keratoderma in diseases classified elsewhere***
     Code first underlying disease, such as:
     Reiter's disease (M02.3-)

     EXCLUDES 1 *gonococcal keratoderma (A54.89)*
                 gonococcal keratosis (A54.89)
                 keratoderma due to vitamin A deficiency (E50.8)
                 keratosis due to vitamin A deficiency (E50.8)
                 xeroderma due to vitamin A deficiency (E50.8)

√4ᵗʰ **L87** **Transepidermal elimination disorders**

     EXCLUDES 1 *granuloma annulare (perforating) (L92.0)*

     L87.0 **Keratosis follicularis et parafollicularis in cutem penetrans**
        Hyperkeratosis follicularis penetrans
        Kyrle disease

     L87.1 **Reactive perforating collagenosis**

     L87.2 **Elastosis perforans serpiginosa**

     L87.8 **Other transepidermal elimination disorders**

     L87.9 **Transepidermal elimination disorder, unspecified**

L88 **Pyoderma gangrenosum**   CC
     Phagedenic pyoderma
     EXCLUDES 1 *dermatitis gangrenosa (L08.0)*
     CC Excl: L08.0, L08.81, L88

√4ᵗʰ **L89** **Pressure ulcer**
     Bed sore   Pressure area
     Decubitus ulcer   Pressure sore
     Plaster ulcer
     Code first any associated gangrene (I96)

     EXCLUDES 2 *decubitus (trophic) ulcer of cervix (uteri) (N86)*
                 diabetic ulcers (E08.621, E08.622, E09.621, E09.622, E10.621,
                    E10.622, E11.621, E11.622, E13.621, E13.622)
                 non-pressure chronic ulcer of skin (L97.-)
                 skin infections (L00-L08)
                 varicose ulcer (I83.0, I83.2)

     CC Excl: For MCC codes in category L89, unless otherwise noted:
     L89.000-L89.95, L97.101-L97.929, L98.411-L98.499

√5ᵗʰ **L89.0** **Pressure ulcer of** elbow

     √6ᵗʰ **L89.00** **Pressure ulcer of** unspecified elbow

        L89.000 **Pressure ulcer of unspecified elbow, unstageable**

        L89.001 **Pressure ulcer of unspecified elbow, stage 1**
            Healing pressure ulcer of unspecified elbow, stage 1
            Pressure pre-ulcer skin changes limited to persistent focal edema, unspecified elbow

        L89.002 **Pressure ulcer of unspecified elbow, stage 2**
            Healing pressure ulcer of unspecified elbow, stage 2
            Pressure ulcer with abrasion, blister, partial thickness skin loss involving epidermis and/or dermis, unspecified elbow

        L89.003 **Pressure ulcer of unspecified elbow, stage 3**   PDx MCC   MCC
            Healing pressure ulcer of unspecified elbow, stage 3
            Pressure ulcer with full thickness skin loss involving damage or necrosis of subcutaneous tissue, unspecified elbow

---

L89.004 **Pressure ulcer of unspecified elbow, stage 4** `PDx MCC` `MCC`
Healing pressure ulcer of unspecified elbow, stage 4
Pressure ulcer with necrosis of soft tissues through to underlying muscle, tendon, or bone, unspecified elbow

L89.009 **Pressure ulcer of unspecified elbow, unspecified stage**
Healing pressure ulcer of elbow NOS
Healing pressure ulcer of unspecified elbow, unspecified stage

✓6th **L89.01** **Pressure ulcer of right elbow**

L89.010 **Pressure ulcer of right elbow, unstageable**

L89.011 **Pressure ulcer of right elbow, stage 1**
Healing pressure ulcer of right elbow, stage 1
Pressure pre-ulcer skin changes limited to persistent focal edema, right elbow

L89.012 **Pressure ulcer of right elbow, stage 2**
Healing pressure ulcer of right elbow, stage 2
Pressure ulcer with abrasion, blister, partial thickness skin loss involving epidermis and/or dermis, right elbow

L89.013 **Pressure ulcer of right elbow, stage 3** `PDx MCC` `MCC`
Healing pressure ulcer of right elbow, stage 3
Pressure ulcer with full thickness skin loss involving damage or necrosis of subcutaneous tissue, right elbow

L89.014 **Pressure ulcer of right elbow, stage 4** `PDx MCC` `MCC`
Healing pressure ulcer of right elbow, stage 4
Pressure ulcer with necrosis of soft tissues through to underlying muscle, tendon, or bone, right elbow

L89.019 **Pressure ulcer of right elbow, unspecified stage**
Healing pressure right of elbow NOS
Healing pressure ulcer of unspecified elbow, unspecified stage

✓6th **L89.02** **Pressure ulcer of left elbow**

L89.020 **Pressure ulcer of left elbow, unstageable**

L89.021 **Pressure ulcer of left elbow, stage 1**
Healing pressure ulcer of left elbow, stage 1
Pressure pre-ulcer skin changes limited to persistent focal edema, left elbow

L89.022 **Pressure ulcer of left elbow, stage 2**
Healing pressure ulcer of left elbow, stage 2
Pressure ulcer with abrasion, blister, partial thickness skin loss involving epidermis and/or dermis, left elbow

L89.023 **Pressure ulcer of left elbow, stage 3** `PDx MCC` `MCC`
Healing pressure ulcer of left elbow, stage 3
Pressure ulcer with full thickness skin loss involving damage or necrosis of subcutaneous tissue, left elbow

L89.024 **Pressure ulcer of left elbow, stage 4** `PDx MCC` `MCC`
Healing pressure ulcer of left elbow, stage 4
Pressure ulcer with necrosis of soft tissues through to underlying muscle, tendon, or bone, left elbow

L89.029 **Pressure ulcer of left elbow, unspecified stage**
Healing pressure ulcer of left of elbow NOS
Healing pressure ulcer of unspecified elbow, unspecified stage

✓5th **L89.1** **Pressure ulcer of back**

✓6th **L89.10** **Pressure ulcer of unspecified part of back**

L89.100 **Pressure ulcer of unspecified part of back, unstageable**

L89.101 **Pressure ulcer of unspecified part of back, stage 1**
Healing pressure ulcer of unspecified part of back, stage 1
Pressure pre-ulcer skin changes limited to persistent focal edema, unspecified part of back

L89.102 **Pressure ulcer of unspecified part of back, stage 2**
Healing pressure ulcer of unspecified part of back, stage 2
Pressure ulcer with abrasion, blister, partial thickness skin loss involving epidermis and/or dermis, unspecified part of back

L89.103 **Pressure ulcer of unspecified part of back, stage 3** `PDx MCC` `MCC`
Healing pressure ulcer of unspecified part of back, stage 3
Pressure ulcer with full thickness skin loss involving damage or necrosis of subcutaneous tissue, unspecified part of back

L89.104 **Pressure ulcer of unspecified part of back, stage 4** `PDx MCC` `MCC`
Healing pressure ulcer of unspecified part of back, stage 4
Pressure ulcer with necrosis of soft tissues through to underlying muscle, tendon, or bone, unspecified part of back

L89.109 **Pressure ulcer of unspecified part of back, unspecified stage**
Healing pressure ulcer of unspecified part of back NOS
Healing pressure ulcer of unspecified part of back, unspecified stage

✓6th **L89.11** **Pressure ulcer of right upper back**
Pressure ulcer of right shoulder blade

L89.110 **Pressure ulcer of right upper back, unstageable**

L89.111 **Pressure ulcer of right upper back, stage 1**
Healing pressure ulcer of right upper back, stage 1
Pressure pre-ulcer skin changes limited to persistent focal edema, right upper back

L89.112 **Pressure ulcer of right upper back, stage 2**
Healing pressure ulcer of right upper back, stage 2
Pressure ulcer with abrasion, blister, partial thickness skin loss involving epidermis and/or dermis, right upper back

L89.113 **Pressure ulcer of right upper back, stage 3** `PDx MCC` `MCC`
Healing pressure ulcer of right upper back, stage 3
Pressure ulcer with full thickness skin loss involving damage or necrosis of subcutaneous tissue, right upper back

L89.114 **Pressure ulcer of right upper back, stage 4** `PDx MCC` `MCC`
Healing pressure ulcer of right upper back, stage 4
Pressure ulcer with necrosis of soft tissues through to underlying muscle, tendon, or bone, right upper back

L89.119 **Pressure ulcer of right upper back, unspecified stage**
Healing pressure ulcer of right upper back NOS
Healing pressure ulcer of right upper back, unspecified stage

✓6th **L89.12** **Pressure ulcer of left upper back**
Pressure ulcer of left shoulder blade

L89.120 **Pressure ulcer of left upper back, unstageable**

L89.121 **Pressure ulcer of left upper back, stage 1**
Healing pressure ulcer of left upper back, stage 1
Pressure pre-ulcer skin changes limited to persistent focal edema, left upper back

L89.122 **Pressure ulcer of left upper back, stage 2**
Healing pressure ulcer of left upper back, stage 2
Pressure ulcer with abrasion, blister, partial thickness skin loss involving epidermis and/or dermis, left upper back

---

✓ Additional Character Required   ✓7th Xtension Alert   Unacceptable PDx   Manifestation   Hospital Acquired Condition   EXCLUDES1 Not Coded Here   EXCLUDES2 Not Included Here

Diseases of the Skin and Subcutaneous Tissue

L89.123–L89.210

L89.123 **Pressure ulcer of left upper back, stage 3** `PDx MCC` `MCC`
  Healing pressure ulcer of left upper back, stage 3
  Pressure ulcer with full thickness skin loss involving damage or necrosis of subcutaneous tissue, left upper back

L89.124 **Pressure ulcer of left upper back, stage 4** `PDx MCC` `MCC`
  Healing pressure ulcer of left upper back, stage 4
  Pressure ulcer with necrosis of soft tissues through to underlying muscle, tendon, or bone, left upper back

L89.129 **Pressure ulcer of left upper back, unspecified stage**
  Healing pressure ulcer of left upper back NOS
  Healing pressure ulcer of left upper back, unspecified stage

√6th **L89.13** **Pressure ulcer of right lower back**

L89.130 **Pressure ulcer of right lower back, unstageable**

L89.131 **Pressure ulcer of right lower back, stage 1**
  Healing pressure ulcer of right lower back, stage 1
  Pressure pre-ulcer skin changes limited to persistent focal edema, right lower back

L89.132 **Pressure ulcer of right lower back, stage 2**
  Healing pressure ulcer of right lower back, stage 2
  Pressure ulcer with abrasion, blister, partial thickness skin loss involving epidermis and/or dermis, right lower back

L89.133 **Pressure ulcer of right lower back, stage 3** `PDx MCC` `MCC`
  Healing pressure ulcer of right lower back, stage 3
  Pressure ulcer with full thickness skin loss involving damage or necrosis of subcutaneous tissue, right lower back

L89.134 **Pressure ulcer of right lower back, stage 4** `PDx MCC` `MCC`
  Healing pressure ulcer of right lower back, stage 4
  Pressure ulcer with necrosis of soft tissues through to underlying muscle, tendon, or bone, right lower back

L89.139 **Pressure ulcer of right lower back, unspecified stage**
  Healing pressure ulcer of right lower back NOS
  Healing pressure ulcer of right lower back, unspecified stage

√6th **L89.14** **Pressure ulcer of left lower back**

L89.140 **Pressure ulcer of left lower back, unstageable**

L89.141 **Pressure ulcer of left lower back, stage 1**
  Healing pressure ulcer of left lower back, stage 1
  Pressure pre-ulcer skin changes limited to persistent focal edema, left lower back

L89.142 **Pressure ulcer of left lower back, stage 2**
  Healing pressure ulcer of left lower back, stage 2
  Pressure ulcer with abrasion, blister, partial thickness skin loss involving epidermis and/or dermis, left lower back

L89.143 **Pressure ulcer of left lower back, stage 3** `PDx MCC` `MCC`
  Healing pressure ulcer of left lower back, stage 3
  Pressure ulcer with full thickness skin loss involving damage or necrosis of subcutaneous tissue, left lower back

L89.144 **Pressure ulcer of left lower back, stage 4** `PDx MCC` `MCC`
  Healing pressure ulcer of left lower back, stage 4
  Pressure ulcer with necrosis of soft tissues through to underlying muscle, tendon, or bone, left lower back

L89.149 **Pressure ulcer of left lower back, unspecified stage**
  Healing pressure ulcer of left lower back NOS
  Healing pressure ulcer of left lower back, unspecified stage

√6th **L89.15** **Pressure ulcer of sacral region**
  Pressure ulcer of coccyx
  Pressure ulcer of tailbone

L89.150 **Pressure ulcer of sacral region, unstageable**

L89.151 **Pressure ulcer of sacral region, stage 1**
  Healing pressure ulcer of sacral region, stage 1
  Pressure pre-ulcer skin changes limited to persistent focal edema, sacral region

L89.152 **Pressure ulcer of sacral region, stage 2**
  Healing pressure ulcer of sacral region, stage 2
  Pressure ulcer with abrasion, blister, partial thickness skin loss involving epidermis and/or dermis, sacral region

L89.153 **Pressure ulcer of sacral region, stage 3** `PDx MCC` `MCC`
  Healing pressure ulcer of sacral region, stage 3
  Pressure ulcer with full thickness skin loss involving damage or necrosis of subcutaneous tissue, sacral region

L89.154 **Pressure ulcer of sacral region, stage 4** `PDx MCC` `MCC`
  Healing pressure ulcer of sacral region, stage 4
  Pressure ulcer with necrosis of soft tissues through to underlying muscle, tendon, or bone, sacral region

L89.159 **Pressure ulcer of sacral region, unspecified stage**
  Healing pressure ulcer of sacral region NOS
  Healing pressure ulcer of sacral region, unspecified stage

√5th **L89.2** **Pressure ulcer of hip**

√6th **L89.20** **Pressure ulcer of unspecified hip**

L89.200 **Pressure ulcer of unspecified hip, unstageable**

L89.201 **Pressure ulcer of unspecified hip, stage 1**
  Healing pressure ulcer of unspecified hip back, stage 1
  Pressure pre-ulcer skin changes limited to persistent focal edema, unspecified hip

L89.202 **Pressure ulcer of unspecified hip, stage 2**
  Healing pressure ulcer of unspecified hip, stage 2
  Pressure ulcer with abrasion, blister, partial thickness skin loss involving epidermis and/or dermis, unspecified hip

L89.203 **Pressure ulcer of unspecified hip, stage 3** `PDx MCC` `MCC`
  Healing pressure ulcer of unspecified hip, stage 3
  Pressure ulcer with full thickness skin loss involving damage or necrosis of subcutaneous tissue, unspecified hip

L89.204 **Pressure ulcer of unspecified hip, stage 4** `PDx MCC` `MCC`
  Healing pressure ulcer of unspecified hip, stage 4
  Pressure ulcer with necrosis of soft tissues through to underlying muscle, tendon, or bone, unspecified hip

L89.209 **Pressure ulcer of unspecified hip, unspecified stage**
  Healing pressure ulcer of unspecified hip NOS
  Healing pressure ulcer of unspecified hip, unspecified stage

√6th **L89.21** **Pressure ulcer of right hip**

L89.210 **Pressure ulcer of right hip, unstageable**

N Newborn: 0   P Pediatric: 0-17   M Maternity: 12-55   A Adult: 15-124   MCC Major CC Condition   PDx MCC PDx acts as own MCC   CC CC Condition   PDx CC PDx acts as own CC

670   ICD-10-CM Draft (2015)

L89.211 Pressure ulcer of right hip, stage 1
  Healing pressure ulcer of right hip back,
    stage 1
  Pressure pre-ulcer skin changes limited to
    persistent focal edema, right hip

L89.212 Pressure ulcer of right hip, stage 2
  Healing pressure ulcer of right hip, stage 2
  Pressure ulcer with abrasion, blister, partial
    thickness skin loss involving epidermis
    and/or dermis, right hip

L89.213 Pressure ulcer of right hip, `PDx MCC` `MCC`
stage 3
  Healing pressure ulcer of right hip, stage 3
  Pressure ulcer with full thickness skin loss
    involving damage or necrosis of
    subcutaneous tissue, right hip

L89.214 Pressure ulcer of right hip, `PDx MCC` `MCC`
stage 4
  Healing pressure ulcer of right hip, stage 4
  Pressure ulcer with necrosis of soft tissues
    through to underlying muscle,
    tendon, or bone, right hip

L89.219 Pressure ulcer of right hip, unspecified
stage
  Healing pressure ulcer of right hip NOS
  Healing pressure ulcer of right hip,
    unspecified stage

✓6th **L89.22 Pressure ulcer of** left hip
L89.220 Pressure ulcer of left hip, unstageable
L89.221 Pressure ulcer of left hip, stage 1
  Healing pressure ulcer of left hip back,
    stage 1
  Pressure pre-ulcer skin changes limited to
    persistent focal edema, left hip

L89.222 Pressure ulcer of left hip, stage 2
  Healing pressure ulcer of left hip, stage 2
  Pressure ulcer with abrasion, blister, partial
    thickness skin loss involving epidermis
    and/or dermis, left hip

L89.223 Pressure ulcer of left hip, `PDx MCC` `MCC`
stage 3
  Healing pressure ulcer of left hip, stage 3
  Pressure ulcer with full thickness skin loss
    involving damage or necrosis of
    subcutaneous tissue, left hip

L89.224 Pressure ulcer of left hip, `PDx MCC` `MCC`
stage 4
  Healing pressure ulcer of left hip, stage 4
  Pressure ulcer with necrosis of soft tissues
    through to underlying muscle,
    tendon, or bone, left hip

L89.229 Pressure ulcer of left hip, unspecified
stage
  Healing pressure ulcer of left hip NOS
  Healing pressure ulcer of left hip,
    unspecified stage

✓5th **L89.3 Pressure ulcer of** buttock
✓6th **L89.30 Pressure ulcer of** unspecified buttock
L89.300 Pressure ulcer of unspecified buttock,
unstageable
L89.301 Pressure ulcer of unspecified buttock,
stage 1
  Healing pressure ulcer of unspecified
    buttock, stage 1
  Pressure pre-ulcer skin changes limited to
    persistent focal edema, unspecified
    buttock

L89.302 Pressure ulcer of unspecified buttock,
stage 2
  Healing pressure ulcer of unspecified
    buttock, stage 2
  Pressure ulcer with abrasion, blister, partial
    thickness skin loss involving epidermis
    and/or dermis, unspecified buttock

L89.303 Pressure ulcer of unspecified `PDx MCC` `MCC`
buttock, stage 3
  Healing pressure ulcer of unspecified
    buttock, stage 3
  Pressure ulcer with full thickness skin loss
    involving damage or necrosis of
    subcutaneous tissue, unspecified
    buttock

L89.304 Pressure ulcer of unspecified `PDx MCC` `MCC`
buttock, stage 4
  Healing pressure ulcer of unspecified
    buttock, stage 4
  Pressure ulcer with necrosis of soft tissues
    through to underlying muscle,
    tendon, or bone, unspecified buttock

L89.309 Pressure ulcer of unspecified buttock,
unspecified stage
  Healing pressure ulcer of unspecified
    buttock NOS
  Healing pressure ulcer of unspecified
    buttock, unspecified stage

✓6th **L89.31 Pressure ulcer of** right buttock
L89.310 Pressure ulcer of right buttock,
unstageable
L89.311 Pressure ulcer of right buttock, stage 1
  Healing pressure ulcer of right buttock,
    stage 1
  Pressure pre-ulcer skin changes limited to
    persistent focal edema, right buttock

L89.312 Pressure ulcer of right buttock, stage 2
  Healing pressure ulcer of right buttock,
    stage 2
  Pressure ulcer with abrasion, blister, partial
    thickness skin loss involving epidermis
    and/or dermis, right buttock

L89.313 Pressure ulcer of right buttock, `PDx MCC` `MCC`
stage 3
  Healing pressure ulcer of right buttock,
    stage 3
  Pressure ulcer with full thickness skin loss
    involving damage or necrosis of
    subcutaneous tissue, right buttock

L89.314 Pressure ulcer of right buttock, `PDx MCC` `MCC`
stage 4
  Healing pressure ulcer of right buttock,
    stage 4
  Pressure ulcer with necrosis of soft tissues
    through to underlying muscle,
    tendon, or bone, right buttock

L89.319 Pressure ulcer of right buttock,
unspecified stage
  Healing pressure ulcer of right buttock NOS
  Healing pressure ulcer of right buttock,
    unspecified stage

✓6th **L89.32 Pressure ulcer of** left buttock
L89.320 Pressure ulcer of left buttock, unstageable
L89.321 Pressure ulcer of left buttock, stage 1
  Healing pressure ulcer of left buttock,
    stage 1
  Pressure pre-ulcer skin changes limited to
    persistent focal edema, left buttock

L89.322 Pressure ulcer of left buttock, stage 2
  Healing pressure ulcer of left buttock,
    stage 2
  Pressure ulcer with abrasion, blister, partial
    thickness skin loss involving epidermis
    and/or dermis, left buttock

L89.323 Pressure ulcer of left buttock, `PDx MCC` `MCC`
stage 3
  Healing pressure ulcer of left buttock,
    stage 3
  Pressure ulcer with full thickness skin loss
    involving damage or necrosis of
    subcutaneous tissue, left buttock

L89.324 Pressure ulcer of left buttock, `PDx MCC` `MCC`
stage 4
  Healing pressure ulcer of left buttock,
    stage 4
  Pressure ulcer with necrosis of soft tissues
    through to underlying muscle,
    tendon, or bone, left buttock

L89.329 Pressure ulcer of left buttock, unspecified
stage
  Healing pressure ulcer of left buttock NOS
  Healing pressure ulcer of left buttock,
    unspecified stage

Diseases of the Skin and Subcutaneous Tissue

L89.4–L89.604

✓5th **L89.4** **Pressure ulcer of contiguous site of** back, buttock and hip

  L89.40 **Pressure ulcer of contiguous site of back, buttock and hip,** unspecified stage
    Healing pressure ulcer of contiguous site of back, buttock and hip NOS
    Healing pressure ulcer of contiguous site of back, buttock and hip, unspecified stage

  L89.41 **Pressure ulcer of contiguous site of back, buttock and hip,** stage 1
    Healing pressure ulcer of contiguous site of back, buttock and hip, stage 1
    Pressure pre-ulcer skin changes limited to persistent focal edema, contiguous site of back, buttock and hip

  L89.42 **Pressure ulcer of contiguous site of back, buttock and hip,** stage 2
    Healing pressure ulcer of contiguous site of back, buttock and hip, stage 2
    Pressure ulcer with abrasion, blister, partial thickness skin loss involving epidermis and/or dermis, contiguous site of back, buttock and hip

  L89.43 **Pressure ulcer of contiguous site of back, buttock and hip,** stage 3 PDx MCC | MCC
    Healing pressure ulcer of contiguous site of back, buttock and hip, stage 3
    Pressure ulcer with full thickness skin loss involving damage or necrosis of subcutaneous tissue, contiguous site of back, buttock and hip

  L89.44 **Pressure ulcer of contiguous site of back,** PDx MCC | MCC **buttock and hip,** stage 4
    Healing pressure ulcer of contiguous site of back, buttock and hip, stage 4
    Pressure ulcer with necrosis of soft tissues through to underlying muscle, tendon, or bone, contiguous site of back, buttock and hip

  L89.45 **Pressure ulcer of contiguous site of back, buttock and hip,** unstageable

✓5th **L89.5** **Pressure ulcer of** ankle

  ✓6th **L89.50** **Pressure ulcer of** unspecified ankle

    L89.500 **Pressure ulcer of unspecified ankle,** unstageable

    L89.501 **Pressure ulcer of unspecified ankle,** stage 1
      Healing pressure ulcer of unspecified ankle, stage 1
      Pressure pre-ulcer skin changes limited to persistent focal edema, unspecified ankle

    L89.502 **Pressure ulcer of unspecified ankle,** stage 2
      Healing pressure ulcer of unspecified ankle, stage 2
      Pressure ulcer with abrasion, blister, partial thickness skin loss involving epidermis and/or dermis, unspecified ankle

    L89.503 **Pressure ulcer of unspecified ankle,** stage 3 PDx MCC | MCC
      Healing pressure ulcer of unspecified ankle, stage 3
      Pressure ulcer with full thickness skin loss involving damage or necrosis of subcutaneous tissue, unspecified ankle

    L89.504 **Pressure ulcer of unspecified ankle,** stage 4 PDx MCC | MCC
      Healing pressure ulcer of unspecified ankle, stage 4
      Pressure ulcer with necrosis of soft tissues through to underlying muscle, tendon, or bone, unspecified ankle

    L89.509 **Pressure ulcer of unspecified ankle,** unspecified stage
      Healing pressure ulcer of unspecified ankle NOS
      Healing pressure ulcer of unspecified ankle, unspecified stage

  ✓6th **L89.51** **Pressure ulcer of** right ankle

    L89.510 **Pressure ulcer of right ankle,** unstageable

    L89.511 **Pressure ulcer of right ankle,** stage 1
      Healing pressure ulcer of right ankle, stage 1
      Pressure pre-ulcer skin changes limited to persistent focal edema, right ankle

    L89.512 **Pressure ulcer of right ankle,** stage 2
      Healing pressure ulcer of right ankle, stage 2
      Pressure ulcer with abrasion, blister, partial thickness skin loss involving epidermis and/or dermis, right ankle

    L89.513 **Pressure ulcer of right ankle,** PDx MCC | MCC **stage 3**
      Healing pressure ulcer of right ankle, stage 3
      Pressure ulcer with full thickness skin loss involving damage or necrosis of subcutaneous tissue, right ankle

    L89.514 **Pressure ulcer of right ankle,** PDx MCC | MCC **stage 4**
      Healing pressure ulcer of right ankle, stage 4
      Pressure ulcer with necrosis of soft tissues through to underlying muscle, tendon, or bone, right ankle

    L89.519 **Pressure ulcer of right ankle,** unspecified stage
      Healing pressure ulcer of right ankle NOS
      Healing pressure ulcer of right ankle, unspecified stage

  ✓6th **L89.52** **Pressure ulcer of** left ankle

    L89.520 **Pressure ulcer of left ankle,** unstageable

    L89.521 **Pressure ulcer of left ankle,** stage 1
      Healing pressure ulcer of left ankle, stage 1
      Pressure pre-ulcer skin changes limited to persistnt focal edema, left ankle

    L89.522 **Pressure ulcer of left ankle,** stage 2
      Healing pressure ulcer of left ankle, stage 2
      Pressure ulcer with abrasion, blister, partial thickness skin loss involving epidermis and/or dermis, left ankle

    L89.523 **Pressure ulcer of left ankle,** PDx MCC | MCC **stage 3**
      Healing pressure ulcer of left ankle, stage 3
      Pressure ulcer with full thickness skin loss involving damage or necrosis of subcutaneous tissue, left ankle

    L89.524 **Pressure ulcer of left ankle,** PDx MCC | MCC **stage 4**
      Healing pressure ulcer of left ankle, stage 4
      Pressure ulcer with necrosis of soft tissues through to underlying muscle, tendon, or bone, left ankle

    L89.529 **Pressure ulcer of left ankle,** unspecified stage
      Healing pressure ulcer of left ankle NOS
      Healing pressure ulcer of left ankle, unspecified stage

✓5th **L89.6** **Pressure ulcer of** heel

  ✓6th **L89.60** **Pressure ulcer of** unspecified heel

    L89.600 **Pressure ulcer of unspecified heel,** unstageable

    L89.601 **Pressure ulcer of unspecified heel,** stage 1
      Healing pressure ulcer of unspecified heel, stage 1
      Pressure pre-ulcer skin changes limited to persistent focal edema, unspecified heel

    L89.602 **Pressure ulcer of unspecified heel,** stage 2
      Healing pressure ulcer of unspecified heel, stage 2
      Pressure ulcer with abrasion, blister, partial thickness skin loss involving epidermis and/or dermis, unspecified heel

    L89.603 **Pressure ulcer of unspecified** PDx MCC | MCC **heel,** stage 3
      Healing pressure ulcer of unspecified heel, stage 3
      Pressure ulcer with full thickness skin loss involving damage or necrosis of subcutaneous tissue, unspecified heel

    L89.604 **Pressure ulcer of unspecified** PDx MCC | MCC **heel,** stage 4
      Healing pressure ulcer of unspecified heel, stage 4
      Pressure ulcer with necrosis of soft tissues through to underlying muscle, tendon, or bone, unspecified heel

N Newborn: 0   P Pediatric: 0-17   M Maternity: 12-55   A Adult: 15-124   MCC Major CC Condition   PDx MCC PDx acts as own MCC   CC CC Condition   PDx CC PDx acts as own CC

672   ICD-10-CM Draft (2015)

L89.609 Pressure ulcer of unspecified heel, unspecified stage
　Healing pressure ulcer of unspecified heel NOS
　Healing pressure ulcer of unspecified heel, unspecified stage

✓6th **L89.61** Pressure ulcer of right heel
　L89.610 Pressure ulcer of right heel, unstageable
　L89.611 Pressure ulcer of right heel, stage 1
　　Healing pressure ulcer of right heel, stage 1
　　Pressure pre-ulcer skin changes limited to persistent focal edema, right heel
　L89.612 Pressure ulcer of right heel, stage 2
　　Healing pressure ulcer of right heel, stage 2
　　Pressure ulcer with abrasion, blister, partial thickness skin loss involving epidermis and/or dermis, right heel
　L89.613 Pressure ulcer of right heel, stage 3 `PDx MCC` `MCC`
　　Healing pressure ulcer of right heel, stage 3
　　Pressure ulcer with full thickness skin loss involving damage or necrosis of subcutaneous tissue, right heel
　L89.614 Pressure ulcer of right heel, stage 4 `PDx MCC` `MCC`
　　Healing pressure ulcer of right heel, stage 4
　　Pressure ulcer with necrosis of soft tissues through to underlying muscle, tendon, or bone, right heel
　L89.619 Pressure ulcer of right heel, unspecified stage
　　Healing pressure ulcer of right heel NOS
　　Healing pressure ulcer of unspecified heel, right stage

✓6th **L89.62** Pressure ulcer of left heel
　L89.620 Pressure ulcer of left heel, unstageable
　L89.621 Pressure ulcer of left heel, stage 1
　　Healing pressure ulcer of left heel, stage 1
　　Pressure pre-ulcer skin changes limited to persistent focal edema, left heel
　L89.622 Pressure ulcer of left heel, stage 2
　　Healing pressure ulcer of left heel, stage 2
　　Pressure ulcer with abrasion, blister, partial thickness skin loss involving epidermis and/or dermis, left heel
　L89.623 Pressure ulcer of left heel, stage 3 `PDx MCC` `MCC`
　　Healing pressure ulcer of left heel, stage 3
　　Pressure ulcer with full thickness skin loss involving damage or necrosis of subcutaneous tissue, left heel
　L89.624 Pressure ulcer of left heel, stage 4 `PDx MCC` `MCC`
　　Healing pressure ulcer of left heel, stage 4
　　Pressure ulcer with necrosis of soft tissues through to underlying muscle, tendon, or bone, left heel
　L89.629 Pressure ulcer of left heel, unspecified stage
　　Healing pressure ulcer of left heel NOS
　　Healing pressure ulcer of left heel, unspecified stage

✓5th **L89.8** Pressure ulcer of other site
　✓6th **L89.81** Pressure ulcer of head
　　Pressure ulcer of face
　　L89.810 Pressure ulcer of head, unstageable
　　L89.811 Pressure ulcer of head, stage 1
　　　Healing pressure ulcer of head, stage 1
　　　Pressure pre-ulcer skin changes limited to persistent focal edema, head
　　L89.812 Pressure ulcer of head, stage 2
　　　Healing pressure ulcer of head, stage 2
　　　Pressure ulcer with abrasion, blister, partial thickness skin loss involving epidermis and/or dermis, head
　　L89.813 Pressure ulcer of head, stage 3 `PDx MCC` `MCC`
　　　Healing pressure ulcer of head, stage 3
　　　Pressure ulcer with full thickness skin loss involving damage or necrosis of subcutaneous tissue, head

　　L89.814 Pressure ulcer of head, stage 4 `PDx MCC` `MCC`
　　　Healing pressure ulcer of head, stage 4
　　　Pressure ulcer with necrosis of soft tissues through to underlying muscle, tendon, or bone, head
　　L89.819 Pressure ulcer of head, unspecified stage
　　　Healing pressure ulcer of head NOS
　　　Healing pressure ulcer of head, unspecified stage

　✓6th **L89.89** Pressure ulcer of other site
　　L89.890 Pressure ulcer of other site, unstageable
　　L89.891 Pressure ulcer of other site, stage 1
　　　Healing pressure ulcer of other site, stage 1
　　　Pressure pre-ulcer skin changes limited to persistent focal edema, other site
　　L89.892 Pressure ulcer of other site, stage 2
　　　Healing pressure ulcer of other site, stage 2
　　　Pressure ulcer with abrasion, blister, partial thickness skin loss involving epidermis and/or dermis, other site
　　L89.893 Pressure ulcer of other site, stage 3 `PDx MCC` `MCC`
　　　Healing pressure ulcer of other site, stage 3
　　　Pressure ulcer with full thickness skin loss involving damage or necrosis of subcutaneous tissue, other site
　　L89.894 Pressure ulcer of other site, stage 4 `PDx MCC` `MCC`
　　　Healing pressure ulcer of other site, stage 4
　　　Pressure ulcer with necrosis of soft tissues through to underlying muscle, tendon, or bone, other site
　　L89.899 Pressure ulcer of other site, unspecified stage
　　　Healing pressure ulcer of other site NOS
　　　Healing pressure ulcer of other site, unspecified stage

✓5th **L89.9** Pressure ulcer of unspecified site
　L89.90 Pressure ulcer of unspecified site, unspecified stage
　　Healing pressure ulcer of unspecified site NOS
　　Healing pressure ulcer of unspecified site, unspecified stage
　L89.91 Pressure ulcer of unspecified site, stage 1
　　Healing pressure ulcer of unspecified site, stage 1
　　Pressure pre-ulcer skin changes limited to persistent focal edema, unspecified site
　L89.92 Pressure ulcer of unspecified site, stage 2
　　Healing pressure ulcer of unspecified site, stage 2
　　Pressure ulcer with abrasion, blister, partial thickness skin loss involving epidermis and/or dermis, unspecified site
　L89.93 Pressure ulcer of unspecified site, stage 3 `PDx MCC` `MCC`
　　Healing pressure ulcer of unspecified site, stage 3
　　Pressure ulcer with full thickness skin loss involving damage or necrosis of subcutaneous tissue, unspecified site
　L89.94 Pressure ulcer of unspecified site, stage 4 `PDx MCC` `MCC`
　　Healing pressure ulcer of unspecified site, stage 4
　　Pressure ulcer with necrosis of soft tissues through to underlying muscle, tendon, or bone, unspecified site
　L89.95 Pressure ulcer of unspecified site, unstageable

✓4th **L90** Atrophic disorders of skin
　L90.0 Lichen sclerosus et atrophicus
　　EXCLUDES 2　lichen sclerosus of external female genital organs (N90.4)
　　　　　lichen sclerosus of external male genital organs (N48.0)
　L90.1 Anetoderma of Schweninger-Buzzi
　L90.2 Anetoderma of Jadassohn-Pellizzari
　L90.3 Atrophoderma of Pasini and Pierini
　L90.4 Acrodermatitis chronica atrophicans
　L90.5 Scar conditions and fibrosis of skin
　　Adherent scar (skin)　　　　Fibrosis of skin NOS
　　Cicatrix　　　　　　　　　Scar NOS
　　Disfigurement of skin due to scar
　　EXCLUDES 2　hypertrophic scar (L91.0)
　　　　　keloid scar (L91.0)
　L90.6 Striae atrophicae
　L90.8 Other atrophic disorders of skin
　L90.9 Atrophic disorder of skin, unspecified

✓ Additional Character Required　✓x7th Xtension Alert　Unacceptable PDx　Manifestation　Hospital Acquired Condition　EXCLUDES 1 Not Coded Here　EXCLUDES 2 Not Included Here

Diseases of the Skin and Subcutaneous Tissue

L91–L97.212

✓4th **L91 Hypertrophic disorders of skin**

L91.0 Hypertrophic scar
    Keloid   Keloid scar
    EXCLUDES 2 *acne keloid (L73.0)*
                  scar NOS (L90.5)

L91.8 Other hypertrophic disorders of the skin

L91.9 Hypertrophic disorder of the skin, unspecified

✓4th **L92 Granulomatous disorders of skin and subcutaneous tissue**
    EXCLUDES 2 *actinic granuloma (L57.5)*

L92.0 Granuloma annulare
    Perforating granuloma annulare

L92.1 Necrobiosis lipoidica, not elsewhere classified
    EXCLUDES 1 *necrobiosis lipoidica associated with diabetes mellitus (E08-E13 with .620)*

L92.2 Granuloma faciale [eosinophilic granuloma of skin]

L92.3 Foreign body granuloma of the skin and subcutaneous tissue
    Use additional code to identify the type of retained foreign body (Z18.-)

L92.8 Other granulomatous disorders of the skin and subcutaneous tissue

L92.9 Granulomatous disorder of the skin and subcutaneous tissue, unspecified

✓4th **L93 Lupus erythematosus**
    Use additional code for adverse effect, if applicable, to identify drug (T36-T50 with fifth or sixth character 5)
    EXCLUDES 1 *lupus exedens (A18.4)*
                  lupus vulgaris (A18.4)
                  scleroderma (M34.-)
                  systemic lupus erythematosus (M32.-)

L93.0 Discoid lupus erythematosus
    Lupus erythematosus NOS

L93.1 Subacute cutaneous lupus erythematosus

L93.2 Other local lupus erythematosus
    Lupus erythematosus profundus
    Lupus panniculitis

✓4th **L94 Other localized connective tissue disorders**
    EXCLUDES 1 *systemic connective tissue disorders (M30-M36)*

L94.0 Localized scleroderma [morphea]
    Circumscribed scleroderma

L94.1 Linear scleroderma
    En coup de sabre lesion

L94.2 Calcinosis cutis

L94.3 Sclerodactyly

L94.4 Gottron's papules

L94.5 Poikiloderma vasculare atrophicans

L94.6 Ainhum

L94.8 Other specified localized connective tissue disorders

L94.9 Localized connective tissue disorder, unspecified

✓4th **L95 Vasculitis limited to skin, not elsewhere classified**
    EXCLUDES 1 *angioma serpiginosum (L81.7)*
                  Henoch(-Schönlein) purpura (D69.0)
                  hypersensitivity angiitis (M31.0)
                  lupus panniculitis (L93.2)
                  panniculitis NOS (M79.3)
                  panniculitis of neck and back (M54.0-)
                  polyarteritis nodosa (M30.0)
                  relapsing panniculitis (M35.6)
                  rheumatoid vasculitis (M05.2)
                  serum sickness (T80.6-)
                  urticaria (L50.-)
                  Wegener's granulomatosis (M31.3-)

L95.0 Livedoid vasculitis
    Atrophie blanche (en plaque)

L95.1 Erythema elevatum diutinum

L95.8 Other vasculitis limited to the skin

L95.9 Vasculitis limited to the skin, unspecified

✓4th **L97 Non-pressure chronic ulcer of lower limb, not elsewhere classified**
    INCLUDES chronic ulcer of skin of lower limb NOS
                non-healing ulcer of skin
                non-infected sinus of skin
                trophic ulcer NOS
                tropical ulcer NOS
                ulcer of skin of lower limb NOS

    Code first any associated underlying condition, such as:
        atherosclerosis of the lower extremities (I70.23-, I70.24-, I70.33-, I70.34-, I70.43-, I70.44-, I70.53-, I70.54-, I70.63-, I70.64-, I70.73-, I70.74-)
        chronic venous hypertension (I87.31-, I87.33-)
        diabetic ulcers (E08.621, E08.622, E09.621, E09.622, E10.621, E10.622, E11.621, E11.622, E13.621, E13.622)
        postphlebitic syndrome (I87.01-, I87.03-)
        postthrombotic syndrome (I87.01-, I87.03-)
        varicose ulcer (I83.0-, I83.2-)
    Code first any associated gangrene (I96)
    EXCLUDES 2 *pressure ulcer (pressure area) (L89.-)*
                  skin infections (L00-L08)
                  specific infections classified to A00-B99

> **CC Excl:** For CC codes in category L97, unless otherwise noted: I70.231-I70.25, L44.8-L45, L94.2, L94.4, L97.101-L97.929, L98.411-L98.499, L98.8, L99

✓5th **L97.1 Non-pressure chronic ulcer of thigh**

    ✓6th **L97.10 Non-pressure chronic ulcer of unspecified thigh**

        L97.101 Non-pressure chronic ulcer of unspecified thigh limited to breakdown of skin `CC`

        L97.102 Non-pressure chronic ulcer of unspecified thigh with fat layer exposed `CC`

        L97.103 Non-pressure chronic ulcer of unspecified thigh with necrosis of muscle `CC`

        L97.104 Non-pressure chronic ulcer of unspecified thigh with necrosis of bone `CC`

        L97.109 Non-pressure chronic ulcer of unspecified thigh with unspecified severity `CC`

    ✓6th **L97.11 Non-pressure chronic ulcer of right thigh**

        L97.111 Non-pressure chronic ulcer of right thigh limited to breakdown of skin `CC`

        L97.112 Non-pressure chronic ulcer of right thigh with fat layer exposed `CC`

        L97.113 Non-pressure chronic ulcer of right thigh with necrosis of muscle `CC`

        L97.114 Non-pressure chronic ulcer of right thigh with necrosis of bone `CC`

        L97.119 Non-pressure chronic ulcer of right thigh with unspecified severity `CC`

    ✓6th **L97.12 Non-pressure chronic ulcer of left thigh**

        L97.121 Non-pressure chronic ulcer of left thigh limited to breakdown of skin `CC`

        L97.122 Non-pressure chronic ulcer of left thigh with fat layer exposed `CC`

        L97.123 Non-pressure chronic ulcer of left thigh with necrosis of muscle `CC`

        L97.124 Non-pressure chronic ulcer of left thigh with necrosis of bone `CC`

        L97.129 Non-pressure chronic ulcer of left thigh with unspecified severity `CC`

✓5th **L97.2 Non-pressure chronic ulcer of calf**

    ✓6th **L97.20 Non-pressure chronic ulcer of unspecified calf**

        L97.201 Non-pressure chronic ulcer of unspecified calf limited to breakdown of skin `CC`

        L97.202 Non-pressure chronic ulcer of unspecified calf with fat layer exposed `CC`

        L97.203 Non-pressure chronic ulcer of unspecified calf with necrosis of muscle `CC`

        L97.204 Non-pressure chronic ulcer of unspecified calf with necrosis of bone `CC`

        L97.209 Non-pressure chronic ulcer of unspecified calf with unspecified severity `CC`

    ✓6th **L97.21 Non-pressure chronic ulcer of right calf**

        L97.211 Non-pressure chronic ulcer of right calf limited to breakdown of skin `CC`

        L97.212 Non-pressure chronic ulcer of right calf with fat layer exposed `CC`

N Newborn: 0   P Pediatric: 0-17   M Maternity: 12-55   A Adult: 15-124   MCC Major CC Condition   PDx MCC PDx acts as own MCC   CC CC Condition   PDx CC PDx acts as own CC

674   ICD-10-CM Draft (2015)

L97.213 **Non-pressure chronic ulcer of right calf** with necrosis of muscle `cc`

L97.214 **Non-pressure chronic ulcer of right calf** with necrosis of bone `cc`

L97.219 **Non-pressure chronic ulcer of right calf** with unspecified severity `cc`

√6ᵗʰ **L97.22 Non-pressure chronic ulcer of left calf**

L97.221 **Non-pressure chronic ulcer of left calf** limited to breakdown of skin `cc`

L97.222 **Non-pressure chronic ulcer of left calf** with fat layer exposed `cc`

L97.223 **Non-pressure chronic ulcer of left calf** with necrosis of muscle `cc`

L97.224 **Non-pressure chronic ulcer of left calf** with necrosis of bone `cc`

L97.229 **Non-pressure chronic ulcer of left calf** with unspecified severity `cc`

√5ᵗʰ **L97.3 Non-pressure chronic ulcer of ankle**

√6ᵗʰ **L97.30 Non-pressure chronic ulcer of unspecified ankle**

L97.301 **Non-pressure chronic ulcer of unspecified ankle** limited to breakdown of skin `cc`

L97.302 **Non-pressure chronic ulcer of unspecified ankle** with fat layer exposed `cc`

L97.303 **Non-pressure chronic ulcer of unspecified ankle** with necrosis of muscle `cc`

L97.304 **Non-pressure chronic ulcer of unspecified ankle** with necrosis of bone `cc`

L97.309 **Non-pressure chronic ulcer of unspecified ankle** with unspecified severity `cc`

√6ᵗʰ **L97.31 Non-pressure chronic ulcer of right ankle**

L97.311 **Non-pressure chronic ulcer of right ankle** limited to breakdown of skin `cc`

L97.312 **Non-pressure chronic ulcer of right ankle** with fat layer exposed `cc`

L97.313 **Non-pressure chronic ulcer of right ankle** with necrosis of muscle `cc`

L97.314 **Non-pressure chronic ulcer of right ankle** with necrosis of bone `cc`

L97.319 **Non-pressure chronic ulcer of right ankle** with unspecified severity `cc`

√6ᵗʰ **L97.32 Non-pressure chronic ulcer of left ankle**

L97.321 **Non-pressure chronic ulcer of left ankle** limited to breakdown of skin `cc`

L97.322 **Non-pressure chronic ulcer of left ankle** with fat layer exposed `cc`

L97.323 **Non-pressure chronic ulcer of left ankle** with necrosis of muscle `cc`

L97.324 **Non-pressure chronic ulcer of left ankle** with necrosis of bone `cc`

L97.329 **Non-pressure chronic ulcer of left ankle** with unspecified severity `cc`

√5ᵗʰ **L97.4 Non-pressure chronic ulcer of heel and midfoot**
Non-pressure chronic ulcer of plantar surface of midfoot

√6ᵗʰ **L97.40 Non-pressure chronic ulcer of unspecified heel and midfoot**

L97.401 **Non-pressure chronic ulcer of unspecified heel and midfoot** limited to breakdown of skin `cc`

L97.402 **Non-pressure chronic ulcer of unspecified heel and midfoot** with fat layer exposed `cc`

L97.403 **Non-pressure chronic ulcer of unspecified heel and midfoot** with necrosis of muscle `cc`

L97.404 **Non-pressure chronic ulcer of unspecified heel and midfoot** with necrosis of bone `cc`

L97.409 **Non-pressure chronic ulcer of unspecified heel and midfoot** with unspecified severity `cc`

√6ᵗʰ **L97.41 Non-pressure chronic ulcer of right heel and midfoot**

L97.411 **Non-pressure chronic ulcer of right heel and midfoot** limited to breakdown of skin `cc`

L97.412 **Non-pressure chronic ulcer of right heel and midfoot** with fat layer exposed `cc`

L97.413 **Non-pressure chronic ulcer of right heel and midfoot** with necrosis of muscle `cc`

L97.414 **Non-pressure chronic ulcer of right heel and midfoot** with necrosis of bone `cc`

L97.419 **Non-pressure chronic ulcer of right heel and midfoot** with unspecified severity `cc`

√6ᵗʰ **L97.42 Non-pressure chronic ulcer of left heel and midfoot**

L97.421 **Non-pressure chronic ulcer of left heel and midfoot** limited to breakdown of skin `cc`

L97.422 **Non-pressure chronic ulcer of left heel and midfoot** with fat layer exposed `cc`

L97.423 **Non-pressure chronic ulcer of left heel and midfoot** with necrosis of muscle `cc`

L97.424 **Non-pressure chronic ulcer of left heel and midfoot** with necrosis of bone `cc`

L97.429 **Non-pressure chronic ulcer of left heel and midfoot** with unspecified severity `cc`

√5ᵗʰ **L97.5 Non-pressure chronic ulcer of other part of foot**
Non-pressure chronic ulcer of toe

√6ᵗʰ **L97.50 Non-pressure chronic ulcer of other part of unspecified foot**

L97.501 **Non-pressure chronic ulcer of other part of unspecified foot** limited to breakdown of skin

L97.502 **Non-pressure chronic ulcer of other part of unspecified foot** with fat layer exposed

L97.503 **Non-pressure chronic ulcer of other part of unspecified foot** with necrosis of muscle

L97.504 **Non-pressure chronic ulcer of other part of unspecified foot** with necrosis of bone

L97.509 **Non-pressure chronic ulcer of other part of unspecified foot** with unspecified severity

√6ᵗʰ **L97.51 Non-pressure chronic ulcer of other part of right foot**

L97.511 **Non-pressure chronic ulcer of other part of right foot** limited to breakdown of skin

L97.512 **Non-pressure chronic ulcer of other part of right foot** with fat layer exposed

L97.513 **Non-pressure chronic ulcer of other part of right foot** with necrosis of muscle

L97.514 **Non-pressure chronic ulcer of other part of right foot** with necrosis of bone

L97.519 **Non-pressure chronic ulcer of other part of right foot** with unspecified severity

√6ᵗʰ **L97.52 Non-pressure chronic ulcer of other part of left foot**

L97.521 **Non-pressure chronic ulcer of other part of left foot** limited to breakdown of skin

L97.522 **Non-pressure chronic ulcer of other part of left foot** with fat layer exposed

L97.523 **Non-pressure chronic ulcer of other part of left foot** with necrosis of muscle

L97.524 **Non-pressure chronic ulcer of other part of left foot** with necrosis of bone

L97.529 **Non-pressure chronic ulcer of other part of left foot** with unspecified severity

√5ᵗʰ **L97.8 Non-pressure chronic ulcer of other part of lower leg**

√6ᵗʰ **L97.80 Non-pressure chronic ulcer of other part of unspecified lower leg**

L97.801 **Non-pressure chronic ulcer of other part of unspecified lower leg** limited to breakdown of skin `cc`

L97.802 **Non-pressure chronic ulcer of other part of unspecified lower leg** with fat layer exposed `cc`

L97.803 **Non-pressure chronic ulcer of other part of unspecified lower leg** with necrosis of muscle `cc`

L97.804 **Non-pressure chronic ulcer of other part of unspecified lower leg** with necrosis of bone `cc`

L97.809 **Non-pressure chronic ulcer of other part of unspecified lower leg** with unspecified severity `cc`

√6ᵗʰ **L97.81 Non-pressure chronic ulcer of other part of right lower leg**

L97.811 **Non-pressure chronic ulcer of other part of right lower leg** limited to breakdown of skin `cc`

Diseases of the Skin and Subcutaneous Tissue

L97.812–L99

L97.812 Non-pressure chronic ulcer of other part of right lower leg with fat layer exposed `CC`

L97.813 Non-pressure chronic ulcer of other part of right lower leg with necrosis of muscle `CC`

L97.814 Non-pressure chronic ulcer of other part of right lower leg with necrosis of bone `CC`

L97.819 Non-pressure chronic ulcer of other part of right lower leg with unspecified severity `CC`

✓6ᵗʰ **L97.82 Non-pressure chronic ulcer of other part of left lower leg**

L97.821 Non-pressure chronic ulcer of other part of left lower leg limited to breakdown of skin `CC`

L97.822 Non-pressure chronic ulcer of other part of left lower leg with fat layer exposed `CC`

L97.823 Non-pressure chronic ulcer of other part of left lower leg with necrosis of muscle `CC`

L97.824 Non-pressure chronic ulcer of other part of left lower leg with necrosis of bone `CC`

L97.829 Non-pressure chronic ulcer of other part of left lower leg with unspecified severity `CC`

✓5ᵗʰ **L97.9 Non-pressure chronic ulcer of unspecified part of lower leg**

✓6ᵗʰ **L97.90 Non-pressure chronic ulcer of unspecified lower leg**

L97.901 Non-pressure chronic ulcer of unspecified part of unspecified lower leg limited to breakdown of skin `CC`

L97.902 Non-pressure chronic ulcer of unspecified part of unspecified lower leg with fat layer exposed `CC`

L97.903 Non-pressure chronic ulcer of unspecified part of unspecified lower leg with necrosis of muscle `CC`

L97.904 Non-pressure chronic ulcer of unspecified part of unspecified lower leg with necrosis of bone `CC`

L97.909 Non-pressure chronic ulcer of unspecified part of unspecified lower leg with unspecified severity `CC`

✓6ᵗʰ **L97.91 Non-pressure chronic ulcer of unspecified part of right lower leg**

L97.911 Non-pressure chronic ulcer of unspecified part of right lower leg limited to breakdown of skin `CC`

L97.912 Non-pressure chronic ulcer of unspecified part of right lower leg with fat layer exposed `CC`

L97.913 Non-pressure chronic ulcer of unspecified part of right lower leg with necrosis of muscle `CC`

L97.914 Non-pressure chronic ulcer of unspecified part of right lower leg with necrosis of bone `CC`

L97.919 Non-pressure chronic ulcer of unspecified part of right lower leg with unspecified severity `CC`

✓6ᵗʰ **L97.92 Non-pressure chronic ulcer of unspecified part of left lower leg**

L97.921 Non-pressure chronic ulcer of unspecified part of left lower leg limited to breakdown of skin `CC`

L97.922 Non-pressure chronic ulcer of unspecified part of left lower leg with fat layer exposed `CC`

L97.923 Non-pressure chronic ulcer of unspecified part of left lower leg with necrosis of muscle `CC`

L97.924 Non-pressure chronic ulcer of unspecified part of left lower leg with necrosis of bone `CC`

L97.929 Non-pressure chronic ulcer of unspecified part of left lower leg with unspecified severity `CC`

✓4ᵗʰ **L98 Other disorders of skin and subcutaneous tissue, not elsewhere classified**

L98.0 Pyogenic granuloma
> EXCLUDES 2   pyogenic granuloma of gingiva (K06.8)
> pyogenic granuloma of maxillary alveolar ridge (K04.5)
> pyogenic granuloma of oral mucosa (K13.4)

L98.1 Factitial dermatitis
Neurotic excoriation

L98.2 Febrile neutrophilic dermatosis [Sweet]

L98.3 Eosinophilic cellulitis [Wells] `CC`
CC Excl: A17.9, A18.4, A18.82, A18.84, A18.89, A48.2-A48.4, A48.8-A49.9, B78.1, B95.0-B96.89, E83.2, L02.811-L02.818, L02.91, L03.811-L03.91, L08.0, L08.81-L08.9, L44.8-L45, L73.2, L88, L92.8, L94.2, L94.4, L98.0, L98.3, L98.8, L99, M00.011-M00.012, M00.021-M00.022, M00.031-M00.032, M00.041-M00.042, M00.051-M00.052, M00.061-M00.062, M00.071-M00.072, Z16.10-Z16.39

✓5ᵗʰ **L98.4 Non-pressure chronic ulcer of skin, not elsewhere classified**
Chronic ulcer of skin NOS   Ulcer of skin NOS
Tropical ulcer NOS
> EXCLUDES 2   pressure ulcer (pressure area) (L89.-)
> gangrene (I96)
> skin infections (L00-L08)
> specific infections classified to A00-B99
> ulcer of lower limb NEC (L97.-)
> varicose ulcer (I83.0-I82.2)

✓6ᵗʰ **L98.41 Non-pressure chronic ulcer of buttock**

L98.411 Non-pressure chronic ulcer of buttock limited to breakdown of skin

L98.412 Non-pressure chronic ulcer of buttock with fat layer exposed

L98.413 Non-pressure chronic ulcer of buttock with necrosis of muscle

L98.414 Non-pressure chronic ulcer of buttock with necrosis of bone

L98.419 Non-pressure chronic ulcer of buttock with unspecified severity

✓6ᵗʰ **L98.42 Non-pressure chronic ulcer of back**

L98.421 Non-pressure chronic ulcer of back limited to breakdown of skin

L98.422 Non-pressure chronic ulcer of back with fat layer exposed

L98.423 Non-pressure chronic ulcer of back with necrosis of muscle

L98.424 Non-pressure chronic ulcer of back with necrosis of bone

L98.429 Non-pressure chronic ulcer of back with unspecified severity

✓6ᵗʰ **L98.49 Non-pressure chronic ulcer of skin of other sites**
Non-pressure chronic ulcer of skin NOS

L98.491 Non-pressure chronic ulcer of skin of other sites limited to breakdown of skin

L98.492 Non-pressure chronic ulcer of skin of other sites with fat layer exposed

L98.493 Non-pressure chronic ulcer of skin of other sites with necrosis of muscle

L98.494 Non-pressure chronic ulcer of skin of other sites with necrosis of bone

L98.499 Non-pressure chronic ulcer of skin of other sites with unspecified severity

L98.5 Mucinosis of the skin
Focal mucinosis   Reticular erythematous mucinosis
Lichen myxedematosus
> EXCLUDES 1   focal oral mucinosis (K13.79)
> myxedema (E03.9)

L98.6 Other infiltrative disorders of the skin and subcutaneous tissue
> EXCLUDES 1   hyalinosis cutis et mucosae (E78.89)

L98.8 Other specified disorders of the skin and subcutaneous tissue
AHA: 2013, 2Q, 32

L98.9 Disorder of the skin and subcutaneous tissue, unspecified

L99 *Other disorders of skin and subcutaneous tissue in diseases classified elsewhere*
Code first underlying disease, such as:
amyloidosis (E85.-)
> EXCLUDES 1   skin disorders in diabetes (E08-E13 with .62)
> skin disorders in gonorrhea (A54.89)
> skin disorders in syphilis (A51.31, A52.79)

N Newborn: 0   P Pediatric: 0-17   M Maternity: 12-55   A Adult: 15-124   MCC Major CC Condition   PDx MCC PDx acts as own MCC   CC CC Condition   PDx CC PDx acts as own CC

676   ICD-10-CM Draft (2015)

Chapter 13. Diseases of the Musculoskeletal System and Connective Tissue (M00-M99)

NOTE Use an external cause code following the code for the musculoskeletal condition, if applicable, to identify the cause of the musculoskeletal condition.

EXCLUDES 2 *arthropathic psoriasis (L40.5-)*
certain conditions originating in the perinatal period (P04-P96)
certain infectious and parasitic diseases (A00-B99)
compartment syndrome (traumatic) (T79.A-)
complications of pregnancy, childbirth and the puerperium (O00-O9A)
congenital malformations, deformations, and chromosomal abnormalities (Q00-Q99)
endocrine, nutritional and metabolic diseases (E00-E88)
injury, poisoning and certain other consequences of external causes (S00-T88)
neoplasms (C00-D49)
symptoms, signs and abnormal clinical and laboratory findings, not elsewhere classified (R00-R94)

This chapter contains the following blocks:

M00-M02   Infectious arthropathies
M05-M14   Inflammatory polyarthropathies
M15-M19   Osteoarthritis
M20-M25   Other joint disorders
M26-M27   Dentofacial anomalies [including malocclusion] and other disorders of jaw
M30-M36   Systemic connective tissue disorders
M40-M43   Deforming dorsopathies
M45-M49   Spondylopathies
M50-M54   Other dorsopathies
M60-M63   Disorders of muscles
M65-M67   Disorders of synovium and tendon
M70-M79   Other soft tissue disorders
M80-M85   Disorders of bone density and structure
M86-M90   Other osteopathies
M91-M94   Chondropathies
M95   Other disorders of the musculoskeletal system and connective tissue
M96   Intraoperative and postprocedural complications and disorders of musculoskeletal system, not elsewhere classified
M99   Biomechanical lesions, not elsewhere classified

ARTHROPATHIES (M00-M25)

INCLUDES disorders affecting predominantly peripheral (limb) joints

Infectious arthropathies (M00-M02)

NOTE This block comprises arthropathies due to microbiological agents. Distinction is made between the following types of etiological relationship:
a) direct infection of joint, where organisms invade synovial tissue and microbial antigen is present in the joint;
b) indirect infection, which may be of two types: a reactive arthropathy, where microbial infection of the body is established but neither organisms nor antigens can be identified in the joint, and a postinfective arthropathy, where microbial antigen is present but recovery of an organism is inconstant and evidence of local multiplication is lacking.

√4ᵗʰ **M00 Pyogenic arthritis**

√5ᵗʰ **M00.0 Staphylococcal arthritis and polyarthritis**
Use additional code (B95.61-B95.8) to identify bacterial agent
EXCLUDES 2 *infection and inflammatory reaction due to internal joint prosthesis (T84.5-)*

M00.00 Staphylococcal arthritis, unspecified joint **CC**
CC Excl: A17.9, A18.02, A18.09, A18.82, A18.84, A18.89, A39.83-A39.84, A54.40, A54.42-A54.43, A54.82, A54.84, A54.89-A54.9, B06.82, M00.00, M00.019, M00.029, M00.039, M00.049, M00.059, M00.069, M00.079, M00.08-M02.30, M02.319, M02.329, M02.339, M02.349, M02.359, M02.369, M02.379-M02.9, M05.40-M05.59, M05.70-M06.09, M06.20-M06.39, M06.80-M07.69, M11.00-M11.9, M12.10-M15.0, M15.3-M15.9, M16.2-M16.9, M17.2-M17.9, M18.2-M18.9, M19.111-M19.93, M24.10-M24.176, M25.00, M25.08-M25.18, M25.40-M25.676, M25.80-M25.9, M35.2, M36.1-M36.4, R26.2, R29.4

√6ᵗʰ **M00.01 Staphylococcal arthritis, shoulder**
M00.011 Staphylococcal arthritis, right shoulder
M00.012 Staphylococcal arthritis, left shoulder
M00.019 Staphylococcal arthritis, unspecified shoulder **CC**
CC Excl: A17.9, A18.02, A18.09, A18.82, A18.84, A18.89, A39.83-A39.84, A54.40, A54.42-A54.43, A54.82, A54.84, A54.89-A54.9, B06.82, M00.00, M00.019, M00.08-M00.119, M00.18-M00.219, M00.28-M00.819, M00.88-M01.X19, M01.X8-M02.119, M02.18-M02.30, M02.319, M02.38-M02.819, M02.88-M02.9, M05.40-M05.59, M05.70-M06.09, M06.20-M06.39, M06.80-M07.619, M07.68-M07.69, M11.00-M11.019, M11.08-M11.119, M11.18-M11.219, M11.28-M11.819, M11.88-M11.9, M12.10-M12.119, M12.18-M12.219, M12.28-M12.319, M12.38-M12.419, M12.48-M12.519, M12.58-M12.819, M12.88-M13.119, M13.80-M13.819, M13.88-M15.0, M15.3-M15.9, M19.011-M19.019, M19.111-M19.119, M19.211-M19.219, M19.90-M19.93, M24.10-M24.119, M25.00-M25.019, M25.08-M25.119, M25.18, M25.40-M25.419, M25.48-M25.519, M25.60-M25.619, M25.80-M25.819, M25.9, M35.2, M36.1-M36.4, R26.2

√6ᵗʰ **M00.02 Staphylococcal arthritis, elbow**
M00.021 Staphylococcal arthritis, right elbow
M00.022 Staphylococcal arthritis, left elbow
M00.029 Staphylococcal arthritis, unspecified elbow **CC**
CC Excl: A17.9, A18.02, A18.09, A18.82, A18.84, A18.89, A39.83-A39.84, A54.40, A54.42-A54.43, A54.82, A54.84, A54.89-A54.9, B06.82, M00.00, M00.029, M00.08-M00.10, M00.121-M00.129, M00.18-M00.20, M00.221-M00.229, M00.28-M00.80, M00.821-M00.829, M00.88-M01.X0, M01.X21-M01.X29, M01.X8, M01.X9, M02.00-M02.1, M02.121-M02.129, M02.18-M02.30, M02.329, M02.38-M02.80, M02.821-M02.829, M02.88-M02.9, M05.40-M05.59, M05.70-M06.09, M06.20-M06.39, M06.80-M07.60, M07.621-M07.629, M07.68-M07.69, M11.00, M11.021-M11.029, M11.08-M11.10, M11.121-M11.129, M11.18-M11.20, M11.221-M11.229, M11.28-M11.80, M11.821-M11.829, M11.88-M11.9, M12.10, M12.121-M12.129, M12.18-M12.20, M12.221-M12.229, M12.28-M12.30, M12.321-M12.329, M12.38-M12.40, M12.421-M12.429, M12.48-M12.50, M12.521-M12.529, M12.58-M12.80, M12.821-M12.829, M12.88-M13.10, M13.121-M13.129, M13.80, M13.821-M13.829, M13.88-M15.0, M15.3-M15.9, M19.021-M19.029, M19.121-M19.129, M19.221-M19.229, M19.90-M19.93, M24.10, M24.121-M24.129, M25.00, M25.021-M25.029, M25.08-M25.10, M25.121-M25.129, M25.18, M25.40, M25.421-M25.429, M25.48-M25.50, M25.521-M25.529, M25.60, M25.621-M25.629, M25.80, M25.821-M25.829, M25.9, M35.2, M36.1-M36.4, R26.2

√ Additional Character Required   √x7ᵗʰ Xtension Alert   Unacceptable PDx   Manifestation   Hospital Acquired Condition   **EXCLUDES 1** Not Coded Here   **EXCLUDES 2** Not Included Here

Diseases of the Musculoskeletal System and Connective Tissue

M00.03–M00.069

✓6th **M00.03 Staphylococcal arthritis, wrist**
Staphylococcal arthritis of carpal bones

M00.031 Staphylococcal arthritis, right wrist

M00.032 Staphylococcal arthritis, left wrist

M00.039 Staphylococcal arthritis, unspecified CC
wrist

CC Excl: A17.9, A18.02, A18.09, A18.82,
A18.84, A18.89, A39.83-A39.84, A54.40,
A54.42-A54.43, A54.82, A54.84, A54.89-
A54.9, B06.82, M00.00, M00.039, M00.08-
M00.10, M00.131-M00.139, M00.18-M00.20,
M00.231-M00.239, M00.28-M00.80,
M00.831-M00.839, M00.88-M01.X0,
M01.X31-M01.X39, M01.X8-M02.10,
M02.131-M02.139, M02.18-M02.30,
M02.339, M02.38-M02.80, M02.831-
M02.839, M02.88-M02.9, M05.40-M05.59,
M05.70-M06.09, M06.20-M06.39, M06.80 -
M07.60, M07.631-M07.639, M07.68-M07.69,
M11.00, M11.031-M11.039, M11.08-M11.10,
M11.131-M11.139, M11.18-M11.20,
M11.231-M11.239, M11.28-M11.80,
M11.831-M11.839, M11.88-M11.9, M12.10,
M12.131-M12.139, M12.18-M12.20,
M12.231-M12.239, M12.28-M12.30,
M12.331-M12.339, M12.38-M12.40,
M12.431-M12.439, M12.48-M12.50,
M12.531-M12.539, M12.58-M12.80,
M12.831-M12.839, M12.88-M13.10,
M13.131-M13.139, M13.80, M13.831-
M13.839, M13.88-M15.0, M15.3-M15.9,
M19.031-M19.039, M19.131-M19.139,
M19.231-M19.239, M19.90-M19.93, M24.10,
M24.131-M24.139, M25.00, M25.031-
M25.039, M25.08-M25.10, M25.131-
M25.139, M25.18, M25.40, M25.431-
M25.439, M25.48-M25.50, M25.531-
M25.539, M25.60, M25.631-M25.639,
M25.80, M25.831-M25.839, M25.9, M35.2,
M36.1-M36.4, R26.2

✓6th **M00.04 Staphylococcal arthritis, hand**
Staphylococcal arthritis of metacarpus and phalanges

M00.041 Staphylococcal arthritis, right hand

M00.042 Staphylococcal arthritis, left hand

M00.049 Staphylococcal arthritis, unspecified CC
hand

CC Excl: A17.9, A18.02, A18.09, A18.82,
A18.84, A18.89, A39.83-A39.84, A54.40,
A54.42-A54.43, A54.82, A54.84, A54.89-
A54.9, B06.82, M00.00, M00.049, M00.08-
M00.10, M00.141-M00.149, M00.18-M00.20,
M00.241-M00.249, M00.28-M00.80,
M00.841-M00.849, M00.88-M01.X0,
M01.X41-M01.X49, M01.X8-M02.10,
M02.141-M02.149, M02.18-M02.30,
M02.349, M02.38-M02.80, M02.841-
M02.849, M02.88-M02.9, M05.40-M05.59,
M05.70-M06.09, M06.20-M06.39, M06.80-
M07.60, M07.641-M07.649, M07.68-M07.69,
M11.00, M11.041-M11.049, M11.08-M11.10,
M11.141-M11.149, M11.18-M11.20,
M11.241-M11.249, M11.28-M11.80,
M11.841-M11.849, M11.88-M11.9, M12.10,
M12.141-M12.149, M12.18-M12.20,
M12.241-M12.249, M12.28-M12.30,
M12.341-M12.349, M12.38-M12.40,
M12.441-M12.449, M12.48-M12.50,
M12.541-M12.549, M12.58-M12.80,
M12.841-M12.849, M12.88-M13.10,
M13.141-M13.149, M13.80, M13.841-
M13.849, M13.88-M15.9, M18.0-M18.9,
M19.041-M19.049, M19.141-M19.149,
M19.241-M19.249, M19.90-M19.93, M24.10,
M24.141-M24.149, M25.00, M25.041-
M25.049, M25.08-M25.10, M25.141-
M25.149, M25.18, M25.40, M25.441-
M25.449, M25.48-M25.50, M25.60, M25.641-
M25.649, M25.80, M25.841-M25.849, M25.9,
M35.2, M36.1-M36.4, R26.2

✓6th **M00.05 Staphylococcal arthritis, hip**

M00.051 Staphylococcal arthritis, right hip

M00.052 Staphylococcal arthritis, left hip

M00.059 Staphylococcal arthritis, unspecified CC
hip

CC Excl: A17.9, A18.02, A18.09, A18.82,
A18.84, A18.89, A39.83-A39.84, A54.40,
A54.42-A54.43, A54.82, A54.84, A54.89-
A54.9, B06.82, M00.00, M00.059, M00.08-
M00.10, M00.151-M00.159, M00.18-M00.20,
M00.251-M00.259, M00.28-M00.80,
M00.851-M00.859, M00.88-M01.X0,
M01.X51-M01.X59, M01.X8-M02.10,
M02.151-M02.159, M02.18-M02.30,
M02.359, M02.38-M02.80, M02.851-
M02.859, M02.88-M02.9, M05.40-M05.59,
M05.70-M06.09, M06.20-M06.39, M06.80-
M07.60, M07.651-M07.659, M07.68-M07.69,
M11.00, M11.051-M11.059, M11.08-M11.10,
M11.151-M11.159, M11.18-M11.20,
M11.251-M11.259, M11.28-M11.80,
M11.851-M11.859, M11.88-M11.9, M12.10,
M12.151-M12.159, M12.18-M12.20,
M12.251-M12.259, M12.28-M12.30,
M12.351-M12.359, M12.38-M12.40,
M12.451-M12.459, M12.48-M12.50,
M12.551-M12.559, M12.58-M12.80,
M12.851-M12.859, M12.88-M13.10,
M13.151-M13.159, M13.80, M13.851-
M13.859, M13.88-M15.0, M15.3-M16.9,
M19.90-M19.93, M24.10, M24.151-M24.159,
M25.00, M25.051-M25.059, M25.08-M25.10,
M25.151-M25.159, M25.18, M25.40,
M25.451-M25.459, M25.48-M25.50,
M25.551-M25.559, M25.60, M25.651-
M25.659, M25.80, M25.851-M25.859, M25.9,
M35.2, M36.1-M36.4, R26.2, R29.4

✓6th **M00.06 Staphylococcal arthritis, knee**

M00.061 Staphylococcal arthritis, right knee

M00.062 Staphylococcal arthritis, left knee

M00.069 Staphylococcal arthritis, unspecified CC
knee

CC Excl: A17.9, A18.02, A18.09, A18.82,
A18.84, A18.89, A39.83-A39.84, A54.40,
A54.42-A54.43, A54.82, A54.84, A54.89-
A54.9, B06.82, M00.00, M00.069, M00.08-
M00.10, M00.161-M00.169, M00.18-M00.20,
M00.261-M00.269, M00.28-M00.80,
M00.861-M00.869, M00.88-M01.X0,
M01.X61-M01.X69, M01.X8-M02.10,
M02.161-M02.169, M02.18-M02.30,
M02.369, M02.38-M02.80, M02.861-
M02.869, M02.88-M02.9, M05.40-M05.59,
M05.70-M06.09, M06.20-M06.39, M06.80-
M07.60, M07.661-M07.669, M07.68-M07.69,
M11.00, M11.061-M11.069, M11.08-M11.10,
M11.161-M11.169, M11.18-M11.20,
M11.261-M11.269, M11.28-M11.80,
M11.861-M11.869, M11.88-M11.9, M12.10,
M12.161-M12.169, M12.18-M12.20,
M12.261-M12.269, M12.28-M12.30,
M12.361-M12.369, M12.38-M12.40,
M12.461-M12.469, M12.48-M12.50,
M12.561-M12.569, M12.58-M12.80,
M12.861-M12.869, M12.88-M13.10,
M13.161-M13.169, M13.80, M13.861-
M13.869, M13.88-M15.0, M15.3-M15.9,
M17.0-M17.9, M19.90-M19.93, M24.10,
M25.00, M25.061-M25.069, M25.08-M25.10,
M25.161-M25.169, M25.18, M25.40,
M25.461-M25.469, M25.48-M25.50,
M25.561-M25.569, M25.60, M25.661-
M25.669, M25.80, M25.861-M25.869, M25.9,
M35.2, M36.1-M36.4, R26.2

N Newborn: 0   P Pediatric: 0-17   M Maternity: 12-55   A Adult: 15-124   MCC Major CC Condition   PDx MCC PDx acts as own MCC   CC CC Condition   PDx CC PDx acts as own CC

678   ICD-10-CM Draft (2015)

☑6ᵗʰ **M00.07** **Staphylococcal arthritis, ankle and foot**
Staphylococcal arthritis, tarsus, metatarsus and phalanges

M00.071 **Staphylococcal arthritis, right ankle and foot**

M00.072 **Staphylococcal arthritis, left ankle and foot**

M00.079 **Staphylococcal arthritis, unspecified ankle and foot** `CC`
CC Excl: A17.9, A18.02, A18.09, A18.82, A18.84, A18.89, A39.83-A39.84, A54.40, A54.42-A54.43, A54.82, A54.84, A54.89-A54.9, B06.82, M00.00, M00.10, M00.171-M00.20, M00.271-M00.80, M00.871-M01.X0, M01.X71-M02.10, M02.171-M02.30, M02.379-M02.80, M02.871-M2.9, M05.40-M05.59, M05.70-M06.09, M06.20-M06.39, M06.80-M07.60, M07.671-M07.69, M11.00, M11.071-M11.10, M11.171-M11.20, M11.271-M11.80, M11.871-M11.9, M12.10, M12.171-M12.20, M12.271-M12.30, M12.371-M12.40, M12.471-M12.50, M12.571-M12.80, M12.871-M13.10, M13.171-M13.80, M13.871-M15.0, M15.3-M15.9, M19.071-M19.079, M19.171-M19.179, M19.271-M19.93, M24.10, M24.171-M24.176, M25.00, M25.071-M25.10, M25.171-M25.18, M25.40, M25.471-M25.50, M25.571-M25.60, M25.671-M25.676, M25.80, M25.871-M25.9, M35.2, M36.1-M36.4, R26.2

M00.08 **Staphylococcal arthritis, vertebrae** `CC`
CC Excl: A17.9, A18.02, A18.09, A18.82, A18.84, A18.89, A39.83-A39.84, A54.40, A54.42-A54.43, A54.82, A54.84, A54.89-A54.9, B06.82, M00.00, M00.019, M00.029, M00.039, M00.049, M00.059, M00.069, M00.079, M00.08-M02.30, M02.319, M02.329, M02.339, M02.349, M02.359, M02.369, M02.379-M2.9, M05.40-M05.59, M05.70-M06.09, M06.20-M06.39, M06.80-M07.69, M11.00-M11.9, M12.10-M15.0, M15.3-M15.9, M16.2-M16.9, M17.2-M17.9, M18.2-M18.9, M19.111-M19.93, M24.10-M24.176, M25.00, M25.08-M25.18, M25.40-M25.676, M25.80-M25.9, M35.2, M36.1-M36.4, R26.2, R29.4

M00.09 **Staphylococcal polyarthritis** `CC`
CC Excl: See code: M00.08

☑5ᵗʰ **M00.1** **Pneumococcal arthritis and polyarthritis**

M00.10 **Pneumococcal arthritis, unspecified joint** `CC`
CC Excl: See code: M00.08

☑6ᵗʰ **M00.11** **Pneumococcal arthritis, shoulder**

M00.111 **Pneumococcal arthritis, right shoulder** `CC`
CC Excl: A17.9, A18.02, A18.09, A18.82, A18.84, A18.89, A39.83-A39.84, A54.40, A54.42-A54.43, A54.82, A54.84, A54.89-A54.9, B06.82, M00.00, M00.019, M00.08-M00.119, M00.18-M00.219, M00.28-M00.819, M00.88-M01.X19, M01.X8-M02.119, M02.18-M02.211

M00.112 **Pneumococcal arthritis, left shoulder** `CC`
CC Excl: See code: M00.111

M00.119 **Pneumococcal arthritis, unspecified shoulder** `CC`
CC Excl: See code: M00.111

☑6ᵗʰ **M00.12** **Pneumococcal arthritis, elbow**

M00.121 **Pneumococcal arthritis, right elbow** `CC`
CC Excl: A17.9, A18.02, A18.09, A18.82, A18.84, A18.89, A39.83-A39.84, A54.40, A54.42-A54.43, A54.82, A54.84, A54.89-A54.9, B06.82, M00.00, M00.029, M00.08-M00.10, M00.121-M00.129, M00.18-M00.20, M00.221-M00.229, M00.28-M00.80, M00.821-M00.829, M00.88-M01.X0, M01.X21-M01.X29, M01.X8-M02.10, M02.121-M02.129, M02.18-M02.30, M02.329, M02.38-M02.80, M02.821-M02.829, M02.88-M02.9, M05.40-M05.59, M05.70-M06.09, M06.20-M06.39, M06.80-M07.60, M07.621-M07.629, M07.68-M07.69, M11.00, M11.021-M11.029, M11.08-M11.10, M11.121-M11.129, M11.18-M11.20, M11.221-M11.229, M11.28-M11.80, M11.821-M11.829, M11.88-M11.9, M12.10, M12.121-M12.129, M12.18-M12.20, M12.221-M12.229, M12.28-M12.30, M12.321-M12.329, M12.38-M12.40, M12.421-M12.429, M12.48-M12.50, M12.521-M12.529, M12.58-M12.80, M12.821-M12.829, M12.88-M13.10, M13.121-M13.129, M13.18-M13.80, M13.821-M13.829, M13.88-M15.0, M15.3-M15.9, M19.021-M19.029, M19.121-M19.129, M19.221-M19.229, M19.90-M19.93, M24.10, M24.121-M24.129, M25.00, M25.021-M25.029, M25.08-M25.10, M25.121-M25.129, M25.18, M25.40, M25.421-M25.429, M25.48-M25.50, M25.521-M25.529, M25.60, M25.621-M25.629, M25.80, M25.821-M25.829, M25.9, M35.2, M36.1-M36.4, R26.2

M00.122 **Pneumococcal arthritis, left elbow** `CC`
CC Excl: See code: M00.121

M00.129 **Pneumococcal arthritis, unspecified elbow** `CC`
CC Excl: See code: M00.121

☑6ᵗʰ **M00.13** **Pneumococcal arthritis, wrist**
Pneumococcal arthritis of carpal bones

M00.131 **Pneumococcal arthritis, right wrist** `CC`
CC Excl: A17.9, A18.02, A18.09, A18.82, A18.84, A18.89, A39.83-A39.84, A54.40, A54.42-A54.43, A54.82, A54.84, A54.89-A54.9, B06.82, M00.00, M00.039, M00.08-M00.10, M00.131-M00.139, M00.18-M00.20, M00.231-M00.239, M00.28-M00.80, M00.831-M00.839, M00.88-M01.X0, M01.X31-M01.X39, M01.X8-M02.10, M02.131-M02.139, M02.18-M02.30, M02.339, M02.38-M02.80, M02.831-M02.839, M02.88-M02.9, M05.40-M05.59, M05.70-M06.09, M06.20-M06.39, M06.80-M07.60, M07.631-M07.639, M07.68-M07.69, M11.00, M11.031-M11.039, M11.08-M11.10, M11.131-M11.139, M11.18-M11.20, M11.231-M11.239, M11.28-M11.80, M11.831-M11.839, M11.88-M11.9, M12.10, M12.131-M12.139, M12.18-M12.20, M12.231-M12.239, M12.28-M12.30, M12.331-M12.339, M12.38-M12.40, M12.431-M12.439, M12.48-M12.50, M12.531-M12.539, M12.58-M12.80, M12.831-M12.839, M12.88-M13.10, M13.131-M13.139, M13.80, M13.831-M13.839, M13.88-M15.0, M15.3-M15.9, M19.031-M19.039, M19.131-M19.139, M19.231-M19.239, M19.90-M19.93, M24.10, M24.131-M24.139, M25.00, M25.031-M25.039, M25.08-M25.10, M25.131-M25.139, M25.18, M25.40, M25.431-M25.439, M25.48-M25.50, M25.531-M25.539, M25.60, M25.631-M25.639, M25.80, M25.831-M25.839, M25.9, M35.2, M36.1-M36.4, R26.2

M00.132 **Pneumococcal arthritis, left wrist** `CC`
CC Excl: See code: M00.131

M00.139 **Pneumococcal arthritis, unspecified wrist** `CC`
CC Excl: See code: M00.131

☑ Additional Character Required   ☑x7ᵗʰ Xtension Alert   Unacceptable PDx   Manifestation   Hospital Acquired Condition   **EXCLUDES 1** Not Coded Here   **EXCLUDES 2** Not Included Here

✓6th **M00.14 Pneumococcal arthritis, hand**
Pneumococcal arthritis of metacarpus and phalanges

M00.141 Pneumococcal arthritis, right hand CC
CC Excl: A17.9, A18.02, A18.09, A18.82, A18.84, A18.89, A39.83-A39.84, A54.40, A54.42-A54.43, A54.82, A54.84, A54.89-A54.9, B06.82, M00.00, M00.049, M00.08-M00.10, M00.141-M00.149, M00.18-M00.20, M00.241-M00.249, M00.28-M00.80, M00.841-M00.849, M00.88-M01.X0, M01.X41-M01.X49, M01.X8-M02.10, M02.141-M02.149, M02.18-M02.30, M02.349, M02.38-M02.80, M02.841-M02.849, M02.88-M02.9, M05.40-M05.59, M05.70-M06.09, M06.20-M06.39, M07.60-M07.60, M07.641-M07.649, M07.68-M07.69, M11.00, M11.041-M11.049, M11.08-M11.10, M11.141-M11.149, M11.18-M11.20, M11.241-M11.249, M11.28-M11.80, M11.841-M11.849, M11.88-M11.9, M12.10, M12.141-M12.149, M12.18-M12.20, M12.241-M12.249, M12.28-M12.30, M12.341-M12.349, M12.38-M12.40, M12.441-M12.449, M12.48-M12.50, M12.541-M12.549, M12.58-M12.80, M12.841-M12.849, M12.88-M13.10, M13.141-M13.149, M13.80, M13.841-M13.849, M13.88-M15.9, M18.0-M18.9, M19.041-M19.049, M19.141-M19.149, M19.241-M19.249, M19.90-M19.93, M24.10, M24.141-M24.149, M25.00, M25.041-M25.049, M25.08-M25.10, M25.141-M25.149, M25.18, M25.40, M25.441-M25.449, M25.48-M25.50, M25.60, M25.641-M25.649, M25.80, M25.841-M25.849, M25.9, M35.2, M36.1-M36.4, R26.2

M00.142 Pneumococcal arthritis, left hand CC
CC Excl: See code: M00.141

M00.149 Pneumococcal arthritis, unspecified hand CC
CC Excl: See code: M00.141

✓6th **M00.15 Pneumococcal arthritis, hip**

M00.151 Pneumococcal arthritis, right hip CC
CC Excl: A17.9, A18.02, A18.09, A18.82, A18.84, A18.89, A39.83-A39.84, A54.40, A54.42-A54.43, A54.82, A54.84, A54.89-A54.9, B06.82, M00.00, M00.059, M00.08-M00.10, M00.151-M00.159, M00.18-M00.20, M00.251-M00.259, M00.28-M00.80, M00.851-M00.859, M00.88-M01.X0, M01.X51-M01.X59, M01.X8-M02.10, M02.151-M02.159, M02.18-M02.30, M02.359, M02.38-M02.80, M02.851-M02.859, M02.88-M02.9, M05.40-M05.59, M05.70-M06.09, M06.20-M06.39, M06.80-M07.60, M07.651-M07.659, M07.68-M07.69, M11.00, M11.051-M11.059, M11.08-M11.10, M11.151-M11.159, M11.18-M11.20, M11.251-M11.259, M11.28-M11.80, M11.851-M11.859, M11.88-M11.9, M12.10, M12.151-M12.159, M12.18-M12.20, M12.251-M12.259, M12.28-M12.30, M12.351-M12.359, M12.38-M12.40, M12.451-M12.459, M12.48-M12.50, M12.551-M12.559, M12.58-M12.80, M12.851-M12.859, M12.88-M13.10, M13.151-M13.159, M13.80, M13.851-M13.859, M13.88-M15.0, M15.3-M16.9, M19.90-M19.93, M24.10, M24.151-M24.159, M25.00, M25.051-M25.059, M25.08-M25.10, M25.151-M25.159, M25.18, M25.40, M25.451-M25.459, M25.48-M25.50, M25.551-M25.559, M25.60, M25.651-M25.659, M25.80, M25.851-M25.859, M25.9, M35.2, M36.1-M36.4, R26.2, R29.4

M00.152 Pneumococcal arthritis, left hip CC
CC Excl: See code: M00.151

M00.159 Pneumococcal arthritis, unspecified hip CC
CC Excl: See code: M00.151

✓6th **M00.16 Pneumococcal arthritis, knee**

M00.161 Pneumococcal arthritis, right knee CC
CC Excl: A17.9, A18.02, A18.09, A18.82, A18.84, A18.89, A39.83-A39.84, A54.40, A54.42-A54.43, A54.82, A54.84, A54.89-A54.9, B06.82, M00.00, M00.069, M00.08-M00.10, M00.161-M00.169, M00.18-M00.20, M00.261-M00.269, M00.28-M00.80, M00.861-M00.869, M00.88-M01.X0, M01.X61-M01.X69, M01.X8-M02.10, M02.161-M02.169, M02.18-M02.30, M02.369, M02.38-M02.80, M02.861-M02.869, M02.88-M02.9, M05.40-M05.59, M05.70-M06.09, M06.20-M06.39, M06.80-M07.60, M07.661-M07.669, M07.68-M07.69, M11.00, M11.061-M11.069, M11.08-M11.10, M11.161-M11.169, M11.18-M11.20, M11.261-M11.269, M11.28-M11.80, M11.861-M11.869, M11.88-M11.9, M12.10, M12.161-M12.169, M12.18-M12.20, M12.261-M12.269, M12.28-M12.30, M12.361-M12.369, M12.38-M12.40, M12.461-M12.469, M12.48-M12.50, M12.561-M12.569, M12.58-M12.80, M12.861-M12.869, M12.88-M13.10, M13.161-M13.169, M13.80, M13.861-M13.869, M13.88-M15.0, M15.3-M15.9, M17.0-M17.9, M19.90-M19.93, M24.10, M25.00, M25.061-M25.069, M25.08-M25.10, M25.161-M25.169, M25.18, M25.40, M25.461-M25.469, M25.48-M25.50, M25.561-M25.569, M25.60, M25.661-M25.669, M25.80, M25.861-M25.869, M25.9, M35.2, M36.1-M36.4, R26.2

M00.162 Pneumococcal arthritis, left knee CC
CC Excl: See code: M00.161

M00.169 Pneumococcal arthritis, unspecified knee CC
CC Excl: See code: M00.161

✓6th **M00.17 Pneumococcal arthritis, ankle and foot**
Pneumococcal arthritis, tarsus, metatarsus and phalanges

M00.171 Pneumococcal arthritis, right ankle and foot CC
CC Excl: A17.9, A18.02, A18.09, A18.82, A18.84, A18.89, A39.83-A39.84, A54.40, A54.42-A54.43, A54.82, A54.84, A54.89-A54.9, B06.82, M00.00, M00.079-M00.20, M00.271-M00.80, M00.871-M01.X0, M01.X71-M02.10, M02.171-M02.30, M02.379-M02.80, M02.871-M02.9, M05.40-M05.59, M05.70-M06.09, M06.20-M06.39, M06.80-M07.60, M07.671-M07.69, M11.00, M11.071-M11.10, M11.171-M11.20, M11.271-M11.80, M11.871-M11.9, M12.10, M12.171-M12.20, M12.271-M12.30, M12.371-M12.40, M12.471-M12.50, M12.571-M12.80, M12.871-M13.10, M13.171-M13.80, M13.871-M15.0, M15.3-M15.9, M19.071-M19.079, M19.171-M19.179, M19.271-M19.93, M24.10, M24.171-M24.176, M25.00, M25.071-M25.10, M25.171-M25.18, M25.40, M25.471-M25.50, M25.571-M25.60, M25.671-M25.676, M25.80, M25.871-M25.9, M35.2, M36.1-M36.4, R26.2

M00.172 Pneumococcal arthritis, left ankle and foot CC
CC Excl: See code: M00.171

M00.179 Pneumococcal arthritis, unspecified ankle and foot CC
CC Excl: See code: M00.171

M00.18 Pneumococcal arthritis, vertebrae CC
CC Excl: A17.9, A18.02, A18.09, A18.82, A18.84, A18.89, A39.83-A39.84, A54.40, A54.42-A54.43, A54.82, A54.84, A54.89-A54.9, B06.82, M00.00, M00.019, M00.029, M00.039, M00.049, M00.059, M00.069, M00.079, M00.08-M02.30, M02.319, M02.329, M02.339, M02.349, M02.359, M02.379-M02.9, M05.40-M05.59, M05.70-M06.09, M06.20-M06.39, M06.80-M07.69, M11.00-M11.9, M12.10-M15.0, M15.3-M15.9, M16.2-M16.9, M17.2-M17.9, M18.2-M18.9, M19.111-M19.93, M24.10-M24.176, M25.00, M25.08-M25.18, M25.40-M25.676, M25.80-M25.9, M35.2, M36.1-M36.4, R26.2, R29.4

M00.19 Pneumococcal polyarthritis CC
CC Excl: See code: M00.18

✓5th **M00.2 Other streptococcal arthritis and polyarthritis**
Use additional code (B95.0-B95.2, B95.4-B95.5) to identify bacterial agent

M00.20 Other streptococcal arthritis, unspecified joint CC
CC Excl: See code: M00.18

N Newborn: 0   P Pediatric: 0-17   M Maternity: 12-55   A Adult: 15-124   MCC Major CC Condition   PDx MCC PDx acts as own MCC   CC CC Condition   PDx CC PDx acts as own CC

680   ICD-10-CM Draft (2015)

✓6ᵗʰ **M00.21** Other streptococcal arthritis, shoulder

M00.211 Other streptococcal arthritis, right shoulder   CC
CC Excl: A17.9, A18.02, A18.09, A18.82, A18.84, A18.89, A39.83-A39.84, A54.40, A54.42-A54.43, A54.82, A54.84, A54.89-A54.9, B06.82, M00.00, M00.019, M00.08-M00.119, M00.18-M00.219, M00.28-M00.819, M00.88-M01.X19, M01.X8-M02.119, M02.18-M02.211

M00.212 Other streptococcal arthritis, left shoulder   CC
CC Excl: See code: M00.211

M00.219 Other streptococcal arthritis, unspecified shoulder   CC
CC Excl: See code: M00.211

✓6ᵗʰ **M00.22** Other streptococcal arthritis, elbow

M00.221 Other streptococcal arthritis, right elbow   CC
CC Excl: A17.9, A18.02, A18.09, A18.82, A18.84, A18.89, A39.83-A39.84, A54.40, A54.42-A54.43, A54.82, A54.84, A54.89-A54.9, B06.82, M00.00, M00.029, M00.08-M00.10, M00.121-M00.129, M00.18-M00.20, M00.221-M00.229, M00.28-M00.80, M00.821-M00.829, M00.88-M01.X0, M01.X21-M01.X29, M01.X8-M02.10, M02.121-M02.129, M02.18-M02.30, M02.329, M02.38-M02.80, M02.821-M02.829, M02.88-M02.9, M05.40-M05.59, M05.70-M06.09, M06.20-M06.39, M06.80-M07.60, M07.621-M07.629, M07.68-M07.69, M11.00, M11.021-M11.029, M11.08-M11.10, M11.121-M11.129, M11.18-M11.20, M11.221-M11.229, M11.28-M11.80, M11.821-M11.829, M11.88-M11.9, M12.10, M12.121-M12.129, M12.18-M12.20, M12.221-M12.229, M12.28-M12.30, M12.321-M12.329, M12.38-M12.40, M12.421-M12.429, M12.48-M12.50, M12.521-M12.529, M12.58-M12.80, M12.821-M12.829, M12.88-M13.10, M13.121-M13.129, M13.80, M13.821-M13.829, M13.88-M15.0, M15.3-M15.9, M19.021-M19.029, M19.121-M19.129, M19.221-M19.229, M19.90-M19.93, M24.10, M24.121-M24.129, M25.00, M25.021-M25.029, M25.08-M25.10, M25.121-M25.129, M25.18, M25.40, M25.421-M25.429, M25.48-M25.50, M25.521-M25.529, M25.60, M25.621-M25.629, M25.80, M25.821-M25.829, M25.9, M35.2, M36.1-M36.4, R26.2

M00.222 Other streptococcal arthritis, left elbow   CC
CC Excl: See code: M00.221

M00.229 Other streptococcal arthritis, unspecified elbow   CC
CC Excl: See code: M00.221

✓6ᵗʰ **M00.23** Other streptococcal arthritis, wrist
Other streptococcal arthritis of carpal bones

M00.231 Other streptococcal arthritis, right wrist   CC
CC Excl: A17.9, A18.02, A18.09, A18.82, A18.84, A18.89, A39.83-A39.84, A54.40, A54.42-A54.43, A54.82, A54.84, A54.89-A54.9, B06.82, M00.00, M00.039, M00.08-M00.10, M00.131-M00.139, M00.18-M00.20, M00.231-M00.239, M00.28-M00.80, M00.831-M00.839, M00.88-M01.X0, M01.X31-M01.X39, M01.X8-M02.10, M02.131-M02.139, M02.18-M02.30, M02.339, M02.38-M02.80, M02.831-M02.839, M02.88-M02.9, M05.40-M05.59, M05.70-M06.09, M06.20-M06.39, M06.80-M07.60, M07.631-M07.639, M07.68-M07.69, M11.00, M11.031-M11.039, M11.08-M11.10, M11.131-M11.139, M11.18-M11.20, M11.231-M11.239, M11.28-M11.80, M11.831-M11.839, M11.88-M11.9, M12.10, M12.131-M12.139, M12.18-M12.20, M12.231-M12.239, M12.28-M12.30, M12.331-M12.339, M12.38-M12.40, M12.431-M12.439, M12.48-M12.50, M12.531-M12.539, M12.58-M12.80, M12.831-M12.839, M12.88-M13.10, M13.131-M13.139, M13.80, M13.831-M13.839, M13.88-M15.0, M15.3-M15.9, M19.031-M19.039, M19.131-M19.139, M19.231-M19.239, M19.90-M19.93, M24.10, M24.131-M24.139, M25.00, M25.031-M25.039, M25.08-M25.10, M25.131-M25.139, M25.18, M25.40, M25.431-M25.439, M25.48-M25.50, M25.531-M25.539, M25.60, M25.631-M25.639, M25.80, M25.831-M25.839, M25.9, M35.2, M36.1-M36.4, R26.2

M00.232 Other streptococcal arthritis, left wrist   CC
CC Excl: See code: M00.231

M00.239 Other streptococcal arthritis, unspecified wrist   CC
CC Excl: See code: M00.231

✓6ᵗʰ **M00.24** Other streptococcal arthritis, hand
Other streptococcal arthritis metacarpus and phalanges

M00.241 Other streptococcal arthritis, right hand   CC
CC Excl: A17.9, A18.02, A18.09, A18.82, A18.84, A18.89, A39.83-A39.84, A54.40, A54.42-A54.43, A54.82, A54.84, A54.89-A54.9, B06.82, M00.00, M00.049, M00.08-M00.10, M00.141-M00.149, M00.18-M00.20, M00.241-M00.249, M00.28-M00.80, M00.841-M00.849, M00.88-M01.X0, M01.X41-M01.X49, M01.X8-M02.10, M02.141-M02.149, M02.18-M02.30, M02.349, M02.38-M02.80, M02.841-M02.849, M02.88-M02.9, M05.40-M05.59, M05.70-M06.09, M06.20-M06.39, M06.80-M07.60, M07.641-M07.649, M07.68-M07.69, M11.00, M11.041-M11.049, M11.08-M11.10, M11.141-M11.149, M11.18-M11.20, M11.241-M11.249, M11.28-M11.80, M11.841-M11.849, M11.88-M11.9, M12.10, M12.141-M12.149, M12.18-M12.20, M12.241-M12.249, M12.28-M12.30, M12.341-M12.349, M12.38-M12.40, M12.441-M12.449, M12.48-M12.50, M12.541-M12.549, M12.58-M12.80, M12.841-M12.849, M12.88-M13.10, M13.141-M13.149, M13.80, M13.841-M13.849, M13.88-M15.9, M18.0-M18.9, M19.041-M19.049, M19.141-M19.149, M19.241-M19.249, M19.90-M19.93, M24.10, M24.141-M24.149, M25.00, M25.041-M25.049, M25.08-M25.10, M25.141-M25.149, M25.18, M25.40, M25.441-M25.449, M25.48-M25.50, M25.60, M25.641-M25.649, M25.80, M25.841-M25.849, M25.9, M35.2, M36.1-M36.4, R26.2

M00.242 Other streptococcal arthritis, left hand   CC
CC Excl: See code: M00.241

M00.249 Other streptococcal arthritis, unspecified hand   CC
CC Excl: See code: M00.241

✓6ᵗʰ **M00.25** Other streptococcal arthritis, hip

M00.251 Other streptococcal arthritis, right hip   CC
CC Excl: A17.9, A18.02, A18.09, A18.82, A18.84, A18.89, A39.83-A39.84, A54.40, A54.42-A54.43, A54.82, A54.84, A54.89-A54.9, B06.82, M00.00, M00.059, M00.08-M00.10, M00.151-M00.159, M00.18-M00.20, M00.251-M00.259, M00.28-M00.80, M00.851-M00.859, M00.88-M01.X0, M01.X51-M01.X59, M01.X8-M02.10, M02.151-M02.159, M02.18-M02.30, M02.359, M02.38-M02.80, M02.851-M02.859, M02.88-M02.9, M05.40-M05.59, M05.70-M06.09, M06.20-M06.39, M06.80-M07.60, M07.651-M07.659, M07.68-M07.69, M11.00, M11.051-M11.059, M11.08-M11.10, M11.151-M11.159, M11.18-M11.20, M11.251-M11.259, M11.28-M11.80, M11.851-M11.859, M11.88-M11.9, M12.10, M12.151-M12.159, M12.18-M12.20, M12.251-M12.259, M12.28-M12.30, M12.351-M12.359, M12.38-M12.40, M12.451-M12.459, M12.48-M12.50, M12.551-M12.559, M12.58-M12.80, M12.851-M12.859, M12.88-M13.10, M13.151-M13.159, M13.80, M13.851-M13.859, M13.88-M15.0, M15.3-M16.9, M19.90-M19.93, M24.10, M24.151-M24.159, M25.00, M25.051-M25.059, M25.08-M25.10, M25.151-M25.159, M25.18, M25.40, M25.451-M25.459, M25.48-M25.50, M25.551-M25.559, M25.60, M25.651-M25.659, M25.80, M25.851-M25.859, M25.9, M35.2, M36.1-M36.4, R26.2, R29.4

M00.252 Other streptococcal arthritis, left hip   CC
CC Excl: See code: M00.251

M00.259 Other streptococcal arthritis, unspecified hip   CC
CC Excl: See code: M00.251

✓ Additional Character Required   ✓x7ᵗʰ Xtension Alert   Unacceptable PDx   Manifestation   Hospital Acquired Condition   EXCLUDES 1 Not Coded Here   EXCLUDES 2 Not Included Here

✓6th **M00.26 Other streptococcal arthritis, knee**

M00.261 Other streptococcal arthritis, right knee CC
CC Excl: A17.9, A18.02, A18.09, A18.82, A18.84, A18.89, A39.83-A39.84, A54.40, A54.42-A54.43, A54.82, A54.84, A54.89-A54.9, B06.82, M00.00, M00.069, M00.08-M00.10, M00.161-M00.169, M00.18-M00.20, M00.261-M00.269, M00.28-M00.80, M00.861-M00.869, M00.88-M01.X0, M01.X61-M01.X69, M01.X8-M02.10, M02.161-M02.169, M02.18-M02.30, M02.369, M02.38-M02.80, M02.861-M02.869, M02.88-M02.9, M05.40-M05.59, M05.70-M06.09, M06.20-M06.39, M06.80-M07.60, M07.661-M07.669, M07.68-M07.69, M11.00, M11.061-M11.069, M11.08-M11.10, M11.161-M11.169, M11.18-M11.20, M11.261-M11.269, M11.28-M11.80, M11.861-M11.869, M11.88-M11.9, M12.10, M12.161-M12.169, M12.18-M12.20, M12.261-M12.269, M12.28-M12.30, M12.361-M12.369, M12.38-M12.40, M12.461-M12.469, M12.48-M12.50, M12.561-M12.569, M12.58-M12.80, M12.861-M12.869, M12.88-M13.10, M13.161-M13.169, M13.80, M13.861-M13.869, M13.88-M15.0, M15.3-M15.9, M17.0-M17.9, M19.90-M19.93, M24.10, M25.00, M25.061-M25.069, M25.08-M25.10, M25.161-M25.169, M25.18, M25.40, M25.461-M25.469, M25.48-M25.50, M25.561-M25.569, M25.60, M25.661-M25.669, M25.80, M25.861-M25.869, M25.9, M35.2, M36.1-M36.4, R26.2

M00.262 Other streptococcal arthritis, left knee CC
CC Excl: See code: M00.261

M00.269 Other streptococcal arthritis, unspecified knee CC
CC Excl: See code: M00.261

✓6th **M00.27 Other streptococcal arthritis, ankle and foot**
Other streptococcal arthritis, tarsus, metatarsus and phalanges

M00.271 Other streptococcal arthritis, right ankle and foot CC
CC Excl: A17.9, A18.02, A18.09, A18.82, A18.84, A18.89, A39.83-A39.84, A54.40, A54.42-A54.43, A54.82, A54.84, A54.89-A54.9, B06.82, M00.00, M00.079-M00.10, M00.171-M00.20, M00.271-M00.80, M00.871-M01.X0, M01.X71-M02.10, M02.171-M02.30, M02.379-M02.80, M02.871-M02.9, M05.40-M05.59, M05.70-M06.09, M06.20-M06.39, M06.80-M07.60, M07.671-M07.69, M11.00, M11.071-M11.10, M11.171-M11.20, M11.271-M11.80, M11.871-M11.9, M12.10, M12.171-M12.20, M12.271-M12.30, M12.371-M12.40, M12.471-M12.50, M12.571-M12.80, M12.871-M13.10, M13.171-M13.80, M13.871-M15.0, M15.3-M15.9, M19.071-M19.079, M19.171-M19.179, M19.271-M19.93, M24.10, M24.171-M24.176, M25.00, M25.071-M25.10, M25.171-M25.18, M25.40, M25.471-M25.50, M25.571-M25.60, M25.671-M25.676, M25.80, M25.871-M25.9, M35.2, M36.1-M36.4, R26.2

M00.272 Other streptococcal arthritis, left ankle and foot CC
CC Excl: See code: M00.271

M00.279 Other streptococcal arthritis, unspecified ankle and foot CC
CC Excl: See code: M00.271

M00.28 Other streptococcal arthritis, vertebrae CC
CC Excl: A17.9, A18.02, A18.09, A18.82, A18.84, A18.89, A39.83-A39.84, A54.40, A54.42-A54.43, A54.82, A54.84, A54.89-A54.9, B06.82, M00.00, M00.019, M00.029, M00.039, M00.049, M00.059, M00.069, M00.079, M00.08-M02.30, M02.319, M02.329, M02.339, M02.349, M02.359, M02.369, M02.379-M02.9, M05.40-M05.59, M05.70-M06.09, M06.20-M06.39, M06.80-M07.69, M11.00-M11.9, M12.10-M15.0, M15.3-M15.9, M16.2-M16.9, M17.2-M17.9, M18.2-M18.9, M19.111-M19.93, M24.10-M24.176, M25.00, M25.08-M25.18, M25.40-M25.676, M25.80-M25.9, M35.2, M36.1-M36.4, R26.2, R29.4

M00.29 Other streptococcal polyarthritis CC
CC Excl: See code: M00.28

✓5th **M00.8 Arthritis and polyarthritis due to other bacteria**
Use additional code (B96) to identify bacteria

M00.80 Arthritis due to other bacteria, unspecified joint CC
CC Excl: See code: M00.28

✓6th **M00.81 Arthritis due to other bacteria, shoulder**

M00.811 Arthritis due to other bacteria, right shoulder CC
CC Excl: A17.9, A18.02, A18.09, A18.82, A18.84, A18.89, A39.83-A39.84, A54.40, A54.42-A54.43, A54.82, A54.84, A54.89-A54.9, B06.82, M00.00, M00.019, M00.08-M00.119, M00.18-M00.219, M00.28-M00.819, M00.88-M01.X19, M01.X8-M02.119, M02.18-M02.211

M00.812 Arthritis due to other bacteria, left shoulder CC
CC Excl: See code: M00.811

M00.819 Arthritis due to other bacteria, unspecified shoulder CC
CC Excl: See code: M00.811

✓6th **M00.82 Arthritis due to other bacteria, elbow**

M00.821 Arthritis due to other bacteria, right elbow CC
CC Excl: A17.9, A18.02, A18.09, A18.82, A18.84, A18.89, A39.83-A39.84, A54.40, A54.42-A54.43, A54.82, A54.84, A54.89-A54.9, B06.82, M00.00, M00.029, M00.08-M00.10, M00.121-M00.129, M00.18-M00.20, M00.221-M00.229, M00.28-M00.80, M00.821-M00.829, M00.88-M01.X0, M01.X21-M01.X29, M01.X8-M02.10, M02.121-M02.129, M02.18-M02.30, M02.329, M02.38-M02.80, M02.821-M02.829, M02.88-M02.9, M05.40-M05.59, M05.70-M06.09, M06.20-M06.39, M06.80-M07.60, M07.621-M07.629, M07.68-M07.69, M11.00, M11.021-M11.029, M11.08-M11.10, M11.121-M11.129, M11.18-M11.20, M11.221-M11.229, M11.28-M11.80, M11.821-M11.829, M11.88-M11.9, M12.10, M12.121-M12.129, M12.18-M12.20, M12.221-M12.229, M12.28-M12.30, M12.321-M12.329, M12.38-M12.40, M12.421-M12.429, M12.48-M12.50, M12.521-M12.529, M12.58-M12.80, M12.821-M12.829, M12.88-M13.10, M13.121-M13.129, M13.80, M13.821-M13.829, M13.88-M15.0, M15.3-M15.9, M19.021-M19.029, M19.121-M19.129, M19.221-M19.229, M19.90-M19.93, M24.10, M24.121-M24.129, M25.00, M25.021-M25.029, M25.08-M25.10, M25.121-M25.129, M25.18, M25.40, M25.421-M25.429, M25.48-M25.50, M25.521-M25.529, M25.60, M25.621-M25.629, M25.80, M25.821-M25.829, M25.9, M35.2, M36.1-M36.4, R26.2

M00.822 Arthritis due to other bacteria, left elbow CC
CC Excl: See code: M00.821

M00.829 Arthritis due to other bacteria, unspecified elbow CC
CC Excl: See code: M00.821

✓6th **M00.83 Arthritis due to other bacteria, wrist**
Arthritis due to other bacteria, carpal bones

M00.831 Arthritis due to other bacteria, right wrist CC
CC Excl: A17.9, A18.02, A18.09, A18.82, A18.84, A18.89, A39.83-A39.84, A54.40, A54.42-A54.43, A54.82, A54.84, A54.89-A54.9, B06.82, M00.00, M00.039, M00.08-M00.10, M00.131-M00.139, M00.18-M00.20, M00.231-M00.239, M00.28-M00.80, M00.831-M00.839, M00.88-M01.X0, M01.X31-M01.X39, M01.X8-M02.10, M02.131-M02.139, M02.18-M02.30, M02.339, M02.38-M02.80, M02.831-M02.839, M02.88-M02.9, M05.40-M05.59, M05.70-M06.09, M06.20-M06.39, M06.80-M07.60, M07.631-M07.639, M07.68-M07.69, M11.00, M11.031-M11.039, M11.08-M11.10, M11.131-M11.139, M11.18-M11.20, M11.231-M11.239, M11.28-M11.80, M11.831-M11.839, M11.88-M11.9, M12.10, M12.131-M12.139, M12.18-M12.20, M12.231-M12.239, M12.28-M12.30, M12.331-M12.339, M12.38-M12.40, M12.431-M12.439, M12.48-M12.50, M12.531-M12.539, M12.58-M12.80, M12.831-M12.839, M12.88-M13.10, M13.131-M13.139, M13.80, M13.831-M13.839, M13.88-M15.0, M15.3-M15.9, M19.031-M19.039, M19.131-M19.139, M19.231-M19.239, M19.90-M19.93, M24.10, M24.131-M24.139, M25.00, M25.031-M25.039, M25.08-M25.10, M25.131-M25.139, M25.18, M25.40, M25.431-M25.439, M25.48-M25.50, M25.531-M25.539, M25.60, M25.631-M25.639, M25.80, M25.831-M25.839, M25.9, M35.2, M36.1-M36.4, R26.2

Ⓝ Newborn: 0   Ⓟ Pediatric: 0-17   Ⓜ Maternity: 12-55   Ⓐ Adult: 15-124   MCC Major CC Condition   PDx MCC PDx acts as own MCC   CC CC Condition   PDx CC PDx acts as own CC

682   ICD-10-CM Draft (2015)

M00.832 Arthritis due to other bacteria, left wrist `cc`
CC Excl: See code: M00.831

M00.839 Arthritis due to other bacteria, unspecified wrist `cc`
CC Excl: See code: M00.831

✓6th **M00.84** Arthritis due to other bacteria, hand
Arthritis due to other bacteria, metacarpus and phalanges

M00.841 Arthritis due to other bacteria, right hand `cc`
CC Excl: A17.9, A18.02, A18.09, A18.82, A18.84, A18.89, A39.83-A39.84, A54.40, A54.42-A54.43, A54.82, A54.84, A54.89-A54.9, B06.82, M00.00, M00.049, M00.08-M00.10, M00.141-M00.149, M00.18-M00.20, M00.241-M00.249, M00.28-M00.80, M00.841-M00.849, M00.88-M01.X0, M01.X41-M01.X49, M01.X8-M02.10, M02.141-M02.149, M02.18-M02.30, M02.349, M02.38-M02.80, M02.841-M02.849, M02.88-M02.9, M05.40-M05.59, M05.70-M06.09, M06.20-M06.39, M06.80-M07.60, M07.641-M07.649, M07.68-M07.69, M11.00, M11.041-M11.049, M11.08-M11.10, M11.141-M11.149, M11.18-M11.20, M11.241-M11.249, M11.28-M11.80, M11.841-M11.849, M11.88-M11.9, M12.10, M12.141-M12.149, M12.18-M12.20, M12.241-M12.249, M12.28-M12.30, M12.341-M12.349, M12.38-M12.40, M12.441-M12.449, M12.48-M12.50, M12.541-M12.549, M12.58-M12.80, M12.841-M12.849, M12.88-M13.10, M13.141-M13.149, M13.80, M13.841-M13.849, M13.88-M15.9, M18.0-M18.9, M19.041-M19.049, M19.141-M19.149, M19.241-M19.249, M19.90-M19.93, M24.10, M24.141-M24.149, M25.00, M25.041-M25.049, M25.08-M25.10, M25.141-M25.149, M25.18, M25.40, M25.441-M25.449, M25.48-M25.50, M25.60, M25.641-M25.649, M25.80, M25.841-M25.849, M25.9, M35.2, M36.1-M36.4, R26.2

M00.842 Arthritis due to other bacteria, left hand `cc`
CC Excl: See code: M00.841

M00.849 Arthritis due to other bacteria, unspecified hand `cc`
CC Excl: See code: M00.841

✓6th **M00.85** Arthritis due to other bacteria, hip

M00.851 Arthritis due to other bacteria, right hip `cc`
CC Excl: A17.9, A18.02, A18.09, A18.82, A18.84, A18.89, A39.83-A39.84, A54.40, A54.42-A54.43, A54.82, A54.84, A54.89-A54.9, B06.82, M00.00, M00.059, M00.08-M00.10, M00.151-M00.159, M00.18-M00.20, M00.251-M00.259, M00.28-M00.80, M00.851-M00.859, M00.88-M01.X0, M01.X51-M01.X59, M01.X8-M02.10, M02.151-M02.159, M02.18-M02.30, M02.359, M02.38-M02.80, M02.851-M02.859, M02.88-M02.9, M05.40-M05.59, M05.70-M06.09, M06.20-M06.39, M06.80-M07.60, M07.651-M07.659, M07.68-M07.69, M11.00, M11.051-M11.059, M11.08-M11.10, M11.151-M11.159, M11.18-M11.20, M11.251-M11.259, M11.28-M11.80, M11.851-M11.859, M11.88-M11.9, M12.10, M12.151-M12.159, M12.18-M12.20, M12.251-M12.259, M12.28-M12.30, M12.351-M12.359, M12.38-M12.40, M12.451-M12.459, M12.48-M12.50, M12.551-M12.559, M12.58-M12.80, M12.851-M12.859, M12.88-M13.10, M13.151-M13.159, M13.80, M13.851-M13.859, M13.88-M15.0, M15.3-M16.9, M19.90-M19.93, M24.10, M24.151-M24.159, M25.00, M25.051-M25.059, M25.08-M25.10, M25.151-M25.159, M25.18, M25.40, M25.451-M25.459, M25.48-M25.50, M25.551-M25.559, M25.60, M25.651-M25.659, M25.80, M25.851-M25.859, M25.9, M35.2, M36.1-M36.4, R26.2, R29.4

M00.852 Arthritis due to other bacteria, left hip `cc`
CC Excl: See code: M00.851

M00.859 Arthritis due to other bacteria, unspecified hip `cc`
CC Excl: See code: M00.851

✓6th **M00.86** Arthritis due to other bacteria, knee

M00.861 Arthritis due to other bacteria, right knee `cc`
CC Excl: A17.9, A18.02, A18.09, A18.82, A18.84, A18.89, A39.83-A39.84, A54.40, A54.42-A54.43, A54.82, A54.84, A54.89-A54.9, B06.82, M00.00, M00.069, M00.08-M00.10, M00.161-M00.169, M00.18-M00.20, M00.261-M00.269, M00.28-M00.80, M00.861-M00.869, M00.88-M01.X0, M01.X61-M01.X69, M01.X8-M02.10, M02.161-M02.169, M02.18-M02.30, M02.369, M02.38-M02.80, M02.861-M02.869, M02.88-M02.9, M05.40-M05.59, M05.70-M06.09, M06.20-M06.39, M06.80-M07.60, M07.661-M07.669, M07.68-M07.69, M11.00, M11.061-M11.069, M11.08-M11.10, M11.161-M11.169, M11.18-M11.20, M11.261-M11.269, M11.28-M11.80, M11.861-M11.869, M11.88-M11.9, M12.10, M12.161-M12.169, M12.18-M12.20, M12.261-M12.269, M12.28-M12.30, M12.361-M12.369, M12.38-M12.40, M12.461-M12.469, M12.48-M12.50, M12.561-M12.569, M12.58-M12.80, M12.861-M12.869, M12.88-M13.10, M13.161-M13.169, M13.80, M13.861-M13.869, M13.88-M15.0, M15.3-M15.9, M17.0-M17.9, M19.90-M19.93, M24.10, M25.00, M25.061-M25.069, M25.08-M25.10, M25.161-M25.169, M25.18, M25.40, M25.461-M25.469, M25.48-M25.50, M25.561-M25.569, M25.60, M25.661-M25.669, M25.80, M25.861-M25.869, M25.9, M35.2, M36.1-M36.4, R26.2

M00.862 Arthritis due to other bacteria, left knee `cc`
CC Excl: See code: M00.861

M00.869 Arthritis due to other bacteria, unspecified knee `cc`
CC Excl: See code: M00.861

✓6th **M00.87** Arthritis due to other bacteria, ankle and foot
Arthritis due to other bacteria, tarsus, metatarsus, and phalanges

M00.871 Arthritis due to other bacteria, right ankle and foot `cc`
CC Excl: A17.9, A18.02, A18.09, A18.82, A18.84, A18.89, A39.83-A39.84, A54.40, A54.42-A54.43, A54.82, A54.84, A54.89-A54.9, B06.82, M00.00, M00.071-M00.10, M00.171-M00.20, M00.271-M00.80, M00.871-M01.X0, M01.X71-M02.10, M02.171-M02.30, M02.379-M02.80, M02.871-M02.9, M05.40-M05.59, M05.70-M06.09, M06.20-M06.39, M06.80-M07.60, M07.671-M07.69, M11.00, M11.071-M11.10, M11.171-M11.20, M11.271-M11.80, M11.871-M11.9, M12.10, M12.171-M12.20, M12.271-M12.30, M12.371-M12.40, M12.471-M12.50, M12.571-M12.80, M12.871-M13.10, M13.171-M13.80, M13.871-M15.0, M15.3-M15.9, M19.071-M19.079, M19.171-M19.179, M19.271-M19.93, M24.10, M24.171-M24.176, M25.00, M25.071-M25.10, M25.171-M25.18, M25.40, M25.471-M25.50, M25.571-M25.60, M25.671-M25.676, M25.80, M25.871-M25.9, M35.2, M36.1-M36.4, R26.2

M00.872 Arthritis due to other bacteria, left ankle and foot `cc`
CC Excl: See code: M00.871

M00.879 Arthritis due to other bacteria, unspecified ankle and foot `cc`
CC Excl: See code: M00.871

M00.88 Arthritis due to other bacteria, vertebrae `cc`
CC Excl: A17.9, A18.02, A18.09, A18.82, A18.84, A18.89, A39.83-A39.84, A54.40, A54.42-A54.43, A54.82, A54.84, A54.89-A54.9, B06.82, M00.00, M00.019, M00.029, M00.039, M00.049, M00.059, M00.069, M00.079, M00.08-M02.30, M02.319, M02.329, M02.339, M02.349, M02.359, M02.369, M02.379-M02.9, M05.40-M05.59, M05.70-M06.09, M06.20-M06.39, M06.80-M07.69, M11.00-M11.9, M12.10-M15.0, M15.3-M15.9, M16.2-M16.9, M17.2-M17.9, M18.2-M18.9, M19.111-M19.93, M24.10-M24.176, M25.00, M25.08-M25.18, M25.40-M25.676, M25.80-M25.9, M35.2, M36.1-M36.4, R26.2, R29.4

M00.89 Polyarthritis due to other bacteria `cc`
CC Excl: See code: M00.88

M00.9 Pyogenic arthritis, unspecified `cc`
Infective arthritis NOS
CC Excl: See code: M00.88

M01 Direct infections of joint in infectious and parasitic diseases classified elsewhere

Code first underlying disease, such as:
leprosy [Hansen's disease] (A30.-)
mycoses (B35-B49)
O'nyong-nyong fever (A92.1)
paratyphoid fever (A01.1-A01.4)

EXCLUDES 1   arthropathy in Lyme disease (A69.23)
gonococcal arthritis (A54.42)
meningococcal arthritis (A39.83)
mumps arthritis (B26.85)
postinfective arthropathy (M02.-)
postmeningococcal arthritis (A39.84)
reactive arthritis (M02.3)
rubella arthritis (B06.82)
sarcoidosis arthritis (D86.86)
typhoid fever arthritis (A01.04)
tuberculosis arthritis (A18.01-A18.02)

M01.X Direct infection of joint in infectious and parasitic diseases classified elsewhere

M01.X0 Direct infection of unspecified joint in infectious and parasitic diseases classified elsewhere CC

CC Excl: A02.23, A17.9, A18.02, A18.09, A18.82, A18.84, A18.89, A39.83-A39.84, A54.40, A54.42-A54.43, A54.82, A54.84, A54.89-A54.9, B06.82, M00.00, M00.019, M00.029, M00.039, M00.049, M00.059, M00.069, M00.079, M00.08-M02.30, M02.319, M02.329, M02.339, M02.349, M02.359, M02.369, M02.379-M02.9, M05.40-M05.59, M05.70-M06.09, M06.20-M06.39, M06.80-M07.69, M11.00-M11.9, M12.10-M15.0, M15.3-M15.9, M16.2-M16.9, M17.2-M17.9, M18.2-M18.9, M19.111-M19.93, M24.10-M24.176, M25.00, M25.08-M25.18, M25.40-M25.676, M25.80-M25.9, M35.2, M36.1-M36.4, R29.4

M01.X1 Direct infection of shoulder joint in infectious and parasitic diseases classified elsewhere

M01.X11 Direct infection of right shoulder in infectious and parasitic diseases classified elsewhere CC

CC Excl: A02.23, A17.9, A18.02, A18.09, A18.82, A18.84, A18.89, A39.83-A39.84, A54.40, A54.42-A54.43, A54.82, A54.84, A54.89-A54.9, B06.82, M00.00, M00.019, M00.029, M00.039, M00.049, M00.059, M00.069, M00.079, M00.08-M02.30, M02.319, M02.329, M02.339, M02.349, M02.359, M02.369, M02.379-M02.9, M05.40-M05.59, M05.70-M06.09, M06.20-M06.39, M06.80-M07.69, M11.00-M11.9, M12.10-M12.419

M01.X12 Direct infection of left shoulder in infectious and parasitic diseases classified elsewhere CC
CC Excl: See code: M01.X11

M01.X19 Direct infection of unspecified shoulder in infectious and parasitic diseases classified elsewhere CC
CC Excl: See code: M01.X11

M01.X2 Direct infection of elbow in infectious and parasitic diseases classified elsewhere

M01.X21 Direct infection of right elbow in infectious and parasitic diseases classified elsewhere CC
CC Excl: See code: M01.X0

M01.X22 Direct infection of left elbow in infectious and parasitic diseases classified elsewhere CC
CC Excl: See code: M01.X0

M01.X29 Direct infection of unspecified elbow in infectious and parasitic diseases classified elsewhere CC
CC Excl: See code: M01.X0

M01.X3 Direct infection of wrist in infectious and parasitic diseases classified elsewhere
Direct infection of carpal bones in infectious and parasitic diseases classified elsewhere

M01.X31 Direct infection of right wrist in infectious and parasitic diseases classified elsewhere CC
CC Excl: See code: M01.X0

M01.X32 Direct infection of left wrist in infectious and parasitic diseases classified elsewhere CC
CC Excl: See code: M01.X0

M01.X39 Direct infection of unspecified wrist in infectious and parasitic diseases classified elsewhere CC
CC Excl: See code: M01.X0

M01.X4 Direct infection of hand in infectious and parasitic diseases classified elsewhere
Direct infection of metacarpus and phalanges in infectious and parasitic diseases classified elsewhere

M01.X41 Direct infection of right hand in infectious and parasitic diseases classified elsewhere CC
CC Excl: See code: M01.X0

M01.X42 Direct infection of left hand in infectious and parasitic diseases classified elsewhere CC
CC Excl: See code: M01.X0

M01.X49 Direct infection of unspecified hand in infectious and parasitic diseases classified elsewhere CC
CC Excl: See code: M01.X0

M01.X5 Direct infection of hip in infectious and parasitic diseases classified elsewhere

M01.X51 Direct infection of right hip in infectious and parasitic diseases classified elsewhere CC
CC Excl: See code: M01.X0

M01.X52 Direct infection of left hip in infectious and parasitic diseases classified elsewhere CC
CC Excl: See code: M01.X0

M01.X59 Direct infection of unspecified hip in infectious and parasitic diseases classified elsewhere CC
CC Excl: See code: M01.X0

M01.X6 Direct infection of knee in infectious and parasitic diseases classified elsewhere

M01.X61 Direct infection of right knee in infectious and parasitic diseases classified elsewhere CC
CC Excl: See code: M01.X0

M01.X62 Direct infection of left knee in infectious and parasitic diseases classified elsewhere CC
CC Excl: See code: M01.X0

M01.X69 Direct infection of unspecified knee in infectious and parasitic diseases classified elsewhere CC
CC Excl: See code: M01.X0

M01.X7 Direct infection of ankle and foot in infectious and parasitic diseases classified elsewhere
Direct infection of tarsus, metatarsus and phalanges in infectious and parasitic diseases classified elsewhere

M01.X71 Direct infection of right ankle and foot in infectious and parasitic diseases classified elsewhere CC
CC Excl: See code: M01.X0

M01.X72 Direct infection of left ankle and foot in infectious and parasitic diseases classified elsewhere CC
CC Excl: See code: M01.X0

M01.X79 Direct infection of unspecified ankle and foot in infectious and parasitic diseases classified elsewhere CC
CC Excl: See code: M01.X0

M01.X8 Direct infection of vertebrae in infectious and parasitic diseases classified elsewhere CC
CC Excl: See code: M01.X0

M01.X9 Direct infection of multiple joints in infectious and parasitic diseases classified elsewhere CC
CC Excl: See code: M01.X0

N Newborn: 0   P Pediatric: 0-17   M Maternity: 12-55   A Adult: 15-124   MCC Major CC Condition   PDx MCC PDx acts as own MCC   CC CC Condition   PDx CC PDx acts as own CC

684   ICD-10-CM Draft (2015)

✓4th **M02　Postinfective and reactive arthropathies**

Code first underlying disease, such as:
congenital syphilis [Clutton's joints] (A50.5)
enteritis due to Yersinia enterocolitica (A04.6)
infective endocarditis (I33.0)
viral hepatitis (B15-B19)

　EXCLUDES 1　Behçet's disease (M35.2)
direct infections of joint in infectious and parasitic diseases classified elsewhere (M01.-)
mumps arthritis (B26.85)
postmeningococcal arthritis (A39.84)
rheumatic fever (I00)
rubella arthritis (B06.82)
syphilis arthritis (late) (A52.77)
tabetic arthropathy [Charcôt's] (A52.16)

✓5th **M02.0　Arthropathy following intestinal bypass**

　M02.00　Arthropathy following intestinal bypass, unspecified site

✓6th 　**M02.01　Arthropathy following intestinal bypass, shoulder**
　　M02.011　Arthropathy following intestinal bypass, right shoulder
　　M02.012　Arthropathy following intestinal bypass, left shoulder
　　M02.019　Arthropathy following intestinal bypass, unspecified shoulder

✓6th 　**M02.02　Arthropathy following intestinal bypass, elbow**
　　M02.021　Arthropathy following intestinal bypass, right elbow
　　M02.022　Arthropathy following intestinal bypass, left elbow
　　M02.029　Arthropathy following intestinal bypass, unspecified elbow

✓6th 　**M02.03　Arthropathy following intestinal bypass, wrist**
　　Arthropathy following intestinal bypass, carpal bones
　　M02.031　Arthropathy following intestinal bypass, right wrist
　　M02.032　Arthropathy following intestinal bypass, left wrist
　　M02.039　Arthropathy following intestinal bypass, unspecified wrist

✓6th 　**M02.04　Arthropathy following intestinal bypass, hand**
　　Arthropathy following intestinal bypass, metacarpals and phalanges
　　M02.041　Arthropathy following intestinal bypass, right hand
　　M02.042　Arthropathy following intestinal bypass, left hand
　　M02.049　Arthropathy following intestinal bypass, unspecified hand

✓6th 　**M02.05　Arthropathy following intestinal bypass, hip**
　　M02.051　Arthropathy following intestinal bypass, right hip
　　M02.052　Arthropathy following intestinal bypass, left hip
　　M02.059　Arthropathy following intestinal bypass, unspecified hip

✓6th 　**M02.06　Arthropathy following intestinal bypass, knee**
　　M02.061　Arthropathy following intestinal bypass, right knee
　　M02.062　Arthropathy following intestinal bypass, left knee
　　M02.069　Arthropathy following intestinal bypass, unspecified knee

✓6th 　**M02.07　Arthropathy following intestinal bypass, ankle and foot**
　　Arthropathy following intestinal bypass, tarsus, metatarsus and phalanges
　　M02.071　Arthropathy following intestinal bypass, right ankle and foot
　　M02.072　Arthropathy following intestinal bypass, left ankle and foot
　　M02.079　Arthropathy following intestinal bypass, unspecified ankle and foot

　M02.08　Arthropathy following intestinal bypass, vertebrae
　M02.09　Arthropathy following intestinal bypass, multiple sites

✓5th **M02.1　Postdysenteric arthropathy**

　M02.10　Postdysenteric arthropathy, unspecified site　cc
　　CC Excl: A02.23, A17.9, A18.02, A18.09, A18.82, A18.84, A18.89, A39.83-A39.84, A54.40, A54.42-A54.43, A54.82, A54.84, A54.89-A54.9, B06.82, M00.00, M00.019, M00.029, M00.039, M00.049, M00.059, M00.069, M00.079, M00.08-M02.30, M02.319, M02.329, M02.339, M02.349, M02.359, M02.369, M02.379-M02.9, M05.40-M05.59, M05.70-M06.09, M06.20-M06.39, M06.80-M07.69, M11.00-M11.9, M12.10-M15.0, M15.3-M15.9, M16.2-M16.9, M17.2-M17.9, M18.2-M18.9, M19.111-M19.93, M24.10-M24.176, M25.00, M25.08-M25.18, M25.40-M25.676, M25.80-M25.9, M35.2, M36.1-M36.4, R29.4

✓6th 　**M02.11　Postdysenteric arthropathy, shoulder**
　　M02.111　Postdysenteric arthropathy, right shoulder　cc
　　　CC Excl: See code: M02.10
　　M02.112　Postdysenteric arthropathy, left shoulder　cc
　　　CC Excl: See code: M02.10
　　M02.119　Postdysenteric arthropathy, unspecified shoulder　cc
　　　CC Excl: See code: M02.10

✓6th 　**M02.12　Postdysenteric arthropathy, elbow**
　　M02.121　Postdysenteric arthropathy, right elbow　cc
　　　CC Excl: See code: M02.10
　　M02.122　Postdysenteric arthropathy, left elbow　cc
　　　CC Excl: See code: M02.10
　　M02.129　Postdysenteric arthropathy, unspecified elbow　cc
　　　CC Excl: See code: M02.10

✓6th 　**M02.13　Postdysenteric arthropathy, wrist**
　　Postdysenteric arthropathy, carpal bones
　　M02.131　Postdysenteric arthropathy, right wrist　cc
　　　CC Excl: See code: M02.10
　　M02.132　Postdysenteric arthropathy, left wrist　cc
　　　CC Excl: See code: M02.10
　　M02.139　Postdysenteric arthropathy, unspecified wrist　cc
　　　CC Excl: See code: M02.10

✓6th 　**M02.14　Postdysenteric arthropathy, hand**
　　Postdysenteric arthropathy, metacarpus and phalanges
　　M02.141　Postdysenteric arthropathy, right hand　cc
　　　CC Excl: See code: M02.10
　　M02.142　Postdysenteric arthropathy, left hand　cc
　　　CC Excl: See code: M02.10
　　M02.149　Postdysenteric arthropathy, unspecified hand　cc
　　　CC Excl: See code: M02.10

✓6th 　**M02.15　Postdysenteric arthropathy, hip**
　　M02.151　Postdysenteric arthropathy, right hip　cc
　　　CC Excl: See code: M02.10
　　M02.152　Postdysenteric arthropathy, left hip　cc
　　　CC Excl: See code: M02.10
　　M02.159　Postdysenteric arthropathy, unspecified hip　cc
　　　CC Excl: See code: M02.10

✓6th 　**M02.16　Postdysenteric arthropathy, knee**
　　M02.161　Postdysenteric arthropathy, right knee　cc
　　　CC Excl: A02.23, A17.9, A18.02, A18.09, A18.82, A18.84, A18.89, A39.83-A39.84, A54.40, A54.42-A54.43, A54.82, A54.84, A54.89-A54.9, B06.82, M00.00, M00.019, M00.029, M00.039, M00.049, M00.059, M00.069, M00.079, M00.08-M02.30, M02.319, M02.329, M02.339, M02.349, M02.359, M02.369, M02.379-M02.9, M05.40-M05.59, M05.70-M06.09, M06.20-M06.39, M06.80-M07.69, M11.00-M11.9, M12.10-M12.179, M12.19-M15.0, M15.3-M15.9, M16.2-M16.9, M17.2-M17.9, M18.2-M18.9, M19.111-M19.93, M24.10-M24.176, M25.00, M25.08-M25.18, M25.40-M25.676, M25.80-M25.9, M35.2, M36.1-M36.4, R29.4
　　M02.162　Postdysenteric arthropathy, left knee　cc
　　　CC Excl: See code: M02.161
　　M02.169　Postdysenteric arthropathy, unspecified knee　cc
　　　CC Excl: See code: M02.161

✓ Additional Character Required　　✓x7th Xtension Alert　　Unacceptable PDx　　Manifestation　　Hospital Acquired Condition　　*EXCLUDES 1* Not Coded Here　　*EXCLUDES 2* Not Included Here

✓6th **M02.17 Postdysenteric arthropathy, ankle and foot**
Postdysenteric arthropathy, tarsus, metatarsus and phalanges

    M02.171 Postdysenteric arthropathy, right ankle and foot `CC`
        CC Excl: See code: M02.10

    M02.172 Postdysenteric arthropathy, left ankle and foot `CC`
        CC Excl: See code: M02.10

    M02.179 Postdysenteric arthropathy, unspecified ankle and foot `CC`
        CC Excl: See code: M02.10

  M02.18 Postdysenteric arthropathy, vertebrae `CC`
    CC Excl: See code: M02.10

  M02.19 Postdysenteric arthropathy, multiple sites `CC`
    CC Excl: See code: M02.10

✓5th **M02.2 Postimmunization arthropathy**

  M02.20 Postimmunization arthropathy, unspecified site

✓6th **M02.21 Postimmunization arthropathy, shoulder**

    M02.211 Postimmunization arthropathy, right shoulder

    M02.212 Postimmunization arthropathy, left shoulder

    M02.219 Postimmunization arthropathy, unspecified shoulder

✓6th **M02.22 Postimmunization arthropathy, elbow**

    M02.221 Postimmunization arthropathy, right elbow

    M02.222 Postimmunization arthropathy, left elbow

    M02.229 Postimmunization arthropathy, unspecified elbow

✓6th **M02.23 Postimmunization arthropathy, wrist**
Postimmunization arthropathy, carpal bones

    M02.231 Postimmunization arthropathy, right wrist

    M02.232 Postimmunization arthropathy, left wrist

    M02.239 Postimmunization arthropathy, unspecified wrist

✓6th **M02.24 Postimmunization arthropathy, hand**
Postimmunization arthropathy, metacarpus and phalanges

    M02.241 Postimmunization arthropathy, right hand

    M02.242 Postimmunization arthropathy, left hand

    M02.249 Postimmunization arthropathy, unspecified hand

✓6th **M02.25 Postimmunization arthropathy, hip**

    M02.251 Postimmunization arthropathy, right hip

    M02.252 Postimmunization arthropathy, left hip

    M02.259 Postimmunization arthropathy, unspecified hip

✓6th **M02.26 Postimmunization arthropathy, knee**

    M02.261 Postimmunization arthropathy, right knee

    M02.262 Postimmunization arthropathy, left knee

    M02.269 Postimmunization arthropathy, unspecified knee

✓6th **M02.27 Postimmunization arthropathy, ankle and foot**
Postimmunization arthropathy, tarsus, metatarsus and phalanges

    M02.271 Postimmunization arthropathy, right ankle and foot

    M02.272 Postimmunization arthropathy, left ankle and foot

    M02.279 Postimmunization arthropathy, unspecified ankle and foot

  M02.28 Postimmunization arthropathy, vertebrae

  M02.29 Postimmunization arthropathy, multiple sites

✓5th **M02.3 Reiter's disease**
Reactive arthritis

  M02.30 Reiter's disease, unspecified site `PDx` `CC`
    CC Excl: A02.23, A17.9, A18.02, A18.09, A18.82, A18.84, A18.89, A39.83-A39.84, A54.40, A54.42-A54.43, A54.82, A54.84, A54.89-A54.9, B06.82, M00.00, M00.019, M00.029, M00.039, M00.049, M00.059, M00.069, M00.079, M00.08-M02.30, M02.319, M02.329, M02.339, M02.349, M02.359, M02.369, M02.379-M02.9, M05.40-M05.59, M05.70-M06.09, M06.20-M06.39, M06.80-M07.69, M11.00-M11.9, M12.10-M15.0, M15.3-M15.9, M16.2-M16.9, M17.2-M17.9, M18.2-M18.9, M19.111-M19.93, M24.10-M24.176, M25.00, M25.08-M25.18, M25.40-M25.676, M25.80-M25.9, M35.2, M36.1-M36.4, R29.4

✓6th **M02.31 Reiter's disease, shoulder**

    M02.311 Reiter's disease, right shoulder `PDx CC` `CC`
        CC Excl: See code: M02.30

    M02.312 Reiter's disease, left shoulder `PDx CC` `CC`
        CC Excl: See code: M02.30

    M02.319 Reiter's disease, unspecified shoulder `PDx CC` `CC`
        CC Excl: See code: M02.30

✓6th **M02.32 Reiter's disease, elbow**

    M02.321 Reiter's disease, right elbow `PDx CC` `CC`
        CC Excl: See code: M02.30

    M02.322 Reiter's disease, left elbow `PDx CC` `CC`
        CC Excl: See code: M02.30

    M02.329 Reiter's disease, unspecified elbow `PDx CC` `CC`
        CC Excl: See code: M02.30

✓6th **M02.33 Reiter's disease, wrist**
Reiter's disease, carpal bones

    M02.331 Reiter's disease, right wrist `PDx CC` `CC`
        CC Excl: See code: M02.30

    M02.332 Reiter's disease, left wrist `PDx CC` `CC`
        CC Excl: See code: M02.30

    M02.339 Reiter's disease, unspecified wrist `PDx CC` `CC`
        CC Excl: See code: M02.30

✓6th **M02.34 Reiter's disease, hand**
Reiter's disease, metacarpus and phalanges

    M02.341 Reiter's disease, right hand `PDx CC` `CC`
        CC Excl: See code: M02.30

    M02.342 Reiter's disease, left hand `PDx CC` `CC`
        CC Excl: See code: M02.30

    M02.349 Reiter's disease, unspecified hand `PDx CC` `CC`
        CC Excl: See code: M02.30

✓6th **M02.35 Reiter's disease, hip**

    M02.351 Reiter's disease, right hip `PDx CC` `CC`
        CC Excl: See code: M02.30

    M02.352 Reiter's disease, left hip `PDx CC` `CC`
        CC Excl: See code: M02.30

    M02.359 Reiter's disease, unspecified hip `PDx CC` `CC`
        CC Excl: See code: M02.30

✓6th **M02.36 Reiter's disease, knee**

    M02.361 Reiter's disease, right knee `PDx CC` `CC`
        CC Excl: See code: M02.30

    M02.362 Reiter's disease, left knee `PDx CC` `CC`
        CC Excl: See code: M02.30

    M02.369 Reiter's disease, unspecified knee `PDx CC` `CC`
        CC Excl: See code: M02.30

✓6th **M02.37 Reiter's disease, ankle and foot**
Reiter's disease, tarsus, metatarsus and phalanges

    M02.371 Reiter's disease, right ankle and foot `PDx CC` `CC`
        CC Excl: See code: M02.30

    M02.372 Reiter's disease, left ankle and foot `PDx CC` `CC`
        CC Excl: See code: M02.30

    M02.379 Reiter's disease, unspecified ankle and foot `PDx CC` `CC`
        CC Excl: See code: M02.30

  M02.38 Reiter's disease, vertebrae `PDx CC` `CC`
    CC Excl: See code: M02.30

  M02.39 Reiter's disease, multiple sites `PDx CC` `CC`
    CC Excl: See code: M02.30

N Newborn: 0   P Pediatric: 0-17   M Maternity: 12-55   A Adult: 15-124   MCC Major CC Condition   PDx MCC PDx acts as own MCC   CC CC Condition   PDx CC PDx acts as own CC

686   ICD-10-CM Draft (2015)

✓5ᵗʰ **M02.8** Other reactive arthropathies

    M02.80 **Other reactive arthropathies, unspecified site** CC
        CC Excl: See code: M02.30

  ✓6ᵗʰ **M02.81** **Other reactive arthropathies, shoulder**

      M02.811 **Other reactive arthropathies, right** CC
          shoulder
          CC Excl: A02.23, A17.9, A18.02, A18.09,
          A18.82, A18.84, A18.89, A39.83-A39.84,
          A54.40, A54.42-A54.43, A54.82, A54.84,
          A54.89-A54.9, B06.82, M00.00, M00.019,
          M00.029, M00.039, M00.049, M00.059,
          M00.069, M00.079, M00.08-M02.30,
          M02.319, M02.329, M02.339, M02.349,
          M02.359, M02.369, M02.379-M02.9, M05.40-
          M05.59, M05.70-M06.09, M06.20-M06.39,
          M06.80-M07.69, M11.00-M11.9, M12.10-
          M12.419

      M02.812 **Other reactive arthropathies, left** CC
          shoulder
          CC Excl: See code: M02.811

      M02.819 **Other reactive arthropathies,** CC
          unspecified shoulder
          CC Excl: See code: M02.811

  ✓6ᵗʰ **M02.82** **Other reactive arthropathies, elbow**

      M02.821 **Other reactive arthropathies, right** CC
          elbow
          CC Excl: A02.23, A17.9, A18.02, A18.09,
          A18.82, A18.84, A18.89, A39.83-A39.84,
          A54.40, A54.42-A54.43, A54.82, A54.84,
          A54.89-A54.9, B06.82, M00.00, M00.019,
          M00.029, M00.039, M00.049, M00.059,
          M00.069, M00.079, M00.08-M02.30,
          M02.319, M02.329, M02.339, M02.349,
          M02.359, M02.369, M02.379-M02.9, M05.40-
          M05.59, M05.70-M06.09, M06.20-M06.39,
          M06.80-M07.69, M11.00-M11.9, M12.10-
          M15.0, M15.3-M15.9, M16.2-M16.9, M17.2-
          M17.9, M18.2-M18.9, M19.111-M19.93,
          M24.10-M24.176, M25.00, M25.08-M25.18,
          M25.40-M25.676, M25.80-M25.9, M35.2,
          M36.1-M36.4, R29.4

      M02.822 **Other reactive arthropathies,** CC
          left elbow
          CC Excl: See code: M02.821

      M02.829 **Other reactive arthropathies,** CC
          unspecified elbow
          CC Excl: See code: M02.821

  ✓6ᵗʰ **M02.83** **Other reactive arthropathies, wrist**
        Other reactive arthropathies, carpal bones

      M02.831 **Other reactive arthropathies,** CC
          right wrist
          CC Excl: See code: M02.821

      M02.832 **Other reactive arthropathies,** CC
          left wrist
          CC Excl: See code: M02.821

      M02.839 **Other reactive arthropathies,** CC
          unspecified wrist
          CC Excl: See code: M02.821

  ✓6ᵗʰ **M02.84** **Other reactive arthropathies, hand**
        Other reactive arthropathies, metacarpus and
        phalanges

      M02.841 **Other reactive arthropathies, right** CC
          hand
          CC Excl: See code: M02.821

      M02.842 **Other reactive arthropathies, left** CC
          hand
          CC Excl: See code: M02.821

      M02.849 **Other reactive arthropathies,** CC
          unspecified hand
          CC Excl: See code: M02.821

  ✓6ᵗʰ **M02.85** **Other reactive arthropathies, hip**

      M02.851 **Other reactive arthropathies, right hip** CC
          CC Excl: See code: M02.821

      M02.852 **Other reactive arthropathies, left hip** CC
          CC Excl: See code: M02.821

      M02.859 **Other reactive arthropathies,** CC
          unspecified hip
          CC Excl: See code: M02.821

  ✓6ᵗʰ **M02.86** **Other reactive arthropathies, knee**

      M02.861 **Other reactive arthropathies,** CC
          right knee

      M02.862 **Other reactive arthropathies,** CC
          left knee
          CC Excl: See code: M02.821

      M02.869 **Other reactive arthropathies,** CC
          unspecified knee
          CC Excl: See code: M02.821

  ✓6ᵗʰ **M02.87** **Other reactive arthropathies, ankle and foot**
        Other reactive arthropathies, tarsus, metatarsus and
        phalanges

      M02.871 **Other reactive arthropathies, right** CC
          ankle and foot
          CC Excl: See code: M02.821

      M02.872 **Other reactive arthropathies, left** CC
          ankle and foot
          CC Excl: See code: M02.821

      M02.879 **Other reactive arthropathies,** CC
          unspecified ankle and foot
          CC Excl: See code: M02.821

    M02.88 *Other reactive arthropathies, vertebrae* CC
        CC Excl: See code: M02.821

    M02.89 *Other reactive arthropathies, multiple sites* CC
        CC Excl: See code: M02.821

  M02.9 *Reactive arthropathy, unspecified*

Inflammatory polyarthropathies (M05-M14)

✓4ᵗʰ **M05** **Rheumatoid arthritis with rheumatoid factor**
    EXCLUDES 1   rheumatic fever (I00)
                juvenile rheumatoid arthritis (M08.-)
                rheumatoid arthritis of spine (M45.-)

  ✓5ᵗʰ **M05.0** **Felty's syndrome**
        Rheumatoid arthritis with splenoadenomegaly and leukopenia

    M05.00 **Felty's syndrome, unspecified site**

    ✓6ᵗʰ **M05.01** **Felty's syndrome, shoulder**
      M05.011 **Felty's syndrome, right shoulder**
      M05.012 **Felty's syndrome, left shoulder**
      M05.019 **Felty's syndrome, unspecified shoulder**

    ✓6ᵗʰ **M05.02** **Felty's syndrome, elbow**
      M05.021 **Felty's syndrome, right elbow**
      M05.022 **Felty's syndrome, left elbow**
      M05.029 **Felty's syndrome, unspecified elbow**

    ✓6ᵗʰ **M05.03** **Felty's syndrome, wrist**
        Felty's syndrome, carpal bones
      M05.031 **Felty's syndrome, right wrist**
      M05.032 **Felty's syndrome, left wrist**
      M05.039 **Felty's syndrome, unspecified wrist**

    ✓6ᵗʰ **M05.04** **Felty's syndrome, hand**
        Felty's syndrome, metacarpus and phalanges
      M05.041 **Felty's syndrome, right hand**
      M05.042 **Felty's syndrome, left hand**
      M05.049 **Felty's syndrome, unspecified hand**

    ✓6ᵗʰ **M05.05** **Felty's syndrome, hip**
      M05.051 **Felty's syndrome, right hip**
      M05.052 **Felty's syndrome, left hip**
      M05.059 **Felty's syndrome, unspecified hip**

    ✓6ᵗʰ **M05.06** **Felty's syndrome, knee**
      M05.061 **Felty's syndrome, right knee**
      M05.062 **Felty's syndrome, left knee**
      M05.069 **Felty's syndrome, unspecified knee**

    ✓6ᵗʰ **M05.07** **Felty's syndrome, ankle and foot**
        Felty's syndrome, tarsus, metatarsus and phalanges
      M05.071 **Felty's syndrome, right ankle and foot**
      M05.072 **Felty's syndrome, left ankle and foot**
      M05.079 **Felty's syndrome, unspecified ankle and
          foot**

    M05.09 **Felty's syndrome, multiple sites**

  ✓5ᵗʰ **M05.1** **Rheumatoid lung disease with rheumatoid arthritis**

    M05.10 **Rheumatoid lung disease with rheumatoid arthritis
        of unspecified site**

    ✓6ᵗʰ **M05.11** **Rheumatoid lung disease with rheumatoid arthritis
        of shoulder**
      M05.111 **Rheumatoid lung disease with
          rheumatoid arthritis of right shoulder**
      M05.112 **Rheumatoid lung disease with
          rheumatoid arthritis of left shoulder**

✓ Additional Character Required   ✓x7ᵗʰ Xtension Alert   Unacceptable PDx   Manifestation   Hospital Acquired Condition   EXCLUDES 1 Not Coded Here   EXCLUDES 2 Not Included Here

Diseases of the Musculoskeletal System and Connective Tissue

M05.119–M05.331

M05.119 Rheumatoid lung disease with rheumatoid arthritis of unspecified shoulder

✓6ᵗʰ **M05.12** Rheumatoid lung disease with rheumatoid arthritis of elbow

  M05.121 Rheumatoid lung disease with rheumatoid arthritis of right elbow

  M05.122 Rheumatoid lung disease with rheumatoid arthritis of left elbow

  M05.129 Rheumatoid lung disease with rheumatoid arthritis of unspecified elbow

✓6ᵗʰ **M05.13** Rheumatoid lung disease with rheumatoid arthritis of wrist
  Rheumatoid lung disease with rheumatoid arthritis, carpal bones

  M05.131 Rheumatoid lung disease with rheumatoid arthritis of right wrist

  M05.132 Rheumatoid lung disease with rheumatoid arthritis of left wrist

  M05.139 Rheumatoid lung disease with rheumatoid arthritis of unspecified wrist

✓6ᵗʰ **M05.14** Rheumatoid lung disease with rheumatoid arthritis of hand
  Rheumatoid lung disease with rheumatoid arthritis, metacarpus and phalanges

  M05.141 Rheumatoid lung disease with rheumatoid arthritis of right hand

  M05.142 Rheumatoid lung disease with rheumatoid arthritis of left hand

  M05.149 Rheumatoid lung disease with rheumatoid arthritis of unspecified hand

✓6ᵗʰ **M05.15** Rheumatoid lung disease with rheumatoid arthritis of hip

  M05.151 Rheumatoid lung disease with rheumatoid arthritis of right hip

  M05.152 Rheumatoid lung disease with rheumatoid arthritis of left hip

  M05.159 Rheumatoid lung disease with rheumatoid arthritis of unspecified hip

✓6ᵗʰ **M05.16** Rheumatoid lung disease with rheumatoid arthritis of knee

  M05.161 Rheumatoid lung disease with rheumatoid arthritis of right knee

  M05.162 Rheumatoid lung disease with rheumatoid arthritis of left knee

  M05.169 Rheumatoid lung disease with rheumatoid arthritis of unspecified knee

✓6ᵗʰ **M05.17** Rheumatoid lung disease with rheumatoid arthritis of ankle and foot
  Rheumatoid lung disease with rheumatoid arthritis, tarsus, metatarsus and phalanges

  M05.171 Rheumatoid lung disease with rheumatoid arthritis of right ankle and foot

  M05.172 Rheumatoid lung disease with rheumatoid arthritis of left ankle and foot

  M05.179 Rheumatoid lung disease with rheumatoid arthritis of unspecified ankle and foot

M05.19 Rheumatoid lung disease with rheumatoid arthritis of multiple sites

✓5ᵗʰ **M05.2** Rheumatoid vasculitis with rheumatoid arthritis

  M05.20 Rheumatoid vasculitis with rheumatoid arthritis of unspecified site

✓6ᵗʰ **M05.21** Rheumatoid vasculitis with rheumatoid arthritis of shoulder

  M05.211 Rheumatoid vasculitis with rheumatoid arthritis of right shoulder

  M05.212 Rheumatoid vasculitis with rheumatoid arthritis of left shoulder

  M05.219 Rheumatoid vasculitis with rheumatoid arthritis of unspecified shoulder

✓6ᵗʰ **M05.22** Rheumatoid vasculitis with rheumatoid arthritis of elbow

  M05.221 Rheumatoid vasculitis with rheumatoid arthritis of right elbow

  M05.222 Rheumatoid vasculitis with rheumatoid arthritis of left elbow

  M05.229 Rheumatoid vasculitis with rheumatoid arthritis of unspecified elbow

✓6ᵗʰ **M05.23** Rheumatoid vasculitis with rheumatoid arthritis of wrist
  Rheumatoid vasculitis with rheumatoid arthritis, carpal bones

  M05.231 Rheumatoid vasculitis with rheumatoid arthritis of right wrist

  M05.232 Rheumatoid vasculitis with rheumatoid arthritis of left wrist

  M05.239 Rheumatoid vasculitis with rheumatoid arthritis of unspecified wrist

✓6ᵗʰ **M05.24** Rheumatoid vasculitis with rheumatoid arthritis of hand
  Rheumatoid vasculitis with rheumatoid arthritis, metacarpus and phalanges

  M05.241 Rheumatoid vasculitis with rheumatoid arthritis of right hand

  M05.242 Rheumatoid vasculitis with rheumatoid arthritis of left hand

  M05.249 Rheumatoid vasculitis with rheumatoid arthritis of unspecified hand

✓6ᵗʰ **M05.25** Rheumatoid vasculitis with rheumatoid arthritis of hip

  M05.251 Rheumatoid vasculitis with rheumatoid arthritis of right hip

  M05.252 Rheumatoid vasculitis with rheumatoid arthritis of left hip

  M05.259 Rheumatoid vasculitis with rheumatoid arthritis of unspecified hip

✓6ᵗʰ **M05.26** Rheumatoid vasculitis with rheumatoid arthritis of knee

  M05.261 Rheumatoid vasculitis with rheumatoid arthritis of right knee

  M05.262 Rheumatoid vasculitis with rheumatoid arthritis of left knee

  M05.269 Rheumatoid vasculitis with rheumatoid arthritis of unspecified knee

✓6ᵗʰ **M05.27** Rheumatoid vasculitis with rheumatoid arthritis of ankle and foot
  Rheumatoid vasculitis with rheumatoid arthritis, tarsus, metatarsus and phalanges

  M05.271 Rheumatoid vasculitis with rheumatoid arthritis of right ankle and foot

  M05.272 Rheumatoid vasculitis with rheumatoid arthritis of left ankle and foot

  M05.279 Rheumatoid vasculitis with rheumatoid arthritis of unspecified ankle and foot

M05.29 Rheumatoid vasculitis with rheumatoid arthritis of multiple sites

✓5ᵗʰ **M05.3** Rheumatoid heart disease with rheumatoid arthritis
  Rheumatoid carditis   Rheumatoid myocarditis
  Rheumatoid endocarditis   Rheumatoid pericarditis

  M05.30 Rheumatoid heart disease with rheumatoid arthritis of unspecified site

✓6ᵗʰ **M05.31** Rheumatoid heart disease with rheumatoid arthritis of shoulder

  M05.311 Rheumatoid heart disease with rheumatoid arthritis of right shoulder

  M05.312 Rheumatoid heart disease with rheumatoid arthritis of left shoulder

  M05.319 Rheumatoid heart disease with rheumatoid arthritis of unspecified shoulder

✓6ᵗʰ **M05.32** Rheumatoid heart disease with rheumatoid arthritis of elbow

  M05.321 Rheumatoid heart disease with rheumatoid arthritis of right elbow

  M05.322 Rheumatoid heart disease with rheumatoid arthritis of left elbow

  M05.329 Rheumatoid heart disease with rheumatoid arthritis of unspecified elbow

✓6ᵗʰ **M05.33** Rheumatoid heart disease with rheumatoid arthritis of wrist
  Rheumatoid heart disease with rheumatoid arthritis, carpal bones

  M05.331 Rheumatoid heart disease with rheumatoid arthritis of right wrist

Ⓝ Newborn: 0   Ⓟ Pediatric: 0-17   Ⓜ Maternity: 12-55   Ⓐ Adult: 15-124   MCC Major CC Condition   PDx MCC PDx acts as own MCC   CC CC Condition   PDx CC PDx acts as own CC

688   ICD-10-CM Draft (2015)

M05.332 **Rheumatoid heart disease with rheumatoid arthritis of** left **wrist**

M05.339 **Rheumatoid heart disease with rheumatoid arthritis of** unspecified **wrist**

√6th M05.34 **Rheumatoid heart disease with rheumatoid arthritis of** hand

Rheumatoid heart disease with rheumatoid arthritis, metacarpus and phalanges

M05.341 **Rheumatoid heart disease with rheumatoid arthritis of** right **hand**

M05.342 **Rheumatoid heart disease with rheumatoid arthritis of** left **hand**

M05.349 **Rheumatoid heart disease with rheumatoid arthritis of** unspecified **hand**

√6th M05.35 **Rheumatoid heart disease with rheumatoid arthritis of** hip

M05.351 **Rheumatoid heart disease with rheumatoid arthritis of** right **hip**

M05.352 **Rheumatoid heart disease with rheumatoid arthritis of** left **hip**

M05.359 **Rheumatoid heart disease with rheumatoid arthritis of** unspecified **hip**

√6th M05.36 **Rheumatoid heart disease with rheumatoid arthritis of** knee

M05.361 **Rheumatoid heart disease with rheumatoid arthritis of** right **knee**

M05.362 **Rheumatoid heart disease with rheumatoid arthritis of** left **knee**

M05.369 **Rheumatoid heart disease with rheumatoid arthritis of** unspecified **knee**

√6th M05.37 **Rheumatoid heart disease with rheumatoid arthritis of** ankle and foot

Rheumatoid heart disease with rheumatoid arthritis, tarsus, metatarsus and phalanges

M05.371 **Rheumatoid heart disease with rheumatoid arthritis of** right **ankle and foot**

M05.372 **Rheumatoid heart disease with rheumatoid arthritis of** left **ankle and foot**

M05.379 **Rheumatoid heart disease with rheumatoid arthritis of** unspecified **ankle and foot**

M05.39 **Rheumatoid heart disease with rheumatoid arthritis of** multiple sites

√5th M05.4 **Rheumatoid** myopathy with rheumatoid arthritis

CC Excl: For all CC codes in subcategory M05.4, unless otherwise noted: E08.40-E08.49, E08.618-E08.638, E08.649-E08.8, E09.40-E09.49, E09.618-E09.638, E09.649-E09.8, E10.40-E10.49, E10.618-E10.638, E10.649, E10.69-E10.8, E11.40-E11.49, E11.618-E11.638, E11.649, E11.69-E11.8, E13.40-E13.49, E13.618-E13.638, E13.649-E13.8, G32.89, G70.00-G72.3, G72.81-G73.7, G96.8-G96.9, G98.0-G98.8, G99.8

M05.40 **Rheumatoid myopathy with rheumatoid arthritis of** unspecified **site** `PDx CC CC`

√6th M05.41 **Rheumatoid myopathy with rheumatoid arthritis of** shoulder

M05.411 **Rheumatoid myopathy with rheumatoid arthritis of** right **shoulder** `PDx CC CC`

M05.412 **Rheumatoid myopathy with rheumatoid arthritis of** left **shoulder** `PDx CC CC`

M05.419 **Rheumatoid myopathy with rheumatoid arthritis of** unspecified **shoulder** `PDx CC CC`

√6th M05.42 **Rheumatoid myopathy with rheumatoid arthritis of** elbow

M05.421 **Rheumatoid myopathy with rheumatoid arthritis of** right **elbow** `PDx CC CC`

M05.422 **Rheumatoid myopathy with rheumatoid arthritis of** left **elbow** `PDx CC CC`

M05.429 **Rheumatoid myopathy with rheumatoid arthritis of** unspecified **elbow** `PDx CC CC`

√6th M05.43 **Rheumatoid myopathy with rheumatoid arthritis of** wrist

Rheumatoid myopathy with rheumatoid arthritis, carpal bones

M05.431 **Rheumatoid myopathy with rheumatoid arthritis of** right **wrist** `PDx CC CC`

M05.432 **Rheumatoid myopathy with rheumatoid arthritis of** left **wrist** `PDx CC CC`

M05.439 **Rheumatoid myopathy with rheumatoid arthritis of** unspecified **wrist** `PDx CC CC`

√6th M05.44 **Rheumatoid myopathy with rheumatoid arthritis of** hand

Rheumatoid myopathy with rheumatoid arthritis, metacarpus and phalanges

M05.441 **Rheumatoid myopathy with rheumatoid arthritis of** right **hand** `PDx CC CC`

M05.442 **Rheumatoid myopathy with rheumatoid arthritis of** left **hand** `PDx CC CC`

M05.449 **Rheumatoid myopathy with rheumatoid arthritis of** unspecified **hand** `PDx CC CC`

√6th M05.45 **Rheumatoid myopathy with rheumatoid arthritis of** hip

M05.451 **Rheumatoid myopathy with rheumatoid arthritis of** right **hip** `PDx CC CC`

M05.452 **Rheumatoid myopathy with rheumatoid arthritis of** left **hip** `PDx CC CC`

M05.459 **Rheumatoid myopathy with rheumatoid arthritis of** unspecified **hip** `PDx CC CC`

√6th M05.46 **Rheumatoid myopathy with rheumatoid arthritis of** knee

M05.461 **Rheumatoid myopathy with rheumatoid arthritis of** right **knee** `PDx CC CC`

M05.462 **Rheumatoid myopathy with rheumatoid arthritis of** left **knee** `PDx CC CC`

M05.469 **Rheumatoid myopathy with rheumatoid arthritis of** unspecified **knee** `PDx CC CC`

√6th M05.47 **Rheumatoid myopathy with rheumatoid arthritis of** ankle and foot

Rheumatoid myopathy with rheumatoid arthritis, tarsus, metatarsus and phalanges

M05.471 **Rheumatoid myopathy with rheumatoid arthritis of** right **ankle and foot** `PDx CC CC`

M05.472 **Rheumatoid myopathy with rheumatoid arthritis of** left **ankle and foot** `PDx CC CC`

M05.479 **Rheumatoid myopathy with rheumatoid arthritis of** unspecified **ankle and foot** `PDx CC CC`

M05.49 **Rheumatoid myopathy with rheumatoid arthritis of** multiple sites `PDx CC CC`

√5th M05.5 **Rheumatoid** polyneuropathy with rheumatoid arthritis

M05.50 **Rheumatoid polyneuropathy with rheumatoid arthritis of** unspecified **site**

√6th M05.51 **Rheumatoid polyneuropathy with rheumatoid arthritis of** shoulder

M05.511 **Rheumatoid polyneuropathy with rheumatoid arthritis of** right **shoulder**

M05.512 **Rheumatoid polyneuropathy with rheumatoid arthritis of** left **shoulder**

M05.519 **Rheumatoid polyneuropathy with rheumatoid arthritis of** unspecified **shoulder**

√6th M05.52 **Rheumatoid polyneuropathy with rheumatoid arthritis of** elbow

M05.521 **Rheumatoid polyneuropathy with rheumatoid arthritis of** right **elbow**

M05.522 **Rheumatoid polyneuropathy with rheumatoid arthritis of** left **elbow**

M05.529 **Rheumatoid polyneuropathy with rheumatoid arthritis of** unspecified **elbow**

√6th M05.53 **Rheumatoid polyneuropathy with rheumatoid arthritis of** wrist

Rheumatoid polyneuropathy with rheumatoid arthritis, carpal bones

M05.531 **Rheumatoid polyneuropathy with rheumatoid arthritis of** right **wrist**

M05.532 **Rheumatoid polyneuropathy with rheumatoid arthritis of** left **wrist**

M05.539 **Rheumatoid polyneuropathy with rheumatoid arthritis of** unspecified **wrist**

✔ Additional Character Required   √x7th Xtension Alert   Unacceptable PDx   Manifestation   Hospital Acquired Condition   EXCLUDES 1 Not Coded Here   EXCLUDES 2 Not Included Here

ICD-10-CM Draft (2015)   689

Diseases of the Musculoskeletal System and Connective Tissue

M05.54–M05.732

√6ᵗʰ **M05.54 Rheumatoid polyneuropathy with rheumatoid arthritis of hand**
Rheumatoid polyneuropathy with rheumatoid arthritis, metacarpus and phalanges

- **M05.541 Rheumatoid polyneuropathy with rheumatoid arthritis of right hand**
- **M05.542 Rheumatoid polyneuropathy with rheumatoid arthritis of left hand**
- **M05.549 Rheumatoid polyneuropathy with rheumatoid arthritis of unspecified hand**

√6ᵗʰ **M05.55 Rheumatoid polyneuropathy with rheumatoid arthritis of hip**

- **M05.551 Rheumatoid polyneuropathy with rheumatoid arthritis of right hip**
- **M05.552 Rheumatoid polyneuropathy with rheumatoid arthritis of left hip**
- **M05.559 Rheumatoid polyneuropathy with rheumatoid arthritis of unspecified hip**

√6ᵗʰ **M05.56 Rheumatoid polyneuropathy with rheumatoid arthritis of knee**

- **M05.561 Rheumatoid polyneuropathy with rheumatoid arthritis of right knee**
- **M05.562 Rheumatoid polyneuropathy with rheumatoid arthritis of left knee**
- **M05.569 Rheumatoid polyneuropathy with rheumatoid arthritis of unspecified knee**

√6ᵗʰ **M05.57 Rheumatoid polyneuropathy with rheumatoid arthritis of ankle and foot**
Rheumatoid polyneuropathy with rheumatoid arthritis, tarsus, metatarsus and phalanges

- **M05.571 Rheumatoid polyneuropathy with rheumatoid arthritis of right ankle and foot**
- **M05.572 Rheumatoid polyneuropathy with rheumatoid arthritis of left ankle and foot**
- **M05.579 Rheumatoid polyneuropathy with rheumatoid arthritis of unspecified ankle and foot**

M05.59 Rheumatoid polyneuropathy with rheumatoid arthritis of multiple sites

√5ᵗʰ **M05.6 Rheumatoid arthritis with involvement of other organs and systems**

- **M05.60 Rheumatoid arthritis of unspecified site with involvement of other organs and systems**

√6ᵗʰ **M05.61 Rheumatoid arthritis of shoulder with involvement of other organs and systems**

- **M05.611 Rheumatoid arthritis of right shoulder with involvement of other organs and systems**
- **M05.612 Rheumatoid arthritis of left shoulder with involvement of other organs and systems**
- **M05.619 Rheumatoid arthritis of unspecified shoulder with involvement of other organs and systems**

√6ᵗʰ **M05.62 Rheumatoid arthritis of elbow with involvement of other organs and systems**

- **M05.621 Rheumatoid arthritis of right elbow with involvement of other organs and systems**
- **M05.622 Rheumatoid arthritis of left elbow with involvement of other organs and systems**
- **M05.629 Rheumatoid arthritis of unspecified elbow with involvement of other organs and systems**

√6ᵗʰ **M05.63 Rheumatoid arthritis of wrist with involvement of other organs and systems**
Rheumatoid arthritis of carpal bones with involvement of other organs and systems

- **M05.631 Rheumatoid arthritis of right wrist with involvement of other organs and systems**
- **M05.632 Rheumatoid arthritis of left wrist with involvement of other organs and systems**
- **M05.639 Rheumatoid arthritis of unspecified wrist with involvement of other organs and systems**

√6ᵗʰ **M05.64 Rheumatoid arthritis of hand with involvement of other organs and systems**
Rheumatoid arthritis of metacarpus and phalanges with involvement of other organs and systems

- **M05.641 Rheumatoid arthritis of right hand with involvement of other organs and systems**
- **M05.642 Rheumatoid arthritis of left hand with involvement of other organs and systems**
- **M05.649 Rheumatoid arthritis of unspecified hand with involvement of other organs and systems**

√6ᵗʰ **M05.65 Rheumatoid arthritis of hip with involvement of other organs and systems**

- **M05.651 Rheumatoid arthritis of right hip with involvement of other organs and systems**
- **M05.652 Rheumatoid arthritis of left hip with involvement of other organs and systems**
- **M05.659 Rheumatoid arthritis of unspecified hip with involvement of other organs and systems**

√6ᵗʰ **M05.66 Rheumatoid arthritis of knee with involvement of other organs and systems**

- **M05.661 Rheumatoid arthritis of right knee with involvement of other organs and systems**
- **M05.662 Rheumatoid arthritis of left knee with involvement of other organs and systems**
- **M05.669 Rheumatoid arthritis of unspecified knee with involvement of other organs and systems**

√6ᵗʰ **M05.67 Rheumatoid arthritis of ankle and foot with involvement of other organs and systems**
Rheumatoid arthritis of tarsus, metatarsus and phalanges with involvement of other organs and systems

- **M05.671 Rheumatoid arthritis of right ankle and foot with involvement of other organs and systems**
- **M05.672 Rheumatoid arthritis of left ankle and foot with involvement of other organs and systems**
- **M05.679 Rheumatoid arthritis of unspecified ankle and foot with involvement of other organs and systems**

M05.69 Rheumatoid arthritis of multiple sites with involvement of other organs and systems

√5ᵗʰ **M05.7 Rheumatoid arthritis with rheumatoid factor without organ or systems involvement**

- **M05.70 Rheumatoid arthritis with rheumatoid factor of unspecified site without organ or systems involvement**

√6ᵗʰ **M05.71 Rheumatoid arthritis with rheumatoid factor of shoulder without organ or systems involvement**

- **M05.711 Rheumatoid arthritis with rheumatoid factor of right shoulder without organ or systems involvement**
- **M05.712 Rheumatoid arthritis with rheumatoid factor of left shoulder without organ or systems involvement**
- **M05.719 Rheumatoid arthritis with rheumatoid factor of unspecified shoulder without organ or systems involvement**

√6ᵗʰ **M05.72 Rheumatoid arthritis with rheumatoid factor of elbow without organ or systems involvement**

- **M05.721 Rheumatoid arthritis with rheumatoid factor of right elbow without organ or systems involvement**
- **M05.722 Rheumatoid arthritis with rheumatoid factor of left elbow without organ or systems involvement**
- **M05.729 Rheumatoid arthritis with rheumatoid factor of unspecified elbow without organ or systems involvement**

√6ᵗʰ **M05.73 Rheumatoid arthritis with rheumatoid factor of wrist without organ or systems involvement**

- **M05.731 Rheumatoid arthritis with rheumatoid factor of right wrist without organ or systems involvement**
- **M05.732 Rheumatoid arthritis with rheumatoid factor of left wrist without organ or systems involvement**

Ⓝ Newborn: 0   Ⓟ Pediatric: 0-17   Ⓜ Maternity: 12-55   Ⓐ Adult: 15-124   **MCC** Major CC Condition   **PDx MCC** PDx acts as own MCC   **CC** CC Condition   **PDx CC** PDx acts as own CC

690   ICD-10-CM Draft (2015)

M05.739   Rheumatoid arthritis with rheumatoid factor of unspecified wrist without organ or systems involvement

✓6th **M05.74**   Rheumatoid arthritis with rheumatoid factor of hand without organ or systems involvement

    M05.741   Rheumatoid arthritis with rheumatoid factor of right hand without organ or systems involvement

    M05.742   Rheumatoid arthritis with rheumatoid factor of left hand without organ or systems involvement

    M05.749   Rheumatoid arthritis with rheumatoid factor of unspecified hand without organ or systems involvement

✓6th **M05.75**   Rheumatoid arthritis with rheumatoid factor of hip without organ or systems involvement

    M05.751   Rheumatoid arthritis with rheumatoid factor of right hip without organ or systems involvement

    M05.752   Rheumatoid arthritis with rheumatoid factor of left hip without organ or systems involvement

    M05.759   Rheumatoid arthritis with rheumatoid factor of unspecified hip without organ or systems involvement

✓6th **M05.76**   Rheumatoid arthritis with rheumatoid factor of knee without organ or systems involvement

    M05.761   Rheumatoid arthritis with rheumatoid factor of right knee without organ or systems involvement

    M05.762   Rheumatoid arthritis with rheumatoid factor of left knee without organ or systems involvement

    M05.769   Rheumatoid arthritis with rheumatoid factor of unspecified knee without organ or systems involvement

✓6th **M05.77**   Rheumatoid arthritis with rheumatoid factor of ankle and foot without organ or systems involvement

    M05.771   Rheumatoid arthritis with rheumatoid factor of right ankle and foot without organ or systems involvement

    M05.772   Rheumatoid arthritis with rheumatoid factor of left ankle and foot without organ or systems involvement

    M05.779   Rheumatoid arthritis with rheumatoid factor of unspecified ankle and foot without organ or systems involvement

   M05.79   Rheumatoid arthritis with rheumatoid factor of multiple sites without organ or systems involvement

✓5th **M05.8**   Other rheumatoid arthritis with rheumatoid factor

   M05.80   Other rheumatoid arthritis with rheumatoid factor of unspecified site

✓6th **M05.81**   Other rheumatoid arthritis with rheumatoid factor of shoulder

    M05.811   Other rheumatoid arthritis with rheumatoid factor of right shoulder

    M05.812   Other rheumatoid arthritis with rheumatoid factor of left shoulder

    M05.819   Other rheumatoid arthritis with rheumatoid factor of unspecified shoulder

✓6th **M05.82**   Other rheumatoid arthritis with rheumatoid factor of elbow

    M05.821   Other rheumatoid arthritis with rheumatoid factor of right elbow

    M05.822   Other rheumatoid arthritis with rheumatoid factor of left elbow

    M05.829   Other rheumatoid arthritis with rheumatoid factor of unspecified elbow

✓6th **M05.83**   Other rheumatoid arthritis with rheumatoid factor of wrist

    M05.831   Other rheumatoid arthritis with rheumatoid factor of right wrist

    M05.832   Other rheumatoid arthritis with rheumatoid factor of left wrist

    M05.839   Other rheumatoid arthritis with rheumatoid factor of unspecified wrist

✓6th **M05.84**   Other rheumatoid arthritis with rheumatoid factor of hand

    M05.841   Other rheumatoid arthritis with rheumatoid factor of right hand

    M05.842   Other rheumatoid arthritis with rheumatoid factor of left hand

    M05.849   Other rheumatoid arthritis with rheumatoid factor of unspecified hand

✓6th **M05.85**   Other rheumatoid arthritis with rheumatoid factor of hip

    M05.851   Other rheumatoid arthritis with rheumatoid factor of right hip

    M05.852   Other rheumatoid arthritis with rheumatoid factor of left hip

    M05.859   Other rheumatoid arthritis with rheumatoid factor of unspecified hip

✓6th **M05.86**   Other rheumatoid arthritis with rheumatoid factor of knee

    M05.861   Other rheumatoid arthritis with rheumatoid factor of right knee

    M05.862   Other rheumatoid arthritis with rheumatoid factor of left knee

    M05.869   Other rheumatoid arthritis with rheumatoid factor of unspecified knee

✓6th **M05.87**   Other rheumatoid arthritis with rheumatoid factor of ankle and foot

    M05.871   Other rheumatoid arthritis with rheumatoid factor of right ankle and foot

    M05.872   Other rheumatoid arthritis with rheumatoid factor of left ankle and foot

    M05.879   Other rheumatoid arthritis with rheumatoid factor of unspecified ankle and foot

   M05.89   Other rheumatoid arthritis with rheumatoid factor of multiple sites

  M05.9   Rheumatoid arthritis with rheumatoid factor, unspecified

✓4th **M06**   Other rheumatoid arthritis

✓5th **M06.0**   Rheumatoid arthritis without rheumatoid factor

   M06.00   Rheumatoid arthritis without rheumatoid factor, unspecified site

✓6th **M06.01**   Rheumatoid arthritis without rheumatoid factor, shoulder

    M06.011   Rheumatoid arthritis without rheumatoid factor, right shoulder

    M06.012   Rheumatoid arthritis without rheumatoid factor, left shoulder

    M06.019   Rheumatoid arthritis without rheumatoid factor, unspecified shoulder

✓6th **M06.02**   Rheumatoid arthritis without rheumatoid factor, elbow

    M06.021   Rheumatoid arthritis without rheumatoid factor, right elbow

    M06.022   Rheumatoid arthritis without rheumatoid factor, left elbow

    M06.029   Rheumatoid arthritis without rheumatoid factor, unspecified elbow

✓6th **M06.03**   Rheumatoid arthritis without rheumatoid factor, wrist

    M06.031   Rheumatoid arthritis without rheumatoid factor, right wrist

    M06.032   Rheumatoid arthritis without rheumatoid factor, left wrist

    M06.039   Rheumatoid arthritis without rheumatoid factor, unspecified wrist

✓6th **M06.04**   Rheumatoid arthritis without rheumatoid factor, hand

    M06.041   Rheumatoid arthritis without rheumatoid factor, right hand

    M06.042   Rheumatoid arthritis without rheumatoid factor, left hand

    M06.049   Rheumatoid arthritis without rheumatoid factor, unspecified hand

✓6th **M06.05**   Rheumatoid arthritis without rheumatoid factor, hip

    M06.051   Rheumatoid arthritis without rheumatoid factor, right hip

    M06.052   Rheumatoid arthritis without rheumatoid factor, left hip

✓ Additional Character Required   ✓x7th Xtension Alert   Unacceptable PDx   Manifestation   Hospital Acquired Condition   EXCLUDES 1 Not Coded Here   EXCLUDES 2 Not Included Here

ICD-10-CM Draft (2015)   691

M06.059 **Rheumatoid arthritis without rheumatoid factor, unspecified hip**

✓6ᵗʰ **M06.06 Rheumatoid arthritis without rheumatoid factor, knee**

M06.061 **Rheumatoid arthritis without rheumatoid factor, right knee**

M06.062 **Rheumatoid arthritis without rheumatoid factor, left knee**

M06.069 **Rheumatoid arthritis without rheumatoid factor, unspecified knee**

✓6ᵗʰ **M06.07 Rheumatoid arthritis without rheumatoid factor, ankle and foot**

M06.071 **Rheumatoid arthritis without rheumatoid factor, right ankle and foot**

M06.072 **Rheumatoid arthritis without rheumatoid factor, left ankle and foot**

M06.079 **Rheumatoid arthritis without rheumatoid factor, unspecified ankle and foot**

M06.08 Rheumatoid arthritis without rheumatoid factor, vertebrae

M06.09 Rheumatoid arthritis without rheumatoid factor, multiple sites

M06.1 Adult-onset Still's disease   **A**
    EXCLUDES 1 *Still's disease NOS (M08.2-)*

✓5ᵗʰ **M06.2 Rheumatoid bursitis**

M06.20 Rheumatoid bursitis, unspecified site

✓6ᵗʰ **M06.21 Rheumatoid bursitis, shoulder**

M06.211 **Rheumatoid bursitis, right shoulder**

M06.212 **Rheumatoid bursitis, left shoulder**

M06.219 **Rheumatoid bursitis, unspecified shoulder**

✓6ᵗʰ **M06.22 Rheumatoid bursitis, elbow**

M06.221 **Rheumatoid bursitis, right elbow**

M06.222 **Rheumatoid bursitis, left elbow**

M06.229 **Rheumatoid bursitis, unspecified elbow**

✓6ᵗʰ **M06.23 Rheumatoid bursitis, wrist**

M06.231 **Rheumatoid bursitis, right wrist**

M06.232 **Rheumatoid bursitis, left wrist**

M06.239 **Rheumatoid bursitis, unspecified wrist**

✓6ᵗʰ **M06.24 Rheumatoid bursitis, hand**

M06.241 **Rheumatoid bursitis, right hand**

M06.242 **Rheumatoid bursitis, left hand**

M06.249 **Rheumatoid bursitis, unspecified hand**

✓6ᵗʰ **M06.25 Rheumatoid bursitis, hip**

M06.251 **Rheumatoid bursitis, right hip**

M06.252 **Rheumatoid bursitis, left hip**

M06.259 **Rheumatoid bursitis, unspecified hip**

✓6ᵗʰ **M06.26 Rheumatoid bursitis, knee**

M06.261 **Rheumatoid bursitis, right knee**

M06.262 **Rheumatoid bursitis, left knee**

M06.269 **Rheumatoid bursitis, unspecified knee**

✓6ᵗʰ **M06.27 Rheumatoid bursitis, ankle and foot**

M06.271 **Rheumatoid bursitis, right ankle and foot**

M06.272 **Rheumatoid bursitis, left ankle and foot**

M06.279 **Rheumatoid bursitis, unspecified ankle and foot**

M06.28 Rheumatoid bursitis, vertebrae

M06.29 Rheumatoid bursitis, multiple sites

✓5ᵗʰ **M06.3 Rheumatoid nodule**

M06.30 Rheumatoid nodule, unspecified site

✓6ᵗʰ **M06.31 Rheumatoid nodule, shoulder**

M06.311 **Rheumatoid nodule, right shoulder**

M06.312 **Rheumatoid nodule, left shoulder**

M06.319 **Rheumatoid nodule, unspecified shoulder**

✓6ᵗʰ **M06.32 Rheumatoid nodule, elbow**

M06.321 **Rheumatoid nodule, right elbow**

M06.322 **Rheumatoid nodule, left elbow**

M06.329 **Rheumatoid nodule, unspecified elbow**

✓6ᵗʰ **M06.33 Rheumatoid nodule, wrist**

M06.331 **Rheumatoid nodule, right wrist**

M06.332 **Rheumatoid nodule, left wrist**

M06.339 **Rheumatoid nodule, unspecified wrist**

✓6ᵗʰ **M06.34 Rheumatoid nodule, hand**

M06.341 **Rheumatoid nodule, right hand**

M06.342 **Rheumatoid nodule, left hand**

M06.349 **Rheumatoid nodule, unspecified hand**

✓6ᵗʰ **M06.35 Rheumatoid nodule, hip**

M06.351 **Rheumatoid nodule, right hip**

M06.352 **Rheumatoid nodule, left hip**

M06.359 **Rheumatoid nodule, unspecified hip**

✓6ᵗʰ **M06.36 Rheumatoid nodule, knee**

M06.361 **Rheumatoid nodule, right knee**

M06.362 **Rheumatoid nodule, left knee**

M06.369 **Rheumatoid nodule, unspecified knee**

✓6ᵗʰ **M06.37 Rheumatoid nodule, ankle and foot**

M06.371 **Rheumatoid nodule, right ankle and foot**

M06.372 **Rheumatoid nodule, left ankle and foot**

M06.379 **Rheumatoid nodule, unspecified ankle and foot**

M06.38 Rheumatoid nodule, vertebrae

M06.39 Rheumatoid nodule, multiple sites

M06.4 Inflammatory polyarthropathy
    EXCLUDES 1 *polyarthritis NOS (M13.0)*

✓5ᵗʰ **M06.8 Other specified rheumatoid arthritis**

M06.80 Other specified rheumatoid arthritis, unspecified site

✓6ᵗʰ **M06.81 Other specified rheumatoid arthritis, shoulder**

M06.811 **Other specified rheumatoid arthritis, right shoulder**

M06.812 **Other specified rheumatoid arthritis, left shoulder**

M06.819 **Other specified rheumatoid arthritis, unspecified shoulder**

✓6ᵗʰ **M06.82 Other specified rheumatoid arthritis, elbow**

M06.821 **Other specified rheumatoid arthritis, right elbow**

M06.822 **Other specified rheumatoid arthritis, left elbow**

M06.829 **Other specified rheumatoid arthritis, unspecified elbow**

✓6ᵗʰ **M06.83 Other specified rheumatoid arthritis, wrist**

M06.831 **Other specified rheumatoid arthritis, right wrist**

M06.832 **Other specified rheumatoid arthritis, left wrist**

M06.839 **Other specified rheumatoid arthritis, unspecified wrist**

✓6ᵗʰ **M06.84 Other specified rheumatoid arthritis, hand**

M06.841 **Other specified rheumatoid arthritis, right hand**

M06.842 **Other specified rheumatoid arthritis, left hand**

M06.849 **Other specified rheumatoid arthritis, unspecified hand**

✓6ᵗʰ **M06.85 Other specified rheumatoid arthritis, hip**

M06.851 **Other specified rheumatoid arthritis, right hip**

M06.852 **Other specified rheumatoid arthritis, left hip**

M06.859 **Other specified rheumatoid arthritis, unspecified hip**

✓6ᵗʰ **M06.86 Other specified rheumatoid arthritis, knee**

M06.861 **Other specified rheumatoid arthritis, right knee**

M06.862 **Other specified rheumatoid arthritis, left knee**

M06.869 **Other specified rheumatoid arthritis, unspecified knee**

✓6ᵗʰ **M06.87 Other specified rheumatoid arthritis, ankle and foot**

M06.871 **Other specified rheumatoid arthritis, right ankle and foot**

M06.872 **Other specified rheumatoid arthritis, left ankle and foot**

M06.879 **Other specified rheumatoid arthritis, unspecified ankle and foot**

M06.88 Other specified rheumatoid arthritis, vertebrae

M06.89 Other specified rheumatoid arthritis, multiple sites

M06.9 Rheumatoid arthritis, unspecified

N Newborn: 0   P Pediatric: 0-17   M Maternity: 12-55   A Adult: 15-124   MCC Major CC Condition   PDx MCC PDx acts as own MCC   CC CC Condition   PDx CC PDx acts as own CC

692   ICD-10-CM Draft (2015)

☑4ᵗʰ M07 Enteropathic arthropathies

Code also associated enteropathy, such as:
regional enteritis [Crohn's disease] (K50.-)
ulcerative colitis (K51.-)
EXCLUDES 1 psoriatic arthropathies (L40.5-)

☑5ᵗʰ M07.6 Enteropathic arthropathies

M07.60 Enteropathic arthropathies, unspecified site

☑6ᵗʰ M07.61 Enteropathic arthropathies, shoulder
M07.611 Enteropathic arthropathies, right shoulder
M07.612 Enteropathic arthropathies, left shoulder
M07.619 Enteropathic arthropathies, unspecified shoulder

☑6ᵗʰ M07.62 Enteropathic arthropathies, elbow
M07.621 Enteropathic arthropathies, right elbow
M07.622 Enteropathic arthropathies, left elbow
M07.629 Enteropathic arthropathies, unspecified elbow

☑6ᵗʰ M07.63 Enteropathic arthropathies, wrist
M07.631 Enteropathic arthropathies, right wrist
M07.632 Enteropathic arthropathies, left wrist
M07.639 Enteropathic arthropathies, unspecified wrist

☑6ᵗʰ M07.64 Enteropathic arthropathies, hand
M07.641 Enteropathic arthropathies, right hand
M07.642 Enteropathic arthropathies, left hand
M07.649 Enteropathic arthropathies, unspecified hand

☑6ᵗʰ M07.65 Enteropathic arthropathies, hip
M07.651 Enteropathic arthropathies, right hip
M07.652 Enteropathic arthropathies, left hip
M07.659 Enteropathic arthropathies, unspecified hip

☑6ᵗʰ M07.66 Enteropathic arthropathies, knee
M07.661 Enteropathic arthropathies, right knee
M07.662 Enteropathic arthropathies, left knee
M07.669 Enteropathic arthropathies, unspecified knee

☑6ᵗʰ M07.67 Enteropathic arthropathies, ankle and foot
M07.671 Enteropathic arthropathies, right ankle and foot
M07.672 Enteropathic arthropathies, left ankle and foot
M07.679 Enteropathic arthropathies, unspecified ankle and foot

M07.68 Enteropathic arthropathies, vertebrae
M07.69 Enteropathic arthropathies, multiple sites

☑4ᵗʰ M08 Juvenile arthritis

Code also any associated underlying condition, such as:
regional enteritis [Crohn's disease] (K50.-)
ulcerative colitis (K51.-)
EXCLUDES 1 arthropathy in Whipple's disease (M14.8)
Felty's syndrome (M05.0)
juvenile dermatomyositis (M33.0-)
psoriatic juvenile arthropathy (L40.54)

☑5ᵗʰ M08.0 Unspecified juvenile rheumatoid arthritis
Juvenile rheumatoid arthritis with or without rheumatoid factor

M08.00 Unspecified juvenile rheumatoid arthritis of unspecified site

☑6ᵗʰ M08.01 Unspecified juvenile rheumatoid arthritis, shoulder
M08.011 Unspecified juvenile rheumatoid arthritis, right shoulder
M08.012 Unspecified juvenile rheumatoid arthritis, left shoulder
M08.019 Unspecified juvenile rheumatoid arthritis, unspecified shoulder

☑6ᵗʰ M08.02 Unspecified juvenile rheumatoid arthritis of elbow
M08.021 Unspecified juvenile rheumatoid arthritis, right elbow
M08.022 Unspecified juvenile rheumatoid arthritis, left elbow
M08.029 Unspecified juvenile rheumatoid arthritis, unspecified elbow

☑6ᵗʰ M08.03 Unspecified juvenile rheumatoid arthritis, wrist
M08.031 Unspecified juvenile rheumatoid arthritis, right wrist
M08.032 Unspecified juvenile rheumatoid arthritis, left wrist
M08.039 Unspecified juvenile rheumatoid arthritis, unspecified wrist

☑6ᵗʰ M08.04 Unspecified juvenile rheumatoid arthritis, hand
M08.041 Unspecified juvenile rheumatoid arthritis, right hand
M08.042 Unspecified juvenile rheumatoid arthritis, left hand
M08.049 Unspecified juvenile rheumatoid arthritis, unspecified hand

☑6ᵗʰ M08.05 Unspecified juvenile rheumatoid arthritis, hip
M08.051 Unspecified juvenile rheumatoid arthritis, right hip
M08.052 Unspecified juvenile rheumatoid arthritis, left hip
M08.059 Unspecified juvenile rheumatoid arthritis, unspecified hip

☑6ᵗʰ M08.06 Unspecified juvenile rheumatoid arthritis, knee
M08.061 Unspecified juvenile rheumatoid arthritis, right knee
M08.062 Unspecified juvenile rheumatoid arthritis, left knee
M08.069 Unspecified juvenile rheumatoid arthritis, unspecified knee

☑6ᵗʰ M08.07 Unspecified juvenile rheumatoid arthritis, ankle and foot
M08.071 Unspecified juvenile rheumatoid arthritis, right ankle and foot
M08.072 Unspecified juvenile rheumatoid arthritis, left ankle and foot
M08.079 Unspecified juvenile rheumatoid arthritis, unspecified ankle and foot

M08.08 Unspecified juvenile rheumatoid arthritis, vertebrae
M08.09 Unspecified juvenile rheumatoid arthritis, multiple sites

M08.1 Juvenile ankylosing spondylitis
EXCLUDES 1 ankylosing spondylitis in adults (M45.0-)

☑5ᵗʰ M08.2 Juvenile rheumatoid arthritis with systemic onset
Still's disease NOS
EXCLUDES 1 adult-onset Still's disease (M06.1-)

M08.20 Juvenile rheumatoid arthritis with systemic onset, unspecified site

☑6ᵗʰ M08.21 Juvenile rheumatoid arthritis with systemic onset, shoulder
M08.211 Juvenile rheumatoid arthritis with systemic onset, right shoulder
M08.212 Juvenile rheumatoid arthritis with systemic onset, left shoulder
M08.219 Juvenile rheumatoid arthritis with systemic onset, unspecified shoulder

☑6ᵗʰ M08.22 Juvenile rheumatoid arthritis with systemic onset, elbow
M08.221 Juvenile rheumatoid arthritis with systemic onset, right elbow
M08.222 Juvenile rheumatoid arthritis with systemic onset, left elbow
M08.229 Juvenile rheumatoid arthritis with systemic onset, unspecified elbow

☑6ᵗʰ M08.23 Juvenile rheumatoid arthritis with systemic onset, wrist
M08.231 Juvenile rheumatoid arthritis with systemic onset, right wrist
M08.232 Juvenile rheumatoid arthritis with systemic onset, left wrist
M08.239 Juvenile rheumatoid arthritis with systemic onset, unspecified wrist

☑6ᵗʰ M08.24 Juvenile rheumatoid arthritis with systemic onset, hand
M08.241 Juvenile rheumatoid arthritis with systemic onset, right hand
M08.242 Juvenile rheumatoid arthritis with systemic onset, left hand

☑ Additional Character Required   ✔x7ᵗʰ Xtension Alert   Unacceptable PDx   Manifestation   Hospital Acquired Condition   **EXCLUDES 1** Not Coded Here   **EXCLUDES 2** Not Included Here

ICD-10-CM Draft (2015)   693

M08.249   Juvenile rheumatoid arthritis with systemic onset, unspecified hand

✓6ᵗʰ   M08.25   Juvenile rheumatoid arthritis with systemic onset, hip

    M08.251   Juvenile rheumatoid arthritis with systemic onset, right hip

    M08.252   Juvenile rheumatoid arthritis with systemic onset, left hip

    M08.259   Juvenile rheumatoid arthritis with systemic onset, unspecified hip

✓6ᵗʰ   M08.26   Juvenile rheumatoid arthritis with systemic onset, knee

    M08.261   Juvenile rheumatoid arthritis with systemic onset, right knee

    M08.262   Juvenile rheumatoid arthritis with systemic onset, left knee

    M08.269   Juvenile rheumatoid arthritis with systemic onset, unspecified knee

✓6ᵗʰ   M08.27   Juvenile rheumatoid arthritis with systemic onset, ankle and foot

    M08.271   Juvenile rheumatoid arthritis with systemic onset, right ankle and foot

    M08.272   Juvenile rheumatoid arthritis with systemic onset, left ankle and foot

    M08.279   Juvenile rheumatoid arthritis with systemic onset, unspecified ankle and foot

M08.28   Juvenile rheumatoid arthritis with systemic onset, vertebrae

M08.29   Juvenile rheumatoid arthritis with systemic onset, multiple sites

M08.3   Juvenile rheumatoid polyarthritis (seronegative)

✓5ᵗʰ   M08.4   Pauciarticular juvenile rheumatoid arthritis

M08.40   Pauciarticular juvenile rheumatoid arthritis, unspecified site

✓6ᵗʰ   M08.41   Pauciarticular juvenile rheumatoid arthritis, shoulder

    M08.411   Pauciarticular juvenile rheumatoid arthritis, right shoulder

    M08.412   Pauciarticular juvenile rheumatoid arthritis, left shoulder

    M08.419   Pauciarticular juvenile rheumatoid arthritis, unspecified shoulder

✓6ᵗʰ   M08.42   Pauciarticular juvenile rheumatoid arthritis, elbow

    M08.421   Pauciarticular juvenile rheumatoid arthritis, right elbow

    M08.422   Pauciarticular juvenile rheumatoid arthritis, left elbow

    M08.429   Pauciarticular juvenile rheumatoid arthritis, unspecified elbow

✓6ᵗʰ   M08.43   Pauciarticular juvenile rheumatoid arthritis, wrist

    M08.431   Pauciarticular juvenile rheumatoid arthritis, right wrist

    M08.432   Pauciarticular juvenile rheumatoid arthritis, left wrist

    M08.439   Pauciarticular juvenile rheumatoid arthritis, unspecified wrist

✓6ᵗʰ   M08.44   Pauciarticular juvenile rheumatoid arthritis, hand

    M08.441   Pauciarticular juvenile rheumatoid arthritis, right hand

    M08.442   Pauciarticular juvenile rheumatoid arthritis, left hand

    M08.449   Pauciarticular juvenile rheumatoid arthritis, unspecified hand

✓6ᵗʰ   M08.45   Pauciarticular juvenile rheumatoid arthritis, hip

    M08.451   Pauciarticular juvenile rheumatoid arthritis, right hip

    M08.452   Pauciarticular juvenile rheumatoid arthritis, left hip

    M08.459   Pauciarticular juvenile rheumatoid arthritis, unspecified hip

✓6ᵗʰ   M08.46   Pauciarticular juvenile rheumatoid arthritis, knee

    M08.461   Pauciarticular juvenile rheumatoid arthritis, right knee

    M08.462   Pauciarticular juvenile rheumatoid arthritis, left knee

    M08.469   Pauciarticular juvenile rheumatoid arthritis, unspecified knee

✓6ᵗʰ   M08.47   Pauciarticular juvenile rheumatoid arthritis, ankle and foot

    M08.471   Pauciarticular juvenile rheumatoid arthritis, right ankle and foot

    M08.472   Pauciarticular juvenile rheumatoid arthritis, left ankle and foot

    M08.479   Pauciarticular juvenile rheumatoid arthritis, unspecified ankle and foot

M08.48   Pauciarticular juvenile rheumatoid arthritis, vertebrae

✓5ᵗʰ   M08.8   Other juvenile arthritis

M08.80   Other juvenile arthritis, unspecified site

✓6ᵗʰ   M08.81   Other juvenile arthritis, shoulder

    M08.811   Other juvenile arthritis, right shoulder

    M08.812   Other juvenile arthritis, left shoulder

    M08.819   Other juvenile arthritis, unspecified shoulder

✓6ᵗʰ   M08.82   Other juvenile arthritis, elbow

    M08.821   Other juvenile arthritis, right elbow

    M08.822   Other juvenile arthritis, left elbow

    M08.829   Other juvenile arthritis, unspecified elbow

✓6ᵗʰ   M08.83   Other juvenile arthritis, wrist

    M08.831   Other juvenile arthritis, right wrist

    M08.832   Other juvenile arthritis, left wrist

    M08.839   Other juvenile arthritis, unspecified wrist

✓6ᵗʰ   M08.84   Other juvenile arthritis, hand

    M08.841   Other juvenile arthritis, right hand

    M08.842   Other juvenile arthritis, left hand

    M08.849   Other juvenile arthritis, unspecified hand

✓6ᵗʰ   M08.85   Other juvenile arthritis, hip

    M08.851   Other juvenile arthritis, right hip

    M08.852   Other juvenile arthritis, left hip

    M08.859   Other juvenile arthritis, unspecified hip

✓6ᵗʰ   M08.86   Other juvenile arthritis, knee

    M08.861   Other juvenile arthritis, right knee

    M08.862   Other juvenile arthritis, left knee

    M08.869   Other juvenile arthritis, unspecified knee

✓6ᵗʰ   M08.87   Other juvenile arthritis, ankle and foot

    M08.871   Other juvenile arthritis, right ankle and foot

    M08.872   Other juvenile arthritis, left ankle and foot

    M08.879   Other juvenile arthritis, unspecified ankle and foot

M08.88   Other juvenile arthritis, other specified site

    Other juvenile arthritis, vertebrae

M08.89   Other juvenile arthritis, multiple sites

✓5ᵗʰ   M08.9   Juvenile arthritis, unspecified

    EXCLUDES 1   juvenile rheumatoid arthritis, unspecified (M08.0-)

M08.90   Juvenile arthritis, unspecified, unspecified site

✓6ᵗʰ   M08.91   Juvenile arthritis, unspecified, shoulder

    M08.911   Juvenile arthritis, unspecified, right shoulder

    M08.912   Juvenile arthritis, unspecified, left shoulder

    M08.919   Juvenile arthritis, unspecified, unspecified shoulder

✓6ᵗʰ   M08.92   Juvenile arthritis, unspecified, elbow

    M08.921   Juvenile arthritis, unspecified, right elbow

    M08.922   Juvenile arthritis, unspecified, left elbow

    M08.929   Juvenile arthritis, unspecified, unspecified elbow

✓6ᵗʰ   M08.93   Juvenile arthritis, unspecified, wrist

    M08.931   Juvenile arthritis, unspecified, right wrist

    M08.932   Juvenile arthritis, unspecified, left wrist

    M08.939   Juvenile arthritis, unspecified, unspecified wrist

✓6ᵗʰ   M08.94   Juvenile arthritis, unspecified, hand

    M08.941   Juvenile arthritis, unspecified, right hand

    M08.942   Juvenile arthritis, unspecified, left hand

    M08.949   Juvenile arthritis, unspecified, unspecified hand

✓6ᵗʰ   M08.95   Juvenile arthritis, unspecified, hip

    M08.951   Juvenile arthritis, unspecified, right hip

N Newborn: 0   P Pediatric: 0-17   M Maternity: 12-55   A Adult: 15-124   MCC Major CC Condition   PDx MCC PDx acts as own MCC   CC CC Condition   PDx CC PDx acts as own CC

694   ICD-10-CM Draft (2015)

M08.952   Juvenile arthritis, unspecified, left hip
M08.959   Juvenile arthritis, unspecified, unspecified hip

✓6ᵗʰ M08.96   Juvenile arthritis, unspecified, knee
M08.961   Juvenile arthritis, unspecified, right knee
M08.962   Juvenile arthritis, unspecified, left knee
M08.969   Juvenile arthritis, unspecified, unspecified knee

✓6ᵗʰ M08.97   Juvenile arthritis, unspecified, ankle and foot
M08.971   Juvenile arthritis, unspecified, right ankle and foot
M08.972   Juvenile arthritis, unspecified, left ankle and foot
M08.979   Juvenile arthritis, unspecified, unspecified ankle and foot

M08.98   Juvenile arthritis, unspecified, vertebrae
M08.99   Juvenile arthritis, unspecified, multiple sites

✓4ᵗʰ **M1A   Chronic gout**
Use additional code to identify:
autonomic neuropathy in diseases classified elsewhere (G99.0)
calculus of urinary tract in diseases classified elsewhere (N22)
cardiomyopathy in diseases classified elsewhere (I43)
disorders of external ear in diseases classified elsewhere (H61.1-, H62.8-)
disorders of iris and ciliary body in diseases classified elsewhere (H22)
glomerular disorders in diseases classified elsewhere (N08)

EXCLUDES 1   acute gout (M10.-)
gout NOS (M10.-)

The appropriate 7th character is to be added to each code from category M1A.
0   without tophus (tophi)
1   with tophus (tophi)

✓5ᵗʰ **M1A.0   Idiopathic chronic gout**
Chronic gouty bursitis
Primary chronic gout

✓x7ᵗʰ M1A.00   Idiopathic chronic gout, unspecified site
✓6ᵗʰ M1A.01   Idiopathic chronic gout, shoulder
✓7ᵗʰ   M1A.011   Idiopathic chronic gout, right shoulder
✓7ᵗʰ   M1A.012   Idiopathic chronic gout, left shoulder
✓7ᵗʰ   M1A.019   Idiopathic chronic gout, unspecified shoulder

✓6ᵗʰ M1A.02   Idiopathic chronic gout, elbow
✓7ᵗʰ   M1A.021   Idiopathic chronic gout, right elbow
✓7ᵗʰ   M1A.022   Idiopathic chronic gout, left elbow
✓7ᵗʰ   M1A.029   Idiopathic chronic gout, unspecified elbow

✓6ᵗʰ M1A.03   Idiopathic chronic gout, wrist
✓7ᵗʰ   M1A.031   Idiopathic chronic gout, right wrist
✓7ᵗʰ   M1A.032   Idiopathic chronic gout, left wrist
✓7ᵗʰ   M1A.039   Idiopathic chronic gout, unspecified wrist

✓6ᵗʰ M1A.04   Idiopathic chronic gout, hand
✓7ᵗʰ   M1A.041   Idiopathic chronic gout, right hand
✓7ᵗʰ   M1A.042   Idiopathic chronic gout, left hand
✓7ᵗʰ   M1A.049   Idiopathic chronic gout, unspecified hand

✓6ᵗʰ M1A.05   Idiopathic chronic gout, hip
✓7ᵗʰ   M1A.051   Idiopathic chronic gout, right hip
✓7ᵗʰ   M1A.052   Idiopathic chronic gout, left hip
✓7ᵗʰ   M1A.059   Idiopathic chronic gout, unspecified hip

✓6ᵗʰ M1A.06   Idiopathic chronic gout, knee
✓7ᵗʰ   M1A.061   Idiopathic chronic gout, right knee
✓7ᵗʰ   M1A.062   Idiopathic chronic gout, left knee
✓7ᵗʰ   M1A.069   Idiopathic chronic gout, unspecified knee

✓6ᵗʰ M1A.07   Idiopathic chronic gout, ankle and foot
✓7ᵗʰ   M1A.071   Idiopathic chronic gout, right ankle and foot
✓7ᵗʰ   M1A.072   Idiopathic chronic gout, left ankle and foot
✓7ᵗʰ   M1A.079   Idiopathic chronic gout, unspecified ankle and foot

✓x7ᵗʰ M1A.08   Idiopathic chronic gout, vertebrae
✓x7ᵗʰ M1A.09   Idiopathic chronic gout, multiple sites

✓5ᵗʰ **M1A.1   Lead-induced chronic gout**
Code first toxic effects of lead and its compounds (T56.0-)

✓x7ᵗʰ M1A.10   Lead-induced chronic gout, unspecified site
✓6ᵗʰ M1A.11   Lead-induced chronic gout, shoulder
✓7ᵗʰ   M1A.111   Lead-induced chronic gout, right shoulder
✓7ᵗʰ   M1A.112   Lead-induced chronic gout, left shoulder
✓7ᵗʰ   M1A.119   Lead-induced chronic gout, unspecified shoulder

✓6ᵗʰ M1A.12   Lead-induced chronic gout, elbow
✓7ᵗʰ   M1A.121   Lead-induced chronic gout, right elbow
✓7ᵗʰ   M1A.122   Lead-induced chronic gout, left elbow
✓7ᵗʰ   M1A.129   Lead-induced chronic gout, unspecified elbow

✓6ᵗʰ M1A.13   Lead-induced chronic gout, wrist
✓7ᵗʰ   M1A.131   Lead-induced chronic gout, right wrist
✓7ᵗʰ   M1A.132   Lead-induced chronic gout, left wrist
✓7ᵗʰ   M1A.139   Lead-induced chronic gout, unspecified wrist

✓6ᵗʰ M1A.14   Lead-induced chronic gout, hand
✓7ᵗʰ   M1A.141   Lead-induced chronic gout, right hand
✓7ᵗʰ   M1A.142   Lead-induced chronic gout, left hand
✓7ᵗʰ   M1A.149   Lead-induced chronic gout, unspecified hand

✓6ᵗʰ M1A.15   Lead-induced chronic gout, hip
✓7ᵗʰ   M1A.151   Lead-induced chronic gout, right hip
✓7ᵗʰ   M1A.152   Lead-induced chronic gout, left hip
✓7ᵗʰ   M1A.159   Lead-induced chronic gout, unspecified hip

✓6ᵗʰ M1A.16   Lead-induced chronic gout, knee
✓7ᵗʰ   M1A.161   Lead-induced chronic gout, right knee
✓7ᵗʰ   M1A.162   Lead-induced chronic gout, left knee
✓7ᵗʰ   M1A.169   Lead-induced chronic gout, unspecified knee

✓6ᵗʰ M1A.17   Lead-induced chronic gout, ankle and foot
✓7ᵗʰ   M1A.171   Lead-induced chronic gout, right ankle and foot
✓7ᵗʰ   M1A.172   Lead-induced chronic gout, left ankle and foot
✓7ᵗʰ   M1A.179   Lead-induced chronic gout, unspecified ankle and foot

✓x7ᵗʰ M1A.18   Lead-induced chronic gout, vertebrae
✓x7ᵗʰ M1A.19   Lead-induced chronic gout, multiple sites

✓5ᵗʰ **M1A.2   Drug-induced chronic gout**
Use additional code for adverse effect, if applicable, to identify drug (T36-T50 with fifth or sixth character 5)

✓x7ᵗʰ M1A.20   Drug-induced chronic gout, unspecified site
✓6ᵗʰ M1A.21   Drug-induced chronic gout, shoulder
✓7ᵗʰ   M1A.211   Drug-induced chronic gout, right shoulder
✓7ᵗʰ   M1A.212   Drug-induced chronic gout, left shoulder
✓7ᵗʰ   M1A.219   Drug-induced chronic gout, unspecified shoulder

✓6ᵗʰ M1A.22   Drug-induced chronic gout, elbow
✓7ᵗʰ   M1A.221   Drug-induced chronic gout, right elbow
✓7ᵗʰ   M1A.222   Drug-induced chronic gout, left elbow
✓7ᵗʰ   M1A.229   Drug-induced chronic gout, unspecified elbow

✓6ᵗʰ M1A.23   Drug-induced chronic gout, wrist
✓7ᵗʰ   M1A.231   Drug-induced chronic gout, right wrist
✓7ᵗʰ   M1A.232   Drug-induced chronic gout, left wrist
✓7ᵗʰ   M1A.239   Drug-induced chronic gout, unspecified wrist

✓6ᵗʰ M1A.24   Drug-induced chronic gout, hand
✓7ᵗʰ   M1A.241   Drug-induced chronic gout, right hand
✓7ᵗʰ   M1A.242   Drug-induced chronic gout, left hand
✓7ᵗʰ   M1A.249   Drug-induced chronic gout, unspecified hand

✓6ᵗʰ M1A.25   Drug-induced chronic gout, hip
✓7ᵗʰ   M1A.251   Drug-induced chronic gout, right hip
✓7ᵗʰ   M1A.252   Drug-induced chronic gout, left hip

√7th **M1A.259 Drug-induced chronic gout,** unspecified hip

√6th **M1A.26 Drug-induced chronic gout,** knee

  √7th **M1A.261 Drug-induced chronic gout,** right knee

  √7th **M1A.262 Drug-induced chronic gout,** left knee

  √7th **M1A.269 Drug-induced chronic gout,** unspecified knee

√6th **M1A.27 Drug-induced chronic gout,** ankle and foot

  √7th **M1A.271 Drug-induced chronic gout,** right ankle and foot

  √7th **M1A.272 Drug-induced chronic gout,** left ankle and foot

  √7th **M1A.279 Drug-induced chronic gout,** unspecified ankle and foot

√x7th **M1A.28 Drug-induced chronic gout,** vertebrae

√x7th **M1A.29 Drug-induced chronic gout,** multiple sites

√5th **M1A.3 Chronic gout** due to renal impairment
  Code first associated renal disease

√x7th **M1A.30 Chronic gout due to renal impairment,** unspecified site

√6th **M1A.31 Chronic gout due to renal impairment,** shoulder

  √7th **M1A.311 Chronic gout due to renal impairment,** right shoulder

  √7th **M1A.312 Chronic gout due to renal impairment,** left shoulder

  √7th **M1A.319 Chronic gout due to renal impairment,** unspecified shoulder

√6th **M1A.32 Chronic gout due to renal impairment,** elbow

  √7th **M1A.321 Chronic gout due to renal impairment,** right elbow

  √7th **M1A.322 Chronic gout due to renal impairment,** left elbow

  √7th **M1A.329 Chronic gout due to renal impairment,** unspecified elbow

√6th **M1A.33 Chronic gout due to renal impairment,** wrist

  √7th **M1A.331 Chronic gout due to renal impairment,** right wrist

  √7th **M1A.332 Chronic gout due to renal impairment,** left wrist

  √7th **M1A.339 Chronic gout due to renal impairment,** unspecified wrist

√6th **M1A.34 Chronic gout due to renal impairment,** hand

  √7th **M1A.341 Chronic gout due to renal impairment,** right hand

  √7th **M1A.342 Chronic gout due to renal impairment,** left hand

  √7th **M1A.349 Chronic gout due to renal impairment,** unspecified hand

√6th **M1A.35 Chronic gout due to renal impairment,** hip

  √7th **M1A.351 Chronic gout due to renal impairment,** right hip

  √7th **M1A.352 Chronic gout due to renal impairment,** left hip

  √7th **M1A.359 Chronic gout due to renal impairment,** unspecified hip

√6th **M1A.36 Chronic gout due to renal impairment,** knee

  √7th **M1A.361 Chronic gout due to renal impairment,** right knee

  √7th **M1A.362 Chronic gout due to renal impairment,** left knee

  √7th **M1A.369 Chronic gout due to renal impairment,** unspecified knee

√6th **M1A.37 Chronic gout due to renal impairment,** ankle and foot

  √7th **M1A.371 Chronic gout due to renal impairment,** right ankle and foot

  √7th **M1A.372 Chronic gout due to renal impairment,** left ankle and foot

  √7th **M1A.379 Chronic gout due to renal impairment,** unspecified ankle and foot

√x7th **M1A.38 Chronic gout due to renal impairment,** vertebrae

√x7th **M1A.39 Chronic gout due to renal impairment,** multiple sites

√5th **M1A.4 Other secondary chronic gout**
  Code first associated condition

√x7th **M1A.40 Other secondary chronic gout,** unspecified site

√6th **M1A.41 Other secondary chronic gout,** shoulder

  √7th **M1A.411 Other secondary chronic gout,** right shoulder

  √7th **M1A.412 Other secondary chronic gout,** left shoulder

  √7th **M1A.419 Other secondary chronic gout,** unspecified shoulder

√6th **M1A.42 Other secondary chronic gout,** elbow

  √7th **M1A.421 Other secondary chronic gout,** right elbow

  √7th **M1A.422 Other secondary chronic gout,** left elbow

  √7th **M1A.429 Other secondary chronic gout,** unspecified elbow

√6th **M1A.43 Other secondary chronic gout,** wrist

  √7th **M1A.431 Other secondary chronic gout,** right wrist

  √7th **M1A.432 Other secondary chronic gout,** left wrist

  √7th **M1A.439 Other secondary chronic gout,** unspecified wrist

√6th **M1A.44 Other secondary chronic gout,** hand

  √7th **M1A.441 Other secondary chronic gout,** right hand

  √7th **M1A.442 Other secondary chronic gout,** left hand

  √7th **M1A.449 Other secondary chronic gout,** unspecified hand

√6th **M1A.45 Other secondary chronic gout,** hip

  √7th **M1A.451 Other secondary chronic gout,** right hip

  √7th **M1A.452 Other secondary chronic gout,** left hip

  √7th **M1A.459 Other secondary chronic gout,** unspecified hip

√6th **M1A.46 Other secondary chronic gout,** knee

  √7th **M1A.461 Other secondary chronic gout,** right knee

  √7th **M1A.462 Other secondary chronic gout,** left knee

  √7th **M1A.469 Other secondary chronic gout,** unspecified knee

√6th **M1A.47 Other secondary chronic gout,** ankle and foot

  √7th **M1A.471 Other secondary chronic gout,** right ankle and foot

  √7th **M1A.472 Other secondary chronic gout,** left ankle and foot

  √7th **M1A.479 Other secondary chronic gout,** unspecified ankle and foot

√x7th **M1A.48 Other secondary chronic gout,** vertebrae

√x7th **M1A.49 Other secondary chronic gout,** multiple sites

√x7th **M1A.9 Chronic gout,** unspecified

√4th **M10 Gout**

Acute gout	Gout NOS
Gout attack	Podagra
Gout flare	

Use additional code to identify:
  autonomic neuropathy in diseases classified elsewhere (G99.0)
  calculus of urinary tract in diseases classified elsewhere (N22)
  cardiomyopathy in diseases classified elsewhere (I43)
  disorders of external ear in diseases classified elsewhere (H61.1-, H62.8-)
  disorders of iris and ciliary body in diseases classified elsewhere (H22)
  glomerular disorders in diseases classified elsewhere (N08)

  EXCLUDES 1 chronic gout (M1A.-)

√5th **M10.0 Idiopathic gout**
  Gouty bursitis
  Primary gout

  M10.00 Idiopathic gout, unspecified site

  √6th **M10.01 Idiopathic gout,** shoulder

    M10.011 Idiopathic gout, right shoulder

    M10.012 Idiopathic gout, left shoulder

    M10.019 Idiopathic gout, unspecified shoulder

  √6th **M10.02 Idiopathic gout,** elbow

    M10.021 Idiopathic gout, right elbow

    M10.022 Idiopathic gout, left elbow

    M10.029 Idiopathic gout, unspecified elbow

  √6th **M10.03 Idiopathic gout,** wrist

    M10.031 Idiopathic gout, right wrist

    M10.032 Idiopathic gout, left wrist

N Newborn: 0   P Pediatric: 0-17   M Maternity: 12-55   A Adult: 15-124   MCC Major CC Condition   PDx MCC PDx acts as own MCC   CC CC Condition   PDx CC PDx acts as own CC

696   ICD-10-CM Draft (2015)

M10.039 Idiopathic gout, unspecified wrist
√6ᵗʰ M10.04 Idiopathic gout, hand
  M10.041 Idiopathic gout, right hand
  M10.042 Idiopathic gout, left hand
  M10.049 Idiopathic gout, unspecified hand
√6ᵗʰ M10.05 Idiopathic gout, hip
  M10.051 Idiopathic gout, right hip
  M10.052 Idiopathic gout, left hip
  M10.059 Idiopathic gout, unspecified hip
√6ᵗʰ M10.06 Idiopathic gout, knee
  M10.061 Idiopathic gout, right knee
  M10.062 Idiopathic gout, left knee
  M10.069 Idiopathic gout, unspecified knee
√6ᵗʰ M10.07 Idiopathic gout, ankle and foot
  M10.071 Idiopathic gout, right ankle and foot
  M10.072 Idiopathic gout, left ankle and foot
  M10.079 Idiopathic gout, unspecified ankle and foot
  M10.08 Idiopathic gout, vertebrae
  M10.09 Idiopathic gout, multiple sites
√5ᵗʰ M10.1 Lead-induced gout
    Code first toxic effects of lead and its compounds (T56.0-)
  M10.10 Lead-induced gout, unspecified site
√6ᵗʰ M10.11 Lead-induced gout, shoulder
  M10.111 Lead-induced gout, right shoulder
  M10.112 Lead-induced gout, left shoulder
  M10.119 Lead-induced gout, unspecified shoulder
√6ᵗʰ M10.12 Lead-induced gout, elbow
  M10.121 Lead-induced gout, right elbow
  M10.122 Lead-induced gout, left elbow
  M10.129 Lead-induced gout, unspecified elbow
√6ᵗʰ M10.13 Lead-induced gout, wrist
  M10.131 Lead-induced gout, right wrist
  M10.132 Lead-induced gout, left wrist
  M10.139 Lead-induced gout, unspecified wrist
√6ᵗʰ M10.14 Lead-induced gout, hand
  M10.141 Lead-induced gout, right hand
  M10.142 Lead-induced gout, left hand
  M10.149 Lead-induced gout, unspecified hand
√6ᵗʰ M10.15 Lead-induced gout, hip
  M10.151 Lead-induced gout, right hip
  M10.152 Lead-induced gout, left hip
  M10.159 Lead-induced gout, unspecified hip
√6ᵗʰ M10.16 Lead-induced gout, knee
  M10.161 Lead-induced gout, right knee
  M10.162 Lead-induced gout, left knee
  M10.169 Lead-induced gout, unspecified knee
√6ᵗʰ M10.17 Lead-induced gout, ankle and foot
  M10.171 Lead-induced gout, right ankle and foot
  M10.172 Lead-induced gout, left ankle and foot
  M10.179 Lead-induced gout, unspecified ankle and foot
  M10.18 Lead-induced gout, vertebrae
  M10.19 Lead-induced gout, multiple sites
√5ᵗʰ M10.2 Drug-induced gout
    Use additional code for adverse effect, if applicable, to identify drug (T36-T50 with fifth or sixth character 5)
  M10.20 Drug-induced gout, unspecified site
√6ᵗʰ M10.21 Drug-induced gout, shoulder
  M10.211 Drug-induced gout, right shoulder
  M10.212 Drug-induced gout, left shoulder
  M10.219 Drug-induced gout, unspecified shoulder
√6ᵗʰ M10.22 Drug-induced gout, elbow
  M10.221 Drug-induced gout, right elbow
  M10.222 Drug-induced gout, left elbow
  M10.229 Drug-induced gout, unspecified elbow
√6ᵗʰ M10.23 Drug-induced gout, wrist
  M10.231 Drug-induced gout, right wrist
  M10.232 Drug-induced gout, left wrist
  M10.239 Drug-induced gout, unspecified wrist

√6ᵗʰ M10.24 Drug-induced gout, hand
  M10.241 Drug-induced gout, right hand
  M10.242 Drug-induced gout, left hand
  M10.249 Drug-induced gout, unspecified hand
√6ᵗʰ M10.25 Drug-induced gout, hip
  M10.251 Drug-induced gout, right hip
  M10.252 Drug-induced gout, left hip
  M10.259 Drug-induced gout, unspecified hip
√6ᵗʰ M10.26 Drug-induced gout, knee
  M10.261 Drug-induced gout, right knee
  M10.262 Drug-induced gout, left knee
  M10.269 Drug-induced gout, unspecified knee
√6ᵗʰ M10.27 Drug-induced gout, ankle and foot
  M10.271 Drug-induced gout, right ankle and foot
  M10.272 Drug-induced gout, left ankle and foot
  M10.279 Drug-induced gout, unspecified ankle and foot
  M10.28 Drug-induced gout, vertebrae
  M10.29 Drug-induced gout, multiple sites
√5ᵗʰ M10.3 Gout due to renal impairment
    Code first associated renal disease
  M10.30 Gout due to renal impairment, unspecified site
√6ᵗʰ M10.31 Gout due to renal impairment, shoulder
  M10.311 Gout due to renal impairment, right shoulder
  M10.312 Gout due to renal impairment, left shoulder
  M10.319 Gout due to renal impairment, unspecified shoulder
√6ᵗʰ M10.32 Gout due to renal impairment, elbow
  M10.321 Gout due to renal impairment, right elbow
  M10.322 Gout due to renal impairment, left elbow
  M10.329 Gout due to renal impairment, unspecified elbow
√6ᵗʰ M10.33 Gout due to renal impairment, wrist
  M10.331 Gout due to renal impairment, right wrist
  M10.332 Gout due to renal impairment, left wrist
  M10.339 Gout due to renal impairment, unspecified wrist
√6ᵗʰ M10.34 Gout due to renal impairment, hand
  M10.341 Gout due to renal impairment, right hand
  M10.342 Gout due to renal impairment, left hand
  M10.349 Gout due to renal impairment, unspecified hand
√6ᵗʰ M10.35 Gout due to renal impairment, hip
  M10.351 Gout due to renal impairment, right hip
  M10.352 Gout due to renal impairment, left hip
  M10.359 Gout due to renal impairment, unspecified hip
√6ᵗʰ M10.36 Gout due to renal impairment, knee
  M10.361 Gout due to renal impairment, right knee
  M10.362 Gout due to renal impairment, left knee
  M10.369 Gout due to renal impairment, unspecified knee
√6ᵗʰ M10.37 Gout due to renal impairment, ankle and foot
  M10.371 Gout due to renal impairment, right ankle and foot
  M10.372 Gout due to renal impairment, left ankle and foot
  M10.379 Gout due to renal impairment, unspecified ankle and foot
  M10.38 Gout due to renal impairment, vertebrae
  M10.39 Gout due to renal impairment, multiple sites
√5ᵗʰ M10.4 Other secondary gout
    Code first associated condition
  M10.40 Other secondary gout, unspecified site
√6ᵗʰ M10.41 Other secondary gout, shoulder
  M10.411 Other secondary gout, right shoulder
  M10.412 Other secondary gout, left shoulder
  M10.419 Other secondary gout, unspecified shoulder
√6ᵗʰ M10.42 Other secondary gout, elbow
  M10.421 Other secondary gout, right elbow

M10.422   Other secondary gout, left elbow
M10.429   Other secondary gout, unspecified elbow

✓6th   **M10.43**   Other secondary gout, wrist
M10.431   Other secondary gout, right wrist
M10.432   Other secondary gout, left wrist
M10.439   Other secondary gout, unspecified wrist

✓6th   **M10.44**   Other secondary gout, hand
M10.441   Other secondary gout, right hand
M10.442   Other secondary gout, left hand
M10.449   Other secondary gout, unspecified hand

✓6th   **M10.45**   Other secondary gout, hip
M10.451   Other secondary gout, right hip
M10.452   Other secondary gout, left hip
M10.459   Other secondary gout, unspecified hip

✓6th   **M10.46**   Other secondary gout, knee
M10.461   Other secondary gout, right knee
M10.462   Other secondary gout, left knee
M10.469   Other secondary gout, unspecified knee

✓6th   **M10.47**   Other secondary gout, ankle and foot
M10.471   Other secondary gout, right ankle and foot
M10.472   Other secondary gout, left ankle and foot
M10.479   Other secondary gout, unspecified ankle and foot

M10.48   Other secondary gout, vertebrae
M10.49   Other secondary gout, multiple sites

M10.9   Gout, unspecified
Gout NOS

✓4th   **M11**   **Other crystal arthropathies**

✓5th   **M11.0**   Hydroxyapatite deposition disease
M11.00   Hydroxyapatite deposition disease, unspecified site

✓6th   **M11.01**   Hydroxyapatite deposition disease, shoulder
M11.011   Hydroxyapatite deposition disease, right shoulder
M11.012   Hydroxyapatite deposition disease, left shoulder
M11.019   Hydroxyapatite deposition disease, unspecified shoulder

✓6th   **M11.02**   Hydroxyapatite deposition disease, elbow
M11.021   Hydroxyapatite deposition disease, right elbow
M11.022   Hydroxyapatite deposition disease, left elbow
M11.029   Hydroxyapatite deposition disease, unspecified elbow

✓6th   **M11.03**   Hydroxyapatite deposition disease, wrist
M11.031   Hydroxyapatite deposition disease, right wrist
M11.032   Hydroxyapatite deposition disease, left wrist
M11.039   Hydroxyapatite deposition disease, unspecified wrist

✓6th   **M11.04**   Hydroxyapatite deposition disease, hand
M11.041   Hydroxyapatite deposition disease, right hand
M11.042   Hydroxyapatite deposition disease, left hand
M11.049   Hydroxyapatite deposition disease, unspecified hand

✓6th   **M11.05**   Hydroxyapatite deposition disease, hip
M11.051   Hydroxyapatite deposition disease, right hip
M11.052   Hydroxyapatite deposition disease, left hip
M11.059   Hydroxyapatite deposition disease, unspecified hip

✓6th   **M11.06**   Hydroxyapatite deposition disease, knee
M11.061   Hydroxyapatite deposition disease, right knee
M11.062   Hydroxyapatite deposition disease, left knee
M11.069   Hydroxyapatite deposition disease, unspecified knee

✓6th   **M11.07**   Hydroxyapatite deposition disease, ankle and foot
M11.071   Hydroxyapatite deposition disease, right ankle and foot
M11.072   Hydroxyapatite deposition disease, left ankle and foot
M11.079   Hydroxyapatite deposition disease, unspecified ankle and foot

M11.08   Hydroxyapatite deposition disease, vertebrae
M11.09   Hydroxyapatite deposition disease, multiple sites

✓5th   **M11.1**   Familial chondrocalcinosis
M11.10   Familial chondrocalcinosis, unspecified site

✓6th   **M11.11**   Familial chondrocalcinosis, shoulder
M11.111   Familial chondrocalcinosis, right shoulder
M11.112   Familial chondrocalcinosis, left shoulder
M11.119   Familial chondrocalcinosis, unspecified shoulder

✓6th   **M11.12**   Familial chondrocalcinosis, elbow
M11.121   Familial chondrocalcinosis, right elbow
M11.122   Familial chondrocalcinosis, left elbow
M11.129   Familial chondrocalcinosis, unspecified elbow

✓6th   **M11.13**   Familial chondrocalcinosis, wrist
M11.131   Familial chondrocalcinosis, right wrist
M11.132   Familial chondrocalcinosis, left wrist
M11.139   Familial chondrocalcinosis, unspecified wrist

✓6th   **M11.14**   Familial chondrocalcinosis, hand
M11.141   Familial chondrocalcinosis, right hand
M11.142   Familial chondrocalcinosis, left hand
M11.149   Familial chondrocalcinosis, unspecified hand

✓6th   **M11.15**   Familial chondrocalcinosis, hip
M11.151   Familial chondrocalcinosis, right hip
M11.152   Familial chondrocalcinosis, left hip
M11.159   Familial chondrocalcinosis, unspecified hip

✓6th   **M11.16**   Familial chondrocalcinosis, knee
M11.161   Familial chondrocalcinosis, right knee
M11.162   Familial chondrocalcinosis, left knee
M11.169   Familial chondrocalcinosis, unspecified knee

✓6th   **M11.17**   Familial chondrocalcinosis, ankle and foot
M11.171   Familial chondrocalcinosis, right ankle and foot
M11.172   Familial chondrocalcinosis, left ankle and foot
M11.179   Familial chondrocalcinosis, unspecified ankle and foot

M11.18   Familial chondrocalcinosis, vertebrae
M11.19   Familial chondrocalcinosis, multiple sites

✓5th   **M11.2**   Other chondrocalcinosis
Chondrocalcinosis NOS
M11.20   Other chondrocalcinosis, unspecified site

✓6th   **M11.21**   Other chondrocalcinosis, shoulder
M11.211   Other chondrocalcinosis, right shoulder
M11.212   Other chondrocalcinosis, left shoulder
M11.219   Other chondrocalcinosis, unspecified shoulder

✓6th   **M11.22**   Other chondrocalcinosis, elbow
M11.221   Other chondrocalcinosis, right elbow
M11.222   Other chondrocalcinosis, left elbow
M11.229   Other chondrocalcinosis, unspecified elbow

✓6th   **M11.23**   Other chondrocalcinosis, wrist
M11.231   Other chondrocalcinosis, right wrist
M11.232   Other chondrocalcinosis, left wrist
M11.239   Other chondrocalcinosis, unspecified wrist

✓6th   **M11.24**   Other chondrocalcinosis, hand
M11.241   Other chondrocalcinosis, right hand
M11.242   Other chondrocalcinosis, left hand
M11.249   Other chondrocalcinosis, unspecified hand

N Newborn: 0   P Pediatric: 0-17   M Maternity: 12-55   A Adult: 15-124   MCC Major CC Condition   PDx MCC PDx acts as own MCC   CC CC Condition   PDx CC PDx acts as own CC

698   ICD-10-CM Draft (2015)

√6th **M11.25** Other chondrocalcinosis, hip
    M11.251 Other chondrocalcinosis, right hip
    M11.252 Other chondrocalcinosis, left hip
    M11.259 Other chondrocalcinosis, unspecified hip

√6th **M11.26** Other chondrocalcinosis, knee
    M11.261 Other chondrocalcinosis, right knee
    M11.262 Other chondrocalcinosis, left knee
    M11.269 Other chondrocalcinosis, unspecified knee

√6th **M11.27** Other chondrocalcinosis, ankle and foot
    M11.271 Other chondrocalcinosis, right ankle and foot
    M11.272 Other chondrocalcinosis, left ankle and foot
    M11.279 Other chondrocalcinosis, unspecified ankle and foot

M11.28 Other chondrocalcinosis, vertebrae

M11.29 Other chondrocalcinosis, multiple sites

√5th **M11.8** Other specified crystal arthropathies

M11.80 Other specified crystal arthropathies, unspecified site

√6th **M11.81** Other specified crystal arthropathies, shoulder
    M11.811 Other specified crystal arthropathies, right shoulder
    M11.812 Other specified crystal arthropathies, left shoulder
    M11.819 Other specified crystal arthropathies, unspecified shoulder

√6th **M11.82** Other specified crystal arthropathies, elbow
    M11.821 Other specified crystal arthropathies, right elbow
    M11.822 Other specified crystal arthropathies, left elbow
    M11.829 Other specified crystal arthropathies, unspecified elbow

√6th **M11.83** Other specified crystal arthropathies, wrist
    M11.831 Other specified crystal arthropathies, right wrist
    M11.832 Other specified crystal arthropathies, left wrist
    M11.839 Other specified crystal arthropathies, unspecified wrist

√6th **M11.84** Other specified crystal arthropathies, hand
    M11.841 Other specified crystal arthropathies, right hand
    M11.842 Other specified crystal arthropathies, left hand
    M11.849 Other specified crystal arthropathies, unspecified hand

√6th **M11.85** Other specified crystal arthropathies, hip
    M11.851 Other specified crystal arthropathies, right hip
    M11.852 Other specified crystal arthropathies, left hip
    M11.859 Other specified crystal arthropathies, unspecified hip

√6th **M11.86** Other specified crystal arthropathies, knee
    M11.861 Other specified crystal arthropathies, right knee
    M11.862 Other specified crystal arthropathies, left knee
    M11.869 Other specified crystal arthropathies, unspecified knee

√6th **M11.87** Other specified crystal arthropathies, ankle and foot
    M11.871 Other specified crystal arthropathies, right ankle and foot
    M11.872 Other specified crystal arthropathies, left ankle and foot
    M11.879 Other specified crystal arthropathies, unspecified ankle and foot

M11.88 Other specified crystal arthropathies, vertebrae

M11.89 Other specified crystal arthropathies, multiple sites

M11.9 Crystal arthropathy, unspecified

√4th **M12** Other and unspecified arthropathy
    EXCLUDES 1   arthrosis (M15-M19)
           cricoarytenoid arthropathy (J38.7)

√5th **M12.0** Chronic postrheumatic arthropathy [Jaccoud]

M12.00 Chronic postrheumatic arthropathy [Jaccoud], unspecified site

√6th **M12.01** Chronic postrheumatic arthropathy [Jaccoud], shoulder
    M12.011 Chronic postrheumatic arthropathy [Jaccoud], right shoulder
    M12.012 Chronic postrheumatic arthropathy [Jaccoud], left shoulder
    M12.019 Chronic postrheumatic arthropathy [Jaccoud], unspecified shoulder

√6th **M12.02** Chronic postrheumatic arthropathy [Jaccoud], elbow
    M12.021 Chronic postrheumatic arthropathy [Jaccoud], right elbow
    M12.022 Chronic postrheumatic arthropathy [Jaccoud], left elbow
    M12.029 Chronic postrheumatic arthropathy [Jaccoud], unspecified elbow

√6th **M12.03** Chronic postrheumatic arthropathy [Jaccoud], wrist
    M12.031 Chronic postrheumatic arthropathy [Jaccoud], right wrist
    M12.032 Chronic postrheumatic arthropathy [Jaccoud], left wrist
    M12.039 Chronic postrheumatic arthropathy [Jaccoud], unspecified wrist

√6th **M12.04** Chronic postrheumatic arthropathy [Jaccoud], hand
    M12.041 Chronic postrheumatic arthropathy [Jaccoud], right hand
    M12.042 Chronic postrheumatic arthropathy [Jaccoud], left hand
    M12.049 Chronic postrheumatic arthropathy [Jaccoud], unspecified hand

√6th **M12.05** Chronic postrheumatic arthropathy [Jaccoud], hip
    M12.051 Chronic postrheumatic arthropathy [Jaccoud], right hip
    M12.052 Chronic postrheumatic arthropathy [Jaccoud], left hip
    M12.059 Chronic postrheumatic arthropathy [Jaccoud], unspecified hip

√6th **M12.06** Chronic postrheumatic arthropathy [Jaccoud], knee
    M12.061 Chronic postrheumatic arthropathy [Jaccoud], right knee
    M12.062 Chronic postrheumatic arthropathy [Jaccoud], left knee
    M12.069 Chronic postrheumatic arthropathy [Jaccoud], unspecified knee

√6th **M12.07** Chronic postrheumatic arthropathy [Jaccoud], ankle and foot
    M12.071 Chronic postrheumatic arthropathy [Jaccoud], right ankle and foot
    M12.072 Chronic postrheumatic arthropathy [Jaccoud], left ankle and foot
    M12.079 Chronic postrheumatic arthropathy [Jaccoud], unspecified ankle and foot

M12.08 Chronic postrheumatic arthropathy [Jaccoud], other specified site
    Chronic postrheumatic arthropathy [Jaccoud], vertebrae

M12.09 Chronic postrheumatic arthropathy [Jaccoud], multiple sites

√5th **M12.1** Kaschin-Beck disease
    Osteochondroarthrosis deformans endemica

M12.10 Kaschin-Beck disease, unspecified site

√6th **M12.11** Kaschin-Beck disease, shoulder
    M12.111 Kaschin-Beck disease, right shoulder
    M12.112 Kaschin-Beck disease, left shoulder
    M12.119 Kaschin-Beck disease, unspecified shoulder

√6th **M12.12** Kaschin-Beck disease, elbow
    M12.121 Kaschin-Beck disease, right elbow
    M12.122 Kaschin-Beck disease, left elbow
    M12.129 Kaschin-Beck disease, unspecified elbow

✔ Additional Character Required   x7th Xtension Alert   Unacceptable PDx   Manifestation   Hospital Acquired Condition   EXCLUDES 1 Not Coded Here   EXCLUDES 2 Not Included Here

√6th **M12.13 Kaschin-Beck disease,** wrist
- **M12.131 Kaschin-Beck disease,** right **wrist**
- **M12.132 Kaschin-Beck disease,** left **wrist**
- **M12.139 Kaschin-Beck disease,** unspecified **wrist**

√6th **M12.14 Kaschin-Beck disease,** hand
- **M12.141 Kaschin-Beck disease,** right **hand**
- **M12.142 Kaschin-Beck disease,** left **hand**
- **M12.149 Kaschin-Beck disease,** unspecified **hand**

√6th **M12.15 Kaschin-Beck disease,** hip
- **M12.151 Kaschin-Beck disease,** right **hip**
- **M12.152 Kaschin-Beck disease,** left **hip**
- **M12.159 Kaschin-Beck disease,** unspecified **hip**

√6th **M12.16 Kaschin-Beck disease,** knee
- **M12.161 Kaschin-Beck disease,** right **knee**
- **M12.162 Kaschin-Beck disease,** left **knee**
- **M12.169 Kaschin-Beck disease,** unspecified **knee**

√6th **M12.17 Kaschin-Beck disease,** ankle and foot
- **M12.171 Kaschin-Beck disease,** right **ankle and foot**
- **M12.172 Kaschin-Beck disease,** left **ankle and foot**
- **M12.179 Kaschin-Beck disease,** unspecified **ankle and foot**

M12.18 Kaschin-Beck disease, vertebrae

M12.19 Kaschin-Beck disease, multiple sites

√5th **M12.2 Villonodular synovitis (pigmented)**

M12.20 Villonodular synovitis (pigmented), unspecified site

√6th **M12.21 Villonodular synovitis (pigmented),** shoulder
- **M12.211 Villonodular synovitis (pigmented),** right **shoulder**
- **M12.212 Villonodular synovitis (pigmented),** left **shoulder**
- **M12.219 Villonodular synovitis (pigmented),** unspecified **shoulder**

√6th **M12.22 Villonodular synovitis (pigmented),** elbow
- **M12.221 Villonodular synovitis (pigmented),** right **elbow**
- **M12.222 Villonodular synovitis (pigmented),** left **elbow**
- **M12.229 Villonodular synovitis (pigmented),** unspecified **elbow**

√6th **M12.23 Villonodular synovitis (pigmented),** wrist
- **M12.231 Villonodular synovitis (pigmented),** right **wrist**
- **M12.232 Villonodular synovitis (pigmented),** left **wrist**
- **M12.239 Villonodular synovitis (pigmented),** unspecified **wrist**

√6th **M12.24 Villonodular synovitis (pigmented),** hand
- **M12.241 Villonodular synovitis (pigmented),** right **hand**
- **M12.242 Villonodular synovitis (pigmented),** left **hand**
- **M12.249 Villonodular synovitis (pigmented),** unspecified **hand**

√6th **M12.25 Villonodular synovitis (pigmented),** hip
- **M12.251 Villonodular synovitis (pigmented),** right **hip**
- **M12.252 Villonodular synovitis (pigmented),** left **hip**
- **M12.259 Villonodular synovitis (pigmented),** unspecified **hip**

√6th **M12.26 Villonodular synovitis (pigmented),** knee
- **M12.261 Villonodular synovitis (pigmented),** right **knee**
- **M12.262 Villonodular synovitis (pigmented),** left **knee**
- **M12.269 Villonodular synovitis (pigmented),** unspecified **knee**

√6th **M12.27 Villonodular synovitis (pigmented),** ankle and foot
- **M12.271 Villonodular synovitis (pigmented),** right **ankle and foot**
- **M12.272 Villonodular synovitis (pigmented),** left **ankle and foot**
- **M12.279 Villonodular synovitis (pigmented),** unspecified **ankle and foot**

M12.28 Villonodular synovitis (pigmented), other specified site
    Villonodular synovitis (pigmented), vertebrae

M12.29 Villonodular synovitis (pigmented), multiple sites

√5th **M12.3 Palindromic rheumatism**

M12.30 Palindromic rheumatism, unspecified site

√6th **M12.31 Palindromic rheumatism,** shoulder
- **M12.311 Palindromic rheumatism,** right **shoulder**
- **M12.312 Palindromic rheumatism,** left **shoulder**
- **M12.319 Palindromic rheumatism,** unspecified **shoulder**

√6th **M12.32 Palindromic rheumatism,** elbow
- **M12.321 Palindromic rheumatism,** right **elbow**
- **M12.322 Palindromic rheumatism,** left **elbow**
- **M12.329 Palindromic rheumatism,** unspecified **elbow**

√6th **M12.33 Palindromic rheumatism,** wrist
- **M12.331 Palindromic rheumatism,** right **wrist**
- **M12.332 Palindromic rheumatism,** left **wrist**
- **M12.339 Palindromic rheumatism,** unspecified **wrist**

√6th **M12.34 Palindromic rheumatism,** hand
- **M12.341 Palindromic rheumatism,** right **hand**
- **M12.342 Palindromic rheumatism,** left **hand**
- **M12.349 Palindromic rheumatism,** unspecified **hand**

√6th **M12.35 Palindromic rheumatism,** hip
- **M12.351 Palindromic rheumatism,** right **hip**
- **M12.352 Palindromic rheumatism,** left **hip**
- **M12.359 Palindromic rheumatism,** unspecified **hip**

√6th **M12.36 Palindromic rheumatism,** knee
- **M12.361 Palindromic rheumatism,** right **knee**
- **M12.362 Palindromic rheumatism,** left **knee**
- **M12.369 Palindromic rheumatism,** unspecified **knee**

√6th **M12.37 Palindromic rheumatism,** ankle and foot
- **M12.371 Palindromic rheumatism,** right **ankle and foot**
- **M12.372 Palindromic rheumatism,** left **ankle and foot**
- **M12.379 Palindromic rheumatism,** unspecified **ankle and foot**

M12.38 Palindromic rheumatism, other specified site
    Palindromic rheumatism, vertebrae

M12.39 Palindromic rheumatism, multiple sites

√5th **M12.4 Intermittent hydrarthrosis**

M12.40 Intermittent hydrarthrosis, unspecified site

√6th **M12.41 Intermittent hydrarthrosis,** shoulder
- **M12.411 Intermittent hydrarthrosis,** right **shoulder**
- **M12.412 Intermittent hydrarthrosis,** left **shoulder**
- **M12.419 Intermittent hydrarthrosis,** unspecified **shoulder**

√6th **M12.42 Intermittent hydrarthrosis,** elbow
- **M12.421 Intermittent hydrarthrosis,** right **elbow**
- **M12.422 Intermittent hydrarthrosis,** left **elbow**
- **M12.429 Intermittent hydrarthrosis,** unspecified **elbow**

√6th **M12.43 Intermittent hydrarthrosis,** wrist
- **M12.431 Intermittent hydrarthrosis,** right **wrist**
- **M12.432 Intermittent hydrarthrosis,** left **wrist**
- **M12.439 Intermittent hydrarthrosis,** unspecified **wrist**

√6th **M12.44 Intermittent hydrarthrosis,** hand
- **M12.441 Intermittent hydrarthrosis,** right **hand**
- **M12.442 Intermittent hydrarthrosis,** left **hand**
- **M12.449 Intermittent hydrarthrosis,** unspecified **hand**

√6th **M12.45 Intermittent hydrarthrosis,** hip
- **M12.451 Intermittent hydrarthrosis,** right **hip**
- **M12.452 Intermittent hydrarthrosis,** left **hip**
- **M12.459 Intermittent hydrarthrosis,** unspecified **hip**

N Newborn: 0   P Pediatric: 0-17   M Maternity: 12-55   A Adult: 15-124   MCC Major CC Condition   PDx MCC PDx acts as own MCC   CC CC Condition   PDx CC PDx acts as own CC

700   ICD-10-CM Draft (2015)

√6ᵗʰ **M12.46 Intermittent hydrarthrosis,** knee
 M12.461 Intermittent hydrarthrosis, right knee
 M12.462 Intermittent hydrarthrosis, left knee
 M12.469 Intermittent hydrarthrosis, unspecified knee

√6ᵗʰ **M12.47 Intermittent hydrarthrosis,** ankle and foot
 M12.471 Intermittent hydrarthrosis, right ankle and foot
 M12.472 Intermittent hydrarthrosis, left ankle and foot
 M12.479 Intermittent hydrarthrosis, unspecified ankle and foot

M12.48 Intermittent hydrarthrosis, other site

M12.49 Intermittent hydrarthrosis, multiple sites

√5ᵗʰ **M12.5 Traumatic arthropathy**
 EXCLUDES 1 *current injury-see Alphabetic Index*
  post-traumatic osteoarthritis NOS (M19.1-)
  post-traumatic osteoarthritis of first carpometacarpal joint (M18.2-M18.3)
  post-traumatic osteoarthritis of hip (M16.4-M16.5)
  post-traumatic osteoarthritis of knee (M17.2-M17.3)
  post-traumatic osteoarthritis of other single joints (M19.1-)

M12.50 Traumatic arthropathy, unspecified site

√6ᵗʰ **M12.51 Traumatic arthropathy,** shoulder
 M12.511 Traumatic arthropathy, right shoulder
 M12.512 Traumatic arthropathy, left shoulder
 M12.519 Traumatic arthropathy, unspecified shoulder

√6ᵗʰ **M12.52 Traumatic arthropathy,** elbow
 M12.521 Traumatic arthropathy, right elbow
 M12.522 Traumatic arthropathy, left elbow
 M12.529 Traumatic arthropathy, unspecified elbow

√6ᵗʰ **M12.53 Traumatic arthropathy,** wrist
 M12.531 Traumatic arthropathy, right wrist
 M12.532 Traumatic arthropathy, left wrist
 M12.539 Traumatic arthropathy, unspecified wrist

√6ᵗʰ **M12.54 Traumatic arthropathy,** hand
 M12.541 Traumatic arthropathy, right hand
 M12.542 Traumatic arthropathy, left hand
 M12.549 Traumatic arthropathy, unspecified hand

√6ᵗʰ **M12.55 Traumatic arthropathy,** hip
 M12.551 Traumatic arthropathy, right hip
 M12.552 Traumatic arthropathy, left hip
 M12.559 Traumatic arthropathy, unspecified hip

√6ᵗʰ **M12.56 Traumatic arthropathy,** knee
 M12.561 Traumatic arthropathy, right knee
 M12.562 Traumatic arthropathy, left knee
 M12.569 Traumatic arthropathy, unspecified knee

√6ᵗʰ **M12.57 Traumatic arthropathy,** ankle and foot
 M12.571 Traumatic arthropathy, right ankle and foot
 M12.572 Traumatic arthropathy, left ankle and foot
 M12.579 Traumatic arthropathy, unspecified ankle and foot

M12.58 Traumatic arthropathy, other specified site
 Traumatic arthropathy, vertebrae

M12.59 Traumatic arthropathy, multiple sites

√5ᵗʰ **M12.8 Other specific arthropathies, not elsewhere classified**
 Transient arthropathy

M12.80 Other specific arthropathies, not elsewhere classified, unspecified site

√6ᵗʰ **M12.81 Other specific arthropathies, not elsewhere classified,** shoulder
 M12.811 Other specific arthropathies, not elsewhere classified, right shoulder
 M12.812 Other specific arthropathies, not elsewhere classified, left shoulder
 M12.819 Other specific arthropathies, not elsewhere classified, unspecified shoulder

√6ᵗʰ **M12.82 Other specific arthropathies, not elsewhere classified,** elbow
 M12.821 Other specific arthropathies, not elsewhere classified, right elbow
 M12.822 Other specific arthropathies, not elsewhere classified, left elbow
 M12.829 Other specific arthropathies, not elsewhere classified, unspecified elbow

√6ᵗʰ **M12.83 Other specific arthropathies, not elsewhere classified,** wrist
 M12.831 Other specific arthropathies, not elsewhere classified, right wrist
 M12.832 Other specific arthropathies, not elsewhere classified, left wrist
 M12.839 Other specific arthropathies, not elsewhere classified, unspecified wrist

√6ᵗʰ **M12.84 Other specific arthropathies, not elsewhere classified,** hand
 M12.841 Other specific arthropathies, not elsewhere classified, right hand
 M12.842 Other specific arthropathies, not elsewhere classified, left hand
 M12.849 Other specific arthropathies, not elsewhere classified, unspecified hand

√6ᵗʰ **M12.85 Other specific arthropathies, not elsewhere classified,** hip
 M12.851 Other specific arthropathies, not elsewhere classified, right hip
 M12.852 Other specific arthropathies, not elsewhere classified, left hip
 M12.859 Other specific arthropathies, not elsewhere classified, unspecified hip

√6ᵗʰ **M12.86 Other specific arthropathies, not elsewhere classified,** knee
 M12.861 Other specific arthropathies, not elsewhere classified, right knee
 M12.862 Other specific arthropathies, not elsewhere classified, left knee
 M12.869 Other specific arthropathies, not elsewhere classified, unspecified knee

√6ᵗʰ **M12.87 Other specific arthropathies, not elsewhere classified,** ankle and foot
 M12.871 Other specific arthropathies, not elsewhere classified, right ankle and foot
 M12.872 Other specific arthropathies, not elsewhere classified, left ankle and foot
 M12.879 Other specific arthropathies, not elsewhere classified, unspecified ankle and foot

M12.88 Other specific arthropathies, not elsewhere classified, other specified site
 Other specific arthropathies, not elsewhere classified, vertebrae

M12.89 Other specific arthropathies, not elsewhere classified, multiple sites

M12.9 Arthropathy, unspecified

√4ᵗʰ **M13 Other arthritis**
 EXCLUDES 1 *arthrosis (M15-M19)*
  osteoarthritis (M15-M19)

M13.0 Polyarthritis, unspecified

√5ᵗʰ **M13.1 Monoarthritis, not elsewhere classified**
 M13.10 Monoarthritis, not elsewhere classified, unspecified site

√6ᵗʰ **M13.11 Monoarthritis, not elsewhere classified,** shoulder
 M13.111 Monoarthritis, not elsewhere classified, right shoulder
 M13.112 Monoarthritis, not elsewhere classified, left shoulder
 M13.119 Monoarthritis, not elsewhere classified, unspecified shoulder

√6ᵗʰ **M13.12 Monoarthritis, not elsewhere classified,** elbow
 M13.121 Monoarthritis, not elsewhere classified, right elbow
 M13.122 Monoarthritis, not elsewhere classified, left elbow
 M13.129 Monoarthritis, not elsewhere classified, unspecified elbow

√6ᵗʰ **M13.13 Monoarthritis, not elsewhere classified,** wrist
 M13.131 Monoarthritis, not elsewhere classified, right wrist

✓ Additional Character Required √x7ᵗʰ Xtension Alert Unacceptable PDx Manifestation Hospital Acquired Condition EXCLUDES 1 Not Coded Here EXCLUDES 2 Not Included Here

ICD-10-CM Draft (2015) 701

M13.132 **Monoarthritis, not elsewhere classified, left wrist**

M13.139 **Monoarthritis, not elsewhere classified, unspecified wrist**

√6th M13.14 **Monoarthritis, not elsewhere classified, hand**

M13.141 **Monoarthritis, not elsewhere classified, right hand**

M13.142 **Monoarthritis, not elsewhere classified, left hand**

M13.149 **Monoarthritis, not elsewhere classified, unspecified hand**

√6th M13.15 **Monoarthritis, not elsewhere classified, hip**

M13.151 **Monoarthritis, not elsewhere classified, right hip**

M13.152 **Monoarthritis, not elsewhere classified, left hip**

M13.159 **Monoarthritis, not elsewhere classified, unspecified hip**

√6th M13.16 **Monoarthritis, not elsewhere classified, knee**

M13.161 **Monoarthritis, not elsewhere classified, right knee**

M13.162 **Monoarthritis, not elsewhere classified, left knee**

M13.169 **Monoarthritis, not elsewhere classified, unspecified knee**

√6th M13.17 **Monoarthritis, not elsewhere classified, ankle and foot**

M13.171 **Monoarthritis, not elsewhere classified, right ankle and foot**

M13.172 **Monoarthritis, not elsewhere classified, left ankle and foot**

M13.179 **Monoarthritis, not elsewhere classified, unspecified ankle and foot**

√5th M13.8 **Other specified arthritis**
Allergic arthritis
EXCLUDES 1 *osteoarthritis (M15-M19)*

M13.80 **Other specified arthritis, unspecified site**

√6th M13.81 **Other specified arthritis, shoulder**

M13.811 **Other specified arthritis, right shoulder**

M13.812 **Other specified arthritis, left shoulder**

M13.819 **Other specified arthritis, unspecified shoulder**

√6th M13.82 **Other specified arthritis, elbow**

M13.821 **Other specified arthritis, right elbow**

M13.822 **Other specified arthritis, left elbow**

M13.829 **Other specified arthritis, unspecified elbow**

√6th M13.83 **Other specified arthritis, wrist**

M13.831 **Other specified arthritis, right wrist**

M13.832 **Other specified arthritis, left wrist**

M13.839 **Other specified arthritis, unspecified wrist**

√6th M13.84 **Other specified arthritis, hand**

M13.841 **Other specified arthritis, right hand**

M13.842 **Other specified arthritis, left hand**

M13.849 **Other specified arthritis, unspecified hand**

√6th M13.85 **Other specified arthritis, hip**

M13.851 **Other specified arthritis, right hip**

M13.852 **Other specified arthritis, left hip**

M13.859 **Other specified arthritis, unspecified hip**

√6th M13.86 **Other specified arthritis, knee**

M13.861 **Other specified arthritis, right knee**

M13.862 **Other specified arthritis, left knee**

M13.869 **Other specified arthritis, unspecified knee**

√6th M13.87 **Other specified arthritis, ankle and foot**

M13.871 **Other specified arthritis, right ankle and foot**

M13.872 **Other specified arthritis, left ankle and foot**

M13.879 **Other specified arthritis, unspecified ankle and foot**

M13.88 **Other specified arthritis, other site**

M13.89 **Other specified arthritis, multiple sites**

√4th M14 **Arthropathies in other diseases classified elsewhere**
EXCLUDES 1 arthropathy in:
diabetes mellitus (E08-E13 with .61-)
hematological disorders (M36.2-M36.3)
hypersensitivity reactions (M36.4)
neoplastic disease (M36.1)
neurosyphillis (A52.16)
sarcoidosis (D86.86)
enteropathic arthropathies (M07.-)
juvenile psoriatic arthropathy (L40.54)
lipoid dermatoarthritis (E78.81)

√5th M14.6 **Charcôt's joint**
Neuropathic arthropathy
EXCLUDES 1 *Charcôt's joint in diabetes mellitus (E08-E13 with .610-)*
Charcôt's joint in tabes dorsalis (A52.16)

M14.60 **Charcôt's joint, unspecified site**

√6th M14.61 **Charcôt's joint, shoulder**

M14.611 **Charcôt's joint, right shoulder**

M14.612 **Charcôt's joint, left shoulder**

M14.619 **Charcôt's joint, unspecified shoulder**

√6th M14.62 **Charcôt's joint, elbow**

M14.621 **Charcôt's joint, right elbow**

M14.622 **Charcôt's joint, left elbow**

M14.629 **Charcôt's joint, unspecified elbow**

√6th M14.63 **Charcôt's joint, wrist**

M14.631 **Charcôt's joint, right wrist**

M14.632 **Charcôt's joint, left wrist**

M14.639 **Charcôt's joint, unspecified wrist**

√6th M14.64 **Charcôt's joint, hand**

M14.641 **Charcôt's joint, right hand**

M14.642 **Charcôt's joint, left hand**

M14.649 **Charcôt's joint, unspecified hand**

√6th M14.65 **Charcôt's joint, hip**

M14.651 **Charcôt's joint, right hip**

M14.652 **Charcôt's joint, left hip**

M14.659 **Charcôt's joint, unspecified hip**

√6th M14.66 **Charcôt's joint, knee**

M14.661 **Charcôt's joint, right knee**

M14.662 **Charcôt's joint, left knee**

M14.669 **Charcôt's joint, unspecified knee**

√6th M14.67 **Charcôt's joint, ankle and foot**

M14.671 **Charcôt's joint, right ankle and foot**

M14.672 **Charcôt's joint, left ankle and foot**

M14.679 **Charcôt's joint, unspecified ankle and foot**

M14.68 **Charcôt's joint, vertebrae**

M14.69 **Charcôt's joint, multiple sites**

√5th M14.8 **Arthropathies in other specified diseases classified elsewhere**
Code first underlying disease, such as:
amyloidosis (E85.-)
erythema multiforme (L51.-)
erythema nodosum (L52)
hemochromatosis (E83.11-)
hyperparathyroidism (E21.-)
hypothyroidism (E00-E03)
sickle-cell disorders (D57.-)
thyrotoxicosis [hyperthyroidism] (E05.-)
Whipple's disease (K90.81)

M14.80 ***Arthropathies in other specified diseases classified elsewhere, unspecified site***

√6th M14.81 **Arthropathies in other specified diseases classified elsewhere, shoulder**

M14.811 ***Arthropathies in other specified diseases classified elsewhere, right shoulder***

M14.812 ***Arthropathies in other specified diseases classified elsewhere, left shoulder***

M14.819 ***Arthropathies in other specified diseases classified elsewhere, unspecified shoulder***

√6th M14.82 **Arthropathies in other specified diseases classified elsewhere, elbow**

M14.821 ***Arthropathies in other specified diseases classified elsewhere, right elbow***

M14.822 ***Arthropathies in other specified diseases classified elsewhere, left elbow***

M14.829 ***Arthropathies in other specified diseases classified elsewhere, unspecified elbow***

N Newborn: 0   P Pediatric: 0-17   M Maternity: 12-55   A Adult: 15-124   MCC Major CC Condition   PDx MCC PDx acts as own MCC   CC CC Condition   PDx CC PDx acts as own CC

702   ICD-10-CM Draft (2015)

√6ᵗʰ **M14.83 Arthropathies in other specified diseases classified elsewhere, wrist**
- *M14.831 Arthropathies in other specified diseases classified elsewhere, right wrist*
- *M14.832 Arthropathies in other specified diseases classified elsewhere, left wrist*
- *M14.839 Arthropathies in other specified diseases classified elsewhere, unspecified wrist*

√6ᵗʰ **M14.84 Arthropathies in other specified diseases classified elsewhere, hand**
- *M14.841 Arthropathies in other specified diseases classified elsewhere, right hand*
- *M14.842 Arthropathies in other specified diseases classified elsewhere, left hand*
- *M14.849 Arthropathies in other specified diseases classified elsewhere, unspecified hand*

√6ᵗʰ **M14.85 Arthropathies in other specified diseases classified elsewhere, hip**
- *M14.851 Arthropathies in other specified diseases classified elsewhere, right hip*
- *M14.852 Arthropathies in other specified diseases classified elsewhere, left hip*
- *M14.859 Arthropathies in other specified diseases classified elsewhere, unspecified hip*

√6ᵗʰ **M14.86 Arthropathies in other specified diseases classified elsewhere, knee**
- *M14.861 Arthropathies in other specified diseases classified elsewhere, right knee*
- *M14.862 Arthropathies in other specified diseases classified elsewhere, left knee*
- *M14.869 Arthropathies in other specified diseases classified elsewhere, unspecified knee*

√6ᵗʰ **M14.87 Arthropathies in other specified diseases classified elsewhere, ankle and foot**
- *M14.871 Arthropathies in other specified diseases classified elsewhere, right ankle and foot*
- *M14.872 Arthropathies in other specified diseases classified elsewhere, left ankle and foot*
- *M14.879 Arthropathies in other specified diseases classified elsewhere, unspecified ankle and foot*

M14.88 Arthropathies in other specified diseases classified elsewhere, vertebrae

M14.89 Arthropathies in other specified diseases classified elsewhere, multiple sites

Osteoarthritis (M15-M19)

EXCLUDES 2 osteoarthritis of spine (M47.-)

√4ᵗʰ **M15 Polyosteoarthritis**

INCLUDES arthritis of multiple sites

EXCLUDES 1 bilateral involvement of single joint (M16-M19)

M15.0 Primary generalized (osteo)arthritis

M15.1 Heberden's nodes (with arthropathy)
Interphalangeal distal osteoarthritis

M15.2 Bouchard's nodes (with arthropathy)
Juxtaphalangeal distal osteoarthritis

M15.3 Secondary multiple arthritis
Post-traumatic polyosteoarthritis

M15.4 Erosive (osteo)arthritis

M15.8 Other polyosteoarthritis

M15.9 Polyosteoarthritis, unspecified
Generalized osteoarthritis NOS

√4ᵗʰ **M16 Osteoarthritis of hip**

M16.0 Bilateral primary osteoarthritis of hip ✓

√5ᵗʰ **M16.1 Unilateral primary osteoarthritis of hip**
Primary osteoarthritis of hip NOS
- **M16.10 Unilateral primary osteoarthritis, unspecified hip**
- **M16.11 Unilateral primary osteoarthritis, right hip**
- **M16.12 Unilateral primary osteoarthritis, left hip**

M16.2 Bilateral osteoarthritis resulting from hip dysplasia

√5ᵗʰ **M16.3 Unilateral osteoarthritis resulting from hip dysplasia**
Dysplastic osteoarthritis of hip NOS
- **M16.30 Unilateral osteoarthritis resulting from hip dysplasia, unspecified hip**
- **M16.31 Unilateral osteoarthritis resulting from hip dysplasia, right hip**

M16.32 Unilateral osteoarthritis resulting from hip dysplasia, left hip

M16.4 Bilateral post-traumatic osteoarthritis of hip

√5ᵗʰ **M16.5 Unilateral post-traumatic osteoarthritis of hip**
Post-traumatic osteoarthritis of hip NOS
- **M16.50 Unilateral post-traumatic osteoarthritis, unspecified hip**
- **M16.51 Unilateral post-traumatic osteoarthritis, right hip**
- **M16.52 Unilateral post-traumatic osteoarthritis, left hip**

M16.6 Other bilateral secondary osteoarthritis of hip

M16.7 Other unilateral secondary osteoarthritis of hip
Secondary osteoarthritis of hip NOS

M16.9 Osteoarthritis of hip, unspecified

√4ᵗʰ **M17 Osteoarthritis of knee**

M17.0 Bilateral primary osteoarthritis of knee

√5ᵗʰ **M17.1 Unilateral primary osteoarthritis of knee**
Primary osteoarthritis of knee NOS
- **M17.10 Unilateral primary osteoarthritis, unspecified knee**
- **M17.11 Unilateral primary osteoarthritis, right knee**
- **M17.12 Unilateral primary osteoarthritis, left knee**

M17.2 Bilateral post-traumatic osteoarthritis of knee

√5ᵗʰ **M17.3 Unilateral post-traumatic osteoarthritis of knee**
Post-traumatic osteoarthritis of knee NOS
- **M17.30 Unilateral post-traumatic osteoarthritis, unspecified knee**
- **M17.31 Unilateral post-traumatic osteoarthritis, right knee**
- **M17.32 Unilateral post-traumatic osteoarthritis, left knee**

M17.4 Other bilateral secondary osteoarthritis of knee

M17.5 Other unilateral secondary osteoarthritis of knee
Secondary osteoarthritis of knee NOS

M17.9 Osteoarthritis of knee, unspecified

√4ᵗʰ **M18 Osteoarthritis of first carpometacarpal joint**

M18.0 Bilateral primary osteoarthritis of first carpometacarpal joints

√5ᵗʰ **M18.1 Unilateral primary osteoarthritis of first carpometacarpal joint**
Primary osteoarthritis of first carpometacarpal joint NOS
- **M18.10 Unilateral primary osteoarthritis of first carpometacarpal joint, unspecified hand**
- **M18.11 Unilateral primary osteoarthritis of first carpometacarpal joint, right hand**
- **M18.12 Unilateral primary osteoarthritis of first carpometacarpal joint, left hand**

M18.2 Bilateral post-traumatic osteoarthritis of first carpometacarpal joints

√5ᵗʰ **M18.3 Unilateral post-traumatic osteoarthritis of first carpometacarpal joint**
Post-traumatic osteoarthritis of first carpometacarpal joint NOS
- **M18.30 Unilateral post-traumatic osteoarthritis of first carpometacarpal joint, unspecified hand**
- **M18.31 Unilateral post-traumatic osteoarthritis of first carpometacarpal joint, right hand**
- **M18.32 Unilateral post-traumatic osteoarthritis of first carpometacarpal joint, left hand**

M18.4 Other bilateral secondary osteoarthritis of first carpometacarpal joints

√5ᵗʰ **M18.5 Other unilateral secondary osteoarthritis of first carpometacarpal joint**
Secondary osteoarthritis of first carpometacarpal joint NOS
- **M18.50 Other unilateral secondary osteoarthritis of first carpometacarpal joint, unspecified hand**
- **M18.51 Other unilateral secondary osteoarthritis of first carpometacarpal joint, right hand**
- **M18.52 Other unilateral secondary osteoarthritis of first carpometacarpal joint, left hand**

M18.9 Osteoarthritis of first carpometacarpal joint, unspecified

√4ᵗʰ **M19 Other and unspecified osteoarthritis**

EXCLUDES 1 polyarthritis (M15.-)

EXCLUDES 2 arthrosis of spine (M47.-)
hallux rigidus (M20.2)
osteoarthritis of spine (M47.-)

√5ᵗʰ **M19.0 Primary osteoarthritis of other joints**

√6ᵗʰ **M19.01 Primary osteoarthritis, shoulder**

M19.011 Primary osteoarthritis, right shoulder

✓ Additional Character Required   √x7ᵗʰ Xtension Alert   Unacceptable PDx   Manifestation   Hospital Acquired Condition   *EXCLUDES 1* Not Coded Here   *EXCLUDES 2* Not Included Here

M19.012 **Primary** osteoarthritis, **left shoulder**
M19.019 **Primary** osteoarthritis, **unspecified** shoulder

✓6ᵗʰ M19.02 **Primary** osteoarthritis, **elbow**
    M19.021 **Primary** osteoarthritis, **right elbow**
    M19.022 **Primary** osteoarthritis, **left elbow**
    M19.029 **Primary** osteoarthritis, **unspecified elbow**

✓6ᵗʰ M19.03 **Primary** osteoarthritis, **wrist**
    M19.031 **Primary** osteoarthritis, **right wrist**
    M19.032 **Primary** osteoarthritis, **left wrist**
    M19.039 **Primary** osteoarthritis, **unspecified wrist**

✓6ᵗʰ M19.04 **Primary** osteoarthritis, **hand**
    EXCLUDES 2 *primary osteoarthritis of first carpometacarpal joint (M18.0-, M18.1-)*
    M19.041 **Primary** osteoarthritis, **right hand**
    M19.042 **Primary** osteoarthritis, **left hand**
    M19.049 **Primary** osteoarthritis, **unspecified hand**

✓6ᵗʰ M19.07 **Primary** osteoarthritis **ankle and foot**
    M19.071 **Primary** osteoarthritis, **right ankle and foot**
    M19.072 **Primary** osteoarthritis, **left ankle and foot**
    M19.079 **Primary** osteoarthritis, **unspecified ankle and foot**

✓5ᵗʰ M19.1 **Post-traumatic** osteoarthritis of other joints

✓6ᵗʰ M19.11 **Post-traumatic** osteoarthritis, **shoulder**
    M19.111 **Post-traumatic** osteoarthritis, **right shoulder**
    M19.112 **Post-traumatic** osteoarthritis, **left shoulder**
    M19.119 **Post-traumatic** osteoarthritis, **unspecified shoulder**

✓6ᵗʰ M19.12 **Post-traumatic** osteoarthritis, **elbow**
    M19.121 **Post-traumatic** osteoarthritis, **right elbow**
    M19.122 **Post-traumatic** osteoarthritis, **left elbow**
    M19.129 **Post-traumatic** osteoarthritis, **unspecified elbow**

✓6ᵗʰ M19.13 **Post-traumatic** osteoarthritis, **wrist**
    M19.131 **Post-traumatic** osteoarthritis, **right wrist**
    M19.132 **Post-traumatic** osteoarthritis, **left wrist**
    M19.139 **Post-traumatic** osteoarthritis, **unspecified wrist**

✓6ᵗʰ M19.14 **Post-traumatic** osteoarthritis, **hand**
    EXCLUDES 2 *post-traumatic osteoarthritis of first carpometacarpal joint (M18.2-, M18.3-)*
    M19.141 **Post-traumatic** osteoarthritis, **right hand**
    M19.142 **Post-traumatic** osteoarthritis, **left hand**
    M19.149 **Post-traumatic** osteoarthritis, **unspecified hand**

✓6ᵗʰ M19.17 **Post-traumatic** osteoarthritis, **ankle and foot**
    M19.171 **Post-traumatic** osteoarthritis, **right ankle and foot**
    M19.172 **Post-traumatic** osteoarthritis, **left ankle and foot**
    M19.179 **Post-traumatic** osteoarthritis, **unspecified ankle and foot**

✓5ᵗʰ M19.2 **Secondary** osteoarthritis of other joints

✓6ᵗʰ M19.21 **Secondary** osteoarthritis, **shoulder**
    M19.211 **Secondary** osteoarthritis, **right shoulder**
    M19.212 **Secondary** osteoarthritis, **left shoulder**
    M19.219 **Secondary** osteoarthritis, **unspecified shoulder**

✓6ᵗʰ M19.22 **Secondary** osteoarthritis, **elbow**
    M19.221 **Secondary** osteoarthritis, **right elbow**
    M19.222 **Secondary** osteoarthritis, **left elbow**
    M19.229 **Secondary** osteoarthritis, **unspecified elbow**

✓6ᵗʰ M19.23 **Secondary** osteoarthritis, **wrist**
    M19.231 **Secondary** osteoarthritis, **right wrist**
    M19.232 **Secondary** osteoarthritis, **left wrist**
    M19.239 **Secondary** osteoarthritis, **unspecified wrist**

✓6ᵗʰ M19.24 **Secondary** osteoarthritis, **hand**
    M19.241 **Secondary** osteoarthritis, **right hand**
    M19.242 **Secondary** osteoarthritis, **left hand**

M19.249 **Secondary** osteoarthritis, **unspecified hand**

✓6ᵗʰ M19.27 **Secondary** osteoarthritis, **ankle and foot**
    M19.271 **Secondary** osteoarthritis, **right ankle and foot**
    M19.272 **Secondary** osteoarthritis, **left ankle and foot**
    M19.279 **Secondary** osteoarthritis, **unspecified ankle and foot**

✓5ᵗʰ M19.9 **Osteoarthritis, unspecified site**

M19.90 **Unspecified** osteoarthritis, **unspecified site**
    Arthrosis NOS
    Arthritis NOS
    Osteoarthritis NOS

M19.91 **Primary** osteoarthritis, **unspecified site**
    Primary osteoarthritis NOS

M19.92 **Post-traumatic** osteoarthritis, **unspecified site**
    Post-traumatic osteoarthritis NOS

M19.93 **Secondary** osteoarthritis, **unspecified site**
    Secondary osteoarthritis NOS

Other joint disorders (M20-M25)
EXCLUDES 2 *joints of the spine (M40-M54)*

✓4ᵗʰ **M20 Acquired deformities of fingers and toes**
    EXCLUDES 1 *acquired absence of fingers and toes (Z89.-)*
    congenital absence of fingers and toes (Q71.3-, Q72.3-)
    congenital deformities and malformations of fingers and toes (Q66-, Q68-Q70, Q74-)

✓5ᵗʰ M20.0 **Deformity of finger(s)**
    EXCLUDES 1 *clubbing of fingers (R68.3)*
    palmar fascial fibromatosis [Dupuytren] (M72.0)
    trigger finger (M65.3)

✓6ᵗʰ M20.00 **Unspecified deformity of finger(s)**
    M20.001 **Unspecified deformity of right finger(s)**
    M20.002 **Unspecified deformity of left finger(s)**
    M20.009 **Unspecified deformity of unspecified finger(s)**

✓6ᵗʰ M20.01 **Mallet finger**
    M20.011 **Mallet finger of right finger(s)**
    M20.012 **Mallet finger of left finger(s)**
    M20.019 **Mallet finger of unspecified finger(s)**

✓6ᵗʰ M20.02 **Boutonnière deformity**
    M20.021 **Boutonnière deformity of right finger(s)**
    M20.022 **Boutonnière deformity of left finger(s)**
    M20.029 **Boutonnière deformity of unspecified finger(s)**

✓6ᵗʰ M20.03 **Swan-neck deformity**
    M20.031 **Swan-neck deformity of right finger(s)**
    M20.032 **Swan-neck deformity of left finger(s)**
    M20.039 **Swan-neck deformity of unspecified finger(s)**

✓6ᵗʰ M20.09 **Other deformity of finger(s)**
    M20.091 **Other deformity of right finger(s)**
    M20.092 **Other deformity of left finger(s)**
    M20.099 **Other deformity of finger(s), unspecified finger(s)**

✓5ᵗʰ M20.1 **Hallux valgus (acquired)**
    Bunion
    M20.10 **Hallux valgus (acquired), unspecified foot**
    M20.11 **Hallux valgus (acquired), right foot**
    M20.12 **Hallux valgus (acquired), left foot**

✓5ᵗʰ M20.2 **Hallux rigidus**
    M20.20 **Hallux rigidus, unspecified foot**
    M20.21 **Hallux rigidus, right foot**
    M20.22 **Hallux rigidus, left foot**

✓5ᵗʰ M20.3 **Hallux varus (acquired)**
    M20.30 **Hallux varus (acquired), unspecified foot**
    M20.31 **Hallux varus (acquired), right foot**
    M20.32 **Hallux varus (acquired), left foot**

✓5ᵗʰ M20.4 **Other hammer toe(s) (acquired)**
    M20.40 **Other hammer toe(s) (acquired), unspecified foot**
    M20.41 **Other hammer toe(s) (acquired), right foot**
    M20.42 **Other hammer toe(s) (acquired), left foot**

✓5th M20.5 Other deformities of toe(s) (acquired)

    ✓6th M20.5X Other deformities of toe(s) (acquired)

        M20.5X1 Other deformities of toe(s) (acquired), right foot

        M20.5X2 Other deformities of toe(s) (acquired), left foot

        M20.5X9 Other deformities of toe(s) (acquired), unspecified foot

✓5th M20.6 Acquired deformities of toe(s), unspecified

    M20.60 Acquired deformities of toe(s), unspecified, unspecified foot

    M20.61 Acquired deformities of toe(s), unspecified, right foot

    M20.62 Acquired deformities of toe(s), unspecified, left foot

✓4th M21 Other acquired deformities of limbs

    EXCLUDES 1 acquired absence of limb (Z89.-)
                  congenital absence of limbs (Q71-Q73)
                  congenital deformities and malformations of limbs (Q65-Q66, Q68-Q74)
    EXCLUDES 2 acquired deformities of fingers or toes (M20.-)
                  coxa plana (M91.2)

✓5th M21.0 Valgus deformity, not elsewhere classified

    EXCLUDES 1 metatarsus valgus (Q66.6)
                  talipes calcaneovalgus (Q66.4)

    M21.00 Valgus deformity, not elsewhere classified, unspecified site

    ✓6th M21.02 Valgus deformity, not elsewhere classified, elbow
        Cubitus valgus

        M21.021 Valgus deformity, not elsewhere classified, right elbow

        M21.022 Valgus deformity, not elsewhere classified, left elbow

        M21.029 Valgus deformity, not elsewhere classified, unspecified elbow

    ✓6th M21.05 Valgus deformity, not elsewhere classified, hip

        M21.051 Valgus deformity, not elsewhere classified, right hip

        M21.052 Valgus deformity, not elsewhere classified, left hip

        M21.059 Valgus deformity, not elsewhere classified, unspecified hip

    ✓6th M21.06 Valgus deformity, not elsewhere classified, knee
        Genu valgum
        Knock knee

        M21.061 Valgus deformity, not elsewhere classified, right knee

        M21.062 Valgus deformity, not elsewhere classified, left knee

        M21.069 Valgus deformity, not elsewhere classified, unspecified knee

    ✓6th M21.07 Valgus deformity, not elsewhere classified, ankle

        M21.071 Valgus deformity, not elsewhere classified, right ankle

        M21.072 Valgus deformity, not elsewhere classified, left ankle

        M21.079 Valgus deformity, not elsewhere classified, unspecified ankle

✓5th M21.1 Varus deformity, not elsewhere classified

    EXCLUDES 1 metatarsus varus (Q66.2)
                  tibia vara (M92.5)

    M21.10 Varus deformity, not elsewhere classified, unspecified site

    ✓6th M21.12 Varus deformity, not elsewhere classified, elbow
        Cubitus varus, elbow

        M21.121 Varus deformity, not elsewhere classified, right elbow

        M21.122 Varus deformity, not elsewhere classified, left elbow

        M21.129 Varus deformity, not elsewhere classified, unspecified elbow

    ✓6th M21.15 Varus deformity, not elsewhere classified, hip

        M21.151 Varus deformity, not elsewhere classified, right hip

        M21.152 Varus deformity, not elsewhere classified, left hip

        M21.159 Varus deformity, not elsewhere classified, unspecified

✓6th M21.16 Varus deformity, not elsewhere classified, knee
    Bow leg
    Genu varum

    M21.161 Varus deformity, not elsewhere classified, right knee

    M21.162 Varus deformity, not elsewhere classified, left knee

    M21.169 Varus deformity, not elsewhere classified, unspecified knee

✓6th M21.17 Varus deformity, not elsewhere classified, ankle

    M21.171 Varus deformity, not elsewhere classified, right ankle

    M21.172 Varus deformity, not elsewhere classified, left ankle

    M21.179 Varus deformity, not elsewhere classified, unspecified ankle

✓5th M21.2 Flexion deformity

    M21.20 Flexion deformity, unspecified site

    ✓6th M21.21 Flexion deformity, shoulder

        M21.211 Flexion deformity, right shoulder

        M21.212 Flexion deformity, left shoulder

        M21.219 Flexion deformity, unspecified shoulder

    ✓6th M21.22 Flexion deformity, elbow

        M21.221 Flexion deformity, right elbow

        M21.222 Flexion deformity, left elbow

        M21.229 Flexion deformity, unspecified elbow

    ✓6th M21.23 Flexion deformity, wrist

        M21.231 Flexion deformity, right wrist

        M21.232 Flexion deformity, left wrist

        M21.239 Flexion deformity, unspecified wrist

    ✓6th M21.24 Flexion deformity, finger joints

        M21.241 Flexion deformity, right finger joints

        M21.242 Flexion deformity, left finger joints

        M21.249 Flexion deformity, unspecified finger joints

    ✓6th M21.25 Flexion deformity, hip

        M21.251 Flexion deformity, right hip

        M21.252 Flexion deformity, left hip

        M21.259 Flexion deformity, unspecified hip

    ✓6th M21.26 Flexion deformity, knee

        M21.261 Flexion deformity, right knee

        M21.262 Flexion deformity, left knee

        M21.269 Flexion deformity, unspecified knee

    ✓6th M21.27 Flexion deformity, ankle and toes

        M21.271 Flexion deformity, right ankle and toes

        M21.272 Flexion deformity, left ankle and toes

        M21.279 Flexion deformity, unspecified ankle and toes

✓5th M21.3 Wrist or foot drop (acquired)

    ✓6th M21.33 Wrist drop (acquired)

        M21.331 Wrist drop, right wrist

        M21.332 Wrist drop, left wrist

        M21.339 Wrist drop, unspecified wrist

    ✓6th M21.37 Foot drop (acquired)

        M21.371 Foot drop, right foot

        M21.372 Foot drop, left foot

        M21.379 Foot drop, unspecified foot

✓5th M21.4 Flat foot [pes planus] (acquired)

    EXCLUDES 1 congenital pes planus (Q66.5-)

    M21.40 Flat foot [pes planus] (acquired), unspecified foot

    M21.41 Flat foot [pes planus] (acquired), right foot

    M21.42 Flat foot [pes planus] (acquired), left foot

✓5th M21.5 Acquired clawhand, clubhand, clawfoot and clubfoot

    EXCLUDES 1 clubfoot, not specified as acquired (Q66.89)

    ✓6th M21.51 Acquired clawhand

        M21.511 Acquired clawhand, right hand

        M21.512 Acquired clawhand, left hand

        M21.519 Acquired clawhand, unspecified hand

    ✓6th M21.52 Acquired clubhand

        M21.521 Acquired clubhand, right hand

        M21.522 Acquired clubhand, left hand

        M21.529 Acquired clubhand, unspecified hand

✓ Additional Character Required   ✓x7th Xtension Alert   Unacceptable PDx   Manifestation   Hospital Acquired Condition   *EXCLUDES 1* Not Coded Here   *EXCLUDES 2* Not Included Here

ICD-10-CM Draft (2015)   705

√6ᵗʰ **M21.53** **Acquired** clawfoot
     M21.531 **Acquired clawfoot,** right **foot**
     M21.532 **Acquired clawfoot,** left **foot**
     M21.539 **Acquired clawfoot,** unspecified **foot**

√6ᵗʰ **M21.54** **Acquired** clubfoot
     M21.541 **Acquired clubfoot,** right **foot**
     M21.542 **Acquired clubfoot,** left **foot**
     M21.549 **Acquired clubfoot,** unspecified **foot**

√5ᵗʰ **M21.6** **Other acquired deformities of foot**
     EXCLUDES 2   *deformities of toe (acquired) (M20.1-M20.6)*

√6ᵗʰ **M21.6X** **Other acquired deformities of** foot
     M21.6X1 **Other acquired deformities of** right **foot**
     M21.6X2 **Other acquired deformities of** left **foot**
     M21.6X9 **Other acquired deformities of** unspecified **foot**

√5ᵗʰ **M21.7** **Unequal limb length (acquired)**
     NOTE   The site used should correspond to the shorter limb.
     M21.70 **Unequal limb length (acquired),** unspecified **site**

√6ᵗʰ **M21.72** **Unequal limb length (acquired),** humerus
     M21.721 **Unequal limb length (acquired),** right **humerus**
     M21.722 **Unequal limb length (acquired),** left **humerus**
     M21.729 **Unequal limb length (acquired),** unspecified **humerus**

√6ᵗʰ **M21.73** **Unequal limb length (acquired),** ulna and radius
     M21.731 **Unequal limb length (acquired),** right **ulna**
     M21.732 **Unequal limb length (acquired),** left **ulna**
     M21.733 **Unequal limb length (acquired),** right **radius**
     M21.734 **Unequal limb length (acquired),** left **radius**
     M21.739 **Unequal limb length (acquired),** unspecified **ulna and radius**

√6ᵗʰ **M21.75** **Unequal limb length (acquired),** femur
     M21.751 **Unequal limb length (acquired),** right **femur**
     M21.752 **Unequal limb length (acquired),** left **femur**
     M21.759 **Unequal limb length (acquired),** unspecified **femur**

√6ᵗʰ **M21.76** **Unequal limb length (acquired),** tibia and fibula
     M21.761 **Unequal limb length (acquired),** right **tibia**
     M21.762 **Unequal limb length (acquired),** left **tibia**
     M21.763 **Unequal limb length (acquired),** right **fibula**
     M21.764 **Unequal limb length (acquired),** left **fibula**
     M21.769 **Unequal limb length (acquired),** unspecified **tibia and fibula**

√5ᵗʰ **M21.8** **Other specified acquired deformities of limbs**
     EXCLUDES 2   *coxa plana (M91.2)*
     M21.80 **Other specified acquired deformities of** unspecified **limb**

√6ᵗʰ **M21.82** **Other specified acquired deformities of** upper arm
     M21.821 **Other specified acquired deformities of** right **upper arm**
     M21.822 **Other specified acquired deformities of** left **upper arm**
     M21.829 **Other specified acquired deformities of** unspecified **upper arm**

√6ᵗʰ **M21.83** **Other specified acquired deformities of** forearm
     M21.831 **Other specified acquired deformities of** right **forearm**
     M21.832 **Other specified acquired deformities of** left **forearm**
     M21.839 **Other specified acquired deformities of** unspecified **forearm**

√6ᵗʰ **M21.85** **Other specified acquired deformities of** thigh
     M21.851 **Other specified acquired deformities of** right **thigh**
     M21.852 **Other specified acquired deformities of** left **thigh**
     M21.859 **Other specified acquired deformities of** unspecified **thigh**

√6ᵗʰ **M21.86** **Other specified acquired deformities of** lower leg
     M21.861 **Other specified acquired deformities of** right **lower leg**

     M21.862 **Other specified acquired deformities of** left **lower leg**
     M21.869 **Other specified acquired deformities of** unspecified **lower leg**

√5ᵗʰ **M21.9** **Unspecified acquired deformity of limb and hand**
     M21.90 **Unspecified acquired deformity of** unspecified **limb**

√6ᵗʰ **M21.92** **Unspecified acquired deformity of** upper arm
     M21.921 **Unspecified acquired deformity of** right **upper arm**
     M21.922 **Unspecified acquired deformity of** left **upper arm**
     M21.929 **Unspecified acquired deformity of** unspecified **upper arm**

√6ᵗʰ **M21.93** **Unspecified acquired deformity of** forearm
     M21.931 **Unspecified acquired deformity of** right **forearm**
     M21.932 **Unspecified acquired deformity of** left **forearm**
     M21.939 **Unspecified acquired deformity of** unspecified **forearm**

√6ᵗʰ **M21.94** **Unspecified acquired deformity of** hand
     M21.941 **Unspecified acquired deformity of hand,** right **hand**
     M21.942 **Unspecified acquired deformity of hand,** left **hand**
     M21.949 **Unspecified acquired deformity of hand,** unspecified **hand**

√6ᵗʰ **M21.95** **Unspecified acquired deformity of** thigh
     M21.951 **Unspecified acquired deformity of** right **thigh**
     M21.952 **Unspecified acquired deformity of** left **thigh**
     M21.959 **Unspecified acquired deformity of** unspecified **thigh**

√6ᵗʰ **M21.96** **Unspecified acquired deformity of** lower leg
     M21.961 **Unspecified acquired deformity of** right **lower leg**
     M21.962 **Unspecified acquired deformity of** left **lower leg**
     M21.969 **Unspecified acquired deformity of** unspecified **lower leg**

√4ᵗʰ **M22** **Disorder of patella**
     EXCLUDES 1   *traumatic dislocation of patella (S83.0-)*

√5ᵗʰ **M22.0** **Recurrent dislocation** of patella
     M22.00 **Recurrent dislocation of patella,** unspecified **knee**
     M22.01 **Recurrent dislocation of patella,** right **knee**
     M22.02 **Recurrent dislocation of patella,** left **knee**

√5ᵗʰ **M22.1** **Recurrent subluxation** of patella
     Incomplete dislocation of patella
     M22.10 **Recurrent subluxation of patella,** unspecified **knee**
     M22.11 **Recurrent subluxation of patella,** right **knee**
     M22.12 **Recurrent subluxation of patella,** left **knee**

√5ᵗʰ **M22.2** **Patellofemoral disorders**
√6ᵗʰ   **M22.2X** **Patellofemoral disorders**
     M22.2X1 **Patellofemoral disorders,** right **knee**
     M22.2X2 **Patellofemoral disorders,** left **knee**
     M22.2X9 **Patellofemoral disorders,** unspecified **knee**

√5ᵗʰ **M22.3** **Other derangements** of patella
√6ᵗʰ   **M22.3X** **Other derangements of patella**
     M22.3X1 **Other derangements of patella,** right **knee**
     M22.3X2 **Other derangements of patella,** left **knee**
     M22.3X9 **Other derangements of patella,** unspecified **knee**

√5ᵗʰ **M22.4** **Chondromalacia patellae**
     M22.40 **Chondromalacia patellae,** unspecified **knee**
     M22.41 **Chondromalacia patellae,** right **knee**
     M22.42 **Chondromalacia patellae,** left **knee**

√5ᵗʰ **M22.8** **Other disorders of patella**
√6ᵗʰ   **M22.8X** **Other disorders of patella**
     M22.8X1 **Other disorders of patella,** right **knee**
     M22.8X2 **Other disorders of patella,** left **knee**
     M22.8X9 **Other disorders of patella,** unspecified **knee**

✓5ᵗʰ **M22.9** Unspecified disorder of patella

    M22.90 Unspecified disorder of patella, unspecified knee

    M22.91 Unspecified disorder of patella, right knee

    M22.92 Unspecified disorder of patella, left knee

✓4ᵗʰ **M23 Internal derangement of knee**

    EXCLUDES 1   *ankylosis (M24.66)*
        current injury—see injury of knee and lower leg (S80-S89)
        deformity of knee (M21.-)
        osteochondritis dissecans (M93.2)
        recurrent dislocation or subluxation of joints (M24.4)
        recurrent dislocation or subluxation of patella (M22.0-M22.1)

✓5ᵗʰ **M23.0 Cystic meniscus**

  ✓6ᵗʰ **M23.00** Cystic meniscus, unspecified meniscus
     Cystic meniscus, unspecified lateral meniscus
     Cystic meniscus, unspecified medial meniscus

    M23.000 Cystic meniscus, unspecified lateral meniscus, right knee

    M23.001 Cystic meniscus, unspecified lateral meniscus, left knee

    M23.002 Cystic meniscus, unspecified lateral meniscus, unspecified knee

    M23.003 Cystic meniscus, unspecified medial meniscus, right knee

    M23.004 Cystic meniscus, unspecified medial meniscus, left knee

    M23.005 Cystic meniscus, unspecified medial meniscus, unspecified knee

    M23.006 Cystic meniscus, unspecified meniscus, right knee

    M23.007 Cystic meniscus, unspecified meniscus, left knee

    M23.009 Cystic meniscus, unspecified meniscus, unspecified knee

  ✓6ᵗʰ **M23.01** Cystic meniscus, anterior horn of medial meniscus

    M23.011 Cystic meniscus, anterior horn of medial meniscus, right knee

    M23.012 Cystic meniscus, anterior horn of medial meniscus, left knee

    M23.019 Cystic meniscus, anterior horn of medial meniscus, unspecified knee

  ✓6ᵗʰ **M23.02** Cystic meniscus, posterior horn of medial meniscus

    M23.021 Cystic meniscus, posterior horn of medial meniscus, right knee

    M23.022 Cystic meniscus, posterior horn of medial meniscus, left knee

    M23.029 Cystic meniscus, posterior horn of medial meniscus, unspecified knee

  ✓6ᵗʰ **M23.03** Cystic meniscus, other medial meniscus

    M23.031 Cystic meniscus, other medial meniscus, right knee

    M23.032 Cystic meniscus, other medial meniscus, left knee

    M23.039 Cystic meniscus, other medial meniscus, unspecified knee

  ✓6ᵗʰ **M23.04** Cystic meniscus, anterior horn of lateral meniscus

    M23.041 Cystic meniscus, anterior horn of lateral meniscus, right knee

    M23.042 Cystic meniscus, anterior horn of lateral meniscus, left knee

    M23.049 Cystic meniscus, anterior horn of lateral meniscus, unspecified knee

  ✓6ᵗʰ **M23.05** Cystic meniscus, posterior horn of lateral meniscus

    M23.051 Cystic meniscus, posterior horn of lateral meniscus, right knee

    M23.052 Cystic meniscus, posterior horn of lateral meniscus, left knee

    M23.059 Cystic meniscus, posterior horn of lateral meniscus, unspecified knee

  ✓6ᵗʰ **M23.06** Cystic meniscus, other lateral meniscus

    M23.061 Cystic meniscus, other lateral meniscus, right knee

    M23.062 Cystic meniscus, other lateral meniscus, left knee

    M23.069 Cystic meniscus, other lateral meniscus, unspecified knee

✓5ᵗʰ **M23.2 Derangement of meniscus due to old tear or injury**
    Old bucket-handle tear

  ✓6ᵗʰ **M23.20** Derangement of unspecified meniscus due to old tear or injury
     Derangement of unspecified lateral meniscus due to old tear or injury
     Derangement of unspecified medial meniscus due to old tear or injury

    M23.200 Derangement of unspecified lateral meniscus due to old tear or injury, right knee

    M23.201 Derangement of unspecified lateral meniscus due to old tear or injury, left knee

    M23.202 Derangement of unspecified lateral meniscus due to old tear or injury, unspecified knee

    M23.203 Derangement of unspecified medial meniscus due to old tear or injury, right knee

    M23.204 Derangement of unspecified medial meniscus due to old tear or injury, left knee

    M23.205 Derangement of unspecified medial meniscus due to old tear or injury, unspecified knee

    M23.206 Derangement of unspecified meniscus due to old tear or injury, right knee

    M23.207 Derangement of unspecified meniscus due to old tear or injury, left knee

    M23.209 Derangement of unspecified meniscus due to old tear or injury, unspecified knee

  ✓6ᵗʰ **M23.21** Derangement of anterior horn of medial meniscus due to old tear or injury

    M23.211 Derangement of anterior horn of medial meniscus due to old tear or injury, right knee

    M23.212 Derangement of anterior horn of medial meniscus due to old tear or injury, left knee

    M23.219 Derangement of anterior horn of medial meniscus due to old tear or injury, unspecified knee

  ✓6ᵗʰ **M23.22** Derangement of posterior horn of medial meniscus due to old tear or injury

    M23.221 Derangement of posterior horn of medial meniscus due to old tear or injury, right knee

    M23.222 Derangement of posterior horn of medial meniscus due to old tear or injury, left knee

    M23.229 Derangement of posterior horn of medial meniscus due to old tear or injury, unspecified knee

  ✓6ᵗʰ **M23.23** Derangement of other medial meniscus due to old tear or injury

    M23.231 Derangement of other medial meniscus due to old tear or injury, right knee

    M23.232 Derangement of other medial meniscus due to old tear or injury, left knee

    M23.239 Derangement of other medial meniscus due to old tear or injury, unspecified knee

  ✓6ᵗʰ **M23.24** Derangement of anterior horn of lateral meniscus due to old tear or injury

    M23.241 Derangement of anterior horn of lateral meniscus due to old tear or injury, right knee

    M23.242 Derangement of anterior horn of lateral meniscus due to old tear or injury, left knee

    M23.249 Derangement of anterior horn of lateral meniscus due to old tear or injury, unspecified knee

  ✓6ᵗʰ **M23.25** Derangement of posterior horn of lateral meniscus due to old tear or injury

    M23.251 Derangement of posterior horn of lateral meniscus due to old tear or injury, right knee

---

✓ Additional Character Required   ✓x7ᵗʰ Xtension Alert   Unacceptable PDx   Manifestation   Hospital Acquired Condition   **EXCLUDES 1** Not Coded Here   **EXCLUDES 2** Not Included Here

M23.252 Derangement of posterior horn of lateral meniscus due to old tear or injury, left knee

M23.259 Derangement of posterior horn of lateral meniscus due to old tear or injury, unspecified knee

√6ᵗʰ **M23.26** Derangement of other lateral meniscus due to old tear or injury

M23.261 Derangement of other lateral meniscus due to old tear or injury, right knee

M23.262 Derangement of other lateral meniscus due to old tear or injury, left knee

M23.269 Derangement of other lateral meniscus due to old tear or injury, unspecified knee

√5ᵗʰ **M23.3** Other meniscus derangements
     Degenerate meniscus
     Detached meniscus
     Retained meniscus

√6ᵗʰ **M23.30** Other meniscus derangements, unspecified meniscus
     Other meniscus derangements, unspecified lateral meniscus
     Other meniscus derangements, unspecified medial meniscus

M23.300 Other meniscus derangements, unspecified lateral meniscus, right knee

M23.301 Other meniscus derangements, unspecified lateral meniscus, left knee

M23.302 Other meniscus derangements, unspecified lateral meniscus, unspecified knee

M23.303 Other meniscus derangements, unspecified medial meniscus, right knee

M23.304 Other meniscus derangements, unspecified medial meniscus, left knee

M23.305 Other meniscus derangements, unspecified medial meniscus, unspecified knee

M23.306 Other meniscus derangements, unspecified meniscus, right knee

M23.307 Other meniscus derangements, unspecified meniscus, left knee

M23.309 Other meniscus derangements, unspecified meniscus, unspecified knee

√6ᵗʰ **M23.31** Other meniscus derangements, anterior horn of medial meniscus

M23.311 Other meniscus derangements, anterior horn of medial meniscus, right knee

M23.312 Other meniscus derangements, anterior horn of medial meniscus, left knee

M23.319 Other meniscus derangements, anterior horn of medial meniscus, unspecified knee

√6ᵗʰ **M23.32** Other meniscus derangements, posterior horn of medial meniscus

M23.321 Other meniscus derangements, posterior horn of medial meniscus, right knee

M23.322 Other meniscus derangements, posterior horn of medial meniscus, left knee

M23.329 Other meniscus derangements, posterior horn of medial meniscus, unspecified knee

√6ᵗʰ **M23.33** Other meniscus derangements, other medial meniscus

M23.331 Other meniscus derangements, other medial meniscus, right knee

M23.332 Other meniscus derangements, other medial meniscus, left knee

M23.339 Other meniscus derangements, other medial meniscus, unspecified knee

√6ᵗʰ **M23.34** Other meniscus derangements, anterior horn of lateral meniscus

M23.341 Other meniscus derangements, anterior horn of lateral meniscus, right knee

M23.342 Other meniscus derangements, anterior horn of lateral meniscus, left knee

M23.349 Other meniscus derangements, anterior horn of lateral meniscus, unspecified knee

√6ᵗʰ **M23.35** Other meniscus derangements, posterior horn of lateral meniscus

M23.351 Other meniscus derangements, posterior horn of lateral meniscus, right knee

M23.352 Other meniscus derangements, posterior horn of lateral meniscus, left knee

M23.359 Other meniscus derangements, posterior horn of lateral meniscus, unspecified knee

√6ᵗʰ **M23.36** Other meniscus derangements, other lateral meniscus

M23.361 Other meniscus derangements, other lateral meniscus, right knee

M23.362 Other meniscus derangements, other lateral meniscus, left knee

M23.369 Other meniscus derangements, other lateral meniscus, unspecified knee

√5ᵗʰ **M23.4** Loose body in knee

M23.40 Loose body in knee, unspecified knee

M23.41 Loose body in knee, right knee

M23.42 Loose body in knee, left knee

√5ᵗʰ **M23.5** Chronic instability of knee

M23.50 Chronic instability of knee, unspecified knee

M23.51 Chronic instability of knee, right knee

M23.52 Chronic instability of knee, left knee

√5ᵗʰ **M23.6** Other spontaneous disruption of ligament(s) of knee

√6ᵗʰ **M23.60** Other spontaneous disruption of unspecified ligament of knee

M23.601 Other spontaneous disruption of unspecified ligament of right knee

M23.602 Other spontaneous disruption of unspecified ligament of left knee

M23.609 Other spontaneous disruption of unspecified ligament of unspecified knee

√6ᵗʰ **M23.61** Other spontaneous disruption of anterior cruciate ligament of knee

M23.611 Other spontaneous disruption of anterior cruciate ligament of right knee

M23.612 Other spontaneous disruption of anterior cruciate ligament of left knee

M23.619 Other spontaneous disruption of anterior cruciate ligament of unspecified knee

√6ᵗʰ **M23.62** Other spontaneous disruption of posterior cruciate ligament of knee

M23.621 Other spontaneous disruption of posterior cruciate ligament of right knee

M23.622 Other spontaneous disruption of posterior cruciate ligament of left knee

M23.629 Other spontaneous disruption of posterior cruciate ligament of unspecified knee

√6ᵗʰ **M23.63** Other spontaneous disruption of medial collateral ligament of knee

M23.631 Other spontaneous disruption of medial collateral ligament of right knee

M23.632 Other spontaneous disruption of medial collateral ligament of left knee

M23.639 Other spontaneous disruption of medial collateral ligament of unspecified knee

√6ᵗʰ **M23.64** Other spontaneous disruption of lateral collateral ligament of knee

M23.641 Other spontaneous disruption of lateral collateral ligament of right knee

M23.642 Other spontaneous disruption of lateral collateral ligament of left knee

M23.649 Other spontaneous disruption of lateral collateral ligament of unspecified knee

√6ᵗʰ **M23.67** Other spontaneous disruption of capsular ligament of knee

M23.671 Other spontaneous disruption of capsular ligament of right knee

M23.672 Other spontaneous disruption of capsular ligament of left knee

M23.679 Other spontaneous disruption of capsular ligament of unspecified knee

Ⓝ Newborn: 0   Ⓟ Pediatric: 0-17   Ⓜ Maternity: 12-55   Ⓐ Adult: 15-124   **MCC** Major CC Condition   **PDx MCC** PDx acts as own MCC   **CC** CC Condition   **PDx CC** PDx acts as own CC

708   ICD-10-CM Draft (2015)

✓5th **M23.8 Other internal derangements of knee**
Laxity of ligament of knee
Snapping knee

    ✓6th **M23.8X Other internal derangements of knee**
      M23.8X1 Other internal derangements of right knee
      M23.8X2 Other internal derangements of left knee
      M23.8X9 Other internal derangements of unspecified knee

✓5th **M23.9 Unspecified internal derangement of knee**
    M23.90 Unspecified internal derangement of unspecified knee
    M23.91 Unspecified internal derangement of right knee
    M23.92 Unspecified internal derangement of left knee

✓4th **M24 Other specific joint derangements**
    EXCLUDES 1 *current injury—see injury of joint by body region*
    EXCLUDES 2 *ganglion (M67.4)*
      snapping knee (M23.8-)
      temporomandibular joint disorders (M26.6-)

✓5th **M24.0 Loose body in joint**
    EXCLUDES 2 *loose body in knee (M23.4)*

    M24.00 Loose body in unspecified joint

    ✓6th **M24.01 Loose body in shoulder**
      M24.011 Loose body in right shoulder
      M24.012 Loose body in left shoulder
      M24.019 Loose body in unspecified shoulder

    ✓6th **M24.02 Loose body in elbow**
      M24.021 Loose body in right elbow
      M24.022 Loose body in left elbow
      M24.029 Loose body in unspecified elbow

    ✓6th **M24.03 Loose body in wrist**
      M24.031 Loose body in right wrist
      M24.032 Loose body in left wrist
      M24.039 Loose body in unspecified wrist

    ✓6th **M24.04 Loose body in finger joints**
      M24.041 Loose body in right finger joint(s)
      M24.042 Loose body in left finger joint(s)
      M24.049 Loose body in unspecified finger joint(s)

    ✓6th **M24.05 Loose body in hip**
      M24.051 Loose body in right hip
      M24.052 Loose body in left hip
      M24.059 Loose body in unspecified hip

    ✓6th **M24.07 Loose body in ankle and toe joints**
      M24.071 Loose body in right ankle
      M24.072 Loose body in left ankle
      M24.073 Loose body in unspecified ankle
      M24.074 Loose body in right toe joint(s)
      M24.075 Loose body in left toe joint(s)
      M24.076 Loose body in unspecified toe joints

    M24.08 Loose body, other site

✓5th **M24.1 Other articular cartilage disorders**
    EXCLUDES 2 *chondrocalcinosis (M11.1, M11.2-)*
      internal derangement of knee (M23.-)
      metastatic calcification (E83.5)
      ochronosis (E70.2)

    M24.10 Other articular cartilage disorders, unspecified site

    ✓6th **M24.11 Other articular cartilage disorders, shoulder**
      M24.111 Other articular cartilage disorders, right shoulder
      M24.112 Other articular cartilage disorders, left shoulder
      M24.119 Other articular cartilage disorders, unspecified shoulder

    ✓6th **M24.12 Other articular cartilage disorders, elbow**
      M24.121 Other articular cartilage disorders, right elbow
      M24.122 Other articular cartilage disorders, left elbow
      M24.129 Other articular cartilage disorders, unspecified elbow

    ✓6th **M24.13 Other articular cartilage disorders, wrist**
      M24.131 Other articular cartilage disorders, right wrist

      M24.132 Other articular cartilage disorders, left wrist
      M24.139 Other articular cartilage disorders, unspecified wrist

    ✓6th **M24.14 Other articular cartilage disorders, hand**
      M24.141 Other articular cartilage disorders, right hand
      M24.142 Other articular cartilage disorders, left hand
      M24.149 Other articular cartilage disorders, unspecified hand

    ✓6th **M24.15 Other articular cartilage disorders, hip**
      M24.151 Other articular cartilage disorders, right hip
      M24.152 Other articular cartilage disorders, left hip
      M24.159 Other articular cartilage disorders, unspecified hip

    ✓6th **M24.17 Other articular cartilage disorders, ankle and foot**
      M24.171 Other articular cartilage disorders, right ankle
      M24.172 Other articular cartilage disorders, left ankle
      M24.173 Other articular cartilage disorders, unspecified ankle
      M24.174 Other articular cartilage disorders, right foot
      M24.175 Other articular cartilage disorders, left foot
      M24.176 Other articular cartilage disorders, unspecified foot

✓5th **M24.2 Disorder of ligament**
Instability secondary to old ligament injury
Ligamentous laxity NOS
    EXCLUDES 1 *familial ligamentous laxity (M35.7)*
    EXCLUDES 2 *internal derangement of knee (M23.5-M23.89)*

    M24.20 Disorder of ligament, unspecified site

    ✓6th **M24.21 Disorder of ligament, shoulder**
      M24.211 Disorder of ligament, right shoulder
      M24.212 Disorder of ligament, left shoulder
      M24.219 Disorder of ligament, unspecified shoulder

    ✓6th **M24.22 Disorder of ligament, elbow**
      M24.221 Disorder of ligament, right elbow
      M24.222 Disorder of ligament, left elbow
      M24.229 Disorder of ligament, unspecified elbow

    ✓6th **M24.23 Disorder of ligament, wrist**
      M24.231 Disorder of ligament, right wrist
      M24.232 Disorder of ligament, left wrist
      M24.239 Disorder of ligament, unspecified wrist

    ✓6th **M24.24 Disorder of ligament, hand**
      M24.241 Disorder of ligament, right hand
      M24.242 Disorder of ligament, left hand
      M24.249 Disorder of ligament, unspecified hand

    ✓6th **M24.25 Disorder of ligament, hip**
      M24.251 Disorder of ligament, right hip
      M24.252 Disorder of ligament, left hip
      M24.259 Disorder of ligament, unspecified hip

    ✓6th **M24.27 Disorder of ligament, ankle and foot**
      M24.271 Disorder of ligament, right ankle
      M24.272 Disorder of ligament, left ankle
      M24.273 Disorder of ligament, unspecified ankle
      M24.274 Disorder of ligament, right foot
      M24.275 Disorder of ligament, left foot
      M24.276 Disorder of ligament, unspecified foot

    M24.28 Disorder of ligament, vertebrae

✓5th **M24.3 Pathological dislocation of joint, not elsewhere classified**
    EXCLUDES 1 *congenital dislocation or displacement of joint—see congenital malformations and deformations of the musculoskeletal system (Q65-Q79)*
      current injury—see injury of joints and ligaments by body region
      recurrent dislocation of joint (M24.4-)

    M24.30 Pathological dislocation of unspecified joint, not elsewhere classified

✓ Additional Character Required   ✓x7th Xtension Alert   Unacceptable PDx   Manifestation   Hospital Acquired Condition   EXCLUDES 1 Not Coded Here   EXCLUDES 2 Not Included Here

ICD-10-CM Draft (2015)   709

✓6ᵗʰ **M24.31 Pathological dislocation of shoulder, not elsewhere classified**
    M24.311 Pathological dislocation of right shoulder, not elsewhere classified
    M24.312 Pathological dislocation of left shoulder, not elsewhere classified
    M24.319 Pathological dislocation of unspecified shoulder, not elsewhere classified

✓6ᵗʰ **M24.32 Pathological dislocation of elbow, not elsewhere classified**
    M24.321 Pathological dislocation of right elbow, not elsewhere classified
    M24.322 Pathological dislocation of left elbow, not elsewhere classified
    M24.329 Pathological dislocation of unspecified elbow, not elsewhere classified

✓6ᵗʰ **M24.33 Pathological dislocation of wrist, not elsewhere classified**
    M24.331 Pathological dislocation of right wrist, not elsewhere classified
    M24.332 Pathological dislocation of left wrist, not elsewhere classified
    M24.339 Pathological dislocation of unspecified wrist, not elsewhere classified

✓6ᵗʰ **M24.34 Pathological dislocation of hand, not elsewhere classified**
    M24.341 Pathological dislocation of right hand, not elsewhere classified
    M24.342 Pathological dislocation of left hand, not elsewhere classified
    M24.349 Pathological dislocation of unspecified hand, not elsewhere classified

✓6ᵗʰ **M24.35 Pathological dislocation of hip, not elsewhere classified**
    M24.351 Pathological dislocation of right hip, not elsewhere classified
    M24.352 Pathological dislocation of left hip, not elsewhere classified
    M24.359 Pathological dislocation of unspecified hip, not elsewhere classified

✓6ᵗʰ **M24.36 Pathological dislocation of knee, not elsewhere classified**
    M24.361 Pathological dislocation of right knee, not elsewhere classified
    M24.362 Pathological dislocation of left knee, not elsewhere classified
    M24.369 Pathological dislocation of unspecified knee, not elsewhere classified

✓6ᵗʰ **M24.37 Pathological dislocation of ankle and foot, not elsewhere classified**
    M24.371 Pathological dislocation of right ankle, not elsewhere classified
    M24.372 Pathological dislocation of left ankle, not elsewhere classified
    M24.373 Pathological dislocation of unspecified ankle, not elsewhere classified
    M24.374 Pathological dislocation of right foot, not elsewhere classified
    M24.375 Pathological dislocation of left foot, not elsewhere classified
    M24.376 Pathological dislocation of unspecified foot, not elsewhere classified

✓5ᵗʰ **M24.4 Recurrent dislocation of joint**
    Recurrent subluxation of joint
    EXCLUDES 2   recurrent dislocation of patella (M22.0-M22.1)
           recurrent vertebral dislocation (M43.3-, M43.4, M43.5-)
    M24.40 Recurrent dislocation, unspecified joint
✓6ᵗʰ   M24.41 Recurrent dislocation, shoulder
    M24.411 Recurrent dislocation, right shoulder
    M24.412 Recurrent dislocation, left shoulder
    M24.419 Recurrent dislocation, unspecified shoulder
✓6ᵗʰ   M24.42 Recurrent dislocation, elbow
    M24.421 Recurrent dislocation, right elbow
    M24.422 Recurrent dislocation, left elbow
    M24.429 Recurrent dislocation, unspecified elbow

✓6ᵗʰ **M24.43 Recurrent dislocation, wrist**
    M24.431 Recurrent dislocation, right wrist
    M24.432 Recurrent dislocation, left wrist
    M24.439 Recurrent dislocation, unspecified wrist

✓6ᵗʰ **M24.44 Recurrent dislocation, hand and finger(s)**
    M24.441 Recurrent dislocation, right hand
    M24.442 Recurrent dislocation, left hand
    M24.443 Recurrent dislocation, unspecified hand
    M24.444 Recurrent dislocation, right finger
    M24.445 Recurrent dislocation, left finger
    M24.446 Recurrent dislocation, unspecified finger

✓6ᵗʰ **M24.45 Recurrent dislocation, hip**
    M24.451 Recurrent dislocation, right hip
    M24.452 Recurrent dislocation, left hip
    M24.459 Recurrent dislocation, unspecified hip

✓6ᵗʰ **M24.46 Recurrent dislocation, knee**
    M24.461 Recurrent dislocation, right knee
    M24.462 Recurrent dislocation, left knee
    M24.469 Recurrent dislocation, unspecified knee

✓6ᵗʰ **M24.47 Recurrent dislocation, ankle, foot and toes**
    M24.471 Recurrent dislocation, right ankle
    M24.472 Recurrent dislocation, left ankle
    M24.473 Recurrent dislocation, unspecified ankle
    M24.474 Recurrent dislocation, right foot
    M24.475 Recurrent dislocation, left foot
    M24.476 Recurrent dislocation, unspecified foot
    M24.477 Recurrent dislocation, right toe(s)
    M24.478 Recurrent dislocation, left toe(s)
    M24.479 Recurrent dislocation, unspecified toe(s)

✓5ᵗʰ **M24.5 Contracture of joint**
    EXCLUDES 1   contracture of muscle without contracture of joint (M62.4-)
           contracture of tendon (sheath) without contracture of joint (M62.4-)
           Dupuytren's contracture (M72.0)
    EXCLUDES 2   acquired deformities of limbs (M20-M21)
    M24.50 Contracture, unspecified joint
✓6ᵗʰ   M24.51 Contracture, shoulder
    M24.511 Contracture, right shoulder
    M24.512 Contracture, left shoulder
    M24.519 Contracture, unspecified shoulder
✓6ᵗʰ   M24.52 Contracture, elbow
    M24.521 Contracture, right elbow
    M24.522 Contracture, left elbow
    M24.529 Contracture, unspecified elbow
✓6ᵗʰ   M24.53 Contracture, wrist
    M24.531 Contracture, right wrist
    M24.532 Contracture, left wrist
    M24.539 Contracture, unspecified wrist
✓6ᵗʰ   M24.54 Contracture, hand
    M24.541 Contracture, right hand
    M24.542 Contracture, left hand
    M24.549 Contracture, unspecified hand
✓6ᵗʰ   M24.55 Contracture, hip
    M24.551 Contracture, right hip
    M24.552 Contracture, left hip
    M24.559 Contracture, unspecified hip
✓6ᵗʰ   M24.56 Contracture, knee
    M24.561 Contracture, right knee
    M24.562 Contracture, left knee
    M24.569 Contracture, unspecified knee
✓6ᵗʰ   M24.57 Contracture, ankle and foot
    M24.571 Contracture, right ankle
    M24.572 Contracture, left ankle
    M24.573 Contracture, unspecified ankle
    M24.574 Contracture, right foot
    M24.575 Contracture, left foot
    M24.576 Contracture, unspecified foot

✓5ᵗʰ **M24.6 Ankylosis of joint**
    EXCLUDES 1   stiffness of joint without ankylosis (M25.6-)
    EXCLUDES 2   spine (M43.2-)
    M24.60 Ankylosis, unspecified joint

N Newborn: 0   P Pediatric: 0-17   M Maternity: 12-55   A Adult: 15-124   MCC Major CC Condition   PDx MCC PDx acts as own MCC   CC CC Condition   PDx CC PDx acts as own CC

710   ICD-10-CM Draft (2015)

✓6th **M24.61 Ankylosis, shoulder**
    M24.611 Ankylosis, right shoulder
    M24.612 Ankylosis, left shoulder
    M24.619 Ankylosis, unspecified shoulder

✓6th **M24.62 Ankylosis, elbow**
    M24.621 Ankylosis, right elbow
    M24.622 Ankylosis, left elbow
    M24.629 Ankylosis, unspecified elbow

✓6th **M24.63 Ankylosis, wrist**
    M24.631 Ankylosis, right wrist
    M24.632 Ankylosis, left wrist
    M24.639 Ankylosis, unspecified wrist

✓6th **M24.64 Ankylosis, hand**
    M24.641 Ankylosis, right hand
    M24.642 Ankylosis, left hand
    M24.649 Ankylosis, unspecified hand

✓6th **M24.65 Ankylosis, hip**
    M24.651 Ankylosis, right hip
    M24.652 Ankylosis, left hip
    M24.659 Ankylosis, unspecified hip

✓6th **M24.66 Ankylosis, knee**
    M24.661 Ankylosis, right knee
    M24.662 Ankylosis, left knee
    M24.669 Ankylosis, unspecified knee

✓6th **M24.67 Ankylosis, ankle and foot**
    M24.671 Ankylosis, right ankle
    M24.672 Ankylosis, left ankle
    M24.673 Ankylosis, unspecified ankle
    M24.674 Ankylosis, right foot
    M24.675 Ankylosis, left foot
    M24.676 Ankylosis, unspecified foot

M24.7 Protrusio acetabuli

✓5th **M24.8 Other specific joint derangements, not elsewhere classified**
  EXCLUDES 2 *iliotibial band syndrome (M76.3)*

  M24.80 Other specific joint derangements of unspecified joint, not elsewhere classified

✓6th **M24.81 Other specific joint derangements of shoulder, not elsewhere classified**
    M24.811 Other specific joint derangements of right shoulder, not elsewhere classified
    M24.812 Other specific joint derangements of left shoulder, not elsewhere classified
    M24.819 Other specific joint derangements of unspecified shoulder, not elsewhere classified

✓6th **M24.82 Other specific joint derangements of elbow, not elsewhere classified**
    M24.821 Other specific joint derangements of right elbow, not elsewhere classified
    M24.822 Other specific joint derangements of left elbow, not elsewhere classified
    M24.829 Other specific joint derangements of unspecified elbow, not elsewhere classified

✓6th **M24.83 Other specific joint derangements of wrist, not elsewhere classified**
    M24.831 Other specific joint derangements of right wrist, not elsewhere classified
    M24.832 Other specific joint derangements of left wrist, not elsewhere classified
    M24.839 Other specific joint derangements of unspecified wrist, not elsewhere classified

✓6th **M24.84 Other specific joint derangements of hand, not elsewhere classified**
    M24.841 Other specific joint derangements of right hand, not elsewhere classified
    M24.842 Other specific joint derangements of left hand, not elsewhere classified
    M24.849 Other specific joint derangements of unspecified hand, not elsewhere classified

✓6th **M24.85 Other specific joint derangements of hip, not elsewhere classified**
    Irritable hip
    M24.851 Other specific joint derangements of right hip, not elsewhere classified

    M24.852 Other specific joint derangements of left hip, not elsewhere classified
    M24.859 Other specific joint derangements of unspecified hip, not elsewhere classified

✓6th **M24.87 Other specific joint derangements of ankle and foot, not elsewhere classified**
    M24.871 Other specific joint derangements of right ankle, not elsewhere classified
    M24.872 Other specific joint derangements of left ankle, not elsewhere classified
    M24.873 Other specific joint derangements of unspecified ankle, not elsewhere classified
    M24.874 Other specific joint derangements of right foot, not elsewhere classified
    M24.875 Other specific joint derangements left foot, not elsewhere classified
    M24.876 Other specific joint derangements of unspecified foot, not elsewhere classified

M24.9 Joint derangement, unspecified

M25 Other joint disorder, not elsewhere classified
  EXCLUDES 2 *abnormality of gait and mobility (R26.-)*
      acquired deformities of limb (M20-M21)
      calcification of bursa (M71.4-)
      calcification of shoulder (joint) (M75.3)
      calcification of tendon (M65.2-)
      difficulty in walking (R26.2)
      temporomandibular joint disorder (M26.6-)

✓5th **M25.0 Hemarthrosis**
  EXCLUDES 1 *current injury—see injury of joint by body region*
      hemophilic arthropathy (M36.2)

  M25.00 Hemarthrosis, unspecified joint CC
    CC Excl: M25.00-M25.08, T79.A11A, T79.A12A, T79.A19A, T79.A21A, T79.A22A, T79.A29A

✓6th **M25.01 Hemarthrosis, shoulder**
    M25.011 Hemarthrosis, right shoulder CC
      CC Excl: M25.00-M25.039, M25.08, T79.A11A, T79.A12A, T79.A19A
    M25.012 Hemarthrosis, left shoulder CC
      CC Excl: See code: M25.011
    M25.019 Hemarthrosis, unspecified shoulder CC
      CC Excl: See code: M25.011

✓6th **M25.02 Hemarthrosis, elbow**
    M25.021 Hemarthrosis, right elbow CC
      CC Excl: M25.00-M25.029, M25.08, T79.A11A, T79.A12A, T79.A19A
    M25.022 Hemarthrosis, left elbow CC
      CC Excl: See code: M25.022
    M25.029 Hemarthrosis, unspecified elbow CC
      CC Excl: See code: M25.022

✓6th **M25.03 Hemarthrosis, wrist**
    M25.031 Hemarthrosis, right wrist CC
      CC Excl: M25.00, M25.021-M25.049, M25.08, T79.A11-T79.A19 with 7th character A
    M25.032 Hemarthrosis, left wrist CC
      CC Excl: See code: M25.031
    M25.039 Hemarthrosis, unspecified wrist CC
      CC Excl: See code: M25.031

✓6th **M25.04 Hemarthrosis, hand**
    M25.041 Hemarthrosis, right hand CC
      CC Excl: M25.00, M25.031-M25.049, M25.08, T79.A11-T79.A19 with 7th character A
    M25.042 Hemarthrosis, left hand CC
      CC Excl: See code: M25.041
    M25.049 Hemarthrosis, unspecified hand CC
      CC Excl: See code: M25.041

✓6th **M25.05 Hemarthrosis, hip**
    M25.051 Hemarthrosis, right hip CC
      CC Excl: M25.00-M25.08, T79.A11A, T79.A12A, T79.A19A, T79.A21A, T79.A22A, T79.A29A
    M25.052 Hemarthrosis, left hip CC
      CC Excl: See code: M25.051
    M25.059 Hemarthrosis, unspecified hip CC
      CC Excl: See code: M25.051

✓6th **M25.06 Hemarthrosis, knee**
    M25.061 Hemarthrosis, right knee CC
      CC Excl: M25.00, M25.061-M25.08, T79.A21-T79.A29 with 7th character A

✓ Additional Character Required ✓x7th Xtension Alert Unacceptable PDx Manifestation Hospital Acquired Condition EXCLUDES 1 Not Coded Here EXCLUDES 2 Not Included Here

ICD-10-CM Draft (2015)   711

M25.062 **Hemarthrosis,** left knee `CC`
　　CC Excl: See code: M25.061
M25.069 **Hemarthrosis,** unspecified knee `CC`
　　CC Excl: See code: M25.061
√6ᵗʰ M25.07 **Hemarthrosis,** ankle and foot
M25.071 **Hemarthrosis,** right ankle `CC`
　　CC Excl: See code: M25.061
M25.072 **Hemarthrosis,** left ankle `CC`
　　CC Excl: See code: M25.061
M25.073 **Hemarthrosis,** unspecified ankle `CC`
　　CC Excl: See code: M25.061
M25.074 **Hemarthrosis,** right foot `CC`
　　CC Excl: See code: M25.061
M25.075 **Hemarthrosis,** left foot `CC`
　　CC Excl: See code: M25.061
M25.076 **Hemarthrosis,** unspecified foot `CC`
　　CC Excl: See code: M25.061
M25.08 **Hemarthrosis,** other specified site
　　Hemarthrosis, vertebrae
　　CC Excl: M25.00-M25.08, T79.A11A, T79.A12A,
　　T79.A19A, T79.A21A, T79.A22A, T79.A29A
√5ᵗʰ M25.1 **Fistula of joint**
M25.10 **Fistula,** unspecified joint
√6ᵗʰ M25.11 **Fistula,** shoulder
M25.111 **Fistula,** right shoulder
M25.112 **Fistula,** left shoulder
M25.119 **Fistula,** unspecified shoulder
√6ᵗʰ M25.12 **Fistula,** elbow
M25.121 **Fistula,** right elbow
M25.122 **Fistula,** left elbow
M25.129 **Fistula,** unspecified elbow
√6ᵗʰ M25.13 **Fistula,** wrist
M25.131 **Fistula,** right wrist
M25.132 **Fistula,** left wrist
M25.139 **Fistula,** unspecified wrist
√6ᵗʰ M25.14 **Fistula,** hand
M25.141 **Fistula,** right hand
M25.142 **Fistula,** left hand
M25.149 **Fistula,** unspecified hand
√6ᵗʰ M25.15 **Fistula,** hip
M25.151 **Fistula,** right hip
M25.152 **Fistula,** left hip
M25.159 **Fistula,** unspecified hip
√6ᵗʰ M25.16 **Fistula,** knee
M25.161 **Fistula,** right knee
M25.162 **Fistula,** left knee
M25.169 **Fistula,** unspecified knee
√6ᵗʰ M25.17 **Fistula,** ankle and foot
M25.171 **Fistula,** right ankle
M25.172 **Fistula,** left ankle
M25.173 **Fistula,** unspecified ankle
M25.174 **Fistula,** right foot
M25.175 **Fistula,** left foot
M25.176 **Fistula,** unspecified foot
M25.18 **Fistula,** other specified site
　　Fistula, vertebrae
√5ᵗʰ M25.2 **Flail joint**
M25.20 **Flail joint,** unspecified joint
√6ᵗʰ M25.21 **Flail joint,** shoulder
M25.211 **Flail joint,** right shoulder
M25.212 **Flail joint,** left shoulder
M25.219 **Flail joint,** unspecified shoulder
√6ᵗʰ M25.22 **Flail joint,** elbow
M25.221 **Flail joint,** right elbow
M25.222 **Flail joint,** left elbow
M25.229 **Flail joint,** unspecified elbow
√6ᵗʰ M25.23 **Flail joint,** wrist
M25.231 **Flail joint,** right wrist
M25.232 **Flail joint,** left wrist
M25.239 **Flail joint,** unspecified wrist
√6ᵗʰ M25.24 **Flail joint,** hand
M25.241 **Flail joint,** right hand
M25.242 **Flail joint,** left hand

M25.249 **Flail joint,** unspecified hand
√6ᵗʰ M25.25 **Flail joint,** hip
M25.251 **Flail joint,** right hip
M25.252 **Flail joint,** left hip
M25.259 **Flail joint,** unspecified hip
√6ᵗʰ M25.26 **Flail joint,** knee
M25.261 **Flail joint,** right knee
M25.262 **Flail joint,** left knee
M25.269 **Flail joint,** unspecified knee
√6ᵗʰ M25.27 **Flail joint,** ankle and foot
M25.271 **Flail joint,** right ankle and foot
M25.272 **Flail joint,** left ankle and foot
M25.279 **Flail joint,** unspecified ankle and foot
M25.28 **Flail joint,** other site
√5ᵗʰ M25.3 **Other instability of joint**
　　EXCLUDES 1　instability of joint secondary to old ligament injury
　　　(M24.2-)
　　　instability of joint secondary to removal of joint
　　　prosthesis (M96.8-)
　　EXCLUDES 2　spinal instabilities (M53.2-)
M25.30 **Other instability,** unspecified joint
√6ᵗʰ M25.31 **Other instability,** shoulder
M25.311 **Other instability,** right shoulder
M25.312 **Other instability,** left shoulder
M25.319 **Other instability,** unspecified shoulder
√6ᵗʰ M25.32 **Other instability,** elbow
M25.321 **Other instability,** right elbow
M25.322 **Other instability,** left elbow
M25.329 **Other instability,** unspecified elbow
√6ᵗʰ M25.33 **Other instability,** wrist
M25.331 **Other instability,** right wrist
M25.332 **Other instability,** left wrist
M25.339 **Other instability,** unspecified wrist
√6ᵗʰ M25.34 **Other instability,** hand
M25.341 **Other instability,** right hand
M25.342 **Other instability,** left hand
M25.349 **Other instability,** unspecified hand
√6ᵗʰ M25.35 **Other instability,** hip
M25.351 **Other instability,** right hip
M25.352 **Other instability,** left hip
M25.359 **Other instability,** unspecified hip
√6ᵗʰ M25.36 **Other instability,** knee
M25.361 **Other instability,** right knee
M25.362 **Other instability,** left knee
M25.369 **Other instability,** unspecified knee
√6ᵗʰ M25.37 **Other instability,** ankle and foot
M25.371 **Other instability,** right ankle
M25.372 **Other instability,** left ankle
M25.373 **Other instability,** unspecified ankle
M25.374 **Other instability,** right foot
M25.375 **Other instability,** left foot
M25.376 **Other instability,** unspecified foot
√5ᵗʰ M25.4 **Effusion of joint**
　　EXCLUDES 1　hydrarthrosis in yaws (A66.6)
　　　intermittent hydrarthrosis (M12.4-)
　　　other infective (teno)synovitis (M65.1-)
M25.40 **Effusion,** unspecified joint
√6ᵗʰ M25.41 **Effusion,** shoulder
M25.411 **Effusion,** right shoulder
M25.412 **Effusion,** left shoulder
M25.419 **Effusion,** unspecified shoulder
√6ᵗʰ M25.42 **Effusion,** elbow
M25.421 **Effusion,** right elbow
M25.422 **Effusion,** left elbow
M25.429 **Effusion,** unspecified elbow
√6ᵗʰ M25.43 **Effusion,** wrist
M25.431 **Effusion,** right wrist
M25.432 **Effusion,** left wrist
M25.439 **Effusion,** unspecified wrist
√6ᵗʰ M25.44 **Effusion,** hand
M25.441 **Effusion,** right hand
M25.442 **Effusion,** left hand

M25.449 Effusion, unspecified hand

√6th **M25.45 Effusion, hip**
    M25.451 Effusion, right hip
    M25.452 Effusion, left hip
    M25.459 Effusion, unspecified hip

√6th **M25.46 Effusion, knee**
    M25.461 Effusion, right knee
    M25.462 Effusion, left knee
    M25.469 Effusion, unspecified knee

√6th **M25.47 Effusion, ankle and foot**
    M25.471 Effusion, right ankle
    M25.472 Effusion, left ankle
    M25.473 Effusion, unspecified ankle
    M25.474 Effusion, right foot
    M25.475 Effusion, left foot
    M25.476 Effusion, unspecified foot

    M25.48 Effusion, other site

√5th **M25.5 Pain in joint**
    EXCLUDES 2   pain in hand (M79.64-)
                  pain in fingers (M79.64-)
                  pain in foot (M79.67-)
                  pain in limb (M79.6-)
                  pain in toes (M79.67-)

    M25.50 Pain in unspecified joint

√6th **M25.51 Pain in shoulder**
    M25.511 Pain in right shoulder
    M25.512 Pain in left shoulder
    M25.519 Pain in unspecified shoulder

√6th **M25.52 Pain in elbow**
    M25.521 Pain in right elbow
    M25.522 Pain in left elbow
    M25.529 Pain in unspecified elbow

√6th **M25.53 Pain in wrist**
    M25.531 Pain in right wrist
    M25.532 Pain in left wrist
    M25.539 Pain in unspecified wrist

√6th **M25.55 Pain in hip**
    M25.551 Pain in right hip
    M25.552 Pain in left hip
    M25.559 Pain in unspecified hip

√6th **M25.56 Pain in knee**
    M25.561 Pain in right knee
    M25.562 Pain in left knee
    M25.569 Pain in unspecified knee

√6th **M25.57 Pain in ankle and joints of foot**
    M25.571 Pain in right ankle and joints of right foot
    M25.572 Pain in left ankle and joints of left foot
    M25.579 Pain in unspecified ankle and joints of unspecified foot

√5th **M25.6 Stiffness of joint, not elsewhere classified**
    EXCLUDES 1   ankylosis of joint (M24.6-)
                  contracture of joint (M24.5-)

    M25.60 Stiffness of unspecified joint, not elsewhere classified

√6th **M25.61 Stiffness of shoulder, not elsewhere classified**
    M25.611 Stiffness of right shoulder, not elsewhere classified
    M25.612 Stiffness of left shoulder, not elsewhere classified
    M25.619 Stiffness of unspecified shoulder, not elsewhere classified

√6th **M25.62 Stiffness of elbow, not elsewhere classified**
    M25.621 Stiffness of right elbow, not elsewhere classified
    M25.622 Stiffness of left elbow, not elsewhere classified
    M25.629 Stiffness of unspecified elbow, not elsewhere classified

√6th **M25.63 Stiffness of wrist, not elsewhere classified**
    M25.631 Stiffness of right wrist, not elsewhere classified
    M25.632 Stiffness of left wrist, not elsewhere classified

M25.639 Stiffness of unspecified wrist, not elsewhere classified

√6th **M25.64 Stiffness of hand, not elsewhere classified**
    M25.641 Stiffness of right hand, not elsewhere classified
    M25.642 Stiffness of left hand, not elsewhere classified
    M25.649 Stiffness of unspecified hand, not elsewhere classified

√6th **M25.65 Stiffness of hip, not elsewhere classified**
    M25.651 Stiffness of right hip, not elsewhere classified
    M25.652 Stiffness of left hip, not elsewhere classified
    M25.659 Stiffness of unspecified hip, not elsewhere classified

√6th **M25.66 Stiffness of knee, not elsewhere classified**
    M25.661 Stiffness of right knee, not elsewhere classified
    M25.662 Stiffness of left knee, not elsewhere classified
    M25.669 Stiffness of unspecified knee, not elsewhere classified

√6th **M25.67 Stiffness of ankle and foot, not elsewhere classified**
    M25.671 Stiffness of right ankle, not elsewhere classified
    M25.672 Stiffness of left ankle, not elsewhere classified
    M25.673 Stiffness of unspecified ankle, not elsewhere classified
    M25.674 Stiffness of right foot, not elsewhere classified
    M25.675 Stiffness of left foot, not elsewhere classified
    M25.676 Stiffness of unspecified foot, not elsewhere classified

√5th **M25.7 Osteophyte**
    M25.70 Osteophyte, unspecified joint

√6th **M25.71 Osteophyte, shoulder**
    M25.711 Osteophyte, right shoulder
    M25.712 Osteophyte, left shoulder
    M25.719 Osteophyte, unspecified shoulder

√6th **M25.72 Osteophyte, elbow**
    M25.721 Osteophyte, right elbow
    M25.722 Osteophyte, left elbow
    M25.729 Osteophyte, unspecified elbow

√6th **M25.73 Osteophyte, wrist**
    M25.731 Osteophyte, right wrist
    M25.732 Osteophyte, left wrist
    M25.739 Osteophyte, unspecified wrist

√6th **M25.74 Osteophyte, hand**
    M25.741 Osteophyte, right hand
    M25.742 Osteophyte, left hand
    M25.749 Osteophyte, unspecified hand

√6th **M25.75 Osteophyte, hip**
    M25.751 Osteophyte, right hip
    M25.752 Osteophyte, left hip
    M25.759 Osteophyte, unspecified hip

√6th **M25.76 Osteophyte, knee**
    M25.761 Osteophyte, right knee
    M25.762 Osteophyte, left knee
    M25.769 Osteophyte, unspecified knee

√6th **M25.77 Osteophyte, ankle and foot**
    M25.771 Osteophyte, right ankle
    M25.772 Osteophyte, left ankle
    M25.773 Osteophyte, unspecified ankle
    M25.774 Osteophyte, right foot
    M25.775 Osteophyte, left foot
    M25.776 Osteophyte, unspecified foot

    M25.78 Osteophyte, vertebrae

√5th **M25.8 Other specified joint disorders**
    M25.80 Other specified joint disorders, unspecified joint

☑ Additional Character Required   √x7th Xtension Alert   Unacceptable PDx   Manifestation   Hospital Acquired Condition   EXCLUDES 1 Not Coded Here   EXCLUDES 2 Not Included Here

ICD-10-CM Draft (2015)   713

✓6ᵗʰ **M25.81** Other specified joint disorders, shoulder
  M25.811 Other specified joint disorders, right shoulder
  M25.812 Other specified joint disorders, left shoulder
  M25.819 Other specified joint disorders, unspecified shoulder

✓6ᵗʰ **M25.82** Other specified joint disorders, elbow
  M25.821 Other specified joint disorders, right elbow
  M25.822 Other specified joint disorders, left elbow
  M25.829 Other specified joint disorders, unspecified elbow

✓6ᵗʰ **M25.83** Other specified joint disorders, wrist
  M25.831 Other specified joint disorders, right wrist
  M25.832 Other specified joint disorders, left wrist
  M25.839 Other specified joint disorders, unspecified wrist

✓6ᵗʰ **M25.84** Other specified joint disorders, hand
  M25.841 Other specified joint disorders, right hand
  M25.842 Other specified joint disorders, left hand
  M25.849 Other specified joint disorders, unspecified hand

✓6ᵗʰ **M25.85** Other specified joint disorders, hip
  M25.851 Other specified joint disorders, right hip
  M25.852 Other specified joint disorders, left hip
  M25.859 Other specified joint disorders, unspecified hip

✓6ᵗʰ **M25.86** Other specified joint disorders, knee
  M25.861 Other specified joint disorders, right knee
  M25.862 Other specified joint disorders, left knee
  M25.869 Other specified joint disorders, unspecified knee

✓6ᵗʰ **M25.87** Other specified joint disorders, ankle and foot
  M25.871 Other specified joint disorders, right ankle and foot
  M25.872 Other specified joint disorders, left ankle and foot
  M25.879 Other specified joint disorders, unspecified ankle and foot

M25.9 Joint disorder, unspecified

Dentofacial anomalies [including malocclusion] and other disorders of jaw (M26-M27)

EXCLUDES 1   hemifacial atrophy or hypertrophy (Q67.4)
    unilateral condylar hyperplasia or hypoplasia (M27.8)

✓4ᵗʰ **M26 Dentofacial anomalies [including malocclusion]**

✓5ᵗʰ **M26.0 Major anomalies of jaw size**
  EXCLUDES 1   acromegaly (E22.0)
      Robin's syndrome (Q87.0)

  M26.00 Unspecified anomaly of jaw size
  M26.01 Maxillary hyperplasia
  M26.02 Maxillary hypoplasia
  M26.03 Mandibular hyperplasia
  M26.04 Mandibular hypoplasia
  M26.05 Macrogenia
  M26.06 Microgenia
  M26.07 Excessive tuberosity of jaw
      Entire maxillary tuberosity
  M26.09 Other specified anomalies of jaw size

✓5ᵗʰ **M26.1 Anomalies of jaw-cranial base relationship**
  M26.10 Unspecified anomaly of jaw-cranial base relationship
  M26.11 Maxillary asymmetry
  M26.12 Other jaw asymmetry
  M26.19 Other specified anomalies of jaw-cranial base relationship

✓5ᵗʰ **M26.2 Anomalies of dental arch relationship**
  M26.20 Unspecified anomaly of dental arch relationship
  ✓6ᵗʰ **M26.21** Malocclusion, Angle's class
      M26.211 Malocclusion, Angle's class I
          Neutro-occlusion

  M26.212 Malocclusion, Angle's class II
      Disto-occlusion Division I
      Disto-occlusion Division II
  M26.213 Malocclusion, Angle's class III
      Mesio-occlusion
  M26.219 Malocclusion, Angle's class, unspecified

✓6ᵗʰ **M26.22** Open occlusal relationship
  M26.220 Open anterior occlusal relationship
      Anterior openbite
  M26.221 Open posterior occlusal relationship
      Posterior openbite

M26.23 Excessive horizontal overlap
    Excessive horizontal overjet

M26.24 Reverse articulation
    Crossbite (anterior) (posterior)

M26.25 Anomalies of interarch distance

M26.29 Other anomalies of dental arch relationship
    Midline deviation of dental arch
    Overbite (excessive) deep
    Overbite (excessive) horizontal
    Overbite (excessive) vertical
    Posterior lingual occlusion of mandibular teeth

✓5ᵗʰ **M26.3 Anomalies of tooth position of fully erupted tooth or teeth**
  EXCLUDES 2   embedded and impacted teeth (K01.-)

  M26.30 Unspecified anomaly of tooth position of fully erupted tooth or teeth
      Abnormal spacing of fully erupted tooth or teeth NOS
      Displacement of fully erupted tooth or teeth NOS
      Transposition of fully erupted tooth or teeth NOS
  M26.31 Crowding of fully erupted teeth
  M26.32 Excessive spacing of fully erupted teeth
      Diastema of fully erupted tooth or teeth NOS
  M26.33 Horizontal displacement of fully erupted tooth or teeth
      Tipped tooth or teeth
      Tipping of fully erupted tooth
  M26.34 Vertical displacement of fully erupted tooth or teeth
      Extruded tooth
      Infraeruption of tooth or teeth
      Supraeruption of tooth or teeth
  M26.35 Rotation of fully erupted tooth or teeth
  M26.36 Insufficient interocclusal distance of fully erupted teeth (ridge)
      Lack of adequate intermaxillary vertical dimension of fully erupted teeth
  M26.37 Excessive interocclusal distance of fully erupted teeth
      Excessive intermaxillary vertical dimension of fully erupted teeth
      Loss of occlusal vertical dimension of fully erupted teeth
  M26.39 Other anomalies of tooth position of fully erupted tooth or teeth

M26.4 Malocclusion, unspecified

✓5ᵗʰ **M26.5 Dentofacial functional abnormalities**
  EXCLUDES 1   bruxism (F45.8)
      teeth-grinding NOS (F45.8)

  M26.50 Dentofacial functional abnormalities, unspecified
  M26.51 Abnormal jaw closure
  M26.52 Limited mandibular range of motion
  M26.53 Deviation in opening and closing of the mandible
  M26.54 Insufficient anterior guidance
      Insufficient anterior occlusal guidance
  M26.55 Centric occlusion maximum intercuspation discrepancy
      EXCLUDES 1   centric occlusion NOS (M26.59)
  M26.56 Non-working side interference
      Balancing side interference
  M26.57 Lack of posterior occlusal support
  M26.59 Other dentofacial functional abnormalities
      Centric occlusion (of teeth) NOS
      Malocclusion due to abnormal swallowing
      Malocclusion due to mouth breathing
      Malocclusion due to tongue, lip or finger habits

✓5ᵗʰ **M26.6 Temporomandibular joint disorders**
  EXCLUDES 2   current temporomandibular joint dislocation (S03.0)
      current temporomandibular joint sprain (S03.4)

  M26.60 Temporomandibular joint disorder, unspecified

N Newborn: 0   P Pediatric: 0-17   M Maternity: 12-55   A Adult: 15-124   MCC Major CC Condition   PDx MCC PDx acts as own MCC   CC CC Condition   PDx CC PDx acts as own CC

714   ICD-10-CM Draft (2015)

M26.61 Adhesions and ankylosis of temporomandibular joint

M26.62 Arthralgia of temporomandibular joint

M26.63 Articular disc disorder of temporomandibular joint

M26.69 Other specified disorders of temporomandibular joint

√5th **M26.7** Dental alveolar anomalies

M26.70 Unspecified alveolar anomaly

M26.71 Alveolar maxillary hyperplasia

M26.72 Alveolar mandibular hyperplasia

M26.73 Alveolar maxillary hypoplasia

M26.74 Alveolar mandibular hypoplasia

M26.79 Other specified alveolar anomalies

√5th **M26.8** Other dentofacial anomalies

M26.81 Anterior soft tissue impingement
Anterior soft tissue impingement on teeth

M26.82 Posterior soft tissue impingement
Posterior soft tissue impingement on teeth

M26.89 Other dentofacial anomalies

M26.9 Dentofacial anomaly, unspecified

√4th **M27** Other diseases of jaws

M27.0 Developmental disorders of jaws
Latent bone cyst of jaw   Torus mandibularis
Stafne's cyst   Torus palatinus

M27.1 Giant cell granuloma, central
Giant cell granuloma NOS
EXCLUDES1 *peripheral giant cell granuloma (K06.8)*

M27.2 Inflammatory conditions of jaws
Osteitis of jaw(s)
Osteomyelitis (neonatal) jaw(s)
Osteoradionecrosis jaw(s)
Periostitis jaw(s)
Sequestrum of jaw bone
Use additional code (W88-W90, X39.0) to identify radiation, if radiation-induced
EXCLUDES2 *osteonecrosis of jaw due to drug (M87.180)*

M27.3 Alveolitis of jaws
Alveolar osteitis
Dry socket

√5th **M27.4** Other and unspecified cysts of jaw
EXCLUDES1 *cysts of oral region (K09.-)*
latent bone cyst of jaw (M27.0)
Stafne's cyst (M27.0)

M27.40 Unspecified cyst of jaw
Cyst of jaw NOS

M27.49 Other cysts of jaw
Aneurysmal cyst of jaw
Hemorrhagic cyst of jaw
Traumatic cyst of jaw

√5th **M27.5** Periradicular pathology associated with previous endodontic treatment

M27.51 Perforation of root canal space due to endodontic treatment

M27.52 Endodontic overfill

M27.53 Endodontic underfill

M27.59 Other periradicular pathology associated with previous endodontic treatment

√5th **M27.6** Endosseous dental implant failure

M27.61 Osseointegration failure of dental implant
Hemorrhagic complications of dental implant placement
Iatrogenic osseointegration failure of dental implant
Osseointegration failure of dental implant due to complications of systemic disease
Osseointegration failure of dental implant due to poor bone quality
Pre-integration failure of dental implant NOS
Pre-osseointegration failure of dental implant

M27.62 Post-osseointegration biological failure of dental implant
Failure of dental implant due to lack of attached gingiva
Failure of dental implant due to occlusal trauma (caused by poor prosthetic design)
Failure of dental implant due to parafunctional habits
Failure of dental implant due to periodontal infection (peri-implantitis)
Failure of dental implant due to poor oral hygiene
Iatrogenic post-osseointegration failure of dental implant
Post-osseointegration failure of dental implant due to complications of systemic disease

M27.63 Post-osseointegration mechanical failure of dental implant
Failure of dental prosthesis causing loss of dental implant
Fracture of dental implant
EXCLUDES2 *cracked tooth (K03.81)*
fractured dental restorative material with loss of material (K08.531)
fractured dental restorative material without loss of material (K08.530)
fractured tooth (S02.5)

M27.69 Other endosseous dental implant failure
Dental implant failure NOS

M27.8 Other specified diseases of jaws
Cherubism
Exostosis
Fibrous dysplasia
Unilateral condylar hyperplasia
Unilateral condylar hypoplasia
EXCLUDES1 *jaw pain (R68.84)*

M27.9 Disease of jaws, unspecified

Systemic connective tissue disorders (M30-M36)

INCLUDES autoimmune disease NOS
collagen (vascular) disease NOS
systemic autoimmune disease
systemic collagen (vascular) disease

EXCLUDES1 *autoimmune disease, single organ or single cell-type—code to relevant condition category*

√4th **M30** Polyarteritis nodosa and related conditions
EXCLUDES1 *microscopic polyarteritis (M31.7)*

M30.0 Polyarteritis nodosa   CC
CC Excl: E08.51-E08.59, E08.618-E08.638, E08.649-E08.8, E09.51-E09.59, E09.618-E09.638, E09.649-E09.8, E10.51-E10.59, E10.618-E10.638, E10.649, E10.69-E10.8, E11.51-E11.59, E11.618-E11.638, E11.649, E11.69-E11.8, E13.51-E13.59, E13.618-E13.638, E13.649-E13.8, I87.8, I99.8-I99.9, M30.0-M31.7

M30.1 Polyarteritis with lung involvement [Churg-Strauss]   CC
Allergic granulomatous angiitis
CC Excl: See code: M30.0

M30.2 Juvenile polyarteritis   CC
CC Excl: See code: M30.0

M30.3 Mucocutaneous lymph node syndrome [Kawasaki]   CC
CC Excl: I87.8, I99.8-I99.9, M30.0-M31.1, M31.30-M31.7

M30.8 Other conditions related to polyarteritis nodosa   CC
Polyangiitis overlap syndrome
CC Excl: See code: M30.0

√4th **M31** Other necrotizing vasculopathies

M31.0 Hypersensitivity angiitis   CC
Goodpasture's syndrome
CC Excl: See code: M30.0

M31.1 Thrombotic microangiopathy   MCC
Thrombotic thrombocytopenic purpura
CC Excl: See code: M30.0

M31.2 Lethal midline granuloma   CC
CC Excl: See code: M30.0

√5th **M31.3** Wegener's granulomatosis
Necrotizing respiratory granulomatosis

M31.30 Wegener's granulomatosis without renal involvement   CC
Wegener's granulomatosis NOS
CC Excl: See code: M30.0

M31.31 Wegener's granulomatosis with renal involvement   CC
CC Excl: See code: M30.0

M31.4 Aortic arch syndrome [Takayasu]   CC
CC Excl: See code: M30.0

M31.5 Giant cell arteritis with polymyalgia rheumatica

M31.6 Other giant cell arteritis

M31.7 Microscopic polyangiitis `CC`
Microscopic polyarteritis
EXCLUDES 1 polyarteritis nodosa (M30.0)
CC Excl: See code: M30.0

M31.8 Other specified necrotizing vasculopathies `CC`
Hypocomplementemic vasculitis
Septic vasculitis
CC Excl: I77.5, M31.8-M31.9

M31.9 Necrotizing vasculopathy, unspecified `CC`
CC Excl: See code: M31.8

√4th **M32 Systemic lupus erythematosus (SLE)**
EXCLUDES 1 lupus erythematosus (discoid) (NOS) (L93.0)

M32.0 Drug-induced systemic lupus erythematosus
Use additional code for adverse effect, if applicable, to identify drug (T36-T50 with fifth or sixth character 5)

√5th **M32.1 Systemic lupus erythematosus with organ or system involvement**

M32.10 Systemic lupus erythematosus, organ or system involvement unspecified

M32.11 Endocarditis in systemic lupus erythematosus `PDx CC` `CC`
Libman-Sacks disease
CC Excl: I38-I39, I87.8, I99.8-I99.9

M32.12 Pericarditis in systemic lupus erythematosus `PDx CC` `CC`
Lupus pericarditis
CC Excl: I01.0, I09.2, I30.0-I30.9, I31.3-I32, I87.8, I99.8-I99.9

M32.13 Lung involvement in systemic lupus erythematosus
Pleural effusion due to systemic lupus erythematosus

M32.14 Glomerular disease in systemic lupus erythematosus
Lupus renal disease NOS
AHA: 2013, 4Q, 125

M32.15 Tubulo-interstitial nephropathy in systemic lupus erythematosus

M32.19 Other organ or system involvement in systemic lupus erythematosus

M32.8 Other forms of systemic lupus erythematosus

M32.9 Systemic lupus erythematosus, unspecified
SLE NOS
Systemic lupus erythematosus NOS
Systemic lupus erythematosus without organ involvement

√4th **M33 Dermatopolymyositis**

√5th **M33.0 Juvenile dermatopolymyositis**

M33.00 Juvenile dermatopolymyositis, organ involvement unspecified `CC`
CC Excl: M33.00-M33.19, M33.90-M33.99, M36.0

M33.01 Juvenile dermatopolymyositis with respiratory involvement `CC`
CC Excl: See code: M33.00

M33.02 Juvenile dermatopolymyositis with myopathy `PDx CC` `CC`
CC Excl: E08.40-E08.49, E08.618-E08.638, E08.649-E08.8, E09.40-E09.49, E09.618-E09.638, E09.649-E09.8, E10.40-E10.49, E10.618-E10.638, E10.649, E10.69-E10.8, E11.40-E11.49, E11.618-E11.638, E11.649, E11.69-E11.8, E13.40-E13.49, E13.618-E13.638, E13.649-E13.8, G32.89, G70.00-G72.3, G72.81-G73.7, G96.8-G96.9, G98.0-G98.8, G99.8, M33.00-M33.19, M33.90-M33.99, M36.0

M33.09 Juvenile dermatopolymyositis with other organ involvement `CC`
CC Excl: See code: M33.00

√5th **M33.1 Other dermatopolymyositis**

M33.10 Other dermatopolymyositis, organ involvement unspecified `CC`
CC Excl: See code: M33.00

M33.11 Other dermatopolymyositis with respiratory involvement `CC`
CC Excl: See code: M33.00

M33.12 Other dermatopolymyositis with myopathy `PDx CC` `CC`
CC Excl: See code: M33.02

M33.19 Other dermatopolymyositis with other organ involvement `CC`
CC Excl: See code: M33.00

√5th **M33.2 Polymyositis**

M33.20 Polymyositis, organ involvement unspecified `CC`
CC Excl: M33.20-M33.29

M33.21 Polymyositis with respiratory involvement `CC`
CC Excl: See code: M33.20

M33.22 Polymyositis with myopathy `PDx CC` `CC`
CC Excl: E08.40-E08.49, E08.618-E08.638, E08.649-E08.8, E09.40-E09.49, E09.618-E09.638, E09.649-E09.8, E10.40-E10.49, E10.618-E10.638, E10.649, E10.69-E10.8, E11.40-E11.49, E11.618-E11.638, E11.649, E11.69-E11.8, E13.40-E13.49, E13.618-E13.638, E13.649-E13.8, G32.89, G70.00-G72.3, G72.81-G73.7, G96.8-G96.9, G98.0-G98.8, G99.8, M33.20-M33.29

M33.29 Polymyositis with other organ involvement `CC`
CC Excl: See code: M33.20

√5th **M33.9 Dermatopolymyositis, unspecified**

M33.90 Dermatopolymyositis, unspecified, organ involvement unspecified `CC`
CC Excl: See code: M33.19

M33.91 Dermatopolymyositis, unspecified with respiratory involvement `CC`
CC Excl: See code: M33.19

M33.92 Dermatopolymyositis, unspecified with myopathy `PDx CC` `CC`
CC Excl: See code: M33.12

M33.99 Dermatopolymyositis, unspecified with other organ involvement `CC`
CC Excl: See code: M33.19

√4th **M34 Systemic sclerosis [scleroderma]**
EXCLUDES 1 circumscribed scleroderma (L94.0)
neonatal scleroderma (P83.8)

M34.0 Progressive systemic sclerosis

M34.1 CR(E)ST syndrome
Combination of calcinosis, Raynaud's phenomenon, esophageal dysfunction, sclerodactyly, telangiectasia

M34.2 Systemic sclerosis induced by drug and chemical
Code first poisoning due to drug or toxin, if applicable (T36-T65 with fifth or sixth character 1-4 or 6)
Use additional code for adverse effect, if applicable, to identify drug (T36-T50 with fifth or sixth character 5)

√5th **M34.8 Other forms of systemic sclerosis**

M34.81 Systemic sclerosis with lung involvement `PDx CC` `CC`
CC Excl: No excl

M34.82 Systemic sclerosis with myopathy `PDx CC` `CC`
CC Excl: E08.40-E08.49, E08.618-E08.638, E08.649-E08.8, E09.40-E09.49, E09.618-E09.638, E09.649-E09.8, E10.40-E10.49, E10.618-E10.638, E10.649, E10.69-E10.8, E11.40-E11.49, E11.618-E11.638, E11.649, E11.69-E11.8, E13.40-E13.49, E13.618-E13.638, E13.649-E13.8, G32.89, G70.00-G72.3, G72.81-G73.7, G96.8-G96.9, G98.0-G98.8, G99.8

M34.83 Systemic sclerosis with polyneuropathy

M34.89 Other systemic sclerosis

M34.9 Systemic sclerosis, unspecified

√4th **M35 Other systemic involvement of connective tissue**
EXCLUDES 1 reactive perforating collagenosis (L87.1)

√5th **M35.0 Sicca syndrome [Sjögren]**

M35.00 Sicca syndrome, unspecified

M35.01 Sicca syndrome with keratoconjunctivitis

M35.02 Sicca syndrome with lung involvement

M35.03 Sicca syndrome with myopathy `PDx CC` `CC`
CC Excl: See code M34.82

M35.04 Sicca syndrome with tubulo-interstitial nephropathy
Renal tubular acidosis in sicca syndrome

M35.09 Sicca syndrome with other organ involvement

M35.1 Other overlap syndromes `CC`
Mixed connective tissue disease
EXCLUDES 1 polyangiitis overlap syndrome (M30.8)
CC Excl: G72.41-G72.49, M35.1, M35.5, M35.8

M35.2 Behçet's disease `CC`
CC Excl: A02.23, A17.9, A18.02, A18.09, A18.82, A18.84, A18.89, A39.83-A39.84, A54.40, A54.42-A54.43, A54.82, A54.84, A54.89-A54.9, B06.82, M00.00, M00.019, M00.029, M00.039, M00.049, M00.059, M00.069, M00.079, M00.08-M02.30, M02.319, M02.329, M02.339, M02.349, M02.359, M02.369, M02.379-M02.9, M05.40-M05.59, M05.70-M06.09, M06.20-M06.39, M06.80-M07.69, M11.00-M11.9, M12.10-M15.0, M15.3-M15.9, M16.2-M16.9, M17.2-M17.9, M18.2-M18.9, M19.111-M19.93, M24.10-M24.176, M25.00, M25.08-M25.18, M25.40-M25.676, M25.80-M25.9, M35.2, M36.1-M36.4, R29.4

M35.3 Polymyalgia rheumatica
EXCLUDES 1 polymyalgia rheumatica with giant cell arteritis (M31.5)

M35.4 Diffuse (eosinophilic) fasciitis

M35.5 Multifocal fibrosclerosis `CC`
  CC Excl: G72.41-G72.49, M35.1, M35.5, M35.8

M35.6 Relapsing panniculitis [Weber-Christian]
  EXCLUDES 1 *lupus panniculitis (L93.2)*
              panniculitis NOS (M79.3-)

M35.7 Hypermobility syndrome
  Familial ligamentous laxity
  EXCLUDES 1 *Ehlers-Danlos syndrome (Q79.6)*
              ligamentous laxity, NOS (M24.2-)

M35.8 Other specified systemic involvement of connective tissue `CC`
  CC Excl: G72.41-G72.49, M35.1, M35.5, M35.8

M35.9 Systemic involvement of connective tissue, unspecified
  Autoimmune disease (systemic) NOS
  Collagen (vascular) disease NOS

✓4th **M36 Systemic disorders of connective tissue in diseases classified elsewhere**
  EXCLUDES 2 *arthropathies in diseases classified elsewhere (M14.-)*

M36.0 Dermato(poly)myositis in neoplastic disease `CC`
  Code first underlying neoplasm (C00-D49)
  CC Excl: M33.00-M33.19, M33.90-M33.99, M36.0

M36.1 Arthropathy in neoplastic disease
  Code first underlying neoplasm, such as:
    leukemia (C91-C95)
    malignant histiocytosis (C96.A)
    multiple myeloma (C90.0)

M36.2 Hemophilic arthropathy
  Hemarthrosis in hemophilic arthropathy
  Code first underlying disease, such as:
    factor VIII deficiency (D66)
      with vascular defect (D68.0)
    factor IX deficiency (D67)
    hemophilia (classical) (D66)
    hemophilia B (D67)
    hemophilia C (D68.1)

M36.3 Arthropathy in other blood disorders

M36.4 Arthropathy in hypersensitivity reactions classified elsewhere
  Code first underlying disease, such as:
    Henoch (-Schönlein) purpura (D69.0)
    serum sickness (T80.6-)

M36.8 Systemic disorders of connective tissue in other diseases classified elsewhere
  Code first underlying disease, such as:
    alkaptonuria (E70.2)
    hypogammaglobulinemia (D80.-)
    ochronosis (E70.2)

DORSOPATHIES (M40-M54)

Deforming dorsopathies (M40-M43)

✓4th **M40 Kyphosis and lordosis**
  EXCLUDES 1 *congenital kyphosis and lordosis (Q76.4)*
              kyphoscoliosis (M41.-)
              postprocedural kyphosis and lordosis (M96.-)

✓5th **M40.0 Postural kyphosis**
  EXCLUDES 1 *osteochondrosis of spine (M42.-)*
  M40.00 Postural kyphosis, site unspecified
  M40.03 Postural kyphosis, cervicothoracic region
  M40.04 Postural kyphosis, thoracic region
  M40.05 Postural kyphosis, thoracolumbar region

✓5th **M40.1 Other secondary kyphosis**
  M40.10 Other secondary kyphosis, site unspecified
  M40.12 Other secondary kyphosis, cervical region
  M40.13 Other secondary kyphosis, cervicothoracic region
  M40.14 Other secondary kyphosis, thoracic region
  M40.15 Other secondary kyphosis, thoracolumbar region

✓5th **M40.2 Other and unspecified kyphosis**
  ✓6th **M40.20 Unspecified kyphosis**
    M40.202 Unspecified kyphosis, cervical region
    M40.203 Unspecified kyphosis, cervicothoracic region
    M40.204 Unspecified kyphosis, thoracic region
    M40.205 Unspecified kyphosis, thoracolumbar region
    M40.209 Unspecified kyphosis, site unspecified

  ✓6th **M40.29 Other kyphosis**
    M40.292 Other kyphosis, cervical region
    M40.293 Other kyphosis, cervicothoracic region
    M40.294 Other kyphosis, thoracic region
    M40.295 Other kyphosis, thoracolumbar region
    M40.299 Other kyphosis, site unspecified

✓5th **M40.3 Flatback syndrome**
  M40.30 Flatback syndrome, site unspecified
  M40.35 Flatback syndrome, thoracolumbar region
  M40.36 Flatback syndrome, lumbar region
  M40.37 Flatback syndrome, lumbosacral region

✓5th **M40.4 Postural lordosis**
  Acquired lordosis
  M40.40 Postural lordosis, site unspecified
  M40.45 Postural lordosis, thoracolumbar region
  M40.46 Postural lordosis, lumbar region
  M40.47 Postural lordosis, lumbosacral region

✓5th **M40.5 Lordosis, unspecified**
  M40.50 Lordosis, unspecified, site unspecified
  M40.55 Lordosis, unspecified, thoracolumbar region
  M40.56 Lordosis, unspecified, lumbar region
  M40.57 Lordosis, unspecified, lumbosacral region

✓4th **M41 Scoliosis**
  INCLUDES kyphoscoliosis
  EXCLUDES 1 *congenital scoliosis due to bony malformation (Q76.3)*
              congenital scoliosis NOS (Q67.5)
              kyphoscoliotic heart disease (I27.1)
              postprocedural scoliosis (M96.-)
              postural congenital scoliosis (Q67.5)

✓5th **M41.0 Infantile idiopathic scoliosis**
  M41.00 Infantile idiopathic scoliosis, site unspecified
  M41.02 Infantile idiopathic scoliosis, cervical region
  M41.03 Infantile idiopathic scoliosis, cervicothoracic region
  M41.04 Infantile idiopathic scoliosis, thoracic region
  M41.05 Infantile idiopathic scoliosis, thoracolumbar region
  M41.06 Infantile idiopathic scoliosis, lumbar region
  M41.07 Infantile idiopathic scoliosis, lumbosacral region
  M41.08 Infantile idiopathic scoliosis, sacral and sacrococcygeal region

✓5th **M41.1 Juvenile and adolescent idiopathic scoliosis**
  ✓6th **M41.11 Juvenile idiopathic scoliosis**
    M41.112 Juvenile idiopathic scoliosis, cervical region
    M41.113 Juvenile idiopathic scoliosis, cervicothoracic region
    M41.114 Juvenile idiopathic scoliosis, thoracic region
    M41.115 Juvenile idiopathic scoliosis, thoracolumbar region
    M41.116 Juvenile idiopathic scoliosis, lumbar region
    M41.117 Juvenile idiopathic scoliosis, lumbosacral region
    M41.119 Juvenile idiopathic scoliosis, site unspecified

  ✓6th **M41.12 Adolescent scoliosis**
    M41.122 Adolescent idiopathic scoliosis, cervical region
    M41.123 Adolescent idiopathic scoliosis, cervicothoracic region
    M41.124 Adolescent idiopathic scoliosis, thoracic region
    M41.125 Adolescent idiopathic scoliosis, thoracolumbar region
    M41.126 Adolescent idiopathic scoliosis, lumbar region
    M41.127 Adolescent idiopathic scoliosis, lumbosacral region
    M41.129 Adolescent idiopathic scoliosis, site unspecified

✓5th **M41.2 Other idiopathic scoliosis**
  M41.20 Other idiopathic scoliosis, site unspecified
  M41.22 Other idiopathic scoliosis, cervical region
  M41.23 Other idiopathic scoliosis, cervicothoracic region

M41.24　**Other idiopathic scoliosis, thoracic region**
M41.25　**Other idiopathic scoliosis, thoracolumbar region**
M41.26　**Other idiopathic scoliosis, lumbar region**
M41.27　**Other idiopathic scoliosis, lumbosacral region**

✓5ᵗʰ **M41.3　Thoracogenic scoliosis**
M41.30　**Thoracogenic scoliosis, site unspecified**
M41.34　**Thoracogenic scoliosis, thoracic region**
M41.35　**Thoracogenic scoliosis, thoracolumbar region**

✓5ᵗʰ **M41.4　Neuromuscular scoliosis**
Scoliosis secondary to cerebral palsy, Friedreich's ataxia, poliomyelitis and other neuromuscular disorders
Code also underlying condition
M41.40　**Neuromuscular scoliosis, site unspecified**
M41.41　**Neuromuscular scoliosis, occipito-atlanto-axial region**
M41.42　**Neuromuscular scoliosis, cervical region**
M41.43　**Neuromuscular scoliosis, cervicothoracic region**
M41.44　**Neuromuscular scoliosis, thoracic region**
M41.45　**Neuromuscular scoliosis, thoracolumbar region**
M41.46　**Neuromuscular scoliosis, lumbar region**
M41.47　**Neuromuscular scoliosis, lumbosacral region**

✓5ᵗʰ **M41.5　Other secondary scoliosis**
M41.50　**Other secondary scoliosis, site unspecified**
M41.52　**Other secondary scoliosis, cervical region**
M41.53　**Other secondary scoliosis, cervicothoracic region**
M41.54　**Other secondary scoliosis, thoracic region**
M41.55　**Other secondary scoliosis, thoracolumbar region**
M41.56　**Other secondary scoliosis, lumbar region**
M41.57　**Other secondary scoliosis, lumbosacral region**

✓5ᵗʰ **M41.8　Other forms of scoliosis**
M41.80　**Other forms of scoliosis, site unspecified**
M41.82　**Other forms of scoliosis, cervical region**
M41.83　**Other forms of scoliosis, cervicothoracic region**
M41.84　**Other forms of scoliosis, thoracic region**
M41.85　**Other forms of scoliosis, thoracolumbar region**
M41.86　**Other forms of scoliosis, lumbar region**
M41.87　**Other forms of scoliosis, lumbosacral region**

M41.9　**Scoliosis, unspecified**

✓4ᵗʰ **M42　Spinal osteochondrosis**

✓5ᵗʰ **M42.0　Juvenile osteochondrosis of spine**
Calvé's disease
Scheuermann's disease
EXCLUDES 1　postural kyphosis (M40.0)
M42.00　**Juvenile osteochondrosis of spine, site unspecified**
M42.01　**Juvenile osteochondrosis of spine, occipito-atlanto-axial region**
M42.02　**Juvenile osteochondrosis of spine, cervical region**
M42.03　**Juvenile osteochondrosis of spine, cervicothoracic region**
M42.04　**Juvenile osteochondrosis of spine, thoracic region**
M42.05　**Juvenile osteochondrosis of spine, thoracolumbar region**
M42.06　**Juvenile osteochondrosis of spine, lumbar region**
M42.07　**Juvenile osteochondrosis of spine, lumbosacral region**
M42.08　**Juvenile osteochondrosis of spine, sacral and sacrococcygeal region**
M42.09　**Juvenile osteochondrosis of spine, multiple sites in spine**

✓5ᵗʰ **M42.1　Adult osteochondrosis of spine**
M42.10　**Adult osteochondrosis of spine, site unspecified**　Ⓐ
M42.11　**Adult osteochondrosis of spine, occipito-atlanto-axial region**　Ⓐ
M42.12　**Adult osteochondrosis of spine, cervical region**　Ⓐ
M42.13　**Adult osteochondrosis of spine, cervicothoracic region**　Ⓐ
M42.14　**Adult osteochondrosis of spine, thoracic region**　Ⓐ
M42.15　**Adult osteochondrosis of spine, thoracolumbar region**　Ⓐ
M42.16　**Adult osteochondrosis of spine, lumbar region**　Ⓐ
M42.17　**Adult osteochondrosis of spine, lumbosacral region**　Ⓐ

M42.18　**Adult osteochondrosis of spine, sacral and sacrococcygeal region**　Ⓐ
M42.19　**Adult osteochondrosis of spine, multiple sites in spine**　Ⓐ

M42.9　**Spinal osteochondrosis, unspecified**

✓4ᵗʰ **M43　Other deforming dorsopathies**
EXCLUDES 1　congenital spondylolysis and spondylolisthesis (Q76.2)
hemivertebra (Q76.3-Q76.4)
Klippel-Feil syndrome (Q76.1)
lumbarization and sacralization (Q76.4)
platyspondylisis (Q76.4)
spina bifida occulta (Q76.0)
spinal curvature in osteoporosis (M80.-)
spinal curvature in Paget's disease of bone [osteitis deformans] (M88.-)

✓5ᵗʰ **M43.0　Spondylolysis**
EXCLUDES 1　congenital spondylolysis (Q76.2)
spondylolisthesis (M43.1)
M43.00　**Spondylolysis, site unspecified**
M43.01　**Spondylolysis, occipito-atlanto-axial region**
M43.02　**Spondylolysis, cervical region**
M43.03　**Spondylolysis, cervicothoracic region**
M43.04　**Spondylolysis, thoracic region**
M43.05　**Spondylolysis, thoracolumbar region**
M43.06　**Spondylolysis, lumbar region**
M43.07　**Spondylolysis, lumbosacral region**
M43.08　**Spondylolysis, sacral and sacrococcygeal region**
M43.09　**Spondylolysis, multiple sites in spine**

✓5ᵗʰ **M43.1　Spondylolisthesis**
EXCLUDES 1　acute traumatic of lumbosacral region (S33.1)
acute traumatic of sites other than lumbosacral— code to Fracture, vertebra, by region
congenital spondylolisthesis (Q76.2)
M43.10　**Spondylolisthesis, site unspecified**
M43.11　**Spondylolisthesis, occipito-atlanto-axial region**
M43.12　**Spondylolisthesis, cervical region**
M43.13　**Spondylolisthesis, cervicothoracic region**
M43.14　**Spondylolisthesis, thoracic region**
M43.15　**Spondylolisthesis, thoracolumbar region**
M43.16　**Spondylolisthesis, lumbar region**
M43.17　**Spondylolisthesis, lumbosacral region**
M43.18　**Spondylolisthesis, sacral and sacrococcygeal region**
M43.19　**Spondylolisthesis, multiple sites in spine**

✓5ᵗʰ **M43.2　Fusion of spine**
Ankylosis of spinal joint
EXCLUDES 1　ankylosing spondylitis (M45.0-)
congenital fusion of spine (Q76.4)
EXCLUDES 2　arthrodesis status (Z98.1)
pseudoarthrosis after fusion or arthrodesis (M96.0)
M43.20　**Fusion of spine, site unspecified**
M43.21　**Fusion of spine, occipito-atlanto-axial region**
M43.22　**Fusion of spine, cervical region**
M43.23　**Fusion of spine, cervicothoracic region**
M43.24　**Fusion of spine, thoracic region**
M43.25　**Fusion of spine, thoracolumbar region**
M43.26　**Fusion of spine, lumbar region**
M43.27　**Fusion of spine, lumbosacral region**
M43.28　**Fusion of spine, sacral and sacrococcygeal region**

M43.3　**Recurrent atlantoaxial dislocation with myelopathy**
M43.4　**Other recurrent atlantoaxial dislocation**

✓5ᵗʰ **M43.5　Other recurrent vertebral dislocation**
EXCLUDES 1　biomechanical lesions NEC (M99.-)

✓6ᵗʰ **M43.5X　Other recurrent vertebral dislocation**
M43.5X2　**Other recurrent vertebral dislocation, cervical region**
M43.5X3　**Other recurrent vertebral dislocation, cervicothoracic region**
M43.5X4　**Other recurrent vertebral dislocation, thoracic region**
M43.5X5　**Other recurrent vertebral dislocation, thoracolumbar region**
M43.5X6　**Other recurrent vertebral dislocation, lumbar region**

M43.5X7   Other recurrent vertebral dislocation, lumbosacral **region**

M43.5X8   Other recurrent vertebral dislocation, sacral and sacrococcygeal **region**

M43.5X9   Other recurrent vertebral dislocation, site unspecified

M43.6   Torticollis

EXCLUDES 1   congenital (sternomastoid) torticollis (Q68.0)
current injury—see Injury, of spine, by body region
ocular torticollis (R29.891)
psychogenic torticollis (F45.8)
spasmodic torticollis (G24.3)
torticollis due to birth injury (P15.2)

✓5th M43.8   Other specified deforming dorsopathies

EXCLUDES 2   kyphosis and lordosis (M40.-)
scoliosis (M41.-)

✓6th M43.8X   Other specified deforming dorsopathies

M43.8X1   Other specified deforming dorsopathies, occipito-atlanto-axial **region**

M43.8X2   Other specified deforming dorsopathies, cervical **region**

M43.8X3   Other specified deforming dorsopathies, cervicothoracic **region**

M43.8X4   Other specified deforming dorsopathies, thoracic **region**

M43.8X5   Other specified deforming dorsopathies, thoracolumbar **region**

M43.8X6   Other specified deforming dorsopathies, lumbar **region**

M43.8X7   Other specified deforming dorsopathies, lumbosacral **region**

M43.8X8   Other specified deforming dorsopathies, sacral and sacrococcygeal **region**

M43.8X9   Other specified deforming dorsopathies, site unspecified

M43.9   Deforming dorsopathy, unspecified
Curvature of spine NOS

Spondylopathies (M45-M49)

✓4th M45   Ankylosing spondylitis
Rheumatoid arthritis of spine

EXCLUDES 1   arthropathy in Reiter's disease (M02.3-)
juvenile (ankylosing) spondylitis (M08.1)

EXCLUDES 2   Behçet's disease (M35.2)

M45.0   Ankylosing spondylitis of multiple sites in spine

M45.1   Ankylosing spondylitis of occipito-atlanto-axial **region**

M45.2   Ankylosing spondylitis of cervical **region**

M45.3   Ankylosing spondylitis of cervicothoracic **region**

M45.4   Ankylosing spondylitis of thoracic **region**

M45.5   Ankylosing spondylitis of thoracolumbar **region**

M45.6   Ankylosing spondylitis lumbar **region**

M45.7   Ankylosing spondylitis of lumbosacral **region**

M45.8   Ankylosing spondylitis sacral and sacrococcygeal **region**

M45.9   Ankylosing spondylitis of unspecified sites in spine

✓4th M46   Other inflammatory spondylopathies

✓5th M46.0   Spinal enthesopathy
Disorder of ligamentous or muscular attachments of spine

M46.00   Spinal enthesopathy, site unspecified

M46.01   Spinal enthesopathy, occipito-atlanto-axial **region**

M46.02   Spinal enthesopathy, cervical **region**

M46.03   Spinal enthesopathy, cervicothoracic **region**

M46.04   Spinal enthesopathy, thoracic **region**

M46.05   Spinal enthesopathy, thoracolumbar **region**

M46.06   Spinal enthesopathy, lumbar **region**

M46.07   Spinal enthesopathy, lumbosacral **region**

M46.08   Spinal enthesopathy, sacral and sacrococcygeal **region**

M46.09   Spinal enthesopathy, multiple sites in spine

M46.1   Sacroiliitis, not elsewhere classified

✓5th M46.2   Osteomyelitis of vertebra

CC Excl: For CC codes in subcategory M46.20, unless otherwise noted: A02.24, A17.9, A18.03-A18.09, A18.82, A18.84, A18.89, M46.20-M46.39, M86.00-M86.9

M46.20   Osteomyelitis of vertebra, site unspecified   `CC`

M46.21   Osteomyelitis of vertebra, occipito-atlanto-axial **region**   `CC`

M46.22   Osteomyelitis of vertebra, cervical **region**   `CC`

M46.23   Osteomyelitis of vertebra, cervicothoracic **region**   `CC`

M46.24   Osteomyelitis of vertebra, thoracic **region**   `CC`

M46.25   Osteomyelitis of vertebra, thoracolumbar **region**   `CC`

M46.26   Osteomyelitis of vertebra, lumbar **region**   `CC`

M46.27   Osteomyelitis of vertebra, lumbosacral **region**   `CC`

M46.28   Osteomyelitis of vertebra, sacral and sacrococcygeal **region**   `CC`

✓5th M46.3   Infection of intervertebral disc (pyogenic)
Use additional code (B95-B97) to identify infectious agent

M46.30   Infection of intervertebral disc (pyogenic), site unspecified   `CC`
CC Excl: A17.9-A18.01, A18.03-A18.09, A18.82, A18.84, A18.89, M46.20-M46.39, M86.00-M86.9

M46.31   Infection of intervertebral disc (pyogenic), occipito-atlanto-axial **region**   `CC`
CC Excl: See code: M46.30

M46.32   Infection of intervertebral disc (pyogenic), cervical **region**   `CC`
CC Excl: See code: M46.30

M46.33   Infection of intervertebral disc (pyogenic), cervicothoracic **region**   `CC`
CC Excl: See code: M46.30

M46.34   Infection of intervertebral disc (pyogenic), thoracic **region**   `CC`
CC Excl: See code: M46.30

M46.35   Infection of intervertebral disc (pyogenic), thoracolumbar **region**   `CC`
CC Excl: See code: M46.30

M46.36   Infection of intervertebral disc (pyogenic), lumbar **region**   `CC`
CC Excl: See code: M46.30

M46.37   Infection of intervertebral disc (pyogenic), lumbosacral **region**   `CC`
CC Excl: See code: M46.30

M46.38   Infection of intervertebral disc (pyogenic), sacral and sacrococcygeal **region**   `CC`
CC Excl: See code: M46.30

M46.39   Infection of intervertebral disc (pyogenic), multiple sites in spine   `CC`
CC Excl: See code: M46.30

✓5th M46.4   Discitis, unspecified

M46.40   Discitis, unspecified, site unspecified

M46.41   Discitis, unspecified, occipito-atlanto-axial **region**

M46.42   Discitis, unspecified, cervical **region**

M46.43   Discitis, unspecified, cervicothoracic **region**

M46.44   Discitis, unspecified, thoracic **region**

M46.45   Discitis, unspecified, thoracolumbar **region**

M46.46   Discitis, unspecified, lumbar **region**

M46.47   Discitis, unspecified, lumbosacral **region**

M46.48   Discitis, unspecified, sacral and sacrococcygeal **region**

M46.49   Discitis, unspecified, multiple sites in spine

✓5th M46.5   Other infective spondylopathies

M46.50   Other infective spondylopathies, site unspecified

M46.51   Other infective spondylopathies, occipito-atlanto-axial **region**

M46.52   Other infective spondylopathies, cervical **region**

M46.53   Other infective spondylopathies, cervicothoracic **region**

M46.54   Other infective spondylopathies, thoracic **region**

M46.55   Other infective spondylopathies, thoracolumbar **region**

M46.56   Other infective spondylopathies, lumbar **region**

M46.57   Other infective spondylopathies, lumbosacral **region**

M46.58   Other infective spondylopathies, sacral and sacrococcygeal **region**

M46.59   Other infective spondylopathies, multiple sites in spine

✓5th M46.8   Other specified inflammatory spondylopathies

M46.80   Other specified inflammatory spondylopathies, site unspecified

✓ Additional Character Required   ✓x7th Xtension Alert   Unacceptable PDx   Manifestation   Hospital Acquired Condition   *EXCLUDES 1* Not Coded Here   *EXCLUDES 2* Not Included Here

ICD-10-CM Draft (2015)   719

Diseases of the Musculoskeletal System and Connective Tissue

M46.81–M47.897

M46.81 Other specified inflammatory spondylopathies, occipito-atlanto-axial region

M46.82 Other specified inflammatory spondylopathies, cervical region

M46.83 Other specified inflammatory spondylopathies, cervicothoracic region

M46.84 Other specified inflammatory spondylopathies, thoracic region

M46.85 Other specified inflammatory spondylopathies, thoracolumbar region

M46.86 Other specified inflammatory spondylopathies, lumbar region

M46.87 Other specified inflammatory spondylopathies, lumbosacral region

M46.88 Other specified inflammatory spondylopathies, sacral and sacrococcygeal region

M46.89 Other specified inflammatory spondylopathies, multiple sites in spine

✓5th **M46.9** Unspecified inflammatory spondylopathy

M46.90 Unspecified inflammatory spondylopathy, site unspecified

M46.91 Unspecified inflammatory spondylopathy, occipito-atlanto-axial region

M46.92 Unspecified inflammatory spondylopathy, cervical region

M46.93 Unspecified inflammatory spondylopathy, cervicothoracic region

M46.94 Unspecified inflammatory spondylopathy, thoracic region

M46.95 Unspecified inflammatory spondylopathy, thoracolumbar region

M46.96 Unspecified inflammatory spondylopathy, lumbar region

M46.97 Unspecified inflammatory spondylopathy, lumbosacral region

M46.98 Unspecified inflammatory spondylopathy, sacral and sacrococcygeal region

M46.99 Unspecified inflammatory spondylopathy, multiple sites in spine

✓4th **M47 Spondylosis**

INCLUDES arthrosis or osteoarthritis of spine
degeneration of facet joints

✓5th **M47.0** Anterior spinal and vertebral artery compression syndromes

✓6th **M47.01** Anterior spinal artery compression syndromes

CC Excl: For CC codes in subcategory M47.01, unless otherwise noted: M47.011–M47.029, M47.11–M47.13, M47.21–M47.23, M47.811–M47.813, M47.891–M47.893

M47.011 Anterior spinal artery compression syndromes, occipito-atlanto-axial region   CC

M47.012 Anterior spinal artery compression syndromes, cervical region   CC

M47.013 Anterior spinal artery compression syndromes, cervicothoracic region   CC

M47.014 Anterior spinal artery compression syndromes, thoracic region   CC

M47.015 Anterior spinal artery compression syndromes, thoracolumbar region   CC

M47.016 Anterior spinal artery compression syndromes, lumbar region   CC

M47.019 Anterior spinal artery compression syndromes, site unspecified   CC

✓6th **M47.02** Vertebral artery compression syndromes

M47.021 Vertebral artery compression syndromes, occipito-atlanto-axial region   CC

M47.022 Vertebral artery compression syndromes, cervical region   CC

M47.029 Vertebral artery compression syndromes, site unspecified   CC

✓5th **M47.1** Other spondylosis with myelopathy

Spondylogenic compression of spinal cord

EXCLUDES 1 vertebral subluxation (M43.3-M43.5X9)

M47.10 Other spondylosis with myelopathy, site unspecified   CC
CC Excl: M25.78, M47.011–M47.9, M48.10–M48.38, M48.9

M47.11 Other spondylosis with myelopathy, occipito-atlanto-axial region   CC
CC Excl: M47.011–M47.029, M47.11–M47.13, M47.21–M47.23, M47.811–M47.813, M47.891–M47.893

M47.12 Other spondylosis with myelopathy, cervical region   CC
CC Excl: See code: M47.11

M47.13 Other spondylosis with myelopathy, cervicothoracic region   CC
CC Excl: See code: M47.11

M47.14 Other spondylosis with myelopathy, thoracic region   CC
CC Excl: M47.14–M47.15

M47.15 Other spondylosis with myelopathy, thoracolumbar region   CC
CC Excl: See code: M47.14

M47.16 Other spondylosis with myelopathy, lumbar region   CC
CC Excl: M46.40, M46.46–M46.49, M47.16–M47.18, M47.26–M47.28, M47.816–M47.818, M47.896–M47.898, M51.06–M51.07, M51.26–M51.27, M51.36–M51.37, M51.46–M51.47, M51.86–M51.9

✓5th **M47.2** Other spondylosis with radiculopathy

M47.20 Other spondylosis with radiculopathy, site unspecified

M47.21 Other spondylosis with radiculopathy, occipito-atlanto-axial region

M47.22 Other spondylosis with radiculopathy, cervical region

M47.23 Other spondylosis with radiculopathy, cervicothoracic region

M47.24 Other spondylosis with radiculopathy, thoracic region

M47.25 Other spondylosis with radiculopathy, thoracolumbar region

M47.26 Other spondylosis with radiculopathy, lumbar region

M47.27 Other spondylosis with radiculopathy, lumbosacral region

M47.28 Other spondylosis with radiculopathy, sacral and sacrococcygeal region

✓5th **M47.8** Other spondylosis

✓6th **M47.81** Spondylosis without myelopathy or radiculopathy

M47.811 Spondylosis without myelopathy or radiculopathy, occipito-atlanto-axial region

M47.812 Spondylosis without myelopathy or radiculopathy, cervical region

M47.813 Spondylosis without myelopathy or radiculopathy, cervicothoracic region

M47.814 Spondylosis without myelopathy or radiculopathy, thoracic region

M47.815 Spondylosis without myelopathy or radiculopathy, thoracolumbar region

M47.816 Spondylosis without myelopathy or radiculopathy, lumbar region

M47.817 Spondylosis without myelopathy or radiculopathy, lumbosacral region

M47.818 Spondylosis without myelopathy or radiculopathy, sacral and sacrococcygeal region

M47.819 Spondylosis without myelopathy or radiculopathy, site unspecified

✓6th **M47.89** Other spondylosis

M47.891 Other spondylosis, occipito-atlanto-axial region

M47.892 Other spondylosis, cervical region

M47.893 Other spondylosis, cervicothoracic region

M47.894 Other spondylosis, thoracic region

M47.895 Other spondylosis, thoracolumbar region

M47.896 Other spondylosis, lumbar region

M47.897 Other spondylosis, lumbosacral region

N Newborn: 0   P Pediatric: 0-17   M Maternity: 12-55   A Adult: 15-124   MCC Major CC Condition   PDx MCC PDx acts as own MCC   CC CC Condition   PDx CC PDx acts as own CC

720   ICD-10-CM Draft (2015)

M47.898   **Other spondylosis,** sacral and sacrococcygeal **region**

M47.899   **Other spondylosis,** site unspecified

M47.9   Spondylosis, unspecified

√4ᵗʰ **M48   Other spondylopathies**

√5ᵗʰ **M48.0   Spinal stenosis**
Caudal stenosis

M48.00   **Spinal stenosis,** site unspecified

M48.01   **Spinal stenosis,** occipito-atlanto-axial **region**

M48.02   **Spinal stenosis,** cervical **region**

M48.03   **Spinal stenosis,** cervicothoracic **region**

M48.04   **Spinal stenosis,** thoracic **region**

M48.05   **Spinal stenosis,** thoracolumbar **region**

M48.06   **Spinal stenosis,** lumbar **region**

M48.07   **Spinal stenosis,** lumbosacral **region**

M48.08   **Spinal stenosis,** sacral and sacrococcygeal **region**

√5ᵗʰ **M48.1   Ankylosing hyperostosis [Forestier]**
Diffuse idiopathic skeletal hyperostosis [DISH]

M48.10   **Ankylosing hyperostosis [Forestier],** site unspecified

M48.11   **Ankylosing hyperostosis [Forestier],** occipito-atlanto-axial **region**

M48.12   **Ankylosing hyperostosis [Forestier],** cervical **region**

M48.13   **Ankylosing hyperostosis [Forestier],** cervicothoracic **region**

M48.14   **Ankylosing hyperostosis [Forestier],** thoracic **region**

M48.15   **Ankylosing hyperostosis [Forestier],** thoracolumbar **region**

M48.16   **Ankylosing hyperostosis [Forestier],** lumbar **region**

M48.17   **Ankylosing hyperostosis [Forestier],** lumbosacral **region**

M48.18   **Ankylosing hyperostosis [Forestier],** sacral and sacrococcygeal **region**

M48.19   **Ankylosing hyperostosis [Forestier],** multiple sites **in spine**

√5ᵗʰ **M48.2   Kissing spine**

M48.20   **Kissing spine,** site unspecified

M48.21   **Kissing spine,** occipito-atlanto-axial **region**

M48.22   **Kissing spine,** cervical **region**

M48.23   **Kissing spine,** cervicothoracic **region**

M48.24   **Kissing spine,** thoracic **region**

M48.25   **Kissing spine,** thoracolumbar **region**

M48.26   **Kissing spine,** lumbar **region**

M48.27   **Kissing spine,** lumbosacral **region**

√5ᵗʰ **M48.3   Traumatic spondylopathy**

> **CC Excl:** For CC codes in subcategory M48.3, unless otherwise noted: M48.30–M48.38

M48.30   **Traumatic spondylopathy,** site unspecified   CC

M48.31   **Traumatic spondylopathy,** occipito-atlanto-axial **region**   CC

M48.32   **Traumatic spondylopathy,** cervical **region**   CC

M48.33   **Traumatic spondylopathy,** cervicothoracic **region**   CC

M48.34   **Traumatic spondylopathy,** thoracic **region**   CC

M48.35   **Traumatic spondylopathy,** thoracolumbar **region**   CC

M48.36   **Traumatic spondylopathy,** lumbar **region**   CC

M48.37   **Traumatic spondylopathy,** lumbosacral **region**   CC

M48.38   **Traumatic spondylopathy,** sacral and sacrococcygeal **region**   CC

√5ᵗʰ **M48.4   Fatigue fracture of vertebra**
Stress fracture of vertebra
> EXCLUDES 1   *pathological fracture NOS (M84.4-)*
> *pathological fracture of vertebra due to neoplasm (M84.58)*
> *pathological fracture of vertebra due to other diagnosis (M84.68)*
> *pathological fracture of vertebra due to osteoporosis (M80.-)*
> *traumatic fracture of vertebrae (S12.0-S12.3-, S22.0-, S32.0-)*

> The appropriate 7th character is to be added to each code from subcategory M48.4.
> A   initial encounter for fracture
> D   subsequent encounter for fracture with routine healing
> G   subsequent encounter for fracture with delayed healing
> S   sequela of fracture

√x7ᵗʰ   M48.40   **Fatigue fracture of vertebra,** site unspecified

√x7ᵗʰ   M48.41   **Fatigue fracture of vertebra,** occipito-atlanto-axial **region**

√x7ᵗʰ   M48.42   **Fatigue fracture of vertebra,** cervical **region**

√x7ᵗʰ   M48.43   **Fatigue fracture of vertebra,** cervicothoracic **region**

√x7ᵗʰ   M48.44   **Fatigue fracture of vertebra,** thoracic **region**

√x7ᵗʰ   M48.45   **Fatigue fracture of vertebra,** thoracolumbar **region**

√x7ᵗʰ   M48.46   **Fatigue fracture of vertebra,** lumbar **region**

√x7ᵗʰ   M48.47   **Fatigue fracture of vertebra,** lumbosacral **region**

√x7ᵗʰ   M48.48   **Fatigue fracture of vertebra,** sacral and sacrococcygeal **region**

√5ᵗʰ **M48.5   Collapsed vertebra, not elsewhere classified**
Collapsed vertebra NOS
Wedging of vertebra NOS
> EXCLUDES 1   *current injury—see Injury of spine, by body region*
> *fatigue fracture of vertebra (M48.4)*
> *pathological fracture of vertebra due to neoplasm (M84.58)*
> *pathological fracture of vertebra due to other diagnosis (M84.68)*
> *pathological fracture of vertebra due to osteoporosis (M80.-)*
> *pathological fracture NOS (M84.4-)*
> *stress fracture of vertebra (M48.4-)*
> *traumatic fracture of vertebra (S12-, S22-, S32-)*

> The appropriate 7th character is to be added to each code from subcategory M48.5.
> A   initial encounter for fracture
> D   subsequent encounter for fracture with routine healing
> G   subsequent encounter for fracture with delayed healing
> S   sequela of fracture

> **CC Excl:** For CC codes in subcategory M48.5 with 7th character A, unless otherwise noted: M48.40X–M48.58X with 7th A, M80.00X–M84.68X with 7th A

√x7ᵗʰ   M48.50   **Collapsed vertebra, not elsewhere classified,** site unspecified   CC

√x7ᵗʰ   M48.51   **Collapsed vertebra, not elsewhere classified,** occipito-atlanto-axial **region**   CC

√x7ᵗʰ   M48.52   **Collapsed vertebra, not elsewhere classified,** cervical **region**   CC

√x7ᵗʰ   M48.53   **Collapsed vertebra, not elsewhere classified,** cervicothoracic **region**   CC

√x7ᵗʰ   M48.54   **Collapsed vertebra, not elsewhere classified,** thoracic **region**   CC

√x7ᵗʰ   M48.55   **Collapsed vertebra, not elsewhere classified,** thoracolumbar **region**   CC

√x7ᵗʰ   M48.56   **Collapsed vertebra, not elsewhere classified,** lumbar **region**   CC

√x7ᵗʰ   M48.57   **Collapsed vertebra, not elsewhere classified,** lumbosacral **region**   CC

√x7ᵗʰ   M48.58   **Collapsed vertebra, not elsewhere classified,** sacral and sacrococcygeal **region**   CC

☑ Additional Character Required   √x7ᵗʰ Xtension Alert   Unacceptable PDx   Manifestation   Hospital Acquired Condition   EXCLUDES 1 Not Coded Here   EXCLUDES 2 Not Included Here

ICD-10-CM Draft (2015)   721

Diseases of the Musculoskeletal System and Connective Tissue

M48.8–M50.83

☑5ᵗʰ **M48.8 Other specified spondylopathies**
Ossification of posterior longitudinal ligament

    ☑6ᵗʰ **M48.8X Other specified spondylopathies**

      M48.8X1 Other specified spondylopathies, occipito-atlanto-axial region

      M48.8X2 Other specified spondylopathies, cervical region

      M48.8X3 Other specified spondylopathies, cervicothoracic region

      M48.8X4 Other specified spondylopathies, thoracic region

      M48.8X5 Other specified spondylopathies, thoracolumbar region

      M48.8X6 Other specified spondylopathies, lumbar region

      M48.8X7 Other specified spondylopathies, lumbosacral region

      M48.8X8 Other specified spondylopathies, sacral and sacrococcygeal region

      M48.8X9 Other specified spondylopathies, site unspecified

    M48.9 Spondylopathy, unspecified

☑4ᵗʰ **M49 Spondylopathies in diseases classified elsewhere**

   INCLUDES curvature of spine in diseases classified elsewhere
deformity of spine in diseases classified elsewhere
kyphosis in diseases classified elsewhere
scoliosis in diseases classified elsewhere
spondylopathy in diseases classified elsewhere

   Code first underlying disease, such as:
brucellosis (A23.-)
Charcôt-Marie-Tooth disease (G60.0)
enterobacterial infections (A01-A04)
osteitis fibrosa cystica (E21.0)

   EXCLUDES 1 curvature of spine in tuberculosis [Pott's] (A18.01)
enteropathic arthropathies (M07.-)
gonococcal spondylitis (A54.41)
neuropathic [tabes dorsalis] spondylitis (A52.11)
neuropathic spondylopathy in syringomyelia (G95.0)
neuropathic spondylopathy in tabes dorsalis (A52.11)
nonsyphilitic neuropathic spondylopathy NEC (G98.0)
spondylitis in syphilis (acquired) (A52.77)
tuberculous spondylitis (A18.01)
typhoid fever spondylitis (A01.05)

☑5ᵗʰ **M49.8 Spondylopathy in diseases classified elsewhere**

    M49.80 Spondylopathy in diseases classified elsewhere, site unspecified

    M49.81 Spondylopathy in diseases classified elsewhere, occipito-atlanto-axial region

    M49.82 Spondylopathy in diseases classified elsewhere, cervical region

    M49.83 Spondylopathy in diseases classified elsewhere, cervicothoracic region

    M49.84 Spondylopathy in diseases classified elsewhere, thoracic region

    M49.85 Spondylopathy in diseases classified elsewhere, thoracolumbar region

    M49.86 Spondylopathy in diseases classified elsewhere, lumbar region

    M49.87 Spondylopathy in diseases classified elsewhere, lumbosacral region

    M49.88 Spondylopathy in diseases classified elsewhere, sacral and sacrococcygeal region

    M49.89 Spondylopathy in diseases classified elsewhere, multiple sites in spine

Other dorsopathies (M50-M54)

   EXCLUDES 1 current injury—see injury of spine by body region
discitis NOS (M46.4-)

☑4ᵗʰ **M50 Cervical disc disorders**

   NOTE Code to the most superior level of disorder.
   INCLUDES cervicothoracic disc disorders with cervicalgia
cervicothoracic disc disorders

☑5ᵗʰ **M50.0 Cervical disc disorder with myelopathy**

    M50.00 Cervical disc disorder with myelopathy, unspecified cervical region `CC`
CC Excl: M50.00-M50.03, M50.20-M50.23

    M50.01 Cervical disc disorder with myelopathy, high cervical region `CC`
C2-C3 disc disorder with myelopathy
C3-C4 disc disorder with myelopathy
CC Excl: See code: M50.00

    M50.02 Cervical disc disorder with myelopathy, mid-cervical region `CC`
C4-C5 disc disorder with myelopathy
C5-C6 disc disorder with myelopathy
C6-C7 disc disorder with myelopathy
CC Excl: See code: M50.00

    M50.03 Cervical disc disorder with myelopathy, cervicothoracic region `CC`
C7-T1 disc disorder with myelopathy
CC Excl: See code: M50.00

☑5ᵗʰ **M50.1 Cervical disc disorder with radiculopathy**

   EXCLUDES 2 brachial radiculitis NOS (M54.13)

    M50.10 Cervical disc disorder with radiculopathy, unspecified cervical region

    M50.11 Cervical disc disorder with radiculopathy, high cervical region
C2-C3 disc disorder with radiculopathy
C3 radiculopathy due to disc disorder
C3-C4 disc disorder with radiculopathy
C4 radiculopathy due to disc disorder

    M50.12 Cervical disc disorder with radiculopathy, mid-cervical region
C4-C5 disc disorder with radiculopathy
C5 radiculopathy due to disc disorder
C5-C6 disc disorder with radiculopathy
C6 radiculopathy due to disc disorder
C6-C7 disc disorder with radiculopathy
C7 radiculopathy due to disc disorder

    M50.13 Cervical disc disorder with radiculopathy, cervicothoracic region
C7-T1 disc disorder with radiculopathy
C8 radiculopathy due to disc disorder

☑5ᵗʰ **M50.2 Other cervical disc displacement**

    M50.20 Other cervical disc displacement, unspecified cervical region

    M50.21 Other cervical disc displacement, high cervical region
Other C2-C3 cervical disc displacement
Other C3-C4 cervical disc displacement

    M50.22 Other cervical disc displacement, mid-cervical region
Other C4-C5 cervical disc displacement
Other C5-C6 cervical disc displacement
Other C6-C7 cervical disc displacement

    M50.23 Other cervical disc displacement, cervicothoracic region
Other C7-T1 cervical disc displacement

☑5ᵗʰ **M50.3 Other cervical disc degeneration**

    M50.30 Other cervical disc degeneration, unspecified cervical region

    M50.31 Other cervical disc degeneration, high cervical region
Other C2-C3 cervical disc degeneration
Other C3-C4 cervical disc degeneration

    M50.32 Other cervical disc degeneration, mid-cervical region
Other C4-C5 cervical disc degeneration
Other C5-C6 cervical disc degeneration
Other C6-C7 cervical disc degeneration

    M50.33 Other cervical disc degeneration, cervicothoracic region
Other C7-T1 cervical disc degeneration

☑5ᵗʰ **M50.8 Other cervical disc disorders**

    M50.80 Other cervical disc disorders, unspecified cervical region

    M50.81 Other cervical disc disorders, high cervical region
Other C2-C3 cervical disc disorders
Other C3-C4 cervical disc disorders

    M50.82 Other cervical disc disorders, mid-cervical region
Other C4-C5 cervical disc disorders
Other C5-C6 cervical disc disorders
Other C6-C7 cervical disc disorders

    M50.83 Other cervical disc disorders, cervicothoracic region
Other C7-T1 cervical disc disorders

N Newborn: 0   **P** Pediatric: 0-17   **M** Maternity: 12-55   **A** Adult: 15-124   **MCC** Major CC Condition   **PDx MCC** PDx acts as own MCC   **CC** CC Condition   **PDx CC** PDx acts as own CC

722   ICD-10-CM Draft (2015)

✓5ᵗʰ **M50.9 Cervical disc disorder,** unspecified

M50.90 Cervical disc disorder, unspecified, unspecified cervical region

M50.91 Cervical disc disorder, unspecified, high cervical region
C2-C3 cervical disc disorder, unspecified
C3-C4 cervical disc disorder, unspecified

M50.92 Cervical disc disorder, unspecified, mid-cervical region
C4-C5 cervical disc disorder, unspecified
C5-C6 cervical disc disorder, unspecified
C6-C7 cervical disc disorder, unspecified

M50.93 Cervical disc disorder, unspecified, cervicothoracic region
C7-T1 cervical disc disorder, unspecified

✓4ᵗʰ **M51 Thoracic, thoracolumbar, and lumbosacral intervertebral disc disorders**
EXCLUDES 2 *cervical and cervicothoracic disc disorders (M50.-)*
sacral and sacrococcygeal disorders (M53.3)

✓5ᵗʰ **M51.0 Thoracic, thoracolumbar and lumbosacral intervertebral disc disorders** with myelopathy

M51.04 Intervertebral disc disorders with myelopathy, thoracic region   CC
CC Excl: M51.04-M51.05, M51.24-M51.25

M51.05 Intervertebral disc disorders with myelopathy, thoracolumbar region   CC
CC Excl: See code: M51.04

M51.06 Intervertebral disc disorders with myelopathy, lumbar region   CC
CC Excl: M51.06-M51.07, M51.24-M51.25

✓5ᵗʰ **M51.1 Thoracic, thoracolumbar and lumbosacral intervertebral disc disorders** with radiculopathy
Sciatica due to intervertebral disc disorder
EXCLUDES 1 *lumbar radiculitis NOS (M54.16)*
sciatica NOS (M54.3)

M51.14 Intervertebral disc disorders with radiculopathy, thoracic region

M51.15 Intervertebral disc disorders with radiculopathy, thoracolumbar region

M51.16 Intervertebral disc disorders with radiculopathy, lumbar region

M51.17 Intervertebral disc disorders with radiculopathy, lumbosacral region

✓5ᵗʰ **M51.2 Other thoracic, thoracolumbar and lumbosacral intervertebral disc** displacement
Lumbago due to displacement of intervertebral disc

M51.24 Other intervertebral disc displacement, thoracic region

M51.25 Other intervertebral disc displacement, thoracolumbar region

M51.26 Other intervertebral disc displacement, lumbar region

M51.27 Other intervertebral disc displacement, lumbosacral region

✓5ᵗʰ **M51.3 Other thoracic, thoracolumbar and lumbosacral intervertebral disc** degeneration
AHA: 2013, 3Q, 22

M51.34 Other intervertebral disc degeneration, thoracic region

M51.35 Other intervertebral disc degeneration, thoracolumbar region

M51.36 Other intervertebral disc degeneration, lumbar region

M51.37 Other intervertebral disc degeneration, lumbosacral region

✓5ᵗʰ **M51.4 Schmorl's nodes**

M51.44 Schmorl's nodes, thoracic region
M51.45 Schmorl's nodes, thoracolumbar region
M51.46 Schmorl's nodes, lumbar region
M51.47 Schmorl's nodes, lumbosacral region

✓5ᵗʰ **M51.8 Other thoracic, thoracolumbar and lumbosacral intervertebral** disc disorders

M51.84 Other intervertebral disc disorders, thoracic region
M51.85 Other intervertebral disc disorders, thoracolumbar region
M51.86 Other intervertebral disc disorders, lumbar region

M51.87 Other intervertebral disc disorders, lumbosacral region

M51.9 Unspecified thoracic, thoracolumbar and lumbosacral intervertebral disc disorder

✓4ᵗʰ **M53 Other and unspecified dorsopathies, not elsewhere classified**

M53.0 Cervicocranial syndrome
Posterior cervical sympathetic syndrome

M53.1 Cervicobrachial syndrome
EXCLUDES 2 *cervical disc disorder (M50.-)*
thoracic outlet syndrome (G54.0)

✓5ᵗʰ **M53.2 Spinal instabilities**

✓6ᵗʰ **M53.2X Spinal** instabilities

M53.2X1 Spinal instabilities, occipito-atlanto-axial region
M53.2X2 Spinal instabilities, cervical region
M53.2X3 Spinal instabilities, cervicothoracic region
M53.2X4 Spinal instabilities, thoracic region
M53.2X5 Spinal instabilities, thoracolumbar region
M53.2X6 Spinal instabilities, lumbar region
M53.2X7 Spinal instabilities, lumbosacral region
M53.2X8 Spinal instabilities, sacral and sacrococcygeal region
M53.2X9 Spinal instabilities, site unspecified

M53.3 Sacrococcygeal disorders, not elsewhere classified
Coccygodynia

✓5ᵗʰ **M53.8 Other specified dorsopathies**

M53.80 Other specified dorsopathies, site unspecified
M53.81 Other specified dorsopathies, occipito-atlanto-axial region
M53.82 Other specified dorsopathies, cervical region
M53.83 Other specified dorsopathies, cervicothoracic region
M53.84 Other specified dorsopathies, thoracic region
M53.85 Other specified dorsopathies, thoracolumbar region
M53.86 Other specified dorsopathies, lumbar region
M53.87 Other specified dorsopathies, lumbosacral region
M53.88 Other specified dorsopathies, sacral and sacrococcygeal region

M53.9 Dorsopathy, unspecified

✓4ᵗʰ **M54 Dorsalgia**
EXCLUDES 1 *psychogenic dorsalgia (F45.41)*

✓5ᵗʰ **M54.0 Panniculitis affecting regions of neck and back**
EXCLUDES 1 *lupus panniculitis (L93.2)*
panniculitis NOS (M79.3)
relapsing [Weber-Christian] panniculitis (M35.6)

M54.00 Panniculitis affecting regions of neck and back, site unspecified

M54.01 Panniculitis affecting regions of neck and back, occipito-atlanto-axial region

M54.02 Panniculitis affecting regions of neck and back, cervical region

M54.03 Panniculitis affecting regions of neck and back, cervicothoracic region

M54.04 Panniculitis affecting regions of neck and back, thoracic region

M54.05 Panniculitis affecting regions of neck and back, thoracolumbar region

M54.06 Panniculitis affecting regions of neck and back, lumbar region

M54.07 Panniculitis affecting regions of neck and back, lumbosacral region

M54.08 Panniculitis affecting regions of neck and back, sacral and sacrococcygeal region

M54.09 Panniculitis affecting regions, neck and back, multiple sites in spine

✓ Additional Character Required   ✓x7ᵗʰ Xtension Alert   Unacceptable PDx   Manifestation   Hospital Acquired Condition   EXCLUDES 1 Not Coded Here   EXCLUDES 2 Not Included Here

ICD-10-CM Draft (2015)   723

✓5ᵗʰ **M54.1 Radiculopathy**
Brachial neuritis or radiculitis NOS
Lumbar neuritis or radiculitis NOS
Lumbosacral neuritis or radiculitis NOS
Thoracic neuritis or radiculitis NOS
Radiculitis NOS
EXCLUDES 1   *neuralgia and neuritis NOS (M79.2)*
radiculopathy with cervical disc disorder (M50.1)
radiculopathy with lumbar and other intervertebral disc disorder (M51.1-)
radiculopathy with spondylosis (M47.2-)

     M54.10 Radiculopathy, site unspecified
     M54.11 Radiculopathy, occipito-atlanto-axial region
     M54.12 Radiculopathy, cervical region
     M54.13 Radiculopathy, cervicothoracic region
     M54.14 Radiculopathy, thoracic region
     M54.15 Radiculopathy, thoracolumbar region
     M54.16 Radiculopathy, lumbar region
     M54.17 Radiculopathy, lumbosacral region
     M54.18 Radiculopathy, sacral and sacrococcygeal region

M54.2 Cervicalgia
EXCLUDES 1   *cervicalgia due to intervertebral cervical disc disorder (M50.-)*

✓5ᵗʰ **M54.3 Sciatica**
EXCLUDES 1   *lesion of sciatic nerve (G57.0)*
sciatica due to intervertebral disc disorder (M51.1-)
sciatica with lumbago (M54.4-)

     M54.30 Sciatica, unspecified side
     M54.31 Sciatica, right side
     M54.32 Sciatica, left side

✓5ᵗʰ **M54.4 Lumbago with sciatica**
EXCLUDES 1   *lumbago with sciatica due to intervertebral disc disorder (M51.1-)*

     M54.40 Lumbago with sciatica, unspecified side
     M54.41 Lumbago with sciatica, right side
     M54.42 Lumbago with sciatica, left side

M54.5 Low back pain
Loin pain
Lumbago NOS
EXCLUDES 1   *low back strain (S39.012)*
lumbago due to intervertebral disc displacement (M51.2-)
lumbago with sciatica (M54.4-)

M54.6 Pain in thoracic spine
EXCLUDES 1   *pain in thoracic spine due to intervertebral disc disorder (M51.-)*

✓5ᵗʰ **M54.8 Other dorsalgia**
EXCLUDES 1   *dorsalgia in thoracic region (M54.6)*
low back pain (M54.5)

     M54.81 Occipital neuralgia
     M54.89 Other dorsalgia

M54.9 Dorsalgia, unspecified
Backache NOS
Back pain NOS

SOFT TISSUE DISORDERS (M60-M79)

Disorders of muscles (M60-M63)

EXCLUDES 1   *dermatopolymyositis (M33.-)*
muscular dystrophies and myopathies (G71-G72)
myopathy in amyloidosis (E85.-)
myopathy in polyarteritis nodosa (M30.0)
myopathy in rheumatoid arthritis (M05.32)
myopathy in scleroderma (M34.-)
myopathy in Sjögren's syndrome (M35.03)
myopathy in systemic lupus erythematosus (M32.-)

✓4ᵗʰ **M60 Myositis**
EXCLUDES 2   *inclusion body myositis [IBM] (G72.41)*

✓5ᵗʰ **M60.0 Infective myositis**
Tropical pyomyositis
Use additional code (B95-B97) to identify infectious agent

> **CC Excl: For CC codes in subcategory M60.0, unless otherwise noted:** K68.12, M60.000-M60.19, M61.00-M61.19, M61.30-M61.59, M62.3, M62.50-M62.59, M62.89, M72.6

✓6ᵗʰ **M60.00 Infective myositis, unspecified site**
     M60.000 Infective myositis, unspecified right arm   CC
       Infective myositis, right upper limb NOS
     M60.001 Infective myositis, unspecified left arm   CC
       Infective myositis, left upper limb NOS
     M60.002 Infective myositis, unspecified arm   CC
       Infective myositis, upper limb NOS
     M60.003 Infective myositis, unspecified right leg   CC
       Infective myositis, right lower limb NOS
     M60.004 Infective myositis, unspecified left leg   CC
       Infective myositis, left lower limb NOS
     M60.005 Infective myositis, unspecified leg   CC
       Infective myositis, lower limb NOS
     M60.009 Infective myositis, unspecified site   CC

✓6ᵗʰ **M60.01 Infective myositis, shoulder**
     M60.011 Infective myositis, right shoulder   CC
     M60.012 Infective myositis, left shoulder   CC
     M60.019 Infective myositis, unspecified shoulder   CC

✓6ᵗʰ **M60.02 Infective myositis, upper arm**
     M60.021 Infective myositis, right upper arm   CC
     M60.022 Infective myositis, left upper arm   CC
     M60.029 Infective myositis, unspecified upper arm   CC

✓6ᵗʰ **M60.03 Infective myositis, forearm**
     M60.031 Infective myositis, right forearm   CC
     M60.032 Infective myositis, left forearm   CC
     M60.039 Infective myositis, unspecified forearm   CC

✓6ᵗʰ **M60.04 Infective myositis, hand and fingers**
     M60.041 Infective myositis, right hand   CC
     M60.042 Infective myositis, left hand   CC
     M60.043 Infective myositis, unspecified hand   CC
     M60.044 Infective myositis, right finger(s)   CC
     M60.045 Infective myositis, left finger(s)   CC
     M60.046 Infective myositis, unspecified finger(s)   CC

✓6ᵗʰ **M60.05 Infective myositis, thigh**
     M60.051 Infective myositis, right thigh   CC
     M60.052 Infective myositis, left thigh   CC
     M60.059 Infective myositis, unspecified thigh   CC

✓6ᵗʰ **M60.06 Infective myositis, lower leg**
     M60.061 Infective myositis, right lower leg   CC
     M60.062 Infective myositis, left lower leg   CC
     M60.069 Infective myositis, unspecified lower leg   CC

✓6ᵗʰ **M60.07 Infective myositis, ankle, foot and toes**
     M60.070 Infective myositis, right ankle   CC
     M60.071 Infective myositis, left ankle   CC
     M60.072 Infective myositis, unspecified ankle   CC
     M60.073 Infective myositis, right foot   CC
     M60.074 Infective myositis, left foot   CC
     M60.075 Infective myositis, unspecified foot   CC
     M60.076 Infective myositis, right toe(s)   CC
     M60.077 Infective myositis, left toe(s)   CC
     M60.078 Infective myositis, unspecified toe(s)   CC

     M60.08 Infective myositis, other site   CC
     M60.09 Infective myositis, multiple sites   CC

M60.1 Interstitial myositis
     M60.10 Interstitial myositis of unspecified site

✓6ᵗʰ **M60.11 Interstitial myositis, shoulder**
     M60.111 Interstitial myositis, right shoulder
     M60.112 Interstitial myositis, left shoulder
     M60.119 Interstitial myositis, unspecified shoulder

✓6ᵗʰ **M60.12 Interstitial myositis, upper arm**
     M60.121 Interstitial myositis, right upper arm
     M60.122 Interstitial myositis, left upper arm
     M60.129 Interstitial myositis, unspecified upper arm

✓6ᵗʰ **M60.13 Interstitial myositis, forearm**
     M60.131 Interstitial myositis, right forearm

N Newborn: 0   P Pediatric: 0-17   M Maternity: 12-55   A Adult: 15-124   MCC Major CC Condition   PDx MCC PDx acts as own MCC   CC CC Condition   PDx CC PDx acts as own CC

724   ICD-10-CM Draft (2015)

Diseases of the Musculoskeletal System and Connective Tissue

M60.132–M61.042

M60.132 Interstitial myositis, left forearm
M60.139 Interstitial myositis, unspecified forearm
✓6th M60.14 Interstitial myositis, hand
M60.141 Interstitial myositis, right hand
M60.142 Interstitial myositis, left hand
M60.149 Interstitial myositis, unspecified hand
✓6th M60.15 Interstitial myositis, thigh
M60.151 Interstitial myositis, right thigh
M60.152 Interstitial myositis, left thigh
M60.159 Interstitial myositis, unspecified thigh
✓6th M60.16 Interstitial myositis, lower leg
M60.161 Interstitial myositis, right lower leg
M60.162 Interstitial myositis, left lower leg
M60.169 Interstitial myositis, unspecified lower leg
✓6th M60.17 Interstitial myositis, ankle and foot
M60.171 Interstitial myositis, right ankle and foot
M60.172 Interstitial myositis, left ankle and foot
M60.179 Interstitial myositis, unspecified ankle and foot
M60.18 Interstitial myositis, other site
M60.19 Interstitial myositis, multiple sites
✓5th M60.2 Foreign body granuloma of soft tissue, not elsewhere classified
Use additional code to identify the type of retained foreign body (Z18.-)
EXCLUDES 1 foreign body granuloma of skin and subcutaneous tissue (L92.3)
M60.20 Foreign body granuloma of soft tissue, not elsewhere classified, unspecified site
✓6th M60.21 Foreign body granuloma of soft tissue, not elsewhere classified, shoulder
M60.211 Foreign body granuloma of soft tissue, not elsewhere classified, right shoulder
M60.212 Foreign body granuloma of soft tissue, not elsewhere classified, left shoulder
M60.219 Foreign body granuloma of soft tissue, not elsewhere classified, unspecified shoulder
✓6th M60.22 Foreign body granuloma of soft tissue, not elsewhere classified, upper arm
M60.221 Foreign body granuloma of soft tissue, not elsewhere classified, right upper arm
M60.222 Foreign body granuloma of soft tissue, not elsewhere classified, left upper arm
M60.229 Foreign body granuloma of soft tissue, not elsewhere classified, unspecified upper arm
✓6th M60.23 Foreign body granuloma of soft tissue, not elsewhere classified, forearm
M60.231 Foreign body granuloma of soft tissue, not elsewhere classified, right forearm
M60.232 Foreign body granuloma of soft tissue, not elsewhere classified, left forearm
M60.239 Foreign body granuloma of soft tissue, not elsewhere classified, unspecified forearm
✓6th M60.24 Foreign body granuloma of soft tissue, not elsewhere classified, hand
M60.241 Foreign body granuloma of soft tissue, not elsewhere classified, right hand
M60.242 Foreign body granuloma of soft tissue, not elsewhere classified, left hand
M60.249 Foreign body granuloma of soft tissue, not elsewhere classified, unspecified hand
✓6th M60.25 Foreign body granuloma of soft tissue, not elsewhere classified, thigh
M60.251 Foreign body granuloma of soft tissue, not elsewhere classified, right thigh
M60.252 Foreign body granuloma of soft tissue, not elsewhere classified, left thigh
M60.259 Foreign body granuloma of soft tissue, not elsewhere classified, unspecified thigh
✓6th M60.26 Foreign body granuloma of soft tissue, not elsewhere classified, lower leg
M60.261 Foreign body granuloma of soft tissue, not elsewhere classified, right lower leg
M60.262 Foreign body granuloma of soft tissue, not elsewhere classified, left lower leg

M60.269 Foreign body granuloma of soft tissue, not elsewhere classified, unspecified lower leg
✓6th M60.27 Foreign body granuloma of soft tissue, not elsewhere classified, ankle and foot
M60.271 Foreign body granuloma of soft tissue, not elsewhere classified, right ankle and foot
M60.272 Foreign body granuloma of soft tissue, not elsewhere classified, left ankle and foot
M60.279 Foreign body granuloma of soft tissue, not elsewhere classified, unspecified ankle and foot
M60.28 Foreign body granuloma of soft tissue, not elsewhere classified, other site
✓5th M60.8 Other myositis
M60.80 Other myositis, unspecified site
✓6th M60.81 Other myositis shoulder
M60.811 Other myositis, right shoulder
M60.812 Other myositis, left shoulder
M60.819 Other myositis, unspecified shoulder
✓6th M60.82 Other myositis, upper arm
M60.821 Other myositis, right upper arm
M60.822 Other myositis, left upper arm
M60.829 Other myositis, unspecified upper arm
✓6th M60.83 Other myositis, forearm
M60.831 Other myositis, right forearm
M60.832 Other myositis, left forearm
M60.839 Other myositis, unspecified forearm
✓6th M60.84 Other myositis, hand
M60.841 Other myositis, right hand
M60.842 Other myositis, left hand
M60.849 Other myositis, unspecified hand
✓6th M60.85 Other myositis, thigh
M60.851 Other myositis, right thigh
M60.852 Other myositis, left thigh
M60.859 Other myositis, unspecified thigh
✓6th M60.86 Other myositis, lower leg
M60.861 Other myositis, right lower leg
M60.862 Other myositis, left lower leg
M60.869 Other myositis, unspecified lower leg
✓6th M60.87 Other myositis, ankle and foot
M60.871 Other myositis, right ankle and foot
M60.872 Other myositis, left ankle and foot
M60.879 Other myositis, unspecified ankle and foot
M60.88 Other myositis, other site
M60.89 Other myositis, multiple sites
M60.9 Myositis, unspecified
✓4th M61 Calcification and ossification of muscle
✓5th M61.0 Myositis ossificans traumatica
M61.00 Myositis ossificans traumatica, unspecified site
✓6th M61.01 Myositis ossificans traumatica, shoulder
M61.011 Myositis ossificans traumatica, right shoulder
M61.012 Myositis ossificans traumatica, left shoulder
M61.019 Myositis ossificans traumatica, unspecified shoulder
✓6th M61.02 Myositis ossificans traumatica, upper arm
M61.021 Myositis ossificans traumatica, right upper arm
M61.022 Myositis ossificans traumatica, left upper arm
M61.029 Myositis ossificans traumatica, unspecified upper arm
✓6th M61.03 Myositis ossificans traumatica, forearm
M61.031 Myositis ossificans traumatica, right forearm
M61.032 Myositis ossificans traumatica, left forearm
M61.039 Myositis ossificans traumatica, unspecified forearm
✓6th M61.04 Myositis ossificans traumatica, hand
M61.041 Myositis ossificans traumatica, right hand
M61.042 Myositis ossificans traumatica, left hand

M61.049　Myositis ossificans traumatica, unspecified **hand**

✓6ᵗʰ **M61.05** Myositis ossificans traumatica, thigh

M61.051　Myositis ossificans traumatica, **right thigh**

M61.052　Myositis ossificans traumatica, **left thigh**

M61.059　Myositis ossificans traumatica, unspecified **thigh**

✓6ᵗʰ **M61.06** Myositis ossificans traumatica, lower leg

M61.061　Myositis ossificans traumatica, **right lower leg**

M61.062　Myositis ossificans traumatica, **left lower leg**

M61.069　Myositis ossificans traumatica, unspecified **lower leg**

✓6ᵗʰ **M61.07** Myositis ossificans traumatica, ankle and foot

M61.071　Myositis ossificans traumatica, **right ankle and foot**

M61.072　Myositis ossificans traumatica, **left ankle and foot**

M61.079　Myositis ossificans traumatica, unspecified **ankle and foot**

M61.08　Myositis ossificans traumatica, other site

M61.09　Myositis ossificans traumatica, multiple sites

✓5ᵗʰ **M61.1** Myositis ossificans progressiva
Fibrodysplasia ossificans progressiva

M61.10　Myositis ossificans progressiva, unspecified site

✓6ᵗʰ **M61.11** Myositis ossificans progressiva, shoulder

M61.111　Myositis ossificans progressiva, **right shoulder**

M61.112　Myositis ossificans progressiva, **left shoulder**

M61.119　Myositis ossificans progressiva, unspecified **shoulder**

✓6ᵗʰ **M61.12** Myositis ossificans progressiva, upper arm

M61.121　Myositis ossificans progressiva, **right upper arm**

M61.122　Myositis ossificans progressiva, **left upper arm**

M61.129　Myositis ossificans progressiva, unspecified **arm**

✓6ᵗʰ **M61.13** Myositis ossificans progressiva, forearm

M61.131　Myositis ossificans progressiva, **right forearm**

M61.132　Myositis ossificans progressiva, **left forearm**

M61.139　Myositis ossificans progressiva, unspecified **forearm**

✓6ᵗʰ **M61.14** Myositis ossificans progressiva, hand and finger(s)

M61.141　Myositis ossificans progressiva, **right hand**

M61.142　Myositis ossificans progressiva, **left hand**

M61.143　Myositis ossificans progressiva, unspecified **hand**

M61.144　Myositis ossificans progressiva, **right finger(s)**

M61.145　Myositis ossificans progressiva, **left finger(s)**

M61.146　Myositis ossificans progressiva, unspecified **finger(s)**

✓6ᵗʰ **M61.15** Myositis ossificans progressiva, thigh

M61.151　Myositis ossificans progressiva, **right thigh**

M61.152　Myositis ossificans progressiva, **left thigh**

M61.159　Myositis ossificans progressiva, unspecified **thigh**

✓6ᵗʰ **M61.16** Myositis ossificans progressiva, lower leg

M61.161　Myositis ossificans progressiva, **right lower leg**

M61.162　Myositis ossificans progressiva, **left lower leg**

M61.169　Myositis ossificans progressiva, unspecified **lower leg**

✓6ᵗʰ **M61.17** Myositis ossificans progressiva, ankle, foot and toe(s)

M61.171　Myositis ossificans progressiva, **right ankle**

M61.172　Myositis ossificans progressiva, **left ankle**

M61.173　Myositis ossificans progressiva, unspecified **ankle**

M61.174　Myositis ossificans progressiva, **right foot**

M61.175　Myositis ossificans progressiva, **left foot**

M61.176　Myositis ossificans progressiva, unspecified **foot**

M61.177　Myositis ossificans progressiva, **right toe(s)**

M61.178　Myositis ossificans progressiva, **left toe(s)**

M61.179　Myositis ossificans progressiva, unspecified **toe(s)**

M61.18　Myositis ossificans progressiva, other site

M61.19　Myositis ossificans progressiva, multiple sites

✓5ᵗʰ **M61.2** Paralytic calcification and ossification of muscle
Myositis ossificans associated with quadriplegia or paraplegia

M61.20　Paralytic calcification and ossification of muscle, unspecified site

✓6ᵗʰ **M61.21** Paralytic calcification and ossification of muscle, shoulder

M61.211　Paralytic calcification and ossification of muscle, **right shoulder**

M61.212　Paralytic calcification and ossification of muscle, **left shoulder**

M61.219　Paralytic calcification and ossification of muscle, unspecified **shoulder**

✓6ᵗʰ **M61.22** Paralytic calcification and ossification of muscle, upper arm

M61.221　Paralytic calcification and ossification of muscle, **right upper arm**

M61.222　Paralytic calcification and ossification of muscle, **left upper arm**

M61.229　Paralytic calcification and ossification of muscle, unspecified **upper arm**

✓6ᵗʰ **M61.23** Paralytic calcification and ossification of muscle, forearm

M61.231　Paralytic calcification and ossification of muscle, **right forearm**

M61.232　Paralytic calcification and ossification of muscle, **left forearm**

M61.239　Paralytic calcification and ossification of muscle, unspecified **forearm**

✓6ᵗʰ **M61.24** Paralytic calcification and ossification of muscle, hand

M61.241　Paralytic calcification and ossification of muscle, **right hand**

M61.242　Paralytic calcification and ossification of muscle, **left hand**

M61.249　Paralytic calcification and ossification of muscle, unspecified **hand**

✓6ᵗʰ **M61.25** Paralytic calcification and ossification of muscle, thigh

M61.251　Paralytic calcification and ossification of muscle, **right thigh**

M61.252　Paralytic calcification and ossification of muscle, **left thigh**

M61.259　Paralytic calcification and ossification of muscle, unspecified **thigh**

✓6ᵗʰ **M61.26** Paralytic calcification and ossification of muscle, lower leg

M61.261　Paralytic calcification and ossification of muscle, **right lower leg**

M61.262　Paralytic calcification and ossification of muscle, **left lower leg**

M61.269　Paralytic calcification and ossification of muscle, unspecified **lower leg**

✓6ᵗʰ **M61.27** Paralytic calcification and ossification of muscle, ankle and foot

M61.271　Paralytic calcification and ossification of muscle, **right ankle and foot**

M61.272　Paralytic calcification and ossification of muscle, **left ankle and foot**

M61.279　Paralytic calcification and ossification of muscle, unspecified **ankle and foot**

M61.28　Paralytic calcification and ossification of muscle, other site

M61.29　Paralytic calcification and ossification of muscle, multiple sites

Ⓝ Newborn: 0　Ⓟ Pediatric: 0-17　Ⓜ Maternity: 12-55　Ⓐ Adult: 15-124　ᴹᶜᶜ Major CC Condition　ᴾᴰˣ ᴹᶜᶜ PDx acts as own MCC　ᶜᶜ CC Condition　ᴾᴰˣ ᶜᶜ PDx acts as own CC

726　ICD-10-CM Draft (2015)

√5th **M61.3 Calcification and ossification of muscles** associated with burns
    Myositis ossificans associated with burns

    M61.30 Calcification and ossification of muscles associated with burns, unspecified site

√6th **M61.31 Calcification and ossification of muscles associated with burns,** shoulder
    M61.311 Calcification and ossification of muscles associated with burns, right shoulder
    M61.312 Calcification and ossification of muscles associated with burns, left shoulder
    M61.319 Calcification and ossification of muscles associated with burns, unspecified shoulder

√6th **M61.32 Calcification and ossification of muscles associated with burns,** upper arm
    M61.321 Calcification and ossification of muscles associated with burns, right upper arm
    M61.322 Calcification and ossification of muscles associated with burns, left upper arm
    M61.329 Calcification and ossification of muscles associated with burns, unspecified upper arm

√6th **M61.33 Calcification and ossification of muscles associated with burns,** forearm
    M61.331 Calcification and ossification of muscles associated with burns, right forearm
    M61.332 Calcification and ossification of muscles associated with burns, left forearm
    M61.339 Calcification and ossification of muscles associated with burns, unspecified forearm

√6th **M61.34 Calcification and ossification of muscles associated with burns,** hand
    M61.341 Calcification and ossification of muscles associated with burns, right hand
    M61.342 Calcification and ossification of muscles associated with burns, left hand
    M61.349 Calcification and ossification of muscles associated with burns, unspecified hand

√6th **M61.35 Calcification and ossification of muscles associated with burns,** thigh
    M61.351 Calcification and ossification of muscles associated with burns, right thigh
    M61.352 Calcification and ossification of muscles associated with burns, left thigh
    M61.359 Calcification and ossification of muscles associated with burns, unspecified thigh

√6th **M61.36 Calcification and ossification of muscles associated with burns,** lower leg
    M61.361 Calcification and ossification of muscles associated with burns, right lower leg
    M61.362 Calcification and ossification of muscles associated with burns, left lower leg
    M61.369 Calcification and ossification of muscles associated with burns, unspecified lower leg

√6th **M61.37 Calcification and ossification of muscles associated with burns,** ankle and foot
    M61.371 Calcification and ossification of muscles associated with burns, right ankle and foot
    M61.372 Calcification and ossification of muscles associated with burns, left ankle and foot
    M61.379 Calcification and ossification of muscles associated with burns, unspecified ankle and foot

    M61.38 Calcification and ossification of muscles associated with burns, other site

    M61.39 Calcification and ossification of muscles associated with burns, multiple sites

√5th **M61.4 Other calcification** of muscle
    EXCLUDES 1 *calcific tendinitis NOS (M65.2-)*
                 calcific tendinitis of shoulder (M75.3)

    M61.40 Other calcification of muscle, unspecified site

√6th **M61.41 Other calcification of muscle,** shoulder
    M61.411 Other calcification of muscle, right shoulder

    M61.412 Other calcification of muscle, left shoulder
    M61.419 Other calcification of muscle, unspecified shoulder

√6th **M61.42 Other calcification of muscle,** upper arm
    M61.421 Other calcification of muscle, right upper arm
    M61.422 Other calcification of muscle, left upper arm
    M61.429 Other calcification of muscle, unspecified upper arm

√6th **M61.43 Other calcification of muscle,** forearm
    M61.431 Other calcification of muscle, right forearm
    M61.432 Other calcification of muscle, left forearm
    M61.439 Other calcification of muscle, unspecified forearm

√6th **M61.44 Other calcification of muscle,** hand
    M61.441 Other calcification of muscle, right hand
    M61.442 Other calcification of muscle, left hand
    M61.449 Other calcification of muscle, unspecified hand

√6th **M61.45 Other calcification of muscle,** thigh
    M61.451 Other calcification of muscle, right thigh
    M61.452 Other calcification of muscle, left thigh
    M61.459 Other calcification of muscle, unspecified thigh

√6th **M61.46 Other calcification of muscle,** lower leg
    M61.461 Other calcification of muscle, right lower leg
    M61.462 Other calcification of muscle, left lower leg
    M61.469 Other calcification of muscle, unspecified lower leg

√6th **M61.47 Other calcification of muscle,** ankle and foot
    M61.471 Other calcification of muscle, right ankle and foot
    M61.472 Other calcification of muscle, left ankle and foot
    M61.479 Other calcification of muscle, unspecified ankle and foot

    M61.48 Other calcification of muscle, other site

    M61.49 Other calcification of muscle, multiple sites

√5th **M61.5 Other ossification** of muscle

    M61.50 Other ossification of muscle, unspecified site

√6th **M61.51 Other ossification of muscle,** shoulder
    M61.511 Other ossification of muscle, right shoulder
    M61.512 Other ossification of muscle, left shoulder
    M61.519 Other ossification of muscle, unspecified shoulder

√6th **M61.52 Other ossification of muscle,** upper arm
    M61.521 Other ossification of muscle, right upper arm
    M61.522 Other ossification of muscle, left upper arm
    M61.529 Other ossification of muscle, unspecified upper arm

√6th **M61.53 Other ossification of muscle,** forearm
    M61.531 Other ossification of muscle, right forearm
    M61.532 Other ossification of muscle, left forearm
    M61.539 Other ossification of muscle, unspecified forearm

√6th **M61.54 Other ossification of muscle,** hand
    M61.541 Other ossification of muscle, right hand
    M61.542 Other ossification of muscle, left hand
    M61.549 Other ossification of muscle, unspecified hand

√6th **M61.55 Other ossification of muscle,** thigh
    M61.551 Other ossification of muscle, right thigh
    M61.552 Other ossification of muscle, left thigh
    M61.559 Other ossification of muscle, unspecified thigh

√6th **M61.56 Other ossification of muscle,** lower leg
    M61.561 Other ossification of muscle, right lower leg
    M61.562 Other ossification of muscle, left lower leg

√ Additional Character Required   √x7th Xtension Alert   Unacceptable PDx   Manifestation   Hospital Acquired Condition   EXCLUDES 1 Not Coded Here   EXCLUDES 2 Not Included Here

M61.569 Other ossification of muscle, unspecified lower leg

☑6ᵗʰ **M61.57** Other ossification of muscle, ankle and foot

    M61.571 Other ossification of muscle, right ankle and foot

    M61.572 Other ossification of muscle, left ankle and foot

    M61.579 Other ossification of muscle, unspecified ankle and foot

M61.58 Other ossification of muscle, other site

M61.59 Other ossification of muscle, multiple sites

M61.9 Calcification and ossification of muscle, unspecified

☑4ᵗʰ **M62 Other disorders of muscle**

    EXCLUDES 1   *alcoholic myopathy (G72.1)*
           cramp and spasm (R25.2)
           drug-induced myopathy (G72.0)
           myalgia (M79.1)
           stiff-man syndrome (G25.82)

    EXCLUDES 2   *nontraumatic hematoma of muscle (M79.81)*

☑5ᵗʰ **M62.0** Separation of muscle (nontraumatic)
    Diastasis of muscle

    EXCLUDES 1   *diastasis recti complicating pregnancy, labor and delivery (O71.8)*
           traumatic separation of muscle—see strain of muscle by body region

    M62.00 Separation of muscle (nontraumatic), unspecified site

☑6ᵗʰ **M62.01** Separation of muscle (nontraumatic), shoulder

    M62.011 Separation of muscle (nontraumatic), right shoulder

    M62.012 Separation of muscle (nontraumatic), left shoulder

    M62.019 Separation of muscle (nontraumatic), unspecified shoulder

☑6ᵗʰ **M62.02** Separation of muscle (nontraumatic), upper arm

    M62.021 Separation of muscle (nontraumatic), right upper arm

    M62.022 Separation of muscle (nontraumatic), left upper arm

    M62.029 Separation of muscle (nontraumatic), unspecified upper arm

☑6ᵗʰ **M62.03** Separation of muscle (nontraumatic), forearm

    M62.031 Separation of muscle (nontraumatic), right forearm

    M62.032 Separation of muscle (nontraumatic), left forearm

    M62.039 Separation of muscle (nontraumatic), unspecified forearm

☑6ᵗʰ **M62.04** Separation of muscle (nontraumatic), hand

    M62.041 Separation of muscle (nontraumatic), right hand

    M62.042 Separation of muscle (nontraumatic), left hand

    M62.049 Separation of muscle (nontraumatic), unspecified hand

☑6ᵗʰ **M62.05** Separation of muscle (nontraumatic), thigh

    M62.051 Separation of muscle (nontraumatic), right thigh

    M62.052 Separation of muscle (nontraumatic), left thigh

    M62.059 Separation of muscle (nontraumatic), unspecified thigh

☑6ᵗʰ **M62.06** Separation of muscle (nontraumatic), lower leg

    M62.061 Separation of muscle (nontraumatic), right lower leg

    M62.062 Separation of muscle (nontraumatic), left lower leg

    M62.069 Separation of muscle (nontraumatic), unspecified lower leg

☑6ᵗʰ **M62.07** Separation of muscle (nontraumatic), ankle and foot

    M62.071 Separation of muscle (nontraumatic), right ankle and foot

    M62.072 Separation of muscle (nontraumatic), left ankle and foot

    M62.079 Separation of muscle (nontraumatic), unspecified ankle and foot

M62.08 Separation of muscle (nontraumatic), other site

☑5ᵗʰ **M62.1** Other rupture of muscle (nontraumatic)

    EXCLUDES 1   *traumatic rupture of muscle—see strain of muscle by body region*

    EXCLUDES 2   *rupture of tendon (M66.-)*

    M62.10 Other rupture of muscle (nontraumatic), unspecified site

☑6ᵗʰ **M62.11** Other rupture of muscle (nontraumatic), shoulder

    M62.111 Other rupture of muscle (nontraumatic), right shoulder

    M62.112 Other rupture of muscle (nontraumatic), left shoulder

    M62.119 Other rupture of muscle (nontraumatic), unspecified shoulder

☑6ᵗʰ **M62.12** Other rupture of muscle (nontraumatic), upper arm

    M62.121 Other rupture of muscle (nontraumatic), right upper arm

    M62.122 Other rupture of muscle (nontraumatic), left upper arm

    M62.129 Other rupture of muscle (nontraumatic), unspecified upper arm

☑6ᵗʰ **M62.13** Other rupture of muscle (nontraumatic), forearm

    M62.131 Other rupture of muscle (nontraumatic), right forearm

    M62.132 Other rupture of muscle (nontraumatic), left forearm

    M62.139 Other rupture of muscle (nontraumatic), unspecified forearm

☑6ᵗʰ **M62.14** Other rupture of muscle (nontraumatic), hand

    M62.141 Other rupture of muscle (nontraumatic), right hand

    M62.142 Other rupture of muscle (nontraumatic), left hand

    M62.149 Other rupture of muscle (nontraumatic), unspecified hand

☑6ᵗʰ **M62.15** Other rupture of muscle (nontraumatic), thigh

    M62.151 Other rupture of muscle (nontraumatic), right thigh

    M62.152 Other rupture of muscle (nontraumatic), left thigh

    M62.159 Other rupture of muscle (nontraumatic), unspecified thigh

☑6ᵗʰ **M62.16** Other rupture of muscle (nontraumatic), lower leg

    M62.161 Other rupture of muscle (nontraumatic), right lower leg

    M62.162 Other rupture of muscle (nontraumatic), left lower leg

    M62.169 Other rupture of muscle (nontraumatic), unspecified lower leg

☑6ᵗʰ **M62.17** Other rupture of muscle (nontraumatic), ankle and foot

    M62.171 Other rupture of muscle (nontraumatic), right ankle and foot

    M62.172 Other rupture of muscle (nontraumatic), left ankle and foot

    M62.179 Other rupture of muscle (nontraumatic), unspecified ankle and foot

M62.18 Other rupture of muscle (nontraumatic), other site

☑5ᵗʰ **M62.2** Nontraumatic ischemic infarction of muscle

    EXCLUDES 1   *compartment syndrome (traumatic) (T79.A-)*
           nontraumatic compartment syndrome (M79.A-)
           rhabdomyolysis (M62.82)
           traumatic ischemia of muscle (T79.6)
           Volkmann's ischemic contracture (T79.6)

    M62.20 Nontraumatic ischemic infarction of muscle, unspecified site

☑6ᵗʰ **M62.21** Nontraumatic ischemic infarction of muscle, shoulder

    M62.211 Nontraumatic ischemic infarction of muscle, right shoulder

    M62.212 Nontraumatic ischemic infarction of muscle, left shoulder

    M62.219 Nontraumatic ischemic infarction of muscle, unspecified shoulder

☑6ᵗʰ **M62.22** Nontraumatic ischemic infarction of muscle, upper arm

    M62.221 Nontraumatic ischemic infarction of muscle, right upper arm

Ⓝ Newborn: 0   Ⓟ Pediatric: 0-17   Ⓜ Maternity: 12-55   Ⓐ Adult: 15-124   **MCC** Major CC Condition   **PDx MCC** PDx acts as own MCC   **CC** CC Condition   **PDx CC** PDx acts as own CC

728   ICD-10-CM Draft (2015)

M62.222 Nontraumatic ischemic infarction of muscle, left upper arm

M62.229 Nontraumatic ischemic infarction of muscle, unspecified upper arm

√6th M62.23 Nontraumatic ischemic infarction of muscle, forearm

M62.231 Nontraumatic ischemic infarction of muscle, right forearm

M62.232 Nontraumatic ischemic infarction of muscle, left forearm

M62.239 Nontraumatic ischemic infarction of muscle, unspecified forearm

√6th M62.24 Nontraumatic ischemic infarction of muscle, hand

M62.241 Nontraumatic ischemic infarction of muscle, right hand

M62.242 Nontraumatic ischemic infarction of muscle, left hand

M62.249 Nontraumatic ischemic infarction of muscle, unspecified hand

√6th M62.25 Nontraumatic ischemic infarction of muscle, thigh

M62.251 Nontraumatic ischemic infarction of muscle, right thigh

M62.252 Nontraumatic ischemic infarction of muscle, left thigh

M62.259 Nontraumatic ischemic infarction of muscle, unspecified thigh

√6th M62.26 Nontraumatic ischemic infarction of muscle, lower leg

M62.261 Nontraumatic ischemic infarction of muscle, right lower leg

M62.262 Nontraumatic ischemic infarction of muscle, left lower leg

M62.269 Nontraumatic ischemic infarction of muscle, unspecified lower leg

√6th M62.27 Nontraumatic ischemic infarction of muscle, ankle and foot

M62.271 Nontraumatic ischemic infarction of muscle, right ankle and foot

M62.272 Nontraumatic ischemic infarction of muscle, left ankle and foot

M62.279 Nontraumatic ischemic infarction of muscle, unspecified ankle and foot

M62.28 Nontraumatic ischemic infarction of muscle, other site

M62.3 Immobility syndrome (paraplegic)

√5th M62.4 Contracture of muscle
Contracture of tendon (sheath)
EXCLUDES 1 contracture of joint (M24.5-)

M62.40 Contracture of muscle, unspecified site

√6th M62.41 Contracture of muscle, shoulder
M62.411 Contracture of muscle, right shoulder
M62.412 Contracture of muscle, left shoulder
M62.419 Contracture of muscle, unspecified shoulder

√6th M62.42 Contracture of muscle, upper arm
M62.421 Contracture of muscle, right upper arm
M62.422 Contracture of muscle, left upper arm
M62.429 Contracture of muscle, unspecified upper arm

√6th M62.43 Contracture of muscle, forearm
M62.431 Contracture of muscle, right forearm
M62.432 Contracture of muscle, left forearm
M62.439 Contracture of muscle, unspecified forearm

√6th M62.44 Contracture of muscle, hand
M62.441 Contracture of muscle, right hand
M62.442 Contracture of muscle, left hand
M62.449 Contracture of muscle, unspecified hand

√6th M62.45 Contracture of muscle, thigh
M62.451 Contracture of muscle, right thigh
M62.452 Contracture of muscle, left thigh
M62.459 Contracture of muscle, unspecified thigh

√6th M62.46 Contracture of muscle, lower leg
M62.461 Contracture of muscle, right lower leg
M62.462 Contracture of muscle, left lower leg

M62.469 Contracture of muscle, unspecified lower leg

√6th M62.47 Contracture of muscle, ankle and foot
M62.471 Contracture of muscle, right ankle and foot
M62.472 Contracture of muscle, left ankle and foot
M62.479 Contracture of muscle, unspecified ankle and foot

M62.48 Contracture of muscle, other site

M62.49 Contracture of muscle, multiple sites

√5th M62.5 Muscle wasting and atrophy, not elsewhere classified
Disuse atrophy NEC
EXCLUDES 1 neuralgic amyotrophy (G54.5)
progressive muscular atrophy (G12.29)
EXCLUDES 2 pelvic muscle wasting (N81.84)

M62.50 Muscle wasting and atrophy, not elsewhere classified, unspecified site

√6th M62.51 Muscle wasting and atrophy, not elsewhere classified, shoulder
M62.511 Muscle wasting and atrophy, not elsewhere classified, right shoulder
M62.512 Muscle wasting and atrophy, not elsewhere classified, left shoulder
M62.519 Muscle wasting and atrophy, not elsewhere classified, unspecified shoulder

√6th M62.52 Muscle wasting and atrophy, not elsewhere classified, upper arm
M62.521 Muscle wasting and atrophy, not elsewhere classified, right upper arm
M62.522 Muscle wasting and atrophy, not elsewhere classified, left upper arm
M62.529 Muscle wasting and atrophy, not elsewhere classified, unspecified upper arm

√6th M62.53 Muscle wasting and atrophy, not elsewhere classified, forearm
M62.531 Muscle wasting and atrophy, not elsewhere classified, right forearm
M62.532 Muscle wasting and atrophy, not elsewhere classified, left forearm
M62.539 Muscle wasting and atrophy, not elsewhere classified, unspecified forearm

√6th M62.54 Muscle wasting and atrophy, not elsewhere classified, hand
M62.541 Muscle wasting and atrophy, not elsewhere classified, right hand
M62.542 Muscle wasting and atrophy, not elsewhere classified, left hand
M62.549 Muscle wasting and atrophy, not elsewhere classified, unspecified hand

√6th M62.55 Muscle wasting and atrophy, not elsewhere classified, thigh
M62.551 Muscle wasting and atrophy, not elsewhere classified, right thigh
M62.552 Muscle wasting and atrophy, not elsewhere classified, left thigh
M62.559 Muscle wasting and atrophy, not elsewhere classified, unspecified thigh

√6th M62.56 Muscle wasting and atrophy, not elsewhere classified, lower leg
M62.561 Muscle wasting and atrophy, not elsewhere classified, right lower leg
M62.562 Muscle wasting and atrophy, not elsewhere classified, left lower leg
M62.569 Muscle wasting and atrophy, not elsewhere classified, unspecified lower leg

√6th M62.57 Muscle wasting and atrophy, not elsewhere classified, ankle and foot
M62.571 Muscle wasting and atrophy, not elsewhere classified, right ankle and foot
M62.572 Muscle wasting and atrophy, not elsewhere classified, left ankle and foot
M62.579 Muscle wasting and atrophy, not elsewhere classified, unspecified ankle and foot

M62.58 Muscle wasting and atrophy, not elsewhere classified, other site

M62.59 Muscle wasting and atrophy, not elsewhere classified, multiple sites

√5ᵗʰ **M62.8 Other specified disorders of muscle**
EXCLUDES 2 nontraumatic hematoma of muscle (M79.81)

M62.81 Muscle weakness (generalized)

M62.82 Rhabdomyolysis CC
EXCLUDES 1 traumatic rhabdomyolysis (T79.6)
CC Excl: K68.12, M60.000-M60.19, M61.00-M61.19, M61.30-M61.59, M62.3, M62.50-M62.59, M62.82, M62.89, M72.6

√6ᵗʰ **M62.83 Muscle spasm**
M62.830 Muscle spasm of back
M62.831 Muscle spasm of calf
Charley-horse
M62.838 Other muscle spasm

M62.89 Other specified disorders of muscle
Muscle (sheath) hernia

M62.9 Disorder of muscle, unspecified

√4ᵗʰ **M63 Disorders of muscle in diseases classified elsewhere**
Code first underlying disease, such as:
leprosy (A30.-)
neoplasm (C49-, C79.89, D21-, D48.1)
schistosomiasis (B65.-)
trichinellosis (B75)
EXCLUDES 1 myopathy in cysticercosis (B69.81)
myopathy in endocrine diseases (G73.7)
myopathy in metabolic diseases (G73.7)
myopathy in sarcoidosis (D86.87)
myopathy in secondary syphilis (A51.49)
myopathy in syphilis (late) (A52.78)
myopathy in toxoplasmosis (B58.82)
myopathy in tuberculosis (A18.09)

√5ᵗʰ **M63.8 Disorders of muscle in diseases classified elsewhere**
M63.80 Disorders of muscle in diseases classified elsewhere, unspecified site
√6ᵗʰ **M63.81 Disorders of muscle in diseases classified elsewhere, shoulder**
M63.811 Disorders of muscle in diseases classified elsewhere, right shoulder
M63.812 Disorders of muscle in diseases classified elsewhere, left shoulder
M63.819 Disorders of muscle in diseases classified elsewhere, unspecified shoulder
√6ᵗʰ **M63.82 Disorders of muscle in diseases classified elsewhere, upper arm**
M63.821 Disorders of muscle in diseases classified elsewhere, right upper arm
M63.822 Disorders of muscle in diseases classified elsewhere, left upper arm
M63.829 Disorders of muscle in diseases classified elsewhere, unspecified upper arm
√6ᵗʰ **M63.83 Disorders of muscle in diseases classified elsewhere, forearm**
M63.831 Disorders of muscle in diseases classified elsewhere, right forearm
M63.832 Disorders of muscle in diseases classified elsewhere, left forearm
M63.839 Disorders of muscle in diseases classified elsewhere, unspecified forearm
√6ᵗʰ **M63.84 Disorders of muscle in diseases classified elsewhere, hand**
M63.841 Disorders of muscle in diseases classified elsewhere, right hand
M63.842 Disorders of muscle in diseases classified elsewhere, left hand
M63.849 Disorders of muscle in diseases classified elsewhere, unspecified hand
√6ᵗʰ **M63.85 Disorders of muscle in diseases classified elsewhere, thigh**
M63.851 Disorders of muscle in diseases classified elsewhere, right thigh
M63.852 Disorders of muscle in diseases classified elsewhere, left thigh
M63.859 Disorders of muscle in diseases classified elsewhere, unspecified thigh

√6ᵗʰ **M63.86 Disorders of muscle in diseases classified elsewhere, lower leg**
M63.861 Disorders of muscle in diseases classified elsewhere, right lower leg
M63.862 Disorders of muscle in diseases classified elsewhere, left lower leg
M63.869 Disorders of muscle in diseases classified elsewhere, unspecified lower leg
√6ᵗʰ **M63.87 Disorders of muscle in diseases classified elsewhere, ankle and foot**
M63.871 Disorders of muscle in diseases classified elsewhere, right ankle and foot
M63.872 Disorders of muscle in diseases classified elsewhere, left ankle and foot
M63.879 Disorders of muscle in diseases classified elsewhere, unspecified ankle and foot
M63.88 Disorders of muscle in diseases classified elsewhere, other site
M63.89 Disorders of muscle in diseases classified elsewhere, multiple sites

Disorders of synovium and tendon (M65-M67)

√4ᵗʰ **M65 Synovitis and tenosynovitis**
EXCLUDES 1 chronic crepitant synovitis of hand and wrist (M70.0-)
current injury—see injury of ligament or tendon by body region
soft tissue disorders related to use, overuse and pressure (M70.-)

√5ᵗʰ **M65.0 Abscess of tendon sheath**
Use additional code (B95-B96) to identify bacterial agent.
M65.00 Abscess of tendon sheath, unspecified site
√6ᵗʰ **M65.01 Abscess of tendon sheath, shoulder**
M65.011 Abscess of tendon sheath, right shoulder
M65.012 Abscess of tendon sheath, left shoulder
M65.019 Abscess of tendon sheath, unspecified shoulder
√6ᵗʰ **M65.02 Abscess of tendon sheath, upper arm**
M65.021 Abscess of tendon sheath, right upper arm
M65.022 Abscess of tendon sheath, left upper arm
M65.029 Abscess of tendon sheath, unspecified upper arm
√6ᵗʰ **M65.03 Abscess of tendon sheath, forearm**
M65.031 Abscess of tendon sheath, right forearm
M65.032 Abscess of tendon sheath, left forearm
M65.039 Abscess of tendon sheath, unspecified forearm
√6ᵗʰ **M65.04 Abscess of tendon sheath, hand**
M65.041 Abscess of tendon sheath, right hand
M65.042 Abscess of tendon sheath, left hand
M65.049 Abscess of tendon sheath, unspecified hand
√6ᵗʰ **M65.05 Abscess of tendon sheath, thigh**
M65.051 Abscess of tendon sheath, right thigh
M65.052 Abscess of tendon sheath, left thigh
M65.059 Abscess of tendon sheath, unspecified thigh
√6ᵗʰ **M65.06 Abscess of tendon sheath, lower leg**
M65.061 Abscess of tendon sheath, right lower leg
M65.062 Abscess of tendon sheath, left lower leg
M65.069 Abscess of tendon sheath, unspecified lower leg
√6ᵗʰ **M65.07 Abscess of tendon sheath, ankle and foot**
M65.071 Abscess of tendon sheath, right ankle and foot
M65.072 Abscess of tendon sheath, left ankle and foot
M65.079 Abscess of tendon sheath, unspecified ankle and foot
M65.08 Abscess of tendon sheath, other site
√5ᵗʰ **M65.1 Other infective (teno)synovitis**
M65.10 Other infective (teno)synovitis, unspecified site
√6ᵗʰ **M65.11 Other infective (teno)synovitis, shoulder**
M65.111 Other infective (teno)synovitis, right shoulder
M65.112 Other infective (teno)synovitis, left shoulder

M65.119 Other infective (teno)synovitis, **unspecified shoulder**

√6th **M65.12 Other infective (teno)synovitis, elbow**
M65.121 Other infective (teno)synovitis, **right elbow**
M65.122 Other infective (teno)synovitis, **left elbow**
M65.129 Other infective (teno)synovitis, **unspecified elbow**

√6th **M65.13 Other infective (teno)synovitis, wrist**
M65.131 Other infective (teno)synovitis, **right wrist**
M65.132 Other infective (teno)synovitis, **left wrist**
M65.139 Other infective (teno)synovitis, **unspecified wrist**

√6th **M65.14 Other infective (teno)synovitis, hand**
M65.141 Other infective (teno)synovitis, **right hand**
M65.142 Other infective (teno)synovitis, **left hand**
M65.149 Other infective (teno)synovitis, **unspecified hand**

√6th **M65.15 Other infective (teno)synovitis, hip**
M65.151 Other infective (teno)synovitis, **right hip**
M65.152 Other infective (teno)synovitis, **left hip**
M65.159 Other infective (teno)synovitis, **unspecified hip**

√6th **M65.16 Other infective (teno)synovitis, knee**
M65.161 Other infective (teno)synovitis, **right knee**
M65.162 Other infective (teno)synovitis, **left knee**
M65.169 Other infective (teno)synovitis, **unspecified knee**

√6th **M65.17 Other infective (teno)synovitis, ankle and foot**
M65.171 Other infective (teno)synovitis, **right ankle and foot**
M65.172 Other infective (teno)synovitis, **left ankle and foot**
M65.179 Other infective (teno)synovitis, **unspecified ankle and foot**

M65.18 Other infective (teno)synovitis, **other site**
M65.19 Other infective (teno)synovitis, **multiple sites**

√5th **M65.2 Calcific tendinitis**
    EXCLUDES 1   tendinitis as classified in M75-M77
                  calcified tendinitis of shoulder (M75.3)
M65.20 Calcific tendinitis, **unspecified site**

√6th **M65.22 Calcific tendinitis, upper arm**
M65.221 Calcific tendinitis, **right upper arm**
M65.222 Calcific tendinitis, **left upper arm**
M65.229 Calcific tendinitis, **unspecified upper arm**

√6th **M65.23 Calcific tendinitis, forearm**
M65.231 Calcific tendinitis, **right forearm**
M65.232 Calcific tendinitis, **left forearm**
M65.239 Calcific tendinitis, **unspecified forearm**

√6th **M65.24 Calcific tendinitis, hand**
M65.241 Calcific tendinitis, **right hand**
M65.242 Calcific tendinitis, **left hand**
M65.249 Calcific tendinitis, **unspecified hand**

√6th **M65.25 Calcific tendinitis, thigh**
M65.251 Calcific tendinitis, **right thigh**
M65.252 Calcific tendinitis, **left thigh**
M65.259 Calcific tendinitis, **unspecified thigh**

√6th **M65.26 Calcific tendinitis, lower leg**
M65.261 Calcific tendinitis, **right lower leg**
M65.262 Calcific tendinitis, **left lower leg**
M65.269 Calcific tendinitis, **unspecified lower leg**

√6th **M65.27 Calcific tendinitis, ankle and foot**
M65.271 Calcific tendinitis, **right ankle and foot**
M65.272 Calcific tendinitis, **left ankle and foot**
M65.279 Calcific tendinitis, **unspecified ankle and foot**

M65.28 Calcific tendinitis, **other site**
M65.29 Calcific tendinitis, **multiple sites**

M65.3 Trigger finger
    Nodular tendinous disease
M65.30 Trigger finger, **unspecified finger**

√6th **M65.31 Trigger thumb**
M65.311 Trigger thumb, **right thumb**

M65.312 Trigger thumb, **left thumb**
M65.319 Trigger thumb, **unspecified thumb**

√6th **M65.32 Trigger finger, index finger**
M65.321 Trigger finger, **right index finger**
M65.322 Trigger finger, **left index finger**
M65.329 Trigger finger, **unspecified index finger**

√6th **M65.33 Trigger finger, middle finger**
M65.331 Trigger finger, **right middle finger**
M65.332 Trigger finger, **left middle finger**
M65.339 Trigger finger, **unspecified middle finger**

√6th **M65.34 Trigger finger, ring finger**
M65.341 Trigger finger, **right ring finger**
M65.342 Trigger finger, **left ring finger**
M65.349 Trigger finger, **unspecified ring finger**

√6th **M65.35 Trigger finger, little finger**
M65.351 Trigger finger, **right little finger**
M65.352 Trigger finger, **left little finger**
M65.359 Trigger finger, **unspecified little finger**

M65.4 Radial styloid tenosynovitis [de Quervain]

√5th **M65.8 Other synovitis and tenosynovitis**
M65.80 Other synovitis and tenosynovitis, **unspecified site**

√6th **M65.81 Other synovitis and tenosynovitis, shoulder**
M65.811 Other synovitis and tenosynovitis, **right shoulder**
M65.812 Other synovitis and tenosynovitis, **left shoulder**
M65.819 Other synovitis and tenosynovitis, **unspecified shoulder**

√6th **M65.82 Other synovitis and tenosynovitis, upper arm**
M65.821 Other synovitis and tenosynovitis, **right upper arm**
M65.822 Other synovitis and tenosynovitis, **left upper arm**
M65.829 Other synovitis and tenosynovitis, **unspecified upper arm**

√6th **M65.83 Other synovitis and tenosynovitis, forearm**
M65.831 Other synovitis and tenosynovitis, **right forearm**
M65.832 Other synovitis and tenosynovitis, **left forearm**
M65.839 Other synovitis and tenosynovitis, **unspecified forearm**

√6th **M65.84 Other synovitis and tenosynovitis, hand**
M65.841 Other synovitis and tenosynovitis, **right hand**
M65.842 Other synovitis and tenosynovitis, **left hand**
M65.849 Other synovitis and tenosynovitis, **unspecified hand**

√6th **M65.85 Other synovitis and tenosynovitis, thigh**
M65.851 Other synovitis and tenosynovitis, **right thigh**
M65.852 Other synovitis and tenosynovitis, **left thigh**
M65.859 Other synovitis and tenosynovitis, **unspecified thigh**

√6th **M65.86 Other synovitis and tenosynovitis, lower leg**
M65.861 Other synovitis and tenosynovitis, **right lower leg**
M65.862 Other synovitis and tenosynovitis, **left lower leg**
M65.869 Other synovitis and tenosynovitis, **unspecified lower leg**

√6th **M65.87 Other synovitis and tenosynovitis, ankle and foot**
M65.871 Other synovitis and tenosynovitis, **right ankle and foot**
M65.872 Other synovitis and tenosynovitis, **left ankle and foot**
M65.879 Other synovitis and tenosynovitis, **unspecified ankle and foot**

M65.88 Other synovitis and tenosynovitis, **other site**
M65.89 Other synovitis and tenosynovitis, **multiple sites**
M65.9 Synovitis and tenosynovitis, unspecified

☑ Additional Character Required   √x7th Xtension Alert   Unacceptable PDx   Manifestation   Hospital Acquired Condition   EXCLUDES 1 Not Coded Here   EXCLUDES 2 Not Included Here

Diseases of the Musculoskeletal System and Connective Tissue

M66–M66.369

☑4th **M66 Spontaneous rupture of synovium and tendon**
     INCLUDES   rupture that occurs when a normal force is applied to tissues that are inferred to have less than normal strength
     EXCLUDES 2   rotator cuff syndrome (M75.1-)
         rupture where an abnormal force is applied to normal tissue—see injury of tendon by body region

     M66.0 Rupture of popliteal cyst

☑5th **M66.1 Rupture of synovium**
         Rupture of synovial cyst
         EXCLUDES 2   rupture of popliteal cyst (M66.0)

         M66.10 Rupture of synovium, unspecified joint

☑6th   **M66.11 Rupture of synovium, shoulder**
         M66.111 Rupture of synovium, right shoulder
         M66.112 Rupture of synovium, left shoulder
         M66.119 Rupture of synovium, unspecified shoulder

☑6th   **M66.12 Rupture of synovium, elbow**
         M66.121 Rupture of synovium, right elbow
         M66.122 Rupture of synovium, left elbow
         M66.129 Rupture of synovium, unspecified elbow

☑6th   **M66.13 Rupture of synovium, wrist**
         M66.131 Rupture of synovium, right wrist
         M66.132 Rupture of synovium, left wrist
         M66.139 Rupture of synovium, unspecified wrist

☑6th   **M66.14 Rupture of synovium, hand and fingers**
         M66.141 Rupture of synovium, right hand
         M66.142 Rupture of synovium, left hand
         M66.143 Rupture of synovium, unspecified hand
         M66.144 Rupture of synovium, right finger(s)
         M66.145 Rupture of synovium, left finger(s)
         M66.146 Rupture of synovium, unspecified finger(s)

☑6th   **M66.15 Rupture of synovium, hip**
         M66.151 Rupture of synovium, right hip
         M66.152 Rupture of synovium, left hip
         M66.159 Rupture of synovium, unspecified hip

☑6th   **M66.17 Rupture of synovium, ankle, foot and toes**
         M66.171 Rupture of synovium, right ankle
         M66.172 Rupture of synovium, left ankle
         M66.173 Rupture of synovium, unspecified ankle
         M66.174 Rupture of synovium, right foot
         M66.175 Rupture of synovium, left foot
         M66.176 Rupture of synovium, unspecified foot
         M66.177 Rupture of synovium, right toe(s)
         M66.178 Rupture of synovium, left toe(s)
         M66.179 Rupture of synovium, unspecified toe(s)

         M66.18 Rupture of synovium, other site

☑5th **M66.2 Spontaneous rupture of extensor tendons**
         M66.20 Spontaneous rupture of extensor tendons, unspecified site

☑6th   **M66.21 Spontaneous rupture of extensor tendons, shoulder**
         M66.211 Spontaneous rupture of extensor tendons, right shoulder
         M66.212 Spontaneous rupture of extensor tendons, left shoulder
         M66.219 Spontaneous rupture of extensor tendons, unspecified shoulder

☑6th   **M66.22 Spontaneous rupture of extensor tendons, upper arm**
         M66.221 Spontaneous rupture of extensor tendons, right upper arm
         M66.222 Spontaneous rupture of extensor tendons, left upper arm
         M66.229 Spontaneous rupture of extensor tendons, unspecified upper arm

☑6th   **M66.23 Spontaneous rupture of extensor tendons, forearm**
         M66.231 Spontaneous rupture of extensor tendons, right forearm
         M66.232 Spontaneous rupture of extensor tendons, left forearm
         M66.239 Spontaneous rupture of extensor tendons, unspecified forearm

☑6th   **M66.24 Spontaneous rupture of extensor tendons, hand**
         M66.241 Spontaneous rupture of extensor tendons, right hand
         M66.242 Spontaneous rupture of extensor tendons, left hand
         M66.249 Spontaneous rupture of extensor tendons, unspecified hand

☑6th   **M66.25 Spontaneous rupture of extensor tendons, thigh**
         M66.251 Spontaneous rupture of extensor tendons, right thigh
         M66.252 Spontaneous rupture of extensor tendons, left thigh
         M66.259 Spontaneous rupture of extensor tendons, unspecified thigh

☑6th   **M66.26 Spontaneous rupture of extensor tendons, lower leg**
         M66.261 Spontaneous rupture of extensor tendons, right lower leg
         M66.262 Spontaneous rupture of extensor tendons, left lower leg
         M66.269 Spontaneous rupture of extensor tendons, unspecified lower leg

☑6th   **M66.27 Spontaneous rupture of extensor tendons, ankle and foot**
         M66.271 Spontaneous rupture of extensor tendons, right ankle and foot
         M66.272 Spontaneous rupture of extensor tendons, left ankle and foot
         M66.279 Spontaneous rupture of extensor tendons, unspecified ankle and foot

         M66.28 Spontaneous rupture of extensor tendons, other site
         M66.29 Spontaneous rupture of extensor tendons, multiple sites

☑5th **M66.3 Spontaneous rupture of flexor tendons**
         M66.30 Spontaneous rupture of flexor tendons, unspecified site

☑6th   **M66.31 Spontaneous rupture of flexor tendons, shoulder**
         M66.311 Spontaneous rupture of flexor tendons, right shoulder
         M66.312 Spontaneous rupture of flexor tendons, left shoulder
         M66.319 Spontaneous rupture of flexor tendons, unspecified shoulder

☑6th   **M66.32 Spontaneous rupture of flexor tendons, upper arm**
         M66.321 Spontaneous rupture of flexor tendons, right upper arm
         M66.322 Spontaneous rupture of flexor tendons, left upper arm
         M66.329 Spontaneous rupture of flexor tendons, unspecified upper arm

☑6th   **M66.33 Spontaneous rupture of flexor tendons, forearm**
         M66.331 Spontaneous rupture of flexor tendons, right forearm
         M66.332 Spontaneous rupture of flexor tendons, left forearm
         M66.339 Spontaneous rupture of flexor tendons, unspecified forearm

☑6th   **M66.34 Spontaneous rupture of flexor tendons, hand**
         M66.341 Spontaneous rupture of flexor tendons, right hand
         M66.342 Spontaneous rupture of flexor tendons, left hand
         M66.349 Spontaneous rupture of flexor tendons, unspecified hand

☑6th   **M66.35 Spontaneous rupture of flexor tendons, thigh**
         M66.351 Spontaneous rupture of flexor tendons, right thigh
         M66.352 Spontaneous rupture of flexor tendons, left thigh
         M66.359 Spontaneous rupture of flexor tendons, unspecified thigh

☑6th   **M66.36 Spontaneous rupture of flexor tendons, lower leg**
         M66.361 Spontaneous rupture of flexor tendons, right lower leg
         M66.362 Spontaneous rupture of flexor tendons, left lower leg
         M66.369 Spontaneous rupture of flexor tendons, unspecified lower leg

√6th **M66.37** **Spontaneous rupture of flexor tendons,** ankle and foot

    M66.371 **Spontaneous rupture of flexor tendons,** right ankle and foot

    M66.372 **Spontaneous rupture of flexor tendons,** left ankle and foot

    M66.379 **Spontaneous rupture of flexor tendons,** unspecified ankle and foot

M66.38 **Spontaneous rupture of flexor tendons,** other site

M66.39 **Spontaneous rupture of flexor tendons,** multiple sites

√5th **M66.8** **Spontaneous rupture of** other tendons

M66.80 **Spontaneous rupture of other tendons,** unspecified site

√6th **M66.81** **Spontaneous rupture of other tendons,** shoulder

    M66.811 **Spontaneous rupture of other tendons,** right shoulder

    M66.812 **Spontaneous rupture of other tendons,** left shoulder

    M66.819 **Spontaneous rupture of other tendons,** unspecified shoulder

√6th **M66.82** **Spontaneous rupture of other tendons,** upper arm

    M66.821 **Spontaneous rupture of other tendons,** right upper arm

    M66.822 **Spontaneous rupture of other tendons,** left upper arm

    M66.829 **Spontaneous rupture of other tendons,** unspecified upper arm

√6th **M66.83** **Spontaneous rupture of other tendons,** forearm

    M66.831 **Spontaneous rupture of other tendons,** right forearm

    M66.832 **Spontaneous rupture of other tendons,** left forearm

    M66.839 **Spontaneous rupture of other tendons,** unspecified forearm

√6th **M66.84** **Spontaneous rupture of other tendons,** hand

    M66.841 **Spontaneous rupture of other tendons,** right hand

    M66.842 **Spontaneous rupture of other tendons,** left hand

    M66.849 **Spontaneous rupture of other tendons,** unspecified hand

√6th **M66.85** **Spontaneous rupture of other tendons,** thigh

    M66.851 **Spontaneous rupture of other tendons,** right thigh

    M66.852 **Spontaneous rupture of other tendons,** left thigh

    M66.859 **Spontaneous rupture of other tendons,** unspecified thigh

√6th **M66.86** **Spontaneous rupture of other tendons,** lower leg

    M66.861 **Spontaneous rupture of other tendons,** right lower leg

    M66.862 **Spontaneous rupture of other tendons,** left lower leg

    M66.869 **Spontaneous rupture of other tendons,** unspecified lower leg

√6th **M66.87** **Spontaneous rupture of other tendons,** ankle and foot

    M66.871 **Spontaneous rupture of other tendons,** right ankle and foot

    M66.872 **Spontaneous rupture of other tendons,** left ankle and foot

    M66.879 **Spontaneous rupture of other tendons,** unspecified ankle and foot

M66.88 **Spontaneous rupture of other tendons,** other

M66.89 **Spontaneous rupture of other tendons,** multiple sites

M66.9 **Spontaneous rupture of** unspecified tendon
Rupture at musculotendinous junction, nontraumatic

√4th **M67** **Other disorders of synovium and tendon**
    EXCLUDES 1 *palmar fascial fibromatosis [Dupuytren] (M72.0)*
    tendinitis NOS (M77.9-)
    xanthomatosis localized to tendons (E78.2)

√5th **M67.0** **Short Achilles tendon (acquired)**

M67.00 **Short Achilles tendon (acquired),** unspecified ankle

M67.01 **Short Achilles tendon (acquired),** right ankle

M67.02 **Short Achilles tendon (acquired),** left ankle

√5th **M67.2** **Synovial hypertrophy, not elsewhere classified**
    EXCLUDES 1 *villonodular synovitis (pigmented) (M12.2-)*

M67.20 **Synovial hypertrophy, not elsewhere classified,** unspecified site

√6th **M67.21** **Synovial hypertrophy, not elsewhere classified,** shoulder

    M67.211 **Synovial hypertrophy, not elsewhere classified,** right shoulder

    M67.212 **Synovial hypertrophy, not elsewhere classified,** left shoulder

    M67.219 **Synovial hypertrophy, not elsewhere classified,** unspecified shoulder

√6th **M67.22** **Synovial hypertrophy, not elsewhere classified,** upper arm

    M67.221 **Synovial hypertrophy, not elsewhere classified,** right upper arm

    M67.222 **Synovial hypertrophy, not elsewhere classified,** left upper arm

    M67.229 **Synovial hypertrophy, not elsewhere classified,** unspecified upper arm

√6th **M67.23** **Synovial hypertrophy, not elsewhere classified,** forearm

    M67.231 **Synovial hypertrophy, not elsewhere classified,** right forearm

    M67.232 **Synovial hypertrophy, not elsewhere classified,** left forearm

    M67.239 **Synovial hypertrophy, not elsewhere classified,** unspecified forearm

√6th **M67.24** **Synovial hypertrophy, not elsewhere classified,** hand

    M67.241 **Synovial hypertrophy, not elsewhere classified,** right hand

    M67.242 **Synovial hypertrophy, not elsewhere classified,** left hand

    M67.249 **Synovial hypertrophy, not elsewhere classified,** unspecified hand

√6th **M67.25** **Synovial hypertrophy, not elsewhere classified,** thigh

    M67.251 **Synovial hypertrophy, not elsewhere classified,** right thigh

    M67.252 **Synovial hypertrophy, not elsewhere classified,** left thigh

    M67.259 **Synovial hypertrophy, not elsewhere classified,** unspecified thigh

√6th **M67.26** **Synovial hypertrophy, not elsewhere classified,** lower leg

    M67.261 **Synovial hypertrophy, not elsewhere classified,** right lower leg

    M67.262 **Synovial hypertrophy, not elsewhere classified,** left lower leg

    M67.269 **Synovial hypertrophy, not elsewhere classified,** unspecified lower leg

√6th **M67.27** **Synovial hypertrophy, not elsewhere classified,** ankle and foot

    M67.271 **Synovial hypertrophy, not elsewhere classified,** right ankle and foot

    M67.272 **Synovial hypertrophy, not elsewhere classified,** left ankle and foot

    M67.279 **Synovial hypertrophy, not elsewhere classified,** unspecified ankle and foot

M67.28 **Synovial hypertrophy, not elsewhere classified,** other site

M67.29 **Synovial hypertrophy, not elsewhere classified,** multiple sites

√5th **M67.3** **Transient synovitis**
Toxic synovitis
    EXCLUDES 1 *palindromic rheumatism (M12.3-)*

M67.30 **Transient synovitis,** unspecified site

√6th **M67.31** **Transient synovitis,** shoulder

    M67.311 **Transient synovitis,** right shoulder

    M67.312 **Transient synovitis,** left shoulder

    M67.319 **Transient synovitis,** unspecified shoulder

√6th **M67.32** **Transient synovitis,** elbow

    M67.321 **Transient synovitis,** right elbow

    M67.322 **Transient synovitis,** left elbow

    M67.329 **Transient synovitis,** unspecified elbow

✓ Additional Character Required √x7th Xtension Alert Unacceptable PDx Manifestation Hospital Acquired Condition EXCLUDES 1 Not Coded Here EXCLUDES 2 Not Included Here

√6th **M67.33 Transient synovitis, wrist**
- M67.331 Transient synovitis, right wrist
- M67.332 Transient synovitis, left wrist
- M67.339 Transient synovitis, unspecified wrist

√6th **M67.34 Transient synovitis, hand**
- M67.341 Transient synovitis, right hand
- M67.342 Transient synovitis, left hand
- M67.349 Transient synovitis, unspecified hand

√6th **M67.35 Transient synovitis, hip**
- M67.351 Transient synovitis, right hip
- M67.352 Transient synovitis, left hip
- M67.359 Transient synovitis, unspecified hip

√6th **M67.36 Transient synovitis, knee**
- M67.361 Transient synovitis, right knee
- M67.362 Transient synovitis, left knee
- M67.369 Transient synovitis, unspecified knee

√6th **M67.37 Transient synovitis, ankle and foot**
- M67.371 Transient synovitis, right ankle and foot
- M67.372 Transient synovitis, left ankle and foot
- M67.379 Transient synovitis, unspecified ankle and foot

M67.38 Transient synovitis, other site

M67.39 Transient synovitis, multiple sites

√5th **M67.4 Ganglion**
Ganglion of joint or tendon (sheath)
EXCLUDES 1   *ganglion in yaws (A66.6)*
EXCLUDES 2   *cyst of bursa (M71.2-M71.3)*
               cyst of synovium (M71.2-M71.3)

M67.40 Ganglion, unspecified site

√6th **M67.41 Ganglion, shoulder**
- M67.411 Ganglion, right shoulder
- M67.412 Ganglion, left shoulder
- M67.419 Ganglion, unspecified shoulder

√6th **M67.42 Ganglion, elbow**
- M67.421 Ganglion, right elbow
- M67.422 Ganglion, left elbow
- M67.429 Ganglion, unspecified elbow

√6th **M67.43 Ganglion, wrist**
- M67.431 Ganglion, right wrist
- M67.432 Ganglion, left wrist
- M67.439 Ganglion, unspecified wrist

√6th **M67.44 Ganglion, hand**
- M67.441 Ganglion, right hand
- M67.442 Ganglion, left hand
- M67.449 Ganglion, unspecified hand

√6th **M67.45 Ganglion, hip**
- M67.451 Ganglion, right hip
- M67.452 Ganglion, left hip
- M67.459 Ganglion, unspecified hip

√6th **M67.46 Ganglion, knee**
- M67.461 Ganglion, right knee
- M67.462 Ganglion, left knee
- M67.469 Ganglion, unspecified knee

√6th **M67.47 Ganglion, ankle and foot**
- M67.471 Ganglion, right ankle and foot
- M67.472 Ganglion, left ankle and foot
- M67.479 Ganglion, unspecified ankle and foot

M67.48 Ganglion, other site

M67.49 Ganglion, multiple sites

√5th **M67.5 Plica syndrome**
Plica knee
- **M67.50 Plica syndrome, unspecified knee**
- **M67.51 Plica syndrome, right knee**
- **M67.52 Plica syndrome, left knee**

√5th **M67.8 Other specified disorders of synovium and tendon**
- **M67.80 Other specified disorders of synovium and tendon, unspecified site**

√6th **M67.81 Other specified disorders of synovium and tendon, shoulder**
- M67.811 Other specified disorders of synovium, right shoulder

M67.812 Other specified disorders of synovium, left shoulder

M67.813 Other specified disorders of tendon, right shoulder

M67.814 Other specified disorders of tendon, left shoulder

M67.819 Other specified disorders of synovium and tendon, unspecified shoulder

√6th **M67.82 Other specified disorders of synovium and tendon, elbow**
- M67.821 Other specified disorders of synovium, right elbow
- M67.822 Other specified disorders of synovium, left elbow
- M67.823 Other specified disorders of tendon, right elbow
- M67.824 Other specified disorders of tendon, left elbow
- M67.829 Other specified disorders of synovium and tendon, unspecified elbow

√6th **M67.83 Other specified disorders of synovium and tendon, wrist**
- M67.831 Other specified disorders of synovium, right wrist
- M67.832 Other specified disorders of synovium, left wrist
- M67.833 Other specified disorders of tendon, right wrist
- M67.834 Other specified disorders of tendon, left wrist
- M67.839 Other specified disorders of synovium and tendon, unspecified forearm

√6th **M67.84 Other specified disorders of synovium and tendon, hand**
- M67.841 Other specified disorders of synovium, right hand
- M67.842 Other specified disorders of synovium, left hand
- M67.843 Other specified disorders of tendon, right hand
- M67.844 Other specified disorders of tendon, left hand
- M67.849 Other specified disorders of synovium and tendon, unspecified hand

√6th **M67.85 Other specified disorders of synovium and tendon, hip**
- M67.851 Other specified disorders of synovium, right hip
- M67.852 Other specified disorders of synovium, left hip
- M67.853 Other specified disorders of tendon, right hip
- M67.854 Other specified disorders of tendon, left hip
- M67.859 Other specified disorders of synovium and tendon, unspecified hip

√6th **M67.86 Other specified disorders of synovium and tendon, knee**
- M67.861 Other specified disorders of synovium, right knee
- M67.862 Other specified disorders of synovium, left knee
- M67.863 Other specified disorders of tendon, right knee
- M67.864 Other specified disorders of tendon, left knee
- M67.869 Other specified disorders of synovium and tendon, unspecified knee

√6th **M67.87 Other specified disorders of synovium and tendon, ankle and foot**
- M67.871 Other specified disorders of synovium, right ankle and foot
- M67.872 Other specified disorders of synovium, left ankle and foot
- M67.873 Other specified disorders of tendon, right ankle and foot
- M67.874 Other specified disorders of tendon, left ankle and foot

N Newborn: 0   P Pediatric: 0-17   M Maternity: 12-55   A Adult: 15-124   MCC Major CC Condition   PDx MCC PDx acts as own MCC   CC CC Condition   PDx CC PDx acts as own CC

734   ICD-10-CM Draft (2015)

M67.879 Other specified disorders of synovium and tendon, unspecified ankle and foot

M67.88 Other specified disorders of synovium and tendon, other site

M67.89 Other specified disorders of synovium and tendon, multiple sites

√5th M67.9 Unspecified disorder of synovium and tendon

M67.90 Unspecified disorder of synovium and tendon, unspecified site

√6th M67.91 Unspecified disorder of synovium and tendon, shoulder

M67.911 Unspecified disorder of synovium and tendon, right shoulder

M67.912 Unspecified disorder of synovium and tendon, left shoulder

M67.919 Unspecified disorder of synovium and tendon, unspecified shoulder

√6th M67.92 Unspecified disorder of synovium and tendon, upper arm

M67.921 Unspecified disorder of synovium and tendon, right upper arm

M67.922 Unspecified disorder of synovium and tendon, left upper arm

M67.929 Unspecified disorder of synovium and tendon, unspecified upper arm

√6th M67.93 Unspecified disorder of synovium and tendon, forearm

M67.931 Unspecified disorder of synovium and tendon, right forearm

M67.932 Unspecified disorder of synovium and tendon, left forearm

M67.939 Unspecified disorder of synovium and tendon, unspecified forearm

√6th M67.94 Unspecified disorder of synovium and tendon, hand

M67.941 Unspecified disorder of synovium and tendon, right hand

M67.942 Unspecified disorder of synovium and tendon, left hand

M67.949 Unspecified disorder of synovium and tendon, unspecified hand

√6th M67.95 Unspecified disorder of synovium and tendon, thigh

M67.951 Unspecified disorder of synovium and tendon, right thigh

M67.952 Unspecified disorder of synovium and tendon, left thigh

M67.959 Unspecified disorder of synovium and tendon, unspecified thigh

√6th M67.96 Unspecified disorder of synovium and tendon, lower leg

M67.961 Unspecified disorder of synovium and tendon, right lower leg

M67.962 Unspecified disorder of synovium and tendon, left lower leg

M67.969 Unspecified disorder of synovium and tendon, unspecified lower leg

√6th M67.97 Unspecified disorder of synovium and tendon, ankle and foot

M67.971 Unspecified disorder of synovium and tendon, right ankle and foot

M67.972 Unspecified disorder of synovium and tendon, left ankle and foot

M67.979 Unspecified disorder of synovium and tendon, unspecified ankle and foot

M67.98 Unspecified disorder of synovium and tendon, other site

M67.99 Unspecified disorder of synovium and tendon, multiple sites

Other soft tissue disorders (M70-M79)

√4th M70 Soft tissue disorders related to use, overuse and pressure

INCLUDES soft tissue disorders of occupational origin

Use additional external cause code to identify activity causing disorder (Y93.-)

EXCLUDES 1 bursitis NOS (M71.9-)

EXCLUDES 2 bursitis of shoulder (M75.5)
enthesopathies (M76-M77)
pressure ulcer (pressure area) (L89.-)

√5th M70.0 Crepitant synovitis (acute) (chronic) of hand and wrist

√6th M70.03 Crepitant synovitis (acute) (chronic), wrist

M70.031 Crepitant synovitis (acute) (chronic), right wrist

M70.032 Crepitant synovitis (acute) (chronic), left wrist

M70.039 Crepitant synovitis (acute) (chronic), unspecified wrist

√6th M70.04 Crepitant synovitis (acute) (chronic), hand

M70.041 Crepitant synovitis (acute) (chronic), right hand

M70.042 Crepitant synovitis (acute) (chronic), left hand

M70.049 Crepitant synovitis (acute) (chronic), unspecified hand

√5th M70.1 Bursitis of hand

M70.10 Bursitis, unspecified hand

M70.11 Bursitis, right hand

M70.12 Bursitis, left hand

√5th M70.2 Olecranon bursitis

M70.20 Olecranon bursitis, unspecified elbow

M70.21 Olecranon bursitis, right elbow

M70.22 Olecranon bursitis, left elbow

√5th M70.3 Other bursitis of elbow

M70.30 Other bursitis of elbow, unspecified elbow

M70.31 Other bursitis of elbow, right elbow

M70.32 Other bursitis of elbow, left elbow

√5th M70.4 Prepatellar bursitis

M70.40 Prepatellar bursitis, unspecified knee

M70.41 Prepatellar bursitis, right knee

M70.42 Prepatellar bursitis, left knee

√5th M70.5 Other bursitis of knee

M70.50 Other bursitis of knee, unspecified knee

M70.51 Other bursitis of knee, right knee

M70.52 Other bursitis of knee, left knee

√5th M70.6 Trochanteric bursitis
Trochanteric tendinitis

M70.60 Trochanteric bursitis, unspecified hip

M70.61 Trochanteric bursitis, right hip

M70.62 Trochanteric bursitis, left hip

√5th M70.7 Other bursitis of hip
Ischial bursitis

M70.70 Other bursitis of hip, unspecified hip

M70.71 Other bursitis of hip, right hip

M70.72 Other bursitis of hip, left hip

√5th M70.8 Other soft tissue disorders related to use, overuse and pressure

M70.80 Other soft tissue disorders related to use, overuse and pressure of unspecified site

√6th M70.81 Other soft tissue disorders related to use, overuse and pressure of shoulder

M70.811 Other soft tissue disorders related to use, overuse and pressure, right shoulder

M70.812 Other soft tissue disorders related to use, overuse and pressure, left shoulder

M70.819 Other soft tissue disorders related to use, overuse and pressure, unspecified shoulder

√6th M70.82 Other soft tissue disorders related to use, overuse and pressure of upper arm

M70.821 Other soft tissue disorders related to use, overuse and pressure, right upper arm

M70.822 Other soft tissue disorders related to use, overuse and pressure, left upper arm

M70.829 Other soft tissue disorders related to use, overuse and pressure, unspecified upper arms

√6th M70.83 Other soft tissue disorders related to use, overuse and pressure of forearm

M70.831 Other soft tissue disorders related to use, overuse and pressure, right forearm

M70.832 Other soft tissue disorders related to use, overuse and pressure, left forearm

✓ Additional Character Required   √x7th Xtension Alert   Unacceptable PDx   Manifestation   Hospital Acquired Condition   EXCLUDES 1 Not Coded Here   EXCLUDES 2 Not Included Here

ICD-10-CM Draft (2015)   735

Diseases of the Musculoskeletal System and Connective Tissue

M70.839–M71.09

     M70.839   Other soft tissue disorders related to use, overuse and pressure, unspecified forearm

√6ᵗʰ M70.84   Other soft tissue disorders related to use, overuse and pressure of hand
     M70.841   Other soft tissue disorders related to use, overuse and pressure, right hand
     M70.842   Other soft tissue disorders related to use, overuse and pressure, left hand
     M70.849   Other soft tissue disorders related to use, overuse and pressure, unspecified hand

√6ᵗʰ M70.85   Other soft tissue disorders related to use, overuse and pressure of thigh
     M70.851   Other soft tissue disorders related to use, overuse and pressure, right thigh
     M70.852   Other soft tissue disorders related to use, overuse and pressure, left thigh
     M70.859   Other soft tissue disorders related to use, overuse and pressure, unspecified thigh

√6ᵗʰ M70.86   Other soft tissue disorders related to use, overuse and pressure lower leg
     M70.861   Other soft tissue disorders related to use, overuse and pressure, right lower leg
     M70.862   Other soft tissue disorders related to use, overuse and pressure, left lower leg
     M70.869   Other soft tissue disorders related to use, overuse and pressure, unspecified leg

√6ᵗʰ M70.87   Other soft tissue disorders related to use, overuse and pressure of ankle and foot
     M70.871   Other soft tissue disorders related to use, overuse and pressure, right ankle and foot
     M70.872   Other soft tissue disorders related to use, overuse and pressure, left ankle and foot
     M70.879   Other soft tissue disorders related to use, overuse and pressure, unspecified ankle and foot

     M70.88   Other soft tissue disorders related to use, overuse and pressure other site

     M70.89   Other soft tissue disorders related to use, overuse and pressure multiple sites

√5ᵗʰ M70.9   Unspecified soft tissue disorder related to use, overuse and pressure

     M70.90   Unspecified soft tissue disorder related to use, overuse and pressure of unspecified site

√6ᵗʰ M70.91   Unspecified soft tissue disorder related to use, overuse and pressure of shoulder
     M70.911   Unspecified soft tissue disorder related to use, overuse and pressure, right shoulder
     M70.912   Unspecified soft tissue disorder related to use, overuse and pressure, left shoulder
     M70.919   Unspecified soft tissue disorder related to use, overuse and pressure, unspecified shoulder

√6ᵗʰ M70.92   Unspecified soft tissue disorder related to use, overuse and pressure of upper arm
     M70.921   Unspecified soft tissue disorder related to use, overuse and pressure, right upper arm
     M70.922   Unspecified soft tissue disorder related to use, overuse and pressure, left upper arm
     M70.929   Unspecified soft tissue disorder related to use, overuse and pressure, unspecified upper arm

√6ᵗʰ M70.93   Unspecified soft tissue disorder related to use, overuse and pressure of forearm
     M70.931   Unspecified soft tissue disorder related to use, overuse and pressure, right forearm
     M70.932   Unspecified soft tissue disorder related to use, overuse and pressure, left forearm
     M70.939   Unspecified soft tissue disorder related to use, overuse and pressure, unspecified forearm

√6ᵗʰ M70.94   Unspecified soft tissue disorder related to use, overuse and pressure of hand
     M70.941   Unspecified soft tissue disorder related to use, overuse and pressure, right hand
     M70.942   Unspecified soft tissue disorder related to use, overuse and pressure, left hand

     M70.949   Unspecified soft tissue disorder related to use, overuse and pressure, unspecified hand

√6ᵗʰ M70.95   Unspecified soft tissue disorder related to use, overuse and pressure of thigh
     M70.951   Unspecified soft tissue disorder related to use, overuse and pressure, right thigh
     M70.952   Unspecified soft tissue disorder related to use, overuse and pressure, left thigh
     M70.959   Unspecified soft tissue disorder related to use, overuse and pressure, unspecified thigh

√6ᵗʰ M70.96   Unspecified soft tissue disorder related to use, overuse and pressure lower leg
     M70.961   Unspecified soft tissue disorder related to use, overuse and pressure, right lower leg
     M70.962   Unspecified soft tissue disorder related to use, overuse and pressure, left lower leg
     M70.969   Unspecified soft tissue disorder related to use, overuse and pressure, unspecified lower leg

√6ᵗʰ M70.97   Unspecified soft tissue disorder related to use, overuse and pressure of ankle and foot
     M70.971   Unspecified soft tissue disorder related to use, overuse and pressure, right ankle and foot
     M70.972   Unspecified soft tissue disorder related to use, overuse and pressure, left ankle and foot
     M70.979   Unspecified soft tissue disorder related to use, overuse and pressure, unspecified ankle and foot

     M70.98   Unspecified soft tissue disorder related to use, overuse and pressure other

     M70.99   Unspecified soft tissue disorder related to use, overuse and pressure multiple sites

√4ᵗʰ **M71 Other bursopathies**
     EXCLUDES 1   bunion (M20.1)
         bursitis related to use, overuse or pressure (M70.-)
         enthesopathies (M76-M77)

√5ᵗʰ M71.0   Abscess of bursa
     Use additional code (B95.-, B96.-) to identify causative organism

     M71.00   Abscess of bursa, unspecified site

√6ᵗʰ M71.01   Abscess of bursa, shoulder
     M71.011   Abscess of bursa, right shoulder
     M71.012   Abscess of bursa, left shoulder
     M71.019   Abscess of bursa, unspecified shoulder

√6ᵗʰ M71.02   Abscess of bursa, elbow
     M71.021   Abscess of bursa, right elbow
     M71.022   Abscess of bursa, left elbow
     M71.029   Abscess of bursa, unspecified elbow

√6ᵗʰ M71.03   Abscess of bursa, wrist
     M71.031   Abscess of bursa, right wrist
     M71.032   Abscess of bursa, left wrist
     M71.039   Abscess of bursa, unspecified wrist

√6ᵗʰ M71.04   Abscess of bursa, hand
     M71.041   Abscess of bursa, right hand
     M71.042   Abscess of bursa, left hand
     M71.049   Abscess of bursa, unspecified hand

√6ᵗʰ M71.05   Abscess of bursa, hip
     M71.051   Abscess of bursa, right hip
     M71.052   Abscess of bursa, left hip
     M71.059   Abscess of bursa, unspecified hip

√6ᵗʰ M71.06   Abscess of bursa, knee
     M71.061   Abscess of bursa, right knee
     M71.062   Abscess of bursa, left knee
     M71.069   Abscess of bursa, unspecified knee

√6ᵗʰ M71.07   Abscess of bursa, ankle and foot
     M71.071   Abscess of bursa, right ankle and foot
     M71.072   Abscess of bursa, left ankle and foot
     M71.079   Abscess of bursa, unspecified ankle and foot

     M71.08   Abscess of bursa, other site

     M71.09   Abscess of bursa, multiple sites

N Newborn: 0   **P** Pediatric: 0-17   **M** Maternity: 12-55   **A** Adult: 15-124   **MCC** Major CC Condition   **PDx MCC** PDx acts as own MCC   **CC** CC Condition   **PDx CC** PDx acts as own CC

736   ICD-10-CM Draft (2015)

✓5th **M71.1 Other infective bursitis**

> Use additional code (B95.-, B96.-) to identify causative organism

    M71.10 Other infective bursitis, unspecified site

✓6th **M71.11 Other infective bursitis, shoulder**

    M71.111 Other infective bursitis, right shoulder
    M71.112 Other infective bursitis, left shoulder
    M71.119 Other infective bursitis, unspecified shoulder

✓6th **M71.12 Other infective bursitis, elbow**

    M71.121 Other infective bursitis, right elbow
    M71.122 Other infective bursitis, left elbow
    M71.129 Other infective bursitis, unspecified elbow

✓6th **M71.13 Other infective bursitis, wrist**

    M71.131 Other infective bursitis, right wrist
    M71.132 Other infective bursitis, left wrist
    M71.139 Other infective bursitis, unspecified wrist

✓6th **M71.14 Other infective bursitis, hand**

    M71.141 Other infective bursitis, right hand
    M71.142 Other infective bursitis, left hand
    M71.149 Other infective bursitis, unspecified hand

✓6th **M71.15 Other infective bursitis, hip**

    M71.151 Other infective bursitis, right hip
    M71.152 Other infective bursitis, left hip
    M71.159 Other infective bursitis, unspecified hip

✓6th **M71.16 Other infective bursitis, knee**

    M71.161 Other infective bursitis, right knee
    M71.162 Other infective bursitis, left knee
    M71.169 Other infective bursitis, unspecified knee

✓6th **M71.17 Other infective bursitis, ankle and foot**

    M71.171 Other infective bursitis, right ankle and foot
    M71.172 Other infective bursitis, left ankle and foot
    M71.179 Other infective bursitis, unspecified ankle and foot

    M71.18 Other infective bursitis, other site

    M71.19 Other infective bursitis, multiple sites

✓5th **M71.2 Synovial cyst of popliteal space [Baker]**

> EXCLUDES 1   synovial cyst of popliteal space with rupture (M66.0)

    M71.20 Synovial cyst of popliteal space [Baker], unspecified knee

    M71.21 Synovial cyst of popliteal space [Baker], right knee

    M71.22 Synovial cyst of popliteal space [Baker], left knee

✓5th **M71.3 Other bursal cyst**

> Synovial cyst NOS
>
> EXCLUDES 1   synovial cyst with rupture (M66.1-)

    M71.30 Other bursal cyst, unspecified site

✓6th **M71.31 Other bursal cyst, shoulder**

    M71.311 Other bursal cyst, right shoulder
    M71.312 Other bursal cyst, left shoulder
    M71.319 Other bursal cyst, unspecified shoulder

✓6th **M71.32 Other bursal cyst, elbow**

    M71.321 Other bursal cyst, right elbow
    M71.322 Other bursal cyst, left elbow
    M71.329 Other bursal cyst, unspecified elbow

✓6th **M71.33 Other bursal cyst, wrist**

    M71.331 Other bursal cyst, right wrist
    M71.332 Other bursal cyst, left wrist
    M71.339 Other bursal cyst, unspecified wrist

✓6th **M71.34 Other bursal cyst, hand**

    M71.341 Other bursal cyst, right hand
    M71.342 Other bursal cyst, left hand
    M71.349 Other bursal cyst, unspecified hand

✓6th **M71.35 Other bursal cyst, hip**

    M71.351 Other bursal cyst, right hip
    M71.352 Other bursal cyst, left hip
    M71.359 Other bursal cyst, unspecified hip

✓6th **M71.37 Other bursal cyst, ankle and foot**

    M71.371 Other bursal cyst, right ankle and foot
    M71.372 Other bursal cyst, left ankle and foot
    M71.379 Other bursal cyst, unspecified ankle and foot

    M71.38 Other bursal cyst, other site

    M71.39 Other bursal cyst, multiple sites

✓5th **M71.4 Calcium deposit in bursa**

> EXCLUDES 2   calcium deposit in bursa of shoulder (M75.3)

    M71.40 Calcium deposit in bursa, unspecified site

✓6th **M71.42 Calcium deposit in bursa, elbow**

    M71.421 Calcium deposit in bursa, right elbow
    M71.422 Calcium deposit in bursa, left elbow
    M71.429 Calcium deposit in bursa, unspecified elbow

✓6th **M71.43 Calcium deposit in bursa, wrist**

    M71.431 Calcium deposit in bursa, right wrist
    M71.432 Calcium deposit in bursa, left wrist
    M71.439 Calcium deposit in bursa, unspecified wrist

✓6th **M71.44 Calcium deposit in bursa, hand**

    M71.441 Calcium deposit in bursa, right hand
    M71.442 Calcium deposit in bursa, left hand
    M71.449 Calcium deposit in bursa, unspecified hand

✓6th **M71.45 Calcium deposit in bursa, hip**

    M71.451 Calcium deposit in bursa, right hip
    M71.452 Calcium deposit in bursa, left hip
    M71.459 Calcium deposit in bursa, unspecified hip

✓6th **M71.46 Calcium deposit in bursa, knee**

    M71.461 Calcium deposit in bursa, right knee
    M71.462 Calcium deposit in bursa, left knee
    M71.469 Calcium deposit in bursa, unspecified knee

✓6th **M71.47 Calcium deposit in bursa, ankle and foot**

    M71.471 Calcium deposit in bursa, right ankle and foot
    M71.472 Calcium deposit in bursa, left ankle and foot
    M71.479 Calcium deposit in bursa, unspecified ankle and foot

    M71.48 Calcium deposit in bursa, other site

    M71.49 Calcium deposit in bursa, multiple sites

✓5th **M71.5 Other bursitis, not elsewhere classified**

> EXCLUDES 1   bursitis NOS (M71.9-)
>
> EXCLUDES 2   bursitis of shoulder (M75.5)
>   bursitis of tibial collateral [Pellegrini-Stieda] (M76.4)

    M71.50 Other bursitis, not elsewhere classified, unspecified site

✓6th **M71.52 Other bursitis, not elsewhere classified, elbow**

    M71.521 Other bursitis, not elsewhere classified, right elbow
    M71.522 Other bursitis, not elsewhere classified, left elbow
    M71.529 Other bursitis, not elsewhere classified, unspecified elbow

✓6th **M71.53 Other bursitis, not elsewhere classified, wrist**

    M71.531 Other bursitis, not elsewhere classified, right wrist
    M71.532 Other bursitis, not elsewhere classified, left wrist
    M71.539 Other bursitis, not elsewhere classified, unspecified wrist

✓6th **M71.54 Other bursitis, not elsewhere classified, hand**

    M71.541 Other bursitis, not elsewhere classified, right hand
    M71.542 Other bursitis, not elsewhere classified, left hand
    M71.549 Other bursitis, not elsewhere classified, unspecified hand

✓6th **M71.55 Other bursitis, not elsewhere classified, hip**

    M71.551 Other bursitis, not elsewhere classified, right hip
    M71.552 Other bursitis, not elsewhere classified, left hip
    M71.559 Other bursitis, not elsewhere classified, unspecified hip

✓6th **M71.56 Other bursitis, not elsewhere classified, knee**

    M71.561 Other bursitis, not elsewhere classified, right knee

✓ Additional Character Required   ✓x7th Xtension Alert   Unacceptable PDx   Manifestation   Hospital Acquired Condition   EXCLUDES 1 Not Coded Here   EXCLUDES 2 Not Included Here

ICD-10-CM Draft (2015)   737

M71.562   Other bursitis, not elsewhere classified, left knee

M71.569   Other bursitis, not elsewhere classified, unspecified knee

✓6th **M71.57**   Other bursitis, not elsewhere classified, ankle and foot

M71.571   Other bursitis, not elsewhere classified, right ankle and foot

M71.572   Other bursitis, not elsewhere classified, left ankle and foot

M71.579   Other bursitis, not elsewhere classified, unspecified ankle and foot

M71.58   Other bursitis, not elsewhere classified, other site

✓5th **M71.8**   **Other specified bursopathies**

M71.80   Other specified bursopathies, unspecified site

✓6th **M71.81**   Other specified bursopathies, shoulder

M71.811   Other specified bursopathies, right shoulder

M71.812   Other specified bursopathies, left shoulder

M71.819   Other specified bursopathies, unspecified shoulder

✓6th **M71.82**   Other specified bursopathies, elbow

M71.821   Other specified bursopathies, right elbow

M71.822   Other specified bursopathies, left elbow

M71.829   Other specified bursopathies, unspecified elbow

✓6th **M71.83**   Other specified bursopathies, wrist

M71.831   Other specified bursopathies, right wrist

M71.832   Other specified bursopathies, left wrist

M71.839   Other specified bursopathies, unspecified wrist

✓6th **M71.84**   Other specified bursopathies, hand

M71.841   Other specified bursopathies, right hand

M71.842   Other specified bursopathies, left hand

M71.849   Other specified bursopathies, unspecified hand

✓6th **M71.85**   Other specified bursopathies, hip

M71.851   Other specified bursopathies, right hip

M71.852   Other specified bursopathies, left hip

M71.859   Other specified bursopathies, unspecified hip

✓6th **M71.86**   Other specified bursopathies, knee

M71.861   Other specified bursopathies, right knee

M71.862   Other specified bursopathies, left knee

M71.869   Other specified bursopathies, unspecified knee

✓6th **M71.87**   Other specified bursopathies, ankle and foot

M71.871   Other specified bursopathies, right ankle and foot

M71.872   Other specified bursopathies, left ankle and foot

M71.879   Other specified bursopathies, unspecified ankle and foot

M71.88   Other specified bursopathies, other site

M71.89   Other specified bursopathies, multiple sites

M71.9   **Bursopathy, unspecified**
Bursitis NOS

✓4th **M72**   **Fibroblastic disorders**
EXCLUDES 2   retroperitoneal fibromatosis (D48.3)

M72.0   **Palmar fascial fibromatosis [Dupuytren]**   A

M72.1   **Knuckle pads**

M72.2   **Plantar fascial fibromatosis**
Plantar fasciitis

M72.4   **Pseudosarcomatous fibromatosis**
Nodular fasciitis

M72.6   **Necrotizing fasciitis**   MCC
Use additional code (B95.-, B96.-) to identify causative organism
CC Excl: K68.12, M60.000-M60.19, M61.00-M61.19, M61.30-M61.59, M62.3, M62.50-M62.59, M62.89, M72.6

M72.8   **Other fibroblastic disorders**
Abscess of fascia
Fasciitis NEC
Other infective fasciitis
Use additional code to (B95.-, B96.-) identify causative organism
EXCLUDES 1   diffuse (eosinophilic) fasciitis (M35.4)
necrotizing fasciitis (M72.6)
nodular fasciitis (M72.4)
perirenal fasciitis NOS (N13.5)
perirenal fasciitis with infection (N13.6)
plantar fasciitis (M72.2)

M72.9   **Fibroblastic disorder, unspecified**
Fasciitis NOS   Fibromatosis NOS

✓4th **M75**   **Shoulder lesions**
EXCLUDES 2   shoulder-hand syndrome (M89.0-)

✓5th **M75.0**   **Adhesive capsulitis of shoulder**
Frozen shoulder
Periarthritis of shoulder

M75.00   Adhesive capsulitis of unspecified shoulder

M75.01   Adhesive capsulitis of right shoulder

M75.02   Adhesive capsulitis of left shoulder

✓5th **M75.1**   **Rotator cuff tear or rupture, not specified as traumatic**
Rotator cuff syndrome
Supraspinatus syndrome
Supraspinatus tear or rupture, not specified as traumatic
EXCLUDES 1   tear of rotator cuff, traumatic (S46.01-)

✓6th **M75.10**   Unspecified rotator cuff tear or rupture, not specified as traumatic

M75.100   Unspecified rotator cuff tear or rupture of unspecified shoulder, not specified as traumatic

M75.101   Unspecified rotator cuff tear or rupture of right shoulder, not specified as traumatic

M75.102   Unspecified rotator cuff tear or rupture of left shoulder, not specified as traumatic

✓6th **M75.11**   Incomplete rotator cuff tear or rupture not specified as traumatic

M75.110   Incomplete rotator cuff tear or rupture of unspecified shoulder, not specified as traumatic

M75.111   Incomplete rotator cuff tear or rupture of right shoulder, not specified as traumatic

M75.112   Incomplete rotator cuff tear or rupture of left shoulder, not specified as traumatic

✓6th **M75.12**   Complete rotator cuff tear or rupture not specified as traumatic

M75.120   Complete rotator cuff tear or rupture of unspecified shoulder, not specified as traumatic

M75.121   Complete rotator cuff tear or rupture of right shoulder, not specified as traumatic

M75.122   Complete rotator cuff tear or rupture of left shoulder, not specified as traumatic

✓5th **M75.2**   **Bicipital tendinitis**

M75.20   Bicipital tendinitis, unspecified shoulder

M75.21   Bicipital tendinitis, right shoulder

M75.22   Bicipital tendinitis, left shoulder

✓5th **M75.3**   **Calcific tendinitis of shoulder**
Calcified bursa of shoulder

M75.30   Calcific tendinitis of unspecified shoulder

M75.31   Calcific tendinitis of right shoulder

M75.32   Calcific tendinitis of left shoulder

✓5th **M75.4**   **Impingement syndrome of shoulder**

M75.40   Impingement syndrome of unspecified shoulder

M75.41   Impingement syndrome of right shoulder

M75.42   Impingement syndrome of left shoulder

✓5th **M75.5**   **Bursitis of shoulder**

M75.50   Bursitis of unspecified shoulder

M75.51   Bursitis of right shoulder

M75.52   Bursitis of left shoulder

✓5th **M75.8**   **Other shoulder lesions**

M75.80   Other shoulder lesions, unspecified shoulder

M75.81   Other shoulder lesions, right shoulder

M75.82   Other shoulder lesions, left shoulder

N Newborn: 0   P Pediatric: 0-17   M Maternity: 12-55   A Adult: 15-124   MCC Major CC Condition   PDx MCC PDx acts as own MCC   CC CC Condition   PDx CC PDx acts as own CC

738   ICD-10-CM Draft (2015)

✓5ᵗʰ **M75.9 Shoulder lesion, unspecified**
    M75.90 Shoulder lesion, unspecified, unspecified shoulder
    M75.91 Shoulder lesion, unspecified, right shoulder
    M75.92 Shoulder lesion, unspecified, left shoulder

✓4ᵗʰ **M76 Enthesopathies, lower limb, excluding foot**
    EXCLUDES 2 bursitis due to use, overuse and pressure (M70.-)
      enthesopathies of ankle and foot (M77.5-)

✓5ᵗʰ **M76.0 Gluteal tendinitis**
    M76.00 Gluteal tendinitis, unspecified hip
    M76.01 Gluteal tendinitis, right hip
    M76.02 Gluteal tendinitis, left hip

✓5ᵗʰ **M76.1 Psoas tendinitis**
    M76.10 Psoas tendinitis, unspecified hip
    M76.11 Psoas tendinitis, right hip
    M76.12 Psoas tendinitis, left hip

✓5ᵗʰ **M76.2 Iliac crest spur**
    M76.20 Iliac crest spur, unspecified hip
    M76.21 Iliac crest spur, right hip
    M76.22 Iliac crest spur, left hip

✓5ᵗʰ **M76.3 Iliotibial band syndrome**
    M76.30 Iliotibial band syndrome, unspecified leg
    M76.31 Iliotibial band syndrome, right leg
    M76.32 Iliotibial band syndrome, left leg

✓5ᵗʰ **M76.4 Tibial collateral bursitis [Pellegrini-Stieda]**
    M76.40 Tibial collateral bursitis [Pellegrini-Stieda], unspecified leg
    M76.41 Tibial collateral bursitis [Pellegrini-Stieda], right leg
    M76.42 Tibial collateral bursitis [Pellegrini-Stieda], left leg

✓5ᵗʰ **M76.5 Patellar tendinitis**
    M76.50 Patellar tendinitis, unspecified knee
    M76.51 Patellar tendinitis, right knee
    M76.52 Patellar tendinitis, left knee

✓5ᵗʰ **M76.6 Achilles tendinitis**
    Achilles bursitis
    M76.60 Achilles tendinitis, unspecified leg
    M76.61 Achilles tendinitis, right leg
    M76.62 Achilles tendinitis, left leg

✓5ᵗʰ **M76.7 Peroneal tendinitis**
    M76.70 Peroneal tendinitis, unspecified leg
    M76.71 Peroneal tendinitis, right leg
    M76.72 Peroneal tendinitis, left leg

✓5ᵗʰ **M76.8 Other specified enthesopathies of lower limb, excluding foot**
    ✓6ᵗʰ M76.81 Anterior tibial syndrome
      M76.811 Anterior tibial syndrome, right leg
      M76.812 Anterior tibial syndrome, left leg
      M76.819 Anterior tibial syndrome, unspecified leg
    ✓6ᵗʰ M76.82 Posterior tibial tendinitis
      M76.821 Posterior tibial tendinitis, right leg
      M76.822 Posterior tibial tendinitis, left leg
      M76.829 Posterior tibial tendinitis, unspecified leg
    ✓6ᵗʰ M76.89 Other specified enthesopathies of lower limb, excluding foot
      M76.891 Other specified enthesopathies of right lower limb, excluding foot
      M76.892 Other specified enthesopathies of left lower limb, excluding foot
      M76.899 Other specified enthesopathies of unspecified lower limb, excluding foot

M76.9 Unspecified enthesopathy, lower limb, excluding foot

✓4ᵗʰ **M77 Other enthesopathies**
    EXCLUDES 1 bursitis NOS (M71.9-)
    EXCLUDES 2 bursitis due to use, overuse and pressure (M70.-)
      osteophyte (M25.7)
      spinal enthesopathy (M46.0-)

✓5ᵗʰ **M77.0 Medial epicondylitis**
    M77.00 Medial epicondylitis, unspecified elbow
    M77.01 Medial epicondylitis, right elbow
    M77.02 Medial epicondylitis, left elbow

✓5ᵗʰ **M77.1 Lateral epicondylitis**
    Tennis elbow
    M77.10 Lateral epicondylitis, unspecified elbow
    M77.11 Lateral epicondylitis, right elbow
    M77.12 Lateral epicondylitis, left elbow

✓5ᵗʰ **M77.2 Periarthritis of wrist**
    M77.20 Periarthritis, unspecified wrist
    M77.21 Periarthritis, right wrist
    M77.22 Periarthritis, left wrist

✓5ᵗʰ **M77.3 Calcaneal spur**
    M77.30 Calcaneal spur, unspecified foot
    M77.31 Calcaneal spur, right foot
    M77.32 Calcaneal spur, left foot

✓5ᵗʰ **M77.4 Metatarsalgia**
    EXCLUDES 1 Morton's metatarsalgia (G57.6)
    M77.40 Metatarsalgia, unspecified foot
    M77.41 Metatarsalgia, right foot
    M77.42 Metatarsalgia, left foot

✓5ᵗʰ **M77.5 Other enthesopathy of foot**
    M77.50 Other enthesopathy of unspecified foot
    M77.51 Other enthesopathy of right foot
    M77.52 Other enthesopathy of left foot

M77.8 Other enthesopathies, not elsewhere classified

M77.9 Enthesopathy, unspecified
    Bone spur NOS   Periarthritis NOS
    Capsulitis NOS   Tendinitis NOS

✓4ᵗʰ **M79 Other and unspecified soft tissue disorders, not elsewhere classified**
    EXCLUDES 1 psychogenic rheumatism (F45.8)
      soft tissue pain, psychogenic (F45.41)

M79.0 Rheumatism, unspecified
    EXCLUDES 1 fibromyalgia (M79.7)
      palindromic rheumatism (M12.3-)

M79.1 Myalgia
    Myofascial pain syndrome
    EXCLUDES 1 fibromyalgia (M79.7)
      myositis (M60.-)

M79.2 Neuralgia and neuritis, unspecified
    EXCLUDES 1 brachial radiculitis NOS (M54.1)
      lumbosacral radiculitis NOS (M54.1)
      mononeuropathies (G56-G58)
      radiculitis NOS (M54.1)
      sciatica (M54.3-M54.4)

M79.3 Panniculitis, unspecified
    EXCLUDES 1 lupus panniculitis (L93.2)
      neck and back panniculitis (M54.0-)
      relapsing [Weber-Christian] panniculitis (M35.6)

M79.4 Hypertrophy of (infrapatellar) fat pad

M79.5 Residual foreign body in soft tissue
    EXCLUDES 1 foreign body granuloma of skin and subcutaneous tissue (L92.3)
      foreign body granuloma of soft tissue (M60.2-)

✓5ᵗʰ **M79.6 Pain in limb, hand, foot, fingers and toes**
    EXCLUDES 2 pain in joint (M25.5-)
    ✓6ᵗʰ M79.60 Pain in limb, unspecified
      M79.601 Pain in right arm
      Pain in right upper limb NOS
      M79.602 Pain in left arm
      Pain in left upper limb NOS
      M79.603 Pain in arm, unspecified
      Pain in upper limb NOS
      M79.604 Pain in right leg
      Pain in right lower limb NOS
      M79.605 Pain in left leg
      Pain in left lower limb NOS
      M79.606 Pain in leg, unspecified
      Pain in lower limb NOS
      M79.609 Pain in unspecified limb
      Pain in limb NOS
    ✓6ᵗʰ M79.62 Pain in upper arm
      Pain in axillary region
      M79.621 Pain in right upper arm
      M79.622 Pain in left upper arm
      M79.629 Pain in unspecified upper arm

Diseases of the Musculoskeletal System and Connective Tissue

M79.63–M80.032

✓6th **M79.63 Pain in forearm**
    M79.631 Pain in right forearm
    M79.632 Pain in left forearm
    M79.639 Pain in unspecified forearm

✓6th **M79.64 Pain in hand and fingers**
    M79.641 Pain in right hand
    M79.642 Pain in left hand
    M79.643 Pain in unspecified hand
    M79.644 Pain in right finger(s)
    M79.645 Pain in left finger(s)
    M79.646 Pain in unspecified finger(s)

✓6th **M79.65 Pain in thigh**
    M79.651 Pain in right thigh
    M79.652 Pain in left thigh
    M79.659 Pain in unspecified thigh

✓6th **M79.66 Pain in lower leg**
    M79.661 Pain in right lower leg
    M79.662 Pain in left lower leg
    M79.669 Pain in unspecified lower leg

✓6th **M79.67 Pain in foot and toes**
    M79.671 Pain in right foot
    M79.672 Pain in left foot
    M79.673 Pain in unspecified foot
    M79.674 Pain in right toe(s)
    M79.675 Pain in left toe(s)
    M79.676 Pain in unspecified toe(s)

M79.7 Fibromyalgia
    Fibromyositis   Myofibrositis
    Fibrositis

✓5th **M79.A Nontraumatic compartment syndrome**
    Code first, if applicable, associated postprocedural complication
    EXCLUDES 1   compartment syndrome NOS (T79.A-)
       fibromyalgia (M79.7)
       nontraumatic ischemic infarction of muscle (M62.2-)
       traumatic compartment syndrome (T79.A-)

✓6th **M79.A1 Nontraumatic compartment syndrome of upper extremity**
    Nontraumatic compartment syndrome of shoulder, arm, forearm, wrist, hand, and fingers

    CC Excl: M70.80-M70.99, M79.81-M79.9, R29.898, S45.301-S45.899 with 7th A, S55.201-S55.899 with 7th A, S65.801-S65.899 with 7th A

    M79.A11 Nontraumatic compartment syndrome CC **of right upper extremity**
    M79.A12 Nontraumatic compartment syndrome CC **of left upper extremity**
    M79.A19 Nontraumatic compartment syndrome CC **of unspecified upper extremity**

✓6th **M79.A2 Nontraumatic compartment syndrome of lower extremity**
    Nontraumatic compartment syndrome of hip, buttock, thigh, leg, foot, and toes

    CC Excl: M70.80-M70.99, M79.81-M79.9, R29.898, S75.801-S75.899 with 7th A, S85.201-S85.299 with 7th A, S85.801-S85.899 with 7th A, S95.001-S95.099 with 7th A, S95.201-S95.899 with 7th A

    M79.A21 Nontraumatic compartment syndrome CC **of right lower extremity**
    M79.A22 Nontraumatic compartment syndrome CC **of left lower extremity**
    M79.A29 Nontraumatic compartment syndrome CC **of unspecified lower extremity**

M79.A3 Nontraumatic compartment syndrome of CC **abdomen**
    CC Excl: S31.001 with 7th A, S31.011 with 7th A, S31.021 with 7th A, S31.031 with 7th A, S31.041 with 7th A, S31.051-S31.159 with 7th A, S31.600-S31.659 with 7th A, S31.831-S31.839 with 7th A, S36.00-S37.99 with 7th A, S38.3XX-S39.023 with 7th A, T14.8-T14.91, T79.8XX-T79.9XX with 7th A

M79.A9 Nontraumatic compartment syndrome of other CC **sites**
    CC Excl: S31.001 with 7th A, S31.011 with 7th A, S31.021 with 7th A, S31.031 with 7th A, S31.041 with 7th A, S31.051 with 7th A, S31.600-S31.659 with 7th A, S36.81X-S36.899 with 7th A

✓5th **M79.8 Other specified soft tissue disorders**

M79.81 Nontraumatic hematoma of soft tissue
    Nontraumatic hematoma of muscle
    Nontraumatic seroma of muscle and soft tissue

M79.89 Other specified soft tissue disorders
    Polyalgia

M79.9 Soft tissue disorder, unspecified

OSTEOPATHIES AND CHONDROPATHIES (M80-M94)

Disorders of bone density and structure (M80-M85)

✓4th **M80 Osteoporosis with current pathological fracture**
    INCLUDES   osteoporosis with current fragility fracture
    Use additional code to identify major osseous defect, if applicable (M89.7-)
    EXCLUDES 1   collapsed vertebra NOS (M48.5)
       pathological fracture NOS (M84.4)
       wedging of vertebra NOS (M48.5)
    EXCLUDES 2   personal history of (healed) osteoporosis fracture (Z87.310)

    The appropriate 7th character is to be added to each code from category M80.
    A   initial encounter for fracture
    D   subsequent encounter for fracture with routine healing
    G   subsequent encounter for fracture with delayed healing
    K   subsequent encounter for fracture with nonunion
    P   subsequent encounter for fracture with malunion
    S   sequela

    CC Excl: For codes M80, CC with 7th character A, unless otherwise noted: M48.40X-M48.58X with 7th A, M80.00X-M84.68X with 7th A
    CC codes with 7th character K or P: M80.00X-M84.68X with 7th [K, P], S02.0XX-S02.92X with 7th K, S12.000-S12.691 with 7th K, S22.000-S22.9XX with 7th K, S32.000-S32.9XX with 7th K, S42.001-S42.92 with 7th [K, P], S49.001-S49.199 with 7th [K, P], S52.001-S52.92X with 7th [K, M, N, P, Q, R], S59.001-S59.299 with 7th [K, P], S62.001-S62.92X with 7th [K, P], S72.001-S72.92X with 7th [K, M, N, P, Q, R], S79.001-S79.199 with 7th [K, P], S82.001-S82.92X with 7th [K, M, N, P, Q, R], S89.001-S89.399 with 7th [K, P], S92.001-S92.919 with 7th [K, P]

✓5th **M80.0 Age-related osteoporosis with current pathological fracture**
    Involutional osteoporosis with current pathological fracture
    Osteoporosis NOS with current pathological fracture
    Postmenopausal osteoporosis with current pathological fracture
    Senile osteoporosis with current pathological fracture

✓x7th **M80.00 Age-related osteoporosis with current pathological fracture, unspecified site** CC A

✓6th **M80.01 Age-related osteoporosis with current pathological fracture, shoulder**
    ✓7th **M80.011 Age-related osteoporosis with current pathological fracture, right shoulder** CC A
    ✓7th **M80.012 Age-related osteoporosis with current pathological fracture, left shoulder** CC A
    ✓7th **M80.019 Age-related osteoporosis with current pathological fracture, unspecified shoulder** CC A

✓6th **M80.02 Age-related osteoporosis with current pathological fracture, humerus**
    ✓7th **M80.021 Age-related osteoporosis with current pathological fracture, right humerus** CC A
    ✓7th **M80.022 Age-related osteoporosis with current pathological fracture, left humerus** CC A
    ✓7th **M80.029 Age-related osteoporosis with current pathological fracture, unspecified humerus** CC A

✓6th **M80.03 Age-related osteoporosis with current pathological fracture, forearm**
    Age-related osteoporosis with current pathological fracture of wrist
    ✓7th **M80.031 Age-related osteoporosis with current pathological fracture, right forearm** CC A
    ✓7th **M80.032 Age-related osteoporosis with current pathological fracture, left forearm** CC A

✓7th **M80.039** Age-related osteoporosis with current pathological fracture, **unspecified forearm**   `cc` `A`

✓6th **M80.04** Age-related osteoporosis with current pathological fracture, **hand**

✓7th **M80.041** Age-related osteoporosis with current pathological fracture, **right hand**   `cc` `A`

✓7th **M80.042** Age-related osteoporosis with current pathological fracture, **left hand**   `cc` `A`

✓7th **M80.049** Age-related osteoporosis with current pathological fracture, **unspecified hand**   `cc` `A`

✓6th **M80.05** Age-related osteoporosis with current pathological fracture, **femur**
Age-related osteoporosis with current pathological fracture of hip

✓7th **M80.051** Age-related osteoporosis with current pathological fracture, **right femur**   `cc` `A`

✓7th **M80.052** Age-related osteoporosis with current pathological fracture, **left femur**   `cc` `A`

✓7th **M80.059** Age-related osteoporosis with current pathological fracture, **unspecified femur**   `cc` `A`

✓6th **M80.06** Age-related osteoporosis with current pathological fracture, **lower leg**

✓7th **M80.061** Age-related osteoporosis with current pathological fracture, **right lower leg**   `cc` `A`

✓7th **M80.062** Age-related osteoporosis with current pathological fracture, **left lower leg**   `cc` `A`

✓7th **M80.069** Age-related osteoporosis with current pathological fracture, **unspecified lower leg**   `cc` `A`

✓6th **M80.07** Age-related osteoporosis with current pathological fracture, **ankle and foot**

✓7th **M80.071** Age-related osteoporosis with current pathological fracture, **right ankle and foot**   `cc` `A`

✓7th **M80.072** Age-related osteoporosis with current pathological fracture, **left ankle and foot**   `cc` `A`

✓7th **M80.079** Age-related osteoporosis with current pathological fracture, **unspecified ankle and foot**   `cc` `A`

✓x7th **M80.08** Age-related osteoporosis with current pathological fracture, **vertebra(e)**   `cc` `A`

✓5th **M80.8** Other osteoporosis with current pathological fracture
Drug-induced osteoporosis with current pathological fracture
Idiopathic osteoporosis with current pathological fracture
Osteoporosis of disuse with current pathological fracture
Postoophorectomy osteoporosis with current pathological fracture
Postsurgical malabsorption osteoporosis with current pathological fracture
Post-traumatic osteoporosis with current pathological fracture
Use additional code for adverse effect, if applicable, to identify drug (T36-T50 with fifth or sixth character 5)

✓x7th **M80.80** Other osteoporosis with current pathological fracture, **unspecified site**   `cc`

✓6th **M80.81** Other osteoporosis with pathological fracture, **shoulder**

✓7th **M80.811** Other osteoporosis with current pathological fracture, **right shoulder**   `cc`

✓7th **M80.812** Other osteoporosis with current pathological fracture, **left shoulder**   `cc`

✓7th **M80.819** Other osteoporosis with current pathological fracture, **unspecified shoulder**   `cc`

✓6th **M80.82** Other osteoporosis with current pathological fracture, **humerus**

✓7th **M80.821** Other osteoporosis with current pathological fracture, **right humerus**   `cc`

✓7th **M80.822** Other osteoporosis with current pathological fracture, **left humerus**   `cc`

✓7th **M80.829** Other osteoporosis with current pathological fracture, **unspecified humerus**   `cc`

✓6th **M80.83** Other osteoporosis with current pathological fracture, **forearm**
Other osteoporosis with current pathological fracture of wrist

✓7th **M80.831** Other osteoporosis with current pathological fracture, **right forearm**   `cc`

✓7th **M80.832** Other osteoporosis with current pathological fracture, **left forearm**   `cc`

✓7th **M80.839** Other osteoporosis with current pathological fracture, **unspecified forearm**   `cc`

✓6th **M80.84** Other osteoporosis with current pathological fracture, **hand**

✓7th **M80.841** Other osteoporosis with current pathological fracture, **right hand**   `cc`

✓7th **M80.842** Other osteoporosis with current pathological fracture, **left hand**   `cc`

✓7th **M80.849** Other osteoporosis with current pathological fracture, **unspecified hand**   `cc`

✓6th **M80.85** Other osteoporosis with current pathological fracture, **femur**
Other osteoporosis with current pathological fracture of hip

✓7th **M80.851** Other osteoporosis with current pathological fracture, **right femur**   `cc`

✓7th **M80.852** Other osteoporosis with current pathological fracture, **left femur**   `cc`

✓7th **M80.859** Other osteoporosis with current pathological fracture, **unspecified femur**   `cc`

✓6th **M80.86** Other osteoporosis with current pathological fracture, **lower leg**

✓7th **M80.861** Other osteoporosis with current pathological fracture, **right lower leg**   `cc`

✓7th **M80.862** Other osteoporosis with current pathological fracture, **left lower leg**   `cc`

✓7th **M80.869** Other osteoporosis with current pathological fracture, **unspecified lower leg**   `cc`

✓6th **M80.87** Other osteoporosis with current pathological fracture, **ankle and foot**

✓7th **M80.871** Other osteoporosis with current pathological fracture, **right ankle and foot**   `cc`

✓7th **M80.872** Other osteoporosis with current pathological fracture, **left ankle and foot**   `cc`

✓7th **M80.879** Other osteoporosis with current pathological fracture, **unspecified ankle and foot**   `cc`

✓x7th **M80.88** Other osteoporosis with current pathological fracture, **vertebra(e)**   `cc`

✓4th **M81** Osteoporosis **without current pathological fracture**
Use additional code to identify:
major osseous defect, if applicable (M89.7-)
personal history of (healed) osteoporosis fracture, if applicable (Z87.310)
EXCLUDES 1 *osteoporosis with current pathological fracture (M80.-)*
Sudeck's atrophy (M89.0)

M81.0 Age-related osteoporosis **without current pathological fracture**   `A`
Involutional osteoporosis without current pathological fracture
Osteoporosis NOS
Postmenopausal osteoporosis without current pathological fracture
Senile osteoporosis without current pathological fracture

M81.6 Localized **osteoporosis [Lequesne]**
EXCLUDES 1 *Sudeck's atrophy (M89.0)*

✓ Additional Character Required   ✓x7th Xtension Alert   Unacceptable PDx   Manifestation   Hospital Acquired Condition   **EXCLUDES 1** Not Coded Here   **EXCLUDES 2** Not Included Here

ICD-10-CM Draft (2015)   741

Diseases of the Musculoskeletal System and Connective Tissue

M81.8–M84.412

M81.8 Other osteoporosis without current pathological fracture
Drug-induced osteoporosis without current pathological fracture
Idiopathic osteoporosis without current pathological fracture
Osteoporosis of disuse without current pathological fracture
Postoophorectomy osteoporosis without current pathological fracture
Postsurgical malabsorption osteoporosis without current pathological fracture
Post-traumatic osteoporosis without current pathological fracture
Use additional code for adverse effect, if applicable, to identify drug (T36-T50 with fifth or sixth character 5)

✓4th **M83 Adult osteomalacia**
> EXCLUDES 1   infantile and juvenile osteomalacia (E55.0)
> renal osteodystrophy (N25.0)
> rickets (active) (E55.0)
> rickets (active) sequelae (E64.3)
> vitamin D-resistant osteomalacia (E83.3)
> vitamin D-resistant rickets (active) (E83.3)

M83.0 Puerperal osteomalacia   M♀

M83.1 Senile osteomalacia   A

M83.2 Adult osteomalacia due to malabsorption   A
Postsurgical malabsorption osteomalacia in adults

M83.3 Adult osteomalacia due to malnutrition   A

M83.4 Aluminum bone disease

M83.5 Other drug-induced osteomalacia in adults   A
Use additional code for adverse effect, if applicable, to identify drug (T36-T50 with fifth or sixth character 5)

M83.8 Other adult osteomalacia   A

M83.9 Adult osteomalacia, unspecified   A

✓4th **M84 Disorder of continuity of bone**
> EXCLUDES 2   traumatic fracture of bone-see fracture, by site

✓5th **M84.3 Stress fracture**
Fatigue fracture   Stress fracture NOS
March fracture   Stress reaction
Use additional external cause code(s) to identify the cause of the stress fracture
> EXCLUDES 1   pathological fracture NOS (M84.4-)
> pathological fracture due to osteoporosis (M80.-)
> traumatic fracture (S12-, S22-, S32-, S42-, S52-, S62-, S72-, S82-, S92-)
> EXCLUDES 2   personal history of (healed) stress (fatigue) fracture (Z87.312)
> stress fracture of vertebra (M48.4-)

The appropriate 7th character is to be added to each code from subcategory M84.3.
A   initial encounter for fracture
D   subsequent encounter for fracture with routine healing
G   subsequent encounter for fracture with delayed healing
K   subsequent encounter for fracture with nonunion
P   subsequent encounter for fracture with malunion
S   sequela

CC Excl: For CC codes in subcatagory M84.3, unless otherwise noted: For CC codes with 7th character K or P: M80.00X-M84.68X with 7th [K, P], S02.0XX-S02.92X with 7th K, S12.000-S12.691 with 7th K, S22.000-S22.9XX with 7th K, S32000-S32.9XX with 7th K, S42.001-S42.92X with 7th [K, P], S49.001-S49.199 with 7th [K, P], S52.001-S52.92X with 7th [K, M, N, P, Q, R], S59.001-S59.299 with 7th [K, P], S62.001-S62.92X with 7th [K, P], S72.001-S72.92X with 7th [K, M, N, P, Q, R], S79.001-S79.199 with 7th [K, P], S82.001-S82.92X with 7th [K, M, N, P, Q, R], S89.001-S89.399 with 7th [K, P], S92.001-S92.919 with 7th [K, P]

✓x7th **M84.30 Stress fracture, unspecified site**   CC

✓6th **M84.31 Stress fracture, shoulder**
   ✓7th **M84.311 Stress fracture, right shoulder**   CC
   ✓7th **M84.312 Stress fracture, left shoulder**   CC
   ✓7th **M84.319 Stress fracture, unspecified shoulder**   CC

✓6th **M84.32 Stress fracture, humerus**
   ✓7th **M84.321 Stress fracture, right humerus**   CC
   ✓7th **M84.322 Stress fracture, left humerus**   CC
   ✓7th **M84.329 Stress fracture, unspecified humerus**   CC

✓6th **M84.33 Stress fracture, ulna and radius**
   ✓7th **M84.331 Stress fracture, right ulna**   CC
   ✓7th **M84.332 Stress fracture, left ulna**   CC
   ✓7th **M84.333 Stress fracture, right radius**   CC

   ✓7th **M84.334 Stress fracture, left radius**   CC
   ✓7th **M84.339 Stress fracture, unspecified ulna and radius**   CC

✓6th **M84.34 Stress fracture, hand and fingers**
   ✓7th **M84.341 Stress fracture, right hand**   CC
   ✓7th **M84.342 Stress fracture, left hand**   CC
   ✓7th **M84.343 Stress fracture, unspecified hand**   CC
   ✓7th **M84.344 Stress fracture, right finger(s)**   CC
   ✓7th **M84.345 Stress fracture, left finger(s)**   CC
   ✓7th **M84.346 Stress fracture, unspecified finger(s)**   CC

✓6th **M84.35 Stress fracture, pelvis and femur**
Stress fracture, hip
   ✓7th **M84.350 Stress fracture, pelvis**   CC
   ✓7th **M84.351 Stress fracture, right femur**   CC
   ✓7th **M84.352 Stress fracture, left femur**   CC
   ✓7th **M84.353 Stress fracture, unspecified femur**   CC
   ✓7th **M84.359 Stress fracture, hip, unspecified**   CC

✓6th **M84.36 Stress fracture, tibia and fibula**
   ✓7th **M84.361 Stress fracture, right tibia**   CC
   ✓7th **M84.362 Stress fracture, left tibia**   CC
   ✓7th **M84.363 Stress fracture, right fibula**   CC
   ✓7th **M84.364 Stress fracture, left fibula**   CC
   ✓7th **M84.369 Stress fracture, unspecified tibia and fibula**   CC

✓6th **M84.37 Stress fracture, ankle, foot and toes**
   ✓7th **M84.371 Stress fracture, right ankle**   CC
   ✓7th **M84.372 Stress fracture, left ankle**   CC
   ✓7th **M84.373 Stress fracture, unspecified ankle**   CC
   ✓7th **M84.374 Stress fracture, right foot**   CC
   ✓7th **M84.375 Stress fracture, left foot**   CC
   ✓7th **M84.376 Stress fracture, unspecified foot**   CC
   ✓7th **M84.377 Stress fracture, right toe(s)**   CC
   ✓7th **M84.378 Stress fracture, left toe(s)**   CC
   ✓7th **M84.379 Stress fracture, unspecified toe(s)**   CC

✓x7th **M84.38 Stress fracture, other site**   CC
> EXCLUDES 2   stress fracture of vertebra (M48.4-)

✓5th **M84.4 Pathological fracture, not elsewhere classified**
Chronic fracture
Pathological fracture NOS
> EXCLUDES 1   collapsed vertebra NEC (M48.5)
> pathological fracture in neoplastic disease (M84.5-)
> pathological fracture in osteoporosis (M80.-)
> pathological fracture in other disease (M84.6-)
> stress fracture (M84.3-)
> traumatic fracture (S12.-, S22.-, S32.-, S42.-, S52.-, S62.-, S72.-, S82.-, S92.-)
> EXCLUDES 2   personal history of (healed) pathological fracture (Z87.311)

The appropriate 7th character is to be added to each code from subcategory M84.4.
A   initial encounter for fracture
D   subsequent encounter for fracture with routine healing
G   subsequent encounter for fracture with delayed healing
K   subsequent encounter for fracture with nonunion
P   subsequent encounter for fracture with malunion
S   sequela

CC Excl: For codes M84.4, CC with 7th character A, unless otherwise noted: M48.40X-M48.58X with 7th A, M80.00X-M84.68X with 7th A
CC with 7th character K or P: M80.00X-M84.68X with 7th [K, P], S02.0XX-S02.92Xwith 7th K, S12.000-S12.691 with 7th K, S22.000-S22.9XX with 7th K, S32.000-S32.9XX with 7th K, S42.001-S42.92X with 7th [K, P], S49.001-S49.199 with 7th [K, P], S52.001-S52.92X with 7th [K, M, N, P, Q, R], S59.001-S59.299 with 7th [K, P], S62.001-S62.92X with 7th [K, P], S72.001-S72.92X with 7th [K, M, N, P, Q, R], S79.001-S79.199 with 7th [K, P], S82.001-S82.92X with 7th [K, M, N, P, Q, R], S89.001-S89.399 with 7th [K, P], S92.001-S92.919 with 7th [K, P]

✓x7th **M84.40 Pathological fracture, unspecified site**   CC

✓6th **M84.41 Pathological fracture, shoulder**
   ✓7th **M84.411 Pathological fracture, right shoulder**   CC
   ✓7th **M84.412 Pathological fracture, left shoulder**   CC

✓7ᵗʰ **M84.419** Pathological fracture, unspecified shoulder **CC**

✓6ᵗʰ **M84.42** Pathological fracture, humerus

  ✓7ᵗʰ **M84.421** Pathological fracture, right humerus **CC**

  ✓7ᵗʰ **M84.422** Pathological fracture, left humerus **CC**

  ✓7ᵗʰ **M84.429** Pathological fracture, unspecified humerus **CC**

✓6ᵗʰ **M84.43** Pathological fracture, ulna and radius

  ✓7ᵗʰ **M84.431** Pathological fracture, right ulna **CC**

  ✓7ᵗʰ **M84.432** Pathological fracture, left ulna **CC**

  ✓7ᵗʰ **M84.433** Pathological fracture, right radius **CC**

  ✓7ᵗʰ **M84.434** Pathological fracture, left radius **CC**

  ✓7ᵗʰ **M84.439** Pathological fracture, unspecified ulna and radius **CC**

✓6ᵗʰ **M84.44** Pathological fracture, hand and fingers

  ✓7ᵗʰ **M84.441** Pathological fracture, right hand **CC**

  ✓7ᵗʰ **M84.442** Pathological fracture, left hand **CC**

  ✓7ᵗʰ **M84.443** Pathological fracture, unspecified hand **CC**

  ✓7ᵗʰ **M84.444** Pathological fracture, right finger(s) **CC**

  ✓7ᵗʰ **M84.445** Pathological fracture, left finger(s) **CC**

  ✓7ᵗʰ **M84.446** Pathological fracture, unspecified finger(s) **CC**

✓6ᵗʰ **M84.45** Pathological fracture, femur and pelvis

  ✓7ᵗʰ **M84.451** Pathological fracture, right femur **CC**

  ✓7ᵗʰ **M84.452** Pathological fracture, left femur **CC**

  ✓7ᵗʰ **M84.453** Pathological fracture, unspecified femur **CC**

  ✓7ᵗʰ **M84.454** Pathological fracture, pelvis **CC**

  ✓7ᵗʰ **M84.459** Pathological fracture, hip, unspecified **CC**

✓6ᵗʰ **M84.46** Pathological fracture, tibia and fibula

  ✓7ᵗʰ **M84.461** Pathological fracture, right tibia **CC**

  ✓7ᵗʰ **M84.462** Pathological fracture, left tibia **CC**

  ✓7ᵗʰ **M84.463** Pathological fracture, right fibula **CC**

  ✓7ᵗʰ **M84.464** Pathological fracture, left fibula **CC**

  ✓7ᵗʰ **M84.469** Pathological fracture, unspecified tibia and fibula

✓6ᵗʰ **M84.47** Pathological fracture, ankle, foot and toes

  ✓7ᵗʰ **M84.471** Pathological fracture, right ankle **CC**

  ✓7ᵗʰ **M84.472** Pathological fracture, left ankle **CC**

  ✓7ᵗʰ **M84.473** Pathological fracture, unspecified ankle **CC**

  ✓7ᵗʰ **M84.474** Pathological fracture, right foot **CC**

  ✓7ᵗʰ **M84.475** Pathological fracture, left foot **CC**

  ✓7ᵗʰ **M84.476** Pathological fracture, unspecified foot **CC**

  ✓7ᵗʰ **M84.477** Pathological fracture, right toe(s) **CC**

  ✓7ᵗʰ **M84.478** Pathological fracture, left toe(s) **CC**

  ✓7ᵗʰ **M84.479** Pathological fracture, unspecified toe(s) **CC**

✓x7ᵗʰ **M84.48** Pathological fracture, other site **CC**

✓5ᵗʰ **M84.5** Pathological fracture in neoplastic disease

Code also underlying neoplasm

> The appropriate 7th character is to be added to each code from subcategory M84.5.
> A   initial encounter for fracture
> D   subsequent encounter for fracture with routine healing
> G   subsequent encounter for fracture with delayed healing
> K   subsequent encounter for fracture with nonunion
> P   subsequent encounter for fracture with malunion
> S   sequela

CC Excl: For codes M84.5, CC with 7th character A, unless otherwise noted: M48.40X-M48.58X with 7th A, M80.00X-M84.68X with 7th A
CC with 7th character K or P: M80.00X-M84.68X with 7th [K, P], S02.0XX-S02.92X with 7th K, S12.000-S12.691 with 7th K, S22.000-S22.9XX with 7th K, S32.000-S32.9XX with 7th K, S42.001-S42.92X with 7th [K, P], S49.001-S49.199 with 7th [K, P], S52.001-S52.92X with 7th [K, M, N, P, Q, R], S59.001-S59.299 with 7th [K, P], S62.001-S62.92X with 7th [K, P], S72.001-S72.92X with 7th [K, M, N, P, Q, R], S79.001-S79.199 with 7th [K, P], S82.001-S82.92X with 7th [K, M, N, P, Q, R], S89.001-S89.399 with 7th [K, P], S92.001-S92.919 with 7th [K, P]

✓x7ᵗʰ **M84.50** Pathological fracture in neoplastic disease, unspecified site **CC**

✓6ᵗʰ **M84.51** Pathological fracture in neoplastic disease, shoulder

  ✓7ᵗʰ **M84.511** Pathological fracture in neoplastic disease, right shoulder **CC**

  ✓7ᵗʰ **M84.512** Pathological fracture in neoplastic disease, left shoulder **CC**

  ✓7ᵗʰ **M84.519** Pathological fracture in neoplastic disease, unspecified shoulder **CC**

✓6ᵗʰ **M84.52** Pathological fracture in neoplastic disease, humerus

  ✓7ᵗʰ **M84.521** Pathological fracture in neoplastic disease, right humerus **CC**

  ✓7ᵗʰ **M84.522** Pathological fracture in neoplastic disease, left humerus **CC**

  ✓7ᵗʰ **M84.529** Pathological fracture in neoplastic disease, unspecified humerus **CC**

✓6ᵗʰ **M84.53** Pathological fracture in neoplastic disease, ulna and radius

  ✓7ᵗʰ **M84.531** Pathological fracture in neoplastic disease, right ulna **CC**

  ✓7ᵗʰ **M84.532** Pathological fracture in neoplastic disease, left ulna **CC**

  ✓7ᵗʰ **M84.533** Pathological fracture in neoplastic disease, right radius **CC**

  ✓7ᵗʰ **M84.534** Pathological fracture in neoplastic disease, left radius **CC**

  ✓7ᵗʰ **M84.539** Pathunspecifiedological fracture in neoplastic disease, ulna and radius **CC**

✓6ᵗʰ **M84.54** Pathological fracture in neoplastic disease, hand

  ✓7ᵗʰ **M84.541** Pathological fracture in neoplastic disease, right hand **CC**

  ✓7ᵗʰ **M84.542** Pathological fracture in neoplastic disease, left hand **CC**

  ✓7ᵗʰ **M84.549** Pathological fracture in neoplastic disease, unspecified hand **CC**

✓6ᵗʰ **M84.55** Pathological fracture in neoplastic disease, pelvis and femur

  ✓7ᵗʰ **M84.550** Pathological fracture in neoplastic disease, pelvis **CC**

  ✓7ᵗʰ **M84.551** Pathological fracture in neoplastic disease, right femur **CC**

  ✓7ᵗʰ **M84.552** Pathological fracture in neoplastic disease, left femur **CC**

  ✓7ᵗʰ **M84.553** Pathological fracture in neoplastic disease, unspecified femur **CC**

  ✓7ᵗʰ **M84.559** Pathological fracture in neoplastic disease, hip, unspecified **CC**

✓6ᵗʰ **M84.56** Pathological fracture in neoplastic disease, tibia and fibula

  ✓7ᵗʰ **M84.561** Pathological fracture in neoplastic disease, right tibia **CC**

  ✓7ᵗʰ **M84.562** Pathological fracture in neoplastic disease, left tibia **CC**

☑ Additional Character Required   ✓x7ᵗʰ Xtension Alert   Unacceptable PDx   Manifestation   Hospital Acquired Condition   *EXCLUDES 1* Not Coded Here   *EXCLUDES 2* Not Included Here

Diseases of the Musculoskeletal System and Connective Tissue

M84.563–M84.839

√7th **M84.563** Pathological fracture in neoplastic disease, **right fibula** CC

√7th **M84.564** Pathological fracture in neoplastic disease, **left fibula** CC

√7th **M84.569** Pathological fracture in neoplastic disease, **unspecified** tibia and fibula CC

√6th **M84.57** Pathological fracture in neoplastic disease, **ankle and foot**

√7th **M84.571** Pathological fracture in neoplastic disease, **right ankle** CC

√7th **M84.572** Pathological fracture in neoplastic disease, **left ankle** CC

√7th **M84.573** Pathological fracture in neoplastic disease, **unspecified ankle** CC

√7th **M84.574** Pathological fracture in neoplastic disease, **right foot** CC

√7th **M84.575** Pathological fracture in neoplastic disease, **left foot** CC

√7th **M84.576** Pathological fracture in neoplastic disease, **unspecified foot** CC

√x7th **M84.58** Pathological fracture in neoplastic disease, **other specified site** CC
Pathological fracture in neoplastic disease, vertebrae

√5th **M84.6** Pathological fracture in other disease
Code also underlying condition
EXCLUDES 1   *pathological fracture in osteoporosis (M80.-)*

> The appropriate 7th character is to be added to each code from subcategory M84.6.
> A   initial encounter for fracture
> D   subsequent encounter for fracture with routine healing
> G   subsequent encounter for fracture with delayed healing
> K   subsequent encounter for fracture with nonunion
> P   subsequent encounter for fracture with malunion
> S   sequela

> **CC Excl: For codes M84.6, CC with 7th character A, unless otherwise noted:** M48.40X-M48.58X with 7th A, M80.00X-M84.68X with 7th A.
> **CC with 7th character K or P:** M80.00X-M84.68X with 7th [K, P], S02.0XX-S02.92X with 7th K, S12.000-S12.691 with 7th K, S22.000-S22.9XX with 7th K, S32.000-S32.9XX with 7th K, S42.001-S42.92X with 7th [K, P], S49.001-S49.199 with 7th [K, P], S52.001-S52.92X with 7th [K, M, N, P, Q, R], S59.001-S59.299 with 7th [K, P], S62.001-S62.92X with 7th [K, P], S72.001-S72.92X with 7th [K, M, N, P, Q, R], S79.001-S79.199 with 7th [K, P], S82.001-S82.92X with 7th [K, M, N, P, Q, R], S89.001-S89.399 with 7th [K, P], S92.001-S92.919 with 7th [K, P]

√x7th **M84.60** Pathological fracture in other disease, **unspecified site** CC

√6th **M84.61** Pathological fracture in other disease, **shoulder**

√7th **M84.611** Pathological fracture in other disease, **right shoulder** CC

√7th **M84.612** Pathological fracture in other disease, **left shoulder** CC

√7th **M84.619** Pathological fracture in other disease, **unspecified shoulder** CC

√6th **M84.62** Pathological fracture in other disease, **humerus**

√7th **M84.621** Pathological fracture in other disease, **right humerus** CC

√7th **M84.622** Pathological fracture in other disease, **left humerus** CC

√7th **M84.629** Pathological fracture in other disease, **unspecified humerus** CC

√6th **M84.63** Pathological fracture in other disease, **ulna and radius**

√7th **M84.631** Pathological fracture in other disease, **right ulna** CC

√7th **M84.632** Pathological fracture in other disease, **left ulna** CC

√7th **M84.633** Pathological fracture in other disease, **right radius** CC

√7th **M84.634** Pathological fracture in other disease, **left radius** CC

√7th **M84.639** Pathological fracture in other disease, **unspecified ulna and radius** CC

√6th **M84.64** Pathological fracture in other disease, **hand**

√7th **M84.641** Pathological fracture in other disease, **right hand** CC

√7th **M84.642** Pathological fracture in other disease, **left hand** CC

√7th **M84.649** Pathological fracture in other disease, **unspecified hand** CC

√6th **M84.65** Pathological fracture in other disease, **pelvis and femur**

√7th **M84.650** Pathological fracture in other disease, **pelvis** CC

√7th **M84.651** Pathological fracture in other disease, **right femur** CC

√7th **M84.652** Pathological fracture in other disease, **left femur** CC

√7th **M84.653** Pathological fracture in other disease, **unspecified femur** CC

√7th **M84.659** Pathological fracture in other disease, **hip, unspecified** CC

√6th **M84.66** Pathological fracture in other disease, **tibia and fibula**

√7th **M84.661** Pathological fracture in other disease, **right tibia** CC

√7th **M84.662** Pathological fracture in other disease, **left tibia** CC

√7th **M84.663** Pathological fracture in other disease, **right fibula** CC

√7th **M84.664** Pathological fracture in other disease, **left fibula** CC

√7th **M84.669** Pathological fracture in other disease, **unspecified tibia and fibula** CC

√6th **M84.67** Pathological fracture in other disease, **ankle and foot**

√7th **M84.671** Pathological fracture in other disease, **right ankle** CC

√7th **M84.672** Pathological fracture in other disease, **left ankle** CC

√7th **M84.673** Pathological fracture in other disease, **unspecified ankle** CC

√7th **M84.674** Pathological fracture in other disease, **right foot** CC

√7th **M84.675** Pathological fracture in other disease, **left foot** CC

√7th **M84.676** Pathological fracture in other disease, **unspecified foot** CC

√x7th **M84.68** Pathological fracture in other disease, **other site** CC

√5th **M84.8** Other disorders of continuity of bone

M84.80 Other disorders of continuity of bone, **unspecified site**

√6th **M84.81** Other disorders of continuity of bone, **shoulder**

M84.811 Other disorders of continuity of bone, **right shoulder**

M84.812 Other disorders of continuity of bone, **left shoulder**

M84.819 Other disorders of continuity of bone, **unspecified shoulder**

√6th **M84.82** Other disorders of continuity of bone, **humerus**

M84.821 Other disorders of continuity of bone, **right humerus**

M84.822 Other disorders of continuity of bone, **left humerus**

M84.829 Other disorders of continuity of bone, **unspecified humerus**

√6th **M84.83** Other disorders of continuity of bone, **ulna and radius**

M84.831 Other disorders of continuity of bone, **right ulna**

M84.832 Other disorders of continuity of bone, **left ulna**

M84.833 Other disorders of continuity of bone, **right radius**

M84.834 Other disorders of continuity of bone, **left radius**

M84.839 Other disorders of continuity of bone, **unspecified ulna and radius**

✓6th **M84.84 Other disorders of continuity of bone,** hand
    M84.841 Other disorders of continuity of bone, right hand
    M84.842 Other disorders of continuity of bone, left hand
    M84.849 Other disorders of continuity of bone, unspecified hand

✓6th **M84.85 Other disorders of continuity of bone,** pelvic region and thigh
    M84.851 Other disorders of continuity of bone, right pelvic region and thigh
    M84.852 Other disorders of continuity of bone, left pelvic region and thigh
    M84.859 Other disorders of continuity of bone, unspecified pelvic region and thigh

✓6th **M84.86 Other disorders of continuity of bone,** tibia and fibula
    M84.861 Other disorders of continuity of bone, right tibia
    M84.862 Other disorders of continuity of bone, left tibia
    M84.863 Other disorders of continuity of bone, right fibula
    M84.864 Other disorders of continuity of bone, left fibula
    M84.869 Other disorders of continuity of bone, unspecified tibia and fibula

✓6th **M84.87 Other disorders of continuity of bone,** ankle and foot
    M84.871 Other disorders of continuity of bone, right ankle and foot
    M84.872 Other disorders of continuity of bone, left ankle and foot
    M84.879 Other disorders of continuity of bone, unspecified ankle and foot

M84.88 Other disorders of continuity of bone, other site
M84.9 Disorder of continuity of bone, unspecified

✓4th **M85 Other disorders of bone density and structure**
  EXCLUDES 1 osteogenesis imperfecta (Q78.0)
    osteopetrosis (Q78.2)
    osteopoikilosis (Q78.8)
    polyostotic fibrous dysplasia (Q78.1)

✓5th **M85.0 Fibrous dysplasia (monostotic)**
  EXCLUDES 2 fibrous dysplasia of jaw (M27.8)
  M85.00 Fibrous dysplasia (monostotic), unspecified site
✓6th **M85.01 Fibrous dysplasia (monostotic),** shoulder
    M85.011 Fibrous dysplasia (monostotic), right shoulder
    M85.012 Fibrous dysplasia (monostotic), left shoulder
    M85.019 Fibrous dysplasia (monostotic), unspecified shoulder
✓6th **M85.02 Fibrous dysplasia (monostotic),** upper arm
    M85.021 Fibrous dysplasia (monostotic), right upper arm
    M85.022 Fibrous dysplasia (monostotic), left upper arm
    M85.029 Fibrous dysplasia (monostotic), unspecified upper arm
✓6th **M85.03 Fibrous dysplasia (monostotic),** forearm
    M85.031 Fibrous dysplasia (monostotic), right forearm
    M85.032 Fibrous dysplasia (monostotic), left forearm
    M85.039 Fibrous dysplasia (monostotic), unspecified forearm
✓6th **M85.04 Fibrous dysplasia (monostotic),** hand
    M85.041 Fibrous dysplasia (monostotic), right hand
    M85.042 Fibrous dysplasia (monostotic), left hand
    M85.049 Fibrous dysplasia (monostotic), unspecified hand
✓6th **M85.05 Fibrous dysplasia (monostotic),** thigh
    M85.051 Fibrous dysplasia (monostotic), right thigh
    M85.052 Fibrous dysplasia (monostotic), left thigh
    M85.059 Fibrous dysplasia (monostotic), unspecified thigh

✓6th **M85.06 Fibrous dysplasia (monostotic),** lower leg
    M85.061 Fibrous dysplasia (monostotic), right lower leg
    M85.062 Fibrous dysplasia (monostotic), left lower leg
    M85.069 Fibrous dysplasia (monostotic), unspecified lower leg
✓6th **M85.07 Fibrous dysplasia (monostotic),** ankle and foot
    M85.071 Fibrous dysplasia (monostotic), right ankle and foot
    M85.072 Fibrous dysplasia (monostotic), left ankle and foot
    M85.079 Fibrous dysplasia (monostotic), unspecified ankle and foot
M85.08 Fibrous dysplasia (monostotic), other site
M85.09 Fibrous dysplasia (monostotic), multiple sites

✓5th **M85.1 Skeletal fluorosis**
  M85.10 Skeletal fluorosis, unspecified site
✓6th **M85.11 Skeletal fluorosis,** shoulder
    M85.111 Skeletal fluorosis, right shoulder
    M85.112 Skeletal fluorosis, left shoulder
    M85.119 Skeletal fluorosis, unspecified shoulder
✓6th **M85.12 Skeletal fluorosis,** upper arm
    M85.121 Skeletal fluorosis, right upper arm
    M85.122 Skeletal fluorosis, left upper arm
    M85.129 Skeletal fluorosis, unspecified upper arm
✓6th **M85.13 Skeletal fluorosis,** forearm
    M85.131 Skeletal fluorosis, right forearm
    M85.132 Skeletal fluorosis, left forearm
    M85.139 Skeletal fluorosis, unspecified forearm
✓6th **M85.14 Skeletal fluorosis,** hand
    M85.141 Skeletal fluorosis, right hand
    M85.142 Skeletal fluorosis, left hand
    M85.149 Skeletal fluorosis, unspecified hand
✓6th **M85.15 Skeletal fluorosis,** thigh
    M85.151 Skeletal fluorosis, right thigh
    M85.152 Skeletal fluorosis, left thigh
    M85.159 Skeletal fluorosis, unspecified thigh
✓6th **M85.16 Skeletal fluorosis,** lower leg
    M85.161 Skeletal fluorosis, right lower leg
    M85.162 Skeletal fluorosis, left lower leg
    M85.169 Skeletal fluorosis, unspecified lower leg
✓6th **M85.17 Skeletal fluorosis,** ankle and foot
    M85.171 Skeletal fluorosis, right ankle and foot
    M85.172 Skeletal fluorosis, left ankle and foot
    M85.179 Skeletal fluorosis, unspecified ankle and foot
M85.18 Skeletal fluorosis, other site
M85.19 Skeletal fluorosis, multiple sites
M85.2 Hyperostosis of skull
✓5th **M85.3 Osteitis condensans**
  M85.30 Osteitis condensans, unspecified site
✓6th **M85.31 Osteitis condensans,** shoulder
    M85.311 Osteitis condensans, right shoulder
    M85.312 Osteitis condensans, left shoulder
    M85.319 Osteitis condensans, unspecified shoulder
✓6th **M85.32 Osteitis condensans,** upper arm
    M85.321 Osteitis condensans, right upper arm
    M85.322 Osteitis condensans, left upper arm
    M85.329 Osteitis condensans, unspecified upper arm
✓6th **M85.33 Osteitis condensans,** forearm
    M85.331 Osteitis condensans, right forearm
    M85.332 Osteitis condensans, left forearm
    M85.339 Osteitis condensans, unspecified forearm
✓6th **M85.34 Osteitis condensans,** hand
    M85.341 Osteitis condensans, right hand
    M85.342 Osteitis condensans, left hand
    M85.349 Osteitis condensans, unspecified hand
✓6th **M85.35 Osteitis condensans,** thigh
    M85.351 Osteitis condensans, right thigh
    M85.352 Osteitis condensans, left thigh

          M85.359   Osteitis condensans, unspecified thigh

✓6ᵗʰ   M85.36   Osteitis condensans, lower leg
          M85.361   Osteitis condensans, right lower leg
          M85.362   Osteitis condensans, left lower leg
          M85.369   Osteitis condensans, unspecified lower leg

✓6ᵗʰ   M85.37   Osteitis condensans, ankle and foot
          M85.371   Osteitis condensans, right ankle and foot
          M85.372   Osteitis condensans, left ankle and foot
          M85.379   Osteitis condensans, unspecified ankle and foot

    M85.38   Osteitis condensans, other site
    M85.39   Osteitis condensans, multiple sites

✓5ᵗʰ   **M85.4   Solitary bone cyst**
    EXCLUDES 2   solitary cyst of jaw (M27.4)

    M85.40   Solitary bone cyst, unspecified site

✓6ᵗʰ   M85.41   Solitary bone cyst, shoulder
          M85.411   Solitary bone cyst, right shoulder
          M85.412   Solitary bone cyst, left shoulder
          M85.419   Solitary bone cyst, unspecified shoulder

✓6ᵗʰ   M85.42   Solitary bone cyst, humerus
          M85.421   Solitary bone cyst, right humerus
          M85.422   Solitary bone cyst, left humerus
          M85.429   Solitary bone cyst, unspecified humerus

✓6ᵗʰ   M85.43   Solitary bone cyst, ulna and radius
          M85.431   Solitary bone cyst, right ulna and radius
          M85.432   Solitary bone cyst, left ulna and radius
          M85.439   Solitary bone cyst, unspecified ulna and radius

✓6ᵗʰ   M85.44   Solitary bone cyst, hand
          M85.441   Solitary bone cyst, right hand
          M85.442   Solitary bone cyst, left hand
          M85.449   Solitary bone cyst, unspecified hand

✓6ᵗʰ   M85.45   Solitary bone cyst, pelvis
          M85.451   Solitary bone cyst, right pelvis
          M85.452   Solitary bone cyst, left pelvis
          M85.459   Solitary bone cyst, unspecified pelvis

✓6ᵗʰ   M85.46   Solitary bone cyst, tibia and fibula
          M85.461   Solitary bone cyst, right tibia and fibula
          M85.462   Solitary bone cyst, left tibia and fibula
          M85.469   Solitary bone cyst, unspecified tibia and fibula

✓6ᵗʰ   M85.47   Solitary bone cyst, ankle and foot
          M85.471   Solitary bone cyst, right ankle and foot
          M85.472   Solitary bone cyst, left ankle and foot
          M85.479   Solitary bone cyst, unspecified ankle and foot

    M85.48   Solitary bone cyst, other site

✓5ᵗʰ   **M85.5   Aneurysmal bone cyst**
    EXCLUDES 2   aneurysmal cyst of jaw (M27.4)

    M85.50   Aneurysmal bone cyst, unspecified site

✓6ᵗʰ   M85.51   Aneurysmal bone cyst, shoulder
          M85.511   Aneurysmal bone cyst, right shoulder
          M85.512   Aneurysmal bone cyst, left shoulder
          M85.519   Aneurysmal bone cyst, unspecified shoulder

✓6ᵗʰ   M85.52   Aneurysmal bone cyst, upper arm
          M85.521   Aneurysmal bone cyst, right upper arm
          M85.522   Aneurysmal bone cyst, left upper arm
          M85.529   Aneurysmal bone cyst, unspecified upper arm

✓6ᵗʰ   M85.53   Aneurysmal bone cyst, forearm
          M85.531   Aneurysmal bone cyst, right forearm
          M85.532   Aneurysmal bone cyst, left forearm
          M85.539   Aneurysmal bone cyst, unspecified forearm

✓6ᵗʰ   M85.54   Aneurysmal bone cyst, hand
          M85.541   Aneurysmal bone cyst, right hand
          M85.542   Aneurysmal bone cyst, left hand
          M85.549   Aneurysmal bone cyst, unspecified hand

✓6ᵗʰ   M85.55   Aneurysmal bone cyst, thigh
          M85.551   Aneurysmal bone cyst, right thigh
          M85.552   Aneurysmal bone cyst, left thigh

          M85.559   Aneurysmal bone cyst, unspecified thigh

✓6ᵗʰ   M85.56   Aneurysmal bone cyst, lower leg
          M85.561   Aneurysmal bone cyst, right lower leg
          M85.562   Aneurysmal bone cyst, left lower leg
          M85.569   Aneurysmal bone cyst, unspecified lower leg

✓6ᵗʰ   M85.57   Aneurysmal bone cyst, ankle and foot
          M85.571   Aneurysmal bone cyst, right ankle and foot
          M85.572   Aneurysmal bone cyst, left ankle and foot
          M85.579   Aneurysmal bone cyst, unspecified ankle and foot

    M85.58   Aneurysmal bone cyst, other site
    M85.59   Aneurysmal bone cyst, multiple sites

✓5ᵗʰ   **M85.6   Other cyst of bone**
    EXCLUDES 1   cyst of jaw NEC (M27.4)
                osteitis fibrosa cystica generalisata [von Recklinghausen's disease of bone] (E21.0)

    M85.60   Other cyst of bone, unspecified site

✓6ᵗʰ   M85.61   Other cyst of bone, shoulder
          M85.611   Other cyst of bone, right shoulder
          M85.612   Other cyst of bone, left shoulder
          M85.619   Other cyst of bone, unspecified shoulder

✓6ᵗʰ   M85.62   Other cyst of bone, upper arm
          M85.621   Other cyst of bone, right upper arm
          M85.622   Other cyst of bone, left upper arm
          M85.629   Other cyst of bone, unspecified upper arm

✓6ᵗʰ   M85.63   Other cyst of bone, forearm
          M85.631   Other cyst of bone, right forearm
          M85.632   Other cyst of bone, left forearm
          M85.639   Other cyst of bone, unspecified forearm

✓6ᵗʰ   M85.64   Other cyst of bone, hand
          M85.641   Other cyst of bone, right hand
          M85.642   Other cyst of bone, left hand
          M85.649   Other cyst of bone, unspecified hand

✓6ᵗʰ   M85.65   Other cyst of bone, thigh
          M85.651   Other cyst of bone, right thigh
          M85.652   Other cyst of bone, left thigh
          M85.659   Other cyst of bone, unspecified thigh

✓6ᵗʰ   M85.66   Other cyst of bone, lower leg
          M85.661   Other cyst of bone, right lower leg
          M85.662   Other cyst of bone, left lower leg
          M85.669   Other cyst of bone, unspecified lower leg

✓6ᵗʰ   M85.67   Other cyst of bone, ankle and foot
          M85.671   Other cyst of bone, right ankle and foot
          M85.672   Other cyst of bone, left ankle and foot
          M85.679   Other cyst of bone, unspecified ankle and foot

    M85.68   Other cyst of bone, other site
    M85.69   Other cyst of bone, multiple sites

✓5ᵗʰ   **M85.8   Other specified disorders of bone density and structure**
    Hyperostosis of bones, except skull
    Osteosclerosis, acquired
    EXCLUDES 1   diffuse idiopathic skeletal hyperostosis [DISH] (M48.1)
                osteosclerosis congenita (Q77.4)
                osteosclerosis fragilitas (generalista) (Q78.2)
                osteosclerosis myelofibrosis (D75.81)

    M85.80   Other specified disorders of bone density and structure, unspecified site

✓6ᵗʰ   M85.81   Other specified disorders of bone density and structure, shoulder
          M85.811   Other specified disorders of bone density and structure, right shoulder
          M85.812   Other specified disorders of bone density and structure, left shoulder
          M85.819   Other specified disorders of bone density and structure, unspecified shoulder

✓6ᵗʰ   M85.82   Other specified disorders of bone density and structure, upper arm
          M85.821   Other specified disorders of bone density and structure, right upper arm
          M85.822   Other specified disorders of bone density and structure, left upper arm

N Newborn: 0   P Pediatric: 0-17   M Maternity: 12-55   A Adult: 15-124   MCC Major CC Condition   PDx MCC PDx acts as own MCC   CC CC Condition   PDx CC PDx acts as own CC

746   ICD-10-CM Draft (2015)

M85.829 Other specified disorders of bone density and structure, unspecified upper arm

✓6th **M85.83 Other specified disorders of bone density and structure, forearm**

    M85.831 Other specified disorders of bone density and structure, right forearm

    M85.832 Other specified disorders of bone density and structure, left forearm

    M85.839 Other specified disorders of bone density and structure, unspecified forearm

✓6th **M85.84 Other specified disorders of bone density and structure, hand**

    M85.841 Other specified disorders of bone density and structure, right hand

    M85.842 Other specified disorders of bone density and structure, left hand

    M85.849 Other specified disorders of bone density and structure, unspecified hand

✓6th **M85.85 Other specified disorders of bone density and structure, thigh**

    M85.851 Other specified disorders of bone density and structure, right thigh

    M85.852 Other specified disorders of bone density and structure, left thigh

    M85.859 Other specified disorders of bone density and structure, unspecified thigh

✓6th **M85.86 Other specified disorders of bone density and structure, lower leg**

    M85.861 Other specified disorders of bone density and structure, right lower leg

    M85.862 Other specified disorders of bone density and structure, left lower leg

    M85.869 Other specified disorders of bone density and structure, unspecified lower leg

✓6th **M85.87 Other specified disorders of bone density and structure, ankle and foot**

    M85.871 Other specified disorders of bone density and structure, right ankle and foot

    M85.872 Other specified disorders of bone density and structure, left ankle and foot

    M85.879 Other specified disorders of bone density and structure, unspecified ankle and foot

M85.88 Other specified disorders of bone density and structure, other site

M85.89 Other specified disorders of bone density and structure, multiple sites

M85.9 Disorder of bone density and structure, unspecified

Other osteopathies (M86-M90)

EXCLUDES 1 postprocedural osteopathies (M96.-)

✓4th **M86 Osteomyelitis**

Use additional code (B95-B97) to identify infectious agent

Use additional code to identify major osseous defect, if applicable (M89.7-)

EXCLUDES 1 osteomyelitis due to:
    echinococcus (B67.2)
    gonococcus (A54.43)
    salmonella (A02.24)

EXCLUDES 2 ostemyelitis of:
    orbit (H05.0-)
    petrous bone (H70.2-)
    vertebra (M46.2-)

✓5th **M86.0 Acute hematogenous osteomyelitis**

M86.00 Acute hematogenous osteomyelitis, unspecified site CC
    CC Excl: A17.9, A18.03-A18.09, A18.82, A18.84, A18.89, M46.20-M46.39, M86.00-M86.9

✓6th **M86.01 Acute hematogenous osteomyelitis, shoulder**

    M86.011 Acute hematogenous osteomyelitis, right shoulder CC
        CC Excl: A17.9, A18.03-A18.09, A18.82, A18.84, A18.89, M46.20-M46.39, M86.00, M86.08-M86.10, M86.18-M86.20, M86.28-M86.319, M86.38-M86.419, M86.48-M86.519, M86.58-M86.619, M86.68-M86.8X1, M86.8X8-M86.9

    M86.012 Acute hematogenous osteomyelitis, left shoulder CC
        CC Excl: See code: M86.011

M86.019 Acute hematogenous osteomyelitis, unspecified shoulder CC
    CC Excl: See code: M86.011

✓6th **M86.02 Acute hematogenous osteomyelitis, humerus**

    M86.021 Acute hematogenous osteomyelitis, right humerus CC
        CC Excl: A17.9, A18.03-A18.09, A18.82, A18.84, A18.89, M46.20-M46.39, M86.00, M86.08-M86.10, M86.18-M86.20, M86.28-M86.30, M86.321-M86.329, M86.38-M86.40, M86.421-M86.429, M86.48-M86.50, M86.521-M86.529, M86.58-M86.60, M86.621-M86.629, M86.68-M86.8X0, M86.8X2, M86.8X8-M86.9

    M86.022 Acute hematogenous osteomyelitis, left humerus CC
        CC Excl: See code: M86.021

    M86.029 Acute hematogenous osteomyelitis, unspecified humerus CC
        CC Excl: See code: M86.021

✓6th **M86.03 Acute hematogenous osteomyelitis, radius and ulna**

    M86.031 Acute hematogenous osteomyelitis, right radius and ulna CC
        CC Excl: A17.9, A18.03-A18.09, A18.82, A18.84, A18.89, M46.20-M46.39, M86.00, M86.08-M86.10, M86.18-M86.20, M86.28-M86.30, M86.331-M86.339, M86.38-M86.40, M86.431-M86.439, M86.48-M86.50, M86.531-M86.539, M86.58-M86.60, M86.631-M86.639, M86.68-M86.8X0, M86.8X3, M86.8X8-M86.9

    M86.032 Acute hematogenous osteomyelitis, left radius and ulna CC
        CC Excl: See code: M86.031

    M86.039 Acute hematogenous osteomyelitis, unspecified radius and ulna CC
        CC Excl: See code: M86.031

✓6th **M86.04 Acute hematogenous osteomyelitis, hand**

    M86.041 Acute hematogenous osteomyelitis, right hand CC
        CC Excl: A17.9, A18.03-A18.09, A18.82, A18.84, A18.89, M46.20-M46.39, M86.00, M86.08-M86.10, M86.18-M86.20, M86.28-M86.30, M86.341-M86.349, M86.38-M86.40, M86.441-M86.449, M86.48-M86.50, M86.541-M86.549, M86.58-M86.60, M86.641-M86.649, M86.68-M86.8X0, M86.8X4, M86.8X8-M86.9

    M86.042 Acute hematogenous osteomyelitis, left hand CC
        CC Excl: See code: M86.041

    M86.049 Acute hematogenous osteomyelitis, unspecified hand CC
        CC Excl: See code: M86.041

✓6th **M86.05 Acute hematogenous osteomyelitis, femur**

    M86.051 Acute hematogenous osteomyelitis, right femur CC
        CC Excl: A17.9, A18.03-A18.09, A18.82, A18.84, A18.89, M46.20-M46.39, M86.00, M86.08-M86.10, M86.18-M86.20, M86.28-M86.30, M86.351-M86.359, M86.38-M86.40, M86.451-M86.459, M86.48-M86.50, M86.551-M86.559, M86.58-M86.60, M86.651-M86.659, M86.68-M86.8X0, M86.8X5, M86.8X8-M86.9

    M86.052 Acute hematogenous osteomyelitis, left femur CC
        CC Excl: See code: M86.051

    M86.059 Acute hematogenous osteomyelitis, unspecified femur CC
        CC Excl: See code: M86.051

✓6th **M86.06 Acute hematogenous osteomyelitis, tibia and fibula**

    M86.061 Acute hematogenous osteomyelitis, right tibia and fibula CC
        CC Excl: A17.9, A18.03-A18.09, A18.82, A18.84, A18.89, M46.20-M46.39, M86.00, M86.08-M86.10, M86.18-M86.20, M86.28-M86.30, M86.361-M86.369, M86.38-M86.40, M86.461-M86.469, M86.48-M86.50, M86.561-M86.569, M86.58-M86.60, M86.661-M86.669, M86.68-M86.8X0, M86.8X6, M86.8X8-M86.9

    M86.062 Acute hematogenous osteomyelitis, left tibia and fibula CC
        CC Excl: See code: M86.061

✓ Additional Character Required ✓x7th Xtension Alert Unacceptable PDx Manifestation Hospital Acquired Condition EXCLUDES 1 Not Coded Here EXCLUDES 2 Not Included Here

M86.069 Acute hematogenous osteomyelitis, unspecified **tibia and fibula** `CC`
CC Excl: See code: M86.061

✓6th **M86.07** Acute hematogenous osteomyelitis, **ankle and foot**

M86.071 Acute hematogenous osteomyelitis, **right ankle and foot** `CC`
CC Excl: A17.9, A18.03-A18.09, A18.82, A18.84, A18.89, M46.20-M46.39, M86.00, M86.08-M86.10, M86.18-M86.20, M86.28-M86.30, M86.371-M86.40, M86.471-M86.50, M86.571-M86.60, M86.671-M86.8X0, M86.8X7-M86.9

M86.072 Acute hematogenous osteomyelitis, **left ankle and foot** `CC`
CC Excl: See code: M86.071

M86.079 Acute hematogenous osteomyelitis, unspecified **ankle and foot** `CC`
CC Excl: See code: M86.071

M86.08 Acute hematogenous osteomyelitis, **other sites** `CC`
CC Excl: A17.9-A18.01, A18.03-A18.09, A18.82, A18.84, A18.89, M46.20-M46.39, M86.00-M86.9

M86.09 Acute hematogenous osteomyelitis, **multiple sites** `CC`
CC Excl: A17.9, A18.03-A18.09, A18.82, A18.84, A18.89, M46.20-M46.39, M86.00-M86.9

✓5th **M86.1** Other acute **osteomyelitis**

M86.10 Other acute osteomyelitis, unspecified site `CC`
CC Excl: See code: 86.09

✓6th **M86.11** Other acute osteomyelitis, **shoulder**

M86.111 Other acute osteomyelitis, **right shoulder** `CC`
CC Excl: See code: M86.071

M86.112 Other acute osteomyelitis, **left shoulder** `CC`
CC Excl: See code: M86.071

M86.119 Other acute osteomyelitis, unspecified **shoulder** `CC`
CC Excl: See code: M86.071

✓6th **M86.12** Other acute osteomyelitis, **humerus**

M86.121 Other acute osteomyelitis, **right humerus** `CC`
CC Excl: See code: M86.021

M86.122 Other acute osteomyelitis, **left humerus** `CC`
CC Excl: See code: M86.021

M86.129 Other acute osteomyelitis, unspecified **humerus** `CC`
CC Excl: See code: M86.021

✓6th **M86.13** Other acute osteomyelitis, **radius and ulna**

M86.131 Other acute osteomyelitis, **right radius and ulna** `CC`
CC Excl: See code: M86.031

M86.132 Other acute osteomyelitis, **left radius and ulna** `CC`
CC Excl: See code: M86.031

M86.139 Other acute osteomyelitis, unspecified **radius and ulna** `CC`
CC Excl: See code: M86.031

✓6th **M86.14** Other acute osteomyelitis, **hand**

M86.141 Other acute osteomyelitis, **right hand** `CC`
CC Excl: See code: M86.041

M86.142 Other acute osteomyelitis, **left hand** `CC`
CC Excl: See code: M86.041

M86.149 Other acute osteomyelitis, unspecified **hand** `CC`
CC Excl: See code: M86.041

✓6th **M86.15** Other acute osteomyelitis, **femur**

M86.151 Other acute osteomyelitis, **right femur** `CC`
CC Excl: See code: M86.051

M86.152 Other acute osteomyelitis, **left femur** `CC`
CC Excl: See code: M86.051

M86.159 Other acute osteomyelitis, unspecified **femur** `CC`
CC Excl: See code: M86.051

✓6th **M86.16** Other acute osteomyelitis, **tibia and fibula**

M86.161 Other acute osteomyelitis, **right tibia and fibula** `CC`
CC Excl: See code: M86.061

M86.162 Other acute osteomyelitis, **left tibia and fibula** `CC`
CC Excl: See code: M86.061

M86.169 Other acute osteomyelitis, unspecified **tibia and fibula** `CC`
CC Excl: See code: M86.061

✓6th **M86.17** Other acute osteomyelitis, **ankle and foot**

M86.171 Other acute osteomyelitis, **right ankle and foot** `CC`
CC Excl: See code: M86.071

M86.172 Other acute osteomyelitis, **left ankle and foot** `CC`
CC Excl: See code: M86.071

M86.179 Other acute osteomyelitis, unspecified **ankle and foot** `CC`
CC Excl: See code: M86.071

M86.18 Other acute osteomyelitis, **other site** `CC`
CC Excl: A17.9-A18.01, A18.03-A18.09, A18.82, A18.84, A18.89, M46.20-M46.39, M86.00-M86.9

M86.19 Other acute osteomyelitis, **multiple sites** `CC`
CC Excl: A17.9, A18.03-A18.09, A18.82, A18.84, A18.89, M46.20-M46.39, M86.00-M86.9

✓5th **M86.2** Subacute **osteomyelitis**

M86.20 Subacute osteomyelitis, unspecified site `CC`
CC Excl: See code: M86.19

✓6th **M86.21** Subacute osteomyelitis, **shoulder**

M86.211 Subacute osteomyelitis, **right shoulder** `CC`
CC Excl: A17.9, A18.03-A18.09, A18.82, A18.84, A18.89, M46.20-M46.39, M86.00, M86.08-M86.10, M86.18-M86.20, M86.28-M86.319, M86.38-M86.419, M86.48-M86.519, M86.58-M86.619, M86.68-M86.8X1, M86.8X8-M86.9

M86.212 Subacute osteomyelitis, **left shoulder** `CC`
CC Excl: See code: M86.211

M86.219 Subacute osteomyelitis, unspecified **shoulder** `CC`
CC Excl: See code: M86.211

✓6th **M86.22** Subacute osteomyelitis, **humerus**

M86.221 Subacute osteomyelitis, **right humerus** `CC`
CC Excl: A17.9, A18.03-A18.09, A18.82, A18.84, A18.89, M46.20-M46.39, M86.00, M86.08-M86.10, M86.18-M86.20, M86.28-M86.30, M86.321-M86.329, M86.38-M86.40, M86.421-M86.429, M86.48-M86.50, M86.521-M86.529, M86.58-M86.60, M86.621-M86.629, M86.68-M86.8X0, M86.8X2, M86.8X8-M86.9

M86.222 Subacute osteomyelitis, **left humerus** `CC`
CC Excl: See code: M86.221

M86.229 Subacute osteomyelitis, unspecified **humerus** `CC`
CC Excl: See code: M86.221

✓6th **M86.23** Subacute osteomyelitis, **radius and ulna**

M86.231 Subacute osteomyelitis, **right radius and ulna** `CC`
CC Excl: A17.9, A18.03-A18.09, A18.82, A18.84, A18.89, M46.20-M46.39, M86.00, M86.08-M86.10, M86.18-M86.20, M86.28-M86.30, M86.331-M86.339, M86.38-M86.40, M86.431-M86.439, M86.48-M86.50, M86.531-M86.539, M86.58-M86.60, M86.631-M86.639, M86.68-M86.8X0, M86.8X3, M86.8X8-M86.9

M86.232 Subacute osteomyelitis, **left radius and ulna** `CC`
CC Excl: See code: M86.231

M86.239 Subacute osteomyelitis, unspecified **radius and ulna** `CC`
CC Excl: See code: M86.231

✓6th **M86.24** Subacute osteomyelitis, **hand**

M86.241 Subacute osteomyelitis, **right hand** `CC`
CC Excl: A17.9, A18.03-A18.09, A18.82, A18.84, A18.89, M46.20-M46.39, M86.00, M86.08-M86.10, M86.18-M86.20, M86.28-M86.30, M86.341-M86.349, M86.38-M86.40, M86.441-M86.449, M86.48-M86.50, M86.541-M86.549, M86.58-M86.60, M86.641-M86.649, M86.68-M86.8X0, M86.8X4, M86.8X8-M86.9

M86.242 Subacute osteomyelitis, **left hand** `CC`
CC Excl: See code: M86.241

M86.249 Subacute osteomyelitis, unspecified **hand** `CC`
CC Excl: See code: M86.241

N Newborn: 0   P Pediatric: 0-17   M Maternity: 12-55   A Adult: 15-124   MCC Major CC Condition   PDx MCC PDx acts as own MCC   CC CC Condition   PDx CC PDx acts as own CC

748   ICD-10-CM Draft (2015)

✓6ᵗʰ **M86.25 Subacute osteomyelitis, femur**

M86.251 Subacute osteomyelitis, right femur `CC`
CC Excl: A17.9, A18.03-A18.09, A18.82, A18.84, A18.89, M46.20-M46.39, M86.00, M86.08-M86.10, M86.18-M86.20, M86.28-M86.30, M86.351-M86.359, M86.38-M86.40, M86.451-M86.459, M86.48-M86.50, M86.551-M86.559, M86.58-M86.60, M86.651-M86.659, M86.68-M86.8X0, M86.8X5, M86.8X8-M86.9

M86.252 Subacute osteomyelitis, left femur `CC`
CC Excl: See code: M86.251

M86.259 Subacute osteomyelitis, unspecified femur `CC`
CC Excl: See code: M86.251

✓6ᵗʰ **M86.26 Subacute osteomyelitis, tibia and fibula**

M86.261 Subacute osteomyelitis, right tibia and fibula `CC`
CC Excl: A17.9, A18.03-A18.09, A18.82, A18.84, A18.89, M46.20-M46.39, M86.00, M86.08-M86.10, M86.18-M86.20, M86.28-M86.30, M86.361-M86.369, M86.38-M86.40, M86.461-M86.469, M86.48-M86.50, M86.561-M86.569, M86.58-M86.60, M86.661-M86.669, M86.68-M86.8X0, M86.8X6, M86.8X8-M86.9

M86.262 Subacute osteomyelitis, left tibia and fibula `CC`
CC Excl: See code: M86.261

M86.269 Subacute osteomyelitis, unspecified tibia and fibula `CC`
CC Excl: See code: M86.261

✓6ᵗʰ **M86.27 Subacute osteomyelitis, ankle and foot**

M86.271 Subacute osteomyelitis, right ankle and foot `CC`
CC Excl: A17.9, A18.03-A18.09, A18.82, A18.84, A18.89, M46.20-M46.39, M86.00, M86.08-M86.10, M86.18-M86.20, M86.28-M86.30, M86.371-M86.40, M86.471-M86.50, M86.571-M86.60, M86.671-M86.8X0, M86.8X7-M86.9

M86.272 Subacute osteomyelitis, left ankle and foot `CC`
CC Excl: See code: M86.271

M86.279 Subacute osteomyelitis, unspecified ankle and foot `CC`
CC Excl: See code: M86.271

M86.28 Subacute osteomyelitis, other site `CC`
CC Excl: A17.9-A18.01, A18.03-A18.09, A18.82, A18.84, A18.89, M46.20-M46.39, M86.00-M86.9

M86.29 Subacute osteomyelitis, multiple sites `CC`
CC Excl: A17.9, A18.03-A18.09, A18.82, A18.84, A18.89, M46.20-M46.39, M86.00-M86.9

✓5ᵗʰ **M86.3 Chronic multifocal osteomyelitis**

M86.30 Chronic multifocal osteomyelitis, unspecified site `CC`
CC Excl: M46.20-M46.39, M86.30-M86.9, M88.0-M88.9, M90.60-M90.69

✓6ᵗʰ **M86.31 Chronic multifocal osteomyelitis, shoulder**

M86.311 Chronic multifocal osteomyelitis, right shoulder `CC`
CC Excl: A02.24, A17.9, A18.03-A18.09, A18.82, A18.84, A18.89, M46.20-M46.39, M86.00-M86.9

M86.312 Chronic multifocal osteomyelitis, left shoulder `CC`
CC Excl: See code: M86.311

M86.319 Chronic multifocal osteomyelitis, unspecified shoulder `CC`
CC Excl: See code: M86.311

✓6ᵗʰ **M86.32 Chronic multifocal osteomyelitis, humerus**

M86.321 Chronic multifocal osteomyelitis, right humerus `CC`
CC Excl: See code: M86.311

M86.322 Chronic multifocal osteomyelitis, left humerus `CC`
CC Excl: See code: M86.311

M86.329 Chronic multifocal osteomyelitis, unspecified humerus `CC`
CC Excl: See code: M86.311

✓6ᵗʰ **M86.33 Chronic multifocal osteomyelitis, radius and ulna**

M86.331 Chronic multifocal osteomyelitis, right radius and ulna `CC`
CC Excl: See code: M86.311

M86.332 Chronic multifocal osteomyelitis, left radius and ulna `CC`
CC Excl: See code: M86.311

M86.339 Chronic multifocal osteomyelitis, unspecified radius and ulna `CC`
CC Excl: See code: M86.311

✓6ᵗʰ **M86.34 Chronic multifocal osteomyelitis, hand**

M86.341 Chronic multifocal osteomyelitis, right hand `CC`
CC Excl: See code: M86.311

M86.342 Chronic multifocal osteomyelitis, left hand `CC`
CC Excl: See code: M86.311

M86.349 Chronic multifocal osteomyelitis, unspecified hand `CC`
CC Excl: See code: M86.311

✓6ᵗʰ **M86.35 Chronic multifocal osteomyelitis, femur**

M86.351 Chronic multifocal osteomyelitis, right femur `CC`
CC Excl: See code: M86.311

M86.352 Chronic multifocal osteomyelitis, left femur `CC`
CC Excl: See code: M86.311

M86.359 Chronic multifocal osteomyelitis, unspecified femur `CC`
CC Excl: See code: M86.311

✓6ᵗʰ **M86.36 Chronic multifocal osteomyelitis, tibia and fibula**

M86.361 Chronic multifocal osteomyelitis, right tibia and fibula `CC`
CC Excl: See code: M86.311

M86.362 Chronic multifocal osteomyelitis, left tibia and fibula `CC`
CC Excl: See code: M86.311

M86.369 Chronic multifocal osteomyelitis, unspecified tibia and fibula `CC`
CC Excl: See code: M86.311

✓6ᵗʰ **M86.37 Chronic multifocal osteomyelitis, ankle and foot**

M86.371 Chronic multifocal osteomyelitis, right ankle and foot `CC`
CC Excl: See code: M86.311

M86.372 Chronic multifocal osteomyelitis, left ankle and foot `CC`
CC Excl: See code: M86.311

M86.379 Chronic multifocal osteomyelitis, unspecified ankle and foot `CC`
CC Excl: See code: M86.311

M86.38 Chronic multifocal osteomyelitis, other site `CC`
CC Excl: See code: 86.311

M86.39 Chronic multifocal osteomyelitis, multiple sites `CC`
CC Excl: See code: 86.311

✓5ᵗʰ **M86.4 Chronic osteomyelitis with draining sinus**

> CC Excl: For CC codes in subcategory M86.4, M86.5, M86.6, M86.8, M86.9, unless otherwise noted: A02.24, A17.9, A18.03-A18.09, A18.82, A18.84, A18.89, M46.20-M46.39, M86.00-M86.9

M86.40 Chronic osteomyelitis with draining sinus, unspecified site `CC`
CC Excl: M46.20-M46.39, M86.30-M86.9, M88.0-M88.9, M90.60-M90.69

✓6ᵗʰ **M86.41 Chronic osteomyelitis with draining sinus, shoulder**

M86.411 Chronic osteomyelitis with draining sinus, right shoulder `CC`

M86.412 Chronic osteomyelitis with draining sinus, left shoulder `CC`

M86.419 Chronic osteomyelitis with draining sinus, unspecified shoulder `CC`

✓6ᵗʰ **M86.42 Chronic osteomyelitis with draining sinus, humerus**

M86.421 Chronic osteomyelitis with draining sinus, right humerus `CC`

M86.422 Chronic osteomyelitis with draining sinus, left humerus `CC`

M86.429 Chronic osteomyelitis with draining sinus, unspecified humerus `CC`

✓6ᵗʰ **M86.43 Chronic osteomyelitis with draining sinus, radius and ulna**

M86.431 Chronic osteomyelitis with draining sinus, right radius and ulna `CC`

M86.432 Chronic osteomyelitis with draining sinus, left radius and ulna `CC`

☑ Additional Character Required   ✓x7ᵗʰ Xtension Alert   Unacceptable PDx   Manifestation   Hospital Acquired Condition   **EXCLUDES 1** Not Coded Here   **EXCLUDES 2** Not Included Here

M86.439 Chronic osteomyelitis with draining sinus, unspecified radius and ulna   CC

✓6th **M86.44** Chronic osteomyelitis with draining sinus, hand

   M86.441 Chronic osteomyelitis with draining sinus, right hand   CC

   M86.442 Chronic osteomyelitis with draining sinus, left hand   CC

   M86.449 Chronic osteomyelitis with draining sinus, unspecified hand   CC

✓6th **M86.45** Chronic osteomyelitis with draining sinus, femur

   M86.451 Chronic osteomyelitis with draining sinus, right femur   CC

   M86.452 Chronic osteomyelitis with draining sinus, left femur   CC

   M86.459 Chronic osteomyelitis with draining sinus, unspecified femur   CC

✓6th **M86.46** Chronic osteomyelitis with draining sinus, tibia and fibula

   M86.461 Chronic osteomyelitis with draining sinus, right tibia and fibula   CC

   M86.462 Chronic osteomyelitis with draining sinus, left tibia and fibula   CC

   M86.469 Chronic osteomyelitis with draining sinus, unspecified tibia and fibula   CC

✓6th **M86.47** Chronic osteomyelitis with draining sinus, ankle and foot

   M86.471 Chronic osteomyelitis with draining sinus, right ankle and foot   CC

   M86.472 Chronic osteomyelitis with draining sinus, left ankle and foot   CC

   M86.479 Chronic osteomyelitis with draining sinus, unspecified ankle and foot   CC

M86.48 Chronic osteomyelitis with draining sinus, other site   CC

M86.49 Chronic osteomyelitis with draining sinus, multiple sites   CC

✓5th **M86.5** Other chronic hematogenous osteomyelitis

M86.50 Other chronic hematogenous osteomyelitis, unspecified site   CC
    CC Excl: M46.20-M46.39, M86.30-M86.9, M88.0-M88.9, M90.60-M90.69

✓6th **M86.51** Other chronic hematogenous osteomyelitis, shoulder

   M86.511 Other chronic hematogenous osteomyelitis, right shoulder   CC

   M86.512 Other chronic hematogenous osteomyelitis, left shoulder   CC

   M86.519 Other chronic hematogenous osteomyelitis, unspecified shoulder   CC

✓6th **M86.52** Other chronic hematogenous osteomyelitis, humerus

   M86.521 Other chronic hematogenous osteomyelitis, right humerus   CC

   M86.522 Other chronic hematogenous osteomyelitis, left humerus   CC

   M86.529 Other chronic hematogenous osteomyelitis, unspecified humerus   CC

✓6th **M86.53** Other chronic hematogenous osteomyelitis, radius and ulna

   M86.531 Other chronic hematogenous osteomyelitis, right radius and ulna   CC

   M86.532 Other chronic hematogenous osteomyelitis, left radius and ulna   CC

   M86.539 Other chronic hematogenous osteomyelitis, unspecified radius and ulna   CC

✓6th **M86.54** Other chronic hematogenous osteomyelitis, hand

   M86.541 Other chronic hematogenous osteomyelitis, right hand   CC

   M86.542 Other chronic hematogenous osteomyelitis, left hand   CC

   M86.549 Other chronic hematogenous osteomyelitis, unspecified hand   CC

✓6th **M86.55** Other chronic hematogenous osteomyelitis, femur

   M86.551 Other chronic hematogenous osteomyelitis, right femur   CC

   M86.552 Other chronic hematogenous osteomyelitis, left femur   CC

M86.559 Other chronic hematogenous osteomyelitis, unspecified femur   CC

✓6th **M86.56** Other chronic hematogenous osteomyelitis, tibia and fibula

   M86.561 Other chronic hematogenous osteomyelitis, right tibia and fibula   CC

   M86.562 Other chronic hematogenous osteomyelitis, left tibia and fibula   CC

   M86.569 Other chronic hematogenous osteomyelitis, unspecified tibia and fibula   CC

✓6th **M86.57** Other chronic hematogenous osteomyelitis, ankle and foot

   M86.571 Other chronic hematogenous osteomyelitis, right ankle and foot   CC

   M86.572 Other chronic hematogenous osteomyelitis, left ankle and foot   CC

   M86.579 Other chronic hematogenous osteomyelitis, unspecified ankle and foot   CC

M86.58 Other chronic hematogenous osteomyelitis, other site   CC

M86.59 Other chronic hematogenous osteomyelitis, multiple sites   CC

✓5th **M86.6** Other chronic osteomyelitis

M86.60 Other chronic osteomyelitis, unspecified site   CC
    CC Excl: M46.20-M46.39, M86.30-M86.9, M88.0-M88.9, M90.60-M90.69

✓6th **M86.61** Other chronic osteomyelitis, shoulder

   M86.611 Other chronic osteomyelitis, right shoulder   CC

   M86.612 Other chronic osteomyelitis, left shoulder   CC

   M86.619 Other chronic osteomyelitis, unspecified shoulder   CC

✓6th **M86.62** Other chronic osteomyelitis, humerus

   M86.621 Other chronic osteomyelitis, right humerus   CC

   M86.622 Other chronic osteomyelitis, left humerus   CC

   M86.629 Other chronic osteomyelitis, unspecified humerus   CC

✓6th **M86.63** Other chronic osteomyelitis, radius and ulna

   M86.631 Other chronic osteomyelitis, right radius and ulna   CC

   M86.632 Other chronic osteomyelitis, left radius and ulna   CC

   M86.639 Other chronic osteomyelitis, unspecified radius and ulna   CC

✓6th **M86.64** Other chronic osteomyelitis, hand

   M86.641 Other chronic osteomyelitis, right hand   CC

   M86.642 Other chronic osteomyelitis, left hand   CC

   M86.649 Other chronic osteomyelitis, unspecified hand   CC

✓6th **M86.65** Other chronic osteomyelitis, thigh

   M86.651 Other chronic osteomyelitis, right thigh   CC

   M86.652 Other chronic osteomyelitis, left thigh   CC

   M86.659 Other chronic osteomyelitis, unspecified thigh   CC

✓6th **M86.66** Other chronic osteomyelitis, tibia and fibula

   M86.661 Other chronic osteomyelitis, right tibia and fibula   CC

   M86.662 Other chronic osteomyelitis, left tibia and fibula   CC

   M86.669 Other chronic osteomyelitis, unspecified tibia and fibula   CC

✓6th **M86.67** Other chronic osteomyelitis, ankle and foot

   M86.671 Other chronic osteomyelitis, right ankle and foot   CC

   M86.672 Other chronic osteomyelitis, left ankle and foot   CC

   M86.679 Other chronic osteomyelitis, unspecified ankle and foot   CC

M86.68 Other chronic osteomyelitis, other site   CC

M86.69 Other chronic osteomyelitis, multiple sites   CC

✓5th **M86.8** Other **osteomyelitis**
Brodie's abscess

✓6th **M86.8X** Other **osteomyelitis**

M86.8X0 Other osteomyelitis, **multiple sites** `cc`

M86.8X1 Other osteomyelitis, **shoulder** `cc`

M86.8X2 Other osteomyelitis, **upper arm** `cc`

M86.8X3 Other osteomyelitis, **forearm** `cc`

M86.8X4 Other osteomyelitis, **hand** `cc`

M86.8X5 Other osteomyelitis, **thigh** `cc`

M86.8X6 Other osteomyelitis, **lower leg** `cc`

M86.8X7 Other osteomyelitis, **ankle and foot** `cc`

M86.8X8 Other osteomyelitis, **other site** `cc`

M86.8X9 Other osteomyelitis, **unspecified sites** `cc`
CC Excl: M46.20–M46.39, M86.30–M86.9, M88.0–M88.9, M90.60–M90.69

M86.9 Osteomyelitis, unspecified `cc`
Infection of bone NOS
Periostitis without osteomyelitis
CC Excl: See code: M86.8X9

✓4th **M87** **Osteonecrosis**
INCLUDES avascular necrosis of bone
Use additional code to identify major osseous defect, if applicable (M89.7-)
EXCLUDES 1 juvenile osteonecrosis (M91-M92)
osteochondropathies (M90-M93)

✓5th **M87.0** Idiopathic aseptic necrosis of bone

M87.00 Idiopathic aseptic necrosis of **unspecified bone** `cc`
CC Excl: M87.00–M87.9, M90.50–M90.59

✓6th **M87.01** Idiopathic aseptic necrosis of **shoulder**
Idiopathic aseptic necrosis of clavicle and scapula

M87.011 Idiopathic aseptic necrosis of **right shoulder** `cc`
CC Excl: M87.00–M87.050, M87.061–M87.073, M87.077–M87.146, M87.161–M87.173, M87.177–M87.250, M87.261–M87.273, M87.277–M87.346, M87.361–M87.373, M87.377–M87.849, M87.861–M87.873, M87.877–M87.9, M90.50–M90.549, M90.561–M90.59

M87.012 Idiopathic aseptic necrosis of **left shoulder** `cc`
CC Excl: See code: M87.011

M87.019 Idiopathic aseptic necrosis of **unspecified shoulder** `cc`
CC Excl: See code: M87.011

✓6th **M87.02** Idiopathic aseptic necrosis of **humerus**

M87.021 Idiopathic aseptic necrosis of **right humerus** `cc`
CC Excl: See code: M87.011

M87.022 Idiopathic aseptic necrosis of **left humerus** `cc`
CC Excl: See code: M87.011

M87.029 Idiopathic aseptic necrosis of **unspecified humerus** `cc`
CC Excl: See code: M87.011

✓6th **M87.03** Idiopathic aseptic necrosis of **radius, ulna and carpus**

M87.031 Idiopathic aseptic necrosis of **right radius** `cc`
CC Excl: M87.00–M87.9, M90.50–M90.59

M87.032 Idiopathic aseptic necrosis of **left radius** `cc`
CC Excl: See code: M87.31

M87.033 Idiopathic aseptic necrosis of **unspecified radius** `cc`
CC Excl: See code: M87.31

M87.034 Idiopathic aseptic necrosis of **right ulna** `cc`
CC Excl: See code: M87.31

M87.035 Idiopathic aseptic necrosis of **left ulna** `cc`
CC Excl: See code: M87.31

M87.036 Idiopathic aseptic necrosis of **unspecified ulna** `cc`
CC Excl: See code: M87.31

M87.037 Idiopathic aseptic necrosis of **right carpus** `cc`
CC Excl: See code: M87.31

M87.038 Idiopathic aseptic necrosis of **left carpus** `cc`
CC Excl: See code: M87.31

M87.039 Idiopathic aseptic necrosis of **unspecified carpus** `cc`
CC Excl: See code: M87.31

✓6th **M87.04** Idiopathic aseptic necrosis of **hand and fingers**
Idiopathic aseptic necrosis of metacarpals and phalanges of hands

M87.041 Idiopathic aseptic necrosis of **right hand** `cc`
CC Excl: See code: M87.31

M87.042 Idiopathic aseptic necrosis of **left hand** `cc`
CC Excl: See code: M87.31

M87.043 Idiopathic aseptic necrosis of **unspecified hand** `cc`
CC Excl: See code: M87.31

M87.044 Idiopathic aseptic necrosis of **right finger(s)** `cc`
CC Excl: See code: M87.31

M87.045 Idiopathic aseptic necrosis of **left finger(s)** `cc`
CC Excl: See code: M87.31

M87.046 Idiopathic aseptic necrosis of **unspecified finger(s)** `cc`
CC Excl: See code: M87.31

✓6th **M87.05** Idiopathic aseptic necrosis of **pelvis and femur**

M87.050 Idiopathic aseptic necrosis of **pelvis** `cc`
CC Excl: See code: M87.31

M87.051 Idiopathic aseptic necrosis of **right femur** `cc`
CC Excl: M87.00, M87.031–M87.073, M87.077–M87.119, M87.131–M87.173, M87.177–M87.219, M87.231–M87.273, M87.277–M87.319, M87.331–M87.373, M87.377–M87.819, M87.831–M87.873, M87.877–M87.9, M90.50, M90.521–M90.59

M87.052 Idiopathic aseptic necrosis of **left femur** `cc`
CC Excl: See code: M87.051

M87.059 Idiopathic aseptic necrosis of **unspecified femur** `cc`
Idiopathic aseptic necrosis of hip NOS
CC Excl: See code: M87.051

✓6th **M87.06** Idiopathic aseptic necrosis of **tibia and fibula**

M87.061 Idiopathic aseptic necrosis of **right tibia** `cc`
CC Excl: M87.00–M87.9, M90.50–M90.59

M87.062 Idiopathic aseptic necrosis of **left tibia** `cc`
CC Excl: See code: M87.61

M87.063 Idiopathic aseptic necrosis of **unspecified tibia** `cc`
CC Excl: See code: M87.61

M87.064 Idiopathic aseptic necrosis of **right fibula** `cc`
CC Excl: See code: M87.61

M87.065 Idiopathic aseptic necrosis of **left fibula** `cc`
CC Excl: See code: M87.61

M87.066 Idiopathic aseptic necrosis of **unspecified fibula** `cc`
CC Excl: See code: M87.61

✓6th **M87.07** Idiopathic aseptic necrosis of **ankle, foot and toes**
Idiopathic aseptic necrosis of metatarsus, tarsus, and phalanges of toes

M87.071 Idiopathic aseptic necrosis of **right ankle** `cc`
CC Excl: See code: M87.61

M87.072 Idiopathic aseptic necrosis of **left ankle** `cc`
CC Excl: See code: M87.61

M87.073 Idiopathic aseptic necrosis of **unspecified ankle** `cc`
CC Excl: See code: M87.61

M87.074 Idiopathic aseptic necrosis of **right foot** `cc`
CC Excl: M87.00, M87.031–M87.050, M87.061–M87.119, M87.131–M87.146, M87.161–M87.219, M87.231–M87.250, M87.261–M87.319, M87.331–M87.346, M87.361–M87.819, M87.831–M87.849, M87.861–M87.9, M90.50, M90.521–M90.549, M90.561–M90.59

M87.075 Idiopathic aseptic necrosis of **left foot** `cc`
CC Excl: See code: M87.074

M87.076 Idiopathic aseptic necrosis of unspecified foot `CC`
CC Excl: See code: M87.074

M87.077 Idiopathic aseptic necrosis of right toe(s) `CC`
CC Excl: M87.00-M87.9, M90.50-M90.59

M87.078 Idiopathic aseptic necrosis of left toe(s) `CC`
CC Excl: See code: M87.077

M87.079 Idiopathic aseptic necrosis of unspecified toe(s) `CC`
CC Excl: See code: M87.077

M87.08 Idiopathic aseptic necrosis of bone, other site `CC`
CC Excl: See code: M87.077

M87.09 Idiopathic aseptic necrosis of bone, multiple sites `CC`
CC Excl: See code: M87.077

✓5ᵗʰ **M87.1 Osteonecrosis due to drugs**
Use additional code for adverse effect, if applicable, to identify drug (T36-T50 with fifth or sixth character 5)

M87.10 Osteonecrosis due to drugs, unspecified bone `CC`
CC Excl: See code: M87.00

✓6ᵗʰ **M87.11 Osteonecrosis due to drugs, shoulder**

M87.111 Osteonecrosis due to drugs, right shoulder `CC`
CC Excl: See code: M87.77

M87.112 Osteonecrosis due to drugs, left shoulder `CC`
CC Excl: See code: M87.77

M87.119 Osteonecrosis due to drugs, unspecified shoulder `CC`
CC Excl: See code: M87.77

✓6ᵗʰ **M87.12 Osteonecrosis due to drugs, humerus**

M87.121 Osteonecrosis due to drugs, right humerus `CC`
CC Excl: M87.00-M87.050, M87.061-M87.073, M87.077-M87.146, M87.161-M87.173, M87.177-M87.250, M87.261-M87.273, M87.277-M87.346, M87.361-M87.373, M87.377-M87.849, M87.861-M87.873, M87.877-M87.9, M90.50-M90.549, M90.561-M90.59

M87.122 Osteonecrosis due to drugs, left humerus `CC`
CC Excl: See code: M87.121

M87.129 Osteonecrosis due to drugs, unspecified humerus `CC`
CC Excl: See code: M87.121

✓6ᵗʰ **M87.13 Osteonecrosis due to drugs of radius, ulna and carpus**

M87.131 Osteonecrosis due to drugs of right radius `CC`
CC Excl: See code: M87.077

M87.132 Osteonecrosis due to drugs of left radius `CC`
CC Excl: See code: M87.077

M87.133 Osteonecrosis due to drugs of unspecified radius `CC`
CC Excl: See code: M87.077

M87.134 Osteonecrosis due to drugs of right ulna `CC`
CC Excl: See code: M87.077

M87.135 Osteonecrosis due to drugs of left ulna `CC`
CC Excl: See code: M87.077

M87.136 Osteonecrosis due to drugs of unspecified ulna `CC`
CC Excl: See code: M87.077

M87.137 Osteonecrosis due to drugs of right carpus `CC`
CC Excl: See code: M87.077

M87.138 Osteonecrosis due to drugs of left carpus `CC`
CC Excl: See code: M87.077

M87.139 Osteonecrosis due to drugs of unspecified carpus `CC`
CC Excl: See code: M87.077

✓6ᵗʰ **M87.14 Osteonecrosis due to drugs, hand and fingers**

M87.141 Osteonecrosis due to drugs, right hand `CC`
CC Excl: See code: M87.077

M87.142 Osteonecrosis due to drugs, left hand `CC`
CC Excl: See code: M87.077

M87.143 Osteonecrosis due to drugs, unspecified hand `CC`
CC Excl: See code: M87.077

M87.144 Osteonecrosis due to drugs, right finger(s) `CC`
CC Excl: See code: M87.077

M87.145 Osteonecrosis due to drugs, left finger(s) `CC`
CC Excl: See code: M87.077

M87.146 Osteonecrosis due to drugs, unspecified finger(s) `CC`
CC Excl: See code: M87.077

✓6ᵗʰ **M87.15 Osteonecrosis due to drugs, pelvis and femur**

M87.150 Osteonecrosis due to drugs, pelvis `CC`
CC Excl: M87.00, M87.031-M87.073, M87.077-M87.119, M87.131-M87.173, M87.177-M87.219, M87.231-M87.273, M87.277-M87.319, M87.331-M87.373, M87.377-M87.819, M87.831-M87.873, M87.877-M87.9, M90.50, M90.521-M90.59

M87.151 Osteonecrosis due to drugs, right femur `CC`
CC Excl: See code: M87.150

M87.152 Osteonecrosis due to drugs, left femur `CC`
CC Excl: See code: M87.150

M87.159 Osteonecrosis due to drugs, unspecified femur `CC`
CC Excl: See code: M87.150

✓6ᵗʰ **M87.16 Osteonecrosis due to drugs, tibia and fibula**

M87.161 Osteonecrosis due to drugs, right tibia `CC`
CC Excl: M87.00-M87.9, M90.50-M90.59

M87.162 Osteonecrosis due to drugs, left tibia `CC`
CC Excl: See code: M87.161

M87.163 Osteonecrosis due to drugs, unspecified tibia `CC`
CC Excl: See code: M87.161

M87.164 Osteonecrosis due to drugs, right fibula `CC`
CC Excl: See code: M87.161

M87.165 Osteonecrosis due to drugs, left fibula `CC`
CC Excl: See code: M87.161

M87.166 Osteonecrosis due to drugs, unspecified fibula `CC`
CC Excl: See code: M87.161

✓6ᵗʰ **M87.17 Osteonecrosis due to drugs, ankle, foot and toes**

M87.171 Osteonecrosis due to drugs, right ankle `CC`
CC Excl: See code: M87.161

M87.172 Osteonecrosis due to drugs, left ankle `CC`
CC Excl: See code: M87.161

M87.173 Osteonecrosis due to drugs, unspecified ankle `CC`
CC Excl: See code: M87.161

M87.174 Osteonecrosis due to drugs, right foot `CC`
CC Excl: M87.00, M87.031-M87.050, M87.061-M87.119, M87.131-M87.146, M87.161-M87.219, M87.231-M87.250, M87.261-M87.319, M87.331-M87.346, M87.361-M87.819, M87.831-M87.849, M87.861-M87.9, M90.50, M90.521-M90.549, M90.561-M90.59

M87.175 Osteonecrosis due to drugs, left foot `CC`
CC Excl: See code: M87.174

M87.176 Osteonecrosis due to drugs, unspecified foot `CC`
CC Excl: See code: M87.174

M87.177 Osteonecrosis due to drugs, right toe(s) `CC`
CC Excl: See code: M87.161

M87.178 Osteonecrosis due to drugs, left toe(s) `CC`
CC Excl: See code: M87.161

M87.179 Osteonecrosis due to drugs, unspecified toe(s) `CC`
CC Excl: See code: M87.161

✓6ᵗʰ **M87.18 Osteonecrosis due to drugs, other site**

M87.180 Osteonecrosis due to drugs, jaw `CC`
CC Excl: See code: M87.161

M87.188 Osteonecrosis due to drugs, other site `CC`
CC Excl: See code: M87.161

M87.19 Osteonecrosis due to drugs, multiple sites `CC`
CC Excl: See code: M87.161

Ⓝ Newborn: 0   Ⓟ Pediatric: 0-17   Ⓜ Maternity: 12-55   Ⓐ Adult: 15-124   `MCC` Major CC Condition   `PDx MCC` PDx acts as own MCC   `CC` CC Condition   `PDx CC` PDx acts as own CC

752   ICD-10-CM Draft (2015)

✓5th **M87.2 Osteonecrosis** due to previous trauma

     M87.20 Osteonecrosis due to previous trauma, `CC`
           unspecified bone
           CC Excl: See code: M87.161

  ✓6th **M87.21 Osteonecrosis due to previous trauma,** shoulder

       M87.211 Osteonecrosis due to previous `CC`
            trauma, right shoulder
            CC Excl: See code: M87.161

       M87.212 Osteonecrosis due to previous `CC`
            trauma, left shoulder
            CC Excl: See code: M87.161

       M87.219 Osteonecrosis due to previous trauma, `CC`
            unspecified shoulder
            CC Excl: See code: M87.161

  ✓6th **M87.22 Osteonecrosis due to previous trauma,** humerus

       M87.221 Osteonecrosis due to previous trauma, `CC`
            right humerus
            CC Excl: M87.00–M87.050, M87.061–
            M87.073, M87.077–M87.146, M87.161–
            M87.173, M87.177–M87.250, M87.261–
            M87.273, M87.277–M87.346, M87.361–
            M87.373, M87.377–M87.849, M87.861–
            M87.873, M87.877–M87.9, M90.50–M90.549,
            M90.561–M90.59

       M87.222 Osteonecrosis due to previous trauma, `CC`
            left humerus
            CC Excl: See code: M87.221

       M87.229 Osteonecrosis due to previous trauma, `CC`
            unspecified humerus
            CC Excl: See code: M87.221

  ✓6th **M87.23 Osteonecrosis due to previous trauma of** radius, ulna and carpus

       M87.231 Osteonecrosis due to previous trauma `CC`
            of right radius
            CC Excl: See code: M87.161

       M87.232 Osteonecrosis due to previous trauma `CC`
            of left radius
            CC Excl: See code: M87.161

       M87.233 Osteonecrosis due to previous trauma `CC`
            of unspecified radius
            CC Excl: See code: M87.161

       M87.234 Osteonecrosis due to previous trauma `CC`
            of right ulna
            CC Excl: See code: M87.161

       M87.235 Osteonecrosis due to previous trauma `CC`
            of left ulna
            CC Excl: See code: M87.161

       M87.236 Osteonecrosis due to previous trauma `CC`
            of unspecified ulna
            CC Excl: See code: M87.161

       M87.237 Osteonecrosis due to previous trauma `CC`
            of right carpus
            CC Excl: See code: M87.161

       M87.238 Osteonecrosis due to previous trauma `CC`
            of left carpus
            CC Excl: See code: M87.161

       M87.239 Osteonecrosis due to previous `CC`
            trauma of unspecified carpus
            CC Excl: See code: M87.161

  ✓6th **M87.24 Osteonecrosis due to previous trauma,** hand and fingers

       M87.241 Osteonecrosis due to previous trauma, `CC`
            right hand
            CC Excl: See code: M87.161

       M87.242 Osteonecrosis due to previous trauma, `CC`
            left hand
            CC Excl: See code: M87.161

       M87.243 Osteonecrosis due to previous trauma, `CC`
            unspecified hand
            CC Excl: See code: M87.161

       M87.244 Osteonecrosis due to previous trauma, `CC`
            right finger(s)
            CC Excl: See code: M87.161

       M87.245 Osteonecrosis due to previous trauma, `CC`
            left finger(s)
            CC Excl: See code: M87.161

       M87.246 Osteonecrosis due to previous trauma, `CC`
            unspecified finger(s)
            CC Excl: See code: M87.161

  ✓6th **M87.25 Osteonecrosis due to previous trauma,** pelvis and femur

       M87.250 Osteonecrosis due to previous trauma, `CC`
            pelvis
            CC Excl: M87.00–M87.9, M90.50–M90.59

       M87.251 Osteonecrosis due to previous trauma, `CC`
            right femur
            CC Excl: M87.00, M87.031–M87.073,
            M87.077–M87.119, M87.131–M87.173,
            M87.177–M87.219, M87.231–M87.273,
            M87.277–M87.319, M87.331–M87.373,
            M87.377–M87.819, M87.831–M87.873,
            M87.877–M87.9, M90.50, M90.521–M90.59

       M87.252 Osteonecrosis due to previous trauma, `CC`
            left femur
            CC Excl: See code: M87.251

       M87.256 Osteonecrosis due to previous trauma, `CC`
            unspecified femur
            CC Excl: See code: M87.251

  ✓6th **M87.26 Osteonecrosis due to previous trauma,** tibia and fibula

       M87.261 Osteonecrosis due to previous trauma, `CC`
            right tibia
            CC Excl: See code: M87.250

       M87.262 Osteonecrosis due to previous trauma, `CC`
            left tibia
            CC Excl: See code: M87.250

       M87.263 Osteonecrosis due to previous trauma, `CC`
            unspecified tibia
            CC Excl: See code: M87.250

       M87.264 Osteonecrosis due to previous trauma, `CC`
            right fibula
            CC Excl: See code: M87.250

       M87.265 Osteonecrosis due to previous trauma, `CC`
            left fibula
            CC Excl: See code: M87.250

       M87.266 Osteonecrosis due to previous trauma, `CC`
            unspecified fibula
            CC Excl: See code: M87.250

  ✓6th **M87.27 Osteonecrosis due to previous trauma,** ankle, foot and toes

       M87.271 Osteonecrosis due to previous trauma, `CC`
            right ankle
            CC Excl: See code: M87.250

       M87.272 Osteonecrosis due to previous trauma, `CC`
            left ankle
            CC Excl: See code: M87.250

       M87.273 Osteonecrosis due to previous trauma, `CC`
            unspecified ankle
            CC Excl: See code: M87.250

       M87.274 Osteonecrosis due to previous trauma, `CC`
            right foot
            CC Excl: M87.00, M87.031–M87.050,
            M87.061–M87.119, M87.131–M87.146,
            M87.161–M87.219, M87.231–M87.250,
            M87.261–M87.319, M87.331–M87.346,
            M87.361–M87.819, M87.831–M87.849,
            M87.861–M87.9, M90.50, M90.521–M90.549,
            M90.561–M90.59

       M87.275 Osteonecrosis due to previous trauma, `CC`
            left foot
            CC Excl: See code: M87.274

       M87.276 Osteonecrosis due to previous trauma, `CC`
            unspecified foot
            CC Excl: See code: M87.274

       M87.277 Osteonecrosis due to previous trauma, `CC`
            right toe(s)
            CC Excl: See code: M87.250

       M87.278 Osteonecrosis due to previous trauma, `CC`
            left toe(s)
            CC Excl: See code: M87.250

       M87.279 Osteonecrosis due to previous trauma, `CC`
            unspecified toe(s)
            CC Excl: See code: M87.250

     M87.28 Osteonecrosis due to previous trauma, other site `CC`
           CC Excl: See code: M87.250

     M87.29 Osteonecrosis due to previous trauma, multiple `CC`
           sites
           CC Excl: See code: M87.250

✓ Additional Character Required   ✓x7th Xtension Alert   Unacceptable PDx   Manifestation   Hospital Acquired Condition   `EXCLUDES 1` Not Coded Here   `EXCLUDES 2` Not Included Here

ICD-10-CM Draft (2015)   753

√5th **M87.3** Other secondary osteonecrosis

    M87.30 Other secondary osteonecrosis, unspecified bone CC
       CC Excl: M87.00–M87.9, M90.50–M90.59

   √6th **M87.31** Other secondary osteonecrosis, shoulder

    M87.311 Other secondary osteonecrosis, right shoulder CC
       CC Excl: See code: M87.30

    M87.312 Other secondary osteonecrosis, left shoulder CC
       CC Excl: See code: M87.30

    M87.319 Other secondary osteonecrosis, unspecified shoulder CC
       CC Excl: See code: M87.30

   √6th **M87.32** Other secondary osteonecrosis, humerus

    M87.321 Other secondary osteonecrosis, right humerus CC
       CC Excl: M87.00–M87.050, M87.061–M87.073, M87.077–M87.146, M87.161–M87.173, M87.177–M87.250, M87.261–M87.273, M87.277–M87.346, M87.361–M87.373, M87.377–M87.849, M87.861–M87.873, M87.877–M87.9, M90.50–M90.549, M90.561–M90.59

    M87.322 Other secondary osteonecrosis, left humerus CC
       CC Excl: See code: M87.321

    M87.329 Other secondary osteonecrosis, unspecified humerus CC
       CC Excl: See code: M87.321

   √6th **M87.33** Other secondary osteonecrosis of radius, ulna and carpus

    M87.331 Other secondary osteonecrosis of right radius CC
       CC Excl: See code: M87.30

    M87.332 Other secondary osteonecrosis of left radius CC
       CC Excl: See code: M87.30

    M87.333 Other secondary osteonecrosis of unspecified radius CC
       CC Excl: See code: M87.30

    M87.334 Other secondary osteonecrosis of right ulna CC
       CC Excl: See code: M87.30

    M87.335 Other secondary osteonecrosis of left ulna CC
       CC Excl: See code: M87.30

    M87.336 Other secondary osteonecrosis of unspecified ulna CC
       CC Excl: See code: M87.30

    M87.337 Other secondary osteonecrosis of right carpus CC
       CC Excl: See code: M87.30

    M87.338 Other secondary osteonecrosis of left carpus CC
       CC Excl: See code: M87.30

    M87.339 Other secondary osteonecrosis of unspecified carpus CC
       CC Excl: See code: M87.30

   √6th **M87.34** Other secondary osteonecrosis, hand and fingers

    M87.341 Other secondary osteonecrosis, right hand CC
       CC Excl: See code: M87.30

    M87.342 Other secondary osteonecrosis, left hand CC
       CC Excl: See code: M87.30

    M87.343 Other secondary osteonecrosis, unspecified hand CC
       CC Excl: See code: M87.30

    M87.344 Other secondary osteonecrosis, right finger(s) CC
       CC Excl: See code: M87.30

    M87.345 Other secondary osteonecrosis, left finger(s) CC
       CC Excl: See code: M87.30

    M87.346 Other secondary osteonecrosis, unspecified finger(s) CC
       CC Excl: See code: M87.30

   √6th **M87.35** Other secondary osteonecrosis, pelvis and femur

    M87.350 Other secondary osteonecrosis, pelvis CC
       CC Excl: M87.00, M87.031–M87.073, M87.077–M87.119, M87.131–M87.173, M87.177–M87.219, M87.231–M87.273, M87.277–M87.319, M87.331–M87.373, M87.377–M87.819, M87.831–M87.873, M87.877–M87.9, M90.50, M90.521–M90.59

    M87.351 Other secondary osteonecrosis, right femur CC
       CC Excl: See code: M87.350

    M87.352 Other secondary osteonecrosis, left femur CC
       CC Excl: See code: M87.350

    M87.353 Other secondary osteonecrosis, unspecified femur CC
       CC Excl: See code: M87.350

   √6th **M87.36** Other secondary osteonecrosis, tibia and fibula

    M87.361 Other secondary osteonecrosis, right tibia CC
       CC Excl: M87.00–M87.9, M90.50–M90.59

    M87.362 Other secondary osteonecrosis, left tibia CC
       CC Excl: See code: M87.361

    M87.363 Other secondary osteonecrosis, unspecified tibia CC
       CC Excl: See code: M87.361

    M87.364 Other secondary osteonecrosis, right fibula CC
       CC Excl: See code: M87.361

    M87.365 Other secondary osteonecrosis, left fibula CC
       CC Excl: See code: M87.361

    M87.366 Other secondary osteonecrosis, unspecified fibula CC
       CC Excl: See code: M87.361

   √6th **M87.37** Other secondary osteonecrosis, ankle and foot

    M87.371 Other secondary osteonecrosis, right ankle CC
       CC Excl: See code: M87.361

    M87.372 Other secondary osteonecrosis, left ankle CC
       CC Excl: See code: M87.361

    M87.373 Other secondary osteonecrosis, unspecified ankle CC
       CC Excl: See code: M87.361

    M87.374 Other secondary osteonecrosis, right foot CC
       CC Excl: M87.00, M87.031–M87.050, M87.061–M87.119, M87.131–M87.146, M87.161–M87.219, M87.231–M87.250, M87.261–M87.319, M87.331–M87.346, M87.361–M87.819, M87.831–M87.849, M87.861–M87.9, M90.50, M90.521–M90.549, M90.561–M90.59

    M87.375 Other secondary osteonecrosis, left foot CC
       CC Excl: See code: M87.374

    M87.376 Other secondary osteonecrosis, unspecified foot CC
       CC Excl: See code: M87.374

    M87.377 Other secondary osteonecrosis, right toe(s) CC
       CC Excl: See code: M87.361

    M87.378 Other secondary osteonecrosis, left toe(s) CC
       CC Excl: See code: M87.361

    M87.379 Other secondary osteonecrosis, unspecified toe(s) CC
       CC Excl: See code: M87.361

    M87.38 Other secondary osteonecrosis, other site CC
       CC Excl: See code: M87.361

    M87.39 Other secondary osteonecrosis, multiple sites CC
       CC Excl: See code: M87.361

√5th **M87.8** Other osteonecrosis

    M87.80 Other osteonecrosis, unspecified bone CC
       CC Excl: See code: M87.361

   √6th **M87.81** Other osteonecrosis, shoulder

    M87.811 Other osteonecrosis, right shoulder CC
       CC Excl: See code: M87.361

    M87.812 Other osteonecrosis, left shoulder CC
       CC Excl: See code: M87.361

N Newborn: 0   P Pediatric: 0-17   M Maternity: 12-55   A Adult: 15-124   MCC Major CC Condition   PDx MCC PDx acts as own MCC   CC CC Condition   PDx CC PDx acts as own CC

754   ICD-10-CM Draft (2015)

M87.819 **Other osteonecrosis, unspecified shoulder** `CC`
CC Excl: See code: M87.361

✓6ᵗʰ **M87.82 Other osteonecrosis, humerus**

M87.821 **Other osteonecrosis, right humerus** `CC`
CC Excl: M87.00-M87.050, M87.061-M87.073, M87.077-M87.146, M87.161-M87.173, M87.177-M87.250, M87.261-M87.273, M87.277-M87.346, M87.361-M87.373, M87.377-M87.849, M87.861-M87.873, M87.877-M87.9, M90.50-M90.549, M90.561-M90.59

M87.822 **Other osteonecrosis, left humerus** `CC`
CC Excl: See code: M87.821

M87.829 **Other osteonecrosis, unspecified humerus** `CC`
CC Excl: See code: M87.821

✓6ᵗʰ **M87.83 Other osteonecrosis of radius, ulna and carpus**

M87.831 **Other osteonecrosis of right radius** `CC`
CC Excl: See code: M87.361

M87.832 **Other osteonecrosis of left radius** `CC`
CC Excl: See code: M87.361

M87.833 **Other osteonecrosis of unspecified radius** `CC`
CC Excl: See code: M87.361

M87.834 **Other osteonecrosis of right ulna** `CC`
CC Excl: See code: M87.361

M87.835 **Other osteonecrosis of left ulna** `CC`
CC Excl: See code: M87.361

M87.836 **Other osteonecrosis of unspecified ulna** `CC`
CC Excl: See code: M87.361

M87.837 **Other osteonecrosis of right carpus** `CC`
CC Excl: See code: M87.361

M87.838 **Other osteonecrosis of left carpus** `CC`
CC Excl: See code: M87.361

M87.839 **Other osteonecrosis of unspecified carpus** `CC`
CC Excl: See code: M87.361

✓6ᵗʰ **M87.84 Other osteonecrosis, hand and fingers**

M87.841 **Other osteonecrosis, right hand** `CC`
CC Excl: See code: M87.361

M87.842 **Other osteonecrosis, left hand** `CC`
CC Excl: See code: M87.361

M87.843 **Other osteonecrosis, unspecified hand** `CC`

M87.844 **Other osteonecrosis, right finger(s)** `CC`
CC Excl: See code: M87.361

M87.845 **Other osteonecrosis, left finger(s)** `CC`
CC Excl: See code: M87.361

M87.849 **Other osteonecrosis, unspecified finger(s)** `CC`
CC Excl: See code: M87.361

✓6ᵗʰ **M87.85 Other osteonecrosis, pelvis and femur**

M87.850 **Other osteonecrosis, pelvis** `CC`
CC Excl: M87.00, M87.031-M87.073, M87.077-M87.119, M87.131-M87.173, M87.177-M87.219, M87.231-M87.273, M87.277-M87.319, M87.331-M87.373, M87.377-M87.819, M87.831-M87.873, M87.877-M87.9, M90.50, M90.521-M90.59

M87.851 **Other osteonecrosis, right femur** `CC`
CC Excl: See code: M87.850

M87.852 **Other osteonecrosis, left femur** `CC`
CC Excl: See code: M87.850

M87.859 **Other osteonecrosis, unspecified femur** `CC`
CC Excl: See code: M87.850

✓6ᵗʰ **M87.86 Other osteonecrosis, tibia and fibula**

M87.861 **Other osteonecrosis, right tibia** `CC`
CC Excl: See code: M87.361

M87.862 **Other osteonecrosis, left tibia** `CC`
CC Excl: See code: M87.361

M87.863 **Other osteonecrosis, unspecified tibia** `CC`
CC Excl: See code: M87.361

M87.864 **Other osteonecrosis, right fibula** `CC`
CC Excl: See code: M87.361

M87.865 **Other osteonecrosis, left fibula** `CC`
CC Excl: See code: M87.361

M87.869 **Other osteonecrosis, unspecified fibula** `CC`

✓6ᵗʰ **M87.87 Other osteonecrosis, ankle, foot and toes**

M87.871 **Other osteonecrosis, right ankle** `CC`
CC Excl: See code: M87.361

M87.872 **Other osteonecrosis, left ankle** `CC`
CC Excl: See code: M87.361

M87.873 **Other osteonecrosis, unspecified ankle** `CC`
CC Excl: See code: M87.361

M87.874 **Other osteonecrosis, right foot** `CC`
CC Excl: M87.00, M87.031-M87.050, M87.061-M87.119, M87.131-M87.146, M87.161-M87.219, M87.231-M87.250, M87.261-M87.319, M87.331-M87.346, M87.361-M87.819, M87.831-M87.849, M87.861-M87.9, M90.50, M90.521-M90.549, M90.561-M90.59

M87.875 **Other osteonecrosis, left foot** `CC`
CC Excl: See code: M87.874

M87.876 **Other osteonecrosis, unspecified foot** `CC`
CC Excl: See code: M87.874

M87.877 **Other osteonecrosis, right toe(s)** `CC`
CC Excl: See code: M87.361

M87.878 **Other osteonecrosis, left toe(s)** `CC`
CC Excl: See code: M87.361

M87.879 **Other osteonecrosis, unspecified toe(s)** `CC`
CC Excl: See code: M87.361

M87.88 Other osteonecrosis, other site `CC`
CC Excl: See code: M87.361

M87.89 Other osteonecrosis, multiple sites `CC`
CC Excl: See code: M87.361

M87.9 Osteonecrosis, unspecified `CC`
Necrosis of bone NOS
CC Excl: See code: M87.361

✓4ᵗʰ **M88 Osteitis deformans [Paget's disease of bone]**
EXCLUDES 1 osteitis deformans in neoplastic disease (M90.6)

M88.0 Osteitis deformans of skull

M88.1 Osteitis deformans of vertebrae

✓5ᵗʰ **M88.8 Osteitis deformans of other bones**

✓6ᵗʰ **M88.81 Osteitis deformans of shoulder**

M88.811 **Osteitis deformans of right shoulder**

M88.812 **Osteitis deformans of left shoulder**

M88.819 **Osteitis deformans of unspecified shoulder**

✓6ᵗʰ **M88.82 Osteitis deformans of upper arm**

M88.821 **Osteitis deformans of right upper arm**

M88.822 **Osteitis deformans of left upper arm**

M88.829 **Osteitis deformans of unspecified upper arm**

✓6ᵗʰ **M88.83 Osteitis deformans of forearm**

M88.831 **Osteitis deformans of right forearm**

M88.832 **Osteitis deformans of left forearm**

M88.839 **Osteitis deformans of unspecified forearm**

✓6ᵗʰ **M88.84 Osteitis deformans of hand**

M88.841 **Osteitis deformans of right hand**

M88.842 **Osteitis deformans of left hand**

M88.849 **Osteitis deformans of unspecified hand**

✓6ᵗʰ **M88.85 Osteitis deformans of thigh**

M88.851 **Osteitis deformans of right thigh**

M88.852 **Osteitis deformans of left thigh**

M88.859 **Osteitis deformans of unspecified thigh**

✓6ᵗʰ **M88.86 Osteitis deformans of lower leg**

M88.861 **Osteitis deformans of right lower leg**

M88.862 **Osteitis deformans of left lower leg**

M88.869 **Osteitis deformans of unspecified lower leg**

✓6ᵗʰ **M88.87 Osteitis deformans of ankle and foot**

M88.871 **Osteitis deformans of right ankle and foot**

M88.872 **Osteitis deformans of left ankle and foot**

M88.879 **Osteitis deformans of unspecified ankle and foot**

M88.88 Osteitis deformans of other bones
EXCLUDES 2 osteitis deformans of skull (M88.0)
osteitis deformans of vertebrae (M88.1)

M88.89 Osteitis deformans of multiple sites

M88.9 Osteitis deformans of unspecified bone

✓4th M89 Other disorders of bone

✓5th M89.0 Algoneurodystrophy

Shoulder-hand syndrome
Sudeck's atrophy

EXCLUDES 1   causalgia, lower limb (G57.7-)
causalgia, upper limb (G56.4-)
complex regional pain syndrome II, lower limb (G57.7-)
complex regional pain syndrome II, upper limb (G56.4-)
reflex sympathetic dystrophy (G90.5-)

M89.00 Algoneurodystrophy, unspecified site

✓6th M89.01 Algoneurodystrophy, shoulder
- M89.011 Algoneurodystrophy, right shoulder
- M89.012 Algoneurodystrophy, left shoulder
- M89.019 Algoneurodystrophy, unspecified shoulder

✓6th M89.02 Algoneurodystrophy, upper arm
- M89.021 Algoneurodystrophy, right upper arm
- M89.022 Algoneurodystrophy, left upper arm
- M89.029 Algoneurodystrophy, unspecified upper arm

✓6th M89.03 Algoneurodystrophy, forearm
- M89.031 Algoneurodystrophy, right forearm
- M89.032 Algoneurodystrophy, left forearm
- M89.039 Algoneurodystrophy, unspecified forearm

✓6th M89.04 Algoneurodystrophy, hand
- M89.041 Algoneurodystrophy, right hand
- M89.042 Algoneurodystrophy, left hand
- M89.049 Algoneurodystrophy, unspecified hand

✓6th M89.05 Algoneurodystrophy, thigh
- M89.051 Algoneurodystrophy, right thigh
- M89.052 Algoneurodystrophy, left thigh
- M89.059 Algoneurodystrophy, unspecified thigh

✓6th M89.06 Algoneurodystrophy, lower leg
- M89.061 Algoneurodystrophy, right lower leg
- M89.062 Algoneurodystrophy, left lower leg
- M89.069 Algoneurodystrophy, unspecified lower leg

✓6th M89.07 Algoneurodystrophy, ankle and foot
- M89.071 Algoneurodystrophy, right ankle and foot
- M89.072 Algoneurodystrophy, left ankle and foot
- M89.079 Algoneurodystrophy, unspecified ankle and foot

M89.08 Algoneurodystrophy, other site

M89.09 Algoneurodystrophy, multiple sites

✓5th M89.1 Physeal arrest

Arrest of growth plate
Epiphyseal arrest
Growth plate arrest

✓6th M89.12 Physeal arrest, humerus
- M89.121 Complete physeal arrest, right proximal humerus
- M89.122 Complete physeal arrest, left proximal humerus
- M89.123 Partial physeal arrest, right proximal humerus
- M89.124 Partial physeal arrest, left proximal humerus
- M89.125 Complete physeal arrest, right distal humerus
- M89.126 Complete physeal arrest, left distal humerus
- M89.127 Partial physeal arrest, right distal humerus
- M89.128 Partial physeal arrest, left distal humerus
- M89.129 Physeal arrest, humerus, unspecified

✓6th M89.13 Physeal arrest, forearm
- M89.131 Complete physeal arrest, right distal radius
- M89.132 Complete physeal arrest, left distal radius
- M89.133 Partial physeal arrest, right distal radius
- M89.134 Partial physeal arrest, left distal radius
- M89.138 Other physeal arrest of forearm
- M89.139 Physeal arrest, forearm, unspecified

✓6th M89.15 Physeal arrest, femur
- M89.151 Complete physeal arrest, right proximal femur
- M89.152 Complete physeal arrest, left proximal femur
- M89.153 Partial physeal arrest, right proximal femur
- M89.154 Partial physeal arrest, left proximal femur
- M89.155 Complete physeal arrest, right distal femur
- M89.156 Complete physeal arrest, left distal femur
- M89.157 Partial physeal arrest, right distal femur
- M89.158 Partial physeal arrest, left distal femur
- M89.159 Physeal arrest, femur, unspecified

✓6th M89.16 Physeal arrest, lower leg
- M89.160 Complete physeal arrest, right proximal tibia
- M89.161 Complete physeal arrest, left proximal tibia
- M89.162 Partial physeal arrest, right proximal tibia
- M89.163 Partial physeal arrest, left proximal tibia
- M89.164 Complete physeal arrest, right distal tibia
- M89.165 Complete physeal arrest, left distal tibia
- M89.166 Partial physeal arrest, right distal tibia
- M89.167 Partial physeal arrest, left distal tibia
- M89.168 Other physeal arrest of lower leg
- M89.169 Physeal arrest, lower leg, unspecified

M89.18 Physeal arrest, other site

✓5th M89.2 Other disorders of bone development and growth

M89.20 Other disorders of bone development and growth, unspecified site

✓6th M89.21 Other disorders of bone development and growth, shoulder
- M89.211 Other disorders of bone development and growth, right shoulder
- M89.212 Other disorders of bone development and growth, left shoulder
- M89.219 Other disorders of bone development and growth, unspecified shoulder

✓6th M89.22 Other disorders of bone development and growth, humerus
- M89.221 Other disorders of bone development and growth, right humerus
- M89.222 Other disorders of bone development and growth, left humerus
- M89.229 Other disorders of bone development and growth, unspecified humerus

✓6th M89.23 Other disorders of bone development and growth, ulna and radius
- M89.231 Other disorders of bone development and growth, right ulna
- M89.232 Other disorders of bone development and growth, left ulna
- M89.233 Other disorders of bone development and growth, right radius
- M89.234 Other disorders of bone development and growth, left radius
- M89.239 Other disorders of bone development and growth, unspecified ulna and radius

✓6th M89.24 Other disorders of bone development and growth, hand
- M89.241 Other disorders of bone development and growth, right hand
- M89.242 Other disorders of bone development and growth, left hand
- M89.249 Other disorders of bone development and growth, unspecified hand

✓6th M89.25 Other disorders of bone development and growth, femur
- M89.251 Other disorders of bone development and growth, right femur
- M89.252 Other disorders of bone development and growth, left femur
- M89.259 Other disorders of bone development and growth, unspecified femur

N Newborn: 0   P Pediatric: 0-17   M Maternity: 12-55   A Adult: 15-124   MCC Major CC Condition   PDx MCC PDx acts as own MCC   CC CC Condition   PDx CC PDx acts as own CC

756   ICD-10-CM Draft (2015)

✓6ᵗʰ **M89.26 Other disorders of bone development and growth, tibia and fibula**
    M89.261 Other disorders of bone development and growth, right tibia
    M89.262 Other disorders of bone development and growth, left tibia
    M89.263 Other disorders of bone development and growth, right fibula
    M89.264 Other disorders of bone development and growth, left fibula
    M89.269 Other disorders of bone development and growth, unspecified lower leg

✓6ᵗʰ **M89.27 Other disorders of bone development and growth, ankle and foot**
    M89.271 Other disorders of bone development and growth, right ankle and foot
    M89.272 Other disorders of bone development and growth, left ankle and foot
    M89.279 Other disorders of bone development and growth, unspecified ankle and foot

M89.28 Other disorders of bone development and growth, other site

M89.29 Other disorders of bone development and growth, multiple sites

✓5ᵗʰ **M89.3 Hypertrophy of bone**
    M89.30 Hypertrophy of bone, unspecified site

✓6ᵗʰ **M89.31 Hypertrophy of bone, shoulder**
    M89.311 Hypertrophy of bone, right shoulder
    M89.312 Hypertrophy of bone, left shoulder
    M89.319 Hypertrophy of bone, unspecified shoulder

✓6ᵗʰ **M89.32 Hypertrophy of bone, humerus**
    M89.321 Hypertrophy of bone, right humerus
    M89.322 Hypertrophy of bone, left humerus
    M89.329 Hypertrophy of bone, unspecified humerus

✓6ᵗʰ **M89.33 Hypertrophy of bone, ulna and radius**
    M89.331 Hypertrophy of bone, right ulna
    M89.332 Hypertrophy of bone, left ulna
    M89.333 Hypertrophy of bone, right radius
    M89.334 Hypertrophy of bone, left radius
    M89.339 Hypertrophy of bone, unspecified ulna and radius

✓6ᵗʰ **M89.34 Hypertrophy of bone, hand**
    M89.341 Hypertrophy of bone, right hand
    M89.342 Hypertrophy of bone, left hand
    M89.349 Hypertrophy of bone, unspecified hand

✓6ᵗʰ **M89.35 Hypertrophy of bone, femur**
    M89.351 Hypertrophy of bone, right femur
    M89.352 Hypertrophy of bone, left femur
    M89.359 Hypertrophy of bone, unspecified femur

✓6ᵗʰ **M89.36 Hypertrophy of bone, tibia and fibula**
    M89.361 Hypertrophy of bone, right tibia
    M89.362 Hypertrophy of bone, left tibia
    M89.363 Hypertrophy of bone, right fibula
    M89.364 Hypertrophy of bone, left fibula
    M89.369 Hypertrophy of bone, unspecified tibia and fibula

✓6ᵗʰ **M89.37 Hypertrophy of bone, ankle and foot**
    M89.371 Hypertrophy of bone, right ankle and foot
    M89.372 Hypertrophy of bone, left ankle and foot
    M89.379 Hypertrophy of bone, unspecified ankle and foot

M89.38 Hypertrophy of bone, other site

M89.39 Hypertrophy of bone, multiple sites

✓5ᵗʰ **M89.4 Other hypertrophic osteoarthropathy**
    Marie-Bamberger disease
    Pachydermoperiostosis
    M89.40 Other hypertrophic osteoarthropathy, unspecified site

✓6ᵗʰ **M89.41 Other hypertrophic osteoarthropathy, shoulder**
    M89.411 Other hypertrophic osteoarthropathy, right shoulder
    M89.412 Other hypertrophic osteoarthropathy, left shoulder
    M89.419 Other hypertrophic osteoarthropathy, unspecified shoulder

✓6ᵗʰ **M89.42 Other hypertrophic osteoarthropathy, upper arm**
    M89.421 Other hypertrophic osteoarthropathy, right upper arm
    M89.422 Other hypertrophic osteoarthropathy, left upper arm
    M89.429 Other hypertrophic osteoarthropathy, unspecified upper arm

✓6ᵗʰ **M89.43 Other hypertrophic osteoarthropathy, forearm**
    M89.431 Other hypertrophic osteoarthropathy, right forearm
    M89.432 Other hypertrophic osteoarthropathy, left forearm
    M89.439 Other hypertrophic osteoarthropathy, unspecified forearm

✓6ᵗʰ **M89.44 Other hypertrophic osteoarthropathy, hand**
    M89.441 Other hypertrophic osteoarthropathy, right hand
    M89.442 Other hypertrophic osteoarthropathy, left hand
    M89.449 Other hypertrophic osteoarthropathy, unspecified hand

✓6ᵗʰ **M89.45 Other hypertrophic osteoarthropathy, thigh**
    M89.451 Other hypertrophic osteoarthropathy, right thigh
    M89.452 Other hypertrophic osteoarthropathy, left thigh
    M89.459 Other hypertrophic osteoarthropathy, unspecified thigh

✓6ᵗʰ **M89.46 Other hypertrophic osteoarthropathy, lower leg**
    M89.461 Other hypertrophic osteoarthropathy, right lower leg
    M89.462 Other hypertrophic osteoarthropathy, left lower leg
    M89.469 Other hypertrophic osteoarthropathy, unspecified lower leg

✓6ᵗʰ **M89.47 Other hypertrophic osteoarthropathy, ankle and foot**
    M89.471 Other hypertrophic osteoarthropathy, right ankle and foot
    M89.472 Other hypertrophic osteoarthropathy, left ankle and foot
    M89.479 Other hypertrophic osteoarthropathy, unspecified ankle and foot

M89.48 Other hypertrophic osteoarthropathy, other site

M89.49 Other hypertrophic osteoarthropathy, multiple sites

✓5ᵗʰ **M89.5 Osteolysis**
    Use additional code to identify major osseous defect, if applicable (M89.7-)
    EXCLUDES 2 *periprosthetic osteolysis of internal prosthetic joint (T84.05-)*

    M89.50 Osteolysis, unspecified site

✓6ᵗʰ **M89.51 Osteolysis, shoulder**
    M89.511 Osteolysis, right shoulder
    M89.512 Osteolysis, left shoulder
    M89.519 Osteolysis, unspecified shoulder

✓6ᵗʰ **M89.52 Osteolysis, upper arm**
    M89.521 Osteolysis, right upper arm
    M89.522 Osteolysis, left upper arm
    M89.529 Osteolysis, unspecified upper arm

✓6ᵗʰ **M89.53 Osteolysis, forearm**
    M89.531 Osteolysis, right forearm
    M89.532 Osteolysis, left forearm
    M89.539 Osteolysis, unspecified forearm

✓6ᵗʰ **M89.54 Osteolysis, hand**
    M89.541 Osteolysis, right hand
    M89.542 Osteolysis, left hand
    M89.549 Osteolysis, unspecified hand

✓6ᵗʰ **M89.55 Osteolysis, thigh**
    M89.551 Osteolysis, right thigh
    M89.552 Osteolysis, left thigh
    M89.559 Osteolysis, unspecified thigh

✓ Additional Character Required ✓x7ᵗʰ Xtension Alert Unacceptable PDx Manifestation Hospital Acquired Condition **EXCLUDES 1** Not Coded Here **EXCLUDES 2** Not Included Here

ICD-10-CM Draft (2015)   757

√6th **M89.56 Osteolysis,** lower leg
   M89.561 Osteolysis, right **lower leg**
   M89.562 Osteolysis, left **lower leg**
   M89.569 Osteolysis, unspecified **lower leg**

√6th **M89.57 Osteolysis,** ankle and foot
   M89.571 Osteolysis, right **ankle and foot**
   M89.572 Osteolysis, left **ankle and foot**
   M89.579 Osteolysis, unspecified **ankle and foot**

  M89.58 Osteolysis, other site
  M89.59 Osteolysis, multiple sites

√5th **M89.6 Osteopathy after poliomyelitis**
  Use additional code (B91) to identify previous poliomyelitis
  EXCLUDES 1 *postpolio syndrome (G14)*

  M89.60 Osteopathy after poliomyelitis, unspecified site

√6th **M89.61 Osteopathy after poliomyelitis,** shoulder
   M89.611 Osteopathy after poliomyelitis, right **shoulder**
   M89.612 Osteopathy after poliomyelitis, left **shoulder**
   M89.619 Osteopathy after poliomyelitis, unspecified **shoulder**

√6th **M89.62 Osteopathy after poliomyelitis,** upper arm
   M89.621 Osteopathy after poliomyelitis, right **upper arm**
   M89.622 Osteopathy after poliomyelitis, left **upper arm**
   M89.629 Osteopathy after poliomyelitis, unspecified **upper arm**

√6th **M89.63 Osteopathy after poliomyelitis,** forearm
   M89.631 Osteopathy after poliomyelitis, right **forearm**
   M89.632 Osteopathy after poliomyelitis, left **forearm**
   M89.639 Osteopathy after poliomyelitis, unspecified **forearm**

√6th **M89.64 Osteopathy after poliomyelitis,** hand
   M89.641 Osteopathy after poliomyelitis, right **hand**
   M89.642 Osteopathy after poliomyelitis, left **hand**
   M89.649 Osteopathy after poliomyelitis, unspecified **hand**

√6th **M89.65 Osteopathy after poliomyelitis,** thigh
   M89.651 Osteopathy after poliomyelitis, right **thigh**
   M89.652 Osteopathy after poliomyelitis, left **thigh**
   M89.659 Osteopathy after poliomyelitis, unspecified **thigh**

√6th **M89.66 Osteopathy after poliomyelitis,** lower leg
   M89.661 Osteopathy after poliomyelitis, right **lower leg**
   M89.662 Osteopathy after poliomyelitis, left **lower leg**
   M89.669 Osteopathy after poliomyelitis, unspecified **lower leg**

√6th **M89.67 Osteopathy after poliomyelitis,** ankle and foot
   M89.671 Osteopathy after poliomyelitis, right **ankle and foot**
   M89.672 Osteopathy after poliomyelitis, left **ankle and foot**
   M89.679 Osteopathy after poliomyelitis, unspecified **ankle and foot**

  M89.68 Osteopathy after poliomyelitis, other site
  M89.69 Osteopathy after poliomyelitis, multiple sites

√5th **M89.7 Major osseous defect**
  Code first underlying disease, if known, such as:
   aseptic necrosis of bone (M87.-)
   malignant neoplasm of bone (C40.-)
   osteolysis (M89.5)
   osteomyelitis (M86.-)
   osteonecrosis (M87.-)
   osteoporosis (M80.-, M81.-)
   periprosthetic osteolysis (T84.05-)

  M89.70 Major osseous defect, unspecified site

√6th **M89.71 Major osseous defect,** shoulder **region**
   Major osseous defect clavicle or scapula
   M89.711 Major osseous defect, right **shoulder region**
   M89.712 Major osseous defect, left **shoulder region**
   M89.719 Major osseous defect, unspecified **shoulder region**

√6th **M89.72 Major osseous defect,** humerus
   M89.721 Major osseous defect, right **humerus**
   M89.722 Major osseous defect, left **humerus**
   M89.729 Major osseous defect, unspecified **humerus**

√6th **M89.73 Major osseous defect,** forearm
   Major osseous defect of radius and ulna
   M89.731 Major osseous defect, right **forearm**
   M89.732 Major osseous defect, left **forearm**
   M89.739 Major osseous defect, unspecified **forearm**

√6th **M89.74 Major osseous defect,** hand
   Major osseous defect of carpus, fingers, metacarpus
   M89.741 Major osseous defect, right **hand**
   M89.742 Major osseous defect, left **hand**
   M89.749 Major osseous defect, unspecified **hand**

√6th **M89.75 Major osseous defect,** pelvic region and thigh
   Major osseous defect of femur and pelvis
   M89.751 Major osseous defect, right **pelvic region and thigh**
   M89.752 Major osseous defect, left **pelvic region and thigh**
   M89.759 Major osseous defect, unspecified **pelvic region and thigh**

√6th **M89.76 Major osseous defect,** lower leg
   Major osseous defect of fibula and tibia
   M89.761 Major osseous defect, right **lower leg**
   M89.762 Major osseous defect, left **lower leg**
   M89.769 Major osseous defect, unspecified **lower leg**

√6th **M89.77 Major osseous defect,** ankle and foot
   Major osseous defect of metatarsus, tarsus, toes
   M89.771 Major osseous defect, right **ankle and foot**
   M89.772 Major osseous defect, left **ankle and foot**
   M89.779 Major osseous defect, unspecified **ankle and foot**

  M89.78 Major osseous defect, other site
  M89.79 Major osseous defect, multiple sites

√5th **M89.8 Other specified disorders of bone**
  Infantile cortical hyperostoses
  Post-traumatic subperiosteal ossification

√6th **M89.8X Other specified disorders of bone**
   M89.8X0 Other specified disorders of bone, multiple sites
   M89.8X1 Other specified disorders of bone, shoulder
   M89.8X2 Other specified disorders of bone, upper arm
   M89.8X3 Other specified disorders of bone, forearm
   M89.8X4 Other specified disorders of bone, hand
   M89.8X5 Other specified disorders of bone, thigh
   M89.8X6 Other specified disorders of bone, lower leg
   M89.8X7 Other specified disorders of bone, ankle and foot
   M89.8X8 Other specified disorders of bone, other site
   M89.8X9 Other specified disorders of bone, unspecified site

M89.9 Disorder of bone, unspecified

N Newborn: 0 P Pediatric: 0-17 M Maternity: 12-55 A Adult: 15-124 MCC Major CC Condition PDx MCC PDx acts as own MCC CC CC Condition PDx CC PDx acts as own CC

758   ICD-10-CM Draft (2015)

☑4ᵗʰ **M90 Osteopathies in diseases classified elsewhere**

　　EXCLUDES 1　osteochondritis, osteomyelitis, and osteopathy (in):
　　　　cryptococcosis (B45.3)
　　　　diabetes mellitus (E08-E13 with .61-)
　　　　gonococcal (A54.43)
　　　　neurogenic syphilis (A52.11)
　　　　renal osteodystrophy (N25.0)
　　　　salmonellosis (A02.24)
　　　　secondary syphilis (A51.46)
　　　　syphilis (late) (A52.77)

☑5ᵗʰ **M90.5 Osteonecrosis in diseases classified elsewhere**

　　Code first underlying disease, such as:
　　　caisson disease (T70.3)
　　　hemoglobinopathy (D50-D64)

　　CC Excl: For CC codes in subcategory M90.5, unless otherwise noted: M87.00-M87.9, M90.50-M90.59

　　M90.50 Osteonecrosis in diseases classified elsewhere, *unspecified site*　　PDx CC | CC

☑6ᵗʰ **M90.51 Osteonecrosis in diseases classified elsewhere, shoulder**

　　　M90.511 Osteonecrosis in diseases classified elsewhere, *right* **shoulder**　　PDx CC | CC
　　　　CC Excl: M87.00-M87.050, M87.061-M87.073, M87.077-M87.146, M87.161-M87.173, M87.177-M87.250, M87.261-M87.273, M87.277-M87.346, M87.361-M87.373, M87.377-M87.849, M87.861-M87.873, M87.877-M87.9, M90.50-M90.549, M90.561-M90.59

　　　M90.512 Osteonecrosis in diseases classified elsewhere, *left* **shoulder**　　PDx CC | CC
　　　　CC Excl: See code: M90.511

　　　M90.519 Osteonecrosis in diseases classified elsewhere, *unspecified* **shoulder**　　PDx CC | CC
　　　　CC Excl: See code: M90.511

☑6ᵗʰ **M90.52 Osteonecrosis in diseases classified elsewhere, upper arm**

　　　M90.521 Osteonecrosis in diseases classified elsewhere, *right* **upper arm**　　PDx CC | CC

　　　M90.522 Osteonecrosis in diseases classified elsewhere, *left* **upper arm**　　PDx CC | CC

　　　M90.529 Osteonecrosis in diseases classified elsewhere, *unspecified* **upper arm**　　PDx CC | CC

☑6ᵗʰ **M90.53 Osteonecrosis in diseases classified elsewhere, forearm**

　　　M90.531 Osteonecrosis in diseases classified elsewhere, *right* **forearm**　　PDx CC | CC

　　　M90.532 Osteonecrosis in diseases classified elsewhere, *left* **forearm**　　PDx CC | CC

　　　M90.539 Osteonecrosis in diseases classified elsewhere, *unspecified* **forearm**　　PDx CC | CC

☑6ᵗʰ **M90.54 Osteonecrosis in diseases classified elsewhere, hand**

　　　M90.541 Osteonecrosis in diseases classified elsewhere, *right* **hand**　　PDx CC | CC

　　　M90.542 Osteonecrosis in diseases classified elsewhere, *left* **hand**　　PDx CC | CC

　　　M90.549 Osteonecrosis in diseases classified elsewhere, *unspecified* **hand**　　PDx CC | CC

☑6ᵗʰ **M90.55 Osteonecrosis in diseases classified elsewhere, thigh**

　　　M90.551 Osteonecrosis in diseases classified elsewhere, *right* **thigh**　　PDx CC | CC
　　　　CC Excl: M87.00, M87.031-M87.073, M87.077-M87.119, M87.131-M87.173, M87.177-M87.219, M87.231-M87.273, M87.277-M87.319, M87.331-M87.373, M87.377-M87.819, M87.831-M87.873, M87.877-M87.9, M90.50, M90.521-M90.59

　　　M90.552 Osteonecrosis in diseases classified elsewhere, *left* **thigh**　　PDx CC | CC
　　　　CC Excl: See code: M90.551

　　　M90.559 Osteonecrosis in diseases classified elsewhere, *unspecified* **thigh**　　PDx CC | CC
　　　　CC Excl: See code: M90.551

☑6ᵗʰ **M90.56 Osteonecrosis in diseases classified elsewhere,** *lower leg*

　　　M90.561 Osteonecrosis in diseases classified elsewhere, *right* **lower leg**　　PDx CC | CC

　　　M90.562 Osteonecrosis in diseases classified elsewhere, *left* **lower leg**　　PDx CC | CC

　　　M90.569 Osteonecrosis in diseases classified elsewhere, *unspecified* **lower leg**　　PDx CC | CC

☑6ᵗʰ **M90.57 Osteonecrosis in diseases classified elsewhere, ankle and foot**

　　　M90.571 Osteonecrosis in diseases classified elsewhere, *right* **ankle and foot**　　PDx CC | CC

　　　M90.572 Osteonecrosis in diseases classified elsewhere, *left* **ankle and foot**　　PDx CC | CC

　　　M90.579 Osteonecrosis in diseases classified elsewhere, *unspecified* **ankle and foot**　　PDx CC | CC

　　M90.58 Osteonecrosis in diseases classified elsewhere, *other site*　　PDx CC | CC

　　M90.59 Osteonecrosis in diseases classified elsewhere, *multiple sites*　　PDx CC | CC

☑5ᵗʰ **M90.6 Osteitis deformans in neoplastic diseases**

　　Osteitis deformans in malignant neoplasm of bone
　　Code first the neoplasm (C40-, C41-)
　　　EXCLUDES 1　osteitis deformans [Paget's disease of bone] (M88.-)

　　M90.60 Osteitis deformans in neoplastic diseases, *unspecified site*

☑6ᵗʰ **M90.61 Osteitis deformans in neoplastic diseases,** *shoulder*

　　　M90.611 Osteitis deformans in neoplastic diseases, *right* **shoulder**

　　　M90.612 Osteitis deformans in neoplastic diseases, *left* **shoulder**

　　　M90.619 Osteitis deformans in neoplastic diseases, *unspecified* **shoulder**

☑6ᵗʰ **M90.62 Osteitis deformans in neoplastic diseases,** *upper arm*

　　　M90.621 Osteitis deformans in neoplastic diseases, *right* **upper arm**

　　　M90.622 Osteitis deformans in neoplastic diseases, *left* **upper arm**

　　　M90.629 Osteitis deformans in neoplastic diseases, *unspecified* **upper arm**

☑6ᵗʰ **M90.63 Osteitis deformans in neoplastic diseases,** *forearm*

　　　M90.631 Osteitis deformans in neoplastic diseases, *right* **forearm**

　　　M90.632 Osteitis deformans in neoplastic diseases, *left* **forearm**

　　　M90.639 Osteitis deformans in neoplastic diseases, *unspecified* **forearm**

☑6ᵗʰ **M90.64 Osteitis deformans in neoplastic diseases,** *hand*

　　　M90.641 Osteitis deformans in neoplastic diseases, *right* **hand**

　　　M90.642 Osteitis deformans in neoplastic diseases, *left* **hand**

　　　M90.649 Osteitis deformans in neoplastic diseases, *unspecified* **hand**

☑6ᵗʰ **M90.65 Osteitis deformans in neoplastic diseases,** *thigh*

　　　M90.651 Osteitis deformans in neoplastic diseases, *right* **thigh**

　　　M90.652 Osteitis deformans in neoplastic diseases, *left* **thigh**

　　　M90.659 Osteitis deformans in neoplastic diseases, *unspecified* **thigh**

☑6ᵗʰ **M90.66 Osteitis deformans in neoplastic diseases,** *lower leg*

　　　M90.661 Osteitis deformans in neoplastic diseases, *right* **lower leg**

　　　M90.662 Osteitis deformans in neoplastic diseases, *left* **lower leg**

　　　M90.669 Osteitis deformans in neoplastic diseases, *unspecified* **lower leg**

☑6ᵗʰ **M90.67 Osteitis deformans in neoplastic diseases,** *ankle and foot*

　　　M90.671 Osteitis deformans in neoplastic diseases, *right* **ankle and foot**

　　　M90.672 Osteitis deformans in neoplastic diseases, *left* **ankle and foot**

　　　M90.679 Osteitis deformans in neoplastic diseases, *unspecified* **ankle and foot**

M90.68 *Osteitis deformans in neoplastic diseases, other site*

M90.69 *Osteitis deformans in neoplastic diseases, multiple sites*

✓5th **M90.8 Osteopathy in diseases classified elsewhere**
Code first underlying disease, such as:
rickets (E55.0)
vitamin-D-resistant rickets (E83.3)

M90.80 *Osteopathy in diseases classified elsewhere, unspecified site*

✓6th **M90.81 Osteopathy in diseases classified elsewhere, shoulder**

     M90.811 *Osteopathy in diseases classified elsewhere, right shoulder*

     M90.812 *Osteopathy in diseases classified elsewhere, left shoulder*

     M90.819 *Osteopathy in diseases classified elsewhere, unspecified shoulder*

✓6th **M90.82 Osteopathy in diseases classified elsewhere, upper arm**

     M90.821 *Osteopathy in diseases classified elsewhere, right upper arm*

     M90.822 *Osteopathy in diseases classified elsewhere, left upper arm*

     M90.829 *Osteopathy in diseases classified elsewhere, unspecified upper arm*

✓6th **M90.83 Osteopathy in diseases classified elsewhere, forearm**

     M90.831 *Osteopathy in diseases classified elsewhere, right forearm*

     M90.832 *Osteopathy in diseases classified elsewhere, left forearm*

     M90.839 *Osteopathy in diseases classified elsewhere, unspecified forearm*

✓6th **M90.84 Osteopathy in diseases classified elsewhere, hand**

     M90.841 *Osteopathy in diseases classified elsewhere, right hand*

     M90.842 *Osteopathy in diseases classified elsewhere, left hand*

     M90.849 *Osteopathy in diseases classified elsewhere, unspecified hand*

✓6th **M90.85 Osteopathy in diseases classified elsewhere, thigh**

     M90.851 *Osteopathy in diseases classified elsewhere, right thigh*

     M90.852 *Osteopathy in diseases classified elsewhere, left thigh*

     M90.859 *Osteopathy in diseases classified elsewhere, unspecified thigh*

✓6th **M90.86 Osteopathy in diseases classified elsewhere, lower leg**

     M90.861 *Osteopathy in diseases classified elsewhere, right lower leg*

     M90.862 *Osteopathy in diseases classified elsewhere, left lower leg*

     M90.869 *Osteopathy in diseases classified elsewhere, unspecified lower leg*

✓6th **M90.87 Osteopathy in diseases classified elsewhere, ankle and foot**

     M90.871 *Osteopathy in diseases classified elsewhere, right ankle and foot*

     M90.872 *Osteopathy in diseases classified elsewhere, left ankle and foot*

     M90.879 *Osteopathy in diseases classified elsewhere, unspecified ankle and foot*

M90.88 *Osteopathy in diseases classified elsewhere, other site*

M90.89 *Osteopathy in diseases classified elsewhere, multiple sites*

Chondropathies (M91-M94)

EXCLUDES 1   *postprocedural chondropathies (M96.-)*

✓4th **M91 Juvenile osteochondrosis of hip and pelvis**
EXCLUDES 1   *slipped upper femoral epiphysis (nontraumatic) (M93.0)*

M91.0 Juvenile osteochondrosis of pelvis
Osteochondrosis (juvenile) of acetabulum
Osteochondrosis (juvenile) of iliac crest [Buchanan]
Osteochondrosis (juvenile) of ischiopubic synchondrosis [van Neck]
Osteochondrosis (juvenile) of symphysis pubis [Pierson]

✓5th **M91.1 Juvenile osteochondrosis of head of femur [Legg-Calvé-Perthes]**

     M91.10 Juvenile osteochondrosis of head of femur [Legg-Calvé-Perthes], unspecified leg

     M91.11 Juvenile osteochondrosis of head of femur [Legg-Calvé-Perthes], right leg

     M91.12 Juvenile osteochondrosis of head of femur [Legg-Calvé-Perthes], left leg

✓5th **M91.2 Coxa plana**
Hip deformity due to previous juvenile osteochondrosis

     M91.20 Coxa plana, unspecified hip

     M91.21 Coxa plana, right hip

     M91.22 Coxa plana, left hip

✓5th **M91.3 Pseudocoxalgia**

     M91.30 Pseudocoxalgia, unspecified hip

     M91.31 Pseudocoxalgia, right hip

     M91.32 Pseudocoxalgia, left hip

✓5th **M91.4 Coxa magna**

     M91.40 Coxa magna, unspecified hip

     M91.41 Coxa magna, right hip

     M91.42 Coxa magna, left hip

✓5th **M91.8 Other juvenile osteochondrosis of hip and pelvis**
Juvenile osteochondrosis after reduction of congenital dislocation of hip

     M91.80 Other juvenile osteochondrosis of hip and pelvis, unspecified leg

     M91.81 Other juvenile osteochondrosis of hip and pelvis, right leg

     M91.82 Other juvenile osteochondrosis of hip and pelvis, left leg

✓5th **M91.9 Juvenile osteochondrosis of hip and pelvis, unspecified**

     M91.90 Juvenile osteochondrosis of hip and pelvis, unspecified, unspecified leg

     M91.91 Juvenile osteochondrosis of hip and pelvis, unspecified, right leg

     M91.92 Juvenile osteochondrosis of hip and pelvis, unspecified, left leg

✓4th **M92 Other juvenile osteochondrosis**

✓5th **M92.0 Juvenile osteochondrosis of humerus**
Osteochondrosis (juvenile) of capitulum of humerus [Panner]
Osteochondrosis (juvenile) of head of humerus [Haas]

     M92.00 Juvenile osteochondrosis of humerus, unspecified arm

     M92.01 Juvenile osteochondrosis of humerus, right arm

     M92.02 Juvenile osteochondrosis of humerus, left arm

✓5th **M92.1 Juvenile osteochondrosis of radius and ulna**
Osteochondrosis (juvenile) of lower ulna [Burns]
Osteochondrosis (juvenile) of radial head [Brailsford]

     M92.10 Juvenile osteochondrosis of radius and ulna, unspecified arm

     M92.11 Juvenile osteochondrosis of radius and ulna, right arm

     M92.12 Juvenile osteochondrosis of radius and ulna, left arm

✓5th **M92.2 Juvenile osteochondrosis, hand**

     ✓6th **M92.20 Unspecified juvenile osteochondrosis, hand**

         M92.201 Unspecified juvenile osteochondrosis, right hand

         M92.202 Unspecified juvenile osteochondrosis, left hand

         M92.209 Unspecified juvenile osteochondrosis, unspecified hand

N Newborn: 0   P Pediatric: 0-17   M Maternity: 12-55   A Adult: 15-124   MCC Major CC Condition   PDx MCC PDx acts as own MCC   CC CC Condition   PDx CC PDx acts as own CC

760   ICD-10-CM Draft (2015)

☑6ᵗʰ **M92.21** Osteochondrosis (juvenile) of carpal lunate [Kienböck]

    M92.211 Osteochondrosis (juvenile) of carpal lunate [Kienböck], right hand

    M92.212 Osteochondrosis (juvenile) of carpal lunate [Kienböck], left hand

    M92.219 Osteochondrosis (juvenile) of carpal lunate [Kienböck], unspecified hand

☑6ᵗʰ **M92.22** Osteochondrosis (juvenile) of metacarpal heads [Mauclaire]

    M92.221 Osteochondrosis (juvenile) of metacarpal heads [Mauclaire], right hand

    M92.222 Osteochondrosis (juvenile) of metacarpal heads [Mauclaire], left hand

    M92.229 Osteochondrosis (juvenile) of metacarpal heads [Mauclaire], unspecified hand

☑6ᵗʰ **M92.29** Other juvenile osteochondrosis, hand

    M92.291 Other juvenile osteochondrosis, right hand

    M92.292 Other juvenile osteochondrosis, left hand

    M92.299 Other juvenile osteochondrosis, unspecified hand

☑5ᵗʰ **M92.3** Other juvenile osteochondrosis, upper limb

    M92.30 Other juvenile osteochondrosis, unspecified upper limb

    M92.31 Other juvenile osteochondrosis, right upper limb

    M92.32 Other juvenile osteochondrosis, left upper limb

☑5ᵗʰ **M92.4** Juvenile osteochondrosis of patella

    Osteochondrosis (juvenile) of primary patellar center [Köhler]

    Osteochondrosis (juvenile) of secondary patellar centre [Sinding Larsen]

    M92.40 Juvenile osteochondrosis of patella, unspecified knee

    M92.41 Juvenile osteochondrosis of patella, right knee

    M92.42 Juvenile osteochondrosis of patella, left knee

☑5ᵗʰ **M92.5** Juvenile osteochondrosis of tibia and fibula

    Osteochondrosis (juvenile) of proximal tibia [Blount]

    Osteochondrosis (juvenile) of tibial tubercle [Osgood-Schlatter]

    Tibia vara

    M92.50 Juvenile osteochondrosis of tibia and fibula, unspecified leg

    M92.51 Juvenile osteochondrosis of tibia and fibula, right leg

    M92.52 Juvenile osteochondrosis of tibia and fibula, left leg

☑5ᵗʰ **M92.6** Juvenile osteochondrosis of tarsus

    Osteochondrosis (juvenile) of calcaneum [Sever]

    Osteochondrosis (juvenile) of os tibiale externum [Haglund]

    Osteochondrosis (juvenile) of talus [Diaz]

    Osteochondrosis (juvenile) of tarsal navicular [Köhler]

    M92.60 Juvenile osteochondrosis of tarsus, unspecified ankle

    M92.61 Juvenile osteochondrosis of tarsus, right ankle

    M92.62 Juvenile osteochondrosis of tarsus, left ankle

☑5ᵗʰ **M92.7** Juvenile osteochondrosis of metatarsus

    Osteochondrosis (juvenile) of fifth metatarsus [Iselin]

    Osteochondrosis (juvenile) of second metatarsus [Freiberg]

    M92.70 Juvenile osteochondrosis of metatarsus, unspecified foot

    M92.71 Juvenile osteochondrosis of metatarsus, right foot

    M92.72 Juvenile osteochondrosis of metatarsus, left foot

M92.8 Other specified juvenile osteochondrosis

    Calcaneal apophysitis

M92.9 Juvenile osteochondrosis, unspecified

    Juvenile apophysitis NOS   Juvenile osteochondritis NOS

    Juvenile epiphysitis NOS   Juvenile osteochondrosis NOS

☑4ᵗʰ **M93 Other osteochondropathies**

    EXCLUDES 2   osteochondrosis of spine (M42.-)

☑5ᵗʰ **M93.0** Slipped upper femoral epiphysis (nontraumatic)

    Use additional code for associated chondrolysis (M94.3)

☑6ᵗʰ **M93.00** Unspecified slipped upper femoral epiphysis (nontraumatic)

    M93.001 Unspecified slipped upper femoral epiphysis (nontraumatic), right hip

    M93.002 Unspecified slipped upper femoral epiphysis (nontraumatic), left hip

    M93.003 Unspecified slipped upper femoral epiphysis (nontraumatic), unspecified hip

☑6ᵗʰ **M93.01** Acute slipped upper femoral epiphysis (nontraumatic)

    M93.011 Acute slipped upper femoral epiphysis (nontraumatic), right hip

    M93.012 Acute slipped upper femoral epiphysis (nontraumatic), left hip

    M93.013 Acute slipped upper femoral epiphysis (nontraumatic), unspecified hip

☑6ᵗʰ **M93.02** Chronic slipped upper femoral epiphysis (nontraumatic)

    M93.021 Chronic slipped upper femoral epiphysis (nontraumatic), right hip

    M93.022 Chronic slipped upper femoral epiphysis (nontraumatic), left hip

    M93.023 Chronic slipped upper femoral epiphysis (nontraumatic), unspecified hip

☑6ᵗʰ **M93.03** Acute on chronic slipped upper femoral epiphysis (nontraumatic)

    M93.031 Acute on chronic slipped upper femoral epiphysis (nontraumatic), right hip

    M93.032 Acute on chronic slipped upper femoral epiphysis (nontraumatic), left hip

    M93.033 Acute on chronic slipped upper femoral epiphysis (nontraumatic), unspecified hip

M93.1 Kienböck's disease of adults   Ⓐ

    Adult osteochondrosis of carpal lunates

☑5ᵗʰ **M93.2** Osteochondritis dissecans

    M93.20 Osteochondritis dissecans of unspecified site

☑6ᵗʰ **M93.21** Osteochondritis dissecans of shoulder

    M93.211 Osteochondritis dissecans, right shoulder

    M93.212 Osteochondritis dissecans, left shoulder

    M93.219 Osteochondritis dissecans, unspecified shoulder

☑6ᵗʰ **M93.22** Osteochondritis dissecans of elbow

    M93.221 Osteochondritis dissecans, right elbow

    M93.222 Osteochondritis dissecans, left elbow

    M93.229 Osteochondritis dissecans, unspecified elbow

☑6ᵗʰ **M93.23** Osteochondritis dissecans of wrist

    M93.231 Osteochondritis dissecans, right wrist

    M93.232 Osteochondritis dissecans, left wrist

    M93.239 Osteochondritis dissecans, unspecified wrist

☑6ᵗʰ **M93.24** Osteochondritis dissecans of joints of hand

    M93.241 Osteochondritis dissecans, joints of right hand

    M93.242 Osteochondritis dissecans, joints of left hand

    M93.249 Osteochondritis dissecans, joints of unspecified hand

☑6ᵗʰ **M93.25** Osteochondritis dissecans of hip

    M93.251 Osteochondritis dissecans, right hip

    M93.252 Osteochondritis dissecans, left hip

    M93.259 Osteochondritis dissecans, unspecified hip

☑6ᵗʰ **M93.26** Osteochondritis dissecans knee

    M93.261 Osteochondritis dissecans, right knee

    M93.262 Osteochondritis dissecans, left knee

    M93.269 Osteochondritis dissecans, unspecified knee

☑6ᵗʰ **M93.27** Osteochondritis dissecans of ankle and joints of foot

    M93.271 Osteochondritis dissecans, right ankle and joints of right foot

    M93.272 Osteochondritis dissecans, left ankle and joints of left foot

    M93.279 Osteochondritis dissecans, unspecified ankle and joints of foot

    M93.28 Osteochondritis dissecans other site

    M93.29 Osteochondritis dissecans multiple sites

☑5ᵗʰ **M93.8** Other specified osteochondropathies

    M93.80 Other specified osteochondropathies of unspecified site

☑ Additional Character Required   ☑x7ᵗʰ Xtension Alert   <u>Unacceptable PDx</u>   Manifestation   Hospital Acquired Condition   **EXCLUDES 1** Not Coded Here   **EXCLUDES 2** Not Included Here

ICD-10-CM Draft (2015)   761

✓6ᵗʰ **M93.81 Other specified osteochondropathies of** shoulder
- **M93.811** Other specified osteochondropathies, right shoulder
- **M93.812** Other specified osteochondropathies, left shoulder
- **M93.819** Other specified osteochondropathies, unspecified shoulder

✓6ᵗʰ **M93.82 Other specified osteochondropathies of** upper arm
- **M93.821** Other specified osteochondropathies, right upper arm
- **M93.822** Other specified osteochondropathies, left upper arm
- **M93.829** Other specified osteochondropathies, unspecified upper arm

✓6ᵗʰ **M93.83 Other specified osteochondropathies of** forearm
- **M93.831** Other specified osteochondropathies, right forearm
- **M93.832** Other specified osteochondropathies, left forearm
- **M93.839** Other specified osteochondropathies, unspecified forearm

✓6ᵗʰ **M93.84 Other specified osteochondropathies of** hand
- **M93.841** Other specified osteochondropathies, right hand
- **M93.842** Other specified osteochondropathies, left hand
- **M93.849** Other specified osteochondropathies, unspecified hand

✓6ᵗʰ **M93.85 Other specified osteochondropathies of** thigh
- **M93.851** Other specified osteochondropathies, right thigh
- **M93.852** Other specified osteochondropathies, left thigh
- **M93.859** Other specified osteochondropathies, unspecified thigh

✓6ᵗʰ **M93.86 Other specified osteochondropathies** lower leg
- **M93.861** Other specified osteochondropathies, right lower leg
- **M93.862** Other specified osteochondropathies, left lower leg
- **M93.869** Other specified osteochondropathies, unspecified lower leg

✓6ᵗʰ **M93.87 Other specified osteochondropathies of** ankle and foot
- **M93.871** Other specified osteochondropathies, right ankle and foot
- **M93.872** Other specified osteochondropathies, left ankle and foot
- **M93.879** Other specified osteochondropathies, unspecified ankle and foot

M93.88 Other specified osteochondropathies other site
M93.89 Other specified osteochondropathies multiple sites

✓5ᵗʰ **M93.9 Osteochondropathy, unspecified**
Apophysitis NOS   Osteochondritis NOS
Epiphysitis NOS   Osteochondrosis NOS
M93.90 Osteochondropathy, unspecified of unspecified site

✓6ᵗʰ **M93.91 Osteochondropathy, unspecified of** shoulder
- **M93.911** Osteochondropathy, unspecified, right shoulder
- **M93.912** Osteochondropathy, unspecified, left shoulder
- **M93.919** Osteochondropathy, unspecified, unspecified shoulder

✓6ᵗʰ **M93.92 Osteochondropathy, unspecified of** upper arm
- **M93.921** Osteochondropathy, unspecified, right upper arm
- **M93.922** Osteochondropathy, unspecified, left upper arm
- **M93.929** Osteochondropathy, unspecified, unspecified upper arm

✓6ᵗʰ **M93.93 Osteochondropathy, unspecified of** forearm
- **M93.931** Osteochondropathy, unspecified, right forearm
- **M93.932** Osteochondropathy, unspecified, left forearm
- **M93.939** Osteochondropathy, unspecified, unspecified forearm

✓6ᵗʰ **M93.94 Osteochondropathy, unspecified of** hand
- **M93.941** Osteochondropathy, unspecified, right hand
- **M93.942** Osteochondropathy, unspecified, left hand
- **M93.949** Osteochondropathy, unspecified, unspecified hand

✓6ᵗʰ **M93.95 Osteochondropathy, unspecified of** thigh
- **M93.951** Osteochondropathy, unspecified, right thigh
- **M93.952** Osteochondropathy, unspecified, left thigh
- **M93.959** Osteochondropathy, unspecified, unspecified thigh

✓6ᵗʰ **M93.96 Osteochondropathy, unspecified** lower leg
- **M93.961** Osteochondropathy, unspecified, right lower leg
- **M93.962** Osteochondropathy, unspecified, left lower leg
- **M93.969** Osteochondropathy, unspecified, unspecified lower leg

✓6ᵗʰ **M93.97 Osteochondropathy, unspecified of** ankle and foot
- **M93.971** Osteochondropathy, unspecified, right ankle and foot
- **M93.972** Osteochondropathy, unspecified, left ankle and foot
- **M93.979** Osteochondropathy, unspecified, unspecified ankle and foot

M93.98 Osteochondropathy, unspecified other site
M93.99 Osteochondropathy, unspecified multiple sites

✓4ᵗʰ **M94 Other disorders of cartilage**
M94.0 Chondrocostal junction syndrome [Tietze]
Costochondritis
M94.1 Relapsing polychondritis
✓5ᵗʰ **M94.2 Chondromalacia**
EXCLUDES 1 chondromalacia patellae (M22.4)
M94.20 Chondromalacia, unspecified site
✓6ᵗʰ **M94.21 Chondromalacia, shoulder**
- **M94.211 Chondromalacia, right shoulder**
- **M94.212 Chondromalacia, left shoulder**
- **M94.219 Chondromalacia, unspecified shoulder**
✓6ᵗʰ **M94.22 Chondromalacia, elbow**
- **M94.221 Chondromalacia, right elbow**
- **M94.222 Chondromalacia, left elbow**
- **M94.229 Chondromalacia, unspecified elbow**
✓6ᵗʰ **M94.23 Chondromalacia, wrist**
- **M94.231 Chondromalacia, right wrist**
- **M94.232 Chondromalacia, left wrist**
- **M94.239 Chondromalacia, unspecified wrist**
✓6ᵗʰ **M94.24 Chondromalacia, joints of hand**
- **M94.241 Chondromalacia, joints of right hand**
- **M94.242 Chondromalacia, joints of left hand**
- **M94.249 Chondromalacia, joints of unspecified hand**
✓6ᵗʰ **M94.25 Chondromalacia, hip**
- **M94.251 Chondromalacia, right hip**
- **M94.252 Chondromalacia, left hip**
- **M94.259 Chondromalacia, unspecified hip**
✓6ᵗʰ **M94.26 Chondromalacia, knee**
- **M94.261 Chondromalacia, right knee**
- **M94.262 Chondromalacia, left knee**
- **M94.269 Chondromalacia, unspecified knee**
✓6ᵗʰ **M94.27 Chondromalacia, ankle and joints of foot**
- **M94.271 Chondromalacia, right ankle and joints of foot**
- **M94.272 Chondromalacia, left ankle and joints of foot**
- **M94.279 Chondromalacia, unspecified ankle and joints of foot**
M94.28 Chondromalacia, other site
M94.29 Chondromalacia, multiple sites

N Newborn: 0   P Pediatric: 0-17   M Maternity: 12-55   A Adult: 15-124   MCC Major CC Condition   PDx MCC PDx acts as own MCC   CC CC Condition   PDx CC PDx acts as own CC

762   ICD-10-CM Draft (2015)

✓5ᵗʰ **M94.3 Chondrolysis**

Code first any associated slipped upper femoral epiphysis (nontraumatic) (M93.0-)

   ✓6ᵗʰ **M94.35 Chondrolysis, hip**

      M94.351 Chondrolysis, right hip

      M94.352 Chondrolysis, left hip

      M94.359 Chondrolysis, unspecified hip

✓5ᵗʰ **M94.8 Other specified disorders of cartilage**

   ✓6ᵗʰ **M94.8X Other specified disorders of cartilage**

      M94.8X0 Other specified disorders of cartilage, multiple sites

      M94.8X1 Other specified disorders of cartilage, shoulder

      M94.8X2 Other specified disorders of cartilage, upper arm

      M94.8X3 Other specified disorders of cartilage, forearm

      M94.8X4 Other specified disorders of cartilage, hand

      M94.8X5 Other specified disorders of cartilage, thigh

      M94.8X6 Other specified disorders of cartilage, lower leg

      M94.8X7 Other specified disorders of cartilage, ankle and foot

      M94.8X8 Other specified disorders of cartilage, other site

      M94.8X9 Other specified disorders of cartilage, unspecified sites

M94.9 Disorder of cartilage, unspecified

Other disorders of the musculoskeletal system and connective tissue (M95)

✓4ᵗʰ **M95 Other acquired deformities of musculoskeletal system and connective tissue**

   EXCLUDES 2   acquired absence of limbs and organs (Z89-Z90)
       acquired deformities of limbs (M20-M21)
       congenital malformations and deformations of the musculoskeletal system (Q65-Q79)
       deforming dorsopathies (M40-M43)
       dentofacial anomalies [including malocclusion] (M26.-)
       postprocedural musculoskeletal disorders (M96.-)

M95.0 Acquired deformity of nose

   EXCLUDES 2   deviated nasal septum (J34.2)

✓5ᵗʰ **M95.1 Cauliflower ear**

   EXCLUDES 2   other acquired deformities of ear (H61.1)

   M95.10 Cauliflower ear, unspecified ear

   M95.11 Cauliflower ear, right ear

   M95.12 Cauliflower ear, left ear

M95.2 Other acquired deformity of head

M95.3 Acquired deformity of neck

M95.4 Acquired deformity of chest and rib

M95.5 Acquired deformity of pelvis

   EXCLUDES 1   maternal care for known or suspected disproportion (O33.-)

M95.8 Other specified acquired deformities of musculoskeletal system

M95.9 Acquired deformity of musculoskeletal system, unspecified

Intraoperative and postprocedural complications and disorders of musculoskeletal system, not elsewhere classified (M96)

✓4ᵗʰ **M96 Intraoperative and postprocedural complications and disorders of musculoskeletal system, not elsewhere classified**

   EXCLUDES 2   arthropathy following intestinal bypass (M02.0-)
       complications of internal orthopedic prosthetic devices, implants and grafts (T84.-)
       disorders associated with osteoporosis (M80)
       presence of functional implants and other devices (Z96-Z97)

M96.0 Pseudarthrosis after fusion or arthrodesis   CC

M96.1 Postlaminectomy syndrome, not elsewhere classified

M96.2 Postradiation kyphosis

M96.3 Postlaminectomy kyphosis

M96.4 Postsurgical lordosis

M96.5 Postradiation scoliosis

✓5ᵗʰ **M96.6 Fracture of bone following insertion of orthopedic implant, joint prosthesis, or bone plate**

Intraoperative fracture of bone during insertion of orthopedic implant, joint prosthesis, or bone plate

   EXCLUDES 2   complication of internal orthopedic devices, implants or grafts (T84.-)

   ✓6ᵗʰ **M96.62 Fracture of humerus following insertion of orthopedic implant, joint prosthesis, or bone plate**

      M96.621 Fracture of humerus following insertion of orthopedic implant, joint prosthesis, or bone plate, right arm   CC

        CC Excl: D78.81-D78.89, E36.8, E89.810-E89.89, H59.011-H59.019, H59.031-H59.099, H59.811-H59.89, H95.811-H95.89, I97.3, L76.81-L76.82, M96.621-M96.69, M96.89, N98.1-N98.9, T84.010-T84.9XX with 7th A; T81.82XA, T81.89XA, T81.9XXA, T84.9

      M96.622 Fracture of humerus following insertion of orthopedic implant, joint prosthesis, or bone plate, left arm   CC
        CC Excl: See code: M96.621

      M96.629 Fracture of humerus following insertion of orthopedic implant, joint prosthesis, or bone plate, unspecified arm   CC
        CC Excl: See code: M96.621

   ✓6ᵗʰ **M96.63 Fracture of radius or ulna following insertion of orthopedic implant, joint prosthesis, or bone plate**

      M96.631 Fracture of radius or ulna following insertion of orthopedic implant, joint prosthesis, or bone plate, right arm   CC
        CC Excl: See code: M96.621

      M96.632 Fracture of radius or ulna following insertion of orthopedic implant, joint prosthesis, or bone plate, left arm   CC
        CC Excl: See code: M96.621

      M96.639 Fracture of radius or ulna following insertion of orthopedic implant, joint prosthesis, or bone plate, unspecified arm   CC
        CC Excl: See code: M96.621

   M96.65 Fracture of pelvis following insertion of orthopedic implant, joint prosthesis, or bone plate   CC
      CC Excl: See code: M96.621

   ✓6ᵗʰ **M96.66 Fracture of femur following insertion of orthopedic implant, joint prosthesis, or bone plate**

      M96.661 Fracture of femur following insertion of orthopedic implant, joint prosthesis, or bone plate, right leg   CC
        CC Excl: See code: M96.621

      M96.662 Fracture of femur following insertion of orthopedic implant, joint prosthesis, or bone plate, left leg   CC
        CC Excl: See code: M96.621

      M96.669 Fracture of femur following insertion of orthopedic implant, joint prosthesis, or bone plate, unspecified leg   CC
        CC Excl: See code: M96.621

   ✓6ᵗʰ **M96.67 Fracture of tibia or fibula following insertion of orthopedic implant, joint prosthesis, or bone plate**

      M96.671 Fracture of tibia or fibula following insertion of orthopedic implant, joint prosthesis, or bone plate, right leg   CC
        CC Excl: See code: M96.621

      M96.672 Fracture of tibia or fibula following insertion of orthopedic implant, joint prosthesis, or bone plate, left leg   CC
        CC Excl: See code: M96.621

      M96.679 Fracture of tibia or fibula following insertion of orthopedic implant, joint prosthesis, or bone plate, unspecified leg   CC
        CC Excl: See code: M96.621

   M96.69 Fracture of other bone following insertion of orthopedic implant, joint prosthesis, or bone plate   CC
      CC Excl: See code: M96.621

✓ Additional Character Required   ✓x7ᵗʰ Xtension Alert   Unacceptable PDx   Manifestation   Hospital Acquired Condition   *EXCLUDES 1* Not Coded Here   *EXCLUDES 2* Not Included Here

Diseases of the Musculoskeletal System and Connective Tissue

M96.8–M99.46

✓5ᵗʰ **M96.8 Other intraoperative and postprocedural complications and disorders of musculoskeletal system, not elsewhere classified**

   ✓6ᵗʰ **M96.81 Intraoperative hemorrhage and hematoma of a musculoskeletal structure complicating a procedure**

       EXCLUDES 1 *intraoperative hemorrhage and hematoma of a musculoskeletal structure due to accidental puncture and laceration during a procedure (M96.82-)*

       M96.810 Intraoperative hemorrhage and hematoma of a musculoskeletal structure complicating a musculoskeletal system procedure CC

         CC Excl: H95.811-H95.89, I85.01, I85.11, I97.3, K21.9, K22.8, K23-K25.0, K25.2, K25.4, K25.6, K26.0, K26.2, K26.4, K26.6, K27.0, K27.2, K27.4, K27.6, K28.0, K28.2, K28.4, K28.6, K29.01, K29.21, K29.31, K29.41, K29.51, K29.61, K29.71, K29.81, K29.91, K31.811, K55.21, K57.01, K57.11, K57.13, K57.21, K57.31, K57.33, K57.41, K57.51, K57.53, K57.81, K57.91, K57.93, K62.5, K92.0-K92.2, M96.810-M96.811, M96.830-M96.89, N98.1-N98.9, P54.1-P54.3, T81.10XA, T81.11XA, T81.12XA, T81.19XA, T81.82XA, T81.89XA, T81.9XXA

       M96.811 Intraoperative hemorrhage and hematoma of a musculoskeletal structure complicating other procedure CC

         CC Excl: See code: M96.810

   ✓6ᵗʰ **M96.82 Accidental puncture and laceration of a musculoskeletal structure during a procedure**

       M96.820 Accidental puncture and laceration of a musculoskeletal structure during a musculoskeletal system procedure CC

         CC Excl: D78.11-D78.12, D78.81-D78.89, E36.11-E36.8, E89.810-E89.89, G96.11, G97.41-G97.49, H59.011-H59.019, H59.031-H59.099, H59.211-H59.229, H59.811-H59.89, H95.31-H95.32, H95.811-H95.89, I97.3, I97.51-I97.52, J95.71-J95.72, K91.71-K91.72, L76.11-L76.12, L76.81-L76.82, M96.820-M96.821, M96.89, N98.1-N98.9, N99.71-N99.72, T81.82XA, T81.89XA, T81.9XXA

       M96.821 Accidental puncture and laceration of a musculoskeletal structure during other procedure CC

         CC Excl: See code: M96.820

   ✓6ᵗʰ **M96.83 Postprocedural hemorrhage and hematoma of a musculoskeletal structure following a procedure**

       M96.830 Postprocedural hemorrhage and hematoma of a musculoskeletal structure following a musculoskeletal system procedure CC

         CC Excl: See code: M96.810

       M96.831 Postprocedural hemorrhage and hematoma of a musculoskeletal structure following other procedure CC

         CC Excl: See code: M96.810

    M96.89 Other intraoperative and postprocedural complications and disorders of the musculoskeletal system CC

       Instability of joint secondary to removal of joint prosthesis

       Use additional code, if applicable, to further specify disorder

       CC Excl: D78.81-D78.89, E36.8, E89.810-E89.89, H59.011-H59.019, H59.031-H59.099, H59.811-H59.89, H95.811-H95.89, I97.3, L76.81-L76.82, M96.89, N98.1-N98.9, T81.82XA, T81.89XA, T81.9XXA

Biomechanical lesions, not elsewhere classified (M99)

✓4ᵗʰ **M99 Biomechanical lesions, not elsewhere classified**

    NOTE This category should not be used if the condition can be classified elsewhere.

   ✓5ᵗʰ **M99.0 Segmental and somatic dysfunction**

       M99.00 Segmental and somatic dysfunction of head region

       M99.01 Segmental and somatic dysfunction of cervical region

       M99.02 Segmental and somatic dysfunction of thoracic region

       M99.03 Segmental and somatic dysfunction of lumbar region

       M99.04 Segmental and somatic dysfunction of sacral region

       M99.05 Segmental and somatic dysfunction of pelvic region

       M99.06 Segmental and somatic dysfunction of lower extremity

       M99.07 Segmental and somatic dysfunction of upper extremity

       M99.08 Segmental and somatic dysfunction of rib cage

       M99.09 Segmental and somatic dysfunction of abdomen and other regions

   ✓5ᵗʰ **M99.1 Subluxation complex (vertebral)**

       CC Excl: For CC codes in subcategory M99.1, unless otherwise noted: M99.10-M99.11, S03.8XX-S03.9XX with 7th A, S12.000-S12.691 with 7th [A, B], S12.9XX-S13.4XX with 7th A, S13.8XXA, S14.0XX-S14.108 with 7th A, S14.111-S14.118 with 7th A, S14.121-S14.128 with 7th A, S14.131-S14.138 with 7th A, S14.141-S14.148 with 7th A, S14.151-S14.158 with 7th A, S16.1XX A, S29.011-S29.019 with 7th A, S38.3XX-S39.013 with 7th A, T14.8-T14.91, T79.A0X-T79.9XX with 7th A

       M99.10 Subluxation complex (vertebral) of head region CC

       M99.11 Subluxation complex (vertebral) of cervical region CC

       M99.12 Subluxation complex (vertebral) of thoracic region

       M99.13 Subluxation complex (vertebral) of lumbar region

       M99.14 Subluxation complex (vertebral) of sacral region

       M99.15 Subluxation complex (vertebral) of pelvic region

       M99.16 Subluxation complex (vertebral) of lower extremity

       M99.17 Subluxation complex (vertebral) of upper extremity

       M99.18 Subluxation complex (vertebral) of rib cage CC

         CC Excl: M99.18, S43.201-S43.226 with 7th character A

       M99.19 Subluxation complex (vertebral) of abdomen and other regions

   ✓5ᵗʰ **M99.2 Subluxation stenosis of neural canal**

       M99.20 Subluxation stenosis of neural canal of head region

       M99.21 Subluxation stenosis of neural canal of cervical region

       M99.22 Subluxation stenosis of neural canal of thoracic region

       M99.23 Subluxation stenosis of neural canal of lumbar region

       M99.24 Subluxation stenosis of neural canal of sacral region

       M99.25 Subluxation stenosis of neural canal of pelvic region

       M99.26 Subluxation stenosis of neural canal of lower extremity

       M99.27 Subluxation stenosis of neural canal of upper extremity

       M99.28 Subluxation stenosis of neural canal of rib cage

       M99.29 Subluxation stenosis of neural canal of abdomen and other regions

   ✓5ᵗʰ **M99.3 Osseous stenosis of neural canal**

       M99.30 Osseous stenosis of neural canal of head region

       M99.31 Osseous stenosis of neural canal of cervical region

       M99.32 Osseous stenosis of neural canal of thoracic region

       M99.33 Osseous stenosis of neural canal of lumbar region

       M99.34 Osseous stenosis of neural canal of sacral region

       M99.35 Osseous stenosis of neural canal of pelvic region

       M99.36 Osseous stenosis of neural canal of lower extremity

       M99.37 Osseous stenosis of neural canal of upper extremity

       M99.38 Osseous stenosis of neural canal of rib cage

       M99.39 Osseous stenosis of neural canal of abdomen and other regions

   ✓5ᵗʰ **M99.4 Connective tissue stenosis of neural canal**

       M99.40 Connective tissue stenosis of neural canal of head region

       M99.41 Connective tissue stenosis of neural canal of cervical region

       M99.42 Connective tissue stenosis of neural canal of thoracic region

       M99.43 Connective tissue stenosis of neural canal of lumbar region

       M99.44 Connective tissue stenosis of neural canal of sacral region

       M99.45 Connective tissue stenosis of neural canal of pelvic region

       M99.46 Connective tissue stenosis of neural canal of lower extremity

N Newborn: 0   P Pediatric: 0-17   M Maternity: 12-55   A Adult: 15-124   MCC Major CC Condition   PDx MCC PDx acts as own MCC   CC CC Condition   PDx CC PDx acts as own CC

764   ICD-10-CM Draft (2015)

M99.47　Connective tissue stenosis of neural canal of upper extremity

M99.48　Connective tissue stenosis of neural canal of rib cage

M99.49　Connective tissue stenosis of neural canal of abdomen and other regions

✓5ᵗʰ　M99.5　Intervertebral disc stenosis of neural canal

M99.50　Intervertebral disc stenosis of neural canal of head region

M99.51　Intervertebral disc stenosis of neural canal of cervical region

M99.52　Intervertebral disc stenosis of neural canal of thoracic region

M99.53　Intervertebral disc stenosis of neural canal of lumbar region

M99.54　Intervertebral disc stenosis of neural canal of sacral region

M99.55　Intervertebral disc stenosis of neural canal of pelvic region

M99.56　Intervertebral disc stenosis of neural canal of lower extremity

M99.57　Intervertebral disc stenosis of neural canal of upper extremity

M99.58　Intervertebral disc stenosis of neural canal of rib cage

M99.59　Intervertebral disc stenosis of neural canal of abdomen and other regions

✓5ᵗʰ　M99.6　Osseous and subluxation stenosis of intervertebral foramina

M99.60　Osseous and subluxation stenosis of intervertebral foramina of head region

M99.61　Osseous and subluxation stenosis of intervertebral foramina of cervical region

M99.62　Osseous and subluxation stenosis of intervertebral foramina of thoracic region

M99.63　Osseous and subluxation stenosis of intervertebral foramina of lumbar region

M99.64　Osseous and subluxation stenosis of intervertebral foramina of sacral region

M99.65　Osseous and subluxation stenosis of intervertebral foramina of pelvic region

M99.66　Osseous and subluxation stenosis of intervertebral foramina of lower extremity

M99.67　Osseous and subluxation stenosis of intervertebral foramina of upper extremity

M99.68　Osseous and subluxation stenosis of intervertebral foramina of rib cage

M99.69　Osseous and subluxation stenosis of intervertebral foramina of abdomen and other regions

✓5ᵗʰ　M99.7　Connective tissue and disc stenosis of intervertebral foramina

M99.70　Connective tissue and disc stenosis of intervertebral foramina of head region

M99.71　Connective tissue and disc stenosis of intervertebral foramina of cervical region

M99.72　Connective tissue and disc stenosis of intervertebral foramina of thoracic region

M99.73　Connective tissue and disc stenosis of intervertebral foramina of lumbar region

M99.74　Connective tissue and disc stenosis of intervertebral foramina of sacral region

M99.75　Connective tissue and disc stenosis of intervertebral foramina of pelvic region

M99.76　Connective tissue and disc stenosis of intervertebral foramina of lower extremity

M99.77　Connective tissue and disc stenosis of intervertebral foramina of upper extremity

M99.78　Connective tissue and disc stenosis of intervertebral foramina of rib cage

M99.79　Connective tissue and disc stenosis of intervertebral foramina of abdomen and other regions

✓5ᵗʰ　M99.8　Other biomechanical lesions

M99.80　Other biomechanical lesions of head region

M99.81　Other biomechanical lesions of cervical region

M99.82　Other biomechanical lesions of thoracic region

M99.83　Other biomechanical lesions of lumbar region

M99.84　Other biomechanical lesions of sacral region

M99.85　Other biomechanical lesions of pelvic region

M99.86　Other biomechanical lesions of lower extremity

M99.87　Other biomechanical lesions of upper extremity

M99.88　Other biomechanical lesions of rib cage

M99.89　Other biomechanical lesions of abdomen and other regions

M99.9　Biomechanical lesion, unspecified

Diseases of the Genitourinary System

N00–N02.5

Chapter 14. Diseases of the Genitourinary System (N00–N99)

EXCLUDES 2

certain conditions originating in the perinatal period (P04-P96)
certain infectious and parasitic diseases (A00-B99)
complications of pregnancy, childbirth and the puerperium (O00-O9A)
congenital malformations, deformations and chromosomal abnormalities (Q00-Q99)
endocrine, nutritional and metabolic diseases (E00-E88)
injury, poisoning and certain other consequences of external causes (S00-T88)
neoplasms (C00-D49)
symptoms, signs and abnormal clinical and laboratory findings, not elsewhere classified (R00-R94)

This chapter contains the following blocks:

N00-N08   Glomerular diseases
N10-N16   Renal tubulo-interstitial diseases
N17-N19   Acute kidney failure and chronic kidney disease
N20-N23   Urolithiasis
N25-N29   Other disorders of kidney and ureter
N30-N39   Other diseases of the urinary system
N40-N53   Diseases of male genital organs
N60-N65   Disorders of breast
N70-N77   Inflammatory diseases of female pelvic organs
N80-N98   Noninflammatory disorders of female genital tract
N99   Intraoperative and postprocedural complications and disorders of genitourinary system, not elsewhere classified

Glomerular diseases (N00-N08)

Code also any associated kidney failure (N17-N19).

EXCLUDES 1   hypertensive chronic kidney disease (I12.-)

✓4ᵗʰ N00   Acute nephritic syndrome

INCLUDES   acute glomerular disease
acute glomerulonephritis
acute nephritis

EXCLUDES 1   acute tubulo-interstitial nephritis (N10)
nephritic syndrome NOS (N05.-)

CC Excl: For MCC codes in category N00, unless otherwise noted:
A17.9, A18.10-A18.11, A18.13, A18.82, A18.84, A18.89, A54.21, A54.29, A54.82, A54.84, A54.89-A54.9, A59.00, A59.8-A59.9, B37.41-B37.49, E08.21-E08.29, E08.618-E08.638, E08.649-E08.8, E09.21-E09.29, E09.618-E09.638, E09.649-E09.8, E10.21-E10.29, E10.618-E10.638, E10.649, E10.69-E10.8, E11.21-E11.29, E11.618-E11.638, E11.649, E11.69-E11.8, E13.21-E13.29, E13.618-E13.638, E13.649-E13.8, E88.3, M10.30-M10.39, N00.0-N11.0, N11.8-N13.39, N13.6, N14.0-N19, N25.0-N26.1, N26.9-N27.9, N28.1-N29, N36.41-N36.43, N36.8-N36.9, N39.8-N39.9, R31.0-R31.9

N00.0   Acute nephritic syndrome with minor glomerular abnormality   MCC
Acute nephritic syndrome with minimal change lesion

N00.1   Acute nephritic syndrome with focal and segmental glomerular lesions   MCC
Acute nephritic syndrome with focal and segmental hyalinosis
Acute nephritic syndrome with focal and segmental sclerosis
Acute nephritic syndrome with focal glomerulonephritis

N00.2   Acute nephritic syndrome with diffuse membranous glomerulonephritis   MCC

N00.3   Acute nephritic syndrome with diffuse mesangial proliferative glomerulonephritis   MCC

N00.4   Acute nephritic syndrome with diffuse endocapillary proliferative glomerulonephritis   MCC

N00.5   Acute nephritic syndrome with diffuse mesangiocapillary glomerulonephritis   MCC
Acute nephritic syndrome with membranoproliferative glomerulonephritis, types 1 and 3, or NOS

N00.6   Acute nephritic syndrome with dense deposit disease   MCC
Acute nephritic syndrome with membranoproliferative glomerulonephritis, type 2

N00.7   Acute nephritic syndrome with diffuse crescentic glomerulonephritis   MCC
Acute nephritic syndrome with extracapillary glomerulonephritis

N00.8   Acute nephritic syndrome with other morphologic changes   MCC
Acute nephritic syndrome with proliferative glomerulonephritis NOS
CC Excl: A17.9, A18.10-A18.11, A18.13, A18.82, A18.84, A18.89, A54.21, A54.29, A54.82, A54.84, A54.89-A54.9, A59.00, A59.8-A59.9, B37.41-B37.49, E08.21-E08.29, E09.21-E09.29, E88.3, M10.30-M10.39, N00.0-N11.0, N11.8-N13.39, N13.6, N14.0-N19,

N25.0-N26.1, N26.9-N27.9, N28.1-N29, N36.41-N36.43, N36.8-N36.9, N39.8-N39.9, R31.0-R31.9

N00.9   Acute nephritic syndrome with unspecified morphologic changes   MCC

✓4ᵗʰ N01   Rapidly progressive nephritic syndrome

INCLUDES   rapidly progressive glomerular disease
rapidly progressive glomerulonephritis
rapidly progressive nephritis

EXCLUDES 1   nephritic syndrome NOS (N05.-)

CC Excl: For MCC codes in category N01, unless otherwise noted:
See code: N00

N01.0   Rapidly progressive nephritic syndrome with minor glomerular abnormality   MCC
Rapidly progressive nephritic syndrome with minimal change lesion

N01.1   Rapidly progressive nephritic syndrome with focal and segmental glomerular lesions   MCC
Rapidly progressive nephritic syndrome with focal and segmental hyalinosis
Rapidly progressive nephritic syndrome with focal and segmental sclerosis
Rapidly progressive nephritic syndrome with focal glomerulonephritis

N01.2   Rapidly progressive nephritic syndrome with diffuse membranous glomerulonephritis   MCC

N01.3   Rapidly progressive nephritic syndrome with diffuse mesangial proliferative glomerulonephritis   MCC

N01.4   Rapidly progressive nephritic syndrome with diffuse endocapillary proliferative glomerulonephritis   MCC

N01.5   Rapidly progressive nephritic syndrome with diffuse mesangiocapillary glomerulonephritis   MCC
Rapidly progressive nephritic syndrome with membranoproliferative glomerulonephritis, types 1 and 3, or NOS

N01.6   Rapidly progressive nephritic syndrome with dense deposit disease   MCC
Rapidly progressive nephritic syndrome with membranoproliferative glomerulonephritis, type 2

N01.7   Rapidly progressive nephritic syndrome with diffuse crescentic glomerulonephritis   MCC
Rapidly progressive nephritic syndrome with extracapillary glomerulonephritis

N01.8   Rapidly progressive nephritic syndrome with other morphologic changes   MCC
Rapidly progressive nephritic syndrome with proliferative glomerulonephritis NOS

N01.9   Rapidly progressive nephritic syndrome with unspecified morphologic changes   MCC

✓4ᵗʰ N02   Recurrent and persistent hematuria

EXCLUDES 1   acute cystitis with hematuria (N30.01)
hematuria NOS (R31.9)
hematuria not associated with specified morphologic lesions (R31.-)

CC Excl: For CC codes in category N02, unless otherwise noted:
See code: N00

N02.0   Recurrent and persistent hematuria with minor glomerular abnormality   CC
Recurrent and persistent hematuria with minimal change lesion

N02.1   Recurrent and persistent hematuria with focal and segmental glomerular lesions   CC
Recurrent and persistent hematuria with focal and segmental hyalinosis
Recurrent and persistent hematuria with focal and segmental sclerosis
Recurrent and persistent hematuria with focal glomerulonephritis

N02.2   Recurrent and persistent hematuria with diffuse membranous glomerulonephritis   CC

N02.3   Recurrent and persistent hematuria with diffuse mesangial proliferative glomerulonephritis   CC

N02.4   Recurrent and persistent hematuria with diffuse endocapillary proliferative glomerulonephritis   CC

N02.5   Recurrent and persistent hematuria with diffuse mesangiocapillary glomerulonephritis   CC
Recurrent and persistent hematuria with membranoproliferative glomerulonephritis, types 1 and 3, or NOS

N Newborn: 0   P Pediatric: 0-17   M Maternity: 12-55   A Adult: 15-124   MCC Major CC Condition   PDx MCC PDx acts as own MCC   CC CC Condition   PDx CC PDx acts as own CC

766   ICD-10-CM Draft (2015)

N02.6 **Recurrent and persistent hematuria with** dense deposit disease `CC`
Recurrent and persistent hematuria with membranoproliferative glomerulonephritis, type 2

N02.7 **Recurrent and persistent hematuria with** diffuse crescentic glomerulonephritis `CC`
Recurrent and persistent hematuria with extracapillary glomerulonephritis

N02.8 **Recurrent and persistent hematuria with** other morphologic changes `CC`
Recurrent and persistent hematuria with proliferative glomerulonephritis NOS
CC Excl: A17.9, A18.10-A18.11, A18.13, A18.82, A18.84, A18.89, A54.21, A54.29, A54.82, A54.84, A54.89-A54.9, A59.00, A59.8-A59.9, B37.41-B37.49, E08.21-E08.29, E08.618-E08.638, E08.649-E08.8, E09.21-E09.29, E09.618-E09.638, E09.649-E09.8, E10.21-E10.29, E10.618-E10.638, E10.649, E10.69-E10.8, E11.21-E11.29, E11.618-E11.638, E11.649, E11.69-E11.8, E13.21-E13.29, E13.618-E13.638, E13.649-E13.8, E88.3, M10.30-M10.39, N00.0-N11.0, N11.8-N13.39, N13.6, N14.0-N19, N25.0-N26.1, N26.9-N27.9, N28.1-N29, N36.41-N36.43, N36.8-N36.9, N39.8-N39.9, R31.0-R31.9

N02.9 **Recurrent and persistent hematuria with** unspecified morphologic changes `CC`

✓4ᵗʰ **N03 Chronic** nephritic syndrome
INCLUDES chronic glomerular disease
chronic glomerulonephritis
chronic nephritis

EXCLUDES 1 chronic tubulo-interstitial nephritis (N11.-)
diffuse sclerosing glomerulonephritis (N05.8-)
nephritic syndrome NOS (N05.-)

CC Excl: For CC codes in category N03, unless otherwise noted:
A17.9, A18.10-A18.11, A18.13, A18.82, A18.84, A18.89, A54.21, A54.29, A54.82, A54.84, A54.89-A54.9, A59.00, A59.8-A59.9, A98.5, B37.41-B37.49, E08.21-E08.29, E08.618-E08.638, E08.649-E08.8, E09.21-E09.29, E09.618-E09.638, E09.649-E09.8, E10.21-E10.29, E10.618-E10.638, E10.649, E10.69-E10.8, E11.21-E11.29, E11.618-E11.638, E11.649, E11.69-E11.8, E13.21-E13.29, E13.618-E13.638, E13.649-E13.8, M10.30-M10.39, N00.0-N11.0, N11.8-N13.39, N13.6, N14.0-N17.9, N19, N25.0-N26.1, N26.9-N27.9, N28.1-N29, N36.41-N36.43, N36.8-N36.9, N39.8-N39.9, R31.0-R31.9

N03.0 **Chronic nephritic syndrome with** minor glomerular abnormality `CC`
Chronic nephritic syndrome with minimal change lesion

N03.1 **Chronic nephritic syndrome with** focal and segmental glomerular lesions `CC`
Chronic nephritic syndrome with focal and segmental hyalinosis
Chronic nephritic syndrome with focal and segmental sclerosis
Chronic nephritic syndrome with focal glomerulonephritis

N03.2 **Chronic nephritic syndrome with** diffuse membranous glomerulonephritis `CC`

N03.3 **Chronic nephritic syndrome with** diffuse mesangial proliferative glomerulonephritis `CC`

N03.4 **Chronic nephritic syndrome with** diffuse endocapillary proliferative glomerulonephritis `CC`

N03.5 **Chronic nephritic syndrome with** diffuse mesangiocapillary glomerulonephritis `CC`
Chronic nephritic syndrome with membranoproliferative glomerulonephritis, types 1 and 3, or NOS

N03.6 **Chronic nephritic syndrome with** dense deposit disease `CC`
Chronic nephritic syndrome with membranoproliferative glomerulonephritis, type 2

N03.7 **Chronic nephritic syndrome with** diffuse crescentic glomerulonephritis `CC`
Chronic nephritic syndrome with extracapillary glomerulonephritis

N03.8 **Chronic nephritic syndrome with** other morphologic changes `CC`
Chronic nephritic syndrome with proliferative glomerulonephritis NOS

N03.9 **Chronic nephritic syndrome with** unspecified morphologic changes `CC`

✓4ᵗʰ **N04 Nephrotic syndrome**
INCLUDES congenital nephrotic syndrome
lipoid nephrosis

CC Excl: For CC codes in category N04, unless otherwise noted:
A17.9, A18.10-A18.11, A18.13, A18.82, A18.84, A18.89, A54.21, A54.29, A54.82, A54.84, A54.89-A54.9, A59.00, A59.8-A59.9, B37.41-B37.49, E08.21-E08.29, E08.618-E08.638, E08.649-E08.8, E09.21-E09.29, E09.618-E09.638, E09.649-E09.8, E10.21-E10.29, E10.618-E10.638, E10.649, E10.69-E10.8, E11.21-E11.29, E11.618-E11.638, E11.649, E11.69-E11.8, E13.21-E13.29, E13.618-E13.638, E13.649-E13.8, M10.30-M10.39, N00.0-N11.0, N11.8-N13.39, N13.6, N14.0-N19, N25.0-N26.1, N26.9-N27.9, N28.1-N29, N36.41-N36.43, N36.8-N36.9, N39.8-N39.9, R31.0-R31.9

N04.0 **Nephrotic syndrome with** minor glomerular abnormality `CC`
Nephrotic syndrome with minimal change lesion

N04.1 **Nephrotic syndrome with** focal and segmental glomerular lesions `CC`
Nephrotic syndrome with focal and segmental hyalinosis
Nephrotic syndrome with focal and segmental sclerosis
Nephrotic syndrome with focal glomerulonephritis

N04.2 **Nephrotic syndrome with** diffuse membranous glomerulonephritis `CC`

N04.3 **Nephrotic syndrome with** diffuse mesangial proliferative glomerulonephritis `CC`

N04.4 **Nephrotic syndrome with** diffuse endocapillary proliferative glomerulonephritis `CC`

N04.5 **Nephrotic syndrome with** diffuse mesangiocapillary glomerulonephritis `CC`
Nephrotic syndrome with membranoproliferative glomerulonephritis, types 1 and 3, or NOS

N04.6 **Nephrotic syndrome with** dense deposit disease `CC`
Nephrotic syndrome with membranoproliferative glomerulonephritis, type 2

N04.7 **Nephrotic syndrome with** diffuse crescentic glomerulonephritis `CC`
Nephrotic syndrome with extracapillary glomerulonephritis
CC Excl: A17.9, A18.10-A18.11, A18.13, A18.82, A18.84, A18.89, A54.21, A54.29, A54.82, A54.84, A54.89-A54.9, A59.00, A59.8-A59.9, B37.41-B37.49, E08.21-E08.29, E08.618-E08.638, E08.649-E08.8, E09.21-E09.29, E09.618-E09.638, E09.649-E09.8, E10.21-E10.29, E10.618-E10.638, E10.649, E10.69-E10.8, E11.21-E11.29, E11.618-E11.638, E11.649, E11.69-E11.8, E13.21-E13.29, E13.618-E13.638, E13.649-E13.8, E88.3, M10.30-M10.39, N00.0-N11.0, N11.8-N13.39, N13.6, N14.0-N19, N25.0-N26.1, N26.9-N27.9, N28.1-N29, N36.41-N36.43, N36.8-N36.9, N39.8-N39.9, R31.0-R31.9

N04.8 **Nephrotic syndrome with** other morphologic changes `CC`
Nephrotic syndrome with proliferative glomerulonephritis NOS
CC Excl: See code: N04.7

N04.9 **Nephrotic syndrome with** unspecified morphologic changes `CC`
CC Excl: See code: N04.7

✓4ᵗʰ **N05 Unspecified** nephritic syndrome
INCLUDES glomerular disease NOS
glomerulonephritis NOS
nephritis NOS
nephropathy NOS and renal disease NOS with morphological lesion specified in .0-.8

EXCLUDES 1 nephropathy NOS with no stated morphological lesion (N28.9)
renal disease NOS with no stated morphological lesion (N28.9)
tubulo-interstitial nephritis NOS (N12)

CC Excl: For CC codes in category N05, unless otherwise noted:
A17.9, A18.10-A18.11, A18.13, A18.82, A18.84, A18.89, A54.21, A54.29, A54.82, A54.84, A54.89-A54.9, A59.00, A59.8-A59.9, A98.5, B37.41-B37.49, E08.21-E08.29, E08.618-E08.638, E08.649-E08.8, E09.21-E09.29, E09.618-E09.638, E09.649-E09.8, E10.21-E10.29, E10.618-E10.638, E10.649, E10.69-E10.8, E11.21-E11.29, E11.618-E11.638, E11.649, E11.69-E11.8, E13.21-E13.29, E13.618-E13.638, E13.649-E13.8, M10.30-M10.39, N00.0-N11.0, N11.8-N13.39, N13.6, N14.0-N17.9, N19, N25.0-N26.1, N26.9-N27.9, N28.1-N29, N36.41-N36.43, N36.8-N36.9, N39.8-N39.9, R31.0-R31.9

N05.0 **Unspecified nephritic syndrome with** minor glomerular abnormality
Unspecified nephritic syndrome with minimal change lesion

N05.1 **Unspecified nephritic syndrome with** focal and segmental glomerular lesions
Unspecified nephritic syndrome with focal and segmental hyalinosis
Unspecified nephritic syndrome with focal and segmental sclerosis
Unspecified nephritic syndrome with focal glomerulonephritis

N05.2 **Unspecified nephritic syndrome with** diffuse membranous glomerulonephritis `CC`

✓ Additional Character Required   √x7ᵗʰ Xtension Alert   Unacceptable PDx   Manifestation   Hospital Acquired Condition   **EXCLUDES 1** Not Coded Here   **EXCLUDES 2** Not Included Here

N05.3 Unspecified nephritic syndrome with diffuse mesangial proliferative glomerulonephritis CC

N05.4 Unspecified nephritic syndrome with diffuse endocapillary proliferative glomerulonephritis CC

N05.5 Unspecified nephritic syndrome with diffuse mesangiocapillary glomerulonephritis CC
Unspecified nephritic syndrome with membranoproliferative glomerulonephritis, types 1 and 3, or NOS

N05.6 Unspecified nephritic syndrome with dense deposit disease
Unspecified nephritic syndrome with membranoproliferative glomerulonephritis, type 2

N05.7 Unspecified nephritic syndrome with diffuse crescentic glomerulonephritis
Unspecified nephritic syndrome with extracapillary glomerulonephritis

N05.8 Unspecified nephritic syndrome with other morphologic changes
Unspecified nephritic syndrome with proliferative glomerulonephritis NOS

N05.9 Unspecified nephritic syndrome with unspecified morphologic changes

N06 Isolated proteinuria with specified morphological lesion
EXCLUDES1 proteinuria not associated with specific morphologic lesions (R80.0)

CC Excl: For CC codes in category N06, unless otherwise noted: See code: N03

N06.0 Isolated proteinuria with minor glomerular abnormality
Isolated proteinuria with minimal change lesion

N06.1 Isolated proteinuria with focal and segmental glomerular lesions
Isolated proteinuria with focal and segmental hyalinosis
Isolated proteinuria with focal and segmental sclerosis
Isolated proteinuria with focal glomerulonephritis

N06.2 Isolated proteinuria with diffuse membranous glomerulonephritis CC

N06.3 Isolated proteinuria with diffuse mesangial proliferative glomerulonephritis CC

N06.4 Isolated proteinuria with diffuse endocapillary proliferative glomerulonephritis CC

N06.5 Isolated proteinuria with diffuse mesangiocapillary glomerulonephritis CC
Isolated proteinuria with membranoproliferative glomerulonephritis, types 1 and 3, or NOS

N06.6 Isolated proteinuria with dense deposit disease
Isolated proteinuria with membranoproliferative glomerulonephritis, type 2

N06.7 Isolated proteinuria with diffuse crescentic glomerulonephritis
Isolated proteinuria with extracapillary glomerulonephritis

N06.8 Isolated proteinuria with other morphologic lesion
Isolated proteinuria with proliferative glomerulonephritis NOS

N06.9 Isolated proteinuria with unspecified morphologic lesion

N07 Hereditary nephropathy, not elsewhere classified
EXCLUDES2 Alport's syndrome (Q87.81-)
hereditary amyloid nephropathy (E85.-)
nail patella syndrome (Q87.2)
non-neuropathic heredofamilial amyloidosis (E85.-)

CC Excl: For CC codes in category N07, unless otherwise noted: A17.9, A18.10-A18.11, A18.13, A18.82, A18.84, A18.89, A54.21, A54.29, A54.82, A54.84, A54.89-A54.9, A59.00, A59.8-A59.9, A98.5, B37.41-B37.49, E08.21-E08.29, E08.618-E08.638, E08.649-E08.8, E09.21-E09.29, E09.618-E09.638, E09.649-E09.8, E10.21-E10.29, E10.618-E10.638, E10.649, E10.69-E10.8, E11.21-E11.29, E11.618-E11.638, E11.649, E11.69-E11.8, E13.21-E13.29, E13.618-E13.638, E13.649-E13.8, M10.30-M10.39, N00.0-N11.0, N11.8-N13.39, N13.6, N14.0-N17.9, N19, N25.0-N26.1, N26.9-N27.9, N28.1-N29, N36.41-N36.43, N36.8-N36.9, N39.8-N39.9, R31.0-R31.9

N07.0 Hereditary nephropathy, not elsewhere classified with minor glomerular abnormality
Hereditary nephropathy, not elsewhere classified with minimal change lesion

N07.1 Hereditary nephropathy, not elsewhere classified with focal and segmental glomerular lesions
Hereditary nephropathy, not elsewhere classified with focal and segmental hyalinosis
Hereditary nephropathy, not elsewhere classified with focal and segmental sclerosis
Hereditary nephropathy, not elsewhere classified with focal glomerulonephritis

N07.2 Hereditary nephropathy, not elsewhere classified with diffuse membranous glomerulonephritis CC

N07.3 Hereditary nephropathy, not elsewhere classified with diffuse mesangial proliferative glomerulonephritis CC

N07.4 Hereditary nephropathy, not elsewhere classified with diffuse endocapillary proliferative glomerulonephritis CC

N07.5 Hereditary nephropathy, not elsewhere classified with diffuse mesangiocapillary glomerulonephritis CC
Hereditary nephropathy, not elsewhere classified with membranoproliferative glomerulonephritis, types 1 and 3, or NOS

N07.6 Hereditary nephropathy, not elsewhere classified with dense deposit disease
Hereditary nephropathy, not elsewhere classified with membranoproliferative glomerulonephritis, type 2

N07.7 Hereditary nephropathy, not elsewhere classified with diffuse crescentic glomerulonephritis
Hereditary nephropathy, not elsewhere classified with extracapillary glomerulonephritis

N07.8 Hereditary nephropathy, not elsewhere classified with other morphologic lesions
Hereditary nephropathy, not elsewhere classified with proliferative glomerulonephritis NOS

N07.9 Hereditary nephropathy, not elsewhere classified with unspecified morphologic lesions

N08 Glomerular disorders in diseases classified elsewhere
Glomerulonephritis   Nephropathy
Nephritis
Code first underlying disease, such as:
amyloidosis (E85.-)
congenital syphilis (A50.5)
cryoglobulinemia (D89.1)
disseminated intravascular coagulation (D65)
gout (M1A.-, M10.-)
microscopic polyangiitis (M31.7)
multiple myeloma (C90.0-)
sepsis (A40.0-A41.9)
sickle-cell disease (D57.0-D57.8)
EXCLUDES1 glomerulonephritis, nephritis and nephropathy (in):
antiglomerular basement membrane disease (M31.0)
diabetes (E08-E13 with .21)
gonococcal (A54.21)
Goodpasture's syndrome (M31.0)
hemolytic-uremic syndrome (D59.3)
lupus (M32.14)
mumps (B26.83)
syphilis (A52.75)
systemic lupus erythematosus (M32.14)
Wegener's granulomatosis (M31.31)
pyelonephritis in diseases classified elsewhere (N16)
renal tubulo-interstitial disorders classified elsewhere (N16)

Renal tubulo-interstitial diseases (N10-N16)

INCLUDES pyelonephritis
EXCLUDES1 pyeloureteritis cystica (N28.85)

[1] N10 Acute tubulo-interstitial nephritis CC
Acute infectious interstitial nephritis   Acute pyelonephritis
Acute pyelitis   Hemoglobin nephrosis
    Myoglobin nephrosis
Use additional code (B95-B97), to identify infectious agent
CC Excl: A17.9, A18.10-A18.11, A18.13, A18.82, A18.84, A18.89, A54.21, A54.29, A54.82, A54.84, A54.89-A54.9, A59.00, A59.8-A59.9, B37.41-B37.49, E08.21-E08.29, E08.618-E08.638, E08.649-E08.8, E09.21-E09.29, E09.618-E09.638, E09.649-E09.8, E10.21-E10.29, E10.618-E10.638, E10.649, E10.69-E10.8, E11.21-E11.29, E11.618-E11.638, E11.649, E11.69-E11.8, E13.21-E13.29, E13.618-E13.638, E13.649-E13.8, M10.30-M10.39, N00.0-N11.0, N11.8-N13.39, N13.6, N14.0-N19, N25.0-N26.1, N26.9-N27.9, N28.1-N29, N36.41-N36.43, N36.8-N36.9, N39.0, N39.8-N39.9, R31.0-R31.9

1 HAC = as SDx not POA, in combination with SDx code T83.51XA also not POA.

N Newborn: 0 P Pediatric: 0-17 M Maternity: 12-55 A Adult: 15-124 MCC Major CC Condition PDx MCC PDx acts as own MCC CC CC Condition PDx CC PDx acts as own CC

☑4ᵗʰ **N11** **Chronic tubulo-interstitial nephritis**
     INCLUDES   chronic infectious interstitial nephritis
                chronic pyelitis
                chronic pyelonephritis
     Use additional code (B95-B97), to identify infectious agent

     N11.0 **Nonobstructive reflux-associated chronic pyelonephritis**
         Pyelonephritis (chronic) associated with (vesicoureteral) reflux
         EXCLUDES 1   *vesicoureteral reflux NOS (N13.70)*

     N11.1 **Chronic obstructive pyelonephritis**   PDx CC | CC
         Pyelonephritis (chronic) associated with anomaly of
            pelviureteric junction
         Pyelonephritis (chronic) associated with anomaly of
            pyeloureteric junction
         Pyelonephritis (chronic) associated with crossing of vessel
         Pyelonephritis (chronic) associated with kinking of ureter
         Pyelonephritis (chronic) associated with obstruction of ureter
         Pyelonephritis (chronic) associated with stricture of pelviureteric
            junction
         Pyelonephritis (chronic) associated with stricture of ureter
         EXCLUDES 1   *calculous pyelonephritis (N20.9)*
                 obstructive uropathy (N13.-)
         CC Excl: N11.1, N13.4-N13.5, N13.8-N13.9, N28.82, N28.89-N30.91,
         N32.89-N33, N36.41-N36.43, N36.8-N36.9, N39.0, N39.8-N39.9,
         Q62.4-Q62.8, Q64.10-Q64.19, Q64.8-Q64.9, R31.0-R31.9, Z90.6

     N11.8 **Other chronic tubulo-interstitial nephritis**   CC
         Nonobstructive chronic pyelonephritis NOS
         CC Excl: A17.9, A18.10-A18.11, A18.13, A18.82, A18.84, A18.89,
         A54.21, A54.29, A54.82, A54.84, A54.89-A54.9, A59.00, A59.8-
         A59.9, A98.5, B37.41-B37.49, E08.21-E08.29, E08.618-E08.638,
         E08.649-E08.8, E09.21-E09.29, E09.618-E09.638, E09.649-E09.8,
         E10.21-E10.29, E10.618-E10.638, E10.649, E10.69-E10.8, E11.21-
         E11.29, E11.618-E11.638, E11.649, E11.69-E11.8, E13.21-E13.29,
         E13.618-E13.638, E13.649-E13.8, M10.30-M10.39, N00.0-N11.0,
         N11.8-N13.39, N13.6, N14.0-N17.9, N19, N25.0-N26.1, N26.9-
         N27.9, N28.1-N29, N36.41-N36.43, N36.8-N36.9, N39.8-N39.9,
         O23.01-O23.03, O23.11-O23.13, O23.21-O23.23, O23.31-O23.33,
         O23.41-O23.513, O23.521-O23.523, O23.591-O23.593, O23.91-
         O23.93, O86.11, O86.13-O86.29, R31.0-R31.9

    1 **N11.9** **Chronic tubulo-interstitial nephritis, unspecified**   CC
         Chronic interstitial nephritis NOS
         Chronic pyelitis NOS
         Chronic pyelonephritis NOS
         CC Excl: A17.9, A18.10-A18.11, A18.13, A18.82, A18.84, A18.89,
         A54.21, A54.29, A54.82, A54.84, A54.89-A54.9, A59.00, A59.8-
         A59.9, B37.41-B37.49, E08.21-E08.29, E09.21-E09.29, M10.30-
         M10.39, N00.0-N11.0, N11.8-N13.39, N13.6, N14.0-N19, N25.0-
         N26.1, N26.9-N27.9, N28.1-N29, N36.41-N36.43, N36.8-N36.9,
         N39.0, N39.8-N39.9, R31.0-R31.9

    1 **N12** **Tubulo-interstitial nephritis, not specified as acute or chronic**   CC
         Interstitial nephritis NOS
         Pyelitis NOS
         Pyelonephritis NOS
         EXCLUDES 1   *calculous pyelonephritis (N20.9)*
         CC Excl: See code: N11.9

☑4ᵗʰ **N13** **Obstructive and reflux uropathy**
     EXCLUDES 2   *calculus of kidney and ureter without hydronephrosis (N20.-)*
               congenital obstructive defects of renal pelvis and ureter (Q62.0-
                Q62.3)
               hydronephrosis with ureteropelvic junction obstruction (Q62.1)
               obstructive pyelonephritis (N11.1)

     CC Excl: For CC codes in category N13, unless otherwise noted:
     See code: N11.9

     N13.1 **Hydronephrosis with ureteral stricture, not elsewhere**   CC
         classified
         EXCLUDES 1   *hydronephrosis with ureteral stricture with infection*
                  (N13.6)

     N13.2 **Hydronephrosis with renal and ureteral calculous**   CC
         obstruction
         EXCLUDES 1   *hydronephrosis with renal and ureteral calculous*
                  obstruction with infection (N13.6)

   ☑5ᵗʰ **N13.3** **Other and unspecified hydronephrosis**
         EXCLUDES 1   *hydronephrosis with infection (N13.6)*
         N13.30   **Unspecified hydronephrosis**   CC
         N13.39   **Other hydronephrosis**   CC

     N13.4 **Hydroureter**   CC
         EXCLUDES 1   *congenital hydroureter (Q62.3-)*
                  hydroureter with infection (N13.6)
                  vesicoureteral-reflux with hydroureter (N13.73-)
         CC Excl: N11.1, N13.4-N13.5, N13.8-N13.9, N28.82, N28.89-N30.91,
         N32.89-N33, N36.41-N36.43, N36.8-N36.9, N39.0, N39.8-N39.9,
         Q62.4-Q62.8, Q64.10-Q64.19, Q64.8-Q64.9, R31.0-R31.9

     N13.5 **Crossing vessel and stricture of ureter without**
         hydronephrosis
         Kinking and stricture of ureter without hydronephrosis
         EXCLUDES 1   *crossing vessel and stricture of ureter without*
                  hydronephrosis with infection (N13.6)

    1 **N13.6** **Pyonephrosis**   CC
         Conditions in N13.1-N13.5 with infection
         Obstructive uropathy with infection
         Use additional code (B95-B97), to identify infectious agent

   ☑5ᵗʰ **N13.7** **Vesicoureteral-reflux**
         EXCLUDES 1   *reflux-associated pyelonephritis (N11.0)*
         N13.70   **Vesicoureteral-reflux, unspecified**
                Vesicoureteral-reflux NOS
         N13.71   **Vesicoureteral-reflux without reflux nephropathy**
     ☑6ᵗʰ **N13.72**   **Vesicoureteral-reflux with reflux nephropathy**
                without hydroureter
            N13.721   **Vesicoureteral-reflux with reflux**
                   nephropathy without hydroureter,
                   unilateral
            N13.722   **Vesicoureteral-reflux with reflux**
                   nephropathy without hydroureter,
                   bilateral
            N13.729   **Vesicoureteral-reflux with reflux**
                   nephropathy without hydroureter,
                   unspecified
     ☑6ᵗʰ **N13.73**   **Vesicoureteral-reflux with reflux nephropathy with**
                hydroureter
            N13.731   **Vesicoureteral-reflux with reflux**
                   nephropathy with hydroureter, unilateral
            N13.732   **Vesicoureteral-reflux with reflux**
                   nephropathy with hydroureter, bilateral
            N13.739   **Vesicoureteral-reflux with reflux**
                   nephropathy with hydroureter,
                   unspecified

     N13.8 **Other obstructive and reflux uropathy**   CC
         Urinary tract obstruction due to specified cause
         Code first, if applicable, any causal condition, such as:
            enlarged prostate (N40.1)
         CC Excl: See code: N11.1

     N13.9 **Obstructive and reflux uropathy, unspecified**
         Urinary tract obstruction NOS

☑4ᵗʰ **N14** **Drug- and heavy-metal-induced tubulo-interstitial and tubular conditions**
     Code first poisoning due to drug or toxin, if applicable (T36-T65 with
         fifth or sixth character 1-4 or 6)
     Use additional code for adverse effect, if applicable, to identify drug
         (T36-T50 with fifth or sixth character 5)

     N14.0 **Analgesic nephropathy**
     N14.1 **Nephropathy induced by other drugs, medicaments and**
         biological substances
     N14.2 **Nephropathy induced by unspecified drug, medicament or**
         biological substance
     N14.3 **Nephropathy induced by heavy metals**
     N14.4 **Toxic nephropathy, not elsewhere classified**

☑4ᵗʰ **N15** **Other renal tubulo-interstitial diseases**
     N15.0 **Balkan nephropathy**
         Balkan endemic nephropathy
    1 **N15.1** **Renal and perinephric abscess**   MCC
         CC Excl: A17.9, A18.10-A18.11, A18.13, A18.82, A18.84, A18.89,
         A54.21, A54.29, A54.82, A54.84, A54.89-A54.9, A59.00, A59.8-
         A59.9, B37.41-B37.49, E08.21-E08.29, E08.618-E08.638, E08.649-
         E08.8, E09.21-E09.29, E09.618-E09.638, E09.649-E09.8, E10.21-
         E10.29, E10.618-E10.638, E10.649, E10.69-E10.8, E11.21-E11.29,
         E11.618-E11.638, E11.649, E11.69-E11.8, E13.21-E13.29, E13.618-
         E13.638, E13.649-E13.8, M10.30-M10.39, N00.0-N11.0, N11.8-
         N13.39, N13.6, N14.0-N19, N25.0-N26.1, N26.9-N27.9, N28.1-N29,
         N36.41-N36.43, N36.8-N36.9, N39.0, N39.8-N39.9, R31.0-R31.9

     N15.8 **Other specified renal tubulo-interstitial diseases**
     N15.9 **Renal tubulo-interstitial disease, unspecified**
         Infection of kidney NOS
         EXCLUDES 1   *urinary tract infection NOS (N39.0)*

---

1 HAC = as SDx not POA, in combination with SDx code T83.51XA also not POA.

☑ Additional Character Required   ☑x7ᵗʰ *X*tension Alert   Unacceptable PDx   Manifestation   Hospital Acquired Condition   **EXCLUDES 1** Not Coded Here   **EXCLUDES 2** Not Included Here

ICD-10-CM Draft (2015)   769

Diseases of the Genitourinary System

N16–N22

handwritten: N 20.0 Calculus of Kidney

N16 *Renal tubulo-interstitial disorders in diseases classified elsewhere*
Pyelonephritis
Tubulo-interstitial nephritis
Code first underlying disease, such as:
brucellosis (A23.0-A23.9)
cryoglobulinemia (D89.1)
glycogen storage disease (E74.0)
leukemia (C91-C95)
lymphoma (C81.0-C85.9, C96.0-C96.9)
multiple myeloma (C90.0-)
sepsis (A40.0-A41.9)
Wilson's disease (E83.0)

EXCLUDES 1   diphtheritic pyelonephritis and tubulo-interstitial nephritis (A36.84)
pyelonephritis and tubulo-interstitial nephritis in candidiasis (B37.49)
pyelonephritis and tubulo-interstitial nephritis in cystinosis (E72.04)
pyelonephritis and tubulo-interstitial nephritis in salmonella infection (A02.25)
pyelonephritis and tubulo-interstitial nephritis in sarcoidosis (D86.84)
pyelonephritis and tubulo-interstitial nephritis in sicca syndrome [Sjogren's] (M35.04)
pyelonephritis and tubulo-interstitial nephritis in systemic lupus erythematosus (M32.15)
pyelonephritis and tubulo-interstitial nephritis in toxoplasmosis (B58.83)
renal tubular degeneration in diabetes (E08-E13 with .29)
syphilitic pyelonephritis and tubulo-interstitial nephritis (A52.75)

Acute kidney failure and chronic kidney disease (N17-N19)

EXCLUDES 2   congenital renal failure (P96.0)
drug- and heavy-metal-induced tubulo-interstitial and tubular conditions (N14.-)
extrarenal uremia (R39.2)
hemolytic-uremic syndrome (D59.3)
hepatorenal syndrome (K76.7)
postpartum hepatorenal syndrome (O90.4)
posttraumatic renal failure (T79.5)
prerenal uremia (R39.2)
renal failure complicating abortion or ectopic or molar pregnancy (O00-O07, O08.4)
renal failure following labor and delivery (O90.4)
renal failure postprocedural (N99.0)

✓4th N17   **Acute kidney failure**
Code also associated underlying condition
EXCLUDES 1   posttraumatic renal failure (T79.5)
AHA: 2013, 4Q, 124

CC Excl: For CC/MCC codes in category N17, unless otherwise noted: E08.21-E08.29, E08.618-E08.638, E08.649-E08.8, E09.21-E09.29, E09.618-E09.638, E09.649-E09.8, E10.21-E10.29, E10.618-E10.638, E10.649, E10.69-E10.8, E11.21-E11.29, E11.618-E11.638, E11.649, E11.69-E11.8, E13.21-E13.29, E13.618-E13.638, E13.649-E13.8, E88.3, M10.30-M10.39, N00.0-N11.0, N11.8-N13.39, N13.6, N14.0-N19, N25.0-N26.1, N26.9-N27.9, N28.1-N29, N36.41-N36.43, N36.8-N36.9, N39.8-N39.9, Q60.0-Q62.39, Q63.0-Q63.9, Q64.8-Q64.9, R31.0-R31.9

N17.0   **Acute kidney failure with tubular necrosis**   MCC
Acute tubular necrosis
Renal tubular necrosis
Tubular necrosis NOS

N17.1   **Acute kidney failure with acute cortical necrosis**   MCC
Acute cortical necrosis
Cortical necrosis NOS
Renal cortical necrosis

N17.2   **Acute kidney failure with medullary necrosis**   MCC
Medullary [papillary] necrosis NOS
Acute medullary [papillary] necrosis
Renal medullary [papillary] necrosis

N17.8   **Other acute kidney failure**   CC
CC Excl: E08.21-E08.29, E08.618-E08.638, E08.649-E08.8, E09.21-E09.29, E09.618-E09.638, E09.649-E09.8, E10.21-E10.29, E10.618-E10.638, E10.649, E10.69-E10.8, E11.21-E11.29, E11.618-E11.638, E11.649, E11.69-E11.8, E13.21-E13.29, E13.618-E13.638, E13.649-E13.8, E88.3, M10.30-M10.39, N00.0-N11.0, N11.8-N13.39, N13.6, N14.0-N19, N25.0-N26.1, N26.9-N27.9, N28.1-N29, N36.41-N36.43, N36.8-N36.9, N39.8-N39.9, R31.0-R31.9

N17.9   **Acute kidney failure, unspecified**   CC
Acute kidney injury (nontraumatic)
EXCLUDES 2   traumatic kidney injury (S37.0-)

✓4th N18   **Chronic kidney disease (CKD)**
Code first any associated:
diabetic chronic kidney disease (E08.22, E09.22, E10.22, E11.22, E13.22)
hypertensive chronic kidney disease (I12-, I13-)
Use additional code to identify kidney transplant status, if applicable, (Z94.0)
AHA: 2013, 1Q, 24

N18.1   **Chronic kidney disease, stage 1**

N18.2   **Chronic kidney disease, stage 2 (mild)**

N18.3   **Chronic kidney disease, stage 3 (moderate)**

N18.4   **Chronic kidney disease, stage 4 (severe)**   CC
CC Excl: E08.21-E08.29, E08.618-E08.638, E08.649-E08.8, E09.21-E09.29, E09.618-E09.638, E09.649-E09.8, E10.21-E10.29, E10.618-E10.638, E10.649, E10.69-E10.8, E11.21-E11.29, E11.618-E11.638, E11.649, E11.69-E11.8, E13.21-E13.29, E13.618-E13.638, E13.649-E13.8, M10.30-M10.39, N00.0-N11.0, N11.8-N13.39, N13.6, N14.0-N19, N25.0-N26.1, N26.9-N27.9, N28.1-N29, N36.41-N36.43, N36.8-N36.9, N39.8-N39.9, Q60.0-Q62.39, Q63.0-Q63.9, Q64.8-Q64.9, R31.0-R31.9

N18.5   **Chronic kidney disease, stage 5**   CC
EXCLUDES 1   chronic kidney disease, stage 5 requiring chronic dialysis (N18.6)
CC Excl: See code: N18.4

N18.6   **End stage renal disease**   MCC
Chronic kidney disease requiring chronic dialysis
Use additional code to identify dialysis status (Z99.2)
AHA: 2013, 4Q, 124-125
CC Excl: E08.21-E08.29, E08.618-E08.638, E08.649-E08.8, E09.21-E09.29, E09.618-E09.638, E09.649-E09.8, E10.21-E10.29, E10.618-E10.638, E10.649, E10.69-E10.8, E11.21-E11.29, E11.618-E11.638, E11.649, E11.69-E11.8, E13.21-E13.29, E13.618-E13.638, E13.649-E13.8, I12.9, M10.30-M10.39, N00.0-N11.0, N11.8-N13.39, N13.6, N14.0-N19, N25.0-N26.1, N26.9-N27.9, N28.1-N29, N36.41-N36.43, N36.8-N36.9, N39.8-N39.9, Q60.0-Q62.39, Q63.0-Q63.9, Q64.8-Q64.9, R31.0-R31.9

N18.9   **Chronic kidney disease, unspecified**
Chronic renal disease   Chronic renal insufficiency
Chronic renal failure NOS   Chronic uremia

N19   **Unspecified kidney failure**
Uremia NOS
EXCLUDES 1   acute kidney failure (N17.-)
chronic kidney disease (N18.-)
chronic uremia (N18.9)
extrarenal uremia (R39.2)
prerenal uremia (R39.2)
renal insufficiency (acute) (N28.9)
uremia of newborn (P96.0)

Urolithiasis (N20-N23)

✓4th N20   **Calculus of kidney and ureter**
Calculous pyelonephritis
EXCLUDES 1   nephrocalcinosis (E83.5)
that with hydronephrosis (N13.2)

N20.0   **Calculus of kidney**
Nephrolithiasis NOS   Staghorn calculus
Renal calculus   Stone in kidney
Renal stone

N20.1   **Calculus of ureter**   CC
Ureteric stone
CC Excl: N11.1, N13.4-N13.5, N13.8-N13.9, N20.0-N22, N28.82, N28.89-N29, N36.41-N36.43, N36.8-N36.9, N39.8-N39.9, R31.0-R31.9

N20.2   **Calculus of kidney with calculus of ureter**   CC

N20.9   **Urinary calculus, unspecified**

✓4th N21   **Calculus of lower urinary tract**
Calculus of lower urinary tract with cystitis and urethritis

N21.0   **Calculus in bladder**
Calculus in diverticulum of bladder
Urinary bladder stone
EXCLUDES 2   staghorn calculus (N20.0)

N21.1   **Calculus in urethra**
EXCLUDES 2   calculus of prostate (N42.0)

N21.8   **Other lower urinary tract calculus**

N21.9   **Calculus of lower urinary tract, unspecified**
EXCLUDES 1   calculus of urinary tract NOS (N20.9)

N22   *Calculus of urinary tract in diseases classified elsewhere*
Code first underlying disease, such as:
gout (M1A.-, M10.-)
schistosomiasis (B65.0-B65.9)

N Newborn: 0   P Pediatric: 0-17   M Maternity: 12-55   A Adult: 15-124   MCC Major CC Condition   PDx MCC PDx acts as own MCC   CC CC Condition   PDx CC PDx acts as own CC

770   ICD-10-CM Draft (2015)

N23 Unspecified **renal colic**

Other disorders of kidney and ureter (N25-N29)

EXCLUDES 2   *disorders of kidney and ureter with urolithiasis (N20-N23)*

☑4ᵗʰ **N25** **Disorders resulting from impaired renal tubular function**
    EXCLUDES 1   *metabolic disorders classifiable to E70-E88*

N25.0 **Renal osteodystrophy**
    Azotemic osteodystrophy   Renal rickets
    Phosphate-losing tubular disorders   Renal short stature

N25.1 **Nephrogenic diabetes insipidus**   CC
    EXCLUDES 1   *diabetes insipidus NOS (E23.2)*
    CC Excl: A17.9, A18.10-A18.11, A18.13, A18.82, A18.84, A18.89,
    A54.21, A54.29, A54.82, A54.84, A54.89-A54.9, A59.00, A59.8-
    A59.9, A98.5, B37.41-B37.49, E08.21-E08.29, E08.618-E08.638,
    E08.649-E08.8, E09.21-E09.29, E09.618-E09.638, E09.649-E09.8,
    E10.21-E10.29, E10.618-E10.638, E10.649, E10.69-E10.8, E11.21-
    E11.29, E11.618-E11.638, E11.649, E11.69-E11.8, E13.21-E13.29,
    E13.618-E13.638, E13.649-E13.8, M10.30-M10.39, N00.0-N11.0,
    N11.8-N13.39, N13.6, N14.0-N17.9, N18.3-N18.6, N19, N25.0-
    N26.1, N26.9-N27.9, N28.1-N29, N36.41-N36.43, N36.8-N36.9,
    N39.8-N39.9, R31.0-R31.9

☑5ᵗʰ **N25.8** **Other disorders resulting from impaired renal tubular function**

N25.81 **Secondary hyperparathyroidism of renal origin** CC
    EXCLUDES 1   *secondary hyperparathyroidism, non-renal (E21.1)*
    CC Excl: A17.9, A18.10-A18.11, A18.13, A18.82, A18.84, A18.89,
    A54.21, A54.29, A54.82, A54.84, A54.89-A54.9, A59.00, A59.8-
    A59.9, A98.5, B37.41-B37.49, E08.21-E08.29, E08.618-E08.638,
    E08.649-E08.8, E09.21-E09.29, E09.618-E09.638, E09.649-E09.8,
    E10.21-E10.29, E10.618-E10.638, E10.649, E10.69-E10.8, E11.21-
    E11.29, E11.618-E11.638, E11.649, E11.69-E11.8, E13.21-E13.29,
    E13.618-E13.638, E13.649-E13.8, M10.30-M10.39, N00.0-N11.0,
    N11.8-N13.39, N13.6, N14.0-N17.9, N19, N25.0-N25.1, N25.89-
    N26.1, N26.9-N27.9, N28.1-N29, N36.41-N36.43, N36.8-N36.9,
    N39.8-N39.9, R31.0-R31.9

N25.89 **Other disorders resulting from impaired renal tubular function**
    Hypokalemic nephropathy
    Lightwood-Albright syndrome
    Renal tubular acidosis NOS

N25.9 **Disorder resulting from impaired renal tubular function, unspecified**

☑4ᵗʰ **N26** **Unspecified contracted kidney**
    EXCLUDES 1   *contracted kidney due to hypertension (I12.-)*
          diffuse sclerosing glomerulonephritis (N05.8-)
          hypertensive nephrosclerosis (arteriolar) (arteriosclerotic) (I12.-)
          small kidney of unknown cause (N27.-)

N26.1 **Atrophy of kidney (terminal)**

N26.2 **Page kidney**

N26.9 **Renal sclerosis, unspecified**

☑4ᵗʰ **N27** **Small kidney of unknown cause**
    INCLUDES   oligonephronia

N27.0 **Small kidney,** unilateral

N27.1 **Small kidney,** bilateral

N27.9 **Small kidney,** unspecified

☑4ᵗʰ **N28** **Other disorders of kidney and ureter, not elsewhere classified**

N28.0 **Ischemia and infarction of kidney** CC
    Renal artery embolism   Renal artery thrombosis
    Renal artery obstruction   Renal infarct
    Renal artery occlusion
    EXCLUDES 1   *atherosclerosis of renal artery (extrarenal part) (I70.1)*
          congenital stenosis of renal artery (Q27.1)
          Goldblatt's kidney (I70.1)
    CC Excl: N13.70-N13.739, N28.0, N28.9-N29

N28.1 **Cyst of kidney, acquired**
    Cyst (multiple)(solitary) of kidney, acquired
    EXCLUDES 1   *cystic kidney disease (congenital) (Q61.-)*

☑5ᵗʰ **N28.8** **Other specified disorders of kidney and ureter**
    EXCLUDES 1   *hydroureter (N13.4)*
          ureteric stricture with hydronephrosis (N13.1)
          ureteric stricture without hydronephrosis (N13.5)

    CC Excl: For CC codes in subcategory N28.8, unless otherwise noted: A17.9, A18.10-A18.11, A18.13, A18.82, A18.84, A18.89, A54.21, A54.29, A54.82, A54.84, A54.89-A54.9, A59.00, A59.8-A59.9, B37.41-B37.49, E08.21-E08.29, E09.21-E09.29, M10.30-M10.39, N00.0-N11.0, N11.8-N13.39, N13.6, N14.0-N19, N25.0-N26.1, N26.9-N27.9, N28.1-N29, N36.41-N36.43, N36.8-N36.9, N39.0, N39.8-N39.9, R31.0-R31.9

N28.81 **Hypertrophy of kidney**

N28.82 **Megaloureter**

N28.83 **Nephroptosis**

¹ **N28.84** **Pyelitis cystica** CC

¹ **N28.85** **Pyeloureteritis cystica** CC

¹ **N28.86** **Ureteritis cystica** CC

N28.89 **Other specified disorders of kidney and ureter**

N28.9 **Disorder of kidney and ureter, unspecified**
    Nephropathy NOS
    Renal disease (acute) NOS
    Renal insufficiency (acute)
    EXCLUDES 1   *chronic renal insufficiency (N18.9)*
          unspecified nephritic syndrome (N05.-)

N29 *Other disorders of kidney and ureter in diseases classified elsewhere*
    Code first underlying disease, such as:
        amyloidosis (E85.-)
        nephrocalcinosis (E83.5)
        schistosomiasis (B65.0-B65.9)
    EXCLUDES 1   *disorders of kidney and ureter in:*
          cystinosis (E72.0)
          gonorrhea (A54.21)
          syphilis (A52.75)
          tuberculosis (A18.11)

Other diseases of the urinary system (N30-N39)

EXCLUDES 1   *urinary infection (complicating):*
    abortion or ectopic or molar pregnancy (O00-O07, O08.8)
    pregnancy, childbirth and the puerperium (O23-, O75.3, O86.2-)

☑4ᵗʰ **N30** **Cystitis**
    Use additional code to identify infectious agent (B95-B97)
    EXCLUDES 1   *prostatocystitis (N41.3)*

    CC Excl: For CC codes in category N30, unless otherwise noted: A17.9, A18.10, A18.12-A18.13, A18.82, A18.84, A18.89, A54.00-A54.02, A54.09-A54.1, A54.82, A54.84, A54.89-A54.9, A59.00, A59.8-A59.9, B37.41-B37.49, N11.1, N13.4-N13.5, N13.8-N13.9, N28.82, N28.89-N30.91, N32.89-N33, N36.41-N36.43, N36.8-N36.9, N39.0, N39.8-N39.9, R31.0-R31.9

☑5ᵗʰ **N30.0** **Acute cystitis**
    EXCLUDES 1   *irradiation cystitis (N30.4-)*
          trigonitis (N30.3-)

¹ **N30.00** **Acute cystitis** without hematuria CC

¹ **N30.01** **Acute cystitis** with hematuria CC

☑5ᵗʰ **N30.1** **Interstitial cystitis (chronic)**

N30.10 **Interstitial cystitis (chronic)** without hematuria

N30.11 **Interstitial cystitis (chronic)** with hematuria

☑5ᵗʰ **N30.2** **Other chronic cystitis**

N30.20 **Other chronic cystitis** without hematuria

N30.21 **Other chronic cystitis** with hematuria

☑5ᵗʰ **N30.3** **Trigonitis**
    Urethrotrigonitis

N30.30 **Trigonitis** without hematuria

N30.31 **Trigonitis** with hematuria

☑5ᵗʰ **N30.4** **Irradiation cystitis**

N30.40 **Irradiation cystitis** without hematuria CC

N30.41 **Irradiation cystitis** with hematuria CC

☑5ᵗʰ **N30.8** **Other cystitis**
    Abscess of bladder

N30.80 **Other cystitis** without hematuria

N30.81 **Other cystitis** with hematuria

☑5ᵗʰ **N30.9** **Cystitis,** unspecified

N30.90 **Cystitis, unspecified** without hematuria

---

¹ HAC = as SDx not POA, in combination with SDx code T83.51XA also not POA.

☑ Additional Character Required   ☑x7ᵗʰ Xtension Alert   Unacceptable PDx   Manifestation   Hospital Acquired Condition   EXCLUDES 1 Not Coded Here   EXCLUDES 2 Not Included Here

Diseases of the Genitourinary System

N30.91–N36.9

(margin handwriting: N39.8 Urinary incontinence)

    N30.91   Cystitis, unspecified with hematuria

✓4ᵗʰ **N31**   **Neuromuscular dysfunction of bladder, not elsewhere classified**
    Use additional code to identify any associated urinary incontinence (N39.3-N39.4-)
    EXCLUDES 1   cord bladder NOS (G95.89)
              neurogenic bladder due to cauda equina syndrome (G83.4)
              neuromuscular dysfunction due to spinal cord lesion (G95.89)

  N31.0   **Uninhibited neuropathic bladder, not elsewhere classified**

  N31.1   **Reflex neuropathic bladder, not elsewhere classified**

  N31.2   **Flaccid neuropathic bladder, not elsewhere classified**
       Atonic (motor) (sensory) neuropathic bladder
       Autonomous neuropathic bladder
       Nonreflex neuropathic bladder

  N31.8   **Other neuromuscular dysfunction of bladder**

  N31.9   **Neuromuscular dysfunction of bladder, unspecified**
       Neurogenic bladder dysfunction NOS

✓4ᵗʰ **N32**   **Other disorders of bladder**
    EXCLUDES 2   calculus of bladder (N21.0)
              cystocele (N81.1-)
              hernia or prolapse of bladder, female (N81.1-)

  N32.0   **Bladder-neck obstruction**
       Bladder-neck stenosis (acquired)
       EXCLUDES 1   congenital bladder-neck obstruction (Q64.3-)

  N32.1   **Vesicointestinal fistula**   CC
       Vesicorectal fistula
       CC Excl: A54.00, A54.02, A54.09-A54.1, A54.82, A54.84, A54.89-A54.9, N32.1-N32.2, N32.89-N33, N36.41-N36.43, N36.8-N36.9, N39.8-N39.9, R30.0, R30.9-R31.9

  N32.2   **Vesical fistula, not elsewhere classified**   CC
       EXCLUDES 1   fistula between bladder and female genital tract (N82.0-N82.1)
       CC Excl: See code: N32.1

  N32.3   **Diverticulum of bladder**
       EXCLUDES 1   congenital diverticulum of bladder (Q64.6)
               diverticulitis of bladder (N30.8-)

✓5ᵗʰ **N32.8**   **Other specified disorders of bladder**
    N32.81   **Overactive bladder**
         Detrusor muscle hyperactivity
         EXCLUDES 1   frequent urination due to specified bladder condition—code to condition

    N32.89   **Other specified disorders of bladder**
         Bladder hemorrhage   Calcified bladder
         Bladder hypertrophy   Contracted bladder

  N32.9   **Bladder disorder, unspecified**

N33   *Bladder disorders in diseases classified elsewhere*
    Code first underlying disease, such as:
    schistosomiasis (B65.0-B65.9)
    EXCLUDES 1   bladder disorder in syphilis (A52.76)
              bladder disorder in tuberculosis (A18.12)
              candidal cystitis (B37.41)
              chlamydial cystitis (A56.01)
              cystitis in gonorrhea (A54.01)
              cystitis in neurogenic bladder (N31.-)
              diphtheritic cystitis (A36.85)
              neurogenic bladder (N31.-)
              syphilitic cystitis (A52.76)
              trichomonal cystitis (A59.03)

✓4ᵗʰ **N34**   **Urethritis and urethral syndrome**
    Use additional code (B95-B97), to identify infectious agent
    EXCLUDES 2   Reiter's disease (M02.3-)
              urethritis in diseases with a predominantly sexual mode of transmission (A50-A64)
              urethrotrigonitis (N30.3-)

  ¹ **N34.0**   **Urethral abscess**   CC
       Abscess (of) Cowper's gland
       Abscess (of) Littrés gland
       Abscess (of) urethral (gland)
       Periurethral abscess
       EXCLUDES 1   urethral caruncle (N36.2)
       CC Excl: A54.00, A54.02, A54.09-A54.1, A54.82, A54.84, A54.89-A54.9, A59.00, A59.03, A59.8-A59.9, B37.41-B37.49, N13.9, N34.0-N34.3, N35.111-N35.9, N36.41-N36.43, N36.8-N39.0, N39.8-N39.9, N44.1-N44.8, N47.6, N48.1-N48.9, N49.1-N49.9, N50.3-N50.8, N51, N53.11-N53.9, Q54.0-Q55.21, Q55.23-Q55.9, Q64.0, Q64.2-Q64.9, R30.0, R30.9-R31.9

  N34.1   **Nonspecific urethritis**
       Nongonococcal urethritis
       Nonvenereal urethritis

  N34.2   **Other urethritis**
       Meatitis, urethral   Ulcer of urethra (meatus)
       Postmenopausal urethritis   Urethritis NOS

  N34.3   **Urethral syndrome, unspecified**

✓4ᵗʰ **N35**   **Urethral stricture**
    EXCLUDES 1   congenital urethral stricture (Q64.3-)
              postprocedural urethral stricture (N99.1-)

✓5ᵗʰ **N35.0**   **Post-traumatic urethral stricture**
       Urethral stricture due to injury
       EXCLUDES 1   postprocedural urethral stricture (N99.1-)

    ✓6ᵗʰ **N35.01**   **Post-traumatic urethral stricture, male**
        N35.010   **Post-traumatic urethral stricture, male, meatal** ♂
        N35.011   **Post-traumatic bulbous urethral stricture**
        N35.012   **Post-traumatic membranous urethral stricture**
        N35.013   **Post-traumatic anterior urethral stricture**
        N35.014   **Post-traumatic urethral stricture, male, unspecified** ♂

    ✓6ᵗʰ **N35.02**   **Post-traumatic urethral stricture, female**
        N35.021   **Urethral stricture due to childbirth** ♀
        N35.028   **Other post-traumatic urethral stricture, female** ♀

✓5ᵗʰ **N35.1**   **Postinfective urethral stricture, not elsewhere classified**
       EXCLUDES 1   urethral stricture associated with schistosomiasis (B65-, N29)
              gonococcal urethral stricture (A54.01)
              syphilitic urethral stricture (A52.76)

    ✓6ᵗʰ **N35.11**   **Postinfective urethral stricture, not elsewhere classified, male**
        N35.111   **Postinfective urethral stricture, not elsewhere classified, male, meatal** ♂
        N35.112   **Postinfective bulbous urethral stricture, not elsewhere classified**
        N35.113   **Postinfective membranous urethral stricture, not elsewhere classified**
        N35.114   **Postinfective anterior urethral stricture, not elsewhere classified**
        N35.119   **Postinfective urethral stricture, not elsewhere classified, male, unspecified** ♂

    N35.12   **Postinfective urethral stricture, not elsewhere classified, female** ♀

  N35.8   **Other urethral stricture**
       EXCLUDES 1   postprocedural urethral stricture (N99.1-)

  N35.9   **Urethral stricture, unspecified**

✓4ᵗʰ **N36**   **Other disorders of urethra**
  N36.0   **Urethral fistula**   CC
       Urethroperineal fistula   Urinary fistula NOS
       Urethrorectal fistula
       EXCLUDES 1   urethroscrotal fistula (N50.8)
              urethrovaginal fistula (N82.1)
              urethrovesicovaginal fistula (N82.1)
       CC Excl: N13.9, N34.0, N34.2-N36.43, N36.5-N37, N39.8-N39.9, N44.1-N44.8, N47.6, N48.1-N48.9, N49.1-N49.9, N50.3-N50.8, N51, N53.11-N53.9, N99.110-N99.12, Q54.0-Q55.21, Q55.23-Q55.9, Q64.0, Q64.8-Q64.9, R30.0, R30.9-R31.9

  N36.1   **Urethral diverticulum**

  N36.2   **Urethral caruncle**

✓5ᵗʰ **N36.4**   **Urethral functional and muscular disorders**
       Use additional code to identify associated urinary stress incontinence (N39.3)

    N36.41   **Hypermobility of urethra**
    N36.42   **Intrinsic sphincter deficiency (ISD)**
    N36.43   **Combined hypermobility of urethra and intrinsic sphincter deficiency**
    N36.44   **Muscular disorders of urethra**
         Bladder sphincter dyssynergy

  N36.5   **Urethral false passage**

  N36.8   **Other specified disorders of urethra**

  N36.9   **Urethral disorder, unspecified**

---

¹ HAC = as SDx not POA, in combination with SDx code T83.51XA also not POA.

N37   Urethral disorders in diseases classified elsewhere
Code first underlying disease
EXCLUDES 1   urethritis (in):
candidal infection (B37.41)
chlamydial (A56.01)
gonorrhea (A54.01)
syphilis (A52.76)
trichomonal infection (A59.03)
tuberculosis (A18.13)

✓4th **N39   Other disorders of urinary system**
EXCLUDES 2   hematuria NOS (R31.-)
recurrent or persistent hematuria (N02.-)
recurrent or persistent hematuria with specified morphological lesion (N02.-)
proteinuria NOS (R80.-)

[1] **N39.0   Urinary tract infection, site not specified**   CC
Use additional code (B95-B97), to identify infectious agent
EXCLUDES 1   candidiasis of urinary tract (B37.4-)
neonatal urinary tract infection (P39.3)
urinary tract infection of specified site, such as:
cystitis (N30.-)
urethritis (N34.-)
(handwritten: due to E coli)   *(handwritten: * Read this add.)*
AHA: 2012, 4Q, 94
CC Excl: A54.82, A54.84, A54.89-A54.9, A59.00, A59.8-A59.9, B37.41-B37.49, N10, N11.9-N13.39, N13.6, N13.9, N15.1, N28.82, N28.84-N30.91, N34.1, N36.41-N36.43, N36.8-N36.9, N39.0, N39.8-N39.9, N99.511, R30.0, R30.9-R31.9, T83.51XA

N39.3   Stress incontinence (female) (male)
Code also any associated overactive bladder (N32.81)
EXCLUDES 1   mixed incontinence (N39.46)

✓5th **N39.4   Other specified urinary incontinence**
Code also any associated overactive bladder (N32.81)
EXCLUDES 1   enuresis NOS (R32)
functional urinary incontinence (R39.81)
urinary incontinence associated with cognitive impairment (R39.81)
urinary incontinence NOS (R32)
urinary incontinence of nonorganic origin (F98.0)

N39.41   Urge incontinence
EXCLUDES 1   mixed incontinence (N39.46)
N39.42   Incontinence without sensory awareness
N39.43   Post-void dribbling
N39.44   Nocturnal enuresis
N39.45   Continuous leakage
N39.46   Mixed incontinence
Urge and stress incontinence
✓6th **N39.49   Other specified urinary incontinence**
N39.490   Overflow incontinence
N39.498   Other specified urinary incontinence
Reflex incontinence
Total incontinence
N39.8   Other specified disorders of urinary system
N39.9   Disorder of urinary system, unspecified

Diseases of male genital organs (N40-N53)

✓4th **N40   Enlarged prostate**
Adenofibromatous hypertrophy of prostate
Benign hypertrophy of the prostate
Benign prostatic hyperplasia
Benign prostatic hypertrophy
BPH
Nodular prostate
Polyp of prostate
EXCLUDES 1   benign neoplasms of prostate (adenoma, benign) (fibroadenoma) (fibroma) (myoma) (D29.1)
EXCLUDES 2   malignant neoplasm of prostate (C61)

N40.0   Enlarged prostate without lower urinary tract symptoms   A ♂
Enlarged prostate NOS   Enlarged prostate without LUTS
N40.1   Enlarged prostate with lower urinary tract symptoms   A ♂
Enlarged prostate with LUTS
Use additional code for associated symptoms, when specified:
incomplete bladder emptying (R39.14)
nocturia (R35.1)
straining on urination (R39.16)
urinary frequency (R35.0)
urinary hesitancy (R39.11)
urinary incontinence (N39.4-)
urinary obstruction (N13.8)
urinary retention (R33.8)
urinary urgency (R39.15)
weak urinary stream (R39.12)

N40.2   Nodular prostate without lower urinary tract symptoms   A ♂
Nodular prostate without LUTS
N40.3   Nodular prostate with lower urinary tract symptoms   A ♂
Use additional code for associated symptoms, when specified:
incomplete bladder emptying (R39.14)
nocturia (R35.1)
straining on urination (R39.16)
urinary frequency (R35.0)
urinary hesitancy (R39.11)
urinary incontinence (N39.4-)
urinary obstruction (N13.8)
urinary retention (R33.8)
urinary urgency (R39.15)
weak urinary stream (R39.12)

✓4th **N41   Inflammatory diseases of prostate**
Use additional code (B95-B97), to identify infectious agent
N41.0   Acute prostatitis   CC A ♂
CC Excl: A18.14, A54.22, A54.82, A54.84, A54.89-A54.9, A59.00, A59.02, A59.8-A59.9, B37.41-B37.49, N40.0-N41.0, N41.1, N41.2-N42.9
N41.1   Chronic prostatitis   A ♂
N41.2   Abscess of prostate   CC A ♂
CC Excl: See code: N41.0
N41.3   Prostatocystitis   A ♂
N41.4   Granulomatous prostatitis   A ♂
N41.8   Other inflammatory diseases of prostate   A ♂
N41.9   Inflammatory disease of prostate, unspecified   A ♂
Prostatitis NOS

✓4th **N42   Other and unspecified disorders of prostate**
N42.0   Calculus of prostate   A ♂
Prostatic stone
N42.1   Congestion and hemorrhage of prostate   A ♂
EXCLUDES 1   enlarged prostate (N40.-)
hematuria (R31.-)
hyperplasia of prostate (N40.-)
inflammatory diseases of prostate (N41.-)
N42.3   Dysplasia of prostate   ♂
Prostatic intraepithelial neoplasia I (PIN I)
Prostatic intraepithelial neoplasia II (PIN II)
EXCLUDES 1   prostatic intraepithelial neoplasia III (PIN III) (D07.5)
✓5th **N42.8   Other specified disorders of prostate**
N42.81   Prostatodynia syndrome   A ♂
Painful prostate syndrome
N42.82   Prostatosis syndrome   A ♂
N42.83   Cyst of prostate   A ♂
N42.89   Other specified disorders of prostate   A ♂
N42.9   Disorder of prostate, unspecified   A ♂

✓4th **N43   Hydrocele and spermatocele**
INCLUDES   hydrocele of spermatic cord, testis or tunica vaginalis
EXCLUDES 1   congenital hydrocele (P83.5)
N43.0   Encysted hydrocele   ♂
N43.1   Infected hydrocele   CC ♂
Use additional code (B95-B97), to identify infectious agent
CC Excl: A59.00, A59.8-A59.9, B37.41-B37.49, N43.0-N43.3
N43.2   Other hydrocele   ♂
N43.3   Hydrocele, unspecified   ♂
✓5th **N43.4   Spermatocele of epididymis**
Spermatic cyst
N43.40   Spermatocele of epididymis, unspecified   ♂
N43.41   Spermatocele of epididymis, single   ♂
N43.42   Spermatocele of epididymis, multiple   ♂

✓4th **N44   Noninflammatory disorders of testis**

CC Excl: For CC codes in category N44, unless otherwise noted: N44.00-N44.04

✓5th **N44.0   Torsion of testis**
N44.00   Torsion of testis, unspecified   CC ♂
N44.01   Extravaginal torsion of spermatic cord   CC ♂
N44.02   Intravaginal torsion of spermatic cord   CC ♂
Torsion of spermatic cord NOS
N44.03   Torsion of appendix testis   CC ♂
N44.04   Torsion of appendix epididymis   CC ♂
N44.1   Cyst of tunica albuginea testis   ♂
N44.2   Benign cyst of testis   ♂

---

1 HAC = as SDx not POA, in combination with SDx code T83.51XA also not POA.

✓ Additional Character Required   ✓x7th Xtension Alert   Unacceptable PDx   Manifestation   Hospital Acquired Condition   EXCLUDES 1 Not Coded Here   EXCLUDES 2 Not Included Here

Diseases of the Genitourinary System

N44.8–N50.9

N44.8   **Other** noninflammatory disorders of the testis   ♂

✓4ᵗʰ N45   Orchitis and epididymitis
Use additional code (B95-B97), to identify infectious agent

N45.1   **Epididymitis**   ♂

N45.2   **Orchitis**   ♂

N45.3   **Epididymo-orchitis**   ♂

N45.4   **Abscess of epididymis or testis**   CC
CC Excl: A54.23, A54.82, A54.84, A54.89-A54.9, A59.00, A59.8-A59.9, B26.0, B37.41-B37.49, N45.1-N45.4

✓4ᵗʰ N46   Male infertility
EXCLUDES 1   vasectomy status (Z98.52)

✓5ᵗʰ **N46.0   Azoospermia**
Absolute male infertility
Male infertility due to germinal (cell) aplasia
Male infertility due to spermatogenic arrest (complete)

    N46.01   **Organic** azoospermia   A♂
        Azoospermia NOS

    ✓6ᵗʰ N46.02   **Azoospermia due to** extratesticular causes
        Code also associated cause

        N46.021   **Azoospermia due to** drug therapy   A♂
        N46.022   **Azoospermia due to** infection   A♂
        N46.023   **Azoospermia due to** obstruction of efferent ducts   A♂
        N46.024   **Azoospermia due to** radiation   A♂
        N46.025   **Azoospermia due to** systemic disease   A♂
        N46.029   **Azoospermia due to** other extratesticular causes   A♂

✓5ᵗʰ **N46.1   Oligospermia**
Male infertility due to germinal cell desquamation
Male infertility due to hypospermatogenesis
Male infertility due to incomplete spermatogenic arrest

    N46.11   **Organic** oligospermia   A♂
        Oligospermia NOS

    ✓6ᵗʰ N46.12   **Oligospermia due to** extratesticular causes
        Code also associated cause

        N46.121   **Oligospermia due to** drug therapy   A♂
        N46.122   **Oligospermia due to** infection   A♂
        N46.123   **Oligospermia due to** obstruction of efferent ducts   A♂
        N46.124   **Oligospermia due to** radiation   A♂
        N46.125   **Oligospermia due to** systemic disease   A♂
        N46.129   **Oligospermia due to** other extratesticular causes   A♂

N46.8   **Other male infertility**   A♂

N46.9   **Male infertility, unspecified**   A♂

✓4ᵗʰ N47   Disorders of prepuce
N47.0   **Adherent prepuce, newborn**   N♂

N47.1   **Phimosis**   ♂

N47.2   **Paraphimosis**   ♂

N47.3   **Deficient foreskin**   ♂

N47.4   **Benign cyst of prepuce**   ♂

N47.5   **Adhesions of prepuce and glans penis**   ♂

N47.6   **Balanoposthitis**   ♂
Use additional code (B95-B97), to identify infectious agent
EXCLUDES 1   balanitis (N48.1)

N47.7   **Other inflammatory diseases of prepuce**   ♂
Use additional code (B95-B97), to identify infectious agent

N47.8   **Other disorders of prepuce**   ♂

✓4ᵗʰ N48   Other disorders of penis
N48.0   **Leukoplakia of penis**   ♂
Balanitis xerotica obliterans
Kraurosis of penis
Lichen sclerosus of external male genital organs
EXCLUDES 1   carcinoma in situ of penis (D07.4)

N48.1   **Balanitis**   ♂
Use additional code (B95-B97), to identify infectious agent
EXCLUDES 1   amebic balanitis (A06.8)
        balanitis xerotica obliterans (N48.0)
        candidal balanitis (B37.42)
        gonococcal balanitis (A54.23)
        herpesviral [herpes simplex] balanitis (A60.01)

✓5ᵗʰ **N48.2   Other inflammatory disorders of penis**
Use additional code (B95-B97), to identify infectious agent
EXCLUDES 1   balanitis (N48.1)
        balanitis xerotica obliterans (N48.0)
        balanoposthitis (N47.6)

    N48.21   **Abscess of corpus cavernosum and penis**   ♂
    N48.22   **Cellulitis of corpus cavernosum and penis**   ♂
    N48.29   **Other inflammatory disorders of penis**   ♂

✓5ᵗʰ **N48.3   Priapism**
Painful erection
Code first underlying cause

> CC Excl: For CC codes in subcategory N48.3, unless otherwise noted: N47.6, N48.0-N48.9, N52.01-N52.9

    N48.30   **Priapism, unspecified**   CC♂
    N48.31   **Priapism** due to trauma   CC♂
    N48.32   Priapism due to disease classified elsewhere   CC♂
    N48.33   **Priapism,** drug-induced   CC♂
    N48.39   **Other** priapism   CC♂

N48.5   **Ulcer of penis**   ♂

N48.6   **Induration penis plastica**   ♂
Peyronie's disease
Plastic induration of penis

✓5ᵗʰ **N48.8   Other specified disorders of penis**
    N48.81   **Thrombosis of superficial vein of penis**   ♂
    N48.82   **Acquired torsion of penis**   ♂
        Acquired torsion of penis NOS
        EXCLUDES 1   congenital torsion of penis (Q55.63)
    N48.83   **Acquired buried penis**   ♂
        EXCLUDES 1   congenital hidden penis (Q55.64)
    N48.89   **Other specified disorders of penis**   ♂

N48.9   **Disorder of penis, unspecified**   ♂

✓4ᵗʰ N49   Inflammatory disorders of male genital organs, not elsewhere classified
Use additional code (B95-B97), to identify infectious agent
EXCLUDES 1   inflammation of penis (N48.1, N48.2-)
        orchitis and epididymitis (N45.-)

N49.0   **Inflammatory disorders of** seminal vesicle   ♂
Vesiculitis NOS

N49.1   **Inflammatory disorders of** spermatic cord, tunica vaginalis and vas deferens   ♂
Vasitis

N49.2   **Inflammatory disorders of** scrotum   ♂

N49.3   **Fournier gangrene**   ♂

N49.8   **Inflammatory disorders of** other specified male genital organs   ♂
Inflammation of multiple sites in male genital organs

N49.9   **Inflammatory disorder of** unspecified male genital organ   ♂
Abscess of unspecified male genital organ
Boil of unspecified male genital organ
Carbuncle of unspecified male genital organ
Cellulitis of unspecified male genital organ

✓4ᵗʰ N50   Other and unspecified disorders of male genital organs
EXCLUDES 2   torsion of testis (N44.0-)

N50.0   **Atrophy of testis**   ♂

N50.1   **Vascular disorders of male genital organs**   ♂
Hematocele, NOS, of male genital organs
Hemorrhage of male genital organs
Thrombosis of male genital organs

N50.3   **Cyst of epididymis**   ♂

N50.8   **Other specified disorders of male genital organs**   ♂
Atrophy of scrotum, seminal vesicle, spermatic cord, tunica vaginalis and vas deferens
Chylocele, tunica vaginalis (nonfilarial) NOS
Edema of scrotum, seminal vesicle, spermatic cord, testis, tunica vaginalis and vas deferens
Hypertrophy of scrotum, seminal vesicle, spermatic cord, testis, tunica vaginalis and vas deferens
Stricture of spermatic cord, tunica vaginalis, and vas deferens
Ulcer of scrotum, seminal vesicle, spermatic cord, testis, tunica vaginalis and vas deferens
Urethroscrotal fistula

N50.9   **Disorder of male genital organs, unspecified**   ♂

N Newborn: 0   P Pediatric: 0-17   M Maternity: 12-55   A Adult: 15-124   MCC Major CC Condition   PDx MCC PDx acts as own MCC   CC CC Condition   PDx CC PDx acts as own CC

774   ICD-10-CM Draft (2015)

N51 Disorders of male genital organs in diseases classified elsewhere ♂

Code first underlying disease, such as:
filariasis (B74.0-B74.9)
EXCLUDES 1 amebic balanitis (A06.8)
candidal balanitis (B37.42)
gonococcal balanitis (A54.23)
gonococcal prostatitis (A54.22)
herpesviral [herpes simplex] balanitis (A60.01)
trichomonal prostatitis (A59.02)
tuberculous prostatitis (A18.14)

☑4ᵗʰ **N52 Male erectile dysfunction**
EXCLUDES 1 psychogenic impotence (F52.21)

☑5ᵗʰ **N52.0 Vasculogenic erectile dysfunction**
N52.01 Erectile dysfunction due to arterial insufficiency Ⓐ♂
N52.02 Corporo-venous occlusive erectile dysfunction Ⓐ♂
N52.03 Combined arterial insufficiency and corporo-venous occlusive erectile dysfunction Ⓐ♂

N52.1 Erectile dysfunction due to diseases classified elsewhere Ⓐ♂
Code first underlying disease

N52.2 Drug-induced erectile dysfunction Ⓐ♂

☑5ᵗʰ **N52.3 Post-surgical erectile dysfunction**
N52.31 Erectile dysfunction following radical prostatectomy Ⓐ♂
N52.32 Erectile dysfunction following radical cystectomy Ⓐ♂
N52.33 Erectile dysfunction following urethral surgery Ⓐ♂
N52.34 Erectile dysfunction following simple prostatectomy Ⓐ♂
N52.39 Other post-surgical erectile dysfunction Ⓐ♂

N52.8 Other male erectile dysfunction Ⓐ♂

N52.9 Male erectile dysfunction, unspecified Ⓐ♂
Impotence NOS

☑4ᵗʰ **N53 Other male sexual dysfunction**
EXCLUDES 1 psychogenic sexual dysfunction (F52.-)

☑5ᵗʰ **N53.1 Ejaculatory dysfunction**
EXCLUDES 1 premature ejaculation (F52.4)
N53.11 Retarded ejaculation ♂
N53.12 Painful ejaculation ♂
N53.13 Anejaculatory orgasm ♂
N53.14 Retrograde ejaculation ♂
N53.19 Other ejaculatory dysfunction ♂
Ejaculatory dysfunction NOS

N53.8 Other male sexual dysfunction ♂

N53.9 Unspecified male sexual dysfunction ♂

Disorders of breast (N60-N65)

EXCLUDES 1 disorders of breast associated with childbirth (O91-O92)

☑4ᵗʰ **N60 Benign mammary dysplasia**
INCLUDES fibrocystic mastopathy

☑5ᵗʰ **N60.0 Solitary cyst of breast**
Cyst of breast
N60.01 Solitary cyst of right breast
N60.02 Solitary cyst of left breast
N60.09 Solitary cyst of unspecified breast

☑5ᵗʰ **N60.1 Diffuse cystic mastopathy**
Cystic breast
Fibrocystic disease of breast
EXCLUDES 1 diffuse cystic mastopathy with epithelial proliferation (N60.3-)
N60.11 Diffuse cystic mastopathy of right breast Ⓐ
N60.12 Diffuse cystic mastopathy of left breast Ⓐ
N60.19 Diffuse cystic mastopathy of unspecified breast Ⓐ

☑5ᵗʰ **N60.2 Fibroadenosis of breast**
Adenofibrosis of breast
EXCLUDES 2 fibroadenoma of breast (D24.-)
N60.21 Fibroadenosis of right breast
N60.22 Fibroadenosis of left breast
N60.29 Fibroadenosis of unspecified breast

☑5ᵗʰ **N60.3 Fibrosclerosis of breast**
Cystic mastopathy with epithelial proliferation
N60.31 Fibrosclerosis of right breast
N60.32 Fibrosclerosis of left breast

N60.39 Fibrosclerosis of unspecified breast

☑5ᵗʰ **N60.4 Mammary duct ectasia**
N60.41 Mammary duct ectasia of right breast
N60.42 Mammary duct ectasia of left breast
N60.49 Mammary duct ectasia of unspecified breast

☑5ᵗʰ **N60.8 Other benign mammary dysplasias**
N60.81 Other benign mammary dysplasias of right breast
N60.82 Other benign mammary dysplasias of left breast
N60.89 Other benign mammary dysplasias of unspecified breast

☑5ᵗʰ **N60.9 Unspecified benign mammary dysplasia**
N60.91 Unspecified benign mammary dysplasia of right breast
N60.92 Unspecified benign mammary dysplasia of left breast
N60.99 Unspecified benign mammary dysplasia of unspecified breast

N61 Inflammatory disorders of breast
Abscess (acute) (chronic) (nonpuerperal) of areola
Abscess (acute) (chronic) (nonpuerperal) of breast
Carbuncle of breast
Infective mastitis (acute) (subacute) (nonpuerperal)
Mastitis (acute) (subacute) (nonpuerperal) NOS
EXCLUDES 1 inflammatory carcinoma of breast (C50.9)
inflammatory disorder of breast associated with childbirth (O91.-)
neonatal infective mastitis (P39.0)
thrombophlebitis of breast [Mondor's disease] (I80.8)

N62 Hypertrophy of breast
Gynecomastia
Hypertrophy of breast NOS
Massive pubertal hypertrophy of breast
EXCLUDES 1 breast engorgement of newborn (P83.4)
disproportion of reconstructed breast (N65.1)

N63 Unspecified lump in breast
Nodule(s) NOS in breast

☑4ᵗʰ **N64 Other disorders of breast**
EXCLUDES 2 mechanical complication of breast prosthesis and implant (T85.4-)

N64.0 Fissure and fistula of nipple

N64.1 Fat necrosis of breast
Fat necrosis (segmental) of breast
Code first breast necrosis due to breast graft (T85.89)

N64.2 Atrophy of breast

N64.3 Galactorrhea not associated with childbirth

N64.4 Mastodynia

☑5ᵗʰ **N64.5 Other signs and symptoms in breast**
EXCLUDES 2 abnormal findings on diagnostic imaging of breast (R92.-)
N64.51 Induration of breast
N64.52 Nipple discharge
EXCLUDES 1 abnormal findings in nipple discharge (R89.-)
N64.53 Retraction of nipple
N64.59 Other signs and symptoms in breast

☑5ᵗʰ **N64.8 Other specified disorders of breast**
N64.81 Ptosis of breast Ⓐ
EXCLUDES 1 ptosis of native breast in relation to reconstructed breast (N65.1)
N64.82 Hypoplasia of breast Ⓐ
Micromastia
EXCLUDES 1 congenital absence of breast (Q83.0)
hypoplasia of native breast in relation to reconstructed breast (N65.1)
N64.89 Other specified disorders of breast
Galactocele
Subinvolution of breast (postlactational)

N64.9 Disorder of breast, unspecified

☑4ᵗʰ **N65 Deformity and disproportion of reconstructed breast**
N65.0 Deformity of reconstructed breast Ⓐ
Contour irregularity in reconstructed breast
Excess tissue in reconstructed breast
Misshapen reconstructed breast

☑ Additional Character Required ☑7ᵗʰ Xtension Alert Unacceptable PDx Manifestation Hospital Acquired Condition *EXCLUDES 1* Not Coded Here *EXCLUDES 2* Not Included Here

Diseases of the Genitourinary System

N65.1   **Disproportion of reconstructed breast**   A
     Breast asymmetry between native breast and reconstructed breast
     Disproportion between native breast and reconstructed breast

Inflammatory diseases of female pelvic organs (N70-N77)

EXCLUDES 1   *inflammatory diseases of female pelvic organs complicating:*
     abortion or ectopic or molar pregnancy (O00-O07, O08.0)
     pregnancy, childbirth and the puerperium (O23-, O75.3, O85, O86-)

☑4th **N70**   **Salpingitis and oophoritis**
     INCLUDES   abscess (of) fallopian tube
         abscess (of) ovary
         pyosalpinx
         salpingo-oophoritis
         tubo-ovarian abscess
         tubo-ovarian inflammatory disease
     Use additional code (B95-B97), to identify infectious agent
     EXCLUDES 1   *gonococcal infection (A54.24)*
         tuberculous infection (A18.17)

> **CC Excl: For CC codes in subcategory N70.0, unless otherwise noted:** A17.9, A18.10, A18.16-A18.18, A18.82, A18.84, A18.89, A54.03, A54.24, A54.82, A54.84, A54.89-A54.9, A59.00, A59.8-A59.9, B37.41-B37.49, N70.01-N71.9, N73.0-N74, N75.9, N76.5, N76.81-N76.89, N90.810-N90.818, N94.818-N94.9, N96, Q55.0-Q55.21, Q55.23-Q55.4, Q55.7-Q55.9

   ☑5th **N70.0**   **Acute salpingitis and oophoritis**
       N70.01   **Acute salpingitis**   CC ♀
       N70.02   **Acute oophoritis**   CC ♀
       N70.03   **Acute salpingitis and oophoritis**   CC ♀

   ☑5th **N70.1**   **Chronic salpingitis and oophoritis**
       Hydrosalpinx
       N70.11   **Chronic salpingitis**   ♀
       N70.12   **Chronic oophoritis**   ♀
       N70.13   **Chronic salpingitis and oophoritis**   ♀

   ☑5th **N70.9**   **Salpingitis and oophoritis, unspecified**
       N70.91   **Salpingitis, unspecified**   ♀
       N70.92   **Oophoritis, unspecified**   ♀
       N70.93   **Salpingitis and oophoritis, unspecified**   ♀

☑4th **N71**   **Inflammatory disease of uterus, except cervix**
     Endo (myo) metritis   Pyometra
     Metritis   Uterine abscess
     Myometritis
     Use additional code (B95-B97), to identify infectious agent
     EXCLUDES 1   *hyperplastic endometritis (N85.0-)*
         infection of uterus following delivery (O85, O86.-)

   N71.0   **Acute inflammatory disease of uterus**   CC ♀
       CC Excl: A17.9, A18.10, A18.16-A18.18, A18.82, A18.84, A18.89, A54.03, A54.24, A54.82, A54.84, A54.89-A54.9, A59.00, A59.8-A59.9, B37.41-B37.49, N70.01-N74, N75.9, N76.5, N76.81-N76.89, N85.8-N85.9, N90.810-N90.818, N94.818-N94.9, N96, Q55.0-Q55.21, Q55.23-Q55.4, Q55.7-Q55.9

   N71.1   **Chronic inflammatory disease of uterus**   ♀
   N71.9   **Inflammatory disease of uterus, unspecified**   ♀

N72   **Inflammatory disease of cervix uteri**   ♀
     Cervicitis (with or without erosion or ectropion)
     Endocervicitis (with or without erosion or ectropion)
     Exocervicitis (with or without erosion or ectropion)
     Use additional code (B95-B97), to identify infectious agent
     EXCLUDES 1   *erosion and ectropion of cervix without cervicitis (N86)*

☑4th **N73**   **Other female pelvic inflammatory diseases**
     Use additional code (B95-B97), to identify infectious agent

> **CC Excl: For CC/MCC codes in category N73, unless otherwise noted:** A17.9, A18.10, A18.16-A18.18, A18.82, A18.84, A18.89, A54.03, A54.24, A54.82, A54.84, A54.89-A54.9, A59.00, A59.8-A59.9, B37.41-B37.49, N70.01-N71.9, N73.0-N74, N75.9, N76.5, N76.81-N76.89, N90.810-N90.818, N94.818-N94.9, N96, Q55.0-Q55.21, Q55.23-Q55.4, Q55.7-Q55.9

   N73.0   **Acute parametritis and pelvic cellulitis**   CC ♀
       Abscess of broad ligament
       Abscess of parametrium
       Pelvic cellulitis, female

   N73.1   **Chronic parametritis and pelvic cellulitis**   ♀
       Any condition in N73.0 specified as chronic
       EXCLUDES 1   *tuberculous parametritis and pelvic cellultis (A18.17)*

   N73.2   **Unspecified parametritis and pelvic cellulitis**   ♀
       Any condition in N73.0 unspecified whether acute or chronic

   N73.3   **Female acute pelvic peritonitis**   MCC

   N73.4   **Female chronic pelvic peritonitis**   CC ♀
       EXCLUDES 1   *tuberculous pelvic (female) peritonitis (A18.17)*

   N73.5   **Female pelvic peritonitis, unspecified**   ♀

   N73.6   **Female pelvic peritoneal adhesions (postinfective)**   ♀
       EXCLUDES 2   *postprocedural pelvic peritoneal adhesions (N99.4)*
       AHA: 2014, 1Q, 6

   N73.8   **Other specified female pelvic inflammatory diseases**   ♀

   N73.9   **Female pelvic inflammatory disease, unspecified**   ♀
       Female pelvic infection or inflammation NOS

N74   *Female pelvic inflammatory disorders in diseases classified elsewhere*   ♀
     Code first underlying disease
     EXCLUDES 1   *chlamydial cervicitis (A56.02)*
         chlamydial pelvic inflammatory disease (A56.11)
         gonococcal cervicitis (A54.03)
         gonococcal pelvic inflammatory disease (A54.24)
         herpesviral [herpes simplex] cervicitis (A60.03)
         herpesviral [herpes simplex] pelvic inflammatory disease (A60.09)
         syphilitic cervicitis (A52.76)
         syphilitic pelvic inflammatory disease (A52.76)
         trichomonal cervicitis (A59.09)
         tuberculous cervicitis (A18.16)
         tuberculous pelvic inflammatory disease (A18.17)

☑4th **N75**   **Diseases of Bartholin's gland**

   N75.0   **Cyst of Bartholin's gland**   ♀

   N75.1   **Abscess of Bartholin's gland**   CC ♀
       CC Excl: A17.9, A18.10, A18.16-A18.18, A18.82, A18.84, A18.89, A59.00-A59.01, A59.8-A59.9, B37.3-B37.49, N75.0-N77.1, N84.3, N90.3, N90.6-N90.9, N94.810-N94.9, N96, Q55.0-Q55.21, Q55.23-Q55.4, Q55.7-Q55.9

   N75.8   **Other diseases of Bartholin's gland**   ♀
       Bartholinitis

   N75.9   **Disease of Bartholin's gland, unspecified**   ♀

☑4th **N76**   **Other inflammation of vagina and vulva**
     Use additional code (B95-B97), to identify infectious agent
     EXCLUDES 2   *senile (atrophic) vaginitis (N95.2)*
         vulvar vestibulitis (N94.810)

   N76.0   **Acute vaginitis**   ♀
       Acute vulvovaginitis
       Vaginitis NOS
       Vulvovaginitis NOS

   N76.1   **Subacute and chronic vaginitis**   ♀
       Chronic vulvovaginitis
       Subacute vulvovaginitis

   N76.2   **Acute vulvitis**   ♀
       Vulvitis NOS

   N76.3   **Subacute and chronic vulvitis**   ♀

   N76.4   **Abscess of vulva**   CC ♀
       Furuncle of vulva
       CC Excl: See code: N75.1

   N76.5   **Ulceration of vagina**   ♀

   N76.6   **Ulceration of vulva**   ♀

   ☑5th **N76.8**   **Other specified inflammation of vagina and vulva**
       N76.81   **Mucositis (ulcerative) of vagina and vulva**   CC ♀
           Code also type of associated therapy, such as:
           antineoplastic and immunosuppressive drugs (T45.1X-)
           radiological procedure and radiotherapy (Y84.2)
           EXCLUDES 2   *gastrointestinal mucositis (ulcerative) (K92.81)*
              nasal mucositis (ulcerative) (J34.81)
              oral mucositis (ulcerative) (K12.3-)
           CC Excl: N72, N75.9, N76.5, N76.81-N76.89
       N76.89   **Other specified inflammation of vagina and vulva**   ♀

☑4th **N77**   **Vulvovaginal ulceration and inflammation in diseases classified elsewhere**

   N77.0   *Ulceration of vulva in diseases classified elsewhere*   ♀
       Code first underlying disease, such as:
       Behçet's disease (M35.2)
       EXCLUDES 1   *ulceration of vulva in gonococcal infection (A54.02)*
         ulceration of vulva in herpesviral [herpes simplex] infection (A60.04)
         ulceration of vulva in syphilis (A51.0)
         ulceration of vulva in tuberculosis (A18.18)

N Newborn: 0   P Pediatric: 0-17   M Maternity: 12-55   A Adult: 15-124   MCC Major CC Condition   PDx MCC PDx acts as own MCC   CC CC Condition   PDx CC PDx acts as own CC

776   ICD-10-CM Draft (2015)

N77.1 *Vaginitis, vulvitis and vulvovaginitis in diseases classified elsewhere* ♀

Code first underlying disease, such as:
pinworm (B80)

EXCLUDES 1　candidal vulvovaginitis (B37.3)
chlamydial vulvovaginitis (A56.02)
gonococcal vulvovaginitis (A54.02)
herpesviral [herpes simplex] vulvovaginitis (A60.04)
trichomonal vulvovaginitis (A59.01)
tuberculous vulvovaginitis (A18.18)
vulvovaginitis in early syphilis (A51.0)
vulvovaginitis in late syphilis (A52.76)

Noninflammatory disorders of female genital tract (N80-N98)

✓4th N80　Endometriosis

N80.0 **Endometriosis of** uterus ♀
Adenomyosis
EXCLUDES 1　stromal endometriosis (D39.0)

N80.1 **Endometriosis of** ovary ♀

N80.2 **Endometriosis of** fallopian tube ♀

N80.3 **Endometriosis of** pelvic peritoneum ♀

N80.4 **Endometriosis of** rectovaginal septum and vagina ♀

N80.5 **Endometriosis of** intestine ♀

N80.6 **Endometriosis in** cutaneous scar ♀

N80.8 **Other** endometriosis ♀

N80.9 **Endometriosis,** unspecified ♀

✓4th N81　Female genital prolapse

EXCLUDES 1　genital prolapse complicating pregnancy, labor or delivery (O34.5-)
prolapse and hernia of ovary and fallopian tube (N83.4)
prolapse of vaginal vault after hysterectomy (N99.3)

N81.0 **Urethrocele** ♀
EXCLUDES 1　urethrocele with cystocele (N81.1-)
urethrocele with prolapse of uterus (N81.2-N81.4)

✓5th N81.1　Cystocele
Cystocele with urethrocele
Cystourethrocele
EXCLUDES 1　cystocele with prolapse of uterus (N81.2-N81.4)

N81.10 **Cystocele,** unspecified
Prolapse of (anterior) vaginal wall NOS

N81.11 **Cystocele,** midline

N81.12 **Cystocele,** lateral
Paravaginal cystocele

N81.2 **Incomplete** uterovaginal prolapse ♀
First degree uterine prolapse
Prolapse of cervix NOS
Second degree uterine prolapse
EXCLUDES 1　cervical stump prolaspe (N81.85)

N81.3 **Complete** uterovaginal prolapse ♀
Procidentia (uteri) NOS
Third degree uterine prolapse

N81.4 **Uterovaginal prolapse,** unspecified ♀
Prolapse of uterus NOS

N81.5 **Vaginal enterocele** ♀
EXCLUDES 1　enterocele with prolapse of uterus (N81.2-N81.4)

N81.6 **Rectocele** ♀
Prolapse of posterior vaginal wall
Use additional code for any associated fecal incontinence, if applicable (R15.-)
EXCLUDES 2　perineocele (N81.81)
rectal prolapse (K62.3)
rectocele with prolapse of uterus (N81.2-N81.4)

✓5th N81.8　Other female genital prolapse

N81.81 **Perineocele** ♀

N81.82 **Incompetence or weakening of** pubocervical ♀
tissue

N81.83 **Incompetence or weakening of** rectovaginal ♀
tissue

N81.84 **Pelvic muscle wasting** ♀
Disuse atrophy of pelvic muscles and anal sphincter

N81.85 **Cervical stump prolapse** ♀

N81.89 **Other female genital prolapse** ♀
Deficient perineum
Old laceration of muscles of pelvic floor

N81.9 **Female genital prolapse, unspecified** ♀

✓4th N82　Fistulae involving female genital tract
EXCLUDES 1　vesicointestinal fistulae (N32.1)

CC Excl: For CC codes in category N82, unless otherwise noted:
N82.0-N82.9

N82.0 **Vesicovaginal fistula** CC ♀

N82.1 **Other female** urinary-genital tract **fistulae** CC ♀
Cervicovesical fistula　　Uteroureteric fistula
Ureterovaginal fistula　　Uterovesical fistula
Urethrovaginal fistula

N82.2 **Fistula of vagina to** small **intestine** CC ♀

N82.3 **Fistula of vagina to** large **intestine** CC ♀
Rectovaginal fistula

N82.4 **Other female** intestinal-genital tract **fistulae** CC ♀
Intestinouterine fistula

N82.5 **Female** genital tract-skin **fistulae** CC ♀
Uterus to abdominal wall fistula
Vaginoperineal fistula

N82.8 **Other** female genital tract fistulae CC ♀

N82.9 **Female genital tract fistula,** unspecified CC ♀

✓4th N83　Noninflammatory disorders of ovary, fallopian tube and broad ligament
EXCLUDES 2　hydrosalpinx (N70.1-)

N83.0 **Follicular cyst of ovary** ♀
Cyst of graafian follicle
Hemorrhagic follicular cyst (of ovary)

N83.1 **Corpus luteum cyst** ♀
Hemorrhagic corpus luteum cyst

✓5th N83.2　Other and unspecified ovarian cysts
EXCLUDES 1　developmental ovarian cyst (Q50.1)
neoplastic ovarian cyst (D27.-)
polycystic ovarian syndrome (E28.2)
Stein-Leventhal syndrome (E28.2)

N83.20 **Unspecified ovarian cysts** ♀

N83.29 **Other ovarian cysts** ♀
Retention cyst of ovary
Simple cyst of ovary

✓5th N83.3　Acquired atrophy of ovary and fallopian tube

N83.31 **Acquired atrophy of** ovary ♀

N83.32 **Acquired atrophy of** fallopian tube ♀

N83.33 **Acquired atrophy of** ovary and fallopian tube ♀

N83.4 **Prolapse and hernia of ovary and fallopian tube** ♀

✓5th N83.5　Torsion of ovary, ovarian pedicle and fallopian tube
Torsion of accessory tube

CC Excl: For CC codes in subcategory N83.5, unless otherwise noted: N83.0-N83.9, N99.83

N83.51 **Torsion of** ovary and ovarian pedicle CC ♀

N83.52 **Torsion of** fallopian tube CC ♀
Torsion of hydatid of Morgagni

N83.53 **Torsion of** ovary, ovarian pedicle and fallopian CC ♀
tube

N83.6 **Hematosalpinx** ♀
EXCLUDES 1　hematosalpinx (with) (in):
hematocolpos (N89.7)
hematometra (N85.7)
tubal pregnancy (O00.1)

N83.7 **Hematoma of broad ligament** ♀

N83.8 **Other noninflammatory disorders of ovary,** ♀
tube and broad ligament
Broad ligament laceration syndrome [Allen-Masters]

N83.9 **Noninflammatory disorder of ovary, fallopian tube** ♀
and broad ligament, unspecified

✓4th N84　Polyp of female genital tract
EXCLUDES 1　adenomatous polyp (D28.-)
placental polyp (O90.89)

N84.0 **Polyp of** corpus uteri ♀
Polyp of endometrium
Polyp of uterus NOS
EXCLUDES 1　polypoid endometrial hyperplasia (N85.0-)

N84.1 **Polyp of** cervix uteri ♀
Mucous polyp of cervix

N84.2 **Polyp of** vagina ♀

N84.3 **Polyp of** vulva ♀
Polyp of labia

N84.8 **Polyp of** other parts **of female genital tract** ♀

N84.9 **Polyp of female genital tract,** unspecified ♀

✓ Additional Character Required　　✓x7th Xtension Alert　　Unacceptable PDx　　Manifestation　　Hospital Acquired Condition　　EXCLUDES 1 Not Coded Here　　EXCLUDES 2 Not Included Here

Diseases of the Genitourinary System

N85–N90.818

✓4ᵗʰ **N85 Other noninflammatory disorders of uterus, except cervix**

EXCLUDES 1   *endometriosis (N80.-)*
inflammatory diseases of uterus (N71.-)
noninflammatory disorders of cervix, except malposition (N86-N88)
polyp of corpus uteri (N84.0)
uterine prolapse (N81.-)

✓5ᵗʰ **N85.0 Endometrial hyperplasia**

N85.00 Endometrial hyperplasia, unspecified ♀
Hyperplasia (adenomatous) (cystic) (glandular) of endometrium
Hyperplastic endometritis

N85.01 Benign endometrial hyperplasia ♀
Endometrial hyperplasia (complex) (simple) without atypia

N85.02 Endometrial intraepithelial neoplasia [EIN] ♀
Endometrial hyperplasia with atypia
EXCLUDES 1   *malignant neoplasm of endometrium (with endometrial intraepithelial neoplasia [EIN]) (C54.1)*

N85.2 Hypertrophy of uterus ♀
Bulky or enlarged uterus
EXCLUDES 1   *puerperal hypertrophy of uterus (O90.89)*

N85.3 Subinvolution of uterus ♀
EXCLUDES 1   *puerperal subinvolution of uterus (O90.89)*

N85.4 Malposition of uterus ♀
Anteversion of uterus
Retroflexion of uterus
Retroversion of uterus
EXCLUDES 1   *malposition of uterus complicating pregnancy, labor or delivery (O34.5-, O65.5)*

N85.5 Inversion of uterus ♀
EXCLUDES 1   *current obstetric trauma (O71.2)*
postpartum inversion of uterus (O71.2)

N85.6 Intrauterine synechiae ♀

N85.7 Hematometra ♀
Hematosalpinx with hematometra
EXCLUDES 1   *hematometra with hematocolpos (N89.7)*

N85.8 Other specified noninflammatory disorders of uterus ♀
Atrophy of uterus, acquired
Fibrosis of uterus NOS

N85.9 Noninflammatory disorder of uterus, unspecified ♀
Disorder of uterus NOS

N86 Erosion and ectropion of cervix uteri ♀
Decubitus (trophic) ulcer of cervix
Eversion of cervix
EXCLUDES 1   *erosion and ectropion of cervix with cervicitis (N72)*

✓4ᵗʰ **N87 Dysplasia of cervix uteri**
EXCLUDES 1   *abnormal results from cervical cytologic examination without histologic confirmation (R87.61-)*
carcinoma in situ of cervix uteri (D06.-)
cervical intraepithelial neoplasia III [CIN III] (D06.-)
HGSIL of cervix (R87.613)
severe dysplasia of cervix uteri (D06.-)

N87.0 Mild cervical dysplasia ♀
Cervical intraepithelial neoplasia I [CIN I]

N87.1 Moderate cervical dysplasia ♀
Cervical intraepithelial neoplasia II [CIN II]

N87.9 Dysplasia of cervix uteri, unspecified ♀
Anaplasia of cervix
Cervical atypism
Cervical dysplasia NOS

✓4ᵗʰ **N88 Other noninflammatory disorders of cervix uteri**
EXCLUDES 2   *inflammatory disease of cervix (N72)*
polyp of cervix (N84.1)

N88.0 Leukoplakia of cervix uteri ♀

N88.1 Old laceration of cervix uteri ♀
Adhesions of cervix
EXCLUDES 1   *current obstetric trauma (O71.3)*

N88.2 Stricture and stenosis of cervix uteri ♀
EXCLUDES 1   *stricture and stenosis of cervix uteri complicating labor (O65.5)*

N88.3 Incompetence of cervix uteri ♀
Investigation and management of (suspected) cervical incompetence in a nonpregnant woman
EXCLUDES 1   *cervical incompetence complicating pregnancy (O34.3-)*

N88.4 Hypertrophic elongation of cervix uteri ♀

N88.8 Other specified noninflammatory disorders of cervix uteri ♀
EXCLUDES 1   *current obstetric trauma (O71.3)*

N88.9 Noninflammatory disorder of cervix uteri, unspecified ♀

✓4ᵗʰ **N89 Other noninflammatory disorders of vagina**
EXCLUDES 1   *abnormal results from vaginal cytologic examination without histologic confirmation (R87.62-)*
carcinoma in situ of vagina (D07.2)
HGSIL of vagina (R87.623)
inflammation of vagina (N76.-)
senile (atrophic) vaginitis (N95.2)
severe dysplasia of vagina (D07.2)
trichomonal leukorrhea (A59.00)
vaginal intraepithelial neoplasia [VAIN], grade III (D07.2)

N89.0 Mild vaginal dysplasia ♀
Vaginal intraepithelial neoplasia [VAIN], grade I

N89.1 Moderate vaginal dysplasia ♀
Vaginal intraepithelial neoplasia [VAIN], grade II

N89.3 Dysplasia of vagina, unspecified ♀

N89.4 Leukoplakia of vagina ♀

N89.5 Stricture and atresia of vagina ♀
Vaginal adhesions   Vaginal stenosis
EXCLUDES 1   *congenital atresia or stricture (Q52.4)*
postprocedural adhesions of vagina (N99.2)

N89.6 Tight hymenal ring ♀
Rigid hymen
Tight introitus
EXCLUDES 1   *imperforate hymen (Q52.3)*

N89.7 Hematocolpos ♀
Hematocolpos with hematometra or hematosalpinx

N89.8 Other specified noninflammatory disorders of vagina ♀
Leukorrhea NOS
Old vaginal laceration
Pessary ulcer of vagina
EXCLUDES 1   *current obstetric trauma (O70-, O71.4, O71.7-O71.8)*
old laceration involving muscles of pelvic floor (N81.8)

N89.9 Noninflammatory disorder of vagina, unspecified ♀

✓4ᵗʰ **N90 Other noninflammatory disorders of vulva and perineum**
EXCLUDES 1   *anogenital (venereal) warts (A63.0)*
carcinoma in situ of vulva (D07.1)
condyloma acuminatum (A63.0)
current obstetric trauma (O70-, O71.7-O71.8)
inflammation of vulva (N76.-)
severe dysplasia of vulva (D07.1)
vulvar intraepithelial neoplasm III [VIN III] (D07.1)

N90.0 Mild vulvar dysplasia ♀
Vulvar intraepithelial neoplasia [VIN], grade I

N90.1 Moderate vulvar dysplasia ♀
Vulvar intraepithelial neoplasia [VIN], grade II

N90.3 Dysplasia of vulva, unspecified ♀

N90.4 Leukoplakia of vulva ♀
Dystrophy of vulva   Lichen sclerosus of external female
Kraurosis of vulva   genital organs

N90.5 Atrophy of vulva ♀
Stenosis of vulva

N90.6 Hypertrophy of vulva ♀
Hypertrophy of labia

N90.7 Vulvar cyst ♀

✓5ᵗʰ **N90.8 Other specified noninflammatory disorders of vulva and perineum**

✓6ᵗʰ **N90.81 Female genital mutilation status**
Female genital cutting status

N90.810 Female genital mutilation status, unspecified ♀
Female genital cutting status, unspecified
Female genital mutilation status NOS

N90.811 Female genital mutilation Type I status ♀
Clitorectomy status
Female genital cutting Type I status

N90.812 Female genital mutilation Type II status ♀
Clitorectomy with excision of labia minora status
Female genital cutting Type II status

N90.813 Female genital mutilation Type III status ♀
Female genital cutting Type III status
Infibulation status

N90.818 Other female genital mutilation status ♀
Female genital cutting Type IV status
Female genital mutilation Type IV status
Other female genital cutting status

N̄ Newborn: 0   P̄ Pediatric: 0-17   M̄ Maternity: 12-55   Ā Adult: 15-124   MCC Major CC Condition   PDx MCC PDx acts as own MCC   CC CC Condition   PDx CC PDx acts as own CC

778   ICD-10-CM Draft (2015)

N90.89 **Other specified noninflammatory disorders of vulva and perineum** ♀
Adhesions of vulva
Hypertrophy of clitoris

N90.9 **Noninflammatory disorder of vulva and perineum, unspecified** ♀

✓4th **N91 Absent, scanty and rare menstruation**
EXCLUDES1 *ovarian dysfunction (E28.-)*

N91.0 **Primary amenorrhea** ♀

N91.1 **Secondary amenorrhea** ♀

N91.2 **Amenorrhea, unspecified** ♀

N91.3 **Primary oligomenorrhea** ♀

N91.4 **Secondary oligomenorrhea** ♀

N91.5 **Oligomenorrhea, unspecified** ♀
Hypomenorrhea NOS

✓4th **N92 Excessive, frequent and irregular menstruation**
EXCLUDES1 *postmenopausal bleeding (N95.0)*
precocious puberty (menstruation) (E30.1)

N92.0 **Excessive and frequent menstruation** with regular cycle ♀
Heavy periods NOS
Menorrhagia NOS
Polymenorrhea

N92.1 **Excessive and frequent menstruation** with irregular cycle ♀
Irregular intermenstrual bleeding
Irregular, shortened intervals between menstrual bleeding
Menometrorrhagia
Metrorrhagia

N92.2 **Excessive menstruation at puberty** P♀
Excessive bleeding associated with onset of menstrual periods
Pubertal menorrhagia
Puberty bleeding

N92.3 **Ovulation bleeding** ♀
Regular intermenstrual bleeding

N92.4 **Excessive bleeding in the premenopausal period** ♀
Climacteric menorrhagia or metrorrhagia
Menopausal menorrhagia or metrorrhagia
Preclimacteric menorrhagia or metrorrhagia
Premenopausal menorrhagia or metrorrhagia

N92.5 **Other specified irregular menstruation** ♀

N92.6 **Irregular menstruation, unspecified** ♀
Irregular bleeding NOS
Irregular periods NOS
EXCLUDES1 *irregular menstruation with:*
lengthened intervals or scanty bleeding (N91.3-N91.5)
shortened intervals or excessive bleeding (N92.1)

✓4th **N93 Other abnormal uterine and vaginal bleeding**
EXCLUDES1 *neonatal vaginal hemorrhage (P54.6)*
precocious puberty (menstruation) (E30.1)
pseudomenses (P54.6)

N93.0 **Postcoital and contact bleeding** ♀

N93.8 **Other specified abnormal uterine and vaginal bleeding** ♀
Dysfunctional or functional uterine or vaginal bleeding NOS

N93.9 **Abnormal uterine and vaginal bleeding, unspecified** ♀

✓4th **N94 Pain and other conditions associated with female genital organs and menstrual cycle**

N94.0 **Mittelschmerz** ♀

N94.1 **Dyspareunia** ♀
EXCLUDES1 *psychogenic dyspareunia (F52.6)*

N94.2 **Vaginismus** ♀
EXCLUDES1 *psychogenic vaginismus (F52.5)*

N94.3 **Premenstrual tension syndrome** ♀
Premenstrual dysphoric disorder
Code also associated menstrual migraine (G43.82-, G43.83-)

N94.4 **Primary dysmenorrhea** ♀

N94.5 **Secondary dysmenorrhea** ♀

N94.6 **Dysmenorrhea, unspecified** ♀
EXCLUDES1 *psychogenic dysmenorrhea (F45.8)*

✓5th N94.8 **Other specified conditions associated with female genital organs and menstrual cycle** ♀

✓6th N94.81 **Vulvodynia**

N94.810 **Vulvar vestibulitis** ♀

N94.818 **Other vulvodynia** ♀

N94.819 **Vulvodynia, unspecified** ♀
Vulvodynia NOS

N94.89 **Other specified conditions associated with female genital organs and menstrual cycle** ♀

N94.9 **Unspecified condition associated with female genital organs and menstrual cycle** ♀

✓4th **N95 Menopausal and other perimenopausal disorders**
Menopausal and other perimenopausal disorders due to naturally occurring (age-related) menopause and perimenopause
EXCLUDES1 *excessive bleeding in the premenopausal period (N92.4)*
menopausal and perimenopausal disorders due to artificial or premature menopause (E89.4-, E28.31-)
premature menopause (E28.31-)
EXCLUDES2 *postmenopausal osteoporosis (M81.0-)*
postmenopausal osteoporosis with current pathological fracture (M80.0-)
postmenopausal urethritis (N34.2)

N95.0 **Postmenopausal bleeding** ♀

N95.1 **Menopausal and female climacteric states** ♀
Symptoms such as flushing, sleeplessness, headache, lack of concentration, associated with natural (age-related) menopause
Use additional code for associated symptoms
EXCLUDES1 *asymptomatic menopausal state (Z78.0)*
symptoms associated with artificial menopause (E89.41)
symptoms associated with premature menopause (E28.310)

N95.2 **Postmenopausal atrophic vaginitis** ♀
Senile (atrophic) vaginitis

N95.8 **Other specified menopausal and perimenopausal disorders** ♀

N95.9 **Unspecified menopausal and perimenopausal disorder** ♀

N96 Recurrent pregnancy loss ♀
Investigation or care in a nonpregnant woman with history of recurrent pregnancy loss
EXCLUDES1 *recurrent pregnancy loss with current pregnancy (O26.2-)*

✓4th **N97 Female infertility**
INCLUDES inability to achieve a pregnancy
sterility, female NOS
EXCLUDES1 *female infertility associated with:*
hypopituitarism (E23.0)
Stein-Leventhal syndrome (E28.2)
EXCLUDES2 *incompetence of cervix uteri (N88.3)*

N97.0 **Female infertility** associated with anovulation ♀

N97.1 **Female infertility of** tubal origin ♀
Female infertility associated with congenital anomaly of tube
Female infertility due to tubal block
Female infertility due to tubal occlusion
Female infertility due to tubal stenosis

N97.2 **Female infertility of** uterine origin ♀
Female infertility associated with congenital anomaly of uterus
Female infertility due to nonimplantation of ovum

N97.8 **Female infertility of** other origin ♀

N97.9 **Female infertility,** unspecified ♀

✓4th **N98 Complications associated with artificial fertilization**

N98.0 **Infection associated with artificial insemination** cc♀
CC Excl: N98.0, T80.211A, T80.212A, T80.218A, T80.219A, T80.22XA, T80.29XA, T82.7XXA, T88.0XXA

N98.1 **Hyperstimulation of ovaries** cc♀
Hyperstimulation of ovaries NOS
Hyperstimulation of ovaries associated with induced ovulation
CC Excl: D78.81-D78.89, E36.8, E89.810-E89.89, H59.011-H59.019, H59.031-H59.099, H59.811-H59.89, H95.811-H95.89, I97.3, L76.81-L76.82, M96.89, N98.1-N98.9, T81.8[2,9]XA, T81.9XXA

N98.2 **Complications of attempted introduction of fertilized ovum following in vitro fertilization** cc♀
CC Excl: See code: N98.1

N98.3 **Complications of attempted introduction of embryo in embryo transfer** cc♀
CC Excl: See code: N98.1

N98.8 **Other complications associated with artificial fertilization** cc♀
CC Excl: See code: N98.1

N98.9 **Complication associated with artificial fertilization, unspecified** cc♀
CC Excl: See code: N98.1

✓ Additional Character Required   ✓x7th Xtension Alert   Unacceptable PDx   Manifestation   Hospital Acquired Condition   EXCLUDES1 Not Coded Here   EXCLUDES2 Not Included Here

ICD-10-CM Draft (2015)   779

Diseases of the Genitourinary System *(side margin)*

N99–N99.89 *(side margin)*

Intraoperative and postprocedural complications and disorders of genitourinary system, not elsewhere classified (N99)

✓4ᵗʰ **N99 Intraoperative and postprocedural complications and disorders of genitourinary system, not elsewhere classified**

     EXCLUDES 2   irradiation cystitis (N30.4-)
       postoophorectomy osteoporosis with current pathological fracture (M80.8-)
       postoophorectomy osteoporosis without current pathological fracture (M81.8)

N99.0 Postprocedural (acute) (chronic) kidney failure
     Use additional code for type of kidney disease

✓5ᵗʰ **N99.1 Postprocedural urethral stricture**
     Postcatheterization urethral stricture

   ✓6ᵗʰ **N99.11 Postprocedural urethral stricture, male**
     N99.110 Postprocedural urethral stricture, male, ♂ meatal
     N99.111 Postprocedural bulbous urethral stricture
     N99.112 Postprocedural membranous urethral stricture
     N99.113 Postprocedural anterior urethral stricture
     N99.114 Postprocedural urethral stricture, male, ♂ unspecified

   N99.12 Postprocedural urethral stricture, female ♀

N99.2 Postprocedural adhesions of vagina ♀
N99.3 Prolapse of vaginal vault after hysterectomy ♀
N99.4 Postprocedural pelvic peritoneal adhesions
     EXCLUDES 2   pelvic peritoneal adhesions NOS (N73.6)
       postinfective pelvic peritoneal adhesions (N73.6)

✓5ᵗʰ **N99.5 Complications of stoma of urinary tract**
     EXCLUDES 2   mechanical complication of urinary (indwelling) catheter (T83.0-)

   ✓6ᵗʰ **N99.51 Complication of cystostomy**
     N99.510 Cystostomy hemorrhage CC
     CC Excl: D78.81-D78.89, E36.8, E89.810-E89.89, H59.011-H59.019, H59.031-H59.099, H59.811-H59.89, H95.811-H95.89, I97.3, L76.81-L76.82, M96.89, N32.89, N33, N98.1-N98.9, N99.510-N99.518, T81.82A, T81.89X-T81.9XX with 7th A, T83.010A, T83.020A, T83.030A, T83.090A, T83.110-T83.29X with 7th A, T83.410-T83.718 with 7th A, T83.728-T83.9XX with 7th A, T85.310-T85.311 with 7th A, T85.320-T85.321 with 7th A, T85.390-T85.391 with 7th A, T85.510-T85.9XX with 7th A, T86.820-T86.829, T86.842-T86.849

     N99.511 Cystostomy infection CC
     CC Excl: D78.81-D78.89, E36.8, E89.810-E89.89, H59.011-H59.019, H59.031-H59.099, H59.811-H59.89, H95.811-H95.89, I97.3, L76.81-L76.82, M96.89, N32.89, N33, N39.0, N98.1-N98.9, N99.510-N99.518, T81.82A, T81.89X-T81.9XX with 7th A, T83.010A, T83.020A, T83.030A, T83.090A, T83.110-T83.29X with 7th A, T83.410-T83.718 with 7th A, T83.728-T83.9XX with 7th A, T85.310-T85.311 with 7th A, T85.320-T85.321 with 7th A, T85.390-T85.391 with 7th A, T85.510-T85.612 with 7th A, T85.614-T85.622 with 7th A, T85.624-T85.692 with 7th A, T85.694-T85.9XX with 7th A, T86.842-T86.849

     N99.512 Cystostomy malfunction CC
     CC Excl: D78.81-D78.89, E36.8, E89.810-E89.89, H59.011-H59.019, H59.031-H59.099, H59.811-H59.89, H95.811-H95.89, I97.3, L76.81-L76.82, M96.89, N32.89, N33, N98.1-N98.9, N99.510-N99.518, T81.82A, T81.89A, T81.9XXA, T83.010A, T83.020A, T83.030A, T83.090A, T83.110A, T83.111A, T83.112A, T83.118A, T83.120A, T83.121A, T83.122A, T83.128A, T83.190A, T83.191A, T83.192A, T83.198A, T83.21XA, T83.22XA, T83.23XA, T83.29XA, T83.410A, T83.418A, T83.420A, T83.428A, T83.490A, T83.498A, T83.51XA, T83.59XA, T83.6XXA, T83.718A, T83.728A, T83.81XA, T83.82XA, T83.83XA, T83.84XA, T83.85XA, T83.86XA, T83.89XA, T83.9XXA

     N99.518 Other cystostomy complication CC
     CC Excl: See code: N99.510

   ✓6ᵗʰ **N99.52 Complication of other external stoma of urinary tract**
     N99.520 Hemorrhage of other external stoma of urinary tract
     N99.521 Infection of other external stoma of urinary tract
     N99.522 Malfunction of other external stoma of urinary tract
     N99.528 Other complication of other external stoma of urinary tract

   ✓6ᵗʰ **N99.53 Complication of other stoma of urinary tract**
     N99.530 Hemorrhage of other stoma of urinary tract
     N99.531 Infection of other stoma of urinary tract
     N99.532 Malfunction of other stoma of urinary tract
     N99.538 Other complication of other stoma of urinary tract

✓5ᵗʰ **N99.6 Intraoperative hemorrhage and hematoma of a genitourinary system organ or structure complicating a procedure**
     EXCLUDES 1   intraoperative hemorrhage and hematoma of a genitourinary system organ or structure due to accidental puncture or laceration during a procedure (N99.7-)

   N99.61 Intraoperative hemorrhage and hematoma of a genitourinary system organ or structure complicating a genitourinary system procedure CC
     CC Excl: H95.811-H95.89, I85.01, I85.11, I97.3, K21.9, K22.8, K23-K25.0, K25.2, K25.4, K25.6, K26.0, K26.2, K26.4, K26.6, K27.0, K27.2, K27.4, K27.6, K28.0, K28.2, K28.4, K28.6, K29.01, K29.21, K29.31, K29.41, K29.51, K29.61, K29.71, K29.81, K29.91, K31.811, K55.21, K57.01, K57.11, K57.13, K57.21, K57.31, K57.33, K57.41, K57.51, K57.53, K57.81, K57.91, K57.93, K62.5, K92.0-K92.2, M96.89, N98.1-N98.9, N99.61-N99.62, N99.820-N99.821, P54.1-P54.3, T81.10XA, T81.11XA, T81.12XA, T81.19XA, T81.82XA, T81.89XA, T81.9XXA

   N99.62 Intraoperative hemorrhage and hematoma of a genitourinary system organ or structure complicating other procedure CC
     CC Excl: See code: N99.61

✓5ᵗʰ **N99.7 Accidental puncture and laceration of a genitourinary system organ or structure during a procedure**

   N99.71 Accidental puncture and laceration of a genitourinary system organ or structure during a genitourinary system procedure CC
     CC Excl: D78.11-D78.12, D78.81-D78.89, E36.11-E36.8, E89.810-E89.89, G96.11, G97.41, G97.48-G97.49, H59.011-H59.019, H59.031-H59.099, H59.211-H59.229, H59.811-H59.89, H95.31-H95.32, H95.811-H95.89, I97.3, I97.51-I97.52, J95.71-J95.72, K91.71-K91.72, L76.11-L76.12, L76.81-L76.82, M96.820-M96.821, M96.89, N98.1-N98.9, N99.71-N99.72, T81.8[2,9]XA, T81.9XXA

   N99.72 Accidental puncture and laceration of a genitourinary system organ or structure during other procedure CC
     CC Excl: See code: N99.71

✓5ᵗʰ **N99.8 Other intraoperative and postprocedural complications and disorders of genitourinary system**

   N99.81 Other intraoperative complications of genitourinary system

   ✓6ᵗʰ **N99.82 Postprocedural hemorrhage and hematoma of a genitourinary system organ or structure following a procedure**
     N99.820 Postprocedural hemorrhage and hematoma of a genitourinary system organ or structure following a genitourinary system procedure CC
     CC Excl: See code: N99.61
     N99.821 Postprocedural hemorrhage and hematoma of a genitourinary system organ or structure following other procedure CC
     CC Excl: See code: N99.61

   N99.83 Residual ovary syndrome ♀
   N99.89 Other postprocedural complications and disorders of genitourinary system

---

N Newborn: 0   P Pediatric: 0-17   M Maternity: 12-55   A Adult: 15-124   MCC Major CC Condition   PDx MCC PDx acts as own MCC   CC CC Condition   PDx CC PDx acts as own CC

Chapter 15. Pregnancy, Childbirth and the Puerperium (O00-O9A)

NOTE   CODES FROM THIS CHAPTER ARE FOR USE ONLY ON MATERNAL RECORDS, NEVER ON NEWBORN RECORDS.

Codes from this chapter are for use for conditions related to or aggravated by the pregnancy, childbirth, or by the puerperium (maternal causes or obstetric causes).

NOTE   Trimesters are counted from the first day of the last menstrual period. They are defined as follows:

1st trimester- less than 14 weeks 0 days
2nd trimester- 14 weeks 0 days to less than 28 weeks 0 days
3rd trimester- 28 weeks 0 days until delivery

Use additional code from category Z3A, Weeks of gestation, to identify the specific week of the pregnancy

EXCLUDES 1   supervision of normal pregnancy (Z34.-)
EXCLUDES 2   mental and behavioral disorders associated with the puerperium (F53)
dobstetrical tetanus (A34)
postpartum necrosis of pituitary gland (E23.0)
puerperal osteomalacia (M83.0)

This chapter contains the following blocks:

O00-O08	Pregnancy with abortive outcome
O09	Supervision of high risk pregnancy
O10-O16	Edema, proteinuria and hypertensive disorders in pregnancy, childbirth and the puerperium
O20-O29	Other maternal disorders predominantly related to pregnancy
O30-O48	Maternal care related to the fetus and amniotic cavity and possible delivery problems
O60-O77	Complications of labor and delivery
O80, O82	Encounter for delivery
O85-O92	Complications predominantly related to the puerperium
O94-O9A	Other obstetric conditions, not elsewhere classified

Pregnancy with abortive outcome (O00-O08)

EXCLUDES 1   continuing pregnancy in multiple gestation after abortion of one fetus or more (O31.1-, O31.3-)

✓4ᵗʰ **O00 Ectopic pregnancy**
INCLUDES   ruptured ectopic pregnancy
Use additional code from category O08 to identify any associated complication

CC Excl: For CC codes in category O00, unless otherwise noted: O00.0-O00.9

O00.0 Abdominal pregnancy   CC M♀
EXCLUDES 1   maternal care for viable fetus in abdominal pregnancy (O36.7-)

O00.1 Tubal pregnancy   CC M♀
Fallopian pregnancy
Rupture of (fallopian) tube due to pregnancy
Tubal abortion

O00.2 Ovarian pregnancy   CC M♀

O00.8 Other ectopic pregnancy   CC M♀
Cervical pregnancy
Cornual pregnancy
Intraligamentous pregnancy
Mural pregnancy

O00.9 Ectopic pregnancy, unspecified   CC M♀

✓4ᵗʰ **O01 Hydatidiform mole**
Use additional code from category O08 to identify any associated complication
EXCLUDES 1   chorioadenoma (destruens) (D39.2)
malignant hydatidiform mole (D39.2)

O01.0 Classical hydatidiform mole   M♀
Complete hydatidiform mole

O01.1 Incomplete and partial hydatidiform mole   M♀

O01.9 Hydatidiform mole, unspecified   M♀
Trophoblastic disease NOS
Vesicular mole NOS

✓4ᵗʰ **O02 Other abnormal products of conception**
Use additional code from category O08 to identify any associated complication
EXCLUDES 1   papyraceous fetus (O31.0-)

O02.0 Blighted ovum and nonhydatidiform mole   M♀
Carneous mole
Fleshy mole
Intrauterine mole NOS
Molar pregnancy NEC
Pathological ovum

O02.1 Missed abortion   M♀
Early fetal death, before completion of 20 weeks of gestation, with retention of dead fetus
EXCLUDES 1   failed induced abortion (O07.-)
fetal death (intrauterine) (late) (O36.4)
missed abortion with blighted ovum (O02.0)
missed abortion with hydatidiform mole (O01.-)
missed abortion with nonhydatidiform (O02.0)
missed abortion with other abnormal products of conception (O02.8-)
missed delivery (O36.4)
stillbirth (P95)

✓5ᵗʰ **O02.8 Other specified abnormal products of conception**
EXCLUDES 1   abnormal products of conception with blighted ovum (O02.0)
abnormal products of conception with hydatidiform mole (O01.-)
abnormal products of conception with nonhydatidiform mole (O02.0)

O02.81 Inappropriate change in quantitative human chorionic gonadotropin (hCG) in early pregnancy   M♀
Biochemical pregnancy
Chemical pregnancy
Inappropriate level of quantitative human chorionic gonadotropin (hCG) for gestational age in early pregnancy

O02.89 Other abnormal products of conception   M♀

O02.9 Abnormal product of conception, unspecified   M♀

✓4ᵗʰ **O03 Spontaneous abortion**
NOTE   Incomplete abortion includes retained products of conception following spontaneous abortion.
INCLUDES   miscarriage

CC Excl: For CC/MCC codes in category O03, unless otherwise noted: O03.0-O07.4, O20.0-O20.9, O25.10-O25.3, O26.10-O26.13, O26.30-O26.43, O26.63-O26.819, O26.841-O26.86, O26.891-O26.93, O29.011-O29.93, O35.7XX0-O35.7XX9, O44.00-O44.13, O45.8X1-O45.93, O75.4, O75.81, O75.89-O75.9, O80, O90.89, O99.111-O99.285, O99.330-O99.335, O99.350-O99.355, O99.511-O99.73, O99.820-O99.825, O99.840-O9A.53, Z33.2

O03.0 Genital tract and pelvic infection following incomplete spontaneous abortion   CC M♀
Endometritis following incomplete spontaneous abortion
Oophoritis following incomplete spontaneous abortion
Parametritis following incomplete spontaneous abortion
Pelvic peritonitis following incomplete spontaneous abortion
Salpingitis following incomplete spontaneous abortion
Salpingo-oophoritis following incomplete spontaneous abortion
EXCLUDES 1   sepsis following incomplete spontaneous abortion (O03.37)
urinary tract infection following incomplete spontaneous abortion (O03.38)

O03.1 Delayed or excessive hemorrhage following incomplete spontaneous abortion   M♀
Afibrinogenemia following incomplete spontaneous abortion
Defibrination syndrome following incomplete spontaneous abortion
Hemolysis following incomplete spontaneous abortion
Intravascular coagulation following incomplete spontaneous abortion

O03.2 Embolism following incomplete spontaneous abortion   MCC M♀
Air embolism following incomplete spontaneous abortion
Amniotic fluid embolism following incomplete spontaneous abortion
Blood-clot embolism following incomplete spontaneous abortion
Embolism NOS following incomplete spontaneous abortion
Fat embolism following incomplete spontaneous abortion
Pulmonary embolism following incomplete spontaneous abortion
Pyemic embolism following incomplete spontaneous abortion
Septic or septicopyemic embolism following incomplete spontaneous abortion
Soap embolism following incomplete spontaneous abortion

✓5ᵗʰ **O03.3 Other and unspecified complications following incomplete spontaneous abortion**

O03.30 Unspecified complication following incomplete spontaneous abortion   CC M♀

✓ Additional Character Required   ✓x7ᵗʰ Xtension Alert   Unacceptable PDx   Manifestation   Hospital Acquired Condition   EXCLUDES 1 Not Coded Here   EXCLUDES 2 Not Included Here

O03.31 Shock following incomplete spontaneous abortion MCC M♀
Circulatory collapse following incomplete spontaneous abortion
Shock (postprocedural) following incomplete spontaneous abortion
EXCLUDES 1 *shock due to infection following incomplete spontaneous abortion (O03.37)*

O03.32 Renal failure following incomplete spontaneous abortion MCC M♀
Kidney failure (acute) following incomplete spontaneous abortion
Oliguria following incomplete spontaneous abortion
Renal shutdown following incomplete spontaneous abortion
Renal tubular necrosis following incomplete spontaneous abortion
Uremia following incomplete spontaneous abortion

O03.33 Metabolic disorder following incomplete spontaneous abortion CC M♀

O03.34 Damage to pelvic organs following incompletespontaneous abortion CC M♀
Laceration, perforation, tear or chemical damage of bladder following incomplete spontaneous abortion
Laceration, perforation, tear or chemical damage of bowel following incomplete spontaneous abortion
Laceration, perforation, tear or chemical damage of broad ligament following incomplete spontaneous abortion
Laceration, perforation, tear or chemical damage of cervix following incomplete spontaneous abortion
Laceration, perforation, tear or chemical damage of periurethral tissue following incomplete spontaneous abortion
Laceration, perforation, tear or chemical damage of uterus following incomplete spontaneous abortion
Laceration, perforation, tear or chemical damage of vagina following incomplete spontaneous abortion

O03.35 Other venous complications following incomplete spontaneous abortion CC M♀

O03.36 Cardiac arrest following incomplete spontaneous abortion CC M♀

O03.37 Sepsis following incomplete spontaneous abortion CC M♀
Use additional code to identify infectious agent (B95-B97)
Use additional code to identify severe sepsis, if applicable (R65.2-)
EXCLUDES 1 *septic or septicopyemic embolism following incomplete spontaneous abortion (O03.2)*

O03.38 Urinary tract infection following incomplete spontaneous abortion CC M♀
Cystitis following incomplete spontaneous abortion

O03.39 Incomplete spontaneous abortion with other complications CC M♀

O03.4 Incomplete spontaneous abortion without complication M♀

O03.5 Genital tract and pelvic infection following complete or unspecified spontaneous abortion CC M♀
Endometritis following complete or unspecified spontaneous abortion
Oophoritis following complete or unspecified spontaneous abortion
Parametritis following complete or unspecified spontaneous abortion
Pelvic peritonitis following complete or unspecified spontaneous abortion
Salpingitis following complete or unspecified spontaneous abortion
Salpingo-oophoritis following complete or unspecified spontaneous abortion
EXCLUDES 1 *sepsis following complete or unspecified spontaneous abortion (O03.87)*
urinary tract infection following complete or unspecified spontaneous abortion (O03.88)

O03.6 Delayed or excessive hemorrhage following complete or unspecified spontaneous abortion M♀
Afibrinogenemia following complete or unspecified spontaneous abortion
Defibrination syndrome following complete or unspecified spontaneous abortion
Hemolysis following complete or unspecified spontaneous abortion
Intravascular coagulation following complete or unspecified spontaneous abortion

O03.7 Embolism following complete or unspecified spontaneous abortion CC M♀
Air embolism following complete or unspecified spontaneous abortion
Amniotic fluid embolism following complete or unspecified spontaneous abortion
Blood-clot embolism following complete or unspecified spontaneous abortion
Embolism NOS following complete or unspecified spontaneous abortion
Fat embolism following complete or unspecified spontaneous abortion
Pulmonary embolism following complete or unspecified spontaneous abortion
Pyemic embolism following complete or unspecified spontaneous abortion
Septic or septicopyemic embolism following complete or unspecified spontaneous abortion
Soap embolism following complete or unspecified spontaneous abortion

✓5ᵗʰ O03.8 Other and unspecified complications following complete or unspecified spontaneous abortion

O03.80 Unspecified complication following complete or unspecified spontaneous abortion CC M♀

O03.81 Shock following complete or unspecified spontaneous abortion MCC M♀
Circulatory collapse following complete or unspecified spontaneous abortion
Shock (postprocedural) following complete or unspecified spontaneous abortion
EXCLUDES 1 *shock due to infection following complete or unspecified spontaneous abortion (O03.87)*

O03.82 Renal failure following complete or unspecified spontaneous abortion MCC M♀
Kidney failure (acute) following complete or unspecified spontaneous abortion
Oliguria following complete or unspecified spontaneous abortion
Renal shutdown following complete or unspecified spontaneous abortion
Renal tubular necrosis following complete or unspecified spontaneous abortion
Uremia following complete or unspecified spontaneous abortion

O03.83 Metabolic disorder following complete or unspecified spontaneous abortion CC M♀

O03.84 Damage to pelvic organs following complete or unspecified spontaneous abortion CC M♀
Laceration, perforation, tear or chemical damage of bladder following complete or unspecified spontaneous abortion
Laceration, perforation, tear or chemical damage of bowel following complete or unspecified spontaneous abortion
Laceration, perforation, tear or chemical damage of broad ligament following complete or unspecified spontaneous abortion
Laceration, perforation, tear or chemical damage of cervix following complete or unspecified spontaneous abortion
Laceration, perforation, tear or chemical damage of periurethral tissue following complete or unspecified spontaneous abortion
Laceration, perforation, tear or chemical damage of uterus following complete or unspecified spontaneous abortion
Laceration, perforation, tear or chemical damage of vagina following complete or unspecified spontaneous abortion

O03.85 Other venous complications following complete or unspecified spontaneous abortion CC M♀

O03.86 Cardiac arrest following complete or unspecified spontaneous abortion CC M♀

O03.87   **Sepsis following complete or unspecified**   `CC` `M♀`
spontaneous abortion
> Use additional code to identify infectious agent (B95-B97)
> Use additional code to identify severe sepsis, if applicable (R65.2-)
> *EXCLUDES 1*   *septic or septicopyemic embolism following complete or unspecified spontaneous abortion (O03.7)*

O03.88   **Urinary tract infection following complete or**   `CC` `M♀`
unspecified spontaneous abortion
> Cystitis following complete or unspecified spontaneous abortion

O03.89   **Complete or unspecified spontaneous**   `CC` `M♀`
abortion with other complications

O03.9   **Complete or unspecified spontaneous abortion without**   `M♀`
complication
> Miscarriage NOS
> Spontaneous abortion NOS

`✓4th` **O04**   **Complications following (induced) termination of pregnancy**
> INCLUDES   complications following (induced) termination of pregnancy
> *EXCLUDES 1*   *encounter for elective termination of pregnancy, uncomplicated (Z33.2)*
> *failed attempted termination of pregnancy (O07.-)*

> **CC Excl: For CC/MCC codes in category O04, unless otherwise noted: See code: O03**

O04.5   **Genital tract and pelvic infection following (induced)**   `CC` `M♀`
termination of pregnancy
> Endometritis following (induced) termination of pregnancy
> Oophoritis following (induced) termination of pregnancy
> Parametritis following (induced) termination of pregnancy
> Pelvic peritonitis following (induced) termination of pregnancy
> Salpingitis following (induced) termination of pregnancy
> Salpingo-oophoritis following (induced) termination of pregnancy
> *EXCLUDES 1*   *sepsis following (induced) termination of pregnancy (O04.87)*
> *urinary tract infection following (induced) termination of pregnancy (O04.88)*

O04.6   **Delayed or excessive hemorrhage following (induced)**   `M♀`
termination of pregnancy
> Afibrinogenemia following (induced) termination of pregnancy
> Defibrination syndrome following (induced) termination of pregnancy
> Hemolysis following (induced) termination of pregnancy
> Intravascular coagulation following (induced) termination of pregnancy

O04.7   **Embolism following (induced) termination of**   `MCC` `M♀`
pregnancy
> Air embolism following (induced) termination of pregnancy
> Amniotic fluid embolism following (induced) termination of pregnancy
> Blood-clot embolism following (induced) termination of pregnancy
> Embolism NOS following (induced) termination of pregnancy
> Fat embolism following (induced) termination of pregnancy
> Pulmonary embolism following (induced) termination of pregnancy
> Pyemic embolism following (induced) termination of pregnancy
> Septic or septicopyemic embolism following (induced) termination of pregnancy
> Soap embolism following (induced) termination of pregnancy

`✓5th` **O04.8**   **(Induced) termination of pregnancy with other and unspecified complications**

O04.80   **(Induced) termination of pregnancy with**   `CC` `M♀`
unspecified complications

O04.81   **Shock following (induced) termination of**   `MCC` `M♀`
pregnancy
> Circulatory collapse following (induced) termination of pregnancy
> Shock (postprocedural) following (induced) termination of pregnancy
> *EXCLUDES 1*   *shock due to infection following (induced) termination of pregnancy (O04.87)*

O04.82   **Renal failure following (induced)**   `MCC` `M♀`
termination of pregnancy
> Kidney failure (acute) following (induced) termination of pregnancy
> Oliguria following (induced) termination of pregnancy
> Renal shutdown following (induced) termination of pregnancy
> Renal tubular necrosis following (induced) termination of pregnancy
> Uremia following (induced) termination of pregnancy

O04.83   **Metabolic disorder following (induced)**   `CC` `M♀`
termination of pregnancy

O04.84   **Damage to pelvic organs following (induced)**   `CC` `M♀`
termination of pregnancy
> Laceration, perforation, tear or chemical damage of bladder following (induced) termination of pregnancy
> Laceration, perforation, tear or chemical damage of bowel following (induced) termination of pregnancy
> Laceration, perforation, tear or chemical damage of broad ligament following (induced) termination of pregnancy
> Laceration, perforation, tear or chemical damage of cervix following (induced) termination of pregnancy
> Laceration, perforation, tear or chemical damage of periurethral tissue following (induced) termination of pregnancy
> Laceration, perforation, tear or chemical damage of uterus following (induced) termination of pregnancy
> Laceration, perforation, tear or chemical damage of vagina following (induced) termination of pregnancy

O04.85   **Other venous complications following**   `CC` `M♀`
(induced) termination of pregnancy

O04.86   **Cardiac arrest following (induced)**   `CC` `M♀`
**termination
of pregnancy**

O04.87   **Sepsis following (induced) termination of**   `CC` `M♀`
pregnancy
> Use additional code to identify infectious agent (B95-B97)
> Use additional code to identify severe sepsis, if applicable (R65.2-)
> *EXCLUDES 1*   *septic or septicopyemic embolism following (induced) termination of pregnancy (O04.7)*
> **CC Excl:** O03.0-O07.4, O20.0-O20.9, O25.10-O25.3, O26.10-O26.13, O26.30-O26.43, O26.63-O26.819, O26.841-O26.86, O26.891-O26.93, O29.011-O29.93, O35.7X-O35.7X, O44.00-O44.13, O45.8X1-O45.93, O75.4, O75.81, O75.89-O75.9, O80, O90.89, O99.111-O99.285, O99.330-O99.335, O99.350-O99.355, O99.511-O99.73, O99.820-O99.825, O99.840-O9A.53, Z33.2

O04.88   **Urinary tract infection following (induced)**   `CC` `M♀`
termination of pregnancy
> Cystitis following (induced) termination of pregnancy
> **CC Excl:** O03.0-O07.4, O20.0-O20.9, O25.10-O25.3, O26.10-O26.13, O26.30-O26.43, O26.63-O26.819, O26.841-O26.86, O26.891-O26.93, O29.011-O29.93, O35.7X-O35.7X, O44.00-O44.13, O45.8X1-O45.93, O75.4, O75.81, O75.89-O75.9, O80, O90.89, O99.111-O99.285, O99.330-O99.335, O99.350-O99.355, O99.511-O99.73, O99.820-O99.825, O99.840-O9A.53, Z33.2

O04.89   **(Induced) termination of pregnancy with**   `CC` `M♀`
other complications
> **CC Excl:** See code O04.88

✓ Additional Character Required   `✓x7th` Xtension Alert   Unacceptable PDx   Manifestation   Hospital Acquired Condition   *EXCLUDES 1* Not Coded Here   *EXCLUDES 2* Not Included Here

ICD-10-CM Draft (2015)   783

✓4ᵗʰ **O07**   **Failed attempted termination of pregnancy**
> INCLUDES   failure of attempted induction of termination of pregnancy
> incomplete elective abortion
> EXCLUDES 1   *incomplete spontaneous abortion (O03.0-)*

O07.0   **Genital tract and pelvic infection following failed**   CC M ♀
attempted termination of pregnancy
> Endometritis following failed attempted termination of pregnancy
> Oophoritis following failed attempted termination of pregnancy
> Parametritis following failed attempted termination of pregnancy
> Pelvic peritonitis following failed attempted termination of pregnancy
> Salpingitis following failed attempted termination of pregnancy
> Salpingo-oophoritis following failed attempted termination of pregnancy
> EXCLUDES 1   *sepsis following failed attempted termination of pregnancy (O07.37)*
> *urinary tract infection following failed attempted termination of pregnancy (O07.38)*
>
> **CC Excl:** O03.0-O04.89, O07.1, O07.30, O07.35-O07.36, O07.38-O07.4, O20.0-O20.9, O25.10-O25.3, O26.10-O26.13, O26.30-O26.43, O26.63-O26.819, O26.841-O26.86, O26.891-O26.93, O29.011-O29.93, O35.7XX0-O35.7XX9, O44.00-O44.13, O45.8X1-O45.93, O75.4, O75.81, O75.89-O75.9, O80, O90.89, O99.111-O99.285, O99.330-O99.335, O99.350-O99.355, O99.511-O99.73, O99.820-O99.825, O99.840-O9A.53, Z33.2

O07.1   **Delayed or excessive hemorrhage following failed**   CC M ♀
attempted termination of pregnancy
> Afibrinogenemia following failed attempted termination of pregnancy
> Defibrination syndrome following failed attempted termination of pregnancy
> Hemolysis following failed attempted termination of pregnancy
> Intravascular coagulation following failed attempted termination of pregnancy
>
> **CC Excl:** O03.0-O04.89, O07.1, O07.30, O07.35-O07.36, O07.38-O07.4, O20.0-O20.9, O25.10-O25.3, O26.10-O26.13, O26.30-O26.43, O26.63-O26.819, O26.841-O26.86, O26.891-O26.93, O29.011-O29.93, O35.7XX0-O35.7XX9, O44.00-O44.13, O45.8X1-O45.93, O75.4, O75.81, O75.89-O75.9, O80, O90.89, O99.111-O99.285, O99.330-O99.335, O99.350-O99.355, O99.511-O99.73, O99.820-O99.825, O99.840-O9A.53, Z33.2

O07.2   **Embolism following failed attempted termination of**   MCC M ♀
pregnancy
> Air embolism following failed attempted termination of pregnancy
> Amniotic fluid embolism following failed attempted termination of pregnancy
> Blood-clot embolism following failed attempted termination of pregnancy
> Embolism NOS following failed attempted termination of pregnancy
> Fat embolism following failed attempted termination of pregnancy
> Pulmonary embolism following failed attempted termination of pregnancy
> Pyemic embolism following failed attempted termination of pregnancy
> Septic or septicopyemic embolism following failed attempted termination of pregnancy
> Soap embolism following failed attempted termination of pregnancy
>
> **CC Excl:** O03.0-O04.89, O07.2-O07.30, O07.35-O07.36, O07.38-O07.4, O20.0-O20.9, O25.10-O25.3, O26.10-O26.13, O26.30-O26.43, O26.63-O26.819, O26.841-O26.86, O26.891-O26.93, O29.011-O29.93, O35.7XX0-O35.7XX9, O44.00-O44.13, O45.8X1-O45.93, O75.4, O75.81, O75.89-O75.9, O80, O90.89, O99.111-O99.285, O99.330-O99.335, O99.350-O99.355, O99.511-O99.73, O99.820-O99.825, O99.840-O9A.53, Z33.2

✓5ᵗʰ **O07.3**   **Failed attempted termination of pregnancy with other and unspecified complications**

     O07.30   **Failed attempted termination of pregnancy**   CC M ♀
with unspecified complications
> **CC Excl:** O03.0-O07.4, O20.0-O20.9, O25.10-O25.3, O26.10-O26.13, O26.30-O26.43, O26.63-O26.819, O26.841-O26.86, O26.891-O26.93, O29.011-O29.93, O35.7X-O35.7X, O44.00-O44.13, O45.8X1-O45.93, O75.4, O75.81, O75.89-O75.9, O80, O90.89, O99.111-O99.285, O99.330-O99.335, O99.350-O99.355, O99.511-O99.73, O99.820-O99.825, O99.840-O9A.53, Z33.2

O07.31   **Shock following failed attempted**   MCC M ♀
termination of pregnancy
> Circulatory collapse following failed attempted termination of pregnancy
> Shock (postprocedural) following failed attempted termination of pregnancy
> EXCLUDES 1   *shock due to infection following failed attempted termination of pregnancy (O07.37)*
>
> **CC Excl:** O03.0-O04.89, O07.30-O07.31, O07.33, O07.35-O07.36, O07.38-O07.4, O20.0-O20.9, O25.10-O25.3, O26.10-O26.13, O26.30-O26.43, O26.63-O26.819, O26.841-O26.86, O26.891-O26.93, O29.011-O29.93, O35.7XX0-O35.7XX9, O44.00-O44.13, O45.8X1-O45.93, O75.4, O75.81, O75.89-O75.9, O80, O90.89, O99.111-O99.285, O99.330-O99.335, O99.350-O99.355, O99.511-O99.73, O99.820-O99.825, O99.840-O9A.53, Z33.2

O07.32   **Renal failure following failed attempted**   MCC M ♀
termination of pregnancy
> Kidney failure (acute) following failed attempted termination of pregnancy
> Oliguria following failed attempted termination of pregnancy
> Renal shutdown following failed attempted termination of pregnancy
> Renal tubular necrosis following failed attempted termination of pregnancy
> Uremia following failed attempted termination of pregnancy
>
> **CC Excl:** O03.0-O04.89, O07.30, O07.32, O07.35-O07.36, O07.38-O07.4, O20.0-O20.9, O25.10-O25.3, O26.10-O26.13, O26.30-O26.43, O26.63-O26.819, O26.841-O26.86, O26.891-O26.93, O29.011-O29.93, O35.7XX0-O35.7XX9, O44.00-O44.13, O45.8X1-O45.93, O75.4, O75.81, O75.89-O75.9, O80, O90.89, O99.111-O99.285, O99.330-O99.335, O99.350-O99.355, O99.511-O99.73, O99.820-O99.825, O99.840-O9A.53, Z33.2

O07.33   **Metabolic disorder following failed**   CC M ♀
attempted termination of pregnancy
> **CC Excl:** See code: O07.30

O07.34   **Damage to pelvic organs following failed**   CC M ♀
attempted termination of pregnancy
> Laceration, perforation, tear or chemical damage of bladder following failed attempted termination of pregnancy
> Laceration, perforation, tear or chemical damage of bowel following failed attempted termination of pregnancy
> Laceration, perforation, tear or chemical damage of broad ligament following failed attempted termination of pregnancy
> Laceration, perforation, tear or chemical damage of cervix following failed attempted termination of pregnancy
> Laceration, perforation, tear or chemical damage of periurethral tissue following failed attempted termination of pregnancy
> Laceration, perforation, tear or chemical damage of uterus following failed attempted termination of pregnancy
> Laceration, perforation, tear or chemical damage of vagina following failed attempted termination of pregnancy
>
> **CC Excl:** O03.0-O04.89, O07.30, O07.34-O07.36, O07.38-O07.4, O20.0-O20.9, O25.10-O25.3, O26.10-O26.13, O26.30-O26.43, O26.63-O26.819, O26.841-O26.86, O26.891-O26.93, O29.011-O29.93, O35.7XX0-O35.7XX9, O44.00-O44.13, O45.8X1-O45.93, O75.4, O75.81, O75.89-O75.9, O80, O90.89, O99.111-O99.285, O99.330-O99.335, O99.350-O99.355, O99.511-O99.73, O99.820-O99.825, O99.840-O9A.53, Z33.2

O07.35   **Other venous complications following failed**   CC M ♀
attempted termination of pregnancy
> **CC Excl:** See code: O07.30

O07.36   **Cardiac arrest following failed attempted**   CC M ♀
termination of pregnancy
> **CC Excl:** See code: O07.30

N Newborn: 0   P Pediatric: 0-17   M Maternity: 12-55   A Adult: 15-124   MCC Major CC Condition   PDx MCC PDx acts as own MCC   CC CC Condition   PDx CC PDx acts as own CC

784   ICD-10-CM Draft (2015)

O07.37 **Sepsis following failed attempted termination of pregnancy** `cc` `M` ♀

Use additional code to identify infectious agent (B95-B97)

Use additional code to identify severe sepsis, if applicable (R65.2-)

EXCLUDES 1 *septic or septicopyemic embolism following failed attempted termination of pregnancy (O07.2)*

CC Excl: O03.0-O07.0, O07.30, O07.35-O07.4, O20.0-O20.9, O25.10-O25.3, O26.10-O26.13, O26.30-O26.43, O26.63-O26.819, O26.841-O26.86, O26.891-O26.93, O29.011-O29.93, O35.7X-O35.7X, O44.00-O44.13, O45.8X1-O45.93, O75.4, O75.81, O75.89-O75.9, O80, O90.89, O99.111-O99.285, O99.330-O99.335, O99.350-O99.355, O99.511-O99.73, O99.820-O99.825, O99.840-O9A.53, Z33.2

O07.38 **Urinary tract infection following failed attempted termination of pregnancy** `cc` `M` ♀

Cystitis following failed attempted termination of pregnancy

CC Excl: See code: O07.30

O07.39 **Failed attempted termination of pregnancy with other complications** `cc` `M` ♀

CC Excl: See code: O07.30

O07.4 **Failed attempted termination of pregnancy without complication** `M` ♀

`✓4ᵗʰ` **O08** **Complications following ectopic and molar pregnancy**

This category is for use with categories O00-O02 to identify any associated complications

CC Excl: For CC/MCC codes in category O08, unless otherwise noted: O08.2-O08.81, O08.83-O08.9, O20.0-O20.9, O25.10-O25.3, O26.10-O26.13, O26.30-O26.43, O26.63-O26.819, O26.841-O26.86, O26.891-O26.93, O29.011-O29.93, O35.7XX0-O35.7XX9, O44.00-O44.13, O45.8X1-O45.93, O75.4, O75.81, O75.89-O75.9, O80, O90.89, O99.111-O99.285, O99.330-O99.335, O99.350-O99.355, O99.511-O99.73, O99.820-O99.825, O99.840-O9A.53

O08.0 **Genital tract and pelvic infection following ectopic and molar pregnancy** `cc` `M` ♀

Endometritis following ectopic and molar pregnancy
Oophoritis following ectopic and molar pregnancy
Parametritis following ectopic and molar pregnancy
Pelvic peritonitis following ectopic and molar pregnancy
Salpingitis following ectopic and molar pregnancy
Salpingo-oophoritis following ectopic and molar pregnancy

EXCLUDES 1 *sepsis following ectopic and molar pregnancy (O08.82)*
urinary tract infection (O08.83)

CC Excl: A34, O08.0, O08.2-O08.9, O20.0-O20.9, O25.10-O25.3, O26.10-O26.13, O26.30-O26.43, O26.63-O26.819, O26.841-O26.86, O26.891-O26.93, O29.011-O29.93, O35.7XX0-O35.7XX9, O44.00-O44.13, O45.8X1-O45.93, O75.4, O75.81, O75.89-O75.9, O80, O90.89, O99.111-O99.285, O99.330-O99.335, O99.350-O99.355, O99.511-O99.73, O99.820-O99.825, O99.840-O9A.53

O08.1 **Delayed or excessive hemorrhage following ectopic and molar pregnancy** `cc` `M` ♀

Afibrinogenemia following ectopic and molar pregnancy
Defibrination syndrome following ectopic and molar pregnancy
Hemolysis following ectopic and molar pregnancy
Intravascular coagulation following ectopic and molar pregnancy

EXCLUDES 1 *delayed or excessive hemorrhage due to incomplete abortion (O03.1)*

CC Excl: O08.1-O08.81, O08.83-O08.9, O20.0-O20.9, O25.10-O25.3, O26.10-O26.13, O26.30-O26.43, O26.63-O26.819, O26.841-O26.86, O26.891-O26.93, O29.011-O29.93, O35.7XX0-O35.7XX9, O44.00-O44.13, O45.8X1-O45.93, O75.4, O75.81, O75.89-O75.9, O80, O90.89, O99.111-O99.285, O99.330-O99.335, O99.350-O99.355, O99.511-O99.73, O99.820-O99.825, O99.840-O9A.53

O08.2 **Embolism following ectopic and molar pregnancy** `mcc` `M` ♀

Air embolism following ectopic and molar pregnancy
Amniotic fluid embolism following ectopic and molar pregnancy
Blood-clot embolism following ectopic and molar pregnancy
Embolism NOS following ectopic and molar pregnancy
Fat embolism following ectopic and molar pregnancy
Pulmonary embolism following ectopic and molar pregnancy
Pyemic embolism following ectopic and molar pregnancy
Septic or septicopyemic embolism following ectopic and molar pregnancy
Soap embolism following ectopic and molar pregnancy

O08.3 **Shock following ectopic and molar pregnancy** `mcc` `M` ♀

Circulatory collapse following ectopic and molar pregnancy
Shock (postprocedural) following ectopic and molar pregnancy

EXCLUDES 1 *shock due to infection following ectopic and molar pregnancy (O08.82)*

O08.4 **Renal failure following ectopic and molar pregnancy** `mcc` `M` ♀

Kidney failure (acute) following ectopic and molar pregnancy
Oliguria following ectopic and molar pregnancy
Renal shutdown following ectopic and molar pregnancy
Renal tubular necrosis following ectopic and molar pregnancy
Uremia following ectopic and molar pregnancy

O08.5 **Metabolic disorders following an ectopic and molar pregnancy** `cc` `M` ♀

O08.6 **Damage to pelvic organs and tissues following an ectopic and molar pregnancy** `cc` `M` ♀

Laceration, perforation, tear or chemical damage of bladder following an ectopic and molar pregnancy
Laceration, perforation, tear or chemical damage of bowel following an ectopic and molar pregnancy
Laceration, perforation, tear or chemical damage of broad ligament following an ectopic and molar pregnancy
Laceration, perforation, tear or chemical damage of cervix following an ectopic and molar pregnancy
Laceration, perforation, tear or chemical damage of periurethral tissue following an ectopic and molar pregnancy
Laceration, perforation, tear or chemical damage of uterus following an ectopic and molar pregnancy
Laceration, perforation, tear or chemical damage of vagina following an ectopic and molar pregnancy

O08.7 **Other venous complications following an ectopic and molar pregnancy** `cc` `M` ♀

`✓5ᵗʰ` **O08.8** **Other complications following an ectopic and molar pregnancy**

O08.81 **Cardiac arrest following an ectopic and molar pregnancy** `cc` `M` ♀

O08.82 **Sepsis following ectopic and molar pregnancy** `cc` `M` ♀

Use additional code to identify infectious agent (B95-B97)

Use additional code to identify severe sepsis, if applicable (R65.2-)

EXCLUDES 1 *septic or septicopyemic embolism following ectopic and molar pregnancy (O08.2)*

CC Excl: See code: O08.0

O08.83 **Urinary tract infection following an ectopic and molar pregnancy** `cc` `M` ♀

Cystitis following an ectopic and molar pregnancy

CC Excl: O08.2-O08.81, O08.83-O08.9, O20.0-O20.9, O25.10-O25.3, O26.10-O26.13, O26.30-O26.43, O26.63-O26.819, O26.841-O26.86, O26.891-O26.93, O29.011-O29.93, O35.7XX0-O35.7XX9, O44.00-O44.13, O45.8X1-O45.93, O75.4, O75.81, O75.89-O75.9, O80, O90.89, O99.111-O99.285, O99.330-O99.335, O99.350-O99.355, O99.511-O99.73, O99.820-O99.825, O99.840-O9A.53

O08.89 **Other complications following an ectopic and molar pregnancy** `cc` `M` ♀

CC Excl: See code: O08.83

O08.9 **Unspecified complication following an ectopic and molar pregnancy** `cc` `M` ♀

CC Excl: See code: O08.83

Supervision of high risk pregnancy (O09)

`✓4ᵗʰ` **O09** **Supervision of high risk pregnancy**

`✓5ᵗʰ` **O09.0** **Supervision of pregnancy with history of infertility**

O09.00 **Supervision of pregnancy with history of infertility, unspecified trimester** `M` ♀

O09.01 **Supervision of pregnancy with history of infertility, first trimester** `M` ♀

O09.02 **Supervision of pregnancy with history of infertility, second trimester** `M` ♀

O09.03 **Supervision of pregnancy with history of infertility, third trimester** `M` ♀

`✓5ᵗʰ` **O09.1** **Supervision of pregnancy with history of ectopic or molar pregnancy**

O09.10 **Supervision of pregnancy with history of ectopic or molar pregnancy, unspecified trimester** `M` ♀

O09.11 **Supervision of pregnancy with history of ectopic or molar pregnancy, first trimester** `M` ♀

O09.12 **Supervision of pregnancy with history of ectopic or molar pregnancy, second trimester** `M` ♀

O09.13 **Supervision of pregnancy with history of ectopic or molar pregnancy, third trimester** `M` ♀

`✓` Additional Character Required `✓x7ᵗʰ` Xtension Alert Unacceptable PDx Manifestation Hospital Acquired Condition *EXCLUDES 1* Not Coded Here *EXCLUDES 2* Not Included Here

✓5th **O09.2 Supervision of pregnancy with** other poor reproductive or obstetric history
  EXCLUDES 2 *pregnancy care for patient with history of recurrent pregnancy loss (O26.2-)*

✓6th **O09.21 Supervision of pregnancy with history of** pre-term labor
  O09.211 **Supervision of pregnancy with history of pre-term labor, first trimester** Ⓜ♀
  O09.212 **Supervision of pregnancy with history of pre-term labor, second trimester** Ⓜ♀
  O09.213 **Supervision of pregnancy with history of pre-term labor, third trimester** Ⓜ♀
  O09.219 **Supervision of pregnancy with history of pre-term labor, unspecified trimester** Ⓜ♀

✓6th **O09.29 Supervision of pregnancy with** other poor reproductive or obstetric history
  Supervision of pregnancy with history of neonatal death
  Supervision of pregnancy with history of stillbirth
  O09.291 **Supervision of pregnancy with other poor reproductive or obstetric history, first trimester** Ⓜ♀
  O09.292 **Supervision of pregnancy with other poor reproductive or obstetric history, second trimester** Ⓜ♀
  O09.293 **Supervision of pregnancy with other poor reproductive or obstetric history, third trimester** Ⓜ♀
  O09.299 **Supervision of pregnancy with other poor reproductive or obstetric history, unspecified trimester** Ⓜ♀

✓5th **O09.3 Supervision of pregnancy with** insufficient antenatal care
  Supervision of concealed pregnancy
  Supervision of hidden pregnancy
  O09.30 **Supervision of pregnancy with insufficient antenatal care, unspecified trimester** Ⓜ♀
  O09.31 **Supervision of pregnancy with insufficient antenatal care, first trimester** Ⓜ♀
  O09.32 **Supervision of pregnancy with insufficient antenatal care, second trimester** Ⓜ♀
  O09.33 **Supervision of pregnancy with insufficient antenatal care, third trimester** Ⓜ♀

✓5th **O09.4 Supervision of pregnancy with** grand multiparity
  O09.40 **Supervision of pregnancy with grand multiparity, unspecified trimester** Ⓜ♀
  O09.41 **Supervision of pregnancy with grand multiparity, first trimester** Ⓜ♀
  O09.42 **Supervision of pregnancy with grand multiparity, second trimester** Ⓜ♀
  O09.43 **Supervision of pregnancy with grand multiparity, third trimester** Ⓜ♀

✓5th **O09.5 Supervision of** elderly primigravida and multigravida
  Pregnancy for a female 35 years and older at expected date of delivery
  ✓6th **O09.51 Supervision of** elderly primigravida
    O09.511 **Supervision of elderly primigravida, first trimester** Ⓜ♀
    O09.512 **Supervision of elderly primigravida, second trimester** Ⓜ♀
    O09.513 **Supervision of elderly primigravida, third trimester** Ⓜ♀
    O09.519 **Supervision of elderly primigravida, unspecified trimester** Ⓜ♀
  ✓6th **O09.52 Supervision of** elderly multigravida
    O09.521 **Supervision of elderly multigravida, first trimester** Ⓜ♀
    O09.522 **Supervision of elderly multigravida, second trimester** Ⓜ♀
    O09.523 **Supervision of elderly multigravida, third trimester** Ⓜ♀
    O09.529 **Supervision of elderly multigravida, unspecified trimester** Ⓜ♀

✓5th **O09.6 Supervision of** young primigravida and multigravida
  Supervision of pregnancy for a female less than 16 years old at expected date of delivery
  ✓6th **O09.61 Supervision of young** primigravida
    O09.611 **Supervision of young primigravida, first trimester** Ⓜ♀
    O09.612 **Supervision of young primigravida, second trimester** Ⓜ♀
    O09.613 **Supervision of young primigravida, third trimester** Ⓜ♀
    O09.619 **Supervision of young primigravida, unspecified trimester** Ⓜ♀
  ✓6th **O09.62 Supervision of young** multigravida
    O09.621 **Supervision of young multigravida, first trimester** Ⓜ♀
    O09.622 **Supervision of young multigravida, second trimester** Ⓜ♀
    O09.623 **Supervision of young multigravida, third trimester** Ⓜ♀
    O09.629 **Supervision of young multigravida, unspecified trimester** Ⓜ♀

✓5th **O09.7 Supervision of high risk pregnancy due to** social problems
  O09.70 **Supervision of high risk pregnancy due to social problems, unspecified trimester** Ⓜ♀
  O09.71 **Supervision of high risk pregnancy due to social problems, first trimester** Ⓜ♀
  O09.72 **Supervision of high risk pregnancy due to social problems, second trimester** Ⓜ♀
  O09.73 **Supervision of high risk pregnancy due to social problems, third trimester** Ⓜ♀

✓5th **O09.8 Supervision of** other high risk pregnancies
  ✓6th **O09.81 Supervision of pregnancy** resulting from assisted reproductive technology
    Supervision of pregnancy resulting from in-vitro fertilization
    O09.811 **Supervision of pregnancy resulting from assisted reproductive technology, first trimester** Ⓜ♀
    O09.812 **Supervision of pregnancy resulting from assisted reproductive technology, second trimester** Ⓜ♀
    O09.813 **Supervision of pregnancy resulting from assisted reproductive technology, third trimester** Ⓜ♀
    O09.819 **Supervision of pregnancy resulting from assisted reproductive technology, unspecified trimester** Ⓜ♀
  ✓6th **O09.82 Supervision of pregnancy with** history of in utero procedure during previous pregnancy
    O09.821 **Supervision of pregnancy with history of in utero procedure during previous pregnancy, first trimester** Ⓜ♀
    O09.822 **Supervision of pregnancy with history of in utero procedure during previous pregnancy, second trimester** Ⓜ♀
    O09.823 **Supervision of pregnancy with history of in utero procedure during previous pregnancy, third trimester** Ⓜ♀
    O09.829 **Supervision of pregnancy with history of in utero procedure during previous pregnancy, unspecified trimester** Ⓜ♀
      EXCLUDES 1 *supervision of pregnancy affected by in utero procedure during current pregnancy (O35.7)*
  ✓6th **O09.89 Supervision of** other high risk pregnancies
    O09.891 **Supervision of other high risk pregnancies, first trimester** Ⓜ♀
    O09.892 **Supervision of other high risk pregnancies, second trimester** Ⓜ♀
    O09.893 **Supervision of other high risk pregnancies, third trimester** Ⓜ♀
    O09.899 **Supervision of other high risk pregnancies, unspecified trimester** Ⓜ♀

✓5th **O09.9 Supervision of high risk pregnancy,** unspecified
  O09.90 **Supervision of high risk pregnancy, unspecified, unspecified trimester** Ⓜ♀
  O09.91 **Supervision of high risk pregnancy, unspecified, first trimester** Ⓜ♀
  O09.92 **Supervision of high risk pregnancy, unspecified, second trimester** Ⓜ♀
  O09.93 **Supervision of high risk pregnancy, unspecified, third trimester** Ⓜ♀

Ⓝ Newborn: 0   Ⓟ Pediatric: 0-17   Ⓜ Maternity: 12-55   Ⓐ Adult: 15-124   MCC Major CC Condition   PDx MCC PDx acts as own MCC   CC CC Condition   PDx CC PDx acts as own CC

786   ICD-10-CM Draft (2015)

Edema, proteinuria and hypertensive disorders in pregnancy, childbirth and the puerperium (O10–O16)

✓4th O10 Pre-existing hypertension complicating pregnancy, childbirth and the puerperium

Pre-existing hypertension with pre-existing proteinuria complicating pregnancy, childbirth and the puerperium

EXCLUDES 2   pre-existing hypertension with superimposed pre-eclampsia complicating pregnancy, childbirth and the puerperium (O11.-)

CC Excl: For CC/MCC codes in category O10, unless otherwise noted: O10.011-O12.03, O12.20-O16.9, O25.10-O26.13, O26.30-O26.43, O26.63-O26.819, O26.841-O26.86, O26.891-O26.93, O29.011-O29.93, O35.7XX0-O35.7XX9, O75.4, O75.81, O75.89-O75.9, O80, O90.89, O99.111-O99.285, O99.330-O99.335, O99.350-O99.355, O99.511-O99.73, O99.820-O99.825, O99.840-O9A.53

✓5th O10.0 Pre-existing essential hypertension complicating pregnancy, childbirth and the puerperium

Any condition in I10 specified as a reason for obstetric care during pregnancy, childbirth or the puerperium

✓6th O10.01 Pre-existing essential hypertension complicating pregnancy

O10.011   Pre-existing essential hypertension complicating pregnancy, **first** trimester   CC M♀

O10.012   Pre-existing essential hypertension complicating pregnancy, **second** trimester   CC M♀

O10.013   Pre-existing essential hypertension complicating pregnancy, **third** trimester   CC M♀

O10.019   Pre-existing essential hypertension complicating pregnancy, **unspecified** trimester   M♀

O10.02   Pre-existing essential hypertension complicating **childbirth**   CC M♀

O10.03   Pre-existing essential hypertension complicating the **puerperium**   M♀

✓5th O10.1 Pre-existing hypertensive heart disease complicating pregnancy, childbirth and the puerperium

Any condition in I11 specified as a reason for obstetric care during pregnancy, childbirth or the puerperium

Use additional code from I11 to identify the type of hypertensive heart disease

✓6th O10.11 Pre-existing hypertensive heart disease complicating pregnancy

O10.111   Pre-existing hypertensive heart disease complicating pregnancy, **first trimester**   M♀

O10.112   Pre-existing hypertensive heart disease complicating pregnancy, **second trimester**   M♀

O10.113   Pre-existing hypertensive heart disease complicating pregnancy, **third trimester**   M♀

O10.119   Pre-existing hypertensive heart disease complicating pregnancy, **unspecified trimester**   M♀

O10.12   Pre-existing hypertensive heart disease complicating **childbirth**   M♀

O10.13   Pre-existing hypertensive heart disease complicating the **puerperium**   M♀

✓5th O10.2 Pre-existing hypertensive chronic kidney disease complicating pregnancy, childbirth and the puerperium

Any condition in I12 specified as a reason for obstetric care during pregnancy, childbirth or the puerperium

Use additional code from I12 to identify the type of hypertensive chronic kidney disease

✓6th O10.21 Pre-existing hypertensive chronic kidney disease complicating pregnancy

O10.211   Pre-existing hypertensive chronic kidney disease complicating pregnancy, **first trimester**   M♀

O10.212   Pre-existing hypertensive chronic kidney disease complicating pregnancy, **second trimester**   M♀

O10.213   Pre-existing hypertensive chronic kidney disease complicating pregnancy, **third trimester**   M♀

O10.219   Pre-existing hypertensive chronic kidney disease complicating pregnancy, **unspecified trimester**   M♀

O10.22   Pre-existing hypertensive chronic kidney disease complicating **childbirth**   M♀

O10.23   Pre-existing hypertensive chronic kidney disease complicating the **puerperium**   M♀

✓5th O10.3 Pre-existing hypertensive heart and chronic kidney disease complicating pregnancy, childbirth and the puerperium

Any condition in I13 specified as a reason for obstetric care during pregnancy, childbirth or the puerperium

Use additional code from I13 to identify the type of hypertensive heart and chronic kidney disease

✓6th O10.31 Pre-existing hypertensive heart and chronic kidney disease complicating pregnancy

O10.311   Pre-existing hypertensive heart and chronic kidney disease complicating pregnancy, **first trimester**   M♀

O10.312   Pre-existing hypertensive heart and chronic kidney disease complicating pregnancy, **second trimester**   M♀

O10.313   Pre-existing hypertensive heart and chronic kidney disease complicating pregnancy, **third trimester**   M♀

O10.319   Pre-existing hypertensive heart and chronic kidney disease complicating pregnancy, **unspecified trimester**   M♀

O10.32   Pre-existing hypertensive heart and chronic kidney disease complicating **childbirth**   M♀

O10.33   Pre-existing hypertensive heart and chronic kidney disease complicating the **puerperium**   M♀

✓5th O10.4 Pre-existing secondary hypertension complicating pregnancy, childbirth and the puerperium

Any condition in I15 specified as a reason for obstetric care during pregnancy, childbirth or the puerperium

Use additional code from I15 to identify the type of secondary hypertension

✓6th O10.41 Pre-existing secondary hypertension complicating pregnancy

O10.411   Pre-existing secondary hypertension complicating pregnancy, **first trimester**   CC M♀

O10.412   Pre-existing secondary hypertension complicating pregnancy, **second trimester**   CC M♀

O10.413   Pre-existing secondary hypertension complicating pregnancy, **third trimester**   CC M♀

O10.419   Pre-existing secondary hypertension complicating pregnancy, **unspecified trimester**   M♀

O10.42   Pre-existing secondary hypertension complicating **childbirth**   MCC M♀

O10.43   Pre-existing secondary hypertension complicating the **puerperium**   CC M♀

✓5th O10.9 Unspecified pre-existing hypertension complicating pregnancy, childbirth and the puerperium

✓6th O10.91 Unspecified pre-existing hypertension complicating pregnancy

O10.911   Unspecified pre-existing hypertension complicating pregnancy, **first trimester**   CC M♀

O10.912   Unspecified pre-existing hypertension complicating pregnancy, **second trimester**   CC M♀

O10.913   Unspecified pre-existing hypertension complicating pregnancy, **third trimester**   CC M♀

O10.919   Unspecified pre-existing hypertension complicating pregnancy, **unspecified trimester**   M♀

O10.92   Unspecified pre-existing hypertension complicating **childbirth**   CC M♀

O10.93   Unspecified pre-existing hypertension complicating the **puerperium**   M♀

✓ Additional Character Required   ✗X7th Xtension Alert   Unacceptable PDx   Manifestation   Hospital Acquired Condition   *EXCLUDES 1* Not Coded Here   *EXCLUDES 2* Not Included Here

ICD-10-CM Draft (2015)   787

Pregnancy, Childbirth and the Puerperium

O11–O21.9

✓4th **O11 Pre-existing hypertension with pre-eclampsia**
Conditions in O10 complicated by pre-eclampsia
Pre-eclampsia superimposed pre-existing hypertension
Use additional code from O10 to identify the type of hypertension

CC Excl: For MCC codes in category O11, unless otherwise noted:
See code: O10

O11.1 Pre-existing hypertension with pre-eclampsia, first trimester MCC M♀

O11.2 Pre-existing hypertension with pre-eclampsia, second trimester MCC M♀

O11.3 Pre-existing hypertension with pre-eclampsia, third trimester MCC M♀

O11.9 Pre-existing hypertension with pre-eclampsia, unspecified trimester M♀

✓4th **O12 Gestational [pregnancy-induced] edema and proteinuria without hypertension**

CC Excl: For CC codes in category O12, unless otherwise noted:
O12.11–O12.13, O12.21–O12.23, O26.831–O26.833, O90.89

✓5th **O12.0 Gestational edema**
- **O12.00 Gestational edema, unspecified trimester** M♀
- **O12.01 Gestational edema, first trimester** M♀
- **O12.02 Gestational edema, second trimester** M♀
- **O12.03 Gestational edema, third trimester** M♀

✓5th **O12.1 Gestational proteinuria**
- **O12.10 Gestational proteinuria, unspecified trimester** M♀
- **O12.11 Gestational proteinuria, first trimester** CC M♀
- **O12.12 Gestational proteinuria, second trimester** CC M♀
- **O12.13 Gestational proteinuria, third trimester** CC M♀

✓5th **O12.2 Gestational edema with proteinuria**
- **O12.20 Gestational edema with proteinuria, unspecified trimester** M♀
- **O12.21 Gestational edema with proteinuria, first trimester** PDx CC CC M♀
- **O12.22 Gestational edema with proteinuria, second trimester** PDx CC CC M♀
- **O12.23 Gestational edema with proteinuria, third trimester** PDx CC CC M♀

✓4th **O13 Gestational [pregnancy-induced] hypertension without significant proteinuria**
INCLUDES gestational hypertension NOS

CC Excl: For CC codes in category O13, unless otherwise noted:
See code: O10

O13.1 Gestational [pregnancy-induced] hypertension without significant proteinuria, first trimester M♀

O13.2 Gestational [pregnancy-induced] hypertension without significant proteinuria, second trimester M♀

O13.3 Gestational [pregnancy-induced] hypertension without significant proteinuria, third trimester M♀

O13.9 Gestational [pregnancy-induced] hypertension without significant proteinuria, unspecified trimester ♀

✓4th **O14 Pre-eclampsia**
EXCLUDES 1 pre-existing hypertension with pre-eclampsia (O11)

CC Excl: For CC codes in category O14, unless otherwise noted:
See code: O10

✓5th **O14.0 Mild to moderate pre-eclampsia**
- **O14.00 Mild to moderate pre-eclampsia, unspecified trimester** M♀
- **O14.02 Mild to moderate pre-eclampsia, second trimester** CC M♀
- **O14.03 Mild to moderate pre-eclampsia, third trimester** CC M♀

✓5th **O14.1 Severe pre-eclampsia**
EXCLUDES 1 HELLP syndrome (O14.2-)
- **O14.10 Severe pre-eclampsia, unspecified trimester** M♀
- **O14.12 Severe pre-eclampsia, second trimester** MCC ♀
- **O14.13 Severe pre-eclampsia, third trimester** MCC ♀

✓5th **O14.2 HELLP syndrome**
Severe pre-eclampsia with hemolysis, elevated liver enzymes and low platelet count (HELLP)
- **O14.20 HELLP syndrome (HELLP), unspecified trimester** M♀
- **O14.22 HELLP syndrome (HELLP), second trimester** MCC M♀
- **O14.23 HELLP syndrome (HELLP), third trimester** MCC M♀

✓5th **O14.9 Unspecified pre-eclampsia**
- **O14.90 Unspecified pre-eclampsia, unspecified trimester** M♀
- **O14.92 Unspecified pre-eclampsia, second trimester** CC M♀
- **O14.93 Unspecified pre-eclampsia, third trimester** CC M♀

✓4th **O15 Eclampsia**
INCLUDES convulsions following conditions in O10-O14 and O16

CC Excl: For MCC codes in category O15, unless otherwise noted:
See code: O10

✓5th **O15.0 Eclampsia in pregnancy**
- **O15.00 Eclampsia in pregnancy, unspecified trimester** M♀
- **O15.02 Eclampsia in pregnancy, second trimester** MCC M♀
- **O15.03 Eclampsia in pregnancy, third trimester** MCC M♀

O15.1 Eclampsia in labor MCC M♀

O15.2 Eclampsia in the puerperium MCC M♀

O15.9 Eclampsia, unspecified as to time period M♀
Eclampsia NOS

✓4th **O16 Unspecified maternal hypertension**

CC Excl: For CC codes in category O16, unless otherwise noted:
See code: O10

O16.1 Unspecified maternal hypertension, first trimester CC M♀

O16.2 Unspecified maternal hypertension, second trimester CC M♀

O16.3 Unspecified maternal hypertension, third trimester CC M♀

O16.9 Unspecified maternal hypertension, unspecified trimester M♀

Other maternal disorders predominantly related to pregnancy (O20-O29)

EXCLUDES 2 maternal care related to the fetus and amniotic cavity and possible delivery problems (O30-O48)
maternal diseases classifiable elsewhere but complicating pregnancy, labor and delivery, and the puerperium (O98-O99)

✓4th **O20 Hemorrhage in early pregnancy**
Hemorrhage before completion of 20 weeks gestation
EXCLUDES 1 pregnancy with abortive outcome (O00-O08)

O20.0 Threatened abortion CC M♀
Hemorrhage specified as due to threatened abortion
CC Excl: O20.0-O20.9, O25.10-O25.3, O26.10-O26.13, O26.30-O26.43, O26.63-O26.819, O26.841-O26.86, O26.891-O26.93, O29.011-O29.93, O35.7XX0-O35.7XX9, O44.00-O44.13, O75.4, O75.81, O75.89-O75.9, O80, O90.89, O99.111-O99.285, O99.330-O99.335, O99.350-O99.355, O99.511-O99.73, O99.820-O99.825, O99.840-O9A.53

O20.8 Other hemorrhage in early pregnancy M♀

O20.9 Hemorrhage in early pregnancy, unspecified CC M♀
CC Excl: See code: O20.0

✓4th **O21 Excessive vomiting in pregnancy**

O21.0 Mild hyperemesis gravidarum M♀
Hyperemesis gravidarum, mild or unspecified, starting before the end of the 20th week of gestation

O21.1 Hyperemesis gravidarum with metabolic disturbance M♀
Hyperemesis gravidarum, starting before the end of the 20th week of gestation, with metabolic disturbance such as carbohydrate depletion
Hyperemesis gravidarum, starting before the end of the 20th week of gestation, with metabolic disturbance such as dehydration
Hyperemesis gravidarum, starting before the end of the 20th week of gestation, with metabolic disturbance such as electrolyte imbalance

O21.2 Late vomiting of pregnancy M♀
Excessive vomiting starting after 20 completed weeks of gestation

O21.8 Other vomiting complicating pregnancy M♀
Vomiting due to diseases classified elsewhere, complicating pregnancy
Use additional code to identify cause

O21.9 Vomiting of pregnancy, unspecified M♀

N Newborn: 0   P Pediatric: 0-17   M Maternity: 12-55   A Adult: 15-124   MCC Major CC Condition   PDx MCC PDx acts as own MCC   CC CC Condition   PDx CC PDx acts as own CC

788   ICD-10-CM Draft (2015)

✓4ᵗʰ **O22 Venous complications and hemorrhoids in pregnancy**

> **EXCLUDES 1** venous complications of:
> abortion NOS (O03.9)
> ectopic or molar pregnancy (O08.7)
> failed attempted abortion (O07.35)
> induced abortion (O04.85)
> spontaneous abortion (O03.89)
>
> **EXCLUDES 2** obstetric pulmonary embolism (O88.-)
> venous complications and hemorrhoids of childbirth and the
> puerperium (O87.-)

> **CC Excl: For CC/MCC codes in category O22, unless otherwise noted:** O22.20–O22.93, O25.10–O25.3, O26.10–O26.13, O26.30–O26.43, O26.63–O26.819, O26.841–O26.86, O26.891–O26.93, O29.011–O29.93, O35.7XX0–O35.7XX9, O75.4, O75.81, O75.89–O75.9, O80, O87.0–O87.3, O87.8–O87.9, O90.89, O99.111–O99.285, O99.330–O99.335, O99.350–O99.355, O99.511–O99.73, O99.820–O99.825, O99.840–O9A.53

✓5ᵗʰ **O22.0 Varicose veins of lower extremity in pregnancy**
Varicose veins NOS in pregnancy

    O22.00 Varicose veins of lower extremity in pregnancy, unspecified trimester MQ

    O22.01 Varicose veins of lower extremity in pregnancy, first trimester MQ

    O22.02 Varicose veins of lower extremity in pregnancy, second trimester MQ

    O22.03 Varicose veins of lower extremity in pregnancy, third trimester MQ

✓5ᵗʰ **O22.1 Genital varices in pregnancy**
Perineal varices in pregnancy
Vaginal varices in pregnancy
Vulval varices in pregnancy

    O22.10 Genital varices in pregnancy, unspecified trimester MQ

    O22.11 Genital varices in pregnancy, first trimester MQ

    O22.12 Genital varices in pregnancy, second trimester MQ

    O22.13 Genital varices in pregnancy, third trimester MQ

✓5ᵗʰ **O22.2 Superficial thrombophlebitis in pregnancy**
Phlebitis in pregnancy NOS
Thrombophlebitis of legs in pregnancy
Thrombosis in pregnancy NOS
Use additional code to identify the superficial thrombophlebitis (I80.0-)

    O22.20 Superficial thrombophlebitis in pregnancy, unspecified trimester CC MQ

    O22.21 Superficial thrombophlebitis in pregnancy, first trimester CC MQ

    O22.22 Superficial thrombophlebitis in pregnancy, second trimester CC MQ

    O22.23 Superficial thrombophlebitis in pregnancy, third trimester CC MQ

✓5ᵗʰ **O22.3 Deep phlebothrombosis in pregnancy**
Deep vein thrombosis, antepartum
Use additional code to identify the deep vein thrombosis (I82.4-, I82.5-, I82.62-, I82.72-)
Use additional code, if applicable, for associated long-term (current) use of anticoagulants (Z79.01)

    O22.30 Deep phlebothrombosis in pregnancy, unspecified trimester CC MQ

    O22.31 Deep phlebothrombosis in pregnancy, first trimester MCC MQ

    O22.32 Deep phlebothrombosis in pregnancy, second trimester MCC MQ

    O22.33 Deep phlebothrombosis in pregnancy, third trimester MCC MQ

✓5ᵗʰ **O22.4 Hemorrhoids in pregnancy**

    O22.40 Hemorrhoids in pregnancy, unspecified trimester CC MQ

    O22.41 Hemorrhoids in pregnancy, first trimester CC MQ

    O22.42 Hemorrhoids in pregnancy, second trimester CC MQ

    O22.43 Hemorrhoids in pregnancy, third trimester CC MQ

✓5ᵗʰ **O22.5 Cerebral venous thrombosis in pregnancy**
Cerebrovenous sinus thrombosis in pregnancy

    O22.50 Cerebral venous thrombosis in pregnancy, unspecified trimester CC MQ

    O22.51 Cerebral venous thrombosis in pregnancy, first trimester CC MQ

    O22.52 Cerebral venous thrombosis in pregnancy, second trimester CC MQ

    O22.53 Cerebral venous thrombosis in pregnancy, third trimester CC MQ

✓5ᵗʰ **O22.8 Other venous complications in pregnancy**

    ✓6ᵗʰ **O22.8X Other venous complications in pregnancy**

       O22.8X1 Other venous complications in pregnancy, first trimester CC MQ

       O22.8X2 Other venous complications in pregnancy, second trimester CC MQ

       O22.8X3 Other venous complications in pregnancy, third trimester CC MQ

       O22.8X9 Other venous complications in pregnancy, unspecified trimester CC MQ

✓5ᵗʰ **O22.9 Venous complication in pregnancy, unspecified**
Gestational phlebitis NOS
Gestational phlebopathy NOS
Gestational thrombosis NOS

    O22.90 Venous complication in pregnancy, unspecified, unspecified trimester CC MQ

    O22.91 Venous complication in pregnancy, unspecified, first trimester MQ

    O22.92 Venous complication in pregnancy, unspecified, second trimester MQ

    O22.93 Venous complication in pregnancy, unspecified, third trimester MQ

✓4ᵗʰ **O23 Infections of genitourinary tract in pregnancy**
Use additional code to identify organism (B95.-, B96.-)

> **EXCLUDES 2** gonococcal infections complicating pregnancy, childbirth and the puerperium (O98.2)
> infections with a predominantly sexual mode of transmission NOS complicating pregnancy, childbirth and the puerperium (O98.3)
> syphilis complicating pregnancy, childbirth and the puerperium (O98.1)
> tuberculosis of genitourinary system complicating pregnancy, childbirth and the puerperium (O98.0)
> venereal disease NOS complicating pregnancy, childbirth and the puerperium (O98.3)

> **CC Excl: For CC codes in category O23, unless otherwise noted:** O23.00–O23.93, O25.10–O25.3, O26.10–O26.13, O26.30–O26.43, O26.63–O26.819, O26.841–O26.86, O26.891–O26.93, O29.011–O29.93, O35.7XX0–O35.7XX9, O75.4, O75.81, O75.89–O75.9, O80, O86.11, O86.13–O86.29, O90.89, O99.111–O99.285, O99.330–O99.335, O99.350–O99.355, O99.511–O99.73, O99.820–O99.825, O99.840–O9A.53

✓5ᵗʰ **O23.0 Infections of kidney in pregnancy**
Pyelonephritis in pregnancy

    O23.00 Infections of kidney in pregnancy, unspecified trimester MQ

    O23.01 Infections of kidney in pregnancy, first trimester CC MQ

    O23.02 Infections of kidney in pregnancy, second trimester CC MQ

    O23.03 Infections of kidney in pregnancy, third trimester CC MQ

✓5ᵗʰ **O23.1 Infections of bladder in pregnancy**

    O23.10 Infections of bladder in pregnancy, unspecified trimester MQ

    O23.11 Infections of bladder in pregnancy, first trimester CC MQ

    O23.12 Infections of bladder in pregnancy, second trimester CC MQ

    O23.13 Infections of bladder in pregnancy, third trimester CC MQ

✓5ᵗʰ **O23.2 Infections of urethra in pregnancy**

    O23.20 Infections of urethra in pregnancy, unspecified trimester MQ

    O23.21 Infections of urethra in pregnancy, first trimester CC MQ

    O23.22 Infections of urethra in pregnancy, second trimester CC MQ

    O23.23 Infections of urethra in pregnancy, third trimester CC MQ

✓5ᵗʰ **O23.3 Infections of other parts of urinary tract in pregnancy**

    O23.30 Infections of other parts of urinary tract in pregnancy, unspecified trimester MQ

    O23.31 Infections of other parts of urinary tract in pregnancy, first trimester CC MQ

✓ Additional Character Required   ✓x7ᵗʰ Xtension Alert   Unacceptable PDx   Manifestation   Hospital Acquired Condition   EXCLUDES 1 Not Coded Here   EXCLUDES 2 Not Included Here

ICD-10-CM Draft (2015)   789

Pregnancy, Childbirth and the Puerperium

O23.32–O24.8

O23.32   Infections of other parts of urinary tract in pregnancy, **second trimester**   CC M ♀

O23.33   Infections of other parts of urinary tract in pregnancy, **third trimester**   CC M ♀

✓5th **O23.4**   **Unspecified** infection of urinary tract in pregnancy

O23.40   Unspecified infection of urinary tract in pregnancy, **unspecified trimester**   M ♀

O23.41   Unspecified infection of urinary tract in pregnancy, **first trimester**   CC M ♀

O23.42   Unspecified infection of urinary tract in pregnancy, **second trimester**   CC M ♀

O23.43   Unspecified infection of urinary tract in pregnancy, **third trimester**   CC M ♀

✓5th **O23.5**   Infections of the **genital tract** in pregnancy

✓6th **O23.51**   Infection of **cervix** in pregnancy

O23.511   Infections of cervix in pregnancy, **first trimester**   CC M ♀

O23.512   Infections of cervix in pregnancy, **second trimester**   CC M ♀

O23.513   Infections of cervix in pregnancy, **third trimester**   CC M ♀

O23.519   Infections of cervix in pregnancy, **unspecified trimester**   M ♀

✓6th **O23.52**   **Salpingo-oophoritis** in pregnancy
Oophoritis in pregnancy
Salpingitis in pregnancy

O23.521   Salpingo-oophoritis in pregnancy, **first trimester**   CC M ♀

O23.522   Salpingo-oophoritis in pregnancy, **second trimester**   CC M ♀

O23.523   Salpingo-oophoritis in pregnancy, **third trimester**   CC M ♀

O23.529   Salpingo-oophoritis in pregnancy, **unspecified trimester**   M ♀

✓6th **O23.59**   Infection of **other part** of genital tract in pregnancy

O23.591   Infection of other part of genital tract in pregnancy, **first trimester**   CC M ♀

O23.592   Infection of other part of genital tract in pregnancy, **second trimester**   CC M ♀

O23.593   Infection of other part of genital tract in pregnancy, **third trimester**   CC M ♀

O23.599   Infection of other part of genital tract in pregnancy, **unspecified trimester**   M ♀

✓5th **O23.9**   **Unspecified** genitourinary tract infection in pregnancy
Genitourinary tract infection in pregnancy NOS

O23.90   Unspecified genitourinary tract infection in pregnancy, **unspecified trimester**   M ♀

O23.91   Unspecified genitourinary tract infection in pregnancy, **first trimester**   CC M ♀

O23.92   Unspecified genitourinary tract infection in pregnancy, **second trimester**   CC M ♀

O23.93   Unspecified genitourinary tract infection in pregnancy, **third trimester**   CC M ♀

✓4th **O24**   **Diabetes mellitus** in pregnancy, childbirth, and the puerperium

> **CC Excl:** For CC/MCC codes in category O24, unless otherwise noted: O24.011-O24.33, O24.811-O25.3, O26.10-O26.13, O26.30-O26.43, O26.63-O26.819, O26.841-O26.86, O26.891-O26.93, O29.011-O29.93, O35.7XX0-O35.7XX9, O75.4, O75.81, O75.89-O75.9, O80, O90.89, O99.111-O99.285, O99.330-O99.335, O99.350-O99.355, O99.511-O99.73, O99.820-O99.825, O99.840-O9A.53

✓5th **O24.0**   **Pre-existing** diabetes mellitus, type 1, in pregnancy, childbirth and the puerperium
Juvenile onset diabetes mellitus, in pregnancy, childbirth and the puerperium
Ketosis-prone diabetes mellitus in pregnancy, childbirth and the puerperium
Use additional code from category E10 to further identify any manifestations

✓6th **O24.01**   Pre-existing diabetes mellitus, type 1, in **pregnancy**

O24.011   Pre-existing diabetes mellitus, type 1, in pregnancy, **first trimester**   CC M ♀

O24.012   Pre-existing diabetes mellitus, type 1, in pregnancy, **second trimester**   CC M ♀

O24.013   Pre-existing diabetes mellitus, type 1, in pregnancy, **third trimester**   CC M ♀

O24.019   Pre-existing diabetes mellitus, type 1, in pregnancy, **unspecified trimester**   CC M ♀

O24.02   Pre-existing diabetes mellitus, type 1, in **childbirth**   MCC M ♀

O24.03   Pre-existing diabetes mellitus, type 1, in the **puerperium**   CC M ♀

✓5th **O24.1**   **Pre-existing** diabetes mellitus, type 2, in pregnancy, childbirth and the puerperium
Insulin-resistant diabetes mellitus in pregnancy, childbirth and the puerperium
Use additional code (for):
from category E11 to further identify any manifestations
long-term (current) use of insulin (Z79.4)

✓6th **O24.11**   Pre-existing diabetes mellitus, type 2, in **pregnancy**

O24.111   Pre-existing diabetes mellitus, type 2, in pregnancy, **first trimester**   CC M ♀

O24.112   Pre-existing diabetes mellitus, type 2, in pregnancy, **second trimester**   CC M ♀

O24.113   Pre-existing diabetes mellitus, type 2, in pregnancy, **third trimester**   CC M ♀

O24.119   Pre-existing diabetes mellitus, type 2, in pregnancy, **unspecified trimester**   CC M ♀

O24.12   Pre-existing diabetes mellitus, type 2, in **childbirth**   MCC M ♀

O24.13   Pre-existing diabetes mellitus, type 2, in the **puerperium**   CC M ♀

✓5th **O24.3**   Unspecified pre-existing **diabetes mellitus** in pregnancy, childbirth and the puerperium
Use additional code (for):
from category E11 to further identify any manifestation
long-term (current) use of insulin (Z79.4)

✓6th **O24.31**   Unspecified pre-existing diabetes mellitus in **pregnancy**

O24.311   Unspecified pre-existing diabetes mellitus in pregnancy, **first trimester**   CC M ♀

O24.312   Unspecified pre-existing diabetes mellitus in pregnancy, **second trimester**   CC M ♀

O24.313   Unspecified pre-existing diabetes mellitus in pregnancy, **third trimester**   CC M ♀

O24.319   Unspecified pre-existing diabetes mellitus in pregnancy, **unspecified trimester**   CC M ♀

O24.32   Unspecified pre-existing diabetes mellitus in **childbirth**   MCC M ♀

O24.33   Unspecified pre-existing diabetes mellitus in the **puerperium**   CC M ♀

✓5th **O24.4**   Gestational **diabetes mellitus**
Diabetes mellitus arising in pregnancy
Gestational diabetes mellitus NOS

✓6th **O24.41**   Gestational diabetes mellitus in **pregnancy**

O24.410   Gestational diabetes mellitus in pregnancy, **diet controlled**   M ♀

O24.414   Gestational diabetes mellitus in pregnancy, **insulin controlled**   M ♀

O24.419   Gestational diabetes mellitus in pregnancy, **unspecified control**   M ♀

✓6th **O24.42**   Gestational diabetes mellitus in **childbirth**

O24.420   Gestational diabetes mellitus in childbirth, **diet controlled**   M ♀

O24.424   Gestational diabetes mellitus in childbirth, **insulin controlled**   M ♀

O24.429   Gestational diabetes mellitus in childbirth, **unspecified control**   M ♀

✓6th **O24.43**   Gestational diabetes mellitus in the **puerperium**

O24.430   Gestational diabetes mellitus in the puerperium, **diet controlled**   M ♀

O24.434   Gestational diabetes mellitus in the puerperium, **insulin controlled**   M ♀

O24.439   Gestational diabetes mellitus in the puerperium, **unspecified control**   M ♀

✓5th **O24.8**   Other pre-existing **diabetes mellitus** in pregnancy, childbirth, and the puerperium
Use additional code (for):
from categories E08, E09 and E13 to further identify any manifestation
long-term (current) use of insulin (Z79.4)

N Newborn: 0   P Pediatric: 0-17   M Maternity: 12-55   A Adult: 15-124   MCC Major CC Condition   PDx MCC PDx acts as own MCC   CC CC Condition   PDx CC PDx acts as own CC

✓6ᵗʰ **O24.81 Other pre-existing diabetes mellitus in** pregnancy
- **O24.811 Other pre-existing diabetes mellitus in pregnancy, first trimester** CC MQ
- **O24.812 Other pre-existing diabetes mellitus in pregnancy, second trimester** CC Q
- **O24.813 Other pre-existing diabetes mellitus in pregnancy, third trimester** CC MQ
- **O24.819 Other pre-existing diabetes mellitus in pregnancy, unspecified trimester** CC MQ

O24.82 Other pre-existing diabetes mellitus in childbirth MCC MQ

O24.83 Other pre-existing diabetes mellitus in the puerperium CC MQ

✓5ᵗʰ **O24.9 Unspecified diabetes mellitus in pregnancy, childbirth and the puerperium**
Use additional code for long-term (current) use of insulin (Z79.4)

✓6ᵗʰ **O24.91 Unspecified diabetes mellitus in** pregnancy
- **O24.911 Unspecified diabetes mellitus in pregnancy, first trimester** CC MQ
- **O24.912 Unspecified diabetes mellitus in pregnancy, second trimester** CC MQ
- **O24.913 Unspecified diabetes mellitus in pregnancy, third trimester** CC MQ
- **O24.919 Unspecified diabetes mellitus in pregnancy, unspecified trimester** CC MQ

O24.92 Unspecified diabetes mellitus in childbirth MQ

O24.93 Unspecified diabetes mellitus in the puerperium CC MQ

✓4ᵗʰ **O25 Malnutrition in pregnancy, childbirth and the puerperium**

✓5ᵗʰ **O25.1 Malnutrition in** pregnancy
- **O25.1Ø Malnutrition in pregnancy,** unspecified trimester MQ
- **O25.11 Malnutrition in pregnancy,** first trimester MQ
- **O25.12 Malnutrition in pregnancy,** second trimester MQ
- **O25.13 Malnutrition in pregnancy,** third trimester MQ

O25.2 Malnutrition in childbirth MQ

O25.3 Malnutrition in the puerperium MQ

✓4ᵗʰ **O26 Maternal care for other conditions predominantly related to pregnancy**

✓5ᵗʰ **O26.Ø Excessive weight gain in pregnancy**
EXCLUDES 2 gestational edema (O12.Ø, O12.2)
- **O26.ØØ Excessive weight gain in pregnancy, unspecified trimester** MQ
- **O26.Ø1 Excessive weight gain in pregnancy,** first trimester MQ
- **O26.Ø2 Excessive weight gain in pregnancy,** second trimester MQ
- **O26.Ø3 Excessive weight gain in pregnancy,** third trimester MQ

✓5ᵗʰ **O26.1 Low weight gain in pregnancy**
- **O26.1Ø Low weight gain in pregnancy,** unspecified trimester MQ
- **O26.11 Low weight gain in pregnancy,** first trimester MQ
- **O26.12 Low weight gain in pregnancy,** second trimester MQ
- **O26.13 Low weight gain in pregnancy,** third trimester MQ

✓5ᵗʰ **O26.2 Pregnancy care for patient with recurrent pregnancy loss**

CC Excl: For CC codes in subcategory O26.2, unless otherwise noted: O26.21-O26.23

- **O26.2Ø Pregnancy care for patient with recurrent pregnancy loss,** unspecified trimester MQ
- **O26.21 Pregnancy care for patient with recurrent pregnancy loss,** first trimester MQ
- **O26.22 Pregnancy care for patient with recurrent pregnancy loss,** second trimester MQ
- **O26.23 Pregnancy care for patient with recurrent pregnancy loss,** third trimester MQ

✓5ᵗʰ **O26.3 Retained intrauterine contraceptive device in pregnancy**
- **O26.3Ø Retained intrauterine contraceptive device in pregnancy,** unspecified trimester MQ
- **O26.31 Retained intrauterine contraceptive device in pregnancy,** first trimester MQ
- **O26.32 Retained intrauterine contraceptive device in pregnancy,** second trimester MQ
- **O26.33 Retained intrauterine contraceptive device in pregnancy,** third trimester MQ

✓5ᵗʰ **O26.4 Herpes gestationis**
- **O26.4Ø Herpes gestationis,** unspecified trimester MQ
- **O26.41 Herpes gestationis,** first trimester MQ
- **O26.42 Herpes gestationis,** second trimester Q
- **O26.43 Herpes gestationis,** third trimester MQ

✓5ᵗʰ **O26.5 Maternal hypotension syndrome**
Supine hypotensive syndrome

CC Excl: For MCC codes in subcategory O26.5, unless otherwise noted: O25.1Ø-O25.3, O26.1Ø-O26.13, O26.3Ø-O26.43, O26.51-O26.53, O26.63-O26.819, O26.841-O26.86, O26.891-O26.93, O29.Ø11-O29.93, O35.7XXØ-O35.7XX9, O75.1, O75.4, O75.81, O75.89-O75.9, O8Ø, O9Ø.89, O99.111-O99.285, O99.33Ø-O99.335, O99.35Ø-O99.355, O99.511-O99.73, O99.82Ø-O99.825, O99.84Ø-O9A.53

- **O26.5Ø Maternal hypotension syndrome,** unspecified trimester MQ
- **O26.51 Maternal hypotension syndrome,** first trimester MQ
- **O26.52 Maternal hypotension syndrome,** second trimester MQ
- **O26.53 Maternal hypotension syndrome,** third trimester MQ

✓5ᵗʰ **O26.6 Liver and biliary tract disorders in pregnancy, childbirth and the puerperium**
Use additional code to identify the specific disorder
EXCLUDES 2 hepatorenal syndrome following labor and delivery (O9Ø.4)

CC Excl: For CC codes in subcategory O26.6, unless otherwise noted: O25.1Ø-O25.3, O26.1Ø-O26.13, O26.3Ø-O26.43, O26.611-O26.819, O26.841-O26.86, O26.891-O26.93, O29.Ø11-O29.93, O35.7XXØ-O35.7XX9, O75.4, O75.81, O75.89-O75.9, O8Ø, O9Ø.89, O99.111-O99.285, O99.33Ø-O99.335, O99.35Ø-O99.355, O99.511-O99.73, O99.82Ø-O99.825, O99.84Ø-O9A.53

✓6ᵗʰ **O26.61 Liver and biliary tract disorders in** pregnancy
- **O26.611 Liver and biliary tract disorders in pregnancy, first trimester** CC MQ
- **O26.612 Liver and biliary tract disorders in pregnancy, second trimester** CC MQ
- **O26.613 Liver and biliary tract disorders in pregnancy, third trimester** CC MQ
- **O26.619 Liver and biliary tract disorders in pregnancy, unspecified trimester** MQ

O26.62 Liver and biliary tract disorders in childbirth CC MQ

O26.63 Liver and biliary tract disorders in the puerperium MQ

✓5ᵗʰ **O26.7 Subluxation of symphysis (pubis) in pregnancy, childbirth and the puerperium**
EXCLUDES 1 traumatic separation of symphysis (pubis) during childbirth (O71.6)

✓6ᵗʰ **O26.71 Subluxation of symphysis (pubis) in pregnancy**
- **O26.711 Subluxation of symphysis (pubis) in pregnancy, first trimester** MQ
- **O26.712 Subluxation of symphysis (pubis) in pregnancy, second trimester** MQ
- **O26.713 Subluxation of symphysis (pubis) in pregnancy, third trimester** MQ
- **O26.719 Subluxation of symphysis (pubis) in pregnancy, unspecified trimester** MQ

O26.72 Subluxation of symphysis (pubis) in childbirth MQ

O26.73 Subluxation of symphysis (pubis) in the puerperium MQ

✓5ᵗʰ **O26.8 Other specified pregnancy related conditions**
✓6ᵗʰ **O26.81 Pregnancy related exhaustion and fatigue**
- **O26.811 Pregnancy related exhaustion and fatigue,** first trimester MQ
- **O26.812 Pregnancy related exhaustion and fatigue,** second trimester MQ
- **O26.813 Pregnancy related exhaustion and fatigue,** third trimester MQ
- **O26.819 Pregnancy related exhaustion and fatigue,** unspecified trimester MQ

✓6ᵗʰ **O26.82 Pregnancy related peripheral neuritis**
- **O26.821 Pregnancy related peripheral neuritis,** first trimester MQ

☑ Additional Character Required   ✓x7ᵗʰ Xtension Alert   Unacceptable PDx   Manifestation   Hospital Acquired Condition   *EXCLUDES 1* Not Coded Here   *EXCLUDES 2* Not Included Here

O26.822 **Pregnancy related peripheral neuritis,** Ⓜ♀ **second trimester**

O26.823 **Pregnancy related peripheral neuritis,** Ⓜ♀ **third trimester**

O26.829 **Pregnancy related peripheral neuritis,** Ⓜ♀ **unspecified trimester**

✓6ᵗʰ O26.83 **Pregnancy related renal disease**
Use additional code to identify the specific disorder

> **CC Excl: For CC codes in subcategory O26.83, unless otherwise noted:** O12.11-O12.13, O12.21-O12.23, O26.831-O26.833, O90.89

O26.831 **Pregnancy related renal disease,** CC Ⓜ♀ **first trimester**

O26.832 **Pregnancy related renal disease,** CC Ⓜ♀ **second trimester**

O26.833 **Pregnancy related renal disease,** CC Ⓜ♀ **third trimester**

O26.839 **Pregnancy related renal disease,** Ⓜ♀ **unspecified trimester**

✓6ᵗʰ O26.84 **Uterine size-date discrepancy complicating pregnancy**
EXCLUDES 1 *encounter for suspected problem with fetal growth ruled out (Z03.74)*

O26.841 **Uterine size-date discrepancy, first** Ⓜ♀ **trimester**

O26.842 **Uterine size-date discrepancy, second** Ⓜ♀ **trimester**

O26.843 **Uterine size-date discrepancy, third** Ⓜ♀ **trimester**

O26.849 **Uterine size-date discrepancy,** Ⓜ♀ **unspecified trimester**

✓6ᵗʰ O26.85 **Spotting complicating pregnancy**

O26.851 **Spotting complicating pregnancy,** Ⓜ♀ **first trimester**

O26.852 **Spotting complicating pregnancy,** Ⓜ♀ **second trimester**

O26.853 **Spotting complicating pregnancy,** Ⓜ♀ **third trimester**

O26.859 **Spotting complicating pregnancy,** Ⓜ♀ **unspecified trimester**

O26.86 **Pruritic urticarial papules and plaques of** Ⓜ♀ **pregnancy (PUPPP)**
Polymorphic eruption of pregnancy

✓6ᵗʰ O26.87 **Cervical shortening**
EXCLUDES 1 *encounter for suspected cervical shortening ruled out (Z03.75)*

> **CC Excl: For CC codes in subcategory O26.87, unless otherwise noted:** O26.872-O26.879, O34.31-O34.33

O26.872 **Cervical shortening, second** CC Ⓜ♀ **trimester**

O26.873 **Cervical shortening, third trimester** CC Ⓜ♀

O26.879 **Cervical shortening, unspecified** CC Ⓜ♀ **trimester**

✓6ᵗʰ O26.89 **Other specified pregnancy related conditions**

O26.891 **Other specified pregnancy related** Ⓜ♀ **conditions, first trimester**

O26.892 **Other specified pregnancy related** Ⓜ♀ **conditions, second trimester**

O26.893 **Other specified pregnancy related** Ⓜ♀ **conditions, third trimester**

O26.899 **Other specified pregnancy related** Ⓜ♀ **conditions, unspecified trimester**

✓5ᵗʰ O26.9 **Pregnancy related conditions, unspecified**

O26.90 **Pregnancy related conditions, unspecified,** Ⓜ♀ **unspecified trimester**

O26.91 **Pregnancy related conditions, unspecified,** Ⓜ♀ **first trimester**

O26.92 **Pregnancy related conditions, unspecified,** Ⓜ♀ **second trimester**

O26.93 **Pregnancy related conditions, unspecified,** Ⓜ♀ **third trimester**

✓4ᵗʰ **O28 Abnormal findings on antenatal screening of mother**
EXCLUDES 1 *diagnostic findings classified elsewhere—see Alphabetical Index*

O28.0 **Abnormal hematological finding on antenatal screening** Ⓜ♀ **of mother**

O28.1 **Abnormal biochemical finding on antenatal screening of** Ⓜ♀ **mother**

O28.2 **Abnormal cytological finding on antenatal screening** Ⓜ♀ **of mother**

O28.3 **Abnormal ultrasonic finding on antenatal screening** Ⓜ♀ **of mother**

O28.4 **Abnormal radiological finding on antenatal screening** Ⓜ♀ **of mother**

O28.5 **Abnormal chromosomal and genetic finding on** Ⓜ♀ **antenatal screening of mother**

O28.8 **Other abnormal findings on antenatal screening of** Ⓜ♀ **mother**

O28.9 **Unspecified abnormal findings on antenatal screening** Ⓜ♀ **of mother**

✓4ᵗʰ **O29 Complications of anesthesia during pregnancy**
INCLUDES maternal complications arising from the administration of a general, regional or local anesthetic, analgesic or other sedation during pregnancy
Use additional code, if necessary, to identify the complication
EXCLUDES 2 *complications of anesthesia during labor and delivery (O74.-)*
complications of anesthesia during the puerperium (O89.-)

✓5ᵗʰ O29.0 **Pulmonary complications of anesthesia during pregnancy**

✓6ᵗʰ O29.01 **Aspiration pneumonitis due to anesthesia during pregnancy**
Inhalation of stomach contents or secretions NOS due to anesthesia during pregnancy
Mendelson's syndrome due to anesthesia during pregnancy

O29.011 **Aspiration pneumonitis due to** Ⓜ♀ **anesthesia during pregnancy, first trimester**

O29.012 **Aspiration pneumonitis due to** Ⓜ♀ **anesthesia during pregnancy, second trimester**

O29.013 **Aspiration pneumonitis due to** Ⓜ♀ **anesthesia during pregnancy, third trimester**

O29.019 **Aspiration pneumonitis due to** Ⓜ♀ **anesthesia during pregnancy, unspecified trimester**

✓6ᵗʰ O29.02 **Pressure collapse of lung due to anesthesia during pregnancy**

O29.021 **Pressure collapse of lung due to** Ⓜ♀ **anesthesia during pregnancy, first trimester**

O29.022 **Pressure collapse of lung due to** Ⓜ♀ **anesthesia during pregnancy, second trimester**

O29.023 **Pressure collapse of lung due to** Ⓜ♀ **anesthesia during pregnancy, third trimester**

O29.029 **Pressure collapse of lung due to** Ⓜ♀ **anesthesia during pregnancy, unspecified trimester**

✓6ᵗʰ O29.09 **Other pulmonary complications of anesthesia during pregnancy**

O29.091 **Other pulmonary complications of** Ⓜ♀ **anesthesia during pregnancy, first trimester**

O29.092 **Other pulmonary complications of** Ⓜ♀ **anesthesia during pregnancy, second trimester**

O29.093 **Other pulmonary complications of** Ⓜ♀ **anesthesia during pregnancy, third trimester**

O29.099 **Other pulmonary complications of** Ⓜ♀ **anesthesia during pregnancy, unspecified trimester**

✓5ᵗʰ O29.1 **Cardiac complications of anesthesia during pregnancy**

✓6ᵗʰ O29.11 **Cardiac arrest due to anesthesia during pregnancy**

O29.111 **Cardiac arrest due to anesthesia** Ⓜ♀ **during pregnancy, first trimester**

O29.112 **Cardiac arrest due to anesthesia** Ⓜ♀ **during pregnancy, second trimester**

O29.113 **Cardiac arrest due to anesthesia** Ⓜ♀ **during pregnancy, third trimester**

Ⓝ Newborn: 0   Ⓟ Pediatric: 0-17   Ⓜ Maternity: 12-55   Ⓐ Adult: 15-124   MCC Major CC Condition   PDx MCC PDx acts as own MCC   CC CC Condition   PDx CC PDx acts as own CC

792   ICD-10-CM Draft (2015)

O29.119   Cardiac arrest due to anesthesia during pregnancy, unspecified trimester   Ⓜ♀

✓6th **O29.12**   Cardiac failure due to anesthesia during pregnancy

     O29.121   Cardiac failure due to anesthesia during pregnancy, first trimester   Ⓜ♀

     O29.122   Cardiac failure due to anesthesia during pregnancy, second trimester   Ⓜ♀

     O29.123   Cardiac failure due to anesthesia during pregnancy, third trimester   Ⓜ♀

     O29.129   Cardiac failure due to anesthesia during pregnancy, unspecified trimester   Ⓜ♀

✓6th **O29.19**   Other cardiac complications of anesthesia during pregnancy

     O29.191   Other cardiac complications of anesthesia during pregnancy, first trimester   Ⓜ♀

     O29.192   Other cardiac complications of anesthesia during pregnancy, second trimester   Ⓜ♀

     O29.193   Other cardiac complications of anesthesia during pregnancy, third trimester   Ⓜ♀

     O29.199   Other cardiac complications of anesthesia during pregnancy, unspecified trimester   Ⓜ♀

✓5th **O29.2**   Central nervous system complications of anesthesia during pregnancy

✓6th **O29.21**   Cerebral anoxia due to anesthesia during pregnancy

     O29.211   Cerebral anoxia due to anesthesia during pregnancy, first trimester   Ⓜ♀

     O29.212   Cerebral anoxia due to anesthesia during pregnancy, second trimester   Ⓜ♀

     O29.213   Cerebral anoxia due to anesthesia during pregnancy, third trimester   Ⓜ♀

     O29.219   Cerebral anoxia due to anesthesia during pregnancy, unspecified trimester   Ⓜ♀

✓6th **O29.29**   Other central nervous system complications of anesthesia during pregnancy

     O29.291   Other central nervous system complications of anesthesia during pregnancy, first trimester   Ⓜ♀

     O29.292   Other central nervous system complications of anesthesia during pregnancy, second trimester   Ⓜ♀

     O29.293   Other central nervous system complications of anesthesia during pregnancy, third trimester   Ⓜ♀

     O29.299   Other central nervous system complications of anesthesia during pregnancy, unspecified trimester   Ⓜ♀

✓5th **O29.3**   Toxic reaction to local anesthesia during pregnancy

✓6th **O29.3X**   Toxic reaction to local anesthesia during pregnancy

     O29.3X1   Toxic reaction to local anesthesia during pregnancy, first trimester   Ⓜ♀

     O29.3X2   Toxic reaction to local anesthesia during pregnancy, second trimester   Ⓜ♀

     O29.3X3   Toxic reaction to local anesthesia during pregnancy, third trimester   Ⓜ♀

     O29.3X9   Toxic reaction to local anesthesia during pregnancy, unspecified trimester   Ⓜ♀

✓5th **O29.4**   Spinal and epidural anesthesia induced headache during pregnancy

     O29.40   Spinal and epidural anesthesia induced headache during pregnancy, unspecified trimester   Ⓜ♀

     O29.41   Spinal and epidural anesthesia induced headache during pregnancy, first trimester   Ⓜ♀

     O29.42   Spinal and epidural anesthesia induced headache during pregnancy, second trimester   Ⓜ♀

     O29.43   Spinal and epidural anesthesia induced headache during pregnancy, third trimester   Ⓜ♀

✓5th **O29.5**   Other complications of spinal and epidural anesthesia during pregnancy

✓6th **O29.5X**   Other complications of spinal and epidural anesthesia during pregnancy

     O29.5X1   Other complications of spinal and epidural anesthesia during pregnancy, first trimester   Ⓜ♀

     O29.5X2   Other complications of spinal and epidural anesthesia during pregnancy, second trimester   Ⓜ♀

     O29.5X3   Other complications of spinal and epidural anesthesia during pregnancy, third trimester   Ⓜ♀

     O29.5X9   Other complications of spinal and epidural anesthesia during pregnancy, unspecified trimester   Ⓜ♀

✓5th **O29.6**   Failed or difficult intubation for anesthesia during pregnancy

     O29.60   Failed or difficult intubation for anesthesia during pregnancy, unspecified trimester   Ⓜ♀

     O29.61   Failed or difficult intubation for anesthesia during pregnancy, first trimester   Ⓜ♀

     O29.62   Failed or difficult intubation for anesthesia during pregnancy, second trimester   Ⓜ♀

     O29.63   Failed or difficult intubation for anesthesia during pregnancy, third trimester   Ⓜ♀

✓5th **O29.8**   Other complications of anesthesia during pregnancy

✓6th **O29.8X**   Other complications of anesthesia during pregnancy

     O29.8X1   Other complications of anesthesia during pregnancy, first trimester   Ⓜ♀

     O29.8X2   Other complications of anesthesia during pregnancy, second trimester   Ⓜ♀

     O29.8X3   Other complications of anesthesia during pregnancy, third trimester   Ⓜ♀

     O29.8X9   Other complications of anesthesia during pregnancy, unspecified trimester   Ⓜ♀

✓5th **O29.9**   Unspecified complication of anesthesia during pregnancy

     O29.90   Unspecified complication of anesthesia during pregnancy, unspecified trimester   Ⓜ♀

     O29.91   Unspecified complication of anesthesia during pregnancy, first trimester   Ⓜ♀

     O29.92   Unspecified complication of anesthesia during pregnancy, second trimester   Ⓜ♀

     O29.93   Unspecified complication of anesthesia during pregnancy, third trimester   Ⓜ♀

Maternal care related to the fetus and amniotic cavity and possible delivery problems (O30-O48)

✓4th **O30**   **Multiple gestation**

     Code also any complications specific to multiple gestation

     CC Excl: For CC codes in category O30, unless otherwise noted: O30.001-O30.019, O30.031-O30.93, O31.10X0-O31.23X9, O31.31X0-O32.9XX9, O80

✓5th **O30.0**   Twin pregnancy

✓6th **O30.00**   Twin pregnancy, unspecified number of placenta and unspecified number of amniotic sacs

     O30.001   Twin pregnancy, unspecified number of placenta and unspecified number of amniotic sacs, first trimester   Ⓜ♀

     O30.002   Twin pregnancy, unspecified number of placenta and unspecified number of amniotic sacs, second trimester   Ⓜ♀

     O30.003   Twin pregnancy, unspecified number of placenta and unspecified number of amniotic sacs, third trimester   Ⓜ♀

     O30.009   Twin pregnancy, unspecified number of placenta and unspecified number of amniotic sacs, unspecified trimester   Ⓜ♀

✓6th **O30.01**   Twin pregnancy, monochorionic/monoamniotic

     Twin pregnancy, one placenta, one amniotic sac

     EXCLUDES 1   conjoined twins (O30.02-)

     O30.011   Twin pregnancy, monochorionic/monoamniotic, first trimester   Ⓜ♀

     O30.012   Twin pregnancy, monochorionic/monoamniotic, second trimester   Ⓜ♀

     O30.013   Twin pregnancy, monochorionic/monoamniotic, third trimester   Ⓜ♀

     O30.019   Twin pregnancy, monochorionic/monoamniotic, unspecified trimester   Ⓜ♀

✓6th **O30.02**   Conjoined twin pregnancy

     O30.021   Conjoined twin pregnancy, first trimester   Ⓜ♀

     O30.022   Conjoined twin pregnancy, second trimester   Ⓜ♀

✓ Additional Character Required   ✓x7th Xtension Alert   Unacceptable PDx   Manifestation   Hospital Acquired Condition   **EXCLUDES 1** Not Coded Here   **EXCLUDES 2** Not Included Here

ICD-10-CM Draft (2015)   793

O30.023   **Conjoined twin pregnancy,** third trimester   M♀

O30.029   **Conjoined twin pregnancy,** unspecified trimester   M♀

√6ᵗʰ   O30.03   **Twin pregnancy,** monochorionic/diamniotic
Twin pregnancy, one placenta, two amniotic sacs

O30.031   **Twin pregnancy, monochorionic/ diamniotic,** first trimester   M♀

O30.032   **Twin pregnancy, monochorionic/ diamniotic,** second trimester   M♀

O30.033   **Twin pregnancy, monochorionic/ diamniotic,** third trimester   M♀

O30.039   **Twin pregnancy, monochorionic/ diamniotic,** unspecified trimester   M♀

√6ᵗʰ   O30.04   **Twin pregnancy,** dichorionic/diamniotic
Twin pregnancy, two placentae, two amniotic sacs

O30.041   **Twin pregnancy, dichorionic/ diamniotic,** first trimester   M♀

O30.042   **Twin pregnancy, dichorionic/ diamniotic,** second trimester   M♀

O30.043   **Twin pregnancy, dichorionic/ diamniotic,** third trimester   M♀

O30.049   **Twin pregnancy, dichorionic/ diamniotic,** unspecified trimester   M♀

√6ᵗʰ   O30.09   **Twin pregnancy,** unable to determine number of placenta and number of amniotic sacs

O30.091   **Twin pregnancy, unable to determine number of placenta and number of amniotic sacs,** first trimester   M♀

O30.092   **Twin pregnancy, unable to determine number of placenta and number of amniotic sacs,** second trimester   M♀

O30.093   **Twin pregnancy, unable to determine number of placenta and number of amniotic sacs,** third trimester   M♀

O30.099   **Twin pregnancy, unable to determine number of placenta and number of amniotic sacs,** unspecified trimester   M♀

√5ᵗʰ   O30.1   Triplet pregnancy

√6ᵗʰ   O30.10   **Triplet pregnancy,** unspecified number of placenta and unspecified number of amniotic sacs

O30.101   **Triplet pregnancy, unspecified number of placenta and unspecified number of amniotic sacs,** first trimester   CC M♀

O30.102   **Triplet pregnancy, unspecified number of placenta and unspecified number of amniotic sacs,** second trimester   CC M♀

O30.103   **Triplet pregnancy, unspecified number of placenta and unspecified number of amniotic sacs,** third trimester   CC M♀

O30.109   **Triplet pregnancy, unspecified number of placenta and unspecified number of amniotic sacs,** unspecified trimester   M♀

√6ᵗʰ   O30.11   **Triplet pregnancy with** two or more monochorionic fetuses

O30.111   **Triplet pregnancy with two or more monochorionic fetuses,** first trimester   CC M♀

O30.112   **Triplet pregnancy with two or more monochorionic fetuses,** second trimester   CC M♀

O30.113   **Triplet pregnancy with two or more monochorionic fetuses,** third trimester   CC M♀

O30.119   **Triplet pregnancy with two or more monochorionic fetuses,** unspecified trimester   M♀

√6ᵗʰ   O30.12   **Triplet pregnancy with** two or more monoamniotic fetuses

O30.121   **Triplet pregnancy with two or more monoamniotic fetuses,** first trimester   CC M♀

O30.122   **Triplet pregnancy with two or more monoamniotic fetuses,** second trimester   CC M♀

O30.123   **Triplet pregnancy with two or more monoamniotic fetuses,** third trimester   CC M♀

O30.129   **Triplet pregnancy with two or more monoamniotic fetuses,** unspecified trimester   CC M♀

√6ᵗʰ   O30.19   **Triplet pregnancy,** unable to determine number of placenta and number of amniotic sacs

O30.191   **Triplet pregnancy, unable to determine number of placenta and number of amniotic sacs,** first trimester   CC M♀

O30.192   **Triplet pregnancy, unable to determine number of placenta and number of amniotic sacs,** second trimester   CC M♀

O30.193   **Triplet pregnancy, unable to determine number of placenta and number of amniotic sacs,** third trimester   CC M♀

O30.199   **Triplet pregnancy, unable to determine number of placenta and number of amniotic sacs,** unspecified trimester   M♀

√6ᵗʰ   O30.2   Quadruplet pregnancy

√6ᵗʰ   O30.20   **Quadruplet pregnancy,** unspecified number of placenta and unspecified number of amniotic sacs

O30.201   **Quadruplet pregnancy, unspecified number of placenta and unspecified number of amniotic sacs,** first trimester   CC M♀

O30.202   **Quadruplet pregnancy, unspecified number of placenta and unspecified number of amniotic sacs,** second trimester   CC M♀

O30.203   **Quadruplet pregnancy, unspecified number of placenta and unspecified number of amniotic sacs,** third trimester   CC M♀

O30.209   **Quadruplet pregnancy, unspecified number of placenta and unspecified number of amniotic sacs,** unspecified trimester   M♀

√6ᵗʰ   O30.21   **Quadruplet pregnancy with** two or more monochorionic fetuses

O30.211   **Quadruplet pregnancy with two or more monochorionic fetuses,** first trimester   CC M♀

O30.212   **Quadruplet pregnancy with two or more monochorionic fetuses,** second trimester   CC M♀

O30.213   **Quadruplet pregnancy with two or more monochorionic fetuses,** third trimester   CC M♀

O30.219   **Quadruplet pregnancy with two or more monochorionic fetuses,** unspecified trimester   M♀

√6ᵗʰ   O30.22   **Quadruplet pregnancy with** two or more monoamniotic fetuses

O30.221   **Quadruplet pregnancy with two or more monoamniotic fetuses,** first trimester   CC M♀

O30.222   **Quadruplet pregnancy with two or more monoamniotic fetuses,** second trimester   CC M♀

O30.223   **Quadruplet pregnancy with two or more monoamniotic fetuses,** third trimester   CC M♀

O30.229   **Quadruplet pregnancy with two or more monoamniotic fetuses,** unspecified trimester   M♀

√6ᵗʰ   O30.29   **Quadruplet pregnancy,** unable to determine number of placenta and number of amniotic sacs

O30.291   **Quadruplet pregnancy, unable to determine number of placenta and number of amniotic sacs,** first trimester   CC M♀

N Newborn: 0   P Pediatric: 0-17   M Maternity: 12-55   A Adult: 15-124   MCC Major CC Condition   PDx MCC PDx acts as own MCC   CC CC Condition   PDx CC PDx acts as own CC

794   ICD-10-CM Draft (2015)

O30.292 Quadruplet pregnancy, unable to determine number of placenta and number of amniotic sacs, second trimester CC MQ

O30.293 Quadruplet pregnancy, unable to determine number of placenta and number of amniotic sacs, third trimester CC MQ

O30.299 Quadruplet pregnancy, unable to determine number of placenta and number of amniotic sacs, unspecified trimester MQ

√5th **O30.8** Other specified multiple gestation
Multiple gestation pregnancy greater than quadruplets

√6th **O30.80** Other specified multiple gestation, unspecified number of placenta and unspecified number of amniotic sacs

O30.801 Other specified multiple gestation, unspecified number of placenta and unspecified number of amniotic sacs, first trimester CC MQ

O30.802 Other specified multiple gestation, unspecified number of placenta and unspecified number of amniotic sacs, second trimester CC MQ

O30.803 Other specified multiple gestation, unspecified number of placenta and unspecified number of amniotic sacs, third trimester CC MQ

O30.809 Other specified multiple gestation, unspecified number of placenta and unspecified number of amniotic sacs, unspecified trimester MQ

√6th **O30.81** Other specified multiple gestation with two or more monochorionic fetuses

O30.811 Other specified multiple gestation with two or more monochorionic fetuses, first trimester CC MQ

O30.812 Other specified multiple gestation with two or more monochorionic fetuses, second trimester CC MQ

O30.813 Other specified multiple gestation with two or more monochorionic fetuses, third trimester CC MQ

O30.819 Other specified multiple gestation with two or more monochorionic fetuses, unspecified trimester MQ

√6th **O30.82** Other specified multiple gestation with two or more monoamniotic fetuses

O30.821 Other specified multiple gestation with two or more monoamniotic fetuses, first trimester CC MQ

O30.822 Other specified multiple gestation with two or more monoamniotic fetuses, second trimester CC MQ

O30.823 Other specified multiple gestation with two or more monoamniotic fetuses, third trimester CC MQ

O30.829 Other specified multiple gestation with two or more monoamniotic fetuses, unspecified trimester MQ

√6th **O30.89** Other specified multiple gestation, unable to determine number of placenta and number of amniotic sacs

O30.891 Other specified multiple gestation, unable to determine number of placenta and number of amniotic sacs, first trimester CC MQ

O30.892 Other specified multiple gestation, unable to determine number of placenta and number of amniotic sacs, second trimester CC MQ

O30.893 Other specified multiple gestation, unable to determine number of placenta and number of amniotic sacs, third trimester CC MQ

O30.899 Other specified multiple gestation, unable to determine number of placenta and number of amniotic sacs, unspecified trimester MQ

√5th **O30.9** Multiple gestation, unspecified
Multiple pregnancy NOS

O30.90 Multiple gestation, unspecified, unspecified trimester MQ

O30.91 Multiple gestation, unspecified, first trimester MQ

O30.92 Multiple gestation, unspecified, second trimester MQ

O30.93 Multiple gestation, unspecified, third trimester MQ

√4th **O31** Complications specific to multiple gestation
EXCLUDES 2 delayed delivery of second twin, triplet, etc. (O63.2)
malpresentation of one fetus or more (O32.9)
placental transfusion syndromes (O43.0-)
AHA: 2012, 4Q, 107

One of the following 7th characters is to be assigned to each code under category O31. 7th character 0 is for single gestations and multiple gestations where the fetus is unspecified. 7th characters 1 through 9 are for cases of multiple gestations to identify the fetus for which the code applies. The appropriate code from category O30, Multiple gestation, must also be assigned when assigning a code from category O31 that has a 7th character of 1 through 9.

0	not applicable or unspecified	3	fetus 3
		4	fetus 4
1	fetus 1	5	fetus 5
2	fetus 2	9	other fetus

√5th **O31.0** Papyraceous fetus
Fetus compressus

√x7th **O31.00** Papyraceous fetus, unspecified trimester MQ

√x7th **O31.01** Papyraceous fetus, first trimester MQ

√x7th **O31.02** Papyraceous fetus, second trimester MQ

√x7th **O31.03** Papyraceous fetus, third trimester MQ

√5th **O31.1** Continuing pregnancy after spontaneous abortion of one fetus or more

√x7th **O31.10** Continuing pregnancy after spontaneous abortion of one fetus or more, unspecified trimester MQ

√x7th **O31.11** Continuing pregnancy after spontaneous abortion of one fetus or more, first trimester MQ

√x7th **O31.12** Continuing pregnancy after spontaneous abortion of one fetus or more, second trimester MQ

√x7th **O31.13** Continuing pregnancy after spontaneous abortion of one fetus or more, third trimester MQ

√5th **O31.2** Continuing pregnancy after intrauterine death of one fetus or more

√x7th **O31.20** Continuing pregnancy after intrauterine death of one fetus or more, unspecified trimester MQ

√x7th **O31.21** Continuing pregnancy after intrauterine death of one fetus or more, first trimester MQ

√x7th **O31.22** Continuing pregnancy after intrauterine death of one fetus or more, second trimester MQ

√x7th **O31.23** Continuing pregnancy after intrauterine death of one fetus or more, third trimester MQ

√5th **O31.3** Continuing pregnancy after elective fetal reduction of one fetus or more
Continuing pregnancy after selective termination of one fetus or more

√x7th **O31.30** Continuing pregnancy after elective fetal reduction of one fetus or more, unspecified trimester MQ

√x7th **O31.31** Continuing pregnancy after elective fetal reduction of one fetus or more, first trimester MQ

√x7th **O31.32** Continuing pregnancy after elective fetal reduction of one fetus or more, second trimester MQ

√x7th **O31.33** Continuing pregnancy after elective fetal reduction of one fetus or more, third trimester MQ

√5th **O31.8** Other complications specific to multiple gestation

√6th **O31.8X** Other complications specific to multiple gestation

CC Excl: For CC codes in subcategory O31.8X, unless otherwise noted: See code: O30

√7th **O31.8X1** Other complications specific to multiple gestation, first trimester CC MQ

√7th **O31.8X2** Other complications specific to multiple gestation, second trimester CC MQ

Pregnancy, Childbirth and the Puerperium

O31.8X3–O34.01

√7ᵗʰ   **O31.8X3**   **Other complications specific to multiple gestation, third trimester**   CC M♀

√7ᵗʰ   **O31.8X9**   **Other complications specific to multiple gestation, unspecified trimester**   M♀

√4ᵗʰ   **O32**   **Maternal care for malpresentation of fetus**

INCLUDES the listed conditions as a reason for observation, hospitalization or other obstetric care of the mother, or for cesarean delivery before onset of labor

EXCLUDES1 malpresentation of fetus with obstructed labor (O64.-)

AHA: 2012, 4Q, 107

One of the following 7th characters is to be assigned to each code under category O32. 7th character Ø is for single gestations and multiple gestations where the fetus is unspecified. 7th characters 1 through 9 are for cases of multiple gestations to identify the fetus for which the code applies. The appropriate code from category O30, Multiple gestation, must also be assigned when assigning a code from category O32 that has a 7th character of 1 through 9.

Ø	not applicable or unspecified	3	fetus 3
		4	fetus 4
1	fetus 1	5	fetus 5
2	fetus 2	9	other fetus

√x7ᵗʰ   **O32.0**   **Maternal care for unstable lie**   M♀

√x7ᵗʰ   **O32.1**   **Maternal care for breech presentation**   M♀
Maternal care for buttocks presentation
Maternal care for complete breech
Maternal care for frank breech
EXCLUDES1 footling presentation (O32.8)
incomplete breech (O32.8)

√x7ᵗʰ   **O32.2**   **Maternal care for transverse and oblique lie**   M♀
Maternal care for oblique presentation
Maternal care for transverse presentation

√x7ᵗʰ   **O32.3**   **Maternal care for face, brow and chin presentation**   M♀

√x7ᵗʰ   **O32.4**   **Maternal care for high head at term**   M♀
Maternal care for failure of head to enter pelvic brim

√x7ᵗʰ   **O32.6**   **Maternal care for compound presentation**   M♀

√x7ᵗʰ   **O32.8**   **Maternal care for other malpresentation of fetus**   M♀
Maternal care for footling presentation
Maternal care for incomplete breech

√x7ᵗʰ   **O32.9**   **Maternal care for malpresentation of fetus, unspecified**   M♀

√4ᵗʰ   **O33**   **Maternal care for disproportion**

INCLUDES the listed conditions as a reason for observation, hospitalization or other obstetric care of the mother, or for cesarean delivery before onset of labor

EXCLUDES1 disproportion with obstructed labor (O65-O66)

O33.0   **Maternal care for disproportion due to deformity of maternal pelvic bones**   CC M♀
Maternal care for disproportion due to pelvic deformity causing disproportion NOS
CC Excl: O33.0

O33.1   **Maternal care for disproportion due to generally contracted pelvis**   M♀
Maternal care for disproportion due to contracted pelvis NOS causing disproportion

O33.2   **Maternal care for disproportion due to inlet contraction of pelvis**   M♀
Maternal care for disproportion due to inlet contraction (pelvis) causing disproportion

√x7ᵗʰ   **O33.3**   **Maternal care for disproportion due to outlet contraction of pelvis**   M♀
Maternal care for disproportion due to mid-cavity contraction (pelvis)
Maternal care for disproportion due to outlet contraction (pelvis)

One of the following 7th characters is to be assigned to code O33.3. 7th character Ø is for single gestations and multiple gestations where the fetus is unspecified. 7th characters 1 through 9 are for cases of multiple gestations to identify the fetus for which the code applies. The appropriate code from category O30, Multiple gestation, must also be assigned when assigning code O33.3 with a 7th character of 1 through 9.

Ø	not applicable or unspecified	3	fetus 3
		4	fetus 4
1	fetus 1	5	fetus 5
2	fetus 2	9	other fetus

√x7ᵗʰ   **O33.4**   **Maternal care for disproportion of mixed maternal and fetal origin**   M♀

One of the following 7th characters is to be assigned to code O33.4. 7th character Ø is for single gestations and multiple gestations where the fetus is unspecified. 7th characters 1 through 9 are for cases of multiple gestations to identify the fetus for which the code applies. The appropriate code from category O30, Multiple gestation, must also be assigned when assigning code O33.4 with a 7th character of 1 through 9.

Ø	not applicable or unspecified	3	fetus 3
		4	fetus 4
1	fetus 1	5	fetus 5
2	fetus 2	9	other fetus

√x7ᵗʰ   **O33.5**   **Maternal care for disproportion due to unusually large fetus**   M♀
Maternal care for disproportion due to disproportion of fetal origin with normally formed fetus
Maternal care for disproportion due to fetal disproportion NOS

One of the following 7th characters is to be assigned to code O33.5. 7th character Ø is for single gestations and multiple gestations where the fetus is unspecified. 7th characters 1 through 9 are for cases of multiple gestations to identify the fetus for which the code applies. The appropriate code from category O30, Multiple gestation, must also be assigned when assigning code O33.5 with a 7th character of 1 through 9.

Ø	not applicable or unspecified	3	fetus 3
		4	fetus 4
1	fetus 1	5	fetus 5
2	fetus 2	9	other fetus

√x7ᵗʰ   **O33.6**   **Maternal care for disproportion due to hydrocephalic fetus**   M♀

One of the following 7th characters is to be assigned to code O33.6. 7th character Ø is for single gestations and multiple gestations where the fetus is unspecified. 7th characters 1 through 9 are for cases of multiple gestations to identify the fetus for which the code applies. The appropriate code from category O30, Multiple gestation, must also be assigned when assigning code O33.6 with a 7th character of 1 through 9.

Ø	not applicable or unspecified	3	fetus 3
		4	fetus 4
1	fetus 1	5	fetus 5
2	fetus 2	9	other fetus

O33.7   **Maternal care for disproportion due to other fetal deformities**   M♀
Maternal care for disproportion due to fetal ascites
Maternal care for disproportion due to fetal hydrops
Maternal care for disproportion due to fetal meningomyelocele
Maternal care for disproportion due to fetal sacral teratoma
Maternal care for disproportion due to fetal tumor
EXCLUDES1 obstructed labor due to other fetal deformities (O66.3)

O33.8   **Maternal care for disproportion of other origin**   M♀

O33.9   **Maternal care for disproportion, unspecified**   M♀
Maternal care for disproportion due to cephalopelvic disproportion NOS
Maternal care for disproportion due to fetopelvic disproportion NOS

√4ᵗʰ   **O34**   **Maternal care for abnormality of pelvic organs**

INCLUDES the listed conditions as a reason for hospitalization or other obstetric care of the mother, or for cesarean delivery before onset of labor

Code first any associated obstructed labor (O65.5)
Use additional code for specific condition

√5ᵗʰ   **O34.0**   **Maternal care for congenital malformation of uterus**

O34.00   **Maternal care for unspecified congenital malformation of uterus, unspecified trimester**   M♀

O34.01   **Maternal care for unspecified congenital malformation of uterus, first trimester**   M♀

N Newborn: 0   P Pediatric: 0-17   M Maternity: 12-55   A Adult: 15-124   MCC Major CC Condition   PDx MCC PDx acts as own MCC   CC CC Condition   PDx CC PDx acts as own CC

796   ICD-10-CM Draft (2015)

O34.02 Maternal care for unspecified congenital malformation of uterus, **second trimester** ♂♀

O34.03 Maternal care for unspecified congenital malformation of uterus, **third trimester** ♂♀

✓5th **O34.1** Maternal care for benign tumor of corpus uteri
    EXCLUDES 2 maternal care for benign tumor of cervix (O34.4-)
         maternal care for malignant neoplasm of uterus (O9A.1-)

O34.10 Maternal care for benign tumor of corpus uteri, **unspecified trimester** ♂♀

O34.11 Maternal care for benign tumor of corpus uteri, **first trimester** ♂♀

O34.12 Maternal care for benign tumor of corpus uteri, **second trimester** ♂♀

O34.13 Maternal care for benign tumor of corpus uteri, **third trimester** ♂♀

✓5th **O34.2** Maternal care due to uterine scar from previous surgery ♂♀

O34.21 Maternal care for scar from previous cesarean delivery ♂♀

O34.29 Maternal care due to uterine scar from other previous surgery ♂♀

✓5th **O34.3** Maternal care for cervical incompetence
    Maternal care for cerclage with or without cervical incompetence
    Maternal care for Shirodkar suture with or without cervical incompetence

    CC Excl: For MCC codes in subcategory O34.3, unless otherwise noted: O26.872-O26.879, O34.31-O34.33

O34.30 Maternal care for cervical incompetence, **unspecified trimester** ♂♀

O34.31 Maternal care for cervical incompetence, **first trimester** MCC ♂♀

O34.32 Maternal care for cervical incompetence, **second trimester** MCC ♂♀

O34.33 Maternal care for cervical incompetence, **third trimester** MCC ♂♀

✓5th **O34.4** Maternal care for other abnormalities of cervix

O34.40 Maternal care for other abnormalities of cervix, **unspecified trimester** ♂♀

O34.41 Maternal care for other abnormalities of cervix, **first trimester** ♂♀

O34.42 Maternal care for other abnormalities of cervix, **second trimester** ♂♀

O34.43 Maternal care for other abnormalities of cervix, **third trimester** ♂♀

✓5th **O34.5** Maternal care for other abnormalities of gravid uterus

✓6th **O34.51** Maternal care for incarceration of gravid uterus

O34.511 Maternal care for incarceration of gravid uterus, **first trimester** ♂♀

O34.512 Maternal care for incarceration of gravid uterus, **second trimester** ♂♀

O34.513 Maternal care for incarceration of gravid uterus, **third trimester** ♂♀

O34.519 Maternal care for incarceration of gravid uterus, **unspecified trimester** ♂♀

✓6th **O34.52** Maternal care for prolapse of gravid uterus

O34.521 Maternal care for prolapse of gravid uterus, **first trimester** ♂♀

O34.522 Maternal care for prolapse of gravid uterus, **second trimester** ♂♀

O34.523 Maternal care for prolapse of gravid uterus, **third trimester** ♂♀

O34.529 Maternal care for prolapse of gravid uterus, **unspecified trimester** ♂♀

✓6th **O34.53** Maternal care for retroversion of gravid uterus

O34.531 Maternal care for retroversion of gravid uterus, **first trimester** ♂♀

O34.532 Maternal care for retroversion of gravid uterus, **second trimester** ♂♀

O34.533 Maternal care for retroversion of gravid uterus, **third trimester** ♂♀

O34.539 Maternal care for retroversion of gravid uterus, **unspecified trimester** ♂♀

✓6th **O34.59** Maternal care for other abnormalities of gravid uterus

O34.591 Maternal care for other abnormalities of gravid uterus, **first trimester** ♂♀

O34.592 Maternal care for other abnormalities of gravid uterus, **second trimester** ♂♀

O34.593 Maternal care for other abnormalities of gravid uterus, **third trimester** ♂♀

O34.599 Maternal care for other abnormalities of gravid uterus, **unspecified trimester** ♂♀

✓5th **O34.6** Maternal care for abnormality of vagina
    EXCLUDES 2 maternal care for vaginal varices in pregnancy (O22.1-)

O34.60 Maternal care for abnormality of vagina, **unspecified trimester** ♂♀

O34.61 Maternal care for abnormality of vagina, **first trimester** ♂♀

O34.62 Maternal care for abnormality of vagina, **second trimester** ♂♀

O34.63 Maternal care for abnormality of vagina, **third trimester** ♂♀

✓5th **O34.7** Maternal care for abnormality of vulva and perineum
    EXCLUDES 2 maternal care for perineal and vulval varices in pregnancy (O22.1-)

O34.70 Maternal care for abnormality of vulva and perineum, **unspecified trimester** ♂♀

O34.71 Maternal care for abnormality of vulva and perineum, **first trimester** ♂♀

O34.72 Maternal care for abnormality of vulva and perineum, **second trimester** ♂♀

O34.73 Maternal care for abnormality of vulva and perineum, **third trimester** ♂♀

✓5th **O34.8** Maternal care for other abnormalities of pelvic organs

O34.80 Maternal care for other abnormalities of pelvic organs, **unspecified trimester** ♂♀

O34.81 Maternal care for other abnormalities of pelvic organs, **first trimester** ♂♀

O34.82 Maternal care for other abnormalities of pelvic organs, **second trimester** ♂♀

O34.83 Maternal care for other abnormalities of pelvic organs, **third trimester** ♂♀

✓5th **O34.9** Maternal care for abnormality of pelvic organ, unspecified

O34.90 Maternal care for abnormality of pelvic organ, unspecified, **unspecified trimester** ♂♀

O34.91 Maternal care for abnormality of pelvic organ, unspecified, **first trimester** ♂♀

O34.92 Maternal care for abnormality of pelvic organ, unspecified, **second trimester** ♂♀

O34.93 Maternal care for abnormality of pelvic organ, unspecified, **third trimester** ♂♀

✓4th **O35** Maternal care for known or suspected fetal abnormality and damage
    INCLUDES the listed conditions in the fetus as a reason for hospitalization or other obstetric care to the mother, or for termination of pregnancy
    Code also any associated maternal condition
    EXCLUDES 1 encounter for suspected maternal and fetal conditions ruled out (Z03.7-)

    One of the following 7th characters is to be assigned to each code under category O35. 7th character Ø is for single gestations and multiple gestations where the fetus is unspecified. 7th characters 1 through 9 are for cases of multiple gestations to identify the fetus for which the code applies. The appropriate code from category O30, Multiple gestation, must also be assigned when assigning a code from category O35 that has a 7th character of 1 through 9.
    Ø not applicable or unspecified   3 fetus 3
                                 4 fetus 4
    1 fetus 1   5 fetus 5
    2 fetus 2   9 other fetus

✓x7th **O35.0** Maternal care for (suspected) central nervous system malformation in fetus ♂♀
    Maternal care for fetal anencephaly
    Maternal care for fetal hydrocephalus
    Maternal care for fetal spina bifida
    EXCLUDES 2 chromosomal abnormality in fetus (O35.1)

✓x7th **O35.1** Maternal care for (suspected) chromosomal abnormality in fetus ♂♀

Pregnancy, Childbirth and the Puerperium

O35.2–O36.599

√x7ᵗʰ **O35.2 Maternal care for (suspected)** hereditary disease in fetus Ⓜ♀
    EXCLUDES 2   *chromosomal abnormality in fetus (O35.1)*

√x7ᵗʰ **O35.3 Maternal care for (suspected)** damage to fetus from viral Ⓜ♀
disease in mother
    Maternal care for damage to fetus from maternal
      cytomegalovirus infection
    Maternal care for damage to fetus from maternal rubella

√x7ᵗʰ **O35.4 Maternal care for (suspected)** damage to fetus from Ⓜ♀
alcohol

√x7ᵗʰ **O35.5 Maternal care for (suspected)** damage to fetus by drugs Ⓜ♀
    Maternal care for damage to fetus from drug addiction

√x7ᵗʰ **O35.6 Maternal care for (suspected)** damage to fetus by Ⓜ♀
radiation

√x7ᵗʰ **O35.7 Maternal care for (suspected)** damage to fetus by other Ⓜ♀
medical procedures
    Maternal care for damage to fetus by amniocentesis
    Maternal care for damage to fetus by biopsy procedures
    Maternal care for damage to fetus by hematological
      investigation
    Maternal care for damage to fetus by intrauterine contraceptive
      device
    Maternal care for damage to fetus by intrauterine surgery

√x7ᵗʰ **O35.8 Maternal care for other (suspected)** fetal abnormality Ⓜ♀
and damage
    Maternal care for damage to fetus from maternal listeriosis
    Maternal care for damage to fetus from maternal toxoplasmosis

√x7ᵗʰ **O35.9 Maternal care for (suspected)** fetal abnormality and Ⓜ♀
damage, unspecified

√4ᵗʰ **O36 Maternal care for other fetal problems**
    INCLUDES   the listed conditions in the fetus as a reason for
      hospitalization or other obstetric care of the mother, or
      for termination of pregnancy
    EXCLUDES 1   *encounter for suspected maternal and fetal conditions ruled out*
      (Z03.7-)
      placental transfusion syndromes (O43.0-)
    EXCLUDES 2   *labor and delivery complicated by fetal stress (O77.-)*

> One of the following 7th characters is to be assigned to each code
> under category O36. 7th character Ø is for single gestations and
> multiple gestations where the fetus is unspecified. 7th characters 1
> through 9 are for cases of multiple gestations to identify the fetus for
> which the code applies. The appropriate code from category O30,
> Multiple gestation, must also be assigned when assigning a code
> from category O36 that has a 7th character of 1 through 9.
>
> | | | | |
> |---|---|---|---|
> | Ø | not applicable or | 3 | fetus 3 |
> | | unspecified | 4 | fetus 4 |
> | 1 | fetus 1 | 5 | fetus 5 |
> | 2 | fetus 2 | 9 | other fetus |

√5ᵗʰ **O36.Ø Maternal care for rhesus isoimmunization**
    Maternal care for Rh incompatibility (with hydrops fetalis)

> **CC Excl: For CC codes in subcategory O36.Ø, unless
> otherwise noted:** O36.Ø11Ø–O36.Ø139, O36.Ø91Ø–
> O36.Ø939

√6ᵗʰ **O36.Ø1 Maternal care for** anti-D [Rh] antibodies
    √7ᵗʰ **O36.Ø11 Maternal care for anti-D [Rh]** ⒸⒸⓂ♀
      antibodies, first trimester
    √7ᵗʰ **O36.Ø12 Maternal care for anti-D [Rh]** ⒸⒸⓂ♀
      antibodies, second trimester
    √7ᵗʰ **O36.Ø13 Maternal care for anti-D [Rh]** ⒸⒸⓂ♀
      antibodies, third trimester
    √7ᵗʰ **O36.Ø19 Maternal care for anti-D [Rh]** Ⓜ♀
      antibodies, unspecified trimester

√6ᵗʰ **O36.Ø9 Maternal care for** other rhesus isoimmunization
    √7ᵗʰ **O36.Ø91 Maternal care for other rhesus** ⒸⒸⓂ♀
      isoimmunization, first trimester
    √7ᵗʰ **O36.Ø92 Maternal care for other rhesus** ⒸⒸⓂ♀
      isoimmunization, second trimester
    √7ᵗʰ **O36.Ø93 Maternal care for other rhesus** ⒸⒸⓂ♀
      isoimmunization, third trimester
    √7ᵗʰ **O36.Ø99 Maternal care for other rhesus** Ⓜ♀
      isoimmunization, unspecified trimester

√5ᵗʰ **O36.1 Maternal care for other isoimmunization**
    Maternal care for ABO isoimmunization
    √6ᵗʰ **O36.11 Maternal care for** Anti-A sensitization
      Maternal care for isoimmunization NOS (with hydrops
       fetalis)
      √7ᵗʰ **O36.111 Maternal care for Anti-A sensitization,** Ⓜ♀
        first trimester

√7ᵗʰ **O36.112 Maternal care for Anti-A sensitization,** Ⓜ♀
    second trimester

√7ᵗʰ **O36.113 Maternal care for Anti-A sensitization,** Ⓜ♀
    third trimester

√7ᵗʰ **O36.119 Maternal care for Anti-A sensitization,** Ⓜ♀
    unspecified trimester

√6ᵗʰ **O36.19 Maternal care for** other isoimmunization
    Maternal care for Anti-B sensitization
    √7ᵗʰ **O36.191 Maternal care for other** Ⓜ♀
      isoimmunization, first trimester
    √7ᵗʰ **O36.192 Maternal care for other** Ⓜ♀
      isoimmunization, second trimester
    √7ᵗʰ **O36.193 Maternal care for other** Ⓜ♀
      isoimmunization, third trimester
    √7ᵗʰ **O36.199 Maternal care for other** Ⓜ♀
      isoimmunization, unspecified trimester

√5ᵗʰ **O36.2 Maternal care for hydrops fetalis**
    Maternal care for hydrops fetalis NOS
    Maternal care for hydrops fetalis not associated with
      isoimmunization
    EXCLUDES 1   *hydrops fetalis associated with ABO isoimmunization*
      (O36.1-)
      hydrops fetalis associated with rhesus isoimmunization
      (O36.Ø-)

√x7ᵗʰ **O36.2Ø Maternal care for hydrops fetalis, unspecified** Ⓜ♀
    trimester

√x7ᵗʰ **O36.21 Maternal care for hydrops fetalis, first** Ⓜ♀
    trimester

√x7ᵗʰ **O36.22 Maternal care for hydrops fetalis, second** Ⓜ♀
    trimester

√x7ᵗʰ **O36.23 Maternal care for hydrops fetalis, third** Ⓜ♀
    trimester

√x7ᵗʰ **O36.4 Maternal care for intrauterine death** ⒸⒸⓂ♀
    Maternal care for intrauterine fetal death NOS
    Maternal care for intrauterine fetal death after completion of 2Ø
      weeks of gestation
    Maternal care for late fetal death
    Maternal care for missed delivery
    EXCLUDES 1   *missed abortion (O02.1)*
      stillbirth (P95)
    CC Excl: O36.4XXØ–O36.4XX9

√5ᵗʰ **O36.5 Maternal care for known or suspected poor fetal growth**

> **CC Excl: For CC codes in subcategory O36.5, unless
> otherwise noted:** O36.511Ø–O36.5139, O36.591Ø–
> O36.5939

√6ᵗʰ **O36.51 Maternal care for known or suspected placental**
insufficiency
    √7ᵗʰ **O36.511 Maternal care for known or** Ⓜ♀
      suspected placental insufficiency, first
      trimester
    √7ᵗʰ **O36.512 Maternal care for known or** Ⓜ♀
      suspected placental insufficiency, second
      trimester
    √7ᵗʰ **O36.513 Maternal care for known or** Ⓜ♀
      suspected placental insufficiency, third
      trimester
    √7ᵗʰ **O36.519 Maternal care for known or suspected** Ⓜ♀
      placental insufficiency, unspecified
      trimester

√6ᵗʰ **O36.59 Maternal care for other known or suspected poor**
fetal growth
    Maternal care for known or suspected light-for-dates
      NOS
    Maternal care for known or suspected small-for-dates
      NOS
    √7ᵗʰ **O36.591 Maternal care for other known or** Ⓜ♀
      suspected poor fetal growth, first
      trimester
    √7ᵗʰ **O36.592 Maternal care for other known or** Ⓜ♀
      suspected poor fetal growth, second
      trimester
    √7ᵗʰ **O36.593 Maternal care for other known or** Ⓜ♀
      suspected poor fetal growth, third
      trimester
    √7ᵗʰ **O36.599 Maternal care for other known or** Ⓜ♀
      suspected poor fetal growth,
      unspecified trimester

Ⓝ Newborn: Ø   Ⓟ Pediatric: Ø-17   Ⓜ Maternity: 12-55   Ⓐ Adult: 15-124   ᴹᶜᶜ Major CC Condition   ᴾᴰˣ ᴹᶜᶜ PDx acts as own MCC   ⒸⒸ CC Condition   ᴾᴰˣ ᶜᶜ PDx acts as own CC

798   ICD-10-CM Draft (2015)

√5ᵗʰ **O36.6 Maternal care for excessive fetal growth**
Maternal care for known or suspected large-for-dates

√x7ᵗʰ **O36.60 Maternal care for excessive fetal growth, unspecified trimester**   M ♀

√x7ᵗʰ **O36.61 Maternal care for excessive fetal growth, first trimester**   M ♀

√x7ᵗʰ **O36.62 Maternal care for excessive fetal growth, second trimester**   M ♀

√x7ᵗʰ **O36.63 Maternal care for excessive fetal growth, third trimester**   M ♀

√5ᵗʰ **O36.7 Maternal care for viable fetus in abdominal pregnancy**

√x7ᵗʰ **O36.70 Maternal care for viable fetus in abdominal pregnancy, unspecified trimester**   M ♀

√x7ᵗʰ **O36.71 Maternal care for viable fetus in abdominal pregnancy, first trimester**   M ♀

√x7ᵗʰ **O36.72 Maternal care for viable fetus in abdominal pregnancy, second trimester**   M ♀

√x7ᵗʰ **O36.73 Maternal care for viable fetus in abdominal pregnancy, third trimester**   M ♀

√5ᵗʰ **O36.8 Maternal care for other specified fetal problems**

√x7ᵗʰ **O36.80 Pregnancy with inconclusive fetal viability**   M ♀
Encounter to determine fetal viability of pregnancy

√6ᵗʰ **O36.81 Decreased fetal movements**

√7ᵗʰ **O36.812 Decreased fetal movements, second trimester**   M ♀

√7ᵗʰ **O36.813 Decreased fetal movements, third trimester**   M ♀

√7ᵗʰ **O36.819 Decreased fetal movements, unspecified trimester**   M ♀

√6ᵗʰ **O36.82 Fetal anemia and thrombocytopenia**

√7ᵗʰ **O36.821 Fetal anemia and thrombocytopenia, first trimester**   M ♀

√7ᵗʰ **O36.822 Fetal anemia and thrombocytopenia, second trimester**   M ♀

√7ᵗʰ **O36.823 Fetal anemia and thrombocytopenia, third trimester**   M ♀

√7ᵗʰ **O36.829 Fetal anemia and thrombocytopenia, unspecified trimester**   M ♀

√6ᵗʰ **O36.89 Maternal care for other specified fetal problems**

√7ᵗʰ **O36.891 Maternal care for other specified fetal problems, first trimester**   M ♀

√7ᵗʰ **O36.892 Maternal care for other specified fetal problems, second trimester**   M ♀

√7ᵗʰ **O36.893 Maternal care for other specified fetal problems, third trimester**   M ♀

√7ᵗʰ **O36.899 Maternal care for other specified fetal problems, unspecified trimester**   M ♀

√5ᵗʰ **O36.9 Maternal care for fetal problem, unspecified**

√x7ᵗʰ **O36.90 Maternal care for fetal problem, unspecified, unspecified trimester**   M ♀

√x7ᵗʰ **O36.91 Maternal care for fetal problem, unspecified, first trimester**   M ♀

√x7ᵗʰ **O36.92 Maternal care for fetal problem, unspecified, second trimester**   M ♀

√x7ᵗʰ **O36.93 Maternal care for fetal problem, unspecified, third trimester**   M ♀

√4ᵗʰ **O40 Polyhydramnios**
Hydramnios
EXCLUDES1 encounter for suspected maternal and fetal conditions ruled out (Z03.7-)

One of the following 7th characters is to be assigned to each code under category O40. 7th character 0 is for single gestations and multiple gestations where the fetus is unspecified. 7th characters 1 through 9 are for cases of multiple gestations to identify the fetus for which the code applies. The appropriate code from category O30, Multiple gestation, must also be assigned when assigning a code from category O40 that has a 7th character of 1 through 9.
0	not applicable or unspecified	3	fetus 3
		4	fetus 4
1	fetus 1	5	fetus 5
2	fetus 2	9	other fetus

√x7ᵗʰ **O40.1 Polyhydramnios, first trimester**   M ♀

√x7ᵗʰ **O40.2 Polyhydramnios, second trimester**   M ♀

√x7ᵗʰ **O40.3 Polyhydramnios, third trimester**   M ♀

√x7ᵗʰ **O40.9 Polyhydramnios, unspecified trimester**   M ♀

√4ᵗʰ **O41 Other disorders of amniotic fluid and membranes**
EXCLUDES1 encounter for suspected maternal and fetal conditions ruled out (Z03.7-)

One of the following 7th characters is to be assigned to each code under category O41. 7th character 0 is for single gestations and multiple gestations where the fetus is unspecified. 7th characters 1 through 9 are for cases of multiple gestations to identify the fetus for which the code applies. The appropriate code from category O30, Multiple gestation, must also be assigned when assigning a code from category O41 that has a 7th character of 1 through 9.
0	not applicable or unspecified	3	fetus 3
		4	fetus 4
1	fetus 1	5	fetus 5
2	fetus 2	9	other fetus

√5ᵗʰ **O41.0 Oligohydramnios**
Oligohydramnios without rupture of membranes

CC Excl: For CC codes in subcategory O41.0, unless otherwise noted: O41.01X0-O41.03X9

√x7ᵗʰ **O41.00 Oligohydramnios, unspecified trimester**   M ♀

√x7ᵗʰ **O41.01 Oligohydramnios, first trimester**   CC M ♀

√x7ᵗʰ **O41.02 Oligohydramnios, second trimester**   CC M ♀

√x7ᵗʰ **O41.03 Oligohydramnios, third trimester**   CC M ♀

√5ᵗʰ **O41.1 Infection of amniotic sac and membranes**

CC Excl: For MCC codes in subcategory O41.1, unless otherwise noted: O41.1010-O41.1039, O41.1210-O41.1239, O41.1410-O41.1439

√6ᵗʰ **O41.10 Infection of amniotic sac and membranes, unspecified**

√7ᵗʰ **O41.101 Infection of amniotic sac and membranes, unspecified, first trimester**   MCC M ♀

√7ᵗʰ **O41.102 Infection of amniotic sac and membranes, unspecified, second trimester**   MCC M ♀

√7ᵗʰ **O41.103 Infection of amniotic sac and membranes, unspecified, third trimester**   MCC M ♀

√7ᵗʰ **O41.109 Infection of amniotic sac and membranes, unspecified, unspecified trimester**   M ♀

√6ᵗʰ **O41.12 Chorioamnionitis**

√7ᵗʰ **O41.121 Chorioamnionitis, first trimester**   MCC M ♀

√7ᵗʰ **O41.122 Chorioamnionitis, second trimester**   MCC M ♀

√7ᵗʰ **O41.123 Chorioamnionitis, third trimester**   MCC M ♀

√7ᵗʰ **O41.129 Chorioamnionitis, unspecified trimester**   M ♀

√6ᵗʰ **O41.14 Placentitis**

√7ᵗʰ **O41.141 Placentitis, first trimester**   MCC M ♀

√7ᵗʰ **O41.142 Placentitis, second trimester**   MCC M ♀

√7ᵗʰ **O41.143 Placentitis, third trimester**   MCC M ♀

√7ᵗʰ **O41.149 Placentitis, unspecified trimester**   M ♀

√5ᵗʰ **O41.8 Other specified disorders of amniotic fluid and membranes**

CC Excl: For CC codes in subcategory O41.8, unless otherwise noted: O41.8X10-O41.8X39

√6ᵗʰ **O41.8X Other specified disorders of amniotic fluid and membranes**

√7ᵗʰ **O41.8X1 Other specified disorders of amniotic fluid and membranes, first trimester**   M ♀

√7ᵗʰ **O41.8X2 Other specified disorders of amniotic fluid and membranes, second trimester**   M ♀

√7ᵗʰ **O41.8X3 Other specified disorders of amniotic fluid and membranes, third trimester**   M ♀

√7ᵗʰ **O41.8X9 Other specified disorders of amniotic fluid and membranes, unspecified trimester**   M ♀

√5ᵗʰ **O41.9 Disorder of amniotic fluid and membranes, unspecified**

√x7ᵗʰ **O41.90 Disorder of amniotic fluid and membranes, unspecified, unspecified trimester**   M ♀

√ Additional Character Required   √x7ᵗʰ Xtension Alert   Unacceptable PDx   Manifestation   Hospital Acquired Condition   EXCLUDES1 Not Coded Here   EXCLUDES2 Not Included Here

Pregnancy, Childbirth and the Puerperium

O41.91–O43.199

√x7ᵗʰ **O41.91** **Disorder of amniotic fluid and membranes, unspecified, first trimester** Ⓜ♀

√x7ᵗʰ **O41.92** **Disorder of amniotic fluid and membranes, unspecified, second trimester** Ⓜ♀

√x7ᵗʰ **O41.93** **Disorder of amniotic fluid and membranes, unspecified, third trimester** Ⓜ♀

√4ᵗʰ **O42** **Premature rupture of membranes**

√5ᵗʰ **O42.0** **Premature rupture of membranes, onset of labor within 24 hours of rupture**

O42.00 **Premature rupture of membranes, onset of labor within 24 hours of rupture, unspecified weeks of gestation** Ⓜ♀

√6ᵗʰ **O42.01** **Preterm premature rupture of membranes, onset of labor within 24 hours of rupture**
Premature rupture of membranes before 37 completed weeks of gestation

O42.011 **Preterm premature rupture of membranes, onset of labor within 24 hours of rupture, first trimester** Ⓜ♀

O42.012 **Preterm premature rupture of membranes, onset of labor within 24 hours of rupture, second trimester** Ⓜ♀

O42.013 **Preterm premature rupture of membranes, onset of labor within 24 hours of rupture, third trimester** Ⓜ♀

O42.019 **Preterm premature rupture of membranes, onset of labor within 24 hours of rupture, unspecified trimester** Ⓜ♀

O42.02 **Full-term premature rupture of membranes, onset of labor within 24 hours of rupture** Ⓜ♀
Premature rupture of membranes after 37 completed weeks of gestation

√5ᵗʰ **O42.1** **Premature rupture of membranes, onset of labor more than 24 hours following rupture**

O42.10 **Premature rupture of membranes, onset of labor more than 24 hours following rupture, unspecified weeks of gestation** Ⓜ♀

√6ᵗʰ **O42.11** **Preterm premature rupture of membranes, onset of labor more than 24 hours following rupture**
Premature rupture of membranes before 37 completed weeks of gestation

O42.111 **Preterm premature rupture of membranes, onset of labor more than 24 hours following rupture, first trimester** Ⓜ♀

O42.112 **Preterm premature rupture of membranes, onset of labor more than 24 hours following rupture, second trimester** Ⓜ♀

O42.113 **Preterm premature rupture of membranes, onset of labor more than 24 hours following rupture, third trimester** Ⓜ♀

O42.119 **Preterm premature rupture of membranes, onset of labor more than 24 hours following rupture, unspecified trimester** Ⓜ♀

O42.12 **Full-term premature rupture of membranes, onset of labor more than 24 hours following rupture** Ⓜ♀
Premature rupture of membranes after 37 completed weeks of gestation

√5ᵗʰ **O42.9** **Premature rupture of membranes, unspecified as to length of time between rupture and onset of labor**

O42.90 **Premature rupture of membranes, unspecified as to length of time between rupture and onset of labor, unspecified weeks of gestation** Ⓜ♀

√6ᵗʰ **O42.91** **Preterm premature rupture of membranes, unspecified as to length of time between rupture and onset of labor**
Premature rupture of membranes before 37 completed weeks of gestation

O42.911 **Preterm premature rupture of membranes, unspecified as to length of time between rupture and onset of labor, first trimester** Ⓜ♀

O42.912 **Preterm premature rupture of membranes, unspecified as to length of time between rupture and onset of abor, second trimester** Ⓜ♀

O42.913 **Preterm premature rupture of membranes, unspecified as to length of time between rupture and onset of labor, third trimester** Ⓜ♀

O42.919 **Preterm premature rupture of membranes, unspecified as to length of time between rupture and onset of labor, unspecified trimester** Ⓜ♀

O42.92 **Full-term premature rupture of membranes, unspecified as to length of time between rupture and onset of labor** Ⓜ♀
Premature rupture of membranes after 37 completed weeks of gestation

√4ᵗʰ **O43** **Placental disorders**

EXCLUDES 2   maternal care for poor fetal growth due to placental insufficiency (O36.5-)
placenta previa (O44.-)
placental polyp (O90.89)
placentitis (O41.14-)
premature separation of placenta [abruptio placentae] (O45.-)

√5ᵗʰ **O43.0** **Placental transfusion syndromes**

√6ᵗʰ **O43.01** **Fetomaternal placental transfusion syndrome**
Maternofetal placental transfusion syndrome

O43.011 **Fetomaternal placental transfusion syndrome, first trimester** Ⓜ♀

O43.012 **Fetomaternal placental transfusion syndrome, second trimester** Ⓜ♀

O43.013 **Fetomaternal placental transfusion syndrome, third trimester** Ⓜ♀

O43.019 **Fetomaternal placental transfusion syndrome, unspecified trimester** Ⓜ♀

√6ᵗʰ **O43.02** **Fetus-to-fetus placental transfusion syndrome**

O43.021 **Fetus-to-fetus placental transfusion syndrome, first trimester** Ⓜ♀

O43.022 **Fetus-to-fetus placental transfusion syndrome, second trimester** Ⓜ♀

O43.023 **Fetus-to-fetus placental transfusion syndrome, third trimester** Ⓜ♀

O43.029 **Fetus-to-fetus placental transfusion syndrome, unspecified trimester** Ⓜ♀

√5ᵗʰ **O43.1** **Malformation of placenta**

√6ᵗʰ **O43.10** **Malformation of placenta, unspecified**
Abnormal placenta NOS

O43.101 **Malformation of placenta, unspecified, first trimester** Ⓜ♀

O43.102 **Malformation of placenta, unspecified, second trimester** Ⓜ♀

O43.103 **Malformation of placenta, unspecified, third trimester** Ⓜ♀

O43.109 **Malformation of placenta, unspecified, unspecified trimester** Ⓜ♀

√6ᵗʰ **O43.11** **Circumvallate placenta**

O43.111 **Circumvallate placenta, first trimester** Ⓜ♀

O43.112 **Circumvallate placenta, second trimester** Ⓜ♀

O43.113 **Circumvallate placenta, third trimester** Ⓜ♀

O43.119 **Circumvallate placenta, unspecified trimester** Ⓜ♀

√6ᵗʰ **O43.12** **Velamentous insertion of umbilical cord**

O43.121 **Velamentous insertion of umbilical cord, first trimester** Ⓜ♀

O43.122 **Velamentous insertion of umbilical cord, second trimester** Ⓜ♀

O43.123 **Velamentous insertion of umbilical cord, third trimester** Ⓜ♀

O43.129 **Velamentous insertion of umbilical cord, unspecified trimester** Ⓜ♀

√6ᵗʰ **O43.19** **Other malformation of placenta**

O43.191 **Other malformation of placenta, first trimester** Ⓜ♀

O43.192 **Other malformation of placenta, second trimester** Ⓜ♀

O43.193 **Other malformation of placenta, third trimester** Ⓜ♀

O43.199 **Other malformation of placenta, unspecified trimester** Ⓜ♀

√5ᵗʰ **O43.2 Morbidly adherent placenta**
Code also associated third stage postpartum hemorrhage, if applicable (O72.0)
EXCLUDES 1 retained placenta (O73.-)

√6ᵗʰ **O43.21 Placenta accreta**
O43.211 **Placenta accreta, first trimester** M♀
O43.212 **Placenta accreta, second trimester** M♀
O43.213 **Placenta accreta, third trimester** M♀
O43.219 **Placenta accreta, unspecified trimester** M♀

√6ᵗʰ **O43.22 Placenta increta**
O43.221 **Placenta increta, first trimester** M♀
O43.222 **Placenta increta, second trimester** M♀
O43.223 **Placenta increta, third trimester** M♀
O43.229 **Placenta increta, unspecified trimester** M♀

√6ᵗʰ **O43.23 Placenta percreta**
O43.231 **Placenta percreta, first trimester** M♀
O43.232 **Placenta percreta, second trimester** M♀
O43.233 **Placenta percreta, third trimester** M♀
O43.239 **Placenta percreta, unspecified trimester** M♀

√5ᵗʰ **O43.8 Other placental disorders**

√6ᵗʰ **O43.81 Placental infarction**
O43.811 **Placental infarction, first trimester** M♀
O43.812 **Placental infarction, second trimester** M♀
O43.813 **Placental infarction, third trimester** M♀
O43.819 **Placental infarction, unspecified trimester** M♀

√6ᵗʰ **O43.89 Other placental disorders**
Placental dysfunction
O43.891 **Other placental disorders, first trimester** M♀
O43.892 **Other placental disorders, second trimester** M♀
O43.893 **Other placental disorders, third trimester** M♀
O43.899 **Other placental disorders, unspecified trimester** M♀

√5ᵗʰ **O43.9 Unspecified placental disorder**
O43.90 **Unspecified placental disorder, unspecified trimester** M♀
O43.91 **Unspecified placental disorder, first trimester** M♀
O43.92 **Unspecified placental disorder, second trimester** M♀
O43.93 **Unspecified placental disorder, third trimester** M♀

√4ᵗʰ **O44 Placenta previa**

CC Excl: For CC/MCC codes in category O44, unless otherwise noted: O20.0-O20.9, O25.10-O25.3, O26.10-O26.13, O26.30-O26.43, O26.63-O26.819, O26.841-O26.86, O26.891-O26.93, O29.011-O29.93, O35.7XX0-O35.7XX9, O44.00-O44.13, O75.4, O75.81, O75.89-O75.9, O80, O90.89, O99.111-O99.285, O99.330-O99.335, O99.350-O99.355, O99.511-O99.73, O99.820-O99.825, O99.840-O9A.53

√5ᵗʰ **O44.0 Placenta previa specified as without hemorrhage**
Low implantation of placenta specified as without hemorrhage
O44.00 **Placenta previa specified as without hemorrhage, unspecified trimester** M♀
O44.01 **Placenta previa specified as without hemorrhage, first trimester** CC M♀
O44.02 **Placenta previa specified as without hemorrhage, second trimester** CC M♀
O44.03 **Placenta previa specified as without hemorrhage, third trimester** CC M♀

√5ᵗʰ **O44.1 Placenta previa with hemorrhage**
Low implantation of placenta, NOS or with hemorrhage
Marginal placenta previa, NOS or with hemorrhage
Partial placenta previa, NOS or with hemorrhage
Total placenta previa, NOS or with hemorrhage
EXCLUDES 1 labor and delivery complicated by hemorrhage from vasa previa (O69.4)
O44.10 **Placenta previa with hemorrhage, unspecified trimester** M♀
O44.11 **Placenta previa with hemorrhage, first trimester** MCC M♀

O44.12 **Placenta previa with hemorrhage, second trimester** MCC M♀
O44.13 **Placenta previa with hemorrhage, third trimester** MCC M♀

√4ᵗʰ **O45 Premature separation of placenta [abruptio placentae]**

√5ᵗʰ **O45.0 Premature separation of placenta with coagulation defect**

CC Excl: For MCC codes in subcategory O45.0, unless otherwise noted: O25.10-O25.3, O26.10-O26.13, O26.30-O26.43, O26.63-O26.819, O26.841-O26.86, O26.891-O26.93, O29.011-O29.93, O35.7XX0-O35.7XX9, O45.001-O45.099, O46.001-O46.93, O67.0-O67.9, O75.4, O75.81, O75.89-O75.9, O80, O90.89, O99.111-O99.285, O99.330-O99.335, O99.350-O99.355, O99.511-O99.73, O99.820-O99.825, O99.840-O9A.53

√6ᵗʰ **O45.00 Premature separation of placenta with coagulation defect, unspecified**
O45.001 **Premature separation of placenta with coagulation defect, unspecified, first trimester** MCC M♀
O45.002 **Premature separation of placenta with coagulation defect, unspecified, second trimester** MCC M♀
O45.003 **Premature separation of placenta with coagulation defect, unspecified, third trimester** MCC M♀
O45.009 **Premature separation of placenta with coagulation defect, unspecified, unspecified trimester** M♀

√6ᵗʰ **O45.01 Premature separation of placenta with afibrinogenemia**
Premature separation of placenta with hypofibrinogenemia
O45.011 **Premature separation of placenta with afibrinogenemia, first trimester** MCC M♀
O45.012 **Premature separation of placenta with afibrinogenemia, second trimester** MCC M♀
O45.013 **Premature separation of placenta with afibrinogenemia, third trimester** MCC M♀
O45.019 **Premature separation of placenta with afibrinogenemia, unspecified trimester** M♀

√6ᵗʰ **O45.02 Premature separation of placenta with disseminated intravascular coagulation**
O45.021 **Premature separation of placenta with disseminated intravascular coagulation, first trimester** MCC M♀
O45.022 **Premature separation of placenta with disseminated intravascular coagulation, second trimester** MCC M♀
O45.023 **Premature separation of placenta with disseminated intravascular coagulation, third trimester** MCC M♀
O45.029 **Premature separation of placenta with disseminated intravascular coagulation, unspecified trimester** M♀

√6ᵗʰ **O45.09 Premature separation of placenta with other coagulation defect**
O45.091 **Premature separation of placenta with other coagulation defect, first trimester** MCC M♀
O45.092 **Premature separation of placenta with other coagulation defect, second trimester** MCC M♀
O45.093 **Premature separation of placenta with other coagulation defect, third trimester** MCC M♀
O45.099 **Premature separation of placenta with other coagulation defect, unspecified trimester** M♀

√ Additional Character Required   √x7ᵗʰ Xtension Alert   Unacceptable PDx   Manifestation   Hospital Acquired Condition   EXCLUDES 1 Not Coded Here   EXCLUDES 2 Not Included Here

Pregnancy, Childbirth and the Puerperium

O45.8–O60.03

✓5th **O45.8** Other premature separation of placenta

> CC Excl: For MCC codes in subcategory O45.8, unless otherwise noted: O20.0–O20.9, O25.10–O25.3, O26.10–O26.13, O26.30–O26.43, O26.63–O26.819, O26.841–O26.86, O26.891–O26.93, O29.011–O29.93, O35.7XX0–O35.7XX9, O44.00–O44.13, O45.8X1–O45.8X3, O45.91–O45.93, O75.4, O75.81, O75.89–O75.9, O80, O90.89, O99.111–O99.285, O99.330–O99.335, O99.350–O99.355, O99.511–O99.73, O99.820–O99.825, O99.840–O9A.53

   ✓6th **O45.8X** Other premature separation of placenta

     O45.8X1 Other premature separation of placenta, **first trimester**   MCC M♀

     O45.8X2 Other premature separation of placenta, **second trimester**   MCC M♀

     O45.8X3 Other premature separation of placenta, **third trimester**   MCC M♀

     O45.8X9 Other premature separation of placenta, **unspecified trimester**   M♀

✓5th **O45.9** Premature separation of placenta, **unspecified**
     Abruptio placentae NOS

> CC Excl: For MCC codes in subcategory O45.9, unless otherwise noted: See code: O45.8

   O45.90 Premature separation of placenta, unspecified, **unspecified trimester**   M♀

   O45.91 Premature separation of placenta, unspecified, **first trimester**   MCC M♀

   O45.92 Premature separation of placenta, unspecified, **second trimester**   MCC M♀

   O45.93 Premature separation of placenta, unspecified, **third trimester**   MCC M♀

✓4th **O46** Antepartum hemorrhage, not elsewhere classified

> EXCLUDES 1   hemorrhage in early pregnancy (O20.-)
> intrapartum hemorrhage NEC (O67.-)
> placenta previa (O44.-)
> premature separation of placenta [abruptio placentae] (O45.-)

✓5th **O46.0** Antepartum hemorrhage with **coagulation defect**

> CC Excl: For MCC codes in subcategory O46.0, unless otherwise noted: See code: O45.0

   ✓6th **O46.00** Antepartum hemorrhage with coagulation defect, **unspecified**

     O46.001 Antepartum hemorrhage with coagulation defect, unspecified, **first trimester**   MCC M♀

     O46.002 Antepartum hemorrhage with coagulation defect, unspecified, **second trimester**   MCC M♀

     O46.003 Antepartum hemorrhage with coagulation defect, unspecified, **third trimester**   MCC M♀

     O46.009 Antepartum hemorrhage with coagulation defect, unspecified, **unspecified trimester**   M♀

   ✓6th **O46.01** Antepartum hemorrhage with **afibrinogenemia**
     Antepartum hemorrhage with hypofibrinogenemia

     O46.011 Antepartum hemorrhage with **afibrinogenemia, first trimester**   MCC M♀

     O46.012 Antepartum hemorrhage with **afibrinogenemia, second trimester**   MCC M♀

     O46.013 Antepartum hemorrhage with **afibrinogenemia, third trimester**   MCC M♀

     O46.019 Antepartum hemorrhage with **afibrinogenemia, unspecified trimester**   M♀

   ✓6th **O46.02** Antepartum hemorrhage with **disseminated intravascular coagulation**

     O46.021 Antepartum hemorrhage with **disseminated intravascular coagulation, first trimester**   MCC M♀

     O46.022 Antepartum hemorrhage with **disseminated intravascular coagulation, second trimester**   MCC M♀

     O46.023 Antepartum hemorrhage with **disseminated intravascular coagulation, third trimester**   MCC M♀

     O46.029 Antepartum hemorrhage with **disseminated intravascular coagulation, unspecified trimester**   M♀

✓6th **O46.09** Antepartum hemorrhage with **other coagulation defect**

   O46.091 Antepartum hemorrhage with other coagulation defect, **first trimester**   MCC M♀

   O46.092 Antepartum hemorrhage with other coagulation defect, **second trimester**   MCC M♀

   O46.093 Antepartum hemorrhage with other coagulation defect, **third trimester**   MCC M♀

   O46.099 Antepartum hemorrhage with other coagulation defect, **unspecified trimester**   M♀

✓5th **O46.8** Other antepartum hemorrhage

   ✓6th **O46.8X** Other antepartum hemorrhage

     O46.8X1 Other antepartum hemorrhage, **first trimester**   M♀

     O46.8X2 Other antepartum hemorrhage, **second trimester**   M♀

     O46.8X3 Other antepartum hemorrhage, **third trimester**   M♀

     O46.8X9 Other antepartum hemorrhage, **unspecified trimester**   M♀

✓5th **O46.9** Antepartum hemorrhage, **unspecified**

   O46.90 Antepartum hemorrhage, unspecified, **unspecified trimester**   M♀

   O46.91 Antepartum hemorrhage, unspecified, **first trimester**   M♀

   O46.92 Antepartum hemorrhage, unspecified, **second trimester**   M♀

   O46.93 Antepartum hemorrhage, unspecified, **third trimester**   M♀

✓4th **O47** False labor

   Braxton Hicks contractions   Threatened labor
> EXCLUDES 1   preterm labor (O60.-)

> CC Excl: For CC codes in catagory O47, unless otherwise noted: O25.10–O25.3, O26.10–O26.13, O26.30–O26.43, O26.63–O26.819, O26.841–O26.86, O26.891–O26.93, O29.011–O29.93, O35.7XX0–O35.7XX9, O47.00–O47.9, O60.00–O60.23, O75.4, O75.81, O75.89–O75.9, O80, O90.89, O99.111–O99.285, O99.330–O99.335, O99.350–O99.355, O99.511–O99.73, O99.820–O99.825, O99.840–O9A.53

   ✓5th **O47.0** False labor before 37 completed weeks of gestation

     O47.00 False labor before 37 completed weeks of gestation, **unspecified trimester**   M♀

     O47.02 False labor before 37 completed weeks of gestation, **second trimester**   CC M♀

     O47.03 False labor before 37 completed weeks of gestation, **third trimester**   CC M♀

   O47.1 False labor at or after 37 completed weeks of gestation   CC M♀

   O47.9 False labor, **unspecified**   M♀

✓4th **O48** Late pregnancy

   O48.0 Post-term pregnancy   M♀
     Pregnancy over 40 completed weeks to 42 completed weeks gestation

   O48.1 Prolonged pregnancy   M♀
     Pregnancy which has advanced beyond 42 completed weeks gestation

Complications of labor and delivery (O60-O77)

✓4th **O60** Preterm labor

> INCLUDES   onset (spontaneous) of labor before 37 completed weeks of gestation
> EXCLUDES 1   false labor (O47.0-)
> threatened labor NOS (O47.0-)

> CC Excl: For CC/MCC codes in category O60, unless otherwise noted: See code: O47

   ✓5th **O60.0** Preterm labor without delivery

     O60.00 Preterm labor without delivery, **unspecified trimester**   M♀

     O60.02 Preterm labor without delivery, **second trimester**   MCC M♀

     O60.03 Preterm labor without delivery, **third trimester**   MCC M♀

N Newborn: 0   P Pediatric: 0-17   M Maternity: 12-55   A Adult: 15-124   MCC Major CC Condition   PDx MCC PDx acts as own MCC   CC CC Condition   PDx CC PDx acts as own CC

802   ICD-10-CM Draft (2015)

☑5ᵗʰ **O60.1 Preterm labor with preterm delivery**

> One of the following 7th characters is to be assigned to each code under subcategory O60.1. 7th character Ø is for single gestations and multiple gestations where the fetus is unspecified. 7th characters 1 through 9 are for cases of multiple gestations to identify the fetus for which the code applies. The appropriate code from category O30, Multiple gestation, must also be assigned when assigning a code from subcategory O60.1 that has a 7th character of 1 through 9.
>
> | Ø | not applicable or | 3 | fetus 3 |
> |---|---|---|---|
> | | unspecified | 4 | fetus 4 |
> | 1 | fetus 1 | 5 | fetus 5 |
> | 2 | fetus 2 | 9 | other fetus |

  ☑x7ᵗʰ **O60.10 Preterm labor with preterm delivery,**   cc M♀
        unspecified trimester
        Preterm labor with delivery NOS

  ☑x7ᵗʰ **O60.12 Preterm labor second trimester with**   mcc M♀
        preterm delivery second trimester

  ☑x7ᵗʰ **O60.13 Preterm labor second trimester with**   mcc M♀
        preterm delivery third trimester

  ☑x7ᵗʰ **O60.14 Preterm labor third trimester with preterm**   mcc M♀
        delivery third trimester

☑5ᵗʰ **O60.2 Term delivery with preterm labor**

> One of the following 7th characters is to be assigned to each code under subcategory O60.2. 7th character Ø is for single gestations and multiple gestations where the fetus is unspecified. 7th characters 1 through 9 are for cases of multiple gestations to identify the fetus for which the code applies. The appropriate code from category O30, Multiple gestation, must also be assigned when assigning a code from subcategory O60.2 that has a 7th character of 1 through 9.
>
> | Ø | not applicable or | 3 | fetus 3 |
> |---|---|---|---|
> | | unspecified | 4 | fetus 4 |
> | 1 | fetus 1 | 5 | fetus 5 |
> | 2 | fetus 2 | 9 | other fetus |

  ☑x7ᵗʰ **O60.20 Term delivery with preterm labor,**   cc M♀
        unspecified trimester

  ☑x7ᵗʰ **O60.22 Term delivery with preterm labor, second**   mcc M♀
        trimester

  ☑x7ᵗʰ **O60.23 Term delivery with preterm labor, third**   mcc M♀
        trimester

☑4ᵗʰ **O61 Failed induction of labor**

  O61.0 Failed medical induction of labor   M♀
      Failed induction (of labor) by oxytocin
      Failed induction (of labor) by prostaglandins

  O61.1 Failed instrumental induction of labor   M♀
      Failed mechanical induction (of labor)
      Failed surgical induction (of labor)

  O61.8 Other failed induction of labor   M♀

  O61.9 Failed induction of labor, unspecified   M♀

☑4ᵗʰ **O62 Abnormalities of forces of labor**

  O62.0 Primary inadequate contractions   M♀
      Failure of cervical dilatation
      Primary hypotonic uterine dysfunction
      Uterine inertia during latent phase of labor

  O62.1 Secondary uterine inertia
      Arrested active phase of labor
      Secondary hypotonic uterine dysfunction

  O62.2 Other uterine inertia   M♀
      Atony of uterus without hemorrhage   Poor contractions
      Atony of uterus NOS   Slow slope active phase
      Desultory labor   of labor
      Hypotonic uterine dysfunction NOS   Uterine inertia NOS
      Irregular labor
      EXCLUDES 1 *atony of uterus with hemorrhage (postpartum) (O72.1)*
             postpartum atony of uterus without hemorrhage
             (O75.89)

  O62.3 Precipitate labor   M♀

  O62.4 Hypertonic, incoordinate, and prolonged uterine   M♀
      contractions
      Cervical spasm   Incoordinate uterine action
      Contraction ring dystocia   Tetanic contractions
      Dyscoordinate labor   Uterine dystocia NOS
      Hour-glass contraction of uterus   Uterine spasm
      Hypertonic uterine dysfunction
      EXCLUDES 1 *dystocia (fetal) (maternal) NOS (O66.9)*

  O62.8 Other abnormalities of forces of labor   M♀

  O62.9 Abnormality of forces of labor, unspecified   M♀

☑4ᵗʰ **O63 Long labor**

  O63.Ø Prolonged first stage (of labor)   M♀
  O63.1 Prolonged second stage (of labor)   M♀
  O63.2 Delayed delivery of second twin, triplet, etc.   M♀
  O63.9 Long labor, unspecified   cc M♀
      Prolonged labor NOS
      CC Excl: O25.10-O25.3, O26.10-O26.13, O26.30-O26.43, O26.63-
      O26.819, O26.841-O26.86, O26.891-O26.93, O29.011-O29.93,
      O35.7XXØ-O35.7XX9, O36.8120-O36.8199, O63.9, O71.00-O71.1,
      O71.5, O71.81, O71.89-O71.9, O75.4, O75.81, O75.89-O75.9, O8Ø,
      O9Ø.89, O99.111-O99.285, O99.330-O99.335, O99.350-O99.355,
      O99.511-O99.73, O99.820-O99.825, O99.840-O9A.53

☑4ᵗʰ **O64 Obstructed labor due to malposition and malpresentation of fetus**

> One of the following 7th characters is to be assigned to each code under category O64. 7th character Ø is for single gestations and multiple gestations where the fetus is unspecified. 7th characters 1 through 9 are for cases of multiple gestations to identify the fetus for which the code applies. The appropriate code from category O30, Multiple gestation, must also be assigned when assigning a code from category O64 that has a 7th character of 1 through 9.
>
> | Ø | not applicable or | 3 | fetus 3 |
> |---|---|---|---|
> | | unspecified | 4 | fetus 4 |
> | 1 | fetus 1 | 5 | fetus 5 |
> | 2 | fetus 2 | 9 | other fetus |

  ☑x7ᵗʰ **O64.Ø Obstructed labor due to incomplete rotation of**   M♀
        fetal head
      Deep transverse arrest
      Obstructed labor due to persistent occipitoiliac (position)
      Obstructed labor due to persistent occipitoposterior (position)
      Obstructed labor due to persistent occipitosacral (position)
      Obstructed labor due to persistent occipitotransverse (position)

  ☑x7ᵗʰ **O64.1 Obstructed labor due to breech presentation**   M♀
      Obstructed labor due to buttocks presentation
      Obstructed labor due to complete breech presentation
      Obstructed labor due to frank breech presentation

  ☑x7ᵗʰ **O64.2 Obstructed labor due to face presentation**   M♀
      Obstructed labor due to chin presentation

  ☑x7ᵗʰ **O64.3 Obstructed labor due to brow presentation**   M♀

  ☑x7ᵗʰ **O64.4 Obstructed labor due to shoulder presentation**   M♀
      Prolapsed arm
      EXCLUDES 1 *impacted shoulders (O66.Ø)*
             shoulder dystocia (O66.Ø)

  ☑x7ᵗʰ **O64.5 Obstructed labor due to compound presentation**   M♀

  ☑x7ᵗʰ **O64.8 Obstructed labor due to other malposition and**   M♀
      malpresentation
      Obstructed labor due to footling presentation
      Obstructed labor due to incomplete breech presentation

  ☑x7ᵗʰ **O64.9 Obstructed labor due to malposition and**   M♀
      malpresentation, unspecified

☑4ᵗʰ **O65 Obstructed labor due to maternal pelvic abnormality**

  O65.Ø Obstructed labor due to deformed pelvis   M♀
  O65.1 Obstructed labor due to generally contracted pelvis   M♀
  O65.2 Obstructed labor due to pelvic inlet contraction   M♀
  O65.3 Obstructed labor due to pelvic outlet and mid-cavity   M♀
      contraction
  O65.4 Obstructed labor due to fetopelvic disproportion,   M♀
      unspecified
      EXCLUDES 1 *dystocia due to abnormality of fetus (O66.2-O66.3)*
  O65.5 Obstructed labor due to abnormality of maternal   M♀
      pelvic organs
      Obstructed labor due to conditions listed in O34-
      Use additional code to identify abnormality of pelvic organs
      (O34.-)
  O65.8 Obstructed labor due to other maternal pelvic   M♀
      abnormalities
  O65.9 Obstructed labor due to maternal pelvic abnormality,   M♀
      unspecified

☑4ᵗʰ **O66 Other obstructed labor**

  O66.Ø Obstructed labor due to shoulder dystocia   M♀
      Impacted shoulders
  O66.1 Obstructed labor due to locked twins   M♀
  O66.2 Obstructed labor due to unusually large fetus   M♀

☑ Additional Character Required   ☑x7ᵗʰ Xtension Alert   Unacceptable PDx   Manifestation   Hospital Acquired Condition   EXCLUDES 1 Not Coded Here   EXCLUDES 2 Not Included Here

O62.0 – poor cervical dilation (handwritten)

Pregnancy, Childbirth and the Puerperium (side margin)

O60.1–O66.2 (side margin)

O66.3 Obstructed labor due to other abnormalities of fetus   M♀
Dystocia due to fetal ascites
Dystocia due to fetal hydrops
Dystocia due to fetal meningomyelocele
Dystocia due to fetal sacral teratoma
Dystocia due to fetal tumor
Dystocia due to hydrocephalic fetus
Use additional code to identify cause of obstruction

√5ᵗʰ **O66.4 Failed trial of labor**

    O66.40 Failed trial of labor, unspecified   M♀

    O66.41 Failed attempted vaginal birth after previous   M♀
    cesarean delivery
      Code first rupture of uterus, if applicable (O71.0-,
      O71.1)

O66.5 Attempted application of vacuum extractor and forceps   M♀
Attempted application of vacuum or forceps, with subsequent
delivery by forceps or cesarean delivery

O66.6 Obstructed labor due to other multiple fetuses   M♀

O66.8 Other specified obstructed labor   M♀
Use additional code to identify cause of obstruction

O66.9 Obstructed labor, unspecified   M♀
Dystocia NOS   Maternal dystocia NOS
Fetal dystocia NOS

√4ᵗʰ **O67 Labor and delivery complicated by intrapartum hemorrhage, not elsewhere classified**
    EXCLUDES 1   *antepartum hemorrhage NEC (O46.-)*
       placenta previa (O44.-)
       premature separation of placenta [abruptio placentae] (O45.-)
    EXCLUDES 2   *postpartum hemorrhage (O72.-)*

    O67.0 Intrapartum hemorrhage with coagulation defect   MCC M♀
    Intrapartum hemorrhage (excessive) associated with
    afibrinogenemia
    Intrapartum hemorrhage (excessive) associated with
    disseminated intravascular coagulation
    Intrapartum hemorrhage (excessive) associated with
    hyperfibrinolysis
    Intrapartum hemorrhage (excessive) associated with
    hypofibrinogenemia
    CC Excl: O25.10-O25.3, O26.10-O26.13, O26.30-O26.43, O26.63-
    O26.819, O26.841-O26.86, O26.891-O26.93, O29.011-O29.93,
    O35.7X-O35.7X, O45.001-O45.099, O46.001-O46.93, O67.0-O67.9,
    O75.4, O75.81, O75.89-O75.9, O80, O90.89, O99.111-O99.285,
    O99.330-O99.335, O99.350-O99.355, O99.511-O99.73, O99.820-
    O99.825, O99.840-O9A.53

    O67.8 Other intrapartum hemorrhage   M♀
    Excessive intrapartum hemorrhage

    O67.9 Intrapartum hemorrhage, unspecified   M♀

O68 Labor and delivery complicated by abnormality of fetal acid-base balance   CC M♀
Fetal acidemia complicating labor and delivery
Fetal acidosis complicating labor and delivery
Fetal alkalosis complicating labor and delivery
Fetal metabolic acidemia complicating labor and delivery
    EXCLUDES 1   *fetal stress NOS (O77.9)*
       labor and delivery complicated by electrocardiographic
       evidence of fetal stress (O77.8)
       labor and delivery complicated by ultrasonic evidence of fetal
       stress (O77.8)
    EXCLUDES 2   *abnormality in fetal heart rate or rhythm (O76)*
       labor and delivery complicated by meconium in amniotic fluid
       (O77.0)
    CC Excl: O68-O76, P03.811

√4ᵗʰ **O69 Labor and delivery complicated by umbilical cord complications**

> One of the following 7th characters is to be assigned to each code
> under category O69. 7th character 0 is for single gestations and
> multiple gestations where the fetus is unspecified. 7th characters 1
> through 9 are for cases of multiple gestations to identify the fetus for
> which the code applies. The appropriate code from category O30,
> Multiple gestation, must also be assigned when assigning a code
> from category O69 that has a 7th character of 1 through 9.
> | | | | |
> |---|---|---|---|
> | 0 | not applicable or | 3 | fetus 3 |
> | | unspecified | 4 | fetus 4 |
> | 1 | fetus 1 | 5 | fetus 5 |
> | 2 | fetus 2 | 9 | other fetus |

√x7ᵗʰ **O69.0 Labor and delivery complicated by** prolapse of cord   M♀

√x7ᵗʰ **O69.1 Labor and delivery complicated by** cord around neck,   M♀
with compression
    EXCLUDES 1   *labor and delivery complicated by cord around neck,*
       without compression (O69.81)

√x7ᵗʰ **O69.2 Labor and delivery complicated by** other cord   M♀
entanglement, with compression
Labor and delivery complicated by compression of cord NOS
Labor and delivery complicated by entanglement of cords of
twins in monoamniotic sac
Labor and delivery complicated by knot in cord
    EXCLUDES 1   *labor and delivery complicated by other cord*
       entanglement, without compression (O69.82)

√x7ᵗʰ **O69.3 Labor and delivery complicated by** short cord   M♀

√x7ᵗʰ **O69.4 Labor and delivery complicated by** vasa previa   M♀
Labor and delivery complicated by hemorrhage from vasa
previa

√x7ᵗʰ **O69.5 Labor and delivery complicated by** vascular lesion of cord   M♀
Labor and delivery complicated by cord bruising
Labor and delivery complicated by cord hematoma
Labor and delivery complicated by thrombosis of umbilical
vessels

√5ᵗʰ **O69.8 Labor and delivery complicated by** other cord complications

    √x7ᵗʰ **O69.81 Labor and delivery complicated by cord** around   M♀
    neck, without compression

    √x7ᵗʰ **O69.82 Labor and delivery complicated by other cord**   M♀
    entanglement, without compression

    √x7ᵗʰ **O69.89 Labor and delivery complicated by** other cord   M♀
    complications

√x7ᵗʰ **O69.9 Labor and delivery complicated by cord complication,**   M♀
unspecified

√4ᵗʰ **O70 Perineal laceration during delivery**
Episiotomy extended by laceration
    EXCLUDES 1   *obstetric high vaginal laceration alone (O71.4)*

    O70.0 First degree perineal laceration during delivery   M♀
    Perineal laceration, rupture or tear involving fourchette during
    delivery
    Perineal laceration, rupture or tear involving labia during
    delivery
    Perineal laceration, rupture or tear involving skin during delivery
    Perineal laceration, rupture or tear involving vagina during
    delivery
    Perineal laceration, rupture or tear involving vulva during
    delivery
    Slight perineal laceration, rupture or tear during delivery

    O70.1 Second degree perineal laceration during delivery   M♀
    Perineal laceration, rupture or tear during delivery as in O70.0,
    also involving pelvic floor
    Perineal laceration, rupture or tear during delivery as in O70.0,
    also involving perineal muscles
    Perineal laceration, rupture or tear during delivery as in O70.0,
    also involving vaginal muscles
    EXCLUDES 1   *perineal laceration involving anal sphincter (O70.2)*

    O70.2 Third degree perineal laceration during delivery   CC M♀
    Perineal laceration, rupture or tear during delivery as in O70.1,
    also involving anal sphincter
    Perineal laceration, rupture or tear during delivery as in O70.1,
    also involving rectovaginal septum
    Perineal laceration, rupture or tear during delivery as in O70.1,
    also involving sphincter NOS
    EXCLUDES 1   *anal sphincter tear during delivery without third degree*
       perineal laceration (O70.4)
       perineal laceration involving anal or rectal mucosa
       (O70.3)
    CC Excl: O25.10-O25.3, O26.10-O26.13, O26.30-O26.43, O26.63-
    O26.819, O26.841-O26.86, O26.891-O26.93, O29.011-O29.93,
    O35.7XX0-O35.7XX9, O36.8120-O36.8199, O70.2, O70.4, O71.00-
    O71.1, O71.5, O71.81, O71.89-O71.9, O75.4, O75.81, O75.89-O75.9,
    O80, O90.89, O99.111-O99.285, O99.330-O99.335, O99.350-
    O99.355, O99.511-O99.73, O99.820-O99.825, O99.840-O9A.53

    O70.3 Fourth degree perineal laceration during delivery   CC M♀
    Perineal laceration, rupture or tear during delivery as in O70.2,
    also involving anal mucosa
    Perineal laceration, rupture or tear during delivery as in O70.2,
    also involving rectal mucosa
    CC Excl: O25.10-O25.3, O26.10-O26.13, O26.30-O26.43, O26.63-
    O26.819, O26.841-O26.86, O26.891-O26.93, O29.011-O29.93,
    O35.7XX0-O35.7XX9, O36.8120-O36.8199, O70.3, O71.00-O71.1,
    O71.5, O71.81, O71.89-O71.9, O75.4, O75.81, O75.89-O75.9, O80,
    O90.89, O99.111-O99.285, O99.330-O99.335, O99.350-O99.355,
    O99.511-O99.73, O99.820-O99.825, O99.840-O9A.53

    O70.4 Anal sphincter tear complicating delivery, not   CC M♀
    associated with third degree laceration
      EXCLUDES 1   *anal sphincter tear with third degree perineal*
       laceration (O70.2)
    CC Excl: See code: O70.2

    O70.9 Perineal laceration during delivery, unspecified   M♀

N Newborn: 0   **P** Pediatric: 0-17   **M** Maternity: 12-55   **A** Adult: 15-124   **MCC** Major CC Condition   **PDx MCC** PDx acts as own MCC   **CC** CC Condition   **PDx CC** PDx acts as own CC

804   ICD-10-CM Draft (2015)

✓4ᵗʰ **O71　Other obstetric trauma**
Obstetric damage from instruments

✓5ᵗʰ **O71.0　Rupture of uterus (spontaneous) before onset of labor**
*EXCLUDES 1　disruption of (current) cesarean delivery wound (O90.0)
laceration of uterus, NEC (O71.81)*

O71.00　Rupture of uterus before onset of labor,　M♀
unspecified trimester

O71.02　Rupture of uterus before onset of labor,　MCC M♀
second trimester
CC Excl: O25.10-O25.3, O26.10-O26.13, O26.30-O26.43,
O26.63-O26.819, O26.841-O26.86, O26.891-O26.93,
O29.011-O29.93, O35.7XX0-O35.7XX9, O36.8120-
O36.8199, O71.00-O71.1, O71.5, O71.81, O71.89-O71.9,
O75.4, O75.81, O75.89-O75.9, O80, O90.89, O99.111-
O99.285, O99.330-O99.335, O99.350-O99.355, O99.511-
O99.73, O99.820-O99.825, O99.840-O9A.53

O71.03　Rupture of uterus before onset of labor,　MCC M♀
third trimester
CC Excl: See code: O71.02

O71.1　Rupture of uterus during labor　MCC M♀
Rupture of uterus not stated as occurring before onset of labor
*EXCLUDES 1　disruption of cesarean delivery wound (O90.0)
laceration of uterus, NEC (O71.81)*
CC Excl: See code: O71.02

O71.2　Postpartum inversion of uterus　CC M♀
CC Excl: O25.10-O25.3, O26.10-O26.13, O26.30-O26.43, O26.63-
O26.819, O26.841-O26.86, O26.891-O26.93, O29.011-O29.93,
O35.7XX0-O35.7XX9, O36.8120-O36.8199, O71.00-O71.2, O71.5,
O71.81, O71.89-O71.9, O75.4, O75.81, O75.89-O75.9, O80, O90.89,
O99.111-O99.285, O99.330-O99.335, O99.350-O99.355, O99.511-
O99.73, O99.820-O99.825, O99.840-O9A.53

O71.3　Obstetric laceration of cervix　CC M♀
Annular detachment of cervix
CC Excl: O25.10-O25.3, O26.10-O26.13, O26.30-O26.43, O26.63-
O26.819, O26.841-O26.86, O26.891-O26.93, O29.011-O29.93,
O35.7XX0-O35.7XX9, O36.8120-O36.8199, O71.00-O71.1, O71.3,
O71.5, O71.81, O71.89-O71.9, O75.4, O75.81, O75.89-O75.9, O80,
O90.89, O99.111-O99.285, O99.330-O99.335, O99.350-O99.355,
O99.511-O99.73, O99.820-O99.825, O99.840-O9A.53

O71.4　Obstetric high vaginal laceration alone　CC M♀
Laceration of vaginal wall without perineal laceration
*EXCLUDES 1　obstetric high vaginal laceration with perineal
laceration (O70.-)*
CC Excl: O25.10-O25.3, O26.10-O26.13, O26.30-O26.43, O26.63-
O26.819, O26.841-O26.86, O26.891-O26.93, O29.011-O29.93,
O35.7XX0-O35.7XX9, O36.8120-O36.8199, O71.00-O71.1, O71.4-
O71.5, O71.81, O71.89-O71.9, O75.4, O75.81, O75.89-O75.9, O80,
O90.89, O99.111-O99.285, O99.330-O99.335, O99.350-O99.355,
O99.511-O99.73, O99.820-O99.825, O99.840-O9A.53

O71.5　Other obstetric injury to pelvic organs　CC M♀
Obstetric injury to bladder
Obstetric injury to urethra
EXCLUDES 2　obstetric periurethral trauma (O71.82)
CC Excl: O25.10-O25.3, O26.10-O26.13, O26.30-O26.43, O26.63-
O26.819, O26.841-O26.86, O26.891-O26.93, O29.011-O29.93,
O35.7XX0-O35.7XX9, O36.8120-O36.8199, O71.00-O71.1, O71.5,
O71.81, O71.89-O71.9, O75.4, O75.81, O75.89-O75.9, O80, O90.89,
O99.111-O99.285, O99.330-O99.335, O99.350-O99.355, O99.511-
O99.73, O99.820-O99.825, O99.840-O9A.53

O71.6　Obstetric damage to pelvic joints and ligaments　CC M♀
Obstetric avulsion of inner symphyseal cartilage
Obstetric damage to coccyx
Obstetric traumatic separation of symphysis (pubis)
CC Excl: O25.10-O25.3, O26.10-O26.13, O26.30-O26.43, O26.63-
O26.819, O26.841-O26.86, O26.891-O26.93, O29.011-O29.93,
O35.7XX0-O35.7XX9, O36.8120-O36.8199, O71.00-O71.1, O71.5-
O71.6, O71.81, O71.89-O71.9, O75.4, O75.81, O75.89-O75.9, O80,
O90.89, O99.111-O99.285, O99.330-O99.335, O99.350-O99.355,
O99.511-O99.73, O99.820-O99.825, O99.840-O9A.53

O71.7　Obstetric hematoma of pelvis　CC M♀
Obstetric hematoma of perineum
Obstetric hematoma of vagina
Obstetric hematoma of vulva
CC Excl: O25.10-O25.3, O26.10-O26.13, O26.30-O26.43, O26.63-
O26.819, O26.841-O26.86, O26.891-O26.93, O29.011-O29.93,
O35.7XX0-O35.7XX9, O36.8120-O36.8199, O71.00-O71.1, O71.5,
O71.7-O71.81, O71.89-O71.9, O75.4, O75.81, O75.89-O75.9, O80,
O90.89, O99.111-O99.285, O99.330-O99.335, O99.350-O99.355,
O99.511-O99.73, O99.820-O99.825, O99.840-O9A.53

✓5ᵗʰ **O71.8　Other specified obstetric trauma**

O71.81　Laceration of uterus, not elsewhere classified　M♀

O71.82　Other specified trauma to perineum and vulva　M♀
Obstetric periurethral trauma

O71.89　Other specified obstetric trauma　M♀

O71.9　Obstetric trauma, unspecified　M♀

✓4ᵗʰ **O72　Postpartum hemorrhage**
INCLUDES　hemorrhage after delivery of fetus or infant

O72.0　Third-stage hemorrhage　CC M♀
Hemorrhage associated with retained, trapped or adherent
placenta
Retained placenta NOS
Code also type of adherent placenta (O43.2-)
CC Excl: O25.10-O25.3, O26.10-O26.13, O26.30-O26.43, O26.63-
O26.819, O26.841-O26.86, O26.891-O26.93, O29.011-O29.93,
O35.7XX0-O35.7XX9, O36.8120-O36.8199, O71.00-O71.1, O71.5,
O71.81, O71.89-O72.0, O75.4, O75.81, O75.89-O75.9, O80, O90.89,
O99.111-O99.285, O99.330-O99.335, O99.350-O99.355, O99.511-
O99.73, O99.820-O99.825, O99.840-O9A.12

O72.1　Other immediate postpartum hemorrhage　CC M♀
Hemorrhage following delivery of placenta
Postpartum hemorrhage (atonic) NOS
Uterine atony with hemorrhage
*EXCLUDES 1　uterine atony NOS (O62.2)
uterine atony without hemorrhage (O62.2)
postpartum atony of uterus without hemorrhage
(O75.89)*
CC Excl: O25.10-O25.3, O26.10-O26.13, O26.30-O26.43, O26.63-
O26.819, O26.841-O26.86, O26.891-O26.93, O29.011-O29.93,
O35.7XX0-O35.7XX9, O36.8120-O36.8199, O71.00-O71.1, O71.5,
O71.81, O71.89-O71.9, O72.1, O75.4, O75.81, O75.89-O75.9, O80,
O90.89, O99.111-O99.285, O99.330-O99.335, O99.350-O99.355,
O99.511-O99.73, O99.820-O99.825, O99.840-O9A.53

O72.2　Delayed and secondary postpartum hemorrhage　CC M♀
Hemorrhage associated with retained portions of placenta or
membranes after the first 24 hours following delivery of
placenta
Retained products of conception NOS, following delivery
CC Excl: O25.10-O25.3, O26.10-O26.13, O26.30-O26.43, O26.63-
O26.819, O26.841-O26.86, O26.891-O26.93, O29.011-O29.93,
O35.7XX0-O35.7XX9, O36.8120-O36.8199, O71.00-O71.1, O71.5,
O71.81, O71.89-O71.9, O72.2, O75.4, O75.81, O75.89-O75.9, O80,
O90.89, O99.111-O99.285, O99.330-O99.335, O99.350-O99.355,
O99.511-O99.73, O99.820-O99.825, O99.840-O9A.53

O72.3　Postpartum coagulation defects　M♀
Postpartum afibrinogenemia
Postpartum fibrinolysis

✓4ᵗʰ **O73　Retained placenta and membranes, without hemorrhage**
*EXCLUDES 1　placenta accreta (O43.21-)
placenta increta (O43.22-)
placenta percreta (O43.23-)*

O73.0　Retained placenta without hemorrhage　M♀
Adherent placenta, without hemorrhage
Trapped placenta without hemorrhage

O73.1　Retained portions of placenta and membranes, without　M♀
hemorrhage
Retained products of conception following delivery, without
hemorrhage

✓4ᵗʰ **O74　Complications of anesthesia during labor and delivery**
INCLUDES　maternal complications arising from the administration of a
general, regional or local anesthetic, analgesic or other
sedation during labor and delivery
Use additional code, if applicable, to identify specific complication

O74.0　Aspiration pneumonitis due to anesthesia during labor　M♀
and delivery
Inhalation of stomach contents or secretions NOS due to
anesthesia during labor and delivery
Mendelson's syndrome due to anesthesia during labor and
delivery

O74.1　Other pulmonary complications of anesthesia during　M♀
labor and delivery

O74.2　Cardiac complications of anesthesia during labor and　M♀
delivery

O74.3　Central nervous system complications of anesthesia　M♀
during labor and delivery

O74.4　Toxic reaction to local anesthesia during labor and　M♀
delivery

O74.5　Spinal and epidural anesthesia-induced headache　M♀
during labor and delivery

O74.6　Other complications of spinal and epidural anesthesia　M♀
during labor and delivery

O74.7　Failed or difficult intubation for anesthesia during　M♀
labor and delivery

O74.8　Other complications of anesthesia during labor and　M♀
delivery

O74.9　Complication of anesthesia during labor and delivery,　M♀
unspecified

✓ Additional Character Required　　✓x7ᵗʰ Xtension Alert　　Unacceptable PDx　　Manifestation　　　　Hospital Acquired Condition　　*EXCLUDES 1* Not Coded Here　　*EXCLUDES 2* Not Included Here

Pregnancy, Childbirth and the Puerperium

075–086.19

✓4ᵗʰ **O75 Other complications of labor and delivery, not elsewhere classified**

> EXCLUDES 2   *puerperal (postpartum) infection (O86.-)*
> *puerperal (postpartum) sepsis (O85)*

O75.0 Maternal distress during labor and delivery   M♀

O75.1 Shock during or following labor and delivery   MCC M♀
> Obstetric shock following labor and delivery
> **CC Excl:** O25.10-O25.3, O26.10-O26.13, O26.30-O26.43, O26.63-
> O26.819, O26.841-O26.86, O26.891-O26.93, O29.011-O29.93,
> O35.7XX0-O35.7XX9, O75.1, O75.4, O75.81, O75.89-O75.9, O80,
> O90.89, O99.111-O99.285, O99.330-O99.335, O99.350-O99.355,
> O99.511-O99.73, O99.820-O99.825, O99.840-O9A.53

O75.2 Pyrexia during labor, not elsewhere classified   CC M♀
> **CC Excl:** O75.2

O75.3 Other infection during labor   MCC M♀
> Sepsis during labor
> Use additional code (B95-B97), to identify infectious agent
> **CC Excl:** O25.10-O25.3, O26.10-O26.13, O26.30-O26.43, O26.63-
> O26.819, O26.841-O26.86, O26.891-O26.93, O29.011-O29.93,
> O35.7XX0-O35.7XX9, O75.3-O75.4, O75.81, O75.89-O75.9, O80,
> O90.89, O99.111-O99.285, O99.330-O99.335, O99.350-O99.355,
> O99.511-O99.73, O99.820-O99.825, O99.840-O9A.53

O75.4 Other complications of obstetric surgery and procedures   M♀
> Cardiac arrest following obstetric surgery or procedures
> Cardiac failure following obstetric surgery or procedures
> Cerebral anoxia following obstetric surgery or procedures
> Pulmonary edema following obstetric surgery or procedures
> Use additional code to identify specific complication
> EXCLUDES 2   *complications of anesthesia during labor and delivery (O74.-)*
> *disruption of obstetrical (surgical) wound (O90.0-O90.1)*
> *hematoma of obstetrical (surgical) wound (O90.2)*
> *infection of obstetrical (surgical) wound (O86.0)*

O75.5 Delayed delivery after artificial rupture of membranes   M♀

✓5ᵗʰ **O75.8 Other specified complications of labor and delivery**

O75.81 Maternal exhaustion complicating labor and delivery   M♀

O75.82 Onset (spontaneous) of labor after 37 completed weeks of gestation but before 39 completed weeks gestation, with delivery by (planned) cesarean section   M♀
> Delivery by (planned) cesarean section occurring after 37 completed weeks of gestation but before 39 completed weeks gestation due to (spontaneous) onset of labor
> Code first to specify reason for planned cesarean section such as:
> cephalopelvic disproportion (normally formed fetus) (O33.9)
> previous cesarean delivery (O34.21)

O75.89 Other specified complications of labor and delivery   M♀

O75.9 Complication of labor and delivery, unspecified   M♀

O76 Abnormality in fetal heart rate and rhythm complicating labor and delivery   M♀
> Depressed fetal heart rate tones complicating labor and delivery
> Fetal bradycardia complicating labor and delivery
> Fetal heart rate abnormal variability complicating labor and delivery
> Fetal heart rate decelerations complicating labor and delivery
> Fetal heart rate irregularity complicating labor and delivery
> Fetal tachycardia complicating labor and delivery
> Non-reassuring fetal heart rate or rhythm complicating labor and delivery
> EXCLUDES 1   *fetal stress NOS (O77.9)*
> *labor and delivery complicated by electrocardiographic evidence of fetal stress (O77.8)*
> *labor and delivery complicated by ultrasonic evidence of fetal stress (O77.8)*
> EXCLUDES 2   *fetal metabolic acidemia (O68)*
> *other fetal stress (O77.0-O77.1)*
> **AHA:** 2013, 4Q, 118

✓4ᵗʰ **O77 Other fetal stress complicating labor and delivery**

O77.0 Labor and delivery complicated by meconium in amniotic fluid   M♀
> **AHA:** 2013, 4Q, 117-118

O77.1 Fetal stress in labor or delivery due to drug administration   M♀

O77.8 Labor and delivery complicated by other evidence of fetal stress   M♀
> Labor and delivery complicated by electrocardiographic evidence of fetal stress
> Labor and delivery complicated by ultrasonic evidence of fetal stress
> EXCLUDES 1   *abnormality in fetal heart rate or rhythm (O76)*
> *abnormality of fetal acid-base balance (O68)*
> *fetal metabolic acidemia (O68)*

O77.9 Labor and delivery complicated by fetal stress, unspecified   M♀
> EXCLUDES 1   *abnormality in fetal heart rate or rhythm (O76)*
> *abnormality of fetal acid-base balance (O68)*
> *fetal metabolic acidemia (O68)*

Encounter for delivery (O80, O82)

O80 Encounter for full-term uncomplicated delivery   M♀
> NOTE   Delivery requiring minimal or no assistance, with or without episiotomy, without fetal manipulation [e.g., rotation version] or instrumentation [forceps] of a spontaneous, cephalic, vaginal, full-term, single, live-born infant. This code is for use as a single diagnosis code and is not to be used with any other code from chapter 15.
> Use additional code to indicate outcome of delivery (Z37.0)
> **AHA:** 2014, 2Q, 9

O82 Encounter for cesarean delivery without indication   M♀
> Use additional code to indicate outcome of delivery (Z37.0)

Complications predominantly related to the puerperium (O85-O92)

> EXCLUDES 2   *mental and behavioral disorders associated with the puerperium (F53)*
> *obstetrical tetanus (A34)*
> *puerperal osteomalacia (M83.0)*

O85 Puerperal sepsis   MCC M♀
> Postpartum sepsis
> Puerperal peritonitis
> Puerperal pyemia
> Use additional code (B95-B97), to identify infectious agent
> Use additional code (R65.2-) to identify severe sepsis, if applicable
> EXCLUDES 1   *fever of unknown origin following delivery (O86.4)*
> *genital tract infection following delivery (O86.1-)*
> *obstetric pyemic and septic embolism (O88.3-)*
> *puerperal septic thrombophlebitis (O86.81)*
> *urinary tract infection following delivery (O86.2-)*
> EXCLUDES 2   *sepsis during labor (O75.3)*
> **CC Excl:** O25.10-O25.3, O26.10-O26.13, O26.30-O26.43, O26.63-O26.819,
> O26.841-O26.86, O26.891-O26.93, O29.011-O29.93, O35.7XX0-O35.7XX9,
> O75.4, O75.81, O75.89-O75.9, O80, O85, O86.12, O86.81-O86.89, O90.89,
> O99.111-O99.285, O99.330-O99.335, O99.350-O99.355, O99.511-O99.73,
> O99.820-O99.825, O99.840-O9A.53

✓4ᵗʰ **O86 Other puerperal infections**
> Use additional code (B95-B97), to identify infectious agent
> EXCLUDES 2   *infection during labor (O75.3)*
> *obstetrical tetanus (A34)*

> **CC Excl: For CC/MCC codes in category O86, unless otherwise noted:** O23.00-O23.93, O25.10-O25.3, O26.10-O26.13, O26.30-O26.43, O26.63-O26.819, O26.841-O26.86, O26.891-O26.93, O29.011-O29.93, O35.7XX0-O35.7XX9, O75.4, O75.81, O75.89-O75.9, O80, O86.11, O86.13-O86.29, O90.89, O99.111-O99.285, O99.330-O99.335, O99.350-O99.355, O99.511-O99.73, O99.820-O99.825, O99.840-O9A.53

O86.0 Infection of obstetric surgical wound   M♀
> Infected cesarean delivery wound following delivery
> Infected perineal repair following delivery

✓5ᵗʰ **O86.1 Other infection of genital tract following delivery**

O86.11 Cervicitis following delivery   CC M♀

O86.12 Endometritis following delivery   CC M♀
> **CC Excl:** O25.10-O25.3, O26.10-O26.13, O26.30-O26.43,
> O26.63-O26.819, O26.841-O26.86, O26.891-O26.93,
> O29.011-O29.93, O35.7XX0-O35.7XX9, O75.4, O75.81,
> O75.89-O75.9, O80, O85, O86.12, O86.81-O86.89,
> O90.89, O99.111-O99.285, O99.330-O99.335, O99.350-
> O99.355, O99.511-O99.73, O99.820-O99.825, O99.840-
> O9A.53

O86.13 Vaginitis following delivery   CC M♀

O86.19 Other infection of genital tract following delivery   CC M♀

N Newborn: 0   P Pediatric: 0-17   M Maternity: 12-55   A Adult: 15-124   MCC Major CC Condition   PDx MCC PDx acts as own MCC   CC CC Condition   PDx CC PDx acts as own CC

806   ICD-10-CM Draft (2015)

Pregnancy, Childbirth and the Puerperium

✓5ᵗʰ **O86.2 Urinary tract infection following delivery**

    O86.20 Urinary tract infection following delivery, unspecified `CC` `M` ♀
        Puerperal urinary tract infection NOS

    O86.21 Infection of kidney following delivery `CC` `M` ♀

    O86.22 Infection of bladder following delivery `CC` `M` ♀
        Infection of urethra following delivery

    O86.29 Other urinary tract infection following delivery `CC` `M` ♀

  O86.4 Pyrexia of unknown origin following delivery `CC` `M` ♀
    Puerperal infection NOS following delivery
    Puerperal pyrexia NOS following delivery
    EXCLUDES 2 *pyrexia during labor (O75.2)*
    CC Excl: O22.20-O22.93, O25.10-O25.3, O26.10-O26.13, O26.30-O26.43, O26.63-O26.819, O26.841-O26.86, O26.891-O26.93, O29.011-O29.93, O35.7XX0-O35.7XX9, O75.4, O75.81, O75.89-O75.9, O80, O86.4, O87.0-O87.3, O87.8-O87.9, O90.89, O99.111-O99.285, O99.330-O99.335, O99.350-O99.355, O99.511-O99.73, O99.820-O99.825, O99.840-O9A.53

✓5ᵗʰ **O86.8 Other specified puerperal infections**

    O86.81 Puerperal septic thrombophlebitis `MCC` `M` ♀
        CC Excl: See code: O85

    O86.89 Other specified puerperal infections `MCC` `M` ♀
        CC Excl: See code: O85

✓4ᵗʰ **O87 Venous complications and hemorrhoids in the puerperium**
  Venous complications in labor, delivery and the puerperium
  EXCLUDES 2 *obstetric embolism (O88.-)*
    puerperal septic thrombophlebitis (O86.81)
    venous complications in pregnancy (O22.-)

  CC Excl: For CC/MCC codes in category O87, unless otherwise noted: O22.20-O22.93, O25.10-O25.3, O26.10-O26.13, O26.30-O26.43, O26.63-O26.819, O26.841-O26.86, O26.891-O26.93, O29.011-O29.93, O35.7XX0-O35.7XX9, O75.4, O75.81, O75.89-O75.9, O80, O87.0-O87.3, O87.8-O87.9, O90.89, O99.111-O99.285, O99.330-O99.335, O99.350-O99.355, O99.511-O99.73, O99.820-O99.825, O99.840-O9A.53

  O87.0 Superficial thrombophlebitis in the puerperium `CC` `M` ♀
    Puerperal phlebitis NOS
    Puerperal thrombosis NOS

  O87.1 Deep phlebothrombosis in the puerperium `MCC` `M` ♀
    Deep vein thrombosis, postpartum
    Pelvic thrombophlebitis, postpartum
    Use additional code to identify the deep vein thrombosis (I82.4-, I82.5-, I82.62-. I82.72-)
    Use additional code, if applicable, for associated long-term (current) use of anticoagulants (Z79.01)

  O87.2 Hemorrhoids in the puerperium `CC` `M` ♀

  O87.3 Cerebral venous thrombosis in the puerperium `CC` `M` ♀
    Cerebrovenous sinus thrombosis in the puerperium

  O87.4 Varicose veins of lower extremity in the puerperium `M` ♀

  O87.8 Other venous complications in the puerperium `CC` `M` ♀
    Genital varices in the puerperium

  O87.9 Venous complication in the puerperium, unspecified `M` ♀
    Puerperal phlebopathy NOS

✓4ᵗʰ **O88 Obstetric embolism**
  EXCLUDES 1 *embolism complicating abortion NOS (O03.2)*
    embolism complicating ectopic or molar pregnancy (O08.2)
    embolism complicating failed attempted abortion (O07.2)
    embolism complicating induced abortion (O04.7)
    embolism complicating spontaneous abortion (O03.2, O03.7)

  CC Excl: For CC/MCC codes in category O88, unless otherwise noted: O25.10-O25.3, O26.10-O26.13, O26.30-O26.43, O26.63-O26.819, O26.841-O26.86, O26.891-O26.93, O29.011-O29.93, O35.7XX0-O35.7XX9, O75.4, O75.81, O75.89-O75.9, O80, O88.011-O88.83, O90.89, O99.111-O99.285, O99.330-O99.335, O99.350-O99.355, O99.511-O99.73, O99.820-O99.825, O99.840-O9A.53

✓5ᵗʰ **O88.0 Obstetric air embolism**

  ✓6ᵗʰ **O88.01 Obstetric air embolism in pregnancy**

    O88.011 Air embolism in pregnancy, first trimester `MCC` `M` ♀

    O88.012 Air embolism in pregnancy, second trimester `MCC` `M` ♀

    O88.013 Air embolism in pregnancy, third trimester `MCC` `M` ♀

    O88.019 Air embolism in pregnancy, unspecified trimester `M` ♀

  O88.02 Air embolism in childbirth `MCC` `M` ♀

  O88.03 Air embolism in the puerperium `MCC` `M` ♀

✓5ᵗʰ **O88.1 Amniotic fluid embolism**
  Anaphylactoid syndrome in pregnancy

  ✓6ᵗʰ **O88.11 Amniotic fluid embolism in pregnancy**

    O88.111 Amniotic fluid embolism in pregnancy, first trimester `MCC` `M` ♀

    O88.112 Amniotic fluid embolism in pregnancy, second trimester `MCC` `M` ♀

    O88.113 Amniotic fluid embolism in pregnancy, third trimester `MCC` `M` ♀

    O88.119 Amniotic fluid embolism in pregnancy, unspecified trimester `M` ♀

  O88.12 Amniotic fluid embolism in childbirth `MCC` `M` ♀

  O88.13 Amniotic fluid embolism in the puerperium `MCC` `M` ♀

✓5ᵗʰ **O88.2 Obstetric thromboembolism**

  ✓6ᵗʰ **O88.21 Thromboembolism in pregnancy**
    Obstetric (pulmonary) embolism NOS

    O88.211 Thromboembolism in pregnancy, first trimester `MCC` `M` ♀

    O88.212 Thromboembolism in pregnancy, second trimester `MCC` `M` ♀

    O88.213 Thromboembolism in pregnancy, third trimester `MCC` `M` ♀

    O88.219 Thromboembolism in pregnancy, unspecified trimester `M` ♀

  O88.22 Thromboembolism in childbirth `MCC` `M` ♀

  O88.23 Thromboembolism in the puerperium `MCC` `M` ♀
    Puerperal (pulmonary) embolism NOS

✓5ᵗʰ **O88.3 Obstetric pyemic and septic embolism**

  ✓6ᵗʰ **O88.31 Pyemic and septic embolism in pregnancy**

    O88.311 Pyemic and septic embolism in pregnancy, first trimester `MCC` `M` ♀

    O88.312 Pyemic and septic embolism in pregnancy, second trimester `MCC` `M` ♀

    O88.313 Pyemic and septic embolism in pregnancy, third trimester `MCC` `M` ♀

    O88.319 Pyemic and septic embolism in pregnancy, unspecified trimester `CC` `M` ♀

  O88.32 Pyemic and septic embolism in childbirth `MCC` `M` ♀

  O88.33 Pyemic and septic embolism in the puerperium `MCC` `M` ♀

✓5ᵗʰ **O88.8 Other obstetric embolism**
  Obstetric fat embolism

  ✓6ᵗʰ **O88.81 Other embolism in pregnancy**

    O88.811 Other embolism in pregnancy, first trimester `MCC` `M` ♀

    O88.812 Other embolism in pregnancy, second trimester `MCC` `M` ♀

    O88.813 Other embolism in pregnancy, third trimester `MCC` `M` ♀

    O88.819 Other embolism in pregnancy, unspecified trimester `M` ♀

  O88.82 Other embolism in childbirth `MCC` `M` ♀

  O88.83 Other embolism in the puerperium `MCC` `M` ♀

✓4ᵗʰ **O89 Complications of anesthesia during the puerperium**
  INCLUDES maternal complications arising from the administration of a general, regional or local anesthetic, analgesic or other sedation during the puerperium
  Use additional code, if applicable, to identify specific complication

✓5ᵗʰ **O89.0 Pulmonary complications of anesthesia during the puerperium**

  O89.01 Aspiration pneumonitis due to anesthesia during the puerperium `M` ♀
    Inhalation of stomach contents or secretions NOS due to anesthesia during the puerperium
    Mendelson's syndrome due to anesthesia during the puerperium

  O89.09 Other pulmonary complications of anesthesia during the puerperium `M` ♀

  O89.1 Cardiac complications of anesthesia during the puerperium `M` ♀

  O89.2 Central nervous system complications of anesthesia during the puerperium `M` ♀

  O89.3 Toxic reaction to local anesthesia during the puerperium `M` ♀

  O89.4 Spinal and epidural anesthesia-induced headache during the puerperium `M` ♀

✔ Additional Character Required   ✔x7ᵗʰ Xtension Alert   Unacceptable PDx   Manifestation   Hospital Acquired Condition   **EXCLUDES 1** Not Coded Here   **EXCLUDES 2** Not Included Here

Pregnancy, Childbirth and the Puerperium   O89.5–O92.29

O89.5   Other complications of spinal and epidural anesthesia during the puerperium   Ⓜ♀

O89.6   Failed or difficult intubation for anesthesia during the puerperium   Ⓜ♀

O89.8   Other complications of anesthesia during the puerperium   Ⓜ♀

O89.9   Complication of anesthesia during the puerperium, unspecified   Ⓜ♀

✓4ᵗʰ **O90**   **Complications of the puerperium, not elsewhere classified**

  O90.0   Disruption of cesarean delivery wound   Ⓜ♀
     Dehiscence of cesarean delivery wound
     EXCLUDES 1   *rupture of uterus (spontaneous) before onset of labor (O71.0-)*
            rupture of uterus during labor (O71.1)

  O90.1   Disruption of perineal obstetric wound   Ⓜ♀
     Disruption of wound of episiotomy
     Disruption of wound of perineal laceration
     Secondary perineal tear

  O90.2   Hematoma of obstetric wound   Ⓜ♀

  O90.3   Peripartum cardiomyopathy   ᴹᶜᶜ Ⓜ♀
     Conditions in I42- arising during pregnancy and the puerperium
     EXCLUDES 1   *pre-existing heart disease complicating pregnancy and the puerperium (O99.4-)*
     CC Excl: O25.10-O25.3, O26.10-O26.13, O26.30-O26.43, O26.63-O26.819, O26.841-O26.86, O26.891-O26.93, O29.011-O29.93, O35.7XX0-O35.7XX9, O75.4, O75.81, O75.89-O75.9, O80, O90.3, O90.89, O99.111-O99.285, O99.330-O99.335, O99.350-O99.73, O99.820-O99.825, O99.840-O9A.53

  O90.4   Postpartum acute kidney failure   ᴹᶜᶜ Ⓜ♀
     Hepatorenal syndrome following labor and delivery
     CC Excl: O25.10-O25.3, O26.10-O26.13, O26.30-O26.43, O26.63-O26.819, O26.841-O26.86, O26.891-O26.93, O29.011-O29.93, O35.7XX0-O35.7XX9, O75.4, O75.81, O75.89-O75.9, O80, O90.4, O90.89, O99.111-O99.285, O99.330-O99.335, O99.350-O99.355, O99.511-O99.73, O99.820-O99.825, O99.840-O9A.53

  O90.5   Postpartum thyroiditis   ⓂⓆ

  O90.6   Postpartum mood disturbance   ⓂⓆ
     Postpartum blues
     Postpartum dysphoria
     Postpartum sadness
     EXCLUDES 1   *postpartum depression (F53)*
            puerperal psychosis (F53)

✓5ᵗʰ **O90.8**   Other complications of the puerperium, not elsewhere classified

    O90.81   Anemia of the puerperium   ⓂⓆ
       Postpartum anemia NOS
       EXCLUDES 1   *pre-existing anemia complicating the puerperium (O99.03)*

    O90.89   Other complications of the puerperium, not elsewhere classified   ⓂⓆ
       Placental polyp

  O90.9   Complication of the puerperium, unspecified   ⓂⓆ

✓4ᵗʰ **O91**   **Infections of breast associated with pregnancy, the puerperium and lactation**
     Use additional code to identify infection

✓5ᵗʰ **O91.0**   Infection of nipple associated with pregnancy, the puerperium and lactation

    ✓6ᵗʰ **O91.01**   Infection of nipple associated with pregnancy
       Gestational abscess of nipple

      O91.011   Infection of nipple associated with pregnancy, first trimester   ⓂⓆ

      O91.012   Infection of nipple associated with pregnancy, second trimester   ⓂⓆ

      O91.013   Infection of nipple associated with pregnancy, third trimester   ⓂⓆ

      O91.019   Infection of nipple associated with pregnancy, unspecified trimester   ⓂⓆ

    O91.02   Infection of nipple associated with the puerperium   ⓂⓆ
       Puerperal abscess of nipple

    O91.03   Infection of nipple associated with lactation   ⓂⓆ
       Abscess of nipple associated with lactation

✓5ᵗʰ **O91.1**   Abscess of breast associated with pregnancy, the puerperium and lactation

    ✓6ᵗʰ **O91.11**   Abscess of breast associated with pregnancy
       Gestational mammary abscess
       Gestational purulent mastitis
       Gestational subareolar abscess

      O91.111   Abscess of breast associated with pregnancy, first trimester   ⓂⓆ

      O91.112   Abscess of breast associated with pregnancy, second trimester   ⓂⓆ

      O91.113   Abscess of breast associated with pregnancy, third trimester   ⓂⓆ

      O91.119   Abscess of breast associated with pregnancy, unspecified trimester   ⓂⓆ

    O91.12   Abscess of breast associated with the puerperium   ⓂⓆ
       Puerperal mammary abscess
       Puerperal purulent mastitis
       Puerperal subareolar abscess

    O91.13   Abscess of breast associated with lactation   ⓂⓆ
       Mammary abscess associated with lactation
       Purulent mastitis associated with lactation
       Subareolar abscess associated with lactation

✓5ᵗʰ **O91.2**   Nonpurulent mastitis associated with pregnancy, the puerperium and lactation

    ✓6ᵗʰ **O91.21**   Nonpurulent mastitis associated with pregnancy
       Gestational interstitial mastitis
       Gestational lymphangitis of breast
       Gestational mastitis NOS
       Gestational parenchymatous mastitis

      O91.211   Nonpurulent mastitis associated with pregnancy, first trimester   ⓂⓆ

      O91.212   Nonpurulent mastitis associated with pregnancy, second trimester   ⓂⓆ

      O91.213   Nonpurulent mastitis associated with pregnancy, third trimester   ⓂⓆ

      O91.219   Nonpurulent mastitis associated with pregnancy, unspecified trimester   ⓂⓆ

    O91.22   Nonpurulent mastitis associated with the puerperium   ⓂⓆ
       Puerperal interstitial mastitis
       Puerperal lymphangitis of breast
       Puerperal mastitis NOS
       Puerperal parenchymatous mastitis

    O91.23   Nonpurulent mastitis associated with lactation   ⓂⓆ
       Interstitial mastitis associated with lactation
       Lymphangitis of breast associated with lactation
       Mastitis NOS associated with lactation
       Parenchymatous mastitis associated with lactation

✓4ᵗʰ **O92**   **Other disorders of breast and disorders of lactation associated with pregnancy and the puerperium**

✓5ᵗʰ **O92.0**   Retracted nipple associated with pregnancy, the puerperium, and lactation

    ✓6ᵗʰ **O92.01**   Retracted nipple associated with pregnancy

      O92.011   Retracted nipple associated with pregnancy, first trimester   ⓂⓆ

      O92.012   Retracted nipple associated with pregnancy, second trimester   ⓂⓆ

      O92.013   Retracted nipple associated with pregnancy, third trimester   ⓂⓆ

      O92.019   Retracted nipple associated with pregnancy, unspecified trimester   ⓂⓆ

    O92.02   Retracted nipple associated with the puerperium   ⓂⓆ

    O92.03   Retracted nipple associated with lactation   ⓂⓆ

✓5ᵗʰ **O92.1**   Cracked nipple associated with pregnancy, the puerperium, and lactation
     Fissure of nipple, gestational or puerperal

    ✓6ᵗʰ **O92.11**   Cracked nipple associated with pregnancy

      O92.111   Cracked nipple associated with pregnancy, first trimester   ⓂⓆ

      O92.112   Cracked nipple associated with pregnancy, second trimester   ⓂⓆ

      O92.113   Cracked nipple associated with pregnancy, third trimester   ⓂⓆ

      O92.119   Cracked nipple associated with pregnancy, unspecified trimester   ⓂⓆ

    O92.12   Cracked nipple associated with the puerperium   ⓂⓆ

    O92.13   Cracked nipple associated with lactation   ⓂⓆ

✓5ᵗʰ **O92.2**   Other and unspecified disorders of breast associated with pregnancy and the puerperium

    O92.20   Unspecified disorder of breast associated with pregnancy and the puerperium   ⓂⓆ

    O92.29   Other disorders of breast associated with pregnancy and the puerperium   ⓂⓆ

Ⓝ Newborn: 0   Ⓟ Pediatric: 0-17   Ⓜ Maternity: 12-55   Ⓐ Adult: 15-124   ᴹᶜᶜ Major CC Condition   ᴾᴰˣᴹᶜᶜ PDx acts as own MCC   ᶜᶜ CC Condition   ᴾᴰˣᶜᶜ PDx acts as own CC

808   ICD-10-CM Draft (2015)

O92.3 **Agalactia** Ⓜ♀
Primary agalactia
EXCLUDES 1 *elective agalactia (O92.5)*
secondary agalactia (O92.5)
therapeutic agalactia (O92.5)

O92.4 **Hypogalactia** Ⓜ♀

O92.5 **Suppressed lactation** Ⓜ♀
Elective agalactia   Therapeutic agalactia
Secondary agalactia
EXCLUDES 1 *primary agalactia (O92.3)*

O92.6 **Galactorrhea** Ⓜ♀

√5ᵗʰ **O92.7** **Other and unspecified disorders of lactation**

O92.70 **Unspecified disorders of lactation** Ⓜ♀

O92.79 **Other disorders of lactation** Ⓜ♀
Puerperal galactocele

Other obstetric conditions, not elsewhere classified (O94-O9A)

O94 **Sequelae of complication of pregnancy, childbirth, and the puerperium** Ⓜ♀
NOTE   This category is to be used to indicate conditions in O00-O77.-, O85-O94 and O98-O9A.- as the cause of late effects. The sequelae include conditions specified as such, or as late effects, which may occur at any time after the puerperium.
Code first condition resulting from (sequela) of complication of pregnancy, childbirth, and the puerperium

√4ᵗʰ **O98** **Maternal infectious and parasitic diseases classifiable elsewhere but complicating pregnancy, childbirth and the puerperium**
INCLUDES   the listed conditions when complicating the pregnant state, when aggravated by the pregnancy, or as a reason for obstetric care
Use additional code (Chapter 1), to identify specific infectious or parasitic disease
EXCLUDES 2 *herpes gestationis (O26.4-)*
infectious carrier state (O99.82-, O99.83-)
obstetrical tetanus (A34)
puerperal infection (O86.-)
puerperal sepsis (O85)
when the reason for maternal care is that the disease is known or suspected to have affected the fetus (O35-O36)

√5ᵗʰ **O98.0** **Tuberculosis complicating pregnancy, childbirth and the puerperium**
Conditions in A15-A19

CC Excl: For CC codes in subcategory O98.0, unless otherwise noted: O25.10-O25.3, O26.10-O26.13, O26.30-O26.43, O26.63-O26.819, O26.841-O26.86, O26.891-O26.93, O29.011-O29.93, O35.7XX0-O35.7XX9, O75.4, O75.81, O75.89-O75.9, O80, O90.89, O98.011-O98.03, O99.111-O99.285, O99.330-O99.335, O99.350-O99.355, O99.511-O99.73, O99.820-O99.825, O99.840-O9A.53

√6ᵗʰ **O98.01** **Tuberculosis complicating pregnancy**

O98.011 **Tuberculosis complicating pregnancy, first trimester** ⒸⒸ Ⓜ♀

O98.012 **Tuberculosis complicating pregnancy, second trimester** ⒸⒸ Ⓜ♀

O98.013 **Tuberculosis complicating pregnancy, third trimester** ⒸⒸ Ⓜ♀

O98.019 **Tuberculosis complicating pregnancy, unspecified trimester** Ⓜ♀

O98.02 **Tuberculosis complicating childbirth** ⒸⒸ Ⓜ♀

O98.03 **Tuberculosis complicating the puerperium** ⒸⒸ Ⓜ♀

√5ᵗʰ **O98.1** **Syphilis complicating pregnancy, childbirth and the puerperium**
Conditions in A50-A53

CC Excl: For CC codes in subcategory O98.1, unless otherwise noted: O26.11-O26.13, O26.31-O26.33, O26.41-O26.43, O26.63-O26.713, O26.72-O26.813, O26.86, O26.891-O26.893, O26.90-O26.93, O29.011-O29.013, O29.021-O29.023, O29.091-O29.093, O29.111-O29.113, O29.121-O29.123, O29.191-O29.193, O29.211-O29.213, O29.291-O29.293, O29.3X1-O29.3X3, O29.41-O29.5X3, O29.61-O29.8X3, O29.91-O29.93, O35.7XX0-O35.7XX9, O98.111-O98.33, O99.351-O99.353, O99.355, O99.89

√6ᵗʰ **O98.11** **Syphilis complicating pregnancy**

O98.111 **Syphilis complicating pregnancy, first trimester** ⒸⒸ Ⓜ♀

O98.112 **Syphilis complicating pregnancy, second trimester** ⒸⒸ Ⓜ♀

O98.113 **Syphilis complicating pregnancy, third trimester** ⒸⒸ Ⓜ♀

O98.119 **Syphilis complicating pregnancy, unspecified trimester** Ⓜ♀

O98.12 **Syphilis complicating childbirth** ⒸⒸ Ⓜ♀

O98.13 **Syphilis complicating the puerperium** ⒸⒸ Ⓜ♀

√5ᵗʰ **O98.2** **Gonorrhea complicating pregnancy, childbirth and the puerperium**
Conditions in A54-

CC Excl: For CC codes in subcategory O98.2, unless otherwise noted: See code: O98.1

√6ᵗʰ **O98.21** **Gonorrhea complicating pregnancy**

O98.211 **Gonorrhea complicating pregnancy, first trimester** ⒸⒸ Ⓜ♀

O98.212 **Gonorrhea complicating pregnancy, second trimester** ⒸⒸ Ⓜ♀

O98.213 **Gonorrhea complicating pregnancy, third trimester** ⒸⒸ Ⓜ♀

O98.219 **Gonorrhea complicating pregnancy, unspecified trimester** Ⓜ♀

O98.22 **Gonorrhea complicating childbirth** ⒸⒸ Ⓜ♀

O98.23 **Gonorrhea complicating the puerperium** ⒸⒸ Ⓜ♀

√5ᵗʰ **O98.3** **Other infections with a predominantly sexual mode of transmission complicating pregnancy, childbirth and the puerperium**
Conditions in A55-A64

CC Excl: For CC codes in subcategory O98.3, unless otherwise noted: See code: O98.1

√6ᵗʰ **O98.31** **Other infections with a predominantly sexual mode of transmission complicating pregnancy**

O98.311 **Other infections with a predominantly sexual mode of transmission complicating pregnancy, first trimester** ⒸⒸ Ⓜ♀

O98.312 **Other infections with a predominantly sexual mode of transmission complicating pregnancy, second trimester** ⒸⒸ Ⓜ♀

O98.313 **Other infections with a predominantly sexual mode of transmission complicating pregnancy, third trimester** ⒸⒸ Ⓜ♀

O98.319 **Other infections with a predominantly sexual mode of transmission complicating pregnancy, unspecified trimester** Ⓜ♀

O98.32 **Other infections with a predominantly sexual mode of transmission complicating childbirth** ⒸⒸ Ⓜ♀

O98.33 **Other infections with a predominantly sexual mode of transmission complicating the puerperium** ⒸⒸ Ⓜ♀

√5ᵗʰ **O98.4** **Viral hepatitis complicating pregnancy, childbirth and the puerperium**
Conditions in B15-B19

CC Excl: For CC codes in subcategory O98.4, unless otherwise noted: O98.411-O98.613, O98.711-O98.93, O99.830-O99.835

√6ᵗʰ **O98.41** **Viral hepatitis complicating pregnancy**

O98.411 **Viral hepatitis complicating pregnancy, first trimester** ⒸⒸ Ⓜ♀

O98.412 **Viral hepatitis complicating pregnancy, second trimester** ⒸⒸ Ⓜ♀

O98.413 **Viral hepatitis complicating pregnancy, third trimester** ⒸⒸ Ⓜ♀

O98.419 **Viral hepatitis complicating pregnancy, unspecified trimester** Ⓜ♀

O98.42 **Viral hepatitis complicating childbirth** ⒸⒸ Ⓜ♀

O98.43 **Viral hepatitis complicating the puerperium** ⒸⒸ Ⓜ♀

√5ᵗʰ **O98.5** **Other viral diseases complicating pregnancy, childbirth and the puerperium**
Conditions in A80-B09, B25-B34, R87.81-, R87.82-
EXCLUDES 1 *human immunodeficiency virus [HIV] disease complicating pregnancy, childbirth and the puerperium (O98.7-)*

CC Excl: For CC codes in subcategory O98.5, unless otherwise noted: See code: O98.4

√6ᵗʰ **O98.51** **Other viral diseases complicating pregnancy**

O98.511 **Other viral diseases complicating pregnancy, first trimester** ⒸⒸ Ⓜ♀

Pregnancy, Childbirth and the Puerperium

O98.512–O99.111

O98.512   Other viral diseases complicating pregnancy, second trimester   CC MQ

O98.513   Other viral diseases complicating pregnancy, third trimester   CC MQ

O98.519   Other viral diseases complicating pregnancy, unspecified trimester   MQ

O98.52   Other viral diseases complicating childbirth   CC MQ

O98.53   Other viral diseases complicating the puerperium   CC MQ

✓5th **O98.6**   Protozoal diseases complicating pregnancy, childbirth and the puerperium
Conditions in B50-B64

> **CC Excl: For CC codes in subcategory O98.6, unless otherwise noted:** O25.10-O25.3, O26.10-O26.13, O26.30-O26.43, O26.63-O26.819, O26.841-O26.86, O26.891-O26.93, O29.011-O29.93, O35.7XX0-O35.7XX9, O75.4, O75.81, O75.89-O75.9, O80, O90.89, O98.411-O98.93, O99.111-O99.285, O99.330-O99.335, O99.350-O99.355, O99.511-O99.73, O99.820-O9A.53

✓6th **O98.61**   Protozoal diseases complicating pregnancy

O98.611   Protozoal diseases complicating pregnancy, first trimester   CC MQ

O98.612   Protozoal diseases complicating pregnancy, second trimester   CC MQ

O98.613   Protozoal diseases complicating pregnancy, third trimester   CC MQ

O98.619   Protozoal diseases complicating pregnancy, unspecified trimester   MQ

O98.62   Protozoal diseases complicating childbirth   CC MQ
CC Excl: O25.10-O25.3, O26.10-O26.13, O26.30-O26.43, O26.63-O26.819, O26.841-O26.86, O26.891-O26.93, O29.011-O29.93, O35.7XX0-O35.7XX9, O75.4, O75.81, O75.89-O75.9, O80, O90.89, O98.611-O98.63, O99.111-O99.285, O99.330-O99.335, O99.350-O99.355, O99.511-O99.73, O99.820-O99.825, O99.840-O9A.53

O98.63   Protozoal diseases complicating the puerperium   CC MQ
CC Excl: See code: O98.62

✓5th **O98.7**   Human immunodeficiency virus [HIV] disease complicating pregnancy, childbirth and the puerperium
Use additional code to identify the type of HIV disease:
acquired immune deficiency syndrome (AIDS) (B20)
asymptomatic HIV status (Z21)
HIV positive NOS (Z21)
symptomatic HIV disease (B20)

> **CC Excl: For CC codes in subcategory O98.7, unless otherwise noted:** O98.411-O98.613, O98.711-O98.93, O99.830-O99.835

✓6th **O98.71**   Human immunodeficiency virus [HIV] disease complicating pregnancy

O98.711   Human immunodeficiency virus [HIV] disease complicating pregnancy, first trimester   CC MQ

O98.712   Human immunodeficiency virus [HIV] disease complicating pregnancy, second trimester   CC MQ

O98.713   Human immunodeficiency virus [HIV] disease complicating pregnancy, third trimester   CC MQ

O98.719   Human immunodeficiency virus [HIV] disease complicating pregnancy, unspecified trimester   MQ

O98.72   Human immunodeficiency virus [HIV] disease complicating childbirth   CC MQ

O98.73   Human immunodeficiency virus [HIV] disease complicating the puerperium   CC MQ

✓5th **O98.8**   Other maternal infectious and parasitic diseases complicating pregnancy, childbirth and the puerperium

> **CC Excl: For CC codes in subcategory O98.8, unless otherwise noted:** See code: O98.7

✓6th **O98.81**   Other maternal infectious and parasitic diseases complicating pregnancy

O98.811   Other maternal infectious and parasitic diseases complicating pregnancy, first trimester   CC MQ

O98.812   Other maternal infectious and parasitic diseases complicating pregnancy, second trimester   CC MQ

O98.813   Other maternal infectious and parasitic diseases complicating pregnancy, third trimester   CC MQ

O98.819   Other maternal infectious and parasitic diseases complicating pregnancy, unspecified trimester   MQ

O98.82   Other maternal infectious and parasitic diseases complicating childbirth   CC MQ

O98.83   Other maternal infectious and parasitic diseases complicating the puerperium   CC MQ

✓5th **O98.9**   Unspecified maternal infectious and parasitic disease complicating pregnancy, childbirth and the puerperium

> **CC Excl: For CC codes in subcategory O98.9, unless otherwise noted:** See code: O98.7

✓6th **O98.91**   Unspecified maternal infectious and parasitic disease complicating pregnancy

O98.911   Unspecified maternal infectious and parasitic disease complicating pregnancy, first trimester   CC MQ

O98.912   Unspecified maternal infectious and parasitic disease complicating pregnancy, second trimester   CC MQ

O98.913   Unspecified maternal infectious and parasitic disease complicating pregnancy, third trimester   CC MQ

O98.919   Unspecified maternal infectious and parasitic disease complicating pregnancy, unspecified trimester   MQ

O98.92   Unspecified maternal infectious and parasitic disease complicating childbirth   CC MQ

O98.93   Unspecified maternal infectious and parasitic disease complicating the puerperium   CC MQ

✓4th **O99**   Other maternal diseases classifiable elsewhere but complicating pregnancy, childbirth and the puerperium
INCLUDES conditions which complicate the pregnant state, are aggravated by the pregnancy or are a main reason for obstetric care
Use additional code to identify specific condition
EXCLUDES 2 when the reason for maternal care is that the condition is known or suspected to have affected the fetus (O35-O36)

✓5th **O99.0**   Anemia complicating pregnancy, childbirth and the puerperium
Conditions in D50-D64
EXCLUDES 1 anemia arising in the puerperium (O90.81)
postpartum anemia NOS (O90.81)

✓6th **O99.01**   Anemia complicating pregnancy

O99.011   Anemia complicating pregnancy, first trimester   MQ

O99.012   Anemia complicating pregnancy, second trimester   MQ

O99.013   Anemia complicating pregnancy, third trimester   MQ

O99.019   Anemia complicating pregnancy, unspecified trimester   MQ

O99.02   Anemia complicating childbirth   MQ

O99.03   Anemia complicating the puerperium   MQ
EXCLUDES 1 postpartum anemia not pre-existing prior to delivery (O90.81)

✓5th **O99.1**   Other diseases of the blood and blood-forming organs and certain disorders involving the immune mechanism complicating pregnancy, childbirth and the puerperium
Conditions in D65-D89
EXCLUDES 2 hemorrhage with coagulation defects (O45.-, O46.0-, O67.0, O72.3)

> **CC Excl: For CC codes in subcategory O99.1, unless otherwise noted:** O25.11-O25.3, O99.281-O99.285, O99.511-O99.513, O99.52-O99.613, O99.62-O99.713, O99.72-O99.73, O99.820-O99.825, O9A.111-O9A.113, O9A.12-O9A.213, O9A.22-O9A.313, O9A.32-O9A.413, O9A.42-O9A.513, O9A.52-O9A.53

✓6th **O99.11**   Other diseases of the blood and blood-forming organs and certain disorders involving the immune mechanism complicating pregnancy

O99.111   Other diseases of the blood and blood-forming organs and certain disorders involving the immune mechanism complicating pregnancy, first trimester   CC MQ

O99.112 Other diseases of the blood and blood-forming organs and certain disorders involving the immune mechanism complicating pregnancy, second trimester　CC M♀

O99.113 Other diseases of the blood and blood-forming organs and certain disorders involving the immune mechanism complicating pregnancy, third trimester　CC M♀

O99.119 Other diseases of the blood and blood-forming organs and certain disorders involving the immune mechanism complicating pregnancy, unspecified trimester　CC M♀
　　CC Excl: O25.10-O99.280, O99.519, O99.619, O99.719, O9A.119, O9A.219, O9A.319, O9A.419, O9A.519

O99.12 Other diseases of the blood and blood-forming organs and certain disorders involving the immune mechanism complicating childbirth　CC M♀

O99.13 Other diseases of the blood and blood-forming organs and certain disorders involving the immune mechanism complicating the puerperium　CC M♀

✓5th **O99.2** Endocrine, nutritional and metabolic diseases complicating pregnancy, childbirth and the puerperium
　　Conditions in E00-E88
　　EXCLUDES 2　diabetes mellitus (O24.-)
　　　　malnutrition (O25.-)
　　　　postpartum thyroiditis (O90.5)

✓6th **O99.21** Obesity complicating pregnancy, childbirth, and the puerperium
　　Use additional code to identify the type of obesity (E66.-)

O99.210 Obesity complicating pregnancy, unspecified trimester　M♀

O99.211 Obesity complicating pregnancy, first trimester　M♀

O99.212 Obesity complicating pregnancy, second trimester　M♀

O99.213 Obesity complicating pregnancy, third trimester　♀

O99.214 Obesity complicating childbirth　M♀

O99.215 Obesity complicating the puerperium　M♀

✓6th **O99.28** Other endocrine, nutritional and metabolic diseases complicating pregnancy, childbirth and the puerperium

O99.280 Endocrine, nutritional and metabolic diseases complicating pregnancy, unspecified trimester　M♀

O99.281 Endocrine, nutritional and metabolic diseases complicating pregnancy, first trimester　M♀

O99.282 Endocrine, nutritional and metabolic diseases complicating pregnancy, second trimester　M♀

O99.283 Endocrine, nutritional and metabolic diseases complicating pregnancy, third trimester　M♀

O99.284 Endocrine, nutritional and metabolic diseases complicating childbirth　M♀

O99.285 Endocrine, nutritional and metabolic diseases complicating the puerperium　M♀

✓5th **O99.3** Mental disorders and diseases of the nervous system complicating pregnancy, childbirth and the puerperium

　　CC Excl: For CC codes in subcategory O99.3, unless otherwise noted: O25.10-O25.3, O26.10-O26.13, O26.30-O26.43, O26.63-O26.819, O26.841-O26.86, O26.891-O26.93, O29.011-O29.93, O35.7XX0-O35.7XX9, O75.4, O75.81, O75.89-O75.9, O80, O90.89, O99.111-O99.285, O99.320-O99.335, O99.350-O99.355, O99.511-O99.73, O99.820-O99.825, O99.840-O9A.53

✓6th **O99.31** Alcohol use complicating pregnancy, childbirth, and the puerperium
　　Use additional code(s) from F10 to identify manifestations of the alcohol use

O99.310 Alcohol use complicating pregnancy, unspecified trimester　M♀

O99.311 Alcohol use complicating pregnancy, first trimester　M♀

O99.312 Alcohol use complicating pregnancy, second trimester　M♀

O99.313 Alcohol use complicating pregnancy, third trimester　M♀

O99.314 Alcohol use complicating childbirth　M♀

O99.315 Alcohol use complicating the puerperium　M♀

✓6th **O99.32** Drug use complicating pregnancy, childbirth, and the puerperium
　　Use additional code(s) from F11-F16 and F18-F19 to identify manifestations of the drug use

O99.320 Drug use complicating pregnancy, unspecified trimester　M♀

O99.321 Drug use complicating pregnancy, first trimester　CC M♀

O99.322 Drug use complicating pregnancy, second trimester　CC M♀

O99.323 Drug use complicating pregnancy, third trimester　CC M♀

O99.324 Drug use complicating childbirth　CC M♀

O99.325 Drug use complicating the puerperium　CC M♀

✓6th **O99.33** Smoking (tobacco) complicating pregnancy, childbirth, and the puerperium
　　Use additional code from F17 to identify type of tobacco

O99.330 Smoking (tobacco) complicating pregnancy, unspecified trimester　M♀

O99.331 Smoking (tobacco) complicating pregnancy, first trimester　M♀

O99.332 Smoking (tobacco) complicating pregnancy, second trimester　M♀

O99.333 Smoking (tobacco) complicating pregnancy, third trimester　M♀

O99.334 Smoking (tobacco) complicating childbirth　M♀

O99.335 Smoking (tobacco) complicating the puerperium　M♀

✓6th **O99.34** Other mental disorders complicating pregnancy, childbirth, and the puerperium
　　Conditions in F01-F09 and F20-F99
　　EXCLUDES 2　postpartum mood disturbance (O90.6)
　　　　postnatal psychosis (F53)
　　　　puerperal psychosis (F53)

O99.340 Other mental disorders complicating pregnancy, unspecified trimester　M♀

O99.341 Other mental disorders complicating pregnancy, first trimester　M♀

O99.342 Other mental disorders complicating pregnancy, second trimester　M♀

O99.343 Other mental disorders complicating pregnancy, third trimester　M♀

O99.344 Other mental disorders complicating childbirth　M♀

O99.345 Other mental disorders complicating the puerperium　M♀

✓6th **O99.35** Diseases of the nervous system complicating pregnancy, childbirth, and the puerperium
　　Conditions in G00-G99
　　EXCLUDES 2　pregnancy related peripheral neuritis (O26.8-)

O99.350 Diseases of the nervous system complicating pregnancy, unspecified trimester　M♀

O99.351 Diseases of the nervous system complicating pregnancy, first trimester　M♀

O99.352 Diseases of the nervous system complicating pregnancy, second trimester　M♀

O99.353 Diseases of the nervous system complicating pregnancy, third trimester　M♀

O99.354 Diseases of the nervous system complicating childbirth　CC M♀
　　CC Excl: See code: O99.1

✓ Additional Character Required　✓x7th Xtension Alert　Unacceptable PDx　Manifestation　Hospital Acquired Condition　EXCLUDES 1 Not Coded Here　EXCLUDES 2 Not Included Here

Pregnancy, Childbirth and the Puerperium

O99.355–O99.840

O99.355   **Diseases of the nervous system complicating the puerperium**   cc Mφ
CC Excl: See code: O99.1

√5ᵗʰ **O99.4**   **Diseases of the circulatory system complicating pregnancy, childbirth and the puerperium**
Conditions in I00-I99
EXCLUDES 1   peripartum cardiomyopathy (O90.3)
EXCLUDES 2   hypertensive disorders (O10-O16)
obstetric embolism (O88.-)
venous complications and cerebrovenous sinus thrombosis in labor, childbirth and the puerperium (O87.-)
venous complications and cerebrovenous sinus thrombosis in pregnancy (O22.-)

CC Excl: For CC codes in subcategory O99.4, unless otherwise noted: O25.10-O25.3, O26.10-O26.13, O26.30-O26.43, O26.63-O26.819, O26.841-O26.86, O26.891-O26.93, O29.011-O29.93, O35.7XX0-O35.7XX9, O75.4, O75.81, O75.89-O75.9, O80, O90.3, O90.89, O99.111-O99.285, O99.330-O99.335, O99.350-O99.73, O99.820-O99.825, O99.840-O9A.53

√6ᵗʰ **O99.41**   **Diseases of the circulatory system complicating pregnancy**

O99.411   **Diseases of the circulatory system complicating pregnancy, first trimester**   cc Mφ

O99.412   **Diseases of the circulatory system complicating pregnancy, second trimester**   cc Mφ

O99.413   **Diseases of the circulatory system complicating pregnancy, third trimester**   cc Mφ

O99.419   **Diseases of the circulatory system complicating pregnancy, unspecified trimester**   Mφ

O99.42   **Diseases of the circulatory system complicating childbirth**   MCC Mφ
CC Excl: See code: O90.3

O99.43   **Diseases of the circulatory system complicating the puerperium**   cc Mφ

√5ᵗʰ **O99.5**   **Diseases of the respiratory system complicating pregnancy, childbirth and the puerperium**
Conditions in J00-J99

√6ᵗʰ **O99.51**   **Diseases of the respiratory system complicating pregnancy**

O99.511   **Diseases of the respiratory system complicating pregnancy, first trimester**   Mφ

O99.512   **Diseases of the respiratory system complicating pregnancy, second trimester**   Mφ

O99.513   **Diseases of the respiratory system complicating pregnancy, third trimester**   Mφ

O99.519   **Diseases of the respiratory system complicating pregnancy, unspecified trimester**   Mφ

O99.52   **Diseases of the respiratory system complicating childbirth**   Mφ

O99.53   **Diseases of the respiratory system complicating the puerperium**   Mφ

√5ᵗʰ **O99.6**   **Diseases of the digestive system complicating pregnancy, childbirth and the puerperium**
Conditions in K00-K93
EXCLUDES 2   liver and biliary tract disorders in pregnancy, childbirth and the puerperium (O26.6-)

√6ᵗʰ **O99.61**   **Diseases of the digestive system complicating pregnancy**

O99.611   **Diseases of the digestive system complicating pregnancy, first trimester**   Mφ

O99.612   **Diseases of the digestive system complicating pregnancy, second trimester**   Mφ

O99.613   **Diseases of the digestive system complicating pregnancy, third trimester**   Mφ

O99.619   **Diseases of the digestive system complicating pregnancy, unspecified trimester**   Mφ

O99.62   **Diseases of the digestive system complicating childbirth**   Mφ

O99.63   **Diseases of the digestive system complicating the puerperium**   Mφ

√5ᵗʰ **O99.7**   **Diseases of the skin and subcutaneous tissue complicating pregnancy, childbirth and the puerperium**
Conditions in L00-L99
EXCLUDES 2   herpes gestationis (O26.4)
pruritic urticarial papules and plaques of pregnancy (PUPPP) (O26.86)

√6ᵗʰ **O99.71**   **Diseases of the skin and subcutaneous tissue complicating pregnancy**

O99.711   **Diseases of the skin and subcutaneous tissue complicating pregnancy, first trimester**   Mφ

O99.712   **Diseases of the skin and subcutaneous tissue complicating pregnancy, second trimester**   Mφ

O99.713   **Diseases of the skin and subcutaneous tissue complicating pregnancy, third trimester**   Mφ

O99.719   **Diseases of the skin and subcutaneous tissue complicating pregnancy, unspecified trimester**   Mφ

O99.72   **Diseases of the skin and subcutaneous tissue complicating childbirth**   Mφ

O99.73   **Diseases of the skin and subcutaneous tissue complicating the puerperium**   Mφ

√5ᵗʰ **O99.8**   **Other specified diseases and conditions complicating pregnancy, childbirth and the puerperium**
Conditions in D00-D48, H00-H95, M00-N99, and Q00-Q99
Use additional code to identify condition
EXCLUDES 2   genitourinary infections in pregnancy (O23.-)
infection of genitourinary tract following delivery (O86.1-O86.3)
malignant neoplasm complicating pregnancy, childbirth and the puerperium (O9A.1-)
maternal care for known or suspected abnormality of maternal pelvic organs (O34.-)
postpartum acute kidney failure (O90.4)
traumatic injuries in pregnancy (O9A.2)

CC Excl: For CC codes in subcategory O99.8, unless otherwise noted: O98.411-O98.613, O98.711-O98.93, O99.830-O99.835

√6ᵗʰ **O99.81**   **Abnormal glucose complicating pregnancy, childbirth and the puerperium**
EXCLUDES 1   gestational diabetes (O24.4-)

O99.810   **Abnormal glucose complicating pregnancy**   Mφ

O99.814   **Abnormal glucose complicating childbirth**   Mφ

O99.815   **Abnormal glucose complicating the puerperium**   Mφ

√6ᵗʰ **O99.82**   **Streptococcus B carrier state complicating pregnancy, childbirth and the puerperium**

O99.820   **Streptococcus B carrier state complicating pregnancy**   Mφ

O99.824   **Streptococcus B carrier state complicating childbirth**   Mφ

O99.825   **Streptococcus B carrier state complicating the puerperium**   Mφ

√6ᵗʰ **O99.83**   **Other infection carrier state complicating pregnancy, childbirth and the puerperium**
Use additional code to identify the carrier state (Z22.-)

O99.830   **Other infection carrier state complicating pregnancy**   cc Mφ

O99.834   **Other infection carrier state complicating childbirth**   cc Mφ

O99.835   **Other infection carrier state complicating the puerperium**   cc Mφ

√6ᵗʰ **O99.84**   **Bariatric surgery status complicating pregnancy, childbirth and the puerperium**
Gastric banding status complicating pregnancy, childbirth and the puerperium
Gastric bypass status for obesity complicating pregnancy, childbirth and the puerperium
Obesity surgery status complicating pregnancy, childbirth and the puerperium

O99.840   **Bariatric surgery status complicating pregnancy, unspecified trimester**   Mφ

N Newborn: 0   P Pediatric: 0-17   M Maternity: 12-55   A Adult: 15-124   MCC Major CC Condition   PDx MCC PDx acts as own MCC   cc CC Condition   PDx CC PDx acts as own CC

O99.841 **Bariatric surgery status complicating** Ⓜ♀
         pregnancy, first trimester

O99.842 **Bariatric surgery status complicating** Ⓜ♀
         pregnancy, second trimester

O99.843 **Bariatric surgery status complicating** Ⓜ♀
         pregnancy, third trimester

O99.844 **Bariatric surgery status complicating** Ⓜ♀
         childbirth

O99.845 **Bariatric surgery status complicating** Ⓜ♀
         the puerperium

O99.89 **Other specified diseases and conditions** Ⓜ♀
        complicating pregnancy, childbirth and the
        puerperium

✓4ᵗʰ **O9A Maternal malignant neoplasms, traumatic injuries and abuse**
     classifiable elsewhere but complicating pregnancy, childbirth
     and the puerperium

✓5ᵗʰ **O9A.1 Malignant neoplasm complicating pregnancy, childbirth and**
     the puerperium
     Conditions in C00-C96
     Use additional code to identify neoplasm
     EXCLUDES 2 *maternal care for benign tumor of corpus uteri (O34.1-)*
               maternal care for benign tumor of cervix (O34.4-)

✓6ᵗʰ **O9A.11 Malignant neoplasm complicating pregnancy**

O9A.111 **Malignant neoplasm complicating** Ⓜ♀
         pregnancy, first trimester

O9A.112 **Malignant neoplasm complicating** Ⓜ♀
         pregnancy, second trimester

O9A.113 **Malignant neoplasm complicating** Ⓜ♀
         pregnancy, third trimester

O9A.119 **Malignant neoplasm complicating** Ⓜ♀
         pregnancy, unspecified trimester

O9A.12 **Malignant neoplasm complicating childbirth** Ⓜ♀

O9A.13 **Malignant neoplasm complicating the** Ⓜ♀
        puerperium

✓5ᵗʰ **O9A.2 Injury, poisoning and certain other consequences of external**
     causes complicating pregnancy, childbirth and the
     puerperium
     Conditions in S00-T88, except T74 and T76
     Use additional code(s) to identify the injury or poisoning
     EXCLUDES 2 *physical, sexual and psychological abuse complicating*
               pregnancy, childbirth and the puerperium
               (O9A.3-, O9A.4-, O9A.5-)

✓6ᵗʰ **O9A.21 Injury, poisoning and certain other consequences of**
     external causes complicating pregnancy

O9A.211 **Injury, poisoning and certain other** Ⓜ♀
         consequences of external causes
         complicating pregnancy,
         first trimester

O9A.212 **Injury, poisoning and certain other** Ⓜ♀
         consequences of external causes
         complicating pregnancy,
         second trimester

O9A.213 **Injury, poisoning and certain other** Ⓜ♀
         consequences of external causes
         complicating pregnancy,
         third trimester

O9A.219 **Injury, poisoning and certain other** Ⓜ♀
         consequences of external causes
         complicating pregnancy, unspecified
         trimester

O9A.22 **Injury, poisoning and certain other** Ⓜ♀
        consequences of external causes complicating
        childbirth

O9A.23 **Injury, poisoning and certain other** Ⓜ♀
        consequences of external causes complicating the
        puerperium

✓5ᵗʰ **O9A.3 Physical abuse complicating pregnancy, childbirth and the**
     puerperium
     Conditions in T74.11 or T76.11
     Use additional code (if applicable):
       to identify any associated current injury due to physical abuse
       to identify the perpetrator of abuse (Y07.-)
     EXCLUDES 2 *sexual abuse complicating pregnancy, childbirth and*
               the puerperium (O9A.4)

✓6ᵗʰ **O9A.31 Physical abuse complicating pregnancy**

O9A.311 **Physical abuse complicating** Ⓜ♀
         pregnancy, first trimester

O9A.312 **Physical abuse complicating** Ⓜ♀
         pregnancy, second trimester

O9A.313 **Physical abuse complicating** Ⓜ♀
         pregnancy, third trimester

O9A.319 **Physical abuse complicating** Ⓜ♀
         pregnancy, unspecified trimester

O9A.32 **Physical abuse complicating childbirth** Ⓜ♀

O9A.33 **Physical abuse complicating the puerperium** Ⓜ♀

✓5ᵗʰ **O9A.4 Sexual abuse complicating pregnancy, childbirth and the**
     puerperium
     Conditions in T74.21 or T76.21
     Use additional code (if applicable):
       to identify any associated current injury due to sexual abuse
       to identify the perpetrator of abuse (Y07.-)

✓6ᵗʰ **O9A.41 Sexual abuse complicating pregnancy**

O9A.411 **Sexual abuse complicating** Ⓜ♀
         pregnancy, first trimester

O9A.412 **Sexual abuse complicating** Ⓜ♀
         pregnancy, second trimester

O9A.413 **Sexual abuse complicating** Ⓜ♀
         pregnancy, third trimester

O9A.419 **Sexual abuse complicating** Ⓜ♀
         pregnancy, unspecified trimester

O9A.42 **Sexual abuse complicating childbirth** Ⓜ♀

O9A.43 **Sexual abuse complicating the puerperium** Ⓜ♀

✓5ᵗʰ **O9A.5 Psychological abuse complicating pregnancy, childbirth and**
     the puerperium
     Conditions in T74.31 or T76.31
     Use additional code to identify the perpetrator of abuse (Y07.-)

✓6ᵗʰ **O9A.51 Psychological abuse complicating pregnancy**

O9A.511 **Psychological abuse complicating** Ⓜ♀
         pregnancy, first trimester

O9A.512 **Psychological abuse complicating** Ⓜ♀
         pregnancy, second trimester

O9A.513 **Psychological abuse complicating** Ⓜ♀
         pregnancy, third trimester

O9A.519 **Psychological abuse complicating** Ⓜ♀
         pregnancy, unspecified trimester

O9A.52 **Psychological abuse complicating childbirth** Ⓜ♀

O9A.53 **Psychological abuse complicating the** Ⓜ♀
        puerperium

✓ Additional Character Required   ✓ₓ7ᵗʰ *X*tension Alert   Unacceptable PDx   Manifestation   Hospital Acquired Condition   EXCLUDES 1 Not Coded Here   EXCLUDES 2 Not Included Here

Certain Conditions Originating in the Perinatal Period

P00–P02.1

Chapter 16. Certain Conditions Originating in the Perinatal Period (P00-P96)

NOTE   Codes from this chapter are for use on newborn records only, never on maternal records.

INCLUDES   conditions that have their origin in the fetal or perinatal period (before birth through the first 28 days after birth) even if morbidity occurs later

EXCLUDES 2   congenital malformations, deformations and chromosomal abnormalities (Q00-Q99)
endocrine, nutritional and metabolic diseases (E00-E88)
injury, poisoning and certain other consequences of external causes (S00-T88)
neoplasms (C00-D49)
tetanus neonatorum (A33)

This chapter contains the following blocks:

P00-P04	Newborn affected by maternal factors and by complications of pregnancy, labor, and delivery
P05-P08	Disorders of newborn related to length of gestation and fetal growth
P09	Abnormal findings on neonatal screening
P10-P15	Birth trauma
P19-P29	Respiratory and cardiovascular disorders specific to the perinatal period
P35-P39	Infections specific to the perinatal period
P50-P61	Hemorrhagic and hematological disorders of newborn
P70-P74	Transitory endocrine and metabolic disorders specific to newborn
P76-P78	Digestive system disorders of newborn
P80-P83	Conditions involving the integument and temperature regulation of newborn
P84	Other problems with newborn
P90-P96	Other disorders originating in the perinatal period

Newborn affected by maternal factors and by complications of pregnancy, labor, and delivery (P00-P04)

NOTE   These codes are for use when the listed maternal conditions are specified as the cause of confirmed morbidity or potential morbidity which have their origin in the perinatal period (before birth through the first 28 days after birth). Codes from these categories are also for use for newborns who are suspected of having an abnormal condition resulting from exposure from the mother or the birth process, but without signs or symptoms, and, which after examination and observation, is found not to exist. These codes may be used even if treatment is begun for a suspected condition that is ruled out.

√4ᵗʰ P00   **Newborn (suspected to be) affected by maternal conditions that may be unrelated to present pregnancy**
Code first any current condition in newborn
EXCLUDES 2   newborn (suspected to be) affected by maternal complications of pregnancy (P01.-)
newborn affected by maternal endocrine and metabolic disorders (P70-P74)
newborn affected by noxious substances transmitted via placenta or breast milk (P04.-)

P00.0   **Newborn (suspected to be) affected by maternal hypertensive disorders**   N
Newborn (suspected to be) affected by maternal conditions classifiable to O10-O11, O13-O16

P00.1   **Newborn (suspected to be) affected by maternal renal and urinary tract diseases**   N
Newborn (suspected to be) affected by maternal conditions classifiable to N00-N39

P00.2   **Newborn (suspected to be) affected by maternal infectious and parasitic diseases**   N
Newborn (suspected to be) affected by maternal infectious disease classifiable to A00-B99, J09 and J10
EXCLUDES 1   infections specific to the perinatal period (P35-P39)
maternal genital tract or other localized infections (P00.8)

P00.3   **Newborn (suspected to be) affected by other maternal circulatory and respiratory diseases**   N
Newborn (suspected to be) affected by maternal conditions classifiable to I00-I99, J00-J99, Q20-Q34 and not included in P00.0, P00.2

P00.4   **Newborn (suspected to be) affected by maternal nutritional disorders**   N
Newborn (suspected to be) affected by maternal disorders classifiable to E40-E64
Maternal malnutrition NOS

P00.5   **Newborn (suspected to be) affected by maternal injury**   N
Newborn (suspected to be) affected by maternal conditions classifiable to O9A.2-

P00.6   **Newborn (suspected to be) affected by surgical procedure on mother**   N
Newborn (suspected to be) affected by amniocentesis
EXCLUDES 1   Cesarean delivery for present delivery (P03.4)
damage to placenta from amniocentesis, Cesarean delivery or surgical induction (P02.1)
previous surgery to uterus or pelvic organs (P03.89)
EXCLUDES 2   newborn affected by complication of (fetal) intrauterine procedure (P96.5)

P00.7   **Newborn (suspected to be) affected by other medical procedures on mother, not elsewhere classified**   N
Newborn (suspected to be) affected by radiation to mother
EXCLUDES 1   damage to placenta from amniocentesis, cesarean delivery or surgical induction (P02.1)
newborn affected by other complications of labor and delivery (P03.-)

√5ᵗʰ P00.8   **Newborn (suspected to be) affected by other maternal conditions**

P00.81   **Newborn (suspected to be) affected by periodontal disease in mother**   N

P00.89   **Newborn (suspected to be) affected by other maternal conditions**   N
Newborn (suspected to be) affected by conditions classifiable to T80-T88
Newborn (suspected to be) affected by maternal genital tract or other localized infections
Newborn (suspected to be) affected by maternal systemic lupus erythematosus

P00.9   **Newborn (suspected to be) affected by unspecified maternal condition**   N

√4ᵗʰ P01   **Newborn (suspected to be) affected by maternal complications of pregnancy**
Code first any current condition in newborn

P01.0   **Newborn (suspected to be) affected by incompetent cervix**   N

P01.1   **Newborn (suspected to be) affected by premature rupture of membranes**   N

P01.2   **Newborn (suspected to be) affected by oligohydramnios**   N
EXCLUDES 1   oligohydramnios due to premature rupture of membranes (P01.1)

P01.3   **Newborn (suspected to be) affected by polyhydramnios**   N
Newborn (suspected to be) affected by hydramnios

P01.4   **Newborn (suspected to be) affected by ectopic pregnancy**   N
Newborn (suspected to be) affected by abdominal pregnancy

P01.5   **Newborn (suspected to be) affected by multiple pregnancy**   N
Newborn (suspected to be) affected by triplet (pregnancy)
Newborn (suspected to be) affected by twin (pregnancy)

P01.6   **Newborn (suspected to be) affected by maternal death**   N

P01.7   **Newborn (suspected to be) affected by malpresentation before labor**   N
Newborn (suspected to be) affected by breech presentation before labor
Newborn (suspected to be) affected by external version before labor
Newborn (suspected to be) affected by face presentation before labor
Newborn (suspected to be) affected by transverse lie before labor
Newborn (suspected to be) affected by unstable lie before labor

P01.8   **Newborn (suspected to be) affected by other maternal complications of pregnancy**   N

P01.9   **Newborn (suspected to be) affected by maternal complication of pregnancy, unspecified**   N

√4ᵗʰ P02   **Newborn (suspected to be) affected by complications of placenta, cord and membranes**
Code first any current condition in newborn

P02.0   **Newborn (suspected to be) affected by placenta previa**   N

P02.1   **Newborn (suspected to be) affected by other forms of placental separation and hemorrhage**   N
Newborn (suspected to be) affected by abruptio placenta
Newborn (suspected to be) affected by accidental hemorrhage
Newborn (suspected to be) affected by antepartum hemorrhage
Newborn (suspected to be) affected by damage to placenta from amniocentesis, cesarean delivery or surgical induction
Newborn (suspected to be) affected by maternal blood loss
Newborn (suspected to be) affected by premature separation of placenta

---

N Newborn: 0   **P** Pediatric: 0-17   **M** Maternity: 12-55   **A** Adult: 15-124   **MCC** Major CC Condition   **PDx MCC** PDx acts as own MCC   **CC** CC Condition   **PDx CC** PDx acts as own CC

814   ICD-10-CM Draft (2015)

✓5th **P02.2 Newborn (suspected to be) affected by other and unspecified morphological and functional abnormalities of placenta**

    P02.20 Newborn (suspected to be) affected by unspecified morphological and functional abnormalities of placenta   N

    P02.29 Newborn (suspected to be) affected by other morphological and functional abnormalities of placenta   N

      Newborn (suspected to be) affected by placental dysfunction

      Newborn (suspected to be) affected by placental infarction

      Newborn (suspected to be) affected by placental insufficiency

P02.3 Newborn (suspected to be) affected by placental transfusion syndromes   N

    Newborn (suspected to be) affected by placental and cord abnormalities resulting in twin-to-twin or other transplacental transfusion

P02.4 Newborn (suspected to be) affected by prolapsed cord   N

P02.5 Newborn (suspected to be) affected by other compression of umbilical cord   N

    Newborn (suspected to be) affected by umbilical cord (tightly) around neck

    Newborn (suspected to be) affected by entanglement of umbilical cord

    Newborn (suspected to be) affected by knot in umbilical cord

✓5th **P02.6 Newborn (suspected to be) affected by other and unspecified conditions of umbilical cord**

    P02.60 Newborn (suspected to be) affected by unspecified conditions of umbilical cord   N

    P02.69 Newborn (suspected to be) affected by other conditions of umbilical cord   N

      Newborn (suspected to be) affected by short umbilical cord

      Newborn (suspected to be) affected by vasa previa

      EXCLUDES 1 *newborn affected by single umbilical artery (Q27.0)*

P02.7 Newborn (suspected to be) affected by chorioamnionitis   N

    Newborn (suspected to be) affected by amnionitis

    Newborn (suspected to be) affected by membranitis

    Newborn (suspected to be) affected by placentitis

P02.8 Newborn (suspected to be) affected by other abnormalities of membranes   N

P02.9 Newborn (suspected to be) affected by abnormality of membranes, unspecified   N

✓4th **P03 Newborn (suspected to be) affected by other complications of labor and delivery**

    Code first any current condition in newborn

P03.0 Newborn (suspected to be) affected by breech delivery and extraction   N

P03.1 Newborn (suspected to be) affected by other malpresentation, malposition and disproportion during labor and delivery   N

    Newborn (suspected to be) affected by contracted pelvis

    Newborn (suspected to be) affected by conditions classifiable to O64-O66

    Newborn (suspected to be) affected by persistent occipitoposterior

    Newborn (suspected to be) affected by transverse lie

P03.2 Newborn (suspected to be) affected by forceps delivery   N

P03.3 Newborn (suspected to be) affected by delivery by vacuum extractor [ventouse]   N

P03.4 Newborn (suspected to be) affected by Cesarean delivery   N

P03.5 Newborn (suspected to be) affected by precipitate delivery   N

    Newborn (suspected to be) affected by rapid second stage

P03.6 Newborn (suspected to be) affected by abnormal uterine contractions   N

    Newborn (suspected to be) affected by conditions classifiable to O62-, except O62.3

    Newborn (suspected to be) affected by hypertonic labor

    Newborn (suspected to be) affected by uterine inertia

✓5th **P03.8 Newborn (suspected to be) affected by other specified complications of labor and delivery**

    ✓6th **P03.81 Newborn (suspected to be) affected by abnormality in fetal (intrauterine) heart rate or rhythm**

      EXCLUDES 1 *neonatal cardiac dysrhythmia (P29.1-)*

      P03.810 Newborn (suspected to be) affected by abnormality in fetal (intrauterine) heart rate or rhythm before the onset of labor   N

      P03.811 Newborn (suspected to be) affected by abnormality in fetal (intrauterine) heart rate or rhythm during labor   N

      P03.819 Newborn (suspected to be) affected by abnormality in fetal (intrauterine) heart rate or rhythm, unspecified as to time of onset   N

    P03.82 Meconium passage during delivery   N

      EXCLUDES 1 *meconium aspiration (P24.00, P24.01)*

      meconium staining (P96.83)

    P03.89 Newborn (suspected to be) affected by other specified complications of labor and delivery   N

      Newborn (suspected to be) affected by abnormality of maternal soft tissues

      Newborn (suspected to be) affected by conditions classifiable to O60-O75 and by procedures used in labor and delivery not included in P02- and P03.0-P03.6

      Newborn (suspected to be) affected by induction of labor

P03.9 Newborn (suspected to be) affected by complication of labor and delivery, unspecified   N

✓4th **P04 Newborn (suspected to be) affected by noxious substances transmitted via placenta or breast milk**

    INCLUDES nonteratogenic effects of substances transmitted via placenta

    EXCLUDES 2 *congenital malformations (Q00-Q99)*

    neonatal jaundice from excessive hemolysis due to drugs or toxins transmitted from mother (P58.4)

    newborn in contact with and (suspected) exposures hazardous to health not transmitted via placenta or breast milk (Z77.-)

P04.0 Newborn (suspected to be) affected by maternal anesthesia and analgesia in pregnancy, labor and delivery   N

    Newborn (suspected to be) affected by reactions and intoxications from maternal opiates and tranquilizers administered during labor and delivery

P04.1 Newborn (suspected to be) affected by other maternal medication   N

    Newborn (suspected to be) affected by cancer chemotherapy

    Newborn (suspected to be) affected by cytotoxic drugs

    EXCLUDES 1 *dysmorphism due to warfarin (Q86.2)*

    fetal hydantoin syndrome (Q86.1)

    maternal use of drugs of addiction (P04.4-)

P04.2 Newborn (suspected to be) affected by maternal use of tobacco   N

    Newborn (suspected to be) affected by exposure in utero to tobacco smoke

    EXCLUDES 2 *newborn exposure to environmental tobacco smoke (P96.81)*

P04.3 Newborn (suspected to be) affected by maternal use of alcohol   N

    EXCLUDES 1 *fetal alcohol syndrome (Q86.0)*

✓5th **P04.4 Newborn (suspected to be) affected by maternal use of drugs of addiction**

    P04.41 Newborn (suspected to be) affected by maternal use of cocaine   N

      "Crack baby"

    P04.49 Newborn (suspected to be) affected by maternal use of other drugs of addiction   N

      EXCLUDES 2 *newborn (suspected to be) affected by maternal anesthesia and analgesia (P04.0)*

      withdrawal symptoms from maternal use of drugs of addiction (P96.1)

P04.5 Newborn (suspected to be) affected by maternal use of nutritional chemical substances   N

P04.6 Newborn (suspected to be) affected by maternal exposure to environmental chemical substances   N

P04.8 Newborn (suspected to be) affected by other maternal noxious substances   N

P04.9 Newborn (suspected to be) affected by maternal noxious substance, unspecified   N

✓ Additional Character Required   ✓x7th Xtension Alert   Unacceptable PDx   Manifestation   Hospital Acquired Condition   EXCLUDES 1 Not Coded Here   EXCLUDES 2 Not Included Here

ICD-10-CM Draft (2015)   815

Disorders of newborn related to length of gestation and fetal growth (P05-P08)

✓4ᵗʰ P05　Disorders of newborn related to slow fetal growth and fetal malnutrition

✓5ᵗʰ **P05.0**　**Newborn light for gestational age**
Newborn light-for-dates

P05.00　Newborn light for gestational age, unspecified weight　N

P05.01　Newborn light for gestational age, less than 500 grams　N

P05.02　Newborn light for gestational age, 500-749 grams　N

P05.03　Newborn light for gestational age, 750-999 grams　N

P05.04　Newborn light for gestational age, 1000-1249 grams　N

P05.05　Newborn light for gestational age, 1250-1499 grams　N

P05.06　Newborn light for gestational age, 1500-1749 grams　N

P05.07　Newborn light for gestational age, 1750-1999 grams　N

P05.08　Newborn light for gestational age, 2000-2499 grams　N

✓5ᵗʰ **P05.1**　**Newborn small for gestational age**
Newborn small-and-light-for-dates
Newborn small-for-dates

P05.10　Newborn small for gestational age, unspecified weight　N

P05.11　Newborn small for gestational age, less than 500 grams　N

P05.12　Newborn small for gestational age, 500-749 grams　N

P05.13　Newborn small for gestational age, 750-999 grams　N

P05.14　Newborn small for gestational age, 1000-1249 grams　N

P05.15　Newborn small for gestational age, 1250-1499 grams　N

P05.16　Newborn small for gestational age, 1500-1749 grams　N

P05.17　Newborn small for gestational age, 1750-1999 grams　N

P05.18　Newborn small for gestational age, 2000-2499 grams　N

P05.2　**Newborn affected by fetal (intrauterine) malnutrition not light or small for gestational age**　N
Infant, not light or small for gestational age, showing signs of fetal malnutrition, such as dry, peeling skin and loss of subcutaneous tissue

> EXCLUDES 1　*newborn affected by fetal malnutrition with light for gestational age (P05.0-)*
> *newborn affected by fetal malnutrition with small for gestational age (P05.1-)*

P05.9　**Newborn affected by slow intrauterine growth, unspecified**　N
Newborn affected by fetal growth retardation NOS

✓4ᵗʰ P07　Disorders of newborn related to short gestation and low birth weight, not elsewhere classified

> NOTE　When both birth weight and gestational age of the newborn are available, both should be coded with birth weight sequenced before gestational age
>
> INCLUDES　the listed conditions, without further specification, as the cause of morbidity or additional care, in newborn
>
> EXCLUDES 1　*low birth weight due to slow fetal growth and fetal malnutrition (P05.-)*

✓5ᵗʰ **P07.0**　**Extremely low birth weight newborn**
Newborn birth weight 999 g. or less

P07.00　Extremely low birth weight newborn, unspecified weight　N

P07.01　Extremely low birth weight newborn, less than 500 grams　N

P07.02　Extremely low birth weight newborn, 500-749 grams　N

P07.03　Extremely low birth weight newborn, 750-999 grams　N

✓5ᵗʰ **P07.1**　**Other low birth weight newborn**
Newborn birth weight 1000-2499 g.

P07.10　Other low birth weight newborn, unspecified weight　N

P07.14　Other low birth weight newborn, 1000-1249 grams　N

P07.15　Other low birth weight newborn, 1250-1499 grams　N

P07.16　Other low birth weight newborn, 1500-1749 grams　N

P07.17　Other low birth weight newborn, 1750-1999 grams　N

P07.18　Other low birth weight newborn, 2000-2499 grams　N

✓5ᵗʰ **P07.2**　**Extreme immaturity of newborn**
Less than 28 completed weeks (less than 196 completed days) of gestation.

P07.20　Extreme immaturity of newborn, unspecified weeks of gestation　N
Gestational age less than 28 completed weeks NOS

P07.21　Extreme immaturity of newborn, gestational age less than 23 completed weeks　N
Extreme immaturity of newborn, gestational age less than 23 weeks, 0 days

P07.22　Extreme immaturity of newborn, gestational age 23 completed weeks　N
Extreme immaturity of newborn, gestational age 23 weeks, 0 days through 23 weeks, 6 days

P07.23　Extreme immaturity of newborn, gestational age 24 completed weeks　N
Extreme immaturity of newborn, gestational age 24 weeks, 0 days through 24 weeks, 6 days

P07.24　Extreme immaturity of newborn, gestational age 25 completed weeks　N
Extreme immaturity of newborn, gestational age 25 weeks, 0 days through 25 weeks, 6 days

P07.25　Extreme immaturity of newborn, gestational age 26 completed weeks　N
Extreme immaturity of newborn, gestational age 26 weeks, 0 days through 26 weeks, 6 days

P07.26　Extreme immaturity of newborn, gestational age 27 completed weeks　N
Extreme immaturity of newborn, gestational age 27 weeks, 0 days through 27 weeks, 6 days

✓5ᵗʰ **P07.3**　**Preterm [premature] newborn [other]**
28 completed weeks or more but less than 37 completed weeks (196 completed days but less than 259 completed days) of gestation
Prematurity NOS

P07.30　Preterm newborn, unspecified weeks of gestation　N

P07.31　Preterm newborn, gestational age 28 completed weeks　N
Preterm newborn, gestational age 28 weeks, 0 days through 28 weeks, 6 days

P07.32　Preterm newborn, gestational age 29 completed weeks　N
Preterm newborn, gestational age 29 weeks, 0 days through 29 weeks, 6 days

P07.33　Preterm newborn, gestational age 30 completed weeks　N
Preterm newborn, gestational age 30 weeks, 0 days through 30 weeks, 6 days

P07.34　Preterm newborn, gestational age 31 completed weeks　N
Preterm newborn, gestational age 31 weeks, 0 days through 31 weeks, 6 days

P07.35　Preterm newborn, gestational age 32 completed weeks　N
Preterm newborn, gestational age 32 weeks, 0 days through 32 weeks, 6 days

P07.36　Preterm newborn, gestational age 33 completed weeks　N
Preterm newborn, gestational age 33 weeks, 0 days through 33 weeks, 6 days

P07.37　Preterm newborn, gestational age 34 completed weeks　N
Preterm newborn, gestational age 34 weeks, 0 days through 34 weeks, 6 days

N Newborn: 0　P Pediatric: 0-17　M Maternity: 12-55　A Adult: 15-124　MCC Major CC Condition　PDx MCC PDx acts as own MCC　CC CC Condition　PDx CC PDx acts as own CC

816　　　ICD-10-CM Draft (2015)

P07.38 **Preterm newborn, gestational age 35 completed weeks** N

Preterm newborn, gestational age 35 weeks, 0 days through 35 weeks, 6 days

P07.39 **Preterm newborn, gestational age 36 completed weeks** N

Preterm newborn, gestational age 36 weeks, 0 days through 36 weeks, 6 days

✓4th **P08** **Disorders of newborn related to long gestation and high birth weight**

NOTE When both birth weight and gestational age of the newborn are available, priority of assignment should be given to birth weight

INCLUDES the listed conditions, without further specification, as causes of morbidity or additional care, in newborn

P08.0 **Exceptionally large newborn baby** N

Usually implies a birth weight of 4500 g. or more

EXCLUDES 1 syndrome of infant of diabetic mother (P70.1)
syndrome of infant of mother with gestational diabetes (P70.0)

P08.1 **Other heavy for gestational age newborn** N

Other newborn heavy- or large-for-dates regardless of period of gestation
Usually implies a birth weight of 4000 g. to 4499 g.

EXCLUDES 1 newborn with a birth weight of 4500 or more (P08.0)
syndrome of infant of diabetic mother (P70.1)
syndrome of infant of mother with gestational diabetes (P70.0).

✓5th **P08.2** **Late newborn, not heavy for gestational age**

AHA: 2014, 1Q, 14

P08.21 **Post-term newborn** N

Newborn with gestation period over 40 completed weeks to 42 completed weeks

P08.22 **Prolonged gestation of newborn** N

Newborn with gestation period over 42 completed weeks (294 days or more), not heavy- or large-for-dates.
Postmaturity NOS

Abnormal findings on neonatal screening (P09)

P09 **Abnormal findings on neonatal screening** N

Use additional code to identify signs, symptoms and conditions associated with the screening

EXCLUDES 2 nonspecific serologic evidence of human immunodeficiency virus [HIV] (R75)

Birth trauma (P10-P15)

✓4th **P10** **Intracranial laceration and hemorrhage due to birth injury**

EXCLUDES 1 intracranial hemorrhage of newborn NOS (P52.9)
intracranial hemorrhage of newborn due to anoxia or hypoxia (P52.-)
nontraumatic intracranial hemorrhage of newborn (P52.-)

P10.0 **Subdural hemorrhage due to birth injury** MCC N

Subdural hematoma (localized) due to birth injury

EXCLUDES 1 subdural hemorrhage accompanying tentorial tear (P10.4)

CC Excl: P10.0-P10.1, P10.4-P11.2, P11.9, P15.0-P15.9, P29.0-P29.2, P29.4, P29.89-P29.9, P52.4, P52.6-P52.9, P94.1-P94.9, P96.0, P96.3-P96.5, P96.82-P96.89

P10.1 **Cerebral hemorrhage due to birth injury** MCC N

CC Excl: See code P10.0

P10.2 **Intraventricular hemorrhage due to birth injury** CC N

CC Excl: P10.2-P10.3, P29.0-P29.2, P29.4, P29.89-P29.9, P50.0-P50.9, P52.0-P52.3, P52.5, P53-P54.0, P54.6-P54.9, P60-P61.9, P94.1-P94.9, P96.0, P96.3-P96.5, P96.82-P96.89

P10.3 **Subarachnoid hemorrhage due to birth injury** MCC N

CC Excl: P10.2-P10.3, P29.0-P29.2, P29.4, P29.89-P29.9, P50.0-P50.9, P52.0-P52.3, P52.5, P53-P54.0, P54.6-P54.9, P60-P61.9, P91.2, P94.1-P94.9, P96.0, P96.3-P96.5, P96.82-P96.89

P10.4 **Tentorial tear due to birth injury** MCC N

CC Excl: See code P10.0

P10.8 **Other intracranial lacerations and hemorrhages due to birth injury** MCC N

CC Excl: See code P10.0

P10.9 **Unspecified intracranial laceration and hemorrhage due to birth injury** MCC N

CC Excl: See code P10.0

✓4th **P11** **Other birth injuries to central nervous system**

P11.0 **Cerebral edema due to birth injury** MCC N

CC Excl: See code P10.0

P11.1 **Other specified brain damage due to birth injury** N

P11.2 **Unspecified brain damage due to birth injury** MCC N

CC Excl: See code P10.0

P11.3 **Birth injury to facial nerve** N

Facial palsy due to birth injury

P11.4 **Birth injury to other cranial nerves** N

P11.5 **Birth injury to spine and spinal cord** N

Fracture of spine due to birth injury

P11.9 **Birth injury to central nervous system, unspecified** MCC N

CC Excl: See code P10.0

✓4th **P12** **Birth injury to scalp**

P12.0 **Cephalhematoma due to birth injury** N

P12.1 **Chignon (from vacuum extraction) due to birth injury** N

P12.2 **Epicranial subaponeurotic hemorrhage due to birth injury** CC N

Subgaleal hemorrhage

CC Excl: P10.0-P10.1, P10.4-P11.2, P11.9, P12.2, P15.0-P15.9, P29.0-P29.2, P29.4, P29.89-P29.9, P52.4, P52.6-P52.9, P94.1-P94.9, P96.0, P96.3-P96.5, P96.82-P96.89

P12.3 **Bruising of scalp due to birth injury** N

P12.4 **Injury of scalp of newborn due to monitoring equipment** N

Sampling incision of scalp of newborn
Scalp clip (electrode) injury of newborn

✓5th **P12.8** **Other birth injuries to scalp**

P12.81 **Caput succedaneum** N

P12.89 **Other birth injuries to scalp** N

P12.9 **Birth injury to scalp, unspecified** N

✓4th **P13** **Birth injury to skeleton**

EXCLUDES 2 birth injury to spine (P11.5)

P13.0 **Fracture of skull due to birth injury** N

P13.1 **Other birth injuries to skull** N

EXCLUDES 1 cephalhematoma (P12.0)

P13.2 **Birth injury to femur** N

P13.3 **Birth injury to other long bones** N

P13.4 **Fracture of clavicle due to birth injury** N

P13.8 **Birth injuries to other parts of skeleton** N

P13.9 **Birth injury to skeleton, unspecified** N

✓4th **P14** **Birth injury to peripheral nervous system**

P14.0 **Erb's paralysis due to birth injury** N

P14.1 **Klumpke's paralysis due to birth injury** N

P14.2 **Phrenic nerve paralysis due to birth injury** N

P14.3 **Other brachial plexus birth injuries** N

P14.8 **Birth injuries to other parts of peripheral nervous system** N

P14.9 **Birth injury to peripheral nervous system, unspecified** N

✓4th **P15** **Other birth injuries**

P15.0 **Birth injury to liver** N

Rupture of liver due to birth injury

P15.1 **Birth injury to spleen** N

Rupture of spleen due to birth injury

P15.2 **Sternomastoid injury due to birth injury** N

P15.3 **Birth injury to eye** N

Subconjunctival hemorrhage due to birth injury
Traumatic glaucoma due to birth injury

P15.4 **Birth injury to face** N

Facial congestion due to birth injury

P15.5 **Birth injury to external genitalia** N

P15.6 **Subcutaneous fat necrosis due to birth injury** N

P15.8 **Other specified birth injuries** N

P15.9 **Birth injury, unspecified** N

Respiratory and cardiovascular disorders specific to the perinatal period (P19-P29)

✓4th **P19** **Metabolic acidemia in newborn**

Metabolic acidemia in newborn

P19.0 **Metabolic acidemia in newborn first noted before onset of labor** N

P19.1 **Metabolic acidemia in newborn first noted during labor** N

P19.2 **Metabolic acidemia noted at birth** N

P19.9 **Metabolic acidemia, unspecified** N

✓ Additional Character Required   ✓x7th Xtension Alert   Unacceptable PDx   Manifestation   Hospital Acquired Condition   EXCLUDES 1 Not Coded Here   EXCLUDES 2 Not Included Here

Certain Conditions Originating in the Perinatal Period

P22-P27.8

✓4th P22 Respiratory distress of newborn

EXCLUDES 1   respiratory arrest of newborn (P28.81)
       respiratory failure of newborn NOS (P28.5)

P22.0 Respiratory distress syndrome of newborn   MCC N

Cardiorespiratory distress syndrome of newborn
Hyaline membrane disease
Idiopathic respiratory distress syndrome [IRDS or RDS] of newborn
Pulmonary hypoperfusion syndrome
Respiratory distress syndrome, type I
CC Excl: J84.83-J84.848, P22.0-P28.5, P28.89-P29.2, P29.4, P29.89-P29.9, P84, P94.1-P94.9, P96.0, P96.3-P96.5, P96.82-P96.89

P22.1 Transient tachypnea of newborn   N

Idiopathic tachypnea of newborn
Respiratory distress syndrome, type II
Wet lung syndrome

P22.8 Other respiratory distress of newborn   N

P22.9 Respiratory distress of newborn, unspecified   N

✓4th P23 Congenital pneumonia

INCLUDES   infective pneumonia acquired in utero or during birth
EXCLUDES 1   neonatal pneumonia resulting from aspiration (P24.-)

CC Excl: For MCC codes in subcategory P23, unless otherwise noted: J84.83-J84.848, P22.0-P28.5, P28.89-P29.2, P29.4, P29.89-P29.9, P84, P94.1-P94.9, P96.0, P96.3-P96.5, P96.82-P96.89

P23.0 Congenital pneumonia due to viral agent   MCC N

Use additional code (B97) to identify organism
EXCLUDES 1   congenital rubella pneumonitis (P35.0)

P23.1 Congenital pneumonia due to Chlamydia   MCC N

P23.2 Congenital pneumonia due to staphylococcus   MCC N

P23.3 Congenital pneumonia due to streptococcus, group B   MCC N

P23.4 Congenital pneumonia due to Escherichia coli   MCC N

P23.5 Congenital pneumonia due to Pseudomonas   MCC N

P23.6 Congenital pneumonia due to other bacterial agents   MCC N

Congenital pneumonia due to Hemophilus influenzae
Congenital pneumonia due to Klebsiella pneumoniae
Congenital pneumonia due to Mycoplasma
Congenital pneumonia due to Streptococcus, except group B
Use additional code (B95-B96) to identify organism

P23.8 Congenital pneumonia due to other organisms   MCC N

P23.9 Congenital pneumonia, unspecified   MCC N

✓4th P24 Neonatal aspiration

INCLUDES   aspiration in utero and during delivery

✓5th P24.0 Meconium aspiration

EXCLUDES 1   meconium passage (without aspiration) during delivery (P03.82)
      meconium staining (P96.83)

P24.00 Meconium aspiration without respiratory symptoms   N

Meconium aspiration NOS

P24.01 Meconium aspiration with respiratory symptoms   MCC N

Meconium aspiration pneumonia
Meconium aspiration pneumonitis
Meconium aspiration syndrome NOS
Use additional code to identify any secondary pulmonary hypertension, if applicable (I27.2)
CC Excl: See code P23

✓5th P24.1 Neonatal aspiration of (clear) amniotic fluid and mucus

Neonatal aspiration of liquor (amnii)

P24.10 Neonatal aspiration of (clear) amniotic fluid and mucus without respiratory symptoms   N

Neonatal aspiration of amniotic fluid and mucus NOS

P24.11 Neonatal aspiration of (clear) amniotic fluid and mucus with respiratory symptoms   MCC N

Neonatal aspiration of amniotic fluid and mucus with pneumonia
Neonatal aspiration of amniotic fluid and mucus with pneumonitis
Use additional code to identify any secondary pulmonary hypertension, if applicable (I27.2)
CC Excl: See code P23

✓5th P24.2 Neonatal aspiration of blood

P24.20 Neonatal aspiration of blood without respiratory symptoms   N

Neonatal aspiration of blood NOS

P24.21 Neonatal aspiration of blood with respiratory symptoms   MCC N

Neonatal aspiration of blood with pneumonia
Neonatal aspiration of blood with pneumonitis
Use additional code to identify any secondary pulmonary hypertension, if applicable (I27.2)
CC Excl: See code P23

✓5th P24.3 Neonatal aspiration of milk and regurgitated food

Neonatal aspiration of stomach contents

P24.30 Neonatal aspiration of milk and regurgitated food without respiratory symptoms   N

Neonatal aspiration of milk and regurgitated food NOS

P24.31 Neonatal aspiration of milk and regurgitated food with respiratory symptoms   MCC N

Neonatal aspiration of milk and regurgitated food with pneumonia
Neonatal aspiration of milk and regurgitated food with pneumonitis
Use additional code to identify any secondary pulmonary hypertension, if applicable (I27.2)
CC Excl: See code P23

✓5th P24.8 Other neonatal aspiration

P24.80 Other neonatal aspiration without respiratory symptoms   N

Neonatal aspiration NEC

P24.81 Other neonatal aspiration with respiratory symptoms   MCC N

Neonatal aspiration pneumonia NEC
Neonatal aspiration with pneumonitis NEC
Neonatal aspiration with pneumonia NOS
Neonatal aspiration with pneumonitis NOS
Use additional code to identify any secondary pulmonary hypertension, if applicable (I27.2)
CC Excl: See code P23

P24.9 Neonatal aspiration, unspecified   N

✓4th P25 Interstitial emphysema and related conditions originating in the perinatal period

CC Excl: For MCC codes in subcategory P25, unless otherwise noted: J84.83-J84.848, P22.0-P28.5, P28.89-P29.2, P29.4, P29.89-P29.9, P84, P94.1-P94.9, P96.0, P96.3-P96.5, P96.82-P96.89

P25.0 Interstitial emphysema originating in the perinatal period   MCC N

P25.1 Pneumothorax originating in the perinatal period   MCC N

P25.2 Pneumomediastinum originating in the perinatal period   MCC N

P25.3 Pneumopericardium originating in the perinatal period   MCC N

P25.8 Other conditions related to interstitial emphysema originating in the perinatal period   MCC N

✓4th P26 Pulmonary hemorrhage originating in the perinatal period

EXCLUDES 1   acute idiopathic hemorrhage in infants over 28 days old (R04.81)

CC Excl: For MCC codes in subcategory P26, unless otherwise noted: J84.83-J84.848, P22.0-P28.5, P28.89-P29.2, P29.4, P29.89-P29.9, P84, P94.1-P94.9, P96.0, P96.3-P96.5, P96.82-P96.89

P26.0 Tracheobronchial hemorrhage originating in the perinatal period   MCC N

P26.1 Massive pulmonary hemorrhage originating in the perinatal period   MCC N

P26.8 Other pulmonary hemorrhages originating in the perinatal period   MCC N

P26.9 Unspecified pulmonary hemorrhage originating in the perinatal period   MCC N

✓4th P27 Chronic respiratory disease originating in the perinatal period

EXCLUDES 1   respiratory distress of newborn (P22.0-P22.9)

CC Excl: For MCC codes in subcategory P27, unless otherwise noted: J84.83-J84.848, P22.0-P28.5, P28.89-P29.2, P29.4, P29.89-P29.9, P84, P94.1-P94.9, P96.0, P96.3-P96.5, P96.82-P96.89

P27.0 Wilson-Mikity syndrome   MCC

Pulmonary dysmaturity

P27.1 Bronchopulmonary dysplasia originating in the perinatal period   MCC

P27.8 Other chronic respiratory diseases originating in the perinatal period   MCC

Congenital pulmonary fibrosis
Ventilator lung in newborn

N Newborn: 0   P Pediatric: 0-17   M Maternity: 12-55   A Adult: 15-124   MCC Major CC Condition   PDx MCC PDx acts as own MCC   CC CC Condition   PDx CC PDx acts as own CC

818   ICD-10-CM Draft (2015)

P27.9 Unspecified chronic respiratory disease originating in the perinatal period `MCC`

✓4ᵗʰ P28 Other respiratory conditions originating in the perinatal period
EXCLUDES 1 *congenital malformations of the respiratory system (Q30-Q34)*

P28.0 Primary atelectasis of newborn `CC` `N`
Primary failure to expand terminal respiratory units
Pulmonary hypoplasia associated with short gestation
Pulmonary immaturity NOS
CC Excl: See code P27

✓5ᵗʰ P28.1 Other and unspecified atelectasis of newborn

P28.10 Unspecified atelectasis of newborn `CC` `N`
Atelectasis of newborn NOS
CC Excl: See code P27

P28.11 Resorption atelectasis without respiratory distress syndrome `CC` `N`
EXCLUDES 1 *resorption atelectasis with respiratory distress syndrome (P22.0)*
CC Excl: See code P27

P28.19 Other atelectasis of newborn `CC` `N`
Partial atelectasis of newborn
Secondary atelectasis of newborn
CC Excl: See code P27

P28.2 Cyanotic attacks of newborn `CC` `N`
EXCLUDES 1 *apnea of newborn (P28.3-P28.4)*
CC Excl: P22.8-P22.9, P28.2-P28.4, P28.81-P28.9, R06.81, R23.0

P28.3 Primary sleep apnea of newborn `CC` `N`
Central sleep apnea of newborn
Obstructive sleep apnea of newborn
Sleep apnea of newborn NOS
CC Excl: P22.8-P22.9, P28.2, P28.4, P28.81-P28.9, R06.81

P28.4 Other apnea of newborn `CC` `N`
Apnea of prematurity
Obstructive apnea of newborn
EXCLUDES 1 *obstructive sleep apnea of newborn (P28.3)*
CC Excl: P22.8-P22.9, P28.2-P28.4, P28.81-P28.9, R06.81

P28.5 Respiratory failure of newborn `MCC` `N`
EXCLUDES 1 *respiratory arrest of newborn (P28.81)*
respiratory distress of newborn (P22.0-)
CC Excl: See code P27

✓5ᵗʰ P28.8 Other specified respiratory conditions of newborn

P28.81 Respiratory arrest of newborn `MCC` `N`
CC Excl: P22.1-P22.9, P24.00, P24.10, P24.20, P24.30, P24.80, Code P28.2-P28.5, P28.89-P28.9, P29.81, R06.81, R09.2

P28.89 Other specified respiratory conditions of newborn `N`
Congenital laryngeal stridor
Sniffles in newborn
Snuffles in newborn
EXCLUDES 1 *early congenital syphilitic rhinitis (A50.05)*

P28.9 Respiratory condition of newborn, unspecified `N`
Respiratory depression in newborn

✓4ᵗʰ P29 Cardiovascular disorders originating in the perinatal period
EXCLUDES 1 *congenital malformations of the circulatory system (Q20-Q28)*

P29.0 Neonatal cardiac failure `N`

✓5ᵗʰ P29.1 Neonatal cardiac dysrhythmia
P29.11 Neonatal tachycardia `N`
P29.12 Neonatal bradycardia `N`

P29.2 Neonatal hypertension `N`

P29.3 Persistent fetal circulation `MCC` `N`
Delayed closure of ductus arteriosus
(Persistent) pulmonary hypertension of newborn
CC Excl: I27.0, I27.2-I27.81, I27.89-I27.9

P29.4 Transient myocardial ischemia in newborn `N`

✓5ᵗʰ P29.8 Other cardiovascular disorders originating in the perinatal period
P29.81 Cardiac arrest of newborn `MCC` `N`
CC Excl: P29.81

P29.89 Other cardiovascular disorders originating in the perinatal period `N`

P29.9 Cardiovascular disorder originating in the perinatal period, unspecified `N`

Infections specific to the perinatal period (P35-P39)

Infections acquired in utero, during birth via the umbilicus, or during the first 28 days after birth
EXCLUDES 2 *asymptomatic human immunodeficiency virus [HIV] infection status (Z21)*
congenital gonococcal infection (A54.-)
congenital pneumonia (P23.-)
congenital syphilis (A50.-)
human immunodeficiency virus [HIV] disease (B20)
infant botulism (A48.51)
infectious diseases not specific to the perinatal period (A00-B99, J09, J10.-)
intestinal infectious disease (A00-A09)
laboratory evidence of human immunodeficiency virus [HIV] (R75)
tetanus neonatorum (A33)

✓4ᵗʰ P35 Congenital viral diseases
INCLUDES *infections acquired in utero or during birth*

P35.0 Congenital rubella syndrome `CC` `N`
Congenital rubella pneumonitis
CC Excl: P29.0-P29.2, P29.4, P29.89-P35.9, P37.0-P37.4, P37.8-P37.9, P94.1-P94.9, P96.0, P96.3-P96.5, P96.82-P96.89

P35.1 Congenital cytomegalovirus infection `MCC` `N`
CC Excl: See code P35.0

P35.2 Congenital herpesviral [herpes simplex] infection `MCC` `N`
CC Excl: A17.82, A28.1, A50.42, A52.14, A75.9, A79.9, A81.1, A81.82-A81.89, A83.0-A85.8, A87.2, A88.0, A88.8, A92.1-A92.8, A93.0, B00.4, B00.82, B01.11-B01.12, B04, B06.01, B08.09, B08.20-B08.22, B08.60-B08.79, B09-B10.09, B26.2, B27.00-B27.99, B33.1, B45.0, B45.2-B45.9, B54, B58.2, B75, B97.10, B97.21, G04.00-G04.01, G04.31, G04.81-G05.4, G37.0, G37.4-G37.5, H66.40-H66.43, J09.X3-J09.X9, J10.2-J10.89, J11.2-J11.89, L44.4, M1A.10X0-M1A.19X1, M32.0-M32.9, P35.2-P35.9, P37.0-P37.4, P37.8-P37.9, T56.0X1A, T56.0X2A, T56.0X3A, T56.0X4A

P35.3 Congenital viral hepatitis `MCC` `N`
CC Excl: See code P35.2

P35.8 Other congenital viral diseases `MCC` `N`
Congenital varicella [chickenpox]
CC Excl: See code P35.2

P35.9 Congenital viral disease, unspecified `MCC` `N`
CC Excl: See code P35.2

✓4ᵗʰ P36 Bacterial sepsis of newborn
INCLUDES *congenital sepsis*
Use additional code(s), if applicable, to identify severe sepsis (R65.2-) and associated acute organ dysfunction(s)

CC Excl: For MCC codes in subcategory P36, unless otherwise noted: P29.0-P29.2, P29.4, P29.89-P29.9, P36.0-P36.9, P37.5, P38.1-P39.9, P53, P60-P61.9, P94.1-P94.9, P96.0, P96.3-P96.5, P96.82-P96.89

P36.0 Sepsis of newborn due to streptococcus, group B `MCC` `N`

✓5ᵗʰ P36.1 Sepsis of newborn due to other and unspecified streptococci
P36.10 Sepsis of newborn due to unspecified streptococci `MCC` `N`
P36.19 Sepsis of newborn due to other streptococci `MCC` `N`

P36.2 Sepsis of newborn due to Staphylococcus aureus `MCC` `N`

✓5ᵗʰ P36.3 Sepsis of newborn due to other and unspecified staphylococci
P36.30 Sepsis of newborn due to unspecified staphylococci `MCC` `N`
P36.39 Sepsis of newborn due to other staphylococci `MCC` `N`

P36.4 Sepsis of newborn due to Escherichia coli `MCC` `N`

P36.5 Sepsis of newborn due to anaerobes `MCC` `N`

P36.8 Other bacterial sepsis of newborn `MCC` `N`
Use additional code from category B96 to identify organism

P36.9 Bacterial sepsis of newborn, unspecified `MCC` `N`

Certain Conditions Originating in the Perinatal Period

P37–P54.Ø

✓4ᵗʰ **P37 Other congenital infectious and parasitic diseases**

    EXCLUDES 2   congenital syphilis (A5Ø.-)
          infectious neonatal diarrhea (AØØ-AØ9)
          necrotizing enterocolitis in newborn (P77.-)
          noninfectious neonatal diarrhea (P78.3)
          ophthalmia neonatorum due to gonococcus (A54.31)
          tetanus neonatorum (A33)

> **CC Excl: For MCC codes in subcategory P37, unless otherwise noted:** A17.82, A28.1, A5Ø.42, A52.14, A75.9, A79.9, A81.1, A81.82-A81.89, A83.Ø-A85.8, A87.2, A88.Ø, A88.8, A92.1-A92.8, A93.Ø, BØØ.4, BØØ.82, BØ1.11-BØ1.12, BØ4, BØ6.Ø1, BØ8.Ø9, BØ8.2Ø-BØ8.22, BØ8.6Ø-BØ8.79, BØ9-B1Ø.Ø9, B26.2, B27.ØØ-B27.99, B33.1, B45.Ø, B45.2-B45.9, B54, B58.2, B75, B97.1Ø, B97.21, GØ4.ØØ-GØ4.Ø1, GØ4.31, GØ4.81-GØ5.4, G37.Ø, G37.4-G37.5, H66.4Ø-H66.43, JØ9.X3-JØ9.X9, J1Ø.2-J1Ø.89, J11.2-J11.89, L44.4, M1A.1ØXØ-M1A.19X1, M32.Ø-M32.9, P35.2-P35.9, P37.Ø-P37.4, P37.8-P37.9, T56.ØX1A, T56.ØX2A, T56.ØX3A, T56.ØX4A

    P37.Ø Congenital tuberculosis   MCC N
    P37.1 Congenital toxoplasmosis   MCC N
         Hydrocephalus due to congenital toxoplasmosis
    P37.2 Neonatal (disseminated) listeriosis   MCC N
    P37.3 Congenital falciparum malaria   MCC N
    P37.4 Other congenital malaria   N
    P37.5 Neonatal candidiasis   N
    P37.8 Other specified congenital infectious and parasitic diseases   MCC N
    P37.9 Congenital infectious or parasitic disease, unspecified   MCC N

✓4ᵗʰ **P38 Omphalitis of newborn**

    EXCLUDES 1   omphalitis not of newborn (LØ8.82)
          tetanus omphalitis (A33)
          umbilical hemorrhage of newborn (P51.-)

    P38.1 Omphalitis with mild hemorrhage   CC N
         CC Excl: P39.2-P39.9
    P38.9 Omphalitis without hemorrhage   CC N
         Omphalitis of newborn NOS
         CC Excl: See code P38.1

✓4ᵗʰ **P39 Other infections specific to the perinatal period**

    Use additional code to identify organism or specific infection

    P39.Ø Neonatal infective mastitis   CC N
         EXCLUDES 1   breast engorgement of newborn (P83.4)
                 noninfective mastitis of newborn (P83.4)
         CC Excl: See code P38.1
    P39.1 Neonatal conjunctivitis and dacryocystitis   N
         Neonatal chlamydial conjunctivitis
         Ophthalmia neonatorum NOS
         EXCLUDES 1   gonococcal conjunctivitis (A54.31)
    P39.2 Intra-amniotic infection affecting newborn, not elsewhere classified   CC N
         CC Excl: AØ2.1, A2Ø.7, A22.7, A39.2-A39.4, A4Ø.9-A41.9, A42.7, A48.2, A48.4, A48.8-A49.9, BØØ.7, B92, B94.2-B96.89, MØØ.Ø11-MØØ.Ø12, MØØ.Ø21-MØØ.Ø22, MØØ.Ø31- MØØ.Ø32, MØØ.Ø41-MØØ.Ø42, MØØ.Ø51- MØØ.Ø52, MØØ.Ø61-MØØ.Ø62, MØØ.Ø71-MØØ.Ø72, P39.2-P39.9, P95, P96.9, R78.81
    P39.3 Neonatal urinary tract infection   CC N
         CC Excl: A49.9, N1Ø-N11.Ø, N11.8-N12, N13.6, N15.1, N28.82, N28.84-N3Ø.31, N3Ø.8Ø-N3Ø.91, N36.9, N39.Ø, N39.9, N99.511, P39.2, P39.4-P39.9, R3Ø.Ø, R3Ø.9, T83.51XA
    P39.4 Neonatal skin infection   CC N
         Neonatal pyoderma
         EXCLUDES 1   pemphigus neonatorum (LØØ)
                 staphylococcal scalded skin syndrome (LØØ)
         CC Excl: See code P39.2
    P39.8 Other specified infections specific to the perinatal period   CC N
         CC Excl: See code P39.2
    P39.9 Infection specific to the perinatal period, unspecified   CC N
         CC Excl: See code P39.2

Hemorrhagic and hematological disorders of newborn (P5Ø-P61)

    EXCLUDES 1   congenital stenosis and stricture of bile ducts (Q44.3)
          Crigler-Najjar syndrome (E8Ø.5)
          Dubin-Johnson syndrome (E8Ø.6)
          Gilbert syndrome (E8Ø.4)
          hereditary hemolytic anemias (D55-D58)

✓4ᵗʰ **P5Ø Newborn affected by intrauterine (fetal) blood loss**

    EXCLUDES 1   congenital anemia from intrauterine (fetal) blood loss (P61.3)

    P5Ø.Ø Newborn affected by intrauterine (fetal) blood loss from vasa previa   N

    P5Ø.1 Newborn affected by intrauterine (fetal) blood loss from ruptured cord   N
    P5Ø.2 Newborn affected by intrauterine (fetal) blood loss from placenta   N
    P5Ø.3 Newborn affected by hemorrhage into co-twin   N
    P5Ø.4 Newborn affected by hemorrhage into maternal circulation   N
    P5Ø.5 Newborn affected by intrauterine (fetal) blood loss from cut end of co-twin's cord   N
    P5Ø.8 Newborn affected by other intrauterine (fetal) blood loss   N
    P5Ø.9 Newborn affected by intrauterine (fetal) blood loss, unspecified   N
         Newborn affected by fetal hemorrhage NOS

✓4ᵗʰ **P51 Umbilical hemorrhage of newborn**

    EXCLUDES 1   omphalitis with mild hemorrhage (P38.1)
          umbilical hemorrhage from cut end of co-twins cord (P5Ø.5)

    P51.Ø Massive umbilical hemorrhage of newborn   N
    P51.8 Other umbilical hemorrhages of newborn   N
         Slipped umbilical ligature NOS
    P51.9 Umbilical hemorrhage of newborn, unspecified   N

✓4ᵗʰ **P52 Intracranial nontraumatic hemorrhage of newborn**

    Intracranial hemorrhage due to anoxia or hypoxia
    EXCLUDES 1   intracranial hemorrhage due to birth injury (P1Ø.-)
          intracranial hemorrhage due to other injury (SØ6.-)

    P52.Ø Intraventricular (nontraumatic) hemorrhage, grade 1, of newborn   CC N
         Subependymal hemorrhage (without intraventricular extension)
         Bleeding into germinal matrix
         CC Excl: P1Ø.2-P1Ø.3, P29.Ø-P29.2, P29.4, P29.89-P29.9, P5Ø.Ø-P5Ø.9, P52.Ø-P52.3, P52.5, P53-P54.Ø, P54.6-P54.9, P6Ø-P61.9, P94.1-P94.9, P96.Ø, P96.3-P96.5, P96.82-P96.89
    P52.1 Intraventricular (nontraumatic) hemorrhage, grade 2, of newborn   CC N
         Subependymal hemorrhage with intraventricular extension
         Bleeding into ventricle
         CC Excl: See code P52.Ø
    ✓5ᵗʰ **P52.2 Intraventricular (nontraumatic) hemorrhage, grade 3 and grade 4, of newborn**
         P52.21 Intraventricular (nontraumatic) hemorrhage, grade 3, of newborn   MCC N
              Subependymal hemorrhage with intraventricular extension with enlargement of ventricle
              CC Excl: See code P52.Ø
         P52.22 Intraventricular (nontraumatic) hemorrhage, grade 4, of newborn   MCC N
              Bleeding into cerebral cortex
              Subependymal hemorrhage with intracerebral extension
              CC Excl: See code P52.Ø
    P52.3 Unspecified intraventricular (nontraumatic) hemorrhage of newborn   CC N
         CC Excl: See code P52.Ø
    P52.4 Intracerebral (nontraumatic) hemorrhage of newborn   MCC N
         CC Excl: P1Ø.Ø-P1Ø.1, P1Ø.4-P11.2, P11.9, P15.Ø-P15.9, P29.Ø-P29.2, P29.4, P29.89-P29.9, P52.4, P52.6-P52.9, P94.1-P94.9, P96.Ø, P96.3-P96.5, P96.82-P96.89
    P52.5 Subarachnoid (nontraumatic) hemorrhage of newborn   MCC N
         CC Excl: P1Ø.2-P1Ø.3, P29.Ø-P29.2, P29.4, P29.89-P29.9, P5Ø.Ø-P5Ø.9, P52.Ø-P52.3, P52.5, P53-P54.Ø, P54.6-P54.9, P6Ø-P61.9, P91.2, P94.1-P94.9, P96.Ø, P96.3-P96.5, P96.82-P96.89
    P52.6 Cerebellar (nontraumatic) and posterior fossa hemorrhage of newborn   MCC N
         CC Excl: See code P52.4
    P52.8 Other intracranial (nontraumatic) hemorrhages of newborn   MCC N
         CC Excl: See code P52.4
    P52.9 Intracranial (nontraumatic) hemorrhage of newborn, unspecified   MCC N
         CC Excl: See code P52.4

    P53 Hemorrhagic disease of newborn   CC N
         Vitamin K deficiency of newborn
         CC Excl: P29.Ø-P29.2, P29.4, P29.89-P29.9, P53, P6Ø-P61.9, P94.1-P94.9, P96.Ø, P96.3-P96.5, P96.82-P96.89

✓4ᵗʰ **P54 Other neonatal hemorrhages**

    EXCLUDES 1   newborn affected by (intrauterine) blood loss (P5Ø.-)
          pulmonary hemorrhage originating in the perinatal period (P26.-)

    P54.Ø Neonatal hematemesis   N
         EXCLUDES 1   neonatal hematemesis due to swallowed maternal blood (P78.2)

N Newborn: Ø   P Pediatric: Ø-17   M Maternity: 12-55   A Adult: 15-124   MCC Major CC Condition   PDx MCC PDx acts as own MCC   CC CC Condition   PDx CC PDx acts as own CC

82Ø   ICD-10-CM Draft (2Ø15)

P54.1 Neonatal melena `MCC` `N`
> EXCLUDES 1   *neonatal melena due to swallowed maternal blood (P78.2)*
> **CC Excl:** P29.0-P29.2, P29.4, P29.89-P29.9, P50.0-P50.9, P53-P54.4, P54.6-P54.9, P60-P61.9, P94.1-P94.9, P96.0, P96.3-P96.5, P96.82-P96.89

P54.2 Neonatal rectal hemorrhage `MCC` `N`
> **CC Excl:** See code P54.1

P54.3 Other neonatal gastrointestinal hemorrhage `MCC` `N`
> **CC Excl:** See code P54.1

P54.4 Neonatal adrenal hemorrhage `CC` `N`
> **CC Excl:** See code P54.1

P54.5 Neonatal cutaneous hemorrhage `N`
> Neonatal bruising
> Neonatal ecchymoses
> Neonatal petechiae
> Neonatal superficial hematomata
> EXCLUDES 2   *bruising of scalp due to birth injury (P12.3)*
>   *cephalhematoma due to birth injury (P12.0)*

P54.6 Neonatal vaginal hemorrhage `N` ♀
> Neonatal pseudomenses

P54.8 Other specified neonatal hemorrhages `N`

P54.9 Neonatal hemorrhage, unspecified `N`

✓4th **P55 Hemolytic disease of newborn**

P55.0 Rh isoimmunization of newborn `N`

P55.1 ABO isoimmunization of newborn `N`

P55.8 Other hemolytic diseases of newborn `N`

P55.9 Hemolytic disease of newborn, unspecified `N`

✓4th **P56 Hydrops fetalis due to hemolytic disease**
> EXCLUDES 1   *hydrops fetalis NOS (P83.2)*

P56.0 Hydrops fetalis due to isoimmunization `MCC` `N`
> **CC Excl:** P29.0-P29.2, P29.4, P29.89-P29.9, P55.0-P57.0, P94.1-P94.9, P96.0, P96.3-P96.5, P96.82-P96.89

✓5th **P56.9 Hydrops fetalis due to other and unspecified hemolytic disease**

     P56.90 Hydrops fetalis due to unspecified hemolytic disease `MCC` `N`
>   **CC Excl:** See code P56.0

     P56.99 Hydrops fetalis due to other hemolytic disease `MCC` `N`
>   **CC Excl:** See code P56.0

✓4th **P57 Kernicterus**

P57.0 Kernicterus due to isoimmunization `MCC` `N`
> **CC Excl:** See code P56.0

P57.8 Other specified kernicterus `MCC` `N`
> EXCLUDES 1   *Crigler-Najjar syndrome (E80.5)*
> **CC Excl:** P29.0-P29.2, P29.4, P29.89-P29.9, P57.8-P59.9, P94.1-P94.9, P96.0, P96.3-P96.5, P96.82-P96.89

P57.9 Kernicterus, unspecified `MCC` `N`
> **CC Excl:** See code P57.8

✓4th **P58 Neonatal jaundice due to other excessive hemolysis**
> EXCLUDES 1   *jaundice due to isoimmunization (P55-P57)*

P58.0 Neonatal jaundice due to bruising `N`

P58.1 Neonatal jaundice due to bleeding `N`

P58.2 Neonatal jaundice due to infection `N`

P58.3 Neonatal jaundice due to polycythemia `N`

✓5th **P58.4 Neonatal jaundice due to drugs or toxins transmitted from mother or given to newborn**
> Code first poisoning due to drug or toxin, if applicable (T36-T65 with fifth or sixth character 1-4 or 6)
> Use additional code for adverse effect, if applicable, to identify drug (T36-T50 with fifth or sixth character 5)

     P58.41 Neonatal jaundice due to drugs or toxins transmitted from mother `N`

     P58.42 Neonatal jaundice due to drugs or toxins given to newborn `N`

P58.5 Neonatal jaundice due to swallowed maternal blood `N`

P58.8 Neonatal jaundice due to other specified excessive hemolysis `N`

P58.9 Neonatal jaundice due to excessive hemolysis, unspecified `N`

✓4th **P59 Neonatal jaundice from other and unspecified causes**
> EXCLUDES 1   *jaundice due to inborn errors of metabolism (E70-E88)*
>   *kernicterus (P57.-)*

P59.0 Neonatal jaundice associated with preterm delivery `N`
> Hyperbilirubinemia of prematurity
> Jaundice due to delayed conjugation associated with preterm delivery

P59.1 Inspissated bile syndrome `MCC` `N`
> **CC Excl:** See code P57.8

✓5th **P59.2 Neonatal jaundice from other and unspecified hepatocellular damage**
> EXCLUDES 1   *congenital viral hepatitis (P35.3)*

     P59.20 Neonatal jaundice from unspecified hepatocellular damage `MCC` `N`
>   **CC Excl:** See code P57.8

     P59.29 Neonatal jaundice from other hepatocellular damage `MCC` `N`
>   Neonatal giant cell hepatitis
>   Neonatal (idiopathic) hepatitis
>   **CC Excl:** See code P57.8

P59.3 Neonatal jaundice from breast milk inhibitor `N`

P59.8 Neonatal jaundice from other specified causes `N`

P59.9 Neonatal jaundice, unspecified `N`
> Neonatal physiological jaundice (intense)(prolonged) NOS

P60 Disseminated intravascular coagulation of newborn `MCC` `N`
> Defibrination syndrome of newborn
> **CC Excl:** P29.0-P29.2, P29.4, P29.89-P29.9, P53, P60-P61.9, P94.1-P94.9, P96.0, P96.3-P96.5, P96.82-P96.89

✓4th **P61 Other perinatal hematological disorders**
> EXCLUDES 1   *transient hypogammaglobulinemia of infancy (D80.7)*

P61.0 Transient neonatal thrombocytopenia `MCC` `N`
> Neonatal thrombocytopenia due to exchange transfusion
> Neonatal thrombocytopenia due to idiopathic maternal thrombocytopenia
> Neonatal thrombocytopenia due to isoimmunization
> **CC Excl:** See code P60

P61.1 Polycythemia neonatorum `N`

P61.2 Anemia of prematurity `CC` `N`
> **CC Excl:** D50.0-D55.9, D56.4, D57.00-D57.3, D57.80-D64.9, D75.9, P61.2-P61.4

P61.3 Congenital anemia from fetal blood loss `CC` `N`
> **CC Excl:** See code P61.2

P61.4 Other congenital anemias, not elsewhere classified `CC` `N`
> Congenital anemia NOS
> **CC Excl:** See code P61.2

P61.5 Transient neonatal neutropenia `MCC` `N`
> EXCLUDES 1   *congenital neutropenia (nontransient) (D70.0)*
> **CC Excl:** D50.1-D53.9, D56.4, D57.00-D57.20, D57.3, D57.811-D57.819, D58.2, D59.0-D59.1, D59.3, D60.0-D61.9, D63.0-D64.9, D75.9, P61.5, P61.8-P61.9

P61.6 Other transient neonatal disorders of coagulation `CC` `N`
> **CC Excl:** P29.0-P29.2, P29.4, P29.89-P29.9, P53, P60-P61.9, P94.1-P94.9, P96.0, P96.3-P96.5, P96.82-P96.89

P61.8 Other specified perinatal hematological disorders `N`

P61.9 Perinatal hematological disorder, unspecified `N`

Transitory endocrine and metabolic disorders specific to newborn (P70-P74)

> INCLUDES   transitory endocrine and metabolic disturbances caused by the infant's response to maternal endocrine and metabolic factors, or its adjustment to extrauterine environment

✓4th **P70 Transitory disorders of carbohydrate metabolism specific to newborn**

P70.0 Syndrome of infant of mother with gestational diabetes `N`
> Newborn (with hypoglycemia) affected by maternal gestational diabetes
> EXCLUDES 1   *newborn (with hypoglycemia) affected by maternal (pre-existing) diabetes mellitus (P70.1)*
>   *syndrome of infant of a diabetic mother (P70.1)*

P70.1 Syndrome of infant of a diabetic mother `N`
> Newborn (with hypoglycemia) affected by maternal (pre-existing) diabetes mellitus
> EXCLUDES 1   *newborn (with hypoglycemia) affected by maternal gestational diabetes (P70.0)*
>   *syndrome of infant of mother with gestational diabetes (P70.0)*

☑ Additional Character Required   ✓x7th Xtension Alert   <u>Unacceptable PDx</u>   Manifestation   Hospital Acquired Condition   EXCLUDES 1 Not Coded Here   EXCLUDES 2 Not Included Here

P70.2   **Neonatal** diabetes mellitus   CC N
     CC Excl: P29.0-P29.2, P29.4, P29.89-P29.9, P70.0-P70.4, P70.9-P71.9, P72.1, P72.9-P74.4, P74.9, P94.0-P94.9, P96.0, P96.3-P96.5, P96.82-P96.89

P70.3   **Iatrogenic** neonatal hypoglycemia   N

P70.4   **Other** neonatal hypoglycemia   N
     Transitory neonatal hypoglycemia

P70.8   **Other** transitory disorders of carbohydrate metabolism   CC N
     of newborn
     CC Excl: P70.0-P70.4, P70.9-P71.9, P72.1, P72.9-P74.4, P74.9, P94.0

P70.9   **Transitory disorder of carbohydrate metabolism of**   N
     newborn, unspecified

✓4ᵗʰ **P71**   **Transitory neonatal disorders of** calcium and magnesium metabolism

> CC Excl: For CC codes in subcategory P71, unless otherwise noted: P29.0-P29.2, P29.4, P29.89-P29.9, P70.0-P70.4, P70.9-P71.9, P72.1, P72.9-P74.4, P74.9, P94.0-P94.9, P96.0, P96.3-P96.5, P96.82-P96.89

P71.0   **Cow's milk hypocalcemia in newborn**   CC N

P71.1   **Other** neonatal hypocalcemia   CC N
     EXCLUDES1   neonatal hypoparathyroidism (P71.4)

P71.2   **Neonatal** hypomagnesemia   CC N

P71.3   **Neonatal** tetany without calcium or magnesium   CC N
     deficiency
     Neonatal tetany NOS

P71.4   **Transitory neonatal** hypoparathyroidism   CC N

P71.8   **Other** transitory neonatal disorders of calcium and   CC N
     magnesium metabolism

P71.9   **Transitory neonatal disorder of calcium and magnesium**   CC N
     metabolism, unspecified

✓4ᵗʰ **P72**   **Other transitory neonatal** endocrine disorders
     EXCLUDES1   congenital hypothyroidism with or without goiter (E03.0-E03.1)
                dyshormogenetic goiter (E07.1)
                Pendred's syndrome (E07.1)

> CC Excl: For CC codes in subcategory P72, unless otherwise noted: P70.0-P70.4, P70.9-P71.9, P72.1, P72.9-P74.4, P74.9, P94.0

P72.0   **Neonatal goiter, not elsewhere classified**   CC N
     Transitory congenital goiter with normal functioning

P72.1   **Transitory** neonatal hyperthyroidism   CC N
     Neonatal thyrotoxicosis
     CC Excl: P29.0-P29.2, P29.4, P29.89-P29.9, P70.0-P70.4, P70.9-P71.9, P72.1, P72.9-P74.4, P74.9, P94.0-P94.9, P96.0, P96.3-P96.5, P96.82-P96.89

P72.2   **Other** transitory neonatal disorders of thyroid function,   CC N
     not elsewhere classified
     Transitory neonatal hypothyroidism

P72.8   **Other specified transitory neonatal endocrine disorders**   CC N

P72.9   **Transitory neonatal endocrine disorder,** unspecified   N

✓4ᵗʰ **P74**   **Other transitory neonatal** electrolyte and metabolic disturbances

P74.0   **Late metabolic acidosis** of newborn   MCC N
     EXCLUDES1   (fetal) metabolic acidosis of newborn (P19)
     CC Excl: P29.0-P29.2, P29.4, P29.89-P29.9, P70.0-P70.4, P70.9-P71.9, P72.1, P72.9-P74.4, P74.9, P94.0-P94.9, P96.0, P96.3-P96.5, P96.82-P96.89

P74.1   **Dehydration** of newborn   N

P74.2   **Disturbances of** sodium balance of newborn   N

P74.3   **Disturbances of** potassium balance of newborn   N

P74.4   **Other transitory electrolyte disturbances of newborn**   N

P74.5   **Transitory** tyrosinemia of newborn   CC N
     CC Excl: P70.0-P70.4, P70.9-P71.9, P72.1, P72.9-P74.4, P74.9, P94.0

P74.6   **Transitory** hyperammonemia of newborn   CC N
     CC Excl: See code: P70.8

P74.8   **Other transitory metabolic disturbances of newborn**   CC N
     Amino-acid metabolic disorders described as transitory
     CC Excl: See code: P70.8

P74.9   **Transitory metabolic disturbance of newborn,** unspecified   N

Digestive system disorders of newborn (P76-P78)

✓4ᵗʰ **P76**   **Other intestinal obstruction of newborn**

P76.0   **Meconium plug syndrome**   N
     Meconium ileus NOS
     EXCLUDES1   meconium ileus in cystic fibrosis (E84.11)

P76.1   **Transitory ileus of newborn**   CC N
     EXCLUDES1   Hirschsprung's disease (Q43.1)
     CC Excl: P76.0-P78.9

P76.2   **Intestinal obstruction due to inspissated milk**   N

P76.8   **Other specified intestinal obstruction of newborn**   N
     EXCLUDES1   intestinal obstruction classifiable to K56-

P76.9   **Intestinal obstruction of newborn, unspecified**   N

✓4ᵗʰ **P77**   **Necrotizing enterocolitis of newborn**

P77.1   **Stage 1 necrotizing enterocolitis in newborn**   MCC N
     Necrotizing enterocolitis without pneumatosis, without perforation
     CC Excl: P29.0-P29.2, P29.4, P29.89-P29.9, P76.0-P78.9, P94.1-P94.9, P96.0, P96.3-P96.5, P96.82-P96.89

P77.2   **Stage 2 necrotizing enterocolitis in newborn**   MCC N
     Necrotizing enterocolitis with pneumatosis, without perforation
     CC Excl: See code P77.1

P77.3   **Stage 3 necrotizing enterocolitis in newborn**   MCC N
     Necrotizing enterocolitis with perforation
     Necrotizing enterocolitis with pneumatosis and perforation
     CC Excl: See code P77.1

P77.9   **Necrotizing enterocolitis in newborn,** unspecified   MCC N
     Necrotizing enterocolitis in newborn, NOS
     CC Excl: See code P77.1

✓4ᵗʰ **P78**   **Other perinatal digestive system disorders**
     EXCLUDES1   cystic fibrosis (E84.0-E84.9)
                neonatal gastrointestinal hemorrhages (P54.0-P54.3)

P78.0   **Perinatal intestinal perforation**   MCC N
     Meconium peritonitis
     CC Excl: See code P77.1

P78.1   **Other neonatal peritonitis**   N
     Neonatal peritonitis NOS

P78.2   **Neonatal hematemesis and melena due to swallowed**   N
     maternal blood

P78.3   **Noninfective neonatal diarrhea**   N
     Neonatal diarrhea NOS

✓5ᵗʰ **P78.8**   **Other specified perinatal digestive system disorders**

P78.81   **Congenital cirrhosis (of liver)**   N

P78.82   **Peptic ulcer of newborn**   N

P78.83   **Newborn esophageal reflux**   N
     Neonatal esophageal reflux

P78.89   **Other specified perinatal digestive system**   N
     disorders

P78.9   **Perinatal digestive system disorder, unspecified**   N

Conditions involving the integument and temperature regulation of newborn (P80-P83)

✓4ᵗʰ **P80**   **Hypothermia of newborn**

P80.0   **Cold injury syndrome**   N
     Severe and usually chronic hypothermia associated with a pink flushed appearance, edema and neurological and biochemical abnormalities.
     EXCLUDES1   mild hypothermia of newborn (P80.8)

P80.8   **Other hypothermia of newborn**   N
     Mild hypothermia of newborn

P80.9   **Hypothermia of newborn, unspecified**   N

✓4ᵗʰ **P81**   **Other disturbances of temperature regulation of newborn**

P81.0   **Environmental hyperthermia of newborn**   N

P81.8   **Other specified disturbances of temperature**   N
     regulation of newborn

P81.9   **Disturbance of temperature regulation of newborn,**   N
     unspecified
     Fever of newborn NOS

N Newborn: 0   P Pediatric: 0-17   M Maternity: 12-55   A Adult: 15-124   MCC Major CC Condition   PDx MCC PDx acts as own MCC   CC CC Condition   PDx CC PDx acts as own CC

822   ICD-10-CM Draft (2015)

✓4th **P83 Other conditions of integument specific to newborn**
    EXCLUDES 1   *congenital malformations of skin and integument (Q80-Q84)*
               hydrops fetalis due to hemolytic disease (P56.-)
               neonatal skin infection (P39.4)
               staphylococcal scalded skin syndrome (L00)
    EXCLUDES 2   *cradle cap (L21.0)*
               diaper [napkin] dermatitis (L22)

    P83.0 Sclerema neonatorum   CC N
       CC Excl: P83.0, P83.30-P83.39

    P83.1 Neonatal erythema toxicum   N

    P83.2 Hydrops fetalis not due to hemolytic disease   MCC N
       Hydrops fetalis NOS
       CC Excl: P29.0-P29.2, P29.4, P29.89-P29.9, P83.2, P94.1-P94.9,
       P96.0, P96.3-P96.5, P96.82-P96.89

  ✓5th **P83.3 Other and unspecified edema specific to newborn**

        P83.30 Unspecified edema specific to newborn   CC N
           CC Excl: P80.0-P83.0, P83.30-P83.39

        P83.39 Other edema specific to newborn   CC N
           CC Excl: See code P83.30

    P83.4 Breast engorgement of newborn   N
       Noninfective mastitis of newborn

    P83.5 Congenital hydrocele   ♂

    P83.6 Umbilical polyp of newborn   N

    P83.8 Other specified conditions of integument specific   N
       to newborn
       Bronze baby syndrome
       Neonatal scleroderma
       Urticaria neonatorum

    P83.9 Condition of the integument specific to newborn,   N
       unspecified

Other problems with newborn (P84)

P84 Other problems with newborn   N
    Acidemia of newborn
    Acidosis of newborn
    Anoxia of newborn NOS
    Asphyxia of newborn NOS
    Hypercapnia of newborn
    Hypoxemia of newborn
    Hypoxia of newborn NOS
    Mixed metabolic and respiratory acidosis of newborn
    EXCLUDES 1   *intracranial hemorrhage due to anoxia or hypoxia (P52.-)*
               hypoxic ischemic encephalopathy [HIE] (P91.6-)
               late metabolic acidosis of newborn (P74.0)
    CC Excl: No Excl

Other disorders originating in the perinatal period (P90-P96)

P90 Convulsions of newborn   MCC N
    EXCLUDES 1   *benign myoclonic epilepsy in infancy (G40.3-)*
               benign neonatal convulsions (familial) (G40.3-)
    CC Excl: P29.0-P29.2, P29.4, P29.89-P29.9, P90, P91.8-P91.9, P94.1-P94.9,
    P96.0, P96.3-P96.5, P96.82-P96.89

✓4th **P91 Other disturbances of cerebral status of newborn**

    P91.0 Neonatal cerebral ischemia   MCC N
       CC Excl: P90-P91.1, P91.3-P91.5, P91.8-P91.9

    P91.1 Acquired periventricular cysts of newborn   MCC N
       CC Excl: See code P91.0

    P91.2 Neonatal cerebral leukomalacia   MCC N
       Periventricular leukomalacia
       CC Excl: P10.2-P10.3, P29.0-P29.2, P29.4, P29.89-P29.9, P50.0-
       P50.9, P52.0-P52.3, P52.5, P53-P54.0, P54.6-P54.9, P60-P61.9,
       P91.2, P94.1-P94.9, P96.0, P96.3-P96.5, P96.82-P96.89

    P91.3 Neonatal cerebral irritability   MCC N
       CC Excl: See code P91.0

    P91.4 Neonatal cerebral depression   MCC N
       CC Excl: See code P91.0

    P91.5 Neonatal coma   MCC N
       CC Excl: See code P91.0

  ✓5th **P91.6 Hypoxic ischemic encephalopathy [HIE]**

        P91.60 Hypoxic ischemic encephalopathy [HIE],   CC N
            unspecified
           CC Excl: P84, P91.60-P91.63

        P91.61 Mild hypoxic ischemic encephalopathy [HIE]   CC N
           CC Excl: See code P91.60

        P91.62 Moderate hypoxic ischemic encephalopathy   CC N
           [HIE]
           CC Excl: See code P91.60

        P91.63 Severe hypoxic ischemic encephalopathy   MCC N
           [HIE]
           CC Excl: See code P91.60

    P91.8 Other specified disturbances of cerebral status of newborn   N

    P91.9 Disturbance of cerebral status of newborn, unspecified   N

✓4th **P92 Feeding problems of newborn**
    EXCLUDES 1   *feeding problems in child over 28 days old (R63.3)*

  ✓5th **P92.0 Vomiting of newborn**
      EXCLUDES 1   *vomiting of child over 28 days old (R11.-)*

        P92.01 Bilious vomiting of newborn   MCC N
           EXCLUDES 1   *bilious vomiting in child over 28 days old*
                  (R11.14)
           CC Excl: P92.01-P92.09

        P92.09 Other vomiting of newborn   N
           EXCLUDES 1   *regurgitation of food in newborn (P92.1)*

    P92.1 Regurgitation and rumination of newborn   N

    P92.2 Slow feeding of newborn   N

    P92.3 Underfeeding of newborn   N

    P92.4 Overfeeding of newborn   N

    P92.5 Neonatal difficulty in feeding at breast   N

    P92.6 Failure to thrive in newborn   N
      EXCLUDES 1   *failure to thrive in child over 28 days old (R62.51)*

    P92.8 Other feeding problems of newborn   N

    P92.9 Feeding problem of newborn, unspecified   N

✓4th **P93 Reactions and intoxications due to drugs administered to**
    newborn
    INCLUDES   reactions and intoxications due to drugs administered to
               fetus affecting newborn
    EXCLUDES 1   *jaundice due to drugs or toxins transmitted from mother or*
               given to newborn (P58.4-)
               reactions and intoxications from maternal opiates, tranquilizers
               and other medication (P04.0-P04.1, P04.4)
               withdrawal symptoms from maternal use of drugs of addiction
               (P96.1)
               withdrawal symptoms from therapeutic use of drugs in
               newborn (P96.2)

    P93.0 Grey baby syndrome   CC N
       Grey syndrome from chloramphenicol administration in
       newborn
       CC Excl: P93.0-P93.8, P96.1-P96.2

    P93.8 Other reactions and intoxications due to drugs   CC N
       administered to newborn
       Use additional code for adverse effect, if applicable, to identify
       drug (T36-T50 with fifth or sixth character 5)
       CC Excl: See code P93.0

✓4th **P94 Disorders of muscle tone of newborn**

    P94.0 Transient neonatal myasthenia gravis   CC N
      EXCLUDES 1   *myasthenia gravis (G70.0)*
       CC Excl: P29.0-P29.2, P29.4, P29.89-P29.9, P70.0-P70.4, P70.9-
       P71.9, P72.1, P72.9-P74.4, P74.9, P94.0-P94.9, P96.0, P96.3-P96.5,
       P96.82-P96.89

    P94.1 Congenital hypertonia   N

    P94.2 Congenital hypotonia   N
       Floppy baby syndrome, unspecified

    P94.8 Other disorders of muscle tone of newborn   N

    P94.9 Disorder of muscle tone of newborn, unspecified   N

  P95 Stillbirth   N
    Deadborn fetus NOS
    Fetal death of unspecified cause
    Stillbirth NOS
    EXCLUDES 1   *maternal care for intrauterine death (O36.4)*
               missed abortion (O02.1)
               outcome of delivery, stillbirth (Z37.1, Z37.3, Z37.4, Z37.7)

✓4th **P96 Other conditions originating in the perinatal period**

    P96.0 Congenital renal failure   N
       Uremia of newborn

    P96.1 Neonatal withdrawal symptoms from maternal use   CC N
       of drugs of addiction
       Drug withdrawal syndrome in infant of dependent mother
       Neonatal abstinence syndrome
      EXCLUDES 1   *reactions and intoxications from maternal opiates and*
               tranquilizers administered during labor and
               delivery (P04.0)
       CC Excl: P93.0-P93.8, P96.1-P96.2

    P96.2 Withdrawal symptoms from therapeutic use of drugs in   CC N
       newborn
       CC Excl: See code P96.1

✓ Additional Character Required   ✓x7th *X*tension Alert   Unacceptable PDx   Manifestation   Hospital Acquired Condition   *EXCLUDES 1* Not Coded Here   *EXCLUDES 2* Not Included Here

P96.3   **Wide cranial sutures of newborn**   N
       Neonatal craniotabes

P96.5   **Complication to newborn due to (fetal) intrauterine**   N
       procedure
       EXCLUDES 2   newborn (suspected to be) affected by amniocentesis
                 (P00.6)

✓5ᵗʰ   **P96.8**   **Other specified conditions originating in the perinatal period**

       P96.81   **Exposure to (parental) (environmental) tobacco**
                 smoke in the perinatal period
                 EXCLUDES 2   newborn affected by in utero exposure to
                              tobacco (P04.2)
                          exposure to environmental tobacco smoke
                          after the perinatal period (Z77.22)

P96.82   **Delayed separation of umbilical cord**   N

P96.83   **Meconium staining**   N
       EXCLUDES 1   meconium aspiration (P24.00, P24.01)
                 meconium passage during delivery (P03.82)

P96.89   **Other specified conditions originating in the**   N
       perinatal period
       Use additional code to specify condition

P96.9   **Condition originating in the perinatal period, unspecified**   N
       Congenital debility NOS

DRAFT

N Newborn: 0   P Pediatric: 0-17   M Maternity: 12-55   A Adult: 15-124   MCC Major CC Condition   PDx MCC PDx acts as own MCC   CC CC Condition   PDx CC PDx acts as own CC

824   ICD-10-CM Draft (2015)

Chapter 17. Congenital Malformations, Deformations and Chromosomal Abnormalities(Q00-Q99)

NOTE Codes from this chapter are not for use on maternal or fetal records.

EXCLUDES 2 inborn errors of metabolism (E70-E88)

This chapter contains the following blocks:

Q00-Q07	Congenital malformations of the nervous system
Q10-Q18	Congenital malformations of eye, ear, face and neck
Q20-Q28	Congenital malformations of the circulatory system
Q30-Q34	Congenital malformations of the respiratory system
Q35-Q37	Cleft lip and cleft palate
Q38-Q45	Other congenital malformations of the digestive system
Q50-Q56	Congenital malformations of genital organs
Q60-Q64	Congenital malformations of the urinary system
Q65-Q79	Congenital malformations and deformations of the musculoskeletal system
Q80-Q89	Other congenital malformations
Q90-Q99	Chromosomal abnormalities, not elsewhere classified

Congenital malformations of the nervous system (Q00-Q07)

✓4th Q00 Anencephaly and similar malformations

> **CC Excl: For MCC codes in category Q00, unless otherwise noted:** Q00.0-Q00.2

Q00.0 Anencephaly   MCC
Acephaly
Acrania
Amyelencephaly
Hemianencephaly
Hemicephaly

Q00.1 Craniorachischisis   MCC

Q00.2 Iniencephaly   MCC

✓4th Q01 Encephalocele
INCLUDES Arnold-Chiari syndrome, type III
encephalocystocele
encephalomyelocele
hydroencephalocele
hydromeningocele, cranial
meningocele, cerebral
meningoencephalocele
EXCLUDES 1 Meckel-Gruber syndrome (Q61.9)

> **CC Excl: For CC codes in category Q01, unless otherwise noted:** Q01.0-Q02, Q04.0-Q04.8

Q01.0 Frontal encephalocele   CC
Q01.1 Nasofrontal encephalocele   CC
Q01.2 Occipital encephalocele   CC
Q01.8 Encephalocele of other sites   CC
Q01.9 Encephalocele, unspecified   CC

Q02 Microcephaly
INCLUDES hydromicrocephaly
micrencephalon
EXCLUDES 1 Meckel-Gruber syndrome (Q61.9)

✓4th Q03 Congenital hydrocephalus
INCLUDES hydrocephalus in newborn
EXCLUDES 1 Arnold-Chiari syndrome, type II (Q07.0-)
acquired hydrocephalus (G91.-)
hydrocephalus due to congenital toxoplasmosis (P37.1)
hydrocephalus with spina bifida (Q05.0-Q05.4)

Q03.0 Malformations of aqueduct of Sylvius
Anomaly of aqueduct of Sylvius
Obstruction of aqueduct of Sylvius, congenital
Stenosis of aqueduct of Sylvius

Q03.1 Atresia of foramina of Magendie and Luschka
Dandy-Walker syndrome

Q03.8 Other congenital hydrocephalus

Q03.9 Congenital hydrocephalus, unspecified

✓4th Q04 Other congenital malformations of brain
EXCLUDES 1 cyclopia (Q87.0)
macrocephaly (Q75.3)

> **CC Excl: For MCC codes in category Q04, unless otherwise noted:** See code: Q01

Q04.0 Congenital malformations of corpus callosum   MCC
Agenesis of corpus callosum

Q04.1 Arhinencephaly   MCC

Q04.2 Holoprosencephaly   MCC

Q04.3 Other reduction deformities of brain   MCC
Absence of part of brain
Agenesis of part of brain
Agyria
Aplasia of part of brain
Hydranencephaly
Hypoplasia of part of brain
Lissencephaly
Microgyria
Pachygyria
EXCLUDES 1 congenital malformations of corpus callosum (Q04.0)

Q04.4 Septo-optic dysplasia of brain   CC
CC Excl: Q04.4-Q04.8

Q04.5 Megalencephaly   CC
CC Excl: See code: Q04.4

Q04.6 Congenital cerebral cysts   CC
Porencephaly
Schizencephaly
EXCLUDES 1 acquired porencephalic cyst (G93.0)
CC Excl: See code: Q04.4

Q04.8 Other specified congenital malformations of brain   CC
Arnold-Chiari syndrome, type IV
Macrogyria
CC Excl: See code: Q04.4

Q04.9 Congenital malformation of brain, unspecified
Congenital anomaly NOS of brain
Congenital deformity NOS of brain
Congenital disease or lesion NOS of brain
Multiple anomalies NOS of brain, congenital

✓4th Q05 Spina bifida
Hydromeningocele (spinal)
Meningocele (spinal)
Meningomyelocele
Myelocele
Myelomeningocele
Rachischisis
Spina bifida (aperta)(cystica)
Syringomyelocele
Use additional code for any associated paraplegia (paraparesis) (G82.2-)
EXCLUDES 1 Arnold-Chiari syndrome, type II (Q07.0-)
spina bifida occulta (Q76.0)

> **CC Excl: For CC codes in category Q05, unless otherwise noted:** E78.71-E78.72, G90.1, Q05.0-Q06.1, Q06.3, Q06.8-Q07.9, Q87.1-Q87.89, Q89.7-Q89.8, Q99.2

Q05.0 Cervical spina bifida with hydrocephalus   CC
Q05.1 Thoracic spina bifida with hydrocephalus   CC
Dorsal spina bifida with hydrocephalus
Thoracolumbar spina bifida with hydrocephalus

Q05.2 Lumbar spina bifida with hydrocephalus   CC
Lumbosacral spina bifida with hydrocephalus

Q05.3 Sacral spina bifida with hydrocephalus   CC
Q05.4 Unspecified spina bifida with hydrocephalus   CC
Q05.5 Cervical spina bifida without hydrocephalus
Q05.6 Thoracic spina bifida without hydrocephalus
Dorsal spina bifida NOS
Thoracolumbar spina bifida NOS

Q05.7 Lumbar spina bifida without hydrocephalus
Lumbosacral spina bifida NOS

Q05.8 Sacral spina bifida without hydrocephalus
Q05.9 Spina bifida, unspecified

✓4th Q06 Other congenital malformations of spinal cord

Q06.0 Amyelia

Q06.1 Hypoplasia and dysplasia of spinal cord
Atelomyelia
Myelatelia
Myelodysplasia of spinal cord

Q06.2 Diastematomyelia

Q06.3 Other congenital cauda equina malformations

Q06.4 Hydromyelia
Hydrorachis

Q06.8 Other specified congenital malformations of spinal cord

Q06.9 Congenital malformation of spinal cord, unspecified
Congenital anomaly NOS of spinal cord
Congenital deformity NOS of spinal cord
Congenital disease or lesion NOS of spinal cord

☑ Additional Character Required   ✓x7th Xtension Alert   Unacceptable PDx   Manifestation   Hospital Acquired Condition   **EXCLUDES 1** Not Coded Here   **EXCLUDES 2** Not Included Here

✓4ᵗʰ Q07 Other congenital malformations of nervous system

EXCLUDES 2   congenital central alveolar hypoventilation syndrome (G47.35)
familial dysautonomia [Riley-Day] (G90.1)
neurofibromatosis (nonmalignant) (Q85.0-)

CC Excl: For CC codes in category Q07, unless otherwise noted:
See code: Q05.0

✓5ᵗʰ Q07.0 Arnold-Chiari syndrome
Arnold-Chiari syndrome, type II

EXCLUDES 1   Arnold-Chiari syndrome, type III (Q01.-)
Arnold-Chiari syndrome, type IV (Q04.8)

Q07.00 Arnold-Chiari syndrome without spina bifida or hydrocephalus

Q07.01 Arnold-Chiari syndrome with spina bifida

Q07.02 Arnold-Chiari syndrome with hydrocephalus   CC

Q07.03 Arnold-Chiari syndrome with spina bifida and hydrocephalus   CC

Q07.8 Other specified congenital malformations of nervous system
Agenesis of nerve
Displacement of brachial plexus
Jaw-winking syndrome
Marcus Gunn's syndrome

Q07.9 Congenital malformation of nervous system, unspecified
Congenital anomaly NOS of nervous system
Congenital deformity NOS of nervous system
Congenital disease or lesion NOS of nervous system

Congenital malformations of eye, ear, face and neck (Q10-Q18)

EXCLUDES 2   cleft lip and cleft palate (Q35-Q37)
congenital malformation of cervical spine (Q05.0, Q05.5, Q67.5, Q76.0-Q76.4)
congenital malformation of larynx (Q31.-)
congenital malformation of lip NEC (Q38.0)
congenital malformation of nose (Q30.-)
congenital malformation of parathyroid gland (Q89.2)
congenital malformation of thyroid gland (Q89.2)

✓4ᵗʰ Q10 Congenital malformations of eyelid, lacrimal apparatus and orbit

EXCLUDES 1   cryptophthalmos NOS (Q11.2)
cryptophthalmos syndrome (Q87.0)

Q10.0 Congenital ptosis

Q10.1 Congenital ectropion

Q10.2 Congenital entropion

Q10.3 Other congenital malformations of eyelid
Ablepharon
Blepharophimosis, congenital
Coloboma of eyelid
Congenital absence or agenesis of cilia
Congenital absence or agenesis of eyelid
Congenital accessory eyelid
Congenital accessory eye muscle
Congenital malformation of eyelid NOS

Q10.4 Absence and agenesis of lacrimal apparatus
Congenital absence of punctum lacrimale

Q10.5 Congenital stenosis and stricture of lacrimal duct

Q10.6 Other congenital malformations of lacrimal apparatus
Congenital malformation of lacrimal apparatus NOS

Q10.7 Congenital malformation of orbit

✓4ᵗʰ Q11 Anophthalmos, microphthalmos and macrophthalmos

Q11.0 Cystic eyeball

Q11.1 Other anophthalmos
Anophthalmos NOS
Agenesis of eye
Aplasia of eye

Q11.2 Microphthalmos
Cryptophthalmos NOS
Dysplasia of eye
Hypoplasia of eye
Rudimentary eye

EXCLUDES 1   cryptophthalmos syndrome (Q87.0)

Q11.3 Macrophthalmos

EXCLUDES 1   macrophthalmos in congenital glaucoma (Q15.0)

✓4ᵗʰ Q12 Congenital lens malformations

Q12.0 Congenital cataract

Q12.1 Congenital displaced lens

Q12.2 Coloboma of lens

Q12.3 Congenital aphakia

Q12.4 Spherophakia

Q12.8 Other congenital lens malformations
Microphakia

Q12.9 Congenital lens malformation, unspecified

✓4ᵗʰ Q13 Congenital malformations of anterior segment of eye

Q13.0 Coloboma of iris
Coloboma NOS

Q13.1 Absence of iris
Aniridia
Use additional code for associated glaucoma (H42)

Q13.2 Other congenital malformations of iris
Anisocoria, congenital
Atresia of pupil
Congenital malformation of iris NOS
Corectopia

Q13.3 Congenital corneal opacity

Q13.4 Other congenital corneal malformations
Congenital malformation of cornea NOS
Microcornea
Peter's anomaly

Q13.5 Blue sclera

✓5ᵗʰ Q13.8 Other congenital malformations of anterior segment of eye

Q13.81 Rieger's anomaly
Use additional code for associated glaucoma (H42)

Q13.89 Other congenital malformations of anterior segment of eye

Q13.9 Congenital malformation of anterior segment of eye, unspecified

✓4ᵗʰ Q14 Congenital malformations of posterior segment of eye

EXCLUDES 2   optic nerve hypoplasia (H47.03-)

Q14.0 Congenital malformation of vitreous humor
Congenital vitreous opacity

Q14.1 Congenital malformation of retina
Congenital retinal aneurysm

Q14.2 Congenital malformation of optic disc
Coloboma of optic disc

Q14.3 Congenital malformation of choroid

Q14.8 Other congenital malformations of posterior segment of eye
Coloboma of the fundus

Q14.9 Congenital malformation of posterior segment of eye, unspecified

✓4ᵗʰ Q15 Other congenital malformations of eye

EXCLUDES 1   congenital nystagmus (H55.01)
ocular albinism (E70.31-)
optic nerve hypoplasia (H47.03-)
retinitis pigmentosa (H35.52)

Q15.0 Congenital glaucoma
Axenfeld's anomaly
Buphthalmos
Glaucoma of childhood
Glaucoma of newborn
Hydrophthalmos
Keratoglobus, congenital, with glaucoma
Macrocornea with glaucoma
Macrophthalmos in congenital glaucoma
Megalocornea with glaucoma

Q15.8 Other specified congenital malformations of eye

Q15.9 Congenital malformation of eye, unspecified
Congenital anomaly of eye
Congenital deformity of eye

✓4ᵗʰ Q16 Congenital malformations of ear causing impairment of hearing

EXCLUDES 1   congenital deafness (H90.-)

Q16.0 Congenital absence of (ear) auricle

Q16.1 Congenital absence, atresia and stricture of auditory canal (external)
Congenital atresia or stricture of osseous meatus

Q16.2 Absence of eustachian tube

Q16.3 Congenital malformation of ear ossicles
Congenital fusion of ear ossicles

Q16.4 Other congenital malformations of middle ear
Congenital malformation of middle ear NOS

Q16.5 Congenital malformation of inner ear
Congenital anomaly of membranous labyrinth
Congenital anomaly of organ of Corti

Q16.9 Congenital malformation of ear causing impairment of hearing, unspecified
Congenital absence of ear NOS

✓4ᵗʰ Q17 Other congenital malformations of ear
EXCLUDES1 congenital malformations of ear with impairment of hearing
(Q16.0–Q16.9)
preauricular sinus (Q18.1)

Q17.0 Accessory auricle
Accessory tragus
Polyotia
Preauricular appendage or tag
Supernumerary ear
Supernumerary lobule

Q17.1 Macrotia

Q17.2 Microtia

Q17.3 Other misshapen ear
Pointed ear

Q17.4 Misplaced ear
Low-set ears
EXCLUDES1 cervical auricle (Q18.2)

Q17.5 Prominent ear
Bat ear

Q17.8 Other specified congenital malformations of ear
Congenital absence of lobe of ear

Q17.9 Congenital malformation of ear, unspecified
Congenital anomaly of ear NOS

✓4ᵗʰ Q18 Other congenital malformations of face and neck
EXCLUDES1 cleft lip and cleft palate (Q35-Q37)
conditions classified to Q67.0-Q67.4
congenital malformations of skull and face bones (Q75.-)
cyclopia (Q87.0)
dentofacial anomalies [including malocclusion] (M26.-)
malformation syndromes affecting facial appearance (Q87.0)
persistent thyroglossal duct (Q89.2)

Q18.0 Sinus, fistula and cyst of branchial cleft
Branchial vestige

Q18.1 Preauricular sinus and cyst
Fistula of auricle, congenital
Cervicoaural fistula

Q18.2 Other branchial cleft malformations
Branchial cleft malformation NOS
Cervical auricle
Otocephaly

Q18.3 Webbing of neck
Pterygium colli

Q18.4 Macrostomia

Q18.5 Microstomia

Q18.6 Macrocheilia
Hypertrophy of lip, congenital

Q18.7 Microcheilia

Q18.8 Other specified congenital malformations of face and neck
Medial cyst of face and neck
Medial fistula of face and neck
Medial sinus of face and neck

Q18.9 Congenital malformation of face and neck, unspecified
Congenital anomaly NOS of face and neck

Congenital malformations of the circulatory system (Q20-Q28)

✓4ᵗʰ Q20 Congenital malformations of cardiac chambers and connections
EXCLUDES1 dextrocardia with situs inversus (Q89.3)
mirror-image atrial arrangement with situs inversus (Q89.3)

CC Excl: For CC/MCC codes in category Q20, unless otherwise noted: E78.71-E78.72, I23.0-I23.3, I23.6-I23.8, I51.0, P29.3, Q20.0-Q21.9, Q23.8-Q23.9, Q24.8-Q24.9, Q27.30, Q27.4, Q28.0-Q28.1, Q28.8-Q28.9, Q87.1-Q87.89, Q89.7-Q89.8, Q99.2

Q20.0 Common arterial trunk MCC
Persistent truncus arteriosus
EXCLUDES1 aortic septal defect (Q21.4)

Q20.1 Double outlet right ventricle MCC
Taussig-Bing syndrome

Q20.2 Double outlet left ventricle MCC

Q20.3 Discordant ventriculoarterial connection MCC
Dextrotransposition of aorta
Transposition of great vessels (complete)

Q20.4 Double inlet ventricle MCC
Common ventricle
Cor triloculare biatriatum
Single ventricle

Q20.5 Discordant atrioventricular connection CC
Corrected transposition
Levotransposition
Ventricular inversion

Q20.6 Isomerism of atrial appendages
Isomerism of atrial appendages with asplenia or polysplenia

Q20.8 Other congenital malformations of cardiac chambers and connections
Cor binoculare

Q20.9 Congenital malformation of cardiac chambers and connections, unspecified

✓4ᵗʰ Q21 Congenital malformations of cardiac septa
EXCLUDES1 acquired cardiac septal defect (I51.0)

CC Excl: For CC/MCC codes in category Q 21, unless otherwise noted: See code Q20.0

Q21.0 Ventricular septal defect CC
Roger's disease

Q21.1 Atrial septal defect CC
Coronary sinus defect
Patent or persistent foramen ovale
Patent or persistent ostium secundum defect (type II)
Patent or persistent sinus venosus defect
CC Excl: E78.71-E78.72, I23.0-I23.3, I23.6-I23.8, I51.0, I51.3, Q20.0-Q20.9, Q21.1-Q21.9, Q23.8-Q23.9, Q24.8-Q24.9, Q27.30, Q27.4, Q28.0-Q28.1, Q28.8-Q28.9, Q87.2-Q87.3, Q87.5-Q87.89, Q89.7-Q89.8

Q21.2 Atrioventricular septal defect CC
Common atrioventricular canal
Endocardial cushion defect
Ostium primum atrial septal defect (type I)

Q21.3 Tetralogy of Fallot MCC
Ventricular septal defect with pulmonary stenosis or atresia, dextroposition of aorta and hypertrophy of right ventricle.

Q21.4 Aortopulmonary septal defect
Aortic septal defect
Aortopulmonary window

Q21.8 Other congenital malformations of cardiac septa
Eisenmenger's defect
Pentalogy of Fallot
EXCLUDES1 Eisenmenger's complex (I27.8)
Eisenmenger's syndrome (I27.8)

Q21.9 Congenital malformation of cardiac septum, unspecified
Septal (heart) defect NOS

✓4ᵗʰ Q22 Congenital malformations of pulmonary and tricuspid valves

Q22.0 Pulmonary valve atresia MCC
CC Excl: E78.71-E78.72, P29.3, Q20.9, Q22.0-Q22.3, Q23.8-Q23.9, Q24.8-Q24.9, Q27.30, Q27.4, Q28.0-Q28.1, Q28.8-Q28.9, Q87.1-Q87.89, Q89.7-Q89.8, Q99.2

Q22.1 Congenital pulmonary valve stenosis CC
CC Excl: See code: Q22.0

Q22.2 Congenital pulmonary valve insufficiency CC
Congenital pulmonary valve regurgitation
CC Excl: E78.71-E78.72, Q20.9, Q22.0-Q22.3, Q23.8-Q23.9, Q24.8-Q24.9, Q27.30, Q27.4, Q28.0-Q28.1, Q28.8-Q28.9, Q87.2-Q87.3, Q87.5-Q87.89, Q89.7-Q89.8

Q22.3 Other congenital malformations of pulmonary valve CC
Congenital malformation of pulmonary valve NOS
Supernumerary cusps of pulmonary valve
CC Excl: See code: Q22.2

Q22.4 Congenital tricuspid stenosis MCC
Congenital tricuspid atresia
CC Excl: E78.71-E78.72, P29.3, Q20.9, Q22.4-Q23.9, Q24.8-Q24.9, Q27.30, Q27.4, Q28.0-Q28.1, Q28.8-Q28.9, Q87.1-Q87.89, Q89.7-Q89.8, Q99.2

Q22.5 Ebstein's anomaly MCC
CC Excl: See code: Q22.4

Q22.6 Hypoplastic right heart syndrome MCC
CC Excl: See code: Q22.4

Q22.8 Other congenital malformations of tricuspid valve MCC
CC Excl: See code: Q22.4

Q22.9 Congenital malformation of tricuspid valve, unspecified MCC
CC Excl: See code: Q22.4

Congenital Malformations, Deformations and Chromosomal Abnormalities   Q23–Q27.2

✓4ᵗʰ **Q23 Congenital malformations of aortic and mitral valves**

> **CC Excl:** For CC/MCC codes in category Q23, unless otherwise noted: See code: Q22.4

Q23.0 Congenital stenosis of aortic valve   CC
Congenital aortic atresia
Congenital aortic stenosis NOS
> **EXCLUDES 1**   congenital stenosis of aortic valve in hypoplastic left heart syndrome (Q23.4)
> congenital subaortic stenosis (Q24.4)
> supravalvular aortic stenosis (congenital) (Q25.3)

Q23.1 Congenital insufficiency of aortic valve   CC
Bicuspid aortic valve
Congenital aortic insufficiency

Q23.2 Congenital mitral stenosis   CC
Congenital mitral atresia

Q23.3 Congenital mitral insufficiency   CC

Q23.4 Hypoplastic left heart syndrome   MCC

Q23.8 Other congenital malformations of aortic and mitral valves

Q23.9 Congenital malformation of aortic and mitral valves, unspecified

✓4ᵗʰ **Q24 Other congenital malformations of heart**
> **EXCLUDES 1**   endocardial fibroelastosis (I42.4)

Q24.0 Dextrocardia   CC
> **EXCLUDES 1**   dextrocardia with situs inversus (Q89.3)
> isomerism of atrial appendages (with asplenia or polysplenia) (Q20.6)
> mirror-image atrial arrangement with situs inversus (Q89.3)

  CC Excl: E78.71-E78.72, Q20.9, Q23.8-Q24.4, Q24.8-Q24.9, Q27.30, Q27.4, Q28.0-Q28.1, Q28.8-Q28.9, Q87.2-Q87.3, Q87.5-Q87.89, Q89.7-Q89.8

Q24.1 Levocardia   CC
  CC Excl: See code: Q24.0

Q24.2 Cor triatriatum   MCC
  CC Excl: E78.71-E78.72, P29.3, Q20.9, Q23.8-Q23.9, Q24.2-Q24.4, Q24.8-Q24.9, Q27.30, Q27.4, Q28.0-Q28.1, Q28.8-Q28.9, Q87.1-Q87.89, Q89.7-Q89.8, Q99.2

Q24.3 Pulmonary infundibular stenosis   CC
Subvalvular pulmonic stenosis
  CC Excl: See code: Q24.2

Q24.4 Congenital subaortic stenosis   MCC
  CC Excl: See code: Q24.2

Q24.5 Malformation of coronary vessels   CC
Congenital coronary (artery) aneurysm
  CC Excl: Q20.9-Q23.9, Q24.5, Q24.8-Q24.9

Q24.6 Congenital heart block   MCC
  CC Excl: E78.71-E78.72, P29.3, Q20.9, Q23.8-Q23.9, Q24.6-Q24.9, Q27.30, Q27.4, Q28.0-Q28.1, Q28.8-Q28.9, Q87.1-Q87.89, Q89.7-Q89.8, Q99.2

Q24.8 Other specified congenital malformations of heart
Congenital diverticulum of left ventricle
Congenital malformation of myocardium
Congenital malformation of pericardium
Malposition of heart
Uhl's disease

Q24.9 Congenital malformation of heart, unspecified
Congenital anomaly of heart
Congenital disease of heart

✓4ᵗʰ **Q25 Congenital malformations of great arteries**

Q25.0 Patent ductus arteriosus   CC
Patent ductus Botallo
Persistent ductus arteriosus
  CC Excl: Q25.0, Q27.30, Q27.4, Q28.0-Q28.1, Q28.8

Q25.1 Coarctation of aorta   CC
Coarctation of aorta (preductal) (postductal)
  CC Excl: E78.71-E78.72, Q25.1-Q25.3, Q27.30, Q27.4, Q28.0-Q28.1, Q28.8-Q28.9, Q87.2-Q87.3, Q87.5-Q87.89, Q89.7-Q89.8

Q25.2 Atresia of aorta   CC
  CC Excl: E78.71-E78.72, P29.3, Q25.1-Q25.3, Q27.30, Q27.4, Q28.0-Q28.1, Q28.8-Q28.9, Q87.1-Q87.89, Q89.7-Q89.8, Q99.2

Q25.3 Supravalvular aortic stenosis   CC
> **EXCLUDES 1**   congenital aortic stenosis NOS (Q23.0)
> congenital stenosis of aortic valve (Q23.0)

  CC Excl: See code: Q25.2

Q25.4 Other congenital malformations of aorta   CC
Absence of aorta
Aneurysm of sinus of Valsalva (ruptured)
Aplasia of aorta
Congenital aneurysm of aorta
Congenital malformations of aorta
Congenital dilatation of aorta
Double aortic arch [vascular ring of aorta]
Hypoplasia of aorta
Persistent convolutions of aortic arch
Persistent right aortic arch
> **EXCLUDES 1**   hypoplasia of aorta in hypoplastic left heart syndrome (Q23.4)

  CC Excl: E78.71-E78.72, Q25.1-Q25.4, Q25.8-Q25.9, Q27.30, Q27.4, Q28.0-Q28.1, Q28.8-Q28.9, Q87.2-Q87.3, Q87.5-Q87.89, Q89.7-Q89.8

Q25.5 Atresia of pulmonary artery   MCC
  CC Excl: Q25.5-Q25.79, Q27.30, Q27.4, Q28.0-Q28.1, Q28.8-Q28.9

Q25.6 Stenosis of pulmonary artery   MCC
Supravalvular pulmonary stenosis
  CC Excl: See code: Q25.5

✓5ᵗʰ **Q25.7 Other congenital malformations of pulmonary artery**

> **CC Excl:** For CC codes in subcategory Q25.7, unless otherwise noted: See code: Q25.5

Q25.71 Coarctation of pulmonary artery   MCC

Q25.72 Congenital pulmonary arteriovenous malformation   MCC
Congenital pulmonary arteriovenous aneurysm

Q25.79 Other congenital malformations of pulmonary artery   MCC
Aberrant pulmonary artery
Agenesis of pulmonary artery
Congenital aneurysm of pulmonary artery
Congenital anomaly of pulmonary artery
Hypoplasia of pulmonary artery

Q25.8 Other congenital malformations of other great arteries   CC
  CC Excl: See code: Q25.4

Q25.9 Congenital malformation of great arteries, unspecified   CC
  CC Excl: See code: Q25.4

✓4ᵗʰ **Q26 Congenital malformations of great veins**

Q26.0 Congenital stenosis of vena cava   CC
Congenital stenosis of vena cava (inferior)(superior)
  CC Excl: Q26.0-Q26.1, Q26.8, Q27.30, Q27.4, Q28.0-Q28.1, Q28.8-Q28.9

Q26.1 Persistent left superior vena cava   CC
  CC Excl: See code: Q26.0

Q26.2 Total anomalous pulmonary venous connection   CC
Total anomalous pulmonary venous return [TAPVR], subdiaphragmatic
Total anomalous pulmonary venous return [TAPVR], supradiaphragmatic
  CC Excl: Q26.2, Q27.30, Q27.4, Q28.0-Q28.1, Q28.8-Q28.9

Q26.3 Partial anomalous pulmonary venous connection   CC
Partial anomalous pulmonary venous return
  CC Excl: Q26.3-Q26.4, Q27.30, Q27.4, Q28.0-Q28.1, Q28.8-Q28.9

Q26.4 Anomalous pulmonary venous connection, unspecified   CC
  CC Excl: See code: Q26.3

Q26.5 Anomalous portal venous connection

Q26.6 Portal vein-hepatic artery fistula

Q26.8 Other congenital malformations of great veins   CC
Absence of vena cava (inferior) (superior)
Azygos continuation of inferior vena cava
Persistent left posterior cardinal vein
Scimitar syndrome
  CC Excl: See code: Q26.0

Q26.9 Congenital malformation of great vein, unspecified   CC
Congenital anomaly of vena cava (inferior) (superior) NOS
  CC Excl: Q26.9-Q27.30, Q27.4, Q28.0-Q28.1, Q28.8-Q28.9

✓4ᵗʰ **Q27 Other congenital malformations of peripheral vascular system**
> **EXCLUDES 2**   anomalies of cerebral and precerebral vessels (Q28.0-Q28.3)
> anomalies of coronary vessels (Q24.5)
> anomalies of pulmonary artery (Q25.5-Q25.7)
> congenital retinal aneurysm (Q14.1)
> hemangioma and lymphangioma (D18.-)

Q27.0 Congenital absence and hypoplasia of umbilical artery
Single umbilical artery

Q27.1 Congenital renal artery stenosis

Q27.2 Other congenital malformations of renal artery
Congenital malformation of renal artery NOS
Multiple renal arteries

N Newborn: 0   P Pediatric: 0-17   M Maternity: 12-55   A Adult: 15-124   **MCC** Major CC Condition   **PDx MCC** PDx acts as own MCC   **CC** CC Condition   **PDx CC** PDx acts as own CC

✓5th **Q27.3** **Arteriovenous malformation (peripheral)**
Arteriovenous aneurysm
EXCLUDES 1   *acquired arteriovenous aneurysm (I77.0)*
EXCLUDES 2   *arteriovenous malformation of cerebral vessels (Q28.2)*
arteriovenous malformation of precerebral vessels (Q28.0)

     Q27.30 **Arteriovenous malformation, site unspecified** `CC`
CC Excl: Q20.0-Q20.8, Q21.0-Q21.9, Q27.30, Q27.4, Q28.0-Q28.1, Q28.8

     Q27.31 **Arteriovenous malformation of vessel of upper limb**

     Q27.32 **Arteriovenous malformation of vessel of lower limb**

     Q27.33 **Arteriovenous malformation of digestive system vessel**

     Q27.34 **Arteriovenous malformation of renal vessel**

     Q27.39 **Arteriovenous malformation, other site**

Q27.4 **Congenital phlebectasia** `CC`
CC Excl: See code: Q27.30

Q27.8 **Other specified congenital malformations of peripheral vascular system**
Absence of peripheral vascular system
Atresia of peripheral vascular system
Congenital aneurysm (peripheral)
Congenital stricture, artery
Congenital varix
EXCLUDES 1   *arteriovenous malformation (Q27.3-)*

Q27.9 **Congenital malformation of peripheral vascular system, unspecified**
Anomaly of artery or vein NOS

✓4th **Q28** **Other congenital malformations of circulatory system**
EXCLUDES 1   *congenital aneurysm NOS (Q27.8)*
congenital coronary aneurysm (Q24.5)
ruptured cerebral arteriovenous malformation (I60.8)
ruptured malformation of precerebral vessels (I72.0)
EXCLUDES 2   *congenital peripheral aneurysm (Q27.8)*
congenital pulmonary aneurysm (Q25.79)
congenital retinal aneurysm (Q14.1)

CC Excl: For CC/MCC codes in category Q28, unless otherwise noted: See code: Q27.30

Q28.0 **Arteriovenous malformation of precerebral vessels** `CC`
Congenital arteriovenous precerebral aneurysm (nonruptured)

Q28.1 **Other malformations of precerebral vessels** `CC`
Congenital malformation of precerebral vessels NOS
Congenital precerebral aneurysm (nonruptured)

Q28.2 **Arteriovenous malformation of cerebral vessels** `MCC`
Arteriovenous malformation of brain NOS
Congenital arteriovenous cerebral aneurysm (nonruptured)
CC Excl: Q27.30, Q27.4, Q28.0-Q28.9

Q28.3 **Other malformations of cerebral vessels** `MCC`
Congenital cerebral aneurysm (nonruptured)
Congenital malformation of cerebral vessels NOS
Developmental venous anomaly
CC Excl: See code: Q28.2

Q28.8 **Other specified congenital malformations of circulatory system** `CC`
Congenital aneurysm, specified site NEC
Spinal vessel anomaly
CC Excl: Q20.0-Q20.8, Q21.0-Q21.9, Q27.30, Q27.4, Q28.0-Q28.1, Q28.8

Q28.9 **Congenital malformation of circulatory system, unspecified** `CC`
CC Excl: Q20.0-Q28.9

Congenital malformations of the respiratory system (Q30-Q34)

✓4th **Q30** **Congenital malformations of nose**
EXCLUDES 1   *congenital deviation of nasal septum (Q67.4)*

Q30.0 **Choanal atresia**
Atresia of nares (anterior) (posterior)
Congenital stenosis of nares (anterior) (posterior)

Q30.1 **Agenesis and underdevelopment of nose**
Congenital absent of nose

Q30.2 **Fissured, notched and cleft nose**

Q30.3 **Congenital perforated nasal septum**

Q30.8 **Other congenital malformations of nose**
Accessory nose
Congenital anomaly of nasal sinus wall

Q30.9 **Congenital malformation of nose, unspecified**

✓4th **Q31** **Congenital malformations of larynx**
EXCLUDES 1   *congenital laryngeal stridor NOS (P28.89)*

CC Excl: For CC codes in category Q31, unless otherwise noted:
J39.8, J45.990, J98.09, Q31.1-Q32.4, Q34.0-Q34.9

Q31.0 **Web of larynx**
Glottic web of larynx
Subglottic web of larynx
Web of larynx NOS

Q31.1 **Congenital subglottic stenosis** `CC`

Q31.2 **Laryngeal hypoplasia** `CC`

Q31.3 **Laryngocele** `CC`

Q31.5 **Congenital laryngomalacia** `CC`

Q31.8 **Other congenital malformations of larynx** `CC`
Absence of larynx
Agenesis of larynx
Atresia of larynx
Congenital cleft thyroid cartilage
Congenital fissure of epiglottis
Congenital stenosis of larynx NEC
Posterior cleft of cricoid cartilage

Q31.9 **Congenital malformation of larynx, unspecified** `CC`

✓4th **Q32** **Congenital malformations of trachea and bronchus**
EXCLUDES 1   *congenital bronchiectasis (Q33.4)*

CC Excl: For CC codes in category Q32, unless otherwise noted:
See code: Q31

Q32.0 **Congenital tracheomalacia** `CC`

Q32.1 **Other congenital malformations of trachea** `CC`
Atresia of trachea
Congenital anomaly of tracheal cartilage
Congenital dilatation of trachea
Congenital malformation of trachea
Congenital stenosis of trachea
Congenital tracheocele

Q32.2 **Congenital bronchomalacia** `CC`

Q32.3 **Congenital stenosis of bronchus** `CC`

Q32.4 **Other congenital malformations of bronchus** `CC`
Absence of bronchus
Agenesis of bronchus
Atresia of bronchus
Congenital diverticulum of bronchus
Congenital malformation of bronchus NOS

✓4th **Q33** **Congenital malformations of lung**

CC Excl: For CC/MCC codes in category Q33, unless otherwise noted: Q33.0-Q34.9

Q33.0 **Congenital cystic lung** `CC`
Congenital cystic lung disease
Congenital honeycomb lung
Congenital polycystic lung disease
EXCLUDES 1   *cystic fibrosis (E84.0)*
cystic lung disease, acquired or unspecified (J98.4)

Q33.1 **Accessory lobe of lung**
Azygos lobe (fissured), lung

Q33.2 **Sequestration of lung** `MCC`

Q33.3 **Agenesis of lung** `MCC`
Congenital absence of lung (lobe)

Q33.4 **Congenital bronchiectasis** `CC`
CC Excl: J44.9, J47.0-J47.9, J68.1, J68.4-J68.9, Q33.4

Q33.5 **Ectopic tissue in lung**

Q33.6 **Congenital hypoplasia and dysplasia of lung** `MCC`
EXCLUDES 1   *pulmonary hypoplasia associated with short gestation (P28.0)*
CC Excl: Q33.0-Q34.9

Q33.8 **Other congenital malformations of lung**

Q33.9 **Congenital malformation of lung, unspecified**

✓4th **Q34** **Other congenital malformations of respiratory system**
EXCLUDES 2   *congenital central alveolar hypoventilation syndrome (G47.35)*

Q34.0 **Anomaly of pleura**

Q34.1 **Congenital cyst of mediastinum**

Q34.8 **Other specified congenital malformations of respiratory system**
Atresia of nasopharynx

Q34.9 **Congenital malformation of respiratory system, unspecified**
Congenital absence of respiratory system
Congenital anomaly of respiratory system NOS

Q35–Q41.9   Congenital Malformations, Deformations and Chromosomal Abnormalities

Cleft lip and cleft palate (Q35-Q37)

Use additional code to identify associated malformation of the nose (Q30.2)

EXCLUDES 1   Robin's syndrome (Q87.0)

✓4th Q35   Cleft palate

> **INCLUDES**   fissure of palate
>   palatoschisis
>
> **EXCLUDES 1**   cleft palate with cleft lip (Q37.-)

   Q35.1   Cleft hard palate

   Q35.3   Cleft soft palate

   Q35.5   Cleft hard palate with cleft soft palate

   Q35.7   Cleft uvula

   Q35.9   Cleft palate, unspecified
> Cleft palate NOS

✓4th Q36   Cleft lip

> Cheiloschisis
> Congenital fissure of lip
> Harelip
> Labium leporinum
>
> **EXCLUDES 1**   cleft lip with cleft palate (Q37.-)

   Q36.0   Cleft lip, bilateral

   Q36.1   Cleft lip, median

   Q36.9   Cleft lip, unilateral
> Cleft lip NOS

✓4th Q37   Cleft palate with cleft lip

> Cheilopalatoschisis

   Q37.0   Cleft hard palate with bilateral cleft lip

   Q37.1   Cleft hard palate with unilateral cleft lip
> Cleft hard palate with cleft lip NOS

   Q37.2   Cleft soft palate with bilateral cleft lip

   Q37.3   Cleft soft palate with unilateral cleft lip
> Cleft soft palate with cleft lip NOS

   Q37.4   Cleft hard and soft palate with bilateral cleft lip

   Q37.5   Cleft hard and soft palate with unilateral cleft lip
> Cleft hard and soft palate with cleft lip NOS

   Q37.8   Unspecified cleft palate with bilateral cleft lip

   Q37.9   Unspecified cleft palate with unilateral cleft lip
> Cleft palate with cleft lip NOS

Other congenital malformations of the digestive system (Q38-Q45)

✓4th Q38   Other congenital malformations of tongue, mouth and pharynx

> **EXCLUDES 1**   dentofacial anomalies (M26.-)
>   macrostomia (Q18.4)
>   microstomia (Q18.5)

   Q38.0   Congenital malformations of lips, not elsewhere classified
> Congenital fistula of lip
> Congenital malformation of lip NOS
> Van der Woude's syndrome
>
> **EXCLUDES 1**   cleft lip (Q36.-)
>   cleft lip with cleft palate (Q37.-)
>   macrocheilia (Q18.6)
>   microcheilia (Q18.7)

   Q38.1   Ankyloglossia
> Tongue tie

   Q38.2   Macroglossia
> Congenital hypertrophy of tongue

   Q38.3   Other congenital malformations of tongue
> Aglossia
> Bifid tongue
> Congenital adhesion of tongue
> Congenital fissure of tongue
> Congenital malformation of tongue NOS
> Double tongue
> Hypoglossia
> Hypoplasia of tongue
> Microglossia

   Q38.4   Congenital malformations of salivary glands and ducts
> Atresia of salivary glands and ducts
> Congenital absence of salivary glands and ducts
> Congenital accessory salivary glands and ducts
> Congenital fistula of salivary gland

   Q38.5   Congenital malformations of palate, not elsewhere classified
> Congenital absence of uvula
> Congenital malformation of palate NOS
> Congenital high arched palate
>
> **EXCLUDES 1**   cleft palate (Q35.-)
>   cleft palate with cleft lip (Q37.-)

   Q38.6   Other congenital malformations of mouth
> Congenital malformation of mouth NOS

   Q38.7   Congenital pharyngeal pouch
> Congenital diverticulum of pharynx
>
> **EXCLUDES 1**   pharyngeal pouch syndrome (D82.1)

   Q38.8   Other congenital malformations of pharynx
> Congenital malformation of pharynx NOS
> Imperforate pharynx

✓4th Q39   Congenital malformations of esophagus

> **CC Excl:** For CC/MCC codes in category Q39, unless otherwise noted: Q39.0-Q39.9, Q45.8-Q45.9

   Q39.0   Atresia of esophagus without fistula   `MCC`
> Atresia of esophagus NOS

   Q39.1   Atresia of esophagus with tracheo-esophageal fistula   `MCC`
> Atresia of esophagus with broncho-esophageal fistula

   Q39.2   Congenital tracheo-esophageal fistula without atresia   `MCC`
> Congenital tracheo-esophageal fistula NOS

   Q39.3   Congenital stenosis and stricture of esophagus   `MCC`

   Q39.4   Esophageal web   `MCC`

   Q39.5   Congenital dilatation of esophagus   `CC`
> Congenital cardiospasm
> **CC Excl:** Q39.5-Q39.9, Q45.8-Q45.9

   Q39.6   Congenital diverticulum of esophagus   `CC`
> Congenital esophageal pouch
> **CC Excl:** See code: Q39.5

   Q39.8   Other congenital malformations of esophagus   `CC`
> Congenital absence of esophagus
> Congenital displacement of esophagus
> Congenital duplication of esophagus
> **CC Excl:** See code: Q39.5

   Q39.9   Congenital malformation of esophagus, unspecified   `CC`
> **CC Excl:** See code: Q39.5

✓4th Q40   Other congenital malformations of upper alimentary tract

   Q40.0   Congenital hypertrophic pyloric stenosis
> Congenital or infantile constriction
> Congenital or infantile hypertrophy
> Congenital or infantile spasm
> Congenital or infantile stenosis
> Congenital or infantile stricture

   Q40.1   Congenital hiatus hernia
> Congenital displacement of cardia through esophageal hiatus
>
> **EXCLUDES 1**   congenital diaphragmatic hernia (Q79.0)

   Q40.2   Other specified congenital malformations of stomach
> Congenital displacement of stomach
> Congenital diverticulum of stomach
> Congenital hourglass stomach
> Congenital duplication of stomach
> Megalogastria
> Microgastria

   Q40.3   Congenital malformation of stomach, unspecified

   Q40.8   Other specified congenital malformations of upper alimentary tract

   Q40.9   Congenital malformation of upper alimentary tract, unspecified
> Congenital anomaly of upper alimentary tract
> Congenital deformity of upper alimentary tract

✓4th Q41   Congenital absence, atresia and stenosis of small intestine

> Congenital obstruction, occlusion or stricture of small intestine or intestine NOS
>
> **EXCLUDES 1**   cystic fibrosis with intestinal manifestation (E84.11)
>   meconium ileus NOS (without cystic fibrosis) (P76.0)

> **CC Excl:** For CC codes in category Q41, unless otherwise noted: Q41.0-Q41.9, Q45.8-Q45.9

   Q41.0   Congenital absence, atresia and stenosis of duodenum   `CC`

   Q41.1   Congenital absence, atresia and stenosis of jejunum   `CC`
> Apple peel syndrome
> Imperforate jejunum

   Q41.2   Congenital absence, atresia and stenosis of ileum   `CC`

   Q41.8   Congenital absence, atresia and stenosis of other specified parts of small intestine   `CC`

   Q41.9   Congenital absence, atresia and stenosis of small intestine, part unspecified   `CC`
> Congenital absence, atresia and stenosis of intestine NOS

N Newborn: 0   **P** Pediatric: 0-17   **M** Maternity: 12-55   **A** Adult: 15-124   **MCC** Major CC Condition   **PDx MCC** PDx acts as own MCC   **CC** CC Condition   **PDx CC** PDx acts as own CC

✓4ᵗʰ **Q42** **Congenital absence, atresia and stenosis of large intestine**
Congenital obstruction, occlusion and stricture of large intestine

> **CC Excl: For CC codes in category Q42, unless otherwise noted:**
> Q42.0-Q42.9, Q45.8-Q45.9

Q42.0 **Congenital absence, atresia and stenosis of rectum with fistula** `CC`

Q42.1 **Congenital absence, atresia and stenosis of rectum without fistula** `CC`
Imperforate rectum

Q42.2 **Congenital absence, atresia and stenosis of anus with fistula** `CC`

Q42.3 **Congenital absence, atresia and stenosis of anus without fistula** `CC`
Imperforate anus

Q42.8 **Congenital absence, atresia and stenosis of other parts of large intestine** `CC`

Q42.9 **Congenital absence, atresia and stenosis of large intestine, part unspecified** `CC`

✓4ᵗʰ **Q43** **Other congenital malformations of intestine**

> **CC Excl: For CC codes in category Q43, unless otherwise noted:**
> Q41.0-Q43.9

Q43.0 **Meckel's diverticulum (displaced) (hypertrophic)**
Persistent omphalomesenteric duct
Persistent vitelline duct

Q43.1 **Hirschsprung's disease** `CC`
Aganglionosis
Congenital (aganglionic) megacolon
CC Excl: Q43.1-Q43.2, Q45.8-Q45.9

Q43.2 **Other congenital functional disorders of colon** `CC`
Congenital dilatation of colon
CC Excl: See code: Q43.1

Q43.3 **Congenital malformations of intestinal fixation** `CC`
Congenital omental, anomalous adhesions [bands]
Congenital peritoneal adhesions [bands]
Incomplete rotation of cecum and colon
Insufficient rotation of cecum and colon
Jackson's membrane
Malrotation of colon
Rotation failure of cecum and colon
Universal mesentery
CC Excl: Q43.3-Q43.9

Q43.4 **Duplication of intestine** `CC`

Q43.5 **Ectopic anus** `CC`

Q43.6 **Congenital fistula of rectum and anus** `CC`
> EXCLUDES 1   congenital fistula of anus with absence, atresia and stenosis (Q42.2)
> congenital fistula of rectum with absence, atresia and stenosis (Q42.0)
> congenital rectovaginal fistula (Q52.2)
> congenital urethrorectal fistula (Q64.73)
> pilonidal fistula or sinus (L05.-)

Q43.7 **Persistent cloaca** `CC`
Cloaca NOS

Q43.8 **Other specified congenital malformations of intestine** `CC`
Congenital blind loop syndrome
Congenital diverticulitis, colon
Congenital diverticulum, intestine
Dolichocolon
Megaloappendix
Megaloduodenum
Microcolon
Transposition of appendix
Transposition of colon
Transposition of intestine
AHA: 2013, 2Q, 31

Q43.9 **Congenital malformation of intestine, unspecified** `CC`

✓4ᵗʰ **Q44** **Congenital malformations of gallbladder, bile ducts and liver**

> **CC Excl: For CC/MCC codes in category Q44, unless otherwise noted:** Q44.0-Q44.7

Q44.0 **Agenesis, aplasia and hypoplasia of gallbladder** `CC`
Congenital absence of gallbladder

Q44.1 **Other congenital malformations of gallbladder** `CC`
Congenital malformation of gallbladder NOS
Intrahepatic gallbladder

Q44.2 **Atresia of bile ducts** `MCC`
CC Excl: Q44.2-Q44.3, Q45.8-Q45.9

Q44.3 **Congenital stenosis and stricture of bile ducts** `MCC`
CC Excl: See code: Q44.2

Q44.4 **Choledochal cyst** `CC`

Q44.5 **Other congenital malformations of bile ducts** `CC`
Accessory hepatic duct
Biliary duct duplication
Congenital malformation of bile duct NOS
Cystic duct duplication

Q44.6 **Cystic disease of liver** `CC`
Fibrocystic disease of liver
CC Excl: Q44.0-Q44.1, Q44.4-Q44.7

Q44.7 **Other congenital malformations of liver** `CC`
Accessory liver
Alagille's syndrome
Congenital absence of liver
Congenital hepatomegaly
Congenital malformation of liver NOS

✓4ᵗʰ **Q45** **Other congenital malformations of digestive system**
> EXCLUDES 2   congenital diaphragmatic hernia (Q79.0)
> congenital hiatus hernia (Q40.1)

> **CC Excl: For CC/MCC codes in category Q45, unless otherwise noted:** Q45.0-Q45.9

Q45.0 **Agenesis, aplasia and hypoplasia of pancreas** `CC`
Congenital absence of pancreas

Q45.1 **Annular pancreas** `CC`

Q45.2 **Congenital pancreatic cyst** `CC`

Q45.3 **Other congenital malformations of pancreas and pancreatic duct** `CC`
Accessory pancreas
Congenital malformation of pancreas or pancreatic duct NOS
> EXCLUDES 1   congenital diabetes mellitus (E10.-)
> cystic fibrosis (E84.0-E84.9)
> fibrocystic disease of pancreas (E84.-)
> neonatal diabetes mellitus (P70.2)

Q45.8 **Other specified congenital malformations of digestive system**
Absence (complete) (partial) of alimentary tract NOS
Duplication of digestive system
Malposition, congenital of digestive system

Q45.9 **Congenital malformation of digestive system, unspecified**
Congenital anomaly of digestive system
Congenital deformity of digestive system

Congenital malformations of genital organs (Q50-Q56)

> EXCLUDES 1   androgen insensitivity syndrome (E34.5-)
> syndromes associated with anomalies in the number and form of chromosomes (Q90-Q99)

✓4ᵗʰ **Q50** **Congenital malformations of ovaries, fallopian tubes and broad ligaments**

✓5ᵗʰ **Q50.0** **Congenital absence of ovary**
> EXCLUDES 1   Turner's syndrome (Q96.-)

Q50.01 **Congenital absence of ovary, unilateral** ♀

Q50.02 **Congenital absence of ovary, bilateral** ♀

Q50.1 **Developmental ovarian cyst** ♀

Q50.2 **Congenital torsion of ovary** ♀

✓5ᵗʰ **Q50.3** **Other congenital malformations of ovary**

Q50.31 **Accessory ovary** ♀

Q50.32 **Ovarian streak** ♀
46, XX with streak gonads

Q50.39 **Other congenital malformation of ovary** ♀
Congenital malformation of ovary NOS

Q50.4 **Embryonic cyst of fallopian tube** ♀
Fimbrial cyst

Q50.5 **Embryonic cyst of broad ligament** ♀
Epoophoron cyst
Parovarian cyst

Q50.6 **Other congenital malformations of fallopian tube and broad ligament** ♀
Absence of fallopian tube and broad ligament
Accessory fallopian tube and broad ligament
Atresia of fallopian tube and broad ligament
Congenital malformation of fallopian tube or broad ligament NOS

✓4ᵗʰ **Q51** **Congenital malformations of uterus and cervix**

Q51.0 **Agenesis and aplasia of uterus** ♀
Congenital absence of uterus

✓ Additional Character Required   ✓x7ᵗʰ Xtension Alert   Unacceptable PDx   Manifestation   Hospital Acquired Condition   EXCLUDES 1 Not Coded Here   EXCLUDES 2 Not Included Here

Q51.1–Q56.0   Congenital Malformations, Deformations and Chromosomal Abnormalities

✓5ᵗʰ **Q51.1** Doubling of uterus with doubling of cervix and vagina

    Q51.10 Doubling of uterus with doubling of cervix and vagina without obstruction ♀
         Doubling of uterus with doubling of cervix and vagina NOS

    Q51.11 Doubling of uterus with doubling of cervix and vagina with obstruction ♀

Q51.2 Other doubling of uterus ♀
     Doubling of uterus NOS
     Septate uterus, complete or partial

Q51.3 Bicornate uterus ♀
     Bicornate uterus, complete or partial

Q51.4 Unicornate uterus ♀
     Unicornate uterus with or without a separate uterine horn
     Uterus with only one functioning horn

Q51.5 Agenesis and aplasia of cervix ♀
     Congenital absence of cervix

Q51.6 Embryonic cyst of cervix ♀

Q51.7 Congenital fistulae between uterus and digestive and urinary tracts ♀

✓5ᵗʰ **Q51.8** Other congenital malformations of uterus and cervix

    ✓6ᵗʰ **Q51.81** Other congenital malformations of uterus
        Q51.810 Arcuate uterus ♀
             Arcuatus uterus
        Q51.811 Hypoplasia of uterus ♀
        Q51.818 Other congenital malformations of uterus ♀
             Müllerian anomaly of uterus NEC

    ✓6ᵗʰ **Q51.82** Other congenital malformations of cervix
        Q51.820 Cervical duplication ♀
        Q51.821 Hypoplasia of cervix ♀
        Q51.828 Other congenital malformations of cervix ♀

Q51.9 Congenital malformation of uterus and cervix, unspecified ♀

✓4ᵗʰ **Q52** Other congenital malformations of female genitalia

Q52.0 Congenital absence of vagina ♀
     Vaginal agenesis, total or partial

✓5ᵗʰ **Q52.1** Doubling of vagina
    EXCLUDES 1   doubling of vagina with doubling of uterus and cervix (Q51.1-)

    Q52.10 Doubling of vagina, unspecified ♀
         Septate vagina NOS
    Q52.11 Transverse vaginal septum ♀
    Q52.12 Longitudinal vaginal septum ♀
         Longitudinal vaginal septum with or without obstruction

Q52.2 Congenital rectovaginal fistula ♀
    EXCLUDES 1   cloaca (Q43.7)

Q52.3 Imperforate hymen ♀

Q52.4 Other congenital malformations of vagina ♀
     Canal of Nuck cyst, congenital
     Congenital malformation of vagina NOS
     Embryonic vaginal cyst
     Gartner's duct cyst

Q52.5 Fusion of labia ♀

Q52.6 Congenital malformation of clitoris ♀

✓5ᵗʰ **Q52.7** Other and unspecified congenital malformations of vulva
    Q52.70 Unspecified congenital malformations of vulva ♀
         Congenital malformation of vulva NOS
    Q52.71 Congenital absence of vulva ♀
    Q52.79 Other congenital malformations of vulva ♀
         Congenital cyst of vulva

Q52.8 Other specified congenital malformations of female genitalia ♀

Q52.9 Congenital malformation of female genitalia, unspecified ♀

✓4ᵗʰ **Q53** Undescended and ectopic testicle

✓5ᵗʰ **Q53.0** Ectopic testis
    Q53.00 Ectopic testis, unspecified ♂
    Q53.01 Ectopic testis, unilateral ♂
    Q53.02 Ectopic testes, bilateral ♂

✓5ᵗʰ **Q53.1** Undescended testicle, unilateral
    Q53.10 Unspecified undescended testicle, unilateral ♂
    Q53.11 Abdominal testis, unilateral ♂

    Q53.12 Ectopic perineal testis, unilateral ♂

✓5ᵗʰ **Q53.2** Undescended testicle, bilateral
    Q53.20 Undescended testicle, unspecified, bilateral ♂
    Q53.21 Abdominal testis, bilateral ♂
    Q53.22 Ectopic perineal testis, bilateral ♂

Q53.9 Undescended testicle, unspecified ♂
     Cryptorchism NOS

✓4ᵗʰ **Q54** Hypospadias
    EXCLUDES 1   epispadias (Q64.0)

Q54.0 Hypospadias, balanic ♂
     Hypospadias, coronal
     Hypospadias, glandular

Q54.1 Hypospadias, penile ♂

Q54.2 Hypospadias, penoscrotal ♂

Q54.3 Hypospadias, perineal ♂

Q54.4 Congenital chordee ♂
     Chordee without hypospadias

Q54.8 Other hypospadias ♂
     Hypospadias with intersex state

Q54.9 Hypospadias, unspecified ♂

✓4ᵗʰ **Q55** Other congenital malformations of male genital organs
    EXCLUDES 1   congenital hydrocele (P83.5)
         hypospadias (Q54.-)

Q55.0 Absence and aplasia of testis ♂
     Monorchism

Q55.1 Hypoplasia of testis and scrotum ♂
     Fusion of testes

✓5ᵗʰ **Q55.2** Other and unspecified congenital malformations of testis and scrotum
    Q55.20 Unspecified congenital malformations of testis and scrotum ♂
         Congenital malformation of testis or scrotum NOS
    Q55.21 Polyorchism ♂
    Q55.22 Retractile testis ♂
    Q55.23 Scrotal transposition ♂
    Q55.29 Other congenital malformations of testis and scrotum ♂

Q55.3 Atresia of vas deferens ♂
     Code first any associated cystic fibrosis (E84.-)

Q55.4 Other congenital malformations of vas deferens, epididymis, seminal vesicles and prostate ♂
     Absence or aplasia of prostate
     Absence or aplasia of spermatic cord
     Congenital malformation of vas deferens, epididymis, seminal vesicles or prostate NOS

Q55.5 Congenital absence and aplasia of penis ♂

✓5ᵗʰ **Q55.6** Other congenital malformations of penis
    Q55.61 Curvature of penis (lateral) ♂
    Q55.62 Hypoplasia of penis ♂
         Micropenis
    Q55.63 Congenital torsion of penis ♂
        EXCLUDES 1   acquired torsion of penis (N48.82)
    Q55.64 Hidden penis ♂
         Buried penis
         Concealed penis
        EXCLUDES 1   acquired buried penis (N48.83)
    Q55.69 Other congenital malformation of penis ♂
         Congenital malformation of penis NOS

Q55.7 Congenital vasocutaneous fistula ♂

Q55.8 Other specified congenital malformations of male genital organs ♂

Q55.9 Congenital malformation of male genital organ, unspecified ♂
     Congenital anomaly of male genital organ
     Congenital deformity of male genital organ

✓4ᵗʰ **Q56** Indeterminate sex and pseudohermaphroditism
    EXCLUDES 1   46, XX true hermaphrodite (Q99.1)
         androgen insensitivity syndrome (E34.5-)
         chimera 46, XX/46, XY true hermaphrodite (Q99.0)
         female pseudohermaphroditism with adrenocortical disorder (E25.-)
         pseudohermaphroditism with specified chromosomal anomaly (Q96-Q99)
         pure gonadal dysgenesis (Q99.1)

Q56.0 Hermaphroditism, not elsewhere classified
     Ovotestis

Ⓝ Newborn: 0   Ⓟ Pediatric: 0-17   Ⓜ Maternity: 12-55   Ⓐ Adult: 15-124   **MCC** Major CC Condition   **PDx MCC** PDx acts as own MCC   **CC** CC Condition   **PDx CC** PDx acts as own CC

Q56.1 Male **pseudohermaphroditism, not elsewhere classified** ♂
46, XY with streak gonads
Male pseudohermaphroditism NOS

Q56.2 Female **pseudohermaphroditism, not elsewhere classified** ♀
Female pseudohermaphroditism NOS

Q56.3 **Pseudohermaphroditism, unspecified**

Q56.4 **Indeterminate sex, unspecified**
Ambiguous genitalia

Congenital malformations of the urinary system (Q60-Q64)

✔4ᵗʰ **Q60** **Renal agenesis and other** reduction defects of kidney
Congenital absence of kidney
Congenital atrophy of kidney
Infantile atrophy of kidney

> **CC Excl:** For CC codes in category Q60, unless otherwise noted: N13.9, Q60.0-Q60.6

Q60.0 **Renal** agenesis, unilateral　　CC

Q60.1 **Renal** agenesis, bilateral　　CC

Q60.2 **Renal** agenesis, unspecified　　CC

Q60.3 **Renal** hypoplasia, unilateral　　CC

Q60.4 **Renal** hypoplasia, bilateral　　CC

Q60.5 **Renal** hypoplasia, unspecified　　CC

Q60.6 **Potter's syndrome**　　CC

✔4ᵗʰ **Q61** **Cystic kidney** disease
EXCLUDES1　acquired cyst of kidney (N28.1)
Potter's syndrome (Q60.6)

✔5ᵗʰ **Q61.0** **Congenital renal** cyst

　Q61.00 **Congenital renal cyst, unspecified**　　CC
Cyst of kidney NOS (congenital)
CC Excl: N13.9, Q61.00, Q61.9

　Q61.01 **Congenital single renal cyst**　　CC
CC Excl: N13.9, Q61.01

　Q61.02 **Congenital multiple renal cysts**　　CC
CC Excl: N13.9, Q61.02, Q61.5-Q61.8

✔5ᵗʰ **Q61.1** **Polycystic kidney, infantile type**
Polycystic kidney, autosomal recessive

　Q61.11 **Cystic dilatation of collecting ducts**
CC Excl: N13.9, Q61.11-Q61.3

　Q61.19 **Other polycystic kidney, infantile type**
CC Excl: See code: Q61.11

Q61.2 **Polycystic kidney, adult type**
Polycystic kidney, autosomal dominant
CC Excl: See code: Q61.11

Q61.3 **Polycystic kidney, unspecified**
CC Excl: See code: Q61.11

Q61.4 **Renal** dysplasia　　♂
Multicystic dysplastic kidney
Multicystic kidney (development)
Multicystic kidney disease
Multicystic renal dysplasia
EXCLUDES1　polycystic kidney disease (Q61.11-Q61.3)
CC Excl: N13.9, Q61.4

Q61.5 **Medullary cystic kidney**　　CC
Nephronopthisis
Sponge kidney NOS
CC Excl: See code: Q61.02

Q61.8 **Other cystic kidney diseases**　　CC
Fibrocystic kidney
Fibrocystic renal degeneration or disease
CC Excl: See code: Q61.02

Q61.9 **Cystic kidney disease, unspecified**　　CC
Meckel-Gruber syndrome
CC Excl: See code: Q61.00

✔4ᵗʰ **Q62** **Congenital obstructive defects of** renal pelvis and congenital malformations of ureter

> **CC Excl:** For CC codes in category Q62, unless otherwise noted: N13.9, Q62.0-Q62.2, Q62.39

Q62.0 **Congenital** hydronephrosis　　CC

✔5ᵗʰ **Q62.1** **Congenital** occlusion of ureter
Atresia and stenosis of ureter

　Q62.10 **Congenital occlusion of** ureter, unspecified　　CC

　Q62.11 **Congenital occlusion of** ureteropelvic junction　　CC

　Q62.12 **Congenital occlusion of** ureterovesical orifice　　CC

Q62.2 **Congenital** megaureter　　CC
Congenital dilatation of ureter

✔5ᵗʰ **Q62.3** **Other obstructive defects of renal pelvis and ureter**

　Q62.31 **Congenital** ureterocele, orthotopic　　CC

　Q62.32 **Cecoureterocele**　　CC
Ectopic ureterocele

　Q62.39 **Other obstructive defects of renal pelvis and ureter**　　CC
Ureteropelvic junction obstruction NOS

Q62.4 **Agenesis of ureter**
Congenital absence ureter

Q62.5 **Duplication of ureter**
Accessory ureter
Double ureter

✔5ᵗʰ **Q62.6** **Malposition of ureter**

　Q62.60 **Malposition of ureter, unspecified**

　Q62.61 **Deviation of ureter**

　Q62.62 **Displacement of ureter**

　Q62.63 **Anomalous implantation of ureter**
Ectopia of ureter
Ectopic ureter

　Q62.69 **Other malposition of ureter**

Q62.7 **Congenital vesico-uretero-renal reflux**

Q62.8 **Other** congenital malformations of ureter
Anomaly of ureter NOS

✔4ᵗʰ **Q63** **Other** congenital malformations of kidney
EXCLUDES1　congenital nephrotic syndrome (N04.-)

Q63.0 **Accessory kidney**

Q63.1 **Lobulated, fused and horseshoe kidney**

Q63.2 **Ectopic kidney**
Congenital displaced kidney
Malrotation of kidney

Q63.3 **Hyperplastic and giant kidney**
Compensatory hypertrophy of kidney

Q63.8 **Other specified congenital malformations of kidney**
Congenital renal calculi

Q63.9 **Congenital malformation of kidney, unspecified**

✔4ᵗʰ **Q64** **Other congenital malformations of urinary system**

Q64.0 **Epispadias**　　♂
EXCLUDES1　hypospadias (Q54.-)

✔5ᵗʰ **Q64.1** **Exstrophy of urinary bladder**

> **CC Excl:** For CC codes in subcategory Q64.1, unless otherwise noted: N13.9, Q64.10-Q64.19, Q64.8-Q64.9

　Q64.10 **Exstrophy of urinary bladder, unspecified**　　CC
Ectopia vesicae

　Q64.11 **Supravesical fissure of urinary bladder**　　CC

　Q64.12 **Cloacal extrophy of urinary bladder**　　CC

　Q64.19 **Other exstrophy of urinary bladder**　　CC
Extroversion of bladder

Q64.2 **Congenital posterior urethral valves**　　CC
CC Excl: N13.9, Q64.2-Q64.39, Q64.8-Q64.9

✔5ᵗʰ **Q64.3** **Other atresia and stenosis of urethra and bladder neck**

> **CC Excl:** For CC codes in subcategory Q64.3, unless otherwise noted: See code: Q64.2

　Q64.31 **Congenital bladder neck obstruction**　　CC
Congenital obstruction of vesicourethral orifice

　Q64.32 **Congenital stricture of urethra**　　CC

　Q64.33 **Congenital stricture of urinary meatus**　　CC

　Q64.39 **Other** atresia and stenosis of urethra and bladder neck　　CC
Atresia and stenosis of urethra and bladder neck NOS

Q64.4 **Malformation of urachus**
Cyst of urachus
Patent urachus
Prolapse of urachus

Q64.5 **Congenital absence of bladder and urethra**

Q64.6 **Congenital diverticulum of bladder**

✔5ᵗʰ **Q64.7** **Other and unspecified congenital malformations of bladder and urethra**
EXCLUDES1　congenital prolapse of bladder (mucosa) (Q79.4)

　Q64.70 **Unspecified congenital malformation of bladder and urethra**
Malformation of bladder or urethra NOS

　Q64.71 **Congenital prolapse of urethra**

　Q64.72 **Congenital prolapse of urinary meatus**

✔ Additional Character Required　✔ˣ⁷ᵗʰ Xtension Alert　Unacceptable PDx　Manifestation　　Hospital Acquired Condition　　EXCLUDES1 Not Coded Here　EXCLUDES2 Not Included Here

Congenital Malformations, Deformations and Chromosomal Abnormalities

Q64.73–Q70.22

Q64.73 Congenital urethrorectal fistula

Q64.74 Double urethra

Q64.75 Double urinary meatus

Q64.79 Other congenital malformations of bladder and urethra

Q64.8 Other specified congenital malformations of urinary system

Q64.9 Congenital malformation of urinary system, unspecified
Congenital anomaly NOS of urinary system
Congenital deformity NOS of urinary system

Congenital malformations and deformations of the musculoskeletal system (Q65-Q79)

✓4ᵗʰ **Q65 Congenital deformities of hip**
EXCLUDES 1 clicking hip (R29.4)

✓5ᵗʰ Q65.0 Congenital dislocation of hip, unilateral

    Q65.00 Congenital dislocation of unspecified hip, unilateral

    Q65.01 Congenital dislocation of right hip, unilateral

    Q65.02 Congenital dislocation of left hip, unilateral

Q65.1 Congenital dislocation of hip, bilateral

Q65.2 Congenital dislocation of hip, unspecified

✓5ᵗʰ Q65.3 Congenital partial dislocation of hip, unilateral

    Q65.30 Congenital partial dislocation of unspecified hip, unilateral

    Q65.31 Congenital partial dislocation of right hip, unilateral

    Q65.32 Congenital partial dislocation of left hip, unilateral

Q65.4 Congenital partial dislocation of hip, bilateral

Q65.5 Congenital partial dislocation of hip, unspecified

Q65.6 Congenital unstable hip
Congenital dislocatable hip

✓5ᵗʰ Q65.8 Other congenital deformities of hip

    Q65.81 Congenital coxa valga

    Q65.82 Congenital coxa vara

    Q65.89 Other specified congenital deformities of hip
Anteversion of femoral neck
Congenital acetabular dysplasia

Q65.9 Congenital deformity of hip, unspecified

✓4ᵗʰ **Q66 Congenital deformities of feet**
EXCLUDES 1 reduction defects of feet (Q72.-)
valgus deformities (acquired) (M21.0-)
varus deformities (acquired) (M21.1-)

Q66.0 Congenital talipes equinovarus

Q66.1 Congenital talipes calcaneovarus

Q66.2 Congenital metatarsus (primus) varus

Q66.3 Other congenital varus deformities of feet
Hallux varus, congenital

Q66.4 Congenital talipes calcaneovalgus

✓5ᵗʰ Q66.5 Congenital pes planus
Congenital flat foot
Congenital rigid flat foot
Congenital spastic (everted) flat foot
EXCLUDES 1 pes planus, acquired (M21.4)

    Q66.50 Congenital pes planus, unspecified foot

    Q66.51 Congenital pes planus, right foot

    Q66.52 Congenital pes planus, left foot

Q66.6 Other congenital valgus deformities of feet
Congenital metatarsus valgus

Q66.7 Congenital pes cavus

✓5ᵗʰ Q66.8 Other congenital deformities of feet

    Q66.80 Congenital vertical talus deformity, unspecified foot

    Q66.81 Congenital vertical talus deformity, right foot

    Q66.82 Congenital vertical talus deformity, left foot

    Q66.89 Other specified congenital deformities of feet
Congenital asymmetric talipes
Congenital clubfoot NOS
Congenital talipes NOS
Congenital tarsal coalition
Hammer toe, congenital

Q66.9 Congenital deformity of feet, unspecified

✓4ᵗʰ **Q67 Congenital musculoskeletal deformities of head, face, spine and chest**
EXCLUDES 1 congenital malformation syndromes classified to Q87-
Potter's syndrome (Q60.6)

Q67.0 Congenital facial asymmetry

Q67.1 Congenital compression facies

Q67.2 Dolichocephaly

Q67.3 Plagiocephaly

Q67.4 Other congenital deformities of skull, face and jaw
Congenital depressions in skull
Congenital hemifacial atrophy or hypertrophy
Deviation of nasal septum, congenital
Squashed or bent nose, congenital
EXCLUDES 1 dentofacial anomalies [including malocclusion] (M26.-)
syphilitic saddle nose (A50.5)

Q67.5 Congenital deformity of spine   CC
Congenital postural scoliosis
Congenital scoliosis NOS
EXCLUDES 1 infantile idiopathic scoliosis (M41.0)
scoliosis due to congenital bony malformation (Q76.3)
CC Excl: Q67.5, Q76.3, Q76.425-Q76.429

Q67.6 Pectus excavatum
Congenital funnel chest

Q67.7 Pectus carinatum
Congenital pigeon chest

Q67.8 Other congenital deformities of chest   CC
Congenital deformity of chest wall NOS
CC Excl: Q67.6-Q67.8, Q68.1, Q74.3

✓4ᵗʰ **Q68 Other congenital musculoskeletal deformities**
EXCLUDES 1 reduction defects of limb(s) (Q71-Q73)
EXCLUDES 2 congenital myotonic chondrodystrophy (G71.13)

Q68.0 Congenital deformity of sternocleidomastoid muscle
Congenital contracture of sternocleidomastoid (muscle)
Congenital (sternomastoid) torticollis
Sternomastoid tumor (congenital)

Q68.1 Congenital deformity of finger(s) and hand   CC
Congenital clubfinger
Spade-like hand (congenital)
CC Excl: See code: Q67.8

Q68.2 Congenital deformity of knee
Congenital dislocation of knee
Congenital genu recurvatum

Q68.3 Congenital bowing of femur
EXCLUDES 1 anteversion of femur (neck) (Q65.89)

Q68.4 Congenital bowing of tibia and fibula

Q68.5 Congenital bowing of long bones of leg, unspecified

Q68.6 Discoid meniscus

Q68.8 Other specified congenital musculoskeletal deformities
Congenital deformity of clavicle
Congenital deformity of elbow
Congenital deformity of forearm
Congenital deformity of scapula
Congenital deformity of wrist
Congenital dislocation of elbow
Congenital dislocation of shoulder
Congenital dislocation of wrist

✓4ᵗʰ **Q69 Polydactyly**

Q69.0 Accessory finger(s)

Q69.1 Accessory thumb(s)

Q69.2 Accessory toe(s)
Accessory hallux

Q69.9 Polydactyly, unspecified
Supernumerary digit(s) NOS

✓4ᵗʰ **Q70 Syndactyly**

✓5ᵗʰ Q70.0 Fused fingers
Complex syndactyly of fingers with synostosis

    Q70.00 Fused fingers, unspecified hand

    Q70.01 Fused fingers, right hand

    Q70.02 Fused fingers, left hand

    Q70.03 Fused fingers, bilateral

✓5ᵗʰ Q70.1 Webbed fingers
Simple syndactyly of fingers without synostosis

    Q70.10 Webbed fingers, unspecified hand

    Q70.11 Webbed fingers, right hand

    Q70.12 Webbed fingers, left hand

    Q70.13 Webbed fingers, bilateral

✓5ᵗʰ Q70.2 Fused toes
Complex syndactyly of toes with synostosis

    Q70.20 Fused toes, unspecified foot

    Q70.21 Fused toes, right foot

    Q70.22 Fused toes, left foot

N Newborn: 0   P Pediatric: 0-17   M Maternity: 12-55   A Adult: 15-124   MCC Major CC Condition   PDx MCC PDx acts as own MCC   CC CC Condition   PDx CC PDx acts as own CC

834   ICD-10-CM Draft (2015)

Q70.23   **Fused toes, bilateral**

✓5ᵗʰ Q70.3   **Webbed toes**
Simple syndactyly of toes without synostosis
Q70.30   **Webbed toes, unspecified foot**
Q70.31   **Webbed toes, right foot**
Q70.32   **Webbed toes, left foot**
Q70.33   **Webbed toes, bilateral**

Q70.4   **Polysyndactyly, unspecified**
EXCLUDES 1   specified syndactyly of hand and feet—code to specified conditions (Q70.0-Q70.3-)

Q70.9   **Syndactyly, unspecified**
Symphalangy NOS

✓4ᵗʰ **Q71   Reduction defects of upper limb**

✓5ᵗʰ Q71.0   **Congenital complete absence of upper limb**
Q71.00   **Congenital complete absence of unspecified upper limb**
Q71.01   **Congenital complete absence of right upper limb**
Q71.02   **Congenital complete absence of left upper limb**
Q71.03   **Congenital complete absence of upper limb, bilateral**

✓5ᵗʰ Q71.1   **Congenital absence of upper arm and forearm with hand present**
Q71.10   **Congenital absence of unspecified upper arm and forearm with hand present**
Q71.11   **Congenital absence of right upper arm and forearm with hand present**
Q71.12   **Congenital absence of left upper arm and forearm with hand present**
Q71.13   **Congenital absence of upper arm and forearm with hand present, bilateral**

✓5ᵗʰ Q71.2   **Congenital absence of both forearm and hand**
Q71.20   **Congenital absence of both forearm and hand, unspecified upper limb**
Q71.21   **Congenital absence of both forearm and hand, right upper limb**
Q71.22   **Congenital absence of both forearm and hand, left upper limb**
Q71.23   **Congenital absence of both forearm and hand, bilateral**

✓5ᵗʰ Q71.3   **Congenital absence of hand and finger**
Q71.30   **Congenital absence of unspecified hand and finger**
Q71.31   **Congenital absence of right hand and finger**
Q71.32   **Congenital absence of left hand and finger**
Q71.33   **Congenital absence of hand and finger, bilateral**

✓5ᵗʰ Q71.4   **Longitudinal reduction defect of radius**
Clubhand (congenital)
Radial clubhand
Q71.40   **Longitudinal reduction defect of unspecified radius**
Q71.41   **Longitudinal reduction defect of right radius**
Q71.42   **Longitudinal reduction defect of left radius**
Q71.43   **Longitudinal reduction defect of radius, bilateral**

✓5ᵗʰ Q71.5   **Longitudinal reduction defect of ulna**
Q71.50   **Longitudinal reduction defect of unspecified ulna**
Q71.51   **Longitudinal reduction defect of right ulna**
Q71.52   **Longitudinal reduction defect of left ulna**
Q71.53   **Longitudinal reduction defect of ulna, bilateral**

✓5ᵗʰ Q71.6   **Lobster-claw hand**
Q71.60   **Lobster-claw hand, unspecified hand**
Q71.61   **Lobster-claw right hand**
Q71.62   **Lobster-claw left hand**
Q71.63   **Lobster-claw hand, bilateral**

✓5ᵗʰ Q71.8   **Other reduction defects of upper limb**
✓6ᵗʰ Q71.81   **Congenital shortening of upper limb**
Q71.811   **Congenital shortening of right upper limb**
Q71.812   **Congenital shortening of left upper limb**
Q71.813   **Congenital shortening of upper limb, bilateral**
Q71.819   **Congenital shortening of unspecified upper limb**
✓6ᵗʰ Q71.89   **Other reduction defects of upper limb**
Q71.891   **Other reduction defects of right upper limb**
Q71.892   **Other reduction defects of left upper limb**

Q71.893   **Other reduction defects of upper limb, bilateral**
Q71.899   **Other reduction defects of unspecified upper limb**

✓5ᵗʰ Q71.9   **Unspecified reduction defect of upper limb**
Q71.90   **Unspecified reduction defect of unspecified upper limb**
Q71.91   **Unspecified reduction defect of right upper limb**
Q71.92   **Unspecified reduction defect of left upper limb**
Q71.93   **Unspecified reduction defect of upper limb, bilateral**

✓4ᵗʰ **Q72   Reduction defects of lower limb**

✓5ᵗʰ Q72.0   **Congenital complete absence of lower limb**
Q72.00   **Congenital complete absence of unspecified lower limb**
Q72.01   **Congenital complete absence of right lower limb**
Q72.02   **Congenital complete absence of left lower limb**
Q72.03   **Congenital complete absence of lower limb, bilateral**

✓5ᵗʰ Q72.1   **Congenital absence of thigh and lower leg with foot present**
Q72.10   **Congenital absence of unspecified thigh and lower leg with foot present**
Q72.11   **Congenital absence of right thigh and lower leg with foot present**
Q72.12   **Congenital absence of left thigh and lower leg with foot present**
Q72.13   **Congenital absence of thigh and lower leg with foot present, bilateral**

✓5ᵗʰ Q72.2   **Congenital absence of both lower leg and foot**
Q72.20   **Congenital absence of both lower leg and foot, unspecified lower limb**
Q72.21   **Congenital absence of both lower leg and foot, right lower limb**
Q72.22   **Congenital absence of both lower leg and foot, left lower limb**
Q72.23   **Congenital absence of both lower leg and foot, bilateral**

✓5ᵗʰ Q72.3   **Congenital absence of foot and toe(s)**
Q72.30   **Congenital absence of unspecified foot and toe(s)**
Q72.31   **Congenital absence of right foot and toe(s)**
Q72.32   **Congenital absence of left foot and toe(s)**
Q72.33   **Congenital absence of foot and toe(s), bilateral**

✓5ᵗʰ Q72.4   **Longitudinal reduction defect of femur**
Proximal femoral focal deficiency
Q72.40   **Longitudinal reduction defect of unspecified femur**
Q72.41   **Longitudinal reduction defect of right femur**
Q72.42   **Longitudinal reduction defect of left femur**
Q72.43   **Longitudinal reduction defect of femur, bilateral**

✓5ᵗʰ Q72.5   **Longitudinal reduction defect of tibia**
Q72.50   **Longitudinal reduction defect of unspecified tibia**
Q72.51   **Longitudinal reduction defect of right tibia**
Q72.52   **Longitudinal reduction defect of left tibia**
Q72.53   **Longitudinal reduction defect of tibia, bilateral**

✓5ᵗʰ Q72.6   **Longitudinal reduction defect of fibula**
Q72.60   **Longitudinal reduction defect of unspecified fibula**
Q72.61   **Longitudinal reduction defect of right fibula**
Q72.62   **Longitudinal reduction defect of left fibula**
Q72.63   **Longitudinal reduction defect of fibula, bilateral**

✓5ᵗʰ Q72.7   **Split foot**
Q72.70   **Split foot, unspecified lower limb**
Q72.71   **Split foot, right lower limb**
Q72.72   **Split foot, left lower limb**
Q72.73   **Split foot, bilateral**

✓5ᵗʰ Q72.8   **Other reduction defects of lower limb**
✓6ᵗʰ Q72.81   **Congenital shortening of lower limb**
Q72.811   **Congenital shortening of right lower limb**
Q72.812   **Congenital shortening of left lower limb**
Q72.813   **Congenital shortening of lower limb, bilateral**
Q72.819   **Congenital shortening of unspecified lower limb**
✓6ᵗʰ Q72.89   **Other reduction defects of lower limb**
Q72.891   **Other reduction defects of right lower limb**

✓ Additional Character Required   ✓x7ᵗʰ Xtension Alert   Unacceptable PDx   Manifestation   Hospital Acquired Condition   EXCLUDES 1 Not Coded Here   EXCLUDES 2 Not Included Here

Q72.892   **Other** reduction defects of **left** lower limb

Q72.893   **Other** reduction defects of lower limb, **bilateral**

Q72.899   **Other** reduction defects of **unspecified** lower limb

✓5ᵗʰ   Q72.9   **Unspecified** reduction defect of lower limb

Q72.90   **Unspecified** reduction defect of **unspecified** lower limb

Q72.91   **Unspecified** reduction defect of **right** lower limb

Q72.92   **Unspecified** reduction defect of **left** lower limb

Q72.93   **Unspecified** reduction defect of lower limb, **bilateral**

✓4ᵗʰ   **Q73**   **Reduction defects of unspecified limb**

Q73.0   **Congenital absence of unspecified limb(s)**
Amelia NOS

Q73.1   **Phocomelia, unspecified limb(s)**
Phocomelia NOS

Q73.8   **Other reduction defects of unspecified limb(s)**
Longitudinal reduction deformity of unspecified limb(s)
Ectromelia of limb NOS
Hemimelia of limb NOS
Reduction defect of limb NOS

✓4ᵗʰ   **Q74**   **Other congenital malformations of limb(s)**
EXCLUDES 1   *polydactyly (Q69.-)*
reduction defect of limb (Q71-Q73)
syndactyly (Q70.-)

Q74.0   **Other congenital malformations of upper limb(s), including shoulder girdle**
Accessory carpal bones
Cleidocranial dysostosis
Congenital pseudarthrosis of clavicle
Macrodactylia (fingers)
Madelung's deformity
Radioulnar synostosis
Sprengel's deformity
Triphalangeal thumb

Q74.1   **Congenital malformation of knee**
Congenital absence of patella
Congenital dislocation of patella
Congenital genu valgum
Congenital genu varum
Rudimentary patella
EXCLUDES 1   *congenital dislocation of knee (Q68.2)*
congenital genu recurvatum (Q68.2)
nail patella syndrome (Q87.2)

Q74.2   **Other congenital malformations of lower limb(s), including pelvic girdle**
Congenital fusion of sacroiliac joint
Congenital malformation of ankle joint
Congenital malformation of sacroiliac joint
EXCLUDES 1   *anteversion of femur (neck) (Q65.89)*

Q74.3   **Arthrogryposis multiplex congenita**   CC
CC Excl: Q67.5, Q73, Q76.425-Q76.429

Q74.8   **Other specified congenital malformations of limb(s)**

Q74.9   **Unspecified congenital malformation of limb(s)**
Congenital anomaly of limb(s) NOS

✓4ᵗʰ   **Q75**   **Other congenital malformations of skull and face bones**
EXCLUDES 1   *congenital malformation of face NOS (Q18.-)*
congenital malformation syndromes classified to Q87.-
dentofacial anomalies [including malocclusion] (M26.-)
musculoskeletal deformities of head and face (Q67.0-Q67.4)
skull defects associated with congenital anomalies of brain such as:
anencephaly (Q00.0)
encephalocele (Q01.-)
hydrocephalus (Q03.-)
microcephaly (Q02)

Q75.0   **Craniosynostosis**
Acrocephaly
Imperfect fusion of skull
Oxycephaly
Trigonocephaly

Q75.1   **Craniofacial dysostosis**
Crouzon's disease

Q75.2   **Hypertelorism**

Q75.3   **Macrocephaly**

Q75.4   **Mandibulofacial dysostosis**
Franceschetti syndrome
Treacher Collins syndrome

Q75.5   **Oculomandibular dysostosis**

Q75.8   **Other specified congenital malformations of skull and face bones**
Absence of skull bone, congenital
Congenital deformity of forehead
Platybasia

Q75.9   **Congenital malformation of skull and face bones, unspecified**
Congenital anomaly of face bones NOS
Congenital anomaly of skull NOS

✓4ᵗʰ   **Q76**   **Congenital malformations of spine and bony thorax**
EXCLUDES 1   *congenital musculoskeletal deformities of spine and chest (Q67.5-Q67.8)*

Q76.0   **Spina bifida occulta**
EXCLUDES 1   *meningocele (spinal) (Q05.-)*
spina bifida (aperta) (cystica) (Q05.-)

Q76.1   **Klippel-Feil syndrome**
Cervical fusion syndrome

Q76.2   **Congenital spondylolisthesis**
Congenital spondylolysis
EXCLUDES 1   *spondylolisthesis (acquired) (M43.1-)*
spondylolysis (acquired) (M43.0-)

Q76.3   **Congenital scoliosis due to congenital bony malformation**   CC
Hemivertebra fusion or failure of segmentation with scoliosis
CC Excl: See code: Q67.5

✓5ᵗʰ   **Q76.4**   **Other congenital malformations of spine, not associated with scoliosis**

CC Excl: For CC codes in subcategory Q76.4, unless otherwise noted: Q67.5, Q76.3, Q76.425-Q76.429

✓6ᵗʰ   **Q76.41**   **Congenital kyphosis**

Q76.411   **Congenital kyphosis, occipito-atlanto-axial region**

Q76.412   **Congenital kyphosis, cervical region**

Q76.413   **Congenital kyphosis, cervicothoracic region**

Q76.414   **Congenital kyphosis, thoracic region**

Q76.415   **Congenital kyphosis, thoracolumbar region**

Q76.419   **Congenital kyphosis, unspecified region**

✓6ᵗʰ   **Q76.42**   **Congenital lordosis**

Q76.425   **Congenital lordosis, thoracolumbar region**   CC

Q76.426   **Congenital lordosis, lumbar region**   CC

Q76.427   **Congenital lordosis, lumbosacral region**   CC

Q76.428   **Congenital lordosis, sacral and sacrococcygeal region**   CC

Q76.429   **Congenital lordosis, unspecified region**   CC

Q76.49   **Other congenital malformations of spine, not associated with scoliosis**
Congenital absence of vertebra NOS
Congenital fusion of spine NOS
Congenital malformation of lumbosacral (joint) (region) NOS
Congenital malformation of spine NOS
Hemivertebra NOS
Malformation of spine NOS
Platyspondylisis NOS
Supernumerary vertebra NOS

Q76.5   **Cervical rib**
Supernumerary rib in cervical region

Q76.6   **Other congenital malformations of ribs**   CC
Accessory rib
Congenital absence of rib
Congenital fusion of ribs
Congenital malformation of ribs NOS
EXCLUDES 1   *short rib syndrome (Q77.2)*
CC Excl: Q76.5-Q76.9, Q77.2

Q76.7   **Congenital malformation of sternum**   CC
Congenital absence of sternum
Sternum bifidum
CC Excl: See code: Q76.6

Q76.8   **Other congenital malformations of bony thorax**   CC
CC Excl: See code: Q76.6

Q76.9   **Congenital malformation of bony thorax, unspecified**   CC
CC Excl: See code: Q76.6b

N Newborn: 0   P Pediatric: 0-17   M Maternity: 12-55   A Adult: 15-124   MCC Major CC Condition   PDx MCC PDx acts as own MCC   CC CC Condition   PDx CC PDx acts as own CC

Q77 Osteochondrodysplasia with defects of growth of tubular bones and spine
EXCLUDES 1 mucopolysaccharidosis (E76.0-E76.3)
EXCLUDES 2 congenital myotonic chondrodystrophy (G71.13)

Q77.0 Achondrogenesis
Hypochondrogenesis

Q77.1 Thanatophoric short stature

Q77.2 Short rib syndrome CC
Asphyxiating thoracic dysplasia [Jeune]
CC Excl: Q76.5-Q76.9, Q77.2

Q77.3 Chondrodysplasia punctata
EXCLUDES 1 Rhizomelic chondrodysplasia punctata (E71.43)

Q77.4 Achondroplasia
Hypochondroplasia
Osteosclerosis congenita

Q77.5 Diastrophic dysplasia

Q77.6 Chondroectodermal dysplasia
Ellis-van Creveld syndrome

Q77.7 Spondyloepiphyseal dysplasia

Q77.8 Other osteochondrodysplasia with defects of growth of tubular bones and spine

Q77.9 Osteochondrodysplasia with defects of growth of tubular bones and spine, unspecified

✓4ᵗʰ Q78 Other osteochondrodysplasias
EXCLUDES 2 congenital myotonic chondrodystrophy (G71.13)

Q78.0 Osteogenesis imperfecta CC
Fragilitas ossium
Osteopsathyrosis
CC Excl: Q77.3, Q77.6, Q78.0-Q78.3, Q78.5-Q78.9

Q78.1 Polyostotic fibrous dysplasia
Albright(-McCune)(-Sternberg) syndrome

Q78.2 Osteopetrosis CC
Albers-Schönberg syndrome
Osteosclerosis NOS
CC Excl: See code: Q78.0

Q78.3 Progressive diaphyseal dysplasia
Camurati-Engelmann syndrome

Q78.4 Enchondromatosis
Maffucci's syndrome
Ollier's disease

Q78.5 Metaphyseal dysplasia
Pyle's syndrome

Q78.6 Multiple congenital exostoses
Diaphyseal aclasis

Q78.8 Other specified osteochondrodysplasias
Osteopoikilosis

Q78.9 Osteochondrodysplasia, unspecified
Chondrodystrophy NOS
Osteodystrophy NOS

✓4ᵗʰ Q79 Congenital malformations of musculoskeletal system, not elsewhere classified
EXCLUDES 2 congenital (sternomastoid) torticollis (Q68.0)

CC Excl: For CC/MCC codes in category Q79, unless otherwise noted: Q79.2-Q79.59

Q79.0 Congenital diaphragmatic hernia MCC
EXCLUDES 1 congenital hiatus hernia (Q40.1)
CC Excl: Q40.1-Q79.1

Q79.1 Other congenital malformations of diaphragm MCC
Absence of diaphragm
Congenital malformation of diaphragm NOS
Eventration of diaphragm
CC Excl: See code: Q79.0

Q79.2 Exomphalos MCC
Omphalocele
EXCLUDES 1 umbilical hernia (K42.-)

Q79.3 Gastroschisis MCC

Q79.4 Prune belly syndrome MCC
Congenital prolapse of bladder mucosa
Eagle-Barrett syndrome

✓5ᵗʰ Q79.5 Other congenital malformations of abdominal wall
EXCLUDES 1 umbilical hernia (K42.-)

Q79.51 Congenital hernia of bladder MCC

Q79.59 Other congenital malformations of abdominal wall MCC

Q79.6 Ehlers-Danlos syndrome CC
CC Excl: Q79.6

Q79.8 Other congenital malformations of musculoskeletal system
Absence of muscle
Absence of tendon
Accessory muscle
Amyotrophia congenita
Congenital constricting bands
Congenital shortening of tendon
Poland syndrome

Q79.9 Congenital malformation of musculoskeletal system, unspecified
Congenital anomaly of musculoskeletal system NOS
Congenital deformity of musculoskeletal system NOS

Other congenital malformations (Q80-Q89)

✓4ᵗʰ Q80 Congenital ichthyosis
EXCLUDES 1 Refsum's disease (G60.1)

Q80.0 Ichthyosis vulgaris

Q80.1 X-linked ichthyosis

Q80.2 Lamellar ichthyosis
Collodion baby

Q80.3 Congenital bullous ichthyosiform erythroderma

Q80.4 Harlequin fetus

Q80.8 Other congenital ichthyosis

Q80.9 Congenital ichthyosis, unspecified

✓4ᵗʰ Q81 Epidermolysis bullosa

Q81.0 Epidermolysis bullosa simplex
EXCLUDES 1 Cockayne's syndrome (Q87.1)

Q81.1 Epidermolysis bullosa letalis
Herlitz' syndrome

Q81.2 Epidermolysis bullosa dystrophica

Q81.8 Other epidermolysis bullosa

Q81.9 Epidermolysis bullosa, unspecified

✓4ᵗʰ Q82 Other congenital malformations of skin
EXCLUDES 1 acrodermatitis enteropathica (E83.2)
congenital erythropoietic porphyria (E80.0)
pilonidal cyst or sinus (L05.-)
Sturge-Weber (-Dimitri) syndrome (Q85.8)

Q82.0 Hereditary lymphedema

Q82.1 Xeroderma pigmentosum

Q82.2 Mastocytosis
Urticaria pigmentosa
EXCLUDES 1 malignant mastocytosis (C96.2)

Q82.3 Incontinentia pigmenti

Q82.4 Ectodermal dysplasia (anhidrotic)
EXCLUDES 1 Ellis-van Creveld syndrome (Q77.6)

Q82.5 Congenital non-neoplastic nevus
Birthmark NOS
Flammeus Nevus
Portwine Nevus
Sanguineous Nevus
Strawberry Nevus
Vascular Nevus NOS
Verrucous Nevus
EXCLUDES 2 araneus nevus (I78.1)
café au lait spots (L81.3)
lentigo (L81.4)
melanocytic nevus (D22.-)
nevus NOS (D22.-)
pigmented nevus (D22.-)
spider nevus (I78.1)
stellar nevus (I78.1)

Q82.8 Other specified congenital malformations of skin
Abnormal palmar creases
Accessory skin tags
Benign familial pemphigus [Hailey-Hailey]
Congenital poikiloderma
Cutis laxa (hyperelastica)
Dermatoglyphic anomalies
Inherited keratosis palmaris et plantaris
Keratosis follicularis [Darier-White]
EXCLUDES 1 Ehlers-Danlos syndrome (Q79.6)

Q82.9 Congenital malformation of skin, unspecified

✓4ᵗʰ Q83 Congenital malformations of breast
EXCLUDES 2 absence of pectoral muscle (Q79.8)
hypoplasia of breast (N64.82)
micromastia (N64.82)

Q83.0 Congenital absence of breast with absent nipple

Congenital Malformations, Deformations and Chromosomal Abnormalities

Q83.1–Q89.Ø9

Q83.1 Accessory breast
Supernumerary breast

Q83.2 Absent nipple

Q83.3 Accessory nipple
Supernumerary nipple

Q83.8 Other congenital malformations of breast

Q83.9 Congenital malformation of breast, unspecified

✓4ᵗʰ **Q84 Other congenital malformations of integument**

Q84.Ø Congenital alopecia
Congenital atrichosis

Q84.1 Congenital morphological disturbances of hair, not elsewhere classified
Beaded hair
Monilethrix
Pili annulati
EXCLUDES 1 *Menkes' kinky hair syndrome (E83.Ø)*

Q84.2 Other congenital malformations of hair
Congenital hypertrichosis
Congenital malformation of hair NOS
Persistent lanugo

Q84.3 Anonychia
EXCLUDES 1 *nail patella syndrome (Q87.2)*

Q84.4 Congenital leukonychia

Q84.5 Enlarged and hypertrophic nails
Congenital onychauxis
Pachyonychia

Q84.6 Other congenital malformations of nails
Congenital clubnail
Congenital koilonychia
Congenital malformation of nail NOS

Q84.8 Other specified congenital malformations of integument
Aplasia cutis congenita

Q84.9 Congenital malformation of integument, unspecified
Congenital anomaly of integument NOS
Congenital deformity of integument NOS

✓4ᵗʰ **Q85 Phakomatoses, not elsewhere classified**
EXCLUDES 1 *ataxia telangiectasia [Louis-Bar] (G11.3)*
familial dysautonomia [Riley-Day] (G9Ø.1)

✓5ᵗʰ **Q85.Ø Neurofibromatosis (nonmalignant)**

Q85.ØØ Neurofibromatosis, unspecified

Q85.Ø1 Neurofibromatosis, type 1
Von Recklinghausen disease

Q85.Ø2 Neurofibromatosis, type 2
Acoustic neurofibromatosis

Q85.Ø3 Schwannomatosis

Q85.Ø9 Other neurofibromatosis

Q85.1 Tuberous sclerosis   CC
Bourneville's disease
Epiloia
CC Excl: Q85.1-Q85.9, Q89.7, Q89.9

Q85.8 Other phakomatoses, not elsewhere classified   CC
Peutz-Jeghers Syndrome
Sturge-Weber(-Dimitri) syndrome
von Hippel-Lindau syndrome
EXCLUDES 1 *Meckel-Gruber syndrome (Q61.9)*
CC Excl: Q85.8-Q85.9, Q89.9

Q85.9 Phakomatosis, unspecified   CC
Hamartosis NOS
CC Excl: See code: Q85.8

✓4ᵗʰ **Q86 Congenital malformation syndromes due to known exogenous causes, not elsewhere classified**
EXCLUDES 2 *iodine-deficiency-related hypothyroidism (EØØ-EØ2)*
nonteratogenic effects of substances transmitted via placenta or breast milk (PØ4.-)

Q86.Ø Fetal alcohol syndrome (dysmorphic)

Q86.1 Fetal hydantoin syndrome   N
Meadow's syndrome

Q86.2 Dysmorphism due to warfarin

Q86.8 Other congenital malformation syndromes due to known exogenous causes

✓4ᵗʰ **Q87 Other specified congenital malformation syndromes affecting multiple systems**
Use additional code(s) to identify all associated manifestations

Q87.Ø Congenital malformation syndromes predominantly affecting facial appearance
Acrocephalopolysyndactyly
Acrocephalosyndactyly [Apert]
Cryptophthalmos syndrome
Cyclopia
Goldenhar syndrome
Moebius syndrome
Oro-facial-digital syndrome
Robin syndrome
Whistling face

Q87.1 Congenital malformation syndromes predominantly associated with short stature   CC
Aarskog syndrome
Cockayne syndrome
De Lange syndrome
Dubowitz syndrome
Noonan syndrome
Prader-Willi syndrome
Robinow-Silverman-Smith syndrome
Russell-Silver syndrome
Seckel syndrome
EXCLUDES 1 *Ellis-van Creveld syndrome (Q77.6)*
Smith-Lemli-Opitz syndrome (E78.72)
CC Excl: E78.71-E78.72, Q85.8-Q85.9, Q87.1-Q87.89, Q89.7-Q89.9, Q99.2

Q87.2 Congenital malformation syndromes predominantly involving limbs   CC
Holt-Oram syndrome
Klippel-Trenaunay-Weber syndrome
Nail patella syndrome
Rubinstein-Taybi syndrome
Sirenomelia syndrome
Thrombocytopenia with absent radius [TAR] syndrome
VATER syndrome
CC Excl: E78.71-E78.72, Q87.1-Q87.89, Q89.8, Q99.2

Q87.3 Congenital malformation syndromes involving early overgrowth   CC
Beckwith-Wiedemann syndrome
Sotos syndrome
Weaver syndrome
CC Excl: See code: Q87.2

✓5ᵗʰ **Q87.4 Marfan's syndrome**

CC Excl: For CC codes in subcategory Q87.4, unless otherwise noted: See code: Q87.1

Q87.4Ø Marfan's syndrome, unspecified   CC

✓6ᵗʰ **Q87.41 Marfan's syndrome with cardiovascular manifestations**

Q87.41Ø Marfan's syndrome with aortic dilation   CC

Q87.418 Marfan's syndrome with other cardiovascular manifestations   CC

Q87.42 Marfan's syndrome with ocular manifestations   CC

Q87.43 Marfan's syndrome with skeletal manifestation   CC

Q87.5 Other congenital malformation syndromes with other skeletal changes   CC
CC Excl: See code: Q87.2

✓5ᵗʰ **Q87.8 Other specified congenital malformation syndromes, not elsewhere classified**
EXCLUDES 1 *Zellweger syndrome (E71.51Ø)*

Q87.81 Alport syndrome   CC
Use additional code to identify stage of chronic kidney disease (N18.1-N18.6)
CC Excl: See code: Q87.2

Q87.89 Other specified congenital malformation syndromes, not elsewhere classified   CC
Laurence-Moon (-Bardet)-Biedl syndrome
CC Excl: See code: Q87.2

✓4ᵗʰ **Q89 Other congenital malformations, not elsewhere classified**

✓5ᵗʰ **Q89.Ø Congenital absence and malformations of spleen**
EXCLUDES 1 *isomerism of atrial appendages (with asplenia or polysplenia) (Q2Ø.6)*

Q89.Ø1 Asplenia (congenital)   CC
CC Excl: Q89.Ø1-Q89.Ø9, Q89.9

Q89.Ø9 Congenital malformations of spleen   CC
Congenital splenomegaly
CC Excl: See code: Q89.Ø1

Q89.1 Congenital malformations of adrenal gland
EXCLUDES 1   adrenogenital disorders (E25.-)
congenital adrenal hyperplasia (E25.0)

Q89.2 Congenital malformations of other endocrine glands
Congenital malformation of parathyroid or thyroid gland
Persistent thyroglossal duct
Thyroglossal cyst
EXCLUDES 1   congenital goiter (E03.0)
congenital hypothyroidism (E03.1)

Q89.3 Situs inversus   CC
Dextrocardia with situs inversus
Mirror-image atrial arrangement with situs inversus
Situs inversus or transversus abdominalis
Situs inversus or transversus thoracis
Transposition of abdominal viscera
Transposition of thoracic viscera
EXCLUDES 1   dextrocardia NOS (Q24.0)
CC Excl: Q89.3, Q89.7, Q89.9

Q89.4 Conjoined twins   MCC
Craniopagus
Dicephaly
Pygopagus
Thoracopagus
CC Excl: Q89.4-Q89.7, Q89.9

Q89.7 Multiple congenital malformations, not elsewhere classified   CC
Multiple congenital anomalies NOS
Multiple congenital deformities NOS
EXCLUDES 1   congenital malformation syndromes affecting multiple systems (Q87.-)
CC Excl: See code: Q89.3

Q89.8 Other specified congenital malformations   CC
Use additional code(s) to identify all associated manifestations
CC Excl: E78.71-E78.72, Q87.1-Q87.89, Q89.8, Q99.2

Q89.9 Congenital malformation, unspecified
Congenital anomaly NOS
Congenital deformity NOS

Chromosomal abnormalities, not elsewhere classified (Q90-Q99)
EXCLUDES 2   mitochondrial metabolic disorders (E88.4-)

√4th **Q90 Down syndrome**
Use additional code(s) to identify any associated physical conditions and degree of intellectual disabilities (F70-F79)

Q90.0 Trisomy 21, nonmosaicism (meiotic nondisjunction)
Q90.1 Trisomy 21, mosaicism (mitotic nondisjunction)
Q90.2 Trisomy 21, translocation
Q90.9 Down syndrome, unspecified
Trisomy 21 NOS

√4th **Q91 Trisomy 18 and Trisomy 13**
CC Excl: For CC codes in category Q91, unless otherwise noted: Q90.0-Q99.1, Q99.8-Q99.9

Q91.0 Trisomy 18, nonmosaicism (meiotic nondisjunction)   CC
Q91.1 Trisomy 18, mosaicism (mitotic nondisjunction)   CC
Q91.2 Trisomy 18, translocation   CC
Q91.3 Trisomy 18, unspecified   CC
Q91.4 Trisomy 13, nonmosaicism (meiotic nondisjunction)   CC
Q91.5 Trisomy 13, mosaicism (mitotic nondisjunction)   CC
Q91.6 Trisomy 13, translocation   CC
Q91.7 Trisomy 13, unspecified   CC

√4th **Q92 Other trisomies and partial trisomies of the autosomes, not elsewhere classified**
INCLUDES   unbalanced translocations and insertions
EXCLUDES 1   trisomies of chromosomes 13, 18, 21 (Q90-Q91)

Q92.0 Whole chromosome trisomy, nonmosaicism (meiotic nondisjunction)
Q92.1 Whole chromosome trisomy, mosaicism (mitotic nondisjunction)
Q92.2 Partial trisomy
Less than whole arm duplicated
Whole arm or more duplicated
EXCLUDES 1   partial trisomy due to unbalanced translocation (Q92.5)
Q92.5 Duplications with other complex rearrangements
Partial trisomy due to unbalanced translocations
Code also any associated deletions due to unbalanced translocations, inversions and insertions (Q93.7)

Q92.6 Marker chromosomes   √5th
Trisomies due to dicentrics
Trisomies due to extra rings
Trisomies due to isochromosomes
Individual with marker heterochromatin
Q92.61 Marker chromosomes in normal individual
Q92.62 Marker chromosomes in abnormal individual
Q92.7 Triploidy and polyploidy
Q92.8 Other specified trisomies and partial trisomies of autosomes
Duplications identified by fluorescence in situ hybridization (FISH)
Duplications identified by in situ hybridization (ISH)
Duplications seen only at prometaphase
Q92.9 Trisomy and partial trisomy of autosomes, unspecified

√4th **Q93 Monosomies and deletions from the autosomes, not elsewhere classified**
CC Excl: For CC/MCC codes in category Q93, unless otherwise noted: Q90.0-Q93.2, Q93.4, Q93.81-Q93.88, Q95.0-Q99.1, Q99.8-Q99.9

Q93.0 Whole chromosome monosomy, nonmosaicism (meiotic nondisjunction)
Q93.1 Whole chromosome monosomy, mosaicism (mitotic nondisjunction)
Q93.2 Chromosome replaced with ring, dicentric or isochromosome
Q93.3 Deletion of short arm of chromosome 4   CC
Wolff-Hirschorn syndrome
Q93.4 Deletion of short arm of chromosome 5   CC
Cri-du-chat syndrome
CC Excl: Q90.0-Q93.3, Q93.5-Q99.1, Q99.8-Q99.9
Q93.5 Other deletions of part of a chromosome   CC
Angelman syndrome
Q93.7 Deletions with other complex rearrangements   CC
Deletions due to unbalanced translocations, inversions and insertions
Code also any associated duplications due to unbalanced translocations, inversions and insertions (Q92.5)
Q93.8 Other deletions from the autosomes   √5th
Q93.81 Velo-cardio-facial syndrome   MCC
Deletion 22q11.2
CC Excl: Q90.0-Q93.7, Q93.88-Q99.1, Q99.8-Q99.9
Q93.88 Other microdeletions   CC
Miller-Dieker syndrome
Smith-Magenis syndrome
CC Excl: Q90.0-Q93.81, Q93.89-Q99.1, Q99.8-Q99.9
Q93.89 Other deletions from the autosomes   CC
Deletions identified by fluorescence in situ hybridization (FISH)
Deletions identified by in situ hybridization (ISH)
Deletions seen only at prometaphase
Q93.9 Deletion from autosomes, unspecified   CC

√4th **Q95 Balanced rearrangements and structural markers, not elsewhere classified**
INCLUDES   Robertsonian and balanced reciprocal translocations and insertions
Q95.0 Balanced translocation and insertion in normal individual
Q95.1 Chromosome inversion in normal individual
Q95.2 Balanced autosomal rearrangement in abnormal individual
Q95.3 Balanced sex/autosomal rearrangement in abnormal individual
Q95.5 Individual with autosomal fragile site
Q95.8 Other balanced rearrangements and structural markers
Q95.9 Balanced rearrangement and structural marker, unspecified

√4th **Q96 Turner's syndrome**
EXCLUDES 1   Noonan syndrome (Q87.1)
Q96.0 Karyotype 45, X   ♀
Q96.1 Karyotype 46, X iso (Xq)   ♀
Karyotype 46, isochromosome Xq
Q96.2 Karyotype 46, X with abnormal sex chromosome, except iso (Xq)   ♀
Karyotype 46, X with abnormal sex chromosome, except isochromosome Xq
Q96.3 Mosaicism, 45, X/46, XX or XY   ♀
Q96.4 Mosaicism, 45, X/other cell line(s) with abnormal sex chromosome   ♀
Q96.8 Other variants of Turner's syndrome   ♀
Q96.9 Turner's syndrome, unspecified   ♀

√ Additional Character Required   √x7th X7th Extension Alert   Unacceptable PDx   Manifestation   Hospital Acquired Condition   EXCLUDES 1 Not Coded Here   EXCLUDES 2 Not Included Here

Q97–Q99.9   Congenital Malformations, Deformations and Chromosomal Abnormalities

✓4ᵗʰ Q97 Other sex chromosome abnormalities, female phenotype, not elsewhere classified

> EXCLUDES 1   *Turner's syndrome (Q96.-)*

Q97.0   **Karyotype 47, XXX**   ♀

Q97.1   **Female with more than three X chromosomes**   ♀

Q97.2   **Mosaicism, lines with various numbers of X chromosomes**   ♀

Q97.3   **Female with 46, XY karyotype**   ♀

Q97.8   **Other specified sex chromosome abnormalities, female phenotype**   ♀

Q97.9   **Sex chromosome abnormality, female phenotype, unspecified**   ♀

✓4ᵗʰ Q98 Other sex chromosome abnormalities, male phenotype, not elsewhere classified

Q98.0   **Klinefelter syndrome karyotype 47, XXY**   ♂

Q98.1   **Klinefelter syndrome, male with more than two X chromosomes**   ♂

Q98.3   **Other male with 46, XX karyotype**   ♂

Q98.4   **Klinefelter syndrome, unspecified**   ♂

Q98.5   **Karyotype 47, XYY**

Q98.6   **Male with structurally abnormal sex chromosome**   ♂

Q98.7   **Male with sex chromosome mosaicism**   ♂

Q98.8   **Other specified sex chromosome abnormalities, male phenotype**   ♂

Q98.9   **Sex chromosome abnormality, male phenotype, unspecified**   ♂

✓4ᵗʰ Q99 Other chromosome abnormalities, not elsewhere classified

Q99.0   **Chimera 46, XX/46, XY**
> Chimera 46, XX/46, XY true hermaphrodite

Q99.1   **46, XX true hermaphrodite**
> 46, XX with streak gonads
> 46, XY with streak gonads
> Pure gonadal dysgenesis

Q99.2   **Fragile X chromosome**
> Fragile X syndrome

Q99.8   **Other specified chromosome abnormalities**

Q99.9   **Chromosomal abnormality, unspecified**

Ⓝ Newborn: 0   Ⓟ Pediatric: 0-17   Ⓜ Maternity: 12-55   Ⓐ Adult: 15-124   **MCC** Major CC Condition   **PDx MCC** PDx acts as own MCC   **CC** CC Condition   **PDx CC** PDx acts as own CC

840   ICD-10-CM Draft (2015)

Chapter 18. Symptoms, Signs and Abnormal Clinical and Laboratory Findings, Not Elsewhere Classified (R00-R99)

NOTE   This chapter includes symptoms, signs, abnormal results of clinical or other investigative procedures, and ill-defined conditions regarding which no diagnosis classifiable elsewhere is recorded.

Signs and symptoms that point rather definitely to a given diagnosis have been assigned to a category in other chapters of the classification. In general, categories in this chapter include the less well-defined conditions and symptoms that, without the necessary study of the case to establish a final diagnosis, point perhaps equally to two or more diseases or to two or more systems of the body. Practically all categories in the chapter could be designated "not otherwise specified", "unknown etiology" or "transient". The Alphabetical Index should be consulted to determine which symptoms and signs are to be allocated here and which to other chapters. The residual subcategories, numbered .8, are generally provided for other relevant symptoms that cannot be allocated elsewhere in the classification.

The conditions and signs or symptoms included in categories R00-R94 consist of:

(a)   cases for which no more specific diagnosis can be made even after all the facts bearing on the case have been investigated;

(b)   signs or symptoms existing at the time of initial encounter that proved to be transient and whose causes could not be determined;

(c)   provisional diagnosis in a patient who failed to return for further investigation or care;

(d)   cases referred elsewhere for investigation or treatment before the diagnosis was made;

(e)   cases in which a more precise diagnosis was not available for any other reason;

(f)   certain symptoms, for which supplementary information is provided, that represent important problems in medical care in their own right.

EXCLUDES 2   abnormal findings on antenatal screening of mother (O28.-)
certain conditions originating in the perinatal period (P04-P96)
signs and symptoms classified in the body system chapters
signs and symptoms of breast (N63, N64.5)

This chapter contains the following blocks:

R00-R09   Symptoms and signs involving the circulatory and respiratory systems
R10-R19   Symptoms and signs involving the digestive system and abdomen
R20-R23   Symptoms and signs involving the skin and subcutaneous tissue
R25-R29   Symptoms and signs involving the nervous and musculoskeletal systems
R30-R39   Symptoms and signs involving the genitourinary system
R40-R46   Symptoms and signs involving cognition, perception, emotional state and behavior
R47-R49   Symptoms and signs involving speech and voice
R50-R69   General symptoms and signs
R70-R79   Abnormal findings on examination of blood, without diagnosis
R80-R82   Abnormal findings on examination of urine, without diagnosis
R83-R89   Abnormal findings on examination of other body fluids, substances and tissues, without diagnosis
R90-R94   Abnormal findings on diagnostic imaging and in function studies, without diagnosis
R97   Abnormal tumor markers
R99   Ill-defined and unknown cause of mortality

Symptoms and signs involving the circulatory and respiratory systems (R00-R09)

✓4th R00   Abnormalities of heart beat

EXCLUDES 1   abnormalities originating in the perinatal period (P29.1-)
specified arrhythmias (I47-I49)

R00.0   Tachycardia, unspecified
Rapid heart beat
Sinoauricular tachycardia NOS
Sinus [sinusal] tachycardia NOS
EXCLUDES 1   neonatal tachycardia (P29.11)
paroxysmal tachycardia (I47.-)

R00.1   Bradycardia, unspecified
Sinoatrial bradycardia
Sinus bradycardia
Slow heart beat
Vagal bradycardia
Use additional code for adverse effect, if applicable, to identify drug (T36-T50 with fifth or sixth character 5)
EXCLUDES 1   neonatal bradycardia (P29.12)

R00.2   Palpitations
Awareness of heart beat

R00.8   Other abnormalities of heart beat

R00.9   Unspecified abnormalities of heart beat

✓4th R01   Cardiac murmurs and other cardiac sounds

EXCLUDES 1   cardiac murmurs and sounds originating in the perinatal period (P29.8)

R01.0   Benign and innocent cardiac murmurs
Functional cardiac murmur

R01.1   Cardiac murmur, unspecified
Cardiac bruit NOS
Heart murmur NOS

R01.2   Other cardiac sounds
Cardiac dullness, increased or decreased
Precordial friction

✓4th R03   Abnormal blood-pressure reading, without diagnosis

13 **R03.0   Elevated blood-pressure reading, without diagnosis of hypertension**
NOTE   This category is to be used to record an episode of elevated blood pressure in a patient in whom no formal diagnosis of hypertension has been made, or as an isolated incidental finding.

R03.1   Nonspecific low blood-pressure reading
EXCLUDES 1   hypotension (I95.-)
maternal hypotension syndrome (O26.5-)
neurogenic orthostatic hypotension (G90.3)

✓4th R04   Hemorrhage from respiratory passages

CC Excl: For CC codes in category Q93, unless otherwise noted:
R04.2-R04.9, R09.3, R68.13

R04.0   Epistaxis
Hemorrhage from nose
Nosebleed

R04.1   Hemorrhage from throat
EXCLUDES 2   hemoptysis (R04.2)

R04.2   Hemoptysis   **CC**
Blood-stained sputum
Cough with hemorrhage
AHA: 2013, 4Q, 118

✓5th R04.8   Hemorrhage from other sites in respiratory passages

R04.81   Acute idiopathic pulmonary hemorrhage in infants   **CC P**
AIPHI
Acute idiopathic hemorrhage in infants over 28 days old
EXCLUDES 1   perinatal pulmonary hemorrhage (P26.-)
von Willebrand's disease (D68.0)

R04.89   Hemorrhage from other sites in respiratory passages   **CC**
Pulmonary hemorrhage NOS

R04.9   Hemorrhage from respiratory passages, unspecified   **CC**

R05   Cough
EXCLUDES 1   cough with hemorrhage (R04.2)
smoker's cough (J41.0)

✓4th R06   Abnormalities of breathing
EXCLUDES 1   acute respiratory distress syndrome (J80)
respiratory arrest (R09.2)
respiratory arrest of newborn (P28.81)
respiratory distress syndrome of newborn (P22.-)
respiratory failure (J96.-)
respiratory failure of newborn (P28.5)

✓5th R06.0   Dyspnea
EXCLUDES 1   tachypnea NOS (R06.82)
transient tachypnea of newborn (P22.1)

R06.00   Dyspnea, unspecified
R06.01   Orthopnea
R06.02   Shortness of breath
R06.09   Other forms of dyspnea

---

13 Questionable admission when used as PDx.

✓ Additional Character Required   ✓x7th Xtension Alert   Unacceptable PDx   Manifestation   Hospital Acquired Condition   **EXCLUDES 1** Not Coded Here   **EXCLUDES 2** Not Included Here

Symptoms, Signs and Abnormal Clinical and Laboratory Findings

R06.1–R10.813

R06.1 Stridor
> **EXCLUDES 1** congenital laryngeal stridor (P28.89)
> laryngismus (stridulus) (J38.5)

R06.2 Wheezing
> **EXCLUDES 1** asthma (J45.-)

R06.3 Periodic breathing   CC
> Cheyne-Stokes breathing
> **CC Excl:** J22, J80, J96.00-J96.92, J98.8-J98.9, R06.3, R06.81, R09.2

R06.4 Hyperventilation
> **EXCLUDES 1** psychogenic hyperventilation (F45.8)

R06.5 Mouth breathing
> **EXCLUDES 2** dry mouth NOS (R68.2)

R06.6 Hiccough
> **EXCLUDES 1** psychogenic hiccough (F45.8)

R06.7 Sneezing

✓5ᵗʰ **R06.8 Other abnormalities of breathing**

     R06.81 Apnea, not elsewhere classified
> Apnea NOS
> **EXCLUDES 1** apnea (of) newborn (P28.4)
> sleep apnea (G47.3-)
> sleep apnea of newborn (primary) (P28.3)

     R06.82 Tachypnea, not elsewhere classified
> Tachypnea NOS
> **EXCLUDES 1** transitory tachypnea of newborn (P22.1)

     R06.83 Snoring

     R06.89 Other abnormalities of breathing
> Breath-holding (spells)
> Sighing

R06.9 Unspecified abnormalities of breathing

✓4ᵗʰ **R07 Pain in throat and chest**
> **EXCLUDES 1** epidemic myalgia (B33.0)
> **EXCLUDES 2** jaw pain (R68.84)
> pain in breast (N64.4)

     R07.0 Pain in throat
> **EXCLUDES 1** chronic sore throat (J31.2)
> sore throat (acute) NOS (J02.9)
> **EXCLUDES 2** dysphagia (R13.1-)
> pain in neck (M54.2)

     R07.1 Chest pain on breathing
> Painful respiration

     R07.2 Precordial pain

✓5ᵗʰ **R07.8 Other chest pain**

     R07.81 Pleurodynia
> Pleurodynia NOS
> **EXCLUDES 1** epidemic pleurodynia (B33.0)

     R07.82 Intercostal pain

     R07.89 Other chest pain
> Anterior chest-wall pain NOS

     R07.9 Chest pain, unspecified

✓4ᵗʰ **R09 Other symptoms and signs involving the circulatory and respiratory system**
> **EXCLUDES 1** acute respiratory distress syndrome (J80)
> respiratory arrest of newborn (P28.81)
> respiratory distress syndrome of newborn (P22.0)
> respiratory failure (J96.-)
> respiratory failure of newborn (P28.5)

✓5ᵗʰ **R09.0 Asphyxia and hypoxemia**
> **EXCLUDES 1** asphyxia due to carbon monoxide (T58.-)
> asphyxia due to foreign body in respiratory tract (T17.-)
> birth (intrauterine) asphyxia (P84)
> hypercapnia (R06.4)
> hyperventilation (R06.4)
> traumatic asphyxia (T71.-)

     R09.01 Asphyxia   CC
> **CC Excl:** G89.0-G89.4, J80, J96.00-J96.92, R09.01-R09.02, R09.2, R41.0-R41.3, R41.82, R41.9, R44.8-R44.9, R45.83-R45.84, R46.0-R46.89, R52, R68.0-R68.19, R68.81-R68.83, R68.89-R69

     R09.02 Hypoxemia

R09.1 Pleurisy
> **EXCLUDES 1** pleurisy with effusion (J90)

10 **R09.2 Respiratory arrest**   MCC
> Cardiorespiratory failure
> **EXCLUDES 1** cardiac arrest (I46.-)
> respiratory arrest of newborn (P28.81)
> respiratory distress of newborn (P22.0)
> respiratory failure (J96.-)
> respiratory failure of newborn (P28.5)
> respiratory insufficiency (R06.89)
> respiratory insufficiency of newborn (P28.5)
> **CC Excl:** See code: R09.01

R09.3 Abnormal sputum
> Abnormal amount of sputum
> Abnormal color of sputum
> Abnormal odor of sputum
> Excessive sputum
> **EXCLUDES 1** blood-stained sputum (R04.2)

✓5ᵗʰ **R09.8 Other specified symptoms and signs involving the circulatory and respiratory systems**

     R09.81 Nasal congestion

     R09.82 Postnasal drip

     R09.89 Other specified symptoms and signs involving the circulatory and respiratory systems
> Abnormal chest percussion
> Bruit (arterial)
> Chest tympany
> Choking sensation
> Feeling of foreign body in throat
> Friction sounds in chest
> Rales
> Weak pulse
> **EXCLUDES 2** foreign body in throat (T17.2-)
> wheezing (R06.2)

Symptoms and signs involving the digestive system and abdomen (R10-R19)

> **EXCLUDES 1** congenital or infantile pylorospasm (Q40.0)
> gastrointestinal hemorrhage (K92.0-K92.2)
> intestinal obstruction (K56.-)
> newborn gastrointestinal hemorrhage (P54.0-P54.3)
> newborn intestinal obstruction (P76.-)
> pylorospasm (K31.3)
> signs and symptoms involving the urinary system (R30-R39)
> symptoms referable to female genital organs (N94.-)
> symptoms referable to male genital organs male (N48-N50)

✓4ᵗʰ **R10 Abdominal and pelvic pain**
> **EXCLUDES 1** renal colic (N23)
> **EXCLUDES 2** dorsalgia (M54.-)
> flatulence and related conditions (R14.-)

     R10.0 Acute abdomen
> Severe abdominal pain (generalized) (with abdominal rigidity)
> **EXCLUDES 1** abdominal rigidity NOS (R19.3)
> generalized abdominal pain NOS (R10.84)
> localized abdominal pain (R10.1-R10.3-)

✓5ᵗʰ **R10.1 Pain localized to upper abdomen**

     R10.10 Upper abdominal pain, unspecified

     R10.11 Right upper quadrant pain

     R10.12 Left upper quadrant pain

     R10.13 Epigastric pain
> Dyspepsia
> **EXCLUDES 1** functional dyspepsia (K30)

     R10.2 Pelvic and perineal pain
> **EXCLUDES 1** vulvodynia (N94.81)

✓5ᵗʰ **R10.3 Pain localized to other parts of lower abdomen**

     R10.30 Lower abdominal pain, unspecified

     R10.31 Right lower quadrant pain

     R10.32 Left lower quadrant pain

     R10.33 Periumbilical pain

✓5ᵗʰ **R10.8 Other abdominal pain**

  ✓6ᵗʰ **R10.81 Abdominal tenderness**
> Abdominal tenderness NOS

     R10.811 Right upper quadrant abdominal tenderness

     R10.812 Left upper quadrant abdominal tenderness

     R10.813 Right lower quadrant abdominal tenderness

---

10 MCC only if patient is discharged alive.

N Newborn: 0   P Pediatric: 0-17   M Maternity: 12-55   A Adult: 15-124   MCC Major CC Condition   PDx MCC PDx acts as own MCC   CC CC Condition   PDx CC PDx acts as own CC

842   ICD-10-CM Draft (2015)

R10.814 **Left lower** quadrant abdominal tenderness

R10.815 **Periumbilic** abdominal tenderness

R10.816 **Epigastric** abdominal tenderness

R10.817 **Generalized** abdominal tenderness

R10.819 Abdominal tenderness, **unspecified** site

✓6ᵗʰ R10.82 **Rebound** abdominal tenderness

R10.821 **Right upper** quadrant rebound abdominal tenderness

R10.822 **Left upper** quadrant rebound abdominal tenderness

R10.823 **Right lower** quadrant rebound abdominal tenderness

R10.824 **Left lower** quadrant rebound abdominal tenderness

R10.825 **Periumbilic** rebound abdominal tenderness

R10.826 **Epigastric** rebound abdominal tenderness

R10.827 **Generalized** rebound abdominal tenderness

R10.829 **Rebound** abdominal tenderness, **unspecified** site

R10.83 **Colic**   **P**
Colic NOS
Infantile colic
EXCLUDES 1   *colic in adult and child over 12 months old (R10.84)*

R10.84 **Generalized** abdominal pain
EXCLUDES 1   *generalized abdominal pain associated with acute abdomen (R10.0)*

R10.9 **Unspecified** abdominal pain

✓4ᵗʰ **R11 Nausea and vomiting**
EXCLUDES 1   *cyclical vomiting associated with migraine (G43.A-)*
excessive vomiting in pregnancy (O21.-)
hematemesis (K92.0)
neonatal hematemesis (P54.0)
newborn vomiting (P92.0-)
psychogenic vomiting (F50.8)
vomiting associated with bulimia nervosa (F50.2)
vomiting following gastrointestinal surgery (K91.0)

R11.0 **Nausea**
Nausea NOS   Nausea without vomiting

✓5ᵗʰ R11.1 **Vomiting**

R11.10 **Vomiting, unspecified**
Vomiting NOS

R11.11 **Vomiting without nausea**

R11.12 **Projectile vomiting**

R11.13 **Vomiting of fecal matter**

R11.14 **Bilious vomiting**
Bilious emesis

R11.2 **Nausea with vomiting, unspecified**
Persistent nausea with vomiting NOS

R12 **Heartburn**
EXCLUDES 1   *dyspepsia NOS (R10.13)*
functional dyspepsia (K30)

✓4ᵗʰ **R13 Aphagia and dysphagia**

R13.0 **Aphagia**
Inability to swallow
EXCLUDES 1   *psychogenic aphagia (F50.9)*

✓5ᵗʰ R13.1 **Dysphagia**
Code first, if applicable, dysphagia following cerebrovascular disease (I69. with final characters -91)
EXCLUDES 1   *psychogenic dysphagia (F45.8)*

R13.10 **Dysphagia, unspecified**
Difficulty in swallowing NOS

R13.11 **Dysphagia, oral phase**

R13.12 **Dysphagia, oropharyngeal phase**

R13.13 **Dysphagia, pharyngeal phase**

R13.14 **Dysphagia, pharyngoesophageal phase**

R13.19 **Other dysphagia**
Cervical dysphagia
Neurogenic dysphagia

✓4ᵗʰ **R14 Flatulence and related conditions**
EXCLUDES 1   *psychogenic aerophagy (F45.8)*

R14.0 **Abdominal distension (gaseous)**
Bloating
Tympanites (abdominal) (intestinal)

R14.1 **Gas pain**

R14.2 **Eructation**

R14.3 **Flatulence**

✓4ᵗʰ **R15 Fecal incontinence**
Encopresis NOS
EXCLUDES 1   *fecal incontinence of nonorganic origin (F98.1)*

R15.0 **Incomplete defecation**
EXCLUDES 1   *constipation (K59.0-)*
fecal impaction (K56.41)

R15.1 **Fecal smearing**
Fecal soiling

R15.2 **Fecal urgency**

R15.9 **Full incontinence of feces**
Fecal incontinence NOS

✓4ᵗʰ **R16 Hepatomegaly and splenomegaly, not elsewhere classified**

R16.0 **Hepatomegaly, not elsewhere classified**
Hepatomegaly NOS

R16.1 **Splenomegaly, not elsewhere classified**
Splenomegaly NOS

R16.2 **Hepatomegaly with splenomegaly, not elsewhere classified**
Hepatosplenomegaly NOS

R17 **Unspecified jaundice**   **CC**
EXCLUDES 1   *neonatal jaundice (P55, P57-P59)*
CC Excl: P57.8-P59.9, R17, R23.8-R23.9

✓4ᵗʰ **R18 Ascites**
INCLUDES   fluid in peritoneal cavity
EXCLUDES 1   *ascites in alcoholic cirrhosis (K70.31)*
ascites in alcoholic hepatitis (K70.11)
ascites in toxic liver disease with chronic active hepatitis (K71.51)

R18.0 **Malignant ascites**   **CC**
Code first malignancy, such as:
malignant neoplasm of ovary (C56.-)
secondary malignant neoplasm of retroperitoneum and peritoneum (C78.6)
CC Excl: G89.0-G89.4, R18.0-R19.09, R19.30-R19.37, R41.0-R41.3, R41.82, R41.9, R44.8-R44.9, R45.83-R45.84, R46.0-R46.89, R52, R68.0-R68.19, R68.81-R68.83, R68.89-R69

R18.8 **Other ascites**   **CC**
Ascites NOS
Peritoneal effusion (chronic)
CC Excl: See code: R18.0

✓4ᵗʰ **R19 Other symptoms and signs involving the digestive system and abdomen**
EXCLUDES 1   *acute abdomen (R10.0)*

✓5ᵗʰ R19.0 **Intra-abdominal and pelvic swelling, mass and lump**
EXCLUDES 1   *abdominal distension (gaseous) (R14.-)*
ascites (R18.-)

R19.00 **Intra-abdominal and pelvic swelling, mass and lump, unspecified** site

R19.01 **Right upper quadrant** abdominal swelling, mass and lump

R19.02 **Left upper quadrant** abdominal swelling, mass and lump

R19.03 **Right lower quadrant** abdominal swelling, mass and lump

R19.04 **Left lower quadrant** abdominal swelling, mass and lump

R19.05 **Periumbilic** swelling, mass or lump
Diffuse or generalized umbilical swelling or mass

R19.06 **Epigastric** swelling, mass or lump

R19.07 **Generalized** intra-abdominal and pelvic swelling, mass and lump
Diffuse or generalized intra-abdominal swelling or mass NOS
Diffuse or generalized pelvic swelling or mass NOS

R19.09 **Other** intra-abdominal and pelvic swelling, mass and lump

✓5ᵗʰ R19.1 **Abnormal bowel sounds**

R19.11 **Absent bowel sounds**

R19.12 **Hyperactive bowel sounds**

Symptoms, Signs and Abnormal Clinical and Laboratory Findings

R19.15–R27.0

R19.15 Other **abnormal bowel sounds**
Abnormal bowel sounds NOS

R19.2 **Visible peristalsis**
Hyperperistalsis

✓5th **R19.3** **Abdominal rigidity**
EXCLUDES 1   *abdominal rigidity with severe abdominal pain (R10.0)*

     R19.30 **Abdominal rigidity, unspecified** site
     R19.31 **Right upper quadrant abdominal rigidity**
     R19.32 **Left upper quadrant abdominal rigidity**
     R19.33 **Right lower quadrant abdominal rigidity**
     R19.34 **Left lower quadrant abdominal rigidity**
     R19.35 **Periumbilic abdominal rigidity**
     R19.36 **Epigastric abdominal rigidity**
     R19.37 **Generalized abdominal rigidity**

R19.4 **Change in bowel habit**
EXCLUDES 1   *constipation (K59.0-)*
         functional diarrhea (K59.1)

R19.5 **Other fecal abnormalities**
Abnormal stool color
Bulky stools
Mucus in stools
Occult blood in feces
Occult blood in stools
EXCLUDES 1   *melena (K92.1)*
         neonatal melena (P54.1)

R19.6 **Halitosis**

R19.7 **Diarrhea, unspecified**
Diarrhea NOS
EXCLUDES 1   *functional diarrhea (K59.1)*
         neonatal diarrhea (P78.3)
         psychogenic diarrhea (F45.8)

R19.8 **Other specified symptoms and signs involving the digestive system and abdomen**

Symptoms and signs involving the skin and subcutaneous tissue (R20-R23)
EXCLUDES 2   *symptoms relating to breast (N64.4-N64.5)*

✓4th **R20** **Disturbances of skin sensation**
EXCLUDES 1   *dissociative anesthesia and sensory loss (F44.6)*
         psychogenic disturbances (F45.8)

R20.0 **Anesthesia of skin**
R20.1 **Hypoesthesia of skin**
R20.2 **Paresthesia of skin**
Formication
Pins and needles
Tingling skin
EXCLUDES 1   *acroparesthesia (I73.8)*

R20.3 **Hyperesthesia**
R20.8 **Other disturbances of skin sensation**
R20.9 **Unspecified disturbances of skin sensation**

R21 **Rash and other nonspecific skin eruption**
Rash NOS
EXCLUDES 1   *specified type of rash—code to condition*
         vesicular eruption (R23.8)

✓4th **R22** **Localized swelling, mass and lump of skin and subcutaneous tissue**
Subcutaneous nodules (localized)(superficial)
EXCLUDES 1   *abnormal findings on diagnostic imaging (R90-R93)*
         edema (R60.-)
         enlarged lymph nodes (R59.-)
         localized adiposity (E65)
         swelling of joint (M25.4-)

R22.0 **Localized swelling, mass and lump, head**
R22.1 **Localized swelling, mass and lump, neck**
R22.2 **Localized swelling, mass and lump, trunk**
EXCLUDES 1   *intra-abdominal or pelvic mass and lump (R19.0-)*
         intra-abdominal or pelvic swelling (R19.0-)
EXCLUDES 2   *breast mass and lump (N63)*

✓5th **R22.3** **Localized swelling, mass and lump, upper limb**
     R22.30 **Localized swelling, mass and lump, unspecified upper limb**
     R22.31 **Localized swelling, mass and lump, right upper limb**
     R22.32 **Localized swelling, mass and lump, left upper limb**
     R22.33 **Localized swelling, mass and lump, upper limb, bilateral**

✓5th **R22.4** **Localized swelling, mass and lump, lower limb**
     R22.40 **Localized swelling, mass and lump, unspecified lower limb**
     R22.41 **Localized swelling, mass and lump, right lower limb**
     R22.42 **Localized swelling, mass and lump, left lower limb**
     R22.43 **Localized swelling, mass and lump, lower limb, bilateral**

R22.9 **Localized swelling, mass and lump, unspecified**

✓4th **R23** **Other skin changes**
R23.0 **Cyanosis**
EXCLUDES 1   *acrocyanosis (I73.8)*
         cyanotic attacks of newborn (P28.2)

R23.1 **Pallor**
Clammy skin

R23.2 **Flushing**
Excessive blushing
Code first, if applicable, menopausal and female climacteric states (N95.1)

R23.3 **Spontaneous ecchymoses**
Petechiae
EXCLUDES 1   *ecchymoses of newborn (P54.5)*
         purpura (D69.-)

R23.4 **Changes in skin texture**
Desquamation of skin
Induration of skin
Scaling of skin
EXCLUDES 1   *epidermal thickening NOS (L85.9)*

R23.8 **Other skin changes**
R23.9 **Unspecified skin changes**

Symptoms and signs involving the nervous and musculoskeletal systems (R25-R29)

✓4th **R25** **Abnormal involuntary movements**
EXCLUDES 1   *specific movement disorders (G20-G26)*
         stereotyped movement disorders (F98.4)
         tic disorders (F95.-)

R25.0 **Abnormal head movements**
R25.1 **Tremor, unspecified**
EXCLUDES 1   *chorea NOS (G25.5)*
         essential tremor (G25.0)
         hysterical tremor (F44.4)
         intention tremor (G25.2)

R25.2 **Cramp and spasm**
EXCLUDES 2   *carpopedal spasm (R29.0)*
         charley-horse (M62.831)
         infantile spasms (G40.4-)
         muscle spasm of back (M62.830)
         muscle spasm of calf (M62.831)

R25.3 **Fasciculation**
Twitching NOS

R25.8 **Other abnormal involuntary movements**
R25.9 **Unspecified abnormal involuntary movements**

✓4th **R26** **Abnormalities of gait and mobility**
EXCLUDES 1   *ataxia NOS (R27.0)*
         hereditary ataxia (G11.-)
         locomotor (syphilitic) ataxia (A52.11)
         immobility syndrome (paraplegic) (M62.3)

R26.0 **Ataxic gait**
Staggering gait

R26.1 **Paralytic gait**
Spastic gait

R26.2 **Difficulty in walking, not elsewhere classified**
EXCLUDES 1   *falling (R29.6)*
         unsteadiness on feet (R26.81)

✓5th **R26.8** **Other abnormalities of gait and mobility**
     R26.81 **Unsteadiness on feet**
     R26.89 **Other abnormalities of gait and mobility**

R26.9 **Unspecified abnormalities of gait and mobility**

✓4th **R27** **Other lack of coordination**
EXCLUDES 1   *ataxic gait (R26.0)*
         hereditary ataxia (G11.-)
         vertigo NOS (R42)

R27.0 **Ataxia, unspecified**
EXCLUDES 1   *ataxia following cerebrovascular disease (I69. with final characters -93)*

N Newborn: 0   P Pediatric: 0-17   M Maternity: 12-55   A Adult: 15-124   MCC Major CC Condition   PDx MCC PDx acts as own MCC   CC CC Condition   PDx CC PDx acts as own CC

844   ICD-10-CM Draft (2015)

R27.8 **Other lack of coordination**

R27.9 **Unspecified lack of coordination**

✓4ᵗʰ **R29** **Other symptoms and signs involving the nervous and musculoskeletal systems**

R29.0 **Tetany** CC
Carpopedal spasm
EXCLUDES 1 *hysterical tetany (F44.5)*
neonatal tetany (P71.3)
parathyroid tetany (E20.9)
post-thyroidectomy tetany (E89.2)
CC Excl: A33, A35, G10-G11.2, G11.4, G20-G25.79, G25.82-G26, G32.81, G80.3, G81.10-G81.14, G89.0-G89.4, G90.3, R29.0, R41.0-R41.3, R41.82, R41.9, R44.8-R44.9, R45.83-R45.84, R46.0-R46.89, R52, R68.0-R68.19, R68.81-R68.83, R68.89-R69

R29.1 **Meningismus** CC
CC Excl: R29.1, R29.810

R29.2 **Abnormal reflex**
EXCLUDES 2 *abnormal pupillary reflex (H57.0)*
hyperactive gag reflex (J39.2)
vasovagal reaction or syncope (R55)

R29.3 **Abnormal posture**

R29.4 **Clicking hip**
EXCLUDES 1 *congenital deformities of hip (Q65.-)*

R29.5 **Transient paralysis** CC
Code first any associated spinal cord injury (S14.0, S14.1-, S24.0, S24.1-, S34.0-, S34.1-)
EXCLUDES 1 *transient ischemic attack (G45.9)*
CC Excl: R29.5, R29.810

R29.6 **Repeated falls**
Falling
Tendency to fall
EXCLUDES 2 *at risk for falling (Z91.81)*
history of falling (Z91.81)

✓5ᵗʰ **R29.8** **Other symptoms and signs involving the nervous and musculoskeletal systems**

✓6ᵗʰ **R29.81** **Other symptoms and signs involving the nervous system**

R29.810 **Facial weakness**
Facial droop
EXCLUDES 1 *Bell's palsy (G51.0)*
facial weakness following cerebrovascular disease (I69. with final characters -92)

R29.818 **Other symptoms and signs involving the nervous system**

✓6ᵗʰ **R29.89** **Other symptoms and signs involving the musculoskeletal system**
EXCLUDES 2 *pain in limb (M79.6-)*

R29.890 **Loss of height**
EXCLUDES 1 *osteoporosis (M80-M81)*

R29.891 **Ocular torticollis**
EXCLUDES 1 *congenital (sternomastoid) torticollis Q68.0*
psychogenic torticollis (F45.8)
spasmodic torticollis (G24.3)
torticollis due to birth injury (P15.8)
torticollis NOS M43.6

R29.898 **Other symptoms and signs involving the musculoskeletal system**

✓5ᵗʰ **R29.9** **Unspecified symptoms and signs involving the nervous and musculoskeletal systems**

R29.90 **Unspecified symptoms and signs involving the nervous system**

R29.91 **Unspecified symptoms and signs involving the musculoskeletal system**

Symptoms and signs involving the genitourinary system (R30-R39)

✓4ᵗʰ **R30** **Pain associated with micturition**
EXCLUDES 1 *psychogenic pain associated with micturition (F45.8)*

R30.0 **Dysuria**
Strangury

R30.1 **Vesical tenesmus**

R30.9 **Painful micturition, unspecified**
Painful urination NOS

✓4ᵗʰ **R31** **Hematuria**
EXCLUDES 1 *hematuria included with underlying conditions, such as:*
acute cystitis with hematuria (N30.01)
recurrent and persistent hematuria in glomerular diseases (N02.-)

R31.0 **Gross hematuria**

R31.1 **Benign essential microscopic hematuria**

R31.2 **Other microscopic hematuria**

R31.9 **Hematuria, unspecified**

R32 **Unspecified urinary incontinence**
Enuresis NOS
EXCLUDES 1 *functional urinary incontinence (R39.81)*
nonorganic enuresis (F98.0)
stress incontinence and other specified urinary incontinence (N39.3-N39.4-)
urinary incontinence associated with cognitive impairment (R39.81)

✓4ᵗʰ **R33** **Retention of urine**
EXCLUDES 1 *psychogenic retention of urine (F45.8)*

R33.0 **Drug induced retention of urine**
Use additional code for adverse effect, if applicable, to identify drug (T36-T50 with fifth or sixth character 5)

R33.8 **Other retention of urine**
Code first, if applicable, any causal condition, such as:
enlarged prostate (N40.1)

R33.9 **Retention of urine, unspecified**

R34 **Anuria and oliguria**
EXCLUDES 1 *anuria and oliguria complicating abortion or ectopic or molar pregnancy (O00-O07, O08.4)*
anuria and oliguria complicating pregnancy (O26.83-)
anuria and oliguria complicating the puerperium (O90.4)

✓4ᵗʰ **R35** **Polyuria**
Code first, if applicable, any causal condition, such as:
enlarged prostate (N40.1)
EXCLUDES 1 *psychogenic polyuria (F45.8)*

R35.0 **Frequency of micturition**

R35.1 **Nocturia**

R35.8 **Other polyuria**
Polyuria NOS

✓4ᵗʰ **R36** **Urethral discharge**

R36.0 **Urethral discharge without blood**

R36.1 **Hematospermia** ♂

R36.9 **Urethral discharge, unspecified**
Penile discharge NOS
Urethrorrhea

R37 **Sexual dysfunction, unspecified**

✓4ᵗʰ **R39** **Other and unspecified symptoms and signs involving the genitourinary system**

R39.0 **Extravasation of urine** CC
CC Excl: R30.1, R39.0, R39.2-R39.9

✓5ᵗʰ **R39.1** **Other difficulties with micturition**
Code first, if applicable, any causal condition, such as:
enlarged prostate (N40.1)

R39.11 **Hesitancy of micturition**

R39.12 **Poor urinary stream**
Weak urinary steam

R39.13 **Splitting of urinary stream**

R39.14 **Feeling of incomplete bladder emptying**

R39.15 **Urgency of urination**
EXCLUDES 1 *urge incontinence (N39.41, N39.46)*

R39.16 **Straining to void**

R39.19 **Other difficulties with micturition**

R39.2 **Extrarenal uremia**
Prerenal uremia
EXCLUDES 1 *uremia NOS (N19)*

✓5ᵗʰ **R39.8** **Other symptoms and signs involving the genitourinary system**

R39.81 **Functional urinary incontinence**
Urinary incontinence due to cognitive impairment, or severe physical disability or immobility
EXCLUDES 1 *stress incontinence and other specified urinary incontinence (N39.3-N39.4-)*
urinary incontinence NOS (R32)

✓ Additional Character Required   ✓x7ᵗʰ Xtension Alert   Unacceptable PDx   Manifestation   Hospital Acquired Condition   EXCLUDES 1 Not Coded Here   EXCLUDES 2 Not Included Here

Symptoms, Signs and Abnormal Clinical and Laboratory Findings

R39.89–R41.83

R39.89   **Other symptoms and signs involving the genitourinary system**

R39.9   **Unspecified symptoms and signs involving the genitourinary system**

Symptoms and signs involving cognition, perception, emotional state and behavior (R40-R46)

> EXCLUDES 1   *symptoms and signs constituting part of a pattern of mental disorder (F01-F99)*

✓4ᵗʰ **R40   Somnolence, stupor and coma**

> EXCLUDES 1   *neonatal coma (P91.5)*
> *somnolence, stupor and coma in diabetes (E08-E13)*
> *somnolence, stupor and coma in hepatic failure (K72.-)*
> *somnolence, stupor and coma in hypoglycemia (nondiabetic) (E15)*

R40.0   **Somnolence**
Drowsiness
> EXCLUDES 1   *coma (R40.2-)*

R40.1   **Stupor**
Catatonic stupor
Semicoma
> EXCLUDES 1   *catatonic schizophrenia (F20.2)*
> *coma (R40.2-)*
> *depressive stupor (F31-F33)*
> *dissociative stupor (F44.2)*
> *manic stupor (F30.2)*

✓5ᵗʰ **R40.2   Coma**
Code first any associated:
fracture of skull (S02.-)
intracranial injury (S06.-)
> NOTE   One code from subcategories R40.21-R40.23 is required to complete the coma scale
AHA: 2014, 1Q, 19

> **CC Excl: For MCC codes in subcategory R40.2, unless otherwise noted:** B15.0-B19.9, E03.5, E08.00-E08.59, E08.618-E09.59, E09.618-E10.59, E10.618-E10.649, E10.69-E11.59, E11.618-E11.649, E11.69-E13.59, E13.618-E16.2, E89.1, G32.89, G89.0-G89.4, G93.81-G93.9, G96.8-G96.9, G98.0-G98.8, G99.8, I60.00-I62.9, K72.91, R40.0-R40.2124, R40.2210-R40.2224, R40.2310-R40.2324, R40.2340-R40.2344, R40.3-R41.3, R41.82, R41.9-R42, R44.8-R44.9, R45.83-R45.84, R46.0-R46.89, R52, R55, R68.0-R68.19, R68.81-R68.83, R68.89-R69, S02.0XX-S02.19X with 7th character [A, B], S02.91X-S02.91X with 7th character [A, B], S06.0X0-S06.9X9 with 7th character A

R40.20   **Unspecified coma**   MCC
Coma NOS
Unconsciousness NOS

✓6ᵗʰ **R40.21   Coma scale, eyes open**

> The following appropriate 7th character is to be added to subcategory R40.21-.
> 0   unspecified time
> 1   in the field [EMT or ambulance]
> 2   at arrival to emergency department
> 3   at hospital admission
> 4   24 hours or more after hospital admission

✓7ᵗʰ   **R40.211   Coma scale, eyes open, never**   MCC
✓7ᵗʰ   **R40.212   Coma scale, eyes open, to pain**   MCC
✓7ᵗʰ   **R40.213   Coma scale, eyes open, to sound**
✓7ᵗʰ   **R40.214   Coma scale, eyes open, spontaneous**

✓6ᵗʰ **R40.22   Coma scale, best verbal response**

> The following appropriate 7th character is to be added to subcategory R40.22-.
> 0   unspecified time
> 1   in the field [EMT or ambulance]
> 2   at arrival to emergency department
> 3   at hospital admission
> 4   24 hours or more after hospital admission

✓7ᵗʰ   **R40.221   Coma scale, best verbal response, none**   MCC
✓7ᵗʰ   **R40.222   Coma scale, best verbal response, incomprehensible words**   MCC
✓7ᵗʰ   **R40.223   Coma scale, best verbal response, inappropriate words**
✓7ᵗʰ   **R40.224   Coma scale, best verbal response, confused conversation**

✓7ᵗʰ   **R40.225   Coma scale, best verbal response, oriented**

✓6ᵗʰ **R40.23   Coma scale, best motor response**

> The following appropriate 7th character is to be added to subcategory R40.23-.
> 0   unspecified time
> 1   in the field [EMT or ambulance]
> 2   at arrival to emergency department
> 3   at hospital admission
> 4   24 hours or more after hospital admission

✓7ᵗʰ   **R40.231   Coma scale, best motor response, none**   MCC
✓7ᵗʰ   **R40.232   Coma scale, best motor response, extension**   MCC
✓7ᵗʰ   **R40.233   Coma scale, best motor response, abnormal**
✓7ᵗʰ   **R40.234   Coma scale, best motor response, flexion withdrawal**   MCC
✓7ᵗʰ   **R40.235   Coma scale, best motor response, localizes pain**
✓7ᵗʰ   **R40.236   Coma scale, best motor response, obeys commands**

✓6ᵗʰ **R40.24   Glasgow coma scale, total score**
> Use codes R40.21- through R40.23- only when the individual score(s) are documented

R40.241   **Glasgow coma scale score 13-15**
R40.242   **Glasgow coma scale score 9-12**
R40.243   **Glasgow coma scale score 3-8**
R40.244   **Other coma, without documented Glasgow coma scale score, or with partial score reported**

R40.3   **Persistent vegetative state**   CC
> CC Excl: See code: R40.2

R40.4   **Transient alteration of awareness**

✓4ᵗʰ **R41   Other symptoms and signs involving cognitive functions and awareness**

> EXCLUDES 1   *dissociative [conversion] disorders (F44.-)*
> *mild cognitive impairment, so stated (G31.84)*

R41.0   **Disorientation, unspecified**
Confusion NOS
Delirium NOS

R41.1   **Anterograde amnesia**

R41.2   **Retrograde amnesia**

R41.3   **Other amnesia**
Amnesia NOS
Memory loss NOS
> EXCLUDES 1   *amnestic disorder due to known physiologic condition (F04)*
> *amnestic syndrome due to psychoactive substance use (F10-F19 with 5th character .6)*
> *mild memory disturbance due to known physiological condition (F06.8)*
> *transient global amnesia (G45.4)*

R41.4   **Neurologic neglect syndrome**   CC
Asomatognosia
Hemi-akinesia
Hemi-inattention
Hemispatial neglect
Left-sided neglect
Sensory neglect
Visuospatial neglect
> EXCLUDES 1   *visuospatial deficit (R41.842)*
> CC Excl: R29.3, R29.6-R29.890, R29.90-R29.91, R41.4

✓5ᵗʰ **R41.8   Other symptoms and signs involving cognitive functions and awareness**

R41.81   **Age-related cognitive decline**   A
Senility NOS

R41.82   **Altered mental status, unspecified**
Change in mental status NOS
> EXCLUDES 1   *altered level of consciousness (R40.-)*
> *altered mental status due to known condition—code to condition*
> *delirium NOS (R41.0)*
AHA: 2012, 4Q, 97

R41.83   **Borderline intellectual functioning**
IQ level 71 to 84
> EXCLUDES 1   *intellectual disabilities (F70-F79)*

N Newborn: 0   P Pediatric: 0-17   M Maternity: 12-55   A Adult: 15-124   MCC Major CC Condition   PDx MCC PDx acts as own MCC   CC CC Condition   PDx CC PDx acts as own CC

846   ICD-10-CM Draft (2015)

☑6ᵗʰ **R41.84** **Other specified cognitive deficit**

    R41.840 **Attention and concentration deficit**
        EXCLUDES 1   *attention-deficit hyperactivity disorders (F90.-)*

    R41.841 **Cognitive communication deficit**

    R41.842 **Visuospatial deficit**

    R41.843 **Psychomotor deficit**

    R41.844 **Frontal lobe and executive function deficit**

  R41.89 **Other symptoms and signs involving cognitive functions and awareness**
    Anosognosia

  R41.9 **Unspecified symptoms and signs involving cognitive functions and awareness**

R42 **Dizziness and giddiness**
  Light-headedness
  Vertigo NOS
  EXCLUDES 1   *vertiginous syndromes (H81.-)*
           vertigo from infrasound (T75.23)

☑4ᵗʰ **R43** **Disturbances of smell and taste**

  R43.0 **Anosmia**

  R43.1 **Parosmia**

  R43.2 **Parageusia**

  R43.8 **Other disturbances of smell and taste**
    Mixed disturbance of smell and taste

  R43.9 **Unspecified disturbances of smell and taste**

☑4ᵗʰ **R44** **Other symptoms and signs involving general sensations and perceptions**
  EXCLUDES 1   *alcoholic hallucinations (F1.5)*
         hallucinations in drug psychosis (F11-F19 with .5)
         hallucinations in mood disorders with psychotic symptoms (F30.2, F31.5, F32.3, F33.3)
         hallucinations in schizophrenia, schizotypal and delusional disorders (F20-F29)
  EXCLUDES 2   *disturbances of skin sensation (R20.-)*

  CC Excl: For CC codes in category R44, unless otherwise noted: G89.0-G89.4, R41.0-R41.3, R41.82, R41.9-R42, R44.0, R44.2-R44.9, R45.83-R45.84, R46.0-R46.89, R52, R68.0-R68.19, R68.81-R68.83, R68.89-R69

  R44.0 **Auditory hallucinations**   CC

  R44.1 **Visual hallucinations**

  R44.2 **Other hallucinations**   CC

  R44.3 **Hallucinations, unspecified**   CC

  R44.8 **Other symptoms and signs involving general sensations and perceptions**

  R44.9 **Unspecified symptoms and signs involving general sensations and perceptions**

☑4ᵗʰ **R45** **Symptoms and signs involving emotional state**

  R45.0 **Nervousness**
    Nervous tension

  R45.1 **Restlessness and agitation**

  R45.2 **Unhappiness**

  R45.3 **Demoralization and apathy**
    EXCLUDES 1   *anhedonia (R45.84)*

  R45.4 **Irritability and anger**

  R45.5 **Hostility**

  R45.6 **Violent behavior**

  R45.7 **State of emotional shock and stress, unspecified**

☑5ᵗʰ **R45.8** **Other symptoms and signs involving emotional state**

    R45.81 **Low self-esteem**

    R45.82 **Worries**

    R45.83 **Excessive crying of child, adolescent or adult**
        EXCLUDES 1   *excessive crying of infant (baby) R68.11*

    R45.84 **Anhedonia**

☑6ᵗʰ   **R45.85** **Homicidal and suicidal ideations**
        EXCLUDES 1   *suicide attempt (T14.91)*

    R45.850 **Homicidal ideations**

    R45.851 **Suicidal ideations**   CC
        CC Excl: F05

    R45.86 **Emotional lability**

    R45.87 **Impulsiveness**

    R45.89 **Other symptoms and signs involving emotional state**

☑4ᵗʰ **R46** **Symptoms and signs involving appearance and behavior**
  EXCLUDES 1   *appearance and behavior in schizophrenia, schizotypal and delusional disorders (F20-F29)*
         mental and behavioral disorders (F01-F99)

  R46.0 **Very low level of personal hygiene**

  R46.1 **Bizarre personal appearance**

  R46.2 **Strange and inexplicable behavior**

  R46.3 **Overactivity**

  R46.4 **Slowness and poor responsiveness**
    EXCLUDES 1   *stupor (R40.1)*

  R46.5 **Suspiciousness and marked evasiveness**

  R46.6 **Undue concern and preoccupation with stressful events**

  R46.7 **Verbosity and circumstantial detail obscuring reason for contact**

☑5ᵗʰ **R46.8** **Other symptoms and signs involving appearance and behavior**

    R46.81 **Obsessive-compulsive behavior**
        EXCLUDES 1   *obsessive-compulsive disorder (F42)*

    R46.89 **Other symptoms and signs involving appearance and behavior**

Symptoms and signs involving speech and voice (R47-R49)

☑4ᵗʰ **R47** **Speech disturbances, not elsewhere classified**
  EXCLUDES 1   *autism (F84.0)*
         cluttering (F80.81)
         specific developmental disorders of speech and language (F80.-)
         stuttering (F80.81)

☑5ᵗʰ **R47.0** **Dysphasia and aphasia**

    R47.01 **Aphasia**   CC
        EXCLUDES 1   *aphasia following cerebrovascular disease (I69. with final characters -20)*
            progressive isolated aphasia (G31.01)
        CC Excl: F80.1, F80.81, I62.00-I66.9, R47.01-R47.9, R49.0-R49.9

    R47.02 **Dysphasia**
        EXCLUDES 1   *dysphasia following cerebrovascular disease (I69. with final characters -21)*

  R47.1 **Dysarthria and anarthria**
    EXCLUDES 1   *dysarthria following cerebrovascular disease (I69. with final characters -22)*

☑5ᵗʰ **R47.8** **Other speech disturbances**
    EXCLUDES 1   *dysarthria following cerebrovascular disease (I69. with final characters -28)*

    R47.81 **Slurred speech**

    R47.82 **Fluency disorder in conditions classified elsewhere**
        Stuttering in conditions classified elsewhere
        Code first underlying disease or condition, such as:
        Parkinson's disease (G20)
        EXCLUDES 1   *adult onset fluency disorder (F98.5)*
            childhood onset fluency disorder (F80.81)
            fluency disorder (stuttering) following cerebrovascular disease (I69. with final characters-23)

    R47.89 **Other speech disturbances**

  R47.9 **Unspecified speech disturbances**

☑4ᵗʰ **R48** **Dyslexia and other symbolic dysfunctions, not elsewhere classified**
  EXCLUDES 1   *specific developmental disorders of scholastic skills (F81.-)*

  R48.0 **Dyslexia and alexia**

  R48.1 **Agnosia**
    Astereognosia (astereognosis)
    Autotopagnosia
    EXCLUDES 1   *visual object agnosia (R48.3)*

  R48.2 **Apraxia**
    EXCLUDES 1   *apraxia following cerebrovascular disease (I69. with final characters -90)*

  R48.3 **Visual agnosia**
    Prosopagnosia
    Simultanagnosia (asimultagnosia)

  R48.8 **Other symbolic dysfunctions**
    Acalculia
    Agraphia

  R48.9 **Unspecified symbolic dysfunctions**

☑ Additional Character Required   ☑x7ᵗʰ Xtension Alert   Unacceptable PDx   Manifestation   Hospital Acquired Condition   *EXCLUDES 1* Not Coded Here   *EXCLUDES 2* Not Included Here

Symptoms, Signs and Abnormal Clinical and Laboratory Findings *(left margin)*
R49–R56.00 *(left margin)*

✓4ᵗʰ **R49** **Voice and resonance disorders**
    EXCLUDES 1   *psychogenic voice and resonance disorders (F44.4)*

  R49.0 **Dysphonia**
     Hoarseness

  R49.1 **Aphonia**
     Loss of voice

  ✓5ᵗʰ **R49.2** **Hypernasality and hyponasality**
     R49.21   **Hypernasality**
     R49.22   **Hyponasality**

  R49.8 **Other voice and resonance disorders**

  R49.9 **Unspecified voice and resonance disorder**
     Change in voice NOS
     Resonance disorder NOS

General symptoms and signs (R50-R69)

✓4ᵗʰ **R50** **Fever of other and unknown origin**
    EXCLUDES 1   *chills without fever (R68.83)*
       febrile convulsions (R56.0-)
       fever of unknown origin during labor (O75.2)
       fever of unknown origin in newborn (P81.9)
       hypothermia due to illness (R68.0)
       malignant hyperthermia due to anesthesia (T88.3)
       puerperal pyrexia NOS (O86.4)

  R50.2 **Drug induced fever**
     Use additional code for adverse effect, if applicable, to identify
     drug (T36-T50 with fifth or sixth character 5)
    EXCLUDES 1   *postvaccination (postimmunization) fever (R50.83)*

  ✓5ᵗʰ **R50.8** **Other specified fever**

     R50.81   ***Fever presenting with conditions classified elsewhere***
        Code first underlying condition when associated fever is
        present, such as with:
        leukemia (C91-C95)
        neutropenia (D70.-)
        sickle-cell disease (D57.-)

     R50.82   **Postprocedural fever**
        EXCLUDES 1   *postprocedural infection (T81.4)*
           posttransfusion fever (R50.84)
           postvaccination (postimmunization) fever
             (R50.83)

     R50.83   **Postvaccination fever**
        Postimmunization fever

     R50.84   **Febrile nonhemolytic transfusion reaction**
        FNHTR
        Posttransfusion fever

  R50.9 **Fever, unspecified**
     Fever NOS   Hyperpyrexia NOS
     Fever of unknown origin [FUO]   Persistent fever
     Fever with chills   Pyrexia NOS
     Fever with rigors

R51 **Headache**
    Facial pain NOS
    EXCLUDES 1   *atypical face pain (G50.1)*
       migraine and other headache syndromes (G43-G44)
       trigeminal neuralgia (G50.0)

R52 **Pain, unspecified**
    Acute pain NOS
    Generalized pain NOS
    Pain NOS
    EXCLUDES 1   *acute and chronic pain, not elsewhere classified (G89.-)*
       localized pain, unspecified type—code to pain by site, such as:
         abdomen pain (R10.-)
         back pain (M54.9)
         breast pain (N64.4)
         chest pain (R07.1-R07.9)
         ear pain (H92.0-)
         eye pain (H57.1)
         headache (R51)
         joint pain (M25.5-)
         limb pain (M79.6-)
         lumbar region pain (M54.5)
         pelvic and perineal pain (R10.2)
         renal colic (N23)
         shoulder pain (M25.51-)
         spine pain (M54.-)
         throat pain (R07.0)
         tongue pain (K14.6)
         tooth pain (K08.8)
       pain disorders exclusively related to psychological factors
        (F45.41)

✓4ᵗʰ **R53** **Malaise and fatigue**

  R53.0 **Neoplastic (malignant) related fatigue**
     Code first associated neoplasm

  R53.1 **Weakness**
     Asthenia NOS
    EXCLUDES 1   *age-related weakness (R54)*
       muscle weakness (M62.8-)
       senile asthenia (R54)

  R53.2 **Functional quadriplegia**   **MCC**
     Complete immobility due to severe physical disability or frailty
    EXCLUDES 1   *frailty NOS (R54)*
       hysterical paralysis (F44.4)
       immobility syndrome (M62.3)
       neurologic quadriplegia (G82.5-)
       quadriplegia (G82.50)
    CC Excl: E08.40-E08.49, E08.618-E08.638, E08.649-E08.8, E09.40-
    E09.49, E09.618-E09.638, E09.649-E09.8, E10.40-E10.49, E10.618-
    E10.638, E10.649, E10.69-E10.8, E11.40-E11.49, E11.618-E11.638,
    E11.649, E11.69-E11.8, E13.40-E13.49, E13.618-E13.638, E13.649-
    E13.8, G04.1, G32.89, G80.0-G80.2, G80.4-G83.9, G90.1, G93.81,
    G93.89-G93.9, G96.8-G96.9, G98.0-G98.8, G99.8, Q06.0-Q06.1,
    Q06.3, Q06.8-Q06.9, Q07.8-Q07.9, R53.2

  ✓5ᵗʰ **R53.8** **Other malaise and fatigue**
    EXCLUDES 1   *combat exhaustion and fatigue (F43.0)*
       congenital debility (P96.9)
       exhaustion and fatigue due to depressive episode
         (F32.-)
       exhaustion and fatigue due to excessive exertion
         (T73.3)
       exhaustion and fatigue due to exposure (T73.2)
       exhaustion and fatigue due to heat (T67.-)
       exhaustion and fatigue due to pregnancy (O26.8-)
       exhaustion and fatigue due to recurrent depressive
         episode (F33)
       exhaustion and fatigue due to senile debility (R54)

     R53.81   **Other malaise**
        Chronic debility   Malaise NOS
        Debility NOS   Nervous debility
        General physical deterioration
        EXCLUDES 1   *age-related physical debility (R54)*

     R53.82   **Chronic fatigue, unspecified**
        Chronic fatigue syndrome NOS
        EXCLUDES 1   *postviral fatigue syndrome (G93.3)*

     R53.83   **Other fatigue**
        Fatigue NOS   Lethargy
        Lack of energy   Tiredness

R54 **Age-related physical debility**   **A**
    Frailty   Senile asthenia
    Old age   Senile debility
    Senescence
    EXCLUDES 1   *age-related cognitive decline (R41.81)*
       senile psychosis (F03)
       senility NOS (R41.81)

R55 **Syncope and collapse**
    Blackout   Vasovagal attack
    Fainting
    EXCLUDES 1   *cardiogenic shock (R57.0)*
       carotid sinus syncope (G90.01)
       heat syncope (T67.1)
       neurocirculatory asthenia (F45.8)
       neurogenic orthostatic hypotension (G90.3)
       orthostatic hypotension (I95.1)
       postprocedural shock (T81.1-)
       psychogenic syncope (F48.8)
       shock NOS (R57.9)
       shock complicating or following abortion or ectopic or molar
         pregnancy (O00-O07, O08.3)
       shock complicating or following labor and delivery (O75.1)
       Stokes-Adams attack (I45.9)
       unconsciousness NOS (R40.2-)

(handwritten annotation: near syncope)

✓4ᵗʰ **R56** **Convulsions, not elsewhere classified**
    EXCLUDES 1   *dissociative convulsions and seizures (F44.5)*
       epileptic convulsions and seizures (G40.-)
       newborn convulsions and seizures (P90)

  ✓5ᵗʰ **R56.0** **Febrile convulsions**

     R56.00   **Simple febrile convulsions**   **CC**
        Febrile convulsion NOS
        Febrile seizure NOS
        CC Excl: G32.89, G40.001-G40.919, G89.0-G89.4, G93.81,
        G93.89-G93.9, G96.8-G96.9, G98.0-G98.8, G99.8, P90,
        P91.8-P91.9, R40.0-R41.3, R41.82, R41.9, R44.8-R44.9,

N Newborn: 0   **P** Pediatric: 0-17   **M** Maternity: 12-55   **A** Adult: 15-124   **MCC** Major CC Condition   **PDx MCC** PDx acts as own MCC   **CC** CC Condition   **PDx CC** PDx acts as own CC

848   ICD-10-CM Draft (2015)

R45.83-R45.84, R46.0-R46.89, R52, R56.00-R56.9, R68.0-R68.19, R68.81-R68.83, R68.89-R69

R56.01 Complex febrile convulsions   `CC`
Atypical febrile seizure
Complex febrile seizure
Complicated febrile seizure
EXCLUDES 1 *status epilepticus (G40.901)*
CC Excl: See code: R56.00

R56.1 Post traumatic seizures   `CC`
EXCLUDES 1 *post traumatic epilepsy (G40.-)*
CC Excl: E08.40-E08.49, E09.40-E09.49, E10.40-E10.49, E11.40-E11.49, E13.40-E13.49, G32.89, G40.001-G40.509, G40.801-G40.804, G40.811-G40.814, G40.821-G40.B19, G93.81, G93.89-G93.9, G96.8-G96.9, G98.0-G98.8, G99.8, R56.1

R56.9 Unspecified convulsions
Convulsion disorder
Fit NOS
Recurrent convulsions
Seizure(s) (convulsive) NOS

✓4th R57 Shock, not elsewhere classified
EXCLUDES 1 *anaphylactic shock NOS (T78.2)*
anaphylactic reaction or shock due to adverse food reaction (T78.0-)
anaphylactic shock due to adverse effect of correct drug or medicament properly administered (T88.6)
anaphylactic shock due to serum (T80.5-)
anesthetic shock (T88.3)
electric shock (T75.4)
obstetric shock (O75.1)
postprocedural shock (T81.1-)
psychic shock (F43.0)
septic shock (R65.21)
shock complicating or following ectopic or molar pregnancy (O00-O07, O08.3)
shock due to lightning (T75.01)
traumatic shock (T79.4)
toxic shock syndrome (A48.3)

CC Excl: For CC/MCC codes in category R57, unless otherwise noted: G89.0-G89.4, R09.89, R41.0-R41.3, R41.82, R41.9, R44.8-R44.9, R45.83-R45.84, R46.0-R46.89, R52, R57.0-R57.9, R65.21-R68.19, R68.81-R68.83, R68.89-R69

10 **R57.0 Cardiogenic shock**   `MCC`
10 **R57.1 Hypovolemic shock**   `MCC`
10 **R57.8 Other shock**   `MCC`
R57.9 Shock, unspecified   `CC`
Failure of peripheral circulation NOS

R58 Hemorrhage, not elsewhere classified
Hemorrhage NOS
EXCLUDES 1 *hemorrhage included with underlying conditions, such as:*
acute duodenal ulcer with hemorrhage (K26.0)
acute gastritis with bleeding (K29.01)
ulcerative enterocolitis with rectal bleeding (K51.01)

✓4th R59 Enlarged lymph nodes
INCLUDES swollen glands
EXCLUDES 1 *acute lymphadenitis (L04.-)*
chronic lymphadenitis (I88.1)
lymphadenitis NOS (I88.9)
mesenteric (acute) (chronic) lymphadenitis (I88.0)

R59.0 Localized enlarged lymph nodes
R59.1 Generalized enlarged lymph nodes
Lymphadenopathy NOS
R59.9 Enlarged lymph nodes, unspecified

✓4th R60 Edema, not elsewhere classified
EXCLUDES 1 *angioneurotic edema (T78.3)*
ascites (R18.-)
cerebral edema (G93.6)
cerebral edema due to birth injury (P11.0)
edema of larynx (J38.4)
edema of nasopharynx (J39.2)
edema of pharynx (J39.2)
gestational edema (O12.0-)
hereditary edema (Q82.0)
hydrops fetalis NOS (P83.2)
hydrothorax (J94.8)
nutritional edema (E40-E46)
hydrops fetalis NOS (P83.2)
newborn edema (P83.3)
pulmonary edema (J81.-)

R60.0 Localized edema

R60.1 Generalized edema
R60.9 Edema, unspecified
Fluid retention NOS

R61 Generalized hyperhidrosis
Excessive sweating
Night sweats
Secondary hyperhidrosis
Code first, if applicable, menopausal and female climacteric states (N95.1)
EXCLUDES 1 *focal (primary) (secondary) hyperhidrosis (L74.5-)*
Frey's syndrome (L74.52)
localized (primary) (secondary) hyperhidrosis (L74.5-)

✓4th R62 Lack of expected normal physiological development in childhood and adults
EXCLUDES 1 *delayed puberty (E30.0)*
gonadal dysgenesis (Q99.1)
hypopituitarism (E23.0)

R62.0 Delayed milestone in childhood   `P`
Delayed attainment of expected physiological developmental stage
Late talker
Late walker

✓5th R62.5 Other and unspecified lack of expected normal physiological development in childhood
EXCLUDES 1 *HIV disease resulting in failure to thrive (B20)*
physical retardation due to malnutrition (E45)

R62.50 Unspecified lack of expected normal physiological development in childhood   `P`
Infantilism NOS

R62.51 Failure to thrive (child)   `P`
Failure to gain weight
EXCLUDES 1 *failure to thrive in child under 28 days old (P92.6)*

R62.52 Short stature (child)   `P`
Lack of growth
Physical retardation
Short stature NOS
EXCLUDES 1 *short stature due to endocrine disorder (E34.3)*

R62.59 Other lack of expected normal physiological development in childhood   `P`

R62.7 Adult failure to thrive   `A`

✓4th R63 Symptoms and signs concerning food and fluid intake
EXCLUDES 1 *bulimia NOS (F50.2)*
eating disorders of nonorganic origin (F50.-)
malnutrition (E40-E46)

R63.0 Anorexia
Loss of appetite
EXCLUDES 1 *anorexia nervosa (F50.0-)*
loss of appetite of nonorganic origin (F50.8)

R63.1 Polydipsia
Excessive thirst

R63.2 Polyphagia
Excessive eating
Hyperalimentation NOS

R63.3 Feeding difficulties
Feeding problem (elderly) (infant) NOS
EXCLUDES 1 *feeding problems of newborn (P92.-)*
infant feeding disorder of nonorganic origin (F98.2-)

R63.4 Abnormal weight loss

R63.5 Abnormal weight gain
EXCLUDES 1 *excessive weight gain in pregnancy (O26.0-)*
obesity (E66.-)

R63.6 Underweight
Use additional code to identify body mass index (BMI), if known (Z68.-)
EXCLUDES 1 *abnormal weight loss (R63.4)*
anorexia nervosa (F50.0-)
malnutrition (E40-E46)

R63.8 Other symptoms and signs concerning food and fluid intake

R64 Cachexia   `CC`
Wasting syndrome
Code first underlying condition, if known
EXCLUDES 1 *abnormal weight loss (R63.4)*
nutritional marasmus (E41)
CC Excl: G89.0-G89.4, R41.0-R41.3, R41.82, R41.9, R44.8-R44.9, R45.83-R45.84, R46.0-R46.89, R52, R64, R68.0-R68.19, R68.81-R68.83, R68.89-R69

---

10 MCC = only if patient is discharged alive.

✓ Additional Character Required   ✓x7th Xtension Alert   Unacceptable PDx   Manifestation   Hospital Acquired Condition   **EXCLUDES 1** Not Coded Here   **EXCLUDES 2** Not Included Here

Symptoms, Signs and Abnormal Clinical and Laboratory Findings

R65–R73.01

✓4ᵗʰ **R65 Symptoms and signs specifically associated with systemic inflammation and infection**

> **CC Excl:** For CC/MCC codes in category R65, unless otherwise noted: A02.1, A20.7, A22.7, A26.7, A32.7, A39.2-A39.4, A40.0-A40.1, A40.8-A41.9, A42.7, A48.2-A48.4, A48.8-A49.9, A54.86, B00.7, B37.7, B92, B94.2-B96.89, R65.10-R65.20, M00.011-M00.012, M00.021-M00.022, M00.031-M00.032, M00.041-M00.042, M00.051-M00.052, M00.061-M00.062, M00.071-M00.072, Z16.10-Z16.39

✓5ᵗʰ **R65.1 Systemic inflammatory response syndrome [SIRS] of non-infectious origin**

> Code first underlying condition, such as:
> heatstroke (T67.0)
> injury and trauma (S00-T88)
>
> *EXCLUDES 1*   sepsis—code to infection
> severe sepsis (R65.2)

R65.10 Systemic inflammatory response syndrome [SIRS] of non-infectious origin without acute organ dysfunction   `CC`

> Systemic inflammatory response syndrome (SIRS) NOS

R65.11 Systemic inflammatory response syndrome [SIRS] of non-infectious origin with acute organ dysfunction   `MCC`

> Use additional code to identify specific acute organ dysfunction, such as:
> acute kidney failure (N17.-)
> acute respiratory failure (J96.0-)
> critical illness myopathy (G72.81)
> critical illness polyneuropathy (G62.81)
> disseminated intravascular coagulopathy [DIC] (D65)
> encephalopathy (metabolic) (septic) (G93.41)
> hepatic failure (K72.0-)

✓5ᵗʰ **R65.2 Severe sepsis**

> Infection with associated acute organ dysfunction
> Sepsis with acute organ dysfunction
> Sepsis with multiple organ dysfunction
> Systemic inflammatory response syndrome due to infectious process with acute organ dysfunction
>
> Code first underlying infection, such as:
> infection following a procedure (T81.4)
> infections following infusion, transfusion and therapeutic injection (T80.2-)
> puerperal sepsis (O85)
> sepsis following complete or unspecified spontaneous abortion (O03.87)
> sepsis following ectopic and molar pregnancy (O08.82)
> sepsis following incomplete spontaneous abortion (O03.37)
> sepsis following (induced) termination of pregnancy (O04.87)
> sepsis NOS (A41.9)
>
> Use additional code to identify specific acute organ dysfunction, such as:
> acute kidney failure (N17.-)
> acute respiratory failure (J96.0-)
> critical illness myopathy (G72.81)
> critical illness polyneuropathy (G62.81)
> disseminated intravascular coagulopathy [DIC] (D65)
> encephalopathy (metabolic) (septic) (G93.41)
> hepatic failure (K72.0-)

R65.20 Severe sepsis without septic shock   `MCC`

> Severe sepsis NOS
> **AHA:** 2013, 4Q, 119

R65.21 Severe sepsis with septic shock   `PDx MCC` `MCC`

> **CC Excl:** G89.0-G89.4, R09.89, R41.0-R41.3, R41.82, R41.9, R44.8-R44.9, R45.83-R45.84, R46.0-R46.89, R52, R57.0-R57.9, R65.21-R68.19, R68.81-R68.83, R68.89-R69

✓4ᵗʰ **R68 Other general symptoms and signs**

R68.0 Hypothermia, not associated with low environmental temperature

> *EXCLUDES 1*   hypothermia due to anesthesia (T88.51)
> hypothermia due to low environmental temperature (T68)
> hypothermia NOS (accidental) (T68)
> newborn hypothermia (P80.-)

✓5ᵗʰ **R68.1 Nonspecific symptoms peculiar to infancy**

> *EXCLUDES 1*   colic, infantile (R10.83)
> neonatal cerebral irritability (P91.3)
> teething syndrome (K00.7)

R68.11 Excessive crying of infant (baby)   `P`

> *EXCLUDES 1*   excessive crying of child, adolescent, or adult (R45.83)

R68.12 Fussy infant (baby)   `P`

> Irritable infant

R68.13 Apparent life threatening event in infant [ALTE]   `P`

> Apparent life threatening event in newborn
> Code first confirmed diagnosis, if known
> Use additional code(s) for associated signs and symptoms if no confirmed diagnosis established, or if signs and symptoms are not associated routinely with confirmed diagnosis, or provide additional information for cause of ALTE

R68.19 Other nonspecific symptoms peculiar to infancy   `P`

R68.2 Dry mouth, unspecified

> *EXCLUDES 1*   dry mouth due to dehydration (E86.0)
> dry mouth due to sicca syndrome [Sjögren] (M35.0-)
> salivary gland hyposecretion (K11.7)

R68.3 Clubbing of fingers

> Clubbing of nails
> *EXCLUDES 1*   congenital clubfinger (Q68.1)

✓5ᵗʰ **R68.8 Other general symptoms and signs**

R68.81 Early satiety

R68.82 Decreased libido   `A`

> Decreased sexual desire

R68.83 Chills (without fever)

> Chills NOS
> *EXCLUDES 1*   chills with fever (R50.9)

R68.84 Jaw pain

> Mandibular pain
> Maxilla pain
> *EXCLUDES 1*   temporomandibular joint arthralgia (M26.62)

R68.89 Other general symptoms and signs

R69 Illness, unspecified

> Unknown and unspecified cases of morbidity

Abnormal findings on examination of blood, without diagnosis (R70-R79)

> *EXCLUDES 1*   abnormalities (of)(on):
> abnormal findings on antenatal screening of mother (O28.-)
> coagulation hemorrhagic disorders (D65-D68)
> lipids (E78.-)
> platelets and thrombocytes (D69.-)
> white blood cells classified elsewhere (D70-D72)
> diagnostic abnormal findings classified elsewhere—see Alphabetical Index
> hemorrhagic and hematological disorders of newborn (P50-P61)

✓4ᵗʰ **R70 Elevated erythrocyte sedimentation rate and abnormality of plasma viscosity**

R70.0 Elevated erythrocyte sedimentation rate

R70.1 Abnormal plasma viscosity

✓4ᵗʰ **R71 Abnormality of red blood cells**

> *EXCLUDES 1*   anemias (D50-D64)
> anemia of premature infant (P61.2)
> benign (familial) polycythemia (D75.0)
> congenital anemias (P61.2-P61.4)
> newborn anemia due to isoimmunization (P55.-)
> polycythemia neonatorum (P61.1)
> polycythemia NOS (D75.1)
> polycythemia vera (D45)
> secondary polycythemia (D75.1)

R71.0 Precipitous drop in hematocrit   `CC`

> Drop (precipitous) in hemoglobin
> Drop in hematocrit
> **CC Excl:** D62, D64.4-D64.9

R71.8 Other abnormality of red blood cells

> Abnormal red-cell morphology NOS   Anisocytosis
> Abnormal red-cell volume NOS   Poikilocytosis

✓4ᵗʰ **R73 Elevated blood glucose level**

> *EXCLUDES 1*   diabetes mellitus (E08-E13)
> diabetes mellitus in pregnancy, childbirth and the puerperium (O24.-)
> neonatal disorders (P70.0-P70.2)
> postsurgical hypoinsulinemia (E89.1)

✓5ᵗʰ **R73.0 Abnormal glucose**

> *EXCLUDES 1*   abnormal glucose in pregnancy (O99.81-)
> diabetes mellitus (E08-E13)
> dysmetabolic syndrome X (E88.81)
> gestational diabetes (O24.4-)
> glycosuria (R81)
> hypoglycemia (E16.2)

R73.01 Impaired fasting glucose

> Elevated fasting glucose

`N` Newborn: 0   `P` Pediatric: 0-17   `M` Maternity: 12-55   `A` Adult: 15-124   `MCC` Major CC Condition   `PDx MCC` PDx acts as own MCC   `CC` CC Condition   `PDx CC` PDx acts as own CC

R73.02 Impaired glucose tolerance (oral)
Elevated glucose tolerance

R73.09 Other abnormal glucose
Abnormal glucose NOS
Abnormal non-fasting glucose tolerance
Latent diabetes
Prediabetes

R73.9 Hyperglycemia, unspecified

✓4ᵗʰ R74 Abnormal serum enzyme levels

R74.0 Nonspecific elevation of levels of transaminase and lactic acid dehydrogenase [LDH]

R74.8 Abnormal levels of other serum enzymes
Abnormal level of acid phosphatase
Abnormal level of alkaline phosphatase
Abnormal level of amylase
Abnormal level of lipase [triacylglycerol lipase]

R74.9 Abnormal serum enzyme level, unspecified

R75 Inconclusive laboratory evidence of human immunodeficiency virus [HIV]
Nonconclusive HIV-test finding in infants
EXCLUDES 1 asymptomatic human immunodeficiency virus [HIV] infection status (Z21)
human immunodeficiency virus [HIV] disease (B20)

✓4ᵗʰ R76 Other abnormal immunological findings in serum

R76.0 Raised antibody titer
EXCLUDES 1 isoimmunization in pregnancy (O36.0-O36.1)
isoimmunization affecting newborn (P55.-)

✓5ᵗʰ R76.1 Nonspecific reaction to test for tuberculosis

R76.11 Nonspecific reaction to tuberculin skin test without active tuberculosis
Abnormal result of Mantoux test
PPD positive
Tuberculin (skin test) positive
Tuberculin (skin test) reactor
EXCLUDES 1 nonspecific reaction to cell mediated immunity measurement of gamma interferon antigen response without active tuberculosis (R76.12)

R76.12 Nonspecific reaction to cell mediated immunity measurement of gamma interferon antigen response without active tuberculosis
Nonspecific reaction to QuantiFERON-TB test (QFT) without active tuberculosis
EXCLUDES 1 nonspecific reaction to tuberculin skin test without active tuberculosis (R76.11)
positive tuberculin skin test (R76.11)

R76.8 Other specified abnormal immunological findings in serum
Raised level of immunoglobulins NOS

R76.9 Abnormal immunological finding in serum, unspecified

✓4ᵗʰ R77 Other abnormalities of plasma proteins
EXCLUDES 1 disorders of plasma-protein metabolism (E88.0)

R77.0 Abnormality of albumin

R77.1 Abnormality of globulin
Hyperglobulinemia NOS

R77.2 Abnormality of alphafetoprotein

R77.8 Other specified abnormalities of plasma proteins

R77.9 Abnormality of plasma protein, unspecified

✓4ᵗʰ R78 Findings of drugs and other substances, not normally found in blood
Use additional code to identify any retained foreign body, if applicable (Z18.-)
EXCLUDES 1 mental or behavioral disorders due to psychoactive substance use (F10-F19)

R78.0 Finding of alcohol in blood
Use additional external cause code (Y90.-), for detail regarding alcohol level

R78.1 Finding of opiate drug in blood

R78.2 Finding of cocaine in blood

R78.3 Finding of hallucinogen in blood

R78.4 Finding of other drugs of addictive potential in blood

R78.5 Finding of other psychotropic drug in blood

R78.6 Finding of steroid agent in blood

✓5ᵗʰ R78.7 Finding of abnormal level of heavy metals in blood

R78.71 Abnormal lead level in blood
EXCLUDES 1 lead poisoning (T56.0-)

R78.79 Finding of abnormal level of heavy metals in blood

✓5ᵗʰ R78.8 Finding of other specified substances, not normally found in blood

R78.81 Bacteremia   CC
EXCLUDES 1 sepsis—code to specified infection (A00-B99)
CC Excl: B34.9, E07.81, G89.0-G89.4, R40.0-R41.3, R41.82, R41.9, R44.8-R44.9, R45.83-R45.84, R46.0-R46.89, R52, R68.0-R68.19, R68.81-R68.83, R68.89-R69, R70.1, R77.0-R77.9, R78.1-R78.6, R78.81, R78.9, R79.1-R79.89, R97.2

R78.89 Finding of other specified substances, not normally found in blood
Finding of abnormal level of lithium in blood

R78.9 Finding of unspecified substance, not normally found in blood

✓4ᵗʰ R79 Other abnormal findings of blood chemistry
Use additional code to identify any retained foreign body, if applicable (Z18.-)
EXCLUDES 1 abnormality of fluid, electrolyte or acid-base balance (E86-E87)
asymptomatic hyperuricemia (E79.0)
hyperglycemia NOS (R73.9)
hypoglycemia NOS (E16.2)
neonatal hypoglycemia (P70.3-P70.4)
specific findings indicating disorder of amino-acid metabolism (E70-E72)
specific findings indicating disorder of carbohydrate metabolism (E73-E74)
specific findings indicating disorder of lipid metabolism (E75.-)

R79.0 Abnormal level of blood mineral
Abnormal blood level of cobalt
Abnormal blood level of copper
Abnormal blood level of iron
Abnormal blood level of magnesium
Abnormal blood level of mineral NEC
Abnormal blood level of zinc
EXCLUDES 1 abnormal level of lithium (R78.89)
disorders of mineral metabolism (E83.-)
neonatal hypomagnesemia (P71.2)
nutritional mineral deficiency (E58-E61)

R79.1 Abnormal coagulation profile
Abnormal or prolonged bleeding time
Abnormal or prolonged coagulation time
Abnormal or prolonged partial thromboplastin time [PTT]
Abnormal or prolonged prothrombin time [PT]
EXCLUDES 1 coagulation defects (D68.-)

✓5ᵗʰ R79.8 Other specified abnormal findings of blood chemistry

R79.81 Abnormal blood-gas level

R79.82 Elevated C-reactive protein [CRP]

R79.89 Other specified abnormal findings of blood chemistry

R79.9 Abnormal finding of blood chemistry, unspecified

Abnormal findings on examination of urine, without diagnosis (R80-R82)

EXCLUDES 1 abnormal findings on antenatal screening of mother (O28.-)
diagnostic abnormal findings classified elsewhere—see Alphabetical Index
specific findings indicating disorder of amino-acid metabolism (E70-E72)

✓4ᵗʰ R80 Proteinuria
EXCLUDES 1 gestational proteinuria (O12.1-)

R80.0 Isolated proteinuria
Idiopathic proteinuria
EXCLUDES 1 isolated proteinuria with specific morphological lesion (N06.-)

R80.1 Persistent proteinuria, unspecified

R80.2 Orthostatic proteinuria, unspecified
Postural proteinuria

R80.3 Bence Jones proteinuria

R80.8 Other proteinuria

R80.9 Proteinuria, unspecified
Albuminuria NOS

R81 Glycosuria
EXCLUDES 1 renal glycosuria (E74.8)

Tap – Read more in the Guidelines page for HIV

Symptoms, Signs and Abnormal Clinical and Laboratory Findings

R82–R85.5

✓4ᵗʰ **R82 Other and unspecified abnormal findings in urine**
Chromoabnormalities in urine
Use additional code to identify any retained foreign body, if applicable
(Z18.-)
EXCLUDES 2   *hematuria (R31.-)*

R82.0 Chyluria   CC
EXCLUDES 1   *filarial chyluria (B74.-)*
CC Excl: G89.0-G89.4, R41.0-R41.3, R41.82, R41.9, R44.8-R44.9,
R45.83-R45.84, R46.0-R46.89, R52, R68.0-R68.19, R68.81-R68.83,
R68.89-R69, R82.0, R82.5-R82.99

R82.1 Myoglobinuria   CC
CC Excl: G89.0-G89.4, R41.0-R41.3, R41.82, R41.9, R44.8-R44.9,
R45.83-R45.84, R46.0-R46.89, R52, R68.0-R68.19, R68.81-R68.83,
R68.89-R69, R82.1, R82.3, R82.5-R82.99

R82.2 Biliuria

R82.3 Hemoglobinuria
EXCLUDES 1   *hemoglobinuria due to hemolysis from external causes
NEC (D59.6)*
*hemoglobinuria due to paroxysmal nocturnal
[Marchiafava-Micheli] (D59.5)*

R82.4 Acetonuria
Ketonuria

**R82.5 Elevated urine levels of drugs, medicaments and biological
substances**
Elevated urine levels of catecholamines
Elevated urine levels of indoleacetic acid
Elevated urine levels of 17-ketosteroids
Elevated urine levels of steroids

**R82.6 Abnormal urine levels of substances chiefly nonmedicinal as
to source**
Abnormal urine level of heavy metals

R82.7 Abnormal findings on microbiological examination of urine
Positive culture findings of urine
EXCLUDES 1   *colonization status (Z22.-)*

**R82.8 Abnormal findings on cytological and histological
examination of urine**

✓5ᵗʰ **R82.9 Other and unspecified abnormal findings in urine**
R82.90 Unspecified abnormal findings in urine
R82.91 Other chromoabnormalities of urine
Chromoconversion (dipstick)
Idiopathic dipstick converts positive for blood with no
cellular forms in sediment
EXCLUDES 1   *hemoglobinuria (R82.3)*
myoglobinuria (R82.1)
R82.99 Other abnormal findings in urine
Cells and casts in urine
Crystalluria
Melanuria

**Abnormal findings on examination of other body fluids,
substances and tissues, without diagnosis (R83-R89)**
EXCLUDES 1   *abnormal findings on antenatal screening of mother (O28.-)*
*diagnostic abnormal findings classified elsewhere—see Alphabetical
Index*
EXCLUDES 2   *abnormal findings on examination of blood, without diagnosis (R70-
R79)*
*abnormal findings on examination of urine, without diagnosis (R80-
R82)*
abnormal tumor markers (R97.-)

✓4ᵗʰ **R83 Abnormal findings in cerebrospinal fluid**
R83.0 Abnormal level of enzymes in cerebrospinal fluid
R83.1 Abnormal level of hormones in cerebrospinal fluid
**R83.2 Abnormal level of other drugs, medicaments and biological
substances in cerebrospinal fluid**
**R83.3 Abnormal level of substances chiefly nonmedicinal as to
source in cerebrospinal fluid**
R83.4 Abnormal immunological findings in cerebrospinal fluid
R83.5 Abnormal microbiological findings in cerebrospinal fluid
Positive culture findings in cerebrospinal fluid
EXCLUDES 1   *colonization status (Z22.-)*
R83.6 Abnormal cytological findings in cerebrospinal fluid
R83.8 Other abnormal findings in cerebrospinal fluid
Abnormal chromosomal findings in cerebrospinal fluid
R83.9 Unspecified abnormal finding in cerebrospinal fluid

✓4ᵗʰ **R84 Abnormal findings in specimens from respiratory organs and
thorax**
Abnormal findings in bronchial washings
Abnormal findings in nasal secretions
Abnormal findings in pleural fluid
Abnormal findings in sputum
Abnormal findings in throat scrapings
EXCLUDES 1   *blood-stained sputum (R04.2)*

**R84.0 Abnormal level of enzymes in specimens from respiratory
organs and thorax**

**R84.1 Abnormal level of hormones in specimens from respiratory
organs and thorax**

**R84.2 Abnormal level of other drugs, medicaments and biological
substances in specimens from respiratory organs and thorax**

**R84.3 Abnormal level of substances chiefly nonmedicinal as to
source in specimens from respiratory organs and thorax**

**R84.4 Abnormal immunological findings in specimens from
respiratory organs and thorax**

**R84.5 Abnormal microbiological findings in specimens from
respiratory organs and thorax**
Positive culture findings in specimens from respiratory organs
and thorax
EXCLUDES 1   *colonization status (Z22.-)*

**R84.6 Abnormal cytological findings in specimens from respiratory
organs and thorax**

**R84.7 Abnormal histological findings in specimens from respiratory
organs and thorax**

**R84.8 Other abnormal findings in specimens from respiratory
organs and thorax**
Abnormal chromosomal findings in specimens from respiratory
organs and thorax

**R84.9 Unspecified abnormal finding in specimens from respiratory
organs and thorax**

✓4ᵗʰ **R85 Abnormal findings in specimens from digestive organs and
abdominal cavity**
INCLUDES   abnormal findings in peritoneal fluid
abnormal findings in saliva
EXCLUDES 1   *cloudy peritoneal dialysis effluent (R88.0)*
fecal abnormalities (R19.5)

**R85.0 Abnormal level of enzymes in specimens from digestive
organs and abdominal cavity**

**R85.1 Abnormal level of hormones in specimens from digestive
organs and abdominal cavity**

**R85.2 Abnormal level of other drugs, medicaments and biological
substances in specimens from digestive organs and
abdominal cavity**

**R85.3 Abnormal level of substances chiefly nonmedicinal as to
source in specimens from digestive organs and abdominal
cavity**

**R85.4 Abnormal immunological findings in specimens from
digestive organs and abdominal cavity**

**R85.5 Abnormal microbiological findings in specimens from
digestive organs and abdominal cavity**
Positive culture findings in specimens from digestive organs and
abdominal cavity
EXCLUDES 1   *colonization status (Z22.-)*

☑5ᵗʰ **R85.6** **Abnormal** cytological **findings in specimens from digestive organs and abdominal cavity**

   ☑6ᵗʰ **R85.61** **Abnormal cytologic smear of anus**

      EXCLUDES 1 *abnormal cytological findings in specimens from other digestive organs and abdominal cavity (R85.69)*

           anal intraepithelial neoplasia I [AIN I] (K62.82)

           anal intraepithelial neoplasia II [AIN II] (K62.82)

           anal intraepithelial neoplasia III [AIN III] (D01.3)

           carcinoma in situ of anus (histologically confirmed) (D01.3)

           dysplasia (mild) (moderate) of anus (histologically confirmed) (K62.82)

           severe dysplasia of anus (histologically confirmed) (D01.3)

      EXCLUDES 2 *anal high risk human papillomavirus (HPV) DNA test positive (R85.81)*

           anal low risk human papillomavirus (HPV) DNA test positive (R85.82)

      R85.610 **Atypical** squamous cells of undetermined significance **on cytologic smear of anus [ASC-US]**

      R85.611 **Atypical squamous cells cannot exclude high grade squamous intraepithelial lesion on cytologic smear of anus [ASC-H]**

      R85.612 **Low grade squamous intraepithelial lesion on cytologic smear of anus [LGSIL]**

      R85.613 **High grade squamous intraepithelial lesion on cytologic smear of anus [HGSIL]**

      R85.614 **Cytologic evidence of** malignancy **on smear of anus**

      R85.615 **Unsatisfactory cytologic smear of anus**

          Inadequate sample of cytologic smear of anus

      R85.616 **Satisfactory anal smear but** lacking transformation zone

      R85.618 Other **abnormal cytological findings on specimens from anus**

      R85.619 Unspecified **abnormal cytological findings in specimens from anus**

          Abnormal anal cytology NOS

          Atypical glandular cells of anus NOS

   R85.69 **Abnormal cytological findings in specimens from other digestive organs and abdominal cavity**

 R85.7 **Abnormal** histological **findings in specimens from digestive organs and abdominal cavity**

☑5ᵗʰ **R85.8** Other **abnormal findings in specimens from digestive organs and abdominal cavity**

   R85.81 **Anal** high risk human papillomavirus [HPV] DNA test positive

      EXCLUDES 1 *anogenital warts due to human papillomavirus (HPV) (A63.0)*

          condyloma acuminatum (A63.0)

   R85.82 **Anal** low risk human papillomavirus [HPV] DNA test positive

      Use additional code for associated human papillomavirus (B97.7)

   R85.89 Other **abnormal findings in specimens from digestive organs and abdominal cavity**

      Abnormal chromosomal findings in specimens from digestive organs and abdominal cavity

 R85.9 Unspecified **abnormal finding in specimens from digestive organs and abdominal cavity**

☑4ᵗʰ **R86** **Abnormal findings in specimens from** male genital organs

   INCLUDES abnormal findings in prostatic secretions

        abnormal findings in semen, seminal fluid

        abnormal spermatozoa

   EXCLUDES 1 *azoospermia (N46.0-)*

        oligospermia (N46.1-)

 R86.0 **Abnormal level of** enzymes **in specimens from male genital organs** ♂

 R86.1 **Abnormal level of** hormones **in specimens from male genital organs** ♂

 R86.2 **Abnormal level of** other drugs, medicaments and biological substances **in specimens from male genital organs** ♂

 R86.3 **Abnormal level of** substances chiefly nonmedicinal **as to source in specimens from male genital organs** ♂

 R86.4 **Abnormal** immunological **findings in specimens from male genital organs** ♂

 R86.5 **Abnormal** microbiological **findings in specimens from male genital organs** ♂

     Positive culture findings in specimens from male genital organs

   EXCLUDES 1 *colonization status (Z22.-)*

 R86.6 **Abnormal** cytological **findings in specimens from male genital organs** ♂

 R86.7 **Abnormal** histological **findings in specimens from male genital organs** ♂

 R86.8 Other **abnormal findings in specimens from male genital organs** ♂

     Abnormal chromosomal findings in specimens from male genital organs

 R86.9 Unspecified **abnormal finding in specimens from male genital organs** ♂

☑4ᵗʰ **R87** **Abnormal findings in specimens from** female genital organs

   Abnormal findings in secretion and smears from cervix uteri

   Abnormal findings in secretion and smears from vagina

   Abnormal findings in secretion and smears from vulva

 R87.0 **Abnormal level of** enzymes **in specimens from female genital organs** ♀

 R87.1 **Abnormal level of** hormones **in specimens from female genital organs** ♀

 R87.2 **Abnormal level of** other drugs, medicaments and biological substances **in specimens from female genital organs** ♀

 R87.3 **Abnormal level of** substances chiefly nonmedicinal **as to source in specimens from female genital organs** ♀

 R87.4 **Abnormal** immunological **findings in specimens from female genital organs** ♀

 R87.5 **Abnormal** microbiological **findings in specimens from female genital organs** ♀

     Positive culture findings in specimens from female genital organs

   EXCLUDES 1 *colonization status (Z22.-)*

☑5ᵗʰ **R87.6** **Abnormal** cytological **findings in specimens from female genital organs**

   ☑6ᵗʰ **R87.61** **Abnormal cytological findings in specimens from cervix uteri**

      EXCLUDES 1 *abnormal cytological findings in specimens from other female genital organs (R87.69)*

          abnormal cytological findings in specimens from vagina (R87.62-)

          carcinoma in situ of cervix uteri (histologically confirmed) (D06.-)

          cervical intraepithelial neoplasia I [CIN I] (N87.0)

          cervical intraepithelial neoplasia II [CIN II] (N87.1)

          cervical intraepithelial neoplasia III [CIN III] (D06.-)

          dysplasia (mild) (moderate) of cervix uteri (histologically confirmed) (N87.-)

          severe dysplasia of cervix uteri (histologically confirmed) (D06.-)

      EXCLUDES 2 *cervical high risk human papillomavirus (HPV) DNA test positive (R87.810)*

          cervical low risk human papillomavirus (HPV) DNA test positive (R87.820)

      R87.610 **Atypical** squamous cells of undetermined significance **on cytologic smear of cervix [ASC-US]** ♀

      R87.611 **Atypical** squamous cells cannot exclude high grade squamous intraepithelial lesion on cytologic smear of cervix [ASC-H] ♀

      R87.612 **Low grade** squamous intraepithelial lesion on cytologic smear of cervix [LGSIL] ♀

      R87.613 **High grade** squamous intraepithelial lesion on cytologic smear of cervix [HGSIL] ♀

      R87.614 **Cytologic evidence of** malignancy **on smear of cervix** ♀

      R87.615 **Unsatisfactory cytologic smear of cervix** ♀

          Inadequate sample of cytologic smear of cervix

☑ Additional Character Required   ✓x7ᵗʰ Xtension Alert   Unacceptable PDx   Manifestation   Hospital Acquired Condition   *EXCLUDES 1* Not Coded Here   *EXCLUDES 2* Not Included Here

R87.616   **Satisfactory cervical smear but lacking transformation zone** ♀

R87.618   **Other abnormal cytological findings on specimens from cervix uteri** ♀

R87.619   **Unspecified abnormal cytological findings in specimens from cervix uteri** ♀
Abnormal cervical cytology NOS
Abnormal Papanicolaou smear of cervix NOS
Abnormal thin preparation smear of cervix NOS
Atypical endocervical cells of cervix NOS
Atypical endometrial cells of cervix NOS
Atypical glandular cells of cervix NOS

√6ᵗʰ R87.62   **Abnormal cytological findings in specimens from vagina**
Use additional code to identify acquired absence of uterus and cervix, if applicable (Z90.71-)
EXCLUDES 1   *abnormal cytological findings in specimens from cervix uteri (R87.61-)*
abnormal cytological findings in specimens from other female genital organs (R87.69)
carcinoma in situ of vagina (histologically confirmed) (D07.2)
dysplasia (mild) (moderate) of vagina (histologically confirmed) (N89.-)
severe dysplasia of vagina (histologically confirmed) (D07.2)
vaginal intraepithelial neoplasia I [VAIN I] (N89.0)
vaginal intraepithelial neoplasia II [VAIN II] (N89.1)
vaginal intraepithelial neoplasia III [VAIN III] (D07.2)
EXCLUDES 2   *vaginal high risk human papillomavirus (HPV) DNA test positive (R87.811)*
vaginal low risk human papillomavirus (HPV) DNA test positive (R87.821)

R87.620   **Atypical squamous cells of undetermined significance on cytologic smear of vagina [ASC-US]** ♀

R87.621   **Atypical squamous cells cannot exclude high grade squamous intraepithelial lesion on cytologic smear of vagina [ASC-H]** ♀

R87.622   **Low grade squamous intraepithelial lesion on cytologic smear of vagina [LGSIL]** ♀

R87.623   **High grade squamous intraepithelial lesion on cytologic smear of vagina [HGSIL]** ♀

R87.624   **Cytologic evidence of malignancy on smear of vagina** ♀

R87.625   **Unsatisfactory cytologic smear of vagina** ♀
Inadequate sample of cytologic smear of vagina

R87.628   **Other abnormal cytological findings on specimens from vagina** ♀

R87.629   **Unspecified abnormal cytological findings in specimens from vagina** ♀
Abnormal Papanicolaou smear of vagina NOS
Abnormal thin preparation smear of vagina NOS
Abnormal vaginal cytology NOS
Atypical endocervical cells of vagina NOS
Atypical endometrial cells of vagina NOS
Atypical glandular cells of vagina NOS

R87.69   **Abnormal cytological findings in specimens from other female genital organs** ♀
Abnormal cytological findings in specimens from female genital organs NOS
EXCLUDES 1   *dysplasia of vulva (histologically confirmed) (N90.0-N90.3)*

R87.7   **Abnormal histological findings in specimens from female genital organs** ♀
EXCLUDES 1   *carcinoma in situ (histologically confirmed) of female genital organs (D06-D07.3)*
cervical intraepithelial neoplasia I [CIN I] (N87.0)
cervical intraepithelial neoplasia II [CIN II] (N87.1)
cervical intraepithelial neoplasia III [CIN III] (D06.-)
dysplasia (mild) (moderate) of cervix uteri (histologically confirmed) (N87.-)
dysplasia (mild) (moderate) of vagina (histologically confirmed) (N89.-)
severe dysplasia of cervix uteri (histologically confirmed) (D06.-)
severe dysplasia of vagina (histologically confirmed) (D07.2)
vaginal intraepithelial neoplasia I [VAIN I] (N89.0)
vaginal intraepithelial neoplasia II [VAIN II] (N89.1)
vaginal intraepithelial neoplasia III [VAIN III] (D07.2)

√5ᵗʰ R87.8   **Other abnormal findings in specimens from female genital organs**

√6ᵗʰ R87.81   **High risk human papillomavirus [HPV] DNA test positive from female genital organs**
EXCLUDES 1   *anogenital warts due to human papillomavirus (HPV) (A63.0)*
condyloma acuminatum (A63.0)

R87.810   **Cervical high risk human papillomavirus [HPV] DNA test positive** ♀

R87.811   **Vaginal high risk human papillomavirus [HPV] DNA test positive** ♀

√6ᵗʰ R87.82   **Low risk human papillomavirus [HPV] DNA test positive from female genital organs**
Use additional code for associated human papillomavirus (B97.7)

R87.820   **Cervical low risk human papillomavirus [HPV] DNA test positive** ♀

R87.821   **Vaginal low risk human papillomavirus [HPV] DNA test positive** ♀

R87.89   **Other abnormal findings in specimens from female genital organs** ♀
Abnormal chromosomal findings in specimens from female genital organs

R87.9   **Unspecified abnormal finding in specimens from female genital organs** ♀

√4ᵗʰ R88   **Abnormal findings in other body fluids and substances**

R88.0   **Cloudy (hemodialysis) (peritoneal) dialysis effluent**

R88.8   **Abnormal findings in other body fluids and substances**

√4ᵗʰ R89   **Abnormal findings in specimens from other organs, systems and tissues**
INCLUDES   abnormal findings in nipple discharge
abnormal findings in synovial fluid
abnormal findings in wound secretions

R89.0   **Abnormal level of enzymes in specimens from other organs, systems and tissues**

R89.1   **Abnormal level of hormones in specimens from other organs, systems and tissues**

R89.2   **Abnormal level of other drugs, medicaments and biological substances in specimens from other organs, systems and tissues**

R89.3   **Abnormal level of substances chiefly nonmedicinal as to source in specimens from other organs, systems and tissues**

R89.4   **Abnormal immunological findings in specimens from other organs, systems and tissues**

R89.5   **Abnormal microbiological findings in specimens from other organs, systems and tissues**
Positive culture findings in specimens from other organs, systems and tissues
EXCLUDES 1   *colonization status (Z22.-)*

R89.6   **Abnormal cytological findings in specimens from other organs, systems and tissues**

R89.7   **Abnormal histological findings in specimens from other organs, systems and tissues**

R89.8   **Other abnormal findings in specimens from other organs, systems and tissues**
Abnormal chromosomal findings in specimens from other organs, systems and tissues

N Newborn: 0   P Pediatric: 0-17   M Maternity: 12-55   A Adult: 15-124   MCC Major CC Condition   PDx MCC PDx acts as own MCC   CC CC Condition   PDx CC PDx acts as own CC

854   ICD-10-CM Draft (2015)

R89.9   **Unspecified** abnormal finding in specimens from other **organs, systems and tissues**

Abnormal findings on diagnostic imaging and in function studies, without diagnosis (R90-R94)

INCLUDES   nonspecific abnormal findings on diagnostic imaging by computerized axial tomography [CAT scan]
nonspecific abnormal findings on diagnostic imaging by magnetic resonance imaging [MRI][NMR]
nonspecific abnormal findings on diagnostic imaging by positron emission tomography [PET scan]
nonspecific abnormal findings on diagnostic imaging by thermography
nonspecific abnormal findings on diagnostic imaging by ultrasound [echogram]
nonspecific abnormal findings on diagnostic imaging by X-ray examination

EXCLUDES 1   *abnormal findings on antenatal screening of mother (O28.-)*
diagnostic abnormal findings classified elsewhere—see Alphabetical Index

✓4ᵗʰ **R90   Abnormal findings on** diagnostic imaging of central nervous system

R90.0   **Intracranial** space-occupying lesion found on diagnostic imaging of central nervous system

✓5ᵗʰ R90.8   **Other abnormal findings on diagnostic imaging of** central nervous system

R90.81   **Abnormal echoencephalogram**

R90.82   **White matter disease, unspecified**

R90.89   **Other abnormal findings on diagnostic imaging of central nervous system**
Other cerebrovascular abnormality found on diagnostic imaging of central nervous system

✓4ᵗʰ **R91   Abnormal findings on diagnostic imaging of** lung

R91.1   **Solitary pulmonary nodule**
Coin lesion lung
Solitary pulmonary nodule, subsegmental branch of the bronchial tree

R91.8   **Other nonspecific abnormal finding of lung field**
Lung mass NOS found on diagnostic imaging of lung
Pulmonary infiltrate NOS
Shadow, lung

✓4ᵗʰ **R92   Abnormal and inconclusive findings on diagnostic imaging of** breast

R92.0   **Mammographic** microcalcification **found on diagnostic imaging of breast**
EXCLUDES 2   *mammographic calcification (calculus) found on diagnostic imaging of breast (R92.1)*

R92.1   **Mammographic** calcification **found on diagnostic imaging of breast**
Mammographic calculus found on diagnostic imaging of breast

R92.2   **Inconclusive mammogram**
Dense breasts NOS
Inconclusive mammogram NEC
Inconclusive mammography due to dense breasts
Inconclusive mammography NEC

R92.8   **Other** abnormal and inconclusive findings on diagnostic imaging of breast

✓4ᵗʰ **R93   Abnormal findings on diagnostic imaging of** other body structures

R93.0   **Abnormal findings on diagnostic imaging of** skull and head, **not elsewhere classified**
EXCLUDES 1   *intracranial space-occupying lesion found on diagnostic imaging (R90.0)*

R93.1   **Abnormal findings on diagnostic imaging of** heart and coronary **circulation**
Abnormal echocardiogram NOS
Abnormal heart shadow

R93.2   **Abnormal findings on diagnostic imaging of** liver and biliary **tract**
Nonvisualization of gallbladder

R93.3   **Abnormal findings on diagnostic imaging of** other parts of digestive tract

R93.4   **Abnormal findings on diagnostic imaging of** urinary organs
Filling defect of bladder found on diagnostic imaging
Filling defect of kidney found on diagnostic imaging
Filling defect of ureter found on diagnostic imaging
EXCLUDES 1   *hypertrophy of kidney (N28.81)*

R93.5   **Abnormal findings on diagnostic imaging of** other abdominal regions, including retroperitoneum

R93.6   **Abnormal findings on diagnostic imaging of** limbs
EXCLUDES 2   *abnormal finding in skin and subcutaneous tissue (R93.8)*

R93.7   **Abnormal findings on diagnostic imaging of** other parts of musculoskeletal system
EXCLUDES 2   *abnormal findings on diagnostic imaging of skull (R93.0)*

R93.8   **Abnormal findings on diagnostic imaging of** other specified body structures
Abnormal finding by radioisotope localization of placenta
Abnormal radiological finding in skin and subcutaneous tissue
Mediastinal shift

R93.9   **Diagnostic imaging inconclusive due to** excess body fat of patient

✓4ᵗʰ **R94   Abnormal results of function studies**
INCLUDES   abnormal results of radionuclide [radioisotope] uptake studies
abnormal results of scintigraphy

✓5ᵗʰ R94.0   **Abnormal results of function studies of** central nervous system

R94.01   **Abnormal** electroencephalogram [EEG]

R94.02   **Abnormal** brain scan

R94.09   **Abnormal results of** other function studies **of central nervous system**

✓5ᵗʰ R94.1   **Abnormal results of function studies of** peripheral nervous system and special senses

✓6ᵗʰ R94.11   **Abnormal results of function studies of** eye

R94.110   **Abnormal** electro-oculogram [EOG]

R94.111   **Abnormal** electroretinogram [ERG]
Abnormal retinal function study

R94.112   **Abnormal** visually evoked potential [VEP]

R94.113   **Abnormal** oculomotor study

R94.118   **Abnormal results of** other **function studies of eye**

✓6ᵗʰ R94.12   **Abnormal results of function studies of** ear and other special senses

R94.120   **Abnormal** auditory function study

R94.121   **Abnormal** vestibular function study

R94.128   **Abnormal results of** other **function studies of ear and other special senses**

✓6ᵗʰ R94.13   **Abnormal results of function studies of** peripheral nervous system

R94.130   **Abnormal response to** nerve stimulation, **unspecified**

R94.131   **Abnormal electromyogram [EMG]**
EXCLUDES 1   *electromyogram of eye (R94.113)*

R94.138   **Abnormal results of** other **function studies of peripheral nervous system**

R94.2   **Abnormal results of** pulmonary function studies
Reduced ventilatory capacity
Reduced vital capacity

✓5ᵗʰ R94.3   **Abnormal results of** cardiovascular function studies

R94.30   **Abnormal result of cardiovascular function study, unspecified**

R94.31   **Abnormal** electrocardiogram [ECG] [EKG]
EXCLUDES 1   *long QT syndrome (I45.81)*

R94.39   **Abnormal result of** other cardiovascular function study
Abnormal electrophysiological intracardiac studies
Abnormal phonocardiogram
Abnormal vectorcardiogram

R94.4   **Abnormal results of** kidney function studies
Abnormal renal function test

R94.5   **Abnormal results of** liver function studies

R94.6   **Abnormal results of** thyroid function studies

R94.7   **Abnormal results of** other endocrine function studies
EXCLUDES 2   *abnormal glucose (R73.0-)*

R94.8   **Abnormal results of function studies of** other organs and systems
Abnormal basal metabolic rate [BMR]
Abnormal bladder function test
Abnormal splenic function test

Symptoms, Signs and Abnormal Clinical and Laboratory Findings

R97–R99

Abnormal tumor markers (R97)

R97 ☑4ᵗʰ **Abnormal tumor markers**
Elevated tumor associated antigens [TAA]
Elevated tumor specific antigens [TSA]

     R97.0   **Elevated carcinoembryonic antigen [CEA]**

     R97.1   **Elevated cancer antigen 125 [CA 125]**   ♀

     13 **R97.2**   **Elevated prostate specific antigen [PSA]**   A♂

     R97.8   **Other abnormal tumor markers**

Ill-defined and unknown cause of mortality (R99)

R99   **Ill-defined and unknown cause of mortality**
Death (unexplained) NOS
Unspecified cause of mortality

---

13 Questionable admission when used as PDx.

🅽 Newborn: 0   🅿 Pediatric: 0-17   🅼 Maternity: 12-55   🅰 Adult: 15-124   **MCC** Major CC Condition   **PDx MCC** PDx acts as own MCC   **CC** CC Condition   **PDx CC** PDx acts as own CC

Chapter 19. Injury, Poisoning and Certain Other Consequences of External Causes (S00-T88)

NOTE   Use secondary code(s) from Chapter 20, External causes of morbidity, to indicate cause of injury. Codes within the T section that include the external cause do not require an additional external cause code.

Use additional code to identify any retained foreign body, if applicable (Z18.-)

EXCLUDES 1   birth trauma (P10-P15)
obstetric trauma (O70-O71)

NOTE   The chapter uses the S-section for coding different types of injuries related to single body regions and the T-section to cover injuries to unspecified body regions as well as poisoning and certain other consequences of external causes.

This chapter contains the following blocks:

S00-S09	Injuries to the head
S10-S19	Injuries to the neck
S20-S29	Injuries to the thorax
S30-S39	Injuries to the abdomen, lower back, lumbar spine, pelvis and external genitals
S40-S49	Injuries to the shoulder and upper arm
S50-S59	Injuries to the elbow and forearm
S60-S69	Injuries to the wrist, hand and fingers
S70-S79	Injuries to the hip and thigh
S80-S89	Injuries to the knee and lower leg
S90-S99	Injuries to the ankle and foot
T07	Injuries involving multiple body regions
T14	Injury of unspecified body region
T15-T19	Effects of foreign body entering through natural orifice
T20-T25	Burns and corrosions of external body surface, specified by site
T26-T28	Burns and corrosions confined to eye and internal organs
T30-T32	Burns and corrosions of multiple and unspecified body regions
T33-T34	Frostbite
T36-T50	Poisoning by, adverse effect of and underdosing of drugs, medicaments and biological substances
T51-T65	Toxic effects of substances chiefly nonmedicinal as to source
T66-T78	Other and unspecified effects of external causes
T79	Certain early complications of trauma
T80-T88	Complications of surgical and medical care, not elsewhere classified

Injuries to the head (S00-S09)

INCLUDES   injuries of ear
injuries of eye
injuries of face [any part]
injuries of gum
injuries of jaw
injuries of oral cavity
injuries of palate
injuries of periocular area
injuries of scalp
injuries of temporomandibular joint area
injuries of tongue
injuries of tooth

Code also for any associated infection

EXCLUDES 2   burns and corrosions (T20-T32)
effects of foreign body in ear (T16)
effects of foreign body in larynx (T17.3)
effects of foreign body in mouth NOS (T18.0)
effects of foreign body in nose (T17.0-T17.1)
effects of foreign body in pharynx (T17.2)
effects of foreign body on external eye (T15.-)
frostbite (T33-T34)
insect bite or sting, venomous (T63.4)

√4th **S00**   **Superficial injury of head**

EXCLUDES 1   diffuse cerebral contusion (S06.2-)
focal cerebral contusion (S06.3-)
injury of eye and orbit (S05.-)
open wound of head (S01.-)

The appropriate 7th is to be added to each code from category S00.
A   initial encounter
D   subsequent encounter
S   sequela

√5th **S00.0**   **Superficial injury of scalp**

√x7th **S00.00**   Unspecified superficial injury of scalp

√x7th **S00.01**   Abrasion of scalp

√x7th **S00.02**   Blister (nonthermal) of scalp

√x7th **S00.03**   Contusion of scalp
Bruise of scalp
Hematoma of scalp

√x7th **S00.04**   External constriction of part of scalp

√x7th **S00.05**   Superficial foreign body of scalp
Splinter in the scalp

√x7th **S00.06**   Insect bite (nonvenomous) of scalp

√x7th **S00.07**   Other superficial bite of scalp
EXCLUDES 1   open bite of scalp (S01.05)

√5th **S00.1**   **Contusion of eyelid and periocular area**
Black eye
EXCLUDES 2   contusion of eyeball and orbital tissues (S05.1)

√x7th **S00.10**   Contusion of unspecified eyelid and periocular area

√x7th **S00.11**   Contusion of right eyelid and periocular area

√x7th **S00.12**   Contusion of left eyelid and periocular area

√5th **S00.2**   **Other and unspecified superficial injuries of eyelid and periocular area**
EXCLUDES 2   superficial injury of conjunctiva and cornea (S05.0-)

√6th **S00.20**   Unspecified superficial injury of eyelid and periocular area

√7th **S00.201**   Unspecified superficial injury of right eyelid and periocular area

√7th **S00.202**   Unspecified superficial injury of left eyelid and periocular area

√7th **S00.209**   Unspecified superficial injury of unspecified eyelid and periocular area

√6th **S00.21**   Abrasion of eyelid and periocular area

√7th **S00.211**   Abrasion of right eyelid and periocular area

√7th **S00.212**   Abrasion of left eyelid and periocular area

√7th **S00.219**   Abrasion of unspecified eyelid and periocular area

√6th **S00.22**   Blister (nonthermal) of eyelid and periocular area

√7th **S00.221**   Blister (nonthermal) of right eyelid and periocular area

√7th **S00.222**   Blister (nonthermal) of left eyelid and periocular area

√7th **S00.229**   Blister (nonthermal) of unspecified eyelid and periocular area

√6th **S00.24**   External constriction of eyelid and periocular area

√7th **S00.241**   External constriction of right eyelid and periocular area

√7th **S00.242**   External constriction of left eyelid and periocular area

√7th **S00.249**   External constriction of unspecified eyelid and periocular area

√6th **S00.25**   Superficial foreign body of eyelid and periocular area
Splinter of eyelid and periocular area
EXCLUDES 2   retained foreign body in eyelid (H02.81-)

√7th **S00.251**   Superficial foreign body of right eyelid and periocular area

√7th **S00.252**   Superficial foreign body of left eyelid and periocular area

√7th **S00.259**   Superficial foreign body of unspecified eyelid and periocular area

√6th **S00.26**   Insect bite (nonvenomous) of eyelid and periocular area

√7th **S00.261**   Insect bite (nonvenomous) of right eyelid and periocular area

√7th **S00.262**   Insect bite (nonvenomous) of left eyelid and periocular area

√7th **S00.269**   Insect bite (nonvenomous) of unspecified eyelid and periocular area

√6th **S00.27**   Other superficial bite of eyelid and periocular area
EXCLUDES 1   open bite of eyelid and periocular area (S01.15)

√7th **S00.271**   Other superficial bite of right eyelid and periocular area

√7th **S00.272**   Other superficial bite of left eyelid and periocular area

√7th **S00.279**   Other superficial bite of unspecified eyelid and periocular area

√5th **S00.3**   **Superficial injury of nose**

√x7th **S00.30**   Unspecified superficial injury of nose

√x7th **S00.31**   Abrasion of nose

√ Additional Character Required   √x7th Xtension Alert   Unacceptable PDx   Manifestation   Hospital Acquired Condition   **EXCLUDES 1** Not Coded Here   **EXCLUDES 2** Not Included Here

Injury, Poisoning and Certain Other Consequences of External Causes

S00.32–S01.05

√x7th **S00.32**   Blister (nonthermal) of nose

√x7th **S00.33**   Contusion of nose
    Bruise of nose
    Hematoma of nose

√x7th **S00.34**   External constriction of nose

√x7th **S00.35**   Superficial foreign body of nose
    Splinter in the nose

√x7th **S00.36**   Insect bite (nonvenomous) of nose

√x7th **S00.37**   Other superficial bite of nose
    EXCLUDES 1   *open bite of nose (S01.25)*

√5th **S00.4**   Superficial injury of ear

  √6th **S00.40**   Unspecified superficial injury of ear

    √7th **S00.401**   Unspecified superficial injury of right ear

    √7th **S00.402**   Unspecified superficial injury of left ear

    √7th **S00.409**   Unspecified superficial injury of unspecified ear

  √6th **S00.41**   Abrasion of ear

    √7th **S00.411**   Abrasion of right ear

    √7th **S00.412**   Abrasion of left ear

    √7th **S00.419**   Abrasion of unspecified ear

  √6th **S00.42**   Blister (nonthermal) of ear

    √7th **S00.421**   Blister (nonthermal) of right ear

    √7th **S00.422**   Blister (nonthermal) of left ear

    √7th **S00.429**   Blister (nonthermal) of unspecified ear

  √6th **S00.43**   Contusion of ear
     Bruise of ear
     Hematoma of ear

    √7th **S00.431**   Contusion of right ear

    √7th **S00.432**   Contusion of left ear

    √7th **S00.439**   Contusion of unspecified ear

  √6th **S00.44**   External constriction of ear

    √7th **S00.441**   External constriction of right ear

    √7th **S00.442**   External constriction of left ear

    √7th **S00.449**   External constriction of unspecified ear

  √6th **S00.45**   Superficial foreign body of ear
     Splinter in the ear

    √7th **S00.451**   Superficial foreign body of right ear

    √7th **S00.452**   Superficial foreign body of left ear

    √7th **S00.459**   Superficial foreign body of unspecified ear

  √6th **S00.46**   Insect bite (nonvenomous) of ear

    √7th **S00.461**   Insect bite (nonvenomous) of right ear

    √7th **S00.462**   Insect bite (nonvenomous) of left ear

    √7th **S00.469**   Insect bite (nonvenomous) of unspecified ear

  √6th **S00.47**   Other superficial bite of ear
     EXCLUDES 1   *open bite of ear (S01.35)*

    √7th **S00.471**   Other superficial bite of right ear

    √7th **S00.472**   Other superficial bite of left ear

    √7th **S00.479**   Other superficial bite of unspecified ear

√5th **S00.5**   Superficial injury of lip and oral cavity

  √6th **S00.50**   Unspecified superficial injury of lip and oral cavity

    √7th **S00.501**   Unspecified superficial injury of lip

    √7th **S00.502**   Unspecified superficial injury of oral cavity

  √6th **S00.51**   Abrasion of lip and oral cavity

    √7th **S00.511**   Abrasion of lip

    √7th **S00.512**   Abrasion of oral cavity

  √6th **S00.52**   Blister (nonthermal) of lip and oral cavity

    √7th **S00.521**   Blister (nonthermal) of lip

    √7th **S00.522**   Blister (nonthermal) of oral cavity

  √6th **S00.53**   Contusion of lip and oral cavity

    √7th **S00.531**   Contusion of lip
       Bruise of lip
       Hematoma of oral cavity

    √7th **S00.532**   Contusion of oral cavity
       Bruise of lip
       Hematoma of oral cavity

  √6th **S00.54**   External constriction of lip and oral cavity

    √7th **S00.541**   External constriction of lip

    √7th **S00.542**   External constriction of oral cavity

  √6th **S00.55**   Superficial foreign body of lip and oral cavity

    √7th **S00.551**   Superficial foreign body of lip
       Splinter of lip and oral cavity

    √7th **S00.552**   Superficial foreign body of oral cavity
       Splinter of lip and oral cavity

  √6th **S00.56**   Insect bite (nonvenomous) of lip and oral cavity

    √7th **S00.561**   Insect bite (nonvenomous) of lip

    √7th **S00.562**   Insect bite (nonvenomous) of oral cavity

  √6th **S00.57**   Other superficial bite of lip and oral cavity

    √7th **S00.571**   Other superficial bite of lip
       EXCLUDES 1   *open bite of lip (S01.551)*

    √7th **S00.572**   Other superficial bite of oral cavity
       EXCLUDES 1   *open bite of oral cavity (S01.552)*

√5th **S00.8**   Superficial injury of other parts of head

  √x7th **S00.80**   Unspecified superficial injury of other part of head

  √x7th **S00.81**   Abrasion of other part of head

  √x7th **S00.82**   Blister (nonthermal) of other part of head

  √x7th **S00.83**   Contusion of other part of head
     Bruise of other part of head
     Hematoma of other part of head

  √x7th **S00.84**   External constriction of other part of head

  √x7th **S00.85**   Superficial foreign body of other part of head
     Splinter in other part of head

  √x7th **S00.86**   Insect bite (nonvenomous) of other part of head

  √x7th **S00.87**   Other superficial bite of other part of head
     EXCLUDES 1   *open bite of other part of head (S01.85)*

√5th **S00.9**   Superficial injury of unspecified part of head

  √x7th **S00.90**   Unspecified superficial injury of unspecified part of head

  √x7th **S00.91**   Abrasion of unspecified part of head

  √x7th **S00.92**   Blister (nonthermal) of unspecified part of head

  √x7th **S00.93**   Contusion of unspecified part of head
     Bruise of head
     Hematoma of head

  √x7th **S00.94**   External constriction of unspecified part of head

  √x7th **S00.95**   Superficial foreign body of unspecified part of head
     Splinter of head

  √x7th **S00.96**   Insect bite (nonvenomous) of unspecified part of head

  √x7th **S00.97**   Other superficial bite of unspecified part of head
     EXCLUDES 1   *open bite of head (S01.95)*

√4th **S01**   **Open wound of head**
   Code also any associated:
     injury of cranial nerve (S04.-)
     injury of muscle and tendon of head (S09.1-)
     intracranial injury (S06.-)
     wound infection
   EXCLUDES 1   *open skull fracture (S02- with 7th B)*
   EXCLUDES 2   *injury of eye and orbit (S05.-)*
           traumatic amputation of part of head (S08.-)

   The appropriate 7th is to be added to each code from category S01.
   A   initial encounter
   D   subsequent encounter
   S   sequela

√5th **S01.0**   Open wound of scalp
   EXCLUDES 1   *avulsion of scalp (S08.0)*

  √x7th **S01.00**   Unspecified open wound of scalp

  √x7th **S01.01**   Laceration without foreign body of scalp

  √x7th **S01.02**   Laceration with foreign body of scalp

  √x7th **S01.03**   Puncture wound without foreign body of scalp

  √x7th **S01.04**   Puncture wound with foreign body of scalp

  √x7th **S01.05**   Open bite of scalp
     Bite of scalp NOS
     EXCLUDES 1   *superficial bite of scalp (S00.06, S00.07-)*

N Newborn: 0   **P** Pediatric: 0-17   **M** Maternity: 12-55   **A** Adult: 15-124   **MCC** Major CC Condition   **PDx MCC** PDx acts as own MCC   **CC** CC Condition   **PDx CC** PDx acts as own CC

858   ICD-10-CM Draft (2015)

√5th **S01.1   Open wound of** eyelid and periocular area
Open wound of eyelid and periocular area with or without involvement of lacrimal passages

> **CC Excl:** For CC codes in subcategory S01.1, unless otherwise noted: CC with 7th character A: S01.101-S01.159 with 7th A, S05.20X-S05.8X9 with 7th A, S05.91X-S05.92X with 7th A, S38.3XXA, T14.8-T14.91, T79.A0X-T79.9XX with 7th A

√6th **S01.10   Unspecified open wound of eyelid and periocular area**

  √7th **S01.101   Unspecified open wound of** right eyelid and periocular area   `CC`

  √7th **S01.102   Unspecified open wound of** left eyelid and periocular area   `CC`

  √7th **S01.109   Unspecified open wound of** unspecified eyelid and periocular area   `CC`

√6th **S01.11   Laceration without foreign body of eyelid and periocular area**

  √7th **S01.111   Laceration without foreign body of** right eyelid and periocular area

  √7th **S01.112   Laceration without foreign body of** left eyelid and periocular area

  √7th **S01.119   Laceration without foreign body of** unspecified eyelid and periocular area

√6th **S01.12   Laceration with foreign body of eyelid and periocular area**

  √7th **S01.121   Laceration with foreign body of** right eyelid and periocular area

  √7th **S01.122   Laceration with foreign body of** left eyelid and periocular area

  √7th **S01.129   Laceration with foreign body of** unspecified eyelid and periocular area

√6th **S01.13   Puncture wound without foreign body of eyelid and periocular area**

  √7th **S01.131   Puncture wound without foreign body of** right eyelid and periocular area

  √7th **S01.132   Puncture wound without foreign body of** left eyelid and periocular area

  √7th **S01.139   Puncture wound without foreign body of** unspecified eyelid and periocular area

√6th **S01.14   Puncture wound with foreign body of eyelid and periocular area**

  √7th **S01.141   Puncture wound with foreign body of** right eyelid and periocular area

  √7th **S01.142   Puncture wound with foreign body of** left eyelid and periocular area

  √7th **S01.149   Puncture wound with foreign body of** unspecified eyelid and periocular area

√6th **S01.15   Open bite of eyelid and periocular area**
Bite of eyelid and periocular area NOS
> **EXCLUDES 1**   superficial bite of eyelid and periocular area (S00.26, S00.27)

  √7th **S01.151   Open bite of** right eyelid and periocular area

  √7th **S01.152   Open bite of** left eyelid and periocular area

  √7th **S01.159   Open bite of** unspecified eyelid and periocular area

√5th **S01.2   Open wound of** nose

√x7th **S01.20   Unspecified open wound of** nose

√x7th **S01.21   Laceration without foreign body of** nose

√x7th **S01.22   Laceration with foreign body of** nose

√x7th **S01.23   Puncture wound without foreign body of** nose

√x7th **S01.24   Puncture wound with foreign body of** nose

√x7th **S01.25   Open bite of** nose
Bite of nose NOS
> **EXCLUDES 1**   superficial bite of nose (S00.36, S00.37)

√5th **S01.3   Open wound of** ear

√6th **S01.30   Unspecified open wound of** ear

  √7th **S01.301   Unspecified open wound of** right ear

  √7th **S01.302   Unspecified open wound of** left ear

  √7th **S01.309   Unspecified open wound of** unspecified ear

√6th **S01.31   Laceration without foreign body of** ear

  √7th **S01.311   Laceration without foreign body of** right ear

  √7th **S01.312   Laceration without foreign body of** left ear

  √7th **S01.319   Laceration without foreign body of** unspecified ear

√6th **S01.32   Laceration with foreign body of** ear

  √7th **S01.321   Laceration with foreign body of** right ear

  √7th **S01.322   Laceration with foreign body of** left ear

  √7th **S01.329   Laceration with foreign body of** unspecified ear

√6th **S01.33   Puncture wound without foreign body of** ear

  √7th **S01.331   Puncture wound without foreign body of** right ear

  √7th **S01.332   Puncture wound without foreign body of** left ear

  √7th **S01.339   Puncture wound without foreign body of** unspecified ear

√6th **S01.34   Puncture wound with foreign body of** ear

  √7th **S01.341   Puncture wound with foreign body of** right ear

  √7th **S01.342   Puncture wound with foreign body of** left ear

  √7th **S01.349   Puncture wound with foreign body of** unspecified ear

√6th **S01.35   Open bite of** ear
Bite of ear NOS
> **EXCLUDES 1**   superficial bite of ear (S00.46, S00.47)

  √7th **S01.351   Open bite of** right ear

  √7th **S01.352   Open bite of** left ear

  √7th **S01.359   Open bite of** unspecified ear

√5th **S01.4   Open wound of** cheek and temporomandibular area

√6th **S01.40   Unspecified open wound of cheek and temporomandibular area**

  √7th **S01.401   Unspecified open wound of** right cheek and temporomandibular area

  √7th **S01.402   Unspecified open wound of** left cheek and temporomandibular area

  √7th **S01.409   Unspecified open wound of** unspecified cheek and temporomandibular area

√6th **S01.41   Laceration without foreign body of cheek and temporomandibular area**

  √7th **S01.411   Laceration without foreign body of** right cheek and temporomandibular area

  √7th **S01.412   Laceration without foreign body of** left cheek and temporomandibular area

  √7th **S01.419   Laceration without foreign body of** unspecified cheek and temporomandibular area

√6th **S01.42   Laceration with foreign body of cheek and temporomandibular area**

  √7th **S01.421   Laceration with foreign body of** right cheek and temporomandibular area

  √7th **S01.422   Laceration with foreign body of** left cheek and temporomandibular area

  √7th **S01.429   Laceration with foreign body of** unspecified cheek and temporomandibular area

√6th **S01.43   Puncture wound without foreign body of cheek and temporomandibular area**

  √7th **S01.431   Puncture wound without foreign body of** right cheek and temporomandibular area

  √7th **S01.432   Puncture wound without foreign body of** left cheek and temporomandibular area

  √7th **S01.439   Puncture wound without foreign body of** unspecified cheek and temporomandibular area

√6th **S01.44   Puncture wound with foreign body of cheek and temporomandibular area**

  √7th **S01.441   Puncture wound with foreign body of** right cheek and temporomandibular area

  √7th **S01.442   Puncture wound with foreign body of** left cheek and temporomandibular area

---

√ Additional Character Required   √x7th Xtension Alert   Unacceptable PDx   Manifestation   Hospital Acquired Condition   **EXCLUDES 1** Not Coded Here   **EXCLUDES 2** Not Included Here

✓7ᵗʰ **S01.449** Puncture wound with foreign body of unspecified cheek and temporomandibular area

✓6ᵗʰ **S01.45** Open bite of cheek and temporomandibular area
Bite of cheek and temporomandibular area NOS
EXCLUDES 2 *superficial bite of cheek and temporomandibular area (S00.86, S00.87)*

✓7ᵗʰ **S01.451** Open bite of right cheek and temporomandibular area

✓7ᵗʰ **S01.452** Open bite of left cheek and temporomandibular area

✓7ᵗʰ **S01.459** Open bite of unspecified cheek and temporomandibular area

✓5ᵗʰ **S01.5** Open wound of lip and oral cavity
EXCLUDES 2 *tooth dislocation (S03.2)*
tooth fracture (S02.5)

✓6ᵗʰ **S01.50** Unspecified open wound of lip and oral cavity

✓7ᵗʰ **S01.501** Unspecified open wound of lip

✓7ᵗʰ **S01.502** Unspecified open wound of oral cavity

✓6ᵗʰ **S01.51** Laceration of lip and oral cavity without foreign body

✓7ᵗʰ **S01.511** Laceration without foreign body of lip

✓7ᵗʰ **S01.512** Laceration without foreign body of oral cavity

✓6ᵗʰ **S01.52** Laceration of lip and oral cavity with foreign body

✓7ᵗʰ **S01.521** Laceration with foreign body of lip

✓7ᵗʰ **S01.522** Laceration with foreign body of oral cavity

✓6ᵗʰ **S01.53** Puncture wound of lip and oral cavity without foreign body

✓7ᵗʰ **S01.531** Puncture wound without foreign body of lip

✓7ᵗʰ **S01.532** Puncture wound without foreign body of oral cavity

✓6ᵗʰ **S01.54** Puncture wound of lip and oral cavity with foreign body

✓7ᵗʰ **S01.541** Puncture wound with foreign body of lip

✓7ᵗʰ **S01.542** Puncture wound with foreign body of oral cavity

✓6ᵗʰ **S01.55** Open bite of lip and oral cavity

✓7ᵗʰ **S01.551** Open bite of lip
Bite of lip NOS
EXCLUDES 1 *superficial bite of lip (S00.571)*

✓7ᵗʰ **S01.552** Open bite of oral cavity
Bite of oral cavity NOS
EXCLUDES 1 *superficial bite of oral cavity (S00.572)*

✓5ᵗʰ **S01.8** Open wound of other parts of head

✓x7ᵗʰ **S01.80** Unspecified open wound of other part of head

✓x7ᵗʰ **S01.81** Laceration without foreign body of other part of head

✓x7ᵗʰ **S01.82** Laceration with foreign body of other part of head

✓x7ᵗʰ **S01.83** Puncture wound without foreign body of other part of head

✓x7ᵗʰ **S01.84** Puncture wound with foreign body of other part of head

✓x7ᵗʰ **S01.85** Open bite of other part of head
Bite of other part of head NOS
EXCLUDES 1 *superficial bite of other part of head (S00.85)*

✓5ᵗʰ **S01.9** Open wound of unspecified part of head

✓x7ᵗʰ **S01.90** Unspecified open wound of unspecified part of head

✓x7ᵗʰ **S01.91** Laceration without foreign body of unspecified part of head

✓x7ᵗʰ **S01.92** Laceration with foreign body of unspecified part of head

✓x7ᵗʰ **S01.93** Puncture wound without foreign body of unspecified part of head

✓x7ᵗʰ **S01.94** Puncture wound with foreign body of unspecified part of head

✓x7ᵗʰ **S01.95** Open bite of unspecified part of head
Bite of head NOS
EXCLUDES 1 *superficial bite of head NOS (S00.97)*

✓4ᵗʰ **S02** **Fracture of skull and facial bones**
NOTE A fracture not indicated as open or closed should be coded to closed.
Code also any associated intracranial injury (S06.-).

The appropriate 7th is to be added to each code from category S02.
A   initial encounter for closed fracture
B   initial encounter for open fracture
D   subsequent encounter for fracture with routine healing
G   subsequent encounter for fracture with delayed healing
K   subsequent encounter for fracture with nonunion
S   sequela

7 ✓x7ᵗʰ **S02.0** **Fracture of vault of skull**   MCC CC
Fracture of frontal bone
Fracture of parietal bone

CC Excl: For CC/MCC codes in subcategory S02.0, unless otherwise noted: CC with 7th character A or MCC with 7th character B: S01.90X-S02.92X with 7th A, S06.0X0-S07.9XX with 7th A, S08.89X-S09.19X with 7th A, S09.8XX-S09.90X with 7th A, S09.92X-S09.93X with 7th A, S16.8XX-S19.9XX with 7th A, S38.3XX with 7th A, T14.8-T14.91, T79.A0X-T79.9XX with 7th A
CC with 7th character K: M80.00X-M84.68X with 7th [K, P], S02.0XX-S02.92X with 7th K, S12.000-S12.691 with 7th K, S22.000-S22.9XX with 7th K, S32.000-S32.9XX with 7th K, S42.001-S42.92X with 7th [K, P], S49.001-S49.199 with 7th [K, P], S52.001-S52.92X with 7th [K, M, N, P, Q, R], S59.001-S59.299 with 7th [K, P], S62.001-S62.92X with 7th [K, P], S72.001-S72.92X with 7th [K, M, N, P, Q, R], S79.001-S79.199 with 7th [K, P], S82.001-S82.92X with 7th [K, M, N, P, Q, R], S89.001-S89.399 with 7th [K, P], S92.001-S92.919 with 7th [K, P]

✓5ᵗʰ **S02.1** **Fracture of base of skull**
EXCLUDES 1 *orbit NOS (S02.8)*
EXCLUDES 2 *orbital floor (S02.3-)*

CC Excl: For CC codes in subcategory S02.1, unless otherwise noted: CC with 7th character A or MCC with 7th character B: S01.90X-S02.92X with 7th A, S06.0X0-S07.9XX with 7th A, S08.89X-S09.19X with 7th A, S09.8XX-S09.90X with 7th A, S09.92X-S09.93X with 7th A, S16.8XX-S19.9XX with 7th A, S38.3XXA, T14.8-T14.91, T79.A0X-T79.9XX with 7th A
CC with 7th character K: M80.00X-M84.68X with 7th [K, P], S02.0XX-S02.92X with 7th K, S12.000-S12.691 with 7th K, S22.000-S22.9XX with 7th K, S32.000-S32.9XX with 7th K, S42.001-S42.92X with 7th [K, P], S49.001-S49.199 with 7th [K, P], S52.001-S52.92X with 7th [K, M, N, P, Q, R], S59.001-S59.299 with 7th [K, P], S62.001-S62.92X with 7th [K, P], S72.001-S72.92X with 7th [K, M, N, P, Q, R], S79.001-S79.199 with 7th [K, P], S82.001-S82.92X with 7th [K, M, N, P, Q, R], S89.001-S89.399 with 7th [K, P], S92.001-S92.919 with 7th [K, P]

7 ✓x7ᵗʰ **S02.10** Unspecified fracture of base of skull   MCC CC

✓6ᵗʰ **S02.11** **Fracture of occiput**

7 ✓7ᵗʰ **S02.110** Type I occipital condyle fracture   MCC CC

7 ✓7ᵗʰ **S02.111** Type II occipital condyle fracture   MCC CC

7 ✓7ᵗʰ **S02.112** Type III occipital condyle fracture   MCC CC

7 ✓7ᵗʰ **S02.113** Unspecified occipital condyle fracture   MCC CC

7 ✓7ᵗʰ **S02.118** Other fracture of occiput   MCC CC

7 ✓7ᵗʰ **S02.119** Unspecified fracture of occiput   MCC CC

7 ✓x7ᵗʰ **S02.19** Other fracture of base of skull   MCC CC
Fracture of anterior fossa of base of skull
Fracture of ethmoid sinus
Fracture of frontal sinus
Fracture of middle fossa of base of skull
Fracture of orbital roof
Fracture of posterior fossa of base of skull
Fracture of sphenoid
Fracture of temporal bone

---

7 HAC = Initial encounter only (7th character A, B or C) and not POA.

N Newborn: 0   P Pediatric: 0-17   M Maternity: 12-55   A Adult: 15-124   MCC Major CC Condition   PDx MCC PDx acts as own MCC   CC CC Condition   PDx CC PDx acts as own CC

860   ICD-10-CM Draft (2015)

7 ✓x7th **S02.2**   **Fracture of nasal bones**   `CC`

CC Excl: CC with 7th character B: S01.90X-S02.92X with 7th A, S06.0X0-S07.9XX with 7th A, S08.89-S09.19X with 7th A, S09.8XX-S09.90X with 7th A, S09.92X-S09.93X with 7th A, S16.8XX-S19.9XX with 7th A, S38.3XXA, T14.8-T14.91, T79.A0X-T79.9XX with 7th A

CC Excl: CC with 7th character K: M80.00X-M84.68X with 7th [K, P], S02.0XX-S02.92X with 7th K, S12.000-S12.691 with 7th K, S22.000-S22.9XX with 7th K, S32.000-S32.9XX with 7th K, S42.001-S42.92X with 7th [K, P], S49.001-S49.199 with 7th [K, P], S52.001-S52.92X with 7th [K, M, N, P, Q, R], S59.001-S59.299 with 7th [K, P], S62.001-S62.92X with 7th [K, P], S72.001-S72.92X with 7th [K, M, N, P, Q, R], S79.001-S79.199 with 7th [K, P], S82.001-S82.92X with 7th [K, M, N, P, Q, R], S89.001-S89.399 with 7th [K, P], S92.001-S92.919 with 7th [K, P]

7 ✓x7th **S02.3**   **Fracture of orbital floor**   `CC`

    EXCLUDES 1   orbit NOS (S02.8)
    EXCLUDES 2   orbital roof (S02.1-)

CC Excl: CC with 7th character A or B: S01.90X-S02.92X with 7th A, S06.0X0-S07.9XX with 7th A, S08.89X-S09.19X with 7th A, S09.8XX-S09.90X with 7th A, S09.92X-S09.93X with 7th A, S16.8XX-S19.9XX with 7th A, S38.3XXA, T14.8-T14.91, T79.A0X-T79.9XX with 7th A

CC with 7th character K: M80.00X-M84.68X with 7th [K, P], S02.0XX-S02.92X with 7th K, S12.000-S12.691 with 7th K, S22.000-S22.9XX with 7th K, S32.000-S32.9XX with 7th K, S42.001-S42.92X with 7th [K, P], S49.001-S49.199 with 7th [K, P], S52.001-S52.92X with 7th [K, M, N, P, Q, R], S59.001-S59.299 with 7th [K, P], S62.001-S62.92X with 7th [K, M, N, P, Q, R], S72.001-S72.92X with 7th [K, M, N, P, Q, R], S79.001-S79.199 with 7th [K, P], S82.001-S82.92X with 7th [K, M, N, P, Q, R], S89.001-S89.399 with 7th [K, P], S92.001-S92.919 with 7th [K, P]

✓5th **S02.4**   **Fracture of malar, maxillary and zygoma bones**
    Fracture of superior maxilla
    Fracture of upper jaw (bone)
    Fracture of zygomatic process of temporal bone

CC Excl: For CC codes in subcategory S02.4, unless otherwise noted: CC with 7th character A or B: S01.90X-S03.0XX with 7th A, S06.0X0-S07.9XX with 7th A, S08.89X-S09.19X with 7th A, S09.8XX-S09.90X with 7th A, S09.92X-S09.93X with 7th A, S16.8XX-S19.9XX with 7th A, S38.3XA, T14.8-T14.91, T79.A0X-T79.9XX with 7th A

CC with 7th character K: M80.00X-M84.68X with 7th [K, P], S02.0XX-S02.92X with 7th K, S12.000-S12.691 with 7th K, S22.000-S22.9XX with 7th K, S32.000-S32.9XX with 7th K, S42.001-S42.92X with 7th [K, P], S49.001-S49.199 with 7th [K, P], S52.001-S52.92X with 7th [K, M, N, P, Q, R], S59.001-S59.299 with 7th [K, P], S62.001-S62.92X with 7th [K, P], S72.001-S72.92X with 7th [K, M, N, P, Q, R], S79.001-S79.199 with 7th [K, P], S82.001-S82.92X with 7th [K, M, N, P, Q, R], S89.001-S89.399 with 7th [K, P], S92.001-S92.919 with 7th [K, P]

✓6th **S02.40**   **Fracture of malar, maxillary and zygoma bones, unspecified**

7 ✓7th **S02.400**   **Malar fracture unspecified**   `CC`
7 ✓7th **S02.401**   **Maxillary fracture, unspecified**   `CC`
7 ✓7th **S02.402**   **Zygomatic fracture, unspecified**   `CC`

✓6th **S02.41**   **LeFort fracture**

7 ✓7th **S02.411**   **LeFort I fracture**   `CC`
7 ✓7th **S02.412**   **LeFort II fracture**   `CC`
7 ✓7th **S02.413**   **LeFort III fracture**   `CC`

7 ✓x7th **S02.42**   **Fracture of alveolus of maxilla**   `CC`

CC Excl: CC with 7th character A or B: S01.90X-S02.92X with 7th A, S06.0X0-S07.9XX with 7th A, S08.89X-S09.19X with 7th A, S09.8XX-S09.90X with 7th A, S09.92X-S09.93X with 7th A, S16.8XX-S19.9XX with 7th A, S38.3XXA, T14.8-T14.91, T79.A0X-T79.9XX with 7th A

CC with 7th character K: M80.00X-M84.68X with 7th [K, P], S02.0XX-S02.92X with 7th K, S12.000-S12.691 with 7th K, S22.000-S22.9XX with 7th K, S32.000-S32.9XX with 7th K, S42.001-S42.92X with 7th [K, P], S49.001-S49.199 with 7th [K, P], S52.001-S52.92X with 7th [K, M, N, P, Q, R], S59.001-S59.299 with 7th [K, P], S62.001-S62.92X with 7th [K, P], S72.001-S72.92X with 7th [K, M, N, P, Q, R], S79.001-S79.199 with 7th [K, P], S82.001-S82.92X with 7th [K, M, N, P, Q, R], S89.001-S89.399 with 7th [K, P], S92.001-S92.919 with 7th [K, P]

✓x7th **S02.5**   **Fracture of tooth (traumatic)**   `CC`
    Broken tooth
    EXCLUDES 1   cracked tooth (nontraumatic) (K03.81)
    CC Excl: CC with 7th character K: See Code: S02.42

✓5th **S02.6**   **Fracture of mandible**
    Fracture of lower jaw (bone)

CC Excl: For CC codes in subcategory S02.6, unless otherwise noted: CC with 7th character A or B: S01.90X-S03.0XX with 7th A, S06.0X0-S07.9XX with 7th A, S08.89-S09.19X with 7th A, S09.8XX-S09.90X with 7th A, S09.92X-S09.93X with 7th A, S16.8XX-S19.9XX with 7th A, S38.3XXA, T14.8-T14.91, T79.A0X-T79.9XX with 7th A

CC with 7th character K: M80.00X-M84.68X with 7th [K, P], S02.0XX-S02.92X with 7th K, S12.000-S12.691 with 7th K, S22.000-S22.9XX with 7th K, S32.000-S32.9XX with 7th K, S42.001-S42.92X with 7th [K, P], S49.001-S49.199 with 7th [K, P], S52.001-S52.92X with 7th [K, M, N, P, Q, R], S59.001-S59.299 with 7th [K, P], S62.001-S62.92X with 7th [K, P], S72.001-S72.92X with 7th [K, M, N, P, Q, R], S79.001-S79.199 with 7th [K, M, N, P, Q, R], S82.001-S82.92X with 7th [K, M, N, P, Q, R], S89.001-S89.399 with 7th [K, P], S92.001-S92.919 with 7th [K, P]

✓6th **S02.60**   **Fracture of mandible, unspecified**

7 ✓7th **S02.600**   **Fracture of unspecified part of body of mandible**   `CC`
7 ✓7th **S02.609**   **Fracture of mandible, unspecified**   `CC`

7 ✓x7th **S02.61**   **Fracture of condylar process of mandible**   `CC`
7 ✓x7th **S02.62**   **Fracture of subcondylar process of mandible**   `CC`
7 ✓x7th **S02.63**   **Fracture of coronoid process of mandible**   `CC`
7 ✓x7th **S02.64**   **Fracture of ramus of mandible**   `CC`
7 ✓x7th **S02.65**   **Fracture of angle of mandible**   `CC`
7 ✓x7th **S02.66**   **Fracture of symphysis of mandible**   `CC`
7 ✓x7th **S02.67**   **Fracture of alveolus of mandible**   `CC`
7 ✓x7th **S02.69**   **Fracture of mandible of other specified site**   `CC`

7 ✓x7th **S02.8**   **Fractures of other specified skull and facial bones**   `CC`
    Fracture of orbit NOS
    Fracture of palate
    EXCLUDES 1   fracture of orbital floor (S02.3-)
            fracture of orbital roof (S02.1-)

CC Excl: CC with 7th character A or B: S01.90X-S02.92X with 7th A, S06.0X0-S07.9XX with 7th A, S08.89-S09.19X with 7th A, S09.8XX-S09.90X with 7th A, S09.92X-S09.93X with 7th A, S16.8XX-S19.9XX with 7th A, S38.3XXA, T14.8-T14.91, T79.A0X-T79.9XX with 7th A

CC with 7th character K: M80.00X-M84.68X with 7th [K, P], S02.0XX-S02.92X with 7th K, S12.000-S12.691 with 7th K, S22.000-S22.9XX with 7th K, S32.000-S32.9XX with 7th K, S42.001-S42.92X with 7th [K, P], S49.001-S49.199 with 7th [K, P], S52.001-S52.92X with 7th [K, M, N, P, Q, R], S59.001-S59.299 with 7th [K, P], S62.001-S62.92X with 7th [K, P], S72.001-S72.92X with 7th [K, M, N, P, Q, R], S79.001-S79.199 with 7th [K, P], S82.001-S82.92X with 7th [K, M, N, P, Q, R], S89.001-S89.399 with 7th [K, P], S92.001-S92.919 with 7th [K, P]

✓5th **S02.9**   **Fracture of unspecified skull and facial bones**

CC Excl: For CC codes in subcategory S02.9, unless otherwise noted: CC with 7th character A or MCC with 7th character B: S01.90X-S02.92X with 7th A, S06.0X0-S07.9XXwith 7th A, S08.89X-S09.19X with 7th A, S09.8XX-S09.90X with 7th A, S09.92X-S09.93X with 7th A, S16.8XX-S19.9XX with 7th A, S38.3XXA, T14.8-T14.91, T79.A0X-T79.9XX with 7th A

CC with 7th character K: M80.00X-M84.68X with 7th [K, P], S02.0XX-S02.92X with 7th K, S12.000-S12.691 with 7th K, S22.000-S22.9XX with 7th K, S32.000-S32.9XX with 7th K, S42.001-S42.92X with 7th [K, P], S49.001-S49.199 with 7th [K, P], S52.001-S52.92X with 7th [K, M, N, P, Q, R], S59.001-S59.299 with 7th [K, P], S62.001-S62.92X with 7th [K, P], S72.001-S72.92X with 7th [K, M, N, P, Q, R], S79.001-S79.199 with 7th [K, P], S82.001-S82.92X with 7th [K, M, N, P, Q, R], S89.001-S89.399 with 7th [K, P], S92.001-S92.919 with 7th [K, P]

7 ✓x7th **S02.91**   **Unspecified fracture of skull**   `MCC` `CC`
7 ✓x7th **S02.92**   **Unspecified fracture of facial bones**   `CC`

---

7 HAC = Initial encounter only (7th character A, B or C) and not POA.

✓ Additional Character Required   ✓x7th Xtension Alert   Unacceptable PDx   Manifestation   Hospital Acquired Condition   EXCLUDES 1 Not Coded Here   EXCLUDES 2 Not Included Here

Injury, Poisoning and Certain Other Consequences of External Causes

S03–S04.9

✓4th **S03   Dislocation and sprain of joints and ligaments of head**

    INCLUDES   avulsion of joint (capsule) or ligament of head
                laceration of cartilage, joint (capsule) or ligament of head
                sprain of cartilage, joint (capsule) or ligament of head
                traumatic hemarthrosis of joint or ligament of head
                traumatic rupture of joint or ligament of head
                traumatic subluxation of joint or ligament of head
                traumatic tear of joint or ligament of head

Code also any associated open wound

EXCLUDES 2   strain of muscle or tendon of head (S09.1)

The appropriate 7th is to be added to each code from category S03.
A   initial encounter
D   subsequent encounter
S   sequela

✓x7th **S03.0   Dislocation of jaw**
      Dislocation of jaw (cartilage) (meniscus)
      Dislocation of mandible
      Dislocation of temporomandibular (joint)

✓x7th **S03.1   Dislocation of septal cartilage of nose**

✓x7th **S03.2   Dislocation of tooth**

✓x7th **S03.4   Sprain of jaw**
      Sprain of temporomandibular (joint) (ligament)

✓x7th **S03.8   Sprain of joints and ligaments of other parts of head**

✓x7th **S03.9   Sprain of joints and ligaments of unspecified parts of head**

✓4th **S04   Injury of cranial nerve**
      The selection of side should be based on the side of the body being affected
      Code first any associated intracranial injury (S06.-)
      Code also any associated:
        open wound of head (S01.-)
        skull fracture (S02.-)

The appropriate 7th is to be added to each code from category S04.
A   initial encounter
D   subsequent encounter
S   sequela

✓5th **S04.0   Injury of optic nerve and pathways**
      Use additional code to identify any visual field defect or blindness (H53.4-, H54)

CC Excl: For CC codes in subcategory S04.0, unless otherwise noted: CC with 7th character A: S04.011-S04.9XX with 7th A

   ✓6th **S04.01   Injury of optic nerve**
         Injury of 2nd cranial nerve
     ✓7th **S04.011   Injury of optic nerve, right eye**   CC
     ✓7th **S04.012   Injury of optic nerve, left eye**   CC
     ✓7th **S04.019   Injury of optic nerve, unspecified eye**   CC
            Injury of optic nerve NOS

   ✓x7th **S04.02   Injury of optic chiasm**   CC

   ✓6th **S04.03   Injury of optic tract and pathways**
         Injury of optic radiation
     ✓7th **S04.031   Injury of optic tract and pathways, right eye**   CC
     ✓7th **S04.032   Injury of optic tract and pathways, left eye**   CC
     ✓7th **S04.039   Injury of optic tract and pathways, unspecified eye**
            Injury of optic tract and pathways NOS

   ✓6th **S04.04   Injury of visual cortex**
     ✓7th **S04.041   Injury of visual cortex, right eye**   CC
     ✓7th **S04.042   Injury of visual cortex, left eye**   CC
     ✓7th **S04.049   Injury of visual cortex, unspecified eye**   CC
            Injury of visual cortex NOS

✓5th **S04.1   Injury of oculomotor nerve**
      Injury of 3rd cranial nerve

CC Excl: For CC codes in subcategory S04.1, unless otherwise noted: CC with 7th character A: S04.10X-S04.12X with 7th A, S04.811-S04.9XX with 7th A

   ✓x7th **S04.10   Injury of oculomotor nerve, unspecified side**   CC
   ✓x7th **S04.11   Injury of oculomotor nerve, right side**   CC
   ✓x7th **S04.12   Injury of oculomotor nerve, left side**   CC

✓5th **S04.2   Injury of trochlear nerve**
      Injury of 4th cranial nerve

CC Excl: For CC codes in subcategory S04.2, unless otherwise noted: CC with 7th character A: S04.20X-S04.22X with 7th A, S04.811-S04.9XX with 7th A

   ✓x7th **S04.20   Injury of trochlear nerve, unspecified side**   CC
   ✓x7th **S04.21   Injury of trochlear nerve, right side**   CC
   ✓x7th **S04.22   Injury of trochlear nerve, left side**   CC

✓5th **S04.3   Injury of trigeminal nerve**
      Injury of 5th cranial nerve

CC Excl: For CC codes in subcategory S04.3, unless otherwise noted: CC with 7th character A: S04.30X-S04.32X with 7th A, S04.811-S04.9XX with 7th A

   ✓x7th **S04.30   Injury of trigeminal nerve, unspecified side**   CC
   ✓x7th **S04.31   Injury of trigeminal nerve, right side**   CC
   ✓x7th **S04.32   Injury of trigeminal nerve, left side**   CC

✓5th **S04.4   Injury of abducent nerve**
      Injury of 6th cranial nerve

CC Excl: For CC codes in subcategory S04.4, unless otherwise noted: CC with 7th character A: S04.40X-S04.42X with 7th A, S04.811-S04.9XX with 7th A

   ✓x7th **S04.40   Injury of abducent nerve, unspecified side**   CC
   ✓x7th **S04.41   Injury of abducent nerve, right side**   CC
   ✓x7th **S04.42   Injury of abducent nerve, left side**   CC

✓5th **S04.5   Injury of facial nerve**
      Injury of 7th cranial nerve

CC Excl: For CC codes in subcategory S04.5, unless otherwise noted: CC with 7th character A: S04.50X-S04.52X with 7th A, S04.811-S04.9XX with 7th A

   ✓x7th **S04.50   Injury of facial nerve, unspecified side**   CC
   ✓x7th **S04.51   Injury of facial nerve, right side**   CC
   ✓x7th **S04.52   Injury of facial nerve, left side**   CC

✓5th **S04.6   Injury of acoustic nerve**
      Injury of auditory nerve
      Injury of 8th cranial nerve

CC Excl: For CC codes in subcategory S04.6, unless otherwise noted: CC with 7th character A: S04.60X-S04.62X with 7th A, S04.811-S04.9XX with 7th A

   ✓x7th **S04.60   Injury of acoustic nerve, unspecified side**   CC
   ✓x7th **S04.61   Injury of acoustic nerve, right side**   CC
   ✓x7th **S04.62   Injury of acoustic nerve, left side**   CC

✓5th **S04.7   Injury of accessory nerve**
      Injury of 11th cranial nerve

CC Excl: For CC codes in subcategory S04.7 unless otherwise noted: S04.70X-S04.9XX with 7th A

   ✓x7th **S04.70   Injury of accessory nerve, unspecified side**   CC
   ✓x7th **S04.71   Injury of accessory nerve, right side**   CC
   ✓x7th **S04.72   Injury of accessory nerve, left side**   CC

✓5th **S04.8   Injury of other cranial nerves**

CC Excl: For CC codes in subcategory S04.8, unless otherwise noted: CC with 7th character A: S04.811-S04.9XX with 7th A

   ✓6th **S04.81   Injury of olfactory [1st] nerve**
     ✓7th **S04.811   Injury of olfactory [1st] nerve, right side**   CC
     ✓7th **S04.812   Injury of olfactory [1st] nerve, left side**   CC
     ✓7th **S04.819   Injury of olfactory [1st] nerve, unspecified side**   CC

   ✓6th **S04.89   Injury of other cranial nerves**
         Injury of vagus [10th] nerve
     ✓7th **S04.891   Injury of other cranial nerves, right side**   CC
     ✓7th **S04.892   Injury of other cranial nerves, left side**   CC
     ✓7th **S04.899   Injury of other cranial nerves, unspecified side**   CC

✓x7th **S04.9   Injury of unspecified cranial nerve**
      CC Excl: CC with 7th character A: S04.8[1,9][1,2,9]A, S04.9XXA

N Newborn: 0   P Pediatric: 0-17   M Maternity: 12-55   A Adult: 15-124   MCC Major CC Condition   PDx MCC PDx acts as own MCC   CC CC Condition   PDx CC PDx acts as own CC

862   ICD-10-CM Draft (2015)

✓4ᵗʰ S05　Injury of eye and orbit
Open wound of eye and orbit
EXCLUDES 2 2nd cranial [optic] nerve injury (S04.0-)
3rd cranial [oculomotor] nerve injury (S04.1-)
open wound of eyelid and periocular area (S01.1-)
orbital bone fracture (S02.1-, S02.3-, S02.8-)
superficial injury of eyelid (S00.1-S00.2)

The appropriate 7th is to be added to each code from category S05.
A　initial encounter
D　subsequent encounter
S　sequela

CC Excl: For CC codes in category S05, unless otherwise noted: CC with 7th character A: S01.101-S01.159 with 7th A, S05.20X-S05.8X9 with 7th A, S05.91X-S05.92X with 7th A, S38.3XXA, T14.8-T14.91, T79.A0X-T79.9XX with 7th A

✓5ᵗʰ S05.0　Injury of conjunctiva and corneal abrasion without foreign body
EXCLUDES 1 foreign body in conjunctival sac (T15.1)
foreign body in cornea (T15.0)

✓x7ᵗʰ **S05.00**　Injury of conjunctiva and corneal abrasion without foreign body, unspecified eye

✓x7ᵗʰ **S05.01**　Injury of conjunctiva and corneal abrasion without foreign body, right eye

✓x7ᵗʰ **S05.02**　Injury of conjunctiva and corneal abrasion without foreign body, left eye

✓5ᵗʰ S05.1　Contusion of eyeball and orbital tissues
Traumatic hyphema
EXCLUDES 2 black eye NOS (S00.1)
contusion of eyelid and periocular area (S00.1)

✓x7ᵗʰ **S05.10**　Contusion of eyeball and orbital tissues, unspecified eye

✓x7ᵗʰ **S05.11**　Contusion of eyeball and orbital tissues, right eye

✓x7ᵗʰ **S05.12**　Contusion of eyeball and orbital tissues, left eye

✓5ᵗʰ S05.2　Ocular laceration and rupture with prolapse or loss of intraocular tissue

✓x7ᵗʰ **S05.20**　Ocular laceration and rupture with prolapse or loss of intraocular tissue, unspecified eye　CC

✓x7ᵗʰ **S05.21**　Ocular laceration and rupture with prolapse or loss of intraocular tissue, right eye　CC

✓x7ᵗʰ **S05.22**　Ocular laceration and rupture with prolapse or loss of intraocular tissue, left eye　CC

✓5ᵗʰ S05.3　Ocular laceration without prolapse or loss of intraocular tissue
Laceration of eye NOS

✓x7ᵗʰ **S05.30**　Ocular laceration without prolapse or loss of intraocular tissue, unspecified eye　CC

✓x7ᵗʰ **S05.31**　Ocular laceration without prolapse or loss of intraocular tissue, right eye　CC

✓x7ᵗʰ **S05.32**　Ocular laceration without prolapse or loss of intraocular tissue, left eye　CC

✓5ᵗʰ S05.4　Penetrating wound of orbit with or without foreign body
EXCLUDES 2 retained (old) foreign body following penetrating wound in orbit (H05.5-)

✓x7ᵗʰ **S05.40**　Penetrating wound of orbit with or without foreign body, unspecified eye　CC

✓x7ᵗʰ **S05.41**　Penetrating wound of orbit with or without foreign body, right eye　CC

✓x7ᵗʰ **S05.42**　Penetrating wound of orbit with or without foreign body, left eye　CC

✓5ᵗʰ S05.5　Penetrating wound with foreign body of eyeball
EXCLUDES 2 retained (old) intraocular foreign body (H44.6-, H44.7)

CC Excl: CC with 7th character A: S01.101-S01.159 with 7th A, S05.20X-S05.8X9 with 7th A, S05.91X-S05.92X with 7th A, S38.3XXA, T14.8-T14.91, T79.8XX-T79.9XX with 7th A

✓x7ᵗʰ **S05.50**　Penetrating wound with foreign body of unspecified eyeball　CC

✓x7ᵗʰ **S05.51**　Penetrating wound with foreign body of right eyeball　CC

✓x7ᵗʰ **S05.52**　Penetrating wound with foreign body of left eyeball　CC

✓5ᵗʰ S05.6　Penetrating wound without foreign body of eyeball
Ocular penetration NOS

✓x7ᵗʰ **S05.60**　Penetrating wound without foreign body of unspecified eyeball

✓x7ᵗʰ **S05.61**　Penetrating wound without foreign body of right eyeball

✓x7ᵗʰ **S05.62**　Penetrating wound without foreign body of left eyeball

✓5ᵗʰ S05.7　Avulsion of eye
Traumatic enucleation

✓x7ᵗʰ **S05.70**　Avulsion of unspecified eye　CC

✓x7ᵗʰ **S05.71**　Avulsion of right eye　CC

✓x7ᵗʰ **S05.72**　Avulsion of left eye　CC

✓5ᵗʰ S05.8　Other injuries of eye and orbit
Lacrimal duct injury

✓6ᵗʰ S05.8X　Other injuries of eye and orbit

✓7ᵗʰ **S05.8X1**　Other injuries of right eye and orbit　CC

✓7ᵗʰ **S05.8X2**　Other injuries of left eye and orbit　CC

✓7ᵗʰ **S05.8X9**　Other injuries of unspecified eye and orbit　CC

✓5ᵗʰ S05.9　Unspecified injury of eye and orbit
Injury of eye NOS

✓x7ᵗʰ **S05.90**　Unspecified injury of unspecified eye and orbit

✓x7ᵗʰ **S05.91**　Unspecified injury of right eye and orbit　CC

✓x7ᵗʰ **S05.92**　Unspecified injury of left eye and orbit　CC

✓4ᵗʰ S06　Intracranial injury
Traumatic brain injury
Code also any associated:
open wound of head (S01.-)
skull fracture (S02.-)
EXCLUDES 1 head injury NOS (S09.90)

The appropriate 7th is to be added to each code from category S06.
A　initial encounter
D　subsequent encounter
S　sequela

For CC/MCC codes in category S06, unless otherwise noted: CC or MCC as indicated with 7th A: S01.90X-S02.92X with 7th A, S06.0X0-S07.9XX with 7th A, S08.89X-S09.19X with 7th A, S09.8X-S09.90X with 7th A, S09.92X-S09.93X with 7th A, S16.8XX-S19.9XX with 7th A, S38.3XXA, T14.8-T14.91, T79.A0X-T79.9XX with 7th A

✓5ᵗʰ S06.0　Concussion
Commotio cerebri
EXCLUDES 1 concussion with other intracranial injuries classified in category S06—code to specified intracranial injury

✓6ᵗʰ S06.0X　Concussion

✓7ᵗʰ **S06.0X0**　Concussion without loss of consciousness

7 ✓7ᵗʰ **S06.0X1**　Concussion with loss of consciousness of 30 minutes or less　CC

7 ✓7ᵗʰ **S06.0X2**　Concussion with loss of consciousness of 31 minutes to 59 minutes　CC

7 ✓7ᵗʰ **S06.0X3**　Concussion with loss of consciousness of 1 hour to 5 hours 59 minutes　CC

7 ✓7ᵗʰ **S06.0X4**　Concussion with loss of consciousness of 6 hours to 24 hours　CC

7 ✓7ᵗʰ **S06.0X5**　Concussion with loss of consciousness greater than 24 hours with return to pre-existing conscious level　CC

7 ✓7ᵗʰ **S06.0X6**　Concussion with loss of consciousness greater than 24 hours without return to pre-existing conscious level with patient surviving　MCC

7 ✓7ᵗʰ **S06.0X7**　Concussion with loss of consciousness of any duration with death due to brain injury prior to regaining consciousness　CC

7 ✓7ᵗʰ **S06.0X8**　Concussion with loss of consciousness of any duration with death due to other cause prior to regaining consciousness　CC

7 ✓7ᵗʰ **S06.0X9**　Concussion with loss of consciousness of unspecified duration　CC
Concussion NOS

---

7 HAC = Initial encounter only (7th character A, B or C) and not POA.

✓ Additional Character Required　　✓x7ᵗʰ Xtension Alert　　Unacceptable PDx　　Manifestation　　Hospital Acquired Condition　　**EXCLUDES 1** Not Coded Here　　**EXCLUDES 2** Not Included Here

✓5ᵗʰ **S06.1 Traumatic cerebral edema**
Diffuse traumatic cerebral edema
Focal traumatic cerebral edema

  ✓6ᵗʰ **S06.1X Traumatic cerebral edema**

    ✓7ᵗʰ **S06.1X0 Traumatic cerebral edema** `PDx MCC` `MCC`
without loss of consciousness
CC Excl: CC with 7th character A: G93.6, G93.82

    7 ✓7ᵗʰ **S06.1X1 Traumatic cerebral edema** `PDx MCC` `MCC`
with loss of consciousness of 30 minutes or less

    7 ✓7ᵗʰ **S06.1X2 Traumatic cerebral edema** `PDx MCC` `MCC`
with loss of consciousness of 31 minutes to 59 minutes

    7 ✓7ᵗʰ **S06.1X3 Traumatic cerebral edema** `PDx MCC` `MCC`
with loss of consciousness of 1 hour to 5 hours 59 minutes

    7 ✓7ᵗʰ **S06.1X4 Traumatic cerebral edema** `PDx MCC` `MCC`
with loss of consciousness of 6 hours to 24 hours

    7 ✓7ᵗʰ **S06.1X5 Traumatic cerebral edema** `PDx MCC` `MCC`
with loss of consciousness greater than 24 hours with return to pre-existing conscious level

    7 ✓7ᵗʰ **S06.1X6 Traumatic cerebral edema** `PDx MCC` `MCC`
with loss of consciousness greater than 24 hours without return to pre-existing conscious level with patient surviving

    7 ✓7ᵗʰ **S06.1X7 Traumatic cerebral edema** `PDx MCC` `MCC`
with loss of consciousness of any duration with death due to brain injury prior to regaining consciousness

    7 ✓7ᵗʰ **S06.1X8 Traumatic cerebral edema** `PDx MCC` `MCC`
with loss of consciousness of any duration with death due to other cause prior to regaining consciousness

    7 ✓7ᵗʰ **S06.1X9 Traumatic cerebral edema** `PDx MCC` `MCC`
with loss of consciousness of unspecified duration
Traumatic cerebral edema NOS
CC Excl: CC with 7th character A: G93.6, G93.82, S01.90X-S02.92X with 7th A, S06.0X0-S07.9X with 7th A, S08.89X-S09.19X with 7th A, S09.8XX-S09.90X with 7th A, S09.92X-S09.93XA, S16.8XX-S19.9XX with 7th A, S38.3XXA, T14.8-T14.91, T79.A0X-T79.9XX with 7th A

✓5ᵗʰ **S06.2 Diffuse traumatic brain injury**
Diffuse axonal brain injury
EXCLUDES 1   traumatic diffuse cerebral edema (S06.1X-)

  ✓6ᵗʰ **S06.2X Diffuse traumatic brain injury**

    ✓7ᵗʰ **S06.2X0 Diffuse traumatic brain injury** without loss of consciousness

    7 ✓7ᵗʰ **S06.2X1 Diffuse traumatic brain injury with** `CC`
loss of consciousness of 30 minutes or less

    7 ✓7ᵗʰ **S06.2X2 Diffuse traumatic brain injury with** `CC`
loss of consciousness of 31 minutes to 59 minutes

    7 ✓7ᵗʰ **S06.2X3 Diffuse traumatic brain injury with** `CC`
loss of consciousness of 1 hour to 5 hours 59 minutes

    7 ✓7ᵗʰ **S06.2X4 Diffuse traumatic brain injury with** `CC`
loss of consciousness of 6 hours to 24 hours

    7 ✓7ᵗʰ **S06.2X5 Diffuse traumatic brain injury with** `CC`
loss of consciousness greater than 24 hours with return to pre-existing conscious levels

    7 ✓7ᵗʰ **S06.2X6 Diffuse traumatic brain injury** `MCC`
with loss of consciousness greater than 24 hours without return to pre-existing conscious level with patient surviving

---

    7 ✓7ᵗʰ **S06.2X7 Diffuse traumatic brain injury** `MCC`
with loss of consciousness of any duration with death due to brain injury prior to regaining consciousness

    7 ✓7ᵗʰ **S06.2X8 Diffuse traumatic brain injury** `MCC`
with loss of consciousness of any duration with death due to other cause prior to regaining consciousness

    7 ✓7ᵗʰ **S06.2X9 Diffuse traumatic brain injury with** `CC`
loss of consciousness of unspecified duration
Diffuse traumatic brain injury NOS

✓5ᵗʰ **S06.3 Focal traumatic brain injury**
EXCLUDES 1   any condition classifiable to S06.4-S06.6
focal cerebral edema (S06.1)

  ✓6ᵗʰ **S06.30 Unspecified focal traumatic brain injury**

    ✓7ᵗʰ **S06.300 Unspecified focal traumatic brain injury** without loss of consciousness

    7 ✓7ᵗʰ **S06.301 Unspecified focal traumatic brain injury with loss of consciousness of** `CC`
30 minutes or less

    7 ✓7ᵗʰ **S06.302 Unspecified focal traumatic brain injury with loss of consciousness of** `CC`
31 minutes to 59 minutes

    7 ✓7ᵗʰ **S06.303 Unspecified focal traumatic brain injury with loss of consciousness of** `CC`
1 hour to 5 hours 59 minutes

    7 ✓7ᵗʰ **S06.304 Unspecified focal traumatic brain injury with loss of consciousness of** `CC`
6 hours to 24 hours

    7 ✓7ᵗʰ **S06.305 Unspecified focal traumatic brain injury with loss of consciousness** `CC`
greater than 24 hours with return to pre-existing conscious level

    7 ✓7ᵗʰ **S06.306 Unspecified focal traumatic brain injury with loss of consciousness** `MCC`
greater than 24 hours without return to pre-existing conscious level with patient surviving

    7 ✓7ᵗʰ **S06.307 Unspecified focal traumatic brain injury with loss of consciousness of** `MCC`
any duration with death due to brain injury prior to regaining consciousness

    7 ✓7ᵗʰ **S06.308 Unspecified focal traumatic brain injury with loss of consciousness of** `MCC`
any duration with death due to other cause prior to regaining consciousness

    7 ✓7ᵗʰ **S06.309 Unspecified focal traumatic brain injury with loss of consciousness of** `CC`
unspecified duration
Unspecified focal traumatic brain injury NOS

  ✓6ᵗʰ **S06.31 Contusion and laceration of right cerebrum**

    7 ✓7ᵗʰ **S06.310 Contusion and laceration of right cerebrum without loss of consciousness** `MCC`

    7 ✓7ᵗʰ **(S06.311) Contusion and laceration of right cerebrum with loss of consciousness of 30 minutes or less** `MCC`

    7 ✓7ᵗʰ **S06.312 Contusion and laceration of right cerebrum with loss of consciousness of 31 minutes to 59 minutes** `MCC`

    7 ✓7ᵗʰ **S06.313 Contusion and laceration of right cerebrum with loss of consciousness of 1 hour to 5 hours 59 minutes** `MCC`

    7 ✓7ᵗʰ **S06.314 Contusion and laceration of right cerebrum with loss of consciousness of 6 hours to 24 hours** `MCC`

    7 ✓7ᵗʰ **S06.315 Contusion and laceration of right cerebrum with loss of consciousness greater than 24 hours with return to pre-existing conscious level** `MCC`

    7 ✓7ᵗʰ **S06.316 Contusion and laceration of right cerebrum with loss of consciousness greater than 24 hours without return to pre-existing conscious level with patient surviving** `MCC`

---

7 HAC = Initial encounter only (7th character A, B or C) and not POA.

Ⓝ Newborn: 0   Ⓟ Pediatric: 0-17   Ⓜ Maternity: 12-55   Ⓐ Adult: 15-124   `MCC` Major CC Condition   `PDx MCC` PDx acts as own MCC   `CC` CC Condition   `PDx CC` PDx acts as own CC

7 √7ᵗʰ **S06.317 Contusion and laceration of right cerebrum with loss of consciousness of any duration with death due to brain injury prior to regaining consciousness** MCC

7 √7ᵗʰ **S06.318 Contusion and laceration of right cerebrum with loss of consciousness of any duration with death due to other cause prior to regaining consciousness** MCC

7 √7ᵗʰ **S06.319 Contusion and laceration of right cerebrum with loss of consciousness of unspecified duration** MCC
  Contusion and laceration of right cerebrum NOS

√6ᵗʰ **S06.32 Contusion and laceration of left cerebrum**

7 √7ᵗʰ **S06.320 Contusion and laceration of left cerebrum without loss of consciousness** MCC

7 √7ᵗʰ **S06.321 Contusion and laceration of left cerebrum with loss of consciousness of 30 minutes or less** MCC

7 √7ᵗʰ **S06.322 Contusion and laceration of left cerebrum with loss of consciousness of 31 minutes to 59 minutes** MCC

7 √7ᵗʰ **S06.323 Contusion and laceration of left cerebrum with loss of consciousness of 1 hour to 5 hours 59 minutes** MCC

7 √7ᵗʰ **S06.324 Contusion and laceration of left cerebrum with loss of consciousness of 6 hours to 24 hours** MCC

7 √7ᵗʰ **S06.325 Contusion and laceration of left cerebrum with loss of consciousness greater than 24 hours with return to pre-existing conscious level** MCC

7 √7ᵗʰ **S06.326 Contusion and laceration of left cerebrum with loss of consciousness greater than 24 hours without return to pre-existing conscious level with patient surviving** MCC

7 √7ᵗʰ **S06.327 Contusion and laceration of left cerebrum with loss of consciousness of any duration with death due to brain injury prior to regaining consciousness** MCC

7 √7ᵗʰ **S06.328 Contusion and laceration of left cerebrum with loss of consciousness of any duration with death due to other cause prior to regaining consciousness** MCC

7 √7ᵗʰ **S06.329 Contusion and laceration of left cerebrum with loss of consciousness of unspecified duration** MCC
  Contusion and laceration of left cerebrum NOS

√6ᵗʰ **S06.33 Contusion and laceration of cerebrum, unspecified**

7 √7ᵗʰ **S06.330 Contusion and laceration of cerebrum, unspecified, without loss of consciousness** MCC

7 √7ᵗʰ **S06.331 Contusion and laceration of cerebrum, unspecified, with loss of consciousness of 30 minutes or less** MCC

7 √7ᵗʰ **S06.332 Contusion and laceration of cerebrum, unspecified, with loss of consciousness of 31 minutes to 59 minutes** MCC

7 √7ᵗʰ **S06.333 Contusion and laceration of cerebrum, unspecified, with loss of consciousness of 1 hour to 5 hours 59 minutes** MCC

7 √7ᵗʰ **S06.334 Contusion and laceration of cerebrum, unspecified, with loss of consciousness of 6 hours to 24 hours** MCC

7 √7ᵗʰ **S06.335 Contusion and laceration of cerebrum, unspecified, with loss of consciousness greater than 24 hours with return to pre-existing conscious level** MCC

7 √7ᵗʰ **S06.336 Contusion and laceration of cerebrum, unspecified, with loss of consciousness greater than 24 hours without return to pre-existing conscious level with patient surviving** MCC

7 √7ᵗʰ **S06.337 Contusion and laceration of cerebrum, unspecified, with loss of consciousness of any duration with death due to brain injury prior to regaining consciousness** MCC

7 √7ᵗʰ **S06.338 Contusion and laceration of cerebrum, unspecified, with loss of consciousness of any duration with death due to other cause prior to regaining consciousness** MCC

7 √7ᵗʰ **S06.339 Contusion and laceration of cerebrum, unspecified, with loss of consciousness of unspecified duration** MCC
  Contusion and laceration of cerebrum NOS

√6ᵗʰ **S06.34 Traumatic hemorrhage of right cerebrum**
  Traumatic intracerebral hemorrhage and hematoma of right cerebrum

7 √7ᵗʰ **S06.340 Traumatic hemorrhage of right cerebrum without loss of consciousness** MCC

7 √7ᵗʰ **S06.341 Traumatic hemorrhage of right cerebrum with loss of consciousness of 30 minutes or less** MCC

7 √7ᵗʰ **S06.342 Traumatic hemorrhage of right cerebrum with loss of consciousness of 31 minutes to 59 minutes** MCC

7 √7ᵗʰ **S06.343 Traumatic hemorrhage of right cerebrum with loss of consciousness of 1 hours to 5 hours 59 minutes** MCC

7 √7ᵗʰ **S06.344 Traumatic hemorrhage of right cerebrum with loss of consciousness of 6 hours to 24 hours** MCC

7 √7ᵗʰ **S06.345 Traumatic hemorrhage of right cerebrum with loss of consciousness greater than 24 hours with return to pre-existing conscious level** MCC

7 √7ᵗʰ **S06.346 Traumatic hemorrhage of right cerebrum with loss of consciousness greater than 24 hours without return to pre-existing conscious level with patient surviving** MCC

7 √7ᵗʰ **S06.347 Traumatic hemorrhage of right cerebrum with loss of consciousness of any duration with death due to brain injury prior to regaining consciousness** MCC

7 √7ᵗʰ **S06.348 Traumatic hemorrhage of right cerebrum with loss of consciousness of any duration with death due to other cause prior to regaining consciousness** MCC

7 √7ᵗʰ **S06.349 Traumatic hemorrhage of right cerebrum with loss of consciousness of unspecified duration** MCC
  Traumatic hemorrhage of right cerebrum NOS

√6ᵗʰ **S06.35 Traumatic hemorrhage of left cerebrum**
  Traumatic intracerebral hemorrhage and hematoma of left cerebrum

7 √7ᵗʰ **S06.350 Traumatic hemorrhage of left cerebrum without loss of consciousness** MCC

7 √7ᵗʰ **S06.351 Traumatic hemorrhage of left cerebrum with loss of consciousness of 30 minutes or less** MCC

7 √7ᵗʰ **S06.352 Traumatic hemorrhage of left cerebrum with loss of consciousness of 31 minutes to 59 minutes** MCC

7 √7ᵗʰ **S06.353 Traumatic hemorrhage of left cerebrum with loss of consciousness of 1 hours to 5 hours 59 minutes** MCC

7 √7ᵗʰ **S06.354 Traumatic hemorrhage of left cerebrum with loss of consciousness of 6 hours to 24 hours** MCC

7 √7ᵗʰ **S06.355 Traumatic hemorrhage of left cerebrum with loss of consciousness greater than 24 hours with return to pre-existing conscious level** MCC

---

7 HAC = Initial encounter only (7th character A, B or C) and not POA.

Injury, Poisoning and Certain Other Consequences of External Causes

S06.356–S06.4X0

7 ✓7th **S06.356** Traumatic hemorrhage of left cerebrum with loss of consciousness greater than 24 hours without return to pre-existing conscious level with patient surviving   MCC

7 ✓7th **S06.357** Traumatic hemorrhage of left cerebrum with loss of consciousness of any duration with death due to brain injury prior to regaining consciousness   MCC

7 ✓7th **S06.358** Traumatic hemorrhage of left cerebrum with loss of consciousness of any duration with death due to other cause prior to regaining consciousness   MCC

7 ✓7th **S06.359** Traumatic hemorrhage of left cerebrum with loss of consciousness of unspecified duration   MCC
  Traumatic hemorrhage of left cerebrum NOS

✓6th **S06.36** Traumatic hemorrhage of cerebrum, unspecified
  Traumatic intracerebral hemorrhage and hematoma, unspecified

7 ✓7th **S06.360** Traumatic hemorrhage of cerebrum, unspecified, without loss of consciousness   MCC

7 ✓7th **S06.361** Traumatic hemorrhage of cerebrum, unspecified, with loss of consciousness of 30 minutes or less   MCC

7 ✓7th **S06.362** Traumatic hemorrhage of cerebrum, unspecified, with loss of consciousness of 31 minutes to 59 minutes   MCC

7 ✓7th **S06.363** Traumatic hemorrhage of cerebrum, unspecified, with loss of consciousness of 1 hours to 5 hours 59 minutes   MCC

7 ✓7th **S06.364** Traumatic hemorrhage of cerebrum, unspecified, with loss of consciousness of 6 hours to 24 hours   MCC

7 ✓7th **S06.365** Traumatic hemorrhage of cerebrum, unspecified, with loss of consciousness greater than 24 hours with return to pre-existing conscious level   MCC

7 ✓7th **S06.366** Traumatic hemorrhage of cerebrum, unspecified, with loss of consciousness greater than 24 hours without return to pre-existing conscious level with patient surviving   MCC

7 ✓7th **S06.367** Traumatic hemorrhage of cerebrum, unspecified, with loss of consciousness of any duration with death due to brain injury prior to regaining consciousness   MCC

7 ✓7th **S06.368** Traumatic hemorrhage of cerebrum, unspecified, with loss of consciousness of any duration with death due to other cause prior to regaining consciousness   MCC

7 ✓7th **S06.369** Traumatic hemorrhage of cerebrum, unspecified, with loss of consciousness of unspecified duration   MCC
  Traumatic hemorrhage of cerebrum NOS

✓6th **S06.37** Contusion, laceration, and hemorrhage of cerebellum

7 ✓7th **S06.370** Contusion, laceration, and hemorrhage of cerebellum without loss of consciousness   MCC
  CC Excl: No Excl

7 ✓7th **S06.371** Contusion, laceration, and hemorrhage of cerebellum with loss of consciousness of 30 minutes or less   CC

7 ✓7th **S06.372** Contusion, laceration, and hemorrhage of cerebellum with loss of consciousness of 31 minutes to 59 minutes   CC

7 ✓7th **S06.373** Contusion, laceration, and hemorrhage of cerebellum with loss of consciousness of 1 hour to 5 hours 59 minutes   CC

7 ✓7th **S06.374** Contusion, laceration, and hemorrhage of cerebellum with loss of consciousness of 6 hours to 24 hours   CC

7 ✓7th **S06.375** Contusion, laceration, and hemorrhage of cerebellum with loss of consciousness greater than 24 hours with return to pre-existing conscious level   CC

7 ✓7th **S06.376** Contusion, laceration, and hemorrhage of cerebellum with loss of consciousness greater than 24 hours without return to pre-existing conscious level with patient surviving   MCC

7 ✓7th **S06.377** Contusion, laceration, and hemorrhage of cerebellum with loss of consciousness of any duration with death due to brain injury prior to regaining consciousness   MCC

7 ✓7th **S06.378** Contusion, laceration, and hemorrhage of cerebellum with loss of consciousness of any duration with death due to other cause prior to regaining consciousness   MCC

7 ✓7th **S06.379** Contusion, laceration, and hemorrhage of cerebellum with loss of consciousness of unspecified duration   CC
  Contusion, laceration, and hemorrhage of cerebellum NOS

✓6th **S06.38** Contusion, laceration, and hemorrhage of brainstem

7 ✓7th **S06.380** Contusion, laceration, and hemorrhage of brainstem without loss of consciousness   MCC
  CC Excl: No Excl

7 ✓7th **S06.381** Contusion, laceration, and hemorrhage of brainstem with loss of consciousness of 30 minutes or less   CC

7 ✓7th **S06.382** Contusion, laceration, and hemorrhage of brainstem with loss of consciousness of 31 minutes to 59 minutes   CC

7 ✓7th **S06.383** Contusion, laceration, and hemorrhage of brainstem with loss of consciousness of 1 hour to 5 hours 59 minutes   CC

7 ✓7th **S06.384** Contusion, laceration, and hemorrhage of brainstem with loss of consciousness of 6 hours to 24 hours   CC

7 ✓7th **S06.385** Contusion, laceration, and hemorrhage of brainstem with loss of consciousness greater than 24 hours with return to pre-existing conscious level   CC

7 ✓7th **S06.386** Contusion, laceration, and hemorrhage of brainstem with loss of consciousness greater than 24 hours without return to pre-existing conscious level with patient surviving   MCC

7 ✓7th **S06.387** Contusion, laceration, and hemorrhage of brainstem with loss of consciousness of any duration with death due to brain injury prior to regaining consciousness   MCC

7 ✓7th **S06.388** Contusion, laceration, and hemorrhage of brainstem with loss of consciousness of any duration with death due to other cause prior to regaining consciousness   MCC

7 ✓7th **S06.389** Contusion, laceration, and hemorrhage of brainstem with loss of consciousness of unspecified duration   CC
  Contusion, laceration, and hemorrhage of brainstem NOS

✓5th **S06.4** Epidural hemorrhage
  Extradural hemorrhage NOS
  Extradural hemorrhage (traumatic)

✓6th **S06.4X** Epidural hemorrhage

7 ✓7th **S06.4X0** Epidural hemorrhage without loss of consciousness   MCC

---

7 HAC = Initial encounter only (7th character A, B or C) and not POA.

N Newborn: 0   P Pediatric: 0-17   M Maternity: 12-55   A Adult: 15-124   MCC Major CC Condition   PDx MCC PDx acts as own MCC   CC CC Condition   PDx CC PDx acts as own CC

866   ICD-10-CM Draft (2015)

7 √7ᵗʰ **S06.4X1** **Epidural hemorrhage with loss of consciousness of 30 minutes or less** `MCC`

7 √7ᵗʰ **S06.4X2** **Epidural hemorrhage with loss of consciousness of 31 minutes to 59 minutes** `MCC`

7 √7ᵗʰ **S06.4X3** **Epidural hemorrhage with loss of consciousness of 1 hour to 5 hours 59 minutes** `MCC`

7 √7ᵗʰ **S06.4X4** **Epidural hemorrhage with loss of consciousness of 6 hours to 24 hours** `MCC`

7 √7ᵗʰ **S06.4X5** **Epidural hemorrhage with loss of consciousness greater than 24 hours with return to pre-existing conscious level** `MCC`

7 √7ᵗʰ **S06.4X6** **Epidural hemorrhage with loss of consciousness greater than 24 hours without return to pre-existing conscious level with patient surviving** `MCC`

7 √7ᵗʰ **S06.4X7** **Epidural hemorrhage with loss of consciousness of any duration with death due to brain injury prior to regaining consciousness** `MCC`

7 √7ᵗʰ **S06.4X8** **Epidural hemorrhage with loss of consciousness of any duration with death due to other causes prior to regaining consciousness** `MCC`

7 √7ᵗʰ **S06.4X9** **Epidural hemorrhage with loss of consciousness of unspecified duration** `MCC`
     Epidural hemorrhage NOS

√5ᵗʰ **S06.5** **Traumatic subdural hemorrhage**

   √6ᵗʰ **S06.5X** **Traumatic subdural hemorrhage**

7 √7ᵗʰ **S06.5X0** **Traumatic subdural hemorrhage without loss of consciousness** `MCC`

7 √7ᵗʰ **S06.5X1** **Traumatic subdural hemorrhage with loss of consciousness of 30 minutes or less** `MCC`

7 √7ᵗʰ **S06.5X2** **Traumatic subdural hemorrhage with loss of consciousness of 31 minutes to 59 minutes** `MCC`

7 √7ᵗʰ **S06.5X3** **Traumatic subdural hemorrhage with loss of consciousness of 1 hour to 5 hours 59 minutes** `MCC`

7 √7ᵗʰ **S06.5X4** **Traumatic subdural hemorrhage with loss of consciousness of 6 hours to 24 hours** `MCC`

7 √7ᵗʰ **S06.5X5** **Traumatic subdural hemorrhage with loss of consciousness greater than 24 hours with return to pre-existing conscious level** `MCC`

7 √7ᵗʰ **S06.5X6** **Traumatic subdural hemorrhage with loss of consciousness greater than 24 hours without return to pre-existing conscious level with patient surviving** `MCC`

7 √7ᵗʰ **S06.5X7** **Traumatic subdural hemorrhage with loss of consciousness of any duration with death due to brain injury before regaining consciousness** `MCC`

7 √7ᵗʰ **S06.5X8** **Traumatic subdural hemorrhage with loss of consciousness of any duration with death due to other cause before regaining consciousness** `MCC`

7 √7ᵗʰ **S06.5X9** **Traumatic subdural hemorrhage with loss of consciousness of unspecified duration** `MCC`
     Traumatic subdural hemorrhage NOS

√5ᵗʰ **S06.6** **Traumatic subarachnoid hemorrhage**

   √6ᵗʰ **S06.6X** **Traumatic subarachnoid hemorrhage**

7 √7ᵗʰ **S06.6X0** **Traumatic subarachnoid hemorrhage without loss of consciousness** `MCC`

7 √7ᵗʰ **S06.6X1** **Traumatic subarachnoid hemorrhage with loss of consciousness of 30 minutes or less** `MCC`

7 √7ᵗʰ **S06.6X2** **Traumatic subarachnoid hemorrhage with loss of consciousness of 31 minutes to 59 minutes** `MCC`

7 √7ᵗʰ **S06.6X3** **Traumatic subarachnoid hemorrhage with loss of consciousness of 1 hour to 5 hours 59 minutes** `MCC`

7 √7ᵗʰ **S06.6X4** **Traumatic subarachnoid hemorrhage with loss of consciousness of 6 hours to 24 hours** `MCC`

7 √7ᵗʰ **S06.6X5** **Traumatic subarachnoid hemorrhage with loss of consciousness greater than 24 hours with return to pre-existing conscious level** `MCC`

7 √7ᵗʰ **S06.6X6** **Traumatic subarachnoid hemorrhage with loss of consciousness greater than 24 hours without return to pre-existing conscious level with patient surviving** `MCC`

7 √7ᵗʰ **S06.6X7** **Traumatic subarachnoid hemorrhage with loss of consciousness of any duration with death due to brain injury prior to regaining consciousness** `MCC`

7 √7ᵗʰ **S06.6X8** **Traumatic subarachnoid hemorrhage with loss of consciousness of any duration with death due to other cause prior to regaining consciousness** `MCC`

7 √7ᵗʰ **S06.6X9** **Traumatic subarachnoid hemorrhage with loss of consciousness of unspecified duration** `MCC`
     Traumatic subarachnoid hemorrhage NOS

√5ᵗʰ **S06.8** **Other specified intracranial injuries**

   √6ᵗʰ **S06.81** **Injury of right internal carotid artery, intracranial portion, not elsewhere classified**

7 √7ᵗʰ **S06.810** **Injury of right internal carotid artery, intracranial portion, not elsewhere classified without loss of consciousness**

7 √7ᵗʰ **S06.811** **Injury of right internal carotid artery, intracranial portion, not elsewhere classified with loss of consciousness of 30 minutes or less** `CC`

7 √7ᵗʰ **S06.812** **Injury of right internal carotid artery, intracranial portion, not elsewhere classified with loss of consciousness of 31 minutes to 59 minutes** `CC`

7 √7ᵗʰ **S06.813** **Injury of right internal carotid artery, intracranial portion, not elsewhere classified with loss of consciousness of 1 hour to 5 hours 59 minutes** `CC`

7 √7ᵗʰ **S06.814** **Injury of right internal carotid artery, intracranial portion, not elsewhere classified with loss of consciousness of 6 hours to 24 hours** `CC`

7 √7ᵗʰ **S06.815** **Injury of right internal carotid artery, intracranial portion, not elsewhere classified with loss of consciousness greater than 24 hours with return to pre-existing conscious level** `CC`

7 √7ᵗʰ **S06.816** **Injury of right internal carotid artery, intracranial portion, not elsewhere classified with loss of consciousness greater than 24 hours without return to pre-existing conscious level with patient surviving** `MCC`

7 √7ᵗʰ **S06.817** **Injury of right internal carotid artery, intracranial portion, not elsewhere classified with loss of consciousness of any duration with death due to brain injury prior to regaining consciousness** `MCC`

7 √7ᵗʰ **S06.818** **Injury of right internal carotid artery, intracranial portion, not elsewhere classified with loss of consciousness of any duration with death due to other cause prior to regaining consciousness** `MCC`

7 √7ᵗʰ **S06.819** **Injury of right internal carotid artery, intracranial portion, not elsewhere classified with loss of consciousness of unspecified duration** `CC`
     Injury of right internal carotid artery, intracranial portion, not elsewhere classified NOS

---

7 HAC = Initial encounter only (7th character A, B or C) and not POA.

☑ Additional Character Required   √x7ᵗʰ *X*tension Alert   Unacceptable PDx   Manifestation   Hospital Acquired Condition   *EXCLUDES 1* Not Coded Here   *EXCLUDES 2* Not Included Here

√6ᵗʰ S06.82 Injury of left internal carotid artery, intracranial portion, not elsewhere classified

    √7ᵗʰ S06.820 Injury of left internal carotid artery, intracranial portion, not elsewhere classified without loss of consciousness

    7 √7ᵗʰ S06.821 Injury of left internal carotid artery, intracranial portion, not elsewhere classified with loss of consciousness of 30 minutes or less   CC

    7 √7ᵗʰ S06.822 Injury of left internal carotid artery, intracranial portion, not elsewhere classified with loss of consciousness of 31 minutes to 59 minutes   CC

    7 √7ᵗʰ S06.823 Injury of left internal carotid artery, intracranial portion, not elsewhere classified with loss of consciousness of 1 hour to 5 hours 59 minutes   CC

    7 √7ᵗʰ S06.824 Injury of left internal carotid artery, intracranial portion, not elsewhere classified with loss of consciousness of 6 hours to 24 hours   CC

    7 √7ᵗʰ S06.825 Injury of left internal carotid artery, intracranial portion, not elsewhere classified with loss of consciousness greater than 24 hours with return to pre-existing conscious level   CC

    7 √7ᵗʰ S06.826 Injury of left internal carotid artery, intracranial portion, not elsewhere classified with loss of consciousness greater than 24 hours without return to pre-existing conscious level with patient surviving   MCC

    7 √7ᵗʰ S06.827 Injury of left internal carotid artery, intracranial portion, not elsewhere classified with loss of consciousness of any duration with death due to brain injury prior to regaining consciousness   MCC

    7 √7ᵗʰ S06.828 Injury of left internal carotid artery, intracranial portion, not elsewhere classified with loss of consciousness of any duration with death due to other cause prior to regaining consciousness   MCC

    7 √7ᵗʰ S06.829 Injury of left internal carotid artery, intracranial portion, not elsewhere classified with loss of consciousness of unspecified duration   CC

         Injury of left internal carotid artery, intracranial portion, not elsewhere classified NOS

√6ᵗʰ S06.89 Other specified intracranial injury

    √7ᵗʰ S06.890 Other specified intracranial injury without loss of consciousness

    7 √7ᵗʰ S06.891 Other specified intracranial injury with loss of consciousness of 30 minutes or less   CC

    7 √7ᵗʰ S06.892 Other specified intracranial injury with loss of consciousness of 31 minutes to 59 minutes   CC

    7 √7ᵗʰ S06.893 Other specified intracranial injury with loss of consciousness of 1 hour to 5 hours 59 minutes   CC

    7 √7ᵗʰ S06.894 Other specified intracranial injury with loss of consciousness of 6 hours to 24 hours   CC

    7 √7ᵗʰ S06.895 Other specified intracranial injury with loss of consciousness greater than 24 hours with return to pre-existing conscious level   CC

    7 √7ᵗʰ S06.896 Other specified intracranial injury with loss of consciousness greater than 24 hours without return to pre-existing conscious level with patient surviving   MCC

    7 √7ᵗʰ S06.897 Other specified intracranial injury with loss of consciousness of any duration with death due to brain injury prior to regaining consciousness   MCC

    7 √7ᵗʰ S06.898 Other specified intracranial injury with loss of consciousness of any duration with death due to other cause prior to regaining consciousness   MCC

    7 √7ᵗʰ S06.899 Other specified intracranial injury with loss of consciousness of unspecified duration   CC

√5ᵗʰ S06.9 Unspecified intracranial injury
     Brain injury NOS
     Head injury NOS with loss of consciousness
     EXCLUDES 1   head injury NOS (S09.90)

√6ᵗʰ S06.9X Unspecified intracranial injury

    √7ᵗʰ S06.9X0 Unspecified intracranial injury without loss of consciousness

    7 √7ᵗʰ S06.9X1 Unspecified intracranial injury with loss of consciousness of 30 minutes or less

    7 √7ᵗʰ S06.9X2 Unspecified intracranial injury with loss of consciousness of 31 minutes to 59 minutes

    7 √7ᵗʰ S06.9X3 Unspecified intracranial injury with loss of consciousness of 1 hour to 5 hours 59 minutes   CC

    7 √7ᵗʰ S06.9X4 Unspecified intracranial injury with loss of consciousness of 6 hours to 24 hours   CC

    7 √7ᵗʰ S06.9X5 Unspecified intracranial injury with loss of consciousness greater than 24 hours with return to pre-existing conscious level   CC

    7 √7ᵗʰ S06.9X6 Unspecified intracranial injury with loss of consciousness greater than 24 hours without return to pre-existing conscious level with patient surviving   MCC

    7 √7ᵗʰ S06.9X7 Unspecified intracranial injury with loss of consciousness of any duration with death due to brain injury prior to regaining consciousness   MCC

    7 √7ᵗʰ S06.9X8 Unspecified intracranial injury with loss of consciousness of any duration with death due to other cause prior to regaining consciousness   MCC

    7 √7ᵗʰ S06.9X9 Unspecified intracranial injury with loss of consciousness of unspecified duration   CC

√4ᵗʰ S07 Crushing injury of head
     Use additional code for all associated injuries, such as:
       intracranial injuries (S06.-)
       skull fractures (S02.-)

> The appropriate 7th is to be added to each code from category S07.
> A   initial encounter
> D   subsequent encounter
> S   sequela

> For CC/MCC codes in category S07, unless otherwise noted: CC with 7th character A: S01.90X-S02.92X with 7th A, S07.0XX-S07.9XX with 7th A, S08.89X-S09.19X with 7th A, S09.8XX-S09.90X with 7th A, S09.92X-S09.93X with 7th A, S16.8XX-S19.9XX with 7th A, T14.8-T14.91, T79.A0X-T79.9XX with 7th A

7 √x7ᵗʰ **S07.0 Crushing injury of face**   CC
7 √x7ᵗʰ **S07.1 Crushing injury of skull**   CC
7 √x7ᵗʰ **S07.8 Crushing injury of other parts of head**   CC
7 √x7ᵗʰ **S07.9 Crushing injury of head, part unspecified**   CC

√4ᵗʰ S08 Avulsion and traumatic amputation of part of head
     NOTE   An amputation not identified as partial or complete should be coded to complete

> The appropriate 7th is to be added to each code from category S08.
> A   initial encounter
> D   subsequent encounter
> S   sequela

√x7ᵗʰ **S08.0 Avulsion of scalp**

√5ᵗʰ **S08.1 Traumatic amputation of ear**

7 HAC = Initial encounter only (7th character A, B or C) and not POA.

N Newborn: 0   P Pediatric: 0-17   M Maternity: 12-55   A Adult: 15-124   MCC Major CC Condition   PDx MCC PDx acts as own MCC   CC CC Condition   PDx CC PDx acts as own CC

868   ICD-10-CM Draft (2015)

√6ᵗʰ **S08.11 Complete** traumatic amputation of ear
- √7ᵗʰ **S08.111 Complete** traumatic amputation of **right** ear
- √7ᵗʰ **S08.112 Complete** traumatic amputation of **left** ear
- √7ᵗʰ **S08.119 Complete** traumatic amputation of **unspecified** ear

√6ᵗʰ **S08.12 Partial** traumatic amputation of ear
- √7ᵗʰ **S08.121 Partial** traumatic amputation of **right** ear
- √7ᵗʰ **S08.122 Partial** traumatic amputation of **left** ear
- √7ᵗʰ **S08.129 Partial** traumatic amputation of **unspecified** ear

√5ᵗʰ **S08.8 Traumatic amputation of** other parts of head
- √6ᵗʰ **S08.81 Traumatic amputation of** nose
  - √7ᵗʰ **S08.811 Complete** traumatic amputation of nose
  - √7ᵗʰ **S08.812 Partial** traumatic amputation of nose
- √x7ᵗʰ **S08.89 Traumatic amputation of** other parts of head

√4ᵗʰ **S09 Other and unspecified injuries of head**

> The appropriate 7th is to be added to each code from category S09.
> A   initial encounter
> D   subsequent encounter
> S   sequela

√x7ᵗʰ **S09.0 Injury of** blood vessels **of head, not elsewhere classified** CC
> EXCLUDES 1   injury of cerebral blood vessels (S06.-)
>   injury of precerebral blood vessels (S15.-)
> CC Excl: CC with 7th character A: S09.0XX with 7th A, S15.101-
> S15.199 with 7th A, S15.8XX-S15.9XX with 7th A, T14.8-T14.91,
> T79.A0X-T79.9XX with 7th A

√5ᵗʰ **S09.1 Injury of** muscle and tendon **of head**
> Code also any associated open wound (S01.-)
> EXCLUDES 2   sprain to joints and ligament of head (S03.9)
- √x7ᵗʰ **S09.10 Unspecified** injury of muscle and tendon of head
  Injury of muscle and tendon of head NOS
- √x7ᵗʰ **S09.11 Strain** of muscle and tendon of head
- √x7ᵗʰ **S09.12 Laceration** of muscle and tendon of head
- √x7ᵗʰ **S09.19 Other** specified injury of muscle and tendon of head

√5ᵗʰ **S09.2 Traumatic rupture of** ear drum
> EXCLUDES 1   traumatic rupture of ear drum due to blast injury
>   (S09.31-)
>
> CC Excl: For CC codes in subcategory S09.2, unless
> otherwise noted: CC with 7th character A: S01.301-
> S01.359 with 7th A, S08.111-S08.129 with 7th A, S09.20X-
> S09.399 with 7th A, S09.91XA, S38.3XXA, T14.8-T14.91,
> T79.8XX-T79.9XX with 7th A
- √x7ᵗʰ **S09.20 Traumatic rupture of** unspecified **ear drum** CC
- √x7ᵗʰ **S09.21 Traumatic rupture of** right **ear drum** CC
- √x7ᵗʰ **S09.22 Traumatic rupture of** left **ear drum** CC

√5ᵗʰ **S09.3 Other specified and unspecified injury of middle and inner ear**
> EXCLUDES 1   injury to ear NOS (S09.91-)
> EXCLUDES 2   injury to external ear (S00.4-, S01.3-, S08.1-)
>
> CC Excl: For CC codes in subcategory S09.3, unless
> otherwise noted: CC with 7th character A: S01.301-
> S01.359 with 7th A, S08.111-S08.129 with 7th A, S09.20X-
> S09.399 with 7th A, S09.91X with 7th A, S38.3XXA, T14.8-
> T14.91, T79.8XX-T79.9XX with 7th A
- √6ᵗʰ **S09.30 Unspecified injury of** middle and inner ear
  - √7ᵗʰ **S09.301 Unspecified injury of** right middle and inner ear CC
  - √7ᵗʰ **S09.302 Unspecified injury of** left middle and inner ear CC
  - √7ᵗʰ **S09.309 Unspecified injury of** unspecified middle and inner ear CC
- √6ᵗʰ **S09.31 Primary** blast injury of ear
  Blast injury of ear NOS
  - √7ᵗʰ **S09.311 Primary** blast injury of **right** ear CC
  - √7ᵗʰ **S09.312 Primary** blast injury of **left** ear CC
  - √7ᵗʰ **S09.313 Primary** blast injury of ear, **bilateral** CC
  - √7ᵗʰ **S09.319 Primary** blast injury of **unspecified** ear CC
- √6ᵗʰ **S09.39 Other** specified injury of middle and inner ear
  Secondary blast injury to ear

√7ᵗʰ **S09.391 Other specified injury of** right middle and inner ear CC
√7ᵗʰ **S09.392 Other specified injury of** left middle and inner ear CC
√7ᵗʰ **S09.399 Other specified injury of** unspecified middle and inner ear CC

√x7ᵗʰ **S09.8 Other specified injuries of head** CC
> CC Excl: No excl

√5ᵗʰ **S09.9 Unspecified injury of face and head**
- √x7ᵗʰ **S09.90 Unspecified injury of** head
  Head injury NOS
  > EXCLUDES 1   brain injury NOS (S06.9-)
  >   head injury NOS with loss of consciousness
  >   (S06.9-)
  >   intracranial injury NOS (S06.9-)
- √x7ᵗʰ **S09.91 Unspecified injury of** ear
  Injury of ear NOS
- √x7ᵗʰ **S09.92 Unspecified injury of** nose
  Injury of nose NOS
- √x7ᵗʰ **S09.93 Unspecified injury of** face
  Injury of face NOS

Injuries to the neck (S10-S19)

INCLUDES   injuries of nape
            injuries of supraclavicular region
            injuries of throat
EXCLUDES 2 burns and corrosions (T20-T32)
            effects of foreign body in esophagus (T18.1)
            effects of foreign body in larynx (T17.3)
            effects of foreign body in pharynx (T17.2)
            effects of foreign body in trachea (T17.4)
            frostbite (T33-T34)
            insect bite or sting, venomous (T63.4)

√4ᵗʰ **S10 Superficial injury of neck**

> The appropriate 7th is to be added to each code from category S10.
> A   initial encounter
> D   subsequent encounter
> S   sequela

√x7ᵗʰ **S10.0 Contusion of throat**
> Contusion of cervical esophagus   Contusion of pharynx
> Contusion of larynx   Contusion of trachea

√5ᵗʰ **S10.1 Other and unspecified superficial injuries of throat**
- √x7ᵗʰ **S10.10 Unspecified** superficial injuries of throat
- √x7ᵗʰ **S10.11 Abrasion** of throat
- √x7ᵗʰ **S10.12 Blister (nonthermal)** of throat
- √x7ᵗʰ **S10.14 External constriction** of part of throat
- √x7ᵗʰ **S10.15 Superficial foreign body** of throat
  Splinter in the throat
- √x7ᵗʰ **S10.16 Insect bite (nonvenomous)** of throat
- √x7ᵗʰ **S10.17 Other superficial bite** of throat
  > EXCLUDES 1   open bite of throat (S11.85)

√5ᵗʰ **S10.8 Superficial injury of** other specified parts of neck
- √x7ᵗʰ **S10.80 Unspecified** superficial injury of other specified part of neck
- √x7ᵗʰ **S10.81 Abrasion** of other specified part of neck
- √x7ᵗʰ **S10.82 Blister (nonthermal)** of other specified part of neck
- √x7ᵗʰ **S10.83 Contusion** of other specified part of neck
- √x7ᵗʰ **S10.84 External constriction** of other specified part of neck
- √x7ᵗʰ **S10.85 Superficial foreign body** of other specified part of neck
  Splinter in other specified part of neck
- √x7ᵗʰ **S10.86 Insect bite** of other specified part of neck
- √x7ᵗʰ **S10.87 Other superficial bite** of other specified part of neck
  > EXCLUDES 1   open bite of other specified parts of neck
  >   (S11.85)

√5ᵗʰ **S10.9 Superficial injury of** unspecified part of neck
- √x7ᵗʰ **S10.90 Unspecified** superficial injury of unspecified part of neck
- √x7ᵗʰ **S10.91 Abrasion** of unspecified part of neck
- √x7ᵗʰ **S10.92 Blister (nonthermal)** of unspecified part of neck
- √x7ᵗʰ **S10.93 Contusion** of unspecified part of neck
- √x7ᵗʰ **S10.94 External constriction** of unspecified part of neck

---

√ Additional Character Required   √x7ᵗʰ Xtension Alert   Unacceptable PDx   Manifestation   Hospital Acquired Condition   EXCLUDES 1 Not Coded Here   EXCLUDES 2 Not Included Here

√x 7th **S10.95 Superficial foreign body of unspecified part of neck**

√x 7th **S10.96 Insect bite of unspecified part of neck**

√x 7th **S10.97 Other superficial bite of unspecified part of neck**

√4th **S11 Open wound of neck**

Code also any associated:
spinal cord injury (S14.0, S14.1-)
wound infection

EXCLUDES 2 *open fracture of vertebra (S12- with 7th B)*

The appropriate 7th is to be added to each code from category S11.

A   initial encounter
D   subsequent encounter
S   sequela

√5th **S11.0 Open wound of larynx and trachea**

CC Excl: For MCC codes in subcategory S11.0, unless otherwise noted: MCC with 7th character A: S11.011–S11.039 with 7th A, S13.4XXA, S13.8XXA, S16.1XX–S16.2XX with 7th A, S38.3XXA, T14.8-T14.91, T79.A0X-T79.9XX with 7th A

√6th **S11.01 Open wound of larynx**

EXCLUDES 2 *open wound of vocal cord (S11.03)*

√7th **S11.011 Laceration without foreign body of larynx**   MCC

√7th **S11.012 Laceration with foreign body of larynx**   MCC

√7th **S11.013 Puncture wound without foreign body of larynx**   MCC

√7th **S11.014 Puncture wound with foreign body of larynx**   MCC

√7th **S11.015 Open bite of larynx**   MCC
Bite of larynx NOS

√7th **S11.019 Unspecified open wound of larynx**   MCC

√6th **S11.02 Open wound of trachea**
Open wound of cervical trachea
Open wound of trachea NOS
EXCLUDES 2 *open wound of thoracic trachea (S27.5-)*

√7th **S11.021 Laceration without foreign body of trachea**   MCC

√7th **S11.022 Laceration with foreign body of trachea**   MCC

√7th **S11.023 Puncture wound without foreign body of trachea**   MCC

√7th **S11.024 Puncture wound with foreign body of trachea**   MCC

√7th **S11.025 Open bite of trachea**   MCC
Bite of trachea NOS

√7th **S11.029 Unspecified open wound of trachea**   MCC

√6th **S11.03 Open wound of vocal cord**

√7th **S11.031 Laceration without foreign body of vocal cord**   MCC

√7th **S11.032 Laceration with foreign body of vocal cord**   MCC

√7th **S11.033 Puncture wound without foreign body of vocal cord**   MCC

√7th **S11.034 Puncture wound with foreign body of vocal cord**   MCC

√7th **S11.035 Open bite of vocal cord**   MCC
Bite of vocal cord NOS

√7th **S11.039 Unspecified open wound of vocal cord**   MCC

√5th **S11.1 Open wound of thyroid gland**

CC Excl: For CC codes in subcategory S11.0, unless otherwise noted: CC with 7th character A: S11.10X–S11.15X with 7th A, S11.80X–S11.95X with 7th A, S13.4XXA, S13.8XXA, S16.1XX–S16.2XX with 7th A, S38.3XXA, T14.8-T14.91, T79.8XX-T79.9XX with 7th A

√x 7th **S11.10 Unspecified open wound of thyroid gland**   CC

√x 7th **S11.11 Laceration without foreign body of thyroid gland**   CC

√x 7th **S11.12 Laceration with foreign body of thyroid gland**   CC
CC Excl: CC with 7th character A: S11.10–S11.15 with 7th A, S11.80–S11.95 with 7th A, S13.4XXA, S13.8XXA, S16.1X–S16.2X with 7th A, S38.3XXA, T14.8-T14.91, T79.A0X-T79.9XX with 7th A

√x 7th **S11.13 Puncture wound without foreign body of thyroid gland**   CC

√x 7th **S11.14 Puncture wound with foreign body of thyroid gland**   CC
CC Excl: See code: S11.12

√x 7th **S11.15 Open bite of thyroid gland**   CC
Bite of thyroid gland NOS

√5th **S11.2 Open wound of pharynx and cervical esophagus**
EXCLUDES 1 *open wound of esophagus NOS (S27.8-)*

√x 7th **S11.20 Unspecified open wound of pharynx and cervical esophagus**   CC

CC Excl: For CC codes in subcategory S11.2, unless otherwise noted: CC with 7th character A: S11.20X–S11.95X with 7th A, S13.4XXA, S13.8XXA, S16.1XX–S16.2XX with 7th A, S38.3XXA, T14.8-T14.91, T79.8XX-T79.9XX with 7th A

√x 7th **S11.21 Laceration without foreign body of pharynx and cervical esophagus**   CC

√x 7th **S11.22 Laceration with foreign body of pharynx and cervical esophagus**   CC
CC Excl: CC with 7th character A: S11.20X–S11.95X with 7th A, S13.4XXA, S13.8XXA, S16.1XX–S16.2XX with 7th A, S38.3XXA, T14.8-T14.91, T79.A0X-T79.9XX with 7th A

√x 7th **S11.23 Puncture wound without foreign body of pharynx and cervical esophagus**   CC

√x 7th **S11.24 Puncture wound with foreign body of pharynx and cervical esophagus**   CC
CC Excl: CC with 7th character A: See Code: S11.22

√x 7th **S11.25 Open bite of pharynx and cervical esophagus**   CC
Bite of pharynx and cervical esophagus NOS

√5th **S11.8 Open wound of other specified parts of neck**

√x 7th **S11.80 Unspecified open wound of other specified part of neck**

√x 7th **S11.81 Laceration without foreign body of other specified part of neck**

√x 7th **S11.82 Laceration with foreign body of other specified part of neck**

√x 7th **S11.83 Puncture wound without foreign body of other specified part of neck**

√x 7th **S11.84 Puncture wound with foreign body of other specified part of neck**

√x 7th **S11.85 Open bite of other specified part of neck**
Bite of other specified part of neck NOS
EXCLUDES 1 *superficial bite of other specified part of neck (S10.87)*

√x 7th **S11.89 Other open wound of other specified part of neck**

√5th **S11.9 Open wound of unspecified part of neck**

√x 7th **S11.90 Unspecified open wound of unspecified part of neck**

√x 7th **S11.91 Laceration without foreign body of unspecified part of neck**

√x 7th **S11.92 Laceration with foreign body of unspecified part of neck**

√x 7th **S11.93 Puncture wound without foreign body of unspecified part of neck**

√x 7th **S11.94 Puncture wound with foreign body of unspecified part of neck**

√x 7th **S11.95 Open bite of unspecified part of neck**
Bite of neck NOS
EXCLUDES 1 *superficial bite of neck (S10.97)*

N Newborn: 0   P Pediatric: 0-17   M Maternity: 12-55   A Adult: 15-124   MCC Major CC Condition   PDx MCC PDx acts as own MCC   CC CC Condition   PDx CC PDx acts as own CC

870   ICD-10-CM Draft (2015)

√4th **S12**   **Fracture of cervical vertebra and other parts of neck**

> **NOTE**   A fracture not indicated as nondisplaced or displaced should be classified to displaced.
> A fracture not indicated as open or closed should be coded to closed.
>
> **INCLUDES**   fracture of cervical neural arch
> fracture of cervical spine
> fracture of cervical spinous process
> fracture of cervical transverse process
> fracture of cervical vertebral arch
> fracture of neck

Code first any associated cervical spinal cord injury (S14.0, S14.1-)

> The appropriate 7th is to be added to all codes from subcategories S12.0-S12.6.
> A   initial encounter for closed fracture
> B   initial encounter for open fracture
> D   subsequent encounter for fracture with routine healing
> G   subsequent encounter for fracture with delayed healing
> K   subsequent encounter for fracture with nonunion
> S   sequela

> **For CC/MCC codes in subcategory S12.0, unless otherwise noted: CC with 7th character A or MCC with 7th character B:** M48.40X-M48.58X with 7th S, M80.08XS, M80.88XS, M84.350XS, M84.454S, M84.550S, M84.58XS, M84.650S, M99.10-M99.11, M99.15-M99.17, M99.19, S03.8XX-S03.9XX with 7th A, S12.000-S13.4XX with 7th [A, B, S], S13.8XX-S14.159 with 7th A, S16.1XXA, S22.000-S22.9XX with 7th S, S23.20X-S23.29X with 7th A, S23.9XXA, S24.109A, S24.119A, S24.139A, S24.149A, S24.159A, S29.001-S29.019 with 7th A, S29.091-S29.9XX with 7th A, S32.000-S32.9XX with 7th S, S33.30X-S33.39X with 7th A, S33.9XXA, S38.1XXA, S38.3XX-S39.013 with 7th A, S39.091-S39.94X with 7th A, T79.A0X-T79.9XX with 7th A
> **CC with 7th character K:** M80.00X-M84.68X with 7th [K, P], S02.0XX-S02.92X with 7th K, S12.000-S12.691 with 7th K, S22.000-S22.9XX with 7th K, S32.000-S32.9XX with 7th K, S42.001-S42.92X with 7th [K, P], S49.001-S49.199 with 7th [K, P], S52.001-S52.92X with 7th [K, M, N, P, Q, R], S59.001-S59.299 with 7th [K, P], S62.001-S62.92X with 7th [K, P], S72.001-S72.92X with 7th [K, M, N, P, Q, R], S79.001-S79.199 with 7th [K, P], S82.001-S82.92X with 7th [K, M, N, P, Q, R], S89.001-S89.399 with 7th [K, P], S92.001-S92.919 with 7th [K, P]

√5th   **S12.0**   **Fracture of first cervical vertebra**
Atlas

   √6th   **S12.00**   Unspecified fracture of first cervical vertebra

     7 √7th   **S12.000**   **Unspecified displaced fracture of first cervical vertebra**   MCC CC

     7 √7th   **S12.001**   **Unspecified nondisplaced fracture of first cervical vertebra**   MCC CC

   7 √x7th   **S12.01**   **Stable burst fracture of first cervical vertebra**   MCC CC

   7 √x7th   **S12.02**   **Unstable burst fracture of first cervical vertebra**   MCC CC

   √6th   **S12.03**   **Posterior arch fracture of first cervical vertebra**

     7 √7th   **S12.030**   **Displaced posterior arch fracture of first cervical vertebra**   MCC CC

     7 √7th   **S12.031**   **Nondisplaced posterior arch fracture of first cervical vertebra**   MCC CC

   √6th   **S12.04**   **Lateral mass fracture of first cervical vertebra**

     7 √7th   **S12.040**   **Displaced lateral mass fracture of first cervical vertebra**   MCC CC

     7 √7th   **S12.041**   **Nondisplaced lateral mass fracture of first cervical vertebra**   MCC CC

   √6th   **S12.09**   Other fracture of first cervical vertebra

     7 √7th   **S12.090**   **Other displaced fracture of first cervical vertebra**   MCC CC

     7 √7th   **S12.091**   **Other nondisplaced fracture of first cervical vertebra**   MCC CC

√5th   **S12.1**   **Fracture of second cervical vertebra**
Axis

   √6th   **S12.10**   Unspecified fracture of second cervical vertebra

     7 √7th   **S12.100**   **Unspecified displaced fracture of second cervical vertebra**   MCC CC

     7 √7th   **S12.101**   **Unspecified nondisplaced fracture of second cervical vertebra**   MCC CC

   √6th   **S12.11**   Type II dens fracture

     7 √7th   **S12.110**   **Anterior displaced Type II dens fracture**   MCC CC

     7 √7th   **S12.111**   **Posterior displaced Type II dens fracture**   MCC CC

     7 √7th   **S12.112**   **Nondisplaced Type II dens fracture**   MCC CC

   √6th   **S12.12**   Other dens fracture

     7 √7th   **S12.120**   **Other displaced dens fracture**   MCC CC

     7 √7th   **S12.121**   **Other nondisplaced dens fracture**   MCC CC

   √6th   **S12.13**   Unspecified traumatic spondylolisthesis of second cervical vertebra

     7 √7th   **S12.130**   **Unspecified traumatic displaced spondylolisthesis of second cervical vertebra**   MCC CC

     7 √7th   **S12.131**   **Unspecified traumatic nondisplaced spondylolisthesis of second cervical vertebra**   MCC CC

   7 √x7th   **S12.14**   **Type III traumatic spondylolisthesis of second cervical vertebra**   MCC CC

   √6th   **S12.15**   Other traumatic spondylolisthesis of second cervical vertebra

     7 √7th   **S12.150**   **Other traumatic displaced spondylolisthesis of second cervical vertebra**   MCC CC

     7 √7th   **S12.151**   **Other traumatic nondisplaced spondylolisthesis of second cervical vertebra**   MCC CC

   √6th   **S12.19**   Other fracture of second cervical vertebra

     7 √7th   **S12.190**   **Other displaced fracture of second cervical vertebra**   MCC CC

     7 √7th   **S12.191**   **Other nondisplaced fracture of second cervical vertebra**   MCC CC

√5th   **S12.2**   **Fracture of third cervical vertebra**

   √6th   **S12.20**   Unspecified fracture of third cervical vertebra

     7 √7th   **S12.200**   **Unspecified displaced fracture of third cervical vertebra**   MCC CC

     7 √7th   **S12.201**   **Unspecified nondisplaced fracture of third cervical vertebra**   MCC CC

   √6th   **S12.23**   Unspecified traumatic spondylolisthesis of third cervical vertebra

     7 √7th   **S12.230**   **Unspecified traumatic displaced spondylolisthesis of third cervical vertebra**   MCC CC

     7 √7th   **S12.231**   **Unspecified traumatic nondisplaced spondylolisthesis of third cervical vertebra**   MCC CC

   7 √x7th   **S12.24**   **Type III traumatic spondylolisthesis of third cervical vertebra**   MCC CC

   √6th   **S12.25**   Other traumatic spondylolisthesis of third cervical vertebra

     7 √7th   **S12.250**   **Other traumatic displaced spondylolisthesis of third cervical vertebra**   MCC CC

     7 √7th   **S12.251**   **Other traumatic nondisplaced spondylolisthesis of third cervical vertebra**   MCC CC

   √6th   **S12.29**   Other fracture of third cervical vertebra

     7 √7th   **S12.290**   **Other displaced fracture of third cervical vertebra**   MCC CC

     7 √7th   **S12.291**   **Other nondisplaced fracture of third cervical vertebra**   MCC CC

√5th   **S12.3**   **Fracture of fourth cervical vertebra**

   √6th   **S12.30**   Unspecified fracture of fourth cervical vertebra

     7 √7th   **S12.300**   **Unspecified displaced fracture of fourth cervical vertebra**   MCC CC

     7 √7th   **S12.301**   **Unspecified nondisplaced fracture of fourth cervical vertebra**   MCC CC

   √6th   **S12.33**   Unspecified traumatic spondylolisthesis of fourth cervical vertebra

     7 √7th   **S12.330**   **Unspecified traumatic displaced spondylolisthesis of fourth cervical vertebra**   MCC CC

     7 √7th   **S12.331**   **Unspecified traumatic nondisplaced spondylolisthesis of fourth cervical vertebra**   MCC CC

   7 √x7th   **S12.34**   **Type III traumatic spondylolisthesis of fourth cervical vertebra**   MCC CC

---

7 HAC = Initial encounter only (7th character A, B or C) and not POA.

√ Additional Character Required   √x7th Xtension Alert   Unacceptable PDx   Manifestation   Hospital Acquired Condition   EXCLUDES 1 Not Coded Here   EXCLUDES 2 Not Included Here

✓6ᵗʰ **S12.35** Other traumatic spondylolisthesis of fourth cervical vertebra

   7 ✓7ᵗʰ **S12.350** Other traumatic displaced spondylolisthesis of fourth cervical vertebra   MCC CC

   7 ✓7ᵗʰ **S12.351** Other traumatic nondisplaced spondylolisthesis of fourth cervical vertebra   MCC CC

✓6ᵗʰ **S12.39** Other fracture of fourth cervical vertebra

   7 ✓7ᵗʰ **S12.390** Other displaced fracture of fourth cervical vertebra   MCC CC

   7 ✓7ᵗʰ **S12.391** Other nondisplaced fracture of fourth cervical vertebra   MCC CC

✓5ᵗʰ **S12.4** Fracture of fifth cervical vertebra

   ✓6ᵗʰ **S12.40** Unspecified fracture of fifth cervical vertebra

     7 ✓7ᵗʰ **S12.400** Unspecified displaced fracture of fifth cervical vertebra   MCC CC

     7 ✓7ᵗʰ **S12.401** Unspecified nondisplaced fracture of fifth cervical vertebra   MCC CC

   ✓6ᵗʰ **S12.43** Unspecified traumatic spondylolisthesis of fifth cervical vertebra

     7 ✓7ᵗʰ **S12.430** Unspecified traumatic displaced spondylolisthesis of fifth cervical vertebra   MCC CC

     7 ✓7ᵗʰ **S12.431** Unspecified traumatic nondisplaced spondylolisthesis of fifth cervical vertebra   MCC CC

  7 ✓x7ᵗʰ **S12.44** Type III traumatic spondylolisthesis of fifth cervical vertebra   MCC CC

   ✓6ᵗʰ **S12.45** Other traumatic spondylolisthesis of fifth cervical vertebra

     7 ✓7ᵗʰ **S12.450** Other traumatic displaced spondylolisthesis of fifth cervical vertebra   MCC CC

     7 ✓7ᵗʰ **S12.451** Other traumatic nondisplaced spondylolisthesis of fifth cervical vertebra   MCC CC

   ✓6ᵗʰ **S12.49** Other fracture of fifth cervical vertebra

     7 ✓7ᵗʰ **S12.490** Other displaced fracture of fifth cervical vertebra   MCC CC

     7 ✓7ᵗʰ **S12.491** Other nondisplaced fracture of fifth cervical vertebra   MCC CC

✓5ᵗʰ **S12.5** Fracture of sixth cervical vertebra

   ✓6ᵗʰ **S12.50** Unspecified fracture of sixth cervical vertebra

     7 ✓7ᵗʰ **S12.500** Unspecified displaced fracture of sixth cervical vertebra   MCC CC

     7 ✓7ᵗʰ **S12.501** Unspecified nondisplaced fracture of sixth cervical vertebra   MCC CC

   ✓6ᵗʰ **S12.53** Unspecified traumatic spondylolisthesis of sixth cervical vertebra

     7 ✓7ᵗʰ **S12.530** Unspecified traumatic displaced spondylolisthesis of sixth cervical vertebra   MCC CC

     7 ✓7ᵗʰ **S12.531** Unspecified traumatic nondisplaced spondylolisthesis of sixth cervical vertebra   MCC CC

  7 ✓x7ᵗʰ **S12.54** Type III traumatic spondylolisthesis of sixth cervical vertebra   MCC CC

   ✓6ᵗʰ **S12.55** Other traumatic spondylolisthesis of sixth cervical vertebra

     7 ✓7ᵗʰ **S12.550** Other traumatic displaced spondylolisthesis of sixth cervical vertebra   MCC CC

     7 ✓7ᵗʰ **S12.551** Other traumatic nondisplaced spondylolisthesis of sixth cervical vertebra   MCC CC

   ✓6ᵗʰ **S12.59** Other fracture of sixth cervical vertebra

     7 ✓7ᵗʰ **S12.590** Other displaced fracture of sixth cervical vertebra   MCC CC

     7 ✓7ᵗʰ **S12.591** Other nondisplaced fracture of sixth cervical vertebra   MCC CC

✓5ᵗʰ **S12.6** Fracture of seventh cervical vertebra

   ✓6ᵗʰ **S12.60** Unspecified fracture of seventh cervical vertebra

     7 ✓7ᵗʰ **S12.600** Unspecified displaced fracture of seventh cervical vertebra   MCC CC

     7 ✓7ᵗʰ **S12.601** Unspecified nondisplaced fracture of seventh cervical vertebra   MCC CC

   ✓6ᵗʰ **S12.63** Unspecified traumatic spondylolisthesis of seventh cervical vertebra

     7 ✓7ᵗʰ **S12.630** Unspecified traumatic displaced spondylolisthesis of seventh cervical vertebra   MCC CC

     7 ✓7ᵗʰ **S12.631** Unspecified traumatic nondisplaced spondylolisthesis of seventh cervical vertebra   MCC CC

  7 ✓x7ᵗʰ **S12.64** Type III traumatic spondylolisthesis of seventh cervical vertebra   MCC CC

   ✓6ᵗʰ **S12.65** Other traumatic spondylolisthesis of seventh cervical vertebra

     7 ✓7ᵗʰ **S12.650** Other traumatic displaced spondylolisthesis of seventh cervical vertebra   MCC CC

     7 ✓7ᵗʰ **S12.651** Other traumatic nondisplaced spondylolisthesis of seventh cervical vertebra   MCC CC

   ✓6ᵗʰ **S12.69** Other fracture of seventh cervical vertebra

     7 ✓7ᵗʰ **S12.690** Other displaced fracture of seventh cervical vertebra   MCC CC

     7 ✓7ᵗʰ **S12.691** Other nondisplaced fracture of seventh cervical vertebra   MCC CC

  7 ✓x7ᵗʰ **S12.8** Fracture of other parts of neck   MCC

     Hyoid bone   Thyroid cartilage
     Larynx   Trachea

     The appropriate 7th is to be added to code S12.8.
     A   initial encounter
     D   subsequent encounter
     S   sequela

     CC Excl: MCC with 7th character A: S03.8XX-S03.9XX with 7th A, S12.8XX with 7th A, S29.011-S29.019 with 7th A, S38.3XX-S39.013 with 7th A, T14.8-T14.91, T79.A0X-T79.9XX with 7th A

  7 ✓x7ᵗʰ **S12.9** Fracture of neck, unspecified   CC
     Fracture of cervical spine NOS
     Fracture of cervical vertebra NOS
     Fracture of neck NOS

     The appropriate 7th is to be added to code S12.9.
     A   initial encounter
     D   subsequent encounter
     S   sequela

     CC Excl: M48.40X-M48.58X with 7th S, M80.08XS, M80.88XS, M84.350S, M84.454S, M84.550S, M84.58XS, M84.650S, M99.10-M99.11, M99.15-M99.17, M99.19, S03.8XX-S03.9XX with 7th A, S12.000-S13.4XX with 7th [A, B, S], S13.8XX-S14.159 with 7th A, S16.1XXA, S22.000-S22.9XX with 7th S, S23.20X-S23.29X with 7th A, S23.9XXA, S24.109A, S24.119A, S24.139A, S24.149A, S24.159A, S29.001-S29.019 with 7th A, S29.091-S29.9XX with 7th A, S32.000-S32.9XX with 7th S, S33.30X-S33.39X with 7th A, S33.9XXA, S38.1XXA, S38.3XX-S39.013 with 7th A, S39.091-S39.94X with 7th A, T14.8-T14.91, T79.A0X-T79.9XX with 7th A

✓4ᵗʰ **S13** Dislocation and sprain of joints and ligaments at neck level

     INCLUDES   avulsion of joint or ligament at neck level
                laceration of cartilage, joint or ligament at neck level
                sprain of cartilage, joint or ligament at neck level
                traumatic hemarthrosis of joint or ligament at neck level
                traumatic rupture of joint or ligament at neck level
                traumatic subluxation of joint or ligament at neck level
                traumatic tear of joint or ligament at neck level

     Code also any associated open wound
     EXCLUDES 2   *strain of muscle or tendon at neck level (S16.1)*

     The appropriate 7th is to be added to each code from category S13.
     A   initial encounter
     D   subsequent encounter
     S   sequela

---

7 HAC = Initial encounter only (7th character A, B or C) and not POA.

Ⓝ Newborn: 0   Ⓟ Pediatric: 0-17   Ⓜ Maternity: 12-55   Ⓐ Adult: 15-124   MCC Major CC Condition   PDx MCC PDx acts as own MCC   CC CC Condition   PDx CC PDx acts as own CC

872   ICD-10-CM Draft (2015)

7 ✓x7ᵗʰ **S13.0 Traumatic rupture of cervical intervertebral disc**   CC
     EXCLUDES 1   *rupture or displacement (nontraumatic) of cervical intervertebral disc NOS (M50.-)*
     CC Excl: CC with 7th character A: M99.10-M99.11, S03.8XX-S03.9XX with 7th A, S12.000-S12.691 with 7th [A, B], S12.9XX-S13.4XX with 7th A, S13.8XXA, S14.0XX-S14.108 with 7th A, S14.111-S14.118 with 7th A, S14.121-S14.128 with 7th A, S14.131-S14.138 with 7th A, S14.141-S14.148 with 7th A, S14.151-S14.158 with 7th A, S16.1XXA, S29.011-S29.019 with 7th A, S38.3XX-S39.013 with 7th A, T14.8-T14.91, T79.A0X-T79.9XX with 7th A

✓5ᵗʰ **S13.1 Subluxation and dislocation of cervical vertebrae**
     Code also any associated:
       open wound of neck (S11.-)
       spinal cord injury (S14.1-)
     EXCLUDES 2   *fracture of cervical vertebrae (S12.0--S12.3-)*

   ✓6ᵗʰ **S13.10 Subluxation and dislocation of unspecified cervical vertebrae**
     7 ✓7ᵗʰ **S13.100 Subluxation of unspecified cervical vertebrae**   CC
     7 ✓7ᵗʰ **S13.101 Dislocation of unspecified cervical vertebrae**   CC

   ✓6ᵗʰ **S13.11 Subluxation and dislocation of C0/C1 cervical vertebrae**
     Subluxation and dislocation of atlantooccipital joint
     Subluxation and dislocation of atloidooccipital joint
     Subluxation and dislocation of occipitoatloid joint
     7 ✓7ᵗʰ **S13.110 Subluxation of C0/C1 cervical vertebrae**   CC
     7 ✓7ᵗʰ **S13.111 Dislocation of C0/C1 cervical vertebrae**   CC

   ✓6ᵗʰ **S13.12 Subluxation and dislocation of C1/C2 cervical vertebrae**
     Subluxation and dislocation of atlantoaxial joint
     7 ✓7ᵗʰ **S13.120 Subluxation of C1/C2 cervical vertebrae**   CC
     7 ✓7ᵗʰ **S13.121 Dislocation of C1/C2 cervical vertebrae**   CC

   ✓6ᵗʰ **S13.13 Subluxation and dislocation of C2/C3 cervical vertebrae**
     7 ✓7ᵗʰ **S13.130 Subluxation of C2/C3 cervical vertebrae**   CC
     7 ✓7ᵗʰ **S13.131 Dislocation of C2/C3 cervical vertebrae**   CC

   ✓6ᵗʰ **S13.14 Subluxation and dislocation of C3/C4 cervical vertebrae**
     7 ✓7ᵗʰ **S13.140 Subluxation of C3/C4 cervical vertebrae**   CC
     7 ✓7ᵗʰ **S13.141 Dislocation of C3/C4 cervical vertebrae**   CC

   ✓6ᵗʰ **S13.15 Subluxation and dislocation of C4/C5 cervical vertebrae**
     7 ✓7ᵗʰ **S13.150 Subluxation of C4/C5 cervical vertebrae**   CC
     7 ✓7ᵗʰ **S13.151 Dislocation of C4/C5 cervical vertebrae**   CC

   ✓6ᵗʰ **S13.16 Subluxation and dislocation of C5/C6 cervical vertebrae**
     7 ✓7ᵗʰ **S13.160 Subluxation of C5/C6 cervical vertebrae**   CC
     7 ✓7ᵗʰ **S13.161 Dislocation of C5/C6 cervical vertebrae**   CC

   ✓6ᵗʰ **S13.17 Subluxation and dislocation of C6/C7 cervical vertebrae**
     7 ✓7ᵗʰ **S13.170 Subluxation of C6/C7 cervical vertebrae**   CC
     7 ✓7ᵗʰ **S13.171 Dislocation of C6/C7 cervical vertebrae**   CC

   ✓6ᵗʰ **S13.18 Subluxation and dislocation of C7/T1 cervical vertebrae**
     7 ✓7ᵗʰ **S13.180 Subluxation of C7/T1 cervical vertebrae**   CC
     7 ✓7ᵗʰ **S13.181 Dislocation of C7/T1 cervical vertebrae**   CC

  ✓5ᵗʰ **S13.2 Dislocation of other and unspecified parts of neck**
    7 **S13.20 Dislocation of unspecified parts of neck**   CC
    7 **S13.29 Dislocation of other parts of neck**   CC

✓x7ᵗʰ **S13.4 Sprain of ligaments of cervical spine**
     Sprain of anterior longitudinal (ligament), cervical
     Sprain of atlanto-axial (joints)
     Sprain of atlanto-occipital (joints)
     Whiplash injury of cervical spine

✓x7ᵗʰ **S13.5 Sprain of thyroid region**
     Sprain of cricoarytenoid (joint) (ligament)
     Sprain of cricothyroid (joint) (ligament)
     Sprain of thyroid cartilage

✓x7ᵗʰ **S13.8 Sprain of joints and ligaments of other parts of neck**

✓x7ᵗʰ **S13.9 Sprain of joints and ligaments of unspecified parts of neck**

✓4ᵗʰ **S14 Injury of nerves and spinal cord at neck level**
    NOTE   Code to highest level of cervical cord injury.
    Code also any associated:
      fracture of cervical vertebra (S12.0- – S12.6-)
      open wound of neck (S11.-)
      transient paralysis (R29.5)

    The appropriate 7th is to be added to each code from category S14.
    A   initial encounter
    D   subsequent encounter
    S   sequela

    CC Excl: For MCC codes in category S14, unless otherwise noted: MCC with 7th character A: M48.40X-M48.58X with 7th S, M80.08XS, M80.88XS, M84.350S, M84.454S, M84.550S, M84.58XS, M84.650S, M99.10-M99.11, M99.15-M99.17, M99.19, S12.000-S13.29X with 7th [A, B, S], S13.9XX-S14.159 with 7th A, S22.000-S22.9XX with 7th S, S23.20X-S23.29X with 7th A, S23.9XA, S24.109XA, S24.119A, S24.139A, S24.149A, S24.159A, S29.001-S29.009 with 7th A, S29.091-S29.9XX with 7th A, S32.000-S32.9XX with 7th S, S33.30X-S33.39X with 7th A, S33.9XXA, S38.1XA, S39.001-S39.003 with 7th A, S39.091-S39.94X with 7th A, T14.8-T14.91, T79.A0X-T79.9XX with 7th A

✓x7ᵗʰ **S14.0 Concussion and edema of cervical spinal cord**   MCC

✓5ᵗʰ **S14.1 Other and unspecified injuries of cervical spinal cord**
   ✓6ᵗʰ **S14.10 Unspecified injury of cervical spinal cord**
     7 ✓7ᵗʰ **S14.101 Unspecified injury at C1 level of cervical spinal cord**   MCC
     7 ✓7ᵗʰ **S14.102 Unspecified injury at C2 level of cervical spinal cord**   MCC
     7 ✓7ᵗʰ **S14.103 Unspecified injury at C3 level of cervical spinal cord**   MCC
     7 ✓7ᵗʰ **S14.104 Unspecified injury at C4 level of cervical spinal cord**   MCC
     7 ✓7ᵗʰ **S14.105 Unspecified injury at C5 level of cervical spinal cord**   MCC
     7 ✓7ᵗʰ **S14.106 Unspecified injury at C6 level of cervical spinal cord**   MCC
     7 ✓7ᵗʰ **S14.107 Unspecified injury at C7 level of cervical spinal cord**   MCC
     ✓7ᵗʰ **S14.108 Unspecified injury at C8 level of cervical spinal cord**   MCC
     7 ✓7ᵗʰ **S14.109 Unspecified injury at unspecified level of cervical spinal cord**   MCC
       Injury of cervical spinal cord NOS
       CC Excl: No excl

   ✓6ᵗʰ **S14.11 Complete lesion of cervical spinal cord**
     7 ✓7ᵗʰ **S14.111 Complete lesion at C1 level of cervical spinal cord**   MCC
     7 ✓7ᵗʰ **S14.112 Complete lesion at C2 level of cervical spinal cord**   MCC
     7 ✓7ᵗʰ **S14.113 Complete lesion at C3 level of cervical spinal cord**   MCC
     7 ✓7ᵗʰ **S14.114 Complete lesion at C4 level of cervical spinal cord**   MCC
     7 ✓7ᵗʰ **S14.115 Complete lesion at C5 level of cervical spinal cord**   MCC
     7 ✓7ᵗʰ **S14.116 Complete lesion at C6 level of cervical spinal cord**   MCC
     7 ✓7ᵗʰ **S14.117 Complete lesion at C7 level of cervical spinal cord**   MCC
     ✓7ᵗʰ **S14.118 Complete lesion at C8 level of cervical spinal cord**   MCC
     ✓7ᵗʰ **S14.119 Complete lesion at unspecified level of cervical spinal cord**

---

7 HAC = Initial encounter only (7th character A, B or C) and not POA.

✓ Additional Character Required   ✓x7ᵗʰ Xtension Alert   Unacceptable PDx   Manifestation   Hospital Acquired Condition   EXCLUDES 1 Not Coded Here   EXCLUDES 2 Not Included Here

√6ᵗʰ **S14.12** Central cord syndrome of cervical spinal cord

7 √7ᵗʰ **S14.121** Central cord syndrome at C1 level of cervical spinal cord   MCC

7 √7ᵗʰ **S14.122** Central cord syndrome at C2 level of cervical spinal cord   MCC

7 √7ᵗʰ **S14.123** Central cord syndrome at C3 level of cervical spinal cord   MCC

7 √7ᵗʰ **S14.124** Central cord syndrome at C4 level of cervical spinal cord   MCC

7 √7ᵗʰ **S14.125** Central cord syndrome at C5 level of cervical spinal cord   MCC

7 √7ᵗʰ **S14.126** Central cord syndrome at C6 level of cervical spinal cord   MCC

7 √7ᵗʰ **S14.127** Central cord syndrome at C7 level of cervical spinal cord   MCC

√7ᵗʰ **S14.128** Central cord syndrome at C8 level of cervical spinal cord   MCC

√7ᵗʰ **S14.129** Central cord syndrome at unspecified level of cervical spinal cord

√6ᵗʰ **S14.13** Anterior cord syndrome of cervical spinal cord

7 √7ᵗʰ **S14.131** Anterior cord syndrome at C1 level of cervical spinal cord   MCC

7 √7ᵗʰ **S14.132** Anterior cord syndrome at C2 level of cervical spinal cord   MCC

7 √7ᵗʰ **S14.133** Anterior cord syndrome at C3 level of cervical spinal cord   MCC

7 √7ᵗʰ **S14.134** Anterior cord syndrome at C4 level of cervical spinal cord   MCC

7 √7ᵗʰ **S14.135** Anterior cord syndrome at C5 level of cervical spinal cord   MCC

7 √7ᵗʰ **S14.136** Anterior cord syndrome at C6 level of cervical spinal cord   MCC

7 √7ᵗʰ **S14.137** Anterior cord syndrome at C7 level of cervical spinal cord   MCC

√7ᵗʰ **S14.138** Anterior cord syndrome at C8 level of cervical spinal cord   MCC

√7ᵗʰ **S14.139** Anterior cord syndrome at unspecified level of cervical spinal cord

√6ᵗʰ **S14.14** Brown-Séquard syndrome of cervical spinal cord

√7ᵗʰ **S14.141** Brown-Séquard syndrome at C1 level of cervical spinal cord   MCC

√7ᵗʰ **S14.142** Brown-Séquard syndrome at C2 level of cervical spinal cord   MCC

√7ᵗʰ **S14.143** Brown-Séquard syndrome at C3 level of cervical spinal cord   MCC

√7ᵗʰ **S14.144** Brown-Séquard syndrome at C4 level of cervical spinal cord   MCC

√7ᵗʰ **S14.145** Brown-Séquard syndrome at C5 level of cervical spinal cord   MCC

√7ᵗʰ **S14.146** Brown-Séquard syndrome at C6 level of cervical spinal cord   MCC

√7ᵗʰ **S14.147** Brown-Séquard syndrome at C7 level of cervical spinal cord   MCC

√7ᵗʰ **S14.148** Brown-Séquard syndrome at C8 level of cervical spinal cord   MCC

√7ᵗʰ **S14.149** Brown-Séquard syndrome at unspecified level of cervical spinal cord

√6ᵗʰ **S14.15** Other incomplete lesions of cervical spinal cord
Incomplete lesion of cervical spinal cord NOS
Posterior cord syndrome of cervical spinal cord

7 √7ᵗʰ **S14.151** Other incomplete lesion at C1 level of cervical spinal cord   MCC

7 √7ᵗʰ **S14.152** Other incomplete lesion at C2 level of cervical spinal cord   MCC

7 √7ᵗʰ **S14.153** Other incomplete lesion at C3 level of cervical spinal cord   MCC

7 √7ᵗʰ **S14.154** Other incomplete lesion at C4 level of cervical spinal cord   MCC

7 √7ᵗʰ **S14.155** Other incomplete lesion at C5 level of cervical spinal cord   MCC

7 √7ᵗʰ **S14.156** Other incomplete lesion at C6 level of cervical spinal cord   MCC

7 √7ᵗʰ **S14.157** Other incomplete lesion at C7 level of cervical spinal cord   MCC

√7ᵗʰ **S14.158** Other incomplete lesion at C8 level of cervical spinal cord   MCC

√7ᵗʰ **S14.159** Other incomplete lesion at unspecified level of cervical spinal cord

√x7ᵗʰ **S14.2** Injury of nerve root of cervical spine

√x7ᵗʰ **S14.3** Injury of brachial plexus

√x7ᵗʰ **S14.4** Injury of peripheral nerves of neck

√x7ᵗʰ **S14.5** Injury of cervical sympathetic nerves

√x7ᵗʰ **S14.8** Injury of other specified nerves of neck

√x7ᵗʰ **S14.9** Injury of unspecified nerves of neck

√4ᵗʰ **S15** Injury of blood vessels at neck level
Code also any associated open wound (S11.-)

> The appropriate 7th is to be added to each code from category S15.
> A   initial encounter
> D   subsequent encounter
> S   sequela

√5ᵗʰ **S15.0** Injury of carotid artery of neck
Injury of carotid artery (common) (external) (internal, extracranial portion)
Injury of carotid artery NOS

> **EXCLUDES 1**   injury of internal carotid artery, intracranial portion (S06.8)

> **CC Excl:** For CC codes in subcategory S15, unless otherwise noted: CC with 7th character A: S09.0XXA, S15.009A, S15.029A, S15.099-S15.199 with 7th A, S15.8XX-S15.9XX with 7th A, T14.8-T14.91, T79.A0X-T79.9XX with 7th A

√6ᵗʰ **S15.00** Unspecified injury of carotid artery

√7ᵗʰ **S15.001** Unspecified injury of right carotid artery   CC

√7ᵗʰ **S15.002** Unspecified injury of left carotid artery   CC

√7ᵗʰ **S15.009** Unspecified injury of unspecified carotid artery   CC

√6ᵗʰ **S15.01** Minor laceration of carotid artery
Incomplete transection of carotid artery
Laceration of carotid artery NOS
Superficial laceration of carotid artery

√7ᵗʰ **S15.011** Minor laceration of right carotid artery   CC

√7ᵗʰ **S15.012** Minor laceration of left carotid artery   CC

√7ᵗʰ **S15.019** Minor laceration of unspecified carotid artery   CC

√6ᵗʰ **S15.02** Major laceration of carotid artery
Complete transection of carotid artery
Traumatic rupture of carotid artery

√7ᵗʰ **S15.021** Major laceration of right carotid artery   CC

√7ᵗʰ **S15.022** Major laceration of left carotid artery   CC

√7ᵗʰ **S15.029** Major laceration of unspecified carotid artery   CC

√6ᵗʰ **S15.09** Other specified injury of carotid artery

√7ᵗʰ **S15.091** Other specified injury of right carotid artery   CC

√7ᵗʰ **S15.092** Other specified injury of left carotid artery   CC

√7ᵗʰ **S15.099** Other specified injury of unspecified carotid artery   CC

√5ᵗʰ **S15.1** Injury of vertebral artery

> **CC Excl:** For CC codes in subcategory S15.1, unless otherwise noted: CC with 7th character A: S09.0XXA, S15.101-S15.199 with 7th A, S15.8XX-S15.9XX with 7th A, T14.8-T14.91, T79.A0X-T79.9XX with 7th A

√6ᵗʰ **S15.10** Unspecified injury of vertebral artery

√7ᵗʰ **S15.101** Unspecified injury of right vertebral artery   CC

√7ᵗʰ **S15.102** Unspecified injury of left vertebral artery   CC

√7ᵗʰ **S15.109** Unspecified injury of unspecified vertebral artery   CC

---

7 HAC = Initial encounter only (7th character A, B or C) and not POA.

√6ᵗʰ **S15.11** **Minor laceration** of vertebral artery
    Incomplete transection of vertebral artery
    Laceration of vertebral artery NOS
    Superficial laceration of vertebral artery

    √7ᵗʰ **S15.111** **Minor laceration of right** vertebral artery `cc`

    √7ᵗʰ **S15.112** **Minor laceration of left** vertebral artery `cc`

    √7ᵗʰ **S15.119** **Minor laceration of unspecified** vertebral artery `cc`

√6ᵗʰ **S15.12** **Major laceration** of vertebral artery
    Complete transection of vertebral artery
    Traumatic rupture of vertebral artery

    √7ᵗʰ **S15.121** **Major laceration of right** vertebral artery `cc`

    √7ᵗʰ **S15.122** **Major laceration of left** vertebral artery `cc`

    √7ᵗʰ **S15.129** **Major laceration of unspecified** vertebral artery `cc`

√6ᵗʰ **S15.19** **Other** specified injury of vertebral artery

    √7ᵗʰ **S15.191** **Other specified injury of right** vertebral artery `cc`

    √7ᵗʰ **S15.192** **Other specified injury of left** vertebral artery `cc`

    √7ᵗʰ **S15.199** **Other specified injury of unspecified** vertebral artery `cc`

√5ᵗʰ **S15.2** **Injury of** external jugular vein

> **CC Excl: For CC codes in subcategory S15.2, unless otherwise noted:** See code: S15.1

√6ᵗʰ **S15.20** **Unspecified** injury of external jugular vein

    √7ᵗʰ **S15.201** **Unspecified injury of right** external jugular vein `cc`

    √7ᵗʰ **S15.202** **Unspecified injury of left** external jugular vein `cc`

    √7ᵗʰ **S15.209** **Unspecified injury of unspecified** external jugular vein `cc`

√6ᵗʰ **S15.21** **Minor laceration** of external jugular vein
    Incomplete transection of external jugular vein
    Laceration of external jugular vein NOS
    Superficial laceration of external jugular vein

    √7ᵗʰ **S15.211** **Minor laceration of right** external jugular vein `cc`

    √7ᵗʰ **S15.212** **Minor laceration of left** external jugular vein `cc`

    √7ᵗʰ **S15.219** **Minor laceration of unspecified** external jugular vein `cc`

√6ᵗʰ **S15.22** **Major laceration** of external jugular vein
    Complete transection of external jugular vein
    Traumatic rupture of external jugular vein

    √7ᵗʰ **S15.221** **Major laceration of right** external jugular vein `cc`

    √7ᵗʰ **S15.222** **Major laceration of left** external jugular vein `cc`

    √7ᵗʰ **S15.229** **Major laceration of unspecified** external jugular vein `cc`

√6ᵗʰ **S15.29** **Other** specified injury of external jugular vein

    √7ᵗʰ **S15.291** **Other specified injury of right** external jugular vein `cc`

    √7ᵗʰ **S15.292** **Other specified injury of left** external jugular vein `cc`

    √7ᵗʰ **S15.299** **Other specified injury of unspecified** external jugular vein `cc`

√5ᵗʰ **S15.3** **Injury of** internal jugular vein

> **CC Excl: For CC codes in subcategory S15.3, unless otherwise noted:** See code: S15.1

√6ᵗʰ **S15.30** **Unspecified** injury of internal jugular vein

    √7ᵗʰ **S15.301** **Unspecified injury of right** internal jugular vein `cc`

    √7ᵗʰ **S15.302** **Unspecified injury of left** internal jugular vein `cc`

    √7ᵗʰ **S15.309** **Unspecified injury of unspecified** internal jugular vein `cc`

√6ᵗʰ **S15.31** **Minor laceration** of internal jugular vein
    Incomplete transection of internal jugular vein
    Laceration of internal jugular vein NOS
    Superficial laceration of internal jugular vein

    √7ᵗʰ **S15.311** **Minor laceration of right** internal jugular vein `cc`

    √7ᵗʰ **S15.312** **Minor laceration of left** internal jugular vein `cc`

    √7ᵗʰ **S15.319** **Minor laceration of unspecified** internal jugular vein `cc`

√6ᵗʰ **S15.32** **Major laceration** of internal jugular vein
    Complete transection of internal jugular vein
    Traumatic rupture of internal jugular vein

    √7ᵗʰ **S15.321** **Major laceration of right** internal jugular vein `cc`

    √7ᵗʰ **S15.322** **Major laceration of left** internal jugular vein `cc`

    √7ᵗʰ **S15.329** **Major laceration of unspecified** internal jugular vein `cc`

√6ᵗʰ **S15.39** **Other** specified injury of internal jugular vein

    √7ᵗʰ **S15.391** **Other specified injury of right** internal jugular vein `cc`

    √7ᵗʰ **S15.392** **Other specified injury of left** internal jugular vein `cc`

    √7ᵗʰ **S15.399** **Other specified injury of unspecified** internal jugular vein `cc`

√x7ᵗʰ **S15.8** **Injury of other specified blood vessels at neck level** `cc`
    CC Excl: See code: S15.1

√x7ᵗʰ **S15.9** **Injury of unspecified blood vessel at neck level** `cc`
    CC Excl: See code: S15.1

√4ᵗʰ **S16** **Injury of muscle, fascia and tendon at neck level**
    Code also any associated open wound (S11.-)
    EXCLUDES 2 sprain of joint or ligament at neck level (S13.9)

> The appropriate 7th is to be added to each code from category S16.
> A   initial encounter
> D   subsequent encounter
> S   sequela

√x7ᵗʰ **S16.1** **Strain of muscle, fascia and tendon at neck level**

√x7ᵗʰ **S16.2** **Laceration of muscle, fascia and tendon at neck level**

√x7ᵗʰ **S16.8** **Other specified injury of muscle, fascia and tendon at neck level**

√x7ᵗʰ **S16.9** **Unspecified injury of muscle, fascia and tendon at neck level**

√4ᵗʰ **S17** **Crushing injury of neck**
    Use additional code for all associated injuries, such as:
    injury of blood vessels (S15.-)
    open wound of neck (S11.-)
    spinal cord injury (S14.0, S14.1-)
    vertebral fracture (S12.0- – S12.3-)

> The appropriate 7th is to be added to each code from category S17.
> A   initial encounter
> D   subsequent encounter
> S   sequela

> **CC Excl: For CC codes in category S17, unless otherwise noted: CC with 7th character A:** S01.90X-S02.92X with 7th A, S07.0XX-S07.9XX with 7th A, S08.89X-S09.19X with 7th A, S09.8XX-S09.90X with 7th A, S09.92X-S09.93X with 7th A, S16.8XX-S19.9XX with 7th A, T14.8-T14.91, T79.A0X-T79.9XX with 7th A

7 √x7ᵗʰ **S17.0** **Crushing injury of larynx and trachea** `cc`
7 √x7ᵗʰ **S17.8** **Crushing injury of other specified parts of neck** `cc`
7 √x7ᵗʰ **S17.9** **Crushing injury of neck, part unspecified** `cc`

√4ᵗʰ **S19** **Other specified and unspecified injuries of neck**

> The appropriate 7th is to be added to each code from category S19.
> A   initial encounter
> D   subsequent encounter
> S   sequela

√5ᵗʰ **S19.8** **Other specified injuries of neck**

    √x7ᵗʰ **S19.80** **Other specified injuries of unspecified part of neck**

    √x7ᵗʰ **S19.81** **Other specified injuries of larynx**

---

7 HAC = Initial encounter only (7th character A, B or C) and not POA.

√ Additional Character Required   √x7ᵗʰ Xtension Alert   Unacceptable PDx   Manifestation   Hospital Acquired Condition   *EXCLUDES 1* Not Coded Here   *EXCLUDES 2* Not Included Here

Injury, Poisoning and Certain Other Consequences of External Causes

S19.82–S20.379

√x7th **S19.82** **Other specified injuries of cervical** trachea
     EXCLUDES 2 *other specified injury of thoracic trachea (S27.5-)*

√x7th **S19.83** **Other specified injuries of** vocal cord

√x7th **S19.84** **Other specified injuries of** thyroid gland

√x7th **S19.85** **Other specified injuries of** pharynx and cervical esophagus

√x7th **S19.89** **Other specified injuries of** other specified part of neck

√x7th **S19.9** **Unspecified injury of neck**

Injuries to the thorax (S20-S29)

INCLUDES   injuries of breast
     injuries of chest (wall)
     injuries of interscapular area

EXCLUDES 2   *burns and corrosions (T20-T32)*
     effects of foreign body in bronchus (T17.5)
     effects of foreign body in esophagus (T18.1)
     effects of foreign body in lung (T17.8)
     effects of foreign body in trachea (T17.4)
     frostbite (T33-T34)
     injuries of axilla
     injuries of clavicle
     injuries of scapular region
     injuries of shoulder
     insect bite or sting, venomous (T63.4)

√4th **S20** **Superficial injury of thorax**

> The appropriate 7th is to be added to each code from category S20.
> A   initial encounter
> D   subsequent encounter
> S   sequela

√5th **S20.0** **Contusion of breast**

√x7th **S20.00** **Contusion of breast,** unspecified breast

√x7th **S20.01** **Contusion of** right breast

√x7th **S20.02** **Contusion of** left breast

√5th **S20.1** **Other and unspecified superficial injuries of breast**

√6th **S20.10** Unspecified **superficial injuries of breast**

√7th **S20.101** Unspecified **superficial injuries of breast,** right breast

√7th **S20.102** Unspecified **superficial injuries of breast,** left breast

√7th **S20.109** Unspecified **superficial injuries of breast,** unspecified breast

√6th **S20.11** Abrasion **of breast**

√7th **S20.111** **Abrasion of breast,** right breast

√7th **S20.112** **Abrasion of breast,** left breast

√7th **S20.119** **Abrasion of breast,** unspecified breast

√6th **S20.12** Blister (nonthermal) **of breast**

√7th **S20.121** **Blister (nonthermal) of breast,** right breast

√7th **S20.122** **Blister (nonthermal) of breast,** left breast

√7th **S20.129** **Blister (nonthermal) of breast,** unspecified breast

√6th **S20.14** External constriction **of part of breast**

√7th **S20.141** **External constriction of part of breast,** right breast

√7th **S20.142** **External constriction of part of breast,** left breast

√7th **S20.149** **External constriction of part of breast,** unspecified breast

√6th **S20.15** **Superficial** foreign body **of breast**
     Splinter in the breast

√7th **S20.151** **Superficial foreign body of breast,** right breast

√7th **S20.152** **Superficial foreign body of breast,** left breast

√7th **S20.159** **Superficial foreign body of breast,** unspecified breast

√6th **S20.16** Insect bite (nonvenomous) **of breast**

√7th **S20.161** **Insect bite (nonvenomous) of breast,** right breast

√7th **S20.162** **Insect bite (nonvenomous) of breast,** left breast

√7th **S20.169** **Insect bite (nonvenomous) of breast,** unspecified **breast**

√6th **S20.17** Other **superficial** bite **of breast**
     EXCLUDES 1 *open bite of breast (S21.05-)*

√7th **S20.171** **Other superficial bite of breast,** right breast

√7th **S20.172** **Other superficial bite of breast,** left breast

√7th **S20.179** **Other superficial bite of breast,** unspecified **breast**

√5th **S20.2** **Contusion of thorax**

√x7th **S20.20** **Contusion of thorax,** unspecified

√6th **S20.21** **Contusion of** front wall **of thorax**

√7th **S20.211** **Contusion of** right **front wall of thorax**

√7th **S20.212** **Contusion of** left **front wall of thorax**

√7th **S20.219** **Contusion of** unspecified **front wall of thorax**

√6th **S20.22** **Contusion of** back wall **of thorax**

√7th **S20.221** **Contusion of** right **back wall of thorax**

√7th **S20.222** **Contusion of** left **back wall of thorax**

√7th **S20.229** **Contusion of** unspecified **back wall of thorax**

√5th **S20.3** **Other and unspecified superficial injuries of** front wall **of** thorax

√6th **S20.30** Unspecified **superficial injuries of front wall of** thorax

√7th **S20.301** Unspecified **superficial injuries of** right **front wall of thorax**

√7th **S20.302** Unspecified **superficial injuries of** left **front wall of thorax**

√7th **S20.309** Unspecified **superficial injuries of** unspecified **front wall of thorax**

√6th **S20.31** Abrasion **of front wall of thorax**

√7th **S20.311** **Abrasion of** right **front wall of thorax**

√7th **S20.312** **Abrasion of** left **front wall of thorax**

√7th **S20.319** **Abrasion of** unspecified **front wall of thorax**

√6th **S20.32** Blister (nonthermal) **of front wall of thorax**

√7th **S20.321** **Blister (nonthermal) of** right **front wall of thorax**

√7th **S20.322** **Blister (nonthermal) of** left **front wall of thorax**

√7th **S20.329** **Blister (nonthermal) of** unspecified **front wall of thorax**

√6th **S20.34** External constriction **of front wall of thorax**

√7th **S20.341** **External constriction of** right **front wall of thorax**

√7th **S20.342** **External constriction of** left **front wall of thorax**

√7th **S20.349** **External constriction of** unspecified **front wall of thorax**

√6th **S20.35** **Superficial** foreign body **of front wall of thorax**
     Splinter in front wall of thorax

√7th **S20.351** **Superficial foreign body of** right **front wall of thorax**

√7th **S20.352** **Superficial foreign body of** left **front wall of thorax**

√7th **S20.359** **Superficial foreign body of** unspecified **front wall of thorax**

√6th **S20.36** Insect bite (nonvenomous) **of front wall of thorax**

√7th **S20.361** **Insect bite (nonvenomous) of** right **front wall of thorax**

√7th **S20.362** **Insect bite (nonvenomous) of** left **front wall of thorax**

√7th **S20.369** **Insect bite (nonvenomous) of** unspecified **front wall of thorax**

√6th **S20.37** Other **superficial** bite **of front wall of thorax**
     EXCLUDES 1 *open bite of front wall of thorax (S21.14)*

√7th **S20.371** **Other superficial bite of** right **front wall of thorax**

√7th **S20.372** **Other superficial bite of** left **front wall of thorax**

√7th **S20.379** **Other superficial bite of** unspecified **front wall of thorax**

N Newborn: 0   P Pediatric: 0-17   M Maternity: 12-55   A Adult: 15-124   MCC Major CC Condition   PDx MCC PDx acts as own MCC   CC CC Condition   PDx CC PDx acts as own CC

876   ICD-10-CM Draft (2015)

✓5ᵗʰ **S20.4 Other and unspecified superficial injuries of** back wall of thorax

  ✓6ᵗʰ **S20.40 Unspecified superficial injuries of back wall of** thorax

    ✓7ᵗʰ **S20.401 Unspecified superficial injuries of right back wall of thorax**

    ✓7ᵗʰ **S20.402 Unspecified superficial injuries of left back wall of thorax**

    ✓7ᵗʰ **S20.409 Unspecified superficial injuries of unspecified back wall of thorax**

  ✓6ᵗʰ **S20.41 Abrasion of back wall of thorax**

    ✓7ᵗʰ **S20.411 Abrasion of right back wall of thorax**

    ✓7ᵗʰ **S20.412 Abrasion of left back wall of thorax**

    ✓7ᵗʰ **S20.419 Abrasion of unspecified back wall of thorax**

  ✓6ᵗʰ **S20.42 Blister (nonthermal) of back wall of thorax**

    ✓7ᵗʰ **S20.421 Blister (nonthermal) of right back wall of thorax**

    ✓7ᵗʰ **S20.422 Blister (nonthermal) of left back wall of thorax**

    ✓7ᵗʰ **S20.429 Blister (nonthermal) of unspecified back wall of thorax**

  ✓6ᵗʰ **S20.44 External constriction of back wall of thorax**

    ✓7ᵗʰ **S20.441 External constriction of right back wall of thorax**

    ✓7ᵗʰ **S20.442 External constriction of left back wall of thorax**

    ✓7ᵗʰ **S20.449 External constriction of unspecified back wall of thorax**

  ✓6ᵗʰ **S20.45 Superficial foreign body of back wall of thorax**
    Splinter of back wall of thorax

    ✓7ᵗʰ **S20.451 Superficial foreign body of right back wall of thorax**

    ✓7ᵗʰ **S20.452 Superficial foreign body of left back wall of thorax**

    ✓7ᵗʰ **S20.459 Superficial foreign body of unspecified back wall of thorax**

  ✓6ᵗʰ **S20.46 Insect bite (nonvenomous) of back wall of thorax**

    ✓7ᵗʰ **S20.461 Insect bite (nonvenomous) of right back wall of thorax**

    ✓7ᵗʰ **S20.462 Insect bite (nonvenomous) of left back wall of thorax**

    ✓7ᵗʰ **S20.469 Insect bite (nonvenomous) of unspecified back wall of thorax**

  ✓6ᵗʰ **S20.47 Other superficial bite of back wall of thorax**
    EXCLUDES 1 open bite of back wall of thorax (S21.24)

    ✓7ᵗʰ **S20.471 Other superficial bite of right back wall of thorax**

    ✓7ᵗʰ **S20.472 Other superficial bite of left back wall of thorax**

    ✓7ᵗʰ **S20.479 Other superficial bite of unspecified back wall of thorax**

✓5ᵗʰ **S20.9 Superficial injury of unspecified parts of thorax**
  EXCLUDES 1 contusion of thorax NOS (S20.20)

  ✓x7ᵗʰ **S20.90 Unspecified superficial injury of unspecified parts of thorax**
    Superficial injury of thoracic wall NOS

  ✓x7ᵗʰ **S20.91 Abrasion of unspecified parts of thorax**

  ✓x7ᵗʰ **S20.92 Blister (nonthermal) of unspecified parts of thorax**

  ✓x7ᵗʰ **S20.94 External constriction of unspecified parts of thorax**

  ✓x7ᵗʰ **S20.95 Superficial foreign body of unspecified parts of thorax**
    Splinter in thorax NOS

  ✓x7ᵗʰ **S20.96 Insect bite (nonvenomous) of unspecified parts of thorax**

  ✓x7ᵗʰ **S20.97 Other superficial bite of unspecified parts of thorax**
    EXCLUDES 1 open bite of thorax NOS (S21.95)

✓4ᵗʰ **S21 Open wound of thorax**
  Code also any associated injury, such as:
    injury of heart (S26.-)
    injury of intrathoracic organs (S27.-)
    rib fracture (S22.3-, S22.4-)
    spinal cord injury (S24.0-, S24.1-)
    traumatic hemopneumothorax (S27.3)
    traumatic hemothorax (S27.1)
    traumatic pneumothorax (S27.0)
    wound infection
  EXCLUDES 1 traumatic amputation (partial) of thorax (S28.1)

  The appropriate 7th is to be added to each code from category S21.
  A   initial encounter
  D   subsequent encounter
  S   sequela

  ✓5ᵗʰ **S21.0 Open wound of breast**

    ✓6ᵗʰ **S21.00 Unspecified open wound of breast**

      ✓7ᵗʰ **S21.001 Unspecified open wound of right breast**

      ✓7ᵗʰ **S21.002 Unspecified open wound of left breast**

      ✓7ᵗʰ **S21.009 Unspecified open wound of unspecified breast**

    ✓6ᵗʰ **S21.01 Laceration without foreign body of breast**

      ✓7ᵗʰ **S21.011 Laceration without foreign body of right breast**

      ✓7ᵗʰ **S21.012 Laceration without foreign body of left breast**

      ✓7ᵗʰ **S21.019 Laceration without foreign body of unspecified breast**

    ✓6ᵗʰ **S21.02 Laceration with foreign body of breast**

      ✓7ᵗʰ **S21.021 Laceration with foreign body of right breast**

      ✓7ᵗʰ **S21.022 Laceration with foreign body of left breast**

      ✓7ᵗʰ **S21.029 Laceration with foreign body of unspecified breast**

    ✓6ᵗʰ **S21.03 Puncture wound without foreign body of breast**

      ✓7ᵗʰ **S21.031 Puncture wound without foreign body of right breast**

      ✓7ᵗʰ **S21.032 Puncture wound without foreign body of left breast**

      ✓7ᵗʰ **S21.039 Puncture wound without foreign body of unspecified breast**

    ✓6ᵗʰ **S21.04 Puncture wound with foreign body of breast**

      ✓7ᵗʰ **S21.041 Puncture wound with foreign body of right breast**

      ✓7ᵗʰ **S21.042 Puncture wound with foreign body of left breast**

      ✓7ᵗʰ **S21.049 Puncture wound with foreign body of unspecified breast**

    ✓6ᵗʰ **S21.05 Open bite of breast**
      Bite of breast NOS
      EXCLUDES 1 superficial bite of breast (S20.17)

      ✓7ᵗʰ **S21.051 Open bite of right breast**

      ✓7ᵗʰ **S21.052 Open bite of left breast**

      ✓7ᵗʰ **S21.059 Open bite of unspecified breast**

  ✓5ᵗʰ **S21.1 Open wound of front wall of thorax without penetration into thoracic cavity**
    Open wound of chest without penetration into thoracic cavity

    CC Excl: For CC codes in subcategory S21.1, unless otherwise noted: CC with 7th character A: S21.101-S21.159 with 7th A, S21.301-S21.95 with 7th A, S23.3XXA, S23.8XXA, S27.50X-S27.69X with 7th A, S27.892-S27.9XX with 7th A, S28.1XXA, S29.021A, S29.029A, S38.3XXA, T14.8-T14.91, T79.7XX-T79.9XX with 7th A

    ✓6ᵗʰ **S21.10 Unspecified open wound of front wall of thorax without penetration into thoracic cavity**

      ✓7ᵗʰ **S21.101 Unspecified open wound of right front wall of thorax without penetration into thoracic cavity** CC

      ✓7ᵗʰ **S21.102 Unspecified open wound of left front wall of thorax without penetration into thoracic cavity** CC

      ✓7ᵗʰ **S21.109 Unspecified open wound of unspecified front wall of thorax without penetration into thoracic cavity** CC

☑ Additional Character Required   ✓x7ᵗʰ Xtension Alert   Unacceptable PDx   Manifestation   Hospital Acquired Condition   **EXCLUDES 1** Not Coded Here   **EXCLUDES 2** Not Included Here

Injury, Poisoning and Certain Other Consequences of External Causes

S21.11–S21.311

✓6ᵗʰ **S21.11** Laceration without foreign body of front wall of thorax without penetration into thoracic cavity

  ✓7ᵗʰ **S21.111** Laceration without foreign body of right front wall of thorax without penetration into thoracic cavity **CC**

  ✓7ᵗʰ **S21.112** Laceration without foreign body of left front wall of thorax without penetration into thoracic cavity **CC**

  ✓7ᵗʰ **S21.119** Laceration without foreign body of unspecified front wall of thorax without penetration into thoracic cavity **CC**

✓6ᵗʰ **S21.12** Laceration with foreign body of front wall of thorax without penetration into thoracic cavity

  ✓7ᵗʰ **S21.121** Laceration with foreign body of right front wall of thorax without penetration into thoracic cavity **CC**

  ✓7ᵗʰ **S21.122** Laceration with foreign body of left front wall of thorax without penetration into thoracic cavity **CC**

  ✓7ᵗʰ **S21.129** Laceration with foreign body of unspecified front wall of thorax without penetration into thoracic cavity **CC**

✓6ᵗʰ **S21.13** Puncture wound without foreign body of front wall of thorax without penetration into thoracic cavity

  ✓7ᵗʰ **S21.131** Puncture wound without foreign body of right front wall of thorax without penetration into thoracic cavity **CC**

  ✓7ᵗʰ **S21.132** Puncture wound without foreign body of left front wall of thorax without penetration into thoracic cavity **CC**

  ✓7ᵗʰ **S21.139** Puncture wound without foreign body of unspecified front wall of thorax without penetration into thoracic cavity **CC**

✓6ᵗʰ **S21.14** Puncture wound with foreign body of front wall of thorax without penetration into thoracic cavity

  ✓7ᵗʰ **S21.141** Puncture wound with foreign body of right front wall of thorax without penetration into thoracic cavity **CC**

  ✓7ᵗʰ **S21.142** Puncture wound with foreign body of left front wall of thorax without penetration into thoracic cavity **CC**

  ✓7ᵗʰ **S21.149** Puncture wound with foreign body of unspecified front wall of thorax without penetration into thoracic cavity **CC**

✓6ᵗʰ **S21.15** Open bite of front wall of thorax without penetration into thoracic cavity

  Bite of front wall of thorax NOS

  EXCLUDES 1   superficial bite of front wall of thorax (S20.37)

  ✓7ᵗʰ **S21.151** Open bite of right front wall of thorax without penetration into thoracic cavity **CC**

  ✓7ᵗʰ **S21.152** Open bite of left front wall of thorax without penetration into thoracic cavity **CC**

  ✓7ᵗʰ **S21.159** Open bite of unspecified front wall of thorax without penetration into thoracic cavity **CC**

✓5ᵗʰ **S21.2** Open wound of back wall of thorax without penetration into thoracic cavity

✓6ᵗʰ **S21.20** Unspecified open wound of back wall of thorax without penetration into thoracic cavity

  ✓7ᵗʰ **S21.201** Unspecified open wound of right back wall of thorax without penetration into thoracic cavity

  ✓7ᵗʰ **S21.202** Unspecified open wound of left back wall of thorax without penetration into thoracic cavity

  ✓7ᵗʰ **S21.209** Unspecified open wound of unspecified back wall of thorax without penetration into thoracic cavity

✓6ᵗʰ **S21.21** Laceration without foreign body of back wall of thorax without penetration into thoracic cavity

  ✓7ᵗʰ **S21.211** Laceration without foreign body of right back wall of thorax without penetration into thoracic cavity

  ✓7ᵗʰ **S21.212** Laceration without foreign body of left back wall of thorax without penetration into thoracic cavity

✓7ᵗʰ **S21.219** Laceration without foreign body of unspecified back wall of thorax without penetration into thoracic cavity

✓6ᵗʰ **S21.22** Laceration with foreign body of back wall of thorax without penetration into thoracic cavity

  ✓7ᵗʰ **S21.221** Laceration with foreign body of right back wall of thorax without penetration into thoracic cavity

  ✓7ᵗʰ **S21.222** Laceration with foreign body of left back wall of thorax without penetration into thoracic cavity

  ✓7ᵗʰ **S21.229** Laceration with foreign body of unspecified back wall of thorax without penetration into thoracic cavity

✓6ᵗʰ **S21.23** Puncture wound without foreign body of back wall of thorax without penetration into thoracic cavity

  ✓7ᵗʰ **S21.231** Puncture wound without foreign body of right back wall of thorax without penetration into thoracic cavity

  ✓7ᵗʰ **S21.232** Puncture wound without foreign body of left back wall of thorax without penetration into thoracic cavity

  ✓7ᵗʰ **S21.239** Puncture wound without foreign body of unspecified back wall of thorax without penetration into thoracic cavity

✓6ᵗʰ **S21.24** Puncture wound with foreign body of back wall of thorax without penetration into thoracic cavity

  ✓7ᵗʰ **S21.241** Puncture wound with foreign body of right back wall of thorax without penetration into thoracic cavity

  ✓7ᵗʰ **S21.242** Puncture wound with foreign body of left back wall of thorax without penetration into thoracic cavity

  ✓7ᵗʰ **S21.249** Puncture wound with foreign body of unspecified back wall of thorax without penetration into thoracic cavity

✓6ᵗʰ **S21.25** Open bite of back wall of thorax without penetration into thoracic cavity

  Bite of back wall of thorax NOS

  EXCLUDES 1   superficial bite of back wall of thorax (S20.47)

  ✓7ᵗʰ **S21.251** Open bite of right back wall of thorax without penetration into thoracic cavity

  ✓7ᵗʰ **S21.252** Open bite of left back wall of thorax without penetration into thoracic cavity

  ✓7ᵗʰ **S21.259** Open bite of unspecified back wall of thorax without penetration into thoracic cavity

✓5ᵗʰ **S21.3** Open wound of front wall of thorax with penetration into thoracic cavity

  Open wound of chest with penetration into thoracic cavity

> **CC Excl:** For MCC codes in subcategory S21.1, unless otherwise noted: MCC with 7th character A: S21.101-S21.159 with 7th A, S21.301-S21.95X with 7th A, S27.50X-S27.69X with 7th A, S27.892-S27.9XX with 7th A, S28.1XXA, S29.021A, S29.029A, S38.3XXA, T14.8-T14.91, T79.7XX-T79.9XX with 7th A

✓6ᵗʰ **S21.30** Unspecified open wound of front wall of thorax with penetration into thoracic cavity

  ✓7ᵗʰ **S21.301** Unspecified open wound of right front wall of thorax with penetration into thoracic cavity **MCC**

  ✓7ᵗʰ **S21.302** Unspecified open wound of left front wall of thorax with penetration into thoracic cavity **MCC**

  ✓7ᵗʰ **S21.309** Unspecified open wound of unspecified front wall of thorax with penetration into thoracic cavity **MCC**

    CC Excl: S21.101-S21.159 with 7th A, S21.301-S21.95 with 7th A, S27.0XX-S27.309 with 7th A, S27.329A, S27.339A, S27.409 with 7th A, S27.50X-S27.803 with 7th A, S27.892-S27.9XX with 7th A, S28.1XXA, S29.021A, S29.029A, S38.3XXA, T14.8-T14.91, T79.7XX-T79.9XX with 7th A

✓6ᵗʰ **S21.31** Laceration without foreign body of front wall of thorax with penetration into thoracic cavity

  ✓7ᵗʰ **S21.311** Laceration without foreign body of right front wall of thorax with penetration into thoracic cavity **MCC**

N Newborn: 0   **P** Pediatric: 0-17   **M** Maternity: 12-55   **A** Adult: 15-124   **MCC** Major CC Condition   **PDx MCC** PDx acts as own MCC   **CC** CC Condition   **PDx CC** PDx acts as own CC

878   ICD-10-CM Draft (2015)

√7ᵗʰ **S21.312** Laceration without foreign body of MCC
left front wall of thorax with
penetration into thoracic cavity

√7ᵗʰ **S21.319** Laceration without foreign body of MCC
unspecified front wall of thorax with
penetration into thoracic cavity

√6ᵗʰ **S21.32** Laceration with foreign body of front wall of thorax
with penetration into thoracic cavity

√7ᵗʰ **S21.321** Laceration with foreign body of MCC
right front wall of thorax with
penetration into thoracic cavity

√7ᵗʰ **S21.322** Laceration with foreign body of left MCC
front wall of thorax with penetration
into thoracic cavity

√7ᵗʰ **S21.329** Laceration with foreign body of MCC
unspecified front wall of thorax with
penetration into thoracic cavity

√6ᵗʰ **S21.33** Puncture wound without foreign body of front wall
of thorax with penetration into thoracic cavity

√7ᵗʰ **S21.331** Puncture wound without foreign MCC
body of right front wall of thorax with
penetration into thoracic cavity

√7ᵗʰ **S21.332** Puncture wound without foreign MCC
body of left front wall of thorax with
penetration into thoracic cavity

√7ᵗʰ **S21.339** Puncture wound without foreign MCC
body of unspecified front wall of thorax
with penetration into thoracic cavity

√6ᵗʰ **S21.34** Puncture wound with foreign body of front wall of
thorax with penetration into thoracic cavity

√7ᵗʰ **S21.341** Puncture wound with foreign body of MCC
right front wall of thorax with
penetration into thoracic cavity

√7ᵗʰ **S21.342** Puncture wound with foreign body of MCC
left front wall of thorax with penetration
into thoracic cavity

√7ᵗʰ **S21.349** Puncture wound with foreign body MCC
of unspecified front wall of thorax with
penetration into thoracic cavity

√6ᵗʰ **S21.35** Open bite of front wall of thorax with penetration
into thoracic cavity

EXCLUDES 1 superficial bite of front wall of thorax (S20.37)

√7ᵗʰ **S21.351** Open bite of right front wall of thorax MCC
with penetration into thoracic cavity

√7ᵗʰ **S21.352** Open bite of left front wall of thorax MCC
with penetration into thoracic cavity

√7ᵗʰ **S21.359** Open bite of unspecified front wall of MCC
thorax with penetration into thoracic
cavity

√5ᵗʰ **S21.4** Open wound of back wall of thorax with penetration into
thoracic cavity

CC Excl: For MCC codes in subcategory S21.4, unless
otherwise noted: MCC with 7th character A: See code:
S21.3

√6ᵗʰ **S21.40** Unspecified open wound of back wall of thorax with
penetration into thoracic cavity

√7ᵗʰ **S21.401** Unspecified open wound of right back MCC
wall of thorax with penetration into
thoracic cavity

√7ᵗʰ **S21.402** Unspecified open wound of left back MCC
wall of thorax with penetration into
thoracic cavity

√7ᵗʰ **S21.409** Unspecified open wound of MCC
unspecified back wall of thorax with
penetration into thoracic cavity

√6ᵗʰ **S21.41** Laceration without foreign body of back wall of
thorax with penetration into thoracic cavity

√7ᵗʰ **S21.411** Laceration without foreign body of MCC
right back wall of thorax with
penetration into thoracic cavity

√7ᵗʰ **S21.412** Laceration without foreign body of MCC
left back wall of thorax with
penetration into thoracic cavity

√7ᵗʰ **S21.419** Laceration without foreign body of MCC
unspecified back wall of thorax with
penetration into thoracic cavity

√6ᵗʰ **S21.42** Laceration with foreign body of back wall of thorax
with penetration into thoracic cavity

√7ᵗʰ **S21.421** Laceration with foreign body of right MCC
back wall of thorax with penetration into
thoracic cavity

√7ᵗʰ **S21.422** Laceration with foreign body of left MCC
back wall of thorax with penetration
into thoracic cavity

√7ᵗʰ **S21.429** Laceration with foreign body of MCC
unspecified back wall of thorax with
penetration into thoracic cavity

√6ᵗʰ **S21.43** Puncture wound without foreign body of back wall
of thorax with penetration into thoracic cavity

√7ᵗʰ **S21.431** Puncture wound without foreign MCC
body of right back wall of thorax with
penetration into thoracic cavity

√7ᵗʰ **S21.432** Puncture wound without foreign MCC
body of left back wall of thorax with
penetration into thoracic cavity

√7ᵗʰ **S21.439** Puncture wound without foreign MCC
body of unspecified back wall of thorax
with penetration into thoracic cavity

√6ᵗʰ **S21.44** Puncture wound with foreign body of back wall of
thorax with penetration into thoracic cavity

√7ᵗʰ **S21.441** Puncture wound with foreign body of MCC
right back wall of thorax with
penetration into thoracic cavity

√7ᵗʰ **S21.442** Puncture wound with foreign body of MCC
left back wall of thorax with penetration
into thoracic cavity

√7ᵗʰ **S21.449** Puncture wound with foreign body of MCC
unspecified back wall of thorax with
penetration into thoracic cavity

√6ᵗʰ **S21.45** Open bite of back wall of thorax with penetration
into thoracic cavity

Bite of back wall of thorax NOS

EXCLUDES 1 superficial bite of back wall of thorax (S20.47)

√7ᵗʰ **S21.451** Open bite of right back wall of thorax MCC
with penetration into thoracic cavity

√7ᵗʰ **S21.452** Open bite of left back wall of thorax MCC
with penetration into thoracic cavity

√7ᵗʰ **S21.459** Open bite of unspecified back wall of MCC
thorax with penetration into thoracic
cavity

√5ᵗʰ **S21.9** Open wound of unspecified part of thorax

Open wound of thoracic wall NOS

CC Excl: For CC codes in subcategory S21.9, unless
otherwise noted: CC with 7th character A: S21.101-
S21.159 with 7th A, S21.301-S21.95X with 7th A,
S23.3XXA, S23.8XXA, S27.50X-S27.69X with 7th A,
S27.892-S27.9XX with 7th A, S28.1XXA, S29.021A,
S29.029A, S38.3XXA, T14.8-T14.91, T79.7XX-T79.9XX with
7th A

√x7ᵗʰ **S21.90** Unspecified open wound of unspecified CC
part of thorax

√x7ᵗʰ **S21.91** Laceration without foreign body of unspecified CC
part of thorax

√x7ᵗʰ **S21.92** Laceration with foreign body of unspecified CC
part of thorax

√x7ᵗʰ **S21.93** Puncture wound without foreign body of CC
unspecified part of thorax

√x7ᵗʰ **S21.94** Puncture wound with foreign body of CC
unspecified part of thorax

√x7ᵗʰ **S21.95** Open bite of unspecified part of thorax CC

EXCLUDES 1 superficial bite of thorax (S20.97)

☑ Additional Character Required √ˣ7ᵗʰ Xtension Alert Unacceptable PDx Manifestation Hospital Acquired Condition *EXCLUDES 1* Not Coded Here *EXCLUDES 2* Not Included Here

ICD-10-CM Draft (2015) 879

✓4ᵗʰ **S22 Fracture of rib(s), sternum and thoracic spine**

NOTE   A fracture not indicated as nondisplaced or displaced should be coded to displaced.
A fracture not indicated as open or closed should be coded to closed.

INCLUDES   fracture of thoracic neural arch
fracture of thoracic spinous process
fracture of thoracic transverse process
fracture of thoracic vertebra
fracture of thoracic vertebral arch

Code first any associated:
   injury of intrathoracic organ (S27.-)
   spinal cord injury (S24.0-, S24.1-)

EXCLUDES 1   transection of thorax (S28.1)
EXCLUDES 2   fracture of clavicle (S42.0-)
             fracture of scapula (S42.1-)

The appropriate 7th is to be added to each code from category S22.
A   initial encounter for closed fracture
B   initial encounter for open fracture
D   subsequent encounter for fracture with routine healing
G   subsequent encounter for fracture with delayed healing
K   subsequent encounter for fracture with nonunion
S   sequela

✓5ᵗʰ **S22.0   Fracture of thoracic vertebra**

CC Excl: For CC/MCC codes in subcategory S22.0, unless otherwise noted: CC with 7th character A or MCC with 7th character B: M48.40X-M48.58X with 7th S, M80.08XS, M80.88XS, M84.350S, M84.454S, M84.550S, M84.58S, M84.650S, M99.12, M99.15-M99.17, M99.19, S03.8XX-S03.9XX with 7th A, S12.000-S12.9XX with 7th S, S13.9XXA, S14.109A, S14.119A, S14.129 A, S14.139A, S14.149A, S14.159A, S22.000-S23.3XX with 7th [A, B, S], S23.8XX-S24.159 with 7th A, S29.001-S29.019 with 7th A, S29.091-S29.9XX with 7th A, S32.000-S32.9XX with 7th S, S33.30X-S33.39X with 7th A, S33.9XA, S38.1XXA, S38.3XX-S39.013 with 7th A, S39.091-S39.94X with 7th A, T14.8-T14.91, T79.A0X-T79.9XX with 7th A

CC with 7th character K: M80.00X-M84.68X with 7th [K, P], S02.0XX-S02.92X with 7th K, S12.000-S12.691 with 7th K, S22.000-S22.9XX with 7th K, S32.000-S32.9XX with 7th K, S42.001-S42.92X with 7th [K, P], S49.001-S49.199 with 7th [K, P], S52.001-S52.92X with 7th [K, M, N, P, Q, R], S59.001-S59.299 with 7th [K, P], S62.001-S62.92X with 7th [K, P], S72.001-S72.92X with 7th [K, M, N, P, Q, R], S79.001-S79.199 with 7th [K, P], S82.001-S82.92X with 7th [K, M, N, P, Q, R], S89.001-S89.399 with 7th [K, P], S92.001-S92.919 with 7th [K, P]

✓6ᵗʰ **S22.00   Fracture of unspecified thoracic vertebra**

7 ✓7ᵗʰ   **S22.000**   Wedge compression fracture of unspecified thoracic vertebra   MCC CC

7 ✓7ᵗʰ   **S22.001**   Stable burst fracture of unspecified thoracic vertebra   MCC CC

7 ✓7ᵗʰ   **S22.002**   Unstable burst fracture of unspecified thoracic vertebra   MCC CC

7 ✓7ᵗʰ   **S22.008**   Other fracture of unspecified thoracic vertebra   MCC CC

7 ✓7ᵗʰ   **S22.009**   Unspecified fracture of unspecified thoracic vertebra   MCC CC

✓6ᵗʰ **S22.01   Fracture of first thoracic vertebra**

7 ✓7ᵗʰ   **S22.010**   Wedge compression fracture of first thoracic vertebra   MCC CC

7 ✓7ᵗʰ   **S22.011**   Stable burst fracture of first thoracic vertebra   MCC CC

7 ✓7ᵗʰ   **S22.012**   Unstable burst fracture of first thoracic vertebra   MCC CC

7 ✓7ᵗʰ   **S22.018**   Other fracture of first thoracic vertebra   MCC CC

7 ✓7ᵗʰ   **S22.019**   Unspecified fracture of first thoracic vertebra   MCC CC

✓6ᵗʰ **S22.02   Fracture of second thoracic vertebra**

7 ✓7ᵗʰ   **S22.020**   Wedge compression fracture of second thoracic vertebra   MCC CC

7 ✓7ᵗʰ   **S22.021**   Stable burst fracture of second thoracic vertebra   MCC CC

7 ✓7ᵗʰ   **S22.022**   Unstable burst fracture of second thoracic vertebra   MCC CC

7 ✓7ᵗʰ   **S22.028**   Other fracture of second thoracic vertebra   MCC CC

7 ✓7ᵗʰ   **S22.029**   Unspecified fracture of second thoracic vertebra   MCC CC

✓6ᵗʰ **S22.03   Fracture of third thoracic vertebra**

7 ✓7ᵗʰ   **S22.030**   Wedge compression fracture of third thoracic vertebra   MCC CC

7 ✓7ᵗʰ   **S22.031**   Stable burst fracture of third thoracic vertebra   MCC CC

7 ✓7ᵗʰ   **S22.032**   Unstable burst fracture of third thoracic vertebra   MCC CC

7 ✓7ᵗʰ   **S22.038**   Other fracture of third thoracic vertebra   MCC CC

7 ✓7ᵗʰ   **S22.039**   Unspecified fracture of third thoracic vertebra   MCC CC

✓6ᵗʰ **S22.04   Fracture of fourth thoracic vertebra**

7 ✓7ᵗʰ   **S22.040**   Wedge compression fracture of fourth thoracic vertebra   MCC CC

7 ✓7ᵗʰ   **S22.041**   Stable burst fracture of fourth thoracic vertebra   MCC CC

7 ✓7ᵗʰ   **S22.042**   Unstable burst fracture of fourth thoracic vertebra   MCC CC

7 ✓7ᵗʰ   **S22.048**   Other fracture of fourth thoracic vertebra   MCC CC

7 ✓7ᵗʰ   **S22.049**   Unspecified fracture of fourth thoracic vertebra   MCC CC

✓6ᵗʰ **S22.05   Fracture of T5-T6 vertebra**

7 ✓7ᵗʰ   **S22.050**   Wedge compression fracture of T5-T6 vertebra   MCC CC

7 ✓7ᵗʰ   **S22.051**   Stable burst fracture of T5-T6 vertebra   MCC CC

7 ✓7ᵗʰ   **S22.052**   Unstable burst fracture of T5-T6 vertebra   MCC CC

7 ✓7ᵗʰ   **S22.058**   Other fracture of T5-T6 vertebra   MCC CC

7 ✓7ᵗʰ   **S22.059**   Unspecified fracture of T5-T6 vertebra   MCC CC

✓6ᵗʰ **S22.06   Fracture of T7-T8 vertebra**

7 ✓7ᵗʰ   **S22.060**   Wedge compression fracture of T7-T8 vertebra   MCC CC

7 ✓7ᵗʰ   **S22.061**   Stable burst fracture of T7-T8 vertebra   MCC CC

7 ✓7ᵗʰ   **S22.062**   Unstable burst fracture of T7-T8 vertebra   MCC CC

7 ✓7ᵗʰ   **S22.068**   Other fracture of T7-T8 thoracic vertebra   MCC CC

7 ✓7ᵗʰ   **S22.069**   Unspecified fracture of T7-T8 vertebra   MCC CC

✓6ᵗʰ **S22.07   Fracture of T9-T10 vertebra**

7 ✓7ᵗʰ   **S22.070**   Wedge compression fracture of T9-T10 vertebra   MCC CC

7 ✓7ᵗʰ   **S22.071**   Stable burst fracture of T9-T10 vertebra   MCC CC

7 ✓7ᵗʰ   **S22.072**   Unstable burst fracture of T9-T10 vertebra   MCC CC

7 ✓7ᵗʰ   **S22.078**   Other fracture of T9-T10 vertebra   MCC CC

7 ✓7ᵗʰ   **S22.079**   Unspecified fracture of T9-T10 vertebra   MCC CC

✓6ᵗʰ **S22.08   Fracture of T11-T12 vertebra**

7 ✓7ᵗʰ   **S22.080**   Wedge compression fracture of T11-T12 vertebra   MCC CC

7 ✓7ᵗʰ   **S22.081**   Stable burst fracture of T11-T12 vertebra   MCC CC

7 ✓7ᵗʰ   **S22.082**   Unstable burst fracture of T11-T12 vertebra   MCC CC

7 ✓7ᵗʰ   **S22.088**   Other fracture of T11-T12 vertebra   MCC CC

7 ✓7ᵗʰ   **S22.089**   Unspecified fracture of T11-T12 vertebra   MCC CC

---

7 HAC = Initial encounter only (7th character A, B or C) and not POA.

N Newborn: 0   P Pediatric: 0-17   M Maternity: 12-55   A Adult: 15-124   MCC Major CC Condition   PDx MCC PDx acts as own MCC   CC CC Condition   PDx CC PDx acts as own CC

880   ICD-10-CM Draft (2015)

√5th **S22.2 Fracture of sternum**

CC Excl: For CC/MCC codes in subcategory S22.2, unless otherwise noted: CC with 7th character A or MCC with 7th character B: S03.8XX-S03.9XX with 7th A, S22.20X-S22.24X with 7th [A, B], S22.5XX-S22.5XX with 7th [A, B], S29.011-S29.019 with 7th A, S38.3XX-S39.013 with 7th A, T14.8-T14.91, T79.A0X-T79.9XX with 7th A

CC with 7th character K: M80.00X-M84.68X with 7th [K, P], S02.0XX-S02.92X with 7th K, S12.000-S12.691 with 7th K, S22.000-S22.9XX with 7th K, S32.000-S32.9XX with 7th K, S42.001-S42.92X with 7th [K, P], S49.001-S49.199 with 7th [K, P], S52.001-S52.92X with 7th [K, M, N, P, Q, R], S59.001-S59.299 with 7th [K, P], S62.001-S62.92X with 7th [K, P], S72.001-S72.92X with 7th [K, M, N, P, Q, R], S79.001-S79.199 with 7th [K, P], S82.001-S82.92X with 7th [K, M, N, P, Q, R], S89.001-S89.399 with 7th [K, P], S92.001-S92.919 with 7th [K, P]

7 √x7th **S22.20 Unspecified fracture of sternum** MCC CC
7 √x7th **S22.21 Fracture of manubrium** MCC CC
7 √x7th **S22.22 Fracture of body of sternum** MCC CC
7 √x7th **S22.23 Sternal manubrial dissociation** MCC CC
7 √x7th **S22.24 Fracture of xiphoid process** MCC CC

√5th **S22.3 Fracture of one rib**

CC Excl: For CC/MCC codes in subcategory S22.3, unless otherwise noted: CC with 7th character A or MCC with 7th character B: S03.8XX-S03.9XXwith 7th A, S22.20X-S22.5XX with 7th [A, B], S29.011-S29.019 with 7th A, S38.3XX-S39.013 with 7th A, T14.8-T14.91, T79.A0X-T79.9XX with 7th A

CC with 7th character K: M80.00X-M84.68X with 7th [K, P], S02.0XX-S02.92X with 7th K, S12.000-S12.691 with 7th K, S22.000-S22.9XX with 7th K, S32.000-S32.9XX with 7th K, S42.001-S42.92X with 7th [K, P], S49.001-S49.199 with 7th [K, P], S52.001-S52.92X with 7th [K, M, N, P, Q, R], S59.001-S59.299 with 7th [K, P], S62.001-S62.92X with 7th [K, P], S72.001-S72.92X with 7th [K, M, N, P, Q, R], S79.001-S79.199 with 7th [K, P], S82.001-S82.92X with 7th [K, M, N, P, Q, R], S89.001-S89.399 with 7th [K, P], S92.001-S92.919 with 7th [K, P]

7 √x7th **S22.31 Fracture of one rib, right side** MCC CC
7 √x7th **S22.32 Fracture of one rib, left side** MCC CC
7 √x7th **S22.39 Fracture of one rib, unspecified side** MCC CC

√5th **S22.4 Multiple fractures of ribs**
Fractures of two or more ribs
EXCLUDES 1 *flail chest (S22.5-)*

CC Excl: For CC/MCC codes in subcategory S22.4, unless otherwise noted: CC with 7th character A or MCC with 7th character B: S03.8XX-S03.9XX with 7th A, S22.31X-S22.5XX with 7th [A, B], S29.011-S29.019 with 7th A, S38.3XX-S39.013 with 7th A, T14.8-T14.91, T79.A0X-T79.9XX with 7th A

CC with 7th character K: M80.00X-M84.68X with 7th [K, P], S02.0XX-S02.92X with 7th K, S12.000-S12.691 with 7th K, S22.000-S22.9XX with 7th K, S32.000-S32.9XX with 7th K, S42.001-S42.92X with 7th [K, P], S49.001-S49.199 with 7th [K, P], S52.001-S52.92X with 7th [K, M, N, P, Q, R], S59.001-S59.299 with 7th [K, P], S62.001-S62.92X with 7th [K, P], S72.001-S72.92X with 7th [K, M, N, P, Q, R], S79.001-S79.199 with 7th [K, P], S82.001-S82.92X with 7th [K, M, N, P, Q, R], S89.001-S89.399 with 7th [K, P], S92.001-S92.919 with 7th [K, P]

7 √x7th **S22.41 Multiple fractures of ribs, right side** MCC CC
7 √x7th **S22.42 Multiple fractures of ribs, left side** MCC CC
7 √x7th **S22.43 Multiple fractures of ribs, bilateral** MCC CC
7 √x7th **S22.49 Multiple fractures of ribs, unspecified side** MCC CC
    CC Excl: No excl for codes with 7th B

7 √x7th **S22.5 Flail chest** MCC CC

CC Excl: For CC/MCC codes in subcategory S22.5, unless otherwise noted: CC with 7th character A or MCC with 7th character B: S03.8XX-S03.9XX with 7th A, S22.20X-S22.5XX with 7th [A, B], S29.011-S29.019 with 7th A, S38.3XX-S39.013 with 7th A, T14.8-T14.91, T79.A0X-T79.9XX with 7th A

CC with 7th character K: M80.00X-M80.88X[K,P], M84.30X-M84.68X[K,P], S02.0X-S02.92X[K], S12.000-S12.691[K], S22.000-S22.9X[K], S32.0[0-4][0-2,8-9]K, S32.050K

√x7th **S22.9 Fracture of bony thorax, part unspecified** MCC CC

CC Excl: For CC/MCC codes in subcategory S22.9, unless otherwise noted: CC with 7th character A or MCC with 7th character B: M80.00X-M80.01X9 with 7th A, M80.041-M80.049 with 7th A, M80.80X-M80.819 with 7th A, M80.841-M80.849 with 7th A, M84.40X-M84.419 with 7th A, M84.441-M84.446 with 7th A, M84.454A, M84.474-M84.519 with 7th A, M84.541-M84.550 with 7th A, M84.574-M84.576 with 7th A, M84.60X-M84.619 with 7th A, M84.641-M84.650 with 7th A, M84.674-M84.68X with 7th A, S03.8XX-S03.9XX with 7th A, S22.9XX-S22.9XX with 7th [A, B], S29.011-S29.019 with 7th A, S32.301-S32.811 with 7th [A, B], S32.89X-S32.9XX with 7th [A, B], S33.4XXA, S33.6XX-S33.8XX with 7th A, S38.3XX-S39.013 with 7th A, S73.001-S73.199 with 7th A, S76.001-S76.019 with 7th A, S76.091-S76.119 with 7th A, S76.191-S76.219 with 7th A, S76.291-S76.319 with 7th A, S76.391-S76.819 with 7th A, S76.891-S76.919 with 7th A, S76.991-S76.999 with 7th A, S79.811-S79.929 with 7th A, T14.8-T14.91, T79.A9X-T79.9XX with 7th A

CC with 7th character K: M80.00X-M84.68X with 7th [K, P], S02.0XX-S02.92X with 7th K, S12.000-S12.691 with 7th K, S22.000-S22.9XX with 7th K, S32.000-S32.9XX with 7th K, S42.001-S42.92X with 7th [K, P], S49.001-S49.199 with 7th [K, P], S52.001-S52.92X with 7th [K, M, N, P, Q, R], S59.001-S59.299 with 7th [K, P], S62.001-S62.92X with 7th [K, P], S72.001-S72.92X with 7th [K, M, N, P, Q, R], S79.001-S79.199 with 7th [K, P], S82.001-S82.92X with 7th [K, M, N, P, Q, R], S89.001-S89.399 with 7th [K, P], S92.001-S92.919 with 7th [K, P]

√4th **S23 Dislocation and sprain of joints and ligaments of thorax**
INCLUDES   avulsion of joint or ligament of thorax
     laceration of cartilage, joint or ligament of thorax
     sprain of cartilage, joint or ligament of thorax
     traumatic hemarthrosis of joint or ligament of thorax
     traumatic rupture of joint or ligament of thorax
     traumatic subluxation of joint or ligament of thorax
     traumatic tear of joint or ligament of thorax
Code also any associated open wound
EXCLUDES 2   *dislocation, sprain of sternoclavicular joint (S43.2, S43.6)*
     strain of muscle or tendon of thorax (S29.01-)

The appropriate 7th is to be added to each code from category S23.
A   initial encounter
D   subsequent encounter
S   sequela

√x7th **S23.0 Traumatic rupture of thoracic intervertebral disc**
     EXCLUDES 1   *rupture or displacement (nontraumatic) of thoracic intervertebral disc NOS (M51- with fifth character 4)*

√5th **S23.1 Subluxation and dislocation of thoracic vertebra**
Code also any associated
     open wound of thorax (S21.-)
     spinal cord injury (S24.0-, S24.1-)
     EXCLUDES 2   *fracture of thoracic vertebrae (S22.0-)*

√6th **S23.10 Subluxation and dislocation of unspecified thoracic vertebra**
  √7th **S23.100 Subluxation of unspecified thoracic vertebra**
  √7th **S23.101 Dislocation of unspecified thoracic vertebra**

√6th **S23.11 Subluxation and dislocation of T1/T2 thoracic vertebra**
  √7th **S23.110 Subluxation of T1/T2 thoracic vertebra**
  √7th **S23.111 Dislocation of T1/T2 thoracic vertebra**

√6th **S23.12 Subluxation and dislocation of T2/T3-T3/T4 thoracic vertebra**
  √7th **S23.120 Subluxation of T2/T3 thoracic vertebra**
  √7th **S23.121 Dislocation of T2/T3 thoracic vertebra**
  √7th **S23.122 Subluxation of T3/T4 thoracic vertebra**
  √7th **S23.123 Dislocation of T3/T4 thoracic vertebra**

√6th **S23.13 Subluxation and dislocation of T4/T5-T5/T6 thoracic vertebra**
  √7th **S23.130 Subluxation of T4/T5 thoracic vertebra**
  √7th **S23.131 Dislocation of T4/T5 thoracic vertebra**
  √7th **S23.132 Subluxation of T5/T6 thoracic vertebra**
  √7th **S23.133 Dislocation of T5/T6 thoracic vertebra**

7 HAC = Initial encounter only (7th character A, B or C) and not POA.

✓ Additional Character Required   √x7th *X*tension Alert   Unacceptable PDx   Manifestation   Hospital Acquired Condition   EXCLUDES 1 Not Coded Here   EXCLUDES 2 Not Included Here

ICD-10-CM Draft (2015)   881

✓6th **S23.14** **Subluxation and dislocation of T6/T7-T7/T8 thoracic vertebra**
- ✓7th **S23.140** **Subluxation of T6/T7 thoracic vertebra**
- ✓7th **S23.141** **Dislocation of T6/T7 thoracic vertebra**
- ✓7th **S23.142** **Subluxation of T7/T8 thoracic vertebra**
- ✓7th **S23.143** **Dislocation of T7/T8 thoracic vertebra**

✓6th **S23.15** **Subluxation and dislocation of T8/T9-T9/T10 thoracic vertebra**
- ✓7th **S23.150** **Subluxation of T8/T9 thoracic vertebra**
- ✓7th **S23.151** **Dislocation of T8/T9 thoracic vertebra**
- ✓7th **S23.152** **Subluxation of T9/T10 thoracic vertebra**
- ✓7th **S23.153** **Dislocation of T9/T10 thoracic vertebra**

✓6th **S23.16** **Subluxation and dislocation of T10/T11-T11/T12 thoracic vertebra**
- ✓7th **S23.160** **Subluxation of T10/T11 thoracic vertebra**
- ✓7th **S23.161** **Dislocation of T10/T11 thoracic vertebra**
- ✓7th **S23.162** **Subluxation of T11/T12 thoracic vertebra**
- ✓7th **S23.163** **Dislocation of T11/T12 thoracic vertebra**

✓6th **S23.17** **Subluxation and dislocation of T12/L1 thoracic vertebra**
- ✓7th **S23.170** **Subluxation of T12/L1 thoracic vertebra**
- ✓7th **S23.171** **Dislocation of T12/L1 thoracic vertebra**

✓5th **S23.2** **Dislocation of other and unspecified parts of thorax**
- ✓x7th **S23.20** **Dislocation of unspecified part of thorax**
- ✓x7th **S23.29** **Dislocation of other parts of thorax**

✓x7th **S23.3** **Sprain of ligaments of thoracic spine**

✓5th **S23.4** **Sprain of ribs and sternum**
- ✓x7th **S23.41** **Sprain of ribs**
- ✓6th **S23.42** **Sprain of sternum**
  - ✓7th **S23.420** **Sprain of sternoclavicular (joint) (ligament)**
  - ✓7th **S23.421** **Sprain of chondrosternal joint**
  - ✓7th **S23.428** **Other sprain of sternum**
  - ✓7th **S23.429** **Unspecified sprain of sternum**

✓x7th **S23.8** **Sprain of other specified parts of thorax**

✓x7th **S23.9** **Sprain of unspecified parts of thorax**

✓4th **S24** **Injury of nerves and spinal cord at thorax level**

> NOTE   Code to highest level of thoracic spinal cord injury. Injuries to the spinal cord (S24.0 and S24.1) refer to the cord level and not bone level injury, and can affect nerve roots at and below the level given.

Code also any associated:
> fracture of thoracic vertebra (S22.0-)
> open wound of thorax (S21.-)
> transient paralysis (R29.5)

EXCLUDES 2   *injury of brachial plexus (S14.3)*

The appropriate 7th is to be added to each code from category S24.
A   initial encounter
D   subsequent encounter
S   sequela

CC Excl: For MCC codes in category S24 unless otherwise noted: MCC with 7th character A: M48.40X-M48.58X with 7th S, M80.08XS, M80.88XS, M84.350S, M84.454S, M84.550S, M84.58S, M84.650S, M99.15-M99.17, M99.19, S12.000-S12.9XX with 7th S, S13.9XXA, S14.109A, S14.119A, S14.129A, S14.139A, S14.149A, S14.159A, S22.000-S22.9XX with 7th S, S23.000-S23.29X with 7th A, S23.9XX-S24.159 with 7th A, S29.001-S29.009 with 7th A, S29.091-S29.9XX with 7th A, S32.000-S32.9XX with 7th S, S33.30X-S33.39X with 7th A, S33.9XXA, S38.1XXA, S39.001-S39.003 with 7th A, S39.091-S39.94X with 7th A, T14.8-T14.91, T79.A0X-T79.9XX with 7th A

✓x7th **S24.0** **Concussion and edema of thoracic spinal cord**   MCC

✓5th **S24.1** **Other and unspecified injuries of thoracic spinal cord**
- ✓6th **S24.10** **Unspecified injury of thoracic spinal cord**
  - 7 ✓7th **S24.101** **Unspecified injury at T1 level of thoracic spinal cord**   MCC
  - 7 ✓7th **S24.102** **Unspecified injury at T2-T6 level of thoracic spinal cord**   MCC
  - 7 ✓7th **S24.103** **Unspecified injury at T7-T10 level of thoracic spinal cord**   MCC
  - 7 ✓7th **S24.104** **Unspecified injury at T11-T12 level thoracic spinal cord**   MCC
  - 7 ✓7th **S24.109** **Unspecified injury at unspecified level of thoracic spinal cord**
    Injury of thoracic spinal cord NOS
    CC Excl: No excl

✓6th **S24.11** **Complete lesion of thoracic spinal cord**
- 7 ✓7th **S24.111** **Complete lesion at T1 level of thoracic spinal cord**   MCC
- 7 ✓7th **S24.112** **Complete lesion at T2-T6 level of thoracic spinal cord**   MCC
- 7 ✓7th **S24.113** **Complete lesion at T7-T10 level of thoracic spinal cord**   MCC
- 7 ✓7th **S24.114** **Complete lesion at T11-T12 level of thoracic spinal cord**   MCC
- ✓7th **S24.119** **Complete lesion at unspecified level of thoracic spinal cord**

✓6th **S24.13** **Anterior cord syndrome of thoracic spinal cord**
- 7 ✓7th **S24.131** **Anterior cord syndrome at T1 level of thoracic spinal cord**   MCC
- 7 ✓7th **S24.132** **Anterior cord syndrome at T2-T6 level of thoracic spinal cord**   MCC
- 7 ✓7th **S24.133** **Anterior cord syndrome at T7-T10 level of thoracic spinal cord**   MCC
- 7 ✓7th **S24.134** **Anterior cord syndrome at T11-T12 level of thoracic spinal cord**   MCC
- ✓7th **S24.139** **Anterior cord syndrome at unspecified level of thoracic spinal cord**

✓6th **S24.14** **Brown-Séquard syndrome of thoracic spinal cord**
- ✓7th **S24.141** **Brown-Séquard syndrome at T1 level of thoracic spinal cord**   MCC
- ✓7th **S24.142** **Brown-Séquard syndrome at T2-T6 level of thoracic spinal cord**   MCC
- ✓7th **S24.143** **Brown-Séquard syndrome at T7-T10 level of thoracic spinal cord**   MCC
- ✓7th **S24.144** **Brown-Séquard syndrome at T11-T12 level of thoracic spinal cord**   MCC
- ✓7th **S24.149** **Brown-Séquard syndrome at unspecified level of thoracic spinal cord**

✓6th **S24.15** **Other incomplete lesions of thoracic spinal cord**
Incomplete lesion of thoracic spinal cord NOS
Posterior cord syndrome of thoracic spinal cord
- 7 ✓7th **S24.151** **Other incomplete lesion at T1 level of thoracic spinal cord**   MCC
- 7 ✓7th **S24.152** **Other incomplete lesion at T2-T6 level of thoracic spinal cord**   MCC
- 7 ✓7th **S24.153** **Other incomplete lesion at T7-T10 level of thoracic spinal cord**   MCC
- 7 ✓7th **S24.154** **Other incomplete lesion at T11-T12 level of thoracic spinal cord**   MCC
- ✓7th **S24.159** **Other incomplete lesion at unspecified level of thoracic spinal cord**

✓x7th **S24.2** **Injury of nerve root of thoracic spine**

✓x7th **S24.3** **Injury of peripheral nerves of thorax**

✓x7th **S24.4** **Injury of thoracic sympathetic nervous system**
Injury of cardiac plexus   Injury of stellate ganglion
Injury of esophageal plexus   Injury of thoracic sympathetic
Injury of pulmonary plexus   ganglion

✓x7th **S24.8** **Injury of other specified nerves of thorax**

✓x7th **S24.9** **Injury of unspecified nerve of thorax**

✓4th **S25** **Injury of blood vessels of thorax**
Code also any associated open wound (S21.-)

The appropriate 7th is to be added to each code from category S25.
A   initial encounter
D   subsequent encounter
S   sequela

✓5th **S25.0** **Injury of thoracic aorta**
Injury of aorta NOS

CC Excl: For MCC codes in subcategory S25.0, unless otherwise noted: MCC with 7th character A: S25.00X-S25.09X with 7th A, T14.8-T14.91, T79.A0X-T79.9XX with 7th AA

---

7 HAC = Initial encounter only (7th character A, B or C) and not POA.

N Newborn: 0   P Pediatric: 0-17   M Maternity: 12-55   A Adult: 15-124   MCC Major CC Condition   PDx MCC PDx acts as own MCC   CC CC Condition   PDx CC PDx acts as own CC

882   ICD-10-CM Draft (2015)

√x 7th **S25.00** Unspecified **injury of thoracic aorta** `MCC`

√x 7th **S25.01** Minor laceration **of thoracic aorta** `MCC`
Incomplete transection of thoracic aorta
Laceration of thoracic aorta NOS
Superficial laceration of thoracic aorta

√x 7th **S25.02** Major laceration **of thoracic aorta** `MCC`
Complete transection of thoracic aorta
Traumatic rupture of thoracic aorta

√x 7th **S25.09** Other **specified injury of thoracic aorta** `MCC`

√5th **S25.1** Injury of **innominate or subclavian artery**

> **CC Excl: For MCC codes in subcategory S25.1, unless otherwise noted: MCC with 7th character A:** S25.101–S25.199 with 7th A, T14.8–T14.91, T79.A0X–T79.9XX with 7th A

√6th **S25.10** Unspecified **injury of innominate or subclavian artery**

√7th **S25.101** Unspecified **injury of right innominate or subclavian artery** `MCC`

√7th **S25.102** Unspecified **injury of left innominate or subclavian artery** `MCC`

√7th **S25.109** Unspecified **injury of unspecified innominate or subclavian artery** `MCC`

√6th **S25.11** Minor laceration **of innominate or subclavian artery**
Incomplete transection of innominate or subclavian artery
Laceration of innominate or subclavian artery NOS
Superficial laceration of innominate or subclavian artery

√7th **S25.111** Minor laceration **of right innominate or subclavian artery** `MCC`

√7th **S25.112** Minor laceration **of left innominate or subclavian artery** `MCC`

√7th **S25.119** Minor laceration **of unspecified innominate or subclavian artery** `MCC`

√6th **S25.12** Major laceration **of innominate or subclavian artery**
Complete transection of innominate or subclavian artery
Traumatic rupture of innominate or subclavian artery

√7th **S25.121** Major laceration **of right innominate or subclavian artery** `MCC`

√7th **S25.122** Major laceration **of left innominate or subclavian artery** `MCC`

√7th **S25.129** Major laceration **of unspecified innominate or subclavian artery** `MCC`

√6th **S25.19** Other **specified injury of innominate or subclavian artery**

√7th **S25.191** Other specified injury **of right innominate or subclavian artery** `MCC`

√7th **S25.192** Other specified injury **of left innominate or subclavian artery** `MCC`

√7th **S25.199** Other specified injury **of unspecified innominate or subclavian artery** `MCC`

√5th **S25.2** Injury of **superior vena cava**
Injury of vena cava NOS

> **CC Excl: For MCC codes in subcategory S25.2, unless otherwise noted: MCC with 7th character A:** S25.20X–S25.29X with 7th A, T14.8–T14.91, T79.A0X–T79.9XX with 7th A

√x 7th **S25.20** Unspecified **injury of superior vena cava** `MCC`

√x 7th **S25.21** Minor laceration **of superior vena cava** `MCC`
Incomplete transection of superior vena cava
Laceration of superior vena cava NOS
Superficial laceration of superior vena cava

√x 7th **S25.22** Major laceration **of superior vena cava** `MCC`
Complete transection of superior vena cava
Traumatic rupture of superior vena cava

√x 7th **S25.29** Other **specified injury of superior vena cava** `MCC`

√5th **S25.3** Injury of **innominate or subclavian vein**

> **CC Excl: For MCC codes in subcategory S25.3, unless otherwise noted: MCC with 7th character A:** S25.301–S25.399 with 7th A, T14.8–T14.91, T79.A0X–T79.9XX with 7th A

√6th **S25.30** Unspecified **injury of innominate or subclavian vein**

√7th **S25.301** Unspecified **injury of right innominate or subclavian vein** `MCC`

√7th **S25.302** Unspecified **injury of left innominate or subclavian vein** `MCC`

√7th **S25.309** Unspecified **injury of unspecified innominate or subclavian vein** `MCC`

√6th **S25.31** Minor laceration **of innominate or subclavian vein**
Incomplete transection of innominate or subclavian vein
Laceration of innominate or subclavian vein NOS
Superficial laceration of innominate or subclavian vein

√7th **S25.311** Minor laceration **of right innominate or subclavian vein** `MCC`

√7th **S25.312** Minor laceration **of left innominate or subclavian vein** `MCC`

√7th **S25.319** Minor laceration **of unspecified innominate or subclavian vein** `MCC`

√6th **S25.32** Major laceration **of innominate or subclavian vein**
Complete transection of innominate or subclavian vein
Traumatic rupture of innominate or subclavian vein

√7th **S25.321** Major laceration **of right innominate or subclavian vein** `MCC`

√7th **S25.322** Major laceration **of left innominate or subclavian vein** `MCC`

√7th **S25.329** Major laceration **of unspecified innominate or subclavian vein** `MCC`

√6th **S25.39** Other **specified injury of innominate or subclavian vein**

√7th **S25.391** Other specified injury **of right innominate or subclavian vein** `MCC`

√7th **S25.392** Other specified injury **of left innominate or subclavian vein** `MCC`

√7th **S25.399** Other specified injury **of unspecified innominate or subclavian vein** `MCC`

√5th **S25.4** Injury of **pulmonary blood vessels**

> **CC Excl: For CC/MCC codes in subcategory S25.4, unless otherwise noted: MCC with 7th character A:** S25.401–S25.499 with 7th A, T14.8–T14.91, T79.A0X–T79.9XX with 7th A

√6th **S25.40** Unspecified **injury of pulmonary blood vessels**

√7th **S25.401** Unspecified **injury of right pulmonary blood vessels** `MCC`

√7th **S25.402** Unspecified **injury of left pulmonary blood vessels** `MCC`

√7th **S25.409** Unspecified **injury of unspecified pulmonary blood vessels** `MCC`

√6th **S25.41** Minor laceration **of pulmonary blood vessels**
Incomplete transection of pulmonary blood vessels
Laceration of pulmonary blood vessels NOS
Superficial laceration of pulmonary blood vessels

√7th **S25.411** Minor laceration **of right pulmonary blood vessels** `MCC`

√7th **S25.412** Minor laceration **of left pulmonary blood vessels** `MCC`

√7th **S25.419** Minor laceration **of unspecified pulmonary blood vessels** `MCC`

√6th **S25.42** Major laceration **of pulmonary blood vessels**
Complete transection of pulmonary blood vessels
Traumatic rupture of pulmonary blood vessels

√7th **S25.421** Major laceration **of right pulmonary blood vessels** `MCC`

√7th **S25.422** Major laceration **of left pulmonary blood vessels** `MCC`

√7th **S25.429** Major laceration **of unspecified pulmonary blood vessels** `MCC`

√6th **S25.49** Other **specified injury of pulmonary blood vessels**

√7th **S25.491** Other specified injury **of right pulmonary blood vessels** `MCC`

√7th **S25.492** Other specified injury **of left pulmonary blood vessels** `MCC`

√7th **S25.499** Other specified injury **of unspecified pulmonary blood vessels** `MCC`

✔ Additional Character Required   √7th Xtension Alert   Unacceptable PDx   Manifestation   Hospital Acquired Condition   **EXCLUDES 1** Not Coded Here   **EXCLUDES 2** Not Included Here

ICD-10-CM Draft (2015)   883

√5ᵗʰ S25.5 Injury of intercostal blood vessels

> **CC Excl:** For CC codes in subcategory S25.5, unless otherwise noted: CC with 7th character A: S25.501–S25.899 with 7th A

√6ᵗʰ **S25.50 Unspecified injury of intercostal blood vessels**

√7ᵗʰ **S25.501** Unspecified injury of intercostal blood vessels, **right** side   CC

√7ᵗʰ **S25.502** Unspecified injury of intercostal blood vessels, **left** side   CC

√7ᵗʰ **S25.509** Unspecified injury of intercostal blood vessels, **unspecified** side   CC

√6ᵗʰ **S25.51 Laceration of intercostal blood vessels**

√7ᵗʰ **S25.511** Laceration of intercostal blood vessels, **right** side   CC

√7ᵗʰ **S25.512** Laceration of intercostal blood vessels, **left** side   CC

√7ᵗʰ **S25.519** Laceration of intercostal blood vessels, **unspecified** side   CC

√6ᵗʰ **S25.59 Other specified injury of intercostal blood vessels**

√7ᵗʰ **S25.591** Other specified injury of intercostal blood vessels, **right** side   CC

√7ᵗʰ **S25.592** Other specified injury of intercostal blood vessels, **left** side   CC

√7ᵗʰ **S25.599** Other specified injury of intercostal blood vessels, **unspecified** side   CC

√5ᵗʰ S25.8 Injury of other blood vessels of thorax
Injury of azygos vein
Injury of mammary artery or vein

> **CC Excl:** For CC codes in subcategory S25.8, unless otherwise noted: CC with 7th character A: S25.00X–S25.99X with 7th A

√6ᵗʰ **S25.80 Unspecified injury of other blood vessels of thorax**

√7ᵗʰ **S25.801** Unspecified injury of other blood vessels of thorax, **right** side   CC

√7ᵗʰ **S25.802** Unspecified injury of other blood vessels of thorax, **left** side   CC

√7ᵗʰ **S25.809** Unspecified injury of other blood vessels of thorax, **unspecified** side   CC

√6ᵗʰ **S25.81 Laceration of other blood vessels of thorax**

√7ᵗʰ **S25.811** Laceration of other blood vessels of thorax, **right** side   CC

√7ᵗʰ **S25.812** Laceration of other blood vessels of thorax, **left** side   CC

√7ᵗʰ **S25.819** Laceration of other blood vessels of thorax, **unspecified** side   CC

√6ᵗʰ **S25.89 Other specified injury of other blood vessels of thorax**

√7ᵗʰ **S25.891** Other specified injury of other blood vessels of thorax, **right** side   CC

√7ᵗʰ **S25.892** Other specified injury of other blood vessels of thorax, **left** side   CC

√7ᵗʰ **S25.899** Other specified injury of other blood vessels of thorax, **unspecified** side   CC

√5ᵗʰ S25.9 Injury of unspecified blood vessel of thorax

> **CC Excl:** For CC codes in subcategory S25.9, unless otherwise noted: See code: S25.8

√x7ᵗʰ **S25.90** Unspecified injury of unspecified blood vessel of thorax   CC

√x7ᵗʰ **S25.91** Laceration of unspecified blood vessel of thorax   CC

√x7ᵗʰ **S25.99** Other specified injury of unspecified blood vessel of thorax   CC

√4ᵗʰ S26 Injury of heart
Code also any associated:
  open wound of thorax (S21.-)
  traumatic hemopneumothorax (S27.2)
  traumatic hemothorax (S27.1)
  traumatic pneumothorax (S27.0)

> The appropriate 7th is to be added to each code from category S26.
> A   initial encounter
> D   subsequent encounter
> S   sequela

√5ᵗʰ S26.0 Injury of heart with hemopericardium

√x7ᵗʰ **S26.00 Unspecified injury of heart with hemopericardium**   CC
> **CC Excl:** CC with 7th character A: S21.301–S21.459 with 7th A, S26.00X–S26.99X with 7th A, S27.50X–S27.69X with 7th A, S27.892–S27.9XX with 7th A, T14.8–T14.91

√x7ᵗʰ **S26.01 Contusion of heart with hemopericardium**   CC
> **CC Excl:** CC with 7th character A: S21.101–S21.159 with 7th A, S21.301–S21.95X with 7th A, S26.00X–S26.99X with 7th A, S27.50X–S27.69X with 7th A, S27.892–S27.9XX with 7th A, S28.1XXA, S29.021A, S29.029A, S38.3XXA, T14.8–T14.91, T79.7XX–T79.9XX with 7th A

√6ᵗʰ **S26.02 Laceration of heart with hemopericardium**

√7ᵗʰ **S26.020 Mild laceration of heart with hemopericardium**   MCC
Laceration of heart without penetration of heart chamber
> **CC Excl:** See code: S26.01

√7ᵗʰ **S26.021 Moderate laceration of heart with hemopericardium**   MCC
Laceration of heart with penetration of heart chamber
> **CC Excl:** See code: S26.01

√7ᵗʰ **S26.022 Major laceration of heart with hemopericardium**   MCC
Laceration of heart with penetration of multiple heart chambers
> **CC Excl:** See code: S26.01

√x7ᵗʰ **S26.09 Other injury of heart with hemopericardium**   CC
> **CC Excl:** CC with 7th character A: S21.301–S21.459 with 7th A, S26.00X–S26.99X with 7th A, S27.50X–S27.69X with 7th A, S27.892–S27.9X with 7th A, T14.8–T14.91

√5ᵗʰ S26.1 Injury of heart without hemopericardium

√x7ᵗʰ **S26.10 Unspecified injury of heart without hemopericardium**   CC
> **CC Excl:** See code: S26.09

√x7ᵗʰ **S26.11 Contusion of heart without hemopericardium**   CC
> **CC Excl:** CC with 7th character A: S21.101–S21.159 with 7th A, S21.301–S21.95X with 7th A, S26.00X–S26.99X with 7th A, S27.50X–S27.69X with 7th A, S27.892–S27.9XX with 7th A, S28.1XXA, S29.021A, S29.029A, S38.3XXA, T14.8–T14.91, T79.7XX–T79.9XX with 7th A

√x7ᵗʰ **S26.12 Laceration of heart without hemopericardium**   MCC CC
> **CC Excl:** MCC with 7th character A: See code: S26.11

√x7ᵗʰ **S26.19 Other injury of heart without hemopericardium**   CC
> **CC Excl:** CC with 7th character A: S21.301–S21.459 with 7th A, S26.00X–S26.99X with 7th A, S27.50X–S27.69X with 7th A, S27.892–S27.9XX with 7th A, T14.8–T14.91

√5ᵗʰ S26.9 Injury of heart, unspecified with or without hemopericardium

√x7ᵗʰ **S26.90 Unspecified injury of heart, unspecified with or without hemopericardium**   CC
> **CC Excl:** See code: S26.19

√x7ᵗʰ **S26.91 Contusion of heart, unspecified with or without hemopericardium**   CC
> **CC Excl:** CC with 7th character A: S21.101–S21.159 with 7th A, S21.301–S21.95 with 7th A, S26.00X–S26.99X with 7th A, S27.50X–S27.69X with 7th A, S27.892–S27.9XX with 7th A, S28.1XX with 7th A, S29.021 with 7th A, S29.029A, S38.3XX with 7th A, T14.8–T14.91, T79.7XX–T79.9XX with 7th A

√x7ᵗʰ **S26.92 Laceration of heart, unspecified with or without hemopericardium**   MCC
Laceration of heart NOS
> **CC Excl:** See code: S26.91

√x7ᵗʰ **S26.99 Other injury of heart, unspecified with or without hemopericardium**   CC
> **CC Excl:** CC with 7th character A: S21.301–S21.459 with 7th A, S26.00X–S26.99X with 7th A, S27.50X–S27.69X with 7th A, S27.892–S27.9X with 7th A, T14.8–T14.91

N Newborn: 0   P Pediatric: 0–17   M Maternity: 12–55   A Adult: 15–124   MCC Major CC Condition   PDx MCC PDx acts as own MCC   CC CC Condition   PDx CC PDx acts as own CC

884   ICD-10-CM Draft (2015)

√4ᵗʰ **S27 Injury of other and unspecified intrathoracic organs**

> Code also any associated open wound of thorax (S21.-)
>
> EXCLUDES 2   injury of cervical esophagus (S10-S19)
> injury of trachea (cervical) (S10-S19)

> The appropriate 7th is to be added to each code from category S27.
> A   initial encounter
> D   subsequent encounter
> S   sequela

√x7ᵗʰ **S27.0 Traumatic pneumothorax**   `CC`

> EXCLUDES 1   spontaneous pneumothorax (J93.-)
> **CC Excl: CC with 7th character A:** S21.101-S21.159 with 7th A, S21.301-S21.95X with 7th A, S27.0XX-S27.399 with 7th A, S27.50X-S27.69X with 7th A, S27.892-S27.9XXA, S28.1XXA, S29.021A, S29.029A, S38.3XXA, T14.8-T14.91, T79.7XX-T79.9XX with 7th A

√x7ᵗʰ **S27.1 Traumatic hemothorax**   `MCC`

> **CC Excl: MCC with 7th character A:** See code: S27.0

√x7ᵗʰ **S27.2 Traumatic hemopneumothorax**   `MCC`

> **CC Excl: MCC with 7th character A:** See code: S27.0

√5ᵗʰ **S27.3 Other and unspecified injuries of lung**

> **CC Excl: For CC codes in subcategory S27.3, unless otherwise noted: CC with 7th character A:** S21.101-S21.159 with 7th A, S21.301-S21.95X with 7th A, S27.301-S27.399 with 7th A, S27.50X-S27.69X with 7th A, S27.892-S27.9XX with 7th A, S28.1XXA, S29.021A, S29.029A, S38.3XXA, T14.8-T14.91, T79.7XX-T79.9XX with 7th A

   √6ᵗʰ **S27.30 Unspecified injury of lung**

     √7ᵗʰ **S27.301 Unspecified injury of lung, unilateral**   `CC`

     √7ᵗʰ **S27.302 Unspecified injury of lung, bilateral**   `CC`

     √7ᵗʰ **S27.309 Unspecified injury of lung, unspecified**   `CC`

   √6ᵗʰ **S27.31 Primary blast injury of lung**
Blast injury of lung NOS

     √7ᵗʰ **S27.311 Primary blast injury of lung, unilateral**   `CC`

     √7ᵗʰ **S27.312 Primary blast injury of lung, bilateral**   `CC`

     √7ᵗʰ **S27.319 Primary blast injury of lung, unspecified**   `CC`

   S27.32 Contusion of lung

     √7ᵗʰ **S27.321 Contusion of lung, unilateral**   `CC`

     √7ᵗʰ **S27.322 Contusion of lung, bilateral**   `CC`

     √7ᵗʰ **S27.329 Contusion of lung, unspecified**   `CC`

   √6ᵗʰ **S27.33 Laceration of lung**

     √7ᵗʰ **S27.331 Laceration of lung, unilateral**   `MCC`

> **CC Excl: MCC with 7th character A:** S21.101-S21.159 with 7th A, S21.301-S21.95X with 7th A, S27.301-S27.399 with 7th A, S27.50X-S27.69X with 7th A, S27.892-S27.9XX with 7th A, S28.1XXA, S29.021A, S29.029A, S38.3XXA, T14.8-T14.91, T79.7XX-T79.9XX with 7th AA

     √7ᵗʰ **S27.332 Laceration of lung, bilateral**   `MCC`

> **CC Excl:** See code: S27.331

     √7ᵗʰ **S27.339 Laceration of lung, unspecified**   `MCC`

> **CC Excl:** See code: S27.331

   √6ᵗʰ **S27.39 Other injuries of lung**
Secondary blast injury of lung

     √7ᵗʰ **S27.391 Other injuries of lung, unilateral**   `CC`

     √7ᵗʰ **S27.392 Other injuries of lung, bilateral**   `CC`

     √7ᵗʰ **S27.399 Other injuries of lung, unspecified**   `CC`

√5ᵗʰ **S27.4 Injury of bronchus**

> **CC Excl: For MCC codes in subcategory S27.4, unless otherwise noted: MCC with 7th character A:** S21.101-S21.159 with 7th A, S21.301-S21.95X with 7th A, S27.401-S27.69X with 7th A, S27.892-S27.9XX with 7th A, S28.1XXA, S29.021XA, S29.029XA, S38.3XXA, T14.8-T14.91, T79.7XX-T79.9XX with 7th A

   √6ᵗʰ **S27.40 Unspecified injury of bronchus**

     √7ᵗʰ **S27.401 Unspecified injury of bronchus, unilateral**   `MCC`

     √7ᵗʰ **S27.402 Unspecified injury of bronchus, bilateral**   `MCC`

     √7ᵗʰ **S27.409 Unspecified injury of bronchus, unspecified**   `MCC`

   √6ᵗʰ **S27.41 Primary blast injury of bronchus**
Blast injury of bronchus NOS

     √7ᵗʰ **S27.411 Primary blast injury of bronchus, unilateral**   `MCC`

     √7ᵗʰ **S27.412 Primary blast injury of bronchus, bilateral**   `MCC`

     √7ᵗʰ **S27.419 Primary blast injury of bronchus, unspecified**   `MCC`

   √6ᵗʰ **S27.42 Contusion of bronchus**

     √7ᵗʰ **S27.421 Contusion of bronchus, unilateral**   `MCC`

     √7ᵗʰ **S27.422 Contusion of bronchus, bilateral**   `MCC`

     √7ᵗʰ **S27.429 Contusion of bronchus, unspecified**   `MCC`

   √6ᵗʰ **S27.43 Laceration of bronchus**

     √7ᵗʰ **S27.431 Laceration of bronchus, unilateral**   `MCC`

     √7ᵗʰ **S27.432 Laceration of bronchus, bilateral**   `MCC`

     √7ᵗʰ **S27.439 Laceration of bronchus, unspecified**   `MCC`

   √6ᵗʰ **S27.49 Other injury of bronchus**
Secondary blast injury of bronchus

     √7ᵗʰ **S27.491 Other injury of bronchus, unilateral**   `MCC`

     √7ᵗʰ **S27.492 Other injury of bronchus, bilateral**   `MCC`

     √7ᵗʰ **S27.499 Other injury of bronchus, unspecified**   `MCC`

√5ᵗʰ **S27.5 Injury of thoracic trachea**

> **CC Excl: For CC codes in subcategory S27.5, unless otherwise noted: CC with 7th character A:** S21.101-S21.159 with 7th A, S21.301-S21.95X with 7th A, S27.50X-S27.69X with 7th A, S27.892-S27.9XX with 7th A, S28.1XXA, S29.021 with 7th A, S29.029A, S38.3XXA, T14.8-T14.91, T79.7XX-T79.9XX with 7th A

   √x7ᵗʰ **S27.50 Unspecified injury of thoracic trachea**   `CC`

   √x7ᵗʰ **S27.51 Primary blast injury of thoracic trachea**   `CC`
Blast injury of thoracic trachea NOS

   √x7ᵗʰ **S27.52 Contusion of thoracic trachea**   `CC`

   √x7ᵗʰ **S27.53 Laceration of thoracic trachea**   `CC`

   √x7ᵗʰ **S27.59 Other injury of thoracic trachea**   `CC`
Secondary blast injury of thoracic trachea

√5ᵗʰ **S27.6 Injury of pleura**

> **CC Excl: For CC codes in subcategory S27.6, unless otherwise noted:** See code: S27.5

   √x7ᵗʰ **S27.60 Unspecified injury of pleura**   `CC`

   √x7ᵗʰ **S27.63 Laceration of pleura**   `CC`

   √x7ᵗʰ **S27.69 Other injury of pleura**   `CC`

√5ᵗʰ **S27.8 Injury of other specified intrathoracic organs**

   √6ᵗʰ **S27.80 Injury of diaphragm**

> **CC Excl: For CC/MCC codes in subcategory S27.80, unless otherwise noted: CC with 7th character A:** S21.101-S21.159 with 7th A, S21.301-S21.95 with 7th A, S27.50X-S27.809 with 7th A, S27.892-S27.9XX with 7th A, S28.1XXA, S29.021A, S29.029A, S38.3XXA, T14.8-T14.91, T79.7XX-T79.9XX with 7th A

     √7ᵗʰ **S27.802 Contusion of diaphragm**   `CC`

     √7ᵗʰ **S27.803 Laceration of diaphragm**   `CC`

     √7ᵗʰ **S27.808 Other injury of diaphragm**   `CC`

     √7ᵗʰ **S27.809 Unspecified injury of diaphragm**   `CC`

   √6ᵗʰ **S27.81 Injury of esophagus (thoracic part)**

     √7ᵗʰ **S27.812 Contusion of esophagus (thoracic part)**   `MCC`

> **CC Excl: MCC with 7th character A:** S21.101-S21.159 with 7th A, S21.301-S21.95 with 7th A, S27.50X-S27.69X with 7th A, S27.812-S27.9XX with 7th A, S28.1XXA, S29.021A, S29.029A, S38.3XXA, T14.8-T14.91, T79.7XX-T79.9XX with 7th A

     √7ᵗʰ **S27.813 Laceration of esophagus (thoracic part)**   `MCC`

> **CC Excl:** See code: S27.812

     √7ᵗʰ **S27.818 Other injury of esophagus (thoracic part)**   `MCC`

> **CC Excl:** See code: S27.812

     √7ᵗʰ **S27.819 Unspecified injury of esophagus (thoracic part)**   `MCC`

> **CC Excl:** See code: S27.812

✓ Additional Character Required   √x7ᵗʰ Xtension Alert   Unacceptable PDx   Manifestation   Hospital Acquired Condition   EXCLUDES 1 Not Coded Here   EXCLUDES 2 Not Included Here

ICD-10-CM Draft (2015)   885

✓6ᵗʰ **S27.89** **Injury of** other specified **intrathoracic organs**
Injury of lymphatic thoracic duct
Injury of thymus gland

> **CC Excl: For CC codes in subcategory S27.89,
> unless otherwise noted: CC with 7th character A:**
> S21.101-S21.159 with 7th A, S21.301-S21.95X with
> 7th A, S27.50X-S27.69X with 7th A, S27.892-S27.9X
> with 7th A, S28.1XXA, S29.021A, S29.029A,
> S38.3XXA, T14.8-T14.91, T79.7XX-T79.9XX with 7th A

    ✓7ᵗʰ **S27.892** **Contusion of other specified
intrathoracic organs** `CC`

    ✓7ᵗʰ **S27.893** **Laceration of other specified
intrathoracic organs** `CC`

    ✓7ᵗʰ **S27.898** **Other injury of other specified
intrathoracic organs** `CC`

    ✓7ᵗʰ **S27.899** **Unspecified injury of other specified
intrathoracic organs** `CC`

✓x7ᵗʰ **S27.9** **Injury of** unspecified **intrathoracic organ** `CC`
CC Excl: CC with 7th character A: S21.101-S21.159 with 7th A,
S21.301-S21.95X with 7th A, S27.50X-S27.69X with 7th A, S27.892-
S27.9XX with 7th A, S28.1XXA, S29.021A, S29.029A, S38.3XXA,
T14.8-T14.91, T79.7XX-T79.9XX with 7th A

✓4ᵗʰ **S28** **Crushing injury of thorax, and traumatic amputation of part of
thorax**

> The appropriate 7th is to be added to each code from
> category S28.
> A   initial encounter
> D   subsequent encounter
> S   sequela

✓x7ᵗʰ **S28.0** **Crushed chest**
Use additional code for all associated injuries
EXCLUDES 1 *flail chest (S22.5)*

✓x7ᵗʰ **S28.1** **Traumatic amputation (partial) of** part of thorax,
except breast `CC`
CC Excl: CC with 7th character A: S21.101-S21.159 with 7th A,
S21.301-S21.95X with 7th A, S23.3XA, S23.8XA, S27.50X-S27.69X
with 7th A, S27.892-S27.9XX with 7th A, S28.1XXA, S29.021A,
S29.029A, S38.3XXA, T14.8-T14.91, T79.7XX-T79.9XX with 7th A

✓5ᵗʰ **S28.2** **Traumatic amputation of** breast

  ✓6ᵗʰ **S28.21** **Complete traumatic amputation of breast**
Traumatic amputation of breast NOS

    ✓7ᵗʰ **S28.211** **Complete traumatic amputation of** right
breast

    ✓7ᵗʰ **S28.212** **Complete traumatic amputation of** left
breast

    ✓7ᵗʰ **S28.219** **Complete traumatic amputation of**
unspecified **breast**

  ✓6ᵗʰ **S28.22** **Partial** traumatic amputation **of breast**

    ✓7ᵗʰ **S28.221** **Partial traumatic amputation of** right
breast

    ✓7ᵗʰ **S28.222** **Partial traumatic amputation of** left **breast**

    ✓7ᵗʰ **S28.229** **Partial traumatic amputation of**
unspecified **breast**

✓4ᵗʰ **S29** **Other and unspecified injuries of thorax**
Code also any associated open wound (S21.-)

> The appropriate 7th is to be added to each code from category
> S29.
> A   initial encounter
> D   subsequent encounter
> S   sequela

✓5ᵗʰ **S29.0** **Injury of muscle and tendon at thorax level**

  ✓6ᵗʰ **S29.00** **Unspecified injury of muscle and tendon of thorax**

    ✓7ᵗʰ **S29.001** **Unspecified injury of muscle and tendon
of** front **wall of thorax**

    ✓7ᵗʰ **S29.002** **Unspecified injury of muscle and tendon
of** back **wall of thorax**

    ✓7ᵗʰ **S29.009** **Unspecified injury of muscle and tendon
of** unspecified **wall of thorax**

  ✓6ᵗʰ **S29.01** **Strain of muscle and tendon of thorax**

    ✓7ᵗʰ **S29.011** **Strain of muscle and tendon of** front **wall
of thorax**

    ✓7ᵗʰ **S29.012** **Strain of muscle and tendon of** back **wall
of thorax**

    ✓7ᵗʰ **S29.019** **Strain of muscle and tendon of**
unspecified **wall of thorax**

  ✓6ᵗʰ **S29.02** **Laceration of muscle and tendon of thorax**

    ✓7ᵗʰ **S29.021** **Laceration of muscle and tendon of** `CC`
front **wall of thorax**
CC Excl: See code: S28.1

    ✓7ᵗʰ **S29.022** **Laceration of muscle and tendon of** back
wall of thorax

    ✓7ᵗʰ **S29.029** **Laceration of muscle and tendon of** `CC`
unspecified **wall of thorax**
CC Excl: See code: S28.1

  ✓6ᵗʰ **S29.09** **Other injury of muscle and tendon of thorax**

    ✓7ᵗʰ **S29.091** **Other injury of muscle and tendon of** front
wall of thorax

    ✓7ᵗʰ **S29.092** **Other injury of muscle and tendon of** back
wall of thorax

    ✓7ᵗʰ **S29.099** **Other injury of muscle and tendon of**
unspecified **wall of thorax**

✓x7ᵗʰ **S29.8** **Other specified injuries of thorax**

✓x7ᵗʰ **S29.9** **Unspecified injury of thorax**

Injuries to the abdomen, lower back, lumbar spine, pelvis and external genitals (S30-S39)

INCLUDES injuries to the abdominal wall
injuries to the anus
injuries to the buttock
injuries to the external genitalia
injuries to the flank
injuries to the groin
EXCLUDES 2 *burns and corrosions (T20-T32)*
effects of foreign body in anus and rectum (T18.5)
effects of foreign body in genitourinary tract (T19.-)
*effects of foreign body in stomach, small intestine and colon (T18.2-
T18.4)*
frostbite (T33-T34)
insect bite or sting, venomous (T63.4)

✓4ᵗʰ **S30** **Superficial injury of abdomen, lower back, pelvis and external
genitals**
EXCLUDES 2 *superficial injury of hip (S70.-)*

> The appropriate 7th is to be added to each code from category
> S30.
> A   initial encounter
> D   subsequent encounter
> S   sequela

✓x7ᵗʰ **S30.0** **Contusion of lower back and pelvis**
Contusion of buttock

✓x7ᵗʰ **S30.1** **Contusion of abdominal wall**
Contusion of flank
Contusion of groin

✓5ᵗʰ **S30.2** **Contusion of** external genital organs

  ✓6ᵗʰ **S30.20** **Contusion of** unspecified **external genital organ**

    ✓7ᵗʰ **S30.201** **Contusion of unspecified external** ♂
genital organ, male

    ✓7ᵗʰ **S30.202** **Contusion of unspecified external** ♀
genital organ, female

  ✓x7ᵗʰ **S30.21** **Contusion of** penis ♂

  ✓x7ᵗʰ **S30.22** **Contusion of** scrotum and testes ♂

  ✓x7ᵗʰ **S30.23** **Contusion of** vagina and vulva ♀

✓x7ᵗʰ **S30.3** **Contusion of** anus

✓5ᵗʰ **S30.8** **Other superficial injuries of abdomen, lower back, pelvis and
external genitals**

  ✓6ᵗʰ **S30.81** **Abrasion of abdomen, lower back, pelvis and
external genitals**

    ✓7ᵗʰ **S30.810** **Abrasion of** lower back and pelvis

    ✓7ᵗʰ **S30.811** **Abrasion of** abdominal wall

    ✓7ᵗʰ **S30.812** **Abrasion of** penis ♂

    ✓7ᵗʰ **S30.813** **Abrasion of** scrotum and testes ♂

    ✓7ᵗʰ **S30.814** **Abrasion of** vagina and vulva ♀

    ✓7ᵗʰ **S30.815** **Abrasion of** unspecified external ♂
genital organs, male

    ✓7ᵗʰ **S30.816** **Abrasion of** unspecified external ♀
genital organs, female

    ✓7ᵗʰ **S30.817** **Abrasion of** anus

Ⓝ Newborn: 0   Ⓟ Pediatric: 0-17   Ⓜ Maternity: 12-55   Ⓐ Adult: 15-124   **MCC** Major CC Condition   **PDx MCC** PDx acts as own MCC   **CC** CC Condition   **PDx CC** PDx acts as own CC

886   ICD-10-CM Draft (2015)

✓6ᵗʰ **S30.82** **Blister** (nonthermal) of abdomen, lower back, pelvis and external genitals

✓7ᵗʰ **S30.820** **Blister** (nonthermal) of lower back and pelvis

✓7ᵗʰ **S30.821** **Blister** (nonthermal) of abdominal wall

✓7ᵗʰ **S30.822** **Blister** (nonthermal) of penis ♂

✓7ᵗʰ **S30.823** **Blister** (nonthermal) of scrotum and testes ♂

✓7ᵗʰ **S30.824** **Blister** (nonthermal) of vagina and vulva ♀

✓7ᵗʰ **S30.825** **Blister** (nonthermal) of unspecified external genital organs, male ♂

✓7ᵗʰ **S30.826** **Blister** (nonthermal) of unspecified external genital organs, female ♀

✓7ᵗʰ **S30.827** **Blister** (nonthermal) of anus

✓6ᵗʰ **S30.84** **External constriction** of abdomen, lower back, pelvis and external genitals

✓7ᵗʰ **S30.840** **External constriction** of lower back and pelvis

✓7ᵗʰ **S30.841** **External constriction** of abdominal wall

✓7ᵗʰ **S30.842** **External constriction** of penis ♂
Hair tourniquet syndrome of penis
Use additional cause code to identify the constricting item (W49.0-)

✓7ᵗʰ **S30.843** **External constriction** of scrotum and testes ♂

✓7ᵗʰ **S30.844** **External constriction** of vagina and vulva ♀

✓7ᵗʰ **S30.845** **External constriction** of unspecified external genital organs, male ♂

✓7ᵗʰ **S30.846** **External constriction** of unspecified external genital organs, female ♀

✓6ᵗʰ **S30.85** **Superficial** foreign body of abdomen, lower back, pelvis and external genitals
Splinter in the abdomen, lower back, pelvis and external genitals

✓7ᵗʰ **S30.850** **Superficial foreign body** of lower back and pelvis

✓7ᵗʰ **S30.851** **Superficial foreign body** of abdominal wall

✓7ᵗʰ **S30.852** **Superficial foreign body** of penis ♂

✓7ᵗʰ **S30.853** **Superficial foreign body** of scrotum and testes ♂

✓7ᵗʰ **S30.854** **Superficial foreign body** of vagina and vulva ♀

✓7ᵗʰ **S30.855** **Superficial foreign body** of unspecified external genital organs, male ♂

✓7ᵗʰ **S30.856** **Superficial foreign body** of unspecified external genital organs, female ♀

✓7ᵗʰ **S30.857** **Superficial foreign body** of anus

✓6ᵗʰ **S30.86** **Insect bite** (nonvenomous) of abdomen, lower back, pelvis and external genitals

✓7ᵗʰ **S30.860** **Insect bite** (nonvenomous) of lower back and pelvis

✓7ᵗʰ **S30.861** **Insect bite** (nonvenomous) of abdominal wall

✓7ᵗʰ **S30.862** **Insect bite** (nonvenomous) of penis ♂

✓7ᵗʰ **S30.863** **Insect bite** (nonvenomous) of scrotum and testes ♂

✓7ᵗʰ **S30.864** **Insect bite** (nonvenomous) of vagina and vulva ♀

✓7ᵗʰ **S30.865** **Insect bite** (nonvenomous) of unspecified external genital organs, male ♂

✓7ᵗʰ **S30.866** **Insect bite** (nonvenomous) of unspecified external genital organs, female ♀

✓7ᵗʰ **S30.867** **Insect bite** (nonvenomous) of anus

✓6ᵗʰ **S30.87** **Other superficial bite** of abdomen, lower back, pelvis and external genitals
EXCLUDES 1 open bite of abdomen, lower back, pelvis and external genitals (S31.05, S31.15, S31.25, S31.35, S31.45, S31.55)

✓7ᵗʰ **S30.870** **Other superficial bite** of lower back and pelvis

✓7ᵗʰ **S30.871** **Other superficial bite** of abdominal wall

✓7ᵗʰ **S30.872** **Other superficial bite** of penis ♂

✓7ᵗʰ **S30.873** **Other superficial bite** of scrotum and testes ♂

✓7ᵗʰ **S30.874** **Other superficial bite** of vagina and vulva ♀

✓7ᵗʰ **S30.875** **Other superficial bite** of unspecified external genital organs, male ♂

✓7ᵗʰ **S30.876** **Other superficial bite** of unspecified external genital organs, female ♀

✓7ᵗʰ **S30.877** **Other superficial bite** of anus

✓5ᵗʰ **S30.9** **Unspecified** superficial injury of abdomen, lower back, pelvis and external genitals

✓x7ᵗʰ **S30.91** **Unspecified superficial injury of** lower back and pelvis

✓x7ᵗʰ **S30.92** **Unspecified superficial injury of** abdominal wall

✓x7ᵗʰ **S30.93** **Unspecified superficial injury of** penis ♂

✓x7ᵗʰ **S30.94** **Unspecified superficial injury of** scrotum and testes ♂

✓x7ᵗʰ **S30.95** **Unspecified superficial injury of** vagina and vulva ♀

✓x7ᵗʰ **S30.96** **Unspecified superficial injury of** unspecified external genital organs, male ♂

✓x7ᵗʰ **S30.97** **Unspecified superficial injury of** unspecified external genital organs, female ♀

✓x7ᵗʰ **S30.98** **Unspecified superficial injury of** anus

✓4ᵗʰ **S31** **Open wound of abdomen, lower back, pelvis and external genitals**
Code also any associated:
spinal cord injury (S24.0, S24.1-, S34.0-, S34.1-)
wound infection
EXCLUDES 1 traumatic amputation of part of abdomen, lower back and pelvis (S38.2-, S38.3)
EXCLUDES 2 open wound of hip (S71.00-S71.02)
open fracture of pelvis (S32.1- – S32.9 with 7th B)

The appropriate 7th is to be added to each code from category S31.
A   initial encounter
D   subsequent encounter
S   sequela

✓5ᵗʰ **S31.0** **Open wound of** lower back and pelvis

✓6ᵗʰ **S31.00** **Unspecified open wound** of lower back and pelvis

✓7ᵗʰ **S31.000** **Unspecified open wound of lower back and pelvis** without penetration into retroperitoneum
Unspecified open wound of lower back and pelvis NOS

✓7ᵗʰ **S31.001** **Unspecified open wound of lower back and pelvis** with penetration into retroperitoneum **MCC**
CC Excl: CC with 7th character A: S31.001A, S31.011A, S31.021, S31.031A, S31.041A, S31.051-S31.159 with 7th A, S31.600-S31.659 with 7th A, S31.831-S31.839 with 7th A, S36.81X-S36.99X with 7th A, S38.3XX-S39.023 with 7th A, T14.8-T14.91, T79.A0X-T79.9XX with 7th A

✓6ᵗʰ **S31.01** **Laceration without foreign body** of lower back and pelvis

✓7ᵗʰ **S31.010** **Laceration without foreign body of lower back and pelvis** without penetration into retroperitoneum
Laceration without foreign body of lower back and pelvis NOS

✓7ᵗʰ **S31.011** **Laceration without foreign body of lower back and pelvis** with penetration into retroperitoneum **MCC**
CC Excl: See code: S30.001

✓6ᵗʰ **S31.02** **Laceration with foreign body** of lower back and pelvis

✓7ᵗʰ **S31.020** **Laceration with foreign body of lower back and pelvis** without penetration into retroperitoneum
Laceration with foreign body of lower back and pelvis NOS

Injury, Poisoning and Certain Other Consequences of External Causes

S31.021–S31.145

√7ᵗʰ **S31.021 Laceration with foreign body of lower** MCC **back and pelvis with penetration into retroperitoneum**
    CC Excl: See code: S30.001

√6ᵗʰ **S31.03 Puncture wound without foreign body of lower back and pelvis**

√7ᵗʰ **S31.030 Puncture wound without foreign body of lower back and pelvis without penetration into retroperitoneum**
    Puncture wound without foreign body of lower back and pelvis NOS

√7ᵗʰ **S31.031 Puncture wound without foreign** MCC **body of lower back and pelvis with penetration into retroperitoneum**
    CC Excl: See code: S30.001

√6ᵗʰ **S31.04 Puncture wound with foreign body of lower back and pelvis**

√7ᵗʰ **S31.040 Puncture wound with foreign body of lower back and pelvis without penetration into retroperitoneum**
    Puncture wound with foreign body of lower back and pelvis NOS

√7ᵗʰ **S31.041 Puncture wound with foreign body** MCC **of lower back and pelvis with penetration into retroperitoneum**
    CC Excl: See code: S30.001

√6ᵗʰ **S31.05 Open bite of lower back and pelvis**
    Bite of lower back and pelvis NOS
    EXCLUDES 1 *superficial bite of lower back and pelvis (S30.860, S30.870)*

√7ᵗʰ **S31.050 Open bite of lower back and pelvis without penetration into retroperitoneum**
    Open bite of lower back and pelvis NOS

√7ᵗʰ **S31.051 Open bite of lower back and pelvis** MCC **with penetration into retroperitoneum**
    CC Excl: See code: S30.001

√5ᵗʰ **S31.1 Open wound of abdominal wall without penetration into peritoneal cavity**
    Open wound of abdominal wall NOS
    EXCLUDES 2 *open wound of abdominal wall with penetration into peritoneal cavity (S31.6-)*

√6ᵗʰ **S31.10 Unspecified open wound of abdominal wall without penetration into peritoneal cavity**

√7ᵗʰ **S31.100 Unspecified open wound of abdominal wall, right upper quadrant without penetration into peritoneal cavity**

√7ᵗʰ **S31.101 Unspecified open wound of abdominal wall, left upper quadrant without penetration into peritoneal cavity**

√7ᵗʰ **S31.102 Unspecified open wound of abdominal wall, epigastric region without penetration into peritoneal cavity**

√7ᵗʰ **S31.103 Unspecified open wound of abdominal wall, right lower quadrant without penetration into peritoneal cavity**

√7ᵗʰ **S31.104 Unspecified open wound of abdominal wall, left lower quadrant without penetration into peritoneal cavity**

√7ᵗʰ **S31.105 Unspecified open wound of abdominal wall, periumbilic region without penetration into peritoneal cavity**

√7ᵗʰ **S31.109 Unspecified open wound of abdominal wall, unspecified quadrant without penetration into peritoneal cavity**
    Unspecified open wound of abdominal wall NOS

√6ᵗʰ **S31.11 Laceration without foreign body of abdominal wall without penetration into peritoneal cavity**

√7ᵗʰ **S31.110 Laceration without foreign body of abdominal wall, right upper quadrant without penetration into peritoneal cavity**

√7ᵗʰ **S31.111 Laceration without foreign body of abdominal wall, left upper quadrant without penetration into peritoneal cavity**

√7ᵗʰ **S31.112 Laceration without foreign body of abdominal wall, epigastric region without penetration into peritoneal cavity**

√7ᵗʰ **S31.113 Laceration without foreign body of abdominal wall, right lower quadrant without penetration into peritoneal cavity**

√7ᵗʰ **S31.114 Laceration without foreign body of abdominal wall, left lower quadrant without penetration into peritoneal cavity**

√7ᵗʰ **S31.115 Laceration without foreign body of abdominal wall, periumbilic region without penetration into peritoneal cavity**

√7ᵗʰ **S31.119 Laceration without foreign body of abdominal wall, unspecified quadrant without penetration into peritoneal cavity**

√6ᵗʰ **S31.12 Laceration with foreign body of abdominal wall without penetration into peritoneal cavity**

√7ᵗʰ **S31.120 Laceration of abdominal wall with foreign body, right upper quadrant without penetration into peritoneal cavity**

√7ᵗʰ **S31.121 Laceration of abdominal wall with foreign body, left upper quadrant without penetration into peritoneal cavity**

√7ᵗʰ **S31.122 Laceration of abdominal wall with foreign body, epigastric region without penetration into peritoneal cavity**

√7ᵗʰ **S31.123 Laceration of abdominal wall with foreign body, right lower quadrant without penetration into peritoneal cavity**

√7ᵗʰ **S31.124 Laceration of abdominal wall with foreign body, left lower quadrant without penetration into peritoneal cavity**

√7ᵗʰ **S31.125 Laceration of abdominal wall with foreign body, periumbilic region without penetration into peritoneal cavity**

√7ᵗʰ **S31.129 Laceration of abdominal wall with foreign body, unspecified quadrant without penetration into peritoneal cavity**

√6ᵗʰ **S31.13 Puncture wound of abdominal wall without foreign body without penetration into peritoneal cavity**

√7ᵗʰ **S31.130 Puncture wound of abdominal wall without foreign body, right upper quadrant without penetration into peritoneal cavity**

√7ᵗʰ **S31.131 Puncture wound of abdominal wall without foreign body, left upper quadrant without penetration into peritoneal cavity**

√7ᵗʰ **S31.132 Puncture wound of abdominal wall without foreign body, epigastric region without penetration into peritoneal cavity**

√7ᵗʰ **S31.133 Puncture wound of abdominal wall without foreign body, right lower quadrant without penetration into peritoneal cavity**

√7ᵗʰ **S31.134 Puncture wound of abdominal wall without foreign body, left lower quadrant without penetration into peritoneal cavity**

√7ᵗʰ **S31.135 Puncture wound of abdominal wall without foreign body, periumbilic region without penetration into peritoneal cavity**

√7ᵗʰ **S31.139 Puncture wound of abdominal wall without foreign body, unspecified quadrant without penetration into peritoneal cavity**

√6ᵗʰ **S31.14 Puncture wound of abdominal wall with foreign body without penetration into peritoneal cavity**

√7ᵗʰ **S31.140 Puncture wound of abdominal wall with foreign body, right upper quadrant without penetration into peritoneal cavity**

√7ᵗʰ **S31.141 Puncture wound of abdominal wall with foreign body, left upper quadrant without penetration into peritoneal cavity**

√7ᵗʰ **S31.142 Puncture wound of abdominal wall with foreign body, epigastric region without penetration into peritoneal cavity**

√7ᵗʰ **S31.143 Puncture wound of abdominal wall with foreign body, right lower quadrant without penetration into peritoneal cavity**

√7ᵗʰ **S31.144 Puncture wound of abdominal wall with foreign body, left lower quadrant without penetration into peritoneal cavity**

√7ᵗʰ **S31.145 Puncture wound of abdominal wall with foreign body, periumbilic region without penetration into peritoneal cavity**

N Newborn: 0 P Pediatric: 0-17 M Maternity: 12-55 A Adult: 15-124 MCC Major CC Condition PDx MCC PDx acts as own MCC CC CC Condition PDx CC PDx acts as own CC

888   ICD-10-CM Draft (2015)

√7th **S31.149** **Puncture wound of abdominal wall with foreign body, unspecified quadrant without penetration into peritoneal cavity**

√6th **S31.15** **Open bite of abdominal wall without penetration into peritoneal cavity**
Bite of abdominal wall NOS
EXCLUDES 1 *superficial bite of abdominal wall (S30.871)*

√7th **S31.150** **Open bite of abdominal wall, right upper quadrant without penetration into peritoneal cavity**

√7th **S31.151** **Open bite of abdominal wall, left upper quadrant without penetration into peritoneal cavity**

√7th **S31.152** **Open bite of abdominal wall, epigastric region without penetration into peritoneal cavity**

√7th **S31.153** **Open bite of abdominal wall, right lower quadrant without penetration into peritoneal cavity**

√7th **S31.154** **Open bite of abdominal wall, left lower quadrant without penetration into peritoneal cavity**

√7th **S31.155** **Open bite of abdominal wall, periumbilic region without penetration into peritoneal cavity**

√7th **S31.159** **Open bite of abdominal wall, unspecified quadrant without penetration into peritoneal cavity**

√5th **S31.2** **Open wound of penis**

√x7th **S31.20** **Unspecified open wound of penis** ♂

√x7th **S31.21** **Laceration without foreign body of penis** ♂

√x7th **S31.22** **Laceration with foreign body of penis** ♂

√x7th **S31.23** **Puncture wound without foreign body of penis** ♂

√x7th **S31.24** **Puncture wound with foreign body of penis** ♂

√x7th **S31.25** **Open bite of penis** ♂
Bite of penis NOS
EXCLUDES 1 *superficial bite of penis (S30.862, S30.872)*

√5th **S31.3** **Open wound of scrotum and testes**

√x7th **S31.30** **Unspecified open wound of scrotum and testes** ♂

√x7th **S31.31** **Laceration without foreign body of scrotum and testes** ♂

√x7th **S31.32** **Laceration with foreign body of scrotum and testes** ♂

√x7th **S31.33** **Puncture wound without foreign body of scrotum and testes** ♂

√x7th **S31.34** **Puncture wound with foreign body of scrotum and testes** ♂

√x7th **S31.35** **Open bite of scrotum and testes** ♂
Bite of scrotum and testes NOS
EXCLUDES 1 *superficial bite of scrotum and testes (S30.863, S30.873)*

√5th **S31.4** **Open wound of vagina and vulva**
EXCLUDES 1 *injury to vagina and vulva during delivery (O70-, O71.4)*

√x7th **S31.40** **Unspecified open wound of vagina and vulva** ♀

√x7th **S31.41** **Laceration without foreign body of vagina and vulva** ♀

√x7th **S31.42** **Laceration with foreign body of vagina and vulva** ♀

√x7th **S31.43** **Puncture wound without foreign body of vagina and vulva** ♀

√x7th **S31.44** **Puncture wound with foreign body of vagina and vulva** ♀

√x7th **S31.45** **Open bite of vagina and vulva** ♀
Bite of vagina and vulva NOS
EXCLUDES 1 *superficial bite of vagina and vulva (S30.864, S30.874)*

√5th **S31.5** **Open wound of unspecified external genital organs**
EXCLUDES 1 *traumatic amputation of external genital organs (S38.21, S38.22)*

√6th **S31.50** **Unspecified open wound of unspecified external genital organs**

√7th **S31.501** **Unspecified open wound of unspecified external genital organs, male** ♂

√7th **S31.502** **Unspecified open wound of unspecified external genital organs, female** ♀

√6th **S31.51** **Laceration without foreign body of unspecified external genital organs**

√7th **S31.511** **Laceration without foreign body of unspecified external genital organs, male** ♂

√7th **S31.512** **Laceration without foreign body of unspecified external genital organs, female** ♀

√6th **S31.52** **Laceration with foreign body of unspecified external genital organs**

√7th **S31.521** **Laceration with foreign body of unspecified external genital organs, male** ♂

√7th **S31.522** **Laceration with foreign body of unspecified external genital organs, female** ♀

√6th **S31.53** **Puncture wound without foreign body of unspecified external genital organs**

√7th **S31.531** **Puncture wound without foreign body of unspecified external genital organs, male** ♂

√7th **S31.532** **Puncture wound without foreign body of unspecified external genital organs, female** ♀

√6th **S31.54** **Puncture wound with foreign body of unspecified external genital organs**

√7th **S31.541** **Puncture wound with foreign body of unspecified external genital organs, male** ♂

√7th **S31.542** **Puncture wound with foreign body of unspecified external genital organs, female** ♀

√6th **S31.55** **Open bite of unspecified external genital organs**
Bite of unspecified external genital organs NOS
EXCLUDES 1 *superficial bite of unspecified external genital organs (S30.865, S30.866, S30.875, S30.876)*

√7th **S31.551** **Open bite of unspecified external genital organs, male** ♂

√7th **S31.552** **Open bite of unspecified external genital organs, female** ♀

√5th **S31.6** **Open wound of abdominal wall with penetration into peritoneal cavity**

CC Excl: For MCC codes in category S31.6, unless otherwise noted: MCC with 7th character A: S31.001A, S31.011A, S31.021, S31.031A, S31.041A, S31.051-S31.159 with 7th A, S31.600-S31.659 with 7th A, S31.831-S31.839 with 7th A, S36.81X-S36.99X with 7th A, S38.3XX-S39.023 with 7th A, T14.8-T14.91, T79.A0X-T79.9XX with 7th A

√6th **S31.60** **Unspecified open wound of abdominal wall with penetration into peritoneal cavity**

√7th **S31.600** **Unspecified open wound of abdominal wall, right upper quadrant with penetration into peritoneal cavity** MCC

√7th **S31.601** **Unspecified open wound of abdominal wall, left upper quadrant with penetration into peritoneal cavity** MCC

√7th **S31.602** **Unspecified open wound of abdominal wall, epigastric region with penetration into peritoneal cavity** MCC

√7th **S31.603** **Unspecified open wound of abdominal wall, right lower quadrant with penetration into peritoneal cavity** MCC

√7th **S31.604** **Unspecified open wound of abdominal wall, left lower quadrant with penetration into peritoneal cavity** MCC

√7th **S31.605** **Unspecified open wound of abdominal wall, periumbilic region with penetration into peritoneal cavity** MCC

√7th **S31.609** **Unspecified open wound of abdominal wall, unspecified quadrant with penetration into peritoneal cavity** MCC

√6th **S31.61** **Laceration without foreign body of abdominal wall with penetration into peritoneal cavity**

√7th **S31.610** **Laceration without foreign body of abdominal wall, right upper quadrant with penetration into peritoneal cavity** MCC

S31.611 √7ᵗʰ **Laceration without foreign body of abdominal wall, left upper quadrant with penetration into peritoneal cavity** MCC

S31.612 √7ᵗʰ **Laceration without foreign body of abdominal wall, epigastric region with penetration into peritoneal cavity** MCC

S31.613 √7ᵗʰ **Laceration without foreign body of abdominal wall, right lower quadrant with penetration into peritoneal cavity** MCC

S31.614 √7ᵗʰ **Laceration without foreign body of abdominal wall, left lower quadrant with penetration into peritoneal cavity** MCC

S31.615 √7ᵗʰ **Laceration without foreign body of abdominal wall, periumbilic region with penetration into peritoneal cavity** MCC

S31.619 √7ᵗʰ **Laceration without foreign body of abdominal wall, unspecified quadrant with penetration into peritoneal cavity** MCC

√6ᵗʰ **S31.62 Laceration with foreign body of abdominal wall with penetration into peritoneal cavity**

S31.620 √7ᵗʰ **Laceration with foreign body of abdominal wall, right upper quadrant with penetration into peritoneal cavity** MCC

S31.621 √7ᵗʰ **Laceration with foreign body of abdominal wall, left upper quadrant with penetration into peritoneal cavity** MCC

S31.622 √7ᵗʰ **Laceration with foreign body of abdominal wall, epigastric region with penetration into peritoneal cavity** MCC

S31.623 √7ᵗʰ **Laceration with foreign body of abdominal wall, right lower quadrant with penetration into peritoneal cavity** MCC

S31.624 √7ᵗʰ **Laceration with foreign body of abdominal wall, left lower quadrant with penetration into peritoneal cavity** MCC

S31.625 √7ᵗʰ **Laceration with foreign body of abdominal wall, periumbilic region with penetration into peritoneal cavity** MCC

S31.629 √7ᵗʰ **Laceration with foreign body of abdominal wall, unspecified quadrant with penetration into peritoneal cavity** MCC

√6ᵗʰ **S31.63 Puncture wound without foreign body of abdominal wall with penetration into peritoneal cavity**

S31.630 √7ᵗʰ **Puncture wound without foreign body of abdominal wall, right upper quadrant with penetration into peritoneal cavity** MCC

S31.631 √7ᵗʰ **Puncture wound without foreign body of abdominal wall, left upper quadrant with penetration into peritoneal cavity** MCC

S31.632 √7ᵗʰ **Puncture wound without foreign body of abdominal wall, epigastric region with penetration into peritoneal cavity** MCC

S31.633 √7ᵗʰ **Puncture wound without foreign body of abdominal wall, right lower quadrant with penetration into peritoneal cavity** MCC

S31.634 √7ᵗʰ **Puncture wound without foreign body of abdominal wall, left lower quadrant with penetration into peritoneal cavity** MCC

S31.635 √7ᵗʰ **Puncture wound without foreign body of abdominal wall, periumbilic region with penetration into peritoneal cavity** MCC

S31.639 √7ᵗʰ **Puncture wound without foreign body of abdominal wall, unspecified quadrant with penetration into peritoneal cavity** MCC

√6ᵗʰ **S31.64 Puncture wound with foreign body of abdominal wall with penetration into peritoneal cavity**

S31.640 √7ᵗʰ **Puncture wound with foreign body of abdominal wall, right upper quadrant with penetration into peritoneal cavity** MCC

S31.641 √7ᵗʰ **Puncture wound with foreign body of abdominal wall, left upper quadrant with penetration into peritoneal cavity** MCC

S31.642 √7ᵗʰ **Puncture wound with foreign body of abdominal wall, epigastric region with penetration into peritoneal cavity** MCC

S31.643 √7ᵗʰ **Puncture wound with foreign body of abdominal wall, right lower quadrant with penetration into peritoneal cavity** MCC

S31.644 √7ᵗʰ **Puncture wound with foreign body of abdominal wall, left lower quadrant with penetration into peritoneal cavity** MCC

S31.645 √7ᵗʰ **Puncture wound with foreign body of abdominal wall, periumbilic region with penetration into peritoneal cavity** MCC

S31.649 √7ᵗʰ **Puncture wound with foreign body of abdominal wall, unspecified quadrant with penetration into peritoneal cavity** MCC

√6ᵗʰ **S31.65 Open bite of abdominal wall with penetration into peritoneal cavity**

EXCLUDES 1   *superficial bite of abdominal wall (S30.861, S30.871)*

S31.650 √7ᵗʰ **Open bite of abdominal wall, right upper quadrant with penetration into peritoneal cavity** MCC

S31.651 √7ᵗʰ **Open bite of abdominal wall, left upper quadrant with penetration into peritoneal cavity** MCC

S31.652 √7ᵗʰ **Open bite of abdominal wall, epigastric region with penetration into peritoneal cavity** MCC

S31.653 √7ᵗʰ **Open bite of abdominal wall, right lower quadrant with penetration into peritoneal cavity** MCC

S31.654 √7ᵗʰ **Open bite of abdominal wall, left lower quadrant with penetration into peritoneal cavity** MCC

S31.655 √7ᵗʰ **Open bite of abdominal wall, periumbilic region with penetration into peritoneal cavity** MCC

S31.659 √7ᵗʰ **Open bite of abdominal wall, unspecified quadrant with penetration into peritoneal cavity** MCC

√5ᵗʰ **S31.8 Open wound of other parts of abdomen, lower back and pelvis**

√6ᵗʰ **S31.80 Open wound of unspecified buttock**

S31.801 √7ᵗʰ **Laceration without foreign body of unspecified buttock**

S31.802 √7ᵗʰ **Laceration with foreign body of unspecified buttock**

S31.803 √7ᵗʰ **Puncture wound without foreign body of unspecified buttock**

S31.804 √7ᵗʰ **Puncture wound with foreign body of unspecified buttock**

S31.805 √7ᵗʰ **Open bite of unspecified buttock**
Bite of buttock NOS
EXCLUDES 1   *superficial bite of buttock (S30.870)*

S31.809 √7ᵗʰ **Unspecified open wound of unspecified buttock**

√6ᵗʰ **S31.81 Open wound of right buttock**

S31.811 √7ᵗʰ **Laceration without foreign body of right buttock**

S31.812 √7ᵗʰ **Laceration with foreign body of right buttock**

S31.813 √7ᵗʰ **Puncture wound without foreign body of right buttock**

S31.814 √7ᵗʰ **Puncture wound with foreign body of right buttock**

S31.815 √7ᵗʰ **Open bite of right buttock**
Bite of right buttock NOS
EXCLUDES 1   *superficial bite of buttock (S30.870)*

S31.819 √7ᵗʰ **Unspecified open wound of right buttock**

√6ᵗʰ **S31.82 Open wound of left buttock**

S31.821 √7ᵗʰ **Laceration without foreign body of left buttock**

S31.822 √7ᵗʰ **Laceration with foreign body of left buttock**

Ⓝ Newborn: 0   Ⓟ Pediatric: 0-17   Ⓜ Maternity: 12-55   Ⓐ Adult: 15-124   MCC Major CC Condition   PDx MCC PDx acts as own MCC   CC CC Condition   PDx CC PDx acts as own CC

890   ICD-10-CM Draft (2015)

√7ᵗʰ **S31.823** Puncture wound without foreign body of left buttock

√7ᵗʰ **S31.824** Puncture wound with foreign body of left buttock

√7ᵗʰ **S31.825** Open bite of left buttock
Bite of left buttock NOS
EXCLUDES 1 superficial bite of buttock (S30.870)

√7ᵗʰ **S31.829** Unspecified open wound of left buttock

√6ᵗʰ **S31.83** Open wound of anus

√7ᵗʰ **S31.831** Laceration without foreign body of anus

√7ᵗʰ **S31.832** Laceration with foreign body of anus

√7ᵗʰ **S31.833** Puncture wound without foreign body of anus

√7ᵗʰ **S31.834** Puncture wound with foreign body of anus

√7ᵗʰ **S31.835** Open bite of anus
Bite of anus NOS (S30.877)
EXCLUDES 1 superficial bite of anus (S30.877)

√7ᵗʰ **S31.839** Unspecified open wound of anus

√4ᵗʰ **S32** Fracture of lumbar spine and pelvis

NOTE A fracture not indicated as displaced or nondisplaced should be coded to displaced.
A fracture not indicated as opened or closed should be coded to closed.

INCLUDES fracture of lumbosacral neural arch
fracture of lumbosacral spinous process
fracture of lumbosacral transverse process
fracture of lumbosacral vertebra
fracture of lumbosacral vertebral arch

Code first any associated spinal cord and spinal nerve injury (S34.-)
EXCLUDES 1 transection of abdomen (S38.3)
EXCLUDES 2 fracture of hip NOS (S72.0-)
AHA: 2012, 4Q, 93

The appropriate 7th is to be added to each code from category S32.
A   initial encounter for closed fracture
B   initial encounter for open fracture
D   subsequent encounter for fracture with routine healing
G   subsequent encounter for fracture with delayed healing
K   subsequent encounter for fracture with nonunion
S   sequela

√5ᵗʰ **S32.0** Fracture of lumbar vertebra
Fracture of lumbar spine NOS

CC Excl: For CC/MCC codes in subcategory S32.0, unless otherwise noted: CC with 7th character A or MCC with 7th character B: M48.40X-M48.58X with 7th S, M80.08XS, M80.88XS, M84.350S, M84.454S, M84.550S, M84.58XS, M84.650S, M99.13, M99.15-M99.17, M99.19, S03.8XX-S03.9XX with 7th A, S12.000-S12.9XX with 7th S, S13.9XXA, S14.109A, S14.119A, S14.129A, S14.139A, S14.149A, S14.159A, S22.000-S22.9XX with 7th S, S23.20X-S23.29X with 7th A, S23.9XXA, S24.109A, S24.119A, S24.139A, S24.149A, S24.159A, S29.001-S29.019 with 7th A, S29.091-S29.9XX with 7th A, S32.000-S33.39X with 7th [A, B, S], S33.5XXA, S33.9XX-S34.01X with 7th A, S34.101-S34.129 with 7th A, S38.1XXA, S38.3XX-S39.013 with 7th A, S39.091-S39.94X with 7th A, T14.8-T14.91, T79.A0X-T79.9XX with 7th A

CC with 7th character K: M80.00X-M84.68X with 7th [K, P], S02.0XX-S02.92X with 7th K, S12.000-S12.691 with 7th K, S22.000-S22.9XX with 7th K, S32.000-S32.9XX with 7th K, S42.001-S42.92X with 7th [K, P], S49.001-S49.199 with 7th [K, P], S52.001-S52.92X with 7th [K, M, N, P, Q, R], S59.001-S59.299 with 7th [K, P], S62.001-S62.92X with 7th [K, P], S72.001-S72.92X with 7th [K, M, N, P, Q, R], S79.001-S79.199 with 7th [K, P], S82.001-S82.92X with 7th [K, M, N, P, Q, R], S89.001-S89.399 with 7th [K, P], S92.001-S92.919 with 7th [K, P]

√6ᵗʰ **S32.00** Fracture of unspecified lumbar vertebra

7 √7ᵗʰ **S32.000** Wedge compression fracture of unspecified lumbar vertebra   MCC CC

7 √7ᵗʰ **S32.001** Stable burst fracture of unspecified lumbar vertebra   MCC CC

7 √7ᵗʰ **S32.002** Unstable burst fracture of unspecified lumbar vertebra   MCC CC

7 √7ᵗʰ **S32.008** Other fracture of unspecified lumbar vertebra   MCC CC

7 √7ᵗʰ **S32.009** Unspecified fracture of unspecified lumbar vertebra   MCC CC

√6ᵗʰ **S32.01** Fracture of first lumbar vertebra

7 √7ᵗʰ **S32.010** Wedge compression fracture of first lumbar vertebra   MCC CC

7 √7ᵗʰ **S32.011** Stable burst fracture of first lumbar vertebra   MCC CC

7 √7ᵗʰ **S32.012** Unstable burst fracture of first lumbar vertebra   MCC CC

7 √7ᵗʰ **S32.018** Other fracture of first lumbar vertebra   MCC CC

7 √7ᵗʰ **S32.019** Unspecified fracture of first lumbar vertebra   MCC CC

√6ᵗʰ **S32.02** Fracture of second lumbar vertebra

7 √7ᵗʰ **S32.020** Wedge compression fracture of second lumbar vertebra   MCC CC

7 √7ᵗʰ **S32.021** Stable burst fracture of second lumbar vertebra   MCC CC

7 √7ᵗʰ **S32.022** Unstable burst fracture of second lumbar vertebra   MCC CC

7 √7ᵗʰ **S32.028** Other fracture of second lumbar vertebra   MCC CC

7 √7ᵗʰ **S32.029** Unspecified fracture of second lumbar vertebra   MCC CC

√6ᵗʰ **S32.03** Fracture of third lumbar vertebra

7 √7ᵗʰ **S32.030** Wedge compression fracture of third lumbar vertebra   MCC CC

7 √7ᵗʰ **S32.031** Stable burst fracture of third lumbar vertebra   MCC CC

7 √7ᵗʰ **S32.032** Unstable burst fracture of third lumbar vertebra   MCC CC

7 √7ᵗʰ **S32.038** Other fracture of third lumbar vertebra   MCC CC

7 √7ᵗʰ **S32.039** Unspecified fracture of third lumbar vertebra   MCC CC

√6ᵗʰ **S32.04** Fracture of fourth lumbar vertebra

7 √7ᵗʰ **S32.040** Wedge compression fracture of fourth lumbar vertebra   MCC CC

7 √7ᵗʰ **S32.041** Stable burst fracture of fourth lumbar vertebra   MCC CC

7 √7ᵗʰ **S32.042** Unstable burst fracture of fourth lumbar vertebra   MCC CC

7 √7ᵗʰ **S32.048** Other fracture of fourth lumbar vertebra   MCC CC

7 √7ᵗʰ **S32.049** Unspecified fracture of fourth lumbar vertebra   MCC CC

√6ᵗʰ **S32.05** Fracture of fifth lumbar vertebra

7 √7ᵗʰ **S32.050** Wedge compression fracture of fifth lumbar vertebra   MCC CC

7 √7ᵗʰ **S32.051** Stable burst fracture of fifth lumbar vertebra   MCC CC

7 √7ᵗʰ **S32.052** Unstable burst fracture of fifth lumbar vertebra   MCC CC

7 √7ᵗʰ **S32.058** Other fracture of fifth lumbar vertebra   MCC CC

7 √7ᵗʰ **S32.059** Unspecified fracture of fifth lumbar vertebra   MCC CC

---

7 HAC = Initial encounter only (7th character A, B or C) and not POA.

√ Additional Character Required   √x7ᵗʰ Xtension Alert   Unacceptable PDx   Manifestation   Hospital Acquired Condition   **EXCLUDES 1** Not Coded Here   **EXCLUDES 2** Not Included Here

√5th **S32.1** **Fracture of** sacrum

> NOTE   For vertical fractures, code to most medial fracture extension.
> Use two codes if both a vertical and transverse fracture are present.
>
> Code also any associated fracture of pelvic ring (S32.8-)

> **CC Excl: For CC/MCC codes in subcategory S32.1, unless otherwise noted: CC with 7th character A or MCC with 7th character B:** M48.40X-M48.58X with 7th S, M80.08XS, M80.88XS, M84.350S, M84.454S, M84.550S, M84.58XS, M84.650S, M99.14-M99.17, M99.19, S03.8XX-S03.9XX with 7th A, S12.000-S12.9XX with 7th S, S13.9XXA, S14.109A, S14.119 , S14.129A, S14.139A, S14.149 A, S14.159A, S22.000-S22.9XX with 7th S, S23.20X-S23.29X with 7th A, S23.9XXA, S24.109A, S24.119A, S24.139A, S24.149 A, S24.159A, S29.001-S29.019 with 7th A, S29.091-S29.9XX with 7th A, S32.000-S32.9XX with 7th S, S33.2XX-S33.4XX with 7th A, S33.6XX-S34.02X with 7th A, S34.131-S34.139 with 7th A, S34.3XX with 7th A, S38.1XX with 7th A, S38.3XX-S39.013 with 7th A, S39.091-S39.94X A, T14.8-T14.91, T79.A0X-T79.9XX with 7th A

> **CC with 7th character K:** M80.00X-M84.68X with 7th [K, P], S02.0XX-S02.92X with 7th K, S12.000-S12.691 with 7th K, S22.000-S22.9XX with 7th K, S32.000-S32.9XX with 7th K, S42.001-S42.92X with 7th [K, P], S49.001-S49.199 with 7th [K, P], S52.001-S52.92X with 7th [K, M, N, P, Q, R], S59.001-S59.299 with 7th [K, P], S62.001-S62.92X with 7th [K, P], S72.001-S72.92X with 7th [K, M, N, P, Q, R], S79.001-S79.199 with 7th [K, P], S82.001-S82.92X with 7th [K, M, N, P, Q, R], S89.001-S89.399 with 7th [K, P], S92.001-S92.919 with 7th [K, P]

7 √x5th **S32.10** **Unspecified** fracture of sacrum   MCC CC

√6th **S32.11** **Zone I** fracture of sacrum
   Vertical sacral ala fracture of sacrum

   7 √7th **S32.110** **Nondisplaced** Zone I fracture of sacrum   MCC CC

   7 √7th **S32.111** **Minimally displaced** Zone I fracture of sacrum   MCC CC

   7 √7th **S32.112** **Severely displaced** Zone I fracture of sacrum   MCC CC

   7 √7th **S32.119** **Unspecified** Zone I fracture of sacrum   MCC CC

√6th **S32.12** **Zone II** fracture of sacrum
   Vertical foraminal region fracture of sacrum

   7 √7th **S32.120** **Nondisplaced** Zone II fracture of sacrum   MCC CC

   7 √7th **S32.121** **Minimally displaced** Zone II fracture of sacrum   MCC CC

   7 √7th **S32.122** **Severely displaced** Zone II fracture of sacrum   MCC CC

   7 √7th **S32.129** **Unspecified** Zone II fracture of sacrum   MCC CC

√6th **S32.13** **Zone III** fracture of sacrum
   Vertical fracture into spinal canal region of sacrum

   7 √7th **S32.130** **Nondisplaced** Zone III fracture of sacrum   MCC CC

   7 √7th **S32.131** **Minimally displaced** Zone III fracture of sacrum   MCC CC

   7 √7th **S32.132** **Severely displaced** Zone III fracture of sacrum   MCC CC

   7 √7th **S32.139** **Unspecified** Zone III fracture of sacrum   MCC CC

7 √x7th **S32.14** **Type 1** fracture of sacrum   MCC CC
   Transverse flexion fracture of sacrum without displacement

7 √x7th **S32.15** **Type 2** fracture of sacrum   MCC CC
   Transverse flexion fracture of sacrum with posterior displacement

7 √x7th **S32.16** **Type 3** fracture of sacrum   MCC CC
   Transverse extension fracture of sacrum with anterior displacement

7 √x7th **S32.17** **Type 4** fracture of sacrum   MCC CC
   Transverse segmental comminution of upper sacrum

7 √x7th **S32.19** **Other** fracture of sacrum   MCC CC

7 √x7th **S32.2** **Fracture of** coccyx   MCC CC
   CC Excl: See code: S32.1

√5th **S32.3** **Fracture of** ilium

> EXCLUDES 1   *fracture of ilium with associated disruption of pelvic ring (S32.8-)*

> **CC Excl: For CC/MCC codes in subcategory S32.3, unless otherwise noted: CC with 7th character A:** M80.00X-M80.019 with 7th A, M80.041-M80.049 with 7th A, M80.80X-M80.819 with 7th A, M80.841-M80.849 with 7th A, M84.40X-M84.419 with 7th A, M84.441-M84.446 with 7th A, M84.454-M84.519 with 7th A, M84.541-M84.550 with 7th A, M84.574-M84.576 with 7th A, M84.60X-M84.619 with 7th A, M84.641-M84.650 with 7th A, M84.674-M84.68X with 7th A, S03.8XX-S03.9XX with 7th A, S22.9XX-S22.9XX with 7th [A, B], S29.011-S29.019 with 7th [A, B], S32.301-S32.811 with 7th [A, B], S32.89X-S32.9XX with 7th [A, B], S33.4XX with 7th A, S33.6XX-S33.8XX with 7th A, S38.3XX-S39.013 with 7th A, S73.001-S73.199 with 7th A, S76.001-S76.019 with 7th A, S76.091-S76.119 with 7th A, S76.191-S76.219 with 7th A, S76.291-S76.319 with 7th A, S76.391-S76.819 with 7th A, S76.891-S76.919 with 7th A, S76.991-S76.999 with 7th A, S79.811-S79.929 with 7th A, T14.8-T14.91, T79.A9X-T79.9XX with 7th A

> **MCC with 7th character B:** M48.40X-M48.58X with 7th A, M80.00X-M84.68X with 7th A, S03.8XX-S03.9XX with 7th A, S22.9XX-S22.9XX with 7th [A, B], S29.011-S29.019 with 7th A, S32.301-S32.399 with 7th [A, B], S32.810-S32.811 with 7th [A, B], S32.89X-S32.9XX with 7th [A, B], S33.4XX with 7th A, S33.6XX-S33.8XX with 7th A, S38.3XX-S39.013 with 7th A, S73.001-S73.199 with 7th A, S76.001-S76.019 with 7th A, S76.091-S76.119 with 7th A, S76.191-S76.219 with 7th A, S76.291-S76.319 with 7th A, S76.391-S76.819 with 7th A, S76.891-S76.919 with 7th A, S76.991-S76.999 with 7th A, S79.811-S79.929 with 7th A, T14.8-T14.91, T79.A0X-T79.9XX with 7th A

> **CC with 7th character K:** M80.00X-M84.68X with 7th [K, P], S02.0XX-S02.92X with 7th K, S12.000-S12.691 with 7th K, S22.000-S22.9XX with 7th K, S32.000-S32.9XX with 7th K, S42.001-S42.92X with 7th [K, P], S49.001-S49.199 with 7th [K, P], S52.001-S52.92X with 7th [K, M, N, P, Q, R], S59.001-S59.299 with 7th [K, P], S62.001-S62.92X with 7th [K, P], S72.001-S72.92X with 7th [K, M, N, P, Q, R], S79.001-S79.199 with 7th [K, P], S82.001-S82.92X with 7th [K, M, N, P, Q, R], S89.001-S89.399 with 7th [K, P], S92.001-S92.919 with 7th [K, P]

√6th **S32.30** **Unspecified** fracture of ilium

   7 √7th **S32.301** **Unspecified** fracture of **right** ilium   MCC CC

   7 √7th **S32.302** **Unspecified** fracture of **left** ilium   MCC CC

   7 √7th **S32.309** **Unspecified** fracture of **unspecified** ilium   MCC CC

√6th **S32.31** **Avulsion** fracture of ilium

   7 √7th **S32.311** **Displaced** avulsion fracture of **right** ilium   MCC CC

   7 √7th **S32.312** **Displaced** avulsion fracture of **left** ilium   MCC CC

   7 √7th **S32.313** **Displaced** avulsion fracture of **unspecified** ilium   MCC CC

   7 √7th **S32.314** **Nondisplaced** avulsion fracture of **right** ilium   MCC CC

   7 √7th **S32.315** **Nondisplaced** avulsion fracture of **left** ilium   MCC CC

   7 √7th **S32.316** **Nondisplaced** avulsion fracture of **unspecified** ilium   MCC CC

√6th **S32.39** **Other** fracture of ilium

   7 √7th **S32.391** **Other fracture of right** ilium   MCC CC

   7 √7th **S32.392** **Other fracture of left** ilium   MCC CC

   7 √7th **S32.399** **Other fracture of unspecified** ilium   MCC CC

---

7 HAC = Initial encounter only (7th character A, B or C) and not POA.

N Newborn: 0   P Pediatric: 0-17   M Maternity: 12-55   A Adult: 15-124   MCC Major CC Condition   PDx MCC PDx acts as own MCC   CC CC Condition   PDx CC PDx acts as own CC

892   ICD-10-CM Draft (2015)

√5ᵗʰ **S32.4   Fracture of acetabulum**

Code also any associated fracture of pelvic ring (S32.8-)

CC Excl: For CC/MCC codes in subcategory S32.4, unless otherwise noted: MCC with 7th character A: M48.40X-M48.58X with 7th A, M80.00X-M84.68X with 7th A, S03.8XX-S03.9XX with 7th A, S22.9XX-S22.9XX with 7th [A, B], S29.011-S29.019 with 7th A, S32.401-S32.499 with 7th [A, B], S32.810-S32.811 with 7th [A, B], S32.89X-S32.9XX with 7th [A, B], S33.4XX with 7th A, S33.6XX-S33.8XX with 7th A, S38.3XX-S39.013 with 7th A, S73.001-S73.199 with 7th A, S76.001-S76.019 with 7th A, S76.091-S76.119 with 7th A, S76.191-S76.219 with 7th A, S76.291-S76.319 with 7th A, S76.391-S76.819 with 7th A, S76.891-S76.919 with 7th A, S76.991-S76.999 with 7th A, S79.811-S79.929 with 7th A, T14.8-T14.91, T79.A0X-T79.9XX with 7th A

MCC with 7th character B: S03.8XX-S03.9XX with 7th A, S22.9XX-S22.9XX with 7th A, S29.011-S29.019 with 7th A, S32.401-S32.499 with 7th [A, B], S32.810-S32.811 with 7th [A, B], S32.89X-S32.9XX with 7th [A, B], S33.4XX with 7th A, S33.6XX-S33.8XX with 7th A, S38.3XX-S39.013 with 7th A, S73.001-S73.199 with 7th A, S76.001-S76.019 with 7th A, S76.091-S76.119 with 7th A, S76.191-S76.219 with 7th A, S76.291-S76.319 with 7th A, S76.391-S76.819 with 7th A, S76.891-S76.919 with 7th A, S76.991-S76.999 with 7th A, S79.811-S79.929 with 7th A, T14.8-T14.91, T79.A0X-T79.9XX with 7th A

CC with 7th character K: M80.00X-M84.68X with 7th [K, P], S02.0XX-S02.92X with 7th K, S12.000-S12.691 with 7th K, S22.000-S22.9XX with 7th K, S32.000-S32.9XX with 7th K, S42.001-S42.92X with 7th [K, P], S49.001-S49.199 with 7th [K, P], S52.001-S52.92X with 7th [K, M, N, P, Q, R], S59.001-S59.299 with 7th [K, P], S62.001-S62.92X with 7th [K, P], S72.001-S72.92X with 7th [K, M, N, P, Q, R], S79.001-S79.199 with 7th [K, P], S82.001-S82.92X with 7th [K, M, N, P, Q, R], S89.001-S89.399 with 7th [K, P], S92.001-S92.919 with 7th [K, P]

√6ᵗʰ **S32.40   Unspecified fracture of acetabulum**

7 √7ᵗʰ **S32.401   Unspecified fracture of right acetabulum**   MCC CC

7 √7ᵗʰ **S32.402   Unspecified fracture of left acetabulum**   MCC CC

7 √7ᵗʰ **S32.409   Unspecified fracture of unspecified acetabulum**   MCC CC

√6ᵗʰ **S32.41   Fracture of anterior wall of acetabulum**

7 √7ᵗʰ **S32.411   Displaced fracture of anterior wall of right acetabulum**   MCC CC

7 √7ᵗʰ **S32.412   Displaced fracture of anterior wall of left acetabulum**   MCC CC

7 √7ᵗʰ **S32.413   Displaced fracture of anterior wall of unspecified acetabulum**   MCC CC

7 √7ᵗʰ **S32.414   Nondisplaced fracture of anterior wall of right acetabulum**   MCC CC

7 √7ᵗʰ **S32.415   Nondisplaced fracture of anterior wall of left acetabulum**   MCC CC

7 √7ᵗʰ **S32.416   Nondisplaced fracture of anterior wall of unspecified acetabulum**   MCC CC

√6ᵗʰ **S32.42   Fracture of posterior wall of acetabulum**

7 √7ᵗʰ **S32.421   Displaced fracture of posterior wall of right acetabulum**   MCC CC

7 √7ᵗʰ **S32.422   Displaced fracture of posterior wall of left acetabulum**   MCC CC

7 √7ᵗʰ **S32.423   Displaced fracture of posterior wall of unspecified acetabulum**   MCC CC

7 √7ᵗʰ **S32.424   Nondisplaced fracture of posterior wall of right acetabulum**   MCC CC

7 √7ᵗʰ **S32.425   Nondisplaced fracture of posterior wall of left acetabulum**   MCC CC

7 √7ᵗʰ **S32.426   Nondisplaced fracture of posterior wall of unspecified acetabulum**   MCC CC

√6ᵗʰ **S32.43   Fracture of anterior column [iliopubic] of acetabulum**

7 √7ᵗʰ **S32.431   Displaced fracture of anterior column [iliopubic] of right acetabulum**   MCC CC

7 √7ᵗʰ **S32.432   Displaced fracture of anterior column [iliopubic] of left acetabulum**   MCC CC

7 √7ᵗʰ **S32.433   Displaced fracture of anterior column [iliopubic] of unspecified acetabulum**   MCC CC

7 √7ᵗʰ **S32.434   Nondisplaced fracture of anterior column [iliopubic] of right acetabulum**   MCC CC

7 √7ᵗʰ **S32.435   Nondisplaced fracture of anterior column [iliopubic] of left acetabulum**   MCC CC

7 √7ᵗʰ **S32.436   Nondisplaced fracture of anterior column [iliopubic] of unspecified acetabulum**   MCC CC

√6ᵗʰ **S32.44   Fracture of posterior column [ilioischial] of acetabulum**

7 √7ᵗʰ **S32.441   Displaced fracture of posterior column [ilioischial] of right acetabulum**   MCC CC

7 √7ᵗʰ **S32.442   Displaced fracture of posterior column [ilioischial] of left acetabulum**   MCC CC

7 √7ᵗʰ **S32.443   Displaced fracture of posterior column [ilioischial] of unspecified acetabulum**   MCC CC

7 √7ᵗʰ **S32.444   Nondisplaced fracture of posterior column [ilioischial] of right acetabulum**   MCC CC

7 √7ᵗʰ **S32.445   Nondisplaced fracture of posterior column [ilioischial] of left acetabulum**   MCC CC

7 √7ᵗʰ **S32.446   Nondisplaced fracture of posterior column [ilioischial] of unspecified acetabulum**   MCC CC

√6ᵗʰ **S32.45   Transverse fracture of acetabulum**

7 √7ᵗʰ **S32.451   Displaced transverse fracture of right acetabulum**   MCC CC

7 √7ᵗʰ **S32.452   Displaced transverse fracture of left acetabulum**   MCC CC

7 √7ᵗʰ **S32.453   Displaced transverse fracture of unspecified acetabulum**   MCC CC

7 √7ᵗʰ **S32.454   Nondisplaced transverse fracture of right acetabulum**   MCC CC

7 √7ᵗʰ **S32.455   Nondisplaced transverse fracture of left acetabulum**   MCC CC

7 √7ᵗʰ **S32.456   Nondisplaced transverse fracture of unspecified acetabulum**   MCC CC

√6ᵗʰ **S32.46   Associated transverse-posterior fracture of acetabulum**

7 √7ᵗʰ **S32.461   Displaced associated transverse-posterior fracture of right acetabulum**   MCC CC

7 √7ᵗʰ **S32.462   Displaced associated transverse-posterior fracture of left acetabulum**   MCC CC

7 √7ᵗʰ **S32.463   Displaced associated transverse-posterior fracture of unspecified acetabulum**   MCC CC

7 √7ᵗʰ **S32.464   Nondisplaced associated transverse-posterior fracture of right acetabulum**   MCC CC

7 √7ᵗʰ **S32.465   Nondisplaced associated transverse-posterior fracture of left acetabulum**   MCC CC

7 √7ᵗʰ **S32.466   Nondisplaced associated transverse-posterior fracture of unspecified acetabulum**   MCC CC

√6ᵗʰ **S32.47   Fracture of medial wall of acetabulum**

7 √7ᵗʰ **S32.471   Displaced fracture of medial wall of right acetabulum**   MCC CC

7 √7ᵗʰ **S32.472   Displaced fracture of medial wall of left acetabulum**   MCC CC

7 √7ᵗʰ **S32.473   Displaced fracture of medial wall of unspecified acetabulum**   MCC CC

7 √7ᵗʰ **S32.474   Nondisplaced fracture of medial wall of right acetabulum**   MCC CC

7 √7ᵗʰ **S32.475   Nondisplaced fracture of medial wall of left acetabulum**   MCC CC

7 √7ᵗʰ **S32.476   Nondisplaced fracture of medial wall of unspecified acetabulum**   MCC CC

---

7 HAC = Initial encounter only (7th character A, B or C) and not POA.

√ Additional Character Required   √x7ᵗʰ Xtension Alert   Unacceptable PDx   Manifestation   Hospital Acquired Condition   *EXCLUDES 1* Not Coded Here   *EXCLUDES 2* Not Included Here

√6th **S32.48** Dome fracture of acetabulum

7 √7th **S32.481** Displaced dome fracture of right acetabulum   MCC CC

7 √7th **S32.482** Displaced dome fracture of left acetabulum   MCC CC

7 √7th **S32.483** Displaced dome fracture of unspecified acetabulum   MCC CC

7 √7th **S32.484** Nondisplaced dome fracture of right acetabulum   MCC CC

7 √7th **S32.485** Nondisplaced dome fracture of left acetabulum   MCC CC

7 √7th **S32.486** Nondisplaced dome fracture of unspecified acetabulum   MCC CC

√6th **S32.49** Other specified fracture of acetabulum

7 √7th **S32.491** Other specified fracture of right acetabulum   MCC CC

7 √7th **S32.492** Other specified fracture of left acetabulum   MCC CC

7 √7th **S32.499** Other specified fracture of unspecified acetabulum   MCC CC

√5th **S32.5** Fracture of pubis

EXCLUDES 1   fracture of pubis with associated disruption of pelvic ring (S32.8-)

CC Excl: For CC/MCC codes in subcategory S32.5, unless otherwise noted: CC with 7th character A or MCC with 7th character B: M48.40X-M48.58X with 7th A, M80.00X-M84.68X with 7th A, S03.8XX-S03.9XX with 7th A, S22.9XX-S22.9XX with 7th [A, B], S29.011-S29.019 with 7th A, S32.501-S32.599 with 7th [A, B], S32.810-S32.811 with 7th [A, B], S32.89X-S32.9XX with 7th [A, B], S33.4XXA, S33.6XX-S33.8XX with 7th A, S38.3X-S39.013 with 7th A, S73.001-S73.199 with 7th A, S76.001-S76.019 with 7th A, S76.091-S76.119 with 7th A, S76.191-S76.219 with 7th A, S76.291-S76.319 with 7th A, S76.391-S76.819 with 7th A, S76.891-S76.919 with 7th A, S76.991-S76.999 with 7th A, S79.811-S79.929 with 7th A, T14.8-T14.91, T79.A0X-T79.9XX with 7th A

CC with 7th character K: M80.00X-M84.68X with 7th [K, P], S02.0XX-S02.92X with 7th K, S12.000-S12.691 with 7th K, S22.000-S22.9XX with 7th K, S32.000-S32.9XX with 7th K, S42.001-S42.92X with 7th [K, P], S49.001-S49.199 with 7th [K, P], S52.001-S52.92X with 7th [K, M, N, P, Q, R], S59.001-S59.299 with 7th [K, P], S62.001-S62.92X with 7th [K, P], S72.001-S72.92X with 7th [K, M, N, P, Q, R], S79.001-S79.199 with 7th [K, P], S82.001-S82.92X with 7th [K, M, N, P, Q, R], S89.001-S89.399 with 7th [K, P], S92.001-S92.919 with 7th [K, P]

√6th **S32.50** Unspecified fracture of pubis

7 √7th **S32.501** Unspecified fracture of right pubis   MCC CC

7 √7th **S32.502** Unspecified fracture of left pubis   MCC CC

7 √7th **S32.509** Unspecified fracture of unspecified pubis   MCC CC

√6th **S32.51** Fracture of superior rim of pubis

7 √7th **S32.511** Fracture of superior rim of right pubis   MCC CC

7 √7th **S32.512** Fracture of superior rim of left pubis   MCC CC

7 √7th **S32.519** Fracture of superior rim of unspecified pubis   MCC CC

√6th **S32.59** Other specified fracture of pubis

7 √7th **S32.591** Other specified fracture of right pubis   MCC CC

7 √7th **S32.592** Other specified fracture of left pubis   MCC CC

7 √7th **S32.599** Other specified fracture of unspecified pubis   MCC CC

√5th **S32.6** Fracture of ischium

EXCLUDES 1   fracture of ischium with associated disruption of pelvic ring (S32.8-)

CC Excl: For CC/MCC codes in subcategory S32.6, unless otherwise noted: CC with 7th character A: S32.601-S32.699 with 7th A

MCC with 7th character B: M48.40X-M48.58X with 7th A, M80.00X-M84.68X with 7th A, S03.8XX-S03.9XX with 7th A, S22.9XX-S22.9XX with 7th [A, B], S29.011-S29.019 with 7th A, S32.601-S32.811 with 7th [A, B], S32.89X-S32.9XX with 7th [A, B], S33.4XXA with 7th A, S33.6XX-S33.8XX with 7th A, S38.3XX-S39.013 with 7th A, S73.001-S73.199 with 7th A, S76.001-S76.019 with 7th A, S76.091-S76.119 with 7th A, S76.191-S76.219 with 7th A, S76.291-S76.319 with 7th A, S76.391-S76.819 with 7th A, S76.891-S76.919 with 7th A, S76.991-S76.999 with 7th A, S79.811-S79.929 with 7th A, T14.8-T14.91, T79.A0X-T79.9XX with 7th A

CC with 7th character K: M80.00X-M84.68X with 7th [K, P], S02.0XX-S02.92X with 7th K, S12.000-S12.691 with 7th K, S22.000-S22.9XX with 7th K, S32.000-S32.9XX with 7th K, S42.001-S42.92X with 7th [K, P], S49.001-S49.199 with 7th [K, P], S52.001-S52.92X with 7th [K, M, N, P, Q, R], S59.001-S59.299 with 7th [K, P], S62.001-S62.92X with 7th [K, P], S72.001-S72.92X with 7th [K, M, N, P, Q, R], S79.001-S79.199 with 7th [K, P], S82.001-S82.92X with 7th [K, M, N, P, Q, R], S89.001-S89.399 with 7th [K, P], S92.001-S92.919 with 7th [K, P]

√6th **S32.60** Unspecified fracture of ischium

7 √7th **S32.601** Unspecified fracture of right ischium   MCC CC

7 √7th **S32.602** Unspecified fracture of left ischium   MCC CC

7 √7th **S32.609** Unspecified fracture of unspecified ischium   MCC CC

√6th **S32.61** Avulsion fracture of ischium

7 √7th **S32.611** Displaced avulsion fracture of right ischium   MCC CC

7 √7th **S32.612** Displaced avulsion fracture of left ischium   MCC CC

7 √7th **S32.613** Displaced avulsion fracture of unspecified ischium   MCC CC

7 √7th **S32.614** Nondisplaced avulsion fracture of right ischium   MCC CC

7 √7th **S32.615** Nondisplaced avulsion fracture of left ischium   MCC CC

7 √7th **S32.616** Nondisplaced avulsion fracture of unspecified ischium   MCC CC

√6th **S32.69** Other specified fracture of ischium

7 √7th **S32.691** Other specified fracture of right ischium   MCC CC

7 √7th **S32.692** Other specified fracture of left ischium   MCC CC

7 √7th **S32.699** Other specified fracture of unspecified ischium   MCC CC

√5th **S32.8** Fracture of other parts of pelvis

Code also any associated:
   fracture of acetabulum (S32.4-)
   sacral fracture (S32.1-)

---

7 HAC = Initial encounter only (7th character A, B or C) and not POA.

N Newborn: 0   P Pediatric: 0-17   M Maternity: 12-55   A Adult: 15-124   MCC Major CC Condition   PDx MCC PDx acts as own MCC   CC CC Condition   PDx CC PDx acts as own CC

894   ICD-10-CM Draft (2015)

✓6ᵗʰ **S32.81 Multiple fractures of pelvis with disruption of pelvic ring**

Multiple pelvic fractures with disruption of pelvic circle

CC Excl: For CC/MCC codes in subcategory S32.81, unless otherwise noted: CC with 7th character A or MCC with 7th character B: M48.40X-M48.58X with 7th A, M80.00X-M84.68X with 7th A, S03.8XX-S03.9XX with 7th A, S22.9XX-S22.9XX with 7th [A, B], S29.011-S29.019 with 7th A, S32.301-S32.811 with 7th [A, B], S32.89X-S32.9XX with 7th [A, B], S33.4XX with 7th A, S33.6XX-S33.8XX with 7th A, S38.3XX-S39.013 with 7th A, S73.001-S73.199 with 7th A, S76.001-S76.019 with 7th A, S76.091-S76.119 with 7th A, S76.191-S76.219 with 7th A, S76.291-S76.319 with 7th A, S76.391-S76.819 with 7th A, S76.891-S76.919 with 7th A, S76.991-S76.999 with 7th A, S79.811-S79.929 with 7th A, T14.8-T14.91, T79.A0X-T79.9XX with 7th A

CC with 7th character K: M80.00X-M84.68X with 7th [K, P], S02.0XX-S02.92X with 7th K, S12.000-S12.691 with 7th K, S22.000-S22.9XX with 7th K, S32.000-S32.9XX with 7th K, S42.001-S42.92X with 7th [K, P], S49.001-S49.199 with 7th [K, P], S52.001-S52.92X with 7th [K, M, N, P, Q, R], S59.001-S59.299 with 7th [K, P], S62.001-S62.92X with 7th [K, P], S72.001-S72.92X with 7th [K, M, N, P, Q, R], S79.001-S79.199 with 7th [K, P], S82.001-S82.92X with 7th [K, M, N, P, Q, R], S89.001-S89.399 with 7th [K, P], S92.001-S92.919 with 7th [K, P]

7 ✓7ᵗʰ **S32.810 Multiple fractures of pelvis with stable disruption of pelvic ring** MCC CC

7 ✓7ᵗʰ **S32.811 Multiple fractures of pelvis with unstable disruption of pelvic ring** MCC CC

7 ✓x7ᵗʰ **S32.82 Multiple fractures of pelvis without disruption of pelvic ring** MCC CC

Multiple pelvic fractures without disruption of pelvic circle

CC Excl: CC with 7th character A or MCC with 7th character B: S32.89 with 7th A
CC with 7th character K: M80.00X-M84.68X with 7th [K, P], S02.0XX-S02.92X with 7th K, S12.000-S12.691 with 7th K, S22.000-S22.9XX with 7th K, S32.000-S32.9XX with 7th K, S42.001-S42.92X with 7th [K, P], S49.001-S49.199 with 7th [K, P], S52.001-S52.92X with 7th [K, M, N, P, Q, R], S59.001-S59.299 with 7th [K, P], S62.001-S62.92X with 7th [K, P], S72.001-S72.92X with 7th [K, M, N, P, Q, R], S79.001-S79.199 with 7th [K, P], S82.001-S82.92X with 7th [K, M, N, P, Q, R], S89.001-S89.399 with 7th [K, P], S92.001-S92.919 with 7th [K, P]

7 ✓x7ᵗʰ **S32.89 Fracture of other parts of pelvis** MCC CC

CC Excl: CC with 7th character A or MCC with 7th character B: M48.40X-M48.58X with 7th A, M80.00X-M84.68X with 7th A, S03.8XX-S03.9XX with 7th A, S22.9XX-S22.9XX with 7th [A, B], S29.011-S29.019 with 7th A, S32.301-S32.9XX with 7th [A, B], S33.4XX with 7th A, S33.6XX-S33.8XX with 7th A, S38.3X-S39.013 with 7th A, S73.001-S73.199 with 7th A, S76.001-S76.019 with 7th A, S76.091-S76.119 with 7th A, S76.191-S76.219 with 7th A, S76.291-S76.319 with 7th A, S76.391-S76.819 with 7th A, S76.891-S76.919 with 7th A, S76.991-S76.999 with 7th A, S79.811-S79.929 with 7th A, T14.8-T14.91, T79.A0X-T79.9XX with 7th A

CC with 7th character K: M80.00X-M84.68X with 7th [K, P], S02.0XX-S02.92X with 7th K, S12.000-S12.691 with 7th K, S22.000-S22.9XX with 7th K, S32.000-S32.9XX with 7th K, S42.001-S42.92X with 7th [K, P], S49.001-S49.199 with 7th [K, P], S52.001-S52.92X with 7th [K, M, N, P, Q, R], S59.001-S59.299 with 7th [K, P], S62.001-S62.92X with 7th [K, P], S72.001-S72.92X with 7th [K, M, N, P, Q, R], S79.001-S79.199 with 7th [K, P], S82.001-S82.92X with 7th [K, M, N, P, Q, R], S89.001-S89.399 with 7th [K, P], S92.001-S92.919 with 7th [K, P]

7 ✓x7ᵗʰ **S32.9 Fracture of unspecified parts of lumbosacral spine and pelvis** MCC CC

Fracture of lumbosacral spine NOS
Fracture of pelvis NOS
AHA: 2012, 4Q, 93
CC Excl: See code: S82.81

✓4ᵗʰ **S33 Dislocation and sprain of joints and ligaments of lumbar spine and pelvis**

INCLUDES avulsion of joint or ligament of lumbar spine and pelvis
laceration of cartilage, joint or ligament of lumbar spine and pelvis
sprain of cartilage, joint or ligament of lumbar spine and pelvis
traumatic hemarthrosis of joint or ligament of lumbar spine and pelvis
traumatic rupture of joint or ligament of lumbar spine and pelvis
traumatic subluxation of joint or ligament of lumbar spine and pelvis
traumatic tear of joint or ligament of lumbar spine and pelvis

Code also any associated open wound

EXCLUDES 1 nontraumatic rupture or displacement of lumbar intervertebral disc NOS (M51.-)
obstetric damage to pelvic joints and ligaments (O71.6)

EXCLUDES 2 dislocation and sprain of joints and ligaments of hip (S73.-)
strain of muscle of lower back and pelvis (S39.01-)

The appropriate 7th is to be added to each code from category S33.
A initial encounter
D subsequent encounter
S sequela

✓x7ᵗʰ **S33.0 Traumatic rupture of lumbar intervertebral disc**

EXCLUDES 1 rupture or displacement (nontraumatic) of lumbar intervertebral disc NOS (M51- with fifth character 6)

✓5ᵗʰ **S33.1 Subluxation and dislocation of lumbar vertebra**

Code also any associated:
open wound of abdomen, lower back and pelvis (S31)
spinal cord injury (S24.0, S24.1-, S34.0-, S34.1-)

EXCLUDES 2 fracture of lumbar vertebrae (S32.0-)

✓6ᵗʰ **S33.10 Subluxation and dislocation of unspecified lumbar vertebra**

✓7ᵗʰ **S33.100 Subluxation of unspecified lumbar vertebra**

✓7ᵗʰ **S33.101 Dislocation of unspecified lumbar vertebra**

✓6ᵗʰ **S33.11 Subluxation and dislocation of L1/L2 lumbar vertebra**

✓7ᵗʰ **S33.110 Subluxation of L1/L2 lumbar vertebra**

✓7ᵗʰ **S33.111 Dislocation of L1/L2 lumbar vertebra**

✓6ᵗʰ **S33.12 Subluxation and dislocation of L2/L3 lumbar vertebra**

✓7ᵗʰ **S33.120 Subluxation of L2/L3 lumbar vertebra**

✓7ᵗʰ **S33.121 Dislocation of L2/L3 lumbar vertebra**

✓6ᵗʰ **S33.13 Subluxation and dislocation of L3/L4 lumbar vertebra**

✓7ᵗʰ **S33.130 Subluxation of L3/L4 lumbar vertebra**

✓7ᵗʰ **S33.131 Dislocation of L3/L4 lumbar vertebra**

✓6ᵗʰ **S33.14 Subluxation and dislocation of L4/L5 lumbar vertebra**

✓7ᵗʰ **S33.140 Subluxation of L4/L5 lumbar vertebra**

✓7ᵗʰ **S33.141 Dislocation of L4/L5 lumbar vertebra**

✓x7ᵗʰ **S33.2 Dislocation of sacroiliac and sacrococcygeal joint**

✓5ᵗʰ **S33.3 Dislocation of other and unspecified parts of lumbar spine and pelvis**

✓x7ᵗʰ **S33.30 Dislocation of unspecified parts of lumbar spine and pelvis**

✓x7ᵗʰ **S33.39 Dislocation of other parts of lumbar spine and pelvis**

✓x7ᵗʰ **S33.4 Traumatic rupture of symphysis pubis**

✓x7ᵗʰ **S33.5 Sprain of ligaments of lumbar spine**

✓x7ᵗʰ **S33.6 Sprain of sacroiliac joint**

✓x7ᵗʰ **S33.8 Sprain of other parts of lumbar spine and pelvis**

✓x7ᵗʰ **S33.9 Sprain of unspecified parts of lumbar spine and pelvis**

7 HAC = Initial encounter only (7th character A, B or C) and not POA.

✔ Additional Character Required ✓x7ᵗʰ Xtension Alert Unacceptable PDx Manifestation Hospital Acquired Condition EXCLUDES 1 Not Coded Here EXCLUDES 2 Not Included Here

✓4th **S34 Injury of lumbar and sacral spinal cord and nerves at abdomen, lower back and pelvis level**

> **NOTE**   Code to highest level of lumbar cord injury.
> Injuries to the spinal cord (S34.0 and S34.1) refer to the cord level and not bone level injury, and can affect nerve roots at and below the level given.

Code also any associated:
  fracture of vertebra (S22.0-, S32.0-)
  open wound of abdomen, lower back and pelvis (S31.-)
  transient paralysis (R29.5)

> The appropriate 7th is to be added to each code from category S34.
> A   initial encounter
> D   subsequent encounter
> S   sequela

✓5th **S34.0 Concussion and edema of lumbar and sacral spinal cord**

  ✓x7th **S34.01 Concussion and edema of lumbar spinal cord** MCC
     CC Excl: MCC with 7th character A: M48.40X-M48.58X with 7th S, M80.08XS, M80.88XS, M84.350S, M84.454S, M84.550S, M84.58XS, M84.650S, M99.15-M99.17, M99.19, S12.000-S12.9XX with 7th S, S13.9XXA, S14.109A, S14.119A, S14.129A, S14.139A, S14.149A, S14.159A, S22.000-S22.9X with 7th S, S23.20X-S23.29X with 7th A, S23.9XXA, S24.109A, S24.119A, S24.139A, S24.149A, S24.159A, S29.001-S29.009 with 7th A, S29.091-S29.9XX with 7th A, S32.000-S32.9XX with 7th S, S33.30X-S33.39X with 7th A, S33.9XX-S34.01X with 7th A, S34.101-S34.129 with 7th A, S38.1XA, S39.001-S39.003 with 7th A, S39.091-S39.94X with 7th A, T14.8-T14.91, T79.A0X-T79.9XX with 7th A

  ✓x7th **S34.02 Concussion and edema of sacral spinal cord** MCC
     Concussion and edema of conus medullaris
     CC Excl: MCC with 7th character A: M48.40X-M48.58X with 7th S, M80.08XS, M80.88XS, M84.350S, M84.454S, M84.550S, M84.58XS, M84.650S, M99.15-M99.17, M99.19, S12.000-S12.9XX with 7th S, S13.9XXA, S14.109A, S14.119A, S14.129A, S14.139A, S14.149A, S14.159A, S22.000-S22.9XX with 7th S, S23.20X-S23.29X with 7th A, S23.9XXA, S24.109A, S24.119A, S24.139A, S24.149A, S24.159A, S29.001-S29.009 with 7th A, S29.091-S29.9XX with 7th A, S32.000-S32.9XX with 7th S, S33.30X-S33.39X with 7th A, S33.9XX-S34.02X with 7th A, S34.131-S34.139 with 7th A, S34.3XXA, S38.1XA, S39.001-S39.003 with 7th A, S39.091-S39.94X with 7th A, T14.8-T14.91, T79.A0X-T79.9XX with 7th A

✓5th **S34.1 Other and unspecified injury of lumbar and sacral spinal cord**

  ✓6th **S34.10 Unspecified injury to lumbar spinal cord**

     CC Excl: For MCC codes in subcategory S34.10, unless otherwise noted: MCC with 7th character A: M48.40X-M48.58X with 7th S, M80.08XS, M80.88XS, M84.350S, M84.454S, M84.550S, M84.58XS, M84.650S, M99.15-M99.17, M99.19, S12.000-S12.9XX with 7th S, S13.9XXA, S14.109A, S14.119A, S14.129A, S14.139A, S14.149A, S14.159A, S22.000-S22.9XX with 7th S, S23.20X-S23.29X with 7th A, S23.9XA, S24.109A, S24.119A, S24.139A, S24.149A, S24.159A, S29.001-S29.009 with 7th A, S29.091-S29.9XX with 7th A, S32.000-S32.9XX with 7th S, S33.30X-S33.39X with 7th A, S33.9XX-S34.01X with 7th A, S34.101-S34.129 with 7th A, S38.1XA, S39.001-S39.003 with 7th A, S39.091-S39.94X with 7th A, T14.8-T14.91, T79.A0X-T79.9XX with 7th A

    7 ✓7th **S34.101 Unspecified injury to L1 level of lumbar spinal cord** MCC

    7 ✓7th **S34.102 Unspecified injury to L2 level of lumbar spinal cord** MCC

    7 ✓7th **S34.103 Unspecified injury to L3 level of lumbar spinal cord** MCC

    7 ✓7th **S34.104 Unspecified injury to L4 level of lumbar spinal cord** MCC

    7 ✓7th **S34.105 Unspecified injury to L5 level of lumbar spinal cord** MCC

    7 ✓7th **S34.109 Unspecified injury to unspecified level of lumbar spinal cord** MCC

  ✓6th **S34.11 Complete lesion of lumbar spinal cord**

     CC Excl: For MCC codes in subcategory S34.11, unless otherwise noted: See code: S34.10

    7 ✓7th **S34.111 Complete lesion of L1 level of lumbar spinal cord** MCC

7 ✓7th **S34.112 Complete lesion of L2 level of lumbar spinal cord** MCC

7 ✓7th **S34.113 Complete lesion of L3 level of lumbar spinal cord** MCC

7 ✓7th **S34.114 Complete lesion of L4 level of lumbar spinal cord** MCC

7 ✓7th **S34.115 Complete lesion of L5 level of lumbar spinal cord** MCC

7 ✓7th **S34.119 Complete lesion of unspecified level of lumbar spinal cord** MCC

✓6th **S34.12 Incomplete lesion of lumbar spinal cord**

     CC Excl: For MCC codes in subcategory S34.12, unless otherwise noted: See code: S34.10

7 ✓7th **S34.121 Incomplete lesion of L1 level of lumbar spinal cord** MCC

7 ✓7th **S34.122 Incomplete lesion of L2 level of lumbar spinal cord** MCC

7 ✓7th **S34.123 Incomplete lesion of L3 level of lumbar spinal cord** MCC

7 ✓7th **S34.124 Incomplete lesion of L4 level of lumbar spinal cord** MCC

7 ✓7th **S34.125 Incomplete lesion of L5 level of lumbar spinal cord** MCC

7 ✓7th **S34.129 Incomplete lesion of unspecified level of lumbar spinal cord** MCC

✓6th **S34.13 Other and unspecified injury to sacral spinal cord**
     Other injury to conus medullaris

     CC Excl: For MCC codes in subcategory S34.13, unless otherwise noted: MCC with 7th character A: M48.40X-M48.58X with 7th S, M80.08XS, M80.88XS, M84.350S, M84.454S, M84.550S, M84.58XS, M84.650S, M99.15-M99.17, M99.19, S12.000-S12.9XX with 7th S, S13.9XXA, S14.109A, S14.119A, S14.129A, S14.139A, S14.149A, S14.159A, S22.000-S22.9XX with 7th S, S23.20X-S23.29X with 7th A, S23.9XXA, S24.109A, S24.119A, S24.139A, S24.149A, S24.159A, S29.001-S29.009 with 7th A, S29.091-S29.9XX with 7th A, S32.000-S32.9XX with 7th S, S33.30X-S33.39X with 7th A, S33.9XX-S34.02X with 7th A, S34.131-S34.139 with 7th A, S34.3XXA, S38.1XXA, S39.001-S39.003 with 7th A, S39.091-S39.94X with 7th A, T14.8-T14.91, T79.A0X-T79.9XX with 7th A

7 ✓7th **S34.131 Complete lesion of sacral spinal cord** MCC
     Complete lesion of conus medullaris

7 ✓7th **S34.132 Incomplete lesion of sacral spinal cord** MCC
     Incomplete lesion of conus medullaris

7 ✓7th **S34.139 Unspecified injury to sacral spinal cord** MCC
     Unspecified injury of conus medullaris

✓5th **S34.2 Injury of nerve root of lumbar and sacral spine**

  ✓x7th **S34.21 Injury of nerve root of lumbar spine**

  ✓x7th **S34.22 Injury of nerve root of sacral spine**

7 ✓x7th **S34.3 Injury of cauda equina** MCC
     CC Excl: See code: S34.13

✓x7th **S34.4 Injury of lumbosacral plexus**

✓x7th **S34.5 Injury of lumbar, sacral and pelvic sympathetic nerves**
     Injury of celiac ganglion or plexus
     Injury of hypogastric plexus
     Injury of mesenteric plexus (inferior) (superior)
     Injury of splanchnic nerve

✓x7th **S34.6 Injury of peripheral nerve(s) at abdomen, lower back and pelvis level**

✓x7th **S34.8 Injury of other nerves at abdomen, lower back and pelvis level**

✓x7th **S34.9 Injury of unspecified nerves at abdomen, lower back and pelvis level**

---

7 HAC = Initial encounter only (7th character A, B or C) and not POA.

N Newborn: 0   P Pediatric: 0-17   M Maternity: 12-55   A Adult: 15-124   MCC Major CC Condition   PDx MCC PDx acts as own MCC   CC CC Condition   PDx CC PDx acts as own CC

896   ICD-10-CM Draft (2015)

√4ᵗʰ **S35 Injury of blood vessels at abdomen, lower back and pelvis level**
Code also any associated open wound (S31.-)

The appropriate 7th is to be added to each code from category S35.
A   initial encounter
D   subsequent encounter
S   sequela

√5ᵗʰ **S35.0 Injury of abdominal aorta**
EXCLUDES 1   injury of aorta NOS (S25.0)

CC Excl: For MCC codes in subcategory S35.0, unless otherwise noted: MCC with 7th character A: S35.00X-S35.09X with 7th A, S35.8X1-S35.99X with 7th A, T14.8-T14.91, T79.A0X-T79.9XX with 7th A

√x7ᵗʰ **S35.00 Unspecified injury of abdominal aorta**   MCC

√x7ᵗʰ **S35.01 Minor laceration of abdominal aorta**   MCC
Incomplete transection of abdominal aorta
Laceration of abdominal aorta NOS
Superficial laceration of abdominal aorta

√x7ᵗʰ **S35.02 Major laceration of abdominal aorta**   MCC
Complete transection of abdominal aorta
Traumatic rupture of abdominal aorta

√x7ᵗʰ **S35.09 Other injury of abdominal aorta**   MCC

√5ᵗʰ **S35.1 Injury of inferior vena cava**
Injury of hepatic vein
EXCLUDES 1   injury of vena cava NOS (S25.2)

CC Excl: For MCC codes in subcategory S35.1, unless otherwise noted: MCC with 7th character A: S35.10X-S35.19X with 7th A, S35.8X1-S35.99X with 7th A, T14.8-T14.91, T79.A0X-T79.9XX with 7th A

√x7ᵗʰ **S35.10 Unspecified injury of inferior vena cava**   MCC

√x7ᵗʰ **S35.11 Minor laceration of inferior vena cava**   MCC
Incomplete transection of inferior vena cava
Laceration of inferior vena cava NOS
Superficial laceration of inferior vena cava

√x7ᵗʰ **S35.12 Major laceration of inferior vena cava**   MCC
Complete transection of inferior vena cava
Traumatic rupture of inferior vena cava

√x7ᵗʰ **S35.19 Other injury of inferior vena cava**   MCC

√5ᵗʰ **S35.2 Injury of celiac or mesenteric artery and branches**

√6ᵗʰ **S35.21 Injury of celiac artery**

CC Excl: For MCC codes in subcategory S35.21, unless otherwise noted: MCC with 7th character A: S35.211-S35.219 with 7th A, S35.8X1-S35.99X with 7th A, T14.8-T14.91, T79.A0X-T79.9XX with 7th A

√7ᵗʰ **S35.211 Minor laceration of celiac artery**   MCC
Incomplete transection of celiac artery
Laceration of celiac artery NOS
Superficial laceration of celiac artery

√7ᵗʰ **S35.212 Major laceration of celiac artery**   MCC
Complete transection of celiac artery
Traumatic rupture of celiac artery

√7ᵗʰ **S35.218 Other injury of celiac artery**   MCC

√7ᵗʰ **S35.219 Unspecified injury of celiac artery**   MCC

√6ᵗʰ **S35.22 Injury of superior mesenteric artery**

CC Excl: For MCC codes in subcategory S35.22, unless otherwise noted: MCC with 7th character A: S35.221-S35.229 with 7th A, S35.8X1-S35.99X with 7th A, T14.8-T14.91, T79.A0X-T79.9XX with 7th A

√7ᵗʰ **S35.221 Minor laceration of superior mesenteric artery**   MCC
Incomplete transection of superior mesenteric artery
Laceration of superior mesenteric artery NOS
Superficial laceration of superior mesenteric artery

√7ᵗʰ **S35.222 Major laceration of superior mesenteric artery**   MCC
Complete transection of superior mesenteric artery
Traumatic rupture of superior mesenteric artery

√7ᵗʰ **S35.228 Other injury of superior mesenteric artery**   MCC

√7ᵗʰ **S35.229 Unspecified injury of superior mesenteric artery**   MCC

√6ᵗʰ **S35.23 Injury of inferior mesenteric artery**

CC Excl: For MCC codes in subcategory S35.23, unless otherwise noted: MCC with 7th character A: S35.231-S35.239 with 7th A, S35.8X1-S35.99X with 7th A, T14.8-T14.91, T79.A0X-T79.9XX with 7th A

√7ᵗʰ **S35.231 Minor laceration of inferior mesenteric artery**   MCC
Incomplete transection of inferior mesenteric artery
Laceration of inferior mesenteric artery NOS
Superficial laceration of inferior mesenteric artery

√7ᵗʰ **S35.232 Major laceration of inferior mesenteric artery**   MCC
Complete transection of inferior mesenteric artery
Traumatic rupture of inferior mesenteric artery

√7ᵗʰ **S35.238 Other injury of inferior mesenteric artery**   MCC

√7ᵗʰ **S35.239 Unspecified injury of inferior mesenteric artery**   MCC

√6ᵗʰ **S35.29 Injury of branches of celiac and mesenteric artery**   MCC
Injury of gastric artery
Injury of gastroduodenal artery
Injury of hepatic artery
Injury of splenic artery

√7ᵗʰ **S35.291 Minor laceration of branches of celiac and mesenteric artery**   MCC
Incomplete transection of branches of celiac and mesenteric artery
Laceration of branches of celiac and mesenteric artery NOS
Superficial laceration of branches of celiac and mesenteric artery
CC Excl: MCC with 7th character A: S35.291A, S35.8X1-S35.99X with 7th A, T14.8-T14.91, T79.A0X with 7th A, T79.A3X-T79.9XX with 7th A

√7ᵗʰ **S35.292 Major laceration of branches of celiac and mesenteric artery**   MCC
Complete transection of branches of celiac and mesenteric artery
Traumatic rupture of branches of celiac and mesenteric artery
CC Excl: MCC with 7th character A: S35.292-S35.298 with 7th A, S35.8X1-S35.99X with 7th A, T14.8-T14.91, T79.A0X-T79.9XX with 7th A

√7ᵗʰ **S35.298 Other injury of branches of celiac and mesenteric artery**   MCC
CC Excl: See code: S35.292

√7ᵗʰ **S35.299 Unspecified injury of branches of celiac and mesenteric artery**   MCC
CC Excl: MCC with 7th character A: S35.299A, S35.8X1-S35.99X with 7th A, T14.8-T14.91, T79.A0X-T79.9XX with 7th A

√5ᵗʰ **S35.3 Injury of portal or splenic vein and branches**

√6ᵗʰ **S35.31 Injury of portal vein**

CC Excl: For MCC codes in subcategory S35.31, unless otherwise noted: MCC with 7th character A: S35.311-S35.319 with 7th A, S35.8X1-S35.99X with 7th A, T14.8-T14.91, T79.A0X-T79.9XX with 7th A

√7ᵗʰ **S35.311 Laceration of portal vein**   MCC

√7ᵗʰ **S35.318 Other specified injury of portal vein**   MCC

√7ᵗʰ **S35.319 Unspecified injury of portal vein**   MCC

√6ᵗʰ **S35.32 Injury of splenic vein**

CC Excl: For MCC codes in subcategory S35.32, unless otherwise noted: MCC with 7th character A: S35.321-S35.329 with 7th A, S35.8X1-S35.99X with 7th A, T14.8-T14.91, T79.A0X-T79.9XX with 7th A

√7ᵗʰ **S35.321 Laceration of splenic vein**   MCC

√7ᵗʰ **S35.328 Other specified injury of splenic vein**   MCC

✓ Additional Character Required   √x7ᵗʰ Xtension Alert   Unacceptable PDx   Manifestation   Hospital Acquired Condition   EXCLUDES 1 Not Coded Here   EXCLUDES 2 Not Included Here

Injury, Poisoning and Certain Other Consequences of External Causes

S35.329–S35.8X8

√7ᵗʰ **S35.329** Unspecified **injury of splenic vein** ᴹᶜᶜ

√6ᵗʰ **S35.33** Injury of **superior mesenteric vein**

> **CC Excl:** For MCC codes in subcategory S35.33, unless otherwise noted: MCC with 7th character A: S35.331-S35.339 with 7th A, S35.8X1-S35.99X with 7th A, T14.8-T14.91, T79.A0X-T79.9XX with 7th A

√7ᵗʰ **S35.331** **Laceration** of superior mesenteric vein ᴹᶜᶜ

√7ᵗʰ **S35.338** **Other** specified injury of superior mesenteric vein ᴹᶜᶜ

√7ᵗʰ **S35.339** **Unspecified** injury of superior mesenteric vein ᴹᶜᶜ

√6ᵗʰ **S35.34** Injury of **inferior mesenteric vein**

> **CC Excl:** For MCC codes in subcategory S35.34, unless otherwise noted: MCC with 7th character A: S35.341-S35.349 with 7th A, S35.8X1-S35.99X with 7th A, T14.8-T14.91, T79.A0X-T79.9XX with 7th A

√7ᵗʰ **S35.341** **Laceration** of inferior mesenteric vein ᴹᶜᶜ

√7ᵗʰ **S35.348** **Other** specified injury of inferior mesenteric vein ᴹᶜᶜ

√7ᵗʰ **S35.349** **Unspecified** injury of inferior mesenteric vein ᴹᶜᶜ

√5ᵗʰ **S35.4** Injury of **renal blood vessels**

√6ᵗʰ **S35.40** **Unspecified** injury of renal blood vessel

√7ᵗʰ **S35.401** **Unspecified injury of right renal artery** ᴹᶜᶜ
> **CC Excl:** MCC with 7th character A: S35.401-S35.403 with 7th A, S35.411-S35.413 with 7th A, S35.491-S35.493 with 7th A, S35.8X1-S35.99X with 7th A, T14.8-T14.91, T79.A0X-T79.9XX with 7th A

√7ᵗʰ **S35.402** **Unspecified injury of left renal artery** ᴹᶜᶜ
> **CC Excl:** See code: S35.401

√7ᵗʰ **S35.403** **Unspecified injury of unspecified renal artery** ᴹᶜᶜ
> **CC Excl:** See code: S35.401

√7ᵗʰ **S35.404** **Unspecified injury of right renal vein** ᴹᶜᶜ
> **CC Excl:** MCC with 7th character A: S35.404-S35.406 with 7th A, S35.414-S35.416 with 7th A, S35.494-S35.496 with 7th A, S35.8X1-S35.99X with 7th A, T14.8-T14.91, T79.A0X-T79.9XX with 7th A

√7ᵗʰ **S35.405** **Unspecified injury of left renal vein** ᴹᶜᶜ
> **CC Excl:** See code: S35.404

√7ᵗʰ **S35.406** **Unspecified injury of unspecified renal vein** ᴹᶜᶜ
> **CC Excl:** See code: S35.404

√6ᵗʰ **S35.41** **Laceration** of renal blood vessel

√7ᵗʰ **S35.411** **Laceration of right renal artery** ᴹᶜᶜ
> **CC Excl:** MCC with 7th character A: S35.401-S35.403 with 7th A, S35.411-S35.413 with 7th A, S35.491-S35.493 with 7th A, S35.8X1-S35.99X with 7th A, T14.8-T14.91, T79.A0X-T79.9XX with 7th A

√7ᵗʰ **S35.412** **Laceration of left renal artery** ᴹᶜᶜ
> **CC Excl:** See code: S35.411

√7ᵗʰ **S35.413** **Laceration of unspecified renal artery** ᴹᶜᶜ
> **CC Excl:** See code: S35.411

√7ᵗʰ **S35.414** **Laceration of right renal vein** ᴹᶜᶜ
> **CC Excl:** MCC with 7th character A: S35.404-S35.406 with 7th A, S35.414-S35.416 with 7th A, S35.494-S35.496 with 7th A, S35.8X1-S35.99X with 7th A, T14.8-T14.91, T79.A0X-T79.9XX with 7th A

√7ᵗʰ **S35.415** **Laceration of left renal vein** ᴹᶜᶜ
> **CC Excl:** See code: S35.414

√7ᵗʰ **S35.416** **Laceration of unspecified renal vein** ᴹᶜᶜ
> **CC Excl:** See code: S35.414

√6ᵗʰ **S35.49** **Other** specified injury of renal blood vessel

√7ᵗʰ **S35.491** **Other specified injury of right renal artery** ᴹᶜᶜ
> **CC Excl:** MCC with 7th character A: S35.401-S35.403 with 7th A, S35.411-S35.413 with 7th A, S35.491-S35.493 with 7th A, S35.8X1-S35.99X with 7th A, T14.8-T14.91, T79.A0X-T79.9XX with 7th A

√7ᵗʰ **S35.492** **Other specified injury of left renal artery** ᴹᶜᶜ
> **CC Excl:** See code: S35.491

√7ᵗʰ **S35.493** **Other specified injury of unspecified renal artery** ᴹᶜᶜ
> **CC Excl:** See code: S35.491

√7ᵗʰ **S35.494** **Other specified injury of right renal vein** ᴹᶜᶜ
> **CC Excl:** MCC with 7th character A: S35.404-S35.406 with 7th A, S35.414-S35.416 with 7th A, S35.494-S35.496 with 7th A, S35.8X1-S35.99X with 7th A, T14.8-T14.91, T79.A0X-T79.9XX with 7th A

√7ᵗʰ **S35.495** **Other specified injury of left renal vein** ᴹᶜᶜ
> **CC Excl:** See code: S35.494

√7ᵗʰ **S35.496** **Other specified injury of unspecified renal vein** ᴹᶜᶜ
> **CC Excl:** See code: S35.494

√5ᵗʰ **S35.5** Injury of **iliac blood vessels**

√x7ᵗʰ **S35.50** Injury of **unspecified iliac blood vessel(s)** ᴹᶜᶜ
> **CC Excl:** MCC with 7th character A: S35.50X-S35.516 with 7th A, S35.59X-S35.99X with 7th A, T14.8-T14.91, T79.A0X-T79.9XX with 7th A

√6ᵗʰ **S35.51** Injury of **iliac artery or vein**
Injury of hypogastric artery or vein

√7ᵗʰ **S35.511** **Injury of right iliac artery** ᴹᶜᶜ
> **CC Excl:** MCC with 7th character A: S35.50X-S35.513 with 7th A, S35.59X-S35.99X with 7th A, T14.8-T14.91, T79.A0X-T79.9XX with 7th A

√7ᵗʰ **S35.512** **Injury of left iliac artery** ᴹᶜᶜ
> **CC Excl:** See code: S35.511

√7ᵗʰ **S35.513** **Injury of unspecified iliac artery** ᴹᶜᶜ
> **CC Excl:** See code: S35.511

√7ᵗʰ **S35.514** **Injury of right iliac vein** ᴹᶜᶜ
> **CC Excl:** MCC with 7th character A: S35.50X-S35.516 with 7th A, S35.59X-S35.99X with 7th A, T14.8-T14.91, T79.A0X-T79.9XX with 7th A

√7ᵗʰ **S35.515** **Injury of left iliac vein** ᴹᶜᶜ
> **CC Excl:** See code: S35.514

√7ᵗʰ **S35.516** **Injury of unspecified iliac vein** ᴹᶜᶜ
> **CC Excl:** See code: S35.514

√6ᵗʰ **S35.53** Injury of **uterine artery or vein**

√7ᵗʰ **S35.531** **Injury of right uterine artery** ᶜᶜ♀
> **CC Excl:** CC with 7th character A: S35.50X with 7th A, S35.531-S35.99X with 7th A, T14.8-T14.91, T79.A0X with 7th A, T79.A3X-T79.9XX with 7th A

√7ᵗʰ **S35.532** **Injury of left uterine artery** ᶜᶜ♀
> **CC Excl:** See code: S35.531

√7ᵗʰ **S35.533** **Injury of unspecified uterine artery** ᶜᶜ♀
> **CC Excl:** See code: S35.531

√7ᵗʰ **S35.534** **Injury of right uterine vein** ᶜᶜ♀
> **CC Excl:** MCC with 7th character A: S35.50X with 7th A, S35.534-S35.99X with 7th A, T14.8-T14.91, T79.A0X with 7th A, T79.A3X-T79.9XX with 7th A

√7ᵗʰ **S35.535** **Injury of left uterine vein** ᶜᶜ♀
> **CC Excl:** See code: S35.534

√7ᵗʰ **S35.536** **Injury of unspecified uterine vein** ᶜᶜ♀
> **CC Excl:** See code: S35.534

√x7ᵗʰ **S35.59** Injury of **other iliac blood vessels** ᴹᶜᶜ
> **CC Excl:** MCC with 7th character A: S35.50X-S35.516 with 7th A, S35.59X-S35.99X with 7th A, T14.8-T14.91, T79.A0X-T79.9XX with 7th A

√6ᵗʰ **S35.8** Injury of **other blood vessels at abdomen, lower back and pelvis level**
Injury of ovarian artery or vein

√6ᵗʰ **S35.8X** Injury of **other blood vessels at abdomen, lower back and pelvis level**

> **CC Excl:** For CC codes in subcategory S35.8X, unless otherwise noted: CC with 7th character A: S35.8X1-S35.99X with 7th A, T14.8-T14.91, T79.A0X with 7th A, T79.A3X-T79.9XX with 7th A

√7ᵗʰ **S35.8X1** **Laceration** of other blood vessels at abdomen, lower back and pelvis level ᶜᶜ

√7ᵗʰ **S35.8X8** **Other** specified injury of other blood vessels at abdomen, lower back and pelvis level ᶜᶜ

N Newborn: 0   P Pediatric: 0-17   M Maternity: 12-55   A Adult: 15-124   ᴹᶜᶜ Major CC Condition   ᴾᴰˣᴹᶜᶜ PDx acts as own MCC   ᶜᶜ CC Condition   ᴾᴰˣᶜᶜ PDx acts as own CC

898   ICD-10-CM Draft (2015)

√7th **S35.8X9** Unspecified injury of other blood vessels at abdomen, lower back and pelvis level `CC`

√5th **S35.9** Injury of unspecified blood vessel at abdomen, lower back and pelvis level

    CC Excl: For CC codes in subcategory S35.9: CC with 7th character A: S35.00-S35.99X with 7th A, T14.8-T14.91, T79.A0X with 7th A, T79.A3X-T79.9XX with 7th A

√x7th **S35.90** Unspecified injury of unspecified blood vessel at abdomen, lower back and pelvis level `CC`

√x7th **S35.91** Laceration of unspecified blood vessel at abdomen, lower back and pelvis level `CC`

√x7th **S35.99** Other specified injury of unspecified blood vessel at abdomen, lower back and pelvis level `CC`

√4th **S36** **Injury of intra-abdominal organs**

    Code also any associated open wound (S31.-)

    The appropriate 7th is to be added to each code from category S36.
    A   initial encounter
    D   subsequent encounter
    S   sequela

√5th **S36.0** Injury of spleen

    CC Excl: For CC/MCC codes in subcategory S36.0, unless otherwise noted: CC or MCC as indicated with 7th A: S31.001A, S31.011A, S31.021A, S31.031A, S31.041A, S31.051-S31.159 with 7th A, S31.600-S31.659 with 7th A, S31.831-S31.839 with 7th A, S36.00X-S36.09X with 7th A, S36.81X-S36.99X with 7th A, S38.3XX-S39.023 with 7th A, T14.8-T14.91, T79.A0X-T79.9XX with 7th A

√x7th **S36.00** Unspecified injury of spleen `CC`

√6th **S36.02** Contusion of spleen

    √7th **S36.020** Minor contusion of spleen `CC`
        Contusion of spleen less than 2 cm

    √7th **S36.021** Major contusion of spleen `CC`
        Contusion of spleen greater than 2 cm

    √7th **S36.029** Unspecified contusion of spleen `CC`

√6th **S36.03** Laceration of spleen

    √7th **S36.030** Superficial (capsular) laceration of spleen `CC`
        Laceration of spleen less than 1cm
        Minor laceration of spleen

    √7th **S36.031** Moderate laceration of spleen `MCC`
        Laceration of spleen 1 to 3 cm

    √7th **S36.032** Major laceration of spleen `MCC`
        Avulsion of spleen
        Laceration of spleen greater than 3 cm
        Massive laceration of spleen
        Multiple moderate lacerations of spleen
        Stellate laceration of spleen

    √7th **S36.039** Unspecified laceration of spleen `CC`

√x7th **S36.09** Other injury of spleen `CC`

√5th **S36.1** Injury of liver and gallbladder and bile duct

√6th **S36.11** Injury of liver

    CC Excl: For CC/MCC codes in subcategory S36.11, unless otherwise noted: CC or MCC as indicated with 7th A: S31.001A, S31.011A, S31.021A, S31.031A, S31.041A, S31.051-S31.159 with 7th A, S31.600-S31.659 with 7th A, S31.831-S31.839 with 7th A, S36.112-S36.119 with 7th A, S36.81X-S36.99X with 7th A, S38.3XX-S39.023 with 7th A, T14.8-T14.91, T79.A0X-T79.9XX with 7th A

    √7th **S36.112** Contusion of liver `CC`

    √7th **S36.113** Laceration of liver, unspecified degree `CC`

    √7th **S36.114** Minor laceration of liver `CC`
        Laceration involving capsule only, or, without significant involvement of hepatic parenchyma [i.e., less than 1cm deep]

    √7th **S36.115** Moderate laceration of liver `MCC`
        Laceration involving parenchyma but without major disruption of parenchyma [i.e., less than 10 cm long and less than 3 cm deep]

    √7th **S36.116** Major laceration of liver `MCC`
        Laceration with significant disruption of hepatic parenchyma [i.e., greater than 10 cm long and 3 cm deep]
        Multiple moderate lacerations, with or without hematoma
        Stellate laceration of liver

    √7th **S36.118** Other injury of liver `CC`

    √7th **S36.119** Unspecified injury of liver `CC`

√6th **S36.12** Injury of gallbladder

    CC Excl: For CC codes in subcategory S36.12, unless otherwise noted: CC with 7th character A: S31.001A, S31.011A, S31.021A, S31.031A, S31.041A, S31.051-S31.159 with 7th A, S31.600-S31.659 with 7th A, S31.831-S31.839 with 7th A, S36.122-S36.13X with 7th A, S36.81X-S36.99X with 7th A, S38.3XX-S39.023 with 7th A, T14.8-T14.91, T79.A0X-T79.9XX with 7th A

    √7th **S36.122** Contusion of gallbladder `CC`

    √7th **S36.123** Laceration of gallbladder `CC`

    √7th **S36.128** Other injury of gallbladder `CC`

    √7th **S36.129** Unspecified injury of gallbladder `CC`

√x7th **S36.13** Injury of bile duct `CC`
    CC Excl: See code: S36.12

√5th **S36.2** Injury of pancreas

    CC Excl: For CC codes in subcategory S36.2, unless otherwise noted: CC with 7th character A: M79.A3, S31.001A, S31.011A, S31.021A, S31.031A, S31.041A, S31.051-S31.159 with 7th A, S31.600-S31.659 with 7th A, S31.831-S31.839 with 7th A, S36.200-S36.299 with 7th A, S36.81X-S36.99X with 7th A, S38.3XX-S39.023 with 7th A, T14.8-T14.91, T79.A3X-T79.9XX with 7th A

√6th **S36.20** Unspecified injury of pancreas

    √7th **S36.200** Unspecified injury of head of pancreas `CC`

    √7th **S36.201** Unspecified injury of body of pancreas `CC`

    √7th **S36.202** Unspecified injury of tail of pancreas `CC`

    √7th **S36.209** Unspecified injury of unspecified part of pancreas `CC`

√6th **S36.22** Contusion of pancreas

    √7th **S36.220** Contusion of head of pancreas `CC`

    √7th **S36.221** Contusion of body of pancreas `CC`

    √7th **S36.222** Contusion of tail of pancreas `CC`

    √7th **S36.229** Contusion of unspecified part of pancreas `CC`

√6th **S36.23** Laceration of pancreas, unspecified degree

    √7th **S36.230** Laceration of head of pancreas, unspecified degree `MCC`

    √7th **S36.231** Laceration of body of pancreas, unspecified degree `CC`

    √7th **S36.232** Laceration of tail of pancreas, unspecified degree `CC`

    √7th **S36.239** Laceration of unspecified part of pancreas, unspecified degree `CC`

√6th **S36.24** Minor laceration of pancreas

    √7th **S36.240** Minor laceration of head of pancreas `CC`

    √7th **S36.241** Minor laceration of body of pancreas `CC`

    √7th **S36.242** Minor laceration of tail of pancreas `CC`

    √7th **S36.249** Minor laceration of unspecified part of pancreas `CC`

√6th **S36.25** Moderate laceration of pancreas

    √7th **S36.250** Moderate laceration of head of pancreas `CC`

    √7th **S36.251** Moderate laceration of body of pancreas `CC`

    √7th **S36.252** Moderate laceration of tail of pancreas `CC`

    √7th **S36.259** Moderate laceration of unspecified part of pancreas `CC`

√6th **S36.26** Major laceration of pancreas

    √7th **S36.260** Major laceration of head of pancreas `CC`

    √7th **S36.261** Major laceration of body of pancreas `CC`

    √7th **S36.262** Major laceration of tail of pancreas `CC`

    √7th **S36.269** Major laceration of unspecified part of pancreas `CC`

√6th **S36.29** Other injury of pancreas

√7th **S36.290** Other injury of head of pancreas   CC

√7th **S36.291** Other injury of body of pancreas   CC

√7th **S36.292** Other injury of tail of pancreas   CC

√7th **S36.299** Other injury of unspecified part of pancreas   CC

√5th **S36.3** Injury of stomach

> CC Excl: For CC codes in subcategory S36.3, unless otherwise noted: CC with 7th character A: M79.A3, S31.001A, S31.011A, S31.021A, S31.031A, S31.041A, S31.051-S31.159 with 7th A, S31.600-S31.659 with 7th A, S31.831-S31.839 with 7th A, S36.30X-S36.39X with 7th A, S36.81X-S36.99X with 7th A, S38.3XX-S39.023 with 7th A, T14.8-T14.91, T79.A3X-T79.9XX with 7th A

√x7th **S36.30** Unspecified injury of stomach   CC

√x7th **S36.32** Contusion of stomach   CC

√x7th **S36.33** Laceration of stomach   CC

√x7th **S36.39** Other injury of stomach   CC

√5th **S36.4** Injury of small intestine

> CC Excl: For CC codes in subcategory S36.4, unless otherwise noted: CC with 7th character A: M79.A3, S31.001A, S31.011A, S31.021A, S31.031A, S31.041A, S31.051-S31.159 with 7th A, S31.600-S31.659 with 7th A, S31.831-S31.839 with 7th A, S36.400-S36.499 with 7th A, S36.81X-S36.99X with 7th A, S38.3XX-S39.023 with 7th A, T14.8-T14.91, T79.A3X-T79.9XX with 7th A

√6th **S36.40** Unspecified injury of small intestine

√7th **S36.400** Unspecified injury of duodenum   CC

√7th **S36.408** Unspecified injury of other part of small intestine   CC

√7th **S36.409** Unspecified injury of unspecified part of small intestine   CC

√6th **S36.41** Primary blast injury of small intestine

Blast injury of small intestine NOS

√7th **S36.410** Primary blast injury of duodenum   CC

√7th **S36.418** Primary blast injury of other part of small intestine   CC

√7th **S36.419** Primary blast injury of unspecified part of small intestine   CC

√6th **S36.42** Contusion of small intestine

√7th **S36.420** Contusion of duodenum   CC

√7th **S36.428** Contusion of other part of small intestine   CC

√7th **S36.429** Contusion of unspecified part of small intestine   CC

√6th **S36.43** Laceration of small intestine

√7th **S36.430** Laceration of duodenum   CC

√7th **S36.438** Laceration of other part of small intestine   CC

√7th **S36.439** Laceration of unspecified part of small intestine   CC

√6th **S36.49** Other injury of small intestine

√7th **S36.490** Other injury of duodenum   CC

√7th **S36.498** Other injury of other part of small intestine   CC

√7th **S36.499** Other injury of unspecified part of small intestine   CC

√5th **S36.5** Injury of colon

EXCLUDES 2   injury of rectum (S36.6-)

> CC Excl: For CC/MCC codes in subcategory S36.5, unless otherwise noted: CC with 7th character A: M79.A3, S31.001A, S31.011A, S31.021A, S31.031A, S31.041A, S31.051-S31.159 with 7th A, S31.600-S31.659 with 7th A, S31.831-S31.839 with 7th A, S36.500-S36.99X with 7th A, S38.3XX-S39.023 with 7th A, T14.8-T14.91, T79.A3X-T79.9XX with 7th A

√6th **S36.50** Unspecified injury of colon

√7th **S36.500** Unspecified injury of ascending [right] colon   CC

√7th **S36.501** Unspecified injury of transverse colon   CC

√7th **S36.502** Unspecified injury of descending [left] colon   CC

√7th **S36.503** Unspecified injury of sigmoid colon   CC

√7th **S36.508** Unspecified injury of other part of colon   CC

√7th **S36.509** Unspecified injury of unspecified part of colon   CC

√6th **S36.51** Primary blast injury of colon

Blast injury of colon NOS

√7th **S36.510** Primary blast injury of ascending [right] colon   CC

√7th **S36.511** Primary blast injury of transverse colon   CC

√7th **S36.512** Primary blast injury of descending [left] colon   CC

√7th **S36.513** Primary blast injury of sigmoid colon   CC

√7th **S36.518** Primary blast injury of other part of colon   CC

√7th **S36.519** Primary blast injury of unspecified part of colon   CC

√6th **S36.52** Contusion of colon

√7th **S36.520** Contusion of ascending [right] colon   CC

√7th **S36.521** Contusion of transverse colon   CC

√7th **S36.522** Contusion of descending [left] colon   CC

√7th **S36.523** Contusion of sigmoid colon   CC

√7th **S36.528** Contusion of other part of colon   CC

√7th **S36.529** Contusion of unspecified part of colon   CC

√6th **S36.53** Laceration of colon

√7th **S36.530** Laceration of ascending [right] colon   CC

√7th **S36.531** Laceration of transverse colon   CC

√7th **S36.532** Laceration of descending [left] colon   CC

√7th **S36.533** Laceration of sigmoid colon   CC

√7th **S36.538** Laceration of other part of colon   CC

√7th **S36.539** Laceration of unspecified part of colon   CC

√6th **S36.59** Other injury of colon

Secondary blast injury of colon

√7th **S36.590** Other injury of ascending [right] colon   CC

√7th **S36.591** Other injury of transverse colon   CC

√7th **S36.592** Other injury of descending [left] colon   CC

√7th **S36.593** Other injury of sigmoid colon   CC

√7th **S36.598** Other injury of other part of colon   CC

√7th **S36.599** Other injury of unspecified part of colon   CC

√5th **S36.6** Injury of rectum

> CC Excl: For CC codes in subcategory S36.6, unless otherwise noted: CC with 7th character A: See Code: S86.5

√x7th **S36.60** Unspecified injury of rectum   CC

√x7th **S36.61** Primary blast injury of rectum   CC

Blast injury of rectum NOS

√x7th **S36.62** Contusion of rectum   CC

√x7th **S36.63** Laceration of rectum   CC

√x7th **S36.69** Other injury of rectum   CC

Secondary blast injury of rectum

√5th **S36.8** Injury of other intra-abdominal organs

> CC Excl: For CC codes in subcategory S36.8, unless otherwise noted: CC with 7th character A: S31.001A, S31.011A, S31.021A, S31.031A, S31.041A, S31.051-S31.159 with 7th A, S31.600-S31.659 with 7th A, S31.831-S31.839 with 7th A, S36.81X-S36.99X with 7th A, S38.3XX-S39.023 with 7th A, T14.8-T14.91, T79.A0X-T79.9XX with 7th A

√x7th **S36.81** Injury of peritoneum   CC

√6th **S36.89** Injury of other intra-abdominal organs

Injury of retroperitoneum

√7th **S36.892** Contusion of other intra-abdominal organs   CC

√7th **S36.893** Laceration of other intra-abdominal organs   CC

√7th **S36.898** Other injury of other intra-abdominal organs   CC

√7th **S36.899** Unspecified injury of other intra-abdominal organs   CC

N Newborn: 0   P Pediatric: 0-17   M Maternity: 12-55   A Adult: 15-124   MCC Major CC Condition   PDx MCC PDx acts as own MCC   CC CC Condition   PDx CC PDx acts as own CC

900   ICD-10-CM Draft (2015)

√5ᵗʰ **S36.9** **Injury of unspecified intra-abdominal organ**

> **CC Excl:** For CC codes in subcategory S36.9, unless otherwise noted: CC with 7th character A: See Code: S36.8

√x7ᵗʰ **S36.90** **Unspecified injury of unspecified intra-abdominal organ** `CC`

√x7ᵗʰ **S36.92** **Contusion of unspecified intra-abdominal organ** `CC`

√x7ᵗʰ **S36.93** **Laceration of unspecified intra-abdominal organ** `CC`

√x7ᵗʰ **S36.99** **Other injury of unspecified intra-abdominal organ** `CC`

√4ᵗʰ **S37** **Injury of urinary and pelvic organs**

Code also any associated open wound (S31.-)

EXCLUDES 1   obstetric trauma to pelvic organs (O71.-)

EXCLUDES 2   injury of peritoneum (S36.81)
             injury of retroperitoneum (S36.89-)

> The appropriate 7th is to be added to each code from category S37.
> A   initial encounter
> D   subsequent encounter
> S   sequela

√5ᵗʰ **S37.0** **Injury of kidney**

EXCLUDES 2   acute kidney injury (nontraumatic) (N17.9)

> **CC Excl:** For CC/MCC codes in subcategory S37.0, unless otherwise noted: CC or MCC as indicated with 7th A: S31.001A, S31.011A, S31.021A, S31.031A, S31.041A, S31.051-S31.159 with 7th A, S31.600-S31.659 with 7th A, S31.831-S31.839 with 7th A, S36.81X-S37.099 with 7th A, S38.3XX-S39.023 with 7th A, T14.8-T14.91, T79.A0X-T79.9XX with 7th A

√6ᵗʰ **S37.00** **Unspecified injury of kidney**

√7ᵗʰ **S37.001** **Unspecified injury of right kidney** `CC`

√7ᵗʰ **S37.002** **Unspecified injury of left kidney** `CC`

√7ᵗʰ **S37.009** **Unspecified injury of unspecified kidney** `CC`

√6ᵗʰ **S37.01** **Minor contusion of kidney**
Contusion of kidney less than 2 cm
Contusion of kidney NOS

√7ᵗʰ **S37.011** **Minor contusion of right kidney** `CC`

√7ᵗʰ **S37.012** **Minor contusion of left kidney** `CC`

√7ᵗʰ **S37.019** **Minor contusion of unspecified kidney** `CC`

√6ᵗʰ **S37.02** **Major contusion of kidney**
Contusion of kidney greater than 2 cm

√7ᵗʰ **S37.021** **Major contusion of right kidney** `CC`

√7ᵗʰ **S37.022** **Major contusion of left kidney** `CC`

√7ᵗʰ **S37.029** **Major contusion of unspecified kidney** `CC`

√6ᵗʰ **S37.03** **Laceration of kidney, unspecified degree**

√7ᵗʰ **S37.031** **Laceration of right kidney, unspecified degree** `CC`

√7ᵗʰ **S37.032** **Laceration of left kidney, unspecified degree** `CC`

√7ᵗʰ **S37.039** **Laceration of unspecified kidney, unspecified degree** `CC`

√6ᵗʰ **S37.04** **Minor laceration of kidney**
Laceration of kidney less than 1 cm

√7ᵗʰ **S37.041** **Minor laceration of right kidney** `CC`

√7ᵗʰ **S37.042** **Minor laceration of left kidney** `CC`

√7ᵗʰ **S37.049** **Minor laceration of unspecified kidney** `CC`

√6ᵗʰ **S37.05** **Moderate laceration of kidney**
Laceration of kidney 1 to 3 cm

√7ᵗʰ **S37.051** **Moderate laceration of right kidney** `CC`

√7ᵗʰ **S37.052** **Moderate laceration of left kidney** `CC`

√7ᵗʰ **S37.059** **Moderate laceration of unspecified kidney** `CC`

√6ᵗʰ **S37.06** **Major laceration of kidney**
Avulsion of kidney
Laceration of kidney greater than 3 cm
Massive laceration of kidney
Multiple moderate lacerations of kidney
Stellate laceration of kidney

√7ᵗʰ **S37.061** **Major laceration of right kidney** `MCC`

√7ᵗʰ **S37.062** **Major laceration of left kidney** `MCC`

√7ᵗʰ **S37.069** **Major laceration of unspecified kidney** `MCC`

√6ᵗʰ **S37.09** **Other injury of kidney**

√7ᵗʰ **S37.091** **Other injury of right kidney** `MCC`

√7ᵗʰ **S37.092** **Other injury of left kidney** `MCC`

√7ᵗʰ **S37.099** **Other injury of unspecified kidney** `MCC`

√5ᵗʰ **S37.1** **Injury of ureter**

> **CC Excl:** For CC codes in subcategory S37.1, unless otherwise noted: CC with 7th character A: S31.001A, S31.011A, S31.021A, S31.031A, S31.041A, S31.051-S31.159 with 7th A, S31.600-S31.659 with 7th A, S31.831-S31.839 with 7th A, S36.81X-S37.099 with 7th A, S38.3XX-S39.023 with 7th A, T14.8-T14.91, T79.A0X-T79.9XX with 7th A

√x7ᵗʰ **S37.10** **Unspecified injury of ureter** `CC`

√x7ᵗʰ **S37.12** **Contusion of ureter** `CC`

√x7ᵗʰ **S37.13** **Laceration of ureter** `CC`

√x7ᵗʰ **S37.19** **Other injury of ureter** `CC`

√5ᵗʰ **S37.2** **Injury of bladder**

> **CC Excl:** For CC codes in subcategory S37.2, unless otherwise noted: CC with 7th character A: S31.001A, S31.011A, S31.021A, S31.031A, S31.041A, S31.051-S31.159 with 7th A, S31.600-S31.659 with 7th A, S31.831-S31.839 with 7th A, S36.81X-S36.99X with 7th A, S37.20-S37.599 with 7th A, S37.822-S37.99 with 7th A, S38.3XX-S39.023 with 7th A, T14.8-T14.91, T79.A0X-T79.9XX with 7th A

√x7ᵗʰ **S37.20** **Unspecified injury of bladder** `CC`

√x7ᵗʰ **S37.22** **Contusion of bladder** `CC`

√x7ᵗʰ **S37.23** **Laceration of bladder** `CC`

√x7ᵗʰ **S37.29** **Other injury of bladder** `CC`

√5ᵗʰ **S37.3** **Injury of urethra**

> **CC Excl:** For CC codes in subcategory S37.3, unless otherwise noted: See code: S37.2

√x7ᵗʰ **S37.30** **Unspecified injury of urethra** `CC`

√x7ᵗʰ **S37.32** **Contusion of urethra** `CC`

√x7ᵗʰ **S37.33** **Laceration of urethra** `CC`

√x7ᵗʰ **S37.39** **Other injury of urethra** `CC`

√5ᵗʰ **S37.4** **Injury of ovary**

√6ᵗʰ **S37.40** **Unspecified injury of ovary**

√7ᵗʰ **S37.401** **Unspecified injury of ovary, unilateral** ♀

√7ᵗʰ **S37.402** **Unspecified injury of ovary, bilateral** ♀

√7ᵗʰ **S37.409** **Unspecified injury of ovary, unspecified** ♀

√6ᵗʰ **S37.42** **Contusion of ovary**

√7ᵗʰ **S37.421** **Contusion of ovary, unilateral** ♀

√7ᵗʰ **S37.422** **Contusion of ovary, bilateral** ♀

√7ᵗʰ **S37.429** **Contusion of ovary, unspecified** ♀

√6ᵗʰ **S37.43** **Laceration of ovary**

√7ᵗʰ **S37.431** **Laceration of ovary, unilateral** ♀

√7ᵗʰ **S37.432** **Laceration of ovary, bilateral** ♀

√7ᵗʰ **S37.439** **Laceration of ovary, unspecified** ♀

√6ᵗʰ **S37.49** **Other injury of ovary**

√7ᵗʰ **S37.491** **Other injury of ovary, unilateral** ♀

√7ᵗʰ **S37.492** **Other injury of ovary, bilateral** ♀

√7ᵗʰ **S37.499** **Other injury of ovary, unspecified** ♀

√5ᵗʰ **S37.5** **Injury of fallopian tube**

S37.50 **Unspecified injury of fallopian tube**

√7ᵗʰ **S37.501** **Unspecified injury of fallopian tube, unilateral** ♀

√7ᵗʰ **S37.502** **Unspecified injury of fallopian tube, bilateral** ♀

√7ᵗʰ **S37.509** **Unspecified injury of fallopian tube, unspecified** ♀

√6ᵗʰ **S37.51** **Primary blast injury of fallopian tube**
Blast injury of fallopian tube NOS

√7ᵗʰ **S37.511** **Primary blast injury of fallopian tube, unilateral** ♀

√7ᵗʰ **S37.512** **Primary blast injury of fallopian tube, bilateral** ♀

√7ᵗʰ **S37.519** **Primary blast injury of fallopian tube, unspecified** ♀

☑ Additional Character Required   √x7ᵗʰ Xtension Alert   **Unacceptable PDx**   Manifestation   Hospital Acquired Condition   *EXCLUDES 1* Not Coded Here   *EXCLUDES 2* Not Included Here

Injury, Poisoning and Certain Other Consequences of External Causes

S37.52–S39.003

√6th **S37.52** Contusion **of fallopian tube**
     √7th **S37.521** Contusion of fallopian tube, unilateral ♀
     √7th **S37.522** Contusion of fallopian tube, bilateral ♀
     √7th **S37.529** Contusion of fallopian tube, unspecified ♀

√6th **S37.53** Laceration **of fallopian tube**
     √7th **S37.531** Laceration of fallopian tube, unilateral ♀
     √7th **S37.532** Laceration of fallopian tube, bilateral ♀
     √7th **S37.539** Laceration of fallopian tube, unspecified ♀

√6th **S37.59** Other injury **of fallopian tube**
     Secondary blast injury of fallopian tube
     √7th **S37.591** Other injury of fallopian tube, unilateral ♀
     √7th **S37.592** Other injury of fallopian tube, bilateral ♀
     √7th **S37.599** Other injury of fallopian tube, unspecified ♀

√5th **S37.6** Injury of **uterus**
     EXCLUDES 1   injury to gravid uterus (O9A.2-)
              injury to uterus during delivery (O71.-)

     CC Excl: For CC codes in subcategory S37.6, unless otherwise noted: CC with 7th character A: S31.001A, S31.011A, S31.021A, S31.031A, S31.041A, S31.051-S31.159 with 7th A, S31.600-S31.659 with 7th A, S31.831-S31.839 with 7th A, S36.81X-S36.99X with 7th A, S37.401-S37.69X with 7th A, S37.822-S37.99X with 7th A, S38.3XX-S39.023 with 7th A, T14.8-T14.91, T79.A0X-T79.9XX with 7th A

     √x7th **S37.60** Unspecified injury **of uterus** CC ♀
     √x7th **S37.62** Contusion **of uterus** CC ♀
     √x7th **S37.63** Laceration **of uterus** CC ♀
     √x7th **S37.69** Other injury **of uterus** CC ♀

√5th **S37.8** Injury of other urinary and pelvic organs
     √6th **S37.81** Injury of **adrenal gland**

         CC Excl: For CC codes in subcategory S37.81, unless otherwise noted: CC with 7th character A: S31.001A, S31.011A, S31.021A, S31.031A, S31.041A, S31.051-S31.159 with 7th A, S31.600-S31.659 with 7th A, S31.831-S31.839 with 7th A, S36.81X-S36.99X with 7th A, S37.812-S37.819 with 7th A, S38.3XX-S39.023 with 7th A, T14.8-T14.91, T79.A0X-T79.9XX with 7th A

         √7th **S37.812** Contusion **of adrenal gland** CC
         √7th **S37.813** Laceration **of adrenal gland** CC
         √7th **S37.818** Other injury **of adrenal gland** CC
         √7th **S37.819** Unspecified injury **of adrenal gland** CC

     √6th **S37.82** Injury of **prostate**
         √7th **S37.822** Contusion **of prostate** ♂
         √7th **S37.823** Laceration **of prostate** ♂
         √7th **S37.828** Other injury **of prostate** ♂
         √7th **S37.829** Unspecified injury **of prostate** ♂

     √6th **S37.89** Injury of **other urinary and pelvic organ**

         CC Excl: For CC codes in subcategory S37.89, unless otherwise noted: CC with 7th character A: S31.001A, S31.011A, S31.021A, S31.031A, S31.041A, S31.051-S31.159 with 7th A, S31.600-S31.659 with 7th A, S31.831-S31.839 with 7th A, S36.81X-S36.99X with 7th A, S37.401-S37.599 with 7th A, S37.822-S37.99X with 7th A, S38.3X-S39.023 with 7th A, T14.8-T14.91, T79.A0X-T79.9XX with 7th A

         √7th **S37.892** Contusion **of other urinary and pelvic organ** CC
         √7th **S37.893** Laceration **of other urinary and pelvic organ** CC
         √7th **S37.898** Other injury **of other urinary and pelvic organ** CC
         √7th **S37.899** Unspecified injury **of other urinary and pelvic organ** CC

√5th **S37.9** Injury of unspecified urinary and pelvic organ

     CC Excl: For CC codes in subcategory S37.9, unless otherwise noted: CC with 7th character A: See code: S37.89

     √x7th **S37.90** Unspecified injury **of unspecified urinary and pelvic organ** CC
     √x7th **S37.92** Contusion **of unspecified urinary and pelvic organ** CC

√x7th **S37.93** Laceration **of unspecified urinary and pelvic organ** CC
√x7th **S37.99** Other injury **of unspecified urinary and pelvic organ** CC

√4th **S38** **Crushing injury and traumatic amputation of abdomen, lower back, pelvis and external genitals**
     NOTE   An amputation not identified as partial or complete should be coded to complete.

     The appropriate 7th is to be added to each code from category S38.
     A   initial encounter
     D   subsequent encounter
     S   sequela

√5th **S38.0** Crushing injury of **external genital organs**
     Use additional code for any associated injuries
     √6th **S38.00** Crushing injury of **unspecified** external genital organs
         √7th **S38.001** Crushing injury of unspecified external genital organs, male ♂
         √7th **S38.002** Crushing injury of unspecified external genital organs, female ♀
     √x7th **S38.01** Crushing injury of **penis** ♂
     √x7th **S38.02** Crushing injury of **scrotum and testis** ♂
     √x7th **S38.03** Crushing injury of **vulva** ♀

√x7th **S38.1** Crushing injury of abdomen, lower back, and pelvis
     Use additional code for all associated injuries, such as:
         fracture of thoracic or lumbar spine and pelvis (S22.0-, S32-)
         injury to intra-abdominal organs (S36.-)
         injury to urinary and pelvic organs (S37.-)
         open wound of abdominal wall (S31.-)
         spinal cord injury (S34.0, S34.1-)
     EXCLUDES 2   crushing injury of external genital organs (S38.0-)

√5th **S38.2** Traumatic amputation **of external genital organs**
     √6th **S38.21** Traumatic amputation of **female** external genital organs
         Traumatic amputation of clitoris
         Traumatic amputation of labium (majus) (minus)
         Traumatic amputation of vulva
         √7th **S38.211** Complete traumatic amputation of female external genital organs ♀
         √7th **S38.212** Partial traumatic amputation of female external genital organs ♀
     √6th **S38.22** Traumatic amputation of **penis**
         √7th **S38.221** Complete traumatic amputation of penis ♂
         √7th **S38.222** Partial traumatic amputation of penis ♂
     √6th **S38.23** Traumatic amputation of **scrotum and testis**
         √7th **S38.231** Complete traumatic amputation of scrotum and testis ♂
         √7th **S38.232** Partial traumatic amputation of scrotum and testis ♂

√x7th **S38.3** Transection (partial) of abdomen

√4th **S39** **Other and unspecified injuries of abdomen, lower back, pelvis and external genitals**
     Code also any associated open wound (S31.-)
     EXCLUDES 2   sprain of joints and ligaments of lumbar spine and pelvis (S33.-)

     The appropriate 7th is to be added to each code from category S39.
     A   initial encounter
     D   subsequent encounter
     S   sequela

√5th **S39.0** Injury of muscle, fascia and tendon of abdomen, lower back and pelvis
     √6th **S39.00** Unspecified injury of muscle, fascia and tendon of abdomen, lower back and pelvis
         √7th **S39.001** Unspecified injury of muscle, fascia and tendon of **abdomen**
         √7th **S39.002** Unspecified injury of muscle, fascia and tendon of **lower back**
         √7th **S39.003** Unspecified injury of muscle, fascia and tendon of **pelvis**

N Newborn: 0   P Pediatric: 0-17   M Maternity: 12-55   A Adult: 15-124   MCC Major CC Condition   PDx MCC PDx acts as own MCC   CC CC Condition   PDx CC PDx acts as own CC

902   ICD-10-CM Draft (2015)

√6ᵗʰ **S39.01** Strain of muscle, fascia and tendon of abdomen, lower back and pelvis
- √7ᵗʰ **S39.011** Strain of muscle, fascia and tendon of abdomen
- √7ᵗʰ **S39.012** Strain of muscle, fascia and tendon of lower back
- √7ᵗʰ **S39.013** Strain of muscle, fascia and tendon of pelvis

√6ᵗʰ **S39.02** Laceration of muscle, fascia and tendon of abdomen, lower back and pelvis
- √7ᵗʰ **S39.021** Laceration of muscle, fascia and tendon of abdomen
- √7ᵗʰ **S39.022** Laceration of muscle, fascia and tendon of lower back
- √7ᵗʰ **S39.023** Laceration of muscle, fascia and tendon of pelvis

√6ᵗʰ **S39.09** Other injury of muscle, fascia and tendon of abdomen, lower back and pelvis
- √7ᵗʰ **S39.091** Other injury of muscle, fascia and tendon of abdomen
- √7ᵗʰ **S39.092** Other injury of muscle, fascia and tendon of lower back
- √7ᵗʰ **S39.093** Other injury of muscle, fascia and tendon of pelvis

√5ᵗʰ **S39.8** Other specified injuries of abdomen, lower back, pelvis and external genitals
- √x7ᵗʰ **S39.81** Other specified injuries of abdomen
- √x7ᵗʰ **S39.82** Other specified injuries of lower back
- √x7ᵗʰ **S39.83** Other specified injuries of pelvis
- √6ᵗʰ **S39.84** Other specified injuries of external genitals
  - √7ᵗʰ **S39.840** Fracture of corpus cavernosum penis   ♂
  - √7ᵗʰ **S39.848** Other specified injuries of external genitals

√5ᵗʰ **S39.9** Unspecified injury of abdomen, lower back, pelvis and external genitals
- √x7ᵗʰ **S39.91** Unspecified injury of abdomen
- √x7ᵗʰ **S39.92** Unspecified injury of lower back
- √x7ᵗʰ **S39.93** Unspecified injury of pelvis
- √x7ᵗʰ **S39.94** Unspecified injury of external genitals

Injuries to the shoulder and upper arm (S40-S49)

INCLUDES injuries of axilla
injuries of scapular region
EXCLUDES 2 burns and corrosions (T20-T32)
frostbite (T33-T34)
injuries of elbow (S50-S59)
insect bite or sting, venomous (T63.4)

√4ᵗʰ **S40 Superficial injury of shoulder and upper arm**

The appropriate 7th is to be added to each code from category S40.
A   initial encounter
D   subsequent encounter
S   sequela

√5ᵗʰ **S40.0** Contusion of shoulder and upper arm
- √6ᵗʰ **S40.01** Contusion of shoulder
  - √7ᵗʰ **S40.011** Contusion of right shoulder
  - √7ᵗʰ **S40.012** Contusion of left shoulder
  - √7ᵗʰ **S40.019** Contusion of unspecified shoulder
- √6ᵗʰ **S40.02** Contusion of upper arm
  - √7ᵗʰ **S40.021** Contusion of right upper arm
  - √7ᵗʰ **S40.022** Contusion of left upper arm
  - √7ᵗʰ **S40.029** Contusion of unspecified upper arm

√5ᵗʰ **S40.2** Other superficial injuries of shoulder
- √6ᵗʰ **S40.21** Abrasion of shoulder
  - √7ᵗʰ **S40.211** Abrasion of right shoulder
  - √7ᵗʰ **S40.212** Abrasion of left shoulder
  - √7ᵗʰ **S40.219** Abrasion of unspecified shoulder
- √6ᵗʰ **S40.22** Blister (nonthermal) of shoulder
  - √7ᵗʰ **S40.221** Blister (nonthermal) of right shoulder
  - √7ᵗʰ **S40.222** Blister (nonthermal) of left shoulder
  - √7ᵗʰ **S40.229** Blister (nonthermal) of unspecified shoulder
- √6ᵗʰ **S40.24** External constriction of shoulder
  - √7ᵗʰ **S40.241** External constriction of right shoulder
  - √7ᵗʰ **S40.242** External constriction of left shoulder
  - √7ᵗʰ **S40.249** External constriction of unspecified shoulder
- √6ᵗʰ **S40.25** Superficial foreign body of shoulder
  Splinter in the shoulder
  - √7ᵗʰ **S40.251** Superficial foreign body of right shoulder
  - √7ᵗʰ **S40.252** Superficial foreign body of left shoulder
  - √7ᵗʰ **S40.259** Superficial foreign body of unspecified shoulder
- √6ᵗʰ **S40.26** Insect bite (nonvenomous) of shoulder
  - √7ᵗʰ **S40.261** Insect bite (nonvenomous) of right shoulder
  - √7ᵗʰ **S40.262** Insect bite (nonvenomous) of left shoulder
  - √7ᵗʰ **S40.269** Insect bite (nonvenomous) of unspecified shoulder
- √6ᵗʰ **S40.27** Other superficial bite of shoulder
  EXCLUDES 1 open bite of shoulder (S41.05)
  - √7ᵗʰ **S40.271** Other superficial bite of right shoulder
  - √7ᵗʰ **S40.272** Other superficial bite of left shoulder
  - √7ᵗʰ **S40.279** Other superficial bite of unspecified shoulder

√5ᵗʰ **S40.8** Other superficial injuries of upper arm
- √6ᵗʰ **S40.81** Abrasion of upper arm
  - √7ᵗʰ **S40.811** Abrasion of right upper arm
  - √7ᵗʰ **S40.812** Abrasion of left upper arm
  - √7ᵗʰ **S40.819** Abrasion of unspecified upper arm
- √6ᵗʰ **S40.82** Blister (nonthermal) of upper arm
  - √7ᵗʰ **S40.821** Blister (nonthermal) of right upper arm
  - √7ᵗʰ **S40.822** Blister (nonthermal) of left upper arm
  - √7ᵗʰ **S40.829** Blister (nonthermal) of unspecified upper arm
- √6ᵗʰ **S40.84** External constriction of upper arm
  - √7ᵗʰ **S40.841** External constriction of right upper arm
  - √7ᵗʰ **S40.842** External constriction of left upper arm
  - √7ᵗʰ **S40.849** External constriction of unspecified upper arm
- √6ᵗʰ **S40.85** Superficial foreign body of upper arm
  Splinter in the upper arm
  - √7ᵗʰ **S40.851** Superficial foreign body of right upper arm
  - √7ᵗʰ **S40.852** Superficial foreign body of left upper arm
  - √7ᵗʰ **S40.859** Superficial foreign body of unspecified upper arm
- √6ᵗʰ **S40.86** Insect bite (nonvenomous) of upper arm
  - √7ᵗʰ **S40.861** Insect bite (nonvenomous) of right upper arm
  - √7ᵗʰ **S40.862** Insect bite (nonvenomous) of left upper arm
  - √7ᵗʰ **S40.869** Insect bite (nonvenomous) of unspecified upper arm
- √6ᵗʰ **S40.87** Other superficial bite of upper arm
  EXCLUDES 1 open bite of upper arm (S41.14)
  EXCLUDES 2 other superficial bite of shoulder (S40.27-)
  - √7ᵗʰ **S40.871** Other superficial bite of right upper arm
  - √7ᵗʰ **S40.872** Other superficial bite of left upper arm
  - √7ᵗʰ **S40.879** Other superficial bite of unspecified upper arm

√5ᵗʰ **S40.9** Unspecified superficial injury of shoulder and upper arm
- √6ᵗʰ **S40.91** Unspecified superficial injury of shoulder
  - √7ᵗʰ **S40.911** Unspecified superficial injury of right shoulder
  - √7ᵗʰ **S40.912** Unspecified superficial injury of left shoulder
  - √7ᵗʰ **S40.919** Unspecified superficial injury of unspecified shoulder
- √6ᵗʰ **S40.92** Unspecified superficial injury of upper arm
  - √7ᵗʰ **S40.921** Unspecified superficial injury of right upper arm

---

✓ Additional Character Required   √x7ᵗʰ Xtension Alert   Unacceptable PDx   Manifestation   Hospital Acquired Condition   **EXCLUDES 1** Not Coded Here   **EXCLUDES 2** Not Included Here

√7ᵗʰ   **S40.922**   Unspecified superficial injury of left upper arm

√7ᵗʰ   **S40.929**   Unspecified superficial injury of unspecified upper arm

√4ᵗʰ **S41**   **Open wound of shoulder and upper arm**
Code also any associated wound infection
EXCLUDES 1   traumatic amputation of shoulder and upper arm (S48.-)
EXCLUDES 2   open fracture of shoulder and upper arm (S42.- with 7th chractrer B or C)

The appropriate 7th is to be added to each code from category S41.
A   initial encounter
D   subsequent encounter
S   sequela

√5ᵗʰ **S41.0**   **Open wound of shoulder**

√6ᵗʰ   **S41.00**   Unspecified open wound of shoulder
    √7ᵗʰ   **S41.001**   Unspecified open wound of right shoulder
    √7ᵗʰ   **S41.002**   Unspecified open wound of left shoulder
    √7ᵗʰ   **S41.009**   Unspecified open wound of unspecified shoulder

√6ᵗʰ   **S41.01**   Laceration without foreign body of shoulder
    √7ᵗʰ   **S41.011**   Laceration without foreign body of right shoulder
    √7ᵗʰ   **S41.012**   Laceration without foreign body of left shoulder
    √7ᵗʰ   **S41.019**   Laceration without foreign body of unspecified shoulder

√6ᵗʰ   **S41.02**   Laceration with foreign body of shoulder
    √7ᵗʰ   **S41.021**   Laceration with foreign body of right shoulder
    √7ᵗʰ   **S41.022**   Laceration with foreign body of left shoulder
    √7ᵗʰ   **S41.029**   Laceration with foreign body of unspecified shoulder

√6ᵗʰ   **S41.03**   Puncture wound without foreign body of shoulder
    √7ᵗʰ   **S41.031**   Puncture wound without foreign body of right shoulder
    √7ᵗʰ   **S41.032**   Puncture wound without foreign body of left shoulder
    √7ᵗʰ   **S41.039**   Puncture wound without foreign body of unspecified shoulder

√6ᵗʰ   **S41.04**   Puncture wound with foreign body of shoulder
    √7ᵗʰ   **S41.041**   Puncture wound with foreign body of right shoulder
    √7ᵗʰ   **S41.042**   Puncture wound with foreign body of left shoulder
    √7ᵗʰ   **S41.049**   Puncture wound with foreign body of unspecified shoulder

√6ᵗʰ   **S41.05**   Open bite of shoulder
Bite of shoulder NOS
    EXCLUDES 1   superficial bite of shoulder (S40.27)
    √7ᵗʰ   **S41.051**   Open bite of right shoulder
    √7ᵗʰ   **S41.052**   Open bite of left shoulder
    √7ᵗʰ   **S41.059**   Open bite of unspecified shoulder

√5ᵗʰ **S41.1**   **Open wound of upper arm**

√6ᵗʰ   **S41.10**   Unspecified open wound of upper arm
    √7ᵗʰ   **S41.101**   Unspecified open wound of right upper arm
    √7ᵗʰ   **S41.102**   Unspecified open wound of left upper arm
    √7ᵗʰ   **S41.109**   Unspecified open wound of unspecified upper arm

√6ᵗʰ   **S41.11**   Laceration without foreign body of upper arm
    √7ᵗʰ   **S41.111**   Laceration without foreign body of right upper arm
    √7ᵗʰ   **S41.112**   Laceration without foreign body of left upper arm
    √7ᵗʰ   **S41.119**   Laceration without foreign body of unspecified upper arm

√6ᵗʰ   **S41.12**   Laceration with foreign body of upper arm
    √7ᵗʰ   **S41.121**   Laceration with foreign body of right upper arm

√7ᵗʰ   **S41.122**   Laceration with foreign body of left upper arm

√7ᵗʰ   **S41.129**   Laceration with foreign body of unspecified upper arm

√6ᵗʰ   **S41.13**   Puncture wound without foreign body of upper arm
    √7ᵗʰ   **S41.131**   Puncture wound without foreign body of right upper arm
    √7ᵗʰ   **S41.132**   Puncture wound without foreign body of left upper arm
    √7ᵗʰ   **S41.139**   Puncture wound without foreign body of unspecified upper arm

√6ᵗʰ   **S41.14**   Puncture wound with foreign body of upper arm
    √7ᵗʰ   **S41.141**   Puncture wound with foreign body of right upper arm
    √7ᵗʰ   **S41.142**   Puncture wound with foreign body of left upper arm
    √7ᵗʰ   **S41.149**   Puncture wound with foreign body of unspecified upper arm

√6ᵗʰ   **S41.15**   Open bite of upper arm
Bite of upper arm NOS
    EXCLUDES 1   superficial bite of upper arm (S40.87)
    √7ᵗʰ   **S41.151**   Open bite of right upper arm
    √7ᵗʰ   **S41.152**   Open bite of left upper arm
    √7ᵗʰ   **S41.159**   Open bite of unspecified upper arm

√4ᵗʰ **S42**   **Fracture of shoulder and upper arm**
NOTE   A fracture not indicated as displaced or nondisplaced should be coded to displaced.
A fracture not indicated as open or closed should be coded to closed.
EXCLUDES 1   traumatic amputation of shoulder and upper arm (S48.-)

The appropriate 7th is to be added to all codes from category S42 [unless otherwise indicated].
A   initial encounter for closed fracture
B   initial encounter for open fracture
D   subsequent encounter for fracture with routine healing
G   subsequent encounter for fracture with delayed healing
K   subsequent encounter for fracture with nonunion
P   subsequent encounter for fracture with malunion
S   sequela

√5ᵗʰ **S42.0**   **Fracture of clavicle**

CC Excl: For CC/MCC codes in subcategory S42.0, unless otherwise noted: CC with 7th character B: S42.001–S42.036 with 7th [A, B], S62.90XB
CC with 7th character K or P: M80.00X–M84.68X with 7th [K, P], S02.0XX–S02.92X with 7th K, S12.000–S12.691 with 7th K, S22.000–S22.9XX with 7th K, S32.000–S32.9XX with 7th K, S42.001–S42.92X with 7th [K, P], S49.001–S49.199 with 7th [K, P], S52.001–S52.92X with 7th [K, M, N, P, Q, R], S59.001–S59.299 with 7th [K, P], S62.001–S62.92X with 7th [K, P], S72.001–S72.92X with 7th [K, M, N, P, Q, R], S79.001–S79.199 with 7th [K, P], S82.001–S82.92X with 7th [K, M, N, P, Q, R], S89.001–S89.399 with 7th [K, P], S92.001–S92.919 with 7th [K, P]

√6ᵗʰ   **S42.00**   Fracture of unspecified part of clavicle
    7 √7ᵗʰ   **S42.001**   Fracture of unspecified part of right clavicle   **CC**
    7 √7ᵗʰ   **S42.002**   Fracture of unspecified part of left clavicle   **CC**
    7 √7ᵗʰ   **S42.009**   Fracture of unspecified part of unspecified clavicle   **CC**
      AHA: 2012, 4Q, 93

√6ᵗʰ   **S42.01**   Fracture of sternal end of clavicle
    7 √7ᵗʰ   **S42.011**   Anterior displaced fracture of sternal end of right clavicle   **CC**
    7 √7ᵗʰ   **S42.012**   Anterior displaced fracture of sternal end of left clavicle   **CC**
    7 √7ᵗʰ   **S42.013**   Anterior displaced fracture of sternal end of unspecified clavicle   **CC**
      Displaced fracture of sternal end of clavicle NOS
    7 √7ᵗʰ   **S42.014**   Posterior displaced fracture of sternal end of right clavicle   **CC**
    7 √7ᵗʰ   **S42.015**   Posterior displaced fracture of sternal end of left clavicle   **CC**
    7 √7ᵗʰ   **S42.016**   Posterior displaced fracture of sternal end of unspecified clavicle   **CC**

---

7 HAC = Initial encounter only (7th character A, B or C) and not POA.

N Newborn: 0   **P** Pediatric: 0-17   **M** Maternity: 12-55   **A** Adult: 15-124   **MCC** Major CC Condition   **PDx MCC** PDx acts as own MCC   **CC** CC Condition   **PDx CC** PDx acts as own CC

904   ICD-10-CM Draft (2015)

7 √7ᵗʰ **S42.017** Nondisplaced fracture of sternal end of right clavicle CC

7 √7ᵗʰ **S42.018** Nondisplaced fracture of sternal end of left clavicle CC

7 √7ᵗʰ **S42.019** Nondisplaced fracture of sternal end of unspecified clavicle CC

√6ᵗʰ **S42.02** Fracture of shaft of clavicle

7 √7ᵗʰ **S42.021** Displaced fracture of shaft of right clavicle CC

7 √7ᵗʰ **S42.022** Displaced fracture of shaft of left clavicle CC

7 √7ᵗʰ **S42.023** Displaced fracture of shaft of unspecified clavicle CC

7 √7ᵗʰ **S42.024** Nondisplaced fracture of shaft of right clavicle CC

7 √7ᵗʰ **S42.025** Nondisplaced fracture of shaft of left clavicle CC

7 √7ᵗʰ **S42.026** Nondisplaced fracture of shaft of unspecified clavicle CC

√6ᵗʰ **S42.03** Fracture of lateral end of clavicle
    Fracture of acromial end of clavicle

7 √7ᵗʰ **S42.031** Displaced fracture of lateral end of right clavicle CC

7 √7ᵗʰ **S42.032** Displaced fracture of lateral end of left clavicle CC

7 √7ᵗʰ **S42.033** Displaced fracture of lateral end of unspecified clavicle CC

7 √7ᵗʰ **S42.034** Nondisplaced fracture of lateral end of right clavicle CC

7 √7ᵗʰ **S42.035** Nondisplaced fracture of lateral end of left clavicle CC

7 √7ᵗʰ **S42.036** Nondisplaced fracture of lateral end of unspecified clavicle CC

√5ᵗʰ **S42.1** Fracture of scapula

> **CC Excl:** For CC/MCC codes in subcatagory S42.1, unless otherwise noted: S42.101-S42.199 with 7th [A, B], S62.90XB
> **CC with 7th character K or P:** M80.00X-M84.68X with 7th [K, P], S02.0XX-S02.92X with 7th K, S12.000-S12.691 with 7th K, S22.000-S22.9XX with 7th K, S32.000-S32.9XX with 7th K, S42.001-S42.92X with 7th [K, P], S49.001-S49.199 with 7th [K, P], S52.001-S52.92X with 7th [K, M, N, P, Q, R], S59.001-S59.299 with 7th [K, P], S62.001-S62.92X with 7th [K, P], S72.001-S72.92X with 7th [K, M, N, P, Q, R], S79.001-S79.199 with 7th [K, P], S82.001-S82.92X with 7th [K, M, N, P, Q, R], S89.001-S89.399 with 7th [K, P], S92.001-S92.919 with 7th [K, P]

√6ᵗʰ **S42.10** Fracture of unspecified part of scapula

7 √7ᵗʰ **S42.101** Fracture of unspecified part of scapula, right shoulder CC

7 √7ᵗʰ **S42.102** Fracture of unspecified part of scapula, left shoulder CC

7 √7ᵗʰ **S42.109** Fracture of unspecified part of scapula, unspecified shoulder CC

√6ᵗʰ **S42.11** Fracture of body of scapula

7 √7ᵗʰ **S42.111** Displaced fracture of body of scapula, right shoulder CC

7 √7ᵗʰ **S42.112** Displaced fracture of body of scapula, left shoulder CC

7 √7ᵗʰ **S42.113** Displaced fracture of body of scapula, unspecified shoulder CC

7 √7ᵗʰ **S42.114** Nondisplaced fracture of body of scapula, right shoulder CC

7 √7ᵗʰ **S42.115** Nondisplaced fracture of body of scapula, left shoulder CC

7 √7ᵗʰ **S42.116** Nondisplaced fracture of body of scapula, unspecified shoulder CC

√6ᵗʰ **S42.12** Fracture of acromial process

7 √7ᵗʰ **S42.121** Displaced fracture of acromial process, right shoulder CC

7 √7ᵗʰ **S42.122** Displaced fracture of acromial process, left shoulder CC

7 √7ᵗʰ **S42.123** Displaced fracture of acromial process, unspecified shoulder CC

7 √7ᵗʰ **S42.124** Nondisplaced fracture of acromial process, right shoulder CC

7 √7ᵗʰ **S42.125** Nondisplaced fracture of acromial process, left shoulder CC

7 √7ᵗʰ **S42.126** Nondisplaced fracture of acromial process, unspecified shoulder CC

√6ᵗʰ **S42.13** Fracture of coracoid process

7 √7ᵗʰ **S42.131** Displaced fracture of coracoid process, right shoulder CC

7 √7ᵗʰ **S42.132** Displaced fracture of coracoid process, left shoulder CC

7 √7ᵗʰ **S42.133** Displaced fracture of coracoid process, unspecified shoulder CC

7 √7ᵗʰ **S42.134** Nondisplaced fracture of coracoid process, right shoulder CC

7 √7ᵗʰ **S42.135** Nondisplaced fracture of coracoid process, left shoulder CC

7 √7ᵗʰ **S42.136** Nondisplaced fracture of coracoid process, unspecified shoulder CC

√6ᵗʰ **S42.14** Fracture of glenoid cavity of scapula

7 √7ᵗʰ **S42.141** Displaced fracture of glenoid cavity of scapula, right shoulder CC

7 √7ᵗʰ **S42.142** Displaced fracture of glenoid cavity of scapula, left shoulder CC

7 √7ᵗʰ **S42.143** Displaced fracture of glenoid cavity of scapula, unspecified shoulder CC

7 √7ᵗʰ **S42.144** Nondisplaced fracture of glenoid cavity of scapula, right shoulder CC

7 √7ᵗʰ **S42.145** Nondisplaced fracture of glenoid cavity of scapula, left shoulder CC

7 √7ᵗʰ **S42.146** Nondisplaced fracture of glenoid cavity of scapula, unspecified shoulder CC

√6ᵗʰ **S42.15** Fracture of neck of scapula

7 √7ᵗʰ **S42.151** Displaced fracture of neck of scapula, right shoulder CC

7 √7ᵗʰ **S42.152** Displaced fracture of neck of scapula, left shoulder CC

7 √7ᵗʰ **S42.153** Displaced fracture of neck of scapula, unspecified shoulder CC

7 √7ᵗʰ **S42.154** Nondisplaced fracture of neck of scapula, right shoulder CC

7 √7ᵗʰ **S42.155** Nondisplaced fracture of neck of scapula, left shoulder CC

7 √7ᵗʰ **S42.156** Nondisplaced fracture of neck of scapula, unspecified shoulder CC

√6ᵗʰ **S42.19** Fracture of other part of scapula

7 √7ᵗʰ **S42.191** Fracture of other part of scapula, right shoulder CC

7 √7ᵗʰ **S42.192** Fracture of other part of scapula, left shoulder CC

7 √7ᵗʰ **S42.199** Fracture of other part of scapula, unspecified shoulder CC

---

7 HAC = Initial encounter only (7th character A, B or C) and not POA.

√ Additional Character Required   ✗x7ᵗʰ Xtension Alert   Unacceptable PDx   Manifestation   Hospital Acquired Condition   EXCLUDES 1 Not Coded Here   EXCLUDES 2 Not Included Here

Injury, Poisoning and Certain Other Consequences of External Causes

S42.2–S42.254

✓5ᵗʰ **S42.2** **Fracture of upper end of humerus**
Fracture of proximal end of humerus
EXCLUDES 2   fracture of shaft of humerus (S42.3-)
physeal fracture of upper end of humerus (S49.0-)

✓6ᵗʰ **S42.20** **Unspecified fracture of upper end of humerus**

7 ✓7ᵗʰ **S42.201** **Unspecified fracture of upper end of right humerus** MCC CC
CC Excl: CC with 7th character A: S42.201-S42.271 with 7th [A, B], S42.279-S42.311 with 7th A, S42.319-S42.481 with 7th A, S42.489-S42.92X with 7th A, S49.001 with 7th A, S49.009-S49.011 with 7th A, S49.019-S49.021 with 7th A, S49.029-S49.031 with 7th A, S49.039-S49.041 with 7th A, S49.049-S49.091 with 7th A, S49.099-S49.101 with 7th A, S49.109-S49.111 with 7th A, S49.119-S49.121 with 7th A, S49.129-S49.131 with 7th A, S49.139-S49.141 with 7th A, S49.149-S49.191 with 7th A, S49.199A
MCC with 7th character B: S42.201-S42.266 with 7th B, S42.291-S42.92X with 7th B, S49.101-S49.199 with 7th A, S62.90XB
CC with 7th character K or P: M80.00X-M84.68X with 7th [K, P], S02.0XX-S02.92X with 7th K, S12.000-S12.691 with 7th K, S22.000-S22.9XX with 7th K, S32.000-S32.9XX with 7th K, S42.001-S42.92X with 7th [K, P], S49.001-S49.199 with 7th [K, P], S52.001-S52.92X with 7th [K, M, N, P, Q, R], S59.001-S59.299 with 7th [K, P], S62.001-S62.92X with 7th [K, P], S72.001-S72.92X with 7th [K, M, N, P, Q, R], S79.001-S79.199 with 7th [K, P], S82.001-S82.92X with 7th [K, M, N, P, Q, R], S89.001-S89.399 with 7th [K, P], S92.001-S92.919 with 7th [K, P]

7 ✓7ᵗʰ **S42.202** **Unspecified fracture of upper end of left humerus** MCC CC
CC Excl: CC with 7th character A: S42.201-S42.266 with 7th B, S42.272-S42.309 with 7th A, S42.312-S42.476 with 7th A, S42.482-S42.92X with 7th A, S49.002-S49.009 with 7th A, S49.012-S49.019 with 7th A, S49.022-S49.029 with 7th A, S49.032-S49.039 with 7th A, S49.042-S49.049 with 7th A, S49.092-S49.099 with 7th A, S49.102-S49.109 with 7th A, S49.112-S49.119 with 7th A, S49.122-S49.129 with 7th A, S49.132-S49.139 with 7th A, S49.142-S49.149 with 7th A, S49.192-S49.199 with 7th A
MCC with 7th character B: MCC Excl: S42.201-S42.266 with 7th B, S42.291-S42.92X with 7th B, S49.101-S49.199 with 7th A, S62.90XB
CC with 7th character K or P: CC Excl: M80.00X-M84.68X with 7th [K, P], S02.0XX-S02.92X with 7th K, S12.000-S12.691 with 7th K, S22.000-S22.9XX with 7th K, S32.000-S32.9XX with 7th K, S42.001-S42.92X with 7th [K, P], S49.001-S49.199 with 7th [K, P], S52.001-S52.92X with 7th [K, M, N, P, Q, R], S59.001-S59.299 with 7th [K, P], S62.001-S62.92X with 7th [K, P], S72.001-S72.92X with 7th [K, M, N, P, Q, R], S79.001-S79.199 with 7th [K, P], S82.001-S82.92X with 7th [K, M, N, P, Q, R], S89.001-S89.399 with 7th [K, P], S92.001-S92.919 with 7th [K, P]

7 ✓7ᵗʰ **S42.209** **Unspecified fracture of upper end of unspecified humerus** MCC CC
CC Excl: CC with 7th character A: S42.201-S42.92X with 7th [A, B], S49.001-S49.199 with 7th A
MCC with 7th character B: S42.201-S42.266 with 7th B, S42.291-S42.92X with 7th B, S49.101-S49.199 with 7th A, S62.90XB
CC with 7th character K or P: M80.00X-M84.68X with 7th [K, P], S02.0XX-S02.92X with 7th K, S12.000-S12.691 with 7th K, S22.000-S22.9XX with 7th K, S32.000-S32.9XX with 7th K, S42.001-S42.92X with 7th [K, P], S49.001-S49.199 with 7th [K, P], S52.001-S52.92X with 7th [K, M, N, P, Q, R], S59.001-S59.299 with 7th [K, P], S62.001-S62.92X with 7th [K, P], S72.001-S72.92X with 7th [K, M, N, P, Q, R], S79.001-S79.199 with 7th [K, P], S82.001-S82.92X with 7th [K, M, N, P, Q, R], S89.001-S89.399 with 7th [K, P], S92.001-S92.919 with 7th [K, P]

✓6ᵗʰ **S42.21** **Unspecified fracture of surgical neck of humerus**
Fracture of neck of humerus NOS

7 ✓7ᵗʰ **S42.211** **Unspecified displaced fracture of surgical neck of right humerus** MCC CC
CC Excl: See code: S42.201

7 ✓7ᵗʰ **S42.212** **Unspecified displaced fracture of surgical neck of left humerus** MCC CC
CC Excl: See code: S42.202

7 ✓7ᵗʰ **S42.213** **Unspecified displaced fracture of surgical neck of unspecified humerus** MCC CC
CC Excl: See code: S42.209

7 ✓7ᵗʰ **S42.214** **Unspecified nondisplaced fracture of surgical neck of right humerus** MCC CC
CC Excl: See code: S42.201

7 ✓7ᵗʰ **S42.215** **Unspecified nondisplaced fracture of surgical neck of left humerus** MCC CC
CC Excl: See code: S42.202

7 ✓7ᵗʰ **S42.216** **Unspecified nondisplaced fracture of surgical neck of unspecified humerus** MCC CC
CC Excl: See code: S42.209

✓6ᵗʰ **S42.22** **2-part fracture of surgical neck of humerus**

7 ✓7ᵗʰ **S42.221** **2-part displaced fracture of surgical neck of right humerus** MCC CC
CC Excl: See code: S42.201

7 ✓7ᵗʰ **S42.222** **2-part displaced fracture of surgical neck of left humerus** MCC CC
CC Excl: See code: S42.202

7 ✓7ᵗʰ **S42.223** **2-part displaced fracture of surgical neck of unspecified humerus** MCC CC
CC Excl: See code: S42.209

7 ✓7ᵗʰ **S42.224** **2-part nondisplaced fracture of surgical neck of right humerus** MCC CC
CC Excl: See code: S42.201

7 ✓7ᵗʰ **S42.225** **2-part nondisplaced fracture of surgical neck of left humerus** MCC CC
CC Excl: See code: S42.202

7 ✓7ᵗʰ **S42.226** **2-part nondisplaced fracture of surgical neck of unspecified humerus** MCC CC
CC Excl: See code: S42.209

✓6ᵗʰ **S42.23** **3-part fracture of surgical neck of humerus**

7 ✓7ᵗʰ **S42.231** **3-part fracture of surgical neck of right humerus** MCC CC
CC Excl: See code: S42.201

7 ✓7ᵗʰ **S42.232** **3-part fracture of surgical neck of left humerus** MCC CC
CC Excl: See code: S42.202

7 ✓7ᵗʰ **S42.239** **3-part fracture of surgical neck of unspecified humerus** MCC CC
CC Excl: See code: S42.209

✓6ᵗʰ **S42.24** **4-part fracture of surgical neck of humerus**

7 ✓7ᵗʰ **S42.241** **4-part fracture of surgical neck of right humerus** MCC CC
CC Excl: See code: S42.201

7 ✓7ᵗʰ **S42.242** **4-part fracture of surgical neck of left humerus** MCC CC
CC Excl: See code: S42.202

7 ✓7ᵗʰ **S42.249** **4-part fracture of surgical neck of unspecified humerus** MCC CC
CC Excl: See code: S42.209

✓6ᵗʰ **S42.25** **Fracture of greater tuberosity of humerus**

7 ✓7ᵗʰ **S42.251** **Displaced fracture of greater tuberosity of right humerus** MCC CC
CC Excl: See code: S42.201

7 ✓7ᵗʰ **S42.252** **Displaced fracture of greater tuberosity of left humerus** MCC CC
CC Excl: See code: S42.202

7 ✓7ᵗʰ **S42.253** **Displaced fracture of greater tuberosity of unspecified humerus** MCC CC
CC Excl: See code: S42.209

7 ✓7ᵗʰ **S42.254** **Nondisplaced fracture of greater tuberosity of right humerus** MCC CC
CC Excl: See code: S42.201

---

7 HAC = Initial encounter only (7th character A, B or C) and not POA.

N Newborn: 0   **P** Pediatric: 0-17   **M** Maternity: 12-55   **A** Adult: 15-124   MCC Major CC Condition   PDx MCC PDx acts as own MCC   CC CC Condition   PDx CC PDx acts as own CC

7 √7ᵗʰ **S42.255** Nondisplaced fracture of greater tuberosity of left humerus `MCC` `CC`
CC Excl: See code: S42.202

7 √7ᵗʰ **S42.256** Nondisplaced fracture of greater tuberosity of unspecified humerus `MCC` `CC`
CC Excl: See code: S42.209

√6ᵗʰ **S42.26** Fracture of lesser tuberosity of humerus

7 √7ᵗʰ **S42.261** Displaced fracture of lesser tuberosity of right humerus `MCC` `CC`
CC Excl: See code: S42.201

7 √7ᵗʰ **S42.262** Displaced fracture of lesser tuberosity of left humerus `MCC` `CC`
CC Excl: See code: S42.202

7 √7ᵗʰ **S42.263** Displaced fracture of lesser tuberosity of unspecified humerus `MCC` `CC`
CC Excl: See code: S42.209

7 √7ᵗʰ **S42.264** Nondisplaced fracture of lesser tuberosity of right humerus `MCC` `CC`
CC Excl: See code: S42.201

7 √7ᵗʰ **S42.265** Nondisplaced fracture of lesser tuberosity of left humerus `MCC` `CC`
CC Excl: See code: S42.202

7 √7ᵗʰ **S42.266** Nondisplaced fracture of lesser tuberosity of unspecified humerus `MCC` `CC`
CC Excl: See code: S42.209

√6ᵗʰ **S42.27** Torus fracture of upper end of humerus

The appropriate 7th is to be added to all codes in subcategory S42.27.
A initial encounter for closed fracture
D subsequent encounter for fracture with routine healing
G subsequent encounter for fracture with delayed healing
K subsequent encounter for fracture with nonunion
P subsequent encounter for fracture with malunion
S sequela

7 √7ᵗʰ **S42.271** Torus fracture of upper end of right humerus `CC`
CC Excl: See code: S42.201

7 √7ᵗʰ **S42.272** Torus fracture of upper end of left humerus `CC`
CC Excl: See code: S42.202

7 √7ᵗʰ **S42.279** Torus fracture of upper end of unspecified humerus `CC`
CC Excl: See code: S42.209

√6ᵗʰ **S42.29** Other fracture of upper end of humerus
Fracture of anatomical neck of humerus
Fracture of articular head of humerus

7 √7ᵗʰ **S42.291** Other displaced fracture of upper end of right humerus `MCC` `CC`
CC Excl: See code: S42.201

7 √7ᵗʰ **S42.292** Other displaced fracture of upper end of left humerus `MCC` `CC`
CC Excl: See code: S42.202

7 √7ᵗʰ **S42.293** Other displaced fracture of upper end of unspecified humerus `MCC` `CC`
CC Excl: See code: S42.209

7 √7ᵗʰ **S42.294** Other nondisplaced fracture of upper end of right humerus `MCC` `CC`
CC Excl: See code: S42.201

7 √7ᵗʰ **S42.295** Other nondisplaced fracture of upper end of left humerus `MCC` `CC`
CC Excl: See code: S42.202

7 √7ᵗʰ **S42.296** Other nondisplaced fracture of upper end of unspecified humerus `MCC` `CC`
CC Excl: See code: S42.209

√5ᵗʰ **S42.3** Fracture of shaft of humerus
Fracture of humerus NOS
Fracture of upper arm NOS
EXCLUDES 2 physeal fractures of upper end of humerus (S49.0-)
physeal fractures of lower end of humerus (S49.1-)

√6ᵗʰ **S42.30** Unspecified fracture of shaft of humerus

7 √7ᵗʰ **S42.301** Unspecified fracture of shaft of humerus, right arm `MCC` `CC`
CC Excl: See code: S42.201

7 √7ᵗʰ **S42.302** Unspecified fracture of shaft of humerus, left arm `MCC` `CC`
CC Excl: See code: S42.202

7 √7ᵗʰ **S42.309** Unspecified fracture of shaft of humerus, unspecified arm `MCC` `CC`
CC Excl: See code: S42.209

√6ᵗʰ **S42.31** Greenstick fracture of shaft of humerus

The appropriate 7th is to be added to all codes in subcategory S42.31.
A initial encounter for closed fracture
D subsequent encounter for fracture with routine healing
G subsequent encounter for fracture with delayed healing
K subsequent encounter for fracture with nonunion
P subsequent encounter for fracture with malunion
S sequela

7 √7ᵗʰ **S42.311** Greenstick fracture of shaft of humerus, right arm `CC`
CC Excl: CC with 7th character A: S42.311A, S42.319-S42.321 with 7th A, S42.323-S42.324 with 7th A, S42.326-S42.331 with 7th A, S42.333-S42.334 with 7th A, S42.336-S42.341 with 7th A, S42.343-S42.344 with 7th A, S42.346-S42.351 with 7th A, S42.353-S42.354 with 7th A, S42.356-S42.361 with 7th A, S42.363-S42.364 with 7th A, S42.366-S42.391 with 7th A, S42.399A
CC with 7th character K or P: M80.00X-M84.68X with 7th [K, P], S02.0XX-S02.92X with 7th K, S12.000-S12.691 with 7th K, S22.000-S22.9XX with 7th K, S32.000-S32.9XX with 7th K, S42.001-S42.92X with 7th [K, P], S49.001-S49.199 with 7th [K, P], S52.001-S52.92X with 7th [K, M, N, P, Q, R], S59.001-S59.299 with 7th [K, P], S62.001-S62.92X with 7th [K, P], S72.001-S72.92X with 7th [K, M, N, P, Q, R], S79.001-S79.199 with 7th [K, P], S82.001-S82.92X with 7th [K, M, N, P, Q, R], S89.001-S89.399 with 7th [K, P], S92.001-S92.919 with 7th [K, P]

7 √7ᵗʰ **S42.312** Greenstick fracture of shaft of humerus, left arm `CC`
CC Excl: CC with 7th character A: S42.312-S42.319 with 7th A, S42.322-S42.323 with 7th A, S42.325-S42.326 with 7th A, S42.332-S42.333 with 7th A, S42.335-S42.336 with 7th A, S42.342-S42.343 with 7th A, S42.345-S42.346 with 7th A, S42.352-S42.353 with 7th A, S42.355-S42.356 with 7th A, S42.362-S42.363 with 7th A, S42.365-S42.366 with 7th A, S42.392-S42.399 with 7th A
CC with 7th character K or P: M80.00X-M84.68X with 7th [K, P], S02.0XX-S02.92X with 7th K, S12.000-S12.691 with 7th K, S22.000-S22.9XX with 7th K, S32.000-S32.9XX with 7th K, S42.001-S42.92X with 7th [K, P], S49.001-S49.199 with 7th [K, P], S52.001-S52.92X with 7th [K, M, N, P, Q, R], S59.001-S59.299 with 7th [K, P], S62.001-S62.92X with 7th [K, P], S72.001-S72.92X with 7th [K, M, N, P, Q, R], S79.001-S79.199 with 7th [K, P], S82.001-S82.92X with 7th [K, M, N, P, Q, R], S89.001-S89.399 with 7th [K, P], S92.001-S92.919 with 7th [K, P]

7 √7ᵗʰ **S42.319** Greenstick fracture of shaft of humerus, unspecified arm `CC`
CC Excl: CC with 7th character A: S42.311-S42.399 with 7th A
CC with 7th character K or P: M80.00X-M84.68X with 7th [K, P], S02.0XX-S02.92X with 7th K, S12.000-S12.691 with 7th K, S22.000-S22.9XX with 7th K, S32.000-S32.9XX with 7th K, S42.001-S42.92X with 7th [K, P], S49.001-S49.199 with 7th [K, P], S52.001-S52.92X with 7th [K, M, N, P, Q, R], S59.001-S59.299 with 7th [K, P], S62.001-S62.92X with 7th [K, P], S72.001-S72.92X with 7th [K, M, N, P, Q, R], S79.001-S79.199 with 7th [K, P], S82.001-S82.92X with 7th [K, M, N, P, Q, R], S89.001-S89.399 with 7th [K, P], S92.001-S92.919 with 7th [K, P]

---

7 HAC = Initial encounter only (7th character A, B or C) and not POA.

☑ Additional Character Required √x7ᵗʰ Xtension Alert Unacceptable PDx Manifestation Hospital Acquired Condition EXCLUDES 1 Not Coded Here EXCLUDES 2 Not Included Here

√6ᵗʰ **S42.32** Transverse **fracture of shaft of humerus**

7 √7ᵗʰ **S42.321** Displaced **transverse fracture of shaft of humerus, right arm** MCC CC
CC Excl: CC with 7th character A: S42.311 with 7th A, S42.319-S42.321 with 7th A, S42.323-S42.324 with 7th A, S42.326-S42.331 with 7th A, S42.333-S42.334 with 7th A, S42.336-S42.341 with 7th A, S42.343-S42.344 with 7th A, S42.346-S42.351 with 7th A, S42.353-S42.354 with 7th A, S42.356-S42.361 with 7th A, S42.363-S42.364 with 7th A, S42.366-S42.391 with 7th A, S42.399A
MCC with 7th character B: S42.201-S42.266 with 7th B, S42.291-S42.92X with 7th B, S49.101-S49.199 with 7th A, S62.90XB
CC with 7th character K or P: M80.00X-M84.68X with 7th [K, P], S02.0XX-S02.92X with 7th K, S12.000-S12.691 with 7th K, S22.000-S22.9XX with 7th K, S32.000-S32.9XX with 7th K, S42.001-S42.92X with 7th [K, P], S49.001-S49.199 with 7th [K, P], S52.001-S52.92X with 7th [K, M, N, P, Q, R], S59.001-S59.299 with 7th [K, P], S62.001-S62.92X with 7th [K, P], S72.001-S72.92X with 7th [K, M, N, P, Q, R], S79.001-S79.199 with 7th [K, P], S82.001-S82.92X with 7th [K, M, N, P, Q, R], S89.001-S89.399 with 7th [K, P], S92.001-S92.919 with 7th [K, P]

7 √7ᵗʰ **S42.322** Displaced **transverse fracture of shaft of humerus, left arm** MCC CC
CC Excl: CC with 7th character A: S42.312-S42.319 with 7th A, S42.322-S42.323 with 7th A, S42.325-S42.326 with 7th A, S42.332-S42.333 with 7th A, S42.335-S42.336 with 7th A, S42.342-S42.343 with 7th A, S42.345-S42.346 with 7th A, S42.352-S42.353 with 7th A, S42.355-S42.356 with 7th A, S42.362-S42.363 with 7th A, S42.365-S42.366 with 7th A, S42.392-S42.399 with 7th A
MCC with 7th character B: S42.201-S42.266 with 7th B, S42.291-S42.92X with 7th B, S49.101-S49.199 with 7th A, S62.90XB
CC with 7th character K or P: M80.00X-M84.68X with 7th [K, P], S02.0XX-S02.92X with 7th K, S12.000-S12.691 with 7th K, S22.000-S22.9XX with 7th K, S32.000-S32.9XX with 7th K, S42.001-S42.92X with 7th [K, P], S49.001-S49.199 with 7th [K, P], S52.001-S52.92X with 7th [K, M, N, P, Q, R], S59.001-S59.299 with 7th [K, P], S62.001-S62.92X with 7th [K, P], S72.001-S72.92X with 7th [K, M, N, P, Q, R], S79.001-S79.199 with 7th [K, P], S82.001-S82.92X with 7th [K, M, N, P, Q, R], S89.001-S89.399 with 7th [K, P], S92.001-S92.919 with 7th [K, P]

7 √7ᵗʰ **S42.323** Displaced **transverse fracture of shaft of humerus, unspecified arm** MCC CC
CC Excl: CC with 7th character A: S42.311-S42.399 with 7th A
MCC with 7th character B: S42.201-S42.266 with 7th B, S42.291-S42.92X with 7th B, S49.101-S49.199 with 7th A, S62.90XB

7 √7ᵗʰ **S42.324** Nondisplaced **transverse fracture of shaft of humerus, right arm** MCC CC
CC Excl: See code: S42.321

7 √7ᵗʰ **S42.325** Nondisplaced **transverse fracture of shaft of humerus, left arm** MCC CC
CC Excl: See code: S42.322

7 √7ᵗʰ **S42.326** Nondisplaced **transverse fracture of shaft of humerus, unspecified arm** MCC CC
CC Excl: See code: S42.323

√6ᵗʰ **S42.33** Oblique **fracture of shaft of humerus**

7 √7ᵗʰ **S42.331** Displaced **oblique fracture of shaft of humerus, right arm** MCC CC
CC Excl: See code: S42.321

7 √7ᵗʰ **S42.332** Displaced **oblique fracture of shaft of humerus, left arm** MCC CC
CC Excl: See code: S42.322

7 √7ᵗʰ **S42.333** Displaced **oblique fracture of shaft of humerus, unspecified arm** MCC CC
CC Excl: See code: S42.323

7 √7ᵗʰ **S42.334** Nondisplaced **oblique fracture of shaft of humerus, right arm** MCC CC
CC Excl: See code: S42.321

7 √7ᵗʰ **S42.335** Nondisplaced **oblique fracture of shaft of humerus, left arm** MCC CC
CC Excl: See code: S42.322

7 √7ᵗʰ **S42.336** Nondisplaced **oblique fracture of shaft of humerus, unspecified arm** MCC CC
CC Excl: See code: S42.323

√6ᵗʰ **S42.34** Spiral **fracture of shaft of humerus**

7 √7ᵗʰ **S42.341** Displaced **spiral fracture of shaft of humerus, right arm** MCC CC
CC Excl: See code: S42.321

7 √7ᵗʰ **S42.342** Displaced **spiral fracture of shaft of humerus, left arm** MCC CC
CC Excl: See code: S42.322

7 √7ᵗʰ **S42.343** Displaced **spiral fracture of shaft of humerus, unspecified arm** MCC CC
CC Excl: See code: S42.323

7 √7ᵗʰ **S42.344** Nondisplaced **spiral fracture of shaft of humerus, right arm** MCC CC
CC Excl: See code: S42.321

7 √7ᵗʰ **S42.345** Nondisplaced **spiral fracture of shaft of humerus, left arm** MCC CC
CC Excl: See code: S42.322

7 √7ᵗʰ **S42.346** Nondisplaced **spiral fracture of shaft of humerus, unspecified arm** MCC CC
CC Excl: See code: S42.323

√6ᵗʰ **S42.35** Comminuted **fracture of shaft of humerus**

7 √7ᵗʰ **S42.351** Displaced **comminuted fracture of shaft of humerus, right arm** MCC CC
CC Excl: See code: S42.321

7 √7ᵗʰ **S42.352** Displaced **comminuted fracture of shaft of humerus, left arm** MCC CC
CC Excl: See code: S42.322

7 √7ᵗʰ **S42.353** Displaced **comminuted fracture of shaft of humerus, unspecified arm** MCC CC
CC Excl: See code: S42.323

7 √7ᵗʰ **S42.354** Nondisplaced **comminuted fracture of shaft of humerus, right arm** MCC CC
CC Excl: See code: S42.321

7 √7ᵗʰ **S42.355** Nondisplaced **comminuted fracture of shaft of humerus, left arm** MCC CC
CC Excl: See code: S42.322

7 √7ᵗʰ **S42.356** Nondisplaced **comminuted fracture of shaft of humerus, unspecified arm** MCC CC
CC Excl: See code: S42.323

√6ᵗʰ **S42.36** Segmental **fracture of shaft of humerus**

7 √7ᵗʰ **S42.361** Displaced **segmental fracture of shaft of humerus, right arm** MCC CC
CC Excl: See code: S42.321

7 √7ᵗʰ **S42.362** Displaced **segmental fracture of shaft of humerus, left arm** MCC CC
CC Excl: See code: S42.322

7 √7ᵗʰ **S42.363** Displaced **segmental fracture of shaft of humerus, unspecified arm** MCC CC
CC Excl: See code: S42.323

7 √7ᵗʰ **S42.364** Nondisplaced **segmental fracture of shaft of humerus, right arm** MCC CC
CC Excl: See code: S42.321

7 √7ᵗʰ **S42.365** Nondisplaced **segmental fracture of shaft of humerus, left arm** MCC CC
CC Excl: See code: S42.322

7 √7ᵗʰ **S42.366** Nondisplaced **segmental fracture of shaft of humerus, unspecified arm** MCC CC
CC Excl: See code: S42.323

√6ᵗʰ **S42.39** Other **fracture of shaft of humerus**

7 √7ᵗʰ **S42.391** Other **fracture of shaft of right humerus** MCC CC
CC Excl: See code: S42.321

7 √7ᵗʰ **S42.392** Other **fracture of shaft of left humerus** MCC CC
CC Excl: See code: S42.322

7 √7ᵗʰ **S42.399** Other **fracture of shaft of unspecified humerus** MCC CC
CC Excl: See code: S42.323

---

7 HAC = Initial encounter only (7th character A, B or C) and not POA.

N Newborn: 0   P Pediatric: 0-17   M Maternity: 12-55   A Adult: 15-124   MCC Major CC Condition   PDx MCC PDx acts as own MCC   CC CC Condition   PDx CC PDx acts as own CC

908   ICD-10-CM Draft (2015)

√5ᵗʰ **S42.4 Fracture of lower end of humerus**
Fracture of distal end of humerus
EXCLUDES 2 *fracture of shaft of humerus (S42.3-)*
physeal fracture of lower end of humerus (S49.1-)

√6ᵗʰ **S42.40 Unspecified fracture of lower end of humerus**
Fracture of elbow NOS

7 √7ᵗʰ **S42.401 Unspecified fracture of lower end of right humerus**   MCC CC
CC Excl: CC with 7th character A: S42.201-S42.271 with 7th [A, B], S42.279-S42.311 with 7th A, S42.319-S42.481 with 7th A, S42.489-S42.92X with 7th A, S49.001A, S49.009-S49.011 with 7th A, S49.019-S49.021 with 7th A, S49.029-S49.031 with 7th A, S49.039-S49.041 with 7th A, S49.049-S49.091 with 7th A, S49.099-S49.101 with 7th A, S49.109-S49.111 with 7th A, S49.119-S49.121 with 7th A, S49.129-S49.131 with 7th A, S49.139-S49.141 with 7th A, S49.149-S49.191 with 7th A, S49.199A
MCC with 7th character B: S42.201-S42.266 with 7th B, S42.291-S42.92X with 7th B, S49.101-S49.199 with 7th A, S62.9XB
CC with 7th character K or P: M80.00X-M84.68X with 7th [K, P], S02.0XX-S02.92X with 7th K, S12.000-S12.691 with 7th K, S22.000-S22.9XX with 7th K, S32.000-S32.9XX with 7th K, S42.001-S42.92X with 7th [K, P], S49.001-S49.199 with 7th [K, P], S52.001-S52.92X with 7th [K, M, N, P, Q, R], S59.001-S59.299 with 7th [K, P], S62.001-S62.92X with 7th [K, P], S72.001-S72.92X with 7th [K, M, N, P, Q, R], S79.001-S79.199 with 7th [K, P], S82.001-S82.92X with 7th [K, M, N, P, Q, R], S89.001-S89.399 with 7th [K, P], S92.001-S92.919 with 7th [K, P]

7 √7ᵗʰ **S42.402 Unspecified fracture of lower end of left humerus**   MCC CC
CC Excl: CC with 7th character A: S42.201-S42.266 with 7th B, S42.272-S42.309 with 7th A, S42.312-S42.476 with 7th A, S42.482-S42.92X with 7th A, S49.002-S49.009 with 7th A, S49.012-S49.019 with 7th A, S49.022-S49.029 with 7th A, S49.032-S49.039 with 7th A, S49.042-S49.049 with 7th A, S49.092-S49.099 with 7th A, S49.102-S49.109 with 7th A, S49.112-S49.119 with 7th A, S49.122-S49.129 with 7th A, S49.132-S49.139 with 7th A, S49.142-S49.149 with 7th A, S49.192-S49.199 with 7th A
MCC with 7th character B: S42.201-S42.266 with 7th B, S42.291-S42.92X with 7th B, S49.101-S49.199 with 7th A, S62.90XB
CC with 7th character K or P: M80.00X-M84.68X with 7th [K, P], S02.0XX-S02.92X with 7th K, S12.000-S12.691 with 7th K, S22.000-S22.9XX with 7th K, S32.000-S32.9XX with 7th K, S42.001-S42.92X with 7th [K, P], S49.001-S49.199 with 7th [K, P], S52.001-S52.92X with 7th [K, M, N, P, Q, R], S59.001-S59.299 with 7th [K, P], S62.001-S62.92X with 7th [K, P], S72.001-S72.92X with 7th [K, M, N, P, Q, R], S79.001-S79.199 with 7th [K, P], S82.001-S82.92X with 7th [K, M, N, P, Q, R], S89.001-S89.399 with 7th [K, P], S92.001-S92.919 with 7th [K, P]

7 √7ᵗʰ **S42.409 Unspecified fracture of lower end of unspecified humerus**   MCC CC
CC Excl: CC with 7th character A: S42.201-S42.92X with 7th [A, B], S49.001-S49.199 with 7th A
MCC with 7th character B: S42.201-S42.266 with 7th B, S42.291-S42.92X with 7th B, S49.101-S49.199 with 7th A, S62.90XB
CC with 7th character K or P: M80.00X-M84.68X with 7th [K, P], S02.0XX-S02.92X with 7th K, S12.000-S12.691 with 7th K, S22.000-S22.9XX with 7th K, S32.000-S32.9XX with 7th K, S42.001-S42.92X with 7th [K, P], S49.001-S49.199 with 7th [K, P], S52.001-S52.92X with 7th [K, M, N, P, Q, R], S59.001-S59.299 with 7th [K, P], S62.001-S62.92X with 7th [K, P], S72.001-S72.92X with 7th [K, M, N, P, Q, R], S79.001-S79.199 with 7th [K, P], S82.001-S82.92X with 7th [K, M, N, P, Q, R], S89.001-S89.399 with 7th [K, P], S92.001-S92.919 with 7th [K, P]

√6ᵗʰ **S42.41 Simple supracondylar fracture without intercondylar fracture of humerus**

7 √7ᵗʰ **S42.411 Displaced simple supracondylar fracture without intercondylar fracture of right humerus**   MCC CC
CC Excl: See code: S42.401

7 √7ᵗʰ **S42.412 Displaced simple supracondylar fracture without intercondylar fracture of left humerus**   MCC CC
CC Excl: See code: S42.402

7 √7ᵗʰ **S42.413 Displaced simple supracondylar fracture without intercondylar fracture of unspecified humerus**   MCC CC
CC Excl: See code: S42.409

7 √7ᵗʰ **S42.414 Nondisplaced simple supracondylar fracture without intercondylar fracture of right humerus**   MCC CC
CC Excl: See code: S42.401

7 √7ᵗʰ **S42.415 Nondisplaced simple supracondylar fracture without intercondylar fracture of left humerus**   MCC CC
CC Excl: See code: S42.402

7 √7ᵗʰ **S42.416 Nondisplaced simple supracondylar fracture without intercondylar fracture of unspecified humerus**   MCC CC
CC Excl: See code: S42.409

√6ᵗʰ **S42.42 Comminuted supracondylar fracture without intercondylar fracture of humerus**

7 √7ᵗʰ **S42.421 Displaced comminuted supracondylar fracture without intercondylar fracture of right humerus**   MCC CC
CC Excl: See code: S42.401

7 √7ᵗʰ **S42.422 Displaced comminuted supracondylar fracture without intercondylar fracture of left humerus**   MCC CC
CC Excl: See code: S42.402

7 √7ᵗʰ **S42.423 Displaced comminuted supracondylar fracture without intercondylar fracture of unspecified humerus**   MCC CC
CC Excl: See code: S42.409

7 √7ᵗʰ **S42.424 Nondisplaced comminuted supracondylar fracture without intercondylar fracture of right humerus**   MCC CC
CC Excl: See code: S42.401

7 √7ᵗʰ **S42.425 Nondisplaced comminuted supracondylar fracture without intercondylar fracture of left humerus**   MCC CC
CC Excl: See code: S42.402

7 √7ᵗʰ **S42.426 Nondisplaced comminuted supracondylar fracture without intercondylar fracture of unspecified humerus**   MCC CC
CC Excl: See code: S42.409

√6ᵗʰ **S42.43 Fracture (avulsion) of lateral epicondyle of humerus**

7 √7ᵗʰ **S42.431 Displaced fracture (avulsion) of lateral epicondyle of right humerus**   MCC CC
CC Excl: See code: S42.401

7 √7ᵗʰ **S42.432 Displaced fracture (avulsion) of lateral epicondyle of left humerus**   MCC CC
CC Excl: See code: S42.402

7 √7ᵗʰ **S42.433 Displaced fracture (avulsion) of lateral epicondyle of unspecified humerus**   MCC CC
CC Excl: See code: S42.409

7 √7ᵗʰ **S42.434 Nondisplaced fracture (avulsion) of lateral epicondyle of right humerus**   MCC CC
CC Excl: See code: S42.401

7 √7ᵗʰ **S42.435 Nondisplaced fracture (avulsion) of lateral epicondyle of left humerus**   MCC CC
CC Excl: See code: S42.402

---

7 HAC = Initial encounter only (7th character A, B or C) and not POA.

☑ Additional Character Required   √x7ᵗʰ Xtension Alert   Unacceptable PDx   Manifestation   Hospital Acquired Condition   EXCLUDES 1 Not Coded Here   EXCLUDES 2 Not Included Here

7 ✓7th **S42.436** **Nondisplaced** fracture (avulsion) of lateral epicondyle of **unspecified humerus** MCC CC
CC Excl: See code: S42.409

✓6th **S42.44** Fracture (avulsion) of **medial epicondyle** of humerus

7 ✓7th **S42.441** **Displaced** fracture (avulsion) of medial epicondyle of **right** humerus MCC CC
CC Excl: See code: S42.401

7 ✓7th **S42.442** **Displaced** fracture (avulsion) of medial epicondyle of **left** humerus MCC CC
CC Excl: See code: S42.402

7 ✓7th **S42.443** **Displaced** fracture (avulsion) of medial epicondyle of **unspecified** humerus MCC CC
CC Excl: See code: S42.409

7 ✓7th **S42.444** **Nondisplaced** fracture (avulsion) of medial epicondyle of **right** humerus MCC CC
CC Excl: See code: S42.401

7 ✓7th **S42.445** **Nondisplaced** fracture (avulsion) of medial epicondyle of **left** humerus MCC CC
CC Excl: See code: S42.402

7 ✓7th **S42.446** **Nondisplaced** fracture (avulsion) medial epicondyle of **unspecified** of humerus MCC CC
CC Excl: See code: S42.409

7 ✓7th **S42.447** **Incarcerated** fracture (avulsion) of medial epicondyle of **right** humerus MCC CC
CC Excl: See code: S42.401

7 ✓7th **S42.448** **Incarcerated** fracture (avulsion) of medial epicondyle of **left** humerus MCC CC
CC Excl: See code: S42.402

7 ✓7th **S42.449** **Incarcerated** fracture (avulsion) of medial epicondyle of **unspecified** humerus MCC CC
CC Excl: See code: S42.409

✓6th **S42.45** Fracture of **lateral condyle** of humerus
Fracture of capitellum of humerus

7 ✓7th **S42.451** **Displaced** fracture of lateral condyle of **right** humerus MCC CC
CC Excl: See code: S42.401

7 ✓7th **S42.452** **Displaced** fracture of lateral condyle of **left** humerus MCC CC
CC Excl: See code: S42.402

7 ✓7th **S42.453** **Displaced** fracture of lateral condyle of **unspecified** humerus MCC CC
CC Excl: See code: S42.409

7 ✓7th **S42.454** **Nondisplaced** fracture of lateral condyle of **right** humerus MCC CC
CC Excl: See code: S42.401

7 ✓7th **S42.455** **Nondisplaced** fracture of lateral condyle of **left** humerus MCC CC
CC Excl: See code: S42.402

7 ✓7th **S42.456** **Nondisplaced** fracture of lateral condyle of **unspecified** humerus MCC CC
CC Excl: See code: S42.409

✓6th **S42.46** Fracture of **medial condyle** of humerus
Trochlea fracture of humerus

7 ✓7th **S42.461** **Displaced** fracture of medial condyle of **right** humerus MCC CC
CC Excl: See code: S42.401

7 ✓7th **S42.462** **Displaced** fracture of medial condyle of **left** humerus MCC CC
CC Excl: See code: S42.402

7 ✓7th **S42.463** **Displaced** fracture of medial condyle of **unspecified** humerus MCC CC
CC Excl: See code: S42.409

7 ✓7th **S42.464** **Nondisplaced** fracture of medial condyle of **right** humerus MCC CC
CC Excl: See code: S42.401

7 ✓7th **S42.465** **Nondisplaced** fracture of medial condyle of **left** humerus MCC CC
CC Excl: See code: S42.402

7 ✓7th **S42.466** **Nondisplaced** fracture of medial condyle of **unspecified** humerus MCC CC
CC Excl: See code: S42.409

✓6th **S42.47** **Transcondylar** fracture of humerus

7 ✓7th **S42.471** **Displaced transcondylar fracture of right humerus** MCC CC
CC Excl: See code: S42.401

7 ✓7th **S42.472** **Displaced transcondylar fracture of left humerus** MCC CC
CC Excl: See code: S42.402

7 ✓7th **S42.473** **Displaced transcondylar fracture of unspecified humerus** MCC CC
CC Excl: See code: S42.409

7 ✓7th **S42.474** **Nondisplaced transcondylar fracture of right humerus** MCC CC
CC Excl: See code: S42.401

7 ✓7th **S42.475** **Nondisplaced transcondylar fracture of left humerus** MCC CC
CC Excl: See code: S42.402

7 ✓7th **S42.476** **Nondisplaced transcondylar fracture of unspecified humerus** MCC CC
CC Excl: See code: S42.409

✓6th **S42.48** **Torus** fracture of lower end of humerus

> The appropriate 7th is to be added to all codes in subcategory S42.48.
> A   initial encounter for closed fracture
> D   subsequent encounter for fracture with routine healing
> G   subsequent encounter for fracture with delayed healing
> K   subsequent encounter for fracture with nonunion
> P   subsequent encounter for fracture with malunion
> S   sequela

7 ✓7th **S42.481** **Torus fracture of lower end of right humerus** CC
CC Excl: CC with 7th character A: S42.201-S42.271 with 7th [A, B], S42.279-S42.311 with 7th A, S42.319-S42.481 with 7th A, S42.489-S42.92X with 7th A, S49.001A, S49.009-S49.011 with 7th A, S49.019-S49.021 with 7th A, S49.029-S49.031 with 7th A, S49.039-S49.041 with 7th A, S49.049-S49.091 with 7th A, S49.099-S49.101 with 7th A, S49.109-S49.111 with 7th A, S49.119-S49.121 with 7th A, S49.129-S49.131 with 7th A, S49.139-S49.141 with 7th A, S49.149-S49.191 with 7th A, S49.199A
CC Excl: with 7th K or P: M80.00X-M84.68X with 7th [K, P], S02.0XX-S02.92X with 7th K, S12.000-S12.691 with 7th K, S22.000-S22.9XX with 7th K, S32.000-S32.9XX with 7th K, S42.001-S42.92X with 7th [K, P], S49.001-S49.199 with 7th [K, P], S52.001-S52.92X with 7th [K, M, N, P, Q, R], S59.001-S59.299 with 7th [K, P], S62.001-S62.92X with 7th [K, P], S72.001-S72.92X with 7th [K, M, N, P, Q, R], S79.001-S79.199 with 7th [K, P], S82.001-S82.92X with 7th [K, M, N, P, Q, R], S89.001-S89.399 with 7th [K, P], S92.001-S92.919 with 7th [K, P]

7 ✓7th **S42.482** **Torus fracture of lower end of left humerus** CC
CC Excl: CC with 7th character A: S42.201-S42.266 with 7th B, S42.272-S42.309 with 7th A, S42.312-S42.476 with 7th A, S42.482-S42.92X with 7th A, S49.002-S49.009 with 7th A, S49.012-S49.019 with 7th A, S49.022-S49.029 with 7th A, S49.032-S49.039 with 7th A, S49.042-S49.049 with 7th A, S49.092-S49.099 with 7th A, S49.102-S49.109 with 7th A, S49.112-S49.119 with 7th A, S49.122-S49.129 with 7th A, S49.132-S49.139 with 7th A, S49.142-S49.149 with 7th A, S49.192-S49.199 with 7th A
CC Excl: with 7th K or P: M80.00X-M84.68X with 7th [K, P], S02.0XX-S02.92X with 7th K, S12.000-S12.691 with 7th K, S22.000-S22.9XX with 7th K, S32.000-S32.9XX with 7th K, S42.001-S42.92X with 7th [K, P], S49.001-S49.199 with 7th [K, P], S52.001-S52.92X with 7th [K, M, N, P, Q, R], S59.001-S59.299 with 7th [K, P], S62.001-S62.92X with 7th [K, P], S72.001-S72.92X with 7th [K, M, N, P, Q, R], S79.001-S79.199 with 7th [K, P], S82.001-S82.92X with 7th [K, M, N, P, Q, R],

---

7 HAC = Initial encounter only (7th character A, B or C) and not POA.

N Newborn: 0   P Pediatric: 0-17   M Maternity: 12-55   A Adult: 15-124   MCC Major CC Condition   PDx MCC PDx acts as own MCC   CC CC Condition   PDx CC PDx acts as own CC

910   ICD-10-CM Draft (2015)

S89.001-S89.399 with 7th [K, P], S92.001-
S92.919 with 7th [K, P]

7 ✓7ᵗʰ **S42.489** **Torus fracture of lower end of** `CC`
unspecified humerus
CC Excl: CC with 7th character A: S42.201-
S42.92X with 7th [A, B], S49.001-S49.199
with 7th A
CC Excl: CC with 7th character K or P:
M80.00X-M84.68X with 7th [K, P], S02.0XX-
S02.92X with 7th K, S12.000-S12.691 with
7th K, S22.000-S22.9XX with 7th K, S32.000-
S32.9XX with 7th K, S42.001-S42.92X with
7th [K, P], S49.001-S49.199 with 7th [K, P],
S52.001-S52.92X with 7th [K, M, N, P, Q, R],
S59.001-S59.299 with 7th [K, P], S62.001-
S62.92X with 7th [K, P], S72.001-S72.92X
with 7th [K, M, N, P, Q, R], S79.001-S79.199
with 7th [K, P], S82.001-S82.92X with 7th [K,
M, N, P, Q, R], S89.001-S89.399 with 7th [K, P],
S92.001-S92.919 with 7th [K, P]

✓6ᵗʰ **S42.49** Other fracture of lower end of humerus

7 ✓7ᵗʰ **S42.491** **Other displaced fracture of lower** `MCC` `CC`
end of right humerus
CC Excl: See code: S42.401

7 ✓7ᵗʰ **S42.492** **Other displaced fracture of lower** `MCC` `CC`
end of left humerus
CC Excl: See code: S42.402

7 ✓7ᵗʰ **S42.493** **Other displaced fracture of lower** `MCC` `CC`
end of unspecified humerus
CC Excl: See code: S42.409

7 ✓7ᵗʰ **S42.494** **Other nondisplaced fracture of** `MCC` `CC`
lower end of right humerus
CC Excl: See code: S42.401

7 ✓7ᵗʰ **S42.495** **Other nondisplaced fracture of** `MCC` `CC`
lower end of left humerus
CC Excl: See code: S42.402

7 ✓7ᵗʰ **S42.496** **Other nondisplaced fracture of** `MCC` `CC`
lower end of unspecified humerus
CC Excl: See code: S42.409

✓5ᵗʰ **S42.9** **Fracture of shoulder girdle, part unspecified**
Fracture of shoulder NOS

7 ✓×7ᵗʰ **S42.90** **Fracture of unspecified shoulder girdle,** `MCC` `CC`
part unspecified
CC Excl: See code: S42.409

7 ✓×7ᵗʰ **S42.91** **Fracture of right shoulder girdle, part** `MCC` `CC`
unspecified
CC Excl: See code: S42.409

7 ✓×7ᵗʰ **S42.92** **Fracture of left shoulder girdle, part** `MCC` `CC`
unspecified
CC Excl: See code: S42.409

✓4ᵗʰ **S43** **Dislocation and sprain of joints and ligaments of shoulder girdle**
`INCLUDES` avulsion of joint or ligament of shoulder girdle
laceration of cartilage, joint or ligament of shoulder girdle
sprain of cartilage, joint or ligament of shoulder girdle
traumatic hemarthrosis of joint or ligament of shoulder girdle
traumatic rupture of joint or ligament of shoulder girdle
traumatic subluxation of joint or ligament of shoulder girdle
traumatic tear of joint or ligament of shoulder girdle

Code also any associated open wound
`EXCLUDES 2` strain of muscle, fascia and tendon of shoulder and upper arm
(S46.-)

The appropriate 7th is to be added to each code from category
S43.
A   initial encounter
D   subsequent encounter
S   sequela

✓5ᵗʰ **S43.0** **Subluxation and dislocation of shoulder joint**
Dislocation of glenohumeral joint
Subluxation of glenohumeral joint

✓6ᵗʰ **S43.00** **Unspecified subluxation and dislocation of shoulder**
joint
Dislocation of humerus NOS
Subluxation of humerus NOS

✓7ᵗʰ **S43.001** **Unspecified subluxation of right shoulder**
joint

✓7ᵗʰ **S43.002** **Unspecified subluxation of left shoulder**
joint

✓7ᵗʰ **S43.003** **Unspecified subluxation of unspecified**
shoulder joint

✓7ᵗʰ **S43.004** **Unspecified dislocation of right shoulder**
joint

✓7ᵗʰ **S43.005** **Unspecified dislocation of left shoulder**
joint

✓7ᵗʰ **S43.006** **Unspecified dislocation of unspecified**
shoulder joint

✓6ᵗʰ **S43.01** Anterior subluxation and dislocation of humerus

✓7ᵗʰ **S43.011** **Anterior subluxation of right humerus**

✓7ᵗʰ **S43.012** **Anterior subluxation of left humerus**

✓7ᵗʰ **S43.013** **Anterior subluxation of unspecified**
humerus

✓7ᵗʰ **S43.014** **Anterior dislocation of right humerus**

✓7ᵗʰ **S43.015** **Anterior dislocation of left humerus**

✓7ᵗʰ **S43.016** **Anterior dislocation of unspecified**
humerus

✓6ᵗʰ **S43.02** Posterior subluxation and dislocation of humerus

✓7ᵗʰ **S43.021** **Posterior subluxation of right humerus**

✓7ᵗʰ **S43.022** **Posterior subluxation of left humerus**

✓7ᵗʰ **S43.023** **Posterior subluxation of unspecified**
humerus

✓7ᵗʰ **S43.024** **Posterior dislocation of right humerus**

✓7ᵗʰ **S43.025** **Posterior dislocation of left humerus**

✓7ᵗʰ **S43.026** **Posterior dislocation of unspecified**
humerus

✓6ᵗʰ **S43.03** Inferior subluxation and dislocation of humerus

✓7ᵗʰ **S43.031** **Inferior subluxation of right humerus**

✓7ᵗʰ **S43.032** **Inferior subluxation of left humerus**

✓7ᵗʰ **S43.033** **Inferior subluxation of unspecified**
humerus

✓7ᵗʰ **S43.034** **Inferior dislocation of right humerus**

✓7ᵗʰ **S43.035** **Inferior dislocation of left humerus**

✓7ᵗʰ **S43.036** **Inferior dislocation of unspecified**
humerus

✓6ᵗʰ **S43.08** Other subluxation and dislocation of shoulder joint

✓7ᵗʰ **S43.081** **Other subluxation of right shoulder joint**

✓7ᵗʰ **S43.082** **Other subluxation of left shoulder joint**

✓7ᵗʰ **S43.083** **Other subluxation of unspecified shoulder**
joint

✓7ᵗʰ **S43.084** **Other dislocation of right shoulder joint**

✓7ᵗʰ **S43.085** **Other dislocation of left shoulder joint**

✓7ᵗʰ **S43.086** **Other dislocation of unspecified shoulder**
joint

✓5ᵗʰ **S43.1** **Subluxation and dislocation of acromioclavicular joint**

✓6ᵗʰ **S43.10** **Unspecified dislocation of acromioclavicular joint**

✓7ᵗʰ **S43.101** **Unspecified dislocation of right**
acromioclavicular joint

✓7ᵗʰ **S43.102** **Unspecified dislocation of left**
acromioclavicular joint

✓7ᵗʰ **S43.109** **Unspecified dislocation of unspecified**
acromioclavicular joint

✓6ᵗʰ **S43.11** **Subluxation of acromioclavicular joint**

✓7ᵗʰ **S43.111** **Subluxation of right acromioclavicular**
joint

✓7ᵗʰ **S43.112** **Subluxation of left acromioclavicular joint**

✓7ᵗʰ **S43.119** **Subluxation of unspecified**
acromioclavicular joint

✓6ᵗʰ **S43.12** **Dislocation of acromioclavicular joint, 100%-200%**
displacement

✓7ᵗʰ **S43.121** **Dislocation of right acromioclavicular**
joint, 100%-200% displacement

✓7ᵗʰ **S43.122** **Dislocation of left acromioclavicular joint,**
100%-200% displacement

✓7ᵗʰ **S43.129** **Dislocation of unspecified**
acromioclavicular joint, 100%-200%
displacement

✓6ᵗʰ **S43.13** **Dislocation of acromioclavicular joint, greater than**
200% displacement

✓7ᵗʰ **S43.131** **Dislocation of right acromioclavicular**
joint, greater than 200% displacement

✓7ᵗʰ **S43.132** **Dislocation of left acromioclavicular joint,**
greater than 200% displacement

---

7 HAC = Initial encounter only (7th character A, B or C) and not POA.

✓ Additional Character Required   ✓×7ᵗʰ Xtension Alert   Unacceptable PDx   Manifestation   Hospital Acquired Condition   `EXCLUDES 1` Not Coded Here   `EXCLUDES 2` Not Included Here

✓7ᵗʰ **S43.139** **Dislocation of** unspecified **acromioclavicular joint, greater than 200% displacement**

✓6ᵗʰ **S43.14** **Inferior dislocation of acromioclavicular joint**

✓7ᵗʰ **S43.141** **Inferior dislocation of** right **acromioclavicular joint**

✓7ᵗʰ **S43.142** **Inferior dislocation of** left **acromioclavicular joint**

✓7ᵗʰ **S43.149** **Inferior dislocation of** unspecified **acromioclavicular joint**

✓6ᵗʰ **S43.15** **Posterior dislocation of acromioclavicular joint**

✓7ᵗʰ **S43.151** **Posterior dislocation of** right **acromioclavicular joint**

✓7ᵗʰ **S43.152** **Posterior dislocation of** left **acromioclavicular joint**

✓7ᵗʰ **S43.159** **Posterior dislocation of** unspecified **acromioclavicular joint**

✓5ᵗʰ **S43.2** **Subluxation and dislocation of** sternoclavicular joint

✓6ᵗʰ **S43.20** Unspecified **subluxation and dislocation of sternoclavicular joint**

7 ✓7ᵗʰ **S43.201** **Unspecified** subluxation **of** right **sternoclavicular joint** `CC`
CC Excl: CC with 7th character A: M99.18, S43.201 with 7th A, S43.203-S43.204 with 7th A, S43.206-S43.211 with 7th A, S43.213-S43.214 with 7th A, S43.216-S43.221 with 7th A, S43.223-S43.224 with 7th A, S43.226A

7 ✓7ᵗʰ **S43.202** **Unspecified** subluxation **of** left **sternoclavicular joint** `CC`
CC Excl: CC with 7th character A: M99.18, S43.202-S43.203 with 7th A, S43.205-S43.206 with 7th A, S43.212-S43.213 with 7th A, S43.215-S43.216 with 7th A, S43.222-S43.223 with 7th A, S43.225-S43.226 with 7th A

7 ✓7ᵗʰ **S43.203** **Unspecified** subluxation **of** unspecified **sternoclavicular joint** `CC`
CC Excl: CC with 7th character A: M99.18, S43.201-S43.226 with 7th A

7 ✓7ᵗʰ **S43.204** **Unspecified** dislocation **of** right **sternoclavicular joint** `CC`
CC Excl: See code: S43.201

7 ✓7ᵗʰ **S43.205** **Unspecified** dislocation **of** left **sternoclavicular joint** `CC`
CC Excl: See code: S43.202

7 ✓7ᵗʰ **S43.206** **Unspecified** dislocation **of** unspecified **sternoclavicular joint** `CC`
CC Excl: See code: S43.203

✓6ᵗʰ **S43.21** Anterior **subluxation and dislocation of sternoclavicular joint**

7 ✓7ᵗʰ **S43.211** Anterior subluxation **of** right **sternoclavicular joint** `CC`
CC Excl: See code: S43.201

7 ✓7ᵗʰ **S43.212** Anterior subluxation **of** left **sternoclavicular joint** `CC`
CC Excl: See code: S43.202

7 ✓7ᵗʰ **S43.213** Anterior subluxation **of** unspecified **sternoclavicular joint** `CC`
CC Excl: See code: S43.203

7 ✓7ᵗʰ **S43.214** Anterior dislocation **of** right **sternoclavicular joint** `CC`
CC Excl: See code: S43.201

7 ✓7ᵗʰ **S43.215** Anterior dislocation **of** left **sternoclavicular joint** `CC`
CC Excl: See code: S43.202

7 ✓7ᵗʰ **S43.216** Anterior dislocation **of** unspecified **sternoclavicular joint** `CC`
CC Excl: See code: S43.203

✓6ᵗʰ **S43.22** Posterior **subluxation and dislocation of sternoclavicular joint**

7 ✓7ᵗʰ **S43.221** Posterior subluxation **of** right **sternoclavicular joint** `CC`
CC Excl: See code: S43.201

7 ✓7ᵗʰ **S43.222** Posterior subluxation **of** left **sternoclavicular joint** `CC`
CC Excl: See code: S43.202

7 ✓7ᵗʰ **S43.223** Posterior subluxation **of** unspecified **sternoclavicular joint** `CC`
CC Excl: See code: S43.203

7 ✓7ᵗʰ **S43.224** Posterior dislocation **of** right **sternoclavicular joint** `CC`
CC Excl: See code: S43.201

7 ✓7ᵗʰ **S43.225** Posterior dislocation **of** left **sternoclavicular joint** `CC`
CC Excl: See code: S43.202

7 ✓7ᵗʰ **S43.226** Posterior dislocation **of** unspecified **sternoclavicular joint** `CC`
CC Excl: See code: S43.203

✓5ᵗʰ **S43.3** **Subluxation and dislocation of other and unspecified parts of shoulder girdle**

✓6ᵗʰ **S43.30** **Subluxation and dislocation of** unspecified **parts of shoulder girdle**
Dislocation of shoulder girdle NOS
Subluxation of shoulder girdle NOS

✓7ᵗʰ **S43.301** **Subluxation of unspecified parts of** right **shoulder girdle**

✓7ᵗʰ **S43.302** **Subluxation of unspecified parts of** left **shoulder girdle**

✓7ᵗʰ **S43.303** **Subluxation of unspecified parts of** unspecified **shoulder girdle**

✓7ᵗʰ **S43.304** **Dislocation of unspecified parts of** right **shoulder girdle**

✓7ᵗʰ **S43.305** **Dislocation of unspecified parts of** left **shoulder girdle**

✓7ᵗʰ **S43.306** **Dislocation of unspecified parts of** unspecified **shoulder girdle**

✓6ᵗʰ **S43.31** **Subluxation and dislocation of scapula**

✓7ᵗʰ **S43.311** **Subluxation of** right **scapula**

✓7ᵗʰ **S43.312** **Subluxation of** left **scapula**

✓7ᵗʰ **S43.313** **Subluxation of** unspecified **scapula**

✓7ᵗʰ **S43.314** **Dislocation of** right **scapula**

✓7ᵗʰ **S43.315** **Dislocation of** left **scapula**

✓7ᵗʰ **S43.316** **Dislocation of** unspecified **scapula**

✓6ᵗʰ **S43.39** **Subluxation and dislocation of other parts of shoulder girdle**

✓7ᵗʰ **S43.391** **Subluxation of other parts of** right **shoulder girdle**

✓7ᵗʰ **S43.392** **Subluxation of other parts of** left **shoulder girdle**

✓7ᵗʰ **S43.393** **Subluxation of other parts of** unspecified **shoulder girdle**

✓7ᵗʰ **S43.394** **Dislocation of other parts of** right **shoulder girdle**

✓7ᵗʰ **S43.395** **Dislocation of other parts of** left **shoulder girdle**

✓7ᵗʰ **S43.396** **Dislocation of other parts of** unspecified **shoulder girdle**

✓5ᵗʰ **S43.4** **Sprain of** shoulder joint

✓6ᵗʰ **S43.40** Unspecified **sprain of shoulder joint**

✓7ᵗʰ **S43.401** **Unspecified sprain of** right **shoulder joint**

✓7ᵗʰ **S43.402** **Unspecified sprain of** left **shoulder joint**

✓7ᵗʰ **S43.409** **Unspecified sprain of** unspecified **shoulder joint**

✓6ᵗʰ **S43.41** **Sprain of coracohumeral (ligament)**

✓7ᵗʰ **S43.411** **Sprain of** right **coracohumeral (ligament)**

✓7ᵗʰ **S43.412** **Sprain of** left **coracohumeral (ligament)**

✓7ᵗʰ **S43.419** **Sprain of** unspecified **coracohumeral (ligament)**

✓6ᵗʰ **S43.42** **Sprain of rotator cuff capsule**
EXCLUDES 1 *rotator cuff syndrome (complete) (incomplete), not specified as traumatic (M75.1-)*
EXCLUDES 2 *injury of tendon of rotator cuff (S46.0-)*

✓7ᵗʰ **S43.421** **Sprain of** right **rotator cuff capsule**

✓7ᵗʰ **S43.422** **Sprain of** left **rotator cuff capsule**

✓7ᵗʰ **S43.429** **Sprain of** unspecified **rotator cuff capsule**

✓6ᵗʰ **S43.43** **Superior glenoid labrum lesion**
SLAP lesion

✓7ᵗʰ **S43.431** **Superior glenoid labrum lesion of** right **shoulder**

✓7ᵗʰ **S43.432** **Superior glenoid labrum lesion of** left **shoulder**

7 HAC = Initial encounter only (7th character A, B or C) and not POA.

Ⓝ Newborn: 0   Ⓟ Pediatric: 0-17   Ⓜ Maternity: 12-55   Ⓐ Adult: 15-124   **MCC** Major CC Condition   **PDx MCC** PDx acts as own MCC   **CC** CC Condition   **PDx CC** PDx acts as own CC

912

ICD-10-CM Draft (2015)

√7th **S43.439** Superior glenoid labrum lesion of unspecified shoulder

√6th **S43.49** Other sprain of shoulder joint

    √7th **S43.491** Other sprain of right shoulder joint

    √7th **S43.492** Other sprain of left shoulder joint

    √7th **S43.499** Other sprain of unspecified shoulder joint

√5th **S43.5** Sprain of acromioclavicular joint
Sprain of acromioclavicular ligament

    √x7th **S43.50** Sprain of unspecified acromioclavicular joint

    √x7th **S43.51** Sprain of right acromioclavicular joint

    √x7th **S43.52** Sprain of left acromioclavicular joint

√5th **S43.6** Sprain of sternoclavicular joint

    √x7th **S43.60** Sprain of unspecified sternoclavicular joint

    √x7th **S43.61** Sprain of right sternoclavicular joint

    √x7th **S43.62** Sprain of left sternoclavicular joint

√5th **S43.8** Sprain of other specified parts of shoulder girdle

    √x7th **S43.80** Sprain of other specified parts of unspecified shoulder girdle

    √x7th **S43.81** Sprain of other specified parts of right shoulder girdle

    √x7th **S43.82** Sprain of other specified parts of left shoulder girdle

√5th **S43.9** Sprain of unspecified parts of shoulder girdle

    √x7th **S43.90** Sprain of unspecified parts of unspecified shoulder girdle
         Sprain of shoulder girdle NOS

    √x7th **S43.91** Sprain of unspecified parts of right shoulder girdle

    √x7th **S43.92** Sprain of unspecified parts of left shoulder girdle

√4th **S44** Injury of nerves at shoulder and upper arm level
Code also any associated open wound (S41.-)
EXCLUDES 2 *injury of brachial plexus (S14.3-)*

The appropriate 7th is to be added to each code from category S44.
A   initial encounter
D   subsequent encounter
S   sequela

√5th **S44.0** Injury of ulnar nerve at upper arm level
EXCLUDES 1 *ulnar nerve NOS (S54.0)*

    √x7th **S44.00** Injury of ulnar nerve at upper arm level, unspecified arm

    √x7th **S44.01** Injury of ulnar nerve at upper arm level, right arm

    √x7th **S44.02** Injury of ulnar nerve at upper arm level, left arm

√5th **S44.1** Injury of median nerve at upper arm level
EXCLUDES 1 *median nerve NOS (S54.1)*

    √x7th **S44.10** Injury of median nerve at upper arm level, unspecified arm

    √x7th **S44.11** Injury of median nerve at upper arm level, right arm

    √x7th **S44.12** Injury of median nerve at upper arm level, left arm

√5th **S44.2** Injury of radial nerve at upper arm level
EXCLUDES 1 *radial nerve NOS (S54.2)*

    √x7th **S44.20** Injury of radial nerve at upper arm level, unspecified arm

    √x7th **S44.21** Injury of radial nerve at upper arm level, right arm

    √x7th **S44.22** Injury of radial nerve at upper arm level, left arm

√5th **S44.3** Injury of axillary nerve

    √x7th **S44.30** Injury of axillary nerve, unspecified arm

    √x7th **S44.31** Injury of axillary nerve, right arm

    √x7th **S44.32** Injury of axillary nerve, left arm

√5th **S44.4** Injury of musculocutaneous nerve

    √x7th **S44.40** Injury of musculocutaneous nerve, unspecified arm

    √x7th **S44.41** Injury of musculocutaneous nerve, right arm

    √x7th **S44.42** Injury of musculocutaneous nerve, left arm

√5th **S44.5** Injury of cutaneous sensory nerve at shoulder and upper arm level

    √x7th **S44.50** Injury of cutaneous sensory nerve at shoulder and upper arm level, unspecified arm

    √x7th **S44.51** Injury of cutaneous sensory nerve at shoulder and upper arm level, right arm

    √x7th **S44.52** Injury of cutaneous sensory nerve at shoulder and upper arm level, left arm

√5th **S44.8** Injury of other nerves at shoulder and upper arm level

√6th **S44.8X** Injury of other nerves at shoulder and upper arm level

    √7th **S44.8X1** Injury of other nerves at shoulder and upper arm level, right arm

    √7th **S44.8X2** Injury of other nerves at shoulder and upper arm level, left arm

    √7th **S44.8X9** Injury of other nerves at shoulder and upper arm level, unspecified arm

√5th **S44.9** Injury of unspecified nerve at shoulder and upper arm level

    √x7th **S44.90** Injury of unspecified nerve at shoulder and upper arm level, unspecified arm

    √x7th **S44.91** Injury of unspecified nerve at shoulder and upper arm level, right arm

    √x7th **S44.92** Injury of unspecified nerve at shoulder and upper arm level, left arm

√4th **S45** Injury of blood vessels at shoulder and upper arm level
Code also any associated open wound (S41.-)
EXCLUDES 2 *injury of subclavian artery (S25.1)*
          injury of subclavian vein (S25.3)

The appropriate 7th is to be added to each code from category S45.
A   initial encounter
D   subsequent encounter
S   sequela

√5th **S45.0** Injury of axillary artery

√6th **S45.00** Unspecified injury of axillary artery

    √7th **S45.001** Unspecified injury of axillary artery, right side   MCC
         CC Excl: MCC with 7th character A:
         S45.001A, S45.009-S45.011 with 7th A, S45.019-S45.091 with 7th A, S45.099A, S45.301A, S45.309-S45.311 with 7th A, S45.319-S45.391 with 7th A, S45.399-S45.801 with 7th A, S45.809-S45.811 with 7th A, S45.819-S45.891 with 7th A, S45.899-S45.901 with 7th A, S45.909-S45.911 with 7th A, S45.919-S45.991 with 7th A, S45.999A, S55.201A, S55.209-S55.211 with 7th A, S55.219-S55.291 with 7th A, S55.299-S55.801 with 7th A, S55.809-S55.811 with 7th A, S55.819-S55.891 with 7th A, S55.899-S55.901 with 7th A, S55.909-S55.911 with 7th A, S55.919-S55.991 with 7th A, S55.999A, S65.801A, S65.809-S65.811 with 7th A, S65.819-S65.891 with 7th A, S65.899-S65.901 with 7th A, S65.909-S65.911 with 7th A, S65.919-S65.991 with 7th A, S65.999A

    √7th **S45.002** Unspecified injury of axillary artery, left side   MCC
         CC Excl: MCC with 7th character A:
         S45.002-S45.009 with 7th A, S45.012-S45.019 with 7th A, S45.092-S45.099 with 7th A, S45.302-S45.309 with 7th A, S45.312-S45.319 with 7th A, S45.392-S45.399 with 7th A, S45.802-S45.809 with 7th A, S45.812-S45.819 with 7th A, S45.892-S45.899 with 7th A, S45.902-S45.909 with 7th A, S45.912-S45.919 with 7th A, S45.992-S45.999 with 7th A, S55.202-S55.209 with 7th A, S55.212-S55.219 with 7th A, S55.292-S55.299 with 7th A, S55.802-S55.809 with 7th A, S55.812-S55.819 with 7th A, S55.892-S55.899 with 7th A, S55.902-S55.909 with 7th A, S55.912-S55.919 with 7th A, S55.992-S55.999 with 7th A, S65.802-S65.809 with 7th A, S65.812-S65.819 with 7th A, S65.892-S65.899 with 7th A, S65.902-S65.909 with 7th A, S65.912-S65.919 with 7th A, S65.992-S65.999 with 7th A

    √7th **S45.009** Unspecified injury of axillary artery, unspecified side   MCC
         CC Excl: MCC with 7th character A:
         S45.001-S45.099 with 7th A, S45.301-S45.999 with 7th A, S55.201-S55.999 with 7th A, S65.801-S65.999 with 7th A

✓ Additional Character Required   √x7th Xtension Alert   Unacceptable PDx   Manifestation   Hospital Acquired Condition   EXCLUDES 1 Not Coded Here   EXCLUDES 2 Not Included Here

Injury, Poisoning and Certain Other Consequences of External Causes

S45.01–S45.109

√6th **S45.01** Laceration of axillary artery

√7th **S45.011** **Laceration of axillary artery, right side** MCC
CC Excl: MCC with 7th character A:
S45.001A, S45.009-S45.011 with 7th A,
S45.019-S45.091 with 7th A, S45.099A,
S45.301A, S45.309-S45.311 with 7th A,
S45.319-S45.391 with 7th A, S45.399-
S45.801 with 7th A, S45.809-S45.811 with
7th A, S45.819-S45.891 with 7th A, S45.899-
S45.901 with 7th A, S45.909-S45.911 with
7th A, S45.919-S45.991 with 7th A, S45.999A,
S55.201A, S55.209-S55.211 with 7th A,
S55.219-S55.291 with 7th A, S55.299-
S55.801 with 7th A, S55.809-S55.811 with
7th A, S55.819-S55.891 with 7th A, S55.899-
S55.901 with 7th A, S55.909-S55.911 with
7th A, S55.919-S55.991 with 7th A, S55.999
with 7th A, S65.801A, S65.809-S65.811 with
7th A, S65.819-S65.891 with 7th A, S65.899-
S65.901 with 7th A, S65.909-S65.911 with
7th A, S65.919-S65.991 with 7th A, S65.999A

√7th **S45.012** **Laceration of axillary artery, left side** MCC
CC Excl: MCC with 7th character A:
S45.002-S45.009 with 7th A, S45.012-
S45.019 with 7th A, S45.092-S45.099 with
7th A, S45.302-S45.309 with 7th A, S45.312-
S45.319 with 7th A, S45.392-S45.399 with
7th A, S45.802-S45.809 with 7th A, S45.812-
S45.819 with 7th A, S45.892-S45.899 with
7th A, S45.902-S45.909 with 7th A, S45.912-
S45.919 with 7th A, S45.992-S45.999 with
7th A, S55.202-S55.209 with 7th A, S55.212-
S55.219 with 7th A, S55.292-S55.299 with
7th A, S55.802-S55.809 with 7th A, S55.812-
S55.819 with 7th A, S55.892-S55.899 with
7th A, S55.902-S55.909 with 7th A, S55.912-
S55.919 with 7th A, S55.992-S55.999 with
7th A, S65.802-S65.809 with 7th A, S65.812-
S65.819 with 7th A, S65.892-S65.899 with
7th A, S65.902-S65.909 with 7th A, S65.912-
S65.919 with 7th A, S65.992-S65.999 with
7th A

√7th **S45.019** **Laceration of axillary artery, unspecified side** MCC
CC Excl: MCC with 7th character A:
S45.001-S45.099 with 7th A, S45.301-
S45.999 with 7th A, S55.201-S55.999 with
7th A, S65.801-S65.999 with 7th A

√6th **S45.09** Other specified injury of axillary artery

√7th **S45.091** **Other specified injury of axillary artery, right side** MCC
CC Excl: MCC with 7th character A:
S45.001A, S45.009-S45.011 with 7th A,
S45.019-S45.091 with 7th A, S45.099A,
S45.301A, S45.309-S45.311 with 7th A,
S45.319-S45.391 with 7th A, S45.399-
S45.801 with 7th A, S45.809-S45.811 with
7th A, S45.819-S45.891 with 7th A, S45.899-
S45.901 with 7th A, S45.909-S45.911 with
7th A, S45.919-S45.991 with 7th A, S45.999A,
S55.201A, S55.209-S55.211 with 7th A,
S55.219-S55.291 with 7th A, S55.299-
S55.801 with 7th A, S55.809-S55.811 with
7th A, S55.819-S55.891 with 7th A, S55.899-
S55.901 with 7th A, S55.909-S55.911 with
7th A, S55.919-S55.991 with 7th A, S55.999A,
S65.801A, S65.809-S65.811 with 7th A,
S65.819-S65.891 with 7th A, S65.899-
S65.901 with 7th A, S65.909-S65.911 with
7th A, S65.919-S65.991 with 7th A, S65.999A

√7th **S45.092** **Other specified injury of axillary artery, left side** MCC
CC Excl: MCC with 7th character A:
S45.002-S45.009 with 7th A, S45.012-
S45.019 with 7th A, S45.092-S45.099 with
7th A, S45.302-S45.309 with 7th A, S45.312-
S45.319 with 7th A, S45.392-S45.399 with
7th A, S45.802-S45.809 with 7th A, S45.812-
S45.819 with 7th A, S45.892-S45.899 with
7th A, S45.902-S45.909 with 7th A, S45.912-
S45.919 with 7th A, S45.992-S45.999 with
7th A, S55.202-S55.209 with 7th A, S55.212-
S55.219 with 7th A, S55.292-S55.299 with
7th A, S55.802-S55.809 with 7th A, S55.812-
S55.819 with 7th A, S55.892-S55.899 with
7th A, S55.902-S55.909 with 7th A, S55.912-
S55.919 with 7th A, S55.992-S55.999 with
7th A, S65.802-S65.809 with 7th A, S65.812-
S65.819 with 7th A, S65.892-S65.899 with
7th A, S65.902-S65.909 with 7th A, S65.912-
S65.919 with 7th A, S65.992-S65.999 with
7th A

√7th **S45.099** **Other specified injury of axillary artery, unspecified side** MCC
CC Excl:MCC with 7th character A:
S45.001-S45.099 with 7th A, S45.301-
S45.999 with 7th A, S55.201-S55.999 with
7th A, S65.801-S65.999 with 7th A

√5th **S45.1** Injury of brachial artery

√6th **S45.10** Unspecified injury of brachial artery

√7th **S45.101** **Unspecified injury of brachial artery, right side** CC
CC Excl: CC with 7th character A: S45.101
with 7th A, S45.109-S45.111 with 7th A,
S45.119-S45.191 with 7th A, S45.199-
S45.201 with 7th A, S45.209-S45.211 with
7th A, S45.219-S45.291 with 7th A, S45.299-
S45.301 with 7th A, S45.309-S45.311 with
7th A, S45.319-S45.391 with 7th A, S45.399-
S45.801 with 7th A, S45.809-S45.811 with
7th A, S45.819-S45.891 with 7th A, S45.899-
S45.901 with 7th A, S45.909-S45.911 with
7th A, S45.919-S45.991 with 7th A, S45.999
with 7th A, S55.201 with 7th A, S55.209-
S55.211 with 7th A, S55.219-S55.291 with
7th A, S55.299-S55.801 with 7th A, S55.809-
S55.811 with 7th A, S55.819-S55.891 with
7th A, S55.899-S55.901 with 7th A, S55.909-
S55.911 with 7th A, S55.919-S55.991 with
7th A, S55.999 with 7th A, S65.801 with 7th
A, S65.809-S65.811 with 7th A, S65.819-
S65.891 with 7th A, S65.899-S65.901 with
7th A, S65.909-S65.911 with 7th A, S65.919-
S65.991 with 7th A, S65.999A

√7th **S45.102** **Unspecified injury of brachial artery, left side** CC
CC Excl: CC with 7th character A: S45.102-
S45.109 with 7th A, S45.112-S45.119 with
7th A, S45.192-S45.199 with 7th A, S45.202-
S45.209 with 7th A, S45.212-S45.219 with
7th A, S45.292-S45.299 with 7th A, S45.302-
S45.309 with 7th A, S45.312-S45.319 with
7th A, S45.392-S45.399 with 7th A, S45.802-
S45.809 with 7th A, S45.812-S45.819 with
7th A, S45.892-S45.899 with 7th A, S45.902-
S45.909 with 7th A, S45.912-S45.919 with
7th A, S45.992-S45.999 with 7th A, S55.202-
S55.209 with 7th A, S55.212-S55.219 with
7th A, S55.292-S55.299 with 7th A, S55.802-
S55.809 with 7th A, S55.812-S55.819 with
7th A, S55.892-S55.899 with 7th A, S55.902-
S55.909 with 7th A, S55.912-S55.919 with
7th A, S55.992-S55.999 with 7th A, S65.802-
S65.809 with 7th A, S65.812-S65.819 with
7th A, S65.892-S65.899 with 7th A, S65.902-
S65.909 with 7th A, S65.912-S65.919 with
7th A, S65.992-S65.999 with 7th A

√7th **S45.109** **Unspecified injury of brachial artery, unspecified side** CC
CC Excl: CC with 7th character A: S45.101-
S45.999 with 7th A, S55.201-S55.999 with
7th A, S65.801-S65.999 with 7th A

N Newborn: 0   P Pediatric: 0-17   M Maternity: 12-55   A Adult: 15-124   MCC Major CC Condition   PDx MCC PDx acts as own MCC   CC CC Condition   PDx CC PDx acts as own CC

914   ICD-10-CM Draft (2015)

✓6th **S45.11   Laceration of brachial artery**

✓7th **S45.111   Laceration of brachial artery, right** `CC`
side
CC Excl: See code: S45.101

✓7th **S45.112   Laceration of brachial artery, left side** `CC`
CC Excl: See code: S45.102

✓7th **S45.119   Laceration of brachial artery,** `CC`
unspecified side
CC Excl: See code: S45.109

✓6th **S45.19   Other specified injury of brachial artery**

✓7th **S45.191   Other specified injury of brachial** `CC`
artery, right side
CC Excl: See code: S45.101

✓7th **S45.192   Other specified injury of** `CC`
brachial artery, left side
CC Excl: See code: S45.102

✓7th **S45.199   Other specified injury of brachial** `CC`
artery, unspecified side
CC Excl: See code: S45.109

✓5th **S45.2   Injury of axillary or brachial vein**

✓6th **S45.20   Unspecified injury of axillary or brachial vein**

✓7th **S45.201   Unspecified injury of axillary or** `CC`
brachial vein, right side
CC Excl: See code: S45.101

✓7th **S45.202   Unspecified injury of axillary or** `CC`
brachial vein, left side
CC Excl: See code: S45.102

✓7th **S45.209   Unspecified injury of axillary or** `CC`
brachial vein, unspecified side
CC Excl: See code: S45.109

✓6th **S45.21   Laceration of axillary or brachial vein**

✓7th **S45.211   Laceration of axillary or brachial** `CC`
vein, right side
CC Excl: See code: S45.101

✓7th **S45.212   Laceration of axillary or brachial** `CC`
vein, left side
CC Excl: See code: S45.102

✓7th **S45.219   Laceration of axillary or brachial** `CC`
vein, unspecified side
CC Excl: See code: S45.109

✓6th **S45.29   Other specified injury of axillary or brachial vein**

✓7th **S45.291   Other specified injury of axillary or** `CC`
brachial vein, right side
CC Excl: See code: S45.101

✓7th **S45.292   Other specified injury of axillary or** `CC`
brachial vein, left side
CC Excl: See code: S45.102

✓7th **S45.299   Other specified injury of axillary or** `CC`
brachial vein, unspecified side
CC Excl: See code: S45.109

✓5th **S45.3   Injury of superficial vein at shoulder and upper arm level**

✓6th **S45.30   Unspecified injury of superficial vein at shoulder and upper arm level**

✓7th **S45.301   Unspecified injury of superficial vein** `CC`
at shoulder and upper arm level,
right arm
CC Excl: CC with 7th character A: S45.301A, S45.309-S45.311 with 7th A, S45.319-S45.391 with 7th A, S45.399-S45.801 with 7th A, S45.809-S45.811 with 7th A, S45.819-S45.891 with 7th A, S45.899-S45.901 with 7th A, S45.909-S45.911 with 7th A, S45.919-S45.991 with 7th A, S45.999 with 7th A, S55.001A, S55.009-S55.011 with 7th A, S55.019-S55.091 with 7th A, S55.099 with 7th A, S55.201 with 7th A, S55.209-S55.211 with 7th A, S55.219-S55.291 with 7th A, S55.299-S55.801 with 7th A, S55.809-S55.811 with 7th A, S55.819-S55.891 with 7th A, S55.899-S55.901 with 7th A, S55.909-S55.911 with 7th A, S55.919-S55.991 with 7th A, S55.999 with 7th A, S65.001 with 7th A, S65.009-S65.011 with 7th A, S65.019-S65.091 with 7th A, S65.099 with 7th A, S65.201 with 7th A, S65.209-S65.211 with 7th A, S65.219-S65.291 with 7th A, S65.299-S65.301 with 7th A, S65.309-S65.311 with 7th A, S65.319-S65.391 with 7th A, S65.399-S65.401 with 7th A, S65.409-S65.411 with 7th A, S65.419-S65.491 with 7th A, S65.499-S65.500 with 7th A, S65.502 with 7th A, S65.504 with 7th A, S65.506 with 7th A, S65.508-S65.510 with 7th A, S65.512 with 7th A, S65.514 with 7th A, S65.516 with 7th A, S65.518-S65.590A, S65.592A, S65.594 A, S65.596A, S65.598-S65.801 with 7th A, S65.809-S65.811 with 7th A, S65.819-S65.891 with 7th A, S65.899-S65.901 with 7th A, S65.909-S65.911 with 7th A, S65.919-S65.991 with 7th A, S65.999A

✓7th **S45.302   Unspecified injury of superficial vein** `CC`
at shoulder and upper arm level,
left arm
CC Excl: CC with 7th character A: S45.302-S45.309 with 7th A, S45.312-S45.319 with 7th A, S45.392-S45.399 with 7th A, S45.802-S45.809 with 7th A, S45.812-S45.819 with 7th A, S45.892-S45.899 with 7th A, S45.902-S45.909 with 7th A, S45.912-S45.919 with 7th A, S45.992-S45.999 with 7th A, S55.002-S55.009 with 7th A, S55.012-S55.019 with 7th A, S55.092-S55.099 with 7th A, S55.202-S55.209 with 7th A, S55.212-S55.219 with 7th A, S55.292-S55.299 with 7th A, S55.802-S55.809 with 7th A, S55.812-S55.819 with 7th A, S55.892-S55.899 with 7th A, S55.902-S55.909 with 7th A, S55.912-S55.919 with 7th A, S55.992-S55.999 with 7th A, S65.002-S65.009 with 7th A, S65.012-S65.019 with 7th A, S65.092-S65.099 with 7th A, S65.202-S65.209 with 7th A, S65.212-S65.219 with 7th A, S65.292-S65.299 with 7th A, S65.302-S65.309 with 7th A, S65.312-S65.319 with 7th A, S65.392-S65.399 with 7th A, S65.402-S65.409 with 7th A, S65.412-S65.419 with 7th A, S65.492-S65.499 with 7th A, S65.501A, S65.503A, S65.505A, S65.507-S65.509 with 7th A, S65.511A, S65.513A, S65.515 A, S65.517-S65.519 with 7th A, S65.591A, S65.593 A, S65.595A, S65.597-S65.599 with 7th A, S65.802-S65.809 with 7th A, S65.812-S65.819 with 7th A, S65.892-S65.899 with 7th A, S65.902-S65.909 with 7th A, S65.912-S65.919 with 7th A, S65.992-S65.999 with 7th A

✓7th **S45.309   Unspecified injury of superficial vein** `CC`
at shoulder and upper arm level,
unspecified arm
CC Excl: CC with 7th character A: S45.301-S45.999 with 7th A, S55.001-S55.099 with 7th A, S55.201-S55.999 with 7th A, S65.001-S65.099 with 7th A, S65.201-S65.999 A

✓6th **S45.31   Laceration of superficial vein at shoulder and upper arm level**

✓7th **S45.311   Laceration of superficial vein at** `CC`
shoulder and upper arm level,
right arm
CC Excl: See code: S45.301

Injury, Poisoning and Certain Other Consequences of External Causes

S45.312–S46.029

☑7ᵗʰ **S45.312 Laceration of superficial vein at shoulder and upper arm level, left arm** CC
CC Excl: See code: S45.302

☑7ᵗʰ **S45.319 Laceration of superficial vein at shoulder and upper arm level, unspecified arm** CC
CC Excl: See code: S45.309

☑6ᵗʰ **S45.39 Other specified injury of superficial vein at shoulder and upper arm level**

☑7ᵗʰ **S45.391 Other specified injury of superficial vein at shoulder and upper arm level, right arm** CC
CC Excl: See code: S45.301

☑7ᵗʰ **S45.392 Other specified injury of superficial vein at shoulder and upper arm level, left arm** CC
CC Excl: See code: S45.302

☑7ᵗʰ **S45.399 Other specified injury of superficial vein at shoulder and upper arm level, unspecified arm** CC
CC Excl: See code: S45.309

☑5ᵗʰ **S45.8 Injury of other specified blood vessels at shoulder and upper arm level**

☑6ᵗʰ **S45.80 Unspecified injury of other specified blood vessels at shoulder and upper arm level**

☑7ᵗʰ **S45.801 Unspecified injury of other specified blood vessels at shoulder and upper arm level, right arm** CC
CC Excl: See code: S45.301

☑7ᵗʰ **S45.802 Unspecified injury of other specified blood vessels at shoulder and upper arm level, left arm** CC
CC Excl: See code: S45.302

☑7ᵗʰ **S45.809 Unspecified injury of other specified blood vessels at shoulder and upper arm level, unspecified arm** CC
CC Excl: See code: S45.309

☑6ᵗʰ **S45.81 Laceration of other specified blood vessels at shoulder and upper arm level**

☑7ᵗʰ **S45.811 Laceration of other specified blood vessels at shoulder and upper arm level, right arm** CC
CC Excl: See code: S45.301

☑7ᵗʰ **S45.812 Laceration of other specified blood vessels at shoulder and upper arm level, left arm** CC
CC Excl: See code: S45.302

☑7ᵗʰ **S45.819 Laceration of other specified blood vessels at shoulder and upper arm level, unspecified arm** CC
CC Excl: See code: S45.309

☑6ᵗʰ **S45.89 Other specified injury of other specified blood vessels at shoulder and upper arm level**

☑7ᵗʰ **S45.891 Other specified injury of other specified blood vessels at shoulder and upper arm level, right arm** CC
CC Excl: See code: S45.301

☑7ᵗʰ **S45.892 Other specified injury of other specified blood vessels at shoulder and upper arm level, left arm** CC
CC Excl: See code: S45.302

☑7ᵗʰ **S45.899 Other specified injury of other specified blood vessels at shoulder and upper arm level, unspecified arm** CC
CC Excl: See code: S45.309

☑5ᵗʰ **S45.9 Injury of unspecified blood vessel at shoulder and upper arm level**

☑6ᵗʰ **S45.90 Unspecified injury of unspecified blood vessel at shoulder and upper arm level**

☑7ᵗʰ **S45.901 Unspecified injury of unspecified blood vessel at shoulder and upper arm level, right arm** CC
CC Excl: See code: S45.301

☑7ᵗʰ **S45.902 Unspecified injury of unspecified blood vessel at shoulder and upper arm level, left arm** CC
CC Excl: See code: S45.302

☑7ᵗʰ **S45.909 Unspecified injury of unspecified blood vessel at shoulder and upper arm level, unspecified arm** CC
CC Excl: See code: S45.309

☑6ᵗʰ **S45.91 Laceration of unspecified blood vessel at shoulder and upper arm level**

☑7ᵗʰ **S45.911 Laceration of unspecified blood vessel at shoulder and upper arm level, right arm** CC
CC Excl: See code: S45.301

☑7ᵗʰ **S45.912 Laceration of unspecified blood vessel at shoulder and upper arm level, left arm** CC
CC Excl: See code: S45.302

☑7ᵗʰ **S45.919 Laceration of unspecified blood vessel at shoulder and upper arm level, unspecified arm** CC
CC Excl: See code: S45.309

☑6ᵗʰ **S45.99 Other specified injury of unspecified blood vessel at shoulder and upper arm level**

☑7ᵗʰ **S45.991 Other specified injury of unspecified blood vessel at shoulder and upper arm level, right arm** CC
CC Excl: See code: S45.301

☑7ᵗʰ **S45.992 Other specified injury of unspecified blood vessel at shoulder and upper arm level, left arm** CC
CC Excl: See code: S45.302

☑7ᵗʰ **S45.999 Other specified injury of unspecified blood vessel at shoulder and upper arm level, unspecified arm** CC
CC Excl: See code: S45.309

☑4ᵗʰ **S46 Injury of muscle, fascia and tendon at shoulder and upper arm level**

Code also any associated open wound (S41.-)

EXCLUDES 2   injury of muscle, fascia and tendon at elbow (S56.-)
sprain of joints and ligaments of shoulder girdle (S43.9)

The appropriate 7th is to be added to each code from category S46.
A   initial encounter
D   subsequent encounter
S   sequela

☑5ᵗʰ **S46.0 Injury of muscle(s) and tendon(s) of the rotator cuff of shoulder**
CC Excl: For CC codes in subcategory S46.0, unless otherwise noted: CC with 7th character A: S41.001A, S41.009-S41.011 with 7th A, S41.019-S41.021 with 7th A, S41.029-S41.031 with 7th A, S41.039-S41.041 with 7th A, S41.049-S41.051 with 7th A, S41.059-S41.101 with 7th A, S41.109-S41.111 with 7th A, S41.119-S41.121 with 7th A, S41.129-S41.131 with 7th A, S41.139-S41.141 with 7th A, S41.149-S41.151 with 7th A, S41.159 A, S46.021A, S46.029A, S46.121A, S46.129A, S46.221A, S46.229A, S46.321A, S46.329A, S46.821A, S46.829A, S46.921A, S46.929A

☑6ᵗʰ **S46.00 Unspecified injury of muscle(s) and tendon(s) of the rotator cuff of shoulder**

☑7ᵗʰ **S46.001 Unspecified injury of muscle(s) and tendon(s) of the rotator cuff of right shoulder**

☑7ᵗʰ **S46.002 Unspecified injury of muscle(s) and tendon(s) of the rotator cuff of left shoulder**

☑7ᵗʰ **S46.009 Unspecified injury of muscle(s) and tendon(s) of the rotator cuff of unspecified shoulder**

☑6ᵗʰ **S46.01 Strain of muscle(s) and tendon(s) of the rotator cuff of shoulder**

☑7ᵗʰ **S46.011 Strain of muscle(s) and tendon(s) of the rotator cuff of right shoulder**

☑7ᵗʰ **S46.012 Strain of muscle(s) and tendon(s) of the rotator cuff of left shoulder**

☑7ᵗʰ **S46.019 Strain of muscle(s) and tendon(s) of the rotator cuff of unspecified shoulder**

☑6ᵗʰ **S46.02 Laceration of muscle(s) and tendon(s) of the rotator cuff of shoulder**

☑7ᵗʰ **S46.021 Laceration of muscle(s) and tendon(s) of the rotator cuff of right shoulder** CC

☑7ᵗʰ **S46.022 Laceration of muscle(s) and tendon(s) of the rotator cuff of left shoulder** CC

☑7ᵗʰ **S46.029 Laceration of muscle(s) and tendon(s) of the rotator cuff of unspecified shoulder** CC

Ⓝ Newborn: 0   Ⓟ Pediatric: 0-17   Ⓜ Maternity: 12-55   Ⓐ Adult: 15-124   MCC Major CC Condition   PDx MCC PDx acts as own MCC   CC CC Condition   PDx CC PDx acts as own CC

916   ICD-10-CM Draft (2015)

✓6ᵗʰ **S46.09** Other injury of muscle(s) and tendon(s) of the rotator cuff of shoulder

   ✓7ᵗʰ **S46.091** Other injury of muscle(s) and tendon(s) of the rotator cuff of right shoulder

   ✓7ᵗʰ **S46.092** Other injury of muscle(s) and tendon(s) of the rotator cuff of left shoulder

   ✓7ᵗʰ **S46.099** Other injury of muscle(s) and tendon(s) of the rotator cuff of unspecified shoulder

✓5ᵗʰ **S46.1** Injury of muscle, fascia and tendon of long head of biceps

 ✓6ᵗʰ **S46.10** Unspecified injury of muscle, fascia and tendon of long head of biceps

   ✓7ᵗʰ **S46.101** Unspecified injury of muscle, fascia and tendon of long head of biceps, right arm

   ✓7ᵗʰ **S46.102** Unspecified injury of muscle, fascia and tendon of long head of biceps, left arm

   ✓7ᵗʰ **S46.109** Unspecified injury of muscle, fascia and tendon of long head of biceps, unspecified arm

 ✓6ᵗʰ **S46.11** Strain of muscle, fascia and tendon of long head of biceps

   ✓7ᵗʰ **S46.111** Strain of muscle, fascia and tendon of long head of biceps, right arm

   ✓7ᵗʰ **S46.112** Strain of muscle, fascia and tendon of long head of biceps, left arm

   ✓7ᵗʰ **S46.119** Strain of muscle, fascia and tendon of long head of biceps, unspecified arm

 ✓6ᵗʰ **S46.12** Laceration of muscle, fascia and tendon of long head of biceps

   ✓7ᵗʰ **S46.121** Laceration of muscle, fascia and tendon of long head of biceps, right arm   **CC**
     CC Excl: CC with 7th character A: S41.001A, S41.009-S41.011 with 7th A, S41.019-S41.021 with 7th A, S41.029-S41.031 with 7th A, S41.039-S41.041 with 7th A, S41.049-S41.051 with 7th A, S41.059-S41.101 with 7th A, S41.109-S41.111 with 7th A, S41.119-S41.121 with 7th A, S41.129-S41.131 with 7th A, S41.139-S41.141 with 7th A, S41.149-S41.151 with 7th A, S41.159A, S46.021A, S46.029A, S46.121A, S46.129A, S46.221A, S46.229 A, S46.321A, S46.329A, S46.821A, S46.829A, S46.921A, S46.929A

   ✓7ᵗʰ **S46.122** Laceration of muscle, fascia and tendon of long head of biceps, left arm   **CC**
     CC Excl: CC with 7th character A: S41.002-S41.009 with 7th A, S41.012-S41.019 with 7th A, S41.022-S41.029 with 7th A, S41.032-S41.039 with 7th A, S41.042-S41.049 with 7th A, S41.052-S41.059 with 7th A, S41.102-S41.109 with 7th A, S41.112-S41.119 with 7th A, S41.122-S41.129 with 7th A, S41.132-S41.139 with 7th A, S41.142-S41.149 with 7th A, S41.152-S41.159 with 7th A, S46.022-S46.029 with 7th A, S46.122-S46.129 with 7th A, S46.222-S46.229 with 7th A, S46.322-S46.329 with 7th A, S46.822-S46.829 with 7th A, S46.922-S46.929 with 7th A

   ✓7ᵗʰ **S46.129** Laceration of muscle, fascia and tendon of long head of biceps, unspecified arm   **CC**
     CC Excl: CC with 7th character A: S41.001-S41.159 with 7th A, S46.021-S46.029 with 7th A, S46.121-S46.129 with 7th A, S46.221-S46.229 with 7th A, S46.321-S46.329 with 7th A, S46.821-S46.829 with 7th A, S46.921-S46.929 with 7th A

 ✓6ᵗʰ **S46.19** Other injury of muscle, fascia and tendon of long head of biceps

   ✓7ᵗʰ **S46.191** Other injury of muscle, fascia and tendon of long head of biceps, right arm

   ✓7ᵗʰ **S46.192** Other injury of muscle, fascia and tendon of long head of biceps, left arm

   ✓7ᵗʰ **S46.199** Other injury of muscle, fascia and tendon of long head of biceps, unspecified arm

✓5ᵗʰ **S46.2** Injury of muscle, fascia and tendon of other parts of biceps

 ✓6ᵗʰ **S46.20** Unspecified injury of muscle, fascia and tendon of other parts of biceps

   ✓7ᵗʰ **S46.201** Unspecified injury of muscle, fascia and tendon of other parts of biceps, right arm

   ✓7ᵗʰ **S46.202** Unspecified injury of muscle, fascia and tendon of other parts of biceps, left arm

   ✓7ᵗʰ **S46.209** Unspecified injury of muscle, fascia and tendon of other parts of biceps, unspecified arm

 ✓6ᵗʰ **S46.21** Strain of muscle, fascia and tendon of other parts of biceps

   ✓7ᵗʰ **S46.211** Strain of muscle, fascia and tendon of other parts of biceps, right arm

   ✓7ᵗʰ **S46.212** Strain of muscle, fascia and tendon of other parts of biceps, left arm

   ✓7ᵗʰ **S46.219** Strain of muscle, fascia and tendon of other parts of biceps, unspecified arm

 ✓6ᵗʰ **S46.22** Laceration of muscle, fascia and tendon of other parts of biceps

   ✓7ᵗʰ **S46.221** Laceration of muscle, fascia and tendon of other parts of biceps, right arm   **CC**
     CC Excl: CC with 7th character A: See code: S46.121

   ✓7ᵗʰ **S46.222** Laceration of muscle, fascia and tendon of other parts of biceps, left arm   **CC**
     CC Excl: CC with 7th character A: See code: S46.122

   ✓7ᵗʰ **S46.229** Laceration of muscle, fascia and tendon of other parts of biceps, unspecified arm   **CC**
     CC Excl: CC with 7th character A: See code: S46.129

 ✓6ᵗʰ **S46.29** Other injury of muscle, fascia and tendon of other parts of biceps

   ✓7ᵗʰ **S46.291** Other injury of muscle, fascia and tendon of other parts of biceps, right arm

   ✓7ᵗʰ **S46.292** Other injury of muscle, fascia and tendon of other parts of biceps, left arm

   ✓7ᵗʰ **S46.299** Other injury of muscle, fascia and tendon of other parts of biceps, unspecified arm

✓5ᵗʰ **S46.3** Injury of muscle, fascia and tendon of triceps

 ✓6ᵗʰ **S46.30** Unspecified injury of muscle, fascia and tendon of triceps

   ✓7ᵗʰ **S46.301** Unspecified injury of muscle, fascia and tendon of triceps, right arm

   ✓7ᵗʰ **S46.302** Unspecified injury of muscle, fascia and tendon of triceps, left arm

   ✓7ᵗʰ **S46.309** Unspecified injury of muscle, fascia and tendon of triceps, unspecified arm

 ✓6ᵗʰ **S46.31** Strain of muscle, fascia and tendon of triceps

   ✓7ᵗʰ **S46.311** Strain of muscle, fascia and tendon of triceps, right arm

   ✓7ᵗʰ **S46.312** Strain of muscle, fascia and tendon of triceps, left arm

   ✓7ᵗʰ **S46.319** Strain of muscle, fascia and tendon of triceps, unspecified arm

 ✓6ᵗʰ **S46.32** Laceration of muscle, fascia and tendon of triceps

   ✓7ᵗʰ **S46.321** Laceration of muscle, fascia and tendon of triceps, right arm   **CC**
     CC Excl: CC with 7th character A: See code: S46.121

   ✓7ᵗʰ **S46.322** Laceration of muscle, fascia and tendon of triceps, left arm   **CC**
     CC Excl: CC with 7th character A: See code: S46.122

   ✓7ᵗʰ **S46.329** Laceration of muscle, fascia and tendon of triceps, unspecified arm   **CC**
     CC Excl: CC with 7th character A: See code: S46.129

 ✓6ᵗʰ **S46.39** Other injury of muscle, fascia and tendon of triceps

   ✓7ᵗʰ **S46.391** Other injury of muscle, fascia and tendon of triceps, right arm

   ✓7ᵗʰ **S46.392** Other injury of muscle, fascia and tendon of triceps, left arm

   ✓7ᵗʰ **S46.399** Other injury of muscle, fascia and tendon of triceps, unspecified arm

---

✓ Additional Character Required   ✓ₓ7ᵗʰ Xtension Alert   Unacceptable PDx   Manifestation   Hospital Acquired Condition   EXCLUDES 1 Not Coded Here   EXCLUDES 2 Not Included Here

√5ᵗʰ **S46.8** **Injury of other muscles, fascia and tendons at shoulder and upper arm level**

  √6ᵗʰ **S46.80** Unspecified injury of other muscles, fascia and tendons at shoulder and upper arm level

    √7ᵗʰ **S46.801** Unspecified injury of other muscles, fascia and tendons at shoulder and upper arm level, right arm

    √7ᵗʰ **S46.802** Unspecified injury of other muscles, fascia and tendons at shoulder and upper arm level, left arm

    √7ᵗʰ **S46.809** Unspecified injury of other muscles, fascia and tendons at shoulder and upper arm level, unspecified arm

  √6ᵗʰ **S46.81** Strain of other muscles, fascia and tendons at shoulder and upper arm level

    √7ᵗʰ **S46.811** Strain of other muscles, fascia and tendons at shoulder and upper arm level, right arm

    √7ᵗʰ **S46.812** Strain of other muscles, fascia and tendons at shoulder and upper arm level, left arm

    √7ᵗʰ **S46.819** Strain of other muscles, fascia and tendons at shoulder and upper arm level, unspecified arm

  √6ᵗʰ **S46.82** Laceration of other muscles, fascia and tendons at shoulder and upper arm level

    √7ᵗʰ **S46.821** Laceration of other muscles, fascia and tendons at shoulder and upper arm level, right arm   CC
      CC Excl: CC with 7th character A: See code: S46.121

    √7ᵗʰ **S46.822** Laceration of other muscles, fascia and tendons at shoulder and upper arm level, left arm   CC
      CC Excl: CC with 7th character A: See code: S46.122

    √7ᵗʰ **S46.829** Laceration of other muscles, fascia and tendons at shoulder and upper arm level, unspecified arm   CC
      CC Excl: CC with 7th character A: See code: S46.129

  √6ᵗʰ **S46.89** Other injury of other muscles, fascia and tendons at shoulder and upper arm level

    √7ᵗʰ **S46.891** Other injury of other muscles, fascia and tendons at shoulder and upper arm level, right arm

    √7ᵗʰ **S46.892** Other injury of other muscles, fascia and tendons at shoulder and upper arm level, left arm

    √7ᵗʰ **S46.899** Other injury of other muscles, fascia and tendons at shoulder and upper arm level, unspecified arm

√5ᵗʰ **S46.9** **Injury of unspecified muscle, fascia and tendon at shoulder and upper arm level**

  √6ᵗʰ **S46.90** Unspecified injury of unspecified muscle, fascia and tendon at shoulder and upper arm level

    √7ᵗʰ **S46.901** Unspecified injury of unspecified muscle, fascia and tendon at shoulder and upper arm level, right arm

    √7ᵗʰ **S46.902** Unspecified injury of unspecified muscle, fascia and tendon at shoulder and upper arm level, left arm

    √7ᵗʰ **S46.909** Unspecified injury of unspecified muscle, fascia and tendon at shoulder and upper arm level, unspecified arm

  √6ᵗʰ **S46.91** Strain of unspecified muscle, fascia and tendon at shoulder and upper arm level

    √7ᵗʰ **S46.911** Strain of unspecified muscle, fascia and tendon at shoulder and upper arm level, right arm

    √7ᵗʰ **S46.912** Strain of unspecified muscle, fascia and tendon at shoulder and upper arm level, left arm

    √7ᵗʰ **S46.919** Strain of unspecified muscle, fascia and tendon at shoulder and upper arm level, unspecified arm

√6ᵗʰ **S46.92** Laceration of unspecified muscle, fascia and tendon at shoulder and upper arm level

    √7ᵗʰ **S46.921** Laceration of unspecified muscle, fascia and tendon at shoulder and upper arm level, right arm   CC
      CC Excl: CC with 7th character A: See code: S46.121

    √7ᵗʰ **S46.922** Laceration of unspecified muscle, fascia and tendon at shoulder and upper arm level, left arm   CC
      CC Excl: CC with 7th character A: See code: S46.122

    √7ᵗʰ **S46.929** Laceration of unspecified muscle, fascia and tendon at shoulder and upper arm level, unspecified arm   CC
      CC Excl: CC with 7th character A: See code: S46.129

  √6ᵗʰ **S46.99** Other injury of unspecified muscle, fascia and tendon at shoulder and upper arm level

    √7ᵗʰ **S46.991** Other injury of unspecified muscle, fascia and tendon at shoulder and upper arm level, right arm

    √7ᵗʰ **S46.992** Other injury of unspecified muscle, fascia and tendon at shoulder and upper arm level, left arm

    √7ᵗʰ **S46.999** Other injury of unspecified muscle, fascia and tendon at shoulder and upper arm level, unspecified arm

√4ᵗʰ **S47** **Crushing injury of shoulder and upper arm**
Use additional code for all associated injuries
EXCLUDES 2   crushing injury of elbow (S57.0-)

The appropriate 7th is to be added to each code from category S47.
A   initial encounter
D   subsequent encounter
S   sequela

√xᵗʰ **S47.1** Crushing injury of right shoulder and upper arm

√xᵗʰ **S47.2** Crushing injury of left shoulder and upper arm

√xᵗʰ **S47.9** Crushing injury of shoulder and upper arm, unspecified arm

√4ᵗʰ **S48** **Traumatic amputation of shoulder and upper arm**
NOTE   An amputation not identified as partial or complete should be coded to complete.
EXCLUDES 1   traumatic amputation at elbow level (S58.0)

The appropriate 7th is to be added to each code from category S48.
A   initial encounter
D   subsequent encounter
S   sequela

√5ᵗʰ **S48.0** **Traumatic amputation at shoulder joint**

  √6ᵗʰ **S48.01** Complete traumatic amputation at shoulder joint

    √7ᵗʰ **S48.011** Complete traumatic amputation at right shoulder joint   CC
      CC Excl: CC with 7th character A: S41.001A, S41.009-S41.011 with 7th A, S41.019-S41.021 with 7th A, S41.029-S41.031 with 7th A, S41.039-S41.041 with 7th A, S41.049-S41.051 with 7th A, S41.059-S41.101 with 7th A, S41.109-S41.111 with 7th A, S41.119-S41.121 with 7th A, S41.129-S41.131 with 7th A, S41.139-S41.141 with 7th A, S41.149-S41.151 with 7th A, S41.159A, S46.021A, S46.029A, S46.121A, S46.129A, S46.221 A, S46.229 A, S46.321A, S46.329A, S46.821A, S46.829A, S46.921A, S46.929A, S48.011 A, S48.019-S48.021 with 7th A, S48.029-S48.111 with 7th A, S48.119-S48.121 with 7th A, S48.129-S48.911 with 7th A, S48.919-S48.921 with 7th A, S48.929A, S51.001A, S51.009-S51.011 with 7th A, S51.019-S51.021 with 7th A, S51.029-S51.031 with 7th A, S51.039-S51.041 with 7th A, S51.049-S51.051 with 7th A, S51.059-S51.801 with 7th A, S51.809-S51.811 with 7th A, S51.819-S51.821 with 7th A, S51.829-S51.831 with 7th A, S51.839-S51.841 with 7th A, S51.849-S51.851 with 7th A, S51.859 with 7th A, S56.021A, S56.029A, S56.121A, S56.123A, S56.125A, S56.127A, S56.129A, S56.221A, S56.229A, S56.321A, S56.329A, S56.421A, S56.423A, S56.425A, S56.427A, S56.429A, S56.521A, S56.529A, S56.821A, S56.829A,

N Newborn: 0   P Pediatric: 0-17   M Maternity: 12-55   A Adult: 15-124   MCC Major CC Condition   PDx MCC PDx acts as own MCC   CC CC Condition   PDx CC PDx acts as own CC

918   ICD-10-CM Draft (2015)

S56.921A, S56.929A, S58.011A, S58.019-
S58.021 with 7th A, S58.029-S58.111 with
7th A, S58.119-S58.121 with 7th A, S58.129-
S58.911 with 7th A, S58.919-S58.921 with
7th A, S58.929A, S61.001A, S61.009-S61.011
with 7th A, S61.019-S61.021 with 7th A,
S61.029-S61.031 with 7th A, S61.039-
S61.041 with 7th A, S61.049-S61.051 with
7th A, S61.059-S61.101 with 7th A, S61.109-
S61.111 with 7th A, S61.119-S61.121 with
7th A, S61.129-S61.131 with 7th A, S61.139-
S61.141 with 7th A, S61.149-S61.151 with
7th A, S61.159-S61.200 with 7th A, S61.202A,
S61.204A, S61.206A, S61.208-S61.210 with
7th A, S61.212A, S61.214A, S61.216A,
S61.218-S61.220 with 7th A, S61.222A,
S61.224A, S61.226A, S61.228-S61.230 with
7th A, S61.232A, S61.234A, S61.236 A,
S61.238-S61.240 with 7th A, S61.242A,
S61.244A, S61.246A, S61.248-S61.250 with
7th A, S61.252A, S61.254A, S61.256A,
S61.258-S61.300 with 7th A, S61.302A,
S61.304A, S61.306A, S61.308-S61.310 with
7th A, S61.312A, S61.314A, S61.316A,
S61.318-S61.320 with 7th A, S61.322A,
S61.324 A, S61.326A, S61.328-S61.330 with
7th A, S61.332A, S61.334A, S61.336A,
S61.338-S61.340 with 7th A, S61.342 A,
S61.344A, S61.346A, S61.348-S61.350 with
7th A, S61.352A, S61.354A, S61.356A,
S61.358-S61.401 with 7th A, S61.409-
S61.411 with 7th A, S61.419-S61.421 with
7th A, S61.429-S61.431 with 7th A, S61.439-
S61.441 with 7th A, S61.449-S61.451 with
7th A, S61.459-S61.501 with 7th A, S61.509-
S61.511 with 7th A, S61.519-S61.521 with
7th A, S61.529-S61.531 with 7th A, S61.539-
S61.541 with 7th A, S61.549-S61.551 with
7th A, S61.559A, S66.021A, S66.029A,
S66.120A, S66.122A, S66.124A, S66.126A,
S66.128-S66.129 with 7th A, S66.221A,
S66.229A, S66.320A, S66.322A, S66.324A,
S66.326A, S66.328-S66.329 with 7th A,
S66.421A, S66.429A, S66.520A, S66.521A,
S66.524A, S66.526A, S66.528-S66.529 with
7th A, S66.821A, S66.829A, S66.921A,
S66.929A, S68.011A, S68.019-S68.021 with
7th A, S68.029-S68.110 with 7th A, S68.112A,
S68.114A, S68.116A, S68.118-S68.120 with
7th A, S68.122A, S68.124A, S68.126 A,
S68.128-S68.411 with 7th A, S68.419-
S68.421 with 7th A, S68.429-S68.511 with
7th A, S68.519-S68.521 with 7th A, S68.529-
S68.610 with 7th A, S68.612A, S68.614A,
S68.616A, S68.618-S68.620 with 7th A,
S68.622A, S68.624A, S68.626A, S68.628-
S68.711 with 7th A, S68.719-S68.721 with
7th A, S68.729A, T14.8-T14.91, T79.A0X-
T79.9XX with 7th A

√7ᵗʰ S48.012 Complete traumatic amputation at left shoulder joint `CC`
CC Excl: CC with 7th character A: S41.002-
S41.009 with 7th A, S41.012-S41.019 with
7th A, S41.022-S41.029 with 7th A, S41.032-
S41.039 with 7th A, S41.042-S41.049 with
7th A, S41.052-S41.059 with 7th A, S41.102-
S41.109 with 7th A, S41.112-S41.119 with
7th A, S41.122-S41.129 with 7th A, S41.132-
S41.139 with 7th A, S41.142-S41.149 with
7th A, S41.152-S41.159 with 7th A, S46.022-
S46.029 with 7th A, S46.122-S46.129 with
7th A, S46.222-S46.229 with 7th A, S46.322-
S46.329 with 7th A, S46.822-S46.829 with
7th A, S46.922-S46.929 with 7th A, S48.012-
S48.019 with 7th A, S48.022-S48.029 with
7th A, S48.112-S48.119 with 7th A, S48.122-
S48.129 with 7th A, S48.912-S48.919 with
7th A, S48.922-S48.929 with 7th A, S51.002-
S51.009 with 7th A, S51.012-S51.019 with
7th A, S51.022-S51.029 with 7th A, S51.032-
S51.039 with 7th A, S51.042-S51.049 with
7th A, S51.052-S51.059 with 7th A, S51.802-
S51.809 with 7th A, S51.812-S51.819 with
7th A, S51.822-S51.829 with 7th A, S51.832-
S51.839 with 7th A, S51.842-S51.849 with
7th A, S51.852-S51.859 with 7th A, S56.022-
S56.029A, S56.122A, S56.124A, S56.126A,
S56.128-S56.129 with 7th A, S56.222-
S56.229 with 7th A, S56.322-S56.329 with
7th A, S56.422A, S56.424A, S56.426 A,
S56.428-S56.429 with 7th A, S56.522-
S56.529 with 7th A, S56.822-S56.829 with

7th A, S56.922-S56.929 with 7th A, S58.012-
S58.019 with 7th A, S58.022-S58.029 with
7th A, S58.112-S58.119 with 7th A, S58.122-
S58.129 with 7th A, S58.912-S58.919 with
7th A, S58.922-S58.929 with 7th A, S61.002-
S61.009 with 7th A, S61.012-S61.019 with
7th A, S61.022-S61.029 with 7th A, S61.032-
S61.039 with 7th A, S61.042-S61.049 with
7th A, S61.052-S61.059 with 7th A, S61.102-
S61.109 with 7th A, S61.112-S61.119 with
7th A, S61.122-S61.129 with 7th A, S61.132-
S61.139 with 7th A, S61.142-S61.149 with
7th A, S61.152-S61.159 with 7th A, S61.201
with 7th A, S61.203A, S61.205A, S61.207-
S61.209 with 7th A, S61.211A, S61.213A,
S61.215A, S61.217-S61.219 with 7th A,
S61.221A, S61.223A, S61.225A, S61.227-
S61.229 with 7th A, S61.231A, S61.233A,
S61.235A, S61.237-S61.239 with 7th A,
S61.241A, S61.243A, S61.245A, S61.247-
S61.249 with 7th A, S61.251A, S61.253A,
S61.255A, S61.257-S61.259 with 7th A,
S61.301A, S61.303A, S61.305A, S61.307-
S61.309 with 7th A, S61.311A, S61.313A,
S61.315A, S61.317-S61.319 with 7th A,
S61.321A, S61.323A, S61.325A, S61.327-
S61.329 with 7th A, S61.331A, S61.333A,
S61.335A, S61.337-S61.339 with 7th A,
S61.341 with 7th A, S61.343A, S61.345A,
S61.347-S61.349 with 7th A, S61.351A,
S61.353A, S61.355A, S61.357-S61.359 with
7th A, S61.402-S61.409 with 7th A, S61.412-
S61.419 with 7th A, S61.422-S61.429 with
7th A, S61.432-S61.439 with 7th A, S61.442-
S61.449 with 7th A, S61.452-S61.459 with
7th A, S61.502-S61.509 with 7th A, S61.512-
S61.519 with 7th A, S61.522-S61.529 with
7th A, S61.532-S61.539 with 7th A, S61.542-
S61.549 with 7th A, S61.552-S61.559 with
7th A, S66.022-S66.029 with 7th A, S66.121A,
S66.123A, S66.125A, S66.127-S66.129 with
7th A, S66.222-S66.229 with 7th A, S66.321A,
S66.323A, S66.325A, S66.327-S66.329 with
7th A, S66.422-S66.429 with 7th A, S66.521A,
S66.523A, S66.525A, S66.527-S66.529 with
7th A, S66.822-S66.829 with 7th A, S66.922-
S66.929 with 7th A, S68.012-S68.019 with
7th A, S68.022-S68.029 with 7th A, S68.111A,
S68.113A, S68.115A, S68.117-S68.119 with
7th A, S68.121 A, S68.123A, S68.125A,
S68.127-S68.129 with 7th A, S68.412-
S68.419A, S68.422-S68.429 with 7th A,
S68.512-S68.519 with 7th A, S68.522-
S68.529 with 7th A, S68.611A, S68.613A,
S68.615 with 7th A, S68.617-S68.619 with
7th A, S68.621A, S68.623A, S68.625A,
S68.627-S68.629 with 7th A, S68.712-
S68.719 with 7th A, S68.722-S68.729 with
7th A, T14.8-T14.91, T79.A0X-T79.9XX with
7th A

√7ᵗʰ S48.019 Complete traumatic amputation at unspecified shoulder joint `CC`
CC Excl: CC with 7th character A: S41.001-
S41.159 with 7th A, S46.021-S46.029 with
7th A, S46.121-S46.129 with 7th A, S46.221-
S46.229 with 7th A, S46.321-S46.329 with
7th A, S46.821-S46.829 with 7th A, S46.921-
S46.929 with 7th A, S48.011-S48.929 with
7th A, S51.001-S51.859 with 7th A, S56.021-
S56.029 with 7th A, S56.121-S56.129 with
7th A, S56.221-S56.229 with 7th A, S56.321-
S56.329 with 7th A, S56.421-S56.429 with
7th A, S56.521-S56.529 with 7th A, S56.821-
S56.829 with 7th A, S56.921-S56.929 with
7th A, S58.011-S58.929 with 7th A, S61.001-
S61.559 with 7th A, S66.021-S66.029 with
7th A, S66.120-S66.129 with 7th A, S66.221-
S66.229 with 7th A, S66.320-S66.329 with
7th A, S66.421-S66.429 with 7th A, S66.520-
S66.529 with 7th A, S66.821-S66.829 with
7th A, S66.921-S66.929 with 7th A, S68.011-
S68.729 with 7th A, T14.8-T14.91, T79.A0X-
T79.9XX with 7th A

√6ᵗʰ S48.02 Partial traumatic amputation at shoulder joint

√7ᵗʰ S48.021 Partial traumatic amputation at right shoulder joint `CC`
CC Excl: CC with 7th character A: See code:
S48.011

√7ᵗʰ **S48.022** **Partial traumatic amputation at left** CC
shoulder joint
CC Excl: CC with 7th character A: See code:
S48.012

√7ᵗʰ **S48.029** **Partial traumatic amputation at** CC
unspecified shoulder joint
CC Excl: CC with 7th character A: See code:
S48.019

√5ᵗʰ **S48.1** **Traumatic amputation at level between shoulder and elbow**

√6ᵗʰ **S48.11** **Complete traumatic amputation at level between shoulder and elbow**

√7ᵗʰ **S48.111** **Complete traumatic amputation at** CC
level between right shoulder and elbow
CC Excl: CC with 7th character A: See code:
S48.011

√7ᵗʰ **S48.112** **Complete traumatic amputation at** CC
level between left shoulder and elbow
CC Excl: CC with 7th character A: See code:
S48.012

√7ᵗʰ **S48.119** **Complete traumatic amputation at** CC
level between unspecified shoulder and elbow
CC Excl: CC with 7th character A: See code:
S48.019

√6ᵗʰ **S48.12** **Partial traumatic amputation at level between shoulder and elbow**

√7ᵗʰ **S48.121** **Partial traumatic amputation at level between right shoulder and elbow**

√7ᵗʰ **S48.122** **Partial traumatic amputation at level between left shoulder and elbow**

√7ᵗʰ **S48.129** **Partial traumatic amputation at level between unspecified shoulder and elbow**

√5ᵗʰ **S48.9** **Traumatic amputation of shoulder and upper arm, level unspecified**

√6ᵗʰ **S48.91** **Complete traumatic amputation of shoulder and upper arm, level unspecified**

√7ᵗʰ **S48.911** **Complete traumatic amputation of** CC
right shoulder and upper arm, level unspecified
CC Excl: CC with 7th character A: See code:
S48.011

√7ᵗʰ **S48.912** **Complete traumatic amputation of** CC
left shoulder and upper arm, level unspecified
CC Excl: CC with 7th character A: See code:
S48.012

√7ᵗʰ **S48.919** **Complete traumatic amputation of** CC
unspecified shoulder and upper arm, level unspecified
CC Excl: CC with 7th character A: See code:
S48.019

√6ᵗʰ **S48.92** **Partial traumatic amputation of shoulder and upper arm, level unspecified**

√7ᵗʰ **S48.921** **Partial traumatic amputation of right** CC
shoulder and upper arm, level unspecified
CC Excl: CC with 7th character A: See code:
S48.011

√7ᵗʰ **S48.922** **Partial traumatic amputation of left** CC
shoulder and upper arm, level unspecified
CC Excl: CC with 7th character A: See code:
S48.012

√7ᵗʰ **S48.929** **Partial traumatic amputation of** CC
unspecified shoulder and upper arm, level unspecified
CC Excl: CC with 7th character A: See code:
S48.019

√4ᵗʰ **S49** **Other and unspecified injuries of shoulder and upper arm**

The appropriate 7th is to be added to each code from subcategories S49.0 and S49.1.
A   initial encounter for closed fracture
D   subsequent encounter for fracture with routine healing
G   subsequent encounter for fracture with delayed healing
K   subsequent encounter for fracture with nonunion
P   subsequent encounter for fracture with malunion
S   sequela

√5ᵗʰ **S49.0** **Physeal fracture of upper end of humerus**

√6ᵗʰ **S49.00** **Unspecified physeal fracture of upper end of humerus**

7 √7ᵗʰ **S49.001** **Unspecified physeal fracture of upper** CC
end of humerus, right arm
CC Excl: CC with 7th character A: S42.201-
S42.271 with 7th [A, B], S42.279-S42.311
with 7th A, S42.319-S42.481 with 7th A,
S42.489-S42.92X with 7th A, S49.001A,
S49.009-S49.011 with 7th A, S49.019-
S49.021 with 7th A, S49.029-S49.031 with
7th A, S49.039-S49.041 with 7th A, S49.049-
S49.091 with 7th A, S49.099-S49.101 with
7th A, S49.109-S49.111 with 7th A, S49.119-
S49.121 with 7th A, S49.129-S49.131 with
7th A, S49.139-S49.141 with 7th A, S49.149-S49.191
with 7th A, S49.199A
CC with 7th character K or P: M80.00X-
M84.68X with 7th [K, P], S02.0XX-S02.92X
with 7th K, S12.000-S12.691 with 7th K,
S22.000-S22.9XX with 7th K, S32.000-
S32.9XX with 7th K, S42.001-S42.92X with
7th [K, P], S49.001-S49.199 with 7th [K, P],
S52.001-S52.92X with 7th [K, M, N, P, Q, R],
S59.001-S59.299 with 7th [K, P], S62.001-
S62.92X with 7th [K, P], S72.001-S72.92X
with 7th [K, M, N, P, Q, R], S79.001-S79.199
with 7th [K, P], S82.001-S82.92X with 7th [K,
M, N, P, Q, R], S89.001-S89.399 with 7th [K, P],
S92.001-S92.919 with 7th [K, P]

7 √7ᵗʰ **S49.002** **Unspecified physeal fracture of upper** CC
end of humerus, left arm
CC Excl: CC with 7th character A: S42.201-
S42.266 with 7th B, S42.272-S42.309 with
7th A, S42.312-S42.476 with 7th A, S42.482-
S42.92X with 7th A, S49.002-S49.009 with
7th A, S49.012-S49.019 with 7th A, S49.022-
S49.029 with 7th A, S49.032-S49.039 with
7th A, S49.042-S49.049 with 7th A, S49.092-
S49.099 with 7th A, S49.102-S49.109 with
7th A, S49.112-S49.119 with 7th A, S49.122-
S49.129 with 7th A, S49.132-S49.139 with
7th A, S49.142-S49.149 with 7th A, S49.192-
S49.199 with 7th A
CC with 7th character K or P: M80.00X-
M84.68X with 7th [K, P], S02.0XX-S02.92X
with 7th K, S12.000-S12.691 with 7th K,
S22.000-S22.9XX with 7th K, S32.000-
S32.9XX with 7th K, S42.001-S42.92X with
7th [K, P], S49.001-S49.199 with 7th [K, P],
S52.001-S52.92X with 7th [K, M, N, P, Q, R],
S59.001-S59.299 with 7th [K, P], S62.001-
S62.92X with 7th [K, P], S72.001-S72.92X
with 7th [K, M, N, P, Q, R], S79.001-S79.199
with 7th [K, P], S82.001-S82.92X with 7th [K,
M, N, P, Q, R], S89.001-S89.399 with 7th [K, P],
S92.001-S92.919 with 7th [K, P]

7 √7ᵗʰ **S49.009** **Unspecified physeal fracture of upper** CC
end of humerus, unspecified arm
CC Excl: CC with 7th character A: S42.201-
S42.92X with 7th [A, B], S49.001-S49.199
with 7th A
CC with 7th character K or P: M80.00X-
M84.68X with 7th [K, P], S02.0XX-S02.92X
with 7th K, S12.000-S12.691 with 7th K,
S22.000-S22.9XX with 7th K, S32.000-
S32.9XX with 7th K, S42.001-S42.92X with
7th [K, P], S49.001-S49.199 with 7th [K, P],
S52.001-S52.92X with 7th [K, M, N, P, Q, R],
S59.001-S59.299 with 7th [K, P], S62.001-
S62.92X with 7th [K, P], S72.001-S72.92X
with 7th [K, M, N, P, Q, R], S79.001-S79.199
with 7th [K, P], S82.001-S82.92X with 7th [K,
M, N, P, Q, R], S89.001-S89.399 with 7th [K, P],
S92.001-S92.919 with 7th [K, P]

---

7 HAC = Initial encounter only (7th character A, B or C) and not POA.

N Newborn: 0   P Pediatric: 0-17   M Maternity: 12-55   A Adult: 15-124   MCC Major CC Condition   PDx MCC PDx acts as own MCC   CC CC Condition   PDx CC PDx acts as own CC

920   ICD-10-CM Draft (2015)

√6ᵗʰ **S49.01** Salter-Harris Type I physeal fracture of upper end of humerus

7 √7ᵗʰ **S49.011** Salter-Harris Type I physeal fracture of upper end of humerus, right arm ᶜᶜ
CC Excl: See code: S49.001

7 √7ᵗʰ **S49.012** Salter-Harris Type I physeal fracture of upper end of humerus, left arm ᶜᶜ
CC Excl: See code: S49.002

7 √7ᵗʰ **S49.019** Salter-Harris Type I physeal fracture of upper end of humerus, unspecified arm ᶜᶜ
CC Excl: See code: S49.009

√6ᵗʰ **S49.02** Salter-Harris Type II physeal fracture of upper end of humerus

7 √7ᵗʰ **S49.021** Salter-Harris Type II physeal fracture of upper end of humerus, right arm ᶜᶜ
CC Excl: See code: S49.001

7 √7ᵗʰ **S49.022** Salter-Harris Type II physeal fracture of upper end of humerus, left arm ᶜᶜ
CC Excl: See code: S49.002

7 √7ᵗʰ **S49.029** Salter-Harris Type II physeal fracture of upper end of humerus, unspecified arm ᶜᶜ
CC Excl: See code: S49.009

√6ᵗʰ **S49.03** Salter-Harris Type III physeal fracture of upper end of humerus

7 √7ᵗʰ **S49.031** Salter Harris Type III physeal fracture of upper end of humerus, right arm ᶜᶜ
CC Excl: See code: S49.001

7 √7ᵗʰ **S49.032** Salter Harris Type III physeal fracture of upper end of humerus, left arm ᶜᶜ
CC Excl: See code: S49.002

7 √7ᵗʰ **S49.039** Salter Harris Type III physeal fracture of upper end of humerus, unspecified arm ᶜᶜ
CC Excl: See code: S49.009

√6ᵗʰ **S49.04** Salter-Harris Type IV physeal fracture of upper end of humerus

7 √7ᵗʰ **S49.041** Salter-Harris Type IV physeal fracture of upper end of humerus, right arm ᶜᶜ
CC Excl: See code: S49.001

7 √7ᵗʰ **S49.042** Salter-Harris Type IV physeal fracture of upper end of humerus, left arm ᶜᶜ
CC Excl: See code: S49.002

7 √7ᵗʰ **S49.049** Salter-Harris Type IV physeal fracture of upper end of humerus, unspecified arm ᶜᶜ
CC Excl: See code: S49.009

√6ᵗʰ **S49.09** Other physeal fracture of upper end of humerus

7 √7ᵗʰ **S49.091** Other physeal fracture of upper end of humerus, right arm ᶜᶜ
CC Excl: See code: S49.001

7 √7ᵗʰ **S49.092** Other physeal fracture of upper end of humerus, left arm ᶜᶜ
CC Excl: See code: S49.002

7 √7ᵗʰ **S49.099** Other physeal fracture of upper end of humerus, unspecified arm ᶜᶜ
CC Excl: See code: S49.009

√5ᵗʰ **S49.1** Physeal fracture of lower end of humerus

√6ᵗʰ **S49.10** Unspecified physeal fracture of lower end of humerus

7 √7ᵗʰ **S49.101** Unspecified physeal fracture of lower end of humerus, right arm ᶜᶜ
CC Excl: See code: S49.001

7 √7ᵗʰ **S49.102** Unspecified physeal fracture of lower end of humerus, left arm ᶜᶜ
CC Excl: See code: S49.002

7 √7ᵗʰ **S49.109** Unspecified physeal fracture of lower end of humerus, unspecified arm ᶜᶜ
CC Excl: See code: S49.009

√6ᵗʰ **S49.11** Salter-Harris Type I physeal fracture of lower end of humerus

7 √7ᵗʰ **S49.111** Salter-Harris Type I physeal fracture of lower end of humerus, right arm ᶜᶜ
CC Excl: See code: S49.001

7 √7ᵗʰ **S49.112** Salter-Harris Type I physeal fracture of lower end of humerus, left arm ᶜᶜ
CC Excl: See code: S49.002

7 √7ᵗʰ **S49.119** Salter-Harris Type I physeal fracture of lower end of humerus, unspecified arm ᶜᶜ
CC Excl: See code: S49.009

√6ᵗʰ **S49.12** Salter-Harris Type II physeal fracture of lower end of humerus

7 √7ᵗʰ **S49.121** Salter-Harris Type II physeal fracture of lower end of humerus, right arm ᶜᶜ
CC Excl: See code: S49.001

7 √7ᵗʰ **S49.122** Salter-Harris Type II physeal fracture of lower end of humerus, left arm ᶜᶜ
CC Excl: See code: S49.002

7 √7ᵗʰ **S49.129** Salter-Harris Type II physeal fracture of lower end of humerus, unspecified arm ᶜᶜ
CC Excl: See code: S49.009

√6ᵗʰ **S49.13** Salter Harris Type III physeal fracture of lower end of humerus

7 √7ᵗʰ **S49.131** Salter-Harris Type III physeal fracture of lower end of humerus, right arm ᶜᶜ
CC Excl: See code: S49.001

7 √7ᵗʰ **S49.132** Salter-Harris Type III physeal fracture of lower end of humerus, left arm ᶜᶜ
CC Excl: See code: S49.002

7 √7ᵗʰ **S49.139** Salter-Harris Type III physeal fracture of lower end of humerus, unspecified arm ᶜᶜ
CC Excl: See code: S49.009

√6ᵗʰ **S49.14** Salter-Harris Type IV physeal fracture of lower end of humerus

7 √7ᵗʰ **S49.141** Salter-Harris Type IV physeal fracture of lower end of humerus, right arm ᶜᶜ
CC Excl: See code: S49.001

7 √7ᵗʰ **S49.142** Salter-Harris Type IV physeal fracture of lower end of humerus, left arm ᶜᶜ
CC Excl: See code: S49.002

7 √7ᵗʰ **S49.149** Salter-Harris Type IV physeal fracture of lower end of humerus, unspecified arm ᶜᶜ
CC Excl: See code: S49.009

√6ᵗʰ **S49.19** Other physeal fracture of lower end of humerus

7 √7ᵗʰ **S49.191** Other physeal fracture of lower end of humerus, right arm ᶜᶜ
CC Excl: See code: S49.001

7 √7ᵗʰ **S49.192** Other physeal fracture of lower end of humerus, left arm ᶜᶜ
CC Excl: See code: S49.002

7 √7ᵗʰ **S49.199** Other physeal fracture of lower end of humerus, unspecified arm ᶜᶜ
CC Excl: See code: S49.009

√5ᵗʰ **S49.8** Other specified injuries of shoulder and upper arm

The appropriate 7th is to be added to each code in subcategory S49.8.
A   initial encounter
D   subsequent encounter
S   sequela

√x7ᵗʰ **S49.80** Other specified injuries of shoulder and upper arm, unspecified arm

√x7ᵗʰ **S49.81** Other specified injuries of right shoulder and upper arm

√x7ᵗʰ **S49.82** Other specified injuries of left shoulder and upper arm

√5ᵗʰ **S49.9** Unspecified injury of shoulder and upper arm

The appropriate 7th is to be added to each code in subcategory S49.9.
A   initial encounter
D   subsequent encounter
S   sequela

√x7ᵗʰ **S49.90** Unspecified injury of shoulder and upper arm, unspecified arm

√x7ᵗʰ **S49.91** Unspecified injury of right shoulder and upper arm

√x7ᵗʰ **S49.92** Unspecified injury of left shoulder and upper arm

---

7 HAC = Initial encounter only (7th character A, B or C) and not POA.

☑ Additional Character Required   √x7ᵗʰ Xtension Alert   Unacceptable PDx   Manifestation   Hospital Acquired Condition   *EXCLUDES 1* Not Coded Here   *EXCLUDES 2* Not Included Here

Injury, Poisoning and Certain Other Consequences of External Causes   S50–S51.042

Injuries to the elbow and forearm (S50-S59)

EXCLUDES 2   burns and corrosions (T20-T32)
frostbite (T33-T34)
injuries of wrist and hand (S60-S69)
insect bite or sting, venomous (T63.4)

√4ᵗʰ **S50**   **Superficial injury of elbow and forearm**

> **EXCLUDES 2**   superficial injury of wrist and hand (S60.-)

> The appropriate 7th is to be added to each code from category S50.
> A   initial encounter
> D   subsequent encounter
> S   sequela

√5ᵗʰ   **S50.0**   **Contusion of elbow**

- √x7ᵗʰ   **S50.00**   Contusion of unspecified elbow
- √x7ᵗʰ   **S50.01**   Contusion of right elbow
- √x7ᵗʰ   **S50.02**   Contusion of left elbow

√5ᵗʰ   **S50.1**   **Contusion of forearm**

- √x7ᵗʰ   **S50.10**   Contusion of unspecified forearm
- √x7ᵗʰ   **S50.11**   Contusion of right forearm
- √x7ᵗʰ   **S50.12**   Contusion of left forearm

√5ᵗʰ   **S50.3**   **Other superficial injuries of elbow**

√6ᵗʰ   **S50.31**   **Abrasion of elbow**
- √7ᵗʰ   **S50.311**   Abrasion of right elbow
- √7ᵗʰ   **S50.312**   Abrasion of left elbow
- √7ᵗʰ   **S50.319**   Abrasion of unspecified elbow

√6ᵗʰ   **S50.32**   **Blister (nonthermal) of elbow**
- √7ᵗʰ   **S50.321**   Blister (nonthermal) of right elbow
- √7ᵗʰ   **S50.322**   Blister (nonthermal) of left elbow
- √7ᵗʰ   **S50.329**   Blister (nonthermal) of unspecified elbow

√6ᵗʰ   **S50.34**   **External constriction of elbow**
- √7ᵗʰ   **S50.341**   External constriction of right elbow
- √7ᵗʰ   **S50.342**   External constriction of left elbow
- √7ᵗʰ   **S50.349**   External constriction of unspecified elbow

√6ᵗʰ   **S50.35**   **Superficial foreign body of elbow**
> Splinter in the elbow
- √7ᵗʰ   **S50.351**   Superficial foreign body of right elbow
- √7ᵗʰ   **S50.352**   Superficial foreign body of left elbow
- √7ᵗʰ   **S50.359**   Superficial foreign body of unspecified elbow

√6ᵗʰ   **S50.36**   **Insect bite (nonvenomous) of elbow**
- √7ᵗʰ   **S50.361**   Insect bite (nonvenomous) of right elbow
- √7ᵗʰ   **S50.362**   Insect bite (nonvenomous) of left elbow
- √7ᵗʰ   **S50.369**   Insect bite (nonvenomous) of unspecified elbow

√6ᵗʰ   **S50.37**   **Other superficial bite of elbow**
> **EXCLUDES 1**   open bite of elbow (S51.04)
- √7ᵗʰ   **S50.371**   Other superficial bite of right elbow
- √7ᵗʰ   **S50.372**   Other superficial bite of left elbow
- √7ᵗʰ   **S50.379**   Other superficial bite of unspecified elbow

√5ᵗʰ   **S50.8**   **Other superficial injuries of forearm**

√6ᵗʰ   **S50.81**   **Abrasion of forearm**
- √7ᵗʰ   **S50.811**   Abrasion of right forearm
- √7ᵗʰ   **S50.812**   Abrasion of left forearm
- √7ᵗʰ   **S50.819**   Abrasion of unspecified forearm

√6ᵗʰ   **S50.82**   **Blister (nonthermal) of forearm**
- √7ᵗʰ   **S50.821**   Blister (nonthermal) of right forearm
- √7ᵗʰ   **S50.822**   Blister (nonthermal) of left forearm
- √7ᵗʰ   **S50.829**   Blister (nonthermal) of unspecified forearm

√6ᵗʰ   **S50.84**   **External constriction of forearm**
- √7ᵗʰ   **S50.841**   External constriction of right forearm
- √7ᵗʰ   **S50.842**   External constriction of left forearm
- √7ᵗʰ   **S50.849**   External constriction of unspecified forearm

√6ᵗʰ   **S50.85**   **Superficial foreign body of forearm**
> Splinter in the forearm
- √7ᵗʰ   **S50.851**   Superficial foreign body of right forearm
- √7ᵗʰ   **S50.852**   Superficial foreign body of left forearm

- √7ᵗʰ   **S50.859**   Superficial foreign body of unspecified forearm

√6ᵗʰ   **S50.86**   **Insect bite (nonvenomous) of forearm**
- √7ᵗʰ   **S50.861**   Insect bite (nonvenomous) of right forearm
- √7ᵗʰ   **S50.862**   Insect bite (nonvenomous) of left forearm
- √7ᵗʰ   **S50.869**   Insect bite (nonvenomous) of unspecified forearm

√6ᵗʰ   **S50.87**   **Other superficial bite of forearm**
> **EXCLUDES 1**   open bite of forearm (S51.84)
- √7ᵗʰ   **S50.871**   Other superficial bite of right forearm
- √7ᵗʰ   **S50.872**   Other superficial bite of left forearm
- √7ᵗʰ   **S50.879**   Other superficial bite of unspecified forearm

√5ᵗʰ   **S50.9**   **Unspecified superficial injury of elbow and forearm**

√6ᵗʰ   **S50.90**   **Unspecified superficial injury of elbow**
- √7ᵗʰ   **S50.901**   Unspecified superficial injury of right elbow
- √7ᵗʰ   **S50.902**   Unspecified superficial injury of left elbow
- √7ᵗʰ   **S50.909**   Unspecified superficial injury of unspecified elbow

√6ᵗʰ   **S50.91**   **Unspecified superficial injury of forearm**
- √7ᵗʰ   **S50.911**   Unspecified superficial injury of right forearm
- √7ᵗʰ   **S50.912**   Unspecified superficial injury of left forearm
- √7ᵗʰ   **S50.919**   Unspecified superficial injury of unspecified forearm

√4ᵗʰ   **S51**   **Open wound of elbow and forearm**

> Code also any associated wound infection
> **EXCLUDES 1**   open fracture of elbow and forearm (S52- with open fracture 7th character)
> traumatic amputation of elbow and forearm (S58.-)
> **EXCLUDES 2**   open wound of wrist and hand (S61.-)

> The appropriate 7th is to be added to each code from category S51.
> A   initial encounter
> D   subsequent encounter
> S   sequela

√5ᵗʰ   **S51.0**   **Open wound of elbow**

√6ᵗʰ   **S51.00**   **Unspecified open wound of elbow**
- √7ᵗʰ   **S51.001**   Unspecified open wound of right elbow
  > **AHA:** 2012, 4Q, 108
- √7ᵗʰ   **S51.002**   Unspecified open wound of left elbow
- √7ᵗʰ   **S51.009**   Unspecified open wound of unspecified elbow
  > Open wound of elbow NOS

√6ᵗʰ   **S51.01**   **Laceration without foreign body of elbow**
- √7ᵗʰ   **S51.011**   Laceration without foreign body of right elbow
- √7ᵗʰ   **S51.012**   Laceration without foreign body of left elbow
- √7ᵗʰ   **S51.019**   Laceration without foreign body of unspecified elbow

√6ᵗʰ   **S51.02**   **Laceration with foreign body of elbow**
- √7ᵗʰ   **S51.021**   Laceration with foreign body of right elbow
- √7ᵗʰ   **S51.022**   Laceration with foreign body of left elbow
- √7ᵗʰ   **S51.029**   Laceration with foreign body of unspecified elbow

√6ᵗʰ   **S51.03**   **Puncture wound without foreign body of elbow**
- √7ᵗʰ   **S51.031**   Puncture wound without foreign body of right elbow
- √7ᵗʰ   **S51.032**   Puncture wound without foreign body of left elbow
- √7ᵗʰ   **S51.039**   Puncture wound without foreign body of unspecified elbow

√6ᵗʰ   **S51.04**   **Puncture wound with foreign body of elbow**
- √7ᵗʰ   **S51.041**   Puncture wound with foreign body of right elbow
- √7ᵗʰ   **S51.042**   Puncture wound with foreign body of left elbow

N Newborn: 0   P Pediatric: 0-17   M Maternity: 12-55   A Adult: 15-124   MCC Major CC Condition   PDx MCC PDx acts as own MCC   CC CC Condition   PDx CC PDx acts as own CC

922   ICD-10-CM Draft (2015)

√7th **S51.049** **Puncture wound with foreign body of unspecified elbow**

√6th **S51.05** Open bite of elbow
Bite of elbow NOS
EXCLUDES 1 superficial bite of elbow (S50.36, S50.37)

√7th **S51.051** **Open bite, right elbow**

√7th **S51.052** **Open bite, left elbow**

√7th **S51.059** **Open bite, unspecified elbow**

√5th **S51.8** Open wound of forearm
EXCLUDES 2 open wound of elbow (S51.0-)

√6th **S51.80** Unspecified open wound of forearm

√7th **S51.801** **Unspecified open wound of right forearm**

√7th **S51.802** **Unspecified open wound of left forearm**

√7th **S51.809** **Unspecified open wound of unspecified forearm**
Open wound of forearm NOS

√6th **S51.81** Laceration without foreign body of forearm

√7th **S51.811** **Laceration without foreign body of right forearm**

√7th **S51.812** **Laceration without foreign body of left forearm**

√7th **S51.819** **Laceration without foreign body of unspecified forearm**

√6th **S51.82** Laceration with foreign body of forearm

√7th **S51.821** **Laceration with foreign body of right forearm**

√7th **S51.822** **Laceration with foreign body of left forearm**

√7th **S51.829** **Laceration with foreign body of unspecified forearm**

√6th **S51.83** Puncture wound without foreign body of forearm

√7th **S51.831** **Puncture wound without foreign body of right forearm**

√7th **S51.832** **Puncture wound without foreign body of left forearm**

√7th **S51.839** **Puncture wound without foreign body of unspecified forearm**

√6th **S51.84** Puncture wound with foreign body of forearm

√7th **S51.841** **Puncture wound with foreign body of right forearm**

√7th **S51.842** **Puncture wound with foreign body of left forearm**

√7th **S51.849** **Puncture wound with foreign body of unspecified forearm**

√6th **S51.85** Open bite of forearm
Bite of forearm NOS
EXCLUDES 1 superficial bite of forearm (S50.86, S50.87)

√7th **S51.851** **Open bite of right forearm**

√7th **S51.852** **Open bite of left forearm**

√7th **S51.859** **Open bite of unspecified forearm**

√4th **S52** **Fracture of forearm**
NOTE A fracture not indicated as displaced or nondisplaced should be coded to displaced.
A fracture not indicated as open or closed should be coded to closed.
The open fracture designations are based on the Gustilo open fracture classification.
EXCLUDES 1 traumatic amputation of forearm (S58.-)
EXCLUDES 2 fracture at wrist and hand level (S62.-)

The appropriate 7th is to be added to all codes from category S52 [unless otherwise indicated].
A initial encounter for closed fracture
B initial encounter for open fracture type I or II
initial encounter for open fracture NOS
C initial encounter for open fracture type IIIA, IIIB, or IIIC
D subsequent encounter for closed fracture with routine healing
E subsequent encounter for open fracture type I or II with routine healing
F subsequent encounter for open fracture type IIIA, IIIB, or IIIC with routine healing
G subsequent encounter for closed fracture with delayed healing
H subsequent encounter for open fracture type I or II with delayed healing
J subsequent encounter for open fracture type IIIA, IIIB, or IIIC with delayed healing
K subsequent encounter for closed fracture with nonunion
M subsequent encounter for open fracture type I or II with nonunion
N subsequent encounter for open fracture type IIIA, IIIB, or IIIC with nonunion
P subsequent encounter for closed fracture with malunion
Q subsequent encounter for open fracture type I or II with malunion
R subsequent encounter for open fracture type IIIA, IIIB, or IIIC with malunion
S sequela

√5th **S52.0** Fracture of upper end of ulna
Fracture of proximal end of ulna
EXCLUDES 2 fracture of elbow NOS (S42.40-)
fractures of shaft of ulna (S52.2-)

√6th **S52.00** Unspecified fracture of upper end of ulna
CC Excl: For CC/MCC codes in subcatagory S52.00: MCC with 7th character B or C: S52.001-S52.009 with 7th [B, C], S52.021-S52.109 with 7th [B, C], S52.121-S52.516 with 7th [B, C], S52.531-S52.616 with 7th [A, B, C], S52.691-S52.92X with 7th [A, B, C], S59.001-S59.099 with 7th A, S59.201-S59.299 with 7th A, S62.90XB
CC with 7th character K, M, N, P, Q, or R: M80.00X-M84.68X with 7th [K, P], S02.0XX-S02.92X with 7th K, S12.000-S12.691 with 7th K, S22.000-S22.9XX with 7th K, S32.000-S32.9XX with 7th K, S42.001-S42.92X with 7th [K, P], S49.001-S49.199 with 7th [K, P], S52.001-S52.92X with 7th [K, M, N, P, Q, R], S59.001-S59.299 with 7th [K, P], S62.001-S62.92X with 7th [K, P], S72.001-S72.92X with 7th [K, M, N, P, Q, R], S79.001-S79.199 with 7th [K, P], S82.001-S82.92X with 7th [K, M, N, P, Q, R], S89.001-S89.399 with 7th [K, P], S92.001-S92.919 with 7th [K, P]

7 √7th **S52.001** **Unspecified fracture of upper end of right ulna** MCC CC

7 √7th **S52.002** **Unspecified fracture of upper end of left ulna** MCC CC

7 √7th **S52.009** **Unspecified fracture of upper end of unspecified ulna** MCC CC

7 HAC = Initial encounter only (7th character A, B or C) and not POA.

√ Additional Character Required √x7th Xtension Alert Unacceptable PDx Manifestation Hospital Acquired Condition EXCLUDES 1 Not Coded Here EXCLUDES 2 Not Included Here
ICD-10-CM Draft (2015) 923

√6ᵗʰ **S52.01** **Torus** fracture of upper end of ulna

> The appropriate 7th is to be added to all codes in subcategory S52.01.
> A   initial encounter for closed fracture
> D   subsequent encounter for fracture with routine healing
> G   subsequent encounter for fracture with delayed healing
> K   subsequent encounter for fracture with nonunion
> P   subsequent encounter for fracture with malunion
> S   sequela

7 √7ᵗʰ **S52.011** **Torus fracture of upper end of right ulna** `CC`

CC Excl: CC with 7th character A: S52.001-S52.011 with 7th [A, B, C], S52.019-S52.111 with 7th A, S52.119-S52.211 with 7th A, S52.219-S52.311 with 7th A, S52.319-S52.521 with 7th A, S52.529-S52.621 with 7th A, S52.629-S52.92X with 7th A, S59.001A, S59.009-S59.011 with 7th A, S59.019-S59.021 with 7th A, S59.029-S59.031 with 7th A, S59.039-S59.041 with 7th A, S59.049-S59.091 with 7th A, S59.099-S59.101 with 7th A, S59.109-S59.111 with 7th A, S59.119-S59.121 with 7th A, S59.129-S59.131 with 7th A, S59.139-S59.141 with 7th A, S59.149-S59.191 with 7th A, S59.199-S59.201 with 7th A, S59.209-S59.211 with 7th A, S59.219-S59.221 with 7th A, S59.229-S59.231 with 7th A, S59.239-S59.241 with 7th A, S59.249-S59.291 with 7th A, S59.299A

CC with 7th character K or P: M80.00X-M84.68X with 7th [K, P], S02.0XX-S02.92X with 7th K, S12.000-S12.691 with 7th K, S22.000-S22.9XX with 7th K, S32.000-S32.9XX with 7th K, S42.001-S42.92X with 7th [K, P], S49.001-S49.199 with 7th [K, P], S52.001-S52.92X with 7th [K, M, N, P, Q, R], S59.001-S59.299 with 7th [K, P], S62.001-S62.92X with 7th [K, P], S72.001-S72.92X with 7th [K, M, N, P, Q, R], S79.001-S79.199 with 7th [K, P], S82.001-S82.92X with 7th [K, M, N, P, Q, R], S89.001-S89.399 with 7th [K, P], S92.001-S92.919 with 7th [K, P]

7 √7ᵗʰ **S52.012** **Torus fracture of upper end of left ulna** `CC`

CC Excl: CC with 7th character A: S52.001-S52.009 with 7th [B, C], S52.012-S52.109 with 7th A, S52.112-S52.209 with 7th A, S52.212-S52.309 with 7th A, S52.312-S52.516 with 7th A, S52.522-S52.616 with 7th A, S52.622-S52.92X with 7th A, S59.002-S59.009 with 7th A, S59.012-S59.019 with 7th A, S59.022-S59.029 with 7th A, S59.032-S59.039 with 7th A, S59.042-S59.049 with 7th A, S59.092-S59.099 with 7th A, S59.102-S59.109 with 7th A, S59.112-S59.119 with 7th A, S59.122-S59.129 with 7th A, S59.132-S59.139 with 7th A, S59.142-S59.149 with 7th A, S59.192-S59.199 with 7th A, S59.202-S59.209 with 7th A, S59.212-S59.219 with 7th A, S59.222-S59.229 with 7th A, S59.232-S59.239 with 7th A, S59.242-S59.249 with 7th A, S59.292-S59.299 with 7th A

CC with 7th character K or P: M80.00X-M84.68X with 7th [K, P], S02.0XX-S02.92X with 7th K, S12.000-S12.691 with 7th K, S22.000-S22.9XX with 7th K, S32.000-S32.9XX with 7th K, S42.001-S42.92X with 7th [K, P], S49.001-S49.199 with 7th [K, P], S52.001-S52.92X with 7th [K, M, N, P, Q, R], S59.001-S59.299 with 7th [K, P], S62.001-S62.92X with 7th [K, P], S72.001-S72.92X with 7th [K, M, N, P, Q, R], S79.001-S79.199 with 7th [K, P], S82.001-S82.92X with 7th [K, M, N, P, Q, R], S89.001-S89.399 with 7th [K, P], S92.001-S92.919 with 7th [K, P]

7 √7ᵗʰ **S52.019** **Torus fracture of upper end of unspecified ulna** `CC`

CC Excl: CC with 7th character A: S52.001-S52.92X with 7th [A, B, C], S59.001-S59.299 with 7th A

CC with 7th character K or P: M80.00X-M84.68X with 7th [K, P], S02.0XX-S02.92X with 7th K, S12.000-S12.691 with 7th K, S22.000-S22.9XX with 7th K, S32.000-S32.9XX with 7th K, S42.001-S42.92X with 7th [K, P], S49.001-S49.199 with 7th [K, P], S52.001-S52.92X with 7th [K, M, N, P, Q, R], S59.001-S59.299 with 7th [K, P], S62.001-S62.92X with 7th [K, P], S72.001-S72.92X with 7th [K, M, N, P, Q, R], S79.001-S79.199 with 7th [K, P], S82.001-S82.92X with 7th [K, M, N, P, Q, R], S89.001-S89.399 with 7th [K, P], S92.001-S92.919 with 7th [K, P]

√6ᵗʰ **S52.02** **Fracture of** olecranon process without intraarticular **extension of** ulna

CC Excl: For CC/MCC codes in subcatagory S52.02, unless otherwise noted: MCC with 7th character B or C: S52.001-S52.009 with 7th [B, C], S52.021-S52.109 with 7th [B, C], S52.121-S52.516 with 7th [B, C], S52.531-S52.616 with 7th [B, C], S52.691-S52.92X with 7th [A, B, C], S59.001-S59.099 with 7th A, S59.201-S59.299 with 7th A, S62.90XB

CC with 7th character K, M, N, P, Q, or R: M80.00X-M84.68X with 7th [K, P], S02.0XX-S02.92X with 7th K, S12.000-S12.691 with 7th K, S22.000-S22.9XX with 7th K, S32.000-S32.9XX with 7th K, S42.001-S42.92X with 7th [K, P], S49.001-S49.199 with 7th [K, P], S52.001-S52.92X with 7th [K, M, N, P, Q, R], S59.001-S59.299 with 7th [K, P], S62.001-S62.92X with 7th [K, P], S72.001-S72.92X with 7th [K, M, N, P, Q, R], S79.001-S79.199 with 7th [K, P], S82.001-S82.92X with 7th [K, M, N, P, Q, R], S89.001-S89.399 with 7th [K, P], S92.001-S92.919 with 7th [K, P]

7 √7ᵗʰ **S52.021** **Displaced** fracture of olecranon process without intraarticular extension of **right** ulna `MCC` `CC`

7 √7ᵗʰ **S52.022** **Displaced** fracture of olecranon process without intraarticular extension of **left** ulna `MCC` `CC`

7 √7ᵗʰ **S52.023** **Displaced** fracture of olecranon process without intraarticular extension of **unspecified** ulna `MCC` `CC`

7 √7ᵗʰ **S52.024** **Nondisplaced** fracture of olecranon process without intraarticular extension of **right** ulna `MCC` `CC`

7 √7ᵗʰ **S52.025** **Nondisplaced** fracture of olecranon process without intraarticular extension of **left** ulna `MCC` `CC`

7 √7ᵗʰ **S52.026** **Nondisplaced** fracture of olecranon process without intraarticular extension of **unspecified** ulna `MCC` `CC`

√6ᵗʰ **S52.03** **Fracture of** olecranon process with intraarticular **extension of** ulna

CC Excl: For CC/MCC codes in subcatagory S52.03, unless otherwise noted: MCC with 7th character B or C: S52.001-S52.009 with 7th [B, C], S52.021-S52.109 with 7th [B, C], S52.121-S52.516 with 7th [B, C], S52.531-S52.616 with 7th [B, C], S52.691-S52.92 with 7th [A, B, C], S59.001-S59.099 with 7th A, S59.201-S59.299 with 7th A, S62.90X with 7th B

CC with 7th character K, M, N, P, Q, or R: M80.00X-M84.68X with 7th [K, P], S02.0XX-S02.92X with 7th K, S12.000-S12.691 with 7th K, S22.000-S22.9XX with 7th K, S32.000-S32.9XX with 7th K, S42.001-S42.92X with 7th [K, P], S49.001-S49.199 with 7th [K, P], S52.001-S52.92X with 7th [K, M, N, P, Q, R], S59.001-S59.299 with 7th [K, P], S62.001-S62.92X with 7th [K, P], S72.001-S72.92X with 7th [K, M, N, P, Q, R], S79.001-S79.199 with 7th [K, P], S82.001-S82.92X with 7th [K, M, N, P, Q, R], S89.001-S89.399 with 7th [K, P], S92.001-S92.919 with 7th [K, P]

7 √7ᵗʰ **S52.031** **Displaced** fracture of olecranon process with intraarticular extension of **right** ulna `MCC` `CC`

---

7 HAC = Initial encounter only (7th character A, B or C) and not POA.

Ⓝ Newborn: 0   Ⓟ Pediatric: 0-17   Ⓜ Maternity: 12-55   Ⓐ Adult: 15-124   `MCC` Major CC Condition   `PDx MCC` PDx acts as own MCC   `CC` CC Condition   `PDx CC` PDx acts as own CC

924   ICD-10-CM Draft (2015)

7 **✓7ᵗʰ** **S52.032** Displaced fracture of olecranon process with intraarticular extension of left ulna   MCC CC

7 **✓7ᵗʰ** **S52.033** Displaced fracture of olecranon process with intraarticular extension of unspecified ulna   MCC CC

7 **✓7ᵗʰ** **S52.034** Nondisplaced fracture of olecranon process with intraarticular extension of right ulna   MCC CC

7 **✓7ᵗʰ** **S52.035** Nondisplaced fracture of olecranon process with intraarticular extension of left ulna   MCC CC

7 **✓7ᵗʰ** **S52.036** Nondisplaced fracture of olecranon process with intraarticular extension of unspecified ulna   MCC CC

✓6ᵗʰ **S52.04** Fracture of coronoid process of ulna

> CC Excl: For CC/MCC codes in subcategory S52.04, unless otherwise noted: MCC with 7th character B or C: S52.001-S52.009 with 7th [B, C], S52.021-S52.109 with 7th [B, C], S52.121-S52.516 with 7th [B, C], S52.531-S52.616 with 7th [A, B, C], S52.691-S52.92X with 7th [A, B, C], S59.001-S59.099 with 7th A, S59.201-S59.299 with 7th A, S62.90XB
> CC with 7th character K, M, N, P, Q, or R: M80.00X-M84.68X with 7th [K, P], S02.0XX-S02.92X with 7th K, S12.000-S12.691 with 7th K, S22.000-S22.9XX with 7th K, S32.000-S32.9XX with 7th K, S42.001-S42.92X with 7th [K, P], S49.001-S49.199 with 7th [K, P], S52.001-S52.92X with 7th [K, M, N, P, Q, R], S59.001-S59.299 with 7th [K, P], S62.001-S62.92X with 7th [K, P], S72.001-S72.92X with 7th [K, M, N, P, Q, R], S79.001-S79.199 with 7th [K, P], S82.001-S82.92X with 7th [K, M, N, P, Q, R], S89.001-S89.399 with 7th [K, P], S92.001-S92.919 with 7th [K, P]

7 **✓7ᵗʰ** **S52.041** Displaced fracture of coronoid process of right ulna   MCC CC

7 **✓7ᵗʰ** **S52.042** Displaced fracture of coronoid process of left ulna   MCC CC

7 **✓7ᵗʰ** **S52.043** Displaced fracture of coronoid process of unspecified ulna   MCC CC

7 **✓7ᵗʰ** **S52.044** Nondisplaced fracture of coronoid process of right ulna   MCC CC

7 **✓7ᵗʰ** **S52.045** Nondisplaced fracture of coronoid process of left ulna   MCC CC

7 **✓7ᵗʰ** **S52.046** Nondisplaced fracture of coronoid process of unspecified ulna   MCC CC

✓6ᵗʰ **S52.09** Other fracture of upper end of ulna

> CC Excl: For CC/MCC codes in subcatagory S52.09, unless otherwise noted: MCC with 7th character B or C: S52.001-S52.009 with 7th [B, C], S52.021-S52.109 with 7th [B, C], S52.121-S52.516 with 7th [B, C], S52.531-S52.616 with 7th [A, B, C], S52.691-S52.92X with 7th [A, B, C], S59.001-S59.099 with 7th A, S59.201-S59.299 with 7th A, S62.90XB
> CC with 7th character K, M, N, P, Q, or R: M80.00X-M84.68X with 7th [K, P], S02.0XX-S02.92X with 7th K, S12.000-S12.691 with 7th K, S22.000-S22.9XX with 7th K, S32.000-S32.9XX with 7th K, S42.001-S42.92X with 7th [K, P], S49.001-S49.199 with 7th [K, P], S52.001-S52.92X with 7th [K, M, N, P, Q, R], S59.001-S59.299 with 7th [K, P], S62.001-S62.92X with 7th [K, P], S72.001-S72.92X with 7th [K, M, N, P, Q, R], S79.001-S79.199 with 7th [K, P], S82.001-S82.92X with 7th [K, M, N, P, Q, R], S89.001-S89.399 with 7th [K, P], S92.001-S92.919 with 7th [K, P]

7 **✓7ᵗʰ** **S52.091** Other fracture of upper end of right ulna   MCC CC

7 **✓7ᵗʰ** **S52.092** Other fracture of upper end of left ulna   MCC CC

7 **✓7ᵗʰ** **S52.099** Other fracture of upper end of unspecified ulna   MCC CC

✓5ᵗʰ **S52.1** Fracture of upper end of radius
Fracture of proximal end of radius
> EXCLUDES 2 physeal fractures of upper end of radius (S59.2-)
> fracture of shaft of radius (S52.3-)

✓6ᵗʰ **S52.10** Unspecified fracture of upper end of radius

> CC Excl: For CC/MCC codes in subcatagory S52.10, unless otherwise noted: MCC with 7th character B or C: S52.001-S52.009 with 7th [B, C], S52.021-S52.109 with 7th [B, C], S52.121-S52.516 with 7th [B, C], S52.531-S52.616 with 7th [A, B, C], S52.691-S52.92X with 7th [A, B, C], S59.001-S59.099 with 7th A, S59.201-S59.299 with 7th A, S62.90XB
> CC with 7th character K, M, N, P, Q, or R: M80.00X-M84.68X with 7th [K, P], S02.0XX-S02.92X with 7th K, S12.000-S12.691 with 7th K, S22.000-S22.9XX with 7th K, S32.000-S32.9XX with 7th K, S42.001-S42.92X with 7th [K, P], S49.001-S49.199 with 7th [K, P], S52.001-S52.92X with 7th [K, M, N, P, Q, R], S59.001-S59.299 with 7th [K, P], S62.001-S62.92X with 7th [K, P], S72.001-S72.92X with 7th [K, M, N, P, Q, R], S79.001-S79.199 with 7th [K, P], S82.001-S82.92X with 7th [K, M, N, P, Q, R], S89.001-S89.399 with 7th [K, P], S92.001-S92.919 with 7th [K, P]

7 **✓7ᵗʰ** **S52.101** Unspecified fracture of upper end of right radius   MCC CC

7 **✓7ᵗʰ** **S52.102** Unspecified fracture of upper end of left radius   MCC CC

7 **✓7ᵗʰ** **S52.109** Unspecified fracture of upper end of unspecified radius   MCC CC

✓6ᵗʰ **S52.11** Torus fracture of upper end of radius

> The appropriate 7th is to be added to all codes in subcategory S52.11.
> A   initial encounter for closed fracture
> D   subsequent encounter for fracture with routine healing
> G   subsequent encounter for fracture with delayed healing
> K   subsequent encounter for fracture with nonunion
> P   subsequent encounter for fracture with malunion
> S   sequela

7 **✓7ᵗʰ** **S52.111** Torus fracture of upper end of right radius   CC

> CC Excl: CC with 7th character A: S52.001-S52.011 with 7th [A, B, C], S52.019-S52.111 with 7th A, S52.119-S52.211 with 7th A, S52.219-S52.311 with 7th A, S52.319-S52.521 with 7th A, S52.529-S52.621 with 7th A, S52.629-S52.92X with 7th A, S59.001 with 7th A, S59.009-S59.011 with 7th A, S59.019-S59.021 with 7th A, S59.029-S59.031 with 7th A, S59.039-S59.041 with 7th A, S59.049-S59.091 with 7th A, S59.099-S59.101 with 7th A, S59.109-S59.111 with 7th A, S59.119-S59.121 with 7th A, S59.129-S59.131 with 7th A, S59.139-S59.141 with 7th A, S59.149-S59.191 with 7th A, S59.199-S59.201 with 7th A, S59.209-S59.211 with 7th A, S59.219-S59.221 with 7th A, S59.229-S59.231 with 7th A, S59.239-S59.241 with 7th A, S59.249-S59.291 with 7th A, S59.299A
> CC with 7th character K, P: M80.00X-M84.68X with 7th [K, P], S02.0XX-S02.92X with 7th K, S12.000-S12.691 with 7th K, S22.000-S22.9XX with 7th K, S32.000-S32.9XX with 7th K, S42.001-S42.92X with 7th [K, P], S49.001-S49.199 with 7th [K, P], S52.001-S52.92X with 7th [K, M, N, P, Q, R], S59.001-S59.299 with 7th [K, P], S62.001-S62.92X with 7th [K, P], S72.001-S72.92X with 7th [K, M, N, P, Q, R], S79.001-S79.199 with 7th [K, P], S82.001-S82.92X with 7th [K, M, N, P, Q, R], S89.001-S89.399 with 7th [K, P], S92.001-S92.919 with 7th [K, P]

---

7 HAC = Initial encounter only (7th character A, B or C) and not POA.

✓ Additional Character Required   ✓ˣ⁷ᵗʰ Xtension Alert   Unacceptable PDx   Manifestation   Hospital Acquired Condition   EXCLUDES 1 Not Coded Here   EXCLUDES 2 Not Included Here

ICD-10-CM Draft (2015)   925

7 √7ᵗʰ **S52.112** **Torus fracture of upper end of left radius** `CC`
CC Excl: CC with 7th character A: S52.001-S52.009 with 7th [B, C], S52.012-S52.109 with 7th A, S52.112-S52.209 with 7th A, S52.212-S52.309 with 7th A, S52.312-S52.516 with 7th A, S52.522-S52.616 with 7th A, S52.622-S52.92X with 7th A, S59.002-S59.009 with 7th A, S59.012-S59.019 with 7th A, S59.022-S59.029 with 7th A, S59.032-S59.039 with 7th A, S59.042-S59.049 with 7th A, S59.092-S59.099 with 7th A, S59.102-S59.109 with 7th A, S59.112-S59.119 with 7th A, S59.122-S59.129 with 7th A, S59.132-S59.139 with 7th A, S59.142-S59.149 with 7th A, S59.192-S59.199 with 7th A, S59.202-S59.209 with 7th A, S59.212-S59.219 with 7th A, S59.222-S59.229 with 7th A, S59.232-S59.239 with 7th A, S59.242-S59.249 with 7th A, S59.292-S59.299 with 7th A

CC with 7th character K or P: M80.00X-M84.68X with 7th [K, P], S02.0XX-S02.92X with 7th K, S12.000-S12.691 with 7th K, S22.000-S22.9XX with 7th K, S32.000-S32.9XX with 7th K, S42.001-S42.92X with 7th [K, P], S49.001-S49.199 with 7th [K, P], S52.001-S52.92X with 7th [K, M, N, P, Q, R], S59.001-S59.299 with 7th [K, P], S62.001-S62.92X with 7th [K, P], S72.001-S72.92X with 7th [K, M, N, P, Q, R], S79.001-S79.199 with 7th [K, P], S82.001-S82.92X with 7th [K, M, N, P, Q, R], S89.001-S89.399 with 7th [K, P], S92.001-S92.919 with 7th [K, P]

√7ᵗʰ **S52.119** **Torus fracture of upper end of unspecified radius** `CC`
CC Excl: CC with 7th character A: S52.001-S52.92X with 7th [A, B, C], S59.001-S59.299 with 7th A
CC Excl: CC with 7th character K or P: M80.00X-M84.68X with 7th [K, P], S02.0XX-S02.92X with 7th K, S12.000-S12.691 with 7th K, S22.000-S22.9XX with 7th K, S32.000-S32.9XX with 7th K, S42.001-S42.92X with 7th [K, P], S49.001-S49.199 with 7th [K, P], S52.001-S52.92X with 7th [K, M, N, P, Q, R], S59.001-S59.299 with 7th [K, P], S62.001-S62.92X with 7th [K, P], S72.001-S72.92X with 7th [K, M, N, P, Q, R], S79.001-S79.199 with 7th [K, P], S82.001-S82.92X with 7th [K, M, N, P, Q, R], S89.001-S89.399 with 7th [K, P], S92.001-S92.919 with 7th [K, P]

√6ᵗʰ **S52.12** **Fracture of head of radius**

CC Excl: For CC/MCC codes in subcatagory S52.12: See code: S52.10

7 √7ᵗʰ **S52.121** **Displaced fracture of head of right radius** `MCC` `CC`
7 √7ᵗʰ **S52.122** **Displaced fracture of head of left radius** `MCC` `CC`
7 √7ᵗʰ **S52.123** **Displaced fracture of head of unspecified radius** `MCC` `CC`
7 √7ᵗʰ **S52.124** **Nondisplaced fracture of head of right radius** `MCC` `CC`
7 √7ᵗʰ **S52.125** **Nondisplaced fracture of head of left radius** `MCC` `CC`
7 √7ᵗʰ **S52.126** **Nondisplaced fracture of head of unspecified radius** `MCC` `CC`

√6ᵗʰ **S52.13** **Fracture of neck of radius**

CC Excl: For CC/MCC codes in subcatagory S52.12: See code: S52.10

7 √7ᵗʰ **S52.131** **Displaced fracture of neck of right radius** `MCC` `CC`
7 √7ᵗʰ **S52.132** **Displaced fracture of neck of left radius** `MCC` `CC`
7 √7ᵗʰ **S52.133** **Displaced fracture of neck of unspecified radius** `MCC` `CC`
7 √7ᵗʰ **S52.134** **Nondisplaced fracture of neck of right radius** `MCC` `CC`
7 √7ᵗʰ **S52.135** **Nondisplaced fracture of neck of left radius** `MCC` `CC`
7 √7ᵗʰ **S52.136** **Nondisplaced fracture of neck of unspecified radius** `MCC` `CC`

√6ᵗʰ **S52.18** **Other fracture of upper end of radius**

CC Excl: For CC/MCC codes in subcatagory S52.12: See code: S52.10

7 √7ᵗʰ **S52.181** **Other fracture of upper end of right radius** `MCC` `CC`
7 √7ᵗʰ **S52.182** **Other fracture of upper end of left radius** `MCC` `CC`
7 √7ᵗʰ **S52.189** **Other fracture of upper end of unspecified radius** `MCC` `CC`

√5ᵗʰ **S52.2** **Fracture of shaft of ulna**

√6ᵗʰ **S52.20** **Unspecified fracture of shaft of ulna**
Fracture of ulna NOS

7 √7ᵗʰ **S52.201** **Unspecified fracture of shaft of right ulna** `MCC` `CC`
CC Excl: CC with 7th character A: S52.001-S52.011 with 7th [A, B, C], S52.019-S52.111 with 7th A, S52.119-S52.211 with 7th A, S52.219-S52.311 with 7th A, S52.319-S52.521 with 7th A, S52.529-S52.621 with 7th A, S52.629-S52.92X with 7th A, S59.001A, S59.009-S59.011 with 7th A, S59.019-S59.021 with 7th A, S59.029-S59.031 with 7th A, S59.039-S59.041 with 7th A, S59.049-S59.091 with 7th A, S59.099-S59.101 with 7th A, S59.109-S59.111 with 7th A, S59.119-S59.121 with 7th A, S59.129-S59.131 with 7th A, S59.139-S59.141 with 7th A, S59.149-S59.191 with 7th A, S59.199-S59.201 with 7th A, S59.209-S59.211 with 7th A, S59.219-S59.221 with 7th A, S59.229-S59.231 with 7th A, S59.239-S59.241 with 7th A, S59.249-S59.291 with 7th A, S59.299A

MCC with 7th character B or C: S52.001-S52.009 with 7th [B, C], S52.021-S52.109 with 7th [B, C], S52.121-S52.516 with 7th [B, C], S52.531-S52.616 with 7th [A, B, C], S52.691-S52.92X with 7th [A, B, C], S59.001-S59.099 with 7th A, S59.201-S59.299 with 7th A, S62.90XB

MCC with 7th character K, M, N, P, Q or R: M80.00X-M84.68X with 7th [K, P], S02.0XX-S02.92X with 7th K, S12.000-S12.691 with 7th K, S22.000-S22.9XX with 7th K, S32.000-S32.9XX with 7th K, S42.001-S42.92X with 7th [K, P], S49.001-S49.199 with 7th [K, P], S52.001-S52.92X with 7th [K, M, N, P, Q, R], S59.001-S59.299 with 7th [K, P], S62.001-S62.92X with 7th [K, P], S72.001-S72.92X with 7th [K, M, N, P, Q, R], S79.001-S79.199 with 7th [K, P], S82.001-S82.92X with 7th [K, M, N, P, Q, R], S89.001-S89.399 with 7th [K, P], S92.001-S92.919 with 7th [K, P]

7 √7ᵗʰ **S52.202** **Unspecified fracture of shaft of left ulna** `MCC` `CC`
CC Excl: CC with 7th character A: S52.001-S52.009 with 7th [B, C], S52.012-S52.109 with 7th A, S52.112-S52.209 with 7th A, S52.212-S52.309 with 7th A, S52.312-S52.516 with 7th A, S52.522-S52.616 with 7th A, S52.622-S52.92X with 7th A, S59.002-S59.009 with 7th A, S59.012-S59.019 with 7th A, S59.022-S59.029 with 7th A, S59.032-S59.039 with 7th A, S59.042-S59.049 with 7th A, S59.092-S59.099 with 7th A, S59.102-S59.109 with 7th A, S59.112-S59.119 with 7th A, S59.122-S59.129 with 7th A, S59.132-S59.139 with 7th A, S59.142-S59.149 with 7th A, S59.192-S59.199 with 7th A, S59.202-S59.209 with 7th A, S59.212-S59.219 with 7th A, S59.222-S59.229 with 7th A, S59.232-S59.239 with 7th A, S59.242-S59.249 with 7th A, S59.292-S59.299 with 7th A

MCC with 7th character B or C: S52.001-S52.009 with 7th [B, C], S52.021-S52.109 with 7th [B, C], S52.121-S52.516 with 7th [B, C], S52.531-S52.616 with 7th [A, B, C], S52.691-S52.92X with 7th [A, B, C], S59.001-S59.099 with 7th A, S59.201-S59.299 with 7th A, S62.90X with 7th B

MCC with 7th character K, M, N, P, Q or R: M80.00X-M84.68X with 7th [K, P], S02.0XX-S02.92X with 7th K, S12.000-S12.691 with 7th K, S22.000-S22.9XX with 7th K, S32.000-S32.9XX with 7th K, S42.001-S42.92X with 7th [K, P], S49.001-S49.199 with 7th [K, P], S52.001-S52.92X with 7th [K, M, N, P, Q, R], S59.001-S59.299 with 7th [K, P], S62.001-

7 HAC = Initial encounter only (7th character A, B or C) and not POA.

`N` Newborn: 0   `P` Pediatric: 0-17   `M` Maternity: 12-55   `A` Adult: 15-124   `MCC` Major CC Condition   `PDx MCC` PDx acts as own MCC   `CC` CC Condition   `PDx CC` PDx acts as own CC

926

ICD-10-CM Draft (2015)

S62.92X with 7th [K, P], S72.001-S72.92X with 7th [K, M, N, P, Q, R], S79.001-S79.199 with 7th [K, P], S82.001-S82.92X with 7th [K, M, N, P, Q, R], S89.001-S89.399 with 7th [K, P], S92.001-S92.919 with 7th [K, P]

7 √7th **S52.209 Unspecified fracture of shaft of unspecified ulna** `MCC` `CC`

CC Excl: CC with 7th character A: S52.001-S52.92X with 7th [A, B, C], S59.001-S59.299 with 7th A

MCC with 7th character B or C: S52.001-S52.92X with 7th [B, C], S52.021-S52.109 with 7th [B, C], S52.121-S52.516 with 7th [B, C], S52.531-S52.616 with 7th [A, B, C], S52.691-S52.92X with 7th [A, B, C], S59.001-S59.099 with 7th A, S59.201-S59.299 with 7th A, S62.90XB

MCC with 7th character K, M, N, P, Q or R: M80.00X-M84.68X with 7th [K, P], S02.0XX-S02.92X with 7th K, S12.000-S12.691 with 7th K, S22.000-S22.9XX with 7th K, S32.000-S32.9XX with 7th K, S42.001-S42.92X with 7th [K, P], S49.001-S49.199 with 7th [K, P], S52.001-S52.92X with 7th [K, M, N, P, Q, R], S59.001-S59.299 with 7th [K, P], S62.001-S62.92X with 7th [K, P], S72.001-S72.92X with 7th [K, M, N, P, Q, R], S79.001-S79.199 with 7th [K, P], S82.001-S82.92X with 7th [K, M, N, P, Q, R], S89.001-S89.399 with 7th [K, P], S92.001-S92.919 with 7th [K, P]

√6th **S52.21 Greensrick fracture of shaft of ulna**

The appropriate 7th is to be added to all codes in subcategory S52.21.
A   initial encounter for closed fracture
D   subsequent encounter for fracture with routine healing
G   subsequent encounter for fracture with delayed healing
K   subsequent encounter for fracture with nonunion
P   subsequent encounter for fracture with malunion
S   sequela

7 √7th **S52.211 Greenstick fracture of shaft of right ulna** `CC`

CC Excl: CC with 7th character A: S52.001-S52.011 with 7th [A, B, C], S52.019-S52.111 with 7th A, S52.119-S52.211 with 7th A, S52.219-S52.311 with 7th A, S52.319-S52.521 with 7th A, S52.529-S52.621 with 7th A, S52.629-S52.92X with 7th A, S59.001 with 7th A, S59.009-S59.011 with 7th A, S59.019-S59.021 with 7th A, S59.029-S59.031 with 7th A, S59.039-S59.041 with 7th A, S59.049-S59.091 with 7th A, S59.099-S59.101 with 7th A, S59.109-S59.111 with 7th A, S59.119-S59.121 with 7th A, S59.129-S59.131 with 7th A, S59.139-S59.141 with 7th A, S59.149-S59.191 with 7th A, S59.199-S59.201 with 7th A, S59.209-S59.211 with 7th A, S59.219-S59.221 with 7th A, S59.229-S59.231 with 7th A, S59.239-S59.241 with 7th A, S59.249-S59.291 with 7th A, S59.299A

CC with 7th character K or P: M80.00X-M84.68X with 7th [K, P], S02.0XX-S02.92X with 7th K, S12.000-S12.691 with 7th K, S22.000-S22.9XX with 7th K, S32.000-S32.9XX with 7th K, S42.001-S42.92X with 7th [K, P], S49.001-S49.199 with 7th [K, P], S52.001-S52.92X with 7th [K, M, N, P, Q, R], S59.001-S59.299 with 7th [K, P], S62.001-S62.92X with 7th [K, P], S72.001-S72.92X with 7th [K, M, N, P, Q, R], S79.001-S79.199 with 7th [K, P], S82.001-S82.92X with 7th [K, M, N, P, Q, R], S89.001-S89.399 with 7th [K, P], S92.001-S92.919 with 7th [K, P]

7 √7th **S52.212 Greenstick fracture of shaft of left ulna** `CC`

CC Excl: CC with 7th character A: S52.001-S52.009 with 7th [B, C], S52.012-S52.109 with 7th A, S52.112-S52.209 with 7th A, S52.212-S52.309 with 7th A, S52.312-S52.516 with 7th A, S52.522-S52.616 with 7th A, S52.622-S52.92X with 7th A, S59.002-S59.009 with 7th A, S59.012-S59.019 with 7th A, S59.022-S59.029 with 7th A, S59.032-S59.039 with 7th A, S59.042-S59.049 with 7th A, S59.092-S59.099 with 7th A, S59.102-S59.109 with 7th A, S59.112-S59.119 with 7th A, S59.122-S59.129 with 7th A, S59.132-S59.139 with 7th A, S59.142-S59.149 with 7th A, S59.192-S59.199 with 7th A, S59.202-S59.209 with 7th A, S59.212-S59.219 with 7th A, S59.222-S59.229 with 7th A, S59.232-S59.239 with 7th A, S59.242-S59.249 with 7th A, S59.292-S59.299 with 7th A

CC with 7th character K or P: M80.00X-M84.68X with 7th [K, P], S02.0XX-S02.92X with 7th K, S12.000-S12.691 with 7th K, S22.000-S22.9XX with 7th K, S32.000-S32.9XX with 7th K, S42.001-S42.92X with 7th [K, P], S49.001-S49.199 with 7th [K, P], S52.001-S52.92X with 7th [K, M, N, P, Q, R], S59.001-S59.299 with 7th [K, P], S62.001-S62.92X with 7th [K, P], S72.001-S72.92X with 7th [K, M, N, P, Q, R], S79.001-S79.199 with 7th [K, P], S82.001-S82.92X with 7th [K, M, N, P, Q, R], S89.001-S89.399 with 7th [K, P], S92.001-S92.919 with 7th [K, P]

7 √7th **S52.219 Greenstick fracture of shaft of unspecified ulna** `CC`

CC Excl: CC with 7th character A: S52.001-S52.92X with 7th [A, B, C], S59.001-S59.299 with 7th A

CC with 7th character K or P: M80.00X-M84.68X with 7th [K, P], S02.0XX-S02.92X with 7th K, S12.000-S12.691 with 7th K, S22.000-S22.9XX with 7th K, S32.000-S32.9XX with 7th K, S42.001-S42.92X with 7th [K, P], S49.001-S49.199 with 7th [K, P], S52.001-S52.92X with 7th [K, M, N, P, Q, R], S59.001-S59.299 with 7th [K, P], S62.001-S62.92X with 7th [K, P], S72.001-S72.92X with 7th [K, M, N, P, Q, R], S79.001-S79.199 with 7th [K, P], S82.001-S82.92X with 7th [K, M, N, P, Q, R], S89.001-S89.399 with 7th [K, P], S92.001-S92.919 with 7th [K, P]

√6th **S52.22 Transverse fracture of shaft of ulna**

7 √7th **S52.221 Displaced transverse fracture of shaft of right ulna** `MCC` `CC`
CC Excl: See code: S52.201

7 √7th **S52.222 Displaced transverse fracture of shaft of left ulna** `MCC` `CC`
CC Excl: See code: S52.202

7 √7th **S52.223 Displaced transverse fracture of shaft of unspecified ulna** `MCC` `CC`
CC Excl: See code: S52.209

7 √7th **S52.224 Nondisplaced transverse fracture of shaft of right ulna** `MCC` `CC`
CC Excl: See code: S52.201

7 √7th **S52.225 Nondisplaced transverse fracture of shaft of left ulna** `MCC` `CC`
CC Excl: See code: S52.202

7 √7th **S52.226 Nondisplaced transverse fracture of shaft of unspecified ulna** `MCC` `CC`
CC Excl: See code: S52.209

√6th **S52.23 Oblique fracture of shaft of ulna**

7 √7th **S52.231 Displaced oblique fracture of shaft of right ulna** `MCC` `CC`
CC Excl: See code: S52.201

7 √7th **S52.232 Displaced oblique fracture of shaft of left ulna** `MCC` `CC`
CC Excl: See code: S52.202

7 √7th **S52.233 Displaced oblique fracture of shaft of unspecified ulna** `MCC` `CC`
CC Excl: See code: S52.209

7 √7th **S52.234 Nondisplaced oblique fracture of shaft of right ulna** `MCC` `CC`
CC Excl: See code: S52.201

---

7 HAC = Initial encounter only (7th character A, B or C) and not POA.

√ Additional Character Required   √x7th Xtension Alert   Unacceptable PDx   Manifestation   Hospital Acquired Condition   *EXCLUDES 1* Not Coded Here   *EXCLUDES 2* Not Included Here

7 ✓7ᵗʰ **S52.235** **Nondisplaced** oblique fracture of shaft of **left** ulna `MCC` `CC`
CC Excl: See code: S52.202

7 ✓7ᵗʰ **S52.236** **Nondisplaced** oblique fracture of shaft of **unspecified** ulna `MCC` `CC`
CC Excl: See code: S52.209

✓6ᵗʰ **S52.24** Spiral fracture of shaft of ulna

7 ✓7ᵗʰ **S52.241** **Displaced** spiral fracture of shaft of ulna, **right arm** `MCC` `CC`
CC Excl: See code: S52.201

7 ✓7ᵗʰ **S52.242** **Displaced** spiral fracture of shaft of ulna, **left arm** `MCC` `CC`
CC Excl: See code: S52.202

7 ✓7ᵗʰ **S52.243** **Displaced** spiral fracture of shaft of ulna, **unspecified** arm `MCC` `CC`
CC Excl: See code: S52.209

7 ✓7ᵗʰ **S52.244** **Nondisplaced** spiral fracture of shaft of ulna, **right arm** `MCC` `CC`
CC Excl: See code: S52.201

7 ✓7ᵗʰ **S52.245** **Nondisplaced** spiral fracture of shaft of ulna, **left arm** `MCC` `CC`
CC Excl: See code: S52.202

7 ✓7ᵗʰ **S52.246** **Nondisplaced** spiral fracture of shaft of ulna, **unspecified** arm `MCC` `CC`
CC Excl: See code: S52.209

✓6ᵗʰ **S52.25** Comminuted fracture of shaft of ulna

7 ✓7ᵗʰ **S52.251** **Displaced** comminuted fracture of shaft of ulna, **right arm** `MCC` `CC`
CC Excl: See code: S52.201

7 ✓7ᵗʰ **S52.252** **Displaced** comminuted fracture of shaft of ulna, **left arm** `MCC` `CC`
CC Excl: See code: S52.202

7 ✓7ᵗʰ **S52.253** **Displaced** comminuted fracture of shaft of ulna, **unspecified** arm `MCC` `CC`
CC Excl: See code: S52.209

7 ✓7ᵗʰ **S52.254** **Nondisplaced** comminuted fracture of shaft of ulna, **right arm** `MCC` `CC`
CC Excl: See code: S52.201

7 ✓7ᵗʰ **S52.255** **Nondisplaced** comminuted fracture of shaft of ulna, **left arm** `MCC` `CC`
CC Excl: See code: S52.202

7 ✓7ᵗʰ **S52.256** **Nondisplaced** comminuted fracture of shaft of ulna, **unspecified** arm `MCC` `CC`
CC Excl: See code: S52.209

✓6ᵗʰ **S52.26** Segmental fracture of shaft of ulna

7 ✓7ᵗʰ **S52.261** **Displaced** segmental fracture of shaft of ulna, **right arm** `MCC` `CC`
CC Excl: See code: S52.201

7 ✓7ᵗʰ **S52.262** **Displaced** segmental fracture of shaft of ulna, **left arm** `MCC` `CC`
CC Excl: See code: S52.202

7 ✓7ᵗʰ **S52.263** **Displaced** segmental fracture of shaft of ulna, **unspecified** arm `MCC` `CC`
CC Excl: See code: S52.209

7 ✓7ᵗʰ **S52.264** **Nondisplaced** segmental fracture of shaft of ulna, **right arm** `MCC` `CC`
CC Excl: See code: S52.201

7 ✓7ᵗʰ **S52.265** **Nondisplaced** segmental fracture of shaft of ulna, **left arm** `MCC` `CC`
CC Excl: See code: S52.202

7 ✓7ᵗʰ **S52.266** **Nondisplaced** segmental fracture of shaft of ulna, **unspecified** arm `MCC` `CC`
CC Excl: See code: S52.209

✓6ᵗʰ **S52.27** Monteggia's fracture of ulna
Fracture of upper shaft of ulna with dislocation of radial head

7 ✓7ᵗʰ **S52.271** Monteggia's fracture of **right** ulna `MCC` `CC`
CC Excl: See code: S52.201

7 ✓7ᵗʰ **S52.272** Monteggia's fracture of **left** ulna `MCC` `CC`
CC Excl: See code: S52.202

7 ✓7ᵗʰ **S52.279** Monteggia's fracture of **unspecified** ulna `MCC` `CC`
CC Excl: See code: S52.209

✓6ᵗʰ **S52.28** Bent bone of ulna

7 ✓7ᵗʰ **S52.281** Bent bone of **right** ulna `MCC` `CC`
CC Excl: See code: S52.201

7 ✓7ᵗʰ **S52.282** Bent bone of **left** ulna `MCC` `CC`
CC Excl: See code: S52.202

7 ✓7ᵗʰ **S52.283** Bent bone of **unspecified** ulna `MCC` `CC`
CC Excl: See code: S52.209

✓6ᵗʰ **S52.29** Other fracture of shaft of ulna

7 ✓7ᵗʰ **S52.291** Other fracture of shaft of **right** ulna `MCC` `CC`
CC Excl: See code: S52.201

7 ✓7ᵗʰ **S52.292** Other fracture of shaft of **left** ulna `MCC` `CC`
CC Excl: See code: S52.202

7 ✓7ᵗʰ **S52.299** Other fracture of shaft of **unspecified** ulna `MCC` `CC`
CC Excl: See code: S52.209

✓5ᵗʰ **S52.3** Fracture of shaft of radius

✓6ᵗʰ **S52.30** Unspecified fracture of shaft of radius

7 ✓7ᵗʰ **S52.301** Unspecified fracture of shaft of **right radius** `MCC` `CC`
CC Excl: See Code: S52.201

7 ✓7ᵗʰ **S52.302** Unspecified fracture of shaft of **left radius** `MCC` `CC`
CC Excl: See Code: S52.202

7 ✓7ᵗʰ **S52.309** Unspecified fracture of shaft of **unspecified radius** `MCC` `CC`
CC Excl: See Code: S52.209

✓6ᵗʰ **S52.31** Greenstick fracture of shaft of radius

The appropriate 7th is to be added to all codes in subcategory S52.31.
A initial encounter for closed fracture
D subsequent encounter for fracture with routine healing
G subsequent encounter for fracture with delayed healing
K subsequent encounter for fracture with nonunion
P subsequent encounter for fracture with malunion
S sequela

7 ✓7ᵗʰ **S52.311** Greenstick fracture of shaft of radius, **right arm** `CC`
CC Excl: CC with 7th character A: S52.001-S52.011 with 7th [A, B, C], S52.019-S52.111 with 7th A, S52.119-S52.211 with 7th A, S52.219-S52.311 with 7th A, S52.319-S52.521 with 7th A, S52.529-S52.621 with 7th A, S52.629-S52.92X with 7th A, S59.001 with 7th A, S59.009-S59.011 with 7th A, S59.019-S59.021 with 7th A, S59.029-S59.031 with 7th A, S59.039-S59.041 with 7th A, S59.049-S59.091 with 7th A, S59.099-S59.101 with 7th A, S59.109-S59.111 with 7th A, S59.119-S59.121 with 7th A, S59.129-S59.131 with 7th A, S59.139-S59.141 with 7th A, S59.149-S59.191 with 7th A, S59.199-S59.201 with 7th A, S59.209-S59.211 with 7th A, S59.219-S59.221 with 7th A, S59.229-S59.231 with 7th A, S59.239-S59.241 with 7th A, S59.249-S59.291 with 7th A, S59.299A
CC with 7th character K or P: M80.00X-M84.68X with 7th [K, P], S02.0XX-S02.92X with 7th K, S12.000-S12.691 with 7th K, S22.000-S22.9XX with 7th K, S32.000-S32.9XX with 7th K, S42.001-S42.92X with 7th [K, P], S49.001-S49.199 with 7th [K, P], S52.001-S52.92X with 7th [K, M, N, P, Q, R], S59.001-S59.299 with 7th [K, P], S62.001-S62.92X with 7th [K, P], S72.001-S72.92X with 7th [K, M, N, P, Q, R], S79.001-S79.199 with 7th [K, P], S82.001-S82.92X with 7th [K, M, N, P, Q, R], S89.001-S89.399 with 7th [K, P], S92.001-S92.919 with 7th [K, P]

---

7 HAC = Initial encounter only (7th character A, B or C) and not POA.

`N` Newborn: 0   `P` Pediatric: 0-17   `M` Maternity: 12-55   `A` Adult: 15-124   `MCC` Major CC Condition   `PDx MCC` PDx acts as own MCC   `CC` CC Condition   `PDx CC` PDx acts as own CC

928   ICD-10-CM Draft (2015)

7 ✓7th **S52.312** **Greenstick fracture of shaft of radius, left arm** `CC`
CC Excl: CC with 7th character A: S52.001-S52.009 with 7th [B, C], S52.012-S52.109 with 7th A, S52.112-S52.209 with 7th A, S52.212-S52.309 with 7th A, S52.312-S52.516 with 7th A, S52.522-S52.616 with 7th A, S52.622-S52.92X with 7th A, S59.002-S59.009 with 7th A, S59.012-S59.019 with 7th A, S59.022-S59.029 with 7th A, S59.032-S59.039 with 7th A, S59.042-S59.049 with 7th A, S59.092-S59.099 with 7th A, S59.102-S59.109 with 7th A, S59.112-S59.119 with 7th A, S59.122-S59.129 with 7th A, S59.132-S59.139 with 7th A, S59.142-S59.149 with 7th A, S59.192-S59.199 with 7th A, S59.202-S59.209 with 7th A, S59.212-S59.219 with 7th A, S59.222-S59.229 with 7th A, S59.232-S59.239 with 7th A, S59.242-S59.249 with 7th A, S59.292-S59.299 with 7th A
CC with 7th character K or P: M80.00X-M84.68X with 7th [K, P], S02.0XX-S02.92X with 7th K, S12.000-S12.691 with 7th K, S22.000-S22.9XX with 7th K, S32.000-S32.9XX with 7th K, S42.001-S42.92X with 7th [K, P], S49.001-S49.199 with 7th [K, P], S52.001-S52.92X with 7th [K, M, N, P, Q, R], S59.001-S59.299 with 7th [K, P], S62.001-S62.92X with 7th [K, P], S72.001-S72.92X with 7th [K, M, N, P, Q, R], S79.001-S79.199 with 7th [K, P], S82.001-S82.92X with 7th [K, M, N, P, Q, R], S89.001-S89.399 with 7th [K, P], S92.001-S92.919 with 7th [K, P]

7 ✓7th **S52.319** **Greenstick fracture of shaft of radius, unspecified arm** `CC`
CC Excl: CC with 7th character A: S52.001-S52.92X with 7th [A, B, C], S59.001-S59.299 with 7th A
CC with 7th character K or P: M80.00X-M84.68X with 7th [K, P], S02.0XX-S02.92X with 7th K, S12.000-S12.691 with 7th K, S22.000-S22.9XX with 7th K, S32.000-S32.9XX with 7th K, S42.001-S42.92X with 7th [K, P], S49.001-S49.199 with 7th [K, P], S52.001-S52.92X with 7th [K, M, N, P, Q, R], S59.001-S59.299 with 7th [K, P], S62.001-S62.92X with 7th [K, P], S72.001-S72.92X with 7th [K, M, N, P, Q, R], S79.001-S79.199 with 7th [K, P], S82.001-S82.92X with 7th [K, M, N, P, Q, R], S89.001-S89.399 with 7th [K, P], S92.001-S92.919 with 7th [K, P]

✓6th **S52.32** **Transverse fracture of shaft of radius**

7 ✓7th **S52.321** **Displaced transverse fracture of shaft of right radius** `MCC` `CC`
CC Excl: See code: S52.201

7 ✓7th **S52.322** **Displaced transverse fracture of shaft of left radius** `MCC` `CC`
CC Excl: See code: S52.202

7 ✓7th **S52.323** **Displaced transverse fracture of shaft of unspecified radius** `MCC` `CC`
CC Excl: See code: S52.209

7 ✓7th **S52.324** **Nondisplaced transverse fracture of shaft of right radius** `MCC` `CC`
CC Excl: See code: S52.201

7 ✓7th **S52.325** **Nondisplaced transverse fracture of shaft of left radius** `MCC` `CC`
CC Excl: See code: S52.202

7 ✓7th **S52.326** **Nondisplaced transverse fracture of shaft of unspecified radius** `MCC` `CC`
CC Excl: See code: S52.209

✓6th **S52.33** **Oblique fracture of shaft of radius**

7 ✓7th **S52.331** **Displaced oblique fracture of shaft of right radius** `MCC` `CC`
CC Excl: See code: S52.201

7 ✓7th **S52.332** **Displaced oblique fracture of shaft of left radius** `MCC` `CC`
CC Excl: See code: S52.202

7 ✓7th **S52.333** **Displaced oblique fracture of shaft of unspecified radius** `MCC` `CC`
CC Excl: See code: S52.209

7 ✓7th **S52.334** **Nondisplaced oblique fracture of shaft of right radius** `MCC` `CC`
CC Excl: See code: S52.201

7 ✓7th **S52.335** **Nondisplaced oblique fracture of shaft of left radius** `MCC` `CC`
CC Excl: See code: S52.202

7 ✓7th **S52.336** **Nondisplaced oblique fracture of shaft of unspecified radius** `MCC` `CC`
CC Excl: See code: S52.209

✓6th **S52.34** **Spiral fracture of shaft of radius**

7 ✓7th **S52.341** **Displaced spiral fracture of shaft of radius, right arm** `MCC` `CC`
CC Excl: See code: S52.201

7 ✓7th **S52.342** **Displaced spiral fracture of shaft of radius, left arm** `MCC` `CC`
CC Excl: See code: S52.202

7 ✓7th **S52.343** **Displaced spiral fracture of shaft of radius, unspecified arm** `MCC` `CC`
CC Excl: See code: S52.209

7 ✓7th **S52.344** **Nondisplaced spiral fracture of shaft of radius, right arm** `MCC` `CC`
CC Excl: See code: S52.201

7 ✓7th **S52.345** **Nondisplaced spiral fracture of shaft of radius, left arm** `MCC` `CC`
CC Excl: See code: S52.202

7 ✓7th **S52.346** **Nondisplaced spiral fracture of shaft of radius, unspecified arm** `MCC` `CC`
CC Excl: See code: S52.209

✓6th **S52.35** **Comminuted fracture of shaft of radius**

7 ✓7th **S52.351** **Displaced comminuted fracture of shaft of radius, right arm** `MCC` `CC`
CC Excl: See code: S52.201

7 ✓7th **S52.352** **Displaced comminuted fracture of shaft of radius, left arm** `MCC` `CC`
CC Excl: See code: S52.202

7 ✓7th **S52.353** **Displaced comminuted fracture sof haft of radius, unspecified arm** `MCC` `CC`
CC Excl: See code: S52.209

7 ✓7th **S52.354** **Nondisplaced comminuted fracture of shaft of radius, right arm** `MCC` `CC`
CC Excl: See code: S52.201

7 ✓7th **S52.355** **Nondisplaced comminuted fracture of shaft of radius, left arm** `MCC` `CC`
CC Excl: See code: S52.202

7 ✓7th **S52.356** **Nondisplaced comminuted fracture of shaft of radius, unspecified arm** `MCC` `CC`
CC Excl: See code: S52.209

✓6th **S52.36** **Segmental fracture of shaft of radius**

7 ✓7th **S52.361** **Displaced segmental fracture of shaft of radius, right arm** `MCC` `CC`
CC Excl: See code: S52.201

7 ✓7th **S52.362** **Displaced segmental fracture of shaft of radius, left arm** `MCC` `CC`
CC Excl: See code: S52.202

7 ✓7th **S52.363** **Displaced segmental fracture of shaft of radius, unspecified arm** `MCC` `CC`
CC Excl: See code: S52.209

7 ✓7th **S52.364** **Nondisplaced segmental fracture of shaft of radius, right arm** `MCC` `CC`
CC Excl: See code: S52.201

7 ✓7th **S52.365** **Nondisplaced segmental fracture of shaft of radius, left arm** `MCC` `CC`
CC Excl: See code: S52.202

7 ✓7th **S52.366** **Nondisplaced segmental fracture of shaft of radius, unspecified arm** `MCC` `CC`
CC Excl: See code: S52.209

✓6th **S52.37** **Galeazzi's fracture**
Fracture of lower shaft of radius with radioulnar joint dislocation

7 ✓7th **S52.371** **Galeazzi's fracture of right radius** `MCC` `CC`
CC Excl: See code: S52.201

7 ✓7th **S52.372** **Galeazzi's fracture of left radius** `MCC` `CC`
CC Excl: See code: S52.202

7 ✓7th **S52.379** **Galeazzi's fracture of unspecified radius** `MCC` `CC`
CC Excl: See code: S52.209

---

7 HAC = Initial encounter only (7th character A, B or C) and not POA.

☑ Additional Character Required ✓x7th Xtension Alert Unacceptable PDx Manifestation Hospital Acquired Condition *EXCLUDES 1* Not Coded Here *EXCLUDES 2* Not Included Here

✓6th **S52.38 Bent bone** of radius

   7 ✓7th **S52.381 Bent bone of** right **radius** MCC CC
     CC Excl: See code: S52.201

   7 ✓7th **S52.382 Bent bone of** left **radius** MCC CC
     CC Excl: See code: S52.202

   7 ✓7th **S52.389 Bent bone of** unspecified **radius** MCC CC
     CC Excl: See code: S52.209

✓6th **S52.39 Other fracture of shaft of radius**

   7 ✓7th **S52.391 Other fracture of shaft of radius, right arm** MCC CC
     CC Excl: See code: S52.201

   7 ✓7th **S52.392 Other fracture of shaft of radius, left arm** MCC CC
     CC Excl: See code: S52.202

   7 ✓7th **S52.399 Other fracture of shaft of radius, unspecified arm** MCC CC
     CC Excl: See code: S52.209

✓5th **S52.5 Fracture of** lower end of radius
   Fracture of distal end of radius
   EXCLUDES 2 *physeal fractures of lower end of radius (S59.2-)*

✓6th **S52.50 Unspecified fracture of the lower end of radius**

   7 ✓7th **S52.501 Unspecified fracture of the lower end of** right **radius** MCC CC
     CC Excl: See code: S52.201

   7 ✓7th **S52.502 Unspecified fracture of the lower end of** left **radius** MCC CC
     CC Excl: See code: S52.202

   7 ✓7th **S52.509 Unspecified fracture of the lower end of** unspecified **radius** MCC CC
     CC Excl: See code: S52.209

✓6th **S52.51 Fracture of** radial styloid process

   7 ✓7th **S52.511 Displaced fracture of** right **radial styloid process** MCC CC
     CC Excl: See code: S52.201

   7 ✓7th **S52.512 Displaced fracture of** left **radial styloid process** MCC CC
     CC Excl: See code: S52.202

   7 ✓7th **S52.513 Displaced fracture of** unspecified **radial styloid process** MCC CC
     CC Excl: See code: S52.209

   7 ✓7th **S52.514 Nondisplaced fracture of** right **radial styloid process** MCC CC
     CC Excl: See code: S52.201

   7 ✓7th **S52.515 Nondisplaced fracture of** left **radial styloid process** MCC CC
     CC Excl: See code: S52.202

   7 ✓7th **S52.516 Nondisplaced fracture of** unspecified **radial styloid process** MCC CC
     CC Excl: See code: S52.209

✓6th **S52.52 Torus** fracture of lower end of radius

   The appropriate 7th is to be added to all codes in subcategory S52.52.
   A   initial encounter for closed fracture
   D   subsequent encounter for fracture with routine healing
   G   subsequent encounter for fracture with delayed healing
   K   subsequent encounter for fracture with nonunion
   P   subsequent encounter for fracture with malunion
   S   sequela

   7 ✓7th **S52.521 Torus fracture of lower end of** right **radius** CC
     CC Excl: CC with 7th character A: S52.001-S52.011 with 7th [A, B, C], S52.019-S52.111 with 7th A, S52.119-S52.211 with 7th A, S52.219-S52.311 with 7th A, S52.319-S52.521 with 7th A, S52.529-S52.621 with 7th A, S52.629-S52.92X with 7th A, S59.001 with 7th A, S59.009-S59.011 with 7th A, S59.019-S59.021 with 7th A, S59.029-S59.031 with 7th A, S59.039-S59.041 with 7th A, S59.049-S59.091 with 7th A, S59.099-S59.101 with 7th A, S59.109-S59.111 with 7th A, S59.119-S59.121 with 7th A, S59.129-S59.131 with 7th A, S59.139-S59.141 with 7th A, S59.149-S59.191 with 7th A, S59.199-S59.201 with 7th A, S59.209-S59.211 with 7th A, S59.219-S59.221 with 7th A, S59.229-S59.231 with 7th A, S59.239-S59.241 with 7th A, S59.249-S59.291 with 7th A, S59.299A

     CC with 7th character K or P: M80.00X-M84.68X with 7th [K, P], S02.0XX-S02.92X with 7th K, S12.000-S12.691 with 7th K, S22.000-S22.9XX with 7th K, S32.000-S32.9XX with 7th K, S42.001-S42.92X with 7th [K, P], S49.001-S49.199 with 7th [K, P], S52.001-S52.92X with 7th [K, M, N, P, Q, R], S59.001-S59.299 with 7th [K, P], S62.001-S62.92X with 7th [K, P], S72.001-S72.92X with 7th [K, M, N, P, Q, R], S79.001-S79.199 with 7th [K, P], S82.001-S82.92X with 7th [K, M, N, P, Q, R], S89.001-S89.399 with 7th [K, P], S92.001-S92.919 with 7th [K, P]

   7 ✓7th **S52.522 Torus fracture of lower end of** left **radius** CC
     CC Excl: CC with 7th character A: S52.001-S52.009 with 7th [B, C], S52.012-S52.109 with 7th A, S52.112-S52.209 with 7th A, S52.212-S52.309 with 7th A, S52.312-S52.516 with 7th A, S52.522-S52.616 with 7th A, S52.622-S52.92X with 7th A, S59.002-S59.009 with 7th A, S59.012-S59.019 with 7th A, S59.022-S59.029 with 7th A, S59.032-S59.039 with 7th A, S59.042-S59.049 with 7th A, S59.092-S59.099 with 7th A, S59.102-S59.109 with 7th A, S59.112-S59.119 with 7th A, S59.122-S59.129 with 7th A, S59.132-S59.139 with 7th A, S59.142-S59.149 with 7th A, S59.192-S59.199 with 7th A, S59.202-S59.209 with 7th A, S59.212-S59.219 with 7th A, S59.222-S59.229 with 7th A, S59.232-S59.239 with 7th A, S59.242-S59.249 with 7th A, S59.292-S59.299 with 7th A

     CC with 7th character K or P: M80.00X-M84.68X with 7th [K, P], S02.0XX-S02.92X with 7th K, S12.000-S12.691 with 7th K, S22.000-S22.9XX with 7th K, S32.000-S32.9XX with 7th K, S42.001-S42.92X with 7th [K, P], S49.001-S49.199 with 7th [K, P], S52.001-S52.92X with 7th [K, M, N, P, Q, R], S59.001-S59.299 with 7th [K, P], S62.001-S62.92X with 7th [K, P], S72.001-S72.92X with 7th [K, M, N, P, Q, R], S79.001-S79.199 with 7th [K, P], S82.001-S82.92X with 7th [K, M, N, P, Q, R], S89.001-S89.399 with 7th [K, P], S92.001-S92.919 with 7th [K, P]

   7 ✓7th **S52.529 Torus fracture of lower end of** unspecified **radius** CC
     CC Excl: See code: S52.209

✓6th **S52.53 Colles'** fracture

   7 ✓7th **S52.531 Colles' fracture of** right **radius** MCC CC
     CC Excl: See code: S52.201

   7 ✓7th **S52.532 Colles' fracture of** left **radius** MCC CC
     CC Excl: See code: S52.202

   7 ✓7th **S52.539 Colles' fracture of** unspecified **radius** MCC CC
     CC Excl: See code: S52.209

✓6th **S52.54 Smith's** fracture

   7 ✓7th **S52.541 Smith's fracture of** right **radius** MCC CC
     CC Excl: See code: S52.201

   7 ✓7th **S52.542 Smith's fracture of** left **radius** MCC CC
     CC Excl: See code: S52.202

   7 ✓7th **S52.549 Smith's fracture of** unspecified **radius** MCC CC
     CC Excl: See code: S52.209

✓6th **S52.55 Other extraarticular** fracture of lower end of radius

   7 ✓7th **S52.551 Other extraarticular fracture of lower end of** right **radius** MCC CC
     CC Excl: See code: S52.201

   7 ✓7th **S52.552 Other extraarticular fracture of lower end of** left **radius** MCC CC
     CC Excl: See code: S52.202

   7 ✓7th **S52.559 Other extraarticular fracture of lower end of** unspecified **radius** MCC CC
     CC Excl: See code: S52.209

✓6th **S52.56 Barton's** fracture

   7 ✓7th **S52.561 Barton's fracture of** right **radius** MCC CC
     CC Excl: See code: S52.201

   7 ✓7th **S52.562 Barton's fracture of** left **radius** MCC CC
     CC Excl: See code: S52.202

---

7 HAC = Initial encounter only (7th character A, B or C) and not POA.

N Newborn: 0   P Pediatric: 0-17   M Maternity: 12-55   A Adult: 15-124   MCC Major CC Condition   PDx MCC PDx acts as own MCC   CC CC Condition   PDx CC PDx acts as own CC

930   ICD-10-CM Draft (2015)

7 ✓7ᵗʰ **S52.569** **Barton's fracture of unspecified radius** ᴹᶜᶜ ᶜᶜ
    CC Excl: See code: S52.209

✓6ᵗʰ **S52.57** Other intraarticular fracture of lower end of radius

7 ✓7ᵗʰ **S52.571** **Other intraarticular fracture of lower end of right radius** ᴹᶜᶜ ᶜᶜ
    CC Excl: See code: S52.201

7 ✓7ᵗʰ **S52.572** **Other intraarticular fracture of lower end of left radius** ᴹᶜᶜ ᶜᶜ
    CC Excl: See code: S52.202

7 ✓7ᵗʰ **S52.579** **Other intraarticular fracture of lower end of unspecified radius** ᴹᶜᶜ ᶜᶜ
    CC Excl: See code: S52.209

✓6ᵗʰ **S52.59** Other fractures of lower end of radius

7 ✓7ᵗʰ **S52.591** **Other fractures of lower end of right radius** ᴹᶜᶜ ᶜᶜ
    CC Excl: See code: S52.201

7 ✓7ᵗʰ **S52.592** **Other fractures of lower end of left radius** ᴹᶜᶜ ᶜᶜ
    CC Excl: See code: S52.202

7 ✓7ᵗʰ **S52.599** **Other fractures of lower end of unspecified radius** ᴹᶜᶜ ᶜᶜ
    CC Excl: See code: S52.209

✓5ᵗʰ **S52.6** **Fracture of lower end of ulna**

✓6ᵗʰ **S52.60** Unspecified fracture of lower end of ulna

7 ✓7ᵗʰ **S52.601** **Unspecified fracture of lower end of right ulna** ᴹᶜᶜ ᶜᶜ
    CC Excl: See code: S52.201

7 ✓7ᵗʰ **S52.602** **Unspecified fracture of lower end of left ulna** ᴹᶜᶜ ᶜᶜ
    CC Excl: See code: S52.202

7 ✓7ᵗʰ **S52.609** **Unspecified fracture of lower end of unspecified ulna** ᴹᶜᶜ ᶜᶜ
    CC Excl: See code: S52.209

✓6ᵗʰ **S52.61** Fracture of ulna styloid process

7 ✓7ᵗʰ **S52.611** **Displaced fracture of right ulna styloid process** ᴹᶜᶜ ᶜᶜ
    CC Excl: See code: S52.201

7 ✓7ᵗʰ **S52.612** **Displaced fracture of left ulna styloid process** ᴹᶜᶜ ᶜᶜ
    CC Excl: See code: S52.202

7 ✓7ᵗʰ **S52.613** **Displaced fracture of unspecified ulna styloid process** ᴹᶜᶜ ᶜᶜ
    CC Excl: See code: S52.209

7 ✓7ᵗʰ **S52.614** **Nondisplaced fracture of right ulna styloid process** ᴹᶜᶜ ᶜᶜ
    CC Excl: See code: S52.201

7 ✓7ᵗʰ **S52.615** **Nondisplaced fracture of left ulna styloid process** ᴹᶜᶜ ᶜᶜ
    CC Excl: See code: S52.202

7 ✓7ᵗʰ **S52.616** **Nondisplaced fracture of unspecified ulna styloid process** ᴹᶜᶜ ᶜᶜ
    CC Excl: See code: S52.209

✓6ᵗʰ **S52.62** Torus fracture of lower end of ulna

The appropriate 7th is to be added to all codes in subcategory S52.62.
A   initial encounter for closed fracture
D   subsequent encounter for fracture with routine healing
G   subsequent encounter for fracture with delayed healing
K   subsequent encounter for fracture with nonunion
P   subsequent encounter for fracture with malunion
S   sequela

7 ✓7ᵗʰ **S52.621** **Torus fracture of lower end of right ulna** ᶜᶜ
    CC Excl: CC with 7th character A: S52.001-S52.011 with 7th [A, B, C], S52.019-S52.111 with 7th A, S52.119-S52.211 with 7th A, S52.219-S52.311 with 7th A, S52.319-S52.521 with 7th A, S52.529-S52.621 with 7th A, S52.629-S52.92X with 7th A, S59.001 with 7th A, S59.009-S59.011 with 7th A, S59.019-S59.021 with 7th A, S59.029-S59.031 with 7th A, S59.039-S59.041 with 7th A, S59.049-S59.091 with 7th A, S59.099-S59.101 with 7th A, S59.109-S59.111 with 7th A, S59.119-S59.121 with 7th A, S59.129-S59.131 with 7th A, S59.139-S59.141 with 7th A, S59.149-S59.191 with 7th A, S59.199-S59.201 with 7th A, S59.209-S59.211 with 7th A, S59.219-S59.221 with 7th A, S59.229-S59.231 with 7th A, S59.239-S59.241 with 7th A, S59.249-S59.291 with 7th A, S59.299A
    CC with 7th character K or P: M80.00X-M84.68X with 7th [K, P], S02.0XX-S02.92X with 7th K, S12.000-S12.691 with 7th K, S22.000-S22.9XX with 7th K, S32.000-S32.9XX with 7th K, S42.001-S42.92X with 7th [K, P], S49.001-S49.199 with 7th [K, P], S52.001-S52.92X with 7th [K, M, N, P, Q, R], S59.001-S59.299 with 7th [K, P], S62.001-S62.92X with 7th [K, P], S72.001-S72.92X with 7th [K, M, N, P, Q, R], S79.001-S79.199 with 7th [K, P], S82.001-S82.92X with 7th [K, M, N, P, Q, R], S89.001-S89.399 with 7th [K, P], S92.001-S92.919 with 7th [K, P]

7 ✓7ᵗʰ **S52.622** **Torus fracture of lower end of left ulna** ᶜᶜ
    CC Excl: CC with 7th character A: S52.001-S52.009 with 7th [B, C], S52.012-S52.109 with 7th A, S52.112-S52.209 with 7th A, S52.212-S52.309 with 7th A, S52.312-S52.516 with 7th A, S52.522-S52.616 with 7th A, S52.622-S52.92X with 7th A, S59.002-S59.009 with 7th A, S59.012-S59.019 with 7th A, S59.022-S59.029 with 7th A, S59.032-S59.039 with 7th A, S59.042-S59.049 with 7th A, S59.092-S59.099 with 7th A, S59.102-S59.109 with 7th A, S59.112-S59.119 with 7th A, S59.122-S59.129 with 7th A, S59.132-S59.139 with 7th A, S59.142-S59.149 with 7th A, S59.192-S59.199 with 7th A, S59.202-S59.209 with 7th A, S59.212-S59.219 with 7th A, S59.222-S59.229 with 7th A, S59.232-S59.239 with 7th A, S59.242-S59.249 with 7th A, S59.292-S59.299 with 7th A
    CC with 7th character K or P: M80.00X-M84.68X with 7th [K, P], S02.0XX-S02.92X with 7th K, S12.000-S12.691 with 7th K, S22.000-S22.9XX with 7th K, S32.000-S32.9XX with 7th K, S42.001-S42.92X with 7th [K, P], S49.001-S49.199 with 7th [K, P], S52.001-S52.92X with 7th [K, M, N, P, Q, R], S59.001-S59.299 with 7th [K, P], S62.001-S62.92X with 7th [K, P], S72.001-S72.92X with 7th [K, M, N, P, Q, R], S79.001-S79.199 with 7th [K, P], S82.001-S82.92X with 7th [K, M, N, P, Q, R], S89.001-S89.399 with 7th [K, P], S92.001-S92.919 with 7th [K, P]

7 ✓7ᵗʰ **S52.629** **Torus fracture of lower end of unspecified ulna** ᶜᶜ
    CC Excl: CC with 7th character A: S52.001-S52.92X with 7th [A, B, C], S59.001-S59.299 with 7th A
    CC with 7th character K or P: M80.00X-M84.68X with 7th [K, P], S02.0XX-S02.92X with 7th K, S12.000-S12.691 with 7th K, S22.000-S22.9XX with 7th K, S32.000-S32.9XX with 7th K, S42.001-S42.92X with 7th [K, P], S49.001-S49.199 with 7th [K, P], S52.001-S52.92X with 7th [K, M, N, P, Q, R], S59.001-S59.299 with 7th [K, P], S62.001-S62.92X with 7th [K, P], S72.001-S72.92X with 7th [K, M, N, P, Q, R], S79.001-S79.199 with 7th [K, P], S82.001-S82.92X with 7th [K, M, N, P, Q, R], S89.001-S89.399 with 7th [K, P], S92.001-S92.919 with 7th [K, P]

✓6ᵗʰ **S52.69** Other fracture of lower end of ulna

7 ✓7ᵗʰ **S52.691** **Other fracture of lower end of right ulna** ᴹᶜᶜ ᶜᶜ
    CC Excl: See code: S52.201

---

7 HAC = Initial encounter only (7th character A, B or C) and not POA.

7 ✓7th **S52.692** **Other fracture of lower end of left ulna** MCC CC
     CC Excl: See code: S52.202

7 ✓7th **S52.699** **Other fracture of lower end of unspecified ulna** MCC CC
     CC Excl: See code: S52.209

✓5th **S52.9** **Unspecified fracture of forearm**

7 ✓x 7th **S52.90** **Unspecified fracture of unspecified forearm** MCC CC
     CC Excl: CC with 7th character A: S52.001-S52.92X with 7th [A, B, C], S59.001-S59.299 with 7th A
     MCC with 7th character B or C: S52.001-S52.009 with 7th [B, C], S52.021-S52.109 with 7th [B, C], S52.121-S52.516 with 7th [B, C], S52.531-S52.616 with 7th [A, B, C], S52.691-S52.92X with 7th [A, B, C], S59.001-S59.099 with 7th A, S59.201-S59.299 with 7th A, S62.90XB
     CC with 7th character K, M, N, P, Q or R: M80.00X-M84.68X with 7th [K, P], S02.0XX-S02.92X with 7th K, S12.000-S12.691 with 7th K, S22.000-S22.9XX with 7th K, S32.000-S32.9XX with 7th K, S42.001-S42.92X with 7th [K, P], S49.001-S49.199 with 7th [K, P], S52.001-S52.92X with 7th [K, M, N, P, Q, R], S59.001-S59.299 with 7th [K, P], S62.001-S62.92X with 7th [K, P], S72.001-S72.92X with 7th [K, M, N, P, Q, R], S79.001-S79.199 with 7th [K, P], S82.001-S82.92X with 7th [K, M, N, P, Q, R], S89.001-S89.399 with 7th [K, P], S92.001-S92.919 with 7th [K, P]

7 ✓x 7th **S52.91** **Unspecified fracture of right forearm** MCC CC
     CC Excl: See code: S52.90

7 ✓x 7th **S52.92** **Unspecified fracture of left forearm** MCC CC
     CC Excl: See code: S52.90

✓4th **S53** **Dislocation and sprain of joints and ligaments of elbow**
     INCLUDES avulsion of joint or ligament of elbow
               laceration of cartilage, joint or ligament of elbow
               sprain of cartilage, joint or ligament of elbow
               traumatic hemarthrosis of joint or ligament of elbow
               traumatic rupture of joint or ligament of elbow
               traumatic subluxation of joint or ligament of elbow
               traumatic tear of joint or ligament of elbow
     Code also any associated open wound
     EXCLUDES 2 strain of muscle, fascia and tendon at forearm level (S56.-)

     The appropriate 7th is to be added to each code from category S53.
     A   initial encounter
     D   subsequent encounter
     S   sequela

✓5th **S53.0** **Subluxation and dislocation of radial head**
     Dislocation of radiohumeral joint
     Subluxation of radiohumeral joint
     EXCLUDES 1 Monteggia's fracture-dislocation (S52.27-)

✓6th **S53.00** **Unspecified subluxation and dislocation of radial head**
     ✓7th **S53.001** **Unspecified subluxation of right radial head**
     ✓7th **S53.002** **Unspecified subluxation of left radial head**
     ✓7th **S53.003** **Unspecified subluxation of unspecified radial head**
     ✓7th **S53.004** **Unspecified dislocation of right radial head**
     ✓7th **S53.005** **Unspecified dislocation of left radial head**
     ✓7th **S53.006** **Unspecified dislocation of unspecified radial head**

✓6th **S53.01** **Anterior subluxation and dislocation of radial head**
     Anteriomedial subluxation and dislocation of radial head
     ✓7th **S53.011** **Anterior subluxation of right radial head**
     ✓7th **S53.012** **Anterior subluxation of left radial head**
     ✓7th **S53.013** **Anterior subluxation of unspecified radial head**
     ✓7th **S53.014** **Anterior dislocation of right radial head**
     ✓7th **S53.015** **Anterior dislocation of left radial head**
     ✓7th **S53.016** **Anterior dislocation of unspecified radial head**

✓6th **S53.02** **Posterior subluxation and dislocation of radial head**
     Posteriolateral subluxation and dislocation of radial head
     ✓7th **S53.021** **Posterior subluxation of right radial head**
     ✓7th **S53.022** **Posterior subluxation of left radial head**

✓7th **S53.023** **Posterior subluxation of unspecified radial head**
✓7th **S53.024** **Posterior dislocation of right radial head**
✓7th **S53.025** **Posterior dislocation of left radial head**
✓7th **S53.026** **Posterior dislocation of unspecified radial head**

✓6th **S53.03** **Nursemaid's elbow**
     ✓7th **S53.031** **Nursemaid's elbow, right elbow**
     ✓7th **S53.032** **Nursemaid's elbow, left elbow**
     ✓7th **S53.033** **Nursemaid's elbow, unspecified elbow**

✓6th **S53.09** **Other subluxation and dislocation of radial head**
     ✓7th **S53.091** **Other subluxation of right radial head**
     ✓7th **S53.092** **Other subluxation of left radial head**
     ✓7th **S53.093** **Other subluxation of unspecified radial head**
     ✓7th **S53.094** **Other dislocation of right radial head**
     ✓7th **S53.095** **Other dislocation of left radial head**
     ✓7th **S53.096** **Other dislocation of unspecified radial head**

✓5th **S53.1** **Subluxation and dislocation of ulnohumeral joint**
     Subluxation and dislocation of elbow NOS
     EXCLUDES 1 dislocation of radial head alone (S53.0-)

✓6th **S53.10** **Unspecified subluxation and dislocation of ulnohumeral joint**
     ✓7th **S53.101** **Unspecified subluxation of right ulnohumeral joint**
     ✓7th **S53.102** **Unspecified subluxation of left ulnohumeral joint**
     ✓7th **S53.103** **Unspecified subluxation of unspecified ulnohumeral joint**
     ✓7th **S53.104** **Unspecified dislocation of right ulnohumeral joint**
     ✓7th **S53.105** **Unspecified dislocation of left ulnohumeral joint**
     ✓7th **S53.106** **Unspecified dislocation of unspecified ulnohumeral joint**

✓6th **S53.11** **Anterior subluxation and dislocation of ulnohumeral joint**
     ✓7th **S53.111** **Anterior subluxation of right ulnohumeral joint**
     ✓7th **S53.112** **Anterior subluxation of left ulnohumeral joint**
     ✓7th **S53.113** **Anterior subluxation of unspecified ulnohumeral joint**
     ✓7th **S53.114** **Anterior dislocation of right ulnohumeral joint**
         AHA: 2012, 4Q, 108
     ✓7th **S53.115** **Anterior dislocation of left ulnohumeral joint**
     ✓7th **S53.116** **Anterior dislocation of unspecified ulnohumeral joint**

✓6th **S53.12** **Posterior subluxation and dislocation of ulnohumeral joint**
     ✓7th **S53.121** **Posterior subluxation of right ulnohumeral joint**
     ✓7th **S53.122** **Posterior subluxation of left ulnohumeral joint**
     ✓7th **S53.123** **Posterior subluxation of unspecified ulnohumeral joint**
     ✓7th **S53.124** **Posterior dislocation of right ulnohumeral joint**
     ✓7th **S53.125** **Posterior dislocation of left ulnohumeral joint**
     ✓7th **S53.126** **Posterior dislocation of unspecified ulnohumeral joint**

✓6th **S53.13** **Medial subluxation and dislocation of ulnohumeral joint**
     ✓7th **S53.131** **Medial subluxation of right ulnohumeral joint**
     ✓7th **S53.132** **Medial subluxation of left ulnohumeral joint**
     ✓7th **S53.133** **Medial subluxation of unspecified ulnohumeral joint**

---

7 HAC = Initial encounter only (7th character A, B or C) and not POA.

N Newborn: 0   P Pediatric: 0-17   M Maternity: 12-55   A Adult: 15-124   MCC Major CC Condition   PDx MCC PDx acts as own MCC   CC CC Condition   PDx CC PDx acts as own CC

932   ICD-10-CM Draft (2015)

√7ᵗʰ **S53.134** Medial dislocation of right ulnohumeral joint

√7ᵗʰ **S53.135** Medial dislocation of left ulnohumeral joint

√7ᵗʰ **S53.136** Medial dislocation of unspecified ulnohumeral joint

√6ᵗʰ **S53.14** Lateral subluxation and dislocation of ulnohumeral joint

√7ᵗʰ **S53.141** Lateral subluxation of right ulnohumeral joint

√7ᵗʰ **S53.142** Lateral subluxation of left ulnohumeral joint

√7ᵗʰ **S53.143** Lateral subluxation of unspecified ulnohumeral joint

√7ᵗʰ **S53.144** Lateral dislocation of right ulnohumeral joint

√7ᵗʰ **S53.145** Lateral dislocation of left ulnohumeral joint

√7ᵗʰ **S53.146** Lateral dislocation of unspecified ulnohumeral joint

√6ᵗʰ **S53.19** Other subluxation and dislocation of ulnohumeral joint

√7ᵗʰ **S53.191** Other subluxation of right ulnohumeral joint

√7ᵗʰ **S53.192** Other subluxation of left ulnohumeral joint

√7ᵗʰ **S53.193** Other subluxation of unspecified ulnohumeral joint

√7ᵗʰ **S53.194** Other dislocation of right ulnohumeral joint

√7ᵗʰ **S53.195** Other dislocation of left ulnohumeral joint

√7ᵗʰ **S53.196** Other dislocation of unspecified ulnohumeral joint

√5ᵗʰ **S53.2** Traumatic rupture of radial collateral ligament
EXCLUDES 1 sprain of radial collateral ligament NOS (S53.43-)

√x7ᵗʰ **S53.20** Traumatic rupture of unspecified radial collateral ligament

√x7ᵗʰ **S53.21** Traumatic rupture of right radial collateral ligament

√x7ᵗʰ **S53.22** Traumatic rupture of left radial collateral ligament

√5ᵗʰ **S53.3** Traumatic rupture of ulnar collateral ligament
EXCLUDES 1 sprain of ulnar collateral ligament (S53.44-)

√x7ᵗʰ **S53.30** Traumatic rupture of unspecified ulnar collateral ligament

√x7ᵗʰ **S53.31** Traumatic rupture of right ulnar collateral ligament

√x7ᵗʰ **S53.32** Traumatic rupture of left ulnar collateral ligament

√5ᵗʰ **S53.4** Sprain of elbow
EXCLUDES 2 traumatic rupture of radial collateral ligament (S53.2-)
traumatic rupture of ulnar collateral ligament (S53.3-)

√6ᵗʰ **S53.40** Unspecified sprain of elbow

√7ᵗʰ **S53.401** Unspecified sprain of right elbow

√7ᵗʰ **S53.402** Unspecified sprain of left elbow

√7ᵗʰ **S53.409** Unspecified sprain of unspecified elbow
Sprain of elbow NOS

√6ᵗʰ **S53.41** Radiohumeral (joint) sprain

√7ᵗʰ **S53.411** Radiohumeral (joint) sprain of right elbow

√7ᵗʰ **S53.412** Radiohumeral (joint) sprain of left elbow

√7ᵗʰ **S53.419** Radiohumeral (joint) sprain of unspecified elbow

√6ᵗʰ **S53.42** Ulnohumeral (joint) sprain

√7ᵗʰ **S53.421** Ulnohumeral (joint) sprain of right elbow

√7ᵗʰ **S53.422** Ulnohumeral (joint) sprain of left elbow

√7ᵗʰ **S53.429** Ulnohumeral (joint) sprain of unspecified elbow

√6ᵗʰ **S53.43** Radial collateral ligament sprain

√7ᵗʰ **S53.431** Radial collateral ligament sprain of right elbow

√7ᵗʰ **S53.432** Radial collateral ligament sprain of left elbow

√7ᵗʰ **S53.439** Radial collateral ligament sprain of unspecified elbow

√6ᵗʰ **S53.44** Ulnar collateral ligament sprain

√7ᵗʰ **S53.441** Ulnar collateral ligament sprain of right elbow

√7ᵗʰ **S53.442** Ulnar collateral ligament sprain of left elbow

√7ᵗʰ **S53.449** Ulnar collateral ligament sprain of unspecified elbow

√6ᵗʰ **S53.49** Other sprain of elbow

√7ᵗʰ **S53.491** Other sprain of right elbow

√7ᵗʰ **S53.492** Other sprain of left elbow

√7ᵗʰ **S53.499** Other sprain of unspecified elbow

√4ᵗʰ **S54** Injury of nerves at forearm level
Code also any associated open wound (S51.-)
EXCLUDES 2 injury of nerves at wrist and hand level (S64.-)

The appropriate 7th is to be added to each code from category S54.
A   initial encounter
D   subsequent encounter
S   sequela

√5ᵗʰ **S54.0** Injury of ulnar nerve at forearm level
Injury of ulnar nerve NOS

√x7ᵗʰ **S54.00** Injury of ulnar nerve at forearm level, unspecified arm

√x7ᵗʰ **S54.01** Injury of ulnar nerve at forearm level, right arm

√x7ᵗʰ **S54.02** Injury of ulnar nerve at forearm level, left arm

√5ᵗʰ **S54.1** Injury of median nerve at forearm level
Injury of median nerve NOS

√x7ᵗʰ **S54.10** Injury of median nerve at forearm level, unspecified arm

√x7ᵗʰ **S54.11** Injury of median nerve at forearm level, right arm

√x7ᵗʰ **S54.12** Injury of median nerve at forearm level, left arm

√5ᵗʰ **S54.2** Injury of radial nerve at forearm level
Injury of radial nerve NOS

√x7ᵗʰ **S54.20** Injury of radial nerve at forearm level, unspecified arm

√x7ᵗʰ **S54.21** Injury of radial nerve at forearm level, right arm

√x7ᵗʰ **S54.22** Injury of radial nerve at forearm level, left arm

√5ᵗʰ **S54.3** Injury of cutaneous sensory nerve at forearm level

√x7ᵗʰ **S54.30** Injury of cutaneous sensory nerve at forearm level, unspecified arm

√x7ᵗʰ **S54.31** Injury of cutaneous sensory nerve at forearm level, right arm

√x7ᵗʰ **S54.32** Injury of cutaneous sensory nerve at forearm level, left arm

√5ᵗʰ **S54.8** Injury of other nerves at forearm level

√6ᵗʰ **S54.8X** Unspecified injury of other nerves at forearm level

√7ᵗʰ **S54.8X1** Unspecified injury of other nerves at forearm level, right arm

√7ᵗʰ **S54.8X2** Unspecified injury of other nerves at forearm level, left arm

√7ᵗʰ **S54.8X9** Unspecified injury of other nerves at forearm level, unspecified arm

√5ᵗʰ **S54.9** Injury of unspecified nerve at forearm level

√x7ᵗʰ **S54.90** Injury of unspecified nerve at forearm level, unspecified arm

√x7ᵗʰ **S54.91** Injury of unspecified nerve at forearm level, right arm

√x7ᵗʰ **S54.92** Injury of unspecified nerve at forearm level, left arm

√4ᵗʰ **S55 Injury of blood vessels at forearm level**
Code also any associated open wound (S51.-)
EXCLUDES 2   injury of blood vessels at wrist and hand level (S65.-)
injury of brachial vessels (S45.1-S45.2)

The appropriate 7th is to be added to each code from category S55.
A   initial encounter
D   subsequent encounter
S   sequela

√5ᵗʰ **S55.0 Injury of ulnar artery at forearm level**

√6ᵗʰ   **S55.00 Unspecified injury of ulnar artery at forearm level**

√7ᵗʰ   **S55.001 Unspecified injury of ulnar artery at forearm level, right arm** `CC`
CC Excl: CC with 7th character A: S45.301A, S45.309-S45.311 with 7th A, S45.319-S45.391 with 7th A, S45.399-S45.801 with 7th A, S45.809-S45.811 with 7th A, S45.819-S45.891 with 7th A, S45.899-S45.901 with 7th A, S45.909-S45.911 with 7th A, S45.919-S45.991 with 7th A, S45.999 with 7th A, S55.001A, S55.009-S55.011 with 7th A, S55.019-S55.091 with 7th A, S55.099 A, S55.201 with 7th A, S55.209-S55.211 with 7th A, S55.219-S55.291 with 7th A, S55.299-S55.801 with 7th A, S55.809-S55.811 with 7th A, S55.819-S55.891 with 7th A, S55.899-S55.901 with 7th A, S55.909-S55.911 with 7th A, S55.919-S55.991 with 7th A, S55.999 with 7th A, S65.001 with 7th A, S65.009-S65.011 with 7th A, S65.019-S65.091 with 7th A, S65.099A, S65.801A, S65.809-S65.811 with 7th A, S65.819-S65.891 with 7th A, S65.899-S65.901 with 7th A, S65.909-S65.911 with 7th A, S65.919-S65.991 with 7th A, S65.999A

√7ᵗʰ   **S55.002 Unspecified injury of ulnar artery at forearm level, left arm** `CC`
CC Excl: CC with 7th character A: S45.302-S45.309 with 7th A, S45.312-S45.319 with 7th A, S45.392-S45.399 with 7th A, S45.802-S45.809 with 7th A, S45.812-S45.819 with 7th A, S45.892-S45.899 with 7th A, S45.902-S45.909 with 7th A, S45.912-S45.919 with 7th A, S45.992-S45.999 with 7th A, S55.002-S55.009 with 7th A, S55.012-S55.019 with 7th A, S55.092-S55.099 with 7th A, S55.202-S55.209 with 7th A, S55.212-S55.219 with 7th A, S55.292-S55.299 with 7th A, S55.802-S55.809 with 7th A, S55.812-S55.819 with 7th A, S55.892-S55.899 with 7th A, S55.902-S55.909 with 7th A, S55.912-S55.919 with 7th A, S55.992-S55.999 with 7th A, S65.002-S65.009 with 7th A, S65.012-S65.019 with 7th A, S65.092-S65.099 with 7th A, S65.802-S65.809 with 7th A, S65.812-S65.819 with 7th A, S65.892-S65.899 with 7th A, S65.902-S65.909 with 7th A, S65.912-S65.919 with 7th A, S65.992-S65.999 with 7th A

√7ᵗʰ   **S55.009 Unspecified injury of ulnar artery at forearm level, unspecified arm** `CC`
CC Excl: CC with 7th character A: S45.301-S45.999 with 7th A, S55.001-S55.099 with 7th A, S55.201-S55.999 with 7th A, S65.001-S65.099 with 7th A, S65.801-S65.999 with 7th A

√6ᵗʰ   **S55.01 Laceration of ulnar artery at forearm level**

√7ᵗʰ   **S55.011 Laceration of ulnar artery at forearm level, right arm** `CC`
CC Excl: See code: S55.001

√7ᵗʰ   **S55.012 Laceration of ulnar artery at forearm level, left arm** `CC`
CC Excl: See code: S55.002

√7ᵗʰ   **S55.019 Laceration of ulnar artery at forearm level, unspecified arm** `CC`
CC Excl: See code: S55.009

√6ᵗʰ   **S55.09 Other specified injury of ulnar artery at forearm level**

√7ᵗʰ   **S55.091 Other specified injury of ulnar artery at forearm level, right arm** `CC`
CC Excl: See code: S55.001

√7ᵗʰ   **S55.092 Other specified injury of ulnar artery at forearm level, left arm** `CC`
CC Excl: See code: S55.002

√7ᵗʰ   **S55.099 Other specified injury of ulnar artery at forearm level, unspecified arm** `CC`
CC Excl: See code: S55.009

√5ᵗʰ **S55.1 Injury of radial artery at forearm level**

√6ᵗʰ   **S55.10 Unspecified injury of radial artery at forearm level**

√7ᵗʰ   **S55.101 Unspecified injury of radial artery at forearm level, right arm** `CC`
CC Excl: CC with 7th character A: S45.301 with 7th A, S45.309-S45.311 with 7th A, S45.319-S45.391 with 7th A, S45.399-S45.801 with 7th A, S45.809-S45.811 with 7th A, S45.819-S45.891 with 7th A, S45.899-S45.901 with 7th A, S45.909-S45.911 with 7th A, S45.919-S45.991 with 7th A, S45.999 with 7th A, S55.101 with 7th A, S55.109-S55.111 with 7th A, S55.119-S55.191 with 7th A, S55.199-S55.201 with 7th A, S55.209-S55.211 with 7th A, S55.219-S55.291 with 7th A, S55.299-S55.801 with 7th A, S55.809-S55.811 with 7th A, S55.819-S55.891 with 7th A, S55.899-S55.901 with 7th A, S55.909-S55.911 with 7th A, S55.919-S55.991 with 7th A, S55.999 with 7th A, S65.101 with 7th A, S65.109-S65.111 with 7th A, S65.119-S65.191 with 7th A, S65.199 with 7th A, S65.801 with 7th A, S65.809-S65.811 with 7th A, S65.819-S65.891 with 7th A, S65.899-S65.901 with 7th A, S65.909-S65.911 with 7th A, S65.919-S65.991 with 7th A, S65.999A

√7ᵗʰ   **S55.102 Unspecified injury of radial artery at forearm level, left arm** `CC`
CC Excl: CC with 7th character A: S45.302-S45.309 with 7th A, S45.312-S45.319 with 7th A, S45.392-S45.399 with 7th A, S45.802-S45.809 with 7th A, S45.812-S45.819 with 7th A, S45.892-S45.899 with 7th A, S45.902-S45.909 with 7th A, S45.912-S45.919 with 7th A, S45.992-S45.999 with 7th A, S55.102-S55.109 with 7th A, S55.112-S55.119 with 7th A, S55.192-S55.199 with 7th A, S55.202-S55.209 with 7th A, S55.212-S55.219 with 7th A, S55.292-S55.299 with 7th A, S55.802-S55.809 with 7th A, S55.812-S55.819 with 7th A, S55.892-S55.899 with 7th A, S55.902-S55.909 with 7th A, S55.912-S55.919 with 7th A, S55.992-S55.999 with 7th A, S65.102-S65.109 with 7th A, S65.112-S65.119 with 7th A, S65.192-S65.199 with 7th A, S65.802-S65.809 with 7th A, S65.812-S65.819 with 7th A, S65.892-S65.899 with 7th A, S65.902-S65.909 with 7th A, S65.912-S65.919 with 7th A, S65.992-S65.999 with 7th A

√7ᵗʰ   **S55.109 Unspecified injury of radial artery at forearm level, unspecified arm** `CC`
CC Excl: CC with 7th character A: S45.301-S45.999 with 7th A, S55.101-S55.999 with 7th A, S65.101-S65.199 with 7th A, S65.801-S65.999 with 7th A

√6ᵗʰ   **S55.11 Laceration of radial artery at forearm level**

√7ᵗʰ   **S55.111 Laceration of radial artery at forearm level, right arm** `CC`
CC Excl: See code: S55.101

√7ᵗʰ   **S55.112 Laceration of radial artery at forearm level, left arm** `CC`
CC Excl: See code: S55.102

√7ᵗʰ   **S55.119 Laceration of radial artery at forearm level, unspecified arm** `CC`
CC Excl: See code: S55.109

√6ᵗʰ   **S55.19 Other specified injury of radial artery at forearm level**

√7ᵗʰ   **S55.191 Other specified injury of radial artery at forearm level, right arm** `CC`
CC Excl: See code: S55.101

√7ᵗʰ   **S55.192 Other specified injury of radial artery at forearm level, left arm** `CC`
CC Excl: See code: S55.102

√7ᵗʰ   **S55.199 Other specified injury of radial artery at forearm level, unspecified arm** `CC`
CC Excl: See code: S55.109

Ⓝ Newborn: 0   Ⓟ Pediatric: 0-17   Ⓜ Maternity: 12-55   Ⓐ Adult: 15-124   MCC Major CC Condition   PDx MCC PDx acts as own MCC   CC CC Condition   PDx CC PDx acts as own CC

934   ICD-10-CM Draft (2015)

✓5ᵗʰ **S55.2 Injury of vein at forearm level**

✓6ᵗʰ **S55.20 Unspecified injury of vein at forearm level**

✓7ᵗʰ **S55.201 Unspecified injury of vein at forearm level, right arm** `CC`
CC Excl: CC with 7th character A: S45.301A, S45.309-S45.311 with 7th A, S45.319-S45.391 with 7th A, S45.399-S45.801 with 7th A, S45.809-S45.811 with 7th A, S45.819-S45.891 with 7th A, S45.899-S45.901 with 7th A, S45.909-S45.911 with 7th A, S45.919-S45.991 with 7th A, S45.999 with 7th A, S55.001 with 7th A, S55.009-S55.011 with 7th A, S55.019-S55.091 with 7th A, S55.099A, S55.201A, S55.209-S55.211 with 7th A, S55.219-S55.291 with 7th A, S55.299-S55.801 with 7th A, S55.809-S55.811 with 7th A, S55.819-S55.891 with 7th A, S55.899-S55.901 with 7th A, S55.909-S55.911 with 7th A, S55.919-S55.991 with 7th A, S55.999A, S65.001 A, S65.009-S65.011 with 7th A, S65.019-S65.091 with 7th A, S65.099A, S65.201A, S65.209-S65.211 with 7th A, S65.219-S65.291 with 7th A, S65.299-S65.301 with 7th A, S65.309-S65.311 with 7th A, S65.319-S65.391 with 7th A, S65.399-S65.401 with 7th A, S65.409-S65.411 with 7th A, S65.419-S65.491 with 7th A, S65.499-S65.500A, S65.502A, S65.504A, S65.506A, S65.508-S65.510 with 7th A, S65.512A, S65.514A, S65.516A, S65.518-S65.590 with 7th A, S65.592A, S65.594A, S65.596A, S65.598-S65.801 with 7th A, S65.809-S65.811 with 7th A, S65.819-S65.891 with 7th A, S65.899-S65.901 with 7th A, S65.909-S65.911 with 7th A, S65.919-S65.991 with 7th A, S65.999A

✓7ᵗʰ **S55.202 Unspecified injury of vein at forearm level, left arm** `CC`
CC Excl: CC with 7th character A: S45.302-S45.309 with 7th A, S45.312-S45.319 with 7th A, S45.392-S45.399 with 7th A, S45.802-S45.809 with 7th A, S45.812-S45.819 with 7th A, S45.892-S45.899 with 7th A, S45.902-S45.909 with 7th A, S45.912-S45.919 with 7th A, S45.992-S45.999 with 7th A, S55.002-S55.009 with 7th A, S55.012-S55.019 with 7th A, S55.092-S55.099 with 7th A, S55.202-S55.209 with 7th A, S55.212-S55.219 with 7th A, S55.292-S55.299 with 7th A, S55.802-S55.809 with 7th A, S55.812-S55.819 with 7th A, S55.892-S55.899 with 7th A, S55.902-S55.909 with 7th A, S55.912-S55.919 with 7th A, S55.992-S55.999 with 7th A, S65.002-S65.009 with 7th A, S65.012-S65.019 with 7th A, S65.092-S65.099 with 7th A, S65.202-S65.209 with 7th A, S65.212-S65.219 with 7th A, S65.292-S65.299 with 7th A, S65.302-S65.309 with 7th A, S65.312-S65.319 with 7th A, S65.392-S65.399 with 7th A, S65.402-S65.409 with 7th A, S65.412-S65.419 with 7th A, S65.492-S65.499 with 7th A, S65.501 with 7th A, S65.503 with 7th A, S65.505 with 7th A, S65.507-S65.509 with 7th A, S65.511 with 7th A, S65.513 with 7th A, S65.515 with 7th A, S65.517-S65.519 with 7th A, S65.591 with 7th A, S65.593 with 7th A, S65.595 with 7th A, S65.597-S65.599 with 7th A, S65.802-S65.809 with 7th A, S65.812-S65.819 with 7th A, S65.892-S65.899 with 7th A, S65.902-S65.909 with 7th A, S65.912-S65.919 with 7th A, S65.992-S65.999 with 7th A

✓7ᵗʰ **S55.209 Unspecified injury of vein at forearm level, unspecified arm** `CC`
CC Excl: CC with 7th character A: S45.301-S45.999 with 7th A, S55.001-S55.099 with 7th A, S55.201-S55.999 with 7th A, S65.001-S65.099 with 7th A, S65.201-S65.999 with 7th A

✓6ᵗʰ **S55.21 Laceration of vein at forearm level**

✓7ᵗʰ **S55.211 Laceration of vein at forearm level, right arm** `CC`
CC Excl: See code: S55.201

✓7ᵗʰ **S55.212 Laceration of vein at forearm level, left arm** `CC`
CC Excl: See code: S55.202

✓7ᵗʰ **S55.219 Laceration of vein at forearm level, unspecified arm** `CC`
CC Excl: See code: S55.209

✓6ᵗʰ **S55.29 Other specified injury of vein at forearm level**

✓7ᵗʰ **S55.291 Other specified injury of vein at forearm level, right arm** `CC`
CC Excl: See code: S55.201

✓7ᵗʰ **S55.292 Other specified injury of vein at forearm level, left arm** `CC`
CC Excl: See code: S55.202

✓7ᵗʰ **S55.299 Other specified injury of vein at forearm level, unspecified arm** `CC`
CC Excl: See code: S55.209

✓5ᵗʰ **S55.8 Injury of other blood vessels at forearm level**

✓6ᵗʰ **S55.80 Unspecified injury of other blood vessels at forearm level**

✓7ᵗʰ **S55.801 Unspecified injury of other blood vessels at forearm level, right arm** `CC`
CC Excl: See code: S55.201

✓7ᵗʰ **S55.802 Unspecified injury of other blood vessels at forearm level, left arm** `CC`
CC Excl: See code: S55.202

✓7ᵗʰ **S55.809 Unspecified injury of other blood vessels at forearm level, unspecified arm** `CC`
CC Excl: See code: S55.209

✓6ᵗʰ **S55.81 Laceration of other blood vessels at forearm level**

✓7ᵗʰ **S55.811 Laceration of other blood vessels at forearm level, right arm** `CC`
CC Excl: See code: S55.201

✓7ᵗʰ **S55.812 Laceration of other blood vessels at forearm level, left arm** `CC`
CC Excl: See code: S55.202

✓7ᵗʰ **S55.819 Laceration of other blood vessels at forearm level, unspecified arm** `CC`
CC Excl: See code: S55.209

✓6ᵗʰ **S55.89 Other specified injury of other blood vessels at forearm level**

✓7ᵗʰ **S55.891 Other specified injury of other blood vessels at forearm level, right arm** `CC`
CC Excl: See code: S55.201

✓7ᵗʰ **S55.892 Other specified injury of other blood vessels at forearm level, left arm** `CC`
CC Excl: See code: S55.202

✓7ᵗʰ **S55.899 Other specified injury of other blood vessels at forearm level, unspecified arm** `CC`
CC Excl: See code: S55.209

✓5ᵗʰ **S55.9 Injury of unspecified blood vessel at forearm level**

✓6ᵗʰ **S55.90 Unspecified injury of unspecified blood vessel at forearm level**

✓7ᵗʰ **S55.901 Unspecified injury of unspecified blood vessel at forearm level, right arm** `CC`
CC Excl: See code: S55.201

✓7ᵗʰ **S55.902 Unspecified injury of unspecified blood vessel at forearm level, left arm** `CC`
CC Excl: See code: S55.202

✓7ᵗʰ **S55.909 Unspecified injury of unspecified blood vessel at forearm level, unspecified arm** `CC`
CC Excl: See code: S55.209

✓6ᵗʰ **S55.91 Laceration of unspecified blood vessel at forearm level**

✓7ᵗʰ **S55.911 Laceration of unspecified blood vessel at forearm level, right arm** `CC`
CC Excl: See code: S55.201

✓7ᵗʰ **S55.912 Laceration of unspecified blood vessel at forearm level, left arm** `CC`
CC Excl: See code: S55.202

✓7ᵗʰ **S55.919 Laceration of unspecified blood vessel at forearm level, unspecified arm** `CC`
CC Excl: See code: S55.209

✓6ᵗʰ **S55.99 Other specified injury of unspecified blood vessel at forearm level**

✓7ᵗʰ **S55.991 Other specified injury of unspecified blood vessel at forearm level, right arm** `CC`
CC Excl: See code: S55.201

✓ Additional Character Required   ✓x7ᵗʰ Xtension Alert   Unacceptable PDx   Manifestation   Hospital Acquired Condition   **EXCLUDES 1** Not Coded Here   **EXCLUDES 2** Not Included Here

√7ᵗʰ **S55.992** **Other specified injury of unspecified blood vessel at forearm level, left arm** `CC`
CC Excl: See code: S55.202

√7ᵗʰ **S55.999** **Other specified injury of unspecified blood vessel at forearm level, unspecified arm** `CC`
CC Excl: See code: S55.209

√4ᵗʰ **S56** **Injury of muscle, fascia and tendon at forearm level**
Code also any associated open wound (S51.-)
EXCLUDES 2   injury of muscle, fascia and tendon at or below wrist (S66.-) · sprain of joints and ligaments of elbow (S53.4-)

The appropriate 7th is to be added to each code from category S56.
A   initial encounter
D   subsequent encounter
S   sequela

√5ᵗʰ **S56.0** **Injury of flexor muscle, fascia and tendon of thumb at forearm level**

√6ᵗʰ **S56.00** **Unspecified injury of flexor muscle, fascia and tendon of thumb at forearm level**

√7ᵗʰ **S56.001** **Unspecified injury of flexor muscle, fascia and tendon of right thumb at forearm level**

√7ᵗʰ **S56.002** **Unspecified injury of flexor muscle, fascia and tendon of left thumb at forearm level**

√7ᵗʰ **S56.009** **Unspecified injury of flexor muscle, fascia and tendon of unspecified thumb at forearm level**

√6ᵗʰ **S56.01** **Strain of flexor muscle, fascia and tendon of thumb at forearm level**

√7ᵗʰ **S56.011** **Strain of flexor muscle, fascia and tendon of right thumb at forearm level**

√7ᵗʰ **S56.012** **Strain of flexor muscle, fascia and tendon of left thumb at forearm level**

√7ᵗʰ **S56.019** **Strain of flexor muscle, fascia and tendon of unspecified thumb at forearm level**

√6ᵗʰ **S56.02** **Laceration of flexor muscle, fascia and tendon of thumb at forearm level**

√7ᵗʰ **S56.021** **Laceration of flexor muscle, fascia and tendon of right thumb at forearm level** `CC`
CC Excl: CC with 7th character A: S51.001A, S51.009-S51.011 with 7th A, S51.019-S51.021 with 7th A, S51.029-S51.031 with 7th A, S51.039-S51.041 with 7th A, S51.049-S51.051 with 7th A, S51.059-S51.801 with 7th A, S51.809-S51.811 with 7th A, S51.819-S51.821 with 7th A, S51.829-S51.831 with 7th A, S51.839-S51.841 with 7th A, S51.849-S51.851 with 7th A, S51.859A, S56.021A, S56.029 A, S56.121A, S56.123A, S56.125A, S56.127A, S56.129 A, S56.221 A, S56.229A, S56.321A, S56.329A, S56.421A, S56.423A, S56.425A, S56.427A, S56.429A, S56.521A, S56.529A, S56.821A, S56.829A, S56.921 A, S56.929A, S61.501A, S61.509-S61.511 with 7th A, S61.519-S61.521 with 7th A, S61.529-S61.531 with 7th A, S61.539-S61.541 with 7th A, S61.549-S61.551 with 7th A, S61.559A

√7ᵗʰ **S56.022** **Laceration of flexor muscle, fascia and tendon of left thumb at forearm level** `CC`
CC Excl: CC with 7th character A: S51.002-S51.009 with 7th A, S51.012-S51.019 with 7th A, S51.022-S51.029 with 7th A, S51.032-S51.039 with 7th A, S51.042-S51.049 with 7th A, S51.052-S51.059 with 7th A, S51.802-S51.809 with 7th A, S51.812-S51.819 with 7th A, S51.822-S51.829 with 7th A, S51.832-S51.839 with 7th A, S51.842-S51.849 with 7th A, S51.852-S51.859 with 7th A, S56.022-S56.029 with 7th A, S56.122A, S56.124A, S56.126A, S56.128-S56.129 with 7th A, S56.222-S56.229 with 7th A, S56.322-S56.329 with 7th A, S56.422A, S56.424 A, S56.426A, S56.428-S56.429 with 7th A, S56.522-S56.529 with 7th A, S56.822-S56.829 with 7th A, S56.922-S56.929 with 7th A, S61.502-S61.509 with 7th A, S61.512-S61.519 with 7th A, S61.522-S61.529 with 7th A, S61.532-S61.539 with 7th A, S61.542-S61.549 with 7th A, S61.552-S61.559 with 7th A

√7ᵗʰ **S56.029** **Laceration of flexor muscle, fascia and tendon of unspecified thumb at forearm level** `CC`
CC Excl: CC with 7th character A: S51.001-S51.859 with 7th A, S56.021-S56.029 with 7th A, S56.121-S56.129 with 7th A, S56.221-S56.229 with 7th A, S56.321-S56.329 with 7th A, S56.421-S56.429 with 7th A, S56.521-S56.529 with 7th A, S56.821-S56.829 with 7th A, S56.921-S56.929 with 7th A, S61.501-S61.559 with 7th A

√6ᵗʰ **S56.09** **Other injury of flexor muscle, fascia and tendon of thumb at forearm level**

√7ᵗʰ **S56.091** **Other injury of flexor muscle, fascia and tendon of right thumb at forearm level**

√7ᵗʰ **S56.092** **Other injury of flexor muscle, fascia and tendon of left thumb at forearm level**

√7ᵗʰ **S56.099** **Other injury of flexor muscle, fascia and tendon of unspecified thumb at forearm level**

√5ᵗʰ **S56.1** **Injury of flexor muscle, fascia and tendon of other and unspecified finger at forearm level**

√6ᵗʰ **S56.10** **Unspecified injury of flexor muscle, fascia and tendon of other and unspecified finger at forearm level**

√7ᵗʰ **S56.101** **Unspecified injury of flexor muscle, fascia and tendon of right index finger at forearm level**

√7ᵗʰ **S56.102** **Unspecified injury of flexor muscle, fascia and tendon of left index finger at forearm level**

√7ᵗʰ **S56.103** **Unspecified injury of flexor muscle, fascia and tendon of right middle finger at forearm level**

√7ᵗʰ **S56.104** **Unspecified injury of flexor muscle, fascia and tendon of left middle finger at forearm level**

√7ᵗʰ **S56.105** **Unspecified injury of flexor muscle, fascia and tendon of right ring finger at forearm level**

√7ᵗʰ **S56.106** **Unspecified injury of flexor muscle, fascia and tendon of left ring finger at forearm level**

√7ᵗʰ **S56.107** **Unspecified injury of flexor muscle, fascia and tendon of right little finger at forearm level**

√7ᵗʰ **S56.108** **Unspecified injury of flexor muscle, fascia and tendon of left little finger at forearm level**

√7ᵗʰ **S56.109** **Unspecified injury of flexor muscle, fascia and tendon of unspecified finger at forearm level**

√6ᵗʰ **S56.11** **Strain of flexor muscle, fascia and tendon of other and unspecified finger at forearm level**

√7ᵗʰ **S56.111** **Strain of flexor muscle, fascia and tendon of right index finger at forearm level**

√7ᵗʰ **S56.112** **Strain of flexor muscle, fascia and tendon of left index finger at forearm level**

√7ᵗʰ **S56.113** **Strain of flexor muscle, fascia and tendon of right middle finger at forearm level**

√7ᵗʰ **S56.114** **Strain of flexor muscle, fascia and tendon of left middle finger at forearm level**

√7ᵗʰ **S56.115** **Strain of flexor muscle, fascia and tendon of right ring finger at forearm level**

√7ᵗʰ **S56.116** **Strain of flexor muscle, fascia and tendon of left ring finger at forearm level**

√7ᵗʰ **S56.117** **Strain of flexor muscle, fascia and tendon of right little finger at forearm level**

√7ᵗʰ **S56.118** **Strain of flexor muscle, fascia and tendon of left little finger at forearm level**

√7ᵗʰ **S56.119** **Strain of flexor muscle, fascia and tendon of finger of unspecified finger at forearm level**

√6ᵗʰ **S56.12** **Laceration of flexor muscle, fascia and tendon of other and unspecified finger at forearm level**

√7ᵗʰ **S56.121** **Laceration of flexor muscle, fascia and tendon of right index finger at forearm level** `CC`
CC Excl: See code: S56.021

N Newborn: 0   P Pediatric: 0-17   M Maternity: 12-55   A Adult: 15-124   MCC Major CC Condition   PDx MCC PDx acts as own MCC   CC CC Condition   PDx CC PDx acts as own CC

936   ICD-10-CM Draft (2015)

√7ᵗʰ **S56.122** **Laceration of flexor muscle, fascia and** CC
**tendon of left index finger at forearm
level**
CC Excl: See code: S56.022

√7ᵗʰ **S56.123** **Laceration of flexor muscle, fascia and** CC
**tendon of right middle finger at forearm
level**
CC Excl: See code: S56.021

√7ᵗʰ **S56.124** **Laceration of flexor muscle, fascia and** CC
**tendon of left middle finger at forearm
level**
CC Excl: See code: S56.022

√7ᵗʰ **S56.125** **Laceration of flexor muscle, fascia and** CC
**tendon of right ring finger at forearm
level**
CC Excl: See code: S56.021

√7ᵗʰ **S56.126** **Laceration of flexor muscle, fascia and** CC
**tendon of left ring finger at forearm
level**
CC Excl: See code: S56.022

√7ᵗʰ **S56.127** **Laceration of flexor muscle, fascia and** CC
**tendon of right little finger at forearm
level**
CC Excl: See code: S56.021

√7ᵗʰ **S56.128** **Laceration of flexor muscle, fascia and** CC
**tendon of left little finger at forearm
level**
CC Excl: See code: S56.022

√7ᵗʰ **S56.129** **Laceration of flexor muscle, fascia and** CC
**tendon of unspecified finger at forearm
level**
CC Excl: See code: S56.029

√6ᵗʰ **S56.19** **Other injury of flexor muscle, fascia and tendon of
other and unspecified finger at forearm level**

√7ᵗʰ **S56.191** **Other injury of flexor muscle, fascia and
tendon of right index finger at forearm
level**

√7ᵗʰ **S56.192** **Other injury of flexor muscle, fascia and
tendon of left index finger at forearm
level**

√7ᵗʰ **S56.193** **Other injury of flexor muscle, fascia and
tendon of right middle finger at forearm
level**

√7ᵗʰ **S56.194** **Other injury of flexor muscle, fascia and
tendon of left middle finger at forearm
level**

√7ᵗʰ **S56.195** **Other injury of flexor muscle, fascia and
tendon of right ring finger at forearm level**

√7ᵗʰ **S56.196** **Other injury of flexor muscle, fascia and
tendon of left ring finger at forearm level**

√7ᵗʰ **S56.197** **Other injury of flexor muscle, fascia and
tendon of right little finger at forearm
level**

√7ᵗʰ **S56.198** **Other injury of flexor muscle, fascia and
tendon of left little finger at forearm level**

√7ᵗʰ **S56.199** **Other injury of flexor muscle, fascia and
tendon of unspecified finger at forearm
level**

√5ᵗʰ **S56.2** **Injury of other flexor muscle, fascia and tendon at forearm
level**

√6ᵗʰ **S56.20** **Unspecified injury of other flexor muscle, fascia and
tendon at forearm level**

√7ᵗʰ **S56.201** **Unspecified injury of other flexor muscle,
fascia and tendon at forearm level, right
arm**

√7ᵗʰ **S56.202** **Unspecified injury of other flexor muscle,
fascia and tendon at forearm level, left
arm**

√7ᵗʰ **S56.209** **Unspecified injury of other flexor muscle,
fascia and tendon at forearm level,
unspecified arm**

√6ᵗʰ **S56.21** **Strain of other flexor muscle, fascia and tendon at
forearm level**

√7ᵗʰ **S56.211** **Strain of other flexor muscle, fascia and
tendon at forearm level, right arm**

√7ᵗʰ **S56.212** **Strain of other flexor muscle, fascia and
tendon at forearm level, left arm**

√7ᵗʰ **S56.219** **Strain of other flexor muscle, fascia and
tendon at forearm level, unspecified arm**

√6ᵗʰ **S56.22** **Laceration of other flexor muscle, fascia and tendon
at forearm level**

√7ᵗʰ **S56.221** **Laceration of other flexor muscle,** CC
**fascia and tendon at forearm level,
right arm**
CC Excl: See code: S56.021

√7ᵗʰ **S56.222** **Laceration of other flexor muscle,** CC
**fascia and tendon at forearm level,
left arm**
CC Excl: See code: S56.022

√7ᵗʰ **S56.229** **Laceration of other flexor muscle,** CC
**fascia and tendon at forearm level,
unspecified arm**
CC Excl: See code: S56.029

√6ᵗʰ **S56.29** **Other injury of other flexor muscle, fascia and
tendon at forearm level**

√7ᵗʰ **S56.291** **Other injury of other flexor muscle, fascia
and tendon at forearm level, right arm**

√7ᵗʰ **S56.292** **Other injury of other flexor muscle, fascia
and tendon at forearm level, left arm**

√7ᵗʰ **S56.299** **Other injury of other flexor muscle, fascia
and tendon at forearm level, unspecified
arm**

√5ᵗʰ **S56.3** **Injury of extensor or abductor muscles, fascia and tendons of
thumb at forearm level**

√6ᵗʰ **S56.30** **Unspecified injury of extensor or abductor muscles,
fascia and tendons of thumb at forearm level**

√7ᵗʰ **S56.301** **Unspecified injury of extensor or abductor
muscles, fascia and tendons of right
thumb at forearm level**

√7ᵗʰ **S56.302** **Unspecified injury of extensor or abductor
muscles, fascia and tendons of left thumb
at forearm level**

√7ᵗʰ **S56.309** **Unspecified injury of extensor or abductor
muscles, fascia and tendons of unspecified
thumb at forearm level**

√6ᵗʰ **S56.31** **Strain of extensor or abductor muscles, fascia and
tendons of thumb at forearm level**

√7ᵗʰ **S56.311** **Strain of extensor or abductor muscles,
fascia and tendons of right thumb at
forearm level**

√7ᵗʰ **S56.312** **Strain of extensor or abductor muscles,
fascia and tendons of left thumb at
forearm level**

√7ᵗʰ **S56.319** **Strain of extensor or abductor muscles,
fascia and tendons of unspecified thumb
at forearm level**

√6ᵗʰ **S56.32** **Laceration of extensor or abductor muscles, fascia
and tendons of thumb at forearm level**

√7ᵗʰ **S56.321** **Laceration of extensor or abductor** CC
**muscles, fascia and tendons of right
thumb at forearm level**
CC Excl: See code: S56.021

√7ᵗʰ **S56.322** **Laceration of extensor or abductor** CC
**muscles, fascia and tendons of left
thumb at forearm level**
CC Excl: See code: S56.022

√7ᵗʰ **S56.329** **Laceration of extensor or abductor** CC
**muscles, fascia and tendons of
unspecified thumb at forearm level**
CC Excl: See code: S56.029

√6ᵗʰ **S56.39** **Other injury of extensor or abductor muscles, fascia
and tendons of thumb at forearm level**

√7ᵗʰ **S56.391** **Other injury of extensor or abductor
muscles, fascia and tendons of right
thumb at forearm level**

√7ᵗʰ **S56.392** **Other injury of extensor or abductor
muscles, fascia and tendons of left thumb
at forearm level**

√7ᵗʰ **S56.399** **Other injury of extensor or abductor
muscles, fascia and tendons of unspecified
thumb at forearm level**

√5ᵗʰ **S56.4** **Injury of extensor muscle, fascia and tendon of other and
unspecified finger at forearm level**

√6ᵗʰ **S56.40** **Unspecified injury of extensor muscle, fascia and
tendon of other and unspecified finger at forearm
level**

✔ Additional Character Required   √x7ᵗʰ Xtension Alert   Unacceptable PDx   Manifestation   Hospital Acquired Condition   EXCLUDES 1 Not Coded Here   EXCLUDES 2 Not Included Here

ICD-10-CM Draft (2015)   937

Injury, Poisoning and Certain Other Consequences of External Causes

S56.401–S56.591

√7th **S56.401** Unspecified injury of extensor muscle, fascia and tendon of right index finger at forearm level

√7th **S56.402** Unspecified injury of extensor muscle, fascia and tendon of left index finger at forearm level

√7th **S56.403** Unspecified injury of extensor muscle, fascia and tendon of right middle finger at forearm level

√7th **S56.404** Unspecified injury of extensor muscle, fascia and tendon of left middle finger at forearm level

√7th **S56.405** Unspecified injury of extensor muscle, fascia and tendon of right ring finger at forearm level

√7th **S56.406** Unspecified injury of extensor muscle, fascia and tendon of left ring finger at forearm level

√7th **S56.407** Unspecified injury of extensor muscle, fascia and tendon of right little finger at forearm level

√7th **S56.408** Unspecified injury of extensor muscle, fascia and tendon of left little finger at forearm level

√7th **S56.409** Unspecified injury of extensor muscle, fascia and tendon of unspecified finger at forearm level

√6th **S56.41** Strain of extensor muscle, fascia and tendon of other and unspecified finger at forearm level

√7th **S56.411** Strain of extensor muscle, fascia and tendon of right index finger at forearm level

√7th **S56.412** Strain of extensor muscle, fascia and tendon of left index finger at forearm level

√7th **S56.413** Strain of extensor muscle, fascia and tendon of right middle finger at forearm level

√7th **S56.414** Strain of extensor muscle, fascia and tendon of left middle finger at forearm level

√7th **S56.415** Strain of extensor muscle, fascia and tendon of right ring finger at forearm level

√7th **S56.416** Strain of extensor muscle, fascia and tendon of left ring finger at forearm level

√7th **S56.417** Strain of extensor muscle, fascia and tendon of right little finger at forearm level

√7th **S56.418** Strain of extensor muscle, fascia and tendon of left little finger at forearm level

√7th **S56.419** Strain of extensor muscle, fascia and tendon of finger, unspecified finger at forearm level

√6th **S56.42** Laceration of extensor muscle, fascia and tendon of other and unspecified finger at forearm level

√7th **S56.421** Laceration of extensor muscle, fascia and tendon of right index finger at forearm level   CC
    CC Excl: See code: S56.021

√7th **S56.422** Laceration of extensor muscle, fascia and tendon of left index finger at forearm level   CC
    CC Excl: See code: S56.022

√7th **S56.423** Laceration of extensor muscle, fascia and tendon of right middle finger at forearm level   CC
    CC Excl: See code: S56.021

√7th **S56.424** Laceration of extensor muscle, fascia and tendon of left middle finger at forearm level   CC
    CC Excl: See code: S56.022

√7th **S56.425** Laceration of extensor muscle, fascia and tendon of right ring finger at forearm level   CC
    CC Excl: See code: S56.021

√7th **S56.426** Laceration of extensor muscle, fascia and tendon of left ring finger at forearm level   CC
    CC Excl: See code: S56.022

√7th **S56.427** Laceration of extensor muscle, fascia and tendon of right little finger at forearm level   CC
    CC Excl: See code: S56.021

√7th **S56.428** Laceration of extensor muscle, fascia and tendon of left little finger at forearm level   CC
    CC Excl: See code: S56.022

√7th **S56.429** Laceration of extensor muscle, fascia and tendon of unspecified finger at forearm level   CC
    CC Excl: See code: S56.029

√6th **S56.49** Other injury of extensor muscle, fascia and tendon of other and unspecified finger at forearm level

√7th **S56.491** Other injury of extensor muscle, fascia and tendon of right index finger at forearm level

√7th **S56.492** Other injury of extensor muscle, fascia and tendon of left index finger at forearm level

√7th **S56.493** Other injury of extensor muscle, fascia and tendon of right middle finger at forearm level

√7th **S56.494** Other injury of extensor muscle, fascia and tendon of left middle finger at forearm level

√7th **S56.495** Other injury of extensor muscle, fascia and tendon of right ring finger at forearm level

√7th **S56.496** Other injury of extensor muscle, fascia and tendon of left ring finger at forearm level

√7th **S56.497** Other injury of extensor muscle, fascia and tendon of right little finger at forearm level

√7th **S56.498** Other injury of extensor muscle, fascia and tendon of left little finger at forearm level

√7th **S56.499** Other injury of extensor muscle, fascia and tendon of unspecified finger at forearm level

√5th **S56.5** Injury of other extensor muscle, fascia and tendon at forearm level

√6th **S56.50** Unspecified injury of other extensor muscle, fascia and tendon at forearm level

√7th **S56.501** Unspecified injury of other extensor muscle, fascia and tendon at forearm level, right arm

√7th **S56.502** Unspecified injury of other extensor muscle, fascia and tendon at forearm level, left arm

√7th **S56.509** Unspecified injury of other extensor muscle, fascia and tendon at forearm level, unspecified arm

√6th **S56.51** Strain of other extensor muscle, fascia and tendon at forearm level

√7th **S56.511** Strain of other extensor muscle, fascia and tendon at forearm level, right arm

√7th **S56.512** Strain of other extensor muscle, fascia and tendon at forearm level, left arm

√7th **S56.519** Strain of other extensor muscle, fascia and tendon at forearm level, unspecified arm

√6th **S56.52** Laceration of other extensor muscle, fascia and tendon at forearm level

√7th **S56.521** Laceration of other extensor muscle, fascia and tendon at forearm level, right arm   CC
    CC Excl: See code: S56.021

√7th **S56.522** Laceration of other extensor muscle, fascia and tendon at forearm level, left arm   CC
    CC Excl: See code: S56.022

√7th **S56.529** Laceration of other extensor muscle, fascia and tendon at forearm level, unspecified arm   CC
    CC Excl: See code: S56.029

√6th **S56.59** Other injury of other extensor muscle, fascia and tendon at forearm level

√7th **S56.591** Other injury of other extensor muscle, fascia and tendon at forearm level, right arm

N Newborn: 0   P Pediatric: 0-17   M Maternity: 12-55   A Adult: 15-124   MCC Major CC Condition   PDx MCC PDx acts as own MCC   CC CC Condition   PDx CC PDx acts as own CC

938   ICD-10-CM Draft (2015)

√7ᵗʰ **S56.592** Other injury of other extensor muscle, fascia and tendon at forearm level, left arm

√7ᵗʰ **S56.599** Other injury of other extensor muscle, fascia and tendon at forearm level, unspecified arm

√5ᵗʰ **S56.8** Injury of other muscles, fascia and tendons at forearm level

√6ᵗʰ **S56.80** Unspecified injury of other muscles, fascia and tendons at forearm level

√7ᵗʰ **S56.801** Unspecified injury of other muscles, fascia and tendons at forearm level, right arm

√7ᵗʰ **S56.802** Unspecified injury of other muscles, fascia and tendons at forearm level, left arm

√7ᵗʰ **S56.809** Unspecified injury of other muscles, fascia and tendons at forearm level, unspecified arm

√6ᵗʰ **S56.81** Strain of other muscles, fascia and tendons at forearm level

√7ᵗʰ **S56.811** Strain of other muscles, fascia and tendons at forearm level, right arm

√7ᵗʰ **S56.812** Strain of other muscles, fascia and tendons at forearm level, left arm

√7ᵗʰ **S56.819** Strain of other muscles, fascia and tendons at forearm level, unspecified arm

√6ᵗʰ **S56.82** Laceration of other muscles, fascia and tendons at forearm level

√7ᵗʰ **S56.821** Laceration of other muscles, fascia and tendons at forearm level, right arm   **CC**
    CC Excl: See code: S56.021

√7ᵗʰ **S56.822** Laceration of other muscles, fascia and tendons at forearm level, left arm   **CC**
    CC Excl: See code: S56.022

√7ᵗʰ **S56.829** Laceration of other muscles, fascia and tendons at forearm level, unspecified arm   **CC**
    CC Excl: See code: S56.029

√6ᵗʰ **S56.89** Other injury of other muscles, fascia and tendons at forearm level

√7ᵗʰ **S56.891** Other injury of other muscles, fascia and tendons at forearm level, right arm

√7ᵗʰ **S56.892** Other injury of other muscles, fascia and tendons at forearm level, left arm

√7ᵗʰ **S56.899** Other injury of other muscles, fascia and tendons at forearm level, unspecified arm

√5ᵗʰ **S56.9** Injury of unspecified muscles, fascia and tendons at forearm level

√6ᵗʰ **S56.90** Unspecified injury of unspecified muscles, fascia and tendons at forearm level

√7ᵗʰ **S56.901** Unspecified injury of unspecified muscles, fascia and tendons at forearm level, right arm

√7ᵗʰ **S56.902** Unspecified injury of unspecified muscles, fascia and tendons at forearm level, left arm

√7ᵗʰ **S56.909** Unspecified injury of unspecified muscles, fascia and tendons at forearm level, unspecified arm

√6ᵗʰ **S56.91** Strain of unspecified muscles, fascia and tendons at forearm level

√7ᵗʰ **S56.911** Strain of unspecified muscles, fascia and tendons at forearm level, right arm

√7ᵗʰ **S56.912** Strain of unspecified muscles, fascia and tendons at forearm level, left arm

√7ᵗʰ **S56.919** Strain of unspecified muscles, fascia and tendons at forearm level, unspecified arm

√6ᵗʰ **S56.92** Laceration of unspecified muscles, fascia and tendons at forearm level

√7ᵗʰ **S56.921** Laceration of unspecified muscles, fascia and tendons at forearm level, right arm   **CC**
    CC Excl: See code: S56.021

√7ᵗʰ **S56.922** Laceration of unspecified muscles, fascia and tendons at forearm level, left arm   **CC**
    CC Excl: See code: S56.022

√7ᵗʰ **S56.929** Laceration of unspecified muscles, fascia and tendons at forearm level, unspecified arm   **CC**
    CC Excl: See code: S56.029

√6ᵗʰ **S56.99** Other injury of unspecified muscles, fascia and tendons at forearm level

√7ᵗʰ **S56.991** Other injury of unspecified muscles, fascia and tendons at forearm level, right arm

√7ᵗʰ **S56.992** Other injury of unspecified muscles, fascia and tendons at forearm level, left arm

√7ᵗʰ **S56.999** Other injury of unspecified muscles, fascia and tendons at forearm level, unspecified arm

√4ᵗʰ **S57** Crushing injury of elbow and forearm

Use additional code(s) for all associated injuries

EXCLUDES 2   crushing injury of wrist and hand (S67.-)

> The appropriate 7th is to be added to each code from category S57.
> A   initial encounter
> D   subsequent encounter
> S   sequela

√5ᵗʰ **S57.0** Crushing injury of elbow

√x7ᵗʰ **S57.00** Crushing injury of unspecified elbow

√x7ᵗʰ **S57.01** Crushing injury of right elbow

√x7ᵗʰ **S57.02** Crushing injury of left elbow

√5ᵗʰ **S57.8** Crushing injury of forearm

√x7ᵗʰ **S57.80** Crushing injury of unspecified forearm

√x7ᵗʰ **S57.81** Crushing injury of right forearm

√x7ᵗʰ **S57.82** Crushing injury of left forearm

√4ᵗʰ **S58** Traumatic amputation of elbow and forearm

NOTE   An amputation not identified as partial or complete should be coded to complete.

EXCLUDES 1   traumatic amputation of wrist and hand (S68.-)

> The appropriate 7th is to be added to each code from category S58.
> A   initial encounter
> D   subsequent encounter
> S   sequela

√5ᵗʰ **S58.0** Traumatic amputation at elbow level

√6ᵗʰ **S58.01** Complete traumatic amputation at elbow level

√7ᵗʰ **S58.011** Complete traumatic amputation at elbow level, right arm   **CC**
CC Excl: CC with 7th character A: S41.001 with 7th A, S41.009–S41.011 with 7th A, S41.019–S41.021 with 7th A, S41.029–S41.031 with 7th A, S41.039–S41.041 with 7th A, S41.049–S41.051 with 7th A, S41.059–S41.101 with 7th A, S41.109–S41.111 with 7th A, S41.119–S41.121 with 7th A, S41.129–S41.131 with 7th A, S41.139–S41.141 with 7th A, S41.149–S41.151 with 7th A, S41.159A, S46.021A, S46.029A, S46.121A, S46.129A, S46.221A, S46.229A, S46.321A, S46.329A, S46.821A, S46.829A, S46.921A, S46.929A, S48.011A, S48.019–S48.021 with 7th A, S48.029–S48.111 with 7th A, S48.119–S48.121 with 7th A, S48.129–S48.911 with 7th A, S48.919–S48.921 with 7th A, S48.929A, S51.001A, S51.009–S51.011 with 7th A, S51.019–S51.021 with 7th A, S51.029–S51.031 with 7th A, S51.039–S51.041 with 7th A, S51.049–S51.051 with 7th A, S51.059–S51.801 with 7th A, S51.809–S51.811 with 7th A, S51.819–S51.821 with 7th A, S51.829–S51.831 with 7th A, S51.839–S51.841 with 7th A, S51.849–S51.851 with 7th A, S51.859A, S56.021A, S56.029A, S56.121A, S56.123A, S56.125A, S56.127A, S56.129A, S56.221A, S56.229A, S56.321A, S56.329A, S56.421A, S56.423A, S56.425 with 7th A, S56.427 with 7th A, S56.429 with 7th A, S56.521 with 7th A, S56.529 with 7th A, S56.821 with 7th A, S56.829 with 7th A, S56.921 with 7th A, S56.929 with 7th A, S58.011 with 7th A, S58.019–S58.021 with 7th A, S58.029–S58.111 with 7th A, S58.119–S58.121 with 7th A, S58.129–S58.911 with 7th A, S58.919–S58.921 with 7th A, S58.929 with 7th A, S61.001 with 7th A, S61.009–S61.011 with 7th A, S61.019–S61.021 with 7th A, S61.029–S61.031 with 7th A, S61.039–S61.041 with

√ Additional Character Required   √x7ᵗʰ Xtension Alert   Unacceptable PDx   Manifestation   Hospital Acquired Condition   *EXCLUDES 1* Not Coded Here   *EXCLUDES 2* Not Included Here

ICD-10-CM Draft (2015)   939

7th A, S61.049-S61.051 with 7th A, S61.059-
S61.101 with 7th A, S61.109-S61.111 with
7th A, S61.119-S61.121 with 7th A, S61.129-
S61.131 with 7th A, S61.139-S61.141 with
7th A, S61.149-S61.151 with 7th A, S61.159-
S61.200 with 7th A, S61.202 with 7th A,
S61.204 with 7th A, S61.206 with 7th A,
S61.208-S61.210 with 7th A, S61.212 with
7th A, S61.214 with 7th A, S61.216 with 7th
A, S61.218-S61.220 with 7th A, S61.222 with
7th A, S61.224 with 7th A, S61.226 with 7th
A, S61.228-S61.230 with 7th A, S61.232 with
7th A, S61.234 with 7th A, S61.236 with 7th
A, S61.238-S61.240 with 7th A, S61.242 with
7th A, S61.244 with 7th A, S61.246 with 7th
A, S61.248-S61.250 with 7th A, S61.252 with
7th A, S61.254 with 7th A, S61.256 with 7th
A, S61.258-S61.300 with 7th A, S61.302 with
7th A, S61.304 with 7th A, S61.306 with 7th
A, S61.308-S61.310 with 7th A, S61.312 with
7th A, S61.314 with 7th A, S61.316 with 7th
A, S61.318-S61.320 with 7th A, S61.322 with
7th A, S61.324 with 7th A, S61.326 with 7th
A, S61.328-S61.330 with 7th A, S61.332 with
7th A, S61.334 with 7th A, S61.336 with 7th
A, S61.338-S61.340 with 7th A, S61.342 with
7th A, S61.344 with 7th A, S61.346 with 7th
A, S61.348-S61.350 with 7th A, S61.352 with
7th A, S61.354 with 7th A, S61.356 with 7th
A, S61.358-S61.401 with 7th A, S61.409-
S61.411 with 7th A, S61.419-S61.421 with
7th A, S61.429-S61.431 with 7th A, S61.439-
S61.441 with 7th A, S61.449-S61.451 with
7th A, S61.459-S61.501 with 7th A, S61.509-
S61.511 with 7th A, S61.519-S61.521 with
7th A, S61.529-S61.531 with 7th A, S61.539-
S61.541 with 7th A, S61.549-S61.551 with
7th A, S61.559 with 7th A, S66.021 with 7th
A, S66.029 with 7th A, S66.120 with 7th A,
S66.122 with 7th A, S66.124 with 7th A,
S66.126 with 7th A, S66.128-S66.129 with
7th A, S66.221 with 7th A, S66.229 with 7th
A, S66.320 with 7th A, S66.322 with 7th A,
S66.324 with 7th A, S66.326 with 7th A,
S66.328-S66.329 with 7th A, S66.421 with
7th A, S66.429 with 7th A, S66.520 with 7th
A, S66.522 with 7th A, S66.524 with 7th A,
S66.526 with 7th A, S66.528-S66.529 with
7th A, S66.821 with 7th A, S66.829 with 7th
A, S66.921 with 7th A, S66.929 with 7th A,
S68.011 with 7th A, S68.019-S68.021 with
7th A, S68.029-S68.110 with 7th A, S68.112
with 7th A, S68.114 with 7th A, S68.116 with
7th A, S68.118-S68.120 with 7th A, S68.122
with 7th A, S68.124 with 7th A, S68.126 with
7th A, S68.128-S68.411 with 7th A, S68.419-
S68.421 with 7th A, S68.429-S68.511 with
7th A, S68.519-S68.521 with 7th A, S68.529-
S68.610 with 7th A, S68.612 with 7th A,
S68.614 with 7th A, S68.616 with 7th A,
S68.618-S68.620 with 7th A, S68.622A,
S68.624A, S68.626A, S68.628-S68.711 with
7th A, S68.719-S68.721 with 7th A, S68.729A,
T14.8-T14.91, T79.A0X-T79.9.XX with 7th A

√7ᵗʰ **S58.012** **Complete traumatic amputation at**   **CC**
elbow level, left arm
CC Excl: CC with 7th character A: S41.002-
S41.009 with 7th A, S41.012-S41.019 with
7th A, S41.022-S41.029 with 7th A, S41.032-
S41.039 with 7th A, S41.042-S41.049 with
7th A, S41.052-S41.059 with 7th A, S41.102-
S41.109 with 7th A, S41.112-S41.119 with
7th A, S41.122-S41.129 with 7th A, S41.132-
S41.139 with 7th A, S41.142-S41.149 with
7th A, S41.152-S41.159 with 7th A, S46.022-
S46.029 with 7th A, S46.122-S46.129 with
7th A, S46.222-S46.229 with 7th A, S46.322-
S46.329 with 7th A, S46.822-S46.829 with
7th A, S46.922-S46.929 with 7th A, S48.012-
S48.019 with 7th A, S48.022-S48.029 with
7th A, S48.112-S48.119 with 7th A, S48.122-
S48.129 with 7th A, S48.912-S48.919 with
7th A, S48.922-S48.929 with 7th A, S51.002-
S51.009 with 7th A, S51.012-S51.019 with
7th A, S51.022-S51.029 with 7th A, S51.032-
S51.039 with 7th A, S51.042-S51.049 with
7th A, S51.052-S51.059 with 7th A, S51.802-
S51.809 with 7th A, S51.812-S51.819 with
7th A, S51.822-S51.829 with 7th A, S51.832-
S51.839 with 7th A, S51.842-S51.849 with
7th A, S51.852-S51.859 with 7th A, S56.022-
S56.029 with 7th A, S56.122A, S56.124A,

S56.126A, S56.128-S56.129 with 7th A,
S56.222-S56.229 with 7th A, S56.322-
S56.329 with 7th A, S56.422 with 7th A,
S56.424A, S56.426A, S56.428-S56.429 with
7th A, S56.522-S56.529 with 7th A, S56.822-
S56.829 with 7th A, S56.922-S56.929 with
7th A, S58.012-S58.019 with 7th A, S58.022-
S58.029 with 7th A, S58.112-S58.119 with
7th A, S58.122-S58.129 with 7th A, S58.912-
S58.919 with 7th A, S58.922-S58.929 with
7th A, S61.002-S61.009 with 7th A, S61.012-
S61.019 with 7th A, S61.022-S61.029 with
7th A, S61.032-S61.039 with 7th A, S61.042-
S61.049 with 7th A, S61.052-S61.059 with
7th A, S61.102-S61.109 with 7th A, S61.112-
S61.119 with 7th A, S61.122-S61.129 with
7th A, S61.132-S61.139 with 7th A, S61.142-
S61.149 with 7th A, S61.152-S61.159 with
7th A, S61.201A, S61.203A, S61.205A,
S61.207-S61.209 with 7th A, S61.211A,
S61.213A, S61.215A, S61.217-S61.219 with
7th A, S61.221A, S61.223A, S61.225A,
S61.227-S61.229 with 7th A, S61.231A,
S61.233A, S61.235A, S61.237-S61.239 with
7th A, S61.241A, S61.243A, S61.245A,
S61.247-S61.249 with 7th A, S61.251A,
S61.253A, S61.255 with 7th A, S61.257-
S61.259 with 7th A, S61.301A, S61.303A,
S61.305A, S61.307-S61.309 with 7th A,
S61.311A, S61.313A, S61.315A, S61.317-
S61.319A, S61.321A, S61.323A, S61.325A,
S61.327-S61.329 with 7th A, S61.331A,
S61.333A, S61.335 with 7th A, S61.337-
S61.339 with 7th A, S61.341A, S61.343A,
S61.345A, S61.347-S61.349 with 7th A,
S61.351A, S61.353A, S61.355A, S61.357-
S61.359 with 7th A, S61.402-S61.409 with
7th A, S61.412-S61.419 with 7th A, S61.422-
S61.429 with 7th A, S61.432-S61.439 with
7th A, S61.442-S61.449 with 7th A, S61.452-
S61.459 with 7th A, S61.502-S61.509 with
7th A, S61.512-S61.519 with 7th A, S61.522-
S61.529 with 7th A, S61.532-S61.539 with
7th A, S61.542-S61.549 with 7th A, S61.552-
S61.559 with 7th A, S66.022-S66.029 with
7th A, S66.121 character A, S66.123A,
S66.125A, S66.127-S66.129 with 7th A,
S66.222-S66.229 with 7th A, S66.321A,
S66.323A, S66.325A, S66.327-S66.329 with
7th A, S66.422-S66.429 with 7th A, S66.521A,
S66.523A, S66.525A, S66.527-S66.529 with
7th A, S66.822-S66.829 with 7th A, S66.922-
S66.929 with 7th A, S68.012-S68.019 with
7th A, S68.022-S68.029 with 7th A, S68.111A,
S68.113A, S68.115A, S68.117-S68.119A,
S68.121A, S68.123A, S68.125A, S68.127-
S68.129 with 7th A, S68.412-S68.419 with
7th A, S68.422-S68.429 with 7th A, S68.512-
S68.519 with 7th A, S68.522-S68.529 with
7th A, S68.611A, S68.613 , S68.615A,
S68.617-S68.619 with 7th A, S68.621A,
S68.623A, S68.625A, S68.627-S68.629 with
7th A, S68.712-S68.719 with 7th A, S68.722-
S68.729 with 7th A, T14.8-T14.91, T79.A0X-
T79.9.XX with 7th A

√7ᵗʰ **S58.019** **Complete traumatic amputation at**   **CC**
elbow level, unspecified arm
CC Excl: CC with 7th character A: S41.001-
S41.159 with 7th A, S46.021-S46.029 with
7th A, S46.121-S46.129 with 7th A, S46.221-
S46.229 with 7th A, S46.321-S46.329 with
7th A, S46.821-S46.829 with 7th A, S46.921-
S46.929 with 7th A, S48.011-S48.929 with
7th A, S51.001-S51.859 with 7th A, S56.021-
S56.029 with 7th A, S56.121-S56.129 with
7th A, S56.221-S56.229 with 7th A, S56.321-
S56.329 with 7th A, S56.421-S56.429 with
7th A, S56.521-S56.529 with 7th A, S56.821-
S56.829 with 7th A, S56.921-S56.929 with
7th A, S58.011-S58.929 with 7th A, S61.001-
S61.559 with 7th A, S66.021-S66.029 with
7th A, S66.120-S66.129 with 7th A, S66.221-
S66.229 with 7th A, S66.320-S66.329 with
7th A, S66.421-S66.429 with 7th A, S66.520-
S66.529 with 7th A, S66.821-S66.829 with
7th A, S66.921-S66.929 with 7th A, S68.011-
S68.729 with 7th A, T14.8-T14.91, T79.A0X-
T79.9.XX with 7th A

Ⓝ Newborn: 0   Ⓟ Pediatric: 0-17   Ⓜ Maternity: 12-55   Ⓐ Adult: 15-124   **MCC** Major CC Condition   **PDx MCC** PDx acts as own MCC   **CC** CC Condition   **PDx CC** PDx acts as own CC

940   ICD-10-CM Draft (2015)

✓6ᵗʰ **S58.02** Partial traumatic amputation at elbow level

    ✓7ᵗʰ **S58.021** Partial traumatic amputation at elbow level, **right arm** `CC`
        CC Excl: See code: S58.011

    ✓7ᵗʰ **S58.022** Partial traumatic amputation at elbow level, **left arm** `CC`
        CC Excl: See code: S58.012

    ✓7ᵗʰ **S58.029** Partial traumatic amputation at elbow level, **unspecified arm** `CC`
        CC Excl: See code: S58.019

✓5ᵗʰ **S58.1** Traumatic amputation at level **between elbow and wrist**

  ✓6ᵗʰ **S58.11** **Complete** traumatic amputation at level between elbow and wrist

    ✓7ᵗʰ **S58.111** **Complete** traumatic amputation at level between elbow and wrist, **right arm** `CC`
        CC Excl: See code: S58.011

    ✓7ᵗʰ **S58.112** **Complete** traumatic amputation at level between elbow and wrist, **left arm** `CC`
        CC Excl: See code: S58.012

    ✓7ᵗʰ **S58.119** **Complete** traumatic amputation at level between elbow and wrist, **unspecified arm** `CC`
        CC Excl: See code: S58.019

  ✓6ᵗʰ **S58.12** Partial traumatic amputation at level between elbow and wrist

    ✓7ᵗʰ **S58.121** Partial traumatic amputation at level between elbow and wrist, **right arm** `CC`
        CC Excl: See code: S58.011

    ✓7ᵗʰ **S58.122** Partial traumatic amputation at level between elbow and wrist, **left arm** `CC`
        CC Excl: See code: S58.012

    ✓7ᵗʰ **S58.129** Partial traumatic amputation at level between elbow and wrist, **unspecified arm** `CC`
        CC Excl: See code: S58.019

✓5ᵗʰ **S58.9** Traumatic amputation of **forearm, level unspecified**
    EXCLUDES 1 traumatic amputation of wrist (S68.-)

  ✓6ᵗʰ **S58.91** **Complete** traumatic amputation of forearm, level unspecified

    ✓7ᵗʰ **S58.911** **Complete** traumatic amputation of **right** forearm, level unspecified `CC`
        CC Excl: See code: S58.011

    ✓7ᵗʰ **S58.912** **Complete** traumatic amputation of **left** forearm, level unspecified `CC`
        CC Excl: See code: S58.012

    ✓7ᵗʰ **S58.919** **Complete** traumatic amputation of **unspecified** forearm, level unspecified `CC`
        CC Excl: See code: S58.019

  ✓6ᵗʰ **S58.92** Partial traumatic amputation of forearm, level unspecified

    ✓7ᵗʰ **S58.921** Partial traumatic amputation of **right** forearm, level unspecified

    ✓7ᵗʰ **S58.922** Partial traumatic amputation of **left** forearm, level unspecified

    ✓7ᵗʰ **S58.929** Partial traumatic amputation of **unspecified** forearm, level unspecified

✓4ᵗʰ **S59** **Other and unspecified injuries of elbow and forearm**
    EXCLUDES 2 other and unspecified injuries of wrist and hand (S69.-)

> The appropriate 7th is to be added to each code from subcategories S59.0, S59.1, and S59.2.
> A   initial encounter for closed fracture
> D   subsequent encounter for fracture with routine healing
> G   subsequent encounter for fracture with delayed healing
> K   subsequent encounter for fracture with nonunion
> P   subsequent encounter for fracture with malunion
> S   sequela

✓5ᵗʰ **S59.0** Physeal fracture of **lower end of ulna**

  ✓6ᵗʰ **S59.00** **Unspecified** physeal fracture of lower end of ulna

7 ✓7ᵗʰ **S59.001** **Unspecified physeal fracture of lower end of ulna, right arm** `CC`

    CC Excl: CC with 7th character A: S52.001-S52.011 with 7th [A, B, C], S52.019-S52.111 with 7th A, S52.119-S52.211 with 7th A, S52.219-S52.311 with 7th A, S52.319-S52.521 with 7th A, S52.529-S52.621 with 7th A, S52.629-S52.92X with 7th A, S59.001A, S59.009-S59.011 with 7th A, S59.019-S59.021 with 7th A, S59.029-S59.031 with 7th A, S59.039-S59.041 with 7th A, S59.049-S59.091 with 7th A, S59.099-S59.101 with 7th A, S59.109-S59.111 with 7th A, S59.119-S59.121 with 7th A, S59.129-S59.131 with 7th A, S59.139-S59.141 with 7th A, S59.149-S59.191 with 7th A, S59.199-S59.201 with 7th A, S59.209-S59.211 with 7th A, S59.219-S59.221 with 7th A, S59.229-S59.231 with 7th A, S59.239-S59.241 with 7th A, S59.249-S59.291 with 7th A, S59.299A

    CC with 7th character K or P: M80.00X-M84.68X with 7th [K, P], S02.0XX-S02.92X with 7th K, S12.000-S12.691 with 7th K, S22.000-S22.9XX with 7th K, S32.000-S32.9XX with 7th K, S42.001-S42.92X with 7th [K, P], S49.001-S49.199 with 7th [K, P], S52.001-S52.92X with 7th [K, M, N, P, Q, R], S59.001-S59.299 with 7th [K, P], S62.001-S62.92X with 7th [K, P], S72.001-S72.92X with 7th [K, M, N, P, Q, R], S79.001-S79.199 with 7th [K, P], S82.001-S82.92X with 7th [K, M, N, P, Q, R], S89.001-S89.399 with 7th [K, P], S92.001-S92.919 with 7th [K, P]

7 ✓7ᵗʰ **S59.002** **Unspecified physeal fracture of lower end of ulna, left arm** `CC`

    CC Excl: CC with 7th character A: S52.001-S52.009 with 7th [B, C], S52.012-S52.109 with 7th A, S52.112-S52.209 with 7th A, S52.212-S52.309 with 7th A, S52.312-S52.516 with 7th A, S52.522-S52.616 with 7th A, S52.622-S52.92X with 7th A, S59.002-S59.009 with 7th A, S59.012-S59.019 with 7th A, S59.022-S59.029 with 7th A, S59.032-S59.039 with 7th A, S59.042-S59.049 with 7th A, S59.092-S59.099 with 7th A, S59.102-S59.109 with 7th A, S59.112-S59.119 with 7th A, S59.122-S59.129 with 7th A, S59.132-S59.139 with 7th A, S59.142-S59.149 with 7th A, S59.192-S59.199 with 7th A, S59.202-S59.209 with 7th A, S59.212-S59.219 with 7th A, S59.222-S59.229 with 7th A, S59.232-S59.239 with 7th A, S59.242-S59.249 with 7th A, S59.292-S59.299 with 7th A

    CC with 7th character K or P: M80.00X-M84.68X with 7th [K, P], S02.0XX-S02.92X with 7th K, S12.000-S12.691 with 7th K, S22.000-S22.9XX with 7th K, S32.000-S32.9XX with 7th K, S42.001-S42.92X with 7th [K, P], S49.001-S49.199 with 7th [K, P], S52.001-S52.92X with 7th [K, M, N, P, Q, R], S59.001-S59.299 with 7th [K, P], S62.001-S62.92X with 7th [K, P], S72.001-S72.92X with 7th [K, M, N, P, Q, R], S79.001-S79.199 with 7th [K, P], S82.001-S82.92X with 7th [K, M, N, P, Q, R], S89.001-S89.399 with 7th [K, P], S92.001-S92.919 with 7th [K, P]

7 ✓7ᵗʰ **S59.009** **Unspecified physeal fracture of lower end of ulna, unspecified arm** `CC`

    CC Excl: CC with 7th character A: S52.001-S52.92X with 7th [A, B, C], S59.001-S59.299 with 7th A

    CC with 7th character K or P: M80.00X-M84.68X with 7th [K, P], S02.0XX-S02.92X with 7th K, S12.000-S12.691 with 7th K, S22.000-S22.9XX with 7th K, S32.000-S32.9XX with 7th K, S42.001-S42.92X with 7th [K, P], S49.001-S49.199 with 7th [K, P], S52.001-S52.92X with 7th [K, M, N, P, Q, R], S59.001-S59.299 with 7th [K, P], S62.001-S62.92X with 7th [K, P], S72.001-S72.92X with 7th [K, M, N, P, Q, R], S79.001-S79.199 with 7th [K, P], S82.001-S82.92X with 7th [K, M, N, P, Q, R], S89.001-S89.399 with 7th [K, P], S92.001-S92.919 with 7th [K, P]

  ✓6ᵗʰ **S59.01** **Salter-Harris Type I** physeal fracture of lower end of ulna

    7 ✓7ᵗʰ **S59.011** **Salter-Harris Type I physeal fracture of lower end of ulna, right arm** `CC`
        CC Excl: See code: S59.001

---

7 HAC = Initial encounter only (7th character A, B or C) and not POA.

✓ Additional Character Required   ✓x7ᵗʰ Xtension Alert   Unacceptable PDx   Manifestation   Hospital Acquired Condition   **EXCLUDES 1** Not Coded Here   **EXCLUDES 2** Not Included Here

ICD-10-CM Draft (2015)   **941**

7 ✓7ᵗʰ **S59.Ø12** **Salter-Harris Type I physeal fracture of lower end of ulna, left arm** CC
     CC Excl: See code: S59.ØØ2

7 ✓7ᵗʰ **S59.Ø19** **Salter-Harris Type I physeal fracture of lower end of ulna, unspecified arm** CC
     CC Excl: See code: S59.ØØ9

✓6ᵗʰ **S59.Ø2** Salter-Harris Type II physeal fracture of lower end of ulna

7 ✓7ᵗʰ **S59.Ø21** **Salter-Harris Type II physeal fracture of lower end of ulna, right arm** CC
     CC Excl: See code: S59.ØØ1

7 ✓7ᵗʰ **S59.Ø22** **Salter-Harris Type II physeal fracture of lower end of ulna, left arm** CC
     CC Excl: See code: S59.ØØ2

7 ✓7ᵗʰ **S59.Ø29** **Salter-Harris Type II physeal fracture of lower end of ulna, unspecified arm** CC
     CC Excl: See code: S59.ØØ9

✓6ᵗʰ **S59.Ø3** Salter-Harris Type III physeal fracture of lower end of ulna

7 ✓7ᵗʰ **S59.Ø31** **Salter-Harris Type III physeal fracture of lower end of ulna, right arm** CC
     CC Excl: See code: S59.ØØ1

7 ✓7ᵗʰ **S59.Ø32** **Salter-Harris Type III physeal fracture of lower end of ulna, left arm** CC
     CC Excl: See code: S59.ØØ2

7 ✓7ᵗʰ **S59.Ø39** **Salter-Harris Type III physeal fracture of lower end of ulna, unspecified arm** CC
     CC Excl: See code: S59.ØØ9

✓6ᵗʰ **S59.Ø4** Salter-Harris Type IV physeal fracture of lower end of ulna

7 ✓7ᵗʰ **S59.Ø41** **Salter-Harris Type IV physeal fracture of lower end of ulna, right arm** CC
     CC Excl: See code: S59.ØØ1

7 ✓7ᵗʰ **S59.Ø42** **Salter-Harris Type IV physeal fracture of lower end of ulna, left arm** CC
     CC Excl: See code: S59.ØØ2

7 ✓7ᵗʰ **S59.Ø49** **Salter-Harris Type IV physeal fracture of lower end of ulna, unspecified arm** CC
     CC Excl: See code: S59.ØØ9

✓6ᵗʰ **S59.Ø9** Other physeal fracture of lower end of ulna

7 ✓7ᵗʰ **S59.Ø91** **Other physeal fracture of lower end of ulna, right arm** CC
     CC Excl: See code: S59.ØØ1

7 ✓7ᵗʰ **S59.Ø92** **Other physeal fracture of lower end of ulna, left arm** CC
     CC Excl: See code: S59.ØØ2

7 ✓7ᵗʰ **S59.Ø99** **Other physeal fracture of lower end of ulna, unspecified arm** CC
     CC Excl: See code: S59.ØØ9

✓5ᵗʰ **S59.1** Physeal fracture of upper end of radius

     CC Excl: For CC/MCC codes in subcategory S59.1 with 7th K or P: See Code: S59.ØØ9

✓6ᵗʰ **S59.1Ø** Unspecified physeal fracture of upper end of radius

✓7ᵗʰ **S59.1Ø1** **Unspecified physeal fracture of upper end of radius, right arm** CC

✓7ᵗʰ **S59.1Ø2** **Unspecified physeal fracture of upper end of radius, left arm** CC

✓7ᵗʰ **S59.1Ø9** **Unspecified physeal fracture of upper end of radius, unspecified arm** CC

✓6ᵗʰ **S59.11** Salter-Harris Type I physeal fracture of upper end of radius

✓7ᵗʰ **S59.111** **Salter-Harris Type I physeal fracture of upper end of radius, right arm** CC

✓7ᵗʰ **S59.112** **Salter-Harris Type I physeal fracture of upper end of radius, left arm** CC

✓7ᵗʰ **S59.119** **Salter-Harris Type I physeal fracture of upper end of radius, unspecified arm** CC

✓6ᵗʰ **S59.12** Salter-Harris Type II physeal fracture of upper end of radius

✓7ᵗʰ **S59.121** **Salter-Harris Type II physeal fracture of upper end of radius, right arm** CC

✓7ᵗʰ **S59.122** **Salter-Harris Type II physeal fracture of upper end of radius, left arm** CC

✓7ᵗʰ **S59.129** **Salter-Harris Type II physeal fracture of upper end of radius, unspecified arm** CC

✓6ᵗʰ **S59.13** Salter-Harris Type III physeal fracture of upper end of radius

✓7ᵗʰ **S59.131** **Salter-Harris Type III physeal fracture of upper end of radius, right arm** CC

✓7ᵗʰ **S59.132** **Salter-Harris Type III physeal fracture of upper end of radius, left arm** CC

✓7ᵗʰ **S59.139** **Salter-Harris Type III physeal fracture of upper end of radius, unspecified arm** CC

✓6ᵗʰ **S59.14** Salter-Harris Type IV physeal fracture of upper end of radius

✓7ᵗʰ **S59.141** **Salter-Harris Type IV physeal fracture of upper end of radius, right arm** CC

✓7ᵗʰ **S59.142** **Salter-Harris Type IV physeal fracture of upper end of radius, left arm** CC

✓7ᵗʰ **S59.149** **Salter-Harris Type IV physeal fracture of upper end of radius, unspecified arm** CC

✓6ᵗʰ **S59.19** Other physeal fracture of upper end of radius

✓7ᵗʰ **S59.191** **Other physeal fracture of upper end of radius, right arm** CC

✓7ᵗʰ **S59.192** **Other physeal fracture of upper end of radius, left arm** CC

✓7ᵗʰ **S59.199** **Other physeal fracture of upper end of radius, unspecified arm** CC

✓5ᵗʰ **S59.2** Physeal fracture of lower end of radius

✓6ᵗʰ **S59.2Ø** Unspecified physeal fracture of lower end of radius

7 ✓7ᵗʰ **S59.2Ø1** **Unspecified physeal fracture of lower end of radius, right arm** CC
     CC Excl: CC with 7th character A: S52.ØØ1-S52.Ø11 with 7th [A, B, C], S52.Ø19-S52.111 with 7th A, S52.119-S52.211 with 7th A, S52.219-S52.311 with 7th A, S52.319-S52.521 with 7th A, S52.529-S52.621 with 7th A, S52.629-S52.92X with 7th A, S59.ØØ1A, S59.ØØ9-S59.Ø11 with 7th A, S59.Ø19-S59.Ø21 with 7th A, S59.Ø29-S59.Ø31 with 7th A, S59.Ø39-S59.Ø41 with 7th A, S59.Ø49-S59.Ø91 with 7th A, S59.Ø99-S59.1Ø1 with 7th A, S59.1Ø9-S59.111 with 7th A, S59.119-S59.121 with 7th A, S59.129-S59.131 with 7th A, S59.139-S59.141 with 7th A, S59.149-S59.191 with 7th A, S59.199-S59.2Ø1 with 7th A, S59.2Ø9-S59.211 with 7th A, S59.219-S59.221 with 7th A, S59.229-S59.231 with 7th A, S59.239-S59.241 with 7th A, S59.249-S59.291 with 7th A, S59.299A
     CC with 7th character K or P: M8Ø.ØØX-M84.68X with 7th [K, P], SØ2.ØXX-SØ2.92X with 7th K, S12.ØØØ-S12.691 with 7th K, S22.ØØØ-S22.9XX with 7th K, S32.ØØØ-S32.9XX with 7th K, S42.ØØ1-S42.92X with 7th [K, P], S49.ØØ1-S49.199 with 7th [K, P], S52.ØØ1-S52.92X with 7th [K, M, N, P, Q, R], S59.ØØ1-S59.299 with 7th [K, P], S62.ØØ1-S62.92X with 7th [K, P], S72.ØØ1-S72.92X with 7th [K, M, N, P, Q, R], S79.ØØ1-S79.199 with 7th [K, P], S82.ØØ1-S82.92X with 7th [K, M, N, P, Q, R], S89.ØØ1-S89.399 with 7th [K, P], S92.ØØ1-S92.919 with 7th [K, P]

7 ✓7ᵗʰ **S59.2Ø2** **Unspecified physeal fracture of lower end of radius, left arm** CC
     CC Excl: CC with 7th character A: S52.ØØ1-S52.ØØ9 with 7th [B, C], S52.Ø12-S52.1Ø9 with 7th A, S52.112-S52.2Ø9 with 7th A, S52.212-S52.3Ø9 with 7th A, S52.312-S52.516 with 7th A, S52.522-S52.616 with 7th A, S52.622-S52.92X with 7th A, S59.ØØ2-S59.ØØ9 with 7th A, S59.Ø12-S59.Ø19 with 7th A, S59.Ø22-S59.Ø29 with 7th A, S59.Ø32-S59.Ø39 with 7th A, S59.Ø42-S59.Ø49 with 7th A, S59.Ø92-S59.Ø99 with 7th A, S59.1Ø2-S59.1Ø9 with 7th A, S59.112-S59.119 with 7th A, S59.122-S59.129 with 7th A, S59.132-S59.139 with 7th A, S59.142-S59.149 with 7th A, S59.192-S59.199 with 7th A, S59.2Ø2-S59.2Ø9 with 7th A, S59.212-S59.219 with 7th A, S59.222-S59.229 with 7th A, S59.232-S59.239 with 7th A, S59.242-S59.249 with 7th A, S59.292-S59.299 with 7th A
     CC with 7th character K or P: M8Ø.ØØX-M84.68X with 7th [K, P], SØ2.ØXX-SØ2.92X with 7th K, S12.ØØØ-S12.691 with 7th K, S22.ØØØ-S22.9XX with 7th K, S32.ØØØ-S32.9XX with 7th K, S42.ØØ1-S42.92X with 7th [K, P], S49.ØØ1-S49.199 with 7th [K, P],

---

7 HAC = Initial encounter only (7th character A, B or C) and not POA.

N Newborn: Ø   P Pediatric: Ø-17   M Maternity: 12-55   A Adult: 15-124   MCC Major CC Condition   PDx MCC PDx acts as own MCC   CC CC Condition   PDx CC PDx acts as own CC

942   ICD-1Ø-CM Draft (2Ø15)

S52.001–S52.92X with 7th [K, M, N, P, Q, R], S59.001–S59.299 with 7th [K, P], S62.001–S62.92X with 7th [K, P], S72.001–S72.92X with 7th [K, M, N, P, Q, R], S79.001–S79.199 with 7th [K, P], S82.001–S82.92X with 7th [K, M, N, P, Q, R], S89.001–S89.399 with 7th [K, P], S92.001–S92.919 with 7th [K, P]

7 ✓7ᵗʰ **S59.209** **Unspecified physeal fracture of lower end of radius, unspecified arm** CC
     CC Excl: CC with 7th character A: S52.001–S52.92X with 7th [A, B, C], S59.001–S59.299 with 7th A
     CC with 7th character K or P: M80.00X–M84.68X with 7th [K, P], S02.0XX–S02.92X with 7th K, S12.000–S12.691 with 7th K, S22.000–S22.9XX with 7th K, S32.000–S32.9XX with 7th K, S42.001–S42.92X with 7th [K, P], S49.001–S49.199 with 7th [K, P], S52.001–S52.92X with 7th [K, M, N, P, Q, R], S59.001–S59.299 with 7th [K, P], S62.001–S62.92X with 7th [K, P], S72.001–S72.92X with 7th [K, M, N, P, Q, R], S79.001–S79.199 with 7th [K, P], S82.001–S82.92X with 7th [K, M, N, P, Q, R], S89.001–S89.399 with 7th [K, P], S92.001–S92.919 with 7th [K, P]

✓6ᵗʰ **S59.21** Salter-Harris Type I physeal fracture of lower end of radius

7 ✓7ᵗʰ **S59.211** **Salter-Harris Type I physeal fracture of lower end of radius, right arm** CC
     CC Excl: See code: S59.201

7 ✓7ᵗʰ **S59.212** **Salter-Harris Type I physeal fracture of lower end of radius, left arm** CC
     CC Excl: See code: S59.202

7 ✓7ᵗʰ **S59.219** **Salter-Harris Type I physeal fracture of lower end of radius, unspecified arm** CC
     CC Excl: See code: S59.209

✓6ᵗʰ **S59.22** Salter-Harris Type II physeal fracture of lower end of radius

7 ✓7ᵗʰ **S59.221** **Salter-Harris Type II physeal fracture of lower end of radius, right arm** CC
     CC Excl: See code: S59.201

7 ✓7ᵗʰ **S59.222** **Salter-Harris Type II physeal fracture of lower end of radius, left arm** CC
     CC Excl: See code: S59.202

7 ✓7ᵗʰ **S59.229** **Salter-Harris Type II physeal fracture of lower end of radius, unspecified arm** CC
     CC Excl: See code: S59.209

✓6ᵗʰ **S59.23** Salter-Harris Type III physeal fracture of lower end of radius

7 ✓7ᵗʰ **S59.231** **Salter-Harris Type III physeal fracture of lower end of radius, right arm** CC
     CC Excl: See code: S59.201

7 ✓7ᵗʰ **S59.232** **Salter-Harris Type III physeal fracture of lower end of radius, left arm** CC
     CC Excl: See code: S59.202

7 ✓7ᵗʰ **S59.239** **Salter-Harris Type III physeal fracture of lower end of radius, unspecified arm** CC
     CC Excl: See code: S59.209

✓6ᵗʰ **S59.24** Salter-Harris Type IV physeal fracture of lower end of radius

7 ✓7ᵗʰ **S59.241** **Salter-Harris Type IV physeal fracture of lower end of radius, right arm** CC
     CC Excl: See code: S59.201

7 ✓7ᵗʰ **S59.242** **Salter-Harris Type IV physeal fracture of lower end of radius, left arm** CC
     CC Excl: See code: S59.202

7 ✓7ᵗʰ **S59.249** **Salter-Harris Type IV physeal fracture of lower end of radius, unspecified arm** CC
     CC Excl: See code: S59.209

✓6ᵗʰ **S59.29** Other physeal fracture of lower end of radius

7 ✓7ᵗʰ **S59.291** **Other physeal fracture of lower end of radius, right arm** CC
     CC Excl: See code: S59.201

7 ✓7ᵗʰ **S59.292** **Other physeal fracture of lower end of radius, left arm** CC
     CC Excl: See code: S59.202

7 ✓7ᵗʰ **S59.299** **Other physeal fracture of lower end of radius, unspecified arm** CC
     CC Excl: See code: S59.209

✓5ᵗʰ **S59.8** Other specified injuries of elbow and forearm

The appropriate 7th is to be added to each code in subcategory S59.8.
A   initial encounter
D   subsequent encounter
S   sequela

✓6ᵗʰ **S59.80** Other specified injuries of elbow

✓7ᵗʰ **S59.801** Other specified injuries of right elbow

✓7ᵗʰ **S59.802** Other specified injuries of left elbow

✓7ᵗʰ **S59.809** Other specified injuries of unspecified elbow

✓6ᵗʰ **S59.81** Other specified injuries of forearm

✓7ᵗʰ **S59.811** Other specified injuries right forearm

✓7ᵗʰ **S59.812** Other specified injuries left forearm

✓7ᵗʰ **S59.819** Other specified injuries unspecified forearm

✓5ᵗʰ **S59.9** Unspecified injury of elbow and forearm

The appropriate 7th is to be added to each code in subcategory S59.9.
A   initial encounter
D   subsequent encounter
S   sequela

✓6ᵗʰ **S59.90** Unspecified injury of elbow

✓7ᵗʰ **S59.901** Unspecified injury of right elbow

✓7ᵗʰ **S59.902** Unspecified injury of left elbow

✓7ᵗʰ **S59.909** Unspecified injury of unspecified elbow

✓6ᵗʰ **S59.91** Unspecified injury of forearm

✓7ᵗʰ **S59.911** Unspecified injury of right forearm

✓7ᵗʰ **S59.912** Unspecified injury of left forearm

✓7ᵗʰ **S59.919** Unspecified injury of unspecified forearm

Injuries to the wrist, hand and fingers (S60-S69)

EXCLUDES 2   burns and corrosions (T20-T32)
     frostbite (T33-T34)
     insect bite or sting, venomous (T63.4)

✓4ᵗʰ **S60** **Superficial injury of wrist, hand and fingers**

The appropriate 7th is to be added to each code from category S60.
A   initial encounter
D   subsequent encounter
S   sequela

✓5ᵗʰ **S60.0** Contusion of finger without damage to nail
     EXCLUDES 1   contusion involving nail (matrix) (S60.1)

✓x7ᵗʰ **S60.00** Contusion of unspecified finger without damage to nail
     Contusion of finger(s) NOS

✓6ᵗʰ **S60.01** Contusion of thumb without damage to nail

✓7ᵗʰ **S60.011** Contusion of right thumb without damage to nail

✓7ᵗʰ **S60.012** Contusion of left thumb without damage to nail

✓7ᵗʰ **S60.019** Contusion of unspecified thumb without damage to nail

✓6ᵗʰ **S60.02** Contusion of index finger without damage to nail

✓7ᵗʰ **S60.021** Contusion of right index finger without damage to nail

✓7ᵗʰ **S60.022** Contusion of left index finger without damage to nail

✓7ᵗʰ **S60.029** Contusion of unspecified index finger without damage to nail

✓6ᵗʰ **S60.03** Contusion of middle finger without damage to nail

✓7ᵗʰ **S60.031** Contusion of right middle finger without damage to nail

✓7ᵗʰ **S60.032** Contusion of left middle finger without damage to nail

✓7ᵗʰ **S60.039** Contusion of unspecified middle finger without damage to nail

---

7 HAC = Initial encounter only (7th character A, B or C) and not POA.

✓6ᵗʰ **S60.04** Contusion of ring finger without damage to nail

     ✓7ᵗʰ **S60.041** Contusion of right ring finger without damage to nail

     ✓7ᵗʰ **S60.042** Contusion of left ring finger without damage to nail

     ✓7ᵗʰ **S60.049** Contusion of unspecified ring finger without damage to nail

✓6ᵗʰ **S60.05** Contusion of little finger without damage to nail

     ✓7ᵗʰ **S60.051** Contusion of right little finger without damage to nail

     ✓7ᵗʰ **S60.052** Contusion of left little finger without damage to nail

     ✓7ᵗʰ **S60.059** Contusion of unspecified little finger without damage to nail

✓5ᵗʰ **S60.1** Contusion of finger with damage to nail

     ✓x7ᵗʰ **S60.10** Contusion of unspecified finger with damage to nail

     ✓6ᵗʰ **S60.11** Contusion of thumb with damage to nail

         ✓7ᵗʰ **S60.111** Contusion of right thumb with damage to nail

         ✓7ᵗʰ **S60.112** Contusion of left thumb with damage to nail

         ✓7ᵗʰ **S60.119** Contusion of unspecified thumb with damage to nail

     ✓6ᵗʰ **S60.12** Contusion of index finger with damage to nail

         ✓7ᵗʰ **S60.121** Contusion of right index finger with damage to nail

         ✓7ᵗʰ **S60.122** Contusion of left index finger with damage to nail

         ✓7ᵗʰ **S60.129** Contusion of unspecified index finger with damage to nail

     ✓6ᵗʰ **S60.13** Contusion of middle finger with damage to nail

         ✓7ᵗʰ **S60.131** Contusion of right middle finger with damage to nail

         ✓7ᵗʰ **S60.132** Contusion of left middle finger with damage to nail

         ✓7ᵗʰ **S60.139** Contusion of unspecified middle finger with damage to nail

     ✓6ᵗʰ **S60.14** Contusion of ring finger with damage to nail

         ✓7ᵗʰ **S60.141** Contusion of right ring finger with damage to nail

         ✓7ᵗʰ **S60.142** Contusion of left ring finger with damage to nail

         ✓7ᵗʰ **S60.149** Contusion of unspecified ring finger with damage to nail

     ✓6ᵗʰ **S60.15** Contusion of little finger with damage to nail

         ✓7ᵗʰ **S60.151** Contusion of right little finger with damage to nail

         ✓7ᵗʰ **S60.152** Contusion of left little finger with damage to nail

         ✓7ᵗʰ **S60.159** Contusion of unspecified little finger with damage to nail

✓5ᵗʰ **S60.2** Contusion of wrist and hand

     EXCLUDES 2   contusion of fingers (S60.0-, S60.1-)

     ✓6ᵗʰ **S60.21** Contusion of wrist

         ✓7ᵗʰ **S60.211** Contusion of right wrist

         ✓7ᵗʰ **S60.212** Contusion of left wrist

         ✓7ᵗʰ **S60.219** Contusion of unspecified wrist

     ✓6ᵗʰ **S60.22** Contusion of hand

         ✓7ᵗʰ **S60.221** Contusion of right hand

         ✓7ᵗʰ **S60.222** Contusion of left hand

         ✓7ᵗʰ **S60.229** Contusion of unspecified hand

✓5ᵗʰ **S60.3** Other superficial injuries of thumb

     ✓6ᵗʰ **S60.31** Abrasion of thumb

         ✓7ᵗʰ **S60.311** Abrasion of right thumb

         ✓7ᵗʰ **S60.312** Abrasion of left thumb

         ✓7ᵗʰ **S60.319** Abrasion of unspecified thumb

     ✓6ᵗʰ **S60.32** Blister (nonthermal) of thumb

         ✓7ᵗʰ **S60.321** Blister (nonthermal) of right thumb

         ✓7ᵗʰ **S60.322** Blister (nonthermal) of left thumb

         ✓7ᵗʰ **S60.329** Blister (nonthermal) of unspecified thumb

---

✓6ᵗʰ **S60.34** External constriction of thumb

     Hair tourniquet syndrome of thumb

     Use additional cause code to identify the constricting item (W49.0-)

     ✓7ᵗʰ **S60.341** External constriction of right thumb

     ✓7ᵗʰ **S60.342** External constriction of left thumb

     ✓7ᵗʰ **S60.349** External constriction of unspecified thumb

✓6ᵗʰ **S60.35** Superficial foreign body of thumb

     Splinter in the thumb

     ✓7ᵗʰ **S60.351** Superficial foreign body of right thumb

     ✓7ᵗʰ **S60.352** Superficial foreign body of left thumb

     ✓7ᵗʰ **S60.359** Superficial foreign body of unspecified thumb

✓6ᵗʰ **S60.36** Insect bite (nonvenomous) of thumb

     ✓7ᵗʰ **S60.361** Insect bite (nonvenomous) of right thumb

     ✓7ᵗʰ **S60.362** Insect bite (nonvenomous) of left thumb

     ✓7ᵗʰ **S60.369** Insect bite (nonvenomous) of unspecified thumb

✓6ᵗʰ **S60.37** Other superficial bite of thumb

     EXCLUDES 1   open bite of thumb (S61.05-, S61.15-)

     ✓7ᵗʰ **S60.371** Other superficial bite of right thumb

     ✓7ᵗʰ **S60.372** Other superficial bite of left thumb

     ✓7ᵗʰ **S60.379** Other superficial bite of unspecified thumb

✓6ᵗʰ **S60.39** Other superficial injuries of thumb

     ✓7ᵗʰ **S60.391** Other superficial injuries of right thumb

     ✓7ᵗʰ **S60.392** Other superficial injuries of left thumb

     ✓7ᵗʰ **S60.399** Other superficial injuries of unspecified thumb

✓5ᵗʰ **S60.4** Other superficial injuries of other fingers

     ✓6ᵗʰ **S60.41** Abrasion of fingers

         ✓7ᵗʰ **S60.410** Abrasion of right index finger

         ✓7ᵗʰ **S60.411** Abrasion of left index finger

         ✓7ᵗʰ **S60.412** Abrasion of right middle finger

         ✓7ᵗʰ **S60.413** Abrasion of left middle finger

         ✓7ᵗʰ **S60.414** Abrasion of right ring finger

         ✓7ᵗʰ **S60.415** Abrasion of left ring finger

         ✓7ᵗʰ **S60.416** Abrasion of right little finger

         ✓7ᵗʰ **S60.417** Abrasion of left little finger

         ✓7ᵗʰ **S60.418** Abrasion of other finger

             Abrasion of specified finger with unspecified laterality

         ✓7ᵗʰ **S60.419** Abrasion of unspecified finger

     ✓6ᵗʰ **S60.42** Blister (nonthermal) of fingers

         ✓7ᵗʰ **S60.420** Blister (nonthermal) of right index finger

         ✓7ᵗʰ **S60.421** Blister (nonthermal) of left index finger

         ✓7ᵗʰ **S60.422** Blister (nonthermal) of right middle finger

         ✓7ᵗʰ **S60.423** Blister (nonthermal) of left middle finger

         ✓7ᵗʰ **S60.424** Blister (nonthermal) of right ring finger

         ✓7ᵗʰ **S60.425** Blister (nonthermal) of left ring finger

         ✓7ᵗʰ **S60.426** Blister (nonthermal) of right little finger

         ✓7ᵗʰ **S60.427** Blister (nonthermal) of left little finger

         ✓7ᵗʰ **S60.428** Blister (nonthermal) of other finger

             Blister (nonthermal) of specified finger with unspecified laterality

         ✓7ᵗʰ **S60.429** Blister (nonthermal) of unspecified finger

     ✓6ᵗʰ **S60.44** External constriction of fingers

     Hair tourniquet syndrome of finger

     Use additional cause code to identify the constricting item (W49.0-)

         ✓7ᵗʰ **S60.440** External constriction of right index finger

         ✓7ᵗʰ **S60.441** External constriction of left index finger

         ✓7ᵗʰ **S60.442** External constriction of right middle finger

         ✓7ᵗʰ **S60.443** External constriction of left middle finger

         ✓7ᵗʰ **S60.444** External constriction of right ring finger

         ✓7ᵗʰ **S60.445** External constriction of left ring finger

         ✓7ᵗʰ **S60.446** External constriction of right little finger

         ✓7ᵗʰ **S60.447** External constriction of left little finger

---

N Newborn: 0   P Pediatric: 0-17   M Maternity: 12-55   A Adult: 15-124   MCC Major CC Condition   PDx MCC PDx acts as own MCC   CC CC Condition   PDx CC PDx acts as own CC

944   ICD-10-CM Draft (2015)

✓7ᵗʰ **S60.448** **External constriction of** other **finger**
External constriction of specified finger
with unspecified laterality

✓7ᵗʰ **S60.449** **External constriction of** unspecified **finger**

✓6ᵗʰ **S60.45** **Superficial** foreign body **of fingers**
Splinter in the finger(s)

✓7ᵗʰ **S60.450** **Superficial foreign body of** right index
finger

✓7ᵗʰ **S60.451** **Superficial foreign body of** left index
finger

✓7ᵗʰ **S60.452** **Superficial foreign body of** right middle
finger

✓7ᵗʰ **S60.453** **Superficial foreign body of** left middle
finger

✓7ᵗʰ **S60.454** **Superficial foreign body of** right ring
finger

✓7ᵗʰ **S60.455** **Superficial foreign body of** left ring **finger**

✓7ᵗʰ **S60.456** **Superficial foreign body of** right little
finger

✓7ᵗʰ **S60.457** **Superficial foreign body of** left little **finger**

✓7ᵗʰ **S60.458** **Superficial foreign body of** other **finger**
Superficial foreign body of specified finger
with unspecified laterality

✓7ᵗʰ **S60.459** **Superficial foreign body of** unspecified
finger

✓6ᵗʰ **S60.46** **Insect bite (nonvenomous) of fingers**

✓7ᵗʰ **S60.460** **Insect bite (nonvenomous) of** right index
finger

✓7ᵗʰ **S60.461** **Insect bite (nonvenomous) of** left index
finger

✓7ᵗʰ **S60.462** **Insect bite (nonvenomous) of** right middle
finger

✓7ᵗʰ **S60.463** **Insect bite (nonvenomous) of** left middle
finger

✓7ᵗʰ **S60.464** **Insect bite (nonvenomous) of** right ring
finger

✓7ᵗʰ **S60.465** **Insect bite (nonvenomous) of** left ring
finger

✓7ᵗʰ **S60.466** **Insect bite (nonvenomous) of** right little
finger

✓7ᵗʰ **S60.467** **Insect bite (nonvenomous) of** left little
finger

✓7ᵗʰ **S60.468** **Insect bite (nonvenomous) of** other **finger**
Insect bite (nonvenomous) of specified
finger with unspecified laterality

✓7ᵗʰ **S60.469** **Insect bite (nonvenomous) of** unspecified
finger

✓6ᵗʰ **S60.47** **Other superficial bite of fingers**
EXCLUDES 1 *open bite of fingers (S61.25-, S61.35-)*

✓7ᵗʰ **S60.470** **Other superficial bite of** right index **finger**
✓7ᵗʰ **S60.471** **Other superficial bite of** left index **finger**
✓7ᵗʰ **S60.472** **Other superficial bite of** right middle
finger
✓7ᵗʰ **S60.473** **Other superficial bite of** left middle **finger**
✓7ᵗʰ **S60.474** **Other superficial bite of** right ring **finger**
✓7ᵗʰ **S60.475** **Other superficial bite of** left ring **finger**
✓7ᵗʰ **S60.476** **Other superficial bite of** right little **finger**
✓7ᵗʰ **S60.477** **Other superficial bite of** left little **finger**
✓7ᵗʰ **S60.478** **Other superficial bite of** other **finger**
Other superficial bite of specified finger
with xc vunspecified laterality

✓7ᵗʰ **S60.479** **Other superficial bite of** unspecified **finger**

✓5ᵗʰ **S60.5** **Other superficial injuries of** hand
EXCLUDES 2 *superficial injuries of fingers (S60.3-, S60.4-)*

✓6ᵗʰ **S60.51** **Abrasion of hand**
✓7ᵗʰ **S60.511** **Abrasion of** right **hand**
✓7ᵗʰ **S60.512** **Abrasion of** left **hand**
✓7ᵗʰ **S60.519** **Abrasion of** unspecified **hand**

✓6ᵗʰ **S60.52** **Blister (nonthermal) of hand**
✓7ᵗʰ **S60.521** **Blister (nonthermal) of** right **hand**
✓7ᵗʰ **S60.522** **Blister (nonthermal) of** left **hand**
✓7ᵗʰ **S60.529** **Blister (nonthermal) of** unspecified **hand**

✓6ᵗʰ **S60.54** **External constriction of hand**
✓7ᵗʰ **S60.541** **External constriction of** right **hand**
✓7ᵗʰ **S60.542** **External constriction of** left **hand**
✓7ᵗʰ **S60.549** **External constriction of** unspecified **hand**

✓6ᵗʰ **S60.55** **Superficial** foreign body **of hand**
Splinter in the hand

✓7ᵗʰ **S60.551** **Superficial foreign body of** right **hand**
✓7ᵗʰ **S60.552** **Superficial foreign body of** left **hand**
✓7ᵗʰ **S60.559** **Superficial foreign body of** unspecified
hand

✓6ᵗʰ **S60.56** **Insect bite (nonvenomous) of hand**
✓7ᵗʰ **S60.561** **Insect bite (nonvenomous) of** right **hand**
✓7ᵗʰ **S60.562** **Insect bite (nonvenomous) of** left **hand**
✓7ᵗʰ **S60.569** **Insect bite (nonvenomous) of** unspecified
hand

✓6ᵗʰ **S60.57** **Other superficial bite of hand**
EXCLUDES 1 *open bite of hand (S61.45-)*

✓7ᵗʰ **S60.571** **Other superficial bite of hand of** right
hand
✓7ᵗʰ **S60.572** **Other superficial bite of hand of** left **hand**
✓7ᵗʰ **S60.579** **Other superficial bite of hand of**
unspecified **hand**

✓5ᵗʰ **S60.8** **Other superficial injuries of wrist**

✓6ᵗʰ **S60.81** **Abrasion of wrist**
✓7ᵗʰ **S60.811** **Abrasion of** right **wrist**
✓7ᵗʰ **S60.812** **Abrasion of** left **wrist**
✓7ᵗʰ **S60.819** **Abrasion of** unspecified **wrist**

✓6ᵗʰ **S60.82** **Blister (nonthermal) of wrist**
✓7ᵗʰ **S60.821** **Blister (nonthermal) of** right **wrist**
✓7ᵗʰ **S60.822** **Blister (nonthermal) of** left **wrist**
✓7ᵗʰ **S60.829** **Blister (nonthermal) of** unspecified **wrist**

✓6ᵗʰ **S60.84** **External constriction of wrist**
✓7ᵗʰ **S60.841** **External constriction of** right **wrist**
✓7ᵗʰ **S60.842** **External constriction of** left **wrist**
✓7ᵗʰ **S60.849** **External constriction of** unspecified **wrist**

✓6ᵗʰ **S60.85** **Superficial** foreign body **of wrist**
Splinter in the wrist
✓7ᵗʰ **S60.851** **Superficial foreign body of** right **wrist**
✓7ᵗʰ **S60.852** **Superficial foreign body of** left **wrist**
✓7ᵗʰ **S60.859** **Superficial foreign body of** unspecified
wrist

✓6ᵗʰ **S60.86** **Insect bite (nonvenomous) of wrist**
✓7ᵗʰ **S60.861** **Insect bite (nonvenomous) of** right **wrist**
✓7ᵗʰ **S60.862** **Insect bite (nonvenomous) of** left **wrist**
✓7ᵗʰ **S60.869** **Insect bite (nonvenomous) of** unspecified
wrist

✓6ᵗʰ **S60.87** **Other superficial bite of wrist**
EXCLUDES 1 *open bite of wrist (S61.55)*
✓7ᵗʰ **S60.871** **Other superficial bite of** right **wrist**
✓7ᵗʰ **S60.872** **Other superficial bite of** left **wrist**
✓7ᵗʰ **S60.879** **Other superficial bite of** unspecified **wrist**

✓5ᵗʰ **S60.9** **Unspecified** superficial injury of wrist, hand and fingers

✓6ᵗʰ **S60.91** **Unspecified superficial injury of** wrist
✓7ᵗʰ **S60.911** **Unspecified superficial injury of** right
wrist
✓7ᵗʰ **S60.912** **Unspecified superficial injury of** left **wrist**
✓7ᵗʰ **S60.919** **Unspecified superficial injury of**
unspecified **wrist**

✓6ᵗʰ **S60.92** **Unspecified superficial injury of** hand
✓7ᵗʰ **S60.921** **Unspecified superficial injury of** right
hand
✓7ᵗʰ **S60.922** **Unspecified superficial injury of** left **hand**
✓7ᵗʰ **S60.929** **Unspecified superficial injury of**
unspecified **hand**

✓6ᵗʰ **S60.93** **Unspecified superficial injury of** thumb
✓7ᵗʰ **S60.931** **Unspecified superficial injury of** right
thumb
✓7ᵗʰ **S60.932** **Unspecified superficial injury of** left
thumb

✓ Additional Character Required   ✓x7ᵗʰ Xtension Alert   Unacceptable PDx   Manifestation   Hospital Acquired Condition   **EXCLUDES 1** Not Coded Here   **EXCLUDES 2** Not Included Here

√7ᵗʰ **S60.939** Unspecified superficial injury of unspecified thumb

√6ᵗʰ **S60.94** Unspecified superficial injury of other fingers

√7ᵗʰ **S60.940** Unspecified superficial injury of right index finger

√7ᵗʰ **S60.941** Unspecified superficial injury of left index finger

√7ᵗʰ **S60.942** Unspecified superficial injury of right middle finger

√7ᵗʰ **S60.943** Unspecified superficial injury of left middle finger

√7ᵗʰ **S60.944** Unspecified superficial injury of right ring finger

√7ᵗʰ **S60.945** Unspecified superficial injury of left ring finger

√7ᵗʰ **S60.946** Unspecified superficial injury of right little finger

√7ᵗʰ **S60.947** Unspecified superficial injury of left little finger

√7ᵗʰ **S60.948** Unspecified superficial injury of other finger
     Unspecified superficial injury of specified finger with unspecified laterality

√7ᵗʰ **S60.949** Unspecified superficial injury of unspecified finger

√4ᵗʰ **S61** **Open wound of wrist, hand and fingers**
     Code also any associated wound infection
     EXCLUDES 1   open fracture of wrist, hand and finger (S62- with 7th character B)
         traumatic amputation of wrist and hand (S68.-)

     The appropriate 7th is to be added to each code from category S61.
     A   initial encounter
     D   subsequent encounter
     S   sequela

√5ᵗʰ **S61.0** **Open wound of thumb without damage to nail**
     EXCLUDES 1   open wound of thumb with damage to nail (S61.1-)

√6ᵗʰ **S61.00** Unspecified open wound of thumb without damage to nail

√7ᵗʰ **S61.001** Unspecified open wound of right thumb without damage to nail

√7ᵗʰ **S61.002** Unspecified open wound of left thumb without damage to nail

√7ᵗʰ **S61.009** Unspecified open wound of unspecified thumb without damage to nail

√6ᵗʰ **S61.01** Laceration without foreign body of thumb without damage to nail

√7ᵗʰ **S61.011** Laceration without foreign body of right thumb without damage to nail

√7ᵗʰ **S61.012** Laceration without foreign body of left thumb without damage to nail

√7ᵗʰ **S61.019** Laceration without foreign body of unspecified thumb without damage to nail

√6ᵗʰ **S61.02** Laceration with foreign body of thumb without damage to nail

√7ᵗʰ **S61.021** Laceration with foreign body of right thumb without damage to nail

√7ᵗʰ **S61.022** Laceration with foreign body of left thumb without damage to nail

√7ᵗʰ **S61.029** Laceration with foreign body of unspecified thumb without damage to nail

√6ᵗʰ **S61.03** Puncture wound without foreign body of thumb without damage to nail

√7ᵗʰ **S61.031** Puncture wound without foreign body of right thumb without damage to nail

√7ᵗʰ **S61.032** Puncture wound without foreign body of left thumb without damage to nail

√7ᵗʰ **S61.039** Puncture wound without foreign body of unspecified thumb without damage to nail

√6ᵗʰ **S61.04** Puncture wound with foreign body of thumb without damage to nail

√7ᵗʰ **S61.041** Puncture wound with foreign body of right thumb without damage to nail

√7ᵗʰ **S61.042** Puncture wound with foreign body of left thumb without damage to nail

√7ᵗʰ **S61.049** Puncture wound with foreign body of unspecified thumb without damage to nail

√6ᵗʰ **S61.05** Open bite of thumb without damage to nail
     Bite of thumb NOS
     EXCLUDES 1   superficial bite of thumb (S60.36-, S60.37-)

√7ᵗʰ **S61.051** Open bite of right thumb without damage to nail

√7ᵗʰ **S61.052** Open bite of left thumb without damage to nail

√7ᵗʰ **S61.059** Open bite of unspecified thumb without damage to nail

√5ᵗʰ **S61.1** **Open wound of thumb with damage to nail**

√6ᵗʰ **S61.10** Unspecified open wound of thumb with damage to nail

√7ᵗʰ **S61.101** Unspecified open wound of right thumb with damage to nail

√7ᵗʰ **S61.102** Unspecified open wound of left thumb with damage to nail

√7ᵗʰ **S61.109** Unspecified open wound of unspecified thumb with damage to nail

√6ᵗʰ **S61.11** Laceration without foreign body of thumb with damage to nail

√7ᵗʰ **S61.111** Laceration without foreign body of right thumb with damage to nail

√7ᵗʰ **S61.112** Laceration without foreign body of left thumb with damage to nail

√7ᵗʰ **S61.119** Laceration without foreign body of unspecified thumb with damage to nail

√6ᵗʰ **S61.12** Laceration with foreign body of thumb with damage to nail

√7ᵗʰ **S61.121** Laceration with foreign body of right thumb with damage to nail

√7ᵗʰ **S61.122** Laceration with foreign body of left thumb with damage to nail

√7ᵗʰ **S61.129** Laceration with foreign body of unspecified thumb with damage to nail

√6ᵗʰ **S61.13** Puncture wound without foreign body of thumb with damage to nail

√7ᵗʰ **S61.131** Puncture wound without foreign body of right thumb with damage to nail

√7ᵗʰ **S61.132** Puncture wound without foreign body of left thumb with damage to nail

√7ᵗʰ **S61.139** Puncture wound without foreign body of unspecified thumb with damage to nail

√6ᵗʰ **S61.14** Puncture wound with foreign body of thumb with damage to nail

√7ᵗʰ **S61.141** Puncture wound with foreign body of right thumb with damage to nail

√7ᵗʰ **S61.142** Puncture wound with foreign body of left thumb with damage to nail

√7ᵗʰ **S61.149** Puncture wound with foreign body of unspecified thumb with damage to nail

√6ᵗʰ **S61.15** Open bite of thumb with damage to nail
     Bite of thumb with damage to nail NOS
     EXCLUDES 1   superficial bite of thumb (S60.36-, S60.37-)

√7ᵗʰ **S61.151** Open bite of right thumb with damage to nail

√7ᵗʰ **S61.152** Open bite of left thumb with damage to nail

√7ᵗʰ **S61.159** Open bite of unspecified thumb with damage to nail

√5ᵗʰ **S61.2** **Open wound of other finger without damage to nail**
     EXCLUDES 1   open wound of finger involving nail (matrix) (S61.3-)
     EXCLUDES 2   open wound of thumb without damage to nail (S61.0-)

√6ᵗʰ **S61.20** Unspecified open wound of other finger without damage to nail

√7ᵗʰ **S61.200** Unspecified open wound of right index finger without damage to nail

√7ᵗʰ **S61.201** Unspecified open wound of left index finger without damage to nail

√7ᵗʰ **S61.202** Unspecified open wound of right middle finger without damage to nail

---

☒ Newborn: 0   ☐ Pediatric: 0-17   ☐ Maternity: 12-55   ☐ Adult: 15-124   **MCC** Major CC Condition   **PDx MCC** PDx acts as own MCC   **CC** CC Condition   **PDx CC** PDx acts as own CC

946   ICD-10-CM Draft (2015)

√7ᵗʰ **S61.203**   **Unspecified open wound of** left middle finger **without damage to nail**

√7ᵗʰ **S61.204**   **Unspecified open wound of** right ring finger **without damage to nail**

√7ᵗʰ **S61.205**   **Unspecified open wound of** left ring finger **without damage to nail**

√7ᵗʰ **S61.206**   **Unspecified open wound of** right little finger **without damage to nail**

√7ᵗʰ **S61.207**   **Unspecified open wound of** left little finger **without damage to nail**

√7ᵗʰ **S61.208**   **Unspecified open wound of** other finger **without damage to nail**
> Unspecified open wound of specified finger with unspecified laterality without damage to nail

√7ᵗʰ **S61.209**   **Unspecified open wound of** unspecified finger **without damage to nail**

√6ᵗʰ **S61.21**   **Laceration without foreign body of finger without damage to nail**

√7ᵗʰ **S61.210**   **Laceration without foreign body of** right index finger **without damage to nail**

√7ᵗʰ **S61.211**   **Laceration without foreign body of** left index finger **without damage to nail**

√7ᵗʰ **S61.212**   **Laceration without foreign body of** right middle finger **without damage to nail**

√7ᵗʰ **S61.213**   **Laceration without foreign body of** left middle finger **without damage to nail**

√7ᵗʰ **S61.214**   **Laceration without foreign body of** right ring finger **without damage to nail**

√7ᵗʰ **S61.215**   **Laceration without foreign body of** left ring finger **without damage to nail**

√7ᵗʰ **S61.216**   **Laceration without foreign body of** right little finger **without damage to nail**

√7ᵗʰ **S61.217**   **Laceration without foreign body of** left little finger **without damage to nail**

√7ᵗʰ **S61.218**   **Laceration without foreign body of** other finger **without damage to nail**
> Laceration without foreign body of specified finger with unspecified laterality without damage to nail

√7ᵗʰ **S61.219**   **Laceration without foreign body of** unspecified finger **without damage to nail**

√6ᵗʰ **S61.22**   **Laceration with foreign body of finger without damage to nail**

√7ᵗʰ **S61.220**   **Laceration with foreign body of** right index finger **without damage to nail**

√7ᵗʰ **S61.221**   **Laceration with foreign body of** left index finger **without damage to nail**

√7ᵗʰ **S61.222**   **Laceration with foreign body of** right middle finger **without damage to nail**

√7ᵗʰ **S61.223**   **Laceration with foreign body of** left middle finger **without damage to nail**

√7ᵗʰ **S61.224**   **Laceration with foreign body of** right ring finger **without damage to nail**

√7ᵗʰ **S61.225**   **Laceration with foreign body of** left ring finger **without damage to nail**

√7ᵗʰ **S61.226**   **Laceration with foreign body of** right little finger **without damage to nail**

√7ᵗʰ **S61.227**   **Laceration with foreign body of** left little finger **without damage to nail**

√7ᵗʰ **S61.228**   **Laceration with foreign body of** other finger **without damage to nail**
> Laceration with foreign body of specified finger with unspecified laterality without damage to nail

√7ᵗʰ **S61.229**   **Laceration with foreign body of** unspecified finger **without damage to nail**

√6ᵗʰ **S61.23**   **Puncture wound without foreign body of finger without damage to nail**

√7ᵗʰ **S61.230**   **Puncture wound without foreign body of** right index finger **without damage to nail**

√7ᵗʰ **S61.231**   **Puncture wound without foreign body of** left index finger **without damage to nail**

√7ᵗʰ **S61.232**   **Puncture wound without foreign body of** right middle finger **without damage to nail**

√7ᵗʰ **S61.233**   **Puncture wound without foreign body of** left middle finger **without damage to nail**

√7ᵗʰ **S61.234**   **Puncture wound without foreign body of** right ring finger **without damage to nail**

√7ᵗʰ **S61.235**   **Puncture wound without foreign body of** left ring finger **without damage to nail**

√7ᵗʰ **S61.236**   **Puncture wound without foreign body of** right little finger **without damage to nail**

√7ᵗʰ **S61.237**   **Puncture wound without foreign body of** left little finger **without damage to nail**

√7ᵗʰ **S61.238**   **Puncture wound without foreign body of** other finger **without damage to nail**
> Puncture wound without foreign body of specified finger with unspecified laterality without damage to nail

√7ᵗʰ **S61.239**   **Puncture wound without foreign body of** unspecified finger **without damage to nail**

√6ᵗʰ **S61.24**   **Puncture wound with foreign body of finger without damage to nail**

√7ᵗʰ **S61.240**   **Puncture wound with foreign body of** right index finger **without damage to nail**

√7ᵗʰ **S61.241**   **Puncture wound with foreign body of** left index finger **without damage to nail**

√7ᵗʰ **S61.242**   **Puncture wound with foreign body of** right middle finger **without damage to nail**

√7ᵗʰ **S61.243**   **Puncture wound with foreign body of** left middle finger **without damage to nail**

√7ᵗʰ **S61.244**   **Puncture wound with foreign body of** right ring finger **without damage to nail**

√7ᵗʰ **S61.245**   **Puncture wound with foreign body of** left ring finger **without damage to nail**

√7ᵗʰ **S61.246**   **Puncture wound with foreign body of** right little finger **without damage to nail**

√7ᵗʰ **S61.247**   **Puncture wound with foreign body of** left little finger **without damage to nail**

√7ᵗʰ **S61.248**   **Puncture wound with foreign body of** other finger **without damage to nail**
> Puncture wound with foreign body of specified finger with unspecified laterality without damage to nail

√7ᵗʰ **S61.249**   **Puncture wound with foreign body of** unspecified finger **without damage to nail**

√6ᵗʰ **S61.25**   **Open bite of finger without damage to nail**
> Bite of finger without damage to nail NOS
> **EXCLUDES 1** superficial bite of finger (S60.46-, S60.47-)

√7ᵗʰ **S61.250**   **Open bite of** right index finger **without damage to nail**

√7ᵗʰ **S61.251**   **Open bite of** left index finger **without damage to nail**

√7ᵗʰ **S61.252**   **Open bite of** right middle finger **without damage to nail**

√7ᵗʰ **S61.253**   **Open bite of** left middle finger **without damage to nail**

√7ᵗʰ **S61.254**   **Open bite of** right ring finger **without damage to nail**

√7ᵗʰ **S61.255**   **Open bite of** left ring finger **without damage to nail**

√7ᵗʰ **S61.256**   **Open bite of** right little finger **without damage to nail**

√7ᵗʰ **S61.257**   **Open bite of** left little finger **without damage to nail**

√7ᵗʰ **S61.258**   **Open bite of** other finger **without damage to nail**
> Open bite of specified finger with unspecified laterality without damage to nail

√7ᵗʰ **S61.259**   **Open bite of** unspecified finger **without damage to nail**

√5ᵗʰ **S61.3**   **Open wound of** other finger **with damage to nail**

√6ᵗʰ **S61.30**   **Unspecified open wound of finger with damage to nail**

√7ᵗʰ **S61.300**   **Unspecified open wound of** right index finger **with damage to nail**

√7ᵗʰ **S61.301**   **Unspecified open wound of** left index finger **with damage to nail**

✔ Additional Character Required   ✔ˣ⁷ᵗʰ Xtension Alert   Unacceptable PDx   Manifestation   Hospital Acquired Condition   **EXCLUDES 1** Not Coded Here   **EXCLUDES 2** Not Included Here

ICD-10-CM Draft (2015)   947

✓7ᵗʰ **S61.302** Unspecified open wound of right middle finger with damage to nail

✓7ᵗʰ **S61.303** Unspecified open wound of left middle finger with damage to nail

✓7ᵗʰ **S61.304** Unspecified open wound of right ring finger with damage to nail

✓7ᵗʰ **S61.305** Unspecified open wound of left ring finger with damage to nail

✓7ᵗʰ **S61.306** Unspecified open wound of right little finger with damage to nail

✓7ᵗʰ **S61.307** Unspecified open wound of left little finger with damage to nail

✓7ᵗʰ **S61.308** Unspecified open wound of other finger with damage to nail
　　Unspecified open wound of specified finger with unspecified laterality with damage to nail

✓7ᵗʰ **S61.309** Unspecified open wound of unspecified finger with damage to nail

✓6ᵗʰ **S61.31** Laceration without foreign body of finger with damage to nail

✓7ᵗʰ **S61.310** Laceration without foreign body of right index finger with damage to nail

✓7ᵗʰ **S61.311** Laceration without foreign body of left index finger with damage to nail

✓7ᵗʰ **S61.312** Laceration without foreign body of right middle finger with damage to nail

✓7ᵗʰ **S61.313** Laceration without foreign body of left middle finger with damage to nail

✓7ᵗʰ **S61.314** Laceration without foreign body of right ring finger with damage to nail

✓7ᵗʰ **S61.315** Laceration without foreign body of left ring finger with damage to nail

✓7ᵗʰ **S61.316** Laceration without foreign body of right little finger with damage to nail

✓7ᵗʰ **S61.317** Laceration without foreign body of left little finger with damage to nail

✓7ᵗʰ **S61.318** Laceration without foreign body of other finger with damage to nail
　　Laceration without foreign body of specified finger with unspecified laterality with damage to nail

✓7ᵗʰ **S61.319** Laceration without foreign body of unspecified finger with damage to nail

✓6ᵗʰ **S61.32** Laceration with foreign body of finger with damage to nail

✓7ᵗʰ **S61.320** Laceration with foreign body of right index finger with damage to nail

✓7ᵗʰ **S61.321** Laceration with foreign body of left index finger with damage to nail

✓7ᵗʰ **S61.322** Laceration with foreign body of right middle finger with damage to nail

✓7ᵗʰ **S61.323** Laceration with foreign body of left middle finger with damage to nail

✓7ᵗʰ **S61.324** Laceration with foreign body of right ring finger with damage to nail

✓7ᵗʰ **S61.325** Laceration with foreign body of left ring finger with damage to nail

✓7ᵗʰ **S61.326** Laceration with foreign body of right little finger with damage to nail

✓7ᵗʰ **S61.327** Laceration with foreign body of left little finger with damage to nail

✓7ᵗʰ **S61.328** Laceration with foreign body of other finger with damage to nail
　　Laceration with foreign body of specified finger with unspecified laterality with damage to nail

✓7ᵗʰ **S61.329** Laceration with foreign body of unspecified finger with damage to nail

✓6ᵗʰ **S61.33** Puncture wound without foreign body of finger with damage to nail

✓7ᵗʰ **S61.330** Puncture wound without foreign body of right index finger with damage to nail

✓7ᵗʰ **S61.331** Puncture wound without foreign body of left index finger with damage to nail

✓7ᵗʰ **S61.332** Puncture wound without foreign body of right middle finger with damage to nail

✓7ᵗʰ **S61.333** Puncture wound without foreign body of left middle finger with damage to nail

✓7ᵗʰ **S61.334** Puncture wound without foreign body of right ring finger with damage to nail

✓7ᵗʰ **S61.335** Puncture wound without foreign body of left ring finger with damage to nail

✓7ᵗʰ **S61.336** Puncture wound without foreign body of right little finger with damage to nail

✓7ᵗʰ **S61.337** Puncture wound without foreign body of left little finger with damage to nail

✓7ᵗʰ **S61.338** Puncture wound without foreign body of other finger with damage to nail
　　Puncture wound without foreign body of specified finger with unspecified laterality with damage to nail

✓7ᵗʰ **S61.339** Puncture wound without foreign body of unspecified finger with damage to nail

✓6ᵗʰ **S61.34** Puncture wound with foreign body of finger with damage to nail

✓7ᵗʰ **S61.340** Puncture wound with foreign body of right index finger with damage to nail

✓7ᵗʰ **S61.341** Puncture wound with foreign body of left index finger with damage to nail

✓7ᵗʰ **S61.342** Puncture wound with foreign body of right middle finger with damage to nail

✓7ᵗʰ **S61.343** Puncture wound with foreign body of left middle finger with damage to nail

✓7ᵗʰ **S61.344** Puncture wound with foreign body of right ring finger with damage to nail

✓7ᵗʰ **S61.345** Puncture wound with foreign body of left ring finger with damage to nail

✓7ᵗʰ **S61.346** Puncture wound with foreign body of right little finger with damage to nail

✓7ᵗʰ **S61.347** Puncture wound with foreign body of left little finger with damage to nail

✓7ᵗʰ **S61.348** Puncture wound with foreign body of other finger with damage to nail
　　Puncture wound with foreign body of specified finger with unspecified laterality with damage to nail

✓7ᵗʰ **S61.349** Puncture wound with foreign body of unspecified finger with damage to nail

✓6ᵗʰ **S61.35** Open bite of finger with damage to nail
　　Bite of finger with damage to nail NOS
　　EXCLUDES 1　superficial bite of finger (S60.46-, S60.47-)

✓7ᵗʰ **S61.350** Open bite of right index finger with damage to nail

✓7ᵗʰ **S61.351** Open bite of left index finger with damage to nail

✓7ᵗʰ **S61.352** Open bite of right middle finger with damage to nail

✓7ᵗʰ **S61.353** Open bite of left middle finger with damage to nail

✓7ᵗʰ **S61.354** Open bite of right ring finger with damage to nail

✓7ᵗʰ **S61.355** Open bite of left ring finger with damage to nail

✓7ᵗʰ **S61.356** Open bite of right little finger with damage to nail

✓7ᵗʰ **S61.357** Open bite of left little finger with damage to nail

✓7ᵗʰ **S61.358** Open bite of other finger with damage to nail
　　Open bite of specified finger with unspecified laterality with damage to nail

✓7ᵗʰ **S61.359** Open bite of unspecified finger with damage to nail

✓5ᵗʰ **S61.4** Open wound of hand

✓6ᵗʰ **S61.40** Unspecified open wound of hand

✓7ᵗʰ **S61.401** Unspecified open wound of right hand

✓7ᵗʰ **S61.402** Unspecified open wound of left hand

✓7ᵗʰ **S61.409** Unspecified open wound of unspecified hand

N Newborn: 0　　P Pediatric: 0-17　　M Maternity: 12-55　　A Adult: 15-124　　MCC Major CC Condition　　PDx MCC PDx acts as own MCC　　CC CC Condition　　PDx CC PDx acts as own CC

√6ᵗʰ **S61.41** Laceration without foreign body of hand
- √7ᵗʰ **S61.411** Laceration without foreign body of right hand
- √7ᵗʰ **S61.412** Laceration without foreign body of left hand
- √7ᵗʰ **S61.419** Laceration without foreign body of unspecified hand

√6ᵗʰ **S61.42** Laceration with foreign body of hand
- √7ᵗʰ **S61.421** Laceration with foreign body of right hand
- √7ᵗʰ **S61.422** Laceration with foreign body of left hand
- √7ᵗʰ **S61.429** Laceration with foreign body of unspecified hand

√6ᵗʰ **S61.43** Puncture wound without foreign body of hand
- √7ᵗʰ **S61.431** Puncture wound without foreign body of right hand
- √7ᵗʰ **S61.432** Puncture wound without foreign body of left hand
- √7ᵗʰ **S61.439** Puncture wound without foreign body of unspecified hand

√6ᵗʰ **S61.44** Puncture wound with foreign body of hand
- √7ᵗʰ **S61.441** Puncture wound with foreign body of right hand
- √7ᵗʰ **S61.442** Puncture wound with foreign body of left hand
- √7ᵗʰ **S61.449** Puncture wound with foreign body of unspecified hand

√6ᵗʰ **S61.45** Open bite of hand
Bite of hand NOS
> *EXCLUDES 1* superficial bite of hand (S60.56-, S60.57-)
- √7ᵗʰ **S61.451** Open bite of right hand
- √7ᵗʰ **S61.452** Open bite of left hand
- √7ᵗʰ **S61.459** Open bite of unspecified hand

√5ᵗʰ **S61.5** Open wound of wrist

√6ᵗʰ **S61.50** Unspecified open wound of wrist
- √7ᵗʰ **S61.501** Unspecified open wound of right wrist
- √7ᵗʰ **S61.502** Unspecified open wound of left wrist
- √7ᵗʰ **S61.509** Unspecified open wound of unspecified wrist

√6ᵗʰ **S61.51** Laceration without foreign body of wrist
- √7ᵗʰ **S61.511** Laceration without foreign body of right wrist
- √7ᵗʰ **S61.512** Laceration without foreign body of left wrist
- √7ᵗʰ **S61.519** Laceration without foreign body of unspecified wrist

√6ᵗʰ **S61.52** Laceration with foreign body of wrist
- √7ᵗʰ **S61.521** Laceration with foreign body of right wrist
- √7ᵗʰ **S61.522** Laceration with foreign body of left wrist
- √7ᵗʰ **S61.529** Laceration with foreign body of unspecified wrist

√6ᵗʰ **S61.53** Puncture wound without foreign body of wrist
- √7ᵗʰ **S61.531** Puncture wound without foreign body of right wrist
- √7ᵗʰ **S61.532** Puncture wound without foreign body of left wrist
- √7ᵗʰ **S61.539** Puncture wound without foreign body of unspecified wrist

√6ᵗʰ **S61.54** Puncture wound with foreign body of wrist
- √7ᵗʰ **S61.541** Puncture wound with foreign body of right wrist
- √7ᵗʰ **S61.542** Puncture wound with foreign body of left wrist
- √7ᵗʰ **S61.549** Puncture wound with foreign body of unspecified wrist

√6ᵗʰ **S61.55** Open bite of wrist
Bite of wrist NOS
> *EXCLUDES 1* superficial bite of wrist (S60.86-, S60.87-)
- √7ᵗʰ **S61.551** Open bite of right wrist
- √7ᵗʰ **S61.552** Open bite of left wrist
- √7ᵗʰ **S61.559** Open bite of unspecified wrist

√4ᵗʰ **S62** Fracture at wrist and hand level

NOTE A fracture not indicated as displaced or nondisplaced should be coded to displaced.
A fracture not indicated as open or closed should be coded to closed.

EXCLUDES 1 traumatic amputation of wrist and hand (S68.-)
EXCLUDES 2 fracture of distal parts of ulna and radius (S52.-)

The appropriate 7th is to be added to each code from category S62.
- A   initial encounter for closed fracture
- B   initial encounter for open fracture
- D   subsequent encounter for fracture with routine healing
- G   subsequent encounter for fracture with delayed healing
- K   subsequent encounter for fracture with nonunion
- P   subsequent encounter for fracture with malunion
- S   sequela

√5ᵗʰ **S62.0** Fracture of navicular [scaphoid] bone of wrist

CC Excl: For CC codes in subcategory S62.0, unless otherwise noted: CC with 7th character B: S62.001-S62.186 with 7th [A, B]
CC with 7th character K or P: M80.00X-M84.68X with 7th [K, P], S02.0XX-S02.92X with 7th K, S12.000-S12.691 with 7th K, S22.000-S22.9XX with 7th K, S32.000-S32.9XX with 7th K, S42.001-S42.92X with 7th [K, P], S49.001-S49.199 with 7th [K, P], S52.001-S52.92X with 7th [K, M, N, P, Q, R], S59.001-S59.299 with 7th [K, P], S62.001-S62.92X with 7th [K, P], S72.001-S72.92X with 7th [K, M, N, P, Q, R], S79.001-S79.199 with 7th [K, P], S82.001-S82.92X with 7th [K, M, N, P, Q, R], S89.001-S89.399 with 7th [K, P], S92.001-S92.919 with 7th [K, P]

√6ᵗʰ **S62.00** Unspecified fracture of navicular [scaphoid] bone of wrist
- 7 √7ᵗʰ **S62.001** Unspecified fracture of navicular [scaphoid] bone of right wrist   CC
- 7 √7ᵗʰ **S62.002** Unspecified fracture of navicular [scaphoid] bone of left wrist   CC
  AHA: 2012, 4Q, 106
- 7 √7ᵗʰ **S62.009** Unspecified fracture of navicular [scaphoid] bone of unspecified wrist   CC

√6ᵗʰ **S62.01** Fracture of distal pole of navicular [scaphoid] bone of wrist
Fracture of volar tuberosity of navicular [scaphoid] bone of wrist
- 7 √7ᵗʰ **S62.011** Displaced fracture of distal pole of navicular [scaphoid] bone of right wrist   CC
- 7 √7ᵗʰ **S62.012** Displaced fracture of distal pole of navicular [scaphoid] bone of left wrist   CC
- 7 √7ᵗʰ **S62.013** Displaced fracture of distal pole of navicular [scaphoid] bone of unspecified wrist   CC
- 7 √7ᵗʰ **S62.014** Nondisplaced fracture of distal pole of navicular [scaphoid] bone of right wrist   CC
- 7 √7ᵗʰ **S62.015** Nondisplaced fracture of distal pole of navicular [scaphoid] bone of left wrist   CC
- 7 √7ᵗʰ **S62.016** Nondisplaced fracture of distal pole of navicular [scaphoid] bone of unspecified wrist   CC

√6ᵗʰ **S62.02** Fracture of middle third of navicular [scaphoid] bone of wrist
- 7 √7ᵗʰ **S62.021** Displaced fracture of middle third of navicular [scaphoid] bone of right wrist   CC
- 7 √7ᵗʰ **S62.022** Displaced fracture of middle third of navicular [scaphoid] bone of left wrist   CC
- 7 √7ᵗʰ **S62.023** Displaced fracture of middle third of navicular [scaphoid] bone of unspecified wrist   CC
- 7 √7ᵗʰ **S62.024** Nondisplaced fracture of middle third of navicular [scaphoid] bone of right wrist   CC
- 7 √7ᵗʰ **S62.025** Nondisplaced fracture of middle third of navicular [scaphoid] bone of left wrist   CC
- 7 √7ᵗʰ **S62.026** Nondisplaced fracture of middle third of navicular [scaphoid] bone of unspecified wrist   CC

---

7 HAC = Initial encounter only (7th character A, B or C) and not POA.

S62.03–S62.186

Injury, Poisoning and Certain Other Consequences of External Causes

√6th **S62.03** Fracture of proximal third of navicular [scaphoid] bone of wrist

7 √7th **S62.031** Displaced fracture of proximal third of navicular [scaphoid] bone of right wrist `CC`

7 √7th **S62.032** Displaced fracture of proximal third of navicular [scaphoid] bone of left wrist `CC`

7 √7th **S62.033** Displaced fracture of proximal third of navicular [scaphoid] bone of unspecified wrist `CC`

7 √7th **S62.034** Nondisplaced fracture of proximal third of navicular [scaphoid] bone of right wrist `CC`

7 √7th **S62.035** Nondisplaced fracture of proximal third of navicular [scaphoid] bone of left wrist `CC`

7 √7th **S62.036** Nondisplaced fracture of proximal third of navicular [scaphoid] bone of unspecified wrist `CC`

√5th **S62.1** Fracture of other and unspecified carpal bone(s)

EXCLUDES 2   fracture of scaphoid of wrist (S62.0-)

S62.1 CC Excl: For CC codes in subcategory S62.1, unless otherwise noted: See code: S62.0

√6th **S62.10** Fracture of unspecified carpal bone
Fracture of wrist NOS

7 √7th **S62.101** Fracture of unspecified carpal bone, right wrist `CC`

7 √7th **S62.102** Fracture of unspecified carpal bone, left wrist `CC`
AHA: 2012, 4Q, 95

7 √7th **S62.109** Fracture of unspecified carpal bone, unspecified wrist `CC`

√6th **S62.11** Fracture of triquetrum [cuneiform] bone of wrist

7 √7th **S62.111** Displaced fracture of triquetrum [cuneiform] bone, right wrist `CC`

7 √7th **S62.112** Displaced fracture of triquetrum [cuneiform] bone, left wrist `CC`

7 √7th **S62.113** Displaced fracture of triquetrum [cuneiform] bone, unspecified wrist `CC`

7 √7th **S62.114** Nondisplaced fracture of triquetrum [cuneiform] bone, right wrist `CC`

7 √7th **S62.115** Nondisplaced fracture of triquetrum [cuneiform] bone, left wrist `CC`

7 √7th **S62.116** Nondisplaced fracture of triquetrum [cuneiform] bone, unspecified wrist `CC`

√6th **S62.12** Fracture of lunate [semilunar]

7 √7th **S62.121** Displaced fracture of lunate [semilunar], right wrist `CC`

7 √7th **S62.122** Displaced fracture of lunate [semilunar], left wrist `CC`

7 √7th **S62.123** Displaced fracture of lunate [semilunar], unspecified wrist `CC`

7 √7th **S62.124** Nondisplaced fracture of lunate [semilunar], right wrist `CC`

7 √7th **S62.125** Nondisplaced fracture of lunate [semilunar], left wrist `CC`

7 √7th **S62.126** Nondisplaced fracture of lunate [semilunar], unspecified wrist `CC`

√6th **S62.13** Fracture of capitate [os magnum] bone

7 √7th **S62.131** Displaced fracture of capitate [os magnum] bone, right wrist `CC`

7 √7th **S62.132** Displaced fracture of capitate [os magnum] bone, left wrist `CC`

7 √7th **S62.133** Displaced fracture of capitate [os magnum] bone, unspecified wrist `CC`

7 √7th **S62.134** Nondisplaced fracture of capitate [os magnum] bone, right wrist `CC`

7 √7th **S62.135** Nondisplaced fracture of capitate [os magnum] bone, left wrist `CC`

7 √7th **S62.136** Nondisplaced fracture of capitate [os magnum] bone, unspecified wrist `CC`

√6th **S62.14** Fracture of body of hamate [unciform] bone
Fracture of hamate [unciform] bone NOS

7 √7th **S62.141** Displaced fracture of body of hamate [unciform] bone, right wrist `CC`

7 √7th **S62.142** Displaced fracture of body of hamate [unciform] bone, left wrist `CC`

7 √7th **S62.143** Displaced fracture of body of hamate [unciform] bone, unspecified wrist `CC`

7 √7th **S62.144** Nondisplaced fracture of body of hamate [unciform] bone, right wrist `CC`

7 √7th **S62.145** Nondisplaced fracture of body of hamate [unciform] bone, left wrist `CC`

7 √7th **S62.146** Nondisplaced fracture of body of hamate [unciform] bone, unspecified wrist `CC`

√6th **S62.15** Fracture of hook process of hamate [unciform] bone
Fracture of unciform process of hamate [unciform] bone

7 √7th **S62.151** Displaced fracture of hook process of hamate [unciform] bone, right wrist `CC`

7 √7th **S62.152** Displaced fracture of hook process of hamate [unciform] bone, left wrist `CC`

7 √7th **S62.153** Displaced fracture of hook process of hamate [unciform] bone, unspecified wrist `CC`

7 √7th **S62.154** Nondisplaced fracture of hook process of hamate [unciform] bone, right wrist `CC`

7 √7th **S62.155** Nondisplaced fracture of hook process of hamate [unciform] bone, left wrist `CC`

7 √7th **S62.156** Nondisplaced fracture of hook process of hamate [unciform] bone, unspecified wrist `CC`

√6th **S62.16** Fracture of pisiform

7 √7th **S62.161** Displaced fracture of pisiform, right wrist `CC`

7 √7th **S62.162** Displaced fracture of pisiform, left wrist `CC`

7 √7th **S62.163** Displaced fracture of pisiform, unspecified wrist `CC`

7 √7th **S62.164** Nondisplaced fracture of pisiform, right wrist `CC`

7 √7th **S62.165** Nondisplaced fracture of pisiform, left wrist `CC`

7 √7th **S62.166** Nondisplaced fracture of pisiform, unspecified wrist `CC`

√6th **S62.17** Fracture of trapezium [larger multangular]

7 √7th **S62.171** Displaced fracture of trapezium [larger multangular], right wrist `CC`

7 √7th **S62.172** Displaced fracture of trapezium [larger multangular], left wrist `CC`

7 √7th **S62.173** Displaced fracture of trapezium [larger multangular], unspecified wrist `CC`

7 √7th **S62.174** Nondisplaced fracture of trapezium [larger multangular], right wrist `CC`

7 √7th **S62.175** Nondisplaced fracture of trapezium [larger multangular], left wrist `CC`

7 √7th **S62.176** Nondisplaced fracture of trapezium [larger multangular], unspecified wrist `CC`

√6th **S62.18** Fracture of trapezoid [smaller multangular]

7 √7th **S62.181** Displaced fracture of trapezoid [smaller multangular], right wrist `CC`

7 √7th **S62.182** Displaced fracture of trapezoid [smaller multangular], left wrist `CC`

7 √7th **S62.183** Displaced fracture of trapezoid [smaller multangular], unspecified wrist `CC`

7 √7th **S62.184** Nondisplaced fracture of trapezoid [smaller multangular], right wrist `CC`

7 √7th **S62.185** Nondisplaced fracture of trapezoid [smaller multangular], left wrist `CC`

7 √7th **S62.186** Nondisplaced fracture of trapezoid [smaller multangular], unspecified wrist `CC`

---

7 HAC = Initial encounter only (7th character A, B or C) and not POA.

N Newborn: 0   P Pediatric: 0-17   M Maternity: 12-55   A Adult: 15-124   `MCC` Major CC Condition   `PDx MCC` PDx acts as own MCC   `CC` CC Condition   `PDx CC` PDx acts as own CC

950   ICD-10-CM Draft (2015)

√5ᵗʰ **S62.2**   Fracture of first metacarpal bone

> **S62.2 CC Excl:** For CC codes in subcategory S62.2, unless otherwise noted: **CC with 7th character B:** S62.201-S62.399 with 7th [A, B], S62.90X with 7th A
> **CC with 7th character K or P:** M80.00X-M84.68X with 7th [K, P], S02.0XX-S02.92X with 7th K, S12.000-S12.691 with 7th K, S22.000-S22.9XX with 7th K, S32.000-S32.9XX with 7th K, S42.001-S42.92X with 7th [K, P], S49.001-S49.199 with 7th [K, P], S52.001-S52.92X with 7th [K, M, N, P, Q, R], S59.001-S59.299 with 7th [K, P], S62.001-S62.92X with 7th [K, P], S72.001-S72.92X with 7th [K, M, N, P, Q, R], S79.001-S79.199 with 7th [K, P], S82.001-S82.92X with 7th [K, M, N, P, Q, R], S89.001-S89.399 with 7th [K, P], S92.001-S92.919 with 7th [K, P]

√6ᵗʰ **S62.20**   Unspecified fracture of first metacarpal bone

   7 √7ᵗʰ **S62.201**   Unspecified fracture of first metacarpal bone, **right** hand   CC

   7 √7ᵗʰ **S62.202**   Unspecified fracture of first metacarpal bone, **left** hand   CC

   7 √7ᵗʰ **S62.209**   Unspecified fracture of first metacarpal bone, **unspecified** hand   CC

√6ᵗʰ **S62.21**   Bennett's fracture

   7 √7ᵗʰ **S62.211**   Bennett's fracture, **right** hand   CC

   7 √7ᵗʰ **S62.212**   Bennett's fracture, **left** hand   CC

   7 √7ᵗʰ **S62.213**   Bennett's fracture, **unspecified** hand   CC

√6ᵗʰ **S62.22**   Rolando's fracture

   7 √7ᵗʰ **S62.221**   Displaced Rolando's fracture, **right** hand   CC

   7 √7ᵗʰ **S62.222**   Displaced Rolando's fracture, **left** hand   CC

   7 √7ᵗʰ **S62.223**   Displaced Rolando's fracture, **unspecified** hand   CC

   7 √7ᵗʰ **S62.224**   Nondisplaced Rolando's fracture, **right** hand   CC

   7 √7ᵗʰ **S62.225**   Nondisplaced Rolando's fracture, **left** hand   CC

   7 √7ᵗʰ **S62.226**   Nondisplaced Rolando's fracture, **unspecified** hand   CC

√6ᵗʰ **S62.23**   Other fracture of base of first metacarpal bone

   7 √7ᵗʰ **S62.231**   Other displaced fracture of base of first metacarpal bone, **right** hand   CC

   7 √7ᵗʰ **S62.232**   Other displaced fracture of base of first metacarpal bone, **left** hand   CC

   7 √7ᵗʰ **S62.233**   Other displaced fracture of base of first metacarpal bone, **unspecified** hand   CC

   7 √7ᵗʰ **S62.234**   Other nondisplaced fracture of base of first metacarpal bone, **right** hand   CC

   7 √7ᵗʰ **S62.235**   Other nondisplaced fracture of base of first metacarpal bone, **left** hand   CC

   7 √7ᵗʰ **S62.236**   Other nondisplaced fracture of base of first metacarpal bone, **unspecified** hand   CC

√6ᵗʰ **S62.24**   Fracture of shaft of first metacarpal bone

   7 √7ᵗʰ **S62.241**   Displaced fracture of shaft of first metacarpal bone, **right** hand   CC

   7 √7ᵗʰ **S62.242**   Displaced fracture of shaft of first metacarpal bone, **left** hand   CC

   7 √7ᵗʰ **S62.243**   Displaced fracture of shaft of first metacarpal bone, **unspecified** hand   CC

   7 √7ᵗʰ **S62.244**   Nondisplaced fracture of shaft of first metacarpal bone, **right** hand   CC

   7 √7ᵗʰ **S62.245**   Nondisplaced fracture of shaft of first metacarpal bone, **left** hand   CC

   7 √7ᵗʰ **S62.246**   Nondisplaced fracture of shaft of first metacarpal bone, **unspecified** hand   CC

√6ᵗʰ **S62.25**   Fracture of neck of first metacarpal bone

   7 √7ᵗʰ **S62.251**   Displaced fracture of neck of first metacarpal bone, **right** hand   CC

   7 √7ᵗʰ **S62.252**   Displaced fracture of neck of first metacarpal bone, **left** hand   CC

   7 √7ᵗʰ **S62.253**   Displaced fracture of neck of first metacarpal bone, **unspecified** hand   CC

   7 √7ᵗʰ **S62.254**   Nondisplaced fracture of neck of first metacarpal bone, **right** hand   CC

   7 √7ᵗʰ **S62.255**   Nondisplaced fracture of neck of first metacarpal bone, **left** hand   CC

   7 √7ᵗʰ **S62.256**   Nondisplaced fracture of neck of first metacarpal bone, **unspecified** hand   CC

√6ᵗʰ **S62.29**   Other fracture of first metacarpal bone

   7 √7ᵗʰ **S62.291**   Other fracture of first metacarpal bone, **right** hand   CC

   7 √7ᵗʰ **S62.292**   Other fracture of first metacarpal bone, **left** hand   CC

   7 √7ᵗʰ **S62.299**   Other fracture of first metacarpal bone, **unspecified** hand   CC

√5ᵗʰ **S62.3**   Fracture of other and unspecified metacarpal bone

> *EXCLUDES 2*   fracture of first metacarpal bone (S62.2-)

> **CC Excl:** For CC codes in subcategory S62.3, unless otherwise noted: See code: S62.2

√6ᵗʰ **S62.30**   Unspecified fracture of other metacarpal bone

   7 √7ᵗʰ **S62.300**   Unspecified fracture of second metacarpal bone, **right** hand   CC

   7 √7ᵗʰ **S62.301**   Unspecified fracture of second metacarpal bone, **left** hand   CC

   7 √7ᵗʰ **S62.302**   Unspecified fracture of third metacarpal bone, **right** hand   CC

   7 √7ᵗʰ **S62.303**   Unspecified fracture of third metacarpal bone, **left** hand   CC

   7 √7ᵗʰ **S62.304**   Unspecified fracture of fourth metacarpal bone, **right** hand   CC

   7 √7ᵗʰ **S62.305**   Unspecified fracture of fourth metacarpal bone, **left** hand   CC

   7 √7ᵗʰ **S62.306**   Unspecified fracture of fifth metacarpal bone, **right** hand   CC

   7 √7ᵗʰ **S62.307**   Unspecified fracture of fifth metacarpal bone, **left** hand   CC

   7 √7ᵗʰ **S62.308**   Unspecified fracture of other metacarpal bone
> Unspecified fracture of specified metacarpal bone with unspecified laterality

   7 √7ᵗʰ **S62.309**   Unspecified fracture of unspecified metacarpal bone   CC

√6ᵗʰ **S62.31**   Displaced fracture of base of other metacarpal bone

   7 √7ᵗʰ **S62.310**   Displaced fracture of base of second metacarpal bone, **right** hand   CC

   7 √7ᵗʰ **S62.311**   Displaced fracture of base of second metacarpal bone, **left** hand   CC

   7 √7ᵗʰ **S62.312**   Displaced fracture of base of third metacarpal bone, **right** hand   CC

   7 √7ᵗʰ **S62.313**   Displaced fracture of base of third metacarpal bone, **left** hand   CC

   7 √7ᵗʰ **S62.314**   Displaced fracture of base of fourth metacarpal bone, **right** hand   CC

   7 √7ᵗʰ **S62.315**   Displaced fracture of base of fourth metacarpal bone, **left** hand   CC

   7 √7ᵗʰ **S62.316**   Displaced fracture of base of fifth metacarpal bone, **right** hand   CC

   7 √7ᵗʰ **S62.317**   Displaced fracture of base of fifth metacarpal bone, **left** hand   CC

   7 √7ᵗʰ **S62.318**   Displaced fracture of base of other metacarpal bone
> Displaced fracture of base of specified metacarpal bone with unspecified laterality

   7 √7ᵗʰ **S62.319**   Displaced fracture of base of unspecified metacarpal bone   CC

√6ᵗʰ **S62.32**   Displaced fracture of shaft of other metacarpal bone

   7 √7ᵗʰ **S62.320**   Displaced fracture of shaft of second metacarpal bone, **right** hand   CC

   7 √7ᵗʰ **S62.321**   Displaced fracture of shaft of second metacarpal bone, **left** hand   CC

   7 √7ᵗʰ **S62.322**   Displaced fracture of shaft of third metacarpal bone, **right** hand   CC

   7 √7ᵗʰ **S62.323**   Displaced fracture of shaft of third metacarpal bone, **left** hand   CC

   7 √7ᵗʰ **S62.324**   Displaced fracture of shaft of fourth metacarpal bone, **right** hand   CC

---

7 HAC = Initial encounter only (7th character A, B or C) and not POA.

√ Additional Character Required   √x7ᵗʰ Xtension Alert   Unacceptable PDx   Manifestation   Hospital Acquired Condition   *EXCLUDES 1* Not Coded Here   *EXCLUDES 2* Not Included Here

Injury, Poisoning and Certain Other Consequences of External Causes

S62.325–S62.502

7 ✓7ᵗʰ **S62.325 Displaced fracture of shaft of fourth metacarpal bone, left hand** CC

7 ✓7ᵗʰ **S62.326 Displaced fracture of shaft of fifth metacarpal bone, right hand** CC

7 ✓7ᵗʰ **S62.327 Displaced fracture of shaft of fifth metacarpal bone, left hand** CC

7 ✓7ᵗʰ **S62.328 Displaced fracture of shaft of other metacarpal bone** CC
     Displaced fracture of shaft of specified metacarpal bone with unspecified laterality

7 ✓7ᵗʰ **S62.329 Displaced fracture of shaft of unspecified metacarpal bone** CC

✓6ᵗʰ **S62.33 Displaced fracture of neck of other metacarpal bone**

7 ✓7ᵗʰ **S62.330 Displaced fracture of neck of second metacarpal bone, right hand** CC

7 ✓7ᵗʰ **S62.331 Displaced fracture of neck of second metacarpal bone, left hand** CC

7 ✓7ᵗʰ **S62.332 Displaced fracture of neck of third metacarpal bone, right hand** CC

7 ✓7ᵗʰ **S62.333 Displaced fracture of neck of third metacarpal bone, left hand** CC

7 ✓7ᵗʰ **S62.334 Displaced fracture of neck of fourth metacarpal bone, right hand** CC

7 ✓7ᵗʰ **S62.335 Displaced fracture of neck of fourth metacarpal bone, left hand** CC

7 ✓7ᵗʰ **S62.336 Displaced fracture of neck of fifth metacarpal bone, right hand** CC

7 ✓7ᵗʰ **S62.337 Displaced fracture of neck of fifth metacarpal bone, left hand** CC

7 ✓7ᵗʰ **S62.338 Displaced fracture of neck of other metacarpal bone** CC
     Displaced fracture of neck of specified metacarpal bone with unspecified laterality

7 ✓7ᵗʰ **S62.339 Displaced fracture of neck of unspecified metacarpal bone** CC

✓6ᵗʰ **S62.34 Nondisplaced fracture of base of other metacarpal bone**

7 ✓7ᵗʰ **S62.340 Nondisplaced fracture of base of second metacarpal bone, right hand** CC

7 ✓7ᵗʰ **S62.341 Nondisplaced fracture of base of second metacarpal bone, left hand** CC

7 ✓7ᵗʰ **S62.342 Nondisplaced fracture of base of third metacarpal bone, right hand** CC

7 ✓7ᵗʰ **S62.343 Nondisplaced fracture of base of third metacarpal bone, left hand** CC

7 ✓7ᵗʰ **S62.344 Nondisplaced fracture of base of fourth metacarpal bone, right hand** CC

7 ✓7ᵗʰ **S62.345 Nondisplaced fracture of base of fourth metacarpal bone, left hand** CC

7 ✓7ᵗʰ **S62.346 Nondisplaced fracture of base of fifth metacarpal bone, right hand** CC

7 ✓7ᵗʰ **S62.347 Nondisplaced fracture of base of fifth metacarpal bone, left hand** CC

7 ✓7ᵗʰ **S62.348 Nondisplaced fracture of base of other metacarpal bone** CC
     Nondisplaced fracture of base of specified metacarpal bone with unspecified laterality

7 ✓7ᵗʰ **S62.349 Nondisplaced fracture of base of unspecified metacarpal bone** CC

✓6ᵗʰ **S62.35 Nondisplaced fracture of shaft of other metacarpal bone**

7 ✓7ᵗʰ **S62.350 Nondisplaced fracture of shaft of second metacarpal bone, right hand** CC

7 ✓7ᵗʰ **S62.351 Nondisplaced fracture of shaft of second metacarpal bone, left hand** CC

7 ✓7ᵗʰ **S62.352 Nondisplaced fracture of shaft of third metacarpal bone, right hand** CC

7 ✓7ᵗʰ **S62.353 Nondisplaced fracture of shaft of third metacarpal bone, left hand** CC

7 ✓7ᵗʰ **S62.354 Nondisplaced fracture of shaft of fourth metacarpal bone, right hand** CC

7 ✓7ᵗʰ **S62.355 Nondisplaced fracture of shaft of fourth metacarpal bone, left hand** CC

7 ✓7ᵗʰ **S62.356 Nondisplaced fracture of shaft of fifth metacarpal bone, right hand** CC

7 ✓7ᵗʰ **S62.357 Nondisplaced fracture of shaft of fifth metacarpal bone, left hand** CC

7 ✓7ᵗʰ **S62.358 Nondisplaced fracture of shaft of other metacarpal bone** CC
     Nondisplaced fracture of shaft of specified metacarpal bone with unspecified laterality

7 ✓7ᵗʰ **S62.359 Nondisplaced fracture of shaft of unspecified metacarpal bone** CC

✓6ᵗʰ **S62.36 Nondisplaced fracture of neck of other metacarpal bone**

7 ✓7ᵗʰ **S62.360 Nondisplaced fracture of neck of second metacarpal bone, right hand** CC

7 ✓7ᵗʰ **S62.361 Nondisplaced fracture of neck of second metacarpal bone, left hand** CC

7 ✓7ᵗʰ **S62.362 Nondisplaced fracture of neck of third metacarpal bone, right hand** CC

7 ✓7ᵗʰ **S62.363 Nondisplaced fracture of neck of third metacarpal bone, left hand** CC

7 ✓7ᵗʰ **S62.364 Nondisplaced fracture of neck of fourth metacarpal bone, right hand** CC

7 ✓7ᵗʰ **S62.365 Nondisplaced fracture of neck of fourth metacarpal bone, left hand** CC

7 ✓7ᵗʰ **S62.366 Nondisplaced fracture of neck of fifth metacarpal bone, right hand** CC

7 ✓7ᵗʰ **S62.367 Nondisplaced fracture of neck of fifth metacarpal bone, left hand** CC

7 ✓7ᵗʰ **S62.368 Nondisplaced fracture of neck of other metacarpal bone** CC
     Nondisplaced fracture of neck of specified metacarpal bone with unspecified laterality

7 ✓7ᵗʰ **S62.369 Nondisplaced fracture of neck of unspecified metacarpal bone** CC

✓6ᵗʰ **S62.39 Other fracture of other metacarpal bone**

7 ✓7ᵗʰ **S62.390 Other fracture of second metacarpal bone, right hand**

7 ✓7ᵗʰ **S62.391 Other fracture of second metacarpal bone, left hand**

7 ✓7ᵗʰ **S62.392 Other fracture of third metacarpal bone, right hand**

7 ✓7ᵗʰ **S62.393 Other fracture of third metacarpal bone, left hand**

7 ✓7ᵗʰ **S62.394 Other fracture of fourth metacarpal bone, right hand**

7 ✓7ᵗʰ **S62.395 Other fracture of fourth metacarpal bone, left hand**

7 ✓7ᵗʰ **S62.396 Other fracture of fifth metacarpal bone, right hand**

7 ✓7ᵗʰ **S62.397 Other fracture of fifth metacarpal bone, left hand**

7 ✓7ᵗʰ **S62.398 Other fracture of other metacarpal bone**
     Other fracture of specified metacarpal bone with unspecified laterality

7 ✓7ᵗʰ **S62.399 Other fracture of unspecified metacarpal bone**

✓5ᵗʰ **S62.5 Fracture of thumb**

> **CC Excl:** For CC codes in subcategory S62.5, unless otherwise noted: **CC CC with 7th character B:** S62.501-S62.92X with 7th [A, B]
> **CC CC with 7th character K or P:** M80.00X-M84.68X with 7th [K, P], S02.0XX-S02.92X with 7th K, S12.000-S12.691 with 7th K, S22.000-S22.9XX with 7th K, S32.000-S32.9XX with 7th K, S42.001-S42.92X with 7th [K, P], S49.001-S49.199 with 7th [K, P], S52.001-S52.92X with 7th [K, M, N, P, Q, R], S59.001-S59.299 with 7th [K, P], S62.001-S62.92X with 7th [K, P], S72.001-S72.92X with 7th [K, M, N, P, Q, R], S79.001-S79.199 with 7th [K, P], S82.001-S82.92X with 7th [K, M, N, P, Q, R], S89.001-S89.399 with 7th [K, P], S92.001-S92.919 with 7th [K, P]

✓6ᵗʰ **S62.50 Fracture of unspecified phalanx of thumb**

7 ✓7ᵗʰ **S62.501 Fracture of unspecified phalanx of right thumb** CC

7 ✓7ᵗʰ **S62.502 Fracture of unspecified phalanx of left thumb** CC

---

7 HAC = Initial encounter only (7th character A, B or C) and not POA.

Ⓝ Newborn: 0   Ⓟ Pediatric: 0-17   Ⓜ Maternity: 12-55   Ⓐ Adult: 15-124   **MCC** Major CC Condition   **PDx MCC** PDx acts as own MCC   **CC** CC Condition   **PDx CC** PDx acts as own CC

952   ICD-10-CM Draft (2015)

7 ✓7ᵗʰ **S62.509** **Fracture of unspecified phalanx of unspecified thumb**   CC

✓6ᵗʰ **S62.51** Fracture of proximal phalanx of thumb

7 ✓7ᵗʰ **S62.511** **Displaced fracture of proximal phalanx of right thumb**   CC

7 ✓7ᵗʰ **S62.512** **Displaced fracture of proximal phalanx of left thumb**   CC

7 ✓7ᵗʰ **S62.513** **Displaced fracture of proximal phalanx of unspecified thumb**   CC

7 ✓7ᵗʰ **S62.514** **Nondisplaced fracture of proximal phalanx of right thumb**   CC

7 ✓7ᵗʰ **S62.515** **Nondisplaced fracture of proximal phalanx of left thumb**   CC

7 ✓7ᵗʰ **S62.516** **Nondisplaced fracture of proximal phalanx of unspecified thumb**   CC

✓6ᵗʰ **S62.52** Fracture of distal phalanx of thumb

7 ✓7ᵗʰ **S62.521** **Displaced fracture of distal phalanx of right thumb**   CC

7 ✓7ᵗʰ **S62.522** **Displaced fracture of distal phalanx of left thumb**   CC

7 ✓7ᵗʰ **S62.523** **Displaced fracture of distal phalanx of unspecified thumb**   CC

7 ✓7ᵗʰ **S62.524** **Nondisplaced fracture of distal phalanx of right thumb**   CC

7 ✓7ᵗʰ **S62.525** **Nondisplaced fracture of distal phalanx of left thumb**   CC

7 ✓7ᵗʰ **S62.526** **Nondisplaced fracture of distal phalanx of unspecified thumb**   CC

✓5ᵗʰ **S62.6** Fracture of other and unspecified finger(s)

EXCLUDES 2   fracture of thumb (S62.5-)

CC Excl: For CC codes in subcategory S62.6, unless otherwise noted: See code: S62.2

✓6ᵗʰ **S62.60** Fracture of unspecified phalanx of finger

7 ✓7ᵗʰ **S62.600** **Fracture of unspecified phalanx of right index finger**   CC

7 ✓7ᵗʰ **S62.601** **Fracture of unspecified phalanx of left index finger**   CC

7 ✓7ᵗʰ **S62.602** **Fracture of unspecified phalanx of right middle finger**   CC

7 ✓7ᵗʰ **S62.603** **Fracture of unspecified phalanx of left middle finger**   CC

7 ✓7ᵗʰ **S62.604** **Fracture of unspecified phalanx of right ring finger**   CC

7 ✓7ᵗʰ **S62.605** **Fracture of unspecified phalanx of left ring finger**   CC

7 ✓7ᵗʰ **S62.606** **Fracture of unspecified phalanx of right little finger**   CC

7 ✓7ᵗʰ **S62.607** **Fracture of unspecified phalanx of left little finger**   CC

7 ✓7ᵗʰ **S62.608** **Fracture of unspecified phalanx of other finger**   CC

Fracture of unspecified phalanx of specified finger with unspecified laterality

7 ✓7ᵗʰ **S62.609** **Fracture of unspecified phalanx of unspecified finger**   CC

✓6ᵗʰ **S62.61** Displaced fracture of proximal phalanx of finger

7 ✓7ᵗʰ **S62.610** **Displaced fracture of proximal phalanx of right index finger**   CC

7 ✓7ᵗʰ **S62.611** **Displaced fracture of proximal phalanx of left index finger**   CC

7 ✓7ᵗʰ **S62.612** **Displaced fracture of proximal phalanx of right middle finger**   CC

7 ✓7ᵗʰ **S62.613** **Displaced fracture of proximal phalanx of left middle finger**   CC

7 ✓7ᵗʰ **S62.614** **Displaced fracture of proximal phalanx of right ring finger**   CC

7 ✓7ᵗʰ **S62.615** **Displaced fracture of proximal phalanx of left ring finger**   CC

7 ✓7ᵗʰ **S62.616** **Displaced fracture of proximal phalanx of right little finger**   CC

7 ✓7ᵗʰ **S62.617** **Displaced fracture of proximal phalanx of left little finger**   CC

7 ✓7ᵗʰ **S62.618** **Displaced fracture of proximal phalanx of other finger**   CC

Displaced fracture of proximal phalanx of specified finger with unspecified laterality

7 ✓7ᵗʰ **S62.619** **Displaced fracture of proximal phalanx of unspecified finger**   CC

✓6ᵗʰ **S62.62** Displaced fracture of medial phalanx of finger

7 ✓7ᵗʰ **S62.620** **Displaced fracture of medial phalanx of right index finger**   CC

7 ✓7ᵗʰ **S62.621** **Displaced fracture of medial phalanx of left index finger**   CC

7 ✓7ᵗʰ **S62.622** **Displaced fracture of medial phalanx of right middle finger**   CC

7 ✓7ᵗʰ **S62.623** **Displaced fracture of medial phalanx of left middle finger**   CC

7 ✓7ᵗʰ **S62.624** **Displaced fracture of medial phalanx of right ring finger**   CC

7 ✓7ᵗʰ **S62.625** **Displaced fracture of medial phalanx of left ring finger**   CC

7 ✓7ᵗʰ **S62.626** **Displaced fracture of medial phalanx of right little finger**   CC

7 ✓7ᵗʰ **S62.627** **Displaced fracture of medial phalanx of left little finger**   CC

7 ✓7ᵗʰ **S62.628** **Displaced fracture of medial phalanx of other finger**   CC

Displaced fracture of medial phalanx of specified finger with unspecified laterality

7 ✓7ᵗʰ **S62.629** **Displaced fracture of medial phalanx of unspecified finger**   CC

✓6ᵗʰ **S62.63** Displaced fracture of distal phalanx of finger

7 ✓7ᵗʰ **S62.630** **Displaced fracture of distal phalanx of right index finger**   CC

7 ✓7ᵗʰ **S62.631** **Displaced fracture of distal phalanx of left index finger**   CC

7 ✓7ᵗʰ **S62.632** **Displaced fracture of distal phalanx of right middle finger**   CC

7 ✓7ᵗʰ **S62.633** **Displaced fracture of distal phalanx of left middle finger**   CC

7 ✓7ᵗʰ **S62.634** **Displaced fracture of distal phalanx of right ring finger**   CC

7 ✓7ᵗʰ **S62.635** **Displaced fracture of distal phalanx of left ring finger**   CC

7 ✓7ᵗʰ **S62.636** **Displaced fracture of distal phalanx of right little finger**   CC

7 ✓7ᵗʰ **S62.637** **Displaced fracture of distal phalanx of left little finger**   CC

7 ✓7ᵗʰ **S62.638** **Displaced fracture of distal phalanx of other finger**   CC

Displaced fracture of distal phalanx of specified finger with unspecified laterality

7 ✓7ᵗʰ **S62.639** **Displaced fracture of distal phalanx of unspecified finger**   CC

✓6ᵗʰ **S62.64** Nondisplaced fracture of proximal phalanx of finger

7 ✓7ᵗʰ **S62.640** **Nondisplaced fracture of proximal phalanx of right index finger**   CC

7 ✓7ᵗʰ **S62.641** **Nondisplaced fracture of proximal phalanx of left index finger**   CC

7 ✓7ᵗʰ **S62.642** **Nondisplaced fracture of proximal phalanx of right middle finger**   CC

7 ✓7ᵗʰ **S62.643** **Nondisplaced fracture of proximal phalanx of left middle finger**   CC

7 ✓7ᵗʰ **S62.644** **Nondisplaced fracture of proximal phalanx of right ring finger**   CC

7 ✓7ᵗʰ **S62.645** **Nondisplaced fracture of proximal phalanx of left ring finger**   CC

7 ✓7ᵗʰ **S62.646** **Nondisplaced fracture of proximal phalanx of right little finger**   CC

7 ✓7ᵗʰ **S62.647** **Nondisplaced fracture of proximal phalanx of left little finger**   CC

---

7 HAC = Initial encounter only (7th character A, B or C) and not POA.

✓ Additional Character Required   ✓ˣ7ᵗʰ Xtension Alert   Unacceptable PDx   Manifestation   Hospital Acquired Condition   *EXCLUDES 1* Not Coded Here   *EXCLUDES 2* Not Included Here

7 ✓7ᵗʰ **S62.648** **Nondisplaced fracture of proximal phalanx of other finger**   CC
Nondisplaced fracture of proximal phalanx of specified finger with unspecified laterality

7 ✓7ᵗʰ **S62.649** **Nondisplaced fracture of proximal phalanx of unspecified finger**   CC

✓6ᵗʰ **S62.65** Nondisplaced fracture of medial phalanx of finger

7 ✓7ᵗʰ **S62.650** **Nondisplaced fracture of medial phalanx of right index finger**   CC

7 ✓7ᵗʰ **S62.651** **Nondisplaced fracture of medial phalanx of left index finger**   CC

7 ✓7ᵗʰ **S62.652** **Nondisplaced fracture of medial phalanx of right middle finger**   CC

7 ✓7ᵗʰ **S62.653** **Nondisplaced fracture of medial phalanx of left middle finger**   CC

7 ✓7ᵗʰ **S62.654** **Nondisplaced fracture of medial phalanx of right ring finger**   CC

7 ✓7ᵗʰ **S62.655** **Nondisplaced fracture of medial phalanx of left ring finger**   CC

7 ✓7ᵗʰ **S62.656** **Nondisplaced fracture of medial phalanx of right little finger**   CC

7 ✓7ᵗʰ **S62.657** **Nondisplaced fracture of medial phalanx of left little finger**   CC

7 ✓7ᵗʰ **S62.658** **Nondisplaced fracture of medial phalanx of other finger**   CC
Nondisplaced fracture of medial phalanx of specified finger with unspecified laterality

7 ✓7ᵗʰ **S62.659** **Nondisplaced fracture of medial phalanx of unspecified finger**   CC

✓6ᵗʰ **S62.66** Nondisplaced fracture of distal phalanx of finger

7 ✓7ᵗʰ **S62.660** **Nondisplaced fracture of distal phalanx of right index finger**   CC

7 ✓7ᵗʰ **S62.661** **Nondisplaced fracture of distal phalanx of left index finger**   CC

7 ✓7ᵗʰ **S62.662** **Nondisplaced fracture of distal phalanx of right middle finger**   CC

7 ✓7ᵗʰ **S62.663** **Nondisplaced fracture of distal phalanx of left middle finger**   CC

7 ✓7ᵗʰ **S62.664** **Nondisplaced fracture of distal phalanx of right ring finger**   CC

7 ✓7ᵗʰ **S62.665** **Nondisplaced fracture of distal phalanx of left ring finger**   CC

7 ✓7ᵗʰ **S62.666** **Nondisplaced fracture of distal phalanx of right little finger**   CC

7 ✓7ᵗʰ **S62.667** **Nondisplaced fracture of distal phalanx of left little finger**   CC

7 ✓7ᵗʰ **S62.668** **Nondisplaced fracture of distal phalanx of other finger**   CC
Nondisplaced fracture of distal phalanx of specified finger with unspecified laterality

7 ✓7ᵗʰ **S62.669** **Nondisplaced fracture of distal phalanx of unspecified finger**   CC

✓5ᵗʰ **S62.9** **Unspecified fracture of wrist and hand**

7 ✓x7ᵗʰ **S62.90** **Unspecified fracture of unspecified wrist and hand**   CC
CC Excl: CC CC with 7th character B: S42.201-S42.92X with 7th [A, B], S49.001-S49.199 with 7th A, S52.001-S52.009 with 7th [A, B, C], S52.021-S52.109 with 7th [A, B, C], S52.121-S52.516 with 7th [A, B, C], S52.531-S52.616 with 7th [A, B, C], S52.691-S52.92X with 7th [A, B, C], S59.001-S59.299 with 7th A, S62.001-S62.92X with 7th [A, B]
CC CC with 7th character K or P: M80.00X-M84.68X with 7th [K, P], S02.0XX-S02.92X with 7th K, S12.000-S12.691 with 7th K, S22.000-S22.9XX with 7th K, S32.000-S32.9XX with 7th K, S42.001-S42.92X with 7th [K, P], S49.001-S49.199 with 7th [K, P], S52.001-S52.92X with 7th [K, M, N, P, Q, R], S59.001-S59.299 with 7th [K, P], S62.001-S62.92X with 7th [K, P], S72.001-S72.92X with 7th [K, M, N, P, Q, R], S79.001-S79.199 with 7th [K, P], S82.001-S82.92X with 7th [K, M, N, P, Q, R], S89.001-S89.399 with 7th [K, P], S92.001-S92.919 with 7th [K, P]

7 ✓x7ᵗʰ **S62.91** **Unspecified fracture of right wrist and hand**   CC
CC Excl: CC CC with 7th character B: S62.501-S62.92X with 7th [A, B]
CC CC with 7th character K or P: M80.00X-M84.68X with 7th [K, P], S02.0XX-S02.92X with 7th K, S12.000-S12.691 with 7th K, S22.000-S22.9XX with 7th K, S32.000-S32.9XX with 7th K, S42.001-S42.92X with 7th [K, P], S49.001-S49.199 with 7th [K, P], S52.001-S52.92X with 7th [K, M, N, P, Q, R], S59.001-S59.299 with 7th [K, P], S62.001-S62.92X with 7th [K, P], S72.001-S72.92X with 7th [K, M, N, P, Q, R], S79.001-S79.199 with 7th [K, P], S82.001-S82.92X with 7th [K, M, N, P, Q, R], S89.001-S89.399 with 7th [K, P], S92.001-S92.919 with 7th [K, P]

7 ✓x7ᵗʰ **S62.92** **Unspecified fracture of left wrist and hand**   CC
CC Excl: See code: S62.91

✓4ᵗʰ **S63** **Dislocation and sprain of joints and ligaments at wrist and hand level**
INCLUDES   avulsion of joint or ligament at wrist and hand level
laceration of cartilage, joint or ligament at wrist and hand level
sprain of cartilage, joint or ligament at wrist and hand level
traumatic hemarthrosis of joint or ligament at wrist and hand level
traumatic rupture of joint or ligament at wrist and hand level
traumatic subluxation of joint or ligament at wrist and hand level
traumatic tear of joint or ligament at wrist and hand level
Code also any associated open wound
EXCLUDES 2   strain of muscle, fascia and tendon of wrist and hand (S66.-)

The appropriate 7th character is to be added to each code from category S63.
A   initial encounter
D   subsequent encounter
S   sequela

✓5ᵗʰ **S63.0** **Subluxation and dislocation of wrist and hand joints**

✓6ᵗʰ **S63.00** **Unspecified subluxation and dislocation of wrist and hand**
Dislocation of carpal bone NOS
Dislocation of distal end of radius NOS
Subluxation of carpal bone NOS
Subluxation of distal end of radius NOS

✓7ᵗʰ **S63.001** **Unspecified subluxation of right wrist and hand**

✓7ᵗʰ **S63.002** **Unspecified subluxation of left wrist and hand**

✓7ᵗʰ **S63.003** **Unspecified subluxation of unspecified wrist and hand**

✓7ᵗʰ **S63.004** **Unspecified dislocation of right wrist and hand**

✓7ᵗʰ **S63.005** **Unspecified dislocation of left wrist and hand**

✓7ᵗʰ **S63.006** **Unspecified dislocation of unspecified wrist and hand**

✓6ᵗʰ **S63.01** **Subluxation and dislocation of distal radioulnar joint**

✓7ᵗʰ **S63.011** **Subluxation of distal radioulnar joint of right wrist**

✓7ᵗʰ **S63.012** **Subluxation of distal radioulnar joint of left wrist**

✓7ᵗʰ **S63.013** **Subluxation of distal radioulnar joint of unspecified wrist**

✓7ᵗʰ **S63.014** **Dislocation of distal radioulnar joint of right wrist**

✓7ᵗʰ **S63.015** **Dislocation of distal radioulnar joint of left wrist**

✓7ᵗʰ **S63.016** **Dislocation of distal radioulnar joint of unspecified wrist**

✓6ᵗʰ **S63.02** **Subluxation and dislocation of radiocarpal joint**

✓7ᵗʰ **S63.021** **Subluxation of radiocarpal joint of right wrist**

✓7ᵗʰ **S63.022** **Subluxation of radiocarpal joint of left wrist**

✓7ᵗʰ **S63.023** **Subluxation of radiocarpal joint of unspecified wrist**

✓7ᵗʰ **S63.024** **Dislocation of radiocarpal joint of right wrist**

---

7 HAC = Initial encounter only (7th character A, B or C) and not POA.

N Newborn: 0   P Pediatric: 0-17   M Maternity: 12-55   A Adult: 15-124   MCC Major CC Condition   PDx MCC PDx acts as own MCC   CC CC Condition   PDx CC PDx acts as own CC

954   ICD-10-CM Draft (2015)

√7ᵗʰ **S63.025** Dislocation of radiocarpal joint of left wrist

√7ᵗʰ **S63.026** Dislocation of radiocarpal joint of unspecified wrist

√6ᵗʰ **S63.03** Subluxation and dislocation of midcarpal joint

√7ᵗʰ **S63.031** Subluxation of midcarpal joint of right wrist

√7ᵗʰ **S63.032** Subluxation of midcarpal joint of left wrist

√7ᵗʰ **S63.033** Subluxation of midcarpal joint of unspecified wrist

√7ᵗʰ **S63.034** Dislocation of midcarpal joint of right wrist

√7ᵗʰ **S63.035** Dislocation of midcarpal joint of left wrist

√7ᵗʰ **S63.036** Dislocation of midcarpal joint of unspecified wrist

√6ᵗʰ **S63.04** Subluxation and dislocation of carpometacarpal joint of thumb

> EXCLUDES 2   interphalangeal subluxation and dislocation of thumb (S63.1-)

√7ᵗʰ **S63.041** Subluxation of carpometacarpal joint of right thumb

√7ᵗʰ **S63.042** Subluxation of carpometacarpal joint of left thumb

√7ᵗʰ **S63.043** Subluxation of carpometacarpal joint of unspecified thumb

√7ᵗʰ **S63.044** Dislocation of carpometacarpal joint of right thumb

√7ᵗʰ **S63.045** Dislocation of carpometacarpal joint of left thumb

√7ᵗʰ **S63.046** Dislocation of carpometacarpal joint of unspecified thumb

√6ᵗʰ **S63.05** Subluxation and dislocation of other carpometacarpal joint

> EXCLUDES 2   subluxation and dislocation of carpometacarpal joint of thumb (S63.04-)

√7ᵗʰ **S63.051** Subluxation of other carpometacarpal joint of right hand

√7ᵗʰ **S63.052** Subluxation of other carpometacarpal joint of left hand

√7ᵗʰ **S63.053** Subluxation of other carpometacarpal joint of unspecified hand

√7ᵗʰ **S63.054** Dislocation of other carpometacarpal joint of right hand

√7ᵗʰ **S63.055** Dislocation of other carpometacarpal joint of left hand

√7ᵗʰ **S63.056** Dislocation of other carpometacarpal joint of unspecified hand

√6ᵗʰ **S63.06** Subluxation and dislocation of metacarpal (bone), proximal end

√7ᵗʰ **S63.061** Subluxation of metacarpal (bone), proximal end of right hand

√7ᵗʰ **S63.062** Subluxation of metacarpal (bone), proximal end of left hand

√7ᵗʰ **S63.063** Subluxation of metacarpal (bone), proximal end of unspecified hand

√7ᵗʰ **S63.064** Dislocation of metacarpal (bone), proximal end of right hand

√7ᵗʰ **S63.065** Dislocation of metacarpal (bone), proximal end of left hand

√7ᵗʰ **S63.066** Dislocation of metacarpal (bone), proximal end of unspecified hand

√6ᵗʰ **S63.07** Subluxation and dislocation of distal end of ulna

√7ᵗʰ **S63.071** Subluxation of distal end of right ulna

√7ᵗʰ **S63.072** Subluxation of distal end of left ulna

√7ᵗʰ **S63.073** Subluxation of distal end of unspecified ulna

√7ᵗʰ **S63.074** Dislocation of distal end of right ulna

√7ᵗʰ **S63.075** Dislocation of distal end of left ulna

√7ᵗʰ **S63.076** Dislocation of distal end of unspecified ulna

√6ᵗʰ **S63.09** Other subluxation and dislocation of wrist and hand

√7ᵗʰ **S63.091** Other subluxation of right wrist and hand

√7ᵗʰ **S63.092** Other subluxation of left wrist and hand

√7ᵗʰ **S63.093** Other subluxation of unspecified wrist and hand

√7ᵗʰ **S63.094** Other dislocation of right wrist and hand

√7ᵗʰ **S63.095** Other dislocation of left wrist and hand

√7ᵗʰ **S63.096** Other dislocation of unspecified wrist and hand

√5ᵗʰ **S63.1** Subluxation and dislocation of thumb

√6ᵗʰ **S63.10** Unspecified subluxation and dislocation of thumb

√7ᵗʰ **S63.101** Unspecified subluxation of right thumb

√7ᵗʰ **S63.102** Unspecified subluxation of left thumb

√7ᵗʰ **S63.103** Unspecified subluxation of unspecified thumb

√7ᵗʰ **S63.104** Unspecified dislocation of right thumb

√7ᵗʰ **S63.105** Unspecified dislocation of left thumb

√7ᵗʰ **S63.106** Unspecified dislocation of unspecified thumb

√6ᵗʰ **S63.11** Subluxation and dislocation of metacarpophalangeal joint of thumb

√7ᵗʰ **S63.111** Subluxation of metacarpophalangeal joint of right thumb

√7ᵗʰ **S63.112** Subluxation of metacarpophalangeal joint of left thumb

√7ᵗʰ **S63.113** Subluxation of metacarpophalangeal joint of unspecified thumb

√7ᵗʰ **S63.114** Dislocation of metacarpophalangeal joint of right thumb

√7ᵗʰ **S63.115** Dislocation of metacarpophalangeal joint of left thumb

√7ᵗʰ **S63.116** Dislocation of metacarpophalangeal joint of unspecified thumb

√6ᵗʰ **S63.12** Subluxation and dislocation of unspecified interphalangeal joint of thumb

√7ᵗʰ **S63.121** Subluxation of unspecified interphalangeal joint of right thumb

√7ᵗʰ **S63.122** Subluxation of unspecified interphalangeal joint of left thumb

√7ᵗʰ **S63.123** Subluxation of unspecified interphalangeal joint of unspecified thumb

√7ᵗʰ **S63.124** Dislocation of unspecified interphalangeal joint of right thumb

√7ᵗʰ **S63.125** Dislocation of unspecified interphalangeal joint of left thumb

√7ᵗʰ **S63.126** Dislocation of unspecified interphalangeal joint of unspecified thumb

√6ᵗʰ **S63.13** Subluxation and dislocation of proximal interphalangeal joint of thumb

√7ᵗʰ **S63.131** Subluxation of proximal interphalangeal joint of right thumb

√7ᵗʰ **S63.132** Subluxation of proximal interphalangeal joint of left thumb

√7ᵗʰ **S63.133** Subluxation of proximal interphalangeal joint of unspecified thumb

√7ᵗʰ **S63.134** Dislocation of proximal interphalangeal joint of right thumb

√7ᵗʰ **S63.135** Dislocation of proximal interphalangeal joint of left thumb

√7ᵗʰ **S63.136** Dislocation of proximal interphalangeal joint of unspecified thumb

√6ᵗʰ **S63.14** Subluxation and dislocation of distal interphalangeal joint of thumb

√7ᵗʰ **S63.141** Subluxation of distal interphalangeal joint of right thumb

√7ᵗʰ **S63.142** Subluxation of distal interphalangeal joint of left thumb

√7ᵗʰ **S63.143** Subluxation of distal interphalangeal joint of unspecified thumb

√7ᵗʰ **S63.144** Dislocation of distal interphalangeal joint of right thumb

√7ᵗʰ **S63.145** Dislocation of distal interphalangeal joint of left thumb

√7ᵗʰ **S63.146** Dislocation of distal interphalangeal joint of unspecified thumb

✓5ᵗʰ S63.2 Subluxation and dislocation of other finger(s)
> EXCLUDES 2 subluxation and dislocation of thumb (S63.1-)

✓6ᵗʰ S63.20 Unspecified subluxation of other finger
- ✓7ᵗʰ S63.200 Unspecified subluxation of right index finger
- ✓7ᵗʰ S63.201 Unspecified subluxation of left index finger
- ✓7ᵗʰ S63.202 Unspecified subluxation of right middle finger
- ✓7ᵗʰ S63.203 Unspecified subluxation of left middle finger
- ✓7ᵗʰ S63.204 Unspecified subluxation of right ring finger
- ✓7ᵗʰ S63.205 Unspecified subluxation of left ring finger
- ✓7ᵗʰ S63.206 Unspecified subluxation of right little finger
- ✓7ᵗʰ S63.207 Unspecified subluxation of left little finger
- ✓7ᵗʰ S63.208 Unspecified subluxation of other finger
  Unspecified subluxation of specified finger with unspecified laterality
- ✓7ᵗʰ S63.209 Unspecified subluxation of unspecified finger

✓6ᵗʰ S63.21 Subluxation of metacarpophalangeal joint of finger
- ✓7ᵗʰ S63.210 Subluxation of metacarpophalangeal joint of right index finger
- ✓7ᵗʰ S63.211 Subluxation of metacarpophalangeal joint of left index finger
- ✓7ᵗʰ S63.212 Subluxation of metacarpophalangeal joint of right middle finger
- ✓7ᵗʰ S63.213 Subluxation of metacarpophalangeal joint of left middle finger
- ✓7ᵗʰ S63.214 Subluxation of metacarpophalangeal joint of right ring finger
- ✓7ᵗʰ S63.215 Subluxation of metacarpophalangeal joint of left ring finger
- ✓7ᵗʰ S63.216 Subluxation of metacarpophalangeal joint of right little finger
- ✓7ᵗʰ S63.217 Subluxation of metacarpophalangeal joint of left little finger
- ✓7ᵗʰ S63.218 Subluxation of metacarpophalangeal joint of other finger
  Subluxation of metacarpophalangeal joint of specified finger with unspecified laterality
- ✓7ᵗʰ S63.219 Subluxation of metacarpophalangeal joint of unspecified finger

✓6ᵗʰ S63.22 Subluxation of unspecified interphalangeal joint of finger
- ✓7ᵗʰ S63.220 Subluxation of unspecified interphalangeal joint of right index finger
- ✓7ᵗʰ S63.221 Subluxation of unspecified interphalangeal joint of left index finger
- ✓7ᵗʰ S63.222 Subluxation of unspecified interphalangeal joint of right middle finger
- ✓7ᵗʰ S63.223 Subluxation of unspecified interphalangeal joint of left middle finger
- ✓7ᵗʰ S63.224 Subluxation of unspecified interphalangeal joint of right ring finger
- ✓7ᵗʰ S63.225 Subluxation of unspecified interphalangeal joint of left ring finger
- ✓7ᵗʰ S63.226 Subluxation of unspecified interphalangeal joint of right little finger
- ✓7ᵗʰ S63.227 Subluxation of unspecified interphalangeal joint of left little finger
- ✓7ᵗʰ S63.228 Subluxation of unspecified interphalangeal joint of other finger
  Subluxation of unspecified interphalangeal joint of specified finger with unspecified laterality
- ✓7ᵗʰ S63.229 Subluxation of unspecified interphalangeal joint of unspecified finger

✓6ᵗʰ S63.23 Subluxation of proximal interphalangeal joint of finger
- ✓7ᵗʰ S63.230 Subluxation of proximal interphalangeal joint of right index finger
- ✓7ᵗʰ S63.231 Subluxation of proximal interphalangeal joint of left index finger
- ✓7ᵗʰ S63.232 Subluxation of proximal interphalangeal joint of right middle finger
- ✓7ᵗʰ S63.233 Subluxation of proximal interphalangeal joint of left middle finger
- ✓7ᵗʰ S63.234 Subluxation of proximal interphalangeal joint of right ring finger
- ✓7ᵗʰ S63.235 Subluxation of proximal interphalangeal joint of left ring finger
- ✓7ᵗʰ S63.236 Subluxation of proximal interphalangeal joint of right little finger
- ✓7ᵗʰ S63.237 Subluxation of proximal interphalangeal joint of left little finger
- ✓7ᵗʰ S63.238 Subluxation of proximal interphalangeal joint of other finger
  Subluxation of proximal interphalangeal joint of specified finger with unspecified laterality
- ✓7ᵗʰ S63.239 Subluxation of proximal interphalangeal joint of unspecified finger

✓6ᵗʰ S63.24 Subluxation of distal interphalangeal joint of finger
- ✓7ᵗʰ S63.240 Subluxation of distal interphalangeal joint of right index finger
- ✓7ᵗʰ S63.241 Subluxation of distal interphalangeal joint of left index finger
- ✓7ᵗʰ S63.242 Subluxation of distal interphalangeal joint of right middle finger
- ✓7ᵗʰ S63.243 Subluxation of distal interphalangeal joint of left middle finger
- ✓7ᵗʰ S63.244 Subluxation of distal interphalangeal joint of right ring finger
- ✓7ᵗʰ S63.245 Subluxation of distal interphalangeal joint of left ring finger
- ✓7ᵗʰ S63.246 Subluxation of distal interphalangeal joint of right little finger
- ✓7ᵗʰ S63.247 Subluxation of distal interphalangeal joint of left little finger
- ✓7ᵗʰ S63.248 Subluxation of distal interphalangeal joint of other finger
  Subluxation of distal interphalangeal joint of specified finger with unspecified laterality
- ✓7ᵗʰ S63.249 Subluxation of distal interphalangeal joint of unspecified finger

✓6ᵗʰ S63.25 Unspecified dislocation of other finger
- ✓7ᵗʰ S63.250 Unspecified dislocation of right index finger
- ✓7ᵗʰ S63.251 Unspecified dislocation of left index finger
- ✓7ᵗʰ S63.252 Unspecified dislocation of right middle finger
- ✓7ᵗʰ S63.253 Unspecified dislocation of left middle finger
- ✓7ᵗʰ S63.254 Unspecified dislocation of right ring finger
- ✓7ᵗʰ S63.255 Unspecified dislocation of left ring finger
- ✓7ᵗʰ S63.256 Unspecified dislocation of right little finger
- ✓7ᵗʰ S63.257 Unspecified dislocation of left little finger
- ✓7ᵗʰ S63.258 Unspecified dislocation of other finger
  Unspecified dislocation of specified finger with unspecified laterality
- ✓7ᵗʰ S63.259 Unspecified dislocation of unspecified finger
  Unspecified dislocation of specified finger with unspecified laterality

✓6ᵗʰ S63.26 Dislocation of metacarpophalangeal joint of finger
- ✓7ᵗʰ S63.260 Dislocation of metacarpophalangeal joint of right index finger
- ✓7ᵗʰ S63.261 Dislocation of metacarpophalangeal joint of left index finger
- ✓7ᵗʰ S63.262 Dislocation of metacarpophalangeal joint of right middle finger
- ✓7ᵗʰ S63.263 Dislocation of metacarpophalangeal joint of left middle finger
- ✓7ᵗʰ S63.264 Dislocation of metacarpophalangeal joint of right ring finger

√7ᵗʰ **S63.265** Dislocation of metacarpophalangeal joint of left ring finger

√7ᵗʰ **S63.266** Dislocation of metacarpophalangeal joint of right little finger

√7ᵗʰ **S63.267** Dislocation of metacarpophalangeal joint of left little finger

√7ᵗʰ **S63.268** Dislocation of metacarpophalangeal joint of other finger
> Dislocation of metacarpophalangeal joint of specified finger with unspecified laterality

√7ᵗʰ **S63.269** Dislocation of metacarpophalangeal joint of unspecified finger

√6ᵗʰ **S63.27** Dislocation of unspecified interphalangeal joint of finger

√7ᵗʰ **S63.270** Dislocation of unspecified interphalangeal joint of right index finger

√7ᵗʰ **S63.271** Dislocation of unspecified interphalangeal joint of left index finger

√7ᵗʰ **S63.272** Dislocation of unspecified interphalangeal joint of right middle finger

√7ᵗʰ **S63.273** Dislocation of unspecified interphalangeal joint of left middle finger

√7ᵗʰ **S63.274** Dislocation of unspecified interphalangeal joint of right ring finger

√7ᵗʰ **S63.275** Dislocation of unspecified interphalangeal joint of left ring finger

√7ᵗʰ **S63.276** Dislocation of unspecified interphalangeal joint of right little finger

√7ᵗʰ **S63.277** Dislocation of unspecified interphalangeal joint of left little finger

√7ᵗʰ **S63.278** Dislocation of unspecified interphalangeal joint of other finger
> Dislocation of unspecified interphalangeal joint of specified finger with unspecified laterality

√7ᵗʰ **S63.279** Dislocation of unspecified interphalangeal joint of unspecified finger
> Dislocation of unspecified interphalangeal joint of specified finger without specified laterality

√6ᵗʰ **S63.28** Dislocation of proximal interphalangeal joint of finger

√7ᵗʰ **S63.280** Dislocation of proximal interphalangeal joint of right index finger

√7ᵗʰ **S63.281** Dislocation of proximal interphalangeal joint of left index finger

√7ᵗʰ **S63.282** Dislocation of proximal interphalangeal joint of right middle finger

√7ᵗʰ **S63.283** Dislocation of proximal interphalangeal joint of left middle finger

√7ᵗʰ **S63.284** Dislocation of proximal interphalangeal joint of right ring finger

√7ᵗʰ **S63.285** Dislocation of proximal interphalangeal joint of left ring finger

√7ᵗʰ **S63.286** Dislocation of proximal interphalangeal joint of right little finger

√7ᵗʰ **S63.287** Dislocation of proximal interphalangeal joint of left little finger

√7ᵗʰ **S63.288** Dislocation of proximal interphalangeal joint of other finger
> Dislocation of proximal interphalangeal joint of specified finger with unspecified laterality

√7ᵗʰ **S63.289** Dislocation of proximal interphalangeal joint of unspecified finger

√6ᵗʰ **S63.29** Dislocation of distal interphalangeal joint of finger

√7ᵗʰ **S63.290** Dislocation of distal interphalangeal joint of right index finger

√7ᵗʰ **S63.291** Dislocation of distal interphalangeal joint of left index finger

√7ᵗʰ **S63.292** Dislocation of distal interphalangeal joint of right middle finger

√7ᵗʰ **S63.293** Dislocation of distal interphalangeal joint of left middle finger

√7ᵗʰ **S63.294** Dislocation of distal interphalangeal joint of right ring finger

√7ᵗʰ **S63.295** Dislocation of distal interphalangeal joint of left ring finger

√7ᵗʰ **S63.296** Dislocation of distal interphalangeal joint of right little finger

√7ᵗʰ **S63.297** Dislocation of distal interphalangeal joint of left little finger

√7ᵗʰ **S63.298** Dislocation of distal interphalangeal joint of other finger
> Dislocation of distal interphalangeal joint of specified finger with unspecified laterality

√7ᵗʰ **S63.299** Dislocation of distal interphalangeal joint of unspecified finger

√5ᵗʰ **S63.3** Traumatic rupture of ligament of wrist

√6ᵗʰ **S63.30** Traumatic rupture of unspecified ligament of wrist

√7ᵗʰ **S63.301** Traumatic rupture of unspecified ligament of right wrist

√7ᵗʰ **S63.302** Traumatic rupture of unspecified ligament of left wrist

√7ᵗʰ **S63.309** Traumatic rupture of unspecified ligament of unspecified wrist

√6ᵗʰ **S63.31** Traumatic rupture of collateral ligament of wrist

√7ᵗʰ **S63.311** Traumatic rupture of collateral ligament of right wrist

√7ᵗʰ **S63.312** Traumatic rupture of collateral ligament of left wrist

√7ᵗʰ **S63.319** Traumatic rupture of collateral ligament of unspecified wrist

√6ᵗʰ **S63.32** Traumatic rupture of radiocarpal ligament

√7ᵗʰ **S63.321** Traumatic rupture of right radiocarpal ligament

√7ᵗʰ **S63.322** Traumatic rupture of left radiocarpal ligament

√7ᵗʰ **S63.329** Traumatic rupture of unspecified radiocarpal ligament

√6ᵗʰ **S63.33** Traumatic rupture of ulnocarpal (palmar) ligament

√7ᵗʰ **S63.331** Traumatic rupture of right ulnocarpal (palmar) ligament

√7ᵗʰ **S63.332** Traumatic rupture of left ulnocarpal (palmar) ligament

√7ᵗʰ **S63.339** Traumatic rupture of unspecified ulnocarpal (palmar) ligament

√6ᵗʰ **S63.39** Traumatic rupture of other ligament of wrist

√7ᵗʰ **S63.391** Traumatic rupture of other ligament of right wrist

√7ᵗʰ **S63.392** Traumatic rupture of other ligament of left wrist

√7ᵗʰ **S63.399** Traumatic rupture of other ligament of unspecified wrist

√5ᵗʰ **S63.4** Traumatic rupture of ligament of finger at metacarpophalangeal and interphalangeal joint(s)

√6ᵗʰ **S63.40** Traumatic rupture of unspecified ligament of finger at metacarpophalangeal and interphalangeal joint

√7ᵗʰ **S63.400** Traumatic rupture of unspecified ligament of right index finger at metacarpophalangeal and interphalangeal joint

√7ᵗʰ **S63.401** Traumatic rupture of unspecified ligament of left index finger at metacarpophalangeal and interphalangeal joint

√7ᵗʰ **S63.402** Traumatic rupture of unspecified ligament of right middle finger at metacarpophalangeal and interphalangeal joint

√7ᵗʰ **S63.403** Traumatic rupture of unspecified ligament of left middle finger at metacarpophalangeal and interphalangeal joint

√7ᵗʰ **S63.404** Traumatic rupture of unspecified ligament of right ring finger at metacarpophalangeal and interphalangeal joint

---

☑ Additional Character Required   √x7ᵗʰ Xtension Alert   Unacceptable PDx   Manifestation   Hospital Acquired Condition   **EXCLUDES 1** Not Coded Here   **EXCLUDES 2** Not Included Here

✓7th **S63.405** **Traumatic rupture of unspecified ligament of left ring finger at metacarpophalangeal and interphalangeal joint**

✓7th **S63.406** **Traumatic rupture of unspecified ligament of right little finger at metacarpophalangeal and interphalangeal joint**

✓7th **S63.407** **Traumatic rupture of unspecified ligament of left little finger at metacarpophalangeal and interphalangeal joint**

✓7th **S63.408** **Traumatic rupture of unspecified ligament of other finger at metacarpophalangeal and interphalangeal joint**
> Traumatic rupture of unspecified ligament of specified finger with unspecified laterality at metacarpophalangeal and interphalangeal joint

✓7th **S63.409** **Traumatic rupture of unspecified ligament of unspecified finger at metacarpophalangeal and interphalangeal joint**

✓6th **S63.41** **Traumatic rupture of collateral ligament of finger at metacarpophalangeal and interphalangeal joint**

✓7th **S63.410** **Traumatic rupture of collateral ligament of right index finger at metacarpophalangeal and interphalangeal joint**

✓7th **S63.411** **Traumatic rupture of collateral ligament of left index finger at metacarpophalangeal and interphalangeal joint**

✓7th **S63.412** **Traumatic rupture of collateral ligament of right middle finger at metacarpophalangeal and interphalangeal joint**

✓7th **S63.413** **Traumatic rupture of collateral ligament of left middle finger at metacarpophalangeal and interphalangeal joint**

✓7th **S63.414** **Traumatic rupture of collateral ligament of right ring finger at metacarpophalangeal and interphalangeal joint**

✓7th **S63.415** **Traumatic rupture of collateral ligament of left ring finger at metacarpophalangeal and interphalangeal joint**

✓7th **S63.416** **Traumatic rupture of collateral ligament of right little finger at metacarpophalangeal and interphalangeal joint**

✓7th **S63.417** **Traumatic rupture of collateral ligament of left little finger at metacarpophalangeal and interphalangeal joint**

✓7th **S63.418** **Traumatic rupture of collateral ligament of other finger at metacarpophalangeal and interphalangeal joint**
> Traumatic rupture of collateral ligament of specified finger with unspecified laterality at metacarpophalangeal and interphalangeal joint

✓7th **S63.419** **Traumatic rupture of collateral ligament of unspecified finger at metacarpophalangeal and interphalangeal joint**

✓6th **S63.42** **Traumatic rupture of palmar ligament of finger at metacarpophalangeal and interphalangeal joint**

✓7th **S63.420** **Traumatic rupture of palmar ligament of right index finger at metacarpophalangeal and interphalangeal joint**

✓7th **S63.421** **Traumatic rupture of palmar ligament of left index finger at metacarpophalangeal and interphalangeal joint**

✓7th **S63.422** **Traumatic rupture of palmar ligament of right middle finger at metacarpophalangeal and interphalangeal joint**

✓7th **S63.423** **Traumatic rupture of palmar ligament of left middle finger at metacarpophalangeal and interphalangeal joint**

✓7th **S63.424** **Traumatic rupture of palmar ligament of right ring finger at metacarpophalangeal and interphalangeal joint**

✓7th **S63.425** **Traumatic rupture of palmar ligament of left ring finger at metacarpophalangeal and interphalangeal joint**

✓7th **S63.426** **Traumatic rupture of palmar ligament of right little finger at metacarpophalangeal and interphalangeal joint**

✓7th **S63.427** **Traumatic rupture of palmar ligament of left little finger at metacarpophalangeal and interphalangeal joint**

✓7th **S63.428** **Traumatic rupture of palmar ligament of other finger at metacarpophalangeal and interphalangeal joint**
> Traumatic rupture of palmar ligament of specified finger with unspecified laterality at metacarpophalangeal and interphalangeal joint

✓7th **S63.429** **Traumatic rupture of palmar ligament of unspecified finger at metacarpophalangeal and interphalangeal joint**

✓6th **S63.43** **Traumatic rupture of volar plate of finger at metacarpophalangeal and interphalangeal joint**

✓7th **S63.430** **Traumatic rupture of volar plate of right index finger at metacarpophalangeal and interphalangeal joint**

✓7th **S63.431** **Traumatic rupture of volar plate of left index finger at metacarpophalangeal and interphalangeal joint**

✓7th **S63.432** **Traumatic rupture of volar plate of right middle finger at metacarpophalangeal and interphalangeal joint**

✓7th **S63.433** **Traumatic rupture of volar plate of left middle finger at metacarpophalangeal and interphalangeal joint**

✓7th **S63.434** **Traumatic rupture of volar plate of right ring finger at metacarpophalangeal and interphalangeal joint**

✓7th **S63.435** **Traumatic rupture of volar plate of left ring finger at metacarpophalangeal and interphalangeal joint**

✓7th **S63.436** **Traumatic rupture of volar plate of right little finger at metacarpophalangeal and interphalangeal joint**

✓7th **S63.437** **Traumatic rupture of volar plate of left little finger at metacarpophalangeal and interphalangeal joint**

✓7th **S63.438** **Traumatic rupture of volar plate of other finger at metacarpophalangeal and interphalangeal joint**
> Traumatic rupture of volar plate of specified finger with unspecified laterality at metacarpophalangeal and interphalangeal joint

✓7th **S63.439** **Traumatic rupture of volar plate of unspecified finger at metacarpophalangeal and interphalangeal joint**

✓6th **S63.49** **Traumatic rupture of other ligament of finger at metacarpophalangeal and interphalangeal joint**

✓7th **S63.490** **Traumatic rupture of other ligament of right index finger at metacarpophalangeal and interphalangeal joint**

✓7th **S63.491** **Traumatic rupture of other ligament of left index finger at metacarpophalangeal and interphalangeal joint**

✓7th **S63.492** **Traumatic rupture of other ligament of right middle finger at metacarpophalangeal and interphalangeal joint**

N Newborn: 0   P Pediatric: 0-17   M Maternity: 12-55   A Adult: 15-124   MCC Major CC Condition   PDx MCC PDx acts as own MCC   CC CC Condition   PDx CC PDx acts as own CC

958   ICD-10-CM Draft (2015)

√7ᵗʰ **S63.493** **Traumatic rupture of other ligament of left middle finger at metacarpophalangeal and interphalangeal joint**

√7ᵗʰ **S63.494** **Traumatic rupture of other ligament of right ring finger at metacarpophalangeal and interphalangeal joint**

√7ᵗʰ **S63.495** **Traumatic rupture of other ligament of left ring finger at metacarpophalangeal and interphalangeal joint**

√7ᵗʰ **S63.496** **Traumatic rupture of other ligament of right little finger at metacarpophalangeal and interphalangeal joint**

√7ᵗʰ **S63.497** **Traumatic rupture of other ligament of left little finger at metacarpophalangeal and interphalangeal joint**

√7ᵗʰ **S63.498** **Traumatic rupture of other ligament of other finger at metacarpophalangeal and interphalangeal joint**

Traumatic rupture of ligament of specified finger with unspecified laterality at metacarpophalangeal and interphalangeal joint

√7ᵗʰ **S63.499** **Traumatic rupture of other ligament of unspecified finger at metacarpophalangeal and interphalangeal joint**

√5ᵗʰ **S63.5** **Other and unspecified sprain of wrist**

√6ᵗʰ **S63.50** **Unspecified sprain of wrist**

√7ᵗʰ **S63.501** **Unspecified sprain of right wrist**

√7ᵗʰ **S63.502** **Unspecified sprain of left wrist**

√7ᵗʰ **S63.509** **Unspecified sprain of unspecified wrist**

√6ᵗʰ **S63.51** **Sprain of carpal (joint)**

√7ᵗʰ **S63.511** **Sprain of carpal joint of right wrist**

√7ᵗʰ **S63.512** **Sprain of carpal joint of left wrist**

√7ᵗʰ **S63.519** **Sprain of carpal joint of unspecified wrist**

√6ᵗʰ **S63.52** **Sprain of radiocarpal joint**

EXCLUDES 1 traumatic rupture of radiocarpal ligament (S63.32-)

√7ᵗʰ **S63.521** **Sprain of radiocarpal joint of right wrist**

√7ᵗʰ **S63.522** **Sprain of radiocarpal joint of left wrist**

√7ᵗʰ **S63.529** **Sprain of radiocarpal joint of unspecified wrist**

√6ᵗʰ **S63.59** **Other specified sprain of wrist**

√7ᵗʰ **S63.591** **Other specified sprain of right wrist**

√7ᵗʰ **S63.592** **Other specified sprain of left wrist**

√7ᵗʰ **S63.599** **Other specified sprain of unspecified wrist**

√5ᵗʰ **S63.6** **Other and unspecified sprain of finger(s)**

EXCLUDES 1 traumatic rupture of ligament of finger at metacarpophalangeal and interphalangeal joint(s) (S63.4-)

√6ᵗʰ **S63.60** **Unspecified sprain of thumb**

√7ᵗʰ **S63.601** **Unspecified sprain of right thumb**

√7ᵗʰ **S63.602** **Unspecified sprain of left thumb**

√7ᵗʰ **S63.609** **Unspecified sprain of unspecified thumb**

√6ᵗʰ **S63.61** **Unspecified sprain of other and unspecified finger(s)**

√7ᵗʰ **S63.610** **Unspecified sprain of right index finger**

√7ᵗʰ **S63.611** **Unspecified sprain of left index finger**

√7ᵗʰ **S63.612** **Unspecified sprain of right middle finger**

√7ᵗʰ **S63.613** **Unspecified sprain of left middle finger**

√7ᵗʰ **S63.614** **Unspecified sprain of right ring finger**

√7ᵗʰ **S63.615** **Unspecified sprain of left ring finger**

√7ᵗʰ **S63.616** **Unspecified sprain of right little finger**

√7ᵗʰ **S63.617** **Unspecified sprain of left little finger**

√7ᵗʰ **S63.618** **Unspecified sprain of other finger**

Unspecified sprain of specified finger with unspecified laterality

√7ᵗʰ **S63.619** **Unspecified sprain of unspecified finger**

√6ᵗʰ **S63.62** **Sprain of interphalangeal joint of thumb**

√7ᵗʰ **S63.621** **Sprain of interphalangeal joint of right thumb**

√7ᵗʰ **S63.622** **Sprain of interphalangeal joint of left thumb**

√7ᵗʰ **S63.629** **Sprain of interphalangeal joint of unspecified thumb**

√6ᵗʰ **S63.63** **Sprain of interphalangeal joint of other and unspecified finger(s)**

√7ᵗʰ **S63.630** **Sprain of interphalangeal joint of right index finger**

√7ᵗʰ **S63.631** **Sprain of interphalangeal joint of left index finger**

√7ᵗʰ **S63.632** **Sprain of interphalangeal joint of right middle finger**

√7ᵗʰ **S63.633** **Sprain of interphalangeal joint of left middle finger**

√7ᵗʰ **S63.634** **Sprain of interphalangeal joint of right ring finger**

√7ᵗʰ **S63.635** **Sprain of interphalangeal joint of left ring finger**

√7ᵗʰ **S63.636** **Sprain of interphalangeal joint of right little finger**

√7ᵗʰ **S63.637** **Sprain of interphalangeal joint of left little finger**

√7ᵗʰ **S63.638** **Sprain of interphalangeal joint of other finger**

√7ᵗʰ **S63.639** **Sprain of interphalangeal joint of unspecified finger**

√6ᵗʰ **S63.64** **Sprain of metacarpophalangeal joint of thumb**

√7ᵗʰ **S63.641** **Sprain of metacarpophalangeal joint of right thumb**

√7ᵗʰ **S63.642** **Sprain of metacarpophalangeal joint of left thumb**

√7ᵗʰ **S63.649** **Sprain of metacarpophalangeal joint of unspecified thumb**

√6ᵗʰ **S63.65** **Sprain of metacarpophalangeal joint of other and unspecified finger(s)**

√7ᵗʰ **S63.650** **Sprain of metacarpophalangeal joint of right index finger**

√7ᵗʰ **S63.651** **Sprain of metacarpophalangeal joint of left index finger**

√7ᵗʰ **S63.652** **Sprain of metacarpophalangeal joint of right middle finger**

√7ᵗʰ **S63.653** **Sprain of metacarpophalangeal joint of left middle finger**

√7ᵗʰ **S63.654** **Sprain of metacarpophalangeal joint of right ring finger**

√7ᵗʰ **S63.655** **Sprain of metacarpophalangeal joint of left ring finger**

√7ᵗʰ **S63.656** **Sprain of metacarpophalangeal joint of right little finger**

√7ᵗʰ **S63.657** **Sprain of metacarpophalangeal joint of left little finger**

√7ᵗʰ **S63.658** **Sprain of metacarpophalangeal joint of other finger**

Sprain of metacarpophalangeal joint of specified finger with unspecified laterality

√7ᵗʰ **S63.659** **Sprain of metacarpophalangeal joint of unspecified finger**

√6ᵗʰ **S63.68** **Other sprain of thumb**

√7ᵗʰ **S63.681** **Other sprain of right thumb**

√7ᵗʰ **S63.682** **Other sprain of left thumb**

√7ᵗʰ **S63.689** **Other sprain of unspecified thumb**

√6ᵗʰ **S63.69** **Other sprain of other and unspecified finger(s)**

√7ᵗʰ **S63.690** **Other sprain of right index finger**

√7ᵗʰ **S63.691** **Other sprain of left index finger**

√7ᵗʰ **S63.692** **Other sprain of right middle finger**

√7ᵗʰ **S63.693** **Other sprain of left middle finger**

√7ᵗʰ **S63.694** **Other sprain of right ring finger**

√7ᵗʰ **S63.695** **Other sprain of left ring finger**

√7ᵗʰ **S63.696** **Other sprain of right little finger**

√7ᵗʰ **S63.697** **Other sprain of left little finger**

√7ᵗʰ **S63.698** **Other sprain of other finger**

Other sprain of specified finger with unspecified laterality

√7ᵗʰ **S63.699** **Other sprain of unspecified finger**

✔ Additional Character Required   √x7ᵗʰ Xtension Alert   Unacceptable PDx   Manifestation   Hospital Acquired Condition   EXCLUDES 1 Not Coded Here   EXCLUDES 2 Not Included Here

Injury, Poisoning and Certain Other Consequences of External Causes

S63.8–S65.019

√5ᵗʰ **S63.8** Sprain of other part of wrist and hand

    √6ᵗʰ **S63.8X** Sprain of other part of wrist and hand

       √7ᵗʰ **S63.8X1** Sprain of other part of right wrist and hand

       √7ᵗʰ **S63.8X2** Sprain of other part of left wrist and hand

       √7ᵗʰ **S63.8X9** Sprain of other part of unspecified wrist and hand

√5ᵗʰ **S63.9** Sprain of unspecified part of wrist and hand

    √x7ᵗʰ **S63.90** Sprain of unspecified part of unspecified wrist and hand

    √x7ᵗʰ **S63.91** Sprain of unspecified part of right wrist and hand

    √x7ᵗʰ **S63.92** Sprain of unspecified part of left wrist and hand

√4ᵗʰ **S64** **Injury of nerves at wrist and hand level**

    Code also any associated open wound (S61.-)

> The appropriate 7th character is to be added to each code from category S64.
> A   initial encounter
> D   subsequent encounter
> S   sequela

√5ᵗʰ **S64.0** Injury of ulnar nerve at wrist and hand level

    √x7ᵗʰ **S64.00** Injury of ulnar nerve at wrist and hand level of unspecified arm

    √x7ᵗʰ **S64.01** Injury of ulnar nerve at wrist and hand level of right arm

    √x7ᵗʰ **S64.02** Injury of ulnar nerve at wrist and hand level of left arm

√5ᵗʰ **S64.1** Injury of median nerve at wrist and hand level

    √x7ᵗʰ **S64.10** Injury of median nerve at wrist and hand level of unspecified arm

    √x7ᵗʰ **S64.11** Injury of median nerve at wrist and hand level of right arm

    √x7ᵗʰ **S64.12** Injury of median nerve at wrist and hand level of left arm

√5ᵗʰ **S64.2** Injury of radial nerve at wrist and hand level

    √x7ᵗʰ **S64.20** Injury of radial nerve at wrist and hand level of unspecified arm

    √x7ᵗʰ **S64.21** Injury of radial nerve at wrist and hand level of right arm

    √x7ᵗʰ **S64.22** Injury of radial nerve at wrist and hand level of left arm

√5ᵗʰ **S64.3** Injury of digital nerve of thumb

    √x7ᵗʰ **S64.30** Injury of digital nerve of unspecified thumb

    √x7ᵗʰ **S64.31** Injury of digital nerve of right thumb

    √x7ᵗʰ **S64.32** Injury of digital nerve of left thumb

√5ᵗʰ **S64.4** Injury of digital nerve of other and unspecified finger

    √x7ᵗʰ **S64.40** Injury of digital nerve of unspecified finger

    √6ᵗʰ **S64.49** Injury of digital nerve of other finger

       √7ᵗʰ **S64.490** Injury of digital nerve of right index finger

       √7ᵗʰ **S64.491** Injury of digital nerve of left index finger

       √7ᵗʰ **S64.492** Injury of digital nerve of right middle finger

       √7ᵗʰ **S64.493** Injury of digital nerve of left middle finger

       √7ᵗʰ **S64.494** Injury of digital nerve of right ring finger

       √7ᵗʰ **S64.495** Injury of digital nerve of left ring finger

       √7ᵗʰ **S64.496** Injury of digital nerve of right little finger

       √7ᵗʰ **S64.497** Injury of digital nerve of left little finger

       √7ᵗʰ **S64.498** Injury of digital nerve of other finger
         Injury of digital nerve of specified finger with unspecified laterality

√5ᵗʰ **S64.8** Injury of other nerves at wrist and hand level

    √6ᵗʰ **S64.8X** Injury of other nerves at wrist and hand level

       √7ᵗʰ **S64.8X1** Injury of other nerves at wrist and hand level of right arm

       √7ᵗʰ **S64.8X2** Injury of other nerves at wrist and hand level of left arm

       √7ᵗʰ **S64.8X9** Injury of other nerves at wrist and hand level of unspecified arm

√5ᵗʰ **S64.9** Injury of unspecified nerve at wrist and hand level

    √x7ᵗʰ **S64.90** Injury of unspecified nerve at wrist and hand level of unspecified arm

    √x7ᵗʰ **S64.91** Injury of unspecified nerve at wrist and hand level of right arm

    √x7ᵗʰ **S64.92** Injury of unspecified nerve at wrist and hand level of left arm

√4ᵗʰ **S65** **Injury of blood vessels at wrist and hand level**

    Code also any associated open wound (S61.-)

> The appropriate 7th character is to be added to each code from category S65.
> A   initial encounter
> D   subsequent encounter
> S   sequela

√5ᵗʰ **S65.0** Injury of ulnar artery at wrist and hand level

    √6ᵗʰ **S65.00** Unspecified injury of ulnar artery at wrist and hand level

       √7ᵗʰ **S65.001** Unspecified injury of ulnar artery at wrist and hand level of right arm   **CC**
         CC Excl: CC CC with 7th character A: S45.301A, S45.309-S45.311 with 7th A, S45.319-S45.391 with 7th A, S45.399-S45.801 with 7th A, S45.809-S45.811 with 7th A, S45.819-S45.891 with 7th A, S45.899-S45.901 with 7th A, S45.909-S45.911 with 7th A, S45.919-S45.991 with 7th A, S45.999A, S55.001A, S55.009-S55.011 with 7th A, S55.019-S55.091 with 7th A, S55.099A, S55.201A, S55.209-S55.211 with 7th A, S55.219-S55.291 with 7th A, S55.299-S55.801 with 7th A, S55.809-S55.811 with 7th A, S55.819-S55.891 with 7th A, S55.899-S55.901 with 7th A, S55.909-S55.911 with 7th A, S55.919-S55.991 with 7th A, S55.999A, S65.001A, S65.009-S65.011 with 7th A, S65.019-S65.091 with 7th A, S65.099A, S65.801A, S65.809-S65.811 with 7th A, S65.819-S65.891 with 7th A, S65.899-S65.901 with 7th A, S65.909-S65.911 with 7th A, S65.919-S65.991 with 7th A, S65.999A

       √7ᵗʰ **S65.002** Unspecified injury of ulnar artery at wrist and hand level of left arm   **CC**
         CC Excl: CC CC with 7th character A: S45.302-S45.309 with 7th A, S45.312-S45.319 with 7th A, S45.392-S45.399 with 7th A, S45.802-S45.809 with 7th A, S45.812-S45.819 with 7th A, S45.892-S45.899 with 7th A, S45.902-S45.909 with 7th A, S45.912-S45.919 with 7th A, S45.992-S45.999 with 7th A, S55.002-S55.009 with 7th A, S55.012-S55.019 with 7th A, S55.092-S55.099 with 7th A, S55.202-S55.209 with 7th A, S55.212-S55.219 with 7th A, S55.292-S55.299 with 7th A, S55.802-S55.809 with 7th A, S55.812-S55.819 with 7th A, S55.892-S55.899 with 7th A, S55.902-S55.909 with 7th A, S55.912-S55.919 with 7th A, S55.992-S55.999 with 7th A, S65.002-S65.009 with 7th A, S65.012-S65.019 with 7th A, S65.092-S65.099 with 7th A, S65.802-S65.809 with 7th A, S65.812-S65.819 with 7th A, S65.892-S65.899 with 7th A, S65.902-S65.909 with 7th A, S65.912-S65.919 with 7th A, S65.992-S65.999 with 7th A

       √7ᵗʰ **S65.009** Unspecified injury of ulnar artery at wrist and hand level of unspecified arm   **CC**
         CC Excl: CC CC with 7th character A: S45.301-S45.999 with 7th A, S55.001-S55.099 with 7th A, S55.201-S55.999 with 7th A, S65.001-S65.099 with 7th A, S65.801-S65.999 with 7th A

    √6ᵗʰ **S65.01** Laceration of ulnar artery at wrist and hand level

       √7ᵗʰ **S65.011** Laceration of ulnar artery at wrist and hand level of right arm   **CC**
         CC Excl: CC CC with 7th character A: See code: S65.001

       √7ᵗʰ **S65.012** Laceration of ulnar artery at wrist and hand level of left arm   **CC**
         CC Excl: CC CC with 7th character A: See code: S65.002

       √7ᵗʰ **S65.019** Laceration of ulnar artery at wrist and hand level of unspecified arm   **CC**
         CC Excl: CC CC with 7th character A: See code: S65.009

N Newborn: 0   **P** Pediatric: 0-17   **M** Maternity: 12-55   **A** Adult: 15-124   **MCC** Major CC Condition   **PDx MCC** PDx acts as own MCC   **CC** CC Condition   **PDx CC** PDx acts as own CC

960   ICD-10-CM Draft (2015)

√6ᵗʰ **S65.09** Other specified injury of ulnar artery at wrist and hand level

√7ᵗʰ **S65.091** Other specified injury of ulnar artery at wrist and hand level of right arm `CC`
CC Excl: CC CC with 7th character A: See code: S65.001

√7ᵗʰ **S65.092** Other specified injury of ulnar artery at wrist and hand level of left arm `CC`
CC Excl: CC CC with 7th character A: See code: S65.002

√7ᵗʰ **S65.099** Other specified injury of ulnar artery at wrist and hand level of unspecified arm `CC`
CC Excl: CC CC with 7th character A: See code: S65.009

√5ᵗʰ **S65.1** Injury of radial artery at wrist and hand level

√6ᵗʰ **S65.10** Unspecified injury of radial artery at wrist and hand level

√7ᵗʰ **S65.101** Unspecified injury of radial artery at wrist and hand level of right arm `CC`
CC Excl: CC CC with 7th character A: S45.301 A, S45.309-S45.311 with 7th A, S45.319-S45.391 with 7th A, S45.399-S45.801 with 7th A, S45.809-S45.811 with 7th A, S45.819-S45.891 with 7th A, S45.899-S45.901 with 7th A, S45.909-S45.911 with 7th A, S45.919-S45.991 with 7th A, S45.999A, S55.101A, S55.109-S55.111 with 7th A, S55.119-S55.191 with 7th A, S55.199-S55.201 with 7th A, S55.209-S55.211 with 7th A, S55.219-S55.291 with 7th A, S55.299-S55.801 with 7th A, S55.809-S55.811 with 7th A, S55.819-S55.891 with 7th A, S55.899-S55.901 with 7th A, S55.909-S55.911 with 7th A, S55.919-S55.991 with 7th A, S55.999A, S65.101A, S65.109-S65.111 with 7th A, S65.119-S65.191 with 7th A, S65.199A, S65.801 with 7th A, S65.809-S65.811 with 7th A, S65.819-S65.891 with 7th A, S65.899-S65.901 with 7th A, S65.909-S65.911 with 7th A, S65.919-S65.991 with 7th A, S65.999A

√7ᵗʰ **S65.102** Unspecified injury of radial artery at wrist and hand level of left arm `CC`
CC Excl: CC CC with 7th character A: S45.302-S45.309 with 7th A, S45.312-S45.319 with 7th A, S45.392-S45.399 with 7th A, S45.802-S45.809 with 7th A, S45.812-S45.819 with 7th A, S45.892-S45.899 with 7th A, S45.902-S45.909 with 7th A, S45.912-S45.919 with 7th A, S45.992-S45.999 with 7th A, S55.102-S55.109 with 7th A, S55.112-S55.119 with 7th A, S55.192-S55.199 with 7th A, S55.202-S55.209 with 7th A, S55.212-S55.219 with 7th A, S55.292-S55.299 with 7th A, S55.802-S55.809 with 7th A, S55.812-S55.819 with 7th A, S55.892-S55.899 with 7th A, S55.902-S55.909 with 7th A, S55.912-S55.919 with 7th A, S55.992-S55.999 with 7th A, S65.102-S65.109 with 7th A, S65.112-S65.119 with 7th A, S65.192-S65.199 with 7th A, S65.802-S65.809 with 7th A, S65.812-S65.819 with 7th A, S65.892-S65.899 with 7th A, S65.902-S65.909 with 7th A, S65.912-S65.919 with 7th A, S65.992-S65.999 with 7th A

√7ᵗʰ **S65.109** Unspecified injury of radial artery at wrist and hand level of unspecified arm `CC`
CC Excl: CC CC with 7th character A: S45.301-S45.301-S45.999 with 7th A, S55.101-S55.999 with 7th A, S65.101-S65.199 with 7th A, S65.801-S65.999 with 7th A

√6ᵗʰ **S65.11** Laceration of radial artery at wrist and hand level

√7ᵗʰ **S65.111** Laceration of radial artery at wrist and hand level of right arm `CC`
CC Excl: CC CC with 7th character A: See code: S65.101

√7ᵗʰ **S65.112** Laceration of radial artery at wrist and hand level of left arm `CC`
CC Excl: CC CC with 7th character A: See code: S65.102

√7ᵗʰ **S65.119** Laceration of radial artery at wrist and hand level of unspecified arm `CC`
CC Excl: CC CC with 7th character A: See code: S65.109

√6ᵗʰ **S65.19** Other specified injury of radial artery at wrist and hand level

√7ᵗʰ **S65.191** Other specified injury of radial artery at wrist and hand level of right arm `CC`
CC Excl: CC CC with 7th character A: See code: S65.101

√7ᵗʰ **S65.192** Other specified injury of radial artery at wrist and hand level of left arm `CC`
CC Excl: CC CC with 7th character A: See code: S65.102

√7ᵗʰ **S65.199** Other specified injury of radial artery at wrist and hand level of unspecified arm `CC`
CC Excl: CC CC with 7th character A: See code: S65.109

√5ᵗʰ **S65.2** Injury of superficial palmar arch

√6ᵗʰ **S65.20** Unspecified injury of superficial palmar arch

√7ᵗʰ **S65.201** Unspecified injury of superficial palmar arch of right hand `CC`
CC Excl: CC CC with 7th character A: S45.301A, S45.309-S45.311 with 7th A, S45.319-S45.391 with 7th A, S45.399-S45.801 with 7th A, S45.809-S45.811 with 7th A, S45.819-S45.891 with 7th A, S45.899-S45.901 with 7th A, S45.909-S45.911 with 7th A, S45.919-S45.991 with 7th A, S45.999A, S55.201A, S55.209-S55.211 with 7th A, S55.219-S55.291 with 7th A, S55.299-S55.801 with 7th A, S55.809-S55.811 with 7th A, S55.819-S55.891 with 7th A, S55.899-S55.901 with 7th A, S55.909-S55.911 with 7th A, S55.919-S55.991 with 7th A, S55.999A, S65.201A, S65.209-S65.211 with 7th A, S65.219-S65.291 with 7th A, S65.299-S65.301 with 7th A, S65.309-S65.311 with 7th A, S65.319-S65.391 with 7th A, S65.399A, S65.801A, S65.809-S65.811 with 7th A, S65.819-S65.891 with 7th A, S65.899-S65.901 with 7th A, S65.909-S65.911 with 7th A, S65.919-S65.991 with 7th A, S65.999A

√7ᵗʰ **S65.202** Unspecified injury of superficial palmar arch of left hand `CC`
CC Excl: CC CC with 7th character A: S45.302-S45.309 with 7th A, S45.312-S45.319 with 7th A, S45.392-S45.399 with 7th A, S45.802-S45.809 with 7th A, S45.812-S45.819 with 7th A, S45.892-S45.899 with 7th A, S45.902-S45.909 with 7th A, S45.912-S45.919 with 7th A, S45.992-S45.999 with 7th A, S55.202-S55.209 with 7th A, S55.212-S55.219 with 7th A, S55.292-S55.299 with 7th A, S55.802-S55.809 with 7th A, S55.812-S55.819 with 7th A, S55.892-S55.899 with 7th A, S55.902-S55.909 with 7th A, S55.912-S55.919 with 7th A, S55.992-S55.999 with 7th A, S65.202-S65.209 with 7th A, S65.212-S65.219 with 7th A, S65.292-S65.299 with 7th A, S65.302-S65.309 with 7th A, S65.312-S65.319 with 7th A, S65.392-S65.399 with 7th A, S65.802-S65.809 with 7th A, S65.812-S65.819 with 7th A, S65.892-S65.899 with 7th A, S65.902-S65.909 with 7th A, S65.912-S65.919 with 7th A, S65.992-S65.999 with 7th A

√7ᵗʰ **S65.209** Unspecified injury of superficial palmar arch of unspecified hand `CC`
CC Excl: CC CC with 7th character A: S45.301-S45.999 with 7th A, S55.201-S55.999 with 7th A, S65.201-S65.399 with 7th A, S65.801-S65.999 with 7th A

√6ᵗʰ **S65.21** Laceration of superficial palmar arch

√7ᵗʰ **S65.211** Laceration of superficial palmar arch of right hand `CC`
CC Excl: CC CC with 7th character A: See code: S65.201

√7ᵗʰ **S65.212** Laceration of superficial palmar arch of left hand `CC`
CC Excl: CC CC with 7th character A: See code: S65.202

√7ᵗʰ **S65.219** Laceration of superficial palmar arch of unspecified hand `CC`
CC Excl: CC CC with 7th character A: See code: S65.209

√ Additional Character Required √x7ᵗʰ Xtension Alert Unacceptable PDx Manifestation Hospital Acquired Condition *EXCLUDES 1* Not Coded Here *EXCLUDES 2* Not Included Here

√6ᵗʰ **S65.29** Other specified injury of superficial palmar arch

√7ᵗʰ **S65.291** Other specified injury of superficial palmar arch of right hand   CC
CC Excl: CC CC with 7th character A: See code: S65.201

√7ᵗʰ **S65.292** Other specified injury of superficial palmar arch of left hand   CC
CC Excl: CC CC with 7th character A: See code: S65.202

√7ᵗʰ **S65.299** Other specified injury of superficial palmar arch of unspecified hand   CC
CC Excl: CC CC with 7th character A: See code: S65.209

√5ᵗʰ **S65.3** Injury of deep palmar arch

√6ᵗʰ **S65.30** Unspecified injury of deep palmar arch

√7ᵗʰ **S65.301** Unspecified injury of deep palmar arch of right hand   CC
CC Excl: CC CC with 7th character A: See code: S65.201

√7ᵗʰ **S65.302** Unspecified injury of deep palmar arch of left hand   CC
CC Excl: CC CC with 7th character A: See code: S65.202

√7ᵗʰ **S65.309** Unspecified injury of deep palmar arch of unspecified hand   CC
CC Excl: CC CC with 7th character A: See code: S65.209

√6ᵗʰ **S65.31** Laceration of deep palmar arch

√7ᵗʰ **S65.311** Laceration of deep palmar arch of right hand   CC
CC Excl: CC CC with 7th character A: See code: S65.201

√7ᵗʰ **S65.312** Laceration of deep palmar arch of left hand   CC
CC Excl: CC CC with 7th character A: See code: S65.202

√7ᵗʰ **S65.319** Laceration of deep palmar arch of unspecified hand   CC
CC Excl: CC with 7th character A: See code: S65.209

√6ᵗʰ **S65.39** Other specified injury of deep palmar arch

√7ᵗʰ **S65.391** Other specified injury of deep palmar arch of right hand   CC
CC Excl: CC with 7th character A: See code: S65.201

√7ᵗʰ **S65.392** Other specified injury of deep palmar arch of left hand   CC
CC Excl: CC with 7th character A: See code: S65.202

√7ᵗʰ **S65.399** Other specified injury of deep palmar arch of unspecified hand   CC
CC Excl: CC with 7th character A: See code: S65.209

√5ᵗʰ **S65.4** Injury of blood vessel of thumb

√6ᵗʰ **S65.40** Unspecified injury of blood vessel of thumb

√7ᵗʰ **S65.401** Unspecified injury of blood vessel of right thumb   CC
CC Excl: CC with 7th character A: S45.301A, S45.309-S45.311 with 7th A, S45.319-S45.391 with 7th A, S45.399-S45.801 with 7th A, S45.809-S45.811 with 7th A, S45.819-S45.891 with 7th A, S45.899-S45.901 with 7th A, S45.909-S45.911 with 7th A, S45.919-S45.991 with 7th A, S45.999A, S55.201A, S55.209-S55.211 with 7th A, S55.219-S55.291 with 7th A, S55.299-S55.801 with 7th A, S55.809-S55.811 with 7th A, S55.819-S55.891 with 7th A, S55.899-S55.901 with 7th A, S55.909-S55.911 with 7th A, S55.919-S55.991 with 7th A, S55.999A, S65.401A, S65.409-S65.411 with 7th A, S65.419-S65.491 with 7th A, S65.499-S65.500 with 7th A, S65.502 A, S65.504A, S65.506A, S65.508-S65.510 with 7th A, S65.512A, S65.514A, S65.516A, S65.518-S65.590 with 7th A, S65.592A, S65.594A, S65.596 A, S65.598-S65.801 with 7th A, S65.809-S65.811 with 7th A, S65.819-S65.891 with 7th A, S65.899-S65.901 with 7th A, S65.909-S65.911 with 7th A, S65.919-S65.991 with 7th A, S65.999A

√7ᵗʰ **S65.402** Unspecified injury of blood vessel of left thumb   CC
CC Excl: CC with 7th character A: S45.302-S45.309 with 7th A, S45.312-S45.319 with 7th A, S45.392-S45.399 with 7th A, S45.809 with 7th A, S45.812-S45.819 with 7th A, S45.892-S45.899 with 7th A, S45.902-S45.909 with 7th A, S45.912-S45.919 with 7th A, S45.992-S45.999 with 7th A, S55.202-S55.209 with 7th A, S55.212-S55.219 with 7th A, S55.292-S55.299 with 7th A, S55.802-S55.809 with 7th A, S55.812-S55.819 with 7th A, S55.892-S55.899 with 7th A, S55.902-S55.909 with 7th A, S55.912-S55.919 with 7th A, S55.992-S55.999 with 7th A, S65.402-S65.409 with 7th A, S65.412-S65.419 with 7th A, S65.492-S65.499 with 7th A, S65.501A, S65.503A, S65.505A, S65.507-S65.509 with 7th A, S65.511A, S65.513A, S65.515A, S65.517-S65.519 with 7th A, S65.591A, S65.593A, S65.595A, S65.597-S65.599 with 7th A, S65.802-S65.809 with 7th A, S65.812-S65.819 with 7th A, S65.892-S65.899 with 7th A, S65.902-S65.909 with 7th A, S65.912-S65.919 with 7th A, S65.992-S65.999 with 7th A

√7ᵗʰ **S65.409** Unspecified injury of blood vessel of unspecified thumb   CC
CC Excl: CC with 7th character A: S45.301-S45.999 with 7th A, S55.201-S55.999 with 7th A, S65.401-S65.999 with 7th A

√6ᵗʰ **S65.41** Laceration of blood vessel of thumb

√7ᵗʰ **S65.411** Laceration of blood vessel of right thumb   CC
CC Excl: CC with 7th character A: See code: S65.401

√7ᵗʰ **S65.412** Laceration of blood vessel of left thumb   CC
CC Excl: CC with 7th character A: See code: S65.402

√7ᵗʰ **S65.419** Laceration of blood vessel of unspecified thumb   CC
CC Excl: CC with 7th character A: See code: S65.409

√6ᵗʰ **S65.49** Other specified injury of blood vessel of thumb

√7ᵗʰ **S65.491** Other specified injury of blood vessel of right thumb   CC
CC Excl: CC with 7th character A: See code: S65.401

√7ᵗʰ **S65.492** Other specified injury of blood vessel of left thumb   CC
CC Excl: CC with 7th character A: See code: S65.402

√7ᵗʰ **S65.499** Other specified injury of blood vessel of unspecified thumb   CC
CC Excl: CC with 7th character A: See code: S65.409

√5ᵗʰ **S65.5** Injury of blood vessel of other and unspecified finger

√6ᵗʰ **S65.50** Unspecified injury of blood vessel of other and unspecified finger

√7ᵗʰ **S65.500** Unspecified injury of blood vessel of right index finger   CC
CC Excl: CC with 7th character A: See code: S65.401

√7ᵗʰ **S65.501** Unspecified injury of blood vessel of left index finger   CC
CC Excl: CC with 7th character A: See code: S65.402

√7ᵗʰ **S65.502** Unspecified injury of blood vessel of right middle finger   CC
CC Excl: CC with 7th character A: See code: S65.401

√7ᵗʰ **S65.503** Unspecified injury of blood vessel of left middle finger   CC
CC Excl: CC with 7th character A: See code: S65.402

√7ᵗʰ **S65.504** Unspecified injury of blood vessel of right ring finger   CC
CC Excl: CC with 7th character A: See code: S65.401

√7ᵗʰ **S65.505** Unspecified injury of blood vessel of left ring finger   CC
CC Excl: CC with 7th character A: See code: S65.402

Ⓝ Newborn: 0   Ⓟ Pediatric: 0-17   Ⓜ Maternity: 12-55   Ⓐ Adult: 15-124   MCC Major CC Condition   PDx MCC PDx acts as own MCC   CC CC Condition   PDx CC PDx acts as own CC

962   ICD-10-CM Draft (2015)

√7ᵗʰ **S65.506 Unspecified injury of blood vessel** `CC`
of right little finger
CC Excl: CC with 7th character A: See code:
S65.401

√7ᵗʰ **S65.507 Unspecified injury of blood vessel** `CC`
of left little finger
CC Excl: CC with 7th character A: See code:
S65.402

√7ᵗʰ **S65.508 Unspecified injury of blood vessel** `CC`
of other finger
Unspecified injury of blood vessel of
specified finger with unspecified
laterality
CC Excl: CC with 7th character A: See code:
S65.409

√7ᵗʰ **S65.509 Unspecified injury of blood vessel of** `CC`
unspecified finger
CC Excl: CC with 7th character A: See code:
S65.409

√6ᵗʰ **S65.51 Laceration of blood vessel of other and unspecified**
finger

√7ᵗʰ **S65.510 Laceration of blood vessel of right** `CC`
index finger
CC Excl: CC with 7th character A: See code:
S65.401

√7ᵗʰ **S65.511 Laceration of blood vessel of left** `CC`
index finger
CC Excl: CC with 7th character A: See code:
S65.402

√7ᵗʰ **S65.512 Laceration of blood vessel of right** `CC`
middle finger
CC Excl: CC with 7th character A: See code:
S65.401

√7ᵗʰ **S65.513 Laceration of blood vessel of left** `CC`
middle finger
CC Excl: CC with 7th character A: See code:
S65.402

√7ᵗʰ **S65.514 Laceration of blood vessel of right** `CC`
ring finger
CC Excl: CC with 7th character A: See code:
S65.401

√7ᵗʰ **S65.515 Laceration of blood vessel of left** `CC`
ring finger
CC Excl: CC with 7th character A: See code:
S65.402

√7ᵗʰ **S65.516 Laceration of blood vessel of right** `CC`
little finger
CC Excl: CC with 7th character A: See code:
S65.401

√7ᵗʰ **S65.517 Laceration of blood vessel of left** `CC`
little finger
CC Excl: CC with 7th character A: See code:
S65.402

√7ᵗʰ **S65.518 Laceration of blood vessel of other** `CC`
finger
Laceration of blood vessel of specified
finger with unspecified laterality
CC Excl: CC with 7th character A: See code:
S65.409

√7ᵗʰ **S65.519 Laceration of blood vessel of** `CC`
unspecified finger
CC Excl: CC with 7th character A: See code:
S65.409

√6ᵗʰ **S65.59 Other specified injury of blood vessel of other and**
unspecified finger

√7ᵗʰ **S65.590 Other specified injury of blood** `CC`
vessel of right index finger
CC Excl: CC with 7th character A: See code:
S65.401

√7ᵗʰ **S65.591 Other specified injury of blood** `CC`
vessel of left index finger
CC Excl: CC with 7th character A: See code:
S65.402

√7ᵗʰ **S65.592 Other specified injury of blood** `CC`
vessel of right middle finger
CC Excl: CC with 7th character A: See code:
S65.401

√7ᵗʰ **S65.593 Other specified injury of blood** `CC`
vessel of left middle finger
CC Excl: CC with 7th character A: See code:
S65.402

√7ᵗʰ **S65.594 Other specified injury of blood** `CC`
vessel of right ring finger
CC Excl: CC with 7th character A: See code:
S65.401

√7ᵗʰ **S65.595 Other specified injury of blood** `CC`
vessel of left ring finger
CC Excl: CC with 7th character A: See code:
S65.402

√7ᵗʰ **S65.596 Other specified injury of blood** `CC`
vessel of right little finger
CC Excl: CC with 7th character A: See code:
S65.401

√7ᵗʰ **S65.597 Other specified injury of blood** `CC`
vessel of left little finger
CC Excl: CC with 7th character A: See code:
S65.402

√7ᵗʰ **S65.598 Other specified injury of blood** `CC`
vessel of other finger
Other specified injury of blood vessel of
specified finger with unspecified laterality
CC Excl: CC with 7th character A: See code:
S65.409

√7ᵗʰ **S65.599 Other specified injury of blood** `CC`
vessel of unspecified finger
CC Excl: CC with 7th character A: See code:
S65.409

√5ᵗʰ **S65.8 Injury of other blood vessels at wrist and hand level**

√6ᵗʰ **S65.80 Unspecified injury of other blood vessels at wrist**
and hand level

√7ᵗʰ **S65.801 Unspecified injury of other blood** `CC`
vessels at wrist and hand level of
right arm
CC Excl: CC with 7th character A: S45.301A,
S45.309-S45.311 with 7th A, S45.319-
S45.391 with 7th A, S45.399-S45.801 with
7th A, S45.809-S45.811 with 7th A, S45.819-
S45.891 with 7th A, S45.899-S45.901 with
7th A, S45.909-S45.911 with 7th A, S45.919-
S45.991 with 7th A, S45.999A, S55.001A,
S55.009-S55.011 with 7th A, S55.019-
S55.091 with 7th A, S55.099A, S55.201A,
S55.209-S55.211 with 7th A, S55.219-
S55.291 with 7th A, S55.299-S55.801 with
7th A, S55.809-S55.811 with 7th A, S55.819-
S55.891 with 7th A, S55.899-S55.901 with
7th A, S55.909-S55.911 with 7th A, S55.919-
S55.991 with 7th A, S55.999A, S65.001A,
S65.009-S65.011 with 7th A, S65.019-
S65.091 with 7th A, S65.099A, S65.201A,
S65.209-S65.211 with 7th A, S65.219-
S65.291 with 7th A, S65.299-S65.301 with
7th A, S65.309-S65.311 with 7th A, S65.319-
S65.391 with 7th A, S65.399-S65.401 with
7th A, S65.409-S65.411 with 7th A, S65.419-
S65.491 with 7th A, S65.499-S65.500 with
7th A, S65.502A, S65.504A, S65.506A,
S65.508-S65.510 with 7th A, S65.512A,
S65.514A, S65.516A, S65.518-S65.590 with
7th A, S65.592A, S65.594A, S65.596A,
S65.598-S65.801 with 7th A, S65.809-
S65.811 with 7th A, S65.819-S65.891 with
7th A, S65.899-S65.901 with 7th A, S65.909-
S65.911 with 7th A, S65.919-S65.991 with
7th A, S65.999 with 7th A

√7ᵗʰ **S65.802 Unspecified injury of other blood vessels at wrist and hand level of left arm** CC
CC Excl: CC with 7th character A: S45.302-S45.309 with 7th A, S45.312-S45.319 with 7th A, S45.392-S45.399 with 7th A, S45.809 with 7th A, S45.812-S45.819 with 7th A, S45.892-S45.899 with 7th A, S45.902-S45.909 with 7th A, S45.912-S45.919 with 7th A, S45.992-S45.999 with 7th A, S55.002-S55.009 with 7th A, S55.012-S55.019 with 7th A, S55.092-S55.099 with 7th A, S55.202-S55.209 with 7th A, S55.212-S55.219 with 7th A, S55.292-S55.299 with 7th A, S55.802-S55.809 with 7th A, S55.812-S55.819 with 7th A, S55.892-S55.899 with 7th A, S55.902-S55.909 with 7th A, S55.912-S55.919 with 7th A, S55.992-S55.999 with 7th A, S65.002-S65.009 with 7th A, S65.012-S65.019 with 7th A, S65.092-S65.099 with 7th A, S65.202-S65.209 with 7th A, S65.212-S65.219 with 7th A, S65.292-S65.299 with 7th A, S65.302-S65.309 with 7th A, S65.312-S65.319 with 7th A, S65.392-S65.399 with 7th A, S65.402-S65.409 with 7th A, S65.412-S65.419 with 7th A, S65.492-S65.499 with 7th A, S65.501A, S65.503A, S65.505A, S65.507-S65.509 with 7th A, S65.511A, S65.513A, S65.515A, S65.517-S65.519 with 7th A, S65.591A, S65.593A, S65.595A, S65.597-S65.599 with 7th A, S65.802-S65.809 with 7th A, S65.812-S65.819 with 7th A, S65.892-S65.899 with 7th A, S65.902-S65.909 with 7th A, S65.912-S65.919 with 7th A, S65.992-S65.999 with 7th A

√7ᵗʰ **S65.809 Unspecified injury of other blood vessels at wrist and hand level of unspecified arm** CC
CC Excl: CC with 7th character A: S45.301-S45.999 with 7th A, S55.001-S55.099 with 7th A, S55.201-S55.999 with 7th A, S65.001-S65.099 with 7th A, S65.201-S65.999 with 7th A

√6ᵗʰ **S65.81 Laceration of other blood vessels at wrist and hand level**

√7ᵗʰ **S65.811 Laceration of other blood vessels at wrist and hand level of right arm** CC
CC Excl: CC with 7th character A: See code: S65.801

√7ᵗʰ **S65.812 Laceration of other blood vessels at wrist and hand level of left arm** CC
CC Excl: CC with 7th character A: See code: S65.802

√7ᵗʰ **S65.819 Laceration of other blood vessels at wrist and hand level of unspecified arm** CC
CC Excl: CC with 7th character A: See code: S65.809

√6ᵗʰ **S65.89 Other specified injury of other blood vessels at wrist and hand level**

√7ᵗʰ **S65.891 Other specified injury of other blood vessels at wrist and hand level of right arm** CC
CC Excl: CC with 7th character A: See code: S65.801

√7ᵗʰ **S65.892 Other specified injury of other blood vessels at wrist and hand level of left arm** CC
CC Excl: CC with 7th character A: See code: S65.802

√7ᵗʰ **S65.899 Other specified injury of other blood vessels at wrist and hand level of unspecified arm** CC
CC Excl: CC with 7th character A: See code: S65.809

√5ᵗʰ **S65.9 Injury of unspecified blood vessel at wrist and hand level**

√6ᵗʰ **S65.90 Unspecified injury of unspecified blood vessel at wrist and hand level**

√7ᵗʰ **S65.901 Unspecified injury of unspecified blood vessel at wrist and hand level of right arm** CC
CC Excl: CC with 7th character A: See code: S65.801

√7ᵗʰ **S65.902 Unspecified injury of unspecified blood vessel at wrist and hand level of left arm** CC
CC Excl: CC with 7th character A: See code: S65.802

√7ᵗʰ **S65.909 Unspecified injury of unspecified blood vessel at wrist and hand level of unspecified arm** CC
CC Excl: CC with 7th character A: See code: S65.809

√6ᵗʰ **S65.91 Laceration of unspecified blood vessel at wrist and hand level**

√7ᵗʰ **S65.911 Laceration of unspecified blood vessel at wrist and hand level of right arm** CC
CC Excl: CC with 7th character A: See code: S65.801

√7ᵗʰ **S65.912 Laceration of unspecified blood vessel at wrist and hand level of left arm** CC
CC Excl: CC with 7th character A: See code: S65.802

√7ᵗʰ **S65.919 Laceration of unspecified blood vessel at wrist and hand level of unspecified arm** CC
CC Excl: CC with 7th character A: See code: S65.809

√6ᵗʰ **S65.99 Other specified injury of unspecified blood vessel at wrist and hand level**

√7ᵗʰ **S65.991 Other specified injury of unspecified blood vessel at wrist and hand of right arm** CC
CC Excl: CC with 7th character A: See code: S65.801

√7ᵗʰ **S65.992 Other specified injury of unspecified blood vessel at wrist and hand of left arm** CC
CC Excl: CC with 7th character A: See code: S65.802

√7ᵗʰ **S65.999 Other specified injury of unspecified blood vessel at wrist and hand of unspecified arm** CC
CC Excl: CC with 7th character A: See code: S65.809

√4ᵗʰ **S66 Injury of muscle, fascia and tendon at wrist and hand level**
Code also any associated open wound (S61.-)
EXCLUDES 2 *sprain of joints and ligaments of wrist and hand (S63.-)*

The appropriate 7th character is to be added to each code from category S66.
A   initial encounter
D   subsequent encounter
S   sequela

√5ᵗʰ **S66.0 Injury of long flexor muscle, fascia and tendon of thumb at wrist and hand level**

√6ᵗʰ **S66.00 Unspecified injury of long flexor muscle, fascia and tendon of thumb at wrist and hand level**

√7ᵗʰ **S66.001 Unspecified injury of long flexor muscle, fascia and tendon of right thumb at wrist and hand level**

√7ᵗʰ **S66.002 Unspecified injury of long flexor muscle, fascia and tendon of left thumb at wrist and hand level**

√7ᵗʰ **S66.009 Unspecified injury of long flexor muscle, fascia and tendon of unspecified thumb at wrist and hand level**

√6ᵗʰ **S66.01 Strain of long flexor muscle, fascia and tendon of thumb at wrist and hand level**

√7ᵗʰ **S66.011 Strain of long flexor muscle, fascia and tendon of right thumb at wrist and hand level**

√7ᵗʰ **S66.012 Strain of long flexor muscle, fascia and tendon of left thumb at wrist and hand level**

√7ᵗʰ **S66.019 Strain of long flexor muscle, fascia and tendon of unspecified thumb at wrist and hand level**

N Newborn: 0   P Pediatric: 0-17   M Maternity: 12-55   A Adult: 15-124   MCC Major CC Condition   PDx MCC PDx acts as own MCC   CC CC Condition   PDx CC PDx acts as own CC

964   ICD-10-CM Draft (2015)

✓6th **S66.02** Laceration of long flexor muscle, fascia and tendon of thumb at wrist and hand level

✓7th **S66.021** Laceration of long flexor muscle, fascia and tendon of right thumb at wrist and hand level `CC`
CC Excl: CC with 7th character A: S61.401A, S61.409-S61.411 with 7th A, S61.419-S61.421 with 7th A, S61.429-S61.431 with 7th A, S61.439-S61.441 with 7th A, S61.449-S61.451 with 7th A, S61.459A, S66.021A, S66.029A, S66.120A, S66.122A, S66.124A, S66.126A, S66.128-S66.129 with 7th A, S66.221A, S66.229A, S66.320A, S66.322A, S66.324A, S66.326A, S66.328-S66.329 with 7th A, S66.421A, S66.429A, S66.520A, S66.522A, S66.524A, S66.526A, S66.528-S66.529 with 7th A, S66.821A, S66.829A, S66.921A, S66.929 with 7th A

✓7th **S66.022** Laceration of long flexor muscle, fascia and tendon of left thumb at wrist and hand level `CC`
CC Excl: CC with 7th character A: S61.402-S61.409 with 7th A, S61.412-S61.419 with 7th A, S61.422-S61.429 with 7th A, S61.432-S61.439 with 7th A, S61.442-S61.449 with 7th A, S61.452-S61.459 with 7th A, S66.022-S66.029 with 7th A, S66.121A, S66.123A, S66.125A, S66.127-S66.129 with 7th A, S66.222-S66.229 with 7th A, S66.321A, S66.323A, S66.325A, S66.327-S66.329 with 7th A, S66.422-S66.429 with 7th A, S66.521A, S66.523A, S66.525A, S66.527-S66.529 with 7th A, S66.822-S66.829 with 7th A, S66.922-S66.929 with 7th A

✓7th **S66.029** Laceration of long flexor muscle, fascia and tendon of unspecified thumb at wrist and hand level `CC`
CC Excl: CC with 7th character A: S61.401-S61.459 with 7th A, S66.021-S66.029 with 7th A, S66.120-S66.129 with 7th A, S66.221-S66.229 with 7th A, S66.320-S66.329 with 7th A, S66.421-S66.429 with 7th A, S66.520-S66.529 with 7th A, S66.821-S66.829 with 7th A, S66.921-S66.929 with 7th A

✓6th **S66.09** Other specified injury of long flexor muscle, fascia and tendon of thumb at wrist and hand level

✓7th **S66.091** Other specified injury of long flexor muscle, fascia and tendon of right thumb at wrist and hand level

✓7th **S66.092** Other specified injury of long flexor muscle, fascia and tendon of left thumb at wrist and hand level

✓7th **S66.099** Other specified injury of long flexor muscle, fascia and tendon of unspecified thumb at wrist and hand level

✓5th **S66.1** Injury of flexor muscle, fascia and tendon of other and unspecified finger at wrist and hand level
EXCLUDES 2 Injury of long flexor muscle, fascia and tendon of thumb at wrist and hand level (S66.0-)

✓6th **S66.10** Unspecified injury of flexor muscle, fascia and tendon of other and unspecified finger at wrist and hand level

✓7th **S66.100** Unspecified injury of flexor muscle, fascia and tendon of right index finger at wrist and hand level

✓7th **S66.101** Unspecified injury of flexor muscle, fascia and tendon of left index finger at wrist and hand level

✓7th **S66.102** Unspecified injury of flexor muscle, fascia and tendon of right middle finger at wrist and hand level

✓7th **S66.103** Unspecified injury of flexor muscle, fascia and tendon of left middle finger at wrist and hand level

✓7th **S66.104** Unspecified injury of flexor muscle, fascia and tendon of right ring finger at wrist and hand level

✓7th **S66.105** Unspecified injury of flexor muscle, fascia and tendon of left ring finger at wrist and hand level

✓7th **S66.106** Unspecified injury of flexor muscle, fascia and tendon of right little finger at wrist and hand level

✓7th **S66.107** Unspecified injury of flexor muscle, fascia and tendon of left little finger at wrist and hand level

✓7th **S66.108** Unspecified injury of flexor muscle, fascia and tendon of other finger at wrist and hand level
Unspecified injury of flexor muscle, fascia and tendon of specified finger with unspecified laterality at wrist and hand level

✓7th **S66.109** Unspecified injury of flexor muscle, fascia and tendon of unspecified finger at wrist and hand level

✓6th **S66.11** Strain of flexor muscle, fascia and tendon of other and unspecified finger at wrist and hand level

✓7th **S66.110** Strain of flexor muscle, fascia and tendon of right index finger at wrist and hand level

✓7th **S66.111** Strain of flexor muscle, fascia and tendon of left index finger at wrist and hand level

✓7th **S66.112** Strain of flexor muscle, fascia and tendon of right middle finger at wrist and hand level

✓7th **S66.113** Strain of flexor muscle, fascia and tendon of left middle finger at wrist and hand level

✓7th **S66.114** Strain of flexor muscle, fascia and tendon of right ring finger at wrist and hand level

✓7th **S66.115** Strain of flexor muscle, fascia and tendon of left ring finger at wrist and hand level

✓7th **S66.116** Strain of flexor muscle, fascia and tendon of right little finger at wrist and hand level

✓7th **S66.117** Strain of flexor muscle, fascia and tendon of left little finger at wrist and hand level

✓7th **S66.118** Strain of flexor muscle, fascia and tendon of other finger at wrist and hand level
Strain of flexor muscle, fascia and tendon of specified finger with unspecified laterality at wrist and hand level

✓7th **S66.119** Strain of flexor muscle, fascia and tendon of unspecified finger at wrist and hand level

✓6th **S66.12** Laceration of flexor muscle, fascia and tendon of other and unspecified finger at wrist and hand level

✓7th **S66.120** Laceration of flexor muscle, fascia and tendon of right index finger at wrist and hand level `CC`
CC Excl: CC with 7th character A: See code: S66.021

✓7th **S66.121** Laceration of flexor muscle, fascia and tendon of left index finger at wrist and hand level `CC`
CC Excl: CC with 7th character A: See code: S66.022

✓7th **S66.122** Laceration of flexor muscle, fascia and tendon of right middle finger at wrist and hand level `CC`
CC Excl: CC with 7th character A: See code: S66.021

✓7th **S66.123** Laceration of flexor muscle, fascia and tendon of left middle finger at wrist and hand level `CC`
CC Excl: CC with 7th character A: See code: S66.022

✓7th **S66.124** Laceration of flexor muscle, fascia and tendon of right ring finger at wrist and hand level `CC`
CC Excl: CC with 7th character A: See code: S66.021

✓7th **S66.125** Laceration of flexor muscle, fascia and tendon of left ring finger at wrist and hand level `CC`
CC Excl: CC with 7th character A: See code: S66.022

✓7th **S66.126** Laceration of flexor muscle, fascia and tendon of right little finger at wrist and hand level `CC`
CC Excl: CC with 7th character A: See code: S66.021

✓ Additional Character Required   ✓x7th Xtension Alert   Unacceptable PDx   Manifestation   Hospital Acquired Condition   EXCLUDES 1 Not Coded Here   EXCLUDES 2 Not Included Here

√7ᵗʰ **S66.127 Laceration of flexor muscle, fascia** **CC**
and tendon of left little finger at wrist
and hand level
     CC Excl: CC with 7th character A: See code:
     S66.022

√7ᵗʰ **S66.128 Laceration of flexor muscle, fascia** **CC**
and tendon of other finger at wrist
and hand level
     Laceration of flexor muscle, fascia and
     tendon of specified finger with
     unspecified laterality at wrist and
     hand level
     CC Excl: CC with 7th character A: See code:
     S66.029

√7ᵗʰ **S66.129 Laceration of flexor muscle, fascia** **CC**
and tendon of unspecified finger at
wrist and hand level
     CC Excl: CC with 7th character A: See code:
     S66.029

√6ᵗʰ **S66.19 Other injury of flexor muscle, fascia and tendon of**
other and unspecified finger at wrist and hand level

√7ᵗʰ **S66.190 Other injury of flexor muscle, fascia and**
tendon of right index finger at wrist and
hand level

√7ᵗʰ **S66.191 Other injury of flexor muscle, fascia and**
tendon of left index finger at wrist and
hand level

√7ᵗʰ **S66.192 Other injury of flexor muscle, fascia and**
tendon of right middle finger at wrist and
hand level

√7ᵗʰ **S66.193 Other injury of flexor muscle, fascia and**
tendon of left middle finger at wrist and
hand level

√7ᵗʰ **S66.194 Other injury of flexor muscle, fascia and**
tendon of right ring finger at wrist and
hand level

√7ᵗʰ **S66.195 Other injury of flexor muscle, fascia and**
tendon of left ring finger at wrist and hand
level

√7ᵗʰ **S66.196 Other injury of flexor muscle, fascia and**
tendon of right little finger at wrist and
hand level

√7ᵗʰ **S66.197 Other injury of flexor muscle, fascia and**
tendon of left little finger at wrist and
hand level

√7ᵗʰ **S66.198 Other injury of flexor muscle, fascia and**
tendon of other finger at wrist and hand
level
     Other injury of flexor muscle, fascia and
     tendon of specified finger with
     unspecified laterality at wrist and
     hand level

√7ᵗʰ **S66.199 Other injury of flexor muscle, fascia and**
tendon of unspecified finger at wrist and
hand level

√5ᵗʰ **S66.2 Injury of extensor muscle, fascia and tendon of thumb at wrist**
and hand level

√6ᵗʰ **S66.20 Unspecified injury of extensor muscle, fascia and**
tendon of thumb at wrist and hand level

√7ᵗʰ **S66.201 Unspecified injury of extensor muscle,**
fascia and tendon of right thumb at wrist
and hand level

√7ᵗʰ **S66.202 Unspecified injury of extensor muscle,**
fascia and tendon of left thumb at wrist
and hand level

√7ᵗʰ **S66.209 Unspecified injury of extensor muscle,**
fascia and tendon of unspecified thumb at
wrist and hand level

√6ᵗʰ **S66.21 Strain of extensor muscle, fascia and tendon of**
thumb at wrist and hand level

√7ᵗʰ **S66.211 Strain of extensor muscle, fascia and**
tendon of right thumb at wrist and hand
level

√7ᵗʰ **S66.212 Strain of extensor muscle, fascia and**
tendon of left thumb at wrist and hand
level

√7ᵗʰ **S66.219 Strain of extensor muscle, fascia and**
tendon of unspecified thumb at wrist and
hand level

√6ᵗʰ **S66.22 Laceration of extensor muscle, fascia and tendon of**
thumb at wrist and hand level

√7ᵗʰ **S66.221 Laceration of extensor muscle, fascia** **CC**
and tendon of right thumb at wrist and
hand level
     CC Excl: CC with 7th character A: See code:
     S66.021

√7ᵗʰ **S66.222 Laceration of extensor muscle, fascia** **CC**
and tendon of left thumb at wrist and
hand level
     CC Excl: CC with 7th character A: See code:
     S66.022

√7ᵗʰ **S66.229 Laceration of extensor muscle, fascia** **CC**
and tendon of unspecified thumb at
wrist and hand level
     CC Excl: CC with 7th character A: See code:
     S66.029

√6ᵗʰ **S66.29 Other specified injury of extensor muscle, fascia and**
tendon of thumb at wrist and hand level

√7ᵗʰ **S66.291 Other specified injury of extensor muscle,**
fascia and tendon of right thumb at wrist
and hand level

√7ᵗʰ **S66.292 Other specified injury of extensor muscle,**
fascia and tendon of left thumb at wrist
and hand level

√7ᵗʰ **S66.299 Other specified injury of extensor muscle,**
fascia and tendon of unspecified thumb at
wrist and hand level

√5ᵗʰ **S66.3 Injury of extensor muscle, fascia and tendon of other and**
unspecified finger at wrist and hand level
     EXCLUDES 2 *Injury of extensor muscle, fascia and tendon of thumb*
     at wrist and hand level (S66.2-)

√6ᵗʰ **S66.30 Unspecified injury of extensor muscle, fascia and**
tendon of other and unspecified finger at wrist and
hand level

√7ᵗʰ **S66.300 Unspecified injury of extensor muscle,**
fascia and tendon of right index finger at
wrist and hand level

√7ᵗʰ **S66.301 Unspecified injury of extensor muscle,**
fascia and tendon of left index finger at
wrist and hand level

√7ᵗʰ **S66.302 Unspecified injury of extensor muscle,**
fascia and tendon of right middle finger at
wrist and hand level

√7ᵗʰ **S66.303 Unspecified injury of extensor muscle,**
fascia and tendon of left middle finger at
wrist and hand level

√7ᵗʰ **S66.304 Unspecified injury of extensor muscle,**
fascia and tendon of right ring finger at
wrist and hand level

√7ᵗʰ **S66.305 Unspecified injury of extensor muscle,**
fascia and tendon of left ring finger at
wrist and hand level

√7ᵗʰ **S66.306 Unspecified injury of extensor muscle,**
fascia and tendon of right little finger at
wrist and hand level

√7ᵗʰ **S66.307 Unspecified injury of extensor muscle,**
fascia and tendon of left little finger at
wrist and hand level

√7ᵗʰ **S66.308 Unspecified injury of extensor muscle,**
fascia and tendon of other finger at wrist
and hand level
     Unspecified injury of extensor muscle,
     fascia and tendon of specified finger
     with unspecified laterality at wrist and
     hand level

√7ᵗʰ **S66.309 Unspecified injury of extensor muscle,**
fascia and tendon of unspecified finger at
wrist and hand level

√6ᵗʰ **S66.31 Strain of extensor muscle, fascia and tendon of other**
and unspecified finger at wrist and hand level

√7ᵗʰ **S66.310 Strain of extensor muscle, fascia and**
tendon of right index finger at wrist
and hand level

√7ᵗʰ **S66.311 Strain of extensor muscle, fascia and**
tendon of left index finger at wrist
and hand level

√7ᵗʰ **S66.312 Strain of extensor muscle, fascia and**
tendon of right middle finger at wrist
and hand level

√7th **S66.313** **Strain of extensor muscle, fascia and tendon of left middle finger at wrist and hand level**

√7th **S66.314** **Strain of extensor muscle, fascia and tendon of right ring finger at wrist and hand level**

√7th **S66.315** **Strain of extensor muscle, fascia and tendon of left ring finger at wrist and hand level**

√7th **S66.316** **Strain of extensor muscle, fascia and tendon of right little finger at wrist and hand level**

√7th **S66.317** **Strain of extensor muscle, fascia and tendon of left little finger at wrist and hand level**

√7th **S66.318** **Strain of extensor muscle, fascia and tendon of other finger at wrist and hand level**
Strain of extensor muscle, fascia and tendon of specified finger with unspecified laterality at wrist and hand level

√7th **S66.319** **Strain of extensor muscle, fascia and tendon of unspecified finger at wrist and hand level**

√6th **S66.32** Laceration of extensor muscle, fascia and tendon of other and unspecified finger at wrist and hand level

√7th **S66.320** **Laceration of extensor muscle, fascia and tendon of right index finger at wrist and hand level** CC
CC Excl: CC with 7th character A: See code: S66.021

√7th **S66.321** **Laceration of extensor muscle, fascia and tendon of left index finger at wrist and hand level** CC
CC Excl: CC with 7th character A: See code: S66.022

√7th **S66.322** **Laceration of extensor muscle, fascia and tendon of right middle finger at wrist and hand level** CC
CC Excl: CC with 7th character A: See code: S66.021

√7th **S66.323** **Laceration of extensor muscle, fascia and tendon of left middle finger at wrist and hand level** CC
CC Excl: CC with 7th character A: See code: S66.022

√7th **S66.324** **Laceration of extensor muscle, fascia and tendon of right ring finger at wrist and hand level** CC
CC Excl: CC with 7th character A: See code: S66.021

√7th **S66.325** **Laceration of extensor muscle, fascia and tendon of left ring finger at wrist and hand level** CC
CC Excl: CC with 7th character A: See code: S66.022

√7th **S66.326** **Laceration of extensor muscle, fascia and tendon of right little finger at wrist and hand level** CC
CC Excl: CC with 7th character A: See code: S66.021

√7th **S66.327** **Laceration of extensor muscle, fascia and tendon of left little finger at wrist and hand level** CC
CC Excl: CC with 7th character A: See code: S66.022

√7th **S66.328** **Laceration of extensor muscle, fascia and tendon of other finger at wrist and hand level** CC
Laceration of extensor muscle, fascia and tendon of specified finger with unspecified laterality at wrist and hand level
CC Excl: CC with 7th character A: See code: S66.029

√7th **S66.329** **Laceration of extensor muscle, fascia and tendon of unspecified finger at wrist and hand level** CC
CC Excl: CC with 7th character A: See code: S66.029

√6th **S66.39** Other injury of extensor muscle, fascia and tendon of other and unspecified finger at wrist and hand level

√7th **S66.390** **Other injury of extensor muscle, fascia and tendon of right index finger at wrist and hand level**

√7th **S66.391** **Other injury of extensor muscle, fascia and tendon of left index finger at wrist and hand level**

√7th **S66.392** **Other injury of extensor muscle, fascia and tendon of right middle finger at wrist and hand level**

√7th **S66.393** **Other injury of extensor muscle, fascia and tendon of left middle finger at wrist and hand level**

√7th **S66.394** **Other injury of extensor muscle, fascia and tendon of right ring finger at wrist and hand level**

√7th **S66.395** **Other injury of extensor muscle, fascia and tendon of left ring finger at wrist and hand level**

√7th **S66.396** **Other injury of extensor muscle, fascia and tendon of right little finger at wrist and hand level**

√7th **S66.397** **Other injury of extensor muscle, fascia and tendon of left little finger at wrist and hand level**

√7th **S66.398** **Other injury of extensor muscle, fascia and tendon of other finger at wrist and hand level**
Other injury of extensor muscle, fascia and tendon of specified finger with unspecified laterality at wrist and hand level

√7th **S66.399** **Other injury of extensor muscle, fascia and tendon of unspecified finger at wrist and hand level**

√5th **S66.4** Injury of intrinsic muscle, fascia and tendon of thumb at wrist and hand level

√6th **S66.40** Unspecified injury of intrinsic muscle, fascia and tendon of thumb at wrist and hand level

√7th **S66.401** **Unspecified injury of intrinsic muscle, fascia and tendon of right thumb at wrist and hand level**

√7th **S66.402** **Unspecified injury of intrinsic muscle, fascia and tendon of left thumb at wrist and hand level**

√7th **S66.409** **Unspecified injury of intrinsic muscle, fascia and tendon of unspecified thumb at wrist and hand level**

√6th **S66.41** Strain of intrinsic muscle, fascia and tendon of thumb at wrist and hand level

√7th **S66.411** **Strain of intrinsic muscle, fascia and tendon of right thumb at wrist and hand level**

√7th **S66.412** **Strain of intrinsic muscle, fascia and tendon of left thumb at wrist and hand level**

√7th **S66.419** **Strain of intrinsic muscle, fascia and tendon of unspecified thumb at wrist and hand level**

√6th **S66.42** Laceration of intrinsic muscle, fascia and tendon of thumb at wrist and hand level

√7th **S66.421** **Laceration of intrinsic muscle, fascia and tendon of right thumb at wrist and hand level** CC
CC Excl: CC with 7th character A: See code: S66.021

√7th **S66.422** **Laceration of intrinsic muscle, fascia and tendon of left thumb at wrist and hand level** CC
CC Excl: CC with 7th character A: See code: S66.022

√7th **S66.429** **Laceration of intrinsic muscle, fascia and tendon of unspecified thumb at wrist and hand level** CC
CC Excl: CC with 7th character A: See code: S66.029

✓6ᵗʰ **S66.49** **Other** specified injury of intrinsic muscle, fascia and tendon of thumb at wrist and hand level

✓7ᵗʰ **S66.491** Other specified injury of intrinsic muscle, fascia and tendon of right thumb at wrist and hand level

✓7ᵗʰ **S66.492** Other specified injury of intrinsic muscle, fascia and tendon of left thumb at wrist and hand level

✓7ᵗʰ **S66.499** Other specified injury of intrinsic muscle, fascia and tendon of unspecified thumb at wrist and hand level

✓5ᵗʰ **S66.5** Injury of intrinsic muscle, fascia and tendon of other and unspecified finger at wrist and hand level

EXCLUDES 2   *injury of intrinsic muscle, fascia and tendon of thumb at wrist and hand level (S66.4-)*

✓6ᵗʰ **S66.50** **Unspecified** injury of intrinsic muscle, fascia and tendon of other and unspecified finger at wrist and hand level

✓7ᵗʰ **S66.500** Unspecified injury of intrinsic muscle, fascia and tendon of right index finger at wrist and hand level

✓7ᵗʰ **S66.501** Unspecified injury of intrinsic muscle, fascia and tendon of left index finger at wrist and hand level

✓7ᵗʰ **S66.502** Unspecified injury of intrinsic muscle, fascia and tendon of right middle finger at wrist and hand level

✓7ᵗʰ **S66.503** Unspecified injury of intrinsic muscle, fascia and tendon of left middle finger at wrist and hand level

✓7ᵗʰ **S66.504** Unspecified injury of intrinsic muscle, fascia and tendon of right ring finger at wrist and hand level

✓7ᵗʰ **S66.505** Unspecified injury of intrinsic muscle, fascia and tendon of left ring finger at wrist and hand level

✓7ᵗʰ **S66.506** Unspecified injury of intrinsic muscle, fascia and tendon of right little finger at wrist and hand level

✓7ᵗʰ **S66.507** Unspecified injury of intrinsic muscle, fascia and tendon of left little finger at wrist and hand level

✓7ᵗʰ **S66.508** Unspecified injury of intrinsic muscle, fascia and tendon of other finger at wrist and hand level

Unspecified injury of intrinsic muscle, fascia and tendon of specified finger with unspecified laterality at wrist and hand level

✓7ᵗʰ **S66.509** Unspecified injury of intrinsic muscle, fascia and tendon of unspecified finger at wrist and hand level

✓6ᵗʰ **S66.51** **Strain** of intrinsic muscle, fascia and tendon of other and unspecified finger at wrist and hand level

✓7ᵗʰ **S66.510** Strain of intrinsic muscle, fascia and tendon of right index finger at wrist and hand level

✓7ᵗʰ **S66.511** Strain of intrinsic muscle, fascia and tendon of left index finger at wrist and hand level

✓7ᵗʰ **S66.512** Strain of intrinsic muscle, fascia and tendon of right middle finger at wrist and hand level

✓7ᵗʰ **S66.513** Strain of intrinsic muscle, fascia and tendon of left middle finger at wrist and hand level

✓7ᵗʰ **S66.514** Strain of intrinsic muscle, fascia and tendon of right ring finger at wrist and hand level

✓7ᵗʰ **S66.515** Strain of intrinsic muscle, fascia and tendon of left ring finger at wrist and hand level

✓7ᵗʰ **S66.516** Strain of intrinsic muscle, fascia and tendon of right little finger at wrist and hand level

✓7ᵗʰ **S66.517** Strain of intrinsic muscle, fascia and tendon of left little finger at wrist and hand level

✓7ᵗʰ **S66.518** Strain of intrinsic muscle, fascia and tendon of other finger at wrist and hand level

Strain of intrinsic muscle, fascia and tendon of specified finger with unspecified laterality at wrist and hand level

✓7ᵗʰ **S66.519** Strain of intrinsic muscle, fascia and tendon of unspecified finger at wrist and hand level

✓6ᵗʰ **S66.52** Laceration of intrinsic muscle, fascia and tendon of other and unspecified finger at wrist and hand level

✓7ᵗʰ **S66.520** Laceration of intrinsic muscle, fascia and tendon of right index finger at wrist and hand level CC

CC Excl: CC with 7th character A: See code: S66.021

✓7ᵗʰ **S66.521** Laceration of intrinsic muscle, fascia and tendon of left index finger at wrist and hand level CC

CC Excl: CC with 7th character A: See code: S66.022

✓7ᵗʰ **S66.522** Laceration of intrinsic muscle, fascia and tendon of right middle finger at wrist and hand level CC

CC Excl: CC with 7th character A: See code: S66.021

✓7ᵗʰ **S66.523** Laceration of intrinsic muscle, fascia and tendon of left middle finger at wrist and hand level CC

CC Excl: CC with 7th character A: See code: S66.022

✓7ᵗʰ **S66.524** Laceration of intrinsic muscle, fascia and tendon of right ring finger at wrist and hand level CC

CC Excl: CC with 7th character A: See code: S66.021

✓7ᵗʰ **S66.525** Laceration of intrinsic muscle, fascia and tendon of left ring finger at wrist and hand level CC

CC Excl: CC with 7th character A: See code: S66.022

✓7ᵗʰ **S66.526** Laceration of intrinsic muscle, fascia and tendon of right little finger at wrist and hand level CC

CC Excl: CC with 7th character A: See code: S66.021

✓7ᵗʰ **S66.527** Laceration of intrinsic muscle, fascia and tendon of left little finger at wrist and hand level CC

CC Excl: CC with 7th character A: See code: S66.022

✓7ᵗʰ **S66.528** Laceration of intrinsic muscle, fascia and tendon of other finger at wrist and hand level CC

Laceration of intrinsic muscle, fascia and tendon of specified finger with unspecified laterality at wrist and hand level

CC Excl: CC with 7th character A: See code: S66.029

✓7ᵗʰ **S66.529** Laceration of intrinsic muscle, fascia and tendon of unspecified finger at wrist and hand level CC

CC Excl: CC with 7th character A: See code: S66.029

✓6ᵗʰ **S66.59** Other injury of intrinsic muscle, fascia and tendon of other and unspecified finger at wrist and hand level

✓7ᵗʰ **S66.590** Other injury of intrinsic muscle, fascia and tendon of right index finger at wrist and hand level

✓7ᵗʰ **S66.591** Other injury of intrinsic muscle, fascia and tendon of left index finger at wrist and hand level

✓7ᵗʰ **S66.592** Other injury of intrinsic muscle, fascia and tendon of right middle finger at wrist and hand level

✓7ᵗʰ **S66.593** Other injury of intrinsic muscle, fascia and tendon of left middle finger at wrist and hand level

✓7ᵗʰ **S66.594** Other injury of intrinsic muscle, fascia and tendon of right ring finger at wrist and hand level

N Newborn: 0   P Pediatric: 0-17   M Maternity: 12-55   A Adult: 15-124   MCC Major CC Condition   PDx MCC PDx acts as own MCC   CC CC Condition   PDx CC PDx acts as own CC

968

ICD-10-CM Draft (2015)

√7ᵗʰ **S66.595** Other injury of intrinsic muscle, fascia and tendon of left ring finger at wrist and hand level

√7ᵗʰ **S66.596** Other injury of intrinsic muscle, fascia and tendon of right little finger at wrist and hand level

√7ᵗʰ **S66.597** Other injury of intrinsic muscle, fascia and tendon of left little finger at wrist and hand level

√7ᵗʰ **S66.598** Other injury of intrinsic muscle, fascia and tendon of other finger at wrist and hand level

> Other injury of intrinsic muscle, fascia and tendon of specified finger with unspecified laterality at wrist and hand level

√7ᵗʰ **S66.599** Other injury of intrinsic muscle, fascia and tendon of unspecified finger at wrist and hand level

√5ᵗʰ **S66.8** Injury of other specified muscles, fascia and tendons at wrist and hand level

√6ᵗʰ **S66.80** Unspecified injury of other specified muscles, fascia and tendons at wrist and hand level

√7ᵗʰ **S66.801** Unspecified injury of other specified muscles, fascia and tendons at wrist and hand level, right hand

√7ᵗʰ **S66.802** Unspecified injury of other specified muscles, fascia and tendons at wrist and hand level, left hand

√7ᵗʰ **S66.809** Unspecified injury of other specified muscles, fascia and tendons at wrist and hand level, unspecified hand

√6ᵗʰ **S66.81** Strain of other specified muscles, fascia and tendons at wrist and hand level

√7ᵗʰ **S66.811** Strain of other specified muscles, fascia and tendons at wrist and hand level, right hand

√7ᵗʰ **S66.812** Strain of other specified muscles, fascia and tendons at wrist and hand level, left hand

√7ᵗʰ **S66.819** Strain of other specified muscles, fascia and tendons at wrist and hand level, unspecified hand

√6ᵗʰ **S66.82** Laceration of other specified muscles, fascia and tendons at wrist and hand level

√7ᵗʰ **S66.821** Laceration of other specified muscles, fascia and tendons at wrist and hand level, right hand   CC

> CC Excl: CC with 7th character A: See code: S66.021

√7ᵗʰ **S66.822** Laceration of other specified muscles, fascia and tendons at wrist and hand level, left hand   CC

> CC Excl: CC with 7th character A: See code: S66.022

√7ᵗʰ **S66.829** Laceration of other specified muscles, fascia and tendons at wrist and hand level, unspecified hand   CC

> CC Excl: CC with 7th character A: See code: S66.029

√6ᵗʰ **S66.89** Other injury of other specified muscles, fascia and tendons at wrist and hand level

√7ᵗʰ **S66.891** Other injury of other specified muscles, fascia and tendons at wrist and hand level, right hand

√7ᵗʰ **S66.892** Other injury of other specified muscles, fascia and tendons at wrist and hand level, left hand

√7ᵗʰ **S66.899** Other injury of other specified muscles, fascia and tendons at wrist and hand level, unspecified hand

√5ᵗʰ **S66.9** Injury of unspecified muscle, fascia and tendon at wrist and hand level

√6ᵗʰ **S66.90** Unspecified injury of unspecified muscle, fascia and tendon at wrist and hand level

√7ᵗʰ **S66.901** Unspecified injury of unspecified muscle, fascia and tendon at wrist and hand level, right hand

√7ᵗʰ **S66.902** Unspecified injury of unspecified muscle, fascia and tendon at wrist and hand level, left hand

√7ᵗʰ **S66.909** Unspecified injury of unspecified muscle, fascia and tendon at wrist and hand level, unspecified hand

√6ᵗʰ **S66.91** Strain of unspecified muscle, fascia and tendon at wrist and hand level

√7ᵗʰ **S66.911** Strain of unspecified muscle, fascia and tendon at wrist and hand level, right hand

√7ᵗʰ **S66.912** Strain of unspecified muscle, fascia and tendon at wrist and hand level, left hand

√7ᵗʰ **S66.919** Strain of unspecified muscle, fascia and tendon at wrist and hand level, unspecified hand

√6ᵗʰ **S66.92** Laceration of unspecified muscle, fascia and tendon at wrist and hand level

√7ᵗʰ **S66.921** Laceration of unspecified muscle, fascia and tendon at wrist and hand level, right hand   CC

> CC Excl: CC with 7th character A: See code: S66.021

√7ᵗʰ **S66.922** Laceration of unspecified muscle, fascia and tendon at wrist and hand level, left hand   CC

> CC Excl: CC with 7th character A: See code: S66.022

√7ᵗʰ **S66.929** Laceration of unspecified muscle, fascia and tendon at wrist and hand level, unspecified hand   CC

> CC Excl: CC with 7th character A: See code: S66.029

√6ᵗʰ **S66.99** Other injury of unspecified muscle, fascia and tendon at wrist and hand level

√7ᵗʰ **S66.991** Other injury of unspecified muscle, fascia and tendon at wrist and hand level, right hand

√7ᵗʰ **S66.992** Other injury of unspecified muscle, fascia and tendon at wrist and hand level, left hand

√7ᵗʰ **S66.999** Other injury of unspecified muscle, fascia and tendon at wrist and hand level, unspecified hand

√4ᵗʰ **S67 Crushing injury of wrist, hand and fingers**

> Use additional code for all associated injuries, such as:
> fracture of wrist and hand (S62.-)
> open wound of wrist and hand (S61.-)

> The appropriate 7th character is to be added to each code from category S67.
> A   initial encounter
> D   subsequent encounter
> S   sequela

√5ᵗʰ **S67.0 Crushing injury of thumb**

√x7ᵗʰ **S67.00** Crushing injury of unspecified thumb

√x7ᵗʰ **S67.01** Crushing injury of right thumb

√x7ᵗʰ **S67.02** Crushing injury of left thumb

√5ᵗʰ **S67.1 Crushing injury of other and unspecified finger(s)**

> EXCLUDES 2   crushing injury of thumb (S67.0-)

√x7ᵗʰ **S67.10** Crushing injury of unspecified finger(s)

√6ᵗʰ **S67.19** Crushing injury of other finger(s)

√7ᵗʰ **S67.190** Crushing injury of right index finger

√7ᵗʰ **S67.191** Crushing injury of left index finger

√7ᵗʰ **S67.192** Crushing injury of right middle finger

√7ᵗʰ **S67.193** Crushing injury of left middle finger

√7ᵗʰ **S67.194** Crushing injury of right ring finger

√7ᵗʰ **S67.195** Crushing injury of left ring finger

√7ᵗʰ **S67.196** Crushing injury of right little finger

√7ᵗʰ **S67.197** Crushing injury of left little finger

√7ᵗʰ **S67.198** Crushing injury of other finger

> Crushing injury of specified finger with unspecified laterality

√5ᵗʰ **S67.2 Crushing injury of hand**

> EXCLUDES 2   crushing injury of fingers (S67.1-)
> crushing injury of thumb (S67.0-)

√x7ᵗʰ **S67.20** Crushing injury of unspecified hand

✔ Additional Character Required   √x7ᵗʰ Xtension Alert   Unacceptable PDx   Manifestation   Hospital Acquired Condition   EXCLUDES 1 Not Coded Here   EXCLUDES 2 Not Included Here

ICD-10-CM Draft (2015)   969

Injury, Poisoning and Certain Other Consequences of External Causes

S67.21–S68.411

✓7ᵗʰ **S67.21** **Crushing injury of** right **hand**

✓7ᵗʰ **S67.22** **Crushing injury of** left **hand**

✓5ᵗʰ **S67.3** **Crushing injury of** wrist

    ✓x7ᵗʰ **S67.30** **Crushing injury of** unspecified **wrist**

    ✓x7ᵗʰ **S67.31** **Crushing injury of** right **wrist**

    ✓x7ᵗʰ **S67.32** **Crushing injury of** left **wrist**

✓5ᵗʰ **S67.4** **Crushing injury of** wrist and hand

    EXCLUDES 1 *crushing injury of hand alone (S67.2-)*
    crushing injury of wrist alone (S67.3-)
    EXCLUDES 2 *crushing injury of fingers (S67.1-)*
    crushing injury of thumb (S67.0-)

    ✓x7ᵗʰ **S67.40** **Crushing injury of** unspecified **wrist and hand**

    ✓x7ᵗʰ **S67.41** **Crushing injury of** right **wrist and hand**

    ✓x7ᵗʰ **S67.42** **Crushing injury of** left **wrist and hand**

✓5ᵗʰ **S67.9** **Crushing injury of** unspecified part(s) of wrist, hand and fingers

    ✓x7ᵗʰ **S67.90** **Crushing injury of unspecified part(s) of** unspecified **wrist, hand and fingers**

    ✓x7ᵗʰ **S67.91** **Crushing injury of unspecified part(s) of** right **wrist, hand and fingers**

    ✓x7ᵗʰ **S67.92** **Crushing injury of unspecified part(s) of** left **wrist, hand and fingers**

✓4ᵗʰ **S68** **Traumatic amputation of wrist, hand and fingers**

    NOTE An amputation not identified as partial or complete should be coded to complete.

    The appropriate 7th character is to be added to each code from category S68.
    A   initial encounter
    D   subsequent encounter
    S   sequela

✓5ᵗʰ **S68.0** **Traumatic** metacarpophalangeal amputation of thumb
    Traumatic amputation of thumb NOS

    ✓6ᵗʰ **S68.01** **Complete traumatic metacarpophalangeal amputation of thumb**

        ✓7ᵗʰ **S68.011** **Complete traumatic metacarpophalangeal amputation of** right **thumb**

        ✓7ᵗʰ **S68.012** **Complete traumatic metacarpophalangeal amputation of** left **thumb**

        ✓7ᵗʰ **S68.019** **Complete traumatic metacarpophalangeal amputation of** unspecified **thumb**

    ✓6ᵗʰ **S68.02** Partial **traumatic metacarpophalangeal amputation of thumb**

        ✓7ᵗʰ **S68.021** **Partial traumatic metacarpophalangeal amputation of** right **thumb**

        ✓7ᵗʰ **S68.022** **Partial traumatic metacarpophalangeal amputation of** left **thumb**

        ✓7ᵗʰ **S68.029** **Partial traumatic metacarpophalangeal amputation of** unspecified **thumb**

✓5ᵗʰ **S68.1** **Traumatic** metacarpophalangeal **amputation of** other and unspecified finger
    Traumatic amputation of finger NOS
    EXCLUDES 2 *traumatic metacarpophalangeal amputation of thumb (S68.0-)*

    ✓6ᵗʰ **S68.11** **Complete traumatic metacarpophalangeal amputation of other and unspecified finger**

        ✓7ᵗʰ **S68.110** **Complete traumatic metacarpophalangeal amputation of** right **index finger**

        ✓7ᵗʰ **S68.111** **Complete traumatic metacarpophalangeal amputation of** left **index finger**

        ✓7ᵗʰ **S68.112** **Complete traumatic metacarpophalangeal amputation of** right **middle finger**

        ✓7ᵗʰ **S68.113** **Complete traumatic metacarpophalangeal amputation of** left **middle finger**

        ✓7ᵗʰ **S68.114** **Complete traumatic metacarpophalangeal amputation of** right **ring finger**

        ✓7ᵗʰ **S68.115** **Complete traumatic metacarpophalangeal amputation of** left **ring finger**

        ✓7ᵗʰ **S68.116** **Complete traumatic metacarpophalangeal amputation of** right **little finger**

        ✓7ᵗʰ **S68.117** **Complete traumatic metacarpophalangeal amputation of** left **little finger**

        ✓7ᵗʰ **S68.118** **Complete traumatic metacarpophalangeal amputation of** other **finger**
        Complete traumatic metacarpophalangeal amputation of specified finger with unspecified laterality

        ✓7ᵗʰ **S68.119** **Complete traumatic metacarpophalangeal amputation of** unspecified **finger**

    ✓6ᵗʰ **S68.12** Partial **traumatic metacarpophalangeal amputation of other and unspecified finger**

        ✓7ᵗʰ **S68.120** **Partial traumatic metacarpophalangeal amputation of** right index **finger**

        ✓7ᵗʰ **S68.121** **Partial traumatic metacarpophalangeal amputation of** left index **finger**

        ✓7ᵗʰ **S68.122** **Partial traumatic metacarpophalangeal amputation of** right middle **finger**

        ✓7ᵗʰ **S68.123** **Partial traumatic metacarpophalangeal amputation of** left middle **finger**

        ✓7ᵗʰ **S68.124** **Partial traumatic metacarpophalangeal amputation of** right ring **finger**

        ✓7ᵗʰ **S68.125** **Partial traumatic metacarpophalangeal amputation of** left ring **finger**

        ✓7ᵗʰ **S68.126** **Partial traumatic metacarpophalangeal amputation of** right little **finger**

        ✓7ᵗʰ **S68.127** **Partial traumatic metacarpophalangeal amputation of** left little **finger**

        ✓7ᵗʰ **S68.128** **Partial traumatic metacarpophalangeal amputation of** other **finger**
        Partial traumatic metacarpophalangeal amputation of specified finger with unspecified laterality

        ✓7ᵗʰ **S68.129** **Partial traumatic metacarpophalangeal amputation of** unspecified **finger**

✓5ᵗʰ **S68.4** **Traumatic amputation of** hand at wrist level
    Traumatic amputation of hand NOS
    Traumatic amputation of wrist

    ✓6ᵗʰ **S68.41** **Complete traumatic amputation of hand at wrist level**

        ✓7ᵗʰ **S68.411** **Complete traumatic amputation of** **CC** **right hand at wrist level**
        CC Excl: CC with 7th character A: S41.001A, S41.009-S41.011 with 7th A, S41.019-S41.021 with 7th A, S41.029-S41.031 with 7th A, S41.039-S41.041 with 7th A, S41.049-S41.051 with 7th A, S41.059-S41.101 with 7th A, S41.109-S41.111 with 7th A, S41.119-S41.121 with 7th A, S41.129-S41.131 with 7th A, S41.139-S41.141 with 7th A, S41.149-S41.151 with 7th A, S41.159A, S46.021A, S46.029A, S46.121A, S46.129A, S46.221A, S46.229A, S46.321A, S46.329A, S46.821A, S46.829A, S46.921A, S46.929 A, S48.011A, S48.019-S48.021 with 7th A, S48.029-S48.111 with 7th A, S48.119-S48.121 with 7th A, S48.129-S48.911 with 7th A, S48.919-S48.921 with 7th A, S48.929A, S51.001A, S51.009-S51.011 with 7th A, S51.019-S51.021 with 7th A, S51.029-S51.031 with 7th A, S51.039-S51.041 with 7th A, S51.049-S51.051 with 7th A, S51.059-S51.801 with 7th A, S51.809-S51.811 with 7th A, S51.819-S51.821 with 7th A, S51.829-S51.831 with 7th A, S51.839-S51.841 with 7th A, S51.849-S51.851A, S51.859A, S56.021A, S56.029A, S56.121A, S56.123A, S56.125A, S56.127A, S56.129A, S56.221A, S56.229A, S56.321A, S56.329A, S56.421A, S56.423A, S56.425A, S56.427A, S56.429A, S56.521A, S56.529A, S56.821A, S56.829 with 7th A, S56.921 with 7th A, S56.929 with 7th A, S58.011 with 7th A, S58.019-S58.021 with 7th A, S58.029-S58.111 with 7th A, S58.119-S58.121 with 7th A, S58.129-S58.911 with 7th A, S58.919-S58.921 with 7th A, S58.929 with 7th A, S61.001 with 7th A, S61.009-S61.011 with 7th A, S61.019-S61.021 with 7th A, S61.029-S61.031 with 7th A, S61.039-S61.041 with

N Newborn: 0   P Pediatric: 0-17   M Maternity: 12-55   A Adult: 15-124   MCC Major CC Condition   PDx MCC PDx acts as own MCC   CC CC Condition   PDx CC PDx acts as own CC

970   ICD-10-CM Draft (2015)

7th A, S61.049-S61.051 with 7th A, S61.059-
S61.101 with 7th A, S61.109-S61.111 with
7th A, S61.119-S61.121 with 7th A, S61.129-
S61.131 with 7th A, S61.139-S61.141 with
7th A, S61.149-S61.151 with 7th A, S61.159-
S61.200 with 7th A, S61.202A, S61.204A,
S61.206A, S61.208-S61.210 with 7th A,
S61.212A, S61.214A, S61.216A, S61.218-
S61.220 with 7th A, S61.222A, S61.224A,
S61.226A, S61.228-S61.230 with 7th A,
S61.232A, S61.234A, S61.236A, S61.238-
S61.240 with 7th A, S61.242A, S61.244A,
S61.246A, S61.248-S61.250 with 7th A,
S61.252A, S61.254A, S61.256A, S61.258-
S61.300A, S61.302A, S61.304A, S61.306A,
S61.308-S61.310 with 7th A, S61.312A,
S61.314A, S61.316A, S61.318-S61.320 with
7th A, S61.322A, S61.324A, S61.326A,
S61.328-S61.330 with 7th A, S61.332A,
S61.334A, S61.336A, S61.338-S61.340 with
7th A, S61.342A, S61.344A, S61.346A,
S61.348-S61.350 with 7th A, S61.352A,
S61.354A, S61.356A, S61.358-S61.401 with
7th A, S61.409-S61.411 with 7th A, S61.419-
S61.421 with 7th A, S61.429-S61.431 with
7th A, S61.439-S61.441 with 7th A, S61.449-
S61.451 with 7th A, S61.459-S61.501 with
7th A, S61.509-S61.511 with 7th A, S61.519-
S61.521 with 7th A, S61.529-S61.531 with
7th A, S61.539-S61.541 with 7th A, S61.549-
S61.551 with 7th A, S61.559A, S66.021A,
S66.029A, S66.120A, S66.122A, S66.124A,
S66.126A, S66.128-S66.129 with 7th A,
S66.221A, S66.229A, S66.320A, S66.322A,
S66.324A, S66.326A, S66.328-S66.329 with
7th A, S66.421A, S66.429A, S66.520A,
S66.522A, S66.524A, S66.526A, S66.528-
S66.529 with 7th A, S66.821A, S66.829A,
S66.921A, S66.929A, S68.011A, S68.019-
S68.021 with 7th A, S68.029-S68.110 with
7th A, S68.112A, S68.114A, S68.116A,
S68.118-S68.120 with 7th A, S68.122A,
S68.124A, S68.126A, S68.128-S68.411 with
7th A, S68.419-S68.421 with 7th A, S68.429-
S68.511 with 7th A, S68.519-S68.521 with
7th A, S68.529-S68.610 with 7th A, S68.612A,
S68.614A, S68.616A, S68.618-S68.620 with
7th A, S68.622A, S68.624A, S68.626A,
S68.628-S68.711 with 7th A, S68.719-
S68.721 with 7th A, S68.729A, T14.8-T14.91,
T79.A0X-T79.9XX with 7th A

✓7ᵗʰ S68.412 Complete traumatic amputation of **CC**
left hand at wrist level
CC Excl: CC with 7th character A: S41.002-
S41.009 with 7th A, S41.012-S41.019 with
7th A, S41.022-S41.029 with 7th A, S41.032-
S41.039 with 7th A, S41.042-S41.049 with
7th A, S41.052-S41.059 with 7th A, S41.102-
S41.109 with 7th A, S41.112-S41.119 with
7th A, S41.122-S41.129 with 7th A, S41.132-
S41.139 with 7th A, S41.142-S41.149 with
7th A, S41.152-S41.159 with 7th A, S46.022-
S46.029 with 7th A, S46.122-S46.129 with
7th A, S46.222-S46.229 with 7th A, S46.322-
S46.329 with 7th A, S46.822-S46.829 with
7th A, S46.922-S46.929 with 7th A, S48.012-
S48.019 with 7th A, S48.022-S48.029 with
7th A, S48.112-S48.119 with 7th A, S48.122-
S48.129 with 7th A, S48.912-S48.919 with
7th A, S48.922-S48.929 with 7th A, S51.002-
S51.009 with 7th A, S51.012-S51.019 with
7th A, S51.022-S51.029 with 7th A, S51.032-
S51.039 with 7th A, S51.042-S51.049 with
7th A, S51.052-S51.059 with 7th A, S51.802-
S51.809 with 7th A, S51.812-S51.819 with
7th A, S51.822-S51.829 with 7th A, S51.832-
S51.839 with 7th A, S51.842-S51.849 with
7th A, S51.852-S51.859 with 7th A, S56.022-
S56.029 with 7th A, S56.122A, S56.124 A,
S56.126A, S56.128-S56.129 with 7th A,
S56.222-S56.229 with 7th A, S56.322-
S56.329 with 7th A, S56.422A, S56.424A,
S56.426A, S56.428-S56.429 with 7th A,
S56.522-S56.529 with 7th A, S56.822-
S56.829 with 7th A, S56.922-S56.929 with
7th A, S58.012-S58.019 with 7th A, S58.022-
S58.029 with 7th A, S58.112-S58.119 with
7th A, S58.122-S58.129 with 7th A, S58.912-
S58.919 with 7th A, S58.922-S58.929 with
7th A, S61.002-S61.009 with 7th A, S61.012-
S61.019 with 7th A, S61.022-S61.029 with
7th A, S61.032-S61.039 with 7th A, S61.042-

S61.049 with 7th A, S61.052-S61.059 with
7th A, S61.102-S61.109 with 7th A, S61.112-
S61.119 with 7th A, S61.122-S61.129 with
7th A, S61.132-S61.139 with 7th A, S61.142-
S61.149 with 7th A, S61.152-S61.159 with
7th A, S61.201A, S61.203A, S61.205A,
S61.207-S61.209 with 7th A, S61.211A,
S61.213A, S61.215A, S61.217-S61.219 with
7th A, S61.221A, S61.223A, S61.225A,
S61.227-S61.229 with 7th A, S61.231A,
S61.233A, S61.235A, S61.237-S61.239 with
7th A, S61.241A, S61.243A, S61.245 A,
S61.247-S61.249 with 7th A, S61.251A,
S61.253 A, S61.255A, S61.257-S61.259 with
7th A, S61.301 A, S61.303A, S61.305A,
S61.307-S61.309 with 7th A, S61.311A,
S61.313A, S61.315A, S61.317-S61.319 with
7th A, S61.321A, S61.323A, S61.325 A,
S61.327-S61.329 with 7th A, S61.331A,
S61.333A, S61.335A, S61.337-S61.339 with
7th A, S61.341A, S61.343A, S61.345A,
S61.347-S61.349 with 7th A, S61.351A,
S61.353A, S61.355A, S61.357-S61.359 with
7th A, S61.402-S61.409 with 7th A, S61.412-
S61.419 with 7th A, S61.422-S61.429 with
7th A, S61.432-S61.439 with 7th A, S61.442-
S61.449 with 7th A, S61.452-S61.459 with
7th A, S61.502-S61.509 with 7th A, S61.512-
S61.519 with 7th A, S61.522-S61.529 with
7th A, S61.532-S61.539 with 7th A, S61.542-
S61.549 with 7th A, S61.552-S61.559 with
7th A, S66.022-S66.029 with 7th A, S66.121A,
S66.123A, S66.125A, S66.127-S66.129 with
7th A, S66.222-S66.229 with 7th A, S66.321A,
S66.323A, S66.325A, S66.327-S66.329 with
7th A, S66.422-S66.429 with 7th A, S66.521A,
S66.523A, S66.525A, S66.527-S66.529 with
7th A, S66.822-S66.829 with 7th A, S66.922-
S66.929 with 7th A, S68.012-S68.019 with
7th A, S68.022-S68.029 with 7th A, S68.111A,
S68.113A, S68.115A, S68.117-S68.119 with
7th A, S68.121A, S68.123A, S68.125A,
S68.127-S68.129 with 7th A, S68.412-
S68.419 with 7th A, S68.422-S68.429 with
7th A, S68.512-S68.519 with 7th A, S68.522-
S68.529 with 7th A, S68.611A, S68.613A,
S68.615A, S68.617-S68.619 with 7th A,
S68.621A, S68.623A, S68.625A, S68.627-
S68.629 with 7th A, S68.712-S68.719 with
7th A, S68.722-S68.729 with 7th A, T14.8-
T14.91, T79.A0X-T79.9XX with 7th A

✓7ᵗʰ S68.419 Complete traumatic amputation of **CC**
unspecified hand at wrist level
CC Excl: CC with 7th character A: S41.001-
S41.159 with 7th A, S46.021-S46.029 with
7th A, S46.121-S46.129 with 7th A, S46.221-
S46.229 with 7th A, S46.321-S46.329 with
7th A, S46.821-S46.829 with 7th A, S46.921-
S46.929 with 7th A, S48.011-S48.929 with
7th A, S51.001-S51.859 with 7th A, S56.021-
S56.029 with 7th A, S56.121-S56.129 with
7th A, S56.221-S56.229 with 7th A, S56.321-
S56.329 with 7th A, S56.421-S56.429 with
7th A, S56.521-S56.529 with 7th A, S56.821-
S56.829 with 7th A, S56.921-S56.929 with
7th A, S58.011-S58.929 with 7th A, S61.001-
S61.559 with 7th A, S66.021-S66.029 with
7th A, S66.120-S66.129 with 7th A, S66.221-
S66.229 with 7th A, S66.320-S66.329 with
7th A, S66.421-S66.429 with 7th A, S66.520-
S66.529 with 7th A, S66.821-S66.829 with
7th A, S66.921-S66.929 with 7th A, S68.011-
S68.729 with 7th A, T14.8-T14.91, T79.A0X-
T79.9XX with 7th A

✓6ᵗʰ S68.42 Partial traumatic amputation of hand at wrist level

✓7ᵗʰ S68.421 Partial traumatic amputation of **CC**
right hand at wrist level
CC Excl: CC with 7th character A: See code:
S68.411

✓7ᵗʰ S68.422 Partial traumatic amputation of **CC**
left hand at wrist level
CC Excl: CC with 7th character A: See code:
S68.412

✓7ᵗʰ S68.429 Partial traumatic amputation of **CC**
unspecified hand at wrist level
CC Excl: CC with 7th character A: See code:
S68.419

S68.5 Traumatic transphalangeal amputation of thumb
Traumatic interphalangeal joint amputation of thumb

✓6ᵗʰ **S68.51** Complete traumatic transphalangeal amputation of thumb

     ✓7ᵗʰ **S68.511** Complete traumatic transphalangeal amputation of right thumb

     ✓7ᵗʰ **S68.512** Complete traumatic transphalangeal amputation of left thumb

     ✓7ᵗʰ **S68.519** Complete traumatic transphalangeal amputation of unspecified thumb

✓6ᵗʰ **S68.52** Partial traumatic transphalangeal amputation of thumb

     ✓7ᵗʰ **S68.521** Partial traumatic transphalangeal amputation of right thumb

     ✓7ᵗʰ **S68.522** Partial traumatic transphalangeal amputation of left thumb

     ✓7ᵗʰ **S68.529** Partial traumatic transphalangeal amputation of unspecified thumb

✓5ᵗʰ **S68.6** Traumatic transphalangeal amputation of other and unspecified finger

     ✓6ᵗʰ **S68.61** Complete traumatic transphalangeal amputation of other and unspecified finger(s)

         ✓7ᵗʰ **S68.610** Complete traumatic transphalangeal amputation of right index finger

         ✓7ᵗʰ **S68.611** Complete traumatic transphalangeal amputation of left index finger

         ✓7ᵗʰ **S68.612** Complete traumatic transphalangeal amputation of right middle finger

         ✓7ᵗʰ **S68.613** Complete traumatic transphalangeal amputation of left middle finger

         ✓7ᵗʰ **S68.614** Complete traumatic transphalangeal amputation of right ring finger

         ✓7ᵗʰ **S68.615** Complete traumatic transphalangeal amputation of left ring finger

         ✓7ᵗʰ **S68.616** Complete traumatic transphalangeal amputation of right little finger

         ✓7ᵗʰ **S68.617** Complete traumatic transphalangeal amputation of left little finger

         ✓7ᵗʰ **S68.618** Complete traumatic transphalangeal amputation of other finger
             Complete traumatic transphalangeal amputation of specified finger with unspecified laterality

         ✓7ᵗʰ **S68.619** Complete traumatic transphalangeal amputation of unspecified finger

     ✓6ᵗʰ **S68.62** Partial traumatic transphalangeal amputation of other and unspecified finger

         ✓7ᵗʰ **S68.620** Partial traumatic transphalangeal amputation of right index finger

         ✓7ᵗʰ **S68.621** Partial traumatic transphalangeal amputation of left index finger

         ✓7ᵗʰ **S68.622** Partial traumatic transphalangeal amputation of right middle finger

         ✓7ᵗʰ **S68.623** Partial traumatic transphalangeal amputation of left middle finger

         ✓7ᵗʰ **S68.624** Partial traumatic transphalangeal amputation of right ring finger

         ✓7ᵗʰ **S68.625** Partial traumatic transphalangeal amputation of left ring finger

         ✓7ᵗʰ **S68.626** Partial traumatic transphalangeal amputation of right little finger

         ✓7ᵗʰ **S68.627** Partial traumatic transphalangeal amputation of left little finger

         ✓7ᵗʰ **S68.628** Partial traumatic transphalangeal amputation of other finger
             Partial traumatic transphalangeal amputation of specified finger with unspecified laterality

         ✓7ᵗʰ **S68.629** Partial traumatic transphalangeal amputation of unspecified finger

✓5ᵗʰ **S68.7** Traumatic transmetacarpal amputation of hand

     ✓6ᵗʰ **S68.71** Complete traumatic transmetacarpal amputation of hand

         ✓7ᵗʰ **S68.711** Complete traumatic transmetacarpal amputation of right hand   CC
             CC Excl: CC with 7th character A: See code: S68.411

         ✓7ᵗʰ **S68.712** Complete traumatic transmetacarpal amputation of left hand   CC
             CC Excl: CC with 7th character A: See code: S68.412

         ✓7ᵗʰ **S68.719** Complete traumatic transmetacarpal amputation of unspecified hand   CC
             CC Excl: CC with 7th character A: See code: S68.419

     ✓6ᵗʰ **S68.72** Partial traumatic transmetacarpal amputation of hand

         ✓7ᵗʰ **S68.721** Partial traumatic transmetacarpal amputation of right hand   CC
             CC Excl: CC with 7th character A: See code: S68.411

         ✓7ᵗʰ **S68.722** Partial traumatic transmetacarpal amputation of left hand   CC
             CC Excl: CC with 7th character A: See code: S68.412

         ✓7ᵗʰ **S68.729** Partial traumatic transmetacarpal amputation of unspecified hand   CC
             CC Excl: CC with 7th character A: See code: S68.419

✓4ᵗʰ **S69** Other and unspecified injuries of wrist, hand and finger(s)

> The appropriate 7th character is to be added to each code from category S69.
> A   initial encounter
> D   subsequent encounter
> S   sequela

✓5ᵗʰ **S69.8** Other specified injuries of wrist, hand and finger(s)

     ✓x7ᵗʰ **S69.80** Other specified injuries of unspecified wrist, hand and finger(s)

     ✓x7ᵗʰ **S69.81** Other specified injuries of right wrist, hand and finger(s)

     ✓x7ᵗʰ **S69.82** Other specified injuries of left wrist, hand and finger(s)

✓5ᵗʰ **S69.9** Unspecified injury of wrist, hand and finger(s)

     ✓x7ᵗʰ **S69.90** Unspecified injury of unspecified wrist, hand and finger(s)

     ✓x7ᵗʰ **S69.91** Unspecified injury of right wrist, hand and finger(s)

     ✓x7ᵗʰ **S69.92** Unspecified injury of left wrist, hand and finger(s)

Injuries to the hip and thigh (S70-S79)

EXCLUDES 2   burns and corrosions (T20-T32)
           frostbite (T33-T34)
           snake bite (T63.0-)
           venomous insect bite or sting (T63.4-)

✓4ᵗʰ **S70** Superficial injury of hip and thigh

> The appropriate 7th character is to be added to each code from category S70.
> A   initial encounter
> D   subsequent encounter
> S   sequela

✓5ᵗʰ **S70.0** Contusion of hip

     ✓x7ᵗʰ **S70.00** Contusion of unspecified hip

     ✓x7ᵗʰ **S70.01** Contusion of right hip

     ✓x7ᵗʰ **S70.02** Contusion of left hip

✓5ᵗʰ **S70.1** Contusion of thigh

     ✓x7ᵗʰ **S70.10** Contusion of unspecified thigh

     ✓x7ᵗʰ **S70.11** Contusion of right thigh

     ✓x7ᵗʰ **S70.12** Contusion of left thigh

✓5ᵗʰ **S70.2** Other superficial injuries of hip

     ✓6ᵗʰ **S70.21** Abrasion of hip

         ✓7ᵗʰ **S70.211** Abrasion, right hip

         ✓7ᵗʰ **S70.212** Abrasion, left hip

         ✓7ᵗʰ **S70.219** Abrasion, unspecified hip

     ✓6ᵗʰ **S70.22** Blister (nonthermal) of hip

         ✓7ᵗʰ **S70.221** Blister (nonthermal), right hip

         ✓7ᵗʰ **S70.222** Blister (nonthermal), left hip

         ✓7ᵗʰ **S70.229** Blister (nonthermal), unspecified hip

     ✓6ᵗʰ **S70.24** External constriction of hip

         ✓7ᵗʰ **S70.241** External constriction, right hip

         ✓7ᵗʰ **S70.242** External constriction, left hip

         ✓7ᵗʰ **S70.249** External constriction, unspecified hip

Ⓝ Newborn: 0   Ⓟ Pediatric: 0-17   Ⓜ Maternity: 12-55   Ⓐ Adult: 15-124   MCC Major CC Condition   PDx MCC PDx acts as own MCC   CC CC Condition   PDx CC PDx acts as own CC

972   ICD-10-CM Draft (2015)

✓6ᵗʰ **S70.25** Superficial foreign body of hip
Splinter in the hip
- ✓7ᵗʰ **S70.251** Superficial foreign body, right hip
- ✓7ᵗʰ **S70.252** Superficial foreign body, left hip
- ✓7ᵗʰ **S70.259** Superficial foreign body, unspecified hip

✓6ᵗʰ **S70.26** Insect bite (nonvenomous) of hip
- ✓7ᵗʰ **S70.261** Insect bite (nonvenomous), right hip
- ✓7ᵗʰ **S70.262** Insect bite (nonvenomous), left hip
- ✓7ᵗʰ **S70.269** Insect bite (nonvenomous), unspecified hip

✓6ᵗʰ **S70.27** Other superficial bite of hip
> EXCLUDES 1   open bite of hip (S71.05-)
- ✓7ᵗʰ **S70.271** Other superficial bite of hip, right hip
- ✓7ᵗʰ **S70.272** Other superficial bite of hip, left hip
- ✓7ᵗʰ **S70.279** Other superficial bite of hip, unspecified hip

✓5ᵗʰ **S70.3** Other superficial injuries of thigh

✓6ᵗʰ **S70.31** Abrasion of thigh
- ✓7ᵗʰ **S70.311** Abrasion, right thigh
- ✓7ᵗʰ **S70.312** Abrasion, left thigh
- ✓7ᵗʰ **S70.319** Abrasion, unspecified thigh

✓6ᵗʰ **S70.32** Blister (nonthermal) of thigh
- ✓7ᵗʰ **S70.321** Blister (nonthermal), right thigh
- ✓7ᵗʰ **S70.322** Blister (nonthermal), left thigh
- ✓7ᵗʰ **S70.329** Blister (nonthermal), unspecified thigh

✓6ᵗʰ **S70.34** External constriction of thigh
- ✓7ᵗʰ **S70.341** External constriction, right thigh
- ✓7ᵗʰ **S70.342** External constriction, left thigh
- ✓7ᵗʰ **S70.349** External constriction, unspecified thigh

✓6ᵗʰ **S70.35** Superficial foreign body of thigh
Splinter in the thigh
- ✓7ᵗʰ **S70.351** Superficial foreign body, right thigh
- ✓7ᵗʰ **S70.352** Superficial foreign body, left thigh
- ✓7ᵗʰ **S70.359** Superficial foreign body, unspecified thigh

✓6ᵗʰ **S70.36** Insect bite (nonvenomous) of thigh
- ✓7ᵗʰ **S70.361** Insect bite (nonvenomous), right thigh
- ✓7ᵗʰ **S70.362** Insect bite (nonvenomous), left thigh
- ✓7ᵗʰ **S70.369** Insect bite (nonvenomous), unspecified thigh

✓6ᵗʰ **S70.37** Other superficial bite of thigh
> EXCLUDES 1   open bite of thigh (S71.15)
- ✓7ᵗʰ **S70.371** Other superficial bite of right thigh
- ✓7ᵗʰ **S70.372** Other superficial bite of left thigh
- ✓7ᵗʰ **S70.379** Other superficial bite of unspecified thigh

✓5ᵗʰ **S70.9** Unspecified superficial injury of hip and thigh

✓6ᵗʰ **S70.91** Unspecified superficial injury of hip
- ✓7ᵗʰ **S70.911** Unspecified superficial injury of right hip
- ✓7ᵗʰ **S70.912** Unspecified superficial injury of left hip
- ✓7ᵗʰ **S70.919** Unspecified superficial injury of unspecified hip

✓6ᵗʰ **S70.92** Unspecified superficial injury of thigh
- ✓7ᵗʰ **S70.921** Unspecified superficial injury of right thigh
- ✓7ᵗʰ **S70.922** Unspecified superficial injury of left thigh
- ✓7ᵗʰ **S70.929** Unspecified superficial injury of unspecified thigh

✓4ᵗʰ **S71** Open wound of hip and thigh
Code also any associated wound infection
> EXCLUDES 1   open fracture of hip and thigh (S72.-)
>   traumatic amputation of hip and thigh (S78.-)
> EXCLUDES 2   bite of venomous animal (T63.-)
>   open wound of ankle, foot and toes (S91.-)
>   open wound of knee and lower leg (S81.-)

The appropriate 7th character is to be added to each code from category S71.
- A   initial encounter
- D   subsequent encounter
- S   sequela

✓5ᵗʰ **S71.0** Open wound of hip

✓6ᵗʰ **S71.00** Unspecified open wound of hip
- ✓7ᵗʰ **S71.001** Unspecified open wound, right hip
- ✓7ᵗʰ **S71.002** Unspecified open wound, left hip
- ✓7ᵗʰ **S71.009** Unspecified open wound, unspecified hip

✓6ᵗʰ **S71.01** Laceration without foreign body of hip
- ✓7ᵗʰ **S71.011** Laceration without foreign body, right hip
- ✓7ᵗʰ **S71.012** Laceration without foreign body, left hip
- ✓7ᵗʰ **S71.019** Laceration without foreign body, unspecified hip

✓6ᵗʰ **S71.02** Laceration with foreign body of hip
- ✓7ᵗʰ **S71.021** Laceration with foreign body, right hip
- ✓7ᵗʰ **S71.022** Laceration with foreign body, left hip
- ✓7ᵗʰ **S71.029** Laceration with foreign body, unspecified hip

✓6ᵗʰ **S71.03** Puncture wound without foreign body of hip
- ✓7ᵗʰ **S71.031** Puncture wound without foreign body, right hip
- ✓7ᵗʰ **S71.032** Puncture wound without foreign body, left hip
- ✓7ᵗʰ **S71.039** Puncture wound without foreign body, unspecified hip

✓6ᵗʰ **S71.04** Puncture wound with foreign body of hip
- ✓7ᵗʰ **S71.041** Puncture wound with foreign body, right hip
- ✓7ᵗʰ **S71.042** Puncture wound with foreign body, left hip
- ✓7ᵗʰ **S71.049** Puncture wound with foreign body, unspecified hip

✓6ᵗʰ **S71.05** Open bite of hip
Bite of hip NOS
> EXCLUDES 1   superficial bite of hip (S70.26, S70.27)
- ✓7ᵗʰ **S71.051** Open bite, right hip
- ✓7ᵗʰ **S71.052** Open bite, left hip
- ✓7ᵗʰ **S71.059** Open bite, unspecified hip

✓5ᵗʰ **S71.1** Open wound of thigh

✓6ᵗʰ **S71.10** Unspecified open wound of thigh
- ✓7ᵗʰ **S71.101** Unspecified open wound, right thigh
- ✓7ᵗʰ **S71.102** Unspecified open wound, left thigh
- ✓7ᵗʰ **S71.109** Unspecified open wound, unspecified thigh

✓6ᵗʰ **S71.11** Laceration without foreign body of thigh
- ✓7ᵗʰ **S71.111** Laceration without foreign body, right thigh
- ✓7ᵗʰ **S71.112** Laceration without foreign body, left thigh
- ✓7ᵗʰ **S71.119** Laceration without foreign body, unspecified thigh

✓6ᵗʰ **S71.12** Laceration with foreign body of thigh
- ✓7ᵗʰ **S71.121** Laceration with foreign body, right thigh
- ✓7ᵗʰ **S71.122** Laceration with foreign body, left thigh
- ✓7ᵗʰ **S71.129** Laceration with foreign body, unspecified thigh

✓6ᵗʰ **S71.13** Puncture wound without foreign body of thigh
- ✓7ᵗʰ **S71.131** Puncture wound without foreign body, right thigh
- ✓7ᵗʰ **S71.132** Puncture wound without foreign body, left thigh
- ✓7ᵗʰ **S71.139** Puncture wound without foreign body, unspecified thigh

✓6ᵗʰ **S71.14** Puncture wound with foreign body of thigh
- ✓7ᵗʰ **S71.141** Puncture wound with foreign body, right thigh
- ✓7ᵗʰ **S71.142** Puncture wound with foreign body, left thigh
- ✓7ᵗʰ **S71.149** Puncture wound with foreign body, unspecified thigh

✓6ᵗʰ **S71.15** Open bite of thigh
Bite of thigh NOS
> EXCLUDES 1   superficial bite of thigh (S70.37-)
- ✓7ᵗʰ **S71.151** Open bite, right thigh
- ✓7ᵗʰ **S71.152** Open bite, left thigh

✓ Additional Character Required   ✓x7ᵗʰ Xtension Alert   Unacceptable PDx   Manifestation   Hospital Acquired Condition   EXCLUDES 1 Not Coded Here   EXCLUDES 2 Not Included Here

ICD-10-CM Draft (2015)   973

√7ᵗʰ **S71.159   Open bite, unspecified thigh**

√4ᵗʰ **S72   Fracture of femur**

NOTE   A fracture not indicated as displaced or nondisplaced should be coded to displaced.
The open fracture designations are based on the Gustilo open fracture classification A fracture not indicated as open or closed should be coded to closed.

EXCLUDES 1   traumatic amputation of hip and thigh (S78.-)

EXCLUDES 2   fracture of foot (S92.-)
fracture of lower leg and ankle (S82.-)
periprosthetic fracture of prosthetic implant of hip (T84.040, T84.041)

AHA: 2013, 4Q, 128

The appropriate 7th character is to be added to all codes from category S72 [unless otherwise indicated].

A	initial encounter for closed fracture
B	initial encounter for open fracture type I or II
	initial encounter for open fracture NOS
C	initial encounter for open fracture type IIIA, IIIB, or IIIC
D	subsequent encounter for closed fracture with routine healing
E	subsequent encounter for open fracture type I or II with routine healing
F	subsequent encounter for open fracture type IIIA, IIIB, or IIIC with routine healing
G	subsequent encounter for closed fracture with delayed healing
H	subsequent encounter for open fracture type I or II with delayed healing
J	subsequent encounter for open fracture type IIIA, IIIB, or IIIC with delayed healing
K	subsequent encounter for closed fracture with nonunion
M	subsequent encounter for open fracture type I or II with nonunion
N	subsequent encounter for open fracture type IIIA, IIIB, or IIIC with nonunion
P	subsequent encounter for closed fracture with malunion
Q	subsequent encounter for open fracture type I or II with malunion
R	subsequent encounter for open fracture type IIIA, IIIB, or IIIC with malunion
S	sequela

√5ᵗʰ **S72.0   Fracture of head and neck of femur**

EXCLUDES 2   physeal fracture of upper end of femur (S79.0-)

√6ᵗʰ **S72.00   Fracture of unspecified part of neck of femur**
Fracture of hip NOS
Fracture of neck of femur NOS

7 √7ᵗʰ **S72.001   Fracture of unspecified part of neck of right femur**   MCC CC
CC Excl: MCC with 7th A: M48.40X-M48.58X with 7th A, M80.00X-M84.68X with 7th A, S03.8XX-S03.9XX with 7th A, S29.011-S29.019 with 7th A, S38.3XX-S39.013 with 7th A, S72.001-S72.471 with 7th [A, B, C], S72.479-S72.92X with 7th A, S73.101A, S73.109-S73.111 with 7th A, S73.119-S73.121 with 7th A, S73.129-S73.191 with 7th A, S73.199A, S76.001A, S76.009-S76.011 with 7th A, S76.019A, S76.091A, S76.099-S76.101 with 7th A, S76.109-S76.111 with 7th A, S76.119A, S76.191A, S76.199-S76.201 with 7th A, S76.209-S76.211 with 7th A, S76.219A, S76.291A, S76.299-S76.301 with 7th A, S76.309-S76.311 with 7th A, S76.319A, S76.391A, S76.399-S76.801 with 7th A, S76.809-S76.811 with 7th A, S76.819A, S76.891A, S76.899-S76.901 with 7th A, S76.909-S76.911 with 7th A, S76.919A, S76.991A, S76.999A, S79.001A, S79.009-S79.011 with 7th A, S79.019-S79.091 with 7th A, S79.099-S79.101 with 7th A, S79.109-S79.111 with 7th A, S79.119-S79.121 with 7th A, S79.129-S79.131 with 7th A, S79.139-S79.141 with 7th A, S79.149-S79.191 with 7th A, S79.199-S79.811 with 7th A, S79.819-S79.821 with 7th A, S79.829-S79.911 with 7th A, S79.919-S79.921 with 7th A, S79.929A, S82.90X-S82.92X with 7th [A, B, C], T14.8-T14.91, T79.A0X-T79.9XX with 7th A
MCC with 7th B or C: M48.40X-M48.58X with 7th A, M80.00X-M84.68X with 7th A, S03.8XX-S03.9XX with 7th A, S29.011-S29.019 with 7th A, S38.3XX-S39.013 with 7th A, S72.001-S72.92X with 7th [A, B, C], S73.101-S73.199 with 7th A, S76.001-S76.019 with 7th A, S76.091-S76.119 with

7th A, S76.191-S76.219 with 7th A, S76.291-S76.319 with 7th A, S76.391-S76.819 with 7th A, S76.891-S76.919 with 7th A, S76.991-S76.999 with 7th A, S79.001-S79.929 with 7th A, S82.90X-S82.92X with 7th [A, B, C], T14.8-T14.91, T79.A0X-T79.9XX with 7th A
CC with 7th character K, M, N, P, Q or R: M80.00X-M84.68X with 7th [K, P], S02.0XX-S02.92X with 7th K, S12.000-S12.691 with 7th K, S22.000-S22.9XX with 7th K, S32.000-S32.9XX with 7th K, S42.001-S42.92X with 7th [K, P], S49.001-S49.199 with 7th [K, P], S52.001-S52.92X with 7th [K, M, N, P, Q, R], S59.001-S59.299 with 7th [K, P], S62.001-S62.92X with 7th [K, P], S72.001-S72.92X with 7th [K, M, N, P, Q, R], S79.001-S79.199 with 7th [K, P], S82.001-S82.92X with 7th [K, M, N, P, Q, R], S89.001-S89.399 with 7th [K, P], S92.001-S92.919 with 7th [K, P]

7 √7ᵗʰ **S72.002   Fracture of unspecified part of neck of left femur**   MCC CC
CC Excl: MCC with 7th A: M48.40X-M48.58X with 7th A, M80.00X-M84.68X with 7th A, S03.8XX-S03.9XX with 7th A, S29.011-S29.019 with 7th A, S38.3XX-S39.013 with 7th A, S72.001-S72.466 with 7th [B, C], S72.472-S72.92X with 7th A, S73.102-S73.109 with 7th A, S73.112-S73.119 with 7th A, S73.122-S73.129 with 7th A, S73.192-S73.199 with 7th A, S76.002-S76.009 with 7th A, S76.012-S76.019 with 7th A, S76.092-S76.099 with 7th A, S76.102-S76.109 with 7th A, S76.112-S76.119 with 7th A, S76.192-S76.199 with 7th A, S76.202-S76.209 with 7th A, S76.212-S76.219 with 7th A, S76.292-S76.299 with 7th A, S76.302-S76.309 with 7th A, S76.312-S76.319 with 7th A, S76.392-S76.399 with 7th A, S76.802-S76.809 with 7th A, S76.812-S76.819 with 7th A, S76.892-S76.899 with 7th A, S76.902-S76.909 with 7th A, S76.912-S76.919 with 7th A, S76.992-S76.999 with 7th A, S79.002-S79.009 with 7th A, S79.012-S79.019 with 7th A, S79.092-S79.099 with 7th A, S79.102-S79.109 with 7th A, S79.112-S79.119 with 7th A, S79.122-S79.129 with 7th A, S79.132-S79.139 with 7th A, S79.142-S79.149 with 7th A, S79.192-S79.199 with 7th A, S79.812-S79.819 with 7th A, S79.822-S79.829 with 7th A, S79.912-S79.919 with 7th A, S79.922-S79.929 with 7th A, S82.90-S82.92 with 7th [A, B, C], T14.8-T14.91, T79.A0X-T79.9XX with 7th A
MCC with 7th B or C: M48.40X-M48.58X with 7th A, M80.00X-M84.68X with 7th A, S03.8XX-S03.9XX with 7th A, S29.011-S29.019 with 7th A, S38.3XX-S39.013 with 7th A, S72.001-S72.92X with 7th [A, B, C], S73.101-S73.199 with 7th A, S76.001-S76.019 with 7th A, S76.091-S76.119 with 7th A, S76.191-S76.219 with 7th A, S76.291-S76.319 with 7th A, S76.391-S76.819 with 7th A, S76.891-S76.919 with 7th A, S76.991-S76.999 with 7th A, S79.001-S79.929 with 7th A, S82.90X-S82.92X with 7th [A, B, C], T14.8-T14.91, T79.A0X-T79.9XX with 7th A
CC with 7th character K, M, N, P, Q or R: M80.00X-M84.68X with 7th [K, P], S02.0XX-S02.92X with 7th K, S12.000-S12.691 with 7th K, S22.000-S22.9XX with 7th K, S32.000-S32.9XX with 7th K, S42.001-S42.92X with 7th [K, P], S49.001-S49.199 with 7th [K, P], S52.001-S52.92X with 7th [K, M, N, P, Q, R], S59.001-S59.299 with 7th [K, P], S62.001-S62.92X with 7th [K, P], S72.001-S72.92X with 7th [K, M, N, P, Q, R], S79.001-S79.199 with 7th [K, P], S82.001-S82.92X with 7th [K, M, N, P, Q, R], S89.001-S89.399 with 7th [K, P], S92.001-S92.919 with 7th [K, P]

7 HAC = Initial encounter only (7th character A, B or C) and not POA.

7 √7th **S72.009 Fracture of unspecified part of neck of unspecified femur** `MCC` `CC`
CC Excl: MCC with 7th A, B or C: M48.40X-M48.58X with 7th A, M80.00X-M80.68X with 7th A, S03.8XX-S03.9X with 7th A, S29.011-S29.019 with 7th A, S38.3XX-S39.013 with 7th A, S72.001-S72.92X with 7th [A, B, C], S73.101-S73.199 with 7th A, S76.001-S76.019 with 7th A, S76.091-S76.119 with 7th A, S76.191-S76.219 with 7th A, S76.291-S76.319 with 7th A, S76.391-S76.819 with 7th A, S76.891-S76.919 with 7th A, S76.991-S76.999 with 7th A, S79.001-S79.929 with 7th A, S82.90X-S82.92X with 7th [A, B, C], T14.8-T14.91, T79.A0X-T79.9XX with 7th A
CC with 7th character K, M, N, P, Q or R: M80.00X-M84.68X with 7th [K, P], S02.0XX-S02.92X with 7th K, S12.000-S12.691 with 7th K, S22.000-S22.9XX with 7th K, S32.000-S32.9XX with 7th K, S42.001-S42.92X with 7th [K, P], S49.001-S49.199 with 7th [K, P], S52.001-S52.92X with 7th [K, M, N, P, Q, R], S59.001-S59.299 with 7th [K, P], S62.001-S62.92X with 7th [K, P], S72.001-S72.92X with 7th [K, M, N, P, Q, R], S79.001-S79.199 with 7th [K, P], S82.001-S82.92X with 7th [K, M, N, P, Q, R], S89.001-S89.399 with 7th [K, P], S92.001-S92.919 with 7th [K, P]

√6th **S72.01 Unspecified intracapsular fracture of femur**
Subcapital fracture of femur

7 √7th **S72.011 Unspecified intracapsular fracture of right femur** `MCC` `CC`
CC Excl: See code: S72.001

7 √7th **S72.012 Unspecified intracapsular fracture of left femur** `MCC` `CC`
CC Excl: See code: S72.002

7 √7th **S72.019 Unspecified intracapsular fracture of unspecified femur** `MCC` `CC`
CC Excl: See code: S72.009

√6th **S72.02 Fracture of epiphysis (separation) (upper) of femur**
Transepiphyseal fracture of femur
EXCLUDES 1   capital femoral epiphyseal fracture (pediatric) of femur (S79.01-)
Salter-Harris Type I physeal fracture of upper end of femur (S79.01-)

7 √7th **S72.021 Displaced fracture of epiphysis (separation) (upper) of right femur** `MCC` `CC`
CC Excl: See code: S72.001

7 √7th **S72.022 Displaced fracture of epiphysis (separation) (upper) of left femur** `MCC` `CC`
CC Excl: See code: S72.002

7 √7th **S72.023 Displaced fracture of epiphysis (separation) (upper) of unspecified femur** `MCC` `CC`
CC Excl: See code: S72.009

7 √7th **S72.024 Nondisplaced fracture of epiphysis (separation) (upper) of right femur** `MCC` `CC`
CC Excl: See code: S72.001

7 √7th **S72.025 Nondisplaced fracture of epiphysis (separation) (upper) of left femur** `MCC` `CC`
CC Excl: See code: S72.002

7 √7th **S72.026 Nondisplaced fracture of epiphysis (separation) (upper) of unspecified femur** `MCC` `CC`
CC Excl: See code: S72.009

√6th **S72.03 Midcervical fracture of femur**
Transcervical fracture of femur NOS

7 √7th **S72.031 Displaced midcervical fracture of right femur** `MCC` `CC`
CC Excl: See code: S72.001

7 √7th **S72.032 Displaced midcervical fracture of left femur** `MCC` `CC`
CC Excl: See code: S72.002

7 √7th **S72.033 Displaced midcervical fracture of unspecified femur** `MCC` `CC`
CC Excl: See code: S72.009

7 √7th **S72.034 Nondisplaced midcervical fracture of right femur** `MCC` `CC`
CC Excl: See code: S72.001

7 √7th **S72.035 Nondisplaced midcervical fracture of left femur** `MCC` `CC`
CC Excl: See code: S72.002

7 √7th **S72.036 Nondisplaced midcervical fracture of unspecified femur** `MCC` `CC`
CC Excl: See code: S72.009

√6th **S72.04 Fracture of base of neck of femur**
Cervicotrochanteric fracture of femur

7 √7th **S72.041 Displaced fracture of base of neck of right femur** `MCC` `CC`
CC Excl: See code: S72.001

7 √7th **S72.042 Displaced fracture of base of neck of left femur** `MCC` `CC`
CC Excl: See code: S72.002

7 √7th **S72.043 Displaced fracture of base of neck of unspecified femur** `MCC` `CC`
CC Excl: See code: S72.009

7 √7th **S72.044 Nondisplaced fracture of base of neck of right femur** `MCC` `CC`
CC Excl: See code: S72.001

7 √7th **S72.045 Nondisplaced fracture of base of neck of left femur** `MCC` `CC`
CC Excl: See code: S72.002

7 √7th **S72.046 Nondisplaced fracture of base of neck of unspecified femur** `MCC` `CC`
CC Excl: See code: S72.009

√6th **S72.05 Unspecified fracture of head of femur**
Fracture of head of femur NOS

7 √7th **S72.051 Unspecified fracture of head of right femur** `MCC` `CC`
CC Excl: See code: S72.001

7 √7th **S72.052 Unspecified fracture of head of left femur** `MCC` `CC`
CC Excl: See code: S72.002

7 √7th **S72.059 Unspecified fracture of head of unspecified femur** `MCC` `CC`
CC Excl: See code: S72.009

√6th **S72.06 Articular fracture of head of femur**

7 √7th **S72.061 Displaced articular fracture of head of right femur** `MCC` `CC`
CC Excl: See code: S72.001

7 √7th **S72.062 Displaced articular fracture of head of left femur** `MCC` `CC`
CC Excl: See code: S72.002

7 √7th **S72.063 Displaced articular fracture of head of unspecified femur** `MCC` `CC`
CC Excl: See code: S72.009

7 √7th **S72.064 Nondisplaced articular fracture of head of right femur** `MCC` `CC`
CC Excl: See code: S72.001

7 √7th **S72.065 Nondisplaced articular fracture of head of left femur** `MCC` `CC`
CC Excl: See code: S72.002

7 √7th **S72.066 Nondisplaced articular fracture of head of unspecified femur** `MCC` `CC`
CC Excl: See code: S72.009

√6th **S72.09 Other fracture of head and neck of femur**

7 √7th **S72.091 Other fracture of head and neck of right femur** `MCC` `CC`
CC Excl: See code: S72.001

7 √7th **S72.092 Other fracture of head and neck of left femur** `MCC` `CC`
CC Excl: See code: S72.002

7 √7th **S72.099 Other fracture of head and neck of unspecified femur** `MCC` `CC`
CC Excl: See code: S72.009

√5th **S72.1 Pertrochanteric fracture**

√6th **S72.10 Unspecified trochanteric fracture of femur**
Fracture of trochanter NOS

7 √7th **S72.101 Unspecified trochanteric fracture of right femur** `MCC` `CC`
CC Excl: See code: S72.001

7 √7th **S72.102 Unspecified trochanteric fracture of left femur** `MCC` `CC`
CC Excl: See code: S72.002

7 √7th **S72.109 Unspecified trochanteric fracture of unspecified femur** `MCC` `CC`
CC Excl: See code: S72.009

---

7 HAC = Initial encounter only (7th character A, B or C) and not POA.

Injury, Poisoning and Certain Other Consequences of External Causes

S72.11–S72.342

✓6th **S72.11** Fracture of greater trochanter of femur

7 ✓7th **S72.111** Displaced fracture of greater trochanter of right femur `MCC` `CC`
CC Excl: See code: S72.001

7 ✓7th **S72.112** Displaced fracture of greater trochanter of left femur `MCC` `CC`
CC Excl: See code: S72.002

7 ✓7th **S72.113** Displaced fracture of greater trochanter of unspecified femur `MCC` `CC`
CC Excl: See code: S72.009

7 ✓7th **S72.114** Nondisplaced fracture of greater trochanter of right femur `MCC` `CC`
CC Excl: See code: S72.001

7 ✓7th **S72.115** Nondisplaced fracture of greater trochanter of left femur `MCC` `CC`
CC Excl: See code: S72.002

7 ✓7th **S72.116** Nondisplaced fracture of greater trochanter of unspecified femur `MCC` `CC`
CC Excl: See code: S72.009

✓6th **S72.12** Fracture of lesser trochanter of femur

7 ✓7th **S72.121** Displaced fracture of lesser trochanter of right femur `MCC` `CC`
CC Excl: See code: S72.001

7 ✓7th **S72.122** Displaced fracture of lesser trochanter of left femur `MCC` `CC`
CC Excl: See code: S72.002

7 ✓7th **S72.123** Displaced fracture of lesser trochanter of unspecified femur `MCC` `CC`
CC Excl: See code: S72.009

7 ✓7th **S72.124** Nondisplaced fracture of lesser trochanter of right femur `MCC` `CC`
CC Excl: See code: S72.001

7 ✓7th **S72.125** Nondisplaced fracture of lesser trochanter of left femur `MCC` `CC`
CC Excl: See code: S72.002

7 ✓7th **S72.126** Nondisplaced fracture of lesser trochanter of unspecified femur `MCC` `CC`
CC Excl: See code: S72.009

✓6th **S72.13** Apophyseal fracture of femur
EXCLUDES 1 chronic (nontraumatic) slipped upper femoral epiphysis (M93.0-)

7 ✓7th **S72.131** Displaced apophyseal fracture of right femur `MCC` `CC`
CC Excl: See code: S72.001

7 ✓7th **S72.132** Displaced apophyseal fracture of left femur `MCC` `CC`
CC Excl: See code: S72.002

7 ✓7th **S72.133** Displaced apophyseal fracture of unspecified femur `MCC` `CC`
CC Excl: See code: S72.009

7 ✓7th **S72.134** Nondisplaced apophyseal fracture of right femur `MCC` `CC`
CC Excl: See code: S72.001

7 ✓7th **S72.135** Nondisplaced apophyseal fractureof left femur `MCC` `CC`
CC Excl: See code: S72.002

7 ✓7th **S72.136** Nondisplaced apophyseal fracture of unspecified femur `MCC` `CC`
CC Excl: See code: S72.009

✓6th **S72.14** Intertrochanteric fracture of femur

7 ✓7th **S72.141** Displaced intertrochanteric fracture of right femur `MCC` `CC`
CC Excl: See code: S72.001

7 ✓7th **S72.142** Displaced intertrochanteric fracture of left femur `MCC` `CC`
CC Excl: See code: S72.002

7 ✓7th **S72.143** Displaced intertrochanteric fracture of unspecified femur `MCC` `CC`
CC Excl: See code: S72.009

7 ✓7th **S72.144** Nondisplaced intertrochanteric fracture of right femur `MCC` `CC`
CC Excl: See code: S72.001

7 ✓7th **S72.145** Nondisplaced intertrochanteric fracture of left femur `MCC` `CC`
CC Excl: See code: S72.002

7 ✓7th **S72.146** Nondisplaced intertrochanteric fracture of unspecified femur `MCC` `CC`
CC Excl: See code: S72.009

✓5th **S72.2** Subtrochanteric fracture of femur

7 ✓x7th **S72.21** Displaced subtrochanteric fracture of right femur `MCC` `CC`
CC Excl: See code: S72.001

7 ✓x7th **S72.22** Displaced subtrochanteric fracture of left femur `MCC` `CC`
CC Excl: See code: S72.002

7 ✓x7th **S72.23** Displaced subtrochanteric fracture of unspecified femur `MCC` `CC`
CC Excl: See code: S72.009

7 ✓x7th **S72.24** Nondisplaced subtrochanteric fracture of right femur `MCC` `CC`
CC Excl: See code: S72.001

7 ✓x7th **S72.25** Nondisplaced subtrochanteric fracture of left femur `MCC` `CC`
CC Excl: See code: S72.002

7 ✓x7th **S72.26** Nondisplaced subtrochanteric fracture of unspecified femur `MCC` `CC`
CC Excl: See code: S72.009

✓5th **S72.3** Fracture of shaft of femur

✓6th **S72.30** Unspecified fracture of shaft of femur

7 ✓7th **S72.301** Unspecified fracture of shaft of right femur `MCC` `CC`
CC Excl: See code: S72.001

7 ✓7th **S72.302** Unspecified fracture of shaft of left femur `MCC` `CC`
CC Excl: See code: S72.002

7 ✓7th **S72.309** Unspecified fracture of shaft of unspecified femur `MCC` `CC`
CC Excl: See code: S72.009

✓6th **S72.32** Transverse fracture of shaft of femur

7 ✓7th **S72.321** Displaced transverse fracture of shaft of right femur `MCC` `CC`
CC Excl: See code: S72.001

7 ✓7th **S72.322** Displaced transverse fracture of shaft of left femur `MCC` `CC`
CC Excl: See code: S72.002

7 ✓7th **S72.323** Displaced transverse fracture of shaft of unspecified femur `MCC` `CC`
CC Excl: See code: S72.009

7 ✓7th **S72.324** Nondisplaced transverse fracture of shaft of right femur `MCC` `CC`
CC Excl: See code: S72.001

7 ✓7th **S72.325** Nondisplaced transverse fracture of shaft of left femur `MCC` `CC`
CC Excl: See code: S72.002

7 ✓7th **S72.326** Nondisplaced transverse fracture of shaft of unspecified femur `MCC` `CC`
CC Excl: See code: S72.009

✓6th **S72.33** Oblique fracture of shaft of femur

7 ✓7th **S72.331** Displaced oblique fracture of shaft of right femur `MCC` `CC`
CC Excl: See code: S72.001

7 ✓7th **S72.332** Displaced oblique fracture of shaft of left femur `MCC` `CC`
CC Excl: See code: S72.002

7 ✓7th **S72.333** Displaced oblique fracture of shaft of unspecified femur `MCC` `CC`
CC Excl: See code: S72.009

7 ✓7th **S72.334** Nondisplaced oblique fracture of shaft of right femur `MCC` `CC`
CC Excl: See code: S72.001

7 ✓7th **S72.335** Nondisplaced oblique fracture of shaft of left femur `MCC` `CC`
CC Excl: See code: S72.002

7 ✓7th **S72.336** Nondisplaced oblique fracture of shaft of unspecified femur `MCC` `CC`
CC Excl: See code: S72.009

✓6th **S72.34** Spiral fracture of shaft of femur

7 ✓7th **S72.341** Displaced spiral fracture of shaft of right femur `MCC` `CC`
CC Excl: See code: S72.001

7 ✓7th **S72.342** Displaced spiral fracture of shaft of left femur `MCC` `CC`
CC Excl: See code: S72.002

---

7 HAC = Initial encounter only (7th character A, B or C) and not POA.

7 √7ᵗʰ **S72.343** **Displaced spiral fracture of shaft of unspecified femur** `MCC` `CC`
CC Excl: See code: S72.009

7 √7ᵗʰ **S72.344** **Nondisplaced spiral fracture of shaft of right femur** `MCC` `CC`
CC Excl: See code: S72.001

7 √7ᵗʰ **S72.345** **Nondisplaced spiral fracture of shaft of left femur** `MCC` `CC`
CC Excl: See code: S72.002

7 √7ᵗʰ **S72.346** **Nondisplaced spiral fracture of shaft of unspecified femur** `MCC` `CC`
CC Excl: See code: S72.009

√6ᵗʰ **S72.35** **Comminuted fracture of shaft of femur**

7 √7ᵗʰ **S72.351** **Displaced comminuted fracture of shaft of right femur** `MCC` `CC`
CC Excl: See code: S72.001

7 √7ᵗʰ **S72.352** **Displaced comminuted fracture of shaft of left femur** `MCC` `CC`
CC Excl: See code: S72.002

7 √7ᵗʰ **S72.353** **Displaced comminuted fracture of shaft of unspecified femur** `MCC` `CC`
CC Excl: See code: S72.009

7 √7ᵗʰ **S72.354** **Nondisplaced comminuted fracture of shaft of right femur** `MCC` `CC`
CC Excl: See code: S72.001

7 √7ᵗʰ **S72.355** **Nondisplaced comminuted fracture of shaft of left femur** `MCC` `CC`
CC Excl: See code: S72.002

7 √7ᵗʰ **S72.356** **Nondisplaced comminuted fracture of shaft of unspecified femur** `MCC` `CC`
CC Excl: See code: S72.009

√6ᵗʰ **S72.36** **Segmental fracture of shaft of femur**

7 √7ᵗʰ **S72.361** **Displaced segmental fracture of shaft of right femur** `MCC` `CC`
CC Excl: See code: S72.001

7 √7ᵗʰ **S72.362** **Displaced segmental fracture of shaft of left femur** `MCC` `CC`
CC Excl: See code: S72.002

7 √7ᵗʰ **S72.363** **Displaced segmental fracture of shaft of unspecified femur** `MCC` `CC`
CC Excl: See code: S72.009

7 √7ᵗʰ **S72.364** **Nondisplaced segmental fracture of shaft of right femur** `MCC` `CC`
CC Excl: See code: S72.001

7 √7ᵗʰ **S72.365** **Nondisplaced segmental fracture of shaft of left femur** `MCC` `CC`
CC Excl: See code: S72.002

7 √7ᵗʰ **S72.366** **Nondisplaced segmental fracture of shaft of unspecified femur** `MCC` `CC`
CC Excl: See code: S72.009

√6ᵗʰ **S72.39** **Other fracture of shaft of femur**

7 √7ᵗʰ **S72.391** **Other fracture of shaft of right femur** `MCC` `CC`
CC Excl: See code: S72.001

7 √7ᵗʰ **S72.392** **Other fracture of shaft of left femur** `MCC` `CC`
CC Excl: See code: S72.002

7 √7ᵗʰ **S72.399** **Other fracture of shaft of unspecified femur** `MCC` `CC`
CC Excl: See code: S72.009

√5ᵗʰ **S72.4** **Fracture of lower end of femur**
Fracture of distal end of femur
EXCLUDES 2   fracture of shaft of femur (S72.3-)
    physeal fracture of lower end of femur (S79.1-)

√6ᵗʰ **S72.40** **Unspecified fracture of lower end of femur**

7 √7ᵗʰ **S72.401** **Unspecified fracture of lower end of right femur** `MCC` `CC`

CC Excl: CC with 7th character A: M80.00X-M80.019 with 7th A, M80.041-M80.059 with 7th A, M80.80X-M80.819 with 7th A, M80.841-M80.859 with 7th A, M84.40X-M84.419 with 7th A, M84.441-M84.459 with 7th A, M84.474-M84.519 with 7th A, M84.541-M84.559 with 7th A, M84.574-M84.576 with 7th A, M84.60X-M84.619 with 7th A, M84.641-M84.659 with 7th A, M84.674-M84.68X with 7th A, S03.8XX-S03.9XX with 7th A, S29.011-S29.019 with 7th A, S38.3XX-S39.013 with 7th A, S72.001-S72.471 with 7th [A, B, C], S72.479-S72.92X with 7th A, S73.101A, S73.109-S73.111 with 7th A, S73.119-S73.121 with 7th A, S73.129-S73.191 with 7th A, S73.199A, S76.001A, S76.009-S76.011 with 7th A, S76.019A, S76.091A, S76.099-S76.101 with 7th A, S76.109-S76.111 with 7th A, S76.119A, S76.191A, S76.199-S76.201 with 7th A, S76.209-S76.211 with 7th A, S76.219 with 7th A, S76.291A, S76.299-S76.301 with 7th A, S76.309-S76.311 with 7th A, S76.319A, S76.391A, S76.399-S76.801 with 7th A, S76.809-S76.811 with 7th A, S76.819A, S76.891A, S76.899-S76.901 with 7th A, S76.909-S76.911 with 7th A, S76.919A, S76.991A, S76.999A, S79.001A, S79.009-S79.011 with 7th A, S79.019-S79.091 with 7th A, S79.099-S79.101 with 7th A, S79.109-S79.111 with 7th A, S79.119-S79.121 with 7th A, S79.129-S79.131 with 7th A, S79.139-S79.141 with 7th A, S79.149-S79.191 with 7th A, S79.199-S79.811 with 7th A, S79.819-S79.821 with 7th A, S79.829-S79.911 with 7th A, S79.919-S79.921 with 7th A, S79.929 A, S82.90-S82.92X with 7th [A, B, C], T14.8-T14.91, T79.A9X-T79.9XX with 7th A
MCC with 7th B or C: M80.00X-M80.019 with 7th A, M80.041-M80.059 with 7th A, M80.80X-M80.819 with 7th A, M80.841-M80.859 with 7th A, M84.40X-M84.419 with 7th A, M84.441-M84.459 with 7th A, M84.474-M84.519 with 7th A, M84.541-M84.559 with 7th A, M84.574-M84.576 with 7th A, M84.60X-M84.619 with 7th A, M84.641-M84.659 with 7th A, M84.674-M84.68X with 7th A, S03.8XX-S03.9XX with 7th A, S29.011-S29.019 with 7th A, S38.3XX-S39.013 with 7th A, S72.001-S72.92X with 7th [A, B, C], S73.101-S73.199 with 7th A, S76.001-S76.019 with 7th A, S76.091-S76.119 with 7th A, S76.191-S76.219 with 7th A, S76.291-S76.319 with 7th A, S76.391-S76.819 with 7th A, S76.891-S76.919 with 7th A, S76.991-S76.999 with 7th A, S79.001-S79.929 with 7th A, S82.90X-S82.92X with 7th [A, B, C], T14.8-T14.91, T79.A9X-T79.9XX with 7th A
CC with 7th character K, M, N, P, Q or R: M80.00X-M84.68X with 7th [K, P], S02.0XX-S02.92X with 7th K, S12.000-S12.691 with 7th K, S22.000-S22.9XX with 7th K, S32.000-S32.9XX with 7th K, S42.001-S42.92X with 7th [K, P], S49.001-S49.199 with 7th [K, P], S52.001-S52.92X with 7th [K, M, N, P, Q, R], S59.001-S59.299 with 7th [K, P], S62.001-S62.92X with 7th [K, P], S72.001-S72.92X with 7th [K, M, N, P, Q, R], S79.001-S79.199 with 7th [K, P], S82.001-S82.92X with 7th [K, M, N, P, Q, R], S89.001-S89.399 with 7th [K, P], S92.001-S92.919 with 7th [K, P]

---

7 HAC = Initial encounter only (7th character A, B or C) and not POA.

✔ Additional Character Required   √x7ᵗʰ Xtension Alert   Unacceptable PDx   Manifestation   Hospital Acquired Condition   *EXCLUDES 1* Not Coded Here   *EXCLUDES 2* Not Included Here

7 √7ᵗʰ **S72.402 Unspecified fracture of lower end of left femur** MCC CC

CC Excl: CC with 7th character A: M80.00X-M80.019 with 7th A, M80.041-M80.059 with 7th A, M80.80X-M80.819 with 7th A, M80.841-M80.859 with 7th A, M84.40X-M84.419 with 7th A, M84.441-M84.459 with 7th A, M84.474-M84.519 with 7th A, M84.541-M84.559 with 7th A, M84.574-M84.576 with 7th A, M84.60X-M84.619 with 7th A, M84.641-M84.659 with 7th A, M84.674-M84.68 with 7th A, S03.8XX-S03.9XX with 7th A, S29.011-S29.019 with 7th A, S38.3XX-S39.013 with 7th A, S72.001-S72.466 with 7th [B, C], S72.472-S72.92X with 7th A, S73.102-S73.109 with 7th A, S73.112-S73.119 with 7th A, S73.122-S73.129 with 7th A, S73.192-S73.199 with 7th A, S76.002-S76.009 with 7th A, S76.012-S76.019 with 7th A, S76.092-S76.099 with 7th A, S76.102-S76.109 with 7th A, S76.112-S76.119 with 7th A, S76.192-S76.199 with 7th A, S76.202-S76.209 with 7th A, S76.212-S76.219 with 7th A, S76.292-S76.299 with 7th A, S76.302-S76.309 with 7th A, S76.312-S76.319 with 7th A, S76.392-S76.399 with 7th A, S76.802-S76.809 with 7th A, S76.812-S76.819 with 7th A, S76.892-S76.899 with 7th A, S76.902-S76.909 with 7th A, S76.912-S76.919 with 7th A, S76.992-S76.999 with 7th A, S79.002-S79.009 with 7th A, S79.012-S79.019 with 7th A, S79.092-S79.099 with 7th A, S79.102-S79.109 with 7th A, S79.112-S79.119 with 7th A, S79.122-S79.129 with 7th A, S79.132-S79.139 with 7th A, S79.142-S79.149 with 7th A, S79.192-S79.199 with 7th A, S79.812-S79.819 with 7th A, S79.822-S79.829 with 7th A, S79.912-S79.919 with 7th A, S79.922-S79.929 with 7th A, S82.90X-S82.92X with 7th [A, B, C], T14.8-T14.91, T79.A9X-T79.9XX with 7th A

MCC with 7th B or C: M80.00-M80.019 with 7th A, M80.041-M80.059 with 7th A, M80.80X-M80.819 with 7th A, M80.841-M80.859 with 7th A, M84.40X-M84.419 with 7th A, M84.441-M84.459 with 7th A, M84.474-M84.519 with 7th A, M84.541-M84.559 with 7th A, M84.574-M84.576 with 7th A, M84.60X-M84.619 with 7th A, M84.641-M84.659 with 7th A, M84.674-M84.68X with 7th A, S03.8XX-S03.9XX with 7th A, S29.011-S29.019 with 7th A, S38.3XX-S39.013 with 7th A, S72.001-S72.92X with 7th [A, B, C], S73.101-S73.199 with 7th A, S76.001-S76.019 with 7th A, S76.091-S76.119 with 7th A, S76.191-S76.219 with 7th A, S76.291-S76.319 with 7th A, S76.391-S76.819 with 7th A, S76.891-S76.919 with 7th A, S76.991-S76.999 with 7th A, S79.001-S79.929 with 7th A, S82.90-S82.92X with 7th [A, B, C], T14.8-T14.91, T79.A9X-T79.9XX with 7th A

CC with 7th character K, M, N, P, Q or R: M80.00X-M84.68X with 7th [K, P], S02.0XX-S02.92X with 7th K, S12.000-S12.691 with 7th K, S22.000-S22.9XX with 7th K, S32.000-S32.9XX with 7th K, S42.001-S42.92X with 7th [K, P], S49.001-S49.199 with 7th [K, P], S52.001-S52.92X with 7th [K, M, N, P, Q, R], S59.001-S59.299 with 7th [K, P], S62.001-S62.92X with 7th [K, P], S72.001-S72.92X with 7th [K, M, N, P, Q, R], S79.001-S79.199 with 7th [K, P], S82.001-S82.92X with 7th [K, M, N, P, Q, R], S89.001-S89.399 with 7th [K, P], S92.001-S92.919 with 7th [K, P]

7 √7ᵗʰ **S72.409 Unspecified fracture of lower end of unspecified femur** MCC CC

CC Excl: CC with 7th character A, MCC with 7th B or C: M80.00X-M80.019 with 7th A, M80.041-M80.059 with 7th A, M80.80X-M80.819 with 7th A, M80.841-M80.859 with 7th A, M84.40X-M84.419 with 7th A, M84.441-M84.459 with 7th A, M84.474-M84.519 with 7th A, M84.541-M84.559 with 7th A, M84.574-M84.576 with 7th A, M84.60X-M84.619 with 7th A, M84.641-M84.659 with 7th A, M84.674-M84.68 with 7th A, S03.8XX-S03.9XX with 7th A, S29.011-S29.019 with 7th A, S38.3XX-S39.013 with 7th A, S72.001-S72.92X with 7th [A, B, C], S73.101-S73.199 with 7th A, S76.001-S76.019 with 7th A, S76.091-S76.119 with 7th A, S76.191-S76.219 with 7th A, S76.291-S76.319 with 7th A, S76.391-S76.819 with 7th A, S76.891-S76.919 with 7th A, S76.991-S76.999 with 7th A, S79.001-S79.929 with 7th A, S82.90X-S82.92X with 7th [A, B, C], T14.8-T14.91, T79.A9X-T79.9XX with 7th A

CC with 7th character K, M, N, P, Q or R: M80.00X-M84.68X with 7th [K, P], S02.0XX-S02.92X with 7th K, S12.000-S12.691 with 7th K, S22.000-S22.9XX with 7th K, S32.000-S32.9XX with 7th K, S42.001-S42.92X with 7th [K, P], S49.001-S49.199 with 7th [K, P], S52.001-S52.92X with 7th [K, M, N, P, Q, R], S59.001-S59.299 with 7th [K, P], S62.001-S62.92X with 7th [K, P], S72.001-S72.92X with 7th [K, M, N, P, Q, R], S79.001-S79.199 with 7th [K, P], S82.001-S82.92X with 7th [K, M, N, P, Q, R], S89.001-S89.399 with 7th [K, P], S92.001-S92.919 with 7th [K, P]

√6ᵗʰ **S72.41 Unspecified condyle fracture of lower end of femur**
Condyle fracture of femur NOS

7 √7ᵗʰ **S72.411 Displaced unspecified condyle fracture of lower end of right femur** MCC CC
CC Excl: See code: S72.401

7 √7ᵗʰ **S72.412 Displaced unspecified condyle fracture of lower end of left femur** MCC CC
CC Excl: See code: S72.402

7 √7ᵗʰ **S72.413 Displaced unspecified condyle fracture of lower end of unspecified femur** MCC CC
CC Excl: See code: S72.409

7 √7ᵗʰ **S72.414 Nondisplaced unspecified condyle fracture of lower end of right femur** MCC CC
CC Excl: See code: S72.401

7 √7ᵗʰ **S72.415 Nondisplaced unspecified condyle fracture of lower end of left femur** MCC CC
CC Excl: See code: S72.402

7 √7ᵗʰ **S72.416 Nondisplaced unspecified condyle fracture of lower end of unspecified femur** MCC CC
CC Excl: See code: S72.409

√6ᵗʰ **S72.42 Fracture of lateral condyle of femur**

7 √7ᵗʰ **S72.421 Displaced fracture of lateral condyle of right femur** MCC CC
CC Excl: See code: S72.401

7 √7ᵗʰ **S72.422 Displaced fracture of lateral condyle of left femur** MCC CC
CC Excl: See code: S72.402

7 √7ᵗʰ **S72.423 Displaced fracture of lateral condyle of unspecified femur** MCC CC
CC Excl: See code: S72.409

7 √7ᵗʰ **S72.424 Nondisplaced fracture of lateral condyle of right femur** MCC CC
CC Excl: See code: S72.401

7 √7ᵗʰ **S72.425 Nondisplaced fracture of lateral condyle of left femur** MCC CC
CC Excl: See code: S72.402

7 √7ᵗʰ **S72.426 Nondisplaced fracture of lateral condyle of unspecified femur** MCC CC
CC Excl: See code: S72.409

---

7 HAC = Initial encounter only (7th character A, B or C) and not POA.

N Newborn: 0   P Pediatric: 0-17   M Maternity: 12-55   A Adult: 15-124   MCC Major CC Condition   PDx MCC PDx acts as own MCC   CC CC Condition   PDx CC PDx acts as own CC

978   ICD-10-CM Draft (2015)

✓6th **S72.43** Fracture of medial condyle of femur

7 ✓7th **S72.431** **Displaced fracture of medial condyle of right femur** MCC CC
CC Excl: See code: S72.401

7 ✓7th **S72.432** **Displaced fracture of medial condyle of left femur** MCC CC
CC Excl: See code: S72.402

7 ✓7th **S72.433** **Displaced fracture of medial condyle of unspecified femur** MCC CC
CC Excl: See code: S72.409

7 ✓7th **S72.434** **Nondisplaced fracture of medial condyle of right femur** MCC CC
CC Excl: See code: S72.401

7 ✓7th **S72.435** **Nondisplaced fracture of medial condyle of left femur** MCC CC
CC Excl: See code: S72.402

7 ✓7th **S72.436** **Nondisplaced fracture of medial condyle of unspecified femur** MCC CC
CC Excl: See code: S72.409

✓6th **S72.44** Fracture of lower epiphysis (separation) of femur
EXCLUDES 1 *Salter-Harris Type I physeal fracture of lower end of femur (S79.11-)*

7 ✓7th **S72.441** **Displaced fracture of lower epiphysis (separation) of right femur** MCC CC
CC Excl: See code: S72.401

7 ✓7th **S72.442** **Displaced fracture of lower epiphysis (separation) of left femur** MCC CC
CC Excl: See code: S72.402

7 ✓7th **S72.443** **Displaced fracture of lower epiphysis (separation) of unspecified femur** MCC CC
CC Excl: See code: S72.409

7 ✓7th **S72.444** **Nondisplaced fracture of lower epiphysis (separation) of right femur** MCC CC
CC Excl: See code: S72.401

7 ✓7th **S72.445** **Nondisplaced fracture of lower epiphysis (separation) of left femur** MCC CC
CC Excl: See code: S72.402

7 ✓7th **S72.446** **Nondisplaced fracture of lower epiphysis (separation) of unspecified femur** MCC CC
CC Excl: See code: S72.409

✓6th **S72.45** Supracondylar fracture without intracondylar extension of lower end of femur
Supracondylar fracture of lower end of femur NOS
EXCLUDES 1 *supracondylar fracture with intracondylar extension of lower end of femur (S72.46-)*

7 ✓7th **S72.451** **Displaced supracondylar fracture without intracondylar extension of lower end of right femur** MCC CC
CC Excl: See code: S72.401

7 ✓7th **S72.452** **Displaced supracondylar fracture without intracondylar extension of lower end of left femur** MCC CC
CC Excl: See code: S72.402

7 ✓7th **S72.453** **Displaced supracondylar fracture without intracondylar extension of lower end of unspecified femur** MCC CC
CC Excl: See code: S72.409

7 ✓7th **S72.454** **Nondisplaced supracondylar fracture without intracondylar extension of lower end of right femur** MCC CC
CC Excl: See code: S72.401

7 ✓7th **S72.455** **Nondisplaced supracondylar fracture without intracondylar extension of lower end of left femur** MCC CC
CC Excl: See code: S72.402

7 ✓7th **S72.456** **Nondisplaced supracondylar fracture without intracondylar extension of lower end of unspecified femur** MCC CC
CC Excl: See code: S72.409

✓6th **S72.46** Supracondylar fracture with intracondylar extension of lower end of femur
EXCLUDES 1 *supracondylar fracture without intracondylar extension of lower end of femur (S72.45-)*

7 ✓7th **S72.461** **Displaced supracondylar fracture with intracondylar extension of lower end of right femur** MCC CC
CC Excl: See code: S72.401

7 ✓7th **S72.462** **Displaced supracondylar fracture with intracondylar extension of lower end of left femur** MCC CC
CC Excl: See code: S72.402

7 ✓7th **S72.463** **Displaced supracondylar fracture with intracondylar extension of lower end of unspecified femur** MCC CC
CC Excl: See code: S72.409

7 ✓7th **S72.464** **Nondisplaced supracondylar fracture with intracondylar extension of lower end of right femur** MCC CC
CC Excl: See code: S72.401

7 ✓7th **S72.465** **Nondisplaced supracondylar fracture with intracondylar extension of lower end of left femur** MCC CC
CC Excl: See code: S72.402

7 ✓7th **S72.466** **Nondisplaced supracondylar fracture with intracondylar extension of lower end of unspecified femur** MCC CC
CC Excl: See code: S72.409

✓6th **S72.47** Torus fracture of lower end of femur

The appropriate 7th character is to be added to all codes in subcategory S72.47.
A　initial encounter for closed fracture
D　subsequent encounter for fracture with routine healing
G　subsequent encounter for fracture with delayed healing
K　subsequent encounter for fracture with nonunion
P　subsequent encounter for fracture with malunion
S　sequela

7 ✓7th **S72.471** **Torus fracture of lower end of right femur** CC
CC Excl: CC with 7th character A: M80.00X-M80.019 with 7th A, M80.041-M80.059 with 7th A, M80.80X-M80.819 with 7th A, M80.841-M80.859 with 7th A, M84.40X-M84.419 with 7th A, M84.441-M84.459 with 7th A, M84.474-M84.519 with 7th A, M84.541-M84.559 with 7th A, M84.574-M84.576 with 7th A, M84.60X-M84.619 with 7th A, M84.641-M84.659 with 7th A, M84.674-M84.68X with 7th A, S03.8XX-S03.9XX with 7th A, S29.011-S29.019 with 7th A, S38.3X-S39.013 with 7th A, S72.001-S72.471 with 7th [A, B, C], S72.479-S72.92X with 7th A, S73.101 with 7th A, S73.109-S73.111 with 7th A, S73.119-S73.121 with 7th A, S73.129-S73.191 with 7th A, S73.199 with 7th A, S76.001 with 7th A, S76.009-S76.011 with 7th A, S76.019A, S76.091A, S76.099-S76.101 with 7th A, S76.109-S76.111 with 7th A, S76.119A, S76.191A, S76.199-S76.201 with 7th A, S76.209-S76.211 with 7th A, S76.219A, S76.291 A, S76.299-S76.301 with 7th A, S76.309-S76.311 with 7th A, S76.319A, S76.391A, S76.399-S76.801 with 7th A, S76.809-S76.811 with 7th A, S76.819A, S76.891A, S76.899-S76.901 with 7th A, S76.909-S76.911 with 7th A, S76.919A, S76.991A, S76.999A, S79.001A, S79.009-S79.011 with 7th A, S79.019-S79.091 with 7th A, S79.099-S79.101 with 7th A, S79.109-S79.111 with 7th A, S79.119-S79.121 with 7th A, S79.129-S79.131 with 7th A, S79.139-S79.141 with 7th A, S79.149-S79.191 with 7th A, S79.199-S79.811 with 7th A, S79.819-S79.821 with 7th A, S79.829-S79.911 with 7th A, S79.919-S79.921 with 7th A, S79.929A, S82.90X-S82.92X with 7th [A, B, C], T14.8-T14.91, T79.A9X-T79.9XX with 7th A

---

7 HAC = Initial encounter only (7th character A, B or C) and not POA.

✓ Additional Character Required　✓x7th Xtension Alert　Unacceptable PDx　Manifestation　　Hospital Acquired Condition　EXCLUDES 1 Not Coded Here　EXCLUDES 2 Not Included Here

CC Excl: CC with 7th character K or P: M80.00X-M84.68X with 7th [K, P], S02.0XX-S02.92X with 7th K, S12.000-S12.691 with 7th K, S22.000-S22.9XX with 7th K, S32.000-S32.9XX with 7th K, S42.001-S42.92X with 7th [K, P], S49.001-S49.199 with 7th [K, P], S52.001-S52.92X with 7th [K, M, N, P, Q, R], S59.001-S59.299 with 7th [K, P], S62.001-S62.92X with 7th [K, P], S72.001-S72.92X with 7th [K, M, N, P, Q, R], S79.001-S79.199 with 7th [K, P], S82.001-S82.92X with 7th [K, M, N, P, Q, R], S89.001-S89.399 with 7th [K, P], S92.001-S92.919 with 7th [K, P]

7 √7ᵗʰ **S72.472 Torus fracture of lower end of left femur** `CC`

CC Excl: CC with 7th character A: M80.00X-M80.019 with 7th A, M80.041-M80.059 with 7th A, M80.80X-M80.819 with 7th A, M80.841-M80.859 with 7th A, M84.40X-M84.419 with 7th A, M84.441-M84.459 with 7th A, M84.474-M84.519 with 7th A, M84.541-M84.559 with 7th A, M84.574-M84.576 with 7th A, M84.60X-M84.619 with 7th A, M84.641-M84.659 with 7th A, M84.674-M84.68 with 7th A, S03.8XX-S03.9XX with 7th A, S29.011-S29.019 with 7th A, S38.3XX-S39.013 with 7th A, S72.001-S72.466 with 7th [B, C], S72.472-S72.92X with 7th A, S73.102-S73.109 with 7th A, S73.112-S73.119 with 7th A, S73.122-S73.129 with 7th A, S73.192-S73.199 with 7th A, S76.002-S76.009 with 7th A, S76.012-S76.019 with 7th A, S76.092-S76.099 with 7th A, S76.102-S76.109 with 7th A, S76.112-S76.119 with 7th A, S76.192-S76.199 with 7th A, S76.202-S76.209 with 7th A, S76.212-S76.219 with 7th A, S76.292-S76.299 with 7th A, S76.302-S76.309 with 7th A, S76.312-S76.319 with 7th A, S76.392-S76.399 with 7th A, S76.802-S76.809 with 7th A, S76.812-S76.819 with 7th A, S76.892-S76.899 with 7th A, S76.902-S76.909 with 7th A, S76.912-S76.919 with 7th A, S76.992-S76.999 with 7th A, S79.002-S79.009 with 7th A, S79.012-S79.019 with 7th A, S79.092-S79.099 with 7th A, S79.102-S79.109 with 7th A, S79.112-S79.119 with 7th A, S79.122-S79.129 with 7th A, S79.132-S79.139 with 7th A, S79.142-S79.149 with 7th A, S79.192-S79.199 with 7th A, S79.812-S79.819 with 7th A, S79.822-S79.829 with 7th A, S79.912-S79.919 with 7th A, S79.922-S79.929 with 7th A, S82.90X-S82.92X with 7th [A, B, C], T14.8-T14.91, T79.A9X-T79.9XX with 7th A

CC Excl: CC with 7th character K or P: M80.00X-M84.68X with 7th [K, P], S02.0XX-S02.92X with 7th K, S12.000-S12.691 with 7th K, S22.000-S22.9XX with 7th K, S32.000-S32.9XX with 7th K, S42.001-S42.92X with 7th [K, P], S49.001-S49.199 with 7th [K, P], S52.001-S52.92X with 7th [K, M, N, P, Q, R], S59.001-S59.299 with 7th [K, P], S62.001-S62.92X with 7th [K, P], S72.001-S72.92X with 7th [K, M, N, P, Q, R], S79.001-S79.199 with 7th [K, P], S82.001-S82.92X with 7th [K, M, N, P, Q, R], S89.001-S89.399 with 7th [K, P], S92.001-S92.919 with 7th [K, P]

7 √7ᵗʰ **S72.479 Torus fracture of lower end of unspecified femur** `CC`

CC Excl: CC with 7th character A: M80.00X-M80.019 with 7th A, M80.041-M80.059 with 7th A, M80.80X-M80.819 with 7th A, M80.841-M80.859 with 7th A, M84.40X-M84.419 with 7th A, M84.441-M84.459 with 7th A, M84.474-M84.519 with 7th A, M84.541-M84.559 with 7th A, M84.574-M84.576 with 7th A, M84.60X-M84.619 with 7th A, M84.641-M84.659 with 7th A, M84.674-M84.68X with 7th A, S03.8XX-S03.9XX with 7th A, S29.011-S29.019 with 7th A, S38.3XX-S39.013 with 7th A, S72.001-S72.471 with 7th [A, B, C], S72.479-S72.92X with 7th A, S73.101A, S73.109-S73.111 with 7th A, S73.119-S73.121 with 7th A, S73.129-S73.191 with 7th A, S73.199A, S76.001A, S76.009-S76.011 with 7th A, S76.019A, S76.091A, S76.099-S76.101 with 7th A, S76.109-S76.111 with 7th A, S76.119A, S76.191A, S76.199-S76.201 with 7th A, S76.209-S76.211 with 7th A, S76.219A, S76.291A, S76.299-S76.301 with 7th A, S76.309-S76.311 with 7th A, S76.319A, S76.391A, S76.399-S76.801 with 7th A, S76.809-S76.811 with 7th A, S76.819A, S76.891A, S76.899-S76.901 with 7th A, S76.909-S76.911 with 7th A, S76.919A, S76.991A, S76.999A, S79.001A, S79.009-S79.011 with 7th A, S79.019-S79.091 with 7th A, S79.099-S79.101 with 7th A, S79.109-S79.111 with 7th A, S79.119-S79.121 with 7th A, S79.129-S79.131 with 7th A, S79.139-S79.141 with 7th A, S79.149-S79.191 with 7th A, S79.199-S79.811 with 7th A, S79.819-S79.821 with 7th A, S79.829-S79.911 with 7th A, S79.919-S79.921 with 7th A, S79.929A, S82.90X-S82.92X with 7th [A, B, C], T14.8-T14.91, T79.A9X-T79.9XX with 7th A

CC with 7th character K or P: M80.00X-M84.68X with 7th [K, P], S02.0XX-S02.92X with 7th K, S12.000-S12.691 with 7th K, S22.000-S22.9XX with 7th K, S32.000-S32.9XX with 7th K, S42.001-S42.92X with 7th [K, P], S49.001-S49.199 with 7th [K, P], S52.001-S52.92X with 7th [K, M, N, P, Q, R], S59.001-S59.299 with 7th [K, P], S62.001-S62.92X with 7th [K, P], S72.001-S72.92X with 7th [K, M, N, P, Q, R], S79.001-S79.199 with 7th [K, P], S82.001-S82.92X with 7th [K, M, N, P, Q, R], S89.001-S89.399 with 7th [K, P], S92.001-S92.919 with 7th [K, P]

√6ᵗʰ **S72.49 Other fracture of lower end of femur**

7 √7ᵗʰ **S72.491 Other fracture of lower end of right femur** `MCC` `CC`

CC Excl: CC for codes with 7th A: M80.00X-M80.019 with 7th A, M80.041-M80.059 with 7th A, M80.80X-M80.819 with 7th A, M80.841-M80.859 with 7th A, M84.40X-M84.419 with 7th A, M84.441-M84.459 with 7th A, M84.474-M84.519 with 7th A, M84.541-M84.559 with 7th A, M84.574-M84.576 with 7th A, M84.60X-M84.619 with 7th A, M84.641-M84.659 with 7th A, M84.674-M84.68 with 7th A, S03.8XX-S03.9XX with 7th A, S29.011-S29.019 with 7th A, S38.3XX-S39.013 with 7th A, S72.001-S72.471 with 7th [A, B, C], S72.479-S72.92X with 7th A, S73.101 with 7th A, S73.109-S73.111 with 7th A, S73.119-S73.121 with 7th A, S73.129-S73.191 with 7th A, S73.199A, S76.001A, S76.009-S76.011 with 7th A, S76.019A, S76.091A, S76.099-S76.101 with 7th A, S76.109-S76.111 with 7th A, S76.119A, S76.191A, S76.199-S76.201 with 7th A, S76.209-S76.211 with 7th A, S76.219A, S76.291A, S76.299-S76.301 with 7th A, S76.309-S76.311 with 7th A, S76.319A, S76.391A, S76.399-S76.801 with 7th A, S76.809-S76.811 with 7th A, S76.819A, S76.891A, S76.899-S76.901 with 7th A, S76.909-S76.911 with 7th A, S76.919A, S76.991A, S76.999A, S79.001A, S79.009-S79.011 with 7th A, S79.019-S79.091 with 7th A, S79.099-S79.101 with 7th A, S79.109-S79.111 with 7th A, S79.119-S79.121 with 7th A, S79.129-S79.131 with 7th A, S79.139-S79.141 with 7th A, S79.149-S79.191 with 7th A, S79.199-S79.811 with 7th A, S79.819-

---

7 HAC = Initial encounter only (7th character A, B or C) and not POA.

Ⓝ Newborn: 0   Ⓟ Pediatric: 0-17   Ⓜ Maternity: 12-55   Ⓐ Adult: 15-124   `MCC` Major CC Condition   `PDx MCC` PDx acts as own MCC   `CC` CC Condition   `PDx CC` PDx acts as own CC

980   ICD-10-CM Draft (2015)

S79.821 with 7th A, S79.829-S79.911 with 7th A, S79.919-S79.921 with 7th A, S79.929A, S82.90-S82.92 with 7th [A, B, C], T14.8-T14.91, T79.A9X-T79.9XX with 7th A

MCC for codes with 7th B or C: M80.00X-M80.019 with 7th A, M80.041-M80.059 with 7th A, M80.80X-M80.819 with 7th A, M80.841-M80.859 with 7th A, M84.40X-M84.419 with 7th A, M84.441-M84.459 with 7th A, M84.474-M84.519 with 7th A, M84.541-M84.559 with 7th A, M84.574-M84.576 with 7th A, M84.60X-M84.619 with 7th A, M84.641-M84.659 with 7th A, M84.674-M84.68 with 7th A, S03.8XX-S03.9XX with 7th A, S29.011-S29.019 with 7th A, S38.3XX-S39.013 with 7th A, S72.491-S72.499 with 7th [B, C], S73.101-S73.199 with 7th A, S76.001-S76.019 with 7th A, S76.091-S76.119 with 7th A, S76.191-S76.219 with 7th A, S76.291-S76.319 with 7th A, S76.391-S76.819 with 7th A, S76.891-S76.919 with 7th A, S76.991-S76.999 with 7th A, S79.811-S79.929 with 7th A, S82.001-S82.099 with 7th [A, B, C], S82.90X-S82.92X with 7th [A, B, C], T14.8-T14.91, T79.A9X-T79.9XX with 7th A

CC for codes with 7th K, M, N, P, Q or R: M80.00X-M84.68X with 7th [K, P], S02.0XX-S02.92X with 7th K, S12.000-S12.691 with 7th K, S22.000-S22.9XX with 7th K, S32.000-S32.9XX with 7th K, S42.001-S42.92X with 7th [K, P], S49.001-S49.199 with 7th [K, P], S52.001-S52.92X with 7th [K, M, N, P, Q, R], S59.001-S59.299 with 7th [K, P], S62.001-S62.92X with 7th [K, P], S72.001-S72.92X with 7th [K, M, N, P, Q, R], S79.001-S79.199 with 7th [K, P], S82.001-S82.92X with 7th [K, M, N, P, Q, R], S89.001-S89.399 with 7th [K, P], S92.001-S92.919 with 7th [K, P]

7 ☑ √7ᵗʰ **S72.492** **Other fracture of lower end of left femur** MCC CC

CC Excl: CC for codes with 7th A: M80.00X-M80.019 with 7th A, M80.041-M80.059 with 7th A, M80.80X-M80.819 with 7th A, M80.841-M80.859 with 7th A, M84.40X-M84.419 with 7th A, M84.441-M84.459 with 7th A, M84.474-M84.519 with 7th A, M84.541-M84.559 with 7th A, M84.574-M84.576 with 7th A, M84.60X-M84.619 with 7th A, M84.641-M84.659 with 7th A, M84.674-M84.68 with 7th A, S03.8XX-S03.9XX with 7th A, S29.011-S29.019 with 7th A, S38.3XX-S39.013 with 7th A, S72.001-S72.466 with 7th [B, C], S72.472-S72.92X with 7th A, S73.102-S73.109 with 7th A, S73.112-S73.119 with 7th A, S73.122-S73.129 with 7th A, S73.192-S73.199 with 7th A, S76.002-S76.009 with 7th A, S76.012-S76.019 with 7th A, S76.092-S76.099 with 7th A, S76.102-S76.109 with 7th A, S76.112-S76.119 with 7th A, S76.192-S76.199 with 7th A, S76.202-S76.209 with 7th A, S76.212-S76.219 with 7th A, S76.292-S76.299 with 7th A, S76.302-S76.309 with 7th A, S76.312-S76.319 with 7th A, S76.392-S76.399 with 7th A, S76.802-S76.809 with 7th A, S76.812-S76.819 with 7th A, S76.892-S76.899 with 7th A, S76.902-S76.909 with 7th A, S76.912-S76.919 with 7th A, S76.992-S76.999 with 7th A, S79.002-S79.009 with 7th A, S79.012-S79.019 with 7th A, S79.092-S79.099 with 7th A, S79.102-S79.109 with 7th A, S79.112-S79.119 with 7th A, S79.122-S79.129 with 7th A, S79.132-S79.139 with 7th A, S79.142-S79.149 with 7th A, S79.192-S79.199 with 7th A, S79.812-S79.819 with 7th A, S79.822-S79.829 with 7th A, S79.912-S79.919 with 7th A, S79.922-S79.929 with 7th A, S82.90X-S82.92X with 7th [A, B, C], T14.8-T14.91, T79.A9X-T79.9XX with 7th A

MCC for codes with 7th B or C: M80.00X-M80.019 with 7th A, M80.041-M80.059 with 7th A, M80.80X-M80.819 with 7th A, M80.841-M80.859 with 7th A, M84.40X-M84.419 with 7th A, M84.441-M84.459 with 7th A, M84.474-M84.519 with 7th A, M84.541-M84.559 with 7th A, M84.574-M84.576 with 7th A, M84.60X-M84.619 with 7th A, M84.641-M84.659 with 7th A, M84.674-M84.68 with 7th A, S03.8XX-S03.9XX with 7th A, S29.011-S29.019 with 7th A, S38.3X-S39.013 with 7th A, S72.491-S72.499 with 7th [B, C], S73.101-S73.199 with 7th A, S76.001-S76.019 with 7th A, S76.091-S76.119 with 7th A, S76.191-S76.219 with 7th A, S76.291-S76.319 with 7th A, S76.391-S76.819 with 7th A, S76.891-S76.919 with 7th A, S76.991-S76.999 with 7th A, S79.811-S79.929 with 7th A, S82.001-S82.099 with 7th [A, B, C], S82.90X-S82.92X with 7th [A, B, C], T14.8-T14.91, T79.A9X-T79.9XX with 7th A

CC for codes with 7th K, M, N, P, Q or R: M80.00X-M84.68 with 7th [K, P], S02.0XX-S02.92X with 7th K, S12.000-S12.691 with 7th K, S22.000-S22.9XX with 7th K, S32.000-S32.9XX with 7th K, S42.001-S42.92X with 7th [K, P], S49.001-S49.199 with 7th [K, P], S52.001-S52.92X with 7th [K, M, N, P, Q, R], S59.001-S59.299 with 7th [K, P], S62.001-S62.92X with 7th [K, P], S72.001-S72.92X with 7th [K, M, N, P, Q, R], S79.001-S79.199 with 7th [K, P], S82.001-S82.92X with 7th [K, M, N, P, Q, R], S89.001-S89.399 with 7th [K, P], S92.001-S92.919 with 7th [K, P]

7 ☑ √7ᵗʰ **S72.499** **Other fracture of lower end of unspecified femur** MCC CC

CC Excl: CC for codes with 7th A: M80.00X-M80.019 with 7th A, M80.041-M80.059 with 7th A, M80.80X-M80.819 with 7th A, M80.841-M80.859 with 7th A, M84.40X-M84.419 with 7th A, M84.441-M84.459 with 7th A, M84.474-M84.519 with 7th A, M84.541-M84.559 with 7th A, M84.574-M84.576 with 7th A, M84.60X-M84.619 with 7th A, M84.641-M84.659 with 7th A, M84.674-M84.68 with 7th A, S03.8XX-S03.9XX with 7th A, S29.011-S29.019 with 7th A, S38.3XX-S39.013 with 7th A, S72.001-S72.92X with 7th [A, B, C], S73.101-S73.199 with 7th A, S76.001-S76.019 with 7th A, S76.091-S76.119 with 7th A, S76.191-S76.219 with 7th A, S76.291-S76.319 with 7th A, S76.391-S76.819 with 7th A, S76.891-S76.919 with 7th A, S76.991-S76.999 with 7th A, S79.001-S79.929 with 7th A, S82.90X-S82.92X with 7th [A, B, C], T14.8-T14.91, T79.A9X-T79.9XX with 7th A

MCC for codes with 7th B or C: M80.00X-M80.019 with 7th A, M80.041-M80.059 with 7th A, M80.80X-M80.819 with 7th A, M80.841-M80.859 with 7th A, M84.40X-M84.419 with 7th A, M84.441-M84.459 with 7th A, M84.474-M84.519 with 7th A, M84.541-M84.559 with 7th A, M84.574-M84.576 with 7th A, M84.60X-M84.619 with 7th A, M84.641-M84.659 with 7th A, M84.674-M84.68X with 7th A, S03.8XX-S03.9XX with 7th A, S29.011-S29.019 with 7th A, S38.3XX-S39.013 with 7th A, S72.491-S72.499 with 7th [B, C], S73.101-S73.199 with 7th A, S76.001-S76.019 with 7th A, S76.091-S76.119 with 7th A, S76.191-S76.219 with 7th A, S76.291-S76.319 with 7th A, S76.391-S76.819 with 7th A, S76.891-S76.919 with 7th A, S76.991-S76.999 with 7th A, S79.811-S79.929 with 7th A, S82.001-S82.099 with 7th [A, B, C], S82.90X-S82.92X with 7th [A, B, C], T14.8-T14.91, T79.A9X-T79.9XX with 7th A

CC for codes with 7th K, M, N, P, Q or R: M80.00X-M84.68X with 7th [K, P], S02.0XX-S02.92X with 7th K, S12.000-S12.691 with 7th K, S22.000-S22.9XX with 7th K, S32.000-S32.9XX with 7th K, S42.001-S42.92X with 7th [K, P], S49.001-S49.199 with 7th [K, P], S52.001-S52.92X with 7th [K, M, N, P, Q, R], S59.001-S59.299 with 7th [K, P], S62.001-S62.92X with 7th [K, P], S72.001-S72.92X with 7th [K, M, N, P, Q, R], S79.001-S79.199 with 7th [K, P], S82.001-S82.92X with 7th [K, M, N, P, Q, R], S89.001-S89.399 with 7th [K, P], S92.001-S92.919 with 7th [K, P]

---

7 HAC = Initial encounter only (7th character A, B or C) and not POA.

☑ Additional Character Required   √7ᵗʰ Xtension Alert   Unacceptable PDx   Manifestation   Hospital Acquired Condition   EXCLUDES 1 Not Coded Here   EXCLUDES 2 Not Included Here

☑5ᵗʰ **S72.8**   **Other fracture of femur**

    ☑6ᵗʰ **S72.8X**   **Other fracture of femur**

> **CC Excl: For CC/MCC codes in subcategory S72.8X, unless otherwise noted: MCC with 7th A,B or C:** M48.40X-M48.58X with 7th A, M80.00X-M84.68X with 7th A, S03.8XX-S03.9XX with 7th A, S29.011-S29.019 with 7th A, S38.3XX-S39.013 with 7th A, S72.001-S72.92X with 7th [A, B, C], S73.101-S73.199 with 7th A, S76.001-S76.019 with 7th A, S76.091-S76.119 with 7th A, S76.191-S76.219 with 7th A, S76.291-S76.319 with 7th A, S76.391-S76.819 with 7th A, S76.891-S76.919 with 7th A, S76.991-S76.999 with 7th A, S79.001-S79.929 with 7th A, S82.90X-S82.92X with 7th [A, B, C], T14.8-T14.91, T79.A0X-T79.9XX with 7th A
>
> **CC with 7th character K, M, N, P, Q or R:** M80.00X-M84.68X with 7th [K, P], S02.0XX-S02.92X with 7th K, S12.000-S12.691 with 7th K, S22.000-S22.9XX with 7th K, S32.000-S32.9XX with 7th K, S42.001-S42.92X with 7th [K, P], S49.001-S49.199 with 7th [K, P], S52.001-S52.92X with 7th [K, M, N, P, Q, R], S59.001-S59.299 with 7th [K, P], S62.001-S62.92X with 7th [K, P], S72.001-S72.92X with 7th [K, M, N, P, Q, R], S79.001-S79.199 with 7th [K, P], S82.001-S82.92X with 7th [K, M, N, P, Q, R], S89.001-S89.399 with 7th [K, P], S92.001-S92.919 with 7th [K, P]K

    7 ☑7ᵗʰ **S72.8X1**   **Other fracture of right femur**   MCC CC

    7 ☑7ᵗʰ **S72.8X2**   **Other fracture of left femur**   MCC CC

    7 ☑7ᵗʰ **S72.8X9**   **Other fracture of unspecified femur**   MCC CC

☑5ᵗʰ **S72.9**   **Unspecified fracture of femur**
    Fracture of thigh NOS
    Fracture of upper leg NOS
    EXCLUDES 1   fracture of hip NOS (S72.00-, S72.01-)

    7 ☑×7ᵗʰ **S72.90**   **Unspecified fracture of unspecified femur**   MCC CC
       AHA: 2012, 4Q, 93
       CC Excl: See code: S72.8X

    7 ☑×7ᵗʰ **S72.91**   **Unspecified fracture of right femur**   MCC CC
       CC Excl: See code: S72.8X

    7 ☑×7ᵗʰ **S72.92**   **Unspecified fracture of left femur**   MCC CC
       CC Excl: See code: S72.8X

☑4ᵗʰ **S73**   **Dislocation and sprain of joint and ligaments of hip**
    INCLUDES   avulsion of joint or ligament of hip
           laceration of cartilage, joint or ligament of hip
           sprain of cartilage, joint or ligament of hip
           traumatic hemarthrosis of joint or ligament of hip
           traumatic rupture of joint or ligament of hip
           traumatic subluxation of joint or ligament of hip
           traumatic tear of joint or ligament of hip
    Code also any associated open wound
    EXCLUDES 2   strain of muscle, fascia and tendon of hip and thigh (S76.-)

> The appropriate 7th character is to be added to each code from category S73.
> A   initial encounter
> D   subsequent encounter
> S   sequela

☑5ᵗʰ **S73.0**   **Subluxation and dislocation of hip**
    EXCLUDES 2   dislocation and subluxation of hip prosthesis (T84.020, T84.021)

    ☑6ᵗʰ **S73.00**   **Unspecified subluxation and dislocation of hip**
       Dislocation of hip NOS
       Subluxation of hip NOS

      7 ☑7ᵗʰ **S73.001**   **Unspecified subluxation of right hip**   CC
          CC Excl: CC with 7th character A: M99.16-M99.17, M99.19, S33.30X-S33.39X with 7th A, S73.001A, S73.003-S73.004 with 7th A, S73.006A, S73.041A, S73.043-S73.044 with 7th A, S73.046A

      7 ☑7ᵗʰ **S73.002**   **Unspecified subluxation of left hip**   CC
          CC Excl: CC with 7th character A: M99.16-M99.17, M99.19, S33.30X-S33.39X with 7th A, S73.002-S73.003 with 7th A, S73.005-S73.006 with 7th A, S73.042-S73.043 with 7th A, S73.045-S73.046 with 7th A

      7 ☑7ᵗʰ **S73.003**   **Unspecified subluxation of unspecified hip**   CC
          CC Excl: CC with 7th character A: M99.16-M99.17, M99.19, S33.30X-S33.39X with 7th A, S73.001-S73.006 with 7th A, S73.041-S73.046 with 7th A

7 ☑7ᵗʰ **S73.004**   **Unspecified dislocation of right hip**   CC
       CC Excl: See code: S73.001

7 ☑7ᵗʰ **S73.005**   **Unspecified dislocation of left hip**   CC
       CC Excl: See code: S73.002

7 ☑7ᵗʰ **S73.006**   **Unspecified dislocation of unspecified hip**   CC
       CC Excl: See code: S73.003

☑6ᵗʰ **S73.01**   **Posterior subluxation and dislocation of hip**

    7 ☑7ᵗʰ **S73.011**   **Posterior subluxation of right hip**   CC
       CC Excl: CC with 7th character A: M99.16-M99.17, M99.19, S33.30X-S33.39X with 7th A, S73.011 with 7th A, S73.013-S73.014 with 7th A, S73.016 with 7th A

    7 ☑7ᵗʰ **S73.012**   **Posterior subluxation of left hip**   CC
       CC Excl: CC with 7th character A: M99.16-M99.17, M99.19, S33.30X-S33.39X with 7th A, S73.012-S73.013 with 7th A, S73.015-S73.016 with 7th A

    7 ☑7ᵗʰ **S73.013**   **Posterior subluxation of unspecified hip**   CC
       CC Excl: CC with 7th character A:M99.16-M99.17, M99.19, S33.30X-S33.39X with 7th A, S73.011-S73.016 with 7th A

    7 ☑7ᵗʰ **S73.014**   **Posterior dislocation of right hip**   CC
       CC Excl: See code: S73.011

    7 ☑7ᵗʰ **S73.015**   **Posterior dislocation of left hip**   CC
       CC Excl: See code: S73.012

    7 ☑7ᵗʰ **S73.016**   **Posterior dislocation of unspecified hip**   CC
       CC Excl: See code: S73.013

☑6ᵗʰ **S73.02**   **Obturator subluxation and dislocation of hip**

    7 ☑7ᵗʰ **S73.021**   **Obturator subluxation of right hip**   CC
       CC Excl: CC with 7th character A: M99.16-M99.17, M99.19, S33.30X-S33.39X with 7th A, S73.021A, S73.023-S73.024 with 7th A, S73.026A

    7 ☑7ᵗʰ **S73.022**   **Obturator subluxation of left hip**   CC
       CC Excl: CC with 7th character A: M99.16-M99.17, M99.19, S33.30X-S33.39X with 7th A, S73.022-S73.023 with 7th A, S73.025-S73.026 with 7th A

    7 ☑7ᵗʰ **S73.023**   **Obturator subluxation of unspecified hip**   CC
       CC Excl: CC with 7th character A: M99.16-M99.17, M99.19, S33.30X-S33.39X with 7th A, S73.021-S73.026 with 7th A

    7 ☑7ᵗʰ **S73.024**   **Obturator dislocation of right hip**   CC
       CC Excl:See code: S73.021

    7 ☑7ᵗʰ **S73.025**   **Obturator dislocation of left hip**   CC
       CC Excl: See code: S73.022

    7 ☑7ᵗʰ **S73.026**   **Obturator dislocation of unspecified hip**   CC
       CC Excl: See code: S73.023

☑6ᵗʰ **S73.03**   **Other anterior dislocation of hip**

    7 ☑7ᵗʰ **S73.031**   **Other anterior subluxation of right hip**   CC
       CC Excl: CC with 7th character A: M99.16-M99.17, M99.19, S33.30X-S33.39X with 7th A, S73.031A, S73.033-S73.034 with 7th A, S73.036A

    7 ☑7ᵗʰ **S73.032**   **Other anterior subluxation of left hip**   CC
       CC Excl: CC with 7th character AM99.16-M99.17, M99.19, S33.30X-S33.39X with 7th A, S73.032-S73.033 with 7th A, S73.035-S73.036 with 7th A

    7 ☑7ᵗʰ **S73.033**   **Other anterior subluxation of unspecified hip**   CC
       CC Excl: CC with 7th character A: M99.16-M99.17, M99.19, S33.30X-S33.39X with 7th A, S73.031-S73.036 with 7th A

    7 ☑7ᵗʰ **S73.034**   **Other anterior dislocation of right hip**   CC
       CC Excl:See code: S73.031

    7 ☑7ᵗʰ **S73.035**   **Other anterior dislocation of left hip**   CC
       CC Excl: See code: S73.032

    7 ☑7ᵗʰ **S73.036**   **Other anterior dislocation of unspecified hip**   CC
       CC Excl: See code: S73.033

☑6ᵗʰ **S73.04**   **Central dislocation of hip**

---

7 HAC = Initial encounter only (7th character A, B or C) and not POA.

Ⓝ Newborn: 0   Ⓟ Pediatric: 0-17   Ⓜ Maternity: 12-55   Ⓐ Adult: 15-124   MCC Major CC Condition   PDx MCC PDx acts as own MCC   CC CC Condition   PDx CC PDx acts as own CC

982   ICD-10-CM Draft (2015)

7 ☑7ᵗʰ **S73.041** **Central subluxation of right hip**   CC
CC Excl: See code: S73.001

7 ☑7ᵗʰ **S73.042** **Central subluxation of left hip**   CC
CC Excl: See code: S73.002

7 ☑7ᵗʰ **S73.043** **Central subluxation of unspecified hip**   CC
CC Excl: See code: S73.003

7 ☑7ᵗʰ **S73.044** **Central dislocation of right hip**   CC
CC Excl: See code: S73.001

7 ☑7ᵗʰ **S73.045** **Central dislocation of left hip**   CC
CC Excl: See code: S73.002

7 ☑7ᵗʰ **S73.046** **Central dislocation of unspecified hip**   CC
CC Excl: See code: S73.003

☑5ᵗʰ **S73.1** **Sprain of hip**

☑6ᵗʰ **S73.10** **Unspecified sprain of hip**

☑7ᵗʰ **S73.101** **Unspecified sprain of right hip**

☑7ᵗʰ **S73.102** **Unspecified sprain of left hip**

☑7ᵗʰ **S73.109** **Unspecified sprain of unspecified hip**

☑6ᵗʰ **S73.11** **Iliofemoral ligament sprain of hip**

☑7ᵗʰ **S73.111** **Iliofemoral ligament sprain of right hip**

☑7ᵗʰ **S73.112** **Iliofemoral ligament sprain of left hip**

☑7ᵗʰ **S73.119** **Iliofemoral ligament sprain of unspecified hip**

☑6ᵗʰ **S73.12** **Ischiocapsular (ligament) sprain of hip**

☑7ᵗʰ **S73.121** **Ischiocapsular ligament sprain of right hip**

☑7ᵗʰ **S73.122** **Ischiocapsular ligament sprain of left hip**

☑7ᵗʰ **S73.129** **Ischiocapsular ligament sprain of unspecified hip**

☑6ᵗʰ **S73.19** **Other sprain of hip**

☑7ᵗʰ **S73.191** **Other sprain of right hip**

☑7ᵗʰ **S73.192** **Other sprain of left hip**

☑7ᵗʰ **S73.199** **Other sprain of unspecified hip**

☑4ᵗʰ **S74** **Injury of nerves at hip and thigh level**
Code also any associated open wound (S71.-)
EXCLUDES 2 injury of nerves at ankle and foot level (S94.-)
injury of nerves at lower leg level (S84.-)

The appropriate 7th character is to be added to each code from category S74.
A   initial encounter
D   subsequent encounter
S   sequela

☑5ᵗʰ **S74.0** **Injury of sciatic nerve at hip and thigh level**

☑x7ᵗʰ **S74.00** **Injury of sciatic nerve at hip and thigh level, unspecified leg**

☑x7ᵗʰ **S74.01** **Injury of sciatic nerve at hip and thigh level, right leg**

☑x7ᵗʰ **S74.02** **Injury of sciatic nerve at hip and thigh level, left leg**

☑5ᵗʰ **S74.1** **Injury of femoral nerve at hip and thigh level**

☑x7ᵗʰ **S74.10** **Injury of femoral nerve at hip and thigh level, unspecified leg**

☑x7ᵗʰ **S74.11** **Injury of femoral nerve at hip and thigh level, right leg**

☑x7ᵗʰ **S74.12** **Injury of femoral nerve at hip and thigh level, left leg**

☑5ᵗʰ **S74.2** **Injury of cutaneous sensory nerve at hip and thigh level**

☑x7ᵗʰ **S74.20** **Injury of cutaneous sensory nerve at hip and thigh level, unspecified leg**

☑x7ᵗʰ **S74.21** **Injury of cutaneous sensory nerve at hip and high level, right leg**

☑x7ᵗʰ **S74.22** **Injury of cutaneous sensory nerve at hip and thigh level, left leg**

☑5ᵗʰ **S74.8** **Injury of other nerves at hip and thigh level**

☑6ᵗʰ **S74.8X** **Injury of other nerves at hip and thigh level**

☑7ᵗʰ **S74.8X1** **Injury of other nerves at hip and thigh level, right leg**

☑7ᵗʰ **S74.8X2** **Injury of other nerves at hip and thigh level, left leg**

☑7ᵗʰ **S74.8X9** **Injury of other nerves at hip and thigh level, unspecified leg**

☑5ᵗʰ **S74.9** **Injury of unspecified nerve at hip and thigh level**

☑x7ᵗʰ **S74.90** **Injury of unspecified nerve at hip and thigh level, unspecified leg**

☑x7ᵗʰ **S74.91** **Injury of unspecified nerve at hip and thigh level, right leg**

☑x7ᵗʰ **S74.92** **Injury of unspecified nerve at hip and thigh level, left leg**

☑4ᵗʰ **S75** **Injury of blood vessels at hip and thigh level**
Code also any associated open wound (S71.-)
EXCLUDES 2 injury of blood vessels at lower leg level (S85.-)
injury of popliteal artery (S85.0)

The appropriate 7th character is to be added to each code from category S75.
A   initial encounter
D   subsequent encounter
S   sequela

☑5ᵗʰ **S75.0** **Injury of femoral artery**

☑6ᵗʰ **S75.00** **Unspecified injury of femoral artery**

☑7ᵗʰ **S75.001** **Unspecified injury of femoral artery, right leg**   MCC
CC Excl: MCC with 7th A: S75.001A, S75.009-S75.011 with 7th A, S75.019-S75.021 with 7th A, S75.029-S75.091 with 7th A, S75.099 with 7th A, S75.801A, S75.809-S75.811 with 7th A, S75.819-S75.891 with 7th A, S75.899-S75.901 with 7th A, S75.909-S75.911 with 7th A, S75.919-S75.991 with 7th A, S75.999A, S85.201A, S85.209-S85.211 with 7th A, S85.219-S85.291 with 7th A, S85.299A, S85.801A, S85.809-S85.811 with 7th A, S85.819-S85.891 with 7th A, S85.899-S85.901 with 7th A, S85.909-S85.911 with 7th A, S85.919-S85.991 with 7th A, S85.999A, S95.001A, S95.009-S95.011 with 7th A, S95.019-S95.091 with 7th A, S95.099A, S95.201A, S95.209-S95.211 with 7th A, S95.219-S95.291 with 7th A, S95.299A, S95.801 with 7th A, S95.809-S95.811 with 7th A, S95.819-S95.891 with 7th A, S95.899-S95.901 with 7th A, S95.909-S95.911 with 7th A, S95.919-S95.991 with 7th A, S95.999A

☑7ᵗʰ **S75.002** **Unspecified injury of femoral artery, left leg**   MCC
CC Excl: MCC with 7th A: S75.002-S75.009 with 7th A, S75.012-S75.019 with 7th A, S75.022-S75.029 with 7th A, S75.092-S75.099 with 7th A, S75.802-S75.809 with 7th A, S75.812-S75.819 with 7th A, S75.892-S75.899 with 7th A, S75.902-S75.909 with 7th A, S75.912-S75.919 with 7th A, S75.992-S75.999 with 7th A, S85.202-S85.209 with 7th A, S85.212-S85.219 with 7th A, S85.292-S85.299 with 7th A, S85.802-S85.809 with 7th A, S85.812-S85.819 with 7th A, S85.892-S85.899 with 7th A, S85.902-S85.909 with 7th A, S85.912-S85.919 with 7th A, S85.992-S85.999 with 7th A, S95.002-S95.009 with 7th A, S95.012-S95.019 with 7th A, S95.092-S95.099 with 7th A, S95.202-S95.209 with 7th A, S95.212-S95.219 with 7th A, S95.292-S95.299 with 7th A, S95.802-S95.809 with 7th A, S95.812-S95.819 with 7th A, S95.892-S95.899 with 7th A, S95.902-S95.909 with 7th A, S95.912-S95.919 with 7th A, S95.992-S95.999 with 7th A

☑7ᵗʰ **S75.009** **Unspecified injury of femoral artery, unspecified leg**   MCC
CC Excl: MCC with 7th A: S75.001-S75.099 with 7th A, S75.801-S75.999 with 7th A, S85.201-S85.299 with 7th A, S85.801-S85.999 with 7th A, S95.001-S95.099 with 7th A, S95.201-S95.999 with 7th A

☑6ᵗʰ **S75.01** **Minor laceration of femoral artery**
Incomplete transection of femoral artery
Laceration of femoral artery NOS
Superficial laceration of femoral artery

☑7ᵗʰ **S75.011** **Minor laceration of femoral artery, right leg**   MCC
CC Excl: See code: S75.001

☑7ᵗʰ **S75.012** **Minor laceration of femoral artery, left leg**   MCC
CC Excl: See code: S75.002

---

7 HAC = Initial encounter only (7th character A, B or C) and not POA.

☑ Additional Character Required   ☑x7ᵗʰ Xtension Alert   Unacceptable PDx   Manifestation   Hospital Acquired Condition   EXCLUDES 1 Not Coded Here   EXCLUDES 2 Not Included Here
ICD-10-CM Draft (2015)   983

Injury, Poisoning and Certain Other Consequences of External Causes

S75.019–S75.202

√7ᵗʰ **S75.019** **Minor laceration of femoral artery, unspecified leg** ᴹᶜᶜ
CC Excl: See code: S75.009

√6ᵗʰ **S75.02** **Major laceration of femoral artery**
Complete transection of femoral artery
Traumatic rupture of femoral artery

√7ᵗʰ **S75.021** **Major laceration of femoral artery, right leg** ᴹᶜᶜ
CC Excl: See code: S75.001

√7ᵗʰ **S75.022** **Major laceration of femoral artery, left leg** ᴹᶜᶜ
CC Excl: See code: S75.002

√7ᵗʰ **S75.029** **Major laceration of femoral artery, unspecified leg** ᴹᶜᶜ
CC Excl: See code: S75.009

√6ᵗʰ **S75.09** **Other specified injury of femoral artery**

√7ᵗʰ **S75.091** **Other specified injury of femoral artery, right leg** ᴹᶜᶜ
CC Excl: See code: S75.001

√7ᵗʰ **S75.092** **Other specified injury of femoral artery, left leg** ᴹᶜᶜ
CC Excl: See code: S75.002

√7ᵗʰ **S75.099** **Other specified injury of femoral artery, unspecified leg** ᴹᶜᶜ
CC Excl: See code: S75.009

√5ᵗʰ **S75.1** **Injury of femoral vein at hip and thigh level**

√6ᵗʰ **S75.10** **Unspecified injury of femoral vein at hip and thigh level**

√7ᵗʰ **S75.101** **Unspecified injury of femoral vein at hip and thigh level, right leg** ᴹᶜᶜ
CC Excl: MCC with 7th A: S75.101A, S75.109-S75.111 with 7th A, S75.119-S75.121 with 7th A, S75.129-S75.191 with 7th A, S75.199A, S75.801A, S75.809-S75.811 with 7th A, S75.819-S75.891 with 7th A, S75.899-S75.901 with 7th A, S75.909-S75.911 with 7th A, S75.919-S75.991 with 7th A, S75.999 with 7th A, S85.201A, S85.209-S85.211 with 7th A, S85.219-S85.291 with 7th A, S85.299, S85.801A, S85.809-S85.811 with 7th A, S85.819-S85.891 with 7th A, S85.899-S85.901 with 7th A, S85.909-S85.911 with 7th A, S85.919-S85.991 with 7th A, S85.999A, S95.001A, S95.009-S95.011 with 7th A, S95.019-S95.091 with 7th A, S95.099A, S95.201A, S95.209-S95.211 with 7th A, S95.219-S95.291 with 7th A, S95.299-S95.801 with 7th A, S95.809-S95.811 with 7th A, S95.819-S95.891 with 7th A, S95.899-S95.901 with 7th A, S95.909-S95.911 with 7th A, S95.919-S95.991 with 7th A, S95.999A

√7ᵗʰ **S75.102** **Unspecified injury of femoral vein at hip and thigh level, left leg** ᴹᶜᶜ
CC Excl: MCC with 7th A: S75.102-S75.109 with 7th A, S75.112-S75.119 with 7th A, S75.122-S75.129 with 7th A, S75.192-S75.199 with 7th A, S75.802-S75.809 with 7th A, S75.812-S75.819 with 7th A, S75.892-S75.899 with 7th A, S75.902-S75.909 with 7th A, S75.912-S75.919 with 7th A, S75.992-S75.999 with 7th A, S85.202-S85.209 with 7th A, S85.212-S85.219 with 7th A, S85.292-S85.299 with 7th A, S85.802-S85.809 with 7th A, S85.812-S85.819 with 7th A, S85.892-S85.899 with 7th A, S85.902-S85.909 with 7th A, S85.912-S85.919 with 7th A, S85.992-S85.999 with 7th A, S95.002-S95.009 with 7th A, S95.012-S95.019 with 7th A, S95.092-S95.099 with 7th A, S95.202-S95.209 with 7th A, S95.212-S95.219 with 7th A, S95.292-S95.299 with 7th A, S95.802-S95.809 with 7th A, S95.812-S95.819 with 7th A, S95.892-S95.899 with 7th A, S95.902-S95.909 with 7th A, S95.912-S95.919 with 7th A, S95.992-S95.999 with 7th A

√7ᵗʰ **S75.109** **Unspecified injury of femoral vein at hip and thigh level, unspecified leg** ᴹᶜᶜ
CC Excl: MCC with 7th A: S75.101-S75.199 with 7th A, S75.801-S75.999 with 7th A, S85.201-S85.299 with 7th A, S85.801-S85.999 with 7th A, S95.001-S95.099 with 7th A, S95.201-S95.999 with 7th A

√6ᵗʰ **S75.11** **Minor laceration of femoral vein at hip and thigh level**
Incomplete transection of femoral vein at hip and thigh level
Laceration of femoral vein at hip and thigh level NOS
Superficial laceration of femoral vein at hip and thigh level

√7ᵗʰ **S75.111** **Minor laceration of femoral vein at hip and thigh level, right leg** ᴹᶜᶜ
CC Excl: See code: S75.101

√7ᵗʰ **S75.112** **Minor laceration of femoral vein at hip and thigh level, left leg** ᴹᶜᶜ
CC Excl: See code: S75.102

√7ᵗʰ **S75.119** **Minor laceration of femoral vein at hip and thigh level, unspecified leg** ᴹᶜᶜ
CC Excl: See code: S75.109

√6ᵗʰ **S75.12** **Major laceration of femoral vein at hip and thigh level**
Complete transection of femoral vein at hip and thigh level
Traumatic rupture of femoral vein at hip and thigh level

√7ᵗʰ **S75.121** **Major laceration of femoral vein at hip and thigh level, right leg** ᴹᶜᶜ
CC Excl: See code: S75.101

√7ᵗʰ **S75.122** **Major laceration of femoral vein at hip and thigh level, left leg** ᴹᶜᶜ
CC Excl: See code: S75.102

√7ᵗʰ **S75.129** **Major laceration of femoral vein at hip and thigh level, unspecified leg** ᴹᶜᶜ
CC Excl: See code: S75.109

√6ᵗʰ **S75.19** **Other specified injury of femoral vein at hip and thigh level**

√7ᵗʰ **S75.191** **Other specified injury of femoral vein at hip and thigh level, right leg** ᴹᶜᶜ
CC Excl: See code: S75.101

√7ᵗʰ **S75.192** **Other specified injury of femoral vein at hip and thigh level, left leg** ᴹᶜᶜ
CC Excl: See code: S75.102

√7ᵗʰ **S75.199** **Other specified injury of femoral vein at hip and thigh level, unspecified leg** ᴹᶜᶜ
CC Excl: See code: S75.109

√5ᵗʰ **S75.2** **Injury of greater saphenous vein at hip and thigh level**
EXCLUDES 1 greater saphenous vein NOS (S85.3)

√6ᵗʰ **S75.20** **Unspecified injury of greater saphenous vein at hip and thigh level**

√7ᵗʰ **S75.201** **Unspecified injury of greater saphenous vein at hip and thigh level, right leg** ᶜᶜ
CC Excl: CC with 7th character A: S75.201A, S75.209-S75.211 with 7th A, S75.219-S75.221 with 7th A, S75.229-S75.291 with 7th A, S75.299-S75.801 with 7th A, S75.809-S75.811 with 7th A, S75.819-S75.891 with 7th A, S75.899-S75.901 with 7th A, S75.909-S75.911 with 7th A, S75.919-S75.991 with 7th A, S75.999A, S85.201A, S85.209-S85.211 with 7th A, S85.219-S85.291 with 7th A, S85.299-S85.301 with 7th A, S85.309-S85.311 with 7th A, S85.319-S85.391 with 7th A, S85.399-S85.401 with 7th A, S85.409-S85.411 with 7th A, S85.419-S85.491 with 7th A, S85.499A, S85.801A, S85.809-S85.811 with 7th A, S85.819-S85.891 with 7th A, S85.899-S85.901 with 7th A, S85.909-S85.911 with 7th A, S85.919-S85.991 with 7th A, S85.999A, S95.001A, S95.009-S95.011 with 7th A, S95.019-S95.091 with 7th A, S95.099A, S95.201A, S95.209-S95.211 with 7th A, S95.219-S95.291 with 7th A, S95.299-S95.801 with 7th A, S95.809-S95.811 with 7th A, S95.819-S95.891 with 7th A, S95.899-S95.901 with 7th A, S95.909-S95.911 with 7th A, S95.919-S95.991 with 7th A, S95.999A

√7ᵗʰ **S75.202** **Unspecified injury of greater saphenous vein at hip and thigh level, left leg** ᶜᶜ
CC Excl: CC with 7th character A: S75.202-S75.209 with 7th A, S75.212-S75.219 with 7th A, S75.222-S75.229 with 7th A, S75.292-S75.299 with 7th A, S75.802-S75.809 with 7th A, S75.812-S75.819 with 7th A, S75.892-S75.899 with 7th A, S75.902-S75.909 with 7th A, S75.912-S75.919 with 7th A, S75.992-S75.999 with 7th A, S85.202-S85.209 with

7th A, S85.212-S85.219 with 7th A, S85.292-
S85.299 with 7th A, S85.302-S85.309 with
7th A, S85.312-S85.319 with 7th A, S85.392-
S85.399 with 7th A, S85.402-S85.409 with
7th A, S85.412-S85.419 with 7th A, S85.492-
S85.499 with 7th A, S85.802-S85.809 with
7th A, S85.812-S85.819 with 7th A, S85.892-
S85.899 with 7th A, S85.902-S85.909 with
7th A, S85.912-S85.919 with 7th A, S85.992-
S85.999 with 7th A, S95.002-S95.009 with
7th A, S95.012-S95.019 with 7th A, S95.092-
S95.099 with 7th A, S95.202-S95.209 with
7th A, S95.212-S95.219 with 7th A, S95.292-
S95.299 with 7th A, S95.802-S95.809 with
7th A, S95.812-S95.819 with 7th A, S95.892-
S95.899 with 7th A, S95.902-S95.909 with
7th A, S95.912-S95.919 with 7th A, S95.992-
S95.999 with 7th A

√7th **S75.209   Unspecified injury of greater**   CC
saphenous vein at hip and thigh
level, unspecified leg
CC Excl: CC with 7th character A: S75.201-
S75.999 with 7th A, S85.201-S85.499 with
7th A, S85.801-S85.999 with 7th A, S95.001-
S95.099 with 7th A, S95.201-S95.999 with
7th A

√6th **S75.21   Minor laceration of greater saphenous vein at hip**
and thigh level
Incomplete transection of greater saphenous vein at
hip and thigh level
Laceration of greater saphenous vein at hip and thigh
level NOS
Superficial laceration of greater saphenous vein at hip
and thigh level

√7th **S75.211   Minor laceration of greater saphenous**   CC
vein at hip and thigh level, right leg
CC Excl: See code: S75.201

√7th **S75.212   Minor laceration of greater saphenous**   CC
vein at hip and thigh level, left leg
CC Excl: See code: S75.202

√7th **S75.219   Minor laceration of greater saphenous**   CC
vein at hip and thigh level,
unspecified leg
CC Excl: See code: S75.209

√6th **S75.22   Major laceration of greater saphenous vein at hip**
and thigh level
Complete transection of greater saphenous vein at hip
and thigh level
Traumatic rupture of greater saphenous vein at hip
and thigh level

√7th **S75.221   Major laceration of greater saphenous**   CC
vein at hip and thigh level, right leg
CC Excl: See code: S75.201

√7th **S75.222   Major laceration of greater saphenous**   CC
vein at hip and thigh level, left leg
CC Excl: See code: S75.202

√7th **S75.229   Major laceration of greater saphenous**   CC
vein at hip and thigh level,
unspecified leg
CC Excl: See code: S75.209

√6th **S75.29   Other specified injury of greater saphenous vein at**
hip and thigh level

√7th **S75.291   Other specified injury of greater**   CC
saphenous vein at hip and thigh
level, right leg
CC Excl: See code: S75.201

√7th **S75.292   Other specified injury of greater**   CC
saphenous vein at hip and thigh
level, left leg
CC Excl: See code: S75.202

√7th **S75.299   Other specified injury of greater**   CC
saphenous vein at hip and thigh level,
unspecified leg
CC Excl: See code: S75.209

√5th **S75.8   Injury of other blood vessels at hip and thigh level**

√6th **S75.80   Unspecified injury of other blood vessels at hip and**
thigh level

√7th **S75.801   Unspecified injury of other blood**   CC
vessels at hip and thigh level, right leg
CC Excl: CC with 7th character A: M79.A21-
M79.A29, S75.001 with 7th A, S75.009-
S75.011 with 7th A, S75.019-S75.021 with
7th A, S75.029-S75.091 with 7th A, S75.099-
S75.101 with 7th A, S75.109-S75.111 with

7th A, S75.119-S75.121 with 7th A, S75.129-
S75.191 with 7th A, S75.199-S75.201 with
7th A, S75.209-S75.211 with 7th A, S75.219-
S75.221 with 7th A, S75.229-S75.291 with
7th A, S75.299-S75.801 with 7th A, S75.809-
S75.811 with 7th A, S75.819-S75.891 with
7th A, S75.899-S75.901 with 7th A, S75.909-
S75.911 with 7th A, S75.919-S75.991 with
7th A, S75.999A, S85.001A, S85.009-S85.011
with 7th A, S85.019-S85.091 with 7th A,
S85.099-S85.101 with 7th A, S85.109-
S85.111 with 7th A, S85.119-S85.121 with
7th A, S85.129-S85.131 with 7th A, S85.139-
S85.141 with 7th A, S85.149-S85.151 with
7th A, S85.159-S85.161 with 7th A, S85.169-
S85.171 with 7th A, S85.179-S85.181 with
7th A, S85.189-S85.201 with 7th A, S85.209-
S85.211 with 7th A, S85.219-S85.291 with
7th A, S85.299-S85.301 with 7th A, S85.309-
S85.311 with 7th A, S85.319-S85.391 with
7th A, S85.399-S85.401 with 7th A, S85.409-
S85.411 with 7th A, S85.419-S85.491 with
7th A, S85.499-S85.501 with 7th A, S85.509-
S85.511 with 7th A, S85.519-S85.591 with
7th A, S85.599-S85.801 with 7th A, S85.809-
S85.811 with 7th A, S85.819-S85.891 with
7th A, S85.899-S85.901 with 7th A, S85.909-
S85.911 with 7th A, S85.919-S85.991 with
7th A, S85.999A, S95.001A, S95.009-S95.011
with 7th A, S95.019-S95.091 with 7th A,
S95.099-S95.101 with 7th A, S95.109-
S95.111 with 7th A, S95.119-S95.191 with
7th A, S95.199-S95.201 with 7th A, S95.209-
S95.211 with 7th A, S95.219-S95.291 with
7th A, S95.299-S95.801 with 7th A, S95.809-
S95.811 with 7th A, S95.819-S95.891 with
7th A, S95.899-S95.901 with 7th A, S95.909-
S95.911 with 7th A, S95.919-S95.991 with
7th A, S95.999A

√7th **S75.802   Unspecified injury of other blood**   CC
vessels at hip and thigh level, left leg
CC Excl: CC with 7th character A: M79.A21-
M79.A29, S75.002-S75.009 with 7th A,
S75.012-S75.019 with 7th A, S75.022-
S75.029 with 7th A, S75.092-S75.099 with
7th A, S75.102-S75.109 with 7th A, S75.112-
S75.119 with 7th A, S75.122-S75.129 with
7th A, S75.192-S75.199 with 7th A, S75.202-
S75.209 with 7th A, S75.212-S75.219 with
7th A, S75.222-S75.229 with 7th A, S75.292-
S75.299 with 7th A, S75.802-S75.809 with
7th A, S75.812-S75.819 with 7th A, S75.892-
S75.899 with 7th A, S75.902-S75.909 with
7th A, S75.912-S75.919 with 7th A, S75.992-
S75.999 with 7th A, S85.002-S85.009 with
7th A, S85.012-S85.019 with 7th A, S85.092-
S85.099 with 7th A, S85.102-S85.109 with
7th A, S85.112-S85.119 with 7th A, S85.122-
S85.129 with 7th A, S85.132-S85.139 with
7th A, S85.142-S85.149 with 7th A, S85.152-
S85.159 with 7th A, S85.162-S85.169 with
7th A, S85.172-S85.179 with 7th A, S85.182-
S85.189 with 7th A, S85.202-S85.209 with
7th A, S85.212-S85.219 with 7th A, S85.292-
S85.299 with 7th A, S85.302-S85.309 with
7th A, S85.312-S85.319 with 7th A, S85.392-
S85.399 with 7th A, S85.402-S85.409 with
7th A, S85.412-S85.419 with 7th A, S85.492-
S85.499 with 7th A, S85.502-S85.509 with
7th A, S85.512-S85.519 with 7th A, S85.592-
S85.599 with 7th A, S85.802-S85.809 with
7th A, S85.812-S85.819 with 7th A, S85.892-
S85.899 with 7th A, S85.902-S85.909 with
7th A, S85.912-S85.919 with 7th A, S85.992-
S85.999 with 7th A, S95.002-S95.009 with
7th A, S95.012-S95.019 with 7th A, S95.092-
S95.099 with 7th A, S95.102-S95.109 with
7th A, S95.112-S95.119 with 7th A, S95.192-
S95.199 with 7th A, S95.202-S95.209 with
7th A, S95.212-S95.219 with 7th A, S95.292-
S95.299 with 7th A, S95.802-S95.809 with
7th A, S95.812-S95.819 with 7th A, S95.892-
S95.899 with 7th A, S95.902-S95.909 with
7th A, S95.912-S95.919 with 7th A, S95.992-
S95.999 with 7th A

√7th **S75.809   Unspecified injury of other blood**   CC
vessels at hip and thigh level,
unspecified leg
CC Excl: CC with 7th character A: M79.A21-
M79.A29, S75.001-S75.999 with 7th A,
S85.001-S85.999 with 7th A, S95.001-
S95.999 with 7th A

✔ Additional Character Required   √x7th Xtension Alert   Unacceptable PDx   Manifestation   Hospital Acquired Condition   EXCLUDES 1 Not Coded Here   EXCLUDES 2 Not Included Here

ICD-10-CM Draft (2015)   985

✓6ᵗʰ **S75.81** Laceration of other blood vessels at hip and thigh level

    ✓7ᵗʰ **S75.811** Laceration of other blood vessels at hip and thigh level, right leg   `CC`
       CC Excl: See code: S75.801

    ✓7ᵗʰ **S75.812** Laceration of other blood vessels at hip and thigh level, left leg   `CC`
       CC Excl: See code: S75.802

    ✓7ᵗʰ **S75.819** Laceration of other blood vessels at hip and thigh level, unspecified leg   `CC`
       CC Excl: See code: S75.809

✓6ᵗʰ **S75.89** Other specified injury of other blood vessels at hip and thigh level

    ✓7ᵗʰ **S75.891** Other specified injury of other blood vessels at hip and thigh level, right leg   `CC`
       CC Excl: See code: S75.801

    ✓7ᵗʰ **S75.892** Other specified injury of other blood vessels at hip and thigh level, left leg   `CC`
       CC Excl: See code: S75.802

    ✓7ᵗʰ **S75.899** Other specified injury of other blood vessels at hip and thigh level, unspecified leg   `CC`
       CC Excl: See code: S75.809

✓5ᵗʰ **S75.9** Injury of unspecified blood vessel at hip and thigh level

   ✓6ᵗʰ **S75.90** Unspecified injury of unspecified blood vessel at hip and thigh level

    ✓7ᵗʰ **S75.901** Unspecified injury of unspecified blood vessel at hip and thigh level, right leg   `CC`
       CC Excl: See code: S75.801

    ✓7ᵗʰ **S75.902** Unspecified injury of unspecified blood vessel at hip and thigh level, left leg   `CC`
       CC Excl: See code: S75.802

    ✓7ᵗʰ **S75.909** Unspecified injury of unspecified blood vessel at hip and thigh level, unspecified leg   `CC`
       CC Excl: See code: S75.809

   ✓6ᵗʰ **S75.91** Laceration of unspecified blood vessel at hip and thigh level

    ✓7ᵗʰ **S75.911** Laceration of unspecified blood vessel at hip and thigh level, right leg   `CC`
       CC Excl: See code: S75.801

    ✓7ᵗʰ **S75.912** Laceration of unspecified blood vessel at hip and thigh level, left leg   `CC`
       CC Excl: See code: S75.802

    ✓7ᵗʰ **S75.919** Laceration of unspecified blood vessel at hip and thigh level, unspecified leg   `CC`
       CC Excl: See code: S75.809

   ✓6ᵗʰ **S75.99** Other specified injury of unspecified blood vessel at hip and thigh level

    ✓7ᵗʰ **S75.991** Other specified injury of unspecified blood vessel at hip and thigh level, right leg   `CC`
       CC Excl: See code: S75.801

    ✓7ᵗʰ **S75.992** Other specified injury of unspecified blood vessel at hip and thigh level, left leg   `CC`
       CC Excl: See code: S75.802

    ✓7ᵗʰ **S75.999** Other specified injury of unspecified blood vessel at hip and thigh level, unspecified leg   `CC`
       CC Excl: See code: S75.809

✓4ᵗʰ **S76** Injury of muscle, fascia and tendon at hip and thigh level

    Code also any associated open wound (S71.-)

    EXCLUDES 2   injury of muscle, fascia and tendon at lower leg level (S86)
               sprain of joint and ligament of hip (S73.1)

    The appropriate 7th character is to be added to each code from category S76.
    A   initial encounter
    D   subsequent encounter
    S   sequela

   ✓5ᵗʰ **S76.0** Injury of muscle, fascia and tendon of hip

   ✓6ᵗʰ **S76.00** Unspecified injury of muscle, fascia and tendon of hip

    ✓7ᵗʰ **S76.001** Unspecified injury of muscle, fascia and tendon of right hip

    ✓7ᵗʰ **S76.002** Unspecified injury of muscle, fascia and tendon of left hip

    ✓7ᵗʰ **S76.009** Unspecified injury of muscle, fascia and tendon of unspecified hip

   ✓6ᵗʰ **S76.01** Strain of muscle, fascia and tendon of hip

    ✓7ᵗʰ **S76.011** Strain of muscle, fascia and tendon of right hip

    ✓7ᵗʰ **S76.012** Strain of muscle, fascia and tendon of left hip

    ✓7ᵗʰ **S76.019** Strain of muscle, fascia and tendon of unspecified hip

   ✓6ᵗʰ **S76.02** Laceration of muscle, fascia and tendon of hip

    ✓7ᵗʰ **S76.021** Laceration of muscle, fascia and tendon of right hip   `CC`
       CC Excl: CC with 7th character A: S71.001A, S71.009-S71.011 with 7th A, S71.019-S71.021 with 7th A, S71.029-S71.031 with 7th A, S71.039-S71.041 with 7th A, S71.049-S71.051 with 7th A, S71.059-S71.101 with 7th A, S71.109-S71.111 with 7th A, S71.119-S71.121 with 7th A, S71.129-S71.131 with 7th A, S71.139-S71.141 with 7th A, S71.149-S71.151 with 7th A, S71.159 with 7th A, S76.021 with 7th A, S76.029A, S76.121A, S76.129A, S76.221A, S76.229A, S76.321A, S76.329A, S76.821A, S76.829A, S76.921A, S76.929A

    ✓7ᵗʰ **S76.022** Laceration of muscle, fascia and tendon of left hip   `CC`
       CC Excl: CC with 7th character A: S71.002-S71.009 with 7th A, S71.012-S71.019 with 7th A, S71.022-S71.029 with 7th A, S71.032-S71.039 with 7th A, S71.042-S71.049 with 7th A, S71.052-S71.059 with 7th A, S71.102-S71.109 with 7th A, S71.112-S71.119 with 7th A, S71.122-S71.129 with 7th A, S71.132-S71.139 with 7th A, S71.142-S71.149 with 7th A, S71.152-S71.159 with 7th A, S76.022-S76.029 with 7th A, S76.122-S76.129 with 7th A, S76.222-S76.229 with 7th A, S76.322-S76.329 with 7th A, S76.822-S76.829 with 7th A, S76.922-S76.929 with 7th A

    ✓7ᵗʰ **S76.029** Laceration of muscle, fascia and tendon of unspecified hip   `CC`
       CC Excl: CC with 7th character A: S71.001-S71.159 with 7th A, S76.021-S76.029 with 7th A, S76.121-S76.129 with 7th A, S76.221-S76.229 with 7th A, S76.321-S76.329 with 7th A, S76.821-S76.829 with 7th A, S76.921-S76.929 with 7th A

   ✓6ᵗʰ **S76.09** Other specified injury of muscle, fascia and tendon of hip

    ✓7ᵗʰ **S76.091** Other specified injury of muscle, fascia and tendon of right hip

    ✓7ᵗʰ **S76.092** Other specified injury of muscle, fascia and tendon of left hip

    ✓7ᵗʰ **S76.099** Other specified injury of muscle, fascia and tendon of unspecified hip

   ✓5ᵗʰ **S76.1** Injury of quadriceps muscle, fascia and tendon
     Injury of patellar ligament (tendon)

   ✓6ᵗʰ **S76.10** Unspecified injury of quadriceps muscle, fascia and tendon

    ✓7ᵗʰ **S76.101** Unspecified injury of right quadriceps muscle, fascia and tendon

    ✓7ᵗʰ **S76.102** Unspecified injury of left quadriceps muscle, fascia and tendon

    ✓7ᵗʰ **S76.109** Unspecified injury of unspecified quadriceps muscle, fascia and tendon

   ✓6ᵗʰ **S76.11** Strain of quadriceps muscle, fascia and tendon

    ✓7ᵗʰ **S76.111** Strain of right quadriceps muscle, fascia and tendon

    ✓7ᵗʰ **S76.112** Strain of left quadriceps muscle, fascia and tendon

    ✓7ᵗʰ **S76.119** Strain of unspecified quadriceps muscle, fascia and tendon

   ✓6ᵗʰ **S76.12** Laceration of quadriceps muscle, fascia and tendon

    ✓7ᵗʰ **S76.121** Laceration of right quadriceps muscle, fascia and tendon   `CC`
       CC Excl: See code: S76.021

    ✓7ᵗʰ **S76.122** Laceration of left quadriceps muscle, fascia and tendon   `CC`
       CC Excl: See code: S76.022

Ⓝ Newborn: 0   Ⓟ Pediatric: 0-17   Ⓜ Maternity: 12-55   Ⓐ Adult: 15-124   `MCC` Major CC Condition   `PDx MCC` PDx acts as own MCC   `CC` CC Condition   `PDx CC` PDx acts as own CC

986   ICD-10-CM Draft (2015)

✓7ᵗʰ **S76.129** Laceration of unspecified quadriceps [CC]
muscle, fascia and tendon
CC Excl: See code: S76.029

✓6ᵗʰ **S76.19** Other specified injury of quadriceps muscle, fascia and tendon

✓7ᵗʰ **S76.191** Other specified injury of right quadriceps muscle, fascia and tendon

✓7ᵗʰ **S76.192** Other specified injury of left quadriceps muscle, fascia and tendon

✓7ᵗʰ **S76.199** Other specified injury of unspecified quadriceps muscle, fascia and tendon

✓5ᵗʰ **S76.2** Injury of adductor muscle, fascia and tendon of thigh

✓6ᵗʰ **S76.20** Unspecified injury of adductor muscle, fascia and tendon of thigh

✓7ᵗʰ **S76.201** Unspecified injury of adductor muscle, fascia and tendon of right thigh

✓7ᵗʰ **S76.202** Unspecified injury of adductor muscle, fascia and tendon of left thigh

✓7ᵗʰ **S76.209** Unspecified injury of adductor muscle, fascia and tendon of unspecified thigh

✓6ᵗʰ **S76.21** Strain of adductor muscle, fascia and tendon of thigh

✓7ᵗʰ **S76.211** Strain of adductor muscle, fascia and tendon of right thigh

✓7ᵗʰ **S76.212** Strain of adductor muscle, fascia and tendon of left thigh

✓7ᵗʰ **S76.219** Strain of adductor muscle, fascia and tendon of unspecified thigh

✓6ᵗʰ **S76.22** Laceration of adductor muscle, fascia and tendon of thigh

✓7ᵗʰ **S76.221** Laceration of adductor muscle, fascia [CC]
and tendon of right thigh
CC Excl: See code: S76.021

✓7ᵗʰ **S76.222** Laceration of adductor muscle, fascia [CC]
and tendon of left thigh
CC Excl: See code: S76.022

✓7ᵗʰ **S76.229** Laceration of adductor muscle, fascia [CC]
and tendon of unspecified thigh
CC Excl: See code: S76.029

✓6ᵗʰ **S76.29** Other injury of adductor muscle, fascia and tendon of thigh

✓7ᵗʰ **S76.291** Other injury of adductor muscle, fascia and tendon of right thigh

✓7ᵗʰ **S76.292** Other injury of adductor muscle, fascia and tendon of left thigh

✓7ᵗʰ **S76.299** Other injury of adductor muscle, fascia and tendon of unspecified thigh

✓5ᵗʰ **S76.3** Injury of muscle, fascia and tendon of the posterior muscle group at thigh level

✓6ᵗʰ **S76.30** Unspecified injury of muscle, fascia and tendon of the posterior muscle group at thigh level

✓7ᵗʰ **S76.301** Unspecified injury of muscle, fascia and tendon of the posterior muscle group at thigh level, right thigh

✓7ᵗʰ **S76.302** Unspecified injury of muscle, fascia and tendon of the posterior muscle group at thigh level, left thigh

✓7ᵗʰ **S76.309** Unspecified injury of muscle, fascia and tendon of the posterior muscle group at thigh level, unspecified thigh

✓6ᵗʰ **S76.31** Strain of muscle, fascia and tendon of the posterior muscle group at thigh level

✓7ᵗʰ **S76.311** Strain of muscle, fascia and tendon of the posterior muscle group at thigh level, right thigh

✓7ᵗʰ **S76.312** Strain of muscle, fascia and tendon of the posterior muscle group at thigh level, left thigh

✓7ᵗʰ **S76.319** Strain of muscle, fascia and tendon of the posterior muscle group at thigh level, unspecified thigh

✓6ᵗʰ **S76.32** Laceration of muscle, fascia and tendon of the posterior muscle group at thigh level

✓7ᵗʰ **S76.321** Laceration of muscle, fascia and [CC]
tendon of the posterior muscle group at thigh level, right thigh
CC Excl: See code: S76.021

✓7ᵗʰ **S76.322** Laceration of muscle, fascia and [CC]
tendon of the posterior muscle group at thigh level, left thigh
CC Excl: See code: S76.022

✓7ᵗʰ **S76.329** Laceration of muscle, fascia and [CC]
tendon of the posterior muscle group at thigh level, unspecified thigh
CC Excl: See code: S76.029

✓6ᵗʰ **S76.39** Other specified injury of muscle, fascia and tendon of the posterior muscle group at thigh level

✓7ᵗʰ **S76.391** Other specified injury of muscle, fascia and tendon of the posterior muscle group at thigh level, right thigh

✓7ᵗʰ **S76.392** Other specified injury of muscle, fascia and tendon of the posterior muscle group at thigh level, left thigh

✓7ᵗʰ **S76.399** Other specified injury of muscle, fascia and tendon of the posterior muscle group at thigh level, unspecified thigh

✓5ᵗʰ **S76.8** Injury of other specified muscles, fascia and tendons at thigh level

✓6ᵗʰ **S76.80** Unspecified injury of other specified muscles, fascia and tendons at thigh level

✓7ᵗʰ **S76.801** Unspecified injury of other specified muscles, fascia and tendons at thigh level, right thigh

✓7ᵗʰ **S76.802** Unspecified injury of other specified muscles, fascia and tendons at thigh level, left thigh

✓7ᵗʰ **S76.809** Unspecified injury of other specified muscles, fascia and tendons at thigh level, unspecified thigh

✓6ᵗʰ **S76.81** Strain of other specified muscles, fascia and tendons at thigh level

✓7ᵗʰ **S76.811** Strain of other specified muscles, fascia and tendons at thigh level, right thigh

✓7ᵗʰ **S76.812** Strain of other specified muscles, fascia and tendons at thigh level, left thigh

✓7ᵗʰ **S76.819** Strain of other specified muscles, fascia and tendons at thigh level, unspecified thigh

✓6ᵗʰ **S76.82** Laceration of other specified muscles, fascia and tendons at thigh level

✓7ᵗʰ **S76.821** Laceration of other specified muscles, [CC]
fascia and tendons at thigh level, right thigh
CC Excl: See code: S76.021

✓7ᵗʰ **S76.822** Laceration of other specified muscles, [CC]
fascia and tendons at thigh level, left thigh
CC Excl: See code: S76.022

✓7ᵗʰ **S76.829** Laceration of other specified muscles, [CC]
fascia and tendons at thigh level, unspecified thigh
CC Excl: See code: S76.029

✓6ᵗʰ **S76.89** Other injury of other specified muscles, fascia and tendons at thigh level

✓7ᵗʰ **S76.891** Other injury of other specified muscles, fascia and tendons at thigh level, right thigh

✓7ᵗʰ **S76.892** Other injury of other specified muscles, fascia and tendons at thigh level, left thigh

✓7ᵗʰ **S76.899** Other injury of other specified muscles, fascia and tendons at thigh level, unspecified thigh

✓5ᵗʰ **S76.9** Injury of unspecified muscles, fascia and tendons at thigh level

✓6ᵗʰ **S76.90** Unspecified injury of unspecified muscles, fascia and tendons at thigh level

✓7ᵗʰ **S76.901** Unspecified injury of unspecified muscles, fascia and tendons at thigh level, right thigh

✓7ᵗʰ **S76.902** Unspecified injury of unspecified muscles, fascia and tendons at thigh level, left thigh

✓7ᵗʰ **S76.909** Unspecified injury of unspecified muscles, fascia and tendons at thigh level, unspecified thigh

✓ Additional Character Required   ✓x7ᵗʰ Xtension Alert   Unacceptable PDx   Manifestation   Hospital Acquired Condition   EXCLUDES 1 Not Coded Here   EXCLUDES 2 Not Included Here

ICD-10-CM Draft (2015)   987

√6ᵗʰ **S76.91 Strain** of unspecified muscles, fascia and tendons at thigh level

√7ᵗʰ **S76.911 Strain** of unspecified muscles, fascia and tendons at thigh level, right thigh

√7ᵗʰ **S76.912 Strain** of unspecified muscles, fascia and tendons at thigh level, left thigh

√7ᵗʰ **S76.919 Strain** of unspecified muscles, fascia and tendons at thigh level, unspecified thigh

√6ᵗʰ **S76.92 Laceration** of unspecified muscles, fascia and tendons at thigh level

√7ᵗʰ **S76.921 Laceration** of unspecified muscles, fascia and tendons at thigh level, right thigh `CC`
CC Excl: See code: S76.021

√7ᵗʰ **S76.922 Laceration** of unspecified muscles, fascia and tendons at thigh level, left thigh `CC`
CC Excl: See code: S76.022

√7ᵗʰ **S76.929 Laceration** of unspecified muscles, fascia and tendons at thigh level, unspecified thigh `CC`
CC Excl: See code: S76.029

√6ᵗʰ **S76.99 Other** specified injury of unspecified muscles, fascia and tendons at thigh level

√7ᵗʰ **S76.991 Other** specified injury of unspecified muscles, fascia and tendons at thigh level, right thigh

√7ᵗʰ **S76.992 Other** specified injury of unspecified muscles, fascia and tendons at thigh level, left thigh

√7ᵗʰ **S76.999 Other** specified injury of unspecified muscles, fascia and tendons at thigh level, unspecified thigh

√4ᵗʰ **S77 Crushing injury of hip and thigh**
Use additional code(s) for all associated injuries
EXCLUDES 2 crushing injury of ankle and foot (S97.-)
crushing injury of lower leg (S87.-)

The appropriate 7th character is to be added to each code from category S77.
A   initial encounter
D   subsequent encounter
S   sequela

√5ᵗʰ **S77.0 Crushing injury of hip**

CC Excl: For CC codes in subcategory S77.0, unless otherwise noted: CC with 7th character A: S77.00X-S77.02X with 7th A, S77.20X-S77.22X with 7th A

7 √x7ᵗʰ **S77.00 Crushing injury of unspecified hip** `CC`
7 √x7ᵗʰ **S77.01 Crushing injury of right hip** `CC`
7 √x7ᵗʰ **S77.02 Crushing injury of left hip** `CC`

√5ᵗʰ **S77.1 Crushing injury of thigh**

CC Excl: For CC codes in subcategory S77.1, unless otherwise noted: CC with 7th character A: S77.00X-S77.02X with 7th A, S77.20X-S77.22X with 7th A

7 √x7ᵗʰ **S77.10 Crushing injury of unspecified thigh** `CC`
7 √x7ᵗʰ **S77.11 Crushing injury of right thigh** `CC`
7 √x7ᵗʰ **S77.12 Crushing injury of left thigh** `CC`

√5ᵗʰ **S77.2 Crushing injury of hip with thigh**
√x7ᵗʰ **S77.20 Crushing injury of unspecified hip with thigh**
√x7ᵗʰ **S77.21 Crushing injury of right hip with thigh**
√x7ᵗʰ **S77.22 Crushing injury of left hip with thigh**

√4ᵗʰ **S78 Traumatic amputation of hip and thigh**
NOTE An amputation not identified as partial or complete should be coded to complete.
EXCLUDES 1 traumatic amputation of knee (S88.0-)

The appropriate 7th character is to be added to each code from category S78.
A   initial encounter
D   subsequent encounter
S   sequela

√5ᵗʰ **S78.0 Traumatic amputation at hip joint**

√6ᵗʰ **S78.01 Complete** traumatic amputation at hip joint

√7ᵗʰ **S78.011 Complete** traumatic amputation at right hip joint `CC`
CC Excl: CC with 7th character A: S71.001A, S71.009-S71.011 with 7th A, S71.019-S71.021 with 7th A, S71.029-S71.031 with 7th A, S71.039-S71.041 with 7th A, S71.049-S71.051 with 7th A, S71.059-S71.101 with 7th A, S71.109-S71.111 with 7th A, S71.119-S71.121 with 7th A, S71.129-S71.131 with 7th A, S71.139-S71.141 with 7th A, S71.149-S71.151 with 7th A, S71.159A, S76.021A, S76.029A, S76.121A, S76.129A, S76.221 A, S76.229A, S76.321A, S76.329A, S76.821A, S76.829A, S76.921A, S76.929A, S78.011A, S78.019-S78.021 with 7th A, S78.029-S78.111 with 7th A, S78.119-S78.121 with 7th A, S78.129-S78.911 with 7th A, S78.919-S78.921 with 7th A, S78.929A, S81.001A, S81.009-S81.011 with 7th A, S81.019-S81.021 with 7th A, S81.029-S81.031 with 7th A, S81.039-S81.041 with 7th A, S81.049-S81.051 with 7th A, S81.059-S81.801 with 7th A, S81.809-S81.811 with 7th A, S81.819-S81.821 with 7th A, S81.829-S81.831 with 7th A, S81.839-S81.841 with 7th A, S81.849-S81.851 with 7th A, S81.859A, S98.129-S98.131 with 7th A, S98.139-S98.141 with 7th A, S98.149-S98.211 with 7th A, S98.219-S98.221 with 7th A, S98.229-S98.311 with 7th A, S98.319-S98.321 with 7th A, S98.329-S98.911 with 7th A, S98.919-S98.921 with 7th A, S98.929 A, T14.8-T14.91, T79.A0X-T79.9XX with 7th A

√7ᵗʰ **S78.012 Complete** traumatic amputation at left hip joint `CC`
CC Excl: CC with 7th character A: S71.002-S71.009 with 7th A, S71.012-S71.019 with 7th A, S71.022-S71.029 with 7th A, S71.032-S71.039 with 7th A, S71.042-S71.049 with 7th A, S71.052-S71.059 with 7th A, S71.102-S71.109 with 7th A, S71.112-S71.119 with 7th A, S71.122-S71.129 with 7th A, S71.132-S71.139 with 7th A, S71.142-S71.149 with 7th A, S71.152-S71.159 with 7th A, S76.022-S76.029 with 7th A, S76.122-S76.129 with 7th A, S76.222-S76.229 with 7th A, S76.322-S76.329 with 7th A, S76.822-S76.829 with 7th A, S76.922-S76.929 with 7th A, S78.012-S78.019 with 7th A, S78.022-S78.029 with 7th A, S78.112-S78.119 with 7th A, S78.122-S78.129 with 7th A, S78.912-S78.919 with 7th A, S78.922-S78.929 with 7th A, S81.002-S81.009 with 7th A, S81.012-S81.019 with 7th A, S81.022-S81.029 with 7th A, S81.032-S81.039 with 7th A, S81.042-S81.049 with 7th A, S81.052-S81.059 with 7th A, S81.802-S81.809 with 7th A, S81.812-S81.819 with 7th A, S81.822-S81.829 with 7th A, S81.832-S81.839 with 7th A, S81.842-S81.849 with 7th A, S81.852-S81.859 with 7th A, S86.022-S86.029 with 7th A, S86.122-S86.129 with 7th A, S86.222-S86.229 with 7th A, S86.322-S86.329 with 7th A, S86.822-S86.829 with 7th A, S86.922-S86.929 with 7th A, S88.012-S88.019 with 7th A, S88.022-S88.029 with 7th A, S88.112-S88.119 with 7th A, S88.122-S88.129 with 7th A, S88.912-S88.919 with 7th A, S88.922-S88.929 with 7th A, S91.002-S91.009 with 7th A, S91.012-S91.019 with 7th A, S91.022-S91.029 with 7th A, S91.032-S91.039 with 7th A, S91.042-S91.049 with 7th A, S91.052-S91.059 with 7th A, S91.102-S91.103 with 7th A, S91.105-S91.109 with 7th A, S91.112-S91.113 with 7th A, S91.115-S91.119 with 7th A, S91.122-S91.123 with 7th A, S91.125-S91.129 with 7th A, S91.132-S91.133 with 7th A, S91.135-S91.139 with 7th A, S91.142-S91.143 with 7th A, S91.145-S91.149 with 7th A, S91.152-S91.153 with 7th A, S91.155-S91.159 with 7th A, S91.202-S91.203 with 7th A, S91.205-S91.209 with 7th A, S91.212-S91.213 with 7th A, S91.215-S91.219 with 7th A, S91.222-S91.223 with 7th A, S91.225-S91.229 with 7th A, S91.232-S91.233 with 7th A, S91.235-S91.239 with 7th A, S91.242-S91.243 with 7th A, S91.245-S91.249 with 7th A, S91.252-S91.253 with 7th A, S91.255-S91.259 with 7th A, S91.302-S91.309 with 7th A, S91.312-S91.319 with 7th A, S91.322-S91.329 with 7th A, S91.332-

7 HAC = Initial encounter only (7th character A, B or C) and not POA.

N Newborn: 0 P Pediatric: 0-17 M Maternity: 12-55 A Adult: 15-124 MCC Major CC Condition PDx MCC PDx acts as own MCC CC CC Condition PDx CC PDx acts as own CC

988 ICD-10-CM Draft (2015)

S91.339 with 7th A, S91.342-S91.349 with 7th A, S91.352-S91.359 with 7th A, S96.022-S96.029 with 7th A, S96.122-S96.129 with 7th A, S96.222-S96.229 with 7th A, S96.822-S96.829 with 7th A, S96.922-S96.929 with 7th A, S98.012-S98.019 with 7th A, S98.022-S98.029 with 7th A, S98.112-S98.119 with 7th A, S98.122-S98.129 with 7th A, S98.132-S98.139 with 7th A, S98.142-S98.149 with 7th A, S98.212-S98.219 with 7th A, S98.222-S98.229 with 7th A, S98.312-S98.319 with 7th A, S98.322-S98.329 with 7th A, S98.912-S98.919 with 7th A, S98.922-S98.929 with 7th A, T14.8-T14.91, T79.A0X-T79.9XX with 7th A

☑7ᵗʰ **S78.019 Complete traumatic amputation at unspecified hip joint** CC
 CC Excl: CC with 7th character A: S71.001-S71.159 with 7th A, S76.021-S76.029 with 7th A, S76.121-S76.129 with 7th A, S76.221-S76.229 with 7th A, S76.321-S76.329 with 7th A, S76.821-S76.829 with 7th A, S76.921-S76.929 with 7th A, S78.011-S78.929 with 7th A, S81.001-S81.859 with 7th A, S86.021-S86.029 with 7th A, S86.121-S86.129 with 7th A, S86.221-S86.229 with 7th A, S86.321-S86.329 with 7th A, S86.821-S86.829 with 7th A, S86.921-S86.929 with 7th A, S88.011-S88.929 with 7th A, S91.001-S91.359 with 7th A, S96.021-S96.029 with 7th A, S96.121-S96.129 with 7th A, S96.221-S96.229 with 7th A, S96.821-S96.829 with 7th A, S96.921-S96.929 with 7th A, S98.011-S98.929 with 7th A, T14.8-T14.91, T79.A0X-T79.9XX with 7th A

☑6ᵗʰ **S78.02 Partial traumatic amputation at hip joint**
 ☑7ᵗʰ **S78.021 Partial traumatic amputation at right hip joint** CC
  CC Excl: See code: S78.011
 ☑7ᵗʰ **S78.022 Partial traumatic amputation at left hip joint** CC
  CC Excl: See code: S78.012
 ☑7ᵗʰ **S78.029 Partial traumatic amputation at unspecified hip joint** CC
  CC Excl: See code: S78.019

☑5ᵗʰ **S78.1 Traumatic amputation at level between hip and knee**
 EXCLUDES 1 *traumatic amputation of knee (S88.0-)*
 ☑6ᵗʰ **S78.11 Complete traumatic amputation at level between hip and knee**
  ☑7ᵗʰ **S78.111 Complete traumatic amputation at level between right hip and knee** CC
   CC Excl: See code: S78.011
  ☑7ᵗʰ **S78.112 Complete traumatic amputation at level between left hip and knee** CC
   CC Excl: See code: S78.012
  ☑7ᵗʰ **S78.119 Complete traumatic amputation at level between unspecified hip and knee** CC
   CC Excl: See code: S78.019
 ☑6ᵗʰ **S78.12 Partial traumatic amputation at level between hip and knee**
  ☑7ᵗʰ **S78.121 Partial traumatic amputation at level between right hip and knee** CC
   CC Excl: See code: S78.011
  ☑7ᵗʰ **S78.122 Partial traumatic amputation at level between left hip and knee** CC
   CC Excl: See code: S78.012
  ☑7ᵗʰ **S78.129 Partial traumatic amputation at level between unspecified hip and knee** CC
   CC Excl: See code: S78.019

☑5ᵗʰ **S78.9 Traumatic amputation of hip and thigh, level unspecified**
 ☑6ᵗʰ **S78.91 Complete traumatic amputation of hip and thigh, level unspecified**
  ☑7ᵗʰ **S78.911 Complete traumatic amputation of right hip and thigh, level unspecified** CC
   CC Excl: See code: S78.011
  ☑7ᵗʰ **S78.912 Complete traumatic amputation of left hip and thigh, level unspecified** CC
   CC Excl: See code: S78.012
  ☑7ᵗʰ **S78.919 Complete traumatic amputation of unspecified hip and thigh, level unspecified** CC
   CC Excl: See code: S78.019

☑6ᵗʰ **S78.92 Partial traumatic amputation of hip and thigh, level unspecified**
 ☑7ᵗʰ **S78.921 Partial traumatic amputation of right hip and thigh, level unspecified** CC
  CC Excl: See code: S78.011
 ☑7ᵗʰ **S78.922 Partial traumatic amputation of left hip and thigh, level unspecified** CC
  CC Excl: See code: S78.012
 ☑7ᵗʰ **S78.929 Partial traumatic amputation of unspecified hip and thigh, level unspecified** CC
  CC Excl: See code: S78.019

☑4ᵗʰ **S79 Other and unspecified injuries of hip and thigh**
 ☑5ᵗʰ **S79.0 Physeal fracture of upper end of femur**
  NOTE A fracture not indicated as open or closed should be coded to closed.
  EXCLUDES 1 *apophyseal fracture of upper end of femur (S72.13-) nontraumatic slipped upper femoral epiphysis (M93.0-)*

  The appropriate 7th character is to be added to each code from subcategory S79.0.
  A initial encounter for closed fracture
  D subsequent encounter for fracture with routine healing
  G subsequent encounter for fracture with delayed healing
  K subsequent encounter for fracture with nonunion
  P subsequent encounter for fracture with malunion
  S sequela

 ☑6ᵗʰ **S79.00 Unspecified physeal fracture of upper end of femur**
  7 ☑7ᵗʰ **S79.001 Unspecified physeal fracture of upper end of right femur** MCC CC
   CC Excl: MCC with 7th A: M48.40X-M48.58X with 7th A, M80.00X-M84.68X with 7th A, S03.8XX-S03.9XX with 7th A, S29.011-S29.019 with 7th A, S38.3XX-S39.013 with 7th A, S72.001-S72.471 with 7th [A, B, C], S72.479-S72.92X with 7th A, S73.101A, S73.109-S73.111 with 7th A, S73.119-S73.121 with 7th A, S73.129-S73.191 with 7th A, S73.199A, S76.001 A, S76.009-S76.011 with 7th A, S76.019A, S76.091A, S76.099-S76.101 with 7th A, S76.109-S76.111 with 7th A, S76.119A, S76.191A, S76.199-S76.201 with 7th A, S76.209-S76.211 with 7th A, S76.219A, S76.291A, S76.299-S76.301 with 7th A, S76.309-S76.311 with 7th A, S76.319A, S76.391A, S76.399-S76.801 with 7th A, S76.809-S76.811 with 7th A, S76.819 A, S76.891A, S76.899-S76.901 with 7th A, S76.909-S76.911 with 7th A, S76.919A, S76.991A, S76.999A, S79.001A, S79.009-S79.011 with 7th A, S79.019-S79.091 with 7th A, S79.099-S79.101 with 7th A, S79.109-S79.111 with 7th A, S79.119-S79.121 with 7th A, S79.129-S79.131 with 7th A, S79.139-S79.141 with 7th A, S79.149-S79.191 with 7th A, S79.199-S79.811 with 7th A, S79.819-S79.821 with 7th A, S79.829-S79.911 with 7th A, S79.919-S79.921 with 7th A, S79.929 with 7th A, S82.90X-S82.92X with 7th [A, B, C], T14.8-T14.91, T79.A0X-T79.9XX with 7th A
   CC Excl: CC with 7th character K or P: M80.00X-M84.68X with 7th [K, P], S02.0XX-S02.92X with 7th K, S12.000-S12.691 with 7th K, S22.000-S22.9XX with 7th K, S32.000-S32.9XX with 7th K, S42.001-S42.92X with 7th [K, P], S49.001-S49.199 with 7th [K, P], S52.001-S52.92X with 7th [K, M, N, P, Q, R], S59.001-S59.299 with 7th [K, P], S62.001-S62.92X with 7th [K, P], S72.001-S72.92X with 7th [K, M, N, P, Q, R], S79.001-S79.199 with 7th [K, P], S82.001-S82.92X with 7th [K, M, N, P, Q, R], S89.001-S89.399 with 7th [K, P], S92.001-S92.919 with 7th [K, P]

---

7 HAC = Initial encounter only (7th character A, B or C) and not POA.

7 ✓7ᵗʰ **S79.002 Unspecified physeal fracture of upper end of left femur** MCC CC

CC Excl: MCC with 7th A: M48.40X-M48.58X with 7th A, M80.00X-M84.68X with 7th A, S03.8XX-S03.9XX with 7th A, S29.011-S29.019 with 7th A, S38.3XX-S39.013 with 7th A, S72.001-S72.466 with 7th [B, C], S72.472-S72.92X with 7th A, S73.102-S73.109 with 7th A, S73.112-S73.119 with 7th A, S73.122-S73.129 with 7th A, S73.192-S73.199 with 7th A, S76.002-S76.009 with 7th A, S76.012-S76.019 with 7th A, S76.092-S76.099 with 7th A, S76.102-S76.109 with 7th A, S76.112-S76.119 with 7th A, S76.192-S76.199 with 7th A, S76.202-S76.209 with 7th A, S76.212-S76.219 with 7th A, S76.292-S76.299 with 7th A, S76.302-S76.309 with 7th A, S76.312-S76.319 with 7th A, S76.392-S76.399 with 7th A, S76.802-S76.809 with 7th A, S76.812-S76.819 with 7th A, S76.892-S76.899 with 7th A, S76.902-S76.909 with 7th A, S76.912-S76.919 with 7th A, S76.992-S76.999 with 7th A, S79.002-S79.009 with 7th A, S79.012-S79.019 with 7th A, S79.092-S79.099 with 7th A, S79.102-S79.109 with 7th A, S79.112-S79.119 with 7th A, S79.122-S79.129 with 7th A, S79.132-S79.139 with 7th A, S79.142-S79.149 with 7th A, S79.192-S79.199 with 7th A, S79.812-S79.819 with 7th A, S79.822-S79.829 with 7th A, S79.912-S79.919 with 7th A, S79.922-S79.929 with 7th A, S82.90X-S82.92X with 7th [A, B, C], T14.8-T14.91, T79.A0X-T79.9XX with 7th A

CC Excl: CC with 7th character K or P: M80.00X-M84.68X with 7th [K, P], S02.0XX-S02.92X with 7th K, S12.000-S12.691 with 7th K, S22.000-S22.9XX with 7th K, S32.000-S32.9XX with 7th K, S42.001-S42.92X with 7th [K, P], S49.001-S49.199 with 7th [K, P], S52.001-S52.92X with 7th [K, M, N, P, Q, R], S59.001-S59.299 with 7th [K, P], S62.001-S62.92X with 7th [K, P], S72.001-S72.92X with 7th [K, M, N, P, Q, R], S79.001-S79.199 with 7th [K, P], S82.001-S82.92X with 7th [K, M, N, P, Q, R], S89.001-S89.399 with 7th [K, P], S92.001-S92.919 with 7th [K, P]

7 ✓7ᵗʰ **S79.009 Unspecified physeal fracture of upper end of unspecified femur** MCC CC

CC Excl: MCC with 7th A: M48.40X-M48.58X with 7th A, M80.00X-M84.68X with 7th A, S03.8XX-S03.9XX with 7th A, S29.011-S29.019 with 7th A, S38.3XX-S39.013 with 7th A, S72.001-S72.92X with 7th [A, B, C], S73.101-S73.199 with 7th A, S76.001-S76.019 with 7th A, S76.091-S76.119 with 7th A, S76.191-S76.219 with 7th A, S76.291-S76.319 with 7th A, S76.391-S76.819 with 7th A, S76.891-S76.919 with 7th A, S76.991-S76.999 with 7th A, S79.001-S79.929 with 7th A, S82.90X-S82.92X with 7th [A, B, C], T14.8-T14.91, T79.A0X-T79.9XX with 7th A

CC Excl: CC with 7th character K or P: M80.00X-M84.68X with 7th [K, P], S02.0XX-S02.92X with 7th K, S12.000-S12.691 with 7th K, S22.000-S22.9XX with 7th K, S32.000-S32.9XX with 7th K, S42.001-S42.92X with 7th [K, P], S49.001-S49.199 with 7th [K, P], S52.001-S52.92X with 7th [K, M, N, P, Q, R], S59.001-S59.299 with 7th [K, P], S62.001-S62.92X with 7th [K, P], S72.001-S72.92X with 7th [K, M, N, P, Q, R], S79.001-S79.199 with 7th [K, P], S82.001-S82.92X with 7th [K, M, N, P, Q, R], S89.001-S89.399 with 7th [K, P], S92.001-S92.919 with 7th [K, P]

✓6ᵗʰ **S79.01 Salter-Harris Type I physeal fracture of upper end of femur**

Acute on chronic slipped capital femoral epiphysis (traumatic)
Acute slipped capital femoral epiphysis (traumatic)
Capital femoral epiphyseal fracture

EXCLUDES 1 *chronic slipped upper femoral epiphysis (nontraumatic) (M93.02-)*

7 ✓7ᵗʰ **S79.011 Salter-Harris Type I physeal fracture of upper end of right femur** MCC CC

CC Excl: See code: S79.001

7 ✓7ᵗʰ (**S79.012**) **Salter-Harris Type I physeal fracture of upper end of left femur** MCC CC

CC Excl: See code: S79.002

[handwritten margin note: 7th char D subsequent encounter]

7 ✓7ᵗʰ **S79.019 Salter-Harris Type I physeal fracture of upper end of unspecified femur** MCC CC

CC Excl: See code: S79.009

✓6ᵗʰ **S79.09 Other physeal fracture of upper end of femur**

7 ✓7ᵗʰ **S79.091 Other physeal fracture of upper end of right femur** MCC CC

CC Excl: See code: S79.001

7 ✓7ᵗʰ **S79.092 Other physeal fracture of upper end of left femur** MCC CC

CC Excl: See code: S79.002

7 ✓7ᵗʰ **S79.099 Other physeal fracture of upper end of unspecified femur** MCC CC

CC Excl: See code: S79.009

✓5ᵗʰ **S79.1 Physeal fracture of lower end of femur**

NOTE   A fracture not indicated as open or closed should be coded to closed.

The appropriate 7th character is to be added to each code from subcategory S79.1.
A   initial encounter for closed fracture
D   subsequent encounter for fracture with routine healing
G   subsequent encounter for fracture with delayed healing
K   subsequent encounter for fracture with nonunion
P   subsequent encounter for fracture with malunion
S   sequela

✓6ᵗʰ **S79.10 Unspecified physeal fracture of lower end of femur**

7 ✓7ᵗʰ **S79.101 Unspecified physeal fracture of lower end of right femur** CC

CC Excl: CC with 7th character A: M80.00X-M80.019 with 7th A, M80.041-M80.059 with 7th A, M80.80X-M80.819 with 7th A, M80.841-M80.859 with 7th A, M84.40X-M84.419 with 7th A, M84.441-M84.459 with 7th A, M84.474-M84.519 with 7th A, M84.541-M84.559 with 7th A, M84.574-M84.576 with 7th A, M84.60X-M84.619 with 7th A, M84.641-M84.659 with 7th A, M84.674-M84.68X with 7th A, S03.8XX-S03.9XX with 7th A, S29.011-S29.019 with 7th A, S38.3XX-S39.013 with 7th A, S72.001-S72.471 with 7th [A, B, C], S72.479-S72.92X with 7th A, S73.101A, S73.109-S73.111 with 7th A, S73.119-S73.121 with 7th A, S73.129-S73.191 with 7th A, S73.199A, S76.001A, S76.009-S76.011 with 7th A, S76.019A, S76.091A, S76.099-S76.101 with 7th A, S76.109-S76.111 with 7th A, S76.119 with 7th A, S76.191A, S76.199-S76.201 with 7th A, S76.209-S76.211 with 7th A, S76.219A, S76.291A, S76.299-S76.301 with 7th A, S76.309-S76.311 with 7th A, S76.319A, S76.391A, S76.399-S76.801 with 7th A, S76.809-S76.811 with 7th A, S76.819 with 7th A, S76.891A, S76.899-S76.901 with 7th A, S76.909-S76.911 with 7th A, S76.919A, S76.991A, S76.999A, S79.001A, S79.009-S79.011 with 7th A, S79.019-S79.091 with 7th A, S79.099-S79.101 with 7th A, S79.109-S79.111 with 7th A, S79.119-S79.121 with 7th A, S79.129-S79.131 with 7th A, S79.139-S79.141 with 7th A, S79.149-S79.191 with 7th A, S79.199-S79.811 with 7th A, S79.819-S79.821 with 7th A, S79.829-S79.911 with 7th A, S79.919-S79.921 with 7th A, S79.929 with 7th A, S82.90X-S82.92X with 7th [A, B, C], T14.8-T14.91, T79.A9X-T79.9XX with 7th A

CC Excl: CC with 7th character K or P: M80.00X-M84.68 with 7th [K, P], S02.0XX-S02.92X with 7th K, S12.000-S12.691 with 7th K, S22.000-S22.9XX with 7th K, S32.000-S32.9XX with 7th K, S42.001-S42.92X with 7th [K, P], S49.001-S49.199 with 7th [K, P], S52.001-S52.92X with 7th [K, M, N, P, Q, R], S59.001-S59.299 with 7th [K, P], S62.001-S62.92X with 7th [K, P], S72.001-S72.92X with 7th [K, M, N, P, Q, R], S79.001-S79.199 with 7th [K, P], S82.001-S82.92X with 7th [K, M, N, P, Q, R], S89.001-S89.399 with 7th [K, P], S92.001-S92.919 with 7th [K, P]

---

7 HAC = Initial encounter only (7th character A, B or C) and not POA.

N Newborn: 0   P Pediatric: 0-17   M Maternity: 12-55   A Adult: 15-124   MCC Major CC Condition   PDx MCC PDx acts as own MCC   CC CC Condition   PDx CC PDx acts as own CC

990   ICD-10-CM Draft (2015)

7 √7th **S79.102** **Unspecified physeal fracture of lower end of left femur** CC

CC Excl: CC with 7th character A: M80.00X-M80.019 with 7th A, M80.041-M80.059 with 7th A, M80.80X-M80.819 with 7th A, M80.841-M80.859 with 7th A, M84.40X-M84.419 with 7th A, M84.441-M84.459 with 7th A, M84.474-M84.519 with 7th A, M84.541-M84.559 with 7th A, M84.574-M84.576 with 7th A, M84.60X-M84.619 with 7th A, M84.641-M84.659 with 7th A, M84.674-M84.68X with 7th A, S03.8XX-S03.9XX with 7th A, S29.011-S29.019 with 7th A, S38.3XX-S39.013 with 7th A, S72.001-S72.466 with 7th [B, C], S72.472-S72.92 with 7th A, S73.102-S73.109 with 7th A, S73.112-S73.119 with 7th A, S73.122-S73.129 with 7th A, S73.192-S73.199 with 7th A, S76.002-S76.009 with 7th A, S76.012-S76.019 with 7th A, S76.092-S76.099 with 7th A, S76.102-S76.109 with 7th A, S76.112-S76.119 with 7th A, S76.192-S76.199 with 7th A, S76.202-S76.209 with 7th A, S76.212-S76.219 with 7th A, S76.292-S76.299 with 7th A, S76.302-S76.309 with 7th A, S76.312-S76.319 with 7th A, S76.392-S76.399 with 7th A, S76.802-S76.809 with 7th A, S76.812-S76.819 with 7th A, S76.892-S76.899 with 7th A, S76.902-S76.909 with 7th A, S76.912-S76.919 with 7th A, S76.992-S76.999 with 7th A, S79.002-S79.009 with 7th A, S79.012-S79.019 with 7th A, S79.092-S79.099 with 7th A, S79.102-S79.109 with 7th A, S79.112-S79.119 with 7th A, S79.122-S79.129 with 7th A, S79.132-S79.139 with 7th A, S79.142-S79.149 with 7th A, S79.192-S79.199 with 7th A, S79.812-S79.819 with 7th A, S79.822-S79.829 with 7th A, S79.912-S79.919 with 7th A, S79.922-S79.929 with 7th A, S82.90X-S82.92X with 7th [A, B, C], T14.8-T14.91, T79.A9X-T79.9XX with 7th A

CC Excl: CC with 7th character K or P: M80.00X-M84.68X with 7th [K, P], S02.0XX-S02.92X with 7th K, S12.000-S12.691 with 7th K, S22.000-S22.9XX with 7th K, S32.000-S32.9XX with 7th K, S42.001-S42.92X with 7th [K, P], S49.001-S49.199 with 7th [K, P], S52.001-S52.92X with 7th [K, M, N, P, Q, R], S59.001-S59.299 with 7th [K, P], S62.001-S62.92X with 7th [K, P], S72.001-S72.92X with 7th [K, M, N, P, Q, R], S79.001-S79.199 with 7th [K, P], S82.001-S82.92X with 7th [K, M, N, P, Q, R], S89.001-S89.399 with 7th [K, P], S92.001-S92.919 with 7th [K, P]

7 √7th **S79.109** **Unspecified physeal fracture of lower end of unspecified femur** CC

CC Excl: CC with 7th character A: M80.00X-M80.019 with 7th A, M80.041-M80.059 with 7th A, M80.80X-M80.819 with 7th A, M80.841-M80.859 with 7th A, M84.40X-M84.419 with 7th A, M84.441-M84.459 with 7th A, M84.474-M84.519 with 7th A, M84.541-M84.559 with 7th A, M84.574-M84.576 with 7th A, M84.60X-M84.619 with 7th A, M84.641-M84.659 with 7th A, M84.674-M84.68X with 7th A, S03.8XX-S03.9XX with 7th A, S29.011-S29.019 with 7th A, S38.3XX-S39.013 with 7th A, S72.001-S72.92 with 7th [A, B, C], S73.101-S73.199 with 7th A, S76.001-S76.019 with 7th A, S76.091-S76.119 with 7th A, S76.191-S76.219 with 7th A, S76.291-S76.319 with 7th A, S76.391-S76.819 with 7th A, S76.891-S76.919 with 7th A, S76.991-S76.999 with 7th A, S79.001-S79.929 with 7th A, S82.90X-S82.92X with 7th [A, B, C], T14.8-T14.91, T79.A9X-T79.9XX with 7th A

CC Excl: CC with 7th character K or P: M80.00X-M84.68 with 7th [K, P], S02.0XX-S02.92X with 7th K, S12.000-S12.691 with 7th K, S22.000-S22.9XX with 7th K, S32.000-S32.9XX with 7th K, S42.001-S42.92X with 7th [K, P], S49.001-S49.199 with 7th [K, P], S52.001-S52.92X with 7th [K, M, N, P, Q, R], S59.001-S59.299 with 7th [K, P], S62.001-S62.92X with 7th [K, P], S72.001-S72.92X with 7th [K, M, N, P, Q, R], S79.001-S79.199 with 7th [K, P], S82.001-S82.92X with 7th [K, M, N, P, Q, R], S89.001-S89.399 with 7th [K, P], S92.001-S92.919 with 7th [K, P]

√6th **S79.11** **Salter-Harris Type I physeal fracture of lower end of femur**

7 √7th **S79.111** **Salter-Harris Type I physeal fracture of lower end of right femur** CC
    CC Excl: See code: S79.101

7 √7th **S79.112** **Salter-Harris Type I physeal fracture of lower end of left femur** CC
    CC Excl: See code: S79.102

7 √7th **S79.119** **Salter-Harris Type I physeal fracture of lower end of unspecified femur** CC
    CC Excl: See code: S79.109

√6th **S79.12** **Salter-Harris Type II physeal fracture of lower end of femur**

7 √7th **S79.121** **Salter-Harris Type II physeal fracture of lower end of right femur** CC
    CC Excl: See code: S79.101

7 √7th **S79.122** **Salter-Harris Type II physeal fracture of lower end of left femur** CC
    CC Excl: See code: S79.102

7 √7th **S79.129** **Salter-Harris Type II physeal fracture of lower end of unspecified femur** CC
    CC Excl: See code: S79.109

√6th **S79.13** **Salter-Harris Type III physeal fracture of lower end of femur**

7 √7th **S79.131** **Salter-Harris Type III physeal fracture of lower end of right femur** CC
    CC Excl: See code: S79.101

7 √7th **S79.132** **Salter-Harris Type III physeal fracture of lower end of left femur** CC
    CC Excl: See code: S79.102

7 √7th **S79.139** **Salter-Harris Type III physeal fracture of lower end of unspecified femur** CC
    CC Excl: See code: S79.109

√6th **S79.14** **Salter-Harris Type IV physeal fracture of lower end of femur**

7 √7th **S79.141** **Salter-Harris Type IV physeal fracture of lower end of right femur** CC
    CC Excl: See code: S79.101

7 √7th **S79.142** **Salter-Harris Type IV physeal fracture of lower end of left femur** CC
    CC Excl: See code: S79.102

7 √7th **S79.149** **Salter-Harris Type IV physeal fracture of lower end of unspecified femur** CC
    CC Excl: See code: S79.109

√6th **S79.19** **Other physeal fracture of lower end of femur**

7 √7th **S79.191** **Other physeal fracture of lower end of right femur** CC
    CC Excl: See code: S79.101

7 √7th **S79.192** **Other physeal fracture of lower end of left femur** CC
    CC Excl: See code: S79.102

7 √7th **S79.199** **Other physeal fracture of lower end of unspecified femur** CC
    CC Excl: See code: S79.109

√5th **S79.8** **Other specified injuries of hip and thigh**

> The appropriate 7th character is to be added to each code in subcategory S79.8.
> A   initial encounter
> D   subsequent encounter
> S   sequela

√6th **S79.81** **Other specified injuries of hip**

√7th **S79.811** **Other specified injuries of right hip**

√7th **S79.812** **Other specified injuries of left hip**

√7th **S79.819** **Other specified injuries of unspecified hip**

√6th **S79.82** **Other specified injuries of thigh**

√7th **S79.821** **Other specified injuries of right thigh**

√7th **S79.822** **Other specified injuries of left thigh**

√7th **S79.829** **Other specified injuries of unspecified thigh**

---

7 HAC = Initial encounter only (7th character A, B or C) and not POA.

☑ Additional Character Required   √x7th Xtension Alert   Unacceptable PDx   Manifestation   Hospital Acquired Condition   EXCLUDES 1 Not Coded Here   EXCLUDES 2 Not Included Here

√5ᵗʰ **S79.9** **Unspecified injury of hip and thigh**

> The appropriate 7th character is to be added to each code in subcategory S79.9.
> A   initial encounter
> D   subsequent encounter
> S   sequela

  √6ᵗʰ **S79.91** **Unspecified injury of hip**

    √7ᵗʰ S79.911   Unspecified injury of right hip

    √7ᵗʰ S79.912   Unspecified injury of left hip

    √7ᵗʰ S79.919   Unspecified injury of unspecified hip

  √6ᵗʰ **S79.92** **Unspecified injury of thigh**

    √7ᵗʰ S79.921   Unspecified injury of right thigh

    √7ᵗʰ S79.922   Unspecified injury of left thigh

    √7ᵗʰ S79.929   Unspecified injury of unspecified thigh

Injuries to the knee and lower leg (S80-S89)

EXCLUDES 2   burns and corrosions (T20-T32)
frostbite (T33-T34)
injuries of ankle and foot, except fracture of ankle and malleolus (S90-S99)
insect bite or sting, venomous (T63.4)

√4ᵗʰ **S80** **Superficial injury of knee and lower leg**

EXCLUDES 2   superficial injury of ankle and foot (S90.-)

> The appropriate 7th character is to be added to each code from category S80.
> A   initial encounter
> D   subsequent encounter
> S   sequela

√5ᵗʰ **S80.0** **Contusion of knee**

  √x7ᵗʰ S80.00   Contusion of unspecified knee

  √x7ᵗʰ S80.01   Contusion of right knee

  √x7ᵗʰ S80.02   Contusion of left knee

√5ᵗʰ **S80.1** **Contusion of lower leg**

  √x7ᵗʰ S80.10   Contusion of unspecified lower leg

  √x7ᵗʰ S80.11   Contusion of right lower leg

  √x7ᵗʰ S80.12   Contusion of left lower leg

√5ᵗʰ **S80.2** **Other superficial injuries of knee**

  √6ᵗʰ **S80.21** **Abrasion of knee**

    √7ᵗʰ S80.211   Abrasion, right knee

    √7ᵗʰ S80.212   Abrasion, left knee

    √7ᵗʰ S80.219   Abrasion, unspecified knee

  √6ᵗʰ **S80.22** **Blister (nonthermal) of knee**

    √7ᵗʰ S80.221   Blister (nonthermal), right knee

    √7ᵗʰ S80.222   Blister (nonthermal), left knee

    √7ᵗʰ S80.229   Blister (nonthermal), unspecified knee

  √6ᵗʰ **S80.24** **External constriction of knee**

    √7ᵗʰ S80.241   External constriction, right knee

    √7ᵗʰ S80.242   External constriction, left knee

    √7ᵗʰ S80.249   External constriction, unspecified knee

  √6ᵗʰ **S80.25** **Superficial foreign body of knee**
      Splinter in the knee

    √7ᵗʰ S80.251   Superficial foreign body, right knee

    √7ᵗʰ S80.252   Superficial foreign body, left knee

    √7ᵗʰ S80.259   Superficial foreign body, unspecified knee

  √6ᵗʰ **S80.26** **Insect bite (nonvenomous) of knee**

    √7ᵗʰ S80.261   Insect bite (nonvenomous), right knee

    √7ᵗʰ S80.262   Insect bite (nonvenomous), left knee

    √7ᵗʰ S80.269   Insect bite (nonvenomous), unspecified knee

  √6ᵗʰ **S80.27** **Other superficial bite of knee**

    EXCLUDES 1   open bite of knee (S81.05-)

    √7ᵗʰ S80.271   Other superficial bite of right knee

    √7ᵗʰ S80.272   Other superficial bite of left knee

    √7ᵗʰ S80.279   Other superficial bite of unspecified knee

√5ᵗʰ **S80.8** **Other superficial injuries of lower leg**

  √6ᵗʰ **S80.81** **Abrasion of lower leg**

    √7ᵗʰ S80.811   Abrasion, right lower leg

    √7ᵗʰ S80.812   Abrasion, left lower leg

    √7ᵗʰ S80.819   Abrasion, unspecified lower leg

  √6ᵗʰ **S80.82** **Blister (nonthermal) of lower leg**

    √7ᵗʰ S80.821   Blister (nonthermal), right lower leg

    √7ᵗʰ S80.822   Blister (nonthermal), left lower leg

    √7ᵗʰ S80.829   Blister (nonthermal), unspecified lower leg

  √6ᵗʰ **S80.84** **External constriction of lower leg**

    √7ᵗʰ S80.841   External constriction, right lower leg

    √7ᵗʰ S80.842   External constriction, left lower leg

    √7ᵗʰ S80.849   External constriction, unspecified lower leg

  √6ᵗʰ **S80.85** **Superficial foreign body of lower leg**
      Splinter in the lower leg

    √7ᵗʰ S80.851   Superficial foreign body, right lower leg

    √7ᵗʰ S80.852   Superficial foreign body, left lower leg

    √7ᵗʰ S80.859   Superficial foreign body, unspecified lower leg

  √6ᵗʰ **S80.86** **Insect bite (nonvenomous) of lower leg**

    √7ᵗʰ S80.861   Insect bite (nonvenomous), right lower leg

    √7ᵗʰ S80.862   Insect bite (nonvenomous), left lower leg

    √7ᵗʰ S80.869   Insect bite (nonvenomous), unspecified lower leg

  √6ᵗʰ **S80.87** **Other superficial bite of lower leg**

    EXCLUDES 1   open bite of lower leg (S81.85-)

    √7ᵗʰ S80.871   Other superficial bite, right lower leg

    √7ᵗʰ S80.872   Other superficial bite, left lower leg

    √7ᵗʰ S80.879   Other superficial bite, unspecified lower leg

√5ᵗʰ **S80.9** **Unspecified superficial injury of knee and lower leg**

  √6ᵗʰ **S80.91** **Unspecified superficial injury of knee**

    √7ᵗʰ S80.911   Unspecified superficial injury of right knee

    √7ᵗʰ S80.912   Unspecified superficial injury of left knee

    √7ᵗʰ S80.919   Unspecified superficial injury of unspecified knee

  √6ᵗʰ **S80.92** **Unspecified superficial injury of lower leg**

    √7ᵗʰ S80.921   Unspecified superficial injury of right lower leg

    √7ᵗʰ S80.922   Unspecified superficial injury of left lower leg

    √7ᵗʰ S80.929   Unspecified superficial injury of unspecified lower leg

√4ᵗʰ **S81** **Open wound of knee and lower leg**

Code also any associated wound infection

EXCLUDES 1   open fracture of knee and lower leg (S82.-)
traumatic amputation of lower leg (S88.-)

EXCLUDES 2   open wound of ankle and foot (S91.-)

> The appropriate 7th character is to be added to each code from category S81.
> A   initial encounter
> D   subsequent encounter
> S   sequela

√5ᵗʰ **S81.0** **Open wound of knee**

  √6ᵗʰ **S81.00** **Unspecified open wound of knee**

    √7ᵗʰ S81.001   Unspecified open wound, right knee

    √7ᵗʰ S81.002   Unspecified open wound, left knee

    √7ᵗʰ S81.009   Unspecified open wound, unspecified knee

  √6ᵗʰ **S81.01** **Laceration without foreign body of knee**

    √7ᵗʰ S81.011   Laceration without foreign body, right knee

    √7ᵗʰ S81.012   Laceration without foreign body, left knee

    √7ᵗʰ S81.019   Laceration without foreign body, unspecified knee

  √6ᵗʰ **S81.02** **Laceration with foreign body of knee**

    √7ᵗʰ S81.021   Laceration with foreign body, right knee

    √7ᵗʰ S81.022   Laceration with foreign body, left knee

    √7ᵗʰ S81.029   Laceration with foreign body, unspecified knee

  √6ᵗʰ **S81.03** **Puncture wound without foreign body of knee**

    √7ᵗʰ S81.031   Puncture wound without foreign body, right knee

Ⓝ Newborn: 0   Ⓟ Pediatric: 0-17   Ⓜ Maternity: 12-55   Ⓐ Adult: 15-124   **MCC** Major CC Condition   **PDx MCC** PDx acts as own MCC   **CC** CC Condition   **PDx CC** PDx acts as own CC

992   ICD-10-CM Draft (2015)

√7ᵗʰ **S81.032** Puncture wound without foreign body, left knee

√7ᵗʰ **S81.039** Puncture wound without foreign body, unspecified knee

√6ᵗʰ **S81.04** Puncture wound with foreign body of knee

√7ᵗʰ **S81.041** Puncture wound with foreign body, right knee

√7ᵗʰ **S81.042** Puncture wound with foreign body, left knee

√7ᵗʰ **S81.049** Puncture wound with foreign body, unspecified knee

√6ᵗʰ **S81.05** Open bite of knee
Bite of knee NOS
EXCLUDES 1 superficial bite of knee (S80.27-)

√7ᵗʰ **S81.051** Open bite, right knee

√7ᵗʰ **S81.052** Open bite, left knee

√7ᵗʰ **S81.059** Open bite, unspecified knee

√5ᵗʰ **S81.8** Open wound of lower leg

√6ᵗʰ **S81.80** Unspecified open wound of lower leg

√7ᵗʰ **S81.801** Unspecified open wound, right lower leg

√7ᵗʰ **S81.802** Unspecified open wound, left lower leg

√7ᵗʰ **S81.809** Unspecified open wound, unspecified lower leg

√6ᵗʰ **S81.81** Laceration without foreign body of lower leg

√7ᵗʰ **S81.811** Laceration without foreign body, right lower leg

√7ᵗʰ **S81.812** Laceration without foreign body, left lower leg

√7ᵗʰ **S81.819** Laceration without foreign body, unspecified lower leg

√6ᵗʰ **S81.82** Laceration with foreign body of lower leg

√7ᵗʰ **S81.821** Laceration with foreign body, right lower leg

√7ᵗʰ **S81.822** Laceration with foreign body, left lower leg

√7ᵗʰ **S81.829** Laceration with foreign body, unspecified lower leg

√6ᵗʰ **S81.83** Puncture wound without foreign body of lower leg

√7ᵗʰ **S81.831** Puncture wound without foreign body, right lower leg

√7ᵗʰ **S81.832** Puncture wound without foreign body, left lower leg

√7ᵗʰ **S81.839** Puncture wound without foreign body, unspecified lower leg

√6ᵗʰ **S81.84** Puncture wound with foreign body of lower leg

√7ᵗʰ **S81.841** Puncture wound with foreign body, right lower leg

√7ᵗʰ **S81.842** Puncture wound with foreign body, left lower leg

√7ᵗʰ **S81.849** Puncture wound with foreign body, unspecified lower leg

√6ᵗʰ **S81.85** Open bite of lower leg
Bite of lower leg NOS
EXCLUDES 1 superficial bite of lower leg (S80.86-, S80.87-)

√7ᵗʰ **S81.851** Open bite, right lower leg

√7ᵗʰ **S81.852** Open bite, left lower leg

√7ᵗʰ **S81.859** Open bite, unspecified lower leg

√4ᵗʰ **S82** Fracture of lower leg, including ankle
NOTE A fracture not indicated as displaced or nondisplaced should be coded to displaced.
A fracture not designated as open or closed should be coded to closed.
The open fracture designations are based on the Gustilo open fracture classification.
INCLUDES fracture of malleolus
EXCLUDES 1 traumatic amputation of lower leg (S88.-)
EXCLUDES 2 fracture of foot, except ankle (S92.-)
periprosthetic fracture of prosthetic implant of knee (T84.042, T84.043)

The appropriate 7th character is to be added to all codes from category S82 [unless otherwise indicated].
A   initial encounter for closed fracture
B   initial encounter for open fracture type I or II
    initial encounter for open fracture NOS
C   initial encounter for open fracture type IIIA, IIIB, or IIIC
D   subsequent encounter for closed fracture with routine healing
E   subsequent encounter for open fracture type I or II with routine healing
F   subsequent encounter for open fracture type IIIA, IIIB, or IIIC with routine healing
G   subsequent encounter for closed fracture with delayed healing
H   subsequent encounter for open fracture type I or II with delayed healing
J   subsequent encounter for open fracture type IIIA, IIIB or IIIC with delayed healing
K   subsequent encounter for closed fracture with nonunion
M   subsequent encounter for open fracture type I or II with nonunion
N   subsequent encounter for open fracture type IIIA, IIIB or IIIC with nonunion
P   subsequent encounter for closed fracture with malunion
Q   subsequent encounter for open fracture type I or II with malunion
R   subsequent encounter for open fracture type IIIA, IIIB or IIIC with malunion
S   sequela

√5ᵗʰ **S82.0** Fracture of patella
Knee cap

√6ᵗʰ **S82.00** Unspecified fracture of patella

7 √7ᵗʰ **S82.001** Unspecified fracture of right patella **CC**
CC Excl: CC with 7th character A: S82.001-S82.099 with 7th [A, B, C]
CC with 7th character B or C: M80.00X-M80.019 with 7th A, M80.041-M80.049 with 7th A, M80.80X-M80.819 with 7th A, M80.841-M80.849 with 7th A, M84.40X-M84.419 with 7th A, M84.441-M84.446 with 7th A, M84.454 with 7th A, M84.474-M84.519 with 7th A, M84.541-M84.550 with 7th A, M84.574-M84.576 with 7th A, M84.60X-M84.619 with 7th A, M84.641-M84.650 with 7th A, M84.674-M84.68X with 7th A, S03.8XX-S03.9XX with 7th A, S29.011-S29.019 with 7th A, S38.3XX-S39.013 with 7th A, S73.101-S73.199 with 7th A, S76.001-S76.019 with 7th A, S76.091-S76.119 with 7th A, S76.191-S76.219 with 7th A, S76.291-S76.319 with 7th A, S76.391-S76.819 with 7th A, S76.891-S76.919 with 7th A, S76.991-S76.999 with 7th A, S79.811-S79.929 with 7th A, S82.001-S82.156 with 7th [B, C], S82.191-S82.299 with 7th [A, B, C], S82.401-S82.499 with 7th [A, B, C], S82.831-S82.839 with 7th [A, B, C], S82.861-S82.866 with 7th [A, B, C], S82.90X-S82.92X with 7th [A, B, C], S89.001-S89.099 with 7th A, S89.201-S89.299 with 7th A, T14.8-T14.91, T79.A9X-T79.9XX with 7th A
CC Excl: CC with 7th character K, M, N, P, Q or R: M80.00X-M84.68 with 7th [K, P], S02.0XX-S02.92X with 7th K, S12.000-S12.691 with 7th K, S22.000-S22.9XX with 7th K, S32.000-S32.9XX with 7th K, S42.001-S42.92X with 7th [K, P], S49.001-S49.199 with 7th [K, P], S52.001-S52.92X with 7th [K, M, N, P, Q, R], S59.001-S59.299 with 7th [K, P], S62.001-S62.92X with 7th [K, P], S72.001-S72.92X with 7th [K, M, N, P, Q, R], S79.001-S79.199 with 7th [K, P], S82.001-S82.92X with 7th [K, M, N, P, Q, R], S89.001-S89.399 with 7th [K, P], S92.001-S92.919 with 7th [K, P]

7 HAC = Initial encounter only (7th character A, B or C) and not POA.

√ Additional Character Required   √x7ᵗʰ Xtension Alert   Unacceptable PDx   Manifestation   Hospital Acquired Condition   **EXCLUDES 1** Not Coded Here   **EXCLUDES 2** Not Included Here

ICD-10-CM Draft (2015)   **993**

7 √7th **S82.002** **Unspecified fracture of left patella** `CC`
CC Excl: CC with 7th character A: S82.001-
S82.099 with 7th [B, C]
CC with 7th character B or C: M80.00X-
M80.019 with 7th A, M80.041-M80.049 with
7th A, M80.80X-M80.819 with 7th A,
M80.841-M80.849 with 7th A, M84.40X-
M84.419 with 7th A, M84.441-M84.446 with
7th A, M84.454 with 7th A, M84.474-M84.519
with 7th A, M84.541-M84.550 with 7th A,
M84.574-M84.576 with 7th A, M84.60X-
M84.619 with 7th A, M84.641-M84.650 with
7th A, M84.674-M84.68 with 7th A, S03.8XX-
S03.9XX with 7th A, S29.011-S29.019 with
7th A, S38.3X-S39.013 with 7th A, S73.101-
S73.199 with 7th A, S76.001-S76.019 with
7th A, S76.091-S76.119 with 7th A, S76.191-
S76.219 with 7th A, S76.291-S76.319 with
7th A, S76.391-S76.819 with 7th A, S76.891-
S76.919 with 7th A, S76.991-S76.999 with
7th A, S79.811-S79.929 with 7th A, S82.001-
S82.156 with 7th [B, C], S82.191-S82.299 with
7th [A, B, C], S82.401-S82.499 with 7th [A, B,
C], S82.831-S82.839 with 7th [A, B, C],
S82.861-S82.866 with 7th [A, B, C], S82.90X-
S82.92X with 7th [A, B, C], S89.001-S89.099
with 7th A, S89.201-S89.299 with 7th A,
T14.8-T14.91, T79.A9X-T79.9XX with 7th A
CC Excl: CC with 7th character K, M, N, P, Q
or R: M80.00X-M84.68X with 7th [K, P],
S02.0XX-S02.92X with 7th K, S12.000-
S12.691 with 7th K, S22.000-S22.9XX with
7th K, S32.000-S32.9XX with 7th K, S42.001-
S42.92X with 7th [K, P], S49.001-S49.199 with
7th [K, P], S52.001-S52.92X with 7th [K, M, N,
P, Q, R], S59.001-S59.299 with 7th [K, P],
S62.001-S62.92X with 7th [K, P], S72.001-
S72.92X with 7th [K, M, N, P, Q, R], S79.001-
S79.199 with 7th [K, P], S82.001-S82.92X with
7th [K, M, N, P, Q, R], S89.001-S89.399 with
7th [K, P], S92.001-S92.919 with 7th [K, P]

7 √7th **S82.009** **Unspecified fracture of unspecified patella** `CC`
CC Excl: CC with 7th character A: S82.001-
S82.099 with 7th [A, B, C]
CC with 7th character B or C: M80.00X-
M80.019 with 7th A, M80.041-M80.049 with
7th A, M80.80X-M80.819 with 7th A,
M80.841-M80.849 with 7th A, M84.40X-
M84.419 with 7th A, M84.441-M84.446 with
7th A, M84.454 with 7th A, M84.474-M84.519
with 7th A, M84.541-M84.550 with 7th A,
M84.574-M84.576 with 7th A, M84.60X-
M84.619 with 7th A, M84.641-M84.650 with
7th A, M84.674-M84.68X with 7th A,
S03.8XX-S03.9XX with 7th A, S29.011-
S29.019 with 7th A, S38.3XX-S39.013 with
7th A, S73.101-S73.199 with 7th A, S76.001-
S76.019 with 7th A, S76.091-S76.119 with
7th A, S76.191-S76.219 with 7th A, S76.291-
S76.319 with 7th A, S76.391-S76.819 with
7th A, S76.891-S76.919 with 7th A, S76.991-
S76.999 with 7th A, S79.811-S79.929 with
7th A, S82.001-S82.156 with 7th [B, C],
S82.191-S82.299 with 7th [A, B, C], S82.401-
S82.499 with 7th [A, B, C], S82.831-S82.839
with 7th [A, B, C], S82.861-S82.866 with 7th
[A, B, C], S82.90X-S82.92X with 7th [A, B, C],
S89.001-S89.099 with 7th A, S89.201-
S89.299 with 7th A, T14.8-T14.91, T79.A9X-
T79.9XX with 7th A
CC Excl: CC with 7th character K, M, N, P, Q
or R: M80.00X-M84.68 with 7th [K, P],
S02.0XX-S02.92X with 7th K, S12.000-
S12.691 with 7th K, S22.000-S22.9XX with
7th K, S32.000-S32.9XX with 7th K, S42.001-
S42.92X with 7th [K, P], S49.001-S49.199 with
7th [K, P], S52.001-S52.92X with 7th [K, M, N,
P, Q, R], S59.001-S59.299 with 7th [K, P],
S62.001-S62.92X with 7th [K, P], S72.001-
S72.92X with 7th [K, M, N, P, Q, R], S79.001-
S79.199 with 7th [K, P], S82.001-S82.92X with
7th [K, M, N, P, Q, R], S89.001-S89.399 with
7th [K, P], S92.001-S92.919 with 7th [K, P]

√6th **S82.01** **Osteochondral fracture of patella**
7 √7th **S82.011** **Displaced osteochondral fracture of right patella** `CC`
CC Excl: See code: S82.001

7 √7th **S82.012** **Displaced osteochondral fracture of left patella** `CC`
CC Excl: See code: S82.002

7 √7th **S82.013** **Displaced osteochondral fracture of unspecified patella** `CC`
CC Excl: See code: S82.009

7 √7th **S82.014** **Nondisplaced osteochondral fracture of right patella** `CC`
CC Excl: See code: S82.001

7 √7th **S82.015** **Nondisplaced osteochondral fracture of left patella** `CC`
CC Excl: See code: S82.002

7 √7th **S82.016** **Nondisplaced osteochondral fracture of unspecified patella** `CC`
CC Excl: See code: S82.009

√6th **S82.02** **Longitudinal fracture of patella**
7 √7th **S82.021** **Displaced longitudinal fracture of right patella** `CC`
CC Excl: See code: S82.001

7 √7th **S82.022** **Displaced longitudinal fracture of left patella** `CC`
CC Excl: See code: S82.002

7 √7th **S82.023** **Displaced longitudinal fracture of unspecified patella** `CC`
CC Excl: See code: S82.009

7 √7th **S82.024** **Nondisplaced longitudinal fracture of right patella** `CC`
CC Excl: See code: S82.001

7 √7th **S82.025** **Nondisplaced longitudinal fracture of left patella** `CC`
CC Excl: See code: S82.002

7 √7th **S82.026** **Nondisplaced longitudinal fracture of unspecified patella** `CC`
CC Excl: See code: S82.009

√6th **S82.03** **Transverse fracture of patella**
7 √7th **S82.031** **Displaced transverse fracture of right patella** `CC`
CC Excl: See code: S82.001

7 √7th **S82.032** **Displaced transverse fracture of left patella** `CC`
CC Excl: See code: S82.002

7 √7th **S82.033** **Displaced transverse fracture of unspecified patella** `CC`
CC Excl: See code: S82.009

7 √7th **S82.034** **Nondisplaced transverse fracture of right patella** `CC`
CC Excl: See code: S82.001

7 √7th **S82.035** **Nondisplaced transverse fracture of left patella** `CC`
CC Excl: See code: S82.002

7 √7th **S82.036** **Nondisplaced transverse fracture of unspecified patella** `CC`
CC Excl: See code: S82.009

√6th **S82.04** **Comminuted fracture of patella**
7 √7th **S82.041** **Displaced comminuted fracture of right patella** `CC`
CC Excl: See code: S82.001

7 √7th **S82.042** **Displaced comminuted fracture of left patella** `CC`
CC Excl: See code: S82.002

7 √7th **S82.043** **Displaced comminuted fracture of unspecified patella** `CC`
CC Excl: See code: S82.009

7 √7th **S82.044** **Nondisplaced comminuted fracture of right patella** `CC`
CC Excl: See code: S82.001

7 √7th **S82.045** **Nondisplaced comminuted fracture of left patella** `CC`
CC Excl: See code: S82.002

7 √7th **S82.046** **Nondisplaced comminuted fracture of unspecified patella** `CC`
CC Excl: See code: S82.009

√6th **S82.09** **Other fracture of patella**
7 √7th **S82.091** **Other fracture of right patella** `CC`
CC Excl: See code: S82.001

7 √7th **S82.092** **Other fracture of left patella** `CC`
CC Excl: See code: S82.002

7 √7th **S82.099** **Other fracture of unspecified patella** `CC`
CC Excl: See code: S82.009

---

7 HAC = Initial encounter only (7th character A, B or C) and not POA.

Ⓝ Newborn: 0   Ⓟ Pediatric: 0-17   Ⓜ Maternity: 12-55   Ⓐ Adult: 15-124   `MCC` Major CC Condition   `PDx MCC` PDx acts as own MCC   `CC` CC Condition   `PDx CC` PDx acts as own CC

994   ICD-10-CM Draft (2015)

✓5ᵗʰ **S82.1   Fracture of upper end of tibia**
Fracture of proximal end of tibia
EXCLUDES 2   *fracture of shaft of tibia (S82.2-)*
physeal fracture of upper end of tibia (S89.0-)

✓6ᵗʰ **S82.10   Unspecified fracture of upper end of tibia**

7 ✓7ᵗʰ **S82.101   Unspecified fracture of upper end of right tibia**   MCC CC

CC Excl: CC with 7th character A: M80.00X-M80.019 with 7th A, M80.041-M80.049 with 7th A, M80.061-M80.079 with 7th A, M80.80X-M80.819 with 7th A, M80.841-M80.849 with 7th A, M80.861-M80.879 with 7th A, M84.40X-M84.419 with 7th A, M84.441-M84.446 with 7th A, M84.454 with 7th A, M84.461-M84.519 with 7th A, M84.541-M84.550 with 7th A, M84.561-M84.576 with 7th A, M84.60X-M84.619 with 7th A, M84.641-M84.650 with 7th A, M84.661-M84.68X with 7th A, S03.8XX-S03.9XX with 7th A, S29.011-S29.019 with 7th A, S38.3XX-S39.013 with 7th A, S73.101A, S73.109-S73.111 with 7th A, S73.119-S73.121 with 7th A, S73.129-S73.191 with 7th A, S73.199A, S76.001A, S76.009-S76.011 with 7th A, S76.019A, S76.091A, S76.099-S76.101 with 7th A, S76.109-S76.111 with 7th A, S76.119A, S76.191A, S76.199-S76.201 with 7th A, S76.209-S76.211 with 7th A, S76.219A, S76.291A, S76.299-S76.301 with 7th A, S76.309-S76.311 with 7th A, S76.319A, S76.391A, S76.399-S76.801 with 7th A, S76.809-S76.811 with 7th A, S76.819A, S76.891A, S76.899-S76.901 with 7th A, S76.909-S76.911 with 7th A, S76.919A, S76.991A, S76.999A, S79.811A, S79.819-S79.821 with 7th A, S79.829-S79.911 with 7th A, S79.919-S79.921 with 7th A, S79.929A, S82.101-S82.156 with 7th [A, B, C], S82.191-S82.299 with 7th [A, B, C], S82.401-S82.499 with 7th [A, B, C], S82.831-S82.839 with 7th [A, B, C], S82.861-S82.866 with 7th [A, B, C], S82.90X-S82.92X with 7th [A, B, C], S89.001A, S89.009-S89.011 with 7th A, S89.019-S89.021 with 7th A, S89.029-S89.031 with 7th A, S89.039-S89.041 with 7th A, S89.049-S89.091 with 7th A, S89.099A, S89.201A, S89.209-S89.211 with 7th A, S89.219-S89.221 with 7th A, S89.229-S89.291 with 7th A, S89.299A, T14.8-T14.91, T79.A9X-T79.9XX with 7th A

MCC with 7th B or C: M80.00X-M80.019 with 7th A, M80.041-M80.049 with 7th A, M80.061-M80.079 with 7th A, M80.80X-M80.819 with 7th A, M80.841-M80.849 with 7th A, M80.861-M80.879 with 7th A, M84.40X-M84.419 with 7th A, M84.441-M84.446 with 7th A, M84.454 with 7th A, M84.461-M84.519 with 7th A, M84.541-M84.550 with 7th A, M84.561-M84.576 with 7th A, M84.60X-M84.619 with 7th A, M84.641-M84.650 with 7th A, M84.661-M84.68X with 7th A, S03.8XX-S03.9XX with 7th A, S29.011-S29.019 with 7th A, S38.3X-S39.013 with 7th A, S73.101-S73.199 with 7th A, S76.001-S76.019 with 7th A, S76.091-S76.119 with 7th A, S76.191-S76.219 with 7th A, S76.291-S76.319 with 7th A, S76.391-S76.819 with 7th A, S76.891-S76.919 with 7th A, S76.991-S76.999 with 7th A, S79.811-S79.929 with 7th A, S82.101-S82.156 with 7th [A, B, C], S82.191-S82.299 with 7th [A, B, C], S82.401-S82.499 with 7th [A, B, C], S82.831-S82.839 with 7th [A, B, C], S82.861-S82.866 with 7th [A, B, C], S82.90X-S82.92X with 7th [A, B, C], S89.001-S89.099 with 7th A, S89.201-S89.299 with 7th A, T14.8-T14.91, T79.A9X-T79.9XX with 7th A

CC with 7th character K, M, N, P, Q or R: M80.00X-M84.68X with 7th [K, P], S02.0XX-S02.92X with 7th K, S12.000-S12.691 with 7th K, S22.000-S22.9XX with 7th K, S32.000-S32.9XX with 7th K, S42.001-S42.92X with 7th [K, P], S49.001-S49.199 with 7th [K, P], S52.001-S52.92X with 7th [K, M, N, P, Q, R], S59.001-S59.299 with 7th [K, P], S62.001-S62.92X with 7th [K, P], S72.001-S72.92X with 7th [K, M, N, P, Q, R], S79.001-S79.199 with 7th [K, P], S82.001-S82.92X with 7th [K, M, N, P, Q, R], S89.001-S89.399 with 7th [K, P], S92.001-S92.919 with 7th [K, P]

7 ✓7ᵗʰ **S82.102   Unspecified fracture of upper end of left tibia**   MCC CC

CC Excl: CC with 7th character A: M80.00X-M80.019 with 7th A, M80.041-M80.049 with 7th A, M80.061-M80.079 with 7th A, M80.80X-M80.819 with 7th A, M80.841-M80.849 with 7th A, M80.861-M80.879 with 7th A, M84.40X-M84.419 with 7th A, M84.441-M84.446 with 7th A, M84.454 with 7th A, M84.461-M84.519 with 7th A, M84.541-M84.550 with 7th A, M84.561-M84.576 with 7th A, M84.60X-M84.619 with 7th A, M84.641-M84.650 with 7th A, M84.661-M84.68 with 7th A, S03.8XX-S03.9XX with 7th A, S29.011-S29.019 with 7th A, S38.3XX-S39.013 with 7th A, S73.102-S73.109 with 7th A, S73.112-S73.119 with 7th A, S73.122-S73.129 with 7th A, S73.192-S73.199 with 7th A, S76.002-S76.009 with 7th A, S76.012-S76.019 with 7th A, S76.092-S76.099 with 7th A, S76.102-S76.109 with 7th A, S76.112-S76.119 with 7th A, S76.192-S76.199 with 7th A, S76.202-S76.209 with 7th A, S76.212-S76.219 with 7th A, S76.292-S76.299 with 7th A, S76.302-S76.309 with 7th A, S76.312-S76.319 with 7th A, S76.392-S76.399 with 7th A, S76.802-S76.809 with 7th A, S76.812-S76.819 with 7th A, S76.892-S76.899 with 7th A, S76.902-S76.909 with 7th A, S76.912-S76.919 with 7th A, S76.992-S76.999 with 7th A, S79.812-S79.819 with 7th A, S79.822-S79.829 with 7th A, S79.912-S79.919 with 7th A, S79.922-S79.929 with 7th A, S82.101-S82.156 with 7th [B, C], S82.191-S82.299 with 7th [B, C], S82.401-S82.499 with 7th [B, C], S82.831-S82.839 with 7th [B, C], S82.861-S82.866 with 7th [B, C], S82.90X-S82.92X with 7th [A, B, C], S89.002-S89.009 with 7th A, S89.012-S89.019 with 7th A, S89.022-S89.029 with 7th A, S89.032-S89.039 with 7th A, S89.042-S89.049 with 7th A, S89.092-S89.099 with 7th A, S89.202-S89.209 with 7th A, S89.212-S89.219 with 7th A, S89.222-S89.229 with 7th A, S89.292-S89.299 with 7th A, T14.8-T14.91, T79.A9X-T79.9XX with 7th A

CC with 7th character K, M, N, P, Q or R: M80.00X-M84.68 with 7th [K, P], S02.0XX-S02.92X with 7th K, S12.000-S12.691 with 7th K, S22.000-S22.9XX with 7th K, S32.000-S32.9XX with 7th K, S42.001-S42.92X with 7th [K, P], S49.001-S49.199 with 7th [K, P], S52.001-S52.92X with 7th [K, M, N, P, Q, R], S59.001-S59.299 with 7th [K, P], S62.001-S62.92X with 7th [K, P], S72.001-S72.92X with 7th [K, M, N, P, Q, R], S79.001-S79.199 with 7th [K, P], S82.001-S82.92X with 7th [K, M, N, P, Q, R], S89.001-S89.399 with 7th [K, P], S92.001-S92.919 with 7th [K, P]

---

7 HAC = Initial encounter only (7th character A, B or C) and not POA.

7 √7ᵗʰ **S82.109** **Unspecified fracture of upper end of unspecified tibia** MCC CC
CC Excl: CC with 7th character A: M80.00X-M80.019 with 7th A, M80.041-M80.049 with 7th A, M80.061-M80.079 with 7th A, M80.80X-M80.819 with 7th A, M80.841-M80.849 with 7th A, M80.861-M80.879 with 7th A, M84.40X-M84.419 with 7th A, M84.441-M84.446 with 7th A, M84.454 with 7th A, M84.461-M84.519 with 7th A, M84.541-M84.550 with 7th A, M84.561-M84.576 with 7th A, M84.60X-M84.619 with 7th A, M84.641-M84.650 with 7th A, M84.661-M84.68 with 7th A, S03.8XX-S03.9XX with 7th A, S29.011-S29.019 with 7th A, S38.3XX-S39.013 with 7th A, S73.101-S73.199 with 7th A, S76.001-S76.019 with 7th A, S76.091-S76.119 with 7th A, S76.191-S76.219 with 7th A, S76.291-S76.319 with 7th A, S76.391-S76.819 with 7th A, S76.891-S76.919 with 7th A, S76.991-S76.999 with 7th A, S79.811-S79.929 with 7th A, S82.101-S82.156 with 7th [A, B, C], S82.191-S82.299 with 7th [A, B, C], S82.401-S82.499 with 7th [A, B, C], S82.831-S82.839 with 7th [A, B, C], S82.861-S82.866 with 7th [A, B, C], S82.90X-S82.92X with 7th [A, B, C], S89.001-S89.099 with 7th A, S89.201-S89.299 with 7th A, T14.8-T14.91, T79.A9X-T79.9XX with 7th A
CC with 7th character K, M, N, P, Q or R: M80.00X-M84.68 with 7th [K, P], S02.0XX-S02.92X with 7th K, S12.000-S12.691 with 7th K, S22.000-S22.9XX with 7th K, S32.000-S32.9XX with 7th K, S42.001-S42.92X with 7th [K, P], S49.001-S49.199 with 7th [K, P], S52.001-S52.92X with 7th [K, M, N, P, Q, R], S59.001-S59.299 with 7th [K, P], S62.001-S62.92X with 7th [K, P], S72.001-S72.92X with 7th [K, M, N, P, Q, R], S79.001-S79.199 with 7th [K, P], S82.001-S82.92X with 7th [K, M, N, P, Q, R], S89.001-S89.399 with 7th [K, P], S92.001-S92.919 with 7th [K, P]

√6ᵗʰ **S82.11** **Fracture of tibial spine**

7 √7ᵗʰ **S82.111** **Displaced fracture of right tibial spine** MCC CC
CC Excl: See code: S82.101

7 √7ᵗʰ **S82.112** **Displaced fracture of left tibial spine** MCC CC
CC Excl: See code: S82.102

7 √7ᵗʰ **S82.113** **Displaced fracture of unspecified tibial spine** MCC CC
CC Excl: See code: S82.109

7 √7ᵗʰ **S82.114** **Nondisplaced fracture of right tibial spine** MCC CC
CC Excl: See code: S82.101

7 √7ᵗʰ **S82.115** **Nondisplaced fracture of left tibial spine** MCC CC
CC Excl: See code: S82.102

7 √7ᵗʰ **S82.116** **Nondisplaced fracture of unspecified tibial spine** MCC CC
CC Excl: See code: S82.109

√6ᵗʰ **S82.12** **Fracture of lateral condyle of tibia**

7 √7ᵗʰ **S82.121** **Displaced fracture of lateral condyle of right tibia** MCC CC
CC Excl: See code: S82.101

7 √7ᵗʰ **S82.122** **Displaced fracture of lateral condyle of left tibia** MCC CC
CC Excl: See code: S82.102

7 √7ᵗʰ **S82.123** **Displaced fracture of lateral condyle of unspecified tibia** MCC CC
CC Excl: See code: S82.109

7 √7ᵗʰ **S82.124** **Nondisplaced fracture of lateral condyle of right tibia** MCC CC
CC Excl: See code: S82.101

7 √7ᵗʰ **S82.125** **Nondisplaced fracture of lateral condyle of left tibia** MCC CC
CC Excl: See code: S82.102

7 √7ᵗʰ **S82.126** **Nondisplaced fracture of lateral condyle of unspecified tibia** MCC CC
CC Excl: See code: S82.109

√6ᵗʰ **S82.13** **Fracture of medial condyle of tibia**

7 √7ᵗʰ **S82.131** **Displaced fracture of medial condyle of right tibia** MCC CC
CC Excl: See code: S82.101

7 √7ᵗʰ **S82.132** **Displaced fracture of medial condyle of left tibia** MCC CC
CC Excl: See code: S82.102

7 √7ᵗʰ **S82.133** **Displaced fracture of medial condyle of unspecified tibia** MCC CC
CC Excl: See code: S82.109

7 √7ᵗʰ **S82.134** **Nondisplaced fracture of medial condyle of right tibia** MCC CC
CC Excl: See code: S82.101

7 √7ᵗʰ **S82.135** **Nondisplaced fracture of medial condyle of left tibia** MCC CC
CC Excl: See code: S82.102

7 √7ᵗʰ **S82.136** **Nondisplaced fracture of medial condyle of unspecified tibia** MCC CC
CC Excl: See code: S82.109

√6ᵗʰ **S82.14** **Bicondylar fracture of tibia**
Fracture of tibial plateau NOS

7 √7ᵗʰ **S82.141** **Displaced bicondylar fracture of right tibia** MCC CC
CC Excl: See code: S82.101

7 √7ᵗʰ **S82.142** **Displaced bicondylar fracture of left tibia** MCC CC
CC Excl: See code: S82.102

7 √7ᵗʰ **S82.143** **Displaced bicondylar fracture of unspecified tibia** MCC CC
CC Excl: See code: S82.109

7 √7ᵗʰ **S82.144** **Nondisplaced bicondylar fracture of right tibia** MCC CC
CC Excl: See code: S82.101

7 √7ᵗʰ **S82.145** **Nondisplaced bicondylar fracture of left tibia** MCC CC
CC Excl: See code: S82.102

7 √7ᵗʰ **S82.146** **Nondisplaced bicondylar fracture of unspecified tibia** MCC CC
CC Excl: See code: S82.109

√6ᵗʰ **S82.15** **Fracture of tibial tuberosity**

7 √7ᵗʰ **S82.151** **Displaced fracture of right tibial tuberosity** MCC CC
CC Excl: See code: S82.101

7 √7ᵗʰ **S82.152** **Displaced fracture of left tibial tuberosity** MCC CC
CC Excl: See code: S82.102

7 √7ᵗʰ **S82.153** **Displaced fracture of unspecified tibial tuberosity** MCC CC
CC Excl: See code: S82.109

7 √7ᵗʰ **S82.154** **Nondisplaced fracture of right tibial tuberosity** MCC CC
CC Excl: See code: S82.101

7 √7ᵗʰ **S82.155** **Nondisplaced fracture of left tibial tuberosity** MCC CC
CC Excl: See code: S82.102

7 √7ᵗʰ **S82.156** **Nondisplaced fracture of unspecified tibial tuberosity** MCC CC
CC Excl: See code: S82.109

√6ᵗʰ **S82.16** **Torus fracture of upper end of tibia**

The appropriate 7th character is to be added to all codes in subcategory S82.16.
A   initial encounter for closed fracture
D   subsequent encounter for fracture with routine healing
G   subsequent encounter for fracture with delayed healing
K   subsequent encounter for fracture with nonunion
P   subsequent encounter for fracture with malunion
S   sequela

7 HAC = Initial encounter only (7th character A, B or C) and not POA.

7 √7ᵗʰ **S82.161** **Torus fracture of upper end of right** `CC`
tibia

CC Excl: CC with 7th character A: S82.101-
S82.161 with 7th [A, B, C], S82.169-S82.299
with 7th A, S82.311A, S82.319A, S82.401-
S82.811 with 7th [A, B, C], S82.819-S82.821
with 7th A, S82.829-S82.839 with 7th A,
S82.861-S82.866 with 7th [A, B, C], S89.001A,
S89.009-S89.011 with 7th A, S89.019-
S89.021 with 7th A, S89.029-S89.031 with
7th A, S89.039-S89.041 with 7th A, S89.049-
S89.091 with 7th A, S89.099A, S89.201A,
S89.209-S89.211 with 7th A, S89.219-
S89.221 with 7th A, S89.229-S89.291 with
7th A, S89.299A

CC with 7th character K or P: M80.00X-
M84.68X with 7th [K, P], S02.0XX-S02.92X
with 7th K, S12.000-S12.691 with 7th K,
S22.000-S22.9XX with 7th K, S32.000-
S32.9XX with 7th K, S42.001-S42.92X with 7th
[K, P], S49.001-S49.199 with 7th [K, P],
S52.001-S52.92X with 7th [K, M, N, P, Q, R],
S59.001-S59.299 with 7th [K, P], S62.001-
S62.92X with 7th [K, P], S72.001-S72.92X
with 7th [K, M, N, P, Q, R], S79.001-S79.199
with 7th [K, P], S82.001-S82.92X with 7th [K,
M, N, P, Q, R], S89.001-S89.399 with 7th [K, P],
S92.001-S92.919 with 7th [K, P]

7 √7ᵗʰ **S82.162** **Torus fracture of upper end of left** `CC`
tibia

CC Excl: CC with 7th character A: S82.101-
S82.156 with 7th [B, C], S82.162-S82.299 with
7th A, S82.312-S82.319 with 7th A, S82.401-
S82.499 with 7th [B, C], S82.812-S82.819 with
7th A, S82.822-S82.839 with 7th A, S82.861-
S82.866 with 7th [B, C], S89.002-S89.009 with
7th A, S89.012-S89.019 with 7th A, S89.022-
S89.029 with 7th A, S89.032-S89.039 with
7th A, S89.042-S89.049 with 7th A, S89.092-
S89.099 with 7th A, S89.202-S89.209 with
7th A, S89.212-S89.219 with 7th A, S89.222-
S89.229 with 7th A, S89.292-S89.299 with
7th A

CC with 7th character K or P: M80.00X-
M84.68X with 7th [K, P], S02.0XX-S02.92X
with 7th K, S12.000-S12.691 with 7th K,
S22.000-S22.9XX with 7th K, S32.000-
S32.9XX with 7th K, S42.001-S42.92X with
7th [K, P], S49.001-S49.199 with 7th [K, P],
S52.001-S52.92X with 7th [K, M, N, P, Q, R],
S59.001-S59.299 with 7th [K, P], S62.001-
S62.92X with 7th [K, P], S72.001-S72.92X
with 7th [K, M, N, P, Q, R], S79.001-S79.199
with 7th [K, P], S82.001-S82.92X with 7th [K,
M, N, P, Q, R], S89.001-S89.399 with 7th [K, P],
S92.001-S92.919 with 7th [K, P]

7 √7ᵗʰ **S82.169** **Torus fracture of upper end of** `CC`
unspecified tibia

CC Excl: CC with 7th character A: S82.101-
S82.299 with 7th [A, B, C], S82.311-S82.319
with 7th A, S82.401-S82.839 with 7th [A, B,
C], S82.861-S82.866 with 7th [A, B, C],
S89.001-S89.099 with 7th A, S89.201-
S89.299 with 7th A

CC with 7th character K or P: M80.00X-
M84.68X with 7th [K, P], S02.0XX-S02.92X
with 7th K, S12.000-S12.691 with 7th K,
S22.000-S22.9XX with 7th K, S32.000-
S32.9XX with 7th K, S42.001-S42.92X with
7th [K, P], S49.001-S49.199 with 7th [K, P],
S52.001-S52.92X with 7th [K, M, N, P, Q, R],
S59.001-S59.299 with 7th [K, P], S62.001-
S62.92X with 7th [K, P], S72.001-S72.92X
with 7th [K, M, N, P, Q, R], S79.001-S79.199
with 7th [K, P], S82.001-S82.92X with 7th [K,
M, N, P, Q, R], S89.001-S89.399 with 7th [K, P],
S92.001-S92.919 with 7th [K, P]

√6ᵗʰ **S82.19** Other fracture of upper end of tibia

7 √7ᵗʰ **S82.191** **Other fracture of upper end** `MCC` `CC`
of right tibia
CC Excl: See code: S82.101

7 √7ᵗʰ **S82.192** **Other fracture of upper end** `MCC` `CC`
of left tibia
CC Excl: See code: S82.102

7 √7ᵗʰ **S82.199** **Other fracture of upper end of** `MCC` `CC`
unspecified tibia
CC Excl: See code: S82.109

√5ᵗʰ **S82.2** Fracture of shaft of tibia

√6ᵗʰ **S82.20** **Unspecified fracture of shaft of tibia**
Fracture of tibia NOS

7 √7ᵗʰ **S82.201** **Unspecified fracture of shaft of** `MCC` `CC`
right tibia

CC Excl: CC with 7th character A: M80.00X-
M80.019 with 7th A, M80.041-M80.049 with
7th A, M80.061-M80.079 with 7th A,
M80.80X-M80.819 with 7th A, M80.841-
M80.849 with 7th A, M80.861-M80.879 with
7th A, M84.40X-M84.419 with 7th A,
M84.441-M84.446 with 7th A, M84.454 with
7th A, M84.461-M84.519 with 7th A,
M84.541-M84.550 with 7th A, M84.561-
M84.576 with 7th A, M84.60X-M84.619 with
7th A, M84.641-M84.650 with 7th A,
M84.661-M84.68 with 7th A, S03.8XX-
S03.9XX with 7th A, S29.011-S29.019 with
7th A, S38.3XX-S39.013 with 7th A, S73.101A,
S73.109-S73.111 with 7th A, S73.119-
S73.121 with 7th A, S73.129-S73.191 with
7th A, S73.199A, S76.001A, S76.009-S76.011
with 7th A, S76.019A, S76.091A, S76.099-
S76.101 with 7th A, S76.109-S76.111 with
7th A, S76.119A, S76.191A, S76.199-S76.201
with 7th A, S76.209-S76.211 with 7th A,
S76.219A, S76.291A, S76.299-S76.301 with
7th A, S76.309-S76.311 with 7th A, S76.319A,
S76.391A, S76.399-S76.801 with 7th A,
S76.809-S76.811 with 7th A, S76.819A,
S76.891A, S76.899-S76.901 with 7th A,
S76.909-S76.911 with 7th A, S76.919A,
S76.991A, S76.999A, S79.811A, S79.819-
S79.821 with 7th A, S79.829-S79.911 with
7th A, S79.919-S79.921 with 7th A, S79.929A,
S82.101-S82.161 with 7th [A, B, C], S82.169-
S82.299 with 7th A, S82.311 with 7th A,
S82.319 with 7th A, S82.401-S82.811 with
7th [A, B, C], S82.819-S82.821 with 7th A,
S82.829-S82.839 with 7th A, S82.861-
S82.866 with 7th [A, B, C], S82.90X-S82.92X
with 7th [A, B, C], S89.001A, S89.009-S89.011
with 7th A, S89.019-S89.021 with 7th A,
S89.029-S89.031 with 7th A, S89.039-
S89.041 with 7th A, S89.049-S89.091 with
7th A, S89.099A, S89.201A, S89.209-S89.211
with 7th A, S89.219-S89.221 with 7th A,
S89.229-S89.291 with 7th A, S89.299A,
T14.8-T14.91, T79.A9X-T79.9XX with 7th A

MCC with 7th B or C: M80.00X-M80.019
with 7th A, M80.041-M80.049 with 7th A,
M80.061-M80.079 with 7th A, M80.80X-
M80.819 with 7th A, M80.841-M80.849 with
7th A, M80.861-M80.879 with 7th A,
M84.40X-M84.419 with 7th A, M84.441-
M84.446 with 7th A, M84.454 with 7th A,
M84.461-M84.519 with 7th A, M84.541-
M84.550 with 7th A, M84.561-M84.576 with
7th A, M84.60X-M84.619 with 7th A,
M84.641-M84.650 with 7th A, M84.661-
M84.68 with 7th A, S03.8X-S03.9X with 7th A,
S29.011-S29.019 with 7th A, S38.3XX-
S39.013 with 7th A, S73.101-S73.199 with
7th A, S76.001-S76.019 with 7th A, S76.091-
S76.119 with 7th A, S76.191-S76.219 with
7th A, S76.291-S76.319 with 7th A, S76.391-
S76.819 with 7th A, S76.891-S76.919 with
7th A, S76.991-S76.999 with 7th A, S79.811-
S79.929 with 7th A, S82.101-S82.156 with
7th [A, B, C], S82.191-S82.299 with 7th [A, B,
C], S82.401-S82.499 with 7th [A, B, C],
S82.831-S82.839 with 7th [A, B, C], S82.861-
S82.866 with 7th [A, B, C], S82.90X-S82.92X
with 7th [A, B, C], S89.001-S89.099 with 7th
A, S89.201-S89.299 with 7th A, T14.8-T14.91,
T79.A9X-T79.9XX with 7th A

CC with 7th character K, M, N, P, Q or R:
M80.00X-M84.68X with 7th [K, P], S02.0XX-
S02.92X with 7th K, S12.000-S12.691 with
7th K, S22.000-S22.9XX with 7th K, S32.000-
S32.9XX with 7th K, S42.001-S42.92X with
7th [K, P], S49.001-S49.199 with 7th [K, P],
S52.001-S52.92X with 7th [K, M, N, P, Q, R],
S59.001-S59.299 with 7th [K, P], S62.001-
S62.92X with 7th [K, P], S72.001-S72.92X
with 7th [K, M, N, P, Q, R], S79.001-S79.199
with 7th [K, P], S82.001-S82.92X with 7th [K,
M, N, P, Q, R], S89.001-S89.399 with 7th [K, P],
S92.001-S92.919 with 7th [K, P]

7 HAC = Initial encounter only (7th character A, B or C) and not POA.

✓ Additional Character Required   √x7ᵗʰ *X*tension Alert   Unacceptable PDx   ● Manifestation   Hospital Acquired Condition   `EXCLUDES 1` Not Coded Here   `EXCLUDES 2` Not Included Here

ICD-10-CM Draft (2015)   **997**

Injury, Poisoning and Certain Other Consequences of External Causes

S82.202–S82.301

7 √7th **S82.202** **Unspecified fracture of shaft of left tibia** `MCC` `CC`
CC Excl: See code: S82.192

7 √7th **S82.209** **Unspecified fracture of shaft of unspecified tibia** `MCC` `CC`
CC Excl: See code: S82.199

√6th **S82.22** Transverse fracture of shaft of tibia

7 √7th **S82.221** **Displaced transverse fracture of shaft of right tibia** `MCC` `CC`
CC Excl: See code: S82.191

7 √7th **S82.222** **Displaced transverse fracture of shaft of left tibia** `MCC` `CC`
CC Excl: See code: S82.192

7 √7th **S82.223** **Displaced transverse fracture of shaft of unspecified tibia** `MCC` `CC`
CC Excl: See code: S82.199

7 √7th **S82.224** **Nondisplaced transverse fracture of shaft of right tibia** `MCC` `CC`
CC Excl: See code: S82.191

7 √7th **S82.225** **Nondisplaced transverse fracture of shaft of left tibia** `MCC` `CC`
CC Excl: See code: S82.192

7 √7th **S82.226** **Nondisplaced transverse fracture of shaft of unspecified tibia** `MCC` `CC`
CC Excl: See code: S82.199

√6th **S82.23** Oblique fracture of shaft of tibia

7 √7th **S82.231** **Displaced oblique fracture of shaft of right tibia** `MCC` `CC`
CC Excl: See code: S82.191

7 √7th **S82.232** **Displaced oblique fracture of shaft of left tibia** `MCC` `CC`
CC Excl: See code: S82.192

7 √7th **S82.233** **Displaced oblique fracture of shaft of unspecified tibia** `MCC` `CC`
CC Excl: See code: S82.199

7 √7th **S82.234** **Nondisplaced oblique fracture of shaft of right tibia** `MCC` `CC`
CC Excl: See code: S82.191

7 √7th **S82.235** **Nondisplaced oblique fracture of shaft of left tibia** `MCC` `CC`
CC Excl: See code: S82.192

7 √7th **S82.236** **Nondisplaced oblique fracture of shaft of unspecified tibia** `MCC` `CC`
CC Excl: See code: S82.199

√6th **S82.24** Spiral fracture of shaft of tibia
Toddler fracture

7 √7th **S82.241** **Displaced spiral fracture of shaft of right tibia** `MCC` `CC`
CC Excl: See code: S82.191

7 √7th **S82.242** **Displaced spiral fracture of shaft of left tibia** `MCC` `CC`
CC Excl: See code: S82.192

7 √7th **S82.243** **Displaced spiral fracture of shaft of unspecified tibia** `MCC` `CC`
CC Excl: See code: S82.199

7 √7th **S82.244** **Nondisplaced spiral fracture of shaft of right tibia** `MCC` `CC`
CC Excl: See code: S82.191

7 √7th **S82.245** **Nondisplaced spiral fracture of shaft of left tibia** `MCC` `CC`
CC Excl: See code: S82.192

7 √7th **S82.246** **Nondisplaced spiral fracture of shaft of unspecified tibia** `MCC` `CC`
CC Excl: See code: S82.199

√6th **S82.25** Comminuted fracture of shaft of tibia

7 √7th **S82.251** **Displaced comminuted fracture of shaft of right tibia** `MCC` `CC`
CC Excl: See code: S82.191

7 √7th **S82.252** **Displaced comminuted fracture of shaft of left tibia** `MCC` `CC`
CC Excl: See code: S82.192

7 √7th **S82.253** **Displaced comminuted fracture of shaft of unspecified tibia** `MCC` `CC`
CC Excl: See code: S82.199

7 √7th **S82.254** **Nondisplaced comminuted fracture of shaft of right tibia** `MCC` `CC`
CC Excl: See code: S82.191

7 √7th **S82.255** **Nondisplaced comminuted fracture of shaft of left tibia** `MCC` `CC`
CC Excl: See code: S82.192

7 √7th **S82.256** **Nondisplaced comminuted fracture of shaft of unspecified tibia** `MCC` `CC`
CC Excl: See code: S82.199

√6th **S82.26** Segmental fracture of shaft of tibia

7 √7th **S82.261** **Displaced segmental fracture of shaft of right tibia** `MCC` `CC`
CC Excl: See code: S82.191

7 √7th **S82.262** **Displaced segmental fracture of shaft of left tibia** `MCC` `CC`
CC Excl: See code: S82.192

7 √7th **S82.263** **Displaced segmental fracture of shaft of unspecified tibia** `MCC` `CC`
CC Excl: See code: S82.199

7 √7th **S82.264** **Nondisplaced segmental fracture of shaft of right tibia** `MCC` `CC`
CC Excl: See code: S82.191

7 √7th **S82.265** **Nondisplaced segmental fracture of shaft of left tibia** `MCC` `CC`
CC Excl: See code: S82.192

7 √7th **S82.266** **Nondisplaced segmental fracture of shaft of unspecified tibia** `MCC` `CC`
CC Excl: See code: S82.199

√6th **S82.29** Other fracture of shaft of tibia

7 √7th **S82.291** **Other fracture of shaft of right tibia** `MCC` `CC`
CC Excl: See code: S82.191

7 √7th **S82.292** **Other fracture of shaft of left tibia** `MCC` `CC`
CC Excl: See code: S82.192

7 √7th **S82.299** **Other fracture of shaft of unspecified tibia** `MCC` `CC`
CC Excl: See code: S82.199

√5th **S82.3** Fracture of lower end of tibia
`EXCLUDES 1` bimalleolar fracture of lower leg (S82.84-)
fracture of medial malleolus alone (S82.5-)
Maisonneuve's fracture (S82.86-)
pilon fracture of distal tibia (S82.87-)
trimalleolar fractures of lower leg (S82.85-)

√6th **S82.30** Unspecified fracture of lower end of tibia

CC Excl: For CC codes in subcategory S82.30, unless otherwise noted: CC with 7th character B or C: M80.00X-M80.019 with 7th A, M80.041-M80.049 with 7th A, M80.061-M80.079 with 7th A, M80.80X-M80.819 with 7th A, M80.841-M80.849 with 7th A, M80.861-M80.879 with 7th A, M84.40X-M84.419 with 7th A, M84.441-M84.446 with 7th A, M84.454 with 7th A, M84.461-M84.519 with 7th A, M84.541-M84.550 with 7th A, M84.561-M84.576 with 7th A, M84.60X-M84.619 with 7th A, M84.641-M84.650 with 7th A, M84.661-M84.68 with 7th A, S03.8XX-S03.9XX with 7th A, S29.011-S29.019 with 7th A, S38.3XX-S39.013 with 7th A, S73.101-S73.199 with 7th A, S76.001-S76.019 with 7th A, S76.091-S76.119 with 7th A, S76.191-S76.219 with 7th A, S76.291-S76.319 with 7th A, S76.391-S76.819 with 7th A, S76.891-S76.919 with 7th A, S76.991-S76.999 with 7th A, S79.811-S79.929 with 7th A, S82.301-S82.309 with 7th [A, B, C], S82.391-S82.399 with 7th [A, B, C], S82.51X-S82.66X with 7th [B, C], S82.841-S82.856 with 7th [A, B, C], S82.871-S82.92X with 7th [B, C], S89.101-S89.199 with 7th A, S89.301-S89.399 with 7th A, T14.8-T14.91, T79.A9X-T79.9XX with 7th A
CC with 7th character K, M, N, P, Q or R: M80.00X-M84.68X with 7th [K, P], S02.0XX-S02.92X with 7th K, S12.000-S12.691 with 7th K, S22.000-S22.9XX with 7th K, S32.000-S32.9XX with 7th K, S42.001-S42.92X with 7th [K, P], S49.001-S49.199 with 7th [K, P], S52.001-S52.92X with 7th [K, M, N, P, Q, R], S59.001-S59.299 with 7th [K, P], S62.001-S62.92X with 7th [K, P], S72.001-S72.92X with 7th [K, M, N, P, Q, R], S79.001-S79.199 with 7th [K, P], S82.001-S82.92X with 7th [K, M, N, P, Q, R], S89.001-S89.399 with 7th [K, P], S92.001-S92.919 with 7th [K, P]

7 √7th **S82.301** **Unspecified fracture of lower end of right tibia** `CC`

---

7 HAC = Initial encounter only (7th character A, B or C) and not POA.

7 √7ᵗʰ **S82.302 Unspecified fracture of lower end of left tibia** `CC`

7 √7ᵗʰ **S82.309 Unspecified fracture of lower end of unspecified tibia** `CC`

√6ᵗʰ **S82.31 Torus fracture of lower end of tibia**

> The appropriate 7th character is to be added to all codes in subcategory S82.31.
> A initial encounter for closed fracture
> D subsequent encounter for fracture with routine healing
> G subsequent encounter for fracture with delayed healing
> K subsequent encounter for fracture with nonunion
> P subsequent encounter for fracture with malunion
> S sequela

7 √7ᵗʰ **S82.311 Torus fracture of lower end of right tibia** `CC`

CC Excl: CC with 7th character A: S82.101-S82.161 with 7th [A, B, C], S82.169-S82.299 with 7th A, S82.311 with 7th A, S82.319 with 7th A, S82.401-S82.811 with 7th [A, B, C], S82.819-S82.821 with 7th A, S82.829-S82.839 with 7th A, S82.861-S82.866 with 7th [A, B, C], S89.001 with 7th A, S89.009-S89.011 with 7th A, S89.019-S89.021 with 7th A, S89.029-S89.031 with 7th A, S89.039-S89.041 with 7th A, S89.049-S89.091 with 7th A, S89.099A, S89.201A, S89.209-S89.211 with 7th A, S89.219-S89.221 with 7th A, S89.229-S89.291 with 7th A, S89.299A
CC with 7th character K or P: M80.00X-M84.68X with 7th [K, P], S02.0XX-S02.92X with 7th K, S12.000-S12.691 with 7th K, S22.000-S22.9XX with 7th K, S32.000-S32.9XX with 7th K, S42.001-S42.92X with 7th [K, P], S49.001-S49.199 with 7th [K, P], S52.001-S52.92X with 7th [K, M, N, P, Q, R], S59.001-S59.299 with 7th [K, P], S62.001-S62.92X with 7th [K, P], S72.001-S72.92X with 7th [K, M, N, P, Q, R], S79.001-S79.199 with 7th [K, P], S82.001-S82.92X with 7th [K, M, N, P, Q, R], S89.001-S89.399 with 7th [K, P], S92.001-S92.919 with 7th [K, P]

7 √7ᵗʰ **S82.312 Torus fracture of lower end of left tibia** `CC`

CC Excl: CC with 7th character A: S82.101-S82.156 with 7th [B, C], S82.162-S82.299 with 7th A, S82.312-S82.319 with 7th A, S82.401-S82.499 with 7th [B, C], S82.812-S82.819 with 7th A, S82.822-S82.839 with 7th A, S82.861-S82.866 with 7th [B, C], S89.002-S89.009 with 7th A, S89.012-S89.019 with 7th A, S89.022-S89.029 with 7th A, S89.032-S89.039 with 7th A, S89.042-S89.049 with 7th A, S89.092-S89.099 with 7th A, S89.202-S89.209 with 7th A, S89.212-S89.219 with 7th A, S89.222-S89.229 with 7th A, S89.292-S89.299 with 7th A
CC with 7th character K or P: M80.00X-M84.68X with 7th [K, P], S02.0XX-S02.92X with 7th K, S12.000-S12.691 with 7th K, S22.000-S22.9XX with 7th K, S32.000-S32.9XX with 7th K, S42.001-S42.92X with 7th [K, P], S49.001-S49.199 with 7th [K, P], S52.001-S52.92X with 7th [K, M, N, P, Q, R], S59.001-S59.299 with 7th [K, P], S62.001-S62.92X with 7th [K, P], S72.001-S72.92X with 7th [K, M, N, P, Q, R], S79.001-S79.199 with 7th [K, P], S82.001-S82.92X with 7th [K, M, N, P, Q, R], S89.001-S89.399 with 7th [K, P], S92.001-S92.919 with 7th [K, P]

7 √7ᵗʰ **S82.319 Torus fracture of lower end of unspecified tibia** `CC`

CC Excl: CC with 7th character A: S82.101-S82.299 with 7th [A, B, C], S82.311-S82.319 with 7th A, S82.401-S82.839 with 7th [A, B, C], S82.861-S82.866 with 7th [A, B, C], S89.001-S89.099 with 7th A, S89.201-S89.299 with 7th A
CC with 7th character K or P: M80.00X-M84.68X with 7th [K, P], S02.0XX-S02.92X with 7th K, S12.000-S12.691 with 7th K, S22.000-S22.9XX with 7th K, S32.000-S32.9XX with 7th K, S42.001-S42.92X with 7th [K, P], S49.001-S49.199 with 7th [K, P], S52.001-S52.92X with 7th [K, M, N, P, Q, R], S59.001-S59.299 with 7th [K, P], S62.001-S62.92X with 7th [K, P], S72.001-S72.92X with 7th [K, M, N, P, Q, R], S79.001-S79.199 with 7th [K, P], S82.001-S82.92X with 7th [K, M, N, P, Q, R], S89.001-S89.399 with 7th [K, P], S92.001-S92.919 with 7th [K, P]

√6ᵗʰ **S82.39 Other fracture of lower end of tibia**

> **CC Excl: For CC codes in subcategory S82.39, unless otherwise noted:** See code: S82.30

7 √7ᵗʰ **S82.391 Other fracture of lower end of right tibia** `CC`

7 √7ᵗʰ **S82.392 Other fracture of lower end of left tibia** `CC`

7 √7ᵗʰ **S82.399 Other fracture of lower end of unspecified tibia** `CC`

√5ᵗʰ **S82.4 Fracture of shaft of fibula**

EXCLUDES 2 fracture of lateral malleolus alone (S82.6-)

> **CC Excl: For CC codes in subcategory S82.4, unless otherwise noted: MCC for codes with 7th B or C:** M80.00X-M80.019 with 7th A, M80.041-M80.049 with 7th A, M80.061-M80.079 with 7th A, M80.80X-M80.819 with 7th A, M80.841-M80.849 with 7th A, M80.861-M80.879 with 7th A, M84.40X-M84.419 with 7th A, M84.441-M84.446 with 7th A, M84.454 with 7th A, M84.461-M84.519 with 7th A, M84.541-M84.550 with 7th A, M84.561-M84.576 with 7th A, M84.60X-M84.619 with 7th A, M84.641-M84.650 with 7th A, M84.661-M84.68 with 7th A, S03.8XX-S03.9XX with 7th A, S29.011-S29.019 with 7th A, S38.3XX-S39.013 with 7th A, S73.101-S73.199 with 7th A, S76.001-S76.019 with 7th A, S76.091-S76.119 with 7th A, S76.191-S76.219 with 7th A, S76.291-S76.319 with 7th A, S76.391-S76.819 with 7th A, S76.891-S76.919 with 7th A, S76.991-S76.999 with 7th A, S79.811-S79.929 with 7th A, S82.101-S82.156 with 7th [A, B, C], S82.191-S82.299 with 7th [A, B, C], S82.401-S82.499 with 7th [A, B, C], S82.831-S82.839 with 7th [A, B, C], S82.861-S82.866 with 7th [A, B, C], S82.90X-S82.92X with 7th [A, B, C], S89.001-S89.099 with 7th A, S89.201-S89.299 with 7th A, T14.8-T14.91, T79.A9X-T79.9XX with 7th A
> **CC with 7th character K, M, N, P, Q or R:** M80.00X-M84.68X with 7th [K, P], S02.0XX-S02.92X with 7th K, S12.000-S12.691 with 7th K, S22.000-S22.9XX with 7th K, S32.000-S32.9XX with 7th K, S42.001-S42.92X with 7th [K, P], S49.001-S49.199 with 7th [K, P], S52.001-S52.92X with 7th [K, M, N, P, Q, R], S59.001-S59.299 with 7th [K, P], S62.001-S62.92X with 7th [K, P], S72.001-S72.92X with 7th [K, M, N, P, Q, R], S79.001-S79.199 with 7th [K, P], S82.001-S82.92X with 7th [K, M, N, P, Q, R], S89.001-S89.399 with 7th [K, P], S92.001-S92.919 with 7th [K, P]

√6ᵗʰ **S82.40 Unspecified fracture of shaft of fibula**

7 √7ᵗʰ **S82.401 Unspecified fracture of shaft of right fibula** `MCC` `CC`

7 √7ᵗʰ **S82.402 Unspecified fracture of shaft of left fibula** `MCC` `CC`

7 √7ᵗʰ **S82.409 Unspecified fracture of shaft of unspecified fibula** `MCC` `CC`

√6ᵗʰ **S82.42 Transverse fracture of shaft of fibula**

7 √7ᵗʰ **S82.421 Displaced transverse fracture of shaft of right fibula** `MCC` `CC`

7 √7ᵗʰ **S82.422 Displaced transverse fracture of shaft of left fibula** `MCC` `CC`

7 √7ᵗʰ **S82.423 Displaced transverse fracture of shaft of unspecified fibula** `MCC` `CC`

7 √7ᵗʰ **S82.424 Nondisplaced transverse fracture of shaft of right fibula** `MCC` `CC`

7 √7ᵗʰ **S82.425 Nondisplaced transverse fracture of shaft of left fibula** `MCC` `CC`

7 HAC = Initial encounter only (7th character A, B or C) and not POA.

☑ Additional Character Required √x7ᵗʰ Xtension Alert Unacceptable PDx Manifestation Hospital Acquired Condition *EXCLUDES 1* Not Coded Here *EXCLUDES 2* Not Included Here
ICD-10-CM Draft (2015) 999

7 √7ᵗʰ **S82.426** Nondisplaced transverse fracture of shaft of unspecified fibula `MCC` `CC`

√6ᵗʰ **S82.43** Oblique fracture of shaft of fibula

7 √7ᵗʰ **S82.431** Displaced oblique fracture of shaft of right fibula `MCC` `CC`

7 √7ᵗʰ **S82.432** Displaced oblique fracture of shaft of left fibula `MCC` `CC`

7 √7ᵗʰ **S82.433** Displaced oblique fracture of shaft of unspecified fibula `MCC` `CC`

7 √7ᵗʰ **S82.434** Nondisplaced oblique fracture of shaft of right fibula `MCC` `CC`

7 √7ᵗʰ **S82.435** Nondisplaced oblique fracture of shaft of left fibula `MCC` `CC`

7 √7ᵗʰ **S82.436** Nondisplaced oblique fracture of shaft of unspecified fibula `MCC` `CC`

√6ᵗʰ **S82.44** Spiral fracture of shaft of fibula

7 √7ᵗʰ **S82.441** Displaced spiral fracture of shaft of right fibula `MCC` `CC`

7 √7ᵗʰ **S82.442** Displaced spiral fracture of shaft of left fibula `MCC` `CC`

7 √7ᵗʰ **S82.443** Displaced spiral fracture of shaft of unspecified fibula `MCC` `CC`

7 √7ᵗʰ **S82.444** Nondisplaced spiral fracture of shaft of right fibula `MCC` `CC`

7 √7ᵗʰ **S82.445** Nondisplaced spiral fracture of shaft of left fibula `MCC` `CC`

7 √7ᵗʰ **S82.446** Nondisplaced spiral fracture of sahft of unspecified fibula `MCC` `CC`

√6ᵗʰ **S82.45** Comminuted fracture of shaft of fibula

7 √7ᵗʰ **S82.451** Displaced comminuted fracture of shaft of right fibula `MCC` `CC`

7 √7ᵗʰ **S82.452** Displaced comminuted fracture of shaft of left fibula `MCC` `CC`

7 √7ᵗʰ **S82.453** Displaced comminuted fracture of shaft of unspecified fibula `MCC` `CC`

7 √7ᵗʰ **S82.454** Nondisplaced comminuted fracture of shaft of right fibula `MCC` `CC`

7 √7ᵗʰ **S82.455** Nondisplaced comminuted fracture of shaft of left fibula `MCC` `CC`

7 √7ᵗʰ **S82.456** Nondisplaced comminuted fracture of shaft of unspecified fibula `MCC` `CC`

√6ᵗʰ **S82.46** Segmental fracture of shaft of fibula

7 √7ᵗʰ **S82.461** Displaced segmental fracture of shaft of right fibula `MCC` `CC`

7 √7ᵗʰ **S82.462** Displaced segmental fracture of shaft of left fibula `MCC` `CC`

7 √7ᵗʰ **S82.463** Displaced segmental fracture of shaft of unspecified fibula `MCC` `CC`

7 √7ᵗʰ **S82.464** Nondisplaced segmental fracture of shaft of right fibula `MCC` `CC`

7 √7ᵗʰ **S82.465** Nondisplaced segmental fracture of shaft of left fibula `MCC` `CC`

7 √7ᵗʰ **S82.466** Nondisplaced segmental fracture of shaft of unspecified fibula `MCC` `CC`

√6ᵗʰ **S82.49** Other fracture of shaft of fibula

7 √7ᵗʰ **S82.491** Other fracture of shaft of right fibula `MCC` `CC`

7 √7ᵗʰ **S82.492** Other fracture of shaft of left fibula `MCC` `CC`

7 √7ᵗʰ **S82.499** Other fracture of shaft of unspecified fibula `MCC` `CC`

√5ᵗʰ **S82.5** Fracture of medial malleolus

EXCLUDES 1 pilon fracture of distal tibia (S82.87-)
Salter-Harris type III of lower end of tibia (S89.13-)
Salter-Harris type IV of lower end of tibia (S89.14-)

CC Excl: For CC codes in subcategory S82.5, unless otherwise noted: CC with 7th character B or C: M80.00X-M80.019 with 7th A, M80.041-M80.049 with 7th A, M80.061-M80.079 with 7th A, M80.80X-M80.819 with 7th A, M80.841-M80.849 with 7th A, M80.861-M80.879 with 7th A, M84.40X-M84.419 with 7th A, M84.441-M84.446 with 7th A, M84.454 with 7th A, M84.461-M84.519 with 7th A, M84.541-M84.550 with 7th A, M84.561-M84.576 with 7th A, M84.60X-M84.619 with 7th A, M84.641-M84.650 with 7th A, M84.661-M84.68X with 7th A, S03.8XX-S03.9XX with 7th A, S29.011-S29.019 with 7th A, S38.3XX-S39.013 with 7th A, S73.101-S73.199 with 7th A, S76.001-S76.019 with 7th A, S76.091-S76.119 with 7th A, S76.191-S76.219 with 7th A, S76.291-S76.319 with 7th A, S76.391-S76.819 with 7th A, S76.891-S76.919 with 7th A, S76.991-S76.999 with 7th A, S79.811-S79.929 with 7th A, S82.301-S82.309 with 7th [A, B, C], S82.391-S82.399 with 7th [A, B, C], S82.51X-S82.66X with 7th [B, C], S82.841-S82.856 with 7th [A, B, C], S82.871-S82.92X with 7th [B, C], S89.101-S89.199 with 7th A, S89.301-S89.399 with 7th A, T14.8-T14.91, T79.A9X-T79.9XX with 7th A
CC with 7th character K, M, N, P, Q or R: M80.00X-M84.68X with 7th [K, P], S02.0XX-S02.92X with 7th K, S12.000-S12.691 with 7th K, S22.000-S22.9XX with 7th K, S32.000-S32.9XX with 7th K, S42.001-S42.92X with 7th [K, P], S49.001-S49.199 with 7th [K, P], S52.001-S52.92X with 7th [K, M, N, P, Q, R], S59.001-S59.299 with 7th [K, P], S62.001-S62.92X with 7th [K, P], S72.001-S72.92X with 7th [K, M, N, P, Q, R], S79.001-S79.199 with 7th [K, P], S82.001-S82.92X with 7th [K, M, N, P, Q, R], S89.001-S89.399 with 7th [K, P], S92.001-S92.919 with 7th [K, P]

7 √x 7ᵗʰ **S82.51** Displaced fracture of medial malleolus of right tibia `CC`

7 √x 7ᵗʰ **S82.52** Displaced fracture of medial malleolus of left tibia `CC`

7 √x 7ᵗʰ **S82.53** Displaced fracture of medial malleolus of unspecified tibia `CC`

7 √x 7ᵗʰ **S82.54** Nondisplaced fracture of medial malleolus of right tibia `CC`

7 √x 7ᵗʰ **S82.55** Nondisplaced fracture of medial malleolus of left tibia `CC`

7 √x 7ᵗʰ **S82.56** Nondisplaced fracture of medial malleolus of unspecified tibia `CC`

√5ᵗʰ **S82.6** Fracture of lateral malleolus

EXCLUDES 1 pilon fracture of distal tibia (S82.87-)

CC Excl: For CC codes in subcategory S82.5, unless otherwise noted: CC with 7th character B or C: M80.00X-M80.019 with 7th A, M80.041-M80.049 with 7th A, M80.061-M80.079 with 7th A, M80.80X-M80.819 with 7th A, M80.841-M80.849 with 7th A, M80.861-M80.879 with 7th A, M84.40X-M84.419 with 7th A, M84.441-M84.446 with 7th A, M84.454 with 7th A, M84.461-M84.519 with 7th A, M84.541-M84.550 with 7th A, M84.561-M84.576 with 7th A, M84.60X-M84.619 with 7th A, M84.641-M84.650 with 7th A, M84.661-M84.68X with 7th A, S03.8XX-S03.9XX with 7th A, S29.011-S29.019 with 7th A, S38.3XX-S39.013 with 7th A, S73.101-S73.199 with 7th A, S76.001-S76.019 with 7th A, S76.091-S76.119 with 7th A, S76.191-S76.219 with 7th A, S76.291-S76.319 with 7th A, S76.391-S76.819 with 7th A, S76.891-S76.919 with 7th A, S76.991-S76.999 with 7th A, S79.811-S79.929 with 7th A, S82.301-S82.309 with 7th [A, B, C], S82.391-S82.399 with 7th [A, B, C], S82.51X-S82.66X with 7th [B, C], S82.841-S82.856 with 7th [A, B, C], S82.871-S82.92X with 7th [B, C], S89.101-S89.199 with 7th A, S89.301-S89.399 with 7th A, T14.8-T14.91, T79.A9X-T79.9XX with 7th A
CC with 7th character K, M, N, P, Q or R: M80.00X-M84.68X with 7th [K, P], S02.0XX-S02.92X with 7th K, S12.000-S12.691 with 7th K, S22.000-S22.9XX with 7th K, S32.000-S32.9XX with 7th K, S42.001-S42.92X with 7th [K, P], S49.001-S49.199 with 7th [K, P], S52.001-S52.92X with 7th [K, M, N, P, Q, R], S59.001-S59.299 with 7th [K, P], S62.001-S62.92X with 7th [K, P], S72.001-S72.92X with 7th [K, M, N, P, Q, R], S79.001-S79.199 with 7th [K, P], S82.001-S82.92X with 7th [K, M, N, P, Q, R], S89.001-S89.399 with 7th [K, P], S92.001-S92.919 with 7th [K, P]

7 √x 7ᵗʰ **S82.61** Displaced fracture of lateral malleolus of right fibula `CC`

7 √x 7ᵗʰ **S82.62** Displaced fracture of lateral malleolus of left fibula `CC`

---

7 HAC = Initial encounter only (7th character A, B or C) and not POA.

Ⓝ Newborn: 0   Ⓟ Pediatric: 0-17   Ⓜ Maternity: 12-55   Ⓐ Adult: 15-124   `MCC` Major CC Condition   `PDx MCC` PDx acts as own MCC   `CC` CC Condition   `PDx CC` PDx acts as own CC

1000

ICD-10-CM Draft (2015)

7 ✓x7ᵗʰ **S82.63** Displaced **fracture of lateral malleolus of unspecified** fibula   CC

7 ✓x7ᵗʰ **S82.64** Nondisplaced **fracture of lateral malleolus of right** fibula   CC

7 ✓x7ᵗʰ **S82.65** Nondisplaced **fracture of lateral malleolus of left** fibula   CC

7 ✓x7ᵗʰ **S82.66** Nondisplaced **fracture of lateral malleolus of unspecified** fibula   CC

✓5ᵗʰ **S82.8** Other fractures of **lower leg**

✓6ᵗʰ **S82.81** Torus **fracture of upper end of fibula**

The appropriate 7th character is to be added to all codes in subcategory S82.81.
A   initial encounter for closed fracture
D   subsequent encounter for fracture with routine healing
G   subsequent encounter for fracture with delayed healing
K   subsequent encounter for fracture wit nonunion
P   subsequent encounter for fracture with malunion
S   sequela

CC Excl: For codes in subcatgory S82.81, unless otherwise noted: CC with 7th character K or P: See code S82.6

✓7ᵗʰ **S82.811** Torus **fracture of upper end of right** fibula   CC

✓7ᵗʰ **S82.812** Torus **fracture of upper end of left** fibula   CC

✓7ᵗʰ **S82.819** Torus **fracture of upper end of unspecified** fibula   CC

✓6ᵗʰ **S82.82** Torus **fracture of lower end of fibula**

The appropriate 7th character is to be added to all codes in subcategory S82.82.
A   initial encounter for closed fracture
D   subsequent encounter for fracture with routine healing
G   subsequent encounter for fracture with delayed healing
K   subsequent encounter for fracture with nonunion
P   subsequent encounter for fracture with malunion
S   sequela

CC Excl: For codes in subcatgory S82.82, unless otherwise noted: CC with 7th character K or P: See code S82.6

✓7ᵗʰ **S82.821** Torus **fracture of lower end of right** fibula   CC

✓7ᵗʰ **S82.822** Torus **fracture of lower end of left** fibula   CC

✓7ᵗʰ **S82.829** Torus **fracture of lower end of unspecified** fibula   CC

✓6ᵗʰ **S82.83** Other **fracture of upper and lower end of fibula**

CC Excl: For codes in subcategory S82.83, unless otherwise noted: MCC with 7th B or C: M80.00X-M80.019 with 7th A, M80.041-M80.049 with 7th A, M80.061-M80.079 with 7th A, M80.80X-M80.819 with 7th A, M80.841-M80.849 with 7th A, M80.861-M80.879 with 7th A, M84.40X-M84.419 with 7th A, M84.441-M84.446 with 7th A, M84.454 with 7th A, M84.461-M84.519 with 7th A, M84.541-M84.550 with 7th A, M84.561-M84.576 with 7th A, M84.60X-M84.619 with 7th A, M84.641-M84.650 with 7th A, M84.661-M84.68X with 7th A, S03.8XX-S03.9XX with 7th A, S29.011-S29.019 with 7th A, S38.3XX-S39.013 with 7th A, S73.101-S73.199 with 7th A, S76.001-S76.019 with 7th A, S76.091-S76.119 with 7th A, S76.191-S76.219 with 7th A, S76.291-S76.319 with 7th A, S76.391-S76.819 with 7th A, S76.891-S76.919 with 7th A, S76.991-S76.999 with 7th A, S79.811-S79.929 with 7th A, S82.101-S82.156 with 7th [A, B, C], S82.191-S82.299 with 7th [A, B, C], S82.401-S82.499 with 7th [A, B, C], S82.831-S82.839 with 7th [A, B, C], S82.861-S82.866 with 7th [A, B, C], S82.90X-S82.92X with 7th [A, B, C], S89.001-S89.099 with 7th A, S89.201-S89.299 with 7th A, T14.8-T14.91, T79.A9X-T79.9XX with 7th A
CC with 7th character K, M, N, P, Q or R: M80.00X-M84.68X with 7th [K, P], S02.0XX-S02.92X with 7th K, S12.000-S12.691 with 7th K, S22.000-S22.9XX with 7th K, S32.000-S32.9XX with 7th K, S42.001-S42.92X with 7th [K, P], S49.001-S49.199 with 7th [K, P], S52.001-S52.92X with 7th [K, M, N, P, Q, R], S59.001-S59.299 with 7th [K, P], S62.001-S62.92X with 7th [K, P], S72.001-S72.92X with 7th [K, M, N, P, Q, R], S79.001-S79.199 with 7th [K, P], S82.001-S82.92X with 7th [K, M, N, P, Q, R], S89.001-S89.399 with 7th [K, P], S92.001-S92.919 with 7th [K, P]

7 ✓7ᵗʰ **S82.831** Other **fracture of upper and lower end of right** fibula   MCC CC

7 ✓7ᵗʰ **S82.832** Other **fracture of upper and lower end of left** fibula   MCC CC

7 ✓7ᵗʰ **S82.839** Other **fracture of upper and lower end of unspecified** fibula   MCC CC

✓6ᵗʰ **S82.84** Bimalleolar **fracture of lower leg**

CC Excl: For codes in subcatgory S82.84, unless otherwise noted: CC with 7th character B or C: M80.00X-M80.019 with 7th A, M80.041-M80.049 with 7th A, M80.061-M80.079 with 7th A, M80.80X-M80.819 with 7th A, M80.841-M80.849 with 7th A, M80.861-M80.879 with 7th A, M84.40X-M84.419 with 7th A, M84.441-M84.446 with 7th A, M84.454 with 7th A, M84.461-M84.519 with 7th A, M84.541-M84.550 with 7th A, M84.561-M84.576 with 7th A, M84.60X-M84.619 with 7th A, M84.641-M84.650 with 7th A, M84.661-M84.68 with 7th A, S03.8XX-S03.9XX with 7th A, S29.011-S29.019 with 7th A, S38.3XX-S39.013 with 7th A, S73.101-S73.199 with 7th A, S76.001-S76.019 with 7th A, S76.091-S76.119 with 7th A, S76.191-S76.219 with 7th A, S76.291-S76.319 with 7th A, S76.391-S76.819 with 7th A, S76.891-S76.919 with 7th A, S76.991-S76.999 with 7th A, S79.811-S79.929 with 7th A, S82.301-S82.309 with 7th [A, B, C], S82.391-S82.399 with 7th [A, B, C], S82.51X-S82.66X with 7th [B, C], S82.841-S82.856 with 7th [A, B, C], S82.871-S82.92X with 7th [B, C], S89.101-S89.199 with 7th A, S89.301-S89.399 with 7th A, T14.8-T14.91, T79.A9X-T79.9XX with 7th A
CC with 7th character K, M, N, P, Q or R: M80.00X-M84.68X with 7th [K, P], S02.0XX-S02.92X with 7th K, S12.000-S12.691 with 7th K, S22.000-S22.9XX with 7th K, S32.000-S32.9XX with 7th K, S42.001-S42.92X with 7th [K, P], S49.001-S49.199 with 7th [K, P], S52.001-S52.92X with 7th [K, M, N, P, Q, R], S59.001-S59.299 with 7th [K, P], S62.001-S62.92X with 7th [K, P], S72.001-S72.92X with 7th [K, M, N, P, Q, R], S79.001-S79.199 with 7th [K, P], S82.001-S82.92X with 7th [K, M, N, P, Q, R], S89.001-S89.399 with 7th [K, P], S92.001-S92.919 with 7th [K, P]

7 ✓7ᵗʰ **S82.841** Displaced **bimalleolar fracture of right lower leg**   CC

7 ✓7ᵗʰ **S82.842** Displaced **bimalleolar fracture of left lower leg**   CC

7 ✓7ᵗʰ **S82.843** Displaced **bimalleolar fracture of unspecified lower leg**   CC

7 ✓7ᵗʰ **S82.844** Nondisplaced **bimalleolar fracture of right lower leg**   CC

7 HAC = Initial encounter only (7th character A, B or C) and not POA.

✓ Additional Character Required   ✓x7ᵗʰ Xtension Alert   Unacceptable PDx   Manifestation   Hospital Acquired Condition   EXCLUDES 1 Not Coded Here   EXCLUDES 2 Not Included Here

7 √7ᵗʰ **S82.845 Nondisplaced bimalleolar fracture of left lower leg** CC

7 √7ᵗʰ **S82.846 Nondisplaced bimalleolar fracture of unspecified lower leg** CC

√6ᵗʰ **S82.85 Trimalleolar fracture of lower leg**

> **CC Excl:** For codes in subcatgory S82.85, unless otherwise noted: See code: S82.84

7 √7ᵗʰ **S82.851 Displaced trimalleolar fracture of right lower leg** CC

7 √7ᵗʰ **S82.852 Displaced trimalleolar fracture of left lower leg** CC

7 √7ᵗʰ **S82.853 Displaced trimalleolar fracture of unspecified lower leg** CC

7 √7ᵗʰ **S82.854 Nondisplaced trimalleolar fracture of right lower leg** CC

7 √7ᵗʰ **S82.855 Nondisplaced trimalleolar fracture of left lower leg** CC

7 √7ᵗʰ **S82.856 Nondisplaced trimalleolar fracture of unspecified lower leg** CC

√6ᵗʰ **S82.86 Maisonneuve's fracture**

> **CC Excl:** For codes in subcatgory S82.86, unless otherwise noted: See code: S82.84

7 √7ᵗʰ **S82.861 Displaced Maisonneuve's fracture of right leg** MCC CC

7 √7ᵗʰ **S82.862 Displaced Maisonneuve's fracture of left leg** MCC CC

7 √7ᵗʰ **S82.863 Displaced Maisonneuve's fracture of unspecified leg** MCC CC

7 √7ᵗʰ **S82.864 Nondisplaced Maisonneuve's fracture of right leg** MCC CC

7 √7ᵗʰ **S82.865 Nondisplaced Maisonneuve's fracture of left leg** MCC CC

7 √7ᵗʰ **S82.866 Nondisplaced Maisonneuve's fracture of unspecified leg** MCC CC

√6ᵗʰ **S82.87 Pilon fracture of tibia**

> **CC Excl:** For codes in subcatgory S82.87, unless otherwise noted: See code: S82.85

7 √7ᵗʰ **S82.871 Displaced pilon fracture of right tibia** CC

7 √7ᵗʰ **S82.872 Displaced pilon fracture of left tibia** CC

7 √7ᵗʰ **S82.873 Displaced pilon fracture of unspecified tibia** CC

7 √7ᵗʰ **S82.874 Nondisplaced pilon fracture of right tibia** CC

7 √7ᵗʰ **S82.875 Nondisplaced pilon fracture of left tibia** CC

7 √7ᵗʰ **S82.876 Nondisplaced pilon fracture of unspecified tibia** CC

√6ᵗʰ **S82.89 Other fractures of lower leg**
Fracture of ankle NOS

> **CC Excl:** For codes in subcatgory S82.89, unless otherwise noted: See code: S82.84

7 √7ᵗʰ **S82.891 Other fracture of right lower leg** CC

7 √7ᵗʰ **S82.892 Other fracture of left lower leg** CC

7 √7ᵗʰ **S82.899 Other fracture of unspecified lower leg** CC

√5ᵗʰ **S82.9 Unspecified fracture of lower leg**

> **CC Excl:** For codes in subcatgory S82.9, unless otherwise noted: CC with 7th character B or C: See code: S82.84

7 √x7ᵗʰ **S82.90 Unspecified fracture of unspecified lower leg** CC

7 √x7ᵗʰ **S82.91 Unspecified fracture of right lower leg** CC

7 √x7ᵗʰ **S82.92 Unspecified fracture of left lower leg** CC

√4ᵗʰ **S83 Dislocation and sprain of joints and ligaments of knee**

> **INCLUDES**   avulsion of joint or ligament of knee
> laceration of cartilage, joint or ligament of knee
> sprain of cartilage, joint or ligament of knee
> traumatic hemarthrosis of joint or ligament of knee
> traumatic rupture of joint or ligament of knee
> traumatic subluxation of joint or ligament of knee
> traumatic tear of joint or ligament of knee

Code also any associated open wound

> **EXCLUDES 1**   derangement of patella (M22.0-M22.3)
> injury of patellar ligament (tendon) (S76.1-)
> internal derangement of knee (M23.-)
> old dislocation of knee (M24.36)
> pathological dislocation of knee (M24.36)
> recurrent dislocation of knee (M22.0)

> **EXCLUDES 2**   strain of muscle, fascia and tendon of lower leg (S86.-)

> The appropriate 7th character is to be added to each code from category S83.
> A   initial encounter
> D   subsequent encounter
> S   sequela

√5ᵗʰ **S83.0 Subluxation and dislocation of patella**

√6ᵗʰ **S83.00 Unspecified subluxation and dislocation of patella**

√7ᵗʰ **S83.001 Unspecified subluxation of right patella**

√7ᵗʰ **S83.002 Unspecified subluxation of left patella**

√7ᵗʰ **S83.003 Unspecified subluxation of unspecified patella**

√7ᵗʰ **S83.004 Unspecified dislocation of right patella**

√7ᵗʰ **S83.005 Unspecified dislocation of left patella**

√7ᵗʰ **S83.006 Unspecified dislocation of unspecified patella**

√6ᵗʰ **S83.01 Lateral subluxation and dislocation of patella**

√7ᵗʰ **S83.011 Lateral subluxation of right patella**

√7ᵗʰ **S83.012 Lateral subluxation of left patella**

√7ᵗʰ **S83.013 Lateral subluxation of unspecified patella**

√7ᵗʰ **S83.014 Lateral dislocation of right patella**

√7ᵗʰ **S83.015 Lateral dislocation of left patella**

√7ᵗʰ **S83.016 Lateral dislocation of unspecified patella**

√6ᵗʰ **S83.09 Other subluxation and dislocation of patella**

√7ᵗʰ **S83.091 Other subluxation of right patella**

√7ᵗʰ **S83.092 Other subluxation of left patella**

√7ᵗʰ **S83.093 Other subluxation of unspecified patella**

√7ᵗʰ **S83.094 Other dislocation of right patella**

√7ᵗʰ **S83.095 Other dislocation of left patella**

√7ᵗʰ **S83.096 Other dislocation of unspecified patella**

√5ᵗʰ **S83.1 Subluxation and dislocation of knee**

> **EXCLUDES 2**   instability of knee prosthesis (T84.022, T84.023)

√6ᵗʰ **S83.10 Unspecified subluxation and dislocation of knee**

√7ᵗʰ **S83.101 Unspecified subluxation of right knee**

√7ᵗʰ **S83.102 Unspecified subluxation of left knee**

√7ᵗʰ **S83.103 Unspecified subluxation of unspecified knee**

√7ᵗʰ **S83.104 Unspecified dislocation of right knee**

√7ᵗʰ **S83.105 Unspecified dislocation of left knee**

√7ᵗʰ **S83.106 Unspecified dislocation of unspecified knee**

√6ᵗʰ **S83.11 Anterior subluxation and dislocation of proximal end of tibia**
Posterior subluxation and dislocation of distal end of femur

√7ᵗʰ **S83.111 Anterior subluxation of proximal end of tibia, right knee**

√7ᵗʰ **S83.112 Anterior subluxation of proximal end of tibia, left knee**

√7ᵗʰ **S83.113 Anterior subluxation of proximal end of tibia, unspecified knee**

√7ᵗʰ **S83.114 Anterior dislocation of proximal end of tibia, right knee**

√7ᵗʰ **S83.115 Anterior dislocation of proximal end of tibia, left knee**

√7ᵗʰ **S83.116 Anterior dislocation of proximal end of tibia, unspecified knee**

---

7 HAC = Initial encounter only (7th character A, B or C) and not POA.

N Newborn: 0   P Pediatric: 0-17   M Maternity: 12-55   A Adult: 15-124   MCC Major CC Condition   PDx MCC PDx acts as own MCC   CC CC Condition   PDx CC PDx acts as own CC

1002   ICD-10-CM Draft (2015)

✓6ᵗʰ **S83.12 Posterior subluxation and dislocation of proximal end of tibia**
Anterior dislocation of distal end of femur

    ✓7ᵗʰ **S83.121 Posterior subluxation of proximal end of tibia, right knee**

    ✓7ᵗʰ **S83.122 Posterior subluxation of proximal end of tibia, left knee**

    ✓7ᵗʰ **S83.123 Posterior subluxation of proximal end of tibia, unspecified knee**

    ✓7ᵗʰ **S83.124 Posterior dislocation of proximal end of tibia, right knee**

    ✓7ᵗʰ **S83.125 Posterior dislocation of proximal end of tibia, left knee**

    ✓7ᵗʰ **S83.126 Posterior dislocation of proximal end of tibia, unspecified knee**

✓6ᵗʰ **S83.13 Medial subluxation and dislocation of proximal end of tibia**

    ✓7ᵗʰ **S83.131 Medial subluxation of proximal end of tibia, right knee**

    ✓7ᵗʰ **S83.132 Medial subluxation of proximal end of tibia, left knee**

    ✓7ᵗʰ **S83.133 Medial subluxation of proximal end of tibia, unspecified knee**

    ✓7ᵗʰ **S83.134 Medial dislocation of proximal end of tibia, right knee**

    ✓7ᵗʰ **S83.135 Medial dislocation of proximal end of tibia, left knee**

    ✓7ᵗʰ **S83.136 Medial dislocation of proximal end of tibia, unspecified knee**

✓6ᵗʰ **S83.14 Lateral subluxation and dislocation of proximal end of tibia**

    ✓7ᵗʰ **S83.141 Lateral subluxation of proximal end of tibia, right knee**

    ✓7ᵗʰ **S83.142 Lateral subluxation of proximal end of tibia, left knee**

    ✓7ᵗʰ **S83.143 Lateral subluxation of proximal end of tibia, unspecified knee**

    ✓7ᵗʰ **S83.144 Lateral dislocation of proximal end of tibia, right knee**

    ✓7ᵗʰ **S83.145 Lateral dislocation of proximal end of tibia, left knee**

    ✓7ᵗʰ **S83.146 Lateral dislocation of proximal end of tibia, unspecified knee**

✓6ᵗʰ **S83.19 Other subluxation and dislocation of knee**

    ✓7ᵗʰ **S83.191 Other subluxation of right knee**

    ✓7ᵗʰ **S83.192 Other subluxation of left knee**

    ✓7ᵗʰ **S83.193 Other subluxation of unspecified knee**

    ✓7ᵗʰ **S83.194 Other dislocation of right knee**

    ✓7ᵗʰ **S83.195 Other dislocation of left knee**

    ✓7ᵗʰ **S83.196 Other dislocation of unspecified knee**

✓5ᵗʰ **S83.2 Tear of meniscus, current injury**
EXCLUDES 1   old bucket-handle tear (M23.2)

✓6ᵗʰ **S83.20 Tear of unspecified meniscus, current injury**
Tear of meniscus of knee NOS

    ✓7ᵗʰ **S83.200 Bucket-handle tear of unspecified meniscus, current injury, right knee**

    ✓7ᵗʰ **S83.201 Bucket-handle tear of unspecified meniscus, current injury, left knee**

    ✓7ᵗʰ **S83.202 Bucket-handle tear of unspecified meniscus, current injury, unspecified knee**

    ✓7ᵗʰ **S83.203 Other tear of unspecified meniscus, current injury, right knee**

    ✓7ᵗʰ **S83.204 Other tear of unspecified meniscus, current injury, left knee**

    ✓7ᵗʰ **S83.205 Other tear of unspecified meniscus, current injury, unspecified knee**

    ✓7ᵗʰ **S83.206 Unspecified tear of unspecified meniscus, current injury, right knee**

    ✓7ᵗʰ **S83.207 Unspecified tear of unspecified meniscus, current injury, left knee**

    ✓7ᵗʰ **S83.209 Unspecified tear of unspecified meniscus, current injury, unspecified knee**

✓6ᵗʰ **S83.21 Bucket-handle tear of medial meniscus, current injury**

    ✓7ᵗʰ **S83.211 Bucket-handle tear of medial meniscus, current injury, right knee**

    ✓7ᵗʰ **S83.212 Bucket-handle tear of medial meniscus, current injury, left knee**

    ✓7ᵗʰ **S83.219 Bucket-handle tear of medial meniscus, current injury, unspecified knee**

✓6ᵗʰ **S83.22 Peripheral tear of medial meniscus, current injury**

    ✓7ᵗʰ **S83.221 Peripheral tear of medial meniscus, current injury, right knee**

    ✓7ᵗʰ **S83.222 Peripheral tear of medial meniscus, current injury, left knee**

    ✓7ᵗʰ **S83.229 Peripheral tear of medial meniscus, current injury, unspecified knee**

✓6ᵗʰ **S83.23 Complex tear of medial meniscus, current injury**

    ✓7ᵗʰ **S83.231 Complex tear of medial meniscus, current injury, right knee**

    ✓7ᵗʰ **S83.232 Complex tear of medial meniscus, current injury, left knee**

    ✓7ᵗʰ **S83.239 Complex tear of medial meniscus, current injury, unspecified knee**

✓6ᵗʰ **S83.24 Other tear of medial meniscus, current injury**

    ✓7ᵗʰ **S83.241 Other tear of medial meniscus, current injury, right knee**

    ✓7ᵗʰ **S83.242 Other tear of medial meniscus, current injury, left knee**

    ✓7ᵗʰ **S83.249 Other tear of medial meniscus, current injury, unspecified knee**

✓6ᵗʰ **S83.25 Bucket-handle tear of lateral meniscus, current injury**

    ✓7ᵗʰ **S83.251 Bucket-handle tear of lateral meniscus, current injury, right knee**

    ✓7ᵗʰ **S83.252 Bucket-handle tear of lateral meniscus, current injury, left knee**

    ✓7ᵗʰ **S83.259 Bucket-handle tear of lateral meniscus, current injury, unspecified knee**

✓6ᵗʰ **S83.26 Peripheral tear of lateral meniscus, current injury**

    ✓7ᵗʰ **S83.261 Peripheral tear of lateral meniscus, current injury, right knee**

    ✓7ᵗʰ **S83.262 Peripheral tear of lateral meniscus, current injury, left knee**

    ✓7ᵗʰ **S83.269 Peripheral tear of lateral meniscus, current injury, unspecified knee**

✓6ᵗʰ **S83.27 Complex tear of lateral meniscus, current injury**

    ✓7ᵗʰ **S83.271 Complex tear of lateral meniscus, current injury, right knee**

    ✓7ᵗʰ **S83.272 Complex tear of lateral meniscus, current injury, left knee**

    ✓7ᵗʰ **S83.279 Complex tear of lateral meniscus, current injury, unspecified knee**

✓6ᵗʰ **S83.28 Other tear of lateral meniscus, current injury**

    ✓7ᵗʰ **S83.281 Other tear of lateral meniscus, current injury, right knee**

    ✓7ᵗʰ **S83.282 Other tear of lateral meniscus, current injury, left knee**

    ✓7ᵗʰ **S83.289 Other tear of lateral meniscus, current injury, unspecified knee**

✓5ᵗʰ **S83.3 Tear of articular cartilage of knee, current**

    ✓x7ᵗʰ **S83.30 Tear of articular cartilage of unspecified knee, current**

    ✓x7ᵗʰ **S83.31 Tear of articular cartilage of right knee, current**

    ✓x7ᵗʰ **S83.32 Tear of articular cartilage of left knee, current**

✓5ᵗʰ **S83.4 Sprain of collateral ligament of knee**

✓6ᵗʰ **S83.40 Sprain of unspecified collateral ligament of knee**

    ✓7ᵗʰ **S83.401 Sprain of unspecified collateral ligament of right knee**

    ✓7ᵗʰ **S83.402 Sprain of unspecified collateral ligament of left knee**

    ✓7ᵗʰ **S83.409 Sprain of unspecified collateral ligament of unspecified knee**

✓ Additional Character Required   ✓x7ᵗʰ Xtension Alert   Unacceptable PDx   Manifestation   Hospital Acquired Condition   EXCLUDES 1 Not Coded Here   EXCLUDES 2 Not Included Here

✓6th **S83.41** Sprain of medial collateral ligament of knee
Sprain of tibial collateral ligament

  ✓7th **S83.411** Sprain of medial collateral ligament of right knee

  ✓7th **S83.412** Sprain of medial collateral ligament of left knee

  ✓7th **S83.419** Sprain of medial collateral ligament of unspecified knee

✓6th **S83.42** Sprain of lateral collateral ligament of knee
Sprain of fibular collateral ligament

  ✓7th **S83.421** Sprain of lateral collateral ligament of right knee

  ✓7th **S83.422** Sprain of lateral collateral ligament of left knee

  ✓7th **S83.429** Sprain of lateral collateral ligament of unspecified knee

✓5th **S83.5** Sprain of cruciate ligament of knee

  ✓6th **S83.50** Sprain of unspecified cruciate ligament of knee

    ✓7th **S83.501** Sprain of unspecified cruciate ligament of right knee

    ✓7th **S83.502** Sprain of unspecified cruciate ligament of left knee

    ✓7th **S83.509** Sprain of unspecified cruciate ligament of unspecified knee

  ✓6th **S83.51** Sprain of anterior cruciate ligament of knee

    ✓7th **S83.511** Sprain of anterior cruciate ligament of right knee

    ✓7th **S83.512** Sprain of anterior cruciate ligament of left knee

    ✓7th **S83.519** Sprain of anterior cruciate ligament of unspecified knee

  ✓6th **S83.52** Sprain of posterior cruciate ligament of knee

    ✓7th **S83.521** Sprain of posterior cruciate ligament of right knee

    ✓7th **S83.522** Sprain of posterior cruciate ligament of left knee

    ✓7th **S83.529** Sprain of posterior cruciate ligament of unspecified knee

✓5th **S83.6** Sprain of the superior tibiofibular joint and ligament

  ✓x7th **S83.60** Sprain of the superior tibiofibular joint and ligament, unspecified knee

  ✓x7th **S83.61** Sprain of the superior tibiofibular joint and ligament, right knee

  ✓x7th **S83.62** Sprain of the superior tibiofibular joint and ligament, left knee

✓5th **S83.8** Sprain of other specified parts of knee

  ✓6th **S83.8X** Sprain of other specified parts of knee

    ✓7th **S83.8X1** Sprain of other specified parts of right knee

    ✓7th **S83.8X2** Sprain of other specified parts of left knee

    ✓7th **S83.8X9** Sprain of other specified parts of unspecified knee

✓5th **S83.9** Sprain of unspecified site of knee

  ✓x7th **S83.90** Sprain of unspecified site of unspecified knee

  ✓x7th **S83.91** Sprain of unspecified site of right knee

  ✓x7th **S83.92** Sprain of unspecified site of left knee

✓4th **S84** Injury of nerves at lower leg level
Code also any associated open wound (S81.-)
EXCLUDES 2 *injury of nerves at ankle and foot level (S94.-)*

> The appropriate 7th character is to be added to each code from category S84.
> A   initial encounter
> D   subsequent encounter
> S   sequela

✓5th **S84.0** Injury of tibial nerve at lower leg level

  ✓x7th **S84.00** Injury of tibial nerve at lower leg level, unspecified leg

  ✓x7th **S84.01** Injury of tibial nerve at lower leg level, right leg

  ✓x7th **S84.02** Injury of tibial nerve at lower leg level, left leg

✓5th **S84.1** Injury of peroneal nerve at lower leg level

  ✓x7th **S84.10** Injury of peroneal nerve at lower leg level, unspecified leg

  ✓x7th **S84.11** Injury of peroneal nerve at lower leg level, right leg

  ✓x7th **S84.12** Injury of peroneal nerve at lower leg level, left leg

✓5th **S84.2** Injury of cutaneous sensory nerve at lower leg level

  ✓x7th **S84.20** Injury of cutaneous sensory nerve at lower leg level, unspecified

  ✓x7th **S84.21** Injury of cutaneous sensory nerve at lower leg level, right leg

  ✓x7th **S84.22** Injury of cutaneous sensory nerve at lower leg level, left leg

✓5th **S84.8** Injury of other nerves at lower leg level

  ✓6th **S84.80** Injury of other nerves at lower leg level

    ✓7th **S84.801** Injury of other nerves at lower leg level, right leg

    ✓7th **S84.802** Injury of other nerves at lower leg level, left leg

    ✓7th **S84.809** Injury of other nerves at lower leg level, unspecified leg

✓5th **S84.9** Injury of unspecified nerve at lower leg level

  ✓x7th **S84.90** Injury of unspecified nerve at lower leg level, unspecified leg

  ✓x7th **S84.91** Injury of unspecified nerve at lower leg level, right leg

  ✓x7th **S84.92** Injury of unspecified nerve at lower leg level, left leg

✓4th **S85** Injury of blood vessels at lower leg level
Code also any associated open wound (S81.-)
EXCLUDES 2 *injury of blood vessels at ankle and foot level (S95.-)*

> The appropriate 7th character is to be added to each code from category S85.
> A   initial encounter
> D   subsequent encounter
> S   sequela

✓5th **S85.0** Injury of popliteal artery

  ✓6th **S85.00** Unspecified injury of popliteal artery

    ✓7th **S85.001** Unspecified injury of popliteal artery, MCC right leg

      CC Excl: MCC with 7th character A: S75.801 with 7th A, S75.809-S75.811 with 7th A, S75.819-S75.891 with 7th A, S75.899-S75.901 with 7th A, S75.909-S75.911 with 7th A, S75.919-S75.991 with 7th A, S75.999A, S85.001A, S85.009-S85.011 with 7th A, S85.019-S85.091 with 7th A, S85.099A, S85.201A, S85.209-S85.211 with 7th A, S85.219-S85.291 with 7th A, S85.299A, S85.801A, S85.809-S85.811 with 7th A, S85.819-S85.891 with 7th A, S85.899-S85.901 with 7th A, S85.909-S85.911 with 7th A, S85.919-S85.991 with 7th A, S85.999A, S95.001A, S95.009-S95.011 with 7th A, S95.019-S95.091 with 7th A, S95.099A, S95.201A, S95.209-S95.211 with 7th A, S95.219-S95.291 with 7th A, S95.299-S95.801 with 7th A, S95.809-S95.811 with 7th A, S95.819-S95.891 with 7th A, S95.899-S95.901 with 7th A, S95.909-S95.911 with 7th A, S95.919-S95.991 with 7th A, S95.999 with 7th A

    ✓7th **S85.002** Unspecified injury of popliteal artery, MCC left leg

      CC Excl: MCC with 7th character A: S75.802-S75.809 with 7th A, S75.812-S75.819 with 7th A, S75.892-S75.899 with 7th A, S75.902-S75.909 with 7th A, S75.912-S75.919 with 7th A, S75.992-S75.999 with 7th A, S85.002-S85.009 with 7th A, S85.012-S85.019 with 7th A, S85.092-S85.099 with 7th A, S85.202-S85.209 with 7th A, S85.212-S85.219 with 7th A, S85.292-S85.299 with 7th A, S85.802-S85.809 with 7th A, S85.812-S85.819 with 7th A, S85.892-S85.899 with 7th A, S85.902-S85.909 with 7th A, S85.912-S85.919 with 7th A, S85.992-S85.999 with 7th A, S95.002-S95.009 with 7th A, S95.012-S95.019 with 7th A, S95.092-S95.099 with 7th A, S95.202-S95.209 with 7th A, S95.212-S95.219 with 7th A, S95.292-S95.299 with 7th A, S95.802-S95.809 with 7th A, S95.812-S95.819 with 7th A, S95.892-S95.899 with 7th A, S95.902-S95.909 with 7th A, S95.912-S95.919 with 7th A, S95.992-S95.999 with 7th A

Ⓝ Newborn: 0   Ⓟ Pediatric: 0-17   Ⓜ Maternity: 12-55   Ⓐ Adult: 15-124   MCC Major CC Condition   PDx MCC PDx acts as own MCC   CC CC Condition   PDx CC PDx acts as own CC

1004   ICD-10-CM Draft (2015)

√7ᵗʰ **S85.009** **Unspecified injury of popliteal artery, unspecified leg** MCC
CC Excl: MCC with 7th character A:
S75.801-S75.999 with 7th A, S85.001-
S85.099 with 7th A, S85.201-S85.299 with
7th A, S85.801-S85.999 with 7th A, S95.001-
S95.099 with 7th A, S95.201-S95.999 with
7th A

√6ᵗʰ **S85.01** **Laceration of popliteal artery**

√7ᵗʰ **S85.011** **Laceration of popliteal artery, right leg** MCC
CC Excl: See code: S85.001

√7ᵗʰ **S85.012** **Laceration of popliteal artery, left leg** MCC
CC Excl: See code: S85.002

√7ᵗʰ **S85.019** **Laceration of popliteal artery, unspecified leg** MCC
CC Excl: See code: S85.009

√6ᵗʰ **S85.09** **Other specified injury of popliteal artery**

√7ᵗʰ **S85.091** **Other specified injury of popliteal artery, right leg** MCC
CC Excl: See code: S85.001

√7ᵗʰ **S85.092** **Other specified injury of popliteal artery, left leg** MCC
CC Excl: See code: S85.002

√7ᵗʰ **S85.099** **Other specified injury of popliteal artery, unspecified leg** MCC
CC Excl: See code: S85.009

√5ᵗʰ **S85.1** **Injury of tibial artery**

√6ᵗʰ **S85.10** **Unspecified injury of unspecified tibial artery**
Injury of tibial artery NOS

√7ᵗʰ **S85.101** **Unspecified injury of unspecified tibial artery, right leg** CC
CC Excl: CC with 7th character A: S75.801
with 7th A, S75.809-S75.811 with 7th A,
S75.819-S75.891 with 7th A, S75.899-
S75.901 with 7th A, S75.909-S75.911 with
7th A, S75.919-S75.991 with 7th A, S75.999A,
S85.101-S85.111 with 7th A,
S85.119-S85.121 with 7th A, S85.129A,
S85.201A, S85.209-S85.211 with 7th A,
S85.219-S85.291 with 7th A, S85.299 with
7th A, S85.801A, S85.809-S85.811 with 7th A,
S85.819-S85.891 with 7th A, S85.899-
S85.901 with 7th A, S85.909-S85.911 with
7th A, S85.919-S85.991 with 7th A, S85.999A,
S95.001A, S95.009-S95.011 with 7th A,
S95.019-S95.091 with 7th A, S95.099A,
S95.201A, S95.209-S95.211 with 7th A,
S95.219-S95.291 with 7th A, S95.299-
S95.801 with 7th A, S95.809-S95.811 with
7th A, S95.819-S95.891 with 7th A, S95.899-
S95.901 with 7th A, S95.909-S95.911 with
7th A, S95.919-S95.991 with 7th A, S95.999

√7ᵗʰ **S85.102** **Unspecified injury of unspecified tibial artery, left leg** CC
CC Excl: CC with 7th character A: S75.802-
S75.809 with 7th A, S75.812-S75.819 with
7th A, S75.892-S75.899 with 7th A, S75.902-
S75.909 with 7th A, S75.912-S75.919 with
7th A, S75.992-S75.999 with 7th A, S85.102-
S85.109 with 7th A, S85.112-S85.119 with
7th A, S85.122-S85.129 with 7th A, S85.202-
S85.209 with 7th A, S85.212-S85.219 with
7th A, S85.292-S85.299 with 7th A, S85.802-
S85.809 with 7th A, S85.812-S85.819 with
7th A, S85.892-S85.899 with 7th A, S85.902-
S85.909 with 7th A, S85.912-S85.919 with
7th A, S85.992-S85.999 with 7th A, S95.002-
S95.009 with 7th A, S95.012-S95.019 with
7th A, S95.092-S95.099 with 7th A, S95.202-
S95.209 with 7th A, S95.212-S95.219 with
7th A, S95.292-S95.299 with 7th A, S95.802-
S95.809 with 7th A, S95.812-S95.819 with
7th A, S95.892-S95.899 with 7th A, S95.902-
S95.909 with 7th A, S95.912-S95.919 with
7th A, S95.992-S95.999 with 7th A

√7ᵗʰ **S85.109** **Unspecified injury of unspecified tibial artery, unspecified leg** CC
CC Excl: CC with 7th character A: S75.801-
S75.999 with 7th A, S85.101-S85.129 with
7th A, S85.201-S85.299 with 7th A, S85.801-
S85.999 with 7th A, S95.001-S95.099 with
7th A, S95.201-S95.999 with 7th A

√6ᵗʰ **S85.11** **Laceration of unspecified tibial artery**

√7ᵗʰ **S85.111** **Laceration of unspecified tibial artery, right leg** CC
CC Excl: See code: S85.101

√7ᵗʰ **S85.112** **Laceration of unspecified tibial artery, left leg** CC
CC Excl: See code: S85.102

√7ᵗʰ **S85.119** **Laceration of unspecified tibial artery, unspecified leg** CC
CC Excl: See code: S85.109

√6ᵗʰ **S85.12** **Other specified injury of unspecified tibial artery**

√7ᵗʰ **S85.121** **Other specified injury of unspecified tibial artery, right leg** CC
CC Excl: See code: S85.101

√7ᵗʰ **S85.122** **Other specified injury of unspecified tibial artery, left leg** CC
CC Excl: See code: S85.102

√7ᵗʰ **S85.129** **Other specified injury of unspecified tibial artery, unspecified leg** CC
CC Excl: See code: S85.109

√6ᵗʰ **S85.13** **Unspecified injury of anterior tibial artery**

√7ᵗʰ **S85.131** **Unspecified injury of anterior tibial artery, right leg** CC
CC Excl: CC with 7th character A: S75.801
with 7th A, S75.809-S75.811 with 7th A,
S75.819-S75.891 with 7th A, S75.899-
S75.901 with 7th A, S75.909-S75.911 with
7th A, S75.919-S75.991 with 7th A, S75.999A,
S85.131A, S85.139-S85.141 with 7th A,
S85.149-S85.151 with 7th A, S85.159A,
S85.201A, S85.209-S85.211 with 7th A,
S85.219-S85.291 with 7th A, S85.299A,
S85.801A, S85.809-S85.811 with 7th A,
S85.819-S85.891 with 7th A, S85.899-
S85.901 with 7th A, S85.909-S85.911 with
7th A, S85.919-S85.991 with 7th A, S85.999A,
S95.001A, S95.009-S95.011 with 7th A,
S95.019-S95.091 with 7th A, S95.099A,
S95.201A, S95.209-S95.211 with 7th A,
S95.219-S95.291 with 7th A, S95.299-
S95.801 with 7th A, S95.809-S95.811 with
7th A, S95.819-S95.891 with 7th A, S95.899-
S95.901 with 7th A, S95.909-S95.911 with
7th A, S95.919-S95.991 with 7th A, S95.999
with 7th A

√7ᵗʰ **S85.132** **Unspecified injury of anterior tibial artery, left leg** CC
CC Excl: CC with 7th character A: S75.802-
S75.809 with 7th A, S75.812-S75.819 with
7th A, S75.892-S75.899 with 7th A, S75.902-
S75.909 with 7th A, S75.912-S75.919 with
7th A, S75.992-S75.999 with 7th A, S85.132-
S85.139 with 7th A, S85.142-S85.149 with
7th A, S85.152-S85.159 with 7th A, S85.202-
S85.209 with 7th A, S85.212-S85.219 with
7th A, S85.292-S85.299 with 7th A, S85.802-
S85.809 with 7th A, S85.812-S85.819 with
7th A, S85.892-S85.899 with 7th A, S85.902-
S85.909 with 7th A, S85.912-S85.919 with
7th A, S85.992-S85.999 with 7th A, S95.002-
S95.009 with 7th A, S95.012-S95.019 with
7th A, S95.092-S95.099 with 7th A, S95.202-
S95.209 with 7th A, S95.212-S95.219 with
7th A, S95.292-S95.299 with 7th A, S95.802-
S95.809 with 7th A, S95.812-S95.819 with
7th A, S95.892-S95.899 with 7th A, S95.902-
S95.909 with 7th A, S95.912-S95.919 with
7th A, S95.992-S95.999 with 7th A

√7ᵗʰ **S85.139** **Unspecified injury of anterior tibial artery, unspecified leg** CC
CC Excl: CC with 7th character A: S75.801-
S75.999 with 7th A, S85.131-S85.159 with
7th A, S85.201-S85.299 with 7th A, S85.801-
S85.999 with 7th A, S95.001-S95.099 with
7th A, S95.201-S95.999 with 7th A

√6ᵗʰ **S85.14** Laceration of anterior tibial artery

   √7ᵗʰ **S85.141** Laceration of anterior tibial artery, right leg `CC`
      CC Excl: See code: S85.131

   √7ᵗʰ **S85.142** Laceration of anterior tibial artery, left leg `CC`
      CC Excl: See code: S85.132

   √7ᵗʰ **S85.149** Laceration of anterior tibial artery, unspecified leg `CC`
      CC Excl: See code: S85.139

√6ᵗʰ **S85.15** Other specified injury of anterior tibial artery

   √7ᵗʰ **S85.151** Other specified injury of anterior tibial artery, right leg `CC`
      CC Excl: See code: S85.131

   √7ᵗʰ **S85.152** Other specified injury of anterior tibial artery, left leg `CC`
      CC Excl: See code: S85.132

   √7ᵗʰ **S85.159** Other specified injury of anterior tibial artery, unspecified leg `CC`
      CC Excl: See code: S85.139

√6ᵗʰ **S85.16** Unspecified injury of posterior tibial artery

   √7ᵗʰ **S85.161** Unspecified injury of posterior tibial artery, right leg `CC`
      CC Excl: CC with 7th character A: S75.801 with 7th A, S75.809-S75.811 with 7th A, S75.819-S75.891 with 7th A, S75.899-S75.901 with 7th A, S75.909-S75.911 with 7th A, S75.919-S75.991 with 7th A, S75.999 with 7th A, S85.161 with 7th A, S85.169-S85.171 with 7th A, S85.179-S85.181 with 7th A, S85.189-S85.201 with 7th A, S85.209-S85.211 with 7th A, S85.219-S85.291 with 7th A, S85.299A, S85.801A, S85.809-S85.811 with 7th A, S85.819-S85.891 with 7th A, S85.899-S85.901 with 7th A, S85.909-S85.911 with 7th A, S85.919-S85.991 with 7th A, S85.999A, S95.001A, S95.009-S95.011 with 7th A, S95.019-S95.091 with 7th A, S95.099A, S95.201A, S95.209-S95.211 with 7th A, S95.219-S95.291 with 7th A, S95.299-S95.801 with 7th A, S95.809-S95.811 with 7th A, S95.819-S95.891 with 7th A, S95.899-S95.901 with 7th A, S95.909-S95.911 with 7th A, S95.919-S95.991 with 7th A, S95.999 with 7th A

   √7ᵗʰ **S85.162** Unspecified injury of posterior tibial artery, left leg `CC`
      CC Excl: CC with 7th character A: S75.802-S75.809 with 7th A, S75.812-S75.819 with 7th A, S75.892-S75.899 with 7th A, S75.902-S75.909 with 7th A, S75.912-S75.919 with 7th A, S75.992-S75.999 with 7th A, S85.162-S85.169 with 7th A, S85.172-S85.179 with 7th A, S85.182-S85.189 with 7th A, S85.202-S85.209 with 7th A, S85.212-S85.219 with 7th A, S85.292-S85.299 with 7th A, S85.802-S85.809 with 7th A, S85.812-S85.819 with 7th A, S85.892-S85.899 with 7th A, S85.902-S85.909 with 7th A, S85.912-S85.919 with 7th A, S85.992-S85.999 with 7th A, S95.002-S95.009 with 7th A, S95.012-S95.019 with 7th A, S95.092-S95.099 with 7th A, S95.202-S95.209 with 7th A, S95.212-S95.219 with 7th A, S95.292-S95.299 with 7th A, S95.802-S95.809 with 7th A, S95.812-S95.819 with 7th A, S95.892-S95.899 with 7th A, S95.902-S95.909 with 7th A, S95.912-S95.919 with 7th A, S95.992-S95.999 with 7th A

   √7ᵗʰ **S85.169** Unspecified injury of posterior tibial artery, unspecified leg `CC`
      CC Excl: CC with 7th character A: S75.801-S75.999 with 7th A, S85.161-S85.299 with 7th A, S85.801-S85.999 with 7th A, S95.001-S95.099 with 7th A, S95.201-S95.999 with 7th A

√6ᵗʰ **S85.17** Laceration of posterior tibial artery

   √7ᵗʰ **S85.171** Laceration of posterior tibial artery, right leg `CC`
      CC Excl: See code: S85.161

   √7ᵗʰ **S85.172** Laceration of posterior tibial artery, left leg `CC`
      CC Excl: See code: S85.162

   √7ᵗʰ **S85.179** Laceration of posterior tibial artery, unspecified leg `CC`
      CC Excl: See code: S85.169

√6ᵗʰ **S85.18** Other specified injury of posterior tibial artery

   √7ᵗʰ **S85.181** Other specified injury of posterior tibial artery, right leg `CC`
      CC Excl: See code: S85.161

   √7ᵗʰ **S85.182** Other specified injury of posterior tibial artery, left leg `CC`
      CC Excl: See code: S85.162

   √7ᵗʰ **S85.189** Other specified injury of posterior tibial artery, unspecified leg `CC`
      CC Excl: See code: S85.169

√5ᵗʰ **S85.2** Injury of peroneal artery

  √6ᵗʰ **S85.20** Unspecified injury of peroneal artery

   √7ᵗʰ **S85.201** Unspecified injury of peroneal artery, right leg `CC`
      CC Excl: CC with 7th character A: M79.A21-M79.A29, S75.001 with 7th A, S75.009-S75.011 with 7th A, S75.019-S75.021 with 7th A, S75.029-S75.091 with 7th A, S75.099-S75.101 with 7th A, S75.109-S75.111 with 7th A, S75.119-S75.121 with 7th A, S75.129-S75.191 with 7th A, S75.199-S75.201 with 7th A, S75.209-S75.211 with 7th A, S75.219-S75.221 with 7th A, S75.229-S75.291 with 7th A, S75.299-S75.801 with 7th A, S75.809-S75.811 with 7th A, S75.819-S75.891 with 7th A, S75.899-S75.901 with 7th A, S75.909-S75.911 with 7th A, S75.919-S75.991 with 7th A, S75.999A, S85.001A, S85.009-S85.011 with 7th A, S85.019-S85.091 with 7th A, S85.099-S85.101 with 7th A, S85.109-S85.111 with 7th A, S85.119-S85.121 with 7th A, S85.129-S85.131 with 7th A, S85.139-S85.141 with 7th A, S85.149-S85.151 with 7th A, S85.159-S85.161 with 7th A, S85.169-S85.171 with 7th A, S85.179-S85.181 with 7th A, S85.189-S85.201 with 7th A, S85.209-S85.211 with 7th A, S85.219-S85.291 with 7th A, S85.299-S85.301 with 7th A, S85.309-S85.311 with 7th A, S85.319-S85.391 with 7th A, S85.399-S85.401 with 7th A, S85.409-S85.411 with 7th A, S85.419-S85.491 with 7th A, S85.499-S85.501 with 7th A, S85.509-S85.511 with 7th A, S85.519-S85.591 with 7th A, S85.599-S85.801 with 7th A, S85.809-S85.811 with 7th A, S85.819-S85.891 with 7th A, S85.899-S85.901 with 7th A, S85.909-S85.911 with 7th A, S85.919-S85.991 with 7th A, S85.999 with 7th A, S95.001 with 7th A, S95.009-S95.011 with 7th A, S95.019-S95.091 with 7th A, S95.099-S95.101 with 7th A, S95.109-S95.111 with 7th A, S95.119-S95.191 with 7th A, S95.199-S95.201 with 7th A, S95.209-S95.211 with 7th A, S95.219-S95.291 with 7th A, S95.299-S95.801 with 7th A, S95.809-S95.811 with 7th A, S95.819-S95.891 with 7th A, S95.899-S95.901 with 7th A, S95.909-S95.911 with 7th A, S95.919-S95.991 with 7th A, S95.999 with 7th A

N Newborn: 0   P Pediatric: 0-17   M Maternity: 12-55   A Adult: 15-124   MCC Major CC Condition   PDx MCC PDx acts as own MCC   CC CC Condition   PDx CC PDx acts as own CC

1006   ICD-10-CM Draft (2015)

√7ᵗʰ **S85.202**　**Unspecified injury of peroneal artery, left leg** CC

CC Excl: CC with 7th character A: M79.A21-M79.A29, S75.002-S75.009 with 7th A, S75.012-S75.019 with 7th A, S75.022-S75.029 with 7th A, S75.092-S75.099 with 7th A, S75.102-S75.109 with 7th A, S75.112-S75.119 with 7th A, S75.122-S75.129 with 7th A, S75.192-S75.199 with 7th A, S75.202-S75.209 with 7th A, S75.212-S75.219 with 7th A, S75.222-S75.229 with 7th A, S75.292-S75.299 with 7th A, S75.802-S75.809 with 7th A, S75.812-S75.819 with 7th A, S75.892-S75.899 with 7th A, S75.902-S75.909 with 7th A, S75.912-S75.919 with 7th A, S75.992-S75.999A, S85.002-S85.009 with 7th A, S85.012-S85.019 with 7th A, S85.092-S85.099 with 7th A, S85.102-S85.109 with 7th A, S85.112-S85.119 with 7th A, S85.122-S85.129 with 7th A, S85.132-S85.139 with 7th A, S85.142-S85.149 with 7th A, S85.152-S85.159 with 7th A, S85.162-S85.169 with 7th A, S85.172-S85.179 with 7th A, S85.182-S85.189 with 7th A, S85.202-S85.209 with 7th A, S85.212-S85.219 with 7th A, S85.292-S85.299 with 7th A, S85.302-S85.309 with 7th A, S85.312-S85.319 with 7th A, S85.392-S85.399 with 7th A, S85.402-S85.409 with 7th A, S85.412-S85.419 with 7th A, S85.492-S85.499 with 7th A, S85.502-S85.509 with 7th A, S85.512-S85.519 with 7th A, S85.592-S85.599 with 7th A, S85.802-S85.809 with 7th A, S85.812-S85.819 with 7th A, S85.892-S85.899 with 7th A, S85.902-S85.909 with 7th A, S85.912-S85.919 with 7th A, S85.992-S85.999 with 7th A, S95.002-S95.009 with 7th A, S95.012-S95.019 with 7th A, S95.092-S95.099 with 7th A, S95.102-S95.109 with 7th A, S95.112-S95.119 with 7th A, S95.192-S95.199 with 7th A, S95.202-S95.209 with 7th A, S95.212-S95.219 with 7th A, S95.292-S95.299 with 7th A, S95.802-S95.809 with 7th A, S95.812-S95.819 with 7th A, S95.892-S95.899 with 7th A, S95.902-S95.909 with 7th A, S95.912-S95.919 with 7th A, S95.992-S95.999 with 7th A

√7ᵗʰ **S85.209**　**Unspecified injury of peroneal artery, unspecified leg** CC

CC Excl: CC with 7th character A: M79.A21-M79.A29, S75.001-S75.999 with 7th A, S85.001-S85.999 with 7th A, S95.001-S95.999 with 7th A

√6ᵗʰ **S85.21**　**Laceration of peroneal artery**

√7ᵗʰ **S85.211**　**Laceration of peroneal artery, right leg** CC

CC Excl: See code: S85.201

√7ᵗʰ **S85.212**　**Laceration of peroneal artery, left leg** CC

CC Excl: See code: S85.202

√7ᵗʰ **S85.219**　**Laceration of peroneal artery, unspecified leg** CC

CC Excl: See code: S85.209

√6ᵗʰ **S85.29**　**Other specified injury of peroneal artery**

√7ᵗʰ **S85.291**　**Other specified injury of peroneal artery, right leg** CC

CC Excl: See code: S85.201

√7ᵗʰ **S85.292**　**Other specified injury of peroneal artery, left leg** CC

CC Excl: See code: S85.202

√7ᵗʰ **S85.299**　**Other specified injury of peroneal artery, unspecified leg** CC

CC Excl: See code: S85.209

√5ᵗʰ **S85.3**　**Injury of greater saphenous vein at lower leg level**
Injury of greater saphenous vein NOS
Injury of saphenous vein NOS

√6ᵗʰ **S85.30**　**Unspecified injury of greater saphenous vein at lower leg level**

√7ᵗʰ **S85.301**　**Unspecified injury of greater saphenous vein at lower leg level, right leg** CC

CC Excl: CC with 7th character A: S75.201 with 7th A, S75.209-S75.211 with 7th A, S75.219-S75.221 with 7th A, S75.229-S75.291 with 7th A, S75.299-S75.801 with 7th A, S75.809-S75.811 with 7th A, S75.819-S75.891 with 7th A, S75.899-S75.901 with 7th A, S75.909-S75.911 with 7th A, S75.919-S75.991 with 7th A, S75.999A, S85.201A, S85.209-S85.211 with 7th A, S85.219-S85.291 with 7th A, S85.299-S85.301 with 7th A, S85.309-S85.311 with 7th A, S85.319-S85.391 with 7th A, S85.399-S85.401 with 7th A, S85.409-S85.411 with 7th A, S85.419-S85.491 with 7th A, S85.499 with 7th A, S85.801 with 7th A, S85.809-S85.811 with 7th A, S85.819-S85.891 with 7th A, S85.899-S85.901 with 7th A, S85.909-S85.911 with 7th A, S85.919-S85.991 with 7th A, S85.999A, S95.001A, S95.009-S95.011 with 7th A, S95.019-S95.091 with 7th A, S95.099A, S95.201A, S95.209-S95.211 with 7th A, S95.219-S95.291 with 7th A, S95.299-S95.801 with 7th A, S95.809-S95.811 with 7th A, S95.819-S95.891 with 7th A, S95.899-S95.901 with 7th A, S95.909-S95.911 with 7th A, S95.919-S95.991 with 7th A, S95.999 with 7th A

√7ᵗʰ **S85.302**　**Unspecified injury of greater saphenous vein at lower leg level, left leg** CC

CC Excl: CC with 7th character A: S75.202-S75.209 with 7th A, S75.212-S75.219 with 7th A, S75.222-S75.229 with 7th A, S75.292-S75.299 with 7th A, S75.802-S75.809 with 7th A, S75.812-S75.819 with 7th A, S75.892-S75.899 with 7th A, S75.902-S75.909 with 7th A, S75.912-S75.919 with 7th A, S75.992-S75.999 with 7th A, S85.202-S85.209 with 7th A, S85.212-S85.219 with 7th A, S85.292-S85.299 with 7th A, S85.302-S85.309 with 7th A, S85.312-S85.319 with 7th A, S85.392-S85.399 with 7th A, S85.402-S85.409 with 7th A, S85.412-S85.419 with 7th A, S85.492-S85.499 with 7th A, S85.802-S85.809 with 7th A, S85.812-S85.819 with 7th A, S85.892-S85.899 with 7th A, S85.902-S85.909 with 7th A, S85.912-S85.919 with 7th A, S85.992-S85.999 with 7th A, S95.002-S95.009 with 7th A, S95.012-S95.019 with 7th A, S95.092-S95.099 with 7th A, S95.202-S95.209 with 7th A, S95.212-S95.219 with 7th A, S95.292-S95.299 with 7th A, S95.802-S95.809 with 7th A, S95.812-S95.819 with 7th A, S95.892-S95.899 with 7th A, S95.902-S95.909 with 7th A, S95.912-S95.919 with 7th A, S95.992-S95.999 with 7th A

√7ᵗʰ **S85.309**　**Unspecified injury of greater saphenous vein at lower leg level, unspecified leg** CC

CC Excl: CC with 7th character A: S75.201-S75.999 with 7th A, S85.201-S85.499 with 7th A, S85.801-S85.999 with 7th A, S95.001-S95.099 with 7th A, S95.201-S95.999 with 7th A

√6ᵗʰ **S85.31**　**Laceration of greater saphenous vein at lower leg level**

√7ᵗʰ **S85.311**　**Laceration of greater saphenous vein at lower leg level, right leg** CC

CC Excl: See code: S85.301

√7ᵗʰ **S85.312**　**Laceration of greater saphenous vein at lower leg level, left leg** CC

CC Excl: See code: S85.302

√7ᵗʰ **S85.319**　**Laceration of greater saphenous vein at lower leg level, unspecified leg** CC

CC Excl: See code: S85.309

✓ Additional Character Required　　√x7ᵗʰ Xtension Alert　　Unacceptable PDx　　Manifestation　　Hospital Acquired Condition　　EXCLUDES 1 Not Coded Here　　EXCLUDES 2 Not Included Here

ICD-10-CM Draft (2015)　　　　　　　　　　　　　　　　　　　　　　　　　　　　　　　　　　　　　1007

✓6ᵗʰ **S85.39** Other specified injury of greater saphenous vein at lower leg level

✓7ᵗʰ **S85.391** Other specified injury of greater saphenous vein at lower leg level, right leg   CC
CC Excl: See code: S85.301

✓7ᵗʰ **S85.392** Other specified injury of greater saphenous vein at lower leg level, left leg   CC
CC Excl: See code: S85.302

✓7ᵗʰ **S85.399** Other specified injury of greater saphenous vein at lower leg level, unspecified leg   CC
CC Excl: See code: S85.309

✓5ᵗʰ **S85.4** Injury of lesser saphenous vein at lower leg level

✓6ᵗʰ **S85.40** Unspecified injury of lesser saphenous vein at lower leg level

✓7ᵗʰ **S85.401** Unspecified injury of lesser saphenous vein at lower leg level, right leg   CC
CC Excl: See code: S85.301

✓7ᵗʰ **S85.402** Unspecified injury of lesser saphenous vein at lower leg level, left leg   CC
CC Excl: See code: S85.302

✓7ᵗʰ **S85.409** Unspecified injury of lesser saphenous vein at lower leg level, unspecified leg   CC
CC Excl: See code: S85.309

✓6ᵗʰ **S85.41** Laceration of lesser saphenous vein at lower leg level

✓7ᵗʰ **S85.411** Laceration of lesser saphenous vein at lower leg level, right leg   CC
CC Excl: See code: S85.301

✓7ᵗʰ **S85.412** Laceration of lesser saphenous vein at lower leg level, left leg   CC
CC Excl: See code: S85.302

✓7ᵗʰ **S85.419** Laceration of lesser saphenous vein at lower leg level, unspecified leg   CC
CC Excl: See code: S85.309

✓6ᵗʰ **S85.49** Other specified injury of lesser saphenous vein at lower leg level

✓7ᵗʰ **S85.491** Other specified injury of lesser saphenous vein at lower leg level, right leg   CC
CC Excl: See code: S85.301

✓7ᵗʰ **S85.492** Other specified injury of lesser saphenous vein at lower leg level, left leg   CC
CC Excl: See code: S85.302

✓7ᵗʰ **S85.499** Other specified injury of lesser saphenous vein at lower leg level, unspecified leg   CC
CC Excl: See code: S85.309

✓5ᵗʰ **S85.5** Injury of popliteal vein

✓6ᵗʰ **S85.50** Unspecified injury of popliteal vein

✓7ᵗʰ **S85.501** Unspecified injury of popliteal vein, right leg   MCC
CC Excl: MCC with 7th A: S75.801 with 7th A, S75.809-S75.811 with 7th A, S75.819-S75.891 with 7th A, S75.899-S75.901 with 7th A, S75.909-S75.911 with 7th A, S75.919-S75.991 with 7th A, S75.999 with 7th A, S85.201 with 7th A, S85.209-S85.211 with 7th A, S85.219-S85.291 with 7th A, S85.299A, S85.501A, S85.509-S85.511 with 7th A, S85.519-S85.591 with 7th A, S85.599-S85.801 with 7th A, S85.809-S85.811 with 7th A, S85.819-S85.891 with 7th A, S85.899-S85.901 with 7th A, S85.909-S85.911 with 7th A, S85.919-S85.991 with 7th A, S85.999A, S95.001A, S95.009-S95.011 with 7th A, S95.019-S95.091 with 7th A, S95.099 with 7th A, S95.201 with 7th A, S95.209-S95.211 with 7th A, S95.219-S95.291 with 7th A, S95.299-S95.801 with 7th A, S95.809-S95.811 with 7th A, S95.819-S95.891 with 7th A, S95.899-S95.901 with 7th A, S95.909-S95.911 with 7th A, S95.919-S95.991 with 7th A, S95.999 with 7th A

✓7ᵗʰ **S85.502** Unspecified injury of popliteal vein, left leg   MCC
CC Excl: MCC with 7th A: S75.802-S75.809 with 7th A, S75.812-S75.819 with 7th A, S75.892-S75.899 with 7th A, S75.902-S75.909 with 7th A, S75.912-S75.919 with 7th A, S75.992-S75.999 with 7th A, S85.202-S85.209 with 7th A, S85.212-S85.219 with 7th A, S85.292-S85.299 with 7th A, S85.502-S85.509 with 7th A, S85.512-S85.519 with 7th A, S85.592-S85.599 with 7th A, S85.802-S85.809 with 7th A, S85.812-S85.819 with 7th A, S85.892-S85.899 with 7th A, S85.902-S85.909 with 7th A, S85.912-S85.919 with 7th A, S85.992-S85.999 with 7th A, S95.002-S95.009 with 7th A, S95.012-S95.019 with 7th A, S95.092-S95.099 with 7th A, S95.202-S95.209 with 7th A, S95.212-S95.219 with 7th A, S95.292-S95.299 with 7th A, S95.802-S95.809 with 7th A, S95.812-S95.819 with 7th A, S95.892-S95.899 with 7th A, S95.902-S95.909 with 7th A, S95.912-S95.919 with 7th A, S95.992-S95.999 with 7th A

✓7ᵗʰ **S85.509** Unspecified injury of popliteal vein, unspecified leg   MCC
CC Excl: MCC with 7th A: S75.801-S75.999 with 7th A, S85.201-S85.299 with 7th A, S85.501-S85.999 with 7th A, S95.001-S95.099 with 7th A, S95.201-S95.999 with 7th A

✓6ᵗʰ **S85.51** Laceration of popliteal vein

✓7ᵗʰ **S85.511** Laceration of popliteal vein, right leg   MCC
CC Excl: See code: S85.501

✓7ᵗʰ **S85.512** Laceration of popliteal vein, left leg   MCC
CC Excl: See code: S85.502

✓7ᵗʰ **S85.519** Laceration of popliteal vein, unspecified leg   MCC
CC Excl: See code: S85.509

✓6ᵗʰ **S85.59** Other specified injury of popliteal vein

✓7ᵗʰ **S85.591** Other specified injury of popliteal vein, right leg   MCC
CC Excl: See code: S85.501

✓7ᵗʰ **S85.592** Other specified injury of popliteal vein, left leg   MCC
CC Excl: See code: S85.502

✓7ᵗʰ **S85.599** Other specified injury of popliteal vein, unspecified leg   MCC
CC Excl: See code: S85.509

✓5ᵗʰ **S85.8** Injury of other blood vessels at lower leg level

✓6ᵗʰ **S85.80** Unspecified injury of other blood vessels at lower leg level

✓7ᵗʰ **S85.801** Unspecified injury of other blood vessels at lower leg level, right leg   CC
CC Excl: CC with 7th character A: See code: S85.501

✓7ᵗʰ **S85.802** Unspecified injury of other blood vessels at lower leg level, left leg   CC
CC Excl: CC with 7th character A: See code: S85.502

✓7ᵗʰ **S85.809** Unspecified injury of other blood vessels at lower leg level, unspecified leg   CC
CC Excl: CC with 7th character A: See code: S85.509

✓6ᵗʰ **S85.81** Laceration of other blood vessels at lower leg level

✓7ᵗʰ **S85.811** Laceration of other blood vessels at lower leg level, right leg   CC
CC Excl: CC with 7th character A: See code: S85.501

✓7ᵗʰ **S85.812** Laceration of other blood vessels at lower leg level, left leg   CC
CC Excl: CC with 7th character A: See code: S85.502

✓7ᵗʰ **S85.819** Laceration of other blood vessels at lower leg level, unspecified leg   CC
CC Excl: CC with 7th character A: See code: S85.509

Ⓝ Newborn: 0   Ⓟ Pediatric: 0-17   Ⓜ Maternity: 12-55   Ⓐ Adult: 15-124   MCC Major CC Condition   PDx MCC PDx acts as own MCC   CC CC Condition   PDx CC PDx acts as own CC

1008   ICD-10-CM Draft (2015)

√6th **S85.89** Other specified injury of other blood vessels at lower leg level

   √7th **S85.891** Other specified injury of other blood vessels at lower leg level, right leg `CC`
     CC Excl: CC with 7th character A: See code: S85.501

   √7th **S85.892** Other specified injury of other blood vessels at lower leg level, left leg `CC`
     CC Excl: CC with 7th character A: See code: S85.502

   √7th **S85.899** Other specified injury of other blood vessels at lower leg level, unspecified leg `CC`
     CC Excl: CC with 7th character A: See code: S85.509

√5th **S85.9** Injury of unspecified blood vessel at lower leg level

  √6th **S85.90** Unspecified injury of unspecified blood vessel at lower leg level

   √7th **S85.901** Unspecified injury of unspecified blood vessel at lower leg level, right leg `CC`
     CC Excl: See code: S85.501

   √7th **S85.902** Unspecified injury of unspecified blood vessel at lower leg level, left leg `CC`
     CC Excl: See code: S85.502

   √7th **S85.909** Unspecified injury of unspecified blood vessel at lower leg level, unspecified leg `CC`
     CC Excl: See code: S85.509

  √6th **S85.91** Laceration of unspecified blood vessel at lower leg level

   √7th **S85.911** Laceration of unspecified blood vessel at lower leg level, right leg `CC`
     CC Excl: See code: S85.501

   √7th **S85.912** Laceration of unspecified blood vessel at lower leg level, left leg `CC`
     CC Excl: See code: S85.502

   √7th **S85.919** Laceration of unspecified blood vessel at lower leg level, unspecified leg `CC`
     CC Excl: See code: S85.509

  √6th **S85.99** Other specified injury of unspecified blood vessel at lower leg level

   √7th **S85.991** Other specified injury of unspecified blood vessel at lower leg level, right leg `CC`
     CC Excl: See code: S85.501

   √7th **S85.992** Other specified injury of unspecified blood vessel at lower leg level, left leg `CC`
     CC Excl: See code: S85.502

   √7th **S85.999** Other specified injury of unspecified blood vessel at lower leg level, unspecified leg `CC`
     CC Excl: See code: S85.509

√4th **S86** **Injury of muscle, fascia and tendon at lower leg level**

  Code also any associated open wound (S81.-)

  EXCLUDES 2 injury of muscle, fascia and tendon at ankle (S96.-)
    injury of patellar ligament (tendon) (S76.1-)
    sprain of joints and ligaments of knee (S83.-)

  The appropriate 7th character is to be added to each code from category S86.
  A   initial encounter
  D   subsequent encounter
  S   sequela

√5th **S86.0** Injury of Achilles tendon

  √6th **S86.00** Unspecified injury of Achilles tendon
   √7th **S86.001** Unspecified injury of right Achilles tendon
   √7th **S86.002** Unspecified injury of left Achilles tendon
   √7th **S86.009** Unspecified injury of unspecified Achilles tendon

  √6th **S86.01** Strain of Achilles tendon
   √7th **S86.011** Strain of right Achilles tendon
   √7th **S86.012** Strain of left Achilles tendon
   √7th **S86.019** Strain of unspecified Achilles tendon

  √6th **S86.02** Laceration of Achilles tendon

   √7th **S86.021** Laceration of right Achilles tendon `CC`
     CC Excl: CC with 7th character A: S81.001 with 7th A, S81.009-S81.011 with 7th A, S81.019-S81.021 with 7th A, S81.029-S81.031 with 7th A, S81.039-S81.041 with 7th A, S81.049-S81.051 with 7th A, S81.059-S81.801 with 7th A, S81.809-S81.811 with 7th A, S81.819-S81.821 with 7th A, S81.829-S81.831 with 7th A, S81.839-S81.841 with 7th A, S81.849-S81.851 with 7th A, S81.859A, S86.021A, S86.029A, S86.121A, S86.129A, S86.221A, S86.229A, S86.321A, S86.329A, S86.821A, S86.829A, S86.921A, S86.929A, S91.001A, S91.009-S91.011 with 7th A, S91.019-S91.021 with 7th A, S91.029-S91.031 with 7th A, S91.039-S91.041 with 7th A, S91.049-S91.051 with 7th A, S91.059A, S96.021A, S96.029A, S96.121A, S96.129A, S96.221A, S96.229A, S96.821A, S96.829A, S96.921A, S96.929A

   √7th **S86.022** Laceration of left Achilles tendon `CC`
     CC Excl: CC with 7th character A: S81.002-S81.009 with 7th A, S81.012-S81.019 with 7th A, S81.022-S81.029 with 7th A, S81.032-S81.039 with 7th A, S81.042-S81.049 with 7th A, S81.052-S81.059 with 7th A, S81.802-S81.809 with 7th A, S81.812-S81.819 with 7th A, S81.822-S81.829 with 7th A, S81.832-S81.839 with 7th A, S81.842-S81.849 with 7th A, S81.852-S81.859 with 7th A, S86.022-S86.029 with 7th A, S86.122-S86.129 with 7th A, S86.222-S86.229 with 7th A, S86.322-S86.329 with 7th A, S86.822-S86.829 with 7th A, S86.922-S86.929 with 7th A, S91.002-S91.009 with 7th A, S91.012-S91.019 with 7th A, S91.022-S91.029 with 7th A, S91.032-S91.039 with 7th A, S91.042-S91.049 with 7th A, S91.052-S91.059 with 7th A, S96.022-S96.029 with 7th A, S96.122-S96.129 with 7th A, S96.222-S96.229 with 7th A, S96.822-S96.829 with 7th A, S96.922-S96.929 with 7th A

   √7th **S86.029** Laceration of unspecified Achilles tendon `CC`
     CC Excl: CC with 7th character A: S81.001-S81.859 with 7th A, S86.021-S86.029 with 7th A, S86.121-S86.129 with 7th A, S86.221-S86.229 with 7th A, S86.321-S86.329 with 7th A, S86.821-S86.829 with 7th A, S86.921-S86.929 with 7th A, S91.001-S91.059 with 7th A, S96.021-S96.029 with 7th A, S96.121-S96.129 with 7th A, S96.221-S96.229 with 7th A, S96.821-S96.829 with 7th A, S96.921-S96.929 with 7th A

  √6th **S86.09** Other specified injury of Achilles tendon
   √7th **S86.091** Other specified injury of right Achilles tendon
   √7th **S86.092** Other specified injury of left Achilles tendon
   √7th **S86.099** Other specified injury of unspecified Achilles tendon

√5th **S86.1** Injury of other muscle(s) and tendon(s) of posterior muscle group at lower leg level

  √6th **S86.10** Unspecified injury of other muscle(s) and tendon(s) of posterior muscle group at lower leg level

   √7th **S86.101** Unspecified injury of other muscle(s) and tendon(s) of posterior muscle group at lower leg level, right leg

   √7th **S86.102** Unspecified injury of other muscle(s) and tendon(s) of posterior muscle group at lower leg level, left leg

   √7th **S86.109** Unspecified injury of other muscle(s) and tendon(s) of posterior muscle group at lower leg level, unspecified leg

  √6th **S86.11** Strain of other muscle(s) and tendon(s) of posterior muscle group at lower leg level

   √7th **S86.111** Strain of other muscle(s) and tendon(s) of posterior muscle group at lower leg level, right leg

   √7th **S86.112** Strain of other muscle(s) and tendon(s) of posterior muscle group at lower leg level, left leg

---

✔ Additional Character Required   √x7th Xtension Alert   Unacceptable PDx   Manifestation   Hospital Acquired Condition   **EXCLUDES 1** Not Coded Here   **EXCLUDES 2** Not Included Here

ICD-10-CM Draft (2015)   1009

√7th **S86.119** Strain of other muscle(s) and tendon(s) of posterior muscle group at lower leg level, **unspecified** leg

√6th **S86.12** **Laceration** of other muscle(s) and tendon(s) of posterior muscle group at lower leg level

√7th **S86.121** Laceration of other muscle(s) and tendon(s) of posterior muscle group at lower leg level, **right** leg   `CC`
CC Excl: See code: S86.021

√7th **S86.122** Laceration of other muscle(s) and tendon(s) of posterior muscle group at lower leg level, **left** leg   `CC`
CC Excl: See code: S86.022

√7th **S86.129** Laceration of other muscle(s) and tendon(s) of posterior muscle group at lower leg level, **unspecified** leg   `CC`
CC Excl: See code: S86.029

√6th **S86.19** **Other** injury of other muscle(s) and tendon(s) of posterior muscle group at lower leg level

√7th **S86.191** Other injury of other muscle(s) and tendon(s) of posterior muscle group at lower leg level, **right** leg

√7th **S86.192** Other injury of other muscle(s) and tendon(s) of posterior muscle group at lower leg level, **left** leg

√7th **S86.199** Other injury of other muscle(s) and tendon(s) of posterior muscle group at lower leg level, **unspecified** leg

√5th **S86.2** Injury of muscle(s) and tendon(s) of **anterior muscle group** at lower leg level

√6th **S86.20** **Unspecified** injury of muscle(s) and tendon(s) of anterior muscle group at lower leg level

√7th **S86.201** Unspecified injury of muscle(s) and tendon(s) of anterior muscle group at lower leg level, **right** leg

√7th **S86.202** Unspecified injury of muscle(s) and tendon(s) of anterior muscle group at lower leg level, **left** leg

√7th **S86.209** Unspecified injury of muscle(s) and tendon(s) of anterior muscle group at lower leg level, **unspecified** leg

√6th **S86.21** **Strain** of muscle(s) and tendon(s) of anterior muscle group at lower leg level

√7th **S86.211** Strain of muscle(s) and tendon(s) of anterior muscle group at lower leg level, **right** leg

√7th **S86.212** Strain of muscle(s) and tendon(s) of anterior muscle group at lower leg level, **left** leg

√7th **S86.219** Strain of muscle(s) and tendon(s) of anterior muscle group at lower leg level, **unspecified** leg

√6th **S86.22** **Laceration** of muscle(s) and tendon(s) of anterior muscle group at lower leg level

√7th **S86.221** Laceration of muscle(s) and tendon(s) of anterior muscle group at lower leg level, **right** leg   `CC`
CC Excl: See code: S86.021

√7th **S86.222** Laceration of muscle(s) and tendon(s) of anterior muscle group at lower leg level, **left** leg   `CC`
CC Excl: See code: S86.022

√7th **S86.229** Laceration of muscle(s) and tendon(s) of anterior muscle group at lower leg level, **unspecified** leg   `CC`
CC Excl: See code: S86.029

√6th **S86.29** **Other** injury of muscle(s) and tendon(s) of anterior muscle group at lower leg level

√7th **S86.291** Other injury of muscle(s) and tendon(s) of anterior muscle group at lower leg level, **right** leg

√7th **S86.292** Other injury of muscle(s) and tendon(s) of anterior muscle group at lower leg level, **left** leg

√7th **S86.299** Other injury of muscle(s) and tendon(s) of anterior muscle group at lower leg level, **unspecified** leg

√5th **S86.3** Injury of muscle(s) and tendon(s) of **peroneal muscle group** at lower leg level

√6th **S86.30** **Unspecified** injury of muscle(s) and tendon(s) of peroneal muscle group at lower leg level

√7th **S86.301** Unspecified injury of muscle(s) and tendon(s) of peroneal muscle group at lower leg level, **right** leg

√7th **S86.302** Unspecified injury of muscle(s) and tendon(s) of peroneal muscle group at lower leg level, **left** leg

√7th **S86.309** Unspecified injury of muscle(s) and tendon(s) of peroneal muscle group at lower leg level, **unspecified** leg

√6th **S86.31** **Strain** of muscle(s) and tendon(s) of peroneal muscle group at lower leg level

√7th **S86.311** Strain of muscle(s) and tendon(s) of peroneal muscle group at lower leg level, **right** leg

√7th **S86.312** Strain of muscle(s) and tendon(s) of peroneal muscle group at lower leg level, **left** leg

√7th **S86.319** Strain of muscle(s) and tendon(s) of peroneal muscle group at lower leg level, **unspecified** leg

√6th **S86.32** **Laceration** of muscle(s) and tendon(s) of peroneal muscle group at lower leg level

√7th **S86.321** Laceration of muscle(s) and tendon(s) of peroneal muscle group at lower leg level, **right** leg   `CC`
CC Excl: See code: S86.021

√7th **S86.322** Laceration of muscle(s) and tendon(s) of peroneal muscle group at lower leg level, **left** leg   `CC`
CC Excl: See code: S86.022

√7th **S86.329** Laceration of muscle(s) and tendon(s) of peroneal muscle group at lower leg level, **unspecified** leg   `CC`
CC Excl: See code: S86.029

√6th **S86.39** **Other** injury of muscle(s) and tendon(s) of peroneal muscle group at lower leg level

√7th **S86.391** Other injury of muscle(s) and tendon(s) of peroneal muscle group at lower leg level, **right** leg

√7th **S86.392** Other injury of muscle(s) and tendon(s) of peroneal muscle group at lower leg level, **left** leg

√7th **S86.399** Other injury of muscle(s) and tendon(s) of peroneal muscle group at lower leg level, **unspecified** leg

√5th **S86.8** Injury of **other muscles and tendons** at lower leg level

√6th **S86.80** **Unspecified** injury of other muscles and tendons at lower leg level

√7th **S86.801** Unspecified injury of other muscle(s) and tendon(s) at lower leg level, **right** leg

√7th **S86.802** Unspecified injury of other muscle(s) and tendon(s) at lower leg level, **left** leg

√7th **S86.809** Unspecified injury of other muscle(s) and tendon(s) at lower leg level, **unspecified** leg

√6th **S86.81** **Strain** of other muscles and tendons at lower leg level

√7th **S86.811** Strain of other muscle(s) and tendon(s) at lower leg level, **right** leg

√7th **S86.812** Strain of other muscle(s) and tendon(s) at lower leg level, **left** leg

√7th **S86.819** Strain of other muscle(s) and tendon(s) at lower leg level, **unspecified** leg

√6th **S86.82** **Laceration** of other muscles and tendons at lower leg level

√7th **S86.821** Laceration of other muscle(s) and tendon(s) at lower leg level, **right** leg   `CC`
CC Excl: See code: S86.021

√7th **S86.822** Laceration of other muscle(s) and tendon(s) at lower leg level, **left** leg   `CC`
CC Excl: See code: S86.022

N Newborn: 0   P Pediatric: 0-17   M Maternity: 12-55   A Adult: 15-124   MCC Major CC Condition   PDx MCC PDx acts as own MCC   CC CC Condition   PDx CC PDx acts as own CC

1010   ICD-10-CM Draft (2015)

√7ᵗʰ **S86.829** Laceration of other muscle(s) and tendon(s) at lower leg level, **unspecified leg**   **CC**

CC Excl: See code: S86.029

√6ᵗʰ **S86.89** **Other** injury of other muscles and tendons at lower leg level

√7ᵗʰ **S86.891** Other injury of other muscle(s) and tendon(s) at lower leg level, **right** leg

√7ᵗʰ **S86.892** Other injury of other muscle(s) and tendon(s) at lower leg level, **left** leg

√7ᵗʰ **S86.899** Other injury of other muscle(s) and tendon(s) at lower leg level, **unspecified leg**

√5ᵗʰ **S86.9** Injury of **unspecified** muscle and tendon at lower leg level

√6ᵗʰ **S86.90** **Unspecified** injury of unspecified muscle and tendon at lower leg level

√7ᵗʰ **S86.901** Unspecified injury of unspecified muscle(s) and tendon(s) at lower leg level, **right leg**

√7ᵗʰ **S86.902** Unspecified injury of unspecified muscle(s) and tendon(s) at lower leg level, **left leg**

√7ᵗʰ **S86.909** Unspecified injury of unspecified muscle(s) and tendon(s) at lower leg level, **unspecified** leg

√6ᵗʰ **S86.91** **Strain** of unspecified muscle and tendon at lower leg level

√7ᵗʰ **S86.911** Strain of unspecified muscle(s) and tendon(s) at lower leg level, **right** leg

√7ᵗʰ **S86.912** Strain of unspecified muscle(s) and tendon(s) at lower leg level, **left** leg

√7ᵗʰ **S86.919** Strain of unspecified muscle(s) and tendon(s) at lower leg level, **unspecified leg**

√6ᵗʰ **S86.92** **Laceration** of unspecified muscle and tendon at lower leg level

√7ᵗʰ **S86.921** Laceration of unspecified muscle(s) and tendon(s) at lower leg level, **right leg**   **CC**

CC Excl: See code: S86.021

√7ᵗʰ **S86.922** Laceration of unspecified muscle(s) and tendon(s) at lower leg level, **left leg**   **CC**

CC Excl: See code: S86.022

√7ᵗʰ **S86.929** Laceration of unspecified muscle(s) and tendon(s) at lower leg level, **unspecified leg**   **CC**

CC Excl: See code: S86.029

√6ᵗʰ **S86.99** **Other** injury of unspecified muscle and tendon at lower leg level

√7ᵗʰ **S86.991** Other injury of unspecified muscle(s) and tendon(s) at lower leg level, **right** leg

√7ᵗʰ **S86.992** Other injury of unspecified muscle(s) and tendon(s) at lower leg level, **left** leg

√7ᵗʰ **S86.999** Other injury of unspecified muscle(s) and tendon(s) at lower leg level, **unspecified leg**

√4ᵗʰ **S87** **Crushing injury of lower leg**

Use additional code(s) for all associated injuries

EXCLUDES 2 crushing injury of ankle and foot (S97.-)

The appropriate 7th character is to be added to each code from category S87.
A   initial encounter
D   subsequent encounter
S   sequela

√5ᵗʰ **S87.0** **Crushing injury of knee**

√x7ᵗʰ **S87.00** Crushing injury of **unspecified** knee

√x7ᵗʰ **S87.01** Crushing injury of **right** knee

√x7ᵗʰ **S87.02** Crushing injury of **left** knee

√5ᵗʰ **S87.8** **Crushing injury of lower leg**

√x7ᵗʰ **S87.80** Crushing injury of **unspecified** lower leg

√x7ᵗʰ **S87.81** Crushing injury of **right** lower leg

√x7ᵗʰ **S87.82** Crushing injury of **left** lower leg

√4ᵗʰ **S88** **Traumatic amputation of lower leg**

NOTE   An amputation not identified as partial or complete should be coded to complete.

EXCLUDES 1 traumatic amputation of ankle and foot (S98.-)

The appropriate 7th character is to be added to each code from category S88.
A   initial encounter
D   subsequent encounter
S   sequela

√5ᵗʰ **S88.0** **Traumatic amputation at knee level**

√6ᵗʰ **S88.01** **Complete** traumatic amputation at knee level

√7ᵗʰ **S88.011** **Complete traumatic amputation at knee level, right lower leg**   **CC**

CC Excl: CC with 7th character A: S71.001 with 7th A, S71.009-S71.011 with 7th A, S71.019-S71.021 with 7th A, S71.029-S71.031 with 7th A, S71.039-S71.041 with 7th A, S71.049-S71.051 with 7th A, S71.059-S71.101 with 7th A, S71.109-S71.111 with 7th A, S71.119-S71.121 with 7th A, S71.129-S71.131 with 7th A, S71.139-S71.141 with 7th A, S71.149-S71.151 with 7th A, S71.159A, S76.021A, S76.029A, S76.121 A, S76.129A, S76.221A, S76.229A, S76.321A, S76.329A, S76.821A, S76.829A, S76.921A, S76.929A, S78.011A, S78.019-S78.021 with 7th A, S78.029-S78.111 with 7th A, S78.119-S78.121 with 7th A, S78.129-S78.911 with 7th A, S78.919-S78.921 with 7th A, S78.929A, S81.001A, S81.009-S81.011 with 7th A, S81.019-S81.021 with 7th A, S81.029-S81.031 with 7th A, S81.039-S81.041 with 7th A, S81.049-S81.051 with 7th A, S81.059-S81.801 with 7th A, S81.809-S81.811 with 7th A, S81.819-S81.821 with 7th A, S81.829-S81.831 with 7th A, S81.839-S81.841 with 7th A, S81.849-S81.851 with 7th A, S81.859 with 7th A, S86.021A, S86.029A, S86.121A, S86.129A, S86.221A, S86.229A, S86.321A, S86.329A, S86.821A, S86.829A, S86.921A, S86.929A, S88.011A, S88.019-S88.021 with 7th A, S88.029-S88.111 with 7th A, S88.119-S88.121 with 7th A, S88.129-S88.911 with 7th A, S88.919-S88.921 with 7th A, S88.929A, S91.001A, S91.009-S91.011 with 7th A, S91.019-S91.021 with 7th A, S91.029-S91.031 with 7th A, S91.039-S91.041 with 7th A, S91.049-S91.051 with 7th A, S91.059-S91.101 with 7th A, S91.103-S91.104 with 7th A, S91.106-S91.111 with 7th A, S91.113-S91.114 with 7th A, S91.116-S91.121 with 7th A, S91.123-S91.124 with 7th A, S91.126-S91.131 with 7th A, S91.133-S91.134 with 7th A, S91.136-S91.141 with 7th A, S91.143-S91.144 with 7th A, S91.146-S91.151 with 7th A, S91.153-S91.154 with 7th A, S91.156-S91.201 with 7th A, S91.203-S91.204 with 7th A, S91.206-S91.211 with 7th A, S91.213-S91.214 with 7th A, S91.216-S91.221 with 7th A, S91.223-S91.224 with 7th A, S91.226-S91.231 with 7th A, S91.233-S91.234 with 7th A, S91.236-S91.241 with 7th A, S91.243-S91.244 with 7th A, S91.246-S91.251 with 7th A, S91.253-S91.254 with 7th A, S91.256-S91.301 with 7th A, S91.309-S91.311 with 7th A, S91.319-S91.321 with 7th A, S91.329-S91.331 with 7th A, S91.339-S91.341 with 7th A, S91.349-S91.351 with 7th A, S91.359A, S96.021A, S96.029A, S96.121A, S96.129A, S96.221A, S96.229A, S96.821A, S96.829A, S96.921A, S96.929A, S98.011A, S98.019-S98.021 with 7th A, S98.029-S98.111 with 7th A, S98.119-S98.121 with 7th A, S98.122-S98.129 with 7th A, S98.131-S98.139 with 7th A, S98.142-S98.149 with 7th A, S98.212-S98.219 with 7th A, S98.222-S98.229 with 7th A, S98.312-S98.319 with 7th A, S98.322-S98.329 with 7th A, S98.912-S98.919 with 7th A, S98.922-S98.929 with 7th A, T14.8-T14.91, T79.A0X-T79.9XX with 7th A

√ Additional Character Required   √x7ᵗʰ Xtension Alert   Unacceptable PDx   Manifestation   Hospital Acquired Condition   EXCLUDES 1 Not Coded Here   EXCLUDES 2 Not Included Here

✓7ᵗʰ **S88.012　Complete traumatic amputation at** CC
knee level, left lower leg
CC Excl: CC with 7th character A: S71.002-
S71.009 with 7th A, S71.012-S71.019 with
7th A, S71.022-S71.029 with 7th A, S71.032-
S71.039 with 7th A, S71.042-S71.049 with
7th A, S71.052-S71.059 with 7th A, S71.102-
S71.109 with 7th A, S71.112-S71.119 with
7th A, S71.122-S71.129 with 7th A, S71.132-
S71.139 with 7th A, S71.142-S71.149 with
7th A, S71.152-S71.159 with 7th A, S76.022-
S76.029 with 7th A, S76.122-S76.129 with
7th A, S76.222-S76.229 with 7th A, S76.322-
S76.329 with 7th A, S76.822-S76.829 with
7th A, S76.922-S76.929 with 7th A, S78.012-
S78.019 with 7th A, S78.022-S78.029 with
7th A, S78.112-S78.119 with 7th A, S78.122-
S78.129 with 7th A, S78.912-S78.919 with
7th A, S78.922-S78.929 with 7th A, S81.002-
S81.009 with 7th A, S81.012-S81.019 with
7th A, S81.022-S81.029 with 7th A, S81.032-
S81.039 with 7th A, S81.042-S81.049 with
7th A, S81.052-S81.059 with 7th A, S81.802-
S81.809 with 7th A, S81.812-S81.819 with
7th A, S81.822-S81.829 with 7th A, S81.832-
S81.839 with 7th A, S81.842-S81.849 with
7th A, S81.852-S81.859 with 7th A, S86.022-
S86.029 with 7th A, S86.122-S86.129 with
7th A, S86.222-S86.229 with 7th A, S86.322-
S86.329 with 7th A, S86.822-S86.829 with
7th A, S86.922-S86.929 with 7th A, S88.012-
S88.019 with 7th A, S88.022-S88.029 with
7th A, S88.112-S88.119 with 7th A, S88.122-
S88.129 with 7th A, S88.912-S88.919 with
7th A, S88.922-S88.929 with 7th A, S91.002-
S91.009 with 7th A, S91.012-S91.019 with
7th A, S91.022-S91.029 with 7th A, S91.032-
S91.039 with 7th A, S91.042-S91.049 with
7th A, S91.052-S91.059 with 7th A, S91.102-
S91.103 with 7th A, S91.105-S91.109 with
7th A, S91.112-S91.113 with 7th A, S91.115-
S91.119 with 7th A, S91.122-S91.123 with
7th A, S91.125-S91.129 with 7th A, S91.132-
S91.133 with 7th A, S91.135-S91.139 with
7th A, S91.142-S91.143 with 7th A, S91.145-
S91.149 with 7th A, S91.152-S91.153 with
7th A, S91.155-S91.159 with 7th A, S91.202-
S91.203 with 7th A, S91.205-S91.209 with
7th A, S91.212-S91.213 with 7th A, S91.215-
S91.219 with 7th A, S91.222-S91.223 with
7th A, S91.225-S91.229 with 7th A, S91.232-
S91.233 with 7th A, S91.235-S91.239 with
7th A, S91.242-S91.243 with 7th A, S91.245-
S91.249 with 7th A, S91.252-S91.253 with
7th A, S91.255-S91.259 with 7th A, S91.302-
S91.309 with 7th A, S91.312-S91.319 with
7th A, S91.322-S91.329 with 7th A, S91.332-
S91.339 with 7th A, S91.342-S91.349 with
7th A, S91.352-S91.359 with 7th A, S96.022-
S96.029 with 7th A, S96.122-S96.129 with
7th A, S96.222-S96.229 with 7th A, S96.822-
S96.829 with 7th A, S96.922-S96.929 with
7th A, S98.012-S98.019 with 7th A, S98.022-
S98.029 with 7th A, S98.112-S98.119 with
7th A, S98.122-S98.129 with 7th A, S98.132-
S98.139 with 7th A, S98.142-S98.149 with
7th A, S98.212-S98.219 with 7th A, S98.222-
S98.229 with 7th A, S98.312-S98.319 with
7th A, S98.322-S98.329 with 7th A, S98.912-
S98.919 with 7th A, S98.922-S98.929 with
7th A, T14.8-T14.91, T79.A0X-T79.9XX with
7th A

✓7ᵗʰ **S88.019　Complete traumatic amputation at** CC
knee level, unspecified lower leg
CC Excl: CC with 7th character A: S71.001-
S71.159 with 7th A, S76.021-S76.029 with
7th A, S76.121-S76.129 with 7th A, S76.221-
S76.229 with 7th A, S76.321-S76.329 with
7th A, S76.821-S76.829 with 7th A, S76.921-
S76.929 with 7th A, S78.011-S78.929 with
7th A, S81.001-S81.859 with 7th A, S86.021-
S86.029 with 7th A, S86.121-S86.129 with
7th A, S86.221-S86.229 with 7th A, S86.321-
S86.329 with 7th A, S86.821-S86.829 with
7th A, S86.921-S86.929 with 7th A, S88.011-
S88.929 with 7th A, S91.001-S91.359 with
7th A, S96.021-S96.029 with 7th A, S96.121-
S96.129 with 7th A, S96.221-S96.229 with
7th A, S96.821-S96.829 with 7th A, S96.921-
S96.929 with 7th A, S98.011-S98.929 with
7th A, T14.8-T14.91, T79.A0X-T79.9XX with
7th A

✓6ᵗʰ **S88.02　Partial traumatic amputation at knee level**

✓7ᵗʰ **S88.021　Partial traumatic amputation at knee** CC
level, right lower leg
CC Excl: See code: S88.011

✓7ᵗʰ **S88.022　Partial traumatic amputation at knee** CC
level, left lower leg
CC Excl: See code: S88.012

✓7ᵗʰ **S88.029　Partial traumatic amputation at knee** CC
level, unspecified lower leg
CC Excl: See code: S88.019

✓5ᵗʰ **S88.1　Traumatic amputation at level between knee and ankle**

✓6ᵗʰ **S88.11　Complete traumatic amputation at level between
knee and ankle**

✓7ᵗʰ **S88.111　Complete traumatic amputation at** CC
**levelbetween knee and ankle, right
lower leg**
CC Excl: See code: S88.011

✓7ᵗʰ **S88.112　Complete traumatic amputation at** CC
**level between knee and ankle, left
lower leg**
CC Excl: See code: S88.012

✓7ᵗʰ **S88.119　Complete traumatic amputation at** CC
**level between knee and ankle,
unspecified lower leg**
CC Excl: See code: S88.019

✓6ᵗʰ **S88.12　Partial traumatic amputation at level between knee
and ankle**

✓7ᵗʰ **S88.121　Partial traumatic amputation at** CC
**level between knee and ankle, right
lower leg**
CC Excl: See code: S88.011

✓7ᵗʰ **S88.122　Partial traumatic amputation at** CC
**levelbetween knee and ankle, left
lower leg**
CC Excl: See code: S88.012

✓7ᵗʰ **S88.129　Partial traumatic amputation at level** CC
**between knee and ankle, unspecified
lower leg**
CC Excl: See code: S88.019

✓5ᵗʰ **S88.9　Traumatic amputation of lower leg, level unspecified**

✓6ᵗʰ **S88.91　Complete traumatic amputation of lower leg, level
unspecified**

✓7ᵗʰ **S88.911　Complete traumatic amputation of** CC
right lower leg, level unspecified
CC Excl: See code: S88.011

✓7ᵗʰ **S88.912　Complete traumatic amputation of** CC
left lower leg, level unspecified
CC Excl: See code: S88.012

✓7ᵗʰ **S88.919　Complete traumatic amputation of** CC
unspecified lower leg, level unspecified
CC Excl: See code: S88.019

✓6ᵗʰ **S88.92　Partial traumatic amputation of lower leg, level
unspecified**

✓7ᵗʰ **S88.921　Partial traumatic amputation of** CC
right lower leg, level unspecified
CC Excl: See code: S88.011

✓7ᵗʰ **S88.922　Partial traumatic amputation of left** CC
lower leg, level unspecified
CC Excl: See code: S88.012

✓7ᵗʰ **S88.929　Partial traumatic amputation of** CC
unspecified lower leg, level unspecified
CC Excl: See code: S88.019

✓4th **S89   Other and unspecified injuries of lower leg**

> **NOTE**   A fracture not indicated as open or closed should be coded to closed.

> **EXCLUDES 2**   *other and unspecified injuries of ankle and foot (S99.-)*

The appropriate 7th character is to be added to each code from subcategories S89.0, S89.1, S89.2, and S89.3.
A   initial encounter for closed fracture
D   subsequent encounter for fracture with routine healing
G   subsequent encounter for fracture with delayed healing
K   subsequent encounter for fracture with nonunion
P   subsequent encounter for fracture with malunion
S   sequela

✓5th **S89.0   Physeal fracture of upper end of tibia**

✓6th   **S89.00   Unspecified physeal fracture of upper end of tibia**

7 ✓7th   **S89.001   Unspecified physeal fracture of upper end of right tibia**   CC

CC Excl: CC with 7th character A: M80.00X-M80.019 with 7th A, M80.041-M80.049 with 7th A, M80.061-M80.079 with 7th A, M80.80X-M80.819 with 7th A, M80.841-M80.849 with 7th A, M80.861-M80.879 with 7th A, M84.40X-M84.419 with 7th A, M84.441-M84.446 with 7th A, M84.454 with 7th A, M84.461-M84.519 with 7th A, M84.541-M84.550 with 7th A, M84.561-M84.576 with 7th A, M84.60X-M84.619 with 7th A, M84.641-M84.650 with 7th A, M84.661-M84.68X with 7th A, S03.8XX-S03.9XX with 7th A, S29.011-S29.019 with 7th A, S38.3XX-S39.013 with 7th A, S73.101A, S73.109-S73.111 with 7th A, S73.119-S73.121 with 7th A, S73.129-S73.191 with 7th A, S73.199A, S76.001A, S76.009-S76.011 with 7th A, S76.019A, S76.091A, S76.099-S76.101 with 7th A, S76.109-S76.111 with 7th A, S76.119A, S76.191A, S76.199-S76.201 with 7th A, S76.209-S76.211 with 7th A, S76.219A, S76.291A, S76.299-S76.301 with 7th A, S76.309-S76.311 with 7th A, S76.319A, S76.391A, S76.399-S76.801 with 7th A, S76.809-S76.811 with 7th A, S76.819A, S76.891A, S76.899-S76.901 with 7th A, S76.909-S76.911 with 7th A, S76.919A, S76.991A, S76.999A, S79.811A, S79.819-S79.821 with 7th A, S79.829-S79.911 with 7th A, S79.919-S79.921 with 7th A, S79.929A, S82.101-S82.156 with 7th [A, B, C], S82.191-S82.299 with 7th [A, B, C], S82.401-S82.499 with 7th [A, B, C], S82.831-S82.839 with 7th [A, B, C], S82.861-S82.866 with 7th [A, B, C], S82.90X-S82.92X with 7th [A, B, C], S89.001 with 7th A, S89.009-S89.011 with 7th A, S89.019-S89.021 with 7th A, S89.029-S89.031 with 7th A, S89.039-S89.041 with 7th A, S89.049-S89.091 with 7th A, S89.099A, S89.201A, S89.209-S89.211 with 7th A, S89.219-S89.221 with 7th A, S89.229-S89.291 with 7th A, S89.299A, T14.8-T14.91, T79.A9X-T79.9XX with 7th A

CC with 7th character K or P: M80.00X-M84.68X with 7th [K, P], S02.0XX-S02.92X with 7th K, S12.000-S12.691 with 7th K, S22.000-S22.9XX with 7th K, S32.000-S32.9XX with 7th K, S42.001-S42.92X with 7th [K, P], S49.001-S49.199 with 7th [K, P], S52.001-S52.92X with 7th [K, M, N, P, Q, R], S59.001-S59.299 with 7th [K, P], S62.001-S62.92X with 7th [K, P], S72.001-S72.92X with 7th [K, M, N, P, Q, R], S79.001-S79.199 with 7th [K, P], S82.001-S82.92X with 7th [K, M, N, P, Q, R], S89.001-S89.399 with 7th [K, P], S92.001-S92.919 with 7th [K, P]

7 ✓7th   **S89.002   Unspecified physeal fracture of upper end of left tibia**   CC

CC Excl: CC with 7th character A: M80.00X-M80.019 with 7th A, M80.041-M80.049 with 7th A, M80.061-M80.079 with 7th A, M80.80X-M80.819 with 7th A, M80.841-M80.849 with 7th A, M80.861-M80.879 with 7th A, M84.40X-M84.419 with 7th A, M84.441-M84.446 with 7th A, M84.454 with 7th A, M84.461-M84.519 with 7th A, M84.541-M84.550 with 7th A, M84.561-M84.576 with 7th A, M84.60X-M84.619 with 7th A, M84.641-M84.650 with 7th A, M84.661-M84.68X with 7th A, S03.8XX-S03.9XX with 7th A, S29.011-S29.019 with 7th A, S38.3XX-S39.013 with 7th A, S73.102-S73.109 with 7th A, S73.112-S73.119 with 7th A, S73.122-S73.129 with 7th A, S73.192-S73.199 with 7th A, S76.002-S76.009 with 7th A, S76.012-S76.019 with 7th A, S76.092-S76.099 with 7th A, S76.102-S76.109 with 7th A, S76.112-S76.119 with 7th A, S76.192-S76.199 with 7th A, S76.202-S76.209 with 7th A, S76.212-S76.219 with 7th A, S76.292-S76.299 with 7th A, S76.302-S76.309 with 7th A, S76.312-S76.319 with 7th A, S76.392-S76.399 with 7th A, S76.802-S76.809 with 7th A, S76.812-S76.819 with 7th A, S76.892-S76.899 with 7th A, S76.902-S76.909 with 7th A, S76.912-S76.919 with 7th A, S76.992-S76.999 with 7th A, S79.812-S79.819 with 7th A, S79.822-S79.829 with 7th A, S79.912-S79.919 with 7th A, S79.922-S79.929 with 7th A, S82.101-S82.156 with 7th [B, C], S82.191-S82.299 with 7th [B, C], S82.401-S82.499 with 7th [B, C], S82.831-S82.839 with 7th [B, C], S82.861-S82.866 with 7th [B, C], S82.90X-S82.92X with 7th [A, B, C], S89.002-S89.009 with 7th A, S89.012-S89.019 with 7th A, S89.022-S89.029 with 7th A, S89.032-S89.039 with 7th A, S89.042-S89.049 with 7th A, S89.092-S89.099 with 7th A, S89.202-S89.209 with 7th A, S89.212-S89.219 with 7th A, S89.222-S89.229 with 7th A, S89.292-S89.299 with 7th A, T14.8-T14.91, T79.A9X-T79.9XX with 7th A

CC with 7th character K or P: M80.00X-M84.68X with 7th [K, P], S02.0XX-S02.92X with 7th K, S12.000-S12.691 with 7th K, S22.000-S22.9XX with 7th K, S32.000-S32.9XX with 7th K, S42.001-S42.92X with 7th [K, P], S49.001-S49.199 with 7th [K, P], S52.001-S52.92X with 7th [K, M, N, P, Q, R], S59.001-S59.299 with 7th [K, P], S62.001-S62.92X with 7th [K, P], S72.001-S72.92X with 7th [K, M, N, P, Q, R], S79.001-S79.199 with 7th [K, P], S82.001-S82.92X with 7th [K, M, N, P, Q, R], S89.001-S89.399 with 7th [K, P], S92.001-S92.919 with 7th [K, P]

---

7 HAC = Initial encounter only (7th character A, B or C) and not POA.

✓ Additional Character Required   ✓x7th Xtension Alert   Unacceptable PDx   Manifestation   Hospital Acquired Condition   **EXCLUDES 1** Not Coded Here   **EXCLUDES 2** Not Included Here

7 ✓7ᵗʰ **S89.009 Unspecified physeal fracture of** CC
upper end of unspecified tibia
CC Excl: CC with 7th character A: M80.00X-
M80.019 with 7th A, M80.041-M80.049 with
7th A, M80.061-M80.079 with 7th A,
M80.80X-M80.819 with 7th A, M80.841-
M80.849 with 7th A, M80.861-M80.879 with
7th A, M84.40X-M84.419 with 7th A,
M84.441-M84.446 with 7th A, M84.454 with
7th A, M84.461-M84.519 with 7th A,
M84.541-M84.550 with 7th A, M84.561-
M84.576 with 7th A, M84.60X-M84.619 with
7th A, M84.641-M84.650 with 7th A,
M84.661-M84.68X with 7th A, S03.8XX-
S03.9XX with 7th A, S29.011-S29.019 with
7th A, S38.3XX-S39.013 with 7th A, S73.101-
S73.199 with 7th A, S76.001-S76.019 with
7th A, S76.091-S76.119 with 7th A, S76.191-
S76.219 with 7th A, S76.291-S76.319 with
7th A, S76.391-S76.819 with 7th A, S76.891-
S76.919 with 7th A, S76.991-S76.999 with
7th A, S79.811-S79.929 with 7th A, S82.101-
S82.156 with 7th [A, B, C], S82.191-S82.299
with 7th [A, B, C], S82.401-S82.499 with 7th
[A, B, C], S82.831-S82.839 with 7th [A, B, C],
S82.861-S82.866 with 7th [A, B, C], S82.90X-
S82.92X with 7th [A, B, C], S89.001-S89.099
with 7th A, S89.201-S89.299 with 7th A,
T14.8-T14.91, T79.A9X-T79.9XX with 7th A
CC with 7th character K or P: M80.00X-
M84.68X with 7th [K, P], S02.0XX-S02.92X
with 7th K, S12.000-S12.691 with 7th K,
S22.000-S22.9XX with 7th K, S32.000-
S32.9XX with 7th K, S42.001-S42.92X with
7th [K, P], S49.001-S49.199 with 7th [K, P],
S52.001-S52.92X with 7th [K, M, N, P, Q, R],
S59.001-S59.299 with 7th [K, P], S62.001-
S62.92X with 7th [K, P], S72.001-S72.92X
with 7th [K, M, N, P, Q, R], S79.001-S79.199
with 7th [K, P], S82.001-S82.92X with 7th [K,
M, N, P, Q, R], S89.001-S89.399 with 7th [K, P],
S92.001-S92.919 with 7th [K, P]

✓6ᵗʰ **S89.01 Salter-Harris Type I physeal fracture of upper end of tibia**

7 ✓7ᵗʰ **S89.011 Salter-Harris Type I physeal fracture** CC
of upper end of right tibia
CC Excl: See code: S89.001

7 ✓7ᵗʰ **S89.012 Salter-Harris Type I physeal fracture** CC
of upper end of left tibia
CC Excl: See code: S89.002

7 ✓7ᵗʰ **S89.019 Salter-Harris Type I physeal fracture** CC
of upper end of unspecified tibia
CC Excl: See code: S89.009

✓6ᵗʰ **S89.02 Salter-Harris Type II physeal fracture of upper end of tibia**

7 ✓7ᵗʰ **S89.021 Salter-Harris Type II physeal fracture** CC
of upper end of right tibia
CC Excl: See code: S89.001

7 ✓7ᵗʰ **S89.022 Salter-Harris Type II physeal fracture** CC
of upper end of left tibia
CC Excl: See code: S89.002

7 ✓7ᵗʰ **S89.029 Salter-Harris Type II physeal fracture** CC
of upper end of unspecified tibia
CC Excl: See code: S89.009

✓6ᵗʰ **S89.03 Salter-Harris Type III physeal fracture of upper end of tibia**

7 ✓7ᵗʰ **S89.031 Salter-Harris Type III physeal fracture** CC
of upper end of right tibia
CC Excl: See code: S89.001

7 ✓7ᵗʰ **S89.032 Salter-Harris Type III physeal fracture** CC
of upper end of left tibia
CC Excl: See code: S89.002

7 ✓7ᵗʰ **S89.039 Salter-Harris Type III physeal fracture** CC
of upper end of unspecified tibia
CC Excl: See code: S89.009

✓6ᵗʰ **S89.04 Salter-Harris Type IV physeal fracture of upper end of tibia**

7 ✓7ᵗʰ **S89.041 Salter-Harris Type IV physeal fracture** CC
of upper end of right tibia
CC Excl: See code: S89.001

7 ✓7ᵗʰ **S89.042 Salter-Harris Type IV physeal fracture** CC
of upper end of left tibia
CC Excl: See code: S89.002

7 ✓7ᵗʰ **S89.049 Salter-Harris Type IV physeal fracture** CC
of upper end of unspecified tibia
CC Excl: See code: S89.009

✓6ᵗʰ **S89.09 Other physeal fracture of upper end of tibia**

7 ✓7ᵗʰ **S89.091 Other physeal fracture of upper end** CC
of right tibia
CC Excl: See code: S89.001

7 ✓7ᵗʰ **S89.092 Other physeal fracture of upper end** CC
of left tibia
CC Excl: See code: S89.002

7 ✓7ᵗʰ **S89.099 Other physeal fracture of upper end** CC
of unspecified tibia
CC Excl: See code: S89.009

✓5ᵗʰ **S89.1 Physeal fracture of lower end of tibia**

CC Excl: For CC codes in subcategory S89.1, unless
otherwise noted: CC with 7th character K or P:
M80.00X-M80.019 with 7th A, M80.041-M80.049 with 7th
A, M80.061-M80.079 with 7th A, M80.80X-M80.819 with
7th A, M80.841-M80.849 with 7th A, M80.861-M80.879
with 7th A, M84.40X-M84.419 with 7th A, M84.441-
M84.446 with 7th A, M84.454 with 7th A, M84.461-
M84.519 with 7th A, M84.541-M84.550 with 7th A,
M84.561-M84.576 with 7th A, M84.60X-M84.619 with 7th
A, M84.641-M84.650 with 7th A, M84.661-M84.68X with
7th A, S03.8XX-S03.9XX with 7th A, S29.011-S29.019 with
7th A, S38.3XX-S39.013 with 7th A, S73.101-S73.199 with
7th A, S76.001-S76.019 with 7th A, S76.091-S76.119 with
7th A, S76.191-S76.219 with 7th A, S76.291-S76.319 with
7th A, S76.391-S76.819 with 7th A, S76.891-S76.919 with
7th A, S76.991-S76.999 with 7th A, S79.811-S79.929 with
7th A, S82.101-S82.156 with 7th [A, B, C], S82.191-S82.299
with 7th [A, B, C], S82.401-S82.499 with 7th [A, B, C],
S82.831-S82.839 with 7th [A, B, C], S82.861-S82.866 with
7th [A, B, C], S82.90X-S82.92X with 7th [A, B, C], S89.001-
S89.099 with 7th A, S89.201-S89.299 with 7th A, T14.8-
T14.91, T79.A9X-T79.9XX with 7th A

✓6ᵗʰ **S89.10 Unspecified physeal fracture of lower end of tibia**

✓7ᵗʰ **S89.101 Unspecified physeal fracture of lower** CC
end of right tibia

✓7ᵗʰ **S89.102 Unspecified physeal fracture of lower** CC
end of left tibia

✓7ᵗʰ **S89.109 Unspecified physeal fracture of lower** CC
end of unspecified tibia

✓6ᵗʰ **S89.11 Salter-Harris Type I physeal fracture of ower end of tibia**

✓7ᵗʰ **S89.111 Salter-Harris Type I physeal fracture of** CC
lower end of right tibia

✓7ᵗʰ **S89.112 Salter-Harris Type I physeal fracture** CC
oflower end of left tibia

✓7ᵗʰ **S89.119 Salter-Harris Type I physeal fracture** CC
of lower end of unspecified tibia

✓6ᵗʰ **S89.12 Salter-Harris Type II physeal fracture of lower end of tibia**

✓7ᵗʰ **S89.121 Salter-Harris Type II physeal fracture** CC
of lower end of right tibia

✓7ᵗʰ **S89.122 Salter-Harris Type II physeal fracture** CC
of lower end of left tibia

✓7ᵗʰ **S89.129 Salter-Harris Type II physeal fracture** CC
of lower end of unspecified tibia

✓6ᵗʰ **S89.13 Salter-Harris Type III physeal fracture of lower end of tibia**

EXCLUDES 1 *fracture of medial malleolus (adult) (S82.5-)*

✓7ᵗʰ **S89.131 Salter-Harris Type III physeal fracture** CC
of lower end of right tibia

✓7ᵗʰ **S89.132 Salter-Harris Type III physeal fracture** CC
of lower end of left tibia

✓7ᵗʰ **S89.139 Salter-Harris Type III physeal fracture** CC
of lower end of unspecified tibia

✓6ᵗʰ **S89.14 Salter-Harris Type IV physeal fracture of lower end of tibia**

EXCLUDES 1 *fracture of medial malleolus (adult) (S82.5-)*

✓7ᵗʰ **S89.141 Salter-Harris Type IV physeal fracture** CC
oflower end of right tibia

✓7ᵗʰ **S89.142 Salter-Harris Type IV physeal fracture** CC
of lower end of left tibia

✓7ᵗʰ **S89.149 Salter-Harris Type IV physeal fracture** CC
of lower end of unspecified tibia

---

7 HAC = Initial encounter only (7th character A, B or C) and not POA.

N Newborn: 0   P Pediatric: 0-17   M Maternity: 12-55   A Adult: 15-124   MCC Major CC Condition   PDx MCC PDx acts as own MCC   CC CC Condition   PDx CC PDx acts as own CC

1014   ICD-10-CM Draft (2015)

√6th S89.19   Other physeal fracture of lower end of tibia

    √7th S89.191   Other physeal fracture of lower end of right tibia CC

    √7th S89.192   Other physeal fracture of lower end of left tibia CC

    √7th S89.199   Other physeal fracture of lower end of unspecified tibia CC

√5th S89.2   Physeal fracture of upper end of fibula

> **CC Excl: For CC codes in subcategory S89.2, unless otherwise noted:** See code: S89.1

√6th S89.20   Unspecified physeal fracture of upper end of fibula

    √7th S89.201   Unspecified physeal fracture of upper end of right fibula CC

    √7th S89.202   Unspecified physeal fracture of upper end of left fibula CC

    √7th S89.209   Unspecified physeal fracture of upper end of unspecified fibula CC

√6th S89.21   Salter-Harris Type I physeal fracture of upper end of fibula

    √7th S89.211   Salter-Harris Type I physeal fracture of upper end of right fibula CC

    √7th S89.212   Salter-Harris Type I physeal fracture of upper end of left fibula CC

    √7th S89.219   Salter-Harris Type I physeal fracture of upper end of unspecified fibula CC

√6th S89.22   Salter-Harris Type II physeal fracture of upper end of fibula

    √7th S89.221   Salter-Harris Type II physeal fracture of upper end of right fibula CC

    √7th S89.222   Salter-Harris Type II physeal fracture of upper end of left fibula CC

    √7th S89.229   Salter-Harris Type II physeal fracture of upper end of unspecified fibula CC

√6th S89.29   Other physeal fracture of upper end of fibula

    √7th S89.291   Other physeal fracture of upper end of right fibula CC

    √7th S89.292   Other physeal fracture of upper end of left fibula CC

    √7th S89.299   Other physeal fracture of upper end of unspecified fibula CC

√5th S89.3   Physeal fracture of lower end of fibula

> **CC Excl: For CC codes in subcategory S89.3, unless otherwise noted:** See code: S89.1

√6th S89.30   Unspecified physeal fracture of lower end of fibula

    √7th S89.301   Unspecified physeal fracture of lower end of right fibula CC

    √7th S89.302   Unspecified physeal fracture of lower end of left fibula CC

    √7th S89.309   Unspecified physeal fracture of lower end of unspecified fibula CC

√6th S89.31   Salter-Harris Type I physeal fracture of lower end of fibula

    √7th S89.311   Salter-Harris Type I physeal fracture of lower end of right fibula CC

    √7th S89.312   Salter-Harris Type I physeal fracture of lower end of left fibula CC

    √7th S89.319   Salter-Harris Type I physeal fracture of lower end of unspecified fibula CC

√6th S89.32   Salter-Harris Type II physeal fracture of lower end of fibula

    √7th S89.321   Salter-Harris Type II physeal fracture of lower end of right fibula CC

    √7th S89.322   Salter-Harris Type II physeal fracture of lower end of left fibula CC

    √7th S89.329   Salter-Harris Type II physeal fracture of lower end of unspecified fibula CC

√6th S89.39   Other physeal fracture of lower end of fibula

    √7th S89.391   Other physeal fracture of lower end of right fibula CC

    √7th S89.392   Other physeal fracture of lower end of left fibula CC

    √7th S89.399   Other physeal fracture of lower end of unspecified fibula CC

√5th S89.8   Other specified injuries of lower leg

> The appropriate 7th character is to be added to each code in subcategory S89.8.
> A   initial encounter
> D   subsequent encounter
> S   sequela

√x7th S89.80   Other specified injuries of unspecified lower leg

√x7th S89.81   Other specified injuries of right lower leg

√x7th S89.82   Other specified injuries of left lower leg

√5th S89.9   Unspecified injury of lower leg

> The appropriate 7th character is to be added to each code in subcategory S89.9.
> A   initial encounter
> D   subsequent encounter
> S   sequela

√x7th S89.90   Unspecified injury of unspecified lower leg

√x7th S89.91   Unspecified injury of right lower leg

√x7th S89.92   Unspecified injury of left lower leg

Injuries to the ankle and foot (S90-S99)

EXCLUDES 2   burns and corrosions (T20-T32)
    fracture of ankle and malleolus (S82.-)
    frostbite (T33-T34)
    insect bite or sting, venomous (T63.4)

√4th S90   Superficial injury of ankle, foot and toes

> The appropriate 7th character is to be added to each code from category S90.
> A   initial encounter
> D   subsequent encounter
> S   sequela

√5th S90.0   Contusion of ankle

√x7th S90.00   Contusion of unspecified ankle

√x7th S90.01   Contusion of right ankle

√x7th S90.02   Contusion of left ankle

√5th S90.1   Contusion of toe without damage to nail

√6th S90.11   Contusion of great toe without damage to nail

    √7th S90.111   Contusion of right great toe without damage to nail

    √7th S90.112   Contusion of left great toe without damage to nail

    √7th S90.119   Contusion of unspecified great toe without damage to nail

√6th S90.12   Contusion of lesser toe without damage to nail

    √7th S90.121   Contusion of right lesser toe(s) without damage to nail

    √7th S90.122   Contusion of left lesser toe(s) without damage to nail

    √7th S90.129   Contusion of unspecified lesser toe(s) without damage to nail
        Contusion of toe NOS

√5th S90.2   Contusion of toe with damage to nail

√6th S90.21   Contusion of great toe with damage to nail

    √7th S90.211   Contusion of right great toe with damage to nail

    √7th S90.212   Contusion of left great toe with damage to nail

    √7th S90.219   Contusion of unspecified great toe with damage to nail

√6th S90.22   Contusion of lesser toe with damage to nail

    √7th S90.221   Contusion of right lesser toe(s) with damage to nail

    √7th S90.222   Contusion of left lesser toe(s) with damage to nail

    √7th S90.229   Contusion of unspecified lesser toe(s) with damage to nail

√5th S90.3   Contusion of foot
> EXCLUDES 2   contusion of toes (S90.1-, S90.2-)

√x7th S90.30   Contusion of unspecified foot
    Contusion of foot NOS

√x7th S90.31   Contusion of right foot

√x7th S90.32   Contusion of left foot

☑ Additional Character Required   √x7th Xtension Alert   Unacceptable PDx   Manifestation   Hospital Acquired Condition   EXCLUDES 1 Not Coded Here   EXCLUDES 2 Not Included Here

ICD-10-CM Draft (2015)   1015

√5ᵗʰ **S90.4   Other superficial injuries of toe**

   √6ᵗʰ **S90.41   Abrasion of toe**

     √7ᵗʰ **S90.411   Abrasion, right great toe**
     √7ᵗʰ **S90.412   Abrasion, left great toe**
     √7ᵗʰ **S90.413   Abrasion, unspecified great toe**
     √7ᵗʰ **S90.414   Abrasion, right lesser toe(s)**
     √7ᵗʰ **S90.415   Abrasion, left lesser toe(s)**
     √7ᵗʰ **S90.416   Abrasion, unspecified lesser toe(s)**

   √6ᵗʰ **S90.42   Blister (nonthermal) of toe**

     √7ᵗʰ **S90.421   Blister (nonthermal), right great toe**
     √7ᵗʰ **S90.422   Blister (nonthermal), left great toe**
     √7ᵗʰ **S90.423   Blister (nonthermal), unspecified great toe**
     √7ᵗʰ **S90.424   Blister (nonthermal), right lesser toe(s)**
     √7ᵗʰ **S90.425   Blister (nonthermal), left lesser toe(s)**
     √7ᵗʰ **S90.426   Blister (nonthermal), unspecified lesser toe(s)**

   √6ᵗʰ **S90.44   External constriction of toe**
      Hair tourniquet syndrome of toe

     √7ᵗʰ **S90.441   External constriction, right great toe**
     √7ᵗʰ **S90.442   External constriction, left great toe**
     √7ᵗʰ **S90.443   External constriction, unspecified great toe**
     √7ᵗʰ **S90.444   External constriction, right lesser toe(s)**
     √7ᵗʰ **S90.445   External constriction, left lesser toe(s)**
     √7ᵗʰ **S90.446   External constriction, unspecified lesser toe(s)**

   √6ᵗʰ **S90.45   Superficial foreign body of toe**
      Splinter in the toe

     √7ᵗʰ **S90.451   Superficial foreign body, right great toe**
     √7ᵗʰ **S90.452   Superficial foreign body, left great toe**
     √7ᵗʰ **S90.453   Superficial foreign body, unspecified great toe**
     √7ᵗʰ **S90.454   Superficial foreign body, right lesser toe(s)**
     √7ᵗʰ **S90.455   Superficial foreign body, left lesser toe(s)**
     √7ᵗʰ **S90.456   Superficial foreign body, unspecified lesser toe(s)**

   √6ᵗʰ **S90.46   Insect bite (nonvenomous) of toe**

     √7ᵗʰ **S90.461   Insect bite (nonvenomous), right great toe**
     √7ᵗʰ **S90.462   Insect bite (nonvenomous), left great toe**
     √7ᵗʰ **S90.463   Insect bite (nonvenomous), unspecified great toe**
     √7ᵗʰ **S90.464   Insect bite (nonvenomous), right lesser toe(s)**
     √7ᵗʰ **S90.465   Insect bite (nonvenomous), left lesser toe(s)**
     √7ᵗʰ **S90.466   Insect bite (nonvenomous), unspecified lesser toe(s)**

   √6ᵗʰ **S90.47   Other superficial bite of toe**
      EXCLUDES 1   *open bite of toe (S91.15-, S91.25-)*

     √7ᵗʰ **S90.471   Other superficial bite of right great toe**
     √7ᵗʰ **S90.472   Other superficial bite of left great toe**
     √7ᵗʰ **S90.473   Other superficial bite of unspecified great toe**
     √7ᵗʰ **S90.474   Other superficial bite of right lesser toe(s)**
     √7ᵗʰ **S90.475   Other superficial bite of left lesser toe(s)**
     √7ᵗʰ **S90.476   Other superficial bite of unspecified lesser toe(s)**

√5ᵗʰ **S90.5   Other superficial injuries of ankle**

   √6ᵗʰ **S90.51   Abrasion of ankle**

     √7ᵗʰ **S90.511   Abrasion, right ankle**
     √7ᵗʰ **S90.512   Abrasion, left ankle**
     √7ᵗʰ **S90.519   Abrasion, unspecified ankle**

   √6ᵗʰ **S90.52   Blister (nonthermal) of ankle**

     √7ᵗʰ **S90.521   Blister (nonthermal), right ankle**
     √7ᵗʰ **S90.522   Blister (nonthermal), left ankle**
     √7ᵗʰ **S90.529   Blister (nonthermal), unspecified ankle**

   √6ᵗʰ **S90.54   External constriction of ankle**

     √7ᵗʰ **S90.541   External constriction, right ankle**
     √7ᵗʰ **S90.542   External constriction, left ankle**

     √7ᵗʰ **S90.549   External constriction, unspecified ankle**

   √6ᵗʰ **S90.55   Superficial foreign body of ankle**
      Splinter in the ankle

     √7ᵗʰ **S90.551   Superficial foreign body, right ankle**
     √7ᵗʰ **S90.552   Superficial foreign body, left ankle**
     √7ᵗʰ **S90.559   Superficial foreign body, unspecified ankle**

   √6ᵗʰ **S90.56   Insect bite (nonvenomous) of ankle**

     √7ᵗʰ **S90.561   Insect bite (nonvenomous), right ankle**
     √7ᵗʰ **S90.562   Insect bite (nonvenomous), left ankle**
     √7ᵗʰ **S90.569   Insect bite (nonvenomous), unspecified ankle**

   √6ᵗʰ **S90.57   Other superficial bite of ankle**
      EXCLUDES 1   *open bite of ankle (S91.05-)*

     √7ᵗʰ **S90.571   Other superficial bite of ankle, right ankle**
     √7ᵗʰ **S90.572   Other superficial bite of ankle, left ankle**
     √7ᵗʰ **S90.579   Other superficial bite of ankle, unspecified ankle**

√5ᵗʰ **S90.8   Other superficial injuries of foot**

   √6ᵗʰ **S90.81   Abrasion of foot**

     √7ᵗʰ **S90.811   Abrasion, right foot**
     √7ᵗʰ **S90.812   Abrasion, left foot**
     √7ᵗʰ **S90.819   Abrasion, unspecified foot**

   √6ᵗʰ **S90.82   Blister (nonthermal) of foot**

     √7ᵗʰ **S90.821   Blister (nonthermal), right foot**
     √7ᵗʰ **S90.822   Blister (nonthermal), left foot**
     √7ᵗʰ **S90.829   Blister (nonthermal), unspecified foot**

   √6ᵗʰ **S90.84   External constriction of foot**

     √7ᵗʰ **S90.841   External constriction, right foot**
     √7ᵗʰ **S90.842   External constriction, left foot**
     √7ᵗʰ **S90.849   External constriction, unspecified foot**

   √6ᵗʰ **S90.85   Superficial foreign body of foot**
      Splinter in the foot

     √7ᵗʰ **S90.851   Superficial foreign body, right foot**
     √7ᵗʰ **S90.852   Superficial foreign body, left foot**
     √7ᵗʰ **S90.859   Superficial foreign body, unspecified foot**

   √6ᵗʰ **S90.86   Insect bite (nonvenomous) of foot**

     √7ᵗʰ **S90.861   Insect bite (nonvenomous), right foot**
     √7ᵗʰ **S90.862   Insect bite (nonvenomous), left foot**
     √7ᵗʰ **S90.869   Insect bite (nonvenomous), unspecified foot**

   √6ᵗʰ **S90.87   Other superficial bite of foot**
      EXCLUDES 1   *open bite of foot (S91.35-)*

     √7ᵗʰ **S90.871   Other superficial bite of right foot**
     √7ᵗʰ **S90.872   Other superficial bite of left foot**
     √7ᵗʰ **S90.879   Other superficial bite of unspecified foot**

√5ᵗʰ **S90.9   Unspecified superficial injury of ankle, foot and toe**

   √6ᵗʰ **S90.91   Unspecified superficial injury of ankle**

     √7ᵗʰ **S90.911   Unspecified superficial injury of right ankle**
     √7ᵗʰ **S90.912   Unspecified superficial injury of left ankle**
     √7ᵗʰ **S90.919   Unspecified superficial injury of unspecified ankle**

   √6ᵗʰ **S90.92   Unspecified superficial injury of foot**

     √7ᵗʰ **S90.921   Unspecified superficial injury of right foot**
     √7ᵗʰ **S90.922   Unspecified superficial injury of left foot**
     √7ᵗʰ **S90.929   Unspecified superficial injury of unspecified foot**

   √6ᵗʰ **S90.93   Unspecified superficial injury of toes**

     √7ᵗʰ **S90.931   Unspecified superficial injury of right great toe**
     √7ᵗʰ **S90.932   Unspecified superficial injury of left great toe**
     √7ᵗʰ **S90.933   Unspecified superficial injury of unspecified great toe**
     √7ᵗʰ **S90.934   Unspecified superficial injury of right lesser toe(s)**
     √7ᵗʰ **S90.935   Unspecified superficial injury of left lesser toe(s)**

N Newborn: 0   **P** Pediatric: 0-17   **M** Maternity: 12-55   **A** Adult: 15-124   **MCC** Major CC Condition   **PDx MCC** PDx acts as own MCC   **CC** CC Condition   **PDx CC** PDx acts as own CC

1016   ICD-10-CM Draft (2015)

√7ᵗʰ **S90.936** Unspecified superficial injury of unspecified lesser **toe(s)**

√4ᵗʰ **S91 Open wound of ankle, foot and toes**
Code also any associated wound infection
EXCLUDES 1 open fracture of ankle, foot and toes (S92-with 7th B)
traumatic amputation of ankle and foot (S98.-)

The appropriate 7th character is to be added to each code from category S91.
A   initial encounter
D   subsequent encounter
S   sequela

√5ᵗʰ **S91.0 Open wound of ankle**
√6ᵗʰ **S91.00** Unspecified open wound of ankle
√7ᵗʰ **S91.001** Unspecified open wound, right ankle
√7ᵗʰ **S91.002** Unspecified open wound, left ankle
√7ᵗʰ **S91.009** Unspecified open wound, unspecified ankle
√6ᵗʰ **S91.01** Laceration without foreign body of ankle
√7ᵗʰ **S91.011** Laceration without foreign body, right ankle
√7ᵗʰ **S91.012** Laceration without foreign body, left ankle
√7ᵗʰ **S91.019** Laceration without foreign body, unspecified ankle
√6ᵗʰ **S91.02** Laceration with foreign body of ankle
√7ᵗʰ **S91.021** Laceration with foreign body, right ankle
√7ᵗʰ **S91.022** Laceration with foreign body, left ankle
√7ᵗʰ **S91.029** Laceration with foreign body, unspecified ankle
√6ᵗʰ **S91.03** Puncture wound without foreign body of ankle
√7ᵗʰ **S91.031** Puncture wound without foreign body, right ankle
√7ᵗʰ **S91.032** Puncture wound without foreign body, left ankle
√7ᵗʰ **S91.039** Puncture wound without foreign body, unspecified ankle
√6ᵗʰ **S91.04** Puncture wound with foreign body of ankle
√7ᵗʰ **S91.041** Puncture wound with foreign body, right ankle
√7ᵗʰ **S91.042** Puncture wound with foreign body, left ankle
√7ᵗʰ **S91.049** Puncture wound with foreign body, unspecified ankle
√6ᵗʰ **S91.05** Open bite of ankle
EXCLUDES 1 superficial bite of ankle (S90.56-, S90.57-)
√7ᵗʰ **S91.051** Open bite, right ankle
√7ᵗʰ **S91.052** Open bite, left ankle
√7ᵗʰ **S91.059** Open bite, unspecified ankle
√5ᵗʰ **S91.1 Open wound of toe without damage to nail**
√6ᵗʰ **S91.10** Unspecified open wound of toe without damage to nail
√7ᵗʰ **S91.101** Unspecified open wound of right great toe without damage to nail
√7ᵗʰ **S91.102** Unspecified open wound of left great toe without damage to nail
√7ᵗʰ **S91.103** Unspecified open wound of unspecified great toe without damage to nail
√7ᵗʰ **S91.104** Unspecified open wound of right lesser toe(s) without damage to nail
√7ᵗʰ **S91.105** Unspecified open wound of left lesser toe(s) without damage to nail
√7ᵗʰ **S91.106** Unspecified open wound of unspecified lesser toe(s) without damage to nail
√7ᵗʰ **S91.109** Unspecified open wound of unspecified toe(s) without damage to nail
√6ᵗʰ **S91.11** Laceration without foreign body of toe without damage to nail
√7ᵗʰ **S91.111** Laceration without foreign body of right great toe without damage to nail
√7ᵗʰ **S91.112** Laceration without foreign body of left great toe without damage to nail

√7ᵗʰ **S91.113** Laceration without foreign body of unspecified great toe without damage to nail
√7ᵗʰ **S91.114** Laceration without foreign body of right lesser toe(s) without damage to nail
√7ᵗʰ **S91.115** Laceration without foreign body of left lesser toe(s) without damage to nail
√7ᵗʰ **S91.116** Laceration without foreign body of unspecified lesser toe(s) without damage to nail
√7ᵗʰ **S91.119** Laceration without foreign body of unspecified toe without damage to nail
√6ᵗʰ **S91.12** Laceration with foreign body of toe without damage to nail
√7ᵗʰ **S91.121** Laceration with foreign body of right great toe without damage to nail
√7ᵗʰ **S91.122** Laceration with foreign body of left great toe without damage to nail
√7ᵗʰ **S91.123** Laceration with foreign body of unspecified great toe without damage to nail
√7ᵗʰ **S91.124** Laceration with foreign body of right lesser toe(s) without damage to nail
√7ᵗʰ **S91.125** Laceration with foreign body of left lesser toe(s) without damage to nail
√7ᵗʰ **S91.126** Laceration with foreign body of unspecified lesser toe(s) without damage to nail
√7ᵗʰ **S91.129** Laceration with foreign body of unspecified toe(s) without damage to nail
√6ᵗʰ **S91.13** Puncture wound without foreign body of toe without damage to nail
√7ᵗʰ **S91.131** Puncture wound without foreign body of right great toe without damage to nail
√7ᵗʰ **S91.132** Puncture wound without foreign body of left great toe without damage to nail
√7ᵗʰ **S91.133** Puncture wound without foreign body of unspecified great toe without damage to nail
√7ᵗʰ **S91.134** Puncture wound without foreign body of right lesser toe(s) without damage to nail
√7ᵗʰ **S91.135** Puncture wound without foreign body of left lesser toe(s) without damage to nail
√7ᵗʰ **S91.136** Puncture wound without foreign body of unspecified lesser toe(s) without damage to nail
√7ᵗʰ **S91.139** Puncture wound without foreign body of unspecified toe(s) without damage to nail
√6ᵗʰ **S91.14** Puncture wound with foreign body of toe without damage to nail
√7ᵗʰ **S91.141** Puncture wound with foreign body of right great toe without damage to nail
√7ᵗʰ **S91.142** Puncture wound with foreign body of left great toe without damage to nail
√7ᵗʰ **S91.143** Puncture wound with foreign body of unspecified great toe without damage to nail
√7ᵗʰ **S91.144** Puncture wound with foreign body of right lesser toe(s) without damage to nail
√7ᵗʰ **S91.145** Puncture wound with foreign body of left lesser toe(s) without damage to nail
√7ᵗʰ **S91.146** Puncture wound with foreign body of unspecified lesser toe(s) without damage to nail
√7ᵗʰ **S91.149** Puncture wound with foreign body of unspecified toe(s) without damage to nail
√6ᵗʰ **S91.15** Open bite of toe without damage to nail
Bite of toe NOS
EXCLUDES 1 superficial bite of toe (S90.46-, S90.47-)
√7ᵗʰ **S91.151** Open bite of right great toe without damage to nail
√7ᵗʰ **S91.152** Open bite of left great toe without damage to nail
√7ᵗʰ **S91.153** Open bite of unspecified great toe without damage to nail
√7ᵗʰ **S91.154** Open bite of right lesser toe(s) without damage to nail

√7ᵗʰ S91.155   Open bite of left lesser toe(s) without damage to nail

√7ᵗʰ S91.156   Open bite of unspecified lesser toe(s) without damage to nail

√7ᵗʰ S91.159   Open bite of unspecified toe(s) without damage to nail

√5ᵗʰ **S91.2   Open wound of toe with damage to nail**

√6ᵗʰ S91.20   Unspecified open wound of toe with damage to nail

√7ᵗʰ S91.201   Unspecified open wound of right great toe with damage to nail

√7ᵗʰ S91.202   Unspecified open wound of left great toe with damage to nail

√7ᵗʰ S91.203   Unspecified open wound of unspecified great toe with damage to nail

√7ᵗʰ S91.204   Unspecified open wound of right lesser toe(s) with damage to nail

√7ᵗʰ S91.205   Unspecified open wound of left lesser toe(s) with damage to nail

√7ᵗʰ S91.206   Unspecified open wound of unspecified lesser toe(s) with damage to nail

√7ᵗʰ S91.209   Unspecified open wound of unspecified toe(s) with damage to nail

√6ᵗʰ S91.21   Laceration without foreign body of toe with damage to nail

√7ᵗʰ S91.211   Laceration without foreign body of right great toe with damage to nail

√7ᵗʰ S91.212   Laceration without foreign body of left great toe with damage to nail

√7ᵗʰ S91.213   Laceration without foreign body of unspecified great toe with damage to nail

√7ᵗʰ S91.214   Laceration without foreign body of right lesser toe(s) with damage to nail

√7ᵗʰ S91.215   Laceration without foreign body of left lesser toe(s) with damage to nail

√7ᵗʰ S91.216   Laceration without foreign body of unspecified lesser toe(s) with damage to nail

√7ᵗʰ S91.219   Laceration without foreign body of unspecified toe(s) with damage to nail

√6ᵗʰ S91.22   Laceration with foreign body of toe with damage to nail

√7ᵗʰ S91.221   Laceration with foreign body of right great toe with damage to nail

√7ᵗʰ S91.222   Laceration with foreign body of left great toe with damage to nail

√7ᵗʰ S91.223   Laceration with foreign body of unspecified great toe with damage to nail

√7ᵗʰ S91.224   Laceration with foreign body of right lesser toe(s) with damage to nail

√7ᵗʰ S91.225   Laceration with foreign body of left lesser toe(s) with damage to nail

√7ᵗʰ S91.226   Laceration with foreign body of unspecified lesser toe(s) with damage to nail

√7ᵗʰ S91.229   Laceration with foreign body of unspecified toe(s) with damage to nail

√6ᵗʰ S91.23   Puncture wound without foreign body of toe with damage to nail

√7ᵗʰ S91.231   Puncture wound without foreign body of right great toe with damage to nail

√7ᵗʰ S91.232   Puncture wound without foreign body of left great toe with damage to nail

√7ᵗʰ S91.233   Puncture wound without foreign body of unspecified great toe with damage to nail

√7ᵗʰ S91.234   Puncture wound without foreign body of right lesser toe(s) with damage to nail

√7ᵗʰ S91.235   Puncture wound without foreign body of left lesser toe(s) with damage to nail

√7ᵗʰ S91.236   Puncture wound without foreign body of unspecified lesser toe(s) with damage to nail

√7ᵗʰ S91.239   Puncture wound without foreign body of unspecified toe(s) with damage to nail

√6ᵗʰ S91.24   Puncture wound with foreign body of toe with damage to nail

√7ᵗʰ S91.241   Puncture wound with foreign body of right great toe with damage to nail

√7ᵗʰ S91.242   Puncture wound with foreign body of left great toe with damage to nail

√7ᵗʰ S91.243   Puncture wound with foreign body of unspecified great toe with damage to nail

√7ᵗʰ S91.244   Puncture wound with foreign body of right lesser toe(s) with damage to nail

√7ᵗʰ S91.245   Puncture wound with foreign body of left lesser toe(s) with damage to nail

√7ᵗʰ S91.246   Puncture wound with foreign body of unspecified lesser toe(s) with damage to nail

√7ᵗʰ S91.249   Puncture wound with foreign body of unspecified toe(s) with damage to nail

√6ᵗʰ S91.25   Open bite of toe with damage to nail
     Bite of toe with damage to nail NOS
     EXCLUDES 1 *superficial bite of toe (S90.46-, S90.47-)*

√7ᵗʰ S91.251   Open bite of right great toe with damage to nail

√7ᵗʰ S91.252   Open bite of left great toe with damage to nail

√7ᵗʰ S91.253   Open bite of unspecified great toe with damage to nail

√7ᵗʰ S91.254   Open bite of right lesser toe(s) with damage to nail

√7ᵗʰ S91.255   Open bite of left lesser toe(s) with damage to nail

√7ᵗʰ S91.256   Open bite of unspecified lesser toe(s) with damage to nail

√7ᵗʰ S91.259   Open bite of unspecified toe(s) with damage to nail

√5ᵗʰ **S91.3   Open wound of foot**

√6ᵗʰ S91.30   Unspecified open wound of foot

√7ᵗʰ S91.301   Unspecified open wound, right foot

√7ᵗʰ S91.302   Unspecified open wound, left foot

√7ᵗʰ S91.309   Unspecified open wound, unspecified foot

√6ᵗʰ S91.31   Laceration without foreign body of foot

√7ᵗʰ S91.311   Laceration without foreign body, right foot

√7ᵗʰ S91.312   Laceration without foreign body, left foot

√7ᵗʰ S91.319   Laceration without foreign body, unspecified foot

√6ᵗʰ S91.32   Laceration with foreign body of foot

√7ᵗʰ S91.321   Laceration with foreign body, right foot

√7ᵗʰ S91.322   Laceration with foreign body, left foot

√7ᵗʰ S91.329   Laceration with foreign body, unspecified foot

√6ᵗʰ S91.33   Puncture wound without foreign body of foot

√7ᵗʰ S91.331   Puncture wound without foreign body, right foot

√7ᵗʰ S91.332   Puncture wound without foreign body, left foot

√7ᵗʰ S91.339   Puncture wound without foreign body, unspecified foot

√6ᵗʰ S91.34   Puncture wound with foreign body of foot

√7ᵗʰ S91.341   Puncture wound with foreign body, right foot

√7ᵗʰ S91.342   Puncture wound with foreign body, left foot

√7ᵗʰ S91.349   Puncture wound with foreign body, unspecified foot

√6ᵗʰ S91.35   Open bite of foot
     EXCLUDES 1 *superficial bite of foot (S90.86-, S90.87-)*

√7ᵗʰ S91.351   Open bite, right foot

√7ᵗʰ S91.352   Open bite, left foot

√7ᵗʰ S91.359   Open bite, unspecified foot

N Newborn: 0   P Pediatric: 0-17   M Maternity: 12-55   A Adult: 15-124   MCC Major CC Condition   PDx MCC PDx acts as own MCC   CC CC Condition   PDx CC PDx acts as own CC

1018   ICD-10-CM Draft (2015)

✓4ᵗʰ **S92 Fracture of foot and toe, except ankle**

> **NOTE** A fracture not indicated as displaced or nondisplaced should be coded to displaced.
> A fracture not indicated as open or closed should be coded to closed.
>
> EXCLUDES 1   traumatic amputation of ankle and foot (S98.-)
> EXCLUDES 2   fracture of ankle (S82.-)
>   fracture of malleolus (S82.-)

> The appropriate 7th character is to be added to each code from category S92.
> A   initial encounter for closed fracture
> B   initial encounter for open fracture
> D   subsequent encounter for fracture with routine healing
> G   subsequent encounter for fracture with delayed healing
> K   subsequent encounter for fracture with nonunion
> P   subsequent encounter for fracture with malunion
> S   sequela

✓5ᵗʰ **S92.0 Fracture of calcaneus**
> Heel bone
> Os calcis

> **CC Excl:** For CC codes in subcategory S92.0, unless otherwise noted: CC with 7th character B: M80.00X-M80.019 with 7th A, M80.041-M80.049 with 7th A, M80.061-M80.079 with 7th A, M80.80X-M80.819 with 7th A, M80.841-M80.849 with 7th A, M80.861-M80.879 with 7th A, M84.40X-M84.419 with 7th A, M84.441-M84.446 with 7th A, M84.454 with 7th A, M84.461-M84.519 with 7th A, M84.541-M84.550 with 7th A, M84.561-M84.576 with 7th A, M84.60X-M84.619 with 7th A, M84.641-M84.650 with 7th A, M84.661-M84.68X with 7th A, S03.8XX-S03.9XX with 7th A, S29.011-S29.019 with 7th A, S38.3XX-S39.013 with 7th A, S73.101-S73.199 with 7th A, S76.001-S76.019 with 7th A, S76.091-S76.119 with 7th A, S76.191-S76.219 with 7th A, S76.291-S76.319 with 7th A, S76.391-S76.819 with 7th A, S76.891-S76.919 with 7th A, S76.991-S76.999 with 7th A, S79.811-S79.929 with 7th A, S82.90X-S82.92X with 7th [A, B, C], S92.001-S92.356 with 7th B, S92.901-S92.909 with 7th [A, B], T14.8-T14.91, T79.A9X-T79.9XX with 7th A
> **CC with 7th character K or P:** M80.00X-M84.68X with 7th [K, P], S02.0XX-S02.92X with 7th K, S12.000-S12.691 with 7th K, S22.000-S22.9XX with 7th K, S32.000-S32.9XX with 7th K, S42.001-S42.92X with 7th [K, P], S49.001-S49.199 with 7th [K, P], S52.001-S52.92X with 7th [K, M, N, P, Q, R], S59.001-S59.299 with 7th [K, P], S62.001-S62.92X with 7th [K, P], S72.001-S72.92X with 7th [K, M, N, P, Q, R], S79.001-S79.199 with 7th [K, P], S82.001-S82.92X with 7th [K, M, N, P, Q, R], S89.001-S89.399 with 7th [K, P], S92.001-S92.919 with 7th [K, P]

✓6ᵗʰ **S92.00 Unspecified fracture of calcaneus**
- 7 ✓7ᵗʰ **S92.001 Unspecified fracture of right calcaneus** CC
- 7 ✓7ᵗʰ **S92.002 Unspecified fracture of left calcaneus** CC
- 7 ✓7ᵗʰ **S92.009 Unspecified fracture of unspecified calcaneus** CC

✓6ᵗʰ **S92.01 Fracture of body of calcaneus**
- 7 ✓7ᵗʰ **S92.011 Displaced fracture of body of right calcaneus** CC
- 7 ✓7ᵗʰ **S92.012 Displaced fracture of body of left calcaneus** CC
- 7 ✓7ᵗʰ **S92.013 Displaced fracture of body of unspecified calcaneus** CC
- 7 ✓7ᵗʰ **S92.014 Nondisplaced fracture of body of right calcaneus** CC
- 7 ✓7ᵗʰ **S92.015 Nondisplaced fracture of body of left calcaneus** CC
- 7 ✓7ᵗʰ **S92.016 Nondisplaced fracture of body of unspecified calcaneus** CC

✓6ᵗʰ **S92.02 Fracture of anterior process of calcaneus**
- 7 ✓7ᵗʰ **S92.021 Displaced fracture of anterior process of right calcaneus** CC
- 7 ✓7ᵗʰ **S92.022 Displaced fracture of anterior process of left calcaneus** CC
- 7 ✓7ᵗʰ **S92.023 Displaced fracture of anterior process of unspecified calcaneus** CC
- 7 ✓7ᵗʰ **S92.024 Nondisplaced fracture of anterior process of right calcaneus** CC
- 7 ✓7ᵗʰ **S92.025 Nondisplaced fracture of anterior process of left calcaneus** CC
- 7 ✓7ᵗʰ **S92.026 Nondisplaced fracture of anterior process of unspecified calcaneus** CC

✓6ᵗʰ **S92.03 Avulsion fracture of tuberosity of calcaneus**
- 7 ✓7ᵗʰ **S92.031 Displaced avulsion fracture of tuberosity of right calcaneus** CC
- 7 ✓7ᵗʰ **S92.032 Displaced avulsion fracture of tuberosity of left calcaneus** CC
- 7 ✓7ᵗʰ **S92.033 Displaced avulsion fracture of tuberosity of unspecified calcaneus** CC
- 7 ✓7ᵗʰ **S92.034 Nondisplaced avulsion fracture of tuberosity of right calcaneus** CC
- 7 ✓7ᵗʰ **S92.035 Nondisplaced avulsion fracture of tuberosity of left calcaneus** CC
- 7 ✓7ᵗʰ **S92.036 Nondisplaced avulsion fracture of tuberosity of unspecified calcaneus** CC

✓6ᵗʰ **S92.04 Other fracture of tuberosity of calcaneus**
- 7 ✓7ᵗʰ **S92.041 Displaced other fracture of tuberosity of right calcaneus** CC
- 7 ✓7ᵗʰ **S92.042 Displaced other fracture of tuberosity of left calcaneus** CC
- 7 ✓7ᵗʰ **S92.043 Displaced other fracture of tuberosity of unspecified calcaneus** CC
- 7 ✓7ᵗʰ **S92.044 Nondisplaced other fracture of tuberosity of right calcaneus** CC
- 7 ✓7ᵗʰ **S92.045 Nondisplaced other fracture of tuberosity of left calcaneus** CC
- 7 ✓7ᵗʰ **S92.046 Nondisplaced other fracture of tuberosity of unspecified calcaneus** CC

✓6ᵗʰ **S92.05 Other extraarticular fracture of calcaneus**
- 7 ✓7ᵗʰ **S92.051 Displaced other extraarticular fracture of right calcaneus** CC
- 7 ✓7ᵗʰ **S92.052 Displaced other extraarticular fracture of left calcaneus** CC
- 7 ✓7ᵗʰ **S92.053 Displaced other extraarticular fracture of unspecified calcaneus** CC
- 7 ✓7ᵗʰ **S92.054 Nondisplaced other extraarticular fracture of right calcaneus** CC
- 7 ✓7ᵗʰ **S92.055 Nondisplaced other extraarticular fracture of left calcaneus** CC
- 7 ✓7ᵗʰ **S92.056 Nondisplaced other extraarticular fracture of unspecified calcaneus** CC

✓6ᵗʰ **S92.06 Intraarticular fracture of calcaneus**
- 7 ✓7ᵗʰ **S92.061 Displaced intraarticular fracture of right calcaneus** CC
- 7 ✓7ᵗʰ **S92.062 Displaced intraarticular fracture of left calcaneus** CC
- 7 ✓7ᵗʰ **S92.063 Displaced intraarticular fracture of unspecified calcaneus** CC
- 7 ✓7ᵗʰ **S92.064 Nondisplaced intraarticular fracture of right calcaneus** CC
- 7 ✓7ᵗʰ **S92.065 Nondisplaced intraarticular fracture of left calcaneus** CC
- 7 ✓7ᵗʰ **S92.066 Nondisplaced intraarticular fracture of unspecified calcaneus** CC

---

7 HAC = Initial encounter only (7th character A, B or C) and not POA.

✓ Additional Character Required   ✓x7ᵗʰ Xtension Alert   Unacceptable PDx   Manifestation   Hospital Acquired Condition   EXCLUDES 1 Not Coded Here   EXCLUDES 2 Not Included Here

√5th **S92.1 Fracture of** talus
Astragalus

> **CC Excl:** For CC codes in subcategory S92.1, unless otherwise noted: CC with 7th character B: M80.00X-M80.019 with 7th A, M80.041-M80.049 with 7th A, M80.80X-M80.819 with 7th A, M80.841-M80.849 with 7th A, M84.40X-M84.419 with 7th A, M84.441-M84.446 with 7th A, M84.454 with 7th A, M84.474-M84.519 with 7th A, M84.541-M84.550 with 7th A, M84.574-M84.576 with 7th A, M84.60X-M84.619 with 7th A, M84.641-M84.650 with 7th A, M84.674-M84.68X with 7th A, S03.8XX-S03.9XX with 7th A, S29.011-S29.019 with 7th A, S38.3XX-S39.013 with 7th A, S73.101-S73.199 with 7th A, S76.001-S76.019 with 7th A, S76.091-S76.119 with 7th A, S76.191-S76.219 with 7th A, S76.291-S76.319 with 7th A, S76.391-S76.819 with 7th A, S76.891-S76.919 with 7th A, S76.991-S76.999 with 7th A, S79.811-S79.929 with 7th A, S82.90X-S82.92X with 7th [A, B, C], S92.001-S92.356 with 7th B, S92.901-S92.909 with 7th [A, B], T14.8-T14.91, T79.A9X-T79.9XX with 7th A
> **CC with 7th character K or P:** M80.00X-M84.68X with 7th [K, P], S02.0XX-S02.92X with 7th K, S12.000-S12.691 with 7th K, S22.000-S22.9XX with 7th K, S32.000-S32.9XX with 7th K, S42.001-S42.92X with 7th [K, P], S49.001-S49.199 with 7th [K, P], S52.001-S52.92X with 7th [K, M, N, P, Q, R], S59.001-S59.299 with 7th [K, P], S62.001-S62.92X with 7th [K, P], S72.001-S72.92X with 7th [K, M, N, P, Q, R], S79.001-S79.199 with 7th [K, P], S82.001-S82.92X with 7th [K, M, N, P, Q, R], S89.001-S89.399 with 7th [K, P], S92.001-S92.919 with 7th [K, P]

√6th **S92.10 Unspecified fracture of talus**
   7 √7th **S92.101** Unspecified fracture of right talus   CC
   7 √7th **S92.102** Unspecified fracture of left talus   CC
   7 √7th **S92.109** Unspecified fracture of unspecified talus   CC

√6th **S92.11 Fracture of neck of talus**
   7 √7th **S92.111** Displaced fracture of neck of right talus   CC
   7 √7th **S92.112** Displaced fracture of neck of left talus   CC
   7 √7th **S92.113** Displaced fracture of neck of unspecified talus   CC
   7 √7th **S92.114** Nondisplaced fracture of neck of right talus   CC
   7 √7th **S92.115** Nondisplaced fracture of neck of left talus   CC
   7 √7th **S92.116** Nondisplaced fracture of neck of unspecified talus   CC

√6th **S92.12 Fracture of body of talus**
   7 √7th **S92.121** Displaced fracture of body of right talus   CC
   7 √7th **S92.122** Displaced fracture of body of left talus   CC
   7 √7th **S92.123** Displaced fracture of body of unspecified talus   CC
   7 √7th **S92.124** Nondisplaced fracture of body of right talus   CC
   7 √7th **S92.125** Nondisplaced fracture of body of left talus   CC
   7 √7th **S92.126** Nondisplaced fracture of body of unspecified talus   CC

√6th **S92.13 Fracture of posterior process of talus**
   7 √7th **S92.131** Displaced fracture of posterior process of right talus   CC
   7 √7th **S92.132** Displaced fracture of posterior process of left talus   CC
   7 √7th **S92.133** Displaced fracture of posterior process of unspecified talus   CC
   7 √7th **S92.134** Nondisplaced fracture of posterior process of right talus   CC
   7 √7th **S92.135** Nondisplaced fracture of posterior process of left talus   CC
   7 √7th **S92.136** Nondisplaced fracture of posterior process of unspecified talus   CC

√6th **S92.14 Dome fracture of talus**
   EXCLUDES 1   osteochondritis dissecans (M93.2)
   7 √7th **S92.141** Displaced dome fracture of right talus   CC
   7 √7th **S92.142** Displaced dome fracture of left talus   CC

   7 √7th **S92.143** Displaced dome fracture of unspecified talus   CC
   7 √7th **S92.144** Nondisplaced dome fracture of right talus   CC
   7 √7th **S92.145** Nondisplaced dome fracture of left talus   CC
   7 √7th **S92.146** Nondisplaced dome fracture of unspecified talus   CC

√6th **S92.15 Avulsion fracture (chip fracture) of talus**
   7 √7th **S92.151** Displaced avulsion fracture (chip fracture) of right talus   CC
   7 √7th **S92.152** Displaced avulsion fracture (chip fracture) of left talus   CC
   7 √7th **S92.153** Displaced avulsion fracture (chip fracture) of unspecified talus   CC
   7 √7th **S92.154** Nondisplaced avulsion fracture (chip fracture) of right talus   CC
   7 √7th **S92.155** Nondisplaced avulsion fracture (chip fracture) of left talus   CC
   7 √7th **S92.156** Nondisplaced avulsion fracture (chip fracture) of unspecified talus   CC

√6th **S92.19 Other fracture of talus**
   7 √7th **S92.191** Other fracture of right talus   CC
   7 √7th **S92.192** Other fracture of left talus   CC
   7 √7th **S92.199** Other fracture of unspecified talus   CC

√5th **S92.2 Fracture of other and unspecified tarsal bone(s)**

> **CC Excl:** For CC codes in subcategory S92.2, unless otherwise noted: CC with 7th character B: S92.001-S92.919 with 7th [A, B]
> **CC with 7th character K or P:** M80.00X-M84.68X with 7th [K, P], S02.0XX-S02.92X with 7th K, S12.000-S12.691 with 7th K, S22.000-S22.9XX with 7th K, S32.000-S32.9XX with 7th K, S42.001-S42.92X with 7th [K, P], S49.001-S49.199 with 7th [K, P], S52.001-S52.92X with 7th [K, M, N, P, Q, R], S59.001-S59.299 with 7th [K, P], S62.001-S62.92X with 7th [K, P], S72.001-S72.92X with 7th [K, M, N, P, Q, R], S79.001-S79.199 with 7th [K, P], S82.001-S82.92X with 7th [K, M, N, P, Q, R], S89.001-S89.399 with 7th [K, P], S92.001-S92.919 with 7th [K, P]

√6th **S92.20 Fracture of unspecified tarsal bone(s)**
   7 √7th **S92.201** Fracture of unspecified tarsal bone(s) of right foot   CC
   7 √7th **S92.202** Fracture of unspecified tarsal bone(s) of left foot   CC
   7 √7th **S92.209** Fracture of unspecified tarsal bone(s) of unspecified foot   CC

√6th **S92.21 Fracture of cuboid bone**
   7 √7th **S92.211** Displaced fracture of cuboid bone of right foot   CC
   7 √7th **S92.212** Displaced fracture of cuboid bone of left foot   CC
   7 √7th **S92.213** Displaced fracture of cuboid bone of unspecified foot   CC
   7 √7th **S92.214** Nondisplaced fracture of cuboid bone of right foot   CC
   7 √7th **S92.215** Nondisplaced fracture of cuboid bone of left foot   CC
   7 √7th **S92.216** Nondisplaced fracture of cuboid bone of unspecified foot   CC

√6th **S92.22 Fracture of lateral cuneiform**
   7 √7th **S92.221** Displaced fracture of lateral cuneiform of right foot   CC
   7 √7th **S92.222** Displaced fracture of lateral cuneiform of left foot   CC
   7 √7th **S92.223** Displaced fracture of lateral cuneiform of unspecified foot   CC
   7 √7th **S92.224** Nondisplaced fracture of lateral cuneiform of right foot   CC
   7 √7th **S92.225** Nondisplaced fracture of lateral cuneiform of left foot   CC
   7 √7th **S92.226** Nondisplaced fracture of lateral cuneiform of unspecified foot   CC

√6th **S92.23 Fracture of intermediate cuneiform**
   7 √7th **S92.231** Displaced fracture of intermediate cuneiform of right foot   CC

---

7 HAC = Initial encounter only (7th character A, B or C) and not POA.

N Newborn: 0   P Pediatric: 0-17   M Maternity: 12-55   A Adult: 15-124   MCC Major CC Condition   PDx MCC PDx acts as own MCC   CC CC Condition   PDx CC PDx acts as own CC

7 √7ᵗʰ **S92.232 Displaced** fracture of intermediate cuneiform of **left** foot `CC`

7 √7ᵗʰ **S92.233 Displaced** fracture of intermediate cuneiform of **unspecified** foot `CC`

7 √7ᵗʰ **S92.234 Nondisplaced** fracture of intermediate cuneiform of **right** foot `CC`

7 √7ᵗʰ **S92.235 Nondisplaced** fracture of intermediate cuneiform of **left** foot `CC`

7 √7ᵗʰ **S92.236 Nondisplaced** fracture of intermediate cuneiform of **unspecified** foot `CC`

√6ᵗʰ **S92.24 Fracture of medial cuneiform**

7 √7ᵗʰ **S92.241 Displaced** fracture of medial cuneiform of **right** foot `CC`

7 √7ᵗʰ **S92.242 Displaced** fracture of medial cuneiform of **left** foot `CC`

7 √7ᵗʰ **S92.243 Displaced** fracture of medial cuneiform of **unspecified** foot `CC`

7 √7ᵗʰ **S92.244 Nondisplaced** fracture of medial cuneiform of **right** foot `CC`

7 √7ᵗʰ **S92.245 Nondisplaced** fracture of medial cuneiform of **left** foot `CC`

7 √7ᵗʰ **S92.246 Nondisplaced** fracture of medial cuneiform of **unspecified** foot `CC`

√6ᵗʰ **S92.25 Fracture of navicular [scaphoid] of foot**

7 √7ᵗʰ **S92.251 Displaced** fracture of navicular [scaphoid] of **right** foot `CC`

7 √7ᵗʰ **S92.252 Displaced** fracture of navicular [scaphoid] of **left** foot `CC`

7 √7ᵗʰ **S92.253 Displaced** fracture of navicular [scaphoid] of **unspecified** foot `CC`

7 √7ᵗʰ **S92.254 Nondisplaced** fracture of navicular [scaphoid] of **right** foot `CC`

7 √7ᵗʰ **S92.255 Nondisplaced** fracture of navicular [scaphoid] of **left** foot `CC`

7 √7ᵗʰ **S92.256 Nondisplaced** fracture of navicular [scaphoid] of **unspecified** foot `CC`

√5ᵗʰ **S92.3 Fracture of metatarsal bone(s)**

CC Excl: For CC codes in subcategory S92.3, unless otherwise noted: See code: S92.2

√6ᵗʰ **S92.30 Fracture of unspecified metatarsal bone(s)**

7 √7ᵗʰ **S92.301 Fracture of unspecified metatarsal bone(s), right** foot `CC`

7 √7ᵗʰ **S92.302 Fracture of unspecified metatarsal bone(s), left** foot `CC`

7 √7ᵗʰ **S92.309 Fracture of unspecified metatarsal bone(s), unspecified** foot `CC`

√6ᵗʰ **S92.31 Fracture of first metatarsal bone**

7 √7ᵗʰ **S92.311 Displaced** fracture of first metatarsal bone, **right** foot `CC`

7 √7ᵗʰ **S92.312 Displaced** fracture of first metatarsal bone, **left** foot `CC`

7 √7ᵗʰ **S92.313 Displaced** fracture of first metatarsal bone, **unspecified** foot `CC`

7 √7ᵗʰ **S92.314 Nondisplaced** fracture of first metatarsal bone, **right** foot `CC`

7 √7ᵗʰ **S92.315 Nondisplaced** fracture of first metatarsal bone, **left** foot `CC`

7 √7ᵗʰ **S92.316 Nondisplaced** fracture of first metatarsal bone, **unspecified** foot `CC`

√6ᵗʰ **S92.32 Fracture of second metatarsal bone**

7 √7ᵗʰ **S92.321 Displaced** fracture of second metatarsal bone, **right** foot `CC`

7 √7ᵗʰ **S92.322 Displaced** fracture of second metatarsal bone, **left** foot `CC`

7 √7ᵗʰ **S92.323 Displaced** fracture of second metatarsal bone, **unspecified** foot `CC`

7 √7ᵗʰ **S92.324 Nondisplaced** fracture of second metatarsal bone, **right** foot `CC`

7 √7ᵗʰ **S92.325 Nondisplaced** fracture of second metatarsal bone, **left** foot `CC`

7 √7ᵗʰ **S92.326 Nondisplaced** fracture of second metatarsal bone, **unspecified** foot `CC`

√6ᵗʰ **S92.33 Fracture of third metatarsal bone**

7 √7ᵗʰ **S92.331 Displaced** fracture of third metatarsal bone, **right** foot `CC`

7 √7ᵗʰ **S92.332 Displaced** fracture of third metatarsal bone, **left** foot `CC`

7 √7ᵗʰ **S92.333 Displaced** fracture of third metatarsal bone, **unspecified** foot `CC`

7 √7ᵗʰ **S92.334 Nondisplaced** fracture of third metatarsal bone, **right** foot `CC`

7 √7ᵗʰ **S92.335 Nondisplaced** fracture of third metatarsal bone, **left** foot `CC`

7 √7ᵗʰ **S92.336 Nondisplaced** fracture of third metatarsal bone, **unspecified** foot `CC`

√6ᵗʰ **S92.34 Fracture of fourth metatarsal bone**

7 √7ᵗʰ **S92.341 Displaced** fracture of fourth metatarsal bone, **right** foot `CC`

7 √7ᵗʰ **S92.342 Displaced** fracture of fourth metatarsal bone, **left** foot `CC`

7 √7ᵗʰ **S92.343 Displaced** fracture of fourth metatarsal bone, **unspecified** foot `CC`

7 √7ᵗʰ **S92.344 Nondisplaced** fracture of fourth metatarsal bone, **right** foot `CC`

7 √7ᵗʰ **S92.345 Nondisplaced** fracture of fourth metatarsal bone, **left** foot `CC`

7 √7ᵗʰ **S92.346 Nondisplaced** fracture of fourth metatarsal bone, **unspecified** foot `CC`

√6ᵗʰ **S92.35 Fracture of fifth metatarsal bone**

7 √7ᵗʰ **S92.351 Displaced** fracture of fifth metatarsal bone, **right** foot `CC`

7 √7ᵗʰ **S92.352 Displaced** fracture of fifth metatarsal bone, **left** foot `CC`

7 √7ᵗʰ **S92.353 Displaced** fracture of fifth metatarsal bone, **unspecified** foot `CC`

7 √7ᵗʰ **S92.354 Nondisplaced** fracture of fifth metatarsal bone, **right** foot `CC`

7 √7ᵗʰ **S92.355 Nondisplaced** fracture of fifth metatarsal bone, **left** foot `CC`

7 √7ᵗʰ **S92.356 Nondisplaced** fracture of fifth metatarsal bone, **unspecified** foot `CC`

√5ᵗʰ **S92.4 Fracture of great toe**

CC Excl: For CC codes in subcategory S92.4, unless otherwise noted: CC with 7th character K or P: M80.00X-M84.68X with 7th [K, P], S02.0XX-S02.92X with 7th K, S12.000-S12.691 with 7th K, S22.000-S22.9XX with 7th K, S32.000-S32.9XX with 7th K, S42.001-S42.92X with 7th [K, P], S49.001-S49.199 with 7th [K, P], S52.001-S52.92X with 7th [K, M, N, P, Q, R], S59.001-S59.299 with 7th [K, P], S62.001-S62.92X with 7th [K, P], S72.001-S72.92X with 7th [K, M, N, P, Q, R], S79.001-S79.199 with 7th [K, P], S82.001-S82.92X with 7th [K, M, N, P, Q, R], S89.001-S89.399 with 7th [K, P], S92.001-S92.919 with 7th [K, P]

√6ᵗʰ **S92.40 Unspecified fracture of great toe**

√7ᵗʰ **S92.401 Displaced unspecified** fracture of **right great toe** `CC`

√7ᵗʰ **S92.402 Displaced unspecified** fracture of **left great toe** `CC`

√7ᵗʰ **S92.403 Displaced unspecified** fracture of **unspecified great toe** `CC`

√7ᵗʰ **S92.404 Nondisplaced unspecified** fracture of **right great toe** `CC`

√7ᵗʰ **S92.405 Nondisplaced unspecified** fracture of **left great toe** `CC`

√7ᵗʰ **S92.406 Nondisplaced unspecified** fracture of **unspecified great toe** `CC`

√6ᵗʰ **S92.41 Fracture of proximal phalanx of great toe**

√7ᵗʰ **S92.411 Displaced** fracture of proximal phalanx of **right great toe** `CC`

√7ᵗʰ **S92.412 Displaced** fracture of proximal phalanx of **left great toe** `CC`

√7ᵗʰ **S92.413 Displaced** fracture of proximal phalanx of **unspecified great toe** `CC`

√7ᵗʰ **S92.414 Nondisplaced** fracture of proximal phalanx of **right great toe** `CC`

√7ᵗʰ **S92.415 Nondisplaced** fracture of proximal phalanx of **left great toe** `CC`

---

7 HAC = Initial encounter only (7th character A, B or C) and not POA.

√ Additional Character Required √x7ᵗʰ Xtension Alert Unacceptable PDx Manifestation Hospital Acquired Condition *EXCLUDES 1* Not Coded Here *EXCLUDES 2* Not Included Here

Injury, Poisoning and Certain Other Consequences of External Causes   S92.416–S93.105

√7ᵗʰ **S92.416** Nondisplaced **fracture** of proximal phalanx of unspecified great **toe** ᶜᶜ

√6ᵗʰ **S92.42** **Fracture** of distal phalanx of great toe

√7ᵗʰ **S92.421** Displaced **fracture** of distal phalanx of right great **toe** ᶜᶜ

√7ᵗʰ **S92.422** Displaced **fracture** of distal phalanx of left great **toe** ᶜᶜ

√7ᵗʰ **S92.423** Displaced **fracture** of distal phalanx of unspecified great **toe** ᶜᶜ

√7ᵗʰ **S92.424** Nondisplaced **fracture** of distal phalanx of right great **toe** ᶜᶜ

√7ᵗʰ **S92.425** Nondisplaced **fracture** of distal phalanx of left great **toe** ᶜᶜ

√7ᵗʰ **S92.426** Nondisplaced **fracture** of distal phalanx of unspecified great **toe** ᶜᶜ

√6ᵗʰ **S92.49** Other fracture of great toe

√7ᵗʰ **S92.491** Other fracture of right great **toe** ᶜᶜ

√7ᵗʰ **S92.492** Other fracture of left great **toe** ᶜᶜ

√7ᵗʰ **S92.499** Other fracture of unspecified great **toe** ᶜᶜ

√5ᵗʰ **S92.5** Fracture of lesser toe(s)

> **CC Excl: For CC codes in subcategory S92.5, unless otherwise noted:** See code: S92.4

√6ᵗʰ **S92.50** Unspecified fracture of lesser toe(s)

√7ᵗʰ **S92.501** Displaced unspecified fracture of right lesser **toe(s)** ᶜᶜ

√7ᵗʰ **S92.502** Displaced unspecified fracture of left lesser **toe(s)** ᶜᶜ

√7ᵗʰ **S92.503** Displaced unspecified fracture of unspecified lesser **toe(s)** ᶜᶜ

√7ᵗʰ **S92.504** Nondisplaced unspecified fracture of right lesser **toe(s)** ᶜᶜ

√7ᵗʰ **S92.505** Nondisplaced unspecified fracture of left lesser **toe(s)** ᶜᶜ

√7ᵗʰ **S92.506** Nondisplaced unspecified fracture of unspecified lesser **toe(s)** ᶜᶜ

√6ᵗʰ **S92.51** Fracture of proximal phalanx of lesser toe(s)

√7ᵗʰ **S92.511** Displaced **fracture** of proximal phalanx of right lesser **toe(s)** ᶜᶜ

√7ᵗʰ **S92.512** Displaced **fracture** of proximal phalanx of left lesser **toe(s)** ᶜᶜ

√7ᵗʰ **S92.513** Displaced **fracture** of proximal phalanx of unspecified lesser **toe(s)** ᶜᶜ

√7ᵗʰ **S92.514** Nondisplaced **fracture** of proximal phalanx of right lesser **toe(s)** ᶜᶜ

√7ᵗʰ **S92.515** Nondisplaced **fracture** of proximal phalanx of left lesser **toe(s)** ᶜᶜ

√7ᵗʰ **S92.516** Nondisplaced **fracture** of proximal phalanx of unspecified lesser **toe(s)** ᶜᶜ

√6ᵗʰ **S92.52** Fracture of medial phalanx of lesser toe(s)

√7ᵗʰ **S92.521** Displaced **fracture** of medial phalanx of right lesser **toe(s)** ᶜᶜ

√7ᵗʰ **S92.522** Displaced **fracture** of medial phalanx of left lesser **toe(s)** ᶜᶜ

√7ᵗʰ **S92.523** Displaced **fracture** of medial phalanx of unspecified lesser **toe(s)** ᶜᶜ

√7ᵗʰ **S92.524** Nondisplaced **fracture** of medial phalanx of right lesser **toe(s)** ᶜᶜ

√7ᵗʰ **S92.525** Nondisplaced **fracture** of medial phalanx of left lesser **toe(s)** ᶜᶜ

√7ᵗʰ **S92.526** Nondisplaced **fracture** of medial phalanx of unspecified lesser **toe(s)** ᶜᶜ

√6ᵗʰ **S92.53** Fracture of distal phalanx of lesser toe(s)

√7ᵗʰ **S92.531** Displaced fracture of distal phalanx of right lesser **toe(s)** ᶜᶜ

√7ᵗʰ **S92.532** Displaced fracture of distal phalanx of left lesser **toe(s)** ᶜᶜ

√7ᵗʰ **S92.533** Displaced fracture of distal phalanx of unspecified lesser **toe(s)** ᶜᶜ

√7ᵗʰ **S92.534** Nondisplaced **fracture** of distal phalanx of right lesser **toe(s)** ᶜᶜ

√7ᵗʰ **S92.535** Nondisplaced **fracture** of distal phalanx of left lesser **toe(s)** ᶜᶜ

√7ᵗʰ **S92.536** Nondisplaced **fracture** of distal phalanx of unspecified lesser **toe(s)** ᶜᶜ

√6ᵗʰ **S92.59** Other fracture of lesser toe(s)

√7ᵗʰ **S92.591** Other fracture of right lesser **toe(s)** ᶜᶜ

√7ᵗʰ **S92.592** Other fracture of left lesser **toe(s)** ᶜᶜ

√7ᵗʰ **S92.599** Other fracture of unspecified lesser **toe(s)** ᶜᶜ

√5ᵗʰ **S92.9** Unspecified fracture of foot and toe

√6ᵗʰ **S92.90** Unspecified fracture of foot

> **CC Excl: For CC codes in subcategory S92.90, unless otherwise noted: CC with 7th character B:** S92.001-S92.919 with 7th [A, B] **CC with 7th character K or P:** M80.00X-M84.68X with 7th [K, P], S02.0XX-S02.92X with 7th K, S12.000-S12.691 with 7th K, S22.000-S22.9XX with 7th K, S32.000-S32.9XX with 7th K, S42.001-S42.92X with 7th [K, P], S49.001-S49.199 with 7th [K, P], S52.001-S52.92X with 7th [K, M, N, P, Q, R], S59.001-S59.299 with 7th [K, P], S62.001-S62.92X with 7th [K, P], S72.001-S72.92X with 7th [K, M, N, P, Q, R], S79.001-S79.199 with 7th [K, P], S82.001-S82.92X with 7th [K, M, N, P, Q, R], S89.001-S89.399 with 7th [K, P], S92.001-S92.919 with 7th [K, P]

7 √7ᵗʰ **S92.901** Unspecified fracture of right foot ᶜᶜ

7 √7ᵗʰ **S92.902** Unspecified fracture of left foot ᶜᶜ

7 √7ᵗʰ **S92.909** Unspecified fracture of unspecified foot ᶜᶜ

√6ᵗʰ **S92.91** Unspecified fracture of toe

> **CC Excl: For CC codes in subcategory S92.91, unless otherwise noted:** See code: S92.90

√7ᵗʰ **S92.911** Unspecified fracture of right toe(s) ᶜᶜ

√7ᵗʰ **S92.912** Unspecified fracture of left toe(s) ᶜᶜ

√7ᵗʰ **S92.919** Unspecified fracture of unspecified toe(s) ᶜᶜ

√4ᵗʰ **S93** **Dislocation and sprain of joints and ligaments at ankle, foot and toe level**

> **INCLUDES**   avulsion of joint or ligament of ankle, foot and toe
> laceration of cartilage, joint or ligament of ankle, foot and toe
> sprain of cartilage, joint or ligament of ankle, foot and toe
> traumatic hemarthrosis of joint or ligament of ankle, foot and toe
> traumatic rupture of joint or ligament of ankle, foot and toe
> traumatic subluxation of joint or ligament of ankle, foot and toe
> traumatic tear of joint or ligament of ankle, foot and toe

Code also any associated open wound

> **EXCLUDES 2**   *strain of muscle and tendon of ankle and foot (S96.-)*

> The appropriate 7th character is to be added to each code from category S93.
> A   initial encounter
> D   subsequent encounter
> S   sequela

√5ᵗʰ **S93.0** Subluxation and dislocation of ankle joint
Subluxation and dislocation of astragalus
Subluxation and dislocation of fibula, lower end
Subluxation and dislocation of talus
Subluxation and dislocation of tibia, lower end

√x7ᵗʰ **S93.01** Subluxation of right ankle joint

√x7ᵗʰ **S93.02** Subluxation of left ankle joint

√x7ᵗʰ **S93.03** Subluxation of unspecified ankle joint

√x7ᵗʰ **S93.04** Dislocation of right ankle joint

√x7ᵗʰ **S93.05** Dislocation of left ankle joint

√x7ᵗʰ **S93.06** Dislocation of unspecified ankle joint

√5ᵗʰ **S93.1** Subluxation and dislocation of toe

√6ᵗʰ **S93.10** Unspecified subluxation and dislocation of toe
Dislocation of toe NOS
Subluxation of toe NOS

√7ᵗʰ **S93.101** Unspecified subluxation of right toe(s)

√7ᵗʰ **S93.102** Unspecified subluxation of left toe(s)

√7ᵗʰ **S93.103** Unspecified subluxation of unspecified toe(s)

√7ᵗʰ **S93.104** Unspecified dislocation of right toe(s)

√7ᵗʰ **S93.105** Unspecified dislocation of left toe(s)

---

7 HAC = Initial encounter only (7th character A, B or C) and not POA.

Ⓝ Newborn: Ø   Ⓟ Pediatric: Ø-17   Ⓜ Maternity: 12-55   Ⓐ Adult: 15-124   **MCC** Major CC Condition   **PDx MCC** PDx acts as own MCC   **CC** CC Condition   **PDx CC** PDx acts as own CC

1022   ICD-10-CM Draft (2015)

√7ᵗʰ **S93.106** Unspecified dislocation of unspecified toe(s)

√6ᵗʰ **S93.11** **Dislocation of interphalangeal joint**

√7ᵗʰ **S93.111** Dislocation of interphalangeal joint of right great toe

√7ᵗʰ **S93.112** Dislocation of interphalangeal joint of left great toe

√7ᵗʰ **S93.113** Dislocation of interphalangeal joint of unspecified great toe

√7ᵗʰ **S93.114** Dislocation of interphalangeal joint of right lesser toe(s)

√7ᵗʰ **S93.115** Dislocation of interphalangeal joint of left lesser toe(s)

√7ᵗʰ **S93.116** Dislocation of interphalangeal joint of unspecified lesser toe(s)

√7ᵗʰ **S93.119** Dislocation of interphalangeal joint of unspecified toe(s)

√6ᵗʰ **S93.12** **Dislocation of metatarsophalangeal joint**

√7ᵗʰ **S93.121** Dislocation of metatarsophalangeal joint of right great toe

√7ᵗʰ **S93.122** Dislocation of metatarsophalangeal joint of left great toe

√7ᵗʰ **S93.123** Dislocation of metatarsophalangeal joint of unspecified great toe

√7ᵗʰ **S93.124** Dislocation of metatarsophalangeal joint of right lesser toe(s)

√7ᵗʰ **S93.125** Dislocation of metatarsophalangeal joint of left lesser toe(s)

√7ᵗʰ **S93.126** Dislocation of metatarsophalangeal joint of unspecified lesser toe(s)

√7ᵗʰ **S93.129** Dislocation of metatarsophalangeal joint of unspecified toe(s)

√6ᵗʰ **S93.13** **Subluxation of interphalangeal joint**

√7ᵗʰ **S93.131** Subluxation of interphalangeal joint of right great toe

√7ᵗʰ **S93.132** Subluxation of interphalangeal joint of left great toe

√7ᵗʰ **S93.133** Subluxation of interphalangeal joint of unspecified great toe

√7ᵗʰ **S93.134** Subluxation of interphalangeal joint of right lesser toe(s)

√7ᵗʰ **S93.135** Subluxation of interphalangeal joint of left lesser toe(s)

√7ᵗʰ **S93.136** Subluxation of interphalangeal joint of unspecified lesser toe(s)

√7ᵗʰ **S93.139** Subluxation of interphalangeal joint of unspecified toe(s)

√6ᵗʰ **S93.14** **Subluxation of metatarsophalangeal joint**

√7ᵗʰ **S93.141** Subluxation of metatarsophalangeal joint of right great toe

√7ᵗʰ **S93.142** Subluxation of metatarsophalangeal joint of left great toe

√7ᵗʰ **S93.143** Subluxation of metatarsophalangeal joint of unspecified great toe

√7ᵗʰ **S93.144** Subluxation of metatarsophalangeal joint of right lesser toe(s)

√7ᵗʰ **S93.145** Subluxation of metatarsophalangeal joint of left lesser toe(s)

√7ᵗʰ **S93.146** Subluxation of metatarsophalangeal joint of unspecified lesser toe(s)

√7ᵗʰ **S93.149** Subluxation of metatarsophalangeal joint of unspecified toe(s)

√5ᵗʰ **S93.3** **Subluxation and dislocation of foot**

EXCLUDES 2   dislocation of toe (S93.1-)

√6ᵗʰ **S93.30** Unspecified subluxation and dislocation of foot
Dislocation of foot NOS
Subluxation of foot NOS

√7ᵗʰ **S93.301** Unspecified subluxation of right foot

√7ᵗʰ **S93.302** Unspecified subluxation of left foot

√7ᵗʰ **S93.303** Unspecified subluxation of unspecified foot

√7ᵗʰ **S93.304** Unspecified dislocation of right foot

√7ᵗʰ **S93.305** Unspecified dislocation of left foot

√7ᵗʰ **S93.306** Unspecified dislocation of unspecified foot

√6ᵗʰ **S93.31** **Subluxation and dislocation of tarsal joint**

√7ᵗʰ **S93.311** Subluxation of tarsal joint of right foot

√7ᵗʰ **S93.312** Subluxation of tarsal joint of left foot

√7ᵗʰ **S93.313** Subluxation of tarsal joint of unspecified foot

√7ᵗʰ **S93.314** Dislocation of tarsal joint of right foot

√7ᵗʰ **S93.315** Dislocation of tarsal joint of left foot

√7ᵗʰ **S93.316** Dislocation of tarsal joint of unspecified foot

√6ᵗʰ **S93.32** **Subluxation and dislocation of tarsometatarsal joint**

√7ᵗʰ **S93.321** Subluxation of tarsometatarsal joint of right foot

√7ᵗʰ **S93.322** Subluxation of tarsometatarsal joint of left foot

√7ᵗʰ **S93.323** Subluxation of tarsometatarsal joint of unspecified foot

√7ᵗʰ **S93.324** Dislocation of tarsometatarsal joint of right foot

√7ᵗʰ **S93.325** Dislocation of tarsometatarsal joint of left foot

√7ᵗʰ **S93.326** Dislocation of tarsometatarsal joint of unspecified foot

√6ᵗʰ **S93.33** **Other subluxation and dislocation of foot**

√7ᵗʰ **S93.331** Other subluxation of right foot

√7ᵗʰ **S93.332** Other subluxation of left foot

√7ᵗʰ **S93.333** Other subluxation of unspecified foot

√7ᵗʰ **S93.334** Other dislocation of right foot

√7ᵗʰ **S93.335** Other dislocation of left foot

√7ᵗʰ **S93.336** Other dislocation of unspecified foot

√5ᵗʰ **S93.4** **Sprain of ankle**

EXCLUDES 2   injury of Achilles tendon (S86.0-)

√6ᵗʰ **S93.40** Sprain of unspecified ligament of ankle
Sprain of ankle NOS
Sprained ankle NOS

√7ᵗʰ **S93.401** Sprain of unspecified ligament of right ankle

√7ᵗʰ **S93.402** Sprain of unspecified ligament of left ankle

√7ᵗʰ **S93.409** Sprain of unspecified ligament of unspecified ankle

√6ᵗʰ **S93.41** Sprain of calcaneofibular ligament

√7ᵗʰ **S93.411** Sprain of calcaneofibular ligament of right ankle

√7ᵗʰ **S93.412** Sprain of calcaneofibular ligament of left ankle

√7ᵗʰ **S93.419** Sprain of calcaneofibular ligament of unspecified ankle

√6ᵗʰ **S93.42** Sprain of deltoid ligament

√7ᵗʰ **S93.421** Sprain of deltoid ligament of right ankle

√7ᵗʰ **S93.422** Sprain of deltoid ligament of left ankle

√7ᵗʰ **S93.429** Sprain of deltoid ligament of unspecified ankle

√6ᵗʰ **S93.43** Sprain of tibiofibular ligament

√7ᵗʰ **S93.431** Sprain of tibiofibular ligament of right ankle

√7ᵗʰ **S93.432** Sprain of tibiofibular ligament of left ankle

√7ᵗʰ **S93.439** Sprain of tibiofibular ligament of unspecified ankle

√6ᵗʰ **S93.49** Sprain of other ligament of ankle
Sprain of internal collateral ligament
Sprain of talofibular ligament

√7ᵗʰ **S93.491** Sprain of other ligament of right ankle

√7ᵗʰ **S93.492** Sprain of other ligament of left ankle

√7ᵗʰ **S93.499** Sprain of other ligament of unspecified ankle

√5ᵗʰ **S93.5** **Sprain of toe**

√6ᵗʰ **S93.50** Unspecified sprain of toe

√7ᵗʰ **S93.501** Unspecified sprain of right great toe

√7ᵗʰ **S93.502** Unspecified sprain of left great toe

☑ Additional Character Required   √x7ᵗʰ Xtension Alert   Unacceptable PDx   Manifestation   Hospital Acquired Condition   EXCLUDES 1 Not Coded Here   EXCLUDES 2 Not Included Here

ICD-10-CM Draft (2015)   1023

√7ᵗʰ **S93.503** **Unspecified sprain of** unspecified great toe

√7ᵗʰ **S93.504** **Unspecified sprain of** right lesser toe(s)

√7ᵗʰ **S93.505** **Unspecified sprain of** left lesser toe(s)

√7ᵗʰ **S93.506** **Unspecified sprain of** unspecified lesser toe(s)

√7ᵗʰ **S93.509** **Unspecified sprain of** unspecified toe(s)

√6ᵗʰ **S93.51** **Sprain of** interphalangeal joint **of toe**

√7ᵗʰ **S93.511** **Sprain of interphalangeal joint of** right great toe

√7ᵗʰ **S93.512** **Sprain of interphalangeal joint of** left great toe

√7ᵗʰ **S93.513** **Sprain of interphalangeal joint of** unspecified great toe

√7ᵗʰ **S93.514** **Sprain of interphalangeal joint of** right lesser toe(s)

√7ᵗʰ **S93.515** **Sprain of interphalangeal joint of** left lesser toe(s)

√7ᵗʰ **S93.516** **Sprain of interphalangeal joint of** unspecified lesser toe(s)

√7ᵗʰ **S93.519** **Sprain of interphalangeal joint of** unspecified toe(s)

√6ᵗʰ **S93.52** **Sprain of** metatarsophalangeal joint **of toe**

√7ᵗʰ **S93.521** **Sprain of metatarsophalangeal joint of** right great toe

√7ᵗʰ **S93.522** **Sprain of metatarsophalangeal joint of** left great toe

√7ᵗʰ **S93.523** **Sprain of metatarsophalangeal joint of** unspecified great toe

√7ᵗʰ **S93.524** **Sprain of metatarsophalangeal joint of** right lesser toe(s)

√7ᵗʰ **S93.525** **Sprain of metatarsophalangeal joint of** left lesser toe(s)

√7ᵗʰ **S93.526** **Sprain of metatarsophalangeal joint of** unspecified lesser toe(s)

√7ᵗʰ **S93.529** **Sprain of metatarsophalangeal joint of** unspecified toe(s)

√5ᵗʰ **S93.6** **Sprain of** foot

EXCLUDES 2 sprain of metatarsophalangeal joint of toe (S93.52-)
sprain of toe (S93.5-)

√6ᵗʰ **S93.60** **Unspecified sprain of foot**

√7ᵗʰ **S93.601** **Unspecified sprain of** right foot

√7ᵗʰ **S93.602** **Unspecified sprain of** left foot

√7ᵗʰ **S93.609** **Unspecified sprain of** unspecified foot

√6ᵗʰ **S93.61** **Sprain of** tarsal ligament **of foot**

√7ᵗʰ **S93.611** **Sprain of tarsal ligament of** right foot

√7ᵗʰ **S93.612** **Sprain of tarsal ligament of** left foot

√7ᵗʰ **S93.619** **Sprain of tarsal ligament of** unspecified foot

√6ᵗʰ **S93.62** **Sprain of** tarsometatarsal ligament **of foot**

√7ᵗʰ **S93.621** **Sprain of tarsometatarsal ligament of** right foot

√7ᵗʰ **S93.622** **Sprain of tarsometatarsal ligament of** left foot

√7ᵗʰ **S93.629** **Sprain of tarsometatarsal ligament of** unspecified foot

√6ᵗʰ **S93.69** **Other sprain of foot**

√7ᵗʰ **S93.691** **Other sprain of** right foot

√7ᵗʰ **S93.692** **Other sprain of** left foot

√7ᵗʰ **S93.699** **Other sprain of** unspecified foot

√4ᵗʰ **S94** **Injury of nerves at ankle and foot level**
Code also any associated open wound (S91.-)

The appropriate 7th character is to be added to each code from category S94.
A   initial encounter
D   subsequent encounter
S   sequela

√5ᵗʰ **S94.0** **Injury of** lateral plantar **nerve**

√x7ᵗʰ **S94.00** **Injury of lateral plantar nerve,** unspecified leg

√x7ᵗʰ **S94.01** **Injury of lateral plantar nerve,** right leg

√x7ᵗʰ **S94.02** **Injury of lateral plantar nerve,** left leg

√5ᵗʰ **S94.1** **Injury of** medial plantar **nerve**

√x7ᵗʰ **S94.10** **Injury of medial plantar nerve,** unspecified leg

√x7ᵗʰ **S94.11** **Injury of medial plantar nerve,** right leg

√x7ᵗʰ **S94.12** **Injury of medial plantar nerve,** left leg

√5ᵗʰ **S94.2** **Injury of deep** peroneal **nerve at ankle and foot level**
Injury of terminal, lateral branch of deep peroneal nerve

√x7ᵗʰ **S94.20** **Injury of deep peroneal nerve at ankle and foot level,** unspecified leg

√x7ᵗʰ **S94.21** **Injury of deep peroneal nerve at ankle and foot level,** right leg

√x7ᵗʰ **S94.22** **Injury of deep peroneal nerve at ankle and foot level,** left leg

√5ᵗʰ **S94.3** **Injury of** cutaneous sensory **nerve at ankle and foot level**

√x7ᵗʰ **S94.30** **Injury of cutaneous sensory nerve at ankle and foot level,** unspecified leg

√x7ᵗʰ **S94.31** **Injury of cutaneous sensory nerve at ankle and foot level,** right leg

√x7ᵗʰ **S94.32** **Injury of cutaneous sensory nerve at ankle and foot level,** left leg

√5ᵗʰ **S94.8** **Injury of** other **nerves at ankle and foot level**

√6ᵗʰ **S94.8X** **Injury of other nerves at ankle and foot level**

√7ᵗʰ **S94.8X1** **Injury of other nerves at ankle and foot level,** right leg

√7ᵗʰ **S94.8X2** **Injury of other nerves at ankle and foot level,** left leg

√7ᵗʰ **S94.8X9** **Injury of other nerves at ankle and foot level,** unspecified leg

√5ᵗʰ **S94.9** **Injury of** unspecified **nerve at ankle and foot level**

√x7ᵗʰ **S94.90** **Injury of unspecified nerve at ankle and foot level,** unspecified leg

√x7ᵗʰ **S94.91** **Injury of unspecified nerve at ankle and foot level,** right leg

√x7ᵗʰ **S94.92** **Injury of unspecified nerve at ankle and foot level,** left leg

√4ᵗʰ **S95** **Injury of blood vessels at ankle and foot level**
Code also any associated open wound (S91.-)
EXCLUDES 2 injury of posterior tibial artery and vein (S85.1-, S85.8-)

The appropriate 7th character is to be added to each code from category S95.
A   initial encounter
D   subsequent encounter
S   sequela

√5ᵗʰ **S95.0** **Injury of** dorsal artery **of foot**

√6ᵗʰ **S95.00** **Unspecified injury of dorsal artery of foot**

√7ᵗʰ **S95.001** **Unspecified injury of dorsal artery** CC
of right foot
CC Excl: CC with 7th character A: M79.A21-M79.A29, S75.001 with 7th A, S75.009-S75.011 with 7th A, S75.019-S75.021 with 7th A, S75.029-S75.091 with 7th A, S75.099-S75.101 with 7th A, S75.109-S75.111 with 7th A, S75.119-S75.121 with 7th A, S75.129-S75.191 with 7th A, S75.199-S75.201 with 7th A, S75.209-S75.211 with 7th A, S75.219-S75.221 with 7th A, S75.229-S75.291 with 7th A, S75.299-S75.801 with 7th A, S75.809-S75.811 with 7th A, S75.819-S75.891 with 7th A, S75.899-S75.901 with 7th A, S75.909-S75.911 with 7th A, S75.919-S75.991 with 7th A, S75.999A, S85.001A, S85.009-S85.011 with 7th A, S85.019-S85.091 with 7th A, S85.099-S85.101 with 7th A, S85.109-S85.111 with 7th A, S85.119-S85.121 with

N Newborn: 0   P Pediatric: 0-17   M Maternity: 12-55   A Adult: 15-124   MCC Major CC Condition   PDx MCC PDx acts as own MCC   CC CC Condition   PDx CC PDx acts as own CC

1024   ICD-10-CM Draft (2015)

7th A, S85.129-S85.131 with 7th A, S85.139-
S85.141 with 7th A, S85.149-S85.151 with
7th A, S85.159-S85.161 with 7th A, S85.169-
S85.171 with 7th A, S85.179-S85.181 with
7th A, S85.189-S85.201 with 7th A, S85.209-
S85.211 with 7th A, S85.219-S85.291 with
7th A, S85.299-S85.301 with 7th A, S85.309-
S85.311 with 7th A, S85.319-S85.391 with
7th A, S85.399-S85.401 with 7th A, S85.409-
S85.411 with 7th A, S85.419-S85.491 with
7th A, S85.499-S85.501 with 7th A, S85.509-
S85.511 with 7th A, S85.519-S85.591 with
7th A, S85.599-S85.801 with 7th A, S85.809-
S85.811 with 7th A, S85.819-S85.891 with
7th A, S85.899-S85.901 with 7th A, S85.909-
S85.911 with 7th A, S85.919-S85.991 with
7th A, S85.999A, S95.001A, S95.009-S95.011
with 7th A, S95.019-S95.091 with 7th A,
S95.099-S95.101 with 7th A, S95.109-
S95.111 with 7th A, S95.119-S95.191 with
7th A, S95.199-S95.201 with 7th A, S95.209-
S95.211 with 7th A, S95.219-S95.291 with
7th A, S95.299-S95.801 with 7th A, S95.809-
S95.811 with 7th A, S95.819-S95.891 with
7th A, S95.899-S95.901 with 7th A, S95.909-
S95.911 with 7th A, S95.919-S95.991 with
7th A, S95.999A

✓7ᵗʰ **S95.002 Unspecified injury of dorsal artery** cc
of left foot
CC Excl: CC with 7th character A: M79.A21-
M79.A29, S75.002-S75.009 with 7th A,
S75.012-S75.019 with 7th A, S75.022-
S75.029 with 7th A, S75.092-S75.099 with
7th A, S75.102-S75.109 with 7th A, S75.112-
S75.119 with 7th A, S75.122-S75.129 with
7th A, S75.192-S75.199 with 7th A, S75.202-
S75.209 with 7th A, S75.212-S75.219 with
7th A, S75.222-S75.229 with 7th A, S75.292-
S75.299 with 7th A, S75.802-S75.809 with
7th A, S75.812-S75.819 with 7th A, S75.892-
S75.899 with 7th A, S75.902-S75.909 with
7th A, S75.912-S75.919 with 7th A, S75.992-
S75.999 with 7th A, S85.002-S85.009 with
7th A, S85.012-S85.019 with 7th A, S85.092-
S85.099 with 7th A, S85.102-S85.109 with
7th A, S85.112-S85.119 with 7th A, S85.122-
S85.129 with 7th A, S85.132-S85.139 with
7th A, S85.142-S85.149 with 7th A, S85.152-
S85.159 with 7th A, S85.162-S85.169 with
7th A, S85.172-S85.179 with 7th A, S85.182-
S85.189 with 7th A, S85.202-S85.209 with
7th A, S85.212-S85.219 with 7th A, S85.292-
S85.299 with 7th A, S85.302-S85.309 with
7th A, S85.312-S85.319 with 7th A, S85.392-
S85.399 with 7th A, S85.402-S85.409 with
7th A, S85.412-S85.419 with 7th A, S85.492-
S85.499 with 7th A, S85.502-S85.509 with
7th A, S85.512-S85.519 with 7th A, S85.592-
S85.599 with 7th A, S85.802-S85.809 with
7th A, S85.812-S85.819 with 7th A, S85.892-
S85.899 with 7th A, S85.902-S85.909 with
7th A, S85.912-S85.919 with 7th A, S85.992-
S85.999 with 7th A, S95.002-S95.009 with
7th A, S95.012-S95.019 with 7th A, S95.092-
S95.099 with 7th A, S95.102-S95.109 with
7th A, S95.112-S95.119 with 7th A, S95.192-
S95.199 with 7th A, S95.202-S95.209 with
7th A, S95.212-S95.219 with 7th A, S95.292-
S95.299 with 7th A, S95.802-S95.809 with
7th A, S95.812-S95.819 with 7th A, S95.892-
S95.899 with 7th A, S95.902-S95.909 with
7th A, S95.912-S95.919 with 7th A, S95.992-
S95.999 with 7th A

✓7ᵗʰ **S95.009 Unspecified injury of dorsal artery** cc
of unspecified foot
CC Excl: CC with 7th character A: M79.A21-
M79.A29, S75.001-S75.999 with 7th A,
S85.001-S85.999 with 7th A, S95.001-
S95.999 with 7th A

✓6ᵗʰ **S95.01 Laceration of dorsal artery of foot**

✓7ᵗʰ **S95.011 Laceration of dorsal artery of** cc
right foot
CC Excl: M79.A21-M79.A29, S75.001 with
7th A, S75.009-S75.011 with 7th A, S75.019-
S75.021 with 7th A, S75.029-S75.091 with
7th A, S75.099-S75.101 with 7th A, S75.109-
S75.111 with 7th A, S75.119-S75.121 with
7th A, S75.129-S75.191 with 7th A, S75.199-
S75.201 with 7th A, S75.209-S75.211 with
7th A, S75.219-S75.221 with 7th A, S75.229-
S75.291 with 7th A, S75.299-S75.801 with
7th A, S75.809-S75.811 with 7th A, S75.819-
S75.891 with 7th A, S75.899-S75.901 with
7th A, S75.909-S75.911 with 7th A, S75.919-
S75.991 with 7th A, S75.999 with 7th A,
S85.001 with 7th A, S85.009-S85.011 with
7th A, S85.019-S85.091 with 7th A, S85.099-
S85.101 with 7th A, S85.109-S85.111 with
7th A, S85.119-S85.121 with 7th A, S85.129-
S85.131 with 7th A, S85.139-S85.141 with
7th A, S85.149-S85.151 with 7th A, S85.159-
S85.161 with 7th A, S85.169-S85.171 with
7th A, S85.179-S85.181 with 7th A, S85.189-
S85.201 with 7th A, S85.209-S85.211 with
7th A, S85.219-S85.291 with 7th A, S85.299-
S85.301 with 7th A, S85.309-S85.311 with
7th A, S85.319-S85.391 with 7th A, S85.399-
S85.401 with 7th A, S85.409-S85.411 with
7th A, S85.419-S85.491 with 7th A, S85.499-
S85.501 with 7th A, S85.509-S85.511 with
7th A, S85.519-S85.591 with 7th A, S85.599-
S85.801 with 7th A, S85.809-S85.811 with
7th A, S85.819-S85.891 with 7th A, S85.899-
S85.901 with 7th A, S85.909-S85.911 with
7th A, S85.919-S85.991 with 7th A, S85.999A,
S95.001A, S95.009-S95.011 with 7th A,
S95.019-S95.091 with 7th A, S95.099-
S95.101 with 7th A, S95.109-S95.111 with
7th A, S95.119-S95.191 with 7th A, S95.199-
S95.201 with 7th A, S95.209-S95.211 with
7th A, S95.219-S95.291 with 7th A, S95.299-
S95.801 with 7th A, S95.809-S95.811 with
7th A, S95.819-S95.891 with 7th A, S95.899-
S95.901 with 7th A, S95.909-S95.911 with
7th A, S95.919-S95.991 with 7th A, S95.999
with 7th A

✓7ᵗʰ **S95.012 Laceration of dorsal artery of** cc
left foot
CC Excl: M79.A21-M79.A29, S75.002-S75.009
with 7th A, S75.012-S75.019 with 7th A,
S75.022-S75.029 with 7th A, S75.092-
S75.099 with 7th A, S75.102-S75.109 with
7th A, S75.112-S75.119 with 7th A, S75.122-
S75.129 with 7th A, S75.192-S75.199 with
7th A, S75.202-S75.209 with 7th A, S75.212-
S75.219 with 7th A, S75.222-S75.229 with
7th A, S75.292-S75.299 with 7th A, S75.802-
S75.809 with 7th A, S75.812-S75.819 with
7th A, S75.892-S75.899 with 7th A, S75.902-
S75.909 with 7th A, S75.912-S75.919 with
7th A, S75.992-S75.999 with 7th A, S85.002-
S85.009 with 7th A, S85.012-S85.019 with
7th A, S85.092-S85.099 with 7th A, S85.102-
S85.109 with 7th A, S85.112-S85.119 with
7th A, S85.122-S85.129 with 7th A, S85.132-
S85.139 with 7th A, S85.142-S85.149 with
7th A, S85.152-S85.159 with 7th A, S85.162-
S85.169 with 7th A, S85.172-S85.179 with
7th A, S85.182-S85.189 with 7th A, S85.202-
S85.209 with 7th A, S85.212-S85.219 with
7th A, S85.292-S85.299 with 7th A, S85.302-
S85.309 with 7th A, S85.312-S85.319 with
7th A, S85.392-S85.399 with 7th A, S85.402-
S85.409 with 7th A, S85.412-S85.419 with
7th A, S85.492-S85.499 with 7th A, S85.502-
S85.509 with 7th A, S85.512-S85.519 with
7th A, S85.592-S85.599 with 7th A, S85.802-
S85.809 with 7th A, S85.812-S85.819 with
7th A, S85.892-S85.899 with 7th A, S85.902-
S85.909 with 7th A, S85.912-S85.919 with
7th A, S85.992-S85.999 with 7th A, S95.002-
S95.009 with 7th A, S95.012-S95.019 with
7th A, S95.092-S95.099 with 7th A, S95.102-
S95.109 with 7th A, S95.112-S95.119 with
7th A, S95.192-S95.199 with 7th A, S95.202-
S95.209 with 7th A, S95.212-S95.219 with
7th A, S95.292-S95.299 with 7th A, S95.802-
S95.809 with 7th A, S95.812-S95.819 with
7th A, S95.892-S95.899 with 7th A, S95.902-
S95.909 with 7th A, S95.912-S95.919 with
7th A, S95.992-S95.999 with 7th A

Injury, Poisoning and Certain Other Consequences of External Causes

S95.019–S95.899

√7ᵗʰ **S95.019 Laceration of dorsal artery of unspecified foot**   CC
     CC Excl: M79.A21-M79.A29, S75.001-S75.999 with 7th A, S85.001-S85.999 with 7th A, S95.001-S95.999 with 7th A

√6ᵗʰ **S95.09 Other specified injury of dorsal artery of foot**

√7ᵗʰ **S95.091 Other specified injury of dorsal artery of right foot**   CC
     CC Excl: See code: S95.001

√7ᵗʰ **S95.092 Other specified injury of dorsal artery of left foot**   CC
     CC Excl: See code: S95.002

√7ᵗʰ **S95.099 Other specified injury of dorsal artery of unspecified foot**   CC
     CC Excl: See code: S95.009

√5ᵗʰ **S95.1 Injury of plantar artery of foot**

√6ᵗʰ **S95.10 Unspecified injury of plantar artery of foot**

√7ᵗʰ **S95.101 Unspecified injury of plantar artery of right foot**   CC
     CC Excl: CC with 7th character A: S75.801 with 7th A, S75.809-S75.811 with 7th A, S75.819-S75.891 with 7th A, S75.899-S75.901 with 7th A, S75.909-S75.911 with 7th A, S75.919-S75.991 with 7th A, S75.999 with 7th A, S85.201 with 7th A, S85.209-S85.211 with 7th A, S85.219-S85.291 with 7th A, S85.299 with 7th A, S85.801 with 7th A, S85.809-S85.811 with 7th A, S85.819-S85.891 with 7th A, S85.899-S85.901 with 7th A, S85.909-S85.911 with 7th A, S85.919-S85.991 with 7th A, S85.999 with 7th A, S95.001 with 7th A, S95.009-S95.011 with 7th A, S95.019-S95.091 with 7th A, S95.099-S95.101 with 7th A, S95.109-S95.111 with 7th A, S95.119-S95.191 with 7th A, S95.199-S95.201 with 7th A, S95.209-S95.211 with 7th A, S95.219-S95.291 with 7th A, S95.299-S95.801 with 7th A, S95.809-S95.811 with 7th A, S95.819-S95.891 with 7th A, S95.899-S95.901 with 7th A, S95.909-S95.911 with 7th A, S95.919-S95.991 with 7th A, S95.999 with 7th A

√7ᵗʰ **S95.102 Unspecified injury of plantar artery of left foot**   CC
     CC Excl: CC with 7th character A: S75.802-S75.809 with 7th A, S75.812-S75.819 with 7th A, S75.892-S75.899 with 7th A, S75.902-S75.909 with 7th A, S75.912-S75.919 with 7th A, S75.992-S75.999 with 7th A, S85.202-S85.209 with 7th A, S85.212-S85.219 with 7th A, S85.292-S85.299 with 7th A, S85.802-S85.809 with 7th A, S85.812-S85.819 with 7th A, S85.892-S85.899 with 7th A, S85.902-S85.909 with 7th A, S85.912-S85.919 with 7th A, S85.992-S85.999 with 7th A, S95.002-S95.009 with 7th A, S95.012-S95.019 with 7th A, S95.092-S95.099 with 7th A, S95.102-S95.109 with 7th A, S95.112-S95.119 with 7th A, S95.192-S95.199 with 7th A, S95.202-S95.209 with 7th A, S95.212-S95.219 with 7th A, S95.292-S95.299 with 7th A, S95.802-S95.809 with 7th A, S95.812-S95.819 with 7th A, S95.892-S95.899 with 7th A, S95.902-S95.909 with 7th A, S95.912-S95.919 with 7th A, S95.992-S95.999 with 7th A

√7ᵗʰ **S95.109 Unspecified injury of plantar artery of unspecified foot**   CC
     CC Excl: CC with 7th character A: S75.801-S75.999 with 7th A, S85.201-S85.299 with 7th A, S85.801-S85.999 with 7th A, S95.001-S95.999 with 7th A

√6ᵗʰ **S95.11 Laceration of plantar artery of foot**

√7ᵗʰ **S95.111 Laceration of plantar artery of right foot**   CC
     CC Excl: See code: S95.101

√7ᵗʰ **S95.112 Laceration of plantar artery of left foot**   CC
     CC Excl: See code: S95.102

√7ᵗʰ **S95.119 Laceration of plantar artery of unspecified foot**   CC
     CC Excl: See code: S95.109

√6ᵗʰ **S95.19 Other specified injury of plantar artery of foot**

√7ᵗʰ **S95.191 Other specified injury of plantar artery of right foot**   CC
     CC Excl: See code: S95.101

√7ᵗʰ **S95.192 Other specified injury of plantar artery of left foot**   CC
     CC Excl: See code: S95.102

√7ᵗʰ **S95.199 Other specified injury of plantar artery of unspecified foot**   CC
     CC Excl: See code: S95.109

√5ᵗʰ **S95.2 Injury of dorsal vein of foot**

√6ᵗʰ **S95.20 Unspecified injury of dorsal vein of foot**

√7ᵗʰ **S95.201 Unspecified injury of dorsal vein of right foot**   CC
     CC Excl: See code: S95.001

√7ᵗʰ **S95.202 Unspecified injury of dorsal vein of left foot**   CC
     CC Excl: See code: S95.002

√7ᵗʰ **S95.209 Unspecified injury of dorsal vein of unspecified foot**   CC
     CC Excl: See code: S95.009

√6ᵗʰ **S95.21 Laceration of dorsal vein of foot**

√7ᵗʰ **S95.211 Laceration of dorsal vein of right foot**   CC
     CC Excl: See code: S95.001

√7ᵗʰ **S95.212 Laceration of dorsal vein of left foot**   CC
     CC Excl: See code: S95.002

√7ᵗʰ **S95.219 Laceration of dorsal vein of unspecified foot**   CC
     CC Excl: See code: S95.009

√6ᵗʰ **S95.29 Other specified injury of dorsal vein of foot**

√7ᵗʰ **S95.291 Other specified injury of dorsal vein of right foot**   CC
     CC Excl: See code: S95.001

√7ᵗʰ **S95.292 Other specified injury of dorsal vein of left foot**   CC
     CC Excl: See code: S95.002

√7ᵗʰ **S95.299 Other specified injury of dorsal vein of unspecified foot**   CC
     CC Excl: See code: S95.009

√5ᵗʰ **S95.8 Injury of other blood vessels at ankle and foot level**

√6ᵗʰ **S95.80 Unspecified injury of other blood vessels at ankle and foot level**

√7ᵗʰ **S95.801 Unspecified injury of other blood vessels at ankle and foot level, right leg**   CC
     CC Excl: See code: S95.001

√7ᵗʰ **S95.802 Unspecified injury of other blood vessels at ankle and foot level, left leg**   CC
     CC Excl: See code: S95.002

√7ᵗʰ **S95.809 Unspecified injury of other blood vessels at ankle and foot level, unspecified leg**   CC
     CC Excl: See code: S95.009

√6ᵗʰ **S95.81 Laceration of other blood vessels at ankle and foot level**

√7ᵗʰ **S95.811 Laceration of other blood vessels at ankle and foot level, right leg**   CC
     CC Excl: See code: S95.001

√7ᵗʰ **S95.812 Laceration of other blood vessels at ankle and foot level, left leg**   CC
     CC Excl: See code: S95.002

√7ᵗʰ **S95.819 Laceration of other blood vessels at ankle and foot level, unspecified leg**   CC
     CC Excl: See code: S95.009

√6ᵗʰ **S95.89 Other specified injury of other blood vessels at ankle and foot level**

√7ᵗʰ **S95.891 Other specified injury of other blood vessels at ankle and foot level, right leg**   CC
     CC Excl: See code: S95.001

√7ᵗʰ **S95.892 Other specified injury of other blood vessels at ankle and foot level, left leg**   CC
     CC Excl: See code: S95.002

√7ᵗʰ **S95.899 Other specified injury of other blood vessels at ankle and foot level, unspecified leg**   CC
     CC Excl: See code: S95.009

N Newborn: 0   **P** Pediatric: 0-17   **M** Maternity: 12-55   **A** Adult: 15-124   **MCC** Major CC Condition   **PDx MCC** PDx acts as own MCC   **CC** CC Condition   **PDx CC** PDx acts as own CC

1026

ICD-10-CM Draft (2015)

✓5ᵗʰ **S95.9** Injury of unspecified blood vessel at ankle and foot level

✓6ᵗʰ **S95.90** Unspecified injury of unspecified blood vessel at ankle and foot level

✓7ᵗʰ **S95.901** Unspecified injury of unspecified blood vessel at ankle and foot level, right leg   `CC`
CC Excl: See code: S95.001

✓7ᵗʰ **S95.902** Unspecified injury of unspecified blood vessel at ankle and foot level, left leg   `CC`
CC Excl: See code: S95.002

✓7ᵗʰ **S95.909** Unspecified injury of unspecified blood vessel at ankle and foot level, unspecified leg   `CC`
CC Excl: See code: S95.009

✓6ᵗʰ **S95.91** Laceration of unspecified blood vessel at ankle and foot level

✓7ᵗʰ **S95.911** Laceration of unspecified blood vessel at ankle and foot level, right leg   `CC`
CC Excl: See code: S95.001

✓7ᵗʰ **S95.912** Laceration of unspecified blood vessel at ankle and foot level, left leg   `CC`
CC Excl: See code: S95.002

✓7ᵗʰ **S95.919** Laceration of unspecified blood vessel at ankle and foot level, unspecified leg   `CC`
CC Excl: See code: S95.009

✓6ᵗʰ **S95.99** Other specified injury of unspecified blood vessel at ankle and foot level

✓7ᵗʰ **S95.991** Other specified injury of unspecified blood vessel at ankle and foot level, right leg   `CC`
CC Excl: See code: S95.001

✓7ᵗʰ **S95.992** Other specified injury of unspecified blood vessel at ankle and foot level, left leg   `CC`
CC Excl: See code: S95.002

✓7ᵗʰ **S95.999** Other specified injury of unspecified blood vessel at ankle and foot level, unspecified leg   `CC`
CC Excl: See code: S95.009

✓4ᵗʰ **S96** Injury of muscle and tendon at ankle and foot level

Code also any associated open wound (S91.-)

EXCLUDES 2 injury of Achilles tendon (S86.0-)
sprain of joints and ligaments of ankle and foot (S93.-)

The appropriate 7th character is to be added to each code from category S96.
A   initial encounter
D   subsequent encounter
S   sequela

✓5ᵗʰ **S96.0** Injury of muscle and tendon of long flexor muscle of toe at ankle and foot level

✓6ᵗʰ **S96.00** Unspecified injury of muscle and tendon of long flexor muscle of toe at ankle and foot level

✓7ᵗʰ **S96.001** Unspecified injury of muscle and tendon of long flexor muscle of toe at ankle and foot level, right foot

✓7ᵗʰ **S96.002** Unspecified injury of muscle and tendon of long flexor muscle of toe at ankle and foot level, left foot

✓7ᵗʰ **S96.009** Unspecified injury of muscle and tendon of long flexor muscle of toe at ankle and foot level, unspecified foot

✓6ᵗʰ **S96.01** Strain of muscle and tendon of long flexor muscle of toe at ankle and foot level

✓7ᵗʰ **S96.011** Strain of muscle and tendon of long flexor muscle of toe at ankle and foot level, right foot

✓7ᵗʰ **S96.012** Strain of muscle and tendon of long flexor muscle of toe at ankle and foot level, left foot

✓7ᵗʰ **S96.019** Strain of muscle and tendon of long flexor muscle of toe at ankle and foot level, unspecified foot

✓6ᵗʰ **S96.02** Laceration of muscle and tendon of long flexor muscle of toe at ankle and foot level

✓7ᵗʰ **S96.021** Laceration of muscle and tendon of long flexor muscle of toe at ankle and foot level, right foot   `CC`
CC Excl: CC with 7th character A: S81.001A, S81.009-S81.011 with 7th A, S81.019-S81.021 with 7th A, S81.029-S81.031 with 7th A, S81.039-S81.041 with 7th A, S81.049-S81.051 with 7th A, S81.059-S81.801 with 7th A, S81.809-S81.811 with 7th A, S81.819-S81.821 with 7th A, S81.829-S81.831 with 7th A, S81.839-S81.841 with 7th A, S81.849-S81.851 with 7th A, S81.859A, S86.021 A, S86.029 with 7th A, S86.121A, S86.129A, S86.221A, S86.229A, S86.321A, S86.329A, S86.821A, S86.829A, S86.921A, S86.929A, S91.001A, S91.009-S91.011 with 7th A, S91.019-S91.021 with 7th A, S91.029-S91.031 with 7th A, S91.039-S91.041 with 7th A, S91.049-S91.051 with 7th A, S91.059A, S96.021A, S96.029A, S96.121A, S96.129A, S96.221A, S96.229A, S96.821A, S96.829A, S96.921A, S96.929A

✓7ᵗʰ **S96.022** Laceration of muscle and tendon of long flexor muscle of toe at ankle and foot level, left foot   `CC`
CC Excl: CC with 7th character A: S81.002-S81.009 with 7th A, S81.012-S81.019 with 7th A, S81.022-S81.029 with 7th A, S81.032-S81.039 with 7th A, S81.042-S81.049 with 7th A, S81.052-S81.059 with 7th A, S81.802-S81.809 with 7th A, S81.812-S81.819 with 7th A, S81.822-S81.829 with 7th A, S81.832-S81.839 with 7th A, S81.842-S81.849 with 7th A, S81.852-S81.859 with 7th A, S86.022-S86.029 with 7th A, S86.122-S86.129 with 7th A, S86.222-S86.229 with 7th A, S86.322-S86.329 with 7th A, S86.822-S86.829 with 7th A, S86.922-S86.929 with 7th A, S91.002-S91.009 with 7th A, S91.012-S91.019 with 7th A, S91.022-S91.029 with 7th A, S91.032-S91.039 with 7th A, S91.042-S91.049 with 7th A, S91.052-S91.059 with 7th A, S96.022-S96.029 with 7th A, S96.122-S96.129 with 7th A, S96.222-S96.229 with 7th A, S96.822-S96.829 with 7th A, S96.922-S96.929 with 7th A

✓7ᵗʰ **S96.029** Laceration of muscle and tendon of long flexor muscle of toe at ankle and foot level, unspecified foot   `CC`
CC Excl: CC with 7th character A: S81.001-S81.859 with 7th A, S86.021-S86.029 with 7th A, S86.121-S86.129 with 7th A, S86.221-S86.229 with 7th A, S86.321-S86.329 with 7th A, S86.821-S86.829 with 7th A, S86.921-S86.929 with 7th A, S91.001-S91.059 with 7th A, S96.021-S96.029 with 7th A, S96.121-S96.129 with 7th A, S96.221-S96.229 with 7th A, S96.821-S96.829 with 7th A, S96.921-S96.929 with 7th A

✓6ᵗʰ **S96.09** Other injury of muscle and tendon of long flexor muscle of toe at ankle and foot level

✓7ᵗʰ **S96.091** Other injury of muscle and tendon of long flexor muscle of toe at ankle and foot level, right foot

✓7ᵗʰ **S96.092** Other injury of muscle and tendon of long flexor muscle of toe at ankle and foot level, left foot

✓7ᵗʰ **S96.099** Other injury of muscle and tendon of long flexor muscle of toe at ankle and foot level, unspecified foot

✓5ᵗʰ **S96.1** Injury of muscle and tendon of long extensor muscle of toe at ankle and foot level

✓6ᵗʰ **S96.10** Unspecified injury of muscle and tendon of long extensor muscle of toe at ankle and foot level

✓7ᵗʰ **S96.101** Unspecified injury of muscle and tendon of long extensor muscle of toe at ankle and foot level, right foot

✓7ᵗʰ **S96.102** Unspecified injury of muscle and tendon of long extensor muscle of toe at ankle and foot level, left foot

✓7ᵗʰ **S96.109** Unspecified injury of muscle and tendon of long extensor muscle of toe at ankle and foot level, unspecified foot

---

✓ Additional Character Required   ✓x7ᵗʰ Xtension Alert   Unacceptable PDx   Manifestation   Hospital Acquired Condition   *EXCLUDES 1* Not Coded Here   *EXCLUDES 2* Not Included Here

ICD-10-CM Draft (2015)   1027

✓6ᵗʰ **S96.11** Strain of muscle and tendon of long extensor muscle of toe at ankle and foot level

  ✓7ᵗʰ **S96.111** Strain of muscle and tendon of long extensor muscle of toe at ankle and foot level, right foot

  ✓7ᵗʰ **S96.112** Strain of muscle and tendon of long extensor muscle of toe at ankle and foot level, left foot

  ✓7ᵗʰ **S96.119** Strain of muscle and tendon of long extensor muscle of toe at ankle and foot level, unspecified foot

✓6ᵗʰ **S96.12** Laceration of muscle and tendon of long extensor muscle of toe at ankle and foot level

  ✓7ᵗʰ **S96.121** Laceration of muscle and tendon of long extensor muscle of toe at ankle and foot level, right foot   **CC**
    CC Excl: See code: S95.021

  ✓7ᵗʰ **S96.122** Laceration of muscle and tendon of long extensor muscle of toe at ankle and foot level, left foot   **CC**
    CC Excl: See code: S95.022

  ✓7ᵗʰ **S96.129** Laceration of muscle and tendon of long extensor muscle of toe at ankle and foot level, unspecified foot   **CC**
    CC Excl: See code: S95.029

✓6ᵗʰ **S96.19** Other specified injury of muscle and tendon of long extensor muscle of toe at ankle and foot level

  ✓7ᵗʰ **S96.191** Other specified injury of muscle and tendon of long extensor muscle of toe at ankle and foot level, right foot

  ✓7ᵗʰ **S96.192** Other specified injury of muscle and tendon of long extensor muscle of toe at ankle and foot level, left foot

  ✓7ᵗʰ **S96.199** Other specified injury of muscle and tendon of long extensor muscle of toe at ankle and foot level, unspecified foot

✓5ᵗʰ **S96.2** Injury of intrinsic muscle and tendon at ankle and foot level

  ✓6ᵗʰ **S96.20** Unspecified injury of intrinsic muscle and tendon at ankle and foot level

    ✓7ᵗʰ **S96.201** Unspecified injury of intrinsic muscle and tendon at ankle and foot level, right foot

    ✓7ᵗʰ **S96.202** Unspecified injury of intrinsic muscle and tendon at ankle and foot level, left foot

    ✓7ᵗʰ **S96.209** Unspecified injury of intrinsic muscle and tendon at ankle and foot level, unspecified foot

  ✓6ᵗʰ **S96.21** Strain of intrinsic muscle and tendon at ankle and foot level

    ✓7ᵗʰ **S96.211** Strain of intrinsic muscle and tendon at ankle and foot level, right foot

    ✓7ᵗʰ **S96.212** Strain of intrinsic muscle and tendon at ankle and foot level, left foot

    ✓7ᵗʰ **S96.219** Strain of intrinsic muscle and tendon at ankle and foot level, unspecified foot

  ✓6ᵗʰ **S96.22** Laceration of intrinsic muscle and tendon at ankle and foot level

    ✓7ᵗʰ **S96.221** Laceration of intrinsic muscle and tendon at ankle and foot level, right foot   **CC**
      CC Excl: See code: S95.021

    ✓7ᵗʰ **S96.222** Laceration of intrinsic muscle and tendon at ankle and foot level, left foot   **CC**
      CC Excl: See code: S95.022

    ✓7ᵗʰ **S96.229** Laceration of intrinsic muscle and tendon at ankle and foot level, unspecified foot   **CC**
      CC Excl: See code: S95.029

  ✓6ᵗʰ **S96.29** Other specified injury of intrinsic muscle and tendon at ankle and foot level

    ✓7ᵗʰ **S96.291** Other specified injury of intrinsic muscle and tendon at ankle and foot level, right foot

    ✓7ᵗʰ **S96.292** Other specified injury of intrinsic muscle and tendon at ankle and foot level, left foot

  ✓7ᵗʰ **S96.299** Other specified injury of intrinsic muscle and tendon at ankle and foot level, unspecified foot

✓5ᵗʰ **S96.8** Injury of other specified muscles and tendons at ankle and foot level

  ✓6ᵗʰ **S96.80** Unspecified injury of other specified muscles and tendons at ankle and foot level

    ✓7ᵗʰ **S96.801** Unspecified injury of other specified muscles and tendons at ankle and foot level, right foot

    ✓7ᵗʰ **S96.802** Unspecified injury of other specified muscles and tendons at ankle and foot level, left foot

    ✓7ᵗʰ **S96.809** Unspecified injury of other specified muscles and tendons at ankle and foot level, unspecified foot

  ✓6ᵗʰ **S96.81** Strain of other specified muscles and tendons at ankle and foot level

    ✓7ᵗʰ **S96.811** Strain of other specified muscles and tendons at ankle and foot level, right foot

    ✓7ᵗʰ **S96.812** Strain of other specified muscles and tendons at ankle and foot level, left foot

    ✓7ᵗʰ **S96.819** Strain of other specified muscles and tendons at ankle and foot level, unspecified foot

  ✓6ᵗʰ **S96.82** Laceration of other specified muscles and tendons at ankle and foot level

    ✓7ᵗʰ **S96.821** Laceration of other specified muscles and tendons at ankle and foot level, right foot   **CC**
      CC Excl: See code: S95.021

    ✓7ᵗʰ **S96.822** Laceration of other specified muscles and tendons at ankle and foot level, left foot   **CC**
      CC Excl: See code: S95.022

    ✓7ᵗʰ **S96.829** Laceration of other specified muscles and tendons at ankle and foot level, unspecified foot   **CC**
      CC Excl: See code: S95.029

  ✓6ᵗʰ **S96.89** Other specified injury of other specified muscles and tendons at ankle and foot level

    ✓7ᵗʰ **S96.891** Other specified injury of other specified muscles and tendons at ankle and foot level, right foot

    ✓7ᵗʰ **S96.892** Other specified injury of other specified muscles and tendons at ankle and foot level, left foot

    ✓7ᵗʰ **S96.899** Other specified injury of other specified muscles and tendons at ankle and foot level, unspecified foot

✓5ᵗʰ **S96.9** Injury of unspecified muscle and tendon at ankle and foot level

  ✓6ᵗʰ **S96.90** Unspecified injury of unspecified muscle and tendon at ankle and foot level

    ✓7ᵗʰ **S96.901** Unspecified injury of unspecified muscle and tendon at ankle and foot level, right foot

    ✓7ᵗʰ **S96.902** Unspecified injury of unspecified muscle and tendon at ankle and foot level, left foot

    ✓7ᵗʰ **S96.909** Unspecified injury of unspecified muscle and tendon at ankle and foot level, unspecified foot

  ✓6ᵗʰ **S96.91** Strain of unspecified muscle and tendon at ankle and foot level

    ✓7ᵗʰ **S96.911** Strain of unspecified muscle and tendon at ankle and foot level, right foot

    ✓7ᵗʰ **S96.912** Strain of unspecified muscle and tendon at ankle and foot level, left foot

    ✓7ᵗʰ **S96.919** Strain of unspecified muscle and tendon at ankle and foot level, unspecified foot

---

N Newborn: 0   **P** Pediatric: 0-17   **M** Maternity: 12-55   **A** Adult: 15-124   **MCC** Major CC Condition   **PDx MCC** PDx acts as own MCC   **CC** CC Condition   **PDx CC** PDx acts as own CC

1028   ICD-10-CM Draft (2015)

☑6ᵗʰ **S96.92** Laceration of unspecified muscle and tendon at ankle and foot level

☑7ᵗʰ **S96.921** Laceration of unspecified muscle and tendon at ankle and foot level, right foot `CC`
CC Excl: See code: S95.021

☑7ᵗʰ **S96.922** Laceration of unspecified muscle and tendon at ankle and foot level, left foot `CC`
CC Excl: See code: S95.022

☑7ᵗʰ **S96.929** Laceration of unspecified muscle and tendon at ankle and foot level, unspecified foot `CC`
CC Excl: See code: S95.029

☑6ᵗʰ **S96.99** Other specified injury of unspecified muscle and tendon at ankle and foot level

☑7ᵗʰ **S96.991** Other specified injury of unspecified muscle and tendon at ankle and foot level, right foot

☑7ᵗʰ **S96.992** Other specified injury of unspecified muscle and tendon at ankle and foot level, left foot

☑7ᵗʰ **S96.999** Other specified injury of unspecified muscle and tendon at ankle and foot level, unspecified foot

☑4ᵗʰ **S97** Crushing injury of ankle and foot
Use additional code(s) for all associated injuries

The appropriate 7th character is to be added to each code from category S97.
A   initial encounter
D   subsequent encounter
S   sequela

☑5ᵗʰ **S97.0** Crushing injury of ankle

☑x7ᵗʰ **S97.00** Crushing injury of unspecified ankle

☑x7ᵗʰ **S97.01** Crushing injury of right ankle

☑x7ᵗʰ **S97.02** Crushing injury of left ankle

☑5ᵗʰ **S97.1** Crushing injury of toe

☑6ᵗʰ **S97.10** Crushing injury of unspecified toe(s)

☑7ᵗʰ **S97.101** Crushing injury of unspecified right toe(s)

☑7ᵗʰ **S97.102** Crushing injury of unspecified left toe(s)

☑7ᵗʰ **S97.109** Crushing injury of unspecified toe(s)
Crushing injury of toe NOS

☑6ᵗʰ **S97.11** Crushing injury of great toe

☑7ᵗʰ **S97.111** Crushing injury of right great toe

☑7ᵗʰ **S97.112** Crushing injury of left great toe

☑7ᵗʰ **S97.119** Crushing injury of unspecified great toe

☑6ᵗʰ **S97.12** Crushing injury of lesser toe(s)

☑7ᵗʰ **S97.121** Crushing injury of right lesser toe(s)

☑7ᵗʰ **S97.122** Crushing injury of left lesser toe(s)

☑7ᵗʰ **S97.129** Crushing injury of unspecified lesser toe(s)

☑5ᵗʰ **S97.8** Crushing injury of foot

☑x7ᵗʰ **S97.80** Crushing injury of unspecified foot
Crushing injury of foot NOS

☑x7ᵗʰ **S97.81** Crushing injury of right foot

☑x7ᵗʰ **S97.82** Crushing injury of left foot

☑4ᵗʰ **S98** Traumatic amputation of ankle and foot
An amputation not identified as partial or complete should be coded to complete

The appropriate 7th character is to be added to each code from category S98.
A   initial encounter
D   subsequent encounter
S   sequela

☑5ᵗʰ **S98.0** Traumatic amputation of foot at ankle level

☑6ᵗʰ **S98.01** Complete traumatic amputation of foot at ankle level

☑7ᵗʰ **S98.011** Complete traumatic amputation of right foot at ankle level `CC`
CC Excl: CC with 7th character A: S71.001 with 7th A, S71.009-S71.011 with 7th A, S71.019-S71.021 with 7th A, S71.029-S71.031 with 7th A, S71.039-S71.041 with 7th A, S71.049-S71.051 with 7th A, S71.059-S71.101 with 7th A, S71.109-S71.111 with 7th A, S71.119-S71.121 with 7th A, S71.129-S71.131 with 7th A, S71.139-S71.141 with 7th A, S71.149-S71.151 with 7th A, S71.159 with 7th A, S76.021 with 7th A, S76.029 with 7th A, S76.121 with 7th A, S76.129 with 7th A, S76.221 with 7th A, S76.229 with 7th A, S76.321 with 7th A, S76.329 with 7th A, S76.821 with 7th A, S76.829 with 7th A, S76.921 with 7th A, S76.929 with 7th A, S78.011 with 7th A, S78.019-S78.021 with 7th A, S78.029-S78.111 with 7th A, S78.119-S78.121 with 7th A, S78.129-S78.911 with 7th A, S78.919-S78.921 with 7th A, S78.929 with 7th A, S81.001 with 7th A, S81.009-S81.011 with 7th A, S81.019-S81.021 with 7th A, S81.029-S81.031 with 7th A, S81.039-S81.041 with 7th A, S81.049-S81.051 with 7th A, S81.059-S81.801 with 7th A, S81.809-S81.811 with 7th A, S81.819-S81.821 with 7th A, S81.829-S81.831 with 7th A, S81.839-S81.841 with 7th A, S81.849-S81.851 with 7th A, S81.859 with 7th A, S86.021 with 7th A, S86.029 with 7th A, S86.121 with 7th A, S86.129 with 7th A, S86.221 with 7th A, S86.229 with 7th A, S86.321 with 7th A, S86.329 with 7th A, S86.821 with 7th A, S86.829 with 7th A, S86.921 with 7th A, S86.929 with 7th A, S88.011 with 7th A, S88.019-S88.021 with 7th A, S88.029-S88.111 with 7th A, S88.119-S88.121 with 7th A, S88.129-S88.911 with 7th A, S88.919-S88.921 with 7th A, S88.929 with 7th A, S91.001 with 7th A, S91.009-S91.011 with 7th A, S91.019-S91.021 with 7th A, S91.029-S91.031 with 7th A, S91.039-S91.041 with 7th A, S91.049-S91.051 with 7th A, S91.059-S91.101 with 7th A, S91.103-S91.104 with 7th A, S91.106-S91.111 with 7th A, S91.113-S91.114 with 7th A, S91.116-S91.121 with 7th A, S91.123-S91.124 with 7th A, S91.126-S91.131 with 7th A, S91.133-S91.134 with 7th A, S91.136-S91.141 with 7th A, S91.143-S91.144 with 7th A, S91.146-S91.151 with 7th A, S91.153-S91.154 with 7th A, S91.156-S91.201 with 7th A, S91.203-S91.204 with 7th A, S91.206-S91.211 with 7th A, S91.213-S91.214 with 7th A, S91.216-S91.221 with 7th A, S91.223-S91.224 with 7th A, S91.226-S91.231 with 7th A, S91.233-S91.234 with 7th A, S91.236-S91.241 with 7th A, S91.243-S91.244 with 7th A, S91.246-S91.251 with 7th A, S91.253-S91.254 with 7th A, S91.256-S91.301 with 7th A, S91.309-S91.311 with 7th A, S91.319-S91.321 with 7th A, S91.329-S91.331 with 7th A, S91.339-S91.341 with 7th A, S91.349-S91.351 with 7th A, S91.359 with 7th A, S96.021 with 7th A, S96.029 with 7th A, S96.121 with 7th A, S96.129 with 7th A, S96.221 with 7th A, S96.229 with 7th A, S96.821 with 7th A, S96.829 with 7th A, S96.921 with 7th A, S96.929 with 7th A, S98.011 with 7th A, S98.019-S98.021 with 7th A, S98.029-S98.111 with 7th A, S98.119-S98.121 with 7th A

√7th **S98.012 Complete traumatic amputation of left foot at ankle level** `CC`
CC Excl: CC with 7th character A: S71.002-S71.009 with 7th A, S71.012-S71.019 with 7th A, S71.022-S71.029 with 7th A, S71.032-S71.039 with 7th A, S71.042-S71.049 with 7th A, S71.052-S71.059 with 7th A, S71.102-S71.109 with 7th A, S71.112-S71.119 with 7th A, S71.122-S71.129 with 7th A, S71.132-S71.139 with 7th A, S71.142-S71.149 with 7th A, S71.152-S71.159 with 7th A, S76.022-S76.029 with 7th A, S76.122-S76.129 with 7th A, S76.222-S76.229 with 7th A, S76.322-S76.329 with 7th A, S76.822-S76.829 with 7th A, S76.922-S76.929 with 7th A, S78.012-S78.019 with 7th A, S78.022-S78.029 with 7th A, S78.112-S78.119 with 7th A, S78.122-S78.129 with 7th A, S78.912-S78.919 with 7th A, S78.922-S78.929 with 7th A, S81.002-S81.009 with 7th A, S81.012-S81.019 with 7th A, S81.022-S81.029 with 7th A, S81.032-S81.039 with 7th A, S81.042-S81.049 with 7th A, S81.052-S81.059 with 7th A, S81.802-S81.809 with 7th A, S81.812-S81.819 with 7th A, S81.822-S81.829 with 7th A, S81.832-S81.839 with 7th A, S81.842-S81.849 with 7th A, S81.852-S81.859 with 7th A, S86.022-S86.029 with 7th A, S86.122-S86.129 with 7th A, S86.222-S86.229 with 7th A, S86.322-S86.329 with 7th A, S86.822-S86.829 with 7th A, S86.922-S86.929 with 7th A, S88.012-S88.019 with 7th A, S88.022-S88.029 with 7th A, S88.112-S88.119 with 7th A, S88.122-S88.129 with 7th A, S88.912-S88.919 with 7th A, S88.922-S88.929 with 7th A, S91.002-S91.009 with 7th A, S91.012-S91.019 with 7th A, S91.022-S91.029 with 7th A, S91.032-S91.039 with 7th A, S91.042-S91.049 with 7th A, S91.052-S91.059 with 7th A, S91.102-S91.103 with 7th A, S91.105-S91.109 with 7th A, S91.112-S91.113 with 7th A, S91.115-S91.119 with 7th A, S91.122-S91.123 with 7th A, S91.125-S91.129 with 7th A, S91.132-S91.133 with 7th A, S91.135-S91.139 with 7th A, S91.142-S91.143 with 7th A, S91.145-S91.149 with 7th A, S91.152-S91.153 with 7th A, S91.155-S91.159 with 7th A, S91.202-S91.203 with 7th A, S91.205-S91.209 with 7th A, S91.212-S91.213 with 7th A, S91.215-S91.219 with 7th A, S91.222-S91.223 with 7th A, S91.225-S91.229 with 7th A, S91.232-S91.233 with 7th A, S91.235-S91.239 with 7th A, S91.242-S91.243 with 7th A, S91.245-S91.249 with 7th A, S91.252-S91.253 with 7th A, S91.255-S91.259 with 7th A, S91.302-S91.309 with 7th A, S91.312-S91.319 with 7th A, S91.322-S91.329 with 7th A, S91.332-S91.339 with 7th A, S91.342-S91.349 with 7th A, S91.352-S91.359 with 7th A, S96.022-S96.029 with 7th A, S96.122-S96.129 with 7th A, S96.222-S96.229 with 7th A, S96.822-S96.829 with 7th A, S96.922-S96.929 with 7th A, S98.012-S98.019 with 7th A, S98.022-S98.029 with 7th A, S98.112-S98.119 with 7th A, S98.122-S98.129 with 7th A, S98.132-S98.139 with 7th A, S98.142-S98.149 with 7th A, S98.212-S98.219 with 7th A, S98.222-S98.229 with 7th A, S98.312-S98.319 with 7th A, S98.322-S98.329 with 7th A, S98.912-S98.919 with 7th A, S98.922-S98.929 with 7th A, T14.8-T14.91, T79.A0X-T79.9XX with 7th A

√7th **S98.019 Complete traumatic amputation of unspecified foot at ankle level** `CC`
CC Excl: CC with 7th character A: S71.001-S71.159 with 7th A, S76.021-S76.029 with 7th A, S76.121-S76.129 with 7th A, S76.221-S76.229 with 7th A, S76.321-S76.329 with 7th A, S76.821-S76.829 with 7th A, S76.921-S76.929 with 7th A, S78.011-S78.929 with 7th A, S81.001-S81.859 with 7th A, S86.021-S86.029 with 7th A, S86.121-S86.129 with 7th A, S86.221-S86.229 with 7th A, S86.321-S86.329 with 7th A, S86.821-S86.829 with 7th A, S86.921-S86.929 with 7th A, S88.011-S88.929 with 7th A, S91.001-S91.359 with 7th A, S96.021-S96.029 with 7th A, S96.121-S96.129 with 7th A, S96.221-S96.229 with 7th A, S96.821-S96.829 with 7th A, S96.921-S96.929 with 7th A, S98.011-S98.929 with 7th A, T14.8-T14.91, T79.A0X-T79.9XX with 7th A

√6th **S98.02 Partial traumatic amputation of foot at ankle level**

√7th **S98.021 Partial traumatic amputation of right foot at ankle level** `CC`
CC Excl: See code: S98.011

√7th **S98.022 Partial traumatic amputation of left foot at ankle level** `CC`
CC Excl: See code: S98.012

√7th **S98.029 Partial traumatic amputation of unspecified foot at ankle level** `CC`
CC Excl: See code: S98.019

√5th **S98.1 Traumatic amputation of one toe**

√6th **S98.11 Complete traumatic amputation of great toe**

√7th **S98.111 Complete traumatic amputation of right great toe**

√7th **S98.112 Complete traumatic amputation of left great toe**

√7th **S98.119 Complete traumatic amputation of unspecified great toe**

√6th **S98.12 Partial traumatic amputation of great toe**

√7th **S98.121 Partial traumatic amputation of right great toe**

√7th **S98.122 Partial traumatic amputation of left great toe**

√7th **S98.129 Partial traumatic amputation of unspecified great toe**

√6th **S98.13 Complete traumatic amputation of one lesser toe**
Traumatic amputation of toe NOS

√7th **S98.131 Complete traumatic amputation of one right lesser toe**

√7th **S98.132 Complete traumatic amputation of one left lesser toe**

√7th **S98.139 Complete traumatic amputation of one unspecified lesser toe**

√6th **S98.14 Partial traumatic amputation of one lesser toe**

√7th **S98.141 Partial traumatic amputation of one right lesser toe**

√7th **S98.142 Partial traumatic amputation of one left lesser toe**

√7th **S98.149 Partial traumatic amputation of one unspecified lesser toe**

√5th **S98.2 Traumatic amputation of two or more lesser toes**

√6th **S98.21 Complete traumatic amputation of two or more lesser toes**

√7th **S98.211 Complete traumatic amputation of two or more right lesser toes**

√7th **S98.212 Complete traumatic amputation of two or more left lesser toes**

√7th **S98.219 Complete traumatic amputation of two or more unspecified lesser toes**

√6th **S98.22 Partial traumatic amputation of two or more lesser toes**

√7th **S98.221 Partial traumatic amputation of two or more right lesser toes**

√7th **S98.222 Partial traumatic amputation of two or more left lesser toes**

√7th **S98.229 Partial traumatic amputation of two or more unspecified lesser toes**

√5th **S98.3 Traumatic amputation of midfoot**

√6th **S98.31 Complete traumatic amputation of midfoot**

√7th **S98.311 Complete traumatic amputation of right midfoot** `CC`
CC Excl: See code: S98.011

√7th **S98.312 Complete traumatic amputation of left midfoot** `CC`
CC Excl: See code: S98.012

√7th **S98.319 Complete traumatic amputation of unspecified midfoot** `CC`
CC Excl: See code: S98.019

√6th **S98.32 Partial traumatic amputation of midfoot**

√7th **S98.321 Partial traumatic amputation of right midfoot** `CC`
CC Excl: See code: S98.011

√7th **S98.322 Partial traumatic amputation of left midfoot** `CC`
CC Excl: See code: S98.012

N Newborn: 0   P Pediatric: 0-17   M Maternity: 12-55   A Adult: 15-124   MCC Major CC Condition   PDx MCC PDx acts as own MCC   CC CC Condition   PDx CC PDx acts as own CC

1030   ICD-10-CM Draft (2015)

✓7ᵗʰ S98.329 **Partial traumatic amputation of** CC
unspecified midfoot
CC Excl: See code: S98.019

✓5ᵗʰ S98.9 **Traumatic amputation of foot, level unspecified**

✓6ᵗʰ S98.91 **Complete traumatic amputation of foot, level unspecified**

✓7ᵗʰ S98.911 **Complete traumatic amputation of right foot, level unspecified** CC
CC Excl: See code: S98.011

✓7ᵗʰ S98.912 **Complete traumatic amputation of left foot, level unspecified** CC
CC Excl: See code: S98.012

✓7ᵗʰ S98.919 **Complete traumatic amputation of unspecified foot, level unspecified** CC
CC Excl: See code: S98.019

✓6ᵗʰ S98.92 **Partial traumatic amputation of foot, level unspecified**

✓7ᵗʰ S98.921 **Partial traumatic amputation of right foot, level unspecified** CC
CC Excl: See code: S98.011

✓7ᵗʰ S98.922 **Partial traumatic amputation of left foot, level unspecified** CC
CC Excl: See code: S98.012

✓7ᵗʰ S98.929 **Partial traumatic amputation of unspecified foot, level unspecified** CC
CC Excl: See code: S98.019

✓4ᵗʰ **S99 Other and unspecified injuries of ankle and foot**

The appropriate 7th character is to be added to each code from category S99.
A   initial encounter
D   subsequent encounter
S   sequela

✓5ᵗʰ S99.8 **Other specified injuries of ankle and foot**

✓6ᵗʰ S99.81 **Other specified injuries of ankle**

✓7ᵗʰ S99.811 **Other specified injuries of right ankle**

✓7ᵗʰ S99.812 **Other specified injuries of left ankle**

✓7ᵗʰ S99.819 **Other specified injuries of unspecified ankle**

✓6ᵗʰ S99.82 **Other specified injuries of foot**

✓7ᵗʰ S99.821 **Other specified injuries of right foot**

✓7ᵗʰ S99.822 **Other specified injuries of left foot**

✓7ᵗʰ S99.829 **Other specified injuries of unspecified foot**

✓5ᵗʰ S99.9 **Unspecified injury of ankle and foot**

✓6ᵗʰ S99.91 **Unspecified injury of ankle**

✓7ᵗʰ S99.911 **Unspecified injury of right ankle**

✓7ᵗʰ S99.912 **Unspecified injury of left ankle**

✓7ᵗʰ S99.919 **Unspecified injury of unspecified ankle**

✓6ᵗʰ S99.92 **Unspecified injury of foot**

✓7ᵗʰ S99.921 **Unspecified injury of right foot**

✓7ᵗʰ S99.922 **Unspecified injury of left foot**

✓7ᵗʰ S99.929 **Unspecified injury of unspecified foot**

Injury, Poisoning And Other Consequences Of External Causes (T07-T88)

Injuries involving multiple body regions (T07)

EXCLUDES 1 *burns and corrosions (T20-T32)*
frostbite (T33-T34)
insect bite or sting, venomous (T63.4)
sunburn (L55.-)

T07 Unspecified multiple injuries
EXCLUDES 1 *injury NOS (T14)*

Injury of unspecified body region (T14)

✓4ᵗʰ **T14 Injury of unspecified body region**
EXCLUDES 1 *multiple unspecified injuries (T07)*

T14.8 **Other injury of unspecified body region**
Abrasion NOS   Fracture NOS
Contusion NOS   Skin injury NOS
Crush injury NOS   Vascular injury NOS

✓5ᵗʰ T14.9 **Unspecified injury**

T14.90 **Injury, unspecified**
Injury NOS

T14.91 **Suicide attempt**
Attempted suicide NOS

Effects of foreign body entering through natural orifice (T15-T19)

EXCLUDES 2 *foreign body accidentally left in operation wound (T81.5-)*
foreign body in penetrating wound—See open wound by body region
residual foreign body in soft tissue (M79.5)
splinter, without open wound—See superficial injury by body region

✓4ᵗʰ **T15 Foreign body on external eye**
EXCLUDES 2 *foreign body in penetrating wound of orbit and eye ball (S05.4-, S05.5-)*
open wound of eyelid and periocular area (S01.1-)
retained foreign body in eyelid (H02.8-)
retained (old) foreign body in penetrating wound of orbit and eye ball (H05.5-, H44.6-, H44.7-)
superficial foreign body of eyelid and periocular area (S00.25-)

The appropriate 7th character is to be added to each code from category T15.
A   initial encounter
D   subsequent encounter
S   sequela

✓5ᵗʰ T15.0 **Foreign body in cornea**
✓x7ᵗʰ T15.00 **Foreign body in cornea, unspecified eye**
✓x7ᵗʰ T15.01 **Foreign body in cornea, right eye**
✓x7ᵗʰ T15.02 **Foreign body in cornea, left eye**

✓5ᵗʰ T15.1 **Foreign body in conjunctival sac**
✓x7ᵗʰ T15.10 **Foreign body in conjunctival sac, unspecified eye**
✓x7ᵗʰ T15.11 **Foreign body in conjunctival sac, right eye**
✓x7ᵗʰ T15.12 **Foreign body in conjunctival sac, left eye**

✓5ᵗʰ T15.8 **Foreign body in other and multiple parts of external eye**
Foreign body in lacrimal punctum
✓x7ᵗʰ T15.80 **Foreign body in other and multiple parts of external eye, unspecified eye**
✓x7ᵗʰ T15.81 **Foreign body in other and multiple parts of external eye, right eye**
✓x7ᵗʰ T15.82 **Foreign body in other and multiple parts of external eye, left eye**

✓5ᵗʰ T15.9 **Foreign body on external eye, part unspecified**
✓x7ᵗʰ T15.90 **Foreign body on external eye, part unspecified, unspecified eye**
✓x7ᵗʰ T15.91 **Foreign body on external eye, part unspecified, right eye**
✓x7ᵗʰ T15.92 **Foreign body on external eye, part unspecified, left eye**

✓4ᵗʰ **T16 Foreign body in ear**
Foreign body in auditory canal

The appropriate 7th character is to be added to each code from category T16.
A   initial encounter
D   subsequent encounter
S   sequela

✓x7ᵗʰ T16.1 **Foreign body in right ear**

Injury, Poisoning and Certain Other Consequences of External Causes

T16.2–T17.900

✓x7ᵗʰ **T16.2**   Foreign body in left ear

✓x7ᵗʰ **T16.9**   Foreign body in ear, unspecified ear

✓4ᵗʰ **T17**   **Foreign body in respiratory tract**

> The appropriate 7th character is to be added to each code from category T17.
> A   initial encounter
> D   subsequent encounter
> S   sequela

✓x7ᵗʰ **T17.0**   Foreign body in nasal sinus

✓x7ᵗʰ **T17.1**   Foreign body in nostril
     Foreign body in nose NOS

✓5ᵗʰ **T17.2**   Foreign body in pharynx
     Foreign body in nasopharynx   Foreign body in throat NOS

   ✓6ᵗʰ **T17.20**   Unspecified foreign body in pharynx

     ✓7ᵗʰ **T17.200**   Unspecified foreign body in pharynx causing asphyxiation

     ✓7ᵗʰ **T17.208**   Unspecified foreign body in pharynx causing other injury

   ✓6ᵗʰ **T17.21**   Gastric contents in pharynx
       Aspiration of gastric contents into pharynx
       Vomitus in pharynx

     ✓7ᵗʰ **T17.210**   Gastric contents in pharynx causing asphyxiation

     ✓7ᵗʰ **T17.218**   Gastric contents in pharynx causing other injury

   ✓6ᵗʰ **T17.22**   Food in pharynx
       Bones in pharynx   Seeds in pharynx

     ✓7ᵗʰ **T17.220**   Food in pharynx causing asphyxiation

     ✓7ᵗʰ **T17.228**   Food in pharynx causing other injury

   ✓6ᵗʰ **T17.29**   Other foreign object in pharynx

     ✓7ᵗʰ **T17.290**   Other foreign object in pharynx causing asphyxiation

     ✓7ᵗʰ **T17.298**   Other foreign object in pharynx causing other injury

✓5ᵗʰ **T17.3**   Foreign body in larynx

   ✓6ᵗʰ **T17.30**   Unspecified foreign body in larynx

     ✓7ᵗʰ **T17.300**   Unspecified foreign body in larynx causing asphyxiation

     ✓7ᵗʰ **T17.308**   Unspecified foreign body in larynx causing other injury

   ✓6ᵗʰ **T17.31**   Gastric contents in larynx
       Aspiration of gastric contents into larynx
       Vomitus in larynx

     ✓7ᵗʰ **T17.310**   Gastric contents in larynx causing asphyxiation

     ✓7ᵗʰ **T17.318**   Gastric contents in larynx causing other injury

   ✓6ᵗʰ **T17.32**   Food in larynx
       Bones in larynx   Seeds in larynx

     ✓7ᵗʰ **T17.320**   Food in larynx causing asphyxiation

     ✓7ᵗʰ **T17.328**   Food in larynx causing other injury

   ✓6ᵗʰ **T17.39**   Other foreign object in larynx

     ✓7ᵗʰ **T17.390**   Other foreign object in larynx causing asphyxiation

     ✓7ᵗʰ **T17.398**   Other foreign object in larynx causing other injury

✓5ᵗʰ **T17.4**   Foreign body in trachea

> **CC Excl: For CC codes in subcategory T17.4: CC with 7th character A, unless otherwise noted:** T17.400-T17.498 with 7th A

   ✓6ᵗʰ **T17.40**   Unspecified foreign body in trachea

     ✓7ᵗʰ **T17.400**   Unspecified foreign body in trachea causing asphyxiation   CC

     ✓7ᵗʰ **T17.408**   Unspecified foreign body in trachea causing other injury   CC

   ✓6ᵗʰ **T17.41**   Gastric contents in trachea
       Aspiration of gastric contents into trachea
       Vomitus in trachea

     ✓7ᵗʰ **T17.410**   Gastric contents in trachea causing asphyxiation   CC

     ✓7ᵗʰ **T17.418**   Gastric contents in trachea causing other injury   CC

   ✓6ᵗʰ **T17.42**   Food in trachea
       Bones in trachea   Seeds in trachea

     ✓7ᵗʰ **T17.420**   Food in trachea causing asphyxiation   CC

     ✓7ᵗʰ **T17.428**   Food in trachea causing other injury   CC

   ✓6ᵗʰ **T17.49**   Other foreign object in trachea

     ✓7ᵗʰ **T17.490**   Other foreign object in trachea causing asphyxiation

     ✓7ᵗʰ **T17.498**   Other foreign object in trachea causing other injury   CC

✓5ᵗʰ **T17.5**   Foreign body in bronchus

> **CC Excl: For CC codes in subcategory T17.5: CC with 7th character A, unless otherwise noted:** T17.400-T17.998 with 7th A

   ✓6ᵗʰ **T17.50**   Unspecified foreign body in bronchus

     ✓7ᵗʰ **T17.500**   Unspecified foreign body in bronchus causing asphyxiation   CC

     ✓7ᵗʰ **T17.508**   Unspecified foreign body in bronchus causing other injury   CC

   ✓6ᵗʰ **T17.51**   Gastric contents in bronchus
       Aspiration of gastric contents into bronchus
       Vomitus in bronchus

     ✓7ᵗʰ **T17.510**   Gastric contents in bronchus causing asphyxiation   CC

     ✓7ᵗʰ **T17.518**   Gastric contents in bronchus causing other injury   CC

   ✓6ᵗʰ **T17.52**   Food in bronchus
       Bones in bronchus   Seeds in bronchus

     ✓7ᵗʰ **T17.520**   Food in bronchus causing asphyxiation   CC

     ✓7ᵗʰ **T17.528**   Food in bronchus causing other injury   CC

   ✓6ᵗʰ **T17.59**   Other foreign object in bronchus

     ✓7ᵗʰ **T17.590**   Other foreign object in bronchus causing asphyxiation   CC

     ✓7ᵗʰ **T17.598**   Other foreign object in bronchus causing other injury   CC

✓5ᵗʰ **T17.8**   Foreign body in other parts of respiratory tract
     Foreign body in bronchioles   Foreign body in lung

> **CC Excl: For CC codes in subcategory T17.8: CC with 7th character A, unless otherwise noted:** See code: T17.5

   ✓6ᵗʰ **T17.80**   Unspecified foreign body in other parts of respiratory tract

     ✓7ᵗʰ **T17.800**   Unspecified foreign body in other parts of respiratory tract causing asphyxiation   CC

     ✓7ᵗʰ **T17.808**   Unspecified foreign body in other parts of respiratory tract causing other injury   CC

   ✓6ᵗʰ **T17.81**   Gastric contents in other parts of respiratory tract
       Aspiration of gastric contents into other parts of respiratory tract
       Vomitus in other parts of respiratory tract

     ✓7ᵗʰ **T17.810**   Gastric contents in other parts of respiratory tract causing asphyxiation   CC

     ✓7ᵗʰ **T17.818**   Gastric contents in other parts of respiratory tract causing other injury   CC

   ✓6ᵗʰ **T17.82**   Food in other parts of respiratory tract
       Bones in other parts of respiratory tract
       Seeds in other parts of respiratory tract

     ✓7ᵗʰ **T17.820**   Food in other parts of respiratory tract causing asphyxiation   CC

     ✓7ᵗʰ **T17.828**   Food in other parts of respiratory tract causing other injury   CC

   ✓6ᵗʰ **T17.89**   Other foreign object in other parts of respiratory tract

     ✓7ᵗʰ **T17.890**   Other foreign object in other parts of respiratory tract causing asphyxiation   CC

     ✓7ᵗʰ **T17.898**   Other foreign object in other parts of respiratory tract causing other injury   CC

✓5ᵗʰ **T17.9**   Foreign body in respiratory tract, part unspecified

   ✓6ᵗʰ **T17.90**   Unspecified foreign body in respiratory tract, part unspecified

     ✓7ᵗʰ **T17.900**   Unspecified foreign body in respiratory tract, part unspecified causing asphyxiation

---

N Newborn: 0   P Pediatric: 0-17   M Maternity: 12-55   A Adult: 15-124   MCC Major CC Condition   PDx MCC PDx acts as own MCC   CC CC Condition   PDx CC PDx acts as own CC

1032   ICD-10-CM Draft (2015)

☑7ᵗʰ **T17.908 Unspecified foreign body in respiratory tract, part unspecified** causing other injury

☑6ᵗʰ **T17.91 Gastric contents in respiratory tract, part unspecified**
Aspiration of gastric contents into respiratory tract, part unspecified
Vomitus in trachea respiratory tract, part unspecified

☑7ᵗʰ **T17.910 Gastric contents in respiratory tract, part unspecified** causing asphyxiation

☑7ᵗʰ **T17.918 Gastric contents in respiratory tract, part unspecified** causing other injury

☑6ᵗʰ **T17.92 Food in respiratory tract, part unspecified**
Bones in respiratory tract, part unspecified
Seeds in respiratory tract, part unspecified

☑7ᵗʰ **T17.920 Food in respiratory tract, part unspecified** causing asphyxiation

☑7ᵗʰ **T17.928 Food in respiratory tract, part unspecified** causing other injury

☑6ᵗʰ **T17.99 Other foreign object in respiratory tract, part unspecified**

☑7ᵗʰ **T17.990 Other foreign object in respiratory tract, part unspecified** in causing asphyxiation

☑7ᵗʰ **T17.998 Other foreign object in respiratory tract, part unspecified** causing other injury

☑4ᵗʰ **T18 Foreign body in alimentary tract**
EXCLUDES 2 *foreign body in pharynx (T17.2-)*

The appropriate 7th character is to be added to each code from category T18.
A   initial encounter
D   subsequent encounter
S   sequela

☑x7ᵗʰ **T18.0 Foreign body in** mouth

☑5ᵗʰ **T18.1 Foreign body in** esophagus
EXCLUDES 2 *foreign body in respiratory tract (T17.-)*

☑6ᵗʰ **T18.10 Unspecified foreign body in esophagus**

☑7ᵗʰ **T18.100 Unspecified foreign body in esophagus causing compression of trachea**
Unspecified foreign body in esophagus causing obstruction of respiration

☑7ᵗʰ **T18.108 Unspecified foreign body in esophagus causing other injury**

☑6ᵗʰ **T18.11 Gastric contents in esophagus**
Vomitus in esophagus

☑7ᵗʰ **T18.110 Gastric contents in esophagus causing compression of trachea**
Gastric contents in esophagus causing obstruction of respiration

☑7ᵗʰ **T18.118 Gastric contents in esophagus causing other injury**

☑6ᵗʰ **T18.12 Food in esophagus**
Bones in esophagus   Seeds in esophagus

☑7ᵗʰ **T18.120 Food in esophagus causing compression of trachea**
Food in esophagus causing obstruction of respiration

☑7ᵗʰ **T18.128 Food in esophagus** causing other injury

☑6ᵗʰ **T18.19 Other foreign object in esophagus**

☑7ᵗʰ **T18.190 Other foreign object in esophagus causing compression of trachea**
Other foreign body in esophagus causing obstruction of respiration

☑7ᵗʰ **T18.198 Other foreign object in esophagus causing other injury**

☑x7ᵗʰ **T18.2 Foreign body in** stomach

☑x7ᵗʰ **T18.3 Foreign body in** small intestine

☑x7ᵗʰ **T18.4 Foreign body in** colon

☑x7ᵗʰ **T18.5 Foreign body in** anus and rectum
Foreign body in rectosigmoid (junction)

☑x7ᵗʰ **T18.8 Foreign body in** other parts of alimentary tract

☑x7ᵗʰ **T18.9 Foreign body of alimentary tract,** part unspecified
Foreign body in digestive system NOS
Swallowed foreign body NOS

☑4ᵗʰ **T19 Foreign body in genitourinary tract**
EXCLUDES 2 *complications due to implanted mesh (T83.7-)*
mechanical complications of contraceptive device (intrauterine) (vaginal) (T83.3-)
presence of contraceptive device (intrauterine) (vaginal) (Z97.5)

The appropriate 7th character is to be added to each code from category T19.
A   initial encounter
D   subsequent encounter
S   sequela

☑x7ᵗʰ **T19.0 Foreign body in** urethra

☑x7ᵗʰ **T19.1 Foreign body in** bladder

☑x7ᵗʰ **T19.2 Foreign body in** vulva and vagina   ♀

☑x7ᵗʰ **T19.3 Foreign body in** uterus   ♀

☑x7ᵗʰ **T19.4 Foreign body in** penis   ♂

☑x7ᵗʰ **T19.8 Foreign body in** other parts of genitourinary tract

☑x7ᵗʰ **T19.9 Foreign body in** genitourinary tract, part unspecified

Burns and corrosions (T20-T32)

INCLUDES   burns (thermal) from electrical heating appliances
burns (thermal) from electricity
burns (thermal) from flame
burns (thermal) from friction
burns (thermal) from hot air and hot gases
burns (thermal) from hot objects
burns (thermal) from lightning
burns (thermal) from radiation
chemical burn [corrosion] (external) (internal)
scalds
EXCLUDES 2 *erythema [dermatitis] ab igne (L59.0)*
radiation-related disorders of the skin and subcutaneous tissue (L55-L59)
sunburn (L55.-)

Burns and corrosions of external body surface, specified by site (T20-T25)

INCLUDES   burns and corrosions of first degree [erythema]
burns and corrosions of second degree [blisters] [epidermal loss]
burns and corrosions of third degree [deep necrosis of underlying tissue] [full-thickness skin loss]
Use additional code from category T31 or T32 to identify extent of body surface involved

☑4ᵗʰ **T20 Burn and corrosion of head, face, and neck**
EXCLUDES 2 *burn and corrosion of ear drum (T28.41, T28.91)*
burn and corrosion of eye and adnexa (T26.-)
burn and corrosion of mouth and pharynx (T28.0)

The appropriate 7th character is to be added to each code from category T20.
A   initial encounter
D   subsequent encounter
S   sequela

☑5ᵗʰ **T20.0 Burn of** unspecified degree of head, face, and neck
Use additional external cause code to identify the source, place and intent of the burn (X00-X19, X75-X77, X96-X98, Y92)

☑7ᵗʰ **T20.00 Burn of unspecified degree of head, face, and neck, unspecified site**

☑6ᵗʰ **T20.01 Burn of unspecified degree of** ear [any part, except ear drum]
EXCLUDES 2 *burn of ear drum (T28.41-)*

☑7ᵗʰ **T20.011 Burn of unspecified degree of** right ear [any part, except ear drum]

☑7ᵗʰ **T20.012 Burn of unspecified degree of** left ear [any part, except ear drum]

☑7ᵗʰ **T20.019 Burn of unspecified degree of** unspecified ear [any part, except ear drum]

☑x7ᵗʰ **T20.02 Burn of unspecified degree of** lip(s)

☑x7ᵗʰ **T20.03 Burn of unspecified degree of** chin

☑x7ᵗʰ **T20.04 Burn of unspecified degree of** nose (septum)

☑x7ᵗʰ **T20.05 Burn of unspecified degree of** scalp [any part]

☑x7ᵗʰ **T20.06 Burn of unspecified degree of** forehead and cheek

☑x7ᵗʰ **T20.07 Burn of unspecified degree of** neck

☑x7ᵗʰ **T20.09 Burn of unspecified degree of** multiple sites of head, face, and neck

Injury, Poisoning and Certain Other Consequences of External Causes

T20.1–T20.619

√5th **T20.1 Burn of first degree of head, face, and neck**
Use additional external cause code to identify the source, place and intent of the burn (X00-X19, X75-X77, X96-X98, Y92)

√7th **T20.10 Burn of first degree of head, face, and neck, unspecified site**

√6th **T20.11 Burn of first degree of ear [any part, except ear drum]**
EXCLUDES 2 burn of ear drum (T28.41-)

√7th **T20.111 Burn of first degree of right ear [any part, except ear drum]**

√7th **T20.112 Burn of first degree of left ear [any part, except ear drum]**

√7th **T20.119 Burn of first degree of unspecified ear [any part, except ear drum]**

√x7th **T20.12 Burn of first degree of lip(s)**

√x7th **T20.13 Burn of first degree of chin**

√x7th **T20.14 Burn of first degree of nose (septum)**

√x7th **T20.15 Burn of first degree of scalp [any part]**

√x7th **T20.16 Burn of first degree of forehead and cheek**

√x7th **T20.17 Burn of first degree of neck**

√x7th **T20.19 Burn of first degree of multiple sites of head, face, and neck**

√5th **T20.2 Burn of second degree of head, face, and neck**
Use additional external cause code to identify the source, place and intent of the burn (X00-X19, X75-X77, X96-X98, Y92)

√x7th **T20.20 Burn of second degree of head, face, and neck, unspecified site**

√6th **T20.21 Burn of second degree of ear [any part, except ear drum]**
EXCLUDES 2 burn of ear drum (T28.41-)

√7th **T20.211 Burn of second degree of right ear [any part, except ear drum]**

√7th **T20.212 Burn of second degree of left ear [any part, except ear drum]**

√7th **T20.219 Burn of second degree of unspecified ear [any part, except ear drum]**

√x7th **T20.22 Burn of second degree of lip(s)**

√x7th **T20.23 Burn of second degree of chin**

√x7th **T20.24 Burn of second degree of nose (septum)**

√x7th **T20.25 Burn of second degree of scalp [any part]**

√x7th **T20.26 Burn of second degree of forehead and cheek**

√x7th **T20.27 Burn of second degree of neck**

√x7th **T20.29 Burn of second degree of multiple sites of head, face, and neck**

√5th **T20.3 Burn of third degree of head, face, and neck**
Use additional external cause code to identify the source, place and intent of the burn (X00-X19, X75-X77, X96-X98, Y92)

7 √x7th **T20.30 Burn of third degree of head, face, and neck, unspecified site** CC
CC Excl: CC with 7th character A: T20.30XA, T20.39XA, T20.70XA, T20.79XA

√6th **T20.31 Burn of third degree of ear [any part, except ear drum]**
EXCLUDES 2 burn of ear drum (T28.41-)

7 √7th **T20.311 Burn of third degree of right ear [any part, except ear drum]** CC
CC Excl: CC with 7th character A: T20.311-T20.319 with 7th A , T20.39XA, T20.711-T20.719 with 7th A, T20.79XA

7 √7th **T20.312 Burn of third degree of left ear [any part, except ear drum]** CC
CC Excl: See code: T20.311

7 √7th **T20.319 Burn of third degree of unspecified ear [any part, except ear drum]** CC
CC Excl: See code: T20.311

7 √x7th **T20.32 Burn of third degree of lip(s)** CC
CC Excl: CC with 7th character A: T20.32XA, T20.39XA, T20.72XA, T20.79XA

7 √x7th **T20.33 Burn of third degree of chin** CC
CC Excl: CC with 7th character A:T20.33XA, T20.39XA, T20.73XA, T20.79XA

7 √x7th **T20.34 Burn of third degree of nose (septum)** CC
CC Excl: CC with 7th character A: T20.34XA, T20.39XA, T20.74XA, T20.79XA

7 √x7th **T20.35 Burn of third degree of scalp [any part]** CC
CC Excl: CC with 7th character A: T20.35XA, T20.39XA, T20.75XA, T20.79XA

7 √x7th **T20.36 Burn of third degree of forehead and cheek** CC
CC Excl: CC with 7th character A: T20.36XA, T20.39XA, T20.76XA, T20.79XA

7 √x7th **T20.37 Burn of third degree of neck** CC
CC Excl: CC with 7th character A:T20.37XA, T20.39XA, T20.77XA, T20.79XA

7 √x7th **T20.39 Burn of third degree of multiple sites of head, face, and neck** CC
CC Excl: CC with 7th character A:T20.30X-T20.39X with 7th A, T20.70X-T20.79X with 7th A

√5th **T20.4 Corrosion of unspecified degree of head, face, and neck**
Code first (T51-T65) to identify chemical and intent
Use additional external cause code to identify place (Y92)

√x7th **T20.40 Corrosion of unspecified degree of head, face, and neck, unspecified site**

√6th **T20.41 Corrosion of unspecified degree of ear [any part, except ear drum]**
EXCLUDES 2 corrosion of ear drum (T28.91-)

√7th **T20.411 Corrosion of unspecified degree of right ear [any part, except ear drum]**

√7th **T20.412 Corrosion of unspecified degree of left ear [any part, except ear drum]**

√7th **T20.419 Corrosion of unspecified degree of unspecified ear [any part, except ear drum]**

√x7th **T20.42 Corrosion of unspecified degree of lip(s)**

√x7th **T20.43 Corrosion of unspecified degree of chin**

√x7th **T20.44 Corrosion of unspecified degree of nose (septum)**

√x7th **T20.45 Corrosion of unspecified degree of scalp [any part]**

√x7th **T20.46 Corrosion of unspecified degree of forehead and cheek**

√x7th **T20.47 Corrosion of unspecified degree of neck**

√x7th **T20.49 Corrosion of unspecified degree of multiple sites of head, face, and neck**

√5th **T20.5 Corrosion of first degree of head, face, and neck**
Code first (T51-T65) to identify chemical and intent
Use additional external cause code to identify place (Y92)

√x7th **T20.50 Corrosion of first degree of head, face, and neck, unspecified site**

√6th **T20.51 Corrosion of first degree of ear [any part, except ear drum]**
EXCLUDES 2 corrosion of ear drum (T28.91-)

√7th **T20.511 Corrosion of first degree of right ear [any part, except ear drum]**

√7th **T20.512 Corrosion of first degree of left ear [any part, except ear drum]**

√7th **T20.519 Corrosion of first degree of unspecified ear [any part, except ear drum]**

√x7th **T20.52 Corrosion of first degree of lip(s)**

√x7th **T20.53 Corrosion of first degree of chin**

√x7th **T20.54 Corrosion of first degree of nose (septum)**

√x7th **T20.55 Corrosion of first degree of scalp [any part]**

√x7th **T20.56 Corrosion of first degree of forehead and cheek**

√x7th **T20.57 Corrosion of first degree of neck**

√x7th **T20.59 Corrosion of first degree of multiple sites of head, face, and neck**

√5th **T20.6 Corrosion of second degree of head, face, and neck**
Code first (T51-T65) to identify chemical and intent
Use additional external cause code to identify place (Y92)

√x7th **T20.60 Corrosion of second degree of head, face, and neck, unspecified site**

√6th **T20.61 Corrosion of second degree of ear [any part, except ear drum]**
EXCLUDES 2 corrosion of ear drum (T28.91-)

√7th **T20.611 Corrosion of second degree of right ear [any part, except ear drum]**

√7th **T20.612 Corrosion of second degree of left ear [any part, except ear drum]**

√7th **T20.619 Corrosion of second degree of unspecified ear [any part, except ear drum]**

---

7 HAC = Initial encounter only (7th character A, B or C) and not POA.

N Newborn: 0   P Pediatric: 0-17   M Maternity: 12-55   A Adult: 15-124   MCC Major CC Condition   PDx MCC PDx acts as own MCC   CC CC Condition   PDx CC PDx acts as own CC

1034   ICD-10-CM Draft (2015)

√x7th **T20.62** **Corrosion of second degree of** lip(s)

√x7th **T20.63** **Corrosion of second degree of** chin

√x7th **T20.64** **Corrosion of second degree of** nose (septum)

√x7th **T20.65** **Corrosion of second degree of** scalp [any part]

√x7th **T20.66** **Corrosion of second degree of** forehead and cheek

√x7th **T20.67** **Corrosion of second degree of** neck

√x7th **T20.69** **Corrosion of second degree of** multiple sites of head, face, and neck

√5th **T20.7** **Corrosion of** third degree **of head, face, and neck**
Code first (T51-T65) to identify chemical and intent
Use additional external cause code to identify place (Y92)

7 √x7th **T20.70** **Corrosion of third degree of head, face, and neck, unspecified site**   CC
CC Excl: CC with 7th character A:T20.30XA, T20.39XA, T20.70XA, T20.79XA

√6th **T20.71** **Corrosion of third degree of** ear [any part, except ear drum]
EXCLUDES 2   corrosion of ear drum (T28.91-)

7 √7th **T20.711** **Corrosion of third degree of** right **ear [any part, except ear drum]**   CC
CC Excl: CC with 7th character A: T20.311-T20.319 with 7th A, T20.39XA, T20.711-T20.719 with 7th A, T20.79XA

7 √7th **T20.712** **Corrosion of third degree of** left **ear [any part, except ear drum]**   CC
CC Excl: See code: T20.711

7 √7th **T20.719** **Corrosion of third degree of** unspecified **ear [any part, except ear drum]**   CC
CC Excl: See code: T20.711

7 √x7th **T20.72** **Corrosion of third degree of** lip(s)   CC
CC Excl: CC with 7th character A: See code: T20.32

7 √x7th **T20.73** **Corrosion of third degree of** chin   CC
CC Excl: CC with 7th character A: See code: T20.33

7 √x7th **T20.74** **Corrosion of third degree of** nose (septum)   CC
CC Excl: CC with 7th character A: See code: T20.34

7 √x7th **T20.75** **Corrosion of third degree of** scalp [any part]   CC
CC Excl: CC with 7th character A: See code: T20.35

7 √x7th **T20.76** **Corrosion of third degree of** forehead and cheek   CC
CC Excl: CC with 7th character A: See code: T20.36

7 √x7th **T20.77** **Corrosion of third degree of** neck   CC
CC Excl: CC with 7th character A: See code: T20.37

7 √x7th **T20.79** **Corrosion of third degree of** multiple sites of head, face, and neck   CC
CC Excl: CC with 7th character A: See code: T20.39

√4th **T21** **Burn and corrosion of trunk**
Burns and corrosion of hip region
EXCLUDES 2   burns and corrosion of:
axilla (T22- with fifth character 4)
scapular region (T22- with fifth character 6)
shoulder (T22.- with fifth character 5)

The appropriate 7th character is to be added to each code from category T21.
A   initial encounter
D   subsequent encounter
S   sequela

√5th **T21.0** **Burn of** unspecified degree **of trunk**
Use additional external cause code to identify the source, place and intent of the burn (X00-X19, X75-X77, X96-X98, Y92)

√x7th **T21.00** **Burn of unspecified degree of trunk,** unspecified site

√x7th **T21.01** **Burn of unspecified degree of** chest wall
Burn of of unspecified degree of breast

√x7th **T21.02** **Burn of unspecified degree of** abdominal wall
Burn of unspecified degree of flank
Burn of unspecified degree of groin

√x7th **T21.03** **Burn of unspecified degree of** upper back
Burn of unspecified degree of interscapular region

√x7th **T21.04** **Burn of unspecified degree of** lower back

√x7th **T21.05** **Burn of unspecified degree of** buttock
Burn of unspecified degree of anus

√x7th **T21.06** **Burn of unspecified degree of** male genital region ♂
Burn of unspecified degree of penis
Burn of unspecified degree of scrotum
Burn of unspecified degree of testis

√x7th **T21.07** **Burn of unspecified degree of** female genital region ♀
Burn of unspecified degree of labium (majus) (minus)
Burn of unspecified degree of perineum
Burn of unspecified degree of vulva
EXCLUDES 2   burn of vagina (T28.3)

√x7th **T21.09** **Burn of unspecified degree of** other site **of trunk**

√5th **T21.1** **Burn of** first degree **of trunk**
Use additional external cause code to identify the source, place and intent of the burn (X00-X19, X75-X77, X96-X98, Y92)

√x7th **T21.10** **Burn of first degree of trunk,** unspecified site

√x7th **T21.11** **Burn of first degree of** chest wall
Burn of first degree of breast

√x7th **T21.12** **Burn of first degree of** abdominal wall
Burn of first degree of flank
Burn of first degree of groin

√x7th **T21.13** **Burn of first degree of** upper back
Burn of first degree of interscapular region

√x7th **T21.14** **Burn of first degree of** lower back

√x7th **T21.15** **Burn of first degree of** buttock
Burn of first degree of anus

√x7th **T21.16** **Burn of first degree of** male genital region ♂
Burn of first degree of penis
Burn of first degree of scrotum
Burn of first degree of testis

√x7th **T21.17** **Burn of first degree of** female genital region ♀
Burn of first degree of labium (majus) (minus)
Burn of first degree of perineum
Burn of first degree of vulva
EXCLUDES 2   burn of vagina (T28.3)

√x7th **T21.19** **Burn of first degree of** other site **of trunk**

√5th **T21.2** **Burn of** second degree **of trunk**
Use additional external cause code to identify the source, place and intent of the burn (X00-X19, X75-X77, X96-X98, Y92)

√x7th **T21.20** **Burn of second degree of trunk,** unspecified site

√x7th **T21.21** **Burn of second degree of** chest wall
Burn of second degree of breast

√x7th **T21.22** **Burn of second degree of** abdominal wall
Burn of second degree of flank
Burn of second degree of groin

√x7th **T21.23** **Burn of second degree of** upper back
Burn of second degree of interscapular region

√x7th **T21.24** **Burn of second degree of** lower back

√x7th **T21.25** **Burn of second degree of** buttock
Burn of second degree of anus

√x7th **T21.26** **Burn of second degree of** male genital region ♂
Burn of second degree of penis
Burn of second degree of scrotum
Burn of second degree of testis

√x7th **T21.27** **Burn of second degree of** female genital region ♀
Burn of second degree of labium (majus) (minus)
Burn of second degree of perineum
Burn of second degree of vulva
EXCLUDES 2   burn of vagina (T28.3)

√x7th **T21.29** **Burn of second degree of** other site **of trunk**

√5th **T21.3** **Burn of** third degree **of trunk**
Use additional external cause code to identify the source, place and intent of the burn (X00-X19, X75-X77, X96-X98, Y92)

7 √x7th **T21.30** **Burn of third degree of trunk,** unspecified site   CC
CC Excl: CC with 7th character A:
T21.30XA,T21.39XA,T21.70XA,T21.79XA

7 √x7th **T21.31** **Burn of third degree of** chest wall   CC
Burn of third degree of breast
CC Excl: CC with 7th character A:
T21.30XA,T21.31XA,T21.39XA,T21.71XA,T21.79XA

7 √x7th **T21.32** **Burn of third degree of** abdominal wall   CC
Burn of third degree of flank
Burn of third degree of groin
CC Excl: CC with 7th character A:
T21.30XA,T21.32XA,T21.39XA,T21.72XA,T21.79XA

7 √x7th **T21.33** **Burn of third degree of** upper back   CC
Burn of third degree of interscapular region
CC Excl: CC with 7th character A: T2130XA,T2133-T2135 with 7th A, T2139XA,T2170XA,T2173-T2175 with 7th A,T2179XA

7 HAC = Initial encounter only (7th character A, B or C) and not POA.

7 √x7ᵗʰ **T21.34 Burn of third degree of lower back**   CC
CC Excl: See code: T21.133

7 √x7ᵗʰ **T21.35 Burn of third degree of buttock**   CC
Burn of third degree of anus
CC Excl: See code: T21.133

7 √x7ᵗʰ **T21.36 Burn of third degree of male genital region**   CC♂
Burn of third degree of penis
Burn of third degree of scrotum
Burn of third degree of testis
CC Excl: CC with 7th character A:
T21.30XA,T21.36XA,T21.37XA,T21.39XA,T21.70XA,T21.76XA,T21.77XA,T21.79XA

7 √x7ᵗʰ **T21.37 Burn of third degree of female genital region**   CC♀
Burn of third degree of labium (majus) (minus)
Burn of third degree of perineum
Burn of third degree of vulva
EXCLUDES 2   burn of vagina (T28.3)
CC Excl: See code: T21.136

7 √x7ᵗʰ **T21.39 Burn of third degree of other site of trunk**   CC
CC Excl: CC with 7th character A: T22.30X-T22.312
with 7th A, T22.319A, T22.391-T22.399 with 7th A,
T22.70X-T22.719 with 7th A, T22.791-T22.799 with 7th A

√5ᵗʰ **T21.4 Corrosion of unspecified degree of trunk**
Code first (T51-T65) to identify chemical and intent
Use additional external cause code to identify place (Y92)

√x7ᵗʰ **T21.40 Corrosion of unspecified degree of trunk, unspecified site**

√x7ᵗʰ **T21.41 Corrosion of unspecified degree of chest wall**
Corrosion of unspecified degree of breast

√x7ᵗʰ **T21.42 Corrosion of unspecified degree of abdominal wall**
Corrosion of unspecified degree of flank
Corrosion of unspecified degree of groin

√x7ᵗʰ **T21.43 Corrosion of unspecified degree of upper back**
Corrosion of unspecified degree of interscapular region

√x7ᵗʰ **T21.44 Corrosion of unspecified degree of lower back**

√x7ᵗʰ **T21.45 Corrosion of unspecified degree of buttock**
Corrosion of unspecified degree of anus

√x7ᵗʰ **T21.46 Corrosion of unspecified degree of male genital region**   ♂
Corrosion of unspecified degree of penis
Corrosion of unspecified degree of scrotum
Corrosion of unspecified degree of testis

√x7ᵗʰ **T21.47 Corrosion of unspecified degree of female genital region**   ♀
Corrosion of unspecified degree of labium (majus) (minus)
Corrosion of unspecified degree of perineum
Corrosion of unspecified degree of vulva
EXCLUDES 2   corrosion of vagina (T28.8)

√x7ᵗʰ **T21.49 Corrosion of unspecified degree of other site of trunk**

√5ᵗʰ **T21.5 Corrosion of first degree of trunk**
Code first (T51-T65) to identify chemical and intent
Use additional external cause code to identify place (Y92)

√x7ᵗʰ **T21.50 Corrosion of first degree of trunk, unspecified site**

√x7ᵗʰ **T21.51 Corrosion of first degree of chest wall**
Corrosion of first degree of breast

√x7ᵗʰ **T21.52 Corrosion of first degree of abdominal wall**
Corrosion of first degree of flank
Corrosion of first degree of groin

√x7ᵗʰ **T21.53 Corrosion of first degree of upper back**
Corrosion of first degree of interscapular region

√x7ᵗʰ **T21.54 Corrosion of first degree of lower back**

√x7ᵗʰ **T21.55 Corrosion of first degree of buttock**
Corrosion of first degree of anus

√x7ᵗʰ **T21.56 Corrosion of first degree of male genital region**   ♂
Corrosion of first degree of penis
Corrosion of first degree of scrotum
Corrosion of first degree of testis

√x7ᵗʰ **T21.57 Corrosion of first degree of female genital region**   ♀
Corrosion of first degree of labium (majus) (minus)
Corrosion of first degree of perineum
Corrosion of first degree of vulva
EXCLUDES 2   corrosion of vagina (T28.8)

√x7ᵗʰ **T21.59 Corrosion of first degree of other site of trunk**

√5ᵗʰ **T21.6 Corrosion of second degree of trunk**
Code first (T51-T65) to identify chemical and intent
Use additional external cause code to identify place (Y92)

√x7ᵗʰ **T21.60 Corrosion of second degree of trunk, unspecified site**

√x7ᵗʰ **T21.61 Corrosion of second degree of chest wall**
Corrosion of second degree of breast

√x7ᵗʰ **T21.62 Corrosion of second degree of abdominal wall**
Corrosion of second degree of flank
Corrosion of second degree of groin

√x7ᵗʰ **T21.63 Corrosion of second degree of upper back**
Corrosion of second degree of interscapular region

√x7ᵗʰ **T21.64 Corrosion of second degree of lower back**

√x7ᵗʰ **T21.65 Corrosion of second degree of buttock**
Corrosion of second degree of anus

√x7ᵗʰ **T21.66 Corrosion of second degree of male genital region**   ♂
Corrosion of second degree of penis
Corrosion of second degree of scrotum
Corrosion of second degree of testis

√x7ᵗʰ **T21.67 Corrosion of second degree of female genital region**   ♀
Corrosion of second degree of labium (majus) (minus)
Corrosion of second degree of perineum
Corrosion of second degree of vulva
EXCLUDES 2   corrosion of vagina (T28.8)

√x7ᵗʰ **T21.69 Corrosion of second degree of other site of trunk**

√5ᵗʰ **T21.7 Corrosion of third degree of trunk**
Code first (T51-T65) to identify chemical and intent
Use additional external cause code to identify place (Y92)

7 √x7ᵗʰ **T21.70 Corrosion of third degree of trunk, unspecified site**   CC
CC Excl: CC with 7th character A: See code: T21.30

7 √x7ᵗʰ **T21.71 Corrosion of third degree of chest wall**   CC
Corrosion of third degree of breast
CC Excl: CC with 7th character A: See code: T21.31

7 √x7ᵗʰ **T21.72 Corrosion of third degree of abdominal wall**   CC
Corrosion of third degree of flank
Corrosion of third degree of groin
CC Excl: CC with 7th character A: See code: T21.32

7 √x7ᵗʰ **T21.73 Corrosion of third degree of upper back**   CC
Corrosion of third degree of interscapular region
CC Excl: CC with 7th character A: See code: T21.33

7 √x7ᵗʰ **T21.74 Corrosion of third degree of lower back**   CC
CC Excl: See code: T21.33

7 √x7ᵗʰ **T21.75 Corrosion of third degree of buttock**   CC
Corrosion of third degree of anus
CC Excl: See code: T21.33

7 √x7ᵗʰ **T21.76 Corrosion of third degree of male genital region**   CC♂
Corrosion of third degree of penis
Corrosion of third degree of scrotum
Corrosion of third degree of testis
CC Excl: CC with 7th character A: See code: T21.36

7 √x7ᵗʰ **T21.77 Corrosion of third degree of female genital region**   CC♀
Corrosion of third degree of labium (majus) (minus)
Corrosion of third degree of perineum
Corrosion of third degree of vulva
EXCLUDES 2   corrosion of vagina (T28.8)
CC Excl: See code: T21.36

7 √x7ᵗʰ **T21.79 Corrosion of third degree of other site of trunk**   CC
CC Excl: CC with 7th character A: See code: T21.30

√4ᵗʰ **T22 Burn and corrosion of shoulder and upper limb, except wrist and hand**
EXCLUDES 2   burn and corrosion of interscapular region (T21.-)
burn and corrosion of wrist and hand (T23.-)

The appropriate 7th character is to be added to each code from category T22.
A   initial encounter
D   subsequent encounter
S   sequela

√5ᵗʰ **T22.0 Burn of unspecified degree of shoulder and upper limb, except wrist and hand**
Use additional external cause code to identify the source, place and intent of the burn (X00-X19, X75-X77, X96-X98, Y92)

√x7ᵗʰ **T22.00 Burn of unspecified degree of shoulder and upper limb, except wrist and hand, unspecified site**

---

7 HAC = Initial encounter only (7th character A, B or C) and not POA.

N Newborn: 0   P Pediatric: 0-17   M Maternity: 12-55   A Adult: 15-124   MCC Major CC Condition   PDx MCC PDx acts as own MCC   CC CC Condition   PDx CC PDx acts as own CC

1036   ICD-10-CM Draft (2015)

☑6ᵗʰ **T22.01** **Burn of unspecified degree of** forearm
    ☑7ᵗʰ **T22.011** Burn of unspecified degree of right forearm
    ☑7ᵗʰ **T22.012** Burn of unspecified degree of left forearm
    ☑7ᵗʰ **T22.019** Burn of unspecified degree of unspecified forearm

☑6ᵗʰ **T22.02** **Burn of unspecified degree of** elbow
    ☑7ᵗʰ **T22.021** Burn of unspecified degree of right elbow
    ☑7ᵗʰ **T22.022** Burn of unspecified degree of left elbow
    ☑7ᵗʰ **T22.029** Burn of unspecified degree of unspecified elbow

☑6ᵗʰ **T22.03** **Burn of unspecified degree of** upper arm
    ☑7ᵗʰ **T22.031** Burn of unspecified degree of right upper arm
    ☑7ᵗʰ **T22.032** Burn of unspecified degree of left upper arm
    ☑7ᵗʰ **T22.039** Burn of unspecified degree of unspecified upper arm

☑6ᵗʰ **T22.04** **Burn of unspecified degree of** axilla
    ☑7ᵗʰ **T22.041** Burn of unspecified degree of right axilla
    ☑7ᵗʰ **T22.042** Burn of unspecified degree of left axilla
    ☑7ᵗʰ **T22.049** Burn of unspecified degree of unspecified axilla

☑6ᵗʰ **T22.05** **Burn of unspecified degree of** shoulder
    ☑7ᵗʰ **T22.051** Burn of unspecified degree of right shoulder
    ☑7ᵗʰ **T22.052** Burn of unspecified degree of left shoulder
    ☑7ᵗʰ **T22.059** Burn of unspecified degree of unspecified shoulder

☑6ᵗʰ **T22.06** **Burn of unspecified degree of** scapular region
    ☑7ᵗʰ **T22.061** Burn of unspecified degree of right scapular region
    ☑7ᵗʰ **T22.062** Burn of unspecified degree of left scapular region
    ☑7ᵗʰ **T22.069** Burn of unspecified degree of unspecified scapular region

☑6ᵗʰ **T22.09** **Burn of unspecified degree of** multiple sites of shoulder and upper limb, except wrist and hand
    ☑7ᵗʰ **T22.091** Burn of unspecified degree of multiple sites of right shoulder and upper limb, except wrist and hand
    ☑7ᵗʰ **T22.092** Burn of unspecified degree of multiple sites of left shoulder and upper limb, except wrist and hand
    ☑7ᵗʰ **T22.099** Burn of unspecified degree of multiple sites of unspecified shoulder and upper limb, except wrist and hand

☑5ᵗʰ **T22.1** **Burn of** first degree of shoulder and upper limb, except wrist and hand
    Use additional external cause code to identify the source, place and intent of the burn (X00-X19, X75-X77, X96-X98, Y92)

☑x7ᵗʰ **T22.10** **Burn of first degree of shoulder and upper limb, except wrist and hand,** unspecified site

☑6ᵗʰ **T22.11** **Burn of first degree of** forearm
    ☑7ᵗʰ **T22.111** Burn of first degree of right forearm
    ☑7ᵗʰ **T22.112** Burn of first degree of left forearm
    ☑7ᵗʰ **T22.119** Burn of first degree of unspecified forearm

☑6ᵗʰ **T22.12** **Burn of first degree of** elbow
    ☑7ᵗʰ **T22.121** Burn of first degree of right elbow
    ☑7ᵗʰ **T22.122** Burn of first degree of left elbow
    ☑7ᵗʰ **T22.129** Burn of first degree of unspecified elbow

☑6ᵗʰ **T22.13** **Burn of first degree of** upper arm
    ☑7ᵗʰ **T22.131** Burn of first degree of right upper arm
    ☑7ᵗʰ **T22.132** Burn of first degree of left upper arm
    ☑7ᵗʰ **T22.139** Burn of first degree of unspecified upper arm

☑6ᵗʰ **T22.14** **Burn of first degree of** axilla
    ☑7ᵗʰ **T22.141** Burn of first degree of right axilla
    ☑7ᵗʰ **T22.142** Burn of first degree of left axilla
    ☑7ᵗʰ **T22.149** Burn of first degree of unspecified axilla

☑6ᵗʰ **T22.15** **Burn of first degree of** shoulder
    ☑7ᵗʰ **T22.151** Burn of first degree of right shoulder
    ☑7ᵗʰ **T22.152** Burn of first degree of left shoulder
    ☑7ᵗʰ **T22.159** Burn of first degree of unspecified shoulder

☑6ᵗʰ **T22.16** **Burn of first degree of** scapular region
    ☑7ᵗʰ **T22.161** Burn of first degree of right scapular region
    ☑7ᵗʰ **T22.162** Burn of first degree of left scapular region
    ☑7ᵗʰ **T22.169** Burn of first degree of unspecified scapular region

☑6ᵗʰ **T22.19** **Burn of first degree of** multiple sites of shoulder and upper limb, except wrist and hand
    ☑7ᵗʰ **T22.191** Burn of first degree of multiple sites of right shoulder and upper limb, except wrist and hand
    ☑7ᵗʰ **T22.192** Burn of first degree of multiple sites of left shoulder and upper limb, except wrist and hand
    ☑7ᵗʰ **T22.199** Burn of first degree of multiple sites of unspecified shoulder and upper limb, except wrist and hand

☑5ᵗʰ **T22.2** **Burn of** second degree of shoulder and upper limb, except wrist and hand
    Use additional external cause code to identify the source, place and intent of the burn (X00-X19, X75-X77, X96-X98, Y92)

☑x7ᵗʰ **T22.20** **Burn of second degree of shoulder and upper limb, except wrist and hand,** unspecified site

☑6ᵗʰ **T22.21** **Burn of second degree of** forearm
    ☑7ᵗʰ **T22.211** Burn of second degree of right forearm
    ☑7ᵗʰ **T22.212** Burn of second degree of left forearm
    ☑7ᵗʰ **T22.219** Burn of second degree of unspecified forearm

☑6ᵗʰ **T22.22** **Burn of second degree of** elbow
    ☑7ᵗʰ **T22.221** Burn of second degree of right elbow
    ☑7ᵗʰ **T22.222** Burn of second degree of left elbow
    ☑7ᵗʰ **T22.229** Burn of second degree of unspecified elbow

☑6ᵗʰ **T22.23** **Burn of second degree of** upper arm
    ☑7ᵗʰ **T22.231** Burn of second degree of right upper arm
    ☑7ᵗʰ **T22.232** Burn of second degree of left upper arm
    ☑7ᵗʰ **T22.239** Burn of second degree of unspecified upper arm

☑6ᵗʰ **T22.24** **Burn of second degree of** axilla
    ☑7ᵗʰ **T22.241** Burn of second degree of right axilla
    ☑7ᵗʰ **T22.242** Burn of second degree of left axilla
    ☑7ᵗʰ **T22.249** Burn of second degree of unspecified axilla

☑6ᵗʰ **T22.25** **Burn of second degree of** shoulder
    ☑7ᵗʰ **T22.251** Burn of second degree of right shoulder
    ☑7ᵗʰ **T22.252** Burn of second degree of left shoulder
    ☑7ᵗʰ **T22.259** Burn of second degree of unspecified shoulder

☑6ᵗʰ **T22.26** **Burn of second degree of** scapular region
    ☑7ᵗʰ **T22.261** Burn of second degree of right scapular region
    ☑7ᵗʰ **T22.262** Burn of second degree of left scapular region
    ☑7ᵗʰ **T22.269** Burn of second degree of unspecified scapular region

☑6ᵗʰ **T22.29** **Burn of second degree of** multiple sites of shoulder and upper limb, except wrist and hand
    ☑7ᵗʰ **T22.291** Burn of second degree of multiple sites of right shoulder and upper limb, except wrist and hand
    ☑7ᵗʰ **T22.292** Burn of second degree of multiple sites of left shoulder and upper limb, except wrist and hand
    ☑7ᵗʰ **T22.299** Burn of second degree of multiple sites of unspecified shoulder and upper limb, except wrist and hand

☑ Additional Character Required   ✓x7ᵗʰ Xtension Alert   Unacceptable PDx   Manifestation   Hospital Acquired Condition   *EXCLUDES 1* Not Coded Here   *EXCLUDES 2* Not Included Here

ICD-10-CM Draft (2015)   1037

Injury, Poisoning and Certain Other Consequences of External Causes

T22.3–T22.491

√5ᵗʰ **T22.3** Burn of third degree of shoulder and upper limb, except wrist and hand

       Use additional external cause code to identify the source, place and intent of the burn (X00-X19, X75-X77, X96-X98, Y92)

   7 √x7ᵗʰ **T22.30** Burn of third degree of shoulder and upper limb, except wrist and hand, **unspecified site**   CC
       CC Excl: CC with 7th character A: T22.30XA,T22.391-T22.399 with 7th A,T22.70XA,T22.791-T22.799 with 7th A

   √6ᵗʰ **T22.31** Burn of third degree of **forearm**

     7 √7ᵗʰ **T22.311** **Burn of third degree of right forearm**   CC
       CC Excl: CC with 7th character A: T22.30XA,T22.311-T22.319 with 7th A,T22.391-T22.399 with 7th A,T22.70XA,T22.711-T22.719 with 7th A,T22.791-T22.799 with 7th A

     7 √7ᵗʰ **T22.312** **Burn of third degree of left forearm**   CC
       CC Excl: See code: T22.311

     7 √7ᵗʰ **T22.319** **Burn of third degree of unspecified forearm**   CC
       CC Excl: See code: T22.311

   √6ᵗʰ **T22.32** Burn of third degree of **elbow**

     7 √7ᵗʰ **T22.321** **Burn of third degree of right elbow**   CC
       CC Excl: CC with 7th character A: T22.30XA,T22.321-T22.329 with 7th A, T22.391-T22.399 with 7th A,T22.70XA,T22.721-T22.729 with 7th A, T22.791-T22.799 with 7th A

     7 √7ᵗʰ **T22.322** **Burn of third degree of left elbow**   CC
       CC Excl: See code: T22.321

     7 √7ᵗʰ **T22.329** **Burn of third degree of unspecified elbow**   CC
       CC Excl: See code: T22.321

   √6ᵗʰ **T22.33** Burn of third degree of **upper arm**

     7 √7ᵗʰ **T22.331** **Burn of third degree of right upper arm**   CC
       CC Excl: CC with 7th character A: T22.30XA,T22.331-T22.339 with 7th A,T22.391-T22.399 with 7th A,T22.70XA,T22.731-T22.739 with 7th A,T22.791-T22.799 with 7th A

     7 √7ᵗʰ **T22.332** **Burn of third degree of left upper arm**   CC
       CC Excl: See code: T22.331

     7 √7ᵗʰ **T22.339** **Burn of third degree of unspecified upper arm**   CC
       CC Excl: See code: T22.331

   √6ᵗʰ **T22.34** Burn of third degree of **axilla**

     7 √7ᵗʰ **T22.341** **Burn of third degree of right axilla**   CC
       CC Excl: CC with 7th character A: T22.30XA,T22.341-T22.349 with 7th A,T22.391-T22.399 with 7th A,T22.70XA,T22.741-T22.749 with 7th A,T22.791-T22.799 with 7th A

     7 √7ᵗʰ **T22.342** **Burn of third degree of left axilla**   CC
       CC Excl: See code: T22.341

     7 √7ᵗʰ **T22.349** **Burn of third degree of unspecified axilla**   CC
       CC Excl: See code: T22.341

   √6ᵗʰ **T22.35** Burn of third degree of **shoulder**

     7 √7ᵗʰ **T22.351** **Burn of third degree of right shoulder**   CC
       CC Excl: CC with 7th character A: T22.30XA,T22.351-T22.359 with 7th A, T22.391-T22.399 with 7th A,T22.70XA,T22.751-T22.759 with 7th A, T22.791-T22.799 with 7th A

     7 √7ᵗʰ **T22.352** **Burn of third degree of left shoulder**   CC
       CC Excl: See code: T22.351

     7 √7ᵗʰ **T22.359** **Burn of third degree of unspecified shoulder**   CC
       CC Excl: See code: T22.351

   √6ᵗʰ **T22.36** Burn of third degree of **scapular region**

     7 √7ᵗʰ **T22.361** **Burn of third degree of right scapular region**   CC
       CC Excl: CC with 7th character A: T22.30XA,T22.361-T22.369 with 7th A, T22.391-T22.399 with 7th A,T22.70XA,T22.761-T22.769 with 7th A, T22.791-T22.799 with 7th A

     7 √7ᵗʰ **T22.362** **Burn of third degree of left scapular region**   CC
       CC Excl: See code: T22.361

     7 √7ᵗʰ **T22.369** **Burn of third degree of unspecified scapular region**   CC
       CC Excl: See code: T22.361

   √6ᵗʰ **T22.39** Burn of third degree of **multiple sites** of shoulder and upper limb, except wrist and hand

     7 √7ᵗʰ **T22.391** **Burn of third degree of multiple sites of right shoulder and upper limb, except wrist and hand**   CC
       CC Excl: CC with 7th character A: T22.30XA,T22.391-T22.399 with 7th A,T22.70XA,T22.791-T22.799 with 7th A

     7 √7ᵗʰ **T22.392** **Burn of third degree of multiple sites of left shoulder and upper limb, except wrist and hand**   CC
       CC Excl: See code: T22.391

     7 √7ᵗʰ **T22.399** **Burn of third degree of multiple sites of unspecified shoulder and upper limb, except wrist and hand**   CC
       CC Excl: See code: T22.391

√5ᵗʰ **T22.4** Corrosion of **unspecified degree** of shoulder and upper limb, except wrist and hand

       Code first (T51-T65) to identify chemical and intent
       Use additional external cause code to identify place (Y92)

   √x7ᵗʰ **T22.40** Corrosion of unspecified degree of shoulder and upper limb, except wrist and hand, **unspecified site**

   √6ᵗʰ **T22.41** Corrosion of unspecified degree of **forearm**

     √7ᵗʰ **T22.411** **Corrosion of unspecified degree of right forearm**

     √7ᵗʰ **T22.412** **Corrosion of unspecified degree of left forearm**

     √7ᵗʰ **T22.419** **Corrosion of unspecified degree of unspecified forearm**

   √6ᵗʰ **T22.42** Corrosion of unspecified degree of **elbow**

     √7ᵗʰ **T22.421** **Corrosion of unspecified degree of right elbow**

     √7ᵗʰ **T22.422** **Corrosion of unspecified degree of left elbow**

     √7ᵗʰ **T22.429** **Corrosion of unspecified degree of unspecified elbow**

   √6ᵗʰ **T22.43** Corrosion of unspecified degree of **upper arm**

     √7ᵗʰ **T22.431** **Corrosion of unspecified degree of right upper arm**

     √7ᵗʰ **T22.432** **Corrosion of unspecified degree of left upper arm**

     √7ᵗʰ **T22.439** **Corrosion of unspecified degree of unspecified upper arm**

   √6ᵗʰ **T22.44** Corrosion of unspecified degree of **axilla**

     √7ᵗʰ **T22.441** **Corrosion of unspecified degree of right axilla**

     √7ᵗʰ **T22.442** **Corrosion of unspecified degree of left axilla**

     √7ᵗʰ **T22.449** **Corrosion of unspecified degree of unspecified axilla**

   √6ᵗʰ **T22.45** Corrosion of unspecified degree of **shoulder**

     √7ᵗʰ **T22.451** **Corrosion of unspecified degree of right shoulder**

     √7ᵗʰ **T22.452** **Corrosion of unspecified degree of left shoulder**

     √7ᵗʰ **T22.459** **Corrosion of unspecified degree of unspecified shoulder**

   √6ᵗʰ **T22.46** Corrosion of unspecified degree of **scapular region**

     √7ᵗʰ **T22.461** **Corrosion of unspecified degree of right scapular region**

     √7ᵗʰ **T22.462** **Corrosion of unspecified degree of left scapular region**

     √7ᵗʰ **T22.469** **Corrosion of unspecified degree of unspecified scapular region**

   √6ᵗʰ **T22.49** Corrosion of unspecified degree of **multiple sites** of shoulder and upper limb, except wrist and hand

     √7ᵗʰ **T22.491** **Corrosion of unspecified degree of multiple sites of right shoulder and upper limb, except wrist and hand**

---

7 HAC = Initial encounter only (7th character A, B or C) and not POA.

Ⓝ Newborn: 0   Ⓟ Pediatric: 0-17   Ⓜ Maternity: 12-55   Ⓐ Adult: 15-124   **MCC** Major CC Condition   **PDx MCC** PDx acts as own MCC   **CC** CC Condition   **PDx CC** PDx acts as own CC

1038   ICD-10-CM Draft (2015)

✓7th **T22.492** Corrosion of unspecified degree of multiple sites of left shoulder and upper limb, except wrist and hand

✓7th **T22.499** Corrosion of unspecified degree of multiple sites of unspecified shoulder and upper limb, except wrist and hand

✓5th **T22.5** Corrosion of first degree of shoulder and upper limb, except wrist and hand
　　Code first (T51-T65) to identify chemical and intent
　　Use additional external cause code to identify place (Y92)

✓x7th **T22.50** Corrosion of first degree of shoulder and upper limb, except wrist and hand unspecified site

✓6th **T22.51** Corrosion of first degree of forearm
　　✓7th **T22.511** Corrosion of first degree of right forearm
　　✓7th **T22.512** Corrosion of first degree of left forearm
　　✓7th **T22.519** Corrosion of first degree of unspecified forearm

✓6th **T22.52** Corrosion of first degree of elbow
　　✓7th **T22.521** Corrosion of first degree of right elbow
　　✓7th **T22.522** Corrosion of first degree of left elbow
　　✓7th **T22.529** Corrosion of first degree of unspecified elbow

✓6th **T22.53** Corrosion of first degree of upper arm
　　✓7th **T22.531** Corrosion of first degree of right upper arm
　　✓7th **T22.532** Corrosion of first degree of left upper arm
　　✓7th **T22.539** Corrosion of first degree of unspecified upper arm

✓6th **T22.54** Corrosion of first degree of axilla
　　✓7th **T22.541** Corrosion of first degree of right axilla
　　✓7th **T22.542** Corrosion of first degree of left axilla
　　✓7th **T22.549** Corrosion of first degree of unspecified axilla

✓6th **T22.55** Corrosion of first degree of shoulder
　　✓7th **T22.551** Corrosion of first degree of right shoulder
　　✓7th **T22.552** Corrosion of first degree of left shoulder
　　✓7th **T22.559** Corrosion of first degree of unspecified shoulder

✓6th **T22.56** Corrosion of first degree of scapular region
　　✓7th **T22.561** Corrosion of first degree of right scapular region
　　✓7th **T22.562** Corrosion of first degree of left scapular region
　　✓7th **T22.569** Corrosion of first degree of unspecified scapular region

✓6th **T22.59** Corrosion of first degree of multiple sites of shoulder and upper limb, except wrist and hand
　　✓7th **T22.591** Corrosion of first degree of multiple sites of right shoulder and upper limb, except wrist and hand
　　✓7th **T22.592** Corrosion of first degree of multiple sites of left shoulder and upper limb, except wrist and hand
　　✓7th **T22.599** Corrosion of first degree of multiple sites of unspecified shoulder and upper limb, except wrist and hand

✓5th **T22.6** Corrosion of second degree of shoulder and upper limb, except wrist and hand
　　Code first (T51-T65) to identify chemical and intent
　　Use additional external cause code to identify place (Y92)

✓x7th **T22.60** Corrosion of second degree of shoulder and upper limb, except wrist and hand, unspecified site

✓6th **T22.61** Corrosion of second degree of forearm
　　✓7th **T22.611** Corrosion of second degree of right forearm
　　✓7th **T22.612** Corrosion of second degree of left forearm
　　✓7th **T22.619** Corrosion of second degree of unspecified forearm

✓6th **T22.62** Corrosion of second degree of elbow
　　✓7th **T22.621** Corrosion of second degree of right elbow
　　✓7th **T22.622** Corrosion of second degree of left elbow

✓7th **T22.629** Corrosion of second degree of unspecified elbow

✓6th **T22.63** Corrosion of second degree of upper arm
　　✓7th **T22.631** Corrosion of second degree of right upper arm
　　✓7th **T22.632** Corrosion of second degree of left upper arm
　　✓7th **T22.639** Corrosion of second degree of unspecified upper arm

✓6th **T22.64** Corrosion of second degree of axilla
　　✓7th **T22.641** Corrosion of second degree of right axilla
　　✓7th **T22.642** Corrosion of second degree of left axilla
　　✓7th **T22.649** Corrosion of second degree of unspecified axilla

✓6th **T22.65** Corrosion of second degree of shoulder
　　✓7th **T22.651** Corrosion of second degree of right shoulder
　　✓7th **T22.652** Corrosion of second degree of left shoulder
　　✓7th **T22.659** Corrosion of second degree of unspecified shoulder

✓6th **T22.66** Corrosion of second degree of scapular region
　　✓7th **T22.661** Corrosion of second degree of right scapular region
　　✓7th **T22.662** Corrosion of second degree of left scapular region
　　✓7th **T22.669** Corrosion of second degree of unspecified scapular region

✓6th **T22.69** Corrosion of second degree of multiple sites of shoulder and upper limb, except wrist and hand
　　✓7th **T22.691** Corrosion of second degree of multiple sites of right shoulder and upper limb, except wrist and hand
　　✓7th **T22.692** Corrosion of second degree of multiple sites of left shoulder and upper limb, except wrist and hand
　　✓7th **T22.699** Corrosion of second degree of multiple sites of unspecified shoulder and upper limb, except wrist and hand

✓5th **T22.7** Corrosion of third degree of shoulder and upper limb, except wrist and hand
　　Code first (T51-T65) to identify chemical and intent
　　Use additional external cause code to identify place (Y92)

7 ✓x7th **T22.70** Corrosion of third degree of shoulder and upper limb, except wrist and hand, unspecified site **CC**
　　CC Excl: CC with 7th character A: See code: T22.30

✓6th **T22.71** Corrosion of third degree of forearm
　7 ✓7th **T22.711** Corrosion of third degree of right forearm **CC**
　　　CC Excl: CC with 7th character A: See code: T22.311
　7 ✓7th **T22.712** Corrosion of third degree of left forearm **CC**
　　　CC Excl: See code: T22.311
　7 ✓7th **T22.719** Corrosion of third degree of unspecified forearm **CC**
　　　CC Excl: See code: T22.311

✓6th **T22.72** Corrosion of third degree of elbow
　7 ✓7th **T22.721** Corrosion of third degree of right elbow **CC**
　　　CC Excl: CC with 7th character A: See code: T22.321
　7 ✓7th **T22.722** Corrosion of third degree of left elbow **CC**
　　　CC Excl: See code: T22.321
　7 ✓7th **T22.729** Corrosion of third degree of unspecified elbow **CC**
　　　CC Excl: See code: T22.321

✓6th **T22.73** Corrosion of third degree of upper arm
　7 ✓7th **T22.731** Corrosion of third degree of right upper arm **CC**
　　　CC Excl: CC with 7th character A: See code: T22.331

---

7 HAC = Initial encounter only (7th character A, B or C) and not POA.

✓ Additional Character Required　✓x7th Xtension Alert　Unacceptable PDx　Manifestation　Hospital Acquired Condition　**EXCLUDES 1** Not Coded Here　**EXCLUDES 2** Not Included Here

7 ✓7th **T22.732** **Corrosion of third degree of left upper arm** CC
    CC Excl: See code: T22.331

7 ✓7th **T22.739** **Corrosion of third degree of unspecified upper arm** CC
    CC Excl: See code: T22.331

✓6th **T22.74** **Corrosion of third degree of axilla**

7 ✓7th **T22.741** **Corrosion of third degree of right axilla** CC
    CC Excl: CC with 7th character A: See code: T22.341

7 ✓7th **T22.742** **Corrosion of third degree of left axilla** CC
    CC Excl: See code: T22.341

7 ✓7th **T22.749** **Corrosion of third degree of unspecified axilla** CC
    CC Excl: See code: T22.341

✓6th **T22.75** **Corrosion of third degree of shoulder**

7 ✓7th **T22.751** **Corrosion of third degree of right shoulder** CC
    CC Excl: CC with 7th character A: See code: T22.351

7 ✓7th **T22.752** **Corrosion of third degree of left shoulder** CC
    CC Excl: See code: T22.351

7 ✓7th **T22.759** **Corrosion of third degree of unspecified shoulder** CC
    CC Excl: See code: T22.351

✓6th **T22.76** **Corrosion of third degree of scapular region**

7 ✓7th **T22.761** **Corrosion of third degree of right scapular region** CC
    CC Excl: CC with 7th character A: See code: T22.361

7 ✓7th **T22.762** **Corrosion of third degree of left scapular region** CC
    CC Excl: See code: T22.361

7 ✓7th **T22.769** **Corrosion of third degree of unspecified scapular region** CC
    CC Excl: See code: T22.361

✓6th **T22.79** **Corrosion of third degree of multiple sites of shoulder and upper limb, except wrist and hand**

7 ✓7th **T22.791** **Corrosion of third degree of multiple sites of right shoulder and upper limb, except wrist and hand** CC
    CC Excl: CC with 7th character A: See code: T22.391

7 ✓7th **T22.792** **Corrosion of third degree of multiple sites of left shoulder and upper limb, except wrist and hand** CC
    CC Excl: See code: T22.391

7 ✓7th **T22.799** **Corrosion of third degree of multiple sites of unspecified shoulder and upper limb, except wrist and hand** CC
    CC Excl: See code: T22.391

✓4th **T23** **Burn and corrosion of wrist and hand**

> The appropriate 7th character is to be added to each code from category T23.
> A   initial encounter
> D   subsequent encounter
> S   sequela

✓5th **T23.0** **Burn of unspecified degree of wrist and hand**
    Use additional external cause code to identify the source, place and intent of the burn (X00-X19, X75-X77, X96-X98, Y92)

✓6th **T23.00** **Burn of unspecified degree of hand, unspecified site**

✓7th **T23.001** **Burn of unspecified degree of right hand, unspecified site**

✓7th **T23.002** **Burn of unspecified degree of left hand, unspecified site**

✓7th **T23.009** **Burn of unspecified degree of unspecified hand, unspecified site**

✓6th **T23.01** **Burn of unspecified degree of thumb (nail)**

✓7th **T23.011** **Burn of unspecified degree of right thumb (nail)**

✓7th **T23.012** **Burn of unspecified degree of left thumb (nail)**

✓7th **T23.019** **Burn of unspecified degree of unspecified thumb (nail)**

✓6th **T23.02** **Burn of unspecified degree of single finger (nail) except thumb**

✓7th **T23.021** **Burn of unspecified degree of single right finger (nail) except thumb**

✓7th **T23.022** **Burn of unspecified degree of single left finger (nail) except thumb**

✓7th **T23.029** **Burn of unspecified degree of unspecified single finger (nail) except thumb**

✓6th **T23.03** **Burn of unspecified degree of multiple fingers (nail), not including thumb**

✓7th **T23.031** **Burn of unspecified degree of multiple right fingers (nail), not including thumb**

✓7th **T23.032** **Burn of unspecified degree of multiple left fingers (nail), not including thumb**

✓7th **T23.039** **Burn of unspecified degree of unspecified multiple fingers (nail), not including thumb**

✓6th **T23.04** **Burn of unspecified degree of multiple fingers (nail), including thumb**

✓7th **T23.041** **Burn of unspecified degree of multiple right fingers (nail), including thumb**

✓7th **T23.042** **Burn of unspecified degree of multiple left fingers (nail), including thumb**

✓7th **T23.049** **Burn of unspecified degree of unspecified multiple fingers (nail), including thumb**

✓6th **T23.05** **Burn of unspecified degree of palm**

✓7th **T23.051** **Burn of unspecified degree of right palm**

✓7th **T23.052** **Burn of unspecified degree of left palm**

✓7th **T23.059** **Burn of unspecified degree of unspecified palm**

✓6th **T23.06** **Burn of unspecified degree of back of hand**

✓7th **T23.061** **Burn of unspecified degree of back of right hand**

✓7th **T23.062** **Burn of unspecified degree of back of left hand**

✓7th **T23.069** **Burn of unspecified degree of back of unspecified hand**

✓6th **T23.07** **Burn of unspecified degree of wrist**

✓7th **T23.071** **Burn of unspecified degree of right wrist**

✓7th **T23.072** **Burn of unspecified degree of left wrist**

✓7th **T23.079** **Burn of unspecified degree of unspecified wrist**

✓6th **T23.09** **Burn of unspecified degree of multiple sites of wrist and hand**

✓7th **T23.091** **Burn of unspecified degree of multiple sites of right wrist and hand**

✓7th **T23.092** **Burn of unspecified degree of multiple sites of left wrist and hand**

✓7th **T23.099** **Burn of unspecified degree of multiple sites of unspecified wrist and hand**

✓5th **T23.1** **Burn of first degree of wrist and hand**
    Use additional external cause code to identify the source, place and intent of the burn (X00-X19, X75-X77, X96-X98, Y92)

✓6th **T23.10** **Burn of first degree of hand, unspecified site**

✓7th **T23.101** **Burn of first degree of right hand, unspecified site**

✓7th **T23.102** **Burn of first degree of left hand, unspecified site**

✓7th **T23.109** **Burn of first degree of unspecified hand, unspecified site**

✓6th **T23.11** **Burn of first degree of thumb (nail)**

✓7th **T23.111** **Burn of first degree of right thumb (nail)**

✓7th **T23.112** **Burn of first degree of left thumb (nail)**

✓7th **T23.119** **Burn of first degree of unspecified thumb (nail)**

✓6th **T23.12** **Burn of first degree of single finger (nail) except thumb**

✓7th **T23.121** **Burn of first degree of single right finger (nail) except thumb**

✓7th **T23.122** **Burn of first degree of single left finger (nail) except thumb**

---

7 HAC = Initial encounter only (7th character A, B or C) and not POA.

N Newborn: 0   P Pediatric: 0-17   M Maternity: 12-55   A Adult: 15-124   MCC Major CC Condition   PDx MCC PDx acts as own MCC   CC CC Condition   PDx CC PDx acts as own CC

1040   ICD-10-CM Draft (2015)

√7th **T23.129** Burn of first degree of unspecified single finger (nail) except thumb

√6th **T23.13** Burn of first degree of multiple fingers (nail), not including thumb

√7th **T23.131** Burn of first degree of multiple right fingers (nail), not including thumb

√7th **T23.132** Burn of first degree of multiple left fingers (nail), not including thumb

√7th **T23.139** Burn of first degree of unspecified multiple fingers (nail), not including thumb

√6th **T23.14** Burn of first degree of multiple fingers (nail), including thumb

√7th **T23.141** Burn of first degree of multiple right fingers (nail), including thumb

√7th **T23.142** Burn of first degree of multiple left fingers (nail), including thumb

√7th **T23.149** Burn of first degree of unspecified multiple fingers (nail), including thumb

√6th **T23.15** Burn of first degree of palm

√7th **T23.151** Burn of first degree of right palm

√7th **T23.152** Burn of first degree of left palm

√7th **T23.159** Burn of first degree of unspecified palm

√6th **T23.16** Burn of first degree of back of hand

√7th **T23.161** Burn of first degree of back of right hand

√7th **T23.162** Burn of first degree of back of left hand

√7th **T23.169** Burn of first degree of back of unspecified hand

√6th **T23.17** Burn of first degree of wrist

√7th **T23.171** Burn of first degree of right wrist

√7th **T23.172** Burn of first degree of left wrist

√7th **T23.179** Burn of first degree of unspecified wrist

√6th **T23.19** Burn of first degree of multiple sites of wrist and hand

√7th **T23.191** Burn of first degree of multiple sites of right wrist and hand

√7th **T23.192** Burn of first degree of multiple sites of left wrist and hand

√7th **T23.199** Burn of first degree of multiple sites of unspecified wrist and hand

√5th **T23.2** Burn of second degree of wrist and hand
Use additional external cause code to identify the source, place and intent of the burn (X00-X19, X75-X77, X96-X98, Y92)

√6th **T23.20** Burn of second degree of hand, unspecified site

√7th **T23.201** Burn of second degree of right hand, unspecified site

√7th **T23.202** Burn of second degree of left hand, unspecified site

√7th **T23.209** Burn of second degree of unspecified hand, unspecified site

√6th **T23.21** Burn of second degree of thumb (nail)

√7th **T23.211** Burn of second degree of right thumb (nail)

√7th **T23.212** Burn of second degree of left thumb (nail)

√7th **T23.219** Burn of second degree of unspecified thumb (nail)

√6th **T23.22** Burn of second degree of single finger (nail) except thumb

√7th **T23.221** Burn of second degree of single right finger (nail) except thumb

√7th **T23.222** Burn of second degree of single left finger (nail) except thumb

√7th **T23.229** Burn of second degree of unspecified single finger (nail) except thumb

√6th **T23.23** Burn of second degree of multiple fingers (nail), not including thumb

√7th **T23.231** Burn of second degree of multiple right fingers (nail), not including thumb

√7th **T23.232** Burn of second degree of multiple left fingers (nail), not including thumb

√7th **T23.239** Burn of second degree of unspecified multiple fingers (nail), not including thumb

√6th **T23.24** Burn of second degree of multiple fingers (nail), including thumb

√7th **T23.241** Burn of second degree of multiple right fingers (nail), including thumb

√7th **T23.242** Burn of second degree of multiple left fingers (nail), including thumb

√7th **T23.249** Burn of second degree of unspecified multiple fingers (nail), including thumb

√6th **T23.25** Burn of second degree of palm

√7th **T23.251** Burn of second degree of right palm

√7th **T23.252** Burn of second degree of left palm

√7th **T23.259** Burn of second degree of unspecified palm

√6th **T23.26** Burn of second degree of back of hand

√7th **T23.261** Burn of second degree of back of right hand

√7th **T23.262** Burn of second degree of back of left hand

√7th **T23.269** Burn of second degree of back of unspecified hand

√6th **T23.27** Burn of second degree of wrist

√7th **T23.271** Burn of second degree of right wrist

√7th **T23.272** Burn of second degree of left wrist

√7th **T23.279** Burn of second degree of unspecified wrist

√6th **T23.29** Burn of second degree of multiple sites of wrist and hand

√7th **T23.291** Burn of second degree of multiple sites of right wrist and hand

√7th **T23.292** Burn of second degree of multiple sites of left wrist and hand

√7th **T23.299** Burn of second degree of multiple sites of unspecified wrist and hand

√5th **T23.3** Burn of third degree of wrist and hand
Use additional external cause code to identify the source, place and intent of the burn (X00-X19, X75-X77, X96-X98, Y92)

√6th **T23.30** Burn of third degree of hand, unspecified site

7 √7th **T23.301** Burn of third degree of right hand, unspecified site   CC
CC Excl: CC with 7th character A: T23.30X-T23.319 with 7th A, T23.391-T23.399 with 7th A, T23.701-T23.719 with 7th A, T23.791-T23.799 with 7th A

7 √7th **T23.302** Burn of third degree of left hand, unspecified site   CC
CC Excl: See code: T23.301

7 √7th **T23.309** Burn of third degree of unspecified hand, unspecified site   CC
CC Excl: See code: T23.301

√6th **T23.31** Burn of third degree of thumb (nail)

7 √7th **T23.311** Burn of third degree of right thumb (nail)   CC
CC Excl: CC with 7th character A: T23.301-T23.319 with 7th A, T23.391-T23.399 with 7th A, T23.701-T23.719 with 7th A, T23.791-T23.799 with 7th A

7 √7th **T23.312** Burn of third degree of left thumb (nail)   CC
CC Excl: See code: T23.311

7 √7th **T23.319** Burn of third degree of unspecified thumb (nail)   CC
CC Excl: See code: T23.311

√6th **T23.32** Burn of third degree of single finger (nail) except thumb

7 √7th **T23.321** Burn of third degree of single right finger (nail) except thumb   CC
CC Excl: CC with 7th character A: T23.301-T23.309 with 7th A, T23.321-T23.329 with 7th, A T23.391-T23.399 with 7th A, T23.701-T23.709 with 7th A, T23.721-T23.729 with 7th A, T23.791-T23.799 with 7th A

---

7 HAC = Initial encounter only (7th character A, B or C) and not POA.

☑ Additional Character Required   √7th Xtension Alert   Unacceptable PDx   Manifestation   Hospital Acquired Condition   EXCLUDES 1 Not Coded Here   EXCLUDES 2 Not Included Here

ICD-10-CM Draft (2015)   1041

7 ✓7ᵗʰ **T23.322 Burn of third degree of single left finger (nail) except thumb** CC
CC Excl: See code: T23.321

7 ✓7ᵗʰ **T23.329 Burn of third degree of unspecified single finger (nail) except thumb** CC
CC Excl: See code: T23.321

✓6ᵗʰ **T23.33 Burn of third degree of multiple fingers (nail), not including thumb**

7 ✓7ᵗʰ **T23.331 Burn of third degree of multiple right fingers (nail), not including thumb** CC
CC Excl: CC with 7th character A:
T23.301-T23.309 with 7th A,T23.331-T23.339 with 7th A,T23.391-T23.399 with 7th A, T23.701-T23.709 with 7th A,T23.731-T23.739 with 7th A,T23.791-T23.799 with 7th A

7 ✓7ᵗʰ **T23.332 Burn of third degree of multiple left fingers (nail), not including thumb** CC
CC Excl: See code: T23.331

7 ✓7ᵗʰ **T23.339 Burn of third degree of unspecified multiple fingers (nail), not including thumb** CC
CC Excl: See code: T23.331

✓6ᵗʰ **T23.34 Burn of third degree of multiple fingers (nail), including thumb**

7 ✓7ᵗʰ **T23.341 Burn of third degree of multiple right fingers (nail), including thumb** CC
CC Excl: CC with 7th character A:
T23.301-T23.309 with 7th A, T23.341-T23.349 with 7th A, T23.391-T23.399 with 7th A, T23.701-T23.709 with 7th A, T23.741-T23.749 with 7th A, T23.791-T23.799 with 7th A

7 ✓7ᵗʰ **T23.342 Burn of third degree of multiple left fingers (nail), including thumb** CC
CC Excl: See code: T23.341

7 ✓7ᵗʰ **T23.349 Burn of third degree of unspecified multiple fingers (nail), including thumb** CC
CC Excl: See code: T23.341

✓6ᵗʰ **T23.35 Burn of third degree of palm**

7 ✓7ᵗʰ **T23.351 Burn of third degree of right palm** CC
CC Excl: CC with 7th character A:
T23.301-T23.309 with 7th A,T23.351-T23.359 with 7th A,T23.391-T23.399 with 7th A, T23.701-T23.709 with 7th A, T23.751-T23.759 with 7th A,T23.791-T23.799 with 7th A

7 ✓7ᵗʰ **T23.352 Burn of third degree of left palm** CC
CC Excl: See code: T23.351

7 ✓7ᵗʰ **T23.359 Burn of third degree of unspecified palm** CC
CC Excl: See code: T23.351

✓6ᵗʰ **T23.36 Burn of third degree of back of hand**

7 ✓7ᵗʰ **T23.361 Burn of third degree of back of right hand** CC
CC Excl: CC with 7th character A:
T23.301-T23.309 with 7th A,T23.361-T23.369 with 7th A,T23.391-T23.399 with 7th A, T23.701-T23.709 with 7th A,T23.761-T23.769 with 7th A,T23.791-T23.799 with 7th A

7 ✓7ᵗʰ **T23.362 Burn of third degree of back of left hand** CC
CC Excl: See code: T23.361

7 ✓7ᵗʰ **T23.369 Burn of third degree of back of unspecified hand** CC
CC Excl: See code: T23.361

✓6ᵗʰ **T23.37 Burn of third degree of wrist**

7 ✓7ᵗʰ **T23.371 Burn of third degree of right wrist** CC
CC Excl: CC with 7th character A:
T23.301-T23.309 with 7th A,T23.371-T23.379 with 7th A, T23.391-T23.399 with 7th A, T23.701-T23.709 with 7th A, T23.771-T23.779 with 7th A, T23.791-T23.799 with 7th A

7 ✓7ᵗʰ **T23.372 Burn of third degree of left wrist** CC
CC Excl: See code: T23.371

7 ✓7ᵗʰ **T23.379 Burn of third degree of unspecified wrist** CC
CC Excl: See code: T23.371

✓6ᵗʰ **T23.39 Burn of third degree of multiple sites of wrist and hand**

7 ✓7ᵗʰ **T23.391 Burn of third degree of multiple sites of right wrist and hand** CC
CC Excl: See code: T23.301

7 ✓7ᵗʰ **T23.392 Burn of third degree of multiple sites of left wrist and hand** CC
CC Excl: See code: T23.301

7 ✓7ᵗʰ **T23.399 Burn of third degree of multiple sites of unspecified wrist and hand** CC
CC Excl: See code: T23.301

✓5ᵗʰ **T23.4 Corrosion of unspecified degree of wrist and hand**
Code first (T51-T65) to identify chemical and intent
Use additional external cause code to identify place (Y92)

✓6ᵗʰ **T23.40 Corrosion of unspecified degree of hand, unspecified site**

✓7ᵗʰ **T23.401 Corrosion of unspecified degree of right hand, unspecified site**

✓7ᵗʰ **T23.402 Corrosion of unspecified degree of left hand, unspecified site**

✓7ᵗʰ **T23.409 Corrosion of unspecified degree of unspecified hand, unspecified site**

✓6ᵗʰ **T23.41 Corrosion of unspecified degree of thumb (nail)**

✓7ᵗʰ **T23.411 Corrosion of unspecified degree of right thumb (nail)**

✓7ᵗʰ **T23.412 Corrosion of unspecified degree of left thumb (nail)**

✓7ᵗʰ **T23.419 Corrosion of unspecified degree of unspecified thumb (nail)**

✓6ᵗʰ **T23.42 Corrosion of unspecified degree of single finger (nail) except thumb**

✓7ᵗʰ **T23.421 Corrosion of unspecified degree of single right finger (nail) except thumb**

✓7ᵗʰ **T23.422 Corrosion of unspecified degree of single left finger (nail) except thumb**

✓7ᵗʰ **T23.429 Corrosion of unspecified degree of unspecified single finger (nail) except thumb**

✓6ᵗʰ **T23.43 Corrosion of unspecified degree of multiple fingers (nail), not including thumb**

✓7ᵗʰ **T23.431 Corrosion of unspecified degree of multiple right fingers (nail), not including thumb**

✓7ᵗʰ **T23.432 Corrosion of unspecified degree of multiple left fingers (nail), not including thumb**

✓7ᵗʰ **T23.439 Corrosion of unspecified degree of unspecified multiple fingers (nail), not including thumb**

✓6ᵗʰ **T23.44 Corrosion of unspecified degree of multiple fingers (nail), including thumb**

✓7ᵗʰ **T23.441 Corrosion of unspecified degree of multiple right fingers (nail), including thumb**

✓7ᵗʰ **T23.442 Corrosion of unspecified degree of multiple left fingers (nail), including thumb**

✓7ᵗʰ **T23.449 Corrosion of unspecified degree of unspecified multiple fingers (nail), including thumb**

✓6ᵗʰ **T23.45 Corrosion of unspecified degree of palm**

✓7ᵗʰ **T23.451 Corrosion of unspecified degree of right palm**

✓7ᵗʰ **T23.452 Corrosion of unspecified degree of left palm**

✓7ᵗʰ **T23.459 Corrosion of unspecified degree of unspecified palm**

✓6ᵗʰ **T23.46 Corrosion of unspecified degree of back of hand**

✓7ᵗʰ **T23.461 Corrosion of unspecified degree of back of right hand**

✓7ᵗʰ **T23.462 Corrosion of unspecified degree of back of left hand**

✓7ᵗʰ **T23.469 Corrosion of unspecified degree of back of unspecified hand**

---

7 HAC = Initial encounter only (7th character A, B or C) and not POA.

√6ᵗʰ **T23.47** Corrosion of unspecified degree of wrist

  √7ᵗʰ **T23.471** Corrosion of unspecified degree of right wrist

  √7ᵗʰ **T23.472** Corrosion of unspecified degree of left wrist

  √7ᵗʰ **T23.479** Corrosion of unspecified degree of unspecified wrist

√6ᵗʰ **T23.49** Corrosion of unspecified degree of multiple sites of wrist and hand

  √7ᵗʰ **T23.491** Corrosion of unspecified degree of multiple sites of right wrist and hand

  √7ᵗʰ **T23.492** Corrosion of unspecified degree of multiple sites of left wrist and hand

  √7ᵗʰ **T23.499** Corrosion of unspecified degree of multiple sites of unspecified wrist and hand

√5ᵗʰ **T23.5** Corrosion of first degree of wrist and hand

  Code first (T51-T65) to identify chemical and intent
  Use additional external cause code to identify place (Y92)

√6ᵗʰ **T23.50** Corrosion of first degree of hand, unspecified site

  √7ᵗʰ **T23.501** Corrosion of first degree of right hand, unspecified site

  √7ᵗʰ **T23.502** Corrosion of first degree of left hand, unspecified site

  √7ᵗʰ **T23.509** Corrosion of first degree of unspecified hand, unspecified site

√6ᵗʰ **T23.51** Corrosion of first degree of thumb (nail)

  √7ᵗʰ **T23.511** Corrosion of first degree of right thumb (nail)

  √7ᵗʰ **T23.512** Corrosion of first degree of left thumb (nail)

  √7ᵗʰ **T23.519** Corrosion of first degree of unspecified thumb (nail)

√6ᵗʰ **T23.52** Corrosion of first degree of single finger (nail) except thumb

  √7ᵗʰ **T23.521** Corrosion of first degree of single right finger (nail) except thumb

  √7ᵗʰ **T23.522** Corrosion of first degree of single left finger (nail) except thumb

  √7ᵗʰ **T23.529** Corrosion of first degree of unspecified single finger (nail) except thumb

√6ᵗʰ **T23.53** Corrosion of first degree of multiple fingers (nail), not including thumb

  √7ᵗʰ **T23.531** Corrosion of first degree of multiple right fingers (nail), not including thumb

  √7ᵗʰ **T23.532** Corrosion of first degree of multiple left fingers (nail), not including thumb

  √7ᵗʰ **T23.539** Corrosion of first degree of unspecified multiple fingers (nail), not including thumb

√6ᵗʰ **T23.54** Corrosion of first degree of multiple fingers (nail), including thumb

  √7ᵗʰ **T23.541** Corrosion of first degree of multiple right fingers (nail), including thumb

  √7ᵗʰ **T23.542** Corrosion of first degree of multiple left fingers (nail), including thumb

  √7ᵗʰ **T23.549** Corrosion of first degree of unspecified multiple fingers (nail), including thumb

√6ᵗʰ **T23.55** Corrosion of first degree of palm

  √7ᵗʰ **T23.551** Corrosion of first degree of right palm

  √7ᵗʰ **T23.552** Corrosion of first degree of left palm

  √7ᵗʰ **T23.559** Corrosion of first degree of unspecified palm

√6ᵗʰ **T23.56** Corrosion of first degree of back of hand

  √7ᵗʰ **T23.561** Corrosion of first degree of back of right hand

  √7ᵗʰ **T23.562** Corrosion of first degree of back of left hand

  √7ᵗʰ **T23.569** Corrosion of first degree of back of unspecified hand

√6ᵗʰ **T23.57** Corrosion of first degree of wrist

  √7ᵗʰ **T23.571** Corrosion of first degree of right wrist

  √7ᵗʰ **T23.572** Corrosion of first degree of left wrist

  √7ᵗʰ **T23.579** Corrosion of first degree of unspecified wrist

√6ᵗʰ **T23.59** Corrosion of first degree of multiple sites of wrist and hand

  √7ᵗʰ **T23.591** Corrosion of first degree of multiple sites of right wrist and hand

  √7ᵗʰ **T23.592** Corrosion of first degree of multiple sites of left wrist and hand

  √7ᵗʰ **T23.599** Corrosion of first degree of multiple sites of unspecified wrist and hand

√5ᵗʰ **T23.6** Corrosion of second degree of wrist and hand

  Code first (T51-T65) to identify chemical and intent
  Use additional external cause code to identify place (Y92)

√6ᵗʰ **T23.60** Corrosion of second degree of hand, unspecified site

  √7ᵗʰ **T23.601** Corrosion of second degree of right hand, unspecified site

  √7ᵗʰ **T23.602** Corrosion of second degree of left hand, unspecified site

  √7ᵗʰ **T23.609** Corrosion of second degree of unspecified hand, unspecified site

√6ᵗʰ **T23.61** Corrosion of second degree of thumb (nail)

  √7ᵗʰ **T23.611** Corrosion of second degree of right thumb (nail)

  √7ᵗʰ **T23.612** Corrosion of second degree of left thumb (nail)

  √7ᵗʰ **T23.619** Corrosion of second degree of unspecified thumb (nail)

√6ᵗʰ **T23.62** Corrosion of second degree of single finger (nail) except thumb

  √7ᵗʰ **T23.621** Corrosion of second degree of single right finger (nail) except thumb

  √7ᵗʰ **T23.622** Corrosion of second degree of single left finger (nail) except thumb

  √7ᵗʰ **T23.629** Corrosion of second degree of unspecified single finger (nail) except thumb

√6ᵗʰ **T23.63** Corrosion of second degree of multiple fingers (nail), not including thumb

  √7ᵗʰ **T23.631** Corrosion of second degree of multiple right fingers (nail), not including thumb

  √7ᵗʰ **T23.632** Corrosion of second degree of multiple left fingers (nail), not including thumb

  √7ᵗʰ **T23.639** Corrosion of second degree of unspecified multiple fingers (nail), not including thumb

√6ᵗʰ **T23.64** Corrosion of second degree of multiple fingers (nail), including thumb

  √7ᵗʰ **T23.641** Corrosion of second degree of multiple right fingers (nail), including thumb

  √7ᵗʰ **T23.642** Corrosion of second degree of multiple left fingers (nail), including thumb

  √7ᵗʰ **T23.649** Corrosion of second degree of unspecified multiple fingers (nail), including thumb

√6ᵗʰ **T23.65** Corrosion of second degree of palm

  √7ᵗʰ **T23.651** Corrosion of second degree of right palm

  √7ᵗʰ **T23.652** Corrosion of second degree of left palm

  √7ᵗʰ **T23.659** Corrosion of second degree of unspecified palm

√6ᵗʰ **T23.66** Corrosion of second degree of back of hand

  √7ᵗʰ **T23.661** Corrosion of second degree back of right hand

  √7ᵗʰ **T23.662** Corrosion of second degree back of left hand

  √7ᵗʰ **T23.669** Corrosion of second degree back of unspecified hand

√6ᵗʰ **T23.67** Corrosion of second degree of wrist

  √7ᵗʰ **T23.671** Corrosion of second degree of right wrist

  √7ᵗʰ **T23.672** Corrosion of second degree of left wrist

  √7ᵗʰ **T23.679** Corrosion of second degree of unspecified wrist

√6ᵗʰ **T23.69** Corrosion of second degree of multiple sites of wrist and hand

  √7ᵗʰ **T23.691** Corrosion of second degree of multiple sites of right wrist and hand

---

☑ Additional Character Required √ₓ7ᵗʰ Xtension Alert Unacceptable PDx Manifestation Hospital Acquired Condition EXCLUDES 1 Not Coded Here EXCLUDES 2 Not Included Here

7th✓ T23.692 Corrosion of second degree of multiple sites of **left** wrist and hand

7th✓ T23.699 Corrosion of second degree of multiple sites of **unspecified** wrist and hand

✓5th T23.7 Corrosion of third degree of wrist and hand
Code first (T51-T65) to identify chemical and intent
Use additional external cause code to identify place (Y92)

✓6th T23.70 Corrosion of third degree of hand, unspecified site

7 **7th✓ T23.701** Corrosion of third degree of **right** hand, unspecified site   CC
CC Excl: CC with 7th character A: T23.301-T23.319 with 7th A, T23.391-T23.399 with 7th A, T23.701-T23.719 with 7th A, T23.791-T23.799 with 7th A

7 **7th✓ T23.702** Corrosion of third degree of **left** hand, unspecified site   CC
CC Excl: See code: T23.701

7 **7th✓ T23.709** Corrosion of third degree of **unspecified** hand, unspecified site   CC
CC Excl: See code: T23.701

✓6th T23.71 Corrosion of third degree of thumb (nail)

7 **7th✓ T23.711** Corrosion of third degree of **right** thumb (nail)   CC
CC Excl: CC with 7th character A: T23.301-T23.319 with 7th A, T23.391-T23.399 with 7th A, T23.701-T23.719 with 7th A, T23.791-T23.799 with 7th A

7 **7th✓ T23.712** Corrosion of third degree of **left** thumb (nail)   CC
CC Excl: See code: T23.711

7 **7th✓ T23.719** Corrosion of third degree of **unspecified** thumb (nail)   CC
CC Excl: See code: T23.711

✓6th T23.72 Corrosion of third degree of single finger (nail) except thumb

7 **7th✓ T23.721** Corrosion of third degree of single **right** finger (nail) except thumb   CC
CC Excl: CC with 7th character A: T23.301-T23.309 with 7th A, T23.321-T23.329 with 7th A, T23.391-T23.399 with 7th A, T23.701-T23.709 with 7th A, T23.721-T23.729 with 7th A, T23.791-T23.799 with 7th A

7 **7th✓ T23.722** Corrosion of third degree of single **left** finger (nail) except thumb   CC
CC Excl: See code: T23.721

7 **7th✓ T23.729** Corrosion of third degree of **unspecified** single finger (nail) except thumb   CC
CC Excl: See code: T23.721

✓6th T23.73 Corrosion of third degree of multiple fingers (nail), not including thumb

7 **7th✓ T23.731** Corrosion of third degree of multiple **right** fingers (nail), not including thumb   CC
CC Excl: CC with 7th character A: T23.301-T23.309 with 7th A, T23.331-T23.339 with 7th A, T23.391-T23.399 with 7th A, T23.701-T23.709 with 7th A, T23.731-T23.739 with 7th A, T23.791-T23.799 with 7th A

7 **7th✓ T23.732** Corrosion of third degree of multiple **left** fingers (nail), not including thumb   CC
CC Excl: See code: T23.731

7 **7th✓ T23.739** Corrosion of third degree of **unspecified** multiple fingers (nail), not including thumb   CC
CC Excl: See code: T23.731

✓6th T23.74 Corrosion of third degree of multiple fingers (nail), including thumb

7 **7th✓ T23.741** Corrosion of third degree of multiple **right** fingers (nail), including thumb   CC
CC Excl: CC with 7th character A: T23.301-T23.309 with 7th A, T23.341-T23.349 with 7th A, T23.391-T23.399 with 7th A, T23.701-T23.709 with 7th A, T23.741-T23.749 with 7th A, T23.791-T23.799 with 7th A

7 **7th✓ T23.742** Corrosion of third degree of multiple **left** fingers (nail), including thumb   CC
CC Excl: See code: T23.741

7 **7th✓ T23.749** Corrosion of third degree of **unspecified** multiple fingers (nail), including thumb   CC
CC Excl: See code: T23.741

✓6th T23.75 Corrosion of third degree of palm

7 **7th✓ T23.751** Corrosion of third degree of **right** palm   CC
CC Excl: CC with 7th character A: T23.301-T23.309 with 7th A, T23.351-T23.359 with 7th A, T23.391-T23.399 with 7th A, T23.701-T23.709 with 7th A, T23.751-T23.759 with 7th A, T23.791-T23.799 with 7th A

7 **7th✓ T23.752** Corrosion of third degree of **left** palm   CC
CC Excl: See code: T23.751

7 **7th✓ T23.759** Corrosion of third degree of **unspecified** palm   CC
CC Excl: See code: T23.751

✓6th T23.76 Corrosion of third degree of back of hand

7 **7th✓ T23.761** Corrosion of third degree of back of **right** hand   CC
CC Excl: CC with 7th character A: T23.301-T23.309 with 7th A, T23.361-T23.369 with 7th A, T23.391-T23.399 with 7th A, T23.701-T23.709 with 7th A, T23.761-T23.769 with 7th A, T23.791-T23.799 with 7th A

7 **7th✓ T23.762** Corrosion of third degree of back of **left** hand   CC
CC Excl: See code: T23.761

7 **7th✓ T23.769** Corrosion of third degree back of **unspecified** hand   CC
CC Excl: See code: T23.761

✓6th T23.77 Corrosion of third degree of wrist

7 **7th✓ T23.771** Corrosion of third degree of **right** wrist   CC
CC Excl: CC with 7th character A: T23.301-T23.309 with 7th A, T23.371-T23.379 with 7th A, T23.391-T23.399 with 7th A, T23.701-T23.709 with 7th A, T23.771-T23.779 with 7th A, T23.791-T23.799 with 7th A

7 **7th✓ T23.772** Corrosion of third degree of **left** wrist   CC
CC Excl: See code: T23.771

7 **7th✓ T23.779** Corrosion of third degree of **unspecified** wrist   CC
CC Excl: See code: T23.771

✓6th T23.79 Corrosion of third degree of multiple sites of wrist and hand

7 **7th✓ T23.791** Corrosion of third degree of multiple sites of **right** wrist and hand   CC
CC Excl: See code: T23.702

7 **7th✓ T23.792** Corrosion of third degree of multiple sites of **left** wrist and hand   CC
CC Excl: See code: T23.702

7 **7th✓ T23.799** Corrosion of third degree of multiple sites of **unspecified** wrist and hand   CC
CC Excl: See code: T23.702

✓4th T24 Burn and corrosion of lower limb, except ankle and foot
EXCLUDES 2   burn and corrosion of ankle and foot (T25.-)
burn and corrosion of hip region (T21.-)

The appropriate 7th character is to be added to each code from category T24.
A   initial encounter
D   subsequent encounter
S   sequela

✓5th T24.0 Burn of unspecified degree of lower limb, except ankle and foot
Use additional external cause code to identify the source, place and intent of the burn (X00-X19, X75-X77, X96-X98, Y92)

✓6th T24.00 Burn of unspecified degree of unspecified site of lower limb, except ankle and foot

---

7 HAC = Initial encounter only (7th character A, B or C) and not POA.

N Newborn: 0   P Pediatric: 0-17   M Maternity: 12-55   A Adult: 15-124   MCC Major CC Condition   PDx MCC PDx acts as own MCC   CC CC Condition   PDx CC PDx acts as own CC

1044   ICD-10-CM Draft (2015)

✓7ᵗʰ **T24.001** Burn of unspecified degree of unspecified site of **right** lower limb, except ankle and foot

✓7ᵗʰ **T24.002** Burn of unspecified degree of unspecified site of **left** lower limb, except ankle and foot

✓7ᵗʰ **T24.009** Burn of unspecified degree of unspecified site of **unspecified** lower limb, except ankle and foot

✓6ᵗʰ **T24.01** Burn of unspecified degree of **thigh**

✓7ᵗʰ **T24.011** Burn of unspecified degree of **right** thigh

✓7ᵗʰ **T24.012** Burn of unspecified degree of **left** thigh

✓7ᵗʰ **T24.019** Burn of unspecified degree of **unspecified** thigh

✓6ᵗʰ **T24.02** Burn of unspecified degree of **knee**

✓7ᵗʰ **T24.021** Burn of unspecified degree of **right** knee

✓7ᵗʰ **T24.022** Burn of unspecified degree of **left** knee

✓7ᵗʰ **T24.029** Burn of unspecified degree of **unspecified** knee

✓6ᵗʰ **T24.03** Burn of unspecified degree of **lower leg**

✓7ᵗʰ **T24.031** Burn of unspecified degree of **right** lower leg

✓7ᵗʰ **T24.032** Burn of unspecified degree of **left** lower leg

✓7ᵗʰ **T24.039** Burn of unspecified degree of **unspecified** lower leg

✓6ᵗʰ **T24.09** Burn of unspecified degree of **multiple sites** of lower limb, except ankle and foot

✓7ᵗʰ **T24.091** Burn of unspecified degree of multiple sites of **right** lower limb, except ankle and foot

✓7ᵗʰ **T24.092** Burn of unspecified degree of multiple sites of **left** lower limb, except ankle and foot

✓7ᵗʰ **T24.099** Burn of unspecified degree of multiple sites of **unspecified** lower limb, except ankle and foot

✓5ᵗʰ **T24.1** Burn of **first degree** of lower limb, except ankle and foot
Use additional external cause code to identify the source, place and intent of the burn (X00-X19, X75-X77, X96-X98, Y92)

✓6ᵗʰ **T24.10** Burn of first degree of **unspecified site** of lower limb, except ankle and foot

✓7ᵗʰ **T24.101** Burn of first degree of unspecified site of **right** lower limb, except ankle and foot

✓7ᵗʰ **T24.102** Burn of first degree of unspecified site of **left** lower limb, except ankle and foot

✓7ᵗʰ **T24.109** Burn of first degree of unspecified site of **unspecified** lower limb, except ankle and foot

✓6ᵗʰ **T24.11** Burn of first degree of **thigh**

✓7ᵗʰ **T24.111** Burn of first degree of **right** thigh

✓7ᵗʰ **T24.112** Burn of first degree of **left** thigh

✓7ᵗʰ **T24.119** Burn of first degree of **unspecified** thigh

✓6ᵗʰ **T24.12** Burn of first degree of **knee**

✓7ᵗʰ **T24.121** Burn of first degree of **right** knee

✓7ᵗʰ **T24.122** Burn of first degree of **left** knee

✓7ᵗʰ **T24.129** Burn of first degree of **unspecified** knee

✓6ᵗʰ **T24.13** Burn of first degree of **lower leg**

✓7ᵗʰ **T24.131** Burn of first degree of **right** lower leg

✓7ᵗʰ **T24.132** Burn of first degree of **left** lower leg

✓7ᵗʰ **T24.139** Burn of first degree of **unspecified** lower leg

✓6ᵗʰ **T24.19** Burn of first degree of **multiple sites** of lower limb, except ankle and foot

✓7ᵗʰ **T24.191** Burn of first degree of multiple sites of **right** lower limb, except ankle and foot

✓7ᵗʰ **T24.192** Burn of first degree of multiple sites of **left** lower limb, except ankle and foot

✓7ᵗʰ **T24.199** Burn of first degree of multiple sites of **unspecified** lower limb, except ankle and foot

✓5ᵗʰ **T24.2** Burn of **second degree** of lower limb, except ankle and foot
Use additional external cause code to identify the source, place and intent of the burn (X00-X19, X75-X77, X96-X98, Y92)

✓6ᵗʰ **T24.20** Burn of second degree of **unspecified site** of lower limb, except ankle and foot

✓7ᵗʰ **T24.201** Burn of second degree of unspecified site of **right** lower limb, except ankle and foot

✓7ᵗʰ **T24.202** Burn of second degree of unspecified site of **left** lower limb, except ankle and foot

✓7ᵗʰ **T24.209** Burn of second degree of unspecified site of **unspecified** lower limb, except ankle and foot

✓6ᵗʰ **T24.21** Burn of second degree of **thigh**

✓7ᵗʰ **T24.211** Burn of second degree of **right** thigh

✓7ᵗʰ **T24.212** Burn of second degree of **left** thigh

✓7ᵗʰ **T24.219** Burn of second degree of **unspecified** thigh

✓6ᵗʰ **T24.22** Burn of second degree of **knee**

✓7ᵗʰ **T24.221** Burn of second degree of **right** knee

✓7ᵗʰ **T24.222** Burn of second degree of **left** knee

✓7ᵗʰ **T24.229** Burn of second degree of **unspecified** knee

✓6ᵗʰ **T24.23** Burn of second degree of **lower leg**

✓7ᵗʰ **T24.231** Burn of second degree of **right** lower leg

✓7ᵗʰ **T24.232** Burn of second degree of **left** lower leg

✓7ᵗʰ **T24.239** Burn of second degree of **unspecified** lower leg

✓6ᵗʰ **T24.29** Burn of second degree of **multiple sites** of lower limb, except ankle and foot

✓7ᵗʰ **T24.291** Burn of second degree of multiple sites of **right** lower limb, except ankle and foot

✓7ᵗʰ **T24.292** Burn of second degree of multiple sites of **left** lower limb, except ankle and foot

✓7ᵗʰ **T24.299** Burn of second degree of multiple sites of **unspecified** lower limb, except ankle and foot

✓5ᵗʰ **T24.3** Burn of **third degree** of lower limb, except ankle and foot
Use additional external cause code to identify the source, place and intent of the burn (X00-X19, X75-X77, X96-X98, Y92)

✓6ᵗʰ **T24.30** Burn of third degree of **unspecified site** of lower limb, except ankle and foot

7 ✓7ᵗʰ **T24.301** Burn of third degree of unspecified site of **right** lower limb, except ankle and foot   **CC**
CC Excl: CC with 7th character A: T24.301-T24.309 with 7th A, T24.391-T24.399 with 7th A, T24.701-T24.709 with 7th A, T24.791-T24.799 with 7th A, T25.391-T25.399 with 7th A, T25.791-T25.790 with 7th A

7 ✓7ᵗʰ **T24.302** Burn of third degree of unspecified site of **left** lower limb, except ankle and foot   **CC**
CC Excl: See code: T24.301

7 ✓7ᵗʰ **T24.309** Burn of third degree of unspecified site of **unspecified** lower limb, except ankle and foot   **CC**
CC Excl: See code: T24.301

✓6ᵗʰ **T24.31** Burn of third degree of **thigh**

7 ✓7ᵗʰ **T24.311** Burn of third degree of **right** thigh   **CC**
CC Excl: CC with 7th character A: T24.301-T24.309 with 7th A, T24.311-T24.319 with 7th A, T24.391-T24.399 with 7th A, T24.701-T24.709 with 7th A, T24.711-T24.719 with 7th A, T24.791-T24.799 with 7th A, T25.391-T25.399 with 7th A, T25.791-T25.790 with 7th A

7 ✓7ᵗʰ **T24.312** Burn of third degree of **left** thigh   **CC**
CC Excl: See code: T24.311

7 ✓7ᵗʰ **T24.319** Burn of third degree of **unspecified** thigh   **CC**
CC Excl: See code: T24.311

---

7 HAC = Initial encounter only (7th character A, B or C) and not POA.

Injury, Poisoning and Certain Other Consequences of External Causes

T24.32–T24.611

√6ᵗʰ **T24.32** Burn of third degree of knee
- 7 √7ᵗʰ **T24.321** **Burn of third degree of right knee** CC
  - CC Excl: CC with 7th character A: T24.301-T24.309 with 7th A, T24.321-T24.329 with 7th A, T24.391-T24.399 with 7th A, T24.701-T24.709 with 7th A, T24.721-T24.729 with 7th A, T24.791-T24.799 with 7th A, T25.391-T25.399 with 7th A, T25.791-T25.790 with 7th A
- 7 √7ᵗʰ **T24.322** **Burn of third degree of left knee** CC
  - CC Excl: See code: T24.321
- 7 √7ᵗʰ **T24.329** **Burn of third degree of unspecified knee** CC
  - CC Excl: See code: T24.321

√6ᵗʰ **T24.33** Burn of third degree of lower leg
- 7 √7ᵗʰ **T24.331** **Burn of third degree of right lower leg** CC
  - CC Excl: CC with 7th character A: T24.301-T24.309 with 7th A, T24.331-T24.339 with 7th A, T24.391-T24.399 with 7th A, T24.701-T24.709 with 7th A, T24.731-T24.739 with 7th A, T24.791-T24.799 with 7th A, T25.391-T25.399 with 7th A, T25.791-T25.790 with 7th A
- 7 √7ᵗʰ **T24.332** **Burn of third degree of left lower leg** CC
  - CC Excl: See code: T24.331
- 7 √7ᵗʰ **T24.339** **Burn of third degree of unspecified lower leg** CC
  - CC Excl: See code: T24.331

√6ᵗʰ **T24.39** Burn of third degree of multiple sites of lower limb, except ankle and foot
- 7 √7ᵗʰ **T24.391** **Burn of third degree of multiple sites of right lower limb, except ankle and foot** CC
  - CC Excl: CC with 7th character A: T24.301-T24.309 with 7th A, T24.391-T24.399 with 7th A, T24.701-T24.709 with 7th A, T24.791-T24.799 with 7th A, T25.391-T25.399 with 7th A, T25.791-T25.799 with 7th A
- 7 √7ᵗʰ **T24.392** **Burn of third degree of multiple sites of left lower limb, except ankle and foot** CC
  - CC Excl: See code: T24.301
- 7 √7ᵗʰ **T24.399** **Burn of third degree of multiple sites of unspecified lower limb, except ankle and foot** CC
  - CC Excl: See code: T24.301

√5ᵗʰ **T24.4** Corrosion of unspecified degree of lower limb, except ankle and foot
- Code first (T51-T65) to identify chemical and intent
- Use additional external cause code to identify place (Y92)

√6ᵗʰ **T24.40** Corrosion of unspecified degree of unspecified site of lower limb, except ankle and foot
- √7ᵗʰ **T24.401** Corrosion of unspecified degree of unspecified site of right lower limb, except ankle and foot
- √7ᵗʰ **T24.402** Corrosion of unspecified degree of unspecified site of left lower limb, except ankle and foot
- √7ᵗʰ **T24.409** Corrosion of unspecified degree of unspecified site of unspecified lower limb, except ankle and foot

√6ᵗʰ **T24.41** Corrosion of unspecified degree of thigh
- √7ᵗʰ **T24.411** Corrosion of unspecified degree of right thigh
- √7ᵗʰ **T24.412** Corrosion of unspecified degree of left thigh
- √7ᵗʰ **T24.419** Corrosion of unspecified degree of unspecified thigh

√6ᵗʰ **T24.42** Corrosion of unspecified degree of knee
- √7ᵗʰ **T24.421** Corrosion of unspecified degree of right knee
- √7ᵗʰ **T24.422** Corrosion of unspecified degree of left knee
- √7ᵗʰ **T24.429** Corrosion of unspecified degree of unspecified knee

√6ᵗʰ **T24.43** Corrosion of unspecified degree of lower leg
- √7ᵗʰ **T24.431** Corrosion of unspecified degree of right lower leg
- √7ᵗʰ **T24.432** Corrosion of unspecified degree of left lower leg
- √7ᵗʰ **T24.439** Corrosion of unspecified degree of unspecified lower leg

√6ᵗʰ **T24.49** Corrosion of unspecified degree of multiple sites of lower limb, except ankle and foot
- √7ᵗʰ **T24.491** Corrosion of unspecified degree of multiple sites of right lower limb, except ankle and foot
- √7ᵗʰ **T24.492** Corrosion of unspecified degree of multiple sites of left lower limb, except ankle and foot
- √7ᵗʰ **T24.499** Corrosion of unspecified degree of multiple sites of unspecified lower limb, except ankle and foot

√5ᵗʰ **T24.5** Corrosion of first degree of lower limb, except ankle and foot
- Code first (T51-T65) to identify chemical and intent
- Use additional external cause code to identify place (Y92)

√6ᵗʰ **T24.50** Corrosion of first degree of unspecified site of lower limb, except ankle and foot
- √7ᵗʰ **T24.501** Corrosion of first degree of unspecified site of right lower limb, except ankle and foot
- √7ᵗʰ **T24.502** Corrosion of first degree of unspecified site of left lower limb, except ankle and foot
- √7ᵗʰ **T24.509** Corrosion of first degree of unspecified site of unspecified lower limb, except ankle and foot

√6ᵗʰ **T24.51** Corrosion of first degree of thigh
- √7ᵗʰ **T24.511** Corrosion of first degree of right thigh
- √7ᵗʰ **T24.512** Corrosion of first degree of left thigh
- √7ᵗʰ **T24.519** Corrosion of first degree of unspecified thigh

√6ᵗʰ **T24.52** Corrosion of first degree of knee
- √7ᵗʰ **T24.521** Corrosion of first degree of right knee
- √7ᵗʰ **T24.522** Corrosion of first degree of left knee
- √7ᵗʰ **T24.529** Corrosion of first degree of unspecified knee

√6ᵗʰ **T24.53** Corrosion of first degree of lower leg
- √7ᵗʰ **T24.531** Corrosion of first degree of right lower leg
- √7ᵗʰ **T24.532** Corrosion of first degree of left lower leg
- √7ᵗʰ **T24.539** Corrosion of first degree of unspecified lower leg

√6ᵗʰ **T24.59** Corrosion of first degree of multiple sites of lower limb, except ankle and foot
- √7ᵗʰ **T24.591** Corrosion of first degree of multiple sites of right lower limb, except ankle and foot
- √7ᵗʰ **T24.592** Corrosion of first degree of multiple sites of left lower limb, except ankle and foot
- √7ᵗʰ **T24.599** Corrosion of first degree of multiple sites of unspecified lower limb, except ankle and foot

√5ᵗʰ **T24.6** Corrosion of second degree of lower limb, except ankle and foot
- Code first (T51-T65) to identify chemical and intent
- Use additional external cause code to identify place (Y92)

√6ᵗʰ **T24.60** Corrosion of second degree of unspecified site of lower limb, except ankle and foot
- √7ᵗʰ **T24.601** Corrosion of second degree of unspecified site of right lower limb, except ankle and foot
- √7ᵗʰ **T24.602** Corrosion of second degree of unspecified site of left lower limb, except ankle and foot
- √7ᵗʰ **T24.609** Corrosion of second degree of unspecified site of unspecified lower limb, except ankle and foot

√6ᵗʰ **T24.61** Corrosion of second degree of thigh
- √7ᵗʰ **T24.611** Corrosion of second degree of right thigh

---

7 HAC = Initial encounter only (7th character A, B or C) and not POA.

Ⓝ Newborn: 0   Ⓟ Pediatric: 0-17   Ⓜ Maternity: 12-55   Ⓐ Adult: 15-124   **MCC** Major CC Condition   **PDx MCC** PDx acts as own MCC   **CC** CC Condition   **PDx CC** PDx acts as own CC

√7ᵗʰ **T24.612** Corrosion of second degree of left thigh

√7ᵗʰ **T24.619** Corrosion of second degree of unspecified thigh

√6ᵗʰ **T24.62** Corrosion of second degree of knee

√7ᵗʰ **T24.621** Corrosion of second degree of right knee

√7ᵗʰ **T24.622** Corrosion of second degree of left knee

√7ᵗʰ **T24.629** Corrosion of second degree of unspecified knee

√6ᵗʰ **T24.63** Corrosion of second degree of lower leg

√7ᵗʰ **T24.631** Corrosion of second degree of right lower leg

√7ᵗʰ **T24.632** Corrosion of second degree of left lower leg

√7ᵗʰ **T24.639** Corrosion of second degree of unspecified lower leg

√6ᵗʰ **T24.69** Corrosion of second degree of multiple sites of lower limb, except ankle and foot

√7ᵗʰ **T24.691** Corrosion of second degree of multiple sites of right lower limb, except ankle and foot

√7ᵗʰ **T24.692** Corrosion of second degree of multiple sites of left lower limb, except ankle and foot

√7ᵗʰ **T24.699** Corrosion of second degree of multiple sites of unspecified lower limb, except ankle and foot

√5ᵗʰ **T24.7** Corrosion of third degree of lower limb, except ankle and foot

Code first (T51-T65) to identify chemical and intent

Use additional external cause code to identify place (Y92)

√6ᵗʰ **T24.70** Corrosion of third degree of unspecified site of lower limb, except ankle and foot

7 √7ᵗʰ **T24.701** Corrosion of third degree of unspecified site of right lower limb, except ankle and foot　　CC

CC Excl: CC with 7th character A: See code: T24.301

7 √7ᵗʰ **T24.702** Corrosion of third degree of unspecified site of left lower limb, except ankle and foot　　CC

CC Excl: See code: T24.301

7 √7ᵗʰ **T24.709** Corrosion of third degree of unspecified site of unspecified lower limb, except ankle and foot　　CC

CC Excl: See code: T24.301

√6ᵗʰ **T24.71** Corrosion of third degree of thigh

7 √7ᵗʰ **T24.711** Corrosion of third degree of right thigh　　CC

CC Excl: CC with 7th character A: See code: T24.311

7 √7ᵗʰ **T24.712** Corrosion of third degree of left thigh　　CC

CC Excl: See code: T24.311

7 √7ᵗʰ **T24.719** Corrosion of third degree of unspecified thigh　　CC

CC Excl: See code: T24.311

√6ᵗʰ **T24.72** Corrosion of third degree of knee

7 √7ᵗʰ **T24.721** Corrosion of third degree of right knee　　CC

CC Excl: CC with 7th character A: See code: T24.321

7 √7ᵗʰ **T24.722** Corrosion of third degree of left knee　　CC

CC Excl: See code: T24.321

7 √7ᵗʰ **T24.729** Corrosion of third degree of unspecified knee　　CC

CC Excl: See code: T24.321

√6ᵗʰ **T24.73** Corrosion of third degree of lower leg

7 √7ᵗʰ **T24.731** Corrosion of third degree of right lower leg　　CC

CC Excl: CC with 7th character A: See code: T24.331

7 √7ᵗʰ **T24.732** Corrosion of third degree of left lower leg　　CC

CC Excl: See code: T24.331

7 √7ᵗʰ **T24.739** Corrosion of third degree of unspecified lower leg　　CC

CC Excl: See code: T24.331

√6ᵗʰ **T24.79** Corrosion of third degree of multiple sites of lower limb, except ankle and foot

7 √7ᵗʰ **T24.791** Corrosion of third degree of multiple sites of right lower limb, except ankle and foot　　CC

CC Excl: CC with 7th character A: See code: T24.301

7 √7ᵗʰ **T24.792** Corrosion of third degree of multiple sites of left lower limb, except ankle and foot　　CC

CC Excl: See code: T24.301

7 √7ᵗʰ **T24.799** Corrosion of third degree of multiple sites of unspecified lower limb, except ankle and foot　　CC

CC Excl: See code: T24.301

√4ᵗʰ **T25** Burn and corrosion of ankle and foot

The appropriate 7th character is to be added to each code from category T25.
A　initial encounter
D　subsequent encounter
S　sequela

√5ᵗʰ **T25.0** Burn of unspecified degree of ankle and foot

Use additional external cause code to identify the source, place and intent of the burn (X00-X19, X75-X77, X96-X98, Y92)

√6ᵗʰ **T25.01** Burn of unspecified degree of ankle

√7ᵗʰ **T25.011** Burn of unspecified degree of right ankle

√7ᵗʰ **T25.012** Burn of unspecified degree of left ankle

√7ᵗʰ **T25.019** Burn of unspecified degree of unspecified ankle

√6ᵗʰ **T25.02** Burn of unspecified degree of foot

EXCLUDES 2　*burn of unspecified degree of toe(s) (nail) (T25.03-)*

√7ᵗʰ **T25.021** Burn of unspecified degree of right foot

√7ᵗʰ **T25.022** Burn of unspecified degree of left foot

√7ᵗʰ **T25.029** Burn of unspecified degree of unspecified foot

√6ᵗʰ **T25.03** Burn of unspecified degree of toe(s) (nail)

√7ᵗʰ **T25.031** Burn of unspecified degree of right toe(s) (nail)

√7ᵗʰ **T25.032** Burn of unspecified degree of left toe(s) (nail)

√7ᵗʰ **T25.039** Burn of unspecified degree of unspecified toe(s) (nail)

√6ᵗʰ **T25.09** Burn of unspecified degree of multiple sites of ankle and foot

√7ᵗʰ **T25.091** Burn of unspecified degree of multiple sites of right ankle and foot

√7ᵗʰ **T25.092** Burn of unspecified degree of multiple sites of left ankle and foot

√7ᵗʰ **T25.099** Burn of unspecified degree of multiple sites of unspecified ankle and foot

√5ᵗʰ **T25.1** Burn of first degree of ankle and foot

Use additional external cause code to identify the source, place and intent of the burn (X00-X19, X75-X77, X96-X98, Y92)

√6ᵗʰ **T25.11** Burn of first degree of ankle

√7ᵗʰ **T25.111** Burn of first degree of right ankle

√7ᵗʰ **T25.112** Burn of first degree of left ankle

√7ᵗʰ **T25.119** Burn of first degree of unspecified ankle

√6ᵗʰ **T25.12** Burn of first degree of foot

EXCLUDES 2　*burn of first degree of toe(s) (nail) (T25.13-)*

√7ᵗʰ **T25.121** Burn of first degree of right foot

√7ᵗʰ **T25.122** Burn of first degree of left foot

√7ᵗʰ **T25.129** Burn of first degree of unspecified foot

√6ᵗʰ **T25.13** Burn of first degree of toe(s) (nail)

√7ᵗʰ **T25.131** Burn of first degree of right toe(s) (nail)

√7ᵗʰ **T25.132** Burn of first degree of left toe(s) (nail)

√7ᵗʰ **T25.139** Burn of first degree of unspecified toe(s) (nail)

√6ᵗʰ **T25.19** Burn of first degree of multiple sites of ankle and foot

√7ᵗʰ **T25.191** Burn of first degree of multiple sites of right ankle and foot

---

7 HAC = Initial encounter only (7th character A, B or C) and not POA.

☑ Additional Character Required　　√x7ᵗʰ Xtension Alert　　Unacceptable PDx　　Manifestation　　Hospital Acquired Condition　　EXCLUDES 1 Not Coded Here　　EXCLUDES 2 Not Included Here

Injury, Poisoning and Certain Other Consequences of External Causes

T25.192–T25.539

√7ᵗʰ **T25.192** Burn of first degree of multiple sites of left ankle and foot

√7ᵗʰ **T25.199** Burn of first degree of multiple sites of unspecified ankle and foot

√5ᵗʰ **T25.2** Burn of second degree of ankle and foot
   Use additional external cause code to identify the source, place and intent of the burn (X00-X19, X75-X77, X96-X98, Y92)

   √6ᵗʰ **T25.21** Burn of second degree of ankle
      √7ᵗʰ **T25.211** Burn of second degree of right ankle
      √7ᵗʰ **T25.212** Burn of second degree of left ankle
      √7ᵗʰ **T25.219** Burn of second degree of unspecified ankle

   √6ᵗʰ **T25.22** Burn of second degree of foot
      EXCLUDES 2 burn of second degree of toe(s) (nail) (T25.23-)
      √7ᵗʰ **T25.221** Burn of second degree of right foot
      √7ᵗʰ **T25.222** Burn of second degree of left foot
      √7ᵗʰ **T25.229** Burn of second degree of unspecified foot

   √6ᵗʰ **T25.23** Burn of second degree of toe(s) (nail)
      √7ᵗʰ **T25.231** Burn of second degree of right toe(s) (nail)
      √7ᵗʰ **T25.232** Burn of second degree of left toe(s) (nail)
      √7ᵗʰ **T25.239** Burn of second degree of unspecified toe(s) (nail)

   √6ᵗʰ **T25.29** Burn of second degree of multiple sites of ankle and foot
      √7ᵗʰ **T25.291** Burn of second degree of multiple sites of right ankle and foot
      √7ᵗʰ **T25.292** Burn of second degree of multiple sites of left ankle and foot
      √7ᵗʰ **T25.299** Burn of second degree of multiple sites of unspecified ankle and foot

√5ᵗʰ **T25.3** Burn of third degree of ankle and foot
   Use additional external cause code to identify the source, place and intent of the burn (X00-X19, X75-X77, X96-X98, Y92)

   √6ᵗʰ **T25.31** Burn of third degree of ankle
      7 √7ᵗʰ **T25.311** Burn of third degree of right ankle   CC
         CC Excl: CC with 7th character A: T24.301-T24.309 with 7th A, T24.391-T24.399 with 7th A, T24.701-T24.709 with 7th A, T24.791-T24.799 with 7th A, T25.311-T25.319 with 7th A, T25.391-T25.399 with 7th A, T25.711-T25.719 with 7th A, T25.791-T25.790 with 7th A
      7 √7ᵗʰ **T25.312** Burn of third degree of left ankle   CC
         CC Excl: See code: T25.311
      7 √7ᵗʰ **T25.319** Burn of third degree of unspecified ankle   CC
         CC Excl: See code: T25.311

   √6ᵗʰ **T25.32** Burn of third degree of foot
      EXCLUDES 2 burn of third degree of toe(s) (nail) (T25.33-)
      7 √7ᵗʰ **T25.321** Burn of third degree of right foot   CC
         CC Excl: CC with 7th character A: T24.301-T24.309 with 7th A, T24.391-T24.399 with 7th A, T24.701-T24.709 with 7th A, T24.791-T24.799 with 7th A, T25.321-T25.329 with 7th A, T25.391-T25.399 with 7th A, T25.721-T25.729 with 7th A, T25.791-T25.799 with 7th A
      7 √7ᵗʰ **T25.322** Burn of third degree of left foot   CC
         CC Excl: See code: T25.321
      7 √7ᵗʰ **T25.329** Burn of third degree of unspecified foot   CC
         CC Excl: See code: T25.321

   √6ᵗʰ **T25.33** Burn of third degree of toe(s) (nail)
      7 √7ᵗʰ **T25.331** Burn of third degree of right toe(s) (nail)   CC
         CC Excl: CC with 7th character A: T24.301-T24.309 with 7th A, T24.391-T24.399 with 7th A, T24.701-T24.709 with 7th A, T24.791-T24.799 with 7th A, T25.331-T25.339 with 7th A, T25.391-T25.399 with 7th A, T25.731-T25.739 with 7th A, T25.791-T25.799 with 7th A
      7 √7ᵗʰ **T25.332** Burn of third degree of left toe(s) (nail)   CC
         CC Excl: See code: T25.331

7 √7ᵗʰ **T25.339** Burn of third degree of unspecified toe(s) (nail)   CC
   CC Excl: See code: T25.331

√6ᵗʰ **T25.39** Burn of third degree of multiple sites of ankle and foot
   7 √7ᵗʰ **T25.391** Burn of third degree of multiple sites of right ankle and foot   CC
      CC Excl: CC with 7th character A: See code: T25.331
   7 √7ᵗʰ **T25.392** Burn of third degree of multiple sites of left ankle and foot   CC
      CC Excl: See code: T25.331
   7 √7ᵗʰ **T25.399** Burn of third degree of multiple sites of unspecified ankle and foot   CC
      CC Excl: See code: T25.331

√5ᵗʰ **T25.4** Corrosion of unspecified degree of ankle and foot
   Code first (T51-T65) to identify chemical and intent
   Use additional external cause code to identify place (Y92)

   √6ᵗʰ **T25.41** Corrosion of unspecified degree of ankle
      √7ᵗʰ **T25.411** Corrosion of unspecified degree of right ankle
      √7ᵗʰ **T25.412** Corrosion of unspecified degree of left ankle
      √7ᵗʰ **T25.419** Corrosion of unspecified degree of unspecified ankle

   √6ᵗʰ **T25.42** Corrosion of unspecified degree of foot
      EXCLUDES 2 corrosion of unspecified degree of toe(s) (nail) (T25.43-)
      √7ᵗʰ **T25.421** Corrosion of unspecified degree of right foot
      √7ᵗʰ **T25.422** Corrosion of unspecified degree of left foot
      √7ᵗʰ **T25.429** Corrosion of unspecified degree of unspecified foot

   √6ᵗʰ **T25.43** Corrosion of unspecified degree of toe(s) (nail)
      √7ᵗʰ **T25.431** Corrosion of unspecified degree of right toe(s) (nail)
      √7ᵗʰ **T25.432** Corrosion of unspecified degree of left toe(s) (nail)
      √7ᵗʰ **T25.439** Corrosion of unspecified degree of unspecified toe(s) (nail)

   √6ᵗʰ **T25.49** Corrosion of unspecified degree of multiple sites of ankle and foot
      √7ᵗʰ **T25.491** Corrosion of unspecified degree of multiple sites of right ankle and foot
      √7ᵗʰ **T25.492** Corrosion of unspecified degree of multiple sites of left ankle and foot
      √7ᵗʰ **T25.499** Corrosion of unspecified degree of multiple sites of unspecified ankle and foot

√5ᵗʰ **T25.5** Corrosion of first degree of ankle and foot
   Code first (T51-T65) to identify chemical and intent
   Use additional external cause code to identify place (Y92)

   √6ᵗʰ **T25.51** Corrosion of first degree of ankle
      √7ᵗʰ **T25.511** Corrosion of first degree of right ankle
      √7ᵗʰ **T25.512** Corrosion of first degree of left ankle
      √7ᵗʰ **T25.519** Corrosion of first degree of unspecified ankle

   √6ᵗʰ **T25.52** Corrosion of first degree of foot
      EXCLUDES 2 corrosion of first degree of toe(s) (nail) (T25.53-)
      √7ᵗʰ **T25.521** Corrosion of first degree of right foot
      √7ᵗʰ **T25.522** Corrosion of first degree of left foot
      √7ᵗʰ **T25.529** Corrosion of first degree of unspecified foot

   √6ᵗʰ **T25.53** Corrosion of first degree of toe(s) (nail)
      √7ᵗʰ **T25.531** Corrosion of first degree of right toe(s) (nail)
      √7ᵗʰ **T25.532** Corrosion of first degree of left toe(s) (nail)
      √7ᵗʰ **T25.539** Corrosion of first degree of unspecified toe(s) (nail)

---

7 HAC = Initial encounter only (7th character A, B or C) and not POA.

√6th **T25.59** **Corrosion of first degree of** multiple sites **of ankle and foot**

  7 √7th **T25.591** Corrosion of first degree of multiple sites of right ankle and foot

  √7th **T25.592** Corrosion of first degree of multiple sites of left ankle and foot

  √7th **T25.599** Corrosion of first degree of multiple sites of unspecified ankle and foot

√5th **T25.6** **Corrosion of** second degree **of ankle and foot**

  Code first (T51-T65) to identify chemical and intent
  Use additional external cause code to identify place (Y92)

  √6th **T25.61** **Corrosion of second degree of** ankle

    √7th **T25.611** Corrosion of second degree of right ankle

    √7th **T25.612** Corrosion of second degree of left ankle

    √7th **T25.619** Corrosion of second degree of unspecified ankle

  √6th **T25.62** **Corrosion of second degree of** foot

    EXCLUDES 2 corrosion of second degree of toe(s) (nail) (T25.63-)

    √7th **T25.621** Corrosion of second degree of right foot

    √7th **T25.622** Corrosion of second degree of left foot

    √7th **T25.629** Corrosion of second degree of unspecified foot

  √6th **T25.63** **Corrosion of second degree of** toe(s) (nail)

    √7th **T25.631** Corrosion of second degree of right toe(s) (nail)

    √7th **T25.632** Corrosion of second degree of left toe(s) (nail)

    √7th **T25.639** Corrosion of second degree of unspecified toe(s) (nail)

  √6th **T25.69** **Corrosion of second degree of** multiple sites **of ankle and foot**

    √7th **T25.691** Corrosion of second degree of right ankle and foot

    √7th **T25.692** Corrosion of second degree of left ankle and foot

    √7th **T25.699** Corrosion of second degree of unspecified ankle and foot

√5th **T25.7** **Corrosion of** third degree **of ankle and foot**

  Code first (T51-T65) to identify chemical and intent
  Use additional external cause code to identify place (Y92)

  √6th **T25.71** **Corrosion of third degree of** ankle

    7 √7th **T25.711** **Corrosion of third degree of** right **ankle** CC
      CC Excl: CC with 7th character A:
      T24.301-T24.309 with 7th A, T24.391-
      T24.399 with 7th A, T24.701-T24.709 with
      7th A, T24.791-T24.799 with 7th A, T25.311-
      T25.319 with 7th A, T25.391-T25.399 with
      7th A, T25.711-T25.719 with 7th A, T25.791-
      T25.799 with 7th A

    7 √7th **T25.712** **Corrosion of third degree of** left **ankle** CC
      CC Excl: See code: T25.711

    7 √7th **T25.719** **Corrosion of third degree of** unspecified **ankle** CC
      CC Excl: See code: T25.711

  √6th **T25.72** **Corrosion of third degree of** foot

    EXCLUDES 2 corrosion of third degree of toe(s) (nail) (T25.73-)

    7 √7th **T25.721** **Corrosion of third degree of** right **foot** CC
      CC Excl: CC with 7th character A:
      T24.301-T24.309 with 7th A, T24.391-
      T24.399 with 7th A, T24.701-T24.709 with
      7th A, T24.791-T24.799 with 7th A, T25.321-
      T25.329 with 7th A, T25.391-T25.399 with
      7th A, T25.721-T25.729 with 7th A, T25.791-
      T25.799 with 7th A

    7 √7th **T25.722** **Corrosion of third degree of** left **foot** CC
      CC Excl: See code: T25.721

    7 √7th **T25.729** **Corrosion of third degree of** unspecified **foot** CC
      CC Excl: See code: T25.721

  √6th **T25.73** **Corrosion of third degree of** toe(s) (nail)

    7 √7th **T25.731** **Corrosion of third degree of** right **toe(s) (nail)** CC
      CC Excl: CC with 7th character A:
      T24.301-T24.309 with 7th A, T24.391-
      T24.399 with 7th A, T24.701-T24.709 with
      7th A, T24.791-T24.799 with 7th A, T25.331-
      T25.399 with 7th A, T25.731-T25.799 with
      7th A

    7 √7th **T25.732** **Corrosion of third degree of** left **toe(s) (nail)** CC
      CC Excl: See code: T25.731

    7 √7th **T25.739** **Corrosion of third degree of** unspecified **toe(s) (nail)** CC
      CC Excl: See code: T25.731

  √6th **T25.79** **Corrosion of third degree of** multiple sites **of ankle and foot**

    7 √7th **T25.791** **Corrosion of third degree of multiple sites of** right **ankle and foot** CC
      CC Excl: CC with 7th character A:
      T24.301-T24.309 with 7th A, T24.391-
      T24.399 with 7th A, T24.701-T24.709 with
      7th A, T24.791-T24.799 with 7th A, T25.391-
      T25.399 with 7th A, T25.791-T25.799 with
      7th A

    7 √7th **T25.792** **Corrosion of third degree of multiple sites of** left **ankle and foot** CC
      CC Excl: See code: T25.791

    7 √7th **T25.799** **Corrosion of third degree of multiple sites of** unspecified **ankle and foot** CC
      CC Excl: See code: T25.791

Burns and corrosions confined to eye and internal organs (T26-T28)

√4th **T26** **Burn and corrosion confined to eye and adnexa**

  The appropriate 7th character is to be added to each code from category T26.
  A   initial encounter
  D   subsequent encounter
  S   sequela

  √5th **T26.0** **Burn of** eyelid and periocular area
    Use additional external cause code to identify the source, place and intent of the burn (X00-X19, X75-X77, X96-X98, Y92)

    √x7th **T26.00** Burn of unspecified eyelid and periocular area

    √x7th **T26.01** Burn of right eyelid and periocular area

    √x7th **T26.02** Burn of left eyelid and periocular area

  √5th **T26.1** **Burn of** cornea and conjunctival sac
    Use additional external cause code to identify the source, place and intent of the burn (X00-X19, X75-X77, X96-X98, Y92)

    √x7th **T26.10** Burn of cornea and conjunctival sac, unspecified eye

    √x7th **T26.11** Burn of cornea and conjunctival sac, right eye

    √x7th **T26.12** Burn of cornea and conjunctival sac, left eye

  √5th **T26.2** **Burn with resulting** rupture and destruction of eyeball
    Use additional external cause code to identify the source, place and intent of the burn (X00-X19, X75-X77, X96-X98, Y92)

    7 √x7th **T26.20** **Burn with resulting rupture and destruction of** unspecified **eyeball** CC
      CC Excl: No Excl

    7 √x7th **T26.21** **Burn with resulting rupture and destruction of** right **eyeball** CC
      CC Excl: No Excl

    7 √x7th **T26.22** **Burn with resulting rupture and destruction of** left **eyeball** CC
      CC Excl: No Excl

  √5th **T26.3** **Burns of** other specified parts **of eye and adnexa**
    Use additional external cause code to identify the source, place and intent of the burn (X00-X19, X75-X77, X96-X98, Y92)

    √x7th **T26.30** Burns of other specified parts of unspecified eye and adnexa

    √x7th **T26.31** Burns of other specified parts of right eye and adnexa

    √x7th **T26.32** Burns of other specified parts of left eye and adnexa

7 HAC = Initial encounter only (7th character A, B or C) and not POA.

√ Additional Character Required   √x7th Xtension Alert   Unacceptable PDx   Manifestation   Hospital Acquired Condition   EXCLUDES 1 Not Coded Here   EXCLUDES 2 Not Included Here
ICD-10-CM Draft (2015)   1049

Injury, Poisoning and Certain Other Consequences of External Causes   **T26.4-T31.20**

√5ᵗʰ **T26.4 Burn of eye and adnexa, part unspecified**
Use additional external cause code to identify the source, place and intent of the burn (X00-X19, X75-X77, X96-X98, Y92)

√x7ᵗʰ **T26.40 Burn of unspecified eye and adnexa, part unspecified**

√x7ᵗʰ **T26.41 Burn of right eye and adnexa, part unspecified**

√x7ᵗʰ **T26.42 Burn of left eye and adnexa, part unspecified**

√5ᵗʰ **T26.5 Corrosion of eyelid and periocular area**
Code first (T51-T65) to identify chemical and intent
Use additional external cause code to identify place (Y92)

√x7ᵗʰ **T26.50 Corrosion of unspecified eyelid and periocular area**

√x7ᵗʰ **T26.51 Corrosion of right eyelid and periocular area**

√x7ᵗʰ **T26.52 Corrosion of left eyelid and periocular area**

√5ᵗʰ **T26.6 Corrosion of cornea and conjunctival sac**
Code first (T51-T65) to identify chemical and intent
Use additional external cause code to identify place (Y92)

√x7ᵗʰ **T26.60 Corrosion of cornea and conjunctival sac, unspecified eye**

√x7ᵗʰ **T26.61 Corrosion of cornea and conjunctival sac, right eye**

√x7ᵗʰ **T26.62 Corrosion of cornea and conjunctival sac, left eye**

√5ᵗʰ **T26.7 Corrosion with resulting rupture and destruction of eyeball**
Code first (T51-T65) to identify chemical and intent
Use additional external cause code to identify place (Y92)

7 √x7ᵗʰ **T26.70 Corrosion with resulting rupture and destruction of unspecified eyeball** CC
CC Excl: No Excl

7 √x7ᵗʰ **T26.71 Corrosion with resulting rupture and destruction of right eyeball** CC
CC Excl: No Excl

7 √x7ᵗʰ **T26.72 Corrosion with resulting rupture and destruction of left eyeball** CC
CC Excl: No Excl

√5ᵗʰ **T26.8 Corrosions of other specified parts of eye and adnexa**
Code first (T51-T65) to identify chemical and intent
Use additional external cause code to identify place (Y92)

√x7ᵗʰ **T26.80 Corrosions of other specified parts of unspecified eye and adnexa**

√x7ᵗʰ **T26.81 Corrosions of other specified parts of right eye and adnexa**

√x7ᵗʰ **T26.82 Corrosions of other specified parts of left eye and adnexa**

√5ᵗʰ **T26.9 Corrosion of eye and adnexa, part unspecified**
Code first (T51-T65) to identify chemical and intent
Use additional external cause code to identify place (Y92)

√x7ᵗʰ **T26.90 Corrosion of unspecified eye and adnexa, part unspecified**

√x7ᵗʰ **T26.91 Corrosion of right eye and adnexa, part unspecified**

√x7ᵗʰ **T26.92 Corrosion of left eye and adnexa, part unspecified**

√4ᵗʰ **T27 Burn and corrosion of respiratory tract**
Use additional external cause code to identify the source and intent of the burn (X00-X19, X75-X77, X96-X98)
Use additional external cause code to identify place (Y92)

The appropriate 7th character is to be added to each code from category T27.
A   initial encounter
D   subsequent encounter
S   sequela

CC Excl: For CC codes in subcategory T27: CC with 7th character A: T27.0XX-T27.7XX with 7th A, T28.3XX-T28.49X with 7th A, T28.8XX-T28.99X with 7th A

7 √x7ᵗʰ **T27.0 Burn of larynx and trachea** CC

7 √x7ᵗʰ **T27.1 Burn involving larynx and trachea with lung** CC

7 √x7ᵗʰ **T27.2 Burn of other parts of respiratory tract** CC
Burn of thoracic cavity

7 √x7ᵗʰ **T27.3 Burn of respiratory tract, part unspecified** CC
Code first (T51-T65) to identify chemical and intent for codes T27.4-T27.7

7 √x7ᵗʰ **T27.4 Corrosion of larynx and trachea** CC

7 √x7ᵗʰ **T27.5 Corrosion involving larynx and trachea with lung** CC

7 √x7ᵗʰ **T27.6 Corrosion of other parts of respiratory tract** CC

7 √x7ᵗʰ **T27.7 Corrosion of respiratory tract, part unspecified** CC

√4ᵗʰ **T28 Burn and corrosion of other internal organs**
Use additional external cause code to identify the source and intent of the burn (X00- X19, X75-X77, X96-X98)
Use additional external cause code to identify place (Y92)

The appropriate 7th character is to be added to each code from category T28.
A   initial encounter
D   subsequent encounter
S   sequela

√x7ᵗʰ **T28.0 Burn of mouth and pharynx**

7 √x7ᵗʰ **T28.1 Burn of esophagus** CC
CC Excl: CC with 7th character A: T28.1XXA, T28.3XX-T28.49X with 7th A, T28.6XXA, T28.8XX-T28.99X with 7th A

7 √x7ᵗʰ **T28.2 Burn of other parts of alimentary tract** CC
CC Excl: CC with 7th character A: T28.2XX-T28.49X with 7th A, T28.7XX-T28.99X with 7th A

√x7ᵗʰ **T28.3 Burn of internal genitourinary organs**

√5ᵗʰ **T28.4 Burns of other and unspecified internal organs**

√x7ᵗʰ **T28.40 Burn of unspecified internal organ**

√6ᵗʰ **T28.41 Burn of ear drum**

√7ᵗʰ **T28.411 Burn of right ear drum**

√7ᵗʰ **T28.412 Burn of left ear drum**

√7ᵗʰ **T28.419 Burn of unspecified ear drum**

√x7ᵗʰ **T28.49 Burn of other internal organ**
Code first (T51-T65) to identify chemical and intent for T28.5-T28.9-

√x7ᵗʰ **T28.5 Corrosion of mouth and pharynx**

7 √x7ᵗʰ **T28.6 Corrosion of esophagus** CC
CC Excl: CC with 7th character A: T28.1XXA, T28.3XX-T28.49X with 7th A, T28.6XXA, T28.8XX-T28.99X with 7th A

7 √x7ᵗʰ **T28.7 Corrosion of other parts of alimentary tract** CC
CC Excl: CC with 7th character A: T28.2XX-T28.49X with 7th A, T28.7XX-T28.99X with 7th A

√x7ᵗʰ **T28.8 Corrosion of internal genitourinary organs**

√5ᵗʰ **T28.9 Corrosions of other and unspecified internal organs**

√x7ᵗʰ **T28.90 Corrosions of unspecified internal organs**

√6ᵗʰ **T28.91 Corrosions of ear drum**

√7ᵗʰ **T28.911 Corrosions of right ear drum**

√7ᵗʰ **T28.912 Corrosions of left ear drum**

√7ᵗʰ **T28.919 Corrosions of unspecified ear drum**

√x7ᵗʰ **T28.99 Corrosions of other internal organs**

Burns and corrosions of multiple and unspecified body regions (T30-T32)

√4ᵗʰ **T30 Burn and corrosion, body region unspecified**

T30.0 Burn of unspecified body region, unspecified degree
NOTE This code is not for inpatient use. Code to specified site and degree of burns.
Burn NOS   Multiple burns NOS

T30.4 Corrosion of unspecified body region, unspecified degree
NOTE This code is not for inpatient use. Code to specified site and degree of corrosion.
Corrosion NOS   Multiple corrosion NOS

√4ᵗʰ **T31 Burns classified according to extent of body surface involved**
NOTE This category is to be used as the primary code only when the site of the burn is unspecified. It should be used as a supplementary code with categories T20-T25 when the site is specified.

CC Excl: For CC codes in category T31: CC or MCC as indicated with 7th A, unless otherwise noted: T31.0-T32.99

T31.0 Burns involving less than 10% of body surface

√5ᵗʰ **T31.1 Burns involving 10-19% of body surface**

T31.10 Burns involving 10-19% of body surface with 0% to 9% third degree burns CC
Burns involving 10-19% of body surface NOS

T31.11 Burns involving 10-19% of body surface with 10-19% third degree burns CC

√5ᵗʰ **T31.2 Burns involving 20-29% of body surface**

T31.20 Burns involving 20-29% of body surface with 0% to 9% third degree burns CC
Burns involving 20-29% of body surface NOS

---

7 HAC = Initial encounter only (7th character A, B or C) and not POA.

T31.21 **Burns involving 20-29% of body surface with 10-19% third degree burns** `MCC`

T31.22 **Burns involving 20-29% of body surface with 20-29% third degree burns** `MCC`

√5ᵗʰ T31.3 **Burns involving 30-39% of body surface**

T31.30 **Burns involving 30-39% of body surface with 0% to 9% third degree burns** `CC`
Burns involving 30-39% of body surface NOS

T31.31 **Burns involving 30-39% of body surface with 10-19% third degree burns** `MCC`

T31.32 **Burns involving 30-39% of body surface with 20-29% third degree burns** `MCC`

T31.33 **Burns involving 30-39% of body surface 30-39% third degree burns** `MCC`

√5ᵗʰ T31.4 **Burns involving 40-49% of body surface**

T31.40 **Burns involving 40-49% of body surface with 0% to 9% third degree burns** `CC`
Burns involving 40-49% of body surface NOS

T31.41 **Burns involving 40-49% of body surface with 10-19% third degree burns** `MCC`

T31.42 **Burns involving 40-49% of body surface with 20-29% third degree burns** `MCC`

T31.43 **Burns involving 40-49% of body surface with 30-39% third degree burns** `MCC`

T31.44 **Burns involving 40-49% of body surface with 40-49% third degree burns** `MCC`

√5ᵗʰ T31.5 **Burns involving 50-59% of body surface**

T31.50 **Burns involving 50-59% of body surface with 0% to 9% third degree burns** `CC`
Burns involving 50-59% of body surface NOS

T31.51 **Burns involving 50-59% of body surface with 10-19% third degree burns** `MCC`

T31.52 **Burns involving 50-59% of body surface with 20-29% third degree burns** `MCC`

T31.53 **Burns involving 50-59% of body surface with 30-39% third degree burns** `MCC`

T31.54 **Burns involving 50-59% of body surface with 40-49% third degree burns** `MCC`

T31.55 **Burns involving 50-59% of body surface with 50-59% third degree burns** `MCC`

√5ᵗʰ T31.6 **Burns involving 60-69% of body surface**

T31.60 **Burns involving 60-69% of body surface with 0% to 9% third degree burns** `CC`
Burns involving 60-69% of body surface NOS

T31.61 **Burns involving 60-69% of body surface with 10-19% third degree burns** `MCC`

T31.62 **Burns involving 60-69% of body surface with 20-29% third degree burns** `MCC`

T31.63 **Burns involving 60-69% of body surface with 30-39% third degree burns** `MCC`

T31.64 **Burns involving 60-69% of body surface with 40-49% third degree burns** `MCC`

T31.65 **Burns involving 60-69% of body surface with 50-59% third degree burns** `MCC`

T31.66 **Burns involving 60-69% of body surface with 60-69% third degree burns** `MCC`

√5ᵗʰ T31.7 **Burns involving 70-79% of body surface**

T31.70 **Burns involving 70-79% of body surface with 0% to 9% third degree burns** `CC`
Burns involving 70-79% of body surface NOS

T31.71 **Burns involving 70-79% of body surface with 10-19% third degree burns** `MCC`

T31.72 **Burns involving 70-79% of body surface with 20-29% third degree burns** `MCC`

T31.73 **Burns involving 70-79% of body surface with 30-39% third degree burns** `MCC`

T31.74 **Burns involving 70-79% of body surface with 40-49% third degree burns** `MCC`

T31.75 **Burns involving 70-79% of body surface with 50-59% third degree burns** `MCC`

T31.76 **Burns involving 70-79% of body surface with 60-69% third degree burns** `MCC`

T31.77 **Burns involving 70-79% of body surface with 70-79% third degree burns** `MCC`

√5ᵗʰ T31.8 **Burns involving 80-89% of body surface**

T31.80 **Burns involving 80-89% of body surface with 0% to 9% third degree burns** `CC`
Burns involving 80-89% of body surface NOS

T31.81 **Burns involving 80-89% of body surface with 10-19% third degree burns** `MCC`

T31.82 **Burns involving 80-89% of body surface with 20-29% third degree burns** `MCC`

T31.83 **Burns involving 80-89% of body surface with 30-39% third degree burns** `MCC`

T31.84 **Burns involving 80-89% of body surface with 40-49% third degree burns** `MCC`

T31.85 **Burns involving 80-89% of body surface with 50-59% third degree burns** `MCC`

T31.86 **Burns involving 80-89% of body surface with 60-69% third degree burns** `MCC`

T31.87 **Burns involving 80-89% of body surface with 70-79% third degree burns** `MCC`

T31.88 **Burns involving 80-89% of body surface with 80-89% third degree burns** `MCC`

√5ᵗʰ T31.9 **Burns involving 90% or more of body surface**

T31.90 **Burns involving 90% or more of body surface with 0% to 9% third degree burns** `CC`
Burns involving 90% or more of body surface NOS

T31.91 **Burns involving 90% or more of body surface with 10-19% third degree burns** `MCC`

T31.92 **Burns involving 90% or more of body surface with 20-29% third degree burns** `MCC`

T31.93 **Burns involving 90% or more of body surface with 30-39% third degree burns** `MCC`

T31.94 **Burns involving 90% or more of body surface with 40-49% third degree burns** `MCC`

T31.95 **Burns involving 90% or more of body surface with 50-59% third degree burns** `MCC`

T31.96 **Burns involving 90% or more of body surface with 60-69% third degree burns** `MCC`

T31.97 **Burns involving 90% or more of body surface with 70-79% third degree burns** `MCC`

T31.98 **Burns involving 90% or more of body surface with 80-89% third degree burns** `MCC`

T31.99 **Burns involving 90% or more of body surface with 90% or more third degree burns** `MCC`

√4ᵗʰ **T32 Corrosions classified according to extent of body surface involved**

> **NOTE** This category is to be used as the primary code only when the site of the corrosion is unspecified. It may be used as a supplementary code with categories T20-T25 when the site is specified.

> **CC Excl:** For CC/MCC codes in category T32: CC or MCC as indicated with 7th A, unless otherwise noted:
> See code: T31

T32.0 **Corrosions involving less than 10% of body surface**

√5ᵗʰ T32.1 **Corrosions involving 10-19% of body surface**

T32.10 **Corrosions involving 10-19% of body surface with 0% to 9% third degree corrosion** `CC`
Corrosions involving 10-19% of body surface NOS

T32.11 **Corrosions involving 10-19% of body surface with 10-19% third degree corrosion** `CC`

√5ᵗʰ T32.2 **Corrosions involving 20-29% of body surface**

T32.20 **Corrosions involving 20-29% of body surface with 0% to 9% third degree corrosion** `CC`

T32.21 **Corrosions involving 20-29% of body surface with 10-19% third degree corrosion** `MCC`

T32.22 **Corrosions involving 20-29% of body surface with 20-29% third degree corrosion** `MCC`

√5ᵗʰ T32.3 **Corrosions involving 30-39% of body surface**

T32.30 **Corrosions involving 30-39% of body surface with 0% to 9% third degree corrosion** `CC`

T32.31 **Corrosions involving 30-39% of body surface with 10-19% third degree corrosion** `MCC`

T32.32 **Corrosions involving 30-39% of body surface with 20-29% third degree corrosion** `MCC`

T32.33 **Corrosions involving 30-39% of body surface with 30-39% third degree corrosion** `MCC`

Injury, Poisoning and Certain Other Consequences of External Causes

✓5ᵗʰ T32.4 Corrosions involving 40-49% of body surface

T32.40 Corrosions involving 40-49% of body surface with 0% to 9% third degree corrosion `CC`

T32.41 Corrosions involving 40-49% of body surface with 10-19% third degree corrosion `MCC`

T32.42 Corrosions involving 40-49% of body surface with 20-29% third degree corrosion `MCC`

T32.43 Corrosions involving 40-49% of body surface with 30-39% third degree corrosion `MCC`

T32.44 Corrosions involving 40-49% of body surface with 40-49% third degree corrosion `MCC`

✓5ᵗʰ T32.5 Corrosions involving 50-59% of body surface

T32.50 Corrosions involving 50-59% of body surface with 0% to 9% third degree corrosion `CC`

T32.51 Corrosions involving 50-59% of body surface with 10-19% third degree corrosion `MCC`

T32.52 Corrosions involving 50-59% of body surface with 20-29% third degree corrosion `MCC`

T32.53 Corrosions involving 50-59% of body surface with 30-39% third degree corrosion `MCC`

T32.54 Corrosions involving 50-59% of body surface with 40-49% third degree corrosion `MCC`

T32.55 Corrosions involving 50-59% of body surface with 50-59% third degree corrosion `MCC`

✓5ᵗʰ T32.6 Corrosions involving 60-69% of body surface

T32.60 Corrosions involving 60-69% of body surface with 0% to 9% third degree corrosion `CC`

T32.61 Corrosions involving 60-69% of body surface with 10-19% third degree corrosion `MCC`

T32.62 Corrosions involving 60-69% of body surface with 20-29% third degree corrosion `MCC`

T32.63 Corrosions involving 60-69% of body surface with 30-39% third degree corrosion `MCC`

T32.64 Corrosions involving 60-69% of body surface with 40-49% third degree corrosion `MCC`

T32.65 Corrosions involving 60-69% of body surface with 50-59% third degree corrosion `MCC`

T32.66 Corrosions involving 60-69% of body surface with 60-69% third degree corrosion `MCC`

✓5ᵗʰ T32.7 Corrosions involving 70-79% of body surface

T32.70 Corrosions involving 70-79% of body surface with 0% to 9% third degree corrosion `CC`

T32.71 Corrosions involving 70-79% of body surface with 10-19% third degree corrosion `MCC`

T32.72 Corrosions involving 70-79% of body surface with 20-29% third degree corrosion `MCC`

T32.73 Corrosions involving 70-79% of body surface with 30-39% third degree corrosion `MCC`

T32.74 Corrosions involving 70-79% of body surface with 40-49% third degree corrosion `MCC`

T32.75 Corrosions involving 70-79% of body surface with 50-59% third degree corrosion `MCC`

T32.76 Corrosions involving 70-79% of body surface with 60-69% third degree corrosion `MCC`

T32.77 Corrosions involving 70-79% of body surface with 70-79% third degree corrosion `MCC`

✓5ᵗʰ T32.8 Corrosions involving 80-89% of body surface

T32.80 Corrosions involving 80-89% of body surface with 0% to 9% third degree corrosion `CC`

T32.81 Corrosions involving 80-89% of body surface with 10-19% third degree corrosion `MCC`

T32.82 Corrosions involving 80-89% of body surface with 20-29% third degree corrosion `MCC`

T32.83 Corrosions involving 80-89% of body surface with 30-39% third degree corrosion `MCC`

T32.84 Corrosions involving 80-89% of body surface with 40-49% third degree corrosion `MCC`

T32.85 Corrosions involving 80-89% of body surface with 50-59% third degree corrosion `MCC`

T32.86 Corrosions involving 80-89% of body surface with 60-69% third degree corrosion `MCC`

T32.87 Corrosions involving 80-89% of body surface with 70-79% third degree corrosion `MCC`

T32.88 Corrosions involving 80-89% of body surface with 80-89% third degree corrosion `MCC`

✓5ᵗʰ T32.9 Corrosions involving 90% or more of body surface

T32.90 Corrosions involving 90% or more of body surface with 0% to 9% third degree corrosion `CC`

T32.91 Corrosions involving 90% or more of body surface with 10-19% third degree corrosion `MCC`

T32.92 Corrosions involving 90% or more of body surface with 20-29% third degree corrosion `MCC`

T32.93 Corrosions involving 90% or more of body surface with 30-39% third degree corrosion `MCC`

T32.94 Corrosions involving 90% or more of body surface with 40-49% third degree corrosion `MCC`

T32.95 Corrosions involving 90% or more of body surface with 50-59% third degree corrosion `MCC`

T32.96 Corrosions involving 90% or more of body surface with 60-69% third degree corrosion `MCC`

T32.97 Corrosions involving 90% or more of body surface with 70-79% third degree corrosion `MCC`

T32.98 Corrosions involving 90% or more of body surface with 80-89% third degree corrosion `MCC`

T32.99 Corrosions involving 90% or more of body surface with 90% or more third degree corrosion `MCC`

Frostbite (T33-T34)

EXCLUDES 2   hypothermia and other effects of reduced temperature (T68, T69-)

✓4ᵗʰ T33 Superficial frostbite

INCLUDES   frostbite with partial thickness skin loss

The appropriate 7th character is to be added to each code from category T33.

A   initial encounter
D   subsequent encounter
S   sequela

✓5ᵗʰ T33.0 Superficial frostbite of head

CC Excl: For CC codes in subcategory T33.0 and T33.1: CC with 7th character A, unless otherwise noted:T33.011-T33.42X with 7th A, T33.60X-T33.72X with 7th A, T33.90X-T34.42X with 7th A, T34.60X-T34.72X with 7th A, T34.90X-T34.99X with 7th A

✓6ᵗʰ T33.01 Superficial frostbite of ear

7 ✓7ᵗʰ **T33.011** Superficial frostbite of right ear `CC`

7 ✓7ᵗʰ **T33.012** Superficial frostbite of left ear `CC`

7 ✓7ᵗʰ **T33.019** Superficial frostbite of unspecified ear `CC`

7 ✓x7ᵗʰ **T33.02** Superficial frostbite of nose `CC`

7 ✓x7ᵗʰ **T33.09** Superficial frostbite of other part of head `CC`

7 ✓x7ᵗʰ **T33.1** Superficial frostbite of neck `CC`
CC Excl: T33.011-T34.99X with 7th A, T69.021-T69.029 with 7th A

7 ✓x7ᵗʰ **T33.2** Superficial frostbite of thorax `CC`
CC Excl: For CC codes in subcategory T33.2: CC with 7th character A, unless otherwise noted: T33.011-T34.99X with 7th A, T69.021-T69.029 with 7th A

7 ✓x7ᵗʰ **T33.3** Superficial frostbite of abdominal wall, lower back and pelvis `CC`
CC Excl: See code: T33.2

✓5ᵗʰ T33.4 Superficial frostbite of arm

EXCLUDES 2   superficial frostbite of wrist and hand (T33.5-)

CC Excl: For CC codes in subcategory T33.4: CC with 7th character A, unless otherwise noted: T33.011-T34.99X with 7th A, T69.021-T69.029 with 7th A

7 ✓x7ᵗʰ **T33.40** Superficial frostbite of unspecified arm `CC`

7 ✓x7ᵗʰ **T33.41** Superficial frostbite of right arm `CC`

7 ✓x7ᵗʰ **T33.42** Superficial frostbite of left arm `CC`

✓5ᵗʰ T33.5 Superficial frostbite of wrist, hand, and fingers

CC Excl: For CC codes in subcategory T33.5: CC with 7th character A, unless otherwise noted: T33.2XX-T33.72X with 7th A, T33.90X-T33.99X with 7th A, T34.2XX-T34.72X with 7th A, T34.90X-T34.99X with 7th A

✓6ᵗʰ T33.51 Superficial frostbite of wrist

7 ✓7ᵗʰ **T33.511** Superficial frostbite of right wrist `CC`

7 ✓7ᵗʰ **T33.512** Superficial frostbite of left wrist `CC`

7 ✓7ᵗʰ **T33.519** Superficial frostbite of unspecified wrist `CC`

---

7 HAC = Initial encounter only (7th character A, B or C) and not POA.

√6th **T33.52** Superficial frostbite of hand
  EXCLUDES 2   superficial frostbite of fingers (T33.53-)
    7   √7th   **T33.521**   **Superficial frostbite of right hand**   CC
    7   √7th   **T33.522**   **Superficial frostbite of left hand**   CC
    7   √7th   **T33.529**   **Superficial frostbite of unspecified hand**   CC

√6th **T33.53** Superficial frostbite of finger(s)
    7   √7th   **T33.531**   **Superficial frostbite of right finger(s)**   CC
    7   √7th   **T33.532**   **Superficial frostbite of left finger(s)**   CC
    7   √7th   **T33.539**   **Superficial frostbite of unspecified finger(s)**   CC

√5th **T33.6** Superficial frostbite of hip and thigh

> **CC Excl:** For CC codes in subcategory T33.6: CC with 7th character A, unless otherwise noted: T33.011-T34.99X with 7th A, T69.021-T69.029 with 7th A

    7   √x7th   **T33.60**   **Superficial frostbite of unspecified hip and thigh**   CC
    7   √x7th   **T33.61**   **Superficial frostbite of right hip and thigh**   CC
    7   √x7th   **T33.62**   **Superficial frostbite of left hip and thigh**   CC

√5th **T33.7** Superficial frostbite of knee and lower leg

> **CC Excl:** For CC codes in subcategory T33.7: CC with 7th character A, unless otherwise noted: See code: T33.6

    EXCLUDES 2   superficial frostbite of ankle and foot (T33.8-)
    7   √x7th   **T33.70**   **Superficial frostbite of unspecified knee and lower leg**   CC
    7   √x7th   **T33.71**   **Superficial frostbite of right knee and lower leg**   CC
    7   √x7th   **T33.72**   **Superficial frostbite of left knee and lower leg**   CC

√5th **T33.8** Superficial frostbite of ankle, foot, and toe(s)

> **CC Excl:** For CC codes in subcategory T33.8: CC with 7th character A, unless otherwise noted: T33.2XX-T33.42X with 7th A, T33.60X-T33.99X with 7th A, T34.2XX-T34.42X with 7th A, T34.60X-T34.99X with 7th A

√6th **T33.81** Superficial frostbite of ankle
    7   √7th   **T33.811**   **Superficial frostbite of right ankle**   CC
    7   √7th   **T33.812**   **Superficial frostbite of left ankle**   CC
    7   √7th   **T33.819**   **Superficial frostbite of unspecified ankle**   CC

√6th **T33.82** Superficial frostbite of foot
    7   √7th   **T33.821**   **Superficial frostbite of right foot**   CC
    7   √7th   **T33.822**   **Superficial frostbite of left foot**   CC
    7   √7th   **T33.829**   **Superficial frostbite of unspecified foot**   CC

√6th **T33.83** Superficial frostbite of toe(s)
    7   √7th   **T33.831**   **Superficial frostbite of right toe(s)**   CC
    7   √7th   **T33.832**   **Superficial frostbite of left toe(s)**   CC
    7   √7th   **T33.839**   **Superficial frostbite of unspecified toe(s)**   CC

√5th **T33.9** Superficial frostbite of other and unspecified sites

> **CC Excl:** For CC codes in subcategory T33.9: CC with 7th character A, unless otherwise noted: T33.011-T34.99X with 7th A, T69.021-T69.029 with 7th A

    7   √x7th   **T33.90**   **Superficial frostbite of unspecified sites**   CC
      Superficial frostbite NOS
    7   √x7th   **T33.99**   **Superficial frostbite of other sites**   CC
      Superficial frostbite of leg NOS
      Superficial frostbite of trunk NOS

√4th **T34** **Frostbite with tissue necrosis**

> The appropriate 7th character is to be added to each code from category T34.
> A   initial encounter
> D   subsequent encounter
> S   sequela

√5th **T34.0** Frostbite with tissue necrosis of head

> **CC Excl:** For CC codes in subcategory T34.0: CC with 7th character A, unless otherwise noted: T33.011-T33.42 with 7th A, T33.60X-T33.72X with 7th A, T33.90X-T34.42X with 7th A, T34.60X-T34.72X with 7th A, T34.90X-T34.99X with 7th A

√6th **T34.01** Frostbite with tissue necrosis of ear

    7   √7th   **T34.011**   **Frostbite with tissue necrosis of right ear**   CC
    7   √7th   **T34.012**   **Frostbite with tissue necrosis of left ear**   CC
    7   √7th   **T34.019**   **Frostbite with tissue necrosis of unspecified ear**   CC

    7   √x7th   **T34.02**   **Frostbite with tissue necrosis of nose**   CC
    7   √x7th   **T34.09**   **Frostbite with tissue necrosis of other part of head**   CC

√x7th **T34.1** Frostbite with tissue necrosis of neck   CC
> **CC Excl:** CC with 7th character A: T33.011-T33.42X with 7th A, T33.60X-T33.72X with 7th A, T33.90X-T34.42X with 7th A, T34.60X-T34.72X with 7th A, T34.90X-T34.99X with 7th A

√x7th **T34.2** Frostbite with tissue necrosis of thorax   CC
> **CC Excl:** CC with 7th character A: T33.011-T34.99X with 7th A, T69.021-T69.029 with 7th A

√x7th **T34.3** Frostbite with tissue necrosis of abdominal wall, lower back and pelvis   CC
> **CC Excl:** CC with 7th character A: See code: T34.2

√5th **T34.4** Frostbite with tissue necrosis of arm
    EXCLUDES 2   frostbite with tissue necrosis of wrist and hand (T34.5-)

> **CC Excl:** For CC codes in subcategory T34.4: CC with 7th character A, unless otherwise noted: See code: T34.2

    7   √x7th   **T34.40**   **Frostbite with tissue necrosis of unspecified arm**   CC
    7   √x7th   **T34.41**   **Frostbite with tissue necrosis of right arm**   CC
    7   √x7th   **T34.42**   **Frostbite with tissue necrosis of left arm**   CC

√5th **T34.5** Frostbite with tissue necrosis of wrist, hand, and finger(s)

> **CC Excl:** For CC codes in subcategory T34.5: CC with 7th character A, unless otherwise noted: T33.2XX-T33.72X with 7th A, T33.90X-T33.99X with 7th A, T34.2XX-T34.72X with 7th A, T34.90X-T34.99X with 7th A

√6th **T34.51** Frostbite with tissue necrosis of wrist
    7   √7th   **T34.511**   **Frostbite with tissue necrosis of right wrist**   CC
    7   √7th   **T34.512**   **Frostbite with tissue necrosis of left wrist**   CC
    7   √7th   **T34.519**   **Frostbite with tissue necrosis of unspecified wrist**   CC

√6th **T34.52** Frostbite with tissue necrosis of hand
    EXCLUDES 2   frostbite with tissue necrosis of finger(s) (T34.53-)
    7   √7th   **T34.521**   **Frostbite with tissue necrosis of right hand**   CC
    7   √7th   **T34.522**   **Frostbite with tissue necrosis of left hand**   CC
    7   √7th   **T34.529**   **Frostbite with tissue necrosis of unspecified hand**   CC

√6th **T34.53** Frostbite with tissue necrosis of finger(s)
    7   √7th   **T34.531**   **Frostbite with tissue necrosis of right finger(s)**   CC
    7   √7th   **T34.532**   **Frostbite with tissue necrosis of left finger(s)**   CC
    7   √7th   **T34.539**   **Frostbite with tissue necrosis of unspecified finger(s)**   CC

√5th **T34.6** Frostbite with tissue necrosis of hip and thigh

> **CC Excl:** For CC codes in subcategory T34.6: CC with 7th character A, unless otherwise noted: T33.011-T34.99X with 7th A, T69.021-T69.029 with 7th A

    7   √x7th   **T34.60**   **Frostbite with tissue necrosis of unspecified hip and thigh**   CC
    7   √x7th   **T34.61**   **Frostbite with tissue necrosis of right hip and thigh**   CC
    7   √x7th   **T34.62**   **Frostbite with tissue necrosis of left hip and thigh**   CC

√5th **T34.7** Frostbite with tissue necrosis of knee and lower leg
    EXCLUDES 2   frostbite with tissue necrosis of ankle and foot (T34.8-)

> **CC Excl:** For CC codes in subcategory T34.7: CC with 7th character A, unless otherwise noted: See code: T34.6

    7   √x7th   **T34.70**   **Frostbite with tissue necrosis of unspecified knee and lower leg**   CC
    7   √x7th   **T34.71**   **Frostbite with tissue necrosis of right knee and lower leg**   CC

---

7 HAC = Initial encounter only (7th character A, B or C) and not POA.

✓ Additional Character Required   √x7th Xtension Alert   Unacceptable PDx   Manifestation   Hospital Acquired Condition   EXCLUDES 1 Not Coded Here   EXCLUDES 2 Not Included Here

Injury, Poisoning and Certain Other Consequences of External Causes

T34.72–T36.3X6

7 ✓x7ᵗʰ **T34.72** Frostbite with tissue necrosis of left knee and lower leg   CC

✓5ᵗʰ **T34.8** Frostbite with tissue necrosis of ankle, foot, and toe(s)

> CC Excl: For CC codes in subcategory T34.8: CC with 7th character A, unless otherwise noted: T33.2XX-T33.42X with 7th A, T33.60X-T33.99X with 7th A, T34.2XX-T34.42X with 7th A, T34.60X-T34.99X with 7th A

✓6ᵗʰ **T34.81** Frostbite with tissue necrosis of ankle

7 ✓7ᵗʰ **T34.811** Frostbite with tissue necrosis of right ankle   CC

7 ✓7ᵗʰ **T34.812** Frostbite with tissue necrosis of left ankle   CC

7 ✓7ᵗʰ **T34.819** Frostbite with tissue necrosis of unspecified ankle   CC

✓6ᵗʰ **T34.82** Frostbite with tissue necrosis of foot

7 ✓7ᵗʰ **T34.821** Frostbite with tissue necrosis of right foot   CC

7 ✓7ᵗʰ **T34.822** Frostbite with tissue necrosis of left foot   CC

7 ✓7ᵗʰ **T34.829** Frostbite with tissue necrosis of unspecified foot   CC

✓6ᵗʰ **T34.83** Frostbite with tissue necrosis of toe(s)

7 ✓7ᵗʰ **T34.831** Frostbite with tissue necrosis of right toe(s)   CC

7 ✓7ᵗʰ **T34.832** Frostbite with tissue necrosis of left toe(s)   CC

7 ✓7ᵗʰ **T34.839** Frostbite with tissue necrosis of unspecified toe(s)   CC

✓5ᵗʰ **T34.9** Frostbite with tissue necrosis of other and unspecified sites

> CC Excl: For CC codes in subcategory T34.9: CC with 7th character A, unless otherwise noted: T33.011-T34.99X with 7th A, T69.021-T69.029 with 7th A

7 ✓x7ᵗʰ **T34.90** Frostbite with tissue necrosis of unspecified sites   CC
Frostbite with tissue necrosis NOS

7 ✓x7ᵗʰ **T34.99** Frostbite with tissue necrosis of other sites   CC
Frostbite with tissue necrosis of leg NOS
Frostbite with tissue necrosis of trunk NOS

Poisoning by, adverse effects of and underdosing of drugs, medicaments and biological substances (T36-T50)

INCLUDES adverse effect of correct substance properly administered
poisoning by overdose of substance
poisoning by wrong substance given or taken in error
underdosing by (inadvertently) (deliberately) taking less substance than prescribed or instructed

Code first, for adverse effects, the nature of the adverse effect, such as:
adverse effect NOS (T88.7)
aspirin gastritis (K29.-)
blood disorders (D56-D76)
contact dermatitis (L23-L25)
dermatitis due to substances taken internally (L27.-)
nephropathy (N14.0-N14.2)

NOTE The drug giving rise to the adverse effect should be identified by use of codes from categories T36-T50 with fifth or sixth character 5.

Use additional code(s) to specify:
manifestations of poisoning
underdosing or failure in dosage during medical and surgical care (Y63.6, Y63.8-Y63.9)
underdosing of medication regimen (Z91.12-, Z91.13-)

EXCLUDES 1 toxic reaction to local anesthesia in pregnancy (O29.3-)
EXCLUDES 2 abuse and dependence of psychoactive substances (F10-F19)
abuse of non-dependence-producing substances (F55.-)
drug reaction and poisoning affecting newborn (P00-P96)
pathological drug intoxication (inebriation) (F10-F19)

✓4ᵗʰ **T36** Poisoning by, adverse effect of and underdosing of systemic antibiotics

EXCLUDES 1 antineoplastic antibiotics (T45.1-)
locally applied antibiotic NEC (T49.0)
topically used antibiotic for ear, nose and throat (T49.6)
topically used antibiotic for eye (T49.5)

> The appropriate 7th character is to be added to each code from category T36.
> A   initial encounter
> D   subsequent encounter
> S   sequela

✓5ᵗʰ **T36.0** Poisoning by, adverse effect of and underdosing of penicillins

✓6ᵗʰ **T36.0X** Poisoning by, adverse effect of and underdosing of penicillins

✓7ᵗʰ **T36.0X1** Poisoning by penicillins, accidental (unintentional)
Poisoning by penicillins NOS

✓7ᵗʰ **T36.0X2** Poisoning by penicillins, intentional self-harm

✓7ᵗʰ **T36.0X3** Poisoning by penicillins, assault

✓7ᵗʰ **T36.0X4** Poisoning by penicillins, undetermined

✓7ᵗʰ **T36.0X5** Adverse effect of penicillins

✓7ᵗʰ **T36.0X6** Underdosing of penicillins

✓5ᵗʰ **T36.1** Poisoning by, adverse effect of and underdosing of cephalosporins and other beta-lactam antibiotics

✓6ᵗʰ **T36.1X** Poisoning by, adverse effect of and underdosing of cephalosporins and other beta-lactam antibiotics

✓7ᵗʰ **T36.1X1** Poisoning by cephalosporins and other beta-lactam antibiotics, accidental (unintentional)
Poisoning by cephalosporins and other beta-lactam antibiotics NOS

✓7ᵗʰ **T36.1X2** Poisoning by cephalosporins and other beta-lactam antibiotics, intentional self-harm

✓7ᵗʰ **T36.1X3** Poisoning by cephalosporins and other beta-lactam antibiotics, assault

✓7ᵗʰ **T36.1X4** Poisoning by cephalosporins and other beta-lactam antibiotics, undetermined

✓7ᵗʰ **T36.1X5** Adverse effect of cephalosporins and other beta-lactam antibiotics

✓7ᵗʰ **T36.1X6** Underdosing of cephalosporins and other beta-lactam antibiotics

✓5ᵗʰ **T36.2** Poisoning by, adverse effect of and underdosing of chloramphenicol group

✓6ᵗʰ **T36.2X** Poisoning by, adverse effect of and underdosing of chloramphenicol group

✓7ᵗʰ **T36.2X1** Poisoning by chloramphenicol group, accidental (unintentional)
Poisoning by chloramphenicol group NOS

✓7ᵗʰ **T36.2X2** Poisoning by chloramphenicol group, intentional self-harm

✓7ᵗʰ **T36.2X3** Poisoning by chloramphenicol group, assault

✓7ᵗʰ **T36.2X4** Poisoning by chloramphenicol group, undetermined

✓7ᵗʰ **T36.2X5** Adverse effect of chloramphenicol group

✓7ᵗʰ **T36.2X6** Underdosing of chloramphenicol group

✓5ᵗʰ **T36.3** Poisoning by, adverse effect of and underdosing of macrolides

✓6ᵗʰ **T36.3X** Poisoning by, adverse effect of and underdosing of macrolides

✓7ᵗʰ **T36.3X1** Poisoning by macrolides, accidental (unintentional)
Poisoning by macrolides NOS

✓7ᵗʰ **T36.3X2** Poisoning by macrolides, intentional self-harm

✓7ᵗʰ **T36.3X3** Poisoning by macrolides, assault

✓7ᵗʰ **T36.3X4** Poisoning by macrolides, undetermined

✓7ᵗʰ **T36.3X5** Adverse effect of macrolides

✓7ᵗʰ **T36.3X6** Underdosing of macrolides

---

7 HAC = Initial encounter only (7th character A, B or C) and not POA.

N Newborn: 0   P Pediatric: 0-17   M Maternity: 12-55   A Adult: 15-124   MCC Major CC Condition   PDx MCC PDx acts as own MCC   CC CC Condition   PDx CC PDx acts as own CC

1054   ICD-10-CM Draft (2015)

√5th **T36.4** **Poisoning by, adverse effect of and underdosing of tetracyclines**

√6th **T36.4X** **Poisoning by, adverse effect of and underdosing of tetracyclines**

√7th **T36.4X1** **Poisoning by tetracyclines, accidental (unintentional)**
Poisoning by tetracyclines NOS

√7th **T36.4X2** **Poisoning by tetracyclines, intentional self-harm**

√7th **T36.4X3** **Poisoning by tetracyclines, assault**

√7th **T36.4X4** **Poisoning by tetracyclines, undetermined**

√7th **T36.4X5** **Adverse effect of tetracyclines**

√7th **T36.4X6** **Underdosing of tetracyclines**

√5th **T36.5** **Poisoning by, adverse effect of and underdosing of aminoglycosides**
Poisoning by, adverse effect of and underdosing of streptomycin

√6th **T36.5X** **Poisoning by, adverse effect of and underdosing of aminoglycosides**

√7th **T36.5X1** **Poisoning by aminoglycosides, accidental (unintentional)**
Poisoning by aminoglycosides NOS

√7th **T36.5X2** **Poisoning by aminoglycosides, intentional self-harm**

√7th **T36.5X3** **Poisoning by aminoglycosides, assault**

√7th **T36.5X4** **Poisoning by aminoglycosides, undetermined**

√7th **T36.5X5** **Adverse effect of aminoglycosides**

√7th **T36.5X6** **Underdosing of aminoglycosides**

√5th **T36.6** **Poisoning by, adverse effect of and underdosing of rifampicins**

√6th **T36.6X** **Poisoning by, adverse effect of and underdosing of rifampicins**

√7th **T36.6X1** **Poisoning by rifampicins, accidental (unintentional)**
Poisoning by rifampicins NOS

√7th **T36.6X2** **Poisoning by rifampicins, intentional self-harm**

√7th **T36.6X3** **Poisoning by rifampicins, assault**

√7th **T36.6X4** **Poisoning by rifampicins, undetermined**

√7th **T36.6X5** **Adverse effect of rifampicins**

√7th **T36.6X6** **Underdosing of rifampicins**

√5th **T36.7** **Poisoning by, adverse effect of and underdosing of antifungal antibiotics, systemically used**

√6th **T36.7X** **Poisoning by, adverse effect of and underdosing of antifungal antibiotics, systemically used**

√7th **T36.7X1** **Poisoning by antifungal antibiotics, systemically used, accidental (unintentional)**
Poisoning by antifungal antibiotics, systemically used NOS

√7th **T36.7X2** **Poisoning by antifungal antibiotics, systemically used, intentional self-harm**

√7th **T36.7X3** **Poisoning by antifungal antibiotics, systemically used, assault**

√7th **T36.7X4** **Poisoning by antifungal antibiotics, systemically used, undetermined**

√7th **T36.7X5** **Adverse effect of antifungal antibiotics, systemically used**

√7th **T36.7X6** **Underdosing of antifungal antibiotics, systemically used**

√5th **T36.8** **Poisoning by, adverse effect of and underdosing of other systemic antibiotics**

√6th **T36.8X** **Poisoning by, adverse effect of and underdosing of other systemic antibiotics**

√7th **T36.8X1** **Poisoning by other systemic antibiotics, accidental (unintentional)**
Poisoning by other systemic antibiotics NOS

√7th **T36.8X2** **Poisoning by other systemic antibiotics, intentional self-harm**

√7th **T36.8X3** **Poisoning by other systemic antibiotics, assault**

√7th **T36.8X4** **Poisoning by other systemic antibiotics, undetermined**

√7th **T36.8X5** **Adverse effect of other systemic antibiotics**

√7th **T36.8X6** **Underdosing of other systemic antibiotics**

√5th **T36.9** **Poisoning by, adverse effect of and underdosing of unspecified systemic antibiotic**

√x7th **T36.91** **Poisoning by unspecified systemic antibiotic, accidental (unintentional)**
Poisoning by systemic antibiotic NOS

√x7th **T36.92** **Poisoning by unspecified systemic antibiotic, intentional self-harm**

√x7th **T36.93** **Poisoning by unspecified systemic antibiotic, assault**

√x7th **T36.94** **Poisoning by unspecified systemic antibiotic, undetermined**

√x7th **T36.95** **Adverse effect of unspecified systemic antibiotic**

√x7th **T36.96** **Underdosing of unspecified systemic antibiotic**

√4th **T37** **Poisoning by, adverse effect of and underdosing of other systemic anti- infectives and antiparasitics**

EXCLUDES 1 *anti-infectives topically used for ear, nose and throat (T49.6-)*
anti-infectives topically used for eye (T49.5-)
locally applied anti-infectives NEC (T49.0-)

The appropriate 7th character is to be added to each code from category T37.
A   initial encounter
D   subsequent encounter
S   sequela

√5th **T37.0** **Poisoning by, adverse effect of and underdosing of sulfonamides**

√6th **T37.0X** **Poisoning by, adverse effect of and underdosing of sulfonamides**

√7th **T37.0X1** **Poisoning by sulfonamides, accidental (unintentional)**
Poisoning by sulfonamides NOS

√7th **T37.0X2** **Poisoning by sulfonamides, intentional self-harm**

√7th **T37.0X3** **Poisoning by sulfonamides, assault**

√7th **T37.0X4** **Poisoning by sulfonamides, undetermined**

√7th **T37.0X5** **Adverse effect of sulfonamides**

√7th **T37.0X6** **Underdosing of sulfonamides**

√5th **T37.1** **Poisoning by, adverse effect of and underdosing of antimycobacterial drugs**

EXCLUDES 1 *rifampicins (T36.6-)*
streptomycin (T36.5-)

√6th **T37.1X** **Poisoning by, adverse effect of and underdosing of antimycobacterial drugs**

√7th **T37.1X1** **Poisoning by antimycobacterial drugs, accidental (unintentional)**
Poisoning by antimycobacterial drugs NOS

√7th **T37.1X2** **Poisoning by antimycobacterial drugs, intentional self-harm**

√7th **T37.1X3** **Poisoning by antimycobacterial drugs, assault**

√7th **T37.1X4** **Poisoning by antimycobacterial drugs, undetermined**

√7th **T37.1X5** **Adverse effect of antimycobacterial drugs**

√7th **T37.1X6** **Underdosing of antimycobacterial drugs**

√5th **T37.2** **Poisoning by, adverse effect of and underdosing of antimalarials and drugs acting on other blood protozoa**

EXCLUDES 1 *hydroxyquinoline derivatives (T37.8-)*

√6th **T37.2X** **Poisoning by, adverse effect of and underdosing of antimalarials and drugs acting on other blood protozoa**

√7th **T37.2X1** **Poisoning by antimalarials and drugs acting on other blood protozoa, accidental (unintentional)**
Poisoning by antimalarials and drugs acting on other blood protozoa NOS

√7th **T37.2X2** **Poisoning by antimalarials and drugs acting on other blood protozoa, intentional self-harm**

√7th **T37.2X3** **Poisoning by antimalarials and drugs acting on other blood protozoa, assault**

☑ Additional Character Required   √x7th Xtension Alert   Unacceptable PDx   Manifestation   Hospital Acquired Condition   **EXCLUDES 1** Not Coded Here   **EXCLUDES 2** Not Included Here

ICD-10-CM Draft (2015) 1055

√7ᵗʰ **T37.2X4** **Poisoning by** antimalarials and drugs acting on other blood protozoa, **undetermined**

√7ᵗʰ **T37.2X5** **Adverse effect** of antimalarials and drugs acting on other blood protozoa

√7ᵗʰ **T37.2X6** **Underdosing** of antimalarials and drugs acting on other blood protozoa

√5ᵗʰ **T37.3** **Poisoning by, adverse effect of and underdosing of** other antiprotozoal drugs

    √6ᵗʰ **T37.3X** **Poisoning by, adverse effect of and underdosing of** other antiprotozoal **drugs**

       √7ᵗʰ **T37.3X1** **Poisoning by** other antiprotozoal drugs, **accidental (unintentional)**
          Poisoning by other antiprotozoal drugs NOS

       √7ᵗʰ **T37.3X2** **Poisoning by** other antiprotozoal drugs, **intentional self-harm**

       √7ᵗʰ **T37.3X3** **Poisoning by** other antiprotozoal drugs, **assault**

       √7ᵗʰ **T37.3X4** **Poisoning by** other antiprotozoal drugs, **undetermined**

       √7ᵗʰ **T37.3X5** **Adverse effect** of other antiprotozoal drugs

       √7ᵗʰ **T37.3X6** **Underdosing** of other antiprotozoal drugs

√5ᵗʰ **T37.4** **Poisoning by, adverse effect of and underdosing of** anthelminthics

    √6ᵗʰ **T37.4X** **Poisoning by, adverse effect of and underdosing of** anthelminthics

       √7ᵗʰ **T37.4X1** **Poisoning by** anthelminthics, **accidental (unintentional)**
          Poisoning by anthelminthics NOS

       √7ᵗʰ **T37.4X2** **Poisoning by** anthelminthics, **intentional self-harm**

       √7ᵗʰ **T37.4X3** **Poisoning by** anthelminthics, **assault**

       √7ᵗʰ **T37.4X4** **Poisoning by** anthelminthics, **undetermined**

       √7ᵗʰ **T37.4X5** **Adverse effect** of anthelminthics

       √7ᵗʰ **T37.4X6** **Underdosing** of anthelminthics

√5ᵗʰ **T37.5** **Poisoning by, adverse effect of and underdosing of** antiviral drugs
    EXCLUDES 1   *amantadine (T42.8-)*
                cytarabine (T45.1-)

    √6ᵗʰ **T37.5X** **Poisoning by, adverse effect of and underdosing of** antiviral drugs

       √7ᵗʰ **T37.5X1** **Poisoning by** antiviral drugs, **accidental (unintentional)**
          Poisoning by antiviral drugs NOS

       √7ᵗʰ **T37.5X2** **Poisoning by** antiviral drugs, **intentional self-harm**

       √7ᵗʰ **T37.5X3** **Poisoning by** antiviral drugs, **assault**

       √7ᵗʰ **T37.5X4** **Poisoning by** antiviral drugs, **undetermined**

       √7ᵗʰ **T37.5X5** **Adverse effect** of antiviral drugs

       √7ᵗʰ **T37.5X6** **Underdosing** of antiviral drugs

√5ᵗʰ **T37.8** **Poisoning by, adverse effect of and underdosing of** other specified systemic anti-infectives and antiparasitics
    Poisoning by, adverse effect of and underdosing of hydroxyquinoline derivatives
    EXCLUDES 1   *antimalarial drugs (T37.2-)*

    √6ᵗʰ **T37.8X** **Poisoning by, adverse effect of and underdosing of** other specified systemic anti-infectives and antiparasitics

       √7ᵗʰ **T37.8X1** **Poisoning by** other specified systemic anti-infectives and antiparasitics, **accidental (unintentional)**
          Poisoning by other specified systemic anti-infectives and antiparasitics NOS

       √7ᵗʰ **T37.8X2** **Poisoning by** other specified systemic anti-infectives and antiparasitics, **intentional self-harm**

       √7ᵗʰ **T37.8X3** **Poisoning by** other specified systemic anti-infectives and antiparasitics, **assault**

       √7ᵗʰ **T37.8X4** **Poisoning by** other specified systemic anti-infectives and antiparasitics, **undetermined**

       √7ᵗʰ **T37.8X5** **Adverse effect** of other specified systemic anti-infectives and antiparasitics

       √7ᵗʰ **T37.8X6** **Underdosing** of other specified systemic anti-infectives and antiparasitics

√5ᵗʰ **T37.9** **Poisoning by, adverse effect of and underdosing of** unspecified systemic anti-infective and antiparasitics

    √×7ᵗʰ **T37.91** **Poisoning by** unspecified systemic anti-infective and antiparasitics, **accidental (unintentional)**
       Poisoning by, adverse effect of and underdosing of systemic anti-infective and antiparasitics NOS

    √×7ᵗʰ **T37.92** **Poisoning by** unspecified systemic anti-infective and antiparasitics, **intentional self-harm**

    √×7ᵗʰ **T37.93** **Poisoning by** unspecified systemic anti-infective and antiparasitics, **assault**

    √×7ᵗʰ **T37.94** **Poisoning by** unspecified systemic anti-infective and antiparasitics, **undetermined**

    √×7ᵗʰ **T37.95** **Adverse effect** of unspecified systemic anti-infective and antiparasitic

    √×7ᵗʰ **T37.96** **Underdosing** of unspecified systemic anti-infectives and antiparasitics

√4ᵗʰ **T38** **Poisoning by, adverse effect of and underdosing of hormones and their synthetic substitutes and antagonists, not elsewhere classified**
    EXCLUDES 1   *mineralocorticoids and their antagonists (T50.0-)*
                oxytocic hormones (T48.0-)
                parathyroid hormones and derivatives (T50.9-)

The appropriate 7th character is to be added to each code from category T38.
A   initial encounter
D   subsequent encounter
S   sequela

√5ᵗʰ **T38.0** **Poisoning by, adverse effect of and underdosing of** glucocorticoids and synthetic analogues
    EXCLUDES 1   *glucocorticoids, topically used (T49.-)*

    √6ᵗʰ **T38.0X** **Poisoning by, adverse effect of and underdosing of** glucocorticoids and synthetic analogues

       √7ᵗʰ **T38.0X1** **Poisoning by** glucocorticoids and synthetic analogues, **accidental (unintentional)**
          Poisoning by glucocorticoids and synthetic analogues NOS

       √7ᵗʰ **T38.0X2** **Poisoning by** glucocorticoids and synthetic analogues, **intentional self-harm**

       √7ᵗʰ **T38.0X3** **Poisoning by** glucocorticoids and synthetic analogues, **assault**

       √7ᵗʰ **T38.0X4** **Poisoning by** glucocorticoids and synthetic analogues, **undetermined**

       √7ᵗʰ **T38.0X5** **Adverse effect** of glucocorticoids and synthetic analogues

       √7ᵗʰ **T38.0X6** **Underdosing** of glucocorticoids and synthetic analogues

√5ᵗʰ **T38.1** **Poisoning by, adverse effect of and underdosing of** thyroid hormones and substitutes

    √6ᵗʰ **T38.1X** **Poisoning by, adverse effect of and underdosing of** thyroid hormones and substitutes

       √7ᵗʰ **T38.1X1** **Poisoning by** thyroid hormones and substitutes, **accidental (unintentional)**
          Poisoning by thyroid hormones and substitutes NOS

       √7ᵗʰ **T38.1X2** **Poisoning by** thyroid hormones and substitutes, **intentional self-harm**

       √7ᵗʰ **T38.1X3** **Poisoning by** thyroid hormones and substitutes, **assault**

       √7ᵗʰ **T38.1X4** **Poisoning by** thyroid hormones and substitutes, **undetermined**

       √7ᵗʰ **T38.1X5** **Adverse effect** of thyroid hormones and substitutes

       √7ᵗʰ **T38.1X6** **Underdosing** of thyroid hormones and substitutes

√5ᵗʰ **T38.2** **Poisoning by, adverse effect of and underdosing of** antithyroid drugs

    √6ᵗʰ **T38.2X** **Poisoning by, adverse effect of and underdosing of** antithyroid drugs

       √7ᵗʰ **T38.2X1** **Poisoning by** antithyroid drugs, **accidental (unintentional)**
          Poisoning by antithyroid drugs NOS

N Newborn: 0   **P** Pediatric: 0-17   **M** Maternity: 12-55   **A** Adult: 15-124   **MCC** Major CC Condition   **PDx MCC** PDx acts as own MCC   **CC** CC Condition   **PDx CC** PDx acts as own CC

1056   ICD-10-CM Draft (2015)

☑7ᵗʰ **T38.2X2** Poisoning by antithyroid drugs, intentional self-harm

☑7ᵗʰ **T38.2X3** Poisoning by antithyroid drugs, assault

☑7ᵗʰ **T38.2X4** Poisoning by antithyroid drugs, undetermined

☑7ᵗʰ **T38.2X5** Adverse effect of antithyroid drugs

☑7ᵗʰ **T38.2X6** Underdosing of antithyroid drugs

☑5ᵗʰ **T38.3** Poisoning by, adverse effect of and underdosing of insulin and oral hypoglycemic [antidiabetic] drugs

  ☑6ᵗʰ **T38.3X** Poisoning by, adverse effect of and underdosing of insulin and oral hypoglycemic [antidiabetic] drugs

    ☑7ᵗʰ **T38.3X1** Poisoning by insulin and oral hypoglycemic [antidiabetic] drugs, accidental (unintentional)
      Poisoning by insulin and oral hypoglycemic [antidiabetic] drugs NOS

    ☑7ᵗʰ **T38.3X2** Poisoning by insulin and oral hypoglycemic [antidiabetic] drugs, intentional self-harm

    ☑7ᵗʰ **T38.3X3** Poisoning by insulin and oral hypoglycemic [antidiabetic] drugs, assault

    ☑7ᵗʰ **T38.3X4** Poisoning by insulin and oral hypoglycemic [antidiabetic] drugs, undetermined

    ☑7ᵗʰ **T38.3X5** Adverse effect of insulin and oral hypoglycemic [antidiabetic] drugs

    ☑7ᵗʰ **T38.3X6** Underdosing of insulin and oral hypoglycemic [antidiabetic] drugs

☑5ᵗʰ **T38.4** Poisoning by, adverse effect of and underdosing of oral contraceptives
  Poisoning by, adverse effect of and underdosing of multiple- and single-ingredient oral contraceptive preparations

  ☑6ᵗʰ **T38.4X** Poisoning by, adverse effect of and underdosing of oral contraceptives

    ☑7ᵗʰ **T38.4X1** Poisoning by oral contraceptives, accidental (unintentional)
      Poisoning by oral contraceptives NOS

    ☑7ᵗʰ **T38.4X2** Poisoning by oral contraceptives, intentional self-harm

    ☑7ᵗʰ **T38.4X3** Poisoning by oral contraceptives, assault

    ☑7ᵗʰ **T38.4X4** Poisoning by oral contraceptives, undetermined

    ☑7ᵗʰ **T38.4X5** Adverse effect of oral contraceptives

    ☑7ᵗʰ **T38.4X6** Underdosing of oral contraceptives

☑5ᵗʰ **T38.5** Poisoning by, adverse effect of and underdosing of other estrogens and progestogens
  Poisoning by, adverse effect of and underdosing of estrogens and progestogens mixtures and substitutes

  ☑6ᵗʰ **T38.5X** Poisoning by, adverse effect of and underdosing of other estrogens and progestogens

    ☑7ᵗʰ **T38.5X1** Poisoning by other estrogens and progestogens, accidental (unintentional)
      Poisoning by other estrogens and progestogens NOS

    ☑7ᵗʰ **T38.5X2** Poisoning by other estrogens and progestogens, intentional self-harm

    ☑7ᵗʰ **T38.5X3** Poisoning by other estrogens and progestogens, assault

    ☑7ᵗʰ **T38.5X4** Poisoning by other estrogens and progestogens, undetermined

    ☑7ᵗʰ **T38.5X5** Adverse effect of other estrogens and progestogens

    ☑7ᵗʰ **T38.5X6** Underdosing of other estrogens and progestogens

☑5ᵗʰ **T38.6** Poisoning by, adverse effect of and underdosing of antigonadotrophins, antiestrogens, antiandrogens, not elsewhere classified
  Poisoning by, adverse effect of and underdosing of tamoxifen

  ☑6ᵗʰ **T38.6X** Poisoning by, adverse effect of and underdosing of antigonadotrophins, antiestrogens, antiandrogens, not elsewhere classified

☑7ᵗʰ **T38.6X1** Poisoning by antigonadotrophins, antiestrogens, antiandrogens, not elsewhere classified, accidental (unintentional)
  Poisoning by antigonadotrophins, antiestrogens, antiandrogens, not elsewhere classified NOS

☑7ᵗʰ **T38.6X2** Poisoning by antigonadotrophins, antiestrogens, antiandrogens, not elsewhere classified, intentional self-harm

☑7ᵗʰ **T38.6X3** Poisoning by antigonadotrophins, antiestrogens, antiandrogens, not elsewhere classified, assault

☑7ᵗʰ **T38.6X4** Poisoning by antigonadotrophins, antiestrogens, antiandrogens, not elsewhere classified, undetermined

☑7ᵗʰ **T38.6X5** Adverse effect of antigonadotrophins, antiestrogens, antiandrogens, not elsewhere classified

☑7ᵗʰ **T38.6X6** Underdosing of antigonadotrophins, antiestrogens, antiandrogens, not elsewhere classified

☑5ᵗʰ **T38.7** Poisoning by, adverse effect of and underdosing of androgens and anabolic congeners

  ☑6ᵗʰ **T38.7X** Poisoning by, adverse effect of and underdosing of androgens and anabolic congeners

    ☑7ᵗʰ **T38.7X1** Poisoning by androgens and anabolic congeners, accidental (unintentional)
      Poisoning by androgens and anabolic congeners NOS

    ☑7ᵗʰ **T38.7X2** Poisoning by androgens and anabolic congeners, intentional self-harm

    ☑7ᵗʰ **T38.7X3** Poisoning by androgens and anabolic congeners, assault

    ☑7ᵗʰ **T38.7X4** Poisoning by androgens and anabolic congeners, undetermined

    ☑7ᵗʰ **T38.7X5** Adverse effect of androgens and anabolic congeners

    ☑7ᵗʰ **T38.7X6** Underdosing of androgens and anabolic congeners

☑5ᵗʰ **T38.8** Poisoning by, adverse effect of and underdosing of other and unspecified hormones and synthetic substitutes

  ☑6ᵗʰ **T38.80** Poisoning by, adverse effect of and underdosing of unspecified hormones and synthetic substitutes

    ☑7ᵗʰ **T38.801** Poisoning by unspecified hormones and synthetic substitutes, accidental (unintentional)
      Poisoning by unspecified hormones and synthetic substitutes NOS

    ☑7ᵗʰ **T38.802** Poisoning by unspecified hormones and synthetic substitutes, intentional self-harm

    ☑7ᵗʰ **T38.803** Poisoning by unspecified hormones and synthetic substitutes, assault

    ☑7ᵗʰ **T38.804** Poisoning by unspecified hormones and synthetic substitutes, undetermined

    ☑7ᵗʰ **T38.805** Adverse effect of unspecified hormones and synthetic substitutes

    ☑7ᵗʰ **T38.806** Underdosing of unspecified hormones and synthetic substitutes

  ☑6ᵗʰ **T38.81** Poisoning by, adverse effect of and underdosing of anterior pituitary [adenohypophyseal] hormones

    ☑7ᵗʰ **T38.811** Poisoning by anterior pituitary [adenohypophyseal] hormones, accidental (unintentional)
      Poisoning by anterior pituitary [adenohypophyseal] hormones NOS

    ☑7ᵗʰ **T38.812** Poisoning by anterior pituitary [adenohypophyseal] hormones, intentional self-harm

    ☑7ᵗʰ **T38.813** Poisoning by anterior pituitary [adenohypophyseal] hormones, assault

    ☑7ᵗʰ **T38.814** Poisoning by anterior pituitary [adenohypophyseal] hormones, undetermined

    ☑7ᵗʰ **T38.815** Adverse effect of anterior pituitary [adenohypophyseal] hormones

---

☑ Additional Character Required   ✓x7ᵗʰ Xtension Alert   Unacceptable PDx   Manifestation   Hospital Acquired Condition   EXCLUDES 1 Not Coded Here   EXCLUDES 2 Not Included Here

ICD-10-CM Draft (2015)   1057

✓7th **T38.816** Underdosing of anterior pituitary [adenohypophyseal] hormones

✓6th **T38.89** Poisoning by, adverse effect of and underdosing of other hormones and synthetic substitutes

    ✓7th **T38.891** Poisoning by other hormones and synthetic substitutes, accidental (unintentional)
        Poisoning by other hormones and synthetic substitutes NOS

    ✓7th **T38.892** Poisoning by other hormones and synthetic substitutes, intentional self-harm

    ✓7th **T38.893** Poisoning by other hormones and synthetic substitutes, assault

    ✓7th **T38.894** Poisoning by other hormones and synthetic substitutes, undetermined

    ✓7th **T38.895** Adverse effect of other hormones and synthetic substitutes

    ✓7th **T38.896** Underdosing of other hormones and synthetic substitutes

✓5th **T38.9** Poisoning by, adverse effect of and underdosing of other and unspecified hormone antagonists

    ✓6th **T38.90** Poisoning by, adverse effect of and underdosing of unspecified hormone antagonists

        ✓7th **T38.901** Poisoning by unspecified hormone antagonists, accidental (unintentional)
           Poisoning by unspecified hormone antagonists NOS

        ✓7th **T38.902** Poisoning by unspecified hormone antagonists, intentional self-harm

        ✓7th **T38.903** Poisoning by unspecified hormone antagonists, assault

        ✓7th **T38.904** Poisoning by unspecified hormone antagonists, undetermined

        ✓7th **T38.905** Adverse effect of unspecified hormone antagonists

        ✓7th **T38.906** Underdosing of unspecified hormone antagonists

    ✓6th **T38.99** Poisoning by, adverse effect of and underdosing of other hormone antagonists

        ✓7th **T38.991** Poisoning by other hormone antagonists, accidental (unintentional)
           Poisoning by other hormone antagonists NOS

        ✓7th **T38.992** Poisoning by other hormone antagonists, intentional self-harm

        ✓7th **T38.993** Poisoning by other hormone antagonists, assault

        ✓7th **T38.994** Poisoning by other hormone antagonists, undetermined

        ✓7th **T38.995** Adverse effect of other hormone antagonists

        ✓7th **T38.996** Underdosing of other hormone antagonists

✓4th **T39** Poisoning by, adverse effect of and underdosing of nonopioid analgesics, antipyretics and antirheumatics

> The appropriate 7th character is to be added to each code from category T39.
> A   initial encounter
> D   subsequent encounter
> S   sequela

✓5th **T39.0** Poisoning by, adverse effect of and underdosing of salicylates

    ✓6th **T39.01** Poisoning by, adverse effect of and underdosing of aspirin
        Poisoning by, adverse effect of and underdosing of acetylsalicylic acid

        ✓7th **T39.011** Poisoning by aspirin, accidental (unintentional)

        ✓7th **T39.012** Poisoning by aspirin, intentional self-harm

        ✓7th **T39.013** Poisoning by aspirin, assault

        ✓7th **T39.014** Poisoning by aspirin, undetermined

        ✓7th **T39.015** Adverse effect of aspirin

        ✓7th **T39.016** Underdosing of aspirin

    ✓6th **T39.09** Poisoning by, adverse effect of and underdosing of other salicylates

        ✓7th **T39.091** Poisoning by salicylates, accidental (unintentional)
           Poisoning by salicylates NOS

        ✓7th **T39.092** Poisoning by salicylates, intentional self-harm

        ✓7th **T39.093** Poisoning by salicylates, assault

        ✓7th **T39.094** Poisoning by salicylates, undetermined

        ✓7th **T39.095** Adverse effect of salicylates

        ✓7th **T39.096** Underdosing of salicylates

✓5th **T39.1** Poisoning by, adverse effect of and underdosing of 4-Aminophenol derivatives

    ✓6th **T39.1X** Poisoning by, adverse effect of and underdosing of 4-Aminophenol derivatives

        ✓7th **T39.1X1** Poisoning by 4-Aminophenol derivatives, accidental (unintentional)
           Poisoning by 4-Aminophenol derivatives NOS

        ✓7th **T39.1X2** Poisoning by 4-Aminophenol derivatives, intentional self-harm

        ✓7th **T39.1X3** Poisoning by 4-Aminophenol derivatives, assault

        ✓7th **T39.1X4** Poisoning by 4-Aminophenol derivatives, undetermined

        ✓7th **T39.1X5** Adverse effect of 4-Aminophenol derivatives

        ✓7th **T39.1X6** Underdosing of 4-Aminophenol derivatives

✓5th **T39.2** Poisoning by, adverse effect of and underdosing of pyrazolone derivatives

    ✓6th **T39.2X** Poisoning by, adverse effect of and underdosing of pyrazolone derivatives

        ✓7th **T39.2X1** Poisoning by pyrazolone derivatives, accidental (unintentional)
           Poisoning by pyrazolone derivatives NOS

        ✓7th **T39.2X2** Poisoning by pyrazolone derivatives, intentional self-harm

        ✓7th **T39.2X3** Poisoning by pyrazolone derivatives, assault

        ✓7th **T39.2X4** Poisoning by pyrazolone derivatives, undetermined

        ✓7th **T39.2X5** Adverse effect of pyrazolone derivatives

        ✓7th **T39.2X6** Underdosing of pyrazolone derivatives

✓5th **T39.3** Poisoning by, adverse effect of and underdosing of other nonsteroidal anti-inflammatory drugs [NSAID]

    ✓6th **T39.31** Poisoning by, adverse effect of and underdosing of propionic acid derivatives
        Poisoning by, adverse effect of and underdosing of fenoprofen
        Poisoning by, adverse effect of and underdosing of flurbiprofen
        Poisoning by, adverse effect of and underdosing of ibuprofen
        Poisoning by, adverse effect of and underdosing of ketoprofen
        Poisoning by, adverse effect of and underdosing of naproxen
        Poisoning by, adverse effect of and underdosing of oxaprozin

        ✓7th **T39.311** Poisoning by propionic acid derivatives, accidental (unintentional)

        ✓7th **T39.312** Poisoning by propionic acid derivatives, intentional self-harm

        ✓7th **T39.313** Poisoning by propionic acid derivatives, assault

        ✓7th **T39.314** Poisoning by propionic acid derivatives, undetermined

        ✓7th **T39.315** Adverse effect of propionic acid derivatives

        ✓7th **T39.316** Underdosing of propionic acid derivatives

N Newborn: 0   P Pediatric: 0-17   M Maternity: 12-55   A Adult: 15-124   MCC Major CC Condition   PDx MCC PDx acts as own MCC   CC CC Condition   PDx CC PDx acts as own CC

1058   ICD-10-CM Draft (2015)

√6ᵗʰ **T39.39** Poisoning by, adverse effect of and underdosing of other nonsteroidal anti-inflammatory drugs [NSAID]

    √7ᵗʰ **T39.391** Poisoning by other nonsteroidal anti-inflammatory drugs [NSAID], accidental (unintentional)
        Poisoning by other nonsteroidal anti-inflammatory drugs NOS

    √7ᵗʰ **T39.392** Poisoning by other nonsteroidal anti-inflammatory drugs [NSAID], intentional self-harm

    √7ᵗʰ **T39.393** Poisoning by other nonsteroidal anti-inflammatory drugs [NSAID], assault

    √7ᵗʰ **T39.394** Poisoning by other nonsteroidal anti-inflammatory drugs [NSAID], undetermined

    √7ᵗʰ **T39.395** Adverse effect of other nonsteroidal anti-inflammatory drugs [NSAID]

    √7ᵗʰ **T39.396** Underdosing of other nonsteroidal anti-inflammatory drugs [NSAID]

√5ᵗʰ **T39.4** Poisoning by, adverse effect of and underdosing of antirheumatics, not elsewhere classified

    EXCLUDES 1   poisoning by, adverse effect of and underdosing of glucocorticoids (T38.0-)
        poisoning by, adverse effect of and underdosing of salicylates (T39.0-)

√6ᵗʰ **T39.4X** Poisoning by, adverse effect of and underdosing of antirheumatics, not elsewhere classified

    √7ᵗʰ **T39.4X1** Poisoning by antirheumatics, not elsewhere classified, accidental (unintentional)
        Poisoning by antirheumatics, not elsewhere classified NOS

    √7ᵗʰ **T39.4X2** Poisoning by antirheumatics, not elsewhere classified, intentional self-harm

    √7ᵗʰ **T39.4X3** Poisoning by antirheumatics, not elsewhere classified, assault

    √7ᵗʰ **T39.4X4** Poisoning by antirheumatics, not elsewhere classified, undetermined

    √7ᵗʰ **T39.4X5** Adverse effect of antirheumatics, not elsewhere classified

    √7ᵗʰ **T39.4X6** Underdosing of antirheumatics, not elsewhere classified

√5ᵗʰ **T39.8** Poisoning by, adverse effect of and underdosing of other nonopioid analgesics and antipyretics, not elsewhere classified

√6ᵗʰ **T39.8X** Poisoning by, adverse effect of and underdosing of other nonopioid analgesics and antipyretics, not elsewhere classified

    √7ᵗʰ **T39.8X1** Poisoning by other nonopioid analgesics and antipyretics, not elsewhere classified, accidental (unintentional)
        Poisoning by other nonopioid analgesics and antipyretics, not elsewhere classified NOS

    √7ᵗʰ **T39.8X2** Poisoning by other nonopioid analgesics and antipyretics, not elsewhere classified, intentional self-harm

    √7ᵗʰ **T39.8X3** Poisoning by other nonopioid analgesics and antipyretics, not elsewhere classified, assault

    √7ᵗʰ **T39.8X4** Poisoning by other nonopioid analgesics and antipyretics, not elsewhere classified, undetermined

    √7ᵗʰ **T39.8X5** Adverse effect of other nonopioid analgesics and antipyretics, not elsewhere classified

    √7ᵗʰ **T39.8X6** Underdosing of other nonopioid analgesics and antipyretics, not elsewhere classified

√5ᵗʰ **T39.9** Poisoning by, adverse effect of and underdosing of unspecified nonopioid analgesic, antipyretic and antirheumatic

    √x7ᵗʰ **T39.91** Poisoning by unspecified nonopioid analgesic, antipyretic and antirheumatic, accidental (unintentional)
        Poisoning by nonopioid analgesic, antipyretic and antirheumatic NOS

    √x7ᵗʰ **T39.92** Poisoning by unspecified nonopioid analgesic, antipyretic and antirheumatic, intentional self-harm

    √x7ᵗʰ **T39.93** Poisoning by unspecified nonopioid analgesic, antipyretic and antirheumatic, assault

    √x7ᵗʰ **T39.94** Poisoning by unspecified nonopioid analgesic, antipyretic and antirheumatic, undetermined

    √x7ᵗʰ **T39.95** Adverse effect of unspecified nonopioid analgesic, antipyretic and antirheumatic

    √x7ᵗʰ **T39.96** Underdosing of unspecified nonopioid analgesic, antipyretic and antirheumatic

√4ᵗʰ **T40** Poisoning by, adverse effect of and underdosing of narcotics and psychodysleptics [hallucinogens]

    EXCLUDES 2   drug dependence and related mental and behavioral disorders due to psychoactive substance use (F10-F19-)

    The appropriate 7th character is to be added to each code from category T40.
    A   initial encounter
    D   subsequent encounter
    S   sequela

√5ᵗʰ **T40.0** Poisoning by, adverse effect of and underdosing of opium

√6ᵗʰ **T40.0X** Poisoning by, adverse effect of and underdosing of opium

    √7ᵗʰ **T40.0X1** Poisoning by opium, accidental (unintentional)
        Poisoning by opium NOS

    √7ᵗʰ **T40.0X2** Poisoning by opium, intentional self-harm

    √7ᵗʰ **T40.0X3** Poisoning by opium, assault

    √7ᵗʰ **T40.0X4** Poisoning by opium, undetermined

    √7ᵗʰ **T40.0X5** Adverse effect of opium

    √7ᵗʰ **T40.0X6** Underdosing of opium

√5ᵗʰ **T40.1** Poisoning by and adverse effect of heroin

√6ᵗʰ **T40.1X** Poisoning by and adverse effect of heroin

    √7ᵗʰ **T40.1X1** Poisoning by heroin, accidental (unintentional)
        Poisoning by heroin NOS

    √7ᵗʰ **T40.1X2** Poisoning by heroin, intentional self-harm

    √7ᵗʰ **T40.1X3** Poisoning by heroin, assault

    √7ᵗʰ **T40.1X4** Poisoning by heroin, undetermined

√5ᵗʰ **T40.2** Poisoning by, adverse effect of and underdosing of other opioids

√6ᵗʰ **T40.2X** Poisoning by, adverse effect of and underdosing of other opioids

    √7ᵗʰ **T40.2X1** Poisoning by other opioids, accidental (unintentional)
        Poisoning by other opioids NOS

    √7ᵗʰ **T40.2X2** Poisoning by other opioids, intentional self-harm

    √7ᵗʰ **T40.2X3** Poisoning by other opioids, assault

    √7ᵗʰ **T40.2X4** Poisoning by other opioids, undetermined

    √7ᵗʰ **T40.2X5** Adverse effect of other opioids

    √7ᵗʰ **T40.2X6** Underdosing of other opioids

√5ᵗʰ **T40.3** Poisoning by, adverse effect of and underdosing of methadone

√6ᵗʰ **T40.3X** Poisoning by, adverse effect of and underdosing of methadone

    √7ᵗʰ **T40.3X1** Poisoning by methadone, accidental (unintentional)
        Poisoning by methadone NOS

    √7ᵗʰ **T40.3X2** Poisoning by methadone, intentional self-harm

    √7ᵗʰ **T40.3X3** Poisoning by methadone, assault

    √7ᵗʰ **T40.3X4** Poisoning by methadone, undetermined

    √7ᵗʰ **T40.3X5** Adverse effect of methadone

    √7ᵗʰ **T40.3X6** Underdosing of methadone

√5ᵗʰ **T40.4** Poisoning by, adverse effect of and underdosing of other synthetic narcotics

√6ᵗʰ **T40.4X** Poisoning by, adverse effect of and underdosing of other synthetic narcotics

    √7ᵗʰ **T40.4X1** Poisoning by other synthetic narcotics, accidental (unintentional)
        Poisoning by other synthetic narcotics NOS

    √7ᵗʰ **T40.4X2** Poisoning by other synthetic narcotics, intentional self-harm

√ Additional Character Required   √x7ᵗʰ Xtension Alert   Unacceptable PDx   Manifestation   Hospital Acquired Condition   EXCLUDES 1 Not Coded Here   EXCLUDES 2 Not Included Here

ICD-10-CM Draft (2015)   1059

Injury, Poisoning and Certain Other Consequences of External Causes

T40.4X3–T41.1X3

√7th **T40.4X3** Poisoning by other synthetic narcotics, assault

√7th **T40.4X4** Poisoning by other synthetic narcotics, undetermined

√7th **T40.4X5** Adverse effect of other synthetic narcotics

√7th **T40.4X6** Underdosing of other synthetic narcotics

√5th **T40.5** Poisoning by, adverse effect of and underdosing of cocaine

√6th **T40.5X** Poisoning by, adverse effect of and underdosing of cocaine

√7th **T40.5X1** Poisoning by cocaine, accidental (unintentional)
Poisoning by cocaine NOS

√7th **T40.5X2** Poisoning by cocaine, intentional self-harm

√7th **T40.5X3** Poisoning by cocaine, assault

√7th **T40.5X4** Poisoning by cocaine, undetermined

√7th **T40.5X5** Adverse effect of cocaine

√7th **T40.5X6** Underdosing of cocaine

√5th **T40.6** Poisoning by, adverse effect of and underdosing of other and unspecified narcotics

√6th **T40.60** Poisoning by, adverse effect of and underdosing of unspecified narcotics

√7th **T40.601** Poisoning by unspecified narcotics, accidental (unintentional)
Poisoning by narcotics NOS

√7th **T40.602** Poisoning by unspecified narcotics, intentional self-harm

√7th **T40.603** Poisoning by unspecified narcotics, assault

√7th **T40.604** Poisoning by unspecified narcotics, undetermined

√7th **T40.605** Adverse effect of unspecified narcotics

√7th **T40.606** Underdosing of unspecified narcotics

√6th **T40.69** Poisoning by, adverse effect of and underdosing of other narcotics

√7th **T40.691** Poisoning by other narcotics, accidental (unintentional)
Poisoning by other narcotics NOS

√7th **T40.692** Poisoning by other narcotics, intentional self-harm

√7th **T40.693** Poisoning by other narcotics, assault

√7th **T40.694** Poisoning by other narcotics, undetermined

√7th **T40.695** Adverse effect of other narcotics

√7th **T40.696** Underdosing of other narcotics

√5th **T40.7** Poisoning by, adverse effect of and underdosing of cannabis (derivatives)

√6th **T40.7X** Poisoning by, adverse effect of and underdosing of cannabis (derivatives)

√7th **T40.7X1** Poisoning by cannabis (derivatives), accidental (unintentional)
Poisoning by cannabis NOS

√7th **T40.7X2** Poisoning by cannabis (derivatives), intentional self-harm

√7th **T40.7X3** Poisoning by cannabis (derivatives), assault

√7th **T40.7X4** Poisoning by cannabis (derivatives), undetermined

√7th **T40.7X5** Adverse effect of cannabis (derivatives)

√7th **T40.7X6** Underdosing of cannabis (derivatives)

√5th **T40.8** Poisoning by and adverse effect of lysergide [LSD]

√6th **T40.8X** Poisoning by and adverse effect of lysergide [LSD]

√7th **T40.8X1** Poisoning by lysergide [LSD], accidental (unintentional)
Poisoning by lysergide [LSD]NOS

√7th **T40.8X2** Poisoning by lysergide [LSD], intentional self-harm

√7th **T40.8X3** Poisoning by lysergide [LSD], assault

√7th **T40.8X4** Poisoning by lysergide [LSD], undetermined

√5th **T40.9** Poisoning by, adverse effect of and underdosing of other and unspecified psychodysleptics [hallucinogens]

√6th **T40.90** Poisoning by, adverse effect of and underdosing of unspecified psychodysleptics [hallucinogens]

√7th **T40.901** Poisoning by unspecified psychodysleptics [hallucinogens], accidental (unintentional)

√7th **T40.902** Poisoning by unspecified psychodysleptics [hallucinogens], intentional self-harm

√7th **T40.903** Poisoning by unspecified psychodysleptics [hallucinogens], assault

√7th **T40.904** Poisoning by unspecified psychodysleptics [hallucinogens], undetermined

√7th **T40.905** Adverse effect of unspecified psychodysleptics [hallucinogens]

√7th **T40.906** Underdosing of unspecified psychodysleptics

√6th **T40.99** Poisoning by, adverse effect of and underdosing of other psychodysleptics [hallucinogens]

√7th **T40.991** Poisoning by other psychodysleptics [hallucinogens], accidental (unintentional)
Poisoning by other psychodysleptics [hallucinogens] NOS

√7th **T40.992** Poisoning by other psychodysleptics [hallucinogens], intentional self-harm

√7th **T40.993** Poisoning by other psychodysleptics [hallucinogens], assault

√7th **T40.994** Poisoning by other psychodysleptics [hallucinogens], undetermined

√7th **T40.995** Adverse effect of other psychodysleptics [hallucinogens]

√7th **T40.996** Underdosing of other psychodysleptics

√4th **T41** Poisoning by, adverse effect of and underdosing of anesthetics and therapeutic gases

EXCLUDES 1   benzodiazepines (T42.4-)
cocaine (T40.5-)
complications of anesthesia during labor and delivery (O74.-)
complications of anesthesia during pregnancy (O29.-)
complications of anesthesia during the puerperium (O89.-)
opioids (T40.0-T40.2-)

> The appropriate 7th character is to be added to each code from category T41.
> A   initial encounter
> D   subsequent encounter
> S   sequela

√5th **T41.0** Poisoning by, adverse effect of and underdosing of inhaled anesthetics

EXCLUDES 1   oxygen (T41.5-)

√6th **T41.0X** Poisoning by, adverse effect of and underdosing of inhaled anesthetics

√7th **T41.0X1** Poisoning by inhaled anesthetics, accidental (unintentional)
Poisoning by inhaled anesthetics NOS

√7th **T41.0X2** Poisoning by inhaled anesthetics, intentional self-harm

√7th **T41.0X3** Poisoning by inhaled anesthetics, assault

√7th **T41.0X4** Poisoning by inhaled anesthetics, undetermined

√7th **T41.0X5** Adverse effect of inhaled anesthetics

√7th **T41.0X6** Underdosing of inhaled anesthetics

√5th **T41.1** Poisoning by, adverse effect of and underdosing of intravenous anesthetics
Poisoning by, adverse effect of and underdosing of thiobarbiturates

√6th **T41.1X** Poisoning by, adverse effect of and underdosing of intravenous anesthetics

√7th **T41.1X1** Poisoning by intravenous anesthetics, accidental (unintentional)
Poisoning by intravenous anesthetics NOS

√7th **T41.1X2** Poisoning by intravenous anesthetics, intentional self-harm

√7th **T41.1X3** Poisoning by intravenous anesthetics, assault

N Newborn: 0   P Pediatric: 0-17   M Maternity: 12-55   A Adult: 15-124   MCC Major CC Condition   PDx MCC PDx acts as own MCC   CC CC Condition   PDx CC PDx acts as own CC

1060   ICD-10-CM Draft (2015)

√7ᵗʰ **T41.1X4** Poisoning by intravenous anesthetics, undetermined

√7ᵗʰ **T41.1X5** Adverse effect of intravenous anesthetics

√7ᵗʰ **T41.1X6** Underdosing of intravenous anesthetics

√5ᵗʰ **T41.2** Poisoning by, adverse effect of and underdosing of other and unspecified general anesthetics

√6ᵗʰ **T41.20** Poisoning by, adverse effect of and underdosing of unspecified general anesthetics

√7ᵗʰ **T41.201** Poisoning by unspecified general anesthetics, accidental (unintentional)
Poisoning by general anesthetics NOS

√7ᵗʰ **T41.202** Poisoning by unspecified general anesthetics, intentional self-harm

√7ᵗʰ **T41.203** Poisoning by unspecified general anesthetics, assault

√7ᵗʰ **T41.204** Poisoning by unspecified general anesthetics, undetermined

√7ᵗʰ **T41.205** Adverse effect of unspecified general anesthetics

√7ᵗʰ **T41.206** Underdosing of unspecified general anesthetics

√6ᵗʰ **T41.29** Poisoning by, adverse effect of and underdosing of other general anesthetics

√7ᵗʰ **T41.291** Poisoning by other general anesthetics, accidental (unintentional)
Poisoning by other general anesthetics NOS

√7ᵗʰ **T41.292** Poisoning by other general anesthetics, intentional self-harm

√7ᵗʰ **T41.293** Poisoning by other general anesthetics, assault

√7ᵗʰ **T41.294** Poisoning by other general anesthetics, undetermined

√7ᵗʰ **T41.295** Adverse effect of other general anesthetics

√7ᵗʰ **T41.296** Underdosing of other general anesthetics

√5ᵗʰ **T41.3** Poisoning by, adverse effect of and underdosing of local anesthetics
Cocaine (topical)
EXCLUDES 2 poisoning by cocaine used as a central nervous system stimulant (T40.5X1-T40.5X4)

√6ᵗʰ **T41.3X** Poisoning by, adverse effect of and underdosing of local anesthetics

√7ᵗʰ **T41.3X1** Poisoning by local anesthetics, accidental (unintentional)
Poisoning by local anesthetics NOS

√7ᵗʰ **T41.3X2** Poisoning by local anesthetics, intentional self-harm

√7ᵗʰ **T41.3X3** Poisoning by local anesthetics, assault

√7ᵗʰ **T41.3X4** Poisoning by local anesthetics, undetermined

√7ᵗʰ **T41.3X5** Adverse effect of local anesthetics

√7ᵗʰ **T41.3X6** Underdosing of local anesthetics

√5ᵗʰ **T41.4** Poisoning by, adverse effect of and underdosing of unspecified anesthetic

√x7ᵗʰ **T41.41** Poisoning by unspecified anesthetic, accidental (unintentional)
Poisoning by anesthetic NOS

√x7ᵗʰ **T41.42** Poisoning by unspecified anesthetic, intentional self-harm

√x7ᵗʰ **T41.43** Poisoning by unspecified anesthetic, assault

√x7ᵗʰ **T41.44** Poisoning by unspecified anesthetic, undetermined

√x7ᵗʰ **T41.45** Adverse effect of unspecified anesthetic

√x7ᵗʰ **T41.46** Underdosing of unspecified anesthetics

√5ᵗʰ **T41.5** Poisoning by, adverse effect of and underdosing of therapeutic gases

√6ᵗʰ **T41.5X** Poisoning by, adverse effect of and underdosing of therapeutic gases

√7ᵗʰ **T41.5X1** Poisoning by therapeutic gases, accidental (unintentional)
Poisoning by therapeutic gases NOS

√7ᵗʰ **T41.5X2** Poisoning by therapeutic gases, intentional self-harm

√7ᵗʰ **T41.5X3** Poisoning by therapeutic gases, assault

√7ᵗʰ **T41.5X4** Poisoning by therapeutic gases, undetermined

√7ᵗʰ **T41.5X5** Adverse effect of therapeutic gases

√7ᵗʰ **T41.5X6** Underdosing of therapeutic gases

√4ᵗʰ **T42** Poisoning by, adverse effect of and underdosing of antiepileptic, sedative-hypnotic and antiparkinsonism drugs
EXCLUDES 2 drug dependence and related mental and behavioral disorders due to psychoactive substance use (F10- – F19-)

The appropriate 7th character is to be added to each code from category T42.
A   initial encounter
D   subsequent encounter
S   sequela

√5ᵗʰ **T42.0** Poisoning by, adverse effect of and underdosing of hydantoin derivatives

√6ᵗʰ **T42.0X** Poisoning by, adverse effect of and underdosing of hydantoin derivatives

√7ᵗʰ **T42.0X1** Poisoning by hydantoin derivatives, accidental (unintentional)
Poisoning by hydantoin derivatives NOS

√7ᵗʰ **T42.0X2** Poisoning by hydantoin derivatives, intentional self-harm

√7ᵗʰ **T42.0X3** Poisoning by hydantoin derivatives, assault

√7ᵗʰ **T42.0X4** Poisoning by hydantoin derivatives, undetermined

√7ᵗʰ **T42.0X5** Adverse effect of hydantoin derivatives

√7ᵗʰ **T42.0X6** Underdosing of hydantoin derivatives

√5ᵗʰ **T42.1** Poisoning by, adverse effect of and underdosing of iminostilbenes
Poisoning by, adverse effect of and underdosing of carbamazepine

√6ᵗʰ **T42.1X** Poisoning by, adverse effect of and underdosing of iminostilbenes

√7ᵗʰ **T42.1X1** Poisoning by iminostilbenes, accidental (unintentional)
Poisoning by iminostilbenes NOS

√7ᵗʰ **T42.1X2** Poisoning by iminostilbenes, intentional self-harm

√7ᵗʰ **T42.1X3** Poisoning by iminostilbenes, assault

√7ᵗʰ **T42.1X4** Poisoning by iminostilbenes, undetermined

√7ᵗʰ **T42.1X5** Adverse effect of iminostilbenes

√7ᵗʰ **T42.1X6** Underdosing of iminostilbenes

√5ᵗʰ **T42.2** Poisoning by, adverse effect of and underdosing of succinimides and oxazolidinediones

√6ᵗʰ **T42.2X** Poisoning by, adverse effect of and underdosing of succinimides and oxazolidinediones

√7ᵗʰ **T42.2X1** Poisoning by succinimides and oxazolidinediones, accidental (unintentional)
Poisoning by succinimides and oxazolidinediones NOS

√7ᵗʰ **T42.2X2** Poisoning by succinimides and oxazolidinediones, intentional self-harm

√7ᵗʰ **T42.2X3** Poisoning by succinimides and oxazolidinediones, assault

√7ᵗʰ **T42.2X4** Poisoning by succinimides and oxazolidinediones, undetermined

√7ᵗʰ **T42.2X5** Adverse effect of succinimides and oxazolidinediones

√7ᵗʰ **T42.2X6** Underdosing of succinimides and oxazolidinediones

√5ᵗʰ **T42.3** Poisoning by, adverse effect of and underdosing of barbiturates
EXCLUDES 1 poisoning by, adverse effect of and underdosing of thiobarbiturates (T41.1-)

√6ᵗʰ **T42.3X** Poisoning by, adverse effect of and underdosing of barbiturates

√7ᵗʰ **T42.3X1** Poisoning by barbiturates, accidental (unintentional)
Poisoning by barbiturates NOS

√7ᵗʰ **T42.3X2** Poisoning by barbiturates, intentional self-harm

√7ᵗʰ **T42.3X3** Poisoning by barbiturates, assault

✓ Additional Character Required   √x7ᵗʰ Xtension Alert   Unacceptable PDx   Manifestation   Hospital Acquired Condition   EXCLUDES 1 Not Coded Here   EXCLUDES 2 Not Included Here

ICD-10-CM Draft (2015)   1061

Injury, Poisoning and Certain Other Consequences of External Causes

T42.3X4–T43.026

     ✓7th **T42.3X4** Poisoning by barbiturates, undetermined

     ✓7th **T42.3X5** Adverse effect of barbiturates

     ✓7th **T42.3X6** Underdosing of barbiturates

✓5th **T42.4** Poisoning by, adverse effect of and underdosing of benzodiazepines

     ✓6th **T42.4X** Poisoning by, adverse effect of and underdosing of benzodiazepines

         ✓7th **T42.4X1** Poisoning by benzodiazepines, accidental (unintentional)
             Poisoning by benzodiazepines NOS

         ✓7th **T42.4X2** Poisoning by benzodiazepines, intentional self-harm

         ✓7th **T42.4X3** Poisoning by benzodiazepines, assault

         ✓7th **T42.4X4** Poisoning by benzodiazepines, undetermined

         ✓7th **T42.4X5** Adverse effect of benzodiazepines

         ✓7th **T42.4X6** Underdosing of benzodiazepines

✓5th **T42.5** Poisoning by, adverse effect of and underdosing of mixed antiepileptics

     ✓6th **T42.5X** Poisoning by, adverse effect of and underdosing of antiepileptics

         ✓7th **T42.5X1** Poisoning by mixed antiepileptics, accidental (unintentional)
             Poisoning by mixed antiepileptics NOS

         ✓7th **T42.5X2** Poisoning by mixed antiepileptics, intentional self-harm

         ✓7th **T42.5X3** Poisoning by mixed antiepileptics, assault

         ✓7th **T42.5X4** Poisoning by mixed antiepileptics, undetermined

         ✓7th **T42.5X5** Adverse effect of mixed antiepileptics

         ✓7th **T42.5X6** Underdosing of mixed antiepileptics

✓5th **T42.6** Poisoning by, adverse effect of and underdosing of other antiepileptic and sedative-hypnotic drugs
     Poisoning by, adverse effect of and underdosing of methaqualone
     Poisoning by, adverse effect of and underdosing of valproic acid

     EXCLUDES 1   poisoning by, adverse effect of and underdosing of carbamazepine (T42.1-)

     ✓6th **T42.6X** Poisoning by, adverse effect of and underdosing of other antiepileptic and sedative-hypnotic drugs

         ✓7th **T42.6X1** Poisoning by other antiepileptic and sedative-hypnotic drugs, accidental (unintentional)
             Poisoning by other antiepileptic and sedative-hypnotic drugs NOS

         ✓7th **T42.6X2** Poisoning by other antiepileptic and sedative-hypnotic drugs, intentional self-harm

         ✓7th **T42.6X3** Poisoning by other antiepileptic and sedative-hypnotic drugs, assault

         ✓7th **T42.6X4** Poisoning by other antiepileptic and sedative-hypnotic drugs, undetermined

         ✓7th **T42.6X5** Adverse effect of other antiepileptic and sedative-hypnotic drugs

         ✓7th **T42.6X6** Underdosing of other antiepileptic and sedative-hypnotic drugs

✓5th **T42.7** Poisoning by, adverse effect of and underdosing of unspecified antiepileptic and sedative-hypnotic drugs

     ✓x7th **T42.71** Poisoning by unspecified antiepileptic and sedative-hypnotic drugs, accidental (unintentional)
         Poisoning by antiepileptic and sedative-hypnotic drugs NOS

     ✓x7th **T42.72** Poisoning by unspecified antiepileptic and sedative-hypnotic drugs, intentional self-harm

     ✓x7th **T42.73** Poisoning by unspecified antiepileptic and sedative-hypnotic drugs, assault

     ✓x7th **T42.74** Poisoning by unspecified antiepileptic and sedative-hypnotic drugs, undetermined

     ✓x7th **T42.75** Adverse effect of unspecified antiepileptic and sedative-hypnotic drugs

     ✓x7th **T42.76** Underdosing of unspecified antiepileptic and sedative-hypnotic drugs

✓5th **T42.8** Poisoning by, adverse effect of and underdosing of antiparkinsonism drugs and other central muscle-tone depressants
     Poisoning by, adverse effect of and underdosing of amantadine

     ✓6th **T42.8X** Poisoning by, adverse effect of and underdosing of antiparkinsonism drugs and other central muscle-tone depressants

         ✓7th **T42.8X1** Poisoning by antiparkinsonism drugs and other central muscle-tone depressants, accidental (unintentional)
             Poisoning by antiparkinsonism drugs and other central muscle-tone depressants NOS

         ✓7th **T42.8X2** Poisoning by antiparkinsonism drugs and other central muscle-tone depressants, intentional self-harm

         ✓7th **T42.8X3** Poisoning by antiparkinsonism drugs and other central muscle-tone depressants, assault

         ✓7th **T42.8X4** Poisoning by antiparkinsonism drugs and other central muscle-tone depressants, undetermined

         ✓7th **T42.8X5** Adverse effect of antiparkinsonism drugs and other central muscle-tone depressants

         ✓7th **T42.8X6** Underdosing of antiparkinsonism drugs and other central muscle-tone depressants

✓4th **T43** Poisoning by, adverse effect of and underdosing of psychotropic drugs, not elsewhere classified

     EXCLUDES 1   appetite depressants (T50.5-)
             barbiturates (T42.3-)
             benzodiazepines (T42.4-)
             methaqualone (T42.6-)
             psychodysleptics [hallucinogens] (T40.7-T40.9-)

     EXCLUDES 2   drug dependence and related mental and behavioral disorders due to psychoactive substance use (F10.- – F19.-)

The appropriate 7th character is to be added to each code from category T43.
A   initial encounter
D   subsequent encounter
S   sequela

✓5th **T43.0** Poisoning by, adverse effect of and underdosing of tricyclic and tetracyclic antidepressants

     ✓6th **T43.01** Poisoning by, adverse effect of and underdosing of tricyclic antidepressants

         ✓7th **T43.011** Poisoning by tricyclic antidepressants, accidental (unintentional)
             Poisoning by tricyclic antidepressants NOS

         ✓7th **T43.012** Poisoning by tricyclic antidepressants, intentional self-harm

         ✓7th **T43.013** Poisoning by tricyclic antidepressants, assault

         ✓7th **T43.014** Poisoning by tricyclic antidepressants, undetermined

         ✓7th **T43.015** Adverse effect of tricyclic antidepressants

         ✓7th **T43.016** Underdosing of tricyclic antidepressants

     ✓6th **T43.02** Poisoning by, adverse effect of and underdosing of tetracyclic antidepressants

         ✓7th **T43.021** Poisoning by tetracyclic antidepressants, accidental (unintentional)
             Poisoning by tetracyclic antidepressants NOS

         ✓7th **T43.022** Poisoning by tetracyclic antidepressants, intentional self-harm

         ✓7th **T43.023** Poisoning by tetracyclic antidepressants, assault

         ✓7th **T43.024** Poisoning by tetracyclic antidepressants, undetermined

         ✓7th **T43.025** Adverse effect of tetracyclic antidepressants

         ✓7th **T43.026** Underdosing of tetracyclic antidepressants

√5ᵗʰ **T43.1** Poisoning by, adverse effect of and underdosing of monoamine-oxidase-inhibitor antidepressants

  √6ᵗʰ **T43.1X** Poisoning by, adverse effect of and underdosing of monoamine-oxidase-inhibitor antidepressants

    √7ᵗʰ **T43.1X1** Poisoning by monoamine-oxidase-inhibitor antidepressants, accidental (unintentional)
      Poisoning by monoamine-oxidase-inhibitor antidepressants NOS

    √7ᵗʰ **T43.1X2** Poisoning by monoamine-oxidase-inhibitor antidepressants, intentional self-harm

    √7ᵗʰ **T43.1X3** Poisoning by monoamine-oxidase-inhibitor antidepressants, assault

    √7ᵗʰ **T43.1X4** Poisoning by monoamine-oxidase-inhibitor antidepressants, undetermined

    √7ᵗʰ **T43.1X5** Adverse effect of monoamine-oxidase-inhibitor antidepressants

    √7ᵗʰ **T43.1X6** Underdosing of monoamine-oxidase-inhibitor antidepressants

√5ᵗʰ **T43.2** Poisoning by, adverse effect of and underdosing of other and unspecified antidepressants

  √6ᵗʰ **T43.20** Poisoning by, adverse effect of and underdosing of unspecified antidepressants

    √7ᵗʰ **T43.201** Poisoning by unspecified antidepressants, accidental (unintentional)
      Poisoning by antidepressants NOS

    √7ᵗʰ **T43.202** Poisoning by unspecified antidepressants, intentional self-harm

    √7ᵗʰ **T43.203** Poisoning by unspecified antidepressants, assault

    √7ᵗʰ **T43.204** Poisoning by unspecified antidepressants, undetermined

    √7ᵗʰ **T43.205** Adverse effect of unspecified antidepressants

    √7ᵗʰ **T43.206** Underdosing of unspecified antidepressants

  √6ᵗʰ **T43.21** Poisoning by, adverse effect of and underdosing of selective serotonin and norepinephrine reuptake inhibitors
    Poisoning by, adverse effect of and underdosing of SSNRI antidepressants

    √7ᵗʰ **T43.211** Poisoning by selective serotonin and norepinephrine reuptake inhibitors, accidental (unintentional)

    √7ᵗʰ **T43.212** Poisoning by selective serotonin and norepinephrine reuptake inhibitors, intentional self-harm

    √7ᵗʰ **T43.213** Poisoning by selective serotonin and norepinephrine reuptake inhibitors, assault

    √7ᵗʰ **T43.214** Poisoning by selective serotonin and norepinephrine reuptake inhibitors, undetermined

    √7ᵗʰ **T43.215** Adverse effect of selective serotonin and norepinephrine reuptake inhibitors

    √7ᵗʰ **T43.216** Underdosing of selective serotonin and norepinephrine reuptake inhibitors

  √6ᵗʰ **T43.22** Poisoning by, adverse effect of and underdosing of selective serotonin reuptake inhibitors
    Poisoning by, adverse effect of and underdosing of SSRI antidepressants

    √7ᵗʰ **T43.221** Poisoning by selective serotonin reuptake inhibitors, accidental (unintentional)

    √7ᵗʰ **T43.222** Poisoning by selective serotonin reuptake inhibitors, intentional self-harm

    √7ᵗʰ **T43.223** Poisoning by selective serotonin reuptake inhibitors, assault

    √7ᵗʰ **T43.224** Poisoning by selective serotonin reuptake inhibitors, undetermined

    √7ᵗʰ **T43.225** Adverse effect of selective serotonin reuptake inhibitors

    √7ᵗʰ **T43.226** Underdosing of selective serotonin reuptake inhibitors

√6ᵗʰ **T43.29** Poisoning by, adverse effect of and underdosing of other antidepressants

    √7ᵗʰ **T43.291** Poisoning by other antidepressants, accidental (unintentional)
      Poisoning by other antidepressants NOS

    √7ᵗʰ **T43.292** Poisoning by other antidepressants, intentional self-harm

    √7ᵗʰ **T43.293** Poisoning by other antidepressants, assault

    √7ᵗʰ **T43.294** Poisoning by other antidepressants, undetermined

    √7ᵗʰ **T43.295** Adverse effect of other antidepressants

    √7ᵗʰ **T43.296** Underdosing of other antidepressants

√5ᵗʰ **T43.3** Poisoning by, adverse effect of and underdosing of phenothiazine antipsychotics and neuroleptics

  √6ᵗʰ **T43.3X** Poisoning by, adverse effect of and underdosing of phenothiazine antipsychotics and neuroleptics

    √7ᵗʰ **T43.3X1** Poisoning by phenothiazine antipsychotics and neuroleptics, accidental (unintentional)
      Poisoning by phenothiazine antipsychotics and neuroleptics NOS

    √7ᵗʰ **T43.3X2** Poisoning by phenothiazine antipsychotics and neuroleptics, intentional self-harm

    √7ᵗʰ **T43.3X3** Poisoning by phenothiazine antipsychotics and neuroleptics, assault

    √7ᵗʰ **T43.3X4** Poisoning by phenothiazine antipsychotics and neuroleptics, undetermined

    √7ᵗʰ **T43.3X5** Adverse effect of phenothiazine antipsychotics and neuroleptics

    √7ᵗʰ **T43.3X6** Underdosing of phenothiazine antipsychotics and neuroleptics

√5ᵗʰ **T43.4** Poisoning by, adverse effect of and underdosing of butyrophenone and thiothixene neuroleptics

  √6ᵗʰ **T43.4X** Poisoning by, adverse effect of and underdosing of butyrophenone and thiothixene neuroleptics

    √7ᵗʰ **T43.4X1** Poisoning by butyrophenone and thiothixene neuroleptics, accidental (unintentional)
      Poisoning by butyrophenone and thiothixene neuroleptics NOS

    √7ᵗʰ **T43.4X2** Poisoning by butyrophenone and thiothixene neuroleptics, intentional self-harm

    √7ᵗʰ **T43.4X3** Poisoning by butyrophenone and thiothixene neuroleptics, assault

    √7ᵗʰ **T43.4X4** Poisoning by butyrophenone and thiothixene neuroleptics, undetermined

    √7ᵗʰ **T43.4X5** Adverse effect of butyrophenone and thiothixene neuroleptics

    √7ᵗʰ **T43.4X6** Underdosing of butyrophenone and thiothixene neuroleptics

√5ᵗʰ **T43.5** Poisoning by, adverse effect of and underdosing of other and unspecified antipsychotics and neuroleptics
  EXCLUDES 1 poisoning by, adverse effect of and underdosing of rauwolfia (T46.5-)

  √6ᵗʰ **T43.50** Poisoning by, adverse effect of and underdosing of unspecified antipsychotics and neuroleptics

    √7ᵗʰ **T43.501** Poisoning by unspecified antipsychotics and neuroleptics, accidental (unintentional)
      Poisoning by antipsychotics and neuroleptics NOS

    √7ᵗʰ **T43.502** Poisoning by unspecified antipsychotics and neuroleptics, intentional self-harm

    √7ᵗʰ **T43.503** Poisoning by unspecified antipsychotics and neuroleptics, assault

    √7ᵗʰ **T43.504** Poisoning by unspecified antipsychotics and neuroleptics, undetermined

    √7ᵗʰ **T43.505** Adverse effect of unspecified antipsychotics and neuroleptics

    √7ᵗʰ **T43.506** Underdosing of unspecified antipsychotics and neuroleptics

Injury, Poisoning and Certain Other Consequences of External Causes

T43.59–T44.1X1

√6ᵗʰ **T43.59** **Poisoning by, adverse effect of and underdosing of other antipsychotics and neuroleptics**

√7ᵗʰ **T43.591** **Poisoning by other antipsychotics and neuroleptics, accidental (unintentional)**
Poisoning by other antipsychotics and neuroleptics NOS

√7ᵗʰ **T43.592** **Poisoning by other antipsychotics and neuroleptics, intentional self-harm**

√7ᵗʰ **T43.593** **Poisoning by other antipsychotics and neuroleptics, assault**

√7ᵗʰ **T43.594** **Poisoning by other antipsychotics and neuroleptics, undetermined**

√7ᵗʰ **T43.595** **Adverse effect of other antipsychotics and neuroleptics**

√7ᵗʰ **T43.596** **Underdosing of other antipsychotics and neuroleptics**

√5ᵗʰ **T43.6** **Poisoning by, adverse effect of and underdosing of psychostimulants**

EXCLUDES 1   *poisoning by, adverse effect of and underdosing of cocaine (T40.5-)*

√6ᵗʰ **T43.60** **Poisoning by, adverse effect of and underdosing of unspecified psychostimulant**

√7ᵗʰ **T43.601** **Poisoning by unspecified psychostimulants, accidental (unintentional)**
Poisoning by psychostimulants NOS

√7ᵗʰ **T43.602** **Poisoning by unspecified psychostimulants, intentional self-harm**

√7ᵗʰ **T43.603** **Poisoning by unspecified psychostimulants, assault**

√7ᵗʰ **T43.604** **Poisoning by unspecified psychostimulants, undetermined**

√7ᵗʰ **T43.605** **Adverse effect of unspecified psychostimulants**

√7ᵗʰ **T43.606** **Underdosing of unspecified psychostimulants**

√6ᵗʰ **T43.61** **Poisoning by, adverse effect of and underdosing of caffeine**

√7ᵗʰ **T43.611** **Poisoning by caffeine, accidental (unintentional)**
Poisoning by caffeine NOS

√7ᵗʰ **T43.612** **Poisoning by caffeine, intentional self-harm**

√7ᵗʰ **T43.613** **Poisoning by caffeine, assault**

√7ᵗʰ **T43.614** **Poisoning by caffeine, undetermined**

√7ᵗʰ **T43.615** **Adverse effect of caffeine**

√7ᵗʰ **T43.616** **Underdosing of caffeine**

√6ᵗʰ **T43.62** **Poisoning by, adverse effect of and underdosing of amphetamines**
Poisoning by, adverse effect of and underdosing of methamphetamines

√7ᵗʰ **T43.621** **Poisoning by amphetamines, accidental (unintentional)**
Poisoning by amphetamines NOS

√7ᵗʰ **T43.622** **Poisoning by amphetamines, intentional self-harm**

√7ᵗʰ **T43.623** **Poisoning by amphetamines, assault**

√7ᵗʰ **T43.624** **Poisoning by amphetamines, undetermined**

√7ᵗʰ **T43.625** **Adverse effect of amphetamines**

√7ᵗʰ **T43.626** **Underdosing of amphetamines**

√6ᵗʰ **T43.63** **Poisoning by, adverse effect of and underdosing of methylphenidate**

√7ᵗʰ **T43.631** **Poisoning by methylphenidate, accidental (unintentional)**
Poisoning by methylphenidate NOS

√7ᵗʰ **T43.632** **Poisoning by methylphenidate, intentional self-harm**

√7ᵗʰ **T43.633** **Poisoning by methylphenidate, assault**

√7ᵗʰ **T43.634** **Poisoning by methylphenidate, undetermined**

√7ᵗʰ **T43.635** **Adverse effect of methylphenidate**

√7ᵗʰ **T43.636** **Underdosing of methylphenidate**

√6ᵗʰ **T43.69** **Poisoning by, adverse effect of and underdosing of other psychostimulants**

√7ᵗʰ **T43.691** **Poisoning by other psychostimulants, accidental (unintentional)**
Poisoning by other psychostimulants NOS

√7ᵗʰ **T43.692** **Poisoning by other psychostimulants, intentional self-harm**

√7ᵗʰ **T43.693** **Poisoning by other psychostimulants, assault**

√7ᵗʰ **T43.694** **Poisoning by other psychostimulants, undetermined**

√7ᵗʰ **T43.695** **Adverse effect of other psychostimulants**

√7ᵗʰ **T43.696** **Underdosing of other psychostimulants**

√5ᵗʰ **T43.8** **Poisoning by, adverse effect of and underdosing of other psychotropic drugs**

√6ᵗʰ **T43.8X** **Poisoning by, adverse effect of and underdosing of other psychotropic drugs**

√7ᵗʰ **T43.8X1** **Poisoning by other psychotropic drugs, accidental (unintentional)**
Poisoning by other psychotropic drugs NOS

√7ᵗʰ **T43.8X2** **Poisoning by other psychotropic drugs, intentional self-harm**

√7ᵗʰ **T43.8X3** **Poisoning by other psychotropic drugs, assault**

√7ᵗʰ **T43.8X4** **Poisoning by other psychotropic drugs, undetermined**

√7ᵗʰ **T43.8X5** **Adverse effect of other psychotropic drugs**

√7ᵗʰ **T43.8X6** **Underdosing of other psychotropic drugs**

√5ᵗʰ **T43.9** **Poisoning by, adverse effect of and underdosing of unspecified psychotropic drug**

√x7ᵗʰ **T43.91** **Poisoning by unspecified psychotropic drug, accidental (unintentional)**
Poisoning by psychotropic drug NOS

√x7ᵗʰ **T43.92** **Poisoning by unspecified psychotropic drug, intentional self-harm**

√x7ᵗʰ **T43.93** **Poisoning by unspecified psychotropic drug, assault**

√x7ᵗʰ **T43.94** **Poisoning by unspecified psychotropic drug, undetermined**

√x7ᵗʰ **T43.95** **Adverse effect of unspecified psychotropic drug**

√x7ᵗʰ **T43.96** **Underdosing of unspecified psychotropic drug**

√4ᵗʰ **T44** **Poisoning by, adverse effect of and underdosing of drugs primarily affecting the autonomic nervous system**

The appropriate 7th character is to be added to each code from category T44.
A   initial encounter
D   subsequent encounter
S   sequela

√5ᵗʰ **T44.0** **Poisoning by, adverse effect of and underdosing of anticholinesterase agents**

√6ᵗʰ **T44.0X** **Poisoning by, adverse effect of and underdosing of anticholinesterase agents**

√7ᵗʰ **T44.0X1** **Poisoning by anticholinesterase agents, accidental (unintentional)**
Poisoning by anticholinesterase agents NOS

√7ᵗʰ **T44.0X2** **Poisoning by anticholinesterase agents, intentional self-harm**

√7ᵗʰ **T44.0X3** **Poisoning by anticholinesterase agents, assault**

√7ᵗʰ **T44.0X4** **Poisoning by anticholinesterase agents, undetermined**

√7ᵗʰ **T44.0X5** **Adverse effect of anticholinesterase agents**

√7ᵗʰ **T44.0X6** **Underdosing of anticholinesterase agents**

√5ᵗʰ **T44.1** **Poisoning by, adverse effect of and underdosing of other parasympathomimetics [cholinergics]**

√6ᵗʰ **T44.1X** **Poisoning by, adverse effect of and underdosing of other parasympathomimetics [cholinergics]**

√7ᵗʰ **T44.1X1** **Poisoning by other parasympathomimetics [cholinergics], accidental (unintentional)**
Poisoning by other parasympathomimetics [cholinergics] NOS

Ⓝ Newborn: 0   Ⓟ Pediatric: 0–17   Ⓜ Maternity: 12–55   Ⓐ Adult: 15–124   **MCC** Major CC Condition   **PDx MCC** PDx acts as own MCC   **CC** CC Condition   **PDx CC** PDx acts as own CC

1064   ICD-10-CM Draft (2015)

✓7th **T44.1X2** **Poisoning by other parasympathomimetics [cholinergics], intentional self-harm**

✓7th **T44.1X3** **Poisoning by other parasympathomimetics [cholinergics], assault**

✓7th **T44.1X4** **Poisoning by other parasympathomimetics [cholinergics], undetermined**

✓7th **T44.1X5** Adverse effect of other parasympathomimetics [cholinergics]

✓7th **T44.1X6** Underdosing of other parasympathomimetics

✓5th **T44.2** **Poisoning by, adverse effect of and underdosing of ganglionic blocking drugs**

✓6th **T44.2X** **Poisoning by, adverse effect of and underdosing of ganglionic blocking drugs**

✓7th **T44.2X1** **Poisoning by ganglionic blocking drugs, accidental (unintentional)**
Poisoning by ganglionic blocking drugs NOS

✓7th **T44.2X2** **Poisoning by ganglionic blocking drugs, intentional self-harm**

✓7th **T44.2X3** **Poisoning by ganglionic blocking drugs, assault**

✓7th **T44.2X4** **Poisoning by ganglionic blocking drugs, undetermined**

✓7th **T44.2X5** Adverse effect of ganglionic blocking drugs

✓7th **T44.2X6** Underdosing of ganglionic blocking drugs

T44.3 **Poisoning by, adverse effect of and underdosing of other parasympatholytics [anticholinergics and antimuscarinics] and spasmolytics**
Poisoning by, adverse effect of and underdosing of papaverine

✓6th **T44.3X** **Poisoning by, adverse effect of and underdosing of other parasympatholytics [anticholinergics and antimuscarinics] and spasmolytics**

✓7th **T44.3X1** **Poisoning by other parasympatholytics [anticholinergics and antimuscarinics] and spasmolytics, accidental (unintentional)**
Poisoning by other parasympatholytics [anticholinergics and antimuscarinics] and spasmolytics NOS

✓7th **T44.3X2** **Poisoning by other parasympatholytics [anticholinergics and antimuscarinics] and spasmolytics, intentional self-harm**

✓7th **T44.3X3** **Poisoning by other parasympatholytics [anticholinergics and antimuscarinics] and spasmolytics, assault**

✓7th **T44.3X4** **Poisoning by other parasympatholytics [anticholinergics and antimuscarinics] and spasmolytics, undetermined**

✓7th **T44.3X5** Adverse effect of other parasympatholytics [anticholinergics and antimuscarinics] and spasmolytics

✓7th **T44.3X6** Underdosing of other parasympatholytics [anticholinergics and antimuscarinics] and spasmolytics

✓5th **T44.4** **Poisoning by, adverse effect of and underdosing of predominantly alpha-adrenoreceptor agonists**
Poisoning by, adverse effect of and underdosing of metaraminol

✓6th **T44.4X** **Poisoning by, adverse effect of and underdosing of predominantly alpha-adrenoreceptor agonists**

✓7th **T44.4X1** **Poisoning by predominantly alpha-adrenoreceptor agonists, accidental (unintentional)**
Poisoning by predominantly alpha-adrenoreceptor agonists NOS

✓7th **T44.4X2** **Poisoning by predominantly alpha-adrenoreceptor agonists, intentional self-harm**

✓7th **T44.4X3** **Poisoning by predominantly alpha-adrenoreceptor agonists, assault**

✓7th **T44.4X4** **Poisoning by predominantly alpha-adrenoreceptor agonists, undetermined**

✓7th **T44.4X5** Adverse effect of predominantly alpha-adrenoreceptor agonists

✓7th **T44.4X6** Underdosing of predominantly alpha-adrenoreceptor agonists

✓5th **T44.5** **Poisoning by, adverse effect of and underdosing of predominantly beta-adrenoreceptor agonists**
EXCLUDES 1 *poisoning by, adverse effect of and underdosing of beta-adrenoreceptor agonists used in asthma therapy (T48.6-)*

✓6th **T44.5X** **Poisoning by, adverse effect of and underdosing of predominantly beta-adrenoreceptor agonists**

✓7th **T44.5X1** **Poisoning by predominantly beta-adrenoreceptor agonists, accidental (unintentional)**
Poisoning by predominantly beta-adrenoreceptor agonists NOS

✓7th **T44.5X2** **Poisoning by predominantly beta-adrenoreceptor agonists, intentional self-harm**

✓7th **T44.5X3** **Poisoning by predominantly beta-adrenoreceptor agonists, assault**

✓7th **T44.5X4** **Poisoning by predominantly beta-adrenoreceptor agonists, undetermined**

✓7th **T44.5X5** Adverse effect of predominantly beta-adrenoreceptor agonists

✓7th **T44.5X6** Underdosing of predominantly beta-adrenoreceptor agonists

✓5th **T44.6** **Poisoning by, adverse effect of and underdosing of alpha-adrenoreceptor antagonists**
EXCLUDES 1 *poisoning by, adverse effect of and underdosing of ergot alkaloids (T48.0)*

✓6th **T44.6X** **Poisoning by, adverse effect of and underdosing of alpha-adrenoreceptor antagonists**

✓7th **T44.6X1** **Poisoning by alpha-adrenoreceptor antagonists, accidental (unintentional)**
Poisoning by alpha-adrenoreceptor antagonists NOS

✓7th **T44.6X2** **Poisoning by alpha-adrenoreceptor antagonists, intentional self-harm**

✓7th **T44.6X3** **Poisoning by alpha-adrenoreceptor antagonists, assault**

✓7th **T44.6X4** **Poisoning by alpha-adrenoreceptor antagonists, undetermined**

✓7th **T44.6X5** Adverse effect of alpha-adrenoreceptor antagonists

✓7th **T44.6X6** Underdosing of alpha-adrenoreceptor antagonists

✓5th **T44.7** **Poisoning by, adverse effect of and underdosing of beta-adrenoreceptor antagonists**

✓6th **T44.7X** **Poisoning by, adverse effect of and underdosing of beta-adrenoreceptor antagonists**

✓7th **T44.7X1** **Poisoning by beta-adrenoreceptor antagonists, accidental (unintentional)**
Poisoning by beta-adrenoreceptor antagonists NOS

✓7th **T44.7X2** **Poisoning by beta-adrenoreceptor antagonists, intentional self-harm**

✓7th **T44.7X3** **Poisoning by beta-adrenoreceptor antagonists, assault**

✓7th **T44.7X4** **Poisoning by beta-adrenoreceptor antagonists, undetermined**

✓7th **T44.7X5** Adverse effect of beta-adrenoreceptor antagonists

✓7th **T44.7X6** Underdosing of beta-adrenoreceptor antagonists

✓5th **T44.8** **Poisoning by, adverse effect of and underdosing of centrally-acting and adrenergic-neuron- blocking agents**
EXCLUDES 1 *poisoning by, adverse effect of and underdosing of clonidine (T46.5)*
poisoning by, adverse effect of and underdosing of guanethidine (T46.5)

✓6th **T44.8X** **Poisoning by, adverse effect of and underdosing of centrally-acting and adrenergic-neuron-blocking agents**

✓7th **T44.8X1** **Poisoning by centrally-acting and adrenergic-neuron-blocking agents, accidental (unintentional)**
Poisoning by centrally-acting and adrenergic-neuron-blocking agents NOS

Injury, Poisoning and Certain Other Consequences of External Causes

T44.8X2–T45.4X2

√7ᵗʰ **T44.8X2 Poisoning by centrally-acting and adrenergic-neuron-blocking agents, intentional self-harm**

√7ᵗʰ **T44.8X3 Poisoning by centrally-acting and adrenergic-neuron-blocking agents, assault**

√7ᵗʰ **T44.8X4 Poisoning by centrally-acting and adrenergic-neuron-blocking agents, undetermined**

√7ᵗʰ **T44.8X5 Adverse effect of centrally-acting and adrenergic-neuron-blocking agents**

√7ᵗʰ **T44.8X6 Underdosing of centrally-acting and adrenergic-neuron-blocking agents**

√5ᵗʰ **T44.9 Poisoning by, adverse effect of and underdosing of other and unspecified drugs primarily affecting the autonomic nervous system**
Poisoning by, adverse effect of and underdosing of drug stimulating both alpha and beta-adrenoreceptors

√6ᵗʰ **T44.90 Poisoning by, adverse effect of and underdosing of unspecified drugs primarily affecting the autonomic nervous system**

√7ᵗʰ **T44.901 Poisoning by unspecified drugs primarily affecting the autonomic nervous system, accidental (unintentional)**
Poisoning by unspecified drugs primarily affecting the autonomic nervous system NOS

√7ᵗʰ **T44.902 Poisoning by unspecified drugs primarily affecting the autonomic nervous system, intentional self-harm**

√7ᵗʰ **T44.903 Poisoning by unspecified drugs primarily affecting the autonomic nervous system, assault**

√7ᵗʰ **T44.904 Poisoning by unspecified drugs primarily affecting the autonomic nervous system, undetermined**

√7ᵗʰ **T44.905 Adverse effect of unspecified drugs primarily affecting the autonomic nervous system**

√7ᵗʰ **T44.906 Underdosing of unspecified drugs primarily affecting the autonomic nervous system**

√6ᵗʰ **T44.99 Poisoning by, adverse effect of and underdosing of other drugs primarily affecting the autonomic nervous system**

√7ᵗʰ **T44.991 Poisoning by other drug primarily affecting the autonomic nervous system, accidental (unintentional)**
Poisoning by other drugs primarily affecting the autonomic nervous system NOS

√7ᵗʰ **T44.992 Poisoning by other drug primarily affecting the autonomic nervous system, intentional self-harm**

√7ᵗʰ **T44.993 Poisoning by other drug primarily affecting the autonomic nervous system, assault**

√7ᵗʰ **T44.994 Poisoning by other drug primarily affecting the autonomic nervous system, undetermined**

√7ᵗʰ **T44.995 Adverse effect of other drug primarily affecting the autonomic nervous system**

√7ᵗʰ **T44.996 Underdosing of other drug primarily affecting the autonomic nervous system**

√4ᵗʰ **T45 Poisoning by, adverse effect of and underdosing of primarily systemic and hematological agents, not elsewhere classified**

The appropriate 7th character is to be added to each code from category T45.
A   initial encounter
D   subsequent encounter
S   sequela

√5ᵗʰ **T45.0 Poisoning by, adverse effect of and underdosing of antiallergic and antiemetic drugs**
EXCLUDES 1 poisoning by, adverse effect of and underdosing of phenothiazine-based neuroleptics (T43.3)

√6ᵗʰ **T45.0X Poisoning by, adverse effect of and underdosing of antiallergic and antiemetic drugs**

√7ᵗʰ **T45.0X1 Poisoning by antiallergic and antiemetic drugs, accidental (unintentional)**
Poisoning by antiallergic and antiemetic drugs NOS

√7ᵗʰ **T45.0X2 Poisoning by antiallergic and antiemetic drugs, intentional self-harm**

√7ᵗʰ **T45.0X3 Poisoning by antiallergic and antiemetic drugs, assault**

√7ᵗʰ **T45.0X4 Poisoning by antiallergic and antiemetic drugs, undetermined**

√7ᵗʰ **T45.0X5 Adverse effect of antiallergic and antiemetic drugs**

√7ᵗʰ **T45.0X6 Underdosing of antiallergic and antiemetic drugs**

√5ᵗʰ **T45.1 Poisoning by, adverse effect of and underdosing of antineoplastic and immunosuppressive drugs**
EXCLUDES 1 poisoning by, adverse effect of and underdosing of tamoxifen (T38.6)

√6ᵗʰ **T45.1X Poisoning by, adverse effect of and underdosing of antineoplastic and immunosuppressive drugs**

√7ᵗʰ **T45.1X1 Poisoning by antineoplastic and immunosuppressive drugs, accidental (unintentional)**
Poisoning by antineoplastic and immunosuppressive drugs NOS

√7ᵗʰ **T45.1X2 Poisoning by antineoplastic and immunosuppressive drugs, intentional self-harm**

√7ᵗʰ **T45.1X3 Poisoning by antineoplastic and immunosuppressive drugs, assault**

√7ᵗʰ **T45.1X4 Poisoning by antineoplastic and immunosuppressive drugs, undetermined**

√7ᵗʰ **T45.1X5 Adverse effect of antineoplastic and immunosuppressive drugs**

√7ᵗʰ **T45.1X6 Underdosing of antineoplastic and immunosuppressive drugs**

√5ᵗʰ **T45.2 Poisoning by, adverse effect of and underdosing of vitamins**
EXCLUDES 2 poisoning by, adverse effect of and underdosing of iron (T45.4)
poisoning by, adverse effect of and underdosing of nicotinic acid (derivatives) (T46.7)
poisoning by, adverse effect of and underdosing of vitamin K (T45.7)

√6ᵗʰ **T45.2X Poisoning by, adverse effect of and underdosing of vitamins**

√7ᵗʰ **T45.2X1 Poisoning by vitamins, accidental (unintentional)**
Poisoning by vitamins NOS

√7ᵗʰ **T45.2X2 Poisoning by vitamins, intentional self-harm**

√7ᵗʰ **T45.2X3 Poisoning by vitamins, assault**

√7ᵗʰ **T45.2X4 Poisoning by vitamins, undetermined**

√7ᵗʰ **T45.2X5 Adverse effect of vitamins**

√7ᵗʰ **T45.2X6 Underdosing of vitamins**
EXCLUDES 1 vitamin deficiencies (E50-E56)

√5ᵗʰ **T45.3 Poisoning by, adverse effect of and underdosing of enzymes**

√6ᵗʰ **T45.3X Poisoning by, adverse effect of and underdosing of enzymes**

√7ᵗʰ **T45.3X1 Poisoning by enzymes, accidental (unintentional)**
Poisoning by enzymes NOS

√7ᵗʰ **T45.3X2 Poisoning by enzymes, intentional self-harm**

√7ᵗʰ **T45.3X3 Poisoning by enzymes, assault**

√7ᵗʰ **T45.3X4 Poisoning by enzymes, undetermined**

√7ᵗʰ **T45.3X5 Adverse effect of enzymes**

√7ᵗʰ **T45.3X6 Underdosing of enzymes**

√5ᵗʰ **T45.4 Poisoning by, adverse effect of and underdosing of iron and its compounds**

√6ᵗʰ **T45.4X Poisoning by, adverse effect of and underdosing of iron and its compounds**

T45.4X1 Poisoning by iron and its compounds, accidental (unintentional)
Poisoning by iron and its compounds NOS

√7ᵗʰ **T45.4X2 Poisoning by iron and its compounds, intentional self-harm**

√7th **T45.4X3** **Poisoning by iron and its compounds,** assault

√7th **T45.4X4** **Poisoning by iron and its compounds,** undetermined

√7th **T45.4X5** Adverse effect of iron and its compounds

√7th **T45.4X6** Underdosing of iron and its compounds
EXCLUDES 1 *iron deficiency (E61.1)*

√5th **T45.5** **Poisoning by, adverse effect of and underdosing of anticoagulants and antithrombotic drugs**

√6th **T45.51** **Poisoning by, adverse effect of and underdosing of anticoagulants**

√7th **T45.511** **Poisoning by anticoagulants,** accidental (unintentional)
Poisoning by anticoagulants NOS

√7th **T45.512** **Poisoning by anticoagulants,** intentional self-harm

√7th **T45.513** **Poisoning by anticoagulants,** assault

√7th **T45.514** **Poisoning by anticoagulants,** undetermined

√7th **T45.515** Adverse effect of anticoagulants
AHA: 2013, 2Q, 34

√7th **T45.516** Underdosing of anticoagulants

√6th **T45.52** **Poisoning by, adverse effect of and underdosing of antithrombotic drugs**
Poisoning by, adverse effect of and underdosing of antiplatelet drugs
EXCLUDES 2 *poisoning by, adverse effect of and underdosing of aspirin (T39.01-) poisoning by, adverse effect of and underdosing of acetylsalicylic acid (T39.01-)*

√7th **T45.521** **Poisoning by antithrombotic drugs,** accidental (unintentional)
Poisoning by antithrombotic drug NOS

√7th **T45.522** **Poisoning by antithrombotic drugs,** intentional self-harm

√7th **T45.523** **Poisoning by antithrombotic drugs,** assault

√7th **T45.524** **Poisoning by antithrombotic drugs,** undetermined

√7th **T45.525** Adverse effect of antithrombotic drugs

√7th **T45.526** Underdosing of antithrombotic drugs

√5th **T45.6** **Poisoning by, adverse effect of and underdosing of fibrinolysis-affecting drugs**

√6th **T45.60** **Poisoning by, adverse effect of and underdosing of unspecified fibrinolysis-affecting drugs**

√7th **T45.601** **Poisoning by unspecified fibrinolysis-affecting drugs,** accidental (unintentional)
Poisoning by fibrinolysis-affecting drug NOS

√7th **T45.602** **Poisoning by unspecified fibrinolysis-affecting drugs,** intentional self-harm

√7th **T45.603** **Poisoning by unspecified fibrinolysis-affecting drugs,** assault

√7th **T45.604** **Poisoning by unspecified fibrinolysis-affecting drugs,** undetermined

√7th **T45.605** Adverse effect of unspecified fibrinolysis-affecting drugs

√7th **T45.606** Underdosing of unspecified fibrinolysis-affecting drugs

√6th **T45.61** **Poisoning by, adverse effect of and underdosing of thrombolytic drugs**

√7th **T45.611** **Poisoning by thrombolytic drug,** accidental (unintentional)
Poisoning by thrombolytic drug NOS

√7th **T45.612** **Poisoning by thrombolytic drug,** intentional self-harm

√7th **T45.613** **Poisoning by thrombolytic drug,** assault

√7th **T45.614** **Poisoning by thrombolytic drug,** undetermined

√7th **T45.615** Adverse effect of thrombolytic drugs

√7th **T45.616** Underdosing of thrombolytic drugs

√6th **T45.62** **Poisoning by, adverse effect of and underdosing of hemostatic drugs**

√7th **T45.621** **Poisoning by hemostatic drug,** accidental (unintentional)
Poisoning by hemostatic drug NOS

√7th **T45.622** **Poisoning by hemostatic drug,** intentional self-harm

√7th **T45.623** **Poisoning by hemostatic drug,** assault

√7th **T45.624** **Poisoning by hemostatic drug,** undetermined

√7th **T45.625** Adverse effect of hemostatic drug

√7th **T45.626** Underdosing of hemostatic drugs

√6th **T45.69** **Poisoning by, adverse effect of and underdosing of other fibrinolysis-affecting drugs**

√7th **T45.691** **Poisoning by other fibrinolysis-affecting drugs,** accidental (unintentional)
Poisoning by other fibrinolysis-affecting drug NOS

√7th **T45.692** **Poisoning by other fibrinolysis-affecting drugs,** intentional self-harm

√7th **T45.693** **Poisoning by other fibrinolysis-affecting drugs,** assault

√7th **T45.694** **Poisoning by other fibrinolysis-affecting drugs,** undetermined

√7th **T45.695** Adverse effect of other fibrinolysis-affecting drugs

√7th **T45.696** Underdosing of other fibrinolysis-affecting drugs

√5th **T45.7** **Poisoning by, adverse effect of and underdosing of anticoagulant antagonists, vitamin K and other coagulants**

√6th **T45.7X** **Poisoning by, adverse effect of and underdosing of anticoagulant antagonists, vitamin K and other coagulants**

√7th **T45.7X1** **Poisoning by anticoagulant antagonists, vitamin K and other coagulants,** accidental (unintentional)
Poisoning by anticoagulant antagonists, vitamin K and other coagulants NOS

√7th **T45.7X2** **Poisoning by anticoagulant antagonists, vitamin K and other coagulants,** intentional self-harm

√7th **T45.7X3** **Poisoning by anticoagulant antagonists, vitamin K and other coagulants,** assault

√7th **T45.7X4** **Poisoning by anticoagulant antagonists, vitamin K and other coagulants,** undetermined

√7th **T45.7X5** Adverse effect of anticoagulant antagonists, vitamin K and other coagulants

√7th **T45.7X6** Underdosing of anticoagulant antagonist, vitamin K and other coagulants
EXCLUDES 1 *vitamin K deficiency (E56.1)*

√5th **T45.8** **Poisoning by, adverse effect of and underdosing of other primarily systemic and hematological agents**
Poisoning by, adverse effect of and underdosing of liver preparations and other antianemic agents
Poisoning by, adverse effect of and underdosing of natural blood and blood products
Poisoning by, adverse effect of and underdosing of plasma substitute
EXCLUDES 2 *poisoning by, adverse effect of and underdosing of immunoglobulin (T50.Z1) poisoning by, adverse effect of and underdosing of iron (T45.4) transfusion reactions (T80.-)*

√6th **T45.8X** **Poisoning by, adverse effect of and underdosing of other primarily systemic and hematological agents**

√7th **T45.8X1** **Poisoning by other primarily systemic and hematological agents,** accidental (unintentional)
Poisoning by other primarily systemic and hematological agents NOS

√7th **T45.8X2** **Poisoning by other primarily systemic and hematological agents,** intentional self-harm

√7th **T45.8X3** **Poisoning by other primarily systemic and hematological agents,** assault

√7th **T45.8X4** **Poisoning by other primarily systemic and hematological agents,** undetermined

Injury, Poisoning and Certain Other Consequences of External Causes

T45.8X5–T46.5X6

✓7th **T45.8X5** Adverse effect of other primarily systemic and hematological agents

✓7th **T45.8X6** Underdosing of other primarily systemic and hematological agents

✓5th **T45.9** Poisoning by, adverse effect of and underdosing of unspecified primarily systemic and hematological agent

✓x7th **T45.91** Poisoning by unspecified primarily systemic and hematological agent, accidental (unintentional)
Poisoning by primarily systemic and hematological agent NOS

✓x7th **T45.92** Poisoning by unspecified primarily systemic and hematological agent, intentional self-harm

✓x7th **T45.93** Poisoning by unspecified primarily systemic and hematological agent, assault

✓x7th **T45.94** Poisoning by unspecified primarily systemic and hematological agent, undetermined

✓x7th **T45.95** Adverse effect of unspecified primarily systemic and hematological agent

✓x7th **T45.96** Underdosing of unspecified primarily systemic and hematological agent

✓4th **T46** Poisoning by, adverse effect of and underdosing of agents primarily affecting the cardiovascular system

EXCLUDES 1   poisoning by, adverse effect of and underdosing of metaraminol (T44.4)

The appropriate 7th character is to be added to each code from category T46.
A   initial encounter
D   subsequent encounter
S   sequela

✓5th **T46.0** Poisoning by, adverse effect of and underdosing of cardiac-stimulant glycosides and drugs of similar action

✓6th **T46.0X** Poisoning by, adverse effect of and underdosing of cardiac-stimulant glycosides and drugs of similar action

✓7th **T46.0X1** Poisoning by cardiac-stimulant glycosides and drugs of similar action, accidental (unintentional)
Poisoning by cardiac-stimulant glycosides and drugs of similar action NOS

✓7th **T46.0X2** Poisoning by cardiac-stimulant glycosides and drugs of similar action, intentional self-harm

✓7th **T46.0X3** Poisoning by cardiac-stimulant glycosides and drugs of similar action, assault

✓7th **T46.0X4** Poisoning by cardiac-stimulant glycosides and drugs of similar action, undetermined

✓7th **T46.0X5** Adverse effect of cardiac-stimulant glycosides and drugs of similar action

✓7th **T46.0X6** Underdosing of cardiac-stimulant glycosides and drugs of similar action

T46.1 Poisoning by, adverse effect of and underdosing of calcium-channel blockers

✓6th **T46.1X** Poisoning by, adverse effect of and underdosing of calcium-channel blockers

✓7th **T46.1X1** Poisoning by calcium-channel blockers, accidental (unintentional)
Poisoning by calcium-channel blockers NOS

✓7th **T46.1X2** Poisoning by calcium-channel blockers, intentional self-harm

✓7th **T46.1X3** Poisoning by calcium-channel blockers, assault

✓7th **T46.1X4** Poisoning by calcium-channel blockers, undetermined

✓7th **T46.1X5** Adverse effect of calcium-channel blockers

✓7th **T46.1X6** Underdosing of calcium-channel blockers

✓5th **T46.2** Poisoning by, adverse effect of and underdosing of other antidysrhythmic drugs, not elsewhere classified

EXCLUDES 1   poisoning by, adverse effect of and underdosing of beta-adrenoreceptor antagonists (T44.7-)

✓6th **T46.2X** Poisoning by, adverse effect of and underdosing of other antidysrhythmic drugs

✓7th **T46.2X1** Poisoning by other antidysrhythmic drugs, accidental (unintentional)
Poisoning by other antidysrhythmic drugs NOS

✓7th **T46.2X2** Poisoning by other antidysrhythmic drugs, intentional self-harm

✓7th **T46.2X3** Poisoning by other antidysrhythmic drugs, assault

✓7th **T46.2X4** Poisoning by other antidysrhythmic drugs, undetermined

✓7th **T46.2X5** Adverse effect of other antidysrhythmic drugs

✓7th **T46.2X6** Underdosing of other antidysrhythmic drugs

✓5th **T46.3** Poisoning by, adverse effect of and underdosing of coronary vasodilators
Poisoning by, adverse effect of and underdosing of dipyridamole

EXCLUDES 1   poisoning by, adverse effect of and underdosing of calcium-channel blockers (T46.1)

✓6th **T46.3X** Poisoning by, adverse effect of and underdosing of coronary vasodilators

✓7th **T46.3X1** Poisoning by coronary vasodilators, accidental (unintentional)
Poisoning by coronary vasodilators NOS

✓7th **T46.3X2** Poisoning by coronary vasodilators, intentional self-harm

✓7th **T46.3X3** Poisoning by coronary vasodilators, assault

✓7th **T46.3X4** Poisoning by coronary vasodilators, undetermined

✓7th **T46.3X5** Adverse effect of coronary vasodilators

✓7th **T46.3X6** Underdosing of coronary vasodilators

✓5th **T46.4** Poisoning by, adverse effect of and underdosing of angiotensin-converting-enzyme inhibitors

✓6th **T46.4X** Poisoning by, adverse effect of and underdosing of angiotensin-converting-enzyme inhibitors

✓7th **T46.4X1** Poisoning by angiotensin-converting-enzyme inhibitors, accidental (unintentional)
Poisoning by angiotensin-converting-enzyme inhibitors NOS

✓7th **T46.4X2** Poisoning by angiotensin-converting-enzyme inhibitors, intentional self-harm

✓7th **T46.4X3** Poisoning by angiotensin-converting-enzyme inhibitors, assault

✓7th **T46.4X4** Poisoning by angiotensin-converting-enzyme inhibitors, undetermined

✓7th **T46.4X5** Adverse effect of angiotensin-converting-enzyme inhibitors

✓7th **T46.4X6** Underdosing of angiotensin-converting-enzyme inhibitors

✓5th **T46.5** Poisoning by, adverse effect of and underdosing of other antihypertensive drugs

EXCLUDES 2   poisoning by, adverse effect of and underdosing of beta-adrenoreceptor antagonists (T44.7)
poisoning by, adverse effect of and underdosing of calcium-channel blockers (T46.1)
poisoning by, adverse effect of and underdosing of diuretics (T50.0-T50.2)

✓6th **T46.5X** Poisoning by, adverse effect of and underdosing of other antihypertensive drugs

✓7th **T46.5X1** Poisoning by other antihypertensive drugs, accidental (unintentional)
Poisoning by other antihypertensive drugs NOS

✓7th **T46.5X2** Poisoning by other antihypertensive drugs, intentional self-harm

✓7th **T46.5X3** Poisoning by other antihypertensive drugs, assault

✓7th **T46.5X4** Poisoning by other antihypertensive drugs, undetermined

✓7th **T46.5X5** Adverse effect of other antihypertensive drugs

✓7th **T46.5X6** Underdosing of other antihypertensive drugs

Ⓝ Newborn: 0   Ⓟ Pediatric: 0-17   Ⓜ Maternity: 12-55   Ⓐ Adult: 15-124   MCC Major CC Condition   PDx MCC PDx acts as own MCC   CC CC Condition   PDx CC PDx acts as own CC

1068   ICD-10-CM Draft (2015)

✓5th **T46.6 Poisoning by, adverse effect of and underdosing of antihyperlipidemic and antiarteriosclerotic drugs**

✓6th **T46.6X Poisoning by, adverse effect of and underdosing of** antihyperlipidemic and antiarteriosclerotic **drugs**

✓7th **T46.6X1 Poisoning by antihyperlipidemic and antiarteriosclerotic drugs,** accidental **(unintentional)**
Poisoning by antihyperlipidemic and antiarteriosclerotic drugs NOS

✓7th **T46.6X2 Poisoning by antihyperlipidemic and antiarteriosclerotic drugs,** intentional self-harm

✓7th **T46.6X3 Poisoning by antihyperlipidemic and antiarteriosclerotic drugs,** assault

✓7th **T46.6X4 Poisoning by antihyperlipidemic and antiarteriosclerotic drugs,** undetermined

✓7th **T46.6X5** Adverse effect **of antihyperlipidemic and antiarteriosclerotic drugs**

✓7th **T46.6X6** Underdosing **of antihyperlipidemic and antiarteriosclerotic drugs**

✓5th **T46.7 Poisoning by, adverse effect of and underdosing of peripheral vasodilators**
Poisoning by, adverse effect of and underdosing of nicotinic acid (derivatives)

EXCLUDES 1 *poisoning by, adverse effect of and underdosing of papaverine (T44.3)*

✓6th **T46.7X Poisoning by, adverse effect of and underdosing of** peripheral vasodilators

✓7th **T46.7X1 Poisoning by peripheral vasodilators,** accidental (unintentional)
Poisoning by peripheral vasodilators NOS

✓7th **T46.7X2 Poisoning by peripheral vasodilators,** intentional self-harm

✓7th **T46.7X3 Poisoning by peripheral vasodilators,** assault

✓7th **T46.7X4 Poisoning by peripheral vasodilators,** undetermined

✓7th **T46.7X5** Adverse effect **of peripheral vasodilators**

✓7th **T46.7X6** Underdosing **of peripheral vasodilators**

✓5th **T46.8 Poisoning by, adverse effect of and underdosing of antivaricose drugs, including sclerosing agents**

✓6th **T46.8X Poisoning by, adverse effect of and underdosing of** antivaricose **drugs, including sclerosing agents**

✓7th **T46.8X1 Poisoning by antivaricose drugs, including sclerosing agents,** accidental (unintentional)
Poisoning by antivaricose drugs, including sclerosing agents NOS

✓7th **T46.8X2 Poisoning by antivaricose drugs, including sclerosing agents,** intentional self-harm

✓7th **T46.8X3 Poisoning by antivaricose drugs, including sclerosing agents,** assault

✓7th **T46.8X4 Poisoning by antivaricose drugs, including sclerosing agents,** undetermined

✓7th **T46.8X5** Adverse effect **of antivaricose drugs, including sclerosing agents**

✓7th **T46.8X6** Underdosing **of antivaricose drugs, including sclerosing agents**

✓5th **T46.9 Poisoning by, adverse effect of and underdosing of other and unspecified** agents primarily affecting the cardiovascular system

✓6th **T46.90 Poisoning by, adverse effect of and underdosing of** unspecified **agents primarily affecting the cardiovascular system**

✓7th **T46.901 Poisoning by unspecified agents primarily affecting the cardiovascular system,** accidental (unintentional)

✓7th **T46.902 Poisoning by unspecified agents primarily affecting the cardiovascular system,** intentional self-harm

✓7th **T46.903 Poisoning by unspecified agents primarily affecting the cardiovascular system,** assault

✓7th **T46.904 Poisoning by unspecified agents primarily affecting the cardiovascular system,** undetermined

✓7th **T46.905** Adverse effect **of unspecified agents primarily affecting the cardiovascular system**

✓7th **T46.906** Underdosing **of unspecified agents primarily affecting the cardiovascular system**

✓6th **T46.99 Poisoning by, adverse effect of and underdosing of** other **agents primarily affecting the cardiovascular system**

✓7th **T46.991 Poisoning by other agents primarily affecting the cardiovascular system,** accidental (unintentional)

✓7th **T46.992 Poisoning by other agents primarily affecting the cardiovascular system,** intentional self-harm

✓7th **T46.993 Poisoning by other agents primarily affecting the cardiovascular system,** assault

✓7th **T46.994 Poisoning by other agents primarily affecting the cardiovascular system,** undetermined

✓7th **T46.995** Adverse effect **of other agents primarily affecting the cardiovascular system**

✓7th **T46.996** Underdosing **of other agents primarily affecting the cardiovascular system**

✓4th **T47 Poisoning by, adverse effect of and underdosing of agents primarily affecting the gastrointestinal system**

The appropriate 7th character is to be added to each code from category T47.
A   initial encounter
D   subsequent encounter
S   sequela

✓5th **T47.0 Poisoning by, adverse effect of and underdosing of histamine H2-receptor blockers**

✓6th **T47.0X Poisoning by, adverse effect of and underdosing of** histamine H2-receptor blockers

✓7th **T47.0X1 Poisoning by histamine H2-receptor blockers,** accidental (unintentional)
Poisoning by histamine H2-receptor blockers NOS

✓7th **T47.0X2 Poisoning by histamine H2-receptor blockers,** intentional self-harm

✓7th **T47.0X3 Poisoning by histamine H2-receptor blockers,** assault

✓7th **T47.0X4 Poisoning by histamine H2-receptor blockers,** undetermined

✓7th **T47.0X5** Adverse effect **of histamine H2-receptor blockers**

✓7th **T47.0X6** Underdosing **of histamine H2-receptor blockers**

✓5th **T47.1 Poisoning by, adverse effect of and underdosing of other antacids and anti-gastric-secretion drugs**

✓6th **T47.1X Poisoning by, adverse effect of and underdosing of** other antacids and anti-gastric-secretion **drugs**

✓7th **T47.1X1 Poisoning by other antacids and anti-gastric-secretion drugs,** accidental (unintentional)
Poisoning by other antacids and anti-gastric-secretion drugs NOS

✓7th **T47.1X2 Poisoning by other antacids and anti-gastric-secretion drugs,** intentional self-harm

✓7th **T47.1X3 Poisoning by other antacids and anti-gastric-secretion drugs,** assault

✓7th **T47.1X4 Poisoning by other antacids and anti-gastric-secretion drugs,** undetermined

✓7th **T47.1X5** Adverse effect **of other antacids and anti-gastric-secretion drugs**

✓7th **T47.1X6** Underdosing **of other antacids and anti-gastric-secretion drugs**

✓5th **T47.2 Poisoning by, adverse effect of and underdosing of stimulant laxatives**

✓6th **T47.2X Poisoning by, adverse effect of and underdosing of** stimulant laxatives

✓7th **T47.2X1 Poisoning by stimulant laxatives,** accidental (unintentional)
Poisoning by stimulant laxatives NOS

✓7th **T47.2X2** **Poisoning by stimulant laxatives,** intentional self-harm

✓7th **T47.2X3** **Poisoning by stimulant laxatives,** assault

✓7th **T47.2X4** **Poisoning by stimulant laxatives,** undetermined

✓7th **T47.2X5** Adverse effect of stimulant laxatives

✓7th **T47.2X6** Underdosing of stimulant laxatives

✓5th **T47.3** Poisoning by, adverse effect of and underdosing of saline and osmotic laxatives

✓6th **T47.3X** **Poisoning by and adverse effect of** saline and osmotic laxatives

✓7th **T47.3X1** **Poisoning by saline and osmotic laxatives,** accidental (unintentional)
Poisoning by saline and osmotic laxatives NOS

✓7th **T47.3X2** **Poisoning by saline and osmotic laxatives,** intentional self-harm

✓7th **T47.3X3** **Poisoning by saline and osmotic laxatives,** assault

✓7th **T47.3X4** **Poisoning by saline and osmotic laxatives,** undetermined

✓7th **T47.3X5** Adverse effect of saline and osmotic laxatives

✓7th **T47.3X6** Underdosing of saline and osmotic laxatives

✓5th **T47.4** Poisoning by, adverse effect of and underdosing of other laxatives

✓6th **T47.4X** **Poisoning by, adverse effect of and underdosing of** other laxatives

✓7th **T47.4X1** **Poisoning by other laxatives,** accidental (unintentional)
Poisoning by other laxatives NOS

✓7th **T47.4X2** **Poisoning by other laxatives,** intentional self-harm

✓7th **T47.4X3** **Poisoning by other laxatives,** assault

✓7th **T47.4X4** **Poisoning by other laxatives,** undetermined

✓7th **T47.4X5** Adverse effect of other laxatives

✓7th **T47.4X6** Underdosing of other laxatives

✓5th **T47.5** Poisoning by, adverse effect of and underdosing of digestants

✓6th **T47.5X** **Poisoning by, adverse effect of and underdosing of** digestants

✓7th **T47.5X1** **Poisoning by digestants,** accidental (unintentional)
Poisoning by digestants NOS

✓7th **T47.5X2** **Poisoning by digestants,** intentional self-harm

✓7th **T47.5X3** **Poisoning by digestants,** assault

✓7th **T47.5X4** **Poisoning by digestants,** undetermined

✓7th **T47.5X5** Adverse effect of digestants

✓7th **T47.5X6** Underdosing of digestants

✓5th **T47.6** Poisoning by, adverse effect of and underdosing of antidiarrheal drugs

EXCLUDES 2 *poisoning by, adverse effect of and underdosing of systemic antibiotics and other anti-infectives (T36-T37)*

✓6th **T47.6X** **Poisoning by, adverse effect of and underdosing of** antidiarrheal drugs

✓7th **T47.6X1** **Poisoning by antidiarrheal drugs,** accidental (unintentional)
Poisoning by antidiarrheal drugs NOS

✓7th **T47.6X2** **Poisoning by antidiarrheal drugs,** intentional self-harm

✓7th **T47.6X3** **Poisoning by antidiarrheal drugs,** assault

✓7th **T47.6X4** **Poisoning by antidiarrheal drugs,** undetermined

✓7th **T47.6X5** Adverse effect of antidiarrheal drugs

✓7th **T47.6X6** Underdosing of antidiarrheal drugs

✓5th **T47.7** Poisoning by, adverse effect of and underdosing of emetics

✓6th **T47.7X** **Poisoning by, adverse effect of and underdosing of** emetics

✓7th **T47.7X1** **Poisoning by emetics,** accidental (unintentional)
Poisoning by emetics NOS

✓7th **T47.7X2** **Poisoning by emetics,** intentional self-harm

✓7th **T47.7X3** **Poisoning by emetics,** assault

✓7th **T47.7X4** **Poisoning by emetics,** undetermined

✓7th **T47.7X5** Adverse effect of emetics

✓7th **T47.7X6** Underdosing of emetics

✓5th **T47.8** Poisoning by, adverse effect of and underdosing of other agents primarily affecting gastrointestinal system

✓6th **T47.8X** **Poisoning by, adverse effect of and underdosing of** other agents primarily affecting gastrointestinal system

✓7th **T47.8X1** **Poisoning by other agents primarily affecting gastrointestinal system,** accidental (unintentional)
Poisoning by other agents primarily affecting gastrointestinal system NOS

✓7th **T47.8X2** **Poisoning by other agents primarily affecting gastrointestinal system,** intentional self-harm

✓7th **T47.8X3** **Poisoning by other agents primarily affecting gastrointestinal system,** assault

✓7th **T47.8X4** **Poisoning by other agents primarily affecting gastrointestinal system,** undetermined

✓7th **T47.8X5** Adverse effect of other agents primarily affecting gastrointestinal system

✓7th **T47.8X6** Underdosing of other agents primarily affecting gastrointestinal system

✓5th **T47.9** Poisoning by, adverse effect of and underdosing of unspecified agents primarily affecting the gastrointestinal system

✓x7th **T47.91** **Poisoning by unspecified agents primarily affecting the gastrointestinal system,** accidental (unintentional)
Poisoning by agents primarily affecting the gastrointestinal system NOS

✓x7th **T47.92** **Poisoning by unspecified agents primarily affecting the gastrointestinal system,** intentional self-harm

✓x7th **T47.93** **Poisoning by unspecified agents primarily affecting the gastrointestinal system,** assault

✓x7th **T47.94** **Poisoning by unspecified agents primarily affecting the gastrointestinal system,** undetermined

✓x7th **T47.95** Adverse effect of unspecified agents primarily affecting the gastrointestinal system

✓x7th **T47.96** Underdosing of unspecified agents primarily affecting the gastrointestinal system

✓4th **T48** **Poisoning by, adverse effect of and underdosing of agents primarily acting on smooth and skeletal muscles and the respiratory system**

The appropriate 7th character is to be added to each code from category T48.
A   initial encounter
D   subsequent encounter
S   sequela

✓5th **T48.0** Poisoning by, adverse effect of and underdosing of oxytocic drugs

EXCLUDES 1 *poisoning by, adverse effect of and underdosing of estrogens, progestogens and antagonists (T38.4-T38.6)*

✓6th **T48.0X** **Poisoning by, adverse effect of and underdosing of** oxytocic drugs

✓7th **T48.0X1** **Poisoning by oxytocic drugs,** accidental (unintentional)
Poisoning by oxytocic drugs NOS

✓7th **T48.0X2** **Poisoning by oxytocic drugs,** intentional self-harm

✓7th **T48.0X3** **Poisoning by oxytocic drugs,** assault

✓7th **T48.0X4** **Poisoning by oxytocic drugs,** undetermined

✓7th **T48.0X5** Adverse effect of oxytocic drugs

✓7th **T48.0X6** Underdosing of oxytocic drugs

✓5ᵗʰ **T48.1** **Poisoning by, adverse effect of and underdosing of skeletal muscle relaxants [neuromuscular blocking agents]**

    ✓6ᵗʰ **T48.1X** **Poisoning by, adverse effect of and underdosing of skeletal muscle relaxants [neuromuscular blocking agents]**

       ✓7ᵗʰ **T48.1X1** **Poisoning by skeletal muscle relaxants [neuromuscular blocking agents], accidental (unintentional)**
          Poisoning by skeletal muscle relaxants [neuromuscular blocking agents] NOS

       ✓7ᵗʰ **T48.1X2** **Poisoning by skeletal muscle relaxants [neuromuscular blocking agents], intentional self-harm**

       ✓7ᵗʰ **T48.1X3** **Poisoning by skeletal muscle relaxants [neuromuscular blocking agents], assault**

       ✓7ᵗʰ **T48.1X4** **Poisoning by skeletal muscle relaxants [neuromuscular blocking agents], undetermined**

       ✓7ᵗʰ **T48.1X5** **Adverse effect of skeletal muscle relaxants [neuromuscular blocking agents]**

       ✓7ᵗʰ **T48.1X6** **Underdosing of skeletal muscle relaxants [neuromuscular blocking agents]**

✓5ᵗʰ **T48.2** **Poisoning by, adverse effect of and underdosing of other and unspecified drugs acting on muscles**

    ✓6ᵗʰ **T48.20** **Poisoning by, adverse effect of and underdosing of unspecified drugs acting on muscles**

       ✓7ᵗʰ **T48.201** **Poisoning by unspecified drugs acting on muscles, accidental (unintentional)**
          Poisoning by unspecified drugs acting on muscles NOS

       ✓7ᵗʰ **T48.202** **Poisoning by unspecified drugs acting on muscles, intentional self-harm**

       ✓7ᵗʰ **T48.203** **Poisoning by unspecified drugs acting on muscles, assault**

       ✓7ᵗʰ **T48.204** **Poisoning by unspecified drugs acting on muscles, undetermined**

       ✓7ᵗʰ **T48.205** **Adverse effect of unspecified drugs acting on muscles**

       ✓7ᵗʰ **T48.206** **Underdosing of unspecified drugs acting on muscles**

    ✓6ᵗʰ **T48.29** **Poisoning by, adverse effect of and underdosing of other drugs acting on muscles**

       ✓7ᵗʰ **T48.291** **Poisoning by other drugs acting on muscles, accidental (unintentional)**
          Poisoning by other drugs acting on muscles NOS

       ✓7ᵗʰ **T48.292** **Poisoning by other drugs acting on muscles, intentional self-harm**

       ✓7ᵗʰ **T48.293** **Poisoning by other drugs acting on muscles, assault**

       ✓7ᵗʰ **T48.294** **Poisoning by other drugs acting on muscles, undetermined**

       ✓7ᵗʰ **T48.295** **Adverse effect of other drugs acting on muscles**

       ✓7ᵗʰ **T48.296** **Underdosing of other drugs acting on muscles**

✓5ᵗʰ **T48.3** **Poisoning by, adverse effect of and underdosing of antitussives**

    ✓6ᵗʰ **T48.3X** **Poisoning by, adverse effect of and underdosing of antitussives**

       ✓7ᵗʰ **T48.3X1** **Poisoning by antitussives, accidental (unintentional)**
          Poisoning by antitussives NOS

       ✓7ᵗʰ **T48.3X2** **Poisoning by antitussives, intentional self-harm**

       ✓7ᵗʰ **T48.3X3** **Poisoning by antitussives, assault**

       ✓7ᵗʰ **T48.3X4** **Poisoning by antitussives, undetermined**

       ✓7ᵗʰ **T48.3X5** **Adverse effect of antitussives**

       ✓7ᵗʰ **T48.3X6** **Underdosing of antitussives**

✓5ᵗʰ **T48.4** **Poisoning by, adverse effect of and underdosing of expectorants**

    ✓6ᵗʰ **T48.4X** **Poisoning by, adverse effect of and underdosing of expectorants**

       ✓7ᵗʰ **T48.4X1** **Poisoning by expectorants, accidental (unintentional)**
          Poisoning by expectorants NOS

       ✓7ᵗʰ **T48.4X2** **Poisoning by expectorants, intentional self-harm**

       ✓7ᵗʰ **T48.4X3** **Poisoning by expectorants, assault**

       ✓7ᵗʰ **T48.4X4** **Poisoning by expectorants, undetermined**

       ✓7ᵗʰ **T48.4X5** **Adverse effect of expectorants**

       ✓7ᵗʰ **T48.4X6** **Underdosing of expectorants**

✓5ᵗʰ **T48.5** **Poisoning by, adverse effect of and underdosing of other anti-common-cold drugs**
    Poisoning by, adverse effect of and underdosing of decongestants
    EXCLUDES 2   *poisoning by, adverse effect of and underdosing of antipyretics, NEC (T39.9-)*
       poisoning by, adverse effect of and underdosing of non-steroidal antiinflammatory drugs (T39.3-)
       poisoning by, adverse effect of and underdosing of salicylates (T39.0-)

    ✓6ᵗʰ **T48.5X** **Poisoning by, adverse effect of and underdosing of other anti-common-cold drugs**

       ✓7ᵗʰ **T48.5X1** **Poisoning by other anti-common-cold drugs, accidental (unintentional)**
          Poisoning by other anti-common-cold drugs NOS

       ✓7ᵗʰ **T48.5X2** **Poisoning by other anti-common-cold drugs, intentional self-harm**

       ✓7ᵗʰ **T48.5X3** **Poisoning by other anti-common-cold drugs, assault**

       ✓7ᵗʰ **T48.5X4** **Poisoning by other anti-common-cold drugs, undetermined**

       ✓7ᵗʰ **T48.5X5** **Adverse effect of other anti-common-cold drugs**

       ✓7ᵗʰ **T48.5X6** **Underdosing of other anti-common-cold drugs**

✓5ᵗʰ **T48.6** **Poisoning by, adverse effect of and underdosing of antiasthmatics, not elsewhere classified**
    Poisoning by, adverse effect of and underdosing of beta-adrenoreceptor agonists used in asthma therapy
    EXCLUDES 1   *poisoning by, adverse effect of and underdosing of anterior pituitary [adenohypophyseal] hormones (T38.8)*
       poisoning by, adverse effect of and underdosing of beta-adrenoreceptor agonists not used in asthma therapy (T44.5)

    ✓6ᵗʰ **T48.6X** **Poisoning by, adverse effect of and underdosing of antiasthmatics**

       ✓7ᵗʰ **T48.6X1** **Poisoning by antiasthmatics, accidental (unintentional)**
          Poisoning by antiasthmatics NOS

       ✓7ᵗʰ **T48.6X2** **Poisoning by antiasthmatics, intentional self-harm**

       ✓7ᵗʰ **T48.6X3** **Poisoning by antiasthmatics, assault**

       ✓7ᵗʰ **T48.6X4** **Poisoning by antiasthmatics, undetermined**

       ✓7ᵗʰ **T48.6X5** **Adverse effect of antiasthmatics**

       ✓7ᵗʰ **T48.6X6** **Underdosing of antiasthmatics**

✓5ᵗʰ **T48.9** **Poisoning by, adverse effect of and underdosing of other and unspecified agents primarily acting on the respiratory system**

    ✓6ᵗʰ **T48.90** **Poisoning by, adverse effect of and underdosing of unspecified agents primarily acting on the respiratory system**

       ✓7ᵗʰ **T48.901** **Poisoning by unspecified agents primarily acting on the respiratory system, accidental (unintentional)**

       ✓7ᵗʰ **T48.902** **Poisoning by unspecified agents primarily acting on the respiratory system, intentional self-harm**

       ✓7ᵗʰ **T48.903** **Poisoning by unspecified agents primarily acting on the respiratory system, assault**

       ✓7ᵗʰ **T48.904** **Poisoning by unspecified agents primarily acting on the respiratory system, undetermined**

       ✓7ᵗʰ **T48.905** **Adverse effect of unspecified agents primarily acting on the respiratory system**

       ✓7ᵗʰ **T48.906** **Underdosing of unspecified agents primarily acting on the respiratory system**

✓ Additional Character Required   ✓x7ᵗʰ Xtension Alert   Unacceptable PDx   Manifestation   Hospital Acquired Condition   EXCLUDES 1 Not Coded Here   EXCLUDES 2 Not Included Here

Injury, Poisoning and Certain Other Consequences of External Causes   T48.99–T49.6X1

√6ᵗʰ **T48.99** **Poisoning by, adverse effect of and underdosing of** other **agents primarily acting on the respiratory system**

√7ᵗʰ **T48.991** Poisoning by other agents primarily acting on the respiratory system, accidental (unintentional)

√7ᵗʰ **T48.992** Poisoning by other agents primarily acting on the respiratory system, intentional self-harm

√7ᵗʰ **T48.993** Poisoning by other agents primarily acting on the respiratory system, assault

√7ᵗʰ **T48.994** Poisoning by other agents primarily acting on the respiratory system, undetermined

√7ᵗʰ **T48.995** Adverse effect of other agents primarily acting on the respiratory system

√7ᵗʰ **T48.996** Underdosing of other agents primarily acting on the respiratory system

√4ᵗʰ **T49** **Poisoning by, adverse effect of and underdosing of topical agents primarily affecting skin and mucous membrane and by ophthalmological, otorhinolaryngological and dental drugs**

Poisoning by, adverse effect of and underdosing of glucocorticoids, topically used

> The appropriate 7th character is to be added to each code from category T49.
> A   initial encounter
> D   subsequent encounter
> S   sequela

√5ᵗʰ **T49.Ø** **Poisoning by, adverse effect of and underdosing of local antifungal, anti-infective and anti-inflammatory drugs**

√6ᵗʰ **T49.ØX** **Poisoning by, adverse effect of and underdosing of local antifungal, anti-infective and anti-inflammatory drugs**

√7ᵗʰ **T49.ØX1** Poisoning by local antifungal, anti-infective and anti-inflammatory drugs, accidental (unintentional)

Poisoning by local antifungal, anti-infective and anti-inflammatory drugs NOS

√7ᵗʰ **T49.ØX2** Poisoning by local antifungal, anti-infective and anti-inflammatory drugs, intentional self-harm

√7ᵗʰ **T49.ØX3** Poisoning by local antifungal, anti-infective and anti-inflammatory drugs, assault

√7ᵗʰ **T49.ØX4** Poisoning by local antifungal, anti-infective and anti-inflammatory drugs, undetermined

√7ᵗʰ **T49.ØX5** Adverse effect of local antifungal, anti-infective and anti-inflammatory drugs

√7ᵗʰ **T49.ØX6** Underdosing of local antifungal, anti-infective and anti-inflammatory drugs

√5ᵗʰ **T49.1** **Poisoning by, adverse effect of and underdosing of antipruritics**

√6ᵗʰ **T49.1X** **Poisoning by, adverse effect of and underdosing of antipruritics**

√7ᵗʰ **T49.1X1** Poisoning by antipruritics, accidental (unintentional)

Poisoning by antipruritics NOS

√7ᵗʰ **T49.1X2** Poisoning by antipruritics, intentional self-harm

√7ᵗʰ **T49.1X3** Poisoning by antipruritics, assault

√7ᵗʰ **T49.1X4** Poisoning by antipruritics, undetermined

√7ᵗʰ **T49.1X5** Adverse effect of antipruritics

√7ᵗʰ **T49.1X6** Underdosing of antipruritics

√5ᵗʰ **T49.2** **Poisoning by, adverse effect of and underdosing of local astringents and local detergents**

√6ᵗʰ **T49.2X** **Poisoning by, adverse effect of and underdosing of local astringents and local detergents**

√7ᵗʰ **T49.2X1** Poisoning by local astringents and local detergents, accidental (unintentional)

Poisoning by local astringents and local detergents NOS

√7ᵗʰ **T49.2X2** Poisoning by local astringents and local detergents, intentional self-harm

√7ᵗʰ **T49.2X3** Poisoning by local astringents and local detergents, assault

√7ᵗʰ **T49.2X4** Poisoning by local astringents and local detergents, undetermined

√7ᵗʰ **T49.2X5** Adverse effect of local astringents and local detergents

√7ᵗʰ **T49.2X6** Underdosing of local astringents and local detergents

√5ᵗʰ **T49.3** **Poisoning by, adverse effect of and underdosing of emollients, demulcents and protectants**

√6ᵗʰ **T49.3X** **Poisoning by, adverse effect of and underdosing of** emollients, demulcents and protectants

√7ᵗʰ **T49.3X1** Poisoning by emollients, demulcents and protectants, accidental (unintentional)

Poisoning by emollients, demulcents and protectants NOS

√7ᵗʰ **T49.3X2** Poisoning by emollients, demulcents and protectants, intentional self-harm

√7ᵗʰ **T49.3X3** Poisoning by emollients, demulcents and protectants, assault

√7ᵗʰ **T49.3X4** Poisoning by emollients, demulcents and protectants, undetermined

√7ᵗʰ **T49.3X5** Adverse effect of emollients, demulcents and protectants

√7ᵗʰ **T49.3X6** Underdosing of emollients, demulcents and protectants

√5ᵗʰ **T49.4** **Poisoning by, adverse effect of and underdosing of keratolytics, keratoplastics, and other hair treatment drugs and preparations**

√6ᵗʰ **T49.4X** **Poisoning by, adverse effect of and underdosing of** keratolytics, keratoplastics, and other hair treatment drugs and preparations

√7ᵗʰ **T49.4X1** Poisoning by keratolytics, keratoplastics, and other hair treatment drugs and preparations, accidental (unintentional)

Poisoning by keratolytics, keratoplastics, and other hair treatment drugs and preparations NOS

√7ᵗʰ **T49.4X2** Poisoning by keratolytics, keratoplastics, and other hair treatment drugs and preparations, intentional self-harm

√7ᵗʰ **T49.4X3** Poisoning by keratolytics, keratoplastics, and other hair treatment drugs and preparations, assault

√7ᵗʰ **T49.4X4** Poisoning by keratolytics, keratoplastics, and other hair treatment drugs and preparations, undetermined

√7ᵗʰ **T49.4X5** Adverse effect of keratolytics, keratoplastics, and other hair treatment drugs and preparations

√7ᵗʰ **T49.4X6** Underdosing of keratolytics, keratoplastics, and other hair treatment drugs and preparations

√5ᵗʰ **T49.5** **Poisoning by, adverse effect of and underdosing of ophthalmological drugs and preparations**

√6ᵗʰ **T49.5X** **Poisoning by, adverse effect of and underdosing of** ophthalmological drugs and preparations

√7ᵗʰ **T49.5X1** Poisoning by ophthalmological drugs and preparations, accidental (unintentional)

Poisoning by ophthalmological drugs and preparations NOS

√7ᵗʰ **T49.5X2** Poisoning by ophthalmological drugs and preparations, intentional self-harm

√7ᵗʰ **T49.5X3** Poisoning by ophthalmological drugs and preparations, assault

√7ᵗʰ **T49.5X4** Poisoning by ophthalmological drugs and preparations, undetermined

√7ᵗʰ **T49.5X5** Adverse effect of ophthalmological drugs and preparations

√7ᵗʰ **T49.5X6** Underdosing of ophthalmological drugs and preparations

√5ᵗʰ **T49.6** **Poisoning by, adverse effect of and underdosing of otorhinolaryngological drugs and preparations**

√6ᵗʰ **T49.6X** **Poisoning by, adverse effect of and underdosing of** otorhinolaryngological drugs and preparations

√7ᵗʰ **T49.6X1** Poisoning by otorhinolaryngological drugs and preparations, accidental (unintentional)

Poisoning by otorhinolaryngological drugs and preparations NOS

N Newborn: Ø   P Pediatric: Ø-17   M Maternity: 12-55   A Adult: 15-124   MCC Major CC Condition   PDx MCC PDx acts as own MCC   CC CC Condition   PDx CC PDx acts as own CC

1Ø72   ICD-1Ø-CM Draft (2Ø15)

✓7th **T49.6X2** Poisoning by otorhinolaryngological drugs and preparations, intentional self-harm

✓7th **T49.6X3** Poisoning by otorhinolaryngological drugs and preparations, assault

✓7th **T49.6X4** Poisoning by otorhinolaryngological drugs and preparations, undetermined

✓7th **T49.6X5** Adverse effect of otorhinolaryngological drugs and preparations

✓7th **T49.6X6** Underdosing of otorhinolaryngological drugs and preparations

✓5th **T49.7** Poisoning by, adverse effect of and underdosing of dental drugs, topically applied

✓6th **T49.7X** Poisoning by, adverse effect of and underdosing of dental drugs, topically applied

✓7th **T49.7X1** Poisoning by dental drugs, topically applied, accidental (unintentional)
Poisoning by dental drugs, topically applied NOS

✓7th **T49.7X2** Poisoning by dental drugs, topically applied, intentional self-harm

✓7th **T49.7X3** Poisoning by dental drugs, topically applied, assault

✓7th **T49.7X4** Poisoning by dental drugs, topically applied, undetermined

✓7th **T49.7X5** Adverse effect of dental drugs, topically applied

✓7th **T49.7X6** Underdosing of dental drugs, topically applied

✓5th **T49.8** Poisoning by, adverse effect of and underdosing of other topical agents
Poisoning by, adverse effect of and underdosing of spermicides

✓6th **T49.8X** Poisoning by, adverse effect of and underdosing of other topical agents

✓7th **T49.8X1** Poisoning by other topical agents, accidental (unintentional)
Poisoning by other topical agents NOS

✓7th **T49.8X2** Poisoning by other topical agents, intentional self-harm

✓7th **T49.8X3** Poisoning by other topical agents, assault

✓7th **T49.8X4** Poisoning by other topical agents, undetermined

✓7th **T49.8X5** Adverse effect of other topical agents

✓7th **T49.8X6** Underdosing of other topical agents

✓5th **T49.9** Poisoning by, adverse effect of and underdosing of unspecified topical agent

✓x7th **T49.91** Poisoning by unspecified topical agent, accidental (unintentional)

✓x7th **T49.92** Poisoning by unspecified topical agent, intentional self-harm

✓x7th **T49.93** Poisoning by unspecified topical agent, assault

✓x7th **T49.94** Poisoning by unspecified topical agent, undetermined

✓x7th **T49.95** Adverse effect of unspecified topical agent

✓x7th **T49.96** Underdosing of unspecified topical agent

✓4th **T50** Poisoning by, adverse effect of and underdosing of diuretics and other and unspecified drugs, medicaments and biological substances

> The appropriate 7th character is to be added to each code from category T50.
> A   initial encounter
> D   subsequent encounter
> S   sequela

✓5th **T50.0** Poisoning by, adverse effect of and underdosing of mineralocorticoids and their antagonists

✓6th **T50.0X** Poisoning by, adverse effect of and underdosing of mineralocorticoids and their antagonists

✓7th **T50.0X1** Poisoning by mineralocorticoids and their antagonists, accidental (unintentional)
Poisoning by mineralocorticoids and their antagonists NOS

✓7th **T50.0X2** Poisoning by mineralocorticoids and their antagonists, intentional self-harm

✓7th **T50.0X3** Poisoning by mineralocorticoids and their antagonists, assault

✓7th **T50.0X4** Poisoning by mineralocorticoids and their antagonists, undetermined

✓7th **T50.0X5** Adverse effect of mineralocorticoids and their antagonists

✓7th **T50.0X6** Underdosing of mineralocorticoids and their antagonists

✓5th **T50.1** Poisoning by, adverse effect of and underdosing of loop [high-ceiling] diuretics

✓6th **T50.1X** Poisoning by, adverse effect of and underdosing of loop [high-ceiling] diuretics

✓7th **T50.1X1** Poisoning by loop [high-ceiling] diuretics, accidental (unintentional)
Poisoning by loop [high-ceiling] diuretics NOS

✓7th **T50.1X2** Poisoning by loop [high-ceiling] diuretics, intentional self-harm

✓7th **T50.1X3** Poisoning by loop [high-ceiling] diuretics, assault

✓7th **T50.1X4** Poisoning by loop [high-ceiling] diuretics, undetermined

✓7th **T50.1X5** Adverse effect of loop [high-ceiling] diuretics

✓7th **T50.1X6** Underdosing of loop [high-ceiling] diuretics

✓5th **T50.2** Poisoning by, adverse effect of and underdosing of carbonic-anhydrase inhibitors, benzothiadiazides and other diuretics
Poisoning by, adverse effect of and underdosing of acetazolamide

✓6th **T50.2X** Poisoning by, adverse effect of and underdosing of carbonic-anhydrase inhibitors, benzothiadiazides and other diuretics

✓7th **T50.2X1** Poisoning by carbonic-anhydrase inhibitors, benzothiadiazides and other diuretics, accidental (unintentional)
Poisoning by carbonic-anhydrase inhibitors, benzothiadiazides and other diuretics NOS

✓7th **T50.2X2** Poisoning by carbonic-anhydrase inhibitors, benzothiadiazides and other diuretics, intentional self-harm

✓7th **T50.2X3** Poisoning by carbonic-anhydrase inhibitors, benzothiadiazides and other diuretics, assault

✓7th **T50.2X4** Poisoning by carbonic-anhydrase inhibitors, benzothiadiazides and other diuretics, undetermined

✓7th **T50.2X5** Adverse effect of carbonic-anhydrase inhibitors, benzothiadiazides and other diuretics

✓7th **T50.2X6** Underdosing of carbonic-anhydrase inhibitors, benzothiadiazides and other diuretics

✓5th **T50.3** Poisoning by, adverse effect of and underdosing of electrolytic, caloric and water-balance agents
Poisoning by, adverse effect of and underdosing of oral rehydration salts

✓6th **T50.3X** Poisoning by, adverse effect of and underdosing of electrolytic, caloric and water-balance agents

✓7th **T50.3X1** Poisoning by electrolytic, caloric and water-balance agents, accidental (unintentional)
Poisoning by electrolytic, caloric and water-balance agents NOS

✓7th **T50.3X2** Poisoning by electrolytic, caloric and water-balance agents, intentional self-harm

✓7th **T50.3X3** Poisoning by electrolytic, caloric and water-balance agents, assault

✓7th **T50.3X4** Poisoning by electrolytic, caloric and water-balance agents, undetermined

✓7th **T50.3X5** Adverse effect of electrolytic, caloric and water-balance agents

✓7th **T50.3X6** Underdosing of electrolytic, caloric and water-balance agents

---

✓ Additional Character Required   ✓x7th Xtension Alert   Unacceptable PDx   Manifestation   Hospital Acquired Condition   EXCLUDES 1 Not Coded Here   EXCLUDES 2 Not Included Here

ICD-10-CM Draft (2015)   1073

Injury, Poisoning and Certain Other Consequences of External Causes

T50.4–T50.B13

√5ᵗʰ **T50.4** **Poisoning by, adverse effect of and underdosing of drugs affecting uric acid metabolism**

√6ᵗʰ **T50.4X** **Poisoning by, adverse effect of and underdosing of drugs** affecting uric acid metabolism

√7ᵗʰ **T50.4X1** **Poisoning by drugs affecting uric acid metabolism, accidental (unintentional)**
Poisoning by drugs affecting uric acid metabolism NOS

√7ᵗʰ **T50.4X2** **Poisoning by drugs affecting uric acid metabolism, intentional self-harm**

√7ᵗʰ **T50.4X3** **Poisoning by drugs affecting uric acid metabolism, assault**

√7ᵗʰ **T50.4X4** **Poisoning by drugs affecting uric acid metabolism, undetermined**

√7ᵗʰ **T50.4X5** **Adverse effect** of drugs affecting uric acid metabolism

√7ᵗʰ **T50.4X6** **Underdosing** of drugs affecting uric acid metabolism

√5ᵗʰ **T50.5** **Poisoning by, adverse effect of and underdosing of appetite depressants**

√6ᵗʰ **T50.5X** **Poisoning by, adverse effect of and underdosing of appetite depressants**

√7ᵗʰ **T50.5X1** **Poisoning by appetite depressants, accidental (unintentional)**
Poisoning by appetite depressants NOS

√7ᵗʰ **T50.5X2** **Poisoning by appetite depressants, intentional self-harm**

√7ᵗʰ **T50.5X3** **Poisoning by appetite depressants, assault**

√7ᵗʰ **T50.5X4** **Poisoning by appetite depressants, undetermined**

√7ᵗʰ **T50.5X5** **Adverse effect** of appetite depressants

√7ᵗʰ **T50.5X6** **Underdosing** of appetite depressants

√5ᵗʰ **T50.6** **Poisoning by, adverse effect of and underdosing of antidotes and chelating agents**
Poisoning by, adverse effect of and underdosing of alcohol deterrents

√6ᵗʰ **T50.6X** **Poisoning by, adverse effect of and underdosing of antidotes and chelating agents**

√7ᵗʰ **T50.6X1** **Poisoning by antidotes and chelating agents, accidental (unintentional)**
Poisoning by antidotes and chelating agents NOS

√7ᵗʰ **T50.6X2** **Poisoning by antidotes and chelating agents, intentional self-harm**

√7ᵗʰ **T50.6X3** **Poisoning by antidotes and chelating agents, assault**

√7ᵗʰ **T50.6X4** **Poisoning by antidotes and chelating agents, undetermined**

√7ᵗʰ **T50.6X5** **Adverse effect** of antidotes and chelating agents

√7ᵗʰ **T50.6X6** **Underdosing** of antidotes and chelating agents

√5ᵗʰ **T50.7** **Poisoning by, adverse effect of and underdosing of analeptics and opioid receptor antagonists**

√6ᵗʰ **T50.7X** **Poisoning by, adverse effect of and underdosing of analeptics and opioid receptor antagonists**

√7ᵗʰ **T50.7X1** **Poisoning by analeptics and opioid receptor antagonists, accidental (unintentional)**
Poisoning by analeptics and opioid receptor antagonists NOS

√7ᵗʰ **T50.7X2** **Poisoning by analeptics and opioid receptor antagonists, intentional self-harm**

√7ᵗʰ **T50.7X3** **Poisoning by analeptics and opioid receptor antagonists, assault**

√7ᵗʰ **T50.7X4** **Poisoning by analeptics and opioid receptor antagonists, undetermined**

√7ᵗʰ **T50.7X5** **Adverse effect** of analeptics and opioid receptor antagonists

√7ᵗʰ **T50.7X6** **Underdosing** of analeptics and opioid receptor antagonists

√5ᵗʰ **T50.8** **Poisoning by, adverse effect of and underdosing of diagnostic agents**

√6ᵗʰ **T50.8X** **Poisoning by, adverse effect of and underdosing of diagnostic agents**

√7ᵗʰ **T50.8X1** **Poisoning by diagnostic agents, accidental (unintentional)**
Poisoning by diagnostic agents NOS

√7ᵗʰ **T50.8X2** **Poisoning by diagnostic agents, intentional self-harm**

√7ᵗʰ **T50.8X3** **Poisoning by diagnostic agents, assault**

√7ᵗʰ **T50.8X4** **Poisoning by diagnostic agents, undetermined**

√7ᵗʰ **T50.8X5** **Adverse effect** of diagnostic agents

√7ᵗʰ **T50.8X6** **Underdosing** of diagnostic agents

√5ᵗʰ **T50.A** **Poisoning by, adverse effect of and underdosing of bacterial vaccines**

√6ᵗʰ **T50.A1** **Poisoning by, adverse effect of and underdosing of pertussis vaccine, including combinations with a pertussis component**

√7ᵗʰ **T50.A11** **Poisoning by pertussis vaccine, including combinations with a pertussis component, accidental (unintentional)**

√7ᵗʰ **T50.A12** **Poisoning by pertussis vaccine, including combinations with a pertussis component, intentional self-harm**

√7ᵗʰ **T50.A13** **Poisoning by pertussis vaccine, including combinations with a pertussis component, assault**

√7ᵗʰ **T50.A14** **Poisoning by pertussis vaccine, including combinations with a pertussis component, undetermined**

√7ᵗʰ **T50.A15** **Adverse effect** of pertussis vaccine, including combinations with a pertussis component

√7ᵗʰ **T50.A16** **Underdosing** of pertussis vaccine, including combinations with a pertussis component

√6ᵗʰ **T50.A2** **Poisoning by, adverse effect of and underdosing of mixed bacterial vaccines without a pertussis component**

√7ᵗʰ **T50.A21** **Poisoning by mixed bacterial vaccines without a pertussis component, accidental (unintentional)**

√7ᵗʰ **T50.A22** **Poisoning by mixed bacterial vaccines without a pertussis component, intentional self-harm**

√7ᵗʰ **T50.A23** **Poisoning by mixed bacterial vaccines without a pertussis component, assault**

√7ᵗʰ **T50.A24** **Poisoning by mixed bacterial vaccines without a pertussis component, undetermined**

√7ᵗʰ **T50.A25** **Adverse effect** of mixed bacterial vaccines without a pertussis component

√7ᵗʰ **T50.A26** **Underdosing** of mixed bacterial vaccines without a pertussis component

√6ᵗʰ **T50.A9** **Poisoning by, adverse effect of and underdosing of other bacterial vaccines**

√7ᵗʰ **T50.A91** **Poisoning by other bacterial vaccines, accidental (unintentional)**

√7ᵗʰ **T50.A92** **Poisoning by other bacterial vaccines, intentional self-harm**

√7ᵗʰ **T50.A93** **Poisoning by other bacterial vaccines, assault**

√7ᵗʰ **T50.A94** **Poisoning by other bacterial vaccines, undetermined**

√7ᵗʰ **T50.A95** **Adverse effect** of other bacterial vaccines

√7ᵗʰ **T50.A96** **Underdosing** of other bacterial vaccines

√5ᵗʰ **T50.B** **Poisoning by, adverse effect of and underdosing of viral vaccines**

√6ᵗʰ **T50.B1** **Poisoning by, adverse effect of and underdosing of smallpox vaccines**

√7ᵗʰ **T50.B11** **Poisoning by smallpox vaccines, accidental (unintentional)**

√7ᵗʰ **T50.B12** **Poisoning by smallpox vaccines, intentional self-harm**

√7ᵗʰ **T50.B13** **Poisoning by smallpox vaccines, assault**

Ⓝ Newborn: 0   Ⓟ Pediatric: 0-17   Ⓜ Maternity: 12-55   Ⓐ Adult: 15-124   **MCC** Major CC Condition   **PDx MCC** PDx acts as own MCC   **CC** CC Condition   **PDx CC** PDx acts as own CC

1074   ICD-10-CM Draft (2015)

✓7ᵗʰ **T50.B14** Poisoning by smallpox vaccines, undetermined

✓7ᵗʰ **T50.B15** Adverse effect of smallpox vaccines

✓7ᵗʰ **T50.B16** Underdosing of smallpox vaccines

✓6ᵗʰ **T50.B9** Poisoning by, adverse effect of and underdosing of other viral vaccines

✓7ᵗʰ **T50.B91** Poisoning by other viral vaccines, accidental (unintentional)

✓7ᵗʰ **T50.B92** Poisoning by other viral vaccines, intentional self-harm

✓7ᵗʰ **T50.B93** Poisoning by other viral vaccines, assault

✓7ᵗʰ **T50.B94** Poisoning by other viral vaccines, undetermined

✓7ᵗʰ **T50.B95** Adverse effect of other viral vaccines

✓7ᵗʰ **T50.B96** Underdosing of other viral vaccines

✓5ᵗʰ **T50.Z** Poisoning by, adverse effect of and underdosing of other vaccines and biological substances

✓6ᵗʰ **T50.Z1** Poisoning by, adverse effect of and underdosing of immunoglobulin

✓7ᵗʰ **T50.Z11** Poisoning by immunoglobulin, accidental (unintentional)

✓7ᵗʰ **T50.Z12** Poisoning by immunoglobulin, intentional self-harm

✓7ᵗʰ **T50.Z13** Poisoning by immunoglobulin, assault

✓7ᵗʰ **T50.Z14** Poisoning by immunoglobulin, undetermined

✓7ᵗʰ **T50.Z15** Adverse effect of immunoglobulin

✓7ᵗʰ **T50.Z16** Underdosing of immunoglobulin

✓6ᵗʰ **T50.Z9** Poisoning by, adverse effect of and underdosing of other vaccines and biological substances

✓7ᵗʰ **T50.Z91** Poisoning by other vaccines and biological substances, accidental (unintentional)

✓7ᵗʰ **T50.Z92** Poisoning by other vaccines and biological substances, intentional self-harm

✓7ᵗʰ **T50.Z93** Poisoning by other vaccines and biological substances, assault

✓7ᵗʰ **T50.Z94** Poisoning by other vaccines and biological substances, undetermined

✓7ᵗʰ **T50.Z95** Adverse effect of other vaccines and biological substances

✓7ᵗʰ **T50.Z96** Underdosing of other vaccines and biological substances

✓5ᵗʰ **T50.9** Poisoning by, adverse effect of and underdosing of other and unspecified drugs, medicaments and biological substances

✓6ᵗʰ **T50.90** Poisoning by, adverse effect of and underdosing of unspecified drugs, medicaments and biological substances

✓7ᵗʰ **T50.901** Poisoning by unspecified drugs, medicaments and biological substances, accidental (unintentional)

✓7ᵗʰ **T50.902** Poisoning by unspecified drugs, medicaments and biological substances, intentional self-harm

✓7ᵗʰ **T50.903** Poisoning by unspecified drugs, medicaments and biological substances, assault

✓7ᵗʰ **T50.904** Poisoning by unspecified drugs, medicaments and biological substances, undetermined

✓7ᵗʰ **T50.905** Adverse effect of unspecified drugs, medicaments and biological substances

✓7ᵗʰ **T50.906** Underdosing of unspecified drugs, medicaments and biological substances

✓6ᵗʰ **T50.99** Poisoning by, adverse effect of and underdosing of other drugs, medicaments and biological substances

✓7ᵗʰ **T50.991** Poisoning by other drugs, medicaments and biological substances, accidental (unintentional)

✓7ᵗʰ **T50.992** Poisoning by other drugs, medicaments and biological substances, intentional self-harm

✓7ᵗʰ **T50.993** Poisoning by other drugs, medicaments and biological substances, assault

✓7ᵗʰ **T50.994** Poisoning by other drugs, medicaments and biological substances, undetermined

✓7ᵗʰ **T50.995** Adverse effect of other drugs, medicaments and biological substances

✓7ᵗʰ **T50.996** Underdosing of other drugs, medicaments and biological substances

Toxic effects of substances chiefly nonmedicinal as to source (T51-T65)

NOTE When no intent is indicated code to accidental. Undetermined intent is only for use when there is specific documentation in the record that the intent of the toxic effect cannot be determined.

Use additional code(s) for all associated manifestations of toxic effect, such as:
 personal history of foreign body fully removed (Z87.821)
 respiratory conditions due to external agents (J60-J70)
 to identify any retained foreign body, if applicable (Z18.-)

EXCLUDES 1 contact with and (suspected) exposure to toxic substances (Z77.-)

✓4ᵗʰ **T51** Toxic effect of alcohol

> The appropriate 7th character is to be added to each code from category T51.
> A   initial encounter
> D   subsequent encounter
> S   sequela

✓5ᵗʰ **T51.0** Toxic effect of ethanol
Toxic effect of ethyl alcohol

EXCLUDES 2 acute alcohol intoxication or 'hangover' effects (F10.129, F10.229, F10.929)
drunkenness (F10.129, F10.229, F10.929)
pathological alcohol intoxication (F10.129, F10.229, F10.929)

✓6ᵗʰ **T51.0X** Toxic effect of ethanol

✓7ᵗʰ **T51.0X1** Toxic effect of ethanol, accidental (unintentional)
Toxic effect of ethanol NOS

✓7ᵗʰ **T51.0X2** Toxic effect of ethanol, intentional self-harm

✓7ᵗʰ **T51.0X3** Toxic effect of ethanol, assault

✓7ᵗʰ **T51.0X4** Toxic effect of ethanol, undetermined

✓5ᵗʰ **T51.1** Toxic effect of methanol
Toxic effect of methyl alcohol

✓6ᵗʰ **T51.1X** Toxic effect of methanol

✓7ᵗʰ **T51.1X1** Toxic effect of methanol, accidental (unintentional)
Toxic effect of methanol NOS

✓7ᵗʰ **T51.1X2** Toxic effect of methanol, intentional self-harm

✓7ᵗʰ **T51.1X3** Toxic effect of methanol, assault

✓7ᵗʰ **T51.1X4** Toxic effect of methanol, undetermined

✓5ᵗʰ **T51.2** Toxic effect of 2-Propanol
Toxic effect of isopropyl alcohol

✓6ᵗʰ **T51.2X** Toxic effect of 2-Propanol

✓7ᵗʰ **T51.2X1** Toxic effect of 2-Propanol, accidental (unintentional)
Toxic effect of 2-Propanol NOS

✓7ᵗʰ **T51.2X2** Toxic effect of 2-Propanol, intentional self-harm

✓7ᵗʰ **T51.2X3** Toxic effect of 2-Propanol, assault

✓7ᵗʰ **T51.2X4** Toxic effect of 2-Propanol, undetermined

✓5ᵗʰ **T51.3** Toxic effect of fusel oil
Toxic effect of amyl alcohol
Toxic effect of butyl [1-butanol] alcohol
Toxic effect of propyl [1-propanol] alcohol

✓6ᵗʰ **T51.3X** Toxic effect of fusel oil

✓7ᵗʰ **T51.3X1** Toxic effect of fusel oil, accidental (unintentional)
Toxic effect of fusel oil NOS

✓7ᵗʰ **T51.3X2** Toxic effect of fusel oil, intentional self-harm

✓7ᵗʰ **T51.3X3** Toxic effect of fusel oil, assault

✓7ᵗʰ **T51.3X4** Toxic effect of fusel oil, undetermined

✓5ᵗʰ **T51.8** Toxic effect of other alcohols

✓6ᵗʰ **T51.8X** Toxic effect of other alcohols

✓7ᵗʰ **T51.8X1** Toxic effect of other alcohols, accidental (unintentional)
Toxic effect of other alcohols NOS

✓ Additional Character Required   ✓7ᵗʰ Xtension Alert   Unacceptable PDx   Manifestation   Hospital Acquired Condition   *EXCLUDES 1* Not Coded Here   *EXCLUDES 2* Not Included Here

ICD-10-CM Draft (2015)   1075

✓7ᵗʰ   **T51.8X2**   **Toxic effect of other alcohols,** intentional self-harm

✓7ᵗʰ   **T51.8X3**   **Toxic effect of other alcohols,** assault

✓7ᵗʰ   **T51.8X4**   **Toxic effect of other alcohols,** undetermined

✓5ᵗʰ   **T51.9**   **Toxic effect of** unspecified **alcohol**

    ✓x7ᵗʰ   **T51.91**   **Toxic effect of unspecified alcohol,** accidental (unintentional)

    ✓x7ᵗʰ   **T51.92**   **Toxic effect of unspecified alcohol,** intentional self-harm

    ✓x7ᵗʰ   **T51.93**   **Toxic effect of unspecified alcohol,** assault

    ✓x7ᵗʰ   **T51.94**   **Toxic effect of unspecified alcohol,** undetermined

✓4ᵗʰ   **T52**   **Toxic effect of organic solvents**

    EXCLUDES 1   halogen derivatives of aliphatic and aromatic hydrocarbons (T53.-)

    The appropriate 7th character is to be added to each code from category T52.
    A   initial encounter
    D   subsequent encounter
    S   sequela

✓5ᵗʰ   **T52.0**   **Toxic effects of petroleum products**
    Toxic effects of ether petroleum
    Toxic effects of gasoline [petrol]
    Toxic effects of kerosene [paraffin oil]
    Toxic effects of naphtha petroleum
    Toxic effects of paraffin wax
    Toxic effects of spirit petroleum

    ✓6ᵗʰ   **T52.0X**   **Toxic effects of** petroleum products

       ✓7ᵗʰ   **T52.0X1**   **Toxic effect of petroleum products,** accidental (unintentional)
          Toxic effects of petroleum products NOS

       ✓7ᵗʰ   **T52.0X2**   **Toxic effect of petroleum products,** intentional self-harm

       ✓7ᵗʰ   **T52.0X3**   **Toxic effect of petroleum products,** assault

       ✓7ᵗʰ   **T52.0X4**   **Toxic effect of petroleum products,** undetermined

✓5ᵗʰ   **T52.1**   **Toxic effects of benzene**
    EXCLUDES 1   homologues of benzene (T52.2)
            nitroderivatives and aminoderivatives of benzene and its homologues (T65.3)

    ✓6ᵗʰ   **T52.1X**   **Toxic effects of** benzene

       ✓7ᵗʰ   **T52.1X1**   **Toxic effect of benzene,** accidental (unintentional)
          Toxic effects of benzene NOS

       ✓7ᵗʰ   **T52.1X2**   **Toxic effect of benzene,** intentional self-harm

       ✓7ᵗʰ   **T52.1X3**   **Toxic effect of benzene,** assault

       ✓7ᵗʰ   **T52.1X4**   **Toxic effect of benzene,** undetermined

✓5ᵗʰ   **T52.2**   **Toxic effects of homologues of benzene**
    Toxic effects of toluene [methylbenzene]
    Toxic effects of xylene [dimethylbenzene]

    ✓6ᵗʰ   **T52.2X**   **Toxic effects of** homologues of benzene

       ✓7ᵗʰ   **T52.2X1**   **Toxic effect of homologues of benzene,** accidental (unintentional)
          Toxic effects of homologues of benzene NOS

       ✓7ᵗʰ   **T52.2X2**   **Toxic effect of homologues of benzene,** intentional self-harm

       ✓7ᵗʰ   **T52.2X3**   **Toxic effect of homologues of benzene,** assault

       ✓7ᵗʰ   **T52.2X4**   **Toxic effect of homologues of benzene,** undetermined

✓5ᵗʰ   **T52.3**   **Toxic effects of glycols**

    ✓6ᵗʰ   **T52.3X**   **Toxic effects of** glycols

       ✓7ᵗʰ   **T52.3X1**   **Toxic effect of glycols,** accidental (unintentional)
          Toxic effects of glycols NOS

       ✓7ᵗʰ   **T52.3X2**   **Toxic effect of glycols,** intentional self-harm

       ✓7ᵗʰ   **T52.3X3**   **Toxic effect of glycols,** assault

       ✓7ᵗʰ   **T52.3X4**   **Toxic effect of glycols,** undetermined

✓5ᵗʰ   **T52.4**   **Toxic effects of ketones**

    ✓6ᵗʰ   **T52.4X**   **Toxic effects of** ketones

       ✓7ᵗʰ   **T52.4X1**   **Toxic effect of ketones,** accidental (unintentional)
          Toxic effects of ketones NOS

       ✓7ᵗʰ   **T52.4X2**   **Toxic effect of ketones,** intentional self-harm

       ✓7ᵗʰ   **T52.4X3**   **Toxic effect of ketones,** assault

       ✓7ᵗʰ   **T52.4X4**   **Toxic effect of ketones,** undetermined

✓5ᵗʰ   **T52.8**   **Toxic effects of other organic solvents**

    ✓6ᵗʰ   **T52.8X**   **Toxic effects of** other organic solvents

       ✓7ᵗʰ   **T52.8X1**   **Toxic effect of other organic solvents,** accidental (unintentional)
          Toxic effects of other organic solvents NOS

       ✓7ᵗʰ   **T52.8X2**   **Toxic effect of other organic solvents,** intentional self-harm

       ✓7ᵗʰ   **T52.8X3**   **Toxic effect of other organic solvents,** assault

       ✓7ᵗʰ   **T52.8X4**   **Toxic effect of other organic solvents,** undetermined

✓5ᵗʰ   **T52.9**   **Toxic effects of** unspecified **organic solvent**

    ✓x7ᵗʰ   **T52.91**   **Toxic effect of unspecified organic solvent,** accidental (unintentional)

    ✓x7ᵗʰ   **T52.92**   **Toxic effect of unspecified organic solvent,** intentional self-harm

    ✓x7ᵗʰ   **T52.93**   **Toxic effect of unspecified organic solvent,** assault

    ✓x7ᵗʰ   **T52.94**   **Toxic effect of unspecified organic solvent,** undetermined

✓4ᵗʰ   **T53**   **Toxic effect of halogen derivatives of aliphatic and aromatic hydrocarbons**

    The appropriate 7th character is to be added to each code from category T53.
    A   initial encounter
    D   subsequent encounter
    S   sequela

✓5ᵗʰ   **T53.0**   **Toxic effects of** carbon tetrachloride
    Toxic effects of tetrachloromethane

    ✓6ᵗʰ   **T53.0X**   **Toxic effects of** carbon tetrachloride

       ✓7ᵗʰ   **T53.0X1**   **Toxic effect of carbon tetrachloride,** accidental (unintentional)
          Toxic effects of carbon tetrachloride NOS

       ✓7ᵗʰ   **T53.0X2**   **Toxic effect of carbon tetrachloride,** intentional self-harm

       ✓7ᵗʰ   **T53.0X3**   **Toxic effect of carbon tetrachloride,** assault

       ✓7ᵗʰ   **T53.0X4**   **Toxic effect of carbon tetrachloride,** undetermined

✓5ᵗʰ   **T53.1**   **Toxic effects of chloroform**
    Toxic effects of trichloromethane

    ✓6ᵗʰ   **T53.1X**   **Toxic effects of** chloroform

       ✓7ᵗʰ   **T53.1X1**   **Toxic effect of chloroform,** accidental (unintentional)
          Toxic effects of chloroform NOS

       ✓7ᵗʰ   **T53.1X2**   **Toxic effect of chloroform,** intentional self-harm

       ✓7ᵗʰ   **T53.1X3**   **Toxic effect of chloroform,** assault

       ✓7ᵗʰ   **T53.1X4**   **Toxic effect of chloroform,** undetermined

✓5ᵗʰ   **T53.2**   **Toxic effects of trichloroethylene**
    Toxic effects of trichloroethene

    ✓6ᵗʰ   **T53.2X**   **Toxic effects of** trichloroethylene

       ✓7ᵗʰ   **T53.2X1**   **Toxic effect of trichloroethylene,** accidental (unintentional)
          Toxic effects of trichloroethylene NOS

       ✓7ᵗʰ   **T53.2X2**   **Toxic effect of trichloroethylene,** intentional self-harm

       ✓7ᵗʰ   **T53.2X3**   **Toxic effect of trichloroethylene,** assault

       ✓7ᵗʰ   **T53.2X4**   **Toxic effect of trichloroethylene,** undetermined

Ⓝ Newborn: 0   Ⓟ Pediatric: 0-17   Ⓜ Maternity: 12-55   Ⓐ Adult: 15-124   **MCC** Major CC Condition   **PDx MCC** PDx acts as own MCC   **CC** CC Condition   **PDx CC** PDx acts as own CC

1076   ICD-10-CM Draft (2015)

√5ᵗʰ **T53.3** **Toxic effects of tetrachloroethylene**
Toxic effects of perchloroethylene
Toxic effect of tetrachloroethene

√6ᵗʰ **T53.3X** **Toxic effects of** tetrachloroethylene

√7ᵗʰ **T53.3X1** **Toxic effect of tetrachloroethylene, accidental (unintentional)**
Toxic effects of tetrachloroethylene NOS

√7ᵗʰ **T53.3X2** **Toxic effect of tetrachloroethylene, intentional self-harm**

√7ᵗʰ **T53.3X3** **Toxic effect of tetrachloroethylene, assault**

√7ᵗʰ **T53.3X4** **Toxic effect of tetrachloroethylene, undetermined**

√5ᵗʰ **T53.4** **Toxic effects of dichloromethane**
Toxic effects of methylene chloride

√6ᵗʰ **T53.4X** **Toxic effects of** dichloromethane

√7ᵗʰ **T53.4X1** **Toxic effect of dichloromethane, accidental (unintentional)**
Toxic effects of dichloromethane NOS

√7ᵗʰ **T53.4X2** **Toxic effect of dichloromethane, intentional self-harm**

√7ᵗʰ **T53.4X3** **Toxic effect of dichloromethane,** assault

√7ᵗʰ **T53.4X4** **Toxic effect of dichloromethane, undetermined**

√5ᵗʰ **T53.5** **Toxic effects of chlorofluorocarbons**

√6ᵗʰ **T53.5X** **Toxic effects of** chlorofluorocarbons

√7ᵗʰ **T53.5X1** **Toxic effect of chlorofluorocarbons, accidental (unintentional)**
Toxic effects of chlorofluorocarbons NOS

√7ᵗʰ **T53.5X2** **Toxic effect of chlorofluorocarbons, intentional self-harm**

√7ᵗʰ **T53.5X3** **Toxic effect of chlorofluorocarbons, assault**

√7ᵗʰ **T53.5X4** **Toxic effect of chlorofluorocarbons, undetermined**

√5ᵗʰ **T53.6** **Toxic effects of other halogen derivatives of aliphatic hydrocarbons**

√6ᵗʰ **T53.6X** **Toxic effects of other** halogen derivatives of aliphatic hydrocarbons

√7ᵗʰ **T53.6X1** **Toxic effect of other halogen derivatives of aliphatic hydrocarbons, accidental (unintentional)**
Toxic effects of other halogen derivatives of aliphatic hydrocarbons NOS

√7ᵗʰ **T53.6X2** **Toxic effect of other halogen derivatives of aliphatic hydrocarbons,** intentional self-harm

√7ᵗʰ **T53.6X3** **Toxic effect of other halogen derivatives of aliphatic hydrocarbons, assault**

√7ᵗʰ **T53.6X4** **Toxic effect of other halogen derivatives of aliphatic hydrocarbons, undetermined**

√5ᵗʰ **T53.7** **Toxic effects of other halogen derivatives of aromatic hydrocarbons**

√6ᵗʰ **T53.7X** **Toxic effects of other** halogen derivatives of aromatic hydrocarbons

√7ᵗʰ **T53.7X1** **Toxic effect of other halogen derivatives of aromatic hydrocarbons, accidental (unintentional)**
Toxic effects of other halogen derivatives of aromatic hydrocarbons NOS

√7ᵗʰ **T53.7X2** **Toxic effect of other halogen derivatives of aromatic hydrocarbons,** intentional self-harm

√7ᵗʰ **T53.7X3** **Toxic effect of other halogen derivatives of aromatic hydrocarbons, assault**

√7ᵗʰ **T53.7X4** **Toxic effect of other halogen derivatives of aromatic hydrocarbons, undetermined**

√5ᵗʰ **T53.9** **Toxic effects of** unspecified halogen derivatives of aliphatic and aromatic hydrocarbons

√x7ᵗʰ **T53.91** **Toxic effect of unspecified halogen derivatives of aliphatic and aromatic hydrocarbons, accidental (unintentional)**

√x7ᵗʰ **T53.92** **Toxic effect of unspecified halogen derivatives of aliphatic and aromatic hydrocarbons, intentional self-harm**

√x7ᵗʰ **T53.93** **Toxic effect of unspecified halogen derivatives of aliphatic and aromatic hydrocarbons,** assault

√x7ᵗʰ **T53.94** **Toxic effect of unspecified halogen derivatives of aliphatic and aromatic hydrocarbons,** undetermined

√4ᵗʰ **T54** **Toxic effect of corrosive substances**

> The appropriate 7th character is to be added to each code from category T54.
> A   initial encounter
> D   subsequent encounter
> S   sequela

√5ᵗʰ **T54.0** **Toxic effects of phenol and phenol homologues**

√6ᵗʰ **T54.0X** **Toxic effects of** phenol and phenol homologues

√7ᵗʰ **T54.0X1** **Toxic effect of phenol and phenol homologues, accidental (unintentional)**
Toxic effects of phenol and phenol homologues NOS

√7ᵗʰ **T54.0X2** **Toxic effect of phenol and phenol homologues, intentional self-harm**

√7ᵗʰ **T54.0X3** **Toxic effect of phenol and phenol homologues, assault**

√7ᵗʰ **T54.0X4** **Toxic effect of phenol and phenol homologues, undetermined**

√5ᵗʰ **T54.1** **Toxic effects of other corrosive organic compounds**

√6ᵗʰ **T54.1X** **Toxic effects of** other corrosive organic compounds

√7ᵗʰ **T54.1X1** **Toxic effect of other corrosive organic compounds, accidental (unintentional)**
Toxic effects of other corrosive organic compounds NOS

√7ᵗʰ **T54.1X2** **Toxic effect of other corrosive organic compounds, intentional self-harm**

√7ᵗʰ **T54.1X3** **Toxic effect of other corrosive organic compounds, assault**

√7ᵗʰ **T54.1X4** **Toxic effect of other corrosive organic compounds, undetermined**

√5ᵗʰ **T54.2** **Toxic effects of corrosive acids and acid-like substances**
Toxic effects of hydrochloric acid
Toxic effects of sulfuric acid

√6ᵗʰ **T54.2X** **Toxic effects of corrosive** acids and acid-like substances

√7ᵗʰ **T54.2X1** **Toxic effect of corrosive acids and acid-like substances, accidental (unintentional)**
Toxic effects of corrosive acids and acid-like substances NOS

√7ᵗʰ **T54.2X2** **Toxic effect of corrosive acids and acid-like substances, intentional self-harm**

√7ᵗʰ **T54.2X3** **Toxic effect of corrosive acids and acid-like substances, assault**

√7ᵗʰ **T54.2X4** **Toxic effect of corrosive acids and acid-like substances, undetermined**

√5ᵗʰ **T54.3** **Toxic effects of corrosive alkalis and alkali-like substances**
Toxic effects of potassium hydroxide
Toxic effects of sodium hydroxide

√6ᵗʰ **T54.3X** **Toxic effects of corrosive** alkalis and alkali-like substances

√7ᵗʰ **T54.3X1** **Toxic effect of corrosive alkalis and alkali-like substances, accidental (unintentional)**
Toxic effects of corrosive alkalis and alkali-like substances NOS

√7ᵗʰ **T54.3X2** **Toxic effect of corrosive alkalis and alkali-like substances, intentional self-harm**

√7ᵗʰ **T54.3X3** **Toxic effect of corrosive alkalis and alkali-like substances, assault**

√7ᵗʰ **T54.3X4** **Toxic effect of corrosive alkalis and alkali-like substances, undetermined**

√5ᵗʰ **T54.9** **Toxic effects of** unspecified corrosive substance

√x7ᵗʰ **T54.91** **Toxic effect of unspecified corrosive substance, accidental (unintentional)**

√x7ᵗʰ **T54.92** **Toxic effect of unspecified corrosive substance, intentional self-harm**

√x7ᵗʰ **T54.93** **Toxic effect of unspecified corrosive substance, assault**

√x7ᵗʰ **T54.94** **Toxic effect of unspecified corrosive substance, undetermined**

☑ Additional Character Required   √x7ᵗʰ Xtension Alert   Unacceptable PDx   Manifestation   Hospital Acquired Condition   **EXCLUDES 1** Not Coded Here   **EXCLUDES 2** Not Included Here

Injury, Poisoning and Certain Other Consequences of External Causes

T55–T56.894

✓4th **T55** **Toxic effect of soaps and detergents**

> The appropriate 7th character is to be added to each code from category T55.
> A   initial encounter
> D   subsequent encounter
> S   sequela

    ✓5th **T55.0** **Toxic effect of soaps**

       ✓6th **T55.0X** **Toxic effect of soaps**

         ✓7th **T55.0X1** **Toxic effect of soaps, accidental (unintentional)**
           Toxic effect of soaps NOS

         ✓7th **T55.0X2** **Toxic effect of soaps, intentional self-harm**

         ✓7th **T55.0X3** **Toxic effect of soaps, assault**

         ✓7th **T55.0X4** **Toxic effect of soaps, undetermined**

    ✓5th **T55.1** **Toxic effect of detergents**

       ✓6th **T55.1X** **Toxic effect of detergents**

         ✓7th **T55.1X1** **Toxic effect of detergents, accidental (unintentional)**
           Toxic effect of detergents NOS

         ✓7th **T55.1X2** **Toxic effect of detergents, intentional self-harm**

         ✓7th **T55.1X3** **Toxic effect of detergents, assault**

         ✓7th **T55.1X4** **Toxic effect of detergents, undetermined**

✓4th **T56** **Toxic effect of metals**

> INCLUDES   toxic effects of fumes and vapors of metals
> toxic effects of metals from all sources, except medicinal substances

> Use additional code to identify any retained metal foreign body, if applicable (Z18.0-, T18.1-)

> EXCLUDES 1   arsenic and its compounds (T57.0)
> manganese and its compounds (T57.2)

> The appropriate 7th character is to be added to each code from category T56.
> A   initial encounter
> D   subsequent encounter
> S   sequela

    ✓5th **T56.0** **Toxic effects of lead and its compounds**

       ✓6th **T56.0X** **Toxic effects of lead and its compounds**

         ✓7th **T56.0X1** **Toxic effect of lead and its compounds, accidental (unintentional)**
           Toxic effects of lead and its compounds NOS

         ✓7th **T56.0X2** **Toxic effect of lead and its compounds, intentional self-harm**

         ✓7th **T56.0X3** **Toxic effect of lead and its compounds, assault**

         ✓7th **T56.0X4** **Toxic effect of lead and its compounds, undetermined**

    ✓5th **T56.1** **Toxic effects of mercury and its compounds**

       ✓6th **T56.1X** **Toxic effects of mercury and its compounds**

         ✓7th **T56.1X1** **Toxic effect of mercury and its compounds, accidental (unintentional)**
           Toxic effects of mercury and its compounds NOS

         ✓7th **T56.1X2** **Toxic effect of mercury and its compounds, intentional self-harm**

         ✓7th **T56.1X3** **Toxic effect of mercury and its compounds, assault**

         ✓7th **T56.1X4** **Toxic effect of mercury and its compounds, undetermined**

    ✓5th **T56.2** **Toxic effects of chromium and its compounds**

       ✓6th **T56.2X** **Toxic effects of chromium and its compounds**

         ✓7th **T56.2X1** **Toxic effect of chromium and its compounds, accidental (unintentional)**
           Toxic effects of chromium and its compounds NOS

         ✓7th **T56.2X2** **Toxic effect of chromium and its compounds, intentional self-harm**

         ✓7th **T56.2X3** **Toxic effect of chromium and its compounds, assault**

         ✓7th **T56.2X4** **Toxic effect of chromium and its compounds, undetermined**

    ✓5th **T56.3** **Toxic effects of cadmium and its compounds**

       ✓6th **T56.3X** **Toxic effects of cadmium and its compounds**

         ✓7th **T56.3X1** **Toxic effect of cadmium and its compounds, accidental (unintentional)**
           Toxic effects of cadmium and its compounds NOS

         ✓7th **T56.3X2** **Toxic effect of cadmium and its compounds, intentional self-harm**

         ✓7th **T56.3X3** **Toxic effect of cadmium and its compounds, assault**

         ✓7th **T56.3X4** **Toxic effect of cadmium and its compounds, undetermined**

    ✓5th **T56.4** **Toxic effects of copper and its compounds**

       ✓6th **T56.4X** **Toxic effects of copper and its compounds**

         ✓7th **T56.4X1** **Toxic effect of copper and its compounds, accidental (unintentional)**
           Toxic effects of copper and its compounds NOS

         ✓7th **T56.4X2** **Toxic effect of copper and its compounds, intentional self-harm**

         ✓7th **T56.4X3** **Toxic effect of copper and its compounds, assault**

         ✓7th **T56.4X4** **Toxic effect of copper and its compounds, undetermined**

    ✓5th **T56.5** **Toxic effects of zinc and its compounds**

       ✓6th **T56.5X** **Toxic effects of zinc and its compounds**

         ✓7th **T56.5X1** **Toxic effect of zinc and its compounds, accidental (unintentional)**
           Toxic effects of zinc and its compounds NOS

         ✓7th **T56.5X2** **Toxic effect of zinc and its compounds, intentional self-harm**

         ✓7th **T56.5X3** **Toxic effect of zinc and its compounds, assault**

         ✓7th **T56.5X4** **Toxic effect of zinc and its compounds, undetermined**

    ✓5th **T56.6** **Toxic effects of tin and its compounds**

       ✓6th **T56.6X** **Toxic effects of tin and its compounds**

         ✓7th **T56.6X1** **Toxic effect of tin and its compounds, accidental (unintentional)**
           Toxic effects of tin and its compounds NOS

         ✓7th **T56.6X2** **Toxic effect of tin and its compounds, intentional self-harm**

         ✓7th **T56.6X3** **Toxic effect of tin and its compounds, assault**

         ✓7th **T56.6X4** **Toxic effect of tin and its compounds, undetermined**

    ✓5th **T56.7** **Toxic effects of beryllium and its compounds**

       ✓6th **T56.7X** **Toxic effects of beryllium and its compounds**

         ✓7th **T56.7X1** **Toxic effect of beryllium and its compounds, accidental (unintentional)**
           Toxic effects of beryllium and its compounds NOS

         ✓7th **T56.7X2** **Toxic effect of beryllium and its compounds, intentional self-harm**

         ✓7th **T56.7X3** **Toxic effect of beryllium and its compounds, assault**

         ✓7th **T56.7X4** **Toxic effect of beryllium and its compounds, undetermined**

    ✓5th **T56.8** **Toxic effects of other metals**

       ✓6th **T56.81** **Toxic effect of thallium**

         ✓7th **T56.811** **Toxic effect of thallium, accidental (unintentional)**
           Toxic effect of thallium NOS

         ✓7th **T56.812** **Toxic effect of thallium, intentional self-harm**

         ✓7th **T56.813** **Toxic effect of thallium, assault**

         ✓7th **T56.814** **Toxic effect of thallium, undetermined**

       ✓6th **T56.89** **Toxic effects of other metals**

         ✓7th **T56.891** **Toxic effect of other metals, accidental (unintentional)**
           Toxic effects of other metals NOS

         ✓7th **T56.892** **Toxic effect of other metals, intentional self-harm**

         ✓7th **T56.893** **Toxic effect of other metals, assault**

         ✓7th **T56.894** **Toxic effect of other metals, undetermined**

N Newborn: 0   P Pediatric: 0-17   M Maternity: 12-55   A Adult: 15-124   MCC Major CC Condition   PDx MCC PDx acts as own MCC   CC CC Condition   PDx CC PDx acts as own CC

✓5th **T56.9   Toxic effects of** unspecified metal

   ✓x7th **T56.91   Toxic effect of unspecified metal,** accidental (unintentional)

   ✓x7th **T56.92   Toxic effect of unspecified metal,** intentional self-harm

   ✓x7th **T56.93   Toxic effect of unspecified metal,** assault

   ✓x7th **T56.94   Toxic effect of unspecified metal,** undetermined

✓4th **T57   Toxic effect of other inorganic substances**

> The appropriate 7th character is to be added to each code from category T57.
> A   initial encounter
> D   subsequent encounter
> S   sequela

✓5th **T57.0   Toxic effect of arsenic and its compounds**

   ✓6th **T57.0X   Toxic effect of** arsenic and its compounds

     ✓7th **T57.0X1   Toxic effect of arsenic and its compounds,** accidental (unintentional)
        Toxic effect of arsenic and its compounds NOS

     ✓7th **T57.0X2   Toxic effect of arsenic and its compounds,** intentional self-harm

     ✓7th **T57.0X3   Toxic effect of arsenic and its compounds,** assault

     ✓7th **T57.0X4   Toxic effect of arsenic and its compounds,** undetermined

✓5th **T57.1   Toxic effect of phosphorus and its compounds**

   EXCLUDES 1   organophosphate insecticides (T60.0)

   ✓6th **T57.1X   Toxic effect of** phosphorus and its compounds

     ✓7th **T57.1X1   Toxic effect of phosphorus and its compounds,** accidental (unintentional)
        Toxic effect of phosphorus and its compounds NOS

     ✓7th **T57.1X2   Toxic effect of phosphorus and its compounds,** intentional self-harm

     ✓7th **T57.1X3   Toxic effect of phosphorus and its compounds,** assault

     ✓7th **T57.1X4   Toxic effect of phosphorus and its compounds,** undetermined

✓5th **T57.2   Toxic effect of manganese and its compounds**

   ✓6th **T57.2X   Toxic effect of** manganese and its compounds

     ✓7th **T57.2X1   Toxic effect of** manganese and its **compounds,** accidental (unintentional)
        Toxic effect of manganese and its compounds NOS

     ✓7th **T57.2X2   Toxic effect of manganese and its compounds,** intentional self-harm

     ✓7th **T57.2X3   Toxic effect of manganese and its compounds,** assault

     ✓7th **T57.2X4   Toxic effect of manganese and its compounds,** undetermined

✓5th **T57.3   Toxic effect of hydrogen cyanide**

   ✓6th **T57.3X   Toxic effect of** hydrogen cyanide

     ✓7th **T57.3X1   Toxic effect of hydrogen cyanide,** accidental (unintentional)
        Toxic effect of hydrogen cyanide NOS

     ✓7th **T57.3X2   Toxic effect of hydrogen cyanide,** intentional self-harm

     ✓7th **T57.3X3   Toxic effect of hydrogen cyanide,** assault

     ✓7th **T57.3X4   Toxic effect of hydrogen cyanide,** undetermined

✓5th **T57.8   Toxic effect of other specified inorganic substances**

   ✓6th **T57.8X   Toxic effect of** other specified inorganic substances

     ✓7th **T57.8X1   Toxic effect of other specified inorganic substances,** accidental (unintentional)
        Toxic effect of other specified inorganic substances NOS

     ✓7th **T57.8X2   Toxic effect of other specified inorganic substances,** intentional self-harm

     ✓7th **T57.8X3   Toxic effect of other specified inorganic substances,** assault

     ✓7th **T57.8X4   Toxic effect of other specified inorganic substances,** undetermined

✓5th **T57.9   Toxic effect of** unspecified inorganic substance

   ✓x7th **T57.91   Toxic effect of unspecified inorganic substance,** accidental (unintentional)

   ✓x7th **T57.92   Toxic effect of unspecified inorganic substance,** intentional self-harm

   ✓x7th **T57.93   Toxic effect of unspecified inorganic substance,** assault

   ✓x7th **T57.94   Toxic effect of unspecified inorganic substance,** undetermined

✓4th **T58   Toxic effect of carbon monoxide**

   INCLUDES   asphyxiation from carbon monoxide
            toxic effect of carbon monoxide from all sources

> The appropriate 7th character is to be added to each code from category T58.
> A   initial encounter
> D   subsequent encounter
> S   sequela

✓5th **T58.0   Toxic effect of carbon monoxide** from motor vehicle exhaust
     Toxic effect of exhaust gas from gas engine
     Toxic effect of exhaust gas from motor pump

   ✓x7th **T58.01   Toxic effect of carbon monoxide from motor vehicle exhaust,** accidental (unintentional)

   ✓x7th **T58.02   Toxic effect of carbon monoxide from motor vehicle exhaust,** intentional self-harm

   ✓x7th **T58.03   Toxic effect of carbon monoxide from motor vehicle exhaust,** assault

   ✓x7th **T58.04   Toxic effect of carbon monoxide from motor vehicle exhaust,** undetermined

✓5th **T58.1   Toxic effect of carbon monoxide** from utility gas
     Toxic effect of acetylene
     Toxic effect of gas NOS used for lighting, heating, cooking
     Toxic effect of water gas

   ✓x7th **T58.11   Toxic effect of carbon monoxide from utility gas,** accidental (unintentional)

   ✓x7th **T58.12   Toxic effect of carbon monoxide from utility gas,** intentional self-harm

   ✓x7th **T58.13   Toxic effect of carbon monoxide from utility gas,** assault

   ✓x7th **T58.14   Toxic effect of carbon monoxide from utility gas,** undetermined

✓5th **T58.2   Toxic effect of carbon monoxide** from incomplete combustion of other domestic fuels
     Toxic effect of carbon monoxide from incomplete combustion of coal, coke, kerosene, wood

   ✓6th **T58.2X   Toxic effect of carbon monoxide from incomplete combustion of other domestic fuels**

     ✓7th **T58.2X1   Toxic effect of carbon monoxide from incomplete combustion of other domestic fuels,** accidental (unintentional)

     ✓7th **T58.2X2   Toxic effect of carbon monoxide from incomplete combustion of other domestic fuels,** intentional self-harm

     ✓7th **T58.2X3   Toxic effect of carbon monoxide from incomplete combustion of other domestic fuels,** assault

     ✓7th **T58.2X4   Toxic effect of carbon monoxide from incomplete combustion of other domestic fuels,** undetermined

✓5th **T58.8   Toxic effect of carbon monoxide** from other source
     Toxic effect of carbon monoxide from blast furnace gas
     Toxic effect of carbon monoxide from fuels in industrial use
     Toxic effect of carbon monoxide from kiln vapor

   ✓6th **T58.8X   Toxic effect of carbon monoxide from other source**

     ✓7th **T58.8X1   Toxic effect of carbon monoxide from other source,** accidental (unintentional)

     ✓7th **T58.8X2   Toxic effect of carbon monoxide from other source,** intentional self-harm

     ✓7th **T58.8X3   Toxic effect of carbon monoxide from other source,** assault

     ✓7th **T58.8X4   Toxic effect of carbon monoxide from other source,** undetermined

✓5th **T58.9   Toxic effect of carbon monoxide** from unspecified source

   ✓x7th **T58.91   Toxic effect of carbon monoxide from unspecified source,** accidental (unintentional)

✓ Additional Character Required   ✓x7th Xtension Alert   Unacceptable PDx   Manifestation   Hospital Acquired Condition   EXCLUDES 1 Not Coded Here   EXCLUDES 2 Not Included Here

Injury, Poisoning and Certain Other Consequences of External Causes

T58.92–T60.0X2

√x7ᵗʰ **T58.92** Toxic effect of carbon monoxide from unspecified source, *intentional self-harm*

√x7ᵗʰ **T58.93** Toxic effect of carbon monoxide from unspecified source, *assault*

√x7ᵗʰ **T58.94** Toxic effect of carbon monoxide from unspecified source, *undetermined*

√4ᵗʰ **T59** **Toxic effect of other gases, fumes and vapors**
- INCLUDES aerosol propellants
- EXCLUDES 1 *chlorofluorocarbons (T53.5)*

The appropriate 7th character is to be added to each code from category T59.
- A   initial encounter
- D   subsequent encounter
- S   sequela

√5ᵗʰ **T59.0** **Toxic effect of nitrogen oxides**

√6ᵗʰ **T59.0X** Toxic effect of nitrogen oxides

√7ᵗʰ **T59.0X1** Toxic effect of nitrogen oxides, *accidental (unintentional)*
Toxic effect of nitrogen oxides NOS

√7ᵗʰ **T59.0X2** Toxic effect of nitrogen oxides, *intentional self-harm*

√7ᵗʰ **T59.0X3** Toxic effect of nitrogen oxides, *assault*

√7ᵗʰ **T59.0X4** Toxic effect of nitrogen oxides, *undetermined*

√5ᵗʰ **T59.1** **Toxic effect of sulfur dioxide**

√6ᵗʰ **T59.1X** Toxic effect of sulfur dioxide

√7ᵗʰ **T59.1X1** Toxic effect of sulfur dioxide, *accidental (unintentional)*
Toxic effect of sulfur dioxide NOS

√7ᵗʰ **T59.1X2** Toxic effect of sulfur dioxide, *intentional self-harm*

√7ᵗʰ **T59.1X3** Toxic effect of sulfur dioxide, *assault*

√7ᵗʰ **T59.1X4** Toxic effect of sulfur dioxide, *undetermined*

√5ᵗʰ **T59.2** **Toxic effect of formaldehyde**

√6ᵗʰ **T59.2X** Toxic effect of formaldehyde

√7ᵗʰ **T59.2X1** Toxic effect of formaldehyde, *accidental (unintentional)*
Toxic effect of formaldehyde NOS

√7ᵗʰ **T59.2X2** Toxic effect of formaldehyde, *intentional self-harm*

√7ᵗʰ **T59.2X3** Toxic effect of formaldehyde, *assault*

√7ᵗʰ **T59.2X4** Toxic effect of formaldehyde, *undetermined*

√5ᵗʰ **T59.3** **Toxic effect of lacrimogenic gas**
Toxic effect of tear gas

√6ᵗʰ **T59.3X** Toxic effect of lacrimogenic gas

√7ᵗʰ **T59.3X1** Toxic effect of lacrimogenic gas, *accidental (unintentional)*
Toxic effect of lacrimogenic gas NOS

√7ᵗʰ **T59.3X2** Toxic effect of lacrimogenic gas, *intentional self-harm*

√7ᵗʰ **T59.3X3** Toxic effect of lacrimogenic gas, *assault*

√7ᵗʰ **T59.3X4** Toxic effect of lacrimogenic gas, *undetermined*

√5ᵗʰ **T59.4** **Toxic effect of chlorine gas**

√6ᵗʰ **T59.4X** Toxic effect of chlorine gas

√7ᵗʰ **T59.4X1** Toxic effect of chlorine gas, *accidental (unintentional)*
Toxic effect of chlorine gas NOS

√7ᵗʰ **T59.4X2** Toxic effect of chlorine gas, *intentional self-harm*

√7ᵗʰ **T59.4X3** Toxic effect of chlorine gas, *assault*

√7ᵗʰ **T59.4X4** Toxic effect of chlorine gas, *undetermined*

√5ᵗʰ **T59.5** **Toxic effect of fluorine gas and hydrogen fluoride**

√6ᵗʰ **T59.5X** Toxic effect of fluorine gas and hydrogen fluoride

√7ᵗʰ **T59.5X1** Toxic effect of fluorine gas and hydrogen fluoride, *accidental (unintentional)*
Toxic effect of fluorine gas and hydrogen fluoride NOS

√7ᵗʰ **T59.5X2** Toxic effect of fluorine gas and hydrogen fluoride, *intentional self-harm*

√7ᵗʰ **T59.5X3** Toxic effect of fluorine gas and hydrogen fluoride, *assault*

√7ᵗʰ **T59.5X4** Toxic effect of fluorine gas and hydrogen fluoride, *undetermined*

√5ᵗʰ **T59.6** **Toxic effect of hydrogen sulfide**

√6ᵗʰ **T59.6X** Toxic effect of hydrogen sulfide

√7ᵗʰ **T59.6X1** Toxic effect of hydrogen sulfide, *accidental (unintentional)*
Toxic effect of hydrogen sulfide NOS

√7ᵗʰ **T59.6X2** Toxic effect of hydrogen sulfide, *intentional self-harm*

√7ᵗʰ **T59.6X3** Toxic effect of hydrogen sulfide, *assault*

√7ᵗʰ **T59.6X4** Toxic effect of hydrogen sulfide, *undetermined*

√5ᵗʰ **T59.7** **Toxic effect of carbon dioxide**

√6ᵗʰ **T59.7X** Toxic effect of carbon dioxide

√7ᵗʰ **T59.7X1** Toxic effect of carbon dioxide, *accidental (unintentional)*
Toxic effect of carbon dioxide NOS

√7ᵗʰ **T59.7X2** Toxic effect of carbon dioxide, *intentional self-harm*

√7ᵗʰ **T59.7X3** Toxic effect of carbon dioxide, *assault*

√7ᵗʰ **T59.7X4** Toxic effect of carbon dioxide, *undetermined*

√5ᵗʰ **T59.8** **Toxic effect of other specified gases, fumes and vapors**

√6ᵗʰ **T59.81** Toxic effect of smoke
Smoke inhalation
- EXCLUDES 2 *toxic effect of cigarette (tobacco) smoke (T65.22-)*

√7ᵗʰ **T59.811** Toxic effect of smoke, *accidental (unintentional)*
Toxic effect of smoke NOS
AHA: 2013, 4Q, 121

√7ᵗʰ **T59.812** Toxic effect of smoke, *intentional self-harm*

√7ᵗʰ **T59.813** Toxic effect of smoke, *assault*

√7ᵗʰ **T59.814** Toxic effect of smoke, *undetermined*

√6ᵗʰ **T59.89** Toxic effect of other specified gases, fumes and vapors

√7ᵗʰ **T59.891** Toxic effect of other specified gases, fumes and vapors, *accidental (unintentional)*

√7ᵗʰ **T59.892** Toxic effect of other specified gases, fumes and vapors, *intentional self-harm*

√7ᵗʰ **T59.893** Toxic effect of other specified gases, fumes and vapors, *assault*

√7ᵗʰ **T59.894** Toxic effect of other specified gases, fumes and vapors, *undetermined*

√5ᵗʰ **T59.9** **Toxic effect of unspecified gases, fumes and vapors**

√x7ᵗʰ **T59.91** Toxic effect of unspecified gases, fumes and vapors, *accidental (unintentional)*

√x7ᵗʰ **T59.92** Toxic effect of unspecified gases, fumes and vapors, *intentional self-harm*

√x7ᵗʰ **T59.93** Toxic effect of unspecified gases, fumes and vapors, *assault*

√x7ᵗʰ **T59.94** Toxic effect of unspecified gases, fumes and vapors, *undetermined*

√4ᵗʰ **T60** **Toxic effect of pesticides**
- INCLUDES toxic effect of wood preservatives

The appropriate 7th character is to be added to each code from category T60.
- A   initial encounter
- D   subsequent encounter
- S   sequela

√5ᵗʰ **T60.0** **Toxic effect of organophosphate and carbamate insecticides**

√6ᵗʰ **T60.0X** Toxic effect of organophosphate and carbamate insecticides

√7ᵗʰ **T60.0X1** Toxic effect of organophosphate and carbamate insecticides, *accidental (unintentional)*
Toxic effect of organophosphate and carbamate insecticides NOS

√7ᵗʰ **T60.0X2** Toxic effect of organophosphate and carbamate insecticides, *intentional self-harm*

N Newborn: 0   P Pediatric: 0-17   M Maternity: 12-55   A Adult: 15-124   MCC Major CC Condition   PDx MCC PDx acts as own MCC   CC CC Condition   PDx CC PDx acts as own CC

1080   ICD-10-CM Draft (2015)

√7ᵗʰ **T60.0X3** **Toxic effect of organophosphate and carbamate insecticides,** assault

√7ᵗʰ **T60.0X4** **Toxic effect of organophosphate and carbamate insecticides,** undetermined

√5ᵗʰ **T60.1** **Toxic effect of halogenated insecticides**

EXCLUDES 1 *chlorinated hydrocarbon (T53.-)*

√6ᵗʰ **T60.1X** **Toxic effect of** halogenated insecticides

√7ᵗʰ **T60.1X1** **Toxic effect of halogenated insecticides, accidental (unintentional)**
Toxic effect of halogenated insecticides NOS

√7ᵗʰ **T60.1X2** **Toxic effect of halogenated insecticides, intentional self-harm**

√7ᵗʰ **T60.1X3** **Toxic effect of halogenated insecticides, assault**

√7ᵗʰ **T60.1X4** **Toxic effect of halogenated insecticides, undetermined**

√5ᵗʰ **T60.2** **Toxic effect of other insecticides**

√6ᵗʰ **T60.2X** **Toxic effect of** other insecticides

√7ᵗʰ **T60.2X1** **Toxic effect of other insecticides, accidental (unintentional)**
Toxic effect of other insecticides NOS

√7ᵗʰ **T60.2X2** **Toxic effect of other insecticides, intentional self-harm**

√7ᵗʰ **T60.2X3** **Toxic effect of other insecticides,** assault

√7ᵗʰ **T60.2X4** **Toxic effect of other insecticides, undetermined**

√5ᵗʰ **T60.3** **Toxic effect of herbicides and fungicides**

√6ᵗʰ **T60.3X** **Toxic effect of** herbicides and fungicides

√7ᵗʰ **T60.3X1** **Toxic effect of herbicides and fungicides, accidental (unintentional)**
Toxic effect of herbicides and fungicides NOS

√7ᵗʰ **T60.3X2** **Toxic effect of herbicides and fungicides, intentional self-harm**

√7ᵗʰ **T60.3X3** **Toxic effect of herbicides and fungicides, assault**

√7ᵗʰ **T60.3X4** **Toxic effect of herbicides and fungicides, undetermined**

√5ᵗʰ **T60.4** **Toxic effect of rodenticides**

EXCLUDES 1 *strychnine and its salts (T65.1)*
thallium (T56.81-)

√6ᵗʰ **T60.4X** **Toxic effect of** rodenticides

√7ᵗʰ **T60.4X1** **Toxic effect of rodenticides,** accidental **(unintentional)**
Toxic effect of rodenticides NOS

√7ᵗʰ **T60.4X2** **Toxic effect of rodenticides,** intentional self-harm

√7ᵗʰ **T60.4X3** **Toxic effect of rodenticides,** assault

√7ᵗʰ **T60.4X4** **Toxic effect of rodenticides, undetermined**

√5ᵗʰ **T60.8** **Toxic effect of other pesticides**

√6ᵗʰ **T60.8X** **Toxic effect of** other pesticides

√7ᵗʰ **T60.8X1** **Toxic effect of other pesticides,** accidental **(unintentional)**
Toxic effect of other pesticides NOS

√7ᵗʰ **T60.8X2** **Toxic effect of other pesticides, intentional self-harm**

√7ᵗʰ **T60.8X3** **Toxic effect of other pesticides,** assault

√7ᵗʰ **T60.8X4** **Toxic effect of other pesticides, undetermined**

√5ᵗʰ **T60.9** **Toxic effect of** unspecified pesticide

√x7ᵗʰ **T60.91** **Toxic effect of unspecified pesticide,** accidental **(unintentional)**

√x7ᵗʰ **T60.92** **Toxic effect of unspecified pesticide,** intentional self-harm

√x7ᵗʰ **T60.93** **Toxic effect of unspecified pesticide,** assault

√x7ᵗʰ **T60.94** **Toxic effect of unspecified pesticide,** undetermined

√4ᵗʰ **T61** **Toxic effect of noxious substances eaten as seafood**

EXCLUDES 1 *allergic reaction to food, such as:*
anaphylactic reaction or shock due to adverse food reaction (T78.0-)
dermatitis (L23.6, L25.4, L27.2)
gastroenteritis (noninfective) (K52.2)
bacterial foodborne intoxications (A05.-)
toxic effect of aflatoxin and other mycotoxins (T64)
toxic effect of cyanides (T65.0-)
toxic effect of harmful algae bloom (T65.82-)
toxic effect of hydrogen cyanide (T57.3-)
toxic effect of mercury (T56.1-)
toxic effect of red tide (T65.82-)

The appropriate 7th character is to be added to each code from category T61.
A   initial encounter
D   subsequent encounter
S   sequela

√5ᵗʰ **T61.0** **Ciguatera fish** poisoning

√x7ᵗʰ **T61.01** **Ciguatera fish poisoning,** accidental (unintentional)

√x7ᵗʰ **T61.02** **Ciguatera fish poisoning,** intentional self-harm

√x7ᵗʰ **T61.03** **Ciguatera fish poisoning,** assault

√x7ᵗʰ **T61.04** **Ciguatera fish poisoning,** undetermined

√5ᵗʰ **T61.1** **Scombroid fish** poisoning
Histamine-like syndrome

√x7ᵗʰ **T61.11** **Scombroid fish poisoning,** accidental (unintentional)

√x7ᵗʰ **T61.12** **Scombroid fish poisoning,** intentional self-harm

√x7ᵗʰ **T61.13** **Scombroid fish poisoning,** assault

√x7ᵗʰ **T61.14** **Scombroid fish poisoning,** undetermined

√5ᵗʰ **T61.7** **Other fish and shellfish poisoning**

√6ᵗʰ **T61.77** **Other fish poisoning**

√7ᵗʰ **T61.771** **Other fish poisoning,** accidental (unintentional)

√7ᵗʰ **T61.772** **Other fish poisoning,** intentional self-harm

√7ᵗʰ **T61.773** **Other fish poisoning,** assault

√7ᵗʰ **T61.774** **Other fish poisoning,** undetermined

√6ᵗʰ **T61.78** **Other** shellfish poisoning

√7ᵗʰ **T61.781** **Other shellfish poisoning,** accidental (unintentional)

√7ᵗʰ **T61.782** **Other shellfish poisoning,** intentional self-harm

√7ᵗʰ **T61.783** **Other shellfish poisoning,** assault

√7ᵗʰ **T61.784** **Other shellfish poisoning,** undetermined

√5ᵗʰ **T61.8** **Toxic effect of other seafood**

√6ᵗʰ **T61.8X** **Toxic effect of** other seafood

√7ᵗʰ **T61.8X1** **Toxic effect of other seafood,** accidental (unintentional)

√7ᵗʰ **T61.8X2** **Toxic effect of other seafood,** intentional self-harm

√7ᵗʰ **T61.8X3** **Toxic effect of other seafood,** assault

√7ᵗʰ **T61.8X4** **Toxic effect of other seafood, undetermined**

√5ᵗʰ **T61.9** **Toxic effect of** unspecified seafood

√x7ᵗʰ **T61.91** **Toxic effect of unspecified seafood,** accidental (unintentional)

√x7ᵗʰ **T61.92** **Toxic effect of unspecified seafood,** intentional self-harm

√x7ᵗʰ **T61.93** **Toxic effect of unspecified seafood,** assault

√x7ᵗʰ **T61.94** **Toxic effect of unspecified seafood,** undetermined

✓4ᵗʰ **T62 Toxic effect of other noxious substances eaten as food**

EXCLUDES 1   *allergic reaction to food, such as:*
     anaphylactic shock (reaction) due to adverse food reaction
     (T78.0-)
     dermatitis (L23.6, L25.4, L27.2)
     gastroenteritis (noninfective) (K52.2)
     bacterial food borne intoxications (A05.-)
     toxic effect of aflatoxin and other mycotoxins (T64)
     toxic effect of cyanides (T65.0-)
     toxic effect of hydrogen cyanide (T57.3-)
     toxic effect of mercury (T56.1-)

> The appropriate 7th character is to be added to each code from
> category T62.
> A   initial encounter
> D   subsequent encounter
> S   sequela

✓5ᵗʰ **T62.0 Toxic effect of ingested mushrooms**

    ✓6ᵗʰ **T62.0X Toxic effect of** ingested mushrooms

       ✓7ᵗʰ **T62.0X1 Toxic effect of ingested mushrooms,**
                accidental (unintentional)
                Toxic effect of ingested mushrooms NOS

       ✓7ᵗʰ **T62.0X2 Toxic effect of ingested mushrooms,**
                intentional self-harm

       ✓7ᵗʰ **T62.0X3 Toxic effect of ingested mushrooms,**
                assault

       ✓7ᵗʰ **T62.0X4 Toxic effect of ingested mushrooms,**
                undetermined

✓5ᵗʰ **T62.1 Toxic effect of ingested berries**

    ✓6ᵗʰ **T62.1X Toxic effect of** ingested berries

       ✓7ᵗʰ **T62.1X1 Toxic effect of ingested berries, accidental**
                (unintentional)
                Toxic effect of ingested berries NOS

       ✓7ᵗʰ **T62.1X2 Toxic effect of ingested berries,**
                intentional self-harm

       ✓7ᵗʰ **T62.1X3 Toxic effect of ingested berries, assault**

       ✓7ᵗʰ **T62.1X4 Toxic effect of ingested berries,**
                undetermined

✓5ᵗʰ **T62.2 Toxic effect of other ingested (parts of) plant(s)**

    ✓6ᵗʰ **T62.2X Toxic effect of** other ingested **(parts of)** plant(s)

       ✓7ᵗʰ **T62.2X1 Toxic effect of other ingested (parts of)**
                plant(s), accidental (unintentional)
                Toxic effect of other ingested (parts of)
                plant(s) NOS

       ✓7ᵗʰ **T62.2X2 Toxic effect of other ingested (parts of)**
                plant(s), intentional self-harm

       ✓7ᵗʰ **T62.2X3 Toxic effect of other ingested (parts of)**
                plant(s), assault

       ✓7ᵗʰ **T62.2X4 Toxic effect of other ingested (parts of)**
                plant(s), undetermined

✓5ᵗʰ **T62.8 Toxic effect of other specified** noxious substances eaten as
food

    ✓6ᵗʰ **T62.8X Toxic effect of** other specified noxious substances
eaten as food

       ✓7ᵗʰ **T62.8X1 Toxic effect of other specified noxious**
                substances eaten as food, accidental
                (unintentional)
                Toxic effect of other specified noxious
                substances eaten as food NOS

       ✓7ᵗʰ **T62.8X2 Toxic effect of other specified noxious**
                substances eaten as food, intentional self-
                harm

       ✓7ᵗʰ **T62.8X3 Toxic effect of other specified noxious**
                substances eaten as food, assault

       ✓7ᵗʰ **T62.8X4 Toxic effect of other specified noxious**
                substances eaten as food, undetermined

✓5ᵗʰ **T62.9 Toxic effect of** unspecified noxious substance eaten as food

    ✓x7ᵗʰ **T62.91 Toxic effect of unspecified noxious substance eaten**
            as food, accidental (unintentional)
            Toxic effect of unspecified noxious substance eaten as
            food NOS

    ✓x7ᵗʰ **T62.92 Toxic effect of unspecified noxious substance eaten**
            as food, intentional self-harm

    ✓x7ᵗʰ **T62.93 Toxic effect of unspecified noxious substance eaten**
            as food, assault

    ✓x7ᵗʰ **T62.94 Toxic effect of unspecified noxious substance eaten**
            as food, undetermined

✓4ᵗʰ **T63 Toxic effect of contact with venomous animals and plants**

INCLUDES   bite or touch of venomous animal
           pricked or stuck by thorn or leaf
EXCLUDES 2   *ingestion of toxic animal or plant (T61.-, T62.-)*

> The appropriate 7th character is to be added to each code from
> category T63.
> A   initial encounter
> D   subsequent encounter
> S   sequela

✓5ᵗʰ **T63.0 Toxic effect of** snake venom

    ✓6ᵗʰ **T63.00 Toxic effect of** unspecified **snake venom**

       ✓7ᵗʰ **T63.001 Toxic effect of unspecified snake venom,**
                accidental (unintentional)
                Toxic effect of unspecified snake venom
                NOS

       ✓7ᵗʰ **T63.002 Toxic effect of unspecified snake venom,**
                intentional self-harm

       ✓7ᵗʰ **T63.003 Toxic effect of unspecified snake venom,**
                assault

       ✓7ᵗʰ **T63.004 Toxic effect of unspecified snake venom,**
                undetermined

    ✓6ᵗʰ **T63.01 Toxic effect of** rattlesnake **venom**

       ✓7ᵗʰ **T63.011 Toxic effect of rattlesnake venom,**
                accidental (unintentional)
                Toxic effect of rattlesnake venom NOS

       ✓7ᵗʰ **T63.012 Toxic effect of rattlesnake venom,**
                intentional self-harm

       ✓7ᵗʰ **T63.013 Toxic effect of rattlesnake venom, assault**

       ✓7ᵗʰ **T63.014 Toxic effect of rattlesnake venom,**
                undetermined

    ✓6ᵗʰ **T63.02 Toxic effect of** coral snake **venom**

       ✓7ᵗʰ **T63.021 Toxic effect of coral snake venom,**
                accidental (unintentional)
                Toxic effect of coral snake venom NOS

       ✓7ᵗʰ **T63.022 Toxic effect of coral snake venom,**
                intentional self-harm

       ✓7ᵗʰ **T63.023 Toxic effect of coral snake venom, assault**

       ✓7ᵗʰ **T63.024 Toxic effect of coral snake venom,**
                undetermined

    ✓6ᵗʰ **T63.03 Toxic effect of** taipan **venom**

       ✓7ᵗʰ **T63.031 Toxic effect of taipan venom, accidental**
                (unintentional)
                Toxic effect of taipan venom NOS

       ✓7ᵗʰ **T63.032 Toxic effect of taipan venom, intentional**
                self-harm

       ✓7ᵗʰ **T63.033 Toxic effect of taipan venom, assault**

       ✓7ᵗʰ **T63.034 Toxic effect of taipan venom,**
                undetermined

    ✓6ᵗʰ **T63.04 Toxic effect of** cobra **venom**

       ✓7ᵗʰ **T63.041 Toxic effect of cobra venom, accidental**
                (unintentional)
                Toxic effect of cobra venom NOS

       ✓7ᵗʰ **T63.042 Toxic effect of cobra venom, intentional**
                self-harm

       ✓7ᵗʰ **T63.043 Toxic effect of cobra venom, assault**

       ✓7ᵗʰ **T63.044 Toxic effect of cobra venom,**
                undetermined

    ✓6ᵗʰ **T63.06 Toxic effect of venom of** other North and South
American snake

       ✓7ᵗʰ **T63.061 Toxic effect of venom of other North and**
                South American snake, accidental
                (unintentional)
                Toxic effect of venom of other North and
                South American snake NOS

       ✓7ᵗʰ **T63.062 Toxic effect of venom of other North and**
                South American snake, intentional self-
                harm

       ✓7ᵗʰ **T63.063 Toxic effect of venom of other North and**
                South American snake, assault

       ✓7ᵗʰ **T63.064 Toxic effect of venom of other North and**
                South American snake, undetermined

N Newborn: 0   P Pediatric: 0-17   M Maternity: 12-55   A Adult: 15-124   MCC Major CC Condition   PDx MCC PDx acts as own MCC   CC CC Condition   PDx CC PDx acts as own CC

1082   ICD-10-CM Draft (2015)

✓6th **T63.07 Toxic effect of venom of** other Australian snake

✓7th **T63.071 Toxic effect of venom of other Australian snake,** accidental (unintentional)
Toxic effect of venom of other Australian snake NOS

✓7th **T63.072 Toxic effect of venom of other Australian snake,** intentional self-harm

✓7th **T63.073 Toxic effect of venom of other Australian snake,** assault

✓7th **T63.074 Toxic effect of venom of other Australian snake,** undetermined

✓6th **T63.08 Toxic effect of venom of** other African and Asian snake

✓7th **T63.081 Toxic effect of venom of other African and Asian snake,** accidental (unintentional)
Toxic effect of venom of other African and Asian snake NOS

✓7th **T63.082 Toxic effect of venom of other African and Asian snake,** intentional self-harm

✓7th **T63.083 Toxic effect of venom of other African and Asian snake,** assault

✓7th **T63.084 Toxic effect of venom of other African and Asian snake,** undetermined

✓6th **T63.09 Toxic effect of venom of** other snake

✓7th **T63.091 Toxic effect of venom of other snake,** accidental (unintentional)
Toxic effect of venom of other snake NOS

✓7th **T63.092 Toxic effect of venom of other snake,** intentional self-harm

✓7th **T63.093 Toxic effect of venom of other snake,** assault

✓7th **T63.094 Toxic effect of venom of other snake,** undetermined

✓5th **T63.1 Toxic effect of venom of** other reptiles

✓6th **T63.11 Toxic effect of venom of** gila monster

✓7th **T63.111 Toxic effect of venom of gila monster,** accidental (unintentional)
Toxic effect of venom of gila monster NOS

✓7th **T63.112 Toxic effect of venom of gila monster,** intentional self-harm

✓7th **T63.113 Toxic effect of venom of gila monster,** assault

✓7th **T63.114 Toxic effect of venom of gila monster,** undetermined

✓6th **T63.12 Toxic effect of venom of** other venomous lizard

✓7th **T63.121 Toxic effect of venom of other venomous lizard,** accidental (unintentional)
Toxic effect of venom of other venomous lizard NOS

✓7th **T63.122 Toxic effect of venom of other venomous lizard,** intentional self-harm

✓7th **T63.123 Toxic effect of venom of other venomous lizard,** assault

✓7th **T63.124 Toxic effect of venom of other venomous lizard,** undetermined

✓6th **T63.19 Toxic effect of venom of** other reptiles

✓7th **T63.191 Toxic effect of venom of other reptiles,** accidental (unintentional)
Toxic effect of venom of other reptiles NOS

✓7th **T63.192 Toxic effect of venom of other reptiles,** intentional self-harm

✓7th **T63.193 Toxic effect of venom of other reptiles,** assault

✓7th **T63.194 Toxic effect of venom of other reptiles,** undetermined

✓5th **T63.2 Toxic effect of venom of** scorpion

✓6th **T63.2X Toxic effect of venom of scorpion**

✓7th **T63.2X1 Toxic effect of venom of scorpion,** accidental (unintentional)
Toxic effect of venom of scorpion NOS

✓7th **T63.2X2 Toxic effect of venom of scorpion,** intentional self-harm

✓7th **T63.2X3 Toxic effect of venom of scorpion,** assault

✓7th **T63.2X4 Toxic effect of venom of scorpion,** undetermined

✓5th **T63.3 Toxic effect of venom of** spider

✓6th **T63.30 Toxic effect of** unspecified spider venom

✓7th **T63.301 Toxic effect of unspecified spider venom,** accidental (unintentional)

✓7th **T63.302 Toxic effect of unspecified spider venom,** intentional self-harm

✓7th **T63.303 Toxic effect of unspecified spider venom,** assault

✓7th **T63.304 Toxic effect of unspecified spider venom,** undetermined

✓6th **T63.31 Toxic effect of venom of** black widow spider

✓7th **T63.311 Toxic effect of venom of black widow spider,** accidental (unintentional)

✓7th **T63.312 Toxic effect of venom of black widow spider,** intentional self-harm

✓7th **T63.313 Toxic effect of venom of black widow spider,** assault

✓7th **T63.314 Toxic effect of venom of black widow spider,** undetermined

✓6th **T63.32 Toxic effect of venom of** tarantula

✓7th **T63.321 Toxic effect of venom of tarantula,** accidental (unintentional)

✓7th **T63.322 Toxic effect of venom of tarantula,** intentional self-harm

✓7th **T63.323 Toxic effect of venom of tarantula,** assault

✓7th **T63.324 Toxic effect of venom of tarantula,** undetermined

✓6th **T63.33 Toxic effect of venom of** brown recluse spider

✓7th **T63.331 Toxic effect of venom of brown recluse spider,** accidental (unintentional)

✓7th **T63.332 Toxic effect of venom of brown recluse spider,** intentional self-harm

✓7th **T63.333 Toxic effect of venom of brown recluse spider,** assault

✓7th **T63.334 Toxic effect of venom of brown recluse spider,** undetermined

✓6th **T63.39 Toxic effect of venom of** other spider

✓7th **T63.391 Toxic effect of venom of other spider,** accidental (unintentional)

✓7th **T63.392 Toxic effect of venom of other spider,** intentional self-harm

✓7th **T63.393 Toxic effect of venom of other spider,** assault

✓7th **T63.394 Toxic effect of venom of other spider,** undetermined

✓5th **T63.4 Toxic effect of venom of** other arthropods

✓6th **T63.41 Toxic effect of venom of** centipedes and venomous millipedes

✓7th **T63.411 Toxic effect of venom of centipedes and venomous millipedes,** accidental (unintentional)

✓7th **T63.412 Toxic effect of venom of centipedes and venomous millipedes,** intentional self-harm

✓7th **T63.413 Toxic effect of venom of centipedes and venomous millipedes,** assault

✓7th **T63.414 Toxic effect of venom of centipedes and venomous millipedes,** undetermined

✓6th **T63.42 Toxic effect of venom of** ants

✓7th **T63.421 Toxic effect of venom of ants,** accidental (unintentional)

✓7th **T63.422 Toxic effect of venom of ants,** intentional self-harm

✓7th **T63.423 Toxic effect of venom of ants,** assault

✓7th **T63.424 Toxic effect of venom of ants,** undetermined

✓6th **T63.43 Toxic effect of venom of** caterpillars

✓7th **T63.431 Toxic effect of venom of caterpillars,** accidental (unintentional)

✓7th **T63.432 Toxic effect of venom of caterpillars,** intentional self-harm

✓7th **T63.433 Toxic effect of venom of caterpillars,** assault

√7ᵗʰ **T63.434** **Toxic effect of venom of caterpillars, undetermined**

√6ᵗʰ **T63.44** **Toxic effect of venom of** bees

√7ᵗʰ **T63.441** **Toxic effect of venom of bees, accidental (unintentional)**

√7ᵗʰ **T63.442** **Toxic effect of venom of bees, intentional self-harm**

√7ᵗʰ **T63.443** **Toxic effect of venom of bees, assault**

√7ᵗʰ **T63.444** **Toxic effect of venom of bees, undetermined**

√6ᵗʰ **T63.45** **Toxic effect of venom of** hornets

√7ᵗʰ **T63.451** **Toxic effect of venom of hornets, accidental (unintentional)**

√7ᵗʰ **T63.452** **Toxic effect of venom of hornets, intentional self-harm**

√7ᵗʰ **T63.453** **Toxic effect of venom of hornets, assault**

√7ᵗʰ **T63.454** **Toxic effect of venom of hornets, undetermined**

√6ᵗʰ **T63.46** **Toxic effect of venom of** wasps
Toxic effect of yellow jacket

√7ᵗʰ **T63.461** **Toxic effect of venom of wasps, accidental (unintentional)**

√7ᵗʰ **T63.462** **Toxic effect of venom of wasps, intentional self-harm**

√7ᵗʰ **T63.463** **Toxic effect of venom of wasps, assault**

√7ᵗʰ **T63.464** **Toxic effect of venom of wasps, undetermined**

√6ᵗʰ **T63.48** **Toxic effect of venom of** other arthropod

√7ᵗʰ **T63.481** **Toxic effect of venom of other arthropod, accidental (unintentional)**

√7ᵗʰ **T63.482** **Toxic effect of venom of other arthropod, intentional self-harm**

√7ᵗʰ **T63.483** **Toxic effect of venom of other arthropod, assault**

√7ᵗʰ **T63.484** **Toxic effect of venom of other arthropod, undetermined**

√5ᵗʰ **T63.5** **Toxic effect of contact with** venomous fish

EXCLUDES 2 *poisoning by ingestion of fish (T61.-)*

√6ᵗʰ **T63.51** **Toxic effect of contact with** stingray

√7ᵗʰ **T63.511** **Toxic effect of contact with stingray, accidental (unintentional)**

√7ᵗʰ **T63.512** **Toxic effect of contact with stingray, intentional self-harm**

√7ᵗʰ **T63.513** **Toxic effect of contact with stingray, assault**

√7ᵗʰ **T63.514** **Toxic effect of contact with stingray, undetermined**

√6ᵗʰ **T63.59** **Toxic effect of contact with** other venomous fish

√7ᵗʰ **T63.591** **Toxic effect of contact with other venomous fish, accidental (unintentional)**

√7ᵗʰ **T63.592** **Toxic effect of contact with other venomous fish, intentional self-harm**

√7ᵗʰ **T63.593** **Toxic effect of contact with other venomous fish, assault**

√7ᵗʰ **T63.594** **Toxic effect of contact with other venomous fish, undetermined**

√5ᵗʰ **T63.6** **Toxic effect of contact with other** venomous marine animals

EXCLUDES 1 *sea-snake venom (T63.09)*

EXCLUDES 2 *poisoning by ingestion of shellfish (T61.78-)*

√6ᵗʰ **T63.61** **Toxic effect of contact with** Portugese Man-o-war
Toxic effect of contact with bluebottle

√7ᵗʰ **T63.611** **Toxic effect of contact with Portugese Man-o-war, accidental (unintentional)**

√7ᵗʰ **T63.612** **Toxic effect of contact with Portugese Man-o-war, intentional self-harm**

√7ᵗʰ **T63.613** **Toxic effect of contact with Portugese Man-o-war, assault**

√7ᵗʰ **T63.614** **Toxic effect of contact with Portugese Man-o-war, undetermined**

√6ᵗʰ **T63.62** **Toxic effect of contact with** other jellyfish

√7ᵗʰ **T63.621** **Toxic effect of contact with other jellyfish, accidental (unintentional)**

√7ᵗʰ **T63.622** **Toxic effect of contact with other jellyfish, intentional self-harm**

√7ᵗʰ **T63.623** **Toxic effect of contact with other jellyfish, assault**

√7ᵗʰ **T63.624** **Toxic effect of contact with other jellyfish, undetermined**

√6ᵗʰ **T63.63** **Toxic effect of contact with** sea anemone

√7ᵗʰ **T63.631** **Toxic effect of contact with sea anemone, accidental (unintentional)**

√7ᵗʰ **T63.632** **Toxic effect of contact with sea anemone, intentional self-harm**

√7ᵗʰ **T63.633** **Toxic effect of contact with sea anemone, assault**

√7ᵗʰ **T63.634** **Toxic effect of contact with sea anemone, undetermined**

√6ᵗʰ **T63.69** **Toxic effect of contact with** other venomous marine animals

√7ᵗʰ **T63.691** **Toxic effect of contact with other venomous marine animals, accidental (unintentional)**

√7ᵗʰ **T63.692** **Toxic effect of contact with other venomous marine animals, intentional self-harm**

√7ᵗʰ **T63.693** **Toxic effect of contact with other venomous marine animals, assault**

√7ᵗʰ **T63.694** **Toxic effect of contact with other venomous marine animals, undetermined**

√5ᵗʰ **T63.7** **Toxic effect of contact with** venomous plant

√6ᵗʰ **T63.71** **Toxic effect of contact with venomous** marine plant

√7ᵗʰ **T63.711** **Toxic effect of contact with venomous marine plant, accidental (unintentional)**

√7ᵗʰ **T63.712** **Toxic effect of contact with venomous marine plant, intentional self-harm**

√7ᵗʰ **T63.713** **Toxic effect of contact with venomous marine plant, assault**

√7ᵗʰ **T63.714** **Toxic effect of contact with venomous marine plant, undetermined**

√6ᵗʰ **T63.79** **Toxic effect of contact with** other venomous plant

√7ᵗʰ **T63.791** **Toxic effect of contact with other venomous plant, accidental (unintentional)**

√7ᵗʰ **T63.792** **Toxic effect of contact with other venomous plant, intentional self-harm**

√7ᵗʰ **T63.793** **Toxic effect of contact with other venomous plant, assault**

√7ᵗʰ **T63.794** **Toxic effect of contact with other venomous plant, undetermined**

√5ᵗʰ **T63.8** **Toxic effect of contact with** other venomous animals

√6ᵗʰ **T63.81** **Toxic effect of contact with venomous** frog

EXCLUDES 1 *contact with nonvenomous frog (W62.0)*

√7ᵗʰ **T63.811** **Toxic effect of contact with venomous frog, accidental (unintentional)**

√7ᵗʰ **T63.812** **Toxic effect of contact with venomous frog, intentional self-harm**

√7ᵗʰ **T63.813** **Toxic effect of contact with venomous frog, assault**

√7ᵗʰ **T63.814** **Toxic effect of contact with venomous frog, undetermined**

√6ᵗʰ **T63.82** **Toxic effect of contact with venomous** toad

EXCLUDES 1 *contact with nonvenomous toad (W62.1)*

√7ᵗʰ **T63.821** **Toxic effect of contact with venomous toad, accidental (unintentional)**

√7ᵗʰ **T63.822** **Toxic effect of contact with venomous toad, intentional self-harm**

√7ᵗʰ **T63.823** **Toxic effect of contact with venomous toad, assault**

√7ᵗʰ **T63.824** **Toxic effect of contact with venomous toad, undetermined**

√6ᵗʰ **T63.83** **Toxic effect of contact with** other venomous amphibian

EXCLUDES 1 *contact with nonvenomous amphibian (W62.9)*

√7ᵗʰ **T63.831** **Toxic effect of contact with other venomous amphibian, accidental (unintentional)**

Ⓝ Newborn: 0   Ⓟ Pediatric: 0-17   Ⓜ Maternity: 12-55   Ⓐ Adult: 15-124   **MCC** Major CC Condition   **PDx MCC** PDx acts as own MCC   **CC** CC Condition   **PDx CC** PDx acts as own CC

1084   ICD-10-CM Draft (2015)

√7ᵗʰ **T63.832** Toxic effect of contact with other venomous amphibian, *intentional self-harm*

√7ᵗʰ **T63.833** Toxic effect of contact with other venomous amphibian, *assault*

√7ᵗʰ **T63.834** Toxic effect of contact with other venomous amphibian, *undetermined*

√6ᵗʰ **T63.89** Toxic effect of contact with other venomous animals

√7ᵗʰ **T63.891** Toxic effect of contact with other venomous animals, *accidental (unintentional)*

√7ᵗʰ **T63.892** Toxic effect of contact with other venomous animals, *intentional self-harm*

√7ᵗʰ **T63.893** Toxic effect of contact with other venomous animals, *assault*

√7ᵗʰ **T63.894** Toxic effect of contact with other venomous animals, *undetermined*

√5ᵗʰ **T63.9** Toxic effect of contact with unspecified venomous animal

√x7ᵗʰ **T63.91** Toxic effect of contact with unspecified venomous animal, *accidental (unintentional)*

√x7ᵗʰ **T63.92** Toxic effect of contact with unspecified venomous animal, *intentional self-harm*

√x7ᵗʰ **T63.93** Toxic effect of contact with unspecified venomous animal, *assault*

√x7ᵗʰ **T63.94** Toxic effect of contact with unspecified venomous animal, *undetermined*

√4ᵗʰ **T64** **Toxic effect of aflatoxin and other mycotoxin food contaminants**

> The appropriate 7th character is to be added to each code from category T64.
> A initial encounter
> D subsequent encounter
> S sequela

√5ᵗʰ **T64.0** Toxic effect of aflatoxin

√x7ᵗʰ **T64.01** Toxic effect of aflatoxin, *accidental (unintentional)*

√x7ᵗʰ **T64.02** Toxic effect of aflatoxin, *intentional self-harm*

√x7ᵗʰ **T64.03** Toxic effect of aflatoxin, *assault*

√x7ᵗʰ **T64.04** Toxic effect of aflatoxin, *undetermined*

√5ᵗʰ **T64.8** Toxic effect of other mycotoxin food contaminants

√x7ᵗʰ **T64.81** Toxic effect of other mycotoxin food contaminants, *accidental (unintentional)*

√x7ᵗʰ **T64.82** Toxic effect of other mycotoxin food contaminants, *intentional self-harm*

√x7ᵗʰ **T64.83** Toxic effect of other mycotoxin food contaminants, *assault*

√x7ᵗʰ **T64.84** Toxic effect of other mycotoxin food contaminants, *undetermined*

√4ᵗʰ **T65** **Toxic effect of other and unspecified substances**

> The appropriate 7th character is to be added to each code from category T65.
> A initial encounter
> D subsequent encounter
> S sequela

√5ᵗʰ **T65.0** Toxic effect of cyanides

> **EXCLUDES 1** hydrogen cyanide (T57.3-)

√6ᵗʰ **T65.0X** Toxic effect of cyanides

√7ᵗʰ **T65.0X1** Toxic effect of cyanides, *accidental (unintentional)*
Toxic effect of cyanides NOS

√7ᵗʰ **T65.0X2** Toxic effect of cyanides, *intentional self-harm*

√7ᵗʰ **T65.0X3** Toxic effect of cyanides, *assault*

√7ᵗʰ **T65.0X4** Toxic effect of cyanides, *undetermined*

√5ᵗʰ **T65.1** Toxic effect of strychnine and its salts

√6ᵗʰ **T65.1X** Toxic effect of strychnine and its salts

√7ᵗʰ **T65.1X1** Toxic effect of strychnine and its salts, *accidental (unintentional)*
Toxic effect of strychnine and its salts NOS

√7ᵗʰ **T65.1X2** Toxic effect of strychnine and its salts, *intentional self-harm*

√7ᵗʰ **T65.1X3** Toxic effect of strychnine and its salts, *assault*

√7ᵗʰ **T65.1X4** Toxic effect of strychnine and its salts, *undetermined*

√5ᵗʰ **T65.2** Toxic effect of tobacco and nicotine

> **EXCLUDES 2** *nicotine dependence (F17.-)*

√6ᵗʰ **T65.21** Toxic effect of chewing tobacco

√7ᵗʰ **T65.211** Toxic effect of chewing tobacco, *accidental (unintentional)*
Toxic effect of chewing tobacco NOS

√7ᵗʰ **T65.212** Toxic effect of chewing tobacco, *intentional self-harm*

√7ᵗʰ **T65.213** Toxic effect of chewing tobacco, *assault*

√7ᵗʰ **T65.214** Toxic effect of chewing tobacco, *undetermined*

√6ᵗʰ **T65.22** Toxic effect of tobacco cigarettes
Toxic effect of tobacco smoke
Use additional code for exposure to second hand tobacco smoke (Z57.31, Z77.22)

√7ᵗʰ **T65.221** Toxic effect of tobacco cigarettes, *accidental (unintentional)*
Toxic effect of tobacco cigarettes NOS

√7ᵗʰ **T65.222** Toxic effect of tobacco cigarettes, *intentional self-harm*

√7ᵗʰ **T65.223** Toxic effect of tobacco cigarettes, *assault*

√7ᵗʰ **T65.224** Toxic effect of tobacco cigarettes, *undetermined*

√6ᵗʰ **T65.29** Toxic effect of other tobacco and nicotine

√7ᵗʰ **T65.291** Toxic effect of other tobacco and nicotine, *accidental (unintentional)*
Toxic effect of other tobacco and nicotine NOS

√7ᵗʰ **T65.292** Toxic effect of other tobacco and nicotine, *intentional self-harm*

√7ᵗʰ **T65.293** Toxic effect of other tobacco and nicotine, *assault*

√7ᵗʰ **T65.294** Toxic effect of other tobacco and nicotine, *undetermined*

√5ᵗʰ **T65.3** Toxic effect of nitroderivatives and aminoderivatives of benzene and its homologues
Toxic effect of anilin [benzenamine]
Toxic effect of nitrobenzene
Toxic effect of trinitrotoluene

√6ᵗʰ **T65.3X** Toxic effect of nitroderivatives and aminoderivatives of benzene and its homologues

√7ᵗʰ **T65.3X1** Toxic effect of nitroderivatives and aminoderivatives of benzene and its homologues, *accidental (unintentional)*
Toxic effect of nitroderivatives and aminoderivatives of benzene and its homologues NOS

√7ᵗʰ **T65.3X2** Toxic effect of nitroderivatives and aminoderivatives of benzene and its homologues, *intentional self-harm*

√7ᵗʰ **T65.3X3** Toxic effect of nitroderivatives and aminoderivatives of benzene and its homologues, *assault*

√7ᵗʰ **T65.3X4** Toxic effect of nitroderivatives and aminoderivatives of benzene and its homologues, *undetermined*

√5ᵗʰ **T65.4** Toxic effect of carbon disulfide

√6ᵗʰ **T65.4X** Toxic effect of carbon disulfide

√7ᵗʰ **T65.4X1** Toxic effect of carbon disulfide, *accidental (unintentional)*
Toxic effect of carbon disulfide NOS

√7ᵗʰ **T65.4X2** Toxic effect of carbon disulfide, *intentional self-harm*

√7ᵗʰ **T65.4X3** Toxic effect of carbon disulfide, *assault*

√7ᵗʰ **T65.4X4** Toxic effect of carbon disulfide, *undetermined*

√5ᵗʰ **T65.5** Toxic effect of nitroglycerin and other nitric acids and esters
Toxic effect of 1,2,3-Propanetriol trinitrate

√6ᵗʰ **T65.5X** Toxic effect of nitroglycerin and other nitric acids and esters

√7ᵗʰ **T65.5X1** Toxic effect of nitroglycerin and other nitric acids and esters, *accidental (unintentional)*
Toxic effect of nitroglycerin and other nitric acids and esters NOS

T65.5X2–T68

Injury, Poisoning and Certain Other Consequences of External Causes

√7ᵗʰ **T65.5X2**   **Toxic effect of nitroglycerin and other nitric acids and esters, intentional self-harm**

√7ᵗʰ **T65.5X3**   **Toxic effect of nitroglycerin and other nitric acids and esters, assault**

√7ᵗʰ **T65.5X4**   **Toxic effect of nitroglycerin and other nitric acids and esters, undetermined**

√5ᵗʰ **T65.6**   **Toxic effect of paints and dyes, not elsewhere classified**

√6ᵗʰ **T65.6X**   **Toxic effect of paints and dyes, not elsewhere classified**

√7ᵗʰ **T65.6X1**   **Toxic effect of paints and dyes, not elsewhere classified, accidental (unintentional)**
Toxic effect of paints and dyes NOS

√7ᵗʰ **T65.6X2**   **Toxic effect of paints and dyes, not elsewhere classified, intentional self-harm**

√7ᵗʰ **T65.6X3**   **Toxic effect of paints and dyes, not elsewhere classified, assault**

√7ᵗʰ **T65.6X4**   **Toxic effect of paints and dyes, not elsewhere classified, undetermined**

√5ᵗʰ **T65.8**   **Toxic effect of other specified substances**

√6ᵗʰ **T65.81**   **Toxic effect of latex**

√7ᵗʰ **T65.811**   **Toxic effect of latex, accidental (unintentional)**
Toxic effect of latex NOS

√7ᵗʰ **T65.812**   **Toxic effect of latex, intentional self-harm**

√7ᵗʰ **T65.813**   **Toxic effect of latex, assault**

√7ᵗʰ **T65.814**   **Toxic effect of latex, undetermined**

√6ᵗʰ **T65.82**   **Toxic effect of harmful algae and algae toxins**
Toxic effect of (harmful) algae bloom NOS
Toxic effect of blue-green algae bloom
Toxic effect of brown tide
Toxic effect of cyanobacteria bloom
Toxic effect of Florida red tide
Toxic effect of pfiesteria piscicida
Toxic effect of red tide

√7ᵗʰ **T65.821**   **Toxic effect of harmful algae and algae toxins, accidental (unintentional)**
Toxic effect of harmful algae and algae toxins NOS

√7ᵗʰ **T65.822**   **Toxic effect of harmful algae and algae toxins, intentional self-harm**

√7ᵗʰ **T65.823**   **Toxic effect of harmful algae and algae toxins, assault**

√7ᵗʰ **T65.824**   **Toxic effect of harmful algae and algae toxins, undetermined**

√6ᵗʰ **T65.83**   **Toxic effect of fiberglass**

√7ᵗʰ **T65.831**   **Toxic effect of fiberglass, accidental (unintentional)**
Toxic effect of fiberglass NOS

√7ᵗʰ **T65.832**   **Toxic effect of fiberglass, intentional self-harm**

√7ᵗʰ **T65.833**   **Toxic effect of fiberglass, assault**

√7ᵗʰ **T65.834**   **Toxic effect of fiberglass, undetermined**

√6ᵗʰ **T65.89**   **Toxic effect of other specified substances**

√7ᵗʰ **T65.891**   **Toxic effect of other specified substances, accidental (unintentional)**
Toxic effect of other specified substances NOS

√7ᵗʰ **T65.892**   **Toxic effect of other specified substances, intentional self-harm**

√7ᵗʰ **T65.893**   **Toxic effect of other specified substances, assault**

√7ᵗʰ **T65.894**   **Toxic effect of other specified substances, undetermined**

√5ᵗʰ **T65.9**   **Toxic effect of unspecified substance**

√×7ᵗʰ **T65.91**   **Toxic effect of unspecified substance, accidental (unintentional)**
Poisoning NOS

√×7ᵗʰ **T65.92**   **Toxic effect of unspecified substance, intentional self-harm**

√×7ᵗʰ **T65.93**   **Toxic effect of unspecified substance, assault**

√×7ᵗʰ **T65.94**   **Toxic effect of unspecified substance, undetermined**

Other and unspecified effects of external causes (T66-T78)

√×7ᵗʰ **T66**   **Radiation sickness, unspecified**
EXCLUDES 1   specified adverse effects of radiation, such as:
     burns (T20-T31)
     leukemia (C91-C95)
     radiation gastroenteritis and colitis (K52.0)
     radiation pneumonitis (J70.0)
     radiation related disorders of the skin and subcutaneous tissue (L55-L59)
     radiation sunburn (L55.-)

The appropriate 7th character is to be added to code T66.
A   initial encounter
D   subsequent encounter
S   sequela

√4ᵗʰ **T67**   **Effects of heat and light**
EXCLUDES 1   erythema [dermatitis] ab igne (L59.0)
     malignant hyperpyrexia due to anesthesia (T88.3)
     radiation-related disorders of the skin and subcutaneous tissue (L55-L59)
EXCLUDES 2   burns (T20-T31)
     sunburn (L55.-)
     sweat disorder due to heat (L74-L75)

The appropriate 7th character is to be added to each code from category T67.
A   initial encounter
D   subsequent encounter
S   sequela

7   √×7ᵗʰ **T67.0**   **Heatstroke and sunstroke**   CC
Heat apoplexy   Siriasis
Heat pyrexia   Thermoplegia
Use additional code(s) to identify any associated complications of heatstroke, such as:
     coma and stupor (R40.-)
     systemic inflammatory response syndrome (R65.1-)
CC Excl: CC with 7th character A:T67.[0-9]XXA

√×7ᵗʰ **T67.1**   **Heat syncope**
Heat collapse

√×7ᵗʰ **T67.2**   **Heat cramp**

√×7ᵗʰ **T67.3**   **Heat exhaustion, anhydrotic**
Heat prostration due to water depletion
EXCLUDES 1   heat exhaustion due to salt depletion (T67.4)

√×7ᵗʰ **T67.4**   **Heat exhaustion due to salt depletion**
Heat prostration due to salt (and water) depletion

√×7ᵗʰ **T67.5**   **Heat exhaustion, unspecified**
Heat prostration NOS

√×7ᵗʰ **T67.6**   **Heat fatigue, transient**

√×7ᵗʰ **T67.7**   **Heat edema**

√×7ᵗʰ **T67.8**   **Other effects of heat and light**

√×7ᵗʰ **T67.9**   **Effect of heat and light, unspecified**

√×7ᵗʰ **T68**   **Hypothermia**
Accidental hypothermia
Hypothermia NOS
Use additional code to identify source of exposure:
     exposure to excessive cold of man-made origin (W93)
     exposure to excessive cold of natural origin (X31)
EXCLUDES 1   hypothermia following anesthesia (T88.51)
     hypothermia not associated with low environmental temperature (R68.0)
     hypothermia of newborn (P80.-)
EXCLUDES 2   frostbite (T33-T34)

The appropriate 7th character is to be added to code T68.
A   initial encounter
D   subsequent encounter
S   sequela

---

7 HAC = Initial encounter only (7th character A, B or C) and not POA.

N Newborn: 0   P Pediatric: 0-17   M Maternity: 12-55   A Adult: 15-124   MCC Major CC Condition   PDx MCC PDx acts as own MCC   CC CC Condition   PDx CC PDx acts as own CC

1086   ICD-10-CM Draft (2015)

☑4ᵗʰ **T69 Other effects of reduced temperature**
Use additional code to identify source of exposure:
exposure to excessive cold of man-made origin (W93)
exposure to excessive cold of natural origin (X31)
EXCLUDES 2 *frostbite (T33-T34)*

> The appropriate 7th character is to be added to each code from category T69.
> A   initial encounter
> D   subsequent encounter
> S   sequela

☑5ᵗʰ **T69.0 Immersion hand and foot**

☑6ᵗʰ **T69.01 Immersion hand**

☑7ᵗʰ **T69.011 Immersion hand, right hand**

☑7ᵗʰ **T69.012 Immersion hand, left hand**

☑7ᵗʰ **T69.019 Immersion hand, unspecified hand**

☑6ᵗʰ **T69.02 Immersion foot**
Trench foot

> **CC Excl: For CC codes in subcategory T69.02: CC with 7th character A, unless otherwise noted:** T33.2XX-T33.42X with 7th A, T33.60X-T33.72X with 7th A, T33.90X-T33.99X with 7th A, T34.2XX-T34.42X with 7th A, T34.60X-T34.72X with 7th A, T34.90X-T34.99X with 7th A, T69.021-T69.029 with 7th A

7 ☑7ᵗʰ **T69.021 Immersion foot, right foot**   CC

7 ☑7ᵗʰ **T69.022 Immersion foot, left foot**   CC

7 ☑7ᵗʰ **T69.029 Immersion foot, unspecified foot**   CC

☑x7ᵗʰ **T69.1 Chilblains**

☑x7ᵗʰ **T69.8 Other specified effects of reduced temperature**

☑x7ᵗʰ **T69.9 Effect of reduced temperature, unspecified**

☑4ᵗʰ **T70 Effects of air pressure and water pressure**

> The appropriate 7th character is to be added to each code from category T70.
> A   initial encounter
> D   subsequent encounter
> S   sequela

☑x7ᵗʰ **T70.0 Otitic barotrauma**
Aero-otitis media
Effects of change in ambient atmospheric pressure or water pressure on ears

☑x7ᵗʰ **T70.1 Sinus barotrauma**
Aerosinusitis
Effects of change in ambient atmospheric pressure on sinuses

☑5ᵗʰ **T70.2 Other and unspecified effects of high altitude**
EXCLUDES 2 *polycythemia due to high altitude (D75.1)*

☑x7ᵗʰ **T70.20 Unspecified effects of high altitude**

☑x7ᵗʰ **T70.29 Other effects of high altitude**
Alpine sickness
Anoxia due to high altitude
Barotrauma NOS
Hypobaropathy
Mountain sickness

7 ☑x7ᵗʰ **T70.3 Caisson disease [decompression sickness]**   CC
Compressed-air disease   Diver's palsy or paralysis
CC Excl: CC with 7th character A: T70.3XX-T70.9XX with 7th A

☑x7ᵗʰ **T70.4 Effects of high-pressure fluids**
Hydraulic jet injection (industrial)
Pneumatic jet injection (industrial)
Traumatic jet injection (industrial)

☑x7ᵗʰ **T70.8 Other effects of air pressure and water pressure**

☑x7ᵗʰ **T70.9 Effect of air pressure and water pressure, unspecified**

☑4ᵗʰ **T71 Asphyxiation**
Mechanical suffocation   Traumatic suffocation
EXCLUDES 1 *acute respiratory distress (syndrome) (J80)*
anoxia due to high altitude (T70.2)
asphyxia NOS (R09.01)
asphyxia from carbon monoxide (T58.-)
asphyxia from inhalation of food or foreign body (T17.-)
asphyxia from other gases, fumes and vapors (T59.-)
respiratory distress (syndrome) in newborn (P22.-)

> The appropriate 7th character is to be added to each code from category T71.
> A   initial encounter
> D   subsequent encounter
> S   sequela

> **CC Excl: For CC codes in category T71: CC with 7th character A, unless otherwise noted:** T71.111-T71.9XX with 7th A

☑5ᵗʰ **T71.1 Asphyxiation due to mechanical threat to breathing**
Suffocation due to mechanical threat to breathing

☑6ᵗʰ **T71.11 Asphyxiation due to smothering under pillow**

7 ☑7ᵗʰ **T71.111 Asphyxiation due to smothering under pillow, accidental**   CC
Asphyxiation due to smothering under pillow NOS

7 ☑7ᵗʰ **T71.112 Asphyxiation due to smothering under pillow, intentional self-harm**   CC

7 ☑7ᵗʰ **T71.113 Asphyxiation due to smothering under pillow, assault**   CC

7 ☑7ᵗʰ **T71.114 Asphyxiation due to smothering under pillow, undetermined**   CC

☑6ᵗʰ **T71.12 Asphyxiation due to plastic bag**

7 ☑7ᵗʰ **T71.121 Asphyxiation due to plastic bag, accidental**   CC
Asphyxiation due to plastic bag NOS

7 ☑7ᵗʰ **T71.122 Asphyxiation due to plastic bag, intentional self-harm**   CC

7 ☑7ᵗʰ **T71.123 Asphyxiation due to plastic bag, assault**   CC

7 ☑7ᵗʰ **T71.124 Asphyxiation due to plastic bag, undetermined**   CC

☑6ᵗʰ **T71.13 Asphyxiation due to being trapped in bed linens**

7 ☑7ᵗʰ **T71.131 Asphyxiation due to being trapped in bed linens, accidental**   CC
Asphyxiation due to being trapped in bed linens NOS

7 ☑7ᵗʰ **T71.132 Asphyxiation due to being trapped in bed linens, intentional self-harm**   CC

7 ☑7ᵗʰ **T71.133 Asphyxiation due to being trapped in bed linens, assault**   CC

7 ☑7ᵗʰ **T71.134 Asphyxiation due to being trapped in bed linens, undetermined**   CC

☑6ᵗʰ **T71.14 Asphyxiation due to smothering under another person's body (in bed)**

7 ☑7ᵗʰ **T71.141 Asphyxiation due to smothering under another person's body (in bed), accidental**   CC
Asphyxiation due to smothering under another person's body (in bed) NOS

7 ☑7ᵗʰ **T71.143 Asphyxiation due to smothering under another person's body (in bed), assault**   CC

7 ☑7ᵗʰ **T71.144 Asphyxiation due to smothering under another person's body (in bed), undetermined**   CC

☑6ᵗʰ **T71.15 Asphyxiation due to smothering in furniture**

7 ☑7ᵗʰ **T71.151 Asphyxiation due to smothering in furniture, accidental**   CC
Asphyxiation due to smothering in furniture NOS

7 ☑7ᵗʰ **T71.152 Asphyxiation due to smothering in furniture, intentional self-harm**   CC

7 ☑7ᵗʰ **T71.153 Asphyxiation due to smothering in furniture, assault**   CC

7 ☑7ᵗʰ **T71.154 Asphyxiation due to smothering in furniture, undetermined**   CC

---

7 HAC = Initial encounter only (7th character A, B or C) and not POA.

☑ Additional Character Required   ☑x7ᵗʰ Xtension Alert   Unacceptable PDx   Manifestation   Hospital Acquired Condition   EXCLUDES 1 Not Coded Here   EXCLUDES 2 Not Included Here

Injury, Poisoning and Certain Other Consequences of External Causes

T71.16–T75.09

☑6ᵗʰ **T71.16** **Asphyxiation due to hanging**
Hanging by window shade cord
Use additional code for any associated injuries, such as:
crushing injury of neck (S17.-)
fracture of cervical vertebrae (S12.0-S12.2-)
open wound of neck (S11.-)

⁷ ☑7ᵗʰ **T71.161** **Asphyxiation due to hanging, accidental**   CC
Asphyxiation due to hanging NOS
Hanging NOS

⁷ ☑7ᵗʰ **T71.162** **Asphyxiation due to hanging, intentional self-harm**   CC

⁷ ☑7ᵗʰ **T71.163** **Asphyxiation due to hanging, assault**   CC

⁷ ☑7ᵗʰ **T71.164** **Asphyxiation due to hanging, undetermined**   CC

☑6ᵗʰ **T71.19** **Asphyxiation due to mechanical threat to breathing due to other causes**

⁷ ☑7ᵗʰ **T71.191** **Asphyxiation due to mechanical threat to breathing due to other causes, accidental**   CC
Asphyxiation due to other causes NOS

⁷ ☑7ᵗʰ **T71.192** **Asphyxiation due to mechanical threat to breathing due to other causes, intentional self-harm**   CC

⁷ ☑7ᵗʰ **T71.193** **Asphyxiation due to mechanical threat to breathing due to other causes, assault**   CC

⁷ ☑7ᵗʰ **T71.194** **Asphyxiation due to mechanical threat to breathing due to other causes, undetermined**   CC

☑5ᵗʰ **T71.2** **Asphyxiation due to systemic oxygen deficiency due to low oxygen content in ambient air**
Suffocation due to systemic oxygen deficiency due to low oxygen content in ambient air

⁷ ☑x7ᵗʰ **T71.20** **Asphyxiation due to systemic oxygen deficiency due to low oxygen content in ambient air due to unspecified cause**   CC

⁷ ☑x7ᵗʰ **T71.21** **Asphyxiation due to cave-in or falling earth**   CC
Use additional code for any associated cataclysm (X34-X38)

☑6ᵗʰ **T71.22** **Asphyxiation due to being trapped in a car trunk**

☑7ᵗʰ **T71.221** **Asphyxiation due to being trapped in a car trunk, accidental**   CC

☑7ᵗʰ **T71.222** **Asphyxiation due to being trapped in a car trunk, intentional self-harm**   CC

☑7ᵗʰ **T71.223** **Asphyxiation due to being trapped in a car trunk, assault**   CC

☑7ᵗʰ **T71.224** **Asphyxiation due to being trapped in a car trunk, undetermined**   CC

☑6ᵗʰ **T71.23** **Asphyxiation due to being trapped in a (discarded) refrigerator**

☑7ᵗʰ **T71.231** **Asphyxiation due to being trapped in a (discarded) refrigerator, accidental**   CC

☑7ᵗʰ **T71.232** **Asphyxiation due to being trapped in a (discarded) refrigerator, intentional self-harm**   CC

☑7ᵗʰ **T71.233** **Asphyxiation due to being trapped in a (discarded) refrigerator, assault**   CC

☑7ᵗʰ **T71.234** **Asphyxiation due to being trapped in a (discarded) refrigerator, undetermined**   CC

⁷ ☑x7ᵗʰ **T71.29** **Asphyxiation due to being trapped in other low oxygen environment**   CC

⁷ ☑x7ᵗʰ **T71.9** **Asphyxiation due to unspecified cause**   CC
Suffocation (by strangulation) due to unspecified cause
Suffocation NOS
Systemic oxygen deficiency due to low oxygen content in ambient air due to unspecified cause
Systemic oxygen deficiency due to mechanical threat to breathing due to unspecified cause
Traumatic asphyxia NOS

☑4ᵗʰ **T73** **Effects of other deprivation**

The appropriate 7th character is to be added to each code from category T73.
A   initial encounter
D   subsequent encounter
S   sequela

☑x7ᵗʰ **T73.0** **Starvation**
Deprivation of food

☑x7ᵗʰ **T73.1** **Deprivation of water**

☑x7ᵗʰ **T73.2** **Exhaustion due to exposure**

☑x7ᵗʰ **T73.3** **Exhaustion due to excessive exertion**
Exhaustion due to overexertion

☑x7ᵗʰ **T73.8** **Other effects of deprivation**

☑x7ᵗʰ **T73.9** **Effect of deprivation, unspecified**

☑4ᵗʰ **T74** **Adult and child abuse, neglect and other maltreatment, confirmed**
Use additional code, if applicable, to identify any associated current injury
Use additional external cause code to identify perpetrator, if known (Y07.-)

EXCLUDES 1 *abuse and maltreatment in pregnancy (O9A.3-, O9A.4-, O9A.5-)*
adult and child maltreatment, suspected (T76.-)

The appropriate 7th character is to be added to each code from category T74.
A   initial encounter
D   subsequent encounter
S   sequela

CC Excl: For CC codes in category T74: CC with 7th character A, unless otherwise noted: T74.01X-T74.92X with 7th A, T76.01X-T76.92X with 7th A

☑5ᵗʰ **T74.0** **Neglect or abandonment, confirmed**

☑7ᵗʰ **T74.01** **Adult neglect or abandonment, confirmed**   CC A

☑7ᵗʰ **T74.02** **Child neglect or abandonment, confirmed**   CC P

☑5ᵗʰ **T74.1** **Physical abuse, confirmed**
EXCLUDES 2 *sexual abuse (T74.2-)*

☑7ᵗʰ **T74.11** **Adult physical abuse, confirmed**   CC A

☑7ᵗʰ **T74.12** **Child physical abuse, confirmed**   CC P
EXCLUDES 2 *shaken infant syndrome (T74.4)*

☑5ᵗʰ **T74.2** **Sexual abuse, confirmed**
Rape, confirmed   Sexual assault, confirmed

☑7ᵗʰ **T74.21** **Adult sexual abuse, confirmed**   CC A

☑7ᵗʰ **T74.22** **Child sexual abuse, confirmed**   CC P

☑5ᵗʰ **T74.3** **Psychological abuse, confirmed**

☑7ᵗʰ **T74.31** **Adult psychological abuse, confirmed**   A

☑7ᵗʰ **T74.32** **Child psychological abuse, confirmed**   CC P

☑x7ᵗʰ **T74.4** **Shaken infant syndrome**   CC P

☑5ᵗʰ **T74.9** **Unspecified maltreatment, confirmed**

☑x7ᵗʰ **T74.91** **Unspecified adult maltreatment, confirmed**   CC A
CC Excl: CC with 7th character A: T74.91X A, T76.91XA

☑x7ᵗʰ **T74.92** **Unspecified child maltreatment, confirmed**   CC P
CC Excl: CC with 7th character A: T74.01X-T74.92X with 7th A, T76.01X-T76.92X with 7th A

☑4ᵗʰ **T75** **Other and unspecified effects of other external causes**
EXCLUDES 1 *adverse effects NEC (T78.-)*
EXCLUDES 2 *burns (electric) (T20-T31)*

The appropriate 7th character is to be added to each code from category T75.
A   initial encounter
D   subsequent encounter
S   sequela

☑5ᵗʰ **T75.0** **Effects of lightning**
Struck by lightning

☑x7ᵗʰ **T75.00** **Unspecified effects of lightning**
Struck by lightning NOS

☑x7ᵗʰ **T75.01** **Shock due to being struck by lightning**

☑x7ᵗʰ **T75.09** **Other effects of lightning**
Use additional code for other effects of lightning

---

⁷ HAC = Initial encounter only (7th character A, B or C) and not POA.

N Newborn: 0   P Pediatric: 0-17   M Maternity: 12-55   A Adult: 15-124   **MCC** Major CC Condition   **PDx MCC** PDx acts as own MCC   **CC** CC Condition   **PDx CC** PDx acts as own CC

1088   ICD-10-CM Draft (2015)

7 ✓x7ᵗʰ **T75.1** **Unspecified effects of drowning and nonfatal** CC
    submersion
    Immersion
    EXCLUDES 1 *specified effects of drowning—code to effects*
    CC Excl: CC with 7th character A:T75.1XXA

✓5ᵗʰ **T75.2** **Effects of vibration**

 ✓x7ᵗʰ **T75.20** **Unspecified effects of vibration**

 ✓x7ᵗʰ **T75.21** **Pneumatic hammer syndrome**

 ✓x7ᵗʰ **T75.22** **Traumatic vasospastic syndrome**

 ✓x7ᵗʰ **T75.23** **Vertigo from infrasound**
    EXCLUDES 1 *vertigo NOS (R42)*

 T75.29 **Other effects of vibration**

✓x7ᵗʰ **T75.3** **Motion sickness**
   Airsickness   Travel sickness
   Seasickness
   Use additional external cause code to identify vehicle or type of
    motion (Y92.81-, Y93.5-)

✓x7ᵗʰ **T75.4** **Electrocution**
   Shock from electric current
   Shock from electroshock gun (taser)

✓5ᵗʰ **T75.8** **Other specified effects of external causes**

 ✓x7ᵗʰ **T75.81** **Effects of abnormal gravitation [G] forces**

 ✓x7ᵗʰ **T75.82** **Effects of weightlessness**

 ✓x7ᵗʰ **T75.89** **Other specified effects of external causes**

✓4ᵗʰ **T76** **Adult and child abuse, neglect and other maltreatment,**
   suspected
   Use additional code, if applicable, to identify any associated current
    injury
   EXCLUDES 1 *adult and child maltreatment, confirmed (T74.-)*
     suspected abuse and maltreatment in pregnancy (O9A.3-,
      O9A.4-, O9A.5-)
     suspected adult physical and sexual abuse, ruled out (Z04.71)
     suspected adult sexual abused, ruled out (Z04.41)
     suspected child physical abuse, ruled out (Z04.72)
     suspected child sexual abuse, ruled out (Z04.42)

  The appropriate 7th character is to be added to each code from
  category T76.
  A initial encounter
  D subsequent encounter
  S sequela

  CC Excl: For CC codes in category T76: CC with 7th character A,
  unless otherwise noted: T74.01X-T74.92X with 7th A,
  T76.01X-T76.92X with 7th A

✓5ᵗʰ **T76.0** **Neglect or abandonment, suspected**

 ✓x7ᵗʰ **T76.01** **Adult neglect or abandonment, suspected** CC A

 ✓x7ᵗʰ **T76.02** **Child neglect or abandonment, suspected** CC P

✓5ᵗʰ **T76.1** **Physical abuse, suspected**

 ✓x7ᵗʰ **T76.11** **Adult physical abuse, suspected** CC A

 ✓x7ᵗʰ **T76.12** **Child physical abuse, suspected** CC P

✓5ᵗʰ **T76.2** **Sexual abuse, suspected**
   Rape, suspected Sexual abuse, suspected
   EXCLUDES 1 *alleged abuse, ruled out (Z04.7)*

 ✓x7ᵗʰ **T76.21** **Adult sexual abuse, suspected** CC A

 ✓x7ᵗʰ **T76.22** **Child sexual abuse, suspected** CC P

✓5ᵗʰ **T76.3** **Psychological abuse, suspected**

 ✓x7ᵗʰ **T76.31** **Adult psychological abuse, suspected** A

 ✓x7ᵗʰ **T76.32** **Child psychological abuse, suspected** CC P

✓5ᵗʰ **T76.9** **Unspecified maltreatment, suspected**

 ✓x7ᵗʰ **T76.91** **Unspecified adult maltreatment, suspected** CC A
    CC Excl: CC with 7th character A: T74.91XA, T76.91XA

 ✓x7ᵗʰ **T76.92** **Unspecified child maltreatment, suspected** CC P
    CC Excl: CC with 7th character A: T74.01-T74.92 with
     7th A, T76.01-T76.92 with 7th A

✓4ᵗʰ **T78** **Adverse effects, not elsewhere classified**
   EXCLUDES 2 *complications of surgical and medical care NEC (T80-T88)*

  The appropriate 7th character is to be added to each code from
  category T78.
  A initial encounter
  D subsequent encounter
  S sequela

  CC Excl: For CC codes in category T78: CC with 7th character
  A, unless otherwise noted: T78.00X-T78.09X with 7th A

✓5ᵗʰ **T78.0** **Anaphylactic reaction due to food**
   Anaphylactic reaction due to adverse food reaction
   Anaphylactic shock or reaction due to nonpoisonous foods
   Anaphylactoid reaction due to food

 ✓x7ᵗʰ **T78.00** **Anaphylactic reaction due to unspecified food** CC

 ✓x7ᵗʰ **T78.01** **Anaphylactic reaction due to peanuts** CC

 ✓x7ᵗʰ **T78.02** **Anaphylactic reaction due to shellfish** CC
    (crustaceans)

 ✓x7ᵗʰ **T78.03** **Anaphylactic reaction due to other fish** CC

 ✓x7ᵗʰ **T78.04** **Anaphylactic reaction due to fruits and** CC
    vegetables

 ✓x7ᵗʰ **T78.05** **Anaphylactic reaction due to tree nuts and seeds** CC
    EXCLUDES 1 *anaphylactic reaction due to peanuts*
     (T78.01)

 ✓x7ᵗʰ **T78.06** **Anaphylactic reaction due to food additives** CC

 ✓x7ᵗʰ **T78.07** **Anaphylactic reaction due to milk and dairy** CC
    products

 ✓x7ᵗʰ **T78.08** **Anaphylactic reaction due to eggs** CC

 ✓x7ᵗʰ **T78.09** **Anaphylactic reaction due to other food** CC
    products

✓x7ᵗʰ **T78.1** **Other adverse food reactions, not elsewhere classified**
   Use additional code to identify the type of reaction
   EXCLUDES 1 *anaphylactic reaction or shock due to adverse food*
     reaction (T78.0-)
    anaphylactic reaction due to food (T78.0-)
    bacterial food borne intoxications (A05.-)
   EXCLUDES 2 *allergic and dietetic gastroenteritis and colitis (K52.2)*
    allergic rhinitis due to food (J30.5)
    dermatitis due to food in contact with skin (L23.6, L24.6,
     L25.4)
    dermatitis due to ingested food (L27.2)

✓x7ᵗʰ **T78.2** **Anaphylactic shock, unspecified** CC
   Allergic shock   Anaphylaxis
   Anaphylactic reaction
   EXCLUDES 1 *anaphylactic reaction or shock due to adverse effect of*
     correct medicinal substance properly
     administered (T88.6)
    anaphylactic reaction or shock due to adverse food
     reaction (T78.0-)
    anaphylactic reaction or shock due to serum (T80.5-)

✓x7ᵗʰ **T78.3** **Angioneurotic edema**
   Allergic angioedema   Quincke's edema
   Giant urticaria
   EXCLUDES 1 *serum urticaria (T80.6-)*
    urticaria (L50.-)

✓5ᵗʰ **T78.4** **Other and unspecified allergy**
   EXCLUDES 1 *specified types of allergic reaction such as:*
     allergic diarrhea (K52.2)
     allergic gastroenteritis and colitis (K52.2)
     dermatitis (L23-L25, L27-)
     hay fever (J30.1)

 ✓x7ᵗʰ **T78.40** **Allergy, unspecified**
    Allergic reaction NOS Hypersensitivity NOS

 ✓x7ᵗʰ **T78.41** **Arthus phenomenon**
    Arthus reaction

 ✓x7ᵗʰ **T78.49** **Other allergy**

✓x7ᵗʰ **T78.8** **Other adverse effects, not elsewhere classified**

✓ Additional Character Required ✓x7ᵗʰ Xtension Alert Unacceptable PDx Manifestation Hospital Acquired Condition *EXCLUDES 1* Not Coded Here *EXCLUDES 2* Not Included Here

Injury, Poisoning and Certain Other Consequences of External Causes

Certain early complications of trauma (T79)

✓4th T79   Certain early complications of trauma, not elsewhere classified

EXCLUDES 2   acute respiratory distress syndrome (J80)
complications occurring during or following medical procedures (T80-T88)
complications of surgical and medical care NEC (T80-T88)
newborn respiratory distress syndrome (P22.0)

> The appropriate 7th character is to be added to each code from category T79.
> A   initial encounter
> D   subsequent encounter
> S   sequela

✓x7th T79.0   Air embolism (traumatic)   MCC

EXCLUDES 1   air embolism complicating abortion or ectopic or molar pregnancy (O00-O07, O08.2)
air embolism complicating pregnancy, childbirth and the puerperium (O88.0)
air embolism following infusion, transfusion, and therapeutic injection (T80.0)
air embolism following procedure NEC (T81.7-)

CC Excl: MCC with 7th A: D78.81-D78.89, E36.8, E89.810-E89.89, H59.011-H59.019, H59.031-H59.099, H59.811-H59.89, H95.811-H95.89, I97.3, L76.81-L76.82, M96.89, N98.1-N98.9, T14.8-T14.91, T79.0XXA, T79.A0X-T80.0XX with 7th A, T81.82XA, T81.89X-T81.9XX with 7th A

✓x7th T79.1   Fat embolism (traumatic)   MCC

EXCLUDES 1   fat embolism complicating:
   abortion or ectopic or molar pregnancy (O00-O07, O08.2)
   pregnancy, childbirth and the puerperium (O88.8)

CC Excl: MCC with 7th A: D78.81-D78.89, E36.8, E89.810-E89.89, H59.011-H59.019, H59.031-H59.099, H59.811-H59.89, H95.811-H95.89, I97.3, L76.81-L76.82, M96.89, N98.1-N98.9, T14.8-T14.91, T79.1XXA, T79.A0X-T79.9XX with 7th A, T81.82XA, T81.89X-T81.9XX with 7th A

✓x7th T79.2   Traumatic secondary and recurrent hemorrhage and seroma   CC

CC Excl: CC with 7th character A: D78.81-D78.89, E36.8, E89.810-E89.89, H59.011-H59.019, H59.031-H59.099, H59.811-H59.89, H95.811-H95.89, I97.3, L76.81-L76.82, M96.89, N98.1-N98.9, T14.8-T14.91, T79.2XXA, T79.A0X-T79.9XX with 7th A, T81.82XA, T81.89X-T81.9XX with 7th A

✓x7th T79.4   Traumatic shock   MCC

Shock (immediate) (delayed) following injury

EXCLUDES 1   anaphylactic shock due to adverse food reaction (T78.0-)
anaphylactic shock due to correct medicinal substance properly administered (T88.6)
anaphylactic shock due to serum (T80.5-)
anaphylactic shock NOS (T78.2)
anesthetic shock (T88.2)
electric shock (T75.4)
nontraumatic shock NEC (R57.-)
obstetric shock (O75.1)
postprocedural shock (T81.1-)
septic shock (R65.21)
shock complicating abortion or ectopic or molar pregnancy (O00-O07, O08.3)
shock due to lightning (T75.01)
shock NOS (R57.9)

CC Excl: MCC with 7th A: D78.81-D78.89, E36.8, E89.810-E89.89, H59.011-H59.019, H59.031-H59.099, H59.811-H59.89, H95.811-H95.89, I97.3, L76.81-L76.82, M96.89, N98.1-N98.9, T14.8-T14.91, T79.4XXA, T79.A0X-T79.9XX with 7th A, T81.82XA, T81.89X-T81.9XX with 7th A

✓x7th T79.5   Traumatic anuria   MCC

Crush syndrome
Renal failure following crushing

CC Excl: MCC with 7th A: D78.01-D78.02, D78.21-D78.89, E36.01-E36.02, E36.8, E89.810-E89.89, G97.51-G97.52, H59.011-H59.019, H59.031-H59.129, H59.311-H59.329, H59.811-H59.89, H95.21-H95.22, H95.41-H95.89, I97.3-I97.42, I97.610-I97.62, J95.61-J95.62, J95.830-J95.831, K91.61-K91.62, K91.840-K91.841, L76.01-L76.02, L76.21-L76.82, M96.810-M96.811, M96.830-M96.89, N98.1-N98.9, N99.61-N99.62, N99.820-N99.821, T14.8-T14.91, T79.5XXA, T79.A0X-T79.9XX with 7th A, T81.10X-T81.19X with 7th A, T81.82XA, T81.89X-T81.9XX with 7th A, T88.2XXA

✓x7th T79.6   Traumatic ischemia of muscle

Traumatic rhabdomyolysis
Volkmann's ischemic contracture

EXCLUDES 2   anterior tibial syndrome (M76.8)
compartment syndrome (traumatic) (T79.A-)
nontraumatic ischemia of muscle (M62.2-)

✓x7th T79.7   Traumatic subcutaneous emphysema   CC

EXCLUDES 1   emphysema NOS (J43)
emphysema (subcutaneous) resulting from a procedure (T81.82)

CC Excl: CC with 7th character A: D78.81-D78.89, E36.8, E89.810-E89.89, H59.011-H59.019, H59.031-H59.099, H59.811-H59.89, H95.811-H95.89, I97.3, L76.81-L76.82, M96.89, N98.1-N98.9, S21.101-S21.159 with 7th A, S21.301-S21.95X with 7th A, S27.0XX-S27.399 with 7th A, S27.50X-S27.809 with 7th A, S27.892-S27.9XX with 7th A, S28.1XXA, S29.021A, S29.029A, T14.8-T14.91, T79.7XX-T79.9XX with 7th A, T81.82XA, T81.89X-T81.9XX with 7th A

✓5th T79.A   Traumatic compartment syndrome

EXCLUDES 1   fibromyalgia (M79.7)
nontraumatic compartment syndrome (M79.A-)
traumatic ischemic infarction of muscle (T79.6)

✓x7th T79.A0   Compartment syndrome, unspecified   CC

Compartment syndrome NOS

CC Excl: CC with 7th character A: S31.001A, S31.011A, S31.021A, S31.031A, S31.041A, S31.051A, S31.600-S31.659 with 7th A, S36.81X-S36.899 with 7th A

✓6th T79.A1   Traumatic compartment syndrome of upper extremity

Traumatic compartment syndrome of shoulder, arm, forearm, wrist, hand, and fingers

> CC Excl: For CC codes in category T79.A1: CC with 7th character A, unless otherwise noted: M70.80-M70.99, M79.81-M79.9, R29.898

✓7th T79.A11   Traumatic compartment syndrome of right upper extremity   CC

✓7th T79.A12   Traumatic compartment syndrome of left upper extremity   CC

✓7th T79.A19   Traumatic compartment syndrome of unspecified upper extremity   CC

✓6th T79.A2   Traumatic compartment syndrome of lower extremity

Traumatic compartment syndrome of hip, buttock, thigh, leg, foot, and toes

> CC Excl: For CC codes in category T79.A2 : CC with 7th character A, unless otherwise noted: See code: T79.A1

✓7th T79.A21   Traumatic compartment syndrome of right lower extremity   CC

✓7th T79.A22   Traumatic compartment syndrome of left lower extremity   CC

✓7th T79.A29   Traumatic compartment syndrome of unspecified lower extremity   CC

✓x7th T79.A3   Traumatic compartment syndrome of abdomen   CC

CC Excl: CC with 7th character A: S31.001A, S31.011A, S31.021A, S31.031A, S31.041A, S31.051-S31.159 with 7th A, S31.600-S31.659 with 7th A, S31.831-S31.839 with 7th A, S36.00X-S37.99X with 7th A, S38.3XX-S39.023 with 7th A, T14.8-T14.91, T79.8XX-T79.9XX with 7th A

✓x7th T79.A9   Traumatic compartment syndrome of other sites   CC

CC Excl: CC with 7th character A: S31.001A, S31.011A, S31.021A, S31.031A, S31.041A, S31.051A, S31.600-S31.659 with 7th A, S36.81X-S36.899 with 7th A

✓x7th T79.8   Other early complications of trauma

✓x7th T79.9   Unspecified early complication of trauma

N Newborn: 0   P Pediatric: 0-17   M Maternity: 12-55   A Adult: 15-124   MCC Major CC Condition   PDx MCC PDx acts as own MCC   CC CC Condition   PDx CC PDx acts as own CC

1090   ICD-10-CM Draft (2015)

Complications of surgical and medical care, not elsewhere classified (T80-T88)

Use additional code for adverse effect, if applicable, to identify drug (T36-T50 with fifth or sixth character 5)

Use additional code(s) to identify the specified condition resulting from the complication

Use additional code to identify devices involved and details of circumstances (Y62-Y82)

EXCLUDES 2   any encounters with medical care for postprocedural conditions in which no complications are present, such as:
artificial opening status (Z93.-)
closure of external stoma (Z43.-)
fitting and adjustment of external prosthetic device (Z44.-)
burns and corrosions from local applications and irradiation (T20-T32)
complications of surgical procedures during pregnancy, childbirth and the puerperium (O00-O9A)
mechanical complication of respirator [ventilator] (J95.850)
poisoning and toxic effects of drugs and chemicals (T36-T65 with fifth or sixth character 1-4 or 6)
postprocedural fever (R50.82)
specified complications classified elsewhere, such as:
cerebrospinal fluid leak from spinal puncture (G97.0)
colostomy malfunction (K94.0-)
disorders of fluid and electrolyte imbalance (E86-E87)
functional disturbances following cardiac surgery (I97.0-I97.1)
intraoperative and postprocedural complications of specified body systems (D78.-, E36.-, E89.-, G97.3-, G97.4, H59.3-, H59.-, H95.2-, H95.3, I97.4-, I97.5, J95.6-, J95.7, K91.6-, L76.-, M96.-, N99.-)
ostomy complications (J95.0-, K94-, N99.5-)
postgastric surgery syndromes (K91.1)
postlaminectomy syndrome NEC (M96.1)
postmastectomy lymphedema syndrome (I97.2)
postsurgical blind-loop syndrome (K91.2)
ventilator associated pneumonia (J95.851)

✓4th **T80 Complications following infusion, transfusion and therapeutic injection**
INCLUDES   complications following perfusion
EXCLUDES 2   bone marrow transplant rejection (T86.01)
febrile nonhemolytic transfusion reaction (R50.84)
fluid overload due to transfusion (E87.71)
posttransfusion purpura (D69.51)
transfusion associated circulatory overload (TACO) (E87.71)
transfusion (red blood cell) associated hemochromatosis (E83.111)
transfusion related acute lung injury (TRALI) (J95.84)

The appropriate 7th character is to be added to each code from category T80.
A   initial encounter
D   subsequent encounter
S   sequela

7 ✓x7th **T80.0 Air embolism following infusion, transfusion and therapeutic injection**   MCC
CC Excl: MCC with 7th A: T79.0XXA, T80.0XXA

✓x7th **T80.1 Vascular complications following infusion, transfusion and therapeutic injection**   CC
Use additional code to identify the vascular complication
EXCLUDES 2   extravasation of vesicant agent (T80.81-)
infiltration of vesicant agent (T80.81-)
postprocedural vascular complications (T81.7-)
vascular complications specified as due to prosthetic devices, implants and grafts (T82.8-, T83.8, T84.8-, T85.8)
CC Excl: CC with 7th character A: T80.1XXA, T80.810-T80.818 with 7th A, T80.90XA

✓5th **T80.2 Infections following infusion, transfusion and therapeutic injection**
Use additional code to identify the specific infection, such as:
sepsis (A41.9)
Use additional code (R65.2-) to identify severe sepsis, if applicable
EXCLUDES 2   infections specified as due to prosthetic devices, implants and grafts (T82.6-T82.7, T83.5-T83.6, T84.5-T84.7, T85.7)
postprocedural infections (T81.4)

CC Excl: For CC codes in subcategory T80.2: CC with 7th character A, unless otherwise noted: N98.0, T80.211-T80.29X with 7th A, T82.7XXA, T88.0XXA

✓6th **T80.21 Infection due to central venous catheter**

7 ✓7th **T80.211 Bloodstream infection due to central venous catheter**   CC
Catheter-related bloodstream infection (CRBSI) NOS
Central line-associated bloodstream infection (CLABSI)
Bloodstream infection due to Hickman catheter
Bloodstream infection due to peripherally inserted central catheter (PICC)
Bloodstream infection due to portacath (port-a-cath)
Bloodstream infection due to triple lumen catheter
Bloodstream infection due to umbilical venous catheter

7 ✓7th **T80.212 Local infection due to central venous catheter**   CC
Exit or insertion site infection
Local infection due to Hickman catheter
Local infection due to peripherally inserted central catheter (PICC)
Local infection due to portacath (port-a-cath)
Local infection due to triple lumen catheter
Local infection due to umbilical venous catheter
Port or reservoir infection
Tunnel infection

7 ✓7th **T80.218 Other infection due to central venous catheter**   CC
Other central line-associated infection
Other infection due to Hickman catheter
Other infection due to peripherally inserted central catheter (PICC)
Other infection due to portacath (port-a-cath)
Other infection due to triple lumen catheter
Other infection due to umbilical venous catheter

7 ✓7th **T80.219 Unspecified infection due to central venous catheter**   CC
Central line-associated infection NOS
Unspecified infection due to Hickman catheter
Unspecified infection due to peripherally inserted central catheter (PICC)
Unspecified infection due to portacath (port-a-cath)
Unspecified infection due to triple lumen catheter
Unspecified infection due to umbilical venous catheter

✓x7th **T80.22 Acute infection following transfusion, infusion, or injection of blood and blood products**   CC

✓x7th **T80.29 Infection following other infusion, transfusion and therapeutic injection**   CC

✓5th **T80.3 ABO incompatibility reaction due to transfusion of blood or blood products**
EXCLUDES 1   minor blood group antigens reactions (Duffy) (E) (K(ell)) (Kidd) (Lewis) (M) (N) (P) (S) (T80.A)

CC Excl: CC Excl: For CC/MCC codes in subcategory T80.3: CC with 7th character A, unless otherwise noted: T80.30X-T80.A9X with 7th A, T80.910-T80.92X with 7th A

7 ✓x7th **T80.30 ABO incompatibility reaction due to transfusion of blood or blood products, unspecified**   CC
ABO incompatibility blood transfusion NOS
Reaction to ABO incompatibility from transfusion NOS

✓6th **T80.31 ABO incompatibility with hemolytic transfusion reaction**

7 ✓7th **T80.310 ABO incompatibility with acute hemolytic transfusion reaction**   CC
ABO incompatibility with hemolytic transfusion reaction less than 24 hours after transfusion
Acute hemolytic transfusion reaction (AHTR) due to ABO incompatibility

---

7 HAC = Initial encounter only (7th character A, B or C) and not POA.

Injury, Poisoning and Certain Other Consequences of External Causes   T80.311–T80.818

7 ✓7th **T80.311** **ABO incompatibility with delayed hemolytic transfusion reaction** CC
     ABO incompatibility with hemolytic transfusion reaction 24 hours or more after transfusion
     Delayed hemolytic transfusion reaction (DHTR) due to ABO incompatibility

7 ✓7th **T80.319** **ABO incompatibility with hemolytic transfusion reaction, unspecified** CC
     ABO incompatibility with hemolytic transfusion reaction at unspecified time after transfusion
     Hemolytic transfusion reaction (HTR) due to ABO incompatibility NOS

7 ✓x7th **T80.39** **Other ABO incompatibility reaction due to transfusion of blood or blood products** CC
     Delayed serologic transfusion reaction (DSTR) from ABO incompatibility
     Other ABO incompatible blood transfusion
     Other reaction to ABO incompatible blood transfusion

✓x7th **T80.4** **Rh incompatibility reaction due to transfusion of blood or blood products**
     Reaction due to incompatibility of Rh antigens (C) (c) (D) (E) (e)

     CC Excl: For CC/MCC codes in subcategory T80.4: CC with 7th character A, unless otherwise noted: See code: T80.3

✓x7th **T80.40** **Rh incompatibility reaction due to transfusion of blood or blood products, unspecified** CC
     Reaction due to Rh factor in transfusion NOS
     Rh incompatible blood transfusion NOS

✓6th **T80.41** **Rh incompatibility with hemolytic transfusion reaction**

     ✓7th **T80.410** **Rh incompatibility with acute hemolytic transfusion reaction** CC
       Acute hemolytic transfusion reaction (AHTR) due to Rh incompatibility
       Rh incompatibility with hemolytic transfusion reaction less than 24 hours after transfusion

     ✓7th **T80.411** **Rh incompatibility with delayed hemolytic transfusion reaction** CC
       Delayed hemolytic transfusion reaction (DHTR) due to Rh incompatibility
       Rh incompatibility with hemolytic transfusion reaction 24 hours or more after transfusion

     ✓7th **T80.419** **Rh incompatibility with hemolytic transfusion reaction, unspecified** CC
       Hemolytic transfusion reaction (HTR) due to Rh incompatibility NOS
       Rh incompatibility with hemolytic transfusion reaction at unspecified time after transfusion

✓x7th **T80.49** **Other Rh incompatibility reaction due to transfusion of blood or blood products** CC
     Delayed serologic transfusion reaction (DSTR) from Rh incompatibility
     Other reaction to Rh incompatible blood transfusion
     CC Excl: CC with 7th character A: T80.30X-T80.419 with 7th A, T80.A9XA, T80.910-T80.92X with 7th A

✓5th **T80.A** **Non-ABO incompatibility reaction due to transfusion of blood or blood products**
     Reaction due to incompatibility of minor antigens (Duffy) (Kell) (Kidd) (Lewis) (M) (N) (P) (S)

✓x7th **T80.A0** **Non-ABO incompatibility reaction due to transfusion of blood or blood products, unspecified** CC
     Non-ABO antigen incompatibility reaction from transfusion NOS
     CC Excl: CC with 7th character A, unless otherwise noted: T80.30X-T80.419 with 7th A, T80.A9XA, T80.910-T80.92X with 7th A

✓6th **T80.A1** **Non-ABO incompatibility with hemolytic transfusion reaction**

     CC Excl: For CC codes in subcategory T80.A1: CC with 7th character A, unless otherwise noted: See code: T80.A0

✓7th **T80.A10** **Non-ABO incompatibility with acute hemolytic transfusion reaction** CC
     Acute hemolytic transfusion reaction (AHTR) due to non-ABO incompatibility
     Non-ABO incompatibility with hemolytic transfusion reaction less than 24 hours after transfusion

✓7th **T80.A11** **Non-ABO incompatibility with delayed hemolytic transfusion reaction** CC
     Delayed hemolytic transfusion reaction (DHTR) due to non-ABO incompatibility
     Non-ABO incompatibility with hemolytic transfusion reaction 24 or more hours after transfusion

✓7th **T80.A19** **Non-ABO incompatibility with hemolytic transfusion reaction, unspecified** CC
     Hemolytic transfusion reaction (HTR) due to non-ABO incompatibility NOS
     Non-ABO incompatibility with hemolytic transfusion reaction at unspecified time after transfusion

✓x7th **T80.A9** **Other non-ABO incompatibility reaction due to transfusion of blood or blood products** CC
     Delayed serologic transfusion reaction (DSTR) from non-ABO incompatibility
     Other reaction to non-ABO incompatible blood transfusion
     CC Excl: CC with 7th character A: T80.30X-T80.A9X with 7th A, T80.910-T80.92X with 7th A

✓5th **T80.5** **Anaphylactic reaction due to serum**
     Allergic shock due to serum
     Anaphylactic shock due to serum
     Anaphylactoid reaction due to serum
     Anaphylaxis due to serum
     EXCLUDES 1   *ABO incompatibility reaction due to transfusion of blood or blood products (T80.3-)*
       allergic reaction or shock NOS (T78.2)
       anaphylactic reaction or shock NOS (T78.2)
       anaphylactic reaction or shock due to adverse effect of correct medicinal substance properly administered (T88.6)
       other serum reaction (T80.6-)

     CC Excl: For CC/MCC codes in subcategory T80.5: CC with 7th character A, unless otherwise noted: T80.51X-T80.69X with 7th A

✓x7th **T80.51** **Anaphylactic reaction due to administration of blood and blood products** CC

✓x7th **T80.52** **Anaphylactic reaction due to vaccination** CC

✓x7th **T80.59** **Anaphylactic reaction due to other serum** CC

✓5th **T80.6** **Other serum reactions**
     Intoxication by serum   Serum sickness
     Protein sickness   Serum urticaria
     Serum rash
     EXCLUDES 2   *serum hepatitis (B16.-)*

✓x7th **T80.61** **Other serum reaction due to administration of blood and blood products** CC
     CC Excl: CC with 7th character A: See code: T80.5

✓x7th **T80.62** **Other serum reaction due to vaccination** CC
     CC Excl: CC with 7th character A: See code: T80.5

✓x7th **T80.69** **Other serum reaction due to other serum** CC
     CC Excl: CC with 7th character A: T80.61X-T80.69X with 7th A

✓5th **T80.8** **Other complications following infusion, transfusion and therapeutic injection**

✓6th **T80.81** **Extravasation of vesicant agent**
     Infiltration of vesicant agent

     ✓7th **T80.810** **Extravasation of vesicant antineoplastic chemotherapy** CC
       Infiltration of vesicant antineoplastic chemotherapy
       CC Excl: CC with 7th character A: T80.1XXA, T80.810-T80.818 with 7th A, T80.90XA

     ✓7th **T80.818** **Extravasation of other vesicant agent** CC
       Infiltration of other vesicant agent
       CC Excl: CC with 7th character A: See code: T81.810

---

7 HAC = Initial encounter only (7th character A, B or C) and not POA.

N Newborn: 0   P Pediatric: 0-17   M Maternity: 12-55   A Adult: 15-124   MCC Major CC Condition   PDx MCC PDx acts as own MCC   CC CC Condition   PDx CC PDx acts as own CC

1092   ICD-10-CM Draft (2015)

✓x7ᵗʰ **T80.89** **Other complications following infusion, transfusion and therapeutic injection**
　　　Delayed serologic transfusion reaction (DSTR), unspecified incompatibility
　　　Use additional code to identify graft-versus-host reaction, if applicable, (D89.81-)

✓5ᵗʰ **T80.9** **Unspecified complication following infusion, transfusion and therapeutic injection**

✓x7ᵗʰ **T80.90** **Unspecified complication** following infusion and therapeutic injection

✓6ᵗʰ **T80.91** **Hemolytic transfusion reaction, unspecified incompatibility**
　　　EXCLUDES 1 *ABO incompatibility with hemolytic transfusion reaction (T80.31-)*
　　　　　　Non-ABO incompatibility with hemolytic transfusion reaction (T80.A1-)
　　　　　　Rh incompatibility with hemolytic transfusion reaction (T80.41-)

　　　CC Excl: For CC codes in subcategory T80.91: CC with 7th character A, unless otherwise noted: T80.30X-T80.A9X with 7th A, T80.910-T80.92X with 7th A

✓7ᵗʰ **T80.910** **Acute** hemolytic transfusion reaction, unspecified incompatibility `CC`

✓7ᵗʰ **T80.911** **Delayed** hemolytic transfusion reaction, unspecified incompatibility `CC`

✓7ᵗʰ **T80.919** **Hemolytic transfusion reaction, unspecified** incompatibility, unspecified as acute or delayed `CC`
　　　Hemolytic transfusion reaction NOS

✓x7ᵗʰ **T80.92** **Unspecified transfusion reaction**
　　　Transfusion reaction NOS

✓4ᵗʰ **T81** **Complications of procedures, not elsewhere classified**
　　　Use additional code for adverse effect, if applicable, to identify drug (T36-T50 with fifth or sixth character 5)
　　　EXCLUDES 2 *complications following immunization (T88.0-T88.1)*
　　　　　　complications following infusion, transfusion and therapeutic injection (T80.-)
　　　　　　complications of transplanted organs and tissue (T86.-)
　　　　　　specified complications classified elsewhere, such as:
　　　　　　　complication of prosthetic devices, implants and grafts (T82-T85)
　　　　　　　dermatitis due to drugs and medicaments (L23.3, L24.4, L25.1, L27.0-L27.1)
　　　　　　　endosseous dental implant failure (M27.6-)
　　　　　　　floppy iris syndrome (IFIS) (intraoperative) (H21.81)
　　　　　　　intraoperative and postprocedural complications of specific body system (D78.-, E36.-, E89.-, G97.3-, G97.4, H59.3-, H59.-, H95.2-, H95.3, I97.4-, I97.5, J95., K91.-, L76.-, M96.-, N99.-)
　　　　　　　ostomy complications (J95.0-, K94.-, N99.5-)
　　　　　　　plateau iris syndrome (post-iridectomy) (postprocedural) (H21.82)
　　　　　　　poisoning and toxic effects of drugs and chemicals (T36-T65 with fifth or sixth character 1-4 or 6)

　　　The appropriate 7th character is to be added to each code from category T81.
　　　A　initial encounter
　　　D　subsequent encounter
　　　S　sequela

✓5ᵗʰ **T81.1** **Postprocedural shock**
　　　Shock during or resulting from a procedure, not elsewhere classified
　　　EXCLUDES 1 *anaphylactic shock due to correct substance properly administered (T88.6)*
　　　　　　anaphylactic shock due to serum (T80.5-)
　　　　　　anaphylactic shock NOS (T78.2)
　　　　　　anesthetic shock (T88.2)
　　　　　　electric shock (T75.4)
　　　　　　obstetric shock (O75.1)
　　　　　　septic shock (R65.21)
　　　　　　shock following abortion or ectopic or molar pregnancy (O00-O07, O08.3)
　　　　　　traumatic shock (T79.4)

　　　CC Excl: For CC/MCC codes in subcategory T81.1, MCC with 7th A, unless otherwise noted: D78.01-D78.02, D78.21-D78.89, E36.01-E36.02, E36.8, E89.810-E89.89, G97.51-G97.52, H59.011-H59.019, H59.031-H59.129, H59.311-H59.329, H59.811-H59.89, H95.21-H95.22, H95.41-H95.89, I97.3-I97.42, I97.610-I97.62, J95.61-J95.62, J95.830-J95.831, K91.61-K91.62, K91.840-K91.841, L76.01-L76.02, L76.21-L76.82, M96.810-M96.811, M96.830-M96.89, N98.1-N98.9, N99.61-N99.62, N99.820-N99.821, T79.4XXA, T81.10X-T81.19X with 7th A, T81.82XA, T81.89X-T81.9XX with 7th A, T88.2XXA

✓x7ᵗʰ **T81.10** **Postprocedural shock unspecified** `CC`
　　　Collapse NOS during or resulting from a procedure, not elsewhere classified
　　　Postprocedural failure of peripheral circulation
　　　Postprocedural shock NOS

✓x7ᵗʰ **T81.11** **Postprocedural cardiogenic shock** `MCC`

12 ✓x7ᵗʰ **T81.12** **Postprocedural septic shock** `MCC`
　　　Postprocedural endotoxic shock during or resulting from a procedure, not elsewhere classified
　　　Postprocedural gram-negative shock during or resulting from a procedure, not elsewhere classified
　　　Code first underlying infection
　　　Use additional code, to identify any associated acute organ dysfunction, if applicable

✓x7ᵗʰ **T81.19** **Other postprocedural shock** `MCC`
　　　Postprocedural hypovolemic shock

✓5ᵗʰ **T81.3** **Disruption of wound, not elsewhere classified**
　　　Disruption of any suture materials or other closure methods
　　　EXCLUDES 1 *breakdown (mechanical) of permanent sutures (T85.612)*
　　　　　　displacement of permanent sutures (T85.622)
　　　　　　disruption of cesarean delivery wound (O90.0)
　　　　　　disruption of perineal obstetric wound (O90.1)
　　　　　　mechanical complication of permanent sutures NEC (T85.692)
　　　AHA: 2014, 1Q, 23

　　　CC Excl: For CC/MCC codes in subcategory T81.3: CC with 7th character A, unless otherwise noted: D78.81-D78.89, E36.8, E89.810-E89.89, H59.011-H59.019, H59.031-H59.099, H59.811-H59.89, H95.811-H95.89, I97.3, L76.81-L76.82, M96.89, N98.1-N98.9, T81.30X-T81.33X with 7th A, T81.82A, T81.89X-T81.9XX with 7th A

✓x7ᵗʰ **T81.30** **Disruption of wound, unspecified** `CC`
　　　Disruption of wound NOS

✓x7ᵗʰ **T81.31** **Disruption of external operation (surgical) wound, not elsewhere classified** `CC`
　　　Dehiscence of operation wound NOS
　　　Disruption of operation wound NOS
　　　Disruption or dehiscence of closure of cornea
　　　Disruption or dehiscence of closure of mucosa
　　　Disruption or dehiscence of closure of skin and subcutaneous tissue
　　　Full-thickness skin disruption or dehiscence
　　　Superficial disruption or dehiscence of operation wound
　　　EXCLUDES 1 *dehiscence of amputation stump (T87.81)*

✓ Additional Character Required　✓x7ᵗʰ Xtension Alert　Unacceptable PDx　Manifestation　Hospital Acquired Condition　*EXCLUDES 1* Not Coded Here　*EXCLUDES 2* Not Included Here

√x7ᵗʰ **T81.32 Disruption of internal operation (surgical)** `CC`
wound, not elsewhere classified
Deep disruption or dehiscence of operation wound NOS
Disruption or dehiscence of closure of internal organ or other internal tissue
Disruption or dehiscence of closure of muscle or muscle flap
Disruption or dehiscence of closure of ribs or rib cage
Disruption or dehiscence of closure of skull or craniotomy
Disruption or dehiscence of closure of sternum or sternotomy
Disruption or dehiscence of closure of tendon or ligament
Disruption or dehiscence of closure of superficial or muscular fascia

√x7ᵗʰ **T81.33 Disruption of traumatic injury wound repair** `CC`
Disruption or dehiscence of closure of traumatic laceration (external) (internal)

4,6,7,8 √x7ᵗʰ **T81.4 Infection following a procedure** `CC`
Intra-abdominal abscess following a procedure
Postprocedural infection, not elsewhere classified
Sepsis following a procedure
Stitch abscess following a procedure
Subphrenic abscess following a procedure
Wound abscess following a procedure
Use additional code to identify infection
Use additional code (R65.2-) to identify severe sepsis, if applicable
EXCLUDES 1   obstetric surgical wound infection (O86.0)
postprocedural fever NOS (R50.82)
postprocedural retroperitoneal abscess (K68.11)
EXCLUDES 2   bleb associated endophthalmitis (H59.4-)
infection due to infusion, transfusion and therapeutic injection (T80.2-)
infection due to prosthetic devices, implants and grafts (T82.6-T82.7, T83.5-T83.6, T84.5-T84.7, T85.7)
AHA: 2014, 1Q, 23
CC Excl: CC with 7th character A: D78.81-D78.89, E36.8, E89.810-E89.89, H59.011-H59.019, H59.031-H59.099, H59.811-H59.89, H95.811-H95.89, I97.3, K68.11, L76.81-L76.82, M96.89, N98.1-N98.9, T81.4XXA, T81.82XA, T81.89X-T81.9XX with 7th A

√5ᵗʰ **T81.5 Complications of foreign body accidentally left in body following procedure**

CC Excl: For CC codes in subcategory T81.5: CC with 7th character A, unless otherwise noted: D78.81-D78.89, E36.8, E89.810-E89.89, H59.011-H59.019, H59.031-H59.099, H59.811-H59.89, H95.811-H95.89, I97.3, L76.81-L76.82, M96.89, N98.1-N98.9, T81.500-T81.599 with 7th A, T81.82XA, T81.89X-T81.9XX with 7th A

√6ᵗʰ **T81.50 Unspecified complication of foreign body accidentally left in body following procedure**

7 √7ᵗʰ **T81.500 Unspecified complication of foreign** `CC`
body accidentally left in body following surgical operation

7 √7ᵗʰ **T81.501 Unspecified complication of foreign** `CC`
body accidentally left in body following infusion or transfusion

7 √7ᵗʰ **T81.502 Unspecified complication of foreign** `CC`
body accidentally left in body following kidney dialysis

7 √7ᵗʰ **T81.503 Unspecified complication of foreign** `CC`
body accidentally left in body following injection or immunization

7 √7ᵗʰ **T81.504 Unspecified complication of foreign** `CC`
body accidentally left in body following endoscopic examination

7 √7ᵗʰ **T81.505 Unspecified complication of foreign** `CC`
body accidentally left in body following heart catheterization

7 √7ᵗʰ **T81.506 Unspecified complication of foreign** `CC`
body accidentally left in body following aspiration, puncture or other catheterization

7 √7ᵗʰ **T81.507 Unspecified complication of foreign** `CC`
body accidentally left in body following removal of catheter or packing

7 √7ᵗʰ **T81.508 Unspecified complication of foreign** `CC`
body accidentally left in body following other procedure

7 √7ᵗʰ **T81.509 Unspecified complication of foreign** `CC`
body accidentally left in body following unspecified procedure

√6ᵗʰ **T81.51 Adhesions due to foreign body accidentally left in body following procedure**

7 √7ᵗʰ **T81.510 Adhesions due to foreign body** `CC`
accidentally left in body following surgical operation

7 √7ᵗʰ **T81.511 Adhesions due to foreign body** `CC`
accidentally left in body following infusion or transfusion

7 √7ᵗʰ **T81.512 Adhesions due to foreign body** `CC`
accidentally left in body following kidney dialysis

7 √7ᵗʰ **T81.513 Adhesions due to foreign body** `CC`
accidentally left in body following injection or immunization

7 √7ᵗʰ **T81.514 Adhesions due to foreign body** `CC`
accidentally left in body following endoscopic examination

7 √7ᵗʰ **T81.515 Adhesions due to foreign body** `CC`
accidentally left in body following heart catheterization

7 √7ᵗʰ **T81.516 Adhesions due to foreign body** `CC`
accidentally left in body following aspiration, puncture or other catheterization

7 √7ᵗʰ **T81.517 Adhesions due to foreign body** `CC`
accidentally left in body following removal of catheter or packing

7 √7ᵗʰ **T81.518 Adhesions due to foreign body** `CC`
accidentally left in body following other procedure

7 √7ᵗʰ **T81.519 Adhesions due to foreign body** `CC`
accidentally left in body following unspecified procedure

√6ᵗʰ **T81.52 Obstruction due to foreign body accidentally left in body following procedure**

7 √7ᵗʰ **T81.520 Obstruction due to foreign body** `CC`
accidentally left in body following surgical operation

7 √7ᵗʰ **T81.521 Obstruction due to foreign body** `CC`
accidentally left in body following infusion or transfusion

7 √7ᵗʰ **T81.522 Obstruction due to foreign body** `CC`
accidentally left in body following kidney dialysis

7 √7ᵗʰ **T81.523 Obstruction due to foreign body** `CC`
accidentally left in body following injection or immunization

7 √7ᵗʰ **T81.524 Obstruction due to foreign body** `CC`
accidentally left in body following endoscopic examination

7 √7ᵗʰ **T81.525 Obstruction due to foreign body** `CC`
accidentally left in body following heart catheterization

7 √7ᵗʰ **T81.526 Obstruction due to foreign body** `CC`
accidentally left in body following aspiration, puncture or other catheterization

7 √7ᵗʰ **T81.527 Obstruction due to foreign body** `CC`
accidentally left in body following removal of catheter or packing

7 √7ᵗʰ **T81.528 Obstruction due to foreign body** `CC`
accidentally left in body following other procedure

---

4   HAC = as SDx not POA, in combination with PDx E66.01 **AND** one of the following procedure codes: 0D16[0,4,8][7,J,K,Z][9,A,B,L] or 0DV64CZ.

6   HAC = as SDx not POA, in combination with one of the following procedure codes: 0RG[0,1,2,4,6,7,8,A][0,3,4][7,A,J,K,Z][0,1,J]; 0RG[E,F,G,H,J,K][0,3,4][4,7,J,K,Z]Z; 0RG[L,M][0,3,4][4,5,7,J,K,Z]Z; 0RQ[E,F,G,H,J,K,L,M][0,3,4,X]ZZ; 0RU[E,F,G,H,J,K,L,M][0,3,4][7,J,K]Z; 0SG[0,1,3][0,3,4][7,A,J,K,Z][0,1,J]; 0SG[7,8][0,3,4[4,7,J,K,Z]Z.

7   HAC = Initial encounter only (7th character A, B or C) and not POA.

8   HAC = as SDx not POA, in combination with one of the following procedure codes: 02H43[J,K,M]Z; 02H[6,7]3[J,M]Z; 02H[K,L]3JZ; 02HN[0,3,4][J,M]Z; 02PA[0,3,4]MZ; 02PAXMZ; 02WA[0,3,4]MZ; 0JH[6,8][0,3][4,5,6,7,8,9,P]Z; 0J[P,W]T[0,3]PZ.

N Newborn: 0   P Pediatric: 0-17   M Maternity: 12-55   A Adult: 15-124   MCC Major CC Condition   PDx MCC PDx acts as own MCC   CC CC Condition   PDx CC PDx acts as own CC

1094   ICD-10-CM Draft (2015)

7 ✓7th **T81.529** **Obstruction due to foreign body accidentally left in body following unspecified procedure** `CC`

✓6th **T81.53** Perforation due to foreign body accidentally left in body following procedure

7 ✓7th **T81.530** **Perforation due to foreign body accidentally left in body following surgical operation** `CC`

7 ✓7th **T81.531** **Perforation due to foreign body accidentally left in body following infusion or transfusion** `CC`

7 ✓7th **T81.532** **Perforation due to foreign body accidentally left in body following kidney dialysis** `CC`

7 ✓7th **T81.533** **Perforation due to foreign body accidentally left in body following injection or immunization** `CC`

7 ✓7th **T81.534** **Perforation due to foreign body accidentally left in body following endoscopic examination** `CC`

7 ✓7th **T81.535** **Perforation due to foreign body accidentally left in body following heart catheterization** `CC`

7 ✓7th **T81.536** **Perforation due to foreign body accidentally left in body following aspiration, puncture or other catheterization** `CC`

7 ✓7th **T81.537** **Perforation due to foreign body accidentally left in body following removal of catheter or packing** `CC`

7 ✓7th **T81.538** **Perforation due to foreign body accidentally left in body following other procedure** `CC`

7 ✓7th **T81.539** **Perforation due to foreign body accidentally left in body following unspecified procedure** `CC`

✓6th **T81.59** Other complications of foreign body accidentally left in body following procedure

EXCLUDES 2   *obstruction or perforation due to prosthetic devices and implants intentionally left in body (T82.0-T82.5, T83.0-T83.4, T83.7, T84.0-T84.4, T85.0-T85.6)*

7 ✓7th **T81.590** **Other complications of foreign body accidentally left in body following surgical operation** `CC`

7 ✓7th **T81.591** **Other complications of foreign body accidentally left in body following infusion or transfusion** `CC`

7 ✓7th **T81.592** **Other complications of foreign body accidentally left in body following kidney dialysis** `CC`

7 ✓7th **T81.593** **Other complications of foreign body accidentally left in body following injection or immunization** `CC`

7 ✓7th **T81.594** **Other complications of foreign body accidentally left in body following endoscopic examination** `CC`

7 ✓7th **T81.595** **Other complications of foreign body accidentally left in body following heart catheterization** `CC`

7 ✓7th **T81.596** **Other complications of foreign body accidentally left in body following aspiration, puncture or other catheterization** `CC`

7 ✓7th **T81.597** **Other complications of foreign body accidentally left in body following removal of catheter or packing** `CC`

7 ✓7th **T81.598** **Other complications of foreign body accidentally left in body following other procedure** `CC`

7 ✓7th **T81.599** **Other complications of foreign body accidentally left in body following unspecified procedure** `CC`

✓5th **T81.6** Acute reaction to foreign substance accidentally left during a procedure

EXCLUDES 2   *complications of foreign body accidentally left in body cavity or operation wound following procedure (T81.5-)*

CC Excl: For CC codes in subcategory T81.6: CC with 7th character A, unless otherwise noted: D78.81-D78.89, E36.8, E89.810-E89.89, H59.011-H59.019, H59.031-H59.099, H59.811-H59.89, H95.811-H95.89, I97.3, L76.81-L76.82, M96.89, N98.1-N98.9, T81.60-T81.69 with 7th A, T81.82XA, T81.89X-T81.9XX with 7th A

7 ✓x7th **T81.60** **Unspecified acute reaction to foreign substance accidentally left during a procedure** `CC`

7 ✓x7th **T81.61** **Aseptic peritonitis due to foreign substance accidentally left during a procedure** `CC`
Chemical peritonitis

7 ✓x7th **T81.69** **Other acute reaction to foreign substance accidentally left during a procedure** `CC`

✓5th **T81.7** Vascular complications following a procedure, not elsewhere classified

Air embolism following procedure NEC
Phlebitis or thrombophlebitis resulting from a procedure

EXCLUDES 1   *embolism complicating abortion or ectopic or molar pregnancy (O00-O07, O08.2)*
embolism complicating pregnancy, childbirth and the puerperium (O88.-)
traumatic embolism (T79.0)

EXCLUDES 2   *embolism due to prosthetic devices, implants and grafts (T82.8-, T83.8, T84.8-, T85.8)*
embolism following infusion, transfusion and therapeutic injection (T80.0)

✓6th **T81.71** Complication of artery following a procedure, not elsewhere classified

✓7th **T81.710** **Complication of mesenteric artery following a procedure, not elsewhere classified** `CC`
CC Excl: CC with 7th character A: D78.81-D78.89, E36.8, E89.810-E89.89, H59.011-H59.019, H59.031-H59.099, H59.811-H59.89, H95.811-H95.89, I97.3, L76.81-L76.82, M96.89, N98.1-N98.9, T81.710-T81.72X with 7th A, T81.82XA, T81.89X-T81.9XX with 7th A

✓7th **T81.711** **Complication of renal artery following a procedure, not elsewhere classified** `CC`
CC Excl: See code: T81.710

✓7th **T81.718** **Complication of other artery following a procedure, not elsewhere classified** `CC`
CC Excl: CC with 7th character A: D78.81-D78.89, E36.8, E89.810-E89.89, H59.011-H59.019, H59.031-H59.099, H59.811-H59.89, H95.811-H95.89, I97.3, L76.81-L76.82, M96.89, N98.1-N98.9, T81.718-T81.72X with 7th A, T81.82XA, T81.89X-T81.9XX with 7th A

✓7th **T81.719** **Complication of unspecified artery following a procedure, not elsewhere classified**
CC Excl: See code: T81.718

✓x7th **T81.72** **Complication of vein following a procedure, not elsewhere classified** `CC`
CC Excl: See code: T81.718

✓5th **T81.8** Other complications of procedures, not elsewhere classified

EXCLUDES 2   *hypothermia following anesthesia (T88.51)*
malignant hyperpyrexia due to anesthesia (T88.3)

12 ✓x7th **T81.81** **Complication of inhalation therapy**

✓x7th **T81.82** **Emphysema (subcutaneous) resulting from a procedure**

✓x7th **T81.83** **Persistent postprocedural fistula** `CC`
CC Excl: CC with 7th character A: D78.81-D78.89, E36.8, E89.810-E89.89, H59.011-H59.019, H59.031-H59.099, H59.811-H59.89, H95.811-H95.89, I97.3, L76.81-L76.82, M96.89, N98.1-N98.9, T81.82X-T81.9XX with 7th A

✓x7th **T81.89** **Other complications of procedures, not elsewhere classified**
Use additional code to specify complication, such as:
postprocedural delirium (F05)
AHA: 2014, 1Q, 23

✓x7th **T81.9** Unspecified complication of procedure

---

7 HAC = Initial encounter only (7th character A, B or C) and not POA.
12 Unacceptable PDx = initial encounter only (7th character A).

✓ Additional Character Required   ✓x7th Xtension Alert   Unacceptable PDx   Manifestation   Hospital Acquired Condition   EXCLUDES 1 Not Coded Here   EXCLUDES 2 Not Included Here

✓4ᵗʰ **T82 Complications of cardiac and vascular prosthetic devices, implants and grafts**

EXCLUDES 2 *failure and rejection of transplanted organs and tissue (T86.-)*

The appropriate 7th character is to be added to each code from category T82.
A   initial encounter
D   subsequent encounter
S   sequela

✓5ᵗʰ **T82.0 Mechanical complication of** heart valve prosthesis
Mechanical complication of artificial heart valve

EXCLUDES 1 *mechanical complication of biological heart valve graft (T82.22-)*

CC Excl: For CC codes in subcategory T82.0: CC with 7th character A, unless otherwise noted: D78.81-D78.89, E36.8, E89.810-E89.89, H59.011-H59.019, H59.031-H59.099, H59.811-H59.89, H95.811-H95.89, I97.3, L76.81-L76.82, M96.89, N98.1-N98.9, T81.82XA, T81.89X-T82.09X with 7th A

✓x7ᵗʰ **T82.01 Breakdown (mechanical) of heart valve prosthesis**   CC

✓x7ᵗʰ **T82.02 Displacement of heart valve prosthesis**   CC
Malposition of heart valve prosthesis

✓x7ᵗʰ **T82.03 Leakage of heart valve prosthesis**   CC

✓x7ᵗʰ **T82.09 Other mechanical complication of heart valve prosthesis**   CC
Obstruction (mechanical) of heart valve prosthesis
Perforation of heart valve prosthesis
Protrusion of heart valve prosthesis

✓5ᵗʰ **T82.1 Mechanical complication of** cardiac electronic device

CC Excl: For CC codes in subcategory T82.1: CC with 7th character A, unless otherwise noted: D78.81-D78.89, E36.8, E89.810-E89.89, H59.011-H59.019, H59.031-H59.099, H59.811-H59.89, H95.811-H95.89, I97.3, L76.81-L76.82, M96.89, N98.1-N98.9, T81.82XA, T81.89X-T81.9XX with 7th A, T82.110-T82.111, T82.120, T82.121, T82.190-T82.191 with 7th A

✓6ᵗʰ **T82.11 Breakdown (mechanical) of cardiac electronic device**

✓7ᵗʰ **T82.110 Breakdown (mechanical) of cardiac electrode**   CC

✓7ᵗʰ **T82.111 Breakdown (mechanical) of cardiac pulse generator (battery)**   CC

✓7ᵗʰ **T82.118 Breakdown (mechanical) of other cardiac electronic device**   CC
CC Excl: CC with 7th character A: D78.81-D78.89, E36.8, E89.810-E89.89, H59.011-H59.019, H59.031-H59.099, H59.811-H59.89, H95.811-H95.89, I97.3, L76.81-L76.82, M96.89, N98.1-N98.9, T81.82X, T81.89X-T81.9XX, T82.118, T82.128, T82.198, T82.221-T82.228, T82.512, T82.522, T82.532, T82.592, T82.594, T82.598

✓7ᵗʰ **T82.119 Breakdown (mechanical) of unspecified cardiac electronic device**   CC
CC Excl: No Excl

✓6ᵗʰ **T82.12 Displacement of cardiac electronic device**
Malposition of cardiac electronic device

✓7ᵗʰ **T82.120 Displacement of** cardiac electrode   CC

✓7ᵗʰ **T82.121 Displacement of** cardiac pulse generator (battery)   CC

✓7ᵗʰ **T82.128 Displacement of other cardiac electronic device**   CC
CC Excl: See code: T82.118

✓7ᵗʰ **T82.129 Displacement of** unspecified cardiac electronic device   CC
CC Excl: No Excl

✓6ᵗʰ **T82.19 Other mechanical complication of cardiac electronic device**
Leakage of cardiac electronic device
Obstruction of cardiac electronic device
Perforation of cardiac electronic device
Protrusion of cardiac electronic device

✓7ᵗʰ **T82.190 Other mechanical complication of cardiac electrode**   CC

✓7ᵗʰ **T82.191 Other mechanical complication of cardiac pulse generator (battery)**   CC

✓7ᵗʰ **T82.198 Other mechanical complication of other cardiac electronic device**   CC
CC Excl: See code: T82.118

✓7ᵗʰ **T82.199 Other mechanical complication of unspecified cardiac device**   CC
CC Excl: No Excl

✓5ᵗʰ **T82.2 Mechanical complication of** coronary artery bypass graft and biological heart valve graft

EXCLUDES 1 *mechanical complication of artificial heart valve prosthesis (T82.0-d*

✓6ᵗʰ **T82.21 Mechanical complication of** coronary artery bypass graft)

CC Excl: For CC codes in subcategory T82.21: CC with 7th character A, unless otherwise noted: D78.81-D78.89, E36.8, E89.810-E89.89, H59.011-H59.019, H59.031-H59.099, H59.811-H59.89, H95.811-H95.89, I97.3, L76.81-L76.82, M96.89, N98.1-N98.9, T81.82XA, T81.89X-T81.9XX with 7th A, T82.211-T82.218 with 7th A

✓7ᵗʰ **T82.211 Breakdown (mechanical) of coronary artery bypass graft**   CC

✓7ᵗʰ **T82.212 Displacement of coronary artery bypass graft**   CC
Malposition of coronary artery bypass graft

✓7ᵗʰ **T82.213 Leakage of coronary artery bypass graft**   CC

✓7ᵗʰ **T82.218 Other mechanical complication of coronary artery bypass graft**   CC
Obstruction, mechanical of coronary artery bypass graft
Perforation of coronary artery bypass graft
Protrusion of coronary artery bypass graft

✓6ᵗʰ **T82.22 Mechanical complication of** biological heart valve graft)

CC Excl: For CC codes in subcategory T82.22: CC with 7th character A, unless otherwise noted: D78.81-D78.89, E36.8, E89.810-E89.89, H59.011-H59.019, H59.031-H59.099, H59.811-H59.89, H95.811-H95.89, I97.3, L76.81-L76.82, M96.89, N98.1-N98.9, T81.82XA, T81.89X-T81.9XX with 7th A, T82.118A, T82.128A, T82.198A, T82.221-T82.228 with 7th A, T82.512 with 7th A, T82.522 with 7th A, T82.532 with 7th A, T82.592 with 7th A, T82.594 with 7th A, T82.598 with 7th A

✓7ᵗʰ **T82.221 Breakdown (mechanical) of biological heart valve graft**   CC

✓7ᵗʰ **T82.222 Displacement of biological heart valve graft**   CC
Malposition of biological heart valve graft

✓7ᵗʰ **T82.223 Leakage of biological heart valve graft**   CC

✓7ᵗʰ **T82.228 Other mechanical complication of biological heart valve graft**   CC
Obstruction of biological heart valve graft
Perforation of biological heart valve graft
Protrusion of biological heart valve graft

✓5ᵗʰ **T82.3 Mechanical complication of** other vascular grafts

CC Excl: For CC codes in subcategory T82.3: CC with 7th character A: D78.81-D78.89, E36.8, E89.810-E89.89, H59.011-H59.019, H59.031-H59.099, H59.811-H59.89, H95.811-H95.89, I97.3, L76.81-L76.82, M96.89, N98.1-N98.9, T81.82XA, T81.89X-T81.9XX with 7th A, T82.310-T82.511 with 7th A, T82.513-T82.518 with 7th A, T82.520-T82.521 with 7th A, T82.523-T82.531 with 7th A, T82.533-T82.538 with 7th A, T82.590-T82.591 with 7th A, T82.593A, T82.595A

✓6ᵗʰ **T82.31 Breakdown (mechanical) of other vascular grafts**

✓7ᵗʰ **T82.310 Breakdown (mechanical) of** aortic (bifurcation) graft (replacement)   CC

✓7ᵗʰ **T82.311 Breakdown (mechanical) of** carotid arterial graft (bypass)   CC

✓7ᵗʰ **T82.312 Breakdown (mechanical) of** femoral arterial graft (bypass)   CC

✓7ᵗʰ **T82.318 Breakdown (mechanical) of** other vascular grafts   CC

✓7ᵗʰ **T82.319 Breakdown (mechanical) of** unspecified vascular grafts   CC

✓6ᵗʰ **T82.32 Displacement of other vascular grafts**
Malposition of other vascular grafts

✓7ᵗʰ **T82.320 Displacement of** aortic (bifurcation) graft (replacement)   CC

✓7ᵗʰ **T82.321 Displacement of** carotid arterial graft (bypass)   CC

✓7ᵗʰ **T82.322 Displacement of** femoral arterial graft (bypass)   CC

N Newborn: 0   P Pediatric: 0-17   M Maternity: 12-55   A Adult: 15-124   MCC Major CC Condition   PDx MCC PDx acts as own MCC   CC CC Condition   PDx CC PDx acts as own CC

1096   ICD-10-CM Draft (2015)

√7ᵗʰ **T82.328** Displacement of other vascular grafts `CC`

√7ᵗʰ **T82.329** Displacement of unspecified vascular grafts `CC`

√6ᵗʰ **T82.33** Leakage of other vascular grafts

√7ᵗʰ **T82.330** Leakage of aortic (bifurcation) graft (replacement) `CC`

√7ᵗʰ **T82.331** Leakage of carotid arterial graft (bypass) `CC`

√7ᵗʰ **T82.332** Leakage of femoral arterial graft (bypass) `CC`

√7ᵗʰ **T82.338** Leakage of other vascular grafts `CC`

√7ᵗʰ **T82.339** Leakage of unspecified vascular graft `CC`

√6ᵗʰ **T82.39** Other mechanical complication of other vascular grafts
Obstruction (mechanical) of other vascular grafts
Perforation of other vascular grafts
Protrusion of other vascular grafts

√7ᵗʰ **T82.390** Other mechanical complication of aortic (bifurcation) graft (replacement) `CC`

√7ᵗʰ **T82.391** Other mechanical complication of carotid arterial graft (bypass) `CC`

√7ᵗʰ **T82.392** Other mechanical complication of femoral arterial graft (bypass) `CC`

√7ᵗʰ **T82.398** Other mechanical complication of other vascular grafts `CC`

√7ᵗʰ **T82.399** Other mechanical complication of unspecified vascular grafts `CC`

√5ᵗʰ **T82.4** Mechanical complication of vascular dialysis catheter
Mechanical complication of hemodialysis catheter
EXCLUDES 1 *mechanical complication of intraperitoneal dialysis catheter (T85.62)*

CC Excl: For CC codes in subcategory T82.4: CC with 7th character A, unless otherwise noted: See code: T82.3

√x7ᵗʰ **T82.41** Breakdown (mechanical) of vascular dialysis catheter `CC`

√x7ᵗʰ **T82.42** Displacement of vascular dialysis catheter `CC`
Malposition of vascular dialysis catheter

√x7ᵗʰ **T82.43** Leakage of vascular dialysis catheter `CC`

√x7ᵗʰ **T82.49** Other complication of vascular dialysis catheter `CC`
Obstruction (mechanical) of vascular dialysis catheter
Perforation of vascular dialysis catheter
Protrusion of vascular dialysis catheter

√5ᵗʰ **T82.5** Mechanical complication of other cardiac and vascular devices and implants
EXCLUDES 2 *mechanical complication of epidural and subdural infusion catheter (T85.61)*

CC Excl: For CC codes in subcategory T82.5: CC with 7th character A, unless otherwise noted: D78.81-D78.89, E36.8, E89.810-E89.89, H59.011-H59.019, H59.031-H59.099, H59.811-H59.89, H95.811-H95.89, I97.3, L76.81-L76.82, M96.89, N98.1-N98.9, T81.82XA, T81.89X-T81.9XX with 7th A, T82.310-T82.511 with 7th A, T82.513-T82.518 with 7th A, T82.520-T82.521 with 7th A, T82.523-T82.531 with 7th A, T82.533-T82.538 with 7th A, T82.590-T82.591 with 7th A, T82.593A, T82.595A

√6ᵗʰ **T82.51** Breakdown (mechanical) of other cardiac and vascular devices and implants

√7ᵗʰ **T82.510** Breakdown (mechanical) of surgically created arteriovenous fistula `CC`

√7ᵗʰ **T82.511** Breakdown (mechanical) of surgically created arteriovenous shunt `CC`

√7ᵗʰ **T82.512** Breakdown (mechanical) of artificial heart `CC`
CC Excl: CC with 7th character A: D78.81-D78.89, E36.8, E89.810-E89.89, H59.011-H59.019, H59.031-H59.099, H59.811-H59.89, H95.811-H95.89, I97.3, L76.81-L76.82, M96.89, N98.1-N98.9, T81.82XA, T81.89X-T81.9XX with 7th A, T82.118A, T82.128A, T82.198A, T82.221-T82.228 with 7th A, T82.512A, T82.522A, T82.532A, T82.592A, T82.594A, T82.598A

√7ᵗʰ **T82.513** Breakdown (mechanical) of balloon (counterpulsation) device `CC`

√7ᵗʰ **T82.514** Breakdown (mechanical) of infusion catheter `CC`

√7ᵗʰ **T82.515** Breakdown (mechanical) of umbrella device `CC`

√7ᵗʰ **T82.518** Breakdown (mechanical) of other cardiac and vascular devices and implants `CC`

√7ᵗʰ **T82.519** Breakdown (mechanical) of unspecified cardiac and vascular devices and implants `CC`
CC Excl: CC with 7th character A: D78.81-D78.89, E36.8, E89.810-E89.89, H59.011-H59.019, H59.031-H59.099, H59.811-H59.89, H95.811-H95.89, I97.3, L76.81-L76.82, M96.89, N98.1-N98.9, T81.82XA, T81.89X-T81.9XX with 7th A, T82.519A, T82.539A, T82.599-T82.9XX with 7th character A, T85.9XXA

√6ᵗʰ **T82.52** Displacement of other cardiac and vascular devices and implants
Malposition of other cardiac and vascular devices and implants

√7ᵗʰ **T82.520** Displacement of surgically created arteriovenous fistula `CC`

√7ᵗʰ **T82.521** Displacement of surgically created arteriovenous shunt `CC`

√7ᵗʰ **T82.522** Displacement of artificial heart `CC`
CC Excl: CC with 7th character A: D78.81-D78.89, E36.8, E89.810-E89.89, H59.011-H59.019, H59.031-H59.099, H59.811-H59.89, H95.811-H95.89, I97.3, L76.81-L76.82, M96.89, N98.1-N98.9, T81.82XA, T81.89X-T81.9XX with 7th A, T82.118A, T82.128A, T82.198A, T82.221-T82.228 with 7th A, T82.512A, T82.522A, T82.532A, T82.592A, T82.594A, T82.598A

√7ᵗʰ **T82.523** Displacement of balloon (counterpulsation) device `CC`

√7ᵗʰ **T82.524** Displacement of infusion catheter `CC`

√7ᵗʰ **T82.525** Displacement of umbrella device `CC`

√7ᵗʰ **T82.528** Displacement of other cardiac and vascular devices and implants `CC`

√7ᵗʰ **T82.529** Displacement of unspecified cardiac and vascular devices and implants `CC`

√6ᵗʰ **T82.53** Leakage of other cardiac and vascular devices and implants

√7ᵗʰ **T82.530** Leakage of surgically created arteriovenous fistula `CC`

√7ᵗʰ **T82.531** Leakage of surgically created arteriovenous shunt `CC`

√7ᵗʰ **T82.532** Leakage of artificial heart `CC`
CC Excl: CC with 7th character A: D78.81-D78.89, E36.8, E89.810-E89.89, H59.011-H59.019, H59.031-H59.099, H59.811-H59.89, H95.811-H95.89, I97.3, L76.81-L76.82, M96.89, N98.1-N98.9, T81.82XA, T81.89X-T81.9XX with 7th A, T82.118A, T82.128A, T82.198A, T82.221-T82.228 with 7th A, T82.512A, T82.522A, T82.532A, T82.592A, T82.594A, T82.598A

√7ᵗʰ **T82.533** Leakage of balloon (counterpulsation) device `CC`

√7ᵗʰ **T82.534** Leakage of infusion catheter `CC`

√7ᵗʰ **T82.535** Leakage of umbrella device `CC`

√7ᵗʰ **T82.538** Leakage of other cardiac and vascular devices and implants `CC`

√7ᵗʰ **T82.539** Leakage of unspecified cardiac and vascular devices and implants `CC`
CC Excl: CC with 7th character A: D78.81-D78.89, E36.8, E89.810-E89.89, H59.011-H59.019, H59.031-H59.099, H59.811-H59.89, H95.811-H95.89, I97.3, L76.81-L76.82, M96.89, N98.1-N98.9, T81.82XA, T81.89X-T81.9XX with 7th A, T82.519A, T82.539A, T82.599-T82.9XX with 7th character A, T85.9XXA

√6ᵗʰ **T82.59** Other mechanical complication of other cardiac and vascular devices and implants
Obstruction (mechanical) of other cardiac and vascular devices and implants
Perforation of other cardiac and vascular devices and implants
Protrusion of other cardiac and vascular devices and implants

√7ᵗʰ **T82.590** Other mechanical complication of surgically created arteriovenous fistula `CC`

√7th **T82.591** **Other mechanical complication of surgically created arteriovenous shunt** `CC`

√7th **T82.592** **Other mechanical complication of artificial heart** `CC`
CC Excl: CC with 7th character A: D78.81-D78.89, E36.8, E89.810-E89.89, H59.011-H59.019, H59.031-H59.099, H59.811-H59.89, H95.811-H95.89, I97.3, L76.81-L76.82, M96.89, N98.1-N98.9, T81.82XA, T81.89X-T81.9XX with 7th A, T82.118A, T82.128A, T82.198A,T82.221-T82.228 with 7th A, T82.512A, T82.522A, T82.532A, T82.592A, T82.594A, T82.598 with 7th A

√7th **T82.593** **Other mechanical complication of balloon (counterpulsation) device** `CC`

√7th **T82.594** **Other mechanical complication of infusion catheter** `CC`
CC Excl: CC with 7th character A: D78.81-D78.89, E36.8, E89.810-E89.89, H59.011-H59.019, H59.031-H59.099, H59.811-H59.89, H95.811-H95.89, I97.3, L76.81-L76.82, M96.89, N98.1-N98.9, T81.82XA, T81.89X-T81.9XX with 7th A, T82.118A, T82.128A, T82.198A, T82.310-T82.511 with 7th A, T82.513-T82.518 with 7th A, T82.520-T82.521 with 7th A, T82.523-T82.531 with 7th A, T82.533-T82.538 with 7th A, T82.590-T82.591 with 7th A, T82.593A, T82.595 with 7th A

√7th **T82.595** **Other mechanical complication of umbrella device** `CC`

√7th **T82.598** **Other mechanical complication of other cardiac and vascular devices and implants** `CC`
CC Excl: CC with 7th character A: D78.81-D78.89, E36.8, E89.810-E89.89, H59.011-H59.019, H59.031-H59.099, H59.811-H59.89, H95.811-H95.89, I97.3, L76.81-L76.82, M96.89, N98.1-N98.9, T81.82XA, T81.89X-T81.9XX with 7th A, T82.118A, T82.128A, T82.198A,T82.221-T82.228 with 7th A, T82.512A, T82.522A, T82.532A, T82.592 A, T82.594A, T82.598A

√7th **T82.599** **Other mechanical complication of unspecified cardiac and vascular devices and implants** `CC`
CC Excl: CC with 7th character A: D78.81-D78.89, E36.8, E89.810-E89.89, H59.011-H59.019, H59.031-H59.099, H59.811-H59.89, H95.811-H95.89, I97.3, L76.81-L76.82, M96.89, N98.1-N98.9, T81.82XA, T81.89X-T81.9XX with 7th A, T82.519A, T82.539A, T82.599-T82.9XX with 7th A, T85.9XXA

8 √x7th **T82.6** **Infection and inflammatory reaction due to cardiac valve prosthesis** `CC`
Use additional code to identify infection
CC Excl: CC with 7th character A: D78.81-D78.89, E36.8, E89.810-E89.89, H59.011-H59.019, H59.031-H59.099, H59.811-H59.89, H95.811-H95.89, I97.3, L76.81-L76.82, M96.89, N98.1-N98.9, T81.82XA, T81.89X-T82.09X with 7th A, T82.110-T82.118 with 7th A, T82.120-T82.128 with 7th A, T82.190-T82.198 with 7th A, T82.211-T82.9XX with 7th A, T85.310-T85.311 with 7th A, T85.320-T85.321 with 7th A, T85.390-T85.391 with 7th A, T85.510-T85.9XX with 7th A, T86.820-T86.829, T86.842-T86.849

8 √x7th **T82.7** **Infection and inflammatory reaction due to other cardiac and vascular devices, implants and grafts** `CC`
Use additional code to identify infection
CC Excl: See code: T82.6

√5th **T82.8** **Other specified complications of cardiac and vascular prosthetic devices, implants and grafts**

√6th **T82.81** **Embolism of cardiac and vascular prosthetic devices, implants and grafts**

√7th **T82.817** **Embolism of cardiac prosthetic devices, implants and grafts** `CC`
CC Excl: CC with 7th character A: D78.81-D78.89, E36.8, E89.810-E89.89, H59.011-H59.019, H59.031-H59.099, H59.811-H59.89, H95.811-H95.89, I97.3, L76.81-L76.82, M96.89, N98.1-N98.9, T81.82XA, T81.89X-T82.09X with 7th A, T82.110-T82.118 with 7th A, T82.120-T82.128 with 7th A, T82.190-T82.198 with 7th A, T82.221-T82.9XX with 7th A, T85.310-T85.311 with 7th A, T85.320-T85.321 with 7th A, T85.390-T85.391 with 7th A, T85.510-T85.9XX with 7th A, T86.820-T86.829, T86.842-T86.849

√7th **T82.818** **Embolism of vascular prosthetic devices, implants and grafts** `CC`
CC Excl: CC with 7th character A: D78.81-D78.89, E36.8, E89.810-E89.89, H59.011-H59.019, H59.031-H59.099, H59.811-H59.89, H95.811-H95.89, I97.3, L76.81-L76.82, M96.89, N98.1-N98.9, T81.82XA, T81.89X-T82.09X with 7th A, T82.110-T82.118 with 7th A, T82.120-T82.128 with 7th A, T82.190-T82.198 with 7th A, T82.211-T82.9XX with 7th A, T85.310-T85.311 with 7th A, T85.320-T85.321 with 7th A, T85.390-T85.391 with 7th A, T85.510-T85.9XX with 7th A, T86.820-T86.829, T86.842-T86.849

√6th **T82.82** **Fibrosis of cardiac and vascular prosthetic devices, implants and grafts**

√7th **T82.827** **Fibrosis of cardiac prosthetic devices, implants and grafts** `CC`
CC Excl: See code: T82.817

√7th **T82.828** **Fibrosis of vascular prosthetic devices, implants and grafts** `CC`
CC Excl: See code: T82.818

√6th **T82.83** **Hemorrhage of cardiac and vascular prosthetic devices, implants and grafts**

√7th **T82.837** **Hemorrhage of cardiac prosthetic devices, implants and grafts** `CC`
CC Excl: See code: T82.817

√7th **T82.838** **Hemorrhage of vascular prosthetic devices, implants and grafts** `CC`
CC Excl: See code: T82.818

√6th **T82.84** **Pain from cardiac and vascular prosthetic devices, implants and grafts**

√7th **T82.847** **Pain from cardiac prosthetic devices, implants and grafts** `CC`
CC Excl: See code: T82.817

√7th **T82.848** **Pain from vascular prosthetic devices, implants and grafts** `CC`
CC Excl: See code: T82.818

√6th **T82.85** **Stenosis of cardiac and vascular prosthetic devices, implants and grafts**

√7th **T82.857** **Stenosis of cardiac prosthetic devices, implants and grafts** `CC`
CC Excl: See code: T82.817

√7th **T82.858** **Stenosis of vascular prosthetic devices, implants and grafts** `CC`
CC Excl: See code: T82.818

√6th **T82.86** **Thrombosis of cardiac and vascular prosthetic devices, implants and grafts**

√7th **T82.867** **Thrombosis of cardiac prosthetic devices, implants and grafts** `CC`
CC Excl: See code: T82.817

√7th **T82.868** **Thrombosis of vascular prosthetic devices, implants and grafts** `CC`
CC Excl: See code: T82.818

√6th **T82.89** **Other specified complication of cardiac and vascular prosthetic devices, implants and grafts**

√7th **T82.897** **Other specified complication of cardiac prosthetic devices, implants and grafts** `CC`
CC Excl: See code: T82.817

√7th **T82.898** **Other specified complication of vascular prosthetic devices, implants and grafts** `CC`
CC Excl: See code: T82.818

---

8 HAC = as SDx not POA, in combination with one of the following procedure codes: 02H43[J,K,M]Z; 02H[6,7]3[J,M]Z; 02H[K,L]3JZ; 02HN[0,3,4][J,M]Z; 02PA[0,3,4]MZ; 02PAXMZ; 02WA[0,3,4]MZ; 0JH[6,8][0,3][4,5,6,7,8,9,P]Z; 0J[P,W]T[0,3]PZ.

N Newborn: 0   P Pediatric: 0-17   M Maternity: 12-55   A Adult: 15-124   MCC Major CC Condition   PDx MCC PDx acts as own MCC   CC CC Condition   PDx CC PDx acts as own CC

1098   ICD-10-CM Draft (2015)

√x7ᵗʰ **T82.9** Unspecified complication of cardiac and vascular `CC`
prosthetic device, implant and graft
CC Excl: See code: T82.817

√4ᵗʰ **T83** Complications of genitourinary prosthetic devices, implants and
grafts
EXCLUDES 2 *failure and rejection of transplanted organs and tissue (T86.-)*

The appropriate 7th character is to be added to each code from
category T83.
A   initial encounter
D   subsequent encounter
S   sequela

√5ᵗʰ **T83.0** Mechanical complication of urinary (indwelling) catheter
EXCLUDES 2 *complications of stoma of urinary tract (N99.5-)*

For CC codes in subcategory T83.0: CC with 7th character
A, unless otherwise noted: D78.81-D78.89, E36.8, E89.810-
E89.89, H59.011-H59.019, H59.031-H59.099, H59.811-H59.89,
H95.811-H95.89, I97.3, L76.81-L76.82, M96.89, N98.1-N98.9,
N99.510-N99.518, T81.82XA, T81.89X-T81.9XX with 7th A,
T83.010A, T83.020A, T83.030A, T83.090A, T83.110-T83.29X
with 7th A, T83.410-T83.718 with 7th A, T83.728-T83.9XX with
7th A

√6ᵗʰ **T83.01** Breakdown (mechanical) of urinary (indwelling)
catheter

√7ᵗʰ **T83.010** Breakdown (mechanical) of `CC`
cystostomy catheter

√7ᵗʰ **T83.018** Breakdown (mechanical) of other
indwelling urethral catheter

√6ᵗʰ **T83.02** Displacement of urinary (indwelling) catheter
Malposition of urinary (indwelling) catheter

√7ᵗʰ **T83.020** Displacement of cystostomy catheter `CC`

√7ᵗʰ **T83.028** Displacement of other indwelling
urethral catheter

√6ᵗʰ **T83.03** Leakage of urinary (indwelling) catheter

√7ᵗʰ **T83.030** Leakage of cystostomy catheter `CC`

√7ᵗʰ **T83.038** Leakage of other indwelling urethral
catheter

√6ᵗʰ **T83.09** Other mechanical complication of urinary
(indwelling) catheter
Obstruction (mechanical) of urinary (indwelling)
catheter
Perforation of urinary (indwelling) catheter
Protrusion of urinary (indwelling) catheter

√7ᵗʰ **T83.090** Other mechanical complication of `CC`
cystostomy catheter

√7ᵗʰ **T83.098** Other mechanical complication of other
indwelling urethral catheter

√5ᵗʰ **T83.1** Mechanical complication of other urinary devices and
implants

CC Excl: For CC codes in subcategory T83.0: CC with 7th
character A, unless otherwise noted: See code: T83.0

√6ᵗʰ **T83.11** Breakdown (mechanical) of other urinary devices
and implants

√7ᵗʰ **T83.110** Breakdown (mechanical) of urinary `CC`
electronic stimulator device

√7ᵗʰ **T83.111** Breakdown (mechanical) of urinary `CC`
sphincter implant

√7ᵗʰ **T83.112** Breakdown (mechanical) of urinary `CC`
stent

√7ᵗʰ **T83.118** Breakdown (mechanical) of other `CC`
urinary devices and implants

√6ᵗʰ **T83.12** Displacement of other urinary devices and implants
Malposition of other urinary devices and implants

√7ᵗʰ **T83.120** Displacement of urinary electronic `CC`
stimulator device

√7ᵗʰ **T83.121** Displacement of urinary sphincter `CC`
implant

√7ᵗʰ **T83.122** Displacement of urinary stent `CC`

√7ᵗʰ **T83.128** Displacement of other urinary `CC`
devices and implants

√6ᵗʰ **T83.19** Other mechanical complication of other urinary
devices and implants
Leakage of other urinary devices and implants
Obstruction (mechanical) of other urinary devices and
implants
Perforation of other urinary devices and implants
Protrusion of other urinary devices and implants

√7ᵗʰ **T83.190** Other mechanical complication of `CC`
urinary electronic stimulator device

√7ᵗʰ **T83.191** Other mechanical complication of `CC`
urinary sphincter implant

√7ᵗʰ **T83.192** Other mechanical complication of
urinary stent

√7ᵗʰ **T83.198** Other mechanical complication of `CC`
other urinary devices and implants

√5ᵗʰ **T83.2** Mechanical complication of graft of urinary organ

CC Excl: For CC codes in subcategory T83.0: CC with 7th
character A, unless otherwise noted: See code: T83.0

√x7ᵗʰ **T83.21** Breakdown (mechanical) of graft of urinary `CC`
organ

√x7ᵗʰ **T83.22** Displacement of graft of urinary organ `CC`
Malposition of graft of urinary organ

√x7ᵗʰ **T83.23** Leakage of graft of urinary organ `CC`

√x7ᵗʰ **T83.29** Other mechanical complication of graft of `CC`
urinary organ
Obstruction (mechanical) of graft of urinary organ
Perforation of graft of urinary organ
Protrusion of graft of urinary organ

√5ᵗʰ **T83.3** Mechanical complication of intrauterine contraceptive device
√x7ᵗʰ **T83.31** Breakdown (mechanical) of intrauterine ♀
contraceptive device

√x7ᵗʰ **T83.32** Displacement of intrauterine contraceptive ♀
device
Malposition of intrauterine contraceptive device

√x7ᵗʰ **T83.39** Other mechanical complication of intrauterine ♀
contraceptive device
Leakage of intrauterine contraceptive device
Obstruction (mechanical) of intrauterine contraceptive
device
Perforation of intrauterine contraceptive device
Protrusion of intrauterine contraceptive device

√5ᵗʰ **T83.4** Mechanical complication of other prosthetic devices,
implants and grafts of genital tract

CC Excl: For CC codes in subcategory T83.0: CC with 7th
character A, unless otherwise noted: See code: T83.0

√6ᵗʰ **T83.41** Breakdown (mechanical) of other prosthetic devices,
implants and grafts of genital tract

√7ᵗʰ **T83.410** Breakdown (mechanical) of penile `CC`♂
(implanted) prosthesis

√7ᵗʰ **T83.418** Breakdown (mechanical) of other `CC`
prosthetic devices, implants and grafts
of genital tract

√6ᵗʰ **T83.42** Displacement of other prosthetic devices, implants
and grafts of genital tract
Malposition of other prosthetic devices, implants and
grafts of genital tract

√7ᵗʰ **T83.420** Displacement of penile (implanted) `CC`♂
prosthesis

√7ᵗʰ **T83.428** Displacement of other prosthetic `CC`
devices, implants and grafts of genital
tract

√6ᵗʰ **T83.49** Other mechanical complication of other prosthetic
devices, implants and grafts of genital tract
Leakage of other prosthetic devices, implants and
grafts of genital tract
Obstruction, mechanical of other prosthetic devices,
implants and grafts of genital tract
Perforation of other prosthetic devices, implants and
grafts of genital tract
Protrusion of other prosthetic devices, implants and
grafts of genital tract

√7ᵗʰ **T83.490** Other mechanical complication of `CC`♂
penile (implanted) prosthesis

√7ᵗʰ **T83.498** Other mechanical complication of `CC`
other prosthetic devices, implants and
grafts of genital tract

✓ Additional Character Required   √x7ᵗʰ *X*tension Alert   <u>Unacceptable PDx</u>   Manifestation   Hospital Acquired Condition   *EXCLUDES 1* Not Coded Here   *EXCLUDES 2* Not Included Here

√5ᵗʰ **T83.5** **Infection and inflammatory reaction due to prosthetic device, implant and graft in urinary system**
Use additional code to identify infection

7 √x7ᵗʰ **T83.51** **Infection and inflammatory reaction due to indwelling urinary catheter** `CC`
EXCLUDES 2 *complications of stoma of urinary tract (N99.5-)*
CC Excl: CC with 7th character A: D78.81-D78.89, E36.8, E89.810-E89.89, H59.011-H59.019, H59.031-H59.099, H59.811-H59.89, H95.811-H95.89, I97.3, L76.81-L76.82, M96.89, N39.0, N98.1-N98.9, N99.510-N99.518, T81.82XA, T81.89X-T81.9XX with 7th A, T83.010A, T83.020A, T83.030A, T83.090A, T83.110-T83.29X with 7th A, T83.410-T83.718 with 7th A, T83.728-T83.9XX with 7th A, T85.310-T85.311 with 7th A, T85.320-T85.321 with 7th A, T85.390-T85.391 with 7th A, T85.510-T85.612 with 7th A, T85.614-T85.622 with 7th A, T85.624-T85.692 with 7th A, T85.694-T85.9XX with 7th A, T86.842-T86.849

√x7ᵗʰ **T83.59** **Infection and inflammatory reaction due to prosthetic device, implant and graft in urinary system** `CC`
CC Excl: CC with 7th character A: D78.81-D78.89, E36.8, E89.810-E89.89, H59.011-H59.019, H59.031-H59.099, H59.811-H59.89, H95.811-H95.89, I97.3, L76.81-L76.82, M96.89, N98.1-N98.9, N99.510-N99.518, T81.82XA, T81.89X-T81.9XX with 7th A, T83.010A, T83.020A, T83.030A, T83.090A, T83.110-T83.29X with 7th A, T83.410-T83.718 with 7th A, T83.728-T83.9XX with 7th A, T85.310-T85.311 with 7th A, T85.320-T85.321 with 7th A, T85.390-T85.391 with 7th A, T85.510-T85.9XX with 7th A, T86.820-T86.829, T86.842-T86.849

√x7ᵗʰ **T83.6** **Infection and inflammatory reaction due to prosthetic device, implant and graft in genital tract** `CC`
Use additional code to identify infection
CC Excl: See code: T83.59

√5ᵗʰ **T83.7** **Complications due to implanted mesh and other prosthetic materials**

√6ᵗʰ **T83.71** **Erosion of implanted mesh and other prosthetic materials to surrounding organ or tissue**

√7ᵗʰ **T83.711** **Erosion of implanted vaginal mesh and other prosthetic materials to surrounding organ or tissue** ♀
Erosion of implanted vaginal mesh and other prosthetic materials into pelvic floor muscles

√7ᵗʰ **T83.718** **Erosion of other implanted mesh and other prosthetic materials to surrounding organ or tissue** `CC`
CC Excl: CC with 7th character A: D78.81-D78.89, E36.8, E89.810-E89.89, H59.011-H59.019, H59.031-H59.099, H59.811-H59.89, H95.811-H95.89, I97.3, L76.81-L76.82, M96.89, N98.1-N98.9, N99.510-N99.518, T81.82XA, T81.89X-T81.9XX with 7th A, T83.010A, T83.020A, T83.030A, T83.090A, T83.110-T83.29X with 7th A, T83.410-T83.718 with 7th A, T83.728-T83.9XX with 7th A

√6ᵗʰ **T83.72** **Exposure of implanted mesh and other prosthetic materials into surrounding organ or tissue**

√7ᵗʰ **T83.721** **Exposure of implanted vaginal mesh and other prosthetic materials into vagina** ♀
Exposure of implanted vaginal mesh and other prosthetic materials through vaginal wall

√7ᵗʰ **T83.728** **Exposure of other implanted mesh and other prosthetic materials to surrounding organ or tissue** `CC`
CC Excl: See code: T83.718

√5ᵗʰ **T83.8** **Other specified complications of genitourinary prosthetic devices, implants and grafts**

CC Excl: For CC/MCC codes in subcategory T83.8: CC with 7th character A, unless otherwise noted: D78.81-D78.89, E36.8, E89.810-E89.89, H59.011-H59.019, H59.031-H59.099, H59.811-H59.89, H95.811-H95.89, I97.3, L76.81-L76.82, M96.89, N98.1-N98.9, N99.510-N99.518, T81.82XA, T81.89X-T81.9XX with 7th A, T83.010A, T83.020A, T83.030 A, T83.090A, T83.110-T83.29X with 7th A, T83.410-T83.718 with 7th A, T83.728-T83.9XX with 7th A, T85.310-T85.311 with 7th A, T85.320-T85.321 with 7th A, T85.390-T85.391 with 7th A, T85.510-T85.9XX with 7th A, T86.820-T86.829, T86.842-T86.849

√x7ᵗʰ **T83.81** **Embolism of genitourinary prosthetic devices, implants and grafts** `CC`

√x7ᵗʰ **T83.82** **Fibrosis of genitourinary prosthetic devices, implants and grafts** `CC`

√x7ᵗʰ **T83.83** **Hemorrhage of genitourinary prosthetic devices, implants and grafts** `CC`

√x7ᵗʰ **T83.84** **Pain from genitourinary prosthetic devices, implants and grafts** `CC`

√x7ᵗʰ **T83.85** **Stenosis of genitourinary prosthetic devices, implants and grafts** `CC`

√x7ᵗʰ **T83.86** **Thrombosis of genitourinary prosthetic devices, implants and grafts** `CC`

√x7ᵗʰ **T83.89** **Other specified complication of genitourinary prosthetic devices, implants and grafts** `CC`

√x7ᵗʰ **T83.9** **Unspecified complication of genitourinary prosthetic device, implant and graft** `CC`
CC Excl: See code: T83.8

√4ᵗʰ **T84** **Complications of internal orthopedic prosthetic devices, implants and grafts**
EXCLUDES 2 *failure and rejection of transplanted organs and tissues (T86.-)*
fracture of bone following insertion of orthopedic implant, joint prosthesis or bone plate (M96.6)

The appropriate 7th character is to be added to each code from category T84.
A   initial encounter
D   subsequent encounter
S   sequela

√5ᵗʰ **T84.0** **Mechanical complication of internal joint prosthesis**

CC Excl: For CC codes in subcategory T84.0: CC with 7th character A, unless otherwise noted: D78.81-D78.89, E36.8, E89.810-E89.89, H59.011-H59.019, H59.031-H59.099, H59.811-H59.89, H95.811-H95.89, I97.3, L76.81-L76.82, M96.621-M96.69, M96.89, N98.1-N98.9, T81.82XA, T81.89X-T81.9XX with 7th A, T84.010-T84.9XX with 7th A

√6ᵗʰ **T84.01** **Broken internal joint prosthesis**
Breakage (fracture) of prosthetic joint
Broken prosthetic joint implant
EXCLUDES 1 *periprosthetic joint implant fracture (T84.04)*

√7ᵗʰ **T84.010** **Broken internal right hip prosthesis** `CC`

√7ᵗʰ **T84.011** **Broken internal left hip prosthesis** `CC`

√7ᵗʰ **T84.012** **Broken internal right knee prosthesis** `CC`

√7ᵗʰ **T84.013** **Broken internal left knee prosthesis** `CC`

√7ᵗʰ **T84.018** **Broken internal joint prosthesis, other site** `CC`
Use additional code to identify the joint (Z96.6-)

√7ᵗʰ **T84.019** **Broken internal joint prosthesis, unspecified site** `CC`

√6ᵗʰ **T84.02** **Dislocation of internal joint prosthesis**
Instability of internal joint prosthesis
Subluxation of internal joint prosthesis

√7ᵗʰ **T84.020** **Dislocation of internal right hip prosthesis** `CC`

√7ᵗʰ **T84.021** **Dislocation of internal left hip prosthesis** `CC`

√7ᵗʰ **T84.022** **Instability of internal right knee prosthesis** `CC`

√7ᵗʰ **T84.023** **Instability of internal left knee prosthesis** `CC`

√7ᵗʰ **T84.028** **Dislocation of other internal joint prosthesis** `CC`
Use additional code to identify the joint (Z96.6-)

---

7 HAC = Initial encounter only (7th character A, B or C) and not POA.

√7ᵗʰ **T84.029** **Dislocation of** unspecified **internal joint prosthesis** `CC`

√6ᵗʰ **T84.03** Mechanical loosening **of internal prosthetic joint**
Aseptic loosening of prosthetic joint

√7ᵗʰ **T84.030** **Mechanical loosening of internal** right hip **prosthetic joint** `CC`

√7ᵗʰ **T84.031** **Mechanical loosening of internal** left hip **prosthetic joint** `CC`

√7ᵗʰ **T84.032** **Mechanical loosening of internal** right knee **prosthetic joint** `CC`

√7ᵗʰ **T84.033** **Mechanical loosening of internal** left knee **prosthetic joint** `CC`

√7ᵗʰ **T84.038** **Mechanical loosening of** other **internal prosthetic joint** `CC`
Use additional code to identify the joint (Z96.6-)

√7ᵗʰ **T84.039** **Mechanical loosening of** unspecified **internal prosthetic joint** `CC`

√6ᵗʰ **T84.04** Periprosthetic fracture **around internal prosthetic joint**
EXCLUDES 2   breakage (fracture) of prosthetic joint (T84.01)

√7ᵗʰ **T84.040** **Periprosthetic fracture around internal prosthetic** right hip **joint** `CC`

√7ᵗʰ **T84.041** **Periprosthetic fracture around internal prosthetic** left hip **joint** `CC`

√7ᵗʰ **T84.042** **Periprosthetic fracture around internal prosthetic** right knee **joint** `CC`

√7ᵗʰ **T84.043** **Periprosthetic fracture around internal prosthetic** left knee **joint** `CC`

√7ᵗʰ **T84.048** **Periprosthetic fracture around** other **internal prosthetic joint** `CC`
Use additional code to identify the joint (Z96.6-)

√7ᵗʰ **T84.049** **Periprosthetic fracture around** unspecified **internal prosthetic joint** `CC`

√6ᵗʰ **T84.05** Periprosthetic osteolysis **of internal prosthetic joint**
Use additional code to identify major osseous defect, if applicable (M89.7-)

√7ᵗʰ **T84.050** **Periprosthetic osteolysis of internal prosthetic** right hip **joint** `CC`

√7ᵗʰ **T84.051** **Periprosthetic osteolysis of internal prosthetic** left hip **joint** `CC`

√7ᵗʰ **T84.052** **Periprosthetic osteolysis of internal prosthetic** right knee **joint** `CC`

√7ᵗʰ **T84.053** **Periprosthetic osteolysis of internal prosthetic** left knee **joint** `CC`

√7ᵗʰ **T84.058** **Periprosthetic osteolysis of** other **internal prosthetic joint** `CC`
Use additional code to identify the joint (Z96.6-)

√7ᵗʰ **T84.059** **Periprosthetic osteolysis of** unspecified **internal prosthetic joint** `CC`

√6ᵗʰ **T84.06** Wear of articular bearing surface **of internal prosthetic joint**

√7ᵗʰ **T84.060** **Wear of articular bearing surface of internal prosthetic** right hip **joint** `CC`

√7ᵗʰ **T84.061** **Wear of articular bearing surface of internal prosthetic** left hip **joint** `CC`

√7ᵗʰ **T84.062** **Wear of articular bearing surface of internal prosthetic** right knee **joint** `CC`

√7ᵗʰ **T84.063** **Wear of articular bearing surface of internal prosthetic** left knee **joint** `CC`

√7ᵗʰ **T84.068** **Wear of articular bearing surface of** other **internal prosthetic joint** `CC`
Use additional code to identify the joint (Z96.6-)

√7ᵗʰ **T84.069** **Wear of articular bearing surface of** unspecified **internal prosthetic joint** `CC`

√6ᵗʰ **T84.09** Other mechanical complication of internal joint prosthesis
Prosthetic joint implant failure NOS

√7ᵗʰ **T84.090** **Other mechanical complication of internal** right hip **prosthesis** `CC`

√7ᵗʰ **T84.091** **Other mechanical complication of internal** left hip **prosthesis** `CC`

√7ᵗʰ **T84.092** **Other mechanical complication of internal** right knee **prosthesis** `CC`

√7ᵗʰ **T84.093** **Other mechanical complication of internal** left knee **prosthesis** `CC`

√7ᵗʰ **T84.098** **Other mechanical complication of** other **internal joint prosthesis** `CC`
Use additional code to identify the joint (Z96.6-)

√7ᵗʰ **T84.099** **Other mechanical complication of** unspecified **internal joint prosthesis** `CC`

√5ᵗʰ **T84.1** **Mechanical complication of** internal fixation device **of bones of limb**
EXCLUDES 2   mechanical complication of internal fixation device of bones of feet (T84.2-)
mechanical complication of internal fixation device of bones of fingers (T84.2-)
mechanical complication of internal fixation device of bones of hands (T84.2-)
mechanical complication of internal fixation device of bones of toes (T84.2-)

CC Excl: For CC codes in subcategory T84.1: CC with 7th character A, unless otherwise noted: See code: T84.0

√6ᵗʰ **T84.11** Breakdown (mechanical) **of internal fixation device of bones of limb**

√7ᵗʰ **T84.110** **Breakdown (mechanical) of internal fixation device of** right humerus `CC`

√7ᵗʰ **T84.111** **Breakdown (mechanical) of internal fixation device of** left humerus `CC`

√7ᵗʰ **T84.112** **Breakdown (mechanical) of internal fixation device of bone of** right forearm `CC`

√7ᵗʰ **T84.113** **Breakdown (mechanical) of internal fixation device of bone of** left forearm `CC`

√7ᵗʰ **T84.114** **Breakdown (mechanical) of internal fixation device of** right femur `CC`

√7ᵗʰ **T84.115** **Breakdown (mechanical) of internal fixation device of** left femur `CC`

√7ᵗʰ **T84.116** **Breakdown (mechanical) of internal fixation device of bone of** right lower leg `CC`

√7ᵗʰ **T84.117** **Breakdown (mechanical) of internal fixation device of bone of** left lower leg `CC`

√7ᵗʰ **T84.119** **Breakdown (mechanical) of internal fixation device of** unspecified **bone of limb** `CC`

√6ᵗʰ **T84.12** Displacement **of internal fixation device of bones of limb**
Malposition of internal fixation device of bones of limb

√7ᵗʰ **T84.120** **Displacement of internal fixation device of** right humerus `CC`

√7ᵗʰ **T84.121** **Displacement of internal fixation device of** left humerus `CC`

√7ᵗʰ **T84.122** **Displacement of internal fixation device of bone of** right forearm `CC`

√7ᵗʰ **T84.123** **Displacement of internal fixation device of bone of** left forearm `CC`

√7ᵗʰ **T84.124** **Displacement of internal fixation device of** right femur `CC`

√7ᵗʰ **T84.125** **Displacement of internal fixation device of** left femur `CC`

√7ᵗʰ **T84.126** **Displacement of internal fixation device of bone of** right lower leg `CC`

√7ᵗʰ **T84.127** **Displacement of internal fixation device of bone of** left lower leg `CC`

√7ᵗʰ **T84.129** **Displacement of internal fixation device of** unspecified **bone of limb** `CC`

√6ᵗʰ **T84.19** Other **mechanical complication of internal fixation device of bones of limb**
Obstruction (mechanical) of internal fixation device of bones of limb
Perforation of internal fixation device of bones of limb
Protrusion of internal fixation device of bones of limb

√7ᵗʰ **T84.190** **Other mechanical complication of internal fixation device of** right humerus `CC`

✔ Additional Character Required   √x7ᵗʰ Xtension Alert   Unacceptable PDx   Manifestation   Hospital Acquired Condition   EXCLUDES 1 Not Coded Here   EXCLUDES 2 Not Included Here

ICD-10-CM Draft (2015)   1101

√7ᵗʰ **T84.191** **Other mechanical complication of internal fixation device of** left **humerus** `CC`

√7ᵗʰ **T84.192** **Other mechanical complication of internal fixation device of bone of** right forearm `CC`

√7ᵗʰ **T84.193** **Other mechanical complication of internal fixation device of bone of** left forearm `CC`

√7ᵗʰ **T84.194** **Other mechanical complication of internal fixation device of** right femur `CC`

√7ᵗʰ **T84.195** **Other mechanical complication of internal fixation device of** left femur `CC`

√7ᵗʰ **T84.196** **Other mechanical complication of internal fixation device of bone of** right lower leg `CC`

√7ᵗʰ **T84.197** **Other mechanical complication of internal fixation device of bone of** left lower leg `CC`

√7ᵗʰ **T84.199** **Other mechanical complication of internal fixation device of** unspecified bone of limb `CC`

√5ᵗʰ **T84.2** **Mechanical complication of** internal fixation device **of** other bones

> **CC Excl: For CC codes in subcategory T84.2: CC with 7th character A, unless otherwise noted:** See code: T84.0

√6ᵗʰ **T84.21** Breakdown (mechanical) of internal fixation device of other bones

√7ᵗʰ **T84.210** **Breakdown (mechanical) of internal fixation device of bones of** hand and fingers `CC`

√7ᵗʰ **T84.213** **Breakdown (mechanical) of internal fixation device of bones of** foot and toes `CC`

√7ᵗʰ **T84.216** **Breakdown (mechanical) of internal fixation device of** vertebrae `CC`

√7ᵗʰ **T84.218** **Breakdown (mechanical) of internal fixation device of** other bones `CC`

√6ᵗʰ **T84.22** Displacement **of internal fixation device of other bones**

     Malposition of internal fixation device of other bones

√7ᵗʰ **T84.220** **Displacement of internal fixation device of bones of** hand and fingers `CC`

√7ᵗʰ **T84.223** **Displacement of internal fixation device of bones of** foot and toes `CC`

√7ᵗʰ **T84.226** **Displacement of internal fixation device of** vertebrae `CC`

√7ᵗʰ **T84.228** **Displacement of internal fixation device of** other bones `CC`

√6ᵗʰ **T84.29** Other **mechanical complication of internal fixation device of other bones**

     Obstruction (mechanical) of internal fixation device of other bones
     Perforation of internal fixation device of other bones
     Protrusion of internal fixation device of other bones

√7ᵗʰ **T84.290** **Other mechanical complication of internal fixation device of bones of** hand and fingers `CC`

√7ᵗʰ **T84.293** **Other mechanical complication of internal fixation device of bones of** foot and toes `CC`

√7ᵗʰ **T84.296** **Other mechanical complication of internal fixation device of** vertebrae `CC`

√7ᵗʰ **T84.298** **Other mechanical complication of internal fixation device of** other bones `CC`

√5ᵗʰ **T84.3** **Mechanical complication of** other bone devices, implants **and grafts**

> EXCLUDES 2   *other complications of bone graft (T86.83-)*

> **CC Excl: For CC codes in subcategory T84.3: CC with 7th character A, unless otherwise noted:** See code: T84.0

√6ᵗʰ **T84.31** Breakdown (mechanical) of other bone devices, implants and grafts

√7ᵗʰ **T84.310** **Breakdown (mechanical) of** electronic bone stimulator `CC`

√7ᵗʰ **T84.318** **Breakdown (mechanical) of** other bone devices, implants and grafts `CC`

√6ᵗʰ **T84.32** Displacement **of other bone devices, implants and grafts**

     Malposition of other bone devices, implants and grafts

√7ᵗʰ **T84.320** **Displacement of** electronic bone stimulator `CC`

√7ᵗʰ **T84.328** **Displacement of** other **bone devices, implants and grafts** `CC`

√6ᵗʰ **T84.39** Other **mechanical complication of other bone devices, implants and grafts**

     Obstruction (mechanical) of other bone devices, implants and grafts
     Perforation of other bone devices, implants and grafts
     Protrusion of other bone devices, implants and grafts

√7ᵗʰ **T84.390** **Other mechanical complication of electronic bone stimulator** `CC`

√7ᵗʰ **T84.398** **Other mechanical complication of** other **bone devices, implants and grafts** `CC`

√5ᵗʰ **T84.4** **Mechanical complication of** other internal orthopedic devices, implants and grafts

> **CC Excl: For CC codes in subcategory T84.4: CC with 7th character A, unless otherwise noted:** See code: T84.0

√6ᵗʰ **T84.41** Breakdown (mechanical) of other internal orthopedic devices, implants and grafts

√7ᵗʰ **T84.410** **Breakdown (mechanical) of** muscle and tendon graft `CC`

√7ᵗʰ **T84.418** **Breakdown (mechanical) of** other internal orthopedic devices, implants and grafts `CC`

√6ᵗʰ **T84.42** Displacement **of other internal orthopedic devices, implants and grafts**

     Malposition of other internal orthopedic devices, implants and grafts

√7ᵗʰ **T84.420** **Displacement of** muscle and tendon graft `CC`

√7ᵗʰ **T84.428** **Displacement of** other internal orthopedic devices, implants and grafts `CC`

√6ᵗʰ **T84.49** Other **mechanical complication of other internal orthopedic devices, implants and grafts**

     Mechanical complication of other internal orthopedic devices, implants and grafts NOS
     Obstruction (mechanical) of other internal orthopedic devices, implants and grafts
     Perforation of other internal orthopedic devices, implants and grafts
     Protrusion of other internal orthopedic devices, implants and grafts

√7ᵗʰ **T84.490** **Other mechanical complication of** muscle and tendon graft `CC`

√7ᵗʰ **T84.498** **Other mechanical complication of** other internal orthopedic devices, implants and grafts `CC`

√5ᵗʰ **T84.5** **Infection and inflammatory reaction due to** internal joint prosthesis

     Use additional code to identify infection

> **CC Excl: For CC codes in subcategory T84.5: CC with 7th character A, unless otherwise noted:** D78.81-D78.89, E36.8, E89.810-E89.89, H59.011-H59.019, H59.031-H59.099, H59.811-H59.89, H95.811-H95.89, I97.3, L76.81-L76.82, M96.621-M96.69, M96.89, N98.1-N98.9, T81.82XA, T81.89X-T81.9XX with 7th A, T84.010-T84.9XX with 7th A, T85.310-T85.311 with 7th A, T85.320-T85.321 with 7th A, T85.390-T85.391 with 7th A, T85.510-T85.9XX with 7th A, T86.820-T86.829, T86.842-T86.849

√x7ᵗʰ **T84.50** **Infection and inflammatory reaction due to** unspecified internal joint prosthesis `CC`

√x7ᵗʰ **T84.51** **Infection and inflammatory reaction due to internal** right hip prosthesis `CC`

√x7ᵗʰ **T84.52** **Infection and inflammatory reaction due to internal** left hip prosthesis `CC`

√x7ᵗʰ **T84.53** **Infection and inflammatory reaction due to internal** right knee prosthesis `CC`

√x7ᵗʰ **T84.54** **Infection and inflammatory reaction due to internal** left knee prosthesis `CC`

√x7ᵗʰ **T84.59** **Infection and inflammatory reaction due to** other internal joint prosthesis `CC`

N Newborn: 0   P Pediatric: 0-17   M Maternity: 12-55   A Adult: 15-124   MCC Major CC Condition   PDx MCC PDx acts as own MCC   CC CC Condition   PDx CC PDx acts as own CC

✓5ᵗʰ **T84.6** **Infection and inflammatory reaction due to** internal fixation device

Use additional code to identify infection

CC Excl: For CC codes in subcategory T84.6: CC with 7th character A, unless otherwise noted: See code: T84.5

6 ✓x7ᵗʰ **T84.60** **Infection and inflammatory reaction due to internal fixation device of** unspecified **site**   CC

✓6ᵗʰ **T84.61** **Infection and inflammatory reaction due to internal fixation device of** arm

   6 ✓7ᵗʰ **T84.610** **Infection and inflammatory reaction due to internal fixation device of right humerus**   CC

   6 ✓7ᵗʰ **T84.611** **Infection and inflammatory reaction due to internal fixation device of left humerus**   CC

   6 ✓7ᵗʰ **T84.612** **Infection and inflammatory reaction due to internal fixation device of right radius**   CC

   6 ✓7ᵗʰ **T84.613** **Infection and inflammatory reaction due to internal fixation device of left radius**   CC

   6 ✓7ᵗʰ **T84.614** **Infection and inflammatory reaction due to internal fixation device of right ulna**   CC

   6 ✓7ᵗʰ **T84.615** **Infection and inflammatory reaction due to internal fixation device of left ulna**   CC

   6 ✓7ᵗʰ **T84.619** **Infection and inflammatory reaction due to internal fixation device of unspecified bone of arm**   CC

✓6ᵗʰ **T84.62** **Infection and inflammatory reaction due to internal fixation device of** leg

   ✓7ᵗʰ **T84.620** **Infection and inflammatory reaction due to internal fixation device of** right **femur**   CC

   ✓7ᵗʰ **T84.621** **Infection and inflammatory reaction due to internal fixation device of** left **femur**   CC

   ✓7ᵗʰ **T84.622** **Infection and inflammatory reaction due to internal fixation device of** right **tibia**   CC

   ✓7ᵗʰ **T84.623** **Infection and inflammatory reaction due to internal fixation device of** left **tibia**   CC

   ✓7ᵗʰ **T84.624** **Infection and inflammatory reaction due to internal fixation device of** right **fibula**   CC

   ✓7ᵗʰ **T84.625** **Infection and inflammatory reaction due to internal fixation device of** left **fibula**   CC

   ✓7ᵗʰ **T84.629** **Infection and inflammatory reaction due to internal fixation device of unspecified bone of leg**   CC

6 ✓x7ᵗʰ **T84.63** **Infection and inflammatory reaction due to internal fixation device of** spine   CC

6 ✓x7ᵗʰ **T84.69** **Infection and inflammatory reaction due to internal fixation device of** other **site**   CC

6 ✓x7ᵗʰ **T84.7** **Infection and inflammatory reaction due to** other internal orthopedic prosthetic devices, implants and grafts   CC

Use additional code to identify infection

CC Excl: CC with 7th character A: See code: T84.5

✓5ᵗʰ **T84.8** **Other specified complications of internal orthopedic prosthetic devices, implants and grafts**

CC Excl: For CC codes in subcategory T84.8: CC with 7th character A, unless otherwise noted: See code: T84.5

   ✓x7ᵗʰ **T84.81** **Embolism due to internal orthopedic prosthetic devices, implants and grafts**   CC

   ✓x7ᵗʰ **T84.82** **Fibrosis due to internal orthopedic prosthetic devices, implants and grafts**   CC

   ✓x7ᵗʰ **T84.83** **Hemorrhage due to internal orthopedic prosthetic devices, implants and grafts**   CC

   ✓x7ᵗʰ **T84.84** **Pain due to internal orthopedic prosthetic devices, implants and grafts**

   ✓x7ᵗʰ **T84.85** **Stenosis due to internal orthopedic prosthetic devices, implants and grafts**   CC

   ✓x7ᵗʰ **T84.86** **Thrombosis due to internal orthopedic prosthetic devices, implants and grafts**   CC

   ✓x7ᵗʰ **T84.89** **Other specified complication of internal orthopedic prosthetic devices, implants and grafts**   CC

✓x7ᵗʰ **T84.9** **Unspecified complication of internal orthopedic prosthetic device, implant and graft**   CC

CC Excl: See code: T84.8

✓4ᵗʰ **T85** **Complications of other internal prosthetic devices, implants and grafts**

EXCLUDES 2   failure and rejection of transplanted organs and tissue (T86.-)

The appropriate 7th character is to be added to each code from category T85.
A   initial encounter
D   subsequent encounter
S   sequela

✓5ᵗʰ **T85.0** **Mechanical complication of** ventricular intracranial (communicating) shunt

CC Excl: For CC codes in subcategory T85.0: CC with 7th character A, unless otherwise noted: D78.81-D78.89, E36.8, E89.810-E89.89, H59.011-H59.019, H59.031-H59.099, H59.811-H59.89, H95.811-H95.89, I97.3, L76.81-L76.82, M96.89, N98.1-N98.9, T81.82XA, T81.89X-T81.9XX with 7th A, T85.01X-T85.199 with 7th A

   ✓x7ᵗʰ **T85.01** **Breakdown (mechanical) of ventricular intracranial (communicating) shunt**   CC

   ✓x7ᵗʰ **T85.02** **Displacement of ventricular intracranial (communicating) shunt**   CC

Malposition of ventricular intracranial (communicating) shunt

   ✓x7ᵗʰ **T85.03** **Leakage of ventricular intracranial (communicating) shunt**   CC

   ✓x7ᵗʰ **T85.09** **Other mechanical complication of ventricular intracranial (communicating) shunt**   CC

Obstruction (mechanical) of ventricular intracranial (communicating) shunt
Perforation of ventricular intracranial (communicating) shunt
Protrusion of ventricular intracranial (communicating) shunt

✓5ᵗʰ **T85.1** **Mechanical complication of** implanted electronic stimulator of nervous system

CC Excl: For CC codes in subcategory T85.1: CC with 7th character A, unless otherwise noted: See code: T85.0

   ✓6ᵗʰ **T85.11** **Breakdown (mechanical) of implanted electronic stimulator of nervous system**

     ✓7ᵗʰ **T85.110** **Breakdown (mechanical) of implanted electronic neurostimulator (electrode) of brain**   CC

     ✓7ᵗʰ **T85.111** **Breakdown (mechanical) of implanted electronic neurostimulator (electrode) of peripheral nerve**   CC

     ✓7ᵗʰ **T85.112** **Breakdown (mechanical) of implanted electronic neurostimulator (electrode) of spinal cord**   CC

     ✓7ᵗʰ **T85.118** **Breakdown (mechanical) of other implanted electronic stimulator of nervous system**   CC

   ✓6ᵗʰ **T85.12** **Displacement of implanted electronic stimulator of nervous system**

Malposition of implanted electronic stimulator of nervous system

     ✓7ᵗʰ **T85.120** **Displacement of implanted electronic neurostimulator (electrode) of brain**   CC

     ✓7ᵗʰ **T85.121** **Displacement of implanted electronic neurostimulator (electrode) of peripheral nerve**   CC

     ✓7ᵗʰ **T85.122** **Displacement of implanted electronic neurostimulator (electrode) of spinal cord**   CC

     ✓7ᵗʰ **T85.128** **Displacement of other implanted electronic stimulator of nervous system**   CC

---

6 HAC = as SDx not POA, in combination with one of the following procedure codes: 0RG[0,1,2,4,6,7,8,A][0,3,4][7,A,J,K,Z][0,1,J]; 0RG[E,F,G,H,J,K][0,3,4][4,7,J,K,Z]Z; 0RG[L,M][0,3,4][4,5,7,J,K,Z]Z; 0RQ[E,F,G,H,J,K,L,M][0,3,4,X]ZZ; 0RU[E,F,G,H,J,K,L,M][0,3,4][7,J,K]Z; 0SG[0,1,3][0,3,4][7,A,J,K,Z][0,1,J]; 0SG[7,8]0,3,4[4,7,J,K,Z]Z.

✓ Additional Character Required   ✓x7ᵗʰ Xtension Alert   Unacceptable PDx   Manifestation   Hospital Acquired Condition   EXCLUDES 1 Not Coded Here   EXCLUDES 2 Not Included Here

ICD-10-CM Draft (2015)   1103

√6ᵗʰ **T85.19** Other mechanical complication of implanted electronic stimulator of nervous system
Leakage of implanted electronic stimulator of nervous system
Obstruction (mechanical) of implanted electronic stimulator of nervous system
Perforation of implanted electronic stimulator of nervous system
Protrusion of implanted electronic stimulator of nervous system

√7ᵗʰ **T85.190** Other mechanical complication of implanted electronic neurostimulator (electrode) of brain   CC

√7ᵗʰ **T85.191** Other mechanical complication of implanted electronic neurostimulator (electrode) of peripheral nerve   CC

√7ᵗʰ **T85.192** Other mechanical complication of implanted electronic neurostimulator (electrode) of spinal cord   CC

√7ᵗʰ **T85.199** Other mechanical complication of other implanted electronic stimulator of nervous system   CC

√5ᵗʰ **T85.2** Mechanical complication of intraocular lens

CC Excl: For CC codes in subcategory T85.2: CC with 7th character A, unless otherwise noted: D78.81-D78.89, E89.810-E89.89, H59.011-H59.019, H59.031-H59.099, H59.811-H59.89, H95.811-H95.89, I97.3, M96.89, N98.1-N98.9, T85.21X-T85.29X with 7th A

√x7ᵗʰ **T85.21** Breakdown (mechanical) of intraocular lens   CC

√x7ᵗʰ **T85.22** Displacement of intraocular lens   CC
Malposition of intraocular lens

√x7ᵗʰ **T85.29** Other mechanical complication of intraocular lens   CC
Obstruction (mechanical) of intraocular lens
Perforation of intraocular lens
Protrusion of intraocular lens

√5ᵗʰ **T85.3** Mechanical complication of other ocular prosthetic devices, implants and grafts
EXCLUDES 2   other complications of corneal graft (T86.84-)

CC Excl: For CC codes in subcategory T85.3: CC with 7th character A, unless otherwise noted: H59.011-H59.019, H59.031-H59.099, H59.811-H59.89, H95.811-H95.89, I97.3, M96.89, N98.1-N98.9, T85.310-T85.311 with 7th A, T85.320-T85.321 with 7th A, T85.390-T85.391 with 7th A, T85.612A, T85.618A, T85.622A, T85.628A, T85.638A, T85.692A, T85.698-T85.9XX with 7th A, T86.842-T86.849

√6ᵗʰ **T85.31** Breakdown (mechanical) of other ocular prosthetic devices, implants and grafts

√7ᵗʰ **T85.310** Breakdown (mechanical) of prosthetic orbit of right eye   CC

√7ᵗʰ **T85.311** Breakdown (mechanical) of prosthetic orbit of left eye   CC

√7ᵗʰ **T85.318** Breakdown (mechanical) of other ocular prosthetic devices, implants and grafts

√6ᵗʰ **T85.32** Displacement of other ocular prosthetic devices, implants and grafts
Malposition of other ocular prosthetic devices, implants and grafts

√7ᵗʰ **T85.320** Displacement of prosthetic orbit of right eye   CC

√7ᵗʰ **T85.321** Displacement of prosthetic orbit of left eye   CC

√7ᵗʰ **T85.328** Displacement of other ocular prosthetic devices, implants and grafts

√6ᵗʰ **T85.39** Other mechanical complication of other ocular prosthetic devices, implants and grafts
Obstruction (mechanical) of other ocular prosthetic devices, implants and grafts
Perforation of other ocular prosthetic devices, implants and grafts
Protrusion of other ocular prosthetic devices, implants and grafts

√7ᵗʰ **T85.390** Other mechanical complication of prosthetic orbit of right eye   CC

√7ᵗʰ **T85.391** Other mechanical complication of prosthetic orbit of left eye   CC

√7ᵗʰ **T85.398** Other mechanical complication of other ocular prosthetic devices, implants and grafts

√5ᵗʰ **T85.4** Mechanical complication of breast prosthesis and implant

CC Excl: For CC codes in subcategory T85.4: CC with 7th character A, unless otherwise noted: D78.81-D78.89, E89.810-E89.89, H59.011-H59.019, H59.031-H59.099, H59.811-H59.89, H95.811-H95.89, I97.3, M96.89, N98.1-N98.9, T85.41X-T85.49X with 7th A

√x7ᵗʰ **T85.41** Breakdown (mechanical) of breast prosthesis and implant   CC

√x7ᵗʰ **T85.42** Displacement of breast prosthesis and implant   CC
Malposition of breast prosthesis and implant

√x7ᵗʰ **T85.43** Leakage of breast prosthesis and implant   CC

√x7ᵗʰ **T85.44** Capsular contracture of breast implant   CC

√x7ᵗʰ **T85.49** Other mechanical complication of breast prosthesis and implant   CC
Obstruction (mechanical) of breast prosthesis and implant
Perforation of breast prosthesis and implant
Protrusion of breast prosthesis and implant

√5ᵗʰ **T85.5** Mechanical complication of gastrointestinal prosthetic devices, implants and grafts

CC Excl: For CC codes in subcategory T85.5: CC with 7th character A, unless otherwise noted: H95.811-H95.89, I97.3, M96.89, N98.1-N98.9, T85.510-T85.598 with 7th A, T85.612A, T85.618A, T85.622A, T85.628A, T85.638A, T85.692A, T85.698-T85.9XX with 7th A

√6ᵗʰ **T85.51** Breakdown (mechanical) of gastrointestinal prosthetic devices, implants and grafts

√7ᵗʰ **T85.510** Breakdown (mechanical) of bile duct prosthesis   CC

√7ᵗʰ **T85.511** Breakdown (mechanical) of esophageal anti-reflux device   CC

√7ᵗʰ **T85.518** Breakdown (mechanical) of other gastrointestinal prosthetic devices, implants and grafts   CC

√6ᵗʰ **T85.52** Displacement of gastrointestinal prosthetic devices, implants and grafts
Malposition of gastrointestinal prosthetic devices, implants and grafts

√7ᵗʰ **T85.520** Displacement of bile duct prosthesis   CC

√7ᵗʰ **T85.521** Displacement of esophageal anti-reflux device   CC

√7ᵗʰ **T85.528** Displacement of other gastrointestinal prosthetic devices, implants and grafts   CC

√6ᵗʰ **T85.59** Other mechanical complication of gastrointestinal prosthetic devices, implants and
Obstruction, mechanical of gastrointestinal prosthetic devices, implants and grafts
Perforation of gastrointestinal prosthetic devices, implants and grafts
Protrusion of gastrointestinal prosthetic devices, implants and grafts

√7ᵗʰ **T85.590** Other mechanical complication of bile duct prosthesis   CC

√7ᵗʰ **T85.591** Other mechanical complication of esophageal anti-reflux device   CC

√7ᵗʰ **T85.598** Other mechanical complication of other gastrointestinal prosthetic devices, implants and grafts   CC

√5ᵗʰ **T85.6** Mechanical complication of other specified internal and external prosthetic devices, implants and grafts

√6ᵗʰ **T85.61** Breakdown (mechanical) of other specified internal prosthetic devices, implants and grafts

√7ᵗʰ **T85.610** Breakdown (mechanical) of epidural and subdural infusion catheter   CC
CC Excl: CC with 7th character A: H95.811-H95.89, I97.3, M96.89, N98.1-N98.9, T85.610A, T85.612A, T85.618-T85.620 with 7th A, T85.622A, T85.628-T85.630 with 7th A, T85.638-T85.690 with 7th A, T85.692A, T85.698-T85.9XX with 7th A

N Newborn: 0   P Pediatric: 0-17   M Maternity: 12-55   A Adult: 15-124   MCC Major CC Condition   PDx MCC PDx acts as own MCC   CC CC Condition   PDx CC PDx acts as own CC

1104   ICD-10-CM Draft (2015)

✓7ᵗʰ **T85.611 Breakdown (mechanical) of** `CC`
intraperitoneal dialysis catheter
EXCLUDES 1 *mechanical complication of*
vascular dialysis catheter
(T82.4-)
CC Excl: CC with 7th character A: H95.811-
H95.89, I97.3, M96.89, N98.1-N98.9, T85.611-
T85.612 with 7th A, T85.614-T85.618 with
7th A, T85.621-T85.622 with 7th A, T85.624-
T85.628 with 7th A, T85.631-T85.638 with
7th A, T85.691-T85.692 with 7th A, T85.694-
T85.9XX with 7th A

✓7ᵗʰ **T85.612 Breakdown (mechanical) of** `CC`
permanent sutures
EXCLUDES 1 *mechanical complication of*
permanent (wire) suture
used in bone repair (T84.1-
T84.2)
CC Excl: CC with 7th character A: D78.81-
D78.89, E89.810-E89.89, H59.011-H59.019,
H59.031-H59.099, H59.811-H59.89, H95.811-
H95.89, I97.3, M96.89, N98.1-N98.9, T85.310-
T85.311 with 7th A, T85.320-T85.321 with
7th A, T85.390-T85.391 with 7th A, T85.510-
T85.612 with 7th A, T85.614-T85.622 with
7th A, T85.624-T85.692 with 7th A, T85.694-
T85.9XX with 7th A, T86.842-T86.849

✓7ᵗʰ **T85.613 Breakdown (mechanical) of artificial** `CC`
skin graft and decellularized allodermis
Failure of artificial skin graft and
decellularized allodermis
Non-adherence of artificial skin graft
and decellularized allodermis
Poor incorporation of artificial skin graft
and decellularized allodermis
Shearing of artificial skin graft and
decellularized allodermis
CC Excl: CC with 7th character A: H95.811-
H95.89, I97.3, M96.89, N98.1-N98.9, T85.612-
T85.613 with 7th A, T85.618A, T85.622-
T85.623 with 7th A, T85.628A, T85.638A,
T85.692-T85.693 with 7th A, T85.698-
T85.9XX with 7th A, T86.820-T86.829

✓7ᵗʰ **T85.614 Breakdown (mechanical) of insulin** `CC`
pump
CC Excl: CC with 7th character A: H95.811-
H95.89, I97.3, M96.621-M96.69, M96.89,
N98.1-N98.9, N99.510-N99.518, T81.82X with
7th A, T81.89X-T82.09X with 7th A, T82.110-
T82.118 with 7th A, T82.120-T82.128 with
7th A, T82.190-T82.198 with 7th A, T82.211-
T83.010 with 7th A, T83.020A, T83.030A,
T83.090A, T83.110-T83.29X with 7th A,
T83.410-T83.718 with 7th A, T83.728-
T85.29X with 7th A, T85.41X-T85.49X with
7th A, T85.611-T85.612 with 7th A, T85.614-
T85.618 with 7th A, T85.621-T85.622 with
7th A, T85.624-T85.628 with 7th A, T85.631-
T85.638 with 7th A, T85.691-T85.692 with
7th A, T85.694-T85.9XX with 7th A, T86.820-
T86.829

✓7ᵗʰ **T85.618 Breakdown (mechanical) of other** `CC`
specified internal prosthetic devices,
implants and grafts
CC Excl: CC with 7th character A: D78.81-
D78.89, E89.810-E89.89, H59.011-H59.019,
H59.031-H59.099, H59.811-H59.89, H95.811-
H95.89, I97.3, M96.89, N98.1-N98.9, T85.310-
T85.311 with 7th A, T85.320-T85.321 with
7th A, T85.390-T85.391 with 7th A, T85.510-
T85.612 with 7th A, T85.614-T85.622 with
7th A, T85.624-T85.692 with 7th A, T85.694-
T85.9XX with 7th A, T86.842-T86.849

✓6ᵗʰ **T85.62 Displacement of other specified internal prosthetic**
devices, implants and grafts
Malposition of other specified internal prosthetic
devices, implants and grafts

✓7ᵗʰ **T85.620 Displacement of epidural and** `CC`
subdural infusion catheter
CC Excl: CC with 7th character A:
H95.811-H95.89, I97.3, M96.89, N98.1-N98.9,
T85.610A, T85.612A, T85.618-T85.620
with 7th A, T85.622A, T85.628-T85.630 with 7th A,
T85.638-T85.690 with 7th A, T85.69 A,
T85.698-T85.9XX with 7th A

✓7ᵗʰ **T85.621 Displacement of intraperitoneal** `CC`
dialysis catheter
EXCLUDES 1 *mechanical complication of*
vascular dialysis catheter
(T82.4-)
CC Excl: CC with 7th character A:
H95.811-H95.89, I97.3, M96.89, N98.1-N98.9,
T85.611-T85.612 with 7th A, T85.614-
T85.618 with 7th A, T85.621-T85.622 with
7th A, T85.624-T85.628 with 7th A, T85.631-
T85.638 with 7th A, T85.691-T85.692 with
7th A, T85.694-T85.9XX with 7th A

✓7ᵗʰ **T85.622 Displacement of permanent sutures** `CC`
EXCLUDES 1 *mechanical complication of*
permanent (wire) suture
used in bone repair (T84.1-
T84.2)
CC Excl: CC with 7th character A:
D78.81-D78.89, E89.810-E89.89, H59.011-
H59.019, H59.031-H59.099, H59.811-H59.89,
H95.811-H95.89, I97.3, M96.89, N98.1-N98.9,
T85.310-T85.311 with 7th A, T85.320-
T85.321 with 7th A, T85.390-T85.391 with
7th A, T85.510-T85.612 with 7th A, T85.614-
T85.622 with 7th A, T85.624-T85.692 with
7th A, T85.694-T85.9XX with 7th A, T86.842-
T86.849

✓7ᵗʰ **T85.623 Displacement of artificial skin graft** `CC`
and decellularized allodermis
Dislodgement of artificial skin graft and
decellularized allodermis
Displacement of artificial skin graft and
decellularized allodermis
CC Excl: CC with 7th character A:
H95.811-H95.89, I97.3, M96.89, N98.1-N98.9,
T85.612-T85.613 with 7th A, T85.618 with
7th A, T85.622-T85.623 with 7th A, T85.628A,
T85.638A, T85.692-T85.693 with 7th A,
T85.698-T85.9XX with 7th A, T86.820-
T86.829

✓7ᵗʰ **T85.624 Displacement of insulin pump** `CC`
CC Excl: CC with 7th character A:
H95.811-H95.89, I97.3, M96.621-M96.69,
M96.89, N98.1-N98.9, N99.510-N99.518,
T81.82X with 7th A, T81.89X-T82.09X with
7th A, T82.110-T82.118 with 7th A, T82.120-
T82.128 with 7th A, T82.190-T82.198 with
7th A, T82.211-T83.010 with 7th A, T83.020A,
T83.030 with 7th A, T83.090A, T83.110-
T83.29X with 7th A, T83.410-T83.718 with
7th A, T83.728-T85.29X with 7th A, T85.41X-
T85.49X with 7th A, T85.611-T85.612 with
7th A, T85.614-T85.618 with 7th A, T85.621-
T85.622 with 7th A, T85.624-T85.628 with
7th A, T85.631-T85.638 with 7th A, T85.691-
T85.692 with 7th A, T85.694-T85.9XX with
7th A, T86.820-T86.829

T85.628 Displacement of other specified `CC`
internal prosthetic devices, implants
and grafts
CC Excl: CC with 7th character A: D78.81-
D78.89, E89.810-E89.89, H59.011-H59.019,
H59.031-H59.099, H59.811-H59.89, H95.811-
H95.89, I97.3, M96.89, N98.1-N98.9, T85.310-
T85.311 with 7th A, T85.320-T85.321 with
7th A, T85.390-T85.391 with 7th A, T85.510-
T85.612 with 7th A, T85.614-T85.622 with
7th A, T85.624-T85.692 with 7th A, T85.694-
T85.9XX with 7th A, T86.842-T86.849

✓6ᵗʰ **T85.63 Leakage of other specified internal prosthetic**
devices, implants and grafts

✓7ᵗʰ **T85.630 Leakage of epidural and subdural** `CC`
infusion catheter
CC Excl: CC with 7th character A: See code:
T85.620

✓7ᵗʰ **T85.631 Leakage of intraperitoneal dialysis** `CC`
catheter
EXCLUDES 1 *mechanical complication of*
vascular dialysis catheter
(T82.4)
CC Excl: CC with 7th character A: See code:
T85.621

✓7ᵗʰ **T85.633 Leakage of insulin pump** `CC`
CC Excl: CC with 7th character A: See code:
T86.624

✓7ᵗʰ **T85.638** **Leakage of** other **specified internal** CC
prosthetic devices, implants and grafts
CC Excl: CC with 7th character A: See code:
T85.628

✓6ᵗʰ **T85.69** Other **mechanical** complication **of** other **specified**
internal prosthetic devices, implants and grafts
Obstruction, mechanical of other specified internal
prosthetic devices, implants and grafts
Perforation of other specified internal prosthetic
devices, implants and grafts
Protrusion of other specified internal prosthetic
devices, implants and grafts

    ✓7ᵗʰ **T85.690** **Other mechanical complication of** CC
epidural and subdural infusion catheter
CC Excl: CC with 7th character A: See code:
T85.620

    ✓7ᵗʰ **T85.691** **Other mechanical complication of** CC
intraperitoneal dialysis catheter
EXCLUDES 1 *mechanical complication of*
vascular dialysis catheter
(T82.4)
CC Excl: CC with 7th character A: See code:
T85.621

    T85.692 **Other mechanical complication of** CC
permanent sutures
EXCLUDES 1 *mechanical complication of*
permanent (wire) suture
used in bone repair (T84.1-
T84.2)
CC Excl: CC with 7th character A: See code:
T85.622

    ✓7ᵗʰ **T85.693** **Other mechanical complication of** CC
artificial skin graft and decellularized
allodermis
CC Excl: CC with 7th character A: See code:
T85.623

    ✓7ᵗʰ **T85.694** **Other mechanical complication of** CC
insulin pump
CC Excl: CC with 7th character A: See code:
T85.624

    ✓7ᵗʰ **T85.698** **Other mechanical complication of** CC
other **specified internal prosthetic**
devices, implants and grafts
Mechanical complication of nonabsorbable
surgical material NOS
CC Excl: CC with 7th character A: See code:
T85.628

✓5ᵗʰ **T85.7** **Infection and inflammatory reaction due to** other **internal**
prosthetic devices, implants and grafts
Use additional code to identify infection

    ✓x7ᵗʰ **T85.71** **Infection and inflammatory reaction due to** CC
peritoneal dialysis catheter
CC Excl: CC with 7th character A: See code: T85.628

    ✓x7ᵗʰ **T85.72** **Infection and inflammatory reaction due to** CC
insulin pump
CC Excl: CC with 7th character A: D78.81-D78.89,
E36.8, E89.810-E89.89, H59.011-H59.019, H59.031-
H59.099, H59.811-H59.89, H95.811-H95.89, I97.3,
L76.81-L76.82, M96.621-M96.69, M96.89, N98.1-N98.9,
N99.510-N99.518, T81.82XA, T81.89X-T82.09X with 7th
A, T82.110-T82.118 with 7th A, T82.120-T82.128 with
7th A, T82.190-T82.198 with 7th A, T82.211-T83.010
with 7th A, T83.020A, T83.030A, T83.090A, T83.110-
T83.29X with 7th A, T83.410-T83.718 with 7th A,
T83.728-T85.9XX with 7th A, T86.820-T86.829, T86.840-
T86.849

    ✓x7ᵗʰ **T85.79** **Infection and inflammatory reaction due to** CC
other **internal prosthetic devices, implants and**
grafts
CC Excl: See code: T85.72

✓5ᵗʰ **T85.8** **Other specified complications of internal prosthetic devices,**
implants and grafts, not elsewhere classified

    ✓x7ᵗʰ **T85.81** **Embolism due to internal prosthetic devices,** CC
implants and grafts, not elsewhere classified
CC Excl: See code: T85.72

    ✓x7ᵗʰ **T85.82** **Fibrosis due to internal prosthetic devices,** CC
implants and grafts, not elsewhere classified
CC Excl: See code: T85.72

    ✓x7ᵗʰ **T85.83** **Hemorrhage due to internal prosthetic devices,** CC
implants and grafts, not elsewhere classified
CC Excl: See code: T85.72

    ✓x7ᵗʰ **T85.84** **Pain due to internal prosthetic devices, implants** CC
and grafts, not elsewhere classified
CC Excl: See code: T85.72

    ✓x7ᵗʰ **T85.85** **Stenosis due to internal prosthetic devices,** CC
implants and grafts, not elsewhere classified
CC Excl: See code: T85.72

    ✓x7ᵗʰ **T85.86** **Thrombosis due to internal prosthetic devices,** CC
implants and grafts, not elsewhere classified
CC Excl: See code: T85.72

    ✓x7ᵗʰ **T85.89** **Other specified complication of internal** CC
prosthetic devices, implants and grafts, not
elsewhere classified
CC Excl: See code: T85.72

✓x7ᵗʰ **T85.9** **Unspecified complication of internal prosthetic device,**
implant and graft
Complication of internal prosthetic device, implant and graft
NOS

✓4ᵗʰ **T86** **Complications of transplanted organs and tissue**
Use additional code to identify other transplant complications, such as:
graft-versus-host disease (D89.81-)
malignancy associated with organ transplant (C80.2)
post-transplant lymphoproliferative disorders (PTLD) (D47.Z1)

✓5ᵗʰ **T86.0** **Complications of** bone marrow **transplant**

> CC Excl: For CC codes in subcategory T86.0: CC with 7th
> character A, unless otherwise noted: D78.81-D78.89,
> D89.810-D89.813, E89.810-E89.89, H59.011-H59.019, H59.031-
> H59.099, H59.811-H59.89, H95.811-H95.89, I97.3, M96.89,
> N98.1-N98.9, T86.00-T86.09

    T86.00 **Unspecified complication of bone marrow** CC
transplant

    T86.01 **Bone marrow transplant** rejection CC

    T86.02 **Bone marrow transplant** failure CC

    T86.03 **Bone marrow transplant** infection CC

    T86.09 **Other complications of bone marrow transplant** CC

✓5ᵗʰ **T86.1** **Complications of** kidney **transplant**

> CC Excl: For CC codes in subcategory T86.1: CC with 7th
> character A, unless otherwise noted: D78.81-D78.89,
> E89.810-E89.89, H59.011-H59.019, H59.031-H59.099, H59.811-
> H59.89, H95.811-H95.89, I97.3, M96.89, N98.1-N98.9, T86.10-
> T86.19

    T86.10 **Unspecified complication of kidney transplant** CC

    T86.11 **Kidney transplant** rejection CC

    T86.12 **Kidney transplant** failure CC
AHA: 2013, 1Q, 24

    T86.13 **Kidney transplant** infection CC
Use additional code to specify infection

    T86.19 **Other complication of kidney transplant** CC

✓5ᵗʰ **T86.2** **Complications of** heart **transplant**
EXCLUDES 1 complication of:
artificial heart device (T82.5)
heart-lung transplant (T86.3)

> CC Excl: For CC codes in subcategory T86.2: CC with 7th
> character A, unless otherwise noted: D78.81-D78.89,
> E89.810-E89.89, H59.011-H59.019, H59.031-H59.099, H59.811-
> H59.89, H95.811-H95.89, I97.3, M96.89, N98.1-N98.9, T86.20-
> T86.39

    T86.20 **Unspecified complication of heart transplant** CC

    T86.21 **Heart transplant** rejection CC

    T86.22 **Heart transplant** failure CC

    T86.23 **Heart transplant** infection CC
Use additional code to specify infection

    ✓6ᵗʰ **T86.29** **Other complications of heart transplant**

       T86.290 **Cardiac allograft vasculopathy** CC
EXCLUDES 1 *atherosclerosis of coronary*
arteries (I25.75-, I25.76-,
I25.81-)

       T86.298 **Other complications of heart** CC
transplant

✓5ᵗʰ **T86.3** **Complications of** heart-lung **transplant**

> CC Excl: For CC codes in subcategory T86.3: CC with 7th
> character A, unless otherwise noted: See code: T86.2

    T86.30 **Unspecified complication of heart-lung** PDx CC
transplant

    T86.31 **Heart-lung transplant** rejection PDx CC   CC

    T86.32 **Heart-lung transplant** failure PDx CC   CC

    T86.33 **Heart-lung transplant** infection PDx CC   CC
Use additional code to specify infection

    T86.39 **Other complications of heart-lung** PDx CC
transplant

Ⓝ Newborn: 0   Ⓟ Pediatric: 0-17   Ⓜ Maternity: 12-55   Ⓐ Adult: 15-124   **MCC** Major CC Condition   **PDx MCC** PDx acts as own MCC   **CC** CC Condition   **PDx CC** PDx acts as own CC

1106   ICD-10-CM Draft (2015)

☑5ᵗʰ **T86.4** **Complications of liver transplant**

    T86.40 **Unspecified complication of liver transplant** `CC`

        CC Excl: For CC codes in subcategory T86.4: CC with 7th character A, unless otherwise noted: D78.81-D78.89, E89.810-E89.89, H59.011-H59.019, H59.031-H59.099, H59.811-H59.89, H95.811-H95.89, I97.3, M96.89, N98.1-N98.9, T86.40-T86.49

    T86.41 **Liver transplant rejection** `CC`

    T86.42 **Liver transplant failure** `CC`

    T86.43 **Liver transplant infection** `CC`
        Use additional code to identify infection, such as: cytomegalovirus (CMV) infection (B25.-)

    T86.49 **Other complications of liver transplant** `CC`

☑5ᵗʰ **T86.5** **Complications of stem cell transplant** `CC`
    Complications from stem cells from peripheral blood
    Complications from stem cells from umbilical cord

    CC Excl: For CC codes in subcategory T86.5: CC with 7th character A, unless otherwise noted: D78.81-D78.89, E89.810-E89.89, H59.011-H59.019, H59.031-H59.099, H59.811-H59.89, H95.811-H95.89, I97.3, M96.89, N98.1-N98.9, T86.5, T86.830-T86.839

☑5ᵗʰ **T86.8** **Complications of other transplanted organs and tissues**

  ☑6ᵗʰ **T86.81** **Complications of lung transplant**
    EXCLUDES 1 complication of heart-lung transplant (T86.3-)

    CC Excl: For CC codes in subcategory T86.81: CC with 7th character A, unless otherwise noted: D78.81-D78.89, E89.810-E89.89, H59.011-H59.019, H59.031-H59.099, H59.811-H59.89, H95.811-H95.89, I97.3, M96.89, N98.1-N98.9, T86.810-T86.819

    T86.810 **Lung transplant rejection** `CC`

    T86.811 **Lung transplant failure** `CC`

    T86.812 **Lung transplant infection** `CC`
        Use additional code to specify infection

    T86.818 **Other complications of lung transplant** `CC`

    T86.819 **Unspecified complication of lung transplant** `CC`

  ☑6ᵗʰ **T86.82** **Complications of skin graft (allograft) (autograft)**
    EXCLUDES 2 complication of artificial skin graft (T85.693)

    CC Excl: For CC codes in subcategory T86.82: CC with 7th character A, unless otherwise noted: D78.81-D78.89, E89.810-E89.89, H59.011-H59.019, H59.031-H59.099, H59.811-H59.89, H95.811-H95.89, I97.3, M96.89, N98.1-N98.9, T85.613A, T85.623A, T85.693A, T86.820-T86.829

    T86.820 **Skin graft (allograft) rejection** `CC`

    T86.821 **Skin graft (allograft) (autograft) failure** `CC`

    T86.822 **Skin graft (allograft) (autograft) infection** `CC`
        Use additional code to specify infection

    T86.828 **Other complications of skin graft (allograft) (autograft)** `CC`

    T86.829 **Unspecified complication of skin graft (allograft) (autograft)** `CC`

  ☑6ᵗʰ **T86.83** **Complications of bone graft**
    EXCLUDES 2 mechanical complications of bone graft (T84.3-)

    CC Excl: For CC codes in subcategory T86.83: CC with 7th character A, unless otherwise noted: H95.811-H95.89, I97.3, M96.89, N98.1-N98.9, T86.5, T86.830-T86.839

    T86.830 **Bone graft rejection** `CC`

    T86.831 **Bone graft failure** `CC`

    T86.832 **Bone graft infection** `CC`
        Use additional code to specify infection

    T86.838 **Other complications of bone graft** `CC`

    T86.839 **Unspecified complication of bone graft** `CC`

  ☑6ᵗʰ **T86.84** **Complications of corneal transplant**
    EXCLUDES 2 mechanical complications of corneal graft (T85.3-)

    T86.840 **Corneal transplant rejection** `CC`
        CC Excl: CC with 7th character A: H59.011-H59.019, H59.031-H59.099, H59.811-H59.89, H95.811-H95.89, I97.3, M96.89, N98.1-N98.9, T85.318A, T85.328A, T85.398A, T86.840-T86.841

    T86.841 **Corneal transplant failure** `CC`
        CC Excl: See code: T86.840

    T86.842 **Corneal transplant infection**
        Use additional code to specify infection
        CC Excl: CC with 7th character A: H59.011-H59.019, H59.031-H59.099, H59.811-H59.89, H95.811-H95.89, I97.3, M96.621-M96.69, M96.89, N98.1-N98.9, N99.510-N99.518, T81.82XA, T81.89X-T82.09X with 7th A, T82.110-T82.118 with 7th A, T82.120-T82.128 with 7th A, T82.190-T82.198 with 7th A, T82.211-T83.010 with 7th A, T83.020A, T83.030A, T83.090A, T83.110-T83.29X with 7th A, T83.410-T83.718 with 7th A, T83.728-T85.49X with 7th A, T85.612A, T85.618A, T85.622A, T85.628A, T85.638A, T85.692A, T85.698-T85.9XX with 7th A, T86.820-T86.829, T86.840-T86.849

    T86.848 **Other complications of corneal transplant** `CC`
        CC Excl: See code: T86.842

    T86.849 **Unspecified complication of corneal transplant** `CC`
        CC Excl: See code: T86.842

  ☑6ᵗʰ **T86.85** **Complication of intestine transplant**
    T86.850 **Intestine transplant rejection** `CC`
        CC Excl: CC with 7th character A: D47.Z1, D78.81-D78.89, E89.810-E89.89, H59.011-H59.019, H59.031-H59.099, H59.811-H59.89, H95.811-H95.89, I97.3, M96.89, N98.1-N98.9, T86.850-T86.859, T86.90-T86.99

    T86.851 **Intestine transplant failure** `CC`
        CC Excl: See code: T86.850

    T86.852 **Intestine transplant infection** `CC`
        Use additional code to specify infection
        CC Excl: See code: T86.850

    T86.858 **Other complications of intestine transplant** `CC`
        CC Excl: See code: T86.850

    T86.859 **Unspecified complication of intestine transplant** `CC`
        CC Excl: See code: T86.850

  ☑6ᵗʰ **T86.89** **Complications of other transplanted tissue**
    Transplant failure or rejection of pancreas

    T86.890 **Other transplanted tissue rejection** `CC`
        CC Excl: CC with 7th character A: D78.81-D78.89, E89.810-E89.89, H59.011-H59.019, H59.031-H59.099, H59.811-H59.89, H95.811-H95.89, I97.3, M96.89, N98.1-N98.9, T86.890-T86.899

    T86.891 **Other transplanted tissue failure** `CC`
        CC Excl: See code: T86.890

    T86.892 **Other transplanted tissue infection** `CC`
        Use additional code to specify infection
        CC Excl: See code: T86.890

    T86.898 **Other complications of other transplanted tissue** `CC`
        CC Excl: See code: T86.890

    T86.899 **Unspecified complication of other transplanted tissue** `CC`
        CC Excl: See code: T86.890

☑5ᵗʰ **T86.9** **Complication of unspecified transplanted organ and tissue**

    T86.90 **Unspecified complication of unspecified transplanted organ and tissue** `CC`
        CC Excl: CC with 7th character A: D47.Z1, D78.81-D78.89, E89.810-E89.89, H59.011-H59.019, H59.031-H59.099, H59.811-H59.89, H95.811-H95.89, I97.3, M96.89, N98.1-N98.9, T86.850-T86.859, T86.90-T86.99

    T86.91 **Unspecified transplanted organ and tissue rejection** `CC`
        CC Excl: See code: T86.90

    T86.92 **Unspecified transplanted organ and tissue failure** `CC`
        CC Excl: See code: T86.90

    T86.93 **Unspecified transplanted organ and tissue infection** `CC`
        Use additional code to specify infection
        CC Excl: See code: T86.90

☑ Additional Character Required   ☑x7ᵗʰ Xtension Alert   Unacceptable PDx   Manifestation   Hospital Acquired Condition   *EXCLUDES 1* Not Coded Here   *EXCLUDES 2* Not Included Here

ICD-10-CM Draft (2015)   1107

T86.99   Other complications of unspecified transplanted organ and tissue   `CC`
      CC Excl: See code: T86.90

✓4ᵗʰ **T87**   **Complications peculiar to reattachment and amputation**

✓5ᵗʰ **T87.0**   Complications of reattached (part of) upper extremity

✓6ᵗʰ **T87.0X**   Complications of reattached (part of) upper extremity

     CC Excl: For CC codes in subcategory T87.0X: CC with 7th character A, unless otherwise noted: D78.81-D78.89, E36.8, E89.810-E89.89, H59.011-H59.019, H59.031-H59.099, H59.811-H59.89, H95.811-H95.89, I97.3, L76.81-L76.82, M96.89, N98.1-N98.9, T81.82XA, T81.89X-T81.9XX with 7th A, T87.0X1-T87.0X9

T87.0X1   Complications of reattached (part of) right upper extremity   `CC`

T87.0X2   Complications of reattached (part of) left upper extremity   `CC`

T87.0X9   Complications of reattached (part of) unspecified upper extremity   `CC`

✓5ᵗʰ **T87.1**   Complications of reattached (part of) lower extremity

✓6ᵗʰ **T87.1X**   Complications of reattached (part of) lower extremity

     CC Excl: For CC codes in subcategory T87.1X: CC with 7th character A, unless otherwise noted: D78.81-D78.89, E36.8, E89.810-E89.89, H59.011-H59.019, H59.031-H59.099, H59.811-H59.89, H95.811-H95.89, I97.3, L76.81-L76.82, M96.89, N98.1-N98.9, T81.82XA, T81.89X-T81.9XX with 7th A, T87.1X1-T87.1X9

T87.1X1   Complications of reattached (part of) right lower extremity   `CC`

T87.1X2   Complications of reattached (part of) left lower extremity   `CC`

T87.1X9   Complications of reattached (part of) unspecified lower extremity   `CC`

T87.2   Complications of other reattached body part   `CC`
     CC Excl: CC with 7th character A: D78.81-D78.89, E36.8, E89.810-E89.89, H59.011-H59.019, H59.031-H59.099, H59.811-H59.89, H95.811-H95.89, I97.3, L76.81-L76.82, M96.89, N98.1-N98.9, T81.82XA, T81.89X-T81.9XX with 7th A, T87.2

✓5ᵗʰ **T87.3**   Neuroma of amputation stump

T87.30   Neuroma of amputation stump, unspecified extremity

T87.31   Neuroma of amputation stump, right upper extremity

T87.32   Neuroma of amputation stump, left upper extremity

T87.33   Neuroma of amputation stump, right lower extremity

T87.34   Neuroma of amputation stump, left lower extremity

✓5ᵗʰ **T87.4**   Infection of amputation stump

     CC Excl: For CC codes in subcategory T87.4: CC with 7th character A, unless otherwise noted: D78.81-D78.89, E36.8, E89.810-E89.89, H59.011-H59.019, H59.031-H59.099, H59.811-H59.89, H95.811-H95.89, I97.3, L76.81-L76.82, M96.89, N98.1-N98.9, T81.82XA, T81.89X-T81.9XX with 7th A, T87.40-T87.9

T87.40   Infection of amputation stump, unspecified extremity   `CC`

T87.41   Infection of amputation stump, right upper extremity   `CC`

T87.42   Infection of amputation stump, left upper extremity   `CC`

T87.43   Infection of amputation stump, right lower extremity   `CC`

T87.44   Infection of amputation stump, left lower extremity   `CC`

✓5ᵗʰ **T87.5**   Necrosis of amputation stump

T87.50   Necrosis of amputation stump, unspecified extremity

T87.51   Necrosis of amputation stump, right upper extremity

T87.52   Necrosis of amputation stump, left upper extremity

T87.53   Necrosis of amputation stump, right lower extremity

T87.54   Necrosis of amputation stump, left lower extremity

✓5ᵗʰ **T87.8**   Other complications of amputation stump

T87.81   Dehiscence of amputation stump

T87.89   Other complications of amputation stump
     Amputation stump contracture
     Amputation stump contracture of next proximal joint
     Amputation stump flexion
     Amputation stump edema
     Amputation stump hematoma
     EXCLUDES 2   phantom limb syndrome (G54.6-G54.7)

T87.9   Unspecified complications of amputation stump

✓4ᵗʰ **T88**   **Other complications of surgical and medical care, not elsewhere classified**

     EXCLUDES 2   complication following infusion, transfusion and therapeutic injection (T80.-)
        complication following procedure NEC (T81.-)
        complications of anesthesia in labor and delivery (O74.-)
        complications of anesthesia in pregnancy (O29.-)
        complications of anesthesia in puerperium (O89.-)
        complications of devices, implants and grafts (T82-T85)
        complications of obstetric surgery and procedure (O75.4)
        dermatitis due to drugs and medicaments (L23.3, L24.4, L25.1, L27.0-L27.1)
        poisoning and toxic effects of drugs and chemicals (T36-T65 with fifth or sixth character 1-4 or 6)
        specified complications classified elsewhere

     The appropriate 7th character is to be added to each code from category T88.
     A   initial encounter
     D   subsequent encounter
     S   sequela

✓x7ᵗʰ **T88.0**   Infection following immunization   `CC`
     Sepsis following immunization
     CC Excl: CC with 7th character A: N98.0, T80.211-T80.29X with 7th A, T82.7XXA, T88.0XXA

✓x7ᵗʰ **T88.1**   Other complications following immunization, not elsewhere classified   `CC`
     Generalized vaccinia
     Rash following immunization
     EXCLUDES 1   vaccinia not from vaccine (B08.011)
     EXCLUDES 2   anaphylactic shock due to serum (T80.5-)
        other serum reactions (T80.6-)
        postimmunization arthropathy (M02.2)
        postimmunization encephalitis (G04.02)
        postimmunization fever (R50.83)
     CC Excl: CC with 7th character A: T88.1X

✓x7ᵗʰ **T88.2**   Shock due to anesthesia   `CC`
     Use additional code for adverse effect, if applicable, to identify drug (T41.- with fifth or sixth character 5)
     EXCLUDES 1   complications of anesthesia (in):
        labor and delivery (O74.-)
        postprocedural shock NOS (T81.1-)
        pregnancy (O29.-)
        puerperium (O89.-)
     CC Excl: CC with 7th character A: D78.01-D78.02, D78.21-D78.89, E36.01-E36.02, E36.8, E89.810-E89.89, G97.51-G97.52, H59.011-H59.019, H59.031-H59.129, H59.311-H59.329, H59.811-H59.89, H95.21-H95.22, H95.41-H95.89, I97.3-I97.42, I97.610-I97.62, J95.61-J95.62, J95.830-J95.831, K91.61-K91.62, K91.840-K91.841, L76.01-L76.02, L76.21-L76.82, M96.810-M96.811, M96.830-M96.89, N98.1-N98.9, N99.61-N99.62, N99.820-N99.821, T79.4XXA, T81.10X-T81.19X with 7th A, T81.82XA, T81.89X-T81.9XX with 7th A, T88.2XXA

✓x7ᵗʰ **T88.3**   Malignant hyperthermia due to anesthesia   `CC`
     Use additional code for adverse effect, if applicable, to identify drug (T41.- with fifth or sixth character 5)
     CC Excl: CC with 7th character A: D78.01-D78.02, D78.21-D78.89, E36.01-E36.02, E36.8, E89.810-E89.89, G97.51-G97.52, H59.011-H59.019, H59.031-H59.129, H59.311-H59.329, H59.811-H59.89, H95.21-H95.22, H95.41-H95.89, I97.3-I97.42, I97.610-I97.62, J95.61-J95.62, J95.830-J95.831, K91.61-K91.62, K91.840-K91.841, L76.01-L76.02, L76.21-L76.82, M96.810-M96.811, M96.830-M96.89, N98.1-N98.9, N99.61-N99.62, N99.820-N99.821, T79.4XXA, T81.10X-T81.19X with 7th A, T81.82XA, T81.89X-T81.9XX with 7th A, T88.2XX-T88.3XX with 7th A

12   ✓x7ᵗʰ **T88.4**   **Failed or difficult intubation**

---

12 Unacceptable PDx = initial encounter only (7th character A).

N Newborn: 0   P Pediatric: 0-17   M Maternity: 12-55   A Adult: 15-124   MCC Major CC Condition   PDx MCC PDx acts as own MCC   CC CC Condition   PDx CC PDx acts as own CC

1108   ICD-10-CM Draft (2015)

√5ᵗʰ **T88.5 Other complications of anesthesia**
Use additional code for adverse effect, if applicable, to identify drug (T41.- with fifth or sixth character 5)

√x7ᵗʰ **T88.51 Hypothermia following anesthesia**

√x7ᵗʰ **T88.52 Failed moderate sedation during procedure**
Failed conscious sedation during procedure
EXCLUDES 2 *personal history of failed moderate sedation (Z92.83)*

√x7ᵗʰ **T88.59 Other complications of anesthesia**

√x7ᵗʰ **T88.6 Anaphylactic reaction due to adverse effect of correct drug or medicament properly administered**   CC
Anaphylactic shock due to adverse effect of correct drug or medicament properly administered
Anaphylactoid reaction NOS
Use additional code for adverse effect, if applicable, to identify drug (T41.- with fifth or sixth character 5)
EXCLUDES 1 *anaphylactic reaction due to serum (T80.5-)*
anaphylactic shock or reaction due to adverse food reaction (T78.0-)
CC Excl: CC with 7th character A: T78.00X-T78.09X with 7th A

12 √x7ᵗʰ **T88.7 Unspecified adverse effect of drug or medicament**
Drug hypersensitivity NOS
Drug reaction NOS
Use additional code for adverse effect, if applicable, to identify drug (T41.- with fifth or sixth character 5)
EXCLUDES 1 *specified adverse effects of drugs and medicaments (A00-R94 and T80-T88.6, T88.8)*

12 √x7ᵗʰ **T88.8 Other specified complications of surgical and medical care, not elsewhere classified**
Use additional code to identify the complication

12 √x7ᵗʰ **T88.9 Complication of surgical and medical care, unspecified**

✓ Additional Character Required   √x7ᵗʰ Xtension Alert   Unacceptable PDx   Manifestation   Hospital Acquired Condition   *EXCLUDES 1* Not Coded Here   *EXCLUDES 2* Not Included Here

External Causes of Morbidity

V00–V00.158

Chapter 20. External Causes of Morbidity (V00-Y99)

NOTE This chapter permits the classification of environmental events and circumstances as the cause of injury, and other adverse effects. Where a code from this section is applicable, it is intended that it shall be used secondary to a code from another chapter of the Classification indicating the nature of the condition. Most often, the condition will be classifiable to Chapter 19, Injury, poisoning and certain other consequences of external causes (S00-T88). Other conditions that may be stated to be due to external causes are classified in Chapters I to XVIII. For these conditions, codes from Chapter 20 should be used to provide additional information as to the cause of the condition.

This chapter contains the following blocks:

V00-V09	Pedestrian injured in transport accident
V10-V19	Pedal cycle rider injured in transport accident
V20-V29	Motorcycle rider injured in transport accident
V30-V39	Occupant of three-wheeled motor vehicle injured in transport accident
V40-V49	Car occupant injured in transport accident
V50-V59	Occupant of pick-up truck or van injured in transport accident
V60-V69	Occupant of heavy transport vehicle injured in transport accident
V70-V79	Bus occupant injured in transport accident
V80-V89	Other land transport accidents
V90-V94	Water transport accidents
V95-V97	Air and space transport accidents
V98-V99	Other and unspecified transport accidents
W00-X58	Other external causes of accidental injury
W00-W19	Slipping, tripping, stumbling and falls
W20-W49	Exposure to inanimate mechanical forces
W50-W64	Exposure to animate mechanical forces
W65-W74	Accidental non-transport drowning and submersion
W85-W99	Exposure to electric current, radiation and extreme ambient air temperature and pressure
X00-X08	Exposure to smoke, fire and flames
X10-X19	Contact with heat and hot substances
X30-X39	Exposure to forces of nature
X52, X58	Accidental exposure to other specified factors
X71-X83	Intentional self-harm
X92-Y08	Assault
Y21-Y33	Event of undetermined intent
Y35-Y38	Legal intervention, operations of war, military operations, and terrorism
Y62-Y84	Complications of medical and surgical care
Y62-Y69	Misadventures to patients during surgical and medical care
Y70-Y82	Medical devices associated with adverse incidents in diagnostic and therapeutic use
Y83-Y84	Surgical and other medical procedures as the cause of abnormal reaction of the patient, or of later complication, without mention of misadventure at the time of the procedure
Y90-Y99	Supplementary factors related to causes of morbidity classified elsewhere

Accidents (V00-X58)

Transport accidents (V00-V99)

Use additional code to identify:
    airbag injury (W22.1)
    type of street or road (Y92.4-)
    use of cellular telephone and other electronic equipment at the time of the transport accident (Y93.C-)

EXCLUDES 1 *agricultural vehicles in stationary use or maintenance (W31.-)*
assault by crashing of motor vehicle (Y03.-)
automobile or motor cycle in stationary use or maintenance—code to type of accident
crashing of motor vehicle, undetermined intent (Y32)
intentional self-harm by crashing of motor vehicle (X82)

EXCLUDES 2 *transport accidents due to cataclysm (X34-X38)*

This section is structured in 12 groups. Those relating to land transport accidents (V01-V89) reflect the victim's mode of transport and are subdivided to identify the victim's 'counterpart' or the type of event. The vehicle of which the injured person is an occupant is identified in the first two characters since it is seen as the most important factor to identify for prevention purposes. A transport accident is one in which the vehicle involved must be moving or running or in use for transport purposes at the time of the accident.

Pedestrian injured in transport accident (V00-V09)

INCLUDES person changing tire on transport vehicle
person examining engine of vehicle broken down in (on side of) road

EXCLUDES 1 *fall due to non-transport collision with other person (W03)*
pedestrian on foot falling (slipping) on ice and snow (W00.-)
struck or bumped by another person (W51)

✓4th **V00** **Pedestrian conveyance accident**

Use additional place of occurrence and activity external cause codes, if known (Y92-, Y93-)

EXCLUDES 1 *collision with another person without fall (W51)*
fall due to person on foot colliding with another person on foot (W03)
fall from non-moving wheelchair, nonmotorized scooter and motorized mobility scooter without collision (W05.-)
pedestrian (conveyance) collision with other land transport vehicle (V01-V09)
pedestrian on foot falling (slipping) on ice and snow (W00.-)

The appropriate 7th character is to be added to each code from category V00.
A   initial encounter
D   subsequent encounter
S   sequela

✓5th **V00.0** **Pedestrian on foot injured in collision with pedestrian conveyance**

    ✓x7th **V00.01** **Pedestrian on foot injured in collision with roller-skater**

    ✓x7th **V00.02** **Pedestrian on foot injured in collision with skateboarder**

    ✓x7th **V00.09** **Pedestrian on foot injured in collision with other pedestrian conveyance**

✓5th **V00.1** **Rolling-type pedestrian conveyance accident**

    EXCLUDES 1 *accident with babystroller (V00.82-)*
accident with motorized mobility scooter (V00.83-)
accident with wheelchair (powered) (V00.81-)

    ✓6th **V00.11** **In-line roller-skate accident**

        ✓7th **V00.111** **Fall from in-line roller-skates**

        ✓7th **V00.112** **In-line roller-skater colliding with stationary object**

        ✓7th **V00.118** **Other in-line roller-skate accident**
            EXCLUDES 1 *roller-skater collision with other land transport vehicle (V01-V09 with 5th character 1)*

    ✓6th **V00.12** **Non-in- line roller-skate accident**

        ✓7th **V00.121** **Fall from non-in-line roller-skates**

        ✓7th **V00.122** **Non-in-line roller-skater colliding with stationary object**

        ✓7th **V00.128** **Other non-in-line roller-skating accident**
            EXCLUDES 1 *roller-skater collision with other land transport vehicle (V01-V09 with 5th character 1)*

    ✓6th **V00.13** **Skateboard accident**

        ✓7th **V00.131** **Fall from skateboard**

        ✓7th **V00.132** **Skateboarder colliding with stationary object**

        ✓7th **V00.138** **Other skateboard accident**
            EXCLUDES 1 *skateboarder collision with other land transport vehicle (V01-V09 with 5th character 2)*

    ✓6th **V00.14** **Scooter (nonmotorized) accident**
        EXCLUDES 1 *motorscooter accident (V20-V29)*

        ✓7th **V00.141** **Fall from scooter (nonmotorized)**

        ✓7th **V00.142** **Scooter (nonmotorized) colliding with stationary object**

        ✓7th **V00.148** **Other scooter (nonmotorized) accident**
            EXCLUDES 1 *scooter (nonmotorized) collision with other land transport vehicle (V01-V09 with fifth character 9)*

    ✓6th **V00.15** **Heelies accident**
        Rolling shoe
        Wheeled shoe
        Wheelies accident

        ✓7th **V00.151** **Fall from heelies**

        ✓7th **V00.152** **Heelies colliding with stationary object**

        ✓7th **V00.158** **Other heelies accident**

N Newborn: 0   **P** Pediatric: 0-17   **M** Maternity: 12-55   **A** Adult: 15-124   **MCC** Major CC Condition   **PDx MCC** PDx acts as own MCC   **CC** CC Condition   **PDx CC** PDx acts as own CC

1110   ICD-10-CM Draft (2015)

External Causes of Morbidity
V00.18–V01.12

☑6ᵗʰ V00.18 Accident on other rolling-type pedestrian conveyance
- ☑7ᵗʰ **V00.181** Fall from other rolling-type pedestrian conveyance
- ☑7ᵗʰ **V00.182** Pedestrian on other rolling-type pedestrian conveyance colliding with stationary object
- ☑7ᵗʰ **V00.188** Other accident on other rolling-type pedestrian conveyance

☑5ᵗʰ V00.2 Gliding-type pedestrian conveyance accident

☑6ᵗʰ V00.21 Ice-skates accident
- ☑7ᵗʰ **V00.211** Fall from ice-skates
- ☑7ᵗʰ **V00.212** Ice-skater colliding with stationary object
- ☑7ᵗʰ **V00.218** Other ice-skates accident
  - EXCLUDES 1 ice-skater collision with other land transport vehicle (V01-V09 with 5th digit 9)

☑6ᵗʰ V00.22 Sled accident
- ☑7ᵗʰ **V00.221** Fall from sled
- ☑7ᵗʰ **V00.222** Sledder colliding with stationary object
- ☑7ᵗʰ **V00.228** Other sled accident
  - EXCLUDES 1 sled collision with other land transport vehicle (V01-V09 with 5th digit 9)

☑6ᵗʰ V00.28 Other gliding-type pedestrian conveyance accident
- ☑7ᵗʰ **V00.281** Fall from other gliding-type pedestrian conveyance
- ☑7ᵗʰ **V00.282** Pedestrian on other gliding-type pedestrian conveyance colliding with stationary object
- ☑7ᵗʰ **V00.288** Other accident on other gliding-type pedestrian conveyance
  - EXCLUDES 1 gliding-type pedestrian conveyance collision with other land transport vehicle (V01-V09 with 5th digit 9)

☑5ᵗʰ V00.3 Flat-bottomed pedestrian conveyance accident

☑6ᵗʰ V00.31 Snowboard accident
- ☑7ᵗʰ **V00.311** Fall from snowboard
- ☑7ᵗʰ **V00.312** Snowboarder colliding with stationary object
- ☑7ᵗʰ **V00.318** Other snowboard accident
  - EXCLUDES 1 snowboarder collision with other land transport vehicle (V01-V09 with 5th digit 9)

☑6ᵗʰ V00.32 Snow-ski accident
- ☑7ᵗʰ **V00.321** Fall from snow-skis
- ☑7ᵗʰ **V00.322** Snow-skier colliding with stationary object
- ☑7ᵗʰ **V00.328** Other snow-ski accident
  - EXCLUDES 1 snow-skier collision with other land transport vehicle (V01-V09 with 5th digit 9)

☑6ᵗʰ V00.38 Other flat-bottomed pedestrian conveyance accident
- ☑7ᵗʰ **V00.381** Fall from other flat-bottomed pedestrian conveyance
- ☑7ᵗʰ **V00.382** Pedestrian on other flat-bottomed pedestrian conveyance colliding with stationary object
- ☑7ᵗʰ **V00.388** Other accident on other flat-bottomed pedestrian conveyance

☑5ᵗʰ V00.8 Accident on other pedestrian conveyance

☑6ᵗʰ V00.81 Accident with wheelchair (powered)
- ☑7ᵗʰ **V00.811** Fall from moving wheelchair (powered)
  - EXCLUDES 1 fall from non-moving wheelchair (W05.0)
- ☑7ᵗʰ **V00.812** Wheelchair (powered) colliding with stationary object
- ☑7ᵗʰ **V00.818** Other accident with wheelchair (powered)

☑6ᵗʰ V00.82 Accident with babystroller
- ☑7ᵗʰ **V00.821** Fall from babystroller
- ☑7ᵗʰ **V00.822** Babystroller colliding with stationary object
- ☑7ᵗʰ **V00.828** Other accident with babystroller

☑6ᵗʰ V00.83 Accident with motorized mobility scooter
- **V00.831** Fall from motorized mobility scooter
  - EXCLUDES 1 fall from non-moving motorized mobility scooter (W05.2)
- **V00.832** Motorized mobility scooter colliding with stationary object
- **V00.838** Other accident with motorized mobility scooter

☑6ᵗʰ V00.89 Accident on other pedestrian conveyance
- ☑7ᵗʰ **V00.891** Fall from other pedestrian conveyance
- ☑7ᵗʰ **V00.892** Pedestrian on other pedestrian conveyance colliding with stationary object
- ☑7ᵗʰ **V00.898** Other accident on other pedestrian conveyance
  - EXCLUDES 1 other pedestrian (conveyance) collision with other land transport vehicle (V01-V09 with 5th digit 9)

☑4ᵗʰ V01 Pedestrian injured in collision with pedal cycle

The appropriate 7th character is to be added to each code from category V01.
A   initial encounter
D   subsequent encounter
S   sequela

☑5ᵗʰ V01.0 Pedestrian injured in collision with pedal cycle in nontraffic accident
- ☑x7ᵗʰ **V01.00** Pedestrian on foot injured in collision with pedal cycle in nontraffic accident
  - Pedestrian NOS injured in collision with pedal cycle in nontraffic accident
- ☑x7ᵗʰ **V01.01** Pedestrian on roller-skates injured in collision with pedal cycle in nontraffic accident
- ☑x7ᵗʰ **V01.02** Pedestrian on skateboard injured in collision with pedal cycle in nontraffic accident
- ☑x7ᵗʰ **V01.09** Pedestrian with other conveyance injured in collision with pedal cycle in nontraffic accident
  - Pedestrian with babystroller injured in collision with pedal cycle in nontraffic accident
  - Pedestrian on ice-skates injured in collision with pedal cycle in nontraffic accident
  - Pedestrian on nonmotorized scooter injured in collision with pedal cycle in nontraffic accident
  - Pedestrian on sled injured in collision with pedal cycle in nontraffic accident
  - Pedestrian on snowboard injured in collision with pedal cycle in nontraffic accident
  - Pedestrian on snow-skis injured in collision with pedal cycle in nontraffic accident
  - Pedestrian in wheelchair (powered) injured in collision with pedal cycle in nontraffic accident
  - Pedestrian in motorized mobility scooter injured in collision with pedal cycle in nontraffic accident

☑5ᵗʰ V01.1 Pedestrian injured in collision with pedal cycle in traffic accident
- ☑x7ᵗʰ **V01.10** Pedestrian on foot injured in collision with pedal cycle in traffic accident
  - Pedestrian NOS injured in collision with pedal cycle in traffic accident
- ☑x7ᵗʰ **V01.11** Pedestrian on roller-skates injured in collision with pedal cycle in traffic accident
- ☑x7ᵗʰ **V01.12** Pedestrian on skateboard injured in collision with pedal cycle in traffic accident

External Causes of Morbidity

V01.19–V02.92

√x7ᵗʰ **V01.19 Pedestrian with other conveyance injured in collision with pedal cycle in traffic accident**
Pedestrian with babystroller injured in collision with pedal cycle in traffic accident
Pedestrian on ice-skates injured in collision with pedal cycle in traffic accident
Pedestrian on nonmotorized scooter injured in collision with pedal cycle in traffic accident
Pedestrian on sled injured in collision with pedal cycle in traffic accident
Pedestrian on snowboard injured in collision with pedal cycle in traffic accident
Pedestrian on snow-skis injured in collision with pedal cycle in traffic accident
Pedestrian in wheelchair (powered) injured in collision with pedal cycle in traffic accident
Pedestrian in motorized mobility scooter injured in collision with pedal cycle in traffic accident

√5ᵗʰ **V01.9 Pedestrian injured in collision with pedal cycle, unspecified whether traffic or nontraffic accident**

√x7ᵗʰ **V01.90 Pedestrian on foot injured in collision with pedal cycle, unspecified whether traffic or nontraffic accident**
Pedestrian NOS injured in collision with pedal cycle, unspecified whether traffic or nontraffic accident

√x7ᵗʰ **V01.91 Pedestrian on roller-skates injured in collision with pedal cycle, unspecified whether traffic or nontraffic accident**

√x7ᵗʰ **V01.92 Pedestrian on skateboard injured in collision with pedal cycle, unspecified whether traffic or nontraffic accident**

√x7ᵗʰ **V01.99 Pedestrian with other conveyance injured in collision with pedal cycle, unspecified whether traffic or nontraffic accident**
Pedestrian with babystroller injured in collision with pedal cycle, unspecified whether traffic or nontraffic accident
Pedestrian on ice-skates injured in collision with pedal cycle unspecified, whether traffic or nontraffic accident
Pedestrian on nonmotorized scooter injured in collision with pedal cycle, unspecified whether traffic or nontraffic accident
Pedestrian on sled injured in collision with pedal cycle unspecified, whether traffic or nontraffic accident
Pedestrian on snowboard injured in collision with pedal cycle, unspecified whether traffic or nontraffic accident
Pedestrian on snow-skis injured in collision with pedal cycle, unspecified whether traffic or nontraffic accident
Pedestrian in wheelchair (powered) injured in collision with pedal cycle, unspecified whether traffic or nontraffic accident
Pedestrian in motorized mobility scooter injured in collision with pedal cycle, unspecified whether traffic or nontraffic accident

√4ᵗʰ **V02 Pedestrian injured in collision with two- or three-wheeled motor vehicle**

> The appropriate 7th character is to be added to each code from category V02.
> A   initial encounter
> D   subsequent encounter
> S   sequela

√5ᵗʰ **V02.0 Pedestrian injured in collision with two- or three-wheeled motor vehicle in nontraffic accident**

√x7ᵗʰ **V02.00 Pedestrian on foot injured in collision with two- or three-wheeled motor vehicle in nontraffic accident**
Pedestrian NOS injured in collision with two- or three-wheeled motor vehicle in nontraffic accident

√x7ᵗʰ **V02.01 Pedestrian on roller-skates injured in collision with two- or three-wheeled motor vehicle in nontraffic accident**

√x7ᵗʰ **V02.02 Pedestrian on skateboard injured in collision with two- or three-wheeled motor vehicle in nontraffic accident**

√x7ᵗʰ **V02.09 Pedestrian with other conveyance injured in collision with two- or three-wheeled motor vehicle in nontraffic accident**
Pedestrian with babystroller injured in collision with two- or three-wheeled motor vehicle in nontraffic accident
Pedestrian on ice-skates injured in collision with two- or three-wheeled motor vehicle in nontraffic accident
Pedestrian on nonmotorized scooter injured in collision with two- or three-wheeled motor vehicle in nontraffic accident
Pedestrian on sled injured in collision with two- or three-wheeled motor vehicle in nontraffic accident
Pedestrian on snowboard injured in collision with two- or three-wheeled motor vehicle in nontraffic accident
Pedestrian on snow-skis injured in collision with two- or three-wheeled motor vehicle in nontraffic accident
Pedestrian in wheelchair (powered) injured in collision with two- or three-wheeled motor vehicle in nontraffic accident
Pedestrian in motorized mobility scooter injured in collision with two- or three-wheeled motor vehicle in nontraffic accident

√5ᵗʰ **V02.1 Pedestrian injured in collision with two- or three-wheeled motor vehicle in traffic accident**

√x7ᵗʰ **V02.10 Pedestrian on foot injured in collision with two- or three-wheeled motor vehicle in traffic accident**
Pedestrian NOS injured in collision with two- or three-wheeled motor vehicle in traffic accident

√x7ᵗʰ **V02.11 Pedestrian on roller-skates injured in collision with two- or three-wheeled motor vehicle in traffic accident**

√x7ᵗʰ **V02.12 Pedestrian on skateboard injured in collision with two- or three-wheeled motor vehicle in traffic accident**

√x7ᵗʰ **V02.19 Pedestrian with other conveyance injured in collision with two- or three-wheeled motor vehicle in traffic accident**
Pedestrian with babystroller injured in collision with two- or three-wheeled motor vehicle in traffic accident
Pedestrian on ice-skates injured in collision with two- or three-wheeled motor vehicle in traffic accident
Pedestrian on nonmotorized scooter injured in collision with two- or three-wheeled motor vehicle in traffic accident
Pedestrian on sled injured in collision with two- or three-wheeled motor vehicle in traffic accident
Pedestrian on snowboard injured in collision with two- or three-wheeled motor vehicle in traffic accident
Pedestrian on snow-skis injured in collision with two- or three-wheeled motor vehicle in traffic accident
Pedestrian in wheelchair (powered) injured in collision with two- or three-wheeled motor vehicle in traffic accident
Pedestrian in motorized mobility scooter injured in collision with two- or three-wheeled motor vehicle in traffic accident

√5ᵗʰ **V02.9 Pedestrian injured in collision with two- or three-wheeled motor vehicle, unspecified whether traffic or nontraffic accident**

√x7ᵗʰ **V02.90 Pedestrian on foot injured in collision with two- or three-wheeled motor vehicle, unspecified whether traffic or nontraffic accident**
Pedestrian NOS injured in collision with two- or three-wheeled motor vehicle, unspecified whether traffic or nontraffic accident

√x7ᵗʰ **V02.91 Pedestrian on roller-skates injured in collision with two- or three-wheeled motor vehicle, unspecified whether traffic or nontraffic accident**

√x7ᵗʰ **V02.92 Pedestrian on skateboard injured in collision with two- or three-wheeled motor vehicle, unspecified whether traffic or nontraffic accident**

√x7th **V02.99** **Pedestrian with other conveyance injured in collision with two- or three-wheeled motor vehicle, unspecified whether traffic or nontraffic accident**

Pedestrian with babystroller injured in collision with two- or three-wheeled motor vehicle, unspecified whether traffic or nontraffic accident

Pedestrian on ice-skates injured in collision with two- or three-wheeled motor vehicle, unspecified whether traffic or nontraffic accident

Pedestrian on nonmotorized scooter injured in collision with two- or three-wheeled motor vehicle, unspecified whether traffic or nontraffic accident

Pedestrian on sled injured in collision with two- or three-wheeled motor vehicle, unspecified whether traffic or nontraffic accident

Pedestrian on snowboard injured in collision with two- or three-wheeled motor vehicle, unspecified whether traffic or nontraffic accident

Pedestrian on snow-skis injured in collision with two- or three-wheeled motor vehicle, unspecified whether traffic or nontraffic accident

Pedestrian in wheelchair (powered) injured in collision with two- or three-wheeled motor vehicle, unspecified whether traffic or nontraffic accident

Pedestrian in motorized mobility scooter injured in collision with two- or three-wheeled motor vehicle, unspecified whether traffic or nontraffic accident

√4th **V03** **Pedestrian injured in collision with car, pick-up truck or van**

> The appropriate 7th character is to be added to each code from category V03.
> A   initial encounter
> D   subsequent encounter
> S   sequela

√5th **V03.0** **Pedestrian injured in collision with car, pick-up truck or van in nontraffic accident**

√x7th **V03.00** **Pedestrian on foot injured in collision with car, pick-up truck or van in nontraffic accident**

Pedestrian NOS injured in collision with car, pick-up truck or van in nontraffic accident

√x7th **V03.01** **Pedestrian on roller-skates injured in collision with car, pick-up truck or van in nontraffic accident**

√x7th **V03.02** **Pedestrian on skateboard injured in collision with car, pick-up truck or van in nontraffic accident**

√x7th **V03.09** **Pedestrian with other conveyance injured in collision with car, pick-up truck or van in nontraffic accident**

Pedestrian with babystroller injured in collision with car, pick-up truck or van in nontraffic accident

Pedestrian on ice-skates injured in collision with car, pick-up truck or van in nontraffic accident

Pedestrian on nonmotorized scooter injured in collision with car, pick-up truck or van in nontraffic accident

Pedestrian on sled injured in collision with car, pick-up truck or van in nontraffic accident

Pedestrian on snowboard injured in collision with car, pick-up truck or van in nontraffic accident

Pedestrian on snow-skis injured in collision with car, pick-up truck or van in nontraffic accident

Pedestrian in wheelchair (powered) injured in collision with car, pick-up truck or van in nontraffic accident

Pedestrian in motorized mobility scooter injured in collision with car, pick-up truck or van in nontraffic accident

√5th **V03.1** **Pedestrian injured in collision with car, pick-up truck or van in traffic accident**

√x7th **V03.10** **Pedestrian on foot injured in collision with car, pick-up truck or van in traffic accident**

Pedestrian NOS injured in collision with car, pick-up truck or van in traffic accident

√x7th **V03.11** **Pedestrian on roller-skates injured in collision with car, pick-up truck or van in traffic accident**

√x7th **V03.12** **Pedestrian on skateboard injured in collision with car, pick-up truck or van in traffic accident**

√x7th **V03.19** **Pedestrian with other conveyance injured in collision with car, pick-up truck or van in traffic accident**

Pedestrian with babystroller injured in collision with car, pick-up truck or van in traffic accident

Pedestrian on ice-skates injured in collision with car, pick-up truck or van in traffic accident

Pedestrian on nonmotorized scooter injured in collision with car, pick-up truck or van in traffic accident

Pedestrian on sled injured in collision with car, pick-up truck or van in traffic accident

Pedestrian on snowboard injured in collision with car, pick-up truck or van in traffic accident

Pedestrian on snow-skis injured in collision with car, pick-up truck or van in traffic accident

Pedestrian in wheelchair (powered) injured in collision with car, pick-up truck or van in traffic accident

Pedestrian in motorized mobility scooter injured in collision with car, pick-up truck or van in traffic accident

√5th **V03.9** **Pedestrian injured in collision with car, pick-up truck or van, unspecified whether traffic or nontraffic accident**

√x7th **V03.90** **Pedestrian on foot injured in collision with car, pick-up truck or van, unspecified whether traffic or nontraffic accident**

Pedestrian NOS injured in collision with car, pick-up truck or van, unspecified whether traffic or nontraffic accident

√x7th **V03.91** **Pedestrian on roller-skates injured in collision with car, pick-up truck or van, unspecified whether traffic or nontraffic accident**

√x7th **V03.92** **Pedestrian on skateboard injured in collision with car, pick-up truck or van, unspecified whether traffic or nontraffic accident**

√x7th **V03.99** **Pedestrian with other conveyance injured in collision with car, pick-up truck or van, unspecified whether traffic or nontraffic accident**

Pedestrian with babystroller injured in collision with car, pick-up truck or van, unspecified whether traffic or nontraffic accident

Pedestrian on ice-skates injured in collision with car, pick-up truck or van, unspecified whether traffic or nontraffic accident

Pedestrian on nonmotorized scooter injured in collision with car, pick-up truck or van, unspecified whether traffic or nontraffic accident

Pedestrian on sled injured in collision with car, pick-up truck or van, unspecified whether traffic or nontraffic accident

Pedestrian on snowboard injured in collision with car, pick-up truck or van, unspecified whether traffic or nontraffic accident

Pedestrian on snow-skis injured in collision with car, pick-up truck or van, unspecified whether traffic or nontraffic accident

Pedestrian in wheelchair (powered) injured in collision with car, pick-up truck or van, unspecified whether traffic or nontraffic accident

Pedestrian in motorized mobility scooter injured in collision with car, pick-up truck or van, unspecified whether traffic or nontraffic accident

√4th **V04** **Pedestrian injured in collision with heavy transport vehicle or bus**

> **EXCLUDES 1**   pedestrian injured in collision with military vehicle (V09.01, V09.21)

> The appropriate 7th character is to be added to each code from category V04.
> A   initial encounter
> D   subsequent encounter
> S   sequela

√5th **V04.0** **Pedestrian injured in collision with heavy transport vehicle or bus in nontraffic accident**

√x7th **V04.00** **Pedestrian on foot injured in collision with heavy transport vehicle or bus in nontraffic accident**

Pedestrian NOS injured in collision with heavy transport vehicle or bus in nontraffic accident

√x7th **V04.01** **Pedestrian on roller-skates injured in collision with heavy transport vehicle or bus in nontraffic accident**

√x7th **V04.02** **Pedestrian on skateboard injured in collision with heavy transport vehicle or bus in nontraffic accident**

☑ Additional Character Required   √x7th Xtension Alert   Unacceptable PDx   Manifestation   Hospital Acquired Condition   **EXCLUDES 1** Not Coded Here   **EXCLUDES 2** Not Included Here

√x7th V04.09 **Pedestrian with other conveyance injured in collision with heavy transport vehicle or bus in nontraffic accident**

Pedestrian with babystroller injured in collision with heavy transport vehicle or bus in nontraffic accident

Pedestrian on ice-skates injured in collision with heavy transport vehicle or bus in nontraffic accident

Pedestrian on nonmotorized scooter injured in collision with heavy transport vehicle or bus in nontraffic accident

Pedestrian on sled injured in collision with heavy transport vehicle or bus in nontraffic accident

Pedestrian on snowboard injured in collision with heavy transport vehicle or bus in nontraffic accident

Pedestrian on snow-skis injured in collision with heavy transport vehicle or bus in nontraffic accident

Pedestrian in wheelchair (powered) injured in collision with heavy transport vehicle or bus in nontraffic accident

Pedestrian in motorized mobility scooter injured in collision with heavy transport vehicle or bus in nontraffic accident

√5th V04.1 **Pedestrian injured in collision with heavy transport vehicle or bus in traffic accident**

√x7th V04.10 **Pedestrian on foot injured in collision with heavy transport vehicle or bus in traffic accident**

Pedestrian NOS injured in collision with heavy transport vehicle or bus in traffic accident

√x7th V04.11 **Pedestrian on roller-skates injured in collision with heavy transport vehicle or bus in traffic accident**

√x7th V04.12 **Pedestrian on skateboard injured in collision with heavy transport vehicle or bus in traffic accident**

√x7th V04.19 **Pedestrian with other conveyance injured in collision with heavy transport vehicle or bus in traffic accident**

Pedestrian with babystroller injured in collision with heavy transport vehicle or bus in traffic accident

Pedestrian on ice-skates injured in collision with heavy transport vehicle or bus in traffic accident

Pedestrian on nonmotorized scooter injured in collision with heavy transport vehicle or bus in traffic accident

Pedestrian on sled injured in collision with heavy transport vehicle or bus in traffic accident

Pedestrian on snowboard injured in collision with heavy transport vehicle or bus in traffic accident

Pedestrian on snow-skis injured in collision with heavy transport vehicle or bus in traffic accident

Pedestrian in wheelchair (powered) injured in collision with heavy transport vehicle or bus in traffic accident

Pedestrian in motorized mobility scooter injured in collision with heavy transport vehicle or bus in traffic accident

√5th V04.9 **Pedestrian injured in collision with heavy transport vehicle or bus, unspecified whether traffic or nontraffic accident**

√x7th V04.90 **Pedestrian on foot injured in collision with heavy transport vehicle or bus, unspecified whether traffic or nontraffic accident**

Pedestrian NOS injured in collision with heavy transport vehicle or bus, unspecified whether traffic or nontraffic accident

√x7th V04.91 **Pedestrian on roller-skates injured in collision with heavy transport vehicle or bus, unspecified whether traffic or nontraffic accident**

√x7th V04.92 **Pedestrian on skateboard injured in collision with heavy transport vehicle or bus, unspecified whether traffic or nontraffic accident**

√x7th V04.99 **Pedestrian with other conveyance injured in collision with heavy transport vehicle or bus, unspecified whether traffic or nontraffic accident**

Pedestrian with babystroller injured in collision with heavy transport vehicle or bus, unspecified whether traffic or nontraffic accident

Pedestrian on ice-skates injured in collision with heavy transport vehicle or bus, unspecified whether traffic or nontraffic accident

Pedestrian on nonmotorized scooter injured in collision with heavy transport vehicle or bus, unspecified whether traffic or nontraffic accident

Pedestrian on sled injured in collision with heavy transport vehicle or bus, unspecified whether traffic or nontraffic accident

Pedestrian on snowboard injured in collision with heavy transport vehicle or bus, unspecified whether traffic or nontraffic accident

Pedestrian on snow-skis injured in collision with heavy transport vehicle or bus, unspecified whether traffic or nontraffic accident

Pedestrian in wheelchair (powered) injured in collision with heavy transport vehicle or bus, unspecified whether traffic or nontraffic accident

Pedestrian in motorized mobility scooter injured in collision with heavy transport vehicle or bus, unspecified whether traffic or nontraffic accident

√4th V05 **Pedestrian injured in collision with railway train or railway vehicle**

The appropriate 7th character is to be added to each code from category V05.
A   initial encounter
D   subsequent encounter
S   sequela

√5th V05.0 **Pedestrian injured in collision with railway train or railway vehicle in nontraffic accident**

√x7th V05.00 **Pedestrian on foot injured in collision with railway train or railway vehicle in nontraffic accident**

Pedestrian NOS injured in collision with railway train or railway vehicle in nontraffic accident

√x7th V05.01 **Pedestrian on roller-skates injured in collision with railway train or railway vehicle in nontraffic accident**

√x7th V05.02 **Pedestrian on skateboard injured in collision with railway train or railway vehicle in nontraffic accident**

√x7th V05.09 **Pedestrian with other conveyance injured in collision with railway train or railway vehicle in nontraffic accident**

Pedestrian with babystroller injured in collision with railway train or railway vehicle in nontraffic accident

Pedestrian on ice-skates injured in collision with railway train or railway vehicle in nontraffic accident

Pedestrian on nonmotorized scooter injured in collision with railway train or railway vehicle in nontraffic accident

Pedestrian on sled injured in collision with railway train or railway vehicle in nontraffic accident

Pedestrian on snowboard injured in collision with railway train or railway vehicle in nontraffic accident

Pedestrian on snow-skis injured in collision with railway train or railway vehicle in nontraffic accident

Pedestrian in wheelchair (powered) injured in collision with railway train or railway vehicle in nontraffic accident

Pedestrian in motorized mobility scooter injured in collision with railway train or railway vehicle in nontraffic accident

√5th V05.1 **Pedestrian injured in collision with railway train or railway vehicle in traffic accident**

√x7th V05.10 **Pedestrian on foot injured in collision with railway train or railway vehicle in traffic accident**

Pedestrian NOS injured in collision with railway train or railway vehicle in traffic accident

√x7th V05.11 **Pedestrian on roller-skates injured in collision with railway train or railway vehicle in traffic accident**

√x7th V05.12 **Pedestrian on skateboard injured in collision with railway train or railway vehicle in traffic accident**

√x7ᵗʰ **V05.19　Pedestrian with other conveyance injured in collision with railway train or railway vehicle in traffic accident**

　　Pedestrian with babystroller injured in collision with railway train or railway vehicle in traffic accident

　　Pedestrian on ice-skates injured in collision with railway train or railway vehicle in traffic accident

　　Pedestrian on nonmotorized scooter injured in collision with railway train or railway vehicle in traffic accident

　　Pedestrian on sled injured in collision with railway train or railway vehicle in traffic accident

　　Pedestrian on snowboard injured in collision with railway train or railway vehicle in traffic accident

　　Pedestrian on snow-skis injured in collision with railway train or railway vehicle in traffic accident

　　Pedestrian in wheelchair (powered) injured in collision with railway train or railway vehicle in traffic accident

　　Pedestrian in motorized mobility scooter injured in collision with railway train or railway vehicle in traffic accident

√5ᵗʰ **V05.9　Pedestrian injured in collision with railway train or railway vehicle, unspecified whether traffic or nontraffic accident**

√x7ᵗʰ **V05.90　Pedestrian on foot injured in collision with railway train or railway vehicle, unspecified whether traffic or nontraffic accident**

　　Pedestrian NOS injured in collision with railway train or railway vehicle, unspecified whether traffic or nontraffic accident

√x7ᵗʰ **V05.91　Pedestrian on roller-skates injured in collision with railway train or railway vehicle, unspecified whether traffic or nontraffic accident**

√x7ᵗʰ **V05.92　Pedestrian on skateboard injured in collision with railway train or railway vehicle, unspecified whether traffic or nontraffic accident**

√x7ᵗʰ **V05.99　Pedestrian with other conveyance injured in collision with railway train or railway vehicle, unspecified whether traffic or nontraffic accident**

　　Pedestrian with babystroller injured in collision with railway train or railway vehicle, unspecified whether traffic or nontraffic

　　Pedestrian on ice-skates injured in collision with railway train or railway vehicle, unspecified whether traffic or nontraffic

　　Pedestrian on nonmotorized scooter injured in collision with railway train or railway vehicle, unspecified whether traffic or nontraffic

　　Pedestrian on sled injured in collision with railway train or railway vehicle, unspecified whether traffic or nontraffic

　　Pedestrian on snowboard injured in collision with railway train or railway vehicle, unspecified whether traffic or nontraffic

　　Pedestrian on snow-skis injured in collision with railway train or railway vehicle, unspecified whether traffic or nontraffic

　　Pedestrian in wheelchair (powered) injured in collision with railway train or railway vehicle, unspecified whether traffic or nontraffic

　　Pedestrian in motorized mobility scooter injured in collision with railway train or railway vehicle, unspecified whether traffic or nontraffic

√4ᵗʰ **V06　Pedestrian injured in collision with other nonmotor vehicle**

INCLUDES　collision with animal-drawn vehicle, animal being ridden, nonpowered streetcar

EXCLUDES 1　pedestrian injured in collision with pedestrian conveyance (V00.0-)

> The appropriate 7th character is to be added to each code from category V06.
> A　initial encounter
> D　subsequent encounter
> S　sequela

√5ᵗʰ **V06.0　Pedestrian injured in collision with other nonmotor vehicle in nontraffic accident**

√x7ᵗʰ **V06.00　Pedestrian on foot injured in collision with other nonmotor vehicle in nontraffic accident**

　　Pedestrian NOS injured in collision with other nonmotor vehicle in nontraffic accident

√x7ᵗʰ **V06.01　Pedestrian on roller-skates injured in collision with other nonmotor vehicle in nontraffic accident**

√x7ᵗʰ **V06.02　Pedestrian on skateboard injured in collision with other nonmotor vehicle in nontraffic accident**

√x7ᵗʰ **V06.09　Pedestrian with other conveyance injured in collision with other nonmotor vehicle in nontraffic accident**

　　Pedestrian with babystroller injured in collision with other nonmotor vehicle in nontraffic accident

　　Pedestrian on ice-skates injured in collision with other nonmotor vehicle in nontraffic accident

　　Pedestrian on nonmotorized scooter injured in collision with other nonmotor vehicle in nontraffic accident

　　Pedestrian on sled injured in collision with other nonmotor vehicle in nontraffic accident

　　Pedestrian on snowboard injured in collision with other nonmotor vehicle in nontraffic accident

　　Pedestrian on snow-skis injured in collision with other nonmotor vehicle in nontraffic accident

　　Pedestrian in wheelchair (powered) injured in collision with other nonmotor vehicle in nontraffic accident

　　Pedestrian in motorized mobility scooter injured in collision with other nonmotor vehicle in nontraffic accident

√5ᵗʰ **V06.1　Pedestrian injured in collision with other nonmotor vehicle in traffic accident**

√x7ᵗʰ **V06.10　Pedestrian on foot injured in collision with other nonmotor vehicle in traffic accident**

　　Pedestrian NOS injured in collision with other nonmotor vehicle in traffic accident

√x7ᵗʰ **V06.11　Pedestrian on roller-skates injured in collision with other nonmotor vehicle in traffic accident**

√x7ᵗʰ **V06.12　Pedestrian on skateboard injured in collision with other nonmotor vehicle in traffic accident**

√x7ᵗʰ **V06.19　Pedestrian with other conveyance injured in collision with other nonmotor vehicle in traffic accident**

　　Pedestrian with babystroller injured in collision with other nonmotor vehicle in nontraffic accident

　　Pedestrian on ice-skates injured in collision with other nonmotor vehicle in traffic accident

　　Pedestrian on nonmotorized scooter injured in collision with other nonmotor vehicle in traffic accident

　　Pedestrian on sled injured in collision with other nonmotor vehicle in traffic accident

　　Pedestrian on snowboard injured in collision with other nonmotor vehicle in traffic accident

　　Pedestrian on snow-skis injured in collision with other nonmotor vehicle in traffic accident

　　Pedestrian in wheelchair (powered) injured in collision with other nonmotor vehicle in traffic accident

　　Pedestrian in motorized mobility scooter injured in collision with other nonmotor vehicle in traffic accident

√5ᵗʰ **V06.9　Pedestrian injured in collision with other nonmotor vehicle, unspecified whether traffic or nontraffic accident**

√x7ᵗʰ **V06.90　Pedestrian on foot injured in collision with other nonmotor vehicle, unspecified whether traffic or nontraffic accident**

　　Pedestrian NOS injured in collision with other nonmotor vehicle, unspecified whether traffic or nontraffic accident

√x7ᵗʰ **V06.91　Pedestrian on roller-skates injured in collision with other nonmotor vehicle, unspecified whether traffic or nontraffic accident**

√x7ᵗʰ **V06.92　Pedestrian on skateboard injured in collision with other nonmotor vehicle, unspecified whether traffic or nontraffic accident**

✔ Additional Character Required　√x7ᵗʰ Xtension Alert　Unacceptable PDx　Manifestation　Hospital Acquired Condition　EXCLUDES 1 Not Coded Here　EXCLUDES 2 Not Included Here

✓x7ᵗʰ **V06.99 Pedestrian with other conveyance injured in collision with other nonmotor vehicle, unspecified whether traffic or nontraffic accident**

Pedestrian with babystroller injured in collision with other nonmotor vehicle, unspecified whether traffic or nontraffic accident

Pedestrian on ice-skates injured in collision with other nonmotor vehicle, unspecified whether traffic or nontraffic accident

Pedestrian on nonmotorized scooter injured in collision with other nonmotor vehicle, unspecified whether traffic or nontraffic accident

Pedestrian on sled injured in collision with other nonmotor vehicle, unspecified whether traffic or nontraffic accident

Pedestrian on snowboard injured in collision with other nonmotor vehicle, unspecified whether traffic or nontraffic accident

Pedestrian on snow-skis injured in collision with other nonmotor vehicle, unspecified whether traffic or nontraffic accident

Pedestrian in wheelchair (powered) injured in collision with other nonmotor vehicle, unspecified whether traffic or nontraffic accident

Pedestrian in motorized mobility scooter injured in collision with other nonmotor vehicle, unspecified whether traffic or nontraffic accident

✓4ᵗʰ **V09 Pedestrian injured in other and unspecified transport accidents**

The appropriate 7th character is to be added to each code from category V09.
A   initial encounter
D   subsequent encounter
S   sequela

✓5ᵗʰ **V09.0 Pedestrian injured in nontraffic accident involving other and unspecified motor vehicles**

✓x7ᵗʰ **V09.00 Pedestrian injured in nontraffic accident involving unspecified motor vehicles**

✓x7ᵗʰ **V09.01 Pedestrian injured in nontraffic accident involving military vehicle**

✓x7ᵗʰ **V09.09 Pedestrian injured in nontraffic accident involving other motor vehicles**

Pedestrian injured in nontraffic accident by special vehicle

✓x7ᵗʰ **V09.1 Pedestrian injured in unspecified nontraffic accident**

✓5ᵗʰ **V09.2 Pedestrian injured in traffic accident involving other and unspecified motor vehicles**

✓x7ᵗʰ **V09.20 Pedestrian injured in traffic accident involving unspecified motor vehicles**

✓x7ᵗʰ **V09.21 Pedestrian injured in traffic accident involving military vehicle**

✓x7ᵗʰ **V09.29 Pedestrian injured in traffic accident involving other motor vehicles**

✓x7ᵗʰ **V09.3 Pedestrian injured in unspecified traffic accident**

✓x7ᵗʰ **V09.9 Pedestrian injured in unspecified transport accident**

Pedal cycle rider injured in transport accident (V10-V19)

INCLUDES   any non-motorized vehicle, excluding an animal-drawn vehicle, or a sidecar or trailer attached to the pedal cycle

EXCLUDES 2   *rupture of pedal cycle tire (W37.0)*

✓4ᵗʰ **V10 Pedal cycle rider injured in collision with pedestrian or animal**

EXCLUDES 1   *pedal cycle rider collision with animal-drawn vehicle or animal being ridden (V16.-)*

The appropriate 7th character is to be added to each code from category V10.
A   initial encounter
D   subsequent encounter
S   sequela

✓x7ᵗʰ **V10.0 Pedal cycle driver injured in collision with pedestrian or animal in nontraffic accident**

✓x7ᵗʰ **V10.1 Pedal cycle passenger injured in collision with pedestrian or animal in nontraffic accident**

✓x7ᵗʰ **V10.2 Unspecified pedal cyclist injured in collision with pedestrian or animal in nontraffic accident**

✓x7ᵗʰ **V10.3 Person boarding or alighting a pedal cycle injured in collision with pedestrian or animal**

✓x7ᵗʰ **V10.4 Pedal cycle driver injured in collision with pedestrian or animal in traffic accident**

✓x7ᵗʰ **V10.5 Pedal cycle passenger injured in collision with pedestrian or animal in traffic accident**

✓x7ᵗʰ **V10.9 Unspecified pedal cyclist injured in collision with pedestrian or animal in traffic accident**

✓4ᵗʰ **V11 Pedal cycle rider injured in collision with other pedal cycle**

The appropriate 7th character is to be added to each code from category V11.
A   initial encounter
D   subsequent encounter
S   sequela

✓x7ᵗʰ **V11.0 Pedal cycle driver injured in collision with other pedal cycle in nontraffic accident**

✓x7ᵗʰ **V11.1 Pedal cycle passenger injured in collision with other pedal cycle in nontraffic accident**

✓x7ᵗʰ **V11.2 Unspecified pedal cyclist injured in collision with other pedal cycle in nontraffic accident**

✓x7ᵗʰ **V11.3 Person boarding or alighting a pedal cycle injured in collision with other pedal cycle**

✓x7ᵗʰ **V11.4 Pedal cycle driver injured in collision with other pedal cycle in traffic accident**

✓x7ᵗʰ **V11.5 Pedal cycle passenger injured in collision with other pedal cycle in traffic accident**

✓x7ᵗʰ **V11.9 Unspecified pedal cyclist injured in collision with other pedal cycle in traffic accident**

✓4ᵗʰ **V12 Pedal cycle rider injured in collision with two- or three-wheeled motor vehicle**

The appropriate 7th character is to be added to each code from category V12.
A   initial encounter
D   subsequent encounter
S   sequela

✓x7ᵗʰ **V12.0 Pedal cycle driver injured in collision with two- or three-wheeled motor vehicle in nontraffic accident**

✓x7ᵗʰ **V12.1 Pedal cycle passenger injured in collision with two- or three-wheeled motor vehicle in nontraffic accident**

✓x7ᵗʰ **V12.2 Unspecified pedal cyclist injured in collision with two- or three-wheeled motor vehicle in nontraffic accident**

✓x7ᵗʰ **V12.3 Person boarding or alighting a pedal cycle injured in collision with two- or three-wheeled motor vehicle**

✓x7ᵗʰ **V12.4 Pedal cycle driver injured in collision with two- or three-wheeled motor vehicle in traffic accident**

✓x7ᵗʰ **V12.5 Pedal cycle passenger injured in collision with two- or three-wheeled motor vehicle in traffic accident**

✓x7ᵗʰ **V12.9 Unspecified pedal cyclist injured in collision with two- or three-wheeled motor vehicle in traffic accident**

✓4ᵗʰ **V13 Pedal cycle rider injured in collision with car, pick-up truck or van**

The appropriate 7th character is to be added to each code from category V13.
A   initial encounter
D   subsequent encounter
S   sequela

✓x7ᵗʰ **V13.0 Pedal cycle driver injured in collision with car, pick-up truck or van in nontraffic accident**

✓x7ᵗʰ **V13.1 Pedal cycle passenger injured in collision with car, pick-up truck or van in nontraffic accident**

✓x7ᵗʰ **V13.2 Unspecified pedal cyclist injured in collision with car, pick-up truck or van in nontraffic accident**

✓x7ᵗʰ **V13.3 Person boarding or alighting a pedal cycle injured in collision with car, pick-up truck or van**

✓x7ᵗʰ **V13.4 Pedal cycle driver injured in collision with car, pick-up truck or van in traffic accident**

✓x7ᵗʰ **V13.5 Pedal cycle passenger injured in collision with car, pick-up truck or van in traffic accident**

✓x7ᵗʰ **V13.9 Unspecified pedal cyclist injured in collision with car, pick-up truck or van in traffic accident**

Ⓝ Newborn: 0   Ⓟ Pediatric: 0-17   Ⓜ Maternity: 12-55   Ⓐ Adult: 15-124   MCC Major CC Condition   PDx MCC PDx acts as own MCC   CC CC Condition   PDx CC PDx acts as own CC

1116   ICD-10-CM Draft (2015)

✓4th **V14 Pedal cycle rider injured in collision with heavy transport vehicle or bus**

> *EXCLUDES 1* *pedal cycle rider injured in collision with military vehicle (V19.81)*

> The appropriate 7th character is to be added to each code from category V14.
> A   initial encounter
> D   subsequent encounter
> S   sequela

✓x7th **V14.0 Pedal cycle driver injured in collision with heavy transport vehicle or bus in nontraffic accident**

✓x7th **V14.1 Pedal cycle passenger injured in collision with heavy transport vehicle or bus in nontraffic accident**

✓x7th **V14.2 Unspecified pedal cyclist injured in collision with heavy transport vehicle or bus in nontraffic accident**

✓x7th **V14.3 Person boarding or alighting a pedal cycle injured in collision with heavy transport vehicle or bus**

✓x7th **V14.4 Pedal cycle driver injured in collision with heavy transport vehicle or bus in traffic accident**

✓x7th **V14.5 Pedal cycle passenger injured in collision with heavy transport vehicle or bus in traffic accident**

✓x7th **V14.9 Unspecified pedal cyclist injured in collision with heavy transport vehicle or bus in traffic accident**

✓4th **V15 Pedal cycle rider injured in collision with railway train or railway vehicle**

> The appropriate 7th character is to be added to each code from category V15.
> A   initial encounter
> D   subsequent encounter
> S   sequela

✓x7th **V15.0 Pedal cycle driver injured in collision with railway train or railway vehicle in nontraffic accident**

✓x7th **V15.1 Pedal cycle passenger injured in collision with railway train or railway vehicle in nontraffic accident**

✓x7th **V15.2 Unspecified pedal cyclist injured in collision with railway train or railway vehicle in nontraffic accident**

✓x7th **V15.3 Person boarding or alighting a pedal cycle injured in collision with railway train or railway vehicle**

✓x7th **V15.4 Pedal cycle driver injured in collision with railway train or railway vehicle in traffic accident**

✓x7th **V15.5 Pedal cycle passenger injured in collision with railway train or railway vehicle in traffic accident**

✓x7th **V15.9 Unspecified pedal cyclist injured in collision with railway train or railway vehicle in traffic accident**

✓4th **V16 Pedal cycle rider injured in collision with other nonmotor vehicle**

> *INCLUDES* collision with animal-drawn vehicle, animal being ridden, streetcar

> The appropriate 7th character is to be added to each code from category V16.
> A   initial encounter
> D   subsequent encounter
> S   sequela

✓x7th **V16.0 Pedal cycle driver injured in collision with other nonmotor vehicle in nontraffic accident**

✓x7th **V16.1 Pedal cycle passenger injured in collision with other nonmotor vehicle in nontraffic accident**

✓x7th **V16.2 Unspecified pedal cyclist injured in collision with other nonmotor vehicle in nontraffic accident**

✓x7th **V16.3 Person boarding or alighting a pedal cycle injured in collision with other nonmotor vehicle in nontraffic accident**

✓x7th **V16.4 Pedal cycle driver injured in collision with other nonmotor vehicle in traffic accident**

✓x7th **V16.5 Pedal cycle passenger injured in collision with other nonmotor vehicle in traffic accident**

✓x7th **V16.9 Unspecified pedal cyclist injured in collision with other nonmotor vehicle in traffic accident**

✓4th **V17 Pedal cycle rider injured in collision with fixed or stationary object**

> The appropriate 7th character is to be added to each code from category V17.
> A   initial encounter
> D   subsequent encounter
> S   sequela

✓x7th **V17.0 Pedal cycle driver injured in collision with fixed or stationary object in nontraffic accident**

✓x7th **V17.1 Pedal cycle passenger injured in collision with fixed or stationary object in nontraffic accident**

✓x7th **V17.2 Unspecified pedal cyclist injured in collision with fixed or stationary object in nontraffic accident**

✓x7th **V17.3 Person boarding or alighting a pedal cycle injured in collision with fixed or stationary object**

✓x7th **V17.4 Pedal cycle driver injured in collision with fixed or stationary object in traffic accident**

✓x7th **V17.5 Pedal cycle passenger injured in collision with fixed or stationary object in traffic accident**

✓x7th **V17.9 Unspecified pedal cyclist injured in collision with fixed or stationary object in traffic accident**

✓4th **V18 Pedal cycle rider injured in noncollision transport accident**

> *INCLUDES* fall or thrown from pedal cycle (without antecedent collision)
> overturning pedal cycle NOS
> overturning pedal cycle without collision

> The appropriate 7th character is to be added to each code from category V18.
> A   initial encounter
> D   subsequent encounter
> S   sequela

✓x7th **V18.0 Pedal cycle driver injured in noncollision transport accident in nontraffic accident**

✓x7th **V18.1 Pedal cycle passenger injured in noncollision transport accident in nontraffic accident**

✓x7th **V18.2 Unspecified pedal cyclist injured in noncollision transport accident in nontraffic accident**

✓x7th **V18.3 Person boarding or alighting a pedal cycle injured in noncollision transport accident**

✓x7th **V18.4 Pedal cycle driver injured in noncollision transport accident in traffic accident**

✓x7th **V18.5 Pedal cycle passenger injured in noncollision transport accident in traffic accident**

✓x7th **V18.9 Unspecified pedal cyclist injured in noncollision transport accident in traffic accident**

✓4th **V19 Pedal cycle rider injured in other and unspecified transport accidents**

> The appropriate 7th character is to be added to each code from category V19.
> A   initial encounter
> D   subsequent encounter
> S   sequela

✓5th **V19.0 Pedal cycle driver injured in collision with other and unspecified motor vehicles in nontraffic accident**

> ✓x7th **V19.00 Pedal cycle driver injured in collision with unspecified motor vehicles in nontraffic accident**
> ✓x7th **V19.09 Pedal cycle driver injured in collision with other motor vehicles in nontraffic accident**

✓5th **V19.1 Pedal cycle passenger injured in collision with other and unspecified motor vehicles in nontraffic accident**

> ✓x7th **V19.10 Pedal cycle passenger injured in collision with unspecified motor vehicles in nontraffic accident**
> ✓x7th **V19.19 Pedal cycle passenger injured in collision with other motor vehicles in nontraffic accident**

✓5th **V19.2 Unspecified pedal cyclist injured in collision with other and unspecified motor vehicles in nontraffic accident**

> ✓x7th **V19.20 Unspecified pedal cyclist injured in collision with unspecified motor vehicles in nontraffic accident**
> Pedal cycle collision NOS, nontraffic
> ✓x7th **V19.29 Unspecified pedal cyclist injured in collision with other motor vehicles in nontraffic accident**

✓x7th **V19.3 Pedal cyclist (driver) (passenger) injured in unspecified nontraffic accident**
> Pedal cycle accident NOS, nontraffic
> Pedal cyclist injured in nontraffic accident NOS

✓ Additional Character Required   ✓x7th Xtension Alert   Unacceptable PDx   Manifestation   Hospital Acquired Condition   *EXCLUDES 1* Not Coded Here   *EXCLUDES 2* Not Included Here

External Causes of Morbidity

V19.4–V24.9

√5ᵗʰ **V19.4** Pedal cycle driver injured in collision with other and unspecified motor vehicles in traffic accident

√x7ᵗʰ **V19.40** Pedal cycle driver injured in collision with unspecified motor vehicles in traffic accident

√x7ᵗʰ **V19.49** Pedal cycle driver injured in collision with other motor vehicles in traffic accident

√5ᵗʰ **V19.5** Pedal cycle passenger injured in collision with other and unspecified motor vehicles in traffic accident

√x7ᵗʰ **V19.50** Pedal cycle passenger injured in collision with unspecified motor vehicles in traffic accident

√x7ᵗʰ **V19.59** Pedal cycle passenger injured in collision with other motor vehicles in traffic accident

√5ᵗʰ **V19.6** Unspecified pedal cyclist injured in collision with other and unspecified motor vehicles in traffic accident

√x7ᵗʰ **V19.60** Unspecified pedal cyclist injured in collision with unspecified motor vehicles in traffic accident
Pedal cycle collision NOS (traffic)

√x7ᵗʰ **V19.69** Unspecified pedal cyclist injured in collision with other motor vehicles in traffic accident

√5ᵗʰ **V19.8** Pedal cyclist (driver) (passenger) injured in other specified transport accidents

√x7ᵗʰ **V19.81** Pedal cyclist (driver) (passenger) injured in transport accident with military vehicle

√x7ᵗʰ **V19.88** Pedal cyclist (driver) (passenger) injured in other specified transport accidents

√x7ᵗʰ **V19.9** Pedal cyclist (driver) (passenger) injured in unspecified traffic accident
Pedal cycle accident NOS

Motorcycle rider injured in transport accident (V20-V29)

INCLUDES   moped
motorcycle with sidecar
motorized bicycle
motor scooter
EXCLUDES 1   three-wheeled motor vehicle (V30-V39)

√4ᵗʰ **V20** Motorcycle rider injured in collision with pedestrian or animal
EXCLUDES 1   motorcycle rider collision with animal-drawn vehicle or animal being ridden (V26.-)

The appropriate 7th character is to be added to each code from category V20.
A   initial encounter
D   subsequent encounter
S   sequela

√x7ᵗʰ **V20.0** Motorcycle driver injured in collision with pedestrian or animal in nontraffic accident

√x7ᵗʰ **V20.1** Motorcycle passenger injured in collision with pedestrian or animal in nontraffic accident

√x7ᵗʰ **V20.2** Unspecified motorcycle rider injured in collision with pedestrian or animal in nontraffic accident

√x7ᵗʰ **V20.3** Person boarding or alighting a motorcycle injured in collision with pedestrian or animal

√x7ᵗʰ **V20.4** Motorcycle driver injured in collision with pedestrian or animal in traffic accident

√x7ᵗʰ **V20.5** Motorcycle passenger injured in collision with pedestrian or animal in traffic accident

√x7ᵗʰ **V20.9** Unspecified motorcycle rider injured in collision with pedestrian or animal in traffic accident

√4ᵗʰ **V21** Motorcycle rider injured in collision with pedal cycle

The appropriate 7th character is to be added to each code from category V21.
A   initial encounter
D   subsequent encounter
S   sequela

√x7ᵗʰ **V21.0** Motorcycle driver injured in collision with pedal cycle in nontraffic accident

√x7ᵗʰ **V21.1** Motorcycle passenger injured in collision with pedal cycle in nontraffic accident

√x7ᵗʰ **V21.2** Unspecified motorcycle rider injured in collision with pedal cycle in nontraffic accident

√x7ᵗʰ **V21.3** Person boarding or alighting a motorcycle injured in collision with pedal cycle

√x7ᵗʰ **V21.4** Motorcycle driver injured in collision with pedal cycle in traffic accident

√x7ᵗʰ **V21.5** Motorcycle passenger injured in collision with pedal cycle in traffic accident

√x7ᵗʰ **V21.9** Unspecified motorcycle rider injured in collision with pedal cycle in traffic accident

√4ᵗʰ **V22** Motorcycle rider injured in collision with two- or three-wheeled motor vehicle

The appropriate 7th character is to be added to each code from category V22.
A   initial encounter
D   subsequent encounter
S   sequela

√x7ᵗʰ **V22.0** Motorcycle driver injured in collision with two- or three-wheeled motor vehicle in nontraffic accident

√x7ᵗʰ **V22.1** Motorcycle passenger injured in collision with two- or three-wheeled motor vehicle in nontraffic accident

√x7ᵗʰ **V22.2** Unspecified motorcycle rider injured in collision with two- or three-wheeled motor vehicle in nontraffic accident

√x7ᵗʰ **V22.3** Person boarding or alighting a motorcycle injured in collision with two- or three-wheeled motor vehicle

√x7ᵗʰ **V22.4** Motorcycle driver injured in collision with two- or three-wheeled motor vehicle in traffic accident

√x7ᵗʰ **V22.5** Motorcycle passenger injured in collision with two- or three-wheeled motor vehicle in traffic accident

√x7ᵗʰ **V22.9** Unspecified motorcycle rider injured in collision with two- or three-wheeled motor vehicle in traffic accident

√4ᵗʰ **V23** Motorcycle rider injured in collision with car, pick-up truck or van

The appropriate 7th character is to be added to each code from category V23.
A   initial encounter
D   subsequent encounter
S   sequela

√x7ᵗʰ **V23.0** Motorcycle driver injured in collision with car, pick-up truck or van in nontraffic accident

√x7ᵗʰ **V23.1** Motorcycle passenger injured in collision with car, pick-up truck or van in nontraffic accident

√x7ᵗʰ **V23.2** Unspecified motorcycle rider injured in collision with car, pick-up truck or van in nontraffic accident

√x7ᵗʰ **V23.3** Person boarding or alighting a motorcycle injured in collision with car, pick-up truck or van

√x7ᵗʰ **V23.4** Motorcycle driver injured in collision with car, pick-up truck or van in traffic accident

√x7ᵗʰ **V23.5** Motorcycle passenger injured in collision with car, pick-up truck or van in traffic accident

√x7ᵗʰ **V23.9** Unspecified motorcycle rider injured in collision with car, pick-up truck or van in traffic accident

√4ᵗʰ **V24** Motorcycle rider injured in collision with heavy transport vehicle or bus
EXCLUDES 1   motorcycle rider injured in collision with military vehicle (V29.81)

The appropriate 7th character is to be added to each code from category V24.
A   initial encounter
D   subsequent encounter
S   sequela

√x7ᵗʰ **V24.0** Motorcycle driver injured in collision with heavy transport vehicle or bus in nontraffic accident

√x7ᵗʰ **V24.1** Motorcycle passenger injured in collision with heavy transport vehicle or bus in nontraffic accident

√x7ᵗʰ **V24.2** Unspecified motorcycle rider injured in collision with heavy transport vehicle or bus in nontraffic accident

√x7ᵗʰ **V24.3** Person boarding or alighting a motorcycle injured in collision with heavy transport vehicle or bus

√x7ᵗʰ **V24.4** Motorcycle driver injured in collision with heavy transport vehicle or bus in traffic accident

√x7ᵗʰ **V24.5** Motorcycle passenger injured in collision with heavy transport vehicle or bus in traffic accident

√x7ᵗʰ **V24.9** Unspecified motorcycle rider injured in collision with heavy transport vehicle or bus in traffic accident

N Newborn: 0   P Pediatric: 0-17   M Maternity: 12-55   A Adult: 15-124   MCC Major CC Condition   PDx MCC PDx acts as own MCC   CC CC Condition   PDx CC PDx acts as own CC

1118   ICD-10-CM Draft (2015)

☑4ᵗʰ **V25　Motorcycle rider injured in collision with railway train or railway vehicle**

> The appropriate 7th character is to be added to each code from category V25.
> A　initial encounter
> D　subsequent encounter
> S　sequela

√x7ᵗʰ **V25.0　Motorcycle driver injured in collision with railway train or railway vehicle in nontraffic accident**

√x7ᵗʰ **V25.1　Motorcycle passenger injured in collision with railway train or railway vehicle in nontraffic accident**

√x7ᵗʰ **V25.2　Unspecified motorcycle rider injured in collision with railway train or railway vehicle in nontraffic accident**

√x7ᵗʰ **V25.3　Person boarding or alighting a motorcycle injured in collision with railway train or railway vehicle**

√x7ᵗʰ **V25.4　Motorcycle driver injured in collision with railway train or railway vehicle in traffic accident**

√x7ᵗʰ **V25.5　Motorcycle passenger injured in collision with railway train or railway vehicle in traffic accident**

√x7ᵗʰ **V25.9　Unspecified motorcycle rider injured in collision with railway train or railway vehicle in traffic accident**

☑4ᵗʰ **V26　Motorcycle rider injured in collision with other nonmotor vehicle**
> INCLUDES　collision with animal-drawn vehicle, animal being ridden, streetcar

> The appropriate 7th character is to be added to each code from category V26.
> A　initial encounter
> D　subsequent encounter
> S　sequela

√x7ᵗʰ **V26.0　Motorcycle driver injured in collision with other nonmotor vehicle in nontraffic accident**

√x7ᵗʰ **V26.1　Motorcycle passenger injured in collision with other nonmotor vehicle in nontraffic accident**

√x7ᵗʰ **V26.2　Unspecified motorcycle rider injured in collision with other nonmotor vehicle in nontraffic accident**

√x7ᵗʰ **V26.3　Person boarding or alighting a motorcycle injured in collision with other nonmotor vehicle**

√x7ᵗʰ **V26.4　Motorcycle driver injured in collision with other nonmotor vehicle in traffic accident**

√x7ᵗʰ **V26.5　Motorcycle passenger injured in collision with other nonmotor vehicle in traffic accident**

√x7ᵗʰ **V26.9　Unspecified motorcycle rider injured in collision with other nonmotor vehicle in traffic accident**

☑4ᵗʰ **V27　Motorcycle rider injured in collision with fixed or stationary object**

> The appropriate 7th character is to be added to each code from category V27.
> A　initial encounter
> D　subsequent encounter
> S　sequela

√x7ᵗʰ **V27.0　Motorcycle driver injured in collision with fixed or stationary object in nontraffic accident**

√x7ᵗʰ **V27.1　Motorcycle passenger injured in collision with fixed or stationary object in nontraffic accident**

√x7ᵗʰ **V27.2　Unspecified motorcycle rider injured in collision with fixed or stationary object in nontraffic accident**

√x7ᵗʰ **V27.3　Person boarding or alighting a motorcycle injured in collision with fixed or stationary object**

√x7ᵗʰ **V27.4　Motorcycle driver injured in collision with fixed or stationary object in traffic accident**

√x7ᵗʰ **V27.5　Motorcycle passenger injured in collision with fixed or stationary object in traffic accident**

√x7ᵗʰ **V27.9　Unspecified motorcycle rider injured in collision with fixed or stationary object in traffic accident**

☑4ᵗʰ **V28　Motorcycle rider injured in noncollision transport accident**
> INCLUDES　fall or thrown from motorcycle (without antecedent collision)
> overturning motorcycle NOS
> overturning motorcycle without collision

> The appropriate 7th character is to be added to each code from category V28.
> A　initial encounter
> D　subsequent encounter
> S　sequela

√x7ᵗʰ **V28.0　Motorcycle driver injured in noncollision transport accident in nontraffic accident**

√x7ᵗʰ **V28.1　Motorcycle passenger injured in noncollision transport accident in nontraffic accident**

√x7ᵗʰ **V28.2　Unspecified motorcycle rider injured in noncollision transport accident in nontraffic accident**

√x7ᵗʰ **V28.3　Person boarding or alighting a motorcycle injured in noncollision transport accident**

√x7ᵗʰ **V28.4　Motorcycle driver injured in noncollision transport accident in traffic accident**

√x7ᵗʰ **V28.5　Motorcycle passenger injured in noncollision transport accident in traffic accident**

√x7ᵗʰ **V28.9　Unspecified motorcycle rider injured in noncollision transport accident in traffic accident**

☑4ᵗʰ **V29　Motorcycle rider injured in other and unspecified transport accidents**

> The appropriate 7th character is to be added to each code from category V29.
> A　initial encounter
> D　subsequent encounter
> S　sequela

√5ᵗʰ **V29.0　Motorcycle driver injured in collision with other and unspecified motor vehicles in nontraffic accident**

> √x7ᵗʰ **V29.00　Motorcycle driver injured in collision with unspecified motor vehicles in nontraffic accident**
> √x7ᵗʰ **V29.09　Motorcycle driver injured in collision with other motor vehicles in nontraffic accident**

√5ᵗʰ **V29.1　Motorcycle passenger injured in collision with other and unspecified motor vehicles in nontraffic accident**

> √x7ᵗʰ **V29.10　Motorcycle passenger injured in collision with unspecified motor vehicles in nontraffic accident**
> √x7ᵗʰ **V29.19　Motorcycle passenger injured in collision with other motor vehicles in nontraffic accident**

√5ᵗʰ **V29.2　Unspecified motorcycle rider injured in collision with other and unspecified motor vehicles in nontraffic accident**

> √x7ᵗʰ **V29.20　Unspecified motorcycle rider injured in collision with unspecified motor vehicles in nontraffic accident**
> Motorcycle collision NOS, nontraffic
> √x7ᵗʰ **V29.29　Unspecified motorcycle rider injured in collision with other motor vehicles in nontraffic accident**

√x7ᵗʰ **V29.3　Motorcycle rider (driver) (passenger) injured in unspecified nontraffic accident**
> Motorcycle accident NOS, nontraffic
> Motorcycle rider injured in nontraffic accident NOS

√5ᵗʰ **V29.4　Motorcycle driver injured in collision with other and unspecified motor vehicles in traffic accident**

> √x7ᵗʰ **V29.40　Motorcycle driver injured in collision with unspecified motor vehicles in traffic accident**
> √x7ᵗʰ **V29.49　Motorcycle driver injured in collision with other motor vehicles in traffic accident**

√5ᵗʰ **V29.5　Motorcycle passenger injured in collision with other and unspecified motor vehicles in traffic accident**

> √x7ᵗʰ **V29.50　Motorcycle passenger injured in collision with unspecified motor vehicles in traffic accident**
> √x7ᵗʰ **V29.59　Motorcycle passenger injured in collision with other motor vehicles in traffic accident**

√5ᵗʰ **V29.6　Unspecified motorcycle rider injured in collision with other and unspecified motor vehicles in traffic accident**

> √x7ᵗʰ **V29.60　Unspecified motorcycle rider injured in collision with unspecified motor vehicles in traffic accident**
> Motorcycle collision NOS (traffic)
> √x7ᵗʰ **V29.69　Unspecified motorcycle rider injured in collision with other motor vehicles in traffic accident**

√5ᵗʰ **V29.8　Motorcycle rider (driver) (passenger) injured in other specified transport accidents**

> √x7ᵗʰ **V29.81　Motorcycle rider (driver) (passenger) injured in transport accident with military vehicle**

☑ Additional Character Required　　√x7ᵗʰ Xtension Alert　　Unacceptable PDx　　Manifestation　　Hospital Acquired Condition　　EXCLUDES 1 Not Coded Here　　EXCLUDES 2 Not Included Here

√x7ᵗʰ **V29.88** Motorcycle rider (driver) (passenger) injured in other specified transport accidents

√x7ᵗʰ **V29.9** Motorcycle rider (driver) (passenger) injured in unspecified traffic accident

Motorcycle accident NOS

Occupant of three-wheeled motor vehicle injured in transport accident (V30-V39)

INCLUDES   motorized tricycle
motorized rickshaw
three-wheeled motor car

EXCLUDES 1   all-terrain vehicles (V86.-)
motorcycle with sidecar (V20-V29)
vehicle designed primarily for off-road use (V86.-)

√4ᵗʰ **V30 Occupant of three-wheeled motor vehicle injured in collision with pedestrian or animal**

EXCLUDES 1   three-wheeled motor vehicle collision with animal-drawn vehicle or animal being ridden (V36.-)

The appropriate 7th character is to be added to each code from category V30.
A   initial encounter
D   subsequent encounter
S   sequela

√x7ᵗʰ **V30.0** Driver of three-wheeled motor vehicle injured in collision with pedestrian or animal in nontraffic accident

√x7ᵗʰ **V30.1** Passenger in three-wheeled motor vehicle injured in collision with pedestrian or animal in nontraffic accident

√x7ᵗʰ **V30.2** Person on outside of three-wheeled motor vehicle injured in collision with pedestrian or animal in nontraffic accident

√x7ᵗʰ **V30.3** Unspecified occupant of three-wheeled motor vehicle injured in collision with pedestrian or animal in nontraffic accident

√x7ᵗʰ **V30.4** Person boarding or alighting a three-wheeled motor vehicle injured in collision with pedestrian or animal

√x7ᵗʰ **V30.5** Driver of three-wheeled motor vehicle injured in collision with pedestrian or animal in traffic accident

√x7ᵗʰ **V30.6** Passenger in three-wheeled motor vehicle injured in collision with pedestrian or animal in traffic accident

√x7ᵗʰ **V30.7** Person on outside of three-wheeled motor vehicle injured in collision with pedestrian or animal in traffic accident

√x7ᵗʰ **V30.9** Unspecified occupant of three-wheeled motor vehicle injured in collision with pedestrian or animal in traffic accident

√4ᵗʰ **V31 Occupant of three-wheeled motor vehicle injured in collision with pedal cycle**

The appropriate 7th character is to be added to each code from category V31.
A   initial encounter
D   subsequent encounter
S   sequela

√x7ᵗʰ **V31.0** Driver of three-wheeled motor vehicle injured in collision with pedal cycle in nontraffic accident

√x7ᵗʰ **V31.1** Passenger in three-wheeled motor vehicle injured in collision with pedal cycle in nontraffic accident

√x7ᵗʰ **V31.2** Person on outside of three-wheeled motor vehicle injured in collision with pedal cycle in nontraffic accident

√x7ᵗʰ **V31.3** Unspecified occupant of three-wheeled motor vehicle injured in collision with pedal cycle in nontraffic accident

√x7ᵗʰ **V31.4** Person boarding or alighting a three-wheeled motor vehicle injured in collision with pedal cycle

√x7ᵗʰ **V31.5** Driver of three-wheeled motor vehicle injured in collision with pedal cycle in traffic accident

√x7ᵗʰ **V31.6** Passenger in three-wheeled motor vehicle injured in collision with pedal cycle in traffic accident

√x7ᵗʰ **V31.7** Person on outside of three-wheeled motor vehicle injured in collision with pedal cycle in traffic accident

√x7ᵗʰ **V31.9** Unspecified occupant of three-wheeled motor vehicle injured in collision with pedal cycle in traffic accident

√4ᵗʰ **V32 Occupant of three-wheeled motor vehicle injured in collision with two- or three-wheeled motor vehicle**

The appropriate 7th character is to be added to each code from category V32.
A   initial encounter
D   subsequent encounter
S   sequela

√x7ᵗʰ **V32.0** Driver of three-wheeled motor vehicle injured in collision with two- or three-wheeled motor vehicle in nontraffic accident

√x7ᵗʰ **V32.1** Passenger in three-wheeled motor vehicle injured in collision with two- or three-wheeled motor vehicle in nontraffic accident

√x7ᵗʰ **V32.2** Person on outside of three-wheeled motor vehicle injured in collision with two- or three-wheeled motor vehicle in nontraffic accident

√x7ᵗʰ **V32.3** Unspecified occupant of three-wheeled motor vehicle injured in collision with two- or three-wheeled motor vehicle in nontraffic accident

√x7ᵗʰ **V32.4** Person boarding or alighting a three-wheeled motor vehicle injured in collision with two- or three-wheeled motor vehicle

√x7ᵗʰ **V32.5** Driver of three-wheeled motor vehicle injured in collision with two- or three-wheeled motor vehicle in traffic accident

√x7ᵗʰ **V32.6** Passenger in three-wheeled motor vehicle injured in collision with two- or three-wheeled motor vehicle in traffic accident

√x7ᵗʰ **V32.7** Person on outside of three-wheeled motor vehicle injured in collision with two- or three-wheeled motor vehicle in traffic accident

√x7ᵗʰ **V32.9** Unspecified occupant of three-wheeled motor vehicle injured in collision with two- or three-wheeled motor vehicle in traffic accident

√4ᵗʰ **V33 Occupant of three-wheeled motor vehicle injured in collision with car, pick-up truck or van**

The appropriate 7th character is to be added to each code from category V33.
A   initial encounter
D   subsequent encounter
S   sequela

√x7ᵗʰ **V33.0** Driver of three-wheeled motor vehicle injured in collision with car, pick-up truck or van in nontraffic accident

√x7ᵗʰ **V33.1** Passenger in three-wheeled motor vehicle injured in collision with car, pick-up truck or van in nontraffic accident

√x7ᵗʰ **V33.2** Person on outside of three-wheeled motor vehicle injured in collision with car, pick-up truck or van in nontraffic accident

√x7ᵗʰ **V33.3** Unspecified occupant of three-wheeled motor vehicle injured in collision with car, pick-up truck or van in nontraffic accident

√x7ᵗʰ **V33.4** Person boarding or alighting a three-wheeled motor vehicle injured in collision with car, pick-up truck or van

√x7ᵗʰ **V33.5** Driver of three-wheeled motor vehicle injured in collision with car, pick-up truck or van in traffic accident

√x7ᵗʰ **V33.6** Passenger in three-wheeled motor vehicle injured in collision with car, pick-up truck or van in traffic accident

√x7ᵗʰ **V33.7** Person on outside of three-wheeled motor vehicle injured in collision with car, pick-up truck or van in traffic accident

√x7ᵗʰ **V33.9** Unspecified occupant of three-wheeled motor vehicle injured in collision with car, pick-up truck or van in traffic accident

√4ᵗʰ **V34 Occupant of three-wheeled motor vehicle injured in collision with heavy transport vehicle or bus**

EXCLUDES 1   occupant of three-wheeled motor vehicle injured in collision with military vehicle (V39.81)

The appropriate 7th character is to be added to each code from category V34.
A   initial encounter
D   subsequent encounter
S   sequela

√x7ᵗʰ **V34.0** Driver of three-wheeled motor vehicle injured in collision with heavy transport vehicle or bus in nontraffic accident

√x7ᵗʰ **V34.1** Passenger in three-wheeled motor vehicle injured in collision with heavy transport vehicle or bus in nontraffic accident

√x7ᵗʰ **V34.2** Person on outside of three-wheeled motor vehicle injured in collision with heavy transport vehicle or bus in nontraffic accident

N Newborn: 0   P Pediatric: 0-17   M Maternity: 12-55   A Adult: 15-124   MCC Major CC Condition   PDx MCC PDx acts as own MCC   CC CC Condition   PDx CC PDx acts as own CC

1120   ICD-10-CM Draft (2015)

✓x7ᵗʰ **V34.3** Unspecified occupant of three-wheeled motor vehicle injured in collision with heavy transport vehicle or bus in nontraffic accident

✓x7ᵗʰ **V34.4** **Person boarding or alighting** a three-wheeled motor vehicle injured in collision with heavy transport vehicle or bus

✓x7ᵗʰ **V34.5** **Driver** of three-wheeled motor vehicle injured in collision with heavy transport vehicle or bus in traffic accident

✓x7ᵗʰ **V34.6** **Passenger** in three-wheeled motor vehicle injured in collision with heavy transport vehicle or bus in traffic accident

✓x7ᵗʰ **V34.7** **Person on outside** of three-wheeled motor vehicle injured in collision with heavy transport vehicle or bus in traffic accident

✓x7ᵗʰ **V34.9** Unspecified occupant of three-wheeled motor vehicle injured in collision with heavy transport vehicle or bus in traffic accident

✓4ᵗʰ **V35** **Occupant of three-wheeled motor vehicle injured in collision with railway train or railway vehicle**

> The appropriate 7th character is to be added to each code from category V35.
> A   initial encounter
> D   subsequent encounter
> S   sequela

✓x7ᵗʰ **V35.0** **Driver** of three-wheeled motor vehicle injured in collision with railway train or railway vehicle in nontraffic accident

✓x7ᵗʰ **V35.1** **Passenger** in three-wheeled motor vehicle injured in collision with railway train or railway vehicle in nontraffic accident

✓x7ᵗʰ **V35.2** **Person on outside** of three-wheeled motor vehicle injured in collision with railway train or railway vehicle in nontraffic accident

✓x7ᵗʰ **V35.3** Unspecified occupant of three-wheeled motor vehicle injured in collision with railway train or railway vehicle in nontraffic accident

✓x7ᵗʰ **V35.4** **Person boarding or alighting** a three-wheeled motor vehicle injured in collision with railway train or railway vehicle

✓x7ᵗʰ **V35.5** **Driver** of three-wheeled motor vehicle injured in collision with railway train or railway vehicle in traffic accident

✓x7ᵗʰ **V35.6** **Passenger** in three-wheeled motor vehicle injured in collision with railway train or railway vehicle in traffic accident

✓x7ᵗʰ **V35.7** **Person on outside** of three-wheeled motor vehicle injured in collision with railway train or railway vehicle in traffic accident

✓x7ᵗʰ **V35.9** Unspecified occupant of three-wheeled motor vehicle injured in collision with railway train or railway vehicle in traffic accident

✓4ᵗʰ **V36** **Occupant of three-wheeled motor vehicle injured in collision with other nonmotor vehicle**
> INCLUDES   collision with animal-drawn vehicle, animal being ridden, streetcar

> The appropriate 7th character is to be added to each code from category V36.
> A   initial encounter
> D   subsequent encounter
> S   sequela

✓x7ᵗʰ **V36.0** **Driver** of three-wheeled motor vehicle injured in collision with other nonmotor vehicle in nontraffic accident

✓x7ᵗʰ **V36.1** **Passenger** in three-wheeled motor vehicle injured in collision with other nonmotor vehicle in nontraffic accident

✓x7ᵗʰ **V36.2** **Person on outside** of three-wheeled motor vehicle injured in collision with other nonmotor vehicle in nontraffic accident

✓x7ᵗʰ **V36.3** Unspecified occupant of three-wheeled motor vehicle injured in collision with other nonmotor vehicle in nontraffic accident

✓x7ᵗʰ **V36.4** **Person boarding or alighting** a three-wheeled motor vehicle injured in collision with other nonmotor vehicle

✓x7ᵗʰ **V36.5** **Driver** of three-wheeled motor vehicle injured in collision with other nonmotor vehicle in traffic accident

✓x7ᵗʰ **V36.6** **Passenger** in three-wheeled motor vehicle injured in collision with other nonmotor vehicle in traffic accident

✓x7ᵗʰ **V36.7** **Person on outside** of three-wheeled motor vehicle injured in collision with other nonmotor vehicle in traffic accident

✓x7ᵗʰ **V36.9** Unspecified occupant of three-wheeled motor vehicle injured in collision with other nonmotor vehicle in traffic accident

✓4ᵗʰ **V37** **Occupant of three-wheeled motor vehicle injured in collision with fixed or stationary object**

> The appropriate 7th character is to be added to each code from category V37.
> A   initial encounter
> D   subsequent encounter
> S   sequela

✓x7ᵗʰ **V37.0** **Driver** of three-wheeled motor vehicle injured in collision with fixed or stationary object in nontraffic accident

✓x7ᵗʰ **V37.1** **Passenger** in three-wheeled motor vehicle injured in collision with fixed or stationary object in nontraffic accident

✓x7ᵗʰ **V37.2** **Person on outside** of three-wheeled motor vehicle injured in collision with fixed or stationary object in nontraffic accident

✓x7ᵗʰ **V37.3** Unspecified occupant of three-wheeled motor vehicle injured in collision with fixed or stationary object in nontraffic accident

✓x7ᵗʰ **V37.4** **Person boarding or alighting** a three-wheeled motor vehicle injured in collision with fixed or stationary object

✓x7ᵗʰ **V37.5** **Driver** of three-wheeled motor vehicle injured in collision with fixed or stationary object in traffic accident

✓x7ᵗʰ **V37.6** **Passenger** in three-wheeled motor vehicle injured in collision with fixed or stationary object in traffic accident

✓x7ᵗʰ **V37.7** **Person on outside** of three-wheeled motor vehicle injured in collision with fixed or stationary object in traffic accident

✓x7ᵗʰ **V37.9** Unspecified occupant of three-wheeled motor vehicle injured in collision with fixed or stationary object in traffic accident

V38 **Occupant of three-wheeled motor vehicle injured in noncollision transport accident**
> INCLUDES   fall or thrown from three-wheeled motor vehicle
> overturning of three-wheeled motor vehicle NOS
> overturning of three-wheeled motor vehicle without collision

> The appropriate 7th character is to be added to each code from category V38.
> A   initial encounter
> D   subsequent encounter
> S   sequela

✓x7ᵗʰ **V38.0** **Driver** of three-wheeled motor vehicle injured in noncollision transport accident in nontraffic accident

✓x7ᵗʰ **V38.1** **Passenger** in three-wheeled motor vehicle injured in noncollision transport accident in nontraffic accident

✓x7ᵗʰ **V38.2** **Person on outside** of three-wheeled motor vehicle injured in noncollision transport accident in nontraffic accident

✓x7ᵗʰ **V38.3** Unspecified occupant of three-wheeled motor vehicle injured in noncollision transport accident in nontraffic accident

✓x7ᵗʰ **V38.4** **Person boarding or alighting** a three-wheeled motor vehicle injured in noncollision transport accident

✓x7ᵗʰ **V38.5** **Driver** of three-wheeled motor vehicle injured in noncollision transport accident in traffic accident

✓x7ᵗʰ **V38.6** **Passenger** in three-wheeled motor vehicle injured in noncollision transport accident in traffic accident

✓x7ᵗʰ **V38.7** **Person on outside** of three-wheeled motor vehicle injured in noncollision transport accident in traffic accident

✓x7ᵗʰ **V38.9** Unspecified occupant of three-wheeled motor vehicle injured in noncollision transport accident in traffic accident

✓4ᵗʰ **V39** **Occupant of three-wheeled motor vehicle injured in other and unspecified transport accidents**

> The appropriate 7th character is to be added to each code from category V39.
> A   initial encounter
> D   subsequent encounter
> S   sequela

✓5ᵗʰ **V39.0** **Driver** of three-wheeled motor vehicle injured in collision with other and unspecified motor vehicles in nontraffic accident

✓x7ᵗʰ **V39.00** Driver of three-wheeled motor vehicle injured in collision with unspecified motor vehicles in nontraffic accident

✓x7ᵗʰ **V39.09** Driver of three-wheeled motor vehicle injured in collision with other motor vehicles in nontraffic accident

✓ Additional Character Required   ✓x7ᵗʰ Xtension Alert   Unacceptable PDx   Manifestation   Hospital Acquired Condition   EXCLUDES 1 Not Coded Here   EXCLUDES 2 Not Included Here

ICD-10-CM Draft (2015)   1121

External Causes of Morbidity

V39.1–V42.9

√5ᵗʰ **V39.1** **Passenger** in three-wheeled motor vehicle injured in collision with other and unspecified motor vehicles in nontraffic accident

√x7ᵗʰ **V39.10** Passenger in three-wheeled motor vehicle injured in collision with unspecified motor vehicles in nontraffic accident

√x7ᵗʰ **V39.19** Passenger in three-wheeled motor vehicle injured in collision with other motor vehicles in nontraffic accident

√5ᵗʰ **V39.2** Unspecified occupant of three-wheeled motor vehicle injured in collision with other and unspecified motor vehicles in nontraffic accident

√x7ᵗʰ **V39.20** Unspecified occupant of three-wheeled motor vehicle injured in collision with unspecified motor vehicles in nontraffic accident
Collision NOS involving three-wheeled motor vehicle, nontraffic

√x7ᵗʰ **V39.29** Unspecified occupant of three-wheeled motor vehicle injured in collision with other motor vehicles in nontraffic accident

√x7ᵗʰ **V39.3** Occupant (driver) (passenger) of three-wheeled motor vehicle injured in unspecified nontraffic accident
Accident NOS involving three-wheeled motor vehicle, nontraffic
Occupant of three-wheeled motor vehicle injured in nontraffic accident NOS

√5ᵗʰ **V39.4** Driver of three-wheeled motor vehicle injured in collision with other and unspecified motor vehicles in traffic accident

√x7ᵗʰ **V39.40** Driver of three-wheeled motor vehicle injured in collision with unspecified motor vehicles in traffic accident

√x7ᵗʰ **V39.49** Driver of three-wheeled motor vehicle injured in collision with other motor vehicles in traffic accident

√5ᵗʰ **V39.5** Passenger in three-wheeled motor vehicle injured in collision with other and unspecified motor vehicles in traffic accident

√x7ᵗʰ **V39.50** Passenger in three-wheeled motor vehicle injured in collision with unspecified motor vehicles in traffic accident

√x7ᵗʰ **V39.59** Passenger in three-wheeled motor vehicle injured in collision with other motor vehicles in traffic accident

√5ᵗʰ **V39.6** Unspecified occupant of three-wheeled motor vehicle injured in collision with other and unspecified motor vehicles in traffic accident

√x7ᵗʰ **V39.60** Unspecified occupant of three-wheeled motor vehicle injured in collision with unspecified motor vehicles in traffic accident
Collision NOS involving three-wheeled motor vehicle (traffic)

√x7ᵗʰ **V39.69** Unspecified occupant of three-wheeled motor vehicle injured in collision with other motor vehicles in traffic accident

√5ᵗʰ **V39.8** Occupant (driver) (passenger) of three-wheeled motor vehicle injured in other specified transport accidents

√x7ᵗʰ **V39.81** Occupant (driver) (passenger) of three-wheeled motor vehicle injured in transport accident with military vehicle

√x7ᵗʰ **V39.89** Occupant (driver) (passenger) of three-wheeled motor vehicle injured in other specified transport accidents

√x7ᵗʰ **V39.9** Occupant (driver) (passenger) of three-wheeled motor vehicle injured in unspecified traffic accident
Accident NOS involving three-wheeled motor vehicle

Car occupant injured in transport accident (V40-V49)

INCLUDES   a four-wheeled motor vehicle designed primarily for carrying passengers
automobile (pulling a trailer or camper)

EXCLUDES 1   bus (V50-V59)
minibus (V50-V59)
minivan (V50-V59)
motorcoach (V70-V79)
pick-up truck (V50-V59)
sport utility vehicle (SUV) (V50-V59)

√4ᵗʰ **V40** Car occupant injured in collision with pedestrian or animal
EXCLUDES 1   car collision with animal-drawn vehicle or animal being ridden (V46.-)

The appropriate 7th character is to be added to each code from category V40.
A   initial encounter
D   subsequent encounter
S   sequela

√x7ᵗʰ **V40.0** Car driver injured in collision with pedestrian or animal in nontraffic accident

√x7ᵗʰ **V40.1** Car passenger injured in collision with pedestrian or animal in nontraffic accident

√x7ᵗʰ **V40.2** Person on outside of car injured in collision with pedestrian or animal in nontraffic accident

√x7ᵗʰ **V40.3** Unspecified car occupant injured in collision with pedestrian or animal in nontraffic accident

√x7ᵗʰ **V40.4** Person boarding or alighting a car injured in collision with pedestrian or animal

√x7ᵗʰ **V40.5** Car driver injured in collision with pedestrian or animal in traffic accident

√x7ᵗʰ **V40.6** Car passenger injured in collision with pedestrian or animal in traffic accident

√x7ᵗʰ **V40.7** Person on outside of car injured in collision with pedestrian or animal in traffic accident

√x7ᵗʰ **V40.9** Unspecified car occupant injured in collision with pedestrian or animal in traffic accident

√4ᵗʰ **V41** Car occupant injured in collision with pedal cycle

The appropriate 7th character is to be added to each code from category V41.
A   initial encounter
D   subsequent encounter
S   sequela

√x7ᵗʰ **V41.0** Car driver injured in collision with pedal cycle in nontraffic accident

√x7ᵗʰ **V41.1** Car passenger injured in collision with pedal cycle in nontraffic accident

√x7ᵗʰ **V41.2** Person on outside of car injured in collision with pedal cycle in nontraffic accident

√x7ᵗʰ **V41.3** Unspecified car occupant injured in collision with pedal cycle in nontraffic accident

√x7ᵗʰ **V41.4** Person boarding or alighting a car injured in collision with pedal cycle

√x7ᵗʰ **V41.5** Car driver injured in collision with pedal cycle in traffic accident

√x7ᵗʰ **V41.6** Car passenger injured in collision with pedal cycle in traffic accident

√x7ᵗʰ **V41.7** Person on outside of car injured in collision with pedal cycle in traffic accident

√x7ᵗʰ **V41.9** Unspecified car occupant injured in collision with pedal cycle in traffic accident

√4ᵗʰ **V42** Car occupant injured in collision with two- or three-wheeled motor vehicle

The appropriate 7th character is to be added to each code from category V42.
A   initial encounter
D   subsequent encounter
S   sequela

√x7ᵗʰ **V42.0** Car driver injured in collision with two- or three-wheeled motor vehicle in nontraffic accident

√x7ᵗʰ **V42.1** Car passenger injured in collision with two- or three-wheeled motor vehicle in nontraffic accident

√x7ᵗʰ **V42.2** Person on outside of car injured in collision with two- or three-wheeled motor vehicle in nontraffic accident

√x7ᵗʰ **V42.3** Unspecified car occupant injured in collision with two- or three-wheeled motor vehicle in nontraffic accident

√x7ᵗʰ **V42.4** Person boarding or alighting a car injured in collision with two- or three-wheeled motor vehicle

√x7ᵗʰ **V42.5** Car driver injured in collision with two- or three-wheeled motor vehicle in traffic accident

√x7ᵗʰ **V42.6** Car passenger injured in collision with two- or three-wheeled motor vehicle in traffic accident

√x7ᵗʰ **V42.7** Person on outside of car injured in collision with two- or three-wheeled motor vehicle in traffic accident

√x7ᵗʰ **V42.9** Unspecified car occupant injured in collision with two- or three-wheeled motor vehicle in traffic accident

✓4th V43 Car occupant injured in collision with car, pick-up truck or van

> The appropriate 7th character is to be added to each code from category V43.
> A   initial encounter
> D   subsequent encounter
> S   sequela

✓5th V43.0 Car driver injured in collision with car, pick-up truck or van in nontraffic accident

- **✓x7th V43.01** Car driver injured in collision with sport utility vehicle in nontraffic accident
- **✓x7th V43.02** Car driver injured in collision with other type car in nontraffic accident
- **✓x7th V43.03** Car driver injured in collision with pick-up truck in nontraffic accident
- **✓x7th V43.04** Car driver injured in collision with van in nontraffic accident

✓5th V43.1 Car passenger injured in collision with car, pick-up truck or van in nontraffic accident

- **✓x7th V43.11** Car passenger injured in collision with sport utility vehicle in nontraffic accident
- **✓x7th V43.12** Car passenger injured in collision with other type car in nontraffic accident
- **✓x7th V43.13** Car passenger injured in collision with pick-up in nontraffic accident
- **✓x7th V43.14** Car passenger injured in collision with van in nontraffic accident

✓5th V43.2 Person on outside of car injured in collision with car, pick-up truck or van in nontraffic accident

- **✓x7th V43.21** Person on outside of car injured in collision with sport utility vehicle in nontraffic accident
- **✓x7th V43.22** Person on outside of car injured in collision with other type car in nontraffic accident
- **✓x7th V43.23** Person on outside of car injured in collision with pick-up truck in nontraffic accident
- **✓x7th V43.24** Person on outside of car injured in collision with van in nontraffic accident

✓5th V43.3 Unspecified car occupant injured in collision with car, pick-up truck or van in nontraffic accident

- **✓x7th V43.31** Unspecified car occupant injured in collision with sport utility vehicle in nontraffic accident
- **✓x7th V43.32** Unspecified car occupant injured in collision with other type car in nontraffic accident
- **✓x7th V43.33** Unspecified car occupant injured in collision with pick-up truck in nontraffic accident
- **✓x7th V43.34** Unspecified car occupant injured in collision with van in nontraffic accident

✓5th V43.4 Person boarding or alighting a car injured in collision with car, pick-up truck or van

- **✓x7th V43.41** Person boarding or alighting a car injured in collision with sport utility vehicle
- **✓x7th V43.42** Person boarding or alighting a car injured in collision with other type car
- **✓x7th V43.43** Person boarding or alighting a car injured in collision with pick-up truck
- **✓x7th V43.44** Person boarding or alighting a car injured in collision with van

✓5th V43.5 Car driver injured in collision with car, pick-up truck or van in traffic accident

- **✓x7th V43.51** Car driver injured in collision with sport utility vehicle in traffic accident
- **✓x7th V43.52** Car driver injured in collision with other type car in traffic accident
- **✓x7th V43.53** Car driver injured in collision with pick-up truck in traffic accident
- **✓x7th V43.54** Car driver injured in collision with van in traffic accident

✓5th V43.6 Car passenger injured in collision with car, pick-up truck or van in traffic accident

- **✓x7th V43.61** Car passenger injured in collision with sport utility vehicle in traffic accident
- **✓x7th V43.62** Car passenger injured in collision with other type car in traffic accident
- **✓x7th V43.63** Car passenger injured in collision with pick-up truck in traffic accident
- **✓x7th V43.64** Car passenger injured in collision with van in traffic accident

✓5th V43.7 Person on outside of car injured in collision with car, pick-up truck or van in traffic accident

- **✓x7th V43.71** Person on outside of car injured in collision with sport utility vehicle in traffic accident
- **✓x7th V43.72** Person on outside of car injured in collision with other type car in traffic accident
- **✓x7th V43.73** Person on outside of car injured in collision with pick-up truck in traffic accident
- **✓x7th V43.74** Person on outside of car injured in collision with van in traffic accident

✓5th V43.9 Unspecified car occupant injured in collision with car, pick-up truck or van in traffic accident

- **✓x7th V43.91** Unspecified car occupant injured in collision with sport utility vehicle in traffic accident
- **✓x7th V43.92** Unspecified car occupant injured in collision with other type car in traffic accident
- **✓x7th V43.93** Unspecified car occupant injured in collision with pick-up truck in traffic accident
- **✓x7th V43.94** Unspecified car occupant injured in collision with van in traffic accident

✓4th V44 Car occupant injured in collision with heavy transport vehicle or bus

> **EXCLUDES 1**   car occupant injured in collision with military vehicle (V49.81)

> The appropriate 7th character is to be added to each code from category V44.
> A   initial encounter
> D   subsequent encounter
> S   sequela

- **✓x7th V44.0** Car driver injured in collision with heavy transport vehicle or bus in nontraffic accident
- **✓x7th V44.1** Car passenger injured in collision with heavy transport vehicle or bus in nontraffic accident
- **✓x7th V44.2** Person on outside of car injured in collision with heavy transport vehicle or bus in nontraffic accident
- **✓x7th V44.3** Unspecified car occupant injured in collision with heavy transport vehicle or bus in nontraffic accident
- **✓x7th V44.4** Person boarding or alighting a car injured in collision with heavy transport vehicle or bus
- **✓x7th V44.5** Car driver injured in collision with heavy transport vehicle or bus in traffic accident
- **✓x7th V44.6** Car passenger injured in collision with heavy transport vehicle or bus in traffic accident
- **✓x7th V44.7** Person on outside of car injured in collision with heavy transport vehicle or bus in traffic accident
- **✓x7th V44.9** Unspecified car occupant injured in collision with heavy transport vehicle or bus in traffic accident

✓4th V45 Car occupant injured in collision with railway train or railway vehicle

> The appropriate 7th character is to be added to each code from category V45.
> A   initial encounter
> D   subsequent encounter
> S   sequela

- **✓x7th V45.0** Car driver injured in collision with railway train or railway vehicle in nontraffic accident
- **✓x7th V45.1** Car passenger injured in collision with railway train or railway vehicle in nontraffic accident
- **✓x7th V45.2** Person on outside of car injured in collision with railway train or railway vehicle in nontraffic accident
- **✓x7th V45.3** Unspecified car occupant injured in collision with railway train or railway vehicle in nontraffic accident
- **✓x7th V45.4** Person boarding or alighting a car injured in collision with railway train or railway vehicle
- **✓x7th V45.5** Car driver injured in collision with railway train or railway vehicle in traffic accident
- **✓x7th V45.6** Car passenger injured in collision with railway train or railway vehicle in traffic accident
- **✓x7th V45.7** Person on outside of car injured in collision with railway train or railway vehicle in traffic accident
- **✓x7th V45.9** Unspecified car occupant injured in collision with railway train or railway vehicle in traffic accident

✓ Additional Character Required   ✓x7th Xtension Alert   Unacceptable PDx   Manifestation   Hospital Acquired Condition   **EXCLUDES 1** Not Coded Here   **EXCLUDES 2** Not Included Here

ICD-10-CM Draft (2015)   1123

External Causes of Morbidity

V46–V49.60

✓4ᵗʰ V46 Car occupant injured in collision with other nonmotor vehicle

INCLUDES   collision with animal-drawn vehicle, animal being ridden, streetcar

The appropriate 7th character is to be added to each code from category V46.
A   initial encounter
D   subsequent encounter
S   sequela

✓x7ᵗʰ **V46.0** Car driver injured in collision with other nonmotor vehicle in nontraffic accident

✓x7ᵗʰ **V46.1** Car passenger injured in collision with other nonmotor vehicle in nontraffic accident

✓x7ᵗʰ **V46.2** Person on outside of car injured in collision with other nonmotor vehicle in nontraffic accident

✓x7ᵗʰ **V46.3** Unspecified car occupant injured in collision with other nonmotor vehicle in nontraffic accident

✓x7ᵗʰ **V46.4** Person boarding or alighting a car injured in collision with other nonmotor vehicle

✓x7ᵗʰ **V46.5** Car driver injured in collision with other nonmotor vehicle in traffic accident

✓x7ᵗʰ **V46.6** Car passenger injured in collision with other nonmotor vehicle in traffic accident

✓x7ᵗʰ **V46.7** Person on outside of car injured in collision with other nonmotor vehicle in traffic accident

✓x7ᵗʰ **V46.9** Unspecified car occupant injured in collision with other nonmotor vehicle in traffic accident

✓4ᵗʰ V47 Car occupant injured in collision with fixed or stationary object

The appropriate 7th character is to be added to each code from category V47.
A   initial encounter
D   subsequent encounter
S   sequela

✓5ᵗʰ **V47.0** Car driver injured in collision with fixed or stationary object in nontraffic accident

    ✓x7ᵗʰ **V47.01** Driver of sport utility vehicle injured in collision with fixed or stationary object in nontraffic accident

    ✓x7ᵗʰ **V47.02** Driver of other type car injured in collision with fixed or stationary object in nontraffic accident

✓5ᵗʰ **V47.1** Car passenger injured in collision with fixed or stationary object in nontraffic accident

    ✓x7ᵗʰ **V47.11** Passenger of sport utility vehicle injured in collision with fixed or stationary object in nontraffic accident

    ✓x7ᵗʰ **V47.12** Passenger of other type car injured in collision with fixed or stationary object in nontraffic accident

✓5ᵗʰ **V47.2** Person on outside of car injured in collision with fixed or stationary object in nontraffic accident

✓5ᵗʰ **V47.3** Unspecified car occupant injured in collision with fixed or stationary object in nontraffic accident

    ✓x7ᵗʰ **V47.31** Unspecified occupant of sport utility vehicle injured in collision with fixed or stationary object in nontraffic accident

    ✓x7ᵗʰ **V47.32** Unspecified occupant of other type car injured in collision with fixed or stationary object in nontraffic accident

✓x7ᵗʰ **V47.4** Person boarding or alighting a car injured in collision with fixed or stationary object

✓5ᵗʰ **V47.5** Car driver injured in collision with fixed or stationary object in traffic accident

    ✓x7ᵗʰ **V47.51** Driver of sport utility vehicle injured in collision with fixed or stationary object in traffic accident

    ✓x7ᵗʰ **V47.52** Driver of other type car injured in collision with fixed or stationary object in traffic accident

✓5ᵗʰ **V47.6** Car passenger injured in collision with fixed or stationary object in traffic accident

    ✓x7ᵗʰ **V47.61** Passenger of sport utility vehicle injured in collision with fixed or stationary object in traffic accident

    ✓x7ᵗʰ **V47.62** Passenger of other type car injured in collision with fixed or stationary object in traffic accident

✓x7ᵗʰ **V47.7** Person on outside of car injured in collision with fixed or stationary object in traffic accident

✓5ᵗʰ **V47.9** Unspecified car occupant injured in collision with fixed or stationary object in traffic accident

    ✓x7ᵗʰ **V47.91** Unspecified occupant of sport utility vehicle injured in collision with fixed or stationary object in traffic accident

✓x7ᵗʰ **V47.92** Unspecified occupant of other type car injured in collision with fixed or stationary object in traffic accident

✓4ᵗʰ V48 Car occupant injured in noncollision transport accident

INCLUDES   overturning car NOS
            overturning car without collision

The appropriate 7th character is to be added to each code from category V48.
A   initial encounter
D   subsequent encounter
S   sequela

✓x7ᵗʰ **V48.0** Car driver injured in noncollision transport accident in nontraffic accident

✓x7ᵗʰ **V48.1** Car passenger injured in noncollision transport accident in nontraffic accident

✓x7ᵗʰ **V48.2** Person on outside of car injured in noncollision transport accident in nontraffic accident

✓x7ᵗʰ **V48.3** Unspecified car occupant injured in noncollision transport accident in nontraffic accident

✓x7ᵗʰ **V48.4** Person boarding or alighting a car injured in noncollision transport accident

✓x7ᵗʰ **V48.5** Car driver injured in noncollision transport accident in traffic accident

✓x7ᵗʰ **V48.6** Car passenger injured in noncollision transport accident in traffic accident

✓x7ᵗʰ **V48.7** Person on outside of car injured in noncollision transport accident in traffic accident

✓x7ᵗʰ **V48.9** Unspecified car occupant injured in noncollision transport accident in traffic accident

✓4ᵗʰ V49 Car occupant injured in other and unspecified transport accidents

The appropriate 7th character is to be added to each code from category V49.
A   initial encounter
D   subsequent encounter
S   sequela

✓5ᵗʰ **V49.0** Driver injured in collision with other and unspecified motor vehicles in nontraffic accident

    ✓x7ᵗʰ **V49.00** Driver injured in collision with unspecified motor vehicles in nontraffic accident

    ✓x7ᵗʰ **V49.09** Driver injured in collision with other motor vehicles in nontraffic accident

✓5ᵗʰ **V49.1** Passenger injured in collision with other and unspecified motor vehicles in nontraffic accident

    ✓x7ᵗʰ **V49.10** Passenger injured in collision with unspecified motor vehicles in nontraffic accident

    ✓x7ᵗʰ **V49.19** Passenger injured in collision with other motor vehicles in nontraffic accident

✓5ᵗʰ **V49.2** Unspecified car occupant injured in collision with other and unspecified motor vehicles in nontraffic accident

    ✓x7ᵗʰ **V49.20** Unspecified car occupant injured in collision with unspecified motor vehicles in nontraffic accident
       Car collision NOS, nontraffic

    ✓x7ᵗʰ **V49.29** Unspecified car occupant injured in collision with other motor vehicles in nontraffic accident

✓x7ᵗʰ **V49.3** Car occupant (driver) (passenger) injured in unspecified nontraffic accident
       Car accident NOS, nontraffic
       Car occupant injured in nontraffic accident NOS

✓5ᵗʰ **V49.4** Driver injured in collision with other and unspecified motor vehicles in traffic accident

    ✓x7ᵗʰ **V49.40** Driver injured in collision with unspecified motor vehicles in traffic accident

    ✓x7ᵗʰ **V49.49** Driver injured in collision with other motor vehicles in traffic accident

✓5ᵗʰ **V49.5** Passenger injured in collision with other and unspecified motor vehicles in traffic accident

    ✓x7ᵗʰ **V49.50** Passenger injured in collision with unspecified motor vehicles in traffic accident

    ✓x7ᵗʰ **V49.59** Passenger injured in collision with other motor vehicles in traffic accident

✓5ᵗʰ **V49.6** Unspecified car occupant injured in collision with other and unspecified motor vehicles in traffic accident

    ✓x7ᵗʰ **V49.60** Unspecified car occupant injured in collision with unspecified motor vehicles in traffic accident
       Car collision NOS (traffic)

N Newborn: 0   **P** Pediatric: 0-17   **M** Maternity: 12-55   **A** Adult: 15-124   **MCC** Major CC Condition   **PDx MCC** PDx acts as own MCC   **CC** CC Condition   **PDx CC** PDx acts as own CC

✓x7ᵗʰ **V49.69** Unspecified car occupant injured in collision with other motor vehicles in traffic accident

✓5ᵗʰ **V49.8** Car occupant (driver) (passenger) injured in other specified transport accidents

✓x7ᵗʰ **V49.81** Car occupant (driver) (passenger) injured in transport accident with military vehicle

✓x7ᵗʰ **V49.88** Car occupant (driver) (passenger) injured in other specified transport accidents

✓x7ᵗʰ **V49.9** Car occupant (driver) (passenger) injured in unspecified traffic accident
Car accident NOS

Occupant of pick-up truck or van injured in transport accident (V50-V59)

INCLUDES   a four or six wheel motor vehicle designed primarily for carrying passengers and property but weighing less than the local limit for classification as a heavy goods vehicle
minibus
minivan
sport utility vehicle (SUV)
truck
van
EXCLUDES 1   heavy transport vehicle (V60-V69)

✓4ᵗʰ **V50** Occupant of pick-up truck or van injured in collision with pedestrian or animal
EXCLUDES 1   pick-up truck or van collision with animal-drawn vehicle or animal being ridden (V56.-)

The appropriate 7th character is to be added to each code from category V50.
A   initial encounter
D   subsequent encounter
S   sequela

✓x7ᵗʰ **V50.0** Driver of pick-up truck or van injured in collision with pedestrian or animal in nontraffic accident

✓x7ᵗʰ **V50.1** Passenger in pick-up truck or van injured in collision with pedestrian or animal in nontraffic accident

✓x7ᵗʰ **V50.2** Person on outside of pick-up truck or van injured in collision with pedestrian or animal in nontraffic accident

✓x7ᵗʰ **V50.3** Unspecified occupant of pick-up truck or van injured in collision with pedestrian or animal in nontraffic accident

✓x7ᵗʰ **V50.4** Person boarding or alighting a pick-up truck or van injured in collision with pedestrian or animal

✓x7ᵗʰ **V50.5** Driver of pick-up truck or van injured in collision with pedestrian or animal in traffic accident

✓x7ᵗʰ **V50.6** Passenger in pick-up truck or van injured in collision with pedestrian or animal in traffic accident

✓x7ᵗʰ **V50.7** Person on outside of pick-up truck or van injured in collision with pedestrian or animal in traffic accident

✓x7ᵗʰ **V50.9** Unspecified occupant of pick-up truck or van injured in collision with pedestrian or animal in traffic accident

✓4ᵗʰ **V51** Occupant of pick-up truck or van injured in collision with pedal cycle

The appropriate 7th character is to be added to each code from category V51.
A   initial encounter
D   subsequent encounter
S   sequela

✓x7ᵗʰ **V51.0** Driver of pick-up truck or van injured in collision with pedal cycle in nontraffic accident

✓x7ᵗʰ **V51.1** Passenger in pick-up truck or van injured in collision with pedal cycle in nontraffic accident

✓x7ᵗʰ **V51.2** Person on outside of pick-up truck or van injured in collision with pedal cycle in nontraffic accident

✓x7ᵗʰ **V51.3** Unspecified occupant of pick-up truck or van injured in collision with pedal cycle in nontraffic accident

✓x7ᵗʰ **V51.4** Person boarding or alighting a pick-up truck or van injured in collision with pedal cycle

✓x7ᵗʰ **V51.5** Driver of pick-up truck or van injured in collision with pedal cycle in traffic accident

✓x7ᵗʰ **V51.6** Passenger in pick-up truck or van injured in collision with pedal cycle in traffic accident

✓x7ᵗʰ **V51.7** Person on outside of pick-up truck or van injured in collision with pedal cycle in traffic accident

✓x7ᵗʰ **V51.9** Unspecified occupant of pick-up truck or van injured in collision with pedal cycle in traffic accident

✓4ᵗʰ **V52** Occupant of pick-up truck or van injured in collision with two- or three-wheeled motor vehicle

The appropriate 7th character is to be added to each code from category V52.
A   initial encounter
D   subsequent encounter
S   sequela

✓x7ᵗʰ **V52.0** Driver of pick-up truck or van injured in collision with two- or three-wheeled motor vehicle in nontraffic accident

✓x7ᵗʰ **V52.1** Passenger in pick-up truck or van injured in collision with two- or three-wheeled motor vehicle in nontraffic accident

✓x7ᵗʰ **V52.2** Person on outside of pick-up truck or van injured in collision with two- or three-wheeled motor vehicle in nontraffic accident

✓x7ᵗʰ **V52.3** Unspecified occupant of pick-up truck or van injured in collision with two- or three-wheeled motor vehicle in nontraffic accident

✓x7ᵗʰ **V52.4** Person boarding or alighting a pick-up truck or van injured in collision with two- or three-wheeled motor vehicle

✓x7ᵗʰ **V52.5** Driver of pick-up truck or van injured in collision with two- or three-wheeled motor vehicle in traffic accident

✓x7ᵗʰ **V52.6** Passenger in pick-up truck or van injured in collision with two- or three-wheeled motor vehicle in traffic accident

✓x7ᵗʰ **V52.7** Person on outside of pick-up truck or van injured in collision with two- or three-wheeled motor vehicle in traffic accident

✓x7ᵗʰ **V52.9** Unspecified occupant of pick-up truck or van injured in collision with two- or three-wheeled motor vehicle in traffic accident

✓4ᵗʰ **V53** Occupant of pick-up truck or van injured in collision with car, pick-up truck or van

The appropriate 7th character is to be added to each code from category V53.
A   initial encounter
D   subsequent encounter
S   sequela

✓x7ᵗʰ **V53.0** Driver of pick-up truck or van injured in collision with car, pick-up truck or van in nontraffic accident

✓x7ᵗʰ **V53.1** Passenger in pick-up truck or van injured in collision with car, pick-up truck or van in nontraffic accident

✓x7ᵗʰ **V53.2** Person on outside of pick-up truck or van injured in collision with car, pick-up truck or van in nontraffic accident

✓x7ᵗʰ **V53.3** Unspecified occupant of pick-up truck or van injured in collision with car, pick-up truck or van in nontraffic accident

✓x7ᵗʰ **V53.4** Person boarding or alighting a pick-up truck or van injured in collision with car, pick-up truck or van

✓x7ᵗʰ **V53.5** Driver of pick-up truck or van injured in collision with car, pick-up truck or van in traffic accident

✓x7ᵗʰ **V53.6** Passenger in pick-up truck or van injured in collision with car, pick-up truck or van in traffic accident

✓x7ᵗʰ **V53.7** Person on outside of pick-up truck or van injured in collision with car, pick-up truck or van in traffic accident

✓x7ᵗʰ **V53.9** Unspecified occupant of pick-up truck or van injured in collision with car, pick-up truck or van in traffic accident

✓4ᵗʰ **V54** Occupant of pick-up truck or van injured in collision with heavy transport vehicle or bus
EXCLUDES 1   occupant of pick-up truck or van injured in collision with military vehicle (V59.81)

The appropriate 7th character is to be added to each code from category V54.
A   initial encounter
D   subsequent encounter
S   sequela

✓x7ᵗʰ **V54.0** Driver of pick-up truck or van injured in collision with heavy transport vehicle or bus in nontraffic accident

✓x7ᵗʰ **V54.1** Passenger in pick-up truck or van injured in collision with heavy transport vehicle or bus in nontraffic accident

✓x7ᵗʰ **V54.2** Person on outside of pick-up truck or van injured in collision with heavy transport vehicle or bus in nontraffic accident

✓x7ᵗʰ **V54.3** Unspecified occupant of pick-up truck or van injured in collision with heavy transport vehicle or bus in nontraffic accident

✓x7ᵗʰ **V54.4** Person boarding or alighting a pick-up truck or van injured in collision with heavy transport vehicle or bus

---

✓ Additional Character Required   ✓x7ᵗʰ Xtension Alert   Unacceptable PDx   Manifestation   Hospital Acquired Condition   EXCLUDES 1 Not Coded Here   EXCLUDES 2 Not Included Here

External Causes of Morbidity

V54.5–V59.29

√x7th **V54.5** **Driver** of pick-up truck or van injured in collision with heavy transport vehicle or bus in traffic accident

√x7th **V54.6** **Passenger** in pick-up truck or van injured in collision with heavy transport vehicle or bus in traffic accident

√x7th **V54.7** **Person on outside** of pick-up truck or van injured in collision with heavy transport vehicle or bus in traffic accident

√x7th **V54.9** **Unspecified** occupant of pick-up truck or van injured in collision with heavy transport vehicle or bus in traffic accident

√4th **V55** **Occupant of pick-up truck or van injured in collision with railway train or railway vehicle**

The appropriate 7th character is to be added to each code from category V55.
A   initial encounter
D   subsequent encounter
S   sequela

√x7th **V55.0** **Driver** of pick-up truck or van injured in collision with railway train or railway vehicle in nontraffic accident

√x7th **V55.1** **Passenger** in pick-up truck or van injured in collision with railway train or railway vehicle in nontraffic accident

√x7th **V55.2** **Person on outside** of pick-up truck or van injured in collision with railway train or railway vehicle in nontraffic accident

√x7th **V55.3** **Unspecified** occupant of pick-up truck or van injured in collision with railway train or railway vehicle in nontraffic accident

√x7th **V55.4** **Person boarding or alighting** a pick-up truck or van injured in collision with railway train or railway vehicle

√x7th **V55.5** **Driver** of pick-up truck or van injured in collision with railway train or railway vehicle in traffic accident

√x7th **V55.6** **Passenger** in pick-up truck or van injured in collision with railway train or railway vehicle in traffic accident

√x7th **V55.7** **Person on outside** of pick-up truck or van injured in collision with railway train or railway vehicle in traffic accident

√x7th **V55.9** **Unspecified** occupant of pick-up truck or van injured in collision with railway train or railway vehicle in traffic accident

√4th **V56** **Occupant of pick-up truck or van injured in collision with other nonmotor vehicle**
INCLUDES   collision with animal-drawn vehicle, animal being ridden, streetcar

The appropriate 7th character is to be added to each code from category V56.
A   initial encounter
D   subsequent encounter
S   sequela

√x7th **V56.0** **Driver** of pick-up truck or van injured in collision with other nonmotor vehicle in nontraffic accident

√x7th **V56.1** **Passenger** in pick-up truck or van injured in collision with other nonmotor vehicle in nontraffic accident

√x7th **V56.2** **Person on outside** of pick-up truck or van injured in collision with other nonmotor vehicle in nontraffic accident

√x7th **V56.3** **Unspecified** occupant of pick-up truck or van injured in collision with other nonmotor vehicle in nontraffic accident

√x7th **V56.4** **Person boarding or alighting** a pick-up truck or van injured in collision with other nonmotor vehicle

√x7th **V56.5** **Driver** of pick-up truck or van injured in collision with other nonmotor vehicle in traffic accident

√x7th **V56.6** **Passenger** in pick-up truck or van injured in collision with other nonmotor vehicle in traffic accident

√x7th **V56.7** **Person on outside** of pick-up truck or van injured in collision with other nonmotor vehicle in traffic accident

√x7th **V56.9** **Unspecified** occupant of pick-up truck or van injured in collision with other nonmotor vehicle in traffic accident

√4th **V57** **Occupant of pick-up truck or van injured in collision with fixed or stationary object**

The appropriate 7th character is to be added to each code from category V57.
A   initial encounter
D   subsequent encounter
S   sequela

√x7th **V57.0** **Driver** of pick-up truck or van injured in collision with fixed or stationary object in nontraffic accident

√x7th **V57.1** **Passenger** in pick-up truck or van injured in collision with fixed or stationary object in nontraffic accident

√x7th **V57.2** **Person on outside** of pick-up truck or van injured in collision with fixed or stationary object in nontraffic accident

√x7th **V57.3** **Unspecified** occupant of pick-up truck or van injured in collision with fixed or stationary object in nontraffic accident

√x7th **V57.4** **Person boarding or alighting** a pick-up truck or van injured in collision with fixed or stationary object

√x7th **V57.5** **Driver** of pick-up truck or van injured in collision with fixed or stationary object in traffic accident

√x7th **V57.6** **Passenger** in pick-up truck or van injured in collision with fixed or stationary object in traffic accident

√x7th **V57.7** **Person on outside** of pick-up truck or van injured in collision with fixed or stationary object in traffic accident

√x7th **V57.9** **Unspecified** occupant of pick-up truck or van injured in collision with fixed or stationary object in traffic accident

√4th **V58** **Occupant of pick-up truck or van injured in noncollision transport accident**
INCLUDES   overturning pick-up truck or van NOS
             overturning pick-up truck or van without collision

The appropriate 7th character is to be added to each code from category V58.
A   initial encounter
D   subsequent encounter
S   sequela

√x7th **V58.0** **Driver** of pick-up truck or van injured in noncollision transport accident in nontraffic accident

√x7th **V58.1** **Passenger** in pick-up truck or van injured in noncollision transport accident in nontraffic accident

√x7th **V58.2** **Person on outside** of pick-up truck or van injured in noncollision transport accident in nontraffic accident

√x7th **V58.3** **Unspecified** occupant of pick-up truck or van injured in noncollision transport accident in nontraffic accident

√x7th **V58.4** **Person boarding or alighting** a pick-up truck or van injured in noncollision transport accident

√x7th **V58.5** **Driver** of pick-up truck or van injured in noncollision transport accident in traffic accident

√x7th **V58.6** **Passenger** in pick-up truck or van injured in noncollision transport accident in traffic accident

√x7th **V58.7** **Person on outside** of pick-up truck or van injured in noncollision transport accident in traffic accident

√x7th **V58.9** **Unspecified** occupant of pick-up truck or van injured in noncollision transport accident in traffic accident

√4th **V59** **Occupant of pick-up truck or van injured in other and unspecified transport accidents**

The appropriate 7th character is to be added to each code from category V59.
A   initial encounter
D   subsequent encounter
S   sequela

√5th **V59.0** **Driver** of pick-up truck or van injured in collision with other and unspecified motor vehicles in nontraffic accident

√x7th   **V59.00** **Driver** of pick-up truck or van injured in collision with unspecified motor vehicles in nontraffic accident

√x7th   **V59.09** **Driver** of pick-up truck or van injured in collision with other motor vehicles in nontraffic accident

√5th **V59.1** **Passenger** in pick-up truck or van injured in collision with other and unspecified motor vehicles in nontraffic accident

√x7th   **V59.10** **Passenger** in pick-up truck or van injured in collision with unspecified motor vehicles in nontraffic accident

√x7th   **V59.19** **Passenger** in pick-up truck or van injured in collision with other motor vehicles in nontraffic accident

√5th **V59.2** **Unspecified** occupant of pick-up truck or van injured in collision with other and unspecified motor vehicles in nontraffic accident

√x7th   **V59.20** **Unspecified** occupant of pick-up truck or van injured in collision with unspecified motor vehicles in nontraffic accident
        Collision NOS involving pick-up truck or van, nontraffic

√x7th   **V59.29** **Unspecified** occupant of pick-up truck or van injured in collision with other motor vehicles in nontraffic accident

N Newborn: 0   P Pediatric: 0-17   M Maternity: 12-55   A Adult: 15-124   MCC Major CC Condition   PDx MCC PDx acts as own MCC   CC CC Condition   PDx CC PDx acts as own CC

1126   ICD-10-CM Draft (2015)

✓x7ᵗʰ **V59.3** **Occupant (driver) (passenger) of pick-up truck or van injured in unspecified nontraffic accident**
Accident NOS involving pick-up truck or van, nontraffic
Occupant of pick-up truck or van injured in nontraffic accident NOS

✓5ᵗʰ **V59.4** Driver of pick-up truck or van injured in collision with other and unspecified motor vehicles in traffic accident

  ✓x7ᵗʰ **V59.40** Driver of pick-up truck or van injured in collision with unspecified motor vehicles in traffic accident

  ✓x7ᵗʰ **V59.49** Driver of pick-up truck or van injured in collision with other motor vehicles in traffic accident

✓5ᵗʰ **V59.5** Passenger in pick-up truck or van injured in collision with other and unspecified motor vehicles in traffic accident

  ✓x7ᵗʰ **V59.50** Passenger in pick-up truck or van injured in collision with unspecified motor vehicles in traffic accident

  ✓x7ᵗʰ **V59.59** Passenger in pick-up truck or van injured in collision with other motor vehicles in traffic accident

✓5ᵗʰ **V59.6** Unspecified occupant of pick-up truck or van injured in collision with other and unspecified motor vehicles in traffic accident

  ✓x7ᵗʰ **V59.60** Unspecified occupant of pick-up truck or van injured in collision with unspecified motor vehicles in traffic accident
Collision NOS involving pick-up truck or van (traffic)

  ✓x7ᵗʰ **V59.69** Unspecified occupant of pick-up truck or van injured in collision with other motor vehicles in traffic accident

✓5ᵗʰ **V59.8** Occupant (driver) (passenger) of pick-up truck or van injured in other specified transport accidents

  ✓x7ᵗʰ **V59.81** Occupant (driver) (passenger) of pick-up truck or van injured in transport accident with military vehicle

  ✓x7ᵗʰ **V59.88** Occupant (driver) (passenger) of pick-up truck or van injured in other specified transport accidents

✓x7ᵗʰ **V59.9** Occupant (driver) (passenger) of pick-up truck or van injured in unspecified traffic accident
Accident NOS involving pick-up truck or van

Occupant of heavy transport vehicle injured in transport accident (V60-V69)

INCLUDES 18 wheeler
armored car
panel truck

EXCLUDES 1 *bus*
motorcoach

✓4ᵗʰ **V60** **Occupant of heavy transport vehicle injured in collision with pedestrian or animal**

EXCLUDES 1 *heavy transport vehicle collision with animal-drawn vehicle or animal being ridden (V66.-)*

The appropriate 7th character is to be added to each code from category V60.
A   initial encounter
D   subsequent encounter
S   sequela

✓x7ᵗʰ **V60.0** Driver of heavy transport vehicle injured in collision with pedestrian or animal in nontraffic accident

✓x7ᵗʰ **V60.1** Passenger in heavy transport vehicle injured in collision with pedestrian or animal in nontraffic accident

✓x7ᵗʰ **V60.2** Person on outside of heavy transport vehicle injured in collision with pedestrian or animal in nontraffic accident

✓x7ᵗʰ **V60.3** Unspecified occupant of heavy transport vehicle injured in collision with pedestrian or animal in nontraffic accident

✓x7ᵗʰ **V60.4** Person boarding or alighting a heavy transport vehicle injured in collision with pedestrian or animal

✓x7ᵗʰ **V60.5** Driver of heavy transport vehicle injured in collision with pedestrian or animal in traffic accident

✓x7ᵗʰ **V60.6** Passenger in heavy transport vehicle injured in collision with pedestrian or animal in traffic accident

✓x7ᵗʰ **V60.7** Person on outside of heavy transport vehicle injured in collision with pedestrian or animal in traffic accident

✓x7ᵗʰ **V60.9** Unspecified occupant of heavy transport vehicle injured in collision with pedestrian or animal in traffic accident

✓4ᵗʰ **V61** **Occupant of heavy transport vehicle injured in collision with pedal cycle**

The appropriate 7th character is to be added to each code from category V61.
A   initial encounter
D   subsequent encounter
S   sequela

✓x7ᵗʰ **V61.0** Driver of heavy transport vehicle injured in collision with pedal cycle in nontraffic accident

✓x7ᵗʰ **V61.1** Passenger in heavy transport vehicle injured in collision with pedal cycle in nontraffic accident

✓x7ᵗʰ **V61.2** Person on outside of heavy transport vehicle injured in collision with pedal cycle in nontraffic accident

✓x7ᵗʰ **V61.3** Unspecified occupant of heavy transport vehicle injured in collision with pedal cycle in nontraffic accident

✓x7ᵗʰ **V61.4** Person boarding or alighting a heavy transport vehicle injured in collision with pedal cycle while boarding or alighting

✓x7ᵗʰ **V61.5** Driver of heavy transport vehicle injured in collision with pedal cycle in traffic accident

✓x7ᵗʰ **V61.6** Passenger in heavy transport vehicle injured in collision with pedal cycle in traffic accident

✓x7ᵗʰ **V61.7** Person on outside of heavy transport vehicle injured in collision with pedal cycle in traffic accident

✓x7ᵗʰ **V61.9** Unspecified occupant of heavy transport vehicle injured in collision with pedal cycle in traffic accident

✓4ᵗʰ **V62** **Occupant of heavy transport vehicle injured in collision with two- or three-wheeled motor vehicle**

The appropriate 7th character is to be added to each code from category V62.
A   initial encounter
D   subsequent encounter
S   sequela

✓x7ᵗʰ **V62.0** Driver of heavy transport vehicle injured in collision with two- or three-wheeled motor vehicle in nontraffic accident

✓x7ᵗʰ **V62.1** Passenger in heavy transport vehicle injured in collision with two- or three-wheeled motor vehicle in nontraffic accident

✓x7ᵗʰ **V62.2** Person on outside of heavy transport vehicle injured in collision with two- or three-wheeled motor vehicle in nontraffic accident

✓x7ᵗʰ **V62.3** Unspecified occupant of heavy transport vehicle injured in collision with two- or three-wheeled motor vehicle in nontraffic accident

✓x7ᵗʰ **V62.4** Person boarding or alighting a heavy transport vehicle injured in collision with two- or three-wheeled motor vehicle

✓x7ᵗʰ **V62.5** Driver of heavy transport vehicle injured in collision with two- or three-wheeled motor vehicle in traffic accident

✓x7ᵗʰ **V62.6** Passenger in heavy transport vehicle injured in collision with two- or three-wheeled motor vehicle in traffic accident

✓x7ᵗʰ **V62.7** Person on outside of heavy transport vehicle injured in collision with two- or three-wheeled motor vehicle in traffic accident

✓x7ᵗʰ **V62.9** Unspecified occupant of heavy transport vehicle injured in collision with two- or three-wheeled motor vehicle in traffic accident

✓4ᵗʰ **V63** **Occupant of heavy transport vehicle injured in collision with car, pick-up truck or van**

The appropriate 7th character is to be added to each code from category V63.
A   initial encounter
D   subsequent encounter
S   sequela

✓x7ᵗʰ **V63.0** Driver of heavy transport vehicle injured in collision with car, pick-up truck or van in nontraffic accident

✓x7ᵗʰ **V63.1** Passenger in heavy transport vehicle injured in collision with car, pick-up truck or van in nontraffic accident

✓x7ᵗʰ **V63.2** Person on outside of heavy transport vehicle injured in collision with car, pick-up truck or van in nontraffic accident

✓x7ᵗʰ **V63.3** Unspecified occupant of heavy transport vehicle injured in collision with car, pick-up truck or van in nontraffic accident

✓x7ᵗʰ **V63.4** Person boarding or alighting a heavy transport vehicle injured in collision with car, pick-up truck or van

✓x7ᵗʰ **V63.5** Driver of heavy transport vehicle injured in collision with car, pick-up truck or van in traffic accident

External Causes of Morbidity

V63.6–V68.5

√x7th **V63.6** Passenger in heavy transport vehicle injured in collision with car, pick-up truck or van in traffic accident

√x7th **V63.7** Person on outside of heavy transport vehicle injured in collision with car, pick-up truck or van in traffic accident

√x7th **V63.9** Unspecified occupant of heavy transport vehicle injured in collision with car, pick-up truck or van in traffic accident

√4th **V64** Occupant of heavy transport vehicle injured in collision with heavy transport vehicle or bus

> EXCLUDES 1   occupant of heavy transport vehicle injured in collision with military vehicle (V69.81)

> The appropriate 7th character is to be added to each code from category V64.
> A   initial encounter
> D   subsequent encounter
> S   sequela

√x7th **V64.0** Driver of heavy transport vehicle injured in collision with heavy transport vehicle or bus in nontraffic accident

√x7th **V64.1** Passenger in heavy transport vehicle injured in collision with heavy transport vehicle or bus in nontraffic accident

√x7th **V64.2** Person on outside of heavy transport vehicle injured in collision with heavy transport vehicle or bus in nontraffic accident

√x7th **V64.3** Unspecified occupant of heavy transport vehicle injured in collision with heavy transport vehicle or bus in nontraffic accident

√x7th **V64.4** Person boarding or alighting a heavy transport vehicle injured in collision with heavy transport vehicle or bus while boarding or alighting

√x7th **V64.5** Driver of heavy transport vehicle injured in collision with heavy transport vehicle or bus in traffic accident

√x7th **V64.6** Passenger in heavy transport vehicle injured in collision with heavy transport vehicle or bus in traffic accident

√x7th **V64.7** Person on outside of heavy transport vehicle injured in collision with heavy transport vehicle or bus in traffic accident

√x7th **V64.9** Unspecified occupant of heavy transport vehicle injured in collision with heavy transport vehicle or bus in traffic accident

√4th **V65** Occupant of heavy transport vehicle injured in collision with railway train or railway vehicle

> The appropriate 7th character is to be added to each code from category V65.
> A   initial encounter
> D   subsequent encounter
> S   sequela

√x7th **V65.0** Driver of heavy transport vehicle injured in collision with railway train or railway vehicle in nontraffic accident

√x7th **V65.1** Passenger in heavy transport vehicle injured in collision with railway train or railway vehicle in nontraffic accident

√x7th **V65.2** Person on outside of heavy transport vehicle injured in collision with railway train or railway vehicle in nontraffic accident

√x7th **V65.3** Unspecified occupant of heavy transport vehicle injured in collision with railway train or railway vehicle in nontraffic accident

√x7th **V65.4** Person boarding or alighting a heavy transport vehicle injured in collision with railway train or railway vehicle

√x7th **V65.5** Driver of heavy transport vehicle injured in collision with railway train or railway vehicle in traffic accident

√x7th **V65.6** Passenger in heavy transport vehicle injured in collision with railway train or railway vehicle in traffic accident

√x7th **V65.7** Person on outside of heavy transport vehicle injured in collision with railway train or railway vehicle in traffic accident

√x7th **V65.9** Unspecified occupant of heavy transport vehicle injured in collision with railway train or railway vehicle in traffic accident

√4th **V66** Occupant of heavy transport vehicle injured in collision with other nonmotor vehicle

> INCLUDES   collision with animal-drawn vehicle, animal being ridden, streetcar

> The appropriate 7th character is to be added to each code from category V66.
> A   initial encounter
> D   subsequent encounter
> S   sequela

√x7th **V66.0** Driver of heavy transport vehicle injured in collision with other nonmotor vehicle in nontraffic accident

√x7th **V66.1** Passenger in heavy transport vehicle injured in collision with other nonmotor vehicle in nontraffic accident

√x7th **V66.2** Person on outside of heavy transport vehicle injured in collision with other nonmotor vehicle in nontraffic accident

√x7th **V66.3** Unspecified occupant of heavy transport vehicle injured in collision with other nonmotor vehicle in nontraffic accident

√x7th **V66.4** Person boarding or alighting a heavy transport vehicle injured in collision with other nonmotor vehicle

√x7th **V66.5** Driver of heavy transport vehicle injured in collision with other nonmotor vehicle in traffic accident

√x7th **V66.6** Passenger in heavy transport vehicle injured in collision with other nonmotor vehicle in traffic accident

√x7th **V66.7** Person on outside of heavy transport vehicle injured in collision with other nonmotor vehicle in traffic accident

√x7th **V66.9** Unspecified occupant of heavy transport vehicle injured in collision with other nonmotor vehicle in traffic accident

√4th **V67** Occupant of heavy transport vehicle injured in collision with fixed or stationary object

> The appropriate 7th character is to be added to each code from category V67.
> A   initial encounter
> D   subsequent encounter
> S   sequela

√x7th **V67.0** Driver of heavy transport vehicle injured in collision with fixed or stationary object in nontraffic accident

√x7th **V67.1** Passenger in heavy transport vehicle injured in collision with fixed or stationary object in nontraffic accident

√x7th **V67.2** Person on outside of heavy transport vehicle injured in collision with fixed or stationary object in nontraffic accident

√x7th **V67.3** Unspecified occupant of heavy transport vehicle injured in collision with fixed or stationary object in nontraffic accident

√x7th **V67.4** Person boarding or alighting a heavy transport vehicle injured in collision with fixed or stationary object

√x7th **V67.5** Driver of heavy transport vehicle injured in collision with fixed or stationary object in traffic accident

√x7th **V67.6** Passenger in heavy transport vehicle injured in collision with fixed or stationary object in traffic accident

√x7th **V67.7** Person on outside of heavy transport vehicle injured in collision with fixed or stationary object in traffic accident

√x7th **V67.9** Unspecified occupant of heavy transport vehicle injured in collision with fixed or stationary object in traffic accident

√4th **V68** Occupant of heavy transport vehicle injured in noncollision transport accident

> INCLUDES   overturning heavy transport vehicle NOS
> overturning heavy transport vehicle without collision

> The appropriate 7th character is to be added to each code from category V68.
> A   initial encounter
> D   subsequent encounter
> S   sequela

√x7th **V68.0** Driver of heavy transport vehicle injured in noncollision transport accident in nontraffic accident

√x7th **V68.1** Passenger in heavy transport vehicle injured in noncollision transport accident in nontraffic accident

√x7th **V68.2** Person on outside of heavy transport vehicle injured in noncollision transport accident in nontraffic accident

√x7th **V68.3** Unspecified occupant of heavy transport vehicle injured in noncollision transport accident in nontraffic accident

√x7th **V68.4** Person boarding or alighting a heavy transport vehicle injured in noncollision transport accident

√x7th **V68.5** Driver of heavy transport vehicle injured in noncollision transport accident in traffic accident

N Newborn: 0   P Pediatric: 0-17   M Maternity: 12-55   A Adult: 15-124   MCC Major CC Condition   PDx MCC PDx acts as own MCC   CC CC Condition   PDx CC PDx acts as own CC

1128   ICD-10-CM Draft (2015)

✓x7th **V68.6** Passenger in heavy transport vehicle injured in noncollision transport accident in traffic accident

✓x7th **V68.7** Person on outside of heavy transport vehicle injured in noncollision transport accident in traffic accident

✓x7th **V68.9** Unspecified occupant of heavy transport vehicle injured in noncollision transport accident in traffic accident

✓4th **V69** Occupant of heavy transport vehicle injured in other and unspecified transport accidents

> The appropriate 7th character is to be added to each code from category V69.
> A   initial encounter
> D   subsequent encounter
> S   sequela

✓5th **V69.0** Driver of heavy transport vehicle injured in collision with other and unspecified motor vehicles in nontraffic accident

  ✓x7th **V69.00** Driver of heavy transport vehicle injured in collision with unspecified motor vehicles in nontraffic accident

  ✓x7th **V69.09** Driver of heavy transport vehicle injured in collision with other motor vehicles in nontraffic accident

✓5th **V69.1** Passenger in heavy transport vehicle injured in collision with other and unspecified motor vehicles in nontraffic accident

  ✓x7th **V69.10** Passenger in heavy transport vehicle injured in collision with unspecified motor vehicles in nontraffic accident

  ✓x7th **V69.19** Passenger in heavy transport vehicle injured in collision with other motor vehicles in nontraffic accident

✓5th **V69.2** Unspecified occupant of heavy transport vehicle injured in collision with other and unspecified motor vehicles in nontraffic accident

  ✓x7th **V69.20** Unspecified occupant of heavy transport vehicle injured in collision with unspecified motor vehicles in nontraffic accident
  > Collision NOS involving heavy transport vehicle, nontraffic

  ✓x7th **V69.29** Unspecified occupant of heavy transport vehicle injured in collision with other motor vehicles in nontraffic accident

✓x7th **V69.3** Occupant (driver) (passenger) of heavy transport vehicle injured in unspecified nontraffic accident
  > Accident NOS involving heavy transport vehicle, nontraffic
  > Occupant of heavy transport vehicle injured in nontraffic accident NOS

✓5th **V69.4** Driver of heavy transport vehicle injured in collision with other and unspecified motor vehicles in traffic accident

  ✓x7th **V69.40** Driver of heavy transport vehicle injured in collision with unspecified motor vehicles in traffic accident

  ✓x7th **V69.49** Driver of heavy transport vehicle injured in collision with other motor vehicles in traffic accident

✓5th **V69.5** Passenger in heavy transport vehicle injured in collision with other and unspecified motor vehicles in traffic accident

  ✓x7th **V69.50** Passenger in heavy transport vehicle injured in collision with unspecified motor vehicles in traffic accident

  ✓x7th **V69.59** Passenger in heavy transport vehicle injured in collision with other motor vehicles in traffic accident

✓5th **V69.6** Unspecified occupant of heavy transport vehicle injured in collision with other and unspecified motor vehicles in traffic accident

  ✓x7th **V69.60** Unspecified occupant of heavy transport vehicle injured in collision with unspecified motor vehicles in traffic accident
  > Collision NOS involving heavy transport vehicle (traffic)

  ✓x7th **V69.69** Unspecified occupant of heavy transport vehicle injured in collision with other motor vehicles in traffic accident

✓5th **V69.8** Occupant (driver) (passenger) of heavy transport vehicle injured in other specified transport accidents

  ✓x7th **V69.81** Occupant (driver) (passenger) of heavy transport vehicle injured in transport accidents with military vehicle

  ✓x7th **V69.88** Occupant (driver) (passenger) of heavy transport vehicle injured in other specified transport accidents

✓x7th **V69.9** Occupant (driver) (passenger) of heavy transport vehicle injured in unspecified traffic accident
  > Accident NOS involving heavy transport vehicle

Bus occupant injured in transport accident (V70-V79)

INCLUDES motorcoach
EXCLUDES1 minibus (V50-V59)

✓4th **V70** Bus occupant injured in collision with pedestrian or animal

EXCLUDES1 bus collision with animal-drawn vehicle or animal being ridden (V76.-)

> The appropriate 7th character is to be added to each code from category V70.
> A   initial encounter
> D   subsequent encounter
> S   sequela

✓x7th **V70.0** Driver of bus injured in collision with pedestrian or animal in nontraffic accident

✓x7th **V70.1** Passenger on bus injured in collision with pedestrian or animal in nontraffic accident

✓x7th **V70.2** Person on outside of bus injured in collision with pedestrian or animal in nontraffic accident

✓x7th **V70.3** Unspecified occupant of bus injured in collision with pedestrian or animal in nontraffic accident

✓x7th **V70.4** Person boarding or alighting from bus injured in collision with pedestrian or animal

✓x7th **V70.5** Driver of bus injured in collision with pedestrian or animal in traffic accident

✓x7th **V70.6** Passenger on bus injured in collision with pedestrian or animal in traffic accident

✓x7th **V70.7** Person on outside of bus injured in collision with pedestrian or animal in traffic accident

✓x7th **V70.9** Unspecified occupant of bus injured in collision with pedestrian or animal in traffic accident

✓4th **V71** Bus occupant injured in collision with pedal cycle

> The appropriate 7th character is to be added to each code from category V71.
> A   initial encounter
> D   subsequent encounter
> S   sequela

✓x7th **V71.0** Driver of bus injured in collision with pedal cycle in nontraffic accident

✓x7th **V71.1** Passenger on bus injured in collision with pedal cycle in nontraffic accident

✓x7th **V71.2** Person on outside of bus injured in collision with pedal cycle in nontraffic accident

✓x7th **V71.3** Unspecified occupant of bus injured in collision with pedal cycle in nontraffic accident

✓x7th **V71.4** Person boarding or alighting from bus injured in collision with pedal cycle

✓x7th **V71.5** Driver of bus injured in collision with pedal cycle in traffic accident

✓x7th **V71.6** Passenger on bus injured in collision with pedal cycle in traffic accident

✓x7th **V71.7** Person on outside of bus injured in collision with pedal cycle in traffic accident

✓x7th **V71.9** Unspecified occupant of bus injured in collision with pedal cycle in traffic accident

✓4th **V72** Bus occupant injured in collision with two- or three-wheeled motor vehicle

> The appropriate 7th character is to be added to each code from category V72.
> A   initial encounter
> D   subsequent encounter
> S   sequela

✓x7th **V72.0** Driver of bus injured in collision with two- or three-wheeled motor vehicle in nontraffic accident

✓x7th **V72.1** Passenger on bus injured in collision with two- or three-wheeled motor vehicle in nontraffic accident

✓x7th **V72.2** Person on outside of bus injured in collision with two- or three-wheeled motor vehicle in nontraffic accident

✓x7th **V72.3** Unspecified occupant of bus injured in collision with two- or three-wheeled motor vehicle in nontraffic accident

✓x7th **V72.4** Person boarding or alighting from bus injured in collision with two- or three-wheeled motor vehicle

✓x7th **V72.5** Driver of bus injured in collision with two- or three-wheeled motor vehicle in traffic accident

---

✓ Additional Character Required   ✓x7th Xtension Alert   Unacceptable PDx   Manifestation   Hospital Acquired Condition   EXCLUDES1 Not Coded Here   EXCLUDES2 Not Included Here

√x7ᵗʰ **V72.6** Passenger on bus injured in collision with two- or three-wheeled motor vehicle in traffic accident

√x7ᵗʰ **V72.7** Person on outside of bus injured in collision with two- or three-wheeled motor vehicle in traffic accident

√x7ᵗʰ **V72.9** Unspecified occupant of bus injured in collision with two- or three-wheeled motor vehicle in traffic accident

√4ᵗʰ **V73 Bus occupant injured in collision with car, pick-up truck or van**

> The appropriate 7th character is to be added to each code from category V73.
> A   initial encounter
> D   subsequent encounter
> S   sequela

√x7ᵗʰ **V73.0** Driver of bus injured in collision with car, pick-up truck or van in nontraffic accident

√x7ᵗʰ **V73.1** Passenger on bus injured in collision with car, pick-up truck or van in nontraffic accident

√x7ᵗʰ **V73.2** Person on outside of bus injured in collision with car, pick-up truck or van in nontraffic accident

√x7ᵗʰ **V73.3** Unspecified occupant of bus injured in collision with car, pick-up truck or van in nontraffic accident

√x7ᵗʰ **V73.4** Person boarding or alighting from bus injured in collision with car, pick-up truck or van

√x7ᵗʰ **V73.5** Driver of bus injured in collision with car, pick-up truck or van in traffic accident

√x7ᵗʰ **V73.6** Passenger on bus injured in collision with car, pick-up truck or van in traffic accident

√x7ᵗʰ **V73.7** Person on outside of bus injured in collision with car, pick-up truck or van in traffic accident

√x7ᵗʰ **V73.9** Unspecified occupant of bus injured in collision with car, pick-up truck or van in traffic accident

√4ᵗʰ **V74 Bus occupant injured in collision with heavy transport vehicle or bus**

> EXCLUDES 1   bus occupant injured in collision with military vehicle (V79.81)

> The appropriate 7th character is to be added to each code from category V74.
> A   initial encounter
> D   subsequent encounter
> S   sequela

√x7ᵗʰ **V74.0** Driver of bus injured in collision with heavy transport vehicle or bus in nontraffic accident

√x7ᵗʰ **V74.1** Passenger on bus injured in collision with heavy transport vehicle or bus in nontraffic accident

√x7ᵗʰ **V74.2** Person on outside of bus injured in collision with heavy transport vehicle or bus in nontraffic accident

√x7ᵗʰ **V74.3** Unspecified occupant of bus injured in collision with heavy transport vehicle or bus in nontraffic accident

√x7ᵗʰ **V74.4** Person boarding or alighting from bus injured in collision with heavy transport vehicle or bus

√x7ᵗʰ **V74.5** Driver of bus injured in collision with heavy transport vehicle or bus in traffic accident

√x7ᵗʰ **V74.6** Passenger on bus injured in collision with heavy transport vehicle or bus in traffic accident

√x7ᵗʰ **V74.7** Person on outside of bus injured in collision with heavy transport vehicle or bus in traffic accident

√x7ᵗʰ **V74.9** Unspecified occupant of bus injured in collision with heavy transport vehicle or bus in traffic accident

√4ᵗʰ **V75 Bus occupant injured in collision with railway train or railway vehicle**

> The appropriate 7th character is to be added to each code from category V75.
> A   initial encounter
> D   subsequent encounter
> S   sequela

√x7ᵗʰ **V75.0** Driver of bus injured in collision with railway train or railway vehicle in nontraffic accident

√x7ᵗʰ **V75.1** Passenger on bus injured in collision with railway train or railway vehicle in nontraffic accident

√x7ᵗʰ **V75.2** Person on outside of bus injured in collision with railway train or railway vehicle in nontraffic accident

√x7ᵗʰ **V75.3** Unspecified occupant of bus injured in collision with railway train or railway vehicle in nontraffic accident

√x7ᵗʰ **V75.4** Person boarding or alighting from bus injured in collision with railway train or railway vehicle

√x7ᵗʰ **V75.5** Driver of bus injured in collision with railway train or railway vehicle in traffic accident

√x7ᵗʰ **V75.6** Passenger on bus injured in collision with railway train or railway vehicle in traffic accident

√x7ᵗʰ **V75.7** Person on outside of bus injured in collision with railway train or railway vehicle in traffic accident

√x7ᵗʰ **V75.9** Unspecified occupant of bus injured in collision with railway train or railway vehicle in traffic accident

√4ᵗʰ **V76 Bus occupant injured in collision with other nonmotor vehicle**

> INCLUDES   collision with animal-drawn vehicle, animal being ridden, streetcar

> The appropriate 7th character is to be added to each code from category V76.
> A   initial encounter
> D   subsequent encounter
> S   sequela

√x7ᵗʰ **V76.0** Driver of bus injured in collision with other nonmotor vehicle in nontraffic accident

√x7ᵗʰ **V76.1** Passenger on bus injured in collision with other nonmotor vehicle in nontraffic accident

√x7ᵗʰ **V76.2** Person on outside of bus injured in collision with other nonmotor vehicle in nontraffic accident

√x7ᵗʰ **V76.3** Unspecified occupant of bus injured in collision with other nonmotor vehicle in nontraffic accident

√x7ᵗʰ **V76.4** Person boarding or alighting from bus injured in collision with other nonmotor vehicle

√x7ᵗʰ **V76.5** Driver of bus injured in collision with other nonmotor vehicle in traffic accident

√x7ᵗʰ **V76.6** Passenger on bus injured in collision with other nonmotor vehicle in traffic accident

√x7ᵗʰ **V76.7** Person on outside of bus injured in collision with other nonmotor vehicle in traffic accident

√x7ᵗʰ **V76.9** Unspecified occupant of bus injured in collision with other nonmotor vehicle in traffic accident

√4ᵗʰ **V77 Bus occupant injured in collision with fixed or stationary object**

> The appropriate 7th character is to be added to each code from category V77.
> A   initial encounter
> D   subsequent encounter
> S   sequela

√x7ᵗʰ **V77.0** Driver of bus injured in collision with fixed or stationary object in nontraffic accident

√x7ᵗʰ **V77.1** Passenger on bus injured in collision with fixed or stationary object in nontraffic accident

√x7ᵗʰ **V77.2** Person on outside of bus injured in collision with fixed or stationary object in nontraffic accident

√x7ᵗʰ **V77.3** Unspecified occupant of bus injured in collision with fixed or stationary object in nontraffic accident

√x7ᵗʰ **V77.4** Person boarding or alighting from bus injured in collision with fixed or stationary object

√x7ᵗʰ **V77.5** Driver of bus injured in collision with fixed or stationary object in traffic accident

√x7ᵗʰ **V77.6** Passenger on bus injured in collision with fixed or stationary object in traffic accident

√x7ᵗʰ **V77.7** Person on outside of bus injured in collision with fixed or stationary object in traffic accident

√x7ᵗʰ **V77.9** Unspecified occupant of bus injured in collision with fixed or stationary object in traffic accident

√4ᵗʰ **V78 Bus occupant injured in noncollision transport accident**

> INCLUDES   overturning bus NOS
> overturning bus without collision

> The appropriate 7th character is to be added to each code from category V78.
> A   initial encounter
> D   subsequent encounter
> S   sequela

√x7ᵗʰ **V78.0** Driver of bus injured in noncollision transport accident in nontraffic accident

√x7ᵗʰ **V78.1** Passenger on bus injured in noncollision transport accident in nontraffic accident

√x7ᵗʰ **V78.2** Person on outside of bus injured in noncollision transport accident in nontraffic accident

---

N Newborn: 0   P Pediatric: 0-17   M Maternity: 12-55   A Adult: 15-124   MCC Major CC Condition   PDx MCC PDx acts as own MCC   CC CC Condition   PDx CC PDx acts as own CC

1130   ICD-10-CM Draft (2015)

✓x7ᵗʰ **V78.3** Unspecified occupant of bus injured in noncollision transport accident in nontraffic accident

✓x7ᵗʰ **V78.4** Person boarding or alighting from bus injured in noncollision transport accident

✓x7ᵗʰ **V78.5** Driver of bus injured in noncollision transport accident in traffic accident

✓x7ᵗʰ **V78.6** Passenger on bus injured in noncollision transport accident in traffic accident

✓x7ᵗʰ **V78.7** Person on outside of bus injured in noncollision transport accident in traffic accident

✓x7ᵗʰ **V78.9** Unspecified occupant of bus injured in noncollision transport accident in traffic accident

✓4ᵗʰ **V79 Bus occupant injured in other and unspecified transport accidents**

> The appropriate 7th character is to be added to each code from category V79.
> A initial encounter
> D subsequent encounter
> S sequela

✓5ᵗʰ **V79.0** Driver of bus injured in collision with other and unspecified motor vehicles in nontraffic accident

✓x7ᵗʰ **V79.00** Driver of bus injured in collision with unspecified motor vehicles in nontraffic accident

✓x7ᵗʰ **V79.09** Driver of bus injured in collision with other motor vehicles in nontraffic accident

✓5ᵗʰ **V79.1** Passenger on bus injured in collision with other and unspecified motor vehicles in nontraffic accident

✓x7ᵗʰ **V79.10** Passenger on bus injured in collision with unspecified motor vehicles in nontraffic accident

✓x7ᵗʰ **V79.19** Passenger on bus injured in collision with other motor vehicles in nontraffic accident

✓5ᵗʰ **V79.2** Unspecified bus occupant injured in collision with other and unspecified motor vehicles in nontraffic accident

✓x7ᵗʰ **V79.20** Unspecified bus occupant injured in collision with unspecified motor vehicles in nontraffic accident
Bus collision NOS, nontraffic

✓x7ᵗʰ **V79.29** Unspecified bus occupant injured in collision with other motor vehicles in nontraffic accident

✓x7ᵗʰ **V79.3** Bus occupant (driver) (passenger) injured in unspecified nontraffic accident
Bus accident NOS, nontraffic
Bus occupant injured in nontraffic accident NOS

✓5ᵗʰ **V79.4** Driver of bus injured in collision with other and unspecified motor vehicles in traffic accident

✓x7ᵗʰ **V79.40** Driver of bus injured in collision with unspecified motor vehicles in traffic accident

✓x7ᵗʰ **V79.49** Driver of bus injured in collision with other motor vehicles in traffic accident

✓5ᵗʰ **V79.5** Passenger on bus injured in collision with other and unspecified motor vehicles in traffic accident

✓x7ᵗʰ **V79.50** Passenger on bus injured in collision with unspecified motor vehicles in traffic accident

✓x7ᵗʰ **V79.59** Passenger on bus injured in collision with other motor vehicles in traffic accident

✓5ᵗʰ **V79.6** Unspecified bus occupant injured in collision with other and unspecified motor vehicles in traffic accident

✓x7ᵗʰ **V79.60** Unspecified bus occupant injured in collision with unspecified motor vehicles in traffic accident
Bus collision NOS (traffic)

✓x7ᵗʰ **V79.69** Unspecified bus occupant injured in collision with other motor vehicles in traffic accident

✓5ᵗʰ **V79.8** Bus occupant (driver) (passenger) injured in other specified transport accidents

✓x7ᵗʰ **V79.81** Bus occupant (driver) (passenger) injured in transport accidents with military vehicle

✓x7ᵗʰ **V79.88** Bus occupant (driver) (passenger) injured in other specified transport accidents

✓x7ᵗʰ **V79.9** Bus occupant (driver) (passenger) injured in unspecified traffic accident
Bus accident NOS

Other land transport accidents (V80-V89)

✓4ᵗʰ **V80 Animal-rider or occupant of animal-drawn vehicle injured in transport accident**

> The appropriate 7th character is to be added to each code from category V80.
> A initial encounter
> D subsequent encounter
> S sequela

✓5ᵗʰ **V80.0** Animal-rider or occupant of animal drawn vehicle injured by fall from or being thrown from animal or animal-drawn vehicle in noncollision accident

✓6ᵗʰ **V80.01** Animal-rider injured by fall from or being thrown from animal in noncollision accident

✓7ᵗʰ **V80.010** Animal-rider injured by fall from or being thrown from horse in noncollision accident

✓7ᵗʰ **V80.018** Animal-rider injured by fall from or being thrown from other animal in noncollision accident

✓x7ᵗʰ **V80.02** Occupant of animal-drawn vehicle injured by fall from or being thrown from animal-drawn vehicle in noncollision accident
Overturning animal-drawn vehicle NOS
Overturning animal-drawn vehicle without collision

✓5ᵗʰ **V80.1** Animal-rider or occupant of animal-drawn vehicle injured in collision with pedestrian or animal
EXCLUDES 1 animal-rider or animal-drawn vehicle collision with animal-drawn vehicle or animal being ridden (V80.7)

✓x7ᵗʰ **V80.11** Animal-rider injured in collision with pedestrian or animal

✓x7ᵗʰ **V80.12** Occupant of animal-drawn vehicle injured in collision with pedestrian or animal

✓5ᵗʰ **V80.2** Animal-rider or occupant of animal-drawn vehicle injured in collision with pedal cycle

✓x7ᵗʰ **V80.21** Animal-rider injured in collision with pedal cycle

✓x7ᵗʰ **V80.22** Occupant of animal-drawn vehicle injured in collision with pedal cycle

✓5ᵗʰ **V80.3** Animal-rider or occupant of animal-drawn vehicle injured in collision with two- or three-wheeled motor vehicle

✓x7ᵗʰ **V80.31** Animal-rider injured in collision with two- or three-wheeled motor vehicle

✓x7ᵗʰ **V80.32** Occupant of animal-drawn vehicle injured in collision with two- or three-wheeled motor vehicle

✓5ᵗʰ **V80.4** Animal-rider or occupant of animal-drawn vehicle injured in collision with car, pick-up truck, van, heavy transport vehicle or bus
EXCLUDES 1 animal-rider injured in collision with military vehicle (V80.910)
occupant of animal-drawn vehicle injured in collision with military vehicle (V80.920)

✓x7ᵗʰ **V80.41** Animal-rider injured in collision with car, pick-up truck, van, heavy transport vehicle or bus

✓x7ᵗʰ **V80.42** Occupant of animal-drawn vehicle injured in collision with car, pick-up truck, van, heavy transport vehicle or bus

✓5ᵗʰ **V80.5** Animal-rider or occupant of animal-drawn vehicle injured in collision with other specified motor vehicle

✓x7ᵗʰ **V80.51** Animal-rider injured in collision with other specified motor vehicle

✓x7ᵗʰ **V80.52** Occupant of animal-drawn vehicle injured in collision with other specified motor vehicle

✓5ᵗʰ **V80.6** Animal-rider or occupant of animal-drawn vehicle injured in collision with railway train or railway vehicle

✓x7ᵗʰ **V80.61** Animal-rider injured in collision with railway train or railway vehicle

✓x7ᵗʰ **V80.62** Occupant of animal-drawn vehicle injured in collision with railway train or railway vehicle

✓5ᵗʰ **V80.7** Animal-rider or occupant of animal-drawn vehicle injured in collision with other nonmotor vehicles

✓6ᵗʰ **V80.71** Animal-rider or occupant of animal-drawn vehicle injured in collision with animal being ridden

✓7ᵗʰ **V80.710** Animal-rider injured in collision with other animal being ridden

✓7ᵗʰ **V80.711** Occupant of animal-drawn vehicle injured in collision with animal being ridden

---

✓ Additional Character Required ✓x7ᵗʰ Xtension Alert Unacceptable PDx Manifestation Hospital Acquired Condition **EXCLUDES 1** Not Coded Here **EXCLUDES 2** Not Included Here

External Causes of Morbidity

V80.72–V82.9

✓6ᵗʰ V80.72 Animal-rider or occupant of animal-drawn vehicle injured in collision with other animal-drawn vehicle

✓7ᵗʰ V80.720 Animal-rider injured in collision with animal-drawn vehicle

✓7ᵗʰ V80.721 Occupant of animal-drawn vehicle injured in collision with other animal-drawn vehicle

✓6ᵗʰ V80.73 Animal-rider or occupant of animal-drawn vehicle injured in collision with streetcar

✓7ᵗʰ V80.730 Animal-rider injured in collision with streetcar

✓7ᵗʰ V80.731 Occupant of animal-drawn vehicle injured in collision with streetcar

✓6ᵗʰ V80.79 Animal-rider or occupant of animal-drawn vehicle injured in collision with other nonmotor vehicles

✓7ᵗʰ V80.790 Animal-rider injured in collision with other nonmotor vehicles

✓7ᵗʰ V80.791 Occupant of animal-drawn vehicle injured in collision with other nonmotor vehicles

✓5ᵗʰ V80.8 Animal-rider or occupant of animal-drawn vehicle injured in collision with fixed or stationary object

✓x7ᵗʰ V80.81 Animal-rider injured in collision with fixed or stationary object

✓x7ᵗʰ V80.82 Occupant of animal-drawn vehicle injured in collision with fixed or stationary object

✓5ᵗʰ V80.9 Animal-rider or occupant of animal-drawn vehicle injured in other and unspecified transport accidents

✓6ᵗʰ V80.91 Animal-rider injured in other and unspecified transport accidents

✓7ᵗʰ V80.910 Animal-rider injured in transport accident with military vehicle

✓7ᵗʰ V80.918 Animal-rider injured in other transport accident

✓7ᵗʰ V80.919 Animal-rider injured in unspecified transport accident
Animal rider accident NOS

✓6ᵗʰ V80.92 Occupant of animal-drawn vehicle injured in other and unspecified transport accidents

✓7ᵗʰ V80.920 Occupant of animal-drawn vehicle injured in transport accident with military vehicle

✓7ᵗʰ V80.928 Occupant of animal-drawn vehicle injured in other transport accident

✓7ᵗʰ V80.929 Occupant of animal-drawn vehicle injured in unspecified transport accident
Animal-drawn vehicle accident NOS

✓4ᵗʰ V81 Occupant of railway train or railway vehicle injured in transport accident

INCLUDES derailment of railway train or railway vehicle
person on outside of train

EXCLUDES1 streetcar (V82.-)

The appropriate 7th character is to be added to each code from category V81.
A initial encounter
D subsequent encounter
S sequela

✓x7ᵗʰ V81.0 Occupant of railway train or railway vehicle injured in collision with motor vehicle in nontraffic accident

EXCLUDES1 occupant of railway train or railway vehicle injured due to collision with military vehicle (V81.83)

✓x7ᵗʰ V81.1 Occupant of railway train or railway vehicle injured in collision with motor vehicle in traffic accident

EXCLUDES1 occupant of railway train or railway vehicle injured due to collision with military vehicle (V81.83)

✓x7ᵗʰ V81.2 Occupant of railway train or railway vehicle injured in collision with or hit by rolling stock

✓x7ᵗʰ V81.3 Occupant of railway train or railway vehicle injured in collision with other object
Railway collision NOS

✓x7ᵗʰ V81.4 Person injured while boarding or alighting from railway train or railway vehicle

✓x7ᵗʰ V81.5 Occupant of railway train or railway vehicle injured by fall in railway train or railway vehicle

✓x7ᵗʰ V81.6 Occupant of railway train or railway vehicle injured by fall from railway train or railway vehicle

✓x7ᵗʰ V81.7 Occupant of railway train or railway vehicle injured in derailment without antecedent collision

✓5ᵗʰ V81.8 Occupant of railway train or railway vehicle injured in other specified railway accidents

✓x7ᵗʰ V81.81 Occupant of railway train or railway vehicle injured due to explosion or fire on train

✓x7ᵗʰ V81.82 Occupant of railway train or railway vehicle injured due to object falling onto train
Occupant of railway train or railway vehicle injured due to falling earth onto train
Occupant of railway train or railway vehicle injured due to falling rocks onto train
Occupant of railway train or railway vehicle injured due to falling snow onto train
Occupant of railway train or railway vehicle injured due to falling trees onto train

✓x7ᵗʰ V81.83 Occupant of railway train or railway vehicle injured due to collision with military vehicle

✓x7ᵗʰ V81.89 Occupant of railway train or railway vehicle injured due to other specified railway accident

✓x7ᵗʰ V81.9 Occupant of railway train or railway vehicle injured in unspecified railway accident
Railway accident NOS

✓4ᵗʰ V82 Occupant of powered streetcar injured in transport accident

INCLUDES interurban electric car
person on outside of streetcar
tram (car)
trolley (car)

EXCLUDES1 bus (V70-V79)
motorcoach (V70-V79)
nonpowered streetcar (V76.-)
train (V81.-)

The appropriate 7th character is to be added to each code from category V82.
A initial encounter
D subsequent encounter
S sequela

✓x7ᵗʰ V82.0 Occupant of streetcar injured in collision with motor vehicle in nontraffic accident

✓x7ᵗʰ V82.1 Occupant of streetcar injured in collision with motor vehicle in traffic accident

✓x7ᵗʰ V82.2 Occupant of streetcar injured in collision with or hit by rolling stock

✓x7ᵗʰ V82.3 Occupant of streetcar injured in collision with other object

EXCLUDES1 collision with animal-drawn vehicle or animal being ridden (V82.8)

✓x7ᵗʰ V82.4 Person injured while boarding or alighting from streetcar

✓x7ᵗʰ V82.5 Occupant of streetcar injured by fall in streetcar

EXCLUDES1 fall in streetcar:
while boarding or alighting (V82.4)
with antecedent collision (V82.0-V82.3)

✓x7ᵗʰ V82.6 Occupant of streetcar injured by fall from streetcar

EXCLUDES1 fall from streetcar:
while boarding or alighting (V82.4)
with antecedent collision (V82.0-V82.3)

✓x7ᵗʰ V82.7 Occupant of streetcar injured in derailment without antecedent collision

EXCLUDES1 occupant of streetcar injured in derailment with antecedent collision (V82.0-V82.3)

✓x7ᵗʰ V82.8 Occupant of streetcar injured in other specified transport accidents
Streetcar collision with military vehicle
Streetcar collision with train or nonmotor vehicles

✓x7ᵗʰ V82.9 Occupant of streetcar injured in unspecified traffic accident
Streetcar accident NOS

Ⓝ Newborn: 0 Ⓟ Pediatric: 0-17 Ⓜ Maternity: 12-55 Ⓐ Adult: 15-124 MCC Major CC Condition PDx MCC PDx acts as own MCC CC CC Condition PDx CC PDx acts as own CC

1132 ICD-10-CM Draft (2015)

✓4ᵗʰ **V83 Occupant of special vehicle mainly used on industrial premises injured in transport accident**

   INCLUDES battery-powered airport passenger vehicle
          battery-powered truck (baggage) (mail)
          coal-car in mine
          forklift (truck)
          logging car
          self-propelled industrial truck
          station baggage truck (powered)
          tram, truck, or tub (powered) in mine or quarry

   EXCLUDES1 *special construction vehicles (V85.-)*
          special industrial vehicle in stationary use or maintenance (W31.-)

The appropriate 7th character is to be added to each code from category V83.
  A   initial encounter
  D   subsequent encounter
  S   sequela

✓x7ᵗʰ **V83.0 Driver** of special industrial vehicle **injured** in traffic accident

✓x7ᵗʰ **V83.1 Passenger** of special industrial vehicle injured in traffic accident

✓x7ᵗʰ **V83.2 Person on outside** of special industrial vehicle injured in traffic accident

✓x7ᵗʰ **V83.3 Unspecified** occupant of special industrial vehicle injured in traffic accident

✓x7ᵗʰ **V83.4 Person injured while boarding or alighting** from special industrial vehicle

✓x7ᵗʰ **V83.5 Driver** of special industrial vehicle injured in nontraffic accident

✓x7ᵗʰ **V83.6 Passenger** of special industrial vehicle injured in nontraffic accident

✓x7ᵗʰ **V83.7 Person on outside** of special industrial vehicle injured in nontraffic accident

✓x7ᵗʰ **V83.9 Unspecified occupant** of special industrial vehicle injured in nontraffic accident
      Special-industrial-vehicle accident NOS

✓4ᵗʰ **V84 Occupant of special vehicle mainly used in agriculture injured in transport accident**

   INCLUDES self-propelled farm machinery
          tractor (and trailer)

   EXCLUDES1 *animal-powered farm machinery accident (W30.8-)*
          contact with combine harvester (W30.0)
          special agricultural vehicle in stationary use or maintenance (W30.-)

The appropriate 7th character is to be added to each code from category V84.
  A   initial encounter
  D   subsequent encounter
  S   sequela

✓x7ᵗʰ **V84.0 Driver** of special agricultural vehicle **injured** in traffic accident

✓x7ᵗʰ **V84.1 Passenger** of special agricultural vehicle injured in traffic accident

✓x7ᵗʰ **V84.2 Person on outside** of special agricultural vehicle injured in traffic accident

✓x7ᵗʰ **V84.3 Unspecified occupant** of special agricultural vehicle injured in traffic accident

✓x7ᵗʰ **V84.4 Person injured while boarding or alighting** from special agricultural vehicle

✓x7ᵗʰ **V84.5 Driver** of special agricultural vehicle injured in nontraffic accident

✓x7ᵗʰ **V84.6 Passenger** of special agricultural vehicle injured in nontraffic accident

✓x7ᵗʰ **V84.7 Person on outside** of special agricultural vehicle injured in nontraffic accident

✓x7ᵗʰ **V84.9 Unspecified occupant** of special agricultural vehicle injured in nontraffic accident
      Special-agricultural vehicle accident NOS

✓4ᵗʰ **V85 Occupant of special construction vehicle injured in transport accident**

   INCLUDES bulldozer
          digger
          dump truck
          earth-leveller
          mechanical shovel
          road-roller

   EXCLUDES1 *special industrial vehicle (V83.-)*
          special construction vehicle in stationary use or maintenance (W31.-)

The appropriate 7th character is to be added to each code from category V85.
  A   initial encounter
  D   subsequent encounter
  S   sequela

✓x7ᵗʰ **V85.0 Driver** of special construction vehicle injured in traffic accident

✓x7ᵗʰ **V85.1 Passenger** of special construction vehicle injured in traffic accident

✓x7ᵗʰ **V85.2 Person on outside** of special construction vehicle injured in traffic accident

✓x7ᵗʰ **V85.3 Unspecified** occupant of special construction vehicle injured in traffic accident

✓x7ᵗʰ **V85.4 Person injured while boarding or alighting** from special construction vehicle

✓x7ᵗʰ **V85.5 Driver** of special construction vehicle injured in nontraffic accident

✓x7ᵗʰ **V85.6 Passenger** of special construction vehicle injured in nontraffic accident

✓x7ᵗʰ **V85.7 Person on outside** of special construction vehicle injured in nontraffic accident

✓x7ᵗʰ **V85.9 Unspecified** occupant of special construction vehicle injured in nontraffic accident
      Special-construction-vehicle accident NOS

✓4ᵗʰ **V86 Occupant of special all-terrain or other off-road motor vehicle, injured in transport accident**

   EXCLUDES1 *special all-terrain vehicle in stationary use or maintenance (W31.-)*
          sport-utility vehicle (V50-V59)
          three-wheeled motor vehicle designed for on-road use (V30-V39)

The appropriate 7th character is to be added to each code from category V86.
  A   initial encounter
  D   subsequent encounter
  S   sequela

✓5ᵗʰ **V86.0 Driver** of special all-terrain or other off-road motor vehicle injured in traffic accident

  ✓x7ᵗʰ **V86.01 Driver of ambulance or fire engine** injured in traffic accident

  ✓x7ᵗʰ **V86.02 Driver of snowmobile** injured in traffic accident

  ✓x7ᵗʰ **V86.03 Driver of dune buggy** injured in traffic accident

  ✓x7ᵗʰ **V86.04 Driver of military vehicle** injured in traffic accident

  ✓x7ᵗʰ **V86.09 Driver of other** special all-terrain or other off-road motor vehicle injured in traffic accident
        Driver of dirt bike injured in traffic accident
        Driver of go cart injured in traffic accident
        Driver of golf cart injured in traffic accident

✓5ᵗʰ **V86.1 Passenger** of special all-terrain or other off-road motor vehicle injured in traffic accident

  ✓x7ᵗʰ **V86.11 Passenger of ambulance or fire engine** injured in traffic accident

  ✓x7ᵗʰ **V86.12 Passenger of snowmobile** injured in traffic accident

  ✓x7ᵗʰ **V86.13 Passenger of dune buggy** injured in traffic accident

  ✓x7ᵗʰ **V86.14 Passenger of military vehicle** injured in traffic accident

  ✓x7ᵗʰ **V86.19 Passenger of other** special all-terrain or other off-road motor vehicle injured in traffic accident
        Passenger of dirt bike injured in traffic accident
        Passenger of go cart injured in traffic accident
        Passenger of golf cart injured in traffic accident

✓5ᵗʰ **V86.2 Person on outside** of special all-terrain or other off-road motor vehicle injured in traffic accident

  ✓x7ᵗʰ **V86.21 Person on outside of ambulance or fire engine** injured in traffic accident

  ✓x7ᵗʰ **V86.22 Person on outside of snowmobile** injured in traffic accident

√x7th **V86.23** **Person on outside of** dune buggy **injured in traffic accident**

√x7th **V86.24** **Person on outside of** military vehicle **injured in traffic accident**

√x7th **V86.29** **Person on outside of** other special all-terrain or **other off-road motor vehicle injured in traffic accident**

> Person on outside of dirt bike injured in traffic accident
> Person on outside of go cart in traffic accident
> Person on outside of golf cart injured in traffic accident

√5th **V86.3** Unspecified occupant **of special all-terrain or other off-road motor vehicle injured** in traffic accident

√x7th **V86.31** **Unspecified occupant of** ambulance or fire engine **injured in traffic accident**

√x7th **V86.32** **Unspecified occupant of** snowmobile **injured in traffic accident**

√x7th **V86.33** **Unspecified occupant of** dune buggy **injured in traffic accident**

√x7th **V86.34** **Unspecified occupant of** military vehicle **injured in traffic accident**

√x7th **V86.39** **Unspecified occupant of** other special all-terrain or **other off-road motor vehicle injured in traffic accident**

> Unspecified occupant of dirt bike injured in traffic accident
> Unspecified occupant of go cart injured in traffic accident
> Unspecified occupant of golf cart injured in traffic accident

√5th **V86.4** **Person injured while** boarding or alighting **from special all-terrain or other off-road motor vehicle**

√x7th **V86.41** **Person injured while boarding or alighting from** ambulance or fire engine

√x7th **V86.42** **Person injured while boarding or alighting from** snowmobile

√x7th **V86.43** **Person injured while boarding or alighting from** dune buggy

√x7th **V86.44** **Person injured while boarding or alighting from** military vehicle

√x7th **V86.49** **Person injured while boarding or alighting from** other special all-terrain or other off-road motor vehicle

> Person injured while boarding or alighting from dirt bike
> Person injured while boarding or alighting from go cart
> Person injured while boarding or alighting from golf cart

√5th **V86.5** Driver **of special all-terrain or other off-road motor vehicle injured** in nontraffic accident

√x7th **V86.51** **Driver of** ambulance or fire engine **injured in nontraffic accident**

√x7th **V86.52** **Driver of** snowmobile **injured in nontraffic accident**

√x7th **V86.53** **Driver of** dune buggy **injured in nontraffic accident**

√x7th **V86.54** **Driver of** military vehicle **injured in nontraffic accident**

√x7th **V86.59** **Driver of** other special all-terrain or other off-road **motor vehicle injured in nontraffic accident**

> Driver of dirt bike injured in nontraffic accident
> Driver of go cart injured in nontraffic accident
> Driver of golf cart injured in nontraffic accident

√5th **V86.6** Passenger **of special all-terrain or other off-road motor vehicle injured** in nontraffic accident

√x7th **V86.61** **Passenger of** ambulance or fire engine **injured in nontraffic accident**

√x7th **V86.62** **Passenger of** snowmobile **injured in nontraffic accident**

√x7th **V86.63** **Passenger of** dune buggy **injured in nontraffic accident**

√x7th **V86.64** **Passenger of** military vehicle **injured in nontraffic accident**

√x7th **V86.69** **Passenger of** other special all-terrain or other off-road motor vehicle **injured in nontraffic accident**

> Passenger of dirt bike injured in nontraffic accident
> Passenger of go cart injured in nontraffic accident
> Passenger of golf cart injured in nontraffic accident

√5th **V86.7** Person on outside **of special all-terrain or other off-road motor vehicle injured** in nontraffic accident

√x7th **V86.71** **Person on outside of** ambulance or fire engine **injured in nontraffic accident**

√x7th **V86.72** **Person on outside of** snowmobile **injured in nontraffic accident**

√x7th **V86.73** **Person on outside of** dune buggy **injured in nontraffic accident**

√x7th **V86.74** **Person on outside of** military vehicle **injured in nontraffic accident**

√x7th **V86.79** **Person on outside of** other special all-terrain or **other off-road motor vehicles injured in nontraffic accident**

> Person on outside of dirt bike injured in nontraffic accident
> Person on outside of go cart injured in nontraffic accident
> Person on outside of golf cart injured in nontraffic accident

√5th **V86.9** Unspecified occupant **of special all-terrain or other off-road motor vehicle injured** in nontraffic accident

√x7th **V86.91** **Unspecified occupant of** ambulance or fire engine **injured in nontraffic accident**

√x7th **V86.92** **Unspecified occupant of** snowmobile **injured in nontraffic accident**

√x7th **V86.93** **Unspecified occupant of** dune buggy **injured in nontraffic accident**

√x7th **V86.94** **Unspecified occupant of** military vehicle **injured in nontraffic accident**

√x7th **V86.99** **Unspecified occupant of** other special all-terrain or **other off-road motor vehicle injured in nontraffic accident**

> All-terrain motor-vehicle accident NOS
> Off-road motor-vehicle accident NOS
> Other motor-vehicle accident NOS
> Unspecified occupant of dirt bike injured in nontraffic accident
> Unspecified occupant of go cart injured in nontraffic accident
> Unspecified occupant of golf cart injured in nontraffic accident

√4th **V87** **Traffic accident of specified type but victim's mode of transport unknown**

> EXCLUDES 1 *collision involving:*
> *pedal cycle (V10-V19)*
> *pedestrian (V01-V09)*

> The appropriate 7th character is to be added to each code from category V87.
> A   initial encounter
> D   subsequent encounter
> S   sequela

√x7th **V87.0** **Person injured in collision between** car and two- or three-wheeled powered vehicle **(traffic)**

√x7th **V87.1** **Person injured in collision between** other motor vehicle and two- or three-wheeled motor vehicle **(traffic)**

√x7th **V87.2** **Person injured in collision between** car and pick-up truck or van **(traffic)**

√x7th **V87.3** **Person injured in collision between** car and bus **(traffic)**

√x7th **V87.4** **Person injured in collision between** car and heavy transport vehicle **(traffic)**

√x7th **V87.5** **Person injured in collision between** heavy transport vehicle and bus **(traffic)**

√x7th **V87.6** **Person injured in collision between** railway train or railway vehicle and car **(traffic)**

√x7th **V87.7** **Person injured in collision between** other specified motor vehicles **(traffic)**

√x7th **V87.8** **Person injured in** other specified noncollision transport accidents **involving** motor vehicle **(traffic)**

√x7th **V87.9** **Person injured in** other specified (collision)(noncollision) transport accidents **involving** nonmotor vehicle **(traffic)**

√4th **V88** **Nontraffic accident of specified type but victim's mode of transport unknown**

> EXCLUDES 1 *collision involving:*
> *pedal cycle (V10-V19)*
> *pedestrian (V01-V09)*

> The appropriate 7th character is to be added to each code from category V88.
> A   initial encounter
> D   subsequent encounter
> S   sequela

√x7th **V88.0** **Person injured in collision between** car and two- or three-wheeled motor vehicle, **nontraffic**

√x7th **V88.1** **Person injured in collision between** other motor vehicle and two- or three-wheeled motor vehicle, **nontraffic**

N Newborn: 0   P Pediatric: 0-17   M Maternity: 12-55   A Adult: 15-124   MCC Major CC Condition   PDx MCC PDx acts as own MCC   CC CC Condition   PDx CC PDx acts as own CC

1134   ICD-10-CM Draft (2015)

√x7th **V88.2** **Person injured in collision between car and pick-up truck or van, nontraffic**

√x7th **V88.3** **Person injured in collision between car and bus, nontraffic**

√x7th **V88.4** **Person injured in collision between car and heavy transport vehicle, nontraffic**

√x7th **V88.5** **Person injured in collision between heavy transport vehicle and bus, nontraffic**

√x7th **V88.6** **Person injured in collision between railway train or railway vehicle and car, nontraffic**

√x7th **V88.7** **Person injured in collision between other specified motor vehicle, nontraffic**

√x7th **V88.8** **Person injured in other specified noncollision transport accidents involving motor vehicle, nontraffic**

√x7th **V88.9** **Person injured in other specified (collision)(noncollision) transport accidents involving nonmotor vehicle, nontraffic**

√4th **V89** **Motor- or nonmotor-vehicle accident, type of vehicle unspecified**

> The appropriate 7th character is to be added to each code from category V89.
> A   initial encounter
> D   subsequent encounter
> S   sequela

√x7th **V89.0** **Person injured in unspecified motor-vehicle accident, nontraffic**
Motor-vehicle accident NOS, nontraffic

√x7th **V89.1** **Person injured in unspecified nonmotor-vehicle accident, nontraffic**
Nonmotor-vehicle accident NOS (nontraffic)

√x7th **V89.2** **Person injured in unspecified motor-vehicle accident, traffic**
Motor-vehicle accident [MVA] NOS
Road (traffic) accident [RTA] NOS

√x7th **V89.3** **Person injured in unspecified nonmotor-vehicle accident, traffic**
Nonmotor-vehicle traffic accident NOS

√x7th **V89.9** **Person injured in unspecified vehicle accident**
Collision NOS

Water transport accidents (V90-V94)

√4th **V90** **Drowning and submersion due to accident to watercraft**
EXCLUDES1   *civilian water transport accident involving military watercraft (V94.81-)*
fall into water not from watercraft (W16.-)
military watercraft accident in military or war operations (Y36.0-, Y37.0-)
water-transport-related drowning or submersion without accident to watercraft (V92.-)

> The appropriate 7th character is to be added to each code from category V90.
> A   initial encounter
> D   subsequent encounter
> S   sequela

√5th **V90.0** **Drowning and submersion due to watercraft overturning**
√x7th **V90.00** **Drowning and submersion due to merchant ship overturning**
√x7th **V90.01** **Drowning and submersion due to passenger ship overturning**
Drowning and submersion due to Ferry-boat overturning
Drowning and submersion due to Liner overturning
√x7th **V90.02** **Drowning and submersion due to fishing boat overturning**
√x7th **V90.03** **Drowning and submersion due to other powered watercraft overturning**
Drowning and submersion due to Hovercraft (on open water) overturning
Drowning and submersion due to Jet ski overturning
√x7th **V90.04** **Drowning and submersion due to sailboat overturning**
√x7th **V90.05** **Drowning and submersion due to canoe or kayak overturning**
√x7th **V90.06** **Drowning and submersion due to (nonpowered) inflatable craft overturning**
√x7th **V90.08** **Drowning and submersion due to other unpowered watercraft overturning**
Drowning and submersion due to windsurfer overturning

√x7th **V90.09** **Drowning and submersion due to unspecified watercraft overturning**
Drowning and submersion due to boat NOS overturning
Drowning and submersion due to ship NOS overturning
Drowning and submersion due to watercraft NOS overturning

√5th **V90.1** **Drowning and submersion due to watercraft sinking**
√x7th **V90.10** **Drowning and submersion due to merchant ship sinking**
√x7th **V90.11** **Drowning and submersion due to passenger ship sinking**
Drowning and submersion due to Ferry-boat sinking
Drowning and submersion due to Liner sinking
√x7th **V90.12** **Drowning and submersion due to fishing boat sinking**
√x7th **V90.13** **Drowning and submersion due to other powered watercraft sinking**
Drowning and submersion due to Hovercraft (on open water) sinking
Drowning and submersion due to Jet ski sinking
√x7th **V90.14** **Drowning and submersion due to sailboat sinking**
√x7th **V90.15** **Drowning and submersion due to canoe or kayak sinking**
√x7th **V90.16** **Drowning and submersion due to (nonpowered) inflatable craft sinking**
√x7th **V90.18** **Drowning and submersion due to other unpowered watercraft sinking**
√x7th **V90.19** **Drowning and submersion due to unspecified watercraft sinking**
Drowning and submersion due to boat NOS sinking
Drowning and submersion due to ship NOS sinking
Drowning and submersion due to watercraft NOS sinking

√5th **V90.2** **Drowning and submersion due to falling or jumping from burning watercraft**
√x7th **V90.20** **Drowning and submersion due to falling or jumping from burning merchant ship**
√x7th **V90.21** **Drowning and submersion due to falling or jumping from burning passenger ship**
Drowning and submersion due to falling or jumping from burning Ferry-boat
Drowning and submersion due to falling or jumping from burning Liner
√x7th **V90.22** **Drowning and submersion due to falling or jumping from burning fishing boat**
√x7th **V90.23** **Drowning and submersion due to falling or jumping from other burning powered watercraft**
Drowning and submersion due to falling and jumping from burning Hovercraft (on open water)
Drowning and submersion due to falling and jumping from burning Jet ski
√x7th **V90.24** **Drowning and submersion due to falling or jumping from burning sailboat**
√x7th **V90.25** **Drowning and submersion due to falling or jumping from burning canoe or kayak**
√x7th **V90.26** **Drowning and submersion due to falling or jumping from burning (nonpowered) inflatable craft**
√x7th **V90.27** **Drowning and submersion due to falling or jumping from burning water-skis**
√x7th **V90.28** **Drowning and submersion due to falling or jumping from other burning unpowered watercraft**
Drowning and submersion due to falling and jumping from burning surf-board
Drowning and submersion due to falling and jumping from burning windsurfer
√x7th **V90.29** **Drowning and submersion due to falling or jumping from unspecified burning watercraft**
Drowning and submersion due to falling or jumping from burning boat NOS
Drowning and submersion due to falling or jumping from burning ship NOS
Drowning and submersion due to falling or jumping from burning watercraft NOS

√5th **V90.3** **Drowning and submersion due to falling or jumping from crushed watercraft**
√x7th **V90.30** **Drowning and submersion due to falling or jumping from crushed merchant ship**

✓ Additional Character Required   √x7th Xtension Alert   Unacceptable PDx   Manifestation   Hospital Acquired Condition   EXCLUDES1 Not Coded Here   EXCLUDES2 Not Included Here

ICD-10-CM Draft (2015)   1135

External Causes of Morbidity

V88.2–V90.30

External Causes of Morbidity

V90.31–V91.19

√x7ᵗʰ **V90.31** **Drowning and submersion due to falling or jumping from crushed passenger ship**
Drowning and submersion due to falling and jumping from crushed Ferry boat
Drowning and submersion due to falling and jumping from crushed Liner

√x7ᵗʰ **V90.32** **Drowning and submersion due to falling or jumping from crushed fishing boat**

√x7ᵗʰ **V90.33** **Drowning and submersion due to falling or jumping from other crushed powered watercraft**
Drowning and submersion due to falling and jumping from crushed Hovercraft
Drowning and submersion due to falling and jumping from crushed Jet ski

√x7ᵗʰ **V90.34** **Drowning and submersion due to falling or jumping from crushed sailboat**

√x7ᵗʰ **V90.35** **Drowning and submersion due to falling or jumping from crushed canoe or kayak**

√x7ᵗʰ **V90.36** **Drowning and submersion due to falling or jumping from crushed (nonpowered) inflatable craft**

√x7ᵗʰ **V90.37** **Drowning and submersion due to falling or jumping from crushed water-skis**

√x7ᵗʰ **V90.38** **Drowning and submersion due to falling or jumping from other crushed unpowered watercraft**
Drowning and submersion due to falling and jumping from crushed surf-board
Drowning and submersion due to falling and jumping from crushed windsurfer

√x7ᵗʰ **V90.39** **Drowning and submersion due to falling or jumping from crushed unspecified watercraft**
Drowning and submersion due to falling and jumping from crushed boat NOS
Drowning and submersion due to falling and jumping from crushed ship NOS
Drowning and submersion due to falling and jumping from crushed watercraft NOS

√5ᵗʰ **V90.8** **Drowning and submersion due to other accident to watercraft**

√x7ᵗʰ **V90.80** **Drowning and submersion due to other accident to merchant ship**

√x7ᵗʰ **V90.81** **Drowning and submersion due to other accident to passenger ship**
Drowning and submersion due to other accident to Ferry-boat
Drowning and submersion due to other accident to Liner

√x7ᵗʰ **V90.82** **Drowning and submersion due to other accident to fishing boat**

√x7ᵗʰ **V90.83** **Drowning and submersion due to other accident to other powered watercraft**
Drowning and submersion due to other accident to Hovercraft (on open water)
Drowning and submersion due to other accident to Jet ski

√x7ᵗʰ **V90.84** **Drowning and submersion due to other accident to sailboat**

√x7ᵗʰ **V90.85** **Drowning and submersion due to other accident to canoe or kayak**

√x7ᵗʰ **V90.86** **Drowning and submersion due to other accident to (nonpowered) inflatable craft**

√x7ᵗʰ **V90.87** **Drowning and submersion due to other accident to water-skis**

√x7ᵗʰ **V90.88** **Drowning and submersion due to other accident to other unpowered watercraft**
Drowning and submersion due to other accident to surf-board
Drowning and submersion due to other accident to windsurfer

√x7ᵗʰ **V90.89** **Drowning and submersion due to other accident to unspecified watercraft**
Drowning and submersion due to other accident to boat NOS
Drowning and submersion due to other accident to ship NOS
Drowning and submersion due to other accident to watercraft NOS

√4ᵗʰ **V91** **Other injury due to accident to watercraft**
INCLUDES   any injury except drowning and submersion as a result of an accident to watercraft
EXCLUDES 1   civilian water transport accident involving military watercraft (V94.81-)
military watercraft accident in military or war operations (Y36, Y37.-)
EXCLUDES 2   drowning and submersion due to accident to watercraft (V90.-)

The appropriate 7th character is to be added to each code from category V91.
A   initial encounter
D   subsequent encounter
S   sequela

√5ᵗʰ **V91.0** **Burn due to watercraft on fire**
EXCLUDES 1   burn from localized fire or explosion on board ship without accident to watercraft (V93.-)

√x7ᵗʰ **V91.00** **Burn due to merchant ship on fire**

√x7ᵗʰ **V91.01** **Burn due to passenger ship on fire**
Burn due to Ferry-boat on fire
Burn due to Liner on fire

√x7ᵗʰ **V91.02** **Burn due to fishing boat on fire**

√x7ᵗʰ **V91.03** **Burn due to other powered watercraft on fire**
Burn due to Hovercraft (on open water) on fire
Burn due to Jet ski on fire

√x7ᵗʰ **V91.04** **Burn due to sailboat on fire**

√x7ᵗʰ **V91.05** **Burn due to canoe or kayak on fire**

√x7ᵗʰ **V91.06** **Burn due to (nonpowered) inflatable craft on fire**

√x7ᵗʰ **V91.07** **Burn due to water-skis on fire**

√x7ᵗʰ **V91.08** **Burn due to other unpowered watercraft on fire**

√x7ᵗʰ **V91.09** **Burn due to unspecified watercraft on fire**
Burn due to boat NOS on fire
Burn due to ship NOS on fire
Burn due to watercraft NOS on fire

√5ᵗʰ **V91.1** **Crushed between watercraft and other watercraft or other object due to collision**
Crushed by lifeboat after abandoning ship in a collision
NOTE   select the specified type of watercraft that the victim was on at the time of the collision

√x7ᵗʰ **V91.10** **Crushed between merchant ship and other watercraft or other object due to collision**

√x7ᵗʰ **V91.11** **Crushed between passenger ship and other watercraft or other object due to collision**
Crushed between Ferry-boat and other watercraft or other object due to collision
Crushed between Liner and other watercraft or other object due to collision

√x7ᵗʰ **V91.12** **Crushed between fishing boat and other watercraft or other object due to collision**

√x7ᵗʰ **V91.13** **Crushed between other powered watercraft and other watercraft or other object due to collision**
Crushed between Hovercraft (on open water) and other watercraft or other object due to collision
Crushed between Jet ski and other watercraft or other object due to collision

√x7ᵗʰ **V91.14** **Crushed between sailboat and other watercraft or other object due to collision**

√x7ᵗʰ **V91.15** **Crushed between canoe or kayak and other watercraft or other object due to collision**

√x7ᵗʰ **V91.16** **Crushed between (nonpowered) inflatable craft and other watercraft or other object due to collision**

√x7ᵗʰ **V91.18** **Crushed between other unpowered watercraft and other watercraft or other object due to collision**
Crushed between surfboard and other watercraft or other object due to collision
Crushed between windsurfer and other watercraft or other object due to collision

√x7ᵗʰ **V91.19** **Crushed between unspecified watercraft and other watercraft or other object due to collision**
Crushed between boat NOS and other watercraft or other object due to collision
Crushed between ship NOS and other watercraft or other object due to collision
Crushed between watercraft NOS and other watercraft or other object due to collision

---

N Newborn: 0   P Pediatric: 0-17   M Maternity: 12-55   A Adult: 15-124   MCC Major CC Condition   PDx MCC PDx acts as own MCC   CC CC Condition   PDx CC PDx acts as own CC

1136   ICD-10-CM Draft (2015)

✓5ᵗʰ **V91.2** **Fall due to collision between watercraft and other watercraft or other object**
Fall while remaining on watercraft after collision

> **NOTE**   Select the specified type of watercraft that the victim was on at the time of the collision.

> **EXCLUDES 1**   crushed between watercraft and other watercraft and other object due to collision (V91.1-)
> drowning and submersion due to falling from crushed watercraft (V90.3-)

✓x7ᵗʰ **V91.20** **Fall due to collision between merchant ship and other watercraft or other object**

✓x7ᵗʰ **V91.21** **Fall due to collision between passenger ship and other watercraft or other object**
Fall due to collision between Ferry-boat and other watercraft or other object
Fall due to collision between Liner and other watercraft or other object

✓x7ᵗʰ **V91.22** **Fall due to collision between fishing boat and other watercraft or other object**

✓x7ᵗʰ **V91.23** **Fall due to collision between other powered watercraft and other watercraft or other object**
Fall due to collision between Hovercraft (on open water) and other watercraft or other object
Fall due to collision between Jet ski and other watercraft or other object

✓x7ᵗʰ **V91.24** **Fall due to collision between sailboat and other watercraft or other object**

✓x7ᵗʰ **V91.25** **Fall due to collision between canoe or kayak and other watercraft or other object**

✓x7ᵗʰ **V91.26** **Fall due to collision between (nonpowered) inflatable craft and other watercraft or other object**

✓x7ᵗʰ **V91.29** **Fall due to collision between unspecified watercraft and other watercraft or other object**
Fall due to collision between boat NOS and other watercraft or other object
Fall due to collision between ship NOS and other watercraft or other object
Fall due to collision between watercraft NOS and other watercraft or other object

✓5ᵗʰ **V91.3** **Hit or struck by falling object due to accident to watercraft**
Hit or struck by falling object (part of damaged watercraft or other object) after falling or jumping from damaged watercraft

> **EXCLUDES 2**   drowning or submersion due to fall or jumping from damaged watercraft (V90.2-, V90.3-)

✓x7ᵗʰ **V91.30** **Hit or struck by falling object due to accident to merchant ship**

✓x7ᵗʰ **V91.31** **Hit or struck by falling object due to accident to passenger ship**
Hit or struck by falling object due to accident to Ferry-boat
Hit or struck by falling object due to accident to Liner

✓x7ᵗʰ **V91.32** **Hit or struck by falling object due to accident to fishing boat**

✓x7ᵗʰ **V91.33** **Hit or struck by falling object due to accident to other powered watercraft**
Hit or struck by falling object due to accident to Hovercraft (on open water)
Hit or struck by falling object due to accident to Jet ski

✓x7ᵗʰ **V91.34** **Hit or struck by falling object due to accident to sailboat**

✓x7ᵗʰ **V91.35** **Hit or struck by falling object due to accident to canoe or kayak**

✓x7ᵗʰ **V91.36** **Hit or struck by falling object due to accident to (nonpowered) inflatable craft**

✓x7ᵗʰ **V91.37** **Hit or struck by falling object due to accident to water-skis**
Hit by water-skis after jumping off of waterskis

✓x7ᵗʰ **V91.38** **Hit or struck by falling object due to accident to other unpowered watercraft**
Hit or struck by surf-board after falling off damaged surf-board
Hit or struck by object after falling off damaged windsurfer

✓x7ᵗʰ **V91.39** **Hit or struck by falling object due to accident to unspecified watercraft**
Hit or struck by falling object due to accident to boat NOS
Hit or struck by falling object due to accident to ship NOS
Hit or struck by falling object due to accident to watercraft NOS

✓5ᵗʰ **V91.8** **Other injury due to other accident to watercraft**

✓x7ᵗʰ **V91.80** **Other injury due to other accident to merchant ship**

✓x7ᵗʰ **V91.81** **Other injury due to other accident to passenger ship**
Other injury due to other accident to Ferry-boat
Other injury due to other accident to Liner

✓x7ᵗʰ **V91.82** **Other injury due to other accident to fishing boat**

✓x7ᵗʰ **V91.83** **Other injury due to other accident to other powered watercraft**
Other injury due to other accident to Hovercraft (on open water)
Other injury due to other accident to Jet ski

✓x7ᵗʰ **V91.84** **Other injury due to other accident to sailboat**

✓x7ᵗʰ **V91.85** **Other injury due to other accident to canoe or kayak**

✓x7ᵗʰ **V91.86** **Other injury due to other accident to (nonpowered) inflatable craft**

✓x7ᵗʰ **V91.87** **Other injury due to other accident to water-skis**

✓x7ᵗʰ **V91.88** **Other injury due to other accident to other unpowered watercraft**
Other injury due to other accident to surf-board
Other injury due to other accident to windsurfer

✓x7ᵗʰ **V91.89** **Other injury due to other accident to unspecified watercraft**
Other injury due to other accident to boat NOS
Other injury due to other accident to ship NOS
Other injury due to other accident to watercraft NOS

✓4ᵗʰ **V92** **Drowning and submersion due to accident on board watercraft, without accident to watercraft**

> **EXCLUDES 1**   civilian water transport accident involving military watercraft (V94.81-)
> drowning or submersion due to accident to watercraft (V90-V91)
> drowning or submersion of diver who voluntarily jumps from boat not involved in an accident (W16.711, W16.721)
> fall into water without watercraft (W16.-)
> military watercraft accident in military or war operations (Y36, Y37)

The appropriate 7th character is to be added to each code from category V92.
A   initial encounter
D   subsequent encounter
S   sequela

✓5ᵗʰ **V92.0** **Drowning and submersion due to fall off watercraft**
Drowning and submersion due to fall from gangplank of watercraft
Drowning and submersion due to fall overboard watercraft

> **EXCLUDES 2**   hitting head on object or bottom of body of water due to fall from watercraft (V94.0-)

✓x7ᵗʰ **V92.00** **Drowning and submersion due to fall off merchant ship**

✓x7ᵗʰ **V92.01** **Drowning and submersion due to fall off passenger ship**
Drowning and submersion due to fall off Ferry-boat
Drowning and submersion due to fall off Liner

✓x7ᵗʰ **V92.02** **Drowning and submersion due to fall off fishing boat**

✓x7ᵗʰ **V92.03** **Drowning and submersion due to fall off other powered watercraft**
Drowning and submersion due to fall off Hovercraft (on open water)
Drowning and submersion due to fall off Jet ski

✓x7ᵗʰ **V92.04** **Drowning and submersion due to fall off sailboat**

✓x7ᵗʰ **V92.05** **Drowning and submersion due to fall off canoe or kayak**

✓x7ᵗʰ **V92.06** **Drowning and submersion due to fall off (nonpowered) inflatable craft**

✓x7ᵗʰ **V92.07** **Drowning and submersion due to fall off water-skis**

> **EXCLUDES 1**   drowning and submersion due to falling off burning water-skis (V90.27)
> drowning and submersion due to falling off crushed water-skis (V90.37)
> hit by boat while water-skiing NOS (V94.X)

✓ Additional Character Required   ✓x7ᵗʰ Xtension Alert   Unacceptable PDx   Manifestation   Hospital Acquired Condition   **EXCLUDES 1** Not Coded Here   **EXCLUDES 2** Not Included Here

✓x7th **V92.08 Drowning and submersion due to fall off** other unpowered **watercraft**

Drowning and submersion due to fall off surf-board

Drowning and submersion due to fall off windsurfer

> EXCLUDES 1 *drowning and submersion due to fall off burning unpowered watercraft (V90.28)*
>
> *drowning and submersion due to fall off crushed unpowered watercraft (V90.38)*
>
> *drowning and submersion due to fall off damaged unpowered watercraft (V90.88)*
>
> *drowning and submersion due to rider of nonpowered watercraft being hit by other watercraft (V94.-)*
>
> *other injury due to rider of nonpowered watercraft being hit by other watercraft (V94.-)*

✓x7th **V92.09 Drowning and submersion due to fall off** unspecified **watercraft**

Drowning and submersion due to fall off boat NOS

Drowning and submersion due to fall off ship

Drowning and submersion due to fall off watercraft NOS

✓5th **V92.1 Drowning and submersion due to being** thrown overboard **by motion of watercraft**

> EXCLUDES 1 *drowning and submersion due to fall off surf-board (V92.08)*
>
> *drowning and submersion due to fall off water-skis (V92.07)*
>
> *drowning and submersion due to fall off windsurfer (V92.08)*

✓x7th **V92.10 Drowning and submersion due to being thrown overboard by motion of** merchant ship

✓x7th **V92.11 Drowning and submersion due to being thrown overboard by motion of** passenger ship

Drowning and submersion due to being thrown overboard by motion of Ferry-boat

Drowning and submersion due to being thrown overboard by motion of Liner

✓x7th **V92.12 Drowning and submersion due to being thrown overboard by motion of** fishing boat

✓x7th **V92.13 Drowning and submersion due to being thrown overboard by motion of** other powered **watercraft**

Drowning and submersion due to being thrown overboard by motion of Hovercraft

✓x7th **V92.14 Drowning and submersion due to being thrown overboard by motion of** sailboat

✓x7th **V92.15 Drowning and submersion due to being thrown overboard by motion of** canoe or kayak

✓x7th **V92.16 Drowning and submersion due to being thrown overboard by motion of (nonpowered)** inflatable craft

✓x7th **V92.19 Drowning and submersion due to being thrown overboard by motion of** unspecified **watercraft**

Drowning and submersion due to being thrown overboard by motion of boat NOS

Drowning and submersion due to being thrown overboard by motion of ship NOS

Drowning and submersion due to being thrown overboard by motion of watercraft NOS

✓5th **V92.2 Drowning and submersion due to being** washed overboard **from watercraft**

Code first any associated cataclysm (X37.0-)

✓x7th **V92.20 Drowning and submersion due to being washed overboard from** merchant ship

✓x7th **V92.21 Drowning and submersion due to being washed overboard from** passenger ship

Drowning and submersion due to being washed overboard from Ferry-boat

Drowning and submersion due to being washed overboard from Liner

✓x7th **V92.22 Drowning and submersion due to being washed overboard from** fishing boat

✓x7th **V92.23 Drowning and submersion due to being washed overboard from** other powered **watercraft**

Drowning and submersion due to being washed overboard from Hovercraft (on open water)

Drowning and submersion due to being washed overboard from Jet ski

✓x7th **V92.24 Drowning and submersion due to being washed overboard from** sailboat

✓x7th **V92.25 Drowning and submersion due to being washed overboard from** canoe or kayak

✓x7th **V92.26 Drowning and submersion due to being washed overboard from (nonpowered)** inflatable craft

✓x7th **V92.27 Drowning and submersion due to being washed overboard from** water-skis

> EXCLUDES 1 *drowning and submersion due to fall off water-skis (V92.07)*

✓x7th **V92.28 Drowning and submersion due to being washed overboard from** other unpowered **watercraft**

Drowning and submersion due to being washed overboard from surf-board

Drowning and submersion due to being washed overboard from windsurfer

✓x7th **V92.29 Drowning and submersion due to being washed overboard from** unspecified **watercraft**

Drowning and submersion due to being washed overboard from boat NOS

Drowning and submersion due to being washed overboard from ship NOS

Drowning and submersion due to being washed overboard from watercraft NOS

✓4th **V93 Other injury due to accident on board watercraft, without accident to watercraft**

> EXCLUDES 1 *civilian water transport accident involving military watercraft (V94.81-)*
>
> *other injury due to accident to watercraft (V91.-)*
>
> *military watercraft accident in military or war operations (Y36, Y37.-)*
>
> EXCLUDES 2 *drowning and submersion due to accident on board watercraft, without accident to watercraft (V92.-)*

The appropriate 7th character is to be added to each code from category V93.

A   initial encounter

D   subsequent encounter

S   sequela

✓5th **V93.0 Burn due to localized fire on board watercraft**

> EXCLUDES 1 *burn due to watercraft on fire (V91.0-)*

✓x7th **V93.00 Burn due to localized fire on board** merchant vessel

✓x7th **V93.01 Burn due to localized fire on board** passenger vessel

Burn due to localized fire on board Ferry-boat

Burn due to localized fire on board Liner

✓x7th **V93.02 Burn due to localized fire on board** fishing boat

✓x7th **V93.03 Burn due to localized fire on board** other powered **watercraft**

Burn due to localized fire on board Hovercraft

Burn due to localized fire on board Jet ski

✓x7th **V93.04 Burn due to localized fire on board** sailboat

✓x7th **V93.09 Burn due to localized fire on board** unspecified **watercraft**

Burn due to localized fire on board boat NOS

Burn due to localized fire on board ship NOS

Burn due to localized fire on board watercraft NOS

✓5th **V93.1 Other burn on board watercraft**

Burn due to source other than fire on board watercraft

> EXCLUDES 1 *burn due to watercraft on fire (V91.0-)*

✓x7th **V93.10 Other burn on board** merchant vessel

✓x7th **V93.11 Other burn on board** passenger vessel

Other burn on board Ferry-boat

Other burn on board Liner

✓x7th **V93.12 Other burn on board** fishing boat

✓x7th **V93.13 Other burn on board** other powered **watercraft**

Other burn on board Hovercraft

Other burn on board Jet ski

✓x7th **V93.14 Other burn on board** sailboat

✓x7th **V93.19 Other burn on board** unspecified **watercraft**

Other burn on board boat NOS

Other burn on board ship NOS

Other burn on board watercraft NOS

✓5th **V93.2 Heat exposure on board watercraft**

> EXCLUDES 1 *exposure to man-made heat not aboard watercraft (W92)*
>
> *exposure to natural heat while on board watercraft (X30)*
>
> *exposure to sunlight while on board watercraft (X32)*
>
> EXCLUDES 2 *burn due to fire on board watercraft (V93.0-)*

✓x7th **V93.20 Heat exposure on board** merchant ship

✓x7th **V93.21 Heat exposure on board** passenger ship

Heat exposure on board Ferry-boat

Heat exposure on board Liner

✓x7th **V93.22 Heat exposure on board** fishing boat

✓x7th **V93.23 Heat exposure on board** other powered **watercraft**

Heat exposure on board hovercraft

N Newborn: 0   P Pediatric: 0-17   M Maternity: 12-55   A Adult: 15-124   MCC Major CC Condition   PDx MCC PDx acts as own MCC   CC CC Condition   PDx CC PDx acts as own CC

1188   ICD-10-CM Draft (2015)

√x7ᵗʰ **V93.24 Heat exposure on board** sailboat

√x7ᵗʰ **V93.29 Heat exposure on board** unspecified **watercraft**
Heat exposure on board boat NOS
Heat exposure on board ship NOS
Heat exposure on board watercraft NOS

√5ᵗʰ **V93.3 Fall on board watercraft**
EXCLUDES 1 *fall due to collision of watercraft (V91.2-)*

√x7ᵗʰ **V93.30 Fall on board** merchant ship

√x7ᵗʰ **V93.31 Fall on board** passenger ship
Fall on board Ferry-boat
Fall on board Liner

√x7ᵗʰ **V93.32 Fall on board** fishing boat

√x7ᵗʰ **V93.33 Fall on board** other powered **watercraft**
Fall on board Hovercraft (on open water)
Fall on board Jet ski

√x7ᵗʰ **V93.34 Fall on board** sailboat

√x7ᵗʰ **V93.35 Fall on board** canoe or kayak

√x7ᵗʰ **V93.36 Fall on board** (nonpowered) inflatable craft

√x7ᵗʰ **V93.38 Fall on board** other unpowered **watercraft**

√x7ᵗʰ **V93.39 Fall on board** unspecified **watercraft**
Fall on board boat NOS
Fall on board ship NOS
Fall on board watercraft NOS

√5ᵗʰ **V93.4 Struck by falling object on board watercraft**
Hit by falling object on board watercraft
EXCLUDES 1 *struck by falling object due to accident to watercraft (V91.3)*

√x7ᵗʰ **V93.40 Struck by falling object on** merchant ship

√x7ᵗʰ **V93.41 Struck by falling object on** passenger ship
Struck by falling object on Ferry-boat
Struck by falling object on Liner

√x7ᵗʰ **V93.42 Struck by falling object on** fishing boat

√x7ᵗʰ **V93.43 Struck by falling object on** other powered **watercraft**
Struck by falling object on Hovercraft

√x7ᵗʰ **V93.44 Struck by falling object on** sailboat

√x7ᵗʰ **V93.48 Struck by falling object on** other unpowered **watercraft**

√x7ᵗʰ **V93.49 Struck by falling object on** unspecified **watercraft**

√5ᵗʰ **V93.5 Explosion on board watercraft**
Boiler explosion on steamship
EXCLUDES 2 *fire on board watercraft (V93.0-)*

√x7ᵗʰ **V93.50 Explosion on board** merchant ship

√x7ᵗʰ **V93.51 Explosion on board** passenger ship
Explosion on board Ferry-boat
Explosion on board Liner

√x7ᵗʰ **V93.52 Explosion on board** fishing boat

√x7ᵗʰ **V93.53 Explosion on board** other powered **watercraft**
Explosion on board Hovercraft
Explosion on board Jet ski

√x7ᵗʰ **V93.54 Explosion on board** sailboat

√x7ᵗʰ **V93.59 Explosion on board** unspecified **watercraft**
Explosion on board boat NOS
Explosion on board ship NOS
Explosion on board watercraft NOS

√5ᵗʰ **V93.6 Machinery accident on board watercraft**
EXCLUDES 1 *machinery explosion on board watercraft (V93.4-)*
machinery fire on board watercraft (V93.0-)

√x7ᵗʰ **V93.60 Machinery accident on board** merchant ship

√x7ᵗʰ **V93.61 Machinery accident on board** passenger ship
Machinery accident on board Ferry-boat
Machinery accident on board Liner

√x7ᵗʰ **V93.62 Machinery accident on board** fishing boat

√x7ᵗʰ **V93.63 Machinery accident on board** other powered **watercraft**
Machinery accident on board Hovercraft

√x7ᵗʰ **V93.64 Machinery accident on board** sailboat

√x7ᵗʰ **V93.69 Machinery accident on board** unspecified **watercraft**
Machinery accident on board boat NOS
Machinery accident on board ship NOS
Machinery accident on board watercraft NOS

√5ᵗʰ **V93.8 Other injury due to other accident on board watercraft**
Accidental poisoning by gases or fumes on watercraft

√x7ᵗʰ **V93.80 Other injury due to other accident on board** merchant ship

√x7ᵗʰ **V93.81 Other injury due to other accident on board** passenger ship
Other injury due to other accident on board Ferry-boat
Other injury due to other accident on board Liner

√x7ᵗʰ **V93.82 Other injury due to other accident on board** fishing boat

√x7ᵗʰ **V93.83 Other injury due to other accident on board** other powered **watercraft**
Other injury due to other accident on board Hovercraft
Other injury due to other accident on board Jet ski

√x7ᵗʰ **V93.84 Other injury due to other accident on board** sailboat

√x7ᵗʰ **V93.85 Other injury due to other accident on board** canoe or kayak

√x7ᵗʰ **V93.86 Other injury due to other accident on board** (nonpowered) inflatable craft

√x7ᵗʰ **V93.87 Other injury due to other accident on board** water-skis
Hit or struck by object while waterskiing

√x7ᵗʰ **V93.88 Other injury due to other accident on board** other unpowered **watercraft**
Hit or struck by object while surfing
Hit or struck by object while on board windsurfer

√x7ᵗʰ **V93.89 Other injury due to other accident on board** unspecified **watercraft**
Other injury due to other accident on board boat NOS
Other injury due to other accident on board ship NOS
Other injury due to other accident on board watercraft NOS

√4ᵗʰ **V94 Other and unspecified water transport accidents**
EXCLUDES 1 *military watercraft accidents in military or war operations (Y36, Y37)*

The appropriate 7th character is to be added to each code from category V94.
A   initial encounter
D   subsequent encounter
S   sequela

√x7ᵗʰ **V94.0 Hitting object or bottom of body of water due to fall from watercraft**
EXCLUDES 2 *drowning and submersion due to fall from watercraft (V92.0-)*

√5ᵗʰ **V94.1 Bather struck by watercraft**
Swimmer hit by watercraft

√x7ᵗʰ **V94.11 Bather struck by** powered **watercraft**

√x7ᵗʰ **V94.12 Bather struck by** nonpowered **watercraft**

√5ᵗʰ **V94.2 Rider of nonpowered watercraft struck by other watercraft**

√x7ᵗʰ **V94.21 Rider of nonpowered watercraft struck by** other nonpowered **watercraft**
Canoer hit by other nonpowered watercraft
Surfer hit by other nonpowered watercraft
Windsurfer hit by other nonpowered watercraft

√x7ᵗʰ **V94.22 Rider of nonpowered watercraft struck by** powered **watercraft**
Canoer hit by motorboat
Surfer hit by motorboat
Windsurfer hit by motorboat

√5ᵗʰ **V94.3 Injury to rider of (inflatable) watercraft being pulled behind other watercraft**

√x7ᵗʰ **V94.31 Injury to rider of (inflatable)** recreational **watercraft being pulled behind other watercraft**
Injury to rider of inner-tube pulled behind motor boat

√x7ᵗʰ **V94.32 Injury to rider of** non-recreational **watercraft being pulled behind other watercraft**
Injury to occupant of dingy being pulled behind boat or ship
Injury to occupant of life-raft being pulled behind boat or ship

√x7ᵗʰ **V94.4 Injury to barefoot water-skier**
Injury to person being pulled behind boat or ship

√5ᵗʰ **V94.8 Other water transport accident**

√6ᵗʰ **V94.81 Water transport accident involving military watercraft**

√7ᵗʰ **V94.810 Civilian watercraft involved in water transport accident with military watercraft**
Passenger on civilian watercraft injured due to accident with military watercraft

√7ᵗʰ **V94.811 Civilian in water injured by military watercraft**

√7ᵗʰ **V94.818 Other water transport accident involving military watercraft**

√x7ᵗʰ **V94.89 Other water transport accident**

√x7ᵗʰ **V94.9 Unspecified water transport accident**
Water transport accident NOS

☑ Additional Character Required   √x7ᵗʰ Xtension Alert   Unacceptable PDx   Manifestation   Hospital Acquired Condition   *EXCLUDES 1* Not Coded Here   *EXCLUDES 2* Not Included Here

External Causes of Morbidity

V95–V97.39

Air and space transport accidents (V95-V97)

EXCLUDES 1   military aircraft accidents in military or war operations (Y36, Y37)

√4th **V95   Accident to powered aircraft causing injury to occupant**

> The appropriate 7th character is to be added to each code from category V95.
> A   initial encounter
> D   subsequent encounter
> S   sequela

√5th   **V95.0   Helicopter accident injuring occupant**
   √x7th   **V95.00   Unspecified helicopter accident injuring occupant**
   √x7th   **V95.01   Helicopter crash injuring occupant**
   √x7th   **V95.02   Forced landing of helicopter injuring occupant**
   √x7th   **V95.03   Helicopter collision injuring occupant**
      Helicopter collision with any object, fixed, movable or moving
   √x7th   **V95.04   Helicopter fire injuring occupant**
   √x7th   **V95.05   Helicopter explosion injuring occupant**
   √x7th   **V95.09   Other helicopter accident injuring occupant**

√5th   **V95.1   Ultralight, microlight or powered-glider accident injuring occupant**
   √x7th   **V95.10   Unspecified ultralight, microlight or powered-glider accident injuring occupant**
   √x7th   **V95.11   Ultralight, microlight or powered-glider crash injuring occupant**
   √x7th   **V95.12   Forced landing of ultralight, microlight or powered-glider injuring occupant**
   √x7th   **V95.13   Ultralight, microlight or powered-glider collision injuring occupant**
      Ultralight, microlight or powered-glider collision with any object, fixed, movable or moving
   √x7th   **V95.14   Ultralight, microlight or powered-glider fire injuring occupant**
   √x7th   **V95.15   Ultralight, microlight or powered-glider explosion injuring occupant**
   √x7th   **V95.19   Other ultralight, microlight or powered-glider accident injuring occupant**

√5th   **V95.2   Other private fixed-wing aircraft accident injuring occupant**
   √x7th   **V95.20   Unspecified accident to other private fixed-wing aircraft, injuring occupant**
   √x7th   **V95.21   Other private fixed-wing aircraft crash injuring occupant**
   √x7th   **V95.22   Forced landing of other private fixed-wing aircraft injuring occupant**
   √x7th   **V95.23   Other private fixed-wing aircraft collision injuring occupant**
      Other private fixed-wing aircraft collision with any object, fixed, movable or moving
   √x7th   **V95.24   Other private fixed-wing aircraft fire injuring occupant**
   √x7th   **V95.25   Other private fixed-wing aircraft explosion injuring occupant**
   √x7th   **V95.29   Other accident to other private fixed-wing aircraft injuring occupant**

√5th   **V95.3   Commercial fixed-wing aircraft accident injuring occupant**
   √x7th   **V95.30   Unspecified accident to commercial fixed-wing aircraft injuring occupant**
   √x7th   **V95.31   Commercial fixed-wing aircraft crash injuring occupant**
   √x7th   **V95.32   Forced landing of commercial fixed-wing aircraft injuring occupant**
   √x7th   **V95.33   Commercial fixed-wing aircraft collision injuring occupant**
      Commercial fixed-wing aircraft collision with any object, fixed, movable or moving
   √x7th   **V95.34   Commercial fixed-wing aircraft fire injuring occupant**
   √x7th   **V95.35   Commercial fixed-wing aircraft explosion injuring occupant**
   √x7th   **V95.39   Other accident to commercial fixed-wing aircraft injuring occupant**

√5th   **V95.4   Spacecraft accident injuring occupant**
   √x7th   **V95.40   Unspecified spacecraft accident injuring occupant**
   √x7th   **V95.41   Spacecraft crash injuring occupant**
   √x7th   **V95.42   Forced landing of spacecraft injuring occupant**
   √x7th   **V95.43   Spacecraft collision injuring occupant**
      Spacecraft collision with any object, fixed, moveable or moving
   √x7th   **V95.44   Spacecraft fire injuring occupant**
   √x7th   **V95.45   Spacecraft explosion injuring occupant**

   √x7th   **V95.49   Other spacecraft accident injuring occupant**
√x7th   **V95.8   Other powered aircraft accidents injuring occupant**
√x7th   **V95.9   Unspecified aircraft accident injuring occupant**
      Aircraft accident NOS
      Air transport accident NOS

√4th   **V96   Accident to nonpowered aircraft causing injury to occupant**

> The appropriate 7th character is to be added to each code from category V96.
> A   initial encounter
> D   subsequent encounter
> S   sequela

√5th   **V96.0   Balloon accident injuring occupant**
   √x7th   **V96.00   Unspecified balloon accident injuring occupant**
   √x7th   **V96.01   Balloon crash injuring occupant**
   √x7th   **V96.02   Forced landing of balloon injuring occupant**
   √x7th   **V96.03   Balloon collision injuring occupant**
      Balloon collision with any object, fixed, moveable or moving
   √x7th   **V96.04   Balloon fire injuring occupant**
   √x7th   **V96.05   Balloon explosion injuring occupant**
   √x7th   **V96.09   Other balloon accident injuring occupant**

√5th   **V96.1   Hang-glider accident injuring occupant**
   √x7th   **V96.10   Unspecified hang-glider accident injuring occupant**
   √x7th   **V96.11   Hang-glider crash injuring occupant**
   √x7th   **V96.12   Forced landing of hang-glider injuring occupant**
   √x7th   **V96.13   Hang-glider collision injuring occupant**
      Hang-glider collision with any object, fixed, moveable or moving
   √x7th   **V96.14   Hang-glider fire injuring occupant**
   √x7th   **V96.15   Hang-glider explosion injuring occupant**
   √x7th   **V96.19   Other hang-glider accident injuring occupant**

√5th   **V96.2   Glider (nonpowered) accident injuring occupant**
   √x7th   **V96.20   Unspecified glider (nonpowered) accident injuring occupant**
   √x7th   **V96.21   Glider (nonpowered) crash injuring occupant**
   √x7th   **V96.22   Forced landing of glider (nonpowered) injuring occupant**
   √x7th   **V96.23   Glider (nonpowered) collision injuring occupant**
      Glider (nonpowered) collision with any object, fixed, moveable or moving
   √x7th   **V96.24   Glider (nonpowered) fire injuring occupant**
   √x7th   **V96.25   Glider (nonpowered) explosion injuring occupant**
   √x7th   **V96.29   Other glider (nonpowered) accident injuring occupant**

√x7th   **V96.8   Other nonpowered-aircraft accidents injuring occupant**
      Kite carrying a person accident injuring occupant
√x7th   **V96.9   Unspecified nonpowered-aircraft accident injuring occupant**
      Nonpowered-aircraft accident NOS

√4th   **V97   Other specified air transport accidents**

> The appropriate 7th character is to be added to each code from category V97.
> A   initial encounter
> D   subsequent encounter
> S   sequela

√x7th   **V97.0   Occupant of aircraft injured in other specified air transport accidents**
      Fall in, on or from aircraft in air transport accident
      EXCLUDES 1   accident while boarding or alighting aircraft (V97.1)
√x7th   **V97.1   Person injured while boarding or alighting from aircraft**
√5th   **V97.2   Parachutist accident**
   √x7th   **V97.21   Parachutist entangled in object**
      Parachutist landing in tree
   √x7th   **V97.22   Parachutist injured on landing**
   √x7th   **V97.29   Other parachutist accident**
√5th   **V97.3   Person on ground injured in air transport accident**
   √x7th   **V97.31   Hit by object falling from aircraft**
      Hit by crashing aircraft
      Injured by aircraft hitting house
      Injured by aircraft hitting car
   √x7th   **V97.32   Injured by rotating propeller**
   √x7th   **V97.33   Sucked into jet engine**
   √x7th   **V97.39   Other injury to person on ground due to air transport accident**

N Newborn: 0   P Pediatric: 0-17   M Maternity: 12-55   A Adult: 15-124   MCC Major CC Condition   PDx MCC PDx acts as own MCC   CC CC Condition   PDx CC PDx acts as own CC

☑5ᵗʰ **V97.8　Other air transport accidents, not elsewhere classified**
　　　EXCLUDES 1　*aircraft accident NOS (V95.9)*
　　　　　　　　exposure to changes in air pressure during ascent or descent (W94.-)

　　☑6ᵗʰ **V97.81　Air transport accident involving military aircraft**
　　　　☑7ᵗʰ **V97.810　Civilian aircraft involved in air transport accident with military aircraft**
　　　　　　　　Passenger in civilian aircraft injured due to accident with military aircraft
　　　　☑7ᵗʰ **V97.811　Civilian injured by military aircraft**
　　　　☑7ᵗʰ **V97.818　Other air transport accident involving military aircraft**
　　☑x7ᵗʰ **V97.89　Other air transport accidents, not elsewhere classified**
　　　　　　Injury from machinery on aircraft

Other and unspecified transport accidents (V98-V99)

EXCLUDES 1　*vehicle accident, type of vehicle unspecified (V89.-)*

☑4ᵗʰ **V98　Other specified transport accidents**

> The appropriate 7th character is to be added to each code from category V98.
> A　initial encounter
> D　subsequent encounter
> S　sequela

　☑7ᵗʰ **V98.0　Accident to, on or involving cable-car, not on rails**
　　　　Caught or dragged by cable-car, not on rails
　　　　Fall or jump from cable-car, not on rails
　　　　Object thrown from or in cable-car, not on rails
　☑7ᵗʰ **V98.1　Accident to, on or involving land-yacht**
　☑7ᵗʰ **V98.2　Accident to, on or involving ice yacht**
　☑7ᵗʰ **V98.3　Accident to, on or involving ski lift**
　　　　Accident to, on or involving ski chair-lift
　　　　Accident to, on or involving ski-lift with gondola
　☑7ᵗʰ **V98.8　Other specified transport accidents**

☑x7ᵗʰ **V99　Unspecified transport accident**

> The appropriate 7th character is to be added to code V99.
> A　initial encounter
> D　subsequent encounter
> S　sequela

OTHER EXTERNAL CAUSES OF ACCIDENTAL INJURY (W00-X58)

Slipping, tripping, stumbling and falls (W00-W19)

EXCLUDES 1　*assault involving a fall (Y01-Y02)*
　　　　fall from animal (V80.-)
　　　　fall (in) (from) machinery (in operation) (W28-W31)
　　　　fall (in) (from) transport vehicle (V01-V99)
　　　　intentional self-harm involving a fall (X80-X81)
EXCLUDES 2　*at risk for fall (history of fall) Z91.81*
　　　　fall (in) (from) burning building (X00.-)
　　　　fall into fire (X00-X04, X08-X09)

☑4ᵗʰ **W00　Fall due to ice and snow**
　　INCLUDES　pedestrian on foot falling (slipping) on ice and snow
　　EXCLUDES 1　*fall on (from) ice and snow involving pedestrian conveyance (V00.-)*
　　　　　　fall from stairs and steps not due to ice and snow (W10.-)

> The appropriate 7th character is to be added to each code from category W00.
> A　initial encounter
> D　subsequent encounter
> S　sequela

　☑7ᵗʰ **W00.0　Fall on same level due to ice and snow**
　☑7ᵗʰ **W00.1　Fall from stairs and steps due to ice and snow**
　☑7ᵗʰ **W00.2　Other fall from one level to another due to ice and snow**
　☑7ᵗʰ **W00.9　Unspecified fall due to ice and snow**

☑4ᵗʰ **W01　Fall on same level from slipping, tripping and stumbling**
　　INCLUDES　fall on moving sidewalk
　　EXCLUDES 1　*fall due to bumping (striking) against object (W18.0-)*
　　　　　fall in shower or bathtub (W18.2-)
　　　　　fall on same level NOS (W18.30)
　　　　　fall on same level from slipping, tripping and stumbling due to ice or snow (W00.0)
　　　　　fall off or from toilet (W18.1-)
　　　　　slipping, tripping and stumbling NOS (W18.40)
　　　　　slipping, tripping and stumbling without falling (W18.4-)

> The appropriate 7th character is to be added to each code from category W01.
> A　initial encounter
> D　subsequent encounter
> S　sequela

　☑7ᵗʰ **W01.0　Fall on same level from slipping, tripping and stumbling without subsequent striking against object**
　　　　Falling over animal
　☑5ᵗʰ **W01.1　Fall on same level from slipping, tripping and stumbling with subsequent striking against object**
　　☑7ᵗʰ **W01.10　Fall on same level from slipping, tripping and stumbling with subsequent striking against unspecified object**
　　☑6ᵗʰ **W01.11　Fall on same level from slipping, tripping and stumbling with subsequent striking against sharp object**
　　　　☑7ᵗʰ **W01.110　Fall on same level from slipping, tripping and stumbling with subsequent striking against sharp glass**
　　　　☑7ᵗʰ **W01.111　Fall on same level from slipping, tripping and stumbling with subsequent striking against power tool or machine**
　　　　☑7ᵗʰ **W01.118　Fall on same level from slipping, tripping and stumbling with subsequent striking against other sharp object**
　　　　☑7ᵗʰ **W01.119　Fall on same level from slipping, tripping and stumbling with subsequent striking against unspecified sharp object**
　　☑6ᵗʰ **W01.19　Fall on same level from slipping, tripping and stumbling with subsequent striking against other object**
　　　　☑7ᵗʰ **W01.190　Fall on same level from slipping, tripping and stumbling with subsequent striking against furniture**
　　　　☑7ᵗʰ **W01.198　Fall on same level from slipping, tripping and stumbling with subsequent striking against other object**

☑x7ᵗʰ **W03　Other fall on same level due to collision with another person**
　　　Fall due to non-transport collision with other person
　　EXCLUDES 1　*collision with another person without fall (W51)*
　　　　crushed or pushed by a crowd or human stampede (W52)
　　　　fall involving pedestrian conveyance (V00-V09)
　　　　fall due to ice or snow (W00)
　　　　fall on same level NOS (W18.30)
　　AHA: 2012, 4Q, 108

> The appropriate 7th character is to be added to code W03.
> A　initial encounter
> D　subsequent encounter
> S　sequela

☑x7ᵗʰ **W04　Fall while being carried or supported by other persons**
　　　Accidentally dropped while being carried

> The appropriate 7th character is to be added to code W04.
> A　initial encounter
> D　subsequent encounter
> S　sequela

☑4ᵗʰ **W05　Fall from non-moving wheelchair, nonmotorized scooter and motorized mobility scooter**
　　EXCLUDES 1　*fall from moving motorized mobility scooter (V00.831)*
　　　　fall from moving wheelchair (powered) (V00.811)
　　　　fall from nonmotorized scooter (V00.141)

> The appropriate 7th character is to be added to each code from category W05.
> A　initial encounter
> D　subsequent encounter
> S　sequela

　☑7ᵗʰ **W05.0　Fall from non-moving wheelchair**
　☑7ᵗʰ **W05.1　Fall from non-moving nonmotorized scooter**

☑ Additional Character Required　☑x7ᵗʰ Xtension Alert　Unacceptable PDx　Manifestation　Hospital Acquired Condition　**EXCLUDES 1** Not Coded Here　**EXCLUDES 2** Not Included Here

External Causes of Morbidity

W05.2–W16.122

√x7th **W05.2 Fall from non-moving motorized mobility scooter**

√x7th **W06 Fall from bed**

> The appropriate 7th character is to be added to code W06.
> A   initial encounter
> D   subsequent encounter
> S   sequela

√x7th **W07 Fall from chair**

> The appropriate 7th character is to be added to code W07.
> A   initial encounter
> D   subsequent encounter
> S   sequela

√x7th **W08 Fall from other furniture**

> The appropriate 7th character is to be added to code W08.
> A   initial encounter
> D   subsequent encounter
> S   sequela

√4th **W09 Fall on and from playground equipment**

> EXCLUDES1   *fall involving recreational machinery (W31)*

> The appropriate 7th character is to be added to each code from category W09.
> A   initial encounter
> D   subsequent encounter
> S   sequela

√x7th **W09.0 Fall on or from playground slide**

√x7th **W09.1 Fall from playground swing**

√x7th **W09.2 Fall on or from jungle gym**

√x7th **W09.8 Fall on or from other playground equipment**

√4th **W10 Fall on and from stairs and steps**

> EXCLUDES1   *Fall from stairs and steps due to ice and snow (W00.1)*

> The appropriate 7th character is to be added to each code from category W10.
> A   initial encounter
> D   subsequent encounter
> S   sequela

√x7th **W10.0 Fall (on)(from) escalator**

√x7th **W10.1 Fall (on)(from) sidewalk curb**

√x7th **W10.2 Fall (on)(from) incline**
> Fall (on) (from) ramp

√x7th **W10.8 Fall (on) (from) other stairs and steps**

√x7th **W10.9 Fall (on) (from) unspecified stairs and steps**

√x7th **W11 Fall on and from ladder**

> The apprcpriate 7th character is to be added code W11.
> A   initial encounter
> D   subsequent encounter
> S   sequela

√x7th **W12 Fall on and from scaffolding**

> The appropriate 7th character is to be added to code W12.
> A   initial encounter
> D   subsequent encounter
> S   sequela

√4th **W13 Fall from, out of or through building or structure**

> The appropriate 7th character is to be added to each code from category W13.
> A   initial encounter
> D   subsequent encounter
> S   sequela

√x7th **W13.0 Fall from, out of or through balcony**
> Fall from, out of or through railing

√x7th **W13.1 Fall from, out of or through bridge**

√x7th **W13.2 Fall from, out of or through roof**

√x7th **W13.3 Fall through floor**

√x7th **W13.4 Fall from, out of or through window**
> EXCLUDES2   *fall with subsequent striking against sharp glass (W01.110)*

√x7th **W13.8 Fall from, out of or through other building or structure**
> Fall from, out of or through viaduct
> Fall from, out of or through wall
> Fall from, out of or through flag-pole

√x7th **W13.9 Fall from, out of or through building, not otherwise specified**
> EXCLUDES1   *collapse of a building or structure (W20.-)*
> *fall or jump from burning building or structure (X00.-)*

√x7th **W14 Fall from tree**

> The appropriate 7th character is to be added to code W14.
> A   initial encounter
> D   subsequent encounter
> S   sequela

√x7th **W15 Fall from cliff**

> The appropriate 7th character is to be added to code W15.
> A   initial encounter
> D   subsequent encounter
> S   sequela

√4th **W16 Fall, jump or diving into water**
> EXCLUDES1   *accidental non-watercraft drowning and submersion not involving fall (W65-W74)*
> *effects of air pressure from diving (W94.-)*
> *fall into water from watercraft (V90-V94)*
> *hitting an object or against bottom when falling from watercraft (V94.0)*
> EXCLUDES2   *striking or hitting diving board (W21.4)*

> The appropriate 7th character is to be added to each code from category W16.
> A   initial encounter
> D   subsequent encounter
> S   sequela

√5th **W16.0 Fall into swimming pool**
> Fall into swimming pool NOS
> EXCLUDES1   *fall into empty swimming pool (W17.3)*

√6th **W16.01 Fall into swimming pool striking water surface**

√7th **W16.011 Fall into swimming pool striking water surface causing drowning and submersion**
> EXCLUDES1   *drowning and submersion while in swimming pool without fall (W67)*

√7th **W16.012 Fall into swimming pool striking water surface causing other injury**

√6th **W16.02 Fall into swimming pool striking bottom**

√7th **W16.021 Fall into swimming pool striking bottom causing drowning and submersion**
> EXCLUDES1   *drowning and submersion while in swimming pool without fall (W67)*

√7th **W16.022 Fall into swimming pool striking bottom causing other injury**

√6th **W16.03 Fall into swimming pool striking wall**

√7th **W16.031 Fall into swimming pool striking wall causing drowning and submersion**
> EXCLUDES1   *drowning and submersion while in swimming pool without fall (W67)*

√7th **W16.032 Fall into swimming pool striking wall causing other injury**

√5th **W16.1 Fall into natural body of water**
> Fall into lake   Fall into river
> Fall into open sea   Fall into stream

√6th **W16.11 Fall into natural body of water striking water surface**

√7th **W16.111 Fall into natural body of water striking water surface causing drowning and submersion**
> EXCLUDES1   *drowning and submersion while in natural body of water without fall (W69)*

√7th **W16.112 Fall into natural body of water striking water surface causing other injury**

√6th **W16.12 Fall into natural body of water striking bottom**

√7th **W16.121 Fall into natural body of water striking bottom causing drowning and submersion**
> EXCLUDES1   *drowning and submersion while in natural body of water without fall (W69)*

√7th **W16.122 Fall into natural body of water striking bottom causing other injury**

N Newborn: 0   P Pediatric: 0-17   M Maternity: 12-55   A Adult: 15-124   MCC Major CC Condition   PDx MCC PDx acts as own MCC   CC CC Condition   PDx CC PDx acts as own CC

1142   ICD-10-CM Draft (2015)

☑6ᵗʰ **W16.13 Fall into natural body of water** striking side

☑7ᵗʰ **W16.131 Fall into natural body of water striking side causing** drowning **and submersion**

> *EXCLUDES 1* *drowning and submersion while in natural body of water without fall (W69)*

☑7ᵗʰ **W16.132 Fall into natural body of water striking side causing** other injury

☑5ᵗʰ **W16.2 Fall in (into) filled bathtub or bucket of water**

☑6ᵗʰ **W16.21 Fall in (into)** filled bathtub

> *EXCLUDES 1* *fall into empty bathtub (W18.2)*

☑7ᵗʰ **W16.211 Fall in (into) filled bathtub causing** drowning **and submersion**

> *EXCLUDES 1* *drowning and submersion while in filled bathtub without fall (W65)*

☑7ᵗʰ **W16.212 Fall in (into) filled bathtub causing** other injury

☑6ᵗʰ **W16.22 Fall in (into)** bucket of water

☑7ᵗʰ **W16.221 Fall in (into) bucket of water causing** drowning **and submersion**

☑7ᵗʰ **W16.222 Fall in (into) bucket of water causing** other injury

☑5ᵗʰ **W16.3 Fall into other water**

Fall into fountain   Fall into reservoir

☑6ᵗʰ **W16.31 Fall into other water** striking water surface

☑7ᵗʰ **W16.311 Fall into other water striking water surface causing** drowning **and submersion**

> *EXCLUDES 1* *drowning and submersion while in other water without fall (W73)*

☑7ᵗʰ **W16.312 Fall into other water striking water surface causing** other injury

☑6ᵗʰ **W16.32 Fall into other water** striking bottom

☑7ᵗʰ **W16.321 Fall into other water striking bottom causing** drowning **and submersion**

> *EXCLUDES 1* *drowning and submersion while in other water without fall (W73)*

☑7ᵗʰ **W16.322 Fall into other water striking bottom causing** other injury

☑6ᵗʰ **W16.33 Fall into other water** striking wall

☑7ᵗʰ **W16.331 Fall into other water striking wall causing** drowning **and submersion**

> *EXCLUDES 1* *drowning and submersion while in other water without fall (W73)*

☑7ᵗʰ **W16.332 Fall into other water striking wall causing** other injury

☑5ᵗʰ **W16.4 Fall into unspecified water**

☑x7ᵗʰ **W16.41 Fall into unspecified water causing** drowning **and submersion**

☑x7ᵗʰ **W16.42 Fall into unspecified water causing** other injury

☑5ᵗʰ **W16.5 Jumping or diving into swimming pool**

☑6ᵗʰ **W16.51 Jumping or diving into swimming pool** striking water surface

☑7ᵗʰ **W16.511 Jumping or diving into swimming pool striking water surface causing** drowning **and submersion**

> *EXCLUDES 1* *drowning and submersion while in swimming pool without jumping or diving (W67)*

☑7ᵗʰ **W16.512 Jumping or diving into swimming pool striking water surface causing** other injury

☑6ᵗʰ **W16.52 Jumping or diving into swimming pool** striking bottom

☑7ᵗʰ **W16.521 Jumping or diving into swimming pool striking bottom causing** drowning **and submersion**

> *EXCLUDES 1* *drowning and submersion while in swimming pool without jumping or diving (W67)*

☑7ᵗʰ **W16.522 Jumping or diving into swimming pool striking bottom causing** other injury

☑6ᵗʰ **W16.53 Jumping or diving into swimming pool** striking wall

☑7ᵗʰ **W16.531 Jumping or diving into swimming pool striking wall causing** drowning **and submersion**

> *EXCLUDES 1* *drowning and submersion while in swimming pool without jumping or diving (W67)*

☑7ᵗʰ **W16.532 Jumping or diving into swimming pool striking wall causing** other injury

☑5ᵗʰ **W16.6 Jumping or diving into** natural body of water

Jumping or diving into lake
Jumping or diving into open sea
Jumping or diving into river
Jumping or diving into stream

☑6ᵗʰ **W16.61 Jumping or diving into natural body of water** striking water surface

☑7ᵗʰ **W16.611 Jumping or diving into natural body of water striking water surface causing** drowning **and submersion**

> *EXCLUDES 1* *drowning and submersion while in natural body of water without jumping or diving (W69)*

☑7ᵗʰ **W16.612 Jumping or diving into natural body of water striking water surface causing** other injury

☑6ᵗʰ **W16.62 Jumping or diving into natural body of water** striking bottom

☑7ᵗʰ **W16.621 Jumping or diving into natural body of water striking bottom causing** drowning **and submersion**

> *EXCLUDES 1* *drowning and submersion while in natural body of water without jumping or diving (W69)*

☑7ᵗʰ **W16.622 Jumping or diving into natural body of water striking bottom causing** other injury

☑5ᵗʰ **W16.7 Jumping or diving** from boat

> *EXCLUDES 1* *Fall from boat into water—see watercraft accident (V90-V94)*

☑6ᵗʰ **W16.71 Jumping or diving from boat** striking water surface

☑7ᵗʰ **W16.711 Jumping or diving from boat striking water surface causing** drowning **and submersion**

☑7ᵗʰ **W16.712 Jumping or diving from boat striking water surface causing** other injury

☑6ᵗʰ **W16.72 Jumping or diving from boat** striking bottom

☑7ᵗʰ **W16.721 Jumping or diving from boat striking bottom causing** drowning **and submersion**

☑7ᵗʰ **W16.722 Jumping or diving from boat striking bottom causing** other injury

☑5ᵗʰ **W16.8 Jumping or diving** into other water

Jumping or diving into fountain
Jumping or diving into reservoir

☑6ᵗʰ **W16.81 Jumping or diving into other water** striking water surface

☑7ᵗʰ **W16.811 Jumping or diving into other water striking water surface causing** drowning **and submersion**

> *EXCLUDES 1* *drowning and submersion while in other water without jumping or diving (W73)*

☑7ᵗʰ **W16.812 Jumping or diving into other water striking water surface causing** other injury

☑6ᵗʰ **W16.82 Jumping or diving into other water** striking bottom

☑7ᵗʰ **W16.821 Jumping or diving into other water striking bottom causing** drowning **and submersion**

> *EXCLUDES 1* *drowning and submersion while in other water without jumping or diving (W73)*

☑7ᵗʰ **W16.822 Jumping or diving into other water striking bottom causing** other injury

☑6ᵗʰ **W16.83 Jumping or diving into other water** striking wall

☑7ᵗʰ **W16.831 Jumping or diving into other water striking wall causing** drowning **and submersion**

> *EXCLUDES 1* *drowning and submersion while in other water without jumping or diving (W73)*

☑ Additional Character Required   ☑x7ᵗʰ Xtension Alert   Unacceptable PDx   Manifestation   Hospital Acquired Condition   *EXCLUDES 1* Not Coded Here   *EXCLUDES 2* Not Included Here

ICD-10-CM Draft (2015)   1143

√7th **W16.832 Jumping or diving into other water striking wall causing other injury**

√5th **W16.9 Jumping or diving into unspecified water**

√x7th **W16.91 Jumping or diving into unspecified water causing drowning and submersion**

√x7th **W16.92 Jumping or diving into unspecified water causing other injury**

√4th **W17 Other fall from one level to another**

> The appropriate 7th character is to be added to each code from category W17.
> A initial encounter
> D subsequent encounter
> S sequela

√x7th **W17.0 Fall into well**

√x7th **W17.1 Fall into storm drain or manhole**

√x7th **W17.2 Fall into hole**
Fall into pit

√x7th **W17.3 Fall into empty swimming pool**
> EXCLUDES 1 fall into filled swimming pool (W16.0-)

√x7th **W17.4 Fall from dock**

√5th **W17.8 Other fall from one level to another**

√x7th **W17.81 Fall down embankment (hill)**

√x7th **W17.82 Fall from (out of) grocery cart**
Fall due to grocery cart tipping over

√x7th **W17.89 Other fall from one level to another**
Fall from cherry picker
Fall from lifting device
Fall from mobile elevated work platform [MEWP]
Fall from sky lift

√4th **W18 Other slipping, tripping and stumbling and falls**

> The appropriate 7th character is to be added to each code from category W18.
> A initial encounter
> D subsequent encounter
> S sequela

√5th **W18.0 Fall due to bumping against object**
Striking against object with subsequent fall
> EXCLUDES 1 fall on same level due to slipping, tripping, or stumbling with subsequent striking against object (W01.1-)

√x7th **W18.00 Striking against unspecified object with subsequent fall**

√x7th **W18.01 Striking against sports equipment with subsequent fall**

√x7th **W18.02 Striking against glass with subsequent fall**

√x7th **W18.09 Striking against other object with subsequent fall**

√5th **W18.1 Fall from or off toilet**

√x7th **W18.11 Fall from or off toilet without subsequent striking against object**
Fall from (off) toilet NOS

√x7th **W18.12 Fall from or off toilet with subsequent striking against object**

√x7th **W18.2 Fall in (into) shower or empty bathtub**
> EXCLUDES 1 fall in full bathtub causing drowning or submersion (W16.21-)

√5th **W18.3 Other and unspecified fall on same level**

√x7th **W18.30 Fall on same level, unspecified**

√x7th **W18.31 Fall on same level due to stepping on an object**
Fall on same level due to stepping on an animal
> EXCLUDES 1 slipping, tripping and stumbling without fall due to stepping on animal (W18.41)

√x7th **W18.39 Other fall on same level**

√5th **W18.4 Slipping, tripping and stumbling without falling**
> EXCLUDES 1 collision with another person without fall (W51)

√x7th **W18.40 Slipping, tripping and stumbling without falling, unspecified**

√x7th **W18.41 Slipping, tripping and stumbling without falling due to stepping on object**
Slipping, tripping and stumbling without falling due to stepping on animal
> EXCLUDES 1 slipping, tripping and stumbling with fall due to stepping on animal (W18.31)

√x7th **W18.42 Slipping, tripping and stumbling without falling due to stepping into hole or opening**

√x7th **W18.43 Slipping, tripping and stumbling without falling due to stepping from one level to another**

√x7th **W18.49 Other slipping, tripping and stumbling without falling**

√x7th **W19 Unspecified fall**
Accidental fall NOS
AHA: 2012, 4Q, 95

> The appropriate 7th character is to be added to code W19.
> A initial encounter
> D subsequent encounter
> S sequela

Exposure to inanimate mechanical forces (W20-W49)

> EXCLUDES 1 assault (X92-Y08)
> contact or collision with animals or persons (W50-W64)
> exposure to inanimate mechanical forces involving military or war operations (Y36-, Y37-)
> intentional self-harm (X71-X83)

√4th **W20 Struck by thrown, projected or falling object**
Code first any associated:
cataclysm (X34-X39)
lightning strike (T75.00)
> EXCLUDES 1 falling object in machinery accident (W24, W28-W31)
> falling object in transport accident (V01-V99)
> object set in motion by explosion (W35-W40)
> object set in motion by firearm (W32-W34)
> struck by thrown sports equipment (W21.-)

> The appropriate 7th character is to be added to each code from category W20.
> A initial encounter
> D subsequent encounter
> S sequela

√x7th **W20.0 Struck by falling object in cave-in**
> EXCLUDES 2 asphyxiation due to cave-in (T71.21)

√x7th **W20.1 Struck by object due to collapse of building**
> EXCLUDES 1 struck by object due to collapse of burning building (X00.2, X02.2)

√x7th **W20.8 Other cause of strike by thrown, projected or falling object**
> EXCLUDES 1 struck by thrown sports equipment (W21.-)

√4th **W21 Striking against or struck by sports equipment**
> EXCLUDES 1 assault with sports equipment (Y08.0-)
> striking against or struck by sports equipment with subsequent fall (W18.01)

> The appropriate 7th character is to be added to each code from category W21.
> A initial encounter
> D subsequent encounter
> S sequela

√5th **W21.0 Struck by hit or thrown ball**

√x7th **W21.00 Struck by hit or thrown ball, unspecified type**

√x7th **W21.01 Struck by football**

√x7th **W21.02 Struck by soccer ball**

√x7th **W21.03 Struck by baseball**

√x7th **W21.04 Struck by golf ball**

√x7th **W21.05 Struck by basketball**

√x7th **W21.06 Struck by volleyball**

√x7th **W21.07 Struck by softball**

√x7th **W21.09 Struck by other hit or thrown ball**

√5th **W21.1 Struck by bat, racquet or club**

√x7th **W21.11 Struck by baseball bat**

√x7th **W21.12 Struck by tennis racquet**

√x7th **W21.13 Struck by golf club**

√x7th **W21.19 Struck by other bat, racquet or club**

√5th **W21.2 Struck by hockey stick or puck**

√6th **W21.21 Struck by hockey stick**

√7th **W21.210 Struck by ice hockey stick**

√7th **W21.211 Struck by field hockey stick**

√6th **W21.22 Struck by hockey puck**

√7th **W21.220 Struck by ice hockey puck**

√7th **W21.221 Struck by field hockey puck**

√5th **W21.3 Struck by sports foot wear**

√x7th **W21.31 Struck by shoe cleats**
Stepped on by shoe cleats

☑x7ᵗʰ **W21.32 Struck by skate blades**
　　　Skated over by skate blades

☑x7ᵗʰ **W21.39 Struck by other sports foot wear**

☑x7ᵗʰ **W21.4 Striking against diving board**
　　　Use additional code for subsequent falling into water, if
　　　applicable (W16.-)

☑5ᵗʰ **W21.8 Striking against or struck by other sports equipment**

　　☑x7ᵗʰ **W21.81 Striking against or struck by football helmet**

　　☑x7ᵗʰ **W21.89 Striking against or struck by other sports equipment**

☑x7ᵗʰ **W21.9 Striking against or struck by unspecified sports equipment**

☑4ᵗʰ **W22 Striking against or struck by other objects**
　　EXCLUDES 1　striking against or struck by object with subsequent fall
　　　　(W18.09)

　　The appropriate 7th character is to be added to each code from
　　category W22.
　　A　initial encounter
　　D　subsequent encounter
　　S　sequela

☑5ᵗʰ **W22.0 Striking against stationary object**
　　EXCLUDES 1　striking against stationary sports equipment (W21.8)

　　☑x7ᵗʰ **W22.01 Walked into wall**

　　☑x7ᵗʰ **W22.02 Walked into lamppost**

　　☑x7ᵗʰ **W22.03 Walked into furniture**

　　☑6ᵗʰ **W22.04 Striking against wall of swimming pool**

　　　　☑7ᵗʰ **W22.041 Striking against wall of swimming pool
　　　　　　causing drowning and submersion**
　　　　　　EXCLUDES 1　drowning and submersion while
　　　　　　　　swimming without striking
　　　　　　　　against wall (W67)

　　　　☑7ᵗʰ **W22.042 Striking against wall of swimming pool
　　　　　　causing other injury**

　　☑x7ᵗʰ **W22.09 Striking against other stationary object**

☑5ᵗʰ **W22.1 Striking against or struck by automobile airbag**

　　☑x7ᵗʰ **W22.10 Striking against or struck by unspecified automobile
　　　airbag**

　　☑x7ᵗʰ **W22.11 Striking against or struck by driver side automobile
　　　airbag**

　　☑x7ᵗʰ **W22.12 Striking against or struck by front passenger side
　　　automobile airbag**

　　☑x7ᵗʰ **W22.19 Striking against or struck by other automobile
　　　airbag**

☑x7ᵗʰ **W22.8 Striking against or struck by other objects**
　　Striking against or struck by object NOS
　　EXCLUDES 1　struck by thrown, projected or falling object (W20.-)

☑4ᵗʰ **W23 Caught, crushed, jammed or pinched in or between objects**
　　EXCLUDES 1　injury caused by cutting or piercing instruments (W25-W27)
　　　　injury caused by firearms malfunction (W32.1, W33.1-, W34.1-)
　　　　injury caused by lifting and transmission devices (W24.-)
　　　　injury caused by machinery (W28-W31)
　　　　injury caused by nonpowered hand tools (W27.-)
　　　　injury caused by transport vehicle being used as a means of
　　　　　transportation (V01-V99)
　　　　injury caused by struck by thrown, projected or falling object
　　　　　(W20.-)

　　The appropriate 7th character is to be added to each code from
　　category W23.
　　A　initial encounter
　　D　subsequent encounter
　　S　sequela

☑x7ᵗʰ **W23.0 Caught, crushed, jammed, or pinched between moving
　objects**

☑x7ᵗʰ **W23.1 Caught, crushed, jammed, or pinched between stationary
　objects**

☑4ᵗʰ **W24 Contact with lifting and transmission devices, not elsewhere
　classified**
　　EXCLUDES 1　transport accidents (V01-V99)

　　The appropriate 7th character is to be added to each code from
　　category W24.
　　A　initial encounter
　　D　subsequent encounter
　　S　sequela

☑x7ᵗʰ **W24.0 Contact with lifting devices, not elsewhere classified**
　　Contact with chain hoist
　　Contact with drive belt
　　Contact with pulley (block)

☑x7ᵗʰ **W24.1 Contact with transmission devices, not elsewhere classified**
　　Contact with transmission belt or cable

☑x7ᵗʰ **W25 Contact with sharp glass**
　　Code first any associated:
　　　injury due to flying glass from explosion or firearm discharge (W32-
　　　　W40)
　　　transport accident (V00-V99)
　　EXCLUDES 1　fall on same level due to slipping, tripping and stumbling with
　　　　subsequent striking against sharp glass (W01.10)
　　　　striking against sharp glass with subsequent fall (W18.02)

　　The appropriate 7th character is to be added to code W25.
　　A　initial encounter
　　D　subsequent encounter
　　S　sequela

☑4ᵗʰ **W26 Contact with knife, sword or dagger**

　　The appropriate 7th character is to be added to each code from
　　category W26.
　　A　initial encounter
　　D　subsequent encounter
　　S　sequela

☑x7ᵗʰ **W26.0 Contact with knife**
　　EXCLUDES 1　contact with electric knife (W29.1)

☑x7ᵗʰ **W26.1 Contact with sword or dagger**

☑4ᵗʰ **W27 Contact with nonpowered hand tool**

　　The appropriate 7th character is to be added to each code from
　　category W27.
　　A　initial encounter
　　D　subsequent encounter
　　S　sequela

☑x7ᵗʰ **W27.0 Contact with workbench tool**
　　Contact with auger　　　　　Contact with handsaw
　　Contact with axe　　　　　　Contact with screwdriver
　　Contact with chisel

☑x7ᵗʰ **W27.1 Contact with garden tool**
　　Contact with hoe
　　Contact with nonpowered lawn mower
　　Contact with pitchfork
　　Contact with rake

☑x7ᵗʰ **W27.2 Contact with scissors**

☑x7ᵗʰ **W27.3 Contact with needle (sewing)**
　　EXCLUDES 1　contact with hypodermic needle (W46.-)

☑x7ᵗʰ **W27.4 Contact with kitchen utensil**
　　Contact with fork
　　Contact with ice-pick
　　Contact with can-opener NOS

☑x7ᵗʰ **W27.5 Contact with paper-cutter**

☑x7ᵗʰ **W27.8 Contact with other nonpowered hand tool**
　　Contact with nonpowered sewing machine
　　Contact with shovel

☑x7ᵗʰ **W28 Contact with powered lawn mower**
　　Powered lawn mower (commercial) (residential)
　　EXCLUDES 1　contact with nonpowered lawn mower (W27.1)
　　EXCLUDES 2　exposure to electric current (W86.-)

　　The appropriate 7th character is to be added to code W28.
　　A　initial encounter
　　D　subsequent encounter
　　S　sequela

☑4ᵗʰ **W29 Contact with other powered hand tools and household
　machinery**
　　EXCLUDES 1　contact with commercial machinery (W31.82)
　　　　contact with hot household appliance (X15)
　　　　contact with nonpowered hand tool (W27.-)
　　　　exposure to electric current (W86)

　　The appropriate 7th character is to be added to each code from
　　category W29.
　　A　initial encounter
　　D　subsequent encounter
　　S　sequela

☑x7ᵗʰ **W29.0 Contact with powered kitchen appliance**
　　Contact with blender　　　　Contact with garbage disposal
　　Contact with can-opener　　　Contact with mixer

☑x7ᵗʰ **W29.1 Contact with electric knife**

☑ Additional Character Required　　☑x7ᵗʰ Xtension Alert　　Unacceptable PDx　　Manifestation　　Hospital Acquired Condition　　*EXCLUDES 1* Not Coded Here　　*EXCLUDES 2* Not Included Here

External Causes of Morbidity

W29.2 Contact with other powered household machinery
Contact with electric fan
Contact with powered dryer (clothes) (powered) (spin)
Contact with washing-machine
Contact with sewing machine

W29.3 Contact with powered garden and outdoor hand tools and machinery
Contact with chainsaw
Contact with edger
Contact with garden cultivator (tiller)
Contact with hedge trimmer
Contact with other powered garden tool
EXCLUDES 1   *contact with powered lawn mower (W28)*

W29.4 Contact with nail gun

W29.8 Contact with other powered powered hand tools and household machinery
Contact with do-it-yourself tool NOS

W30 Contact with agricultural machinery
INCLUDES   animal-powered farm machine
EXCLUDES 1   *agricultural transport vehicle accident (V01-V99)*
explosion of grain store (W40.8)
exposure to electric current (W86.-)

The appropriate 7th character is to be added to each code from category W30.
A   initial encounter
D   subsequent encounter
S   sequela

W30.0 Contact with combine harvester
Contact with reaper   Contact with thresher

W30.1 Contact with power take-off devices (PTO)

W30.2 Contact with hay derrick

W30.3 Contact with grain storage elevator
EXCLUDES 1   *explosion of grain store (W40.8)*

W30.8 Contact with other specified agricultural machinery

W30.81 Contact with agricultural transport vehicle in stationary use
Contact with agricultural transport vehicle under repair, not on public roadway
EXCLUDES 1   *agricultural transport vehicle accident (V01-V99)*

W30.89 Contact with other specified agricultural machinery

W30.9 Contact with unspecified agricultural machinery
Contact with farm machinery NOS

W31 Contact with other and unspecified machinery
EXCLUDES 1   *contact with agricultural machinery (W30.-)*
contact with machinery in transport under own power or being towed by a vehicle (V01-V99)
exposure to electric current (W86)

The appropriate 7th character is to be added to each code from category W31.
A   initial encounter
D   subsequent encounter
S   sequela

W31.0 Contact with mining and earth-drilling machinery
Contact with bore or drill (land) (seabed)
Contact with shaft hoist
Contact with shaft lift
Contact with undercutter

W31.1 Contact with metalworking machines
Contact with abrasive wheel
Contact with forging machine
Contact with lathe
Contact with mechanical shears
Contact with metal drilling machine
Contact with milling machine
Contact with power press
Contact with rolling-mill
Contact with metal sawing machine

W31.2 Contact with powered woodworking and forming machines
Contact with band saw   Contact with overhead plane
Contact with bench saw   Contact with powered saw
Contact with circular saw   Contact with radial saw
Contact with molding machine   Contact with sander
EXCLUDES 1   *nonpowered woodworking tools (W27.0)*

W31.3 Contact with prime movers
Contact with gas turbine
Contact with internal combustion engine
Contact with steam engine
Contact with water driven turbine

W31.8 Contact with other specified machinery

W31.81 Contact with recreational machinery
Contact with roller coaster

W31.82 Contact with other commercial machinery
Contact with commercial electric fan
Contact with commercial kitchen appliances
Contact with commercial powered dryer (clothes) (powered) (spin)
Contact with commercial washing-machine
Contact with commercial sewing machine
EXCLUDES 1   *contact with household machinery (W29.-)*
contact with powered lawn mower (W28)

W31.83 Contact with special construction vehicle in stationary use
Contact with special construction vehicle under repair, not on public roadway
EXCLUDES 1   *special construction vehicle accident (V01-V99)*

W31.89 Contact with other specified machinery

W31.9 Contact with unspecified machinery
Contact with machinery NOS

W32 Accidental handgun discharge and malfunction
INCLUDES   accidental discharge and malfunction of gun for single hand use
accidental discharge and malfunction of pistol
accidental discharge and malfunction of revolver
handgun discharge and malfunction NOS
EXCLUDES 1   *accidental airgun discharge and malfunction (W34.010, W34.110)*
accidental BB gun discharge and malfunction (W34.010, W34.110)
accidental pellet gun discharge and malfunction (W34.010, W34.110)
accidental shotgun discharge and malfunction (W33.01, W33.11)
assault by handgun discharge (X93)
handgun discharge involving legal intervention (Y35.0-)
handgun discharge involving military or war operations (Y36.4-)
intentional self-harm by handgun discharge (X72)
Very pistol discharge and malfunction (W34.09, W34.19)

The appropriate 7th character is to be added to each code from category W32.
A   initial encounter
D   subsequent encounter
S   sequela

W32.0 Accidental handgun discharge

W32.1 Accidental handgun malfunction
Injury due to explosion of handgun (parts)
Injury due to malfunction of mechanism or component of handgun
Injury due to recoil of handgun
Powder burn from handgun

W33 Accidental rifle, shotgun and larger firearm discharge and malfunction
INCLUDES   rifle, shotgun and larger firearm discharge and malfunction NOS
EXCLUDES 1   *accidental airgun discharge and malfunction (W34.010, W34.110)*
accidental BB gun discharge and malfunction (W34.010, W34.110)
accidental handgun discharge and malfunction (W32.-)
accidental pellet gun discharge and malfunction (W34.010, W34.110)
assault by rifle, shotgun and larger firearm discharge (X94)
firearm discharge involving legal intervention (Y35.0-)
firearm discharge involving military or war operations (Y36.4-)
intentional self-harm by rifle, shotgun and larger firearm discharge (X73)

The appropriate 7th character is to be added to each code from category W33.
A   initial encounter
D   subsequent encounter
S   sequela

√5th **W33.0** **Accidental rifle, shotgun and larger firearm** discharge

  √x7th **W33.00** **Accidental discharge of** unspecified **larger firearm**
    Discharge of unspecified larger firearm NOS

  √x7th **W33.01** **Accidental discharge of** shotgun
    Discharge of shotgun NOS

  √x7th **W33.02** **Accidental discharge of** hunting rifle
    Discharge of hunting rifle NOS

  √x7th **W33.03** **Accidental discharge of** machine gun
    Discharge of machine gun NOS

  √x7th **W33.09** **Accidental discharge of** other **larger firearm**
    Discharge of other larger firearm NOS

√5th **W33.1** **Accidental rifle, shotgun and larger firearm** malfunction
  Injury due to explosion of rifle, shotgun and larger firearm (parts)
  Injury due to malfunction of mechanism or component of rifle, shotgun and larger firearm
  Injury due to piercing, cutting, crushing or pinching due to (by) slide trigger mechanism, scope or other gun part
  Injury due to recoil of rifle, shotgun and larger firearm
  Powder burn from rifle, shotgun and larger firearm

  √x7th **W33.10** **Accidental malfunction of** unspecified **larger firearm**
    Malfunction of unspecified larger firearm NOS

  √x7th **W33.11** **Accidental malfunction of** shotgun
    Malfunction of shotgun NOS

  √x7th **W33.12** **Accidental malfunction of** hunting rifle
    Malfunction of hunting rifle NOS

  √x7th **W33.13** **Accidental malfunction of** machine gun
    Malfunction of machine gun NOS

  √x7th **W33.19** **Accidental malfunction of** other **larger firearm**
    Malfunction of other larger firearm NOS

√4th **W34** **Accidental discharge and malfunction from other and unspecified firearms and guns**

The appropriate 7th character is to be added to each code from category W34.
A   initial encounter
D   subsequent encounter
S   sequela

√5th **W34.0** **Accidental** discharge **from other and unspecified firearms and guns**

  √x7th **W34.00** **Accidental discharge from** unspecified **firearms or gun**
    Discharge from firearm NOS
    Gunshot wound NOS
    Shot NOS

  √6th **W34.01** **Accidental discharge of** gas, air or spring-operated **guns**

    √7th **W34.010** **Accidental discharge of** airgun
      Accidental discharge of BB gun
      Accidental discharge of pellet gun

    √7th **W34.011** **Accidental discharge of** paintball gun
      Accidental injury due to paintball discharge

    √7th **W34.018** **Accidental discharge of** other gas, air or spring-operated gun

  √x7th **W34.09** **Accidental discharge from** other specified firearms
    Accidental discharge from Very pistol [flare]

√5th **W34.1** **Accidental** malfunction **from other and unspecified firearms and guns**

  √x7th **W34.10** **Accidental malfunction from** unspecified **firearms or gun**
    Firearm malfunction NOS

  √6th **W34.11** **Accidental malfunction of** gas, air or spring-operated **guns**

    √7th **W34.110** **Accidental malfunction of** airgun
      Accidental malfunction of BB gun
      Accidental malfunction of pellet gun

    √7th **W34.111** **Accidental malfunction of** paintball gun
      Accidental injury due to paintball gun malfunction

    √7th **W34.118** **Accidental malfunction of** other gas, air or spring-operated gun

  √x7th **W34.19** **Accidental malfunction from** other specified **firearms**
    Accidental malfunction from Very pistol [flare]

√x7th **W35** **Explosion and rupture of boiler**
  EXCLUDES 1   explosion and rupture of boiler on watercraft (V93.4)

The appropriate 7th character is to be added to code W35.
A   initial encounter
D   subsequent encounter
S   sequela

√4th **W36** **Explosion and rupture of** gas cylinder

The appropriate 7th character is to be added to each code from category W36.
A   initial encounter
D   subsequent encounter
S   sequela

√x7th **W36.1** **Explosion and rupture of** aerosol can

√x7th **W36.2** **Explosion and rupture of** air tank

√x7th **W36.3** **Explosion and rupture of** pressurized-gas tank

√x7th **W36.8** **Explosion and rupture of** other **gas cylinder**

√x7th **W36.9** **Explosion and rupture of** unspecified **gas cylinder**

√4th **W37** **Explosion and rupture of** pressurized tire, pipe or hose

The appropriate 7th character is to be added to each code from category W37.
A   initial encounter
D   subsequent encounter
S   sequela

√x7th **W37.0** **Explosion of** bicycle tire

√x7th **W37.8** **Explosion and rupture of** other pressurized tire, pipe or hose

√x7th **W38** **Explosion and rupture of** other specified pressurized devices

The appropriate 7th character is to be added to code W38.
A   initial encounter
D   subsequent encounter
S   sequela

√x7th **W39** **Discharge of** firework

The appropriate 7th character is to be added to code W39.
A   initial encounter
D   subsequent encounter
S   sequela

√4th **W40** **Explosion of** other **materials**
  EXCLUDES 1   assault by explosive material (X96)
    explosion involving legal intervention (Y35.1-)
    explosion involving military or war operations (Y36.0-, Y36.2-)
    intentional self-harm by explosive material (X75)

The appropriate 7th character is to be added to each code from category W40.
A   initial encounter
D   subsequent encounter
S   sequela

√x7th **W40.0** **Explosion of** blasting material
  Explosion of blasting cap
  Explosion of detonator
  Explosion of dynamite
  Explosion of explosive (any) used in blasting operations

√x7th **W40.1** **Explosion of** explosive gases

Explosion of acetylene	Explosion of fire damp
Explosion of butane	Explosion of gasoline fumes
Explosion of coal gas	Explosion of methane
Explosion in mine NOS	Explosion of propane
Explosion of explosive gas	

√x7th **W40.8** **Explosion of** other specified explosive materials

Explosion in dump NOS	Explosion in grain store
Explosion in factory NOS	Explosion in munitions

  EXCLUDES 1   explosion involving legal intervention (Y35.1-)
    explosion involving military or war operations (Y36.0-, Y36.2-)

√x7th **W40.9** **Explosion of** unspecified **explosive materials**
  Explosion NOS

√4th **W42** **Exposure to noise**

The appropriate 7th character is to be added to each code from category W42.
A   initial encounter
D   subsequent encounter
S   sequela

√x7th **W42.0** **Exposure to supersonic waves**

√x7th **W42.9** **Exposure to other noise**
  Exposure to sound waves NOS

√ Additional Character Required   √x7th Xtension Alert   Unacceptable PDx   Manifestation   Hospital Acquired Condition   EXCLUDES 1 Not Coded Here   EXCLUDES 2 Not Included Here

External Causes of Morbidity

W45–W55.51

√4ᵗʰ **W45 Foreign body or object entering through skin**

> EXCLUDES 2   contact with hand tools (nonpowered) (powered) (W27-W29)
> contact with knife, sword or dagger (W26.-)
> contact with sharp glass (W25.-)
> struck by objects (W20-W22)

> The appropriate 7th character is to be added to each code from category W45.
> A   initial encounter
> D   subsequent encounter
> S   sequela

√x7ᵗʰ **W45.0 Nail entering through skin**

√x7ᵗʰ **W45.1 Paper entering through skin**
> Paper cut

√x7ᵗʰ **W45.2 Lid of can entering through skin**

√x7ᵗʰ **W45.8 Other foreign body or object entering through skin**
> Splinter in skin NOS

√4ᵗʰ **W46 Contact with hypodermic needle**

> The appropriate 7th character is to be added to each code from category W46.
> A   initial encounter
> D   subsequent encounter
> S   sequela

√x7ᵗʰ **W46.0 Contact with hypodermic needle**
> Hypodermic needle stick NOS

√x7ᵗʰ **W46.1 Contact with contaminated hypodermic needle**

√4ᵗʰ **W49 Exposure to other inanimate mechanical forces**

> INCLUDES   exposure to abnormal gravitational [G] forces
> exposure to inanimate mechanical forces NEC

> EXCLUDES 1   exposure to inanimate mechanical forces involving military or war operations (Y36.-, Y37.-)

> The appropriate 7th character is to be added to each code from category W49.
> A   initial encounter
> D   subsequent encounter
> S   sequela

√5ᵗʰ **W49.0 Item causing external constriction**
> √x7ᵗʰ **W49.01 Hair causing external constriction**
> √x7ᵗʰ **W49.02 String or thread causing external constriction**
> √x7ᵗʰ **W49.03 Rubber band causing external constriction**
> √x7ᵗʰ **W49.04 Ring or other jewelry causing external constriction**
> √x7ᵗʰ **W49.09 Other specified item causing external constriction**

√x7ᵗʰ **W49.9 Exposure to other inanimate mechanical forces**

Exposure to animate mechanical forces (W50-W64)

> EXCLUDES 1   Toxic effect of contact with venomous animals and plants (T63.-)

√4ᵗʰ **W50 Accidental hit, strike, kick, twist, bite or scratch by another person**
> Hit, strike, kick, twist, bite, or scratch by another person NOS
> EXCLUDES 1   assault by bodily force (Y04)
> struck by objects (W20-W22)

> The appropriate 7th character is to be added to each code from category W50.
> A   initial encounter
> D   subsequent encounter
> S   sequela

√x7ᵗʰ **W50.0 Accidental hit or strike by another person**
> Hit or strike by another person NOS

√x7ᵗʰ **W50.1 Accidental kick by another person**
> Kick by another person NOS

√x7ᵗʰ **W50.2 Accidental twist by another person**
> Twist by another person NOS

√x7ᵗʰ **W50.3 Accidental bite by another person**
> Human bite   Bite by another person NOS

√x7ᵗʰ **W50.4 Accidental scratch by another person**
> Scratch by another person NOS

√x7ᵗʰ **W51 Accidental striking against or bumped into by another person**
> EXCLUDES 1   assault by striking against or bumping into by another person (Y04.2)
> fall due to collision with another person (W03)

> The appropriate 7th character is to be added to code W51.
> A   initial encounter
> D   subsequent encounter
> S   sequela

√x7ᵗʰ **W52 Crushed, pushed or stepped on by crowd or human stampede**
> Crushed, pushed or stepped on by crowd or human stampede with or without fall

> The appropriate 7th character is to be added to code W52.
> A   initial encounter
> D   subsequent encounter
> S   sequela

√4ᵗʰ **W53 Contact with rodent**
> INCLUDES   Contact with saliva, feces or urine of rodent

> The appropriate 7th character is to be added to each code from category W53.
> A   initial encounter
> D   subsequent encounter
> S   sequela

√5ᵗʰ **W53.0 Contact with mouse**
> √x7ᵗʰ **W53.01 Bitten by mouse**
> √x7ᵗʰ **W53.09 Other contact with mouse**

√5ᵗʰ **W53.1 Contact with rat**
> √x7ᵗʰ **W53.11 Bitten by rat**
> √x7ᵗʰ **W53.19 Other contact with rat**

√5ᵗʰ **W53.2 Contact with squirrel**
> √x7ᵗʰ **W53.21 Bitten by squirrel**
> √x7ᵗʰ **W53.29 Other contact with squirrel**

√5ᵗʰ **W53.8 Contact with other rodent**
> √x7ᵗʰ **W53.81 Bitten by other rodent**
> √x7ᵗʰ **W53.89 Other contact with other rodent**

√4ᵗʰ **W54 Contact with dog**
> INCLUDES   Contact with saliva, feces or urine of dog

> The appropriate 7th character is to be added to each code from category W54.
> A   initial encounter
> D   subsequent encounter
> S   sequela

√x7ᵗʰ **W54.0 Bitten by dog**

√x7ᵗʰ **W54.1 Struck by dog**
> Knocked over by dog

√x7ᵗʰ **W54.8 Other contact with dog**

√4ᵗʰ **W55 Contact with other mammals**
> INCLUDES   Contact with saliva, feces or urine of mammal
> EXCLUDES 1   animal being ridden—see transport accidents
> bitten or struck by dog (W54)
> bitten or struck by rodent (W53.-)
> contact with marine mammals (W56.-)

> The appropriate 7th character is to be added to each code from category W55.
> A   initial encounter
> D   subsequent encounter
> S   sequela

√5ᵗʰ **W55.0 Contact with cat**
> √x7ᵗʰ **W55.01 Bitten by cat**
> √x7ᵗʰ **W55.03 Scratched by cat**
> √x7ᵗʰ **W55.09 Other contact with cat**

√5ᵗʰ **W55.1 Contact with horse**
> √x7ᵗʰ **W55.11 Bitten by horse**
> √x7ᵗʰ **W55.12 Struck by horse**
> √x7ᵗʰ **W55.19 Other contact with horse**

√5ᵗʰ **W55.2 Contact with cow**
> Contact with bull
> √x7ᵗʰ **W55.21 Bitten by cow**
> √x7ᵗʰ **W55.22 Struck by cow**
> Gored by bull
> √x7ᵗʰ **W55.29 Other contact with cow**

√5ᵗʰ **W55.3 Contact with other hoof stock**
> Contact with goats   Contact with sheep
> √x7ᵗʰ **W55.31 Bitten by other hoof stock**
> √x7ᵗʰ **W55.32 Struck by other hoof stock**
> Gored by goat   Gored by ram
> √x7ᵗʰ **W55.39 Other contact with other hoof stock**

√5ᵗʰ **W55.4 Contact with pig**
> √x7ᵗʰ **W55.41 Bitten by pig**
> √x7ᵗʰ **W55.42 Struck by pig**
> √x7ᵗʰ **W55.49 Other contact with pig**

√5ᵗʰ **W55.5 Contact with raccoon**
> √x7ᵗʰ **W55.51 Bitten by raccoon**

N Newborn: 0   P Pediatric: 0-17   M Maternity: 12-55   A Adult: 15-124   MCC Major CC Condition   PDx MCC PDx acts as own MCC   CC CC Condition   PDx CC PDx acts as own CC

1148   ICD-10-CM Draft (2015)

√x7th **W55.52** Struck by raccoon

√x7th **W55.59** Other contact with raccoon

√5th **W55.8** Contact with other mammals

  √x7th **W55.81** Bitten by other mammals

  √x7th **W55.82** Struck by other mammals

  √x7th **W55.89** Other contact with other mammals

√4th **W56** **Contact with nonvenomous marine animal**

   EXCLUDES 1 contact with venomous marine animal (T63.-)

   The appropriate 7th character is to be added to each code from category W56.

   A   initial encounter

   D   subsequent encounter

   S   sequela

√5th **W56.0** Contact with dolphin

  √x7th **W56.01** Bitten by dolphin

  √x7th **W56.02** Struck by dolphin

  √x7th **W56.09** Other contact with dolphin

√5th **W56.1** Contact with sea lion

  √x7th **W56.11** Bitten by sea lion

  √x7th **W56.12** Struck by sea lion

  √x7th **W56.19** Other contact with sea lion

√5th **W56.2** Contact with orca

   Contact with killer whale

  √x7th **W56.21** Bitten by orca

  √x7th **W56.22** Struck by orca

  √x7th **W56.29** Other contact with orca

√5th **W56.3** Contact with other marine mammals

  √x7th **W56.31** Bitten by other marine mammals

  √x7th **W56.32** Struck by other marine mammals

  √x7th **W56.39** Other contact with other marine mammals

√5th **W56.4** Contact with shark

  √x7th **W56.41** Bitten by shark

  √x7th **W56.42** Struck by shark

  √x7th **W56.49** Other contact with shark

√5th **W56.5** Contact with other fish

  √x7th **W56.51** Bitten by other fish

  √x7th **W56.52** Struck by other fish

  √x7th **W56.59** Other contact with other fish

√5th **W56.8** Contact with other nonvenomous marine animals

  √x7th **W56.81** Bitten by other nonvenomous marine animals

  √x7th **W56.82** Struck by other nonvenomous marine animals

  √x7th **W56.89** Other contact with other nonvenomous marine animals

√x7th **W57** **Bitten or stung by nonvenomous insect and other nonvenomous arthropods**

   EXCLUDES 1 contact with venomous insects and arthropods (T63.2-, T63.3-, T63.4-)

   The appropriate 7th character is to be added to code W57.

   A   initial encounter

   D   subsequent encounter

   S   sequela

√4th **W58** **Contact with crocodile or alligator**

   The appropriate 7th character is to be added to each code from category W58.

   A   initial encounter

   D   subsequent encounter

   S   sequela

√5th **W58.0** Contact with alligator

  √x7th **W58.01** Bitten by alligator

  √x7th **W58.02** Struck by alligator

  √x7th **W58.03** Crushed by alligator

  √x7th **W58.09** Other contact with alligator

√5th **W58.1** Contact with crocodile

  √x7th **W58.11** Bitten by crocodile

  √x7th **W58.12** Struck by crocodile

  √x7th **W58.13** Crushed by crocodile

  √x7th **W58.19** Other contact with crocodile

√4th **W59** **Contact with other nonvenomous reptiles**

   EXCLUDES 1 contact with venomous reptile (T63.0-, T63.1-)

   The appropriate 7th character is to be added to each code from category W59.

   A   initial encounter

   D   subsequent encounter

   S   sequela

√5th **W59.0** Contact with nonvenomous lizards

  √x7th **W59.01** Bitten by nonvenomous lizards

  √x7th **W59.02** Struck by nonvenomous lizards

  √x7th **W59.09** Other contact with nonvenomous lizards

   Exposure to nonvenomous lizards

√5th **W59.1** Contact with nonvenomous snakes

  √x7th **W59.11** Bitten by nonvenomous snake

  √x7th **W59.12** Struck by nonvenomous snake

  √x7th **W59.13** Crushed by nonvenomous snake

  √x7th **W59.19** Other contact with nonvenomous snake

√5th **W59.2** Contact with turtles

   EXCLUDES 1 contact with tortoises (W59.8-)

  √x7th **W59.21** Bitten by turtle

  √x7th **W59.22** Struck by turtle

  √x7th **W59.29** Other contact with turtle

   Exposure to turtles

√5th **W59.8** Contact with other nonvenomous reptiles

  √x7th **W59.81** Bitten by other nonvenomous reptiles

  √x7th **W59.82** Struck by other nonvenomous reptiles

  √x7th **W59.83** Crushed by other nonvenomous reptiles

  √x7th **W59.89** Other contact with other nonvenomous reptiles

√x7th **W60** **Contact with nonvenomous plant thorns and spines and sharp leaves**

   EXCLUDES 1 contact with venomous plants (T63.7-)

   The appropriate 7th character is to be added to code W60.

   A   initial encounter

   D   subsequent encounter

   S   sequela

√4th **W61** **Contact with birds (domestic) (wild)**

   INCLUDES contact with excreta of birds

   The appropriate 7th character is to be added to each code from category W61.

   A   initial encounter

   D   subsequent encounter

   S   sequela

√5th **W61.0** Contact with parrot

  √x7th **W61.01** Bitten by parrot

  √x7th **W61.02** Struck by parrot

  √x7th **W61.09** Other contact with parrot

   Exposure to parrots

√5th **W61.1** Contact with macaw

  √x7th **W61.11** Bitten by macaw

  √x7th **W61.12** Struck by macaw

  √x7th **W61.19** Other contact with macaw

   Exposure to macaws

√5th **W61.2** Contact with other psittacines

  √x7th **W61.21** Bitten by other psittacines

  √x7th **W61.22** Struck by other psittacines

  √x7th **W61.29** Other contact with other psittacines

   Exposure to other psittacines

√5th **W61.3** Contact with chicken

  √x7th **W61.32** Struck by chicken

  √x7th **W61.33** Pecked by chicken

  √x7th **W61.39** Other contact with chicken

   Exposure to chickens

√5th **W61.4** Contact with turkey

  √x7th **W61.42** Struck by turkey

  √x7th **W61.43** Pecked by turkey

  √x7th **W61.49** Other contact with turkey

√5th **W61.5** Contact with goose

  √x7th **W61.51** Bitten by goose

  √x7th **W61.52** Struck by goose

  √x7th **W61.59** Other contact with goose

√5th **W61.6** Contact with duck

  √x7th **W61.61** Bitten by duck

  √x7th **W61.62** Struck by duck

  √x7th **W61.69** Other contact with duck

✓ Additional Character Required   √x7th Xtension Alert   Unacceptable PDx   Manifestation   Hospital Acquired Condition   **EXCLUDES 1** Not Coded Here   **EXCLUDES 2** Not Included Here

✓5ᵗʰ **W61.9 Contact with other birds**
✓x7ᵗʰ **W61.91 Bitten by other birds**
✓x7ᵗʰ **W61.92 Struck by other birds**
✓x7ᵗʰ **W61.99 Other contact with other birds**
Contact with bird NOS

✓4ᵗʰ **W62 Contact with nonvenomous amphibians**
EXCLUDES 1   *contact with venomous amphibians (T63.81-R63.83)*

The appropriate 7th character is to be added to each code from category W62.
A   initial encounter
D   subsequent encounter
S   sequela

✓x7ᵗʰ **W62.0 Contact with nonvenomous frogs**
✓x7ᵗʰ **W62.1 Contact with nonvenomous toads**
✓x7ᵗʰ **W62.9 Contact with other nonvenomous amphibians**

✓x7ᵗʰ **W64 Exposure to other animate mechanical forces**
INCLUDES   exposure to nonvenomous animal NOS
EXCLUDES 1   *contact with venomous animal (T63.-)*

The appropriate 7th character is to be added to code W64.
A   initial encounter
D   subsequent encounter
S   sequela

Accidental non-transport drowning and submersion (W65-W74)

EXCLUDES 1   *accidental drowning and submersion due to fall into water (W16.-)*
accidental drowning and submersion due to water transport accident (V90.-, V92.-)
EXCLUDES 2   *accidental drowning and submersion due to cataclysm (X34-X39)*

✓x7ᵗʰ **W65 Accidental drowning and submersion while in bath-tub**
EXCLUDES 1   *accidental drowning and submersion due to fall in (into) bathtub (W16.211)*

The appropriate 7th character is to be added to code W65.
A   initial encounter
D   subsequent encounter
S   sequela

✓x7ᵗʰ **W67 Accidental drowning and submersion while in swimming-pool**
EXCLUDES 1   *accidental drowning and submersion due to fall into swimming pool (W16.011, W16.021, W16.031)*
accidental drowning and submersion due to striking into wall of swimming pool (W22.041)

The appropriate 7th character is to be added to code W67.
A   initial encounter
D   subsequent encounter
S   sequela

✓x7ᵗʰ **W69 Accidental drowning and submersion while in natural water**
Accidental drowning and submersion while in lake
Accidental drowning and submersion while in open sea
Accidental drowning and submersion while in river
Accidental drowning and submersion while in stream
EXCLUDES 1   *accidental drowning and submersion due to fall into natural body of water (W16.111, W16.121, W16.131)*

The appropriate 7th character is to be added to code W69.
A   initial encounter
D   subsequent encounter
S   sequela

✓x7ᵗʰ **W73 Other specified cause of accidental non-transport drowning and submersion**
Accidental drowning and submersion while in quenching tank
Accidental drowning and submersion while in reservoir
EXCLUDES 1   *accidental drowning and submersion due to fall into other water (W16.311, W16.321, W16.331)*

The appropriate 7th character is to be added to code W73.
A   initial encounter
D   subsequent encounter
S   sequela

✓x7ᵗʰ **W74 Unspecified cause of accidental drowning and submersion**
Drowning NOS

The appropriate 7th character is to be added to code W74.
A   initial encounter
D   subsequent encounter
S   sequela

Exposure to electric current, radiation and extreme ambient air temperature and pressure (W85-W99)

EXCLUDES 1   *exposure to:*
failure in dosage of radiation or temperature during surgical and medical care (Y63.2-Y63.5)
lightning (T75.0-)
natural cold (X31)
natural heat (X30)
natural radiation NOS (X39)
radiological procedure and radiotherapy (Y84.2)
sunlight (X32)

✓x7ᵗʰ **W85 Exposure to electric transmission lines**
Broken power line

The appropriate 7th character is to be added to code W85.
A   initial encounter
D   subsequent encounter
S   sequela

✓4ᵗʰ **W86 Exposure to other specified electric current**

The appropriate 7th character is to be added to each code from category W86.
A   initial encounter
D   subsequent encounter
S   sequela

✓x7ᵗʰ **W86.0 Exposure to domestic wiring and appliances**
✓x7ᵗʰ **W86.1 Exposure to industrial wiring, appliances and electrical machinery**
Exposure to conductors
Exposure to control apparatus
Exposure to electrical equipment and machinery
Exposure to transformers
✓x7ᵗʰ **W86.8 Exposure to other electric current**
Exposure to wiring and appliances in or on farm (not farmhouse)
Exposure to wiring and appliances outdoors
Exposure to wiring and appliances in or on public building
Exposure to wiring and appliances in or on residential institutions
Exposure to wiring and appliances in or on schools

✓4ᵗʰ **W88 Exposure to ionizing radiation**
EXCLUDES 1   *exposure to sunlight (X32)*

The appropriate 7th character is to be added to each code from category W88.
A   initial encounter
D   subsequent encounter
S   sequela

✓x7ᵗʰ **W88.0 Exposure to X-rays**
✓x7ᵗʰ **W88.1 Exposure to radioactive isotopes**
✓x7ᵗʰ **W88.8 Exposure to other ionizing radiation**

✓4ᵗʰ **W89 Exposure to man-made visible and ultraviolet light**
INCLUDES   exposure to welding light (arc)
EXCLUDES 2   *exposure to sunlight (X32)*

The appropriate 7th character is to be added to each code from category W89.
A   initial encounter
D   subsequent encounter
S   sequela

✓x7ᵗʰ **W89.0 Exposure to welding light (arc)**
✓x7ᵗʰ **W89.1 Exposure to tanning bed**
✓x7ᵗʰ **W89.8 Exposure to other man-made visible and ultraviolet light**
✓x7ᵗʰ **W89.9 Exposure to unspecified man-made visible and ultraviolet light**

✓4ᵗʰ **W90 Exposure to other nonionizing radiation**
EXCLUDES 1   *exposure to sunlight (X32)*

The appropriate 7th character is to be added to each code from category W90.
A   initial encounter
D   subsequent encounter
S   sequela

✓x7ᵗʰ **W90.0 Exposure to radiofrequency**
✓x7ᵗʰ **W90.1 Exposure to infrared radiation**
✓x7ᵗʰ **W90.2 Exposure to laser radiation**
✓x7ᵗʰ **W90.8 Exposure to other nonionizing radiation**

N Newborn: 0   P Pediatric: 0-17   M Maternity: 12-55   A Adult: 15-124   MCC Major CC Condition   PDx MCC PDx acts as own MCC   CC CC Condition   PDx CC PDx acts as own CC

1150   ICD-10-CM Draft (2015)

✓x7th **W92 Exposure to excessive heat of man-made origin**

> The appropriate 7th character is to be added to code W92.
> A　initial encounter
> D　subsequent encounter
> S　sequela

✓4th **W93 Exposure to excessive cold of man-made origin**

> The appropriate 7th character is to be added to each code from category W93.
> A　initial encounter
> D　subsequent encounter
> S　sequela

- ✓5th **W93.0 Contact with or inhalation of** dry ice
  - ✓x7th **W93.01 Contact** with dry ice
  - ✓x7th **W93.02 Inhalation** of dry ice
- ✓5th **W93.1 Contact with or inhalation of** liquid air
  - ✓x7th **W93.11 Contact** with liquid air
    Contact with liquid hydrogen
    Contact with liquid nitrogen
  - ✓x7th **W93.12 Inhalation** of liquid air
    Inhalation of liquid hydrogen
    Inhalation of liquid nitrogen
- ✓x7th **W93.2 Prolonged exposure in deep freeze unit or refrigerator**
- ✓x7th **W93.8 Exposure to other excessive cold of man-made origin**

✓4th **W94 Exposure to high and low air pressure and changes in air pressure**

> The appropriate 7th character is to be added to each code from category W94.
> A　initial encounter
> D　subsequent encounter
> S　sequela

- ✓x7th **W94.0 Exposure to prolonged high air pressure**
- ✓5th **W94.1 Exposure to prolonged low air pressure**
  - ✓x7th **W94.11 Exposure to residence or prolonged visit at high altitude**
  - ✓x7th **W94.12 Exposure to other prolonged low air pressure**
- ✓5th **W94.2 Exposure to rapid changes in air pressure during** ascent
  - ✓x7th **W94.21 Exposure to reduction in atmospheric pressure while surfacing from** deep-water diving
  - ✓x7th **W94.22 Exposure to reduction in atmospheric pressure while surfacing from** underground
  - ✓x7th **W94.23 Exposure to sudden change in air pressure in** aircraft **during ascent**
  - ✓x7th **W94.29 Exposure to** other **rapid changes in air pressure during ascent**
- ✓5th **W94.3 Exposure to rapid changes in air pressure during** descent
  - ✓x7th **W94.31 Exposure to sudden change in air pressure in** aircraft **during descent**
  - ✓x7th **W94.32 Exposure to high air pressure from rapid descent in** water
  - ✓x7th **W94.39 Exposure to** other **rapid changes in air pressure during descent**

✓x7th **W99 Exposure to other man-made environmental factors**

> The appropriate 7th character is to be added to code W99.
> A　initial encounter
> D　subsequent encounter
> S　sequela

Exposure to smoke, fire and flames (X00-X08)

EXCLUDES 1　arson (X97)
EXCLUDES 2　explosions (W35-W40)
lightning (T75.0-)
transport accident (V01-V99)

✓4th **X00 Exposure to** uncontrolled fire **in building or structure**
INCLUDES　conflagration in building or structure
Code first any associated cataclysm
EXCLUDES 2　exposure to ignition or melting of nightwear (X05)
exposure to ignition or melting of other clothing and apparel (X06.-)
exposure to other specified smoke, fire and flames (X08.-)

> The appropriate 7th character is to be added to each code from category X00.
> A　initial encounter
> D　subsequent encounter
> S　sequela

- ✓x7th **X00.0 Exposure to** flames **in uncontrolled fire in building or structure**
- ✓x7th **X00.1 Exposure to** smoke **in uncontrolled fire in building or structure**
- ✓x7th **X00.2 Injury due to collapse of burning building or structure in uncontrolled fire**
  EXCLUDES 1　injury due to collapse of building not on fire (W20.1)
- ✓x7th **X00.3 Fall from burning building or structure in uncontrolled fire**
- ✓x7th **X00.4 Hit by object from burning building or structure in uncontrolled fire**
- ✓x7th **X00.5 Jump from burning building or structure in uncontrolled fire**
- ✓x7th **X00.8 Other exposure to uncontrolled fire in building or structure**

✓4th **X01 Exposure to uncontrolled fire, not in building or structure**
INCLUDES　exposure to forest fire

> The appropriate 7th character is to be added to each code from category X01.
> A　initial encounter
> D　subsequent encounter
> S　sequela

- ✓x7th **X01.0 Exposure to** flames **in uncontrolled fire, not in building or structure**
- ✓x7th **X01.1 Exposure to** smoke **in uncontrolled fire, not in building or structure**
- ✓x7th **X01.3 Fall due to uncontrolled fire, not in building or structure**
- ✓x7th **X01.4 Hit by object due to uncontrolled fire, not in building or structure**
- ✓x7th **X01.8 Other exposure to uncontrolled fire, not in building or structure**

✓4th **X02 Exposure to** controlled fire **in building or structure**
INCLUDES　exposure to fire in fireplace
exposure to fire in stove

> The appropriate 7th character is to be added to each code from category X02.
> A　initial encounter
> D　subsequent encounter
> S　sequela

- ✓x7th **X02.0 Exposure to** flames **in controlled fire in building or structure**
- ✓x7th **X02.1 Exposure to** smoke **in controlled fire in building or structure**
- ✓x7th **X02.2 Injury due to collapse of burning building or structure in controlled fire**
  EXCLUDES 1　injury due to collapse of building not on fire (W20.1)
- ✓x7th **X02.3 Fall from burning building or structure in controlled fire**
- ✓x7th **X02.4 Hit by object from burning building or structure in controlled fire**
- ✓x7th **X02.5 Jump from burning building or structure in controlled fire**
- ✓x7th **X02.8 Other exposure to controlled fire in building or structure**

✓4th **X03 Exposure to** controlled fire, **not in building or structure**
INCLUDES　exposure to bon fire
exposure to camp-fire
exposure to trash fire

> The appropriate 7th character is to be added to each code from category X03.
> A　initial encounter
> D　subsequent encounter
> S　sequela

- ✓x7th **X03.0 Exposure to** flames **in controlled fire, not in building or structure**
- ✓x7th **X03.1 Exposure to** smoke **in controlled fire, not in building or structure**
- ✓x7th **X03.3 Fall due to controlled fire, not in building or structure**
- ✓x7th **X03.4 Hit by object due to controlled fire, not in building or structure**
- ✓x7th **X03.8 Other exposure to controlled fire, not in building or structure**

✓ Additional Character Required　✓x7th Xtension Alert　Unacceptable PDx　Manifestation　　Hospital Acquired Condition　EXCLUDES 1 Not Coded Here　EXCLUDES 2 Not Included Here

External Causes of Morbidity

X04–X16

√x7th **X04 Exposure to ignition of highly flammable material**
Exposure to ignition of gasoline
Exposure to ignition of kerosene
Exposure to ignition of petrol
EXCLUDES 2 *exposure to ignition or melting of nightwear (X05)*
exposure to ignition or melting of other clothing and apparel (X06)

The appropriate 7th character is to be added to code X04.
A   initial encounter
D   subsequent encounter
S   sequela

√x7th **X05 Exposure to ignition or melting of nightwear**
EXCLUDES 2 *exposure to uncontrolled fire in building or structure (X00.-)*
exposure to uncontrolled fire, not in building or structure (X01.-)
exposure to controlled fire in building or structure (X02.-)
exposure to controlled fire, not in building or structure (X03.-)
exposure to ignition of highly flammable materials (X04.-)

The appropriate 7th character is to be added to code X05.
A   initial encounter
D   subsequent encounter
S   sequela

√4th **X06 Exposure to ignition or melting of other clothing and apparel**
EXCLUDES 2 *exposure to uncontrolled fire in building or structure (X00.-)*
exposure to uncontrolled fire, not in building or structure (X01.-)
exposure to controlled fire in building or structure (X02.-)
exposure to controlled fire, not in building or structure (X03.-)
exposure to ignition of highly flammable materials (X04.-)

The appropriate 7th character is to be added to each code from category X06.
A   initial encounter
D   subsequent encounter
S   sequela

√x7th **X06.0 Exposure to ignition of plastic jewelry**
√x7th **X06.1 Exposure to melting of plastic jewelry**
√x7th **X06.2 Exposure to ignition of other clothing and apparel**
√x7th **X06.3 Exposure to melting of other clothing and apparel**

√4th **X08 Exposure to other specified smoke, fire and flames**

The appropriate 7th character is to be added to each code from category X08.
A   initial encounter
D   subsequent encounter
S   sequela

√5th **X08.0 Exposure to bed fire**
Exposure to mattress fire
√x7th **X08.00 Exposure to bed fire due to unspecified burning material**
√x7th **X08.01 Exposure to bed fire due to burning cigarette**
√x7th **X08.09 Exposure to bed fire due to other burning material**
√5th **X08.1 Exposure to sofa fire**
√x7th **X08.10 Exposure to sofa fire due to unspecified burning material**
√x7th **X08.11 Exposure to sofa fire due to burning cigarette**
√x7th **X08.19 Exposure to sofa fire due to other burning material**
√5th **X08.2 Exposure to other furniture fire**
√x7th **X08.20 Exposure to other furniture fire due to unspecified burning material**
√x7th **X08.21 Exposure to other furniture fire due to burning cigarette**
√x7th **X08.29 Exposure to other furniture fire due to other burning material**
√x7th **X08.8 Exposure to other specified smoke, fire and flames**

Contact with heat and hot substances (X10-X19)
EXCLUDES 1 *exposure to excessive natural heat (X30)*
exposure to fire and flames (X00-X09)

√4th **X10 Contact with hot drinks, food, fats and cooking oils**

The appropriate 7th character is to be added to each code from category X10.
A   initial encounter
D   subsequent encounter
S   sequela

√x7th **X10.0 Contact with hot drinks**
√x7th **X10.1 Contact with hot food**
√x7th **X10.2 Contact with fats and cooking oils**

√4th **X11 Contact with hot tap-water**
INCLUDES   contact with boiling tap-water
contact with boiling water NOS
EXCLUDES 1 *contact with water heated on stove (X12)*

The appropriate 7th character is to be added to each code from category X11.
A   initial encounter
D   subsequent encounter
S   sequela

√x7th **X11.0 Contact with hot water in bath or tub**
EXCLUDES 1 *contact with running hot water in bath or tub (X11.1)*

√x7th **X11.1 Contact with running hot water**
Contact with hot water running out of hose
Contact with hot water running out of tap

√x7th **X11.8 Contact with other hot tap-water**
Contact with hot water in bucket
Contact with hot tap-water NOS

√x7th **X12 Contact with other hot fluids**
Contact with water heated on stove
EXCLUDES 1 *hot (liquid) metals (X18)*

The appropriate 7th character is to be added to code X12.
A   initial encounter
D   subsequent encounter
S   sequela

√4th **X13 Contact with steam and other hot vapors**

The appropriate 7th character is to be added to each code from category X13.
A   initial encounter
D   subsequent encounter
S   sequela

√x7th **X13.0 Inhalation of steam and other hot vapors**
√x7th **X13.1 Other contact with steam and other hot vapors**

√4th **X14 Contact with hot air and other hot gases**

The appropriate 7th character is to be added to each code from category X14.
A   initial encounter
D   subsequent encounter
S   sequela

√x7th **X14.0 Inhalation of hot air and gases**
√x7th **X14.1 Other contact with hot air and other hot gases**

√4th **X15 Contact with hot household appliances**
EXCLUDES 1 *contact with heating appliances (X16)*
contact with powered household appliances (W29.-)
exposure to controlled fire in building or structure due to household appliance (X02.8)
exposure to household appliances electrical current (W86.0)

The appropriate 7th character is to be added to each code from category X15.
A   initial encounter
D   subsequent encounter
S   sequela

√x7th **X15.0 Contact with hot stove (kitchen)**
√x7th **X15.1 Contact with hot toaster**
√x7th **X15.2 Contact with hotplate**
√x7th **X15.3 Contact with hot saucepan or skillet**
√x7th **X15.8 Contact with other hot household appliances**
Contact with cooker   Contact with light bulbs
Contact with kettle

√x7th **X16 Contact with hot heating appliances, radiators and pipes**
EXCLUDES 1 *contact with powered appliances (W29.-)*
exposure to controlled fire in building or structure due to appliance (X02.8)
exposure to industrial appliances electrical current (W86.1)

The appropriate 7th character is to be added to code X16.
A   initial encounter
D   subsequent encounter
S   sequela

N Newborn: 0   P Pediatric: 0-17   M Maternity: 12-55   A Adult: 15-124   MCC Major CC Condition   PDx MCC PDx acts as own MCC   CC CC Condition   PDx CC PDx acts as own CC

1152   ICD-10-CM Draft (2015)

√x7ᵗʰ **X17 Contact with hot engines, machinery and tools**
   EXCLUDES 1   contact with hot heating appliances, radiators and pipes (X16)
            contact with hot household appliances (X15)

The appropriate 7th character is to be added to code X17.
A   initial encounter
D   subsequent encounter
S   sequela

√x7ᵗʰ **X18 Contact with other hot metals**
   Contact with liquid metal

The appropriate 7th character is to be added to code X18.
A   initial encounter
D   subsequent encounter
S   sequela

√x7ᵗʰ **X19 Contact with other heat and hot substances**
   EXCLUDES 1   objects that are not normally hot, e.g., an object made hot by a
            house fire (X00-X09)

The appropriate 7th character is to be added to code X19.
A   initial encounter
D   subsequent encounter
S   sequela

Exposure to forces of nature (X30-X39)

√x7ᵗʰ **X30 Exposure to excessive natural heat**
   Exposure to excessive heat as the cause of sunstroke
   Exposure to heat NOS
   EXCLUDES 1   excessive heat of man-made origin (W92)
            exposure to man-made radiation (W89)
            exposure to sunlight (X32)
            exposure to tanning bed (W89)

The appropriate 7th character is to be added to code X30.
A   initial encounter
D   subsequent encounter
S   sequela

√x7ᵗʰ **X31 Exposure to excessive natural cold**
   Excessive cold as the cause of chilblains NOS
   Excessive cold as the cause of immersion foot or hand
   Exposure to cold NOS
   Exposure to weather conditions
   EXCLUDES 1   cold of man-made origin (W93.-)
            contact with or inhalation of dry ice (W93.-)
            contact with or inhalation of liquefied gas (W93.-)

The appropriate 7th character is to be added to code X31.
A   initial encounter
D   subsequent encounter
S   sequela

√x7ᵗʰ **X32 Exposure to sunlight**
   EXCLUDES 1   radiation-related disorders of the skin and subcutaneous tissue
            (L55-L59)
            man-made radiation (tanning bed) (W89)

The appropriate 7th character is to be added to code X32.
A   initial encounter
D   subsequent encounter
S   sequela

√x7ᵗʰ **X34 Earthquake**
   EXCLUDES 2   tidal wave (tsunami) due to earthquake (X37.41)

The appropriate 7th character is to be added to code X34.
A   initial encounter
D   subsequent encounter
S   sequela

√x7ᵗʰ **X35 Volcanic eruption**
   EXCLUDES 2   tidal wave (tsunami) due to volcanic eruption (X37.41)

The appropriate 7th character is to be added to code X35.
A   initial encounter
D   subsequent encounter
S   sequela

√4ᵗʰ **X36 Avalanche, landslide and other earth movements**
   INCLUDES   victim of mudslide of cataclysmic nature
   EXCLUDES 1   earthquake (X34)
   EXCLUDES 2   transport accident involving collision with avalanche or
            landslide not in motion (V01-V99)

The appropriate 7th character is to be added to each code from
category X36.
A   initial encounter
D   subsequent encounter
S   sequela

√x7ᵗʰ **X36.0 Collapse of dam or man-made structure causing earth
   movement**
√x7ᵗʰ **X36.1 Avalanche, landslide, or mudslide**

√4ᵗʰ **X37 Cataclysmic storm**

The appropriate 7th character is to be added to each code from
category X37.
A   initial encounter
D   subsequent encounter
S   sequela

√x7ᵗʰ **X37.0 Hurricane**
   Storm surge   Typhoon
√x7ᵗʰ **X37.1 Tornado**
   Cyclone   Twister
√x7ᵗʰ **X37.2 Blizzard (snow)(ice)**
√x7ᵗʰ **X37.3 Dust storm**
√5ᵗʰ **X37.4 Tidalwave**
   √x7ᵗʰ **X37.41 Tidal wave due to earthquake or volcanic eruption**
            Tidal wave NOS   Tsunami
   √x7ᵗʰ **X37.42 Tidal wave due to storm**
   √x7ᵗʰ **X37.43 Tidal wave due to landslide**
√x7ᵗʰ **X37.8 Other cataclysmic storms**
   Cloudburst   Torrential rain
   EXCLUDES 2   flood (X38)
√x7ᵗʰ **X37.9 Unspecified cataclysmic storm**
   Storm NOS
   EXCLUDES 1   collapse of dam or man-made structure causing earth
            movement (X39.0)

√x7ᵗʰ **X38 Flood**
   Flood arising from remote storm
   Flood of cataclysmic nature arising from melting snow
   Flood resulting directly from storm
   EXCLUDES 1   collapse of dam or man-made structure causing earth
            movement (X39.0)
            tidal wave NOS (X37.41)
            tidal wave caused by storm (X37.2)

The appropriate 7th character is to be added to code X38.
A   initial encounter
D   subsequent encounter
S   sequela

√4ᵗʰ **X39 Exposure to other forces of nature**

The appropriate 7th character is to be added to each code from
category X39.
A   initial encounter
D   subsequent encounter
S   sequela

√5ᵗʰ **X39.0 Exposure to natural radiation**
   EXCLUDES 1   contact with and (suspected) exposure to radon and
            other naturally occuring radiation (Z77.122)
            exposure to man-made radiation (W88-W90)
            exposure to sunlight (X32)
   √x7ᵗʰ **X39.01 Exposure to radon**
   √x7ᵗʰ **X39.08 Exposure to other natural radiation**
√x7ᵗʰ **X39.8 Other exposure to forces of nature**

Accidental exposure to other specified factors (X52, X58)

√x7ᵗʰ **X52 Prolonged stay in weightless environment**
   Weightlessness in spacecraft (simulator)

The appropriate 7th character is to be added to code X52.
A   initial encounter
D   subsequent encounter
S   sequela

✓ Additional Character Required   √x7ᵗʰ Xtension Alert   Unacceptable PDx   Manifestation   Hospital Acquired Condition   EXCLUDES 1 Not Coded Here   EXCLUDES 2 Not Included Here

External Causes of Morbidity

X58–X82.8

√x7th **X58 Exposure to other specified factors**
    Accident NOS   Exposure NOS

> The appropriate 7th character is to be added to code X58.
> A   initial encounter
> D   subsequent encounter
> S   sequela

Intentional self-harm (X71-X83)
Purposely self-inflicted injury
Suicide (attempted)

√4th **X71 Intentional self-harm by drowning and submersion**

> The appropriate 7th character is to be added to each code from category X71.
> A   initial encounter
> D   subsequent encounter
> S   sequela

  √x7th **X71.0 Intentional self-harm by drowning and submersion while in bathtub**

  √x7th **X71.1 Intentional self-harm by drowning and submersion while in swimming pool**

  √x7th **X71.2 Intentional self-harm by drowning and submersion after jump into swimming pool**

  √x7th **X71.3 Intentional self-harm by drowning and submersion in natural water**

  √x7th **X71.8 Other intentional self-harm by drowning and submersion**

  √x7th **X71.9 Intentional self-harm by drowning and submersion, unspecified**

√x7th **X72 Intentional self-harm by handgun discharge**
    Intentional self-harm by gun for single hand use
    Intentional self-harm by pistol
    Intentional self-harm by revolver
    EXCLUDES 1   Very pistol (X74.8)

> The appropriate 7th character is to be added to code X72.
> A   initial encounter
> D   subsequent encounter
> S   sequela

√4th **X73 Intentional self-harm by rifle, shotgun and larger firearm discharge**
    EXCLUDES 1   airgun (X74.01)

> The appropriate 7th character is to be added to each code from category X73.
> A   initial encounter
> D   subsequent encounter
> S   sequela

  √x7th **X73.0 Intentional self-harm by shotgun discharge**

  √x7th **X73.1 Intentional self-harm by hunting rifle discharge**

  √x7th **X73.2 Intentional self-harm by machine gun discharge**

  √x7th **X73.8 Intentional self-harm by other larger firearm discharge**

  √x7th **X73.9 Intentional self-harm by unspecified larger firearm discharge**

√4th **X74 Intentional self-harm by other and unspecified firearm and gun discharge**

> The appropriate 7th character is to be added to each code from category X74.
> A   initial encounter
> D   subsequent encounter
> S   sequela

  √5th **X74.0 Intentional self-harm by gas, air or spring-operated guns**
    √x7th **X74.01 Intentional self-harm by airgun**
        Intentional self-harm by BB gun discharge
        Intentional self-harm by pellet gun discharge
    √x7th **X74.02 Intentional self-harm by paintball gun**
    √x7th **X74.09 Intentional self-harm by other gas, air or spring-operated gun**
  √x7th **X74.8 Intentional self-harm by other firearm discharge**
    Intentional self-harm by Very pistol [flare] discharge
  √x7th **X74.9 Intentional self-harm by unspecified firearm discharge**

√x7th **X75 Intentional self-harm by explosive material**

> The appropriate 7th character is to be added to code X75.
> A   initial encounter
> D   subsequent encounter
> S   sequela

√x7th **X76 Intentional self-harm by smoke, fire and flames**

> The appropriate 7th character is to be added to code X76.
> A   initial encounter
> D   subsequent encounter
> S   sequela

√4th **X77 Intentional self-harm by steam, hot vapors and hot objects**

> The appropriate 7th character is to be added to each code from category X77.
> A   initial encounter
> D   subsequent encounter
> S   sequela

  √x7th **X77.0 Intentional self-harm by steam or hot vapors**

  √x7th **X77.1 Intentional self-harm by hot tap water**

  √x7th **X77.2 Intentional self-harm by other hot fluids**

  √x7th **X77.3 Intentional self-harm by hot household appliances**

  √x7th **X77.8 Intentional self-harm by other hot objects**

  √x7th **X77.9 Intentional self-harm by unspecified hot objects**

√4th **X78 Intentional self-harm by sharp object**

> The appropriate 7th character is to be added to each code from category X78.
> A   initial encounter
> D   subsequent encounter
> S   sequela

  √x7th **X78.0 Intentional self-harm by sharp glass**

  √x7th **X78.1 Intentional self-harm by knife**

  √x7th **X78.2 Intentional self-harm by sword or dagger**

  √x7th **X78.8 Intentional self-harm by other sharp object**

  √x7th **X78.9 Intentional self-harm by unspecified sharp object**

√x7th **X79 Intentional self-harm by blunt object**

> The appropriate 7th character is to be added to code X79.
> A   initial encounter
> D   subsequent encounter
> S   sequela

√x7th **X80 Intentional self-harm by jumping from a high place**
    Intentional fall from one level to another

> The appropriate 7th character is to be added to code X80.
> A   initial encounter
> D   subsequent encounter
> S   sequela

√4th **X81 Intentional self-harm by jumping or lying in front of moving object**

> The appropriate 7th character is to be added to each code from category X81.
> A   initial encounter
> D   subsequent encounter
> S   sequela

  √x7th **X81.0 Intentional self-harm by jumping or lying in front of motor vehicle**

  √x7th **X81.1 Intentional self-harm by jumping or lying in front of (subway) train**

  √x7th **X81.8 Intentional self-harm by jumping or lying in front of other moving object**

√4th **X82 Intentional self-harm by crashing of motor vehicle**

> The appropriate 7th character is to be added to each code from category X82.
> A   initial encounter
> D   subsequent encounter
> S   sequela

  √x7th **X82.0 Intentional collision of motor vehicle with other motor vehicle**

  √x7th **X82.1 Intentional collision of motor vehicle with train**

  √x7th **X82.2 Intentional collision of motor vehicle with tree**

  √x7th **X82.8 Other intentional self-harm by crashing of motor vehicle**

N Newborn: 0   P Pediatric: 0-17   M Maternity: 12-55   A Adult: 15-124   MCC Major CC Condition   PDx MCC PDx acts as own MCC   CC CC Condition   PDx CC PDx acts as own CC

☑4ᵗʰ **X83** **Intentional self-harm by other specified means**
> EXCLUDES 1   intentional self-harm by poisoning or contact with toxic substance—see Table of Drugs and Chemicals

> The appropriate 7th character is to be added to each code from category X83.
> A   initial encounter
> D   subsequent encounter
> S   sequela

☑x7ᵗʰ **X83.Ø** **Intentional self-harm by** crashing of aircraft

☑x7ᵗʰ **X83.1** **Intentional self-harm by** electrocution

☑x7ᵗʰ **X83.2** **Intentional self-harm by** exposure to extremes of cold

☑x7ᵗʰ **X83.8** **Intentional self-harm by** other specified means

Assault (X92-YØ8)

> INCLUDES   homicide
> injuries inflicted by another person with intent to injure or kill, by any means

> EXCLUDES 1   injuries due to legal intervention (Y35.-)
> injuries due to operations of war (Y36.-)
> injuries due to terrorism (Y38.-)

☑4ᵗʰ **X92** **Assault by drowning and submersion**

> The appropriate 7th character is to be added to each code from category X92.
> A   initial encounter
> D   subsequent encounter
> S   sequela

☑x7ᵗʰ **X92.Ø** **Assault by drowning and submersion while in** bathtub

☑x7ᵗʰ **X92.1** **Assault by drowning and submersion while in** swimming pool

☑x7ᵗʰ **X92.2** **Assault by drowning and submersion** after push into swimming pool

☑x7ᵗʰ **X92.3** **Assault by drowning and submersion** in natural water

☑x7ᵗʰ **X92.8** **Other assault by drowning and submersion**

☑x7ᵗʰ **X92.9** **Assault by drowning and submersion,** unspecified

☑x7ᵗʰ **X93** **Assault by handgun discharge**
> Assault by discharge of gun for single hand use
> Assault by discharge of pistol
> Assault by discharge of revolver
> EXCLUDES 1   Very pistol (X95.8)

> The appropriate 7th character is to be added to code X93.
> A   initial encounter
> D   subsequent encounter
> S   sequela

☑4ᵗʰ **X94** **Assault by rifle, shotgun and larger firearm discharge**
> EXCLUDES 1   airgun (X95.Ø1)

> The appropriate 7th character is to be added to each code from category X94.
> A   initial encounter
> D   subsequent encounter
> S   sequela

☑x7ᵗʰ **X94.Ø** **Assault by** shotgun

☑x7ᵗʰ **X94.1** **Assault by** hunting rifle

☑x7ᵗʰ **X94.2** **Assault by** machine gun

☑x7ᵗʰ **X94.8** **Assault by** other larger firearm discharge

☑x7ᵗʰ **X94.9** **Assault by** unspecified larger firearm discharge

☑4ᵗʰ **X95** **Assault by other and unspecified firearm and gun discharge**

> The appropriate 7th character is to be added to each code from category X95.
> A   initial encounter
> D   subsequent encounter
> S   sequela

☑5ᵗʰ **X95.Ø** **Assault by** gas, air or spring-operated guns

    ☑x7ᵗʰ **X95.Ø1** **Assault by** airgun discharge
>   Assault by BB gun discharge
>   Assault by pellet gun discharge

    ☑x7ᵗʰ **X95.Ø2** **Assault by** paintball gun discharge

    ☑x7ᵗʰ **X95.Ø9** **Assault by** other gas, air or spring-operated gun

☑x7ᵗʰ **X95.8** **Assault by** other firearm discharge
>   Assault by Very pistol [flare] discharge

☑x7ᵗʰ **X95.9** **Assault by** unspecified firearm discharge

☑4ᵗʰ **X96** **Assault by explosive material**
> EXCLUDES 1   incendiary device (X97)
> terrorism involving explosive material (Y38.2-)

> The appropriate 7th character is to be added to each code from category X96.
> A   initial encounter
> D   subsequent encounter
> S   sequela

☑x7ᵗʰ **X96.Ø** **Assault by** antipersonnel bomb
> EXCLUDES 1   antipersonnel bomb use in military or war (Y36.2-)

☑x7ᵗʰ **X96.1** **Assault by** gasoline bomb

☑x7ᵗʰ **X96.2** **Assault by** letter bomb

☑x7ᵗʰ **X96.3** **Assault by** fertilizer bomb

☑x7ᵗʰ **X96.4** **Assault by** pipe bomb

☑x7ᵗʰ **X96.8** **Assault by** other specified explosive

☑x7ᵗʰ **X96.9** **Assault by** unspecified explosive

☑x7ᵗʰ **X97** **Assault by smoke, fire and flames**
> Assault by arson   Assault by incendiary device
> Assault by cigarettes

> The appropriate 7th character is to be added to code X97.
> A   initial encounter
> D   subsequent encounter
> S   sequela

☑4ᵗʰ **X98** **Assault by steam, hot vapors and hot objects**

> The appropriate 7th character is to be added to each code from category X98.
> A   initial encounter
> D   subsequent encounter
> S   sequela

☑x7ᵗʰ **X98.Ø** **Assault by** steam or hot vapors

☑x7ᵗʰ **X98.1** **Assault by** hot tap water

☑x7ᵗʰ **X98.2** **Assault by** hot fluids

☑x7ᵗʰ **X98.3** **Assault by** hot household appliances

☑x7ᵗʰ **X98.8** **Assault by** other hot objects

☑x7ᵗʰ **X98.9** **Assault by** unspecified hot objects

☑4ᵗʰ **X99** **Assault by sharp object**
> EXCLUDES 1   assault by strike by sports equipment (YØ8.Ø-)

> The appropriate 7th character is to be added to each code from category X99.
> A   initial encounter
> D   subsequent encounter
> S   sequela

☑x7ᵗʰ **X99.Ø** **Assault by** sharp glass

☑x7ᵗʰ **X99.1** **Assault by** knife

☑x7ᵗʰ **X99.2** **Assault by** sword or dagger

☑x7ᵗʰ **X99.8** **Assault by** other sharp object

☑x7ᵗʰ **X99.9** **Assault by** unspecified sharp object
>   Assault by stabbing NOS

☑x7ᵗʰ **YØØ** **Assault by blunt object**
> EXCLUDES 1   assault by strike by sports equipment (YØ8.Ø-)

> The appropriate 7th character is to be added to code YØØ.
> A   initial encounter
> D   subsequent encounter
> S   sequela

☑x7ᵗʰ **YØ1** **Assault by pushing from high place**

> The appropriate 7th character is to be added to code YØ1.
> A   initial encounter
> D   subsequent encounter
> S   sequela

☑4ᵗʰ **YØ2** **Assault by pushing or placing victim in front of moving object**

> The appropriate 7th character is to be added to each code from category YØ2.
> A   initial encounter
> D   subsequent encounter
> S   sequela

☑x7ᵗʰ **YØ2.Ø** **Assault by pushing or placing victim in front of** motor vehicle

☑x7ᵗʰ **YØ2.1** **Assault by pushing or placing victim in front of** (subway) train

☑x7ᵗʰ **YØ2.8** **Assault by pushing or placing victim in front of** other moving object

---

☑ Additional Character Required   ☑x7ᵗʰ Xtension Alert   Unacceptable PDx   Manifestation   Hospital Acquired Condition   EXCLUDES 1 Not Coded Here   EXCLUDES 2 Not Included Here

External Causes of Morbidity

Y03–Y09

√4ᵗʰ **Y03 Assault by crashing of motor vehicle**

The appropriate 7th character is to be added to each code from category Y03.
A   initial encounter
D   subsequent encounter
S   sequela

√x7ᵗʰ **Y03.0 Assault by being hit or run over by motor vehicle**

√x7ᵗʰ **Y03.8 Other assault by crashing of motor vehicle**

√4ᵗʰ **Y04 Assault by bodily force**

> EXCLUDES 1   *assault by:*
> *submersion (X92.-)*
> *use of weapon (X93-X95, X99, Y00)*

The appropriate 7th character is to be added to each code from category Y04.
A   initial encounter
D   subsequent encounter
S   sequela

√x7ᵗʰ **Y04.0 Assault by unarmed brawl or fight**

√x7ᵗʰ **Y04.1 Assault by human bite**

√x7ᵗʰ **Y04.2 Assault by strike against or bumped into by another person**

√x7ᵗʰ **Y04.8 Assault by other bodily force**
Assault by bodily force NOS

√4ᵗʰ **Y07 Perpetrator of assault, maltreatment and neglect**

> NOTE   Codes from this category are for use only in cases of confirmed abuse (T74.-)
> Selection of the correct perpetrator code is based on the relationship between the perpetrator and the victim
> INCLUDES   perpetrator of abandonment
> perpetrator of emotional neglect
> perpetrator of mental cruelty
> perpetrator of physical abuse
> perpetrator of physical neglect
> perpetrator of sexual abuse
> perpetrator of torture

√5ᵗʰ **Y07.0 Spouse or partner, perpetrator of maltreatment and neglect**

> NOTE   Spouse or partner, perpetrator of maltreatment and neglect against spouse or partner

     Y07.01 Husband, perpetrator of maltreatment and neglect

     Y07.02 Wife, perpetrator of maltreatment and neglect

     Y07.03 Male partner, perpetrator of maltreatment and neglect

     Y07.04 Female partner, perpetrator of maltreatment and neglect

√5ᵗʰ **Y07.1 Parent (adoptive) (biological), perpetrator of maltreatment and neglect**

     Y07.11 Biological father, perpetrator of maltreatment and neglect

     Y07.12 Biological mother, perpetrator of maltreatment and neglect

     Y07.13 Adoptive father, perpetrator of maltreatment and neglect

     Y07.14 Adoptive mother, perpetrator of maltreatment and neglect

√5ᵗʰ **Y07.4 Other family member, perpetrator of maltreatment and neglect**

√6ᵗʰ **Y07.41 Sibling, perpetrator of maltreatment and neglect**

> EXCLUDES 1   *stepsibling, perpetrator of maltreatment and neglect (Y07.435, Y07.436)*

     Y07.410 Brother, perpetrator of maltreatment and neglect

     Y07.411 Sister, perpetrator of maltreatment and neglect

√6ᵗʰ **Y07.42 Foster parent, perpetrator of maltreatment and neglect**

     Y07.420 Foster father, perpetrator of maltreatment and neglect

     Y07.421 Foster mother, perpetrator of maltreatment and neglect

√6ᵗʰ **Y07.43 Stepparent or stepsibling, perpetrator of maltreatment and neglect**

     Y07.430 Stepfather, perpetrator of maltreatment and neglect

     Y07.432 Male friend of parent (co-residing in household), perpetrator of maltreatment and neglect

     Y07.433 Stepmother, perpetrator of maltreatment and neglect

     Y07.434 Female friend of parent (co-residing in household), perpetrator of maltreatment and neglect

     Y07.435 Stepbrother, perpetrator of maltreatment and neglect

     Y07.436 Stepsister, perpetrator of maltreatment and neglect

√6ᵗʰ **Y07.49 Other family member, perpetrator of maltreatment and neglect**

     Y07.490 Male cousin, perpetrator of maltreatment and neglect

     Y07.491 Female cousin, perpetrator of maltreatment and neglect

     Y07.499 Other family member, perpetrator of maltreatment and neglect

√5ᵗʰ **Y07.5 Non-family member, perpetrator of maltreatment and neglect**

     Y07.50 Unspecified non-family member, perpetrator of maltreatment and neglect

√6ᵗʰ **Y07.51 Daycare provider, perpetrator of maltreatment and neglect**

     Y07.510 At-home childcare provider, perpetrator of maltreatment and neglect

     Y07.511 Daycare center childcare provider, perpetrator of maltreatment and neglect

     Y07.512 At-home adultcare provider, perpetrator of maltreatment and neglect

     Y07.513 Adultcare center provider, perpetrator of maltreatment and neglect

     Y07.519 Unspecified daycare provider, perpetrator of maltreatment and neglect

√6ᵗʰ **Y07.52 Healthcare provider, perpetrator of maltreatment and neglect**

     Y07.521 Mental health provider, perpetrator of maltreatment and neglect

     Y07.528 Other therapist or healthcare provider, perpetrator of maltreatment and neglect
Nurse, perpetrator of maltreatment and neglect
Occupational therapist, perpetrator of maltreatment and neglect
Physical therapist, perpetrator of maltreatment and neglect
Speech therapist, perpetrator of maltreatment and neglect

     Y07.529 Unspecified healthcare provider, perpetrator of maltreatment and neglect

     Y07.53 Teacher or instructor, perpetrator of maltreatment and neglect
Coach, perpetrator of maltreatment and neglect

     Y07.59 Other non-family member, perpetrator of maltreatment and neglect

     Y07.9 Unspecified perpetrator of maltreatment and neglect

√4ᵗʰ **Y08 Assault by other specified means**

The appropriate 7th character is to be added to each code from category Y08.
A   initial encounter
D   subsequent encounter
S   sequela

√5ᵗʰ **Y08.0 Assault by strike by sport equipment**
√x7ᵗʰ **Y08.01 Assault by strike by hockey stick**
√x7ᵗʰ **Y08.02 Assault by strike by baseball bat**
√x7ᵗʰ **Y08.09 Assault by strike by other specified type of sport equipment**

√5ᵗʰ **Y08.8 Assault by other specified means**
√x7ᵗʰ **Y08.81 Assault by crashing of aircraft**
√x7ᵗʰ **Y08.89 Assault by other specified means**

Y09 Assault by unspecified means
Assassination (attempted) NOS   Manslaughter (attempted) NOS
Homicide (attempted) NOS   Murder (attempted) NOS

N Newborn: 0   P Pediatric: 0-17   M Maternity: 12-55   A Adult: 15-124   MCC Major CC Condition   PDx MCC PDx acts as own MCC   CC CC Condition   PDx CC PDx acts as own CC

Event of undetermined intent (Y21-Y33)

Undetermined intent is only for use when there is specific documentation in the record that the intent of the injury cannot be determined. If no such documentation is present, code to accidental (unintentional)

✓4ᵗʰ **Y21** **Drowning and submersion, undetermined intent**

> The appropriate 7th character is to be added to each code from category Y21.
> A   initial encounter
> D   subsequent encounter
> S   sequela

✓x7ᵗʰ **Y21.0** **Drowning and submersion while in bathtub, undetermined intent**

✓x7ᵗʰ **Y21.1** **Drowning and submersion after fall into bathtub, undetermined intent**

✓x7ᵗʰ **Y21.2** **Drowning and submersion while in swimming pool, undetermined intent**

✓x7ᵗʰ **Y21.3** **Drowning and submersion after fall into swimming pool, undetermined intent**

✓x7ᵗʰ **Y21.4** **Drowning and submersion in natural water, undetermined intent**

✓x7ᵗʰ **Y21.8** **Other drowning and submersion, undetermined intent**

✓x7ᵗʰ **Y21.9** **Unspecified drowning and submersion, undetermined intent**

✓x7ᵗʰ **Y22** **Handgun discharge, undetermined intent**
Discharge of gun for single hand use, undetermined intent
Discharge of pistol, undetermined intent
Discharge of revolver, undetermined intent
> EXCLUDES 2   Very pistol (Y24.8)

> The appropriate 7th character is to be added to code Y22.
> A   initial encounter
> D   subsequent encounter
> S   sequela

✓4ᵗʰ **Y23** **Rifle, shotgun and larger firearm discharge, undetermined intent**
> EXCLUDES 2   airgun (Y24.0)

> The appropriate 7th character is to be added to each code from category Y23.
> A   initial encounter
> D   subsequent encounter
> S   sequela

✓x7ᵗʰ **Y23.0** **Shotgun discharge, undetermined intent**

✓x7ᵗʰ **Y23.1** **Hunting rifle discharge, undetermined intent**

✓x7ᵗʰ **Y23.2** **Military firearm discharge, undetermined intent**

✓x7ᵗʰ **Y23.3** **Machine gun discharge, undetermined intent**

✓x7ᵗʰ **Y23.8** **Other larger firearm discharge, undetermined intent**

✓x7ᵗʰ **Y23.9** **Unspecified larger firearm discharge, undetermined intent**

✓4ᵗʰ **Y24** **Other and unspecified firearm discharge, undetermined intent**

> The appropriate 7th character is to be added to each code from category Y24.
> A   initial encounter
> D   subsequent encounter
> S   sequela

✓x7ᵗʰ **Y24.0** **Airgun discharge, undetermined intent**
BB gun discharge, undetermined intent
Pellet gun discharge, undetermined intent

✓x7ᵗʰ **Y24.8** **Other firearm discharge, undetermined intent**
Paintball gun discharge, undetermined intent
Very pistol [flare] discharge, undetermined intent

✓x7ᵗʰ **Y24.9** **Unspecified firearm discharge, undetermined intent**

✓x7ᵗʰ **Y25** **Contact with explosive material, undetermined intent**

> The appropriate 7th character is to be added to code Y25.
> A   initial encounter
> D   subsequent encounter
> S   sequela

✓x7ᵗʰ **Y26** **Exposure to smoke, fire and flames, undetermined intent**

> The appropriate 7th character is to be added to code Y26.
> A   initial encounter
> D   subsequent encounter
> S   sequela

✓4ᵗʰ **Y27** **Contact with steam, hot vapors and hot objects, undetermined intent**

> The appropriate 7th character is to be added to each code from category Y27.
> A   initial encounter
> D   subsequent encounter
> S   sequela

✓x7ᵗʰ **Y27.0** **Contact with steam and hot vapors, undetermined intent**

✓x7ᵗʰ **Y27.1** **Contact with hot tap water, undetermined intent**

✓x7ᵗʰ **Y27.2** **Contact with hot fluids, undetermined intent**

✓x7ᵗʰ **Y27.3** **Contact with hot household appliance, undetermined intent**

✓x7ᵗʰ **Y27.8** **Contact with other hot objects, undetermined intent**

✓x7ᵗʰ **Y27.9** **Contact with unspecified hot objects, undetermined intent**

✓4ᵗʰ **Y28** **Contact with sharp object, undetermined intent**

> The appropriate 7th character is to be added to each code from category Y28.
> A   initial encounter
> D   subsequent encounter
> S   sequela

✓x7ᵗʰ **Y28.0** **Contact with sharp glass, undetermined intent**

✓x7ᵗʰ **Y28.1** **Contact with knife, undetermined intent**

✓x7ᵗʰ **Y28.2** **Contact with sword or dagger, undetermined intent**

✓x7ᵗʰ **Y28.8** **Contact with other sharp object, undetermined intent**

✓x7ᵗʰ **Y28.9** **Contact with unspecified sharp object, undetermined intent**

✓x7ᵗʰ **Y29** **Contact with blunt object, undetermined intent**

> The appropriate 7th character is to be added to code Y29.
> A   initial encounter
> D   subsequent encounter
> S   sequela

✓x7ᵗʰ **Y30** **Falling, jumping or pushed from a high place, undetermined intent**
Victim falling from one level to another, undetermined intent

> The appropriate 7th character is to be added to code Y30.
> A   initial encounter
> D   subsequent encounter
> S   sequela

✓x7ᵗʰ **Y31** **Falling, lying or running before or into moving object, undetermined intent**

> The appropriate 7th character is to be added to code Y31.
> A   initial encounter
> D   subsequent encounter
> S   sequela

✓x7ᵗʰ **Y32** **Crashing of motor vehicle, undetermined intent**

> The appropriate 7th character is to be added to code Y32.
> A   initial encounter
> D   subsequent encounter
> S   sequela

✓x7ᵗʰ **Y33** **Other specified events, undetermined intent**

> The appropriate 7th character is to be added to code Y33.
> A   initial encounter
> D   subsequent encounter
> S   sequela

Legal intervention, operations of war, military operations, and terrorism (Y35-Y38)

✓4ᵗʰ **Y35** **Legal intervention**
> INCLUDES   any injury sustained as a result of an encounter with any law enforcement official, serving in any capacity at the time of the encounter, whether on-duty or off-duty. Includes: injury to law enforcement official, suspect and bystander

> The appropriate 7th character is to be added to each code from category Y35.
> A   initial encounter
> D   subsequent encounter
> S   sequela

✓5ᵗʰ **Y35.0** **Legal intervention involving firearm discharge**

✓ Additional Character Required   ✓x7ᵗʰ Xtension Alert   Unacceptable PDx   Manifestation   Hospital Acquired Condition   EXCLUDES 1 Not Coded Here   EXCLUDES 2 Not Included Here

ICD-10-CM Draft (2015)   1157

√6ᵗʰ **Y35.00 Legal intervention involving** unspecified firearm discharge
Legal intervention involving gunshot wound
Legal intervention involving shot NOS

√7ᵗʰ **Y35.001 Legal intervention involving unspecified firearm discharge,** law enforcement **official injured**

√7ᵗʰ **Y35.002 Legal intervention involving unspecified firearm discharge,** bystander **injured**

√7ᵗʰ **Y35.003 Legal intervention involving unspecified firearm discharge,** suspect **injured**

√6ᵗʰ **Y35.01 Legal intervention involving injury by** machine gun

√7ᵗʰ **Y35.011 Legal intervention involving injury by machine gun,** law enforcement **official injured**

√7ᵗʰ **Y35.012 Legal intervention involving injury by machine gun,** bystander **injured**

√7ᵗʰ **Y35.013 Legal intervention involving injury by machine gun,** suspect **injured**

√6ᵗʰ **Y35.02 Legal intervention involving injury by** handgun

√7ᵗʰ **Y35.021 Legal intervention involving injury by handgun,** law enforcement **official injured**

√7ᵗʰ **Y35.022 Legal intervention involving injury by handgun,** bystander **injured**

√7ᵗʰ **Y35.023 Legal intervention involving injury by handgun,** suspect **injured**

√6ᵗʰ **Y35.03 Legal intervention involving injury by** rifle pellet

√7ᵗʰ **Y35.031 Legal intervention involving injury by rifle pellet,** law enforcement **official injured**

√7ᵗʰ **Y35.032 Legal intervention involving injury by rifle pellet,** bystander **injured**

√7ᵗʰ **Y35.033 Legal intervention involving injury by rifle pellet,** suspect **injured**

√6ᵗʰ **Y35.04 Legal intervention involving injury by** rubber bullet

√7ᵗʰ **Y35.041 Legal intervention involving injury by rubber bullet,** law enforcement **official injured**

√7ᵗʰ **Y35.042 Legal intervention involving injury by rubber bullet,** bystander **injured**

√7ᵗʰ **Y35.043 Legal intervention involving injury by rubber bullet,** suspect **injured**

√6ᵗʰ **Y35.09 Legal intervention involving** other firearm discharge

√7ᵗʰ **Y35.091 Legal intervention involving other firearm discharge,** law enforcement **official injured**

√7ᵗʰ **Y35.092 Legal intervention involving other firearm discharge,** bystander **injured**

√7ᵗʰ **Y35.093 Legal intervention involving other firearm discharge,** suspect **injured**

√5ᵗʰ **Y35.1 Legal intervention involving** explosives

√6ᵗʰ **Y35.10 Legal intervention involving** unspecified explosives

√7ᵗʰ **Y35.101 Legal intervention involving unspecified explosives,** law enforcement **official injured**

√7ᵗʰ **Y35.102 Legal intervention involving unspecified explosives,** bystander **injured**

√7ᵗʰ **Y35.103 Legal intervention involving unspecified explosives,** suspect **injured**

√6ᵗʰ **Y35.11 Legal intervention involving injury by** dynamite

√7ᵗʰ **Y35.111 Legal intervention involving injury by dynamite,** law enforcement **official injured**

√7ᵗʰ **Y35.112 Legal intervention involving injury by dynamite,** bystander **injured**

√7ᵗʰ **Y35.113 Legal intervention involving injury by dynamite,** suspect **injured**

√6ᵗʰ **Y35.12 Legal intervention involving injury by** explosive shell

√7ᵗʰ **Y35.121 Legal intervention involving injury by explosive shell,** law enforcement **official injured**

√7ᵗʰ **Y35.122 Legal intervention involving injury by explosive shell,** bystander **injured**

√7ᵗʰ **Y35.123 Legal intervention involving injury by explosive shell,** suspect **injured**

√6ᵗʰ **Y35.19 Legal intervention involving** other explosives
Legal intervention involving injury by grenade
Legal intervention involving injury by mortar bomb

√7ᵗʰ **Y35.191 Legal intervention involving other explosives,** law enforcement **official injured**

√7ᵗʰ **Y35.192 Legal intervention involving other explosives,** bystander **injured**

√7ᵗʰ **Y35.193 Legal intervention involving other explosives,** suspect **injured**

√5ᵗʰ **Y35.2 Legal intervention involving** gas
Legal intervention involving asphyxiation by gas
Legal intervention involving poisoning by gas

√6ᵗʰ **Y35.20 Legal intervention involving** unspecified gas

√7ᵗʰ **Y35.201 Legal intervention involving unspecified gas,** law enforcement **official injured**

√7ᵗʰ **Y35.202 Legal intervention involving unspecified gas,** bystander **injured**

√7ᵗʰ **Y35.203 Legal intervention involving unspecified gas,** suspect **injured**

√6ᵗʰ **Y35.21 Legal intervention involving injury by** tear gas

√7ᵗʰ **Y35.211 Legal intervention involving injury by tear gas,** law enforcement **official injured**

√7ᵗʰ **Y35.212 Legal intervention involving injury by tear gas,** bystander **injured**

√7ᵗʰ **Y35.213 Legal intervention involving injury by tear gas,** suspect **injured**

√6ᵗʰ **Y35.29 Legal intervention involving** other gas

√7ᵗʰ **Y35.291 Legal intervention involving other gas,** law enforcement **official injured**

√7ᵗʰ **Y35.292 Legal intervention involving other gas,** bystander **injured**

√7ᵗʰ **Y35.293 Legal intervention involving other gas,** suspect **injured**

√5ᵗʰ **Y35.3 Legal intervention involving** blunt objects
Legal intervention involving being hit or struck by blunt object

√6ᵗʰ **Y35.30 Legal intervention involving** unspecified blunt objects

√7ᵗʰ **Y35.301 Legal intervention involving unspecified blunt objects,** law enforcement **official injured**

√7ᵗʰ **Y35.302 Legal intervention involving unspecified blunt objects,** bystander **injured**

√7ᵗʰ **Y35.303 Legal intervention involving unspecified blunt objects,** suspect **injured**

√6ᵗʰ **Y35.31 Legal intervention involving** baton

√7ᵗʰ **Y35.311 Legal intervention involving baton,** law enforcement **official injured**

√7ᵗʰ **Y35.312 Legal intervention involving baton,** bystander **injured**

√7ᵗʰ **Y35.313 Legal intervention involving baton,** suspect **injured**

√6ᵗʰ **Y35.39 Legal intervention involving** other blunt objects

√7ᵗʰ **Y35.391 Legal intervention involving other blunt objects,** law enforcement **official injured**

√7ᵗʰ **Y35.392 Legal intervention involving other blunt objects,** bystander **injured**

√7ᵗʰ **Y35.393 Legal intervention involving other blunt objects,** suspect **injured**

√5ᵗʰ **Y35.4 Legal intervention involving** sharp objects
Legal intervention involving being cut by sharp objects
Legal intervention involving being stabbed by sharp objects

√6ᵗʰ **Y35.40 Legal intervention involving** unspecified sharp objects

√7ᵗʰ **Y35.401 Legal intervention involving unspecified sharp objects,** law enforcement **official injured**

√7ᵗʰ **Y35.402 Legal intervention involving unspecified sharp objects,** bystander **injured**

√7ᵗʰ **Y35.403 Legal intervention involving unspecified sharp objects,** suspect **injured**

√6ᵗʰ **Y35.41 Legal intervention involving** bayonet

√7ᵗʰ **Y35.411 Legal intervention involving bayonet,** law enforcement **official injured**

N Newborn: 0   P Pediatric: 0-17   M Maternity: 12-55   A Adult: 15-124   MCC Major CC Condition   PDx MCC PDx acts as own MCC   CC CC Condition   PDx CC PDx acts as own CC

1158   ICD-10-CM Draft (2015)

✓7th **Y35.412** **Legal intervention involving bayonet, bystander injured**

✓7th **Y35.413** **Legal intervention involving bayonet, suspect injured**

✓6th **Y35.49** **Legal intervention involving other sharp objects**

    ✓7th **Y35.491** **Legal intervention involving other sharp objects, law enforcement official injured**

    ✓7th **Y35.492** **Legal intervention involving other sharp objects, bystander injured**

    ✓7th **Y35.493** **Legal intervention involving other sharp objects, suspect injured**

✓5th **Y35.8** **Legal intervention involving other specified means**

  ✓6th **Y35.81** **Legal intervention involving manhandling**

    ✓7th **Y35.811** **Legal intervention involving manhandling, law enforcement official injured**

    ✓7th **Y35.812** **Legal intervention involving manhandling, bystander injured**

    ✓7th **Y35.813** **Legal intervention involving manhandling, suspect injured**

  ✓6th **Y35.89** **Legal intervention involving other specified means**

    ✓7th **Y35.891** **Legal intervention involving other specified means, law enforcement official injured**

    ✓7th **Y35.892** **Legal intervention involving other specified means, bystander injured**

    ✓7th **Y35.893** **Legal intervention involving other specified means, suspect injured**

✓5th **Y35.9** **Legal intervention, means unspecified**

  ✓x7th **Y35.91** **Legal intervention, means unspecified, law enforcement official injured**

  ✓x7th **Y35.92** **Legal intervention, means unspecified, bystander injured**

  ✓x7th **Y35.93** **Legal intervention, means unspecified, suspect injured**

✓4th **Y36** **Operations of war**

  INCLUDES injuries to military personnel and civilians caused by war, civil insurrection, and peacekeeping missions

  EXCLUDES 1 *injury to military personnel occurring during peacetime military operations (Y37.-)*

     military vehicles involved in transport accidents with non-military vehicle during peacetime (V09.01, V09.21, V19.81, V29.81, V39.81, V49.81, V59.81, V69.81, V79.81)

The appropriate 7th character is to be added to each code from category Y36.
A   initial encounter
D   subsequent encounter
S   sequela

✓5th **Y36.0** **War operations involving explosion of marine weapons**

  ✓6th **Y36.00** **War operations involving explosion of unspecified marine weapon**

    War operations involving underwater blast NOS

    ✓7th **Y36.000** **War operations involving explosion of unspecified marine weapon, military personnel**

    ✓7th **Y36.001** **War operations involving explosion of unspecified marine weapon, civilian**

  ✓6th **Y36.01** **War operations involving explosion of depth-charge**

    ✓7th **Y36.010** **War operations involving explosion of depth-charge, military personnel**

    ✓7th **Y36.011** **War operations involving explosion of depth-charge, civilian**

  ✓6th **Y36.02** **War operations involving explosion of marine mine**

    War operations involving explosion of marine mine, at sea or in harbor

    ✓7th **Y36.020** **War operations involving explosion of marine mine, military personnel**

    ✓7th **Y36.021** **War operations involving explosion of marine mine, civilian**

  ✓6th **Y36.03** **War operations involving explosion of sea-based artillery shell**

    ✓7th **Y36.030** **War operations involving explosion of sea-based artillery shell, military personnel**

    ✓7th **Y36.031** **War operations involving explosion of sea-based artillery shell, civilian**

✓6th **Y36.04** **War operations involving explosion of torpedo**

  ✓7th **Y36.040** **War operations involving explosion of torpedo, military personnel**

  ✓7th **Y36.041** **War operations involving explosion of torpedo, civilian**

✓6th **Y36.05** **War operations involving accidental detonation of onboard marine weapons**

  ✓7th **Y36.050** **War operations involving accidental detonation of onboard marine weapons, military personnel**

  ✓7th **Y36.051** **War operations involving accidental detonation of onboard marine weapons, civilian**

✓6th **Y36.09** **War operations involving explosion of other marine weapons**

  ✓7th **Y36.090** **War operations involving explosion of other marine weapons, military personnel**

  ✓7th **Y36.091** **War operations involving explosion of other marine weapons, civilian**

✓5th **Y36.1** **War operations involving destruction of aircraft**

  ✓6th **Y36.10** **War operations involving unspecified destruction of aircraft**

    ✓7th **Y36.100** **War operations involving unspecified destruction of aircraft, military personnel**

    ✓7th **Y36.101** **War operations involving unspecified destruction of aircraft, civilian**

  ✓6th **Y36.11** **War operations involving destruction of aircraft due to enemy fire or explosives**

    War operations involving destruction of aircraft due to air to air missile

    War operations involving destruction of aircraft due to explosive placed on aircraft

    War operations involving destruction of aircraft due to rocket propelled grenade [RPG]

    War operations involving destruction of aircraft due to small arms fire

    War operations involving destruction of aircraft due to surface to air missile

    ✓7th **Y36.110** **War operations involving destruction of aircraft due to enemy fire or explosives, military personnel**

    ✓7th **Y36.111** **War operations involving destruction of aircraft due to enemy fire or explosives, civilian**

  ✓6th **Y36.12** **War operations involving destruction of aircraft due to collision with other aircraft**

    ✓7th **Y36.120** **War operations involving destruction of aircraft due to collision with other aircraft, military personnel**

    ✓7th **Y36.121** **War operations involving destruction of aircraft due to collision with other aircraft, civilian**

  ✓6th **Y36.13** **War operations involving destruction of aircraft due to onboard fire**

    ✓7th **Y36.130** **War operations involving destruction of aircraft due to onboard fire, military personnel**

    ✓7th **Y36.131** **War operations involving destruction of aircraft due to onboard fire, civilian**

  ✓6th **Y36.14** **War operations involving destruction of aircraft due to accidental detonation of onboard munitions and explosives**

    ✓7th **Y36.140** **War operations involving destruction of aircraft due to accidental detonation of onboard munitions and explosives, military personnel**

    ✓7th **Y36.141** **War operations involving destruction of aircraft due to accidental detonation of onboard munitions and explosives, civilian**

  ✓6th **Y36.19** **War operations involving other destruction of aircraft**

    ✓7th **Y36.190** **War operations involving other destruction of aircraft, military personnel**

    ✓7th **Y36.191** **War operations involving other destruction of aircraft, civilian**

✓ Additional Character Required   ✓x7th Xtension Alert   Unacceptable PDx   Manifestation   Hospital Acquired Condition   EXCLUDES 1 Not Coded Here   EXCLUDES 2 Not Included Here

ICD-10-CM Draft (2015)   1159

√5ᵗʰ **Y36.2 War operations involving** other **explosions and fragments**
> EXCLUDES 1 *war operations involving explosion of aircraft (Y36.1-)*
> *war operations involving explosion of marine weapons (Y36.0-)*
> *war operations involving explosion of nuclear weapons (Y36.5-)*
> *war operations involving explosion occurring after cessation of hostilities (Y36.8-)*

√6ᵗʰ **Y36.20 War operations involving** unspecified **explosion and fragments**
> War operations involving air blast NOS
> War operations involving blast NOS
> War operations involving blast fragments NOS
> War operations involving blast wave NOS
> War operations involving blast wind NOS
> War operations involving explosion NOS
> War operations involving explosion of bomb NOS

√7ᵗʰ **Y36.200 War operations involving unspecified explosion and fragments, military personnel**

√7ᵗʰ **Y36.201 War operations involving unspecified explosion and fragments, civilian**

√6ᵗʰ **Y36.21 War operations involving explosion of** aerial bomb

√7ᵗʰ **Y36.210 War operations involving explosion of aerial bomb, military personnel**

√7ᵗʰ **Y36.211 War operations involving explosion of aerial bomb, civilian**

√6ᵗʰ **Y36.22 War operations involving explosion of** guided missile

√7ᵗʰ **Y36.220 War operations involving explosion of guided missile, military personnel**

√7ᵗʰ **Y36.221 War operations involving explosion of guided missile, civilian**

√6ᵗʰ **Y36.23 War operations involving explosion of** improvised explosive device [IED]
> War operations involving explosion of person-borne improvised explosive device [IED]
> War operations involving explosion of vehicle-borne improvised explosive device [IED]
> War operations involving explosion of roadside improvised explosive device [IED]

√7ᵗʰ **Y36.230 War operations involving explosion of improvised explosive device [IED], military personnel**

√7ᵗʰ **Y36.231 War operations involving explosion of improvised explosive device [IED], civilian**

√6ᵗʰ **Y36.24 War operations involving explosion due to** accidental detonation and discharge of own munitions or munitions launch device

√7ᵗʰ **Y36.240 War operations involving explosion due to accidental detonation and discharge of own munitions or munitions launch device, military personnel**

√7ᵗʰ **Y36.241 War operations involving explosion due to accidental detonation and discharge of own munitions or munitions launch device, civilian**

√6ᵗʰ **Y36.25 War operations involving** fragments from munitions

√7ᵗʰ **Y36.250 War operations involving fragments from munitions, military personnel**

√7ᵗʰ **Y36.251 War operations involving fragments from munitions, civilian**

√6ᵗʰ **Y36.26 War operations involving fragments of** improvised explosive device [IED]
> War operations involving fragments of person-borne improvised explosive device [IED]
> War operations involving fragments of vehicle-borne improvised explosive device [IED]
> War operations involving fragments of roadside improvised explosive device [IED]

√7ᵗʰ **Y36.260 War operations involving fragments of improvised explosive device [IED], military personnel**

√7ᵗʰ **Y36.261 War operations involving fragments of improvised explosive device [IED], civilian**

√6ᵗʰ **Y36.27 War operations involving** fragments from weapons

√7ᵗʰ **Y36.270 War operations involving fragments from weapons, military personnel**

√7ᵗʰ **Y36.271 War operations involving fragments from weapons, civilian**

√6ᵗʰ **Y36.29 War operations involving** other **explosions and fragments**
> War operations involving explosion of grenade
> War operations involving explosions of land mine
> War operations involving shrapnel NOS

√7ᵗʰ **Y36.290 War operations involving other explosions and fragments, military personnel**

√7ᵗʰ **Y36.291 War operations involving other explosions and fragments, civilian**

√5ᵗʰ **Y36.3 War operations involving** fires, conflagrations and hot substances
> War operations involving smoke, fumes, and heat from fires, conflagrations and hot substances
> EXCLUDES 1 *war operations involving fires and conflagrations aboard military aircraft (Y36.1-)*
> *war operations involving fires and conflagrations aboard military watercraft (Y36.0-)*
> *war operations involving fires and conflagrations caused indirectly by conventional weapons (Y36.2-)*
> *war operations involving fires and thermal effects of nuclear weapons (Y36.53-)*

√6ᵗʰ **Y36.30 War operations involving** unspecified **fire, conflagration and hot substance**

√7ᵗʰ **Y36.300 War operations involving unspecified fire, conflagration and hot substance, military personnel**

√7ᵗʰ **Y36.301 War operations involving unspecified fire, conflagration and hot substance, civilian**

√6ᵗʰ **Y36.31 War operations involving** gasoline bomb
> War operations involving incendiary bomb
> War operations involving petrol bomb

√7ᵗʰ **Y36.310 War operations involving gasoline bomb, military personnel**

√7ᵗʰ **Y36.311 War operations involving gasoline bomb, civilian**

√6ᵗʰ **Y36.32 War operations involving** incendiary bullet

√7ᵗʰ **Y36.320 War operations involving incendiary bullet, military personnel**

√7ᵗʰ **Y36.321 War operations involving incendiary bullet, civilian**

√6ᵗʰ **Y36.33 War operations involving** flamethrower

√7ᵗʰ **Y36.330 War operations involving flamethrower, military personnel**

√7ᵗʰ **Y36.331 War operations involving flamethrower, civilian**

√6ᵗʰ **Y36.39 War operations involving other fires,** conflagrations and hot substances

√7ᵗʰ **Y36.390 War operations involving other fires, conflagrations and hot substances, military personnel**

√7ᵗʰ **Y36.391 War operations involving other fires, conflagrations and hot substances, civilian**

√5ᵗʰ **Y36.4 War operations involving firearm discharge and other forms of conventional warfare**

√6ᵗʰ **Y36.41 War operations involving** rubber bullets

√7ᵗʰ **Y36.410 War operations involving rubber bullets, military personnel**

√7ᵗʰ **Y36.411 War operations involving rubber bullets, civilian**

√6ᵗʰ **Y36.42 War operations involving** firearms pellets

√7ᵗʰ **Y36.420 War operations involving firearms pellets, military personnel**

√7ᵗʰ **Y36.421 War operations involving firearms pellets, civilian**

√6ᵗʰ **Y36.43 War operations involving** other **firearms discharge**
> War operations involving bullets NOS
> EXCLUDES 1 *war operations involving munitions fragments (Y36.25-)*
> *war operations involving incendiary bullets (Y36.32-)*

√7ᵗʰ **Y36.430 War operations involving other firearms discharge, military personnel**

N Newborn: 0   P Pediatric: 0-17   M Maternity: 12-55   A Adult: 15-124   MCC Major CC Condition   PDx MCC PDx acts as own MCC   CC CC Condition   PDx CC PDx acts as own CC

1160   ICD-10-CM Draft (2015)

☑7th **Y36.431** **War operations involving** other firearms discharge, civilian

☑6th **Y36.44** **War operations involving** unarmed hand to hand combat

> EXCLUDES 1   *war operations involving combat using blunt or piercing object (Y36.45-)*
> *war operations involving intentional restriction of air and airway (Y36.46-)*
> *war operations involving unintentional restriction of air and airway (Y36.47-)*

☑7th **Y36.440** **War operations involving unarmed hand to hand combat,** military personnel

☑7th **Y36.441** **War operations involving unarmed hand to hand combat,** civilian

☑6th **Y36.45** **War operations involving** combat using blunt or piercing object

☑7th **Y36.450** **War operations involving combat using blunt or piercing object,** military personnel

☑7th **Y36.451** **War operations involving combat using blunt or piercing object,** civilian

☑6th **Y36.46** **War operations involving** intentional restriction of air and airway

☑7th **Y36.460** **War operations involving intentional restriction of air and airway,** military personnel

☑7th **Y36.461** **War operations involving intentional restriction of air and airway,** civilian

☑6th **Y36.47** **War operations involving** unintentional restriction of air and airway

☑7th **Y36.470** **War operations involving unintentional restriction of air and airway,** military personnel

☑7th **Y36.471** **War operations involving unintentional restriction of air and airway,** civilian

☑6th **Y36.49** **War operations involving** other forms of conventional warfare

☑7th **Y36.490** **War operations involving other forms of conventional warfare,** military personnel

☑7th **Y36.491** **War operations involving other forms of conventional warfare,** civilian

☑5th **Y36.5** **War operations involving** nuclear weapons
> War operations involving dirty bomb NOS

☑6th **Y36.50** **War operations involving** unspecified effect of nuclear weapon

☑7th **Y36.500** **War operations involving unspecified effect of nuclear weapon,** military personnel

☑7th **Y36.501** **War operations involving unspecified effect of nuclear weapon,** civilian

☑6th **Y36.51** **War operations involving** direct blast effect of nuclear weapon
> War operations involving blast pressure of nuclear weapon

☑7th **Y36.510** **War operations involving direct blast effect of nuclear weapon,** military personnel

☑7th **Y36.511** **War operations involving direct blast effect of nuclear weapon,** civilian

☑6th **Y36.52** **War operations involving** indirect blast effect of nuclear weapon
> War operations involving being thrown by blast of nuclear weapon
> War operations involving being struck or crushed by blast debris of nuclear weapon

☑7th **Y36.520** **War operations involving indirect blast effect of nuclear weapon,** military personnel

☑7th **Y36.521** **War operations involving indirect blast effect of nuclear weapon,** civilian

☑6th **Y36.53** **War operations involving** thermal radiation effect of nuclear weapon
> War operations involving direct heat from nuclear weapon
> War operation involving fireball effects from nuclear weapon

☑7th **Y36.530** **War operations involving thermal radiation effect of nuclear weapon,** military personnel

☑7th **Y36.531** **War operations involving thermal radiation effect of nuclear weapon,** civilian

☑6th **Y36.54** **War operation involving** nuclear radiation effects of nuclear weapon
> War operation involving acute radiation exposure from nuclear weapon
> War operation involving exposure to immediate ionizing radiation from nuclear weapon
> War operation involving fallout exposure from nuclear weapon
> War operation involving secondary effects of nuclear weapons

☑7th **Y36.540** **War operation involving nuclear radiation effects of nuclear weapon,** military personnel

☑7th **Y36.541** **War operation involving nuclear radiation effects of nuclear weapon,** civilian

☑6th **Y36.59** **War operation involving** other effects of nuclear weapons

☑7th **Y36.590** **War operation involving other effects of nuclear weapons,** military personnel

☑7th **Y36.591** **War operation involving other effects of nuclear weapons,** civilian

☑5th **Y36.6** **War operations involving** biological weapons

☑6th **Y36.6X** **War operations involving** biological weapons

☑7th **Y36.6X0** **War operations involving biological weapons,** military personnel

☑7th **Y36.6X1** **War operations involving biological weapons,** civilian

☑5th **Y36.7** **War operations involving chemical weapons and other forms of unconventional warfare**

> EXCLUDES 1   *war operations involving incendiary devices (Y36.3-, Y36.5-)*

☑6th **Y36.7X** **War operations involving** chemical weapons and other forms of unconventional warfare

☑7th **Y36.7X0** **War operations involving chemical weapons and other forms of unconventional warfare,** military personnel

☑7th **Y36.7X1** **War operations involving chemical weapons and other forms of unconventional warfare,** civilian

☑5th **Y36.8** **War operations occurring** after cessation of hostilities
> War operations classifiable to categories Y36.0-Y36.8 but occurring after cessation of hostilities

☑6th **Y36.81** **Explosion of** mine **placed during war operations but exploding after cessation of hostilities**

☑7th **Y36.810** **Explosion of mine placed during war operations but exploding after cessation of hostilities,** military personnel

☑7th **Y36.811** **Explosion of mine placed during war operations but exploding after cessation of hostilities,** civilian

☑6th **Y36.82** **Explosion of** bomb **placed during war operations but exploding after cessation of hostilities**

☑7th **Y36.820** **Explosion of bomb placed during war operations but exploding after cessation of hostilities,** military personnel

☑7th **Y36.821** **Explosion of bomb placed during war operations but exploding after cessation of hostilities,** civilian

☑6th **Y36.88** Other **war operations occurring after cessation of hostilities**

☑7th **Y36.880** **Other war operations occurring after cessation of hostilities,** military personnel

☑7th **Y36.881** **Other war operations occurring after cessation of hostilities,** civilian

☑ Additional Character Required   ☑x7th Xtension Alert   Unacceptable PDx   Manifestation   Hospital Acquired Condition   EXCLUDES 1 Not Coded Here   EXCLUDES 2 Not Included Here

ICD-10-CM Draft (2015)   1161

External Causes of Morbidity

Y36.89–Y37.200

√6ᵗʰ **Y36.89** Unspecified war operations occurring after cessation of hostilities

    √7ᵗʰ **Y36.890** Unspecified war operations occurring after cessation of hostilities, military personnel

    √7ᵗʰ **Y36.891** Unspecified war operations occurring after cessation of hostilities, civilian

√5ᵗʰ **Y36.9 Other and unspecified war operations**

    √x7ᵗʰ **Y36.90** War operations, unspecified

    √x7ᵗʰ **Y36.91** War operations involving unspecified weapon of mass destruction [WMD]

    √x7ᵗʰ **Y36.92** War operations involving friendly fire

√4ᵗʰ **Y37 Military operations**

    INCLUDES injuries to military personnel and civilians occurring during peacetime on military property and during routine military exercises and operations

    EXCLUDES 1 military aircraft involved in aircraft accident with civilian aircraft (V97.81-)
        military vehicles involved in transport accident with civilian vehicle (V09.01, V09.21, V19.81, V29.81, V39.81, V49.81, V59.81, V69.81, V79.81)
        military watercraft involved in water transport accident with civilian watercraft (V94.81-)
        war operations (Y36.-)

> The appropriate 7th character is to be added to each code from category Y37.
> A   initial encounter
> D   subsequent encounter
> S   sequela

√5ᵗʰ **Y37.0 Military operations involving explosion of marine weapons**

    √6ᵗʰ **Y37.00 Military operations involving explosion of unspecified marine weapon**
        Military operations involving underwater blast NOS

        √7ᵗʰ **Y37.000** Military operations involving explosion of unspecified marine weapon, military personnel

        √7ᵗʰ **Y37.001** Military operations involving explosion of unspecified marine weapon, civilian

    √6ᵗʰ **Y37.01 Military operations involving explosion of depth-charge**

        √7ᵗʰ **Y37.010** Military operations involving explosion of depth-charge, military personnel

        √7ᵗʰ **Y37.011** Military operations involving explosion of depth-charge, civilian

    √6ᵗʰ **Y37.02 Military operations involving explosion of marine mine**
        Military operations involving explosion of marine mine, at sea or in harbor

        √7ᵗʰ **Y37.020** Military operations involving explosion of marine mine, military personnel

        √7ᵗʰ **Y37.021** Military operations involving explosion of marine mine, civilian

    √6ᵗʰ **Y37.03 Military operations involving explosion of sea-based artillery shell**

        √7ᵗʰ **Y37.030** Military operations involving explosion of sea-based artillery shell, military personnel

        √7ᵗʰ **Y37.031** Military operations involving explosion of sea-based artillery shell, civilian

    √6ᵗʰ **Y37.04 Military operations involving explosion of torpedo**

        √7ᵗʰ **Y37.040** Military operations involving explosion of torpedo, military personnel

        √7ᵗʰ **Y37.041** Military operations involving explosion of torpedo, civilian

    √6ᵗʰ **Y37.05 Military operations involving accidental detonation of onboard marine weapons**

        √7ᵗʰ **Y37.050** Military operations involving accidental detonation of onboard marine weapons, military personnel

        √7ᵗʰ **Y37.051** Military operations involving accidental detonation of onboard marine weapons, civilian

    √6ᵗʰ **Y37.09 Military operations involving explosion of other marine weapons**

        √7ᵗʰ **Y37.090** Military operations involving explosion of other marine weapons, military personnel

        √7ᵗʰ **Y37.091** Military operations involving explosion of other marine weapons, civilian

√5ᵗʰ **Y37.1 Military operations involving destruction of aircraft**

    √6ᵗʰ **Y37.10 Military operations involving unspecified destruction of aircraft**

        √7ᵗʰ **Y37.100** Military operations involving unspecified destruction of aircraft, military personnel

        √7ᵗʰ **Y37.101** Military operations involving unspecified destruction of aircraft, civilian

    √6ᵗʰ **Y37.11 Military operations involving destruction of aircraft due to enemy fire or explosives**
        Military operations involving destruction of aircraft due to air to air missile
        Military operations involving destruction of aircraft due to explosive placed on aircraft
        Military operations involving destruction of aircraft due to rocket propelled grenade [RPG]
        Military operations involving destruction of aircraft due to small arms fire
        Military operations involving destruction of aircraft due to surface to air missile

        √7ᵗʰ **Y37.110** Military operations involving destruction of aircraft due to enemy fire or explosives, military personnel

        √7ᵗʰ **Y37.111** Military operations involving destruction of aircraft due to enemy fire or explosives, civilian

    √6ᵗʰ **Y37.12 Military operations involving destruction of aircraft due to collision with other aircraft**

        √7ᵗʰ **Y37.120** Military operations involving destruction of aircraft due to collision with other aircraft, military personnel

        √7ᵗʰ **Y37.121** Military operations involving destruction of aircraft due to collision with other aircraft, civilian

    √6ᵗʰ **Y37.13 Military operations involving destruction of aircraft due to onboard fire**

        √7ᵗʰ **Y37.130** Military operations involving destruction of aircraft due to onboard fire, military personnel

        √7ᵗʰ **Y37.131** Military operations involving destruction of aircraft due to onboard fire, civilian

    √6ᵗʰ **Y37.14 Military operations involving destruction of aircraft due to accidental detonation of onboard munitions and explosives**

        √7ᵗʰ **Y37.140** Military operations involving destruction of aircraft due to accidental detonation of onboard munitions and explosives, military personnel

        √7ᵗʰ **Y37.141** Military operations involving destruction of aircraft due to accidental detonation of onboard munitions and explosives, civilian

    √6ᵗʰ **Y37.19 Military operations involving other destruction of aircraft**

        √7ᵗʰ **Y37.190** Military operations involving other destruction of aircraft, military personnel

        √7ᵗʰ **Y37.191** Military operations involving other destruction of aircraft, civilian

√5ᵗʰ **Y37.2 Military operations involving other explosions and fragments**

    EXCLUDES 1 military operations involving explosion of aircraft (Y37.1-)
        military operations involving explosion of marine weapons (Y37.0-)
        military operations involving explosion of nuclear weapons (Y37.5-)

    √6ᵗʰ **Y37.20 Military operations involving unspecified explosion and fragments**
        Military operations involving air blast NOS
        Military operations involving blast NOS
        Military operations involving blast fragments NOS
        Military operations involving blast wave NOS
        Military operations involving blast wind NOS
        Military operations involving explosion NOS
        Military operations involving explosion of bomb NOS

        √7ᵗʰ **Y37.200** Military operations involving unspecified explosion and fragments, military personnel

---

N Newborn: 0   P Pediatric: 0-17   M Maternity: 12-55   A Adult: 15-124   **MCC** Major CC Condition   **PDx MCC** PDx acts as own MCC   **CC** CC Condition   **PDx CC** PDx acts as own CC

1162   ICD-10-CM Draft (2015)

✓7th **Y37.201** Military operations involving unspecified explosion and fragments, civilian

✓6th **Y37.21** Military operations involving explosion of aerial bomb

✓7th **Y37.210** Military operations involving explosion of aerial bomb, military personnel

✓7th **Y37.211** Military operations involving explosion of aerial bomb, civilian

✓6th **Y37.22** Military operations involving explosion of guided missile

✓7th **Y37.220** Military operations involving explosion of guided missile, military personnel

✓7th **Y37.221** Military operations involving explosion of guided missile, civilian

✓6th **Y37.23** Military operations involving explosion of improvised explosive device [IED]
Military operations involving explosion of person-borne improvised explosive device [IED]
Military operations involving explosion of vehicle-borne improvised explosive device [IED]
Military operations involving explosion of roadside improvised explosive device [IED]

✓7th **Y37.230** Military operations involving explosion of improvised explosive device [IED], military personnel

✓7th **Y37.231** Military operations involving explosion of improvised explosive device [IED], civilian

✓6th **Y37.24** Military operations involving explosion due to accidental detonation and discharge of own munitions or munitions launch device

✓7th **Y37.240** Military operations involving explosion due to accidental detonation and discharge of own munitions or munitions launch device, military personnel

✓7th **Y37.241** Military operations involving explosion due to accidental detonation and discharge of own munitions or munitions launch device, civilian

✓6th **Y37.25** Military operations involving fragments from munitions

✓7th **Y37.250** Military operations involving fragments from munitions, military personnel

✓7th **Y37.251** Military operations involving fragments from munitions, civilian

✓6th **Y37.26** Military operations involving fragments of improvised explosive device [IED]
Military operations involving fragments of person-borne improvised explosive device [IED]
Military operations involving fragments of vehicle-borne improvised explosive device [IED]
Military operations involving fragments of roadside improvised explosive device [IED]

✓7th **Y37.260** Military operations involving fragments of improvised explosive device [IED], military personnel

✓7th **Y37.261** Military operations involving fragments of improvised explosive device [IED], civilian

✓6th **Y37.27** Military operations involving fragments from weapons

✓7th **Y37.270** Military operations involving fragments from weapons, military personnel

✓7th **Y37.271** Military operations involving fragments from weapons, civilian

✓6th **Y37.29** Military operations involving other explosions and fragments
Military operations involving explosion of grenade
Military operations involving explosions of land mine
Military operations involving shrapnel NOS

✓7th **Y37.290** Military operations involving other explosions and fragments, military personnel

✓7th **Y37.291** Military operations involving other explosions and fragments, civilian

✓5th **Y37.3** Military operations involving fires, conflagrations and hot substances
Military operations involving smoke, fumes, and heat from fires, conflagrations and hot substances

EXCLUDES 1   military operations involving fires and conflagrations aboard military aircraft (Y37.1-)
military operations involving fires and conflagrations aboard military watercraft (Y37.0-)
military operations involving fires and conflagrations caused indirectly by conventional weapons (Y37.2-)
military operations involving fires and thermal effects of nuclear weapons (Y36.53-)

✓6th **Y37.30** Military operations involving unspecified fire, conflagration and hot substance

✓7th **Y37.300** Military operations involving unspecified fire, conflagration and hot substance, military personnel

✓7th **Y37.301** Military operations involving unspecified fire, conflagration and hot substance, civilian

✓6th **Y37.31** Military operations involving gasoline bomb
Military operations involving incendiary bomb
Military operations involving petrol bomb

✓7th **Y37.310** Military operations involving gasoline bomb, military personnel

✓7th **Y37.311** Military operations involving gasoline bomb, civilian

✓6th **Y37.32** Military operations involving incendiary bullet

✓7th **Y37.320** Military operations involving incendiary bullet, military personnel

✓7th **Y37.321** Military operations involving incendiary bullet, civilian

✓6th **Y37.33** Military operations involving flamethrower

✓7th **Y37.330** Military operations involving flamethrower, military personnel

✓7th **Y37.331** Military operations involving flamethrower, civilian

✓6th **Y37.39** Military operations involving other fires, conflagrations and hot substances

✓7th **Y37.390** Military operations involving other fires, conflagrations and hot substances, military personnel

✓7th **Y37.391** Military operations involving other fires, conflagrations and hot substances, civilian

✓5th **Y37.4** Military operations involving firearm discharge and other forms of conventional warfare

✓6th **Y37.41** Military operations involving rubber bullets

✓7th **Y37.410** Military operations involving rubber bullets, military personnel

✓7th **Y37.411** Military operations involving rubber bullets, civilian

✓6th **Y37.42** Military operations involving firearms pellets

✓7th **Y37.420** Military operations involving firearms pellets, military personnel

✓7th **Y37.421** Military operations involving firearms pellets, civilian

✓6th **Y37.43** Military operations involving other firearms discharge
Military operations involving bullets NOS

EXCLUDES 1   military operations involving munitions fragments (Y37.25-)
military operations involving incendiary bullets (Y37.32-)

✓7th **Y37.430** Military operations involving other firearms discharge, military personnel

✓7th **Y37.431** Military operations involving other firearms discharge, civilian

✓6th **Y37.44** Military operations involving unarmed hand to hand combat

EXCLUDES 1   military operations involving combat using blunt or piercing object (Y37.45-)
military operations involving intentional restriction of air and airway (Y37.46-)
military operations involving unintentional restriction of air and airway (Y37.47-)

☑ Additional Character Required   ✓x7th *X*tension Alert   Unacceptable PDx   Manifestation   Hospital Acquired Condition   *EXCLUDES 1* Not Coded Here   *EXCLUDES 2* Not Included Here

✓7th **Y37.440** Military operations involving unarmed hand to hand combat, **military personnel**

✓7th **Y37.441** Military operations involving unarmed hand to hand combat, **civilian**

✓6th **Y37.45** Military operations involving **combat using blunt or piercing object**

✓7th **Y37.450** Military operations involving combat using blunt or piercing object, **military personnel**

✓7th **Y37.451** Military operations involving combat using blunt or piercing object, **civilian**

✓6th **Y37.46** Military operations involving **intentional restriction of air and airway**

✓7th **Y37.460** Military operations involving intentional restriction of air and airway, **military personnel**

✓7th **Y37.461** Military operations involving intentional restriction of air and airway, **civilian**

✓6th **Y37.47** Military operations involving **unintentional restriction of air and airway**

✓7th **Y37.470** Military operations involving unintentional restriction of air and airway, **military personnel**

✓7th **Y37.471** Military operations involving unintentional restriction of air and airway, **civilian**

✓6th **Y37.49** Military operations involving **other forms of conventional warfare**

✓7th **Y37.490** Military operations involving other forms of conventional warfare, **military personnel**

✓7th **Y37.491** Military operations involving other forms of conventional warfare, **civilian**

✓5th **Y37.5** Military operations involving **nuclear weapons**
Military operation involving dirty bomb NOS

✓6th **Y37.50** Military operations involving **unspecified effect** of nuclear weapon

✓7th **Y37.500** Military operations involving unspecified effect of nuclear weapon, **military personnel**

✓7th **Y37.501** Military operations involving unspecified effect of nuclear weapon, **civilian**

✓6th **Y37.51** Military operations involving **direct blast effect** of nuclear weapon
Military operations involving blast pressure of nuclear weapon

✓7th **Y37.510** Military operations involving direct blast effect of nuclear weapon, **military personnel**

✓7th **Y37.511** Military operations involving direct blast effect of nuclear weapon, **civilian**

✓6th **Y37.52** Military operations involving **indirect blast effect** of nuclear weapon
Military operations involving being thrown by blast of nuclear weapon
Military operations involving being struck or crushed by blast debris of nuclear weapon

✓7th **Y37.520** Military operations involving indirect blast effect of nuclear weapon, **military personnel**

✓7th **Y37.521** Military operations involving indirect blast effect of nuclear weapon, **civilian**

✓6th **Y37.53** Military operations involving **thermal radiation effect** of nuclear weapon
Military operations involving direct heat from nuclear weapon
Military operation involving fireball effects from nuclear weapon

✓7th **Y37.530** Military operations involving thermal radiation effect of nuclear weapon, **military personnel**

✓7th **Y37.531** Military operations involving thermal radiation effect of nuclear weapon, **civilian**

✓6th **Y37.54** Military operation involving **nuclear radiation effects of nuclear weapon**
Military operation involving acute radiation exposure from nuclear weapon
Military operation involving exposure to immediate ionizing radiation from nuclear weapon
Military operation involving fallout exposure from nuclear weapon
Military operation involving secondary effects of nuclear weapons

✓7th **Y37.540** Military operation involving nuclear radiation effects of nuclear weapon, **military personnel**

✓7th **Y37.541** Military operation involving nuclear radiation effects of nuclear weapon, **civilian**

✓6th **Y37.59** Military operation involving **other effects** of nuclear weapons

✓7th **Y37.590** Military operation involving other effects of nuclear weapons, **military personnel**

✓7th **Y37.591** Military operation involving other effects of nuclear weapons, **civilian**

✓5th **Y37.6** Military operations involving **biological weapons**

✓6th **Y37.6X** Military operations involving biological weapons

✓7th **Y37.6X0** Military operations involving biological weapons, **military personnel**

✓7th **Y37.6X1** Military operations involving biological weapons, **civilian**

✓5th **Y37.7** Military operations involving **chemical weapons and other forms of unconventional warfare**

EXCLUDES 1 military operations involving incendiary devices (Y36.3-, Y36.5-)

✓6th **Y37.7X** Military operations involving **chemical weapons and other forms of unconventional warfare**

✓7th **Y37.7X0** Military operations involving chemical weapons and other forms of unconventional warfare, **military personnel**

✓7th **Y37.7X1** Military operations involving chemical weapons and other forms of unconventional warfare, **civilian**

✓5th **Y37.9** Other and unspecified military operations

✓x7th **Y37.90** Military operations, **unspecified**

✓x7th **Y37.91** Military operations **involving unspecified weapon of mass destruction [WMD]**

✓x7th **Y37.92** Military operations involving **friendly fire**

✓4th **Y38 Terrorism**

NOTE These codes are for use to identify injuries resulting from the unlawful use of force or violence against persons or property to intimidate or coerce a Government, the civilian population, or any segment thereof, in furtherance of political or social objective.

Use additional code for place of occurrence (Y92.-)

The appropriate 7th character is to be added to each code from category Y38.
A initial encounter
D subsequent encounter
S sequela

✓5th **Y38.0** Terrorism involving explosion of marine weapons
Terrorism involving depth-charge
Terrorism involving marine mine
Terrorism involving mine NOS, at sea or in harbor
Terrorism involving sea-based artillery shell
Terrorism involving torpedo
Terrorism involving underwater blast

✓6th **Y38.0X** Terrorism involving explosion of **marine weapons**

✓7th **Y38.0X1** Terrorism involving explosion of marine weapons, **public safety official injured**

✓7th **Y38.0X2** Terrorism involving explosion of marine weapons, **civilian injured**

✓7th **Y38.0X3** Terrorism involving explosion of marine weapons, **terrorist injured**

✓5th **Y38.1 Terrorism involving destruction of aircraft**
    Terrorism involving aircraft burned
    Terrorism involving aircraft exploded
    Terrorism involving aircraft being shot down
    Terrorism involving aircraft used as a weapon

    ✓6th **Y38.1X Terrorism involving destruction of aircraft**

        ✓7th **Y38.1X1 Terrorism involving destruction of aircraft, public safety official injured**

        ✓7th **Y38.1X2 Terrorism involving destruction of aircraft, civilian injured**

        ✓7th **Y38.1X3 Terrorism involving destruction of aircraft, terrorist injured**

✓5th **Y38.2 Terrorism involving other explosions and fragments**
    Terrorism involving antipersonnel (fragments) bomb
    Terrorism involving blast NOS
    Terrorism involving explosion NOS
    Terrorism involving explosion of breech block
    Terrorism involving explosion of cannon block
    Terrorism involving explosion (fragments) of artillery shell
    Terrorism involving explosion (fragments) of bomb
    Terrorism involving explosion (fragments) of grenade
    Terrorism involving explosion (fragments) of guided missile
    Terrorism involving explosion (fragments) of land mine
    Terrorism involving explosion of mortar bomb
    Terrorism involving explosion of munitions
    Terrorism involving explosion (fragments) of rocket
    Terrorism involving explosion (fragments) of shell
    Terrorism involving shrapnel
    Terrorism involving mine NOS, on land

    EXCLUDES1 *terrorism involving explosion of nuclear weapon (Y38.5)*
        terrorism involving suicide bomber (Y38.81)

    ✓6th **Y38.2X Terrorism involving other explosions and fragments**

        ✓7th **Y38.2X1 Terrorism involving other explosions and fragments, public safety official injured**

        ✓7th **Y38.2X2 Terrorism involving other explosions and fragments, civilian injured**

        ✓7th **Y38.2X3 Terrorism involving other explosions and fragments, terrorist injured**

✓5th **Y38.3 Terrorism involving fires, conflagration and hot substances**
    Terrorism involving conflagration NOS
    Terrorism involving fire NOS
    Terrorism involving petrol bomb

    EXCLUDES1 *terrorism involving fire or heat of nuclear weapon (Y38.5)*

    ✓6th **Y38.3X Terrorism involving fires, conflagration and hot substances**

        ✓7th **Y38.3X1 Terrorism involving fires, conflagration and hot substances, public safety official injured**

        ✓7th **Y38.3X2 Terrorism involving fires, conflagration and hot substances, civilian injured**

        ✓7th **Y38.3X3 Terrorism involving fires, conflagration and hot substances, terrorist injured**

✓5th **Y38.4 Terrorism involving firearms**
    Terrorism involving carbine bullet
    Terrorism involving machine gun bullet
    Terrorism involving pellets (shotgun)
    Terrorism involving pistol bullet
    Terrorism involving rifle bullet
    Terrorism involving rubber (rifle) bullet

    ✓6th **Y38.4X Terrorism involving firearms**

        ✓7th **Y38.4X1 Terrorism involving firearms, public safety official injured**

        ✓7th **Y38.4X2 Terrorism involving firearms, civilian injured**

        ✓7th **Y38.4X3 Terrorism involving firearms, terrorist injured**

✓5th **Y38.5 Terrorism involving nuclear weapons**
    Terrorism involving blast effects of nuclear weapon
    Terrorism involving exposure to ionizing radiation from nuclear weapon
    Terrorism involving fireball effect of nuclear weapon
    Terrorism involving heat from nuclear weapon

    ✓6th **Y38.5X Terrorism involving nuclear weapons**

        ✓7th **Y38.5X1 Terrorism involving nuclear weapons, public safety official injured**

        ✓7th **Y38.5X2 Terrorism involving nuclear weapons, civilian injured**

        ✓7th **Y38.5X3 Terrorism involving nuclear weapons, terrorist injured**

✓5th **Y38.6 Terrorism involving biological weapons**
    Terrorism involving anthrax   Terrorism involving smallpox
    Terrorism involving cholera

    ✓6th **Y38.6X Terrorism involving biological weapons**

        ✓7th **Y38.6X1 Terrorism involving biological weapons, public safety official injured**

        ✓7th **Y38.6X2 Terrorism involving biological weapons, civilian injured**

        ✓7th **Y38.6X3 Terrorism involving biological weapons, terrorist injured**

✓5th **Y38.7 Terrorism involving chemical weapons**
    Terrorism involving gases, fumes, chemicals
    Terrorism involving hydrogen cyanide
    Terrorism involving phosgene
    Terrorism involving sarin

    ✓6th **Y38.7X Terrorism involving chemical weapons**

        ✓7th **Y38.7X1 Terrorism involving chemical weapons, public safety official injured**

        ✓7th **Y38.7X2 Terrorism involving chemical weapons, civilian injured**

        ✓7th **Y38.7X3 Terrorism involving chemical weapons, terrorist injured**

✓5th **Y38.8 Terrorism involving other and unspecified means**

    Y38.80 Terrorism involving unspecified means
        Terrorism NOS

    ✓6th **Y38.81 Terrorism involving suicide bomber**

        ✓7th **Y38.811 Terrorism involving suicide bomber, public safety official injured**

        Y38.812 Terrorism involving suicide bomber, civilian injured

    ✓6th **Y38.89 Terrorism involving other means**
        Terrorism involving drowning and submersion
        Terrorism involving lasers
        Terrorism involving piercing or stabbing instruments

        ✓7th **Y38.891 Terrorism involving other means, public safety official injured**

        ✓7th **Y38.892 Terrorism involving other means, civilian injured**

        ✓7th **Y38.893 Terrorism involving other means, terrorist injured**

✓5th **Y38.9 Terrorism, secondary effects**
    NOTE   This code is for use to identify injuries occurring subsequent to a terrorist attack, not those that are due to the initial terrorist attack.

    ✓6th **Y38.9X Terrorism, secondary effects**

        ✓7th **Y38.9X1 Terrorism, secondary effects, public safety official injured**

        ✓7th **Y38.9X2 Terrorism, secondary effects, civilian injured**

Complications of medical and surgical care (Y62-Y84)

INCLUDES   complications of medical devices
    surgical and medical procedures as the cause of abnormal reaction of the patient, or of later complication, without mention of misadventure at the time of the procedure

Misadventures to patients during surgical and medical care (Y62-Y69)

EXCLUDES2   *breakdown or malfunctioning of medical device (during procedure) (after implantation) (ongoing use) (Y70-Y82)*
    surgical and medical procedures as the cause of abnormal reaction of the patient, without mention of misadventure at the time of the procedure (Y83-Y84)

✓4th **Y62 Failure of sterile precautions during surgical and medical care**

    Y62.0 Failure of sterile precautions during surgical operation

    Y62.1 Failure of sterile precautions during infusion or transfusion

    Y62.2 Failure of sterile precautions during kidney dialysis and other perfusion

    Y62.3 Failure of sterile precautions during injection or immunization

    Y62.4 Failure of sterile precautions during endoscopic examination

☑ Additional Character Required   ✓x7th Xtension Alert   Unacceptable PDx   Manifestation   Hospital Acquired Condition   EXCLUDES1 Not Coded Here   EXCLUDES2 Not Included Here

ICD-10-CM Draft (2015)   1165

Y62.5   Failure of sterile precautions during heart catheterization

Y62.6   Failure of sterile precautions during aspiration, puncture and other catheterization

Y62.8   Failure of sterile precautions during other surgical and medical care

Y62.9   Failure of sterile precautions during unspecified surgical and medical care

✓4ᵗʰ **Y63**   **Failure in dosage during surgical and medical care**
> EXCLUDES 2   accidental overdose of drug or wrong drug given in error (T36-T50)

Y63.0   Excessive amount of blood or other fluid given during transfusion or infusion

Y63.1   Incorrect dilution of fluid used during infusion

Y63.2   Overdose of radiation given during therapy

Y63.3   Inadvertent exposure of patient to radiation during medical care

Y63.4   Failure in dosage in electroshock or insulin-shock therapy

Y63.5   Inappropriate temperature in local application and packing

Y63.6   Underdosing and nonadministration of necessary drug, medicament or biological substance

Y63.8   Failure in dosage during other surgical and medical care

Y63.9   Failure in dosage during unspecified surgical and medical care

✓4ᵗʰ **Y64**   **Contaminated medical or biological substances**

Y64.0   Contaminated medical or biological substance, transfused or infused

Y64.1   Contaminated medical or biological substance, injected or used for immunization

Y64.8   Contaminated medical or biological substance administered by other means

Y64.9   Contaminated medical or biological substance administered by unspecified means
> Administered contaminated medical or biological substance NOS

✓4ᵗʰ **Y65**   **Other misadventures during surgical and medical care**

Y65.0   Mismatched blood in transfusion

Y65.1   Wrong fluid used in infusion

Y65.2   Failure in suture or ligature during surgical operation

Y65.3   Endotracheal tube wrongly placed during anesthetic procedure

Y65.4   Failure to introduce or to remove other tube or instrument

✓5ᵗʰ **Y65.5**   Performance of wrong procedure (operation)

   11 **Y65.51**   Performance of wrong procedure (operation) on correct patient
> Wrong device implanted into correct surgical site
> EXCLUDES 1   performance of correct procedure (operation) on wrong side or body part (Y65.53)

   11 **Y65.52**   Performance of procedure (operation) on patient not scheduled for surgery
> Performance of procedure (operation) intended for another patient
> Performance of procedure (operation) on wrong patient

   11 **Y65.53**   Performance of correct procedure (operation) on wrong side or body part
> Performance of correct procedure (operation) on wrong side
> Performance of correct procedure (operation) on wrong site

Y65.8   Other specified misadventures during surgical and medical care

Y66   **Nonadministration of surgical and medical care**
> Premature cessation of surgical and medical care
> EXCLUDES 1   DNR status (Z66)
> palliative care (Z51.5)

Y69   **Unspecified misadventure during surgical and medical care**

Medical devices associated with adverse incidents in diagnostic and therapeutic use (Y70-Y82)

> INCLUDES   breakdown or malfunction of medical devices (during use) (after implantation) (ongoing use)
> EXCLUDES 1   misadventure to patients during surgical and medical care, classifiable to (Y62-Y69)
> later complications following use of medical devices without breakdown or malfunctioning of device (Y83-Y84)

✓4ᵗʰ **Y70**   **Anesthesiology devices associated with adverse incidents**

Y70.0   Diagnostic and monitoring anesthesiology devices associated with adverse incidents

Y70.1   Therapeutic (nonsurgical) and rehabilitative anesthesiology devices associated with adverse incidents

Y70.2   Prosthetic and other implants, materials and accessory anesthesiology devices associated with adverse incidents

Y70.3   Surgical instruments, materials and anesthesiology devices (including sutures) associated with adverse incidents

Y70.8   Miscellaneous anesthesiology devices associated with adverse incidents, not elsewhere classified

✓4ᵗʰ **Y71**   **Cardiovascular devices associated with adverse incidents**

Y71.0   Diagnostic and monitoring cardiovascular devices associated with adverse incidents

Y71.1   Therapeutic (nonsurgical) and rehabilitative cardiovascular devices associated with adverse incidents

Y71.2   Prosthetic and other implants, materials and accessory cardiovascular devices associated with adverse incidents

Y71.3   Surgical instruments, materials and cardiovascular devices (including sutures) associated with adverse incidents

Y71.8   Miscellaneous cardiovascular devices associated with adverse incidents, not elsewhere classified

✓4ᵗʰ **Y72**   **Otorhinolaryngological devices associated with adverse incidents**

Y72.0   Diagnostic and monitoring otorhinolaryngological devices associated with adverse incidents

Y72.1   Therapeutic (nonsurgical) and rehabilitative otorhinolaryngological devices associated with adverse incidents

Y72.2   Prosthetic and other implants, materials and accessory otorhinolaryngological devices associated with adverse incidents

Y72.3   Surgical instruments, materials and otorhinolaryngological devices (including sutures) associated with adverse incidents

Y72.8   Miscellaneous otorhinolaryngological devices associated with adverse incidents, not elsewhere classified

✓4ᵗʰ **Y73**   **Gastroenterology and urology devices associated with adverse incidents**

Y73.0   Diagnostic and monitoring gastroenterology and urology devices associated with adverse incidents

Y73.1   Therapeutic (nonsurgical) and rehabilitative gastroenterology and urology devices associated with adverse incidents

Y73.2   Prosthetic and other implants, materials and accessory gastroenterology and urology devices associated with adverse incidents

Y73.3   Surgical instruments, materials and gastroenterology and urology devices (including sutures) associated with adverse incidents

Y73.8   Miscellaneous gastroenterology and urology devices associated with adverse incidents, not elsewhere classified

✓4ᵗʰ **Y74**   **General hospital and personal-use devices associated with adverse incidents**

Y74.0   Diagnostic and monitoring general hospital and personal-use devices associated with adverse incidents

Y74.1   Therapeutic (nonsurgical) and rehabilitative general hospital and personal-use devices associated with adverse incidents

Y74.2   Prosthetic and other implants, materials and accessory general hospital and personal-use devices associated with adverse incidents

Y74.3   Surgical instruments, materials and general hospital and personal-use devices (including sutures) associated with adverse incidents

Y74.8   Miscellaneous general hospital and personal-use devices associated with adverse incidents, not elsewhere classified

---

11 Wrong procedure performed edit applies.

N Newborn: 0   P Pediatric: 0-17   M Maternity: 12-55   A Adult: 15-124   MCC Major CC Condition   PDx MCC PDx acts as own MCC   CC CC Condition   PDx CC PDx acts as own CC

1166   ICD-10-CM Draft (2015)

✓4ᵗʰ **Y75　Neurological devices associated with adverse incidents**

　Y75.0 Diagnostic and monitoring neurological devices associated with adverse incidents

　Y75.1 Therapeutic (nonsurgical) and rehabilitative neurological devices associated with adverse incidents

　Y75.2 Prosthetic and other implants, materials and neurological devices associated with adverse incidents

　Y75.3 Surgical instruments, materials and neurological devices (including sutures) associated with adverse incidents

　Y75.8 Miscellaneous neurological devices associated with adverse incidents, not elsewhere classified

✓4ᵗʰ **Y76　Obstetric and gynecological devices associated with adverse incidents**

　Y76.0 Diagnostic and monitoring obstetric and gynecological devices associated with adverse incidents　♀

　Y76.1 Therapeutic (nonsurgical) and rehabilitative obstetric and gynecological devices associated with adverse incidents　♀

　Y76.2 Prosthetic and other implants, materials and accessory obstetric and gynecological devices associated with adverse incidents　♀

　Y76.3 Surgical instruments, materials and obstetric and gynecological devices (including sutures) associated with adverse incidents　♀

　Y76.8 Miscellaneous obstetric and gynecological devices associated with adverse incidents, not elsewhere classified　♀

✓4ᵗʰ **Y77　Ophthalmic devices associated with adverse incidents**

　Y77.0 Diagnostic and monitoring ophthalmic devices associated with adverse incidents

　Y77.1 Therapeutic (nonsurgical) and rehabilitative ophthalmic devices associated with adverse incidents

　Y77.2 Prosthetic and other implants, materials and accessory ophthalmic devices associated with adverse incidents

　Y77.3 Surgical instruments, materials and ophthalmic devices (including sutures) associated with adverse incidents

　Y77.8 Miscellaneous ophthalmic devices associated with adverse incidents, not elsewhere classified

✓4ᵗʰ **Y78　Radiological devices associated with adverse incidents**

　Y78.0 Diagnostic and monitoring radiological devices associated with adverse incidents

　Y78.1 Therapeutic (nonsurgical) and rehabilitative radiological devices associated with adverse incidents

　Y78.2 Prosthetic and other implants, materials and accessory radiological devices associated with adverse incidents

　Y78.3 Surgical instruments, materials and radiological devices (including sutures) associated with adverse incidents

　Y78.8 Miscellaneous radiological devices associated with adverse incidents, not elsewhere classified

✓4ᵗʰ **Y79　Orthopedic devices associated with adverse incidents**

　Y79.0 Diagnostic and monitoring orthopedic devices associated with adverse incidents

　Y79.1 Therapeutic (nonsurgical) and rehabilitative orthopedic devices associated with adverse incidents

　Y79.2 Prosthetic and other implants, materials and accessory orthopedic devices associated with adverse incidents

　Y79.3 Surgical instruments, materials and orthopedic devices (including sutures) associated with adverse incidents

　Y79.8 Miscellaneous orthopedic devices associated with adverse incidents, not elsewhere classified

✓4ᵗʰ **Y80　Physical medicine devices associated with adverse incidents**

　Y80.0 Diagnostic and monitoring physical medicine devices associated with adverse incidents

　Y80.1 Therapeutic (nonsurgical) and rehabilitative physical medicine devices associated with adverse incidents

　Y80.2 Prosthetic and other implants, materials and accessory physical medicine devices associated with adverse incidents

　Y80.3 Surgical instruments, materials and physical medicine devices (including sutures) associated with adverse incidents

　Y80.8 Miscellaneous physical medicine devices associated with adverse incidents, not elsewhere classified

✓4ᵗʰ **Y81　General- and plastic-surgery devices associated with adverse incidents**

　Y81.0 Diagnostic and monitoring general- and plastic-surgery devices associated with adverse incidents

　Y81.1 Therapeutic (nonsurgical) and rehabilitative general- and plastic-surgery devices associated with adverse incidents

　Y81.2 Prosthetic and other implants, materials and accessory general- and plastic-surgery devices associated with adverse incidents

　Y81.3 Surgical instruments, materials and general- and plastic-surgery devices (including sutures) associated with adverse incidents

　Y81.8 Miscellaneous general- and plastic-surgery devices associated with adverse incidents, not elsewhere classified

✓4ᵗʰ **Y82　Other and unspecified medical devices associated with adverse incidents**

　Y82.8 Other medical devices associated with adverse incidents

　Y82.9 Unspecified medical devices associated with adverse incidents

Surgical and other medical procedures as the cause of abnormal reaction of the patient, or of later complication, without mention of misadventure at the time of the procedure (Y83-Y84)

> *EXCLUDES 1* misadventures to patients during surgical and medical care, classifiable to (Y62-Y69)

✓4ᵗʰ **Y83　Surgical operation and other surgical procedures as the cause of abnormal reaction of the patient, or of later complication, without mention of misadventure at the time of the procedure**

　Y83.0 Surgical operation with transplant of whole organ as the cause of abnormal reaction of the patient, or of later complication, without mention of misadventure at the time of the procedure

　Y83.1 Surgical operation with implant of artificial internal device as the cause of abnormal reaction of the patient, or of later complication, without mention of misadventure at the time of the procedure

　Y83.2 Surgical operation with anastomosis, bypass or graft as the cause of abnormal reaction of the patient, or of later complication, without mention of misadventure at the time of the procedure

　Y83.3 Surgical operation with formation of external stoma as the cause of abnormal reaction of the patient, or of later complication, without mention of misadventure at the time of the procedure

　Y83.4 Other reconstructive surgery as the cause of abnormal reaction of the patient, or of later complication, without mention of misadventure at the time of the procedure

　Y83.5 Amputation of limb(s) as the cause of abnormal reaction of the patient, or of later complication, without mention of misadventure at the time of the procedure

　Y83.6 Removal of other organ (partial) (total) as the cause of abnormal reaction of the patient, or of later complication, without mention of misadventure at the time of the procedure

　Y83.8 Other surgical procedures as the cause of abnormal reaction of the patient, or of later complication, without mention of misadventure at the time of the procedure

　Y83.9 Surgical procedure, unspecified as the cause of abnormal reaction of the patient, or of later complication, without mention of misadventure at the time of the procedure

✓4ᵗʰ **Y84　Other medical procedures as the cause of abnormal reaction of the patient, or of later complication, without mention of misadventure at the time of the procedure**

　Y84.0 Cardiac catheterization as the cause of abnormal reaction of the patient, or of later complication, without mention of misadventure at the time of the procedure

　Y84.1 Kidney dialysis as the cause of abnormal reaction of the patient, or of later complication, without mention of misadventure at the time of the procedure

　Y84.2 Radiological procedure and radiotherapy as the cause of abnormal reaction of the patient, or of later complication, without mention of misadventure at the time of the procedure

　Y84.3 Shock therapy as the cause of abnormal reaction of the patient, or of later complication, without mention of misadventure at the time of the procedure

　Y84.4 Aspiration of fluid as the cause of abnormal reaction of the patient, or of later complication, without mention of misadventure at the time of the procedure

　Y84.5 Insertion of gastric or duodenal sound as the cause of abnormal reaction of the patient, or of later complication, without mention of misadventure at the time of the procedure

---

✓ Additional Character Required　　✓x7ᵗʰ Xtension Alert　　Unacceptable PDx　　Manifestation　　Hospital Acquired Condition　　*EXCLUDES 1* Not Coded Here　　*EXCLUDES 2* Not Included Here

Y84.6 Urinary catheterization as the cause of abnormal reaction of the patient, or of later complication, without mention of misadventure at the time of the procedure

Y84.7 Blood-sampling as the cause of abnormal reaction of the patient, or of later complication, without mention of misadventure at the time of the procedure

Y84.8 Other medical procedures as the cause of abnormal reaction of the patient, or of later complication, without mention of misadventure at the time of the procedure

Y84.9 Medical procedure, unspecified as the cause of abnormal reaction of the patient, or of later complication, without mention of misadventure at the time of the procedure

Supplementary factors related to causes of morbidity classified elsewhere (Y90-Y99)

NOTE These categories may be used to provide supplementary information concerning causes of morbidity. They are not to be used for single-condition coding.

✓4th **Y90** Evidence of alcohol involvement determined by blood alcohol level

Code first any associated alcohol related disorders (F10)

Y90.0 Blood alcohol level of less than 20 mg/100 ml

Y90.1 Blood alcohol level of 20-39 mg/100 ml

Y90.2 Blood alcohol level of 40-59 mg/100 ml

Y90.3 Blood alcohol level of 60-79 mg/100 ml

Y90.4 Blood alcohol level of 80-99 mg/100 ml

Y90.5 Blood alcohol level of 100-119 mg/100 ml

Y90.6 Blood alcohol level of 120-199 mg/100 ml

Y90.7 Blood alcohol level of 200-239 mg/100 ml

Y90.8 Blood alcohol level of 240 mg/100 ml or more

Y90.9 Presence of alcohol in blood, level not specified

✓4th **Y92** Place of occurrence of the external cause

The following category is for use, when relevant, to identify the place of occurrence of the external cause. Use in conjunction with an activity code.

Place of occurrence should be recorded only at the initial encounter for treatment

✓5th **Y92.0** Non-institutional (private) residence as the place of occurrence of the external cause

EXCLUDES 1 abandoned or derelict house (Y92.89)
home under construction but not yet occupied (Y92.6-)
institutional place of residence (Y92.1-)

✓6th **Y92.00** Unspecified non-institutional (private) residence as the place of occurrence of the external cause

Y92.000 Kitchen of unspecified non-institutional (private) residence as the place of occurrence of the external cause

Y92.001 Dining room of unspecified non-institutional (private) residence as the place of occurrence of the external cause

Y92.002 Bathroom of unspecified non-institutional (private) residence single-family (private) house as the place of occurrence of the external cause

Y92.003 Bedroom of unspecified non-institutional (private) residence as the place of occurrence of the external cause

Y92.007 Garden or yard of unspecified non-institutional (private) residence as the place of occurrence of the external cause

Y92.008 Other place in unspecified non-institutional (private) residence as the place of occurrence of the external cause

Y92.009 Unspecified place in unspecified non-institutional (private) residence as the place of occurrence of the external cause
Home (NOS) as the place of occurrence of the external cause

✓6th **Y92.01** Single-family non-institutional (private) house as the place of occurrence of the external cause
Farmhouse as the place of occurrence of the external cause

EXCLUDES 1 barn (Y92.71)
chicken coop or hen house (Y92.72)
farm field (Y92.73)
orchard (Y92.74)
single family mobile home or trailer (Y92.02-)
slaughter house (Y92.86)

Y92.010 Kitchen of single-family (private) house as the place of occurrence of the external cause

Y92.011 Dining room of single-family (private) house as the place of occurrence of the external cause

Y92.012 Bathroom of single-family (private) house as the place of occurrence of the external cause

Y92.013 Bedroom of single-family (private) house as the place of occurrence of the external cause

Y92.014 Private driveway to single-family (private) house as the place of occurrence of the external cause

Y92.015 Private garage of single-family (private) house as the place of occurrence of the external cause

Y92.016 Swimming-pool in single-family (private) house or garden as the place of occurrence of the external cause

Y92.017 Garden or yard in single-family (private) house as the place of occurrence of the external cause

Y92.018 Other place in single-family (private) house as the place of occurrence of the external cause

Y92.019 Unspecified place in single-family (private) house as the place of occurrence of the external cause

✓6th **Y92.02** Mobile home as the place of occurrence of the external cause

Y92.020 Kitchen in mobile home as the place of occurrence of the external cause

Y92.021 Dining room in mobile home as the place of occurrence of the external cause

Y92.022 Bathroom in mobile home as the place of occurrence of the external cause

Y92.023 Bedroom in mobile home as the place of occurrence of the external cause

Y92.024 Driveway of mobile home as the place of occurrence of the external cause

Y92.025 Garage of mobile home as the place of occurrence of the external cause

Y92.026 Swimming-pool of mobile home as the place of occurrence of the external cause

Y92.027 Garden or yard of mobile home as the place of occurrence of the external cause

Y92.028 Other place in mobile home as the place of occurrence of the external cause

Y92.029 Unspecified place in mobile home as the place of occurrence of the external cause

✓6th **Y92.03** Apartment as the place of occurrence of the external cause
Condominium as the place of occurrence of the external cause
Co-op apartment as the place of occurrence of the external cause

Y92.030 Kitchen in apartment as the place of occurrence of the external cause

Y92.031 Bathroom in apartment as the place of occurrence of the external cause

Y92.032 Bedroom in apartment as the place of occurrence of the external cause

Y92.038 Other place in apartment as the place of occurrence of the external cause

Y92.039 Unspecified place in apartment as the place of occurrence of the external cause

✓6th **Y92.04** Boarding-house as the place of occurrence of the external cause

Y92.040 Kitchen in boarding-house as the place of occurrence of the external cause

Y92.041 Bathroom in boarding-house as the place of occurrence of the external cause

Y92.042 Bedroom in boarding-house as the place of occurrence of the external cause

Y92.043 Driveway of boarding-house as the place of occurrence of the external cause

Y92.044 Garage of boarding-house as the place of occurrence of the external cause

N Newborn: 0   P Pediatric: 0-17   M Maternity: 12-55   A Adult: 15-124   MCC Major CC Condition   PDx MCC PDx acts as own MCC   CC CC Condition   PDx CC PDx acts as own CC

1168   ICD-10-CM Draft (2015)

Y92.045 Swimming-pool of boarding-house as the place of occurrence of the external cause

Y92.046 Garden or yard of boarding-house as the place of occurrence of the external cause

Y92.048 Other place in boarding-house as the place of occurrence of the external cause

Y92.049 Unspecified place in boarding-house as the place of occurrence of the external cause

✓6ᵗʰ **Y92.09** Other non-institutional residence as the place of occurrence of the external cause

Y92.090 Kitchen in other non-institutional residence as the place of occurrence of the external cause

Y92.091 Bathroom in other non-institutional residence as the place of occurrence of the external cause

Y92.092 Bedroom in other non-institutional residence as the place of occurrence of the external cause

Y92.093 Driveway of other non-institutional residence as the place of occurrence of the external cause

Y92.094 Garage of other non-institutional residence as the place of occurrence of the external cause

Y92.095 Swimming-pool of other non-institutional residence as the place of occurrence of the external cause

Y92.096 Garden or yard of other non-institutional residence as the place of occurrence of the external cause

Y92.098 Other place in other non-institutional residence as the place of occurrence of the external cause

Y92.099 Unspecified place in other non-institutional residence as the place of occurrence of the external cause

✓5ᵗʰ **Y92.1** Institutional (nonprivate) residence as the place of occurrence of the external cause

Y92.10 Unspecified residential institution as the place of occurrence of the external cause

✓6ᵗʰ **Y92.11** Children's home and orphanage as the place of occurrence of the external cause

Y92.110 Kitchen in children's home and orphanage as the place of occurrence of the external cause

Y92.111 Bathroom in children's home and orphanage as the place of occurrence of the external cause

Y92.112 Bedroom in children's home and orphanage as the place of occurrence of the external cause

Y92.113 Driveway of children's home and orphanage as the place of occurrence of the external cause

Y92.114 Garage of children's home and orphanage as the place of occurrence of the external cause

Y92.115 Swimming-pool of children's home and orphanage as the place of occurrence of the external cause

Y92.116 Garden or yard of children's home and orphanage as the place of occurrence of the external cause

Y92.118 Other place in children's home and orphanage as the place of occurrence of the external cause

Y92.119 Unspecified place in children's home and orphanage as the place of occurrence of the external cause

✓6ᵗʰ **Y92.12** Nursing home as the place of occurrence of the external cause

Home for the sick as the place of occurrence of the external cause

Hospice as the place of occurrence of the external cause

Y92.120 Kitchen in nursing home as the place of occurrence of the external cause

Y92.121 Bathroom in nursing home as the place of occurrence of the external cause

Y92.122 Bedroom in nursing home as the place of occurrence of the external cause

Y92.123 Driveway of nursing home as the place of occurrence of the external cause

Y92.124 Garage of nursing home as the place of occurrence of the external cause

Y92.125 Swimming-pool of nursing home as the place of occurrence of the external cause

Y92.126 Garden or yard of nursing home as the place of occurrence of the external cause

Y92.128 Other place in nursing home as the place of occurrence of the external cause

Y92.129 Unspecified place in nursing home as the place of occurrence of the external cause

✓6ᵗʰ **Y92.13** Military base as the place of occurrence of the external cause

EXCLUDES 1 military training grounds (Y92.83)

Y92.130 Kitchen on military base as the place of occurrence of the external cause

Y92.131 Mess hall on military base as the place of occurrence of the external cause

Y92.133 Barracks on military base as the place of occurrence of the external cause

Y92.135 Garage on military base as the place of occurrence of the external cause

Y92.136 Swimming-pool on military base as the place of occurrence of the external cause

Y92.137 Garden or yard on military base as the place of occurrence of the external cause

Y92.138 Other place on military base as the place of occurrence of the external cause

Y92.139 Unspecified place military base as the place of occurrence of the external cause

✓6ᵗʰ **Y92.14** Prison as the place of occurrence of the external cause

Y92.140 Kitchen in prison as the place of occurrence of the external cause

Y92.141 Dining room in prison as the place of occurrence of the external cause

Y92.142 Bathroom in prison as the place of occurrence of the external cause

Y92.143 Cell of prison as the place of occurrence of the external cause

Y92.146 Swimming-pool of prison as the place of occurrence of the external cause

Y92.147 Courtyard of prison as the place of occurrence of the external cause

Y92.148 Other place in prison as the place of occurrence of the external cause

Y92.149 Unspecified place in prison as the place of occurrence of the external cause

✓6ᵗʰ **Y92.15** Reform school as the place of occurrence of the external cause

Y92.150 Kitchen in reform school as the place of occurrence of the external cause

Y92.151 Dining room in reform school as the place of occurrence of the external cause

Y92.152 Bathroom in reform school as the place of occurrence of the external cause

Y92.153 Bedroom in reform school as the place of occurrence of the external cause

Y92.154 Driveway of reform school as the place of occurrence of the external cause

Y92.155 Garage of reform school as the place of occurrence of the external cause

Y92.156 Swimming-pool of reform school as the place of occurrence of the external cause

Y92.157 Garden or yard of reform school as the place of occurrence of the external cause

Y92.158 Other place in reform school as the place of occurrence of the external cause

Y92.159 Unspecified place in reform school as the place of occurrence of the external cause

✓ Additional Character Required   ✓x7ᵗʰ Xtension Alert   Unacceptable PDx   Manifestation   Hospital Acquired Condition   EXCLUDES 1 Not Coded Here   EXCLUDES 2 Not Included Here

ICD-10-CM Draft (2015)   1169

External Causes of Morbidity

Y92.16–Y92.29

✓6ᵗʰ **Y92.16** **School dormitory** as the place of occurrence of the external cause

     EXCLUDES 1   *reform school as the place of occurrence of the external cause (Y92.15-)*
school buildings and grounds as the place of occurrence of the external cause (Y92.2-)
school sports and athletic areas as the place of occurrence of the external cause (Y92.3-)

     Y92.160 **Kitchen** in school dormitory as the place of occurrence of the external cause

     Y92.161 **Dining room** in school dormitory as the place of occurrence of the external cause

     Y92.162 **Bathroom** in school dormitory as the place of occurrence of the external cause

     Y92.163 **Bedroom** in school dormitory as the place of occurrence of the external cause

     Y92.168 **Other** place in school dormitory as the place of occurrence of the external cause

     Y92.169 **Unspecified** place in school dormitory as the place of occurrence of the external cause

✓6ᵗʰ **Y92.19** **Other specified residential institution** as the place of occurrence of the external cause

     Y92.190 **Kitchen** in other specified residential institution as the place of occurrence of the external cause

     Y92.191 **Dining room** in other specified residential institution as the place of occurrence of the external cause

     Y92.192 **Bathroom** in other specified residential institution as the place of occurrence of the external cause

     Y92.193 **Bedroom** in other specified residential institution as the place of occurrence of the external cause

     Y92.194 **Driveway** of other specified residential institution as the place of occurrence of the external cause

     Y92.195 **Garage** of other specified residential institution as the place of occurrence of the external cause

     Y92.196 **Pool** of other specified residential institution as the place of occurrence of the external cause

     Y92.197 **Garden or yard** of other specified residential institution as the place of occurrence of the external cause

     Y92.198 **Other** place in other specified residential institution as the place of occurrence of the external cause

     Y92.199 **Unspecified** place in other specified residential institution as the place of occurrence of the external cause

✓5ᵗʰ **Y92.2** **School, other institution and public administrative area** as the place of occurrence of the external cause

     Building and adjacent grounds used by the general public or by a particular group of the public

     EXCLUDES 1   *building under construction as the place of occurrence of the external cause (Y92.6)*
residential institution as the place of occurrence of the external cause (Y92.1)
school dormitory as the place of occurrence of the external cause (Y92.16-)
sports and athletics area of schools as the place of occurrence of the external cause (Y92.3-)

✓6ᵗʰ **Y92.21** **School (private) (public) (state)** as the place of occurrence of the external cause

     Y92.210 **Daycare center** as the place of occurrence of the external cause

     Y92.211 **Elementary school** as the place of occurrence of the external cause

        Kindergarten as the place of occurrence of the external cause

     Y92.212 **Middle school** as the place of occurrence of the external cause

     Y92.213 **High school** as the place of occurrence of the external cause

        AHA: 2012, 4Q, 108

     Y92.214 **College** as the place of occurrence of the external cause

        University as the place of occurrence of the external cause

     Y92.215 **Trade school** as the place of occurrence of the external cause

     Y92.218 **Other school** as the place of occurrence of the external cause

     Y92.219 **Unspecified** school as the place of occurrence of the external cause

Y92.22 **Religious institution** as the place of occurrence of the external cause

     Church as the place of occurrence of the external cause
     Mosque as the place of occurrence of the external cause
     Synagogue as the place of occurrence of the external cause

✓6ᵗʰ **Y92.23** **Hospital** as the place of occurrence of the external cause

     EXCLUDES 1   *ambulatory (outpatient) health services establishments (Y92.53-)*
home for the sick as the place of occurrence of the external cause (Y92.12-)
hospice as the place of occurrence of the external cause (Y92.12-)
nursing home as the place of occurrence of the external cause (Y92.12-)

     Y92.230 **Patient room** in hospital as the place of occurrence of the external cause

     Y92.231 **Patient bathroom** in hospital as the place of occurrence of the external cause

     Y92.232 **Corridor** of hospital as the place of occurrence of the external cause

     Y92.233 **Cafeteria** of hospital as the place of occurrence of the external cause

     Y92.234 **Operating room** of hospital as the place of occurrence of the external cause

     Y92.238 **Other** place in hospital as the place of occurrence of the external cause

     Y92.239 **Unspecified** place in hospital as the place of occurrence of the external cause

✓6ᵗʰ **Y92.24** **Public administrative building** as the place of occurrence of the external cause

     Y92.240 **Courthouse** as the place of occurrence of the external cause

     Y92.241 **Library** as the place of occurrence of the external cause

     Y92.242 **Post office** as the place of occurrence of the external cause

     Y92.243 **City hall** as the place of occurrence of the external cause

     Y92.248 **Other** public administrative building as the place of occurrence of the external cause

✓6ᵗʰ **Y92.25** **Cultural building** as the place of occurrence of the external cause

     Y92.250 **Art Gallery** as the place of occurrence of the external cause

     Y92.251 **Museum** as the place of occurrence of the external cause

     Y92.252 **Music hall** as the place of occurrence of the external cause

     Y92.253 **Opera house** as the place of occurrence of the external cause

     Y92.254 **Theater (live)** as the place of occurrence of the external cause

     Y92.258 **Other** cultural public building as the place of occurrence of the external cause

Y92.26 **Movie house or cinema** as the place of occurrence of the external cause

Y92.29 **Other** specified public building as the place of occurrence of the external cause

     Assembly hall as the place of occurrence of the external cause
     Clubhouse as the place of occurrence of the external cause

---

N Newborn: 0   P Pediatric: 0-17   M Maternity: 12-55   A Adult: 15-124   MCC Major CC Condition   PDx MCC PDx acts as own MCC   CC CC Condition   PDx CC PDx acts as own CC

1170   ICD-10-CM Draft (2015)

☑5ᵗʰ **Y92.3** **Sports and athletics area** as the place of occurrence of the external cause

  ☑6ᵗʰ **Y92.31** **Athletic court** as the place of occurrence of the external cause

    EXCLUDES 1 *tennis court in private home or garden (Y92.Ø9)*

    Y92.31Ø **Basketball court** as the place of occurrence of the external cause

    Y92.311 **Squash court** as the place of occurrence of the external cause

    Y92.312 **Tennis court** as the place of occurrence of the external cause

    Y92.318 **Other athletic court** as the place of occurrence of the external cause

  ☑6ᵗʰ **Y92.32** **Athletic field** as the place of occurrence of the external cause

    Y92.32Ø **Baseball field** as the place of occurrence of the external cause

    Y92.321 **Football field** as the place of occurrence of the external cause

    Y92.322 **Soccer field** as the place of occurrence of the external cause

    Y92.328 **Other athletic field** as the place of occurrence of the external cause

      Cricket field as the place of occurrence of the external cause

      Hockey field as the place of occurrence of the external cause

  ☑6ᵗʰ **Y92.33** **Skating rink** as the place of occurrence of the external cause

    Y92.33Ø **Ice skating rink** (indoor) (outdoor) as the place of occurrence of the external cause

    Y92.331 **Roller skating rink** as the place of occurrence of the external cause

  Y92.34 **Swimming pool (public)** as the place of occurrence of the external cause

    EXCLUDES 1 *swimming pool in private home or garden (Y92.Ø16)*

  Y92.39 **Other specified sports and athletic area** as the place of occurrence of the external cause

    Golf-course as the place of occurrence of the external cause

    Gymnasium as the place of occurrence of the external cause

    Riding-school as the place of occurrence of the external cause

    Stadium as the place of occurrence of the external cause

☑5ᵗʰ **Y92.4** **Street, highway and other paved roadways** as the place of occurrence of the external cause

    EXCLUDES 1 *private driveway of residence (Y92.Ø14, Y92.Ø24, Y92.Ø43, Y92.Ø93, Y92.113, Y92.123, Y92.154, Y92.194)*

  ☑6ᵗʰ **Y92.41** **Street and highway** as the place of occurrence of the external cause

    Y92.41Ø **Unspecified street and highway** as the place of occurrence of the external cause

      Road NOS as the place of occurrence of the external cause

    Y92.411 **Interstate highway** as the place of occurrence of the external cause

      Freeway as the place of occurrence of the external cause

      Motorway as the place of occurrence of the external cause

    Y92.412 **Parkway** as the place of occurrence of the external cause

    Y92.413 **State road** as the place of occurrence of the external cause

    Y92.414 **Local residential or business street** as the place of occurrence of the external cause

    Y92.415 **Exit ramp or entrance ramp** of street or highway as the place of occurrence of the external cause

  ☑6ᵗʰ **Y92.48** **Other paved roadways** as the place of occurrence of the external cause

    Y92.48Ø **Sidewalk** as the place of occurrence of the external cause

    Y92.481 **Parking lot** as the place of occurrence of the external cause

    Y92.482 **Bike path** as the place of occurrence of the external cause

    Y92.488 **Other paved roadways** as the place of occurrence of the external cause

☑5ᵗʰ **Y92.5** **Trade and service area** as the place of occurrence of the external cause

    EXCLUDES 1 *garage in private home (Y92.Ø15)*
      schools and other public administration buildings (Y92.2-)

  ☑6ᵗʰ **Y92.51** **Private commercial establishments** as the place of occurrence of the external cause

    Y92.51Ø **Bank** as the place of occurrence of the external cause

    Y92.511 **Restaurant** or **café** as the place of occurrence of the external cause

    Y92.512 **Supermarket**, **store** or **market** as the place of occurrence of the external cause

    Y92.513 **Shop (commercial)** as the place of occurrence of the external cause

  ☑6ᵗʰ **Y92.52** **Service areas** as the place of occurrence of the external cause

    Y92.52Ø **Airport** as the place of occurrence of the external cause

    Y92.521 **Bus station** as the place of occurrence of the external cause

    Y92.522 **Railway station** as the place of occurrence of the external cause

    Y92.523 **Highway rest stop** as the place of occurrence of the external cause

    Y92.524 **Gas station** as the place of occurrence of the external cause

      Petroleum station as the place of occurrence of the external cause

      Service station as the place of occurrence of the external cause

  ☑6ᵗʰ **Y92.53** **Ambulatory health services establishments** as the place of occurrence of the external cause

    Y92.53Ø **Ambulatory surgery center** as the place of occurrence of the external cause

      Outpatient surgery center, including that connected with a hospital as the place of occurrence of the external cause

      Same day surgery center, including that connected with a hospital as the place of occurrence of the external cause

    Y92.531 **Health care provider office** as the place of occurrence of the external cause

      Physician office as the place of occurrence of the external cause

    Y92.532 **Urgent care center** as the place of occurrence of the external cause

    Y92.538 **Other ambulatory health services establishments** as the place of occurrence of the external cause

  Y92.59 **Other trade areas** as the place of occurrence of the external cause

    Office building as the place of occurrence of the external cause

    Casino as the place of occurrence of the external cause

    Garage (commercial) as the place of occurrence of the external cause

    Hotel as the place of occurrence of the external cause

    Radio or television station as the place of occurrence of the external cause

    Shopping mall as the place of occurrence of the external cause

    Warehouse as the place of occurrence of the external cause

☑5ᵗʰ **Y92.6** **Industrial and construction area** as the place of occurrence of the external cause

  Y92.61 **Building [any] under construction** as the place of occurrence of the external cause

  Y92.62 **Dock or shipyard** as the place of occurrence of the external cause

    Dockyard as the place of occurrence of the external cause

    Dry dock as the place of occurrence of the external cause

    Shipyard as the place of occurrence of the external cause

---

☑ Additional Character Required   √x7ᵗʰ Xtension Alert   Unacceptable PDx   Manifestation   Hospital Acquired Condition   EXCLUDES 1 Not Coded Here   EXCLUDES 2 Not Included Here

External Causes of Morbidity

Y92.63–Y93.14

Y92.63   **Factory as the place of occurrence of the external cause**
> Factory building as the place of occurrence of the external cause
> Factory premises as the place of occurrence of the external cause
> Industrial yard as the place of occurrence of the external cause

Y92.64   **Mine or pit as the place of occurrence of the external cause**
> Mine as the place of occurrence of the external cause

Y92.65   **Oil rig as the place of occurrence of the external cause**
> Pit (coal) (gravel) (sand) as the place of occurrence of the external cause

Y92.69   **Other specified industrial and construction area as the place of occurrence of the external cause**
> Gasworks as the place of occurrence of the external cause
> Power-station (coal) (nuclear) (oil) as the place of occurrence of the external cause
> Tunnel under construction as the place of occurrence of the external cause
> Workshop as the place of occurrence of the external cause

✓5th **Y92.7**   **Farm as the place of occurrence of the external cause**
> Ranch as the place of occurrence of the external cause
> EXCLUDES 1   *farmhouse and home premises of farm (Y92.01-)*

Y92.71   **Barn as the place of occurrence of the external cause**

Y92.72   **Chicken coop as the place of occurrence of the external cause**
> Hen house as the place of occurrence of the external cause

Y92.73   **Farm field as the place of occurrence of the external cause**

Y92.74   **Orchard as the place of occurrence of the external cause**

Y92.79   **Other farm location as the place of occurrence of the external cause**

✓5th **Y92.8**   **Other places as the place of occurrence of the external cause**

✓6th **Y92.81**   **Transport vehicle as the place of occurrence of the external cause**
> EXCLUDES 1   *transport accidents (V00-V99)*

Y92.810   **Car as the place of occurrence of the external cause**

Y92.811   **Bus as the place of occurrence of the external cause**

Y92.812   **Truck as the place of occurrence of the external cause**

Y92.813   **Airplane as the place of occurrence of the external cause**

Y92.814   **Boat as the place of occurrence of the external cause**

Y92.815   **Train as the place of occurrence of the external cause**

Y92.816   **Subway car as the place of occurrence of the external cause**

Y92.818   **Other transport vehicle as the place of occurrence of the external cause**

✓6th **Y92.82**   **Wilderness area**

Y92.820   **Desert as the place of occurrence of the external cause**

Y92.821   **Forest as the place of occurrence of the external cause**

Y92.828   **Other wilderness area as the place of occurrence of the external cause**
> Swamp as the place of occurrence of the external cause
> Mountain as the place of occurrence of the external cause
> Marsh as the place of occurrence of the external cause
> Prairie as the place of occurrence of the external cause

✓6th **Y92.83**   **Recreation area as the place of occurrence of the external cause**

Y92.830   **Public park as the place of occurrence of the external cause**

Y92.831   **Amusement park as the place of occurrence of the external cause**

Y92.832   **Beach as the place of occurrence of the external cause**
> Seashore as the place of occurrence of the external cause

Y92.833   **Campsite as the place of occurrence of the external cause**

Y92.834   **Zoological garden (Zoo) as the place of occurrence of the external cause**

Y92.838   **Other recreation area as the place of occurrence of the external cause**

Y92.84   **Military training ground as the place of occurrence of the external cause**

Y92.85   **Railroad track as the place of occurrence of the external cause**

Y92.86   **Slaughter house as the place of occurrence of the external cause**

Y92.89   **Other specified places as the place of occurrence of the external cause**
> Derelict house as the place of occurrence of the external cause

Y92.9   **Unspecified place or not applicable**

✓4th **Y93**   **Activity codes**
> NOTE   Category Y93 is provided for use to indicate the activity of the person seeking healthcare for an injury or health condition, such as a heart attack while shoveling snow, which resulted from, or was contributed to, by the activity. These codes are appropriate for use for both acute injuries, such as those from chapter 19, and conditions that are due to the long-term, cumulative effects of an activity, such as those from chapter 13. They are also appropriate for use with external cause codes for cause and intent if identifying the activity provides additional information on the event. These codes should be used in conjunction with codes for external cause status (Y99) and place of occurrence (Y92).
> This section contains the following broad activity categories:
> Y93.0   Activities involving walking and running
> Y93.1   Activities involving water and water craft
> Y93.2   Activities involving ice and snow
> Y93.3   Activities involving climbing, rappelling, and jumping off
> Y93.4   Activities involving dancing and other rhythmic movement
> Y93.5   Activities involving other sports and athletics played individually
> Y93.6   Activities involving other sports and athletics played as a team or group
> Y93.7   Activities involving other specified sports and athletics
> Y93.A   Activities involving other cardiorespiratory exercise
> Y93.B   Activities involving other muscle strengthening exercises
> Y93.C   Activities involving computer technology and electronic devices
> Y93.D   Activities involving arts and handcrafts
> Y93.E   Activities involving personal hygiene and interior property and clothing maintenance
> Y93.F   Activities involving caregiving
> Y93.G   Activities involving food preparation, cooking and grilling
> Y93.H   Activities involving exterior property and land maintenance, building and construction
> Y93.I   Activities involving roller coasters and other types of external motion
> Y93.J   Activities involving playing musical instrument
> Y93.K   Activities involving animal care
> Y93.8   Activities, other specified
> Y93.9   Activity, unspecified

✓5th **Y93.0**   **Activities involving walking and running**
> EXCLUDES 1   *activity, walking an animal (Y93.K1)*
> *activity, walking or running on a treadmill (Y93.A1)*

Y93.01   **Activity, walking, marching and hiking**
> Activity, walking, marching and hiking on level or elevated terrain
> EXCLUDES 1   *activity, mountain climbing (Y93.31)*

Y93.02   **Activity, running**

✓5th **Y93.1**   **Activities involving water and water craft**
> EXCLUDES 1   *activities involving ice (Y93.2-)*

Y93.11   **Activity, swimming**

Y93.12   **Activity, springboard and platform diving**

Y93.13   **Activity, water polo**

Y93.14   **Activity, water aerobics and water exercise**

N Newborn: 0   P Pediatric: 0-17   M Maternity: 12-55   A Adult: 15-124   MCC Major CC Condition   PDx MCC PDx acts as own MCC   CC CC Condition   PDx CC PDx acts as own CC

1172   ICD-10-CM Draft (2015)

Y93.15   **Activity, underwater diving and snorkeling**
Activity, SCUBA diving

Y93.16   **Activity, rowing, canoeing, kayaking, rafting and tubing**
Activity, canoeing, kayaking, rafting and tubing in calm and turbulent water

Y93.17   **Activity, water skiing and wake boarding**

Y93.18   **Activity, surfing, windsurfing and boogie boarding**
Activity, water sliding

Y93.19   **Activity, other involving water and watercraft**
Activity involving water NOS
Activity, parasailing
Activity, water survival training and testing

√5th **Y93.2   Activities involving ice and snow**
EXCLUDES 1   *activity, shoveling ice and snow (Y93.H1)*

Y93.21   **Activity, ice skating**
Activity, figure skating (singles) (pairs)
Activity, ice dancing
EXCLUDES 1   *activity, ice hockey (Y93.22)*

Y93.22   **Activity, ice hockey**

Y93.23   **Activity, snow (alpine) (downhill) skiing, snow boarding, sledding, tobogganing and snow tubing**
EXCLUDES 1   *activity, cross country skiing (Y93.24)*

Y93.24   **Activity, cross country skiing**
Activity, nordic skiing

Y93.29   **Activity, other involving ice and snow**
Activity involving ice and snow NOS

√5th **Y93.3   Activities involving climbing, rappelling and jumping off**
EXCLUDES 1   *activity, hiking on level or elevated terrain (Y93.01)*
activity, jumping rope (Y93.56)
activity, trampoline jumping (Y93.44)

Y93.31   **Activity, mountain climbing, rock climbing and wall climbing**

Y93.32   **Activity, rappelling**

Y93.33   **Activity, BASE jumping**
Activity, Building, Antenna, Span, Earth jumping

Y93.34   **Activity, bungee jumping**

Y93.35   **Activity, hang gliding**

Y93.39   **Activity, other involving climbing, rappelling and jumping off**

√5th **Y93.4   Activities involving dancing and other rhythmic movement**
EXCLUDES 1   *activity, martial arts (Y93.75)*

Y93.41   **Activity, dancing**
AHA: 2012, 4Q, 108

Y93.42   **Activity, yoga**

Y93.43   **Activity, gymnastics**
Activity, rhythmic gymnastics
EXCLUDES 1   *activity, trampolining (Y93.44)*

Y93.44   **Activity, trampolining**

Y93.45   **Activity, cheerleading**

Y93.49   **Activity, other involving dancing and other rhythmic movements**

√5th **Y93.5   Activities involving other sports and athletics played individually**
EXCLUDES 1   *activity, dancing (Y93.41)*
activity, gymnastic (Y93.43)
activity, trampolining (Y93.44)
activity, yoga (Y93.42)

Y93.51   **Activity, roller skating (inline) and skateboarding**

Y93.52   **Activity, horseback riding**

Y93.53   **Activity, golf**

Y93.54   **Activity, bowling**

Y93.55   **Activity, bike riding**

Y93.56   **Activity, jumping rope**

Y93.57   **Activity, non-running track and field events**
EXCLUDES 1   *activity, running (any form) (Y93.02)*

Y93.59   **Activity, other involving other sports and athletics played individually**
EXCLUDES 1   *activities involving climbing, rappelling, and jumping (Y93.3-)*
activities involving ice and snow (Y93.2-)
activities involving walking and running (Y93.0-)
activities involving water and watercraft (Y93.1-)

√5th **Y93.6   Activities involving other sports and athletics played as a team or group**
EXCLUDES 1   *activity, ice hockey (Y93.22)*
activity, water polo (Y93.13)

Y93.61   **Activity, American tackle football**
Activity, football NOS

Y93.62   **Activity, American flag or touch football**

Y93.63   **Activity, rugby**

Y93.64   **Activity, baseball**
Activity, softball

Y93.65   **Activity, lacrosse and field hockey**

Y93.66   **Activity, soccer**

Y93.67   **Activity, basketball**

Y93.68   **Activity, volleyball (beach) (court)**

Y93.6A   **Activity, physical games generally associated with school recess, summer camp and children** [P]
Activity, capture the flag   Activity, four square
Activity, dodge ball   Activity, kickball

Y93.69   **Activity, other involving other sports and athletics played as a team or group**
Activity, cricket

√5th **Y93.7   Activities involving other specified sports and athletics**

Y93.71   **Activity, boxing**

Y93.72   **Activity, wrestling**

Y93.73   **Activity, racquet and hand sports**
Activity, handball   Activity, squash
Activity, racquetball   Activity, tennis

Y93.74   **Activity, frisbee**
Activity, ultimate frisbee

Y93.75   **Activity, martial arts**
Activity, combatives

Y93.79   **Activity, other specified sports and athletics**
EXCLUDES 1   *sports and athletics activities specified in categories Y93.0-Y93.6*

√5th **Y93.A   Activities involving other cardiorespiratory exercise**
Activities involving physical training

Y93.A1   **Activity, exercise machines primarily for cardiorespiratory conditioning**
Activity, elliptical and stepper machines
Activity, stationary bike
Activity, treadmill

Y93.A2   **Activity, calisthenics**
Activity, jumping jacks
Activity, warm up and cool down

Y93.A3   **Activity, aerobic and step exercise**

Y93.A4   **Activity, circuit training**

Y93.A5   **Activity, obstacle course**
Activity, challenge course
Activity, confidence course

Y93.A6   **Activity, grass drills**
Activity, guerilla drills

Y93.A9   **Activity, other involving cardiorespiratory exercise**
EXCLUDES 1   *activities involving cardiorespiratory exercise specified in categories Y93.0-Y93.7*

√5th **Y93.B   Activities involving other muscle strengthening exercises**

Y93.B1   **Activity, exercise machines primarily for muscle strengthening**

Y93.B2   **Activity, push-ups, pull-ups, sit-ups**

Y93.B3   **Activity, free weights**
Activity, barbells   Activity, dumbbells

Y93.B4   **Activity, pilates**

Y93.B9   **Activity, other involving muscle strengthening exercises**
EXCLUDES 1   *activities involving muscle strengthening specified in categories Y93.0-Y93.A*

√5th **Y93.C   Activities involving computer technology and electronic devices**
EXCLUDES 1   *activity, electronic musical keyboard or instruments (Y93.J-)*

Y93.C1   **Activity, computer keyboarding**
Activity, electronic game playing using keyboard or other stationary device

☑ Additional Character Required   √x7th *X*tension Alert   Unacceptable PDx   Manifestation   Hospital Acquired Condition   EXCLUDES 1 Not Coded Here   EXCLUDES 2 Not Included Here

ICD-10-CM Draft (2015)   1173

External Causes of Morbidity

Y93.C2–Y99.9

Y93.C2 **Activity, hand held interactive electronic device**
Activity, cellular telephone and communication device
Activity, electronic game playing using interactive device
> **EXCLUDES 1** *activity, electronic game playing using keyboard or other stationary device (Y93.C1)*

Y93.C9 **Activity, other involving computer technology and electronic devices**

✓5th **Y93.D** **Activities involving arts and handcrafts**
> **EXCLUDES 1** *activities involving playing musical instrument (Y93.J-)*

Y93.D1 **Activity, knitting and crocheting**

Y93.D2 **Activity, sewing**

Y93.D3 **Activity, furniture building and finishing**
Activity, furniture repair

Y93.D9 **Activity, other involving arts and handcrafts**

✓5th **Y93.E** **Activities involving personal hygiene and interior property and clothing maintenance**
> **EXCLUDES 1** *activities involving cooking and grilling (Y93.G-)*
> *activities involving exterior property and land maintenance, building and construction (Y93.H-)*
> *activities involving caregiving (Y93.F-)*
> *activity, dishwashing (Y93.G1)*
> *activity, food preparation (Y93.G1)*
> *activity, gardening (Y93.H2)*

Y93.E1 **Activity, personal bathing and showering**

Y93.E2 **Activity, laundry**

Y93.E3 **Activity, vacuuming**

Y93.E4 **Activity, ironing**

Y93.E5 **Activity, floor mopping and cleaning**

Y93.E6 **Activity, residential relocation**
Activity, packing up and unpacking involved in moving to a new residence

Y93.E8 **Activity, other personal hygiene**

Y93.E9 **Activity, other interior property and clothing maintenance**

✓5th **Y93.F** **Activities involving caregiving**
Activity involving the provider of caregiving

Y93.F1 **Activity, caregiving, bathing**

Y93.F2 **Activity, caregiving, lifting**

Y93.F9 **Activity, other caregiving**

✓5th **Y93.G** **Activities involving food preparation, cooking and grilling**

Y93.G1 **Activity, food preparation and clean up**
Activity, dishwashing

Y93.G2 **Activity, grilling and smoking food**

Y93.G3 **Activity, cooking and baking**
Activity, use of stove, oven and microwave oven

Y93.G9 **Activity, other involving cooking and grilling**

✓5th **Y93.H** **Activities involving exterior property and land maintenance, building and construction**

Y93.H1 **Activity, digging, shoveling and raking**
Activity, dirt digging
Activity, raking leaves
Activity, snow shoveling

Y93.H2 **Activity, gardening and landscaping**
Activity, pruning, trimming shrubs, weeding

Y93.H3 **Activity, building and construction**

Y93.H9 **Activity, other involving exterior property and land maintenance, building and construction**

✓5th **Y93.I** **Activities involving roller coasters and other types of external motion**

Y93.I1 **Activity, rollercoaster riding**

Y93.I9 **Activity, other involving external motion**

✓5th **Y93.J** **Activities involving playing musical instrument**
Activity involving playing electric musical instrument

Y93.J1 **Activity, piano playing**
Activity, musical keyboard (electronic) playing

Y93.J2 **Activity, drum and other percussion instrument playing**

Y93.J3 **Activity, string instrument playing**

Y93.J4 **Activity, winds and brass instrument playing**

✓5th **Y93.K** **Activities involving animal care**
> **EXCLUDES 1** *activity, horseback riding (Y93.52)*

Y93.K1 **Activity, walking an animal**

Y93.K2 **Activity, milking an animal**

Y93.K3 **Activity, grooming and shearing an animal**

Y93.K9 **Activity, other involving animal care**

✓5th **Y93.8** **Activities, other specified**

Y93.81 **Activity, refereeing a sports activity**

Y93.82 **Activity, spectator at an event**

Y93.83 **Activity, rough housing and horseplay**

Y93.84 **Activity, sleeping**

Y93.89 **Activity, other specified**

Y93.9 **Activity, unspecified**

Y95 **Nosocomial condition**
AHA: 2013, 4Q, 119

✓4th **Y99** **External cause status**
> **NOTE** A single code from category Y99 should be used in conjunction with the external cause code(s) assigned to a record to indicate the status of the person at the time the event occurred.

Y99.0 **Civilian activity done for income or pay**
Civilian activity done for financial or other compensation
> **EXCLUDES 1** *military activity (Y99.1)*
> *volunteer activity (Y99.2)*

Y99.1 **Military activity**
> **EXCLUDES 1** *activity of off duty military personnel (Y99.8)*

Y99.2 **Volunteer activity**
> **EXCLUDES 1** *activity of child or other family member assisting in compensated work of other family member (Y99.8)*

Y99.8 **Other external cause status**
Activity NEC
Activity of child or other family member assisting in compensated work of other family member
Hobby not done for income
Leisure activity
Off-duty activity of military personnel
Recreation or sport not for income or while a student
Student activity
> **EXCLUDES 1** *civilian activity done for income or compensation (Y99.0)*
> *military activity (Y99.1)*
AHA: 2012, 4Q, 108

Y99.9 **Unspecified external cause status**

N Newborn: 0   P Pediatric: 0-17   M Maternity: 12-55   A Adult: 15-124   MCC Major CC Condition   PDx MCC PDx acts as own MCC   CC CC Condition   PDx CC PDx acts as own CC

Chapter 21. Factors Influencing Health Status and Contact With Health Services (Z00-Z99)

NOTE   Z codes represent reasons for encounters. A corresponding procedure code must accompany a Z code if a procedure is performed. Categories Z00-Z99 are provided for occasions when circumstances other than a disease, injury or external cause classifiable to categories A00-Y89 are recorded as "diagnoses" or "problems". This can arise in two main ways:

(a) When a person who may or may not be sick encounters the health services for some specific purpose, such as to receive limited care or service for a current condition, to donate an organ or tissue, to receive prophylactic vaccination (immunization), or to discuss a problem which is in itself not a disease or injury.

(b) When some circumstance or problem is present which influences the person's health status but is not in itself a current illness or injury.

This chapter contains the following blocks:

Z00-Z13	Persons encountering health services for examinations
Z14-Z15	Genetic carrier and genetic susceptibility to disease
Z16	Resistance to antimicrobial drugs
Z17	Estrogen receptor status
Z18	Retained foreign body fragments
Z20-Z28	Persons with potential health hazards related to communicable diseases
Z30-Z39	Persons encountering health services in circumstances related to reproduction
Z40-Z53	Encounters for other specific health care
Z55-Z65	Persons with potential health hazards related to socioeconomic and psychosocial circumstances
Z66	Do not resuscitate status
Z67	Blood type
Z68	Body mass index (BMI)
Z69-Z76	Persons encountering health services in other circumstances
Z77-Z99	Persons with potential health hazards related to family and personal history and certain conditions influencing health status

Persons encountering health services for examinations (Z00-Z13)

NOTE   Nonspecific abnormal findings disclosed at the time of these examinations are classified to categories R70-R94.

EXCLUDES 1   *examinations related to pregnancy and reproduction (Z30-Z36, Z39-)*

✓4ᵗʰ Z00   Encounter for general examination without complaint, suspected or reported diagnosis

     EXCLUDES 1   *encounter for examination for administrative purposes (Z02.-)*
     EXCLUDES 2   *encounter for pre-procedural examinations (Z01.81-)*
          special screening examinations (Z11-Z13)

✓5ᵗʰ Z00.0   Encounter for general adult medical examination

     Encounter for adult periodic examination (annual) (physical) and any associated laboratory and radiologic examinations

     EXCLUDES 1   *encounter for examination of sign or symptom—code to sign or symptom*
          general health check-up of infant or child (Z00.12-)

     Z00.00   Encounter for general adult medical examination without abnormal findings   A

          Encounter for adult health check-up NOS

     Z00.01   Encounter for general adult medical examination with abnormal findings   A

          Use additional code to identify abnormal findings

✓5ᵗʰ Z00.1   Encounter for newborn, infant and child health examinations

     ✓6ᵗʰ Z00.11   Newborn health examination

          Health check for child under 29 days old
          Use additional code to identify any abnormal findings

          EXCLUDES 1   *health check for child over 28 days old (Z00.12-)*

          Z00.110   Health examination for newborn under 8 days old   N

              Health check for newborn under 8 days old

          Z00.111   Health examination for newborn 8 to 28 days old   N

              Health check for newborn 8 to 28 days old
              Newborn weight check

✓6ᵗʰ Z00.12   Encounter for routine child health examination

     Encounter for development testing of infant or child
     Health check (routine) for child over 28 days old

     EXCLUDES 1   *health check for child under 29 days old (Z00.11-)*
          health supervision of foundling or other healthy infant or child (Z76.1-Z76.2)
          newborn health examination (Z00.11-)

     Z00.121   Encounter for routine child health examination with abnormal findings   P

          Use additional code to identify abnormal findings

     Z00.129   Encounter for routine child health examination without abnormal findings   P

          Encounter for routine child health examination NOS

Z00.2   Encounter for examination for period of rapid growth in childhood   P

Z00.3   Encounter for examination for adolescent development state   P

     Encounter for puberty development state

Z00.5   Encounter for examination of potential donor of organ and tissue   P

Z00.6   Encounter for examination for normal comparison and control in clinical research program

     Examination of participant or control in clinical research program

✓5ᵗʰ Z00.7   Encounter for examination for period of delayed growth in childhood

     Z00.70   Encounter for examination for period of delayed growth in childhood without abnormal findings   P

     Z00.71   Encounter for examination for period of delayed growth in childhood with abnormal findings   P

          Use additional code to identify abnormal findings

Z00.8   Encounter for other general examination

     Encounter for health examination in population surveys

✓4ᵗʰ Z01   Encounter for other special examination without complaint, suspected or reported diagnosis

     INCLUDES   routine examination of specific system
     NOTE   Codes from category Z01 represent the reason for the encounter. A separate procedure code is required to identify any examinations or procedures performed.
     EXCLUDES 1   *encounter for examination for administrative purposes (Z02.-)*
          encounter for examination for suspected conditions, proven not to exist (Z03.-)
          encounter for laboratory and radiologic examinations as a component of general medical examinations (Z00.0-)
          encounter for laboratory, radiologic and imaging examinations for sign(s) and symptom(s)—code to the sign(s) or symptom(s)
     EXCLUDES 2   *screening examinations (Z11-Z13)*

✓5ᵗʰ Z01.0   Encounter for examination of eyes and vision

     EXCLUDES 1   *examination for driving license (Z02.4)*

     Z01.00   Encounter for examination of eyes and vision without abnormal findings

          Encounter for examination of eyes and vision NOS

     Z01.01   Encounter for examination of eyes and vision with abnormal findings

          Use additional code to identify abnormal findings

✓5ᵗʰ Z01.1   Encounter for examination of ears and hearing

     Z01.10   Encounter for examination of ears and hearing without abnormal findings

          Encounter for examination of ears and hearing NOS

     ✓6ᵗʰ Z01.11   Encounter for examination of ears and hearing with abnormal findings

          Z01.110   Encounter for hearing examination following failed hearing screening

          Z01.118   Encounter for examination of ears and hearing with other abnormal findings

              Use additional code to identify abnormal findings

     Z01.12   Encounter for hearing conservation and treatment

✓5ᵗʰ Z01.2   Encounter for dental examination and cleaning

     Z01.20   Encounter for dental examination and cleaning without abnormal findings

          Encounter for dental examination and cleaning NOS

     Z01.21   Encounter for dental examination and cleaning with abnormal findings

          Use additional code to identify abnormal findings

✓ Additional Character Required   ✓x7ᵗʰ Xtension Alert   Unacceptable PDx   Manifestation   Hospital Acquired Condition   **EXCLUDES 1** Not Coded Here   **EXCLUDES 2** Not Included Here

ICD-10-CM Draft (2015)   1175

Factors Influencing Health Status and Contact With Health Services   Z01.3–Z03.89

✓5ᵗʰ **Z01.3 Encounter for examination of blood pressure**

     Z01.30 Encounter for examination of blood pressure without abnormal findings
         Encounter for examination of blood pressure NOS

     Z01.31 Encounter for examination of blood pressure with abnormal findings
         Use additional code to identify abnormal findings

✓5ᵗʰ **Z01.4 Encounter for gynecological examination**
     EXCLUDES 2   pregnancy examination or test (Z32.0-)
                routine examination for contraceptive maintenance (Z30.4-)

     ✓6ᵗʰ **Z01.41 Encounter for routine gynecological examination**
         Encounter for general gynecological examination with or without cervical smear
         Encounter for gynecological examination (general) (routine) NOS
         Encounter for pelvic examination (annual) (periodic)
         Use additional code:
            for screening for human papillomavirus, if applicable, (Z11.51)
            for screening vaginal pap smear, if applicable (Z12.72)
            to identify acquired absence of uterus, if applicable (Z90.71-)
         EXCLUDES 1   gynecologic examination status-post hysterectomy for malignant condition (Z08)
                  screening cervical pap smear not a part of a routine gynecological examination (Z12.4)

         Z01.411 Encounter for gynecological examination (general) (routine) with abnormal findings ♀

         Z01.419 Encounter for gynecological examination (general) (routine) without abnormal findings ♀
            Use additional code to identify abnormal findings

     Z01.42 Encounter for cervical smear to confirm findings of recent normal smear following initial abnormal smear ♀

✓5ᵗʰ **Z01.8 Encounter for other specified special examinations**

     ✓6ᵗʰ **Z01.81 Encounter for preprocedural examinations**
         Encounter for preoperative examinations
         Encounter for radiological and imaging examinations as part of preprocedural examination

         Z01.810 Encounter for preprocedural cardiovascular examination

         Z01.811 Encounter for preprocedural respiratory examination

         Z01.812 Encounter for preprocedural laboratory examination
            Blood and urine tests prior to treatment or procedure

         Z01.818 Encounter for other preprocedural examination
            Encounter for preprocedural examination NOS
            Encounter for examinations prior to antineoplastic chemotherapy

     Z01.82 Encounter for allergy testing
         EXCLUDES 1   encounter for antibody response examination (Z01.84)

     Z01.83 Encounter for blood typing
         Encounter for Rh typing

     Z01.84 Encounter for antibody response examination
         Encounter for immunity status testing
         EXCLUDES 1   encounter for allergy testing (Z01.82)

     Z01.89 Encounter for other specified special examinations

✓4ᵗʰ **Z02 Encounter for administrative examination**

     Z02.0 Encounter for examination for admission to educational institution
         Encounter for examination for admission to preschool (education)
         Encounter for examination for re-admission to school following illness or medical treatment

     Z02.1 Encounter for pre-employment examination

     Z02.2 Encounter for examination for admission to residential institution
         EXCLUDES 1   examination for admission to prison (Z02.89)

     Z02.3 Encounter for examination for recruitment to armed forces

     Z02.4 Encounter for examination for driving license

     Z02.5 Encounter for examination for participation in sport
         EXCLUDES 1   blood-alcohol and blood-drug test (Z02.83)

     Z02.6 Encounter for examination for insurance purposes

✓5ᵗʰ **Z02.7 Encounter for issue of medical certificate**
     EXCLUDES 1   encounter for general medical examination (Z00-Z01, Z02.0-Z02.6, Z02.8-Z02.9)

     Z02.71 Encounter for disability determination
         Encounter for issue of medical certificate of incapacity
         Encounter for issue of medical certificate of invalidity

     Z02.79 Encounter for issue of other medical certificate

✓5ᵗʰ **Z02.8 Encounter for other administrative examinations**

     Z02.81 Encounter for paternity testing

     Z02.82 Encounter for adoption services

     Z02.83 Encounter for blood-alcohol and blood-drug test
         Use additional code for findings of alcohol or drugs in blood (R78.-)

     Z02.89 Encounter for other administrative examinations
         Encounter for examination for admission to prison
         Encounter for examination for admission to summer camp
         Encounter for immigration examination
         Encounter for naturalization examination
         Encounter for premarital examination
         EXCLUDES 1   health supervision of foundling or other healthy infant or child (Z76.1-Z76.2)

     Z02.9 Encounter for administrative examinations, unspecified

✓4ᵗʰ **Z03 Encounter for medical observation for suspected diseases and conditions ruled out**
     NOTE   This category is to be used when a person without a diagnosis is suspected of having an abnormal condition, without signs or symptoms, which requires study, but after examination and observation, is ruled out. This category is also for use for administrative and legal observation status.
     EXCLUDES 1   contact with and (suspected) exposures hazardous to health (Z77.-)
                newborn observation for suspected condition, ruled out (P00-P04)
                person with feared complaint in whom no diagnosis is made (Z71.1)
                signs or symptoms under study—code to signs or symptoms

     Z03.6 Encounter for observation for suspected toxic effect from ingested substance ruled out
         Encounter for observation for suspected adverse effect from drug
         Encounter for observation for suspected poisoning

✓5ᵗʰ **Z03.7 Encounter for suspected maternal and fetal conditions ruled out**
     Encounter for suspected maternal and fetal conditions not found
     EXCLUDES 1   known or suspected fetal anomalies affecting management of mother, not ruled out (O26-, O35-, O36-, O40-, O41-)

     Z03.71 Encounter for suspected problem with amniotic cavity and membrane ruled out Ⓜ♀
         Encounter for suspected oligohydramnios ruled out
         Encounter for suspected polyhydramnios ruled out

     Z03.72 Encounter for suspected placental problem ruled out Ⓜ♀

     Z03.73 Encounter for suspected fetal anomaly ruled out Ⓜ♀

     Z03.74 Encounter for suspected problem with fetal growth ruled out Ⓜ♀

     Z03.75 Encounter for suspected cervical shortening ruled out Ⓜ♀

     Z03.79 Encounter for other suspected maternal and fetal conditions ruled out Ⓜ♀

✓5ᵗʰ **Z03.8 Encounter for observation for other suspected diseases and conditions ruled out**

     ✓6ᵗʰ **Z03.81 Encounter for observation for suspected exposure to biological agents ruled out**

         Z03.810 Encounter for observation for suspected exposure to anthrax ruled out

         Z03.818 Encounter for observation for suspected exposure to other biological agents ruled out

     Z03.89 Encounter for observation for other suspected diseases and conditions ruled out

Ⓝ Newborn: 0   Ⓟ Pediatric: 0-17   Ⓜ Maternity: 12-55   Ⓐ Adult: 15-124   MCC Major CC Condition   PDx MCC PDx acts as own MCC   CC CC Condition   PDx CC PDx acts as own CC

1176   ICD-10-CM Draft (2015)

✓4ᵗʰ ZØ4 Encounter for examination and observation for other reasons

> **INCLUDES** encounter for examination for medicolegal reasons
> **NOTE** This category is to be used when a person without a diagnosis is suspected of having an abnormal condition, without signs or symptoms, which requires study, but after examination and observation, is ruled-out. This category is also for use for administrative and legal observation status.

ZØ4.1 Encounter for examination and observation following transport accident

> **EXCLUDES 1** encounter for examination and observation following work accident (ZØ4.2)

ZØ4.2 Encounter for examination and observation following work accident

ZØ4.3 Encounter for examination and observation following other accident

✓5ᵗʰ ZØ4.4 Encounter for examination and observation following alleged rape

> Encounter for examination and observation of victim following alleged rape
> Encounter for examination and observation of victim following alleged sexual abuse

ZØ4.41 Encounter for examination and observation following alleged adult rape Ⓐ

> Suspected adult rape, ruled out
> Suspected adult sexual abuse, ruled out

ZØ4.42 Encounter for examination and observation following alleged child rape Ⓟ

> Suspected child rape, ruled out
> Suspected child sexual abuse, ruled out

ZØ4.6 Encounter for general psychiatric examination, requested by authority

✓5ᵗʰ ZØ4.7 Encounter for examination and observation following alleged physical abuse

ZØ4.71 Encounter for examination and observation following alleged adult physical abuse Ⓐ

> Suspected adult physical abuse, ruled out
> **EXCLUDES 1** confirmed case of adult physical abuse (T74.-)
> encounter for examination and observation following alleged adult sexual abuse (ZØ4.41)
> suspected case of adult physical abuse, not ruled out (T76.-)

ZØ4.72 Encounter for examination and observation following alleged child physical abuse Ⓟ

> Suspected child physical abuse, ruled out
> **EXCLUDES 1** confirmed case of child physical abuse (T74.-)
> encounter for examination and observation following alleged child sexual abuse (ZØ4.42)
> suspected case of child physical abuse, not ruled out (T76.-)

ZØ4.8 Encounter for examination and observation for other specified reasons

> Encounter for examination and observation for request for expert evidence

ZØ4.9 Encounter for examination and observation for unspecified reason

> Encounter for observation NOS

ZØ8 Encounter for follow-up examination after completed treatment for malignant neoplasm

> Medical surveillance following completed treatment
> Use additional code to identify any acquired absence of organs (Z9Ø.-)
> Use additional code to identify the personal history of malignant neoplasm (Z85.-)
> **EXCLUDES 1** aftercare following medical care (Z43-Z49, Z51)

ZØ9 Encounter for follow-up examination after completed treatment for conditions other than malignant neoplasm

> Medical surveillance following completed treatment
> Use additional code to identify any applicable history of disease code (Z86-. Z87-)
> **EXCLUDES 1** aftercare following medical care (Z43-Z49, Z51)
> surveillance of contraception (Z3Ø.4-)
> surveillance of prosthetic and other medical devices (Z44-Z46)

✓4ᵗʰ Z11 Encounter for screening for infectious and parasitic diseases

> **NOTE** Screening is the testing for disease or disease precursors in asymptomatic individuals so that early detection and treatment can be provided for those who test positive for the disease.
> **EXCLUDES 1** encounter for diagnostic examination—code to sign or symptom

Z11.Ø Encounter for screening for intestinal infectious diseases

Z11.1 Encounter for screening for respiratory tuberculosis

Z11.2 Encounter for screening for other bacterial diseases

Z11.3 Encounter for screening for infections with a predominantly sexual mode of transmission

> **EXCLUDES 2** encounter for screening for human immunodeficiency virus [HIV] (Z11.4)
> encounter for screening for human papillomavirus (Z11.51)

Z11.4 Encounter for screening for human immunodeficiency virus [HIV]

✓5ᵗʰ Z11.5 Encounter for screening for other viral diseases

> **EXCLUDES 2** encounter for screening for viral intestinal disease (Z11.Ø)

Z11.51 Encounter for screening for human papillomavirus (HPV)

Z11.59 Encounter for screening for other viral diseases

Z11.6 Encounter for screening for other protozoal diseases and helminthiases

> **EXCLUDES 2** encounter for screening for protozoal intestinal disease (Z11.Ø)

Z11.8 Encounter for screening for other infectious and parasitic diseases

> Encounter for screening for chlamydia
> Encounter for screening for rickettsial
> Encounter for screening for spirochetal
> Encounter for screening for mycoses

Z11.9 Encounter for screening for infectious and parasitic diseases, unspecified

✓4ᵗʰ Z12 Encounter for screening for malignant neoplasms

> **NOTE** Screening is the testing for disease or disease precursors in asymptomatic individuals so that early detection and treatment can be provided for those who test positive for the disease.
> Use additional code to identify any family history of malignant neoplasm (Z8Ø.-)
> **EXCLUDES 1** encounter for diagnostic examination—code to sign or symptom

Z12.Ø Encounter for screening for malignant neoplasm of stomach

✓5ᵗʰ Z12.1 Encounter for screening for malignant neoplasm of intestinal tract

Z12.1Ø Encounter for screening for malignant neoplasm of intestinal tract, unspecified

Z12.11 Encounter for screening for malignant neoplasm of colon

> Encounter for screening colonoscopy NOS

Z12.12 Encounter for screening for malignant neoplasm of rectum

Z12.13 Encounter for screening for malignant neoplasm of small intestine

Z12.2 Encounter for screening for malignant neoplasm of respiratory organs

✓5ᵗʰ Z12.3 Encounter for screening for malignant neoplasm of breast

Z12.31 Encounter for screening mammogram for malignant neoplasm of breast

> **EXCLUDES 1** inconclusive mammogram (R92.2)

Z12.39 Encounter for other screening for malignant neoplasm of breast

Z12.4 Encounter for screening for malignant neoplasm of cervix ♀

> Encounter for screening pap smear for malignant neoplasm of cervix
> **EXCLUDES 1** encounter for screening for human papillomavirus (Z11.51)
> when screening is part of general gynecological examination (ZØ1.4-)

Z12.5 Encounter for screening for malignant neoplasm of prostate ♂

Z12.6 Encounter for screening for malignant neoplasm of bladder

---

✓ Additional Character Required   ✓x7ᵗʰ Xtension Alert   Unacceptable PDx   Manifestation   Hospital Acquired Condition   **EXCLUDES 1** Not Coded Here   **EXCLUDES 2** Not Included Here

√5ᵗʰ **Z12.7** **Encounter for screening for malignant neoplasm of** other genitourinary organs

     Z12.71 **Encounter for screening for malignant neoplasm of** testis   ♂

     Z12.72 **Encounter for screening for malignant neoplasm of** vagina   ♀

         Vaginal pap smear status-post hysterectomy for non-malignant condition

         Use additional code to identify acquired absence of uterus (Z90.71-)

         EXCLUDES 1   *vaginal pap smear status-post hysterectomy for malignant conditions (Z08)*

     Z12.73 **Encounter for screening for malignant neoplasm of** ovary   ♀

     Z12.79 **Encounter for screening for malignant neoplasm of** other genitourinary organs

√5ᵗʰ **Z12.8** **Encounter for screening for malignant neoplasm of** other sites

     Z12.81 **Encounter for screening for malignant neoplasm of** oral cavity

     Z12.82 **Encounter for screening for malignant neoplasm of** nervous system

     Z12.83 **Encounter for screening for malignant neoplasm of** skin

     Z12.89 **Encounter for screening for malignant neoplasm of** other sites

     Z12.9 **Encounter for screening for malignant neoplasm, site unspecified**

√4ᵗʰ **Z13** **Encounter for screening for** other diseases and disorders

     NOTE   Screening is the testing for disease or disease precursors in asymptomatic individuals so that early detection and treatment can be provided for those who test positive for the disease.

     EXCLUDES 1   *encounter for diagnostic examination—code to sign or symptom*

     Z13.0 **Encounter for screening for diseases of the** blood and blood-forming organs **and certain disorders involving the** immune mechanism

     Z13.1 **Encounter for screening for** diabetes mellitus

     Z13.2 **Encounter for screening for nutritional, metabolic and other endocrine disorders**

     Z13.21 **Encounter for screening for** nutritional **disorder**

√6ᵗʰ **Z13.22** **Encounter for screening for** metabolic **disorder**

     Z13.220 **Encounter for screening for** lipoid **disorders**

         Encounter for screening for cholesterol level

         Encounter for screening for hypercholesterolemia

         Encounter for screening for hyperlipidemia

     Z13.228 **Encounter for screening for other metabolic disorders**

     Z13.29 **Encounter for screening for** other **suspected endocrine disorder**

     EXCLUDES 1   *encounter for screening for diabetes mellitus (Z13.1)*

     Z13.4 **Encounter for screening for certain** developmental disorders in childhood   P

         Encounter for screening for developmental handicaps in early childhood

     EXCLUDES 1   *routine development testing of infant or child (Z00.1-)*

     Z13.5 **Encounter for screening for** eye and ear **disorders**

     EXCLUDES 2   *encounter for general hearing examination (Z01.1-)*
         encounter for general vision examination (Z01.0-)

     Z13.6 **Encounter for screening for** cardiovascular **disorders**

√5ᵗʰ **Z13.7** **Encounter for screening for** genetic and chromosomal **anomalies**

     EXCLUDES 1   *genetic testing for procreative management (Z31.4-)*

     Z13.71 **Encounter for nonprocreative screening for genetic** disease carrier status

     Z13.79 **Encounter for** other **screening for genetic and chromosomal anomalies**

√5ᵗʰ **Z13.8** **Encounter for screening for** other specified diseases and disorders

     EXCLUDES 2   *screening for malignant neoplasms (Z12.-)*

√6ᵗʰ **Z13.81** **Encounter for screening for** digestive system **disorders**

     Z13.810 **Encounter for screening for** upper gastrointestinal **disorder**

     Z13.811 **Encounter for screening for** lower gastrointestinal **disorder**

         EXCLUDES 1   *encounter for screening for intestinal infectious disease (Z11.0)*

     Z13.818 **Encounter for screening for** other **digestive system disorders**

√6ᵗʰ **Z13.82** **Encounter for screening for** musculoskeletal **disorder**

     Z13.820 **Encounter for screening for** osteoporosis

     Z13.828 **Encounter for screening for** other **musculoskeletal disorder**

     Z13.83 **Encounter for screening for** respiratory **disorder NEC**

     EXCLUDES 1   *encounter for screening for respiratory tuberculosis (Z11.1)*

     Z13.84 **Encounter for screening for** dental **disorders**

√6ᵗʰ **Z13.85** **Encounter for screening for** nervous system **disorders**

     Z13.850 **Encounter for screening for** traumatic brain injury

     Z13.858 **Encounter for screening for** other nervous system disorders

     Z13.88 **Encounter for screening for disorder** due to exposure to contaminants

     EXCLUDES 1   *those exposed to contaminants without suspected disorders (Z57-Z77-)*

     Z13.89 **Encounter for screening for** other **disorder**

         Encounter for screening for genitourinary disorders

     Z13.9 **Encounter for screening, unspecified**

Genetic carrier and genetic susceptibility to disease (Z14-Z15)

√4ᵗʰ **Z14** **Genetic carrier**

√5ᵗʰ **Z14.0** Hemophilia A **carrier**

     Z14.01 Asymptomatic hemophilia A carrier

     Z14.02 Symptomatic hemophilia A carrier

     Z14.1 Cystic fibrosis **carrier**

     Z14.8 **Genetic carrier of** other **disease**

√4ᵗʰ **Z15** **Genetic susceptibility to disease**

     Confirmed abnormal gene

     Use additional code, if applicable, for any associated family history of the disease (Z80-Z84)

     EXCLUDES 1   *chromosomal anomalies (Q90-Q99)*

√5ᵗʰ **Z15.0** **Genetic susceptibility to** malignant neoplasm

     Code first, if applicable, any current malignant neoplasm (C00-C75, C81-C96)

     Use additional code, if applicable, for any personal history of malignant neoplasm (Z85.-)

     Z15.01 **Genetic susceptibility to malignant neoplasm of** breast

     Z15.02 **Genetic susceptibility to malignant neoplasm of** ovary   ♀

     Z15.03 **Genetic susceptibility to malignant neoplasm of** prostate   ♂

     Z15.04 **Genetic susceptibility to malignant neoplasm of** endometrium   ♀

     Z15.09 **Genetic susceptibility to other malignant neoplasm**

√5ᵗʰ **Z15.8** **Genetic susceptibility to other disease**

     Z15.81 **Genetic susceptibility to** multiple endocrine neoplasia **[MEN]**

     EXCLUDES 1   *multiple endocrine neoplasia [MEN] syndromes (E31.2-)*

     Z15.89 **Genetic susceptibility to** other **disease**

N Newborn: 0   P Pediatric: 0-17   M Maternity: 12-55   A Adult: 15-124   MCC Major CC Condition   PDx MCC PDx acts as own MCC   CC CC Condition   PDx CC PDx acts as own CC

1178   ICD-10-CM Draft (2015)

Resistance to antimicrobial drugs (Z16)

☑4ᵗʰ **Z16 Resistance to antimicrobial drugs**

> **NOTE** The codes in this category are provided for use as additional codes to identify the resistance and non-responsiveness of a condition to antimicrobial drugs.
>
> Code first the infection
>
> **EXCLUDES 1** *Methicillin resistant Staphylococcus aureus infection (A49.02)*
> *Methicillin resistant Staphylococcus aureus infection in diseases classified elsewhere (B95.62)*
> *Methicillin resistant Staphylococcus aureus pneumonia (J15.212)*
> *Sepsis due to Methicillin resistant Staphylococcus aureus (A41.02)*

☑5ᵗʰ **Z16.1 Resistance to beta lactam antibiotics**

   Z16.10 Resistance to unspecified beta lactam antibiotics

   Z16.11 Resistance to penicillins
      Resistance to amoxicillin
      Resistance to ampicillin

   Z16.12 Extended spectrum beta lactamase (ESBL) resistance

   Z16.19 Resistance to other specified beta lactam antibiotics
      Resistance to cephalosporins

☑5ᵗʰ **Z16.2 Resistance to other antibiotics**

   Z16.20 Resistance to unspecified antibiotic
      Resistance to antibiotics NOS

   Z16.21 Resistance to vancomycin

   Z16.22 Resistance to vancomycin related antibiotics

   Z16.23 Resistance to quinolones and fluoroquinolones

   Z16.24 Resistance to multiple antibiotics

   Z16.29 Resistance to other single specified antibiotic
      Resistance to aminoglycosides
      Resistance to macrolides
      Resistance to sulfonamides
      Resistance to tetracyclines

☑5ᵗʰ **Z16.3 Resistance to other antimicrobial drugs**

> **EXCLUDES 1** *resistance to antibiotics (Z16.1-, Z16.2-)*

   Z16.30 Resistance to unspecified antimicrobial drugs
      Drug resistance NOS

   Z16.31 Resistance to antiparasitic drug(s)
      Resistance to quinine and related compounds

   Z16.32 Resistance to antifungal drug(s)

   Z16.33 Resistance to antiviral drug(s)

   ☑6ᵗʰ **Z16.34 Resistance to antimycobacterial drug(s)**
      Resistance to tuberculostatics

      Z16.341 Resistance to single antimycobacterial drug
        Resistance to antimycobacterial drug NOS

      Z16.342 Resistance to multiple antimycobacterial drugs

   Z16.35 Resistance to multiple antimicrobial drugs

> **EXCLUDES 1** *Resistance to multiple antibiotics only (Z16.24)*

   Z16.39 Resistance to other specified antimicrobial drug

Estrogen receptor status (Z17)

☑4ᵗʰ **Z17 Estrogen receptor status**

   Code first malignant neoplasm of breast (C50.-)

   Z17.0 Estrogen receptor positive status [ER+]

   Z17.1 Estrogen receptor negative status [ER-]

Retained foreign body fragment (Z18)

☑4ᵗʰ **Z18 Retained foreign body fragments**

   Embedded fragment (status)
   Embedded splinter (status)
   Retained foreign body status

> **EXCLUDES 1** *artificial joint prosthesis status (Z96.6-)*
> *foreign body accidentally left during a procedure (T81.5-)*
> *foreign body entering through orifice (T15-T19)*
> *in situ cardiac device (Z95.-)*
> *organ or tissue replaced by means other than transplant (Z96.-, Z97.-)*
> *organ or tissue replaced by transplant (Z94.-)*
> *personal history of retained foreign body fully removed (Z87.821)*
> *superficial foreign body (non-embedded splinter)—code to superficial foreign body, by site*

☑5ᵗʰ **Z18.0 Retained radioactive fragments**

   Z18.01 Retained depleted uranium fragments

   Z18.09 Other retained radioactive fragments
      Other retained depleted isotope fragments
      Retained nontherapeutic radioactive fragments

☑5ᵗʰ **Z18.1 Retained metal fragments**

> **EXCLUDES 1** *retained radioactive metal fragments (Z18.01-Z18.09)*

   Z18.10 Retained metal fragments, unspecified
      Retained metal fragment NOS

   Z18.11 Retained magnetic metal fragments

   Z18.12 Retained nonmagnetic metal fragments

   Z18.2 Retained plastic fragments
      Acrylics fragments
      Diethylhexylphthalates fragments
      Isocyanate fragments

☑5ᵗʰ **Z18.3 Retained organic fragments**

   Z18.31 Retained animal quills or spines

   Z18.32 Retained tooth

   Z18.33 Retained wood fragments

   Z18.39 Other retained organic fragments

☑5ᵗʰ **Z18.8 Other specified retained foreign body**

   Z18.81 Retained glass fragments

   Z18.83 Retained stone or crystalline fragments
      Retained concrete or cement fragments

   Z18.89 Other specified retained foreign body fragments

   Z18.9 Retained foreign body fragments, unspecified material

Persons with potential health hazards related to communicable diseases (Z20-Z28)

☑4ᵗʰ **Z20 Contact with and (suspected) exposure to communicable diseases**

> **EXCLUDES 1** *carrier of infectious disease (Z22.-)*
> *diagnosed current infectious or parasitic disease—see Alphabetic Index*
> **EXCLUDES 2** *personal history of infectious and parasitic diseases (Z86.1-)*

☑5ᵗʰ **Z20.0 Contact with and (suspected) exposure to intestinal infectious diseases**

   Z20.01 Contact with and (suspected) exposure to intestinal infectious diseases due to Escherichia coli (E. coli)

   Z20.09 Contact with and (suspected) exposure to other intestinal infectious diseases

   Z20.1 Contact with and (suspected) exposure to tuberculosis

   Z20.2 Contact with and (suspected) exposure to infections with a predominantly sexual mode of transmission

   Z20.3 Contact with and (suspected) exposure to rabies

   Z20.4 Contact with and (suspected) exposure to rubella

   Z20.5 Contact with and (suspected) exposure to viral hepatitis

   Z20.6 Contact with and (suspected) exposure to human immunodeficiency virus [HIV]

> **EXCLUDES 1** *asymptomatic human immunodeficiency virus [HIV] HIV infection status (Z21)*

   Z20.7 Contact with and (suspected) exposure to pediculosis, acariasis and other infestations

☑5ᵗʰ **Z20.8 Contact with and (suspected) exposure to other communicable diseases**

   ☑6ᵗʰ **Z20.81 Contact with and (suspected) exposure to other bacterial communicable diseases**

      Z20.810 Contact with and (suspected) exposure to anthrax

      Z20.811 Contact with and (suspected) exposure to meningococcus

      Z20.818 Contact with and (suspected) exposure to other bacterial communicable diseases

   ☑6ᵗʰ **Z20.82 Contact with and (suspected) exposure to other viral communicable diseases**

      Z20.820 Contact with and (suspected) exposure to varicella

      Z20.828 Contact with and (suspected) exposure to other viral communicable diseases

   Z20.89 Contact with and (suspected) exposure to other communicable diseases

   Z20.9 Contact with and (suspected) exposure to unspecified communicable disease

---

☑ Additional Character Required   ☑x7ᵗʰ Xtension Alert   Unacceptable PDx   Manifestation   Hospital Acquired Condition   **EXCLUDES 1** Not Coded Here   **EXCLUDES 2** Not Included Here

13Z21 Asymptomatic human immunodeficiency virus [HIV] infection status
HIV positive NOS
Code first human immunodeficiency virus [HIV] disease complicating pregnancy, childbirth and the puerperium, if applicable (O98.7-)
EXCLUDES 1 acquired immunodeficiency syndrome (B20)
contact with human immunodeficiency virus [HIV] (Z20.6)
exposure to human immunodeficiency virus [HIV] (Z20.6)
human immunodeficiency virus [HIV] disease (B20)
inconclusive laboratory evidence of human immunodeficiency virus [HIV] (R75)

✓4ᵗʰ **Z22 Carrier of infectious disease**
Colonization status
Suspected carrier

Z22.0 Carrier of typhoid

Z22.1 Carrier of other intestinal infectious diseases

Z22.2 Carrier of diphtheria

✓5ᵗʰ **Z22.3 Carrier of other specified bacterial diseases**

    Z22.31 Carrier of bacterial disease due to meningococci

    ✓6ᵗʰ **Z22.32 Carrier of bacterial disease due to staphylococci**

        Z22.321 Carrier or suspected carrier of Methicillin susceptible Staphylococcus aureus
MSSA colonization

        Z22.322 Carrier or suspected carrier of Methicillin resistant Staphylococcus aureus
MRSA colonization

    ✓6ᵗʰ **Z22.33 Carrier of bacterial disease due to streptococci**

        Z22.330 Carrier of Group B streptococcus

        Z22.338 Carrier of other streptococcus

    Z22.39 Carrier of other specified bacterial diseases

Z22.4 Carrier of infections with a predominantly sexual mode of transmission

✓5ᵗʰ **Z22.5 Carrier of viral hepatitis**

    Z22.50 Carrier of unspecified viral hepatitis

    Z22.51 Carrier of viral hepatitis B
Hepatitis B surface antigen [HBsAg] carrier

    Z22.52 Carrier of viral hepatitis C

    Z22.59 Carrier of other viral hepatitis

Z22.6 Carrier of human T-lymphotropic virus type-1 [HTLV-1] infection

Z22.8 Carrier of other infectious diseases

Z22.9 Carrier of infectious disease, unspecified

Z23 Encounter for immunization
Code first any routine childhood examination
NOTE Procedure codes are required to identify the types of immunizations given

✓4ᵗʰ **Z28 Immunization not carried out and underimmunization status**
Vaccination not carried out

✓5ᵗʰ **Z28.0 Immunization not carried out because of contraindication**

    Z28.01 Immunization not carried out because of acute illness of patient

    Z28.02 Immunization not carried out because of chronic illness or condition of patient

    Z28.03 Immunization not carried out because of immune compromised state of patient

    Z28.04 Immunization not carried out because of patient allergy to vaccine or component

    Z28.09 Immunization not carried out because of other contraindication

Z28.1 Immunization not carried out because of patient decision for reasons of belief or group pressure
Immunization not carried out because of religious belief

✓5ᵗʰ **Z28.2 Immunization not carried out because of patient decision for other and unspecified reason**

    Z28.20 Immunization not carried out because of patient decision for unspecified reason

    Z28.21 Immunization not carried out because of patient refusal

    Z28.29 Immunization not carried out because of patient decision for other reason

Z28.3 Underimmunization status
Delinquent immunization status
Lapsed immunization schedule status

✓5ᵗʰ **Z28.8 Immunization not carried out for other reason**

    Z28.81 Immunization not carried out due to patient having had the disease

    Z28.82 Immunization not carried out because of caregiver refusal
Immunization not carried out because of guardian refusal
Immunization not carried out because of parent refusal
EXCLUDES 1 immunization not carried out because of caregiver refusal because of religious belief (Z28.1)

    Z28.89 Immunization not carried out for other reason

Z28.9 Immunization not carried out for unspecified reason

Persons encountering health services in circumstances related to reproduction (Z30-Z39)

✓4ᵗʰ **Z30 Encounter for contraceptive management**

✓5ᵗʰ **Z30.0 Encounter for general counseling and advice on contraception**

    ✓6ᵗʰ **Z30.01 Encounter for initial prescription of contraceptives**
EXCLUDES 1 encounter for surveillance of contraceptives (Z30.4-)

        Z30.011 Encounter for initial prescription of contraceptive pills ♀

        Z30.012 Encounter for prescription of emergency contraception ♀
Encounter for postcoital contraception

        Z30.013 Encounter for initial prescription of injectable contraceptive ♀

        Z30.014 Encounter for initial prescription of intrauterine contraceptive device ♀
EXCLUDES 1 encounter for insertion of intrauterine contraceptive device (Z30.430, Z30.432)

        Z30.018 Encounter for initial prescription of other contraceptives ♀

        Z30.019 Encounter for initial prescription of contraceptives, unspecified ♀

    Z30.02 Counseling and instruction in natural family planning to avoid pregnancy

    Z30.09 Encounter for other general counseling and advice on contraception
Encounter for family planning advice NOS

Z30.2 Encounter for sterilization

✓5ᵗʰ **Z30.4 Encounter for surveillance of contraceptives**

    Z30.40 Encounter for surveillance of contraceptives, unspecified

    Z30.41 Encounter for surveillance of contraceptive pills ♀
Encounter for repeat prescription for contraceptive pill

    Z30.42 Encounter for surveillance of injectable contraceptive ♀

    ✓6ᵗʰ **Z30.43 Encounter for surveillance of intrauterine contraceptive device**

        Z30.430 Encounter for insertion of intrauterine contraceptive device ♀

        Z30.431 Encounter for routine checking of intrauterine contraceptive device ♀

        Z30.432 Encounter for removal of intrauterine contraceptive device ♀

        Z30.433 Encounter for removal and reinsertion of intrauterine contraceptive device ♀
Encounter for replacement of intrauterine contraceptive device

    Z30.49 Encounter for surveillance of other contraceptives ♀

Z30.8 Encounter for other contraceptive management
Encounter for postvasectomy sperm count
Encounter for routine examination for contraceptive maintenance
EXCLUDES 1 sperm count following sterilization reversal (Z31.42)
sperm count for fertility testing (Z31.41)

---

13 Questionable admission when used as PDx.

Ⓝ Newborn: 0   Ⓟ Pediatric: 0-17   Ⓜ Maternity: 12-55   Ⓐ Adult: 15-124   **MCC** Major CC Condition   **PDx MCC** PDx acts as own MCC   **CC** CC Condition   **PDx CC** PDx acts as own CC

1180   ICD-10-CM Draft (2015)

Z30.9 **Encounter for contraceptive management, unspecified**

✓4th **Z31** **Encounter for procreative management**
    EXCLUDES 1 complications associated with artificial fertilization (N98.-)
        female infertility (N97.-)
        male infertility (N46.-)

    Z31.0 **Encounter for reversal of previous sterilization**

✓5th   Z31.4 **Encounter for procreative investigation and testing**
        EXCLUDES 1 postvasectomy sperm count (Z30.8)

        Z31.41 **Encounter for fertility testing**
            Encounter for fallopian tube patency testing
            Encounter for sperm count for fertility testing

        Z31.42 **Aftercare following sterilization reversal**
            Sperm count following sterilization reversal

      ✓6th Z31.43 **Encounter for genetic testing of female for procreative management**
            Use additional code for recurrent pregnancy loss, if applicable (N96, O26.-)
            EXCLUDES 1 nonprocreative genetic testing (Z13.7-)

        Z31.430 **Encounter of female for testing for genetic disease carrier status for procreative management** ♀

        Z31.438 **Encounter for other genetic testing of female for procreative management** ♀

      ✓6th Z31.44 **Encounter for genetic testing of male for procreative management**
            EXCLUDES 1 nonprocreative genetic testing (Z13.7-)

        Z31.440 **Encounter of male for testing for genetic disease carrier status for procreative management** ♂

        Z31.441 **Encounter for testing of male partner of patient with recurrent pregnancy loss** A♂

        Z31.448 **Encounter for other genetic testing of male for procreative management** A♂

      Z31.49 **Encounter for other procreative investigation and testing**

    Z31.5 **Encounter for genetic counseling**

✓5th   Z31.6 **Encounter for general counseling and advice on procreation**

        Z31.61 **Procreative counseling and advice using natural family planning**

        Z31.62 **Encounter for fertility preservation counseling**
            Encounter for fertility preservation counseling prior to cancer therapy
            Encounter for fertility preservation counseling prior to surgical removal of gonads

        Z31.69 **Encounter for other general counseling and advice on procreation**

✓5th   Z31.8 **Encounter for other procreative management**

        Z31.81 **Encounter for male factor infertility in female patient** ♀

        Z31.82 **Encounter for Rh incompatibility status** ♀

        Z31.83 **Encounter for assisted reproductive fertility procedure cycle** ♀
            Patient undergoing in vitro fertilization cycle
            Use additional code to identify the type of infertility
            EXCLUDES 1 pre-cycle diagnosis and testing—code to reason for encounter

        Z31.84 **Encounter for fertility preservation procedure**
            Encounter for fertility preservation procedure prior to cancer therapy
            Encounter for fertility preservation procedure prior to surgical removal of gonads

        Z31.89 **Encounter for other procreative management**

    Z31.9 **Encounter for procreative management, unspecified**

✓4th **Z32** **Encounter for pregnancy test and childbirth and childcare instruction**

✓5th   Z32.0 **Encounter for pregnancy test**

        Z32.00 **Encounter for pregnancy test, result unknown** ♀
            Encounter for pregnancy test NOS

        Z32.01 **Encounter for pregnancy test, result positive** M♀

        Z32.02 **Encounter for pregnancy test, result negative** ♀

    Z32.2 **Encounter for childbirth instruction**

    Z32.3 **Encounter for childcare instruction**
        Encounter for prenatal or postpartum childcare instruction

✓4th **Z33** **Pregnant state**

    Z33.1 **Pregnant state, incidental** M♀
        Pregnant state NOS
        EXCLUDES 1 complications of pregnancy (O00-O9A)

    Z33.2 **Encounter for elective termination of pregnancy** M♀
        EXCLUDES 1 early fetal death with retention of dead fetus (O02.1)
            late fetal death (O36.4)
            spontaneous abortion (O03)

✓4th **Z34** **Encounter for supervision of normal pregnancy**
    EXCLUDES 1 any complication of pregnancy (O00-O9A)
        encounter for pregnancy test (Z32.0-)
        encounter for supervision of high risk pregnancy (O09.-)

✓5th   Z34.0 **Encounter for supervision of normal first pregnancy**

        Z34.00 **Encounter for supervision of normal first pregnancy, unspecified trimester** M♀

        Z34.01 **Encounter for supervision of normal first pregnancy, first trimester** M♀

        Z34.02 **Encounter for supervision of normal first pregnancy, second trimester** M♀

        Z34.03 **Encounter for supervision of normal first pregnancy, third trimester** M♀

✓5th   Z34.8 **Encounter for supervision of other normal pregnancy**

        Z34.80 **Encounter for supervision of other normal pregnancy, unspecified trimester** M♀

        Z34.81 **Encounter for supervision of other normal pregnancy, first trimester** M♀

        Z34.82 **Encounter for supervision of other normal pregnancy, second trimester** M♀

        Z34.83 **Encounter for supervision of other normal pregnancy, third trimester** M♀

✓5th   Z34.9 **Encounter for supervision of normal pregnancy, unspecified**

        Z34.90 **Encounter for supervision of normal pregnancy, unspecified, unspecified trimester** M♀

        Z34.91 **Encounter for supervision of normal pregnancy, unspecified, first trimester** M♀

        Z34.92 **Encounter for supervision of normal pregnancy, unspecified, second trimester** M♀

        Z34.93 **Encounter for supervision of normal pregnancy, unspecified, third trimester** M♀

  Z36 **Encounter for antenatal screening of mother** M♀
    EXCLUDES 1 abnormal findings on antenatal screening of mother (O28.-)
        diagnostic examination—code to sign or symptom
        encounter for suspected maternal and fetal conditions ruled out (Z03.7-)
        suspected fetal condition affecting management of pregnancy—code to condition in Chapter 15
    EXCLUDES 2 genetic counseling and testing (Z31.43-, Z31.5)
        routine prenatal care (Z34)

✓4th **Z3A** **Weeks of gestation**
    NOTE Codes from category Z3A are for use, only on the maternal record, to indicate the weeks of gestation of the pregnancy.
    Code first complications of pregnancy, childbirth and the puerperium (O00-O9A)
    AHA: 2014, 2Q, 9; 2013, 2Q, 33

✓5th   Z3A.0 **Weeks of gestation of pregnancy, unspecified or less than 10 weeks**

        Z3A.00 **Weeks of gestation of pregnancy not specified** M♀

        Z3A.01 **Less than 8 weeks gestation of pregnancy** M♀

        Z3A.08 **8 weeks gestation of pregnancy** M♀

        Z3A.09 **9 weeks gestation of pregnancy** M♀

✓5th   Z3A.1 **Weeks of gestation of pregnancy, weeks 10-19**

        Z3A.10 **10 weeks gestation of pregnancy** M♀

        Z3A.11 **11 weeks gestation of pregnancy** M♀

        Z3A.12 **12 weeks gestation of pregnancy** M♀

        Z3A.13 **13 weeks gestation of pregnancy** M♀

        Z3A.14 **14 weeks gestation of pregnancy** M♀

        Z3A.15 **15 weeks gestation of pregnancy** M♀

        Z3A.16 **16 weeks gestation of pregnancy** M♀

        Z3A.17 **17 weeks gestation of pregnancy** M♀

        Z3A.18 **18 weeks gestation of pregnancy** M♀

        Z3A.19 **19 weeks gestation of pregnancy** M♀

✓5th   Z3A.2 **Weeks of gestation of pregnancy, weeks 20-29**

        Z3A.20 **20 weeks gestation of pregnancy** M♀

        Z3A.21 **21 weeks gestation of pregnancy** M♀

✓ Additional Character Required ✓x7th Xtension Alert Unacceptable PDx Manifestation Hospital Acquired Condition *EXCLUDES 1* Not Coded Here *EXCLUDES 2* Not Included Here

[handwritten notes: Z3A.1 - not valid code needs another character here. CCA Brit Exam look for this!]

Factors Influencing Health Status and Contact With Health Services

Z3A.22–Z42.1

Z3A.22   22 weeks **gestation of pregnancy**   M♀
Z3A.23   23 weeks **gestation of pregnancy**   M♀
Z3A.24   24 weeks **gestation of pregnancy**   M♀
Z3A.25   25 weeks **gestation of pregnancy**   M♀
Z3A.26   26 weeks **gestation of pregnancy**   M♀
Z3A.27   27 weeks **gestation of pregnancy**   M♀
Z3A.28   28 weeks **gestation of pregnancy**   M♀
Z3A.29   29 weeks **gestation of pregnancy**   M♀

√5th **Z3A.3 Weeks of gestation of pregnancy, weeks** 30-39
Z3A.30   30 weeks **gestation of pregnancy**   M♀
Z3A.31   31 weeks **gestation of pregnancy**   M♀
Z3A.32   32 weeks **gestation of pregnancy**   M♀
Z3A.33   33 weeks **gestation of pregnancy**   M♀
Z3A.34   34 weeks **gestation of pregnancy**   M♀
Z3A.35   35 weeks **gestation of pregnancy**   M♀
Z3A.36   36 weeks **gestation of pregnancy**   M♀
Z3A.37   37 weeks **gestation of pregnancy**   M♀
Z3A.38   38 weeks **gestation of pregnancy**   M♀
Z3A.39   39 weeks **gestation of pregnancy**   M♀

√5th **Z3A.4 Weeks of gestation of pregnancy, weeks** 40 or greater
Z3A.40   40 weeks **gestation of pregnancy**   M♀
Z3A.41   41 weeks **gestation of pregnancy**   M♀
Z3A.42   42 weeks **gestation of pregnancy**   M♀
Z3A.49   Greater than 42 weeks **gestation of pregnancy**   M♀

√4th **Z37 Outcome of delivery**
> **NOTE**   This category is intended for use as an additional code to identify the outcome of delivery on the mother's record. It is not for use on the newborn record.
> **EXCLUDES 1**   stillbirth (P95)

Z37.0 Single live birth   M♀
     AHA: 2014, 2Q, 9
Z37.1 Single stillbirth   M♀
Z37.2 Twins, both liveborn   M♀
Z37.3 Twins, one liveborn and one stillborn   M♀
Z37.4 Twins, both stillborn   M♀
√5th **Z37.5 Other multiple births, all liveborn**
     Z37.50 Multiple births, unspecified, all liveborn   M♀
     Z37.51 Triplets, all liveborn   M♀
     Z37.52 Quadruplets, all liveborn   M♀
     Z37.53 Quintuplets, all liveborn   M♀
     Z37.54 Sextuplets, all liveborn   M♀
     Z37.59 Other multiple births, all liveborn   M♀
√5th **Z37.6 Other multiple births, some liveborn**
     Z37.60 Multiple births, unspecified, some liveborn   M♀
     Z37.61 Triplets, some liveborn   M♀
     Z37.62 Quadruplets, some liveborn   M♀
     Z37.63 Quintuplets, some liveborn   M♀
     Z37.64 Sextuplets, some liveborn   M♀
     Z37.69 Other multiple births, some liveborn   M♀
Z37.7 Other multiple births, all stillborn   M♀
Z37.9 Outcome of delivery, unspecified   M♀
     Multiple birth NOS
     Single birth NOS

√4th **Z38 Liveborn infants according to place of birth and type of delivery**
> **NOTE**   This category is for use as the principal code on the initial record of a newborn baby. It is to be used for the initial birth record only. It is not to be used on the mother's record.

√5th **Z38.0 Single liveborn infant, born in hospital**
     Single liveborn infant, born in birthing center or other health care facility
     Z38.00 Single liveborn infant, delivered vaginally   N
     Z38.01 Single liveborn infant, delivered by cesarean   N
Z38.1 Single liveborn infant, born outside hospital   N
Z38.2 Single liveborn infant, unspecified as to place of birth   N
     Single liveborn infant NOS
√5th **Z38.3 Twin liveborn infant, born in hospital**
     Z38.30 Twin liveborn infant, delivered vaginally   N
     Z38.31 Twin liveborn infant, delivered by cesarean   N
Z38.4 Twin liveborn infant, born outside hospital   N
Z38.5 Twin liveborn infant, unspecified as to place of birth   N

√5th **Z38.6 Other multiple liveborn infant, born in hospital**
     Z38.61 Triplet liveborn infant, delivered vaginally   N
     Z38.62 Triplet liveborn infant, delivered by cesarean   N
     Z38.63 Quadruplet liveborn infant, delivered vaginally   N
     Z38.64 Quadruplet liveborn infant, delivered by cesarean   N
     Z38.65 Quintuplet liveborn infant, delivered vaginally   N
     Z38.66 Quintuplet liveborn infant, delivered by cesarean   N
     Z38.68 Other multiple liveborn infant, delivered vaginally   N
     Z38.69 Other multiple liveborn infant, delivered by cesarean   N
Z38.7 Other multiple liveborn infant, born outside hospital   N
Z38.8 Other multiple liveborn infant, unspecified as to place of birth   N

√4th **Z39 Encounter for maternal postpartum care and examination**
Z39.0 Encounter for care and examination of mother immediately after delivery   M♀
     Care and observation in uncomplicated cases when the delivery occurs outside a healthcare facility
> **EXCLUDES 1**   care for postpartum complication—see Alphabetic index

Z39.1 Encounter for care and examination of lactating mother   M♀
     Encounter for supervision of lactation
> **EXCLUDES 1**   disorders of lactation (O92.-)

Z39.2 Encounter for routine postpartum follow-up   M♀

Encounters for other specific health care (Z40-Z53)

> **NOTE**   Categories Z40-Z53 are intended for use to indicate a reason for care. They may be used for patients who have already been treated for a disease or injury, but who are receiving aftercare or prophylactic care, or care to consolidate the treatment, or to deal with a residual state.
> **EXCLUDES 2**   follow-up examination for medical surveillance after treatment (Z08-Z09)

√4th **Z40 Encounter for prophylactic surgery**
> **EXCLUDES 1**   organ donations (Z52.-)
>   therapeutic organ removal—code to condition

√5th **Z40.0 Encounter for prophylactic surgery for risk factors related to malignant neoplasms**
     Admission for prophylactic organ removal
     Use additional code to identify risk factor
     Z40.00 Encounter for prophylactic removal of unspecified organ
     Z40.01 Encounter for prophylactic removal of breast
     Z40.02 Encounter for prophylactic removal of ovary   ♀
     Z40.09 Encounter for prophylactic removal of other organ
Z40.8 Encounter for other prophylactic surgery
Z40.9 Encounter for prophylactic surgery, unspecified

√4th **Z41 Encounter for procedures for purposes other than remedying health state**
Z41.1 Encounter for cosmetic surgery
     Encounter for cosmetic breast implant
     Encounter for cosmetic procedure
> **EXCLUDES 1**   encounter for plastic and reconstructive surgery following medical procedure or healed injury (Z42.-)
>   encounter for post-mastectomy breast implantation (Z42.1)

Z41.2 Encounter for routine and ritual male circumcision   ♂
Z41.3 Encounter for ear piercing
Z41.8 Encounter for other procedures for purposes other than remedying health state
Z41.9 Encounter for procedure for purposes other than remedying health state, unspecified

√4th **Z42 Encounter for plastic and reconstructive surgery following medical procedure or healed injury**
> **EXCLUDES 1**   encounter for cosmetic plastic surgery (Z41.1)
>   encounter for plastic surgery for treatment of current injury—code to relevent injury

Z42.1 Encounter for breast reconstruction following mastectomy   A
> **EXCLUDES 1**   deformity and disproportion of reconstructed breast (N65.1-)

N Newborn: 0   P Pediatric: 0-17   M Maternity: 12-55   A Adult: 15-124   MCC Major CC Condition   PDx MCC PDx acts as own MCC   CC CC Condition   PDx CC PDx acts as own CC

Z42.8   Encounter for other plastic and reconstructive surgery following medical procedure or healed injury

✓4ᵗʰ **Z43   Encounter for attention to artificial openings**

INCLUDES   closure of artificial openings
passage of sounds or bougies through artificial openings
reforming artificial openings
removal of catheter from artificial openings
toilet or cleansing of artificial openings

EXCLUDES 1   *artificial opening status only, without need for care (Z93.-)*
complications of external stoma (J95.0-, K94.-, N99.5-)

EXCLUDES 2   *fitting and adjustment of prosthetic and other devices (Z44-Z46)*

Z43.0   **Encounter for attention to tracheostomy**

Z43.1   **Encounter for attention to gastrostomy**   CC
CC Excl: Z43.1

Z43.2   **Encounter for attention to ileostomy**

Z43.3   **Encounter for attention to colostomy**

Z43.4   **Encounter for attention to other artificial openings of digestive tract**

Z43.5   **Encounter for attention to cystostomy**

Z43.6   **Encounter for attention to other artificial openings of urinary tract**
Encounter for attention to nephrostomy
Encounter for attention to ureterostomy
Encounter for attention to urethrostomy

Z43.7   **Encounter for attention to artificial vagina**

Z43.8   **Encounter for attention to other artificial openings**

Z43.9   **Encounter for attention to unspecified artificial opening**

✓4ᵗʰ **Z44   Encounter for fitting and adjustment of external prosthetic device**

INCLUDES   removal or replacement of external prosthetic device
EXCLUDES 1   *malfunction or other complications of device—see Alphabetical Index*
presence of prosthetic device (Z97.-)

✓5ᵗʰ **Z44.0   Encounter for fitting and adjustment of artificial arm**

✓6ᵗʰ **Z44.00**   **Encounter for fitting and adjustment of unspecified artificial arm**

Z44.001   **Encounter for fitting and adjustment of unspecified right artificial arm**

Z44.002   **Encounter for fitting and adjustment of unspecified left artificial arm**

Z44.009   **Encounter for fitting and adjustment of unspecified artificial arm, unspecified arm**

✓6ᵗʰ **Z44.01**   **Encounter for fitting and adjustment of complete artificial arm**

Z44.011   **Encounter for fitting and adjustment of complete right artificial arm**

Z44.012   **Encounter for fitting and adjustment of complete left artificial arm**

Z44.019   **Encounter for fitting and adjustment of complete artificial arm, unspecified arm**

✓6ᵗʰ **Z44.02**   **Encounter for fitting and adjustment of partial artificial arm**

Z44.021   **Encounter for fitting and adjustment of partial artificial right arm**

Z44.022   **Encounter for fitting and adjustment of partial artificial left arm**

Z44.029   **Encounter for fitting and adjustment of partial artificial arm, unspecified arm**

✓5ᵗʰ **Z44.1   Encounter for fitting and adjustment of artificial leg**

✓6ᵗʰ **Z44.10**   **Encounter for fitting and adjustment of unspecified artificial leg**

Z44.101   **Encounter for fitting and adjustment of unspecified right artificial leg**

Z44.102   **Encounter for fitting and adjustment of unspecified left artificial leg**

Z44.109   **Encounter for fitting and adjustment of unspecified artificial leg, unspecified leg**

✓6ᵗʰ **Z44.11**   **Encounter for fitting and adjustment of complete artificial leg**

Z44.111   **Encounter for fitting and adjustment of complete right artificial leg**

Z44.112   **Encounter for fitting and adjustment of complete left artificial leg**

Z44.119   **Encounter for fitting and adjustment of complete artificial leg, unspecified leg**

✓6ᵗʰ **Z44.12**   **Encounter for fitting and adjustment of partial artificial leg**

Z44.121   **Encounter for fitting and adjustment of partial artificial right leg**

Z44.122   **Encounter for fitting and adjustment of partial artificial left leg**

Z44.129   **Encounter for fitting and adjustment of partial artificial leg, unspecified leg**

✓5ᵗʰ **Z44.2   Encounter for fitting and adjustment of artificial eye**

EXCLUDES 1   *mechanical complication of ocular prosthesis (T85.3)*

Z44.20   **Encounter for fitting and adjustment of artificial eye, unspecified**

Z44.21   **Encounter for fitting and adjustment of artificial right eye**

Z44.22   **Encounter for fitting and adjustment of artificial left eye**

✓5ᵗʰ **Z44.3   Encounter for fitting and adjustment of external breast prosthesis**

EXCLUDES 1   *complications of breast implant (T85.4-)*
encounter for adjustment or removal of breast implant (Z45.81-)
encounter for initial breast implant insertion for cosmetic breast augmentation (Z41.1)
encounter for breast reconstruction following mastectomy (Z42.1)

Z44.30   **Encounter for fitting and adjustment of external breast prosthesis, unspecified breast**   ♀

Z44.31   **Encounter for fitting and adjustment of external right breast prosthesis**   ♀

Z44.32   **Encounter for fitting and adjustment of external left breast prosthesis**   ♀

Z44.8   **Encounter for fitting and adjustment of other external prosthetic devices**

Z44.9   **Encounter for fitting and adjustment of unspecified external prosthetic device**

✓4ᵗʰ **Z45   Encounter for adjustment and management of implanted device**

INCLUDES   removal or replacement of implanted device
EXCLUDES 1   *malfunction or other complications of device—see Alphabetical Index*
presence of prosthetic and other devices (Z95-Z97)
EXCLUDES 2   *encounter for fitting and adjustment of non-implanted device (Z46.-)*

✓5ᵗʰ **Z45.0   Encounter for adjustment and management of cardiac device**

✓6ᵗʰ **Z45.01**   **Encounter for adjustment and management of cardiac pacemaker**

EXCLUDES 1   *encounter for adjustment and management of automatic implantable cardiac defibrillator with synchronous cardiac pacemaker (Z45.02)*

¹³**Z45.010**   **Encounter for checking and testing of cardiac pacemaker pulse generator [battery]**
Encounter for replacing cardiac pacemaker pulse generator [battery]

¹³**Z45.018**   **Encounter for adjustment and management of other part of cardiac pacemaker**

¹³**Z45.02**   **Encounter for adjustment and management of automatic implantable cardiac defibrillator**
Encounter for adjustment and management of automatic implantable cardiac defibrillator with synchronous cardiac pacemaker

¹³**Z45.09**   **Encounter for adjustment and management of other cardiac device**

Z45.1   **Encounter for adjustment and management of infusion pump**

Z45.2   **Encounter for adjustment and management of vascular access device**
Encounter for adjustment and management of vascular catheters
EXCLUDES 1   *encounter for adjustment and management of renal dialysis catheter (Z49.01)*

✓5ᵗʰ **Z45.3   Encounter for adjustment and management of implanted devices of the special senses**

Z45.31   **Encounter for adjustment and management of implanted visual substitution device**

---

13 Questionable admission when used as PDx.

✓ Additional Character Required   ✓x7ᵗʰ Xtension Alert   Unacceptable PDx   Manifestation   Hospital Acquired Condition   EXCLUDES 1 Not Coded Here   EXCLUDES 2 Not Included Here

√6ᵗʰ **Z45.32 Encounter for adjustment and management of implanted hearing device**
> EXCLUDES 1   *Encounter for fitting and adjustment of hearing aide (Z46.1)*

     Z45.320 Encounter for adjustment and management of bone conduction device

     Z45.321 Encounter for adjustment and management of cochlear device

     Z45.328 Encounter for adjustment and management of other implanted hearing device

√5ᵗʰ **Z45.4 Encounter for adjustment and management of implanted nervous system device**

     Z45.41 Encounter for adjustment and management of cerebrospinal fluid drainage device
        Encounter for adjustment and management of cerebral ventricular (communicating) shunt

     Z45.42 Encounter for adjustment and management of neuropacemaker (brain) (peripheral nerve) (spinal cord)

     Z45.49 Encounter for adjustment and management of other implanted nervous system device

√5ᵗʰ **Z45.8 Encounter for adjustment and management of other implanted devices**

     √6ᵗʰ **Z45.81 Encounter for adjustment or removal of breast implant**
        Encounter for elective implant exchange (different material) (different size)
        Encounter removal of tissue expander without synchronous insertion of permanent implant
> EXCLUDES 1   *complications of breast implant (T85.4-)*
> *encounter for initial breast implant insertion for cosmetic breast augmentation (Z41.1)*
> *encounter for breast reconstruction following mastectomy (Z42.1)*

        Z45.811 Encounter for adjustment or removal of right breast implant ♀

        Z45.812 Encounter for adjustment or removal of left breast implant ♀

        Z45.819 Encounter for adjustment or removal of unspecified breast implant ♀

     Z45.82 Encounter for adjustment or removal of myringotomy device (stent) (tube)

     Z45.89 Encounter for adjustment and management of other implanted devices

Z45.9 Encounter for adjustment and management of unspecified implanted device

√4ᵗʰ **Z46 Encounter for fitting and adjustment of other devices**
> INCLUDES   removal or replacement of other device
> EXCLUDES 1   *malfunction or other complications of device—see Alphabetical Index*
> EXCLUDES 2   *encounter for fitting and management of implanted devices (Z45.-)*
> *issue of repeat prescription only (Z76.0)*
> *presence of prosthetic and other devices (Z95-Z97)*

Z46.0 Encounter for fitting and adjustment of spectacles and contact lenses

Z46.1 Encounter for fitting and adjustment of hearing aid
> EXCLUDES 1   *encounter for adjustment and management of implanted hearing device (Z45.32-)*

Z46.2 Encounter for fitting and adjustment of other devices related to nervous system and special senses
> EXCLUDES 2   *encounter for adjustment and management of implanted nervous system device (Z45.4-)*
> *encounter for adjustment and management of implanted visual substitution device (Z45.31)*

Z46.3 Encounter for fitting and adjustment of dental prosthetic device
     Encounter for fitting and adjustment of dentures

Z46.4 Encounter for fitting and adjustment of orthodontic device

√5ᵗʰ **Z46.5 Encounter for fitting and adjustment of other gastrointestinal appliance and device**
> EXCLUDES 1   *encounter for attention to artificial openings of digestive tract (Z43.1-Z43.4)*

     Z46.51 Encounter for fitting and adjustment of gastric lap band

     Z46.59 Encounter for fitting and adjustment of other gastrointestinal appliance and device

Z46.6 Encounter for fitting and adjustment of urinary device
> EXCLUDES 2   *attention to artificial openings of urinary tract (Z43.5, Z43.6)*

√5ᵗʰ **Z46.8 Encounter for fitting and adjustment of other specified devices**

     Z46.81 Encounter for fitting and adjustment of insulin pump
        Encounter for insulin pump instruction and training
        Encounter for insulin pump titration

     Z46.82 Encounter for fitting and adjustment of non-vascular catheter

     Z46.89 Encounter for fitting and adjustment of other specified devices
        Encounter for fitting and adjustment of wheelchair

Z46.9 Encounter for fitting and adjustment of unspecified device

√4ᵗʰ **Z47 Orthopedic aftercare**
> EXCLUDES 1   *aftercare for healing fracture—code to fracture with 7th character D*

Z47.1 Aftercare following joint replacement surgery
     Use additional code to identify the joint (Z96.6-)

Z47.2 Encounter for removal of internal fixation device
> EXCLUDES 1   *encounter for adjustment of internal fixation device for fracture treatment—code to fracture with appropriate 7th character*
> *encounter for removal of external fixation device—code to fracture with 7th character D*
> *infection or inflammatory reaction to internal fixation device (T84.6-)*
> *mechanical complication of internal fixation device (T84.1-)*

√5ᵗʰ **Z47.3 Aftercare following explanation of joint prosthesis**
     Aftercare following explanation of joint prosthesis, staged procedure
     Encounter for joint prosthesis insertion following prior explanation of joint prosthesis

     Z47.31 Aftercare following explanation of shoulder joint prosthesis
> EXCLUDES 1   *acquired absence of shoulder joint following prior explanation of shoulder joint prosthesis (Z89.23-)*
> *shoulder joint prosthesis explanation status (Z89.23-)*

     Z47.32 Aftercare following explanation of hip joint prosthesis
> EXCLUDES 1   *acquired absence of hip joint following prior explanation of hip joint prosthesis (Z89.62-)*
> *hip joint prosthesis explanation status (Z89.62-)*

     Z47.33 Aftercare following explanation of knee joint prosthesis
> EXCLUDES 1   *acquired absence of knee joint following prior explanation of knee prosthesis (Z89.52-)*
> *knee joint prosthesis explanation status (Z89.52-)*

√5ᵗʰ **Z47.8 Encounter for other orthopedic aftercare**

     Z47.81 Encounter for orthopedic aftercare following surgical amputation
        Use additional code to identify the limb amputated (Z89.-)

     Z47.82 Encounter for orthopedic aftercare following scoliosis surgery

     Z47.89 Encounter for other orthopedic aftercare

√4ᵗʰ **Z48 Encounter for other postprocedural aftercare**
> EXCLUDES 1   *encounter for follow-up examination after completed treatment (Z08-Z09)*
> EXCLUDES 2   *encounter for attention to artificial openings (Z43.-)*
> *encounter for fitting and adjustment of prosthetic and other devices (Z44-Z46)*

√5ᵗʰ **Z48.0 Encounter for attention to dressings, sutures and drains**
> EXCLUDES 1   *encounter for planned postprocedural wound closure (Z48.1)*

     Z48.00 Encounter for change or removal of nonsurgical wound dressing
        Encounter for change or removal of wound dressing NOS

     Z48.01 Encounter for change or removal of surgical wound dressing

---

N Newborn: 0   P Pediatric: 0-17   M Maternity: 12-55   A Adult: 15-124   MCC Major CC Condition   PDx MCC PDx acts as own MCC   CC CC Condition   PDx CC PDx acts as own CC

Z48.02   **Encounter for removal of sutures**
Encounter for removal of staples

Z48.03   **Encounter for change or removal of drains**

Z48.1   **Encounter for planned postprocedural wound closure**
EXCLUDES 1   *encounter for attention to dressings and sutures (Z48.0-)*

✓5th **Z48.2**   **Encounter for aftercare following organ transplant**

Z48.21   **Encounter for aftercare following heart transplant**   PDx CC cc
CC Excl: D47.Z1,T86.20-T86.23,T86.290,T86.298,T86.30-T86.39,T86.850-T86.859,T86.90-T86.99,Z94.1,Z94.3, Z94.89- Z94.9

Z48.22   **Encounter for aftercare following kidney transplant**   PDx CC cc
CC Excl: D47.Z1,T86.10-T86.13, T86.19, T86.850-T86.859,T86.90-T86.99,Z94.0,Z94.89-Z94.9

Z48.23   **Encounter for aftercare following liver transplant**   PDx CC cc
CC Excl: D47.Z1,T86.40-T86.43,T86.49,T86.850-T86.859,T86.90-T86.99, Z94.4,Z94.89-Z94.9

Z48.24   **Encounter for aftercare following lung transplant**   PDx CC cc
CC Excl: D47.Z1, T86.810-T86.819,T86.49,T86.850-T86.859,T86.90-T86.99,Z94.2,Z94.89-Z94.9

✓6th **Z48.28**   **Encounter for aftercare following multiple organ transplant**

Z48.280   **Encounter for aftercare following heart-lung transplant**   PDxCC cc
CC Excl: See Code: Z48.21

Z48.288   **Encounter for aftercare following multiple organ transplant**

✓6th **Z48.29**   **Encounter for aftercare following other organ transplant**

Z48.290   **Encounter for aftercare following bone marrow transplant**   PDx CC cc
CC Excl: D47.Z1, T86.810-T86.813,T86.00-T86.09,T86.850-T86.859,T86.90-T86.99,Z94.9

Z48.298   **Encounter for aftercare following other organ transplant**

Z48.3   **Aftercare following surgery for neoplasm**
Use additional code to identify the neoplasm

✓5th **Z48.8**   **Encounter for other specified postprocedural aftercare**

✓6th **Z48.81**   **Encounter for surgical aftercare following surgery on specified body systems**
NOTE   These codes identify the body system requiring aftercare. They are for use in conjunction with other aftercare codes to fully explain the aftercare encounter. The condition treated should also be coded if still present.
EXCLUDES 1   *aftercare for injury—code the injury with 7th character D*
aftercare following surgery for neoplasm (Z48.3)
EXCLUDES 2   *aftercare following organ transplant (Z48.2-)*
orthopedic aftercare (Z47.-)

Z48.810   **Encounter for surgical aftercare following surgery on the sense organs**

Z48.811   **Encounter for surgical aftercare following surgery on the nervous system**
EXCLUDES 2   *encounter for surgical aftercare following surgery on the sense organs (Z48.810)*

Z48.812   **Encounter for surgical aftercare following surgery on the circulatory system**
AHA: 2012, 4Q, 96

Z48.813   **Encounter for surgical aftercare following surgery on the respiratory system**

Z48.814   **Encounter for surgical aftercare following surgery on the teeth or oral cavity**

Z48.815   **Encounter for surgical aftercare following surgery on the digestive system**

Z48.816   **Encounter for surgical aftercare following surgery on the genitourinary system**
EXCLUDES 1   *encounter for aftercare following sterilization reversal (Z31.42)*

Z48.817   **Encounter for surgical aftercare following surgery on the skin and subcutaneous tissue**

Z48.89   **Encounter for other specified surgical aftercare**

✓4th **Z49**   **Encounter for care involving renal dialysis**
Code also associated end stage renal disease (N18.6)

✓5th **Z49.0**   **Preparatory care for renal dialysis**
Encounter for dialysis instruction and training

Z49.01   **Encounter for fitting and adjustment of extracorporeal dialysis catheter**
Removal or replacement of renal dialysis catheter
Toilet or cleansing of renal dialysis catheter

Z49.02   **Encounter for fitting and adjustment of peritoneal dialysis catheter**

✓5th **Z49.3**   **Encounter for adequacy testing for dialysis**

Z49.31   **Encounter for adequacy testing for hemodialysis**

Z49.32   **Encounter for adequacy testing for peritoneal dialysis**
Encounter for peritoneal equilibration test

✓4th **Z51**   **Encounter for other aftercare**
Code also condition requiring care
EXCLUDES 1   *follow-up examination after treatment (Z08-Z09)*

Z51.0   **Encounter for antineoplastic radiation therapy**

✓5th **Z51.1**   **Encounter for antineoplastic chemotherapy and immunotherapy**
EXCLUDES 2   *encounter for chemotherapy and immunotherapy for nonneoplastic condition—code to condition*

Z51.11   **Encounter for antineoplastic chemotherapy**

Z51.12   **Encounter for antineoplastic immunotherapy**

Z51.5   **Encounter for palliative care**

✓5th **Z51.8**   **Encounter for other specified aftercare**
EXCLUDES 1   *holiday relief care (Z75.5)*

Z51.81   **Encounter for therapeutic drug level monitoring**
Code also any long-term (current) drug therapy (Z79.-)
EXCLUDES 1   *encounter for blood-drug test for administrative or medicolegal reasons (Z02.83)*

Z51.89   **Encounter for other specified aftercare**
AHA: 2012, 4Q, 95-97

✓4th **Z52**   **Donors of organs and tissues**
INCLUDES   autologous and other living donors
EXCLUDES 1   *cadaveric donor—omit code*
examination of potential donor (Z00.5)
AHA: 2012, 4Q, 99

✓5th **Z52.0**   **Blood donor**

✓6th **Z52.00**   **Unspecified blood donor**

Z52.000   **Unspecified donor, whole blood**

Z52.001   **Unspecified donor, stem cells**

Z52.008   **Unspecified donor, other blood**

✓6th **Z52.01**   **Autologous blood donor**

Z52.010   **Autologous donor, whole blood**

Z52.011   **Autologous donor, stem cells**

Z52.018   **Autologous donor, other blood**

✓6th **Z52.09**   **Other blood donor**
Volunteer donor

Z52.090   **Other blood donor, whole blood**

Z52.091   **Other blood donor, stem cells**

Z52.098   **Other blood donor, other blood**

✓5th **Z52.1**   **Skin donor**

Z52.10   **Skin donor, unspecified**

Z52.11   **Skin donor, autologous**

Z52.19   **Skin donor, other**

✓5th **Z52.2**   **Bone donor**

Z52.20   **Bone donor, unspecified**

Z52.21   **Bone donor, autologous**

Z52.29   **Bone donor, other**

Z52.3   **Bone marrow donor**

Z52.4   **Kidney donor**

Z52.5   **Cornea donor**

Z52.6   **Liver donor**

✓5th **Z52.8**   **Donor of other specified organs or tissues**

✓6th **Z52.81**   **Egg (Oocyte) donor**

Z52.810   **Egg (Oocyte) donor under age 35, anonymous recipient**   ♀
Egg donor under age 35 NOS

Z52.811   **Egg (Oocyte) donor under age 35, designated recipient**   ♀

✓ Additional Character Required   √x7th Xtension Alert   Unacceptable PDx   Manifestation   Hospital Acquired Condition   *EXCLUDES 1* Not Coded Here   *EXCLUDES 2* Not Included Here

ICD-10-CM Draft (2015)   1185

Factors Influencing Health Status and Contact With Health Services

Z52.812–Z62.21

Z52.812   **Egg (Oocyte) donor age 35 and over, anonymous recipient** ♀
     Egg donor age 35 and over NOS

Z52.813   **Egg (Oocyte) donor age 35 and over, designated recipient** ♀

Z52.819   **Egg (Oocyte) donor, unspecified** ♀

Z52.89   **Donor of other specified organs or tissues**

Z52.9   **Donor of unspecified organ or tissue**
     Donor NOS

✓4th **Z53**   **Persons encountering health services for specific procedures and treatment, not carried out**

   ✓5th **Z53.0**   **Procedure and treatment not carried out because of contraindication**

     Z53.01   **Procedure and treatment not carried out due to patient smoking**

     Z53.09   **Procedure and treatment not carried out because of other contraindication**

   Z53.1   **Procedure and treatment not carried out because of patient's decision for reasons of belief and group pressure**

   ✓5th **Z53.2**   **Procedure and treatment not carried out because of patient's decision for other and unspecified reasons**

     Z53.20   **Procedure and treatment not carried out because of patient's decision for unspecified reasons**

     Z53.21   **Procedure and treatment not carried out due to patient leaving prior to being seen by health care provider**

     Z53.29   **Procedure and treatment not carried out because of patient's decision for other reasons**

   Z53.8   **Procedure and treatment not carried out for other reasons**

   Z53.9   **Procedure and treatment not carried out, unspecified reason**

Persons with potential health hazards related to socioeconomic and psychosocial circumstances (Z55-Z65)

✓4th **Z55**   **Problems related to education and literacy**
     EXCLUDES1   disorders of psychological development (F80-F89)

   Z55.0   **Illiteracy and low-level literacy**

   Z55.1   **Schooling unavailable and unattainable**

   Z55.2   **Failed school examinations**

   Z55.3   **Underachievement in school**

   Z55.4   **Educational maladjustment and discord with teachers and classmates**

   Z55.8   **Other problems related to education and literacy**
     Problems related to inadequate teaching

   Z55.9   **Problems related to education and literacy, unspecified**
     Academic problems NOS

✓4th **Z56**   **Problems related to employment and unemployment**
     EXCLUDES2   occupational exposure to risk factors (Z57.-)
         problems related to housing and economic circumstances (Z59.-)

   Z56.0   **Unemployment, unspecified**

   Z56.1   **Change of job**   A

   Z56.2   **Threat of job loss**

   Z56.3   **Stressful work schedule**

   Z56.4   **Discord with boss and workmates**

   Z56.5   **Uncongenial work environment**
     Difficult conditions at work

   Z56.6   **Other physical and mental strain related to work**

   ✓5th **Z56.8**   **Other problems related to employment**

     Z56.81   **Sexual harassment on the job**

     Z56.82   **Military deployment status**
         Individual (civilian or military) currently deployed in theater or in support of military war, peacekeeping and humanitarian operations

     Z56.89   **Other problems related to employment**

   Z56.9   **Unspecified problems related to employment**
     Occupational problems NOS

✓4th **Z57**   **Occupational exposure to risk factors**

   Z57.0   **Occupational exposure to noise**

   Z57.1   **Occupational exposure to radiation**

   Z57.2   **Occupational exposure to dust**

   ✓5th **Z57.3**   **Occupational exposure to other air contaminants**

     Z57.31   **Occupational exposure to environmental tobacco smoke**
         EXCLUDES2   exposure to environmental tobacco smoke (Z77.22)

     Z57.39   **Occupational exposure to other air contaminants**

   Z57.4   **Occupational exposure to toxic agents in agriculture**
     Occupational exposure to solids, liquids, gases or vapors in agriculture

   Z57.5   **Occupational exposure to toxic agents in other industries**
     Occupational exposure to solids, liquids, gases or vapors in other industries

   Z57.6   **Occupational exposure to extreme temperature**

   Z57.7   **Occupational exposure to vibration**

   Z57.8   **Occupational exposure to other risk factors**

   Z57.9   **Occupational exposure to unspecified risk factor**

✓4th **Z59**   **Problems related to housing and economic circumstances**
     EXCLUDES2   problems related to upbringing (Z62.-)

   Z59.0   **Homelessness**

   Z59.1   **Inadequate housing**
     Lack of heating
     Restriction of space
     Technical defects in home preventing adequate care
     Unsatisfactory surroundings
     EXCLUDES1   problems related to the natural and physical environment (Z77.1-)

   Z59.2   **Discord with neighbors, lodgers and landlord**

   Z59.3   **Problems related to living in residential institution**
     Boarding-school resident
     EXCLUDES1   institutional upbringing (Z62.2)

   Z59.4   **Lack of adequate food and safe drinking water**
     Inadequate drinking water supply
     EXCLUDES1   effects of hunger (T73.0)
         inappropriate diet or eating habits (Z72.4)
         malnutrition (E40-E46)

   Z59.5   **Extreme poverty**

   Z59.6   **Low income**

   Z59.7   **Insufficient social insurance and welfare support**

   Z59.8   **Other problems related to housing and economic circumstances**
     Foreclosure on loan   Problems with creditors
     Isolated dwelling

   Z59.9   **Problem related to housing and economic circumstances, unspecified**

✓4th **Z60**   **Problems related to social environment**

   Z60.0   **Problems of adjustment to life-cycle transitions**
     Empty nest syndrome   Problem with adjustment
     Phase of life problem   to retirement [pension]

   Z60.2   **Problems related to living alone**

   Z60.3   **Acculturation difficulty**
     Problem with migration
     Problem with social transplantation

   Z60.4   **Social exclusion and rejection**
     Exclusion and rejection on the basis of personal characteristics, such as unusual physical appearance, illness or behavior.
     EXCLUDES1   target of adverse discrimination such as for racial or religious reasons (Z60.5)

   Z60.5   **Target of (perceived) adverse discrimination and persecution**
     EXCLUDES1   social exclusion and rejection (Z60.4)

   Z60.8   **Other problems related to social environment**

   Z60.9   **Problem related to social environment, unspecified**

✓4th **Z62**   **Problems related to upbringing**
     Current and past negative life events in childhood
     Current and past problems of a child related to upbringing
     EXCLUDES2   maltreatment syndrome (T74.-)
         problems related to housing and economic circumstances (Z59.-)

   Z62.0   **Inadequate parental supervision and control**

   Z62.1   **Parental overprotection**

   ✓5th **Z62.2**   **Upbringing away from parents**
     EXCLUDES1   problems with boarding school (Z59.3)

     Z62.21   **Child in welfare custody**   P
         Child in care of non-parental family member
         Child in foster care
         EXCLUDES2   problem for parent due to child in welfare custody (Z63.5)

N Newborn: 0   P Pediatric: 0-17   M Maternity: 12-55   A Adult: 15-124   MCC Major CC Condition   PDx MCC PDx acts as own MCC   CC CC Condition   PDx CC PDx acts as own CC

1186   ICD-10-CM Draft (2015)

Z62.22 Institutional upbringing
Child living in orphanage or group home

Z62.29 Other upbringing away from parents

Z62.3 Hostility towards and scapegoating of child P

Z62.6 Inappropriate (excessive) parental pressure

✓5th **Z62.8 Other specified problems related to upbringing**

✓6th **Z62.81 Personal history of abuse in childhood**

Z62.810 Personal history of physical and sexual abuse in childhood
EXCLUDES 1 current child physical abuse (T74.12, T76.12)
current child sexual abuse (T74.22, T76.22)

Z62.811 Personal history of psychological abuse in childhood
EXCLUDES 1 current child psychological abuse (T74.32, T76.32)

Z62.812 Personal history of neglect in childhood
EXCLUDES 1 current child neglect (T74.02, T76.02)

Z62.819 Personal history of unspecified abuse in childhood
EXCLUDES 1 current child abuse NOS (T74.92, T76.92)

✓6th **Z62.82 Parent-child conflict**

Z62.820 Parent-biological child conflict
Parent-child problem NOS

Z62.821 Parent-adopted child conflict

Z62.822 Parent-foster child conflict

✓6th **Z62.89 Other specified problems related to upbringing**

Z62.890 Parent-child estrangement NEC

Z62.891 Sibling rivalry

Z62.898 Other specified problems related to upbringing

Z62.9 Problem related to upbringing, unspecified

✓4th **Z63 Other problems related to primary support group, including family circumstances**
EXCLUDES 2 maltreatment syndrome (T74-, T76)
parent-child problems (Z62.-)
problems related to negative life events in childhood (Z62.-)
problems related to upbringing (Z62.-)

Z63.0 Problems in relationship with spouse or partner
EXCLUDES 1 counseling for spousal or partner abuse problems (Z69.1)
counseling related to sexual attitude, behavior, and orientation (Z70.-)

Z63.1 Problems in relationship with in-laws

✓5th **Z63.3 Absence of family member**
EXCLUDES 1 absence of family member due to disappearance and death (Z63.4)
absence of family member due to separation and divorce (Z63.5)

Z63.31 Absence of family member due to military deployment
Individual or family affected by other family member being on military deployment
EXCLUDES 1 family disruption due to return of family member from military deployment (Z63.71)

Z63.32 Other absence of family member

Z63.4 Disappearance and death of family member
Assumed death of family member
Bereavement
AHA: 2014, 1Q, 25

Z63.5 Disruption of family by separation and divorce
Marital estrangement

Z63.6 Dependent relative needing care at home

✓5th **Z63.7 Other stressful life events affecting family and household**

Z63.71 Stress on family due to return of family member from military deployment
Individual or family affected by family member having returned from military deployment (current or past conflict)

Z63.72 Alcoholism and drug addiction in family

Z63.79 Other stressful life events affecting family and household
Anxiety (normal) about sick person in family
Health problems within family
Ill or disturbed family member
Isolated family

Z63.8 Other specified problems related to primary support group
Family discord NOS
Family estrangement NOS
High expressed emotional level within family
Inadequate family support NOS
Inadequate or distorted communication within family

Z63.9 Problem related to primary support group, unspecified
Relationship disorder NOS

✓4th **Z64 Problems related to certain psychosocial circumstances**

Z64.0 Problems related to unwanted pregnancy M♀

Z64.1 Problems related to multiparity ♀

Z64.4 Discord with counselors
Discord with probation officer
Discord with social worker

✓4th **Z65 Problems related to other psychosocial circumstances**

Z65.0 Conviction in civil and criminal proceedings without imprisonment

Z65.1 Imprisonment and other incarceration

Z65.2 Problems related to release from prison

Z65.3 Problems related to other legal circumstances
Arrest
Child custody or support proceedings
Litigation
Prosecution

Z65.4 Victim of crime and terrorism
Victim of torture

Z65.5 Exposure to disaster, war and other hostilities
EXCLUDES 1 target of perceived discrimination or persecution (Z60.5)

Z65.8 Other specified problems related to psychosocial circumstances

Z65.9 Problem related to unspecified psychosocial circumstances

Do not resuscitate status (Z66)

Z66 Do not resuscitate
DNR status

Blood type (Z67)

✓4th **Z67 Blood type**

✓5th **Z67.1 Type A blood**
Z67.10 Type A blood, Rh positive
Z67.11 Type A blood, Rh negative

✓5th **Z67.2 Type B blood**
Z67.20 Type B blood, Rh positive
Z67.21 Type B blood, Rh negative

✓5th **Z67.3 Type AB blood**
Z67.30 Type AB blood, Rh positive
Z67.31 Type AB blood, Rh negative

✓5th **Z67.4 Type O blood**
Z67.40 Type O blood, Rh positive
Z67.41 Type O blood, Rh negative

✓5th **Z67.9 Unspecified blood type**
Z67.90 Unspecified blood type, Rh positive
Z67.91 Unspecified blood type, Rh negative

Body mass index [BMI] (Z68)

✓4th **Z68 Body mass index [BMI]**
Kilograms per meters squared
NOTE BMI adult codes are for use for persons 21 years of age or older.
BMI pediatric codes are for use for persons 2-20 years of age. These percentiles are based on the growth charts published by the Centers for Disease Control and Prevention (CDC)

Z68.1 Body mass index [BMI] 19 or less, adult CC A
CC Excl: E66.01-E66.1,E66.8-E66.9, Z68.1,Z68.20-Z68.39, Z68.1-Z68.54

✓5th **Z68.2 Body mass index [BMI] 20-29, adult**
Z68.20 Body mass index [BMI] 20.0-20.9, adult A

Z68.21 Body mass index [BMI] 21.0-21.9, adult   A
Z68.22 Body mass index [BMI] 22.0-22.9, adult   A
Z68.23 Body mass index [BMI] 23.0-23.9, adult   A
Z68.24 Body mass index [BMI] 24.0-24.9, adult   A
Z68.25 Body mass index [BMI] 25.0-25.9, adult   A
Z68.26 Body mass index [BMI] 26.0-26.9, adult   A
Z68.27 Body mass index [BMI] 27.0-27.9, adult   A
Z68.28 Body mass index [BMI] 28.0-28.9, adult   A
Z68.29 Body mass index [BMI] 29.0-29.9, adult   A

✓5th Z68.3 Body mass index [BMI] 30-39, adult
Z68.30 Body mass index [BMI] 30.0-30.9, adult   A
Z68.31 Body mass index [BMI] 31.0-31.9, adult   A
Z68.32 Body mass index [BMI] 32.0-32.9, adult   A
Z68.33 Body mass index [BMI] 33.0-33.9, adult   A
Z68.34 Body mass index [BMI] 34.0-34.9, adult   A
Z68.35 Body mass index [BMI] 35.0-35.9, adult   A
Z68.36 Body mass index [BMI] 36.0-36.9, adult   A
Z68.37 Body mass index [BMI] 37.0-37.9, adult   A
Z68.38 Body mass index [BMI] 38.0-38.9, adult   A
Z68.39 Body mass index [BMI] 39.0-39.9, adult   A

✓5th Z68.4 Body mass index [BMI] 40 or greater, adult

CC Excl: For CC codes in subcategory Z68.4: CC with 7th
character A, unless otherwise noted: E65-E66.1, E66.8-E66.9,
Z68.1-Z68.54

Z68.41 Body mass index [BMI] 40.0-44.9, adult   CC A
Z68.42 Body mass index [BMI] 45.0-49.9, adult   CC A
Z68.43 Body mass index [BMI] 50-59.9, adult   CC A
Z68.44 Body mass index [BMI] 60.0-69.9, adult   CC A
Z68.45 Body mass index [BMI] 70 or greater, adult   CC A

✓5th Z68.5 Body mass index [BMI] pediatric
Z68.51 Body mass index [BMI] pediatric, less than 5th
percentile for age   P
Z68.52 Body mass index [BMI] pediatric, 5th percentile
to less than 85th percentile for age   P
Z68.53 Body mass index [BMI] pediatric, 85th percentile
to less than 95th percentile for age   P
Z68.54 Body mass index [BMI] pediatric, greater than or
equal to 95th percentile for age   P

Persons encountering health services in other circumstances (Z69-Z76)

✓4th Z69 **Encounter for mental health services for victim and perpetrator of abuse**
Counseling for victims and perpetrators of abuse

✓5th Z69.0 **Encounter for mental health services for child abuse problems**

✓6th Z69.01 **Encounter for mental health services for parental child abuse**
Z69.010 Encounter for mental health services for victim of parental child abuse   P
Z69.011 Encounter for mental health services for perpetrator of parental child abuse
EXCLUDES 1 encounter for mental health services for non-parental child abuse (Z69.02-)

✓6th Z69.02 **Encounter for mental health services for non-parental child abuse**
Z69.020 Encounter for mental health services for victim of non-parental child abuse   P
Z69.021 Encounter for mental health services for perpetrator of non-parental child abuse

✓5th Z69.1 **Encounter for mental health services for spousal or partner abuse problems**
Z69.11 Encounter for mental health services for victim of spousal or partner abuse
Z69.12 Encounter for mental health services for perpetrator of spousal or partner abuse

✓5th Z69.8 **Encounter for mental health services for victim or perpetrator of other abuse**
Z69.81 Encounter for mental health services for victim of other abuse
Encounter for rape victim counseling

Z69.82 Encounter for mental health services for perpetrator of other abuse

✓4th Z70 **Counseling related to sexual attitude, behavior and orientation**
Encounter for mental health services for sexual attitude, behavior and orientation
EXCLUDES 2 contraceptive or procreative counseling (Z30-Z31)

Z70.0 **Counseling related to sexual attitude**

Z70.1 **Counseling related to patient's sexual behavior and orientation**
Patient concerned regarding impotence
Patient concerned regarding non-responsiveness
Patient concerned regarding promiscuity
Patient concerned regarding sexual orientation

Z70.2 **Counseling related to sexual behavior and orientation of third party**
Advice sought regarding sexual behavior and orientation of child
Advice sought regarding sexual behavior and orientation of partner
Advice sought regarding sexual behavior and orientation of spouse

Z70.3 **Counseling related to combined concerns regarding sexual attitude, behavior and orientation**

Z70.8 **Other sex counseling**
Encounter for sex education

Z70.9 **Sex counseling, unspecified**

✓4th Z71 **Persons encountering health services for other counseling and medical advice, not elsewhere classified**
EXCLUDES 2 contraceptive or procreation counseling (Z30-Z31)
sex counseling (Z70.-)

Z71.0 **Person encountering health services to consult on behalf of another person**
Person encountering health services to seek advice or treatment for non-attending third party
EXCLUDES 2 anxiety (normal) about sick person in family (Z63.7)
expectant (adoptive) parent(s) pre-birth pediatrician visit (Z76.81)

Z71.1 **Person with feared health complaint in whom no diagnosis is made**
Person encountering health services with feared condition which was not demonstrated
Person encountering health services in which problem was normal state
"Worried well"
EXCLUDES 1 medical observation for suspected diseases and conditions proven not to exist (Z03.-)

Z71.2 **Person consulting for explanation of examination or test findings**

Z71.3 **Dietary counseling and surveillance**
Use additional code for any associated underlying medical condition
Use additional code to identify body mass index (BMI), if known (Z68.-)

✓5th Z71.4 **Alcohol abuse counseling and surveillance**
Use additional code for alcohol abuse or dependence (F10.-)
Z71.41 Alcohol abuse counseling and surveillance of alcoholic
Z71.42 Counseling for family member of alcoholic
Counseling for significant other, partner, or friend of alcoholic

✓5th Z71.5 **Drug abuse counseling and surveillance**
Use additional code for drug abuse or dependence (F11-F16, F18-F19)
Z71.51 Drug abuse counseling and surveillance of drug abuser
Z71.52 Counseling for family member of drug abuser
Counseling for significant other, partner, or friend of drug abuser

Z71.6 **Tobacco abuse counseling**
Use additional code for nicotine dependence (F17.-)

Z71.7 **Human immunodeficiency virus [HIV] counseling**

✓5th Z71.8 **Other specified counseling**
EXCLUDES 2 counseling for contraception (Z30.0-)
counseling for genetics (Z31.5)
counseling for procreative management (Z31.6-)
Z71.81 Spiritual or religious counseling
Z71.89 Other specified counseling

N Newborn: 0   P Pediatric: 0-17   M Maternity: 12-55   A Adult: 15-124   MCC Major CC Condition   PDx MCC PDx acts as own MCC   CC CC Condition   PDx CC PDx acts as own CC

1188

ICD-10-CM Draft (2015)

Z71.9   **Counseling, unspecified**
Encounter for medical advice NOS

✓4ᵗʰ **Z72**   **Problems related to lifestyle**
EXCLUDES 2   *problems related to life-management difficulty (Z73.-)*
problems related to socioeconomic and psychosocial circumstances (Z55-Z65)

Z72.0   **Tobacco use**
Tobacco use NOS
EXCLUDES 1   *history of tobacco dependence (Z87.891)*
nicotine dependence (F17.2-)
tobacco dependence (F17.2-)
tobacco use during pregnancy (O99.33-)

Z72.3   **Lack of physical exercise**

Z72.4   **Inappropriate diet and eating habits**
EXCLUDES 1   *behavioral eating disorders of infancy or childhood (F98.2- F98.3)*
eating disorders (F50.-)
lack of adequate food (Z59.4)
malnutrition and other nutritional deficiencies (E40-E64)

✓5ᵗʰ **Z72.5**   **High risk sexual behavior**
Promiscuity
EXCLUDES 1   *paraphilias (F65)*

Z72.51   **High risk heterosexual behavior**
Z72.52   **High risk homosexual behavior**
Z72.53   **High risk bisexual behavior**

Z72.6   **Gambling and betting**
EXCLUDES 1   *compulsive or pathological gambling (F63.0)*

Z72.8   **Other problems related to lifestyle**

✓6ᵗʰ **Z72.81**   **Antisocial behavior**
EXCLUDES 1   *conduct disorders (F91.-)*

Z72.810   **Child and adolescent antisocial behavior**   P
Antisocial behavior (child) (adolescent) without manifest psychiatric disorder
Delinquency NOS
Group delinquency
Offenses in the context of gang membership
Stealing in company with others
Truancy from school

Z72.811   **Adult antisocial behavior**   A
Adult antisocial behavior without manifest psychiatric disorder

✓6ᵗʰ **Z72.82**   **Problems related to sleep**

Z72.820   **Sleep deprivation**
Lack of adequate sleep
EXCLUDES 1   *insomnia (G47.0-)*

Z72.821   **Inadequate sleep hygiene**
Bad sleep habits
Irregular sleep habits
Unhealthy sleep wake schedule
EXCLUDES 1   *insomnia (F51.0-, G47.0-)*

Z72.89   **Other problems related to lifestyle**
Self-damaging behavior

Z72.9   **Problem related to lifestyle, unspecified**

✓4ᵗʰ **Z73**   **Problems related to life management difficulty**
EXCLUDES 2   *problems related to socioeconomic and psychosocial circumstances (Z55-Z65)*

Z73.0   **Burn-out**

Z73.1   **Type A behavior pattern**

Z73.2   **Lack of relaxation and leisure**

Z73.3   **Stress, not elsewhere classified**
Physical and mental strain NOS
EXCLUDES 1   *stress related to employment or unemployment (Z56.-)*

Z73.4   **Inadequate social skills, not elsewhere classified**

Z73.5   **Social role conflict, not elsewhere classified**

Z73.6   **Limitation of activities due to disability**
EXCLUDES 1   *care-provider dependency (Z74.-)*

✓5ᵗʰ **Z73.8**   **Other problems related to life management difficulty**

✓6ᵗʰ **Z73.81**   **Behavioral insomnia of childhood**

Z73.810   **Behavioral insomnia of childhood, sleep-onset association type**   P

Z73.811   **Behavioral insomnia of childhood, limit setting type**   P

Z73.812   **Behavioral insomnia of childhood, combined type**   P

Z73.819   **Behavioral insomnia of childhood, unspecified type**   P

Z73.82   **Dual sensory impairment**

Z73.89   **Other problems related to life management difficulty**

Z73.9   **Problem related to life management difficulty, unspecified**

✓4ᵗʰ **Z74**   **Problems related to care provider dependency**
EXCLUDES 2   *dependence on enabling machines or devices NEC (Z99.-)*

✓5ᵗʰ **Z74.0**   **Reduced mobility**

Z74.01   **Bed confinement status**
Bedridden

Z74.09   **Other reduced mobility**
Chair ridden
Reduced mobility NOS
EXCLUDES 2   *wheelchair dependence (Z99.3)*

Z74.1   **Need for assistance with personal care**

Z74.2   **Need for assistance at home and no other household member able to render care**

Z74.3   **Need for continuous supervision**

Z74.8   **Other problems related to care provider dependency**

Z74.9   **Problem related to care provider dependency, unspecified**

✓4ᵗʰ **Z75**   **Problems related to medical facilities and other health care**

Z75.0   **Medical services not available in home**
EXCLUDES 1   *no other household member able to render care (Z74.2)*

Z75.1   **Person awaiting admission to adequate facility elsewhere**

Z75.2   **Other waiting period for investigation and treatment**

Z75.3   **Unavailability and inaccessibility of health-care facilities**
EXCLUDES 1   *bed unavailable (Z75.1)*

Z75.4   **Unavailability and inaccessibility of other helping agencies**

Z75.5   **Holiday relief care**

Z75.8   **Other problems related to medical facilities and other health care**

Z75.9   **Unspecified problem related to medical facilities and other health care**

✓4ᵗʰ **Z76**   **Persons encountering health services in other circumstances**

Z76.0   **Encounter for issue of repeat prescription**
Encounter for issue of repeat prescription for appliance
Encounter for issue of repeat prescription for medicaments
Encounter for issue of repeat prescription for spectacles
EXCLUDES 2   *issue of medical certificate (Z02.7)*
repeat prescription for contraceptive (Z30.4-)

Z76.1   **Encounter for health supervision and care of foundling**

Z76.2   **Encounter for health supervision and care of other healthy infant and child**   P
Encounter for medical or nursing care or supervision of healthy infant under circumstances such as adverse socioeconomic conditions at home
Encounter for medical or nursing care or supervision of healthy infant under circumstances such as awaiting foster or adoptive placement
Encounter for medical or nursing care or supervision of healthy infant under circumstances such as maternal illness
Encounter for medical or nursing care or supervision of healthy infant under circumstances such as number of children at home preventing or interfering with normal care

Z76.3   **Healthy person accompanying sick person**

Z76.4   **Other boarder to healthcare facility**
EXCLUDES 1   *homelessness (Z59.0)*

Z76.5   **Malingerer [conscious simulation]**
Person feigning illness (with obvious motivation)
EXCLUDES 1   *factitious disorder (F68.1-)*
peregrinating patient (F68.1-)

✓5ᵗʰ **Z76.8**   **Persons encountering health services in other specified circumstances**

Z76.81   **Expectant parent(s) prebirth pediatrician visit**
Pre-adoption pediatrician visit for adoptive parent(s)

Z76.82   **Awaiting organ transplant status**
Patient waiting for organ availability

Z76.89   **Persons encountering health services in other specified circumstances**
Persons encountering health services NOS
AHA: 2014, 2Q, 10

✓ Additional Character Required   ✗7ᵗʰ Xtension Alert   Unacceptable PDx   Manifestation   Hospital Acquired Condition   EXCLUDES 1 Not Coded Here   EXCLUDES 2 Not Included Here

Persons with potential health hazards related to family and personal history and certain conditions influencing health status (Z77-Z99)

Code also any follow-up examination (Z08-Z09)

✓4th **Z77 Other contact with and (suspected) exposures hazardous to health**

    INCLUDES   contact with and (suspected) exposures to potential hazards to health

    EXCLUDES 2   *contact with and (suspected) exposure to communicable diseases (Z20.-)*
              exposure to (parental) (environmental) tobacco smoke in the perinatal period (P96.81)
              newborn (suspected to be) affected by noxious substances transmitted via placenta or breast milk (P04.-)
              occupational exposure to risk factors (Z57.-)
              retained foreign body (Z18.-)
              retained foreign body fully removed (Z87.821)
              toxic effects of substances chiefly nonmedicinal as to source (T51-T65)

✓5th **Z77.0 Contact with and (suspected) exposure to hazardous, chiefly nonmedicinal, chemicals**

  ✓6th **Z77.01 Contact with and (suspected) exposure to hazardous metals**

       Z77.010 Contact with and (suspected) exposure to arsenic

       Z77.011 Contact with and (suspected) exposure to lead

       Z77.012 Contact with and (suspected) exposure to uranium
            EXCLUDES 1   *retained depleted uranium fragments (Z18.01)*

       Z77.018 Contact with and (suspected) exposure to other hazardous metals
            Contact with and (suspected) exposure to chromium compounds
            Contact with and (suspected) exposure to nickel dust

  ✓6th **Z77.02 Contact with and (suspected) exposure to hazardous aromatic compounds**

       Z77.020 Contact with and (suspected) exposure to aromatic amines

       Z77.021 Contact with and (suspected) exposure to benzene

       Z77.028 Contact with and (suspected) exposure to other hazardous aromatic compounds
            Aromatic dyes NOS
            Polycyclic aromatic hydrocarbons

  ✓6th **Z77.09 Contact with and (suspected) exposure to other hazardous, chiefly nonmedicinal, chemicals**

       Z77.090 Contact with and (suspected) exposure to asbestos

       Z77.098 Contact with and (suspected) exposure to other hazardous, chiefly nonmedicinal, chemicals
            Dyes NOS

✓5th **Z77.1 Contact with and (suspected) exposure to environmental pollution and hazards in the physical environment**

  ✓6th **Z77.11 Contact with and (suspected) exposure to environmental pollution**

       Z77.110 Contact with and (suspected) exposure to air pollution

       Z77.111 Contact with and (suspected) exposure to water pollution

       Z77.112 Contact with and (suspected) exposure to soil pollution

       Z77.118 Contact with and (suspected) exposure to other environmental pollution

  ✓6th **Z77.12 Contact with and (suspected) exposure to hazards in the physical environment**

       Z77.120 Contact with and (suspected) exposure to mold (toxic)

Z77.121 Contact with and (suspected) exposure to harmful algae and algae toxins
     Contact with and (suspected) exposure to (harmful) algae bloom NOS
     Contact with and (suspected) exposure to blue-green algae bloom
     Contact with and (suspected) exposure to brown tide
     Contact with and (suspected) exposure to cyanobacteria bloom
     Contact with and (suspected) exposure to Florida red tide
     Contact with and (suspected) exposure to pfiesteria piscicida
     Contact with and (suspected) exposure to red tide

Z77.122 Contact with and (suspected) exposure to noise

Z77.123 Contact with and (suspected) exposure to radon and other naturally occuring radiation
     EXCLUDES 2   *radiation exposure as the cause of a confirmed condition (W88-W90, X39.0-)*
              radiation sickness NOS (T66)

Z77.128 Contact with and (suspected) exposure to other hazards in the physical environment

✓5th **Z77.2 Contact with and (suspected) exposure to other hazardous substances**

   Z77.21 Contact with and (suspected) exposure to potentially hazardous body fluids

   Z77.22 Contact with and (suspected) exposure to environmental tobacco smoke (acute) (chronic)
     Exposure to second hand tobacco smoke (acute) (chronic)
     Passive smoking (acute) (chronic)
     EXCLUDES 1   *nicotine dependence (F17.-)*
              tobacco use (Z72.0)
     EXCLUDES 2   *occupational exposure to environmental tobacco smoke (Z57.31)*

   Z77.29 Contact with and (suspected) exposure to other hazardous substances

Z77.9 Other contact with and (suspected) exposures hazardous to health

✓4th **Z78 Other specified health status**

     EXCLUDES 2   *asymptomatic human immunodeficiency virus [HIV] infection status (Z21)*
              postprocedural status (Z93- Z99)
              sex reassignment status (Z87.890)

Z78.0 Asymptomatic menopausal state   A♀
     Menopausal state NOS
     Postmenopausal status NOS
     EXCLUDES 2   *symptomatic menopausal state (N95.1)*

Z78.1 Physical restraint status
     EXCLUDES 1   *physical restraint due to a procedure - omit code*

Z78.9 Other specified health status

✓4th **Z79 Long term (current) drug therapy**

     INCLUDES   long term (current) drug use for prophylactic purposes

     Code also any therapeutic drug level monitoring (Z51.81)

     EXCLUDES 2   *drug abuse and dependence (F11-F19)*
              drug use complicating pregnancy, childbirth, and the puerperium (O99.32-)

✓5th **Z79.0 Long term (current) use of anticoagulants and antithrombotics/antiplatelets**
     EXCLUDES 2   *long term (current) use of aspirin (Z79.82)*

   Z79.01 Long term (current) use of anticoagulants

   Z79.02 Long term (current) use of antithrombotics/antiplatelets

Z79.1 Long term (current) use of non-steroidal anti-inflammatories (NSAID)
     EXCLUDES 2   *long term (current) use of aspirin (Z79.82)*

Z79.2 Long term (current) use of antibiotics

Z79.3 Long term (current) use of hormonal contraceptives
     Long term (current) use of birth control pill or patch

Z79.4 Long term (current) use of insulin

✓5th **Z79.5 Long term (current) use of steroids**

   Z79.51 Long term (current) use of inhaled steroids

   Z79.52 Long term (current) use of systemic steroids

✓5th **Z79.8 Other long term (current) drug therapy**

✓6th **Z79.81 Long term (current) use of agents affecting estrogen receptors and estrogen levels**
Code first, if applicable:
malignant neoplasm of breast (C50.-)
malignant neoplasm of prostate (C61)
Use additional code, if applicable, to identify:
estrogen receptor positive status (Z17.0)
family history of breast cancer (Z80.3)
genetic susceptibility to malignant neoplasm (cancer) (Z15.0-)
personal history of breast cancer (Z85.3)
personal history of prostate cancer (Z85.46)
postmenopausal status (Z78.0)
EXCLUDES 1 hormone replacement therapy (postmenopausal) (Z79.890)

Z79.810 Long term (current) use of selective estrogen receptor modulators (SERMs)
Long term (current) use of raloxifene (Evista)
Long term (current) use of tamoxifen (Nolvadex)
Long term (current) use of toremifene (Fareston)

Z79.811 Long term (current) use of aromatase inhibitors
Long term (current) use of anastrozole (Arimidex)
Long term (current) use of exemestane (Aromasin)
Long term (current) use of letrozole (Femara)

Z79.818 Long term (current) use of other agents affecting estrogen receptors and estrogen levels
Long term (current) use of estrogen receptor downregulators
Long term (current) use of fulvestrant (Faslodex)
Long term (current) use of gonadotropin-releasing hormone (GnRH) agonist
Long term (current) use of goserelin acetate (Zoladex)
Long term (current) use of leuprolide acetate (leuprorelin) (Lupron)
Long term (current) use of megestrol acetate (Megace)

Z79.82 Long term (current) use of aspirin

Z79.83 Long term (current) use of bisphosphonates

✓6th **Z79.89 Other long term (current) drug therapy**

Z79.890 Hormone replacement therapy (postmenopausal) ♀

Z79.891 Long term (current) use of opiate analgesic
Long term (current) use of methadone for pain management
EXCLUDES 1 methadone use NOS (F11.2-)
use of methadone for treatment of heroin addiction (F11.2-)

Z79.899 Other long term (current) drug therapy

✓4th **Z80 Family history of primary malignant neoplasm**

Z80.0 Family history of malignant neoplasm of digestive organs
Conditions classifiable to C15-C26

Z80.1 Family history of malignant neoplasm of trachea, bronchus and lung
Conditions classifiable to C33-C34

Z80.2 Family history of malignant neoplasm of other respiratory and intrathoracic organs
Conditions classifiable to C30-C32, C37-C39

Z80.3 Family history of malignant neoplasm of breast
Conditions classifiable to C50-

✓5th **Z80.4 Family history of malignant neoplasm of genital organs**
Conditions classifiable to C51-C63

Z80.41 Family history of malignant neoplasm of ovary ♀

Z80.42 Family history of malignant neoplasm of prostate ♂

Z80.43 Family history of malignant neoplasm of testis ♂

Z80.49 Family history of malignant neoplasm of other genital organs

✓5th **Z80.5 Family history of malignant neoplasm of urinary tract**
Conditions classifiable to C64-C68

Z80.51 Family history of malignant neoplasm of kidney

Z80.52 Family history of malignant neoplasm of bladder

Z80.59 Family history of malignant neoplasm of other urinary tract organ

Z80.6 Family history of leukemia
Conditions classifiable to C91-C95

Z80.7 Family history of other malignant neoplasms of lymphoid, hematopoietic and related tissues
Conditions classifiable to C81-C90, C96-

Z80.8 Family history of malignant neoplasm of other organs or systems
Conditions classifiable to C00-C14, C40-C49, C69-C79

Z80.9 Family history of malignant neoplasm, unspecified
Conditions classifiable to C80.1

✓4th **Z81 Family history of mental and behavioral disorders**

Z81.0 Family history of intellectual disabilities
Conditions classifiable to F70-F79

Z81.1 Family history of alcohol abuse and dependence
Conditions classifiable to F10-

Z81.2 Family history of tobacco abuse and dependence
Conditions classifiable to F17-

Z81.3 Family history of other psychoactive substance abuse and dependence
Conditions classifiable to F11-F16, F18-F19

Z81.4 Family history of other substance abuse and dependence
Conditions classifiable to F55

Z81.8 Family history of other mental and behavioral disorders
Conditions classifiable elsewhere in F01-F99

✓4th **Z82 Family history of certain disabilities and chronic diseases (leading to disablement)**

Z82.0 Family history of epilepsy and other diseases of the nervous system
Conditions classifiable to G00-G99

Z82.1 Family history of blindness and visual loss
Conditions classifiable to H54-

Z82.2 Family history of deafness and hearing loss
Conditions classifiable to H90-H91

Z82.3 Family history of stroke
Conditions classifiable to I60-I64

✓5th **Z82.4 Family history of ischemic heart disease and other diseases of the circulatory system**
Conditions classifiable to I00-I52, I65-I99

Z82.41 Family history of sudden cardiac death

Z82.49 Family history of ischemic heart disease and other diseases of the circulatory system

Z82.5 Family history of asthma and other chronic lower respiratory diseases
Conditions classifiable to J40-J47
EXCLUDES 2 family history of other diseases of the respiratory system (Z83.6)

✓5th **Z82.6 Family history of arthritis and other diseases of the musculoskeletal system and connective tissue**
Conditions classifiable to M00-M99

Z82.61 Family history of arthritis

Z82.62 Family history of osteoporosis

Z82.69 Family history of other diseases of the musculoskeletal system and connective tissue

✓5th **Z82.7 Family history of congenital malformations, deformations and chromosomal abnormalities**
Conditions classifiable to Q00-Q99

Z82.71 Family history of polycystic kidney

Z82.79 Family history of other congenital malformations, deformations and chromosomal abnormalities

Z82.8 Family history of other disabilities and chronic diseases leading to disablement, not elsewhere classified

✓4th **Z83 Family history of other specific disorders**
EXCLUDES 2 contact with and (suspected) exposure to communicable disease in the family (Z20.-)

Z83.0 Family history of human immunodeficiency virus [HIV] disease
Conditions classifiable to B20

Z83.1 Family history of other infectious and parasitic diseases
Conditions classifiable to A00-B19, B25-B94, B99

Z83.2 Family history of diseases of the blood and blood-forming organs and certain disorders involving the immune mechanism
Conditions classifiable to D50-D89

✓ Additional Character Required   ✓x7th Xtension Alert   Unacceptable PDx   Manifestation   Hospital Acquired Condition   **EXCLUDES 1** Not Coded Here   **EXCLUDES 2** Not Included Here

Z83.3 **Family history of** diabetes mellitus
Conditions classifiable to E08-E13

✓5ᵗʰ **Z83.4** **Family history of other endocrine, nutritional and metabolic diseases**
Conditions classifiable to E00-E07, E15-E88

Z83.41 **Family history of** multiple endocrine neoplasia [MEN] syndrome

Z83.49 **Family history of** other endocrine, nutritional and metabolic diseases

✓5ᵗʰ **Z83.5** **Family history of eye and ear disorders**

✓6ᵗʰ **Z83.51** **Family history of** eye disorders
Conditions classifiable to H00-H53, H55-H59
EXCLUDES 2   family history of blindness and visual loss (Z82.1)

Z83.511 **Family history of** glaucoma

Z83.518 **Family history of** other specified eye disorder

Z83.52 **Family history of** ear disorders
Conditions classifiable to H60-H83, H92-H95
EXCLUDES 2   family history of deafness and hearing loss (Z82.2)

Z83.6 **Family history of other diseases of the** respiratory system
Conditions classifiable to J00-J39, J60-J99
EXCLUDES 2   family history of asthma and other chronic lower respiratory diseases (Z82.5)

✓5ᵗʰ **Z83.7** **Family history of diseases of the digestive system**
Conditions classifiable to K00-K93

Z83.71 **Family history of** colonic polyps
EXCLUDES 1   family history of malignant neoplasm of digestive organs (Z80.0)

Z83.79 **Family history of** other diseases of the digestive system

✓4ᵗʰ **Z84** **Family history of other conditions**

Z84.0 **Family history of diseases of the** skin and subcutaneous tissue
Conditions classifiable to L00-L99

Z84.1 **Family history of disorders of** kidney and ureter
Conditions classifiable to N00-N29

Z84.2 **Family history of other diseases of the** genitourinary system
Conditions classifiable to N30-N99

Z84.3 **Family history of** consanguinity

✓5ᵗʰ **Z84.8** **Family history of other specified conditions**

Z84.81 **Family history of carrier of** genetic disease

Z84.89 **Family history of** other specified conditions

✓4ᵗʰ **Z85** **Personal history of malignant neoplasm**
Code first any follow-up examination after treatment of malignant neoplasm (Z08)
Use additional code to identify:
alcohol use and dependence (F10.-)
exposure to environmental tobacco smoke (Z77.22)
history of tobacco use (Z87.891)
occupational exposure to environmental tobacco smoke (Z57.31)
tobacco dependence (F17.-)
tobacco use (Z72.0)
EXCLUDES 2   personal history of benign neoplasm (Z86.01-)
personal history of carcinoma-in-situ (Z86.00-)

✓5ᵗʰ **Z85.0** **Personal history of malignant neoplasm of** digestive organs

Z85.00 **Personal history of malignant neoplasm of** unspecified digestive organ

Z85.01 **Personal history of malignant neoplasm of** esophagus
Conditions classifiable to C15

✓6ᵗʰ **Z85.02** **Personal history of malignant neoplasm of** stomach

Z85.020 **Personal history of malignant** carcinoid tumor of stomach
Conditions classifiable to C7A.092

Z85.028 **Personal history of** other malignant neoplasm of stomach
Conditions classifiable to C16

✓6ᵗʰ **Z85.03** **Personal history of malignant neoplasm of** large intestine

Z85.030 **Personal history of** malignant carcinoid tumor of large intestine
Conditions classifiable to C7A.022-C7A.025, C7A.029

Z85.038 **Personal history of** other malignant neoplasm of large intestine
Conditions classifiable to C18

✓6ᵗʰ **Z85.04** **Personal history of malignant neoplasm of** rectum, rectosigmoid junction, and anus

Z85.040 **Personal history of malignant** carcinoid tumor of rectum
Conditions classifiable to C7A.026

Z85.048 **Personal history of** other malignant neoplasm of rectum, rectosigmoid junction, and anus
Conditions classifiable to C19-C21

Z85.05 **Personal history of malignant neoplasm of** liver
Conditions classifiable to C22

✓6ᵗʰ **Z85.06** **Personal history of malignant neoplasm of** small intestine

Z85.060 **Personal history of malignant** carcinoid tumor of small intestine
Conditions classifiable to C7A.01-

Z85.068 **Personal history of** other malignant neoplasm of small intestine
Conditions classifiable to C17

Z85.07 **Personal history of malignant neoplasm of** pancreas
Conditions classifiable to C25

Z85.09 **Personal history of malignant neoplasm of** other digestive organs

✓5ᵗʰ **Z85.1** **Personal history of malignant neoplasm of** trachea, bronchus and lung

✓6ᵗʰ **Z85.11** **Personal history of malignant neoplasm of** bronchus and lung

Z85.110 **Personal history of malignant** carcinoid tumor of bronchus and lung
Conditions classifiable to C7A.090

Z85.118 **Personal history of** other malignant neoplasm of bronchus and lung
Conditions classifiable to C34

Z85.12 **Personal history of malignant neoplasm of** trachea
Conditions classifiable to C33

✓5ᵗʰ **Z85.2** **Personal history of malignant neoplasm of other** respiratory and intrathoracic organs

Z85.20 **Personal history of malignant neoplasm of** unspecified respiratory organ

Z85.21 **Personal history of malignant neoplasm of** larynx
Conditions classifiable to C32

Z85.22 **Personal history of malignant neoplasm of** nasal cavities, middle ear, and accessory sinuses
Conditions classifiable to C30-C31

✓6ᵗʰ **Z85.23** **Personal history of malignant neoplasm of** thymus

Z85.230 **Personal history of malignant** carcinoid tumor of thymus
Conditions classifiable to C7A.091

Z85.238 **Personal history of** other malignant neoplasm of thymus
Conditions classifiable to C37

Z85.29 **Personal history of malignant neoplasm of** other respiratory and intrathoracic organs

Z85.3 **Personal history of malignant neoplasm of** breast
Conditions classifiable to C50-

✓5ᵗʰ **Z85.4** **Personal history of malignant neoplasm of** genital organs
Conditions classifiable to C51-C63

Z85.40 **Personal history of malignant neoplasm of** unspecified female genital organ   ♀

Z85.41 **Personal history of malignant neoplasm of** cervix uteri   ♀

Z85.42 **Personal history of malignant neoplasm of** other parts of uterus   ♀

Z85.43 **Personal history of malignant neoplasm of** ovary   ♀

Z85.44 **Personal history of malignant neoplasm of** other female genital organs   ♀

Z85.45 **Personal history of malignant neoplasm of** unspecified male genital organ   ♂

Z85.46 **Personal history of malignant neoplasm of** prostate   ♂

Z85.47 **Personal history of malignant neoplasm of** testis   ♂

Z85.48 **Personal history of malignant neoplasm of** epididymis   ♂

Z85.49 **Personal history of malignant neoplasm of** other male genital organs   ♂

N Newborn: 0   P Pediatric: 0-17   M Maternity: 12-55   A Adult: 15-124   MCC Major CC Condition   PDx MCC PDx acts as own MCC   CC CC Condition   PDx CC PDx acts as own CC

1192   ICD-10-CM Draft (2015)

✓5ᵗʰ Z85.5 Personal history of malignant neoplasm of urinary tract
Conditions classifiable to C64-C68

Z85.50 Personal history of malignant neoplasm of unspecified urinary tract organ

Z85.51 Personal history of malignant neoplasm of bladder

✓6ᵗʰ Z85.52 Personal history of malignant neoplasm of kidney
> EXCLUDES 1   *personal history of malignant neoplasm of renal pelvis (Z85.53)*

     Z85.520 Personal history of malignant carcinoid tumor of kidney
     Conditions classifiable to C7A.093

     Z85.528 Personal history of other malignant neoplasm of kidney
     Conditions classifiable to C64

Z85.53 Personal history of malignant neoplasm of renal pelvis

Z85.54 Personal history of malignant neoplasm of ureter

Z85.59 Personal history of malignant neoplasm of other urinary tract organ

Z85.6 Personal history of leukemia
Conditions classifiable to C91-C95
> EXCLUDES 1   *leukemia in remission C91.0-C95.9 with 5th character 1*

✓5ᵗʰ Z85.7 Personal history of other malignant neoplasms of lymphoid, hematopoietic and related tissues

Z85.71 Personal history of Hodgkin lymphoma
Conditions classifiable to C81

Z85.72 Personal history of non-Hodgkin lymphomas
Conditions classifiable to C82-C85

Z85.79 Personal history of other malignant neoplasms of lymphoid, hematopoietic and related tissues
Conditions classifiable to C88-C90, C96
> EXCLUDES 1   *multiple myeloma in remission (C90.01)*
> *plasma cell leukemia in remission (C90.11)*
> *plasmacytoma in remission (C90.21)*

✓5ᵗʰ Z85.8 Personal history of malignant neoplasms of other organs and systems
Conditions classifiable to C00-C14, C40-C49, C69-C79, C7A.098

✓6ᵗʰ Z85.81 Personal history of malignant neoplasm of lip, oral cavity, and pharynx

     Z85.810 Personal history of malignant neoplasm of tongue

     Z85.818 Personal history of malignant neoplasm of other sites of lip, oral cavity, and pharynx

     Z85.819 Personal history of malignant neoplasm of unspecified site of lip, oral cavity, and pharynx

✓6ᵗʰ Z85.82 Personal history of malignant neoplasm of skin

     Z85.820 Personal history of malignant melanoma of skin
     Conditions classifiable to C43

     Z85.821 Personal history of Merkel cell carcinoma
     Conditions classifiable to C4A

     Z85.828 Personal history of other malignant neoplasm of skin
     Conditions classifiable to C44

✓6ᵗʰ Z85.83 Personal history of malignant neoplasm of bone and soft tissue

     Z85.830 Personal history of malignant neoplasm of bone

     Z85.831 Personal history of malignant neoplasm of soft tissue
     > EXCLUDES 2   *personal history of malignant neoplasm of skin (Z85.82-)*

✓6ᵗʰ Z85.84 Personal history of malignant neoplasm of eye and nervous tissue

     Z85.840 Personal history of malignant neoplasm of eye

     Z85.841 Personal history of malignant neoplasm of brain

     Z85.848 Personal history of malignant neoplasm of other parts of nervous tissue

✓6ᵗʰ Z85.85 Personal history of malignant neoplasm of endocrine glands

     Z85.850 Personal history of malignant neoplasm of thyroid

     Z85.858 Personal history of malignant neoplasm of other endocrine glands

Z85.89 Personal history of malignant neoplasm of other organs and systems

Z85.9 Personal history of malignant neoplasm, unspecified
Conditions classifiable to C7A.00, C80.1

✓4ᵗʰ Z86 Personal history of certain other diseases
Code first any follow-up examination after treatment (Z09)

✓5ᵗʰ Z86.0 Personal history of in-situ and benign neoplasms and neoplasms of uncertain behavior
> EXCLUDES 2   *personal history of malignant neoplasms (Z85.-)*

✓6ᵗʰ Z86.00 Personal history of in-situ neoplasm

     Z86.000 Personal history of in-situ neoplasm of breast

     Z86.001 Personal history of in-situ neoplasm of cervix uteri ♀

     Z86.008 Personal history of in-situ neoplasm of other site

✓6ᵗʰ Z86.01 Personal history of benign neoplasm

     Z86.010 Personal history of colonic polyps

     Z86.011 Personal history of benign neoplasm of the brain

     Z86.012 Personal history of benign carcinoid tumor

     Z86.018 Personal history of other benign neoplasm

Z86.03 Personal history of neoplasm of uncertain behavior

✓5ᵗʰ Z86.1 Personal history of infectious and parasitic diseases
Conditions classifiable to A00-B89, B99
> EXCLUDES 1   *personal history of infectious diseases specific to a body system*
> *sequelae of infectious and parasitic diseases (B90-B94)*

Z86.11 Personal history of tuberculosis

Z86.12 Personal history of poliomyelitis

Z86.13 Personal history of malaria

Z86.14 Personal history of Methicillin resistant Staphylococcus aureus infection
Personal history of MRSA infection

Z86.19 Personal history of other infectious and parasitic diseases

Z86.2 Personal history of diseases of the blood and blood-forming organs and certain disorders involving the immune mechanism
Conditions classifiable to D50-D89

✓5ᵗʰ Z86.3 Personal history of endocrine, nutritional and metabolic diseases
Conditions classifiable to E00-E88

Z86.31 Personal history of diabetic foot ulcer
> EXCLUDES 2   *current diabetic foot ulcer (E08.621, E09.621, E10.621, E11.621, E13.621)*

Z86.32 Personal history of gestational diabetes ♀
Personal history of conditions classifiable to O24.4-
> EXCLUDES 1   *gestational diabetes mellitus in current pregnancy (O24.4-)*

Z86.39 Personal history of other endocrine, nutritional and metabolic disease

✓5ᵗʰ Z86.5 Personal history of mental and behavioral disorders
Conditions classifiable to F40-F59

Z86.51 Personal history of combat and operational stress reaction Ⓐ

Z86.59 Personal history of other mental and behavioral disorders

✓5ᵗʰ Z86.6 Personal history of diseases of the nervous system and sense organs
Conditions classifiable to G00-G99, H00-H95
> EXCLUDES 2   *personal history of anaphylactic shock (Z87.892)*

Z86.61 Personal history of infections of the central nervous system
Personal history of encephalitis
Personal history of meningitis

Z86.69 Personal history of other diseases of the nervous system and sense organs

☑ Additional Character Required   ✓x7ᵗʰ Xtension Alert   Unacceptable PDx   Manifestation   Hospital Acquired Condition   EXCLUDES 1 Not Coded Here   EXCLUDES 2 Not Included Here

ICD-10-CM Draft (2015)   1193

✓5ᵗʰ **Z86.7** **Personal history of diseases of the circulatory system**
Conditions classifiable to I00-I99
EXCLUDES 2   old myocardial infarction (I25.2)
    personal history of anaphylactic shock (Z87.892)
    postmyocardial infarction syndrome (I24.1)

✓6ᵗʰ **Z86.71** **Personal history of venous thrombosis and embolism**
    Z86.711 **Personal history of pulmonary embolism**
    Z86.718 **Personal history of other venous thrombosis and embolism**

Z86.72 **Personal history of thrombophlebitis**

Z86.73 **Personal history of transient ischemic attack (TIA), and cerebral infarction without residual deficits**
Personal history of prolonged reversible ischemic neurological deficit (PRIND)
Personal history of stroke NOS without residual deficits
EXCLUDES 1   personal history of traumatic brain injury (Z87.820)
    sequelae of cerebrovascular disease (I69.-)
AHA: 2012, 4Q, 92

Z86.74 **Personal history of sudden cardiac arrest**
Personal history of sudden cardiac death successfully resuscitated

Z86.79 **Personal history of other diseases of the circulatory system**

✓4ᵗʰ **Z87** **Personal history of other diseases and conditions**
Code first any follow-up examination after treatment (Z09)

✓5ᵗʰ **Z87.0** **Personal history of diseases of the respiratory system**
Conditions classifiable to J00-J99
    Z87.01 **Personal history of pneumonia (recurrent)**
    Z87.09 **Personal history of other diseases of the respiratory system**

✓5ᵗʰ **Z87.1** **Personal history of diseases of the digestive system**
Conditions classifiable to K00-K93
    Z87.11 **Personal history of peptic ulcer disease**
    Z87.19 **Personal history of other diseases of the digestive system**

Z87.2 **Personal history of diseases of the skin and subcutaneous tissue**
Conditions classifiable to L00-L99
EXCLUDES 2   personal history of diabetic foot ulcer (Z86.31)

✓5ᵗʰ **Z87.3** **Personal history of diseases of the musculoskeletal system and connective tissue**
Conditions classifiable to M00-M99
EXCLUDES 2   personal history of (healed) traumatic fracture (Z87.81)

✓6ᵗʰ **Z87.31** **Personal history of (healed) nontraumatic fracture**
    Z87.310 **Personal history of (healed) osteoporosis fracture**
       Personal history of (healed) fragility fracture
       Personal history of (healed) collapsed vertebra due to osteoporosis
    Z87.311 **Personal history of (healed) other pathological fracture**
       Personal history of (healed) collapsed vertebra NOS
       EXCLUDES 2   personal history of osteoporosis fracture (Z87.310)
    Z87.312 **Personal history of (healed) stress fracture**
       Personal history of (healed) fatigue fracture

Z87.39 **Personal history of other diseases of the musculoskeletal system and connective tissue**

✓5ᵗʰ **Z87.4** **Personal history of diseases of genitourinary system**
Conditions classifiable to N00-N99

✓6ᵗʰ **Z87.41** **Personal history of dysplasia of the female genital tract**
EXCLUDES 1   personal history of malignant neoplasm of female genital tract (Z85.40-Z85.44)
    Z87.410 **Personal history of cervical dysplasia** ♀
    Z87.411 **Personal history of vaginal dysplasia** ♀
    Z87.412 **Personal history of vulvar dysplasia** ♀

Z87.42 **Personal history of other diseases of the female genital tract** ♀

✓6ᵗʰ **Z87.43** **Personal history of diseases of the male genital organs**
    Z87.430 **Personal history of prostatic dysplasia**
       EXCLUDES 1   personal history of malignant neoplasm of prostate (Z85.46)
    Z87.438 **Personal history of other diseases of male genital organs**

✓6ᵗʰ **Z87.44** **Personal history of diseases of the urinary system**
EXCLUDES 1   personal history of malignant neoplasm of cervix uteri (Z85.41)
    Z87.440 **Personal history of urinary (tract) infections**
    Z87.441 **Personal history of nephrotic syndrome**
    Z87.442 **Personal history of urinary calculi**
       Personal history of kidney stones
    Z87.448 **Personal history of other diseases of urinary system**

✓5ᵗʰ **Z87.5** **Personal history of complications of pregnancy, childbirth and the puerperium**
Conditions classifiable to O00-O9A
EXCLUDES 2   recurrent pregnancy loss (N96)
    Z87.51 **Personal history of pre-term labor** ♀
       EXCLUDES 1   current pregnancy with history of pre-term labor (O09.21-)
    Z87.59 **Personal history of other complications of pregnancy, childbirth and the puerperium** ♀
       Personal history of trophoblastic disease

✓5ᵗʰ **Z87.7** **Personal history of (corrected) congenital malformations**
Conditions classifiable to Q00-Q89 that have been repaired or corrected
EXCLUDES 1   congenital malformations that have been partially corrected or repaired but which still require medical treatment—code to condition
EXCLUDES 2   other postprocedural states (Z98.-)
    personal history of medical treatment (Z92.-)
    presence of cardiac and vascular implants and grafts (Z95.-)
    presence of other devices (Z97.-)
    presence of other functional implants (Z96.-)
    transplanted organ and tissue status (Z94.-)

✓6ᵗʰ **Z87.71** **Personal history of (corrected) congenital malformations of genitourinary system**
    Z87.710 **Personal history of (corrected) hypospadias** ♂
    Z87.718 **Personal history of other specified (corrected) congenital malformations of genitourinary system**

✓6ᵗʰ **Z87.72** **Personal history of (corrected) congenital malformations of nervous system and sense organs**
    Z87.720 **Personal history of (corrected) congenital malformations of eye**
    Z87.721 **Personal history of (corrected) congenital malformations of ear**
    Z87.728 **Personal history of other specified (corrected) congenital malformations of nervous system and sense organs**

✓6ᵗʰ **Z87.73** **Personal history of (corrected) congenital malformations of digestive system**
    Z87.730 **Personal history of (corrected) cleft lip and palate**
    Z87.738 **Personal history of other specified (corrected) congenital malformations of digestive system**

Z87.74 **Personal history of (corrected) congenital malformations of heart and circulatory system**

Z87.75 **Personal history of (corrected) congenital malformations of respiratory system**

Z87.76 **Personal history of (corrected) congenital malformations of integument, limbs and musculoskeletal system**

✓6ᵗʰ **Z87.79** **Personal history of other (corrected) congenital malformations**
    Z87.790 **Personal history of (corrected) congenital malformations of face and neck**
    Z87.798 **Personal history of other (corrected) congenital malformations**

Ⓝ Newborn: 0   Ⓟ Pediatric: 0-17   Ⓜ Maternity: 12-55   Ⓐ Adult: 15-124   **MCC** Major CC Condition   **PDx MCC** PDx acts as own MCC   **CC** CC Condition   **PDx CC** PDx acts as own CC

1194   ICD-10-CM Draft (2015)

√5ᵗʰ Z87.8 Personal history of other specified conditions
EXCLUDES 2 *personal history of self harm (Z91.5)*

Z87.81 Personal history of (healed) traumatic fracture
EXCLUDES 2 *personal history of (healed) nontraumatic fracture (Z87.31-)*

√6ᵗʰ Z87.82 Personal history of other (healed) physical injury and trauma
Conditions classifiable to S00-T88, except traumatic fractures

Z87.820 Personal history of traumatic brain injury
EXCLUDES 1 *personal history of transient ischemic attack (TIA), and cerebral infarction without residual deficits (Z86.73)*

Z87.821 Personal history of retained foreign body fully removed

Z87.828 Personal history of other (healed) physical injury and trauma

√6ᵗʰ Z87.89 Personal history of other specified conditions

Z87.890 Personal history of sex reassignment

Z87.891 Personal history of nicotine dependence
EXCLUDES 1 *current nicotine dependence (F17.2-)*

Z87.892 Personal history of anaphylaxis
Code also allergy status such as:
allergy status to drugs, medicaments and biological substances (Z88.-)
allergy status, other than to drugs and biological substances (Z91.0-)

Z87.898 Personal history of other specified conditions
AHA: 2013, 1Q, 21

√4ᵗʰ Z88 Allergy status to drugs, medicaments and biological substances
EXCLUDES 2 *allergy status, other than to drugs and biological substances (Z91.0-)*

Z88.0 Allergy status to penicillin
Z88.1 Allergy status to other antibiotic agents status
Z88.2 Allergy status to sulfonamides status
Z88.3 Allergy status to other anti-infective agents status
Z88.4 Allergy status to anesthetic agent status
Z88.5 Allergy status to narcotic agent status
Z88.6 Allergy status to analgesic agent status
Z88.7 Allergy status to serum and vaccine status
Z88.8 Allergy status to other drugs, medicaments and biological substances status
Z88.9 Allergy status to unspecified drugs, medicaments and biological substances status

√4ᵗʰ Z89 Acquired absence of limb
INCLUDES amputation status
postprocedural loss of limb
post-traumatic loss of limb
EXCLUDES 1 *acquired deformities of limbs (M20-M21)*
congenital absence of limbs (Q71-Q73)

√5ᵗʰ Z89.0 Acquired absence of thumb and other finger(s)

√6ᵗʰ Z89.01 Acquired absence of thumb
Z89.011 Acquired absence of right thumb
Z89.012 Acquired absence of left thumb
Z89.019 Acquired absence of unspecified thumb

√6ᵗʰ Z89.02 Acquired absence of other finger(s)
EXCLUDES 2 *acquired absence of thumb (Z89.01-)*
Z89.021 Acquired absence of right finger(s)
Z89.022 Acquired absence of left finger(s)
Z89.029 Acquired absence of unspecified finger(s)

√5ᵗʰ Z89.1 Acquired absence of hand and wrist

√6ᵗʰ Z89.11 Acquired absence of hand
Z89.111 Acquired absence of right hand
Z89.112 Acquired absence of left hand
Z89.119 Acquired absence of unspecified hand

√6ᵗʰ Z89.12 Acquired absence of wrist
Disarticulation at wrist
Z89.121 Acquired absence of right wrist
Z89.122 Acquired absence of left wrist
Z89.129 Acquired absence of unspecified wrist

√5ᵗʰ Z89.2 Acquired absence of upper limb above wrist

√6ᵗʰ Z89.20 Acquired absence of upper limb, unspecified level
Z89.201 Acquired absence of right upper limb, unspecified level
Z89.202 Acquired absence of left upper limb, unspecified level
Z89.209 Acquired absence of unspecified upper limb, unspecified level
Acquired absence of arm NOS

√6ᵗʰ Z89.21 Acquired absence of upper limb below elbow
Z89.211 Acquired absence of right upper limb below elbow
Z89.212 Acquired absence of left upper limb below elbow
Z89.219 Acquired absence of unspecified upper limb below elbow

√6ᵗʰ Z89.22 Acquired absence of upper limb above elbow
Disarticulation at elbow
Z89.221 Acquired absence of right upper limb above elbow
Z89.222 Acquired absence of left upper limb above elbow
Z89.229 Acquired absence of unspecified upper limb above elbow

√6ᵗʰ Z89.23 Acquired absence of shoulder
Acquired absence of shoulder joint following explantation of shoulder joint prosthesis, with or without presence of antibiotic-impregnated cement spacer
Z89.231 Acquired absence of right shoulder
Z89.232 Acquired absence of left shoulder
Z89.239 Acquired absence of unspecified shoulder

√5ᵗʰ Z89.4 Acquired absence of toe(s), foot, and ankle

√6ᵗʰ Z89.41 Acquired absence of great toe
Z89.411 Acquired absence of right great toe
Z89.412 Acquired absence of left great toe
Z89.419 Acquired absence of unspecified great toe

√6ᵗʰ Z89.42 Acquired absence of other toe(s)
EXCLUDES 2 *acquired absence of great toe (Z89.41-)*
Z89.421 Acquired absence of other right toe(s)
Z89.422 Acquired absence of other left toe(s)
Z89.429 Acquired absence of other toe(s), unspecified side

√6ᵗʰ Z89.43 Acquired absence of foot
Z89.431 Acquired absence of right foot
Z89.432 Acquired absence of left foot
Z89.439 Acquired absence of unspecified foot

√6ᵗʰ Z89.44 Acquired absence of ankle
Disarticulation of ankle
Z89.441 Acquired absence of right ankle
Z89.442 Acquired absence of left ankle
Z89.449 Acquired absence of unspecified ankle

√5ᵗʰ Z89.5 Acquired absence of leg below knee

√6ᵗʰ Z89.51 Acquired absence of leg below knee
Z89.511 Acquired absence of right leg below knee
Z89.512 Acquired absence of left leg below knee
Z89.519 Acquired absence of unspecified leg below knee

√6ᵗʰ Z89.52 Acquired absence of knee
Acquired absence of knee joint following explantation of knee joint prosthesis, with or without presence of antibiotic-impregnated cement spacer
Z89.521 Acquired absence of right knee
Z89.522 Acquired absence of left knee
Z89.529 Acquired absence of unspecified knee

√5ᵗʰ Z89.6 Acquired absence of leg above knee

√6ᵗʰ Z89.61 Acquired absence of leg above knee
Acquired absence of leg NOS
Disarticulation at knee
Z89.611 Acquired absence of right leg above knee
Z89.612 Acquired absence of left leg above knee
Z89.619 Acquired absence of unspecified leg above knee

Factors Influencing Health Status and Contact With Health Services

Z89.62–Z91.5

✓6ᵗʰ **Z89.62** **Acquired absence of** hip
Acquired absence of hip joint following explantation of hip joint prosthesis, with or without presence of antibiotic-impregnated cement spacer
Disarticulation at hip

    Z89.621 **Acquired absence of** right **hip joint**

    Z89.622 **Acquired absence of** left **hip joint**

    Z89.629 **Acquired absence of** unspecified **hip joint**

Z89.9 **Acquired absence of limb,** unspecified

✓4ᵗʰ **Z90** **Acquired absence of organs, not elsewhere classified**
    INCLUDES postprocedural or post-traumatic loss of body part NEC
    EXCLUDES 1 congenital absence—see Alphabetical Index
    EXCLUDES 2 postprocedural absence of endocrine glands (E89.-)

  ✓5ᵗʰ **Z90.0** **Acquired absence of part of** head and neck

    Z90.01 **Acquired absence of** eye

    Z90.02 **Acquired absence of** larynx

    Z90.09 **Acquired absence of** other **part of head and neck**
       Acquired absence of nose
       EXCLUDES 2 teeth (K08.1)

  ✓5ᵗʰ **Z90.1** **Acquired absence of** breast and nipple

    Z90.10 **Acquired absence of** unspecified **breast and nipple**

    Z90.11 **Acquired absence of** right **breast and nipple**

    Z90.12 **Acquired absence of** left **breast and nipple**

    Z90.13 **Acquired absence of** bilateral **breasts and nipples**

  Z90.2 **Acquired absence of** lung [part of]

  Z90.3 **Acquired absence of** stomach [part of]

  ✓5ᵗʰ **Z90.4** **Acquired absence of** other **specified parts of digestive tract**

    ✓6ᵗʰ **Z90.41** **Acquired absence of** pancreas
      Use additional code to identify any associated:
       insulin use (Z79.4)
       diabetes mellitus, postpancreatectomy (E13.-)

      Z90.410 **Acquired** total absence **of pancreas**
        Acquired absence of pancreas NOS

      Z90.411 **Acquired** partial absence **of pancreas**

    Z90.49 **Acquired absence of** other **specified parts of digestive tract**

  Z90.5 **Acquired absence of** kidney

  Z90.6 **Acquired absence of** other **parts of urinary tract**
    Acquired absence of bladder

  ✓5ᵗʰ **Z90.7** **Acquired absence of** genital organ(s)
    EXCLUDES 1 personal history of sex reassignment (Z87.890)
    EXCLUDES 2 female genital mutilation status (N90.81-)

    ✓6ᵗʰ **Z90.71** **Acquired absence of** cervix and uterus

      Z90.710 **Acquired absence of** both **cervix and uterus** ♀
        Acquired absence of uterus NOS
        Status post total hysterectomy

      Z90.711 **Acquired absence of uterus with** remaining cervical stump ♀
        Status post partial hysterectomy with remaining cervical stump

      Z90.712 **Acquired absence of cervix with** remaining uterus ♀

    ✓6ᵗʰ **Z90.72** **Acquired absence of** ovaries

      Z90.721 **Acquired absence of ovaries,** unilateral ♀

      Z90.722 **Acquired absence of ovaries,** bilateral ♀

    Z90.79 **Acquired absence of** other **genital organ(s)**

  ✓5ᵗʰ **Z90.8** **Acquired absence of** other **organs**

    Z90.81 **Acquired absence of** spleen

    Z90.89 **Acquired absence of** other **organs**

✓4ᵗʰ **Z91** **Personal risk factors, not elsewhere classified**
    EXCLUDES 2 contact with and (suspected) exposures hazardous to health (Z77.-)
      exposure to pollution and other problems related to physical environment (Z77.1-)
      personal history of physical injury and trauma (Z87.81, Z87.82-)
      occupational exposure to risk factors (Z57.-)

  ✓5ᵗʰ **Z91.0** **Allergy status, other than to drugs and biological substances**
    EXCLUDES 2 allergy status to drugs, medicaments, and biological substances (Z88.-)

    ✓6ᵗʰ **Z91.01** **Food allergy status**
      EXCLUDES 2 food additives allergy status (Z91.02)

      Z91.010 **Allergy to** peanuts

      Z91.011 **Allergy to** milk products
        EXCLUDES 1 lactose intolerance (E73.-)

      Z91.012 **Allergy to** eggs

      Z91.013 **Allergy to** seafood
        Allergy to shellfish
        Allergy to octopus or squid ink

      Z91.018 **Allergy to** other **foods**
        Allergy to nuts other than peanuts

    Z91.02 **Food additives allergy status**

    ✓6ᵗʰ **Z91.03** **Insect allergy status**

      Z91.030 **Bee allergy status**

      Z91.038 **Other insect allergy status**

    ✓6ᵗʰ **Z91.04** **Nonmedicinal substance allergy status**

      Z91.040 **Latex allergy status**
        Latex sensitivity status

      Z91.041 **Radiographic dye allergy status**
        Allergy status to contrast media used for diagnostic X-ray procedure

      Z91.048 **Other nonmedicinal substance allergy status**

    Z91.09 **Other allergy status, other than to drugs and biological substances**

  ✓5ᵗʰ **Z91.1** **Patient's noncompliance with medical treatment and regimen**

    Z91.11 **Patient's noncompliance with** dietary regimen

    ✓6ᵗʰ **Z91.12** **Patient's intentional underdosing of medication regimen**
      Code first underdosing of medication (T36-T50) with fifth or sixth character 6
      EXCLUDES 1 adverse effect of prescribed drug taken as directed—code to adverse effect
        poisoning (overdose)—code to poisoning

      Z91.120 **Patient's intentional underdosing of medication regimen due to** financial hardship

      Z91.128 **Patient's intentional underdosing of medication regimen for** other reason

    ✓6ᵗʰ **Z91.13** **Patient's unintentional underdosing of medication regimen**
      Code first underdosing of medication (T36-T50) with fifth or sixth character 6
      EXCLUDES 1 adverse effect of prescribed drug taken as directed—code to adverse effect
        poisoning (overdose)—code to poisoning

      Z91.130 **Patient's unintentional underdosing of medication regimen due to** age-related debility

      Z91.138 **Patient's unintentional underdosing of medication regimen for** other reason

    Z91.14 **Patient's** other **noncompliance with medication regimen**
      Patient's underdosing of medication NOS

    Z91.15 **Patient's noncompliance with** renal dialysis

    Z91.19 **Patient's noncompliance with** other **medical treatment and regimen**

  ✓5ᵗʰ **Z91.4** **Personal history of psychological trauma, not elsewhere classified**

    ✓6ᵗʰ **Z91.41** **Personal history of** adult abuse
      EXCLUDES 2 personal history of abuse in childhood (Z62.81-)

      Z91.410 **Personal history of adult** physical and sexual **abuse** Ⓐ
        EXCLUDES 1 current adult physical abuse (T74.11, T76.11)
          current adult sexual abuse (T74.21, T76.21)

      Z91.411 **Personal history of adult** psychological **abuse** Ⓐ

      Z91.412 **Personal history of** adult neglect Ⓐ
        EXCLUDES 1 current adult neglect (T74.01, T76.01)

      Z91.419 **Personal history of** unspecified **adult abuse** Ⓐ

    Z91.49 **Other personal history of psychological trauma, not elsewhere classified**

  Z91.5 **Personal history of self-harm**
    Personal history of parasuicide
    Personal history of self-poisoning
    Personal history of suicide attempt

Ⓝ Newborn: 0   Ⓟ Pediatric: 0-17   Ⓜ Maternity: 12-55   Ⓐ Adult: 15-124   **MCC** Major CC Condition   **PDx MCC** PDx acts as own MCC   **CC** CC Condition   **PDx CC** PDx acts as own CC

1196   ICD-10-CM Draft (2015)

✓5th **Z91.8 Other specified personal risk factors, not elsewhere classified**

Z91.81 History of falling
At risk for falling

Z91.82 Personal history of military deployment   A
Individual (civilian or military) with past history of military war, peacekeeping and humanitarian deployment (current or past conflict)
Returned from military deployment

Z91.83 Wandering in diseases classified elsewhere
Code first underlying disorder such as:
Alzheimer's disease (G30.-)
autism or pervasive developmental disorder (F84.-)
intellectual disabilities (F70-F79)
unspecified dementia with behavioral disturbance (F03.9-)

Z91.89 Other specified personal risk factors, not elsewhere classified

✓4th **Z92 Personal history of medical treatment**
EXCLUDES 2 postprocedural states (Z98.-)

Z92.0 Personal history of contraception
EXCLUDES 1 counseling or management of current contraceptive practices (Z30.-)
long term (current) use of contraception (Z79.3)
presence of (intrauterine) contraceptive device (Z97.5)

✓5th **Z92.2 Personal history of drug therapy**
EXCLUDES 2 long term (current) drug therapy (Z79.-)

Z92.21 Personal history of antineoplastic chemotherapy

Z92.22 Personal history of monoclonal drug therapy

Z92.23 Personal history of estrogen therapy

✓6th **Z92.24 Personal history of steroid therapy**

Z92.240 Personal history of inhaled steroid therapy

Z92.241 Personal history of systemic steroid therapy
Personal history of steroid therapy NOS

Z92.25 Personal history of immunosupression therapy
EXCLUDES 2 personal history of steroid therapy (Z92.24)

Z92.29 Personal history of other drug therapy

Z92.3 Personal history of irradiation
Personal history of exposure to therapeutic radiation
EXCLUDES 1 exposure to radiation in the physical environment (Z77.12)
occupational exposure to radiation (Z57.1)

✓5th **Z92.8 Personal history of other medical treatment**

Z92.81 Personal history of extracorporeal membrane oxygenation (ECMO)

Z92.82 Status post administration of tPA (rtPA) in a different facility within the last 24 hours prior to admission to current facility
Code first condition requiring tPA administration, such as:
acute cerebral infarction (I63.-)
acute myocardial infarction (I21-, I22-)
AHA: 2013, 4Q, 124

Z92.83 Personal history of failed moderate sedation
Personal history of failed conscious sedation
EXCLUDES 2 failed moderate sedation during procedure (T88.52)

Z92.89 Personal history of other medical treatment

✓4th **Z93 Artificial opening status**
EXCLUDES 1 artificial openings requiring attention or management (Z43.-)
complications of external stoma (J95.0-, K94.-, N99.5-)

Z93.0 Tracheostomy status
AHA: 2013, 4Q, 129

Z93.1 Gastrostomy status

Z93.2 Ileostomy status

Z93.3 Colostomy status

Z93.4 Other artificial openings of gastrointestinal tract status

✓5th **Z93.5 Cystostomy status**

Z93.50 Unspecified cystostomy status

Z93.51 Cutaneous-vesicostomy status

Z93.52 Appendico-vesicostomy status

Z93.59 Other cystostomy status

Z93.6 Other artificial openings of urinary tract status
Nephrostomy status
Ureterostomy status
Urethrostomy status

Z93.8 Other artificial opening status

Z93.9 Artificial opening status, unspecified

✓4th **Z94 Transplanted organ and tissue status**
INCLUDES organ or tissue replaced by heterogenous or homogenous transplant
EXCLUDES 1 complications of transplanted organ or tissue—see Alphabetical Index
EXCLUDES 2 presence of vascular grafts (Z95.-)

Z94.0 Kidney transplant status   CC
CC Excl: D47.Z1,T86.10-T86.13, T86.19, T86.850-T86.859,T86.90-T86.99,Z94.0,Z94.89-Z94.9

Z94.1 Heart transplant status   CC
EXCLUDES 1 artificial heart status (Z95.812)
heart-valve replacement status (Z95.2-Z95.4)
CC Excl: D47.Z1, T86.20-T86.39, T86.850-T86.859, T86.90-T86.99, Z94.1, Z94.3, Z94.89-Z94.9

Z94.2 Lung transplant status   CC
CC Excl: D47.Z1, T86.810-T86.819,T86.850-T86.859,T86.90-T86.99,Z94.2,Z94.89-Z94.9

Z94.3 Heart and lungs transplant status   PDx CC CC
CC Excl: See Code: Z94.1

Z94.4 Liver transplant status   CC
CC Excl: D47.Z1,T86.40-T86.43,T86.49,T86.850-T86.859,T86.90-T86.99, Z94.4,Z94.89-Z94.9

Z94.5 Skin transplant status
Autogenous skin transplant status

Z94.6 Bone transplant status

Z94.7 Corneal transplant status

✓5th **Z94.8 Other transplanted organ and tissue status**

Z94.81 Bone marrow transplant status   CC
CC Excl: D47.Z1, T86.810-T86.813,T86.00-T86.09,T86.850-T86.859,T86.90-T86.99,Z94.9

Z94.82 Intestine transplant status   CC
CC Excl: D47.Z1, T86.830-T86.839, T86.90-T86.99, Z94.82, Z94.89-Z94.9

Z94.83 Pancreas transplant status   CC
CC Excl: D47.Z1,T86.850-T86.99,Z94.83,Z94.9

Z94.84 Stem cells transplant status   CC
CC Excl: D47.Z1,T86.850-T86.859,T86.90-T86.99,Z94.83,Z94.9

Z94.89 Other transplanted organ and tissue status

Z94.9 Transplanted organ and tissue status, unspecified

✓4th **Z95 Presence of cardiac and vascular implants and grafts**
EXCLUDES 1 complications of cardiac and vascular devices, implants and grafts (T82.-)

Z95.0 Presence of cardiac pacemaker
EXCLUDES 1 adjustment or management of cardiac device (Z45.0)
presence of automatic (implantable) cardiac defibrillator with synchronous cardiac pacemaker (Z95.810)

Z95.1 Presence of aortocoronary bypass graft

Z95.2 Presence of prosthetic heart valve
Presence of heart valve NOS

Z95.3 Presence of xenogenic heart valve

Z95.4 Presence of other heart-valve replacement

Z95.5 Presence of coronary angioplasty implant and graft
EXCLUDES 1 coronary angioplasty status without implant and graft (Z98.61)

✓5th **Z95.8 Presence of other cardiac and vascular implants and grafts**

✓6th **Z95.81 Presence of other cardiac implants and grafts**

Z95.810 Presence of automatic (implantable) cardiac defibrillator
Presence of automatic (implantable) cardiac defibrillator with synchronous cardiac pacemaker

Z95.811 Presence of heart assist device   CC
CC Excl: D47.Z1, I46.2-I46.9, I49.01, R09.2, R57.0-R57.8, T86.20-T86.39, T86.850-T86.859, T86.90-T86.99, Z94.1, Z94.3, Z95.811-Z95.812

Z95.812 Presence of fully implantable artificial heart   CC
CC Excl: See code: Z95.811

Z95.818 Presence of other cardiac implants and grafts

✓6ᵗʰ **Z95.82** Presence of other vascular implants and grafts

Z95.820 Peripheral vascular angioplasty status with implants and grafts
EXCLUDES 1 peripheral vascular angioplasty without implant and graft (Z98.62)

Z95.828 Presence of other vascular implants and grafts
Presence of intravascular prosthesis NEC

Z95.9 Presence of cardiac and vascular implant and graft, unspecified

✓4ᵗʰ **Z96** Presence of other functional implants
EXCLUDES 2 complications of internal prosthetic devices, implants and grafts (T82-T85)
fitting and adjustment of prosthetic and other devices (Z44-Z46)

Z96.0 Presence of urogenital implants

Z96.1 Presence of intraocular lens
Presence of pseudophakia

✓5ᵗʰ **Z96.2** Presence of otological and audiological implants

Z96.20 Presence of otological and audiological implant, unspecified

Z96.21 Cochlear implant status

Z96.22 Myringotomy tube(s) status

Z96.29 Presence of other otological and audiological implants
Presence of bone-conduction hearing device
Presence of eustachian tube stent
Stapes replacement

Z96.3 Presence of artificial larynx

✓5ᵗʰ **Z96.4** Presence of endocrine implants

Z96.41 Presence of insulin pump (external) (internal)

Z96.49 Presence of other endocrine implants

Z96.5 Presence of tooth-root and mandibular implants

✓5ᵗʰ **Z96.6** Presence of orthopedic joint implants

Z96.60 Presence of unspecified orthopedic joint implant

✓6ᵗʰ **Z96.61** Presence of artificial shoulder joint

Z96.611 Presence of right artificial shoulder joint

Z96.612 Presence of left artificial shoulder joint

Z96.619 Presence of unspecified artificial shoulder joint

✓6ᵗʰ **Z96.62** Presence of artificial elbow joint

Z96.621 Presence of right artificial elbow joint

Z96.622 Presence of left artificial elbow joint

Z96.629 Presence of unspecified artificial elbow joint

✓6ᵗʰ **Z96.63** Presence of artificial wrist joint

Z96.631 Presence of right artificial wrist joint

Z96.632 Presence of left artificial wrist joint

Z96.639 Presence of unspecified artificial wrist joint

✓6ᵗʰ **Z96.64** Presence of artificial hip joint
Hip-joint replacement (partial) (total)

Z96.641 Presence of right artificial hip joint

Z96.642 Presence of left artificial hip joint

Z96.643 Presence of artificial hip joint, bilateral

Z96.649 Presence of unspecified artificial hip joint

✓6ᵗʰ **Z96.65** Presence of artificial knee joint

Z96.651 Presence of right artificial knee joint

Z96.652 Presence of left artificial knee joint

Z96.653 Presence of artificial knee joint, bilateral

Z96.659 Presence of unspecified artificial knee joint

✓6ᵗʰ **Z96.66** Presence of artificial ankle joint

Z96.661 Presence of right artificial ankle joint

Z96.662 Presence of left artificial ankle joint

Z96.669 Presence of unspecified artificial ankle joint

✓6ᵗʰ **Z96.69** Presence of other orthopedic joint implants

Z96.691 Finger-joint replacement of right hand

Z96.692 Finger-joint replacement of left hand

Z96.693 Finger-joint replacement, bilateral

Z96.698 Presence of other orthopedic joint implants

Z96.7 Presence of other bone and tendon implants
Presence of skull plate

✓5ᵗʰ **Z96.8** Presence of other specified functional implants

Z96.81 Presence of artificial skin

Z96.89 Presence of other specified functional implants

Z96.9 Presence of functional implant, unspecified

✓4ᵗʰ **Z97** Presence of other devices
EXCLUDES 1 complications of internal prosthetic devices, implants and grafts (T82-T85)
fitting and adjustment of prosthetic and other devices (Z44-Z46)
EXCLUDES 2 presence of cerebrospinal fluid drainage device (Z98.2)

Z97.0 Presence of artificial eye

✓5ᵗʰ **Z97.1** Presence of artificial limb (complete) (partial)

Z97.10 Presence of artificial limb (complete) (partial), unspecified

Z97.11 Presence of artificial right arm (complete) (partial)

Z97.12 Presence of artificial left arm (complete) (partial)

Z97.13 Presence of artificial right leg (complete) (partial)

Z97.14 Presence of artificial left leg (complete) (partial)

Z97.15 Presence of artificial arms, bilateral (complete) (partial)

Z97.16 Presence of artificial legs, bilateral (complete) (partial)

Z97.2 Presence of dental prosthetic device (complete) (partial)
Presence of dentures (complete) (partial)

Z97.3 Presence of spectacles and contact lenses

Z97.4 Presence of external hearing-aid

Z97.5 Presence of (intrauterine) contraceptive device   ♀
EXCLUDES 1 checking, reinsertion or removal of contraceptive device (Z30.43)

Z97.8 Presence of other specified devices

✓4ᵗʰ **Z98** Other postprocedural states
EXCLUDES 2 aftercare (Z43-Z49, Z51)
follow-up medical care (Z08- Z09)
postprocedural complication—see Alphabetical Index

Z98.0 Intestinal bypass and anastomosis status
EXCLUDES 2 bariatric surgery status (Z98.84)
gastric bypass status (Z98.84)
obesity surgery status (Z98.84)

Z98.1 Arthrodesis status

Z98.2 Presence of cerebrospinal fluid drainage device
Presence of CSF shunt

Z98.3 Post therapeutic collapse of lung status
Code first underlying disease

✓5ᵗʰ **Z98.4** Cataract extraction status
Use additional code to identify intraocular lens implant status (Z96.1)
EXCLUDES 1 aphakia (H27.0)

Z98.41 Cataract extraction status, right eye

Z98.42 Cataract extraction status, left eye

Z98.49 Cataract extraction status, unspecified eye

✓5ᵗʰ **Z98.5** Sterilization status
EXCLUDES 1 female infertility (N97.-)
male infertility (N46.-)

Z98.51 Tubal ligation status   ♀

Z98.52 Vasectomy status   A♂

✓5ᵗʰ **Z98.6** Angioplasty status

Z98.61 Coronary angioplasty status
EXCLUDES 1 coronary angioplasty status with implant and graft (Z95.5)

Z98.62 Peripheral vascular angioplasty status
EXCLUDES 1 peripheral vascular angioplasty status with implant and graft (Z95.820)

✓5ᵗʰ **Z98.8** Other specified postprocedural states

✓6ᵗʰ **Z98.81** Dental procedure status

Z98.810 Dental sealant status

Z98.811 Dental restoration status
Dental crown status
Dental fillings status

Z98.818 Other dental procedure status

Z98.82 Breast implant status
EXCLUDES 1 breast implant removal status (Z98.86)

Ⓝ Newborn: 0 Ⓟ Pediatric: 0-17 Ⓜ Maternity: 12-55 Ⓐ Adult: 15-124 MCC Major CC Condition PDx MCC PDx acts as own MCC CC CC Condition PDx CC PDx acts as own CC

1198   ICD-10-CM Draft (2015)

Z98.83 **Filtering (vitreous) bleb after glaucoma surgery status**
EXCLUDES 1 *inflammation (infection) of postprocedural bleb (H59.4-)*

Z98.84 **Bariatric surgery status**
Gastric banding status
Gastric bypass status for obesity
Obesity surgery status
EXCLUDES 1 *bariatric surgery status complicating pregnancy, childbirth, or the puerperium (O99.84)*
EXCLUDES 2 *intestinal bypass and anastomosis status (Z98.0)*

Z98.85 **Transplanted organ removal status**
Transplanted organ previously removed due to complication, failure, rejection or infection
EXCLUDES 1 *encounter for removal of transplanted organ—code to complication of transplanted organ (T86.-)*

Z98.86 **Personal history of breast implant removal**

√6th Z98.87 **Personal history of in utero procedure**
Z98.870 **Personal history of in utero procedure during pregnancy** ♀
EXCLUDES 2 *complications from in utero procedure for current pregnancy (O35.7)*
supervision of current pregnancy with history of in utero procedure during previous pregnancy (O09.82-)
Z98.871 **Personal history of in utero procedure while a fetus**

Z98.89 **Other specified postprocedural states**
Personal history of surgery, not elsewhere classified

√4th **Z99 Dependence on enabling machines and devices, not elsewhere classified**
EXCLUDES 1 *cardiac pacemaker status (Z95.0)*

Z99.0 **Dependence on aspirator**

√5th Z99.1 **Dependence on respirator**
Dependence on ventilator

CC Excl: For CC codes in subcategory Z99.1: CC with 7th character A, unless otherwise noted: J95.850, Z99.0-Z99.12, Z99.81- Z99.89

Z99.11 **Dependence on respirator [ventilator] status** `CC`
Z99.12 **Encounter for respirator [ventilator] dependence during power failure** `CC`
EXCLUDES 1 *mechanical complication of respirator [ventilator] (J95.850)*

Z99.2 **Dependence on renal dialysis**
Hemodialysis status
Peritoneal dialysis status
Presence of arteriovenous shunt for dialysis
Renal dialysis status NOS
EXCLUDES 1 *encounter for fitting and adjustment of dialysis catheter (Z49.0-)*
noncompliance with renal dialysis (Z91.15)
AHA: 2013, 4Q, 125

Z99.3 **Dependence on wheelchair**
Wheelchair confinement status
Code first cause of dependence, such as:
muscular dystrophy (G71.0)
obesity (E66.-)

√5th Z99.8 **Dependence on other enabling machines and devices**
Z99.81 **Dependence on supplemental oxygen**
Dependence on long-term oxygen
AHA: 2013, 4Q, 129
Z99.89 **Dependence on other enabling machines and devices**
Dependence on machine or device NOS

☑ Additional Character Required √x7th Xtension Alert Unacceptable PDx Manifestation Hospital Acquired Condition *EXCLUDES 1* Not Coded Here *EXCLUDES 2* Not Included Here

Illustrations

Peripheral Nervous System

Brain

Cranial Nerves

Eye

Globe (Eyeball)

Middle Ear

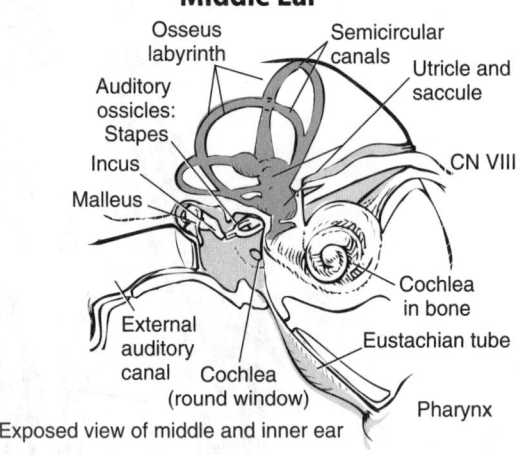

Exposed view of middle and inner ear

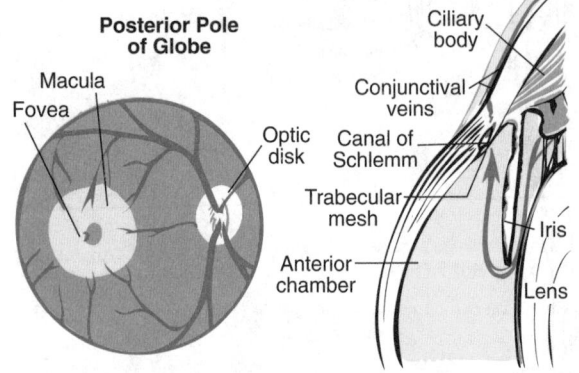

Posterior Pole of Globe

Flow of Aqueous Humor

Lacrimal System

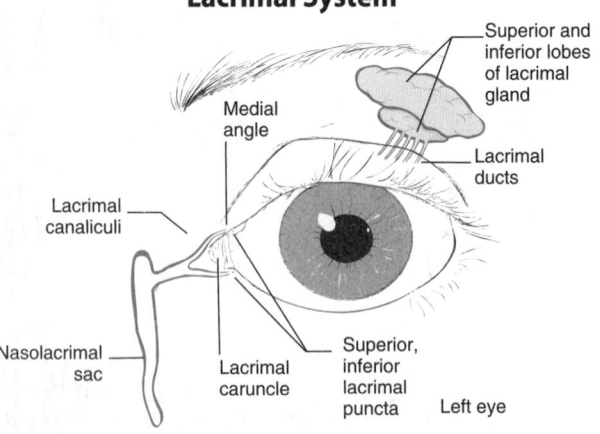

Left eye

Ear and Mastoid

Arteries

Veins

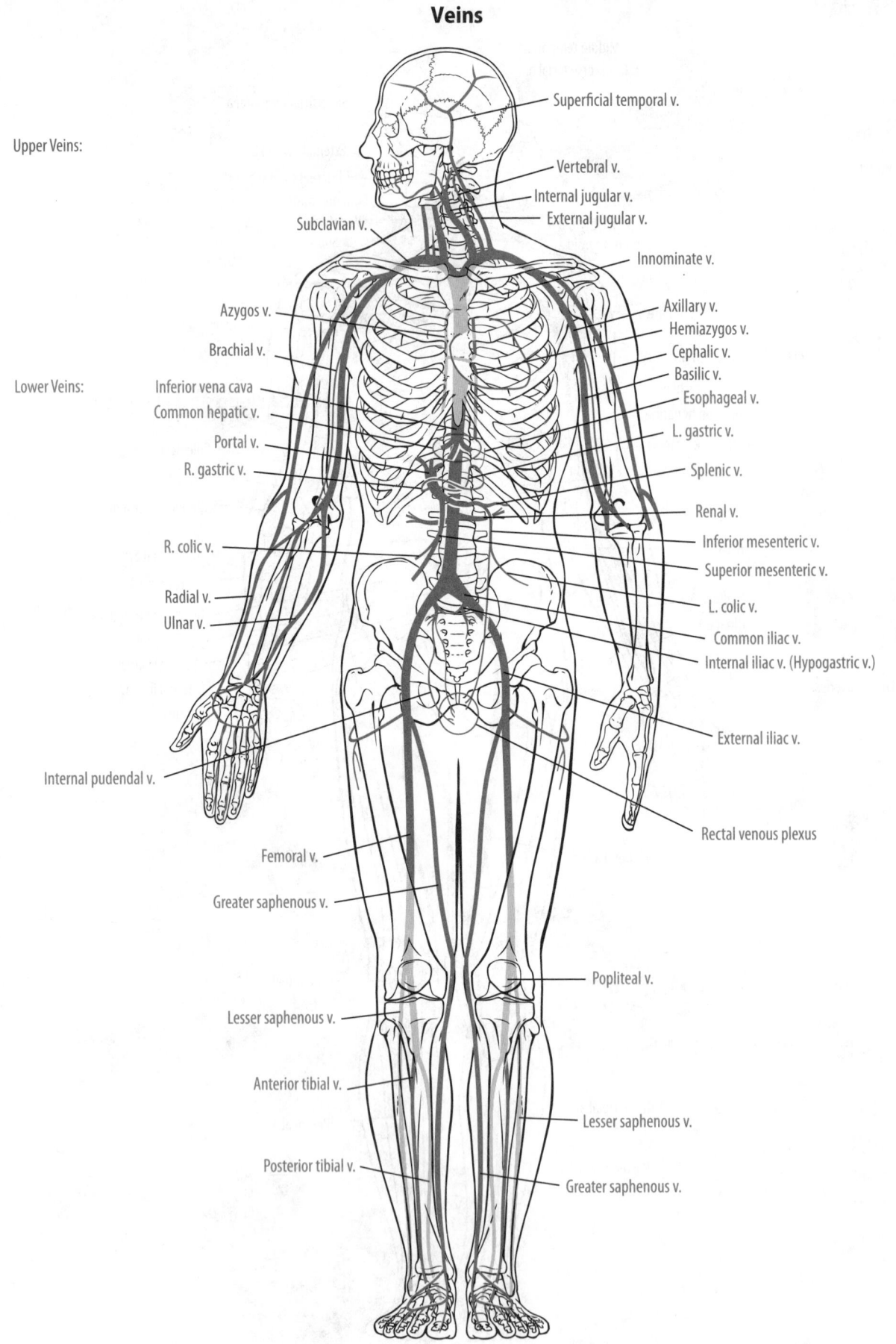

Upper Veins:

Lower Veins:

Superficial temporal v.

Vertebral v.

Internal jugular v.

External jugular v.

Subclavian v.

Innominate v.

Azygos v.

Axillary v.

Hemiazygos v.

Brachial v.

Cephalic v.

Basilic v.

Inferior vena cava

Esophageal v.

Common hepatic v.

L. gastric v.

Portal v.

R. gastric v.

Splenic v.

Renal v.

R. colic v.

Inferior mesenteric v.

Superior mesenteric v.

Radial v.

L. colic v.

Ulnar v.

Common iliac v.

Internal iliac v. (Hypogastric v.)

External iliac v.

Internal pudendal v.

Rectal venous plexus

Femoral v.

Greater saphenous v.

Popliteal v.

Lesser saphenous v.

Anterior tibial v.

Lesser saphenous v.

Posterior tibial v.

Greater saphenous v.

Anatomy of Heart

Arteries of Heart

Cerebrovascular Arteries

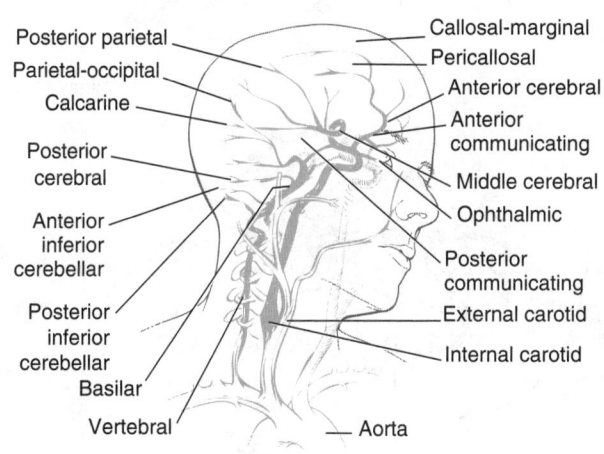

Veins of Head and Neck

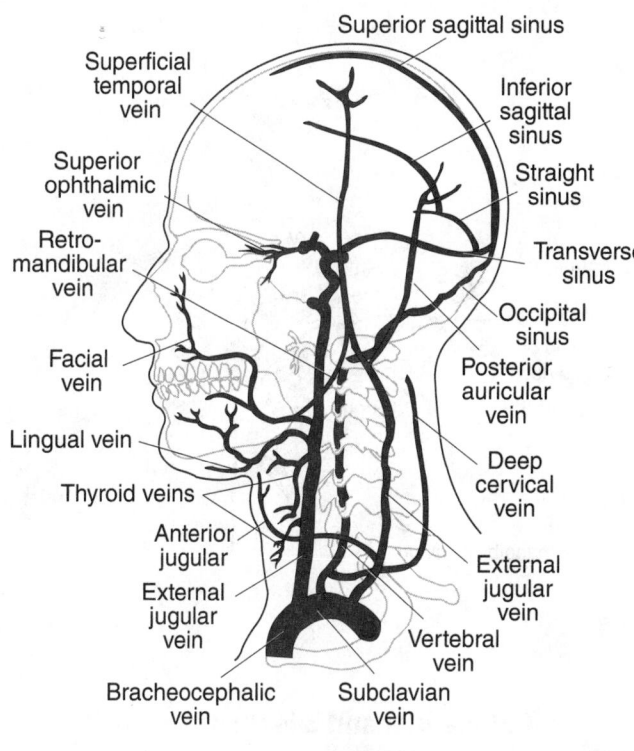

Lymphatic System of Head and Neck

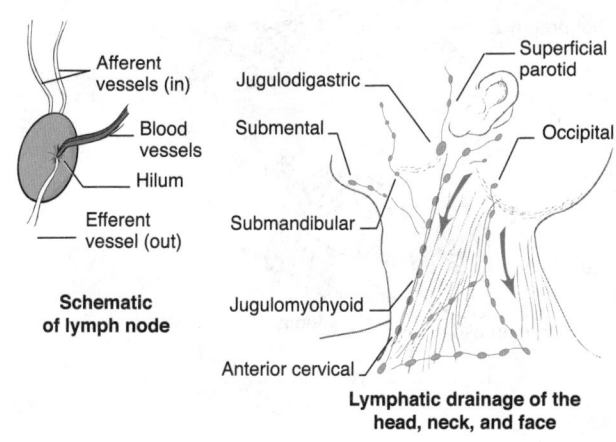

Schematic of lymph node

Lymphatic drainage of the head, neck, and face

Lymph Nodes

Respiratory System

Paranasal Sinuses

Oral Cavity

Pancreas

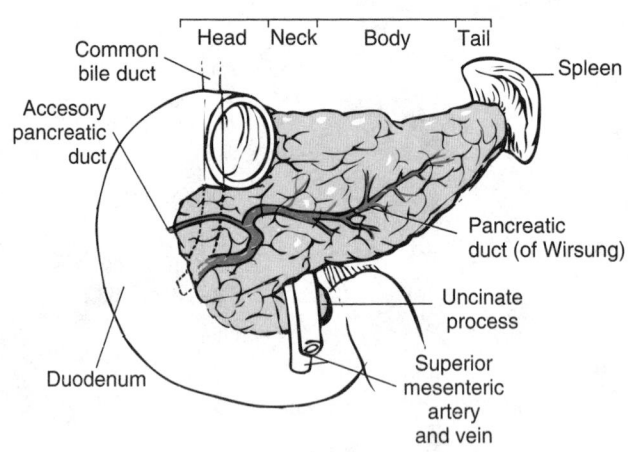

Gallbladder and Bile Ducts

Liver

Gastrointestinal System

Endocrine System

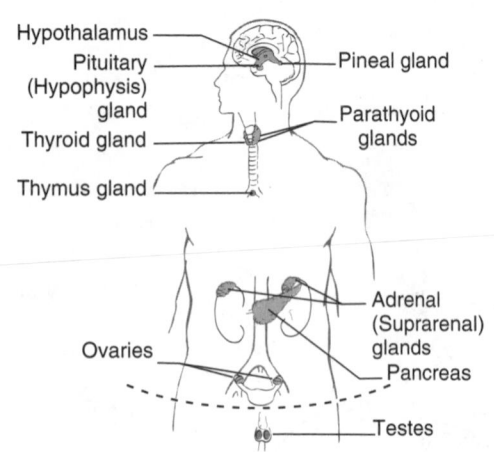

Dorsal View of Parathyroid Gland

Kidney

Urinary System

Male Pelvic Organs

Female Genitourinary System

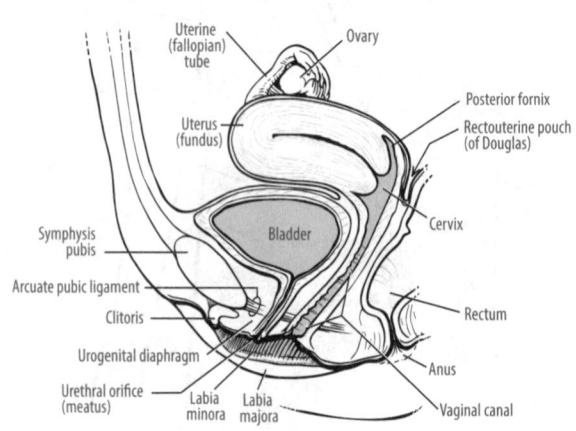

Joints

Shoulder (Anterior View)

Shoulder (Posterior View)

Elbow (Anterior View)

Elbow (Posterior View)

Hand

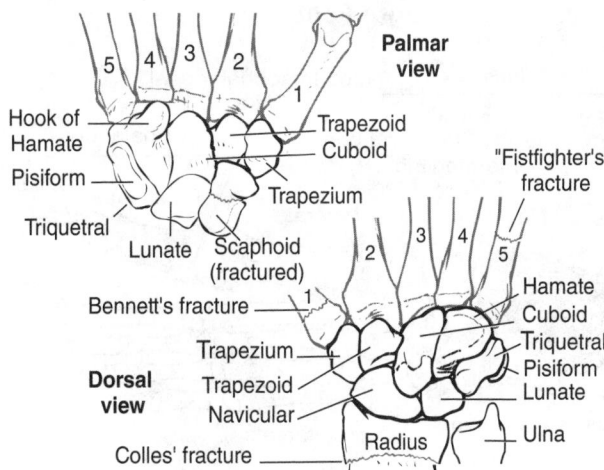

Joints

Hip (Anterior View)

Hip (Posterior View)

Knee (Anterior View)

Knee (Posterior View)

Right Foot

Bones/Joints

Muscles

Temporalis m.
Frontalis m.
Orbicularis oculi m.
Orbicularis oris m.
Depressor labii inferioris m.
Mentalis m.
Sternocleidomastoid m. (Clavicular head)
Sternocleidomastoid m. (Sternal head)
Masseter m.
Zygomaticus major m.
Splenius m.
Omohyoid m.
Levator scapulae m.
Platysma m.
Deltoid m.
Pectoralis major m.
Latissimus dorsi m.
Coracobrachialis m.
Serratus anterior m.
Biceps brachii m. (short head)
Biceps brachii m. (long head)
Biceps brachii m.
Triceps m.
Brachialis m.
Rectus abdominis m.
Linea alba
Brachioradialis m.
Extensor carpi radialis longus m.
Bicipital aponeurosis
External oblique m.
Flexor carpi radialis m.
Palmaris longus m.
Flexor carpi ulnaris m.
Flexor digitorum superficialis m.
Brachioradialis m.
Pronator teres m.
Flexor carpi radialis m.
Extensor carpi radialis longus m.
Extensor carpi radialis brevis m.
Extensor digitorum m.
Extensor retinaculum
Anterior Superior Iliac Spine
Extensor digiti minimi m.
Extensor retinaculum
Iliopsoas m.
Pectineus m.
Adductor longus m.
Sartorius m.
Pudendal n.
Pubic tubercle
Gracilis m.
Tensor fascia latae m.
Vastus lateralis m.
Rectus femoris m.
Tensor fascia latae m.
Vastus medialis m.
Patella
Gastrocnemius m.
Tibia
Tibialis anterior m.
Peroneus longus m.
Soleus m.
Extensor digitorum longus m.
Superior extensor retinaculum
Medial maleolus
Lateral maleolus

Notes